Dedication

We dedicate this edition to all those who advocate to improve the health, enrich the development, and promote the well-being of children and youth throughout the world. Their efforts are essential to achieving these goals and sustaining our hope for a better future.

Preface

The publication of this 17th Edition of *Nelson Textbook of Pediatrics* provides a new and comprehensive update and synthesis of pediatric medicine and related science. It continues to represent the "state of the art" on the broad spectrum of normal and abnormal growth and development and of disorders and diseases that affect children and youth.

This is a time of great opportunity. The promise of medicine, biologic sciences, and technology is greater than ever before. Knowledge of human development, behavior, and disease from molecular to sociologic levels is increasing exponentially. This has led to greater understanding of health and illness in children and youth and substantial improvements in the quality of their care. These advances also hold promise of effectively addressing the new and re-emerging diseases threatening children and their families.

Unfortunately, many children worldwide have not yet benefited from the significant advances in the prevention and treatment of health problems, primarily because of a lack of political will and misplaced priorities. Poverty, war, and bioterrorism present additional substantial risks. In order for our increasing knowledge to benefit all children and youth, good medicine needs to be coupled with effective advocacy.

This edition provides the knowledge that practitioners, house staff, medical students, and others involved in pediatric medicine need to address the enormous range of biopsychosocial problems that children and youth may face. As in previous editions, our goal is to be comprehensive, concise, and reader friendly within a single volume, embracing both the science and the art of pediatrics in our presentation.

The 17th Edition represents a substantial revision and reorganization of the textbook based on a complete review of the field of pediatrics. There are many new chapters and substantial expansion or significant modification of others. Every subject has been scrutinized for possible improvement in its exposition, and no chapter has been left unimproved. Although to an ill child and his or her family and physician even the rarest disorder is of central importance, all health problems cannot be covered with the same degree of detail in one general textbook of pediatrics. Thus, leading articles and subspecialty texts are referenced and should be consulted when more information is desired.

The value of this textbook is due to its expert contributors, and we are indebted to ours for their hard work, knowledge, thoughtfulness, and good judgment. Our sincere appreciation also goes to Judy Fletcher, Deborah Thorp, and Robin Davis at Elsevier and to Carolyn Redman at the Pediatric Department of the Medical College of Wisconsin. All of us have worked hard to produce an edition that will be helpful to those who provide care for children and youth and to those desiring to know more about children's health worldwide.

In this edition we have had informal assistance from many faculty and house staff of the departments of pediatrics at Stanford University, the Medical College of Wisconsin, and Eastern Virginia Medical School. The help of these individuals and of the many practicing pediatricians from around the world who have taken the time to offer thoughtful suggestions is greatly appreciated.

Last and certainly not least, we especially wish to thank our wives for their patience and understanding without which this textbook would not have been possible.

Richard E. Behrman, MD

Robert M. Kliegman, MD

Hal B. Jenson, MD

Contributors

Jon S. Abramson, MD
Professor and Chair, Department of Pediatrics, Wake Forest University School of Medicine; North Carolina Baptist Hospital, Winston-Salem, North Carolina
Streptococcus pneumoniae (Pneumococcus)

Mark J. Abzug, MD
Professor of Pediatrics (Pediatric Infectious Diseases), University of Colorado School of Medicine; The Children's Hospital, Denver, Colorado
Nonpolio Enteroviruses

William G. Adams, MD
Assistant Professor of Pediatrics, Boston University School of Medicine, Boston, Massachusetts
Rabies

John J. Aiken, MD
Assistant Professor of Pediatric Surgery, Medical College of Wisconsin, Milwaukee, Wisconson
Inguinal Hernias

Hassan H. A-Kader, MD
Associate Professor of Pediatrics, University of Arizona, Tucson, Arizona
Cholestasis

Ramin Alemzadeh, MD
Associate Professor of Pediatrics, Section of Endocrinology and Diabetes, Medical College of Wisconsin; Director, Diabetes Program, Children's Hospital of Wisconsin, Milwaukee, Wisconsin
Diabetes Mellitus in Children

Alia Y. Antoon, MD
Assistant Clinical Professor, Harvard Medical School; Chief of Pediatrics, Shriners Burns Hospital; Pediatrician, Massachusetts General Hospital, Boston, Massachusetts
Burn Injuries; Cold Injuries

Carola A. S. Arndt, MD
Associate Professor, Mayo Medical School; Department of Pediatrics, Division of Pediatric Hematology-Oncology, Mayo Clinic and Foundation, Rochester, Minnesota
Soft Tissue Sarcomas; Neoplasms of Bone

Stephen S. Arnon, MD
Senior Investigator and Chief, Infant Botulism Treatment and Prevention Program, California Department of Health Services, Berkeley, California
Botulism (Clostridium botulinum); Tetanus (Clostridium tetani)

Stephen C. Aronoff, MD
Professor and Chair, Department of Pediatrics, Temple University School of Medicine, Philadelphia, Pennsylvania
Candida; Cryptococcus neoformans; Aspergillus; Histoplasmosis (Histoplasma capsulatum); Blastomycosis (Blastomyces dermatitidis); Paracoccidioides brasiliensis; Sporotrichosis (Sporothrix schenckii); Zygomycosis; Primary Amebic Meningoencephalitis; Nonbacterial Food Poisoning

David M. Asher, MD
Chief, Laboratory of Bacterial, Parasitic, and Unconventional Agents, Division of Emerging and Transfusion-Transmitted Diseases, Office of Blood Research and Review, Center for Biologics Evaluation and Research, U.S. Food and Drug Administration, Kensington, Maryland
Transmissible Spongiform Encephalopathies

Joann L. Ater, MD
Associate Professor of Pediatrics, University of Texas M. D. Anderson Cancer Center, Houston, Texas
Brain Tumors in Childhood; Neuroblastoma

Dan Atkins, MD
Associate Professor of Pediatrics, University of Colorado Health Sciences Center; Director, Ambulatory Pediatrics, National Jewish Medical Research Center, Denver, Colorado
Diagnosis of Allergic Disease; Principles of Treatment of Allergic Disease

Marilyn Augustyn, MD
Assistant Professor, Boston University School of Medicine; Boston Medical Center, Boston, Massachusetts
Impact of Violence on Children

Ellis D. Avner, MD
The Gertrude Lee Chandler Tucker Professor and Chair, Department of Pediatrics, Case Western Reserve University School of Medicine; Chief Medical Officer, Rainbow Babies and Children's Hospital, University Hospitals of Cleveland, Cleveland, Ohio
Glomerular Disease; Conditions Particularly Associated with Hematuria; Conditions Particularly Associated with Proteinuria; Tubular Function; Proximal (Type II) Renal Tubular Acidosis; Distal (Type I) Renal Tubular Acidosis; Hyperkalemic (Type IV) Renal Tubular Acidosis; Nephrogenic Diabetes Insipidus; Bartter/Gitelman Syndromes and Other Inherited Tubular Transport Abnormalities; Tubulointerstitial Nephritis; Toxic Nephropathy; Cortical Necrosis; Renal Failure

Parvin Azimi, MD
Clinical Professor of Pediatrics, University of California, San Francisco, School of Medicine; Director, Infectious Diseases, Children's Hospital and Research Center at Oakland, Oakland, California
Chancroid (Haemophilus decreyi); Syphilis (Treponema pallidum); Nonvenereal Treponemal Infections; Leptospira; Relapsing Fever (Borrelia)

William F. Balistreri, MD
Professor of Pediatrics, University of Cincinnati School of Medicine; Director, Division of Gastroenterology, Hepatology, and Nutrition, Children's Hospital Medical Center, Cincinnati, Ohio
Development and Function of the Liver and Biliary System; Manifestations of Liver Disease; Cholestasis; Metabolic Diseases of the Liver; Liver Abscess; Liver Disease Associated with Systemic Disorders; Reye Syndrome and the Mitochondrial Hepatopathies

Robert S. Baltimore, MD
Professor of Pediatrics and of Epidemiology and Public Health, Yale University School of Medicine; Associate Hospital Epidemiologist, Yale-New Haven Hospital; Attending Pediatrician, Yale-New Haven Children's Hospital, New Haven, Connecticut
Listeria monocytogenes; Pseudomonas, Burkholderia, and Stenotrophomonas

Fred F. Barrett, MD
Professor of Pediatrics, University of Tennessee Center for Health Sciences; Associate Medical Director, Le Bonheur Children's Medical Center, Memphis, Tennessee
Infection Associated with Medical Devices

Dorsey M. Bass, MD
Associate Professor of Pediatrics, Stanford University School of Medicine; Attending Physician, Lucile Salter Packard Children's Hospital, Palo Alto, California
Rotavirus and Other Agents of Viral Gastroenteritis

Michael D. Bates, MD, PhD
Assistant Professor of Pediatrics, Division of Gastroenterology, Hepatology, and Nutrition, Division of Developmental Biology, Cincinnati Children's Hospital Medical Center, Cincinnati, Ohio
Development and Function of the Liver and Biliary System

Mark L. Batshaw, MD
Professor and Chair of Pediatrics, George Washington University; Chief Academic Officer, Children's National Medical Center, Washington, DC
Mental Retardation

Howard Bauchner, MD
Professor of Pediatrics and Public Health, Boston University School of Medicine; Director, Division of General Pediatrics, Boston Medical Center, Boston, Massachusetts
Failure to Thrive

Richard E. Behrman, MD
Clinical Professor of Pediatrics, Stanford University School of Medicine and University of California, San Francisco, School of Medicine; Executive Chair, Federation of Pediatric Organizations, Inc., Pediatric Education Steering Committee, Palo Alto, California
Overview of Pediatrics; Children at Special Risk

Daniel Bernstein, MD
Professor of Pediatrics, Stanford University School of Medicine; Chief, Division of Pediatric Cardiology, Co-Director, Children's Heart Center, Lucile Packard Children's Hospital, Palo Alto, California
Developmental Biology of the Cardiovascular System; Evaluation of the Cardiovascular System; Congenital Heart Disease; Acquired Heart Disease; Diseases of the Myocardium and Pericardium; Cardiac Therapeutics; Diseases of the Peripheral Vascular System

Ronald Blanton, MD
Associate Professor of Medicine, Case Western Reserve University School of Medicine; Wade Park Veteran's Administration Hospital, Cleveland, Ohio
Adult Tapeworm Infections; Cysticercosis; Echinococcosis (Echinococcus granulosus and E. multilocularis)

Archie Bleyer, MD
Professor and Mosbacher Chair of Pediatrics, University of Texas; Director, Community Clinical Oncology Program, University of Texas M. D. Anderson Cancer Center, Houston, Texas
Principles of Diagnosis; Principles of Treatment; The Leukemias

Steven Boas, MD
Associate Professor of Pediatrics, Feinberg School of Medicine, Northwestern University; Pediatric Pulmonologist, Children's Memorial Hospital, Chicago, Illinois
Emphysema and Overinflation; α_1-Antitrypsin Deficiency and Emphysema; Other Distal Airway Diseases; Skeletal Diseases Influencing Pulmonary Function

Thomas F. Boat, MD
Professor and Chair, Department of Pediatrics, University of Cincinnati College of Medicine; Director, Research Foundation, Cincinnati Children's Hospital Medical Center, Cincinnati, Ohio
Chronic or Recurrent Respiratory Symptoms; Cystic Fibrosis

Mark Boguniewicz, MD
Professor of Pediatrics, Division of Allergy-Immunology, University of Colorado School of Medicine; National Jewish Medical and Research Center, Denver, Colorado
Adverse Reactions to Drugs; Ocular Allergies

Melissa L. Bondy, PhD
Professor of Epidemiology, University of Texas M. D. Anderson Cancer Center, Houston, Texas
Epidemiology of Childhood and Adolescent Cancer

Robert A. Bonomo, MD
Associate Professor of Medicine, Case Western Reserve University School of Medicine; Section Chief, Division of Infectious Diseases, Veterans Administration Medical Center, Cleveland, Ohio
African Trypanosomiasis (Sleeping Sickness; Trypanosoma brucei complex); American Trypanosomiasis (Chagas Disease; Trypanosoma cruzi)

Neil W. Boris, MD
Assistant Professor of Community Health Sciences, Tulane University School of Public Health and Tropical Medicine; Co-Director, Child Psychiatry Consultation Service, Tulane University Hospital and Medical Center of Louisiana, New Orleans, Louisiana
The Clinical Interview (History); Psychiatric Considerations of Central Nervous System Injury; Psychosomatic Illness; Rumination Disorder; Pica; Enuresis (Bed-wetting); Encopresis; Habit Disorders; Anxiety Disorders; Mood Disorders; Suicide and Attempted Suicide; Disruptive Behavioral Disorders; Pervasive Developmental Disorders and Childhood Psychosis

Laurence A. Boxer, MD
Professor of Pediatrics, University of Michigan School of Medicine; Director, Pediatric Hematology/Oncology, C. S. Mott Children's Hospital, Ann Arbor, Michigan
Neutrophils; Eosinophils; Disorders of Phagocyte Function; Leukopenia; Leukocytosis

David T. Breault, MD, PhD
Clinical Fellow in Pediatrics, Harvard Medical School; Fellow in Endocrinology, Children's Hospital Boston, Boston, Massachusetts
Diabetes Insipidus; Other Abnormalities of Arginine Vasopressin Metabolism and Action

W. Ted Brown, MD, PhD
Chair, Department of Human Genetics, Director, George A. Jervis Clinic, NYS Institute for Basic Research in Developmental Disabilities, Staten Island, New York
Progeria

Rebecca H. Buckley, MD
J. Buren Sidbury Professor of Pediatrics, Professor of
Immunology, Duke University School of Medicine; Chief,
Division of Allergy and Immunology, Department of
Pediatrics, Duke University Medical Center, Durham, North
Carolina
Evaluation of the Immune System; The T-, B- and NK-Cell Systems

Cynthia Budek, MS
Pediatric Nurse Practitioner, Pulmonary Medicine,
Children's Memorial Hospital, Chicago, Illinois
Chronic Severe Respiratory Insufficiency

Brenda Bursch, PhD
Assistant Professor of Psychiatry and Behavioral Sciences,
Assistant Professor of Pediatrics, David Geffen School of
Medicine, University of California, Los Angeles; Associate
Director, Pediatric Pain Program, Mattel Children's Hospital at
UCLA, Los Angeles, California
Pediatric Pain Management

Bruce M. Camitta, MD
Professor of Pediatrics, Medical College of Wisconsin; Children's
Hospital of Wisconsin, Milwaukee, Wisconsin
Polycythemia (Erythrocytosis); The Spleen; The Lymphatic System

James T. Cassidy, MD
Professor of Pediatrics, Department of Child Health;
Chief, Pediatric Rheumatology, University of Missouri,
Columbia, Missouri
Treatment of Rheumatic Diseases; Juvenile Rheumatoid Arthritis;
Postinfectious Arthritis and Related Conditions

Ellen Gould Chadwick, MD
Associate Professor of Pediatrics, Northwestern University
Medical School; Co-Director, Division of Pediatrics, Adolescent
and Maternal HIV Infection, Children's Memorial Hospital,
Chicago, Illinois
Acquired Immunodeficiency Syndrome (Human Immunodeficiency Virus)

Yuan-Tsong Chen, MD, PhD
Professor and Chief, Division of Medical Genetics, Duke
University Medical Center, Durham, North Carolina; Director,
Institute of Biomedical Sciences, Academia Sinica, Taipei,
Taiwan
Glycogen Storage Diseases; Defects in Galactose Metabolism; Defects in
Fructose Metabolism; Defects in Intermediary Carbohydrate Metabolism
Associated with Lactic Acidosis; Deficiency of Xylulose Dehydrogenase
(Essential Benign Pentosuria)

Russell W. Chesney, MD
LeBonheur Professor and Chair of Pediatrics,
University of Tennessee Health Sciences Center;
Senior Vice President for Academic Affairs,
LeBonheur Children's Medical Center, Memphis, Tennessee
Rickets Associated with Renal Tubular Acidosis; Metabolic Bone
Disease

Joseph N. Chorley, MD
Assistant Professor of Pediatrics, Sports Medicine,
Baylor College of Medicine; Staff Member,
Texas Children's Hospital, Houston, Texas
Sports Medicine

Robert D. Christensen, MD
Professor and Chair, Department of Pediatrics, University of
South Florida College of Medicine, St. Petersburg, Florida
Development of the Hematopoietic System

Robin B. Churchill, MD
Assistant Professor of Pediatrics, Eastern Virginia Medical School;
Attending Physician, Pediatric Infectious Diseases Division,
Children's Hospital of The King's Daughters, Norfolk, Virginia
Blastomycosis (*Blastomyces dermatitidis*); *Paracoccidioides brasiliensis*;
Sporotrichosis (*Sporothrix schenckii*); Zygomycosis

Theodore J. Cieslak, MD
Clinical Associate Professor, Uniformed Services University,
Bethesda, Maryland; University of Texas Health Science Center,
San Antonio, Texas; Chairman, San Antonio Military Pediatric
Center, Brooke Army Medical Center, Fort Sam Houston, Texas
Biologic and Chemical Terrorism

Thomas G. Cleary, MD
Professor and Director, Division of Pediatric Infectious Diseases,
University of Texas Health Science Center, Houston; Memorial
Hermann Children's Hospital, Houston, Texas
Salmonella; *Shigella*; *Escherichia coli*

Pinchas Cohen, MD
Professor of Pediatrics, David Geffen School of Medicine,
University of California, Los Angeles; Chief of Endocrinology,
Mattel Children's Hospital, Los Angeles, California
Hyperpituitarism, Tall Stature, and Overgrowth Syndromes

F. Sessions Cole, MD
Park J. White, MD, Professor of Pediatrics, Washington
University School of Medicine; Director, Division of Newborn
Medicine, St. Louis Children's Hospital, St. Louis, Missouri
Pulmonary Alveolar Proteinosis; Inherited Disorders of Surfactant Protein
Metabolism

John L. Colombo, MD
Professor of Pediatrics, Pediatric Pulmonology, University of
Nebraska Medical Center; Attending Physician, Nebraska Health
Systems and Children's Hospital of Omaha, Omaha, Nebraska
Aspiration Syndromes; Chronic Recurrent Aspiration; Gastroesophageal Reflux
and Respiratory Disorders

Kenneth L. Cox, MD
Professor of Pediatrics, Chief, Pediatric Gastroenterology and
Nutrition, Stanford University School of Medicine; Medical
Director, Pediatric Liver Transplant Program, Lucile Salter
Packard Children's Hospital, Palo Alto, California
Liver Transplantation

Richard Dalton, MD
Professor of Child and Adolescent Psychiatry, Clinical Professor
of Pediatrics, Tulane University Health Sciences Center,
New Orleans; Medical Director, East Jefferson Mental Health
Center, Metairie, Louisiana
Psychosocial Problems; Psychosomatic Illness; Rumination Disorder; Pica;
Enuresis (Bed-wetting); Encopresis; Habit Disorders; Anxiety Disorders; Mood
Disorders; Suicide and Attempted Suicide; Disruptive Behavioral Disorders;
Sexual Behavior and Its Variations; Pervasive Developmental Disorders and
Childhood Psychosis; Psychologic Treatment of Children and Adolescents;
Separation and Loss

Alan D. D'Andrea, MD
Professor of Pediatrics, Harvard Medical School;
Dana-Farber Cancer Institute, Boston, Massachusetts
The Constitutional Pancytopenias

Gary L. Darmstadt, MD
Assistant Professor of International Health, Bloomberg School
of Public Health, Johns Hopkins University, Baltimore,
Maryland; Senior Research Advisor, Saving Newborn Lives
Initiative, Save the Children Federation–USA, Washington, DC
The Skin

Jorge H. Daruna, PhD
Associate Professor of Psychiatry, Division of Child and Adolescent Psychiatry, Department of Psychiatry and Neurology, Tulane University School of Medicine, New Orleans, Louisiana
The Clinical Interview (History); Psychiatric Considerations of Central Nervous System Injury

Toni Darville, MD
Associate Professor of Pediatrics and Microbiology/Immunology, University of Arkansas for Medical Sciences, Little Rock, Arkansas
Neisseria gonorrhoeae (Gonococcus)

Robert S. Daum, MD
Professor of Pediatrics, University of Chicago; University of Chicago Children's Hospital, Chicago, Illinois
Haemophilus influenzae

Ira D. Davis, MD
Associate Professor of Pediatrics, Case Western Reserve University School of Medicine; Chief, Division of Pediatric Nephrology, Rainbow Babies and Children's Hospital, Cleveland, Ohio
Glomerular Disease; Conditions Particularly Associated with Hematuria

Peter S. Dayan, MD
Assistant Professor of Clinical Pediatrics, Columbia University College of Physicians and Surgeons; Fellowship Director, Pediatric Emergency Division, Children's Hospital of New York-Presbyterian, New York, New York
Acute Care of the Multiple Trauma Victim

Dorr G. Dearborn, MD, PhD
Professor of Pediatrics, Case Western Reserve University School of Medicine; Attending Pediatrician, Rainbow Babies and Children's Hospital, Cleveland, Ohio
Pulmonary Hemosiderosis

Katherine MacRae Dell, MD
Assistant Professor of Pediatrics, Case Western Reserve University School of Medicine; Attending Pediatric Nephrologist, Rainbow Babies and Children's Hospital, University Hospitals of Cleveland, Cleveland, Ohio
Tubular Function; Proximal (Type II) Renal Tubular Acidosis; Distal (Type I) Renal Tubular Acidosis; Hyperkalemic (Type IV) Renal Tubular Acidosis; Nephrogenic Diabetes Insipidus; Bartter/Gitelman Syndromes and Other Inherited Tubular Transport Abnormalities; Tubulointerstitial Nephritis

Robert J. Desnick, MD, PhD
Professor of Human Genetics and Pediatrics, Mount Sinai School of Medicine; Attending Physician, Pediatrics, Mount Sinai Hospital, New York, New York
Lipidoses; Mucolipidoses; Disorders of Glycoprotein Degradation and Structure

Joseph V. DiCarlo, MD
Assistant Professor of Pediatrics, Stanford University School of Medicine, Palo Alto, California
Scoring Systems and Predictors of Mortality; Renal Stabilization; Nutritional Stabilization; Neurologic Stabilization; Acute (Adult) Respiratory Distress Syndrome (ARDS); Continuous Hemofiltration

Angelo M. DiGeorge, MD
Emeritus Professor of Pediatrics, Temple University School of Medicine, Philadelphia, Pennsylvania
Disorders of the Parathyroid

Patricia A. Donohoue, MD
Professor of Pediatrics, Division of Endocrinology and Diabetes, University of Iowa, Roy J. and Lucille A. Carver College of Medicine, Iowa City, Iowa
Obesity

Mary K. Donovan, RN, MS, PNP
NP Preceptor, Northeastern University; Pediatric Nurse Practitioner, Shriners Burns Hospital, Boston, Massachusetts
Burn Injuries; Cold Injuries

M. Denise Dowd, MD, MPH
Associate Professor of Pediatrics, University of Missouri, Kansas City; Section Chief, Injury Prevention, Children's Memorial Hospital, Kansas City, Missouri
Emergency Medical Services for Children

Daniel A. Doyle, MD
Assistant Professor of Pediatrics, Thomas Jefferson University, Philadelphia, Pennsylvania; A.I. duPont Hospital for Children, Wilmington, Delaware
Disorders of the Parathyroid

Anne Dubin, MD
Associate Professor of Pediatrics, Stanford University School of Medicine; Arrhythmia Service, Lucile Salter Packard Children's Hospital, Palo Alto, California
Cardiac Arrhythmias

J. Stephen Dumler, MD
Associate Professor, Division of Medical Microbiology, Department of Pathology, Graduate Program in Cellular and Molecular Medicine, Department of Molecular Microbiology and Immunology, The Johns Hopkins University School of Medicine, The Bloomsberg School of Public Health; Director, Laboratory of Parasitology, Co-Director, Molecular Microbiology Laboratory, Johns Hopkins Hospital, Baltimore, Maryland
Rickettsial Infections

Paul H. Dworkin, MD
Professor and Chair, Department of Pediatrics, University of Connecticut School of Medicine; Physician-in-Chief, Connecticut Children's Medical Center; Director and Chair, Department of Pediatrics, St. Francis Hospital and Medical Center, Hartford, Connecticut
Child Care

Jack S. Elder, MD
Carter Kissell Professor of Urology, Professor of Pediatrics, Case Western Reserve University School of Medicine; Director, Pediatric Urology, Rainbow Babies and Children's Hospital, Cleveland, Ohio
Urologic Disorders in Infants and Children

Jonathan D. Finder, MD
Assistant Professor of Pediatrics, University of Pittsburgh; Pediatric Pulmonologist, Children's Hospital of Pittsburgh, Pittsburgh, Pennsylvania
Bronchomalacia and Tracheomalacia; Congenital Disorders of the Lung

Margaret C. Fisher, MD
Professor of Pediatrics, Drexel University College of
Medicine, Philadelphia; Chair, Department of Pediatrics,
Monmouth Medical Center, Long Brach,
New Jersey
Clostridium difficile–Associated Diarrhea; Other Anaerobic Infections; Infection
Control and Prophylaxis

Patricia M. Flynn, MD
Professor of Pediatrics, University of Tennessee Center for
Health Sciences; Member, Department of Infectious
Diseases, St. Jude Children's Research Hospital, Memphis,
Tennessee
Infection Associated with Medical Devices; Spore-Forming Intestinal
Protozoa

J. Julio Pérez Fontán, MD
Alumni Endowed Professor of Pediatrics and Professor of
Anesthesiology, Washington University School of Medicine;
Director, Division of Pediatric Critical Care Medicine and
Pediatric Intensive Services, St. Louis Children's Hospital,
St. Louis, Missouri
Development of the Respiratory System; Respiratory Pathophysiology; Defense
Mechanisms and Metabolic Functions of the Lung

Joel A. Forman, MD
Vice-Chair for Education, Assistant Professor of Pediatrics,
Mount Sinai School of Medicine; Director,
Pediatric Residency Program, Mount Sinai Hospital, New York,
New York
Chemical Pollutants

Marc A. Forman, MD
Emeritus Professor of Psychiatry and Pediatrics, Tulane
University School of Medicine, New Orleans; Senior Medical
Consultant for Clinical Research, SARAH Network of Hospitals
of the Locomotor System, Brasilia, Brazil
Assessment and Interviewing; Psychiatric Considerations of Central Nervous
System Injury; Mood Disorders; Pervasive Developmental Disorders and
Childhood Psychosis

Norman Fost, MD, MPH
Professor of Pediatrics and History of Medicine,
University of Wisconsin; Director, Program in Bioethics,
University of Wisconsin Hospital, Madison, Wisconsin
Ethics in Pediatric Care

Lorry R. Frankel, MD
Associate Professor of Pediatrics, Stanford University School of
Medicine; Director, Critical Care Services, Lucile Salter Packard
Children's Hospital, Palo Alto, California
Pediatric Critical Care: An Overview; Interfacility Transfer of the Critically Ill
Infant and Child; Effective Communication with Families in the PICU; Monitoring
Techniques for the Critically Ill Infant and Child; Scoring Systems and Predictors
of Mortality; Pediatric Emergencies and Resuscitation; Shock; Respiratory
Distress and Failure; Mechanical Ventilation; Neurologic Stabilization; Acute
(Adult) Respiratory Distress Syndrome (ARDS); Transplantation Issues in the
PICU; Withdrawal or Withholding of Life Support, Brain Death, and Organ
Procurement

James French, MD
Children's Medical Center, Dayton, Ohio
The Spleen

Madelyn Freundlich, MSW, MPH, JD
Policy Director, Children's Rights, New York, New York
Adoption; Foster Care

Peter Gal, PharmD
Clinical Professor, School of Pharmacy, University of North
Carolina at Chapel Hill; Director, Pharmacy Division,
Greensboro Area Health Education Center, Director, Neonatal
Pharmacotherapy Fellowship, Women's Hospital of Greensboro,
Moses Cone Health System, Greensboro, North Carolina
Principles of Drug Therapy; Medications

Manuel Garcia-Careaga, MD
Assistant Professor of Pediatrics, Stanford University School of
Medicine; Lucile Salter Packard Children's Hospital, Palo Alto,
California
Malabsorptive Disorders

Paula Gardiner, MD
Tufts University School of Medicine, Boston; Resident,
Hallmark Family Health Center, Malden, Massachusetts
Herbal Medicines

Luigi Garibaldi, MD
Director, Pediatric Endocrinology, Saint Barnabas Medical Center,
Livingston, New Jersey; Children's Hospital of New Jersey at
Newark Beth Israel Medical Center, Newark, New Jersey
Physiology of Puberty; Disorders of Pubertal Development

Abraham Gedalia, MD
Professor and Head, Division of Pediatric Rheumatology,
Department of Pediatrics, Louisiana State University Health
Sciences Center; Head, Division of Pediatric Rheumatology,
Children's Hospital, New Orleans, Louisiana
Behçet Disease; Sjögren Syndrome; Familial Mediterranean Fever; Amyloidosis

Michael A. Gerber, MD
Professor of Pediatrics, University of Cincinnati College of
Medicine; Attending Physician, Division of Infectious Diseases,
Cincinnati Children's Hospital Medical Center, Cincinnati, Ohio
Group A Streptococcus; Non–Group A or B Streptococci

Fayez K. Ghishan, MD
Professor of Clinical Pediatrics and Physiology, University of
Arizona; Head, Department of Pediatrics, Director,
Steele Memorial Children's Research Center, Tucson, Arizona
Chronic Diarrhea

Gerald S. Gilchrist, MD
Helen C. Levitt Professor Emeritus, Mayo Foundation, Mayo
Medical School; Formerly Chair, Department of Pediatric and
Adolescent Medicine and Consultant in Pediatric
Hematology/Oncology, Mayo Clinic, Rochester, Minnesota
Lymphoma

Charles M. Ginsburg, MD
Marilyn R. Corrigan Distinguished Chair of Pediatric Research,
Professor of Pediatrics, Associate Dean for Faculty
Development, University of Texas Southwestern Medical
Center, Dallas, Texas
Animal and Human Bites

Bertil Glader, MD, PhD
Professor of Pediatrics, Stanford University School of Medicine;
Attending Hematologist, Lucile Salter Packard Children's
Hospital, Palo Alto, California
The Anemias; Anemias of Inadequate Production

Donald A. Goldmann, MD
Professor of Pediatrics, Harvard Medical School; Epidemiologist,
Children's Hospital Boston, Boston, Massachusetts
Diagnostic Microbiology

Denise Goodman, MD
Assistant Professor, Feinberg School of Medicine of Northwestern University; Attending Physician, Pediatric Intensive Care Unit, Children's Memorial Hospital, Chicago, Illinois
Inflammatory Disorders of the Small Airways

Collin S. Goto, MD
Assistant Clinical Professor of Pediatrics, University of California, San Diego; Attending Physician, Division of Emergency Medicine and Toxicology, Children's Hospital and Health Center, The California Poison Control System, San Diego, California
Heavy Metal Intoxication

David Gozal, MD
Children's Foundation Chair for Pediatric Research, Professor of Pediatrics, Pharmacology, and Toxicology, University of Louisville; Director, Division of Sleep Medicine, Kosair Children's Hospital, Louisville, Kentucky
Neuromuscular Diseases with Pulmonary Consequences

Michael Green, MD, MPH
Professor of Pediatrics and Surgery, University of Pittsburgh School of Medicine; Children's Hospital of Pittsburgh, Pittsburgh, Pennsylvania
Infections in Immunocompromised Persons

Thomas P. Green, MD
Chair, Department of Pediatrics, Women's Board Centennial Professor, Feinberg School of Medicine, Northwestern University; Physician-in-Chief, Children's Memorial Hospital, Chicago, Illinois
Disorders of the Lungs and Lower Airways; Congenital Disorders of the Lungs; Pulmonary Edema; Pulmonary Hemorrhage, Embolism, and Infection

Larry A. Greenbaum, MD, PhD
Associate Professor of Pediatrics, Medical College of Wisconsin; Attending Physician, Children's Hospital of Wisconsin, Milwaukee, Wisconsin
Pathophysiology of Body Fluids and Fluid Therapy

David Grossman, MD, MPH
Professor of Pediatrics, University of Washington; Director, Harborview Injury Prevention and Research Center, Seattle, Washington
Injury Control

Linda Sayler Gudas, PhD
Assistant Clinical Professor, Harvard Medical School; Assistant in Psychiatry, Department of Psychology, Children's Hospital, Boston, Massachusetts
Grief and Bereavement

James G. Gurney, PhD
Associate Professor of Pediatrics, Division of Epidemiology and Clinical Research, University of Minnesota, Minneapolis, Minnesota
Epidemiology of Childhood and Adolescent Cancer

Gabriel G. Haddad, MD
Professor of Pediatrics and Neuroscience, University Chair, Department of Pediatrics, Albert Einstein College of Medicine; Pediatrician-in-Chief, Children's Hospital at Montefiore, Bronx, New York
Development of the Respiratory System; Regulation of Respiration; Respiratory Pathophysiology; Defense Mechanisms and Metabolic Functions of the Lung; Diagnostic Approach to Respiratory Disease; Obstructive Sleep Apnea and Hypoventilation; Primary Ciliary Dyskinesia (Immotile Cilia Syndrome)

Joseph Haddad Jr., MD
Associate Professor and Vice Chair, Department of Otolaryngology/Head and Neck Surgery, Columbia University College of Physicians and Surgeons; Lawrence Savetsky Chair and Director, Pediatric Otolaryngology, Children's Hospital of New York-Presbyterian, New York, New York
Congenital Disorders of the Nose; Acquired Disorders of the Nose; Nasal Polyps; Clinical Manifestations; Hearing Loss; Congenital Malformations; Diseases of the External Ear; The Inner Ear and Diseases of the Bony Labyrinth; Traumatic Injuries of the Ear and Temporal Bone; Tumors of the Ear and Temporal Bone

Judith G. Hall, MD
Professor of Pediatrics and Medical Genetics, University of British Columbia; British Columbia's Children's Hospital, Vancouver, British Columbia, Canada
Chromosomal Clinical Abnormalities; Genetic Counseling

Scott B. Halstead, MD
Adjunct Professor of Preventive Medicine and Biometrics, Uniformed Services University of the Health Sciences, Bethesda, Maryland
Arboviral Encephalitis in North America; Arboviral Encephalitis Outside North America; Dengue Fever and Dengue Hemorrhagic Fever; Yellow Fever; Other Viral Hemorrhagic Fevers; Hantaviruses

Margaret R. Hammerschlag, MD
Professor of Pediatrics and Medicine, Director, Division of Pediatric Infectious Diseases, SUNY Downstate Medical Center, Brooklyn, New York
Chlamydial Infections

Aaron Hamvas, MD
Professor of Pediatrics, Washington University School of Medicine; Medical Director, Neonatal Intensive Care Unit, St. Louis Children's Hospital, St. Louis, Missouri
Pulmonary Alveolar Proteinosis; Inherited Disorders of Surfactant Protein Metabolism

James C. Harris, MD
Professor of Psychiatry and Behavioral Sciences, Professor of Pediatrics, The Johns Hopkins University School of Medicine; Director, Developmental Neuro-Psychiatry, Johns Hopkins University Hospital, Baltimore, Maryland
Disorders of Purine and Pyrimidine Metabolism

Gary E. Hartman, MD
Professor of Surgery and Pediatrics, George Washington University School of Medicine; Chief, Pediatric Surgery, Children's National Medical Center, Washington, DC
Acute Appendicitis; Diaphragmatic Hernia; Epigastric Hernia

David B. Haslam, MD
Assistant Professor of Pediatrics and Molecular Microbiology, Washington University School of Medicine; St. Louis Children's Hospital, St. Louis, Missouri
Enterococcus

Robert H. A. Haslam, MD
Emeritus Professor and Chair, Department of Pediatrics, Professor of Medicine (Neurology), University of Toronto; Emeritus Pediatrician-in-Chief and Staff Neurologist, Hospital for Sick Children, Toronto, Ontario, Canada
Neurologic Evaluation; Headaches; Neurocutaneous Syndromes; Brain Abscess; Pseudotumor Cerebri; Spinal Cord Disorders

Fern R. Hauck, MD
Associate Professor and Director of Research, Department of Family Medicine, University of Virginia Health System, Charlottesville, Virginia
Sudden Infant Death Syndrome

Paul R. Haut, MD
Associate Professor of Pediatrics, Indiana University School of Medicine; Director of Pediatric Stem Cell Transplantation, James Whitcomb Riley Hospital for Children, Indianapolis, Indiana
Pulmonary Tumors

Gregory F. Hayden, MD
Professor of Pediatrics, Director, Center for the Advancement of Generalist Medicine, University of Virginia School of Medicine, Charlottesville, Virginia
The Common Cold; Acute Pharyngitis

Jacqueline T. Hecht, PhD
Professor of Pediatrics, Director, Genetic Counseling Program, University of Texas-Houston, Houston, Texas
General Considerations; Disorders Involving Cartilage Matrix Proteins; Disorders Involving Transmembrane Receptors; Disorders Involving Ion Transporter; Disorders Involving Transcription Factors; Disorders Involving Defective Bone Resorption; Disorders for Which Defects Are Poorly Understood or Unknown

William C. Heird, MD
Professor of Pediatrics, Baylor College of Medicine; Children's Nutrition Research Center, Houston, Texas
Nutritional Requirements; The Feeding of Infants and Children; Food Insecurity, Hunger, and Undernutrition; Vitamin Deficiencies and Excesses

J. Owen Hendley, MD
Professor of Pediatrics, University of Virginia School of Medicine, Charlottesville, Virginia
Sinusitis; Retropharyngeal Abscess, Lateral Pharyngeal (Parapharyngeal) Abscess, and Peritonsillar Cellulitis/Abscess

Fred M. Henretig, MD
Professor of Pediatrics and Emergency Medicine, University of Pennsylvania School of Medicine; Director, Section of Clinical Toxicology, Children's Hospital of Philadelphia, Philadelphia, Pennsylvania
Biologic and Chemical Terrorism

Gloria P. Heresi, MD
Associate Professor of Pediatric Infectious Diseases, University of Texas-Houston Health Science Center; Memorial Hermann Children's Hospital, Houston, Texas
Cholera (*Vibrio cholerae*); *Campylobacter*, *Yersinia*; *Aeromonas* and *Plesiomonas*

Albert C. Hergenroeder, MD
Professor of Pediatrics, Baylor College of Medicine; Chief, Adolescent Medicine Service and Sports Medicine Clinic, Texas Children's Hospital, Houston, Texas
Sports Medicine

Cynthia E. Herzog, MD
Associate Professor, University of Texas M. D. Anderson Cancer Center, Houston, Texas
Retinoblastoma; Gonadal and Germ Cell Neoplasms; Neoplasms of the Liver; Benign Vascular Tumors; Rare Tumors

Lauren D. Holinger, MD
Professor of Otolaryngology/Head and Neck Surgery, Northwestern University; Paul H. Holinger, MD, Professor, Head, Division of Pediatric Otolaryngology and Department of Communicative Disorders, Children's Memorial Hospital, Chicago, Illinois
Congenital Anomalies of the Larynx; Foreign Bodies of the Airway; Laryngotracheal Stenosis, Subglottic Stenosis; Congenital Anomalies of the Trachea and Bronchi; Neoplasms of the Larynx, Trachea, and Bronchi

Steve Holve, MD
Clinical Professor of Pediatrics, The Johns Hopkins University School of Medicine, Baltimore, Maryland; Chief, Department of Pediatrics, Tuba City Indian Medical Center, Tuba City, Arizona
Envenomations

Jeffrey D. Hord, MD
Associate Professor of Pediatrics, Northwestern Ohio Universities College of Medicine; Director, Pediatric Hematology/Oncology, Children's Hospital Medical Center, Akron, Ohio
The Acquired Pancytopenias

William A. Horton, MD
Professor of Molecular and Medical Genetics, Oregon Health Sciences University; Director of Research, Shriners Hospital for Children, Portland, Oregon
General Considerations; Disorders Involving Cartilage Matrix Proteins; Disorders Involving Transmembrane Receptors; Disorders Involving Ion Transporter; Disorders Involving Transcription Factors; Disorders Involving Defective Bone Resorption; Disorders for Which Defects Are Poorly Understood or Unknown

Peter Hotez, MD, PhD
Professor and Chair, Department of Microbiology and Tropical Medicine, The George Washington University Medical Center, Washington, DC
Hookworms (*Ancylostoma* and *Necator americanus*)

Michelle S. Howenstine, MD
Associate Professor of Clinical Pediatrics, Indiana University School of Medicine; James Whitcomb Riley Hospital for Children, Indianapolis, Indiana
Interstitial Lung Diseases

E. Eugene Hoyme, MD
Professor and Chief, Division of Medical Genetics, Department of Pediatrics, Stanford University School of Medicine; Chief, Genetics Service, Lucile Salter Packard Children's Hospital, Stanford, California
The Molecular Basis of Genetic Disorders; Molecular Diagnosis of Genetic Diseases; Patterns of Inheritance

Vicki Huff, PhD
Associate Professor of Molecular Genetics/Cancer Genetics, University of Texas M.D. Anderson Cancer Center, Houston, Texas
Neoplasms of the Kidney

Walter T. Hughes, MD
Professor of Pediatrics, University of Tennessee College of Medicine; Emeritus Member, Department of Infectious Diseases, St. Jude Children's Research Hospital, Memphis, Tennessee
Pneumocystis carinii

Carl E. Hunt, MD
Adjunct Professor of Pediatrics, Uniformed Services University of the Health Sciences; Director, National Center on Sleep Disorders Research, National Heart, Lung, and Blood Institute, National Institutes of Health, Bethesda, Maryland
Sudden Infant Death Syndrome

Sunny Zaheed Hussain, MD
Fellow in Pediatric Gastroenterology, University of Pittsburgh School of Medicine; Children's Hospital of Pittsburgh, Pittsburgh, Pennsylvania
The Esophagus

Jeffrey Hyams, MD
Professor of Pediatrics, University of Connecticut School of Medicine; Head, Division of Digestive Diseases and Nutrition, Connecticut Children's Medical Center, Hartford, Connecticut
Inflammatory Bowel Disease; Food Allergy (Food Hypersensitivity); Eosinophilic Gastroenteritis; Malformations; Ascites; Peritonitis

Richard F. Jacobs, MD
Horace C. Cabe Professor of Pediatrics, University of Arkansas for Medical Sciences; Chief, Pediatric Infectious Diseases, Arkansas Children's Hospital, Little Rock, Arkansas
Actinomyces; *Nocardia*; Tularemia (*Francisella tularensis*); *Brucella*

Norman Jaffe, MD
Professor of Pediatrics, University of Texas M. D. Anderson Cancer Center, Houston, Texas
Neoplasms of the Kidney

Renée R. Jenkins, MD
Professor and Chair of Pediatrics, Howard University College of Medicine; Chair, Department of Pediatrics and Child Health, Howard University Hospital, Washington, DC
The Epidemiology of Adolescent Health Problems; Delivery of Health Care to Adolescents; Depression; Suicide; Violent Behavior; Substance Abuse; The Breast; Menstrual Problems; Contraception; Pregnancy; Sexually Transmitted Diseases

Hal B. Jenson, MD
Professor and Chair, Department of Pediatrics, Director, Center for Pediatric Research, Eastern Virginia Medical School and Children's Hospital of The King's Daughters; Senior Vice President for Academic Affairs, Children's Hospital of The King's Daughters, Norfolk, Virginia
Chronic Fatigue Syndrome; Epstein-Barr Virus; Lymphocytic Choriomeningitis Virus; Polyomaviruses; Human T-Cell Lymphotropic Viruses Types I and II

Chandy C. John, MD
Assistant Professor of Pediatrics, Case Western Reserve University School of Medicine; Division of Pediatric Infectious Diseases, Co-Director, Rainbow Center for International Child Health, Rainbow Babies and Children's Hospital, Cleveland, Ohio
Amebiasis; Trichomoniasis (*Trichomonas vaginalis*); Health Advice for Children Traveling Internationally

Charles F. Johnson, MD
Professor of Pediatrics, The Ohio State University; Children's Hospital, Columbus, Ohio
Abuse and Neglect of Children

Michael V. Johnston, MD
Professor of Neurology and Pediatrics, Kennedy Krieger Institute and The Johns Hopkins University School of Medicine, Baltimore, Maryland
Congenital Anomalies of the Central Nervous System; Seizures in Childhood; Conditions that Mimic Seizures; Movement Disorders; Encephalopathies; Neurodegenerative Disorders of Childhood; Acute Stroke Syndromes

Richard B. Johnston, Jr., MD
Professor of Pediatrics, University of Colorado School of Medicine; National Jewish Medical and Research Center, Denver, Colorado
Monocytes and Macrophages; The Complement System

Kenneth Lyons Jones, MD
Professor of Pediatrics, University of California, San Diego, School of Medicine; UCSD Medical Center, San Diego, California
Dysmorphology

Harry J. Kallas, MD
Associate Professor of Pediatric Critical Care Medicine, Pediatric Medical Director, Life Flight, University of California, Davis, School of Medicine; UC Davis Children's Hospital, Sacramento, California
Drowning and Near-Drowning

Lewis J. Kass, MD
Assistant Professor of Pediatrics, Albert Einstein College of Medicine; Children's Hospital at Montefiore, Bronx, New York
Obstructive Sleep Apnea and Hypoventilation

Mark A. Kay, MD, PhD
Departments of Pediatrics and Genetics, Stanford University, Stanford, California
Gene Therapy

Allesandra N. Kazura, MD
Assistant Professor of Psychiatry and Human Behavior, Brown University School of Medicine; Brown University Centers for Behavioral and Preventive Medicine, Providence, Rhode Island
Psychosomatic Illness

James W. Kazura, MD
Professor of Medicine, International Health, and Pathology, Case Western Reserve University School of Medicine; Attending Physician, University Hospitals of Cleveland, Cleveland, Ohio
Ascariasis (*Ascaris lumbricoides*); Trichuriasis (*Trichuris trichiura*); Enterobiasis (*Enterobius vermicularis*); Strongyloidiasis (*Strongyloides stercoralis*); Lymphatic Filariasis (*Brugia malayi, Brugia timori,* and *Wuchereria bancrofti*); Other Tissue Nematodes; Toxocariasis (Visceral and Ocular Larva Migrans); Trichinosis (*Trichinella spiralis*)

Desmond P. Kelly, MD
Clinical Associate Professor of Pediatrics, University of North Carolina School of Medicine; Director, Clinical Programs, All Kinds of Minds, Chapel Hill, North Carolina
Patterns of Development and Function

Kathi J. Kemper, MD, MPH
Professor of Pediatrics, Wake Forest University School of Medicine; Brenner Children's Hospital
Herbal Medicines

John A. Kerner, MD
Professor of Pediatrics, Director of Nutrition, Director of Pediatric Gastroenterology and Nutrition Fellowship, Stanford University School of Medicine; Director, Nutrition Support Team, Medical Director, Children's Home Pharmacy, Lucile Salter Packard Children's Hospital, Palo Alto, California
Malabsorptive Disorders

Seema Khan, MD
Assistant Professor of Pediatric Gastroenterology, University of Pittsburgh School of Medicine; Children's Hospital of Pittsburgh, Pittsburgh, Pennsylvania
The Esophagus

Charles H. King, MD
Associate Professor of Medicine and International Health, Case Western Reserve School of Medicine; Attending Physician, University Hospitals of Cleveland, Cleveland, Ohio
Schistosomiasis (*Schistosoma*); Flukes (Liver, Lung, and Intestinal)

Stephen Kinsman, MD
Assistant Professor of Pediatrics and Neurology, Director of Pediatric Neurology, University of Maryland School of Medicine, Baltimore, Maryland
Congenital Anomalies of the Central Nervous System

Bruce L. Klein, MD
Associate Professor of Pediatrics and Emergency Medicine, The George Washington University School of Medicine and Health Sciences; Medical Director, Pediatric Transport Service, Children's National Medical Center, Washington, DC
Acute Care of the Multiple Trauma Victim

Marisa S. Klein-Gitelman, MD, MPH
Assistant Professor of Pediatrics, Feinberg School of Medicine, Northwestern University; Interim Head, Division of Immunology/Rheumatology, Children's Memorial Hospital, Chicago, Illinois
Systemic Lupus Erythematosus

Robert M. Kliegman, MD
Professor and Chair, Department of Pediatrics, Medical College of Wisconsin; Pediatrician in Chief, Pam and Les Muma Chair in Pediatrics, Children's Hospital of Wisconsin, Milwaukee, Wisconsin
Mucopolysaccharidoses; Overview of Mortality and Morbidity; The Newborn Infant; High-Risk Pregnancies; The Fetus; The High-Risk Infant; Clinical Manifestations of Diseases in the Newborn Period; Nervous System Disorders; Delivery Room Emergencies; Respiratory Tract Disorders; Digestive System Disorders; Blood Disorders; Genitourinary System; The Umbilicus; Metabolic Disturbances; The Endocrine System

William C. Koch, MD
Associate Professor of Pediatrics, Virginia Commonwealth University; Division of Infectious Diseases, Medical College of Virginia, Richmond, Virginia
Parvovirus B19

Steve Kohl, MD
Clinical Professor of Pediatrics, Oregon Health and Sciences University, Portland, Oregon
Herpes Simplex Virus

Gerald P. Koocher, PhD
Dean, Graduate School for Health Studies, Simmons College, Boston, Massachusetts
Grief and Bereavement

Jill E. Korbin, PhD (Anthropology)
Professor of Anthropology, Associate Dean, College of Arts and Sciences, Case Western Reserve University; Co-Director, Schubert Center for Child Development, Cleveland, Ohio
Cultural Issues in Pediatric Care

Peter J. Krause, MD
Professor of Pediatrics, University of Connecticut School of Medicine; Director, Infectious Diseases, Connecticut Children's Medical Center, Hartford, Connecticut
Malaria (*Plasmodium*); Babesiosis (*Babesia*)

Marzena Krawiec, MD
Assistant Professor of Pediatrics, University of Wisconsin Medical School, Madison, Wisconsin
Wheezing in Infants

John F. Kuttesch, Jr., MD, PhD
Associate Professor of Pediatric Hematology/Oncology, Vanderbilt University Medical Center, Nashville, Tennessee
Brain Tumors in Childhood

Catherine S. Lachenauer, MD
Assistant Professor of Pediatrics, Harvard Medical School; Assistant in Medicine, Children's Hospital, Boston, Massachusetts
Group B Streptococcus

Stephan Ladisch, MD
Professor of Pediatrics and Biochemistry/Molecular Biology, The George Washington University School of Medicine; Scientific Director, Children's Research Institute, Children's National Medical Center, Washington, DC
Histiocytosis Syndromes of Childhood

Stephen LaFranchi, MD
Professor of Pediatrics, Oregon Health and Sciences University; Staff Physician, Doernbecher Children's Hospital, Portland, Oregon
Disorders of the Thyroid Gland

Oren Lakser, MD
Assistant Professor of Pediatrics, Northwestern University; Attending Physician, Division of Pulmonary Medicine, Children's Memorial Hospital, Chicago, Illinois
Parenchymal Disease with Prominent Hypersensitivity, Eosinophilic Infiltration, or Toxin-Mediated Injury; Slowly Resolving Pneumonia; Bronchiectasis; Pulmonary Abscess

Richard M. Lampe, MD
Professor and Chair, Department of Pediatrics, Texas Tech University School of Medicine, Lubbock, Texas
Osteomyelitis and Suppurative Arthritis

Philip J. Landrigan, MD
Ethel H. Wise Professor and Chair, Department of Community and Preventive Medicine, Mount Sinai School of Medicine, New York, New York
Chemical Pollutants

Charles T. Leach, MD
Professor of Pediatrics, Chief, Division of Infectious Diseases, University of Texas Health Science Center at San Antonio; Attending Physician, Christus Santa Rosa Children's Hospital and University Hospital, San Antonio, Texas
Roseola (Human Herpesviruses 6 and 7); Human Herpesvirus 8

Margaret W. Leigh, MD
Professor of Pediatrics, University of North Carolina; Attending Physician, University of North Carolina Hospitals, Chapel Hill, North Carolina
Sarcoidosis

Robert F. Lemanske, Jr., MD
Professor of Pediatrics and Medicine, University of Wisconsin School of Medicine, Madison, Wisconsin
Wheezing in Infants

Steven Lestrud, MD
Professor of Pediatrics, Feinberg School of Medicine, Northwestern University; Attending Physician, Pediatric Pulmonary and Critical Care, Chicago, Illinois
Bronchopulmonary Dysplasia

Donald Y. M. Leung, MD, PhD
Professor of Pediatrics, University of Colorado Health Sciences Center; Head, Division of Pediatric Allergy-Immunology, National Jewish Medical and Research Center, Denver, Colorado
Allergy and the Immunologic Basis of Atopic Disease; Diagnosis of Allergic Disease; Principles of Treatment of Allergic Disease; Allergic Rhinitis; Childhood Asthma; Atopic Dermatitis (Atopic Eczema); Urticaria and Angioedema (Hives); Anaphylaxis; Serum Sickness; Insect Allergy; Adverse Reactions to Foods

Lenore S. Levine, MD
Professor of Pediatrics, College of Physicians and Surgeons, Columbia University; Attending Pediatrician, New York Presbyterian Hospital, New York, New York
Disorders of the Adrenal Glands

Stephen Liben, MD
Associate Professor of Pediatrics, McGill University; Director, Palliative Care Program, The Montreal Children's Hospital of the McGill University Health Center, Montreal, Quebec, Canada
Pediatric Palliative Care: The Care of Children with Life-Limiting Illness

Iris F. Litt, MD
Marron and Mary Elisabeth Kendrick Professor of Pediatrics, Stanford University School of Medicine; Director, Division of Adolescent Medicine, Lucile Salter Packard Children's Hospital, Palo Alto, California
Anorexia Nervosa and Bulimia

Andrew H. Liu, MD
Associate Professor of Pediatric Allergy and Immunology, Training Program Director, National Jewish Medical and Research Center, University of Colorado Health Sciences Center, Denver, Colorado
Childhood Asthma

Sarah S. Long, MD
Professor of Pediatrics, Drexel University College of Medicine; Chief, Section of Infectious Diseases, St. Christopher's Hospital for Children, Philadelphia, Pennsylvania
Diphtheria (*Corynebacterium diphtheriae*); Pertussis (*Bordetella pertussis* and *B. parapertussis*)

Daniel J. Lovell, MD, MPH
Professor of Pediatrics, University of Cincinnati Medical Center; Associate Director, Division of Pediatric Rheumatology, Cincinnati Children's Hospital, Cincinnati, Ohio
Treatment of Rheumatic Diseases

G. Reid Lyon, PhD
Branch Chief, Child Development and Behavior, National Institute of Child Health and Human Development, National Institutes of Health, Rockville, Maryland
Specific Reading Disability (Dyslexia)

Joseph A. Majzoub, MD
Professor of Pediatrics, Harvard Medical School; Chief, Division of Endocrinology, Children's Hospital Boston, Boston, Massachusetts
Diabetes Insipidus; Other Abnormalities of Arginine Vasopressin Metabolism and Action

Yvonne Maldonado, MD
Associate Professor of Pediatrics, Stanford University School of Medicine; Attending Physician, Lucile Salter Packard Children's Hospital, Stanford, California
Measles; Rubella; Mumps

John C. Marini, MD, PhD
Chief, Heritable Disorders Branch, National Institute of Child Health and Human Development, National Institutes of Health, Bethesda, Maryland
Osteogenesis Imperfecta

Morri Markowitz, MD
Professor of Pediatrics, Albert Einstein College of Medicine; Attending Physician, Pediatrics, Division of Environmental Sciences, Children's Hospital at Montefiore, Montefiore Medical Center, Bronx, New York
Lead Poisoning

Reuben K. Matalon, MD
Professor of Pediatrics and Genetics, University of Texas Medical Branch, Galveston, Texas
Aspartic Acid (Canavan Disease)

Lawrence H. Mathers, MD, PhD
Assistant Professor of Pediatrics and Anatomy, Stanford University School of Medicine; Attending Physician, Lucile Salter Packard Children's Hospital, Stanford, California
Effective Communication with Families in the PICU; Pediatric Emergencies and Resuscitation; Shock; Transplantation Issues in the PICU; Withdrawal or Withholding of Life Support, Brain Death, and Organ Procurement

Nancy J. Matyunas, PharmD
Assistant Clinical Professor of Pediatrics, Adjunct Instructor in Pharmacology and Toxicology, University of Louisville, Louisville, Kentucky
Poisonings: Drugs, Chemicals, and Plants

Robert Mazor, MD
Fellow, Department of Pediatrics, Division of Cardiology, Feinberg School of Medicine, Northwestern University; Children's Memorial Hospital, Chicago, Illinois
Pulmonary Edema

Paul L. McCarthy, MD
Professor of Pediatrics, Yale University School of Medicine; Director, Division of General Pediatrics, Children's Hospital at Yale-New Haven, New Haven, Connecticut
The Well Child; Evaluation of the Sick Child in the Office and Clinic

Susanna A. McColley, MD
Associate Professor of Pediatrics, Feinberg School of Medicine, Northwestern University; Director, Cystic Fibrosis Center, Children's Memorial Hospital, Chicago, Illinois
Disorders of the Lungs and Lower Airways; Pulmonary Tumors; Extrapulmonary Diseases with Pulmonary Manifestations

Margaret M. McGovern, MD, PhD
Associate Professor of Human Genetics and Pediatrics, Mount Sinai School of Medicine; Attending Physician, Pediatrics, Mount Sinai Hospital, New York, New York
Lipidoses; Mucolipidoses; Disorders of Glycoprotein Degradation and Structure

Kenneth McIntosh, MD
Professor of Pediatrics, Harvard Medical School; Senior Associate in Medicine, Children's Hospital Boston, Boston, Massachusetts
Respiratory Syncytial Virus; Adenoviruses; Rhinoviruses

Rima McLeod, MD
Jules and Doris Stein Research to Prevent Blindness Professor, University of Chicago, Visual Sciences and Ophthalmology Department, Chicago, Illinois
Toxoplasmosis (*Toxoplasma gondii*)

Peter C. Melby, MD
Associate Professor of Medicine, Division of Infectious Diseases, The University of Texas Health Science Center; Staff Physician, Department of Veterans Affairs Medical Center, South Texas Veterans Health Care System, San Antonio, Texas
Leishmaniasis (*Leishmania*)

Fred A. Mettler, Jr., MD, MPH
Professor and Chair, Department of Radiology, University of New Mexico, Albuquerque, New Mexico
Pediatric Radiation Injuries

Marian G. Michaels, MD, MPH
Associate Professor of Pediatrics and Surgery, University of Pittsburgh School of Medicine; Children's Hospital of Pittsburgh, Pittsburgh, Pennsylvania
Infections in Immunocompromised Persons

Henry Milgrom, MD
Professor of Pediatrics, University of Colorado Health Sciences Center; Senior Faculty Member, National Jewish Medical and Research Center, Denver, Colorado
Allergic Rhinitis

Michael L. Miller, MD
Associate Professor of Pediatrics, Northwestern University Medical School; Children's Memorial Medical Center, Chicago, Illinois
Evaluation of Suspected Rheumatic Disease; Treatment of Rheumatic Diseases; Juvenile Rheumatoid Arthritis; Ankylosing Spondylitis and Other Spondyloarthropathies; Postinfectious Arthritis and Related Conditions; Systemic Lupus Erythematosus; Scleroderma; Vasculitis Syndromes; Musculoskeletal Pain Syndromes; Miscellaneous Conditions Associated with Arthritis

Robert R. Montgomery, MD
Professor of Pediatrics and Vice Chair of Research, Medical College of Wisconsin; Senior Investigator, Blood Center of Southeastern Wisconsin, Milwaukee, Wisconsin
Hemorrhagic and Thrombotic Diseases

Anna-Barbara Moscicki, MD
Professor of Pediatrics, University of California, San Francisco, School of Medicine, San Francisco, California
Human Papillomaviruses

Hugo W. Moser, MD
Professor of Neurology and Pediatrics, Kennedy Krieger Institute, The Johns Hopkins University School of Medicine, Baltimore, Maryland
Disorders of Very Long Chain Fatty Acids

Joseph L. Muenzer, MD
Associate Professor of Pediatrics, University of North Carolina School of Medicine, Chapel Hill, North Carolina
Mucopolysaccharidoses

Flor M. Munoz, MD
Assistant Professor of Pediatrics, Baylor College of Medicine; Texas Children's Hospital, Houston, Texas
Tuberculosis (*Mycobacterium tuberculosis*)

James R. Murphy, PhD
Pediatric Infectious Diseases, University of Texas Health Science Center, Houston, Texas
Cholera (*Vibrio cholerae*); *Campylobacter*, *Yersinia*; *Aeromonas* and *Plesiomonas*

Martin G. Myers, MD
Professor of Pediatrics, University of Texas Medical Branch; Children's Hospital, Galveston, Texas
Varicella-Zoster Virus

Robert D. Needlman, MD
Adjunct Associate Professor of Pediatrics, Case Western Reserve University School of Medicine; Attending Physician, MetroHealth Medical Center, Cleveland, Ohio
Growth and Development

Leonard B. Nelson, MD
Associate Professor of Ophthalmology and Pediatrics, Jefferson Medical College; Co-Director, Department of Pediatric Ophthalmology, Wills Eye Hospital, Philadelphia, Pennsylvania
Disorders of the Eye

Robert M. Nelson, MD, PhD
Associate Professor of Anesthesia and Pediatrics, University of Pennsylvania School of Medicine; Chair, Committees for the Protection of Human Subjects, Children's Hospital of Philadelphia, Philadelphia, Pennsylvania
Ethics in Pediatric Care

Vicky Lee Ng, MD
Assistant Professor of Pediatrics, University of Toronto; Staff Physician, Division of Gastroenterology and Nutrition, Pediatric Academic Multi-Organ Transplant (PAMOT) Program, Hospital for Sick Children, Toronto, Ontario, Canada
Manifestations of Liver Disease

John F. Nicholson, MD
Associate Professor of Pediatrics and Pathology, Columbia University; Associate Attending Pediatrician, Children's Hospital of New York-Presbyterian Hospital, New York, New York
Laboratory Testing in Infants and Children; Reference Ranges for Laboratory Tests and Procedures

Zehava Noah, MD
Associate Professor in Pediatrics, Feinberg School of Medicine, Northwestern University; Attending Physician, Children's Memorial Hospital, Chicago, Illinois
Chronic Severe Respiratory Insufficiency

Lawrence M. Nogee, MD
Associate Professor of Pediatrics, The Johns Hopkins University School of Medicine; Attending Neonatologist, Johns Hopkins Children's Center, Baltimore, Maryland
Pulmonary Alveolar Proteinosis; Inherited Disorders of Surfactant Protein Metabolism

Theresa J. Ochoa, MD
University of Texas-Houston Health Science Center; Pediatric Disease Fellow, Memorial Hermann Children's Hospital, Houston, Texas
Escherichia coli

Robin K. Ohls, MD
Associate Professor of Pediatrics, Division of Neonatology, University of New Mexico School of Medicine; Department of Pediatrics/Neonatology, Children's Hospital of New Mexico, Albuquerque, New Mexico
Development of the Hematopoietic System

Scott E. Olitsky, MD
Associate Professor of Ophthalmology, University of Missouri at Kansas City; Chief of Ophthalmology, The Children's Mercy Hospital, Kansas City, Missouri
Disorders of the Eye

Karen Olness, MD
Professor of Pediatrics, Family Medicine, and International Health, Case Western Reserve University School of Medicine; Director, Rainbow Center for International Child Health, Rainbow Babies and Children's Hospital, Cleveland, Ohio
Child Health in the Developing World

Susan Orenstein, MD
Professor and Chief, Pediatric Gastroenterology, University of Pittsburgh School of Medicine; Children's Hospital of Pittsburgh, Pittsburgh, Pennsylvania
The Esophagus

Gary D. Overturf, MD
Department of Pediatrics, University of New Mexico Medical Center, Albuquerque, New Mexico
Streptococcus pneumoniae (Pneumococcus)

Judith A. Owens, MD, MPH
Associate Professor of Pediatrics, Brown Medical School; Director, Pediatrics Sleep Disorders Clinic, Hasbro Children's Hospital, Providence, Rhode Island
Sleep Disorders

Lauren M. Pachman, MD
Professor of Pediatrics, Division of Immunology/Rheumatology, Feinberg School of Medicine, Northwestern University; Interim Division Head, Disease Pathogenesis Program, Children's Memorial Institute of Education and Research (CMIER), Children's Memorial Hospital, Chicago, Illinois
Juvenile Dermatomyositis; Vasculitis Syndromes

Regina M. Palazzo, MD
Assistant Professor of Pediatrics, Yale University School of Medicine; Director, Cystic Fibrosis Center, Attending Physician, Yale-New Haven Children's Hospital, New Haven, Connecticut
Diagnostic Approach to Respiratory Disease

Demosthenes Pappagianis, MD, PhD
Professor, Department of Medical Microbiology and Immunology, University of California, Davis, School of Medicine, Davis, California
Coccidioidomycosis (*Coccidioides immitis*)

Diane E. Pappas, MD
Associate Professor of Pediatrics, University of Virginia School of Medicine, Charlottesville, Virginia
Sinusitis; Retropharyngeal Abscess, Lateral Pharyngeal (Parapharyngeal) Abscess, and Peritonsillar Cellulitis/Abscess

Jack L. Paradise, MD
Professor of Pediatrics, Family Medicine, and Clinical Epidemiology, Professor of Otolaryngology, University of Pittsburgh School of Medicine; Attending Staff, Children's Hospital of Pittsburgh, Pittsburgh, Pennsylvania
Otitis Media

John S. Parks, MD, PhD
Professor of Pediatrics, Emory University School of Medicine; Director, Pediatric Endocrinology, Egleston Children's Hospital, Atlanta, Georgia
Hormones of the Hypothalamus and Pituitary; Hypopituitarism

Sheral S. Patel, MD
Assistant Professor of Pediatric Infectious Diseases, Case Western Reserve University School of Medicine; Attending Physician, Rainbow Babies and Children's Hospital, University Hospitals of Cleveland, Cleveland, Ohio
Ascariasis (*Ascaris lumbricoides*); Trichuriasis (*Trichuris trichiura*); Enterobiasis (*Enterobius vermicularis*); Strongyloidiasis (*Strongyloides stercoralis*); Lymphatic Filariasis (*Brugia malayi, Brugia timori,* and *Wuchereria bancrofti*); Other Tissue Nematodes; Toxocariasis (Visceral and Ocular Larva Migrans); Trichinosis (*Trichinella spiralis*)

Alberto Peña, MD
Professor of Surgery, Albert Einstein College of Medicine, Bronx, New York; Chief, Pediatric Surgery, Schneider Children's Hospital, North Shore Long Island Jewish Health System, New Hyde Park, New York
Surgical Conditions of the Anus, Rectum, and Colon

James M. Perrin, MD
Professor of Pediatrics, Harvard Medical School; Director, Division of General Pediatrics, Director, Center for Child and Adolescent Health Policy, Massachusetts General Hospital for Children, Boston, Massachusetts
Developmental Disabilities and Chronic Illness; Chronic Illness in Childhood

Michael A. Pesce, PhD
Columbia University College of Physicians and Surgeons; Director, Specialty Laboratory, New York-Presbyterian Hospital at Columbia Medical Center, New York, New York
Laboratory Testing in Infants and Children; Reference Ranges for Laboratory Tests and Procedures

Georges Peter, MD
Professor of Pediatrics, Vice Chair for Faculty Affairs, Brown Medical School; Director, Division of Pediatric Infectious Diseases, Rhode Island Hospital, Providence, Rhode Island
Immunization Practices

John Peters, DO
Assistant Professor of Pediatric Gastroenterology, University of Pittsburgh School of Medicine; Children's Hospital of Pittsburgh, Pittsburgh, Pennsylvania
The Esophagus

Ross E. Petty, MD, PhD
Professor and Head of Pediatrics, University of British Columbia; British Columbia Children's Hospital, Vancouver, Canada
Ankylosing Spondylitis and Other Spondyloarthropathies

Larry K. Pickering, MD
Professor of Pediatrics, Emory University School of Medicine; Senior Advisor to the Director, National Immunization Program, Centers for Disease Control and Prevention, Atlanta, Georgia

Giardiasis and Balantidiasis; Child Care and Communicable Diseases; Gastroenteritis; Viral Hepatitis

Dwight A. Powell, MD
Professor of Pediatrics, The Ohio State University College of Medicine and Public Health; Chief, Section of Pediatric Infectious Diseases, Children's Hospital, Columbus, Ohio

Hansen Disease (*Mycobacterium leprae*); Nontuberculous Mycobacteria; Mycoplasmal Infections

Keith R. Powell, MD
Professor and Chair, Department of Pediatrics, Northeastern Ohio Universities College of Medicine; Vice President and Dr. Noah Miller Chair of Medicine, Children's Hospital Medical Center, Akron, Ohio

Fever; Fever Without a Focus; Sepsis and Shock

Charles G. Prober, MD
Professor of Pediatrics, Medicine, Microbiology, and Immunology, Associate Chair of Pediatrics; Stanford University School of Medicine, Stanford, California

Pneumonia; Central Nervous System Infections

Keith Quirolo, MD
Associate Clinical Professor, Children's Hospital Oakland, Oakland, California

Hemoglobin Disorders

Daniel J. Rader, MD
Associate Professor of Medicine and Pathology, University of Pennsylvania School of Medicine; Director, Preventive Cardiovascular Medicine and Lipid Clinic, Philadelphia, Pennsylvania

Disorders of Lipoprotein Metabolism and Transport

Robert Rapaport, MD
Professor of Pediatrics, Director, Endocrinology and Diabetes, Mount Sinai School of Medicine, New York, New York

Disorders of the Gonads

Michael D. Reed, PharmD
Professor of Pediatrics, Case Western Reserve University School of Medicine; Director, Pediatric Clinical Pharmacology and Toxicology, Rainbow Babies and Children's Hospital, Cleveland, Ohio

Principles of Drug Therapy; Medications

Jack S. Remington, MD
Professor of Medicine, Division of Infectious Diseases and Geographic Medicine, Stanford University School of Medicine; Marcus A. Krupp Research Chair and Chairman, Department of Immunology and Infectious Diseases Research Institute, Palo Alto Medical Foundation, Palo Alto, California

Toxoplasmosis (*Toxoplasma gondii*)

Iraj Rezvani, MD
Professor of Pediatrics, Temple University School of Medicine; Chief, Section of Pediatric Endocrinology and Metabolism, Temple University Children's Medical Center, Philadelphia, Pennsylvania

An Approach to Inborn Errors of Metabolism; Phenylalanine; Tyrosine; Methionine; Cysteine/Cystine; Tryptophan; Valine, Leucine, Isoleucine, and Related Organic Acidemias; Glycine; Serine; Proline and Hydroxyproline; Glutamic Acid; Urea Cycle and Hyperammonemia (Arginine, Citrulline, Ornithine); Histidine; Lysine

Frederick P. Rivara, MD, MPH
George Adkins Professor of Pediatrics, Adjunct Professor of Epidemiology, Head, General Pediatrics, University of Washington, Seattle, Washington

Injury Control; Emergency Medical Services for Children

Kent A. Robertson, MD, PhD
Director, Stem Cell Transplantation, Royal Children's Hospital, Brisbane, Australia

Hematopoietic Stem Cell Transplantation

Luther K. Robinson, MD
Associate Professor of Pediatrics, State University of New York at Buffalo School of Medicine and Biomedical Sciences; Director, Dysmorphology and Clinical Genetics, Buffalo, New York

Marfan Syndrome

George C. Rodgers, Jr., MD, PhD
Professor of Pediatrics and Pharmacology/Toxicology, University of Louisville; Associate Medical Director, Kentucky Regional Poison Center, Kosair Children's Hospital, Louisville, Kentucky

Poisonings: Drugs, Chemicals, and Plants

Genie E. Roosevelt, MD, MPH
Assistant Professor of Pediatrics, University of Colorado Health Sciences; Attending Physician, The Children's Hospital, Denver, Colorado

Acute Inflammatory Upper Airway Obstruction

Carol L. Rosen, MD
Associate Professor of Pediatrics, Divisions of Clinical Epidemiology, Pulmonology, and Neurology, Case Western Reserve University School of Medicine; Director, Pediatric Sleep Services, Rainbow Babies and Children's Hospital, Cleveland, Ohio

Obstructive Sleep Apnea and Hypoventilation

David S. Rosenblatt, MDCM
Professor of Human Genetics, Medicine, Pediatrics, and Biology, McGill University; Royal Victoria Hospital, Montreal, Quebec, Canada

Methionine; Valine, Leucine, Isoleucine, and Related Organic Acidemias

Anne H. Rowley, MD
Professor of Pediatrics and of Microbiology/Immunology, Feinberg School of Medicine, Northwestern University; Attending Physician, Division of Infectious Diseases, Children's Memorial Hospital, Chicago, Illinois

Kawasaki Disease

Ranna A. Rozenfeld, MD
Assistant Professor of Pediatrics, Feinberg School of Medicine, Northwestern University; Attending Physician, Pediatric Critical Care Medicine, Children's Memorial Hospital, Chicago, Illinois

Atelectasis

Jeffrey A. Rudolph, MD
Research Instructor, Cincinnati Children's Hospital Medical Center, Cincinnati, Ohio

Metabolic Diseases of the Liver; Reye Syndrome and the Mitochondrial Hepatopathies

Robert A. Salata, MD
Professor and Vice-Chair, Department of Medicine, Chief, Division of Infectious Diseases, Case Western Reserve University School of Medicine; Attending Physician and Consultant, University Hospitals of Cleveland, Cleveland, Ohio

Amebiasis; Trichomoniasis (*Trichomonas vaginalis*); African Trypanosomiasis (Sleeping Sickness; *Trypanosoma brucei* complex); American Trypanosomiasis (Chagas Disease; *Trypanosoma cruzi*); Health Advice for Children Traveling Internationally

Denise A. Salerno, MD
Assistant Professor of Pediatrics, Temple University School of Medicine; Attending Pediatrician, Temple University Children's Medical Center, Temple University Hospital, Philadelphia, Pennsylvania

Nonbacterial Food Poisoning

Hugh A. Sampson, MD
Professor of Pediatrics and Immunobiology, Mount Sinai School of Medicine; Attending Staff, Mount Sinai Hospital, New York, New York

Anaphylaxis; Adverse Reactions to Foods

Joseph S. Sanfilippo, MD
Professor of Obstetrics, Gynecology, and Reproductive Sciences, Vice-Chair, Reproductive Sciences, University of Pittsburgh School of Medicine; Magee-Women's Hospital, Pittsburgh, Pennsylvania

Gynecologic Problems of Childhood

Harvey B. Sarnat, MD
Professor of Pediatrics (Neurology) and Pathology (Neuropathology), University of California, Los Angeles, School of Medicine; Director, Division of Pediatric Neurology, Neuropathologist, Cedars-Sinai Medical Center, Los Angeles, California

Neuromuscular Disorders

Shigeru Sassa, MD, PhD
Head, Laboratory of Biochemical Hematology, The Rockefeller University, New York, New York

The Porphyrias

Robert Schechter, MD
Clinical Director, Infant Botulism Treatment and Prevention Program, California Department of Health Services, Berkeley; Staff Physician, Children's Hospital, Oakland, California

Botulism (*Clostridium botulinum*)

Gordon E. Schutze, MD
Professor of Pediatrics and Pathology, University of Arkansas for Medical Sciences; Pediatric Residency Program Director, Arkansas Children's Hospital, Little Rock, Arkansas

Actinomyces; *Nocardia*; Tularemia (*Francisella tularensis*); *Brucella*

Jeffrey Schwimmer, MD
Assistant Professor of Pediatrics, Division of Gastroenterology, Hepatology, and Nutrition, University of California, San Diego, School of Medicine; Attending Physician, Gastroenterology, Hepatology, and Nutrition, Children's Hospital and Health Center, San Diego, California

Liver Abscess; Liver Disease Associated with Systemic Disorders

J. Paul Scott, MD
Professor of Pediatrics, Medical College of Wisconsin; Investigator, Blood Center of Southeastern Wisconsin, Milwaukee, Wisconsin

Hemorrhagic and Thrombotic Diseases

Theodore C. Sectish, MD
Assistant Professor of Pediatrics, Stanford University School of Medicine; Director, Residency Training Program in Pediatrics, Director, Pediatric Clerkship, Lucile Salter Packard Children's Hospital, Palo Alto, California

Preventive Pediatrics; Pneumonia

George B. Segel, MD
Professor of Pediatrics and Medicine, Vice-Chair, Department of Pediatrics, University of Rochester Medical Center, Rochester, New York

Definitions and Classification of Hemolytic Anemias; Hereditary Spherocytosis; Hereditary Elliptocytosis; Hereditary Stomatocytosis; Other Membrane Defects; Enzymatic Defects; Hemolytic Anemias Resulting from Extracellular Factors; Hemolytic Anemias Secondary to Other Extracellular Factors

Jane F. Seward, MBBS, MPH
Chief, Viral Vaccine Preventable Diseases Branch, National Immunization Program, Centers for Disease Control and Prevention, Atlanta, Georgia

Varicella-Zoster Virus

Bruce K. Shapiro, MD
Associate Professor of Pediatrics, The Johns Hopkins University School of Medicine; Vice-President, Training, Kennedy Krieger Institute, Baltimore, Maryland

Mental Retardation

Eugene D. Shapiro, MD
Professor of Pediatrics, Epidemiology, and Investigative Medicine, Yale University School of Medicine, Children's Clinical Research Center; Attending Pediatrician, Children's Hospital at Yale-New Haven, New Haven, Connecticut

Lyme Disease (*Borrelia burgdorferi*)

Bennett A. Shaywitz, MD
Professor of Pediatrics, Neurology, and Child Study Center; Co-Director, Yale Center for the Study of Learning and Attention, Department of Pediatrics, New Haven, Connecticut

Specific Reading Disability (Dyslexia)

Sally E. Shaywitz, MD
Professor of Pediatrics and Child Study Center; Co-Director, Yale Center for the Study of Learning and Attention, Department of Pediatrics, New Haven, Connecticut

Specific Reading Disability (Dyslexia)

Joel Shilyansky, MD
Assistant Professor of Surgery, Division of Pediatric Surgery, Medical College of Wisconsin; Pediatric Surgeon, Children's Hospital of Wisconsin, Milwaukee, Wisconsin

Tumors of the Digestive Tract

Benjamin L. Shneider, MD
Associate Professor of Pediatrics, Chief, Division of Pediatric Hepatology, Mount Sinai School of Medicine; Deputy Director, Pediatric Liver Transplantation, Mount Sinai Medical Center, New York, New York

Autoimmune (Chronic) Hepatitis

Stanford T. Shulman, MD
Professor of Pediatrics, Feinberg School of Medicine, Northwestern University; Head, Division of Infectious Diseases, Children's Memorial Hospital, Chicago, Illinois
Kawasaki Disease

Scott H. Sicherer, MD
Assistant Professor of Pediatrics, Jaffe Food Allergy Institute, Division of Pediatric Allergy and Immunology, Mount Sinai School of Medicine, New York, New York
Serum Sickness; Insect Allergy

Robert Sidbury, MD
Assistant Professor of Pediatrics, Division of Dermatology, University of Washington School of Medicine; Children's Hospital and Regional Medical Center, Seattle, Washington
The Skin

Mark D. Simms, MD, MPH
Professor of Pediatrics, Chief, Section of Developmental Pediatrics, Medical College of Wisconsin; Medical Director, Child Development Center, Children's Hospital of Wisconsin, Milwaukee, Wisconsin
Attention-Deficit/Hyperactivity Disorder; Adoption; Foster Care

Eric A. F. Simoes, MD, DCh
Professor of Pediatrics, Section of Infectious Diseases, University of Colorado School of Medicine; Professor of Pediatric Infectious Diseases and Tropical Child Health, Imperial College, London, United Kingdom; The Children's Hospital, Denver, Colorado
Polioviruses

Daniel Sloniewsky, MD
Assistant Professor of Pediatrics, State University of New York, Stony Brook; Stony Brook University Hospital, Stony Brook, New York
Pulmonary Hemorrhage, Embolism, and Infarction

John D. Snyder, MD
Professor of Pediatrics, University of California, San Francisco, School of Medicine, San Francisco, California
Gastroenteritis; Viral Hepatitis

Joseph D. Spahn, MD
Associate Professor of Pediatrics, National Jewish Medical and Research Center, University of Colorado Health Sciences Center; Staff Physician, National Jewish Medical and Research Center, Denver, Colorado
Childhood Asthma

Mark A. Sperling, MD
Professor of Pediatrics, University of Pittsburgh School of Medicine; Division of Endocrinology, Diabetes, and Metabolism, Children's Hospital of Pittsburgh, Pittsburgh, Pennsylvania
Hypoglycemia

Brian Stafford, MD, MPH
Assistant Professor of Psychiatry and Pediatrics, Section of Infant, Child, and Adolescent Psychiatry, Department of Psychiatry and Neurology, Tulane University School of Medicine, New Orleans, Louisiana
Anxiety Disorders

Sergio Stagno, MD
Professor and Chair, Department of Pediatrics, University of Alabama at Birmingham; Physician-in-Chief, Children's Hospital of Alabama, Birmingham, Alabama
Cytomegalovirus

Lawrence R. Stanberry, MD, PhD
Professor and Chair of Pediatrics, University of Texas Medical Branch, Galveston, Texas
Varicella-Zoster Virus

Charles A. Stanley, MD
Professor of Pediatrics, University of Pennsylvania; Chief, Division of Endocrinology/Diabetes, Children's Hospital of Philadelphia, Philadelphia, Pennsylvania
Disorders of Mitochondrial Fatty Acid Oxidation

Jeffrey R. Starke, MD
Professor of Pediatrics, Baylor College of Medicine; Chief, Pediatrics, Ben Taub General Hospital, Houston, Texas
Tuberculosis (*Mycobacterium tuberculosis*)

Madelyn M. Stazzone, MD
Assistant Professor of Pediatric Radiology, University of New Mexico School of Medicine, Albuquerque, New Mexico
Pediatric Radiation Injuries

Barbara W. Stechenberg, MD
Professor of Pediatrics, Tufts University School of Medicine, Boston; Director, Pediatric Infectious Diseases, Baystate Medical Center Children's Hospital, Springfield, Massachusetts
Bartonella

Barbara J. Stoll, MD
Professor of Pediatrics, Emory University School of Medicine, Atlanta, Georgia
Overview of Mortality and Morbidity; The Newborn Infant; High-Risk Pregnancies; The Fetus; The High-Risk Infant; Clinical Manifestations of Diseases in the Newborn Period; Nervous System Disorders; Delivery Room Emergencies; Respiratory Tract Disorders; Digestive System Disorders; Blood Disorders; Genitourinary System; The Umbilicus; Metabolic Disturbances; The Endocrine System; Infections of the Neonatal Infant

Anne Stormorken, MD
Assistant Professor of Pediatrics, Northeastern Ohio Universities College of Medicine; Associate Medical Director, Pediatric Intensive Care Unit, Children's Hospital Medical Center, Akron, Ohio
Sepsis and Shock

Ronald G. Strauss, MD
Professor of Pathology and Pediatrics, University of Iowa College of Medicine; Medical Director, DeGowin Blood Center, University of Iowa Hospitals and Clinics, Iowa City, Iowa
Risks of Blood Component Transfusions

Frederick J. Suchy, MD
Professor and Chair, Department of Pediatrics, Mount Sinai School of Medicine; Pediatrician-in-Chief, Mount Sinai Hospital, New York, New York
Autoimmune (Chronic) Hepatitis; Drug- and Toxin-Induced Liver Injury; Fulminant Hepatic Failure; Cystic Diseases of the Biliary Tract and Liver; Diseases of the Gallbladder; Portal Hypertension and Varices

Francisco A. Sylvester, MD
Assistant Professor, University of Connecticut School of Medicine; Pediatric Gastroenterologist, Connecticut Children's Medical Center, Hartford, Connecticut
Peptic Ulcer Disease

Andrew M. Tershakovec, MD
Associate Professor of Pediatrics, University of Pennsylvania
School of Medicine; Associate Physician, Children's Hospital of
Philadelphia, Philadelphia, Pennsylvania
Disorders of Lipoprotein Metabolism and Transport

George H. Thompson, MD
Professor of Orthopedic Surgery and Pediatrics, Case Western
Reserve University School of Medicine; Director, Pediatric
Orthopedics, Rainbow Babies and Children's Hospital,
Cleveland, Ohio
Growth and Development; Evaluation of the Child; The Foot and Toes;
Torsional and Angular Deformities; Leg-Length Discrepancy; The Knee;
The Hip; The Spine; The Neck; The Upper Limb; Arthrogryposis; Common
Fractures

Norman Tinanoff, DDS
Professor and Chair, Department of Pediatric Dentistry,
University of Maryland Dental School, Baltimore, Maryland
The Oral Cavity

James K. Todd, MD
Professor of Pediatrics, Microbiology, and Preventive
Medicine/Biometrics, University of Colorado School of
Medicine; Children's Hospital of Denver, Denver,
Colorado
Staphylococcus

Lucy Tompkins, MD, PhD
Professor of Medicine (Infectious Diseases) and Microbiology
and Immunology, Chief, Division of Infectious Diseases and
Geographic Medicine, Stanford University School of Medicine;
Director, Hospital Epidemiology and Infection Control Program,
Stanford Hospital and Clinics
Legionella

Kristine Torjesen, MD, MPH
Adjunct Assistant Professor of Pediatrics, Case Western Reserve
University School of Medicine; Program Director, Laos Training
Project, Health Frontiers, Cleveland, Ohio
Child Health in the Developing World

David G. Tubergen, MD
Professor of Pediatrics, University of Texas M. D. Anderson
Cancer Center; Medical Director, M. D. Anderson Physicians
Network, Houston, Texas
The Leukemias

Ronald B. Turner, MD
Professor of Pediatrics, University of Virginia School of
Medicine, Charlottesville, Virginia
The Common Cold; Acute Pharyngitis

Rodrigo E. Urizar, MD
Professor of Pediatrics, Nephrology, Director of Pediatric
Dialysis Services, Albany Medical College, Union University;
Attending Pediatric Nephrologist, Children's Hospital, Albany
Medical Center, Albany, New York
Renal Transplantation

Charles P. Venditti, MD, PhD
Fellow, Human Genetics and Molecular Biology, University of
Pennsylvania School of Medicine; Children's Hospital of
Philadelphia, Philadelphia, Pennsylvania
Disorders of Mitochondrial Fatty Acid Oxidation

Elliott Vichinsky, MD
Adjunct Professor, University of California, San Francisco,
School of Medicine; Director, Hematology/Oncology,
Children's Hospital and Research Center, Oakland,
California
Hemoglobin Disorders

Beth A. Vogt, MD
Associate Professor of Pediatrics, Case Western Reserve
University School of Medicine; Attending Pediatric
Nephrologist, Rainbow Babies and Children's Hospital,
Cleveland, Ohio
Conditions Particularly Associated with Proteinuria; Toxic Nephropathy;
Cortical Necrosis; Renal Failure

Martin E. Weisse, MD
Professor of Pediatrics, Director, Pediatric Residency Program,
Chief, Pediatric Infectious Diseases, West Virginia University,
Morgantown, West Virginia
Candida; Malassezia; Primary Amebic Meningoencephalitis

Steven L. Werlin, MD
Professor of Pediatrics, Medical College of Wisconsin; Children's
Hospital of Wisconsin, Milwaukee, Wisconsin
Exocrine Pancreas

Michael R. Wessels, MD
Professor of Pediatrics, Harvard Medical School; Chief, Division
of Infectious Diseases, Children's Hospital, Boston,
Massachusetts
Group B Streptococcus

Ralph F. Wetmore, MD
Professor of Otorhinolaryngology/Head and Neck Surgery,
University of Pennsylvania School of Medicine; Associate
Surgeon, Children's Hospital of Pennsylvania, Philadelphia,
Pennsylvania
Tonsils and Adenoids

Randall C. Wetzell, MB, BS, MBA
Professor of Pediatrics and Anesthesiology, Keck School of
Medicine, University of Southern California; Chair,
Anesthesiology Critical Care Medicine, Children's Hospital
Los Angeles, Los Angeles, California
Anesthesia and Perioperative Care

Perrin C. White, MD
Professor of Pediatrics, University of Texas Southwestern;
Director, Pediatric Endocrinology, Southwestern Medical
Center at Dallas, Dallas, Texas
Disorders of the Adrenal Glands

Glenna B. Winnie, MD
Associate Professor of Pediatrics, University of Pittsburgh
School of Medicine; Chief, Pulmonary Division, Children's
Hospital of Pittsburgh, Pittsburgh, Pennsylvania
Emphysema and Overinflation; α_1-Antitrypsin Deficiency and Emphysema;
Pleurisy; Pneumothorax; Pneumomediastinum; Hydrothorax; Hemothorax;
Chylothorax

Charles R. Woods, MD
Associate Professor of Pediatrics, Wake Forest University School
of Medicine; Brenner Children's Hospital, Winston-Salem,
North Carolina
Neisseria meningitidis (Meningococcus)

Laura L. Worth, MD, PhD
Assistant Professor of Pediatrics and Cancer Biology, University of Texas M. D. Anderson Cancer Center, Houston, Texas
Molecular and Cellular Biology of Cancer

Peter Wright, MD
Professor of Pediatrics, Microbiology and Immunology, and Pathology, Vanderbilt University School of Medicine, Nashville, Tennessee
Influenza Viruses; Parainfluenza Viruses

David T. Wyatt, MD
Professor of Pediatrics, Section of Endocrinology and Diabetes, Medical College of Wisconsin; Chief, Pediatric Endocrinology, Children's Hospital of Wisconsin, Milwaukee, Wisconsin
Diabetes Mellitus in Children

Robert Wyllie, MD
Chair, Department of Pediatric Gastroenterology, The Cleveland Clinic Foundation, Cleveland, Ohio
Clinical Manifestations of Gastrointestinal Disease; Normal Development, Structure, and Function; Pyloric Stenosis and Congenital Anomalies of the Stomach; Intestinal Atresia, Stenosis, and Malrotation; Intestinal Duplications, Meckel Diverticulum, and Other Remnants of the Omphalomesenteric Duct; Motility Disorders and Hirschsprung Disease; Ileus, Adhesions, Intussusception, and Closed-Loop Obstructions; Foreign Bodies and Bezoars; Recurrent Abdominal Pain of Childhood

Ram Yogev, MD
Professor of Pediatrics, Northwestern University Medical School; Director, Section on Pediatrics, Adolescent and Maternal HIV Infection, Children's Memorial Hospital, Chicago, Illinois
Acquired Immunodeficiency Syndrome (Human Immunodeficiency Virus)

Nader Youssef, MD
Fellow, Pediatric Gastroenterology, University of Pittsburgh School of Medicine; Children's Hospital of Pittsburgh, Pittsburgh, Pennsylvania
The Esophagus

Anita K. M. Zaidi, MBBS, SM
Associate Professor of Pediatrics and Microbiology, Aga Khan University; Consultant, Pediatric Infectious Diseases, Aga Khan University Hospital, Karachi, Pakistan
Diagnostic Microbiology

Lonnie K. Zelter, MD
Professor of Pediatrics, Anesthesiology and Psychiatry and Biobehavioral Sciences, David Geffen School of Medicine, University of California, Los Angeles; Director, Pediatric Pain Program, Mattel Children's Hospital at UCLA, Los Angeles, California
Pediatric Pain Management

Barry Zuckerman, MD
Professor and Chair, Department of Pediatrics, Boston University School of Medicine; Boston Medical Center, Boston, Massachusetts
Impact of Violence on Children

Contents

Part XVI Infectious Diseases 835

Part XVIII   The Respiratory System   1357

Part XXVIII Disorders of the Eye 2083

Scott E. Olitsky and Leonard B. Nelson

Part XXIX The Ear 2127

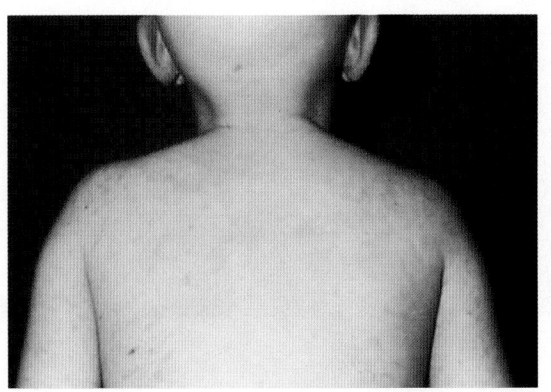

Figure 127–1

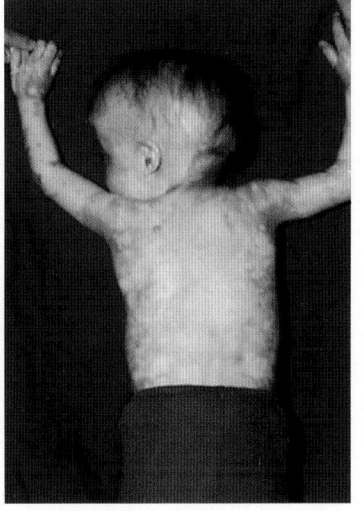

Figure 127–2

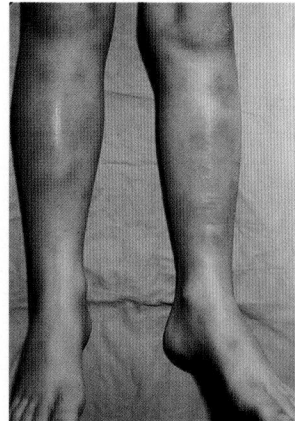

Figure 143–1

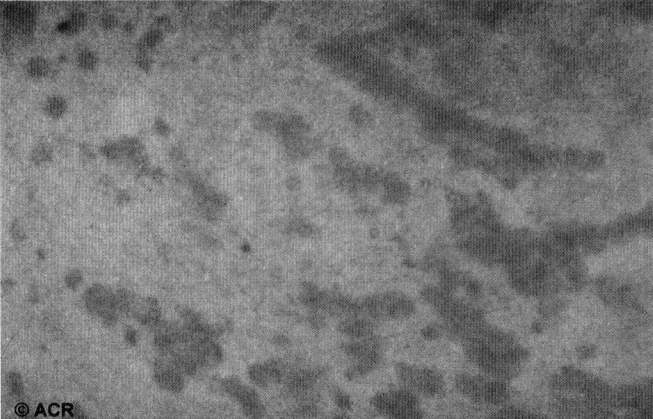

Figure 145–8

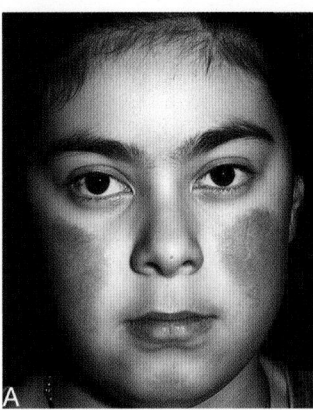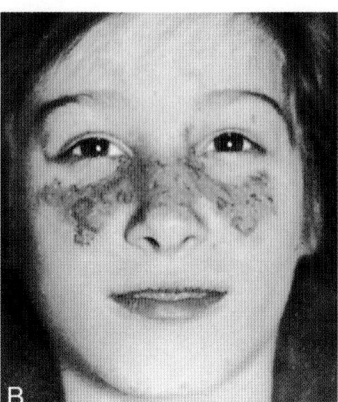

Figure 148–1

FIGURE 127–1. Acute graft versus host disease of the skin with ear, arm, shoulder, and trunk involvement. (Courtesy of Evan Farmer, MD.)

FIGURE 127–2. Chronic graft versus host disease of the skin with sclerodermoid changes. (Courtesy of Evan Farmer, MD.)

FIGURE 143–1. Erythematous nodules and plaques are present over both shins. The skin overlying the lesions is red, smooth, and shiny. The nodules are usually tender. Erythema nodosum is considered a hypersensitivity reaction and can be associated with a variety of diseases, including sarcoidosis, group A streptococcus infection, tuberculosis, coccidioidomycosis, and ulcerative colitis. (Reprinted from the Clinical Slide Collection on the Rheumatic Diseases; Copyright 1991, 1995, 1997. Used by permission of the American College of Rheumatology.)

FIGURE 145–8. The rash of systemic-onset juvenile rheumatoid arthritis. The rash is salmon colored, macular, and nonpruritic. Individual lesions are transient and occur in crops over the trunk and extremities. (Reprinted from the Clinical Slide Collection on the Rheumatic Diseases; Copyright 1991, 1995, 1997. Used by permission of the American College of Rheumatology.)

FIGURE 148–1. The butterfly rash of systemic lupus erythematosus. The rash can vary from an erythematous blush (*A*) to thickened epidermis to scaly patches (*B*).

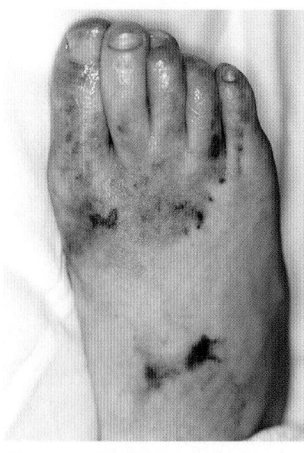

Figure 148–4

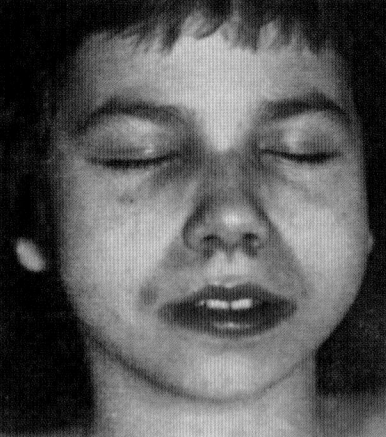

Figure 149–1

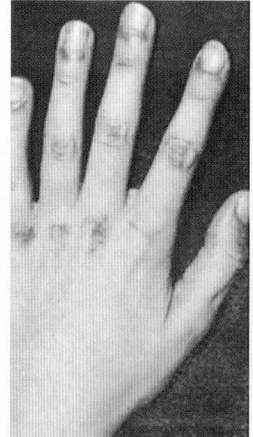

Figure 149–2

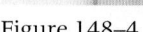

Figure 157–2

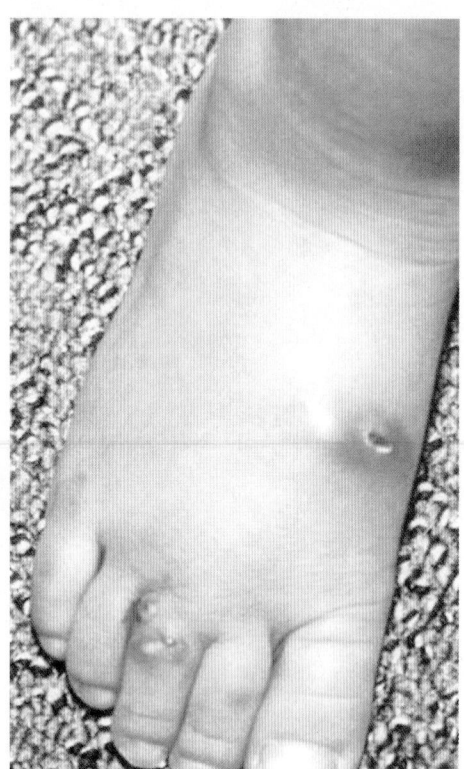

Figure 175–1

FIGURE 148–4. A 12-yr-old girl with systemic lupus erythematosus and antiphospholipid antibodies with painful cutaneous vasculitis of the right foot. Arterial thrombosis documented by angiography resulted in cyanosis of the large toe. Symptoms resolved with treatment with heparin and corticosteroids.

FIGURE 149–1. The facial rash of juvenile dermatomyositis. There is erythema over the bridge of the nose and malar areas, with violaceous (heliotropic) discoloration of the upper eyelids.

FIGURE 149–2. The rash of juvenile dermatomyositis. The skin over the metacarpal and proximal interphalangeal joints may be hypertrophic and pale red (Gottron papules).

FIGURE 157–2. Henoch-Schönlein purpura. (From Korting GW: *Hautkrankheiten bei Kindern und Jugendlichen,* 3rd ed. Stuttgart, FK Schattauer Verlag, 1982.)

FIGURE 175–1. A 2-yr-old female with multiple pustules on the dorsum of the right foot caused by *Nocardia brasiliensis.* (Photograph courtesy of Jaime E. Fergie, MD.)

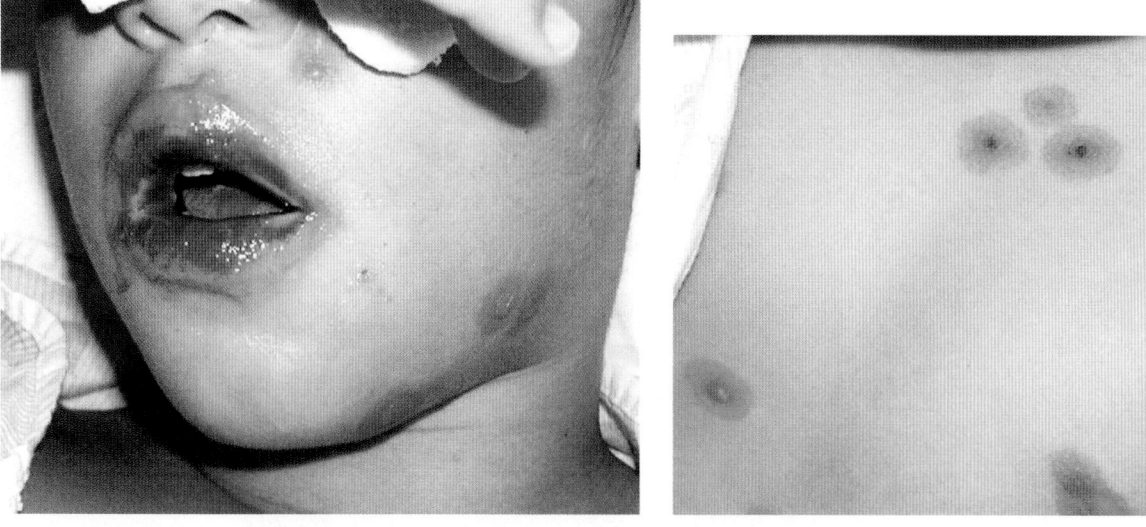

Figure 205–1

Figure 205–2

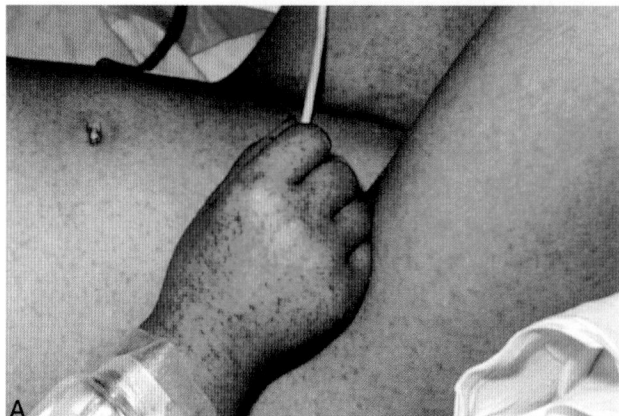
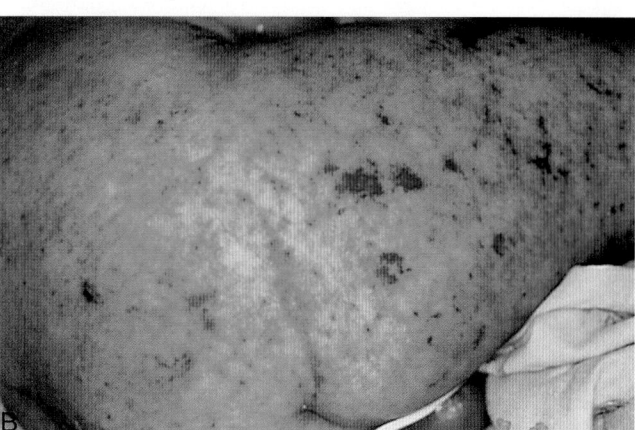

Figure 210–1

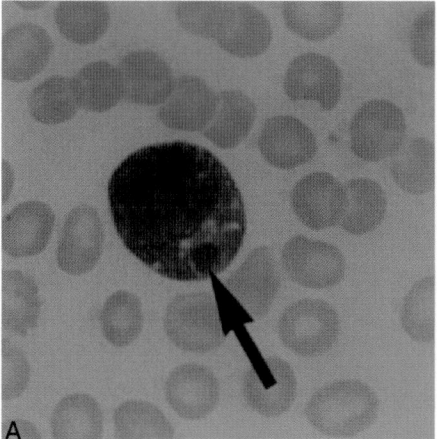
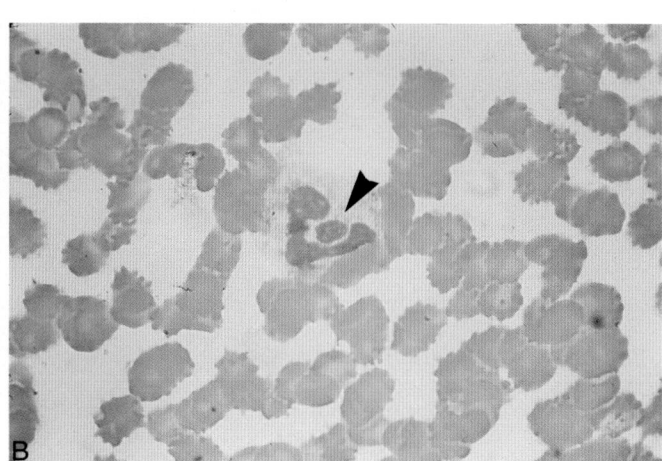

Figure 213–1

FIGURE 205–1. Lip changes found in Stevens-Johnson syndrome associated with *Mycoplasma pneumoniae* infection.

FIGURE 205–2. Classic erythema multiforme skin lesions found in Stevens-Johnson syndrome associated with *Mycoplasma pneumoniae* infection.

FIGURE 210–1. Patient with Rocky Mountain spotted fever. *A*, Rash early in the illness that is prominent on the extremities. *B*, Later in the course of Rocky Mountain spotted fever, the rash may become hemorrhagic or purpuric. (Courtesy of Debra Karp Skopicki, MD.)

FIGURE 213–1. Morulae in peripheral blood leukocytes in patients with HME and anaplasmosis. *A*, A morula *(arrow)* containing *Ehrlichia chaffeensis* in a monocyte. *B*, A morula *(arrowhead)* containing *Anaplasma phagocytophilum* in a neutrophil. Wright stains, original magnifications ×1,200. *Ehrlichia chaffeensis* and *A. phagocytophilum* have similar morphologies but are serologically and genetically distinct.

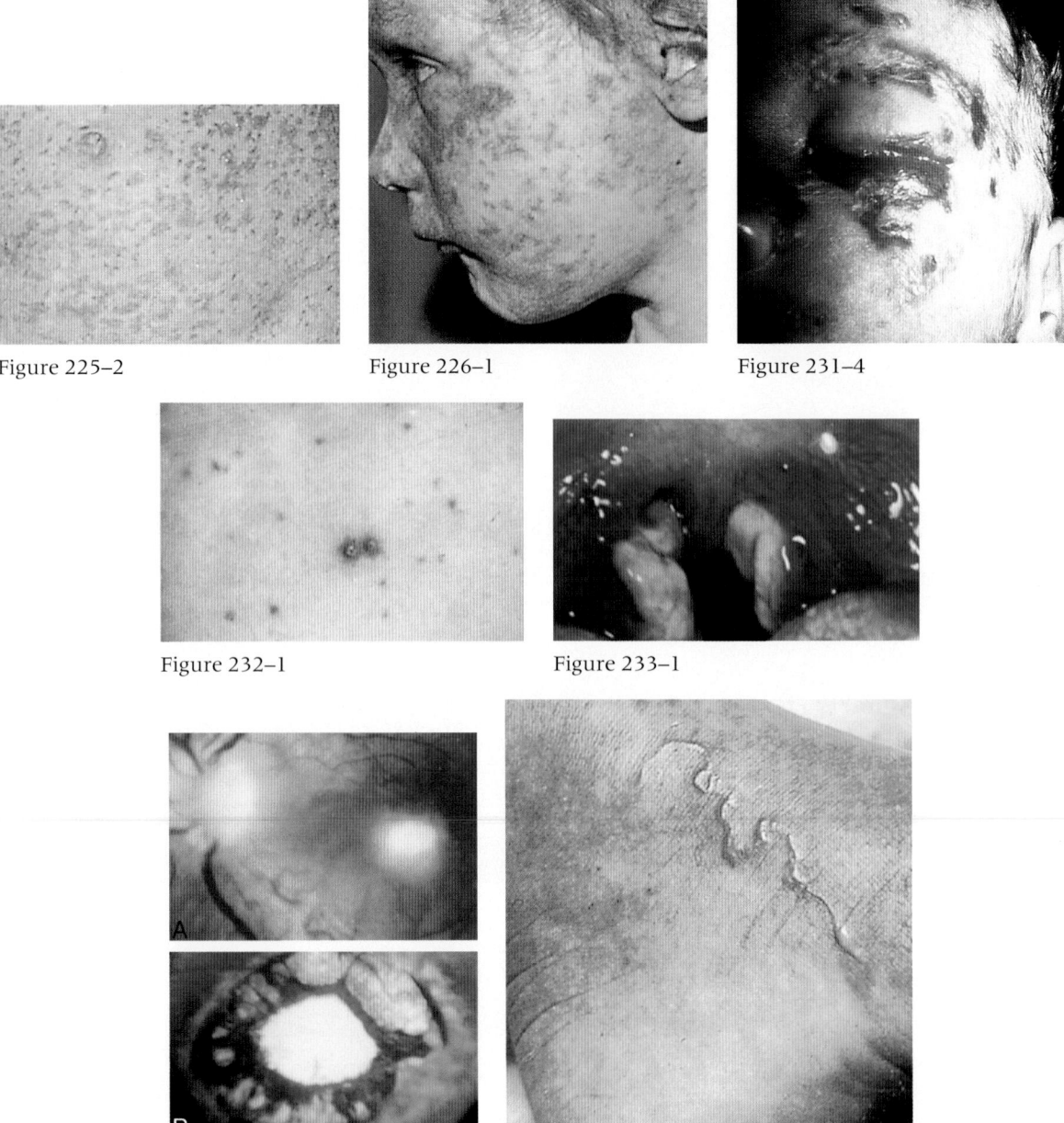

Figure 225–2   Figure 226–1   Figure 231–4

Figure 232–1   Figure 233–1

Figure 266–2   Figure 269–2

FIGURE 225–2. Maculopapular rash of measles. (From Korting GW: *Hautkrankheiten bei Kindern und Jugendlichen*, 3rd ed. Stuttgart, FK Schattauer Verlag, 1982.)

FIGURE 226–1. Rash of rubella (German measles). (From Korting GW: *Hautkrankheiten bei Kindern und Jugendlichen*, 3rd ed. Stuttgart, FK Schattauer Verlag, 1982.)

FIGURE 231–4. Vesicular-pustular lesions on the face of a neonate with herpes simplex virus infection. (From Kohl S: Neonatal herpes simplex virus infection. *Clin Perinatol* 1997;24:129–50.)

FIGURE 232–1. Skin lesions of chickenpox. Note the varying stages of development (macules, papules, and vesicles) present at the same time. (Courtesy of PF Lucchesi.)

FIGURE 233–1. Tonsillitis with membrane formation in infectious mononucleosis. (Courtesy of Alex J. Steigman, MD.)

FIGURE 266–2. Toxoplasmic chorioretinitis. *A,* Active acute lesion by indirect ophthalmoscopy. *B,* The healed foci of toxoplasmic chorioretinitis may resemble a colobomatous defect (macular pseudocoloboma). (*B,* adapted from Desmonts G, Remington J: Congenital toxoplasmosis. In Remington JS, Klein JO [editors]: *Infectious Diseases of the Fetus and Newborn Infant*, 5th ed. Philadelphia, WB Saunders, 2001.)

FIGURE 269–2. Creeping eruption of cutaneous larva migrans. (From Korting GW: *Hautkrankheiten bei Kindern und Jugendlichen*. Stuttgart, FK Schattauer Verlag, 1969.)

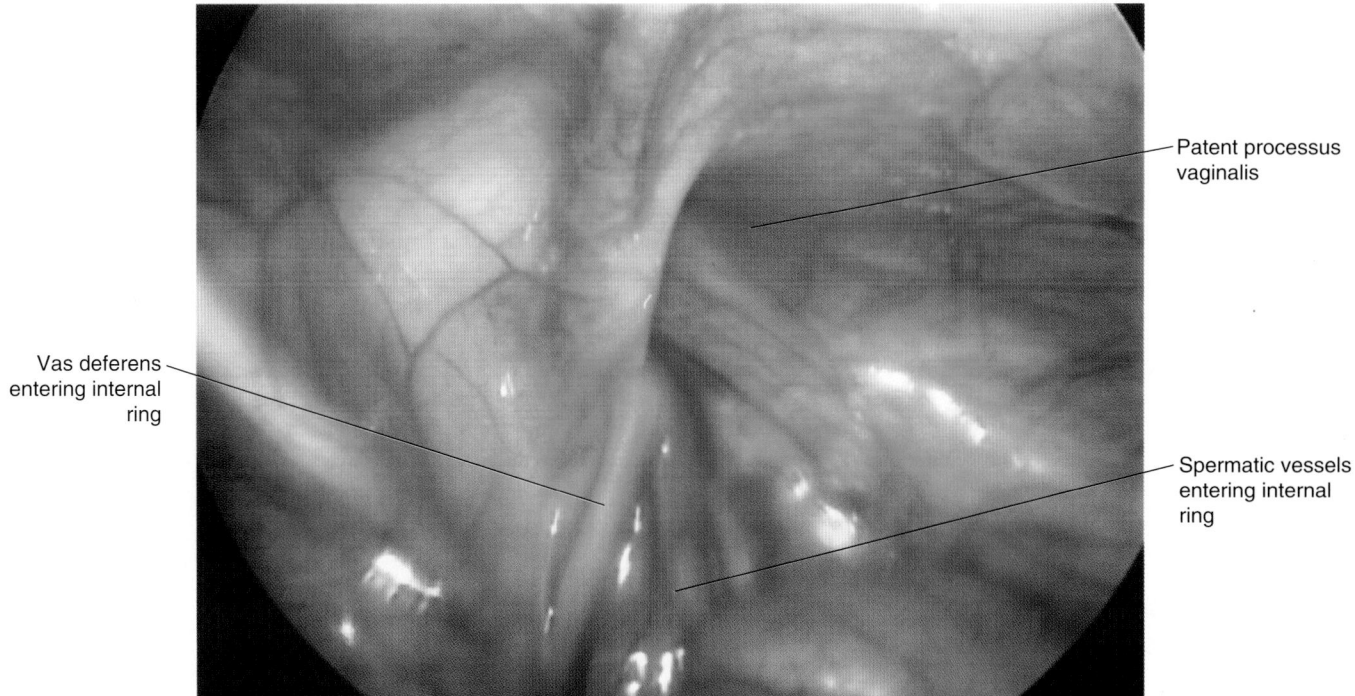

Patent processus
vaginalis

Vas deferens
entering internal
ring

Spermatic vessels
entering internal
ring

Figure 327–2

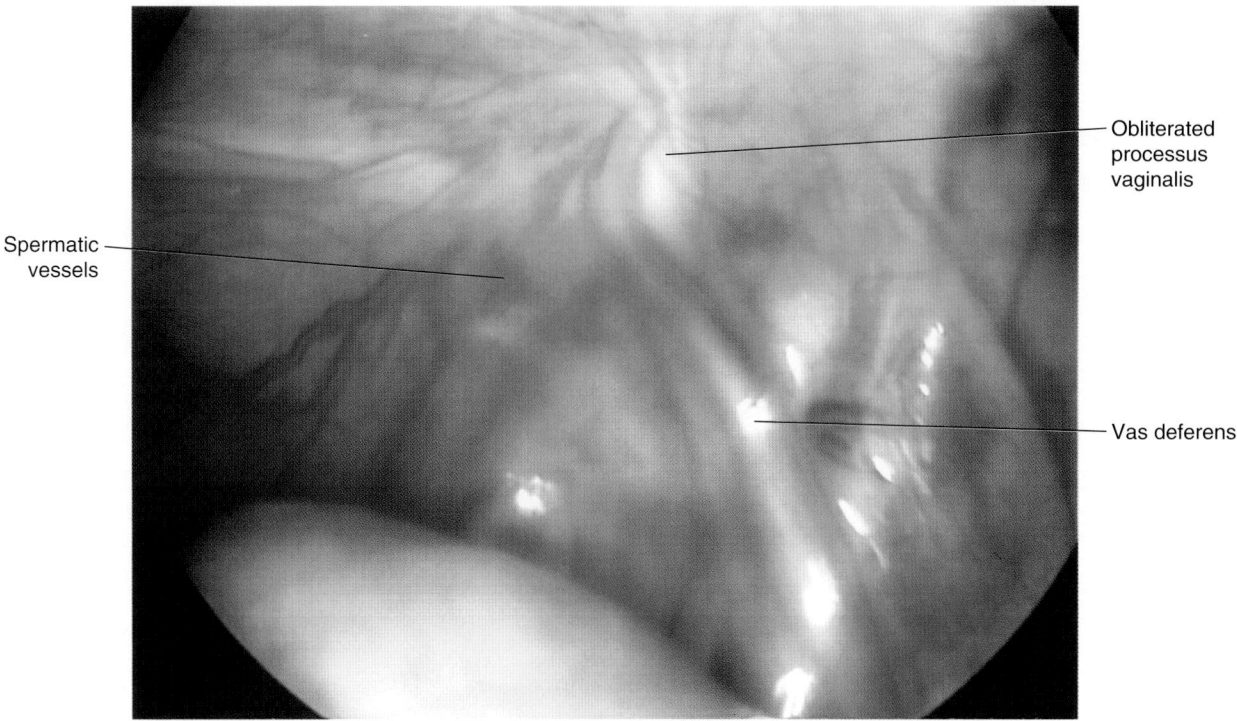

Obliterated
processus
vaginalis

Spermatic
vessels

Vas deferens

Figure 327–3

FIGURE 327–2. Image on laparoscopy of patent processus vaginalis on right side.
FIGURE 327–3. Image on diagnostic laparoscopy of obliterated processus vaginalis on left side.

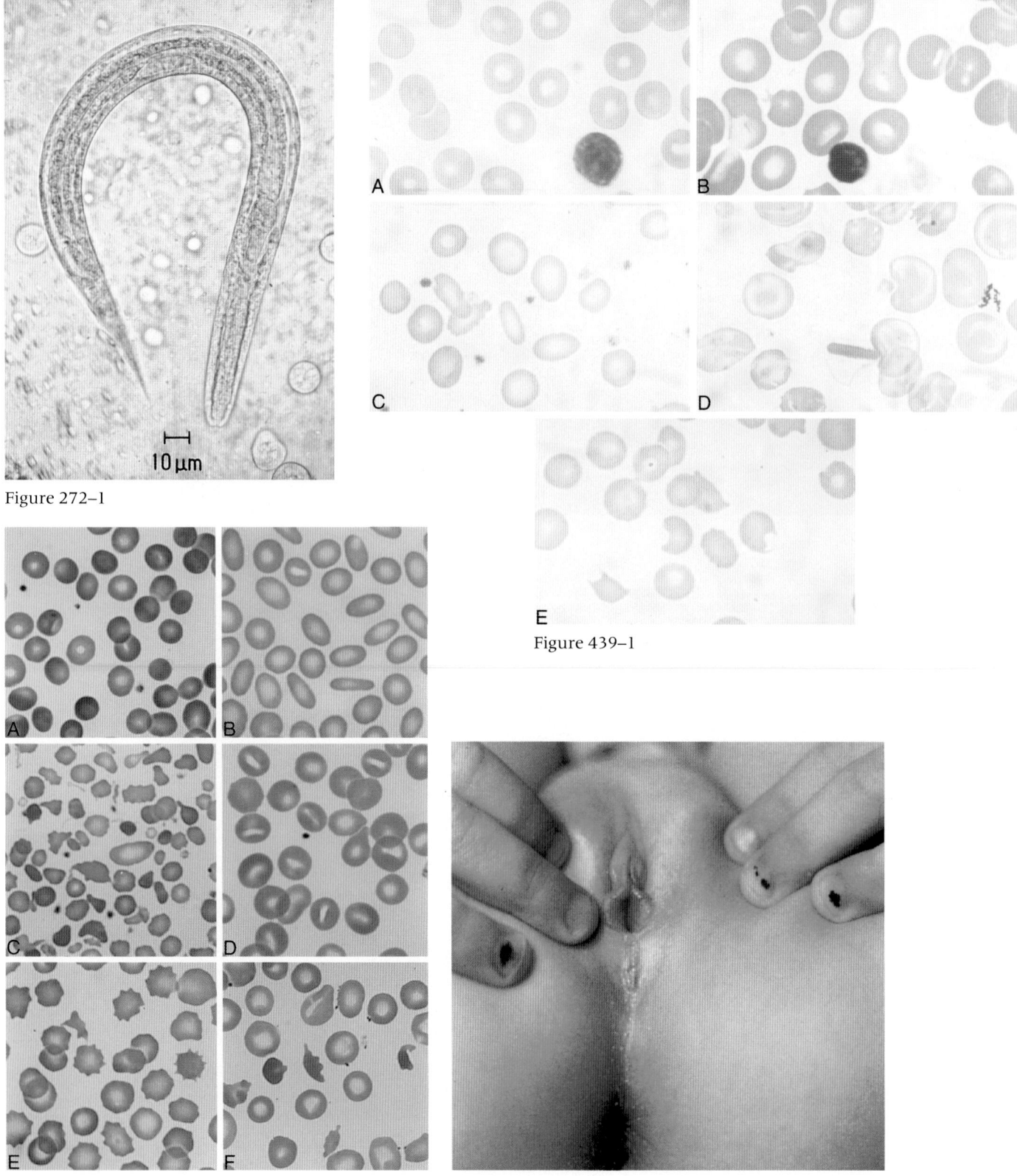

Figure 272–1

Figure 439–1

Figure 450–2

Figure 541–1

FIGURE 272–1. Larvae of intestinal strongyloidiasis.
FIGURE 439–1. Morphologic abnormalities of the red blood cell. *A*, Normal. *B*, Macrocytes (folic acid or vitamin B$_{12}$ deficiency). *C*, Hypochromic microcytes (iron deficiency). *D*, Target cells (Hb CC disease). *E*, Schizocytes (hemolytic-uremic syndrome). (Courtesy of E. Schwartz, MD.)
FIGURE 450–2. Morphology of abnormal red cells. *A*, Hereditary spherocytosis; *B*, hereditary elliptocytosis; *C*, hereditary pyropoikilocytosis; *D*, hereditary stomatocytosis; *E*, acanthocytosis; *F*, fragmentation hemolysis.
FIGURE 541–1. Labial adhesions.

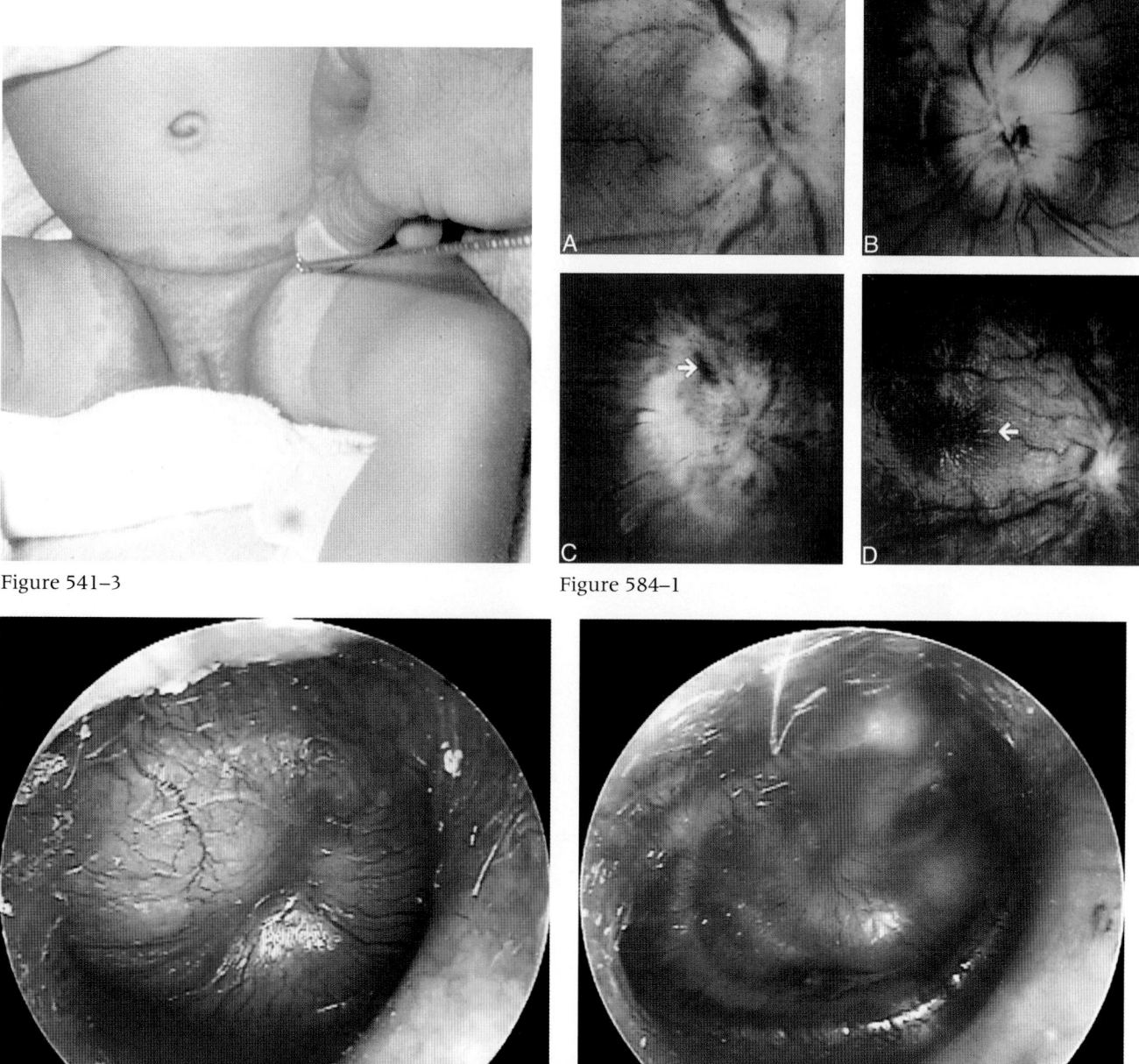

Figure 541–3

Figure 584–1

Figure 630–3

Figure 630–4

FIGURE 541–3. Vulvar psoriasis.
FIGURE 584–1. *A,* Mild papilledema. Blurred disc margins and venous congestion. *B,* Moderate papilledema. Disc edematous and raised. Vessels buried within substance of nerve tissue. *C,* Severe papilledema. Hemorrhages are evident within disc (*arrow*), and there are microinfarcts (soft exudates) in the nerve fiber layer. *D,* Macular star (*arrow*) with edema residues distributed within the Henle layer of the macula.
FIGURE 630–3. Tympanic membrane in acute otitis media (AOM).
FIGURE 630–4. Tympanic membrane in otitis media with effusion (OME).

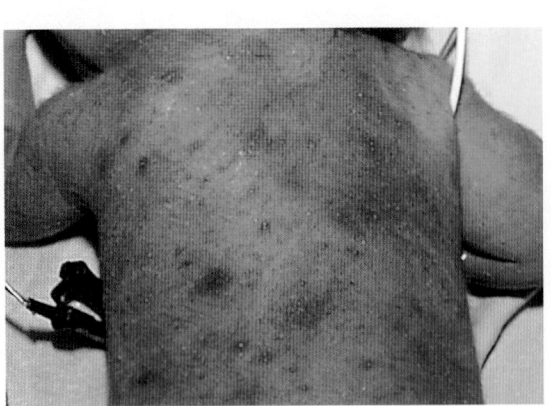

Figure 637–1

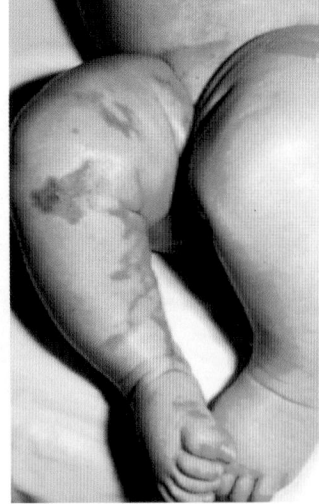

Figure 640–4

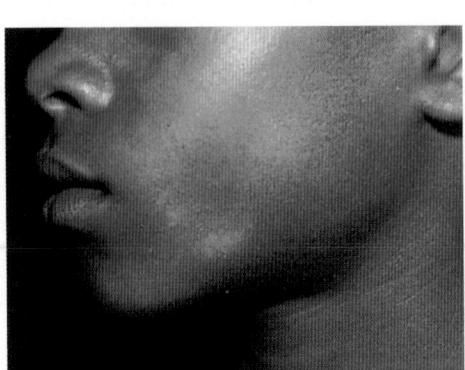

Figure 645–3

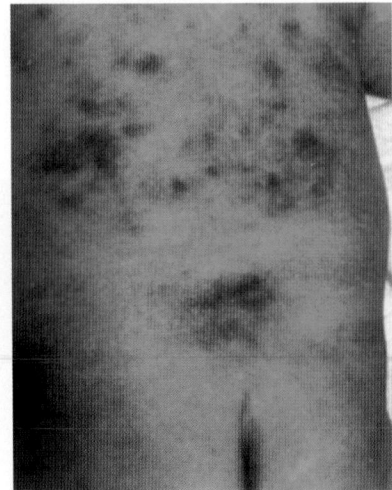

Figure 650–1

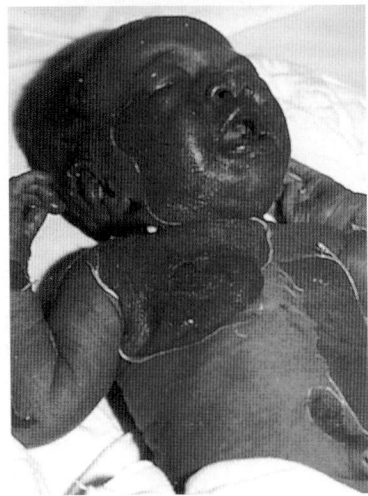

Figure 655–2

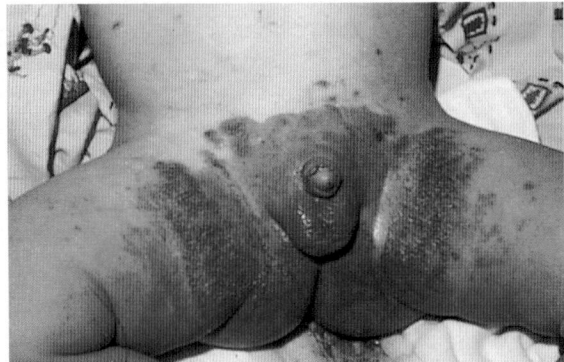

Figure 656–5

FIGURE 637–1. Erythema toxicum on the trunk of a newborn infant.
FIGURE 640–4. Marbled pattern of cutis marmorata telangiectatica congenita on the right leg.
FIGURE 645–3. Patchy hypopigmented lesions with diffuse borders characteristic of pityriasis alba.
FIGURE 650–1. Red-purple nodular infiltration of skin of back caused by subcutaneous fat necrosis.
FIGURE 655–2. Infant with staphylococcal scalded skin syndrome.
FIGURE 656–5. Erythematous confluent plaque with satellite pustules caused by candidal infection.

The Field of Pediatrics

Chapter 1

Overview of Pediatrics

Richard E. Behrman

Pediatrics is concerned with the health of infants, children, and adolescents; their growth and development; and their opportunity to achieve full potential as adults. As physicians who assume a responsibility for children's physical, mental, and emotional progress from conception to maturity, pediatricians must be concerned with social and environmental influences, which have a major impact on the health and well-being of children and their families, as well as with particular organ systems and biologic processes. The young are often among the most vulnerable or disadvantaged in society, and thus their needs require special attention.

SCOPE AND HISTORY OF PEDIATRICS AND VITAL STATISTICS

More than a century ago, pediatrics emerged as a medical specialty in response to increasing awareness that the health problems of children differ from those of adults and that a child's response to illness and stress varies with age. The emphasis and scope of pediatrics continue to change, but these basic observations remain valid.

The health problems of children and youth vary widely among the nations of the world depending on a number of factors, which are often interrelated. These factors include (1) the prevalence and ecology of infectious agents and their hosts; (2) climate and geography; (3) agricultural resources and practices; (4) educational, economic, social, and cultural considerations; (5) stage of industrialization and urbanization; and (6) in many instances, the gene frequencies for some disorders.

Not only do problems differ in various parts of the world, but priorities do also, because they must reflect local concerns, resources, and needs. Assessment of the state of health of any community must begin with a description of the incidence of illness and must continue with studies that show the changes that occur with time and in response to programs of prevention, case finding, therapy, and adequate surveillance. As contemporary problems in any community yield to study and to improved management, new problems become the foci of the attention and efforts of pediatric clinicians and research workers. Accordingly, with time, the relative importance of the various causes of childhood morbidity and mortality may undergo major changes.

In the late 19th century in the United States, of every 1,000 children born alive, 200 might be expected to die before the age of 1 yr of conditions such as dysentery, pneumonia, measles, diphtheria, and whooping cough. The efforts of pediatricians, combined with those of scientists and pioneers in public health, have led to such better understanding of the origin and management of many problems of infants that in the past half century the infant mortality rate in the United States has decreased from around 75/1,000 live births in 1925 to approximately 6.9/1,000

in 2000. Both neonatal (<1 mo) and postneonatal (1–11 mo) mortality have had major reductions. However, most of the decline in infant mortality since 1970 is attributable to a decrease in the birthweight-specific infant mortality rate related to pediatric care, not to the prevention of low-birthweight births. The majority of deaths of infants younger than 1 yr of age occur within the first 28 days of life, most of these within the first 7 days; moreover, a large proportion of those within the first 7 days occur within the 1st day. However, an increasing number of severely ill infants born at very low birthweight survive the neonatal period and die later in infancy of neonatal disease, its sequelae, or its complications. Tables 1–1 and 1–2 show the persistent disproportionately high death rate within the 1st yr, compared with the remainder of childhood.

Postneonatal infant mortality for the United States in 2000 was 2.3/1,000 live births (4.7/1,000 for black infants and 1.9/1,000 for white infants). The leading cause of death in this age group was sudden infant death syndrome, followed in order by congenital anomalies, perinatal conditions, respiratory system diseases, accidents, and infectious diseases. Maternal risk characteristics, such as unmarried status, adolescence, high parity, and less than 12 yr of education, are correlated significantly with increased risk of postneonatal mortality and morbidity and low birthweight.

In developed countries early in the 20th century, efforts at control of infectious disease began to be complemented by better understanding of nutrition. New and continuing discoveries in these areas led to establishment of public well child clinics for low-income families. Along with acute infections and the chronic disturbances associated with deficits of calories, vitamins, minerals, or proteins, the acute nutritional and metabolic disturbances that accompany acute diarrhea received attention.

In the middle years of the 20th century, a profound revolution in child health was brought about by the introduction of antibacterial chemicals and antibiotic agents. With improved control of infectious disease through both prevention and treatment and with other scientific and technical advances, pediatric medicine increasingly turned its attention to a broad spectrum of conditions, each affecting relatively small numbers of children. These included both potentially lethal conditions and temporarily or permanently handicapping conditions; among these disorders were leukemia, cystic fibrosis, diseases of the newborn infant, congenital heart disease, mental retardation, genetic defects, rheumatic diseases, renal diseases, and metabolic and endocrine disorders.

The last two decades of the 20th century were marked by accelerated understanding of and new approaches to the management of many disorders as a consequence of advances in molecular biology, genetics, and immunology. Increasing attention also has been given to behavioral and social aspects of child health, ranging from re-examination of child-rearing practices to creation of major programs aimed at prevention and management of abuse and neglect of infants and children. Developmental psychologists, child psychiatrists, neuroscientists, sociologists, anthropologists, ethnologists, and others have brought us new insights into human potential, including new views of the importance of the environmental circumstances during pregnancy, surrounding

TABLE 1–1.   Death Rates* for All Causes, According to Sex, Race, and Age: United States, Selected Years, 1960–1999

	1960		1970		1980		1990		1999	
	White	*Black*	*White*	*Black*	*White*	*Black*	*White*	*Black*	*White*	*Black*
Male										
<1 yr	2,694	5,307	2,113	4,299	1,230	2,587	896	2,112	658	1,694
1–4 yr	105	209	84	151	66	111	46	86	34	66
5–14 yr	53	75	48	67	35	47	26	41	20	35
15–24 yr	144	212	171	321	167	209	131	252	90	139
Female										
<1 yr	2,008	4,162	1,615	3,369	963	2,124	690	1,736	533	1,403
1–4 yr	85	173	66	129	49	84	36	68	27	52
5–14 yr	35	54	30	44	23	31	18	28	15	23
15–24 yr	55	108	62	112	56	71	46	69	41	46

*Death rates per 100,000 population.
Adapted from Table 119, Statistical Abstract of the United States 1993, 113th ed. Lanham, MD, Berman Press, 1993; Deaths: Final data for 1999. National Vital Statistics Reports 49(8), 2001.

TABLE 1–2.   Death Rates* by Age, Sex, Race, and Hispanic Origin, 1999[†]

	Non-Hispanic White	Non-Hispanic Black	Hispanic	Native American	Asian or Pacific Islander
Male					
<1 yr	637	1,773	655	840	403
1–4 yr	33	70	34	59	27
5–9 yr	17	34	16	19	11
10–14 yr	23	39	23	27	15
15–19 yr	86	145	99	152	53
Female					
<1 yr	506	1,469	566	773	373
1–4 yr	26	54	30	43	19
5–9 yr	14	25	13	25	11
10–14 yr	15	23	17	19	12
15–19 yr	42	48	33	57	26

*Rates per 100,000 population in specified group.
[†]Modified from Deaths: Final data for 1999. National Vital Statistics Reports 49(8), 2001.

birth, and in the early years of child rearing. However, during the latter years of the 20th century there was also a resurgence of some of the infectious diseases previously controlled in developed countries, such as tuberculosis and syphilis; the emergence of new infectious pathogens, such as the human immunodeficiency virus; and the recognition of new disorders related to innovative therapies. In addition, in developing countries, many of the disorders facing children earlier in this century persist, sometimes aggravated by war and famine.

Table 1–3 shows the leading causes of death in various age groups in 1999. The problems of these children have changed significantly in the United States over a generation. Table 1–3 highlights the impact of violent deaths on mortality in older children, adolescents, and young adults.

Tables 1–1, 1–2, and 1–4 show that the nonwhite children and other racial and ethnic groups of children in the United States have not fully benefited from the changes in infant mortality in this century owing to various socioeconomic and other disadvantages that have resisted the efforts of many who have struggled to reduce this disparity, including many pediatricians. Similar disparities between races and ethnic groups occur in several indices of health, such as rates of diseases of the heart and homicides.

In the United States, existing programs for meeting child health problems are not available to all families in need, with gaps between eligibility for public support and parents' ability to pay for services. Needed services are often either nonexistent or fragmented among programs, agencies, or policies. Programs are often poorly coordinated, and the data collection is inadequate. The resources available for maternal and child health care services are also generally inadequate. These findings reflect a need, not just in the United States but in many other parts of the world as well, for continuing re-examination and revision of the system of health care, especially with regard to its impact on the health status of children.

These problems are exacerbated by social and demographic changes in the United States. By 1999, 27% of all children younger than 18 yr of age were living with one parent, more than twice the number of such children in 1970. Of these one-parent families, 85% consisted of children living with their mother. There are substantial differences among children: 56% of black, 32% of Hispanic, 22% of white, and 36% of Native American children live with one parent. Furthermore, in 1997, 57% of women with children younger than 3 yr of age, 64% with children younger than 6 yr, and 74% with children ages 6–17 yr worked full time or part time outside the home. In 1994, children younger than 5 yr with employed mothers were being cared for in a variety of settings: day care center or preschool (29%), non-relative in a home (20%), and relative in a home (43%). In 1996, welfare reform increased incentives for women with low incomes to enter the workforce and provided more support for child care.

Family income is central to the health and well-being of children. Children living in poor families are much more likely than children living in rich or middle-class families to experience material deprivation and poor health, die during childhood, score lower on standardized tests, be retained in grade, drop out of school, have out-of-wedlock births, experience violent crime, end up as poor adults, and suffer other undesirable outcomes. In 1998, 18% of all children in the United States lived in poverty*: white, 14%; black, 36%, Hispanic, 34%. Eight percent of children in the United States live in extreme poverty (in families with incomes less than 50% of the poverty line*). Many of these children live their entire childhood in poverty. Children who live in single-parent families with poorly educated, young, minority (particularly black), or disabled adults are more likely to be poor and live in poverty longer than those who do not live in such families.

The aforementioned findings have generated three sets of goals. The first set includes that all families have access to

---

*Weighted average poverty threshold in 1998 in the United States was $16,530 for four-person families.

TABLE 1–3. Causes of Death at Various Stages

Rank*	Cause	Subrank	Rate†
Under 1 yr: All causes			688
1	Perinatal Conditions		
	Short gestation/low birthweight	1	
	Newborns affected by maternal or placental/cord membranes, complications of pregnancy	2	
	Respiratory distress syndrome	3	
	Infections	4	
	Intrauterine hypoxia/birth asphyxia	5	
2	Congenital malformations, deformations, and chromosomal abnormalities		
3	Sudden infant death syndrome		
4	Injuries and adverse events		
5	Infections/diseases of the circulatory system‡		
1–4 yr: All causes			33
1	Injuries (unintentional)		
2	Congenital malformations, deformations, and chromosomal abnormalities		
3	Malignant neoplasms		
4	Homicide		
5	Diseases of the heart‡		
5–9 yr: All causes			17
1	Injuries (unintentional)		
2	Malignant neoplasms		
3	Congenital malformations, deformations, and chromosomal abnormalities		
4	Homicide		
5	Diseases of the heart‡		
10–14 yr: All causes			21
1	Injuries (unintentional)		
2	Homicide		
3	Suicide		
4	Malignant neoplasms		
5	Diseases of the heart‡		
15–19 yr: All causes			68
1	Injuries (unintentional)		
2	Homicide		
3	Suicide		
4	Malignant neoplasms		
5	Diseases of the heart‡		

*Adapted from Centers for Disease Control and Prevention/National Center for Health Statistics, 1999-2000 National Vital Statistics System, mortality (unlinked file).
†Rate per 100,000 population in specified group.
‡Excludes congenital heart anomalies.

TABLE 1–4. Infant, Neonatal, and Postneonatal Deaths and Mortality Rates by Specified Race or National Origin of Mother: United States, 1999

Race of Mother	Live Births	Number of Deaths			Mortality Rate per 1,000 Live Births		
		Infant	Neonatal	Postneonatal	Infant	Neonatal	Postneonatal
All races	3,959,417	27,864	18,700	9,164	7.0	4.7	2.3
White	3,132,501	18,136	12,186	5,950	5.8	3.9	1.9
Black	605,970	8,480	5,739	2,741	14.0	9.5	4.5
Native American†	40,170	373	202	171	9.3	5.0	4.3
Asian or Pacific Islander	180,776	876	574	302	4.8	3.2	1.7
Chinese	28,853	85	51	34	2.9	1.8	1.2
Japanese	8,722	30	24	6	3.4	2.8	*
Hawaiian	6,093	43	30	13	7.1	4.9	*
Filipino	30,677	179	120	59	5.8	3.9	1.9
Other Asian or Pacific Islander	106,431	539	348	190	5.1	3.3	1.8

*Figure does not meet standard of reliability or precision; based on fewer than 20 deaths in the numerator.
†Includes Aleuts and Eskimos.
Adapted from National Vital Statistics Reports 50(9), 2002.

adequate perinatal, preschool, and family-planning services; that governmental activities be effectively coordinated at national and local levels; that services be so organized that they reach populations at special risk; that there be no insurmountable or inequitable financial barriers to adequate care; that the health care of children have continuity from prenatal through adolescent age periods; and that every family ultimately have access to *all* necessary services, including developmental, dental, genetic, and mental health services. A second set of goals addresses the needs for reducing accidents and environmental risks, for meeting nutritional needs, and for health education aimed at fostering health-promoting lifestyles. A third set of goals covers needs for research in biomedical and behavioral science, in fundamentals of bioscience and human biology, and in the particular problems of mothers and children.

The unfinished business in the quest for physical, mental, and social health in the community is illustrated by the disparities with which deaths due to disease, injuries, and violence are distributed among white, black, and Hispanic children. Homicide has become a major cause of adolescent deaths and has increased in rate also among the very young, in whom the increase may in part represent the more accurate identification of child abuse (Chapter 35); among adolescents it may reflect unresolved social tensions, the epidemic of substance abuse (especially cocaine and crack), and an unhealthy preoccupation with violence in our society. Some of the issues underlying these problems are discussed in Chapters 24, 34, 39, and Part XII.

PATTERNS OF HEALTH CARE

Children (0–21 yr) make up slightly less than one third of the population of the United States. The number of births has been increasing since 1976 and is expected to continue to increase at 1–2% annually. There were 3,959,417 live births in 1999. Table 1–5 indicates the distribution of children in the population by age. The population of children has been increasing since 1950. However, the proportion of children is decreasing relative to the adult population. The racial, ethnic, and cultural diversity among children is increasing significantly.

In 1999, about 117 million visits were made to physicians' offices and 15 million visits were made to hospital outpatient departments by children younger than 15 yr; an additional 60 million and 8 million visits were made by children and young adults (15–24 yr), respectively. The principal diagnoses accounting for almost 40% of these visits were well child visit (15%), middle-ear infection (12%), and injury (10%). The rate of ambulatory visits by children and youth decreases with increasing age. The opposite occurs with adults. In contrast to the large number of children seen in ambulatory settings, 2,258,000 children younger than 15 yr (excluding newborns) were admitted to acute care hospitals in the United States in 1999. Nonwhite children are more likely than white children to use hospital facilities for their ambulatory care, and well child visits are almost 80% higher among white infants than black infants.

Hospitals, particularly in urban areas, are sources of both routine and intensive child care, with medical and surgical services that may range from immunization and developmental counseling to open heart surgery and renal transplantation. Clinical conditions and procedures requiring intensive care are likely to be clustered in university-affiliated centers serving as regional resources. The hospitalization rates for children (excluding newborn infants) are less than those of adults younger than 65 yr of age, except during the first year of life. In 1999, the rates per 1,000 population were as follows: younger than 1 yr, 208.5; 1–4 yr, 46.6; 5–14 yr, 22.2; 15–19 yr, 60.0 (excluding obstetrics). The rate of hospitalization and lengths of hospital stay have declined significantly for children and adults during the past decade. Children represent less than 8% of the total acute hospital discharges, and in children's hospitals about 70% of admissions are for chronic conditions. Ten to 12% of pediatric hospitalizations are related to birth defects and genetic diseases.

PLANNING AND IMPLEMENTING A SYSTEM OF CARE

Physicians caring for children have been increasingly called on to advise in the management of disturbed behavior of children and youth or problematic relationships between child and parent, child and school, or child and community. They are increasingly concerned with problems of mental, social, and societal health. There is also an increasing concern about disparities in how the benefits of what we know about child health reach various groups of children. Just as in many developing countries, so in the United States does the health of children lag far behind what it could be if the means and will to apply current knowledge were focused on the health of children. The medical problems of children are often intimately related to problems of mental and social health. The children most at risk are disproportionately represented among ethnic minority groups. Pediatricians have a responsibility to aggressively address problems such as these.

Linked with these views of the broad scope of pediatric concern is the concept that access to at least a basic level of quality services to promote health and treat illness is a right of every person. Among children in the United States, having health insurance is strongly associated with access to primary care. The failure of health services and health benefits to reach all who need them has led to re-examination of the design of health care systems in many countries, but unresolved problems remain in most health care systems, such as the maldistribution of physicians, institutional unresponsiveness to the perceived needs of the individual, failure of medical services to adjust to the need and convenience of patients, and deficiencies in health education. Efforts to make the delivery of health care more efficient and effective have led imaginative pediatricians to create new categories of health care providers, such as pediatric nurse practitioners, and to participate in new organizations for providing care to children, such as various managed care arrangements.

New insights into the needs of children have reshaped the child health care system in other ways. Growing understanding of the need of infants for certain qualities of stimulation and care has led to restudy and revision of the care of newborn infants (Chapters 9 and 83) and of procedures leading to an adoption or to placement with foster families (Chapters 30 and 31). For handicapped children, the massive centralized institutions of past years are being replaced by community-centered arrangements offering a better opportunity for these children to achieve their maximum potential. Pediatricians have been involved in shaping these and other institutions that provide services to children, and their insights and active contributions will continue to be needed.

TABLE 1–5. Distribution of Children by Age in the United States in 1998 Number (Resident Population in 1000s)

Age (yr)	Total	White	Black	Native American/ Eskimo/Aleut	Asian/Pacific Islander
<1	3,795	3,016	558	41	89
1	3,777	3,015	545	40	87
2	3,771	3,005	522	39	86
3	3,824	3,027	581	40	87
4	3,923	3,090	618	42	85
0–4	19,090	15,153	2,855	201	434
5	3,985	3,137	629	43	85
6	4,022	3,175	631	42	85
7	4,087	3,205	643	46	83
8	3,805	3,002	611	47	71
9	3,960	3,105	648	49	77
5–9	19,838	15,624	3,162	226	400
10	3,902	3,079	622	48	74
11	3,794	3,009	589	47	72
12	3,836	3,036	596	48	77
13	3,775	2,994	575	49	78
14	3,783	2,996	579	49	79
10–14	19,090	15,113	2,960	240	380
15	3,910	3,091	608	49	80
16	3,753	2,978	575	46	75
17	4,029	3,197	629	47	77
18	3,754	2,990	86	41	68
19	3,827	3,044	596	41	72
15–19	19,273	15,300	2,994	224	372
20	3,811	3,042	585	39	72
21	3,580	2,859	533	38	74
0–21	84,682	67,091	13,089	968	1,732
22–85 +	184,500	155,307	1,141	1,374	8,481
Total	269,182	222,398	34,230	2,342	10,213

U.S. Bureau of Census.

COSTS OF HEALTH CARE

The growth of high technology, the increasing number of people older than 65 yr, the redesign of health institutions (particularly with respect to the needs for and the uses of personnel), the public's demand for medical services, and the manner in which the costs of health care are paid have driven the costs of health care in the United States up to a point at which they represent a significant proportion of the gross national product. Although children (0–18 yr) represent about 30% of the population, they account for only about 14% of the personal health care expenditures, or about 60% of adult per capita expenditures. Efforts to contain costs have led to revisions of the way in which physicians and hospitals are paid for services. Limits have been set on the fees for some services, capitated prepayment and various managed care systems flourish, a program of reimbursement (diagnosis-related groups [DRGs]) based on the diagnosis rather than on the particular services rendered to an individual patient has been implemented, and a relative value scale for varying rates of payment among different physician services has been instituted. These and other changes in the system of financing health services raise important ethical and professional issues for pediatricians to address (Chapter 2).

EVALUATION OF HEALTH CARE

The shaping of health care systems to meet the needs of children and their families requires accurate statistical data and difficult decisions in setting priorities. Along with growing concerns about the design and cost of health care systems and the ability to distribute health services equitably has come increasing concern about the quality of health care and about its efficiency and effectiveness. There are large local and regional variations among similar populations of children in the rates of use of procedures and technology and of hospital admissions. These variations require continuing evaluation and explanation in terms of the actual impact of medical and surgical services on health status and the outcome of illness.

GROWTH OF SPECIALIZATION

The amount of information relevant to child health care is rapidly expanding, and no person can become master of it all. Physicians are increasingly dependent on one another for the highest quality of care for their patients; group practices in pediatrics are common in the United States, and although the vast majority of pediatricians are primary care generalists, as many as 25% claim an area of special knowledge and skill.

The growth of specialization within pediatrics has taken a number of different forms: Interests in problems of *age groups* of children have created neonatology and adolescent medicine; interests in *organ systems* have created pediatric cardiology, neurology, child development, allergy, hematology, nephrology, gastroenterology, child psychiatry, pulmonology, endocrinology, and specialization in metabolism and genetics; interests in the *health care system* have created pediatricians devoted to ambulatory care, emergency care, and intensive care; and finally, multidisciplinary subspecialties have grown up around the problems of *handicapped children*, to which pediatrics, neurology, psychiatry, psychology, nursing, physical and occupational therapy, special education, speech therapy, audiology, and nutrition all make essential contributions. This growth of specialization has been most conspicuous in university-affiliated departments of pediatrics and medical centers for children.

NEED FOR CONTINUING SELF-EDUCATION

The explosion of information has also created a need for continuing education, which was felt much less keenly in earlier years, when the new information in any field of medicine was easily accessible through a relatively small number of journals, texts, or monographs. Now, relevant information is so widely scattered among the many published journals that elaborate electronic data systems are necessary to make it accessible. The Internet has dramatically improved access to information by physicians and patients, but judgment about the quality, clinical significance, and appropriate use of such information is a continuing challenge. New auditory and visual aids to learning abound, as do postgraduate courses through which participating physicians can be brought up to date on various aspects of child health care. The American Board of Pediatrics and the American Academy of Pediatrics have arranged for close linkage of continuing education of pediatricians to recertification in pediatrics.

There is no touchstone through which physicians can ensure that the process of their own continuing education will keep them abreast of advancing knowledge in the field, but they must find a way to base their decisions on the best available scientific evidence if they are to discharge their responsibility to their patients. An essential element of this process may be for physicians to take an *active* role, such as participating in medical student and resident education. Efforts in continuing self-education will also be fostered, for example, if clinical problems can be made a stimulus for a review of standard literature, alone or in consultation with an appropriate colleague or consultant. This continuing review will do much to identify those inconsistencies or contradictions that will indicate, in the ultimate best interest of patients, that things are not what they seem or have been said to be. Physicians still learn most from their patients, but this will not be the case if they fall into the easy habit of accepting their patients' problems casually or at face value because the problems appear to be simple.

The tools that physicians must use in dealing with the problems of children and their families fall into three main categories: *cognitive* (up-to-date factual information about diagnostic and therapeutic issues, available on recall or easily found in readily accessible sources, and the ability to relate this information to the pathophysiology of their patients in the context of individual biologic variability); *interpersonal or manual* (e.g., the ability to carry out a productive interview, execute a reliable physical examination, perform a deft venipuncture, or manage cardiac arrest or resuscitation of a depressed newborn infant); and *attitudinal* (the physician's unselfish commitment to the fullest possible implementation of knowledge and skills on behalf of children and their families in an atmosphere of empathic sensitivity and concern). With regard to this last category, it is important that children participate with their families in informed decision-making about their own health care in a manner appropriate to their stage of development and the nature of the particular health problem.

The workaday needs of professional persons for knowledge and skills in care of children vary widely. Primary care physicians need depth in developmental concepts and in the ability to organize an effective system for achieving quality and continuity in assessing and planning for health care during the entire period of growth. They may often have little or no need for immediate recall of esoterica. On the other hand, consultants or subspecialists not only need a comfortable grasp of esoterica within their field and perhaps within related fields but also must be able to cope with controversial issues with flexibility that will permit adaptation of various points of view to the best interest of their unique patient.

At whatever level of care (primary, secondary, or tertiary) or in whatever position (student, pediatric nurse practitioner, resident pediatrician, practitioner of pediatrics or family medicine, or pediatric or other subspecialists), professional persons dealing with children must be able to identify their roles of the moment and their levels of engagement with a child's problem; each must determine whether his or her experience and other resources at hand are adequate to deal with this problem and must be ready to seek other help when they are not. Among the necessary resources are general textbooks, more detailed monographs in subspecialty areas, selected journals, audiovisual and Internet materials, and, above all, colleagues with exceptional or complementary experience and expertise. The intercommunication of all these levels of engagement with medical and health problems of children offers the best hope of bringing us closer to the goal of providing the opportunity for all children to achieve their maximum potential.

1999 National hospital discharge summary with detailed diagnosis and procedure data. *Vital and Health Statistics 2001*, Series 13, Number 151.

Births: Final data for 1999. *National Vital Statistics Reports* 2001;49:1–100.

Deaths: Final data for 1999. *National Vital Statistics Reports* 2001;49:1–116.

Health, United States, 2001. Urban and Rural Health Chartbook. Department of Health and Human Services, 2001, DHHS Publication No. (PHS) 01–1232–1.

Hoyer DL, Freedman MA, Strobino DM, et al: Annual summary of vital statistics: 2000. *Pediatrics* 108:1241–1255, 2001.

McCormick MC, Wernick RM, Elixhauser A, et al: Annual report on access to and utilization of health care for children and youth in the United States–2000. *Ambulatory Pediatrics* 1:3–15, 2001.

National Ambulatory Medical Care Survey: 1999 summary. *Advanced Data* 322:1–36, 2001.

Trends in the well-being of America's children and youth 2001. U.S. Department of Health and Human Services.

Trends in hospital emergency department utilization: United States, 1992–99. *Vital and Health Statistics 2001*, Series 13, Number 150.

Chapter 2
Ethics in Pediatric Care
Robert M. Nelson and Norman Fost

The proper scope of parental decision-making is bounded by the concept of a child's best interest and by the emerging desire and capacity for autonomy or self-determination of an older child or adolescent. In addition, the pediatric clinician has an independent professional obligation to act in a child's "best interest," thus creating the possibility of conflict among child, parent, and clinician. The approach to the ethical issues that arise in pediatric practice must include respect for both a parent's responsibility for the life and health of a child and a child's developing capacity and autonomy. Further complexity is added by the varying social, cultural, and religious views of the role of family, parental authority, appropriate methods for disciplining a child, the age of majority, and alternative approaches to health care.

INFORMED CONSENT, PARENTAL PERMISSION, AND CHILD ASSENT

A competent adult patient has the right to decide, after consultation with a physician, which medical interventions he or she will or will not accept. This right of self-determination (or autonomy) based on personal preferences and values is reflected in the doctrine of voluntary and informed consent. This doctrine, however, has limited direct application to children and adolescents who lack the decisional capacity or legal empowerment to give informed consent to medical care. The capacity for informed decision-making in health care is generally thought to involve the ability to understand and communicate, to reason and deliberate, and to analyze conflicting elements of a decision using a set of personal values. The age at which a competent patient may legally exercise voluntary and informed consent for medical care varies from state to state and may be limited to specific conditions, for example, sexually transmitted diseases, family planning, and drug or alcohol abuse.

In contrast to decisions about one's own care, a parent's right to direct a child's medical care is more limited. It is constrained both by the child's best interest and the independent obligation

of clinicians to act in the child's best interest, even if this places them in conflict with a parent. The concept of parental permission (rather than consent) reflects this shared decision-making involved in pediatric health care. In any given instance, the decision of what is or is not in a child's best interest may be difficult, especially given the diverse views of acceptable child rearing and child welfare. Parents are (and should be) granted wide discretion in raising their children. Nevertheless, in cases involving a substantial risk of harm, the moral focus should be on what is best for the child, not on a parental right to decide.

Respect for children must account for both a child's vulnerability and developing capacity. Thus, this respect encompasses both the protective role of parental permission and the developmental role of child assent. At times, respect for a child requires overriding a child's dissent when a proposed intervention is essential to his or her welfare. Otherwise, assent (i.e., the child's affirmative agreement) should be obtained and dissent honored. In seeking a child's assent, a clinician should help a child understand his or her condition, tell a child what he or she can expect, assess a child's understanding and whether a child feels pressured to assent, and solicit a child's willingness to participate.

TREATMENT OF CRITICALLY ILL CHILDREN

Most children who are critically ill recover and are able to return to an acceptable quality of life. However, some children either respond partially or fail to respond to life-sustaining medical treatment (LSMT), progressing toward death over a time span ranging from minutes to years (see Chapter 38). Under these circumstances, a number of questions arise. Should one initiate or continue LSMT? How does one arrive at this decision? What treatments should be provided as part of palliative care? Is there any difference between starting and stopping a medical intervention? What about specific interventions such as cardiopulmonary resuscitation or artificially provided hydration and nutrition? Should newborn infants and older children be treated differently when considering LSMT?

Transitioning from "Cure" to "Care." The provision of LSMT assumes that the burden of treatment is justified by the anticipated benefit of returning to or sustaining an acceptable quality of life. As the anticipated quality of the outcome deteriorates or becomes increasingly unlikely, or as the burden of treatment becomes intolerable, we ask whether continued LSMT makes sense. Answering this question is difficult, involving a range of possible outcomes, complex estimates of probabilities, differing values of each outcome, and dealing with uncertainty and hope. Medical technology and other treatments should only be used when the benefits for the child outweigh the burdens, especially for children living with life-threatening or terminal conditions.

The concept of *futility* has been invoked in support of the unilateral forgoing of LSMT by health care professionals over the objections of patients and family. Although it seems self-evident that clinicians should not provide futile (or useless) interventions, the application of this principle is problematic if used to justify unilateral professional action based on values that are not shared by the affected patient or family. The concept of futility should be reserved for those interventions that will not in fact achieve a given physiologic outcome. The appeal to futility should not be used to short-circuit the collaborative process by which medical interventions are seen to be disproportionately burdensome.

Life-Sustaining Medical Treatment or Palliative Care? A rigid distinction between LSMT and palliative care (Chapter 38) may be difficult to draw in any given instance, and their integration is often desirable. LSMT can be broadly defined as any intervention that may prolong the life of a patient or alter substantially the expected progression toward death. Examples of LSMT include organ transplantation, ventilator therapy, dialysis, and treatment with vasoactive medications, or more mundane interventions such as antibiotics, chemotherapy, and artificially provided nutrition and hydration. Palliative care interventions focus on the relief of symptoms and conditions that may detract from a child's (and family's) quality of life regardless of the impact on a child's underlying disease process. The control of pain and other symptoms, as well as concern for the psychological or spiritual problems associated with life-threatening or terminal disease, are usually considered palliative and are often appropriate during LSMT. Certain LSMT may also be appropriate in the palliative management of the dying child (see Chapter 38 for full discussion).

Withholding and Withdrawing Life-Sustaining Treatment. (See Chapter 64.) A palliative care plan involves the assessment of available diagnostic and therapeutic interventions based on the goal of improving a child's quality of life while living with a life-threatening or terminal disease. Some interventions that are currently being provided may be withdrawn. Other interventions that are not being provided may be withheld. Although the prevailing view is that there is no moral distinction between withholding or withdrawing interventions that are not medically indicated, the uncertainty inherent in predicting a child's response to treatment suggests that withdrawing treatment based on a child's failure to respond is morally preferable to withholding that same treatment. In addition, withholding treatment out of concern that the withdrawal of that same treatment in the future would be more difficult risks undertreating some children who would in fact respond favorably to that treatment. The withdrawal of LSMT may be psychologically more stressful than withholding LSMT, and may add complexity as the moral values associated with treatment of any given child may shift over time.

The decision to not attempt cardiopulmonary resuscitation is often the initial focus of discussion with parents of children living with life-threatening or terminal conditions. Obtaining a "do not attempt resuscitation" order (DNAR) may become a symbol of a clinician's success at negotiating limits to LSMT with a child's parents and eclipse other interventions that should be considered in providing for a child's comfort. The decision for a DNAR order should not imply a decision to withhold or withdraw other aspects of providing medical treatment, such as oxygen, suctioning, pain medications, and so forth. In addition, the decision is not irrevocable. The DNAR order should be part of a comprehensive plan of care that is periodically reviewed and that should be respected in all aspects of a child's care, including schooling. The extension of DNAR orders for children to the out-of-hospital setting can be an important component of providing comprehensive care. Mechanisms and laws should be in place for DNAR orders to be respected in schools and the prehospital emergency medical system.

One of the more difficult issues in withholding or withdrawing LSMT is the provision of artificial hydration and nutrition. Any person sufficiently dependent on the care of others will die as a result of not receiving hydration and nutrition. Some contend that the artificiality of some methods of providing hydration and nutrition (such as the use of a gastrostomy tube or intravenous hyperalimentation) indicates that they may be withheld or withdrawn as with any LSMT. A more compelling argument is that nutrition and hydration are not in a particular child's best interest regardless of the method of administration. Some states require "clear and convincing evidence" of a patient's prior wishes in order to withdraw such LSMT from patients who are either incompetent or in a permanent vegetative state. This "substituted judgment" is not possible in young children or in patients who became incompetent before expressing such wishes. Although there are legal cases that have allowed the removal of artificial nutrition and hydration based on a patient's "best interests," the rulings are generally in regard to adult patients and are thus of uncertain pediatric applicability.

The decision to withhold or withdraw LSMT does not necessarily imply an intent or choice to hasten a child's death. One can choose how to live while dying without choosing death, even when death is the anticipated outcome of one's choice. The provision of adequate sedation and analgesia to relieve rapidly progressive symptoms such as pain and dyspnea need not be interpreted as causing a child's death.

If a decision has been made that continued survival is not in a patient's best interest, it would seem irrelevant whether he or she died by forgoing LSMT or the administration of a drug. Indeed, the administration of a lethal drug might be preferable because of the opportunity to minimize suffering. However, the reasons for opposition to such decisions are only partly related to concerns for the interests of patients. The objections are based, in part, on the swiftness and irreversibility of action, precluding the possibility of changing course if it is discovered that the decision was wrong. The greater concern, however, has been for "slippery slope" effects: the claim that lowering the barrier against killing will make it easier for physicians to kill others, that boundaries will become less distinct, and that patients without a clear interest in dying will be harmed. Some contend that the current experience in The Netherlands lends some support to this concern. In addition, the backlash against physician-assisted suicide may render the appropriate provision of palliative care more difficult through fear of legal prosecution based simply on the dose of sedatives or narcotics administered.

Disabled Newborns and LSMT. In 1982, an infant with Down syndrome and esophageal atresia was allowed to die at 6 days of age at the parents' request. The case was similar to many others that had occurred during the preceding decade, particularly involving undertreatment of newborns with Down syndrome and spina bifida. Many of these children appeared to have excellent prospects for long, happy lives, suggesting that the decisions were not being made in the best interests of the children. In two large surveys, most pediatricians supported parental control of such decisions; some pediatricians stated that they considered their duty was not to serve the interests of their patient but rather to serve the interests of the family. These problems were compounded by the fact that decisions were often based on erroneous medical assumptions, including inappropriately pessimistic prognoses about quality of life.

As a consequence of concern about this issue in the United States, regulations were eventually promulgated under the authority of a federal child abuse law that prohibited withholding medically beneficial treatment from disabled infants except under certain conditions. These conditions are permanent unconsciousness, "futile" treatment, and "virtually futile" treatment that imposes excessive burdens on an infant. This rule seemed to disqualify one of the most common justifications for forgoing LSMT in children—namely, the likelihood that continued biologic existence would not serve the patients' interests precisely because they would be so disabled that the burden of treatment would be greater than the benefit. One unintended consequence of this rule was an apparent shift from undertreatment to widespread overtreatment, defined as life-prolonging treatment that, in the opinion of the physician, does not serve the interests of the child. However, the regulations address state eligibility for federal child abuse funding and, absent the incorporation of similar language in state statutes, do not dictate the proper scope of medical interventions. A subsequent case involving an infant with spina bifida and other abnormalities upheld the right of a parent to decide to forgo LSMT for their child.

INSTITUTIONAL (HOSPITAL) ETHICS COMMITTEES

The controversy over forgoing LSMT of disabled newborn infants led to the formation of the "infant bioethics committee" as a pediatric forerunner of today's institutional ethics committee (IEC).

An IEC usually provides voluntary consultation, which may involve enhanced communication or conflict resolution. For the vast majority of decisions involving the medical treatment of children (including forgoing LSMT), pediatric clinicians and parents are usually in agreement about the desirability of the proposed intervention. In addition, the views of a child should be given considerable weight, especially when the burden of treatment is great and the potential benefit uncertain or remote.

An IEC typically performs at least three different functions: (1) the drafting and review of institutional policy on such issues as DNAR orders and forgoing LSMT; (2) the education of health care professionals, patients, and families about ethical issues in health care; and (3) case consultation. Although the process of case consultation may vary, ideally the IEC should adopt a collaborative approach that uncovers all the readily available and relevant facts, takes into account the feelings of those involved, and balances the vested interests, while arriving at a recommendation based on a consistent ethical analysis. These committees, or an appropriate alternative, are now required by the Joint Commission on Accreditation of Hospitals, and they often play a consultative role when parents and medical staff cannot agree on the proper course of action. They have acquired considerable influence and are increasingly recognized by state courts as an important factor in decision-making.

SCREENING AND GENETIC TESTING

Screening is the search for asymptomatic illness in a defined population; it is usually performed for the purpose of treatment but it is sometimes done for counseling or research. Several programs, such as newborn screening for inborn errors of metabolism (e.g., phenylketonuria [PKU] and hypothyroidism), are counted among the triumphs of contemporary pediatrics. The success of such programs sometimes obscures serious ethical issues that continue to arise in proposals to screen for other conditions for which the benefits, risks, and costs have not been clearly established. Advances in genetics have led to exponential growth in the number of conditions for which screening tests are available, with insufficient opportunity to study each proposed testing program.

The introduction of screening tests should be done in a carefully controlled manner that allows for the evaluation of the costs (financial, medical, and psychological) and benefits of screening, including the effectiveness of follow-up and treatment protocols. New programs should be considered experimental until the risks and benefits are demonstrated. Screening tests that identify candidates for treatment need to have demonstrated sensitivity, specificity, and high predictive value, lest individuals be falsely labeled and subject to possibly toxic treatments or to psychosocial risks. As these tests are being developed, parents should generally be given the opportunity to exercise informed consent or refusal. These safeguards have not always been systematically applied to screening programs, often resulting in serious harm to many children without compensating benefits. Familiar examples include routine fetal monitoring, which contributed to the rising rate of cesarean sections with little benefit for many infants, and the screening of premature infants for acidosis, resulting in administration of toxic amounts of sodium bicarbonate before its risks were adequately studied.

A persistent ethical issue is whether screening should be voluntary (i.e., "opt in"), routine with the ability to "opt out" or refuse, or mandatory. A voluntary approach entails an informed decision by parents before screening. Concern is often expressed that seeking informed consent is ethically inappropriate for tests of clear benefit, such as PKU screening, because refusal would constitute neglect. Routine testing with an "opt out" approach requires an explicit refusal of screening by parents who object to

this intervention. The principal ethical justification for mandatory screening is the claim that society's obligation to promote child welfare through early detection and treatment of selected conditions supersedes any parental right to refuse this simple medical intervention. However, obtaining informed consent for newborn screening may allow for more prompt and efficient responses to positive results, and for incorporating experimental tests into established screening programs. Although more research is necessary, one study showed that a reasonable attempt at consent could be made on a statewide basis without excessive time or cost and without undue effects on compliance.

These two ethical principles of demonstrated benefit justifying the risks of screening and informed consent can be applied to genetic testing for late-onset disorders. The knowledge of increased risk status may lead to lifestyle changes that can reduce morbidity and the risk of mortality, or may precipitate adverse emotional and psychological responses and discrimination. Because many adults choose not to be tested for late-onset disorders, we cannot assume that a child would want or will benefit from similar testing. Genetic testing of children and adolescents for late-onset disorders is generally inappropriate unless such testing will result in interventions that have been shown to reduce morbidity and mortality when initiated in childhood. Otherwise, such testing should be deferred until the child has the capacity to make an informed and voluntary choice.

ADOLESCENT HEALTH CARE

Many adolescents resemble adults more than they do children in their competence to consent to health care. Competence is not a global quality: teenagers may not be able to support themselves, yet they may still be competent to consent to health care. In addition to competence, there are public health reasons for allowing adolescents to consent to their own health care with regard to reproductive decisions, such as contraception, abortion, and treatment of sexually transmitted diseases. Strict requirements for parental consent may deter many adolescents from seeking health care, with serious implications for their health and other community interests.

Weighed against these arguments are the legitimate interests of parents in maintaining responsibility and authority for child rearing, including the opportunity to influence the sexual attitudes and practices of one's children. Another claim is that public support for access to such treatment, particularly contraception and abortion, implicitly endorses and encourages sexual activity, aggravating rather than ameliorating the problems. Similar concerns underlie the objection to providing sterile needles for intravenous drug abusers for the purpose of reducing the risk of acquiring hepatitis or human immunodeficiency virus. Critics complain that such programs give children the message that illegal drug use is supported by the state as long as it is done safely, even though it is now generally accepted that access to sterile needles results in a decrease in new cases of acquired immunodeficiency syndrome. The pediatrician's role and behavior in these disputes will be influenced by his or her own moral beliefs and by assessments of the competing facts and arguments. Physicians need to consider the possibility that a moralistic position may deter adolescents from seeking health care or counseling.

RESEARCH

The central ethical distinction between research and standard clinical practice is researchers' commitment to generating knowledge, perhaps to the benefit of future patients or society, in addition to their responsibility for patients who are the human subjects of the investigation. Research is defined in the federal regulations as "a systematic investigation designed to develop or contribute to generalizable knowledge." For any research to be performed, the risks should be minimized and reasonable with respect to any anticipated benefits to the subjects and the importance of the resulting knowledge. Because children generally cannot give voluntary and informed consent to their own research participation, there are further restrictions on the research risks to which a child may be exposed. These restrictions specify the conditions under which a parent has the moral and legal authority to permit a child to participate in research.

In *nontherapeutic research,* there is no expected direct benefit for the subject; therefore, any risk may present an unfavorable risk:benefit ratio. Some argue that children, along with other nonconsenting subjects, should never be used in nontherapeutic research, as a person should never be used solely as a means to an end. The more widely held opinion is that children may be exposed to at least *minimal risks,* although the reasons for this exception are disputed. Some argue that children have a duty to contribute to the social welfare, although the federal regulations do not allow competent adults to be used as research subjects for this justification without their consent. Others argue that participation in research can provide an indirect benefit by fostering a sense of altruism or citizenship through a child's assent. The federal regulations allow healthy children to participate in minimal risk research based on an analogy to parental authority to make decisions about risk exposure in everyday life. The regulations also state that children with a condition can be exposed to slightly more than minimal risk in nontherapeutic research if the child's experience is similar to everyday life with that condition and the anticipated knowledge is of vital importance for understanding or benefiting that condition. This "minor increase over minimal risk" category is the most controversial.

Much of the controversy over nontherapeutic research stems from the wide variability in the interpretation of minimal risk. The federal regulations define minimal risks as the risks that are "ordinarily encountered in daily life or during the performance of routine physical or psychological examinations or tests." Some interpret this to include procedures similar to those done in primary care office visits, but others claim that an invasive procedure such as a liver biopsy may be done if the risks, in the hands of a particular investigator, are empirically no higher than those of a routine office visit or if the procedure is routine for a visit to a specialist. When originally proposed, the definition of minimal risk referred to the life of a healthy child. The regulations omitted this phrase out of concern that research would be hindered, thus contributing to the wide range of interpretation. However, many advocate restoring the phrase "of healthy children" to the definition of minimal risk, because valuable research on a condition may still proceed under the "minor increase over minimal risk" category. As originally proposed, the concept of minimal risk serves a moral purpose in limiting a parent's authority to permit nontherapeutic research on a healthy child. To define minimal risk using only statistical considerations (such as the product of probability and magnitude) may overlook this moral purpose. The risks of each intervention or procedure in the research needs to be considered separately and balanced against any direct benefit to the subject or knowledge to be gained.

The term *therapeutic research* is misleading in that not all interventions or procedures included in a research study may offer the prospect of direct benefit to the subject. There are likely to be nontherapeutic aspects of the research, such as an extra blood test or chest radiograph. As discussed above, the nontherapeutic parts of the research need to be no more than a "minor increase over minimal risk" and cannot be justified by the anticipated benefit of other parts of the overall research study. The risks of interventions that offer direct benefit can be more than minimal. However, the risks must be justified by the anticipated benefit, and the balance of anticipated benefit to the risk should be as favorable as that presented by available alternatives. A child should not be disadvantaged by being enrolled in a research study.

Innovative therapy is defined as a new and unproven intervention done primarily for the benefit of the patient, with no intent to gather new information. Such innovations may be more hazardous and ethically more problematic than research, in part because they are not subject to peer review and because toxicity is not being systematically assessed. This kind of therapy is also subject to abuse because its definition is a matter of intent, and thus difficult for others to disprove. Although innovative medical and surgical interventions are not subject to research regulations, some argue that clinicians have a moral obligation to submit innovative therapies to formal evaluation.

The regulations in the United States for the protection of human research subjects rest on two foundations: (1) voluntary and informed consent and (2) the independent review of the research risks. The standard for informed consent in a research setting is higher than for clinical care because the risks and benefits are typically less clear, the investigator has a conflict of interest, and humans have historically been subjected to unauthorized risks when strict requirements for consent were not respected.

Adolescents who are competent may sometimes consent to be research subjects. It is also generally acknowledged that children should be given the opportunity to *dissent,* particularly for nontherapeutic research, when there cannot be a claim that participation is in the child's interest. In the United States, national regulations require that reasonable efforts be made at least to inform children who are capable of understanding that participation is not part of their care and that, therefore, they are free to refuse to participate. In addition to the protection that informed consent is intended to provide, virtually all research involving human subjects in the United States is reviewed by an institutional review board, required by federal regulations for institutions receiving federal research funds and for Food and Drug Administration–regulated drug research. It is uncertain whether such review is legally required for research that is not federally funded or for research in settings that receive no federal funds, such as private clinics. The principles of ethical decision-making that led to the involvement of ethics committees in clinical decisions argue for similar review of research involving children, regardless of the source of funding.

A general ethical principle is that individuals who are capable of voluntary and informed consent be approached first about research participation. An unintended result is that the majority of marketed medications are not labeled for use in children. Pediatricians are left with a difficult choice of using medications "off label" and risking increased toxicity or decreased efficacy, or not using a medication and potentially denying a child an important therapeutic advance. To ameliorate this problem, the United States has granted 6 mo patent extensions for the performance of requested pediatric studies, resulting in new pediatric labeling for many important drugs. New drug applications must include studies in children unless granted a specific waiver. In addition, grants submitted to the National Institutes of Health must include children in the absence of scientific or ethical reasons to the contrary.

FETAL WELL-BEING AND TREATMENT

As our knowledge of factors influencing fetal development and well-being expands, there is increasing discussion about the proper balancing of maternal and fetal interests when a pregnant woman's behavior affects the well-being of her fetus. Interventions can now be directed primarily toward specific medical and surgical conditions of the fetus, rather than toward the general health of the pregnant woman with a secondary impact on the fetus. As a result, questions arise about a clinician's responsibility when the interests of the pregnant woman and her fetus appear to conflict. There are two particularly controversial areas in which this question arises—the provision of fetal medical or surgical treatment and the reporting of pregnant women for drug and alcohol use.

The most dramatic of these conflicts arises when a pregnant woman refuses standard, effective treatment essential for the benefit of a fetus/infant who is at high risk of death or serious disability, such as refusal of cesarean section for placenta previa in a voluntary pregnancy near term involving a presumably normal fetus/infant. Courts in the United States have sometimes decided that a woman can be required to undergo such a procedure when the benefit to the emergent child is clear. A federal court decided that such an order was inappropriate in a case involving a 26-wk-old fetus and, by implication, other cases in which the benefit of intervention was in doubt. In general, a clinician should not oppose a pregnant woman's refusal of a recommended intervention unless (1) the risk to the pregnant woman is negligible, (2) the intervention has been shown effective, and (3) the harm to the fetus is certain, substantial, and irrevocable. When these three conditions exist, a clinician may try to persuade and, if unsuccessful, seek some other avenue of conflict resolution (such as through an IEC). Rarely, and only as a last resort, should a clinician seek judicial authorization to override a pregnant woman's dissent.

Child abuse statutes have also been invoked in attempts to modify the behavior of women who ingest alcohol or illicit drugs during pregnancy and expose the fetus/infant to harm. Pediatricians considering reporting such cases must consider the likelihood of benefit from reporting, the harm to the child as well as to the mother if criminal charges or custody changes are sought, and the possible effects that reporting may have in driving pregnant women away from the health care system, particularly from prenatal care. The US Supreme Court has held that drug testing of pregnant women without consent was in direct violation of the Fourth Amendment, which provides protection from unreasonable searches.

ACCESS TO HEALTH CARE: RATIONING (DISTRIBUTIVE JUSTICE)

The most serious ethical problem in health care in the United States may be the inequality in access to care. No other major industrial country rations basic health care on the basis of ability to pay. Comprising nearly one of every five uninsured persons, more than 9 million children and adolescents lack basic health care coverage. This lack of adequate and affordable health care has serious consequences in terms of death, disability, and suffering. The central ethical principle at stake is fair opportunity to participate in the benefits of society; preventable death and disability undermine the claim that the society is one of equal opportunity. Another aspect of the claim of unfairness is that the present system is maintained by those who are already advantaged because of financial or social status, thereby aggravating existing inequalities.

Rationing of health care can be defined as limiting access to wanted and needed services of known benefit. It is increasingly recognized that no society can provide all beneficial services to all its citizens; rationing is therefore unavoidable. The question is not whether to ration health care services but how to do so fairly. Apart from ability to pay, other ways of rationing could be based on cost:benefit analysis, age, or likely effects on quality of life. Even universal systems of health care coverage effectively ration through limited availability, with the option of purchasing additional desired services using private resources. Some argue that such a multitiered system is fair as long as the basic health care package is appropriately defined and sufficiently funded.

Caplan AL, Blank RH, Merrick JC, eds: *Compelled Compassion: Government Intervention in the Treatment of Critically Ill Newborns*. Totowa, NJ, Humana Press, 1992.

Committee on Bioethics, American Academy of Pediatrics: Informed consent, parental permission, and assent in pediatric practice. *Pediatrics* 1995;95:314.

Committee on Bioethics, American Academy of Pediatrics: Ethics and the care of critically ill infants and children. *Pediatrics* 1996;98:149.

Committee on Bioethics, American Academy of Pediatrics: Religious objections to medical care. *Pediatrics* 1997;99:279.

Committee on Bioethics, American Academy of Pediatrics: Fetal therapy—Ethical considerations. *Pediatrics* 1999;103:1061.

Committee on Bioethics, American Academy of Pediatrics: Institutional ethics committees. *Pediatrics* 2001;107:205.

Committee on Bioethics, American Academy of Pediatrics: Ethical issues with genetic testing in pediatrics. *Pediatrics* 2001;107:1451.

Committee on Bioethics and Committee on Hospital Care, American Academy of Pediatrics: Palliative care for children. *Pediatrics* 2000;106:351.

Helft PR, Siegler M, Lantos J: The rise and fall of the futility movement. *N Engl J Med* 2000;343:293.

Nelson RM: Children as research subjects. In Kahn J, Mastroianni A, Sugarman J (eds): *Beyond Consent: Seeking Justice in Research*. New York: Oxford University Press, 1998, pp 47–66.

Chapter 3
Cultural Issues in Pediatric Care *Jill E. Korbin*

Considering the worldwide diversity of cultures, the diversity of cultures in the United States, and the diversity within any culture, no pediatrician can be expected to be an expert on all cultures that he or she might encounter. What can be expected of the pediatrician, however, is expertise in a set of issues related to understanding how culture impacts the quality of pediatric care and health outcomes. This chapter is directed at facilitating understanding of this complex interaction between culture and pediatric practice.

Culture and ethnicity are relevant to culturally competent clinical care of children and to understanding children and the experience of childhood as relevant to health. The National Academy of Sciences' evaluation of the "current science of early childhood development" made culture the second of 10 core concepts: "Culture influences every aspect of human development and is reflected in childrearing beliefs and practices designed to promote healthy adaptation." However, the complexity of culture and ethnicity in relation to health leaves many questions unanswered.

Current demographic trends in the United States demand a high standard of culturally informed, or culturally competent, health care. As projected, European-Americans will not retain their majority status, and the minority-majority transition will occur at an earlier date for children. Pediatricians can expect to see greater percentages of diverse populations in their practice and research. Demographic trends take on even more importance in pediatric care when coupled with the growing body of evidence on cultural and ethnic disparities in health resulting from a combination of lifestyle issues influenced by socioeconomic disadvantage, biologic and genetic factors, and access to and use of health care. Culture and ethnicity potentially affect all of these matters. Among the most compelling reasons for the tie of culture and ethnicity to pediatrics is that pediatrics, like no other branch of medicine, has the opportunity to shape an individual's lifelong perceptions of health care and use of health services. In addition to enhancing individual health, there is the potential for influence on the health of populations. Children are often at the forefront of societal and cultural change related to health and well-being, such as public health campaigns for smoking cessation and seatbelt use.

CULTURE AND ETHNICITY

Many definitions of culture center on the ideas of culture as a learned, shared, and interpretive force that guides interactions among people. Culture is a broader term encompassing ethnicity. Children are not passive recipients of socialization into their culture, rather they shape and reinterpret it. Culture is experienced variably by different members of a group; it is not static, but dynamic and constantly changing. *Ethnicity*, which is generally used by lay people synonymously with *culture*, refers to group membership by virtue of common ancestry. This membership can be self- or other-identified. The terms *culture*, *ethnicity*, and *race* should not be used interchangeably or synonymously, and care should be taken not to confound culture and ethnicity with religion or socioeconomic class.

The relationship of culture and ethnicity to health care, including pediatrics, has been obscured by the use of major census categories to designate groupings of people, such as Latin-American/Hispanic, Asian/Pacific Islander, Native American, and African-American. There are many distinct groups found within the census categories. The designation European-American similarly encompasses a wide range of cultures and ethnicities. These categories, which have found their way into common parlance, do not reflect cultural reality and may, in fact, mask rather than illuminate culture. At best, these categories can be used as shorthand or a starting point. Geographic considerations also are less frequently noted, such that Puerto Ricans, for example, living in New York may be quite different from Puerto Ricans living in Cleveland. Variability within any cultural or ethnic group often exceeds that between groups, and populations continually adapt to changing circumstances. Furthermore, when culture or ethnicity is identified on the basis of phenotypic characteristics, such as skin color, such groupings may not be meaningful designations of culture or ethnicity, but instead serve as proxies for socioeconomic status.

Both culture and medicine are dynamic and constantly changing. For example, in recent years the extensive use of nonconventional and alternative remedies by the American public, including children, has been recognized (see Chapter 713). The use of complementary and alternative medicine occurs in educated and affluent groups, challenging conventional wisdom that such practices are limited to those culturally different from the dominant society. Such complementary and alternative practices are included in many medical school curriculums.

CULTURAL COMPETENCE AND PEDIATRIC PRACTICE

Cultural "competence" refers to the acquisition of knowledge and skills needed to transcend cultural boundaries; it moves beyond "sensitivity" and "awareness." The need for cultural competence is most obvious among patients who, for example, wear traditional dress or speak another language. In these circumstances, cultural diversity is relatively easy to spot, even if the possible health effects are not always straightforward. On the other hand, even if a patient appears to be culturally similar to the physician, congruence in health beliefs and behaviors cannot be assumed. What might be assumed to be similarities in orientation do not necessarily ensure optimal care, even among physicians. Whereas physicians' children have been found to have better access to pediatricians and increased pediatrician visits if hospitalized, they also experience delays in seeking pediatric care. Furthermore, pediatricians have been found to provide less detailed medical instructions and to be reluctant to discuss children's behavioral problems with fellow physicians than with other parents.

One strategy for achieving cultural competence is to conceptualize illness as a series of unfolding stages. The pediatric visit may not be the first stage but usually comes later in the process after symptom recognition, formulation of etiologic explanations, and lay referral and consultation. Knowledge about each stage obtained during a pediatric visit can diminish the likelihood of cultural conflict or resolve it more quickly if it occurs. In eliciting a narrative account of illness while obtaining a medical history, information on culture can be obtained without adding a burdensome time commitment. Two points in the unfolding process are used here as illustrations: symptom definition and etiologic explanations.

An initial point in an illness episode is the identification of symptoms of ill health. Children may identify these on their own, or they may be identified by a parent or caregiver. Whether or not culturally diverse children, parents or caregivers, and physicians converge on the significance of symptoms is important to the course of subsequent treatment. Folk diagnoses and medical diagnoses may appear divergent, even when they converge in important ways. For example, a Mexican mother's diagnosis of entities such as *susto* (fright sickness), *mal de ojo* (evil eye), or *caida de mollera* (fallen fontanel) may be regarded as being at odds with the physician's diagnosis. Mothers may regard these entities as untreatable by Western physicians, and physicians might dismiss these folk classifications in their diagnosis. However, even though the labels for these conditions and their etiologic attributions differ, the presenting symptoms are likely to be recognized by both parent and physician as significant and potentially life-threatening, thereby establishing more common ground than at first is apparent. Common ground, then, can be found in the seriousness of symptoms, such as fever. Once symptoms are identified as signs of ill health, a process begins to try to explain their cause. Cultural conflict in medical care often emanates from disagreement as to etiology, because discerning the cause is important in formulating the cure. Although there is both intracultural and intercultural variability, there may be more congruence across cultures than was previously thought. Middle-class European-Americans and Latin-Americans, for example, recognize the common cold as a biomedical entity but also attribute its etiology, at least in part, to becoming chilled as part of a hot-cold system of beliefs. Nevertheless, the differences in culture may interfere with care if a pediatrician's planned course of treatment is not presented as related to the family's attribution of the cause of illness.

Cultural knowledge is also empirical knowledge. For example, because remedies have worked in the past, it is assumed that they will work in the future. Middle-class parents in the United States routinely accept a pediatrician prescription for a second course of antibiotics for otitis media if a child's symptoms persist, assuming not that antibiotics are useless, but that a different drug or a longer course of treatment will resolve the problem. The same is true for indigenous treatments that have been proven through the force of custom over time.

EMERGING AREAS IN CULTURE AND PEDIATRICS

One area of interest, termed *evolutionary medicine* or *ethnopediatrics*, looks at cross-cultural variability in child care practices and seeks to understand these practices in the context of human evolution. Sleep problems, a common issue in pediatric practice, serve as an example. Co-sleeping with infants has likely occurred throughout human history, is exceedingly common cross-culturally, and is more common in the United States than was previously thought. While recent years have seen increasing flexibility in pediatric advice in this domain, common pediatric guidance is still that infants and young children should sleep separately from their parents, in a different room, and in their own beds for the night. Some sleep problems, then, may be viewed as rooted in behaviors of child care that may be inconsistent with the biologic needs and capacities of human infants rather than a failure on the part of the parent, child, or both.

Another emerging area is viewing children as active shapers of their social and cultural environment rather than passive recipients of socialization. Even though pediatricians have always relied on children for information, the social sciences are now more supportive of children's viewpoints being included in decisions regarding their lives. The United Nations Convention on the Rights of the Child also includes provisions affirming this position.

A third area involves capitalizing on cultural and ethnic strengths and looking for common ground. Culture and ethnicity have more often been approached as being potential sources of conflict with the health care system rather than recognizing the point of congruence.

American Academy of Pediatrics (1993): Culturally effective pediatric care: Education and training issues. *Pediatrics* 1993;103:167.

Baer R, Bustillo M: Caida de mollera among children of Mexican migrant workers: Implications for the study of folk illnesses. *Med Anthrop Q* 1998;12:241.

Baer R, Weller S, Pachter L, et al: Cross-cultural perspectives on the common cold: Data from five populations. *Hum Organization* 1999;58:251.

Flores D: Culture and the patient-physician relationship: Achieving cultural competency in health care. *J Pediatr* 2000;136:14.

Kemper K: Complementary and alternative medicine for children: Does it work? *Arch Dis Child* 2001;200:84.

Korbin J, Brinkley P, Reebals L, Singh N: Understanding the importance of cultural beliefs and behaviors in clinical practice. In Kliegman R, Neider M, Super D (editors): *Practical Strategies in Pediatric Diagnosis and Therapy.* New York, WB Saunders, 1996, pp 35–39.

Shonkoff J, Phillips D: *From Neurons to Neighborhoods. The Science of Early Childhood Development.* Washington, DC, National Academy Press, 2000.

Sobo E, Rock C: "You ate all that!": Caretaker-child interaction during children's assisted dietary recall interviews. *Med Anthrop Q* 2001;15:222.

Trevathan W, Smith E, McKenna J (editors): *Evolutionary Medicine.* New York, Oxford University Press, 1999.

Chapter 4
Child Health in the Developing World

Kristine Torjesen and Karen Olness

Ninety percent of children in the early 21st century are born into the developing or third world. This chapter reviews the demographics, the health problems of children in the developing world, the larger ramifications of their health problems, the skills needed by individuals and institutions who help them, and future challenges. Fifty years ago, child health leaders such as David Morley and Cicely Williams emphasized the special needs and problems of children in the developing world. Huge population increases in the developing world now mean that there are many more children suffering from the same problems identified by Morley and Williams.

DEMOGRAPHICS

According to current UNICEF data, there are 71 million children younger than 18 yr in the United States and 2.1 billion children younger than 18 yr in the rest of the world. The mortality rate of children younger than 5 yr is 8/1,000 in the United States and 86/1,000 for the overall child population of the world. One thousand infants die each hour; 970 of these deaths occur in developing countries. In addition, human potential is unrealized because of poor health, especially cognitive impairment caused by health problems, with negative effects on individuals, families, communities, and countries in terms of productivity, economics, and politics. Population projections to 2025 show continuing rapid growth in Africa, Western Asia, South Central Asia, Southeast Asia, West Asia, South America, and Latin America, with modest or slowing growth rates in East Asia, North America, and Europe. Hundreds of thousands of children

born in developing countries move into Europe and into North America as refugees, immigrants, or international adoptees. Dr. Robert Haggerty wrote, "Pediatric practice in the next millennium will require greater knowledge of new morbidities...Diversity in ethnic and cultural backgrounds and beliefs will continue to increase, and will need to be understood to prevent and treat diseases of children effectively."

HEALTH PROBLEMS OF CHILDREN IN THE DEVELOPING WORLD

According to the World Health Organization (WHO), 10.5 million children younger than 5 yr died in 1999. Of these, 99% lived in developing countries. Causes of death were attributed to malnutrition (54%), perinatal conditions (20%), pneumonia (19%), diarrhea (15%), measles (8%), malaria (7%), HIV/AIDS (3%), and other (28%). One third of births in the developing world are not registered. Malnutrition among pregnant women leads to stunting of an estimated 182 million children. From 1990 to 2000, at least 20 million were children displaced by disasters at any given time. In 2000, more than 10 million children younger than 15 yr had lost one or both parents to AIDS. There is an increasing number of street children in the world; many suffer infectious diseases such as hepatitis and tuberculosis. In much of the developing world, there are no resources for poor children with conditions such as leukemia, brain tumors, AIDS, head injuries, congenital heart disease, or metabolic disorders.

Between 1980 and 2000, there were dramatic increases in the percentage of children immunized in developing countries and, as a result, diseases such as poliomyelitis and measles are much less common. However, immunizations for diseases such as hepatitis, haemophilus influenza b, and varicella are rarely available in the developing world. The number of children infected with HIV has increased dramatically, as has the number of children suffering from malnutrition associated with disasters. Malaria and tuberculosis also affect greater numbers of children than they did a decade ago. Malaria is the leading cause of hospitalization, mortality, and morbidity in children younger than 5 yr who live in sub-Saharan Africa. Malnutrition, including both calorie and micronutrient deprivation, causes acute and chronic morbidity, contributes to reduced immunity, and increases the likelihood of mortality and morbidity in association with infectious diseases.

IMPAIRED LEARNING

Approximately one third of children younger than 15 yr in developing countries either have or are at risk for impaired learning. Major hazards to early brain development include malnutrition, infectious diseases (e.g., meningitis), prematurity and newborn asphyxia, in utero exposure to alcohol and drugs, lead poisoning, genetic disorders, head injuries, and institutionalization. Malnutrition experienced during the critical periods of brain development from the second trimester of pregnancy until 2 yr of age is most likely to be associated with subsequent cognitive impairment. Galler and others have documented that a few months of malnutrition in the first year of life is associated with learning disabilities, attentional problems, and reduced school performance in 65–70% of children. Iron deficiency, very common among infants in the developing world, is associated with continuing learning problems a decade later. Iodine deficiency is also common, especially in large areas of China, Central Africa, and South America, and is associated with mental impairment in children. Further research indicates that cognitive impairment due to early brain insults may not be apparent until the child is well along in school. Children seem to do fairly well in the early school years but begin to manifest executive dysfunction in middle school years when more goal setting, planning, organizing, and time management are required. Children with learning impairments, especially those without access to special education or training, are likely to drop out of school and to have difficulties finding and maintaining employment, and they are less likely to be contributing citizens in their communities (see Chapter 39).

CHILDREN AND DISASTERS

Most disasters occur in developing countries and are due to natural events such as hurricanes, industrial accidents such as the 1984 chemical disasters in Bhopal, or wars with associated displacement of populations, more than half of whom are children. The number of complex humanitarian emergencies has increased during the past decade. Children involved in such disasters are at risk for infectious diseases, malnutrition, and psychological trauma, which may be lifelong. Children displaced from Southeast Asia, Central Africa, and Bosnia by war have a high prevalence of mental health problems continuing years after resettlement.

INSTITUTIONALIZATION

The number of children institutionalized in developing countries is unknown, but the number of institutions for orphan children has increased in countries of the former Union of Soviet Socialist Republics, Eastern Europe, sub-Saharan Africa, India, and China in the past decade. Reasons include death of parents from AIDS, poverty in families who might ordinarily adopt child relatives, political upheavals, and community chaos. A small percentage of the institutionalized children are adopted by North American or European families. Eighteen thousand children from abroad are adopted into American families each year (see Chapter 30). About half of children adopted from orphanages abroad are malnourished. Rickets is common, as are intestinal parasites. Many children have been infected with tuberculosis, hepatitis B, hepatitis C, or syphilis. Of great concern are the frequent developmental delays and attachment problems, which increase after the first year of life of these orphan children.

APPROACH TO CHILD HEALTH IN THE DEVELOPING WORLD

Traditionally, efforts to improve child health in the developing world have focused on primary health care. This approach concentrates on improving public health and basic health care at the community level, usually by training village health workers to recognize and manage childhood illnesses such as diarrhea and pneumonia. The primary health care approach is essential in developing countries, where access to basic medical facilities and trained health care professionals is often lacking and where the majority of childhood diseases are preventable. However, the primary health care approach includes teaching village health workers to recognize and refer sick patients to acute health care facilities. Currently, there are inadequate resources devoted to training health professionals and establishing such referral centers in most developing countries; they often do not exist and, therefore, sicker children suffer or die. Depending on the resources available and the socioeconomic situation of a given country, these outcomes may be unavoidable. However, as the public health infrastructure improves in a developing country, it becomes increasingly important to train local child health specialists. These child health specialists provide referral care to individual children and serve as the backbone for long-term improvements in child health by providing local expertise and knowledge for the formulation of child health policy in their own countries.

Pediatricians and child health professionals can contribute to improving both primary health care and higher levels of medical care for children in developing countries. The field of pediatrics has excelled at integrating primary health care and preventive care into the practice of curative medicine (Chapter 5). Pediatricians have long recognized the need to provide com-

prehensive care to children and to use any point of contact as an opportunity to assess the overall health of the child and family. These principles are being implemented by WHO on a global level through the program Integrated Management of Childhood Illness (IMCI). In the past, many health programs in developing countries took a single-condition approach (sometimes called a vertical approach), for example, achieving specific immunization goals or eradicating malaria. This very focused approach fails to adequately address the health care needs of children. A visit to the vaccine clinic that does not address a child's malnutrition or diarrhea is a lost opportunity to prevent illness and promote health for that child. IMCI is a positive step toward providing higher-quality, comprehensive care for children in the developing world. The IMCI health care algorithms are written at or slightly above the level of a village health worker, and they target children younger than 5 yr old, the group with the highest death rate from common childhood diseases. However, the broader guideline of integrating curative and preventive care for children is appropriate at all levels of health care provision. For infants 1 wk to 2 mo old, IMCI has as its clinical priorities the assessment of the main signs and symptoms of bacterial infection, diarrhea, feeding problems, low weight, and immunization status. For children 2 mo to 5 yr old, the IMCI priorities of management emphasize cough and breathing difficulties, diarrhea, fever, ear problems, nutritional status, and immunizations.

In most settings, it is difficult to separate the health of the child from that of the family and the broader social context in which the child lives. This is particularly true in the developing world. Maternal health practices strongly impact child health, particularly in the perinatal period. Prenatal care, neonatal resuscitation, maternal nutrition, breast-feeding and weaning practices, and maternal depression all may have profound effects on a child's well-being. Economic conditions and family resources drive health care decision-making. For example, do we pay for our sick child's medication or buy food for our other children? Environmental conditions limit the effective treatment of preventable illnesses, such as diarrhea and malaria. Political instability and violence interfere with the establishment and maintenance of health care systems. Cultural and religious practices may limit or counteract the effectiveness of medical therapies. Child rights abuses may underlie presenting illnesses. Much of the childhood disease burden in developing countries may rightfully be seen as the medical manifestations of social illnesses, such as lack of education, poverty, and other forms of injustice.

HOW CHILD HEALTH PROFESSIONALS CAN HELP THE CHILDREN OF THE WORLD

Depending on their areas of skill and interest, child health professionals can provide service, research, and education in developing countries. The first step is to educate oneself about child health problems in developing countries. Skills are needed for a child health specialist to provide services in developing countries. The concrete skills that improve the likelihood of making a positive contribution toward addressing child health care issues in the developing world include training in pediatrics, public health, epidemiology, infectious diseases, nutrition, and immunizations. Clinical and community outreach experience, even if in an industrialized setting, is also useful. All child health professionals should take training in disaster management and be prepared to help colleagues in their own countries, as well as in other countries, in case of natural disaster, war, or bioterrorism (Chapter 706). There is a great need during disasters for assistance provided by those who understand the special needs and issues of children. Language skills are important, as is prior experience with different cultures and belief systems. Many of the skills required to help children in the developing world are more abstract in nature: flexibility, tolerance for the unexpected, respect for local colleagues and their practice of medicine, ability to function with different and perhaps frustrating cultural norms and communication styles, and ability to triage when faced with limited resources. A particularly difficult dilemma for child health providers in developing countries is balancing the very pressing curative medical needs of children with their more long-term preventive care needs. Children require clean water, food, shelter, warmth, and love to grow healthy; they also need medical treatment for acute illnesses. When faced with limited resources, inadequate public health infrastructure, and many sick children, the individual practitioner can be overwhelmed by a myriad of tasks. With experience, most practitioners in the developing world find a way to prioritize the conflicting and compelling needs before them.

Pediatric research in developing countries has lagged behind that in Western countries. As a result, there is a lack of knowledge in many areas, including, for example, the long-term effects of medications used to treat many parasitic infections, the interactions between traditional herbal therapies and antibiotics, the extent of genetic diseases, the prevalence of iron deficiency, and the neurodevelopmental effects of cerebral malaria. It is appropriate for child health specialists and institutions from wealthier nations to assist colleagues in developing countries to develop research skills, design appropriate projects, find financial support, and implement the research project. The same rules for protection of human subjects should apply everywhere, and it is important that child health researchers assist colleagues in developing countries to develop and use institutional review boards (Chapter 2). Research projects in developing countries should be designed primarily for the benefit of the people in those countries, although information derived may prove to be useful throughout the world. Training child health colleagues in research skills is likely to result in long-term benefits for educational institutions, for trainees, and for children.

For those who cannot donate time and effort, individual financial contributions can be helpful in supporting child health programs managed by others. Child health specialists from wealthier communities can provide education materials, supplies, equipment, and psychological support to colleagues in developing countries. Reciprocal visits and continuing medical education opportunities can be beneficial to both communities. It is important to spend time working with colleagues in the actual setting where any teaching and resources will be applied in order to know what is needed and appropriate for that setting. Building upon personal relationships and contacts can lead to individual efforts to improve child health, or it may open doors for larger collaborations. Developing sister relationships between the pediatric practices of two communities can provide an excellent context for two-way learning experience and for sharing of resources.

FUTURE CHALLENGES

The 1990 United Nations World Summit for Children recommended a 10 year program to achieve basic health and social goals for children. With the exception of the immunization goals, they were not met. The participants could not have anticipated the increased number of children with HIV infection, the increased numbers of disasters, the continuing political upheavals, and burgeoning population numbers. It is important that child health professionals do their best for individual child patients and also participate in the broader public health and community planning on behalf of children. Probably the highest priority for the world should be the prevention of childhood learning problems. Health and human service professionals around the world must foster a global awareness about the impact of early events on the developing brain of a child, on his or her life, on the community, and on the world.

Galler JF, Barrett LR: Children and famine: Long-term impact on development. *Ambulatory Child Health* 2001;7:85–95. *E-mail: ach@blacksci.co.uk*

Jenista JA: The immigrant, refugee or internationally adopted child. *Pediatr Rev* 2001;22(12):419–29.

Mandalakas AM, Torjesen K, Olness K: *Helping the Children: A Practical Manual for Complex Humanitarian Emergencies.* New Brunswick, New Jersey: Johnson and Johnson, 1999.

Morley D, Lovel H: *My Name Is Today.* London, Macmillan, 1986.

Staton D, Harding M, Blackmore L: International child health and the internet. *Ambulatory Child Health* 2001;7(2):127–31. *E-mail: ach@blacksci.co.uk*

TALC: *Teaching-aids at Low Cost.* Centre for International Child Health Institute of Child Health, University of London, United Kingdom. *www.talcuk.org*

UNICEF: *The State of the World's Children 2001.* New York: Oxford University Press, 2001. *www.unicef.org*

Wolf C, Palmer D: *Handbook of Medicine in Developing Countries.* Bristol, TN: Christian Medical and Dental Society, 1999. *www.cmds.org*

World Health Organization (WHO). *www.who.int; www.who.int/child-adolescent-health/; www.who.int/whosis/*

Chapter 5
Preventive Pediatrics
Theodore C. Sectish

Prevention in the health care of infants, children, and adolescents is at the core of the field of pediatrics. During the 20th century, the lifespan of people living in the United States increased by more than 30 yr. Many of the public health measures that contributed to this increased lifespan were aimed at pediatric populations and represent some of the most significant achievements of preventive pediatrics during that century. Key examples include vaccination programs, motor vehicle safety measures, control of infectious diseases, safer and healthier foods, healthier mothers and babies, family planning, fluoridation of drinking water, and recognition of the hazards of tobacco use. Pediatricians have led the way in these and many other scientific, public health, and public policy efforts to address issues that affect populations of children through their professional activities as educators, advocates, scientists, and experts in child health.

At the level of individual patients, pediatricians practice preventive pediatrics with their clinical activities in health supervision. Preventive pediatrics in practice is the focus of this chapter and encompasses (1) health supervision of infants, children, and adolescents, (2) topics of frequent concern during health supervision visits, and (3) unmet needs and future challenges in preventive pediatrics.

HEALTH SUPERVISION OF INFANTS, CHILDREN, AND ADOLESCENTS

Pediatricians have a unique opportunity to improve the lives of children by making effective use of health supervision visits. Guidelines for health supervision address continuing and new morbidities facing children and families. These morbidities include childhood injuries, educational failure, child abuse and neglect, family violence, parental health issues, teenage pregnancy, environmental health concerns, media influences, obesity, and risk-taking behaviors such as the use of tobacco, alcohol, and drugs. Within health supervision visits, pediatricians should assess cognitive development, social competence, and family life in addition to performing traditional well child visits. The effectiveness of health supervision visits depends on the partnership that pediatricians develop with children and families to promote a collaborative effort toward achieving optimal health.

PRINCIPLES OF HEALTH SUPERVISION

Health Promotion. Health is not merely the absence of disease, but includes many dimensions of well-being including physical, mental, social, environmental, and personal. Promoting health requires pediatricians to acknowledge the complex forces that impact health, such as familial, socioeconomic, educational, developmental, and biologic entities. With these complexities in mind, pediatricians tailor health supervision visits to individual children to provide optimal care and promote health.

Partnership. Partnership in health supervision requires an appreciation of the context of each child and family. Children have many unique attributes based on the diversity of family structure, culture, ethnicity, language, socioeconomic status, special health care needs, and educational background. Practitioners who partner with children and families by communication and understanding, educating families about health concerns, acknowledging their strengths, and acquiring their trust may enlist children and families in the process of health supervision. This facilitates early detection of disease during intervals between regularly scheduled visits. Collaboration enables families to establish goals, share responsibility for health care, and develop self-esteem, confidence, and competence.

Communication. (See Chapter 17.1.) Effective communication is at the heart of establishing a therapeutic relationship. In health supervision visits, the roles of pediatricians are expanded beyond diagnosticians to those of healers, educators, and counselors. Effective communication skills include (1) demonstrating respect and empathy for children and families, (2) listening actively to concerns and conveying understanding, (3) using nonjudgmental, open-ended questions to promote dialogue, (4) offering supportive comments to foster self-esteem and confidence, and (5) establishing relationships with children by communicating with them directly.

Continuity and Coordination of Care. Pediatricians spend 25–40% of their time performing health supervision visits throughout infancy, childhood, and adolescence. Although these visits are brief encounters in the lives of children and families, significant relationships are built over time. It is the longitudinal nature of health supervision that allows these brief encounters to have a lasting impact. For children whose lives are affected by chronic conditions, continuity and coordination of care are especially essential to their health care needs (see Chapter 37). The pediatrician should coordinate care, communicate with specialists, collaborate with family and community resources, and co-manage children with chronic illness with subspecialty colleagues. The accessibility of pediatricians in the community and their availability for day-to-day problems promote these important roles. In this context, health supervision evolves into management of chronic conditions, providing patients with a *medical home*.

PERIODIC HEALTH SUPERVISION VISITS

The suggested sequence of health supervision visits is listed in Table 5–1. Beyond history and physical examination, screening, and immunizations, health supervision visits should include surveillance of developmental milestones, observations of parent-child interaction, anticipatory guidance and counseling, and an opportunity to address concerns and questions of children and families. Table 5–2 provides a list of essential elements for health supervision visits at specific ages.

Time devoted to health supervision visits has increased over the last several decades, based in part on the increasing number of potential topics that need to be explored with children and families. To be more time-efficient and ensure complete documentation, pediatricians should consider using *structured encounter forms* or conducting *group well child visits*. Structured encounter forms may improve the delivery of health information, increase parental satisfaction with quality of care, and improve documentation and efficiency. Preprinted forms and downloadable forms from the Internet are available and should be reviewed and adapted for an individual practice setting. *Group well child visits* are effective alternatives or complementary

TABLE 5–1. Suggested Schedule of Health Supervision Visits

Infancy 0–1 yr	Early Childhood 1–4 yr	Middle Childhood 5–10 yr	Adolescence 11–21 yr
Prenatal	15 mo	5 yr	11 yr
Neonatal	18 mo	6 yr	12 yr
First Week	2 yr	8 yr	13 yr
1 mo	3 yr	10 yr	14 yr
2 mo	4 yr		15 yr
4 mo			16 yr
6 mo			17 yr
9 mo			18 yr
12 mo			19 yr
			20 yr
			21 yr

to individual well child visits. Typically, groups of infants and children of similar ages and their families participate in sessions lasting 45–60 min led by primary care pediatric providers. By allowing ample time for discussion about child-rearing issues, group well child visits promote observations of parent-child interactions, facilitate education and interchange, and serve as support groups. Group well child visits for families with infants may improve parental knowledge of parenting and child development, whereas families with adolescents may benefit from sessions that address issues of smoking, drinking alcohol, or nutrition and allow parents to share parenting experiences.

TOPICS OF FREQUENT CONCERN DURING HEALTH SUPERVISION VISITS

In the course of well child visits, pediatricians often provide advice in areas of behavior and parenting and educate families about common issues in growth and development. Information, education, and support provided during health supervision enable parents to feel successful in their roles. Clinics and offices serve as clearinghouses of information by providing patient education materials, such as handouts, brochures, and references, and by training office staff to educate patients and families on the telephone, in the clinic, or in group well child visits. As increasing numbers of families connect to the Internet, pediatricians should be involved in the development, editing, and updating of patient education information and refer families to useful websites like the American Academy of Pediatrics website, *http://www.aap.org*, which provides access to materials and resources. The following topics of parenting and child care, chosen because of their prominence in health supervision visits, are discussed with an emphasis on prevention.

Teething. Most infants have their first teeth erupt at age 6–8 mo of age (Chapter 288). Despite the commonly held parental and professional beliefs about symptoms attributable to teething, there is no evidence to suggest an association of teething with any of the following: fever, mood disturbances, appearance of illness, sleep disturbance, drooling, diarrhea, strong urine, red cheeks, rashes, or flushing of the face or body. During the period of tooth eruption, there are numerous other events that are likely to occur coincidentally, such as the sudden onset of a respiratory or gastrointestinal illness, roseola, or gingivostomatitis. Drooling and sleep disturbances are also common at the time of tooth eruption. Parents should be given advice about common infections and symptoms, normal behaviors, and the lack of association of any of the aforementioned symptoms with teething.

Sleep Problems. Difficulties with transitions to sleep and frequent night awakening are commonly reported in the first year of life. Separation anxiety, which develops in the latter half of the first year of life, is related to difficulty with nighttime settling and night awakening (Chapter 20.5). Pediatricians should educate parents about normal sleep requirements to facilitate their understanding of a child's need for naps, age-related sleep

TABLE 5–2. Essential Elements of Health Supervision Visits at Specific Ages*

Activity	1 wk	1 mo	2 mo	4 mo	6 mo	9 mo	12 mo	15 mo	18 mo	2 yr	3 yr	4 yr	5 yr	6 yr	8 yr	10 yr	11–14 yr	15–17 yr	18–21 yr
Interview (Interview with special attention to family concerns and interval history)																			
Body systems (Review of specific body systems when indicated by interval history or chronic condition)																			
Development	√	√	√	√	√	√	√	√	√	√	√	√	√	√	√	√	√	√	√
Feeding and nutrition	√	√	√	√	√	√	√	√	√	√	√	√	√	√	√	√	√	√	√
Elimination	√	√	√	√	√	√	√	√	√	√		Inquire about constipation, enuresis, encopresis							
Sleep	√	√	√	√	√	√	√	√	√	√		Parasomnias may persist into childhood							
Behavior	√	√	√	√	√	√	√	√	√	√	√	√	√	√	√	√	√	√	√
Family relationships	√	√	√	√	√	√	√	√	√	√	√	√	√	√	√	√	√	√	√
School												√	√	√	√	√	√	√	√
Activities and interests																			
Family history	√ (first visit)									Update periodically									
Pregnancy and newborn history	√ (first visit)																		
Parent-Child Interaction (Observations of parent-child interaction during health supervision visit)																			
Physical Examination (Special attention to elements listed below)																			
Height and weight	√	√	√	√	√	√	√	√	√	√	√	√	√	√	√	√	√	√	√
Head circumference	√	√	√	√	√	√	√	√	√	√									
Blood pressure											√	√	√	√	√	√	√	√	√
Head shape	√	√	√	√	√	√	√	√	√	√	√	√	√	√	√	√	√	√	√
Dental caries	√	√	√	√	√	√	√	√	√	√	√	√	√	√	√	√	√	√	√
Strabismus/nystagmus	√	√	√	√	√	√	√	√	√										
Red reflex	√	√	√	√	√	√	√	√	√	√	√	√	√	√	√	√	√	√	√
Fundoscopic																			
Cardiac murmur	√	√	√	√	√	√	√	√	√	√	√	√	√	√	√	√	√	√	√
Abdominal mass	√	√	√	√	√	√	√	√	√	√	√	√	√	√	√	√	√	√	√
External genitalia	√	√	√	√	√	√	√	√	√	√	√	√	√	√	√	√	√	√	√
Developmental dysplasia of hips	√	√	√	√	√	√	√	√	√										
Abnormal muscle tone	√	√	√	√	√	√	√	√	√										
Scoliosis															√	√	√	√	√
Evidence of abuse or neglect	√	√	√	√	√	√	√	√	√	√	√	√	√	√	√	√	√	√	√

Screening

Hearing screen √ Newborn –3 mo   If at-risk for hearing loss

Newborn metabolic/genetic screen   Prior to 1 mo

Hct/Hgb   At-risk for anemia; females with excessive menstrual bleeding

Urinalysis   √ if not screened by school age

Lead test   If at-risk for lead exposure   Screen high-risk pts

Tuberculin testing   Screen high-risk pts

Lipid screening   If positive family history

STD screening   All sexually active pts

Immunizations

Anticipatory Guidance —Counseling

Suggested areas for discussion

Injury prevention   Car seats, smoke alarms, water temperature, bathing, appropriate caregivers, shaking   Car seats, poisons, falls, safety plugs/locks, hot liquids, sharp/small objects, pools, flames, pets   Seat belts, helmets (bikes, skateboards, skis), crossing streets, strangers, guns   Conflict resolution, drinking, safety

Nutrition and eating behaviors

Developmental expectations

Oral health

Parental health and relationships

Environmental exposures   Passive smoke, direct sunlight, pets, never leave alone in cars   Lead (remodeling, pica), household products, pesticides   Sun exposure, passive smoke, play equipment, neighborhood hazards, workplace exposures (in adolescence)

Media education

School problems

Sexuality and puberty

Family violence and substance abuse

*These suggestions are an abstract of recommendations made by the American Academy of Pediatrics and Bright Futures. They are not intended to be all inclusive but rather serve as reminders of important preventive and health promotion activities that should be considered at specific ages when physician-patient encounters may occur. The content and timing of visits may be altered according to special needs and presence of risk factors. Screening requires a knowledge of specific risk factors for decisions at various age-based visits.

schedules, and regular bedtimes (see Chapter 10). Up to 20% of older infants and children may experience sleep disturbances that include nightmares, restless legs, noisy breathing, or parasomnias such as night terrors, night walking, night talking, or bed-wetting (see Chapter 20.5).

To help a child settle at night, parents should establish a regular bedtime routine starting with a quiet interaction like reading a bedtime story. Transitional objects, such as blankets and teddy bears, are integral elements of bedtime routines and facilitate settling (falling asleep). It is important to allow infants to settle on their own, so that they accomplish a successful independent transition to sleep. If a child protests, parents should use the same consistent approach repeatedly. When parents experience difficulty with a *child who wakes at night*, a similar approach of promoting nighttime settling should be used. It is important to recognize that arousal (awakening from sleep) is a normal phenomenon and hunger is not a common cause for night awakening unless the child has been trained to feed at night (trained nighttime feeder). Parents should delay their response at first so that normal arousal states during sleep do not progress to complete awakening. When parents must respond, they should employ the same approach as they do in their normal bedtime routines.

Nightmares are common in childhood and usually involve vivid, scary, or exciting events, which are easily recalled by children upon awakening. *Night terrors* are less common events lasting 10–15 minutes in duration, during which time the child is not easily aroused and may appear frightened and agitated. On awakening, children who experience night terrors have amnesia, one of the diagnostic features. In advising parents about nightmares and night terrors, it is important to emphasize a calm and soothing approach to relax the child and facilitate settling.

Toilet Training. In the United States, the average age of successful toilet training appears to be increasing: In the 1960s, the mean age was 27–28 mo; in the 1990s, the mean age is 35–39 mo. Causes for this increase are not entirely clear. Factors associated with successful toilet training are older parental age, nonwhite race, female gender, and single parenthood. Early training (before age 2 yr), because of its association with chronic stool retention and encopresis, should be discouraged. A key factor for parents to recognize in successful toilet training is readiness of the child. Readiness is present if a child communicates to his parents before the passage of urine or stool and can withhold elimination for a brief period of time. The process of toilet training includes positive reinforcement and regular toilet times. Minor hurdles in the toilet training process, such as fear of sitting on the toilet or accidents when not wearing diapers, should be met with calm and understanding support.

Temper Tantrums. Temper tantrums are a normal part of child development. However, when children express anger in outbursts of rage it is a significant challenge for parents. Parents may blame their ineffective parenting skills when the problem may relate to individual personality styles of children or triggering situations. Characterizing the type of temper tantrum may help parents to understand, so that they may apply different approaches. Types of temper tantrums include frustration or fatigue-related, attention-seeking or demanding, refusal, disruptive, potentially harmful, or ragelike. If children experience temper tantrums related to excessive fatigue or hunger, the most appropriate response should be to give support, sleep, or food. Positive remarks made at the time of the tantrum may help mitigate feelings of frustration. When a child is insistent and makes unreasonable demands, it is best to ignore him or her and allow time for the child to regain composure. Tantrums manifest by refusal to go to bed or to school should be approached with firmness and consistency. Parents should be clear and consistent in their requests for compliance but they must allow sufficient opportunity and time for children to respond. If this approach fails, it may be necessary to intervene with physical restraint by moving the child into the bedroom or the automobile.

When behavior is disruptive, out of control, and occurring in a public place, such as the grocery store or a parking lot, it is necessary to remove the child from the situation and impose a time-out. A rule of thumb for the length of time-out is approximately 1 min per year of age. When significant rage with the potential for physical injury occurs, the best intervention is holding and physically restraining the child to allow time for the child to become calm and relaxed. Even though temper tantrums are a normal part of childhood and parenting, it is important to assess families to determine if there are contributing factors such as parental depression or family violence that may require other referrals or interventions.

Discipline. This common aspect of parenting is one of the most controversial. Families often have little knowledge about effective techniques of modifying child behavior. Parents have a tendency to apply discipline strategies similar to those used by their parents. Primary care practitioners should inquire about methods of discipline and offer practical advice and alternatives. Well child visits provide observations that may serve as stepping-off points to a discussion about behavior and discipline. The basis of all effective discipline is a positive, supportive, loving parent-child relationship. Key elements include positive role modeling, praise, paying attention and listening to children, and devoting special time to enhance parent-child relationships. Pediatricians should instruct parents to maintain a positive atmosphere within their home and provide clear expectations about desired behaviors. Consistency of parental behavior, open communication within families, and mutual respect form the cornerstones for effective discipline. If there is evidence of marital discord, family dysfunction, substance or alcohol abuse, or family violence, a referral for counseling is the most important priority.

Time-out or *removal of privileges* should be distinguished from *punishment*. *Time-out* involves the removal of positive reinforcement for unacceptable behavior; this technique requires consistency and patience because its effect on behavioral change takes longer to achieve a desired result. Often time-out provokes a reactive emotional response or a tantrum. Parents should remain calm and impassive to avoid prolonging the incident or escalating the level of response. This form of discipline, among the most reliable and enduring in changing child behavior, requires parents to manage their own distress in order to be successful. *Punishment* involves issuing a negative stimulus or verbal reprimand, or inflicting physical pain, to reduce or eliminate an undesired behavior. Behavioral research on corporal punishment is inconclusive and conflicting about the long-term impact of spanking on subsequent behaviors such as antisocial actions and aggression. Clearly, physical punishment may be harsh or abusive. Although verbal reprimands may have marginal short-term benefit by interrupting or eliminating unwanted behaviors, they may interfere with the effectiveness of time-outs when used together. Verbal reprimands may become abusive when reprimands do not address undesired behaviors, but rather assault the character of the child.

Pediatricians must remain empathic, flexible, and committed to their relationship with families so that their roles as educators and child advocates may be fulfilled. Building on the relationship fostered by primary care, pediatricians have an opportunity to guide and educate families through the challenges of parenting and enable them to be successful in their parental roles. Moreover, as future research in behavioral and social science yields insight into the underpinnings of family violence, child abuse, and violence in our society, the application of this research may result in preventive interventions in well child care and recommendations for guiding parents in disciplining their children.

UNMET NEEDS AND FUTURE CHALLENGES IN PREVENTIVE PEDIATRICS

The future of preventive pediatrics will include new immunizations to prevent infections, improved screening tests to provide early diagnosis of disease, unique genetic information to individualize preventive and therapeutic strategies, and enhanced treatments that minimize the impact of chronic conditions on the health of children. The major causes of morbidity and mortality in children, however, will continue to be related to human behavior, society, and the environment (Chapters 4, 34, 50, and Part XXXII). The challenge for pediatricians in practicing preventive pediatrics is to address these threats to the health of children with new approaches to preventive pediatrics. The following topics deserve a place in preventive pediatrics and within health supervision visits.

Tobacco Use. There are 6,000 new young smokers in the United States every day, and the number is rising. Eighty percent of people who smoke had their first cigarette before 18 yr of age. Cigarette smoking is the most preventable cause of mortality and morbidity in the United States today. Pediatricians should become active in all aspects of this public health problem, including health supervision visits. From the time of first meeting a family, especially at the birth of a baby, it is vital to obtain a smoking history and, if necessary, to provide a quit-smoking message. This preventive strategy directed at individual family members who smoke benefits children who will be exposed to passive smoke, which has been shown to increase rates of wheezing and diminish lung function. Parental disapproval of smoking may prevent adolescents from becoming established smokers. Brief educational messages that effectively explain the relationship of smoking to lung cancer, ischemic heart disease, and low birthweight can promote smoking cessation.

Violence. Violence permeates the lives of children (see Chapter 34). Homicide, suicide, child abuse, domestic violence, access to firearms, substance abuse, school shootings, gang participation, media violence, date rape, bullying, and terrorist acts are examples of the daily infiltration of violence into the lives of children. One study demonstrated the pervasive societal effects of violence, finding a relationship between boyhood exposure to physical abuse, sexual abuse, or a battered mother and a significantly increased risk for his later involvement in a teen pregnancy. Pediatricians should assume a clinical role in educating children and families, identifying risk factors, and making referrals for needed services and an advocacy role at the local, regional, and national level in addressing the many issues involved in this complex societal health problem.

Obesity. Childhood obesity is an epidemic in the United States and an important topic for pediatricians to address (also see Chapter 43). Rates of type II diabetes in children have increased significantly and are related to the obesity epidemic (Chapter 583). Growth charts available from the Centers for Disease Control and Prevention(CDC) website at *http://www.cdc.gov/growthcharts/* provide pediatricians with up-to-date information regarding height, weight, head circumference, weight for height, and body mass index (BMI). See Chapter 15. Definitions of overweight (BMI at 85th–95th percentile) and obesity (>95th percentile) are established. In the future, we may be better at predicting which obese children are at greatest risk for long-term side effects based on family history, persistence and severity of obesity, and knowing when to intervene. Pediatricians should use the CDC growth charts to monitor growth status of children. It is recommended that pediatricians calculate and monitor BMI starting at age 2 yr for all children. BMI is very useful in calculating obesity and monitoring growth trends in overweight children and those children who are concerned with their body image.

Media Influences on Behavior. There is growing evidence that demonstrates the impact of media, particularly television, on the health of children. There are untoward effects in terms of violence and aggressive behavior, substance use, sexual activity, body image, school performance, and obesity. This influence is related to content and total viewing time. Within health supervision visits, pediatricians have the opportunity to educate parents and children about these impacts and should recommend limiting television viewing time (and video game time) to 1–2 hr per day and screening its content. Within communities or at the national level, pediatricians may also play an important role as advocates for better programming, alternative leisure activities, and promoting parental involvement.

Parental Health Needs. Health supervision of children is a unique access point to provide guidance and improve the health status of the entire family. Studies have shown the health status of parents, for example, maternal depression, has significant influences on adequacy of preventive health care services for children. There is also evidence that significant health needs exist among women attending well child visits and that they are receptive to having pediatricians play a role in screening and referral for comprehensive health supervision. This role of pediatricians to influence the health of families is consistent with enhanced health supervision guidelines and a natural link to improve the health of children.

Literacy Promotion. The positive effect of early educational interventions on the subsequent cognitive development of children demands that pediatricians play a role in promoting this aspect of family life and early childhood development. *Reach Out and Read,* a program in which books are distributed at well child visits, increases family literacy orientation, particularly for families living in poverty. Pediatricians may easily incorporate educational messages about the importance of reading to infants and children in health supervision visits. Alternatively, they may promote reading within their offices or at a local or community level by establishing and supporting literacy promotion programs.

Reducing Cardiovascular Disease. Pediatricians should refer children who are at risk for cardiovascular disease for appropriate management. Long-term studies of pediatric patients demonstrate that elevated lipids and blood pressure track into adulthood. Obesity is an additional risk. All children should be monitored for obesity and, starting at age 2 yr, educated about appropriate intake of dietary fat (no more than 30% of calories), saturated fat (less than 10% of total calories), and dietary cholesterol (less than 300 mg/day). (See Chapters 43 and 75.3.) Blood pressure measurements should be done at every well child visit starting at age 3 yr. Children with a positive family history for premature cardiovascular disease in a parent (younger than age 55 yr) or grandparent or a parent with high blood cholesterol should be screened with a total blood cholesterol, according to published guidelines (Chapter 75.3). In addition, pediatricians should encourage children to participate in active physical exercise to minimize the cardiovascular risks associated with a sedentary lifestyle.

Overview. Preventive pediatrics requires commitment of pediatricians to constant improvement of the health of children and families. The topics touched upon here are merely a few of the issues that impact children's health and should be included in health supervision visits. The more pediatricians know about their patients and families, their cultural background, and the communities in which they live, the better able they will be to provide quality primary care, including prevention, to children and families.

American Academy of Pediatrics: Tobacco, alcohol, and other drugs: The role of the pediatrician in prevention and management of substance abuse. *Pediatrics* 1998;101:125.

American Academy of Pediatrics Committee on Infectious Disease: *Red Book 2000,* 25th ed. Elk Grove Village, IL, AAP Division of Publications, 2000.

American Academy of Pediatrics Committee on Psychosocial Aspects of Child and Family Health: Guidance for effective discipline. *Pediatrics* 1998;101:723.

American Academy of Pediatrics Committee on Public Education: Children, adolescents, and television. *Pediatrics* 2001;107:423.

American Academy of Pediatrics Committee on Substance Abuse: Tobacco's toll: Implications for the pediatrician. *Pediatrics* 2001;107:794.

American Academy of Pediatrics Task Force on Violence: The role of the pediatrician in youth violence prevention in clinical practice and at the community level. *Pediatrics* 1999;103:173.

Anda RF, Felitti VJ, Chapman DP, et al: Abused boys, battered mothers, and male involvement in teen pregnancy. *Pediatrics* 2001;107:e19.

Centers for Disease Control and Prevention: Ten great public health achievements—United States, 1900–1999. *MMWR* 1999;8:241.

Green M, Pafrey JS (editors): *Bright Futures: Guidelines for Health Supervision of Infants, Children, and Adolescents*, 2nd ed. Arlington, VA, National Center for Education in Maternal and Child Health, 2000. www.brightfutures.org

Kahn RS, Wise PW, Finkelstein JA, et al: The scope of unmet health needs in pediatric settings. *Pediatrics* 1999;103:576.

Mannino DM, Moorman JE, Kingsley B, et al: Health effects related to environmental tobacco smoke exposure in children in the United States. *Arch Pediatr Adolesc Med* 2001;155:36.

McLennan JD, Ketelchuch M: Parental prevention practices for young children in the context of maternal depression. *Pediatrics* 2000;105:1090.

Mendelsohn AL, Mogilner LN, Dreyer BP, et al: The impact of clinic-based literacy intervention on language development in inner-city preschool children. *Pediatrics* 2001;107:130.

Needlman R, Fried LE, Morley DS, et al: Clinic-based intervention to promote literacy. *Am J Dis Child* 1991;145:881.

Regelado M, Halfon N: Primary care promoting optimal child development from birth to age 3 years. *Arch Pediatr Adolesc Med* 2001;155:1311–22.

Sargent JD, Dalton M: Does parental disapproval of smoking prevent adolescents from becoming established smokers? *Pediatrics* 2001;108:1256–62.

Schmidt BD: How to deal with temper tantrums. *Contemp Pediatr* 1989;6:39.

Schum TR, McAuliffe TL, Simms MD, et al: Factors associated with toilet training in the 1990s. *Ambulatory Pediatrics* 2001;1:79.

Stein MT, Wolraich ML, Aceves J, et al: *Guidelines for Health Supervision III*. Elk Grove Village, IL, American Academy of Pediatrics, 1997.

Wake M, Hesketh K, Lucas J: Teething and tooth eruption in infants: A cohort study. *Pediatrics* 2000;106:1374.

Chapter 6
The Well Child *Paul L. McCarthy*

The most powerful diagnostic technology available to pediatricians is the clinical evaluation: the process of observing the child, taking a history, and performing the physical examination. For pediatricians to maximize the benefit of the clinical evaluation, some of the complexities of this process must be appreciated (also see Chapter 5).

UNIQUE CHARACTER OF THE PEDIATRIC CLINICAL EVALUATION

This evaluation involves the physician, the parents, and the child. Historical information is often taken from the parents, and it is not until children reach later developmental stages that they can more actively contribute information about symptoms. These considerations change the manner in which pediatricians gather data about symptoms. Rather than asking, for example, if the child has abdominal pain, physicians ask questions that focus on the manner in which abdominal pain would present to an observer. Thus, questions about loss of appetite, sudden episodes of crying and drawing the legs up in a fetal position, or the child's crying when the parent has placed pressure on the abdomen are appropriate. A 24-mo-old child with a sore throat often does not complain of this but rather is observed by the parents to have more difficulty handling oral secretions, to refuse solids, and to have a foul breath odor. Questions are tailored to elicit this information.

As children become older, they may begin to add historical information that expresses symptoms in unique ways. The information provided by a child at times suggests the diagnosis precisely, but at other times a child's information may reflect a less developed sense of cause-and-effect relationships and may be at variance with the data provided by the parents. Thus, a 4-yr-old child with a urinary tract infection may be observed by the parent to be holding his or her abdomen and to have a subtle change in the frequency of urination. The child, on the other

hand, may perceive that his or her abdominal complaints are related to a specific food that was ingested just before the onset of symptoms. In this instance, the pediatrician may conclude that the parents' history suggests the correct diagnosis (a urinary tract infection) by eliciting further information about, for example, discomfort when urinating.

PARENTS AND CHILD AS PARTICIPANTS IN THE CLINICAL EVALUATION

It is often left to the judgment of parents whether clinical symptoms should be brought to the attention of a physician. Moreover, children's interpretation of symptoms is intimately related to their developmental stage; this also influences the manner in which they transmit clinical information to a physician. Both parents and children must believe that the pediatrician is interested in their concerns and that interactions with the pediatrician will provide them support. This process occurs at both well and sick child visits. At well child visits, the parent or child might describe a specific behavior or symptom. The pediatrician demonstrates concern by listening attentively and by asking follow-up questions demonstrating that the behavior or symptom has been understood. These follow-up questions provide an opportunity for the parent or child to explore his or her own interpretation of these behaviors or symptoms, to understand their emotional response, and to learn from the interpretation provided by the physician. For example, parents reporting that their 9-mo-old child cries when being put to bed and has difficulty falling asleep offers an opportunity for the pediatrician to explore their interpretations of this behavior, to discuss their response to it, and to discuss individual variations in sleeping behavior. Based on this discussion and a more precise appreciation of the meaning of that behavior, strategies to facilitate sleeping can be suggested (Chapters 5 and 20.5).

The same interaction and education process occurs during sick child visits (see Chapter 49). Upper respiratory symptoms may concern parents. In response, the pediatrician may discuss the predominance of nasal breathing in younger children, the related symptoms of nasal stuffiness, and the absence of other evidence of serious pulmonary involvement, such as tachypnea. This enhances parents' abilities to interpret respiratory symptoms during subsequent upper respiratory infections. Similarly, the pediatrician can explain cause-and-effect relationships between infection and symptoms to an older child. Such encounters enhance the confidence of parents and children in their role as participants in the clinical evaluation. Studies have demonstrated the ability of parents to evaluate clinical data reliably and the ability of children, when given developmentally appropriate information, to improve their understanding of clinical causality.

DEVELOPMENTAL DIMENSIONS

The data generated from observation, history, and physical examination are greatly influenced by a child's developmental stage. A portion of the observational assessment of a child focuses on signs related to specific organ systems that are intimately related to age. A child of 1 mo has a more rapid respiratory rate (30 breaths/min) than a 3-yr-old child. An infant's respiratory rate is more sensitive to other influences, such as gastric pressure on the diaphragm caused by the recent ingestion of a meal, than is that of an older child. Other aspects of observational assessment focus on indicators of a child's overall state of well-being or functional status, such as how the child responds visually to the environment. These visual responses undergo developmental change as does the manner in which stimuli should be presented to elicit a child's optimal visual response. A 1-mo-old infant, for example, is more nearsighted and tends to focus on objects held within 1–2 ft of the face; objects presented in the peripheral fields of vision may be ignored. A young infant's ability to maintain attention on a visual stimulus is less developed than that of an older child. Thus, pediatricians must be aware of the developmental dimensions of observing children in order to gather and interpret clinical information accurately.

The data generated during the physical examination are also closely linked to a child's stage of development. Specific findings may be normal in one age group and abnormal in another. For example, a 1-mo-old child normally has a rooting reflex, which facilitates suckling. However, a rooting reflex found in a 2-yr-old child indicates central nervous system abnormalities. The manner in which physical examination findings are elicited also varies from one developmental stage to another. An 8-mo-old child, for example, is beginning to develop a sense of individuality and is aware of strangers and frightened by separation. Therefore, to elicit accurate physical examination data, especially during auscultation of the chest and heart, the examiner should allow the child to remain close to the parent and should approach as unobtrusively as possible. Factors that lessen the strangeness of a situation, such as the warmth of the room, the stethoscope, and the examiner's voice, also help facilitate data gathering. Older children are usually more comfortable with strangers and in separating from the parents; hence, after initial assurances, the physical examination may be done on the examination table.

GUIDELINES FOR EVALUATION

During the clinical encounter, it is often difficult to separate each component of the evaluation. As physicians are taking a history from a parent, they are observing the child and the interaction of the child with the parent; as physicians perform a physical examination, they are evaluating the child's global responses to the specific maneuver being performed. Nevertheless, certain guidelines can be followed during each part of the evaluation.

Observation is best done with a younger child in a comfortable position, usually on the parent's lap. Parental anxiety is easily transmitted to the child; thus, the parent and child must be placed at ease with a greeting and reassuring words. The tone of the examiner's voice is important and should convey a willingness to listen and a sensitivity to concerns being expressed. The manner in which an examiner is oriented to the parent and child is also important: If an examiner sits in one corner of a desk and focuses primarily on the patient's chart, a sense of unwillingness to communicate is conveyed. Sitting close to the parents and child and facing them directly are more effective. An examiner should observe the manner in which the parent and child are interacting: How are the parents responding to the child's needs, and, in turn, how is the child responding to the parents? Pediatricians can modulate the stimuli in this situation to gather important information by observation. The child may initially be clinging to the parent, so the pediatrician should interact with the child, offer the child an object, or attempt some separation of the child and parent to observe the child's response.

A history is best taken with a child in a comfortable position. If the child is quiet and comfortable, the parent can focus better on specific questions. Physicians vary in their amount of note taking during the history. Some prefer to write the history directly to progress notes; others note only key words and, at the end of the examination, transfer the information to the medical record. Whichever technique is used, it is critical that physicians remain responsive to the information being presented. If highly sensitive information is being conveyed and the parent or child is responding emotionally, physicians must convey empathic understanding. This is impossible, however, if note taking continues without interruption. Additional note taking during this critical moment can interfere with important observations about the parent and child and their interaction.

The precision and clarity with which parents and children describe symptoms vary. Ongoing interaction with a family over time enables pediatricians to learn how clinical information is perceived and transmitted within each family. If, for example,

parents perceive their child as vulnerable, minor symptoms may be overemphasized; pediatricians can adjust the assessments accordingly.

The portions of the physical examination that require optimal cooperation are completed first: the blood pressure measurement, pulmonary and cardiac examinations, and evaluations of the eyes and central nervous system. A younger child may be held by the parent or seated on the parent's lap for these parts of the examination. An older child can be seated on the examination table. The pattern and rate of respirations are evaluated initially. Is there tachypnea? Is there increased work of breathing as manifested by subcostal, intercostal, or supraclavicular retractions? Is there an expiratory grunt indicating that the child is expiring against a closed glottis to keep the small airways open longer? What are the colors of the skin, nails, and mucous membranes? After these assessments have been made, the physician may proceed to palpation, percussion (if indicated), and auscultation. It is not uncommon for a younger child to cry as the stethoscope is placed on the chest, but this can usually be overcome by patience and by increasing the child's comfort, such as offering an infant a bottle. The same sequence may be followed for the cardiac examination. The ophthalmologic examination requires that the child be quietly wakeful; ophthalmoscopy can be done with the child in the parent's lap or as the child is being carried over the parent's shoulder. The other parent can sometimes provide visual stimuli; the retina can be seen more easily as the child focuses on such stimuli. Many portions of the neurologic examination, such as eliciting reflexes, also require cooperation and a state of quiet wakefulness. In an older child, this can be accomplished with the child on the examination table, but it is usually more helpful for a younger child to remain on the parent's lap.

After these portions of the examination, the examiner proceeds to the parts of the examination that are usually more bothersome to a child. Abdominal examination requires that a child be on the examination table. It is helpful to have the parent hold a younger patient's hand and speak reassuringly. Thus, the child does not tense the abdominal musculature unnecessarily as might occur during crying. After the abdominal examination, the pulses may be palpated, the genitalia examined, and the hips and extremities evaluated for clinical abnormalities. It is at this time that the examiner proceeds to the most intrusive portions of the examination, evaluation of the ear canals and tympanic membranes and examination of the oropharynx. During the ear examination, the parent may hold the child's head to minimize movement against the otoscope (Chapters 626 and 630). The examiner should recognize that the ear canals are highly sensitive, and the speculum should be introduced gently. The examiner's free hand can be used to put gentle traction on the pinna to straighten the canal. A portion of the hand holding the otoscope, usually the 5th finger, should rest against the head so that the otoscope moves with the head. At times, depending on the amount of cooperation, the ears may be examined with the child in the parent's lap and the head resting against the parent's shoulder. The oropharyngeal examination is performed last, and the tongue blade is introduced gently.

The sequence of performing those portions of the physical examination that require inspection, palpation, percussion, and auscultation (pulmonary, cardiac, and abdominal) varies according to organ system. The most bothersome maneuvers are performed last. For example, during the cardiac examination, inspection can be followed by palpation and percussion and then by auscultation. For the abdominal examination, inspection should be followed by auscultation before percussion and palpation are completed.

With appropriate sensitivity to the child and the parent, an appreciation of the child's developmental stage, and concern for minimizing the discomfort of an examination, pediatricians can almost always obtain accurate clinical information and not cause undue upset to a child.

WELL CHILD EVALUATION

The broad principles of clinical data gathering that have been outlined apply to the well child examination. The recommended schedule of well child visits is outlined in Table 5–1. For children with chronic or intercurrent problems, this sequence may vary (Chapter 37). Certain considerations should be addressed at each visit.

Open-Ended Questions. Physicians should ask general questions that allow a parent or child to voice concerns that might not be raised if questions were too specific (also see Chapter 17). Open-ended questions such as "How are you?" or "How is the baby?" transmit an interest in the general well-being of the child and family. When such open-ended questions are asked, it is important that physicians explore the leads provided by the parents or child; ending the interaction prematurely, without appropriate follow-up questions, is frustrating to the parents and child and sends a mixed message about the physician's interest and concern.

Development. Each well child visit should assess a child's developmental achievements; instruments such as the Denver Developmental Screening Test are helpful, with previous scores serving as reference points for evaluating changes (Chapter 16). As a child matures beyond 5 and 6 yr of age, questions that focus on school performance and talented accomplishments can be substituted for the Denver test. Reviewing developmental milestones with parents provides them with a sense of satisfaction in their child's progress and reinforces the efforts they are making to nurture and teach their children. Reviewing an older child's accomplishments is an important demonstration of support for these activities.

Feeding and Diet. Many changes occur in the dietary intake of children and youth, and these should be reviewed with the parents and children (also see Chapter 41). The transitions from breast milk or infant formula to infant cereals, strained then junior foods, milk, and table foods, and the use of vitamins and fluoride are issues of daily concern for parents. In older children, the intake of excessive salt, carbohydrates, or cholesterol can adversely affect health. The rationale underlying the introduction of certain foods and dietary changes should be discussed with parents and children, so that they can make healthy choices.

Accident Prevention. At each well child care visit, accident prevention should be reviewed (Chapters 5 and 50). Potential hazards around the home are emphasized, as are the importance of car safety measures and proper infant sleep position (on the back). Syrup of ipecac and the telephone number of the local poison control center should be given to the parents at the infant's 6 mo visit. The developmental aspect of accident prevention should be emphasized.

Growth. At each well child visit, the height, weight, and head circumference are measured. These are plotted on standard graphs, such as those provided by the National Center for Health Statistics (see Chapter 15). It is important to review growth parameters with parents and children, because these are objective indicators of a child's progress. If abnormalities in the rate of growth are noted, the clinical evaluation can focus on possible causes. When interpreting these data, the pediatrician must focus on what is normal for this child, given the family background.

Family and Social Relations. To grow and develop normally, children rely on the support and nurturance provided by their family and the social environment. Disturbances in these supports can lead to nonoptimal growth, altered development, and adverse behavioral changes. Pediatricians should assess these supports by observation and questions. Observations should include the hygiene of the child and the child's general level of interest and response to people. How do the parents respond to the child's needs? What is the tone of parents' voices as they discuss the child? In what terms do the parents describe the child? If the child begins crying or is disruptive, how do the parents respond? Do the parents face the young child or do they show lack of interest or concern? Does the child appear depressed or inappropriately anxious? Specific questions from the pediatrician may elucidate other stresses or strengths in the environment. Does the home environment, such as through inclusion of toys and books, nurture the child's developmental potential? Is there an extended network of friends and family that provides support to the children and parents? Is the family under significant stress, such as occurs during illness, moving, or loss of a job? A pediatrician's ability to gather information about these issues and to address them is important in assessing health or dysfunction of a child and family.

A particular challenge is represented by the special needs of children who live in impoverished environments (Chapter 39). Empathizing with the difficulties of raising children in these circumstances, recognizing the obstacles that such children often face in realizing their potential, and assisting parents and children in overcoming some of these adversities are major responsibilities of pediatric care.

Anticipatory Guidance. Based on a developmental orientation, physicians should be aware of issues that may present problems or questions for parents or children between the current and next visits. For example, the rate of growth of a 24-mo-old child lessens compared with that of previous months, and a diminished appetite results. Rather than have the parents be unnecessarily concerned about this, it is prudent to preview the child's rate of growth in the next 6 mo and to discuss its impact on food intake. The developmental achievements that the parents might expect in the next several months and the type of activities that facilitate these developments should also be discussed. For example, a 12-mo-old child's ability to grasp and bring objects to the mouth makes finger foods an option for a child at this age. In addition, this ability points out the need to remove small objects (e.g., peanuts) from the environment to minimize choking and aspiration hazards. The anticipatory guidance that is provided should also review issues in daily caretaking, such as hygiene and sleep patterns. See Chapter 5.

Other Concerns. At the initial well child visit, data about the family medical history and the prenatal and perinatal history should be entered into the medical record. At each well child visit, physicians should record and provide a record of immunizations to parents, notes should be made about any intercurrent illness and laboratory screening tests, and a review of systems should be carried out. After the physical examination is completed, the child's health status should be summarized for the parents. The parents should be complimented on their strengths as caregivers and children complimented about their achievements and progress. It is also important to recognize problems and to express willingness to work on these together with the family. The pediatrician's availability, if problems arise before the next visit, should be stressed to reassure the parents and child about the pediatrician's involvement in ongoing care. Lastly, parents and children should again be given an opportunity to ask questions or raise concerns about any aspect of the well child visit.

Committee on Psychosocial Aspects of Child and Family Health: *Guidelines for Health Supervision III.* Elk Grove Village, IL, American Academy of Pediatrics, 1997.

Green M: Pediatric psychosocial diagnostic interview. In Green M: *Pediatric Diagnosis.* Philadelphia, WB Saunders, 1998, pp 471–82.

McCarthy P, Freudigman K, Cicchetti D, et al: The mother-child interaction and clinical judgment during acute pediatric illnesses *J Pediatr* 2000;136: 809–17.

Growth and Development

Robert D. Needlman

Chapter 7

Overview and Assessment of Variability

Pediatricians need to understand growth and development in order to monitor children's progress, to identify delays or abnormalities in development, and to counsel parents and prescribe treatment. In addition to clinical experience and personal knowledge, effective practice requires familiarity with major theoretical perspectives and evidence-based strategies for optimizing growth and development. In order to target factors that increase or decrease risk, pediatricians need to understand how biologic and social forces interact within the parent-child relationship, within the family, and between the family and the larger society. By monitoring children and families, pediatricians can observe the interrelationships between physical growth and cognitive, motor, and emotional development. At the same time, observation is enhanced by familiarity with developmental theory.

BIOPSYCHOSOCIAL MODELS OF DEVELOPMENT

Development is not determined solely by genetics (nature), nor is the child only a product of the environment (nurture). Rather, biopsychosocial models recognize the importance of both intrinsic and extrinsic forces. Height, for example, is a function of a child's genetic endowment (biologic), personal habits of eating (psychologic), and access to nutritious food (social).

Research demonstrating the profound impact of early experience on the development of the brain has illuminated the interaction of nature and nurture. The brain comprises 100 billion neurons at birth, with each neuron developing on average 15,000 synapses by 3 yr of age. The number of synapses stays roughly constant through the first decade of life, although the number of neurons declines. As some synapses develop, others disappear. Frequently used pathways are preserved, whereas less-used ones are deleted. Thus, experience (nurture) has a direct effect on the physical properties of the brain (nature). Children with different talents and temperaments (nature) also elicit different stimuli from their environment (nurture), and even when environmental inputs are identical, may interpret those inputs differently.

Early experience is particularly important because learning proceeds more efficiently along established synaptic pathways. Traumatic experiences may create enduring alterations in the neurotransmitter and endocrine systems that mediate the stress response, possibly increasing the risk of mental illness later in life. But experiences, positive or negative, rarely *determine* outcomes. Rather, they shift the probabilities one way or another, by influencing the child's ability to respond adaptively to future stimuli. The idea that a child's developmental course is essentially set by 3, 6, or 16 yr of age is not supported by the evidence.

Although biologic, psychologic, and social factors combine to shape development, it is helpful to consider each class of influence separately.

Biologic Influences. Biologic influences on development include genetics, in utero exposure to teratogens, postpartum illnesses, exposure to hazardous substances, and maturation. Adoption and twin studies consistently show that heredity accounts for approximately half of the variance in IQ, and in other personality traits such as sociability and desire for novelty. The specific genes underlying these traits have begun to be identified. The effects on development of prenatal exposure to teratogens such as mercury and alcohol, and of postpartum insults such as meningitis and traumatic brain injury, have been extensively studied. Any chronic illness can affect growth and development, either directly or through changes in parenting or peer experiences.

Physical and neurologic maturation propels children forward and sets lower limits for the emergence of most abilities. The age at which children walk independently is similar around the world, despite great variability in child-rearing practices. Other attainments (e.g., the use of complex sentences) are less tightly bound to a maturational schedule. Maturational changes also generate behavioral challenges at predictable times. For example, decrements in growth rate and sleep requirements around 2 yr of age often generate concerns about poor appetite and refusal to nap. While it is possible to accelerate many developmental milestones—for example, toilet training a 12 mo old or teaching a 3 yr old to read—the long-term benefits of such precocious accomplishments are questionable.

In addition to physical changes in size, body proportions, and strength, maturation brings about hormonal changes. Sexual differentiation, both somatic and neurologic, begins in utero. Behavioral effects of testosterone may be evident even in young children and continue to be salient throughout life. However, correlations between testosterone and such traits as aggression or novelty-seeking have not been consistently demonstrated.

A biologic influence of particular clinical importance is temperament. Temperament refers to a child's characteristic style of responding. The classic theory proposes nine parameters of temperament (Table 7–1). Although temperament is intrinsic to a child and relatively resistant to modification by parenting practices, most temperamental characteristics show only modest stability over time. Active, intense 2-yr-olds, for example, do not necessarily grow into active, intense 22-yr-olds.

The concept of temperament is clinically useful in two ways. First, it can help parents understand and accept the characteristics of their children without feeling responsible for having caused them. Second, behavioral and emotional problems often develop when the temperamental characteristics of children and parents conflict. Active children may be especially problematic for low-key parents; children who are "slow to warm up" may feel especially pressured if their parents are very outgoing; parents who lead highly structured lives may have a hard time meeting the needs of children whose biologic urges occur on an especially irregular schedule. "Goodness of fit" between the child and parents is a powerful predictor of outcome.

Psychologic Influences: Attachment and Contingency. The influence of the child-rearing environment dominates most current models of development. Erik Erikson identified the 1st yr of life as a time when "basic trust" was established through the mother's

TABLE 7–1. **Temperamental Characteristics: Descriptions and Examples**

Characteristic	Description	Example*
Activity level	Amount of gross motor movement	"She ran before she walked." "He would rather sit still than run around."
Rhythmicity	Regularity of biologic cycles	"He is never hungry at the same time each day." "You could set a watch by her nap."
Approach and withdrawal	Typical response to a new stimulus	"She rejects every new food at first." "He loves new people."
Adaptability	How long it takes to adapt to novel stimulus	"Changes upset him." "She adjusts to new people quickly."
Threshold of responsiveness	How intense do stimuli need to be to evoke a response (e.g., feel, sound, light)	"Underwear and socks bother him; he does not like anything touching his skin." "She will eat anything, wear anything, do anything."
Intensity of reaction	How much energy a child expends in emotions and actions	"She shouts when she is happy and wails when she is sad." "He never cries much."
Quality of mood	Usual disposition (e.g., pleasant, glum)	"He does not laugh much." "It seems like she is always happy."
Distractibility	How easily diverted from ongoing activity	"Her mind is always wandering." "He will listen through a whole story."
Attention span and persistence	How long a child pays attention and sticks with difficult tasks	"He goes from toy to toy every minute." "She will keep at a puzzle until she has mastered it."

Typical statements of parents, reflecting the range for each characteristic from very little to very much.

consistent responsiveness to her child's needs. In the 1950s, studies of infants in hospitals and foundling homes documented the devastating effects of maternal deprivation and pointed to the importance of attachment. Attachment refers to a biologically determined tendency of a young child to seek proximity with the parent during times of stress and also to the relationship that allows securely attached children to use their parents to reestablish a sense of well-being after a stressful experience. Insecure attachment may be predictive of later behavioral and learning problems.

At all stages of development children progress optimally when they have adult caregivers who pay attention to their verbal and nonverbal cues and respond accordingly. In early infancy, such contingent responsiveness to signs of overarousal or underarousal helps maintain infants in a state of quiet alertness and fosters autonomic self-regulation. Contingent responses to non-verbal gestures create the groundwork for the shared attention and reciprocity critical for later language and social development. Children learn best when new challenges are just slightly harder than what they have already mastered, a degree of difficulty dubbed the "zone of proximal development."

Social Factors: Family Systems and the Ecologic Model. Contemporary models of child development recognize the critical importance of influences outside of the mother-child dyad. Increasingly, fathers are recognized as playing critical roles, both in their direct relationships with their children, and in supporting mothers. As traditional "nuclear" families become less dominant, the influence of other family members—grandparents, foster and adoptive parents, and nonrelated caregivers—becomes increasingly clear.

Families function as systems, with internal and external boundaries, subsystems, roles, and rules for interaction. In families with rigidly defined parental subsystems, children may be denied any decision-making at all, exacerbating rebelliousness. In families with relatively porous parent-child boundaries, children may be "parentified," required to take on responsibilities beyond their years or recruited to play a spousal role.

Individuals within systems adopt implicit roles. One child is the "troublemaker," another is the "negotiator," another is "quiet." Birth order may have profound effects on personality development, through its influence on family roles and patterns of interaction. Families are also dynamic: Changes in one person's behavior affect every other member of the system; roles shift until a new equilibrium is found. The birth of a new child, attainment of developmental milestones such as independent walking, the onset of nighttime fears, and the death of a grandparent are all changes that require renegotiation of roles within the family and have the potential for healthy adaptation or dysfunction.

The family system, in turn, functions within the larger systems of extended family, subculture, culture, and society (see

Chapters 3 and 4). The ecologic model depicts these relationships as concentric circles, with the parent-child dyad at the center and the larger society at the periphery. Changes at any level are reflected in the levels above and below. The shift from an industrial economy to one based on service and information is an obvious example of societal change with profound effects on families and children.

Unifying Concepts: The Transactional Model, Risk, and Resilience. The transactional model proposes that a child's status at any point in time is a function of the interaction between biologic and social influences. The influences are bidirectional: Biologic factors such as temperament and health status both affect the child-rearing environment and are affected by it. For example, a premature infant may cry little and sleep for long periods; the infant's depressed parent may welcome this "good" behavior, setting up a cycle that leads to poor nutrition and inadequate growth. The child's failure to thrive may reinforce the parent's sense of failure as a parent. At a later stage, impulsivity and inattention associated with early prolonged undernutrition may lead to a referral for aggressive behavior. The "cause" of the aggression in this case is not the prematurity, the undernutrition, or the maternal depression but the interaction of all these factors.

Conversely, children with biologic risk factors may nevertheless do well developmentally if the child-rearing environment is supportive. For example, premature infants with electroencephalographic evidence of neurologic immaturity may be at increased risk of cognitive delay. However, this risk may only be realized when the quality of parent-child interaction is poor. When parent-child interactions are optimal, even moderate prematurity carries a low risk of developmental disability.

Children growing up in poverty are in double developmental jeopardy, because of increased exposure to biologic risk factors such as environmental lead and undernutrition, and decreased access to corrective educational and therapeutic experiences (see Chapters 34 and 39). When early intervention programs provide timely, intensive, comprehensive, and prolonged services (i.e., a level of support that economically advantaged families often take for granted) at-risk children show marked and sustained upswings in their developmental trajectory. Early identification of children at developmental risk, along with early intervention to support parenting, is critically important.

A rough estimate of developmental risk can begin with a tally of risk factors, such as low income, limited parental education, and exposure to community violence. One classic study, for example, documented a nearly linear relationship between developmental outcome at age 13 yr and the number of social and family risk factors at age 4 yr (Fig. 7–1). But protective factors also have to be considered. These factors, like risk factors, may be either biologic (temperamental persistence, athletic talent) or social. In a famous study of children growing up in Hawaii, for

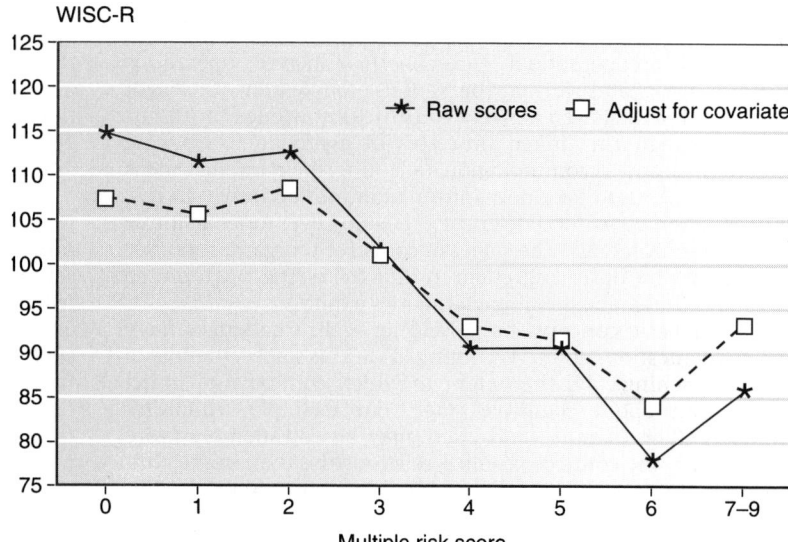

FIGURE 7–1. Relationship between mean IQ scores at 13 yr (both raw and adjusted for covariation of mother's IQ), as related to the number of risk factors. (From Sameroff AJ, Seifer R, Baldwin A, Baldwin C: Stability of intelligence from preschool to adolescence: The influence of social and family risk factors. *Child Dev* 1993;64:80.)

example, the personal histories of children who overcame poverty generally included at least one trusted adult—a parent, grandparent, or teacher—with whom the child had a special, supportive close relationship.

Developmental Domains and Theories of Emotion and Cognition. Another approach to child development tracks development within particular domains such as gross motor, fine motor, social, emotional, language, and cognition. Within each of these categories are developmental lines or sequences of changes leading up to particular attainments. Developmental lines in the gross-motor domain, leading from rolling to creeping to independent walking, are obvious. Others, such as the line leading to the development of conscience, are more subtle.

The concept of a developmental line implies that a child passes though successive stages. The psychoanalytic theories of Sigmund Freud and Erik Erikson and the cognitive theory of Jean Piaget share the idea of stages as qualitatively different epochs in the development of emotion and cognition (Table 7–2). In contrast, the behavioral theory of Skinner relies less on qualitative change and more on the gradual modification of behavior and accumulation of competence.

PSYCHOANALYTIC THEORIES. At the core of *freudian theory* is the idea of body-centered (or broadly "sexual") drives. The focus of the drives shifts with maturation from oral satisfactions (i.e., sucking in the 1st yr of life); to anal sensations (i.e., holding on and letting go during the toddler years); oedipal drives (possessiveness toward a parent in the preschool years), and genital drives (in puberty and beyond) (see Table 7–2). At each stage, the child's drive can potentially conflict with the rules of society. For example, the infant may want to suck longer than his mother wants to nurse; or the toddler may decide he *likes* making a mess. The emotional health of the child and adult depends on adequate resolution of these conflicts. Freud saw middle childhood as a period of *latency*, when the sexual drive is redirected (sublimated) to the achievement of social or external goals.

Freudian ideas have come under broad attack. For example, few believe that the manner of toilet training permanently shapes personality, and middle childhood is no longer seen as conflict-free. Moreover, the effectiveness of psychoanalytic therapy has been difficult to demonstrate empirically. Nonetheless, the freudian legacy includes concepts that are central to an understanding of emotional development: the importance of a child's inner life and sexuality, the normative existence of emotional conflict during childhood, and the possibility that emotional disturbance can have early roots.

Erikson's chief contribution was to recast Freud's stages in terms of the emerging personality (see Table 7–2). For example, the child's sense of *basic trust* develops through the successful negotiation of infantile needs, corresponding to Freud's oral period. As children progress through these psychosocial stages, different issues become salient. Thus, it is predictable that a preschool-age child will be preoccupied with establishing his or her sense of autonomy, whereas a late adolescent may be more focused on establishing meaningful relationships and an occupational identity. Erikson recognized that these stages arise in the context of Western European societal expectations; in other cultures, the salient issues may be quite different.

Erikson's work calls attention to the intrapersonal challenges facing children at different ages in a way that facilitates professional intervention. For example, knowing that the salient issue for school-aged children is industry vs inferiority, pediatricians know to inquire about a child's experiences of mastery and failure and (if necessary) suggest ways to ensure adequate successes.

Piaget is synonymous with the study of cognitive development. A central tenet of piagetian thought is that cognition changes in quality, not just quantity (see Table 7–2). During the sensorimotor stage, an infant's thinking is tied to immediate sensations and a child's ability to manipulate objects. For example, the concept of "in" is embodied in a child's act of putting a block into a cup. With the arrival of language, the nature of thinking changes

TABLE 7–2. Classic Stage Theories

Theory	Infancy (0–1 yr)	Toddlerhood (2–3 yr)	Preschool (3–6 yr)	School Age (6–12 yr)	Adolescence (12–20 yr)
Freud: psychosexual	Oral	Anal	Oedipal	Latency	Adolescence
Erikson: psychosocial	Basic trust	Autonomy vs shame and doubt	Initiative vs guilt	Industry vs inferiority	Identity vs identity diffusion
Piaget: cognitive	Sensorimotor (stages I–IV)	Sensorimotor (stages V, VI)	Preoperational	Concrete operations	Formal operations

dramatically; symbols increasingly take the place of objects and actions. Cognitive stages correspond to the major periods of childhood: preoperational (preschool); concrete operations (school age); and formal operations (adolescence). Piaget described how children actively construct knowledge for themselves through the linked processes of assimilation (seeking experience) and accommodation (adapting their implicit ideas about the world to take new information into account). In this way, children act as "little scientists," creating ever more adaptive and complex theories. The stages of cognitive reorganization can be mapped by observing children and by asking open-ended questions that make the implicit theories explicit.

Piaget's basic concepts have held up well. Challenges have included questions about the timing of various stages, the role of formal teaching, and the extent to which context may affect conclusions about cognitive stage. For example, children's understanding of cause and effect may be considerably more advanced in the context of sibling relationships than in the context of inanimate objects (e.g., various machines); in many children, logical thinking appears well before puberty, the age postulated by Piaget. Of undeniable importance are Piaget's focus on cognition as a subject of empirical study, the universality of the progression of cognitive stages (even if details of timing are controversial), and the image of a child as actively and creatively interpreting the world.

Piaget's work is of special importance to pediatricians for three reasons: (1) It helps make sense of many puzzling behaviors of infancy, such as the common exacerbation of sleep problems at 9 and 18 mo of age; (2) Piagetian observations often lend themselves to quick replication in the office, with little special equipment; and (3) Open-ended questioning, based on Piaget's work, can provide insights into children's understanding of illness and hospitalization.

BEHAVIORAL THEORY. This theoretical perspective distinguishes itself by its lack of concern with a child's inner experience. Its sole focus is on observable behaviors and measurable factors that either increase or decrease the frequency with which these behaviors occur. No stages are implied: Children, adults, and indeed animals all respond the same. In its simplest form, the behaviorist orientation asserts that behaviors that are positively reinforced occur more frequently; behaviors that are negatively reinforced or ignored occur less frequently.

The strengths of this position are its simplicity, wide applicability, and conduciveness to scientific verification. A behavioral approach lends itself to readily taught interventions for various common problems such as temper tantrums and nocturnal enuresis. In cognitively limited children and children with autism spectrum disorders, behavioral interventions utilizing applied behavior analysis (ABA) approaches have demonstrated their ability to teach new, complex behaviors. However, in cases in which misbehavior is symptomatic of an underlying emotional, perceptual, or family problem, an exclusive reliance on behavior therapy risks leaving the cause untreated.

Statistics Used in Describing Growth and Development (see also Chapters 15 and 16). In everyday use, the term *normal* is synonymous with *healthy*. In a statistical sense, *normal* means that a set of values generates a normal (bell-shaped, or gaussian) distribution. This is the case with anthropometric quantities such as height and weight, and with many developmental milestones such as the age of independent standing. For a normally distributed measurement, a histogram with the quantity (e.g., height, or age) on the *x*-axis and the frequency (the number of children of that height, or the number who stand on their own at that age) on the *y*-axis generates a bell-shaped curve. In an ideal bell-shaped curve, the peak corresponds to the arithmetic mean of the sample, and to the median and the mode as well. The median is the value above and below which 50% of the observations lie; the mode is the value having the highest number of observations. Distributions are termed *skewed* if the mean, median, and mode are not the same number.

The extent to which observed values cluster near the mean determines the width of the bell and can be described mathematically by the standard deviation (SD). In the ideal normal curve, a range of values extending from 1 SD below the mean to 1 SD above the mean includes approximately 68% of the values, and each "tail" above and below that range contains 16% of the values. A range encompassing ±2 SD includes 95% of the values (with the upper and lower tails each comprising approximately 2.5% of the values), and ±3 SD encompasses 99.7% of the values (Table 7–3, Fig. 7–2).

TABLE 7–3. Relationship Between SD and Normal Range for Normally Distributed Quantities

Observations Included in Normal Range		Probability of a "Normal" Measurement Deviating from Mean by This Amount	
SD	*%*	*SD*	*%*
±1	68.3	≥1	16.0
±2	95.4	≥2	2.3
±3	99.7	≥3	0.13

SD = standard deviation.

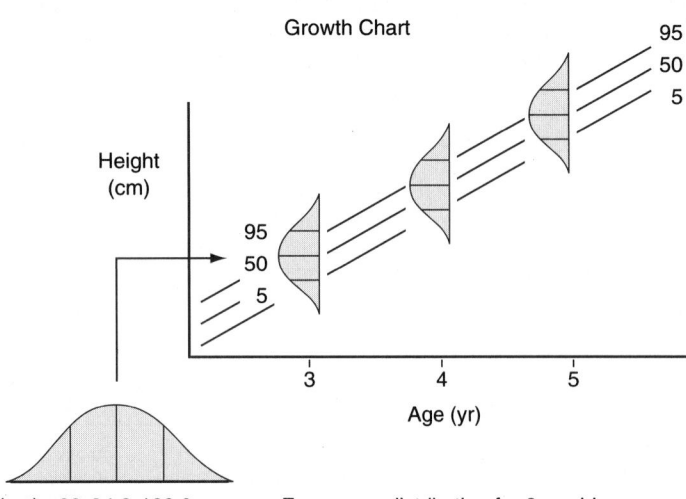

FIGURE 7–2. Relationship between percentile lines on the growth curve and frequency distributions of height at different ages.

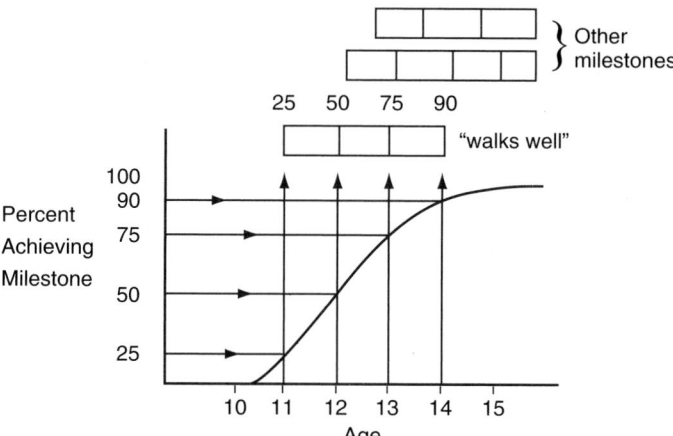

FIGURE 7–3. Method of presenting percentiles for developmental milestones.

For any single measurement, its distance away from the mean can be expressed in terms of the number of SDs (also called a *z score*); one can then consult a table of the normal distribution to find out what percentage of measurements fall within that distance from the mean. Software to convert anthropometric data into z-scores for epidemiologic purposes is readily available. A measurement that falls "outside the normal range"—arbitrarily defined as 2, or sometimes 3 SD on either side of the mean—is atypical, but not necessarily indicative of illness. However, the further a measurement (say, height, weight, or IQ) falls from the mean, the greater the probability that it represents not simply the normal variation, but rather a different, potentially pathologic, condition.

Another way of relating an individual to a group uses percentiles. The percentile is the percentage of individuals in the group who have achieved a certain measured quantity (e.g., a height of 95 cm) or developmental milestone. For anthropometric data, the percentile cutoffs can be calculated from the mean and SD. The 5th, 10th, and 25th percentiles correspond to −1.65 SD, −1.3 SD, and − 0.7 SD, respectively. Figure 7–2 shows conceptually how frequency distributions of a particular parameter (height) at different ages relate to the percentile lines on the growth curve. For developmental milestones, the percentiles are often displayed in boxes, derived from graphs plotting age (*x*-axis) against the percentage of subjects achieving the particular milestone (*y*-axis), as shown in Figure 7–3.

Allmond B, Tanner J: *The Family Is the Patient.* Baltimore, Williams & Wilkins, 1999.
Chess S, Thomas A: *Temperament in Clinical Practice.* New York, Guilford Press, 1986.
Eisenberg L: Experience, brain, and behavior: The importance of a head start. *Pediatrics* 1999;103:1031–5.
Erikson EH: *Childhood and Society,* 2nd ed. New York, WW Norton, 1963.
Rutter M: Nature, nurture and development: From evangelism through science toward policy and practice. *Child Dev* 2002;73:1–21.
Shonkoff J, Phillips D, National Research Council and Institute of Medicine: *From Neurons to Neighborhoods: The Science of Early Childhood Development.* Washington, DC, National Academy Press, 2000.
Werner EE: The children of Kauai: Resiliency and recovery in adolescence and adulthood. *J Adolesc Health* 1992;13:262–8.

Chapter 8
Fetal Growth and Development

The most dramatic events in growth and development occur before birth. This chapter traces the transformation of fertilized egg into embryo and fetus, the elaboration of the nervous sys-tem, and the emergence of behavior in utero. Also important are the psychologic changes occurring in the parents during the period of gestation. With processes so complex, much can go wrong. The uterus is permeable to adverse social and environmental influences such as maternal undernutrition; alcohol, cigarette, and drug use (both legal and illicit); and perhaps psychologic trauma. The complex interplay between these forces and the somatic and neurologic transformations occurring in the fetus influences infants' behavior at birth and may affect parent-child interactions throughout infancy.

Somatic Development

EMBRYONIC PERIOD. Milestones of prenatal development are presented in Table 8–1. By 6 days postconceptual age, as implantation begins, the embryo consists of a spherical mass of cells with a central cavity (the blastocyst). By 2 wk, implantation is complete and the uteroplacental circulation has begun; the embryo has two distinct layers, endoderm and ectoderm, and the amnion has begun to form. By 3 wk, the third primary germ layer (mesoderm) has appeared, along with primitive neural tube and blood vessels. Paired heart tubes have begun to pump.

During wk 4–8, lateral folding of the embryologic plate, followed by growth at the cranial and caudal ends and the budding of arms and legs, produces a human-like shape. Precursors of skeletal muscle and vertebrae (somites) appear, along with the branchial arches that will form the mandible, maxilla, palate, external ear, and other head and neck structures. Lens placodes appear, marking the site of future eyes; the brain grows rapidly. By the end of wk 8, as the embryonic period closes, the rudiments of all major organ systems have developed; the average embryo weighs 9 g and has a crown-rump length of 5 cm.

FETAL PERIOD. From the 9th wk on (the fetal period), somatic changes consist of increases in cell number and size and structural remodeling of several organ systems. Changes in body proportion are depicted in Figure 8–1. By 10 wk, the face is recognizably human. The midgut returns from the umbilical cord into the abdomen, rotating counterclockwise to bring the stomach, small intestine, and large intestine into their normal positions. By 12 wk, the gender of the external genitals becomes clearly distinguishable. Lung development proceeds with the budding of bronchi, bronchioles, and successively smaller divisions. By 20–24 wk, primitive alveoli have formed and surfactant production has begun; before that time, the absence of alveoli renders the lungs useless as organs of gas exchange.

During the 3rd trimester, weight triples and length doubles as body stores of protein, fat, iron, and calcium increase (see Chapter 85). Low birthweight may be due to prematurity,

TABLE 8–1. Milestones of Prenatal Development

Week	Developmental Events
1	Fertilization and implantation; beginning of embryonic period
2	Endoderm and ectoderm appear (bilaminar embryo)
3	First missed menstrual period; mesoderm appears (trilaminar embryo); somites begin to form
4	Neural folds fuse; folding of embryo into human-like shape; arm and leg buds appear; crown-rump length 4–5 mm
5	Lens placodes, primitive mouth, digital rays on hands
6	Primitive nose, philtrum, primary palate; crown-rump length 21–23 mm
7	Eyelids begin
8	Ovaries and testes distinguishable
9	*Fetal* period begins; crown-rump length 5 cm; weight 9 g
10	External genitals distinguishable
20	Usual lower limit of viability; weight 460 g; length 19 cm
25	Third trimester begins; weight 900 g; length 25 cm
28	Eyes open; fetus turns head down; weight 1,300 g
38	Term

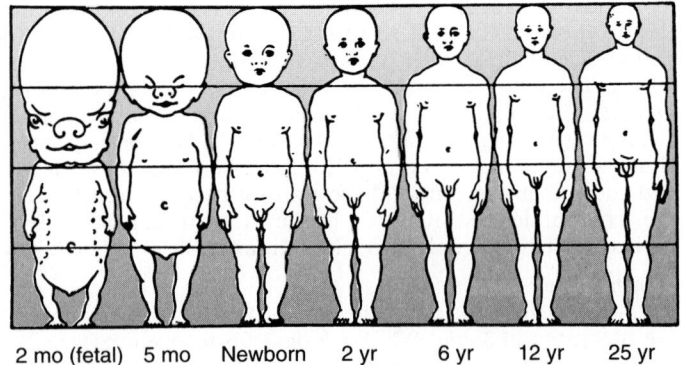

2 mo (fetal) 5 mo Newborn 2 yr 6 yr 12 yr 25 yr

FIGURE 8–1. Changes in body proportions from the 2nd fetal mo to adulthood. (From Robbins WJ, Brody S, Hogan AG, et al: *Growth.* New Haven, Yale University Press, 1928.)

intrauterine growth retardation (small for dates), or both (see Chapter 86).

Neurologic Development. During the 3rd wk, a neural plate appears on the ectodermal surface of the trilaminar embryo. Infolding produces a neural tube that will become the central nervous system (CNS) and a neural crest that will become the peripheral nervous system. Neuroectodermal cells differentiate into neurons, astrocytes, oligodendrocytes, and ependymal cells, whereas microglial cells are derived from mesoderm. By the 5th wk, the three main subdivisions of forebrain, midbrain, and hindbrain are evident. The dorsal and ventral horns of the spinal cord have begun to form, along with the peripheral motor and sensory nerves. Myelinization begins at midgestation and continues throughout the 1st 2 yr of life.

By the end of the embryonic period (wk 8), the gross structure of the nervous system has been established. On a cellular level, the growth of axons and dendrites and the elaboration of synaptic connections continue at a rapid pace, making the CNS vulnerable to teratogenic or hypoxic influences throughout gestation. Rates of increase in DNA (a marker of cell number), overall brain weight, and cholesterol (a marker of myelinization) are shown in Figure 8–2. The prenatal and postnatal peaks of DNA probably represent rapid growth of neurons and glia, respectively.

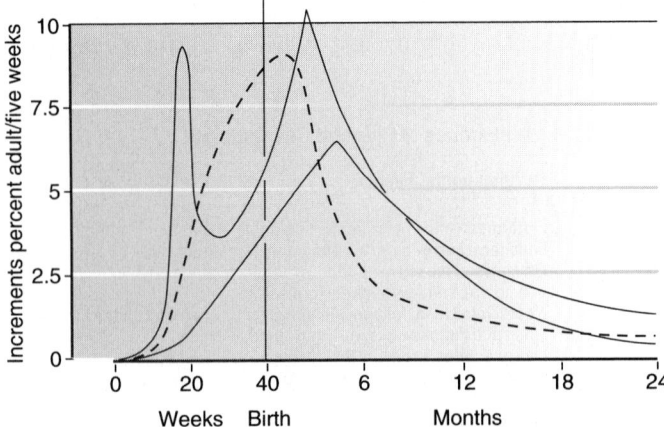

FIGURE 8–2. Velocity curves of the various components of human brain growth. Solid line with two peaks = DNA; dashed line = brain weight; single peak solid line = cholesterol. (From Brasel JA, Gruen RK: In Falkner F, Tanner JM [editors]: *Human Growth: A Comprehensive Treatise.* New York, Plenum Press, 1986, pp 78–95.)

Behavioral Development. Muscle contractions first appear around 8 wk, soon followed by lateral flexion movements. By 13–14 wk, breathing and swallowing motions appear and tactile stimulation elicits graceful movements. The grasp reflex appears at 17 wk and is well developed by 27 wk. Eye opening occurs around 26 wk. By midgestation, the full range of neonatal movements can be observed.

During the 3rd trimester, fetuses respond to external stimuli with heart rate elevation and body movements. As with infants in the postnatal period, reactivity to auditory (vibroacoustic) and visual (bright light) stimuli vary depending on their behavioral state, which can be characterized as quiet sleep, active sleep, and awake. Individual differences in the level of fetal activity are commonly noted by mothers and have been observed ultrasonographically. Fetal behavior is affected by maternal medications and diet, increasing, for example, after ingestion of caffeine, and may be entrained to the mother's diurnal rhythms.

Fetal movement increases in response to a sudden auditory tone, but decreases after several repetitions (habituation). If the tone changes in pitch, the movement increases again, evidence that the fetus distinguishes between a familiar, repeated tone and a novel one. The ability to habituate to repeated stimuli, a form of learning, is diminished in neurologically impaired or physically stressed fetuses. Similar responses to visual and tactile stimuli have been observed.

Psychologic Changes in Parents. The psychologic changes during pregnancy fall roughly into three stages. Stage 1 begins when a woman first learns that she is pregnant. Ambivalent feelings are the norm, whether or not the pregnancy was planned. Elation at the thought of producing a baby and the wish to be the perfect parent compete with fears of inadequacy and of the lifestyle changes that mothering will impose. Old conflicts may resurface as a woman psychologically identifies with her own mother and with herself as a child. The father-to-be faces similar mixed feelings, and problems in the parental relationship may intensify.

Stage 2 begins with awareness of fetal movements, or quickening, at approximately 20 wk or earlier with ultrasonic visualization. This palpable evidence that a fetus exists as a separate being often heightens a woman's feelings, both positive and negative. Parents worry about the fetus's healthy development and mentally rehearse what they will do if the child is malformed. Reassurances based on ultrasound examinations or amniocentesis may not completely allay these fears. During stage 3, toward the end of pregnancy, a woman becomes aware of patterns of fetal activity and reactivity and begins to ascribe to her fetus an individual personality and an ability to survive independently. Appreciation of the psychologic vulnerability of the expectant mother and father and of the powerful contribution of fetal behavior facilitates supportive clinical intervention.

Threats to Fetal Development. Mortality and morbidity are highest during the prenatal period (see Chapter 82). Some 30% of pregnancies end in spontaneous abortion, most often during the 1st trimester as a result of chromosomal or other abnormalities. Major congenital malformations requiring neonatal surgical intervention occur in approximately 2% of live births. Teratogens associated with gross physical and mental abnormalities include various infectious agents (toxoplasmosis, rubella, syphilis), chemical agents (mercury, thalidomide, antiepileptic medications, ethanol), high temperature, and radiation (see Chapters 85 and 700).

For any potential teratogen, the extent and nature of its effects are determined by characteristics of the host as well as the dose and timing of the exposure. Inherited differences in the metabolism of ethanol may predispose certain individuals or groups to fetal alcohol syndrome, for example. Organ systems are most vulnerable during periods of maximum growth and differentiation, generally during the first trimester (organogenesis). Figure 8–3 depicts sensitive periods during gestation for various organ systems.

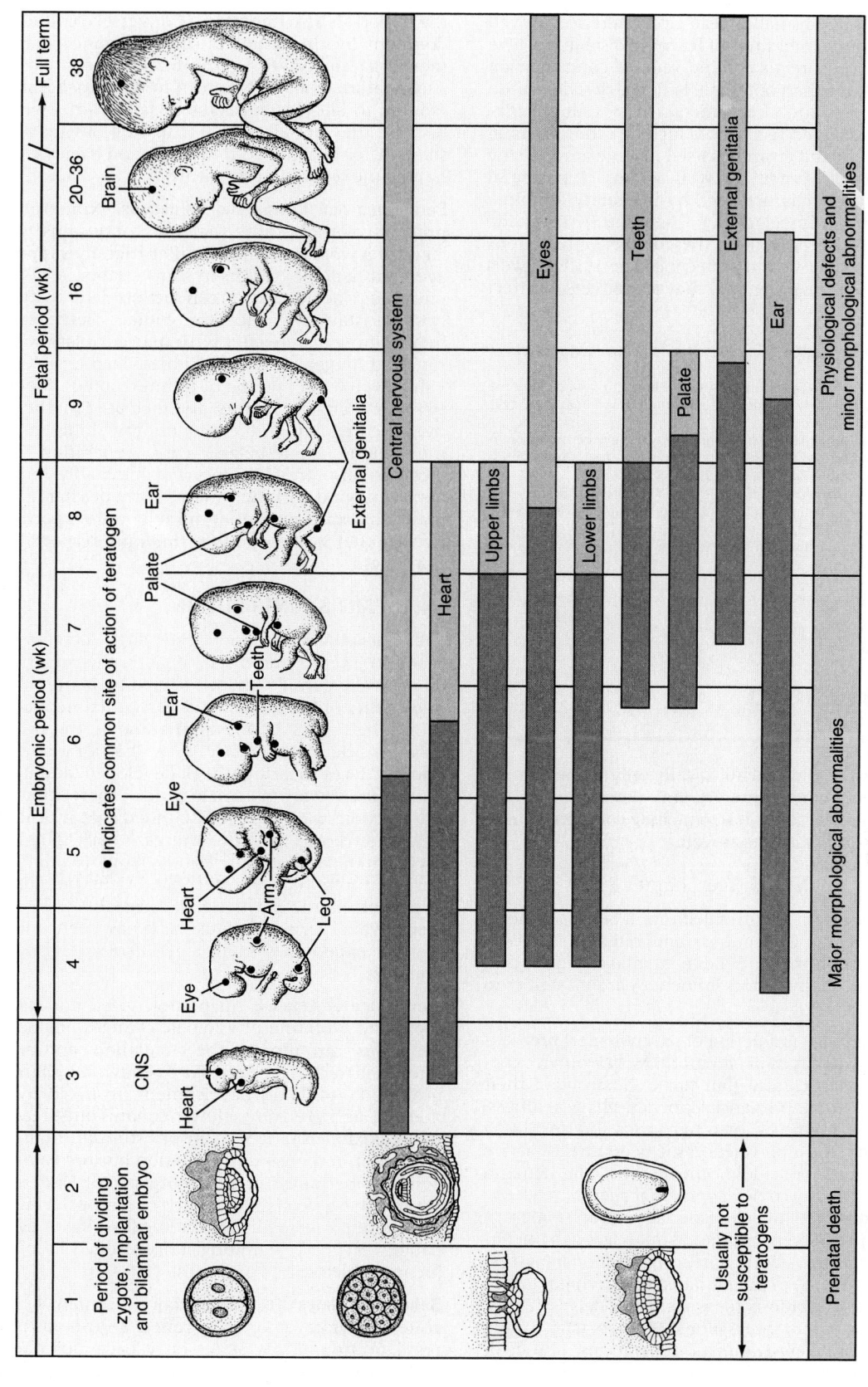

FIGURE 8–3. Schematic illustration of the sensitive or critical periods in prenatal development. Dark boxes denote highly sensitive periods; light boxes indicate states that are less sensitive to teratogens. (From Moore KL: *Before We Are Born: Basic Embryology and Birth Defects*, 2nd ed. Philadelphia, WB Saunders, 1977.)

Teratogenic effects may include not only gross physical malformation but also decreased growth and cognitive or behavioral deficits that only become apparent later in life. Prenatal exposure to cigarette smoke is associated with lower birthweight, shorter length, and smaller head circumference, as well as decreased IQ and increased rates of learning disabilities. The effects of prenatal exposure to cocaine remain controversial, and may be less dramatic than popularly believed. In addition to direct neurotoxic effects and effects mediated by reduced placental blood flow, associated risk factors include other prenatal exposures (e.g., alcohol and cigarettes used in large amounts by many cocaine-addicted women) as well as "toxic" postnatal environments frequently characterized by instability, multiple caregivers, and abuse and neglect (see Chapter 95). The wide range of outcomes observed reflects the complex interactions among biologic and social risk and protective factors. High levels of psychologic stress during pregnancy may also adversely affect fetal development.

Brazelton TB, Cramer BG: *The Earliest Relationship.* Reading, MA, Addison-Wesley Publishing, 1990.

Frank DA, Augustyn M, Knight WG, et al: Growth, development, and behavior in early childhood following prenatal cocaine exposure: A systematic review. *JAMA* 2001;285:1613–25.

Kiuchi M, Nagata N, Ikeno S, et al: The relationship between the response to external light stimulation and behavioral states in the human fetus: How it differs from vibroacoustic stimulation. *Early Hum Dev* 2000;58:153–65.

Koren G, Pastuszak A, Ito S: Drugs in pregnancy. *N Engl J Med* 1998;338:1128–37.

Moore KL: *Before We Are Born: Basic Embryology and Birth Defects,* 5th ed. Philadelphia, WB Saunders, 1998.

Relier JP: Influence of maternal stress on fetal behavior and brain development. *Biol Neonate* 2001;79:168–71.

Chapter 9

The Newborn

Infants thrive physically and psychologically only in the context of their social relationships. Therefore, any description of the newborn's developmental status has to include consideration of the parents' role as social partners as well.

DETERMINANTS OF PARENTING (see Chapter 83)

Parenting a newborn infant requires dedication because a newborn's needs are urgent, continuous, and often unclear. To know what to do, parents must attend to an infant's signals and respond empathically. Many factors influence parents' ability to assume this role.

Prenatal Factors. Pregnancy is a period of psychological preparation for the profound demands of parenting. Most women experience ambivalence, particularly (but not exclusively) if their pregnancy was unplanned. If financial worries, physical illness, prior miscarriages or stillbirths, or other crises interfere with their working through the ambivalence, the neonate may arrive as an unwelcome guest. For adolescent mothers, the demand that they relinquish their own developmental agenda (e.g., the need for an active social life) may be especially burdensome.

The early experience of being mothered may establish unconsciously held expectations about nurturing relationships that permit mothers to "tune in" to their infants. Research has linked the quality of these expectations (or working models) with the quality of later infant-parent interactions. Mothers whose early childhoods were marked by traumatic separations, abuse, or neglect may find it especially difficult to provide consistent, responsive care. Instead, they may re-enact their childhood experiences with their own infants as if unable to conceive of the mother-child relationship in any other way. Maternal

depression, during pregnancy and in the postpartum period, undermines the mother-child relationship, and may threaten the infant's cognitive and emotional development.

Social support during pregnancy—particularly support from the father—is also important. Conversely, conflict with or abandonment by the father during pregnancy may diminish the mother's ability to become absorbed with her infant. Anticipation of an early return to work makes it hard for many women to allow themselves to fall in love with their babies, because they are already anticipating having to separate from them. After 4–6 mo, both mothers and babies are more likely to handle the separation smoothly.

Peripartum and Postpartum Influences. Numerous randomized, prospective trials show that the continuous presence during labor of a woman trained to offer friendly support and encouragement (a doula) results in shorter labor, fewer obstetric complications (including cesarean section), and reduced postpartum hospital stays. Skin-to-skin contact between mothers and infants immediately after birth may correlate with an increased rate and longer duration of breast-feeding. Most new parents value even a brief period of uninterrupted time in which to get to know their new infants, and increased mother-infant contact over the first days of life may improve long-term mother-child interactions. Nonetheless, early separation, although predictably very stressful, does not inevitably impair a mother's ability to bond with her infant. Early discharge home from the maternity ward may undermine bonding, particularly when a new mother is required to resume full responsibility for a busy household.

THE INFANT'S CONTRIBUTION

Interactional Abilities. Soon after birth, neonates are alert and ready to interact and nurse, if given the opportunity. This first alert-awake period may be affected by maternal analgesics and anesthetics or fetal hypoxia. Nearsighted neonates have a fixed focal length of 8–12 in, approximately the distance from the breast to the mother's face, as well as an inborn visual preference for faces. Hearing is well developed, and infants preferentially turn toward a female voice. These innate abilities and predilections increase the likelihood that when a mother gazes at her newborn, the baby will gaze back. The initial period of social interaction, usually lasting about 40 min, is followed by a period of somnolence. After that, briefer periods of alertness or excitation alternate with sleep. If a mother misses her baby's first alert-awake period (because she has been anesthetized), she may not experience as long a period of social interaction for several days.

Modulation of Arousal. Adaptation to extrauterine life requires rapid and profound physiologic changes, including aeration of the lungs, rerouting of the circulation, and activation of the intestinal tract. The necessary behavioral changes are no less profound. To obtain nourishment, to avoid hypo- and hyperthermia, and to ensure safety, neonates must react appropriately to an expanded range of sensory stimuli. Infants must become aroused in response to stimulation but not so overaroused that behavior becomes utterly disorganized. Underaroused infants are not able to feed and interact; overaroused infants show signs of autonomic instability, including flushing or mottling, perioral pallor, hiccuping, vomiting, uncontrolled limb movements, or inconsolable crying.

Behavioral States. The organization of infant behavior into discrete behavioral states may reflect an infant's inborn ability to regulate arousal. Six states have been described: quiet sleep, active sleep, drowsy, alert, fussy, and crying. In the alert state, infants visually fixate on objects or faces and follow them horizontally and (within a month) vertically; they also reliably turn toward a novel sound, as if searching for its source. When overstimulated, they may calm themselves by looking away, yawning, or sucking on their lips or hands, thereby increasing parasympathetic activity and reducing sympathetic nervous activity. The behavioral state determines an infant's muscle tone, spontaneous movement, electroencephalogram pattern, and response to stimuli. In active sleep, for example, an infant may show progressively less reaction to a repeated heel prick (habituation), whereas in the drowsy state the same stimulus may push a child into fussing or crying.

Mutual Regulation. Parents actively participate in an infant's state regulation, alternately stimulating or soothing with the goal of prolonging the social interaction. In turn, the parents are regulated by the infant's signals, for example, responding to cries of hunger with a letdown of milk (or with a bottle). Such interactions constitute a system directed toward furthering the infant's physiologic homeostasis and physical growth. At the same time, they form the basis for the emerging psychologic relationship between parent and child. Infants come to associate the presence of the parent with the pleasurable reduction of tension (as in feeding) and show this preference by calming more quickly for the mother than for a stranger. This response, in turn, strengthens a mother's sense of efficacy and connection with her baby.

CLINICAL IMPLICATIONS: THE PHYSICIAN'S ROLE

Pediatric interventions to support healthy newborn development include (1) promoting optimal medical practices before, during, and after delivery; (2) assessing parent-infant interactions; and (3) teaching parents about their newborn's individual competencies and vulnerabilities.

Optimal Practices. A prenatal pediatric visit allows pediatricians to assess potential threats to bonding (e.g., a tense spousal relationship) and sources of social support and to try to allay unrealistic fears. Supportive hospital policies include the use of birthing rooms rather than operating suite/delivery rooms; encouragement for the father or a trusted relative or friend to remain with the mother during labor or the provision of a professional support person or doula; the practice of giving the newborn infant to the mother immediately after drying and brief assessment; placement of the newborn in the mother's room rather than in a central nursery; and avoiding in-hospital distribution of infant formula. Such policies have been shown to significantly increase breast-feeding rates. After discharge (often within 24 hr of delivery), home visits by nurses and lactation counselors can reduce early feeding problems and identify early-emerging medical conditions. Such family-focused policies may be particularly important for ill infants. Infants requiring transport to another hospital should be brought to see the mother first if at all possible. On discharge home, fathers can shield mothers from unnecessary visits and calls and take over household duties, allowing mothers and infants to get to know each other without distractions.

Assessing Parent-Infant Interactions. During a feeding or when infants are alert and face to face with parents, it is normal for them to appear absorbed in one another. Infants who become overstimulated by the mother's voice or activity may turn away or close their eyes, leading to a premature termination of the encounter. Alternatively, the infant may be ready to interact, whereas the mother may appear preoccupied. Asking a new mother about her own emotional state, and inquiring specifically about a history of depression, facilitates referral for therapy, which may provide long-term benefits to the child.

Teaching About Individual Competencies. The Newborn Behavior Assessment Scale (NBAS) provides a formal measure of an infant's neurodevelopmental competencies, including state control, autonomic reactivity, reflexes, habituation, and orientation toward auditory and visual stimuli. This examination can also be used to demonstrate to parents an infant's capabilities and vulnerabilities. Parents might learn that they need to undress their infant to increase the level of arousal or to swaddle the infant to reduce overstimulation by containing random arm movements. The NBAS can be used to support the development of positive early parent-infant relationships. Demonstration of the NBAS in the 1st wk of life has been shown to correlate with improvements in the caretaking environment months later.

Brazelton TB: *The Neonatal Behavioral Assessment Scale.* Philadelphia, JB Lippincott, 1973.

Crockenberg S, Leerkes E: Infant social and emotional development in family context. In Zeanah CH (editor): *Handbook of Infant Mental Health,* 2nd ed. New York, Guilford Press, 2000, pp 60–91.

Hodnett ED: Caregiver support for women during childbirth. *Cochrane Database Syst Rev* 2002:CD000199.

Kennell JH, Klaus MH: Bonding: Recent observations that alter perinatal care. *Pediatr Rev* 1998;19:4–12.

McLennan JD, Offord DR: Should postpartum depression be targeted to improve child mental health? *J Am Acad Child Adolesc Psychiatry* 2002;41:28–35.

Philipp BL, Merewood A, Miller LW, et al: Baby-friendly hospital initiative improves breastfeeding initiation rates in a US hospital setting. *Pediatrics* 2001;108:677–81.

Chapter 10
The First Year

During the first year of life, physical growth, maturation, acquisition of competence, and psychologic reorganization occur in discontinuous bursts. These changes qualitatively change a child's behavior and social relationships. Children acquire new competences in the gross motor, fine motor, cognitive, and emotional domains. The concept of developmental lines highlights how more complex skills build on simpler ones; but it is also important to realize how development in each domain affects functioning in all of the others. Physical growth parameters and normal ranges for attainable weight, length, and head circumference can be estimated as noted in Tables 10–1 and 10–2. Table 10–3 presents an overview of key milestones by domain, whereas Table 10–4 presents similar information arranged cross-sectionally.

AGE 0–2 MONTHS

The biologic and psychologic challenges facing neonates and their parents were described in Chapter 9. These consist of establishing effective feeding routines and a predictable sleep-wake cycle. The social interactions that occur as parents and infants accomplish these tasks lay the foundation for cognitive and emotional development.

Physical Development. A newborn's weight may decrease 10% below birthweight in the 1st wk as a result of excretion of excess

TABLE 10–1. Formulas for Approximate Average Height and Weight of Normal Infants and Children

Weight	Kilograms	(Pounds)
At birth	3.25	(7)
3–12 mo	$\dfrac{age\ (mo)+9}{2}$	(age [mo] + 11)
1–6 yr	age (yr) × 2 + 8	(age [yr] × 5 + 17)
7–12 yr	$\dfrac{age\ (yr) \times 7 - 5}{2}$	(age [yr] × 7 + 5)

Height	Centimeters	(Inches)
At birth	50	(20)
At 1 yr	75	(30)
2–12 yr	age (yr) × 6 + 77	(age [yr] × 2½ + 30)

TABLE 10–2. Length, Weight, and Head Circumference (C) by Age for Boys and Girls, Birth to 36 Mo

Age	Boys: Percentiles 5th	10th	25th	50th	75th	90th	95th		Girls: Percentiles 5th	10th	25th	50th	75th	90th	95th
	45.6 (18.0)	46.6 (18.4)	48.2 (19.0)	50.0 (19.7)	51.7 (20.4)	53.3 (21.0)	54.2 (21.4)	Length, cm (in)	45.6 (18.0)	46.4 (18.3)	47.7 (18.8)	49.3 (19.4)	51.0 (20.1)	52.6 (20.7)	53.7 (21.1)
birth	2.53 (5.6)	2.77 (6.1)	3.15 (6.9)	3.53 (7.8)	3.88 (8.5)	4.17 (9.2)	4.34 (9.5)	Weight, kg (lb)	2.55 (5.6)	2.75 (6.0)	3.06 (6.7)	3.40 (7.5)	3.72 (8.2)	3.99 (8.8)	4.15 (9.1)
	32.1 (12.7)	33.1 (13.0)	34.5 (13.6)	35.8 (14.1)	37.0 (14.6)	38.0 (15.0)	38.5 (15.2)	Head C, cm (in)	32.3 (12.7)	32.8 (12.9)	33.7 (13.2)	34.7 (13.7)	35.9 (14.1)	37.0 (14.5)	37.7 (14.8)
	52.8 (20.8)	53.6 (21.1)	55.0 (21.7)	56.6 (22.3)	58.3 (23.0)	59.9 (23.6)	60.9 (24.0)	Length, cm (in)	51.5 (20.3)	52.3 (20.6)	53.7 (21.1)	55.3 (21.8)	56.9 (22.4)	58.4 (23.0)	59.3 (23.4)
1 mo	3.77 (8.3)	4.02 (8.8)	4.43 (9.7)	4.88 (10.7)	5.33 (11.7)	5.73 (12.6)	5.97 (13.1)	Weight, kg (lb)	3.55 (7.8)	3.77 (8.3)	4.14 (9.1)	4.54 (10.0)	4.95 (10.9)	5.31 (11.7)	5.52 (12.1)
	36.3 (14.3)	37.0 (14.6)	38.1 (15.0)	39.2 (15.4)	40.2 (15.8)	41.1 (16.2)	41.6 (16.4)	Head C, cm (in)	35.8 (14.1)	36.2 (14.3)	37.0 (14.6)	38.0 (15.0)	39.0 (15.3)	40.0 (15.7)	40.6 (16.0)
	58.3 (22.9)	59.1 (23.3)	60.5 (23.8)	62.1 (24.4)	63.8 (25.1)	65.5 (25.8)	66.5 (26.2)	Length, cm (in)	56.5 (22.2)	57.4 (22.6)	58.8 (23.2)	60.5 (23.8)	62.1 (24.4)	63.6 (25.0)	64.5 (25.4)
3 mo	5.16 (11.3)	5.42 (11.9)	5.87 (12.9)	6.39 (14.1)	6.94 (15.3)	7.46 (16.4)	7.78 (17.1)	Weight, kg (lb)	4.71 (10.4)	4.96 (10.9)	5.38 (11.8)	5.86 (12.9)	6.35 (14.0)	6.80 (15.0)	7.08 (15.6)
	39.3 (15.5)	39.9 (15.7)	40.8 (16.1)	41.8 (16.4)	42.7 (16.8)	43.5 (17.1)	44.0 (17.3)	Head C, cm (in)	38.4 (15.1)	38.8 (15.3)	39.6 (15.6)	40.5 (15.9)	41.4 (16.3)	42.3 (16.6)	42.8 (16.9)
	63.9 (25.2)	64.7 (25.5)	66.2 (26.0)	67.9 (26.7)	71.4 (27.4)	72.5 (28.1)	69.7 (28.5)	Length, cm (in)	61.8 (24.3)	62.8 (24.7)	64.4 (25.3)	66.1 (26.0)	67.8 (26.7)	69.4 (27.3)	70.3 (27.7)
6 mo	6.75 (14.8)	7.04 (15.5)	7.55 (16.6)	8.16 (18.0)	8.83 (19.4)	9.48 (20.8)	9.89 (21.7)	Weight, kg (lb)	6.13 (13.5)	6.41 (14.1)	6.89 (15.2)	7.45 (16.4)	8.05 (17.7)	8.61 (18.9)	8.95 (19.7)
	41.8 (16.5)	42.3 (16.7)	43.1 (17.0)	44.0 (17.3)	44.9 (17.7)	45.7 (18.0)	46.2 (18.2)	Head C, cm (in)	40.7 (16.0)	41.1 (16.2)	41.9 (16.5)	42.7 (16.8)	43.6 (17.2)	44.4 (17.5)	44.9 (17.7)
	68.1 (26.8)	69.0 (27.2)	70.5 (27.8)	72.3 (28.5)	74.3 (29.2)	76.1 (30.0)	77.2 (30.4)	Length, cm (in)	66.0 (26.0)	67.0 (26.4)	68.7 (27.1)	70.6 (27.8)	72.4 (28.5)	74.1 (29.2)	75.0 (29.5)
9 mo	7.90 (17.4)	8.22 (18.1)	8.79 (19.3)	9.48 (20.8)	10.23 (22.5)	10.96 (24.1)	11.43 (25.1)	Weight, kg (lb)	7.25 (15.9)	7.55 (16.6)	8.07 (17.8)	8.69 (19.1)	9.36 (20.6)	10.00 (22.0)	10.40 (22.9)
	43.4 (17.1)	43.9 (17.3)	44.6 (17.6)	45.5 (17.9)	46.3 (18.2)	47.1 (18.6)	47.6 (18.7)	Head C, cm (in)	42.1 (16.6)	42.6 (16.8)	43.3 (17.1)	44.2 (17.4)	45.0 (17.7)	45.8 (18.0)	46.3 (18.2)
	71.6 (28.2)	72.5 (28.6)	74.2 (29.2)	76.1 (30.0)	78.1 (30.8)	80.0 (31.5)	81.2 (32.0)	Length, cm (in)	69.5 (27.4)	70.6 (27.8)	72.4 (28.5)	74.4 (29.3)	76.3 (30.1)	78.1 (30.7)	79.1 (31.1)
12 mo	8.75 (19.3)	9.10 (20.0)	9.71 (21.4)	10.46 (23.0)	11.27 (24.8)	12.07 (26.5)	12.57 (27.7)	Weight, kg (lb)	8.13 (17.9)	8.44 (18.6)	9.00 (19.8)	9.67 (21.3)	10.39 (22.9)	11.10 (24.4)	11.55 (25.4)
	44.4 (17.5)	44.9 (17.7)	45.6 (18.0)	46.5 (18.3)	47.4 (18.6)	48.2 (19.0)	48.6 (19.2)	Head C, cm (in)	43.1 (17.0)	43.6 (17.2)	44.3 (17.5)	45.2 (17.8)	46.1 (18.1)	46.9 (18.4)	47.3 (18.6)
	77.2 (30.4)	78.4 (30.9)	80.3 (31.6)	82.4 (32.4)	84.6 (33.3)	86.6 (34.1)	87.9 (34.6)	Length, cm (in)	75.5 (29.7)	76.7 (30.2)	78.6 (31.0)	80.8 (31.8)	83.0 (32.7)	84.9 (33.4)	86.0 (33.9)
18 mo	9.90 (21.8)	10.29 (22.6)	10.98 (24.2)	11.80 (26.0)	12.70 (28.0)	13.58 (29.9)	14.14 (31.1)	Weight, kg (lb)	9.39 (20.7)	9.73 (21.4)	10.34 (22.8)	11.09 (24.4)	11.92 (26.2)	12.75 (28.0)	13.29 (29.2)
	45.7 (18.0)	46.2 (18.2)	47.0 (18.5)	47.9 (18.8)	48.8 (19.2)	49.6 (19.5)	50.1 (19.7)	Head C, cm (in)	44.4 (17.5)	44.9 (17.7)	45.7 (18.0)	46.6 (18.4)	47.5 (18.7)	48.3 (19.0)	48.8 (19.2)
	81.9 (32.2)	83.2 (32.7)	85.3 (33.6)	87.7 (34.5)	90.0 (35.4)	92.2 (36.3)	93.4 (36.8)	Length, cm (in)	80.4 (31.7)	81.7 (32.2)	83.8 (33.0)	86.2 (33.9)	88.5 (34.9)	90.7 (35.7)	91.9 (36.2)
24 mo	10.70 (23.5)	11.11 (24.5)	11.85 (26.1)	12.74 (28.0)	13.71 (30.2)	14.67 (32.3)	15.28 (33.6)	Weight, kg (lb)	10.27 (22.6)	10.64 (23.4)	11.31 (24.9)	12.13 (26.7)	13.08 (28.8)	14.04 (30.9)	14.68 (32.3)
	46.4 (18.2)	46.9 (18.5)	47.8 (18.8)	48.7 (19.2)	49.7 (19.6)	50.5 (19.9)	51.0 (20.1)	Head C, cm (in)	45.2 (17.8)	45.7 (18.0)	46.6 (18.3)	47.5 (18.7)	48.5 (19.1)	49.3 (19.4)	49.8 (19.6)
	86.1 (33.9)	87.4 (34.4)	89.6 (35.3)	92.1 (36.3)	94.7 (37.3)	97.0 (38.2)	98.5 (38.8)	Length, cm (in)	85.0 (33.5)	86.3 (34.0)	88.6 (34.9)	91.1 (35.9)	93.7 (36.9)	96.0 (37.8)	97.4 (38.3)
30 mo	11.40 (25.1)	11.83 (26.0)	12.61 (27.7)	13.56 (29.8)	14.62 (32.2)	15.66 (34.5)	16.34 (36.0)	Weight, kg (lb)	10.99 (24.2)	11.38 (25.0)	12.12 (26.7)	13.04 (28.7)	14.12 (31.1)	15.24 (33.5)	15.99 (35.2)
	46.7 (18.4)	47.3 (18.6)	48.3 (19.0)	49.3 (19.4)	50.3 (19.8)	51.2 (20.2)	51.7 (20.4)	Head C, cm (in)	45.7 (18.0)	46.3 (18.2)	47.2 (18.6)	48.2 (19.0)	49.2 (19.4)	50.0 (19.7)	50.6 (19.9)
	90.0 (35.4)	91.3 (35.9)	93.5 (36.8)	96.1 (37.8)	98.7 (38.9)	101.2 (39.8)	102.7 (40.4)	Length, cm (in)	88.6 (34.9)	90.0 (35.4)	92.4 (36.4)	95.0 (37.4)	97.7 (38.5)	100.1 (39.4)	101.6 (40.0)
36 mo	12.04 (26.5)	12.49 (27.5)	13.31 (29.3)	14.33 (31.5)	15.48 (34.1)	16.64 (36.6)	17.41 (38.3)	Weight, kg (lb)	11.60 (25.5)	12.03 (26.5)	12.84 (28.2)	13.87 (30.5)	15.08 (33.2)	16.36 (36.0)	17.24 (37.9)
	46.9 (18.5)	47.5 (18.7)	48.6 (19.1)	49.7 (19.6)	50.8 (20.0)	51.7 (20.3)	52.2 (20.6)	Head C, cm (in)	46.0 (18.1)	46.6 (18.3)	47.6 (18.7)	48.6 (19.1)	49.7 (19.6)	50.6 (19.9)	51.1 (20.1)

Data used in creating the 2000 Centers for Disease Control (CDC) growth charts, as described in Chapter 15. English units appear in parentheses, below the corresponding metric units. Data apply to the age range, including the listed age and subsequent month (i.e., "1 mo" represents the average for 1 mo, 0 days through 1 mo, 30 days). Data for additional age points and 3rd and 97th percentiles are available at www.cdc.gov/nchs, along with technical reports.

TABLE 10–3. Developmental Milestones in the First 2 Yr of Life

Milestone	Average Age of Attainment (mo)	Developmental Implications
Gross Motor		
Head steady in sitting	2.0	Allows more visual interaction
Pull to sit, no head lag	3.0	Muscle tone
Hands together in midline	3.0	Self-discovery
Asymmetric tonic neck reflex gone	4.0	Child can inspect hands in midline
Sits without support	6.0	Increasing exploration
Rolls back to stomach	6.5	Truncal flexion, risk of falls
Walks alone	12.0	Exploration, control of proximity to parents
Runs	16.0	Supervision more difficult
Fine Motor		
Grasps rattle	3.5	Object use
Reaches for objects	4.0	Visuomotor coordination
Palmar grasp gone	4.0	Voluntary release
Transfers object hand to hand	5.5	Comparison of objects
Thumb-finger grasp	8.0	Able to explore small objects
Turns pages of book	12.0	Increasing autonomy during book time
Scribbles	13.0	Visuomotor coordination
Builds tower of two cubes	15.0	Uses objects in combination
Builds tower of six cubes	22.0	Requires visual, gross, and fine motor coordination
Communication and Language		
Smiles in response to face, voice	1.5	Child more active social participant
Monosyllabic babble	6.0	Experimentation with sound, tactile sense
Inhibits to "no"	7.0	Response to tone (nonverbal)
Follows one-step command with gesture	7.0	Nonverbal communication
Follows one-step command without gesture (e.g., "Give it to me")	10.0	Verbal receptive language
Speaks first real word	12.0	Beginning of labeling
Speaks 4–6 words	15.0	Acquisition of object and personal names
Speaks 10–15 words	18.0	Acquisition of object and personal names
Speaks two-word sentences (e.g., "Mommy shoe")	19.0	Beginning grammaticization, corresponds with 50+ word vocabulary
Cognitive		
Stares momentarily at spot where object disappeared (e.g., yarn ball dropped)	2.0	Lack of object permanence (out of sight, out of mind)
Stares at own hand	4.0	Self-discovery, cause and effect
Bangs two cubes	8.0	Active comparison of objects
Uncovers toy (after seeing it hidden)	8.0	Object permanence
Egocentric pretend play (e.g., pretends to drink from cup)	12.0	Beginning symbolic thought
Uses stick to reach toy	17.0	Able to link actions to solve problems
Pretend play with doll (gives doll bottle)	17.0	Symbolic thought

extravascular fluid and possibly poor intake. Intake improves as colostrum is replaced by higher-fat milk, as infants learn to latch on and suck more efficiently, and as mothers become more comfortable with feeding techniques. Infants should regain or exceed birthweight by 2 wk of age and should grow at approximately 30 g (1 oz)/day during the 1st mo (Table 10–5). Limb movements consist largely of uncontrolled writhing, with apparently purposeless hand opening and closing. Smiling occurs involuntarily. In contrast, eye gaze, head turning, and sucking are under better control and thus can be used to demonstrate infant perception and cognition. For example, an infant's preferential turning toward the mother's voice is evidence of recognition memory.

Six behavioral states have been described (see Chapter 9). Initially, sleep and wakefulness are evenly distributed throughout the 24 hr (Fig. 10–1). Neurologic maturation accounts for the consolidation of sleep periods into longer and longer blocks. Learning has a role as well. Infants whose parents are consistently more interactive and stimulating during the day learn to concentrate their sleeping during the night. By 2 mo of age, most infants are waking briefly two or three times to feed; some sleep 6 hr or more at a stretch. Crying occurs in response to stimuli that may be obvious (a soiled diaper) but are often obscure. Crying normally peaks at about 6 wk of age, when healthy infants cry up to 3 hr/day, then decreases to 1 hr or less by 3 mo.

Cognitive Development. Caretaking activities provide visual, tactile, olfactory, and auditory stimuli; all of these support the development of cognition. Studies of habituation and gaze preference provide insights into how infants interpret these stimuli. Infants habituate to the familiar, attending less and less to repeated stimuli and increasing their attention when the stimulus changes. Experiments using habituation and renewed attention as outcomes show that infants can differentiate among similar patterns, colors, and consonants. They can recognize facial expressions (smiles) as similar, even when they appear on different faces. They also can match abstract properties of stimuli, such as contour, intensity, or temporal pattern across sensory modalities. For example, 3-wk-old infants can tell whether a spoken voice corresponds to the movements of the lips on a videotape. Blindfolded and given a bumpy pacifier to suck, they subsequently gaze longer at the bumpy pacifier than at a smooth one when both are presented visually.

Such studies suggest that infants are able to perceive objects and events as coherent, even while noting aspects that are discrepant. These abilities allow infants to sort stimuli into meaningful sets: a set of stimuli that correspond to sucking as well as others that correspond to sucking a bottle, sucking a pacifier, and sucking a finger. Infants appear to seek stimuli actively as though satisfying an innate need to make sense of the world.

Emotional Development. Basic trust, the first of Erikson's psychosocial stages, develops as infants learn that their urgent needs are met regularly. The consistent availability of a trusted adult creates the conditions for a secure attachment. Infants who are consistently picked up and held in response to distress cry less at 1 yr and show less aggressive behavior at 2 yr.

TABLE 10–4. Emerging Patterns of Behavior During the 1st Yr of Life

Neonatal Period (1st 4 Wk)

Prone:	Lies in flexed attitude; turns head from side to side; head sags on ventral suspension
Supine:	Generally flexed and a little stiff
Visual:	May fixate face or light in line of vision; "doll's-eye" movement of eyes on turning of the body
Reflex:	Moro response active; stepping and placing reflexes; grasp reflex active
Social:	Visual preference for human face

At 4 Wk

Prone:	Legs more extended; holds chin up; turns head; head lifted momentarily to plane of body on ventral suspension
Supine:	Tonic neck posture predominates; supple and relaxed; head lags on pull to sitting position
Visual:	Watches person; follows moving object
Social:	Body movements in cadence with voice of other in social contact; beginning to smile

At 8 Wk

Prone:	Raises head slightly farther; head sustained in plane of body on ventral suspension
Supine:	Tonic neck posture predominates; head lags on pull to sitting position
Visual:	Follows moving object 180 degrees
Social:	Smiles on social contact; listens to voice and coos

At 12 Wk

Prone:	Lifts head and chest, arms extended; head above plane of body on ventral suspension
Supine:	Tonic neck posture predominates; reaches toward and misses objects; waves at toy
Sitting:	Head lag partially compensated on pull to sitting position; early head control with bobbing motion; back rounded
Reflex:	Typical Moro response has not persisted; makes defensive movements or selective withdrawal reactions
Social:	Sustained social contact; listens to music; says "aah, ngah"

At 16 Wk

Prone:	Lifts head and chest, head in approximately vertical axis; legs extended
Supine:	Symmetric posture predominates, hands in midline; reaches and grasps objects and brings them to mouth
Sitting:	No head lag on pull to sitting position; head steady, tipped forward; enjoys sitting with full truncal support
Standing:	When held erect, pushes with feet
Adaptive:	Sees pellet, but makes no move to it
Social:	Laughs out loud; may show displeasure if social contact is broken; excited at sight of food

At 28 Wk

Prone:	Rolls over; pivots; crawls or creep-crawls (Knobloch)
Supine:	Lifts head; rolls over; squirming movements
Sitting:	Sits briefly, with support of pelvis; leans forward on hands; back rounded
Standing:	May support most of weight; bounces actively
Adaptive:	Reaches out for and grasps large object; transfers objects from hand to hand; grasp uses radial palm; rakes at pellet
Language:	Polysyllabic vowel sounds formed
Social:	Prefers mother; babbles; enjoys mirror; responds to changes in emotional content of social contact

At 40 Wk

Sitting:	Sits up alone and indefinitely without support, back straight
Standing:	Pulls to standing position; "cruises" or walks holding on to furniture
Motor:	Creeps or crawls
Adaptive:	Grasps objects with thumb and forefinger; pokes at things with forefinger; picks up pellet with assisted pincer movement; uncovers hidden toy; attempts to retrieve dropped object; releases object grasped by other person
Language:	Repetitive consonant sounds (mama, dada)
Social:	Responds to sound of name; plays peek-a-boo or pat-a-cake; waves bye-bye

At 52 Wk (1 Yr)

Motor:	Walks with one hand held (48 wk); rises independently, takes several steps (Knobloch)
Adaptive:	Picks up pellet with unassisted pincer movement of forefinger and thumb; releases object to other person on request or gesture
Language:	A few words besides "mama," "dada"
Social:	Plays simple ball game; makes postural adjustment to dressing

Data are derived from those of Gesell (as revised by Knobloch), Shirley, Provence, Wolf, Bailey, and others.

The emotional significance of any experience depends on an individual child's temperament as well as the parent's responses. Consider the impact of different feeding schedules. Hunger generates increasing tension; as the urgency peaks, the infant cries, the parent arrives with a bottle or breast, and the tension dissipates. Infants fed "on demand" consistently experience this link between their distress, the arrival of the parent, and the relief from hunger. Most infants fed on a fixed schedule quickly adapt their hunger cycle to the schedule. Those who cannot because they are temperamentally prone to irregular biologic rhythms experience peri-ods of unrelieved hunger as well as unwanted feedings when they already feel full. Similarly, infants fed at the parents' convenience, with neither attention to the infant's hunger cues nor a fixed schedule, may not consistently experience feeding as the pleasurable reduction of tension. These infants often show increased irritability and physiologic instability (spitting, diarrhea, poor weight gain) as well as later behavioral problems.

Implications for Parents and Pediatricians. Success or failure in establishing feeding and sleep cycles determines parents' feel-

TABLE 10–5. Growth and Caloric Requirements

Age	Approximate Daily Weight Gain (g)	Approximate Monthly Weight Gain	Growth in Length (cm/mo)	Growth in Head Circumference (cm/mo)	Recommended Daily Allowance (kcal/kg/day)
0–3 mo	30	2 lb	3.5	2.00	115
3–6 mo	20	1 1/4 lb	2.0	1.00	110
6–9 mo	15	1 lb	1.5	0.50	100
9–12 mo	12	13 oz	1.2	0.50	100
1–3 yr	8	8 oz	1.0	0.25	100
4–6 yr	6	6 oz	3 cm/yr	1 cm/yr	90–100

Adapted from National Research Council, Food and Nutrition Board: Recommended Daily Allowances. Washington, DC, National Academy of Sciences, 1989; Frank D, Silva M, Needlman R: Failure to thrive: Myth and method. Contemp Pediatr *1993; 10:114.*

ings of efficacy. When things go well, the parents' anxiety and ambivalence, as well as the exhaustion of the early weeks, relent. With physical recovery from delivery and endocrinologic normalization, the mild postpartum depression that affects some 50% of mothers ("baby blues") passes. If sad, overwhelmed, anxious feelings persist, the possibility of moderate to severe postpartum depression needs to be considered. Major depression that arises during pregnancy or in the postpartum period threatens the mother-child relationship and is a risk factor for later cognitive and behavioral problems.

AGE 2–6 MONTHS

At about 2 mo, the emergence of voluntary (social) smiles and increasing eye contact mark a change in the parent-child relationship, heightening the parents' sense of being loved back.

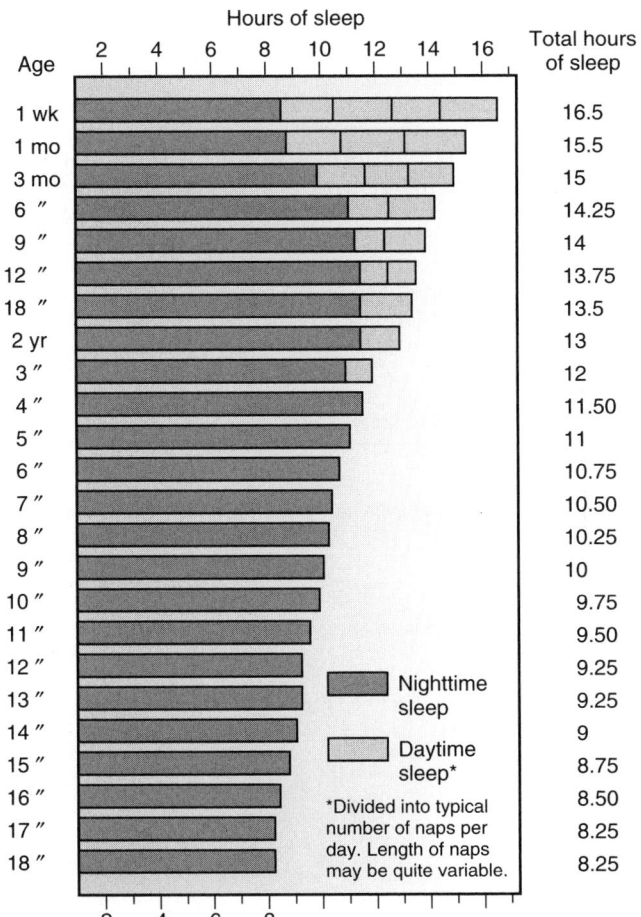

FIGURE 10–1. Typical sleep requirements in children. (From Ferber R: *Solve Your Child's Sleep Problems.* New York, Simon & Schuster, 1985.)

During the next months, an infant's range of motor and social control and cognitive engagement increases dramatically. Mutual regulation takes the form of complex social interchanges.

Physical Development. Between 3 and 4 mo, the rate of growth slows to approximately 20 g/day (see Table 10–5 and Figs. 11–1 and 11–2). Early reflexes that limited voluntary movement recede. Disappearance of the asymmetric tonic neck reflex means that infants can begin to examine objects in the midline and manipulate them with both hands. Waning of the early grasp reflex allows them both to hold objects and voluntarily to let them go. A novel object may elicit purposeful though inefficient reaching. The quality of spontaneous movements also changes, from larger writhing to smaller, circular movements that have been described as "fidgety." Abnormal or absent fidgety movements may constitute a risk factor for later neurologic abnormalities.

Increasing control of truncal flexion makes intentional rolling possible. Infants who routinely sleep on their backs (to prevent sudden infant death syndrome) may learn to roll somewhat later. Once infants can hold their head steady while sitting, they can gaze across at things rather than merely up at them, and can begin taking food from a spoon. At the same time, maturation of the visual system allows greater depth of field.

Total sleep requirements are approximately 14–16 hr/24 hr, with about 9–10 hr concentrated at night; about 70% of infants sleep for a 6- to 8-hr stretch by age 6 mo (see Fig. 10–1). By 4–6 mo, the sleep electroencephalogram shows a mature pattern, with demarcation of rapid eye movement (REM) and four stages of non-REM sleep. The sleep cycle remains shorter than in adults (50–60 min, versus approximately 90). As a result, infants arouse to light sleep or wake frequently during the night, setting the stage for behavioral sleep problems.

Cognitive Development. The overall effect of these developments is a qualitative change in an infant. Four-month-old infants are described as "hatching" socially, becoming interested in a wider world. During feeding, infants no longer focus exclusively on the mother but become distracted. In the mother's arms, the infant may literally turn around, preferring to face outward.

Infants at this age also explore their own bodies, staring intently at their hands, vocalizing, blowing bubbles, and touching their ears, cheeks, and genitals. These explorations represent an early stage in the understanding of cause and effect as infants learn that voluntary muscle movements generate predictable tactile and visual sensations. They also have a role in the emergence of a sense of self. Infants come to associate certain sensations through frequent repetition. For example, the proprioceptive feeling of holding up the hand and wiggling the fingers always accompanies the sight of the fingers moving. Such "self" sensations are consistently linked and reproducible at will. In contrast, sensations that come to be classed as "nonself" occur with less regularity and in varying combinations. The sound, smell, and feel of mother sometimes appears promptly in response to crying but sometimes does not.

Emotional Development and Communication. Outward-looking babies interact with increasing sophistication and range. The primary emotions of anger, joy, interest, fear, disgust, and surprise appear in appropriate contexts as distinct facial expressions. Face to face with a trusted adult, the infant and adult match affective expressions about 30% of the time; the intensity of their smiling, eye widening, and lip puckering rises and falls together. Every few seconds, as excitement builds, the infant turns away, settles, and then returns to the interaction. If the parent turns away, the infant leans forward, reaches, or in other ways tries to get the adult involved again; if that fails, the infant cries angrily.

Infants of depressed parents show a different pattern, spending less time in coordinated movement with their parents and making fewer efforts to re-engage. Rather than anger, they show sadness and a loss of energy when the parents continue to be unavailable. Such face-to-face behavior reveals the infant's ability to share emotional states, the first step in the development of communication; it also shows infants' (and parents') developing expectations about social relationships.

Implications for Parents and Pediatricians. Motor and sensory maturation makes infants at 3–6 mo exciting and interactive, at once cuter and more appealing but also more separate than at a younger age. Some parents experience their 4-mo-old's outward turning as a rejection, secretly fearing that their infants no longer love them. For most parents, however, this is a happy period. Most parents excitedly report that they can hold "conversations" with their infants, taking turns vocalizing and listening. Pediatricians share in the enjoyment, as the baby flirts and coos. If this visit does not feel joyful and relaxed, causes such as social stress, family dysfunction, parental mental illness, or problems in the infant-parent relationship should be considered.

AGE 6–12 MONTHS

Months 6–12 bring increased mobility and exploration of the inanimate world, advances in cognitive understanding and communicative competence, and new tensions around the themes of attachment and separation. Infants develop will and intentions, characteristics that most parents welcome but still find challenging to manage.

Physical Development. Growth slows more (see Table 10–5 and Figs. 11–1 and 11–2). The ability to sit unsupported (about 7 mo) and to pivot while sitting (around 9–10 mo) provides increasing opportunities to manipulate several objects at a time and to experiment with novel combinations of objects. These explorations are aided by the emergence of a pincer grasp (around 9 mo). Many infants begin crawling and pulling to stand around 8 mo and walk before their first birthday either independently or in a walker. Motor achievements correlate with increasing myelinization and cerebellar growth. These ambulatory achievements expand infants' exploratory range and create new physical dangers as well as opportunities for learning. Tooth eruption occurs, usually starting with the mandibular central incisors (Table 10–6). Tooth development also reflects, in part, skeletal maturation and bone age (Table 10–7).

Cognitive Development. At first, everything goes into the mouth; in time, novel objects are picked up, inspected, passed from hand to hand, banged, dropped, and then mouthed. Each action represents a nonverbal idea about what things are for (in piagetian terms, a schema). The complexity of an infant's play, how many different schemata are brought to bear, is a useful index of cognitive development at this age. The pleasure, persistence, and energy with which infants tackle these challenges suggest the existence of an intrinsic drive or mastery motivation. Mastery behavior occurs when infants feel secure; those with less secure attachments show limited experimentation and less competence.

A major milestone is the achievement (about 9 mo) of object constancy, the understanding that objects continue to exist even when not seen. At 4–7 mo, infants look down for a yarn ball that has been dropped but quickly give up if it is not seen. With object constancy, infants persist in searching, finding objects hidden under a cloth or behind the examiner's back.

Emotional Development. The advent of object constancy corresponds with qualitative changes in social and communicative development. Infants look back and forth between an approaching stranger and a parent, as if to contrast known from unknown, and may cling or cry anxiously. Separations often become more difficult. Infants who have been sleeping through the night for months begin to awaken regularly and cry, as though remembering that parents are in the next room.

At the same time, a new demand for autonomy emerges. Infants no longer consent to be fed but turn away as the spoon approaches or insist on holding it themselves. Self-feeding with finger foods allows infants to exercise newly acquired fine

---

TABLE 10–6. Chronology of Human Dentition of Primary or Deciduous and Secondary or Permanent Teeth

	Calcification		Age at Eruption		Age at Shedding	
	Begins at	*Complete at*	*Maxillary*	*Mandibular*	*Maxillary*	*Mandibular*
Primary Teeth						
Central incisors	5th fetal mo	18–24 mo	6–8 mo	5–7 mo	7–8 yr	6–7 yr
Lateral incisors	5th fetal mo	18–24 mo	8–11 mo	7–10 mo	8–9 yr	7–8 yr
Cuspids (canines)	6th fetal mo	30–36 mo	16–20 mo	16–20 mo	11–12 yr	9–11 yr
First molars	5th fetal mo	24–30 mo	10–16 mo	10–16 mo	10–11 yr	10–12 yr
Second molars	6th fetal mo	36 mo	20–30 mo	20–30 mo	10–12 yr	11–13 yr
Secondary Teeth						
Central incisors	3–4 mo	9–10 yr	7–8 yr	6–7 yr		
Lateral incisors	Max, 10–12 mo Mand, 3–4 mo	10–11 yr	8–9 yr	7–8 yr		
Cuspids (canines)	4–5 mo	12–15 yr	11–12 yr	9–11 yr		
First premolars (bicuspids)	18–21 mo	12–13 yr	10–11 yr	10–12 yr		
Second premolars (bicuspids)	24–30 mo	12–14 yr	10–12 yr	11–13 yr		
First molars	Birth	9–10 yr	6–7 yr	6–7 yr		
Second molars	30–36 mo	14–16 yr	12–13 yr	12–13 yr		
Third molars	Max, 7–9 yr Mand, 8–10 yr	18–25 yr	17–22 yr	17–22 yr		

Max = maxillary; Mand = mandibular.
Adapted from chart prepared by PK Losch, Harvard School of Dental Medicine, who provided the data for this table.

TABLE 10–7. **Time of Appearance in Roentgenograms of Centers of Ossification in Infancy and Childhood**

Boys—Age at Appearance*	Bones and Epiphyseal Centers	Girls—Age at Appearance*
3 wk	*Humerus, head*	3 wk
	Carpal bones	
2 mo ± 2 mo	Capitate	2 mo ± 2 mo
3 mo ± 2 mo	Hamate	2 mo ± 2 mo
30 mo ± 16 mo	Triangular†	21 mo ± 14 mo
42 mo ± 19 mo	Lunate†	34 mo ± 13 mo
67 mo ± 19 mo	Trapezium†	47 mo ± 14 mo
69 mo ± 15 mo	Trapezoid†	49 mo ± 12 mo
66 mo ± 15 mo	Scaphoid†	51 mo ± 12 mo
No standards available	Pisiform†	No standards available
	Metacarpal bones	
18 mo ± 5 mo	II	12 mo ± 3 mo
20 mo ± 5 mo	III	13 mo ± 3 mo
23 mo ± 6 mo	IV	15 mo ± 4 mo
26 mo ± 7 mo	V	16 mo ± 5 mo
32 mo ± 9 mo	I	18 mo ± 5 mo
	Fingers (epiphyses)	
16 mo ± 4 mo	Proximal phalanx, 3rd finger	10 mo ± 3 mo
16 mo ± 4 mo	Proximal phalanx, 2nd finger	11 mo ± 3 mo
17 mo ± 5 mo	Proximal phalanx, 4th finger	11 mo ± 3 mo
19 mo ± 7 mo	Distal phalanx, 1st finger	12 mo ± 4 mo
21 mo ± 5 mo	Proximal phalanx, 5th finger	14 mo ± 4 mo
24 mo ± 6 mo	Middle phalanx, 3rd finger	15 mo ± 5 mo
24 mo ± 6 mo	Middle phalanx, 4th finger	15 mo ± 5 mo
26 mo ± 6 mo	Middle phalanx, 2nd finger	16 mo ± 5 mo
28 mo ± 6 mo	Distal phalanx, 3rd finger	18 mo ± 4 mo
28 mo ± 6 mo	Distal phalanx, 4th finger	18 mo ± 5 mo
32 mo ± 7 mo	Proximal phalanx, 1st finger	20 mo ± 5 mo
37 mo ± 9 mo	Distal phalanx, 5th finger	23 mo ± 6 mo
37 mo ± 8 mo	Distal phalanx, 2nd finger	23 mo ± 6 mo
39 mo ± 10 mo	Middle phalanx, 5th finger	22 mo ± 7 mo
152 mo ± 18 mo	Sesamoid (adductor pollicis)	121 mo ± 13 mo
	Hip and knee	
Usually present at birth	Femur, distal	Usually present at birth
Usually present at birth	Tibia, proximal	Usually present at birth
4 mo ± 2 mo	Femur, head	4 mo ± 2 mo
46 mo ± 11 mo	Patella	29 mo ± 7 mo
	Foot and ankle‡	

Values represent mean ± standard deviation, when applicable.
*To nearest month.
†Except for the capitate and hamate bones, the variability of carpal centers is too great to make them very useful clinically.
‡Standards for the foot are available, but normal variation is wide, including some familial variants, so that this area is of little clinical use.
The norms present a composite of published data from the Fels Research Institute, Yellow Springs, OH (Pyle SI, Sontag L: Am J Roentgenol 49:102, 1943), and unpublished data from the Brush Foundation, Case Western Reserve University, Cleveland, OH, and the Harvard School of Public Health, Boston, MA. Compiled by Lieb, Buehl, and Pyle.

motor skills (the pincer grasp); it may be the only way to get a child to eat. Tantrums make their first appearance as the drives for autonomy and mastery come in conflict with parental controls and with the infants' still-limited abilities.

Communication. Infants at 7 mo are adept at nonverbal communication, expressing a range of emotions and responding to vocal tone and facial expressions. Around 9 mo, infants become aware that emotions can be shared between people; they show parents toys gleefully, as if to say, "When you see this thing, you'll be happy, too!" Between 8 and 10 mo, babbling takes on a new complexity, with many syllables ("ba-da-ma") and inflections that mimic the native language. At the same time, infants lose the ability to distinguish between vocal sounds that are undifferentiated in their native language. The first true word—i.e., a sound used consistently to refer to a specific object or person—appears in concert with an infant's discovery of object constancy.

At this age, picture books provide an ideal context for verbal language acquisition. With a familiar book as a shared focus of attention, a parent and child engage in repeated cycles of pointing and labeling, with elaboration and feedback by the parent.

Implications for Parents and Pediatricians. With the developmental reorganization around 9 mo, previously resolved issues of feeding and sleeping re-emerge. Pediatricians can prepare parents at the 6-mo visit so that these problems can be understood as the results of developmental progress and not regression. Parental ambivalence about separation can express itself in a delay in introducing finger foods or drinking from a cup (usually before the 1st birthday) or an intrusive, overly neat approach to meal times. Poor weight gain at this age often reflects a struggle between an infant and parent over control of the infant's eating. Discussions about an infant's drive for autonomy and need for limited choices may avert such problems.

Infants' wariness of strangers often makes the 9-mo examination difficult, particularly if the infant is temperamentally prone to react negatively to unfamiliar situations. Time spent talking with the mother and playing with the child will be rewarded by more cooperation. By using picture books as part of the routine health supervision visit, pediatricians can effectively promote reading aloud while addressing a variety of behavioral issues, including object exploration, autonomy, attention, language, and the continued importance of physical closeness and shared enjoyment.

Brazelton TB: *Touchpoints: The Essential Reference.* Reading, MA, Addison-Wesley Publishing, 1992.
Cohn JF, Tronick EZ: Three-month-old infants' reactions to simulated maternal deprivation. *Child Dev* 1983;54:185.
Mahler MS, Pine S, Bergman A: *The Psychological Birth of the Infant.* London, Hutchinson, 1975.

Needlman R, Klass P, Zuckerman B: Reach out and get your patients to read. *Contemp Pediatr* 2002;19:51–69.

Stern D: *The Interpersonal World of the Infant.* New York, Basic Books, 1985.

Zuckerman BS, Frank DA, Augustyn M: Infancy and toddler years. In Levine MD, Carey WB, Crocker AC (editors): *Developmental-Behavioral Pediatrics*, 3rd ed. Philadelphia, WB Saunders, 1999, pp 24–37.

Chapter 11
The Second Year

At approximately 18 mo of age, the emergence of symbolic thought causes a reorganization of behavior with implications across many developmental domains.

AGE 12–18 MONTHS

Physical Development. The growth rate slows further in the 2nd yr of life (see Table 10–5) and appetite declines. "Baby fat" is burned up by increased mobility; exaggerated lumbar lordosis makes the abdomen protrude. Brain growth continues, with myelinization throughout the 2nd yr (see Fig. 8–2).

Most children begin to walk independently near their first birthday; some do not walk until 15 mo. Highly active, fearless infants tend to walk earlier; less active, more timid infants and those who are preoccupied with exploring objects in detail walk later. Early walking is not associated with advanced development in other domains.

At first, infants toddle with a wide-based gait, knees bent, and arms flexed at the elbow; the entire torso rotates with each stride; the toes may point in or out, and the feet strike the floor flat. Subsequent refinements lead to greater steadiness and energy efficiency. After several months of practice, the center of gravity shifts back and the torso stays more stable, while knees extend and arms swing at the sides for balance. The toes are held in better alignment, and the child is able to stop, pivot, and stoop without toppling over.

Cognitive Development. As toddlers master reaching, grasping, and releasing, and greater mobility gives them access to more and more objects, exploration increases. Toddlers combine objects in novel ways to create interesting effects, such as stacking blocks or putting things into a videocassette recorder slot. Playthings are also more likely to be used for their intended purposes (combs for hair, cups for drinking). Imitation of parents and older children is an important mode of learning. Make-believe play centers on the child's own body (pretending to drink from an empty cup) (Table 11–1; see also Table 10–3).

Emotional Development. Infants developmentally approaching the milestone of their first steps may be irritable. Once they start walking, their predominant mood changes markedly. Toddlers are described as "intoxicated" with their new ability and with the power to control the distance between themselves and their parents. Exploring toddlers orbit around their parents, like comets around the sun, moving away, then returning for a reassuring touch before moving away again. In unfamiliar surroundings, with temperamentally timid children, such orbits might be small or nonexistent; in familiar ones, a bold child might orbit out of sight (see Table 11–1).

A child's ability to use the parent as a secure base for exploration depends on the attachment relationship. Attachment is typically assessed using the so-called "strange situation" procedure, in which the parents temporarily leave the child in an unfamiliar playroom. When their parents leave, most children stop playing, cry, and try to follow. The child's security of attachment is coded based on his or her response upon the parents' return. Securely attached children instantly go to their parents to be picked up, are comforted, and then are able to return to play. Children with ambivalent attachments go to their parents but then may resist being comforted and may hit at their parents in anger. Children categorized as avoidant may not protest when the parents leave and may turn away upon the parents' return. Insecure response patterns may represent strategies infants develop to cope with punitive or unresponsive parenting styles and may predict later cognitive and emotional problems. Controversy continues about how infant temperament and prior experience of separations might affect the interpretation of strange situation results.

Linguistic Development. Receptive language precedes expressive. By the time infants speak their first words, around 12 mo, they already respond appropriately to several simple statements such as "no," "bye-bye," and "give me." By 15 mo, the average child points to major body parts and uses four to six words spontaneously and correctly, including proper nouns. Toddlers also enjoy polysyllabic jargoning (see Tables 10–3 and 11–1) but do not seem upset that no one understands. Most communication of wants and ideas continues to be nonverbal.

Implications for Parents and Pediatricians. Parents who cannot recall any other milestone tend to remember when their child began to walk, perhaps because of the symbolic significance of walking as an act of independence. A child's ability to wander out of sight also obviously increases the risks of injury and need for supervision. When walking is precluded by physical disability, parents and care providers should facilitate exploration and help the child attain greater control over separation and proximity through wheelchairs or other assistance.

Patterns of response similar to those rated in the strange situation procedure may be observable in the pediatric clinic. Many toddlers are comfortable exploring the examination room but cling to the parents under the stress of the examination. Infants who become more, not less, distressed in their parents' arms or who avoid their parents at times of stress may be insecurely attached. Young children who, when distressed, turn to strangers for comfort rather than to parents are particularly worrisome.

AGE 18–24 MONTHS

Physical Development. Motor development is incremental at this age, with improvements in balance and agility and the emergence of running and stair climbing. Height and weight increase at a steady rate, although head growth slows slightly (Figs. 11–1 and 11–2; see also Table 10–5).

Cognitive Development. At approximately 18 mo, several cognitive changes come together to mark the conclusion of the sensorimotor period. Object permanence is firmly established; toddlers anticipate where an object will end up, even though the object was not visible while it was being moved. Cause and effect are better understood, and toddlers demonstrate flexibility in problem solving, for example using a stick to obtain a toy out of reach or figuring out how to wind a mechanical toy. Symbolic transformations in play are no longer tied to the toddler's own body, so that a doll can be "fed" from an empty plate. Like the reorganization at 9 mo, the cognitive changes at 18 mo correlate with important changes in the emotional and linguistic domains (see Table 11–1).

Emotional Development. In many children, the relative independence of the preceding period gives way to increased clinginess around 18 mo. This stage, described as *rapprochement*, may be a reaction to growing awareness of the possibility of separation. Many parents report that they now cannot go anywhere without having a small child attached to them. Separations at bedtime are often difficult, with frequent false starts and tantrums. Many children use a special blanket or stuffed toy as a transi-

TABLE 11–1. **Emerging Patterns of Behavior from 1 to 5 Yr of Age***

	15 Mo
Motor:	Walks alone; crawls up stairs
Adaptive:	Makes tower of 3 cubes; makes a line with crayon; inserts pellet in bottle
Language:	Jargon; follows simple commands; may name a familiar object (ball)
Social:	Indicates some desires or needs by pointing; hugs parents
	18 Mo
Motor:	Runs stiffly; sits on small chair; walks up stairs with one hand held; explores drawers and wastebaskets
Adaptive:	Makes a tower of 4 cubes; imitates scribbling; imitates vertical stroke; dumps pellet from bottle
Language:	10 words (average); names pictures; identifies one or more parts of body
Social:	Feeds self; seeks help when in trouble; may complain when wet or soiled; kisses parent with pucker
	24 Mo
Motor:	Runs well, walks up and down stairs, one step at a time; opens doors; climbs on furniture; jumps
Adaptive:	Tower of 7 cubes (6 at 21 mo); circular scribbling; imitates horizontal stroke; folds paper once imitatively
Language:	Puts 3 words together (subject, verb, object)
Social:	Handles spoon well; often tells immediate experiences; helps to undress; listens to stories with pictures
	30 Mo
Motor:	Goes up stairs alternating feet
Adaptive:	Tower of 9 cubes; makes vertical and horizontal strokes but generally will not join them to make a cross; imitates circular stroke, forming closed figure
Language:	Refers to self by pronoun "I"; knows full name
Social:	Helps put things away; pretends in play
	36 Mo
Motor:	Rides tricycle; stands momentarily on one foot
Adaptive:	Tower of 10 cubes; imitates construction of "bridge" of 3 cubes; copies a circle; imitates a cross
Language:	Knows age and sex; counts 3 objects correctly; repeats 3 numbers or a sentence of 6 syllables
Social:	Plays simple games (in "parallel" with other children); helps in dressing (unbuttons clothing and puts on shoes); washes hands
	48 Mo
Motor:	Hops on one foot; throws ball overhand; uses scissors to cut out pictures; climbs well
Adaptive:	Copies bridge from model; imitates construction of "gate" of 5 cubes; copies cross and square; draws a man with 2 to 4 parts besides head; names longer of 2 lines
Language:	Counts 4 pennies accurately; tells a story
Social:	Plays with several children with beginning of social interaction and role-playing; goes to toilet alone
	60 Mo
Motor:	Skips
Adaptive:	Draws triangle from copy; names heavier of 2 weights
Language:	Names 4 colors; repeats sentence of 10 syllables; counts 10 pennies correctly
Social:	Dresses and undresses; asks questions about meaning of words; domestic role-playing

Data are derived from those of Gesell (as revised by Knobloch), Shirley, Provence, Wolf, Bailey, and others. After 5 yr the Stanford-Binet, Wechsler-Bellevue, and other scales offer the most precise estimates of developmental level. In order to have their greatest value, they should be administered only by an experienced and qualified person.

tional object: something that functions as a symbol of the absent parent (in psychoanalytic terms, the object). The transitional object remains important until the transition to symbolic thought has been completed and the symbolic presence of the parent has been fully internalized. Individual differences in temperament, both in the child and the parents, play a critical role in determining the balance of conflict versus cooperation in the parent-child relationship.

Self-conscious awareness and internalized standards of evaluation first appear at this age. Toddlers looking in a mirror will, for the first time, reach for their own face rather than the mirror image if they notice a red dot on their nose or some other unusual appearance. They begin to recognize when toys are broken and may hand them to parents to fix. When tempted to touch a forbidden object, they may tell themselves "no, no," evidence of internalization of standards of behavior. That they often go on to touch the object anyway demonstrates the relative weakness of internalized inhibitions at this stage (see Table 11–1).

Linguistic Development. Perhaps the most dramatic developments in this period are linguistic. Labeling of objects coincides with the advent of symbolic thought. Children may point at things with their index finger rather than their whole hand as though calling attention to objects not for the purpose of having them but of finding out their names. When this protolinguistic naming is accompanied by the phrase "Whazzat?" the child's intentions are clear. After the realization that words can stand for things, a child's vocabulary balloons from 10–15 words at 18 mo to 100 or more at 2 yr. After acquiring a vocabulary of about 50 words, toddlers begin to combine them to make simple sentences, the beginning of grammar. At this stage, toddlers understand two-step commands, such as "Give me the ball and then get your shoes." The emergence of verbal language marks the end of the sensorimotor period. As toddlers learn to use symbols to express ideas and solve problems, the need for cognition based on direct sensation and motor manipulation wanes (see Table 11–1).

Implications for Parents and Pediatricians. With children's increasing mobility, physical limits on their explorations become less effective; words become increasingly important for behavior control as well as cognition. Children with delayed language

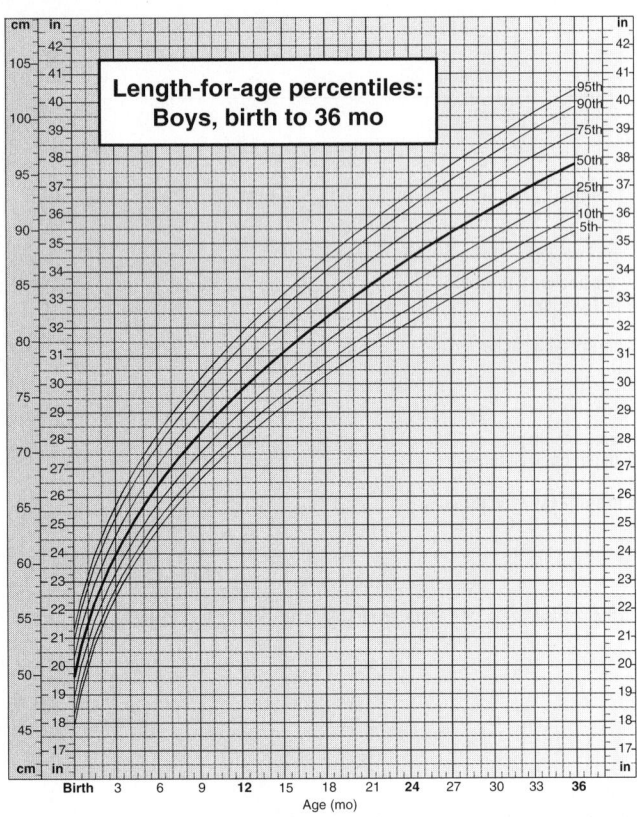

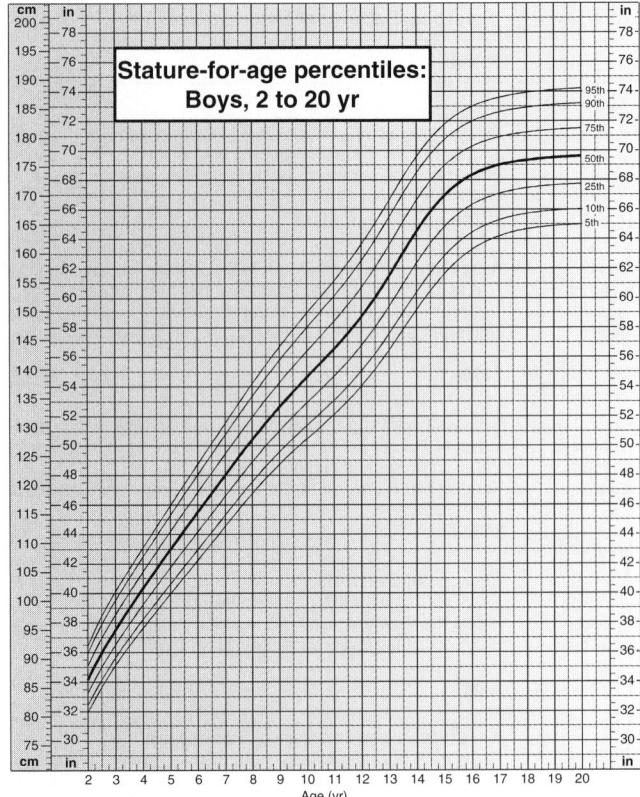

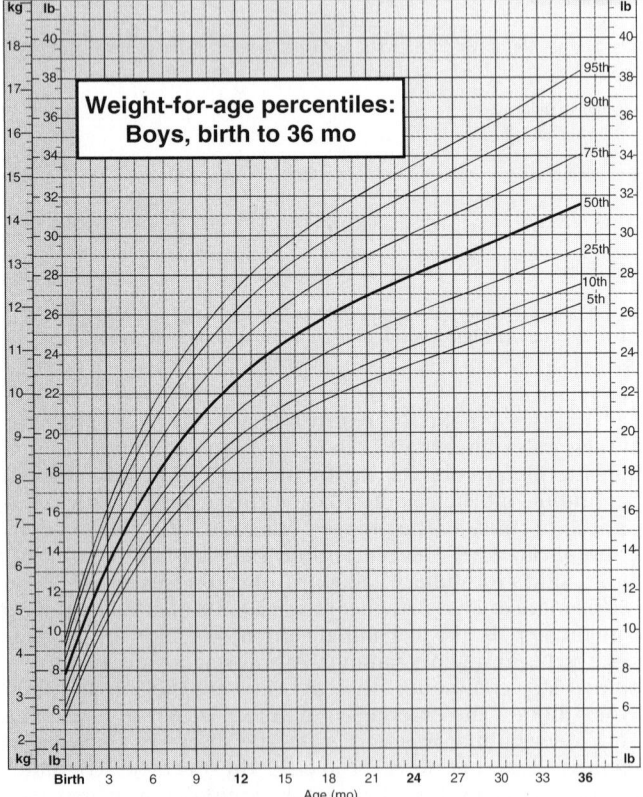

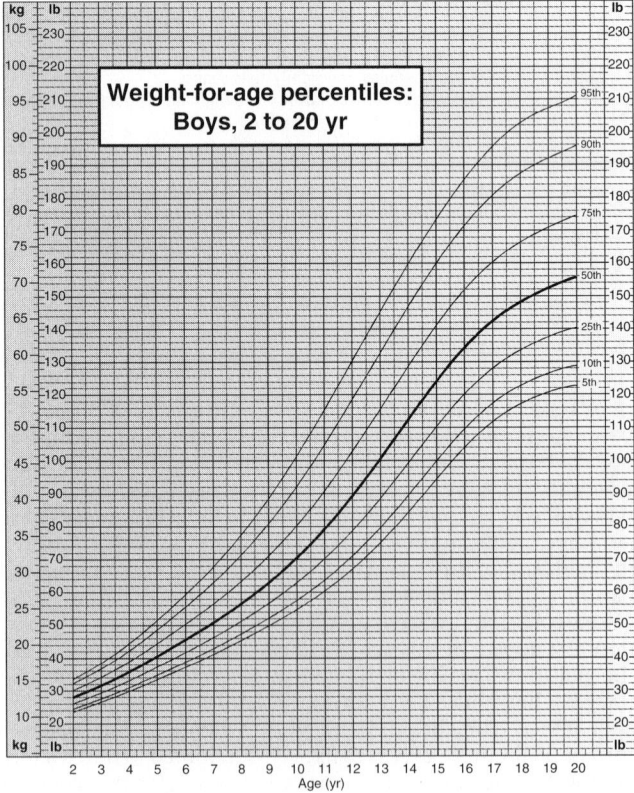

A

FIGURE 11–1. Percentile curves for weight and length/stature by age for boys *(A)* and girls *(B)* birth to 20 yr. (Official 2000 Centers for Disease Control [CDC] growth charts, created by the National Center for Health Statistics [NCHS] [see Chapter 15]. Infant length was measured lying; older children's stature was measured standing. Additional information and technical reports are available at www.cdc.gov/nchs.)

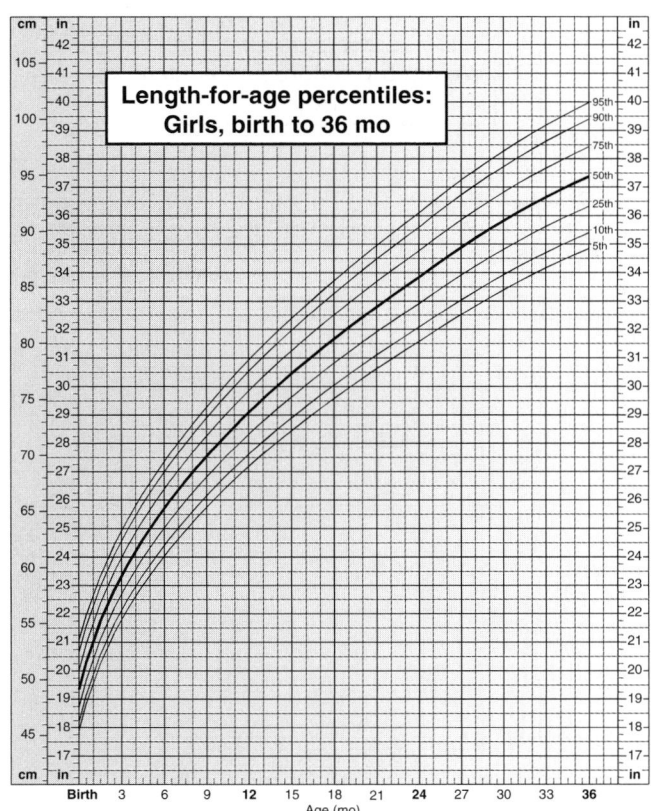

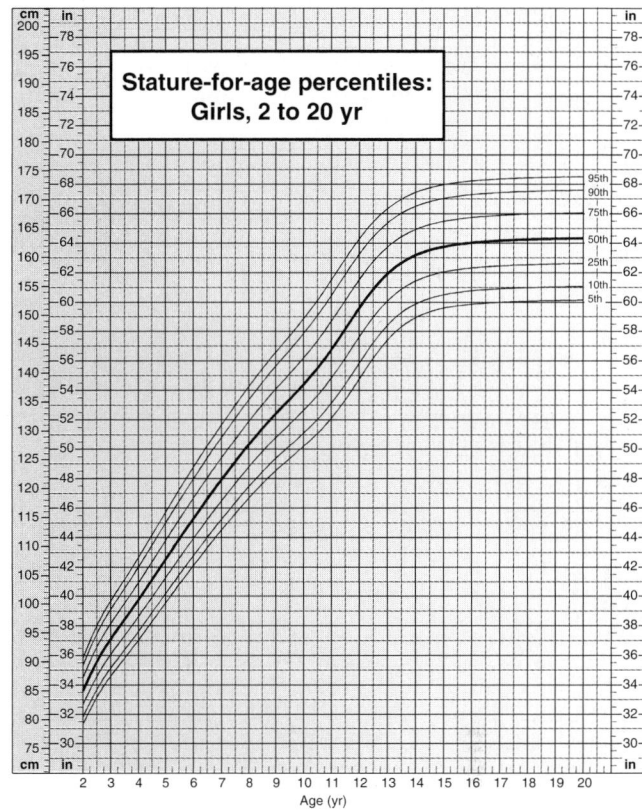

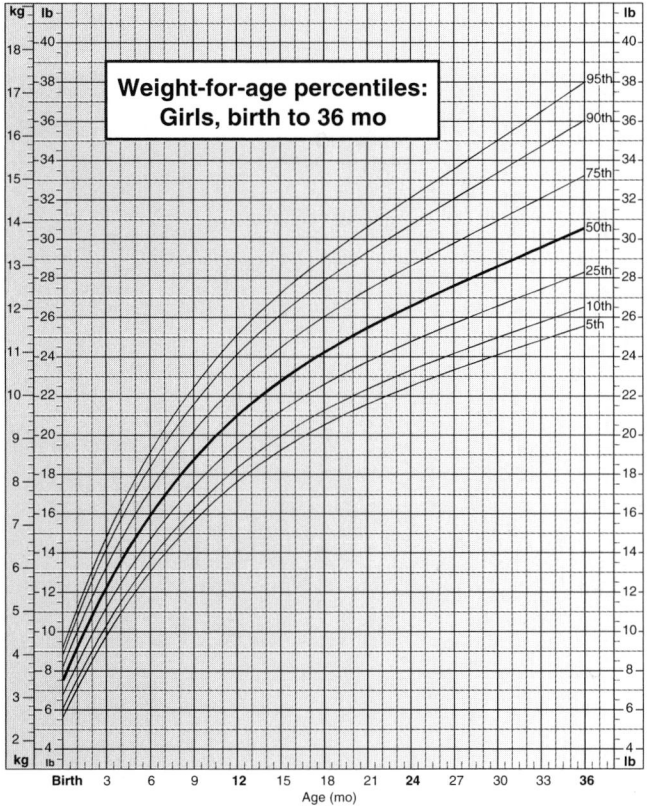

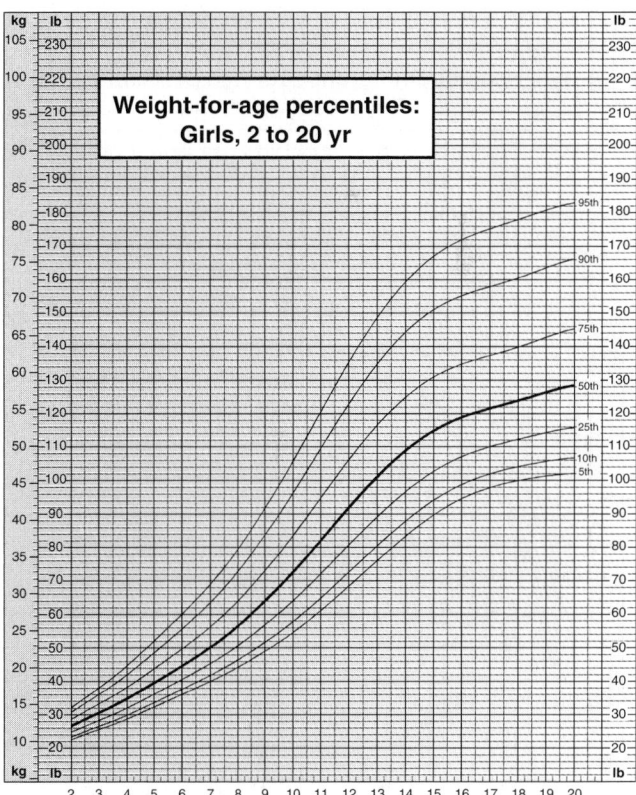

B

FIGURE 11–1. *See legend on opposite page*

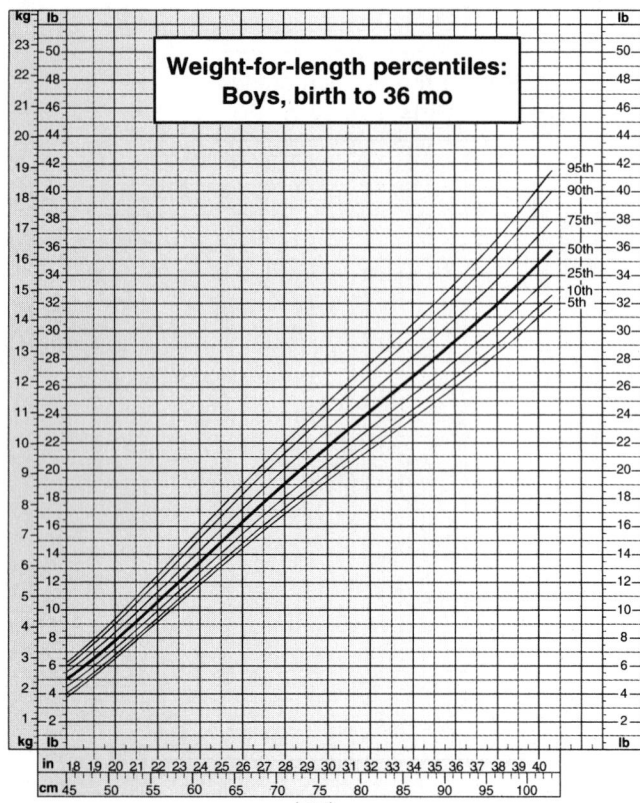

Revised and corrected June 8, 2000.

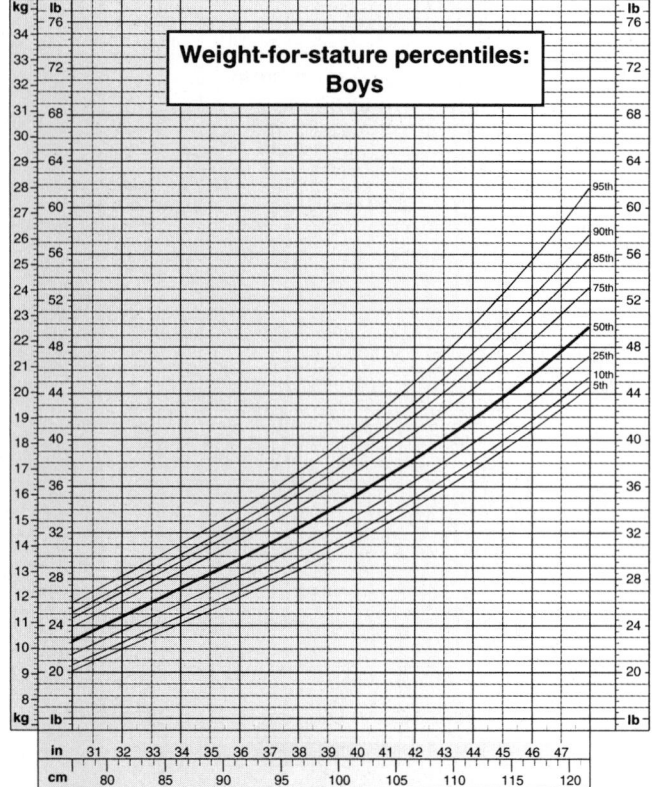

Revised and corrected November 21, 2000.

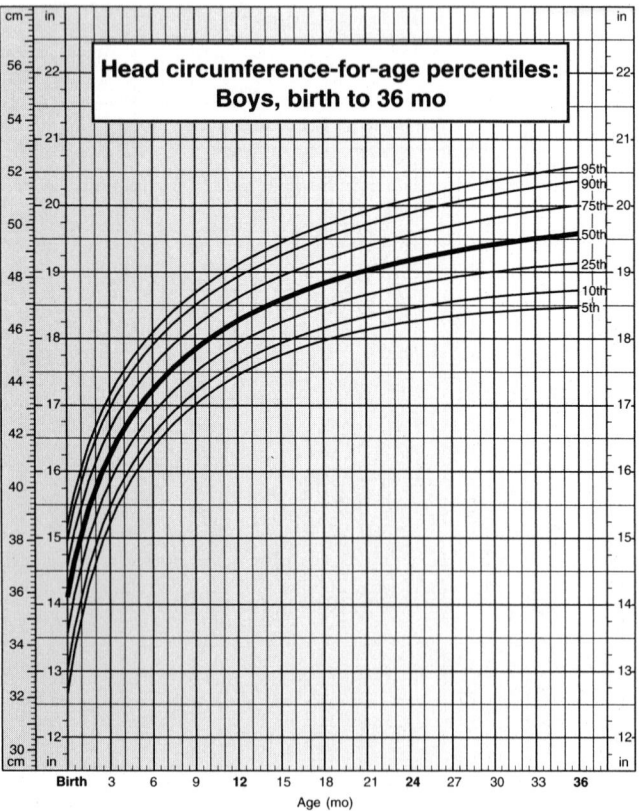

A

FIGURE 11–2. Head circumference and length/stature by weight for boys *(A)* and girls *(B)*.(Official 2000 Centers for Disease Control [CDC] growth charts, created by the National Center for Health Statistics [NCHS] [see Chapter 15]. Additional information and technical reports are available at www.cdc.gov/nchs.)

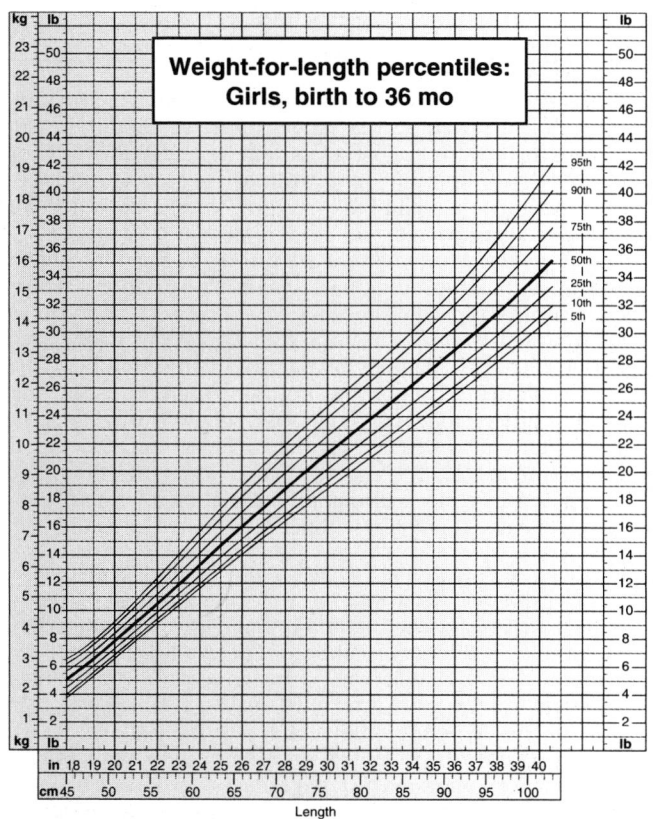

Revised and corrected June 8, 2000.

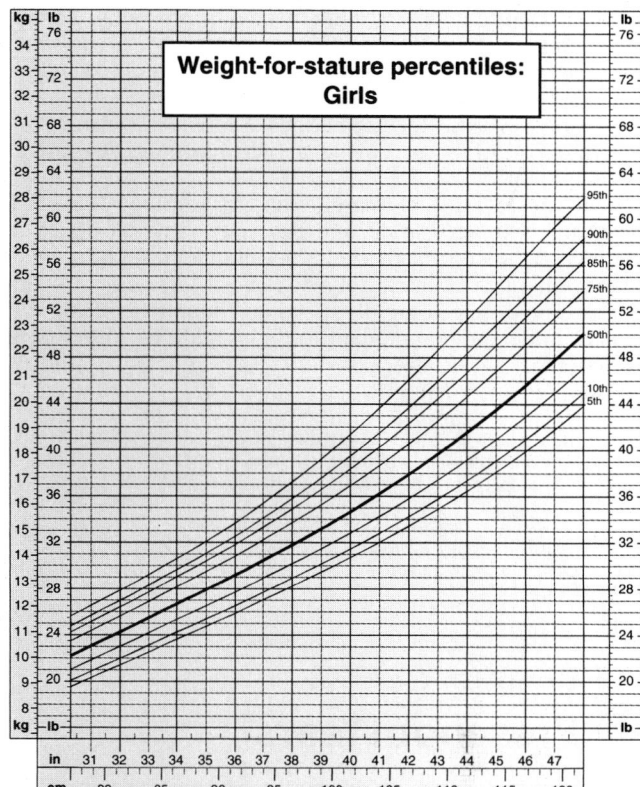

Revised and corrected November 21, 2000.

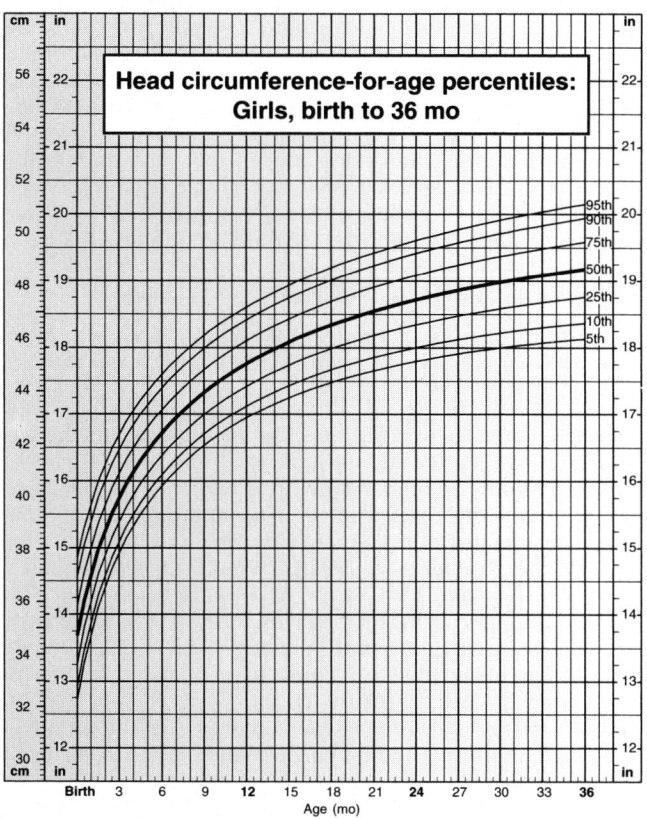

B

FIGURE 11–2. *See legend on opposite page*

acquisition often have greater behavior problems. Language development is facilitated when parents and caregivers use clear, simple sentences, ask questions, and respond to children's incomplete sentences and gestural communication with the appropriate words. Regular periods of looking at picture books together continue to provide an ideal context for language development.

Pediatricians can help parents understand the resurgence of problems with separation and the appearance of a treasured blanket or teddy bear as a developmental phenomenon. Management of difficult behavior and assessment of children with delayed speech are discussed in Chapter 12. Helping parents to understand and adapt to their children's different temperamental styles can constitute an important, and very appreciated, intervention.

Ainsworth MDS, Blehar MC, Waters E, et al: *Patterns of Attachment: A Psychological Study of the Strange Situation.* Hillsdale, NJ, Erlbaum, 1978.

Bates E, Dick F: Language, gesture, and the developing brain. *Dev Psychobiol* 2002;40:293–310.

Fraiberg S: *The Magic Years.* New York, Scribner's, 1959.

Lieberman A: *The Emotional Life of the Toddler.* New York, Free Press, 1993.

Mahler MS, Pine S, Bergman A: *The Psychological Birth of the Infant.* London, Hutchinson, 1975.

Chapter 12
Preschool Years

Between 2 and 5 yr of age, the core issues of attachment and separation are reshaped by the emergence of language and played out in the context of a widening social sphere. As toddlers, children learn to walk away and come back. As preschoolers, they explore emotional separation, alternating between stubborn opposition and cheerful compliance, between bold exploration and clinging dependence. Increasing time spent in classrooms and playgrounds challenges a child's ability to adapt to new rules and relationships. Preschool children know that they can do more than ever before, but they are also very aware of the constraints imposed on them by the adult world, and their own limited abilities.

PHYSICAL DEVELOPMENT (Tables 12–1 and 12–2)

By the end of the 2nd yr, somatic and brain growth slows, with corresponding decreases in nutritional requirements and in appetite (see Table 10–5). Between the ages of 2 and 5 yr, the average child gains approximately 2 kg in weight and 7 cm in height per year. The toddler's prominent abdomen flattens, and the body becomes leaner. Physical energy peaks, and the need for sleep declines to 11–13 hr/24 hr, usually including one nap (see Fig. 10–1). Visual acuity reaches 20/30 by age 3 yr and 20/20 by age 4. All 20 primary teeth have erupted by 3 yr of age (see Table 10–6).

Gross and fine motor milestones are presented in Table 10–4. Most children walk with a mature gait and run steadily before the end of their 3rd yr. Beyond this basic level, there is wide variation in ability as the range of motor activities expands to include throwing, catching, and kicking balls; riding on bicycles; climbing on playground structures; dancing; and other complex pattern behaviors. Stylistic features of gross motor activity, such as tempo, intensity, and cautiousness, also vary significantly because of inborn predilections. Toe walking, if it persists, may be associated with developmental delays, particularly of speech and language.

The effects of such individual differences on cognitive and emotional development depend in part on the demands of the social environment. Energetic, coordinated children may thrive emotionally with parents or teachers who encourage physical activity; lower energy, more cerebral children may thrive with adults who value quiet play.

Handedness is usually established by the 3rd yr. Frustration may result from attempts to change children's hand preference. Variations in fine motor development reflect both individual proclivities and different opportunities for learning. Children who are seldom allowed to use crayons, for example, develop a mature pencil grasp later.

Bowel and bladder control emerge during this period (average age 30 mo, with large individual and cultural variation). Daytime bladder control typically precedes bowel control, and girls precede boys. Bed-wetting is normal up to age 4 yr in girls, 5 yr in boys (see Chapters 20 and 535). Many children master toileting with ease, particularly once they are able to verbalize their bodily needs. For others, toilet training can involve a protracted power struggle. Refusal to defecate in the toilet or potty is relatively common and can lead to constipation and parental frustration. Defusing the issue by a temporary cessation of training (and return to diapers) often allows toilet mastery to proceed.

Implications for Parents and Pediatricians. The normal decrease in appetite at this age often arouses worry about nutrition. For the most part, parents can be reassured that if growth is normal, the child's intake is adequate. Children normally modulate their food intake to match their somatic needs according to feelings of hunger and satiety. Daily intake fluctuates, at times widely, but intake during the period of a week is relatively stable. Parental attempts to control the child's intake interfere with this self-regulatory mechanism as the child must either accede to or rebel against the pressure. The result may be either overeating or undereating.

Motorically precocious, highly active children face increased risks of injury. Parents of such children benefit from early guidance about the need for childproofing the home, constant supervision, and bicycle helmet use (beginning with the tricycle). Parental concerns about possible hyperactivity may reflect inappropriate expectations, heightened fears, or true overactivity. Children who engage in reckless, uncontrollable activity with no apparent regard for personal safety need a safe environment with close supervision. This pattern of indiscriminate activity is sometimes seen among children who have suffered abuse or neglect.

LANGUAGE, COGNITION, AND PLAY

These three domains all involve the symbolic function, a mode of dealing with the world that emerges during the preschool period.

Language. Language development occurs most rapidly between 2 and 5 yr of age. Vocabulary increases from 50–100 words to more than 2,000. Sentence structure advances from telegraphic phrases ("Baby cry") to sentences incorporating all of the major grammatical components. As a rule of thumb, between age 2 and 5 yr, the number of words in a typical sentence equals the child's age (2 by age 2 yr, 3 by age 3 yr, and so on.) By 2½ yr, most children are using possessives ("My ball"), progressives (the "ing" construction, as in "I playing"), questions, and negatives. By 4 yr of age, they can count to 4 and use the past tense; by 5 yr, they can use the future tense.

It is important to distinguish between speech (the production of intelligible sounds) and language, which refers to the underlying mental act. Language includes both expressive and receptive functions. Receptive language (understanding) varies less in its rate of acquisition than does expressive language and therefore has greater prognostic importance. Language assessment is described more fully in Chapters 16 and 29.

Language acquisition depends critically on environmental input. Key determinants include the amount and variety of speech directed toward children and the frequency with which adults ask questions and encourage verbalization. Striking differences in these parameters between upper- and lower-class parents parallel class-related disparities in preschool language development and later school achievement.

Although experience influences the rate of language development, many linguists believe that the basic mechanism for language learning is "hard-wired" in the brain. Children do not simply imitate adult speech. Rather, they abstract the complex rules of grammar from the ambient language, generating implicit hypotheses. Evidence for the existence of such implicit rules comes from analysis of grammatical errors, such as the overgeneralized use of "s" to signify the plural and "ed" to signify the past (e.g., "We seed lots of mouses"). Children have an inborn propensity to create language. For example, deaf orphans raised by nonsigning adults were observed to invent their own sign language, including all of the essential grammar.

Language is a critical barometer of both cognitive and emotional development. Mental retardation may first become apparent with delayed speech at approximately 2 yr. Child abuse and neglect are correlated with delayed language, particularly the ability to convey emotional states. Language plays a critical part in the regulation of behavior through internalized "private speech" in which a child repeats adult prohibitions first audibly and then mentally. Language also allows children to express feelings, such as anger or frustration, without acting them out; consequently, language-delayed children show higher rates of tantrums and other externalizing behaviors.

Preschool language development lays the foundation for later success in school. Approximately 35% of U.S. children may enter school lacking the language skills that are the prerequisites of literacy acquisition. Although children typically learn to read and write in elementary school, critical foundations for literacy are established during the preschool years. Through repeated early exposure to written words, children learn about the uses of writing (telling stories or sending messages) and about its form (left to right, top to bottom). Early errors in writing, like errors in speaking, reveal that literacy acquisition is an active process involving hypothesis generation and revision. One hypothesis is that words that take longer to say ("big words") have more letters in them regardless of what the letters are. At a later stage, letters may be assigned one to a syllable, such as GNYS to spell "genius."

Picture books have a special role not only in familiarizing young children with the printed word but also in the development of verbal language. Reading aloud with a young child is an interactive process in which a parent focuses the child's attention on a particular picture, requests a response (by asking, "What's that?"), and then gives the child feedback ("Right, it's a dog."). This question-feedback routine is repeated many times in the course of reading a book. As a child's sophistication grows, the parent increases the complexity of the task, requesting descriptions ("What color is the dog?") and later projections ("What's that dog going to do?"). The elements of shared attention, active participation, immediate feedback, repetition, and graduated difficulty make such routines ideal for language learning.

The period of rapid language acquisition is also when *developmental dysfluency* and *stuttering* are most likely to emerge. Common difficulties (in about 5% of children) include pauses and repetitions of initial sounds. Stress or excitement exacerbates these difficulties, which generally resolve on their own. About 1% of children continue to have significant stuttering. Indications for referral include whole-word or part-word repetitions, sound prolongations, word blockages, facial tension, avoidance of talking, and persistence of stuttering for longer than 6 mo. Treatment involves guidance to parents to reduce pressures associated with speaking. Specific therapeutic approaches, e.g., use of metronomes, single-syllable speaking, and electronic devices that modify auditory feedback to the child, are controversial.

Cognition. The preschool period corresponds to Piaget's preoperational (prelogical) stage, characterized by magical thinking, egocentrism, and thinking that is dominated by perception (see Table 7–2). Magical thinking includes a confusion of coincidence for causality, animism (attributing motivations to inanimate objects and events), and unrealistic beliefs about the power of wishes. A child might believe that people cause it to rain by carrying umbrellas, that the sun goes down because it is tired, or that feeling resentment toward a sibling can actually make that sibling sick. Egocentrism refers to a child's inability to take another's point of view and does not connote selfishness. For example, a child might try to comfort an upset adult by bringing a favorite stuffed animal.

Piaget demonstrated the dominance of perception over logic by a famous series of so-called conservation experiments. In one, water is poured back and forth from a tall, thin vase to a low, wide dish and children are asked which container has more water. Invariably, they choose the one that looks larger (usually the tall vase), even when the examiner points out that no water has been added or taken away. Such misunderstandings reflect young children's developing hypotheses about the nature of the world as well as their difficulty in attending simultaneously to multiple aspects of a situation.

Play. During the preschool period, play is marked by increasing complexity and imagination, from simple scripts replicating common experiences such as shopping and putting baby to bed (2 or 3 yr of age) to more extended scenarios involving singular events such as going to the zoo or going on a trip (3 or 4 yr of age) to the creation of scenarios that have only been imagined, such as flying to the moon (4 or 5 yr of age). A similar progression in socialization moves from minimal social interaction with peers during play (solo or parallel play, 1 or 2 yr of age) to cooperative play such as building a tower of blocks together (3 or 4 yr of age) to organized group play with distinct role assignments, as in playing house. Play also becomes increasingly rule governed, from early rules about asking (rather than taking) and sharing (2 or 3 yr of age) to rules that change from moment to moment according to the desires of the players (4 and 5 yr of age) to the beginning of the recognition of rules as relatively immutable (5 yr of age and beyond).

Play allows children to experience mastery by solving puzzles, practicing adult roles, assuming the aggressor role rather than the victim (spanking a doll), taking on superpowers (dinosaur and superhero play), and obtaining things that are denied in real life (a make-believe friend or stuffed pet). Creativity, inherent in all play, is particularly apparent in drawing, painting, and other artistic activities. The 4 yr old who chooses to let a big circle with sticks represent a body and limbs knows that real bodies do not actually look like that. The simplicity of the drawing is, at least in part, a matter of choice. Themes and emotions that emerge in a child's drawings often reflect the emotional issues of greatest importance for the child.

Moral thinking mirrors and is constrained by a child's cognitive level. Empathic responses to others' distress arise during the 2nd yr of life, but the ability to cognitively consider another child's point of view remains limited throughout the preschool period. In keeping with a child's inability to focus on more than one aspect of a situation at a time, fairness is taken to mean equal treatment regardless of circumstantial differences. Rules tend to be absolute, with guilt assigned for bad outcomes regardless of intentions.

Implications for Parents and Pediatricians. The significance of language as a target for assessment and intervention cannot be overestimated because of its central role as an indicator of cognitive and emotional development and as a key factor in behavioral regulation and later school success. Detection and assessment of language delays, a critical part of preventive care, is discussed in Chapters 16 and 29. Parents can support emotional development

TABLE 12–1. Percentiles of Stature by Weight and Age, Boys and Girls, 2–20 Yr

	Percentiles													
Age	5th		10th		25th		50th		75th		90th		95th	

Boys: 2–20 Yr

Age	5th		10th		25th		50th		75th		90th		95th	
2.0	81.1	(31.9)	82.4	(32.4)	84.5	(33.3)	86.9	(34.2)	89.2	(35.1)	91.4	(36.0)	92.6	(36.5)
	10.70	(23.5)	11.11	(24.5)	11.85	(26.1)	12.74	(28.0)	13.71	(30.2)	14.67	(32.3)	15.28	(33.6)
2.5	85.3	(33.6)	86.6	(34.1)	88.8	(35.0)	91.3	(36.0)	93.9	(37.0)	96.2	(37.9)	97.7	(38.4)
	11.40	(25.1)	11.83	(26.0)	12.61	(27.7)	13.56	(29.8)	14.62	(32.2)	15.66	(34.5)	16.34	(36.0)
3.0	89.2	(35.1)	90.5	(35.6)	92.7	(36.5)	95.3	(37.5)	97.9	(38.6)	100.4	(39.5)	101.9	(40.1)
	12.10	(26.6)	12.55	(27.6)	13.38	(29.4)	14.40	(31.7)	15.56	(34.2)	16.74	(36.8)	17.51	(38.5)
3.5	92.5	(36.4)	93.9	(37.0)	96.3	(37.9)	99.0	(39.0)	101.8	(40.1)	104.3	(41.1)	105.8	(41.7)
	12.84	(28.2)	13.32	(29.3)	14.20	(31.3)	15.32	(33.7)	16.60	(36.5)	17.93	(39.5)	18.83	(41.4)
4.0	95.6	(37.6)	97.1	(38.2)	99.7	(39.2)	102.5	(40.4)	105.4	(41.5)	108.0	(42.5)	109.5	(43.1)
	13.61	(29.9)	14.13	(31.1)	15.09	(33.2)	16.32	(35.9)	17.75	(39.0)	19.26	(42.4)	20.28	(44.6)
4.5	98.5	(38.8)	100.2	(39.4)	102.9	(40.5)	105.9	(41.7)	108.9	(42.9)	111.6	(43.9)	113.2	(44.5)
	14.41	(31.7)	14.98	(32.9)	16.03	(35.3)	17.38	(38.2)	18.98	(41.7)	20.68	(45.5)	21.85	(48.1)
5.0	101.5	(39.9)	103.2	(40.6)	106.0	(41.7)	109.2	(43.0)	112.3	(44.2)	115.1	(45.3)	116.8	(46.0)
	15.23	(33.5)	15.85	(34.9)	17.00	(37.4)	18.49	(40.7)	20.26	(44.6)	22.18	(48.8)	23.51	(51.7)
5.5	104.4	(41.1)	106.2	(41.8)	109.1	(43.0)	112.4	(44.3)	115.7	(45.5)	118.6	(46.7)	120.3	(47.4)
	16.07	(35.4)	16.74	(36.8)	17.99	(39.6)	19.62	(43.2)	21.59	(47.5)	23.73	(52.2)	25.24	(55.5)
6.0	107.3	(42.2)	109.2	(43.0)	112.2	(44.2)	115.7	(45.5)	119.1	(46.9)	122.1	(48.1)	123.9	(48.8)
	16.94	(37.3)	17.65	(38.8)	19.00	(41.8)	20.78	(45.7)	22.94	(50.5)	25.33	(55.7)	27.03	(59.5)
6.5	110.3	(43.4)	112.2	(44.2)	115.3	(45.4)	118.9	(46.8)	122.4	(48.2)	125.6	(49.4)	127.5	(50.2)
	17.83	(39.2)	18.59	(40.9)	20.03	(44.1)	21.96	(48.3)	24.33	(53.5)	26.99	(59.4)	28.91	(63.6)
7.0	113.2	(44.6)	115.1	(45.3)	118.4	(46.6)	122.0	(48.0)	125.7	(49.5)	129.0	(50.8)	131.0	(51.6)
	18.74	(41.2)	19.55	(43.0)	21.09	(46.4)	23.17	(51.0)	25.76	(56.7)	28.73	(63.2)	30.90	(68.0)
7.5	116.1	(45.7)	118.0	(46.5)	121.4	(47.8)	125.1	(49.3)	128.9	(50.8)	132.4	(52.1)	134.5	(52.9)
	19.69	(43.3)	20.55	(45.2)	22.19	(48.8)	24.43	(53.7)	27.26	(60.0)	30.56	(67.2)	33.02	(72.6)
8.0	118.8	(46.8)	120.8	(47.6)	124.3	(48.9)	128.1	(50.4)	132.1	(52.0)	135.7	(53.4)	137.8	(54.3)
	20.66	(45.5)	21.58	(47.5)	23.34	(51.3)	25.75	(56.7)	28.85	(63.5)	32.51	(71.5)	35.29	(77.6)
8.5	121.4	(47.8)	123.5	(48.6)	127.0	(50.0)	131.0	(51.6)	135.1	(53.2)	138.8	(54.6)	141.0	(55.5)
	21.67	(47.7)	22.65	(49.8)	24.55	(54.0)	27.16	(59.8)	30.55	(67.2)	34.61	(76.2)	37.73	(83.0)
9.0	123.8	(48.7)	126.0	(49.6)	129.6	(51.0)	133.7	(52.7)	137.9	(54.3)	141.8	(55.8)	144.1	(56.7)
	22.71	(50.0)	23.77	(52.3)	25.83	(56.8)	28.68	(63.1)	32.40	(71.3)	36.89	(81.1)	40.36	(88.8)
9.5	126.0	(49.6)	128.3	(50.5)	132.1	(52.0)	136.3	(53.7)	140.7	(55.4)	144.7	(57.0)	147.1	(57.9)
	23.80	(52.4)	24.95	(54.9)	27.20	(59.8)	30.32	(66.7)	34.40	(75.7)	39.34	(86.5)	43.17	(95.0)
10.0	128.2	(50.5)	130.5	(51.4)	134.4	(52.9)	138.8	(54.7)	143.3	(56.4)	147.4	(58.0)	149.9	(59.0)
	24.94	(54.9)	26.21	(57.7)	28.67	(63.1)	32.09	(70.6)	36.56	(80.4)	41.97	(92.3)	46.16	(101.5)
10.5	130.2	(51.3)	132.6	(52.2)	136.7	(53.8)	141.3	(55.6)	145.9	(57.4)	150.1	(59.1)	152.7	(60.1)
	26.17	(57.6)	27.56	(60.6)	30.26	(66.6)	34.00	(74.8)	38.89	(85.6)	44.77	(98.5)	49.30	(108.4)
11.0	132.4	(52.1)	134.9	(53.1)	139.0	(54.7)	143.7	(56.6)	148.5	(58.5)	152.9	(60.2)	155.5	(61.2)
	27.50	(60.5)	29.02	(63.8)	31.98	(70.4)	36.07	(79.4)	41.38	(91.0)	47.73	(105.0)	52.56	(115.6)
11.5	134.7	(53.0)	137.2	(54.0)	141.5	(55.7)	146.4	(57.6)	151.3	(59.6)	155.8	(61.3)	158.6	(62.4)
	28.95	(63.7)	30.62	(67.4)	33.85	(74.5)	38.30	(84.3)	44.03	(96.9)	50.80	(111.8)	55.90	(123.0)
12.0	137.3	(54.1)	139.9	(55.1)	144.3	(56.8)	149.3	(58.8)	154.4	(60.8)	159.0	(62.6)	161.9	(63.7)
	30.55	(67.2)	32.36	(71.2)	35.87	(78.9)	40.67	(89.5)	46.81	(103.0)	53.98	(118.7)	59.30	(130.5)
12.5	140.3	(55.2)	143.0	(56.3)	147.5	(58.1)	152.7	(60.1)	157.9	(62.2)	162.6	(64.0)	165.5	(65.2)
	32.31	(71.1)	34.26	(75.4)	38.04	(83.7)	43.19	(95.0)	49.70	(109.3)	57.20	(125.8)	62.72	(138.0)
13.0	143.6	(56.5)	146.4	(57.6)	151.1	(59.5)	156.4	(61.6)	161.7	(63.7)	166.6	(65.6)	169.5	(66.7)
	34.22	(75.3)	36.32	(79.9)	40.36	(88.8)	45.81	(100.8)	52.66	(115.8)	60.45	(133.0)	66.10	(145.4)
13.5	147.0	(57.9)	150.0	(59.1)	154.9	(61.0)	160.3	(63.1)	165.7	(65.2)	170.5	(67.1)	173.4	(68.3)
	36.29	(79.8)	38.52	(84.7)	42.78	(94.1)	48.51	(106.7)	55.64	(122.4)	63.67	(140.1)	69.44	(152.8)
14.0	150.5	(59.3)	153.6	(60.5)	158.7	(62.5)	164.1	(64.6)	169.5	(66.7)	174.2	(68.6)	177.0	(69.7)
	38.48	(84.6)	40.81	(89.8)	45.27	(99.6)	51.23	(112.7)	58.59	(128.9)	66.82	(147.0)	72.69	(159.9)
14.5	153.8	(60.6)	156.9	(61.8)	162.0	(63.8)	167.5	(65.9)	172.7	(68.0)	177.4	(69.8)	180.1	(70.9)
	40.74	(89.6)	43.16	(95.0)	47.77	(105.1)	53.91	(118.6)	61.46	(135.2)	69.86	(153.7)	75.83	(166.8)
15.0	156.7	(61.7)	159.8	(62.9)	164.8	(64.9)	170.1	(67.0)	175.3	(69.0)	179.8	(70.8)	182.4	(71.8)
	43.02	(94.6)	45.50	(100.1)	50.21	(110.5)	56.49	(124.3)	64.19	(141.2)	72.75	(160.1)	78.83	(173.4)

TABLE 12–1. Percentiles of Stature by Weight and Age, Boys and Girls, 2–20 Yr *Continued*

	Percentiles													
Age	5th		10th		25th		50th		75th		90th		95th	
15.5	159.0	(62.6)	162.0	(63.8)	166.9	(65.7)	172.2	(67.8)	177.2	(69.8)	181.6	(71.5)	184.2	(72.5)
	45.23	(99.5)	47.75	(105.0)	52.53	(115.6)	58.90	(129.6)	66.73	(146.8)	75.45	(166.0)	81.66	(179.7)
16.0	160.8	(63.3)	163.7	(64.5)	168.5	(66.3)	173.6	(68.4)	178.6	(70.3)	182.9	(72.0)	185.5	(73.0)
	47.32	(104.1)	49.85	(109.7)	54.67	(120.3)	61.10	(134.4)	69.03	(151.9)	77.92	(171.4)	84.29	(185.4)
16.5	162.1	(63.8)	165.0	(64.9)	169.6	(66.8)	174.6	(68.8)	179.5	(70.7)	183.8	(72.4)	186.4	(73.4)
	49.19	(108.2)	51.73	(113.8)	56.56	(124.4)	63.03	(138.7)	71.06	(156.3)	80.13	(176.3)	86.68	(190.7)
17.0	163.1	(64.2)	165.8	(65.3)	170.4	(67.1)	175.3	(69.0)	180.2	(70.9)	184.5	(72.6)	187.0	(73.6)
	50.81	(111.8)	53.35	(117.4)	58.19	(128.0)	64.70	(142.3)	72.82	(160.2)	82.07	(180.5)	88.80	(195.3)
17.5	163.8	(64.5)	166.5	(65.5)	170.9	(67.3)	175.8	(69.2)	180.7	(71.1)	184.9	(72.8)	187.5	(73.8)
	52.15	(114.7)	54.69	(120.3)	59.55	(131.0)	66.11	(145.4)	74.32	(163.5)	83.71	(184.2)	90.59	(199.3)
18.0	164.2	(64.7)	166.9	(65.7)	171.3	(67.5)	176.2	(69.4)	181.0	(71.3)	185.3	(72.9)	187.8	(73.9)
	53.23	(117.1)	55.79	(122.7)	60.69	(133.5)	67.29	(148.0)	75.58	(166.3)	85.08	(187.2)	92.05	(202.5)
18.5	164.6	(64.8)	167.2	(65.8)	171.6	(67.6)	176.4	(69.5)	181.2	(71.4)	185.5	(73.0)	188.1	(74.0)
	54.09	(119.0)	56.68	(124.7)	61.63	(135.6)	68.30	(150.3)	76.65	(168.6)	86.19	(189.6)	93.18	(205.0)
19.0	164.8	(64.9)	167.4	(65.9)	171.8	(67.6)	176.6	(69.5)	181.4	(71.4)	185.7	(73.1)	188.3	(74.1)
	54.80	(120.6)	57.43	(126.4)	62.46	(137.4)	69.19	(152.2)	77.59	(170.7)	87.12	(191.7)	94.05	(206.9)
19.5	164.9	(64.9)	167.6	(66.0)	171.9	(67.7)	176.8	(69.6)	181.6	(71.5)	185.9	(73.2)	188.4	(74.2)
	55.36	(121.8)	58.05	(127.7)	63.17	(139.0)	70.00	(154.0)	78.45	(172.6)	87.97	(193.5)	94.83	(208.6)
20.0	165.0	(65.0)	167.7	(66.0)	172.0	(67.7)	176.8	(69.6)	181.7	(71.5)	186.0	(73.2)	188.5	(74.2)
	55.66	(122.5)	58.41	(128.5)	63.64	(140.0)	70.60	(155.3)	79.18	(174.2)	88.81	(195.4)	95.71	(210.6)

Girls: 2–20 Yr

Age	5th		10th		25th		50th		75th		90th		95th	
2.0	79.6	(31.4)	80.9	(31.9)	83.0	(32.7)	85.4	(33.6)	87.7	(34.5)	89.9	(35.4)	91.1	(35.9)
	10.27	(22.6)	10.64	(23.4)	11.31	(24.9)	12.13	(26.7)	13.08	(28.8)	14.04	(30.9)	14.68	(32.3)
2.5	84.2	(33.1)	85.5	(33.7)	87.8	(34.6)	90.3	(35.6)	92.9	(36.6)	95.2	(37.5)	96.6	(38.0)
	10.99	(24.2)	11.38	(25.0)	12.12	(26.7)	13.04	(28.7)	14.12	(31.1)	15.24	(33.5)	15.99	(35.2)
3.0	87.8	(34.6)	89.2	(35.1)	91.6	(36.0)	94.2	(37.1)	96.9	(38.1)	99.3	(39.1)	100.8	(39.7)
	11.66	(25.6)	12.09	(26.6)	12.90	(28.4)	13.94	(30.7)	15.16	(33.4)	16.47	(36.2)	17.36	(38.2)
3.5	91.0	(35.8)	92.4	(36.4)	94.9	(37.3)	97.6	(38.4)	100.5	(39.6)	103.1	(40.6)	104.6	(41.2)
	12.35	(27.2)	12.83	(28.2)	13.72	(30.2)	14.88	(32.7)	16.27	(35.8)	17.78	(39.1)	18.83	(41.4)
4.0	94.0	(37.0)	95.6	(37.6)	98.1	(38.6)	101.0	(39.8)	104.0	(41.0)	106.8	(42.0)	108.4	(42.7)
	13.09	(28.8)	13.61	(29.9)	14.59	(32.1)	15.88	(34.9)	17.44	(38.4)	19.17	(42.2)	20.39	(44.9)
4.5	97.2	(38.3)	98.7	(38.9)	101.4	(39.9)	104.5	(41.1)	107.6	(42.4)	110.5	(43.5)	112.2	(44.2)
	13.88	(30.5)	14.44	(31.8)	15.51	(34.1)	16.93	(37.2)	18.67	(41.1)	20.63	(45.4)	22.04	(48.5)
5.0	100.4	(39.5)	102.0	(40.2)	104.8	(41.3)	108.0	(42.5)	111.2	(43.8)	114.3	(45.0)	116.1	(45.7)
	14.71	(32.4)	15.32	(33.7)	16.47	(36.2)	18.02	(39.7)	19.95	(43.9)	22.15	(48.7)	23.75	(52.3)
5.5	103.6	(40.8)	105.3	(41.5)	108.2	(42.6)	111.5	(43.9)	114.9	(45.2)	118.1	(46.5)	120.0	(47.3)
	15.56	(34.2)	16.22	(35.7)	17.47	(38.4)	19.16	(42.1)	21.28	(46.8)	23.72	(52.2)	25.53	(56.2)
6.0	106.9	(42.1)	108.6	(42.8)	111.6	(43.9)	115.0	(45.3)	118.6	(46.7)	121.9	(48.0)	123.9	(48.8)
	16.44	(36.2)	17.14	(37.7)	18.50	(40.7)	20.34	(44.7)	22.66	(49.9)	25.37	(55.8)	27.39	(60.3)
6.5	110.0	(43.3)	111.8	(44.0)	114.9	(45.2)	118.4	(46.6)	122.1	(48.1)	125.6	(49.4)	127.7	(50.3)
	17.32	(38.1)	18.09	(39.8)	19.56	(43.0)	21.57	(47.4)	24.12	(53.1)	27.11	(59.7)	29.36	(64.6)
7.0	113.1	(44.5)	114.9	(45.2)	118.1	(46.5)	121.8	(47.9)	125.6	(49.4)	129.1	(50.8)	131.3	(51.7)
	18.23	(40.1)	19.06	(41.9)	20.67	(45.5)	22.87	(50.3)	25.68	(56.5)	28.98	(63.8)	31.47	(69.2)
7.5	115.9	(45.6)	117.8	(46.4)	121.1	(47.7)	124.9	(49.2)	128.8	(50.7)	132.5	(52.2)	134.7	(53.0)
	19.16	(42.2)	20.08	(44.2)	21.84	(48.1)	24.26	(53.4)	27.35	(60.2)	31.00	(68.2)	33.75	(74.3)
8.0	118.5	(46.7)	120.5	(47.5)	123.9	(48.8)	127.8	(50.3)	131.9	(51.9)	135.6	(53.4)	137.9	(54.3)
	20.15	(44.3)	21.15	(46.5)	23.09	(50.8)	25.76	(56.7)	29.17	(64.2)	33.19	(73.0)	36.23	(79.7)
8.5	121.0	(47.6)	123.0	(48.4)	126.5	(49.8)	130.6	(51.4)	134.7	(53.0)	138.5	(54.5)	140.9	(55.5)
	21.19	(46.6)	22.30	(49.1)	24.44	(53.8)	27.38	(60.2)	31.15	(68.5)	35.58	(78.3)	38.92	(85.6)
9.0	123.2	(48.5)	125.3	(49.3)	129.0	(50.8)	133.1	(52.4)	137.4	(54.1)	141.4	(55.7)	143.8	(56.6)
	22.32	(49.1)	23.54	(51.8)	25.90	(57.0)	29.14	(64.1)	33.29	(73.2)	38.17	(84.0)	41.82	(92.0)
9.5	125.3	(49.3)	127.6	(50.2)	131.3	(51.7)	135.6	(53.4)	140.1	(55.1)	144.1	(56.7)	146.6	(57.7)
	23.54	(51.8)	24.88	(54.7)	27.48	(60.5)	31.04	(68.3)	35.60	(78.3)	40.93	(90.1)	44.92	(98.8)
10.0	127.5	(50.2)	129.8	(51.1)	133.7	(52.6)	138.2	(54.4)	142.8	(56.2)	147.0	(57.9)	149.6	(58.9)
	24.87	(54.7)	26.33	(57.9)	29.17	(64.2)	33.06	(72.7)	38.04	(83.7)	43.85	(96.5)	48.18	(106.0)

TABLE 12–1. Percentiles of Stature by Weight and Age, Boys and Girls, 2–20 Yr *Continued*

Percentiles

Age	5th		10th		25th		50th		75th		90th		95th	
10.5	129.7	(51.1)	132.2	(52.0)	136.3	(53.7)	141.0	(55.5)	145.8	(57.4)	150.2	(59.1)	152.8	(60.2)
	26.30	(57.9)	27.89	(61.4)	30.97	(68.1)	35.19	(77.4)	40.58	(89.3)	46.87	(103.1)	51.54	(113.4)
11.0	132.4	(52.1)	135.0	(53.1)	139.4	(54.9)	144.3	(56.8)	149.2	(58.7)	153.7	(60.5)	156.4	(61.6)
	27.84	(61.2)	29.54	(65.0)	32.85	(72.3)	37.39	(82.3)	43.19	(95.0)	49.94	(109.9)	54.96	(120.9)
11.5	135.6	(53.4)	138.3	(54.5)	142.8	(56.2)	147.8	(58.2)	152.8	(60.2)	157.3	(61.9)	160.0	(63.0)
	29.46	(64.8)	31.27	(68.8)	34.79	(76.5)	39.62	(87.2)	45.79	(100.7)	52.99	(116.6)	58.34	(128.4)
12.0	139.2	(54.8)	142.0	(55.9)	146.5	(57.7)	151.5	(59.6)	156.4	(61.6)	160.8	(63.3)	163.5	(64.4)
	31.15	(68.5)	33.05	(72.7)	36.75	(80.8)	41.83	(92.0)	48.33	(106.3)	55.95	(123.1)	61.63	(135.6)
12.5	142.8	(56.2)	145.5	(57.3)	149.9	(59.0)	154.8	(60.9)	159.6	(62.8)	163.8	(64.5)	166.4	(65.5)
	32.88	(72.3)	34.85	(76.7)	38.69	(85.1)	43.97	(96.7)	50.76	(111.7)	58.75	(129.2)	64.73	(142.4)
13.0	145.9	(57.4)	148.4	(58.4)	152.7	(60.1)	157.3	(61.9)	162.0	(63.8)	166.1	(65.4)	168.6	(66.4)
	34.61	(76.1)	36.63	(80.6)	40.56	(89.2)	45.98	(101.2)	53.00	(116.6)	61.31	(134.9)	67.59	(148.7)
13.5	148.1	(58.3)	150.6	(59.3)	154.7	(60.9)	159.2	(62.7)	163.7	(64.5)	167.8	(66.1)	170.2	(67.0)
	36.30	(79.9)	38.34	(84.3)	42.32	(93.1)	47.84	(105.2)	55.01	(121.0)	63.60	(139.9)	70.16	(154.4)
14.0	149.7	(58.9)	152.1	(59.9)	156.0	(61.4)	160.5	(63.2)	164.9	(64.9)	168.9	(66.5)	171.3	(67.4)
	37.91	(83.4)	39.95	(87.9)	43.94	(96.7)	49.49	(108.9)	56.76	(124.9)	65.58	(144.3)	72.39	(159.3)
14.5	150.6	(59.3)	153.0	(60.2)	156.9	(61.8)	161.3	(63.5)	165.7	(65.2)	169.7	(66.8)	172.1	(67.7)
	39.41	(86.7)	41.44	(91.2)	45.39	(99.9)	50.93	(112.0)	58.24	(128.1)	67.22	(147.9)	74.28	(163.4)
15.0	151.3	(59.6)	153.6	(60.5)	157.5	(62.0)	161.9	(63.7)	166.3	(65.5)	170.2	(67.0)	172.6	(68.0)
	40.77	(89.7)	42.76	(94.1)	46.65	(102.6)	52.14	(114.7)	59.44	(130.8)	68.55	(150.8)	75.83	(166.8)
15.5	151.7	(59.7)	154.0	(60.6)	157.9	(62.2)	162.3	(63.9)	166.7	(65.6)	170.6	(67.2)	173.0	(68.1)
	41.95	(92.3)	43.90	(96.6)	47.73	(105.0)	53.13	(116.9)	60.40	(132.9)	69.59	(153.1)	77.07	(169.6)
16.0	151.9	(59.8)	154.3	(60.7)	158.2	(62.3)	162.6	(64.0)	166.9	(65.7)	170.9	(67.3)	173.2	(68.2)
	42.96	(94.5)	44.86	(98.7)	48.62	(107.0)	53.95	(118.7)	61.16	(134.6)	70.40	(154.9)	78.05	(171.7)
16.5	152.1	(59.9)	154.5	(60.8)	158.4	(62.4)	162.8	(64.1)	167.1	(65.8)	171.1	(67.4)	173.4	(68.3)
	43.78	(96.3)	45.66	(100.4)	49.35	(108.6)	54.61	(120.1)	61.78	(135.9)	71.06	(156.3)	78.84	(173.5)
17.0	152.3	(60.0)	154.6	(60.9)	158.6	(62.4)	162.9	(64.1)	167.3	(65.9)	171.2	(67.4)	173.6	(68.3)
	44.44	(97.8)	46.29	(101.8)	49.96	(109.9)	55.18	(121.4)	62.33	(137.1)	71.64	(157.6)	79.52	(174.9)
17.5	152.4	(60.0)	154.7	(60.9)	158.7	(62.5)	163.0	(64.2)	167.4	(65.9)	171.3	(67.5)	173.7	(68.4)
	44.95	(98.9)	46.81	(103.0)	50.48	(111.1)	55.71	(122.6)	62.86	(138.3)	72.21	(158.9)	80.13	(176.3)
18.0	152.5	(60.0)	154.8	(61.0)	158.8	(62.5)	163.1	(64.2)	167.5	(65.9)	171.4	(67.5)	173.8	(68.4)
	45.36	(99.8)	47.24	(103.9)	50.95	(112.1)	56.23	(123.7)	63.44	(139.6)	72.83	(160.2)	80.75	(177.7)
18.5	152.5	(60.1)	154.9	(61.0)	158.8	(62.5)	163.2	(64.3)	167.6	(66.0)	171.5	(67.5)	173.8	(68.4)
	45.69	(100.5)	47.62	(104.8)	51.40	(113.1)	56.78	(124.9)	64.09	(141.0)	73.51	(161.7)	81.39	(179.1)
19.0	152.6	(60.1)	154.9	(61.0)	158.9	(62.6)	163.3	(64.3)	167.6	(66.0)	171.5	(67.5)	173.9	(68.5)
	45.97	(101.1)	47.95	(105.5)	51.85	(114.1)	57.35	(126.2)	64.78	(142.5)	74.24	(163.3)	82.02	(180.4)
19.5	152.6	(60.1)	155.0	(61.0)	158.9	(62.6)	163.3	(64.3)	167.7	(66.0)	171.6	(67.6)	173.9	(68.5)
	46.19	(101.6)	48.23	(106.1)	52.24	(114.9)	57.88	(127.3)	65.43	(143.9)	74.91	(164.8)	82.59	(181.7)
20.0	152.7	(60.1)	155.0	(61.0)	159.0	(62.6)	163.3	(64.3)	167.7	(66.0)	171.6	(67.6)	174.0	(68.5)
	46.29	(101.8)	48.38	(106.4)	52.48	(115.5)	58.22	(128.1)	65.85	(144.9)	75.35	(165.8)	82.95	(182.5)

Data used in creating the 2000 Centers for Disease Control (CDC) growth charts, as described in Chapter 15. For each age, stature appears above weight. English units appear in parentheses, to the right of the corresponding metric units. Data for additional age points and 3rd and 97th percentiles are available at www.edc.gov/nchs, along with technical reports.

by using words that describe the child's feeling states ("You sound angry right now") and by urging the child to use words to express feelings rather than acting out the feelings.

Parents should have a regular time each day for reading or looking at books with their children. Programs in which pediatricians give out picture books along with appropriate guidance during primary care visits have been effective in increasing reading aloud and thereby promoting language development, particularly in lower income families.

Preoperational thinking constrains how children understand experiences of illness and treatment. Many children perceive needles as huge objects that threaten to puncture them like a balloon. Verbal explanation is often not as reassuring as giving the child an opportunity to administer make-believe shots to a doll and see, repeatedly, that nothing horrible happens. Explanations that involve several contradictory aspects ("This will hurt a little, but it will keep you from getting sick") will be lost on most preoperational children; the immediate presence of a calm parent is more comforting. Children with precocious language development may elicit overly complex explanations from adults who assume incorrectly that their cognitive sophistication matches their verbal skill.

The imaginative intensity that fuels play and the magical, animist thinking characteristic of preoperational cognition can also generate intense fears. More than 80% of parents report at least one fear in their preschool children, and nearly 50% report

TABLE 12–2. Body Mass Index (BMI) Percentiles for Age, Boys and Girls, 2–20 yr

Boys: Percentiles

Age (Yr)	5th	10th	25th	50th	75th	85th	90th	95th
2.0	14.7	15.1	15.7	16.6	17.6	18.2	18.6	19.3
2.5	14.5	14.9	15.5	16.2	17.1	17.7	18.1	18.7
3.0	14.3	14.7	15.3	16.0	16.8	17.3	17.7	18.2
3.5	14.2	14.5	15.1	15.8	16.6	17.1	17.4	18.0
4.0	14.0	14.3	14.9	15.6	16.4	16.9	17.3	17.8
4.5	13.9	14.2	14.8	15.5	16.3	16.8	17.2	17.8
5.0	13.8	14.1	14.7	15.4	16.3	16.8	17.3	17.9
5.5	13.8	14.1	14.6	15.4	16.3	16.9	17.4	18.1
6.0	13.7	14.0	14.6	15.4	16.4	17.0	17.5	18.4
6.5	13.7	14.0	14.6	15.4	16.5	17.2	17.7	18.8
7.0	13.7	14.0	14.7	15.5	16.6	17.4	18.0	19.2
7.5	13.7	14.1	14.7	15.6	16.8	17.7	18.3	19.6
8.0	13.8	14.1	14.8	15.8	17.1	18.0	18.7	20.1
8.5	13.9	14.2	15.0	16.0	17.3	18.3	19.1	20.6
9.0	14.0	14.3	15.1	16.2	17.6	18.6	19.5	21.1
9.5	14.1	14.5	15.3	16.4	17.9	19.0	19.9	21.6
10.0	14.2	14.6	15.5	16.6	18.2	19.4	20.3	22.2
10.5	14.4	14.8	15.7	16.9	18.6	19.8	20.8	22.7
11.0	14.6	15.0	15.9	17.2	18.9	20.2	21.2	23.2
11.5	14.8	15.2	16.2	17.5	19.3	20.6	21.7	23.7
12.0	15.0	15.5	16.4	17.8	19.7	21.0	22.1	24.2
12.5	15.2	15.7	16.7	18.1	20.1	21.4	22.6	24.7
13.0	15.5	16.0	17.0	18.5	20.4	21.9	23.0	25.2
13.5	15.7	16.3	17.3	18.8	20.8	22.3	23.4	25.6
14.0	16.0	16.5	17.6	19.2	21.2	22.7	23.8	26.0
14.5	16.3	16.8	17.9	19.5	21.6	23.1	24.3	26.5
15.0	16.6	17.1	18.3	19.9	22.0	23.5	24.6	26.8
15.5	16.8	17.4	18.6	20.2	22.4	23.8	25.0	27.2
16.0	17.1	17.7	18.9	20.6	22.7	24.2	25.4	27.6
16.5	17.4	18.0	19.2	20.9	23.1	24.6	25.8	27.9
17.0	17.7	18.3	19.6	21.2	23.4	24.9	26.1	28.3
17.5	18.0	18.6	19.9	21.6	23.8	25.3	26.5	28.6
18.0	18.2	18.9	20.2	21.9	24.1	25.7	26.9	29.0
18.5	18.5	19.2	20.4	22.2	24.5	26.0	27.2	29.3
19.0	18.7	19.4	20.7	22.5	24.8	26.4	27.6	29.7
19.5	18.9	19.6	21.0	22.8	25.1	26.7	28.0	30.2
20.0	19.1	19.8	21.2	23.0	25.4	27.0	28.3	30.6

Girls: Percentiles

Age (Yr)	5th	10th	25th	50th	75th	85th	90th	95th
2.0	14.4	14.8	15.5	16.4	17.4	18.0	18.4	19.1
2.5	14.2	14.5	15.2	16.0	16.9	17.5	17.9	18.6
3.0	14.0	14.3	14.9	15.7	16.6	17.2	17.6	18.3
3.5	13.8	14.2	14.7	15.5	16.4	16.9	17.4	18.1
4.0	13.7	14.0	14.6	15.3	16.2	16.8	17.3	18.0
4.5	13.6	13.9	14.5	15.2	16.1	16.8	17.2	18.1
5.0	13.5	13.8	14.4	15.2	16.1	16.8	17.3	18.3
5.5	13.5	13.8	14.4	15.2	16.2	16.9	17.5	18.5
6.0	13.4	13.7	14.4	15.2	16.3	17.1	17.7	18.8
6.5	13.4	13.8	14.4	15.3	16.5	17.3	18.0	19.2
7.0	13.4	13.8	14.5	15.5	16.7	17.6	18.3	19.7
7.5	13.5	13.9	14.6	15.6	17.0	18.0	18.7	20.2
8.0	13.5	13.9	14.7	15.8	17.3	18.3	19.2	20.7
8.5	13.6	14.1	14.9	16.1	17.6	18.7	19.6	21.2
9.0	13.7	14.2	15.1	16.3	18.0	19.1	20.1	21.8
9.5	13.9	14.4	15.3	16.6	18.3	19.5	20.5	22.4
10.0	14.0	14.5	15.5	16.9	18.7	20.0	21.0	23.0
10.5	14.2	14.7	15.7	17.2	19.1	20.4	21.5	23.6
11.0	14.4	14.9	16.0	17.5	19.5	20.9	22.0	24.1
11.5	14.6	15.2	16.3	17.8	19.9	21.3	22.5	24.7
12.0	14.8	15.4	16.5	18.1	20.2	21.7	23.0	25.3
12.5	15.1	15.7	16.8	18.4	20.6	22.2	23.4	25.8
13.0	15.3	15.9	17.1	18.7	21.0	22.6	23.9	26.3
13.5	15.6	16.2	17.4	19.0	21.3	23.0	24.3	26.8
14.0	15.8	16.4	17.6	19.4	21.7	23.3	24.7	27.3
14.5	16.1	16.7	17.9	19.6	22.0	23.7	25.1	27.7
15.0	16.3	16.9	18.2	19.9	22.3	24.0	25.5	28.1
15.5	16.6	17.2	18.4	20.2	22.6	24.4	25.8	28.5
16.0	16.8	17.4	18.7	20.5	22.9	24.7	26.1	28.9
16.5	17.0	17.6	18.9	20.7	23.2	24.9	26.4	29.3
17.0	17.2	17.8	19.1	20.9	23.4	25.2	26.7	29.6
17.5	17.4	18.0	19.3	21.1	23.6	25.4	27.0	30.0
18.0	17.6	18.2	19.5	21.3	23.8	25.7	27.3	30.3
18.5	17.7	18.3	19.6	21.4	24.0	25.9	27.5	30.7
19.0	17.8	18.4	19.7	21.6	24.2	26.1	27.8	31.0
19.5	17.8	18.5	19.8	21.7	24.3	26.3	28.0	31.4
20.0	17.8	18.5	19.8	21.7	24.4	26.5	28.2	31.8

Data used in creating the 2000 Centers for Disease Control (CDC) growth charts, as described in Chapter 15. Data apply to the age range, including the listed age and subsequent month (i.e., "1 mo" represents the average for 1 mo, 0 days through 1 mo, 30 days). Data for additional age points and 3rd and 97th percentiles are available at www.cdc.gov/nchs, along with technical reports.

seven or more fears. Refusal to take baths or to sit on the toilet may arise from the fear of being washed or flushed down, reflecting a child's immature appreciation of relative size. Attempts to demonstrate rationally that there are no monsters in the closet often fail, inasmuch as the fear arises from prerational thinking, but parents may be able to reassure their children that they can ward off the monsters with "monster spray" or a similar appeal to magical thinking. In general, children's willingness to believe that their parents are large and powerful helps parents provide a sense of safety as children's world view expands.

EMOTIONAL DEVELOPMENT

Emotional challenges facing preschool children include accepting limits while maintaining a sense of self-direction, reining in aggressive and sexual impulses, and interacting with a widening circle of adults and peers. At 2 yr of age, behavioral limits are predominantly external; by 5 yr of age, these controls need to be internalized if a child is to function in a typical classroom. Success in achieving this goal relies on prior emotional development, particularly the ability to use internalized images of trusted adults to provide security in times of stress. Children need to believe themselves worthy of adult approval to be willing to work for it.

Children learn what behaviors are acceptable and how much power they wield vis-à-vis important adults by testing limits. Testing increases when it elicits an exceptional amount of attention, even though that attention is often negative, and when limits are inconsistent. Testing often arouses parental anger or inappropriate solicitude as a child's struggle to separate gives rise to a corresponding challenge for the parents: letting go. Excessively tight limits can undermine a child's sense of initiative, whereas overly loose limits can provoke anxiety in a child who feels that no one is in control.

Control is a central issue. Young children cannot control many aspects of their life—where they go, how long they stay, what they take home from the store. They are also prone to lose internal control as well, that is, to have *temper tantrums*. When a parent occasionally gives in to a child's demands, intermittently reinforcing the tantrum behavior, tantrums can become an entrenched strategy for exerting control. Fear, overtiredness, or physical discomfort also evoke tantrums. Tantrums normally appear toward the end of the 1st yr of life and peak in prevalence between 2 and 4 yr of age. Tantrums lasting more than 15 min or regularly occurring more than three times a day may reflect underlying medical, emotional, or social problems. Frequent tantrums after 5 yr of age tend to persist throughout childhood.

Preschool children normally experience complicated feelings toward their parents that can include possessiveness toward one parent, jealousy and resentment of the other parent, and fear that these negative feelings might lead to abandonment. These emotions, most beyond a child's ability to comprehend or verbalize, often find expression in highly labile moods. The resolution of this crisis (a process extending over years) involves a child's unspoken decision to emulate the parents rather than compete with them. Play and language foster the development of emotional controls by allowing children to express emotions and to enjoy gratifications (such as being big and powerful) that are taboo in real life.

Curiosity about genitals and adult sexual organs is normal, as is *masturbation*. Masturbation that has a compulsive quality or that interferes with a child's normal activities, acting out of sexual intercourse in doll play or with other children, extreme modesty, or mimicry of adult seductive behavior all suggest the possibility of sexual abuse. Modesty appears gradually between 4 and 6 yr of age, with wide variations among cultures and families.

Implications for Parents and Pediatricians. Most parents find it difficult to understand their preschool children at least some

of the time. Rapid shifts between clinging dependence and defiant independence, between sophisticated-sounding language and infantile helplessness, and between angelic joy and uncontrollable rage can erode parents' self-confidence and patience. Guidance emphasizing appropriate expectations for behavioral and emotional development and acknowledging normal parental feelings of anger, guilt, and confusion can help lessen parents' worries both about their children and about themselves. Many parents fail to raise such concerns during pediatric visits because they feel embarrassed or because they do not think the pediatrician can help. Pediatricians need to let parents know that the child's behavior and the parents' reactions are appropriate topics for discussion.

It may be difficult to decide whether a particular child's behavior is normally challenging or indicative of a true problem. Red flags include parents who do not volunteer any positive statements about their children, evidence of threatening or overtly punitive discipline, and the existence of problems (especially tantrums) in daycare or preschool, where most preschool children manage to maintain self-control. The presence of chronic medical problems, developmental delays, or unusual family stresses signal the need for more detailed assessment. Even apparently normal behavior constitutes a problem if it arouses sufficient parental concern. An extended visit devoted to the issue or referral to a mental health professional is appropriate. Reference to *The Classification of Child and Adolescent Mental Diagnoses in Primary Care: Diagnostic and Statistical Manual for Primary Care (DSM-PC)* will help pediatricians distinguish among normal variations, problems, and disorders that may merit referral.

Corporal punishment is accepted in many traditional cultures but may be inappropriate in the modern context in which most families now live (also see Chapter 5). No evidence shows that spanking per se is harmful, but regular use of corporal punishment may reflect an excessive desire for control, as well as a lack of other parenting techniques. Parents usually claim that they do not like spanking but feel that nothing else works. Pediatricians can point out that the spanking is not working either, or it would not have to be used so often. As children habituate to repeated spanking, parents have to spank ever harder to get the desired response, increasing the risk of serious injury. Sufficiently harsh punishment may inhibit undesired behaviors, but at great psychologic cost. Children mimic the corporal punishment they receive, and it is not uncommon for preschool-age children to strike their parents back. Parents may be helped to renounce spanking or at least reserve it for extreme circumstances if they learn more effective discipline techniques, including consistent limit-setting, clear communication, and frequent approval. Time-out for approximately 1 min per year of age is a form of noncorporal punishment backed by extensive research. Parents may require detailed instruction to use time-out effectively.

Dixon SD: Two years: Language emerges. In Dixon SD, Stein MT (editors): *Encounters with Children: Pediatric Behavior and Development.* St Louis, Mosby, 2000, pp 300–26.

Fox NA, Henderson HA, Rubin KH, et al: Continuity and discontinuity of behavioral inhibition and exuberance: Psychophysiological and behavioral influences across the first four years of life. *Child Dev* 2001;72:1–21.

Friedman SB, Schonberg SK (editors): *The Short- and Long-term Consequences of Corporal Punishment.* Supplement to *Pediatrics* 1996;98:803–58.

Ginsburg H, Opper S: *Piaget's Theory of Intellectual Development.* Englewood Cliffs, NJ, Prentice-Hall, 1969.

Schickedanz JA: *Much More than the ABCs: The Early Stages of Reading and Writing.* Washington, DC: National Association for the Education of Young Children (NAEYC), 1999.

Wolraich ML (editor): *The Classification of Child and Adolescent Mental Diagnoses in Primary Care: Diagnostic and Statistical Manual for Primary Care (DSM-PC) Child and Adolescent Version.* Elk Grove Village, IL, American Academy of Pediatrics, 1996.

Chapter 13
Middle Childhood

During middle childhood (6–12 yr), children increasingly separate from parents and seek acceptance from teachers and other adults, and from peers. *Self-esteem* becomes a central issue, as children develop the cognitive ability to consider at the same time their own self-evaluations and their perception of how others see them. For the first time, they are judged according to their ability to produce socially valued outputs, such as good grades or home runs. This focus on accomplishment leads to the central psychosocial issue of this period, as described by Erikson, the crisis between industry and inferiority. Pressure to conform to the style and ideals of the group can be intense, and children who are different, physically or intellectually, are at risk for social isolation and depression.

PHYSICAL DEVELOPMENT

Growth during the period averages 3–3.5 kg (7 lb) and 6 cm (2.5 in) per year (see Figs. 11–1 and 11–2 and Table 12–1). Growth occurs discontinuously, in 3 to 6 irregularly timed spurts each year, each growth spurt lasting on average 8 wk. The head grows only 2–3 cm in circumference throughout the entire period, reflecting slower brain growth than before; myelinization is complete by 7 yr of age. Body habitus (endomorphic, mesomorphic, or ectomorphic) tends to remain relatively stable throughout middle childhood.

Growth of the midface and lower face occurs gradually. Loss of deciduous (baby) teeth is a more dramatic sign of maturation, beginning after eruption of the 1st molars around age 6 yr. Replacement with adult teeth occurs at a rate of about 4/yr. Lymphoid tissues hypertrophy, often giving rise to impressive tonsils and adenoids, which may require surgical removal.

Muscular strength, coordination, and stamina increase progressively, as does the ability to perform complex movements such as dancing, shooting basketballs, or playing the piano. Such higher order motor skills are a result of both maturation and training; the degree of accomplishment reflects wide variability in innate skill, interest, and opportunity. Epidemiologic studies report a general decline in physical fitness among school-age children over the past 15–20 yr. Sedentary habits at this age are associated with increased lifetime risk of obesity and cardiovascular disease.

The sexual organs remain physically immature, but interest in gender differences and sexual behavior remains active in many children and increases progressively until puberty. Masturbation is common, if not universal. In more permissive cultures, sexual experimentation often occurs among prepubertal children.

Implications for Parents and Pediatricians. "Normality" encompasses a wide range of physical sizes, shapes, and abilities in school-age children. Just as importantly, children's feelings about their physical attributes range from pride to shame to apparent nonchalance. Fears of being "defective" can lead to avoidance of situations in which physical differences might be revealed, such as gym class or medical examinations. Children with actual physical disabilities may face special stresses because of their difference. Medical, social, and psychologic risks tend to aggregate in children; multisystem problems are the rule rather than the exception among children at risk for long-term morbidity. The routine physical examination provides an opportunity to elicit concerns and allay fears.

Girls, in particular, often worry that they are overweight, and many engage in unhealthy dieting to achieve an abnormally thin cultural ideal. Shortness, particularly in boys, may be associated with decreased educational attainment and increased risks for behavior problems (although social class remains a more powerful predictor). The availability of recombinant human growth hormone raises the possibility of medical treatment for short children even in the absence of documented hormone deficiency. The decision to treat, with its attendant cost and discomfort, needs to be made in view of the meaning of shortness for the individual child (see Chapter 551).

A child's physical appearance may also evoke strong feelings in parents, leading them to undermine the child's self-esteem inadvertently, or, alternatively, to encourage vanity. Pediatricians can help parents distinguish between true health risks and individual variations that should be accepted. Questions about regular physical activities should be part of the medical history for health supervision visits. Participation in organized *sports* can foster skill, teamwork, and fitness, but excessive pressure to compete often has negative effects. Prepubertal children should not engage in high-stress, high-impact sports such as power lifting or football because skeletal immaturity increases the risk of injury.

COGNITIVE AND LANGUAGE DEVELOPMENT

The thinking of early elementary school-aged children differs qualitatively from that of children just 1 or 2 yr younger. In place of magical, egocentric, and perception-bound cognition, school-aged children increasingly apply rules based on observable phenomena, factor in multiple dimensions and points of view, and interpret their perceptions in view of realistic theories about physical laws. This shift from "preoperational" to "concrete logical operations" was documented by Piaget in a series of "conservation" experiments (see Chapter 12). For example, 5-yr-olds who watch a ball of clay being rolled into a snake might insist that the snake has "more" because it is longer. Seven-year-olds typically reply that the ball and snake must weigh the same because nothing has been added or taken away or because the snake is both longer and thinner. This cognitive reorganization occurs at different rates in different contexts. In the context of social interactions with siblings, young children often demonstrate an ability to understand alternate points of view long before they demonstrate that ability in their thinking about the physical world.

School makes increasing cognitive demands. Mastery of the elementary curriculum requires that a large number of perceptual, cognitive, and language processes work efficiently (Table 13–1). Attention and receptive language affect each other as well as every other aspect of learning. One cannot attend to what one cannot understand or understand without first paying attention. By third grade, children need to be able to sustain attention through a 45-min period.

The first 2 yr of elementary school are devoted to acquiring the fundamentals: reading, writing, and basic mathematics skills. By third or fourth grade, the curriculum requires that children use those fundamentals to learn increasingly complex materials. The goal of reading a paragraph is no longer to decode the words but to understand the content; the goal of writing is no longer spelling or penmanship but composition. The volume of work increases along with the complexity. Children can meet these demands only if they have mastered the basic skills to the point that their execution has become automatic. Children who have to think about how to shape each letter or who have to recalculate basic mathematics facts each time they attempt to solve a word problem fall behind.

Cognitive abilities interact with a wide array of attitudinal and emotional factors in determining classroom performance. A partial list of such factors includes eagerness to please adults, cooperativeness, competitiveness, willingness to work for a delayed reward, belief in one's abilities, and ability to risk trying when success is not ensured. Success predisposes to success, whereas failure undercuts a child's ability to take cognitive-emotional risks in the future.

TABLE 13–1. Selected Perceptual, Cognitive, and Language Processes Required for Elementary School Success

Process	Description	Associated Problems
Perceptual		
Visual analysis	Ability to break a complex figure into components and understand their spatial relationships	Persistent letter confusion (e.g., between *b*, *d*, and *g*); difficulty with basic reading and writing and limited "sight" vocabulary
Proprioception and motor control	Ability to obtain information about body position by feel and unconsciously program complex movements	Poor handwriting, requiring inordinate effort, often with overly tight pencil grasp; special difficulty with timed tasks
Phonologic processing	Ability to perceive differences between similar sounding words and to break down words into constituent sounds	Delayed receptive language skills; attention and behavior problems secondary to not understanding directions; delayed acquisition of letter-sound correlations (phonetics)
Cognitive		
Long-term memory, both storage and recall	Ability to acquire skills that are "automatic" (i.e., accessible without conscious thought)	Delayed mastery of the alphabet (reading and writing letters); slow handwriting; inability to progress beyond basic mathematics
Selective attention	Ability to attend to important stimuli and ignore distractions	Difficulty following multistep instructions, completing assignments, and behaving well; peer interaction problems
Sequencing	Ability to remember things in order; facility with time concepts	Difficulty organizing assignments, planning, spelling, and telling time
Language		
Receptive language	Ability to comprehend complex constructions, function words (e.g., if, when, only, except), nuances of speech, and extended blocks of language (e.g., paragraphs)	Difficulty following directions; wandering attention during lessons and stories; problems with reading comprehension; problems with peer relationships
Expressive language	Ability to recall required words effortlessly (word finding), to control meanings by varying position and word endings, to construct meaningful paragraphs and stories	Difficulty expressing feelings and using words for self-defense, with resulting frustration and physical acting out; struggling during "circle time" and in language-based subjects (e.g., English)

Children's intellectual activity extends beyond the classroom. Beginning in the 3rd or 4th grade, children increasingly enjoy strategy games and word play (puns and insults) that exercise growing cognitive and linguistic mastery. Many become experts on subjects of their own choosing, such as sports trivia or stamps. Others become avid readers.

Implications for Parents and Pediatricians. Children in the cognitive stage of concrete logical operations can understand simple explanations for illnesses and necessary treatments, although they may revert to prelogical thinking under stress (as may adults). A child with pneumonia may be able to explain about white cells fighting the "germs" in the lungs but still secretly harbor the belief that the sickness is a punishment for disobedience.

Academic and classroom behavior problems, like fever, are symptoms that require diagnosis. Among the broad range of possible causes are deficits in specific cognitive, perceptual, or linguistic functions (specific learning disabilities); global cognitive delay (mental retardation); primary attention deficit; and attention deficits secondary to emotional preoccupation, depression, anxiety, or any chronic illness. Commonly, the cause is a combination of several such factors. Assessment of school problems is discussed in Chapters 16 and 29.

Remedial approaches depend on the underlying problem or problems. Children who are inattentive because of receptive language disability will benefit more from language therapy than from stimulant medication. Similarly, psychotherapy is generally less helpful for primary attention deficits than are medication and environmental modifications aimed at increasing structure and decreasing distractions. Simply having a child repeat a failed grade rarely has any beneficial effect and often seriously undercuts the child's self-esteem. See Chapter 29 for a further discussion of learning and behavior problems. Interventions that allow children to exercise their strengths and experience success have beneficial effects that often spill over into problem areas. Educational approaches that value a wide range of talents ("multiple intelligences") beyond the traditional ones of reading, writing, and mathematics promise to allow more children to succeed.

SOCIAL AND EMOTIONAL DEVELOPMENT

Social and emotional development proceeds in three contexts: the home, the school, and the neighborhood. Of these, the home remains the most influential. The parent-child relationship continues to provide a secure base from which children can venture forth. Milestones of a school child's increasing independence include the first sleepover at a friend's house and the first time at overnight camp. Parents should make demands for effort in school and extracurricular activities, celebrate successes, and offer unconditional acceptance when failures occur. Regular chores provide an opportunity for children to contribute to the family in a meaningful way, supporting self-esteem. Siblings have critical roles as competitors, loyal supporters, and role models. Sibling relationships exert lasting effects on personality development, influencing an individual's self-image, approach to conflict resolution, interests, and even career choices.

The beginning of school coincides with a child's further separation from the family and the increasing importance of teacher and peer relationships. In addition to friendships that may persist for months or years, experience with a large number of superficial friendships and antagonisms contributes to a child's growing social competence. Popularity, a central ingredient of self-esteem, may be won through possessions (having the right toys or the right clothes) as well as through personal attractiveness, accomplishments, and actual social skills.

Conformity is rewarded. Some children conform readily and enjoy easy social success; those who adopt individualistic styles or have visible differences may be stigmatized as "weird." Such children may be painfully aware that they are different, or they may be puzzled by their lack of popularity. Children with social skills deficits may go to extreme lengths to win acceptance, only to meet with repeated failure. Attributions conferred by peers, such as funny, stupid, bad, or scary, may become incorporated into a child's self-image. The peer group exerts a profound influence on the child's personality, often including mannerisms, speaking accent, aspirations, and relationship to the law. Parents may have their greatest effect indirectly, through actions that change the peer group (e.g., moving to a new community, or insisting on involvement in structured after-school activities).

In the neighborhood, real dangers such as busy streets, bullies, and strangers tax school-aged children's common sense and resourcefulness. Interactions with peers without close adult supervision call on increasing conflict resolution or pugilistic skills. Observation of older children and adults as well as advertisements in store windows and on television expose children to adult materialism, sexuality, and violence. Many of these experiences reinforce children's feeling of powerlessness in the larger world. Compensatory fantasies of being powerful may fuel the fascination with superheroes. Hero worship and adoption of adult-like dress and mannerisms are "dress rehearsals" for adult roles and represent ways of appropriating adult power. A balance between fantasy and appropriate ability to negotiate real world challenges indicates healthy emotional development.

Implications for Parents and Pediatricians. Children need unconditional support as well as realistic demands as they venture into a world that is often frightening. Children who show unusual difficulty in separating from parents and in facing school and neighborhood challenges may be reacting to their parents' difficulty letting them go. Other parents exert excessive pressure on their children to adopt adult behaviors and achieve academic or competitive success. Children who struggle to meet such expectations may develop behavior problems or somatic symptoms such as headaches or stomachaches as a result (Chapter 19).

Many children face stressors that exceed the normal challenges of separation and "making it" in school and neighborhood. Divorce affects nearly 50% of children. Violence between parents, parental substance abuse, and other mental health problems may also impair a child's ability to use home as a secure base for refueling emotional energies. In many neighborhoods, the threats of gangs and random violence make the normal development of independence extremely dangerous. Children in late elementary and middle school may join gangs as a means of self-protection and a way to appropriate power and belong to a cohesive group. The high prevalence of adjustment disorders among school-aged children attests to the effects of such overwhelming stressors on development.

Pediatricians need to be alert to children's functioning in all contexts (home, school, neighborhood) and consider how each of those environments either supports or overwhelms the child's ability to adapt and grow. Use of the HEADSS mnemonic—*H*ome, *E*ducation and employment, peer *A*ctivities, *D*rugs, *S*exuality, and *S*uicide or depression can help. Originally designed for adolescents, with minor modifications it also works well for school-aged children.

Boyce WT, Essex MJ, Woodward HR, et al: The confluence of mental, physical, social, and academic difficulties in middle childhood. I: Exploring the head waters of early life morbidities. *J Am Acad Child Adolesc Psychiatry* 2002;41:580–7.

Gardner H: *Frames of Mind: The Theory of Multiple Intelligences.* New York, Basic Books, 1983.

Jellinek M, Patel B, Froehle M: *Bright Futures in Practice: Mental Health—Volume I, Practice Guide.* Arlington, VA: National Center for Education in Maternal and Child Health, 2002.

Levine MD: Middle Childhood. In Levine MD, Carey WB, Crocker AC (editors): *Developmental-Behavioral Pediatrics,* 3rd ed. Philadelphia, WB Saunders, 1999, pp 51–68.

Thompson M, Grace C, Cohen L: *Best Friends, Worst Enemies.* New York, Ballantine, 2001.

Wells R, Stein M: Seven to ten years: The world of middle childhood. In Dixon SD, Stein MT (editors): *Encounters with Children: Pediatric Behavior and Development.* St Louis, Mosby, 2000, pp 402–25.

Chapter 14
Adolescence

(See also Part XII and Chapters 555 and 556.)

Between 10 and 20 yr of age, children undergo rapid changes in body size, shape, physiology, and psychologic and social functioning. Hormones set the developmental agenda in conjunction with social structures designed to foster the transition from childhood to adulthood.

Adolescence proceeds across three distinct periods—early, middle, and late—each marked by a characteristic set of salient biologic, psychologic, and social issues (Table 14–1). However,

individual variation is substantial, both in terms of the timing of somatic changes and the quality of the adolescent's experience. Gender and subculture profoundly affect the developmental course, as do physical and social stressors such as cerebral palsy or parental alcoholism.

EARLY ADOLESCENCE

Biologic Development. Adrenal production of androgen (chiefly dehydroepiandrosterone sulfate [DHEAS]) may occur as early as 6 yr of age, with development of underarm odor and faint genital hair (adrenarche). Levels of luteinizing hormone (LH) and follicle-stimulating hormone (FSH) rise progressively throughout middle childhood without dramatic effect. The rapid changes of puberty begin with increased sensitivity of the pituitary to gonadotropin-releasing hormone (GnRH), pulsatile release of GnRH, LH, and FSH during sleep, and corresponding increases in gonadal androgens and estrogens. The triggers for these changes are incompletely understood, but may involve neuronal development that is ongoing throughout middle childhood and adolescence. Contemporary children in the United States may enter puberty earlier than the published norms (although reports of dramatically earlier puberty are controversial), perhaps related to increased weight and adiposity. The resulting sequence of somatic and physiologic changes gives rise to the sexual maturity rating (SMR) or Tanner stages. Figures 14–1 and 14–2 depict the somatic changes used in the SMR scale; Tables 14–2 and 14–3 describe these changes in words. Table 14–4 lists median ages and

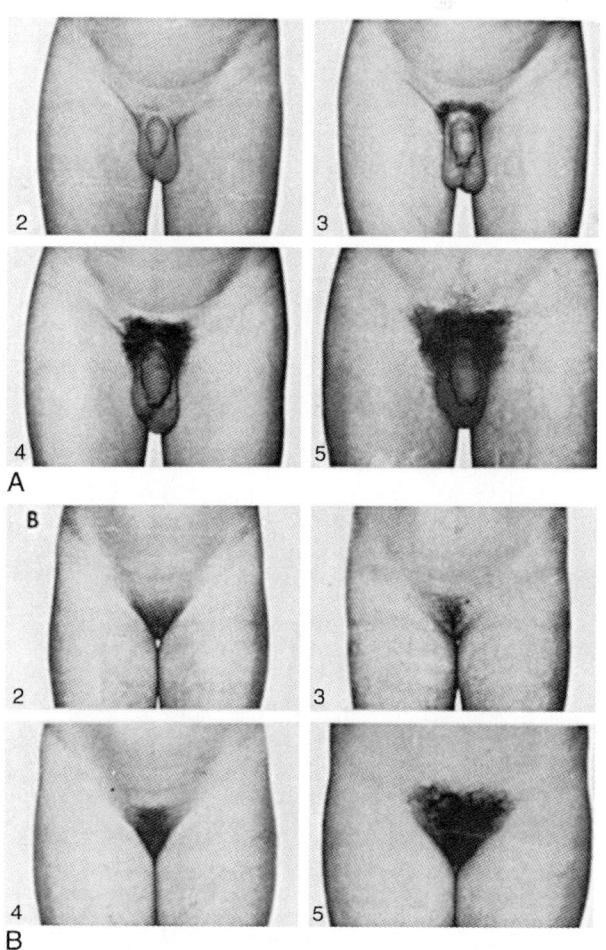

FIGURE 14–1. Sex maturity ratings of pubic hair changes in adolescent boys and girls. (Courtesy of JM Tanner, MD, Institute of Child Health, Department of Growth and Development, University of London, London, England.)

TABLE 14–1. Central Issues in Early, Middle, and Late Adolescence

Variable	Early Adolescence	Middle Adolescence	Late Adolescence
Age (yr)	10–13	14–16	17–20 and beyond
SMR*	1–2	3–5	5
Somatic	Secondary sex characteristics; beginning of rapid growth; awkward	Height growth peaks; body shape and composition change; acne and odor; menarche; spermarche	Slower growth
Sexual	Sexual interest usually exceeds sexual activity	Sexual drive surges; experimentation; questions of sexual orientation	Consolidation of sexual identity
Cognitive and moral	Concrete operations; conventional morality	Emergence of abstract thought; questioning mores; self-centered	Idealism; absolutism
Self-concept	Preoccupation with changing body; self-consciousness	Concern with attractiveness, increasing introspection	Relatively stable body image
Family	Bids for increased independence; ambivalence	Continued struggle for acceptance of greater autonomy	Practical independence; family remains secure base
Peers	Same-sex groups; conformity; cliques	Dating; peer groups less important	Intimacy; possibly commitment
Relationship to society	Middle-school adjustment	Gauging skills and opportunities	Career decisions (e.g., drop out, college, work)

*See text and Figures 14–1 and 14–2.
SMR = sexual maturity rating.

normal ranges for key stages of breast, pubic hair, and penile development. Note that the SMR stages are not perfectly synchronized (e.g., SMR2 penis development precedes SMR2 pubic hair by on average 1.5 years). Figures 14–3 and 14–4 depict the typical sequence of pubertal changes in males and females, respectively. The range of normal for progress through the stages of sexual maturity is wide.

In girls, the first visible sign of puberty is the appearance of breast buds, between 8 and 13 yr. Menses typically begin 2–2$\frac{1}{2}$ yr later (normal range 9–16 yr), around the peak in height

velocity (see Fig. 14–4). Less obvious changes include enlargement of the ovaries, uterus, labia, and clitoris; thickening of endometrium and the vaginal mucosa; and increased vaginal glycogen, predisposing to yeast infections.

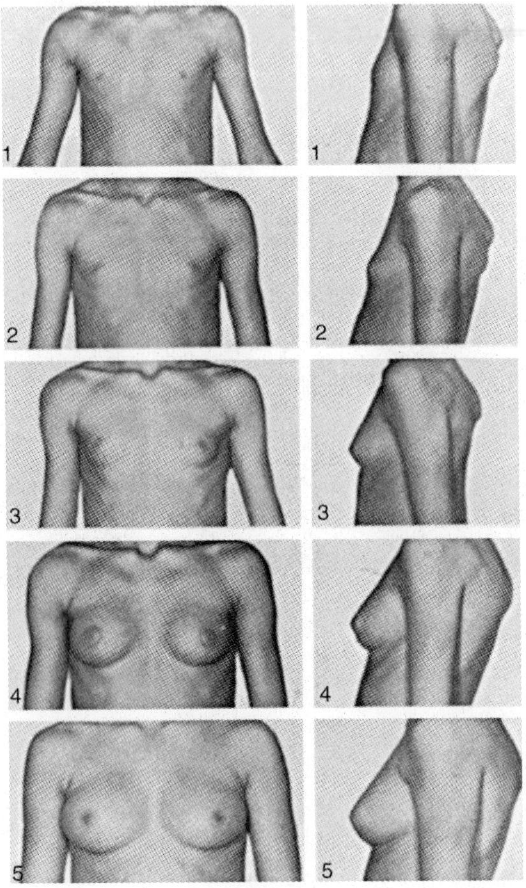

In boys, testicular enlargement begins as early as 9$\frac{1}{2}$ yr. Peak growth occurs when testis volumes reach approximately 9–10 cm^3. Under the influence of LH and testosterone, the seminiferous tubules, epididymis, seminal vesicles, and prostate enlarge. The left testis normally is lower than the right; the opposite may be true in situs inversus. Some degree of breast hypertrophy occurs in 40–65% of pubertal boys as a result of a relative excess of estrogenic stimulation. Gynecomastia sufficient to cause embarrassment and social disability occurs in fewer than 10%. Breast swelling less than 4 cm in diameter has a 90% chance of spontaneous resolution within 3 yr. For greater degrees of enlargement, hormonal or surgical treatment may be indicated. Obesity may exacerbate gynecomastia and should be addressed through diet and exercise.

For both sexes, growth acceleration begins in early adolescence, but peak growth velocities are not reached until SMR3 or 4. Boys typically peak 2–3 yr later than girls (Fig. 14–5) and continue their linear growth for approximately 2–3 yr after girls have stopped. The growth spurt begins distally, with enlargement of hands and feet followed by the arms and legs and finally by the trunk and chest. This asymmetric growth gives young adolescents a gawky look. Rapid enlargement of the larynx, pharynx, and lungs leads to changes in vocal quality, often heralded by a period of vocal instability (voice cracking) or dysphonation. Adrenal androgens stimulate the sebaceous glands, promoting the development of acne. Elongation of the optic

FIGURE 14–2. Sex maturity ratings of breast changes in adolescent girls. (Courtesy of JM Tanner, MD, Institute of Child Health, Department of Growth and Development, University of London, London, England.)

TABLE 14–2. Classification of Sex Maturity Stages in Girls

SMR Stage	Pubic Hair	Breasts
1	Preadolescent	Preadolescent
2	Sparse, lightly pigmented, straight, medial border of labia	Breast and papilla elevated as small mound; areolar diameter increased
3	Darker, beginning to curl, increased amount	Breast and areola enlarged, no contour separation
4	Coarse, curly, abundant but amount less than in adult	Areola and papilla form secondary mound
5	Adult feminine triangle, spread to medial surface of thighs	Mature, nipple projects, areola part of general breast contour

SMR = sexual maturity rating.
From Tanner JM: Growth at Adolescence, 2nd ed. Oxford, England, Blackwell Scientific Publications, 1962.

TABLE 14–3. Classification of Sex Maturity Stages in Boys

SMR Stage	Pubic Hair	Penis	Testes
1	None	Preadolescent	Preadolescent
2	Scanty, long, slightly pigmented	Slight enlargement	Enlarged scrotum, pink, texture altered
3	Darker, starts to curl, small amount	Longer	Larger
4	Resembles adult type but less in quantity; coarse, curly	Larger; glans and breadth increase in size	Larger, scrotum dark
5	Adult distribution, spread to medial surface of thighs	Adult size	Adult size

SMR = sexual maturity rating.
Adapted from Tanner JM: Growth at Adolescence, 2nd ed. Oxford, England, Blackwell Scientific Publications, 1962.

TABLE 14–4. Variability in Timing of Sexual Maturation

SMR	Early (mean − 2 SD Early)	Average (median)	Late (mean + 2 SD Late)
Timing of SMR Stages in Girls			
Pubic Hair			
SMR2	9.0	11.2	13.5
SMR3	9.6	11.9	14.1
SMR4	10.3	12.6	14.8
Breast Development			
SMR2	8.9	10.9	12.9
SMR3	9.8	11.9	13.9
SMR4	10.5	12.9	15.3
Timing of SMR Stages in Boys			
Pubic Hair			
SMR2	9.9	12.0	14.1
SMR3	11.2	13.1	14.9
SMR4	12.0	13.9	15.7
Penis Development			
SMR2	9.2	10.5	13.7
SMR3	10.1	12.4	14.6
SMR4	11.2	13.2	15.4

SMR = sexual maturity rating; SD = Standard deviation.
Data from Tanner JM, Davies PSW: Clinical longitudinal standards for height and height velocity for North American children. J Pediatr 1985; 107:317.

globe often results in nearsightedness. Dental changes include jaw growth, loss of the final deciduous teeth, and eruption of the permanent cuspids, premolars, and finally molars (see Table 10–6). Orthodontic appliances may be needed.

Sexuality. Sexuality includes not only sexual behaviors but also interest and fantasies, sexual orientation, attitudes toward sex and its relationship to emotions, and awareness of socially defined roles and mores.

Interest in sex increases in early puberty. Ejaculation occurs for the first time, usually during masturbation and later spontaneously in sleep. Some boys worry that these emissions are signs of infection. Early adolescents sometimes masturbate socially; mutual sexual exploration is not necessarily a sign of homosexuality (Chapter 26). Sexual behavior, other than masturbation, is less common in early puberty, although 31% of an urban sample reported sexual intercourse before 14 yr of age.

The relationship between hormonal changes and sexual interest and activity is controversial; no consistent links between hormones and sexual arousal, age of first intercourse, or frequency of intercourse have been found.

Cognitive and Moral Development. In piagetian theory, adolescence marks the transition from the concrete operational thinking characteristic of school-aged children (Chapter 13) to formal logical operations. Formal operations include the ability to manipulate abstractions such as algebraic expressions, to reason from known principles, to weigh many points of view according to varying criteria, and to think about the process of thinking itself. Some early adolescents demonstrate formal thinking, others acquire the capability later, and others do not ever fully acquire it. Young adolescents may be able to apply formal operations to schoolwork but not to personal dilemmas. When the emotional stakes are high, magical thinking, such as the conviction of invulnerability, may interfere with higher order cognition. The ability to treat possibilities as real entities may affect critical decisions, such as whether or not to have unprotected intercourse or engage in other risk-taking behavior.

Some theorists argue that the transition from concrete to formal operations follows from quantitative increases in knowledge, experience, and cognitive efficiency rather than a qualitative reorganization of thinking. Consistent with this view are data showing a steady rise in cognitive processing speed from late childhood through early adulthood, associated with a reduction in synaptic number (pruning of less-used pathways) and progressive maturation of electroencephalographic results.

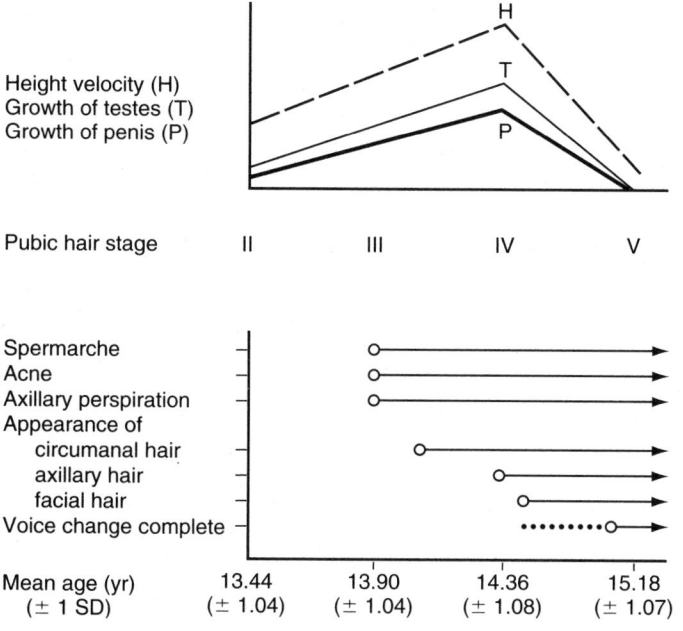

FIGURE 14–3. Sequence of maturational events in males. (Adapted from Marshall WA, Tanner JM: Variations in the pattern of pubertal changes in boys. *Arch Dis Child* 1970;45:13.)

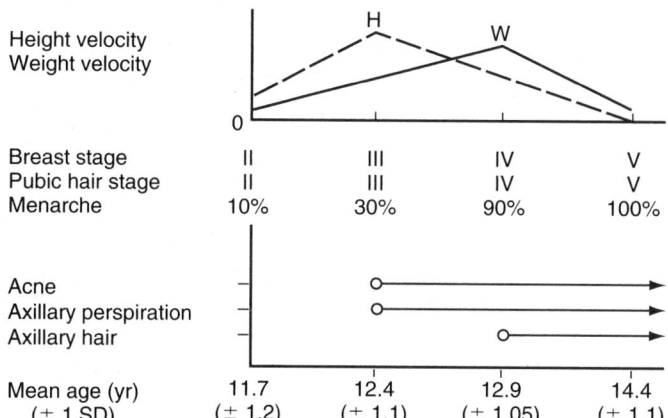

FIGURE 14–4. Sequence of maturational events in females. (Adapted from Marshall WA, Tanner JM: Variations in pattern of pubertal changes in girls. *Arch Dis Child* 1969;44:291.)

TABLE 14–5. Modal Age at Onset and Completion of Fusion in Skeletal Areas in Adolescence

Boys: Modal Age Between (yr)	Area	Girls: Modal Age Between (yr)
	Elbow	
13.0–13.5	Onset in humerus	11.0–11.5
15.0–15.5	Complete in ulna	12.5–13.0
	Foot and Ankle	
14.0–14.5	Onset in great toe	12.5–13.0
15.5–16	Complete in tibia, fibula	14.0–14.5
	Hand and Wrist	
15.0–15.5	Onset in distal phalanges	13.0–13.5
17.5–18.0	Complete in radius	16.0–16.5
	Knee	
15.0–15.5	Onset in tibial tuberosity	13.5–14.0
17.5–18.0	Complete in fibula	16.0–16.5
	Hip and Pelvis	
15.5–16.0	Onset in greater trochanter	14.0–14.5
after 18.0	Complete in symphysis	17.5–18.0
	Shoulder and Clavicle	
15.5–16.0	Onset in greater tubercle of humerus	14.0–14.5
after 18.0	Complete in clavicle	17.5–18.0

It is unclear whether or not the hormonal changes of puberty directly affect cognitive development.

The development of moral thinking roughly parallels general cognitive development. Most preadolescents perceive right and wrong as absolute and unquestionable. Taking a loaf of bread to feed a starving child is wrong because it is "stealing." Adolescents often question received morality, embracing the behavior standards of the peer group. Group membership may allow them to avoid guilt feelings for perceived moral infractions by shifting responsibility from themselves to the group.

Self-Concept. Self-consciousness increases exponentially in response to the somatic transformations of puberty. Self-awareness at this age tends to center on external characteristics in contrast to the introspection of later adolescence. It is normal for early adolescents to scrutinize their appearance and to feel that everyone else is staring at them too. Girls, in particular, are at risk for viewing themselves as overweight. Dieting behavior is common, and girls who rate themselves as fat/out of shape may be at increased risk of depression (Chapter 23). Severe body image distortions, such as anorexia nervosa, also tend to appear at this age (Chapter 104). There is controversy about whether puberty may increase self-esteem in boys but undermine it in girls as both sexes assume gender roles that incorporate societal inequalities in power and prestige.

Relationships with Family, Peers, and Society. In early adolescence, the trend toward separation from family with increasing involvement in peer activities accelerates. A symbolic expression of this shift is the renunciation of family norms of dress and grooming in favor of the peer group "uniform." Such stylistic changes frequently spark conflicts that are truly about power or difficulty accepting separation. Not all adolescents rebel, and not all parents reject such assertions of separateness as signs of insurrection. Most adolescents continue to strive to please their parents even while they disagree on certain issues.

Separation from family often involves selecting adults outside of the family as role models and developing close relationships with particular teachers or the parents of other children. Organizations such as scouting, sports teams, or gangs provide an important sense of extra-familial belonging.

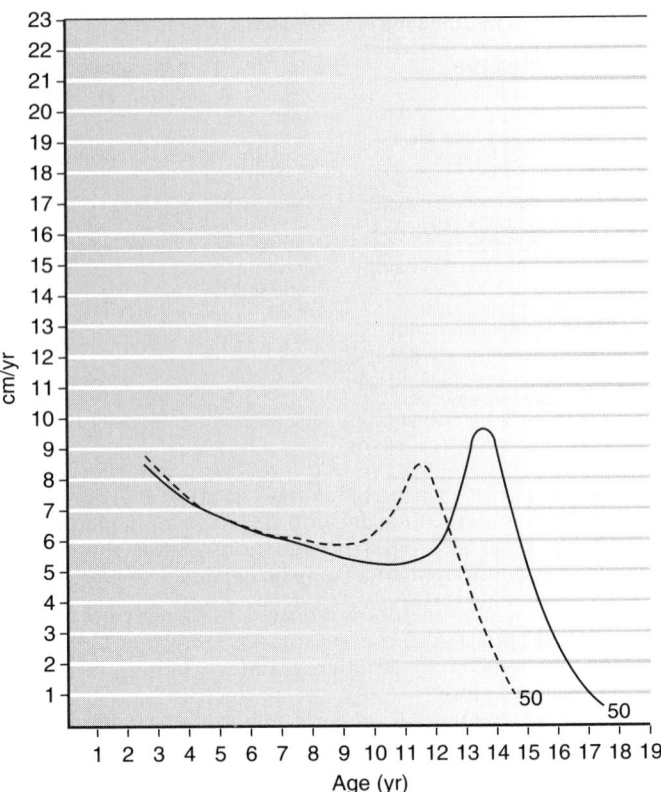

FIGURE 14–5. Height velocity curves for U.S. boys *(solid line)* and girls *(dashed line)* who have their peak height velocity at the average age (i.e., average growth tempo). (From Tanner JM, Davies PSW: Clinical longitudinal standards for height and height velocity for North American children. *J Pediatr* 1985;107: 317.)

Early adolescents often socialize in same-sex peer groups. Scatological jokes, teasing directed against the other gender, and rumor mongering about who likes whom attest to burgeoning sexual interest. Belonging is all important. In one-to-one friendships, boys and girls may differ in important ways. Female friendships may center on sharing confidences, whereas male relationships may focus more on shared activities and competition.

An early adolescent's relationship to society centers on school. The shift from elementary to junior high school entails giving up the protection of the homeroom in exchange for the additional stimulation and responsibility involved in moving from class to class. This change in school structure mirrors and reinforces the changes involved in separating from the family.

The societal preoccupation with youth and sexuality generates constant exposure to sexually suggestive and explicit images. At the same time, reliable information about sexuality in general, and contraception in particular, remains sparse. Ready access to pornography on the Internet may increase the risk of premature sexual activity or exploitation.

Implications for Parents and Pediatricians. Physical growth, body preoccupation, and sexual interest correlate with sexual maturity, whereas cognitive advancement, separation, and changes in social behavior may correlate more closely with chronological age or grade in school. Discordance between chronological age and sexual maturation may increase the stress of early adolescence. As a group, early maturing boys enjoy greater social success and higher self-esteem than do those who mature later. For girls, by contrast, early maturation is associated with poorer school performance and lower self-esteem.

Early adolescents often have questions about the somatic and sexual changes they are experiencing. Among both rural and urban adolescents, the range of sophistication is wide. During a physical examination, a pediatrician can anticipate concerns and volunteer information that the adolescent may have been too uncomfortable to request. Parents, too, may have concerns that they are hesitant to discuss. If the parent is interviewed alone, it is important that this be done first, before the interview with the child, to avoid undermining the adolescent's trust.

The adolescent's level of cognitive sophistication has implications for the sort of explanations that will be most helpful. Open-ended questions about common dilemmas facing young adolescents (e.g., whether or not to join a clique or gang or to abide by family rules that seem unjustified) can provide information about cognitive level and help assess the likelihood of risky behavior (see Chapters 5 and 17).

Parents and children often need help differentiating between the normal discomforts of the age and truly concerning behaviors. Discomfort with one's body is normal; the conviction that one is overweight and needs to diet despite objective evidence to the contrary is concerning. Bids for autonomy in the form of avoidance of family activities, demands for privacy, and increased argumentativeness are normal; extreme withdrawal or antagonism may be a sign of dysfunction. Interest in sex, sometimes heralded by the appearance of pornographic magazines, is normal; sexual intercourse in early adolescence, though fairly common, is usually a sign of developmental dysfunction. Bewilderment and dysphoria at the start of junior high school are normal; continued failure to adapt several weeks to months later suggests a more serious problem.

MIDDLE ADOLESCENCE

Biologic Development. In middle adolescence, growth accelerates above the prepubertal rate of 6–7 cm (3 in) per year. In the average girl, the growth spurt peaks at 11.5 yr at a top velocity of 8.3 cm (3.8 in) per year and then slows to a stop at 16 yr (see Fig. 14–4). In the average boy, the growth spurt starts later, peaks at 13.5 yr at 9.5 cm (4.3 in) per year, and then slows to a stop at 18 yr. Weight gain parallels linear growth, with a delay of several months, so that adolescents seem first to stretch and then fill out. Pubertal weight gains account for approximately 40% of adult weight. Muscle mass also increases, followed several months later by an increase in strength; boys show greater gains in both. Lean body mass, approximately 80% in the average prepubertal child, increases in boys to 90% and decreases in girls to 75% as subcutaneous fat accumulates.

Bone maturation correlates closely with SMR because epiphyseal closure is under androgenic control (Table 14–5). Boys with SMR3 pubic hair and SMR4 genitals normally have their peak growth spurt ahead of them; girls at the same SMR are usually past their peaks (see Figs. 14–3 and 14–4). Widening of the shoulders in boys and of the hips in girls is also hormonally determined. Other physiologic changes include a doubling in heart size and lung vital capacity from preadolescent norms. Blood pressure, blood volume, and hematocrit rise, particularly in boys. Androgenic stimulation of sebaceous and apocrine glands results in acne and body odor. A physiologic increase in sleepiness may be mistaken for laziness.

Sexual maturation in middle adolescence is dramatic, with the achievement of menarche in 30% of girls by SMR3 (mean age 12–14 yr) and in 90% by SMR4 (mean age 13–15 yr). Menarche usually follows approximately 1 yr after the growth spurt begins. The timing of menarche, not completely understood, appears to be determined by genetics as well as such factors as adiposity, chronic illness, and exercise. In developed countries, the average age at menarche has decreased in the past century, perhaps in response to better nutrition and less physical activity. Before menarche, the uterus achieves a mature config-

uration, vaginal lubrication increases, and a clear vaginal discharge appears, sometimes mistaken for a sign of infection. In boys, spermarche occurs and the penis lengthens and widens.

Sexuality. Dating becomes a normative activity during middle adolescence. The degree of sexual activity varies widely. At age 16 yr, approximately 30% of girls and 45% of boys report having sexual intercourse, whereas 17% report petting, and some 22% report kissing as the only sexual behavior.

Biologic maturation and social pressures combine to determine sexual activity. High testosterone and low religiosity together may predict which boys become sexually active. Most parents discourage sexual activity, but some actually encourage it in hopes of boosting the child's popularity or of living vicariously through the child's experiences. *Homosexual experimentation* is common and does not necessarily reflect a child's ultimate sexual orientation. Many adolescents worry that they might be homosexual, and dread being found out. As a result, homosexual dating and sexual activity during adolescence are rare. Homosexual adolescents face increased risk of isolation and depression. Fear of stigmatization may keep them from discussing their concerns with pediatricians or other potentially helpful adults (see Chapter 26).

In addition to sexual orientation, middle adolescents begin to sort out other important aspects of sexual identity, including beliefs about love, honesty, and propriety. Dating relationships are often superficial at this age, emphasizing attractiveness and sexual experimentation rather than intimacy. Adolescents tend to choose one of three sexual paths: celibacy, monogamy, or polygamous experimentation. Most have some knowledge of the risks of pregnancy, acquired immunodeficiency syndrome, and other sexually transmitted diseases, but knowledge does not consistently control behavior. A minority use any contraception at first intercourse, and fewer than 75% consistently use condoms or other effective methods.

Cognitive and Moral Development. With the transition to formal operational thought, middle adolescents question and analyze extensively. Questioning of moral conventions fosters the development of personal codes of ethics. Such codes often appear designed to justify the adolescent's sexual appetite: "Anything I want is right." In other cases, adolescents may embrace a code that is more strict than that of their parents, perhaps in response to the anxiety engendered by the weakening of the conventional limits. An adolescent's new flexibility of thought has pervasive effects on relationships with self and others.

Self-Concept. The peer group exerts less influence over dress, activities, and behavior. Middle adolescents often experiment with different personae, changing styles of dress, groups of friends, and interests from month to month. Many philosophize about the meaning of their lives and wonder, "Who am I?" and "Why am I here?" Intense feelings of inner turmoil and misery are common and may be difficult to differentiate from psychiatric illness. Girls may tend to characterize themselves and their peers according to interpersonal relationships ("I am a girl with close friends"), whereas boys as a group may focus on abilities ("I am good at sports").

Relationships with Family, Peers, and Society. Puberty commonly results in strained relationships between adolescents and their parents. As part of separation, adolescents may become distant from parents, redirecting emotional and sexual energies toward peer relationships. Dating can become a lightning rod for parent-child battles, in which the real issue may be the fact of separation rather than the particulars of "with whom" or "how late."

As dating increases, the need to belong to same-sex groups declines. Physical attractiveness and popularity remain critical factors in both peer relationships and self-esteem. Children with visible differences, such as cleft lip, are at risk for problems developing social skills and confidence and may have more difficulty establishing satisfying relationships.

Middle adolescents often begin thinking seriously about what they want to do as adults, a question that formerly had been comfortably hypothetical. The process involves self-assessment and assessment of the opportunities available. The presence or absence of realistic role models, as opposed to the idealized ones of earlier periods, can be crucial.

Implications for Parents and Pediatricians. Physical and sexual maturation, changes in sexual behavior and identity, emotional distance from parents, waning peer group influence, introspection, and growing cognizance of life after childhood all combine to make middle adolescence a time when the opportunity to talk confidentially with a nonjudgmental, informed adult can be particularly appreciated and helpful.

Adolescents vary greatly in their rate of physical and social progress and in the resolution of central conflicts about autonomy and self-esteem. Questions about family and peer relationships can help locate a child along the developmental continuum and facilitate individualized counseling. In asking about dating and sex, it is important not to convey the assumption of heterosexuality because that will reduce the likelihood that concerns about sexual orientation will surface. In talking to a boy, for example, one might observe that some boys are interested sexually in girls, some boys are interested in other boys, and some are interested in both (or neither).

LATE ADOLESCENCE

Biologic Development. The somatic changes in this period are modest by comparison. The final stages of breast, penile, and pubic hair development occur by 17–18 yr of age in 95% of males and females. Minor changes in hair distribution often continue for several years in males, including the growth of facial and chest hair and the onset of male-pattern baldness in a few.

Psychosocial Development. Sexual experimentation decreases as adolescents adopt more stable sexual identities. Cognition tends to be less self-centered, with increasing thoughts about concepts such as justice, patriotism, and history. Older adolescents are often idealistic but also may be absolutist and intolerant of opposing views. Religious or political groups that promise answers to complex questions may hold great appeal.

Slowing physical changes permit the emergence of a more stable body image. Intimate relationships are also an important component of identity for many older adolescents. In contrast to the often superficial dating relationships of middle adolescence, these relationships increasingly involve love and commitment. Career decisions become pressing because an adolescent's self-concept is increasingly bound up in the emerging role in society (as student, worker, or parent).

Implications for Parents and Pediatricians. Erikson identified the crucial task of adolescence as that of establishing a stable sense of identity, including separation from family of origin, initiation of intimacy, and realistic planning for economic independence. To achieve these milestones, developmental progress is required of both adolescents and their parents. Continued difficulty in any of these areas may constitute an indication for referral for counseling.

Delemarre-van de Waal HA: Regulation of puberty. *Best Pract Res Clin Endocrinol Metab* 2002;16:1–12.

Felice M, Maehr J: Eleven to thirteen years: Early adolescence—age of rapid changes. Fourteen to sixteen years: Mid-adolescence—dating game. In Dixon SD, Stein MT (editors): *Encounters with Children: Pediatric Behavior and Development.* St Louis, Mosby, 2000, pp 426–476.

Ford CA, Coleman WL: Adolescent development and behavior: Implications for the primary care physician. In Levine MD, Carey WB, Crocker AC (editors): *Developmental-Behavioral Pediatrics,* 3rd ed. Philadelphia, WB Saunders, 1999, pp 69–80.

Marshall WA, Tanner JM: Variations in the pattern of pubertal change in girls. *Arch Dis Child* 1969;44:291.

Marshall WA, Tanner JM: Variations in the pattern of pubertal change in boys. *Arch Dis Child* 1970;45:13.

Rutter M, Graham P, Chadwick OFD, et al: Adolescent turmoil: Fact or fiction? *J Child Psychol Psychiatr* 1976;17:35.

Tanner JM, Davies PSW: Clinical longitudinal standards for height and height velocity for North American children. *J Pediatr* 1985;107:317.

Chapter 15
Assessment of Growth

Growth assessment is an essential component of pediatric health surveillance because almost any problem within the physiologic, interpersonal, and social domains can adversely affect growth. The most powerful tool in growth assessment is the growth chart (see Figs. 11–1 and 11–2). Combined with an accurate scale, a length board, stadiometer, and tape measure, the growth chart provides most of the information needed to assess growth. Major concerns are undernutrition and failure to thrive, but in addition obesity is now recognized as a growing epidemic.

GROWTH CHART DERIVATION AND INTERPRETATION

In 2000, the Centers for Disease Control and Prevention (CDC) published revised growth charts, with significant improvements. The new charts contain data from five national surveys conducted between 1963 and 1994. Analyses were done to render the data representative of the United States population, both demographically and in terms of breast-feeding prevalence. Excluded from the charts are data from very low birthweight children, because their growth patterns are different, and also the most recent data for children 6 yr of age and older, so that the recent rapid increase in the prevalence of obesity would not unduly raise the upper limits of normal. Several deficiencies of the older charts have been corrected, such as the over-representation of bottle-fed infants, and the reliance on a local data set for the infant charts. The disjunction between length and height, when moving from the infant curves to those for older children, no longer exists, and z-scores (see Chapter 7) calculated from the curves now match those calculated using the standard CDC software. Most importantly, the new standard provides body mass index (BMI, see below) curves through age 20 yr, facilitating identification of obesity.

It is important to realize that the revised charts do not represent *optimal* growth, because they still incorporate data from many bottle-fed infants. Compared to the current standards, an exclusively breast-fed infant would be expected to plot higher for weight in the first 6 mo of life, but relatively lower in the 2nd half of the 1st year. Awareness of this growth difference should avoid overidentification of growth problems in breast-fed infants. The World Health Organization (WHO) is developing charts based on exclusively breast-fed infants, which will become the international standard for children up to 5 yr of age.

Caution must also be used in applying the charts to adolescents. Growth during adolescence is linked temporally to the onset of puberty, which varies widely (Chapter 14). By using cross-sectional data based on chronological age, the charts lump together subjects who are at different stages of maturation. For example, the data for 12-yr-old boys include both early-maturing boys who are at the peak of their growth spurts and later-maturing ones who are still growing at their prepubertal rate. The net result is to artifactually level off the growth peak, making it seem as though adolescent children grow more gradually and for a longer period than they do. The standard charts may indicate poor or excessive growth when a child is growing normally but happens to be a late or early maturer. Growth charts derived from longitudinal data are recommended for adolescents, when precision is necessary.

For infants, the measure of linear growth is *length*, taken by two examiners (one to position the child) with the child supine on a measuring board. For older children, the measure is *stature*, taken with a child standing on a stadiometer. This technical difference results in children's appearing to shift down in length as they change from the younger to the older chart. The data are presented in five standard charts: (1) weight for age; (2) height (length and stature) for age; (3) head circumference for age; (4) weight for height (length and stature); and (5) BMI. Separate charts are provided for boys and girls (see Figs. 11–1 and 11–2). Charts with lines for the 3rd and 97th percentile are also available.

Each chart is composed of seven or eight percentile curves, representing the distribution of weight, length, stature, or head circumference values at each age. The percentile curve indicates the percentage of children at a given age on the *x*-axis whose measured value falls below the corresponding value on the *y*-axis. For example, on the weight chart for boys 0–36 mo of age (see Fig. 11–1*A*), the 9-mo age line intersects the 25th percentile curve at 8.6 kg, indicating that 25% of the 9-mo-old boys in the National Center for Health Statistics sample weigh less than 8.6 kg (75% weigh more). Similarly, a 9-mo-old boy weighing more than 11.2 kg is heavier than 95% of his peers.

By definition, the 50th percentile is the median, the value above (and below) which 50% of the observed values fall. It is also termed the *standard value* in the sense that the standard height for a 7-mo girl is 67 cm (see Fig. 11–1*B*). The weight-for-height charts (see Fig. 11–2) are constructed in an analogous fashion, with length or stature in place of age on the *x*-axis. According to the chart, the median or standard weight for a girl measuring 110 cm is 18.6 kg.

The numeric data on which the charts are based are presented in Tables 12–1 and 12–2. The charts are useful because they facilitate assessment of growth over time. Specialized charts have also been developed for United States children with various conditions, including Down, Turner, and Klinefelter syndromes and achondroplasia.

ANALYSIS OF GROWTH PATTERNS

Growth is a process rather than a static quality. An infant at the 5th percentile of weight for age may be growing normally, may be failing to grow, or may be recovering from growth failure, depending on the *trajectory* of the growth curve. Typically, infants and children stay within one or two growth channels. This *canalization* attests to the robust control that genes exert over body size.

A normal exception commonly occurs during the 1st 2 yr of life. For full-term infants, size at birth reflects the influence of the uterine environment; size at age 2 yr correlates with mean parental height, reflecting the influence of genes. Between birth and 18 mo, small infants often shift percentiles upward toward their parents' mean percentile. Large neonates with smaller parents often shift downward, with decelerating growth beginning at 3–6 mo and ending as an infant achieves a new growth channel at approximately 13–18 mo.

It is important to correct for various factors in plotting and interpreting growth charts. For premature infants, overdiagnosis of growth failure can be avoided by subtracting the weeks of prematurity from the postnatal age when plotting growth parameters. Very low birthweight (VLBW, <1,500 g) infants may continue to show *catch-up growth* through early school age. The presence of neurologic abnormality (e.g., cerebral palsy) in VLBW infants may limit catch-up growth. Growth standards for premature infants were published in the 1960s and recently updated (in Scandinavia).

For adolescents, normal variations in the timing of the growth spurt can lead to misdiagnosis of growth abnormalities. In general

practice, cognizance of the relationship between sexual maturity and growth suffices (see Chapter 14). Special growth charts have been developed for early-, average-, and late-maturing adolescents that can be used when additional precision is needed. For children with particularly tall or short parents, there is a risk of overdiagnosing growth disorders if parental height is not taken into account or, conversely, of underdiagnosing growth disorders if parental height is accepted uncritically as the explanation. Standards have been developed to allow adjustments on the adolescent height curve based on mean parental height. These charts are based on a small, possibly nonrepresentative sample, which limits the generalizability of these standards.

The analysis of growth patterns provides critical information for the diagnosis of *failure to thrive* (FTT) (see Chapter 36). There is no universally agreed-on criterion for FTT or growth failure; most consider the diagnosis if a child's weight is below the 5th percentile or drops down more than two major percentile lines. Calculation of weight gain in grams per day, using Table 10–5 for age-related standards, allows more precise estimation of growth rate.

Weight-for-height below the 5th percentile remains the single best growth chart indicator of acute undernutrition. Children who have been chronically malnourished may be short as well as thin, so that their weight-for-height curves may appear relatively normal. Chronic, severe undernutrition in infancy can also depress head growth, an ominous predictor of later cognitive disability.

When growth parameters fall below the 5th percentile, it becomes necessary to express the values as percentages of the median or standard value. For example, a 12-mo-old girl weighing 7.1 kg is at 75% of the median weight (9.5 kg) for her age. Using the calculated percentage of standard rather than the percentile, growth failure can be graded from mild to severe according to Table 15–1. These designations correlate with risk of mortality in developing countries; their correlation with short- and long-term sequelae of growth failure in the United States is less well documented. Another way to describe extremes of height is the *height age*, the age at which the standard (median) height equals the child's present height. A 30-mo-old child who is as tall as an average 13 mo old has a height age of 13 mo. The *weight age* is defined analogously.

Nutritional insufficiency must be differentiated from congenital, constitutional, familial, and endocrine causes of decreased linear growth (see also Chapter 42). In the latter cases, the length declines first or at the same time as the weight; weight for height is normal or elevated. In nutritional insufficiency, the weight declines before the length and the weight for height is low (unless there has been chronic stunting). Figure 15–1 depicts typical growth curves for four classes of decreased linear growth. In congenital pathologic short stature, an infant is born small and growth gradually tapers off throughout infancy. Causes include chromosomal abnormalities (Turner syndrome, trisomy 21), infection (TORCH [toxoplasmosis, other infections,

TABLE 15–1. Severity of Malnutrition: Stunting and Wasting

Grade of Malnutrition	Weight for Age* (Wasting)	Height for Age† (Stunting)	Weight for Height‡
0, normal	>90	>95	>90
1, mild	75–90	90–95	81–90
2, moderate	60–74	85–89	70–80
3, severe	<60	<85	<70

Values represent percentage of median for age.

*Data from Gomez F, Galvan RR, Frank S, et al: Mortality in second- and third-degree malnutrition. J Trop Pediatr, 2:77, 1956.

†Data from Waterlow JC: Evolution of kwashiorkor and marasmus. Lancet, 2:712, 1974.

‡Data from Waterlow JC: Classification and definition of protein-calorie malnutrition. BMJ 3:566, 1972.

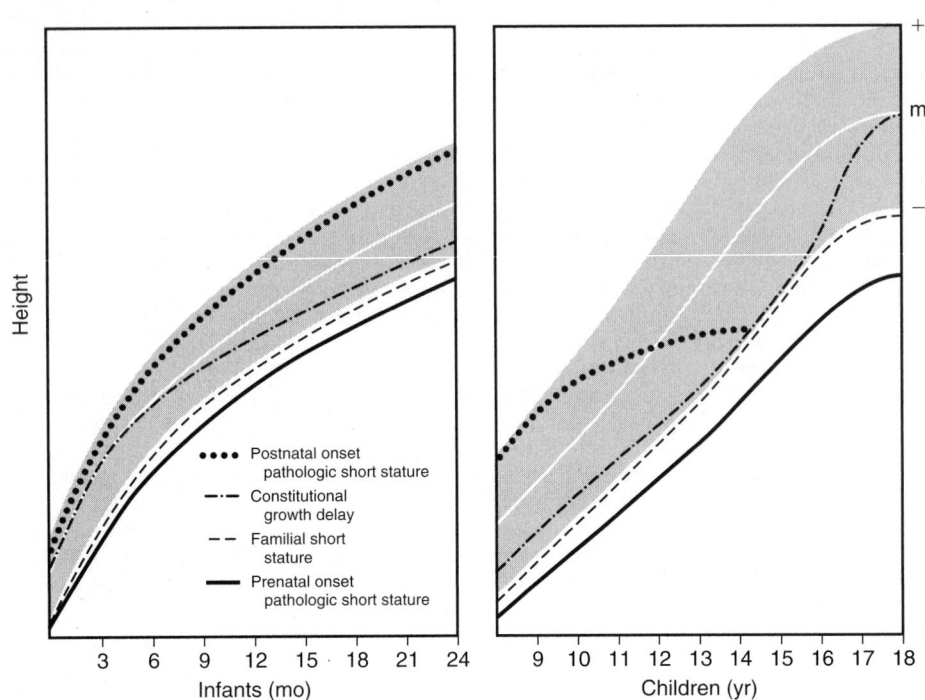

FIGURE 15–1. Height for age curves of the four general causes of proportional short stature: postnatal onset pathologic short stature, constitutional growth delay, familial short stature, and prenatal onset short stature. (From Mahoney CP: Evaluating the child with short stature. *Pediatr Clin North Am* 1987;34:825.)

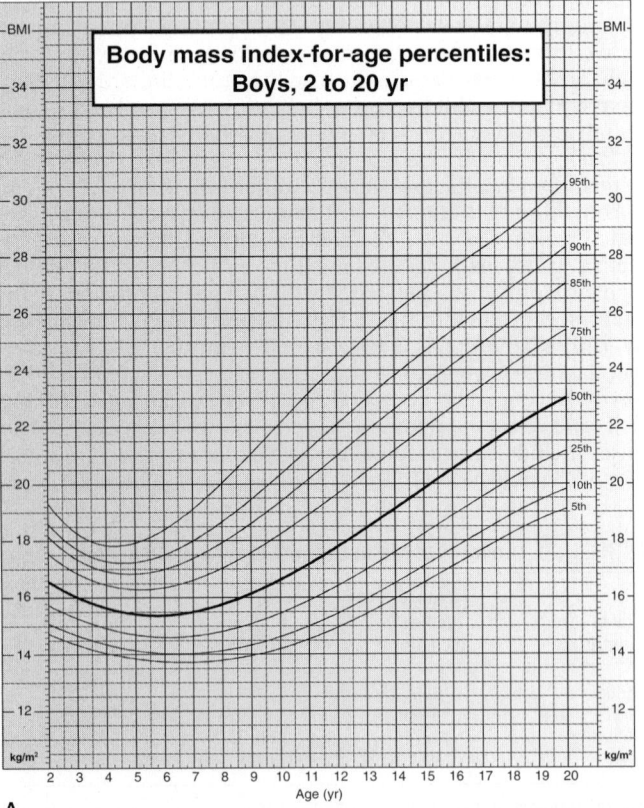

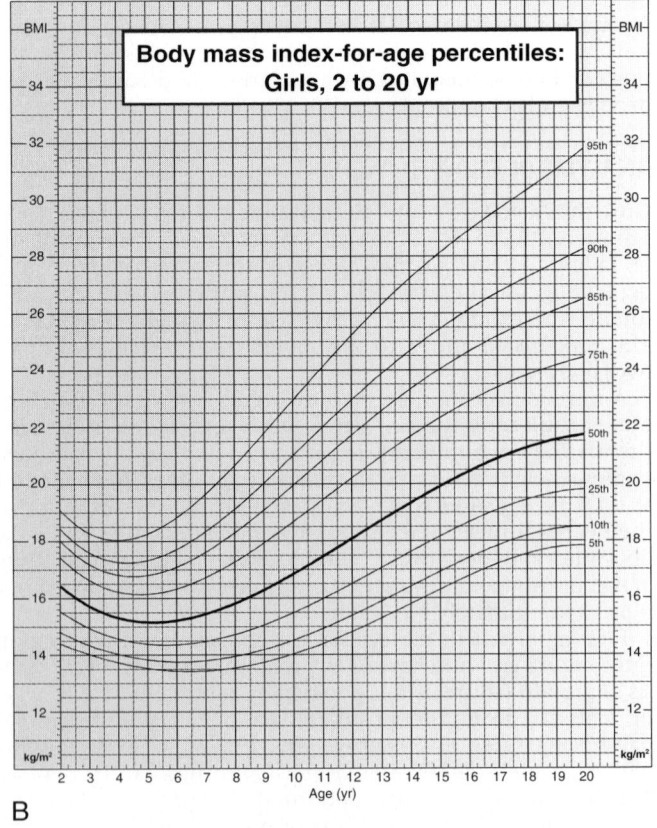

FIGURE 15–2. Body mass index (BMI) percentiles for boys *(A)* and girls *(B)* age 2–20 yr. (Official Centers for Disease Control [CDC] growth charts, as described in this chapter. 85th to 95th percentile is "at risk for overweight"; >95th percentile is "overweight"; <5th percentile is "underweight." Technical information and interpretation and management guides are available at www.cdc.gov/nchs. See also Table 12–2.)

rubella, cytomegalovirus infection, and herpes simplex] infections), teratogens (phenytoin [Dilantin], alcohol), and extreme prematurity. In constitutional growth delay, weight and height decrease near the end of infancy, parallel the norm through middle childhood, and accelerate toward the end of adolescence. Adult size is normal. In familial short stature, both the infant and parents are small; growth runs parallel to and just below the normal curves.

Growth charts can confirm an impression of obesity if the weight for height exceeds 120% of the standard (median) weight for height. The *body mass index* (BMI) can be calculated as weight per height^2 when weight is in kilograms and height is in meters (Fig. 15–2). If measurements are made in pounds and inches, the conversion requires 2 steps: (1) convert fractions to decimals (thus, 32 $^3/_4$ lbs becomes 32.75) and (2) calculate BMI as lbs per inch^2, then multiply by 730 (thus, a BMI of 0.031 lbs/in^2 corresponds to a BMI of 22 kg/m^2, which can then be plotted on standard BMI tables; see Fig. 15–2). According to the CDC, a BMI over the 95th percentile indicates "overweight," between 85th and 95th percentile is "risk of overweight," and below the 5th percentile is "underweight." Although widely accepted as the best clinical measure of under- and overweight, BMI may not provide an accurate index of adiposity, because it does not differentiate lean tissue and bone from fat. Measurement of triceps and subscapular skinfold thickness give a better estimate of adiposity (Fig. 15–3), although considerable experience is needed for accuracy, and variability in fat distribution may confound the measurement.

Accurate measurement of weight and length is of obvious importance. Scales should be calibrated regularly. Supine length should be measured on a board; length measurements using a tape are inaccurate. Stature is best measured using a stadiometer; swing-arm measuring sticks attached to office scales are inaccurate. Head circumference is measured from the supraorbital ridge in front to the farthest point of the occiput in back. Cloth tapes stretch and should be avoided.

OTHER INDICES OF GROWTH

Body Proportions. Body proportions follow a sequence of regular changes with development. The head and trunk are relatively large at birth, with progressive lengthening of the limbs throughout development, particularly during puberty (Chapter 14). Proportionality can be assessed by measuring the *lower body segment,* defined as the length from the symphysis pubis to the floor, and the *upper body segment,* defined as the height minus the lower body segment. The ratio of upper body segment divided by lower body segment (U/L ratio) equals approximately 1.7 at birth, 1.3 at 3 yr of age, and 1.0 after 7 yr of age. Higher U/L ratios are characteristic of short-limb dwarfism or bone disorders such as rickets.

Skeletal Maturation. Reference standards for bone maturation facilitate estimation of bone age (see Tables 10–7 and 14–5). *Bone age* correlates well with stage of pubertal development and can be helpful in predicting adult height in early- or late-maturing adolescents. In familial short stature, the bone age is normal (comparable to chronological age). In constitutional delay, endocrinologic short stature, and undernutrition, the bone age is low and comparable to the height age. The most commonly used standards are those of Gruelich and Pyle, which require radiographs of the left hand and wrist; knee films are sometimes added for younger children. Sontag's method requires radiographs of each major joint on the left side of the body. A method developed by Tanner and colleagues may offer added accuracy. Skeletal maturation is linked more closely to sexual maturity rating than to chronological age. It is more rapid and less variable in girls than in boys.

Dental Development. Dental development includes mineralization, eruption, and exfoliation (see Table 10–6). Initial mineralization begins as early as the second trimester (mean age for central incisors, 14 wk) and continues through 3 yr of age for the primary (deciduous) teeth and 25 yr of age for the permanent teeth. Mineralization begins at the crown and progresses toward the root. Mean ages for eruption of primary teeth are given in Table 10–6. Eruption begins with the central incisors and progresses laterally. Exfoliation begins at about 6 yr of age and continues through 12 yr of age. Eruption of the permanent teeth may follow exfoliation immediately or may lag by 4–5 mo. The timing of dental development is poorly correlated with other processes of growth and maturation.

Delayed eruption is usually considered when there are no teeth by approximately 13 mo of age (mean +3 SD). Common causes include hypothyroid, hypoparathyroid, familial, and (the most common) idiopathic. Individual teeth may fail to erupt because of mechanical blockage (crowding, gum fibrosis). Causes of early exfoliation include histiocytosis X, cyclic neutropenia, trauma, and idiopathic factors. Nutritional and metabolic disturbances, prolonged illness, and certain medications (tetracycline) commonly result in discoloration or malformations of the dental enamel. A discrete line of pitting on the enamel suggests a time-limited insult.

Physiologic and Structural Growth. Virtually every organ and physiologic process undergoes a predictable sequence of structural or functional changes, or both, during development. Reference values for developmental changes in a wide variety of systems (pituitary and renal function, electroencephalogram, electrocardiogram) have been published. Physiologic and structural changes of particular relevance to general pediatrics include the following:

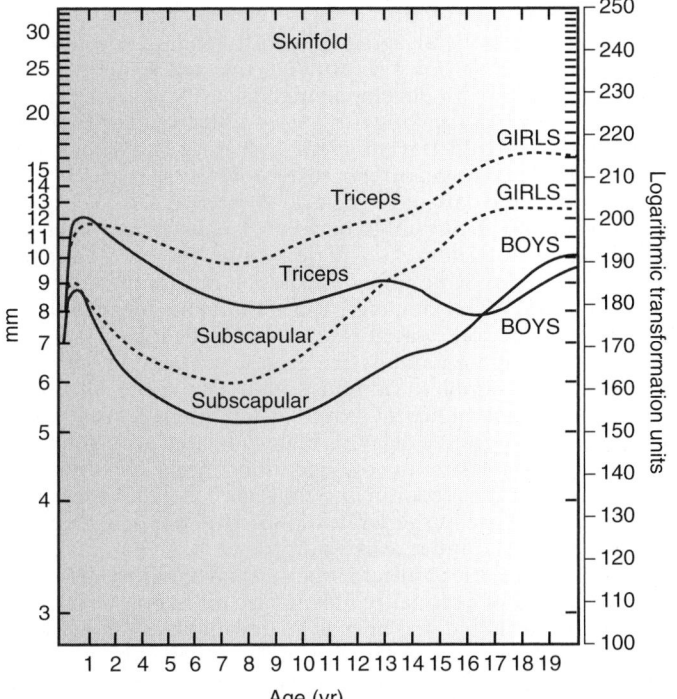

FIGURE 15–3. Skinfold thickness by age and sex, as measured by Harpenden skinfold calipers over triceps and under scapula. Scale is in millimeters on the left side and logarithmic transformation units on the right side. The lines shown are the 50th percentiles for British children. (From Tanner JM: *Fetus into Man: Physical Growth from Conception to Maturity.* Cambridge, MA, Harvard University Press, 1978.)

1. Respiratory rate and pulse rate decrease sharply during the first 2 yr and then more gradually throughout childhood; blood pressure rises steadily beginning at approximately 6 yr of age (Chapters 356 and 415).

2. Development of the paranasal sinuses continues throughout childhood. The ethmoids, maxillary, and sphenoid sinuses are present from birth; the frontal sinuses first appear radiologically around 6 yr of age. The ethmoids reach their maximum size relatively early in childhood (7–14 yr of age); the others reach their maximum size after puberty (also see Chapter 365).

3. Lymphoid tissues develop rapidly, reaching adult size by 6 yr of age and continuing to hypertrophy throughout childhood and early adolescence before receding to adult size (Chapter 480).

4. The metabolism of medications and a child's response to them change rapidly in the 1st mo of life and again under hormonal influences in puberty. No single pattern is characteristic of all medications, and individual variation is the rule. Awareness of the possibility of changes and close monitoring are important (see Chapter 711).

5. Nutritional needs as well as a wide variety of biochemical and hematologic values undergo marked developmental changes. For example, the alkaline phosphatase level increases during periods of rapid bone growth (Chapter 691); hemoglobin has a physiologic nadir at approximately 2 mo of age (see Chapter 445).

Bowers DF: Tooth development and abnormalities of appearance. In Johnson TR, Moore WM, Jeffries JE (editors): *Children Are Different: Developmental Physiology.* Columbus, OH, Ross Laboratories, 1978, pp 64–67.

Ogden CL, Kuczmarski RJ, Flegal KM, et al: Centers for Disease Control and Prevention 2000 growth charts for the United States: Improvements to the 1977 National Center for Health Statistics version. *Pediatrics* 2002;109:45–60.

Skjaerven R, Gjessing HK, Bakketeig LS: New standards for birth weight by gestational age using family data. *Am J Obstet Gynecol* 2000;183:689–96.

Strauss RS: Childhood obesity. *Pediatr Clin North Am* 2002;49:175–201.

Tanner JM, Davies PSW: Clinical longitudinal standards for height and height velocity for North American children. *J Pediatr* 1985;107:317.

Tanner JM, Whitehouse RH, Cameron N, et al: *Assessment of Skeletal Maturity and Prediction of Adult Height (TW2 Method).* London, Academic Press, 1983.

Tillmann V, Thalange NK, Foster PJ, et al: The relationship between stature, growth, and short-term changes in height and weight in normal prepubertal children. *Pediatr Res* 1998;44:882–6.

Chapter 16
Developmental Assessment

Developmental assessment includes early identification of problems through screening and surveillance, and more definitive assessment including both standardized and nonstandardized measures, as well as integration of information from the developmental, social, and family history and the medical history and examination. The goal of developmental assessment is not only to generate a diagnosis, but equally important to analyze the pattern of strengths and weaknesses in the child, family, and available developmental, educational, and social support systems, in order to direct treatment.

The 1990 Individuals with Disabilities Education Act (IDEA) requires that every state in the United States create a system to identify and treat developmental disabilities in children 3–5 yr of age, and all states extend these entitlements to children beginning at birth to children deemed at risk for developmental problems and to those with established delays. Pediatricians should have a central role in early identification, although in practice this is not always the case (Chapters 29, 37, and 39). They are most effective in detecting disabilities associated with congenital or genetic abnormalities. Less dramatic problems in cognition, language, learning, and behavior are often first detected by parents or teachers.

Screening and Surveillance. The ideal screening test must be highly sensitive (detect nearly all children with problems) and reasonably specific (label few healthy children as ill or delayed). It should also measure what it purports to measure (content validity), give similar results on repeat administration and on administration by different examiners (test-retest and inter-rater reliability), and be relatively quick and inexpensive. Table 16–1 lists several of the more common screening tests and their strengths and limitations. The ideal developmental screening test does not exist.

The most widely used and researched test is the Denver Developmental Screening Test-II (Denver II). However, despite its popularity, it does not function well as a screening test, having limited sensitivity for subtle delays and modest predictive validity. It remains of value because it offers clinicians 125 easily administered developmental test items, with age norms (generated from a large Colorado sample) presented in a convenient one-page format. A series of brief parent questionnaires based on the Denver II milestones and a questionnaire assessing the home environment are also available.

Rapid screening with reasonably good sensitivity and specificity is possible using a structured set of 10 questions eliciting parental concerns in various areas of development. The approach has been formalized as the Parents' Evaluation of Developmental Status (PEDS) questionnaire. The approach works because parents are generally accurate observers of their children's development and behavior. Screening efficiency can be further enhanced by using a formal screening test as a second-level screen for any child "flagged" by systematic parent questioning.

The Ages and Stages Questionnaires (ASQ) are a series of 11 questionnaires designed to be completed at home by parents at several time points from 4 to 48 mo. Validity and reliability are established, with overall agreement with standard developmental tests of 76–91%. However, the ASQ may fail to identify up to 13% of children with developmental delays. Scoring and interpretation are quick, making the ASQ especially suitable for busy practices. The Child Development Inventory is another well-standardized parent-report measure.

Screening for language delays is particularly important because of the strong links between language and cognitive development and later school performance. The Early Language Milestone (ELM) Scale provides pass-fail ratings in expressive, receptive, and visual language, using a format similar to that of the Denver. The scale was normed on a racially mixed sample of middle-class children and has been well validated in both low- and high-risk samples. Administration takes 2–3 min; most items can be completed by parental reporting. Sensitivity for language and cognitive delays is high compared with gold standard diagnostic tests; the test identifies many children even before their parents report being concerned. A modified scoring method can be used to generate a numeric score or age equivalent for diagnostic and research purposes.

Like the ELM, the Clinical Linguistic and Auditory Milestone Scale (CLAMS) is a sequence of language milestones that can be quickly administered, has been validated in infants and toddlers suspected of language delay and in those with known motor delays, and correlates well with standard diagnostic language tests. Paired with a similar series of nonverbal adaptive (problem-solving) milestones, the test correlates well with a gold standard test of mental retardation.

Other procedures that can be useful for developmental screening include the draw-a-person test and the kinetic family drawing ("draw your family, with everybody doing something"). A box of eight new crayons is nearly irresistible to most young children. The crayons can be used for counting, identify-

TABLE 16–1. **Instruments and Questionnaires for Brief Developmental Assessment**

Instrument	Age Range	Time (min)	Notes	Source
Denver-II	0–6 yr	30–45	Better sensitivity for language delays than older version	Denver Developmental Materials, PO Box 6169, Denver, CO 80206
Early Screening Inventory	3–6 yr	15–20	A quick, multidomain screen with good sensitivity and specificity compared with McCarthy Scales (a well-accepted test)	Teachers College Press, 1234 Amsterdam Ave, New York, NY 10027
ELM	0–3 yr	5–10	Well-normed, quick screen for expressive, receptive, and visual language; very useful in infancy; does not assess other domains	Pro-Ed, 8700 Shoal Creek Boulevard, Austin, TX 78757–6897
CAT/CLAMS	0–3 yr	10–20	CLAMS alone gives quick language quotient; CAT/CLAMS correlates well with Bayley (traditional gold standard)	Contact Dr. AJ Capute, The Kennedy Institute for Handicapped Children, 707 North Broadway St., Baltimore, MD 21205
Ages and Stages Questionnaires (ASQ)	4–48 mo	15–20	Series of self-administered questionnaires; multiple domains; good sensitivity and specificity; designed for ages that fall *between* usual pediatric schedule (e.g., 4, 8, 16 months)	Paul H Brookes Publishing Co., PO Box 10624, Baltimore, MD 21285
PEDS	0–8 yr	<5	Well-documented psychometrics; can be self-administered by parents	Ellsworth & Vandermeer Press, 4405 Scenic Drive, Nashville, TN 37204
PEER, PEEX, and PEERAMID	4–15 yr (different tests)	45	Rich source of observations and analysis of school-related functions, weak on validation	Educators Publishing Service, 31 Smith Place, Cambridge, MA 02138–9731, www.epsbooks.com

ELM = Early Language Milestone Scale; CAT = Clinical Adaptive Test; CLAMS = Clinical Linguistic and Auditory Milestone Scale; PEDS = Parents' Evaluation of Developmental Status; PEER = Pediatric Examination of Educational Readiness; PEEX = Pediatric Early Elementary Examination; PEERAMID = Pediatric Examination of Educational Readiness at Middle Childhood.

Adapted from Blackman JA: Developmental screening: Infants, toddlers, and preschoolers. In Levine MD, Carey WB, Crocker AC (editors): Developmental-Behavioral Pediatrics. Philadelphia, WB Saunders, 1992, pp 617–623.

---

ing colors, following simple commands ("Put one crayon in the sink and give two to your mom") as well as drawing. Much information can be obtained by asking children about their drawings. Asking a child to identify pictures in a children's book or (at older ages) to describe the action in the pictures is a good way to elicit higher-order thinking.

Behavioral and psychiatric problems are common and often accompany developmental concerns. Screening for behavioral problems using the Pediatric Symptom Checklist (Fig. 16–1) is a simple, well-validated method. *Bright Futures: Guidelines for Health Supervision of Infants, Children and Adolescents* features numerous "trigger questions" that function as informal screens for developmental and behavioral adjustment (also see Chapter 5). The companion volume, *Bright Futures in Practice: Mental Health— Volume II: Toolkit,* provides a wealth of other screening instruments and approaches.

LIMITATIONS OF SCREENING. Screening tests are subject to a number of abuses, including failure to follow the instructions for administration and scoring; overinterpretation of the results (essentially confusing screening with diagnosis); focusing on the screening test to the exclusion of other sources of information; screening too infrequently; using tests that are culturally biased; and failing to follow up with further assessments and treatment when indicated. Community-wide programs of early developmental screening, while of intuitive value, have not been shown to actually improve developmental outcomes at school age. Screening and assessment without effective follow-up may do more harm than good.

DEVELOPMENTAL SURVEILLANCE. Surveillance has been put forward as an antidote to the shortcomings of developmental screening. The transactional nature of development ensures that a child's status at any single point in time can never entirely predict later development. As with physical growth, a series of observations made over time provides much more information than an assessment at a single time point, allowing for estimation of developmental rate. Prediction is more accurate when it makes use of several sources of information, including the medical and social histories. These considerations underlie the concept of developmental surveillance, a process that includes regular elicitation of the developmental history, attention to

parental concerns, careful developmental observations, and promotion of development.

Critics of surveillance have pointed out that a pediatrician's judgment is subject to a host of biases that undermine its accuracy. Pediatricians may overestimate IQ in children they know well or in children who are physically attractive or socially adept.

An approach combining ongoing surveillance with periodic use of screening tests may be the most effective and practical solution. A multidomain battery of milestones, such as the Denver, as well as systematically applied informal observations can be used as a framework for regular observations rather than as a stand-alone test. Parent questionnaires can streamline data collection and may encourage parents to voice their questions and concerns. Early identification of developmental and emotional problems will be maximized by keeping the following five principles in mind:

1. Parents, as a rule, are accurate observers of their children's behaviors; parental concerns about possible developmental delays are often appropriate and need to be taken seriously; conversely, a lack of parental concern should not be relied on as the sole indicator of normal development.

2. No child is too young for formal audiologic testing. In-office audiologic screening cannot rule out clinically significant hearing loss. Hearing-impaired children often use visual cues to "pass" hearing tests. Audiologic testing is indicated by the presence of any of the historic and physical findings listed in Box 16–1.

3. Risk factors are additive. Biologic impairments that may be relatively minor on their own (e.g., recurrent otitis) may have major impacts in the presence of environmental risk factors (e.g., maternal depression). Awareness of problems in one area should trigger increased vigilance in other areas. For example, emotional problems are common causes and consequences of cognitive and language disorders; environmental risk factors, such as maternal depression, frequently coexist with biologic risks, such as prematurity or lead toxicity.

4. Discomfort, fatigue, shyness, and oppositionality may adversely affect a child's performance on developmental

The Pediatric Symptom Checklist*

Please mark under the heading that best fits your child:

	Never	Sometimes	Often
1. Complains of aches or pains	___	___	___
2. Spends more time alone	___	___	___
3. Tires easily, little energy	___	___	___
4. Fidgety, unable to sit still	___	___	___
5. Has trouble with a teacher	___	___	___
6. Less interested in school	___	___	___
7. Acts as if driven by a motor	___	___	___
8. Daydreams too much	___	___	___
9. Distracted easily	___	___	___
10. Is afraid of new situations	___	___	___
11. Feels sad, unhappy	___	___	___
12. Is irritable, angry	___	___	___
13. Feels hopeless	___	___	___
14. Has trouble concentrating	___	___	___
15. Less interest in friends	___	___	___
16. Fights with other children	___	___	___
17. Absent from school	___	___	___
18. School grades dropping	___	___	___
19. Is down on him or herself	___	___	___
20. Visits doctor with doctor finding nothing wrong	___	___	___
21. Has trouble sleeping	___	___	___
22. Worries a lot	___	___	___
23. Wants to be with you more than before	___	___	___
24. Feels he or she is bad	___	___	___
25. Takes unnecessary risks	___	___	___
26. Gets hurt frequently	___	___	___
27. Seems to be having less fun	___	___	___
28. Acts younger than children his or her age	___	___	___
29. Does not listen to rules	___	___	___
30. Does not show feelings	___	___	___
31. Does not understand other people's feelings	___	___	___
32. Teases others	___	___	___
33. Blames others for his or her troubles	___	___	___
34. Takes things that do not belong to him or her	___	___	___
35. Refuses to share	___	___	___

*School items in bold were not counted for the 4–5-yr-old sample.

FIGURE 16–1. The Pediatric Symptom Checklist. (From Little M, Murphy JM, Jellinek MS, et al: Screening 4- and 5-year-old children for psychosocial dysfunction: A preliminary study with the pediatric symptom checklist. *J Dev Behav Pediatr* 1994;15:191.)

testing. Rescreening is appropriate when these factors are suspected but should not be unduly delayed. Caution should be exercised before proclaiming that a child will "grow out of" a problem.

5. Pediatricians and parents may worry about the adverse effects of labeling a child. Screening test results are not diagnoses. Follow-up assessment and intervention are critical. It is a child's progress over time that is important rather than any labels given along the way. In all but the most severe cases, a child's progress cannot be accurately predicted at the outset; an attitude of realistic optimism is appropriate.

DIAGNOSTIC ASSESSMENT

Once a child has been identified as having a potential problem, the next step is diagnostic assessment. The form and content of the assessment depend on the age of the child, the nature of the problem, and the available medical and community resources. Pediatricians function as part of a team that may also include psychologists, educators, social workers, and other professionals. Central to a pediatrician's role is medical evaluation of a developmentally disabled child (also see Chapter 37).

Medical Evaluation of Developmental Delays. The prevalence of more common developmental disabilities is listed in Table 16–2. The medical evaluation includes history, physical examination, and laboratory testing. Taking a thorough family history, including neurologic, psychiatric, and social difficulties (e.g., legal problems), is indispensable. The family history may shed light on the multigenerational origins of family dysfunction and resilience and may illuminate the parents' beliefs about the causes of the child's problem (e.g., "He's just like his uncle") (see Chapter 17).

The prenatal history should include a search for potential teratogenic exposures, including radiation or medications, infectious illnesses, fever, addictive substances, and trauma. The perinatal history includes birthweight, gestational age, Apgar scores, and any medical complications (Chapter 83.1). Postnatal medical factors that are sometimes overlooked include chronic respiratory or allergic illness, recurrent otitis, head trauma, and sleep problems (particularly signs of obstructive sleep apnea [Chapter 369]).

In the physical examination, points of particular importance include growth parameters and head circumference, facial and other dysmorphology, eye findings (e.g., cataracts in various inborn errors of metabolism), and signs of neurocutaneous disorders (café-au-lait spots in neurofibromatosis, hypopigmented macules in tuberous sclerosis).

No single set of laboratory tests is indicated in all cases. Most states screen for phenylketonuria, hypothyroidism, and other metabolic conditions in the neonatal period. Iron deficiency and lead toxicity are common contributors to developmental delays and are easily detected. Electroencephalograms and neuroimaging are not routinely indicated but should be used if there is clinical suspicion of seizure or encephalopathy or in cases of microcephaly or of rapidly expanding head circumference.

The medical evaluation for mental retardation (Chapter 37.2) and autism (Chapter 27.1) should include chromosomal and molecular biologic testing for fragile X, the most commonly

BOX 16–1. Indications for Audiologic Evaluation

Neonatal intensive care
  Birth wt <2,500 g: All cases
  Birth wt >2,500 g: If medical complications (asphyxia, seizures, persistent fetal circulation, intracranial hemorrhage, assisted ventilation, hyperbilirubinemia, ototoxic drugs)
Proven or suspected intrauterine infection
Bacterial meningitis
Anomalies of 1st or 2nd branchial arch (microtia, auricular dysplasia, micrognathia)
Anomalies of neural crest/ectoderm (widely spaced eyes; pigmentary defects)
Family history of hereditary or unexplained deafness
Parental concern about hearing loss
Delayed speech or language development
Other developmental disabilities (mental retardation, cerebral palsy, autism, blindness)

From Coplan J: Deafness: Ever heard of it? Delayed recognition of permanent hearing loss. *Pediatrics* 1987; 79:206.

identified genetic cause of mental retardation (Chapter 70). Classic physical findings in fragile X such as long faces, large ears, and large testes may be absent in infancy. Milder forms of cognitive and behavioral disturbance have been associated with partial mutations and heterozygosity for fragile X in girls as well as boys. A diagnosis of fragile X does not change therapy but has implications for genetic counseling. Ammonia and organic and amino acids may be included to screen for metabolic disease. With progressive loss of milestones, and particularly if there is associated growth delay, human immunodeficiency virus must be considered (Chapter 254).

Developmental Diagnosis for Infants and Preschool-Aged Children. The most widely used newborn behavioral examination is the Brazelton Neonatal Behavioral Assessment Scale (NBAS). The NBAS allows quantitative estimation of an infant's neurologic intactness, adaptation to extrauterine life, primitive reflexes, state organization, self-regulatory ability, and interactive capacities from birth to 1 mo. The examination takes approximately 30–45 min and requires extensive training for an examiner to reach proficiency.

The NBAS is a poor predictor of later development, not surprising given the salience of environmental influences on development. In practice, the assessment functions well as an intervention in its own right (Chapter 9). Demonstrating neonates' behavioral abilities and vulnerabilities to their parents (e.g., their ability to track visually and turn toward sounds and their vulnerability to overstimulation) is consistently associated with improvements in the child-rearing environment months later.

For older infants and preschool-aged children, the diagnostic process may include formal developmental testing, playroom observations, parent and family interviews, home observations, and team meetings. It often involves a multidisciplinary team of educators, psychologists, parents, social workers, therapists, and pediatricians. Pediatricians contribute medical expertise and knowledge of the child and family accumulated over time. Diagnostic and therapeutic services are provided through the federal- and state-mandated early intervention programs and through multidisciplinary child development teams.

For young children, intervention relies on parental participation. The federal Early Intervention law (PL 105-17) mandates family involvement at all stages of the process of assessment, construction of a service plan, and monitoring of a child's progress. Pediatricians can help parents understand their rights and responsibilities under the law, review the process of developmental assessment and service planning to ensure that the parents are comfortable with the plan, and advocate with the early intervention system on behalf of a child.

To monitor a child's progress and advise the parents, a pediatrician needs to have realistic expectations about the effectiveness of early intervention. For children who face predominantly social/environmental risk factors (e.g., poverty), strong evidence shows that early intervention can raise IQ in the short term, as well as rates of school completion, job satisfaction, and social adjustment in the long term. For children at biologic risk because of prematurity, interventions combining direct therapy for a child with family support (home visiting, parent education) have resulted in significant gains in cognitive and emotional development. For children with established disabilities, the findings are more complex and controversial. Gains in IQ are modest overall, with greater gains among less severely affected children. However, improvements in family adjustment and alleviation of parental stress are consistently found. For children with autism-spectrum disorders, intensive language and interpersonal therapy may result in significant gains.

Diagnostic Assessment for School-Aged Children. Pediatricians are often called on to diagnose specific learning disabilities or attention deficit disorder in school-aged children with academic or behavioral problems or both (Chapter 29). The medical evaluation includes the factors discussed in the prior chapters. Vision and hearing deficits, although seldom the sole causes of school problems, must be evaluated. The interview should assess functioning in the home, the school, and the neighborhood and with peers (Chapters 13 and 14).

Definitive diagnosis usually requires a team effort. Educational testing is indicated to define areas of academic strength and weakness. Psychologic evaluation is indicated to assess emotional problems, such as depression or anxiety, that may be either causes or consequences of the school problems. Assessment of family functioning is essential. Neuropsychologic testing may be indicated to assess specific functional deficits (short-term memory, verbal processing) that may cause a child to be inattentive (Chapters 13 and 29). Pediatricians can facilitate these referrals and synthesize the information for parents and the school. Pediatricians with special interest in assessment of learning problems may also choose to use one of a series of neurodevelopmental tests, such as the Pediatric Early Elementary Examination (PEEX), to obtain a better sense of a child's functioning in various school-related cognitive areas (see Table 16–1).

Referrals to psychologic and educational specialists may be expensive and may not be covered by insurance. An alternative is assessment in the school. In the United States, under federal law, each child is entitled to comprehensive educational assessment and the establishment of an individualized educational plan (IEP) as part of free public education. The assessment must be completed within approximately 2–3 mo, and parents must approve the IEP before it can be instituted.

In practice, the quality of these educational assessments varies depending on the skills of the school psychologist, the workload, and the educational resources available within the school system. If the assessment is inadequate, the parents have the right to demand an independent evaluation at the school's expense. The following questions can aid pediatricians in the important task of assessing the assessment:

1. Was sufficient time taken for the child to feel comfortable with the examiner and setting? The anxiety of confronting a stranger in a strange room may lower a child's score considerably.

2. Were a psychologic interview and projective testing as well as the more standard educational tests performed? Some school psychologists ignore the emotional aspects of learning, focusing solely on the cognitive.

3. Was IQ testing done? Were individual or group tests done?

4. Did the testing address all major areas of functioning (e.g., receptive and expressive language, visuomotor skills, short- and long-term memory)?

5. Was an attempt made to synthesize the findings in the report, or were the scores simply reported?

TABLE 16–2. **Prevalence of Developmental Disabilities**

Condition	Prevalence per 1,000
Cerebral palsy	2–3
Visual impairment	0.3–0.6
Hearing impairment	0.8–2
Mental retardation	25
Learning disability	75
ADHD	150
Behavioral disorders	6–13%

ADHD = attention-deficit/hyperactivity disorder.
Adapted from Levy SE, Hyman SL: Pediatric assessment of the child with developmental delay. Pediatr Clin North Am 1993; 40:465.

AAP Committee on Children with Disabilities: Developmental surveillance and screening of infants and young children. *Pediatrics* 2001;108:192–6.

Glascoe FP: Early detection of developmental and behavioral problems. *Pediatr Rev* 2000;21:272–9; quiz 280.

Jellinek M, Patel B, Froehle M: *Bright Futures in Practice: Mental Health—Volume II, Tool Kit.* Arlington, VA, National Center for Education in Maternal and Child Health, 2002.

Kelleher KJ, McInerny TK, Gardner WP, et al: Increasing identification of psychosocial problems: 1979–1996. *Pediatrics* 2000;105:1313–21.

Poduska JM: Parent's perceptions of their first graders' need for mental health and educational services. *J Am Acad Child Adolesc Psychiatry* 2000;39:584–91.

Solomon R: Pediatricians and early intervention: Everything you need to know but are too busy to ask. *Infants Young Children* 1995;7:31.

Psychologic Disorders

Chapter 17

Assessment and Interviewing

17.1 The Clinical Interview (History)

Neil W. Boris, Marc A. Forman, and Jorge H. Daruna

The clinical interview is a major means of engaging patients and their families in active management of their own care (see Chapters 5 and 6). Primary care practitioners must manage both the physical and behavioral health of children. The clinical interview must, therefore, serve as both a tool for gathering information and a means for influencing behavior. One well-practiced part of a clinical interview in most pediatric and general medical settings is the simple collection of medical data related to the signs and symptoms of a presenting illness, the nature and course of past medical illnesses, the family history, and a review of systems. Other aspects of a patient's life, such as psychosocial functioning, often get less or scant attention in interviewing. However, the presence of psychosocial problems can significantly influence the course of a disease, alter compliance with treatment recommendations, or even be the source of a patient or family's "hidden agenda" related to a given visit. Furthermore, managing behavioral concerns without understanding family functioning or the child's emotional state is akin to driving while blind. Pediatricians need to use clinical interviews to assess the emotional states of their patients and uncover clues that might point to psychosocial distress or disturbance within the family context. Understanding developmental issues related to information gathering and principles of family assessment is also central to successful interviewing (see also Chapter 6).

Assessing a child's emotional state or delving into family functioning requires both specific skills and a considered approach consistent with the individual physician's style. The first goal is to build rapport with both family and child. Pediatricians who develop modes of interaction matched to the child's developmental stage will likely have the most success building rapport, and a brief review of developmental issues related to engaging patients and their families follows. However, there are some general principles regarding interviewing and assessment that are useful to consider first.

Efficient communication requires unbroken attention; a closed door and no interruptions promote efficiency. Ensuring privacy, whenever possible, will increase the yield of information generally, and is especially important when psychosocial issues are being discussed. Privacy is not always easily attained (e.g., an open ward) and without it the physician may not be aware that their patient (or the family) has not felt comfortable enough to share relevant information. Setting aside adequate time for an interview is also important. Comprehensively exploring both psychosocial and biomedical aspects of the condition of a child who has just become a new patient needs at least 30–40 min for significant exchange of the most basic relevant information.

The use of time is equally important. Building rapport with parents requires taking time to address their major concerns at each visit. The pediatrician should follow the opening attempt to build rapport with the child by asking open-ended questions to the caregivers about their concerns or questions. Using patient-centered interviewing improves data gathering and increases patient satisfaction, which, in turn, improves compliance. Patient-centered interviewing refers to guiding the patient or parents through the interview by explicitly allowing them to present their foremost concerns. With practice, it takes no longer to focus on the concerns of patient and/or parent, than to "lead" the interview. Centering the dialogue on the patient or family's agenda often results in less time required to undo misunderstandings later. Furthermore, it is typically possible to multi-task, by, for instance, following up on a parent's questions or concerns while finishing the physical examination of the child. Finally, a primary determinant of malpractice claims is poor physician-patient (or family) communication, and, from the patient's perspective, "not being heard" is the central communication problem.

A great deal of interview data can be gathered through careful attention to nonverbal cues. Just as the physician who palpates but does not auscultate may miss important data on a physical examination, the physician who does not actively note information about facial expressions or body language will miss important information related to the patient's mental state. For example, an adolescent who is expressionless and averts his or her eyes is obviously uncomfortable. Unless the physician notes this and inquires gently about what might be bothering the patient, an opportunity to reach that adolescent will be missed. Furthermore, the patient with unmet needs may return or seek care elsewhere, effectively decreasing efficiency. Scanning for nonverbal cues and commenting on them is part of effective interviewing.

Often, the goals of patient encounters go beyond building rapport with the child, incorporating the concerns of the family into the interview, and gathering nonverbal data. Typically, there is some information that the physician must communicate. Again, presenting information should involve more than words. For instance, simply using eye contact and a positive tone of voice when detailing a medication regimen will increase the likelihood that the patient or parent will understand the information. Legible written instructions and a noncondescending explanation of why the patient should comply will further increase compliance. Finally, when necessary, offering a reminder call may prove effective. It may be necessary to provide positive, clear directions repeatedly.

One of the challenges of working with children is that effective interaction requires attention to developmental issues. What works for a child at one developmental stage will not work at another stage. What follows are some considerations and guidelines for interviewing matched to developmental stages.

Infancy and Early Childhood. Infants and toddlers have tremendous capacity for forming memories, though they do not have language available to describe them. This means that the frequent office or clinic visits before 3 yr of age can collectively provide a "positive memory bank" for an individual child, which can then become the building blocks for a positive and meaningful relationship with the child and his or her family. The practitioner who actively makes eye contact with and plays, even briefly, with young children will create these positive relationship building blocks. Furthermore, paying this kind of direct attention to the young child is almost always comforting to parents.

Initial or casual encounters with preschool children are often made easier when introduced in a whisper, which young children may find more personal, private, and reassuring than jollity; they commonly whisper in response. When children are old enough, at 4–5 yr, it is important for the pediatrician to form the habit of discussing with them their symptoms, diagnoses, and treatments in terms they can understand. The use of drawings to illustrate and explain medical problems can be very useful.

Caring for an infant is challenging to most parents. Using a prenatal visit to understand a family's expectations, ways of coping, and level of stress is time well spent. Predicting for new parents what are the common stress points and setting basic ground rules for when and how to call for help will typically decrease calls to the office. Providing web-based or written parent resources is often helpful. Maternal depression has a significant impact on the infant and young child. Infants of depressed mothers have been found to have alterations of in utero physiologic responsiveness and in electroencephalography in the first weeks of life compared with matched controls. Furthermore, inadequate maternal responsiveness to their infants is correlated with the degree of maternal depression and, in time, with insecure child attachment. One or two questions about mood and functioning are, therefore, necessary at the first postnatal visit ("Some parents find the weeks after birth very stressful—how are you doing?" "Have you had periods of sadness or depression since your baby was born?"). Often, depressed mood is evident through nonverbal communication. If the parent admits to significant sadness or just appears sad and overwhelmed, having a depression screening instrument in the office (such as the Beck Depression Inventory) will assist greatly in deciding which parents need referral. The vast majority of parents are relieved to be able to share their difficulties and will readily fill out a screening questionnaire. The pediatrician who recognizes maternal depression and completes a referral may significantly decrease the untoward impact of this depression on their patient.

The School-Aged Child. As children reach school age, asking about their interests directly at the outset of any interaction in developmentally appropriate language is of paramount importance. Noting specific interests or comments in the patient record will allow for follow-up queries at subsequent visits and communicate the physician's attentiveness and caring. School-aged children are largely well, but family or peer-relationship problems and worries or fears are extremely common and should be inquired about. These concerns, when accompanied by learning difficulties, attention or behavioral problems, anxiety, or other like symptoms, may together be very stressful for children and their families. The clinician should ask how everyone gets along at home and which children the child likes to spend time with. Children who do not have a best friend (or friends) or who express concerns about parental fighting may, for instance, require extra support or even referral for counseling. This is especially true if they are performing poorly at school or if the parent reports behavior problems. When this is the case, getting the parent(s) and at least one teacher to fill out a behavioral problems screening instrument (such as the Child Behavior Checklist) may be helpful for identifying and tracking specific problems. Behavioral screening instruments, however, are inadequate for making psychiatric diagnoses.

Parents of school-aged children may be stressed. The pediatrician who inquires about parental concerns and asks open-ended questions about the child's social functioning will allow for useful discussion of stressors. Of particular importance, at all stages of development, is domestic violence (see Chapters 5 and 34). Domestic violence is both common and a source of shame for parents; active questioning of parents is required to uncover it. Furthermore, for the school-aged child, domestic violence is both frightening and confusing—children are unlikely to be able to put their feelings into words spontaneously. Domestic violence is both greatly under-recognized and associated with serious family morbidity and mortality. Many practitioners feel anxious inquiring about domestic violence, but making a query about family discourse need not be off-putting to the family. For instance, first stating: "At this visit, I usually ask about how a child's parents are handling their stress—how are you doing in this regard?" suggests that family concerns are also the concern of the pediatrician. A follow-up question might be: "You know, one issue that really impacts children is parental fighting, especially physical fights—has this ever been a problem in your home?" Avoiding accusation puts parents at ease, and data suggest that, when asked, both victims and victimizers will speak about the issue. However, it is true that parents are sometimes more comfortable talking about these issues outside the child's presence and the pediatrician should offer this option. Unfortunately, there are no simple demographic indicators of families at greatest risk for violence at home: The problem is common for single parents but cuts across social strata. When the pediatrician hears about physical fighting in the home, he or she should ask about the current situation and assess family safety directly. A referral to a shelter for ongoing violence is of paramount importance, though many families will need assistance in following through with this recommendation. At a minimum, both giving shelter numbers and scheduling another appointment with the pediatrician within 2 wk are necessary. Having the parent fill out a behavioral problems screening checklist is also indicated for every domestic violence situation; the impact of this stressor on the child is clearly important and should be documented. Referral may be necessary particularly when aggression, withdrawal, school failure, or role reversal (e.g., the child becomes the parent's caretaker) are evident.

Adolescents. A key developmental milestone for each adolescent is gaining autonomy from his or her parents or caretakers (see Chapter 14 and Part XII). The pediatrician can support the adolescent in gaining autonomy by directing the interview to the adolescent, beginning at the time of puberty. By inviting the parents to leave the room, the physician affords the adolescent a sense of privacy and increases the chance of gaining insight into issues that would not be discussed in front of parents. Confidentiality is important to consider when interviewing adolescents. Though adolescents highly value private consultation with their physicians, a survey of primary care providers revealed that a minority of practitioners ask parents to leave the room during health visits. Physical examinations of adolescents should also be conducted with their parents not present, unless a patient requests otherwise.

Although adolescence has been traditionally viewed as a period of "storm and stress," there is evidence that most adolescents do not experience more stress at this developmental stage than at others. On the other hand, risk-taking behavior is not uncommon among adolescents and most adolescents report peer pressure to take risks. Experimentation with alcohol, tobacco, drugs, and sex are typical. Adolescence is also a period when the incidences of several major mental illnesses increase dramatically. Major depression, bipolar disorder, panic disorder, and schizophrenia are chronic conditions, and there is evidence that early stabilization of these illnesses in adolescents may improve long-term outcome. Finally, adolescence is a stage during which consolidation of sexual orientation generally occurs and this process, especially for many of the youth who self-identify as homosexual, is associated with considerable stress, elevated levels of risk-taking, and higher rates of suicide attempts.

Each adolescent visit requires a careful social history and an opportunity for discussion about how to make choices regarding tobacco use, alcohol use, drug use, and sexual risk-taking. Familiarity with a good psychiatric review of symptoms is necessary for cases in which mental illness is suspected. The adolescent interview requires careful attention to detail, and using a structured format for briefly assessing risk-taking behaviors, social stressors, sexual identity and orientation, and psychologic adjustment is recommended. Suicidal ideation should also be discussed. During adolescence more lives will be saved by a good interview and respectful counseling about behavior than by a thorough physical examination. Inquiring about suicide does not promote suicidal ideation.

With practice, an interview that begins with open-ended questions about social functioning and finishes with an inquiry about suicidal ideation should be possible in a 15-min visit with an adolescent. Good eye contact, a practiced transition statement (e.g., "now I'd like to ask about some issues that I ask all teens about"), and the use of reflection and encouragement will put most adolescents at ease. Even if the pediatrician gets a negative response to questions about suicidal ideation, he or she will have certified that a topic as "personal" as suicide is one that the adolescent can return to talk about. Creating an atmosphere in which the adolescent has "permission" to discuss his or her most private concerns is critical; when the pediatrician takes the lead in opening up topics such as drug use and sexual practices, "permission" is granted.

For the parent, caring for an adolescent can be exasperating. Open communication between parents and their teenage children promotes positive adjustment for the adolescent. However, parents often feel disconnected from their adolescents, in part because peer influence becomes more and more important during adolescence, resulting in a degree of withdrawal from parents. The pediatrician can play the role of "parenting coach" quite effectively at this developmental stage by both modeling (e.g., asking to meet with the adolescent alone to talk about teen issues) and suggesting that the parent routinely do the same. Again, addressing parents' specific concerns is important, and there are a number of web-based and print resources that can provide "backup" for the busy physician; parents typically will value being pointed in the direction of good parenting books and resources.

OTHER SOURCES FOR ASSESSMENT

Institutions or Agencies. School reports are important to the psychosocial assessment, especially if they include both an academic evaluation and a description of the child's relationships with schoolmates and teachers. Requests for school reports should be made only with the written permission of the child's parents or legal guardians. Reports from child-care agencies may also be helpful, especially in the case of adopted children or children in foster care. Such agencies often have extensive background material and may have reports of earlier psychologic examinations.

Psychologic Testing. A number of instruments may be administered to parents by trained pediatric staff to assess development, behavioral problems, family stress, and parenting skills. It is wise to have a set of instruments and their scoring templates and age norms at the office. Some examples of particularly helpful instruments include the Vineland Adaptive Behavior Scales, the Child Behavior Checklist, the Infant-Toddler Social-Emotional Assessment, the Childhood Depression Inventory, and the Parenting Stress Index. Use of these validated checklists can facilitate early identification of problems that may necessitate

referral to a child psychiatrist or other appropriate specialist. Although checklists do not provide diagnoses, they will assist in improving assessment efficiency, tracking symptoms, and deciding whom to refer.

Individual psychologic testing should be conducted by trained psychologists. Comprehensive assessments of sensory-motor development, language, and academic achievement may require additional involvement of occupational therapists, speech/language pathologists, or educational consultants. The major tests used in the psychologic assessment of children can be classified into four groups: (1) tests of general intelligence; (2) tests of academic achievement; (3) tests of specific sensory, motor, or cognitive functions; and (4) tests of behavioral or personality characteristics. Tests that are widely used to assess general cognitive proficiency or intelligence for specific age groups (shown in parentheses) include the following: The Bayley Scales of Infant Development (0–42 mo); Stanford-Binet Intelligence Scale, 4th edition (2 yr–adult); McCarthy Scales of Children's Abilities (2.5–8.5 yr); Kaufman Assessment Battery for Children (2.5–12.5 yr); Wechsler Preschool and Primary Intelligence Scale-Revised (3–7 yr); Wechsler Intelligence Scale for Children, 3rd edition (6–16 yr); and Wechsler Adult Intelligence Scale, 3rd edition (16 yr– adult).

Academic achievement tests are designed to measure competence in specific areas of knowledge or skill (e.g., arithmetic, reading) usually acquired through formal education in schools. Some frequently used tests in this category include the Peabody Individual Achievement Test, Revised; the Wide Range Achievement Test, 3rd edition; and the Woodcock-Johnson Psychoeducational Battery, Revised.

Numerous tests have been developed to measure more circumscribed skills such as auditory perception (e.g., Seashore Rhythms test); language (e.g., Boston Naming Test); verbal memory (e.g., California Verbal Learning Test); abstract reasoning (e.g., Children's Category Test; Wisconsin Card Sorting Test); constructional ability and nonverbal memory (e.g., Rey's Complex Figure test); motor proficiency (e.g., Finger Tapping Test; Purdue Pegboard Test); and sustained attention (e.g., Continuous Performance tests).

Evaluation of behavioral or personality characteristics often relies on questionnaires completed by parents or teachers (e.g., Conners Rating Scales; Child Behavior Checklist) to rate the frequency with which children show various behaviors (e.g., hyperactivity, aggression). In older children and adolescents, it is also possible to assess self-reported feelings and thoughts using questionnaires such as the Youth Self-Report, Piers-Harris Self-Concept Scale, or Reynolds Child Depression Scale. These scales are useful but do not substitute for carefully conducted clinical interviews. Assessments using projective tests, which require a child to report associations provoked by relatively abstract pictures (e.g., Rorschach inkblot test) or make up stories to pictures depicting specific situations (e.g., Children's Apperception Test; Thematic Apperception Test) are useful in uncovering issues or concerns that preoccupy children as well as distortions or idiosyncrasies that characterize their thought processes.

Neuropsychologic testing is synonymous with extensive testing using various instruments from all of the categories listed earlier. However, it should be noted that more testing is not necessarily helpful. Tests should be chosen to address specific questions that will help make decisions about interventions. In choosing tests, it is essential that they have demonstrable reliability and validity. They should also have norms that are relatively recent and representative of the general population. An ongoing collaborative relationship with a psychologist or other specialist facilitates appropriate use of testing in a pediatric practice.

Psychologic tests should not be used to differentiate between so-called organic and functional causes of behavior. All causes of behavior are organic in the sense that behavior is biologically driven. If a question arises about the type of biologic disturbance that may underlie a behavioral impairment, other forms of assessment should be used, such as brain imaging techniques; neurophysiologic, endocrinologic, and immunologic tests; and/ or chromosomal-genetic studies.

Psychiatric Consultation. A psychiatric consultation may be a valuable part of assessment of child symptoms (even "physical" symptoms) or family stress or discord. Physicians should inform both parent and child what the psychiatric consultation is intended to assess. The child's consent is helpful and is usually easily obtained when the reasons for referral are explained and some idea of what to expect is furnished. Helpful information on psychiatric assessment is available to both the physician and parents. In fact, standardized guidelines for psychiatric assessment of infants, children, and adolescents have been published by the American Academy of Child and Adolescent Psychiatry, and free "Facts for Families" sheets on various psychiatric symptoms are available on the web or by phone. The need for a psychiatric consultation or referral can perhaps best be expressed in terms of the joint need of the family and physician for help in areas where the psychiatrist has special expertise, with the understanding that the collaboration of physician and family in management of the other health care needs of the child will remain intact.

Correlation of Data. Physicians must avoid early diagnostic closure even when parents' initial description of their problem gives a reasonably clear idea of what is going on. So long as physicians remain receptive and perceptive listeners, new and important information will emerge, as parents and perhaps patients begin to feel more trusting and as they are educated by a physician's questions. Furthermore, weighing of data must be done in the context of a family's sociocultural pattern (see Chapter 3). It is important that physicians not use their personal value system or style of living as a yardstick against which to measure a family's behavior or their success or failure in coping with their life situation. A family's feelings of anger, frustration, anxiety, failure, or depression are more valid indicators of where they need help.

It is also important that the principal item of concern be accurately identified. Parents may present as the prime concern, for example, a problem such as bed-wetting of many years' duration. Why then have they come for help now? It is important to determine whether there may be important hidden issues the parents do not recognize or acknowledge or cannot face. By the same token, it must be understood that the parents' assessment of the problem is critical for the child. Physicians, having collected and assessed appropriate data, sometimes can only conclude that children presented by their parents as having a problem are functioning within normal limits. In such a case, it must be determined what personal, familial, social, or cultural considerations compel the parents to see their child's behavior as a major problem. It must then be determined what re-education they may need to feel reassured and not be left with the impression that their anxiety has been casually dismissed.

Referral. When problems have not been internalized by the child, it may be sufficient simply to counsel the parents, school personnel, or both. If this has been done and a maladaptive child or situation continues to present problems, the child and family will probably require more intensive or extensive help and should be referred to a child psychiatrist or psychiatric clinic. It is important that pediatricians avoid communicating that psychiatric referral is a last resort. The need for psychiatric consultation or referral should be expressed in terms of the joint need of the family and physician for help in areas where the psychiatrist has special expertise, with the understanding that the collaboration of physician and family in management of the other health care needs of the child remains intact.

Carlat DJ: The psychiatric review of symptoms: A screening tool for family physicians. *Am Fam Physician* 1998;58:1617.

Cole SA: Reducing malpractice risk through more effective communication. *American Journal of Managed Care* 1997;3:649.

McLennan JD, Kotelchuck M: Parental prevention practices for young children in the context of maternal depression. *Pediatrics* 2000;105:1090.

Proimos J: Confidentiality issues in the adolescent population. *Curr Opin Pediatr* 1997;9:325.

Purcell JS, Hergenroeder AC, Kozinetz C, et al: Interviewing techniques with adolescents in primary care. *J Adolesc Health* 1997;20:300.

Rowland-Morin PA, Carroll JG: Verbal communication skills and patient satisfaction. A study of doctor-patient interviews. *Evaluation and the Health Professions* 1990;13:168.

Smith RC, Marshall-Dorsey AA, Osborn GG, et al: Evidence-based guidelines for teaching patient-centered interviewing. *Patient Education and Counseling* 2000;39:27.

Stein MT, Coleman WL, Epstein RM: "We've tried everything and nothing works": Family-centered pediatrics and clinical problem-solving. *J Dev Behav Pediatr* 2001;22:S55.

17.2   Psychosocial Problems

Richard Dalton and Marc A. Forman

A psychosocial disorder in a child may be manifested as a disturbance in feelings (e.g., depression, anxiety), in bodily functions (e.g., psychosomatic disorders), in behavior (e.g., conduct disturbances, passive-aggressive behavior), or in performance (e.g., learning problems). Dysfunction may involve any or all of these areas. Psychosocial problems may be produced by such physical or emotional stresses as birth defects, physical injury, inconsistent and contradictory child-rearing practices, marital conflict, child abuse and neglect, overindulgence, chronic illness, and so on. In general, particular agents do not produce specific symptoms or disorders; rather, children's psychosocial problems are multifactorial in origin, their expression depending on many variables, including temperament, developmental level, the nature and duration of stress, past experiences, and the coping and adaptive abilities of the family. Chronic stresses or a series of stressful events is much more difficult for a child and family to manage than a single acute stressful episode. Children may react immediately to traumatic events or may keep their feelings dormant until maladaptive reactions become apparent during later periods of vulnerability.

Anticipatory guidance during periods of stress may considerably help children and their families to achieve more positive outcomes. Parents should be encouraged to prepare their children in advance for potentially traumatic events that can be anticipated (e.g., elective surgery, separation, or divorce). Children should be allowed or encouraged to express their feelings of dismay, fear, or anger rather than being told to be a "good girl" or "brave boy."

Infants and toddlers tend to react to stressful situations with impairment of physiologic functions, such as disturbances of feeding and sleep, with relatively global expressions of anger or fear, as in temper tantrums, or with withdrawal and avoidance behavior. School-aged children demonstrate their difficulties through altered interpersonal relationships with peers and family members, through impairment of school performance, by the development of specific psychologic syndromes, such as psychosomatic disorders, or by regressing to earlier, more childish modes of functioning.

Parents are frequently concerned whether the particular behaviors of their children are normal or whether they represent problems that require intervention. Some "symptomatic" actions of children may be part of normal development. For example, a temper tantrum may express the normal negativism of a toddler; on the other hand, temper tantrums on slight provocation in a 6-yr-old child may indicate psychosocial disturbance. Whether behavior is judged to be a developmental variation or evidence of a more serious problem depends on the age of the child; on the frequency, intensity, and number of symptoms; and especially on the degree of functional impairment. The decision of parents to seek help is determined, in turn, by the characteristics of their children's behavior; by the amount of distress it causes the children, parents, teachers, and others; and by their past experiences in discussing psychosocial matters with their physicians.

Achenbach TM, Edelbrock CS: *Manual for Child Behavior Checklist and Revised Child Behavior Profile.* Burlington, VT, University of Vermont, Department of Psychiatry, 1993.

Carlat DJ: The psychiatric review of symptoms: A screening tool for family physicians. *Am Fam Physician* 1998;58:1617.

Impara JC, Murphy LJ (editors): *Buros Desk References: Psychological Assessment in the Schools.* Lincoln, NE, Buros Institute, 1994.

Kestenbaum CJ: The clinical interview of the child. In Wiener JM (editor): *Textbook of Child and Adolescent Psychiatry.* Washington, DC, American Psychiatric Press, 1991.

King RA, Work Group on Quality Issues: Practice parameters for the psychiatric assessment of children and adolescents. *J Am Acad Child Adolesc Psychiatry* 1997;36(Suppl):4S.

Purcell JS, Hergenroeder AC, Kozinetz C, et al: Interviewing techniques with adolescents in primary care. *J Adolesc Health* 1997;20:300–5.

Reynolds CR, Kamphaus RW (editors): *Handbook of Psychological and Educational Assessment of Children. Vol I. Intelligence and Achievement. Vol II. Personality, Behavior, and Context.* New York, Guilford Press, 1990.

Rich J: *Interviewing Children and Adolescents.* London, Macmillan, 1968.

Thomas JM, Benham AL, Gean M, et al: Practice parameters for the psychiatric assessment of infants and toddlers (0–36 mo). *J Am Acad Child Adolesc Psychiatry* 1997;36(Suppl):21S.

Stein MT, Coleman WL, Epstein RM: "We've tried everything and nothing works": Family-centered pediatrics and clinical problem-solving. *J Dev Behav Pediatr* 2001;22:S55–60.

Task Force on DSM-IV: *Diagnostic and Statistical Manual of Mental Disorders, 4th ed: DSM-IV.* Washington, DC, American Psychiatric Association, 1991.

Chapter 18

Psychiatric Considerations of Central Nervous System

Injury *Jorge H. Daruna, Marc A. Forman, and Neil W. Boris*

Injury to the central nervous system (CNS) as a result of physical trauma, exposure to toxic substances, or infection may cause psychiatric disturbances.

Epidemiology. *Head injury* is a relatively common event in pediatric populations. Infants and young children may be victims of abuse (see Chapter 35). Children of all ages may be injured in falls or automobile accidents (see Chapter 50). Older children and adolescents may be further affected by sports-related head trauma (see Chapter 677). Severity of injury has been found to predict behavioral disturbance. Although severity can be difficult to gauge in some instances, loss of consciousness exceeding 20–30 min is often associated with serious sequelae.

Injuries early in life may be more generally incapacitating than those that occur later, even though neural plasticity remains high in young children. The immature brain may be more globally affected, even though deficits may not be immediately evident and only gradually manifest as the child develops behaviorally. Brain injury before the age of 3 yr has been associated with later seizures, which independently increase the risk of behavioral disturbance. Early brain injury can also result from inadvertent ingestion of neurotoxic substances such as lead, which causes significant behavioral morbidity (Chapter 703).

Estimates of the frequency of behavioral disturbance after brain injury are variable, but consistently indicate that there is an increased risk of psychiatric disorder. In the case of severe brain injury, the estimates of psychiatric morbidity range from 54% to 76%, though there is great variability in both severity and course of postinjury disturbance.

Clinical Manifestations. Most often the behavioral disturbance resembles attention-deficit/hyperactivity disorder (ADHD) or takes the form of a depressive disorder. Psychosis is not generally seen as a result of brain injury in childhood. Typically, there may be problems with motor function. Cognitive skills, particularly attention and memory, may be compromised. Impairments in the regulation of emotion and social behavior occur frequently. Affected children can seem to lack insight and empathy. Some deficits may not be apparent until late childhood or adolescence, when there is a need for greater efficiency, flexibility, and speed in cognitive processing. Those with the highest risk for significant behavioral disturbance come predominantly from the groups who incurred severe injury, who had prior behavioral problems, and whose family functions poorly. The serious head trauma either gives rise to novel psychiatric disorders or further aggravates a psychiatric disorder that may have arisen originally as a result of genetic and/or psychosocial influences. Even when the head injury has been judged to be mild, there may be educational problems in as many as 25–50% of afflicted children.

Insults to the brain can occur prenatally and have lifelong consequences. Preterm birth may adversely impact the development of neural systems. Very premature infants are at increased risk for severe neurodevelopmental disorders and exhibit cognitive deficits, educational handicaps, and behavioral disturbances, particularly ADHD and anxiety disorders. Another major cause of prenatal brain injury is exposure to toxic substances such as tobacco, alcohol, and a variety of medicines, including illicit drugs. Prenatal exposure to such substances is associated with impairment in growth, cognition, and self-regulation of behavior. However, the initial impression that crack-cocaine is especially devastating has not been supported by research that controls for confounding variables such as harsh psychosocial conditions and use of legal drugs like tobacco and alcohol, although one study reports that cocaine-exposed infants show significant cognitive deficits by 2 yr, even when the previously noted variables are controlled.

Infections during pregnancy also can cause serious behavioral morbidity. In some cases, the behavioral disturbance is not evident until late adolescence. For example, there is evidence that at least some cases of schizophrenia may be attributable to maternal viral infection during pregnancy. Postnatal infections of the CNS, such as encephalitis, also may cause brain injury, with behavioral consequences that resemble the range of disorders seen after physical or toxic trauma to the brain. Behavioral disturbances may also follow infection with organisms such as group A β-hemolytic streptococci as the result of antibodies to the pathogen that may cross react with neural tissue. In particular, obsessive-compulsive disorder and Tourette disorder have been reported to result from such an autoimmune process (see Chapter 21).

Treatment. The most significant factor in a child's adjustment to brain injury is the capacity of the family to cope and adapt. This in turn can be facilitated by access to professional expertise, as well as to educational programs and other resources available in the community. Initially, it is probably best to not give premature reassurance, particularly because what may seem to be minimal early deficits may later manifest as impairments of greater significance. Such children need to be followed and periodically evaluated as they mature. Most children who develop psychiatric disturbances as a result of CNS injury, as well as their families, need appropriate psychosocial support and educational programs designed to remediate specific disorders. A frequently beneficial approach is to assist the child to understand his or her maladaptive behavioral patterns and focus on developing strategies for adequate self-regulation and skill acquisition; coaching and practice are very important. It is also important for the child to have the opportunity to discuss troubling feelings and thoughts that may be provoked by the actions of others who may reject or tease the child.

The parents and other family members have their own concerns and will need guidance and emotional support to deal effectively with the child's behavior both at home and at school. Fair and firm discipline is always useful. Behavior modification techniques can help the child to acquire situation-appropriate behaviors.

Pharmacologic treatments may be helpful as well. Stimulant medications can improve attention, decrease overactivity, and thus improve behavior at school. Affective symptoms may be treated with antidepressants and mood stabilizers. Severe impulsivity and agitation may respond to low doses of atypical neuroleptics. Given the increased risk of seizure in brain-injured children, medicines that lower the seizure threshold should be avoided. It should also be kept in mind that brain-injured children are a heterogeneous group for whom the efficacy of specific pharmacologic agents has not been sufficiently investigated.

Bloom DR, Levin HS, Ewing-Cobbs L, et al: Lifetime and novel psychiatric disorders after pediatric traumatic brain injury. *J Am Acad Child Adolesc Psychiatry* 2001;40:572.

Frank DA, Augustyn M, Knight WG, et al: Growth, development and behavior in early childhood following prenatal cocaine exposure: A systematic review. *JAMA* 2001;285:1613.

Hack M, Taylor HG: Perinatal brain injury in preterm infants and later neurobehavioral function. *JAMA* 2000;284:1973.

Middleton JA: Practitioner review: Psychological sequelae of head injury in children and adolescents. *J Child Psychol Psychiatry* 2001;42:165.

Needleman HL, Reiss JA, Tobin MJ, et al: Bone lead levels and delinquent behavior. *JAMA* 1996;275:363.

Ott D, Caplan R, Guthrie D, et al: Measures of psychopathology in children with complex partial seizures and primary generalized epilepsy with absence. *J Am Acad Child Adolesc Psychiatry* 2001;40:907.

Powell JW, Barber-Foss KD: Traumatic brain injury in high school athletes. *JAMA* 1999;282:958.

Singer LT, Arendt R, Minnes S, et al: Cognitive and Motor Outcome in Cocaine-exposed infants. *JAMA* 2002;287:1952.

Swedo, SE, Lonard HL, Mittleman BB, et al: Identification of children with pediatric autoimmune neuropsychiatric disorders associated with streptococcal infections (PANDAS) as a marker associated with rheumatic fever. *Am J Psychiat* 1997;154:110.

Chapter 19

Psychosomatic Illness

*Alessandra N. Kazura, Neil W. Boris,
and Richard Dalton*

Physiologic regulation is influenced by psychologic state in humans; most organ systems and many medical conditions are stress sensitive. From the bronchial constriction of asthma to the weal and flare skin response, there are many examples of chronic or recurring conditions whose physiologic course is related to psychologic adjustment. The *Diagnostic and Statistical Manual* (DSM) nosology distinguishes three broad categories of psychosomatic disorders:

1. Psychophysiologic disorders occur when psychologic conflict affects the development or recurrence of a physical condition (e.g., asthma, eczema, or irritable bowel syndrome). Though physical symptoms are observable, the course of these disorders is influenced by psychologic function.

2. Somatoform disorders present with somatic complaints and/or dysfunctions that are not under conscious control and for which physical findings are absent or insufficient to explain all complaints. These disorders include body dysmorphic disorder, conversion disorder, hypochondriasis, somatization disorder, and somatoform pain disorder.

3. Factitious disorder presents with somatic and/or psychologic symptoms that are consciously controlled. It is presumed that the benefits associated with assuming a sick role unconsciously motivate the patient to maintain symptoms. Munchausen syndrome is an example of a chronic factitious disorder.

Distinguishing somatoform disorders from factitious disorders can be difficult: In the former, symptoms are associated with unconscious conflict, whereas in the latter the unconscious need to be cared for motivates the falsification of symptoms.

Although there are multiple theories regarding what factors most influence the cause and course of psychosomatic disorders, Engel's biopsychosocial approach to development and psychopathology offers a pragmatic organizational schema. Underlying temperamental factors, environmental stress, family issues, and individual psychodynamics all contribute, some more than others, depending on the situation. The notion of specific personality types leading to particular disorders has not been substantiated, although some studies have demonstrated family clustering of somatization disorder, antisocial personality disorder, and substance use disorders.

It is extremely difficult to document the relative influence of psychologic factors in psychophysiologic conditions, and the mechanisms of influence for most of these disorders are not well studied. For instance, even a disorder such as *reflex sympathetic dystrophy*—which presents with chronic painful swelling in an extremity, decreased skin temperature, cyanosis, and delayed capillary refilling—may require psychotherapy to maximize function. Although there is no substitute for adequate medical evaluation, the pediatrician should have a low threshold for recommending proven adjunctive therapies for children with recurring physical symptoms.

Conversion disorder, the loss or alteration of physical functioning without a demonstrable organic illness, is a type of somatoform disorder that usually presents in adolescence or adulthood. However, numerous childhood cases have occurred. Conversion reactions usually start suddenly, can often be traced to a precipitating environmental event, and may end abruptly after a short duration. Voluntary musculature and organs of special sense are the most frequent target sites for expressions of psychologic conflict. Pseudoseizures are the most common conversion symptom, but such reactions may take many forms, including blindness, paralysis, diplopia, and gait disturbances. Physical examination often fails to reveal objective abnormalities. Histories may reveal a close relationship with a person who exhibited similar symptoms or a recent episode of actual illness. Deep tendon reflexes can be elicited in a paralyzed leg, and pupillary responses to light are noted in patients with hysterical blindness. Video electroencephalography and postictal serum prolactin levels are helpful in distinguishing pseudoseizures from seizures. Although conversion disorder is probably not genetically mediated, anxiety and chaotic disorganization patterns of disturbance are found in family members. Cultural factors affect the expression of illness and distress, and normative cultural behaviors should be ruled out before diagnosing conversion disorder. Follow-up studies suggest that about one third of children diagnosed with conversion disorder are later diagnosed with an explanatory medical disorder.

Hypochondriasis, preoccupation with the fear of having a serious illness, and *somatization disorder*, multiple somatic complaints associated with generalized anxiety, are also somatoform disorders. Hypochondriasis and somatization disorder, like conversion disorder, are characterized by unconscious physiologic and psychologic conflict that is expressed as physical symptoms. Although community samples show that only half of children and adolescents questioned report at least one somatic symptom during the preceding 2 wk, these disorders are characterized by recurring symptoms. Because recurrent abdominal pain accounts for 2–4% of all pediatric visits and headaches account for 1–2%, a comprehensive social history and review of symptoms should be conducted with each case. Prevalence studies suggest that 11% of boys and 15% of girls have ongoing somatic symptoms. Most of these children do well with regular visits and reassurance, though some children and parents insist on unnecessary medical workup. Children with multiple complaints, high levels of anxiety, and family dysfunction will require psychiatric referral.

Munchausen syndrome by proxy is a factitious disorder in which parents induce physical symptoms in their children. It is considered a form of child abuse, sometimes ending in death (also see Chapter 35). The signs and symptoms can be varied, including fractures, poisonings, persistent complaints of apnea, and unusual injuries. Therapy includes separation of the child from the abusing parent and further investigation, as in cases of child abuse.

Body dysmorphic disorder should be considered in patients presenting with preoccupation with imagined or minor abnormalities in physical appearance. The anxious obsession about physical appearance that characterizes body dysmorphic disorder is often associated with social limitations and dysphoria. The prevalence in adolescents and children is not known, although studies of adults with this diagnosis suggest frequent onset of symptoms during adolescence (also see Chapter 104).

Several general principles guide the management of children with psychosomatic disorders:

1. Assessment should include inquiries about past somatic symptoms and family members or acquaintances with similar symptoms because these may provide clues to symptom source. Potential reasons underlying the need for secondary gain can be garnered from a comprehensive social history. In particular, history of maltreatment, bereavement, or mood and anxiety symptoms should be inquired about. Responses to placebo administration are not reliable in differentiating somatoform disorders from organic conditions.

2. Because the symptoms of psychosomatic disorders are not within the child's conscious control, they are not acting or malingering, and attempting to talk them out of their symptoms or confronting them is contraindicated.

3. Early integration of pediatric and mental health assessment and treatment is important to prevent patients from seeking unnecessary work-up.

4. The child and family should be helped to live as normally as possible to avoid crippling psychologic invalidism. Emphasis should be placed on early return to school after acute illness, participation in recreational activities, and normal peer interactions. Parents should be informed that some children unconsciously use their symptoms to maintain dependency and that firm, gentle insistence on the fullest possible range of activities for the child is indicated.

5. Ideally, parents and children should understand the psychologic origins of symptoms; however, functional improvement may be achieved without full insight.

6. Psychotherapy for the child and family is often indicated, in addition to conservative pediatric management.

7. Psychoactive medications may be useful in treating symptoms of anxiety or depression, especially when these symptoms are prominent.

8. The physician should be alert for indications of psychosomatic or physical illness in parents, with which children may unconsciously identify; successful treatment of parental illness may be necessary to ensure a favorable outcome in the child.

American Psychiatric Association: *Diagnostic and Statistical Manual of Mental Disorders*, 4th ed, Text Revision. Washington, DC, American Psychiatric Press, 2000.

Bools CN, Neale BA, Meadow SR: Follow up of victims of fabricated illness (Munchausen syndrome by proxy). *Arch Dis Child* 1993;69:625.

Campo JV, Fritsch SL: Somatization disorder in children and adolescents. *J Am Acad Child Adolesc Psychiatry* 1994;33:1223.

Engel G: The clinical application of the biopsychosocial model. *Am J Psychiatry* 1980;137:535.

Fritz GK, Fritsch SL, Hagino O: Somatoform disorders in children and adolescents: A review of the past 10 years. *J Am Acad Child Adolesc Psychiatry* 1997;36:1329.

Liang S, Boyce WT: The psychobiology of childhood stress. *Curr Opin Pediatr* 1993;5:545.

McGrath P, McAlpine LM: Psychological perspectives on pediatric pain. *J Pediatr* 1993;122:52.

Mitchell I, Brummett J, DeForest J, et al: Apnea and factitious illness (Munchausen syndrome) by proxy. *Pediatrics* 1993;92:810.

Nemzer E: Psychosomatic illnesses in children and adolescents. In Garfinkel B, Carlson G, Weller E (editors): *Psychiatric Disorders in Children and Adolescents.* Philadelphia, WB Saunders, 1990.

Pawl RP: Controversies surrounding reflex sympathetic dystrophy: A review article. *Curr Rev Pain* 2000;4(4):259–67.

Steinhausen HC, von Aster M, Pfeiffer E, et al: Comparative studies of conversion disorders in childhood and adolescence. *J Child Psychol Psychiatry* 1989;30:615.

Taylor DC: Outlandish factitious illness. In David TJ (ed): *Recent Advances in Pediatrics*, No. 10. Edinburgh, Churchill Livingstone, 1992.

Chapter 20
Vegetative Disorders

The five disorders included under this appellation are classified in the *Diagnostic and Statistical Manual of Mental Disorders*, fourth edition, under Eating Disorders (rumination disorder and pica, along with bulimia and anorexia nervosa, which are discussed in Chapter 104), Elimination Disorders (encopresis and enuresis), and Sleep Disorders.

20.1 Rumination Disorder
Neil W. Boris and Richard Dalton

The hallmark of this disorder is a weight loss or failure to gain at the expected level because of repeated regurgitation of food without nausea or associated gastrointestinal illness. This rare disorder occurs more commonly in males and usually appears between 3 and 14 mo of age. It is potentially fatal; some reports indicate that up to one fourth of affected children die. There are psychogenic and self-stimulating ruminators. The former type occurs in infants with otherwise normal development, although there is often a disturbed parent-child relationship and the child may fail to thrive (Chapter 36). The self-stimulating variety is usually seen in mentally retarded individuals of any age and often occurs even in the presence of nurturing parents. The differential diagnosis should include congenital anomalies that affect the development of the gastrointestinal system and pyloric valve.

Behavioral treatment is directed toward positively reinforcing correct eating behavior and negatively reinforcing rumination. Adverse conditioning is often used. Parent counseling and family therapy are often necessary to manage underlying conflicts and to help educate the parents about appropriate approaches to be taken toward the child and the problem.

20.2 Pica
Neil W. Boris and Richard Dalton

This eating disorder involves repeated or chronic ingestion of non-nutritive substances, which may include plaster, charcoal, clay, wool, ashes, paint, and earth. Although tasting or mouthing of objects is normal in infants and toddlers, pica after the 2nd yr of life needs investigation. Mental retardation and lack of parental nurturing (psychologic and nutritional) are predisposing factors, and pica appears to be more common in children with autism and other brain-behavior disorders such as Kleine-Levin syndrome. Persistent pica is also often associated with family disorganization, poor supervision, and psychologic neglect. Pica appears to be more prevalent in the lower socioeconomic classes. It usually remits in childhood but can continue into adolescence and adulthood. In particular, geophagia (eating of earth) is associated with pregnancy and is not seen as abnormal in some cultures. Children with pica are at an increased risk for lead poisoning (Chapter 703), iron-deficiency anemia (Chapter 447), and parasitic infections (see Part XVI, Sections 12 and 13). Screening for lead intoxication, iron-deficiency anemia, and parasitic infestation is always indicated.

20.3　Enuresis (Bed-wetting)

Neil W. Boris and Richard Dalton

Enuresis is defined as the voluntary or involuntary repeated discharge of urine into clothes or bed after a developmental age when bladder control should be established. Most children with a mental age of 5 have obtained bladder control during the day and night. The diagnosis of enuresis is made when urine is voided twice a week for at least 3 consecutive months or clinically significant distress occurs in areas of the child's life as a result of the wetting (see also Chapters 5 and 535). The prevalence of enuresis at age 5 yr is 7% for males and 3% for females. At age 10 yr, it is 3% for males and 2% for females, and at age 18 yr, it is 1% for males and extremely rare in females. Twin studies show that there is a marked familial pattern: A 68% concordance rate in monozygotic twins and a 36% concordance rate in dizygotic twins has been documented. However, linkage studies have implicated multiple chromosomes, particularly chromosome 22, and varying patterns of transmission appear likely.

Etiology. Beyond genetic factors, the cause of enuresis likely involves a complex web of physiologic and, perhaps, psychologic factors. Children with nocturnal enuresis, for instance, may both hyposecrete arginine vasopressin (AVP) generally and be less responsive to the lower urine osmolality associated with fluid loading. Independent evidence suggests that tubular sodium-potassium exchange in the kidney, partly influenced by AVP secretion, is associated with nocturnal enuresis. Evidence also suggests that AVP receptor function in the tubule may be a key factor in the pathophysiology of the disorder. On the other hand, there may also be associations between sleep and enuresis. Although enuresis may occur at any stage of sleep, there is some support for a relationship between sleep architecture, diminished capacity to be aroused from sleep, and abnormal bladder function in enuretics.

The relationship between enuresis and psychologic functioning also appears complex. Large-scale studies reveal that older enuretic children have a higher incidence of psychopathology generally than non-enuretic children, though no single disorder accounts for the group differences. Smaller studies suggest that children with attention-deficit/hyperactivity disorder more commonly are enuretic than age-matched comparison children. Secondary enuresis is associated with life stress and/or traumatic experiences, particularly in children who were late in first achieving nighttime dryness. The pediatrician should inquire about stressful events with all children who present with secondary enuresis.

Clinical Manifestations. Bed-wetting may be divided into the persistent (primary) type, in which the child has never been dry at night, and the regressive (secondary) type, in which a child who has been continent for 6 mo or more then begins to wet the bed. Primary enuresis represents approximately 90% of all cases. Further classification involves *nocturnal* enuresis (voiding urine at night), and *diurnal* enuresis (voiding urine while awake). Primary nocturnal enuresis is the most common and well studied subtype. Diurnal enuresis is more common in girls and rarely occurs after the age of 9 yr. The most common cause of daytime enuresis in the preschool child is waiting until the last minute to void urine (micturition deferral). In addition to micturition deferral, etiologic factors to consider in diurnal enuresis include a urinary tract infection, chemical urethritis, associated constipation, diabetes, and giggle or stress incontinence. Children with both nocturnal and diurnal enuresis, especially in the presence of voiding difficulties, are more likely to have abnormalities of the urinary tract, and ultrasonography or uroflowmetry is indicated for these cases. Otherwise anatomic abnormalities are rarely associated with either nocturnal or diurnal enuresis and invasive or costly studies are contraindicated. A urinalysis and urine culture will rule out both infectious cause and the elevated urine osmolality associated with diabetes.

Treatment. Management of the child with enuresis should begin with behavioral treatment. General guidelines for a first-line approach would be as follows:

1. It is important to enlist the cooperation of the child to deal with the problem. Rewarding the child for being dry at night is a useful step. The child or parent can chart the dry nights, and, with each dry night, a small reward can be given. More substantial rewards should be given for increasing success.
2. The child should void before retiring.
3. Waking the child repeatedly to take him or her to the bathroom is not generally useful and may further engender or aggravate anger in child or parents. Some data indicate that enuretic children are more difficult to awaken than age-matched peers. However, using an alarm clock to wake the child once 2–3 hr after falling asleep is indicated.
4. Punishment or humiliation of the child by parents or others should be strongly discouraged.

One study showed that consistent dry bed training (as earlier) with positive reinforcement has a success rate of 85% or more. The use of conditioning devices (e.g., an alarm that rings when the child wets a special sheet) also is often helpful in training the child to improve bladder capacity and avoid enuresis. In effect, these devices provide a consistent mode for behavioral retraining. Again, consent of the child should be a prerequisite for use of such a device. Bell and pad alarm systems have a success rate of approximately 75% across many studies, with relapse rates that are lower than those with pharmacologic intervention. These devices are simple and cost-effective. However, psychotherapy for traumatized children with secondary enuresis may be indicated, especially when behavioral training has failed and traumatic experiences temporally associated with the onset of enuresis are noted.

Pharmacotherapy for enuresis is second-line treatment and should be reserved for those patients who have failed behavioral treatment. Head-to-head comparison studies of the bell and pad versus imipramine and desmopressin acetate (DDAVP) reveal significantly lower relapse rates for the bell and pad, although the initial response rates are similar. Imipramine (Tofranil) at a maximum dosage of 2.5 mg/kg/24 hr before bedtime has shown a success rate of approximately 50%, with a relapse rate of 30% or more even after 6 mo of treatment. Imipramine is associated with cardiac conduction disturbances and is deadly in overdose. DDAVP can be administered orally or intranasally at bedtime. The fast action of DDAVP suggests a role for special occasions (such as overnights) when rapid control of enuresis is desired. Unfortunately, the relapse rate upon discontinuation of DDAVP is very high, and 1 month of treatment typically costs as much as a bell and pad system (which can be used for several months as necessary). DDAVP is also associated with rare side effects of hyponatremia and water intoxication, with resulting seizures.

20.4 Encopresis

Neil W. Boris and Richard Dalton

Encopresis refers to the passage of feces into inappropriate places after a chronologic age of 4 yr (or equivalent developmental level). Subtypes include encopresis with constipation and overflow incontinence (retentive encopresis) and encopresis without constipation and overflow incontinence (nonretentive). Encopresis may persist from infancy onward (e.g., primary) or may appear after successful toilet training (e.g., secondary). About two thirds of encopresis cases are of the retentive type and associated with chronic constipation; it is less clear what percentage of cases are primary versus secondary. In children younger than 4 yr of age, the male:female ratio for chronic constipation is 1:1. In the school-aged child, however, encopresis is more common in males, though good epidemiologic studies are lacking.

Clinical Manifestations. The first consideration in managing encopresis is assessment of fecal retention. A positive rectal examination is sufficient to document fecal retention, but a negative rectal examination in the presence of encopresis requires plain abdominal roentgenograms. The presence of fecal retention is evidence of chronic constipation, and treatment will require active constipation management (Chapter 287).

Many children with encopresis present with abnormal anal sphincter physiology as documented either by electromyography or difficulty in defecating a rectal balloon. The inability to defecate a balloon at presentation is associated with poorer response to treatment. Abnormal anal sphincter function is a marker for chronic constipation; children with this pathology do not appear to have a higher incidence of behavioral or psychiatric disorders than those without. However, a chart review study suggests that primary encopresis in boys is associated with global developmental delays and enuresis, whereas secondary encopresis is associated with high levels of psychosocial stressors and conduct disorder. Associated behavioral or psychiatric problems obviously may complicate the treatment of encopresis—especially when parents respond to soiling with retaliatory, punitive measures and children become angry, ashamed, and resistant to intervention. School performance and attendance may be secondarily affected as the child becomes the target of scorn and derision from schoolmates because of the offensive odor.

Treatment. The standard treatment approach to encopresis begins with clearance of impacted fecal material and short-term use of mineral oil or laxatives to prevent further constipation. Concomitant behavioral management is also indicated. The focus of behavioral treatment should be on compliance with regular postprandial toilet sitting and adoption of a high-fiber diet. On some occasions, manual disimpaction is required before the treatment can begin; rarely megacolon is observed and referral to a gastroenterologist is required. Several studies suggest that once impacted stool is removed, the combination of constipation management and simple behavior therapy is successful in the majority of cases, though it is often a period of months before soiling stops completely. However, compliance may wane and failure of this standard treatment approach sometimes requires more intensive intervention with a special emphasis on adherence to a high-fiber diet and family support for behavior change. Parents should be actively encouraged to issue rewards for compliance to the child from the outset of treatment and to avoid power struggles with the child. Keeping

records of the child's progress is necessary. In cases where behavioral or psychiatric problems are evident, group or individual psychotherapy may be necessary.

Biofeedback, which is used to train the anal sphincter muscle, has been helpful in some cases but controlled trials do not suggest higher rates of improvement as compared to the standard treatment regimen. Long-term laxative use is contraindicated. Several case reports suggest improvement in some children on tricyclic antidepressants, though there is not enough data to warrant regular use of these drugs, particularly given their narrow therapeutic window and association with cardiac dysrhythmias. Furthermore, tricyclic antidepressants often cause or exacerbate constipation and should be avoided in children with retentive encopresis. The few long-term follow-up studies suggest that encopresis eventually resolves in most children, regardless of treatment approach.

Bernstein SA, Williford SL: Intranasal desmopressin-associated hyponatremia: A case report and literature review. *J Fam Pract* 1997;44:203.

Butler, RJ: Annotation: Night wetting in children: Psychological aspects. *J Child Psychol Psychiatry* 1998;39:453.

Fergusson DM, Horwood LJ: Nocturnal enuresis and behavioral problems in adolescence: A 15 year longitudinal study. *Pediatrics* 1994;94:662.

Foreman DM, Thambirajah MS: Conduct disorder, enuresis and specific developmental delays in two types of encopresis: A case-note study of 63 boys. *Eur Child Adolesc Psychiatry* 1996;5:33.

Loening-Baucke V: Constipation in early childhood: Patient characteristics, treatment and long-term follow-up. *Am Fam Physician* 1994;49:397.

Loening-Baucke V: Encopresis and soiling. *Pediatr Clin North Am* 1996;43:279.

Mikkelsen EJ: Enuresis and encopresis: Ten years of progress. *J Am Acad Child Adolesc Psychiatry* 2001;40:1146.

Robson WL, Leung AKC, Bloom DA: Daytime wetting in childhood. *Clin Pediatr* 1996;35:91.

Rose EA, Porcerelli JH, Neale AV: Pica: Common but commonly missed. *Journal of the American Board of Family Practice* 2000;13:353.

Stark L J, Owens-Stively J, Spirito A, et al: Group behavioral treatment of retentive encopresis. *J Pediatr Psychol* 1990;15:659.

20.5 Sleep Disorders

Judith A. Owens

General Considerations. In order to evaluate sleep problems, it is important to first have an understanding of what constitutes "normal" sleep in children and adolescents. Sleep disturbances, as well as many characteristics of sleep itself, have some distinctly different features in children from sleep and sleep disorders in adults. In addition, sleep architecture and sleep patterns and behaviors change significantly across the age spectrum from infancy to preschool to adolescence. A summary of some of the more important normal developmental changes in children's sleep is found in Table 20–1.

Most sleep problems in children may be broadly conceptualized as resulting from either inadequate duration of sleep for age (insufficient sleep *quantity*) or disruption and fragmentation of sleep (poor sleep *quality*). Insufficient sleep is usually the result of difficulty initiating (delayed sleep onset) and/or maintaining sleep (prolonged night wakings), whereas sleep fragmentation most often results from frequent, repetitive, and brief arousals during sleep. Inadequate sleep duration, especially in older children and adolescents, may also represent a conscious lifestyle decision to sacrifice sleep in favor of competing priorities such as homework and social activities. The underlying causes of sleep onset delay/prolonged night wakings or sleep fragmentation may in turn be related to primarily behavioral factors (e.g., bedtime resistance resulting in shortened sleep duration) and/or medical causes (e.g., obstructive sleep apnea causing frequent brief arousals).

As in adults, both insufficient quantity and poor quality of sleep in children usually result in *excessive daytime sleepiness* and decreased daytime alertness levels. However, sleepiness in children may not be immediately recognizable as drowsiness, yawning, and the other "classic" manifestations of sleepiness

TABLE 20–1. Normal Developmental Changes in Children's Sleep

Age Category	Average Sleep Duration (24 hr)	Sleep Patterns	Additional Variables Impacting on Sleep	Sleep Disorders
Newborns (0–3 mo)	16–20 hr	1 to 4 hr sleep periods followed by 1 to 2 hr awake periods Amount daytime sleep = amount nighttime sleep	Prematurity: few differences in sleep development Birth trauma associated with sleep disruption Breast-fed, shorter sleep periods	Colic Apnea of infancy
Infants (3–12 mo)	14–15 hr total at 4 mo; 13–14 hr total at 6 mo (11 hr/night; 3 hr in 2 naps/day) Nap for 2–4 hr/day at 9 to 12 mo	Sleep periods 3–4 hr first 3 mo; 6–8 hr periods at 4–6 mo; day/night differentiation develops 6 wk to 3 mo 70–80% "settle" (sleep through the night) at 9 mo	Self-soothing skills develop starting at 3 mo; may "signal" night wakings (crying) to parents Settling and night wakings influenced by parenting, feeding practices Co-sleeping common	Sleep onset association disorder/night wakings Rhythmic movement disorders (head banging, body rocking)
Toddlers (1–3 yr)	12–14 hr total Nap 1.5–3.5 hr (1 nap/day)	Night wakings often resume	Nighttime fears develop; transitional objects, bedtime routines important	Sleep onset association disorder Limit setting sleep disorder/bedtime resistance
Preschool (3–6 yr)	11–12 hr Napping declines; most stop by age 5 yr	Night waking in about 20%	Napping patterns influenced by parental, school practices Sleep problems may become chronic	Limit setting sleep disorder Sleepwalking Sleep terrors Obstructive sleep apnea
Middle childhood (6–12 yr)	10 hr	Low levels daytime sleepiness Increased discrepancy school/non-school night sleep amounts	School and behavior problems may be related to sleep problems Stressful events affect sleep; poor sleep affects coping skills	Nightmares Anxiety-related sleep onset delay Insufficient sleep
Adolescence (>12 yr)	9 hr ideal; 7 hr actual	Often irregular; influence of lifestyle; later bedtimes/earlier rise times	Phase delay at puberty; daytime alertness decreases at mid-puberty	Insufficient sleep Delayed sleep phase Narcolepsy Restless legs syndrome/periodic limb movement disorder

that occur in adults. Instead, it often takes the form of mood disturbances, behavioral problems such as hyperactivity and poor impulse control, and neurocognitive dysfunction including inattention and impaired vigilance that, over time, may ultimately result in significant social, school, and learning problems.

Parasomnias (see below), which are episodic sleep behaviors such as sleepwalking and enuresis, constitute another category of sleep disorders occurring in children. *Circadian rhythm disorders*, such as delayed (later sleep onset and rise times) sleep phase, in which normal sleep-wake patterns are disturbed, and *primary disorders of excessive daytime sleepiness*, which are characterized by abnormal regulation of sleep and wakefulness (e.g., narcolepsy), are covered in more detail under adolescent sleep.

Certain pediatric populations are relatively more vulnerable to developing sleep problems on either an acute or chronic basis. These include children with medical problems, including chronic illnesses such as cystic fibrosis and rheumatoid arthritis and acute illnesses such as otitis media; children on medications that have stimulant (e.g., methylphenidate), sleep-disrupting (e.g., some asthma medications), or daytime sedating (e.g., some anticonvulsants) effects; hospitalized children; and children with a variety of psychiatric disorders, including attention-deficit/hyperactivity disorder (ADHD), depression, and anxiety disorders. Children with neurologic disorders may be more prone to nocturnal seizures, as well as other sleep disruptions, and children with blindness and developmental delay syndromes (e.g., autism/pervasive developmental delay) are at increased risk for severe sleep onset difficulty and night wakings, as well as circadian rhythm disturbances.

Health Supervision. Sleep disturbances are one of the most common issues raised by parents during health supervision, and it is estimated that upwards of 25% of children experience a significant sleep problem at some point during childhood. Although

many sleep problems in infants and children are transient and self-limited in nature, certain intrinsic and extrinsic risk factors (difficult temperament, acute or chronic illness, maternal depression, family stress, etc.) may predispose a given child to develop a more chronic sleep disturbance. Inadequate or poor sleep in children may have negative consequences on a host of functional domains, including mood, behavior, learning, and health outcomes. Furthermore, the impact of childhood sleep problems is intensified by their direct effect on parents' sleep, resulting in daytime fatigue, mood disturbances, and a decreased level of effective parenting.

Therefore, it is especially important for pediatricians to both screen for and recognize sleep disorders in children and adolescents during health encounters. In addition, the well child visit is an opportunity to educate parents about normal sleep in children and to teach them strategies to prevent sleep problems from either developing in the first place (primary prevention), or from becoming chronic if problems already exist (secondary prevention). Developmentally appropriate *screening* for sleep disturbances should take place in the context of every well child visit and should include a range of potential sleep problems; one simple sleep screening algorithm, the "BEARS," is outlined in Table 20–2. Because parents may not always be aware of sleep problems, especially in older children and adolescents, it is also important to question the child directly about sleep concerns. The recognition and evaluation of sleep problems in children requires both an understanding of the association between sleep disturbances and daytime consequences, such as irritability, inattention, and poor impulse control, and familiarity with the developmentally appropriate differential diagnoses of common presenting sleep complaints (difficulty initiating and maintaining sleep, episodic nocturnal events, etc.). In particular, an assessment of sleep patterns and possible sleep problems should be part of the initial evaluation of every child presenting with behavioral and/or academic problems, especially ADHD.

TABLE 20–2. BEARS Sleep Screening Algorithm

The "BEARS" instrument is divided into 5 major sleep domains, providing a comprehensive screen for the major sleep disorders affecting children in the 2-18 year old age range. Each sleep domain has a set of age-appropriate "trigger questions" for use in the clinical interview.
B = Bedtime problems
E = Excessive daytime sleepiness
A = Awakenings during the night
R = Regularity and duration of sleep
S = Snoring

Examples of Developmentally Appropriate Trigger Questions

	Toddler/Preschool (2–5 yr)	*School-aged (6–12 yr)*	*Adolescent (13–18 yr)*
1) **B**edtime problems	Does your child have any problems going to bed? Falling asleep?	Does your child have any problems at bedtime? (P) Do you have any problems going to bed? (C)	Do you have any problems falling asleep at bedtime? (C)
2) **E**xcessive daytime sleepiness	Does your child seem over tired or sleepy a lot during the day? Does she still take naps?	Does your child have difficulty waking in the morning, seem sleepy during the day or take naps? (P) Do you feel tired a lot? (C)	Do you feel sleepy a lot during the day? in school? while driving? (C)
3) **A**wakenings during the night	Does your child wake up a lot at night?	Does your child seem to wake up a lot at night? Any sleepwalking or nightmares? (P) Do you wake up a lot at night? Have trouble getting back to sleep? (C)	Do you wake up a lot at night? Have trouble getting back to sleep? (C)
4) **R**egularity and duration of sleep	Does your child have a regular bedtime and wake time? What are they?	What time does your child go to bed and get up on school days? Weekends? Do you think he/she is getting enough sleep? (P)	What time do you usually go to bed on school nights? Weekends? How much sleep do you usually get? (C)
5) **S**noring	Does your child snore a lot or have difficulty breathing at night?	Does your child have loud or nightly snoring or any breathing difficulties at night? (P)	Does your teenager snore loudly or nightly? (P)

P = Parent; C = Child.

Effective *preventative measures* may include educating parents of newborns about normal sleep amounts and patterns; suggesting that parents put their 4–6-month-old infants to bed "drowsy but awake" in order to avoid dependence on parental presence at sleep onset and to foster the infants' ability to "self-soothe," discussing the importance of regular bedtimes, bedtime routines, and transitional objects for toddlers; and providing parents and children with basic information about good "sleep hygiene" (Table 20–3) and adequate sleep amounts.

It is important also to consider the cultural and family context within which sleep problems in children occur (Chapter 3). For example, *co-sleeping* of infants and parents is a common and accepted practice in many ethnic groups, including African-Americans, Hispanics, and Southeast Asians. Therefore, the goal of independent "self-soothing" in young infants may not be shared by these families. On the other hand, the institution of co-sleeping by parents as an attempt to address a child's underlying sleep problem, rather than as a lifestyle choice, is likely to yield only a temporary respite from the problem and may set the stage for more significant sleep issues.

Behavioral Sleep Disorders. Sleep problems, like many behavioral issues in children, are often primarily defined by parental concerns rather than by objective criteria. Many of the behaviorally based sleep disorders are the result of the interaction between normal developmental sleep changes, as outlined above, and parental response to those changes. For example, one of the most common sleep disorders found in infants and toddlers is *sleep onset association disorder*. In this disorder, the child learns to fall asleep only under certain conditions or associations, such as being rocked or fed, and does not develop the ability to self-soothe. During the night, when the child experiences the type of brief arousal that normally occurs at the end of a sleep cycle (every 90–120 min) or awakens for other reasons, he or she is not able to get back to sleep without those same conditions being present. The infant then "signals" the parent by crying (or

coming into the parents' bedroom if the child is no longer in a crib) until the necessary associations are provided. Thus, the problem is one of prolonged night waking resulting in insufficient sleep (for both child and parent!).

The treatment approach to sleep onset association disorder typically involves a program of withdrawal of parental assistance at sleep onset and during the night (systematic ignoring). In older infants, the introduction of more appropriate sleep associations that will be readily available to the child during the night (transitional objects such as a blanket or toy) in addition to positive reinforcement (e.g., stickers for remaining in bed) is often beneficial. The goal is to allow the infant or child to develop skills in self-soothing during the night, as well as at bedtime. "Graduated extinction" is a more gradual process of weaning the child from dependence upon parental presence that utilizes periodic "checks" by the parents at successively longer time intervals during the sleep-wake transition. If the child has become habituated to awaken for nighttime feedings ("learned hunger"), then these feedings should be slowly eliminated. Parents must be consistent in applying behavioral programs to avoid inadvertent, intermittent reinforcement of night wakings; they should also be forewarned that crying behavior frequently temporarily escalates at the beginning of treatment ("post-extinction burst").

In contrast, *limit setting sleep disorder*, a disorder most common in children preschool-aged and older, is characterized by difficulty falling asleep and bedtime resistance ("curtain calls") rather than night wakings. The prolonged sleep onset delay results in inadequate sleep duration. Most commonly, this disorder develops from a parent's inability or unwillingness to set consistent bedtime rules and enforce a regular bedtime, often exacerbated by the child's oppositional behavior. In some cases, however, the child's resistance at bedtime is due to an underlying problem in falling asleep caused by other factors (e.g., medical conditions such as asthma or medication use, a sleep disorder such as Restless Legs syndrome, or anxiety) or a mismatch

TABLE 20–3. Basic Principles of Sleep Hygiene for Children

1. **Have a set bedtime and bedtime routine** for your child.
2. **Bedtime and wake-up time should be about the same time on school nights and non-school nights.** There should not be more than about an hour difference from one day to another.
3. **Make the hour before bed shared quiet time.** Avoid such high-energy activities as rough play, and stimulating activities such as watching TV or playing computer games just before bed.
4. **Don't send your child to bed hungry.** A *light* snack (such as milk and cookies) before bed is a good idea. Heavy meals within an hour or two of bedtime, however, may interfere with sleep.
5. **Avoid products containing caffeine for at least several hours before bedtime.** These include caffeinated sodas, coffee, tea, and chocolate.
6. **Make sure your child spends time outside every day** whenever possible and is involved in regular exercise.
7. **Keep your child's bedroom quiet and dark.** A low-level nightlight is acceptable for children who find completely dark rooms frightening.
8. **Keep your child's bedroom at a comfortable temperature** during the night (less than 75 degrees).
9. **Don't use your child's bedroom for time-out or punishment.**
10. **Keep the television set out of your child's bedroom.** Children can easily develop the bad habit of "needing" the TV to fall asleep. It's also much more difficult to control your child's TV viewing if the set is in the bedroom.

TABLE 20–4. Differentiation of Episodic Nocturnal Phenomena

Characteristics	Sleepwalking	Sleep Terrors	Nightmares	Nocturnal Seizures
Timing During Night	First third	First third	Last third	Variable; often at sleep-wake transition
Sleep Stage	SWS	SWS	REM	Non-REM>REM
Clinical Description				
1. Displacement from bed	Usual during event	May occur during event	Occasional after event	Unusual
2. Autonomic arousal/agitation	Low to mild	High to extreme	Mild to high	Variable
3. Stereotypic/repetitive behavior	Variable; complex behaviors	Variable	None; little motor behavior	Common
4. Arousal threshold	High; agitated if awakened	High; agitated if awakened	Low; awake and agitated after event	High; awake and confused after event
5. Associated daytime sleepiness	None	None	Yes, if night waking prolonged	Probable
Recall of Event	None or fragmentary	None or fragmentary	Frequent, vivid	None
Incidence	Common (20% at least one episode; 1 to 6% chronic)	Rare (1 to 6%); 10% of sleepwalkers	Very common	Infrequent
Family History	Common	Common	No	Variable

REM = rapid eye movement; SWS = slow wave sleep.

between the child's intrinsic circadian rhythm ("night owl") and parental expectations.

Successful treatment of limit setting sleep disorder generally involves a combination of decreased parental attention for bedtime-delaying behavior, establishment of bedtime routines, and positive reinforcement (e.g., sticker charts) for appropriate behavior at bedtime. Older children may benefit from being taught relaxation techniques to help themselves fall asleep more readily.

Parasomnias. *Parasomnias* are defined as episodic nocturnal behaviors that often involve cognitive disorientation and autonomic and skeletal muscle disturbance. Many of the parasomnias are associated with relative central nervous system immaturity and, thus, tend to be much more common in children than adults and to abate with age. The *partial arousal parasomnias*, which include sleepwalking and sleep terrors, have several features in common. Because they typically occur at the transition out of Stage 4 or slow wave sleep (SWS), partial arousal parasomnias have clinical features of both the awake (ambulation, vocalizations) and the sleeping (high arousal threshold, unresponsiveness to the environment) state, and there is usually amnesia for the events. They are more common in preschoolers and school-aged children because of the relatively higher percentage of SWS in younger children. Furthermore, any factors that are associated with an increase in the relative percentage of SWS (certain medications, previous sleep deprivation) may increase the frequency of events in a predisposed child. The typical timing of partial arousal parasomnias during the first 2 hr of sleep is related to the predominance of SWS in the first third of the night. Finally, there appears to be a genetic predisposition for both sleepwalking and night terrors.

In contrast, *nightmares*, which are much more common than the partial arousal parasomnias but are often confused with them, are concentrated in the last third of the night, when rapid eye movement of REM sleep is most prominent. Partial arousal parasomnias may also be difficult to distinguish from nocturnal seizures. Table 20–4 summarizes similarities and differences among these four nocturnal arousal events.

The treatment of partial arousal parasomnias generally involves parental education and reassurance, avoidance of exacerbating factors such as sleep deprivation, and, particularly in the case of sleepwalking, institution of safety precautions. Pharmacotherapy or psychotherapy is rarely indicated. However, frequent and persistent nightmares in a child warrant further investigation regarding possible trauma, such as sexual abuse, and/or evaluation for a more global anxiety disorder.

Rhythmic movement disorders, including body rocking and head banging, are parasomnias that are much more common in the first year of life and generally disappear by age 4 yr. They occur largely during sleep-wake transition, and are characterized by repetitive, stereotypic movements involving large muscle groups. Although occasionally associated with developmental delay, the vast majority occur in normal children and do not result in physical injury to the child. Treatment is generally parental reassurance.

Sleep in Adolescents. Although sleep patterns and the types of sleep disorders most commonly found in adolescents share features with those of both younger children and of adults, the physiologic changes that occur during puberty and the developmental challenges of adolescence contribute to a number of unique aspects of adolescent sleep. In order to appreciate the impact of these physiologic and psychologic changes, it is important first to consider them in the context of human sleep regulation and some of the basic principles that govern sleep and wakefulness. The first principle relates to those factors that determine the relative level of sleepiness or alertness occurring throughout a given 24-hr time period; these include both intrinsic *circadian* factors or rhythms ("biologic time clock") and *homeostatic* factors (duration and quality of previous sleep as well as time awake since the last sleep period). For example, there are two periods of clock-dependent maximum sleepiness ("circadian troughs") and maximum alertness that occur during the course of a 24-hour day. The degree of sleepiness experienced during a given circadian trough period, however, is also influenced by the relative sleep need existing at the time (e.g., is increased in the sleep-deprived individual). Intrinsic circadian rhythms are in turn affected to a degree by external time cues or "zeitgebers" (e.g., timing of meals, alarm clocks, etc.), but they are most sensitive to light/darkness signals, which switch the body's production of the hormone melatonin off (light) or on (dark).

A second important principle of sleep regulation relates to the consequences of the failure to meet basic sleep needs. Individual sleep needs are dependent upon a number of factors, including age and the amount of sleep obtained in the preceding period. Inadequate sleep on a chronic basis results in what is called a *sleep debt*. If the sleep debt becomes large enough and is not voluntarily paid back, the body may respond by overriding voluntary control of wakefulness, resulting in periods of decreased alertness, dozing off, and napping. In addition, the sleep-deprived individual may experience very brief (several seconds) repeated daytime *microsleeps* of which he or she may be completely unaware, but which nonetheless may result in significant lapses in attention and vigilance. This becomes a particularly problematic issue in adolescents, who may be operating motor vehicles ("drowsy driving").

FEATURES OF ADOLESCENT SLEEP. Adolescent sleep needs are not dramatically different from sleep needs of preadolescents, about 9 hours per night. In contrast, most adolescents obtain on the order of 7 to 7½ hr of sleep per night, which results in a considerable sleep debt over time. Part of the reason for this insufficient sleep relates to pubertal influences on melatonin and circadian sleep/wake cycles, which cause a relative *phase delay* (later sleep onset and wake times). Not only are adolescents less likely to fall asleep early, but the start time of many high schools precludes a corresponding later wake time in the morning. In addition, many adolescents have highly irregular sleep/wake patterns from weekday to weekend; when coupled with a physiologic tendency to develop decreased daytime alertness levels in mid to late puberty, this all results in considerable increase in sleepiness levels and consequent impairment in mood, attention, memory, behavioral control, and academic performance.

Adolescents may also suffer from a number of sleep disorders, some of which are detailed in other chapters. Studies have suggested that the prevalence of significant sleep problems in adolescents is high (at least 20%) and that particular groups of adolescents, such as those with chronic medical or psychiatric problems, may be at increased risk. As would be expected, *circadian rhythm* disturbances, especially *delayed sleep phase syndrome*, are prominent in adolescence; these are sometimes treated with a combination of exogenous melatonin and bright light therapy to help "reset" the clock. Teenagers with a severely delayed sleep phase (greater than 3 to 4 hr) may benefit from a technique called chronotherapy, in which the sleep onset and wake times are successively delayed over a period of time until the new sleep onset time coincides with the desired bedtime.

Psychophysiologic insomnia (difficulty initiating and/or maintaining sleep) is also common in adolescents. In this disorder, the individual develops conditioned anxiety around difficulty falling or staying asleep, which leads to heightened arousal and further compromises the ability to sleep. Treatment usually involves educating the adolescent about principles of sleep hygiene (Table 20–5), instructing him or her to use the bed for sleep only and to get out of bed if unable to fall asleep (stimulus control), restricting time-in-bed to the actual time asleep (sleep restriction), and teaching relaxation techniques to reduce anxiety. Hypnotic medications are rarely needed.

Narcolepsy is a primary disorder of excessive daytime sleepiness that affects an estimated 0.05% of Americans. Narcolepsy often presents with symptoms in adolescence, but usually goes unrecognized and undiagnosed until adulthood. In about 25% of cases, there is a family history of narcolepsy; secondary narcolepsy following brain injury or in association with other medical illnesses may also occur. The cardinal and usual initial presenting feature of narcolepsy is repetitive episodes of profound sleepiness that may occur both at rest and during periods of activity (talking, eating, etc.). These "sleep attacks" may be very brief (microsleeps), resulting primarily in lapses in attention and in mood disturbances. Thus, patients with narcolepsy may be initially misdiagnosed with a psychiatric disorder such as ADHD or depression. Other features that may occur in narcolepsy include cataplexy (sudden loss of total body or partial muscle tone, usually in response to an emotional stimulus), hypnogogic (at sleep onset) and/or hypnopompic (on waking) visual, auditory or tactile hallucinations, and sleep paralysis (temporary loss of voluntary muscle control) at sleep onset or offset. The "gold standard" of diagnosis is overnight polysomnography followed by a multiple sleep latency test (MSLT). The MSLT involves a series of opportunities to nap during which narcoleptics demonstrate a pathologically shortened sleep onset latency, as well as periods of REM sleep occurring immediately after sleep onset. The treatment of narcolepsy generally involves a combination of medications to combat daytime sleepiness (stimulants) and REM sleep suppressants to prevent cataleptic attacks.

Restless Legs syndrome (RLS)/periodic limb movement disorder (PLMD) is a sleep disorder that is characterized by what is often described as uncomfortable "creeping" or "crawling" sensations

---

TABLE 20–5. **Basic Principles of Sleep Hygiene for Adolescents**

1. **Wake up and go to bed at about the same time** every night. Bedtime and wake time should not differ from school to non-school nights by more than approximately an hour.
2. **Avoid sleeping in on weekends** to "catch-up" on sleep. This makes it more likely that you will have problems falling asleep.
3. If you take **naps**, they should be **short** (no more than an hour) and **scheduled in the early to mid-afternoon**. However, if you have a problem with falling asleep at night, **napping** during the day may make it worse and should be avoided.
4. **Spend time outside** every day. Exposure to sunlight helps to keep your body's internal clock on track.
5. **Exercise regularly**. Exercise may help you fall asleep and sleep more deeply.
6. **Use your bed for sleeping only**. Don't study, read, listen to music, watch TV, etc., on your bed.
7. Make the 30–60 minutes before bedtime a **quiet or wind-down time**. Relaxing, calm, enjoyable activities such as reading a book or listening to calm music help your body and mind slow down enough to let you get to sleep. Don't study, watch exciting/scary movies, exercise, or get involved in "energizing" activities just before bed.
8. Eat regular meals and **don't go to bed hungry**. A light snack before bed is a good idea; eating a full meal in the hour before bed is not.
9. **Avoid** eating or drinking products containing **caffeine** from dinner time on. These include caffeinated sodas, coffee, tea, and chocolate.
10. **Do not use alcohol**. Alcohol disrupts sleep and may cause you to awaken throughout the night.
11. **Smoking disturbs sleep**. Don't smoke at least one hour before bed (and preferably, not at all!).
12. Don't use **sleeping pills, melatonin**, or other **over-the-counter sleep aids** to help you sleep unless specifically recommended by your doctor. These can be dangerous, and the sleep problems often return when you stop the medicine.

occurring primarily in the lower extremities and during periods of rest or inactivity (e.g., sleep onset), which are relieved by movement. In younger children, these sensations may be manifested as "growing pains." The symptoms often result in significantly delayed sleep onset. RLS appears to have a genetic basis and exacerbating factors include increased caffeine intake, iron deficiency (low ferritin), and pregnancy. Although the prevalence of RLS in adolescents is unknown, approximately 1 in 2000 adults has the disorder. RLS is thought to be related to decreased dopaminergic activity; pharmacologic treatment generally involves dopaminergic agents. Approximately 80% of patients with RLS also have repetitive rhythmic kicking movements of the lower extremities during sleep called periodic limb movements. The sleeper is usually unaware of the leg movements and of the resulting sleep fragmentation. Both RLS and PLMD may result in manifestations of significant daytime sleepiness, including inattention and hyperactivity. RLS is a clinical diagnosis; the diagnosis of PLMD requires polysomnography to detect the characteristic rhythmic movements of the anterior tibialis muscle group and frequent arousals.

Evaluation of Pediatric Sleep Problems. The clinical evaluation of a child presenting with a sleep problem involves a careful medical history to assess for potential medical causes of sleep disturbances, such as allergies, concomitant medications, and acute or chronic pain conditions. A developmental history is important because of the aforementioned frequent association of sleep problems with severe developmental delay. Assessment of the child's current level of functioning (school, home, etc.) is key in evaluating possible mood, behavioral, and neurocognitive sequelae of sleep problems. Current sleep patterns, including usual sleep duration and sleep/wake schedule, are often best assessed with a sleep diary, in which parents record daily sleep behaviors for an extended period. A review of sleep habits, such as bedtime routines, daily caffeine intake, and the sleeping environment (temperature, noise level, etc.) may reveal environmental factors that contribute to the sleep problems.

Nocturnal symptoms that may be indicative of a medically based sleep disorder such as obstructive sleep apnea (loud snoring, choking/gasping, sweating) or periodic limb movements (restless sleep, repetitive kicking movements) should be elicited. However, an overnight sleep study is seldom warranted in the evaluation of a child with sleep problems unless there are symptoms suggestive of obstructive sleep apnea (Chapter 369) or periodic leg movements, unusual features of episodic nocturnal events, or daytime sleepiness that is unexplained.

Carskadon MA, Wolfson AR, Acebo C, et al: Adolescent sleep patterns, circadian timing, and sleepiness at a transition to early school days. *Sleep* 1998;21(8): 871–81.

Dahl RE: Narcolepsy in children and adolescents. *Child Adolesc Psychiatr Clin N Am* 1996;5(3):649–59.

Ferber R: Clinical assessment of child and adolescent sleep disorders. *Child Adolesc Psychiatr Clin N Am* 1996;5(3):569–79.

Ferber R, Kryger M: *Principles and Practice of Sleep Medicine in the Child.* Philadelphia, WB Saunders, 1995.

Mindell JA, Owends JA, Carskadon MA: Developmental features of sleep. *Child Adolesc Psychiatr Clin N Am* 1999;8(4):695–719.

Morrison DN, McGee R, Stanton WR: Sleep problems in adolescence. *J Am Acad Child Adolesc Psychiatry* 1992;31(1):94–9.

National Sleep Foundation: *Adolescent Sleep Needs and Patterns.* Washington DC, 1999; www.sleepfoundation.org.

Picchietti DL, Walters AS: Restless legs syndrome and periodic limb movement disorder in children and adolescents. *Child Adolesc Psychiatr Clin N Am* 1996;5(3):729–40.

Rosen GM, Ferber R, Mahowald MW: Evaluation of parasomnias in children. *Child Adolesc Psychiatr Clin N Am* 1996;5(3):601–14.

Sheldon SH, Spire JP, Levy HB: *Pediatric Sleep Medicine.* Philadelphia, WB Saunders, 1992.

Wise MS: Childhood narcolepsy. *Neurology* 1998;50 (Suppl 1):S37–S42.

Wolfson AR: Sleeping patterns of children and adolescents. *Sleep Disorders* 1996;5(3):549–64.

Chapter 21
Habit Disorders
Neil W. Boris and Richard Dalton

Habit disorders include tension-discharging phenomena, such as head banging, body rocking, thumb sucking, nail biting, hair pulling (trichotillomania), teeth grinding (bruxism), hitting or biting parts of one's own body, body manipulations, repetitive vocalizations, and air swallowing (aerophagia). Tics, which involve the involuntary movement of various muscle groups, are also included. Many children at various developmental points show repetitive patterns of movement that can be described as habits. Whether they are considered disorders depends on the degree to which they interfere with the child's physical, emotional, or social functioning. Some habit patterns may be learned by imitation of adults. Many begin as a purposeful movement that, for some reason, becomes repetitive, with the habit losing its original significance and becoming a means of discharging tension. For example, a child who has an eye irritation or is attempting not to shed tears might try closing the eyelids several times in rapid succession. This activity may become repetitive and incorporated into the child's behavior as an outlet for tension. Such symptoms are often reinforced by attention from parents or others. Other movements, such as rhythmic head banging and rocking in early life, can persist without parental reinforcement, occurring when the child is put to bed or is alone; these movements seem to provide a kind of sensory solace for the child. In many cases, children who exhibit head banging or rocking either have been neglected or have developmental delays. These movements represent a kind of internal stroking. Some children twist their hair or touch or play with parts of their bodies in repetitive ways. As these children become older, they may learn to inhibit some of their rhythmic habit patterns, particularly in social situations. In some cases, however, social anxiety can increase repetitive behaviors. The prevalence of habit disorders is not known. In part, this is because habit disorders are a heterogeneous group of disorders with varying causes. The natural course can vary, though children with mental retardation may be more refractory to treatment.

Teeth grinding, or *bruxism*, is quite common, can begin in the first 5 yr of life, and seems to be associated with daytime anxiety. Untreated bruxism may create problems with dental occlusion. Helping the child find ways to reduce anxiety may relieve the problem, though studies of psychologic treatment for bruxism are rare. Bedtime can be made more enjoyable and relaxed by reading or talking with the child, permitting review of fears or angers experienced during the day. Praise and other emotional support are useful at these times. To what degree bruxism is heritable is not known. Persistent bruxism requires referral to a dentist and may present as muscular or temporomandibular joint pain.

Thumb sucking is normal in infancy and toddlerhood. Older children who thumb suck may eventually affect alignment of the teeth. Like other rhythmic patterns of behavior, thumb sucking can be seen as a way of securing extra self-nurturance. The best strategy for dealing with thumb sucking is to provide the child with praise for substitute behaviors. Parents should ignore thumb sucking, if possible, while giving attention to more positive aspects of the child's behavior. When the child actively tries to restrain thumb sucking, he or she should be given praise and encouragement. The use of noxious agents (e.g., bitter salves) to control thumb sucking is not well studied and should be considered a second-line approach.

Tics involve repetitive movements of muscle groups and represent discharges of tension related to central nervous system electrochemical signals. Parts of the body most frequently involved are the muscles of the face, neck, shoulders, trunk, and hands. There may be lip smacking and grimacing, tongue thrusting, eye blinking, throat clearing, and so on. Tics must be distinguished from petit mal or other nongeneralized seizure disorders. Seizure disorders are characterized both by transient inability to interact during periods of eye blinking or lip smacking or amnesia for the event. An electroencephalogram (EEG) may be necessary in some cases to distinguish tic disorders from seizure disorders. Tics can be distinguished from dyskinetic movements and dystonias by their discontinuation during sleep and by virtue of the conscious control that can be achieved for short periods. However, it is very difficult to continuously and consciously inhibit tics. In some cases, tics are transient; in others, the development of tics is temporally related to the use of dopaminergic agonists such as stimulant medications. When this happens, discontinuing the stimulant will usually, but not always, lead to remission of tics. Clinical experience suggests that about half of patients will not redevelop tics when a stimulant is restarted.

EEG findings and cognitive testing do not differentiate patients with tics from control subjects. Most children with simple motor tics do not require treatment, though some may experience associated problems including neuropsychologic dysfunction, academic underachievement, or low self-esteem. These associated problems may require psychotherapeutic intervention.

Gilles de la Tourette syndrome, which has a lifetime prevalence rate of 0.5/1,000 individuals, commonly presents in childhood. Fifty per cent of patients with Tourette syndrome have symptom onset prior to age 7. Tourette syndrome is characterized by a history of motor *and* vocal tics (though they do not have to be present concurrently for diagnosis). In many cases multiple tics or complex vocal sounds such as barking and grunting are present. Rarely, shouting obscene words is evident. Tourette syndrome is more common in the first-degree relatives of patients with Tourette syndrome than in the general population and affects boys three to four times more often than girls. It is more common in whites than in other races.

Children with Tourette syndrome often suffer from associated behavioral, emotional, and academic problems. In particular, these children have higher rates of obsessive-compulsive disorder (OCD), attention-deficit/hyperactivity disorder (ADHD), and oppositional-defiant disorder. The fact that Tourette disorder is highly co-morbid with these specific psychiatric disorders suggests dysfunction in particular regions of the brain.

Although the etiology of Tourette syndrome is uncertain, an interplay among genetic, neurobiologic, psychologic, and environmental factors is likely. Neuroimaging studies suggest that there is a lack of normal asymmetry within the striatum. The precipitation and worsening of tics by stimulant medication suggests dopaminergic involvement in tic and Tourette disorders. Single photon emission computed tomography scan data implicate dysfunction in dopamine receptor binding in severely affected children. In addition, just as with OCD, there is evidence to suggest that a subgroup of prepubertal children who suddenly develop Tourette syndrome suffer with a *pediatric autoimmune neuropsychiatric disorder associated with streptococcal infection* (PANDAS), in which antibodies to group A streptococcal infections cross react with basal ganglia tissue and subsequently precipitate symptoms. The diagnostic index of suspicion should be raised when symptoms develop precipitously after a streptococcal-like episode of pharyngitis in children. In many cases, tics or obsessions may flare after further episodes of infection. A thorough history and an antistreptolysin O (ASO) titer are indicated to confirm the presence of a PANDAS. Treatment of PANDAS includes acute and prophylactic antibiotic therapy. There may be a role for intravenous immunoglobulin during acute infection or even therapeutic plasma exchange for severely affected children, though data on these treatments are limited. Rarely, Lyme disease may also present with clinical manifestations of Tourette syndrome (see Chapter 204). Many environmental factors serve as emotional stressors, which also precipitate or increase tics and Gilles de la Tourette syndrome. Laboratory studies are nonspecific; up to 80% of patients with Tourette syndrome have nonspecific abnormal EEG findings. Abnormal amounts of various neurotransmitter metabolites as well as lower scores on verbal subscales of psychometric tests have been reported.

Treatment for Gilles de la Tourette syndrome should only occur after careful consideration of the functional limitations associated with each given child's symptoms, associated symptoms (e.g., ADHD, OCD, or oppositional tendencies), and risks and benefits of pharmacotherapy. In many cases, supportive management is all that is indicated. Children and families often gain support from organizations like the Tourette's Syndrome Association. Pharmacotherapy is indicated when tics interfere with social development or classroom function. There is some controversy over what agents are first-line treatments, though neuroleptics have the strongest track record in controlled trials. Haloperidol and pimozide, dopaminergic antagonists, have been shown to reduce the severity of tics by 65%. Because potentially severe side effects attend the use of both medications, most clinicians now use novel neuroleptics such as risperidone and olanzapine. Clonidine, an α_2 agonist, has also been shown to be effective in controlled trials. However, sedation and low blood pressure are associated with clonidine; the role for guanfacine (Tenex), which is less sedating, has not been firmly established (see Chapter 28.2). Botulinum toxin has also recently been shown to be effective for motor tics.

Some children with Tourette syndorme require medications aimed at obsessive-compulsive symptoms or attention and impulsivity problems. Unfortunately, psychostimulants may make tics worse in children with co-morbid Tourette disorder and ADHD. The physician must weigh the benefits of improvement in ADHD symptoms with the potential exacerbation of tics. Tourette disorder may persist throughout life; however, studies have shown a significant diminution in symptoms in adolescence and early adulthood in about two thirds of cases.

Coffey BJ, Biederman J, Geller DA, et al: The course of Tourette's disorder: A literature review. *Harv Rev Psychiatry* 2000;8:192–8.

Cohen D, Leckman J: Developmental psychopathology and neurobiology of Tourette's syndrome. *J Am Acad Child Adolesc Psychiatry* 1994;33:2–15.

Foster LG: Nervous habits and stereotyped behaviors in preschool children. *J Am Acad Child Adolesc Psychiatry* 1998;37:711–7.

Leonard HL, Swedo SE: Paediatric autoimmune neuropsychiatric disorders associated with streptococcal infection (PANDAS). *International Journal of Neuropsychopharmacology* 2001;4:191–8.

March JS, Leonard HL: Obsessive-compulsive disorder in children and adolescents: A review of the past 10 years. *J Am Acad Child Adolesc Psychiatry* 1996;35:1265–73.

Muller-Vahl KR, Berding G, Kolbe H, et al: Dopamine D2 receptor imaging in Gilles de la Tourette syndrome. *Acta Neurol Scand* 2000;101:165–71.

Sallee FR, Nesbitt L, Jackson C, et al: Relative efficacy of haloperidol and pimozide in children and adolescents with Tourette's disorder. *Am J Psychiatry* 1997;154:1057–64.

Scahill L, Chappell PB, King RA, et al: Pharmacologic treatment of tic disorders. *Child Adolesc Psychiatr Clin N Am* 2000;9:99–117.

Chapter 22
Anxiety Disorders
Brian Stafford, Neil W. Boris, and Richard Dalton

Anxiety is a normal phenomenon that has evolutionary value for the species. Anxiety has both a physiologic component, mediated by the autonomic nervous system, and a cognitive and behavioral component, expressed in worrying and wariness. When anxiety becomes disabling, interfering with social interactions and development, a diagnosis should be made and intervention initiated. Separation anxiety disorder, childhood onset social phobia, generalized anxiety disorder, obsessive-compulsive disorder (OCD), phobias, post-traumatic stress disorder (PTSD), and panic disorder are all defined by the occurrence of either diffuse or specific anxiety, often related to predictable situations or "cues." As a group, anxiety disorders are the most common psychiatric disorders of childhood: epidemiologic data suggest that they occur in 5–18% of all children and adolescents. Anxiety disorders are often co-morbid with other psychiatric disorders (including a second anxiety disorder), and significant impairment in day-to-day functioning is not uncommon.

Because anxiety is both a normal phenomenon and, when highly activated, strongly associated with impairment, the pediatrician will be required to differentiate normal from abnormal across development. Fortunately, anxiety has an identifiable developmental progression for most children. For instance, most infants exhibit stranger wariness or anxiety beginning at 7–9 mo of age. Furthermore, studies document that behavioral inhibition to the unfamiliar (e.g., withdrawal/fearfulness to novel stimuli associated with physiologic arousal) is evident in about 10–15% of the population at 12 mo of age and is moderately stable. Most children who display behavioral inhibition do not eventually develop impairing levels of anxiety. However, data from a cohort of behaviorally inhibited infants followed longitudinally revealed that both a family history of anxiety disorders and maternal over-involvement or enmeshment predicted later clinically significant anxiety problems. The infant who is excessively clingy and difficult to calm during pediatric visits should be followed for signs of increasing levels of anxiety.

Preschoolers typically develop specific fears related to the dark, to animals, and to imaginary situations. Preoccupation with orderliness and routines (so-called "just right" phenomena) also often take on an anxious quality for preschool children. Parental reassurance is usually sufficient to help the child through this period. Although most school-aged children give up the imaginary fears of early childhood, some replace them with fears of bodily harm or other worries. In adolescence, both social anxiety and general worrying (about school, friends, and family) are not uncommon.

Genetic or temperamental factors contribute more to the development of some anxiety disorders, whereas environmental factors are closely linked to the cause for others. Specifically, behavioral inhibition appears to be a heritable tendency and is linked with social phobia, generalized anxiety, and selective mutism. OCD and other disorders associated with OCD-like behaviors, such as Tourette and other tic disorders, tend to have high genetic risk as well (see Chapter 21). Environmental factors, such as parent-infant attachment and exposure to trauma, contribute more to separation anxiety disorder and PTSD. Even in those disorders associated with environmental risk, nature and nurture interact to create maladaptive behavior.

Separation anxiety disorder (SAD) is characterized by unrealistic and persistent worries of possible harm befalling primary caregivers, reluctance to go to school or sleep without being near the parents, persistent avoidance of being alone, nightmares involving themes of separation, numerous somatic complaints, and complaints of subjective distress. The first clinical sign of the disorder may not appear until third or fourth grade, typically after holidays, a period where the child has been home because of illness, or the stability of the family structure has been threatened by illness, divorce, or other calamity. In many cases, parents are unable to be assertive in returning the child to school. In these instances, the pediatrician should screen for parental depression or anxiety. Often referral for parental treatment or family therapy is necessary before separation anxiety and concomitant school refusal can be successfully treated.

A large percentage of children with SAD develop feelings of panic when they are coerced to separate from their parents. Children with SAD appear to have a higher than expected likelihood of developing panic disorder in adolescence. When a child reports recurring acute severe anxiety, antidepressant or anxiolytic medication is often necessary. After promising initial data, subsequent controlled studies of tricyclic antidepressants (e.g., imipramine) and benzodiazepines (e.g., clonazepam) have revealed that these agents are not generally effective. Alternatively, data supports the use of selective serotonin reuptake inhibitors (SSRIs; see Chapter 28.2). Individual and/or group cognitive behavioral therapy may also add benefit, though attention to the family context remains necessary.

Childhood-onset *social phobia* (SP) is characterized by excessive anxiety in social settings (including school) leading to social isolation. These children and adolescents often maintain the desire for involvement with family and familiar peers. The long-term course is variable, though good longitudinal studies are lacking. However, some children are very distressed by their inability to engage in meaningful relationships with peers and seek treatment. A family history of social phobia or extreme shyness is not uncommon. SSRIs are considered the treatment of choice. Buspirone, alprazolam, and phenelzine have been shown to be helpful, though they are less well studied and are not considered first-line medications (see Chapter 28.2).

School refusal is associated with both SAD and SP. School refusal occurs in about 1–2% of children and is commonly addressed by pediatricians. Younger children often show reluctance to separate from caregivers with concomitant worries about the caregiver's well-being (SAD), whereas older children demonstrate fear of exposure to unfamiliar or possibly humiliating environments (SP). Somatic complaints, especially abdominal pain and/or headaches, are common. As many as 75% of children who refuse to go to school also suffer from clinical and subclinical depressive symptoms in addition to anxiety. There may be increasing tension in the parent-child relationship or other indices of family disruption (e.g., domestic violence, divorce, or other major stressors) contributing to this disorder. Management of school refusal typically requires parent management or even family therapy. Working with school personnel is almost always indicated; anxious children often require special attention from teachers, counselors, or school nurses. Typically, parents who are coached to calmly send their children to school and to reward the child for each completed day of school will be successful. In cases of ongoing school refusal, referral to a child psychiatrist is indicated. Young children with affective symptoms have a good prognosis, whereas adolescents with more insidious onset or with significant somatic complaints have a more guarded prognosis.

Selective mutism (previously classified as elective mutism) has recently been conceptualized as a disorder that overlaps with social phobia. Children with selective mutism talk almost exclusively at home, though they are reticent to do so in other settings such as school, daycare, or even relatives' homes. Often, one or more stressors—such as a new classroom or parental or sibling conflict—drive an already shy child to become reluctant to speak. Fluoxetine has been shown to be effective for children whose school performance is severely limited by their symptoms (see Chapter 28.2).

Panic disorder is a syndrome of recurrent, discrete episodes of marked fear or discomfort in which individuals experience abrupt onset of physical and psychologic symptoms. The physical symptoms can include palpitations, sweating, shaking, shortness of breath, dizziness, chest pain, and nausea. Children who present with acute respiratory distress, but without fever, wheezing, or stridor also may be experiencing a panic attack. The associated psychologic symptoms include fear of death, impending doom, and loss of control. Panic disorder is uncommon before adolescence, with the peak age of onset being between 15 and 19 yr. Preliminary studies in adults suggest a predisposition to react to autonomic arousal with anxiety is a specific risk factor leading to panic disorder. The increasing rates of panic attack are also directly related to increasing sexual maturity. Some adolescents with panic disorder may develop **agoraphobia**, a subsequent fear that a panic attack may occur in a place where help or escape may be unavailable. Neither panic disorder nor agoraphobia is well studied in children or adolescents. As in the treatment of adults with panic disorder, SSRIs have shown effectiveness in the treatment of adolescents (see Chapter 28.2).

Children who suffer from *generalized anxiety disorder* (GAD) frequently experience unrealistic worries about future events or about the appropriateness of past behavior and their own competence. They frequently present with somatic complaints, are markedly self-conscious, need large amounts of reassurance, and have trouble relaxing. Onset may be gradual or sudden, though GAD does not often become manifest until puberty. Boys and girls are equally affected and the prevalence in adolescence is 2.4%. GAD is characteristically seen in middle and upper middle class white children. Children with GAD are generally good candidates for cognitive-behavioral therapy, though a trial of buspirone or an SSRI may be indicated when symptoms are particularly limiting.

It is important to distinguish children with GAD from those who present with specific repetitive thoughts that invade consciousness (obsessions) or repetitive rituals or movements that are driven by anxiety (compulsions). The most common obsessions are concerned with bodily wastes and secretions, the fear that something calamitous will happen, or the need for sameness. The most common compulsions are handwashing, continual checking of locks, and touching. In times of stress (bedtime, preparing for school), some children touch certain objects, verbalize certain words, or wash their hands repeatedly. *OCD* is diagnosed when the thoughts or rituals cause distress, consume time, or interfere with occupational or social functioning. The children's Yale-Brown Obsessive-Compulsive Scale (C-YBOCS) and the Anxiety Disorders Interview Schedule for Children (ADIS-C) are reliable and valid methods of discriminating individuals with OCD from those without the disorder. The C-YBOCS is very helpful in following progression of symptoms with treatment. Neuroimaging studies of individuals with obsessive-compulsive disorders have documented abnormalities in the frontal lobes, basal ganglia, and their associated pathways. OCD may present in preschoolers or appear suddenly later in development.

Controlled trials of both pharmacotherapy and cognitive-behavioral therapy have shown efficacy for OCD. All of the SSRIs have established efficacy for the treatment of OCD and fluvoxamine and sertraline have Food and Drug Administration (FDA) approval for use in children. Clomipramine (Anafranil), a tricyclic antidepressant, was the first medication to gain FDA approval for childhood OCD but can cause side effects typically associated with tricyclics, such as dry mouth, dizziness, somnolence, fatigue, and tremor. In addition, tricyclic medications have been associated with electrocardiogram (ECG) abnormalities, and pretreatment and periodic ECGs are necessary. Controlled trials suggest that cognitive-behavior therapy may lead to somewhat higher response rates, greater symptom reduction levels, and more durable treatment gains than medication alone. For this reason, many experts recommend completion of a behavioral treatment with crossover to pharmacologic management when response is partial or symptoms are severe.

Ten per cent of children with OCD seem to have their symptoms triggered or exacerbated by group A β-hemolytic streptococcal infections (GABHS). In a process similar to Sydenham's chorea, it appears that GABHS bacteria trigger antineuronal antibodies that cross react with caudate neural tissue in genetically susceptible hosts leading to swelling of this region and obsessions and compulsions. This subtype of OCD, called pediatric autoimmune neuropsychiatric disorders associated with streptococcal infection (PANDAS), is characterized by sudden

and dramatic onset or exacerbation of OCD or tic symptoms, associated neurologic findings, and a recent streptococcal infection. The pediatrician should be aware of the infectious cause of some cases of tic disorders and OCD and follow management guidelines (see Chapter 21).

Children with *phobias* avoid specific objects or situations that reliably trigger physiologic arousal (e.g., dogs or spiders). Neither obsessions nor compulsions are associated with the fear response, and phobias only rarely interfere with social, educational, or interpersonal functioning. The parents of phobic children should remain calm in the face of the child's anxiety or panic. Parents who become anxious themselves may reinforce their children's anxiety, and the pediatrician can usefully interrupt this cycle by calmly noting that phobias are not unusual and rarely cause impairment. The prevalence of specific phobias in childhood is 0.5–2.0%. Systematic desensitization is a form of behavior therapy that gradually exposes the individual to the fear-inducing situation or object while simultaneously teaching relaxation techniques for anxiety management. Successful repeated exposure will lead to extinguishing anxiety for that stimulus.

Post-traumatic stress disorder (PTSD) is an anxiety disorder resulting from the long- and short-term effects of trauma that causes behavioral and physiologic sequelae in toddlers, children, and adolescents. A new diagnostic category, *acute stress disorder*, has been added to the nosology, reflecting the fact that traumatic events often cause acute symptoms, which may or may not resolve. Previous trauma exposure, a history of other psychopathology, and parental symptoms of PTSD predict childhood-onset PTSD. Many adolescent and adult psychopathologic conditions such as conduct disorder, depression, and some personality disorders, have been shown to be related to previous trauma. PTSD also is linked to mood disorders, disruptive behavior, and other diagnoses in childhood. Epidemiologic studies have placed the lifetime prevalence of PTSD by age 18 at 6% in a community sample. Many others—up to 40%—may demonstrate symptoms but not fulfill the diagnostic criteria.

Life-threatening events that pose harm to the child or the caregiver and that produce considerable stress or fear are required to make the diagnosis of PTSD. Three clusters of symptoms are also essential for diagnosis: re-experiencing, avoidance, and hyperarousal. Persistent re-experiencing of the stressor through intrusive recollections, nightmares, and reenactment in play are typical responses in children. Persistent avoidance of reminders and numbing of emotional responsiveness such as isolation, amnesia, and avoidance constitute the second cluster of behaviors. Finally, symptoms of hyperarousal, such as hypervigilance, poor concentration, extreme startle responses, agitation, and sleep problems round out the symptom profile of PTSD. Occasionally, children regress in some of their developmental milestones after a traumatic event. Avoidance symptoms are commonly observable in younger children, whereas older children may be more able to describe re-experiencing and hyperarousal symptoms. Repetitive play involving the event, psychosomatic complaints, and nightmares may also be observed.

Initial interventions after a trauma should focus on reunification with a parent and attending to physical needs in a safe place. Aggressive treatment of pain may decrease the likelihood of PTSD, and facilitating a return to comforting routines, including regular sleep, is indicated. Long-term treatment may include individual, group, school-based, or family therapy as well as pharmacotherapy in selected cases. Individual treatment involves transforming the child's concept of victim to survivor and can occur through play therapy, psychodynamic therapy, and cognitive-behavioral therapy modalities. Group work is also helpful for identifying which children may need more intensive assistance. Goals of family work include helping the child establish a sense of security, validating his or her emotions, and anticipating situations when the child will need more support from the family. Clonidine or guanfacine may be helpful for sleep disturbance, persistent arousal, and exaggerated startle. Co-morbid depression and affective numbing may respond to an SSRI-class of medication, such as sertraline, paroxetine, or nefazodone. Tricyclics may also be effective agents in adolescents, although their efficacy in younger children is questionable (see Chapter 28.2).

Abellarte MJ, Ginsburg GS, Walkup JT, et al: The treatment of anxiety disorders in children and adolescents. *Biol Psychiatry* 1999;46:1567–78.

Anonymous: Fluvoxamine for the treatment of anxiety disorders in children and adolescents. The Research Unit on Pediatric Psychopharmacology Anxiety Study Group. *N Engl J Med* 2001;344:1279–85.

Crawford AM, Manassis K: Familial predictors of treatment outcome in childhood anxiety disorders. *J Am Acad Child Adolesc Psychiatry* 2001;40:1182–9.

Kendall PC, Brady EU, Verduin TL: Comorbidity in childhood anxiety disorders and treatment outcome. *J Am Acad Child Adolesc Psychiatry* 2001;40:787–94.

King NJ, Bernstein GA: School refusal in children and adolescents: A review of the past 10 years. *J Am Acad Child Adolesc Psychiatry* 2001;40:197–205.

Manassis K: Childhood anxiety disorders: Lessons from the literature. *Can J Psychiatry* 2000;45:724–30.

Rapoport JL, Inoff-Germain G: Treatment of obsessive-compulsive disorder in children and adolescents. *J Child Psychol Psychiatry* 2000;41:419–31.

Zahn-Waxler C, Klimes-Dougan B, Slattery MJ: Internalizing problems of childhood and adolescence: Prospects, pitfalls, and progress in understanding the development of anxiety and depression. *Dev Psychopathol* 2000;12:443–56.

Chapter 23
Mood Disorders

Neil W. Boris, Richard Dalton, and Marc A. Forman

Major depressive disorder, dysthymic disorder, and bipolar disorder are the three major types of affective or mood disorders seen in children and adolescents.

23.1 Major Depression

Although in the past there was some doubt as to whether prepubertal children experience depression similar to that seen in adults, this view has been dispelled through the use of structured interviews and rating scales. *Major depression* is characterized by dysphoria (which in children may present as irritability) and an obvious loss of interest and pleasure in usual activities. Diagnostic symptoms also include a significant weight change secondary to decreased or increased food intake, insomnia or hypersomnia, psychomotor agitation or retardation, fatigue or loss of energy on most days, feelings of worthlessness and excessive guilt, diminished ability to concentrate, and recurrent thoughts of death. A melancholic subtype of depression, characterized by marked anhedonia and early morning awakening, has been described in adolescents.

Epidemiology. The prevalence of depression varies based on sampling and measurement: Studies in childhood report rates of 0.4–2.5% and in adolescence, 0.4–8.3%. The lifetime prevalence of depression starting in adolescence is 15–20%, underscoring the fact that depression is a common disorder. At least twice as many girls as boys meet criteria for depression during adolescence; prepubertal depression is equally common among the sexes. Depression is undertreated across the life span, despite available and effective treatments shown to counter the high cost of lost productivity (e.g., school failure in adolescence) associated with ongoing depression.

Etiology. Many factors contribute to causing depression. However, there is strong evidence of a genetic basis for major depressive disorders across the life span. Individuals at high genetic risk appear to be more sensitive to the effects of adverse environmental conditions. Twin studies have shown a 76% concordance for depression among monozygotic twins reared together and 67% for monozygotic twins reared apart compared with 19% for dizygotic twins reared together. There is also an increased rate of depression (3–6 times greater) in first-degree relatives of patients suffering from a major affective disorder. Low functional levels of norepinephrine and serotonin are thought to be important genetic markers for depression and low urinary levels of 3-methoxyhydroxyphenylglycol and 5-hydroxyindoleacetic acid have been described in depressed patients. Positron emission tomography scans reveal altered metabolic activity in specific brain regions associated with mood, sleep, and appetite regulation. Neuroimaging data are reinforced by the fact that antidepressants that block presynaptic reuptake of serotonin are highly effective in treating depression. The development of hopelessness and helplessness secondary to an actual loss or the perception of loss suggests that cognitive factors play a role in the onset and maintenance of depression. Numerous studies confirm that adverse life events clearly play a role in causing depression, and there is even research on the pathophysiology linking experience and mood.

Clinical Manifestations. Depressive symptoms vary according to age and developmental level. Spitz described the *anaclitic depression of infancy,* and Bowlby observed that separation from a primary caregiver after 6–7 mo of age first leads to strong protest (e.g., crying and searching). Eventually, abandoned infants become withdrawn and apathetic, exhibiting hypotonia, lethargy, and an obviously sad facial expression. These infants often cry silently and, when picked up, may cling to a stranger, though they are usually inconsolable.

The clinical picture of depression in children somewhat parallels that of adults, except that children are more likely to present with separation anxiety, phobias, somatic complaints, and behavioral problems. Instead of reporting sadness, children may behave irritably. The hallmark of psychotic depression in children is the occurrence of hallucinations; delusions are more common in adolescents and adults.

The symptoms of a major depressive episode usually develop over a period of many days or weeks. The duration of each episode of depression is variable, though symptoms often persist for 7–9 mo without treatment; 6–10% of episodes are more protracted. Several longitudinal studies show that children and adolescents who are depressed are at risk for the development of later episodes of depression. Other studies have shown that, within 2 yr of the first depressive episode, 40% of children who have had a major depressive disorder experience a relapse. For children, like adults, depression should be considered a chronic disease marked by periods of normal mood. However, 20–40% of teenagers hospitalized with major depression develop a manic episode within 3–4 yr of discharge. Three predictors of later mania in depressed adolescents are (1) a depressive symptom cluster characterized by rapid onset, psychomotor retardation, and mood-congruent psychotic features; (2) a family history of bipolar illness or other affective illness; and (3) induction of hypomania by antidepressant medication. The picture of depression is further complicated by the fact that co-morbidity commonly occurs: 20–50% of depressed children have two or more diagnoses, including an anxiety disorder (30–80%), a disruptive behavior disorder (10–80%), dysthymic disorder (30–80%), or substance abuse disorder (20–30%).

Diagnosis. The Children's Depression Inventory, Children's Depression Scale, Depression Self-Rating Scale, and the Center for Epidemiological Studies Depression Scale for Children have all been shown to be helpful to clinicians in diagnosing depression in children and adolescents. However, clinical interview with the child and multiple adults familiar with the child remains the gold standard. There are no biologic tests specific for depression, though various biologic markers have been studied. For instance, during major depressive episodes, some children have been shown to hyposecrete growth hormone in response to insulin-induced hypoglycemia, whereas others produce higher growth hormone peaks during sleep. However, no test has sufficient sensitivity or specificity to assist in diagnostic assessment.

Treatment. Both psychotherapy and pharmacotherapy are effective in treating depression in childhood and adolescence. Psychotherapy is especially important for patients with multiple diagnoses or precipitants related to family disruption or conflict. Cognitive behavioral therapy (12–16 wk) has been most well studied and is effective in about 70% of cases of adolescent depression. Rigorous studies have also shown that selective serotonin reuptake inhibitors (SSRIs) reduce depressive symptoms in about 70% of cases. However, only 1 of 12 controlled studies of tricyclic antidepressants (TCAs) have demonstrated efficacy, and these agents, which have a narrow therapeutic window and serious side effects, are rarely indicated for depression in childhood. Furthermore, because depression is strongly associated with suicidal ideation and attempts and TCAs are deadly in overdose, the pediatrician should avoid using these drugs for depression.

23.2 Dysthymic Disorder

When compared with major depression, *dysthymic disorder* is a less severe but more protracted syndrome involving depressed mood for at least 1 yr. Poor appetite, sleep problems, decreased energy and self-esteem, and feelings of hopelessness are characteristic of dysthymia. Dysphoria is less intense but more chronic, with only brief periods of normal mood.

Etiology. Although the genetic basis of major depression has been demonstrated, the data regarding the genetic basis for dysthymic disorder are less firm. Dysthymia may be a partial phenotypic expression of an underlying genetic disorder or a different syndrome that has certain symptom clusters in common with major depression. Prevalence in childhood is 0.6–1.7% and in adolescence, 1.6–8.0%.

Clinical Manifestations. With the exception of hallucinations and delusions, other symptoms of major depression may be present, though severe sleep disturbance, appetite loss, or anhedonia suggest evolving major depression. Children who have dysthymia have had frequent disruptions of important relationships, often beginning as early as infancy. There is often a history of depressive illness in both parents. Affected children show more general emotional and social maladjustment. They often present as helpless, passive, clinging, dependent, and lonely children. Others relate in a more hardened, aloof, negativistic manner and are reluctant to invest emotion or trust in relationships. Untreated dysthymic disorder is generally chronic and is associated with increased risk for the subsequent development of major depression (70%), bipolar disorder (13%), and substance abuse disorder (15%). Frequently, children with dysthymia have a co-occurring second psychiatric disorder.

Treatment. Antidepressant pharmacotherapy is useful in the treatment of dysthymic patients, though there are few good studies of dysthymia in children. Antidepressants are especially helpful for those who display vegetative symptoms of depression. When dysthymic symptoms are associated with a second condition (anorexia, somatization disorder, substance abuse disorder, physical illness), both conditions require intervention. Often a full spectrum of therapies, including alliance building and dynamic psychotherapy, family therapy, parent management training, liaison work with the child's school, and pharmacotherapy, is indicated.

23.3 Bipolar Disorder

Bipolar illness is characterized by either alternating depression and mania (a typical adult presentation) or rapid cycling of mood, which may appear as irritable depression and dysregulation of affect. The rapid cycling, mixed variant is more common in children and young adolescents. One per cent of adult bipolar patients report that their symptoms began in early childhood; about 10% report that symptoms began during early adolescence. Epidemiologic studies suggest that the prevalence rate during childhood and adolescence is 1%, though differing diagnostic standards have led to varying estimates of prevalence.

Etiology. Bipolar disorder has genetic roots: a concordance rate of 65% in monozygotic twins and less than 20% in dizygotic twins supports this hypothesis. Further, first-degree relatives of individuals with bipolar disorder are much more likely than the general population to develop a mood disorder. Twenty per cent of adolescents presenting with major depressive symptoms develop manic episodes later.

Clinical Manifestations. The clinical manifestations of bipolar disorder may be different for prepubertal children and early adolescents as compared with older adolescents and adults. Defined episodes of depression alternating with euphoria, grandiose thoughts, high activity levels, pressured speech, distractibility, hypersexuality, hyper-religiosity, overspending, and hallucinations and delusions are characteristic of classic bipolar disorder and represent the typical mid to late adolescent or adult pattern of symptoms. In 70% of these cases, careful history reveals that at least one episode of depression preceded the manic symptoms. Some children and adolescents, however, present with irritability, grandiosity, explosive aggression, hyperactivity, rapid thinking, and cognitive impairment. These children, who often do not fully meet current DSM-IV criteria for bipolar disorder, clearly suffer from symptoms that impair their functioning and require intervention. Rarely, symptoms are evident as early as the preschool period. Because some studies suggest that children with early-onset symptoms are more likely to have first-degree relatives with a mood disorder, they are currently considered by many psychiatrists as suffering from a form of bipolar disorder. These children may fulfill criteria for one or more disruptive behavioral disorders, particularly attention-deficit/hyperactivity disorder and/or conduct disorder. There is considerable controversy about the prevalence and diagnostic features of this early-onset form of bipolar disorder. However, severe early mood instability is associated with high levels of school failure, poor peer relations, and high levels of risk taking and substance abuse in early adolescence.

Treatment. Therapy of bipolar disorder typically requires the use of mood-stabilizing medications (Chapter 28.2). Psychotherapy alone is usually ineffective for bipolar disorder. The pharmacologic management of bipolar disorder is generally best left to child psychiatrists except in unusual circumstances. Lithium carbonate is effective in the treatment of bipolar illness and manic symptoms in about 60% of cases. Lithium is administered orally, followed by measurement of blood levels. The ideal therapeutic range for the initial treatment of acute symptoms is a blood level of 1.0–1.2 mEq/L, and the recommended blood level for maintenance therapy is 0.5–0.8 mEq/L. Lithium is associated with renal impairment and hypothyroidism, and baseline and follow-up renal function and thyroid function tests are imperative. Lithium side effects are the major reason that this medicine is not always useful for maintenance purposes. The antiepileptics, carbamazepine (Tegretol) and valproic acid, are especially effective in rapid cycling adult bipolar disorder. These agents are also now considered first-line agents for bipolar disorder in childhood. Both are potentially toxic to the liver, and baseline and follow-up liver function tests are imperative. Tegretol is also associated with Stevens-Johnson syndrome and leukopenia, though both are rare events. Several new mood-stabilizing agents are also used for bipolar disorder. Lamotrigine is the most promising of these, especially for depression associated with bipolar disorder. However, about 10% of children and adolescents taking lamotrigine develop a rash; because a high percentage of these rashes evolve into Stevens-Johnson syndrome and other life-threatening rashes, the medicine should be discontinued when the rash is first noted. In addition to mood stabilizers, novel antipsychotic medications, especially risperidone and olanzapine, have shown promise. They are especially useful with children from chaotic families who cannot be counted on to comply with difficult dosing requirements and frequent lab visits.

Early onset of symptoms and high levels of aggression appear to be related to treatment failure. Some children require multiple medications. Family conflict is commonly associated with early-onset bipolar disorder, and one of the psychotherapeutic approaches helpful in conduct disorders is typically indicated (see Chapter 28).

American Academy of Child and Adolescent Psychiatry: Practice parameters for the assessment and treatment of children and adolescents with bipolar disorder. *J Am Acad Child Adolesc Psychiatry* 1997;34(Suppl):157S–76S.

American Academy of Child and Adolescent Psychiatry: Practice parameters for the assessment and treatment of children and adolescents with depressive disorders. *J Am Acad Child Adolesc Psychiatry* 1998;37(Suppl):63S–83S.

Angold A, Costello EJ, Erkanli A: Comorbidity. *J Child Psychol Psychiatry* 1999;40:57–87.

Birmaher B, Ryan ND, Williamson DE, et al: Childhood and adolescent depression: A review of the past 10 years. Part I. *J Am Acad Child Adolesc Psychiatry* 1996;35:1427–34.

Bowlby J: *Attachment and Loss, Vol 2. Separation.* New York, Basic Books, 1973.

Carlson GA: Mania and ADHD: Comorbidity or confusion. *J Affect Disord* 1998;51:177–87.

Emslie GJ, Mayes TL: Mood disorders in children and adolescents: Psychopharmacological treatment. *Biol Psychiatry* 2001;49:1082–90.

Geller B, Luby J: Child and adolescent bipolar disorder: A review of the past 10 years. *J Am Acad Child Adolesc Psychiatry* 1997;36:1178–88.

Geller B, Zimerman B, Williams M, et al: Diagnostic characteristics of 93 cases of a prepubertal and early adolescent bipolar disorder phenotype by gender, puberty and comorbid attention deficit hyperactivity disorder. *J Child Adolesc Psychopharmacol* 2000;10:157–64.

Kowatch RA, Bucci JP: Mood stabilizers and anticonvulsants. *Pediatric Clin N Am* 1998;45:1173–86.

Spencer TJ, Biederman J, Wozniak J, et al: Parsing pediatric bipolar disorder from its associated comorbidity with the disruptive behavior disorders. *Biol Psychiatry* 2000;49:1062–70.

Chapter 24
Suicide and Attempted Suicide *Neil W. Boris and Richard Dalton*

See also Chapter 102.

Suicide is the second leading cause of adolescent death, and the rate of completed suicide for males has increased dramatically in the last 4 decades. The vast majority of children and adolescents who complete suicide have some form of psychiatric illness. Pediatricians and primary care providers should ask about suicidal ideation at each adolescent visit and must be comfortable assessing suicide risk and knowing when to refer children and adolescents for mental health care.

Epidemiology. Suicide is extremely rare before puberty. However, rates of completed suicide increase steadily across the teen years and into young adulthood, peaking in the early 20s. Yearly in the United States, about 2,000 13- to 19-yr-olds complete suicide, though underreporting of suicide has been documented. As age increases from prepuberty to late adolescence, the ratio of male to female suicides rises from 3:1 to about 4.5:1. It is estimated that there are 5 to 45 suicide attempts for each completed suicide and in some samples as many as 25% of adolescents admit to suicidal ideation. About 3 times as many females attempt suicide as males. Most suicide attempts among females involve ingestion or superficial cutting, whereas more lethal means are used by males (e.g., hanging, firearms). The increase in suicide rates has been greater in black than in white youth resulting in the rate of suicide among black teens approaching that of whites, especially in late adolescence; as is true for whites, 3–5 times as many black males complete suicide as females.

RISK FACTORS. Perhaps the easiest way to understand the origins of suicidal behavior is by considering a biopsychosocial framework. From the biologic perspective, twin studies that control for life events known to be related to suicidal behavior reveal that suicidal ideation and suicide attempts are significantly more common among monozygotic twin pairs than dizygotic twin pairs. Pedigree analyses further support the influence of genetic factors on suicidal behavior. In addition, a large body of recent research focused on understanding what the genes associated with suicidal behavior might code for suggests that heritable alterations in the serotonin system are associated with suicide completion. The serotonin system is important in regulating impulsivity, aggression, and mood, and these three factors are, in turn, related both to psychiatric diagnoses and to gender. For instance, although adolescent females are more at risk for depression than males, males are generally more aggressive and impulsive than females. There is a strong association between mood disorders and both suicide attempts and completion for both sexes. For males, the addition of conduct disorder or chronic anxiety is also associated with completed suicide, especially when combined with alcohol abuse (which is associated with impulsivity). For females, chronic anxiety, especially panic disorder, is associated with suicide completion. Not surprisingly, children and adolescents with a previous history of suicide attempts are at higher risk for suicide completion regardless of their psychiatric status. These data suggest that there are several interconnected risks, probably mediated primarily by biologic and genetic factors, which predict suicide.

Psychologic and social factors must also be considered to obtain a more complete picture of suicidal behavior. Two thirds of child or adolescent suicide attempters can name a precipitating event for their action. For instance, a remote or recent history of child maltreatment or sexual assault is associated with suicide. Many studies have revealed a more general association between family conflict and suicide attempts, and this association is strongest for children and early adolescents. For older adolescents, life events such as relationship breakups are commonly associated with suicide attempts. Adolescents who identify themselves as homosexual are at increased risk for suicide, and those with gender dysphoria appear also to be at high risk for suicide. When a feeling of hopelessness is associated with an adolescent's current psychologic state, then suicide risk increases. For some recent immigrants, for instance, high levels of acculturative stress, especially in the context of family dysfunction and the perception of limited options in the future, are associated with suicidal ideation.

A major factor predicting death from suicide is lethality of means used by the suicidal child or adolescent. So-called "violent" suicides, those completed by use of firearms or hanging, account for the increased suicide rate among adolescent males. Use of carbon monoxide poisoning in adolescent suicide is uncommon but deadly. Overdoses, on the other hand, are common but do not often kill. Preadolescents attempt suicide most commonly by jumping from heights; self-poisoning, hanging, stabbing, and running into traffic are less common. Still, episodes of self-poisoning that occur after age 6 yr are less likely to be accidental and should be treated as if the behavior had suicidal potential or as a possible case of child abuse and neglect.

Assessment and Management. Assessment of suicidal ideation should be a part of each health visit in adolescence (see Chapter 100). There is no evidence that discussing suicide with individuals increases their likelihood of harming themselves. On the other hand, there is evidence that suicidal persons who seek medical care do not discuss suicidal thoughts, symptoms of depression, or patterns of drug use unless specifically asked. Given that suicide is a leading cause of death in adolescence, the physician will prevent more deaths by asking about suicide than by auscultating the lungs.

The first principle of suicide assessment is that suicidal ideation should be taken seriously. Physicians, parents, and others must scrupulously avoid sarcasm, kidding, daring, or belittling the individual who reveals thoughts of suicide. If a suicidal threat is labeled "manipulative," power or control becomes a major issue influencing behavior, and the risk of suicide may increase. In the case of the child or adolescent seen after a suicide attempt, a thorough history regarding ingestion is necessary, and aggressive management for poisoning implemented as indicated. Alcohol or drug intoxication is not uncommon and may also require acute management.

The second principle of suicide assessment is that the child or adolescent must be understood within the biopsychosocial framework. Box 24–1 lists some guidelines for assessment. The child or adolescent's psychiatric status is a primary concern. A careful psychiatric history and mental status examination are necessary to assess risk for suicide completion. Physicians who are uncomfortable with psychiatric assessment should seek immediate consultation with a mental health professional. Signs and symptoms of mood disorders, conduct problems, chronic anxiety, or substance abuse suggest the need for intervention and indicate risk for eventual suicide completion. Previous suicide attempts should also be documented. In order to identify precipitating events, the physician should carefully explore, in detail, the child's life during the 48–72 hr prior to either the threat or the suicide attempt. The degree of premeditation or impulsivity should be assessed. In most instances, a child or an adolescent will openly discuss how intent they were on harming themselves, their reasons for attempting suicide, and whether they remain suicidal. Furthermore, the physician should be able both to evaluate the response of the immediate family to a child or adolescent's attempt and to assess the degree of ongoing family conflict.

When suicidal patients have been seen in the physician's office, the physician should enter into a no-suicide contract with the patient. The parents should be notified, and a psychiatric consultation should be obtained. Because 50% of suicide attempters do not attend even one outpatient psychiatric session, the physician should procure a specifically arranged appointment within 1 or 2 days. If possible, the patient and family should meet the therapist immediately after the examination by the physician. In most cases, suicide attempters who are seen in the emergency room should be admitted to the hospital for 1 day or more so that a more adequate evaluation can be made of the patient's frame of mind and of the circumstances of the family or environment. Such admissions usually require 2–3 days, unless medical needs require a longer stay or a serious psychiatric disorder, such as depression or psychosis, is found. If social service and psychiatric assessments are adequate and arrangements for appropriate follow-up care can be made, disposition can be made fairly rapidly. The physician must give careful attention to how the family and friends have responded to the patient's act. A hostile and angry family, such as is frequently seen, will necessitate a different disposition or resolution than a family that is supportive, sympathetic, and understanding. The latter supports a decision for the patient to return home. Some families may completely deny the seriousness of the behavior; this can be discouraging and provocative to the patient, whose act has been a desperate attempt to compel a different response. The family members should be helped to examine their roles in the interactions that preceded the attempt, without being made to feel overly guilty.

Psychiatric hospitalization is indicated when the individual continues to be actively suicidal, when major psychiatric disorders are found within the attempter, or when major family problems complicate ongoing protection of the attempter.

BOX 24–1. Checklists for Assessing Child or Adolescent Suicide Attempters in an Emergency Room or Crisis Center

ATTEMPTERS AT GREATER RISK FOR SUICIDE
Suicidal History
  Still thinking of suicide
  Have made a prior suicide attempt
Demographics
  Male
  Live alone
Mental State
  Depressed, manic, hypomanic, severely anxious, or have a mixture of these states
  Substance abuse alone or in association with a mood disorder
  Irritable, agitated, threatening violence to others, delusional, or hallucinating
Do not discharge such patients without psychiatric evaluation.
Look for signs of clinical depression:
  Depressed mood most of the time
  Loss of interest or pleasure in usual activities
  Weight loss or gain
  Can't sleep or sleeps too much
  Restless or slowed-down
  Fatigue, loss of energy
  Feels worthless or guilty
  Low self-esteem, disappointed with self
  Feels hopeless about future
  Can't concentrate, indecisive
  Recurring thoughts of death
  Irritable, upset by little things
Look for signs of mania or hypomania:
  Depressed mood most of the time
  Elated, expansive, or irritable mood
  Inflated self-esteem, grandiosity
  Decreased need for sleep
  More talkative than usual, pressured speech
  Racing thoughts
  Abrupt topic changes when talking
  Distractible
  Excessive participation in multiple activities
  Agitated or restless
  Hypersexual, spends foolishly, uninhibited remarks

From American Foundation for Suicide Prevention: Today's suicide attempter could be tomorrow's suicide (poster). New York, American Foundation for Suicide Prevention, 1999, 1-888-333-AFSP.

American Academy of Child and Adolescent Psychiatry: Practice parameters for the assessment and treatment of children and adolescents with suicidal behavior. *J Am Acad Child Adolesc Psychiatry* 2001;40(Suppl):25S–51S.

Aschkenasy JR, Clark DC, Zinn LD, et al: The non-psychiatric physician's responsibilities for the suicidal adolescent. *N Y State J Med* 1992;92:97–104.

Brent D, Baugher M, Bridge B, et al: Age- and sex-related risk factors for adolescent suicide. *J Am Acad Child Adolesc Psychiatry* 1999;38:1497–505.

Centers for Disease Control: Suicide among black youths—United States, 1980–1995. *MMWR* 1998;47:193–5.

Gross-Isseroff R, Biegon A, Voet H, Weizman A: The suicide brain: A review of postmortem receptor/transporter binding studies. *Neurosci Biobehav Rev* 1998;22:653–61.

Horowitz LM, Wang PS, Koocher GP, et al: Detecting suicide risk in a pediatric emergency department: Development of a brief screening tool. *Pediatrics* 2001;107:1133–7.

Kaplan S, Pelcovitz D, Salzinger S, et al: Adolescent physical abuse and suicide attempts. *J Am Acad Child Adolesc Psychiatry* 1997;36:799–808.

Mann JJ, Brent DA, Arango V: The neurobiology and genetics of suicide and attempted suicide: A focus on the serotonergic system. *Neuropsychopharmacology* 2001;24:467–77.

Ohberg A, Lonnqvist J: Suicides hidden among undetermined deaths. *Acta Psychiatr Scand* 1998;98:214–8.

Russell ST, Joyner K: Adolescent sexual orientation and suicide risk: Evidence from a national study. *Am J Pub Health* 2001;91:1276–81.

Chapter 25
Disruptive Behavioral
Disorders *Neil W. Boris and Richard Dalton*

Numerous behaviors considered appropriate at certain early developmental levels are obviously pathologic when they present at later ages. Lying, impulsiveness, breath holding, defiance, and temper tantrums are frequently noted around the ages of 2–4 yr, when children begin to need autonomy but do not have the motor and social skills necessary for successful independence. These behaviors are typically the result of frustration and anger. About one half of preschoolers in the United States are brought to the attention of physicians at some time because of destructive and disobedient behaviors. Moreover, some studies suggest that disruptive, antisocial behaviors are intermittently committed by one half of this country's adolescents.

Breath holding is not unusual during the first years of life. Breath holding is frequently used by infants and toddlers in an attempt to control their environment and their caregivers. Although some children hold their breath until they lose consciousness, sometimes leading to a seizure, there is no increased risk of their later developing a seizure disorder. Parents are best advised to ignore the behavior. Without sufficient reinforcement, breath holding most often disappears. When breath holding does not respond to parent coaching or is accompanied by head banging or high levels of aggression, referral for developmental evaluation or family counseling is indicated.

Defiance, oppositionalism, and *temper tantrums* are not uncommon in children 18 mo to 3 yr of age, when the struggle to develop a goal-corrected partnership with primary caregivers is paramount. Parental and caregiver response to this behavior is very important. Caregivers who respond to toddler defiance with punitive anger run the risk of reinforcing the defiance and teaching the child that out-of-control emotions are a reasonable response to frustration. In response to tantrums and oppositionalism, parents are advised to give the child time and space to recover by turning away briefly. It is useful to advise parents to tell their child, once he or she is calm, that the reasons for frustration are understandable but that oppositional behavior is not acceptable. If the child presents with escalating oppositionalism, parents should be advised to calmly place the child in time-out for 2–3 minutes (see Chapter 5).

If behavioral measures such as time-out fail, physicians must assess how the parents handle anger before making further recommendations about how to approach the child's problems. Children are often frightened by the strength and intensity of their own angry feelings and by the intensity of the angry feelings they arouse in their parents. It is therefore of prime importance that parents model the anger control that they wish their children to exhibit. Some parents are unable to see that they sometimes lose control themselves; they are not, therefore, helping their children to internalize controls. Advising parents to calmly provide simple choices of activities that a toddler or young child may choose will help the child to feel more in control and to develop a sense of autonomy. Providing the child with options also typically helps reduce the child's feelings of anger and shame. Such negative, internalized feelings may later have adverse effects on interpersonal relationships, intimacy, and personality development.

Lying is often used by 2–4 yr olds as a method of playing with the language. By observing the reactions of parents and caregivers, preschoolers learn about expectations for honesty in communication. Lying is also a form of fantasy for children, who describe things as they wish them to be rather than as they are. For instance, in order to avoid an unpleasant confrontation, a child who has not done something that a parent wanted may say that it has been done to avoid an unpleasant confrontation. The child's sense of time and reason does not permit the realization that this only postpones an even angrier confrontation.

In school-aged children, lying most often is an effort to cover up something that the child does not want to accept in his or her own behavior. The lie is invented, therefore, to achieve temporary good feeling and protect against a loss of self-esteem. Although lying is common in childhood, children with low self-esteem are more prone to habitually lie. In many cases, habitual lying is also promoted by poor adult modeling. For instance, when mothers and fathers accuse each other frequently of lying, the child, drawn into a loyalty conflict, is likely to become distressed and increase defensive lying. Many adolescents lie to avoid parental disapproval. As with other antisocial behaviors, lying may be used as a method of rebellion.

Regardless of age or developmental level, when lying becomes a frequent way of managing conflict and anxiety, intervention is warranted. Initially, the parents should confront the child to give a clear message of what is acceptable. At the same time, sensitivity and support are necessary for a successful intervention, because children and adolescents may react to their shame and embarrassment with angry denial and acting out. If the situation cannot be resolved (i.e., parental understanding of the situation and the child's understanding that lying is not a reasonable alternative), professional intervention is indicated. In some cases, chronic lying occurs in combination with several other antisocial behaviors and is a sign of an underlying psychopathology or family dysfunction.

Almost all children *steal* something at some point in their lives. When preschoolers and school-aged children steal more than once or twice, the behavior may be a response to a sense of internal loss. These children frequently feel neglected and are, in fact, emotionally deprived. Their stealing is impulsive, but the gratification derived does not satisfy the underlying need. In children and adolescents, stealing can sometimes be an expression of anger or revenge for real or imagined frustrations by the parents. In many instances, stealing becomes one way in which the child or adolescent can manipulate and attempt to control interactions with parents. Like lying, stealing can be learned from adults. Parents who boast about outwitting tax laws or exceeding speed limits are implicitly condoning rule breaking as an acceptable behavior.

It is important for parents to help the child undo the theft by returning the stolen articles or by rendering their equivalent either in money that the child can earn or in services. When stealing is part of a pattern of conduct problems, referral to a child psychiatrist is warranted. Both problematic peer influence and lack of supervision by parents may exacerbate stealing and other conduct problems. Interventions as simple as getting a child a Big Brother or Sister have been shown to improve school function and diminish conduct problems. In some cases, however, more intensive intervention may be necessary.

Unlike the previous behaviors, *truancy* and *run-away behavior* are never developmentally appropriate. About half of school refusal incidents result from child and adolescent behavioral problems; the other half is related to mood and anxiety symptoms. Often, truancy represents disorganization within the home or developing personality problems, or both. Whereas younger children often threaten to run away out of frustration or a desire to get back at parents, children who run away with nowhere to go are almost always expressing a serious underlying problem (see Chapter 39). During middle childhood, most runaways are escaping abuse and neglect within the home. In adolescence, disagreements with the parents, developing personality problems, and abuse and neglect all must be considered as possible precipitants. Adolescent runaways are at extremely high risk for substance abuse, intimate partner violence, and other risk-taking behaviors.

Although the interest in fire is ubiquitous in early childhood, unsupervised *fire setting* is always inappropriate. Early school-aged children tend to set fires because of both curiosity and latent hostility secondary to deprivation within a disorganized and neglectful family. These young children set fires by themselves within their homes. In adolescence, fire setting is a sign of delinquency; again, traumatic experiences, often associated with family conflict, are common. Teenagers often set fires in small groups, seeking revenge upon school and community authorities.

At the very least, fire setting requires intervention by the parents. Most often, intervention by mental health professionals is also indicated. A combination of family therapy, alliance-building individual therapy, parent management training, and community involvement is often necessary to effect a reasonable change. The recidivistic young fire setter is very difficult to manage, however. Many adult arsonists were childhood fire setters.

Although there is no totally satisfactory theory about the nature and cause of *antisocial behavior*, risk factors within the individual and family have been identified. Adoption and twin studies strongly suggest that both genetic factors and child-rearing practices contribute to the development of aggressive behaviors. In well-controlled studies, adopted children with antisocial biologic fathers presented later in life with more antisocial behaviors than did those with antisocial adoptive fathers. However, children with both biologic and adoptive antisocial fathers were the most antisocial in later life. Sociocultural factors, temperament, some psychiatric conditions, and cognitive limitations can also predispose individuals to antisocial acting out.

Aggression is a serious symptom and is associated with significant morbidity and mortality in childhood. Data suggest that aggression is often stable over time. Children may not "grow out" of this behavior, and early intervention is indicated for persistent aggressive behavior. Aggressive tendencies are heritable, although environmental factors may promote aggression in susceptible children. Both enduring and temporary risk conditions impacting a family may increase aggressive behavior in children. For instance, aggression in childhood has been correlated with family unemployment, discord, criminality, and psychiatric disorders as well as births to teenage or unmarried mothers. Boys are almost universally reported to be more aggressive than girls. In many animals, administration of male sex hormones to females produces more aggressive behavior. Difficult temperament and later aggressiveness have been shown to be related, though there is evidence that these children may elicit punitive caregiving within the family environment, setting up a cycle of increasing aggression. Aggressive children often misperceive social cues and react with inappropriate hostility toward both peers and parents. Nonetheless, marital discord and aggression within the home certainly contribute to aggression by children.

Clinically, it is important to differentiate the causes and motives for childhood aggression. Intentional aggression may be primarily instrumental, to achieve an end, or primarily hostile, to inflict physical or psychologic pain. Children who are callous and unempathic and who are frequently aggressive require mental health intervention. These children are at high risk for suspension from school and eventual school failure. Learning disorders are commonly evident and should be screened for in aggressive children. Other forms of psychopathology are not uncommon; in particular, aggressive children with attention-deficit/hyperactivity disorder (ADHD) may develop oppositional-defiant disorder and/or conduct disorder. Some aggressive, impulsive children may instead have bipolar disorder; a family history of mood disorders, grandiosity, and cyclic mood disturbance may be evident in the history of these children.

Aggressive behavior in boys is relatively consistent from the preschool period through adolescence; a boy with a high level of aggressive behavior from 3–6 yr of age has a high probability of carrying this behavior into adolescence, especially without effective family-focused intervention. The developmental progression of aggression among girls is less well studied. There are clearly fewer girls with physically aggressive behavior in early childhood. On the other hand, interpersonal coercive behavior, especially in peer relationships, is not uncommon among girls and appears to be related to the development of more physical aggression in adolescence (e.g., fighting, stealing, etc.).

Children exposed to aggressive models on television or in play display more aggressive behavior compared with children not exposed to these models (see Chapter 34). Parents' anger and aggressive or harsh punishment model behavior that children may imitate when they are physically or psychologically hurt. As Lewis has noted, parental abuse may be transmitted to the next generation by several modes: Children imitate aggression that they have witnessed; abuse can cause brain injury (which itself predisposes the child toward violence); and internalized rage more often than not results from abuse.

Conduct disorder is a distinct clinical entity manifested by several different antisocial behaviors: stealing, lying, fire setting, truancy, property destruction, cruelty to animals, rape, use of a weapon while fighting, armed robbery, physical cruelty to others, and repeated attempts to run away from home. A pattern of such behaviors that has existed for at least 6 mo warrants the diagnosis of conduct disorder. One third to one half of adolescent psychiatric clinic patients present with symptoms of conduct disorder. *Oppositional-defiant disorder* is defined by less severe behavior than conduct disorder: temper tantrums, continuous arguing, defiance of rules, continual blaming of others, angry and resentful affect, spiteful and vindictive behavior, and frequent use of obscene language. Some children may present with symptoms of all three disruptive behavior disorders (ADHD, oppositional-defiant disorder, and conduct disorder). For instance, one third of children and adolescents with psychiatric diagnoses seen in community-based clinics are considered oppositional, and children with ADHD are significantly more likely to meet criteria for oppositional-defiant disorder than those with other presenting problems. Still, the majority of children diagnosed with a disruptive behavior disorder meet criteria only for that disorder. The risk factors (from child, parent, and environment) associated with the development of conduct disorder are very similar to those previously mentioned in association with the development of specific antisocial and aggressive behaviors. Aggressive behavior is stable across generations within families. Inconsistent parenting practices as well as overly punitive disciplinary measures have been associated with conduct-disordered children. Parents of conduct-disordered children are less accepting of their children and show less warmth and support for them. However, only about a third of children with conduct disorder go on to have antisocial personality disorder in adulthood. Adult criminality is predicted by an early age of onset of conduct disorder symptoms, numerous episodes and varieties of antisocial behaviors, parental criminality, and marital discord.

In many children, oppositional behavior may appear in the form of *passive-aggressive behaviors*. Prevalence rates of 16–22% have been noted. Children with passive-aggressive behavior express hostility indirectly as procrastination, stubbornness, or resistance. Parents often complain that such children do not hear them and that they fail to respond to repeated requests. Academic underachievement is common. Children may unconsciously adopt passive-aggressive strategies for a variety of motives: to gain independence while maintaining dependence; to counter underlying low self-esteem; to maintain control and autonomy when threatened by anxiety; and to get revenge. These children are fearful of direct expression of assertiveness, aggression, and hostility. The child-rearing styles of their parents are often intimidating, critical, and inconsistent or, on the other hand, indulgent and permissive.

Treatment. Many different approaches have been used in the therapy of children and adolescents with aggressive behavior, conduct disorder, and oppositional-defiant disorder. Individual treatment focusing on alliance building and conflict resolution is sometimes useful in establishing the basic trust necessary for a positive therapeutic outcome; however, individual therapy is not always effective in ameliorating behavioral problems. Group therapy has shown some promise in treating adolescents with behavioral difficulties, and anger management therapy has demonstrated some positive results with younger children. Training in problem-solving skills involves modeling, role playing, and practicing to help children deal more successfully with interpersonal relations; it is somewhat effective in modifying maladaptive styles of relating and behaving. Effective results have been obtained with parent management training, in which parents are trained directly to promote prosocial behaviors within the home and to place reasonable limits on unwanted, destructive behaviors. In the case of passive-aggressive behavior, for instance, parents would be encouraged to set firm limits and expectations for the child and reach agreement with the child on what his or her important tasks and responsibilities are. Compliance and age-appropriate assertiveness and independence are then promoted and rewarded. Multisystemic therapy (MST), an in-home treatment involving the identified patient, parents, siblings, and peers as well as school and neighborhood and other environmental forces, has been shown to be effective with aggressive, conduct-disordered children and adolescents. This multilevel approach is informed by data on the varying ecologic risks that are related to conduct disorder.

Pharmacotherapy for aggression or disruptive and antisocial behavior is generally used as an adjunct to family-based therapy, parent training, or MST. There are little data suggesting that pharmacotherapy alone is effective in reducing persistent aggression, oppositional behavior, or antisocial behavior. However, children with underlying biologic vulnerability (intermittent psychotic disorders, attention deficit disorder) may benefit from judicious use of appropriate medication. There are no medications specifically intended for treatment of antisocial behaviors. Lithium, antipsychotics, anticonvulsants such as valproate, and α_2-agonists such as clonidine may diminish aggressive acting out in selected individuals, though these medications may also have significant side effects (see Chapter 28.2). Some children present with such severe behavioral problems that residential treatment or psychiatric hospitalization is necessary for a successful outcome.

American Academy of Child and Adolescent Psychiatry: Practice parameters for the assessment and treatment of children and adolescents with conduct disorder. *J Am Acad Child Adolesc Psychiatry* 1997;36(Suppl):122S–39S.

August GJ, Realmuto GM, Joyce T, et al: Persistence and desistance of oppositional defiant disorder in a community sample of children with ADHD. *J Am Acad Child Adolesc Psychiatry* 1999;38:1262–70.

Conseur A, Rivara FP, Barnoski R, et al: Maternal and perinatal risk factors for later delinquency. *Pediatrics* 1997;99:785–90.

DiMario FJ Jr: Prospective study of children with cyanotic and pallid breath-holding spells. *Pediatrics* 2001;107:265–9.

Henneggler SW, Schoenwald SK, Pickrel SAG: *Multisystemic Treatment of Antisocial Behavior in Children and Adolescents.* New York, Guilford, 1998.

Kazdin A: Treatment for aggressive and antisocial children. *Child Adolesc Clin N Am* 2000;9:841–58.

Leiberman AF: *The Emotional Life of the Toddler.* New York, Simon and Schuster, 2000.

Lewis DO: Conduct disorders. *In:* Garfinkel B, Carlson G, Weller E (eds): *Psychiatric Disorders in Children and Adolescents.* Philadelphia, WB Saunders, 1990.

Rutter M: Introduction: Concepts of antisocial behaviour, of cause, and of genetic influences. In Bock CT, Goode J (editors): *Genetics of Criminal and Antisocial Behaviour.* Chichester, Wiley, 1996, pp 1–20.

Speltz ML, McClellan J, DeKlyen M, et al: Preschool boys with oppositional defiant disorder: Clinical presentation and diagnostic change. *J Am Acad Child Adolesc Psychiatry* 1999;38:838–45.

Webster-Stratton C, Hammond M: Treating children with early-onset conduct problems: A comparison of child and parent training interventions. *J Consult Clin Psychol* 1997;65:93–109.

Chapter 26

Sexual Behavior and Its Variations *Richard Dalton*

See also Chapters 555 and 556.

Gender identity refers to the individual's sense of self as a male or a female. *Gender role* refers to those behaviors within a culture commonly thought to be associated with maleness or femaleness. Thus, one's gender identity is intact when a biologic male identifies himself as a man and a biologic female identifies herself as a woman. If the male performs the sort of behavior associated with being a man within his culture, he is said to fit comfortably within his gender role. However, if a man is uncomfortable with those behaviors identified with men within his culture, the implication is that he has trouble with his gender role. The same is true for women. However, as society has changed, gender roles have changed. In the past, gender roles were shaped by traditionally defined masculine and feminine roles. As the economics of family life have changed—and both sexes have become potentially self-sufficient economically—gender roles, as they relate to job choices and performance, have changed dramatically or, in some cases, have simply disappeared. Fewer behaviors are specific solely to one gender.

Children identify themselves as boys or girls by about 18 mo of age (i.e., establish a gender identity). Between 18 and 30 mo of age, children establish *gender stability*, the concept that boys become men and girls become women. By 30 mo, gender constancy, the immutability of one's gender, is firmly established and resistant to change. Although there are numerous theories suggesting which environmental and biologic factors are most important to the establishment of a firm gender identity, at this point we still do not understand, in a way that has treatment implications, which factors are most important in any given child.

Children are naturally curious about their bodies. The 2-yr-old child ought to be taught the proper names for the parts of the body, including the genitals. Parents should react calmly when their children explore and manipulate their own bodies with enjoyment, although open masturbation by older children suggests poor awareness of social reality or lack of parental censorship. Parents should inform their children that *masturbation* is not a social activity and should be limited to the bedroom when the child is alone. An overly excited or overly punitive reaction will serve only to excite the child. It is important that masturbation be accepted as a normal aspect of the child's sexual life and that guilt be avoided. By puberty, children should be given explanations of its normality. This can be done in conjunction with explanations of ejaculation, orgasm, and menstruation so that children can understand them, too, as normal bodily functions.

It is quite common for preschool children to hug and kiss each other. More explicit sexual behavior, such as oral contact, attempts at simulated intercourse, or anal stimulation, is probably learned through observation or direct involvement with older children or adults. Intervention designed to uncover the source of the child's knowledge followed by appropriate action is indicated in these situations (Chapter 35).

Especially between the ages of 10 and 12 yr, boys and girls typically explore sexual issues with best friends (same-sex friends) as a means of gathering information. This should not be viewed as a prelude for homosexuality but as a developmental stage in most children. At any age, the compulsive need for sex serves as a defense against underlying dependency, separation, and autonomy issues. It is usually during adolescence that gender object interests are realized. The teenager's actual or perceived sexual experiences and their reinforcements are important in shaping ultimate gender role behaviors.

Transsexualism, the conviction by a person biologically of one gender that he or she is a member of the other gender, is the most obvious example of gender identity confusion. Transsexual adolescents feel discomfort and a sense of inappropriateness about their assigned sex. They spend years trying to figure out how to get rid of the primary and secondary sexual characteristics that define them biologically. Gender roles of the opposite biologic sex are usually adopted.

The prevalence of transsexualism is 1/30,000 for males and 1/100,000 for females. Transsexuals usually have a difficult time with social and occupational functioning. Concurrent psychopathologic conditions and depression are part of the reason; societal consternation is the other part. The natural history of transsexualism is not well understood. A preponderance of adult transsexuals had gender identity disorders as children and adolescents. Extreme femininity in boys is a predisposing factor. Some say that they remember being confused about gender identity as early as 2 yr of age. Which particular effeminate boys will later show transsexual behavior cannot be accurately predicted.

Treatment of transsexualism has taken two directions. Many transsexual adults have opted for hormonal and surgical therapies to produce primary and secondary sexual characteristics of the gender with which they identify. Follow-up studies consistently show continued distress after these treatments. Long-term dynamic and behavioral therapies also have been tried. Although there are anecdotal reports of successful re-identification with the given biologic sex, without statistical controls it is impossible to know whether this represents a response to therapy or a spontaneous change that would have occurred without it. Spontaneous remissions occur.

Transvestism, cross-dressing, may occur transiently in preschool boys who dress up in their mothers' clothing, or it may occur chronically in preschool and school-aged boys who feel genuinely excited when dressed in women's clothing. Cross-dressing in girls is rarely an identified problem. Chronic cross-dressing might represent underlying transsexualism, although that is generally not the case. Transvestism usually indicates that other gender roles may also be problematic for the individual. Physicians consulted by parents should investigate other areas of gender identification and gender behavior. Does the child verbalize a preference to be of the opposite sex? Does the child deny or disparage his or her own sexual anatomy or assert that opposite anatomic structures will develop? Three to 6% of school-aged boys and 10–12% of school-aged girls often behave like the opposite sex, but less than 2% of boys and 2–4% of girls actually wish to be the opposite sex.

26.1 Gender Identity Disorder

Ten or more gender-atypical behaviors (GABs) are exhibited in 22.8% of school-aged boys and 38.6% of girls. Most children exhibit one or more GABs. These behaviors are to be expected in most children and are most often not indicative of gender identity disorder (GID). However, persistent distress about being a particular gender while being preoccupied with cross-gender roles or repudiation of given anatomic genital structures is the hallmark of GID. It encompasses transsexualism, transvestism, and effeminacy in boys. The cause of GID is unknown. Some suggest that GID ought not be considered a psychiatric disturbance. Despite the fact that normative studies consistently show that more girls express the wish to be the opposite sex, clinic samples consistently include many more boys than girls (7 to 1).

Clinical Manifestations. Many GID children develop the disorder prior to 4 yr of age. They are often ostracized by peers and have a difficult social adjustment, sometimes with subsequent depres-

sion. One half or more of the boys develop a homosexual orientation during adolescence and adulthood. GID is associated with numerous other childhood and adolescent disorders. Using the Child Behavior Checklist, it has been shown that 84% of feminine boys display behavioral disturbances similar to those seen within a psychiatric clinic population; 60% endorsed items related to peer difficulties and met the criteria for the diagnosis of separation anxiety disorder. Others have found that GID is unrelated to ethnic background, religion, or educational level. Although the natural history of GID suggests a strong relationship between GID and homosexuality, the fact that many gay men and lesbians do not retrospectively recall a history of cross-gender behavior and that a proportion of individuals with childhood GID (10–30%) later identify as heterosexual indicate that GID is probably not just an early manifestation of homosexuality.

Treatment. The relationship between GID and separation anxiety disorder and other disturbances supports the importance of psychotherapy and possibly pharmacotherapy if behaviors satisfy criteria for separation anxiety disorder or other anxiety disorders. Other approaches are often employed and have been shown to be helpful. Parenting techniques that specify which behaviors are appropriate and what is expected of the child regarding gender role behaviors have shown promise in managing a significant percentage of children with GID. The extent of parental involvement in treatment appears to be correlated with a lessening of cross-gender behaviors. The physician needs to help the parents control their own frustration and disappointment and minimize judgmental, rejecting behavior. Punishment, castigation, or shaming will not support the child's attempts to struggle with whatever intrapsychic, interpersonal, or cultural conflicts exist. Underlying family conflicts and parent-child conflicts need to be managed therapeutically.

26.2 Homosexuality

Homosexuality, the romantic and physical attraction to someone of the same gender, has occurred throughout the ages in about 5% of men and women. Historically, acceptance of homosexuality has waxed and waned within societies. The view is currently held by some that homosexuality is best regarded as an alternative lifestyle. The American Psychiatric Association no longer lists it among mental disorders.

Etiology. This is uncertain. Many view its development as a normal variant of sexual development; others point to problematic parent-child relationships. Numerous psychologic theories have been proffered to explain homosexual development. They include problems of sexual identification with parents; problematic relationships between either parent and the child; abuse; overly eroticized attachment; and underlying anxiety and affective proclivities in the individual who will later present with homosexual behavior. Although each theory has been accompanied by anecdotal reports and case studies, none has been substantiated in well-controlled studies.

Biologic causes have also been proposed. Focusing on the perceived homology between homosexual behavior in humans and lower animals, researchers have proposed the "dual mating center" theory, stating that there are hypothalamic areas that regulate male and female sexual behavior. It is hypothesized that too little androgen production in males during a critical prenatal period causes the female center to overdevelop; conversely, excessive androgen production in females leads to the overdevelopment of the male center. Proponents point to the fact that some homosexual men demonstrate "estrogen feedback responses," in which, because of decreased androgen levels, administration of estrogen causes increased production of luteinizing hormone. Many other investigators dispute this theory because of the lack of consistent findings (e.g., XY males with testicular feminization syndrome do not exhibit this response).

LeVay's finding that heterosexual and homosexual men have differences in hypothalamic structure and size also suggests a biologic substrate for sexual orientation, although the possibility of AIDS in his postmortem specimens may have biased these findings. Other researchers have noted that the anterior commissure in homosexual men is significantly larger than that in heterosexual men. This anatomic difference correlates with both sexual orientation and gender; i.e., the anterior commissure is also larger in heterosexual women than in heterosexual men. Furthermore, Hamer et al. discovered a possible genetic marker for male homosexuality in a small group of individuals and are searching for a gene. Many researchers are skeptical of these biologic findings. Some note that the current evidence that postulates biologic factors in the development of sexual orientation is no more compelling than the current evidence linked to psychologic theories.

There are probably multiple mechanisms leading to homosexuality in adolescence and adulthood, just as there are probably multiple mechanisms leading to heterosexuality; many complex factors contribute to sexual development. Cultural, biologic, and psychologic factors probably contribute to sexual orientation development.

Clinical Manifestations and Diagnosis. If a child is found to be engaging in homosexual behavior, parents should not immediately conclude that this means that the child is already homosexual. Sexual behavior during adolescence does not necessarily predict future sexual orientation. It is estimated that 6% of females and 17% of males have had at least one homosexual experience during adolescence. Children sexually explore in the same way that they explore other parts of their environment. The first task of the physician after discovering that a child has engaged in homosexual activity is to help the younger child feel safe and less guilty. Parents should avoid suspicious, scolding, threatening, shaming, or guilt-inducing attitudes or behaviors toward the child. The physician can serve as a model for the parent through his or her own calm, sensitive, careful exploration of feelings and behavior with the child. The physician should expect denials on the part of the child and avoidance of and embarrassment with the subject, but discussion helps the child understand that sexual behavior is comprehensible and that sexual feelings and curiosity are normal. It is important to know whether the child's information and understanding of sexual matters are appropriate for his or her age.

If the same-sex behavior involves another child in the family, he or she should be treated in the same manner. If an older child is the initiator or seducer, he or she should be told clearly and firmly that such behavior will not be tolerated and that he or she will be expected to act with responsibility and control. The older child should talk with a physician or mental health professional; if concerns about emotional and social adjustment become evident, referral for a psychiatric evaluation is indicated. Physicians must not let their own negative feelings aggravate the negative feelings that parents might have for an older child seen as a perpetrator, especially if the older child is not a member of the younger child's family. The physician may need to help the parents of exploited children refrain from ill-considered acts of revenge against the offenders. On the other hand, if there has been physical violence or psychologic coercion, both psychiatric and legal interventions are indicated.

In taking a history of sexual behavior, the pediatrician should not presume exclusively heterosexual behavior. Confidentiality must be maintained, except in sexual abuse cases. Depending on the patient's prior experience, the physical examination should

include an assessment of possible sexually transmitted diseases (STDs). All sexually active males should have appropriate laboratory testing for STDs. Immunization for hepatitis B is recommended and should be provided for all males who anticipate having sex with another male. Human immunodeficiency virus (HIV) testing with the necessary consent is appropriate in these situations. Counseling before and after HIV testing is also necessary. Homosexual activity between adolescent girls is associated with a far lower risk of STDs. However, both HIV infection and other STDs can be transmitted during lesbian sexual activity, especially if one of the partners has also had sex with a man.

When the social opprobrium is considered, it is not surprising that homosexual feelings and wishes create psychologic conflicts in adolescents. Studies suggest that 3–30% of adolescent suicides are attributed to conflicts regarding sexual orientation. In a Minnesota study, 28.1% of gay/bisexual males (grades 7–12) had attempted suicide at least once, compared with 4.2% of heterosexual males of the same age. Although a greater percentage of lesbian adolescents attempted suicide than heterosexual females (20.5% compared with 14.5%), the difference was not statistically significant (see Chapter 24). Troiden's model of homosexual identity development helps elucidate the stages associated with sexual orientation acceptance. These include sensitization, i.e., the awareness of being different because of same-gender attraction; sexual identity confusion, i.e., turmoil often related to trying to reconcile one's feelings with negative societal stigmatization; sexual identity assumption, i.e., acknowledgment of one's own gay identity; and integration and commitment, i.e., incorporation of sexual identity into a positive self-acceptance.

Treatment. In spite of some anecdotal reports to the contrary, very little can be done to change one's sexual orientation. Even in cases in which individuals have expressed the desire to change, significantly less than half of those who have tried have been able to change sexual orientation with various behavioral and dynamic therapies. Often, attempts to change sexual orientation lead only to additional guilt and further stigmatization. Psychotherapy is more appropriately used for concurrent disorders (separation anxiety disorder, conduct disorder, dysthymic disorder, depression) and to help with the conflict that often ensues as one moves toward sexual orientation acceptance. Families usually need assistance in coping with this knowledge and their attendant anger and disappointment. Children need help in understanding how to cope with the reactions of others.

Allen L, Gorski R: Sexual orientation and the size of the anterior commissure in the human brain. *Proc Natl Acad Sci U S A* 1992;89:7199.

Bailey J, Michael J, Neale M, et al: Heritable factors influencing sexual orientation in women. *Arch Gen Psychiatry* 1993;50:217.

Bradley SJ, Zucker KJ: Gender identity disorder: A review of the past 10 years. *J Am Acad Child Adolesc Psychiatry* 1997;36:872.

Byrne W, Parsons B: Human sexual orientation: The biologic theories reappraised. *Arch Gen Psychiatry* 1993;50:228.

Coates S, Person E: Extreme boyhood femininity: Isolated behavior or pervasive disorder? *J Am Acad Child Adolesc Psychiatry* 1985;24:702.

Committee on Adolescence (American Academy of Pediatrics): Homosexuality and adolescence. *Pediatrics* 1993;92:631.

DuRant RH, Krowchuk DP, Sinal SH: Victimization, use of violence, and drug use at school among male adolescents who engage in same-sex sexual behavior. *J Pediatr* 1998;132:13.

Friedrich WN, Fisher J, Broughton D, et al: Normal sexual behavior in children: A contemporary sample. *Pediatrics* 1998;101:E9.

Hamer D, Magnuson V, Pattatucci A: A linkage between DNA markers on the X chromosome and male sexual orientation. *Science* 1993;261:321.

LeVay S: *The Sexual Brain*. Cambridge, MIT Press, 1993.

Sandberg D, Meyer-Bahlburg H, Ehrhardt A, et al: The prevalence of gender-atypical behavior in elementary school children. *J Am Acad Child Adolesc Psychiatry* 1993;32:306.

Troiden R: Homosexual identity development. *J Adolesc Health Care* 1989;9:105.

Chapter 27
Pervasive Developmental Disorders and Childhood Psychosis *Richard Dalton,*

Marc A. Forman, and Neil W. Boris

Pervasive developmental disorders include autistic disorder, Asperger disorder, childhood disintegrative disorder, and Rett disorder.

27.1 Autistic Disorder

Autism develops before 36 mo of age and is typically diagnosable at 18 mo of age. It is characterized by a qualitative impairment in verbal and nonverbal communication, in imaginative activity, and in reciprocal social interactions.

Epidemiology. Recent studies show prevalence rates ranging from 10 to 20 per 10,000 children. There is controversy regarding whether the incidence of autism is increasing. The disorder is much more common in males than females (3–4:1). Autism can be associated with other neurologic disorders, particularly seizure disorders, and to a lesser extent, tuberous sclerosis and fragile X syndrome.

Etiology. The cause of autism is multifactorial. Genetic factors play a significant role. There is a 60–90% concordance rate for monozygotic twins and less than 5% concordance rate for dizygotic twins. What is actually inherited is not entirely clear; language and cognitive abnormalities are more common in relatives of autistic children than in the general population. In various case reports on autistic children, anomalies have been reported in all but three chromosomes, but most promising may be the findings of deletions and duplications in chromosome 15.

Theories of causation have also centered on a variety of other possibilities, especially pre- or perinatal brain injury. Deficits in the reticular activating system, structural cerebellar changes, forebrain hippocampal lesions, and neuroradiologic abnormalities in the prefrontal and temporal lobe areas have been documented. Autistic children have also been reported to have an increase in brain volume in several regions, and idiopathic infantile macrocephaly has been associated with autism. Studies also demonstrate anatomic changes in the anterior cingulate gyrus, an area of the brain associated with decision-making and the ascription of feelings and thoughts. Abnormal neurochemical findings have also been associated with autism, with dopamine, catecholamine, and serotonin levels or pathways implicated. However, the literature on brain structure and function in autistic children is conflicting and there is no diagnostic imaging or other test for autism.

Contrary to notions in vogue in the past, autism is not induced by parents. A number of excellent epidemiologic studies have established that there is no association between the use of measles-mumps-rubella vaccine and autism.

Clinical Manifestations. Early measurable diagnostic symptoms and signs of autism include poor eye contact, little symbolic play, limited joint attention or orienting to one's name, and reliance on nonverbal communication with delay in use of words. Stereotypical body movements, a marked need for sameness, and a very narrow range of interests, are also common. The autistic child is often withdrawn and spends hours in solitary play. Ritualistic behavior prevails, reflecting the child's need to maintain a consistent, predictable environment. Tantrum-like rages may accompany disruptions of routine. Eye contact is typically minimal or absent. Visual scanning of hand and finger movements, mouthing of objects, and rubbing of surfaces may indicate a heightened awareness and sensitivity to some stimuli, whereas diminished responses to pain and lack of startle responses to sudden loud noises reflect lowered sensitivity to other stimuli. If speech is present, echolalia, pronoun reversal, nonsense rhyming, and other idiosyncratic language forms may predominate. Early diagnosis of children at risk for autism can be facilitated by the use of the Checklist for Autism in Toddlers (CHAT), a screening instrument. Research using home movies of 1-yr birthday parties has shown that children at risk for autistic disorder can be reliably identified at this age. These children do not share affect with caregivers by pointing, communicating interest, or sharing in joint attention.

Intelligence by conventional psychologic testing usually falls in the functionally retarded range; however, the deficits in language and socialization make it difficult to obtain an accurate estimate of the autistic child's intellectual potential. Some autistic children perform adequately in nonverbal tests, and those with developed speech may demonstrate adequate intellectual capacity. Occasionally, an autistic child may have an isolated, remarkable talent, analogous to that of the adult savant.

Although first described as a social illness, subsequent studies have focused on the communicative and cognitive deficits of autism and, particularly, on the types of cognitive processing deficits most apparent in emotional situations. Autistic children also show deficits in their understanding of what the other person might be feeling or thinking, a so-called lack of a "theory of mind." On some psychologic tests, children with autism pay more attention to specific details while overlooking the entire gestalt of the object, demonstrating a "lack of central coherence."

Treatment. Considerable advances have been made in the treatment of autism, especially within the educational, psychosocial, and biologic areas. There is compelling evidence that intensive behavioral therapy, beginning before 3 yr of age and targeted toward speech and language development, is successful both in improving language capacity and later social functioning. Treatment is most successful when geared toward the individual's particular behavior patterns and language function. Parent education, training, and support is always indicated, and pharmacotherapy for certain target symptoms may be helpful.

Working with families of autistic children is vital to the child's overall care. Children with autism require alternate educational approaches even when language capacity is near normal. Such services in general have not yet been sufficiently developed to provide adequate support and continuity of care. One successful educational model is the program for the Treatment and Education of Autistic and Related Communication Handicapped Children (TEACCH). The following treatment principles are emphasized: use of objective measures such as the Childhood Autism Rating Scale (CARS) to measure behavior and behavioral change; enhancement of skills and acceptance by the environment of autism-related deficits; use of interventions based on cognitive and behavioral theories; use of visual structures for optimal education; and multidisciplinary training for all professionals working with autistic children. Educational programming should begin as early as possible, preferably by age 2–4.

Older children and adolescents with relatively higher intelligence but with poor social skills and psychiatric symptoms (e.g., depression, anxiety, obsessive-compulsive symptoms) may require psychotherapy, behavioral or cognitive therapy, and pharmacotherapy. Typically, behavior modification is a major part of the overall treatment for older children with autism. These procedures include enhancement (i.e., rewards emphasizing appropriate choice) and reduction (extinction, time-out, punishment). Ethical concerns about vigorous aversive therapy approaches have led to specific guidelines. Social skills training is also currently used as a treatment modality and appears effective, especially in a group format.

Unfortunately, there are unfounded claims of beneficial results from many unproven therapies for autism, almost all of which have not been subjected to scientific study. Those studies that have been done have discredited the technique of facilitated communication and have shown that auditory integration therapy has no positive effect. Claims of beneficial results from the use of secretin, a peptide hormone that stimulates pancreatic secretion, have not been substantiated by scientific study. Similarly, the dietary supplement N, N-dimethylglycine has no benefit.

Because a subgroup of autistic children present with psychiatric symptoms, pharmacotherapy is sometimes used to ameliorate target behaviors. The behaviors include hyperactivity, tantrums, physical aggression, self-injurious behavior, stereotypes, and anxiety symptoms—especially obsessive-compulsive behaviors. The older neuroleptics were limited in their usefulness because of their tendency to produce extrapyramidal symptoms and tardive dyskinesia. Open label trials of the newer atypical neuroleptics (e.g., risperidone, olanzapine) have shown effectiveness in treating the above behaviors, and in some instances, have also improved social relatedness (see Chapter 28.2).

Naltrexone, an opiate antagonist, was also originally touted as useful, especially for self-injurious behavior, but its utility has not yet been proven. Clomipramine, a tricyclic antidepressant with serotonin reuptake inhibition action, has demonstrated usefulness in reducing compulsions and stereotypes in autistic children. However, it does lower the seizure threshold, can cause agranulocytosis, and has cardiotoxic and behavior toxicity effects. Other medicines used to treat psychiatric symptoms in autistic children include the stimulants, the serotonin reuptake inhibitors (SSRIs), and clonidine. The SSRIs, in particular, appear to be somewhat effective in diminishing hyperactive, agitated, and obsessive-compulsive behaviors, although there have not yet been sufficient, controlled studies regarding their utility (Chapter 28.2).

Prognosis. Some children, especially those with speech, may grow up to live self-sufficient, employed, albeit isolated, lives in the community. Many others remain dependent on family for their everyday lives or require placement in facilities outside the home. Because early, intensive therapy may improve language and social function, delayed diagnosis may lead to worse outcome. There is no increased risk for the development of schizophrenia in adulthood but the cost of delayed diagnosis across the life span is high. A better prognosis is associated with higher intelligence, functional speech, and less bizarre symptoms and behavior. The symptom profile for some children may change as they grow older and seizures or self-injurious behavior becomes more common.

27.2 Asperger Disorder

Children with this disorder have a qualitative impairment in the development of reciprocal social interaction, often demonstrating repetitive behaviors and restricted, obsessional, idiosyncratic interests. They do not, however, have the severe language impairments that characterize autism. Though somewhat socially aware, these children appear to others to be peculiar or eccentric. Prevalence is estimated to be approximately 3/1,000 children. This disorder may represent a higher-functioning form of autism, although this distinction remains controversial. Group social skills training is the hallmark of intervention, although children with Asperger disorder appear to be at high risk for other psychiatric disorders, particularly oppositional-defiant disorder and mood disorders.

27.3 Childhood Disintegrative Disorder

This disorder, also known as Heller dementia, is a rare condition of unknown cause, characterized by normal development up to 2–4 yr followed by severe deterioration of mental and social functioning, with regression to a very impaired "autistic" state. Language, social skills, and imagination are profoundly affected; bowel and bladder control may be lost; and motor stereotypes and seizures are often present. Although this condition may be the result of an underlying neurologic illness, none has been identified. The prognosis is always poor.

27.4 Rett Disorder

This is an X-linked dominant disorder affecting girls almost exclusively; boys affected with the disorder die at birth. It has a prevalence of 1/10,000. Development proceeds normally until approximately 1–2 yr of age, at which time language and motor development regress and acquired microcephaly becomes apparent. These girls present with midline, stereotypic hand-wringing, ataxia, breathing dysfunction, bruxism, scoliosis, and profound intellectual handicap. Autistic behaviors are typical, but over time, social relatedness may improve. Lower limb involvement may progress, leading to wheelchair dependency later in life. Postmortem examinations have revealed greatly reduced brain size and weight as well as number of synapses. A gene that causes Rett syndrome has been identified; it encodes the methyl CpG-binding protein 2 (MeCP2).

27.5 Childhood Schizophrenia

Psychotic reactions in older children tend more closely to resemble the psychoses of adulthood, and the same diagnostic criteria apply. Psychosis associated with a mood disorder, such as bipolar illness, is discussed in Chapter 23.

Clinical Manifestations. In *childhood schizophrenia,* prominent symptoms include thought disorder, disorganized speech, delusions, and hallucinations. The latter two symptoms, in addition to later onset, higher intelligence scores, and fewer perinatal complications, differentiate schizophrenia from autism. As the symptoms imply, schizophrenic children are typically severely impaired. They may have paranoid delusions, aggressive behavior, hebephrenic silliness, social withdrawal, and alternating moods not apparently related to environmental stimuli.

The prevalence of adult schizophrenia is 1%. The typical age of onset is late adolescence to early adulthood. Early-onset schizophrenia (e.g., prepubertal or early adolescence) is very rare. As infants, half of schizophrenic children are said to have had abnormally delayed development, and unusual sensory sensitivities. Schizophrenic children show significant premorbid maladjustments, including social withdrawal, disruptive behaviors, developmental delays, and speech and language problems. The onset of the disorder is usually insidious. Auditory hallucinations are seen in 80% of schizophrenic children. Delusions and formal thought disorders usually do not present until mid-adolescence. Children with early-onset schizophrenia show preliminary evidence of progressive ventricular enlargement, decrease in total cerebral volume, and decline in intellectual functioning. The prognosis is poor. The symptoms in childhood that most predict psychotic adult psychopathology are affective blunting and disturbed interpersonal relationships, as opposed to delusions and hallucinations.

Individuals with various psychotic processes are often misdiagnosed as schizophrenic. In a recent National Institute of Mental Health childhood-onset schizophrenia (COS) study, over 1,300 children were referred with a putative diagnosis of COS. After various screening and evaluation procedures, about 5% were actually labeled with COS and accepted into the research program. The majority of misdiagnosed patients were later noted to suffer with bipolar disorder, major depressive disorder with psychosis, and psychosis, not otherwise specified.

Treatment. A multimodal therapeutic approach is necessary to manage this illness. Parent training is necessary to teach effective techniques to modify the schizophrenic child's behavior to improve social functioning. Individual therapy designed to build a positive alliance is also very important. School and community liaison work can establish and maintain a day-to-day schedule for the patient. Neuroleptic therapy is often effective in managing hallucinations and psychotic delusions. The use of haloperidol has largely been replaced by newer atypical antipsychotics such as risperidone and olanzapine. These medications appear to have lower risks for extrapyramidal symptoms and tardive dyskinesia. However, weight gain is common with atypical neuroleptics. Clozapine appears to be the most effective antipsychotic medication for refractory cases, but the risk of agranulocytosis and seizures limits its use (see Chapter 28.2).

American Academy of Child and Adolescent Psychiatry: Practice parameters for the assessment and treatment of children, adolescents, and adults with autism and other pervasive developmental disorders. *J Am Acad Child Adolesc Psychiatry* 1999;38(Supp):32S–54S.

American Academy of Child and Adolescent Psychiatry: Practice parameters for the assessment and treatment of children and adolescents with schizophrenia. *J Am Acad Child Adolesc Psychiatry* 2001;40(Supp):4S–23S.

American Academy of Neurology: Practice parameter: Screening and diagnosis of autism. *Neurology* 2000;55:468–79.

Amir RE, Van den Veyver IB, Wan M, et al: Rett syndrome is caused by mutations in X-linked MECP2, encoding methyl-CpG-binding protein 2. *Nat Genet* 1999;23:185–90.

Baron-Cohen S, Wheelwright S, Cox A, et al: Early identification of autism by the checklist for autism in toddlers (CHAT). *J R Soc Med* 2000;93:521–5.

Cook EH Jr: Genetics of autism. *Child Adolesc Psychiatr Clin of N Am* 2001;10:333–50.

Dales L, Hammer SJ, Smith NJ: Time trends in autism and in MMR immunization coverage in California. *JAMA* 2001;285:1183–5.

Eliez S, Reiss AL: MRI neuroimaging of childhood psychiatric disorders: A selective review. *J Child Psychol Psychiatry* 2000;41:679–94.

Lombroso PJ: Genetics of childhood disorders: XIV. A gene for Rett syndrome: News flash. *J Am Acad Child Adolesc Psychiatry* 2000;39:671–4.

Posey DJ, McDougle CJ: The pharmacotherapy of target symptoms associated with autistic disorder and other pervasive developmental disorders. *Harv Rev Psychiatry* 2000;8:45–63.

Rapoport JL, Inoff-Germain G: Update on childhood-onset schizophrenia. *Curr Psychiatry Rep* 2000;2:410–5.

Rogers SJ: Interventions that facilitate socialization in children with autism. *J Autism Dev Disord* 2000;30:399–409.

Sandler AD, Sutton KA, DeWeese J, et al: Lack of benefit of a single dose of synthetic human secretin in the treatment of autism and pervasive developmental disorder. *N Engl J Med* 1999;341:1801–6.

Tanguay PE: Pervasive developmental disorders: A 10-year review. *J Am Acad Child Adolesc Psychiatry* 1999;39:1079–95.

Chapter 28
Psychologic Treatment of Children and Adolescents

Richard Dalton

28.1 Illness and Death

All clinical phenomena relate to various organizational levels: molecular, anatomic, physiologic, intrapsychic, interpersonal, familial, and social. Accordingly, physicians should focus on patients' discomfort rather than on a categorization of clinical manifestations as either organically or psychologically determined. The psychologic aspects of illness should be evaluated from the outset, and physicians should act as a model for parents and children by showing interest in a child's feelings and demonstrating that it is possible and appropriate to communicate discomfort in verbal, symbolic language.

For *hospitalized children*, potential challenges include coping with separation (Chapter 33); adapting to a new environment;

adjusting to multiple caregivers; often associating with very sick children; and sometimes experiencing the disorientation of intensive care, anesthesia, and surgery. To help mitigate potential problems, a preadmission visit to the hospital is often important to meet the people who will be offering care and to ask questions about what will happen. For children younger than age 5–6 yr, parents should room with the child if feasible. Creative and active recreational or socialization programs, with liberal visiting hours (including visits from siblings), and chances to act out feared procedures in play with dolls or mannequins all are helpful. Sensitive, sympathetic, and accepting attitudes toward children and parents by the hospital staff are very important. There is often an underlying tension between the hospital caregivers and the parents. Hospital routines and schedules often serve to complicate the relationship between parents and hospital workers. Guilt and anger can result, unnecessarily complicating an already difficult situation (Chapter 54).

Ambulatory care in clinics or offices where patients receive discontinuous care from a series of physicians whose intercommunication is often limited may create a problem. Parents often become confused and unable to verbalize major concerns about their children. Recommendations for care may become inappropriate or irrelevant, and compliance with advice or directions becomes poor. At the end of any initial diagnostic or management activity, physicians should habitually inquire whether there are other things parents or children may wish to talk about during this visit. In busy emergency rooms, conflicting expectations between how the professional staff expects the emergency room to be used and what patients actually need can lead to confusion. When these different expectations are critically examined, ways may be found to deal more effectively with the patterns of use of emergency services.

With *chronically or fatally ill children*, patients and parents experience each symptom as a threat to physical integrity and life. The more serious the clinical state, the greater the intensity of the emotions aroused (see Chapters 33, 37, and 38). In dealing with chronic illness that shortens life, parents need physicians' early support in developing a relatively guilt-free understanding of the disease and how to manage it. They need guidance to help them comfortably answer their child's questions about the disease. Parents of critically or fatally ill children may creatively support each other in group meetings under the professional guidance of physicians, psychologists, or social workers. Young children take most cues from their parents. With older children, especially adolescents, parents must be prepared to deal with the anger of their children because of their fate. Children need both the parents' psychologic strengths and resources and the physician's availability and objectivity. The siblings of an ill child require information about the disease and the support and attention of the parents for their own needs.

Physicians must stand for hope and for relief of discomfort, ready to help parents and children avoid emotionally crippling psychologic handicaps. In potentially *fulminant lethal processes*, the intensity of parental anxiety, guilt, and despair may be greater than it is with more chronic illnesses (Chapters 33, 38, and 54; also see Chapter 60 for discussion of transplant issues). A hospital team approach representing medical, nursing, psychologic, and social work disciplines, among others, should provide support. The primary physician needs to stay involved and close to the child and to the clinical situation.

After *the death of a child*, the parents need opportunities to talk out their feelings with the physician, one of whose goals should be to help them avoid psychologically encapsulating the lost child in an unmourned state (see Chapter 33). Physicians need the patience to listen (both to the stated and to the implied questions and misconceptions), to answer questions, and to help families with funeral arrangements (see Chapters 33, 38, and 64).

28.2 Psychopharmacology

Using drugs to modify children's behavior is controversial. Their effects on behavior are influenced by the maturity of the central nervous system, by intrapsychic and psychosocial factors, by the personality or charisma of the physician prescribing them, by the problem itself, and by the milieu (e.g., patient, parents, time of day given). Although potentially helpful, psychiatric medications can cause very serious side effects. Even though some guidelines for their use are offered in Table 28–1, only clinicians with appropriate training and experience should prescribe the antipsychotics, mood stabilizers, and tricyclic antidepressants.

Neuroleptics are appropriately used for hallucinations, delusions, thought disorders, and severe agitation. They are primarily indicated for children and adolescents suffering with schizophrenic disorders, mood-congruent and mood-incongruent psychotic reactions secondary to major affective disorders, autism presenting with stereotypic and withdrawal symptoms and self-abuse, and Gilles de la Tourette syndrome. This class of medicine is inappropriately used for anxiety, conduct disorder without extreme aggression, and attention deficit disorder.

Neuroleptics can be subdivided into typical (low-potency, mid-potency, and high-potency subtypes) and novel, atypical types (clozapine, risperidone, olanzapine, quetiapine, and ziprasidone). Thioridazine (Mellaril), a low-potency, high-dosage typical antipsychotic is no longer recommended for usage because of potential hepatotoxicity. Low-potency typical antipsychotics usually require a higher dose than the other neuroleptics for symptom remission. They tend to cause sedation, producing numerous anticholinergic side effects but comparatively fewer extrapyramidal symptoms. Mesoridazine is an example of a mid-potency medicine. It produces more extrapyramidal symptoms than the low-potency drugs. Thiothixene and haloperidol are high-potency medicines that produce, comparatively, the greatest number of extrapyramidal symptoms. Clozapine, an atypical neuroleptic, has efficacy in the treatment of negative schizophrenic symptoms. However, threatening side effects include agranulocytosis and seizure development. Although it is often effective when other agents are not, its use is often limited to refractory cases because of its toxicity. The other atypicals are a substantial improvement over the typical antipsychotic medications, not only because they appear to be more effective, but also because they are less likely to cause tardive dyskinesia and extrapyramidal symptoms. However, QTc prolongation on electroencephalographic studies and weight gain can be problematic.

The most worrisome side effect of the typical neuroleptics is the development of **tardive dyskinesia**. This is characterized by choreoathetoid movements of the trunk, limbs, and facial musculature; these movements develop in approximately 20–30% of children treated long term with neuroleptics. Dyskinesia can occur during the treatment with the drug or after it has been discontinued, in which case it is referred to as *withdrawal dyskinesia*. This latter type of dyskinesia, the symptoms of which can include nausea, vomiting, diaphoresis, ataxia, oral dyskinesia, and various dystonic movements, is reversible in most cases, whereas the dyskinesia developing during drug use may not be reversible. The best instrument for the assessment of abnormal movements of children and adolescents is the Abnormal Involuntary Movement Scale (AIMS). Treatment of tardive dyskinesia involves decreasing or discontinuing the medication if possible, despite the fact that it has been noted that increasing the neuroleptic causes a temporary diminution of dyskinetic symptoms. Prophylactic measures involving drug-free holidays and periodic discontinuation of neuroleptics are also advisable to help mitigate the development of tardive dyskinesia.

Extrapyramidal symptoms, a Parkinson-like syndrome (akathisia, bradykinesia, torticollis, drooling, and involuntary hand movements, among others), develop in at least one fourth of children treated with neuroleptics. The imbalance created by the dopaminergic blocking action of the antipsychotic medication disrupts a needed balance between the dopaminergic system and the cholinergic system within the basal ganglia. The high-potency neuroleptics, which contain few anticholinergic properties, are the most likely to produce extrapyramidal symptoms. This syndrome can be treated by decreasing the neuroleptic or adding an anticholinergic agent (trihexyphenidyl HCl [Artane], benztropine mesylate [Cogentin]).

Neuroleptic malignant syndrome, a rare side effect of neuroleptic use, can be fatal. Its development is heralded by a high fever and a "lead pipe" stiffness of the extremities. Patients' creatinine phosphokinase level is also markedly elevated. Immediate discontinuation of the medicine and supportive care are necessary during the early part of the syndrome.

Stimulant medications are used to treat the signs and symptoms of attention-deficit/hyperactivity disorder (see Chapter 29.2). Although the mechanism of action is not entirely clear, these medications increase children's ability to attend, improve classroom behavior, and increase social acceptance of affected children in various situations. These stimulants should be used concurrently with individual, family, and community therapy.

Antidepressants and *mood stabilizers* are useful in the treatment of affective disorders. Antidepressants generally are effective for depression, whereas lithium, carbamazepine, valproate, and lamotrigine have shown efficacy in the treatment of mania. Adult patients with bipolar and unipolar disorders are often treated with long-term pharmacotherapy, and this is becoming more common in childhood and adolescence. Because of the propensity of tricyclic antidepressants to cause heart block, a pretreatment electrocardiogram (ECG) and follow-up ECGs are necessary. Heart block usually takes at least a few weeks to develop. Although deaths in school-aged children taking desipramine have been reported, sudden deaths have not been reported in conjunction with the use of other tricyclics or with other nontricyclic antidepressants. Before prescribing tricyclics in general and desipramine in particular, clinicians must procure a detailed medical history, including examination of a patient's cardiovascular system and ascertainment of any family history of cardiac disease (including unexplained syncope and sudden death). A child with a suspicious history or with abnormal ECG findings should have a pediatric or cardiologic assessment before these medicines are used. The desipramine dose should not exceed 3.5–5.0 mg/kg. A pretreatment lithium evaluation includes thyroid studies, renal function tests, and electrolyte determinations. Lithium blood levels should also be determined while patients are taking the medication. Prolonged use of lithium may cause hypothyroidism.

Serotonin reuptake blockers, especially fluoxetine (Prozac), sertraline (Zoloft), and paroxetine (Paxil), are effective in patients with mild depressive symptoms, anxiety, and compulsions. Paroxetine is especially useful because of its relatively short half-life and lack of side effects. Clonidine has been partially successful in treating children with attention-deficit/hyperactivity disorder and in those who have a personal history of tics (including Gilles de la Tourette syndrome).

Carbamazepine, an *antiepileptic* medicine, is effective in the treatment of mania and episodic dyscontrol syndrome. *β-Blocking agents* (nadolol [Corgard]) appear to decrease aggressiveness in mentally retarded patients. *Opiate antagonists* significantly change some behaviors in autistic children and have promise in the treatment of self-injurious behavior in severely and profoundly mentally retarded individuals. Clomipramine (Anafranil) is efficacious in the treatment of obsessive-compulsive disorder. Seizures have been reported secondary to its use, however.

Some parents are adamantly opposed to the use of psychotropic medications. If drugs are used, they should be used for as short a time as possible. As with any clinical disorder, physicians should

TABLE 28–1. Psychopharmacology

Medication Class	Use	Dosage	Side Effects/ Toxicity/Caution	Pretreatment Work-up
Antipsychotics—Traditional	**All:** severe agitation; psychosis; mania; stereotypic movements; self-abuse; extreme aggressiveness; Tourette		**All Classes:** Sedation, weight gain, anticholinergic effects (dry mouth, blurred vision; constipation); hypersensitivity reactions (hepatic, skin); blood dyscrasias; parkinsonism; neuroleptic malignant syndrome; orthostatic hypotension; agranulocytosis and seizures (especially with clozapine) **N.B.:** Thioridazine (Mellaril) is no longer recommended because of hepatotoxicity **N.B.:** Tardive dyskinesia is a potential side effect	CBC with differential, blood chemistry panel (including hepatic enzymes) Pregnancy test; height and weight measures
Low-Potency/High-Dosage Chlorpromazine (Thorazine)		Initial: 10–30 mg/24 hr in single or divided doses. Maintenance: 100–900 mg/24 hr in divided doses		
Mid-Potency/Mid-Dosage Mesoridazine (Serentil)		10–75 mg/24 hr in divided doses		
High-Potency/Low-Dosage Haloperidol (Haldol)		Initial: 0.5–1 mg/24 hr in single or divided doses		
Trifluoperazine (Stelazine) Thiothixine (Navane)				
Antipsychotics—Novel (Atypical)			Same general side effects as Traditional Antipsychotics	**All:** Cardiovascular history; ECG; Chem 12; electrolytes; pregnancy tests: weight and height measures
Clozapine (Clozaril)		Initial: 12.5–25 mg/24 hr; then increase by 25–50 mg/24 hr; maintenance dose: 250–500 mg/24 hr in divided doses	Seizures, agranulocytosis, weight gain	History of seizures; CBC/differential
Risperidone (Risperdal)		Initial: 0.5 mg bid; then increase by 0.5 mg each 3–4 days to 2–4 mg/24 hr	Weight gain, mild EPS, increase in Prolactin levels, prolongation of QTc	
Quetiapine (Seroquel)		Initial: 25 mg bid; then increase by 50–100 mg every 2–3 days to 50–500 mg/24 hr	Sedation, weight gain	Ophthalmological exam
Olanzapine (Zyprexa)		Initial: 2.5–5 mg hs; if necessary, increase by 2.5 mg every 3–4 days to 5–15 mg/24 hr	Sedation, weight gain, prolongation of QTc	
Ziprasidone (Geodon)		40–80 mg/24 hr in divided doses	Prolongation of QTc	
Stimulants	**All Drugs:** ADHD (with and without behavioral acting out): Narcolepsy (methylphenidate, dextroamphetamine)		Lower seizure threshold; insomnia, decreased appetite, possible weight loss; irritability and tearfulness; abdominal pain, headache; elevated systolic blood pressure; development and worsening of tics; possible subnormal height and weight growth. Possible precipitation of hypomania in bipolar patients; pemoline (Cylert) is no longer recommended because of hepatotoxicity	Medical history, heart rate, blood pressure, CBC with differential (with prolonged use)

Table continued on following page

97

TABLE 28-1. Psychopharmacology *Continued*

Medication Class	Use	Dosage	Side Effects/ Toxicity/Caution	Pretreatment Work-up
Methylphenidate (Ritalin, Concerta, Metadate ER)		Ritalin: 0.3–1.0 mg/kg/24 hr in divided doses; Concerta: 18 mg in single dose, increase to 36 mg if necessary; Metadate ER: 10 mg increased to 60 mg/24 hr if necessary	Possible sudden death in doses >3.5–5 mg/kg; hypertension, orthostatic hypotension, cardiac arrhythmia, lengthening of PR or QRS interval on ECG; overdose leading to death	Thorough individual and family history for cardiologic problems; 12-lead ECG; blood pressure monitoring. Plasma blood levels indicated after therapy has begun only if clinical response is poor
Dextroamphetamine (Dexedrine, Adderall)		Dexedrine: 0.2–0.6 mg/kg/24 hr in divided doses; Adderall: Initial: 2.5–5 mg; increase by 2.5–5 mg/24 hr to 60 mg/24 hr (Narcolepsy)	As above	As above
Antidepressants				
Tricyclics				
Desipramine (Norpramin)	Major depressive disorder in mid to late adolescence; ADHD (12 yr and older); separation anxiety disorder	For major depression disorder and separation anxiety disorder, 2–3 mg/kg/24 hr in divided doses. (Therapeutic blood level, 100–250 mg/mL)	Seizures; overdose leading to death; ST-T wave changes on ECG, conduction abnormalities; psychiatric changes including mania and confusion; weight gain; hyperthermia; vertigo; constipation	As above
Imipramine (Tofranil)	As above; enuresis	As above. For enuresis usually 25–50 mg qhs (continued for at least 4–6 mo after remission of enuresis)		
Clomipramine (Anafranil)	Obsessive-compulsive disorder (OCD)	Starting dose of 25 mg, which is increased slowly (2–3 wk) to either 100 mg or 3 mg/kg (whichever is smaller) in divided doses. Thereafter, increase to a maximum of 250–300 mg		
Selective Serotonin Reuptake Inhibitors				
Fluoxetine (Prozac)	Mild-moderate depression, anxiety, OCD	10–20 mg/24 hr (possibly higher for OCD)	Fluoxetine and its principal metabolite have a long half-life (1–4 days). Can inhibit its own metabolism; thus, an increase in dose may result in a disproportionate increase in side effects. Drug interactions with compounds metabolized by several isoenzymes of the cytochrome P 450 system (especially terfenadine, astemizole, cisapride); gastrointestinal difficulties (nausea, diarrhea, vomiting); CNS effects (agitation, disinhibition, jitteriness, headache, insomnia); tremor; serotonin syndrome (fever, myoclonus, confusion, tachycardia, rigidity…) when taken with MAO inhibitors or L-tryptophan; mania; self-injurious behavior and behavioral activation and dyscontrol	
Paroxetine (Paxil)	As above	10–30 mg/24 hr	As above except shorter half-life (24 hr); withdrawal symptoms if stopped abruptly	
Sertraline (Zoloft)	As above	25–50 mg/24 hr with meals	Similar to paroxetine; fairly inactive metabolite has longer half-life; exhibits linear relationship between dose and side effects	
Fluvoxamine (Luvox)	OCD	Initial: 50 mg each night. Increase slowly to no more than 300 mg/24 hr in divided doses.	Similar to sertraline; less interference with cytochrome P450 system	

Drug	Indications	Dosage	Side Effects	Laboratory/Monitoring
Venlafaxine (Effexor)	Depression	37.5 mg/24 hr increased by no more than 37.5–75 mg/24 hr to a maximum 225 mg/24 hr in divided doses, with meals	As above, except for little interference with cytochrome P450 system	
Aminoketone				
Bupropion (Wellbutrin)	Depression, ADHD	Initial: 75–100 mg/24 hr increased slowly to 200–300 mg/24 hr (bid dosing); total daily dose should not exceed 450 mg	Seizures, restlessness, agitation, weight loss, rashes, nocturia, mania, flulike symptoms	
Mood Stabilizers				
Lithium carbonate	Bipolar cycling typical of older adolescents and adults, some cases of unipolar illness, affective type of aggression	600–1,200 mg/24 hr (therapeutic blood level: 0.6–1.2 mEq/L)	Gastrointestinal disturbance, tremor, ataxia, confusion, coma, death; hypothyroidism. Once discontinued, lithium is often not as effective when restarted. Overdose leading to death	Creatinine clearance, thyroid studies, ECG, electrolytes, calcium, phosphorus, Chem 12, pregnancy test, CBC with differential
Carbamazepine (Tegretol)	Bipolar cycling including rapid cycling; aggressive behavior in organically impaired patients	Initial: 100–200 mg/24 hr increased to 400–1,000 mg/24 hr (therapeutic blood level: 8–12 µg/mL)	Fever, sore throat, hematologic problems (white cell decrease), dizziness, drowsiness, neuromuscular disturbance, blurred vision; overdose leading to death	Physical examination, medical history, CBC with differential, BUN, hepatic enzymes; EKG; pregnancy test
Valproic acid (Depakene)	Rapid cycling bipolar disorder, aggression	Initial: 125–250 mg/24 hr or 10–15 mg/kg; increase by 5–10 mg/kg/24 hr up to 60 mg/kg/24 hr in divided doses (therapeutic blood level: 50–120 µg/mL)	Hepatic failure (usually in the first few months of treatment; younger children (under 10 yr, especially under 2 yr), patients with prior hepatic disease history, those on multiple anticonvulsants, those with severe seizure history plus mental retardation, and those with congenital metabolic disorders are especially vulnerable. Obesity, birth defects in pregnancy; possible clotting problems; depression; nausea, vomiting, indigestion (at initiation of therapy), rashes; overdose leading to coma and possibly death; pancreatitis; polycystic ovary syndrome	Physical examination, medical history, hepatic enzymes; amylase; Chem 12; CBC with differential; EKG; FSH/LH for girls
Lamotrigine (Lamictil)	Bipolar depression, especially Bipolar II depression; dysphoric mania, rapid cycling Bipolar II	Initial: 25 mg/24 hr during first 2 weeks; if necessary, increase by 50 mg/24 hr each week to a maximum of 300–400 mg/24 hr **N.B.:** NOT yet recommended for patients under 18 yr	Sedation, nausea, headache; Rash in 10% of patients (Risk of Stevens-Johnson reaction); Concurrent use with valproic acid doubles the lamotrigine blood level	Same as other mood stabilizers
Antihypertensives				
Clonidine (Catapres)	Hyperactivity; aggression associated with ADHD; secondary use in tic disorder	0.1–0.25 mg/24 hr	Sedating bradycardia, hypotension; withdrawal symptoms; sudden deaths reported when used with stimulants	Physical examination, medical history, blood pressure, ECG
Guanfacine (Tenex)	Aggression associated with ADHD; tic disorder	0.5–1 mg qhs	Sedation, headaches (less hypotension than clonidine)	Blood pressure

ADHD, attention-deficit/hyperactivity disorder; BUN, blood urea nitrogen; CBC, complete blood count; CNS, central nervous system; ECG, electrocardiogram; EPS, extrapyramidal symptoms; MAO, monoamine oxidase; OCD, obsessive-compulsive disorder.

initially avoid using several medications at the same time and should not shift back and forth from one medication to another when no immediate response occurs. Because psychotropic medications have significant biochemical effects on developing children, it is important to give an appropriate explanation to parents and children about the rationale for medication. Parents and children must have an opportunity to discuss their feelings and thoughts about psychotropic medication use in general and the specific drug that is ordered. Even with thought disorders, in which pharmacotherapy has a firmly established place, medication is rarely if ever the sole treatment indicated. The complexity of emotional conditions demands an integrated approach involving various therapies: psychodynamic (individual, family, or group), behavioral, milieu, medication, and the use of resources in the family, school, and community. These factors must be knowledgeably selected, judiciously coordinated, and skillfully applied to ensure maximal benefit for a child.

28.3   Psychotherapy

When it has been determined that psychopathology exists in a child or within a family and that it requires intervention, a pediatrician may develop and implement the therapeutic plan or may refer to a mental health consultant. The choice of treatment should be left to the consultant, with the referring physician reassuring the family and patient that close communication with the consultant will be maintained. The primary physician should continue to evaluate the child's progress throughout the treatment process and to provide medical care for the patient.

There are many types of *individual psychotherapy*. Most involve the development of an alliance with patients that provides an opportunity to look at the problems precipitating therapy. Younger children often express their concerns and developmental issues in *play therapy*, a specific modality designed to foster symbolic and metaphoric individual expression. Older children and adolescents are more likely to participate in talking during therapy. *Dynamic therapy* is designed to understand the psychologic motivations for a child's problems and to develop a therapeutic process based on that understanding. *Behavior therapy* and *cognitive-behavior therapy* are especially useful in treating anxiety, depression, and some behavioral problems.

There are several types of *family therapy:* directive, structural, strategic, and object-relations. In each, the therapist works primarily with the family to impart understanding or to help organize change. A particular directive approach, *parent management training*, is very useful in treating behavioral problems. This approach involves training parents to respond in specific and consistent ways to a child's behavior.

Group therapy is especially useful for children suffering from poorly developed social skills. Group therapy for preadolescents tends to emphasize structured activities through which therapist and children alike can discover how they relate to each other and find ways to change. It is an especially profitable approach for treating the social problems of adolescents.

Barriers to involving the generalist or pediatrician in psychotherapeutic activities with children include a presumed lack of time and lack of adequate conceptual background. Although psychotherapy primarily emphasizes listening and interviewing, two skills important to all fields of medicine, experience is an important and necessary asset for psychotherapists.

28.4   Psychiatric Hospitalization

Psychiatric hospitalization of a disturbed or emotionally ill child in a general, pediatric, or psychiatric hospital is at times helpful or necessary, and it may serve a number of functions. In children with many psychosomatic disorders or in a suicidal or drugged adolescent, indications for hospitalization may be med-

ical as well as psychiatric. If treatment of a child in a psychiatric hospital is thought necessary, consultation with a child psychiatrist is essential for decision-making and planning. The indications for admission include thought, behavior, and affect that are so irrational that they will not respond to less restrictive therapy; complex psychiatric problems that require skilled medical and nursing care; extremely disturbed family interactions that contribute to problematic behavior or interfere with needed care; and dangerous behavior that cannot otherwise be managed. Admission to residential treatment reflects the family's decompensation as often as the child's.

Dalton R, Forman MA: *Psychiatric Hospitalization of School-Age Children*. Washington, DC, American Psychiatric Press, 1992.

Findling R, McNamara N, Gracious B: Paediatric uses of atypical antipsychotics. *Expert Opinion on Pharmacotherapy* 2000;1:1935.

Gadow KD: Pediatric psychopharmacology: A review of recent research. *J Child Psychol Psychiatry* 1992;33:153.

James A, Javaloyes A: Practitioner review: The treatment of bipolar disorder in children and adolescents. *J Child Psychol Psychiatry* 2001;42:439.

Leonard H, March J, Rickler K, et al: Pharmacology of selective serotonin reuptake inhibitors in children and adolescents. *J Am Acad Child Adolesc Psychiatry* 1997;36:725.

Riddle M, Kastelic E, Frosch E: Pediatric psychopharmacology. *J Child Psychol Psychiatry* 2001;42:73.

Schowalter JE: Psychodynamics and medication. *J Am Acad Child Adolesc Psychiatry* 1989;28:681.

Special feature: Rating scales and assessment instruments for use in pediatric psychopharmacology research. *Psychopharmacol Bull* 1985;24:1.

Sporn A, Rapoport J: Childhood onset schizophrenia. *Child and Adolescent Psychopharmacology News* 2001;6:1.

Stallard P, Mastroyannopoulou K, Lewis M, et al: The siblings of children with life-threatening conditions. *Child Psychol Psychiatr Rev* 1997;2:26.

Werry JS, Wollersheim JP: Behavior therapy with children and adolescents: A twenty-year overview. *J Am Acad Child Adolesc Psychiatry* 1989;28:1.

Chapter 29
Neurodevelopmental Dysfunction in the School-Aged Child

29.1   Patterns of Development and Function*

Desmond P. Kelly

A neurodevelopmental function is a basic brain process that may be needed for learning and productivity. Neurodevelopmental variation refers to the differences in neurodevelopmental strengths and weaknesses that exist between individuals and that can change over time. Wide variations exist among individuals, and these differences need not represent pathology or abnormality. Neurodevelopmental dysfunctions reflect disruptions of neuroanatomic structure or psychophysiologic function and may be associated with academic underachievement, behavioral difficulties, and problems with social adjustment.

Etiology. Multiple factors and diverse causes underlie neurodevelopmental dysfunctions. These include genetic, medical, environmental, and sociocultural influences. Molecular genetic studies have identified some of the genes that contribute to

---

* This chapter is a revision of the chapter in the 16th Edition authored by Melvin Levine, MD.

these dysfunctions. It is well established that reading disorders can be both familial and heritable, and investigations have linked some reading disabilities to a specific gene locus on the short arm of chromosome 6. Chromosomal abnormalities can lead to unique patterns of dysfunction such as visual-spatial difficulties in girls with Turner syndrome or language deficits in individuals with fragile X syndrome. Perinatal risk factors that have been associated with subsequent academic problems include very preterm birth, severe intrauterine growth retardation, and prenatal exposure to alcohol. Environmental toxins including lead, infections such as meningitis and AIDS, and brain injury from intraventricular hemorrhage or head trauma increase the risk for disorders of learning and attention. There have been conflicting reports regarding the contribution of persistent otitis media with effusion and conductive hearing loss to subsequent language problems. Environmental and sociocultural deprivation can also lead to, or at least potentiate, neurodevelopmental dysfunction. In individual cases, a definite cause usually cannot be ascertained.

Pathogenesis. Advanced neuroimaging techniques are enabling confirmation of theories on the neurobiologic basis of learning problems. Functional magnetic resonance imaging has indicated decreased left temporoparietal cortical activity during a phonologic task of rhyming and decreased occipitoparietal extrastriate activity during an orthographic task of letter matching in children with reading disorder (dyslexia) compared to children with normal reading abilities. Studies of children with attention deficits have noted structural changes involving the frontal/striatal system and intra- and interhemispheric white matter projections. Quantitative electroencephalograms have been reported to be abnormal in 25–45% of children with learning disorders. However, the heterogeneity of study populations impedes generalization of these findings or clinical application for individual students.

Epidemiology. It could be postulated that all individuals harbor some form of neurodevelopmental dysfunction. A high percentage of children encounter difficulty in a particular academic area during their school careers, although in most cases this is transient. The number of children whose neurodevelopmental dysfunction significantly impedes their academic success is lower. Estimates of the prevalence of learning disorders range from 3–10%, whereas attention deficits have been reported in 4–12% of school-aged children. These estimates are beset by differences in the definitions and criteria used for classification and diagnosis and depend on the method of assessment. Medical classification systems include the *Diagnostic and Statistical Manual of Mental Disorders* of the American Psychiatric Association (DSM) and the *International Classification of Diseases* (ICD) of the World Health Organization. The DSM differentiates *learning disorders* (reading disorder, mathematics disorder, and disorder of written expression) from *motor skills disorder* and *communication disorders.* Neurologists favor diagnostic terms such as dyslexia (reading disorder), dyscalculia (mathematics), or dysgraphia (writing). Within the educational system *specific learning disabilities* are defined by discrepancies between scores on tests of intelligence and tests of academic achievement that are used to determine eligibility for special education services.

Clinical Manifestations. School-aged children with neurodevelopmental dysfunctions vary widely with regard to clinical symptoms. Their specific patterns of academic performance and behavior represent final common pathways, the convergence of many forces, including interacting cognitive strengths and deficits, environmental or cultural factors, temperament, educational experience, and intrinsic resiliency.

Eight areas of *neurodevelopmental function* (so-called neurodevelopmental constructs) are especially germane to understanding an academically delayed child.

ATTENTION. Attention subsumes a series of control mechanisms through which the brain regulates behavior and learning. Children with attentional dysfunction comprise a widely heterogeneous group who show various patterns of impairment of these controls (also see Chapter 29.2). The resulting symptoms may affect learning, behavior, or social interactions. Located in different parts of the brain, including the brain stem and frontal cortex, these controls are responsible for regulating the following:

1. *Mental energy* related to central nervous system (CNS) arousal, and the mobilization and distribution of mental effort: Children with diminished alertness and arousal are likely to exhibit signs of mental fatigue in a classroom. They often yawn, stretch, fidget, and daydream. They sometimes become overactive in an effort to attain a higher level of arousal. They may have difficulties falling asleep or awakening on time. They are apt to have difficulty allocating and sustaining their concentration, and their efforts at work may be erratic and unpredictable. Those affected by this form of weak control may manifest extreme *performance inconsistency.*

2. *Processing* and regulation of incoming stimuli: These children may have difficulty discriminating between important and unimportant information (also known as **selective attention**). Such weaknesses of saliency determination result in focusing on the wrong stimuli at home and in school. Weak saliency determination can make it difficult for a student to take notes, summarize information, or know what to study for a test. More overt forms of weak processing controls result in various types of distractibility, which may take the form of listening to extraneous noises instead of a teacher, staring out the window, or constantly thinking about the future. These children often show evidence of superficial concentration, not focusing with sufficient intensity to capture specific information. As a result, directions and explanations may have to be repeated or they may miss details such as changes in operational signs in mathematics. They may exhibit difficulties with cognitive activation, passively processing and not linking information with prior knowledge and experience, or over-relying on prior experience. Many of these children display insatiability and tend to be restless, to feel bored easily, and to require constant, high levels of stimulation or excitement.

3. *Production*, or the output of work, behavior, and social activity: Children with attention difficulties have a tendency to perform without previewing a likely outcome or thinking through what they are about to do. The consequent *impulsivity* can lead to careless mistakes in academic work and unintended misbehavior. They may show hyperactivity and have difficulty pacing, or doing tasks at the appropriate speed. Such children have difficulty with self-monitoring, not knowing how they are doing during and right after an academic endeavor or a behavior. As a result, they can get into trouble without realizing it. Finally, these children commonly are under-responsive to punishment and reward.

It is important to appreciate that most children with attentional dysfunction also harbor other forms of neurodevelopmental dysfunction. The latter can have a significant impact on the symptoms exhibited by a child. There is also considerable confusion and disagreement about the appropriate terminology to be applied to children with attentional difficulties. The *Diagnostic and Statistical Manual of Mental Disorders*, fourth edition, uses the term *Attention-Deficit/Hyperactivity Disorder* (ADHD) and makes a distinction between individuals who have trouble predominantly with inattention and those who exhibit substantial hyperactivity and impulsivity. It is likely that there are multiple subtypes of attention deficits.

MEMORY. As children proceed through school, demand for the efficient use of memory progressively increases. Students are expected to be selective, systematic, and strategic in entering new procedures and factual data in memory. They must become proficient in their use of both long- and short-term memory to file and retrieve rules, facts, concepts, and skills. By secondary school, rapid and precise recall is heavily emphasized. Not surprisingly, some students experience tremendous frustration when memory dysfunctions prevent them from satisfying academic demands.

Some children have difficulty with the initial registration of information in *short-term memory.* They have trouble quickly determining whether or not new information is relevant and transforming it to fit into short-term memory by condensing or shortening it. In some cases, children with attentional dysfunction have problems being selective and sufficiently alert to register salient information in memory. Others have difficulty registering newly introduced information at the level or depth needed to retain it. Registration weaknesses can be highly specific. Some students may have trouble with registering visual-spatial data in memory, whereas others may be deficient in the registration of language. Still others have a problem putting linear chunks or sequences of data in short-term memory.

Many children experience problems with *active working memory.* They are ineffective at temporarily suspending information in memory while they are working on it. Normally active working memory enables a student to keep in mind all of the different components of a task, such as a mathematics problem, while completing it. A student with an active working memory dysfunction, for example, might carry a number and then forget what it was that he or she intended to do after carrying that number. Active working memory during reading enables children to remember the beginning of a paragraph when they arrive at the end of it. It lets them remember what they intend to express in writing while they are attempting to remember where to place a comma or how to spell a particular word. It also enables the linkage between new incoming information that is held in short-term memory with prior knowledge or skills held in long-term memory.

Other youngsters experience frustration in their efforts at *consolidating* information in *long-term memory.* They are ineffective when filing data for later access. Ordinarily, consolidation in long-term memory is accomplished in one or more of four ways: (1) pairing two bits of information together (such as a group of letters and the English sound it represents), (2) storing procedures (consolidating new skills such as the steps in solving math problems), (3) classifying data in categories (e.g., filing all the insects together in memory), and (4) linking new information to established rules, patterns, or systems of organization (so-called rule-based learning).

Some children can register and consolidate facts and procedures in memory but seem to have inordinate difficulty *accessing or retrieving* these items when they need them. They may have difficulty remembering one half of a paired association such as matching a name with a face or a historical event with a date. They are prone to encounter difficulty with *simultaneous recall,* the frequent need to retrieve several facts or procedures at once. Finally, some students exhibit *delayed automatization.* Not enough of what they have learned in the past is accessible to them instantaneously and with no expenditure of effort. Such skills as letter formation, the mastery of mathematic facts, and word decoding must ultimately become automatic if students are to make good academic progress.

LANGUAGE. All of the basic academic skills are conveyed largely through language and it is not surprising that children with language dysfunctions usually have troubled educational careers.

Language disorder has many forms. Some children have particular problems with *phonology* (see Chapter 29.3). They experience unclear reception of English language sounds and are said to have difficulty with phonologic awareness. They may have trouble discriminating between and forming associations with the sounds of their native language. Language sounds are most often composed of more than one acoustic signal. For example, in English there are stop consonants, such as "puh" and "kuh." For the brain to process these language sounds, it must accommodate the very rapid transition (about 30 msec in duration) from the sound "k" to the "uh" in "kuh." In some cases, affected students may have trouble processing these acoustic signals within language sounds rapidly enough. Commonly, a weak phonologic sense has a negative effect on reading. A student with a poor appreciation of language sounds is likely to form unstable associative linkages between those sounds and visual symbols (i.e., letter combinations). It can be hard for them to conceptualize words as made up of language sound segments (phonemes); thus, their ability to break words down into their constituent sounds and then reblend them into pronounceable words is impeded. They may also have problems manipulating language sounds in their minds and blending them to form a word.

Semantic deficits are also common. Affected children have trouble learning the meaning of new words and using them appropriately. It is especially hard for them to develop a strong enough sense of how words relate to each other in their meanings. Other common language deficiencies include difficulty with *syntax* (word order), problems with *discourse* (paragraphs and passages), an underdeveloped sense of how language works (weak *metalinguistics*), and trouble with drawing appropriate inferences (i.e., supplying missing information) from language. Many adolescents fail to develop higher language functions. They have problems dealing with abstract and symbolic language, highly technical vocabulary, verbal concepts, densely packed verbal information in textbooks, foreign language learning, and figures of speech (including metaphors and similes).

It is common to distinguish between *receptive language dysfunctions* (those affecting understanding) and *expressive language dysfunctions* (those impeding production or communication). Children with primarily receptive language problems may have difficulty following instructions in the classroom, understanding verbal explanations, and interpreting what they have read. Expressive weaknesses include oromotor problems affecting articulation and verbal fluency. Some students experience difficulty with sound sequencing within words. Others find it hard to regulate the rhythm or prosody of their language. Their speech may be dysfluent, hesitant, and somehow inappropriate in its tone. Problems with *word retrieval* can also thwart expressive language fluency. Despite an adequate vocabulary, affected children have problems in finding exact words when they need them (as in a class discussion). They may reveal marked hesitation and keep substituting definitions for words (circumlocution). Still others with expressive impediments have trouble formulating sentences, using grammar acceptably, and organizing spoken (and possibly written) narrative. Some studies have linked expressive language dysfunction to delinquent behavior. This is especially true when an expressive language disorder occurs in a context of environmental deprivation or turmoil.

Students with strong language strengths may make use of their linguistic facility to overcome other learning problems. For example, it may be possible to verbalize one's way through a mathematics curriculum, thereby circumventing a tendency to be confused by predominantly nonverbal concepts (such as ratio, equation, and diameter).

SPATIAL ORDERING. Visual processing abilities entail the appreciation of spatial attributes. Awareness of shape and position, and perception of relative size, foreground and background relationships, and form constancy are among the constituents of spatial ordering. Children with spatial ordering weaknesses may encounter some initial problems with letter and word recognition. Spelling may emerge as a weakness because these children commonly experience trouble recalling the precise visual configurations of words. In general, however, children who are confused about spatial attributes are unlikely to have long-standing or serious academic problems unless their spatial weaknesses are complicated by additional academically relevant neurodevelopmental dysfunctions. At one time, it was thought that visual-spatial processing dysfunctions were a common cause of chronic reading disabilities; research, for the most part, has refuted this opinion.

Children with spatial ordering weaknesses may be late in discriminating between left and right. They may also show signs of gross motor clumsiness because they may be poor at making use of visual-spatial data to program motor responses, or they may have difficulty drawing and engaging in crafts activities.

TEMPORAL-SEQUENTIAL ORDERING. Awareness of time and sequence is an important neurodevelopmental function. Students in school need to be able to manage time, to process and produce multistep explanations and procedures, and to develop memory capacity for extended sequences. The latter includes preservation of serial order in motor procedures, in narrative, and in various mathematical algorithms.

Children who have difficulties with temporal-sequential ordering may be delayed in learning to tell time. They may have great difficulty in following multistep commands, performing acts that necessitate a sequence of steps in the proper order, mastering the months of the year, or organizing narrative. Affected children may also have trouble managing time. They may be frustrated in adhering to schedules, in learning the order of their classes in school, or in meeting deadlines.

NEUROMOTOR FUNCTION. There are three distinct yet related forms of neuromotor ability relating to function in school: fine motor dexterity, graphomotor fluency, and gross motor coordination.

Problems with *fine motor function* can affect a child's ability to excel in artistic and crafts activities. They may also interfere with learning a musical instrument or mastering a computer keyboard. *Eye-hand incoordination* may be prominent because the child has trouble with the rapid and precise integration of visual inputs with specific motor plans for hand movements. Others may encounter difficulty remembering fine motor procedures such as tying shoelaces or playing a musical instrument. The term *dyspraxia* in general relates to difficulty in developing an ideomotor plan and activating coordinated motor actions to complete a task or solve a motor problem such as assembling a model.

Graphomotor function refers to the specific motor aspects of written output. Several subtypes of graphomotor dysfunction significantly impede writing. Some students harbor *weaknesses of visualization* during writing. They have trouble picturing the configurations of letters and words as they write. Their written output tends to be poorly legible with inconsistent spacing between words. Others have weaknesses in *graphomotor memory*, the ability to recall letter and number forms rapidly and accurately. They labor over individual letters and much prefer printing (manuscript) to cursive writing. Some of them exhibit signs of *finger agnosia* or difficulty with *graphomotor feedback;* they have trouble localizing their fingers while they write. As a result, they need to keep their eyes very close to the page and tend to apply excessive pressure to the pencil. Others struggle with *graphomotor production* deficits. Such students have trouble producing the highly coordinated motor sequences needed for writing. Although they may understand and be able to visualize what it is they need to write, they have difficulty assigning writing roles to specific muscle groups in their hands. This phenomenon has also been described as *dyspraxic dysgraphia*. It is important to emphasize that a child may show excellent fine motor dexterity (as revealed in mechanical or artistic domains) but very poor graphomotor fluency (with labored or poorly legible writing).

Some children exhibit *gross motor dysfunction.* They may have problems in processing "outer spatial" information to guide gross motor actions; affected children are inept at catching or throwing a ball because they cannot form accurate judgments about trajectories in space. Still others demonstrate diminished *body position sense.* They do not efficiently receive or interpret proprioceptive and kinesthetic feedback from peripheral joints and muscles. They are likely to be impaired when activities demand balance and the ongoing tracking of body movement. Others are unable to satisfy the motor praxis demands of certain gross motor activities. It is hard for them to recall or plan complex motor procedures (such as those needed for dancing, gymnastics, and swimming). Children with gross motor problems may incur considerable embarrassment in physical education classes. Gross motor weaknesses can lead to social rejection, withdrawal, and generalized feelings of inadequacy.

HIGHER-ORDER COGNITION. This series of functions consists of various sophisticated thinking skills. Included are the formation of concepts, critical thinking, problem-solving skills, understanding and formulation of rules, brainstorming and creativity, and metacognition (i.e., the ability to think about thinking).

Children vary considerably in their capacities to understand the *conceptual bases of skills and content areas.* As students progress through their education, concepts become increasingly abstract and complex. New concepts are likely to contain previously encountered concepts. Some of these youngsters have a pervasive weak grasp of concepts, whereas others have difficulty only with concepts in highly specific domains (e.g., mathematics, social studies, or science). Some students prefer to conceptualize verbally, whereas others are more comfortable in forming concepts without the interposition of language (perhaps using visual imagery). Many of the best students try to solidify concepts both linguistically and nonverbally.

Problem-solving skills are an important part of mathematics and virtually every other subject in school. Children with good problem-solving skills are good strategists. They are excellent at previewing or estimating answers, coming up with several alternative techniques to meet challenges, selecting the best techniques, and monitoring what they are doing so that they can deploy alternative strategies as needed. Poor problem solvers, on the other hand, tend to be rigid or impulsive and fail to undertake challenges in a stepwise fashion. They may then encounter significant difficulties in course work that requires methodical strategy deployment and flexible problem solving.

Brainstorming skills are needed to develop a topic for a report, to think about the best way to undertake a project, and to deal with various other open-ended academic challenges. Some students cannot generate original ideas. They prefer to be told exactly what to do. They balk at having to devise a topic, deploy imagination, develop an argument, or think freely and independently.

Critical thinking skills represent another higher cognitive ability acquired during childhood. Successful students often display a keen ability to evaluate statements, products, and people using objective criteria. They are able to tease out their own personal biases and appreciate the viewpoints of others.

Metacognitive abilities are the capacity to think about thinking. Children with good metacognition are able to observe themselves thinking or studying. They can thereby develop an understanding of thought processes, enabling them to enhance their personal learning strategies and become more efficient and active learners. Those youngsters who lack metacognition tend to perform intellectual tasks the hard way. They are unlikely to appropriate effective techniques to study for a test, to write a report, or to meet other complex academic challenges.

SOCIAL COGNITION. A student's social abilities are stringently tested throughout the school day and in the neighborhood after school. Increasing evidence shows that social cognition exists as a discrete area of neurodevelopmental function. There are multiple subskills within social cognition. These include the ability to enter smoothly into new relationships, the capacity to time and stage interactions effectively, the appropriate degree of sensitivity to social feedback cues, the knowledge of how to resolve social conflict without aggression, the adaptive use of language in social contexts *(verbal pragmatics),* the ability to establish truly reciprocal (sharing) relationships with others (especially peers), and the inclination to overcome one's innate egocentricity to praise or nurture others. In addition to these skills, students need to be conscious of their own image development and to be adept at marketing themselves to peers and adults. Regrettably, some children have no idea of how adversely they are affecting others. Social skill deficits can exert an enduring negative effect on behavioral adjustment, mental health, and, ultimately, success in a career.

ACADEMIC EFFECTS. Neurodevelopmental dysfunctions are likely to occur in varying clusters within individual children. Combinations of dysfunctions commonly result in academic delays, frequently affecting the acquisition of basic skills and subskills in reading, spelling, writing, and mathematics.

Reading. (Also see Chapter 29.3.) Reading disabilities, also termed dyslexia, may stem from many neurodevelopmental factors. Most commonly, language dysfunctions are present in children with significant reading delays. Initially, such children are likely to reveal *poor phonologic awareness,* as observed in their difficulty appreciating and manipulating language sounds (see earlier). They may then have debilitating problems in forming associations in memory between English language sounds and combinations of letters. This gap results in deficiencies at the level of decoding individual words. Affected children may be slow to acquire a *sight vocabulary* (a repertoire of words they can identify instantly). When decoding skills are delayed or overly laborious, reading comprehension is subsequently seriously compromised. Students with visual-spatial dysfunctions may also have trouble learning to read, but this is a relatively rare cause of reading difficulty. Children with weaknesses of temporal-sequential ordering or active working memory may experience difficulty in breaking down words into their component sounds (phonemes) and reblending them into correct sequences. Memory difficulties can cause problems with reading recall and summarization skill, with associative memory for sounds and symbols, and with the acquisition of vocabulary. Some youngsters with higher-order cognitive deficiencies experience trouble in understanding what they read because they lack a strong grasp of the concepts in a text.

Children with reading difficulties commonly avoid reading. Thus, it is not unusual for a child whose reading is deficient to superimpose on this problem a lack of reading practice. Consequently, a delay in reading proficiency becomes increasingly pronounced over time.

Spelling. Impairments in spelling ability take various forms. Those with language disorders may have difficulty in applying a knowledge of phonology to spelling. They may overuse their visual (configurational) sense of words, and thus their attempts at spelling are phonetically poor approximations yet visually comparable to the actual word (e.g., faght for fight). Other youngsters seem to have the opposite problem, trouble with revisualization or the recall of word configurations. When their phonologic abilities are adequate, their spelling efforts are often phonetically correct but visually far afield (e.g., fite for fight). Some children lack a sense of the *morphology* of language, the sense that certain letter combinations impart certain meanings within words. They may be insensitive to suffixes, prefixes, and word roots. This can be reflected in their spelling patterns. For example, a child may spell the word *played* as *plade.*

Children with certain memory disorders can spell words adequately during a spelling bee or on a spelling list, but they misspell the same words when writing a paragraph. They appear to have a memory problem that leads to difficulty in sustaining several different operations simultaneously.

Some students commit *mixed spelling errors,* many of which are orthographically illegal (i.e., they deploy letter combinations never found in English). Such children have the worst prognoses with regard to spelling proficiency. Overall, the analysis of a child's spelling errors can provide valuable insights into the nature of his or her overall neurodevelopmental profile.

Writing. As children proceed through school, demands for large amounts of well-organized written output increase. Writing difficulties have been classified as Disorder of Written Expression or *dysgraphia.* In many cases, writing is laborious because of an underlying graphomotor dysfunction. In such instances, a child's graphomotor fluency does not keep pace with ideation and language production. Thoughts may also be forgotten or underdeveloped during writing because the mechanical effort is so taxing.

Just as students with simultaneous memory deficiencies experience difficulty with spelling in paragraphs, they are also prone to serious problems with writing in general. Their written output is often inconsistent in its legibility, ideation, and use of rules (of punctuation, capitalization, and grammar). Children with sequential ordering problems may have difficulty in organizing their ideas effectively when they write. Those with expressive language dysfunctions may not be able to use language effectively on paper. Students with active working memory dysfunctions have difficulty getting the ideas in a paragraph to cohere because they keep forgetting what they wish to express. Finally, students with attentional dysfunction may find it hard to mobilize and sustain the mental effort, the pacing, and the self-monitoring demands of writing. In fact, writing difficulties are the most frequently encountered academic problems among children with weak attention controls.

Mathematics. Delays in mathematical ability, Mathematics Disorder or Developmental Dyscalculia, can be especially refractory to correction. In one school-based study, it was found that no student who was delayed more than 6 mo in mathematics in 6th grade ever caught up, and a more recent study has shown persistence of severe arithmetic disorder in half of affected preteen children. Factors associated with persistence of difficulties included severity of the disorder and arithmetic problems in siblings of the probands. Thus, significant mathematical weaknesses can become virtually insurmountable, as the subject is so highly cumulative in its structure. Various forms of mathematical disability plague students.

Some children experience mathematics failure because of discrete higher-order cognitive weaknesses. They cannot grasp arithmetic concepts. Good mathematicians are able to deploy both verbal and nonverbal conceptual abilities to understand such concepts as fractions, percentages, equations, and proportion. It may also be hard for them to apply concepts effectively or be systematic in solving word problems or when confronted with practical situations.

Some youngsters show circumscribed memory weaknesses that compromise mathematical ability. Some have trouble in automatizing mathematical facts (such as the multiplication tables). Others have difficulty in recalling appropriate procedural sequences or *algorithms* (such as the steps involved in solving a long division problem). Still others have weak active working memory; thus, when they focus on one portion of a mathematical problem, they are likely to forget other components of the same problem.

Some students with language dysfunctions have difficulty in mathematics because they have trouble understanding their teachers' verbal explanations of quantitative concepts and operations. Such students are likely to experience frustration in solving word problems and in processing the vast network of technical vocabulary in this subject area. Many students with attention deficits falter in mathematics classes because they are poor at focusing on fine detail (such as operational signs). They may take an impulsive approach to mathematical problem solving and engage in little or no self-monitoring. Consequently, they commit frequent careless errors. Mathematics involves a degree of visualization. Children who have difficulty forming and recalling visual imagery to enhance learning may be at a disadvantage in acquiring mathematical skills. It may be hard, for example, for them to picture geometric shapes or to think about fractions.

It is not unusual for individuals with mathematical disabilities to develop superimposed mathematical phobias. Anxiety over mathematics can be especially disheartening and can aggravate an underlying skill delay.

Content Area Subjects. Children with neurodevelopmental dysfunctions may experience difficulty in a wide range of academic content areas. The sciences may be a special problem, especially because they necessitate the processing of dense verbal material in textbooks and the rapid convergent recall of facts. Social studies courses often entail use of sophisticated language and a mastery of verbal abstract concepts (e.g., democracy, liberalism, and taxation with representation). Students with higher cognitive weaknesses may not grasp such concepts.

Foreign language learning can be a serious problem for students with language disorders or memory gaps. In particular, those with even mild trouble with phonologic awareness, semantics, or syntax in their first language may have serious problems adding a second language. Some adolescents require foreign language waivers to graduate from high school and enter college. Younger children with learning problems often need to postpone foreign language learning until well into their high school years.

Some students harbor incapacitating *organizational problems* that adversely affect performance in content area subjects. They often lack effective learning strategies. Some are too impulsive to make use of techniques to facilitate studying and work output. Others struggle because they are unable to maintain a systematized notebook, keep track of assignments, get to places on time, meet deadlines, find things, organize a locker, and remember what books to take home from school. Many disorganized students also have trouble studying for tests. They do not seem to know how and what to study and for how long. They frequently lack self-testing skills.

NONACADEMIC IMPACTS. Neurodevelopmental dysfunctions commonly exert impacts that extend far beyond school. Some nonacademic impacts are closely related to the dysfunctions themselves, whereas other sequelae are secondary to persistent failure and frustration. The impulsivity and lack of effective self-monitoring of children with attention deficits may lead to unacceptable actions that were unintentional. In some cases, children with neurodevelopmental dysfunctions have excessive performance anxiety or clinical depression. Sadness, self-deprecatory comments, declining self-esteem, chronic fatigue, loss of interests, and even suicidal ideation may ensue. Some children lose motivation. They tend to give up and exhibit *learned helplessness*, a sense that they have no personal control over their destinies. Therefore, they feel no need to exert effort. This perspective ultimately can promote depression, pessimism, and a loss of ambition.

Diagnosis (Assessment). A child who is functioning poorly during the school years requires a careful multidisciplinary evaluation. An optimal evaluation team should consist of a pediatrician, a psychologist or psychiatrist, and a psychoeducational specialist (sometimes called an educational diagnostician). The latter is a clinician (usually a special educator or educational psychologist) who can undertake a detailed analysis of academic skills and subskills. Other professionals should become involved, as needed in individual cases, such as a speech and language pathologist, an occupational therapist, a neurologist, and a social worker.

Many children undergo evaluations in school. Such assessments are guaranteed in the United States under Public Law 101–476, the Individuals with Disabilities Education Act (IDEA). In addition, children found to have attentional dysfunc-

tion and other disorders may qualify for educational accommodations under Section 504 of the Rehabilitation Act of 1973.

Multidisciplinary evaluations conducted in schools are usually very helpful, but they are susceptible to biases and conflicts of interest. School budgeting constraints or lack of personnel may also affect the quality of evaluations and the extent of recommended services. Because of such limitations, demand for independent evaluations and for second opinions outside of the school setting is growing. Many pediatricians become involved in such outside assessments.

Pediatricians can be helpful in gathering and organizing data relating to a child with neurodevelopmental dysfunctions. They can obtain such data through the use of questionnaires completed by the parents, the school, and (if old enough) the child. These questionnaires can provide up-to-date information about behavioral adjustment, patterns of academic performance, and traits associated with specific developmental dysfunctions. In addition, questionnaires can elicit relevant data about a child's health history, family background, and demographic variables relevant to a child's learning difficulty. The ANSER System Questionnaires have been developed for this purpose. Standardized behavioral checklists also can aid in evaluation. Among these are the Child Behavior Checklist (CBCL) and the Behavior Assessment System for Children (BASC).

Evaluation of a child with suspected neurodevelopmental dysfunctions should include complete physical, neurologic, and sensory examinations to rule out underlying or associated conditions that could be exacerbating learning difficulties. It is rare that a specific cause is uncovered. A physician may also perform an extended neurologic and developmental assessment. Available pediatric neurodevelopmental examination instruments that facilitate direct sampling of various neurodevelopmental functions, such as attention, memory, and language, include the Pediatric Early Elementary Examination (PEEX II) and the Pediatric Examination of Educational Readiness at Middle Childhood (PEERAMID II). Examinations of this type also include direct behavioral observations and assessment of minor neurologic indicators (sometimes called *soft signs*). The latter include various associated movements and other phenomena frequently associated with neurodevelopmental dysfunction (see also Chapters 16, 17, and 584).

An evaluation commonly includes *intelligence testing* that provides an overall intelligence quotient (IQ). This testing can be useful in relating specific subtest scores to other diagnostic data. Such comparisons can uncover revealing patterns suggestive of specific neurodevelopmental dysfunctions.

Psychoeducational tests yield relevant data, especially when such assessments include careful analyses that pinpoint where breakdowns are occurring in the processes of reading, spelling, writing, and mathematics. A psychoeducational specialist, making use of input from multiple sources, can help a pediatrician formulate specific recommendations for regular and special educational teachers.

A mental health specialist can be valuable in identifying family-based issues or psychiatric disorders that may be complicating or aggravating neurodevelopmental dysfunctions.

Treatment. Treatment of children with neurodevelopmental dysfunctions often also needs to be multidisciplinary. Most children require several of the following forms of intervention.

DEMYSTIFICATION. Many children with neurodevelopmental dysfunctions have little or no understanding of the nature or sources of their difficulties. Once an appropriate descriptive assessment has been performed, it is especially important to explain to children the nature of the dysfunction while at the same time delineating their strengths. This explanation should be provided in nontechnical language, infusing a sense of optimism and communicating a desire to be helpful and supportive in the future.

BYPASS STRATEGIES (ACCOMMODATIONS). Numerous techniques can enable a child to circumvent neurodevelopmental dysfunctions. Such bypass strategies are ordinarily used in the regular classroom; individual forms of intervention in other settings are aimed at strengthening deficient functions. Examples of bypass strategies include using a calculator while solving mathematical problems, writing essays with a word processor, presenting oral instead of written reports, solving fewer mathematical problems, seating a child with attention deficits closer to the teacher to minimize distraction, offering visually presented demonstration models of correctly solved mathematical problems, and granting permission for a student to take scholastic aptitude tests untimed. These bypass strategies do not cure neurodevelopmental dysfunctions but minimize their academic and nonacademic effects.

INTERVENTIONS (REMEDIATION OF SKILLS). Interventions can be used at home and in school to strengthen the weak links in the learning process. Reading specialists, mathematical tutors, and other such professionals can make use of diagnostic data to select techniques that make use of a student's neurodevelopmental strengths in an effort to improve decoding skills, writing ability, or mathematical computation. Remediation need not focus exclusively on specific academic areas. Many students need assistance in acquiring study skills, cognitive strategies, and productive organizational habits.

Remediation may take place in a resource room or learning center at school. To qualify for these services in school, students may need to be labeled or classified as *learning disabled*. To be so designated, testing must document a substantial discrepancy between the child's IQ and his or her academic skill. Unfortunately, some needy students with significant neurodevelopmental dysfunctions do not display such a discrepancy. Fortunately, increasing numbers of schools and regulatory agencies are giving up these arbitrary criteria and providing help to all children who demonstrate an academic delay.

Interventions that can be implemented at home could include drills to aid the automatization of subskills such as arithmetic facts or letter formations.

DEVELOPMENTAL THERAPIES. Considerable controversy exists about the efficacy of treatments to enhance weak developmental functions. It has not been convincingly demonstrated that it is possible to improve substantially a child's fine motor skills, memory, problem-solving proficiency, or temporal-sequential ordering abilities. Nevertheless, some forms of developmental therapy are widely accepted. *Speech and language pathologists* commonly offer intervention for youngsters with various forms of language disability. *Occupational therapists* strive to improve the motor skills of certain students with writing problems or gross motor clumsiness.

CURRICULUM MODIFICATIONS. Many children with neurodevelopmental dysfunctions require alterations in the school curriculum to succeed. This is particularly true as students progress through secondary school. For example, students with memory weaknesses may need to have their courses selected for them so that they do not have an inordinate cumulative memory load in any one semester. The timing of a foreign language, the selection of a mathematical curriculum, and the choice of science courses are critical issues for many of these struggling adolescents.

STRENGTHENING OF STRENGTHS. Affected children need to have their affinities, potentials, and talents identified clearly and exploited widely. It is as important to strengthen strengths as it is to attempt to remedy deficiencies. Athletic skills, artistic inclinations, creative talents, and mechanical aptitudes are among the potential assets of certain students who are underachieving academically. Parents and school personnel need to create opportunities for such students to build on these assets and to achieve respect and praise for their efforts. These well-developed personal assets can ultimately have implications for transitions into young adulthood, including career or college selection.

INDIVIDUAL AND FAMILY COUNSELING. When learning difficulties are complicated by family problems or identifiable psychiatric disorders, psychotherapy may be indicated. Clinical psychologists or child psychiatrists may offer long- or short-term therapy. Such intervention may involve the child alone or the entire family. It is essential, however, that the therapist have a firm understanding of the nature of a child's neurodevelopmental dysfunctions.

CONTROVERSIAL THERAPIES. A variety of treatment methods for neurodevelopmental dysfunctions have been proposed that have no known scientific proof of efficacy. This list includes dietary interventions (vitamins, fatty acids, or elimination of food additives or potential allergens), neuromotor programs or medications to address vestibular dysfunction, eye exercises, filters, tinted lenses, biofeedback, and other technologic devices. Parents should be cautioned against expending the excessive amounts of time and financial resources usually demanded by these remedies. In many cases it is difficult to distinguish the nonspecific beneficial impacts of increased support and attention paid to the child from the supposed target effects of the intervention.

MEDICATION. Certain psychopharmacologic agents may be especially helpful in lessening the toll of neurodevelopmental dysfunctions (see Chapters 28 and 29.2). Most commonly, stimulant medications are used in the treatment of children with attention deficits. They are never a panacea because most youngsters with attention deficits have other associated dysfunctions (such as language disorders, memory problems, motor weaknesses, or social skill deficits). Nevertheless, medications such as methylphenidate (Ritalin or Concerta and Metadate sustained action formulations) and dextroamphetamine (Dexedrine or Adderall) can be important adjuncts to treatment because they seem to help some youngsters focus more selectively and control their impulsivity. Stimulant medication, its indications, administration, and complications are described in Chapter 29.2. When depression or excessive anxiety is a significant component of the clinical picture, antidepressants or antianxiety drugs may be helpful (Chapters 22 and 23). Other drugs may improve behavioral control (Chapter 28). Children receiving medication need regular follow-up visits that include a history to check for side effects, a review of current behavioral checklists, a complete physical examination, and appropriate modifications of medication dose. Periodic trials off medication are recommended, to establish whether the medication is still necessary.

THE ROLE OF THE PEDIATRICIAN

Pediatricians should play a central role in assisting children with neurodevelopmental dysfunctions. Their longitudinal contact with the child and family enables them to critically assess medical, family, and developmental history to identify children at risk. They are well positioned to assess whether early perturbations in developmental progression represent normal variations or warning signs of future learning problems. Regular contact over the course of the school years provides the opportunity to identify and participate in the assessment of learning difficulties, coordinate management, and function as a counselor and advocate.

Key elements are necessary in order for the pediatrician to effectively fill these roles. The pediatrician needs to maintain an accurate base of knowledge regarding the clinical manifestations of neurodevelopmental dysfunction, methods of diagnosis and management, the resources available within the school system as well as other clinicians in the region, and the public laws that entitle eligible students to modifications, accommodations, and interventions. A system of screening and surveillance should be incorporated into routine office visits to promote early identification of learning difficulties. This could include standard screening questionnaires or direct questioning of parents regarding any possible concerns about their child's school performance. If problems emerge, the pediatrician should rule out medical causes and can participate in the assessment process as described earlier. He or she can advise and assist parents in obtaining necessary evaluations through the school or by referral to independent clinicians. Assistance should be provided in the interpretation of the findings, ensuring appropriate demystification of the child and coordinating care if other medical specialists are involved. Pediatricians can also play a critical role in those children who might require medication as a component of a management plan.

Drawing on their relationship with the child and parents, pediatricians can provide helpful advice and counseling in dealing with the stresses associated with learning challenges such as confrontations related to homework, and ensuring students are afforded regular opportunities to pursue their affinities. Children with neurodevelopmental dysfunctions require informed advocacy. They need to have their rights upheld in school and in the community. Pediatricians can be especially helpful in advocating for children in school. Some children, for example, are devastated by being held back in a grade, and the likelihood of benefit may be minimal. A physician may need to represent the rights of the child in opposing such grade retention and other sources of public humiliation. A physician may also need to argue strongly for a child to receive services in school or to benefit from modifications in the curriculum. Pediatricians can also perform advocacy by becoming vocal citizens of their communities. In serving on a school board, for example, a physician can exert a major influence on local policy and on the allocation of resources to school children with special educational needs.

Longitudinal Case Management. All children with neurodevelopmental dysfunctions can benefit from the support and guidance of a case manager or mentor, a professional who can offer advice in a continuing manner and be available to monitor function through the years. Pediatricians may be the ideal professionals to assume this responsibility. With time, new questions inevitably emerge as a child's neurodevelopmental dysfunctions evolve and academic expectations undergo progressive changes. Because children with neurodevelopmental dysfunctions represent an extremely heterogeneous group, no two children require the same management plan, nor is it possible to predict with certainty at age 7 the needs of a youngster when he or she is 14 yr old. Consequently, affected children and their families require vigilant follow-up and individualized objective advice throughout their academic careers.

American Academy of Pediatrics, Committee on Children with Disabilities: The pediatrician's role in development and implementation of an Individual Education Plan (IEP) and/or an Individual Family Service Plan (IFSP). *Pediatrics* 1999;104:124–127.

American Academy of Pediatrics, Committee on Quality Improvement and Subcommittee on Attention-Deficit/Hyperactivity Disorder: Diagnosis and evaluation of the child with Attention-Deficit/Hyperactivity Disorder. *Pediatrics* 2000;105:1158–1170.

Chabot RJ, di Michele F, Prichep L, et al: The clinical role of computerized EEG in the evaluation and treatment of learning and attention disorders in children and adolescents. *J Neuropsychiatry Clin Neuropsychiatry Clin Neurosci* 2001;13:171–186.

Levine MD: *The Pediatric Assessment System for Learning Disorders-Revised* (Questionnaires and Neurodevelopmental Examinations). Cambridge, MA, Educators Publishing Service, 1996.

Levine MD: *Developmental Variation and Learning Disorders*, 2nd ed. Cambridge, MA, Educators Publishing Service, 1999.

Shalev RS, Gross-Tur V: Developmental dyscalculia. *Pediatr Neurol* 2001;24:337–342.

Temple E, Poldrack R, Salidis J, et al: Disrupted neural responses to phonological and orthographic processing in dyslexic children: An fMRI study. *NeuroReport* 2001;12:299–307.

Whitmore K, Hart H, Willems G (eds): *A Neurodevelopmental Approach to Specific Learning Disorders.* Cambridge, UK, MacKeith Press, 1999.

29.2 Attention-Deficit/Hyperactivity Disorder

Mark D. Simms

Attention-deficit/hyperactivity disorder (ADHD) is the most common neurobehavioral disorder of childhood, one of the most prevalent chronic health conditions affecting school-aged children, and the most extensively studied mental disorder of childhood. According to the fourth edition of the American Psychiatric Association's *Diagnostic and Statistical Manual* (DSM-IV), ADHD is characterized by inattention, including increased distractibility and difficulty sustaining attention; poor impulse control and decreased self-inhibitory capacity; and motor overactivity and motor restlessness (Table 29–1). These symptoms are pervasive and interfere with the individual's ability to function under normal circumstances. DSM-IV identifies three types of ADHD: predominantly hyperactive-impulsive symptoms, predominantly inattentive symptoms, and combined type. Affected children commonly experience problems with academic underachievement, interpersonal relationships with family members and peers, and low self-esteem. ADHD frequently co-occurs with other emotional, behavioral, language and learning disorders (Chapter 29.1). Fortunately, a variety of safe and effective psychosocial, behavioral, and pharmacologic therapies are available to treat the disorder's major symptoms.

Etiology. ADHD is a heterogeneous condition for which no single cause has been identified. However, evidence suggests that genetic and environmental factors play a significant role during fetal and postnatal development in the emergence of ADHD during early childhood. Both morphologic and functional brain differences have been identified, including a moderate reduction in the size of the corpus callosum, basal ganglia, and frontal lobes, and hypoperfusion of the frontal-striatal dopamine pathways. Furthermore, ADHD commonly occurs following damage to the CNS (e.g., prematurity or traumatic brain injury), toxic exposure (e.g., fetal alcohol syndrome or lead poisoning), maldevelopment (e.g., mental retardation syndromes), and sequelae of infectious processes affecting the CNS. ADHD also occurs in otherwise physically healthy children. Twin and family studies suggest a strong genetic component to ADHD, and molecular genetic studies have identified abnormalities in the dopamine transporter gene, the D4 receptor gene, and human thyroid receptor beta gene.

Epidemiology. Although the DSM-IV estimates the prevalence to be between 3% and 5% among school-aged children, community samples of school-aged children suggest a prevalence rate ranging from 4% to 12%. The condition is approximately 3 to 4 times more common in males (9.2%) than females (2.9%); however, the inattentive subtype is the most common in females. Environmental factors, such as psychosocial stressors, parenting difficulties, and classroom factors may exacerbate ADHD but do not cause the syndrome. Contrary to common opinion, epidemiologic studies suggest that ADHD is underdiagnosed in the population at large, and children with the disorder are often undertreated with medications.

Clinical Manifestations. DSM-IV criteria were developed in field trials conducted mainly with children 5 to 12 yr of age. These criteria emphasize several factors. Behaviors must be statistically abnormal for the child's age and developmental level, must begin before the age of 7 yr, and must be present for at least 6 mo. Symptoms must also be pervasive in nature (present in at least two or more settings) and impair the child's ability to function normally. Finally, symptoms must not be secondary to another disorder.

TABLE 29–1. DSM-IV Diagnostic Criteria for ADHD

A. Either 1 or 2
    1. Six (or more) of the following symptoms of inattention have persisted for at least 6 mo to a degree that is maladaptive and inconsistent with development level:
      Inattention
      a. Often fails to give close attention to details or makes careless mistakes in school work, work, or other activities
      b. Often has difficulty sustaining attention in tasks or play activities
      c. Often does not seem to listen when spoken to directly
      d. Often does not follow through on instructions and fails to finish schoolwork, chores, or duties in the workplace (not due to oppositional behavior or failure to understand instructions)
      e. Often has difficulty organizing tasks and activities
      f. Often avoids, dislikes, or is reluctant to engage in tasks that require sustained mental effort (such as schoolwork or homework)
      g. Often loses things necessary for tasks or activities (e.g., toys, school assignments, pencils, books, or tools)
      h. Is often easily distracted by extraneous stimuli
      i. Is often forgetful in daily activities

    2. Six (or more) of the following symptoms of hyperactivity-impulsivity have persisted for at least 6 mo to a degree that is maladaptive and inconsistent with developmental level:
      Hyperactivity
      a. Often fidgets with hands or feet or squirms in seat
      b. Often leaves seat in classroom or in other situations in which remaining seated is expected
      c. Often runs about or climbs excessively in situations in which it is inappropriate (in adolescents or adults, may be limited to subjective feelings of restlessness)
      d. Often has difficulty playing or engaging in leisure activities quietly
      e. Is often "on the go" or often acts as if "driven by a motor"
      f. Often talks excessively
      Impulsivity
      g. Often blurts out answers before questions have been completed
      h. Often has difficulty awaiting turn
      i. Often interrupts or intrudes on others (e.g., butts into conversations or games)
B. Some hyperactive-impulsive or inattentive symptoms that caused impairment were present before 7 yr of age.
C. Some impairment from the symptoms is present in 2 or more settings (e.g., at school [or work] or at home).
D. There must be clear evidence of clinically significant impairment in social, academic, or occupational functioning.
E. The symptoms do not occur exclusively during the course of a pervasive developmental disorder, schizophrenia, or other psychotic disorder and are not better accounted for by another mental disorder (e.g., mood disorder, anxiety disorder, dissociative disorder, or personality disorder).

Code based on type:
314.01 Attention-Deficit/Hyperactivity Disorder, Combined Type: if both Criteria A1 and A2 are met for the past 6 months.
314.00 Attention-Deficit/Hyperactivity Disorder, Predominantly Inattentive type: if Criterion A1 is met but Criterion A2 is not met for the past 6 months.
314.01 Attention-Deficit/Hyperactivity Disorder, Predominantly Hyperactive-Impulsive Type: if Criterion A2 is met but Criterion A1 is not met for the past 6 months.

Reprinted with permission from the Diagnostic and Statistical Manual of Mental Disorders, Fourth Edition, Text Revision. Washington, DC, American Psychiatric Association, 2000. Copyright 2000 American Psychiatric Association.

With increasing age, clinical manifestations may change from predominantly motor restlessness, aggressive, and disruptive behavior in preschool children to disorganized, distractible, and inattentive symptoms in older adolescents and adults. In particular, ADHD is more difficult to diagnose in preschool children, who normally tend to be active and restless. The disorder is also difficult to identify in children with cognitive disabilities, who often act in an immature fashion and whose intentions may be difficult to judge.

Diagnosis. Diagnoses of ADHD are made primarily on clinical grounds after a thorough evaluation whose components include behavior rating scales, the clinical interview, physical examination, and neuropsychologic evaluation.

    BEHAVIOR RATING SCALES. Several standardized behavior rating scales are widely available and perform well in discriminating between children with ADHD and controls (e.g., Conner's Rating Scale; ADHD Index; Swanson, Nolan, and Pelham Checklist [SNAP]; ADD-H: Comprehensive Teacher Rating Scale [AcTERS]). Other broad-band checklists, such as the Achenbach Child Behavior Checklist (CBCL) are useful in screening for co-occurring problems in areas other than ADHD (e.g., anxiety, depression, conduct problems, etc.). It is important to gather information from a variety of sources—typically parents, teachers, and, when appropriate, other caretakers—to determine pervasiveness of the symptoms. These scales are useful in establishing the magnitude and pervasiveness of the symptoms but are not sufficient alone to make a diagnosis of ADHD.

    CLINICAL INTERVIEW. A major goal of the clinical interview is exploration of whether symptoms might be the result of other conditions that mimic ADHD. Review of the child's health, development, and social and family history should emphasize factors that might affect the development or integrity of the CNS, or reveal the presence of chronic illness, sensory impairments, or medication use that might affect the child's functioning. Disruptive social factors, such as family discord, situational stresses, abuse, or neglect may result in hyperactive or anxious behaviors. Finally, a family history of first-degree relatives with ADHD, mood or anxiety disorders, learning disability, antisocial disorder, or alcohol or substance abuse may indicate increased risk for ADHD and/or co-morbid conditions.

    PHYSICAL EXAMINATION. No medical screening or laboratory tests are specific to ADHD. However, careful examination may reveal the presence of chronic illnesses, sensory impairments, or genetic/birth defect syndromes that may contribute to behavioral and learning difficulties. The presence of hypertension, motor tics, ataxia, or thyroid disorder may be contraindications for use of stimulant medications to treat ADHD symptoms and should prompt further diagnostic evaluations. Fine motor coordination delays and other "soft signs" are common but are not sufficiently specific to contribute to a diagnosis of ADHD. It is important to note that behavior in a highly structured or novel setting may not reflect typical behavior at home or school. Reliance on observed behavior in a physician's office may result in incorrect diagnosis.

    NEUROPSYCHOLOGIC EXAMINATION. Standardized tests of general intelligence and educational achievement may indicate the presence of mental retardation or specific learning disabilities. Incompatibility between classroom expectations and the child's ability may result in inattentive or inappropriate behaviors. Tests of sustained attention—continuous performance tests—can help corroborate a diagnosis of ADHD but are not adequate by themselves to confirm or deny the diagnosis.

Differential Diagnosis. Chronic illnesses affect up to 20% of children in the United States and may impair children's attention and school performance (e.g., migraine headaches, absence seizures, asthma and allergies, hematologic disorders, juvenile diabetes, childhood cancer, etc.), either because of the disease itself or medications used to treat or control the underlying illness (e.g., medications for asthma, steroids, anticonvulsants, antihistamines). In older children and adolescents, substance abuse may result in declining school performance and inattentive behavior.

Sleep disorders, including those secondary to chronic upper airway obstruction from enlarged tonsils and adenoids, frequently result in behavioral and emotional symptoms. Conversely, behavioral and emotional disorders may cause disrupted sleep patterns.

Depression and anxiety disorders may present many of the same symptoms as ADHD (e.g., inattention, restlessness, inability to focus and concentrate on work, poor organization, forgetfulness) and may be present as co-morbid conditions. Obsessive-compulsive disorder may mimic ADHD, particularly when recurrent and persistent thoughts, impulses, or images are intrusive and interfere with normal daily activities.

Adjustment disorders secondary to major life stresses (e.g., death of a close family member, parental divorce, family violence, parental substance abuse, a move, etc.) or parent-child relationship disorders involving conflicts over discipline, overt child abuse and/or neglect, or overprotection, may result in symptoms similar to ADHD.

Finally, although ADHD is thought to be due to primary impairment of attention, impulse control, and motor activity, other disorders are frequently present as co-morbid conditions: oppositional defiant disorder or conduct disorder (35%), depression and mood disorders (18%), anxiety disorder (25%), and learning disorders (10–25%).

Treatment. Psychosocial interventions, behavior management training, and medication are effective in treating the various components of ADHD. The National Institute of Mental Health Collaborative Multisite Multimodal Treatment Study of Children with Attention-Deficit/Hyperactivity Disorder (MTA study) demonstrated the effectiveness of stimulant medication in treating core symptoms of ADHD, whereas psychosocial interventions and behavior management training were effective in treating many co-morbid disorders frequently seen in children with ADHD.

PSYCHOSOCIAL INTERVENTIONS. Once the diagnosis has been established, parent(s) and child should be educated about the ways in which ADHD can affect learning, behavior, self-esteem, social skills, and family function. Goals should be set to improve the child's relationships with parents, siblings, teachers, and peers; decrease disruptive behaviors; increase independence in completing homework; and improve self-esteem. Behavior therapy should include a broad plan for modifying the physical and social environment, as well as the child's behaviors. For example, school and home settings may be adjusted to accommodate the child's learning style and decrease distractions.

BEHAVIOR MANAGEMENT TRAINING. Training may consist of 8–12 weekly individual or group sessions. Parents learn principles of behavior management with emphasis on consistency, while children work on improving peer relationships and self-esteem. Specific "target" behaviors are identified that impair the child's daily life functions (e.g., violating home or school rules, disruptive behavior, not completing homework assignments, etc.). Next, parents and teachers must implement specific techniques of providing rewards to the child for demonstrating the desired behavior (positive reinforcement) or consequences for failure to meet the goals (negative reinforcement). Family and individual psychotherapy may be necessary in complex situations or to address overt mental health conditions such as depression, anxiety, social withdrawal, school phobia, etc. Psychologists, school personnel, community mental health therapists, or primary care clinicians can provide behavior therapy; however, many clinicians prefer to refer families to community providers because behavior therapy is time-consuming and often requires specific training and skills. National organizations, such as CHADD (Children with Attention Deficit Disorders) and ADDA (Attention Deficit Disorders Association) may also provide valuable support to families and children.

MEDICATION. Stimulants are the most effective psychotropic agents in treating ADHD, but several other types of medications should be considered in management of complex cases. Stimulants have been used for over 60 yr and have an excellent safety record. Research shows that stimulant medications are effective in ameliorating core symptoms of inattention, impulsivity, and hyperactivity. In addition, improvements are seen in noncompliant behaviors, impulsive aggression, social interactions with peers and family members, and academic productivity and accuracy. In contrast, stimulants are not likely to improve reading skills, academic achievement, or antisocial behaviors.

The two main classes of stimulants are methylphenidate and its derivatives (Ritalin, Concerta, Metadate CD, and Methylin) and amphetamine and its derivatives (Dexedrine and Adderall). Both classes are available in short, intermediate, and long-acting forms. All stimulant forms are equally effective, but individual children may respond differently to one or another medication and clinicians may choose one over another to tailor the pharmacologic effect to meet the child's lifestyle needs. When the stimulants are used sequentially, approximately 80% of children will respond favorably to one of them with satisfactory relief of major symptoms of ADHD.

Stimulants have few contraindications and adverse effects are usually predictable and generally mild. Common short-term side effects include loss of appetite, initial weight loss, abdominal discomfort, dysphoria, and difficulty sleeping. A slight increase in heart rate may also be seen. Less often, tics may become evident in children who start stimulant medications. These adverse symptoms usually remit when the dosage is lowered, or when an alternative stimulant preparation or another class of medication is used. Other agents, such as tricyclic antidepressants (imipramine and desipramine) and buproprion (Wellbutrin) are considered second-line agents that have been shown to be effective in treating ADHD, particularly in the presence of co-morbid depression. Alpha-2 adrenergic blocker agents, such as clonidine (Catapres) and guanfacine (Tenex), are also effective and often used alone or in combination with stimulants. See Table 29–2 for doses of stimulants and antidepressants.

Contrary to popular misconceptions, long-term use of stimulants, as recommended, does not result in addiction (i.e., there is no development of tolerance, craving, or withdrawal) and is unlikely to lead individuals with ADHD to abuse drugs. Evidence suggests that adolescents and young adults who take prescribed stimulants for ADHD have a much lower incidence of illicit substance and alcohol abuse than those who do not receive appropriate treatment. Similarly, stimulants do not result in aggressive or assaultive behavior, do not increase the risk of seizures, are not a cause of Tourette syndrome, and do not exacerbate anxiety disorders.

Prognosis. In at least 80% of affected children, symptoms of ADHD persist into adolescence and adulthood. With increasing

TABLE 29–2. Medications Used in the Treatment of Attention-Deficit/Hyperactivity Disorder

Generic Class (Brand Name)	Daily Dosage Schedule	Duration	Prescribing Schedule
Stimulants (First-Line Treatment)			
Methylphenidate			
Short-acting (Ritalin, Methylin)	Twice a day (bid) to 3 times a day (tid)	3–5 hr	5–20 mg bid to tid
Intermediate-acting (Ritalin SR, Metadate ER, Methylin ER)	Once a day (qd) to bid	3–8 hr	20–40 mg qd or 40 mg in the morning and 20 early afternoon
Long-acting (Concerta, Metadate CD, Ritalin LA*)	qd	8–12 hr	18–72 mg qd
Amphetamine			
Short-acting (Dexedrine, Dextrostat)	bid to tid	4–6 hr	5–15 mg bid or 5–10 mg tid
Intermediate-acting (Adderall, Dexedrine spansule)	qd to bid	6–8 hr	5–30 mg qd or 5–15 mg bid
Long-acting (Adderall-XR)	qd		10–30 mg qd
Antidepressants (Second-Line Treatment)			
Tricyclics (TCAs)	bid to tid		2–5 mg/kg/day[†]
Imipramine, Desipramine			
Bupropion			
(Wellbutrin)	qd to tid		50–100 mg tid
(Wellbutrin SR)	bid		100–150 mg bid

*Not FDA approved at time of publication.
[†]Prescribing and monitoring information in Physicians' Desk Reference.

age, hyperactivity tends to decrease while inattention, impulsivity, disorganization, and relationship difficulties often persist and become more prominent. If not properly identified and treated, affected individuals across the age span are at risk for a wide range of unfavorable health and psychosocial outcomes, including accidental injuries, educational under-achievement, employment difficulties, risky sexual behavior, and criminal activity. However, evidence suggests that with a combination of medication and psychosocial and behavioral interventions, most children's symptoms are significantly ameliorated.

American Academy of Child and Adolescent Psychiatry: Summary of the practice parameter for the use of stimulant medication in the treatment of children, adolescents, and adults. *J Am Acad Child Adolesc Psychiatry* 2001;40:1352–5.

American Academy of Pediatrics, Committee on Quality Improvement, Subcommittee on Attention-Deficit/Hyperactivity Disorder: Clinical practice guideline: Diagnosis and evaluation of the child with attention-deficit/hyperactivity disorder. *Pediatrics* 2000;105:1158–70.

American Academy of Pediatrics, Committee on Quality Improvement, Subcommittee on Attention-Deficit/Hyperactivity Disorder: Clinical practice guideline: Treatment of the school-aged child with Attention-Deficit/Hyperactivity Disorder. *Pediatrics* 2001;108:1033–44.

Barkley RA, Murphy KR, Kwasnik D: Motor vehicle driving competencies and risks in teens and young adults with attention deficit hyperactivity disorder. *Pediatrics* 1996;98:1089–95.

Biederman J, Wilens T, Mick E, et al: Pharmacotherapy of attention-deficit/hyperactivity disorder reduces risk for substance use disorder. *Pediatrics* 1999;104:e20.

Jensen PS, Kettle, L, Roper M, et al: Are stimulants overprescribed? Treatment of ADHD in four U.S. communities. *J Am Acad Child Adolesc Psychiatry* 1999;38:797–804.

Liebson CL, Katusic SK, Barbaresi WJ, et al: Use and costs of medical care for children and adolescents with and without attention-deficit/hyperactivity disorder. *JAMA* 2001;285;60–6.

MTA Cooperative Group: A 14-month randomized clinical trial of treatment strategies for attention-deficit/hyperactivity disorder. *Arch Gen Psychiatry* 1999; 56:1073–86.

Pliszka SR, Greenhill LL, Crismon ML, et al: The Texas Children's Medication Algorithm Project: Report of the Texas consensus conference panel on medication treatment of childhood attention-deficit/hyperactivity disorder. Part I. *J Am Acad Child Adolesc Psychiatry* 2000;39:908–19.

Pliszka SR, Greenhill LL, Crismon ML, et al: The Texas Children's Medication Algorithm Project: Report of the Texas consensus conference panel on medication treatment of childhood attention-deficit/hyperactivity disorder. Part II: Tactics. *J Am Acad Child Adolesc Psychiatry* 2000;39:920–7.

Wolraich ML, Greenhill LL, Pelham W, et al: Randomized, controlled trial of OROS Methylphenidate once a day in children with Attention-Deficit/Hyperactivity Disorder. *Pediatrics* 2001;108:883–92.

29.3 Specific Reading Disability (Dyslexia)

G. Reid Lyon, Sally E. Shaywitz, and Bennett A. Shaywitz

Dyslexia is characterized by an unexpected difficulty in reading in children and adults who otherwise possess the intelligence, motivation, and opportunities to learn considered necessary for accurate and fluent reading. Dyslexia is the most common and most comprehensively studied of the learning disabilities (LD), affecting at least 80% of children identified as manifesting LD. When asked to read aloud, most children and adults with dyslexia display a labored approach to decoding and recognizing single words, an approach characterized by hesitations, mispronunciations, and repeated attempts to sound out unfamiliar words. In contrast to the difficulties they experience in decoding single words, individuals with dyslexia have the vocabulary, syntax, and other higher level abilities involved in comprehension.

Etiology. At a cognitive-linguistic level, dyslexia reflects deficits within a specific component of the language system, the phonologic module, which is engaged in processing the sounds of speech. As predicted by this model, dyslexic individuals have difficulty developing an awareness that words, both spoken and written, can be segmented into smaller elemental units of sound—an essential ability given that reading an alphabetic language (i.e., English) requires that the reader map or link printed symbols to sound. Abundant evidence shows that the linguistic abilities related to learning to read involve phonology, with deficits in phonologic awareness best predicting dyslexia. Theories of dyslexia that implicate the visual system or deficits in the temporal processing of auditory and visual stimuli have not been sufficiently substantiated by research.

Dyslexia is both familial and heritable. Family history is one of the most important risk factors; about half of children who have a parent with dyslexia as well as half of the siblings of dyslexics and half of the parents of dyslexics may have the disorder. Linkage studies implicate loci on chromosomes 1, 2, 6, and 15 for the transmission of phonologic awareness deficits and subsequent reading problems. The specific mechanisms by which genetic factors predispose someone to dyslexia are not clear.

A range of neurobiologic investigations using postmortem brain specimens, brain morphometry, and diffusion tensor magnetic resonance imaging suggests that there are differences in the left temporo-parieto-occipital brain regions between dyslexic and nonimpaired readers. Converging evidence using functional brain imaging in both children with dyslexia and adult dyslexic readers shows a failure of left hemisphere posterior brain systems to function properly during reading with increased activation in frontal regions. These data suggest that rather than the smoothly functioning and integrated reading systems observed in nonimpaired children, disruption of the posterior reading systems results in dyslexic children attempting to compensate by shifting to other, ancillary systems, for example, anterior sites such as the inferior frontal gyrus and right hemisphere sites. These data suggest that in dyslexic readers disruption of posterior reading systems underlies the failure of skilled reading to develop, while a shift to ancillary systems supports accurate, but not automatic, word reading.

Epidemiology. Dyslexia may be the most common neurobehavioral disorder affecting children, with prevalence rates ranging from 5–10% in clinic- and school-identified samples to 17.5% in unselected population-based samples. Like hypertension and obesity, dyslexia fits a dimensional model in which reading ability and disability occur along a continuum, with dyslexia representing the lower tail of a normal distribution of reading ability. In contrast to traditional assumptions, several studies indicate similar numbers of affected males and females. Both prospective and retrospective longitudinal studies indicate dyslexia is a persistent, chronic condition rather than a transient developmental lag. Over time, dyslexic and poor readers maintain their relative positions along the distribution of reading ability. However, approaches using focused, early, and intensive intervention provide promise that these trends can be modified.

Clinical Manifestations. Difficulties in decoding and word recognition may vary according to age and developmental level. However, the cardinal signs of dyslexia observed in school-aged children and adults are an inaccurate and labored approach to decoding, word recognition, and text reading. Listening comprehension is typically robust. In several studies, older children have been found to improve reading accuracy over time, albeit without commensurate gains in reading fluency; they remain slow readers. Difficulties in spelling typically reflect the phonologically based difficulties observed in oral reading. A parental history frequently identifies early subtle language difficulties in dyslexic children. Many children identified as dyslexic during the primary grades displayed difficulties playing rhyming games and learning the names for letters and numbers during the preschool and kindergarten years. Indeed, recent longitudinal studies demonstrate that kindergarten assessments of these language skills are highly predictive of later reading skill. Parents also frequently report that although their child relishes the opportunity to be read to, reading aloud to the parent or reading independently is resisted. Dyslexia may co-occur with attention-deficit/hyperactivity disorder (ADHD). Although this co-morbidity has been documented in both referred samples (40% co-morbidity) and nonreferred samples (15% co-morbidity), the two disorders are distinct and separable.

Diagnosis. At all ages, dyslexia is a clinical diagnosis. The clinician seeks to determine through history, observation, and psychometric assessment if there are (1) unexpected difficulties in reading (i.e., difficulties in reading that are unexpected for the person's cognitive capacity as shown by his or her age, intelligence, level of education, or professional status) and (2) associated linguistic problems at the level of phonologic processing. There is no single test score that is pathognomonic of dyslexia. The diagnosis should reflect a thoughtful synthesis of all the clinical data available. Dyslexia is distinguished from other disorders that may prominently feature reading difficulties by the unique, circumscribed nature of the phonologic deficit, one not intruding into other linguistic or cognitive domains. Family history, teacher/classroom observation, and tests of language (particularly phonology), reading, and spelling represent a core assessment for the diagnosis of dyslexia in children; additional tests of intellectual ability, attention, memory, general language skills, and mathematics may be administered as part of a more comprehensive evaluation of cognitive, linguistic, and academic function.

Treatment. The management of dyslexia demands a life-span perspective; early on, the focus is on remediation of the reading problem. Newer knowledge of the importance of early language and phonologic skills may lead to the prevention of significant reading problems, even in predisposed children. As a child matures and enters the more time-demanding setting of secondary school, the emphasis shifts to the important role of providing accommodations. Until very recently school reading intervention was not based on rigorous scientific evidence; overall, it was too little, too general, and too unsystematic. Based on the work of the National Reading Panel, evidence-based reading intervention programs have now been identified. Effective intervention programs are balanced; they provide systematic instruction in phonemic awareness, phonics, fluency, vocabulary, and comprehension strategies and provide ample opportunities for writing, reading, and discussing literature. Taking each component of the reading process in turn, effective interventions improve phonemic awareness (PA): the ability to focus on and manipulate phonemes (speech sounds) in *spoken* syllables and words. The elements found to be most effective in enhancing PA, reading, and spelling skills include teaching children to manipulate phonemes with letters; focusing the instruction on one or two types of phoneme manipulations rather than multiple types; teaching children in small groups; and providing *systematic, explicit* instruction rather than incidental instruction in PA. Providing instruction in PA is necessary but not sufficient to teach children to read. Effective intervention programs include teaching phonics, that is, making sure that the beginning reader understands how letters are linked to sounds (phonemes) to form letter-sound correspondences and spelling patterns. Often overlooked, and critical to effectively teaching phonics, is to make sure that the instruction is explicit and systematic; phonics instruction enhances children's success in learning to read and systematic phonics instruction is more effective than instruction that teaches little or no phonics or teaches phonics haphazardly or in a "by-the-way" approach. The Report of the National Reading Panel also provides information on teaching fluency, vocabulary, and comprehension strategies. The treatment of dyslexia in students in high school, college, and graduate school is typically based on accommodation rather than remediation. College students with a childhood history of dyslexia require extra time in reading and writing assignments as well as examinations. Many adolescent and adult students have been able to improve their reading accuracy, though without commensurate gains in reading speed. Other helpful accommodations include the use of laptop computers with spelling checkers, tape recorders in the classroom, recorded books, access to lecture notes, tutorial services, alternatives to multiple choice tests, and a separate quiet room for taking tests.

Lyon G: Toward a definition of dyslexia. *Annals of Dyslexia* 1995;45:3–27.

Report of the National Reading Panel (2000): *Teaching Children to Read: An Evidence Based Assessment of the Scientific Research Literature on Reading and its Implications for Reading Instruction* (Vol. NIH Pub. No. 00-4754). U.S. Department of Health and Human Services, Public Health Service, National Institutes of Health, National Institute of Child Health and Human Development.

Shaywitz BA, Shaywitz SE, Pugh KR, et al: Disruption of posterior brain systems for reading in children with developmental dyslexia (submitted).

Shaywitz S: Current concepts: Dyslexia. *N Engl J Med* 1998;338(5):307–12.

Shaywitz SE, Fletcher JM, Holahan JM, et al: Persistence of dyslexia: The Connecticut Longitudinal Study at adolescence. *Pediatrics* 1999;104:1351–9.

Torgesen J, Wagner R, Rashotte C, et al: Preventing reading failure in young children with phonological processing disabilities: Group and individual responses to instruction. *Journal of Educational Psychology* 1999;91:579–94.

Chapter 30

Adoption Mark D. Simms and
Madelyn Freundlich

Adoption is a social, emotional, and legal process that provides a new family for children when the birth family is unable or unwilling to parent. Approximately 1 million children in this country are adopted; 2–4% of all American families have adopted. In 1992, the last year for which total adoption statistics are available, 127,441 children of all races and nationalities were adopted in the United States. Of these, 42% were stepparent or relative adoptions, 15.5% were children in foster care, and 5% were children from other countries adopted by United States families. Private agencies or independent practitioners, such as lawyers, handled approximately one third of adoptions.

Over the past several years, there have been significant increases in the number of children adopted from the *foster care system* in this country as well as in the number of children adopted from other countries by United States families. Changes in federal law in 1997 required that children in foster care who could not be safely returned to their families within a reasonable period of time be placed with adoptive families. With the implementation of the Adoption and Safe Families Act, the number of adoptions of children in foster care began to grow from what previously had been about 18,000 adoptions of children in foster care each year. In 1997, approximately 31,000 children were adopted; by 1999, approximately 46,000 children in foster care had been adopted. At the same time, the number of children in foster care who need adoptive families has grown dramatically. In March 2000, an estimated 134,000 children in foster care were waiting to be adopted. Many children in foster care who are waiting to be adopted have "special needs" because they are of school age, part of a sibling group, or members of ethnic or racial minority groups, or because they have physical, emotional, or developmental problems (including HIV infection, AIDS, or prenatal exposure to illicit substances). Federal adoption subsidies, tax credits, special minority recruitment efforts, increased postplacement services, and approval of adoptions by "nontraditional" families (particularly single adults and older couples) are aimed at increasing the adoption opportunities for these children.

International adoptions have increased substantially in the past decade. In 2000, United States families adopted 18,537 children from other countries (compared with 7,093 in 1990). China, Russia, South Korea, and Guatemala have become the primary sending countries for children. Most children placed for international adoption have histories of poverty and social hardship in their home countries, and many are adopted from orphanages and other institutional settings. Children who are adopted internationally may be healthy infants and older children, but they also may have "special needs" that are similar to the needs of children in the United States foster care system. Under a new federal law implementing the Hague Convention on Intercountry Adoption, agencies in the United States that arrange international adoptions must make efforts to obtain accurate and complete health histories on children whom families are considering for adoption.

Role of Pediatricians. Pediatricians can help prospective adoptive parents evaluate the health and developmental history of a child and available background information from birth families in order to assess actual and potential problems or risks that children may have. Adoption agencies increasingly are making efforts to obtain from birth mothers and birth fathers information about their own health and genetic histories and the histories of their children so that this information can be shared with adoptive families. It is likely that more background information will be available in domestic adoptions than in international adoptions. Nevertheless, in international adoptions, pediatricians can assist adoptive families in understanding and evaluating the information that is available about the child's background and current condition (including reviewing any video of the child that has been provided to the family). Assistance in evaluating the child's current status and future health risks should be provided, if possible, before the family travels abroad or the child arrives in the United States. After the child is settled in the new home, pediatricians should encourage adoptive parents to seek a comprehensive assessment of the child's health and development. A significant number of internationally adopted children have acute or chronic medical problems. Routine screening for infectious diseases and disorders of growth and development are recommended for all children arriving in the United States.

Pediatricians also can promote positive adjustment of the child and family by providing guidance and support at all stages of the adoption. Families should be encouraged to speak freely and repeatedly about adoption with the child, beginning in the toddler years and continuing through adolescence. Pediatricians may need to respond to a number of concerns and questions on the part of adoptive parents or adopted adolescents when the adoptee's health and genetic history is incomplete or unknown.

Research shows that most adopted children and families adjust well and lead healthy, productive lives. It is not common that adoptions disrupt. Research, however, shows that disruption rates are higher among children adopted from foster care, which the research associates with their older ages at time of adoption and their histories of multiple placements before their adoptions. As a result of a greater understanding of the needs of families who adopt children from foster care, agencies are placing greater emphasis on the preparation of adoptive parents and ensuring the availability of a full range of postadoption services, including physical health, mental health, and developmental services for their adopted children.

American Academy of Pediatrics, Committee on Early Childhood, Adoption and Dependent Care: *Families and Adoption: The Pediatrician's Role in Supporting Communication.* AAP News, February 1992.

American Academy of Pediatrics, Committee on Early Childhood, Adoption and Dependent Care: Initial medical evaluation of an adopted child. *Pediatrics* 1991;88:642–4.

American Academy of Pediatrics: Medical evaluation of internationally adopted children for infectious diseases. In Pickering LK (editor): *2000 Red Book: Report of The Committee on Infectious Diseases,* 25th ed. Elk Grove Village, IL: American Academy of Pediatrics, 2000, pp 148–52.

Aronson J: Medical evaluation and infectious considerations on arrival. *Pediatr Ann* 2000;29:218–23.

Evan B. Donaldson Adoption Institute: *Adoption in the United States.* http://www.adoptioninstitute.org/research/ressta.html

Holloway JS: Outcome in placements for adoption or long-term fostering. *Arch Dis Child* 1997;76:227–30.

Miller LC: Initial assessment of growth, development, and the effects of institutionalization in internationally adopted children. *Ann Pediatr* 2000;29:224–32.

Saiman L, Aronson J, Zhou J, et al: Prevalence of infectious diseases among internationally adopted children. *Pediatrics* 2001;108:608–12.

Chapter 31

Foster Care *Mark D. Simms and*

Madelyn Freundlich

As of March 2000, there were approximately 588,000 children in state-supported foster care in the United States, compared with 262,000 children in 1982. Over the past 2 decades, efforts to reduce the number of children in foster care have been largely unsuccessful.

Developed as a temporary measure to assist families in crisis, the foster care system became overwhelmed in the 1960s and 1970s as the number of children determined to be abused or neglected and in need of foster care increased dramatically. By the late 1970s, it had become apparent that far too many children were remaining in foster care for extended periods of time without clear plans for their futures. In 1980, the Adoption Assistance and Child Welfare Act (PL 96-272) changed the emphasis of public policy by requiring states to make "reasonable efforts" to prevent children from entering foster care and to reunify children in foster care with their families. The act advanced permanency planning as a process to prevent children from remaining in foster care for indefinite periods of time. It required that children in foster care have clearly defined permanency goals (return home, placement with relatives, adoption) no later than 18 months from the time they entered foster care and that there be periodic court reviews of children's placements and progress toward achieving their permanency goals. Although some progress was realized through the mid-1980s, the drug epidemic that began in the late 1980s set the stage for a new influx of children into foster care. The population of children in foster care has grown steadily since that time in the face of worsening circumstances facing many families (poverty, substance abuse, homelessness, mental health problems). In 1997, the Adoption and Safe Families Act (PL 105-89) was enacted in an effort to prompt more timely permanency planning for children in foster care. Under the new law, a permanency plan must be made for a child in foster care no later than 12 months from the child's entry into care and a petition to terminate parental rights must be filed to free the child for adoption when a child has been in foster care for 15 of the most recent 22 months (with some exceptions). Adoption (see Chapter 30) is now viewed as an important option for children in foster care.

In 1999, there were 3 million reports of child abuse and neglect; of these reports, 868,000 were substantiated for abuse or neglect (see Chapter 35). The vast majority of children in foster care have histories of abuse or neglect. Far fewer children are in care because of the child's own physical or mental health problems or because parents, as a result of a personal or family emergency, voluntarily place their child in foster care. Although foster care has narrowed so that most children and their families can gain access to help only if the child is abused or significantly neglected, new federal programs have been developed to assist families before crises involving child abuse or serious neglect. The Promoting Safe and Stable Families program (under Title IV-B of the Social Security Act), in particular, funds a range of family support and family preservation programs. Although foster care payments under Title IV-E of the Social Security Act continue to far exceed funding for child and family services programs under Title IV-B, greater efforts are being made to address the issues that are associated with child abuse and neglect and the need for children to be placed in foster care: parental substance abuse, domestic abuse, inadequate housing and homelessness, lack of parenting skills, unemployment and underemployment, parental mental and physical health problems, and parental incarceration.

An increasing proportion of children entering foster care are young. Close to half (47%) of the children who entered foster care between October 1999 and March 2000 were younger than 5 yr. Most (42%) were white, but significant percentages were black (29%) and Latino (13%). Children continue to remain in care for significant periods of time, an average of 21 months for children in foster care in March 2000. Importantly, close to half the children in foster care (45%) have been in foster care for 2 or more years.

Children who enter foster care have extraordinarily high rates of medical, developmental, and mental health problems. Most suffer from behavioral and adjustment problems. Nearly 60% of preschoolers are developmentally delayed, and more than half of school-aged children lag behind their peers academically. A disproportionate number of children in foster care have chronic medical conditions (35%), physical growth failure (25%), and congenital abnormalities (15%). Children in foster care have high utilizations rates for all types of care (especially inpatient hospitalization and outpatient mental health services) and, as a group, they incur high health care costs. Both the chances of entering foster care and the likelihood of longer stays in care have been associated with the presence of mental health problems, physical disabilities, and developmental delays. Nonetheless, when children receive needed services, they experience significant improvements in overall health status, stabilization of chronic conditions, and growth and development.

In 1988, the Child Welfare League of America, in collaboration with the American Academy of Pediatrics, published *Standards for the Health Care of Children in Out-of-Home Care* to serve as a blueprint for the effective delivery of services to children in foster care. These standards, in general, have not been implemented. Moreover, despite the availability of comprehensive diagnostic and treatment services under the Medicaid program, known as EPSDT (Early Periodic Screening, Diagnosis, and Treatment), which is mandatory in all states, the majority of children in foster care do not receive these services.

A variety of factors act as barriers to the health care of children in foster care. Most public and private child welfare agencies do not have formal policies or arrangements to provide health care services and, instead, rely on local physicians or health clinics funded by Medicaid. It is often difficult to obtain complete information on the health histories of children who enter foster care because they often have had erratic contact with various health care providers before they enter foster care, and social workers are not always able to obtain detailed information from biological parents at the time children enter care. Once children enter foster care, there is often a diffusion of responsibility regarding obtaining health care services for children. Foster parents often are given very little information about the health care needs of the children for whom they are caring, but they typically are expected to decide when and where children receive health care services. In some cases, social workers may oversee the health care of children in foster care, but coordination with health care providers is often lacking. Uncertainty as to who may make health care treatment decisions for children may further delay health care or result in the denial of health care services.

Recent federal data indicate that the majority of children in foster care for relatively short periods have only one or two placements while they are in care (81% of the children who are in care for less than 12 mo). For children in care for longer periods of time, however, a much smaller percentage have only one or two placements while they are in care (only 39% of the children who have been in care for 48 mo or more). Changes in caregivers and residences are associated with poorer psychological and developmental outcomes for children and often mean changes in children's health care providers. At the same time, regardless of whether children's placements change, children's social workers often change (primarily because of high turnover rates) and, as a result, key aspects of health care planning and coordinating may be disrupted.

The health care of poor children, in general, and of children in foster care, in particular, continues to be a key policy issue. The traditional "safety net" previously provided by federal and state programs for economically distressed families (as represented in the past by the Aid to Families with Dependent Children [AFDC] program, Supplemental Security Income [SSI] program, and food stamps) has been substantially modified or replaced by new time-limited, benefit-limited programs. AFDC was replaced by the Temporary Assistance for Needy Families (TANF) program and the eligibility of children with disabilities under the SSI program was significantly narrowed. The cumulative impact of these policy and program changes may result in even more children entering foster care unless careful attention is paid to meeting the range of needs of vulnerable children and families.

American Academy of Pediatrics, Committee on Early Childhood, Adoption and Dependent Care: Developmental issues for young children in foster care. *Pediatrics* 2000;106:1145–50.

American Academy of Pediatrics, Committee on Early Childhood, Adoption and Dependent Care: Health care of children in foster care. *Pediatrics* 1994;93:335–8.

Child Welfare League of America: *Standards for Health Care Services for Children in Out-of-Home Care.* Washington, DC: Child Welfare League of America, 1988.

Horwitz SM, Balestracci KM, Simms MD: Foster care placement improves children's functioning. *Arch Pediatr Adolesc Med* 2001;155:1255–60.

Horwitz SM, Owens PM, Simms MD: Specialized assessment for children in foster care. *Pediatrics* 2000;106:59–66.

Horwitz SM, Simms MD, Farrington R: Impact of developmental problems on young children's exit from foster care. *J Dev Behav Pediatr* 1994;15:105–10.

Simms MD, Dubowitz H, Szilagyi M: Health care needs of children in the foster care system. *Pediatrics* 2000;106:909–18.

Szilagyi M: The pediatrician and the child in foster care. *Pediatr Rev* 1998;19:39–50.

US General Accounting Office: *Foster Care: Health Needs of Many Young Children Are Unknown and Unmet.* Washington, DC: US General Accounting Office, 1995.

Wyatt DT, Simms MD, Horwitz SM: Widespread growth retardation and variable growth recovery in foster children in the first year after initial placement. *Arch Pediatr Adolesc Med* 1997;151:813–16.

Chapter 32
Child Care *Paul H. Dworkin*

Profound social and demographic changes have resulted in an increasing number of children receiving a portion of their care from someone other than their parents. In the United States, almost two thirds of mothers with children younger than 6 yr are working outside the home, including more than one half of mothers of infants and toddlers. A high divorce rate and increase in births to single women have contributed to approximately one child in four living within a single-parent household headed by the mother. Women work for the same reasons as men—economic necessity and personal choice. The economic climate and changes in family structure have necessitated the availability of child-care services for working parents.

Child care is defined as care provided by an individual outside the nuclear family or in a setting separate from the child's home and is inclusive of such services as baby sitting, daycare, preschool, early childhood program, Head Start, and nursery school. By the mid-1990s, approximately 6 million infants and toddlers in the United States were in some type of child care. Options for families generally include in-home care, family child care, and center child care. Child care is used for children of all ages. Less than 5% of children of working parents receive in-home care, in which a relative or a nonrelative (such as a nanny,

housekeeper, or regular sitter) comes to the child's home to provide care. Approximately 20% of all preschool children who receive supplemental care are in regulated or nonregulated family child care, in which a small group of children, typically six or fewer, receive care in the private home of a caregiver. Nearly one half of employed mothers of 3- and 4-yr-old children report center care as their primary supplemental arrangement. Child-care centers provide care for more than six to 10 children at a time and include for-profit centers, which may be independent or operated by large chains, and nonprofit centers, which may be independent or sponsored by the government (e.g., Head Start), religious organizations, public schools, community agencies, or employers. Most child-care centers are licensed, although standards vary from state to state. Different types of child care have advantages and disadvantages, including cost, familiarity of care provider and environment, convenience, availability, flexibility in scheduling, and reliability. From a developmental perspective, the progression from care in the child's own home to care in another home with a few other children to large-group care may be appropriate. Yet for most families, decisions about child care are based largely on considerations of cost, distance from home, and safety.

The effect of child care on children's development depends on a number of interrelated factors, including the quality and quantity of the child-care experience, as well as characteristics of the child and family. Despite the substantial time spent by children in child-care settings, the predominant influences on children's adjustment and development are the parents and the home environment. The developmental effects of child care are determined by the quality of the interactions and experiences they provide. Child care can protect children from the detrimental effects of maternal depression and poverty. Care provided by insensitive or unresponsive providers can exacerbate difficult family circumstances.

High-quality child care can favorably influence the cognitive and social development of children, especially those from disadvantaged populations. Such children perform better on school entry on standardized tests of intelligence, academic achievement, and measures of accomplishment such as grades and teacher ratings. Conversely, poor-quality child care can adversely affect developmental outcomes. Contrary to popular beliefs, middle-class children are not protected from the effects of poor-quality child care. More time spent in nonmaternal care during the preschool years may be associated with more aggressive, assertive, and defiant behaviors.

Good-quality child care has been associated with a low adult-to-child ratio, small group size, and caregiver training in child development. Other important determinants include a caring and supportive staff that is stable and consistent, a developmentally appropriate curriculum that enables children to learn through a variety of fun activities, and a physical setting that affords cleanliness, sanitation, and adequate space for activities and rest as well as protection from environmental hazards. Unfortunately, child care in the United States is often of poor quality. A study of child-care centers in four states found that only 14% of centers gave good-quality care, with the remaining centers rated as mediocre or poor, often endangering the health and safety of young children. A study of family daycare yielded similar findings, with only 12% of regulated family child-care homes found to provide high-quality care. Only 3% of unregulated family child care was considered high quality, as was only 1% of the care provided by relatives in their own homes.

The lack of national standards for child care and uneven regulation from state to state contribute to the variable quality of child care in the United States. *Licensure* signifies that minimal health, safety, and sanitary practices are being followed, whereas *accreditation* (by the National Association for the Education of Young Children [NAEYC]) suggests a program is of sufficient quality to promote children's development. The American Academy of Pediatrics and the American Public Health Association have published standards for health and safety in child-care programs. The NAEYC also has developed criteria for good child-care practice. Yet a national survey of state regulations for center-based infant and toddler care found that no state regulations fulfill the criteria for good practice, and the majority reflect poor or very poor practice. Efforts to upgrade the quality of child care are likely to require the establishment of federal standards that address such characteristics as staff-to-child ratios, group size, caregiver training, and improved salaries for child-care providers. Additional critical policy issues include parental leave, tax credits for child care, flexible work schedules, and on-site child care provided by employers.

Pediatric providers may assume a number of important roles in promoting successful child-care experiences. Pediatricians can help parents become informed consumers by discussing the advantages and disadvantages of various child-care options, providing accurate information regarding implications for children's health and development, and directing parents to sources of information about child care in the community. The pediatrician can provide guidance to parents regarding a sick child's participation in child care and serve as health consultant to child-care programs. Pediatric advocacy for the availability of high-quality care for all children includes encouraging the implementation of national child-care standards, paid parental infant care leaves, and improved salaries and training for child-care providers.

American Academy of Pediatrics and American Public Health Association: *Caring for Our Children. National Health and Safety Performance Standards: Guidelines for Out-of-Home Child Care Programs.* Elk Grove Village, IL, American Academy of Pediatrics, 1993.

Cost, Quality, Child Outcomes Study Team: *Cost, Quality and Child Outcomes in Child Care Center: Public Report,* 2nd ed. Denver, Department of Economics, University of Colorado, 1995.

Galinsky E, Howes C, Kontos S, et al: *The Study of Children in Family Day Care and Relative Care: Highlights of Findings.* New York, Families & Work Institute, 1994.

NICHD Early Child Care Research Network: The relation of child care to cognitive and language development. *Child Dev* 2000;71:960.

Phillips D, Adams G: Child care and our youngest children. *The Future Child* 2001;11:35.

Saluter AF: *Marital Status and Living Arrangements: March 1993.* US Bureau of the Census, Current Population Reports, Series P20–478. Washington, DC, Government Printing Office, 1994.

Young KT, Marsland KM, Zigler E: The regulatory status of center-based infant and toddler child care. *Am J Orthopsychiatry* 1997;67:535.

Zigler E: School should begin at age 3 years for American children. *J Dev Behav Pediatr* 1998;19:38.

Chapter 33
Separation, Loss, and Bereavement

All children experience involuntary separation from loved ones, think about death, and encounter death in everyday events. Parents and children often turn to their pediatrician and other health care professionals to help them with all types of loss. Relatively brief separations of children from their parents, such as vacations, usually produce minor transient effects, but more enduring and frequent separation may cause significant sequelae. The potential impact of each event must be considered in light of the age and stage of development of the child and the particular relationship with the absent person as well as the nature of the situation. As a trustworthy, familiar resource, pediatricians are uniquely positioned to offer information, support, and guidance and to facilitate coping.

33.1 Separation & Loss

Richard Dalton

The initial reaction of *young children* to separation may involve crying, either of a tantrum-like, protesting type or of a quieter, sadder type. After a few hours or a day or so of separation, children may appear more subdued, withdrawn, and quiet or irritable, fussy, moody, and resistant to authority. Disturbance of appetite may occur, and there may be special difficulties at bedtime, such as reluctance to go to bed and problems in getting to sleep, with a resurgence of old fears and, in younger children, perhaps such regressive behavior as bed-wetting. Children may repeatedly ask where the absent parent is and when he or she will return home. Some children may not refer to parental absence at all. The child may go to the window or door or out into the neighborhood looking for the absent parent; a few may even leave home or their places of temporary placement to search for their parents. This last rather unusual response needs to be considered when a child cannot be found for a while shortly after the separation or departure of a parent.

A child's *response to reunion* may surprise or alarm a parent who is not prepared. A parent who joyfully returns to the family may be met by wary or cautious children, who, after a brief interchange of affection, may move away from the parent and seem indifferent to his or her return. The interpretation of this response depends on the child and his or her style; it may indicate anger at being left and wariness that the event will happen again, or, because children tend to personalize, the child may have felt that he or she caused the parent's departure. For instance, if the mother who frequently says "Stop it, or you'll give me a headache" is hospitalized, the child may unrealistically feel at fault and guilty. As a result of these feelings, children may seem to be more closely attached to the other parent than to the absent one, or even to the grandparent or baby sitter who cared for them during their parent's absence. Immediately after the reunion or after a few days, some children, particularly younger ones, may become more clinging and dependent than they were before separation, while continuing any regressive behavior that had occurred during separation. Such behavior may engage the returned parent more closely and help to re-establish the bond that the child felt was broken. Such reactions are usually transient; within 1–2 wk, children will have recovered their usual behavior and equilibrium. Recurrent separations may tend to make children more wary and guarded about re-establishing the relationship with the repeatedly absent parent, and these traits may affect other personal relationships. Parents should not try to ameliorate a child's behavior by threatening to leave.

Experiences of loss such as *divorce* or *placement in foster care* can give rise to the same kinds of reactions listed earlier, but they are more intense and possibly more lasting. School-aged children may respond with evident depression, seem indifferent, or be markedly angry. Other children appear to deny or avoid the issue, behaviorally or verbally. Most children may cling to the hope or fantasy that the actual placement or separation is not real. Guilt may be generated by the child's feeling that this loss, separation, or placement represents rejection and perhaps punishment for misbehavior. Children may protect a parent at their own expense, believing and asserting that their own badness caused the parent to depart or to place them with relatives or strangers, rather than that the parent has been bad or irresponsible. Besides having their own feelings of guilt, children cannot blame their parents because they sense it may be fairly risky. Parents who discover that a child harbors resentment might punish further for these thoughts or feelings. Children who feel that their misbehavior caused their parents to separate or become divorced have the fantasy that their own trivial or recurrent behavioral patterns have caused their parents to become angry with each other. Some children develop behavioral or psychosomatic symptoms and unwittingly adopt a "sick" role as a strategy for reuniting their parents.

In response to separation and divorce of parents, *older children and adolescents* commonly show more intense anger. Almost all children cling to the magical belief that their parents will reunite after divorce. Wallerstein found that 5 yr after the breakup, about one third of the children studied were "consciously and intensely unhappy and dissatisfied with their life in the postdivorce family." Another one third showed clear evidence of a satisfactory adjustment, and the remaining one third demonstrated a mixed picture with good achievement in some areas and faltering achievement in others. After 10 yr, 45% were doing well, but 41% were poorly adjusted and had academic, social, and emotional problems. As they entered adulthood, many were reluctant to form intimate relationships, fearful of repeating their parents' experience. A large-scale British study indicates that parental divorce had a moderate long-term negative impact on the adult mental health status of children who had experienced it, even after controlling for changes in economic status and problems before divorce. Good adjustment of children after a divorce is related to ongoing involvement with two psychologically healthy parents who minimize conflict and to the support system offered by siblings and other relatives. Divorcing parents should be encouraged to avoid the adversarial process and to use a trained mediator if they cannot resolve disputes on their own. Joint custody arrangements may reduce ongoing parental conflict, but children in joint custody felt overburdened by the demands of maintaining a strong presence in two homes.

Another version of a separation experience occurs when a child's family *moves*. A significant proportion of the population of the United States changes residence each year. The effects of this movement on children and families are frequently overlooked; for children, the move is essentially involuntary. When such changes in family structure as divorce or death precipitate moves, children face the stresses created by both the precipitating events and moving itself. When parents are sad because of the circumstances surrounding the move, this unhappiness will be transmitted to their children. Children who move lose their old friends, the comfort of a familiar bedroom and house, and their ties to school and community. They not only must sever old relationships but also are faced with developing new ones in new neighborhoods and new schools. Children may enter neighborhoods with new and different customs and values, and because academic standards and curricula vary among communities, children who have performed well in one school may find themselves struggling in a new one. Frequent moves during the school years are likely to have adverse consequences on social and academic performance.

Migrant children and families present as a special population (see Chapter 39). Migrant children not only need to adjust to a new community, school, and house but also need to adjust to a new culture and, in many cases, to a new language. Because children have faster language acquisition, they may function as translators for the adults in their families. This powerful position may lead to role reversal and potential conflict within the family. Migrant children are more likely to come from families with low socioeconomic status, live in overcrowded conditions, and have poorly educated parents. All of this, plus the previously mentioned factors, can increase the risk for psychopathologic disorders. In the evaluation of migrant children and families, it is also important to ask about the circumstances of the migration; legal status; conflict of loyalties; and moral, ethical, and religious differences.

Parents should prepare children well in advance of any move and allow them to express any unhappy feelings or misgivings. Parents should acknowledge their own mixed feelings and agree that they will miss their old home while looking forward to a new one. Visits to the new home in advance are often useful preludes to the actual move. Transient periods of regressive behavior may be noted in preschool children after moving, and these should be understood and accepted. Parents should assist the entry of their children into the new community, and exchanges of letters with old friends and visits, whenever possible, should be encouraged.

Ash P: Children in divorce litigation. In Alessi NE, Noshpitz JD (editors): *Basic Handbook of Child and Adolescent Psychiatry, Vol 4: Varieties of Development.* New York, John Wiley & Sons, 1997.

Bolgar R, Zweig-Frank H, Paris J: Childhood antecedents of interpersonal problems in young adult children of divorce. *J Am Acad Child Adolesc Psychiatry* 1995;34:143.

Chase-Lansdale PL, Cherlin AJ, Kiernan KE: The long-term effects of parental divorce on the mental health of young adults: A developmental perspective. *Child Dev* 1995;66:1614.

Dillon PA, Emery RE: Divorce mediation and resolution of child custody disputes: Long-term effects. *Am J Orthopsychiatry* 1996;66:131.

Jensen PS, Lewis RL, Xenakis SN: The military family in review: Context, risk and prevention. *J Am Acad Child Adolesc Psychiatry* 1986;25:225.

Monroe-Blum H, Boyle M, Offord D, et al: Immigrant children: Psychiatric disorder, school performance and service utilization. *Am J Orthopsychiatry* 1989;59:510.

Quinn LS, Behrman RE (editors): Children and divorce. The *Future Child* 1994;4:4.

Steinmann S: The experience of children in a joint custody arrangement: A report of a study. *Am J Orthopsychiatry* 1981;3:220.

Wallerstein JS: The long-term effects of divorce on children: A review. *J Am Acad Child Adolesc Psychiatry* 1991;30:349.

Wallerstein JS, Blakeslee S: *Second Chances: Men, Women and Children a Decade After Divorce.* London, Ticknor & Fields, 1989.

Westermeyer J: *Psychiatric Care of Migrants: A Clinical Guide.* Washington, DC, American Psychiatric Press, 1989.

33.2 Grief and Bereavement

Linda Sayler Gudas and Gerald P. Koocher

Grief is a personal, emotional state of bereavement or an anticipated response to loss. Not all children and families require intensive professional intervention during or following a loss event; and the presence of symptoms such as sadness, yearning, searching, and loneliness are understandable and predictable. Most bereaved families remain socially connected and expect that life will return to some new, albeit different, sense of normalcy. However, the pain and suffering imposed by grief should never be automatically deemed "normal" and thus neglected or ignored. In uncomplicated grief reactions, the steadfast concern of the pediatrician can help promote the family's sense of well-being. In more distressing reactions (such as those seen in traumatic grief), the pediatrician may be a major, first-line force in helping children and families address their loss.

Participation in the care of *a child with a life-threatening or terminal illness* is a profound experience. See Chapter 38 for discussion of palliative and end-of-life care. Withholding of information from children and parents by providers regarding diagnosis and prognosis has generally been abandoned as physicians have learned that protecting patients from the seriousness of their condition does not alleviate concerns and anxieties. Even very young children may have a real understanding of their illness. Children should be told early in their treatment that they have a very serious illness, that people can die of it, but promising treatments and medicines will help.

A death, especially the *death of a family member*, is the most difficult loss for a child. Many secondary losses occur as a result of a family death (e.g., change in income, possible need to relocate, less emotional support from surviving family members, altering of routines, change in status from sibling to only child). The presence of secure and stable adults who can meet the child's needs and who permit discussion about the loss is most important in helping a child grieve. The pediatrician should help the family understand this necessary presence and encourage the protective functioning of the family unit.

Death, separation, and loss as a result of natural and man-made *catastrophes* have become increasingly common events in children's lives. Exposure to such disasters occurs either directly or indirectly, where the event is experienced through the media. The televised scenes of the terrorist attacks in the United States on 9/11/01, subsequent news stories about anthrax, and heightened states of alert exemplify such indirect exposure. Studies have demonstrated that children who experience personal loss in disasters tend to watch more TV coverage than children who do not. However, children without a personal loss watch as a way of participating in the event and may thus experience repetitive exposure to traumatic scenes and stories. The loss and devastation for a child who personally lives through a disaster is significant; the effect of the simultaneous occurrence of disaster and personal loss complicates the bereavement process, as grief reactions become interwoven with post-traumatic stress symptoms (Chapter 22). After a death that occurs as a result of aggressive or traumatic circumstances, access to expert help may be required. Under conditions of threat and fear, children seek proximity to safe, stable, protective figures.

Developmental Perspective. Children's responses to death reflect the family's current culture, past heritage, and sociopolitical environment. Personal experience with terminal illness and dying may also facilitate children's comprehension of death and familiarity with mourning. However, developmental differences in children's efforts to make sense of and master the concept and reality of death do exist and profoundly influence their grief reactions.

Infants and toddlers do not understand all dimensions of death, especially its permanence. However, primitive protest, despair, separation anxiety, and detachment may occur at withdrawal of nurturing caretakers. Very young children also respond in reaction to observing distress in others. Young children also express signs and symptoms of grief in their emotional states, such as irritability or lethargy. In severe cases of grief, failure to thrive may occur. Also see Chapter 36.

The thinking processes of preschool years is prelogical, egocentric, and circular. Preschool children do not show well-established cause and effect reasoning. They typically express magical explanations of death events, sometimes resulting in guilt and self-blame (e.g., "He died because I wouldn't play with him."). Children conceptualize events in the context of their own experiential reality, and therefore consider death in terms of sleep, separation, and injury. In attempts to master the finality and permanence of death, preschoolers frequently ask unrelenting, repeated questions such as "After he finishes getting dead, will Johnny go on vacation with us?" or "When will they put the plane that crashed back together, so Mommy can fly home to make dinner?" Young children will express grief intermittently and show marked affective shifts over brief periods of time. Regression, accompanied by longing, sadness, and anger may accompany grief.

School-aged children think more concretely, recognize the permanence of death, and begin to understand biological processes of the human body (e.g., "You'll die if your body stops working."). Information gathered from the media, peers, and parents form lasting impressions. Consequently, they may ask candid questions about death that adults will have difficulty addressing (e.g., "He must have been blown to pieces, huh?"). Those in middle childhood, the elementary school years, tend to experience more anxiety, more overt symptoms of depression, and more somatic complaints than do younger children. School-aged children are often left with anger focused on the loved one, those who could not save the deceased, or those presumed responsible for the death. Contact with the pediatrician may provide great reassurance, especially for the child with somatic symptoms, and particularly when the death followed medical illness. School and learning problems may also occur, reactions often linked to concentration difficulties or preoccupation with the death. Close collaboration with the child's school may provide important diagnostic information and offer opportunities to mobilize intervention or support.

Around the age of 12 yr, children begin to use symbolic thinking, reason abstractly, and analyze hypothetical or "what if" scenarios systematically. Death and end of life become concepts, rather than events. *Teenagers* begin to understand complex physiologic systems in relationship to death. A developing sense of autonomy and personal identity, coupled with intense physiologic changes, makes adolescents prone to increased interest in bodily functions and focus on themselves. Fascination with dramatic, sensational, or romantic death sometimes occurs and may find expression in copycat behavior (e.g., cluster suicides) as well as competitive behavior to forge emotional links to the deceased person ("He was my best friend."). Somatic expression of grief may revolve around highly complex syndromes (e.g., eating disorders or conversion reactions) as well as symptoms limited to the more immediate perceptions as with younger children (e.g., stomachaches). Quality of life takes on meaning, and the teenager develops a focus on the future. Depression, resentment, mood swings, rage, and risk-taking behaviors can emerge as the adolescent seeks answers to questions of values, safety, evil, and fairness. Alternately, the adolescent may seek philosophical or spiritual explanations (e.g., "being at peace") to ease their sense of loss. Death of a peer may be especially traumatic.

Role of the Pediatrician in Grief. Children often demonstrate that open discussion of their grief provides relief, and they readily share their story with others. Terr and colleagues found that school-aged children often attempt to cope with traumatic loss by seeking out and acquiring information on their own. As a source of accurate and reliable information, the pediatrician should reserve time to meet with the child, parents, and/or entire family to discuss concerns and assess the level of functioning. The pediatrician can perform several preventive roles in such meetings.

The first role is to be an educator about disease, death, and grief. The pediatrician should prepare to address questions such as "Can this happen to me (or someone else I care about)?" "What will happen next?" "Did she suffer?" One need not elaborate on all such questions at one time, but truthful accounts presented in understandable language will help considerably. Even for very young children, clear and honest explanation of what has happened enhances coping. For example, "Dad's heart stopped beating forever because it was damaged in the automobile accident. He doesn't breathe or eat or move anymore. When those things happen, you are dead. Dad can never be alive again." In attempting to make sense of their loss, children and parents often become angry with health care professionals for "letting" their loved one die. School-aged children often concretely believe in the omnipotence of physicians and may also have been told "Dr. Jones will make Mommy better." Questions such as "Why didn't you..." should be answered in a responsive manner and without defensiveness. For example, "We did everything we could for your Mom. I'll be happy to answer any specific questions you have about her care. Sometimes it's hard to understand why someone we love has to die and leave us."

The pediatrician also can offer a safe environment to talk about painful emotions, express fears, and share memories. By giving families permission to talk and by modeling how to address children's concerns, the pediatrician demystifies death. Parents often request practical help. By providing resources, such as literature (both fiction and nonfiction) or referrals to therapeutic services, and offering families tools to learn about illness, loss, and grief, the physician reinforces the sense that other people understand what they are going through and helps normalize their distressing emotions. The pediatrician can also facilitate and demystify the grief process by sharing basic tenets of grief therapy. There is no single right or wrong way to grieve. Everyone grieves differently, and children mourn differently from adults. Grief is not something to "get over" but is a life-long process of adapting, readjusting, and reconnecting.

In addition, the pediatrician should assess routine health and life skills in families affected by loss and coach the family toward a sense of cohesion, moving gradually toward normalcy. Parents and children often report feeling so overwhelmed by grief that they cannot organize and manage such daily tasks as meal preparation or homework. Children cope best with grief in homes where caretakers provide safe, consistent, and predictable routines and life patterns.

The pediatrician's knowledge and understanding of child development can assist in planning age-appropriate solutions and, in a non-authoritarian manner, help families reach decisions about such questions as "How do we tell the children?" "Does he know he's dying?" "Will I get cancer?" "Do I have to tell the kids at school?" "Should Sarah watch TV coverage of the scary event?" "When will things be normal?" "Should Johnny go to the funeral?" For example, the pediatrician might first help parents identify important data to assist in the decision (e.g., "What would Johnny prefer?" "What do you believe you should do?" "What will help him feel most safe and emotionally connected to others at this sad time?"). Second, a review of what might happen and what to tell Johnny might occur (e.g., "There will be a lot of people at the funeral. Some will be crying because they are sad and miss the dead person. A box called a casket will have the body in it."). Finally, adaptive alternatives could be presented to the family (e.g., "Could Johnny have a private showing with just the family present?" "Would Johnny prefer finding ways to remember his brother without attending the service?").

Clinicians must remain vigilant for risk factors in each family member and in the family unit as a whole. Primary care providers, who care for families over time, know bereft patients' premorbid functioning and can identify those at current or future risk for physical and psychiatric morbidity. Providers must focus on symptoms that interfere with a patient's normal activities and compromise a child's attainment of developmental tasks. Symptom duration, intensity, and severity, in context with the family's culture, can help identify complicated grief reactions in need of therapeutic attention. Descriptive words such as *unrelenting, intense, intrusive,* or *prolonged* should raise concern. Total absence of mourning signs, specifically an inability to discuss the loss or express sadness, should also suggest potential problems.

No specific grief sign, symptom, or cluster of behaviors identifies the child or family in need of help. However, further assessment is indicated if the following occur: (1) persistent somatic or psychosomatic complaints of undetermined origin (e.g., headache, stomachache, eating and sleeping disorders, conversion symptoms, symptoms related to the deceased's condition, hypochondriasis); (2) unusual circumstances of death or loss (e.g., sudden, violent, or traumatic death; inexplicable, unbelievable, or particularly senseless death; prolonged, complicated illness; unexpected separation); (3) school/academic/work difficulties (e.g., declining grades or school performance, social withdrawal, aggression); (4) changes in home/family functioning (e.g., multiple family stresses, lack of social support, unavailable or ineffective functioning of caretakers, multiple disruptions in routines, lack of safety); (5) concerning psychologic factors (e.g., persistent guilt or blame, desire to die or talk of suicide, severe separation distress, disturbing hallucinations, self-abuse, risk-taking, symptoms of trauma such as hyperarousal or severe flashbacks, grief from previous or multiple deaths).

Treatment. Suggesting interventions outside the natural support network of family and friends can often prove useful to grieving families. Interventions that enhance or promote attachments and security, as well as give means of expressing and understanding death, help to reduce the likelihood of future or prolonged disturbance, especially in children. Collaboration between pediatric and mental health professionals can help determine timing and appropriateness of services.

Often overlooked interventions for children and families struggling to cope with a loss in the community include positive activities enabling conversation about or active coping with their grief. For example, sending a card or offering food to relatives of the deceased can help children learn the etiquette of behaviors and rituals around bereavement and mutual support. Performing community service or joining charitable organizations, such as fund-raising in memory of the deceased, often prove useful. In the wake of a disaster, parents and older siblings can give blood or volunteer in search and recovery efforts. When a loss does not involve an actual death (e.g., such as parental divorce or geographic relocation), empowering the child to join or start a "divorced kids' club" in school or planning a "new kids in town" party may help. See Chapter 33.1. Participating in constructive activity helps move the family away from a sense of helplessness and hopelessness and facilitates meaning in their loss.

Psychotherapeutic services may benefit the entire family or individual members. Many support or self-help groups focus on specific types of losses (e.g., sudden infant death syndrome, suicide, widow/widowers, or AIDS) and provide an opportunity to talk with other people who have experienced similar losses. Family, couple, or individual counseling may be useful depending on the nature of the residual coping issues. Combinations of approaches may work well for children or parents with evolving needs. For example, a child may participate in family therapy to deal with the loss of a sibling and use individual treatment to address issues of personal ambivalence and guilt feelings related to the death.

The question of pharmacologic intervention for grief reactions often arises in the pediatrician's office. Explaining that medication does not cure grief and often does not reduce the intensity of some symptoms (e.g., separation distress) can help. Although medication can blunt reactions, the psychologic work of grieving still must occur. The pediatrician must consider the patient's premorbid psychiatric vulnerability, current level of functioning, other available supports, and the use of additional therapeutic interventions. Medication, as a first line of defense, rarely proves useful in normal or uncomplicated grief reactions. In certain situations (e.g., severe sleep disruption, incapacitating anxiety, or intense hyperarousal), use of an anxiolytic or antidepressant medication for symptom relief and to provide the patient with the emotional energy to mourn may help. Medication used in conjunction with some form of psychotherapy, and in consultation with a psychopharmacologist, has optimal results. See Chapter 28.

Future Considerations. In recent years, the field of bereavement intervention has faced new challenges, for which scant research and experience exist as guides. One such area involves helping children and families cope in the aftermath of horrific, inexplicable deaths and losses such as terrorist attacks on civilians. The effects of chronic exposure to massive death and destruction, the lack of what Brooks and Siegel refer to as a "geographic safety zone" in which to feel secure, and the identification and management of long-term traumatic grief reactions to such attacks have not been investigated in the pediatric population. Another understudied direction involves addressing help for children and families to cope with grief in nontraditional ways. Health care providers must develop increased sensitivity and cultural awareness to attitudes about death and the rituals surrounding mourning in families of different ethnic and religious beliefs and in multicultural families practicing more pluralistic beliefs (see Chapter 3).

American Academy of Child and Adolescent Psychiatry (2001): *How to Help Children After a Disaster*. From www.aacp.org/publications/facts-fam/disaster/htm

American Academy of Pediatrics and U.S. Center for Mental Health Services (n.d.): *Psychosocial Issues for Children and Families in Disaster: A Guide for the Primary Care Physician*. www.mentalhealth.org/publications/allpubs/SMA95-3022/ SMA3002.htm

American Academy of Pediatrics, Committee on Psychosocial Aspects of Child and Family Health: How Pediatricians Can Respond to the Psychosocial Implications of Disasters. *Pediatrics* 1999;103:521–3.

Boss P: *Ambiguous Loss*. Cambridge, MA, Harvard University Press, 1999.

Brooks B, Siegel PM: *The Scared Child*. New York, Wiley & Sons, 1996.

Gudas LS, Koocher GP: Life-threatening and terminal illness. In Levine MD, Carey WB, Crocker AC (editors): *Developmental-Behavioral Pediatrics*, 3rd ed. Philadelphia, WB Saunders, 1999, pp 346–56.

Gudas LS, Koocher GP: Children with grief. In Walker CE, Roberts MC (editors): *Handbook of Clinical Child Psychology*, 3rd ed. New York, Wiley & Sons, 2001, pp 1046–56.

Melvin D, Lukeman D: Bereavement: A framework for those working with children. *Clin Child Psychol Psychiatry* 2000;5:521–39.

Pfefferbaum B, Gurwitch RH, McDonald NB, et al: Posttraumatic stress among young children after the death of a friend or acquaintance in a terrorist bombing. *Psychiatr Serv* 2000;51:386–8.

Prigerson HG, Jacobs SC: Traumatic grief as a distinct disorder: A rationale, consensus criteria, and a preliminary empirical test. In Stroebe MS, Hansson RO, Stroebe W, et al (editors): *Handbook of Bereavement Research*. Washington, DC, American Psychological Association, 2001, pp 613–37.

Terr L, Bloch DA, Michel BA, et al: Children's thinking in the wake of Challenger. *Am J Psychiatry* 1997;154:744–51.

Urman ML, Funk JB, Elliott R: Children's experiences of traumatic events: The negotiation of normalcy and difference. *Clin Child Psychol Psychiatry* 2001;6:403–24.

Wolfe J, Klar N, Grier HE, et al: Understanding of prognosis among parents of children who died of cancer. *JAMA* 2000;284:2469–74.

Chapter 34

Impact of Violence on Children *Marilyn Augustyn and*

Barry Zuckerman

Violence in the United States is a public health epidemic, affecting victim, witness, and perpetrator. The focus of pediatrics should not be limited to the traditional care of violence-related injury. Exposure to violence disrupts the healthy development of a great many children, and pediatricians need to be aware of this threat. Pediatric providers also have a wider responsibility to advocate on local, state, and national levels for safer environments in which all children can grow and thrive.

The source of first exposure to violence for children is often *domestic violence*. Occasional wife battering is estimated to exist in 16% of all families, and 3.4% (or 1.8 million women) are beaten regularly by their husbands. One study found that 40% of mothers reported violence in their families as a way of "settling disagreements." Family violence is most likely to be perpetrated by those between ages 18 and 30 yr—"the child-rearing years." It is not surprising, then, that the majority of children in these homes have witnessed violence; one study estimated that 3 million children witness domestic violence every year. In a series of 62 domestic incidents, children were *victims* in 15% of domestic violence incidents. Most of the children were injured when they intervened to protect their mother from her partner (see Chapter 35). *Witnessing* violence is only currently being recognized as detrimental to children. Because their scars as bystanders are emotional and not physical, the pediatric clinician may not fully appreciate their distress and thereby miss an opportunity to provide needed interventions.

Another source of witnessed violence is *community violence*. More than one third of New Orleans school-aged children had witnessed severe violence, and 40% had seen a dead body. In inner-city Boston, a study of mothers in a pediatric clinic found

that 10% of children younger than 6 yr had seen a knifing or shooting. In Los Angeles County, the Sheriff's Office estimates that children witness 20% of all murders. Young children living in high crime and violence areas observe death more frequently and at younger ages than children growing up in more secure surroundings.

The most ubiquitous source of exposure to violence for children in the United States is *television*. The average child 2–5 yr of age watches 20 to 30 hr of television a week, hours that are increasingly filled with scenes of violence. More than 3,500 research studies have examined the association between media violence and violent behavior; all but 18 have shown a positive relationship. Perhaps the most significant event that brought home the power and significance of media exposure on children is September 11, 2001. Children watched TV coverage of the attacks for a mean of 3.0 hr on September 11; only 34% of parents reported that they restricted their children's television viewing. Although exposure to media violence cannot be equated to exposure to "real-life" violence, many studies confirm that media violence desensitizes children to the meaning and impact of violent behavior. In the case of September 11th, among children whose parents did not try to restrict television viewing, there was an association between the number of hours of television viewing and the number of reported stress symptoms. Not all children are affected by television violence. Children most at risk from viewing television violence may be children who are also exposed regularly to real-life violence in their homes and communities.

Real-life violence continues to be a major problem in the United States. About 20,000 people in the country die each year as a result of intentional homicide. The leading cause of death in both black and white teenage males in the United States is gunshot wounds. The Massachusetts Department of Education found in a 1995 survey that one in five public high school students carried a weapon on or off school property in the 30 days before the survey. One in 20 had carried a gun. Even more common is bullying, with almost 30% of a large sample of sixth and 10th graders reporting that they have participated in bullying, being bullied, or both.

The violence children experience and witness also has a profound impact on health and development. Beyond injuries, violence affects children psychologically and behaviorally; it may influence how they view the world and their place in it. Children can come to see the world as a dangerous and unpredictable place. This fear may thwart their exploration of the environment, which is essential to learning in childhood. Furthermore, high exposure to violence in children correlates with poorer performances in school, symptoms of anxiety and depression, and lower self-esteem. Violence, particularly domestic violence, also can teach children especially powerful early lessons about the role of violence in relationships. Perhaps the most sobering consequence is that violence may change the way that children view their future—they may believe that they may die at an early age and thus take more risks, such as drinking alcohol, abusing drugs, not wearing seatbelts, and not taking prescribed medication.

Research suggests that high levels of witnessing violence places children at risk for psychologic, social, academic, and physical problems, as well as for engaging in violent acts themselves. (See also Chapter 39.) Mental health effects may include depression, dissociation, aggression, and substance abuse. Some children exposed to severe and/or chronic violence may suffer from post-traumatic stress disorder (PTSD), exhibiting constricted emotions, difficulty concentrating, autonomic disturbances, and re-enactment of the trauma through play or action (see Chapter 22). A particular challenge in treating and diagnosing pediatric PTSD is that a child's caregiver exposed to the same trauma may be suffering from it as well.

The simplest way to recognize whether violence has become a problem in a family is to consistently question both patients (when they are old enough) and parents. This is particularly important during pregnancy and the immediate postpartum period when women may be at highest risk for abuse. It is important to assure families that they are not being singled out but that all families are asked about their exposure to violence. For some families a direct approach is useful: for example, "Violence is a major problem in our world today and one that impacts everyone in our society. Thus I have started asking all my patients and families about violence that they are experiencing in their lives...." In other cases, beginning with general questions and then moving to the specific may be helpful. For example, "Do you feel safe in your home and neighborhood? Has anyone ever hurt you or your child?" When violence has impacted the child, it is important to gather details about symptoms and behaviors.

Many parents and children who have been exposed to violence can be effectively counseled by the pediatrician. Matters to be covered include gathering the facts and details of the event, gaining access to support services, providing information about the symptoms and behaviors common in children exposed to violence, and helping parents talk to their children about the event. When the symptoms are chronic (more than 6 mo) or not improving, if the violent event involved the death or departure of a parent, if the caregivers are unable to empathize with the child, or if the ongoing safety of the child is a concern, it is important that the family be referred to mental health professionals for additional treatment.

American Academy of Pediatrics, Committee on Public Education: Media violence. *Pediatrics* 2001;108:1222–6.

Augustyn M, Parker S, Groves B, et al: Silent victims: Children who witness violence. *Contemp Pediatr* 1995;12:35.

Buka SL, Stichick TL, Birdhistle I, et al: Youth exposure to violence: Prevalence, risks, and consequences. *Am J Orthopsychiatry* 2001;71:298–310.

Eisenstat SA, Bancroft L: Domestic violence. *N Engl J Med* 1999;341:886–92.

Groves B: Witness to violence. In Parker S, Zuckerman B (editors): *Handbook of Developmental and Behavioral Pediatrics*. Boston, Little, Brown, 1995, pp 334–6.

Hurt H, Malmud E, Brodky NL, et al: Exposure to violence. *Arch Pediatr Adolesc Med* 2001;155:1351–6.

Jaffe PG, Hurley DJ, Wolfe D: Children's observations of violence, part 1 and 2: Critical issues in child development and intervention planning. *Can J Psychiatry* 1990;35:466.

Martin SL, Mackie L, Kupper LL, et al: Physical abuse of women before, during, and after pregnancy. *JAMA* 2001;285:1581–4.

Nansel TR, Overpeck M, Pilla RS, et al: Bullying behaviors among US youth: Prevalence and association with psychosocial adjustment. *JAMA* 2001;285:2094–100.

Schuster MA, Stein BD, Jaycox LH, et al: A national survey of stress reactions after the September 11, 2001 terrorist attacks. *N Engl J Med* 2001;345:1507–12.

Stringham P: Violent youth. In Parker S, Zuckerman B (editors): *Handbook of Developmental and Behavioral Pediatrics*. Boston, Little, Brown, 1995, pp 329–31.

Chapter 35
Abuse and Neglect of Children* *Charles F. Johnson*

Child maltreatment encompasses a spectrum of abusive actions, or acts of commission, and lack of action, or acts of omission, that result in morbidity or death (Fig. 35–1). Acts of omission and commission before birth, such as maternal drug abuse and failure to seek appropriate health care during pregnancy, may also have adverse effects on the child. Physical abuse may be narrowly defined as intentional injuries to a child by a caregiver that result in bruises, burns, fractures, lacerations, punctures, or organ damage. A broader definition would include short- and

---

*Some parts of this chapter were adapted from previous sections by B. D. Schmitt and R. D. Krugman.

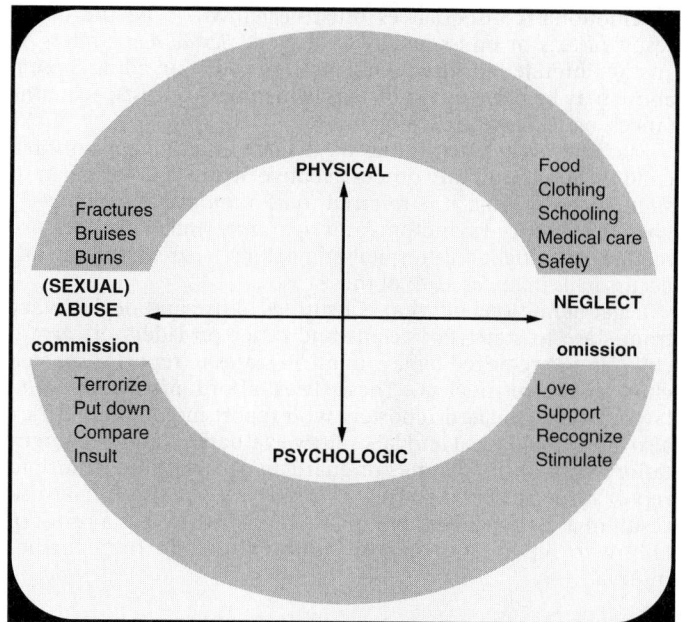

FIGURE 35–1. The spectrum of child maltreatment. Child maltreatment encompasses acts of commission, or abuse, and acts of omission, or neglect, by a caretaker that adversely affect children. The act can be physical or psychologic. The boundaries between these areas are indistinct and psychologic; physical abuse and neglect overlap and may exist at the same time or various times in the child's life. Sexual abuse may be considered a specific type of physical abuse that has strong emotional components. Physical abuse and neglect invariably have short- and long-term psychologic consequences. Psychologic consequences may persist long after the physical wounds heal.

long-term emotional consequences, which can be more debilitating than the physical effects. Physical neglect and other acts of omission may result in failure to thrive, develop, and learn and increased susceptibility to infection. Nutritional neglect is the most common cause of underweight in infancy and may account for more than half the cases of failure to thrive (see Chapter 36). Physicians are most likely to identify medical neglect that results from the failure of a parent to provide appropriate medical care, whereas failure to provide shelter, schooling, adequate clothing, and protection from environmental hazards tends to be observed by neighbors, relatives, teachers, and social workers. Medical neglect of a child with an acute or chronic disease may result in worsening of the condition and death.

Parents may refuse to allow recommended medical treatments because of personal or religious beliefs. The determination of whether this constitutes neglect and, if so, the appropriate action for a physician to take is a difficult decision (see Chapter 2). Neglect of appropriate precautions by caregivers to ensure a child's safety may also involve difficult matters of judgment. Children may be injured despite a variety of protective actions by well-meaning parents.

Psychologic maltreatment includes intentional verbal or behavioral acts or omissions that result in adverse emotional consequences. A caregiver may intentionally fail to provide nurturing verbal and behavioral actions that are necessary for healthy development. Psychologic maltreatment of a child by a caregiver includes spurning, exploiting/corrupting, withholding emotional responsiveness, isolating, or terrorizing. Psychologic maltreatment may be difficult to document when psychopathology or emotional consequences must be shown to be the direct result of acts or omissions by caregivers. *Sexual abuse* refers to any act intended for the sexual gratification of an adult. Sexual abuse may be perpetrated by family members (incest), acquaintances, or, least often, strangers.

Medications and toxins may be given to intentionally poison a child. When this or any other deceptive action is undertaken to simulate a disorder, it is referred to as *Munchausen syndrome by proxy*. The induced symptoms and signs may lead to unnecessary medical investigation, hospital admissions, or treatment; death occurs in as many as 10% of these cases.

Legal definitions of what constitutes abuse and neglect vary from state to state. Physicians and other providers of care to children are required by law in all 50 states to report suspected child abuse or neglect. These laws afford protection from lawsuits to mandated reporters who report in good faith; they also allow for clinical and laboratory evaluations and documentation without the parent's or guardian's permission. Failure to report suspected child abuse may result in a penalty. It may also result in a malpractice claim for damages incurred as a result of failure to report and thereby protect the child from further injury.

Epidemiology. Since 1993, victimization rates per 1,000 children have declined to 11.8. After mandated reporting began in the 1960s, the number of reports to Children's Protective Services (CPS) and law enforcement agencies in the county in which the alleged abuse or neglect occurred had steadily increased. In 1976, there were 669,000 reports of child maltreatment. This number reached 3.0 million in 1995 (1 in every 25 children). The initial increase in reports has been attributed to improved case finding and reporting. In 1995, 36% (1.0 million) reports were "substantiated" by CPS. In 1999, of an estimated 2,974,000 referrals, 39.6% were screened out by CPS agencies. There were an estimated 826,000 victims. An estimated 1,100 children died of abuse in 1999. Children younger than 1 yr accounted for 42.6% of the fatalities. Neglect was the most common cause of death (38.2%). With the advent of child death review teams, it is expected that more child abuse deaths will be revealed. The prevalence of abuse is unknown. A survey of families with children aged 3–18 yr indicated that 140 of 1,000 (14%) were kicked, bitten, punched, hit with an object, beaten up, or threatened with a knife or gun in 1 yr. A 1995 Gallup telephone survey indicated that 49 of every 1,000 children (5%) may have been physically abused. Approximately 10% of injuries to children younger than 5 yr who are seen in emergency departments are due to abuse; 15% of children admitted for burns and 50% of children younger than 1 yr of age with fractures have been abused. In 1999, The National Child Abuse and Neglect Data System (NCANDS) indicated that neglect, physical abuse, and sexual abuse constituted 58.4%, 21.3%, and 11.3%, respectively, of confirmed cases. The rate of maltreatment declined with advancing age. Of perpetrators, 62% were female. Males were the most common perpetrators of sexual abuse.

Although varying definitions and reporting requirements prevent detailed comparisons, parents who abuse their children have been reported from most ethnic, geographic, religious, educational, occupational, and socioeconomic groups. In the 1999 NCANDS report, ethnicity of victims ranged from a low of 4.4/1,000 children for Asian/Pacific Islander victims to 25.2/1,000 of African-American victims. Groups living in poverty have increased reports of physical abuse because of (1) the increased number of crises in their lives (e.g., unemployment or overcrowding), (2) limited access to economic or social resources for support during times of stress, (3) the increased violence in the communities where they live, (4) an association of poverty with other risk factors, such as teenage and single parenthood and substance abuse, and (5) the possi-

bility of more scrutiny by community agencies and neighbors. An increased incidence of physical abuse has been noted on military bases. This may be due to increased surveillance as well as increased risk factors. The presence of spouse abuse increases the likelihood of child abuse (see Chapters 5 and 34). Substance abuse is a common finding in families with abused children. More than 90% of abusing parents have neither psychotic nor criminal personalities. Rather, they tend to be lonely, unhappy, angry, young, single parents who do not plan their closely spaced pregnancies, have little or no knowledge of child development and child health, and have unrealistic expectations for child behavior. Mentally retarded children are more at risk for abuse and neglect. Their parents may injure them in anger after being provoked by what they consider a misbehavior that is actually related to a handicap. From 10–40% of abusive parents have experienced physical abuse as children.

Physical abuse is most likely to occur when a high-risk parent responsible for the care of a high-risk child undergoes stress and reacts to stress with violence. High-risk children include premature infants, infants with chronic medical conditions, colicky babies, and children with learning and behavior problems. The child may be normal but misperceived by an inexperienced parent as difficult, unusual, or abnormal. Normal behavior, such as crying, wetting, soiling, and spilling, may cause the parent to lose control and injure a child. The occasion precipitating the abuse may be associated with a family crisis, such as loss of a job or home, marital strife, death of a sibling, physical exhaustion, or development of an acute or chronic physical or mental illness in the parent or child. Determination of risk factors for abuse and neglect should begin during pregnancy and continue through childhood as part of the routine medical history and in all cases of childhood injury. The presence of risk factors in parents or child should increase the suspicion of abuse; however, when abuse cannot be documented, significant risk factors may necessitate referral for preventive services.

Clinical Manifestations. Physical abuse is suspected when an injury is unexplained, unexplainable, or implausible. If an injury is incompatible with the history given or with the child's development, suspected abuse should be reported. Diagnostic certainty of physical abuse is not required to file a report. It is expected, when children are hurt, that parents will bring them immediately for examination. A delay in seeking medical help should increase suspicion of abuse or neglect. A delay may also be due to a lack of transportation or ignorance about the significance of disease or injury. Before reporting suspected medical neglect, the physician should determine whether the parents have an understanding of disease processes and the intellectual, emotional, economic, and physical resources needed to provide for their children. A report of suspected neglect should bring needed services.

Bruises are the most common manifestation of child abuse and may be found on any body surface. Accidental bruises, from impact trauma, are most likely to be found on thin leading surfaces overlying bone edges, such as the shins, forearms, and brows. Bruises to the buttocks, genitals, back, and back of the hands are less likely to be due to an accident. Children may be struck, thrown, burned, bitten, lacerated, or punctured. The shape of the injury may suggest the object used. Paddles, belts, hands, and other instruments leave specific marks (Fig. 35–2). The most commonly used "instrument" to inflict trauma is the hand. Bilateral, symmetric, or geometric injuries should raise suspicion of child abuse. The color of a bruise is influenced by the time and depth of injury, the body surface involved, and the skin color. A fresh bruise generally appears blue or red-purple. A bruise is older if there is yellow, green, or brown. Bruises of different colors on the same body surface generally are not com-

MARKS from INSTRUMENTS

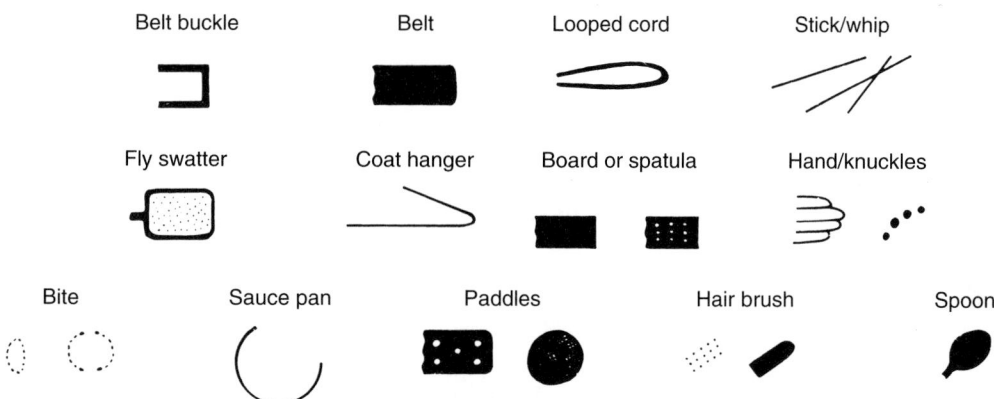

FIGURE 35–2. A variety of instruments may be used to inflict injury on a child. Often the choice of an instrument is a matter of convenience. Marks tend to silhouette or outline the shape of the instrument. The possibility of intentional trauma should prompt a high degree of suspicion when injuries to a child are geometric, paired, mirrored, of various ages or types, or on relatively protected parts of the body. Early recognition of intentional trauma is important to provide therapy and prevent escalation to more serious injury.

patible with a single event. Dark skin may mask bruises. Wrenching or pulling an extremity of an infant may result in a corner chip or "bucket-handle" fracture of the metaphysis. Inflicted fractures of the shaft are more likely to be spiral from twisting rather than transverse from impact. Spiral fractures of the femur before the age of walking are usually inflicted. Cardiopulmonary resuscitation or accidental impact rarely causes rib fractures or retinal hemorrhages in children. The earliest manifestation of fracture healing, manifesting as callus formation, is 7–10 days. Skull fractures cannot be dated.

Hair that is pulled causes alopecia in which the hairs are broken at various lengths. Infants who are left to lie on their backs from neglect or to prevent sudden infant death syndrome (SIDS) may have a flattened occiput with an overlying area of missing hair. Bruises, scars, internal organ damage, and fractures in various stages of healing should suggest the battered child syndrome.

Petechiae of the face and shoulders from intense retching, coughing, crying, or straining may be mistaken for abuse, as may a variety of conditions such as mongolian spots, capillary hemangiomas, pigmented nevi, and other congenital, allergic, self-inflicted, and infectious skin conditions. A single 1-cm, round lesion of impetigo may be difficult to differentiate from a cigarette burn that has become infected. Blood dyscrasias and coagulopathies result in readier bruising. Old and new fractures may be seen in specific chromosomal disorders or rare conditions such as Wilson disease, Schmid-like metaphyseal chondrodysplasia, and osteogenesis imperfecta. Severe monilia of the diaper area may suggest an immersion burn.

Approximately 10% of cases of physical abuse involve *burns*. The shape or pattern of a burn may be diagnostic when it reflects the pattern of an object or method of injury. Cigarette burns produce circular, punched-out lesions of uniform size (Fig. 35–3). An immersion burn occurs when a child is placed in hot water intentionally or unintentionally. Immersion in 147°F water for 1 sec can result in a second-degree burn. Extremity immersions result in glove or stocking burn patterns. When a child's body is placed in hot water, the level of burn demarcation is uniform and distinct. Flexion creases may be spared when the child protectively flexes the extremities. Depending on how the child is held when immersed, the hands and feet may be spared

and splash burns are not expected. The immersion burn pattern is incompatible with falling into a tub or turning on the hot water while in the bathtub. It is necessary to ascertain the developmental skills of the child, water temperature, tub height, and knob type in the investigation of scald burns. Children younger than 24 mo of age may not be able to enter a tub or turn a rotary knob. Immersion burns are most common in infants.

The most common cause of death from physical abuse is *intentional head trauma* (IHT). Twenty-nine per cent of child abuse reports from a children's hospital recorded injuries to the head, face, or cranial contents. More than 95% of serious intracranial injuries during the 1st yr of life are the result of IHT. If an injured infant presents with coma, convulsions, apnea, and increased intracranial pressure, head injury should be considered. A CT scan may reveal intracranial bleeding. An eye exam may reveal retinal hemorrhages. More subtle symptoms of central nervous system (CNS) injury, such as vomiting, irritability, or lethargy, may be misdiagnosed as due to other causes. A missed diagnosis of IHT can lead to further injury, morbidity, and mortality. A bloody spinal tap may not be iatrogenic, particularly if xanthochromia is present. Subdural hematomas in which there are no scalp marks or skull fractures may result from a blow from a hand. The source of injury may be revealed at autopsy when a subgaleal hand print is found. Although grab marks or metaphyseal fractures and rib fractures have been described in association with *shaking* (acceleration-deceleration) and slamming the head against an object, there may be no external marks or fractures. Retinal hemorrhages are seen in 85% of infants who are shaken. They occur commonly with normal birth and rarely with coagulopathies, blood dyscrasias, meningitis, endocarditis, severe hypertension, cardiopulmonary resuscitation, or impact trauma.

Intra-abdominal injuries from impacts are the second most common cause of death in battered children. Affected children may present with recurrent vomiting, abdominal distention, absent bowel sounds, localized tenderness, or shock. Because the abdominal wall is flexible, the overlying skin may be free of bruises. If the child is struck with a fist, a row of three to four 1-cm teardrop-shaped bruises in a slight curve may be seen. The blows may result in a ruptured liver or spleen or perforation or laceration of the small intestine at sites of ligamental support,

BURN MARKS

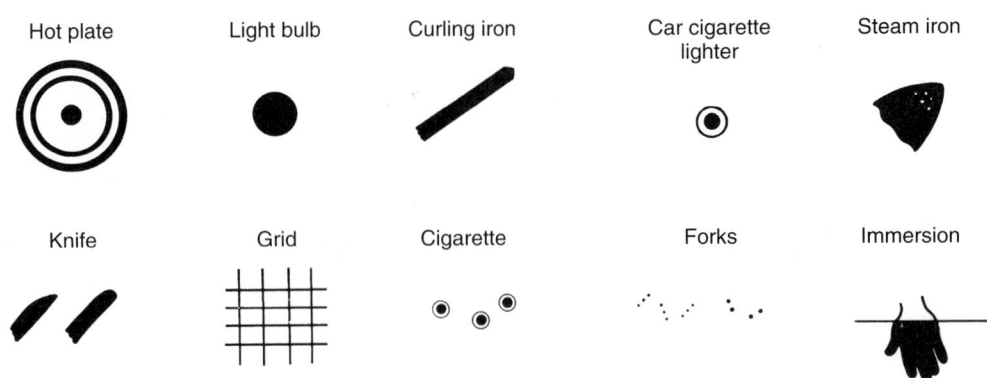

FIGURE 35–3. Marks from heated objects cause burns in a pattern that duplicates that of the object. Familiarity with the common heated objects that are used to traumatize children facilitates recognition of possible intentional injuries. The location of the burn is important in determining its cause. Children tend to explore surfaces with the palmar surface of the hand and rarely touch a heated object repeatedly.

such as the duodenum and proximal jejunum. Intramural hematomas at these sites can lead to temporary obstruction. Chylous ascites and pseudocyst of the pancreas also have been reported from intentional injury.

Laboratory Findings. Screening tests should be obtained in all cases of bruising to rule out a bleeding diathesis. These tests include a prothrombin time, partial thromboplastin time, and platelet count. Abnormal results may follow intracranial bleeding. Children with a hematologic condition, or any chronic condition, may also be abused.

When physical abuse is suspected in a child younger than 2 yr, a *roentgenologic bone survey* consisting of multiple views of the skull, thorax, long bones, hands, feet, pelvis, and spine is necessary. These films should be repeated in 7–10 days to reveal healing of fractures not seen on the initial films. Bone scans may be of value in detecting new fractures of the hands, feet, or ribs. They are not valuable in detecting skull fractures. For children 2–4 yr of age, a bone survey is indicated unless the child is adequately verbal, has very minor injuries, or was in a witnessed and supervised setting (e.g., preschool) when injured. For verbal children older than 4 or 5 yr, roentgenograms need be obtained only if there is bone tenderness or a limited range of motion on physical examination. If films of a tender site are negative, they should be repeated in 7–10 days to detect any calcification, subperiosteal bleeding, or nondisplaced epiphyseal separations that were initially undetected. Bone trauma is found in 10–20% of physically abused children. Fractures considered highly specific for child abuse include metaphyseal, rib, scapular, outer end of clavicle, vertebral, and finger in preambulating children; fractures of different ages; bilateral fractures; and complex skull fractures. Midclavicular, simple linear, and single diaphyseal fractures have a low specificity for abuse. Despite an absence of CNS abnormalities, a head CT scan, ophthalmologic exam, and, if indicated, an MRI study should be obtained when an infant has been severely injured. Fractures, burns, or bruises may be associated with an old or a new head injury. Liver and pancreatic enzyme studies or an abdominal CT scan may uncover damage to these organs. Urine and stool should be screened for blood if abdominal trauma is suspected.

Diagnosis. Suspicion of physical abuse or neglect is usually based on a history that is not in keeping with physical findings or the child's developmental stage. All information should be legibly recorded. All visible lesions should be photographed with a quality analog or digital camera. Color charts, patient identification, and measuring scales should be included in the field. An analysis of the circumstances of the injury is critical. For example, the consequences of a fall depend on (1) child variables, such as surface contacted, age, size, motor skills, motor tone, clothing, and momentum, and (2) environmental variables, such as distance and physical qualities (soft, hard, padded, sharp, dull) of contact surfaces. Data from studies of witnessed falls from hospital beds, bunk beds, windows, and school yard equipment have been used to estimate the force required to cause brain damage and fractures. A fall from 3 ft may rarely result in a simple linear fracture of the skull or clavicle. Falls from 6 ft may rarely result in concussions, subdural hemorrhages, or lacerations. There are no reports of death or severe brain injury from *witnessed* falls of less than 10 ft.

After separation from caretakers, a child older than age 3 yr may be able to tell a sensitive and skillful interviewer that a particular adult hurt him or her. Children may not give a history of intentional injury if they are concerned about retribution from the perpetrator or separation from their home, school, siblings, friends, or nonoffending parent.

The differential diagnosis depends on the particular injuries. For example, roentgenograms of bones in scurvy and syphilis and normally growing bone shafts of infants may resemble nonaccidental bone trauma. The bony changes in these conditions are often symmetric. Children with osteogenesis imperfecta, severe osteomalacia, or sensory deficits (e.g., myelomeningocele or paraplegia) have an increased incidence of pathologic fractures, but rarely of the metaphysis.

Treatment. Appropriate medical, surgical, and psychiatric treatment should be promptly initiated. The law requires that a child *suspected* of being abused or neglected be reported immediately to CPS. Children with suspected abuse should not be discharged from the clinic or office without consulting the county CPS agency. The caseworker confers with the physician to determine whether the child will be safe if released to a parent or whether the child should be taken to an agency office. Ideally a caseworker should come to the hospital or office to evaluate the situation and determine the child's future safety and the need for crisis services. Children and siblings at risk for serious abuse should be placed in homes of appropriate relatives or emergency receiving homes. CPS workers are expected to provide a case plan, which delineates intensive services that lead to the safe return of the child to the home if the plan is followed. CPS should complete its investigation within a reasonable stipulated time. The role of law enforcement is to perform forensic scene investigations, to interview suspects, and, if a criminal act has taken place, to inform the prosecutor's office. In most states, 48 hr after the initial report by telephone or fax by a mandated reporter, a *written* and detailed report is required. The latter is best accomplished using a printed form.

Hospital admission is indicated for children (1) whose medical or surgical condition requires inpatient management, (2) in whom the diagnosis is unclear, and (3) when no alternative safe place for custody is immediately available. If the safety of the child is in doubt, the physician, agency, and court should err on the side of protecting the child. If the parents refuse hospitalization or treatment, an emergency court order must be obtained. The parents should be told by the physician why an inflicted injury is suspected, that the physician is legally obligated to report the circumstance, that the referral is being made to protect the child, that the family will be provided with services, and that a CPS social worker and law enforcement officer will be involved. Siblings and children baby-sat by suspected abusers should have full examinations within 24 hr of the recognition of child abuse. Approximately 20% of them will be found to have signs of physical abuse. Children younger than 2 yr should have skeletal surveys.

Professionals should anticipate anger from abusing or neglectful parents; however, expressing anger in response to parental behavior damages rapport, increases defensiveness, and makes their cooperation less likely. Repeated interrogations, confrontations, and accusations may be avoided by involving CPS workers and law enforcement as a team during the investigation. If the child is hospitalized, the supervised parents should be encouraged to visit, and the hospital staff must be counseled to be courteous, helpful, and observant. The primary physician should maintain contact with the parents. An evaluation by hospital social services and pastoral care should be obtained to determine existing problems, needs, and strengths in the family. An agency caseworker and, when needed, a police officer should visit the home. A psychiatric evaluation of the parents and siblings may be indicated.

Hospitals caring for children should have a team of professionals who are trained and skilled in child abuse recognition, reporting, and services. This team should include a pediatrician, a hospital social worker, a pediatric nurse, a psychologist or psychiatrist, and a data coordinator. Roles of all team members as well as public agencies involved should be formalized in a community plan and clinical pathways. Legal and medical specialty consultants should be available. When evaluations are completed, the team should meet with the child's primary care physician, ward nurse, the CPS representative, and, as appropriate, a law enforcement officer, prosecutor, or any other member of the community agencies involved with the family to share information, clarify medical and social findings, and plan immediate and long-range goals and therapies.

Child welfare agencies are responsible for developing and monitoring a case plan for the child and family. It is important for the pediatrician to coordinate the health care of the abused child. Abused and neglected children require more intensive surveillance and well child care than do nonabused children. Placement in foster care may interrupt preventive care and treatment of acute and chronic illnesses. Because of the number of difficulties experienced by abusive families, no single agency or discipline can provide all the needed services. Services may include parent aides, homemakers, Parents Anonymous groups, telephone hotlines, environmental crisis therapy, substance abuse treatment, Big Brothers and Big Sisters, "foster" grandparents, anger management, and child-rearing counseling. Unless the parent has a serious mental illness, traditional psychotherapy, especially in isolation, may be ineffective.

Prevention. The pediatrician's role in primary abuse prevention includes identifying parents at high risk for being unable to accept, love, and properly discipline and care for their offspring. The history obtained from all parents should include information about pregnancy planning, pregnancy, emotional and physical health, domestic violence, and attitudes about the child and child-rearing experiences and techniques. Parental risks include a history of family violence or child abuse, drug addiction, depression, lack of support, socioeconomic problems, serious psychiatric illness, mental retardation, young parental age, closely spaced pregnancies, single-parent status of the mother, negative parental comments about the newborn infant, lack of evidence of maternal attachment, infrequent visits to a new infant whose discharge is delayed because of prematurity or illness, inappropriate anger toward or spanking of an infant younger than 18 mo or a handicapped child, and neglect of infant hygiene. The use of an instrument on any part of the body, a bruise from corporal punishment, or striking any part of the body aside from the hands or buttocks should be considered inappropriate and reportable. Child risks include mental or physical handicap, chronic illness, prematurity, being a twin, and learning or behavior problems. Abuse and serious neglect may be prevented when at-risk families receive intensive training and support during pregnancy and after delivery. Prevention efforts should include early and frequent contact between mother and baby in the delivery room, rooming-in, increased parental contact with premature infants, extra help calming the crying or "difficult" infant, more frequent office visits for at-risk infants, ongoing counseling regarding discipline and the use of nonphysical responses to behaviors, public health nurse visits or trained home visitors, parenting classes, stress and anger management classes, close follow-up of acute and chronic illnesses, telephone hotlines, arrangement for child care or preschool, and assistance in family planning.

Prognosis. Early studies of abused children returned to their parents without any intervention indicate that about 5% are subsequently killed and that 25% are seriously re-injured. With comprehensive, intensive family treatment, 80–90% of families involved in child maltreatment may be rehabilitated to provide adequate care for their children. Approximately 10–15% of maltreating families, especially those with a history of substance abuse, can only be stabilized and will require an indefinite continuation of supporting services, which may include drug monitoring, until their children are old enough to leave home. Termination of parental rights or continued foster placement is required in 2–3% of cases. If a parent is unable to respond to a treatment plan, this should be documented as soon as possible to afford the child the opportunity to develop in a healthy and permanent home.

Children with injuries to the CNS may develop mental retardation, learning problems, behavior problems, blindness, deafness, motor problems, organic brain syndrome, seizures, hydrocephalus, and ataxia. Common emotional traits of abused children include fearfulness, aggression, hypervigilance, denial, projection, post-traumatic stress disorder (PTSD), a lack of trust, low self-esteem, juvenile delinquency, substance abuse, and hyperactivity. Unsuccessful treatment may result in children who become bullies, juvenile delinquents, violent and antisocial adults, spouse and elderly abusers, and the next generation of child abusers.

35.1 Sexual Abuse

Sexual abuse includes any activity with a child, before the age of legal consent, that is for the sexual gratification of an adult or a significantly older child. Sexual abuse includes oral-genital, genital-genital, genital-rectal, hand-genital, hand-rectal, or hand-breast contact; exposure of sexual anatomy; forced viewing of sexual anatomy; and showing of pornography to a child or using a child in the production of pornography. Sexual intercourse includes vaginal, oral, or rectal penetration. Penetration is entry into an orifice with or without tissue injury. Younger perpetrators tend to have younger victims but are more likely to have intercourse with older victims. Sex acts perpetrated by young children are learned behaviors and are associated with experiencing sexual abuse or exposure to adult sex or pornography. Without detection and intervention, sexual abuse may progress from touching to intercourse. *Sexual play,* on the other hand, may be defined as viewing or touching of the genitals, buttocks, or chest by preadolescent children separated by not more than 4 yr, in which there has been no force or coercion. See Chapter 26 for a discussion of the development of sexual identity and behavior.

Sexual mistreatment of children by family members (incest) and nonrelatives known to the child is the most common type of sexual abuse. The *least common* offender is a stranger. Intrafamilial sexual abuse is difficult to document and manage, because the child must be protected from additional abuse and coercion to not reveal or to deny the abuse while attempts are made to preserve the family unit. Children also may be coerced to recant accusations of abuse by relatives, or they may decide to recant the abuse for fear of ridicule or teasing, retaliation, attendance in court, or loss of contact with needed or loved relatives and friends.

Epidemiology. Most of the increase in child abuse reports through 1992 were due to increased reporting of sexual abuse. The rate of sexual abuse, estimated by the American Association for Protecting Children, went from 1.4/10,000 to 17/10,000 children between 1976 and 1984. Surveys of adult women indicate that from 12–38% were sexually abused by 18 yr of age. The results of one study indicated that the likelihood of extrafamilial and intrafamilial sexual abuse being reported were 8% and 2%, respectively. The incidence of sexual abuse of males ranges from 3–9% of the population, accounting for up to 20% of reports. Because fixed pedophiles show a predilection for boys, it is theorized that the number of males who are sexually abused is higher. Furthermore, boys may refrain from reporting what they might interpret as a homosexual action or a consequence of their failure to protect themselves from assault. From 1992 to 1999, NCANDS data revealed a 39% decline in instances of substantiated cases. State officials cite the following reasons for this decline: (1) increased evidence needed for substantiation, (2) increased caseworker caution due to new legal rights of caregivers, and (3) limitations on cases accepted, effectiveness of prevention programs, and increased prosecution and public awareness. Incarceration of perpetrators and an improved economy are other theories for this decrease.

In 1997, 679 reports (71% of all abuse reports) from a children's hospital were for sexual abuse. Of 744 patients referred to a diagnostic clinic for suspected sexual abuse, 230 (31%) were reported. A lack of substantiation may be due to a child's young age and inability to give a detailed history or a lack of significant physical or laboratory findings. Caregivers may mistake genital erythema, enuresis, masturbation, or nonspecific behaviors as being due to sexual abuse. Suspicion may be increased during divorce proceedings due to distrust of the other parent and changes in the child's behavior caused by the divorce process. Approximately one third of sexual abuse victims are younger than 6 yr of age; one third are 6–12 yr of age; and one third are 12–18 yr of age. Reported offenders are 97% male. Females are more often perpetrators in child-care settings, including baby sitting. The number of female perpetrators may be higher because younger children may confuse sexual abuse by a female with normal hygiene care, and adolescent males may not be trained to recognize sexual activity with an older female as a form of abuse. Sexual abuse by stepfathers is nearly five times higher than by natural fathers. Incest is described in most cultures and is seen at all socioeconomic levels to a greater degree than are physical abuse and neglect.

Etiology. The abuse of daughters by fathers and stepfathers is the most common form of reported incest, although brother-sister incest is considered to be the most common type. Studies of incarcerated adult perpetrators indicate that sexual abuse begins with selection of vulnerable and available victims, innocent physical contact, and seduction through gifts and attention. The propensity for pedophiles to become sexually involved with children often appears in their adolescence. Pedophiles have indicated that they seek positions and opportunities where they can be in contact with potential victims. The vulnerable children they described include those with mental and physical handicaps, unloved and unwanted children, previously abused children, children in single-parent families, children of drug abusers, their own children, and children with low self-esteem and poor achievement. Pornography may be used to initiate sexual activity with a child. Threats and bribes may be used to entice children and keep them from telling. Boys and girls may be told that they are at fault because they did not protect themselves. Care must be exercised when evaluating these data as the characteristics of incarcerated perpetrators or perpetrators in therapy, upon which many study results are based, may be different from those of other perpetrators. Obedience and trust of adults, coupled with a need to maintain family unity, are factors associated with incest. A father's need for sexual gratification and a daughter's need for affection and nurturance may lead to incest when the mother is unavailable and there is a desire to maintain the family unit. These incestuous fathers have been described as rigid, patriarchal, and emotionally immature. They are unlikely to engage in extramarital relationships, and there is a high incidence of alcoholism. The mothers have been described as chronically depressed, unavailable to their husbands because of work or illness, and often the victims of childhood sexual abuse. The child victim tends to be pseudomature and to have taken on many of the adult roles, including housekeeping. The tendency for some of these families to be closely knit and socially isolated prevents detection.

Violence is not common in sexual abuse; however, its incidence increases with the age and size of the victim and specific traits in the perpetrator. Violence is more likely to occur in association with a single incident by a stranger. In cases of violent incest, the father has been described as sociopathic, with sexual abuse extending outside the family circle.

Clinical Manifestations. A child may disclose sexual abuse to the mother and be brought to a physician at that time. If the mother does not believe the child, the child may delay further comment indefinitely or later tell a friend, relative, friend's mother, teacher, or school counselor. Children, given the opportunity, may disclose their abuse to a physician in a private interview or during a physical examination. Sexual abuse should be considered as the cause of physical symptoms such as (1) vaginal, penile, or rectal pain, discharge, bruising, erythema, or bleeding; (2) chronic dysuria, enuresis, constipation, or encopresis; and (3) rarely, premature puberty in a female. Certain behaviors, although more likely to be associated with sexual abuse, have not been found to be diagnostic. They include sexualized activity with peers, animals, or objects; seductive behavior; and age-inappropriate sexual knowledge and curiosity. Nonspecific behaviors include suicide gestures, fear of an individual or place, nightmares, sleep disorders, regression, aggression, withdrawn behavior, PTSD (see Chapter 22), low self-esteem, depression, poor school performance, running away, self-mutilation, anxiety, fire setting, multiple personalities, somatization, phobias, trauma, prostitution, drug abuse, eating disorders, dysmenorrhea, and dyspareunia. Because of secrecy, a desire to protect the abuser or family, or threats by the abuser, the cause of symptoms or behaviors may be denied by the child. When the perpetrator is a breadwinner or is violent, it may also be denied by the nonoffending and dependent parent.

Investigating the possibility of sexual abuse requires supportive, sensitive, and detailed *history* taking. Because of variance in the type of abuse, the ages of the victim and perpetrator, and the time since abuse, less than 15% of cases yield physical or laboratory findings. Ideally, the videotaped forensic interview, which uses open-ended, nonleading questions, should be conducted on one occasion by one or two experienced interviewers in the presence of law enforcement and social service workers who observe behind a one-way mirror. This obviates the need for repeated interviews and possible further trauma to the child. After an initial interview, children who gain trust and comfort may experience a decrease in guilt and fear of reprisal or loss of love and give more detailed information in subsequent interviews. Interviewing should proceed at the child's pace and level of development. It should begin with discussion of general topics and naming of body parts, including "private" parts, and proceed to details about each incident. The sophistication of the information that can be obtained from the child varies with the development of the child and the skill of the interviewer. Anatomic pictures may help clarify the names of body parts and aid in describing the abuse. Anatomically correct dolls, used with young children, may be considered to be suggestive or leading. If a social worker or law enforcement officer has carried out the initial interview, the physician should review this material and decide whether it is necessary to repeat the interview before performing a physical examination. Questions about the abusive actions, including symptoms of trauma, may be asked during the physical examination. Familiarity with the child through participation in the forensic interview, a previous examination, or sick and well child care contacts facilitates a cooperative and nontraumatic physical examination.

PHYSICAL EXAMINATION. Older female and male victims may prefer that a physician of the same sex examine them; when possible, their desires should be respected. A thorough physical *examination* should be conducted, with special attention to the neck and mouth. If present, bite marks should be measured, and wax impressions and wiping for saliva should be done to aid in identification of the perpetrator. The mouth should be examined for redness, abrasions, or purpura that may be due to recent trauma. The abdominal examination should assess the possibility of pregnancy. The rectum should be examined for signs of trauma.

A young female who is resistant despite preparation may be examined while sitting on the parent's lap. Occasionally, the child will be able to separate the labia or buttocks herself. The examination should be explained to the girl; anxiety can be reduced by distracting her. She can be asked to blow on a pinwheel, sing, or count. The female is most easily examined in the supine frog leg position. The hymen is exposed by separation of the labia laterally or by grasping the labia majora with the gloved thumbs and forefingers and gently tugging the labia toward the examiner (Fig. 35–4). This labial traction is best accomplished by an assistant while the genitals are viewed in good lighting and with magnification. If abnormalities are

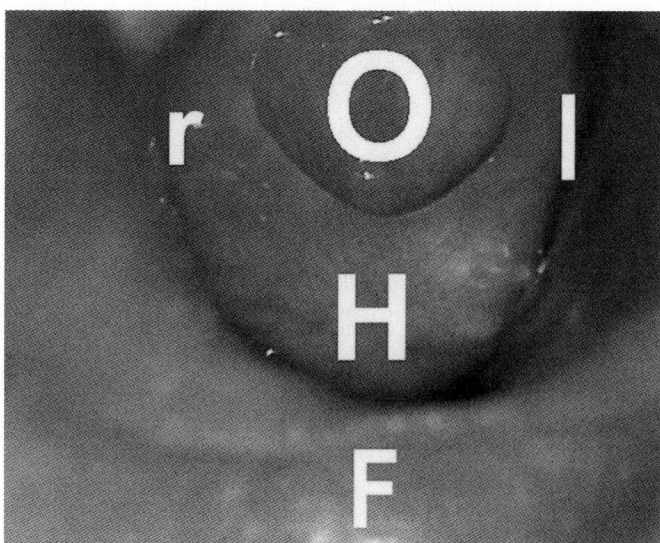

FIGURE 35–4. Normal hymen. This is the hymen of an 8 yr old. The hymen opening (O) has a delicate and almost transparent edge. There is a right (r) and left (l) wall, which may vary in size from 1 to 3 mm. The base of the hymen (H) may vary from 1 to 4 mm. The term *attenuation* is applied to the base when it is less than 1 mm wide. The fourchette (F) is the joining of the labia minora posteriorly. It may be injured from trauma. The vestibule, or space anterior to the hymen which is surrounded by the labia minora, may be penetrated without damage to the hymen.

found on supine examination, the child should be re-examined in the prone knee-chest position. In that position, gravity allows better visualization of the hymen anatomy and confirmation of suspected abnormalities. There are several normal shapes to the hymen. In the infant or prepubertal child, flaps or tabs on the hymen may obscure the opening. This is rectified when drops of sterile saline are used to "float" the tabs, revealing the opening. Maternal hormones thicken the newborn's hymen in a manner similar to the effects of endogenous hormones in adolescence. As this hormone effect wanes, by 1 yr the hymen becomes thin, in some cases to the point of transparency with visible vascularity. As the hymen thickens in adolescence (Fig. 35–5), it folds on itself. This undulation makes the hymen more distendible and the examination of the hymen rim more difficult. A moist cotton swab, a swab covered with a rubber balloon or, less commonly, a Foley catheter may assist in the examination. The Foley is inserted through the hymen opening and then inflated with saline before being drawn against the inner hymen wall. Opening size of the hymen is not considered of diagnostic value. The examination of the hymen, which is facilitated by the use of magnification and proper lighting from a colposcope, should include inspection of the fourchette, the introitus, the urethra, and the edge of the hymen. A speculum examination of the vagina with collection of specimens is indicated when the victim is postpubertal or when nonmenstrual vaginal bleeding or major trauma of the external genitals is present. No child should be forced to have an examination. General anesthesia or sedation may be required if the examination is deemed necessary or if there is bleeding from the rectum or vagina.

Drawings of trauma should be supplemented with photographs or video recordings using the colposcope or photos from a hand-held analog or digital camera with a macro lens. "Suggestive findings" or findings in keeping with a history of

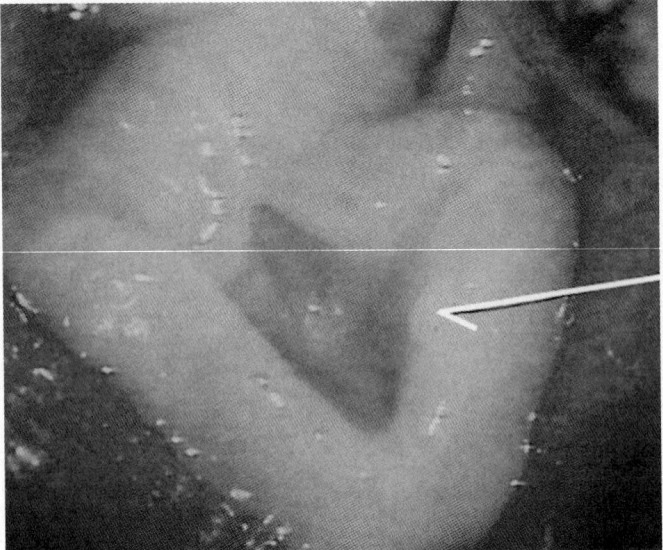

FIGURE 35–5. Hymen with estrogen effects and wart. With the onset of puberty, the hymen becomes thickened, paler in color, and redundant. The resulting folds make it difficult to determine whether there are abnormalities of the edge of the hymen. The *arrow* points to a glistening bump on the left hymen wall. This is a venereal wart. The appearance of these warts varies with location. Other warts on the skin surface were dark in color with an irregular "cauliflower-like" appearance.

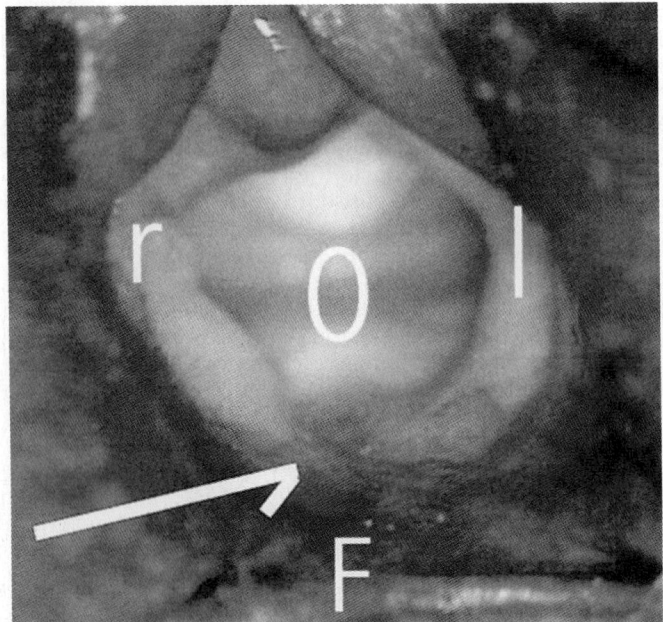

FIGURE 35–6. Hymen tear. The base (*arrow*) of the hymen has been torn to the floor of the vagina. The injury, from finger insertion according to the 8-year-old child, is bleeding. The fourchette (F) has escaped injury. Careful observation may reveal complete healing of the injury over time. The tear also may heal with a V-shaped notch, or remain separated.

sexual abuse include (1) a hymen with new or healed lacerations and transections (Fig. 35–6), remnants, and attenuation; (2) posterior fourchette lacerations; (3) vaginal wall tears; and (4) perianal lacerations. The presence of sperm and semen is "clear evidence" of sexual abuse. Other suggestive findings include bite marks on the genitals or inner thigh or scarring or tears of the labia minora. Straddle injuries usually result in trauma to the labia and clitoris and rarely involve the relatively protected hymen. Accidental penetration of the hymen is unusual and is associated with penetration of underclothing and possibly the wall of the vagina.

Abnormal findings even with a history of repeated anal penetration are unusual. A fissure can result from the insertion of an object larger than the child's normal stool. The use of lubrication may minimize penetration damage. Frequent passage or insertion of a dilating object can result in decreased anal tone and changes in the appearance of anal folds. Examination by an experienced professional, with photo documentation, is necessary if there are any questions about anogenital findings. If immediate dilation of the anus reveals an anterior-posterior diameter greater than 20 mm, with no stool present in the rectal ampulla, that is a strong marker for possible abuse, warranting further investigation. Scar formation, even following an episode of forceful sodomy, is unusual. There are two common, midline, naturally occurring entities that may be confused with scar tissue in the perianal region. The first is a smooth, wedged-shaped area known as *diastasis ani*. This can be found either anterior or posterior to the anus. The second finding is an extension of the median or perineal raphe that has a taglike appearance on the anterior side of the anus. Anal fissures, decreased anal tone, or disruption of folds must be interpreted with caution, because they can be the result of chronic constipation or underlying disease, such as Crohn disease.

Injuries to the male genitals are usually the result of an accident or physical abuse. A bite mark may be found. The forceful retraction of the foreskin may result in a dehiscence of the tissues. Injury from a sexual assault most likely causes a nonspecific, transitory redness of the penis. Routine examination of the genitals of males and females facilitates recognition of normal findings and helps guarantee future cooperation from the child.

Laboratory Findings. Laboratory investigation depends on the history and the time since injury. When a victim is seen within 72 hr of sexual abuse, clothing and skin should be swabbed with a moist cotton applicator. A variety of substances, including urine, fluoresce under a Wood lamp. In addition, specimens of possible offender blood and hair and the victim's nail clippings and clothing should be collected. Tests for rectal blood may be indicated. If there is a history of contact with the perpetrator's genitals, gonorrhea and *Chlamydia* cultures should be obtained from the mouth, anus, and genitals. In the vagina, motile sperm can be found for 6 hr; nonmotile sperm exist for longer than 72 hr. Acid phosphatase is present for 24 hr. Sperm and semen may also be recovered from the mouth, rectum, and clothing. Although the presence of semen substantiates the victim's history of vaginal intercourse, the absence of semen does not contradict it. Less than 5% of victims have positive cultures for gonorrhea or *Chlamydia*. Symptomatic victims, those with positive cultures for other venereal diseases, and children with a history of contact with the perpetrator's genitals should also be tested for syphilis, HIV, and hepatitis B. All specimens should be transferred to the forensic laboratory in sealed, signed, and dated envelopes to ensure an official chain of evidence.

Diagnosis. It is most common for the diagnosis of sexual abuse to depend on the history offered by the victim. False accusations are rare except in unusual cases involving adolescents, emotionally disturbed patients, or patients in custody disputes. Abuse may be revealed during a custody dispute because the child has been separated from an offender and is able to communicate without fear of retaliation or further abuse. The genitals and rectum may heal completely after extensive trauma, and minor trauma, such as abrasions, may heal within 3–4 days. The tear may remain separated, heal to the point where it cannot be easily differentiated from normal, or heal with a V-shaped notch (see Fig. 35–6). Healing depends on the degree of trauma; however, the most severe trauma, requiring surgical repair, may appear normal after a year or less. There may be no observable physical trauma in as many as 85% of children who report sexual abuse. The anus or vagina may not be penetrated, although there is pain experienced. Superficial injuries such as abrasions or erythema heal in days with no lasting signs. Certain types of sexual abuse such as oral or digital stimulation or labial intercourse may not result in tissue damage. If an inserted object is smaller than the expanded size of an opening, no tissue damage would be expected. The data from an interview by a professional trained and experienced in forensic interviewing techniques should not be minimized because there are no physical findings. In one study of 18 victims whose abusers confessed to vaginal penetration, seven children had normal genital examination findings. Abnormal physical or laboratory findings should be reported even if no history is available.

Laboratory findings of pregnancy, sperm, semen, and *nonpregnancy-* or *delivery-related* syphilis, gonorrhea, *Chlamydia*, herpes type II (genital), and HIV may be considered diagnostic of sexual abuse and reported. Condyloma acuminatum appearing after 3 yr of age and *Trichomonas vaginalis* are considered "probably diagnostic." Herpes type I and nonvenereal warts may be autoinoculated to the genitorectal area or transmitted by a perpetrator's mouth or hand. The significance of bacterial vaginosis and genital *Mycoplasma* infection is uncertain. New techniques, such as DNA typing of blood, semen, sperm, or tissue, may positively identify the perpetrator.

Treatment. Sexual abuse is a criminal offense and is investigated by the police. All victims of sexual abuse require psychologic support. Parents, relatives, and siblings may deny the accusation and rebuke or punish the child for reporting the incident. The consequences and appropriate therapy of sexual abuse vary, depending on the type of abuse, the age and other physical and emotional factors in the victim, the frequency of abuse, and the identity of the abuser. Victims of a single nonviolent episode of touching or exposure by a stranger may require reassurance and a chance to express feelings about the event in one or two therapy sessions. Victims may be less distressed by the incident than their parents. In contrast, a single episode of family-related sexual abuse may cause serious, long-term emotional distress and require prolonged individual and group treatment. The therapist may recommend that the victim of incest be returned home if the perpetrator is out of the home or has confessed and is in therapy. The child victim should be placed in foster care if this is his or her desire; if the nonoffending parent is not protective of the child, does not believe the child's story, or is likely to encourage the child to recant; and if family life is chaotic or collection of evidence is not yet complete. Medication to prevent pregnancy may be given to postmenarchal girls in midcycle who have experienced vaginal intercourse within the previous 72 hr. Treatment with antibiotics is initiated to prevent sexually transmitted disease if the perpetrator is known to be infected, if the victim has signs of infection, or if the likelihood of follow-up is poor. All victims should revisit their primary care physicians within 2 wk to ensure that recommended services have been implemented.

Incest offenders may respond to treatment, but success requires a coordinated, multifaceted, multidisciplinary approach. The offending parent and spouse should be referred for psychiatric or psychologic evaluation. The police should investigate offenders, and criminal prosecution should be supported. There is evidence, especially in pedophilia, that incarceration may ensure access to, and efficacy of, simultaneous treatment. Incarceration of a breadwinner may have serious adverse consequences for the family. The behavior of chronic sexual offenders may be resistant to a variety of therapies. All juvenile and prejuvenile offenders should receive therapy to prevent recurrences. In one diagnostic center, 17% of offenders were younger than 17 yr of age.

Prevention. The primary prevention of sexual abuse is related, in part, to normal developmental education and sexual behavior (Chapter 26). Teaching children the proper names of all body parts, including the names, function, and significance of "private parts" (nipples, genitals, and rectum) should begin in the home and continue in the pediatrician's office and school. Children should be taught to say "no" to any action by any person that makes them uncomfortable—but especially actions directed to their "private" areas. They should be given the opportunity to report to a trusted adult any of these actions. Caregivers, including baby sitters and their companions and the boyfriends of single mothers, should be carefully screened. Written permission should be obtained from any caregiver to allow a police screening for offenses. Victim therapy should decrease the potential for re-abuse. Routine family and classroom discussions of uncomfortable events in the lives of children may reveal unsuspected abuse. To improve diagnostic skills, physicians should examine the genitals and rectum routinely, record their findings, become familiar with normal rectal and genital anatomy and the consequences of trauma, listen to and seriously consider what children tell them, and be willing to report and testify when abuse is suspected.

Prognosis. With early and adequate intervention, victims may lead normal adult lives. However, even with intervention, certain adolescent victims may run away from home and fall prey to adolescent prostitution, violence, drug addiction, and unprepared parenthood (see Chapter 39). Others who remain at home may manifest a variety of emotional problems, including depression, suicidal gestures, deterioration in school performance, and conversion reactions. As adults, victims may have difficulties with close relationships; enter abusive relationships; have a variety of somatic complaints of the genitourinary, gastrointestinal, and other systems; and need psychiatric help for depression, anxiety, substance abuse, dissociation, and eating disorders. The risk of untoward effects is greatest for incest victims.

35.2 Nonorganic Failure to Thrive

See Chapter 36 for a full discussion of organic and nonorganic failure to thrive (NOFTT). NOFTT occurs when a child, usually an infant, is not fed adequate calories. The mother may neglect proper feeding because she is involved with external demands and the care of others; is preoccupied with inner problems or depressed; is ignorant about appropriate feeding; is abusing substances; or does not like or understand the infant. Emotional or maternal deprivation is inevitably concurrent with nutritional deprivation. These mothers often feel deprived and unloved themselves and may be acutely or chronically depressed. Multiple and continuing crises, frequently compounded by the physical absence of the father, may overwhelm a mother, who reacts by neglecting her infant. Poverty may also prevent a caregiver from obtaining adequate food for a child. Retarded and emotionally disturbed parents may not have the capacity to provide proper care.

Clinical Manifestations. The dietary history in infants with nutritional neglect may not be accurate because the parent misinforms the physician that the baby is receiving adequate calories. Depending on severity, the infant with NOFTT may exhibit thin extremities, a narrow face, prominent ribs, and wasted buttocks. Neglect of hygiene is evidenced by diaper rash, unwashed skin, untreated impetigo, uncut and dirty fingernails, or unwashed clothing. A flattened occiput with hair loss may indicate that the child has been lying on his or her back. This flattening may be due to being unattended for prolonged periods or positioning to prevent SIDS. Delays in social and speech development are common. Other findings include an avoidance of eye contact, an expressionless face, and the absence of a cuddling response. The amount of time that the mother spends holding, playing with, and talking to her baby is usually reduced or inappropriate. A rejecting or frustrated mother may feed her baby with anger and unnecessary force. This may result in a torn frenulum and an aversion to feeding. Children of all ages may fail to thrive because of intentional or nonintentional malnutrition.

Laboratory Findings. Extensive laboratory evaluation should be delayed until dietary management has been attempted for at least 1 wk and has failed. A skeletal survey is indicated in children younger than 2 yr who have a rejecting parent or evidence of associated physical abuse.

Diagnosis. Children with NOFTT should be hospitalized and given unlimited feedings of a diet appropriate for age for a minimum of 1 wk; this diet usually approaches 150 kcal/kg (ideal weight)/24 hr. Infants with NOFTT usually gain more than 2 oz every 24 hr for 1 wk (approximately 1 lb/wk) or have a gain that is significantly greater than that achieved during a similar period at home. These infants may display a ravenous appetite. A nursing plan should include careful charting of intake, weight, and observations of the mother's feeding style and relationship to the child. The latter may be videotaped for analysis. Deprivational behaviors may improve or resolve in the hospital setting with attention from the staff. Infants who are difficult to feed because of neurologic or mechanical problems may gain weight as a result of the intensive efforts by experienced hospital staff.

Treatment. All cases of NOFTT caused by underfeeding from maternal neglect should be reported to CPS. After appropriate hospital management, approximately 75% of infants are discharged home with added services for the family; 20% go into temporary foster care while the parents receive therapy; and 5% enter long-term foster care with plans for voluntary relinquishment or termination of parental rights. Exercising this last option should be based mainly on the responsiveness of the mother to treatment. Infants who are discharged to their natural home require intensive and long-term intervention. The parents should be provided with clear, written dietary instructions at discharge and be trained to hold the infant close during feedings and to provide frequent and appropriate stimulation. Families may require a homemaker, public health nurse, health visitor, and other types of outreach services. Weekly medical follow-up is necessary to monitor progress.

Prognosis. Without detection and intervention, a small percentage of infants with nutritional neglect die of starvation. Approximately 5–15% of these infants suffer from physical abuse. Weight loss and understature from malnutrition are reversible, but normal head circumference and brain growth may not be achieved if the infant has suffered from NOFTT beyond 6 mo of age. Emotional and educational problems occur in more than half these children.

35.3 Munchausen Syndrome by Proxy (MSBP)

The term *Munchausen syndrome* was used initially to describe situations in which adults falsified their own symptoms. In MSBP, a parent, invariably the mother, simulates or causes disease in a child. The parent may (1) fabricate a medical history; (2) cause symptoms by repeatedly exposing the child to a toxin, medication, infectious agent, or physical trauma, including smothering; or (3) alter laboratory samples or temperature measurements. Depending on the parent's sophistication and secrecy, a variety of convincing, novel, and exotic diseases may be simulated or created. The parent may deny any involvement and, in instances of intentional poisoning, smothering, or trauma, may continue the action while the child is hospitalized. Parents of children hospitalized for evaluation of acute life-threatening events have been videotaped in the process of smothering their children. MSBP is inflicted on children who are either unable or unwilling to identify the true offense and offender. The abusing caregiver gains attention from the relationships formed with health care providers or her own family as a result of the problems created.

Clinical Manifestations. The child's symptoms, their pattern, or the response to treatment may not be compatible with a recognized disease. They may involve any organ system and suggest a panoply of disease processes. Although generally reported in preverbal children, cases have been recognized in children up to 16 yr of age. There may be a history of actual disease in which symptoms persist beyond the time when cure is anticipated. Symptoms in younger children are always associated with the proximity of the mother to the child. The mother may have a background in health care, may be supported by the father who may be unavailable, and may present as a devoted and model parent who forms close relationships with members of the health care team. She may have a history of Munchausen syndrome (MS) and seem relatively unconcerned about the severity of the child's illness.

Apnea and seizures are two common manifestations of MSBP. The observation may be falsified or may be created by partial suffocation. Symptoms also can be created by toxins, medications, water, and salts. Recognition of MSBP requires familiarity with those substances available to families and the wide array of consequences from misuse of these substances. The clinical pattern is variable, depending on the agent. It includes forced ingestion of medications such as ipecac to cause chronic vomiting or laxatives to cause diarrhea, or injection of insulin with consequent seizures. The skin, which is more easily accessible to the perpetrator, may be burned, dyed, tattooed, lacerated, or punctured to simulate acute or chronic skin conditions. Infectious or toxic agents may be administered into any available orifice. Provision of intravenous lines during hospitalization may provide an opportunity for injection of infectious agents from feces, toxins, and pharmacologic agents. Urine and blood samples may be contaminated with foreign blood or stool. Older children may become convinced that they have an illness and dependent on the increased attention attendant upon the situation. This may lead to the child feigning symptoms or to MS.

Diagnosis. Investigations should be based on a high index of suspicion of this diagnosis so that unpleasant, dangerous, or unnecessary tests are not undertaken on the child. Specimens that are carefully collected should be analyzed for potentially harmful agents and for "foreign" blood. All steps in the diagnosis should be carefully documented. Records from other hospitals for the index child and siblings should be obtained and carefully reviewed. Hospitalized children should be under constant surveillance. This may include hidden television monitoring in coordination with law enforcement. Frequent staff meetings with detailed minutes are necessary to ensure that all information is gathered and recorded in a planned and forensic manner.

Treatment. After all laboratory information is collected and the diagnosis is established, the offending parent should be confronted by a nonaccusatory physician and staff who offer help. Any approach may be met with resistance, denial, and threats. All cases should be reported promptly and with careful documentation to CPS. The consequences of MSBP include persistence of abuse, emotional problems, chronic disability in 8% of cases, and death. Other siblings may be, or may have been, at risk; there is an association of this syndrome with unexplained infant deaths.

General

American Humane Association, Children's Division, 63 Inverness Drive East, Englewood, CO 80112-5117. Email http://www.amerhumane.org

American Professional Society Against Child Abuse, 407 South Dearborn, Suite 1300, Chicago, IL 60605. Email http://www.apsac.org

Belsey MA: Child abuse: Measuring a global problem. *World Health Stat Q* 1993;46:69.

Block RW: Child abuse—Controversies and imposters. *Curr Probl Pediatr* 1999;29:253–72.

Committee on Child Abuse and Neglect, 2nd Committee on Children with Disabilities: Assessment of maltreatment of children with disabilities. *Pediatrics* 2001;108:508–11.

Drum PD, Cummings P, Krauss MR, et al: Identified spouse abuse as a risk factor for child abuse. *Child Abuse Negl* 2000;24:1375–81.

Gallup Organization: *Disciplining Children in America. A Gallup Poll Report.* Princeton, NJ, 1995.

Herman-Giddens ME, Brown G, Verblest S, et al: Underascertainment of child abuse mentality in the United States. *JAMA* 1999;282:463–7.

Meyers JEB, Berliner L, Briere J, et al (editors): *The APSAC Handbook on Child Maltreatment*, 2nd ed. Thousand Oaks, CA, Sage Publications, 2002.

Monteleone JA: *Quick-Reference Child Abuse.* St Louis, GW Medical Publishing, 1998.

Monteleone JA, Brodeur AE (editors): *Child Maltreatment: A Clinical Guide and Reference.* St Louis, GW Publishing, 2000 (in press).

Overpeck MD, Brenner RA, Trumble AC, et al: Risk factors for infant homicide in the United States. *N Engl J Med* 1998;339:1211.

Reece RM, Ludwig S (editors): *Child Abuse Medical Diagnosis and Management.* Baltimore, Lippincott Williams & Wilkins, 2001.

Windom MD: *Injury Prevention and Control in Children and Youth.* Elk Grove, IL, American Academy of Pediatrics, 1997.

US Department of Health and Human Services: *10 Years of Reporting Child Maltreatment 1999.* Administration on Children, Youth and Families. Washington, DC, US Government Printing Office, 2001.

Physical Abuse

Boos SC: Constrictive asphyxia: A recognizable form of fatal child abuse. *Child Abuse Negl* 2000;24:1503–7.

Brewster AL, Nelson JP, Hymel KP, et al: Victim, perpetrator, family and incident characteristics of 32 infant maltreatment deaths in the United States Air Force. *Child Abuse Negl* 1998;91:101.

Carpenter RF: The prevalence and distribution of bruising in babies. *Arch Dis Child* 1999;80:363–6.

Carty HM: Fractures caused by child abuse. *J Bone Joint Surg* 1993;75B:849.

Committee on Child Abuse and Neglect: Shaken baby syndrome: Rotational cranial injuries—Technical report. *Pediatrics* 2001;108:206–10.

Duhaime AC, Gennarellia TA, Thibault LE, et al: The shaken baby syndrome: A clinical, pathological, and biomechanical study. *J Neurosurg* 1987;66:409.

Duhaime AC, Lewander WJ, Schut L, et al: Head injury in very young children: Mechanisms, injury types, and ophthalmologic findings in 100 hospitalized patients younger than 2 years of age. *Pediatrics* 1992;9:179.

Gillham B, Tanner G, Cheyne B, et al: Unemployment rates, single parent density and indices of child poverty: Their relationship to different categories of child abuse and neglect. *Child Abuse Negl* 1998;22:79.

Johnson CF: Inflicted injury vs accidental injury: The diagnosis of inflicted injury. *Pediatr Clin North Am* 1990;37:791.

Labbe J, Cauette G: Recent skin injuries in normal children. *Pediatrics* 2001;108:271–6.

Nashelsky MB, Dix JD: The time interval between lethal infant shaking and onset of symptoms: A review of the shaken baby syndrome literature. *Am J Forensic Med Pathol* 1995;16:154.

Raiha HK, Soma D: Victims of child abuse and neglect in the U.S. Army. *Child Abuse Negl* 1997;21:759.

Wilkinson WS, Han DP, Rappley MD, et al: Retinal hemorrhage predicts neurologic injury in the shaken baby syndrome. *Arch Ophthalmol* 1989;107:1472.

Sexual Abuse

Adams J: Evolution of a classification scale: Medical evaluation of suspected child sexual abuse. *Child Maltreatment* 2001;6:31–6.

American Academy of Pediatrics: Guidelines for the evaluation of sexual abuse of children: Subject review. *Pediatrics* 1999;103:186–91.

Bays J, Chadwick D: Medical diagnosis of the sexually abused child. *Child Abuse Negl* 1993;17:91.

Berenson MC, Wiemann C, et al: A case-control study of anatomic changes resulting from sexual abuse. *Am J Obstet Gynecol* 2000;182:820–4.

Budin L, Johnson CF: Sex abuse prevention programs: Offenders' attitudes about their efficacy. *Child Abuse Negl* 1989;13:77–87.

Christian C, Lavelle J, Dejong JL, et al: Forensic evidence findings in prepubertal victims of sexual assault. *Pediatrics* 2000;106:100–4.

Drach KM, Wientzen J, Ricci LR: The diagnostic utility of sexual behavior problems in diagnosing sexual abuse in a forensic child abuse clinic. *Child Abuse Negl* 2001;25:489–503.

Heger A, Emans SJ, Muram D (editors): *Evaluation of the Sexually Abused Child.* New York, Oxford University Press, 2000.

Holmes WC, Slap GB: Sexual abuse of boys. *JAMA* 1998;280:1855.

Ingram DM, Everett VD, Ingram DL: The relationship between the transverse hymenal orifice diameter by the separation technique and other possible markers of sex abuse. *Child Abuse Negl* 2001;25:1109–19.

Jones LM, Finkelhor D, Kopiec K: Why is sexual abuse declining? A survey of state protection administrators, 2001. *Child Abuse Negl* 2001;25:1139–58.

McCann J, Voris J, Simon M, et al: Perianal findings in prepubertal children selected for nonabuse: A descriptive study. *Child Abuse Negl* 1989;13:179.

Swanston HY, Tebbutt JS, O'Toole BI, et al: Sexually abused children 5 years after presentation: A case controlled study. *Pediatrics* 1997;100:600.

Nonorganic Failure to Thrive

Rosenn DW, Loeb LS, Jura MB: Differentiation of organic from non-organic failure to thrive in infancy. *Pediatrics* 1980;66:698.

Schmitt BD, Mauro RD: Nonorganic failure to thrive: An outpatient approach. *Child Abuse Negl* 1989;13:235.

Skuse D, Albanese A, Stanhope R, et al: A new stress-related syndrome of growth failure and hyperphagia in children associated with reversibility of growth-hormone insufficiency. *Lancet* 1996;348:353.

Munchausen Syndrome by Proxy

Hall DE, Eubanks L, Meyyazhagen S, et al: Evaluation of covert video surveillance in the diagnosis of Munchausen syndrome by proxy: Lessons from 41 cases. *Pediatrics* 2000;105:1305–12.

Levin AV, Sheridan MS: *Munchausen Syndrome by Proxy: Issues in Diagnosis and Treatment.* New York, Lexington Books, 1995.

Schreier HA, Libow JA: Munchausen syndrome by proxy: Diagnosis and prevalence. *Am J Orthopsychiatry* 1993;63:318.

Other Types of Child Maltreatment

Eckenrode J, Ganzel B, Henderson C, et al: Preventing child abuse and neglect with a program of nurse home visitation: The limiting effects of domestic violence. *JAMA* 2001;284:1385–91.

Garbarino J: Psychological child maltreatment—A developmental view. *Prim Care* 1993;20:6.

Hebet M, Lavoie F, Piche C, et al: Proximate effects of a child sexual abuse prevention program in elementary school children. *Child Abuse Negl* 2001;25:505–22.

Johnson CF: Physicians and medical neglect: Variables which affect reporting. *Child Abuse Negl* 1993;17:605.

Kairys SW, Johnson CF, Committee on Child Abuse and Neglect: The psychological treatment of children—technical report. *Pediatrics* 2002. www.pediatrics.org/cgi/content/full/109/4/e68

Khamis V: Child psychological maltreatment in Palestinian families. *Child Abuse Negl* 2000;124:1047–59.

Leventhal JM: The prevention of child abuse and neglect: Successfully out of the blocks. *Child Abuse Negl* 2001;25:431–9.

Sidebotham P, Golding J: The ACSPAC Study Team: Child maltreatment in the "children of the nineties." A longitudinal study of parental risk factors. *Child Abuse Negl* 2001;25:1177–200.

PART V

Children with Special Health Needs

Chapter 36
Failure to Thrive *Howard Bauchner*

Failure to thrive (FTT) is diagnosed in an infant or child whose physical growth is significantly less than that of his or her peers, and it is often associated with poor developmental and cognitive functioning. Although there is no clear consensus definition, FTT usually refers to growth below the 3rd or 5th percentile or a change in growth that has crossed two major growth percentiles (i.e., from above the 75th percentile to below the 25th) in a short time. Traditionally, FTT was considered either organic or nonorganic. Organic FTT is marked by an underlying medical condition; nonorganic or psychosocial FTT occurs in a child who is usually younger than age 5 yr and has no known medical condition that causes poor growth (also see Chapter 35.2).

Epidemiology and Etiology. The prevalence of FTT depends on the population sampled. From 5–10% of low-birthweight children and children living in poverty may have FTT. Family dysfunction, neonatal problems other than low birthweight, and maternal depression are also associated with FTT. In the United States, psychosocial FTT is far more common than organic FTT.

The causes of organic FTT are numerous (Table 36–1). Every organ system is represented. Psychosocial FTT is most often due to poverty or poor child-parent interaction. It occasionally occurs with severe stress such as child abuse. Organic and nonorganic etiologic factors may also occur together, for example, in children who are victims of abuse and neglect or temperamentally difficult premature infants.

Clinical Manifestations. The clinical presentation of FTT ranges from failure to meet expected age norms for height and weight, to alopecia, loss of subcutaneous fat, reduced muscle mass, dermatitis, recurrent infections, marasmus, and kwashiorkor. In developed countries, the most common presentation is poor growth detected in an ambulatory setting; in developing countries, recurrent infections, marasmus, and kwashiorkor are more common presentations.

The degree of FTT is usually measured by calculating each growth parameter (weight, height, and weight/height ratio) as a percentage of the median value for age based on appropriate growth charts. Appropriate growth charts are often not available for children with specific medical problems; serial measurements are especially important for these children. For premature infants, correction must be made for the extent of prematurity. Corrected age, rather than chronologic age, should be used in calculations of their growth percentiles until 1–2 yr of corrected age.

For weight, mild, moderate, and severe FTT is equivalent to 75–90%, 60–74%, and less than 60% of standard, respectively. For height, the corresponding values are 90–95%, 85–89%, and less than 85%. For the weight/height ratio, the values are 81–90%, 70–80%, and less than 70%. The weight for age per cent of the standard value traditionally decreases early in the course of FTT, followed by a decrement of height for age. Children with chronic malnutrition often have a normal weight for height because both their weight and height are reduced.

The laboratory evaluation of children with FTT is often not helpful and, therefore, should be used judiciously. A complete blood count, lead level, and urinalysis represent a reasonable initial screen. Bone age is often helpful in distinguishing family short stature (bone age equivalent to chronological age) from endocrine or nutritional abnormalities (bone age is less than chronological age). Other tests, such as thyroid function studies, tests for gastroesophageal reflux and malabsorption, organic and amino acids, or a sweat test, should be performed if indicated by the history or physical examination.

Diagnosis. The history, physical examination, and observation of the parent-child interaction usually suggest the diagnosis. The latter observation, especially with feeding, is often critical to the diagnosis of psychosocial FTT.

The causes of insufficient growth include (1) failure of a parent to offer adequate calories, (2) failure of the child to take sufficient calories, and (3) failure of the child to retain sufficient calories. Reasons why parents or other caregivers may not offer appropriate or sufficient foods include lack of knowledge, parental depression, unusual dietary beliefs, or lack of food. With young infants, it is particularly important to obtain a detailed dietary history, including what the diet consists of, how often the infant is fed, and how the parents respond when the child cries or sleeps for prolonged periods. Children may have difficulty swallowing if they have oral-motor dysfunction, anatomic abnormalities, cardiopulmonary dysfunction, or enlarged and recurrently infected tonsils and adenoids. Vomiting, diarrhea, and malabsorption are general causes of inadequate caloric absorption. It may be helpful to approach the diagnosis in terms of age (Table 36–2) or signs and symptoms (Table 36–3).

Treatment. The treatment of FTT requires an understanding of all the elements that contribute to a child's growth: a child's health and nutritional status, family issues, and the parent-child interaction. Regardless of cause, an appropriate feeding atmosphere at home is important. Children with severe malnutrition must be re-fed carefully.

For children with organic FTT, the underlying medical condition should be treated. The type of caloric supplementation must be based on the severity of FTT and the underlying medical condition. For example, in children with renal failure, the amount of protein in the diet must be carefully monitored. The response to caloric supplementation depends on the specific diagnosis, medical treatment, and severity of FTT.

For older infants and young children with psychosocial FTT, mealtimes should be approximately 20–30 min, solid foods should be offered before liquids, environmental distractions should be minimized, and children should eat with other people and not be force fed. The intake of water, juice, and low-calorie beverages should be limited. High-calorie foods, such as peanut butter, whole milk, cheese, and dried fruits, should be emphasized. High-calorie supplementation, such as Duocal or Polycose, or high-calorie liquids, such as Carnation Instant Breakfast with whole milk, or formulas containing more than 20 calories per ounce (PediaSure, Ensure, and Resource) are sometimes necessary. Weight gain in response to adequate caloric feedings usually establishes the diagnosis of psychosocial FTT.

TABLE 36–1. Major Organic Causes of Failure to Thrive

System	Cause
Gastrointestinal	Gastroesophageal reflux, celiac disease, pyloric stenosis, cleft palate/cleft lip, lactose intolerance, Hirschsprung's disease, milk protein intolerance, hepatitis, cirrhosis, pancreatic insufficiency, biliary disease, inflammatory bowel disease, malabsorption, food alkalines
Renal	Urinary tract infection, renal tubular acidosis, diabetes insipidus, chronic renal insufficiency
Cardiopulmonary	Cardiac diseases leading to congestive heart failure, asthma, bronchopulmonary dysplasia, cystic fibrosis, anatomic abnormalities of the upper airway, obstructive sleep apnea (snoring)
Endocrine	Hypothyroidism, diabetes mellitus, adrenal insufficiency or excess, parathyroid disorders, pituitary disorders, growth hormone deficiency
Neurologic	Mental retardation, cerebral hemorrhages, degenerative disorders
Infectious	Parasitic or bacterial infections of the gastrointestinal tract, tuberculosis, human immunodeficiency virus disease
Metabolic	Inborn errors of metabolism
Congenital	Chromosomal abnormalities, congenital syndromes (fetal alcohol syndrome), perinatal infections
Miscellaneous	Lead poisoning, malignancy, collagen vascular disease, recurrently infected adenoids and tonsils

TABLE 36–2. Approach to Failure to Thrive Based on Age

Age of Onset	Major Diagnostic Consideration
Birth to 3 mo	Psychosocial failure to thrive, perinatal infections, gastroesophageal reflux, inborn errors of metabolism, cystic fibrosis
3–6 mo	Psychosocial failure to thrive, human immunodeficiency virus infection, gastroesophageal reflux, inborn errors of metabolism, milk protein intolerance, cystic fibrosis, renal tubular acidosis
7–12 mo	Psychosocial failure to thrive (autonomy struggles), delayed introduction of solids, gastroesophageal reflux, intestinal parasites, renal tubular acidosis
12 + mo	Psychosocial failure to thrive (coercive feeding, new psychologic stressor), gastroesophageal reflux

Adapted from Frank D, Silva M, Needlman R: Failure to thrive: Mystery, myth and method. Contemporary Pediatrics *1993;10:114.*

TABLE 36–3. Approach to Failure to Thrive Based on Signs and Symptoms

History/Physical Examination	Diagnostic Consideration
Spitting, vomiting, food refusal	Gastroesophageal reflux, chronic tonsillitis, food allergies
Diarrhea, fatty stools	Malabsorption, intestinal parasites, milk protein intolerance
Snoring, mouth breathing, enlarged tonsils	Adenoid hypertrophy, obstructive sleep apnea
Recurrent wheezing, pulmonary infections	Asthma, aspiration
Recurrent infections	Human immunodeficiency virus disease
Travel to/from developing countries	Parasitic or bacterial infections of the gastrointestinal tract

Adapted from Frank D, Silva M, Needlman R: Failure to thrive: Mystery, myth and method. Contemporary Pediatrics *1993;10:114.*

Indications for hospitalization include severe malnutrition, further diagnostic and laboratory evaluation, lack of catch-up growth, and evaluation of the parent-child feeding interaction. Parents of children with organic FTT should be comfortable with the diagnosis and treatment before discharge. For psychosocial FTT, hospitalization often lasts 5–10 days. Caloric intake should be monitored, and the parent-child feeding interaction should be observed (Chapter 35.2). The goals of hospitalization are to obtain sustained catch-up growth and educate parents about appropriate foods and feeding styles. For both organic and psychosocial FTT, the approach to feeding in the hospital should mimic the anticipated treatment at home before discharge.

Prognosis. FTT in the 1st yr of life, regardless of cause, is particularly ominous. Maximal postnatal brain growth occurs during the first 6 mo of life. The brain grows as much during the 1st yr of life as during the rest of a child's life. Approximately one third of children with psychosocial FTT are developmentally delayed and have social and emotional problems. The prognosis for children with organic FTT is more variable, depending on the specific diagnosis and severity of FTT. Ongoing assessment and monitoring of cognitive and emotional development, with appropriate intervention, is necessary for all children with FTT.

Alaimo K, Olson CM, Frongillo EA: Food insufficiency and American school-aged children's cognitive, academic, and psychosocial development. *Pediatrics* 2001;108:44–53.

Berwick DM, Levey JC, Kleinerman R: Failure to thrive: Diagnostic yield of hospitalization. *Arch Dis Child* 1982;57:347.

Bithoney WG, Dubowitz H, Egan H: Failure to thrive/growth deficiency. *Pediatr Rev* 1992;13:453.

Fleishe DR: Comprehensive management of infants with gastroesophageal reflux and failure to thrive. *Curr Probl Pediatr* 1995;25:247.

Frank D, Silva M, Needlman R: Failure to thrive: Mystery, myth and method. *Contemporary Pediatrics* 1993;10:114.

Kelleher KJ, Casey PH, Bradley RH, et al: Risk factors and outcomes for failure to thrive in low birth weight preterm infants. *Pediatrics* 1993;91:941.

Maggion A, Lifshitz F: Nutritional management of failure to thrive. *Pediatr Clin North Am* 1995;42:791.

Wright CM, Waterston A, Aynsley-Green A: Effect of deprivation on weight gain in infancy. *Acta Paediatr* 1994;83:357.

Chapter 37

Developmental Disabilities and Chronic Illness

James M. Perrin

Overview. Children having special health care needs constitute a heterogeneous population that includes youngsters with a wide variety of developmental disabilities and chronic illnesses. A core of basic considerations applies to most children with chronic conditions, and these issues are discussed first.

Early detection of persistent conditions, amelioration of the functional consequences of specific disabilities, and prevention of secondary psychosocial handicaps are central to the provision of care for children with special health needs. Caregivers should recognize the importance of treating the whole child in a family and community context. Physicians occasionally and inappropriately refer to children with chronic conditions by the name of their condition, such as "asthmatics," "sicklers," "leukemics," or "Down's babies." This tendency to characterize children by their disease or disability adversely influences both parental and professional attitudes as well as objective assessments of the child's current abilities and expectations for the future. In general, parents and professionals should work together on behalf of a child who has a disease rather than allowing the disease to define the child.

Most children receive the majority of their health care from a single physician and are educated in regular school settings that require no modifications to meet special developmental or health concerns. Children having special health needs, on the other hand, may see a variety of physician specialists (e.g., neurologists, orthopedists, cardiologists), interact with multiple professionals (e.g., occupational therapists, respiratory therapists, nutritionists, psychologists), and need major adaptive modifications in their school setting (e.g., barrier-free facilities, special education services, and specialized nursing care). Some of these services, especially those of pediatric subspecialists, are provided in hospital-based programs; others, such as home health care and certain supportive therapies, may be offered in community settings. Thus, the pediatrician needs a working knowledge of community services available to families and should help coordinate the subspecialty services received.

An appreciation of the multiple levels at which prevention or treatment efforts can be implemented requires an understanding of the differences inherent in the concepts of disease, functional limitation, and disability or social impact. Disease refers to a specific health condition affecting a child, such as arthritis or congenital cytomegalovirus infection. Functional limitation refers to the problem brought about as a result of the symptoms of the disease, such as a poorly functioning knee or a hearing impairment. Social impact (disability), on the other hand, refers to the social consequences of having the disease, such as the inability to participate competitively in sports or the social isolation that results from difficulty in communicating orally. The child's environment greatly influences these social consequences. Physicians can play a key role in preventing the occurrence of many special health needs and in diminishing their impact on a child's growth and development. Intervention may be targeted at the level of the disease, the functional limitation, or the disability. For the child with arthritis, efforts are directed both toward reducing joint inflammation and toward removing barriers to participation in age-appropriate physical activities.

Several public programs in the United States assist families of children with special health needs. In addition, parent groups in many communities help parents learn effective techniques for caring for children with chronic conditions and for obtaining the necessary health and educational services. Title V Maternal and Child Health Programs for Children with Special Health Needs provide a variety of coordinating and multidisciplinary clinical services for children who have chronic illnesses and developmental disabilities. The Individuals with Disability Education Act (IDEA) supports state-sponsored early intervention and special education programs and mandates an appropriate education in the least restrictive environment for children with disabilities. The Supplemental Security Income (SSI) program provides cash benefits for families whose children have severe physical, mental, or developmental disabilities as well as public health insurance coverage (i.e., Medicaid) in almost every state.

For children younger than age 3 yr, early intervention (EI) programs provide a mechanism for decreasing the impact of special health or developmental needs on children and their families. EI programs that incorporate the best practices offer individualized services designed to strengthen the inherent adaptiveness of participating children and families. Older children also may need special education evaluations and services or special adaptations to maximize their school attendance. Because of their strategic relationship with young children and their parents, pediatricians have an important responsibility with regard to early identification of children at risk and referral to the appropriate services (see also Chapter 5). This responsibility includes maintaining accurate and updated information on all available resources within a community to ensure that families have access to a full range of needed services. Except in the hospital, a child's family provides most care; at times, this involves an extraordinary amount of extra caretaking. Parental health, mental health, and well-being strongly affect child health outcomes in the context of disability. The best predictors of the well-being of children with special health needs include factors that relate to family health and functioning; effective pediatric management should therefore embody a comprehensive approach to the child in the context of the family, addressing the needs of all its members.

Despite the variations among conditions and their clinical requirements, families caring for children with any of these long-term conditions typically face key times of transition when additional community and health services may be necessary to improve child and adolescent functioning. This is especially the case at discharge from hospital to home after a long and complex intensive care experience or other management related to the initial diagnosis. Many families initially rely on hospital-based services to provide a wide range of therapies and now must take on responsibilities for home care, including providing services themselves and coordinating services from a variety of therapists in the home setting. Although discharge plans from hospital-based services may work well in the first few months, as nurses and equipment vendors change and as parents increasingly develop their own skills, the new arrangement needs ongoing monitoring and help. A second period of difficult transition for families is at entry to school, where the management of the child's health condition (medications and other specialized services) and plans for emergencies necessitate cooperation of school personnel. Clinicians can help ensure both the child's integration into school and the availability of school services and plans appropriate to his or her needs. A third time of transition is at adolescence. Many chronic conditions delay onset of puberty or affect cognitive abilities and make many aspects of adolescent life particularly complex. Chronic conditions may influence the ways of approaching risk-taking behaviors, substance and drug use, or the development of healthy sexuality. Families may need support and advice from clinicians during their child's adolescence. Finally, the transition to adulthood of adolescents with disabilities is critical because of difficulties in obtaining health insurance, gaining access to educational and vocational services, shifting from pediatric and adolescent care to adult health services, and achieving personal and economic independence.

37.1 Chronic Illness in Childhood

James M. Perrin

Epidemiology, Severity, and Outcome. The *epidemiology* of chronic illness in childhood differs in important ways from that of long-term illness in adults. Adults face a relatively small number of common chronic conditions (e.g., diabetes, osteoarthritis, coronary artery disease) and few rare diseases. Children, in contrast, face a wide variety of mainly quite rare diseases. Only a few groups of chronic conditions in childhood are common: allergic disorders (mainly asthma, eczema, and hay fever), neurologic disorders (mainly seizure disorders and neuromuscular conditions such as cerebral palsy), obesity, and mental health conditions (especially, attention-deficit/hyperactivity disorder and depression). Other conditions often thought to be common, such as type 1 diabetes, occur in only about 1 in 1,000 children younger than 16 yr, a much lower rate than is seen in adults. Many of the conditions described in this textbook occur with a frequency of much less than 1/1,000.

These epidemiologic distinctions have implications for both physicians and families. The adult pattern means that health care providers for adults have frequent daily experience with the common chronic illnesses of adults, remaining current and knowledgeable about such conditions as hypertension. Similarly, an adult who has been newly diagnosed with high blood pressure probably knows something about the disease and has friends or family members with hypertension. The practicing pediatrician, however, may see a new case of a malignancy only once in a decade and will make the diagnosis of cystic fibrosis or even diabetes infrequently. A family whose child has been newly diagnosed with a rare condition may never even have heard the name of the disease prior to its onset in their child. These epidemiologic facts mean that pediatricians have a difficult task in identifying children with rare conditions and in staying current with applicable technologies.

Although estimates of the size of this population vary greatly (partly because of the wide spectrum of severity of various conditions), data from the 1994–1995 National Health Interview Survey indicate that 15–18% of children and adolescents have some form of chronic condition, including physical conditions, developmental disabilities, disorders of learning, and primary mental health conditions. Adding speech defects, visual and hearing impairments, repeated ear infections, skin allergies, and other common conditions raises the prevalence to over 30%. Approximately 6–7% of all children and adolescents have some limitation of activity owing to a chronic health condition, and 1–2% have conditions severe enough to meet the very restricted definition of disability used by the federal SSI program, which is the main cash support program in the United States for people of all ages with disabling conditions. Within these groups, approximately 40% of children have disorders of development and learning; 35%, chronic physical conditions; and 25%, chronic mental health conditions. With improvements in health care and access to services in the last few decades, almost all these children and adolescents survive to adulthood, although often with major physical or psychologic problems related to their condition.

Severity is difficult to measure in most chronic illnesses. Although new techniques increasingly define the underlying genetic and molecular basis for many conditions, these biologic markers do not commonly correlate well with clinical indicators of severity, likely because a number of other genes and environmental factors affect the expression of the condition. Most measures of severity (e.g., asthma rating scales or hemoglobin A_{1C} in diabetes) reflect the interaction of biologic susceptibility, treatment, and other environmental factors. The effect of the condition on the child's development (cognitive, behavioral, and physical) and on functioning with friends or in school is another aspect of severity. Although this chapter focuses on health conditions that physiologically are relatively severe, many of the issues discussed affect children with milder conditions. Further, one type of severity (e.g., physiologic or clinical) may correlate poorly with others (e.g., psychologic or functional).

The percentage of children with severe, long-term illnesses has more than doubled in the past 2 decades, and at least 90%

of these children survive to young adulthood. Changes in prevalence reflect major advances in the technology of medical and surgical care and substantial improvements in survival as well as marked increase in rates of certain chronic conditions (e.g., asthma, obesity, and mental health conditions). Rates of a few other conditions of much lower prevalence also have increased in recent years, including AIDS, the after-effects of fetal substance exposure, and major pulmonary or neurologic disease in children leaving neonatal intensive care units; however, these increases account for a very small proportion of all chronic illness in children. New genetic techniques have allowed the prenatal and preconception diagnosis of increasing numbers of certain health conditions, and genetic counseling and other interventions have diminished the incidence of other diseases.

Issues Common to Diverse Chronic Conditions. Health care providers typically view each chronic illness as a distinct and separate entity that has its own etiology, natural history, treatment, complications, and physiologic impact. However, families of children with a variety of long-term illnesses face several issues in common, reflecting chronicity itself rather than aspects of the specific disease.

Many chronic childhood illnesses are *high-cost health conditions.* A small percentage of children with major chronic illnesses utilize a large proportion of the child health dollar; 2–4% of children with severe long-term illnesses account for at least 35% of all child health expenditures. These figures reflect only what is paid by public or private insurance. Families face many other expenses, such as the costs of transportation, long-distance phone calls, and special diets, few of which may be reimbursed. Furthermore, chronic illness in a child makes it more difficult for both parents to work outside the home, thereby diminishing the family's financial resources.

The *daily burden of care rests mainly with the families,* and that burden can be extensive, as with a family with two teenagers with muscular dystrophy, both wheelchair-bound and requiring transportation from place to place, or with a youngster with cystic fibrosis who needs time-consuming pulmonary care prior to leaving for school each day. These daily burdens greatly extend the work of families.

Whereas most children require only a single provider for most of their health care and supervision, *children with long-term health conditions frequently have multiple providers and multiple treatments.* A child with hemophilia may have contact with a hematologist, a pediatrician, a specialized dentist, an orthopedist, a hematology nurse, a physical therapist, a psychologist, and a social worker, among others. The recommendations of any member of this group may vary from those of another, and families must often choose among conflicting advice. Clinically, there usually are tradeoffs among the choices, such as the optimal time to do a surgical procedure or the balance between seizure control and alertness. Pediatricians can help families make informed choices.

The comparative rarity of most childhood chronic conditions makes *families feel isolated.* They often wonder why they have been singled out by an unusual condition, and they feel that no other families have had similar experiences. Family programs in specialty centers (e.g., cystic fibrosis or arthritis centers) and parent advocacy programs have worked to break this sense of isolation through groups that help parents learn from each other how to raise children with chronic conditions.

Many of these conditions are unpredictable in their implications, longevity, complications, and developmental impact on the child. The parent whose child has leukemia wonders whether new bleeding signals a relapse that will have a fatal outcome or will be followed by a permanent remission. The parent whose child has mild wheezing at bedtime does not know whether the child will sleep well through the night or awaken severely dyspneic in the middle of the night in need of emergency care. Parents speak frequently of how difficult this unpredictability is for them and how they wish for clear answers to difficult questions, even if the answers may be unfavorable. Many important aspects of chronic disease are unpredictable, both because of great variability in environmental influences and in biologic responsiveness to specific conditions and treatments and because little information is available about many rare diseases.

Many chronic conditions and their treatments cause great *pain*, far in excess of that faced by other children. Sickle cell anemia, hemophilia, arthritis, and leukemia are examples of conditions characterized at times by severe pain.

Chronic illness has a *pervasive influence on a child's daily life*. Frequent interactions with the medical care system, occasional hospitalization, and greater dependence on parents and health care providers characterize their lives. A chronic health impairment may create a sense of "differentness," of being unable to do many things that other children can do.

Finally, a chronic illness creates *additional stresses and demands on families and on children* that apparently healthy children do not face. Perhaps as a result, chronically ill children have about twice the frequency of psychologic or behavioral problems found in healthy control subjects; children with significant neurologic handicaps or sensory deficits have as much as a five times greater risk for these problems. The level of severity correlates poorly with psychologic status. Despite this greater risk of psychologic maladjustment, most children with chronic health conditions are psychologically healthy.

Developmental Aspects of Long-Term Illness. Two issues are central to an understanding of the developmental implications of long-term childhood illness: the development of children's understanding of illness mechanisms and the impact of illness at different stages of child development (also see Chapters 16 and 17).

Clinicians working with children who have long-term illnesses should understand the *developmental stage of their patients' understanding of illness* in order to explain illness and its mechanisms in age-appropriate terms. Because their understanding follows a typical pattern of growth in cognitive abilities, children need different explanations of their continuing disease as they mature. Young children of preschool or early school age tend to have a concrete and relatively superficial understanding of illness. They view illness as a response to their bad behavior or not following the rules (such as wearing a coat to go outside in the cold). Children at this age believe that getting well occurs by adhering to another set of rules. By about the 4th–6th grade, children begin to differentiate themselves from external events that may cause illness. For this age group, germ theory seems very important; with the notion that germs cause almost all illnesses, illness can be prevented by avoiding germs, and better results will be gained from taking medicines, which are seen as fighting germs. This notion of germs can cause confusion or isolation for children of this age who have conditions such as leukemia or diabetes. By 8th grade or even later, children begin to understand the physiologic mechanisms for illness, appreciating the many interrelated causes and the several symptoms of illness. At this age, children usually begin to understand the interaction of body parts, for example, that lungs and hearts are not only near each other but actually work together to maintain body functions.

Physical illness has different effects on children based on their stage of development (see Chapters 7–16). In infancy, the illness may affect the parameters of growth and development by influencing feeding, sleeping, motor abilities (and therefore exploration of the environment), and sensory functions. Physical deformity or fatigue may affect a child's responsiveness to parents, who

may in turn react differently to this child. Frequent hospitalizations may interfere with the normal development of trusting relationships within a family. In later preschool years, when children are developing autonomy, mobility, and self-control, illness may again interfere with these important developmental functions. Early school-aged children may be subject to teasing from classmates; they may need to be absent from school for illness or its treatment and thus miss normal opportunities for early socialization. Middle childhood and adolescence are periods when children expand their areas of competence; responsibility for the care of the child's health condition should shift gradually from the parents to the child. Chronic illness may interfere with this process.

In adolescence, illness may affect the individual's developing independence, greater responsibility for self-care, growing intimacy, and planning for the future. The disease or its treatment may be particularly embarrassing for adolescents and may affect their body image. Adolescence is frequently a time to test the limits of the illness and compliance with recommended therapies. Health conditions that require another person for some care (such as the case of the teenager with cystic fibrosis who needs pulmonary physical therapy before each day of high school) may hinder growth toward independence. With appropriate services, most adolescents with chronic conditions make the transition to adulthood well, with little interference in their finishing education, becoming employed, and entering into significant interpersonal relationships. Sensitivity to the developmental impact of chronic illness will help clinicians provide their patients with appropriate planning and anticipatory guidance and help children and their families find acceptable ways of fulfilling the normal developmental tasks of childhood and adolescence.

Children should take increasing responsibility for the management of their own health condition commensurate with their level of maturity, developmental stage, and understanding of their illness. Areas of responsibility include monitoring the condition, assessing indicators of change and exacerbation, asking for help, and being responsible for self-medication (both at home and at school). Families may need help in learning ways to foster responsibility, and children need education and advice in learning how to become independent in appropriate ways.

Integrating Children with Chronic Conditions into Communities. Changing interests of families, changing notions of the civil rights of people with disabilities, and improved technologies have fostered an increasing emphasis on family-centered services for children with chronic conditions. Parents increasingly take responsibility for monitoring and managing the care of their child, and more care is provided in or near the child's home and less in hospitals. Families want to receive most care in community settings and want to integrate their chronically ill child into community activities, not to limit her or him to services provided mainly for children with special health needs.

Providing services in the community also strengthens early socialization of the child, mainly through participation in child care and, later, social and educational development through participation in school programs. Chronic illness accounts for a sizable number of school absences. Part of that time away from classes reflects the direct effects of illness, such as increased fatigue or necessary hospitalization; however, some represents the need to travel great distances for treatments that are often available only during regular school hours.

Some children with chronic illnesses, especially those with cognitive impairments, need special education services. However, most children with long-term illnesses have no intrinsic cognitive impairment and should be in regular education programs. They may need specialized health services (e.g., access to medicines or planning for emergencies) in order to participate in school, and children who must miss classes frequently need home or hospital instruction to allow them to keep up with their classmates.

Families whose children have long-term health conditions should have access to a wide range of coordinated and comprehensive services. The specific services needed by any one family will vary considerably from those needed by another and will change over time as the child grows and the family changes. The main groups of services that should be available for families include primary and specialized medical and surgical care; nursing services, especially those that will help to strengthen a family's own skills in caring for their child; preventive and therapeutic mental health services; social services; educational planning; and certain special therapies, such as physical therapy, occupational therapy, and nutritional services. Preventive mental health services help diminish the risk of psychologic problems related to the chronicity of the child's condition.

Partly because of the emphasis on specialized medical services and frequent surgeries, hospitalization, or other acute episodes, children with chronic health conditions may lack regular pediatric health supervision. They have lower rates of immunization and screening for common health problems and often lack anticipatory guidance in key areas of growth and development, such as behavior and discipline in the preschool years, preparation for entry to school, and preparation for adolescence, with developing sexuality, growth of independence, and opportunity for substance abuse. Lack of adequate primary care has been associated with greater likelihood of hospitalization for children with some chronic conditions such as asthma, in which preventive use of anti-inflammatory drugs can diminish the number and severity of episodes. The primary care provider should help ensure that children receive services aimed at preventing exacerbation of their condition or diminishing its severity (Chapter 5).

Pediatric Care in the Community. Community pediatricians have a central role in the care of children with chronic illnesses and in supporting their families. Although the pediatrician's involvement may begin with diagnosis and referral to subspecialty services, he or she should also assume responsibility as a continuing advocate for the child and family. This includes continuing communication with specialty providers and helping families make informed choices, especially when advice is conflicting. Along with ongoing primary care, the pediatrician should work with subspecialty services to coordinate medical care and help with efforts to prevent morbidity. Educating parents and children about the disease process and its management, complications, and developmental implications is a central part of the therapeutic effort. Other responsibilities include continued support for children and family members, helping families locate appropriate community resources, and, especially, collaborating with schools and agencies to integrate the child into the community. Tasks with agencies include referral to early intervention services, when appropriate; providing information that may help determine whether a child needs special or regular education services; and helping the child obtain the school services that enhance school attendance. Needed school services typically include appropriate nursing and related services and access to medications or emergency care, although a few children require more extensive services, including personal attendants.

Communication with families is particularly important. Families want clear information, with details that they can understand and information about both positive and negative aspects of the child's condition. They particularly appreciate receiving information and support from a professional familiar to them who provides compassionate and caring services. The child should also participate in developmentally appropriate ways in information sharing.

American Academy of Pediatrics: The role of the pediatrician in transitioning children and adolescents with developmental disabilities and chronic illnesses from school to work or college. *Pediatrics* 2000;106:854.
American Academy of Pediatrics: Provision of educationally-related services for children and adolescents with chronic disease and disabling conditions. *Pediatrics* 2000;105:448.
American Academy of Pediatrics: Care coordination: Integrating health and related systems of care for children with special health care needs. *Pediatrics* 1999;104:978.
American Academy of Pediatrics: The continued importance of Supplemental Security Income (SSI) for children and adolescents with disabilities. *Pediatrics* 2001;107:790.
Dosa NP, Boeing NM, Kanter RK: Excess risk of severe acute illness in children with chronic health conditions. *Pediatrics* 2001;107:499.
Newacheck PW, Strickland B, Shonkoff JP, et al: An epidemiologic profile of children with special health care needs. *Pediatrics* 1998;102:117.
Newacheck PW, Taylor WR: Childhood chronic illness: Prevalence, severity, and impact. *Am J Public Health* 1992;82:364.
Perrin EC, Gerrity PS: Development of children with chronic illness. *Pediatr Clin North Am* 1984;31:19.
Perrin JM, Shayne MW, Bloom SR: *Home and Community Care for Chronically Ill Children.* New York, Oxford University Press, 1993.
Stein REK (editor): *Caring for Children with Chronic Illness.* New York, Springer, 1989.
Strauss D, Ashwal S, Shavelle R, et al: Prognosis for survival and improved function in children with severe developmental disabilities. *J Pediatr* 1997;131:712.
World Health Organization: *International Classification of Functioning.* Geneva 2001. (www3.who.int/icf/icftemplate.cfm)

Chapter 37.2   Mental Retardation

Bruce K. Shapiro and Mark L. Batshaw

Mental retardation refers to a group of disorders that have in common deficits of adaptive and intellectual function and an age of onset before maturity is reached. The designation continues to evolve as a result of new knowledge and changing societal norms.

Definition. The most commonly used definition of mental retardation comes from the American Psychiatric Association's (APA) *Diagnostic and Statistical Manual of Mental Disorders*, Fourth Edition, Text Revision (DSM-IV-TR) (Table 37–1). This classification, although based on previous definitions, has been criticized for depending on IQ test performance rather than adaptive behavior, not taking the standard error of measurement into account, and not being predictive of outcomes for individuals.

The American Association on Mental Retardation (AAMR) has proposed a different classification. Instead of defining degrees of deficit (mild to profound), the AAMR definition substitutes levels of support required (intermittent, limited, extensive, or pervasive) in areas of adaptive function. The reliability of using the "levels of support required" has been challenged. In addition, the AAMR classification system blurs the distinction between mental retardation and other developmental disorders (e.g., communication disorder, autism, specific learning disabilities). As a result, the medical community has generally used the APA definition.

Etiology. There appear to be two overlapping populations of retarded children: mild mental retardation, which is associated with environmental influences, and severe mental retardation, which is linked to biologic causes. Mild mental retardation is four times more likely to be found in the offspring of women who have not completed high school than in women who have graduated. This is presumably a consequence of both genetic (i.e., children may inherit a cognitive impairment) and socioeconomic (i.e., poverty, undernutrition) factors. The specific causes of mild mental retardation, however, are currently identifiable in less than half of affected individuals. The most com-

TABLE 37–1. **Diagnostic Criteria for Mental Retardation**

A. Significantly subaverage intellectual functioning: an IQ score of approximately 70 or below on an individually administered IQ test (for infants, a clinical judgment of significantly subaverage intellectual functioning).
B. Concurrent deficits or impairments in present adaptive functioning (i.e., the person's effectiveness in meeting the standards expected for his or her age by his or her cultural group) in at least two of the following areas: communication, self-care, home living, social/interpersonal skills, use of community resources, self-direction, functional academic skills, work, leisure, health, and safety.
C. The onset is before age 18 years.

Code based on degree of severity reflecting level of intellectual impairment:

317	**Mild Mental Retardation:**	IQ level 50–55 to approximately 70
318.0	**Moderate Mental Retardation:**	IQ level 35–40 to 50–55
318.1	**Severe Mental Retardation:**	IQ level 20–25 to 35–40
318.2	**Profound Mental Retardation:**	IQ level below 20–25
319	**Mental Retardation, Severity Unspecified:**	when there is a strong presumption of mental retardation but the person's intelligence is untestable by standard tests

From American Psychiatric Association: Diagnostic and Statistical Manual of Mental Disorders, *Fourth Edition, Text Revision. Washington, DC, Author, 2000, p 49, reprinted by permission.*

TABLE 37–2. **Identification of Cause in Children with Severe Mental Retardation**

Cause	Percent of Total
Chromosomal disorder	22
Genetic syndrome	21
Developmental brain abnormality	9
Inborn errors of metabolism/neurodegenerative disorder	8
Congenital infections	4
Familial retardation	6
Perinatal causes	4
Postnatal causes	5
Unknown	21
Total	**100**

From Stromme P, Hayberg G: Aetiology in severe and mild mental retardation: A population based study of Norwegian children. Dev Med Child Neurol 2000;42:76–86.

mon biologic causes of mild mental retardation include genetic syndromes with multiple minor congenital anomalies, fetal deprivation, perinatal insults, intrauterine exposure to drugs of abuse, and sex chromosomal abnormalities. Familial clustering is also frequent.

In children with severe mental retardation, a biologic cause (most commonly prenatal) can be identified in over three quarters of cases (Table 37–2). In general, the earlier the problem occurs in development, the more severe its consequences. This is consistent with finding that disorders that affect early embryogenesis are the most common and severe: These include chromosomal (e.g., Down syndrome) and other genetic syndromes (e.g., fragile X syndrome), abnormalities of brain development (e.g., lissencephaly), and inborn errors of metabolism/neurodegenerative disorders (e.g., mucopolysaccharidoses).

Epidemiology. The prevalence of mental retardation depends on the definition used, the method of ascertainment, and the population. According to statistics (based on the APA definition), 2.5% of the population should have mental retardation, and 85% of these individuals should fall into the range of mild mental retardation. In 1997–98, approximately 600,000 children received services for mental retardation in federally supported school programs in the United States. This represented approximately 1.1% of all school-aged children. The reasons for the discrepancy between expected and observed rates of mental retardation is that fewer children than predicted are identified as having mild mental retardation. The following issues influence the identification process: (1) It is more difficult to diagnose mild mental retardation than the more severe forms. Therefore, professionals may defer the diagnosis of mental retardation and "give the benefit of the doubt" to the child. In addition, some instruments (e.g., Stanford-Binet, 4th edition) under-identify young children with mild mental retardation. Further, young children may show cognitive limitations without significant delays in adaptive behavior. As a result, new cases of mild mental retardation continue to be diagnosed until around 9 yr of age. (2) The AAMR and APA classifications of mental retardation use different definitions of significantly sub-average intellectual function. The AAMR definition increases the IQ threshold for mental retardation from 70 to 75 to reflect the standard error of IQ measurement. This definition doubles the prevalence of mental retardation. (3) Children with mental retardation may be incorporated into another diagnosis (e.g., autism, cerebral palsy). (4) It is possible that the number of children with mild mental retardation is actually decreasing as a result of public health programs.

Unlike mild mental retardation, the prevalence of severe mental retardation has not changed appreciably since the 1940s and is approximately 0.3–0.5% of the population. Many of the causes of severe mental retardation involve genetic or congenital brain malformations that can neither be anticipated nor treated at present. In addition, decreases in prevalence of severe mental retardation resulting from improved health care have been offset by new populations with severe deficits. Although prenatal diagnosis has been associated with a decreased prevalence of Down syndrome and early intervention has helped to reduce mental retardation caused by phenylketonuria and congenital hypothyroidism, the increased prevalence of prenatal exposure to drugs of abuse and the improved survival of "micro" premature infants have increased the prevalence of mental retardation.

Overall, mental retardation occurs more frequently in boys than in girls: 2:1 in mild mental retardation and 1.5:1 in severe mental retardation. This may be a consequence of X-linked disorders, the most prominent being fragile X syndrome.

Pathology/Pathogenesis. The limitations in our knowledge of the neuropathology of mental retardation is exemplified by the fact that 10–20% of brains of individuals with severe retardation appear entirely normal by standard neuropathologic study. The majority of brains of these individuals show only mild, nonspecific changes that correlate poorly with the degree of mental retardation. These changes include microcephaly, gray matter heterotopias in the subcortical white matter, unusually regular columnar arrangement of the cortex, and neurons that are more tightly packed than usual. Only a minority of the brains show more specific changes in dendritic and synaptic organization, with dysgenesis of dendritic spines or cortical pyramidal neurons, or impaired growth of dendritic trees.

Since the early 1980s, however, the application of new molecular biologic approaches has improved our understanding of the pathogenesis of mental retardation. The programming of the central nervous system (CNS) is now known to involve a process of induction, and CNS maturation has been defined in terms of genetic, molecular, autocrine, paracrine, and endocrine influences. In addition, several receptors, signaling molecules, and genes have been identified. Furthermore, it is now documented that the maintenance of different neuronal phenotypes in the adult brain involves the same genetic transcripts that play a crucial role during fetal development and activation of similar intracellular signal transduction. The integration of previous embryologic knowledge with this molecular information provides a clearer understanding not only of maturational changes that occur in brain development but also of how and why such changes take place. As an example of this new knowledge, a number of syndromes that were previously thought to involve complex chromosomal abnormalities have been found instead to be caused by single gene mutations involving induction. *Rubinstein-Taybi syndrome*, a disorder marked clinically by broad thumbs and great toes, characteristic facies, and severe mental retardation, has been shown to result from a mutation in the gene encoding for the transcriptional co-activator CREB-binding protein (CBP), a factor important in the control of gene expression during early embryogenesis.

Clinical Manifestations. Early diagnosis of mental retardation facilitates earlier intervention, realistic goal setting, easing of parental anxiety, and greater acceptance of the child in the community. Detecting, identifying, and diagnosing developmental dysfunction is a major justification for well-child care. Most children do not come to the pediatrician's attention because of "failed" screening tests but rather as a result of dysmorphisms, associated dysfunctions, or failure to meet age-appropriate expectations. There are no specific physical characteristics of mental retardation, but dysmorphisms are the earliest signs that bring children to the attention of the pediatrician. They may comprise a genetic syndrome, for example, Down syndrome, or be isolated, as in microcephaly. Associated dysfunctions are neurologic disorders that are seen more frequently in conjunction with mental retardation than in the general population, cerebral palsy and autism being examples. Most children with mental retardation, however, present because they do not keep up with their peers and fail to meet age-expected norms. In early infancy, this failure may include a lack of visual or auditory responsiveness, unusual muscle tone or posture, and feeding difficulties. Between 6 and 18 mo of age, motor delay (i.e., lack of sitting, crawling, walking) is the most common complaint. Language delay and behavior problems are common concerns after 18 mo (Table 37–3). Earlier identification of atypical development is likely to occur with more severe impairments, and mental retardation is usually identifiable by age 3 yr.

Laboratory Findings. The most commonly used medical diagnostic testing for children with mental retardation is neuroimaging; metabolic, molecular, and chromosomal blood testing; and electroencephalography (EEG). These tests should not be used, however, as screening tools for all children with mental retardation. Some children will need multiple tests and others will not require testing. Decisions on diagnostic testing should be based on the medical/family history, physical examination, testing by other disciplines, and the family's wishes. In general, karyotyping is indicated in children with multiple anomalies or positive family histories. Molecular testing for fragile X syndrome is appropriate for a male with moderate mental retardation, unusual physical features, and/or a family history of mental retardation; or a female with more subtle cognitive deficits associated with severe shyness. A child with a progressive neurologic disorder or acute behavioral changes will need metabolic investigation (e.g., urinary organic acids, plasma amino acids, blood lactate, lysosomal enzymes in lymphocytes); and a child with seizure-like episodes should have an EEG performed. Finally, children with abnormal head growth or asymmetric or new neurologic findings should have a neuroimaging procedure.

Although the aforementioned are the most common reasons for performing diagnostic tests, some children with more subtle physical or neurologic findings also can have determinable biologic causes of their mental retardation. About 6% of unexplained mental retardation can be accounted for by "micro" chromosomal abnormalities that can be identified by high resolution chromosomal banding, fluorescent *in situ* hybridization (FISH), or chromosome painting. In addition, magnetic resonance imaging scans have been found to document a significant number of subtle markers of cerebral dysgenesis in children with mental retardation. Formes frustes of amino acid and organic acid disorders have also been associated with mental retardation in addition to the more commonly associated manifestations of behavior change, lethargy, and coma.

How intensively one investigates the cause of a child's mental retardation is based on a number of factors: (1) What is the degree of mental retardation? One is less likely to find a biologic cause in a child with mild mental retardation than in a child with severe retardation. (2) Is there a specific diagnostic path to follow? If there is a medical history, a family history, or physical findings pointing to a specific disorder, a diagnosis is more likely to be made. Conversely, in the absence of these indicators, it is difficult to choose specific tests to perform. (3) Are the parents planning on having additional children? If so, one would be more likely to intensively seek disorders for which prenatal diagnosis or a specific early treatment option is available. (4) What are the parents' wishes? Some parents have little interest in searching for the cause of the retardation and focus exclusively on treatment. Others will be so focused on obtaining a diagnosis that they will have difficulty following through on interventions until a cause has been found. Both extremes and everything in between must be respected, but supportive guidance should be provided in the context of parent education.

Diagnosis/Differential Diagnosis. One of the roles of pediatricians is the early recognition and diagnosis of dysfunction. The developmental surveillance approach to early diagnosis of mental retardation must be multifaceted. Parental concerns and observations about their child's development should be listened to carefully because their observations have been found to be as accurate as developmental screening tests. Medical, genetic, and environmental risk factors should be recognized. Infants at high risk (e.g., history of prematurity, maternal substance abuse, perinatal insult) should be registered in newborn follow-up programs where they are evaluated periodically for developmental lags during the first 2 yr of life and referred to early intervention programs if appropriate. Developmental milestones should be recorded routinely. Abnormal appearance and function should

TABLE 37–3. Common Presentations of Mental Retardation by Age

Age	Area of Concern
Newborn	Dysmorphisms
	Major organ system dysfunction (e.g., feeding and breathing)
Early infancy (2–4 mo)	Failure to interact with the environment
	Concerns about vision and hearing impairments
Later infancy (6–18 mo)	Gross motor delay
Toddlers (2–3 yr)	Language delays or difficulties
Preschool (3–5 yr)	Language difficulties or delays
	Behavior difficulties, including play
	Delays in fine motor skills: cutting, coloring, drawing
School age (over 5 yr)	Academic underachievement
	Behavior difficulties (attention, anxiety, mood, conduct, and so on)

be assessed during health care maintenance visits. Whether developmental surveillance is a more effective technique for identification than recognition of failure to meet age-appropriate expectations (see earlier discussion) has not been established.

Before making the diagnosis of mental retardation, other disorders that affect cognitive abilities and adaptive behavior should be considered. There are conditions that mimic mental retardation and others that include mental retardation as an associated impairment; for example, over half of children with cerebral palsy (Chapter 591) or autism (Chapter 27) also have mental retardation. Differentiation of isolated cerebral palsy from mental retardation relies on motor skills being more affected than cognitive skills and on the presence of pathologic reflexes and tone changes. In autism, language and social adaptive skills are more affected than nonverbal reasoning skills whereas in mental retardation there are usually more equivalent deficits in social, motor, adaptive, and cognitive skills. Sensory deficits (severe hearing and vision loss), communication disorders, and poorly controlled seizure disorders may also mimic mental retardation, and certain progressive neurologic disorders may appear as mental retardation before regression is appreciated.

The formal diagnosis of mental retardation requires the administration of individual tests of intelligence and adaptive functioning. The most commonly used intelligence tests are the Bayley Scales of Infant Development (BSID-II), the Stanford-Binet Intelligence Scale, and the Wechsler Intelligence Scales (also see Chapter 16).

INFANT DEVELOPMENTAL TEST. The BSID-II is used to assess language, visual problem-solving skills, behavior, fine motor skills, and gross motor skills of children between 1 month and 3½ years of age. A Mental Developmental Index (MDI) and a Psychomotor Development Index score (PDI, a measure of motor competence) are derived from the results. This test permits the differentiation of infants with severe mental retardation from typically developing infants but is less helpful in distinguishing between a typical child and one with mild mental retardation.

INTELLIGENCE TESTS IN CHILDREN. The most commonly used psychologic tests for children older than 3 yr of age are the Wechsler Scales. The Wechsler Preschool and Primary Scale of Intelligence-revised (WPPSI-R) is used for children with mental ages of 3–7 yr. The Wechsler Intelligence Scale for Children-3rd edition (WISC-III) is used for children who function above a 6 yr mental age. Both scales contain a number of subtests in the areas of verbal and performance skills. Although children with mental retardation usually score below average on all subscale scores, they occasionally score in the average range in one or more performance areas. The Stanford-Binet Intelligence Scale is an acceptable alternative for school-aged children. It comprises 15 subtests that assess four areas of intelligence: verbal abilities, abstract/visual thinking, quantitative reasoning, and short-term memory. This permits the evaluator to determine, using some caution, areas of relative strength and weakness. The Stanford-Binet, however, tends to underidentify mental retardation in preschool-aged children.

TESTS OF ADAPTIVE FUNCTIONING. The most commonly used test of adaptive behavior is the Vineland Adaptive Behavior Scale (VABS). This test involves parental and/or caregiver/teacher semistructured interviews that assess adaptive behavior in four domains: communication, daily living skills, socialization, and motor skills. Other tests of adaptive behavior include the Woodcock-Johnson Scales of Independent Behavior and the American Association on Mental Retardation Adaptive Behavior Scale (ABS). There is usually (but not always) a good correlation between scores on the intelligence and adaptive scales. Basic adaptive abilities (e.g., feeding, dress-ing, hygiene), however, are more responsive to remedial efforts than is the IQ score. Adaptive abilities are also more variable, which may relate to the underlying condition and to environmental expectations. For example, while individuals with Prader-Willi syndrome have stability of adaptive skills through adulthood, individuals with fragile X syndrome may have increasing deficits over time.

Complications. Children with mental retardation have higher rates of vision, hearing, orthopedic, and behavioral/emotional disorders than do typically developing children. Yet, these disorders generally are detected later in children with mental retardation. If untreated, the associated impairments can potentially adversely affect the individual's outcome more than the intellectual deficit itself.

The most common associated deficits are motor impairments, behavioral/emotional disorders, medical complications, and seizure disorders. In general, the more severe the retardation, the greater are the number and severity of associated impairments. Knowing the cause of the mental retardation can help predict which associated impairments are most likely to occur. For example, fragile X syndrome and fetal alcohol syndrome are associated with a high rate of behavioral disorders, and Down syndrome has many medical complications (e.g., hypothyroidism, atlantoaxial subluxation). If there are associated impairments, they may require ongoing physical therapy, occupational therapy, speech-language therapy, adaptive equipment, glasses, hearing aids, antiepileptic medication, and so forth. Failure to adequately identify and treat these impairments may hinder successful habilitation and result in difficulties in the school, home, and/or neighborhood environment.

Prevention. Prevention of mental retardation can occur at many levels. Examples of primary prevention programs include (1) Heightening the public's awareness of the adverse fetal effects of alcohol and smoking; (2) Promoting maternal folic acid supplements and early prenatal care; (3) Encouraging the use of guards and railings to prevent falls and other accidents in the home; (4) Teaching about locking up medications, potential poisons, and firearms; (5) Ensuring the use of appropriate seat restraints when driving and the wearing of safety helmets when biking/skateboarding; (6) Encouraging safe sexual practices to prevent adolescent pregnancies and the transmission of sexually transmitted diseases, including HIV; and (7) Implementing immunization programs to reduce the prevalence of mental retardation due to encephalitis, meningitis, and congenital infections.

In addition, presymptomatic detection of certain disorders can result in treatment that prevents adverse consequences. State newborn screening for metabolic disorders, newborn hearing screening, and preschool lead poisoning prevention programs are examples. Radiologic screening for atlantoaxial subluxation in a child with Down syndrome is an example of presymptomatic testing in a disorder associated with mental retardation.

Treatment. Although mental retardation is not treatable, many associated impairments are amenable to intervention and may benefit from early identification. Although most children with mental retardation do not have a behavioral or emotional disorder as an associated impairment, challenging behaviors and mental illness occur with a greater frequency in this population than among children with normal development. These disorders are the primary cause for out-of-home placements, reduced employment prospects, and decreased opportunities for social integration. Some behavioral and emotional disorders are difficult to diagnose in children with more severe mental retardation because of their limited abilities to understand, communicate, interpret, or generalize. Other disorders are masked by the mental retardation. For example, the determination of attention-deficit/hyperactivity disorder (ADHD) in the presence of moderate to severe mental retardation is difficult, except in extreme cases. Discerning a thought disorder in someone with autism may be daunting. Finally, some behavioral conditions are unique to mental retardation: e.g., self-stimulatory, self-injurious, and stereotypical behaviors.

Although mental illness is generally of biologic origin and responds to medication, behavioral disorders may result from a mismatch between the child's abilities and the demands of the situation, organic problems, and/or family difficulties. They may also represent attempts by the child to communicate, gain attention, or avoid frustration. In assessing the challenging behavior, one must consider whether it is inappropriate for the child's mental age, rather than for his or her chronological age. When intervention is needed, an environmental change, such as a more appropriate classroom setting, may improve certain behavior problems. Behavior management techniques are also useful and psychopharmacologic agents may be appropriate in certain situations.

Medication is not useful in treating the core symptoms of mental retardation; no agent has been found to improve intellectual function. Medication may be helpful, however, in treating associated behavioral and psychiatric disorders. Psychopharmacology is generally directed at specific symptom complexes including ADHD, self-injurious behavior, aggression, anxiety, and depression. Before long-term therapy with any psychopharmacologic agent is initiated, a short trial should be conducted. Even if a medication proves successful, its use should be re-evaluated at least yearly to assess the need for continued treatment.

Supportive Care and Management. Each child with mental retardation needs a medical home with a pediatrician who is readily accessible to the family to answer questions, help coordinate care, and discuss concerns. The role of the pediatrician includes involvement in prevention efforts, early diagnosis, identification of associated deficits, interdisciplinary management, provision of primary care, and advocacy for the child and family. The management strategies for children with mental retardation should be multi-modal, with efforts directed at all aspects of the child's life: health, education, social and recreational activities, behavior problems, and associated impairments. Support for parents and siblings should also be provided.

PRIMARY CARE. For children with mental retardation, primary care has a number of important components: (1) Provision of the same primary care received by all other children of similar chronological age (see Chapter 5); (2) Anticipatory guidance relevant to the child's functioning: e.g., feeding, toileting, school, accident prevention, sexuality education; and (3) Assessment of issues that are specifically relevant to that child's disorder: e.g., examination of the teeth in children who exhibit bruxism, thyroid function in children with Down syndrome, vision and hearing testing in all children. The American Academy of Pediatrics has published a series of guidelines for children with specific genetic disorders associated with mental retardation (e.g., Down, fragile X, and Williams syndrome). In addition, goals should be considered and programs adjusted as needed during the visit. Decisions should also be made about what additional information is required for future planning or to explain why the child is not meeting expectations. Other evaluations, such as formal psychologic or educational testing, may need to be scheduled.

INTERDISCIPLINARY MANAGEMENT. The pediatrician has the responsibility for consulting with other disciplines to make the diagnosis and coordinate treatment services. Consultant services may include psychology, speech/language pathology, physical therapy, occupational therapy, audiology, nutrition, nursing, social work, as well as medical specialties

such as neurology, genetics, psychiatry, and/or surgical specialties. Contact with early intervention/school personnel is equally important. The family should be an integral part of the planning and direction of this process. Care should be family centered and culturally sensitive; for the older child, his or her participation in planning and decision making should be promoted to whatever extent possible.

PERIODIC RE-EVALUATION. The child's abilities and the family's needs change over time. As the child grows, more information must be provided to parents, goals must be reassessed, and programming needs adjusted. A periodic review should include information about the child's health status as well as his or her functioning at home, school, and in other community settings. Other information, such as formal psychologic or educational testing, may be helpful. Re-evaluation should be undertaken at routine intervals (6–12 mo during early childhood), at any time the child is not meeting expectations, or when he or she is moving from one service delivery system to another. This is especially true during the transition to adulthood, beginning at age 14 yr as mandated by the Individuals with Disabilities Education Act Amendments of 1997 (IDEA '97). This transitioning should include the transfer of care to the adult health care system by age 21.

EDUCATIONAL SERVICES. Education is the single most important discipline involved in the treatment of children with mental retardation. The educational program must be relevant to the child's needs and address the child's individual strengths and weaknesses. The child's developmental level, his or her requirements for support, and goals for independence provide a basis for establishing an Individualized Family Support Plan (IFSP) for early intervention services or an Individualized Education Program (IEP) for school-aged children, as mandated by federal legislation.

LEISURE AND RECREATIONAL ACTIVITIES. The child's social and recreational needs should be addressed. Although young children with mental retardation are generally included in play activities with children who have typical development, adolescents frequently do not have opportunities for appropriate social interactions and are not competitive in extracurricular sports activities. Yet, participation in sports should be encouraged because it offers many benefits, including weight management, development of physical coordination, maintenance of cardiovascular fitness, and improvement of self-image. Social activities are equally important, including dances, trips, dating, and other typical social and recreational events.

FAMILY COUNSELING. Many families adapt well to having a child with mental retardation, but some have emotional/social difficulties. The risks of parental depression and child abuse and neglect are higher in this group of children than in the general population. Among the factors that have been associated with good family coping and parenting skills are stability of the marriage, good parental self-esteem, limited number of siblings, higher socioeconomic status, lower degree of disability/associated impairments, appropriate parental expectations and acceptance of the diagnosis, supportive extended family members, and availability of community programs and respite care services. In those families in which the emotional burden of having a child with mental retardation is great, family counseling, parent support groups, respite care, and home health services should be an integral part of the treatment plan.

ADVOCACY. The pediatrician can play a number of advocacy roles: maintaining close contact with the department of health/local school district to advocate for an appropriate IFSP/IEP; identifying eligibility for financial supports through Supplemental Security Income (SSI) from Social Security; assessing the impact of the Americans with Disabilities Act (ADA) on the adolescent's access to jobs and community activities; referring families to appropriate parental support groups or websites for their specific disorder/syndrome; assuring adequate respite services for the family; becoming involved in the community to help develop educational, recreational, and leisure programs for children with disabilities; and advocating for improved health care coverage by both private and governmental insurers.

Prognosis. Mental retardation is not always a lifelong disorder. Children may meet criteria for mental retardation at an early age but later evolve into a more specific developmental disorder (e.g., communication disorder, autism, slow learner–borderline normal intelligence). Others who are diagnosed with mental retardation during their school years may develop sufficient adaptive behavior skills so that they no longer fit the diagnosis as adolescents, or the effects of maturation and plasticity may result in children moving from one diagnostic category to another (e.g., from moderate to mild retardation). Alternatively some children who are diagnosed with a specific learning disability or communication disorder may not maintain their rate of cognitive growth and fall into the range of mental retardation over time. By adolescence, however, the diagnosis has generally stabilized.

The long-term outcome of individuals with mental retardation depends on the underlying cause, the degree of cognitive and adaptive deficits, the presence of associated medical and developmental impairments, the capabilities of the families, and the school/community supports, services, and training provided to the child and family. As adults, many individuals with mild mental retardation are capable of gaining economic and social independence with functional literacy. They may need periodic supervision, however, especially when under social or economic stress. Most live successfully in the community, either independently or in supervised settings. Life expectancy is not adversely affected by mental retardation itself.

For individuals with moderate mental retardation, the goals of education are to enhance adaptive abilities and "survival" academic and vocational skills so they are better able to live in the adult world. The concept of supported employment has been very beneficial to these individuals; the person is trained by a coach to do a specific job in the setting in which the person is to work. This bypasses the need for a sheltered workshop experience and has resulted in successful work adaptation in the community for many people with mental retardation. These individuals generally live at home or in a supervised setting in the community.

As adults, people with severe-profound mental retardation usually require extensive to pervasive supports. These individuals may have associated impairments, such as cerebral palsy, behavioral disorders, epilepsy, or sensory impairments that further limit their adaptive functioning. They may perform simple tasks in supervised settings, and most people with this level of mental retardation are able to live in the community with appropriate supports.

American Psychiatric Association: *Diagnostic and Statistical Manual of Mental Disorders*, 4th edition (DSM-IV, text revision). Washington, DC, American Psychiatric Association, 2000.

Committee on Children with Disabilities, American Academy of Pediatrics: Pediatrician's role in the development and implementation of an Individualized Education Plan (IEP) and/or an Individual Family Service Plan (IFSP). *Pediatrics* 1999;104:124–7.

Curry CJ, Stevenson RE, Aughton D, et al: Evaluation of mental retardation: Recommendations of a consensus conference. *Am J Med Genet* 1997;72:468–77.

Guralnick MJ: *The Effectiveness of Early Intervention*. Baltimore, Brookes Publishing, 1997.

Luckasson R, Coulter D, Polloway EA, et al: *Mental Retardation: Definition, Classification, and Systems of Supports*, 9th ed. Washington, DC, American Association on Mental Retardation, 1992.

Roeleveld N, Zielhuis GA, Gabreëls F: The prevalence of mental retardation: A critical review of recent literature. *Dev Med Child Neurol* 1997;39:125–32.

Shapiro BK, Batshaw ML: *Mental Retardation. Current Pediatric Therapy 17*. Philadelphia, WB Saunders, 2002.

Shapiro BK, Batshaw ML: Mental retardation. In *Children with Disabilities*, 5th ed. Baltimore, Brookes Publishing, 2002.

Strømme P, Hagberg G. Aetiology in severe and mild mental retardation: A population-based study of Norwegian children. *Dev Med Child Neurol* 2000;42:76–86.

Chapter 38
Pediatric Palliative Care: The Care of Children with Life-Limiting Illness *Stephen Liben*

In the United States more than 50,000 children die every year, resulting in over 250,000 bereaved parents, siblings, and other loved ones having their lives significantly and permanently altered. This chapter focuses on the management of unnecessary suffering of these children as well as how to better support the bereaved they leave behind.

In 1990 the World Health Organization defined palliative care as "The active total care of patients whose disease is not responsive to curative treatment. Control of pain, of other symptoms, and of psychological, social and spiritual problems, is paramount. The goal of palliative care is achievement of the best quality of life for patients and their families." Palliative care is provided in hospitals (some with specialized palliative care units), in the home whenever possible and desired, and in hospices. Hospices provide a structured model of how to finance, maintain, and coordinate a range of palliative care services, often in a freestanding facility. In some countries specialized pediatric hospices (in contrast to adult hospices that may occasionally admit a child) provide an important bridge between hospital care and home care.

Pediatric palliative medicine is that part of palliative care that is practiced by physicians and is involved with the study and medical care of children with life-limiting (or life-threatening) illness. The mandate of pediatricians to oversee children's physical, mental, and emotional health and development from conception to maturity (Chapter 1) includes the practice of palliative medicine for those children in their care who live with a significant possibility of death before reaching adulthood. In addition, many pediatric subspecialties have a responsibility for a unique population of children at high risk for a premature death. Thus, learning the basic knowledge, attitudes, and skills of palliative medicine is integral to the education of both the generalist and subspecialist pediatrician. Such training has the added benefit of improving skills in other areas of care such as communication and symptom control.

Compared with traditional cancer-based adult end-of-life care, pediatric palliative care has:

1. Smaller numbers of dying children. This means that even professionals specializing in the care of children may only rarely encounter the death of a child. The relative infrequency of pediatric deaths has also resulted in chronic underfunding of pediatric end-of-life care services and underrepresentation of children in palliative care research protocols.

2. A broad spectrum of illnesses, including many rare diseases, that often require involvement of a number of disciplines. Although results obtained from adult oncology–based research can have benefits that apply to many palliative care patients, in pediatrics the wide range of often poorly understood disorders

limits the ability to generalize from any one disease-specific research study to another.

3. Unpredictable illness trajectories with significant prognostic uncertainty. It is often impossible to accurately predict the progression of illness for many life-threatening illnesses in pediatrics. This leads to child and family distress from uncertainty coupled with difficulty funding and sustaining pediatric palliative care programs that may need to provide varied amounts of services over years. Palliative care for these children may necessarily involve some overlap with chronic curative care, with palliative care becoming more prominent as the child progresses from being chronically to terminally ill.

4. More uncertainty about whether treatments are supportive/palliative versus those that primarily cure or prolong life. Deciding whether a specific treatment is palliative or life prolonging is not always possible with emerging technologies such as noninvasive respiratory ventilation.

Advances in pediatric medicine have resulted in an increase in the number of children who live longer, often with significant dependence on new (and expensive) technologies. These children have complex chronic conditions across the spectrum of congenital and acquired life-threatening disorders (Chapter 37). Children with complex chronic conditions require a combination of palliative and curative treatments. These children, who may survive frequent near-death crises followed by the renewed need for rehabilitative and life-prolonging treatments, are best served by a system that is flexible and responsive to changing needs.

Care Planning. Although it may not be possible to accurately determine how long a child may live, there is often a delay between the time when a terminal prognosis is first recognized by physicians and when the prognosis is understood by parents. This time delay may impede informed decision-making about how these children spend the end of their lives. Given the inherent prognostic uncertainty of a life-limiting diagnosis, the time when the physician recognizes a significant possibility of patient mortality is probably the best time to initiate discussions concerning resuscitation, symptom control, and end-of-life care planning. Patients and families may be most comfortable continuing with physicians and other care providers with whom they have an established relationship; in most cases the services of a palliative care specialist or *hospice program* can be consultative to the primary or subspecialty care physician and team. Physician discomfort in discussing end-of-life care should not result in the discussion being deferred to others or to a later time. Physician feelings of discomfort are to be expected given the difficult nature and highly charged atmosphere of a child facing death, and physicians may need varying levels of support themselves as they map out a care plan with the child and parents. At times, for a variety of reasons including limited local resources and experience or the need for concurrent respite and care of other family members, transfer to a hospital, or home care, or hospice palliative care program may be necessary.

Home care of the dying child requires 24 hr per day accessibility to experts in pediatric palliative care, a team approach, and an identified coordinator who serves as a link between hospitals, the community, and specialists, and can arrange for hospital admissions and respite care, as needed. Provision of *respite services* is especially important to families caring for children with complex chronic conditions over prolonged periods of time. Such care may involve temporary placement of a child with another family or in an institution such as a hospital or hospice. It is important to plan a respite admission before the family caring for the child feels overwhelmed. The family should be reassured that taking respite is not a personal failure. Although children, when given the choice, prefer to remain at home, a child may need to periodically return to the hospital or hospice even when there is comprehensive home support.

Good end-of-life care can be effectively carried out in a *hospital setting* but only when institutions are flexible enough to modify protocols that may present unnecessary obstacles to the care of dying patients. Within tertiary care hospitals the neonatal and pediatric intensive care units (ICUs) are the locations where most children die (Chapter 64). Many of the children in ICUs die after discussions that lead to the limitation or withdrawal of therapy. Improving the care of these hospitalized children and their families involves liberalizing visiting policies and respecting privacy, as well as removing some of the obstacles inherent in intensive care settings, such as routine testing and monitoring of vital signs. The philosophy of palliative care can be successfully implemented in a hospital setting when the focus of care is maintained on comfort and quality of life. All interventions that affect the child and family need to be assessed in relation to these goals. This proactive approach asks the question "What can we offer that will improve the quality of this child's life?" instead of "What therapies are we no longer going to offer this patient?" Staff who are comfortable and supportive of this approach need to be carefully chosen with consideration given to the fact that pediatric palliative care, like other types of intensive care, is not a skill with which everyone is comfortable. In addition, comprehensive palliative care requires a multidisciplinary approach that may include nurses, physicians, psychologists, psychiatrists, social workers, religious counselors, child-life specialists, and trained volunteers.

Communication Issues and Anticipatory Guidance

THE CHILD. Responding to children's questions about death, such as "What's happening to me? Am I dying?", requires a careful exploration of what is already known by the child, what is really being asked (the question behind the question), and why the question is being asked at this particular time and in this setting. A child's perception of death depends on his or her concepts of universality (the recognition that all things inevitably die), irreversibility (the ability to understand that dead people cannot come back to life), nonfunctionality (the understanding that being dead means that all biologic functions cease), and causality (the ability to understand the objective causes of death). See Chapter 33. Children's fears of death are centered on the concrete fear of being separated from parents and other loved ones, rather than on the existential consequences of an afterlife common to adults. This fear of separation may be responded to in different ways, with some families giving reassurance that loving relatives will be waiting, and others using religious figures or referring to an eternal spiritual connection ("I will always be there for you"). Adolescents have their own unique issues, including risk-taking behavior that seems to challenge their concept of universality ("I am invincible").

It is also important to recognize that a child's expressed question may have different levels of meaning. A child asking, "Am I dying?" may really be testing the honesty of the person being asked. The child asking, "Why is this happening to me?" may be signaling a need to be with someone who is comfortable listening to such unanswerable questions. Many children find nonverbal expression much easier than talking; art, play therapy, and storytelling may be more helpful than direct conversation. Parents have an instinctive duty to protect their children from harm. When facing the death of their child many parents attempt to keep the reality of impending death hidden from their children with the hope that their child can be "protected" from the harsh reality. Although it is important to respect parental wishes to avoid the subject of death with their children, it is also true that many young children already know what is happening to them even when it has been purposely left unspoken. Perpetuating the myth that "everything is going to be all right" takes away the chance to explore fears and provide reassurance. For example, children may blame themselves for their illness and the hardships that it causes for their loved ones. Their guilt can be addressed and resolved only by open, honest communication, requiring a sensitive response that takes into account the child's developmental stage and unique lived experience.

THE SIBLINGS. Brothers and sisters are at special risk both during the course of their sibling's illness and after their death. Because of the extraordinary demands placed on parents to meet the needs of their ill child, healthy siblings may feel that their own needs are not being acknowledged. These feelings of neglect may then trigger guilt about their own good health and resentment towards parents and their ill sibling. Younger siblings may react to the stress by becoming seemingly oblivious to the turmoil around them. Parents need to know that this is a normal response, and siblings should be encouraged to maintain the normal routines of daily living. Siblings who are most involved with their sick brothers or sisters before death usually adjust better both at the time of and after the death. Acknowledging and validating sibling feelings, being honest and open, and appropriately involving them in the life of their sick sibling provide a good foundation for coping with loss.

THE PARENTS. The populations of children who die before reaching adulthood include a disproportionate number of nonverbal and preverbal children who are developmentally unable to make autonomous care decisions. For these children it is parents that take on the role of primary decision-maker. Parents may blame themselves for their child's illness even when logic dictates that they had nothing to do with what is happening to their child ("If only I had taken him to the doctor sooner") and may spend considerable energy and resources looking for "miracle cures." The physician should be sensitive to these possible and not necessarily easily expressed parental concerns. There is potential for physicians to provide much needed support to parents at these times by engaging in active listening while validating the range of concerns that parents may have. Parents also need to know about the availability of home care, respite services, educational books and videotapes, and support groups. It is important to discuss how parents envision their child's death and to address myths surrounding pain control and the benefit of involving siblings. What all parents want to know is that their physician will not abandon them as the goals of care shift primarily from cure to comfort. Physicians should recognize the important role they have in continuing to care for the child and family as the primary goal of treatment changes from prolongation of life to quality of life. Regular meetings between caregivers and the family are essential in order to reassess and manage symptoms, explore the impact of illness on immediate family members, and provide anticipatory guidance. At these meetings, important issues include finding an appropriate physical setting for the meeting (i.e., not a hospital corridor), reviewing what was previously discussed, listening to concerns and issues as they are revealed, having parents repeat back what was said to ensure clarity, and responding with honest, factual answers in areas of uncertainty.

In communications with the child and family, the physician should avoid giving estimates of survival length, even when these are explicitly asked for. These predictions are invariably inaccurate because population-based statistics do not predict the course for individual patients. A more honest approach may be to explore ranges of time in general terms ("weeks to months," "months to years"). At the same time, the physician can ask parents what they might do differently if they knew how long their child would live and then assist them in thinking through the options relating to their specific concerns (e.g., suggest celebrating upcoming holidays/important events earlier in order to take advantage of times when the child may be feeling better). It is

generally wise to suggest that relatives who wish to visit might do so earlier rather than later given the unpredictability of the time course of many illnesses. For the child and family the integration of bad news is a process, not an event. The physician should expect that some issues previously discussed may not be fully resolved for the child and parents (e.g., do not resuscitate orders, artificial feedings) and may need to be revisited over time.

Decision-Making. During the course of a child's life-limiting illness, a series of difficult decisions need to be made in relation to truth telling and disclosure, location of care, medications with risks and benefits (e.g., steroids), the principle of double effect in the beneficent use of analgesics, withholding and or withdrawing life-prolonging technologies, experimental treatments in research protocols, and the use of "alternative" therapies (also see Chapters 2 and 3). Decision-making should remain focused on the goals of therapy rather than on specific limitations of care; e.g., "This is what we can offer," instead of "This is what we can no longer do." Instead of meeting specifically to discuss a do-not-resuscitate order, a more general discussion centered on the goals of therapy will naturally lead to considering which interventions are in the child's best interests. Unclear terms used in doctor's orders in the chart such as "withholding heroic or extraordinary measures" are best replaced by reference to specific interventions that are then documented in a care plan (e.g., "suction airway secretions prn" rather than "do not do lab tests"). It is important to support parents in their decision-making process rather than to make them feel that it is up to them alone to choose what is best. Rather than asking parents if they want to forgo cardiopulmonary resuscitation for their child (placing the full burden of decision-making on them), it might be preferable to discuss why deciding against resuscitation attempts is a reasonable course of action. Once the goals of therapy are agreed upon, the physician may draft a letter that outlines the end-of-life care plan for the child. The letter should be as detailed as possible, including suggestions for medications and the telephone numbers of caregivers who know the patient best. Such a letter, given to the parents, with copies to involved caregivers and institutions, can be a useful aid in communication, especially in times of crisis.

Conflicts in decision-making (see Chapters 2 and 54) can occur within families, within health care teams, between the child and family, and between the family and professional caregivers. For children who are developmentally unable to provide guidance in decision-making (neonates, very young children, neurologically impaired children) parents and health care professionals may come to different conclusions as to what is in the child's best interests. In some families and cultures truth telling and autonomy are much less valued when compared with family integrity (Chapter 3). Although frequently encountered, differences in opinion are often manageable for all involved when lines of communication are kept open and the main goals of care, to provide comfort and quality of life, are agreed upon. Decision-making with adolescents presents specific challenges given the shifting boundary that separates childhood from adulthood (Chapters 2, 14, and 100).

Euthanasia is the intentional, active intervention to terminate a life. The withdrawal of treatments with burdens that outweigh benefits is not euthanasia (Chapters 2 and 64). Providing sufficient analgesia to relieve pain, even if it may have the unintentional effect of shortening life (the principle of double effect), is not the same as intentionally terminating a life. Although controversial, most palliative care professionals would argue against euthanasia and physician-assisted suicide (physicians explicitly providing the means to cause death) because it is unlikely that children or adolescents will actively seek death when they are receiving appropriate pain relief and palliative care.

Symptom Management. Pain control is of paramount importance in reducing the suffering of the child, family, and caregivers, but many dying children do not have their pain successfully treated. See Chapters 66, 87, and 486 for effective management of pain. In 1998 the World Health Organization stated: "Nothing would have a greater impact on the quality of life of children with cancer than the dissemination and implementation of the current principles of palliative care, including pain relief and symptom control."

Pain is a complex sensation influenced by tissue damage as well as by situational factors, including cognitive, behavioral, emotional, social, and cultural issues that are unique to each person. In end-of-life care it is important to form and initiate a pain treatment plan even when the diagnosis may be unclear, the prognosis uncertain, and the ability of the child to communicate limited. Many children with life-limiting illness are unable to verbalize their symptoms and will instead communicate their discomfort nonverbally. Presumptive therapy should be initiated promptly, and treatment plans can then be modified based on the response. For the dying child, in whom accurate assessment of the cause of pain may be difficult, it is important to frequently reassess therapy and to honestly inform parents that it may take several dose and medication adjustments in order to determine optimal analgesic requirements. Guidelines for the treatment of pain and the use of opioids are summarized in Tables 38–1 and 38–2.

Dying children have a multitude of symptoms, in addition to pain, for significant periods before their death. Respiratory symptoms such as *dyspnea* (the subjective sensation of shortness of breath) are common because many children with chronic illnesses have difficulty swallowing and handling their airway secretions. Excessive airway secretions and salivation owing to poor swallowing may sometimes be helped by treatment with oral glycopyrrolate. As death approaches, a buildup of secretions may result in noisy respiration sometimes referred to as a death rattle. Patients at this stage are usually unconscious, and noisy respirations are often more distressing for others than for the child. Pointing out to parents the child's lack of distress and using an anticholinergic drug, such as hyoscine, may be helpful. Pneumonia is a frequent complication in dying children. Dyspnea (as opposed to tachypnea which may not be associated with feelings of distress) can be relieved with the use of regularly scheduled plus as-needed doses of opioids. Oxygen may be helpful in certain cases to relieve hypoxemia-related headaches. As with all medical interventions the question must be asked, "Who is being treated—the child, parents, or staff?" For example, giving oxygen to the cyanotic child who is otherwise quiet and relaxed may serve to relieve only staff discomfort while having no impact on patient distress.

Neurologic symptoms include *seizures* that are often part of the antecedent illness but may increase in frequency and severity toward the end of life. Anticonvulsants should be administered, and parents can be taught to use rectal diazepam at home. Increased *irritability* accompanies some neurodegenerative dis-

---

TABLE 38–1. Pain and Symptom Management

Establish realistic goals of treatment—maintaining comfort is a priority.
Anticipate and plan for symptoms before they occur.
Utilize a stepwise approach to pain management (see Figure 66–1).
Choose the least invasive route for medications—by mouth whenever possible.
Prescribe regular (not PRN) medications for constant pain.
Consider use of adjuvant drugs:

- Antidepressants and anticonvulsants—neuropathic pain
- Neuroleptics—nausea, agitation
- Sedatives and hypnotics—anxiety or muscle spasm
- Steroids—resistant pain
- Stimulants—opioid-induced somnolence

Consider anesthetic blocks for regional pain. Use topical local anesthetics when possible (see Chapter 66).
Always include cognitive (guided imagery, distraction), physical (TENS, physiotherapy, massage), and behavioral (biofeedback, behavior modification) techniques.

TENS = transcutaneous electrical nerve stimulation.

orders; it may be particularly disruptive because of the resultant break in normal sleep-wake patterns and the difficulty in finding respite facilities for children who have prolonged crying. Judicious use of sedatives in the daytime (e.g., benzodiazepines) combined with hypnotics at night (e.g., chloral hydrate) may achieve a balance that can dramatically improve the quality of life for both child and caregivers.

Feeding and *hydration* issues raise ethical questions that include the use of nasogastric and gastrostomy feedings for the child who can no longer feed by mouth (see also Chapter 2). These complex questions require evaluating the risks and benefits of artificial feedings and taking into consideration the child's functional level and prognosis. At times it may be appropriate to initiate a trial of tube feedings with the understanding that they may be discontinued at a later stage of the illness. A commonly held but unsubstantiated belief is that hydration is a "comfort measure," which may result in well-meaning but disruptive and invasive attempts to administer intravenous fluids to a dying child. Studies of dying adults show that the sensation of thirst may be alleviated by careful efforts to keep the mouth moist and clean. There may also be deleterious side effects to artificial hydration in the form of increased secretions, need for frequent urination, and exacerbation of dyspnea.

Nausea demands prompt treatment after a search for common causes (drug effects, constipation, primary disease, metabolic disturbance). Drugs such as metoclopramide, phenothiazines, ondansetron, and steroids may be used depending on the cause and desired secondary effects (e.g., if sedation is desired, a sedating phenothiazine may be used). *Vomiting* may accompany nausea but may also occur without nausea in the presence of bowel obstruction. *Constipation* is common in neurologic disorders, and the first step is to assess stool frequency and quantity. Children with minimal solid food intake may be comfortable with bowel movements as infrequent as weekly. Children on

---

TABLE 38–2. Opioid Use Guidelines

Clarify the differences between tolerance vs. physical dependence vs. addiction.
Dispel the myth that strong medications should be saved for last.
Anticipate and treat/prevent common side effects (constipation, pruritus, nausea, dysphoria, somnolence).
Always start constipation treatment when starting opioids.
Begin with weak opioids for mild pain (e.g., codeine). Replace with strong opioids (e.g., morphine) for unresponsive or persisting pain (see Figure 66–1).
Start with short-acting opioids at regular intervals then convert to long-acting only when dose requirements have stabilized.
Consider switching to a different opioid when limited by side effects (e.g., myoclonus).
Consider subcutaneous infusions when oral/rectal routes are no longer possible.

regular opioids should routinely be placed on stool softeners (docusate) and may also need the addition of laxative agents (senna derivatives, lactulose). *Diarrhea* may be particularly difficult for the child and family and may be treated with loperamide and opioids. Paradoxical diarrhea, a result of overflow resulting from constipation, must also be considered.

Hematologic issues include consideration of transfusions for anemia and thrombocytopenia. Most children in the palliative phase may be managed by intermittent red cell and platelet transfusions for bleeding that interferes with the quality of life. Serious bleeding is disturbing for all concerned, and a plan involving the use of fast-acting sedatives should be prepared in advance.

Skin care issues include the prevention of problems such as bedsores by the early use of inexpensive egg-crate type foam mattresses and careful attention to positioning. Pruritus may be secondary to systemic disorders or drug therapy. Treatment includes avoiding excessive use of soap, using moisturizers, trimming fingernails, and wearing loose-fitting clothing, in addition to administering topical or systemic steroids. Oral antihistamines and other specific therapies may also be indicated (e.g., cholestyramine in biliary disease).

When discussing possible therapies or interventions with adolescent patients or with the parents of any ill child, it is important to raise the issue of complementary or alternative medicine because it has been shown that many patients use some form of alternative medicine therapy but are reluctant to bring it up with their physician (Chapters 3 and 713). Although mostly unproven, some therapies are inexpensive and provide relief to individual patients. Other therapies may be expensive, painful, intrusive, and even dangerous. By initiating conversation and inviting discussion in a nonjudgmental way, the physician can offer advice on the safety of different therapies and may help avoid expensive and dangerous interventions.

The Terminal Phase. As death approaches, the major tasks of the physician are to help prepare the child and family for expected problems and issues and to continue to stay involved in care. If the child is at home, regular phone calls should be made to help manage new symptoms as they occur (e.g., terminal airway secretions, seizures, irritability, myoclonus, vomiting). Legal issues such as who will perform the declaration of death may be addressed, and the necessary documents can be partially filled out and left in a sealed envelope in the child's home. For children in the hospital, the care plan should be clear to all involved professionals and should include an understanding of the specific needs and requests of the child and family.

Initiating a discussion of the options for funeral arrangements may be appropriate inasmuch as some parents prefer to settle these practical issues before the child's death. Attendance of young siblings at the funeral should be discussed and sibling participation encouraged. Excluding siblings from the funeral deprives them of an opportunity for partial closure and may devalue their need to grieve.

In an intensive care setting, where technology can put distance between the child and parent, the physician should discontinue the use of unneeded equipment. While still in the ICU, even children on ventilators can be placed in their parents' arms. Parents who may not have held their infant since birth may be afraid to ask permission to hold their child but will be relieved to be offered the opportunity when it is presented. Hearing and the ability to sense touch is often present until death. Siblings and family members should be encouraged to talk to and touch the child, even if he or she seems unresponsive. It seems that many children who live with prolonged illness die only after their parents have begun the process of "letting go." Some children appear to wait for "permission to die," and their parents' acceptance of the inevitable may play a role in the timing of their death.

For the family, the moment of death is an event that is recalled in detail for years to come. After death, they should be given the option of remaining with their child for as long as they would like. During this time, physicians and other professionals do best by not trying to "do and say too much." Quietly sitting with the family and asking whether they would consider holding the infant may be appropriate in some cultures. Different ethnic and cultural practices should be taken into consideration and facilitated (Chapter 3). In some traditions it is important to have the family take the child to the place of worship directly instead of passing through the hospital morgue. Arranging this and other details in advance will help avoid some stress for both family and staff.

The physician should discuss the option of an autopsy and organ donation, answering questions that parents may be reluctant to ask (e.g., Will the face be disturbed?). Parents might also be reminded that they may have questions later on that can be answered by an autopsy (e.g., "Will present and future siblings and grandchildren be affected?"). The parents can also be offered genetic counseling when appropriate.

The physician's decision to attend the funeral is a personal one. It may serve the dual purpose of showing respect as well as helping him or her cope with a personal sense of loss.

Bereavement involves a complex, individualized process that is only partially understood. What is known is that the death of a child is not something to "get over," and intense feelings of sadness may persist for years. The physician should arrange to meet with the family at a set time after the death, to review autopsy results if applicable, and to answer questions that may remain. When the death occurs after a prolonged hospitalization, a hospital memorial service may be held. These services often serve as an opportunity for closure by staff who were involved in care but who may not have been present at the child's death.

The physician can be proactive in preventing the phenomenon of replacement children. Physicians have in the past suggested to parents, "Get on with your lives," and "Why not have another child as soon as possible?" Instead, parents should be made aware that nothing can replace the uniqueness of their deceased child and that, although their memories will remain forever, the pain for most does subside with time. Physicians should also be aware that the divorce rate for bereaved couples is not necessarily higher than for the general population. Divorce is, therefore, not an inevitable result of the grieving process and couples should be referred for counseling when appropriate.

Because grieving for a deceased child is among the most stressful of life experiences, it is recommended that a professional trained in bereavement counseling be consulted following the death of a child. Long-term follow-up should be the norm, including regular phone calls at significant times such as birthdays, anniversaries of the death, and significant holidays. Other interventions that may be helpful include support groups for bereaved parents and siblings, where those who share common experiences can learn from one another. Such support groups include The Compassionate Friends and Candlelighters/Lamplighters.

The Pediatrician. Care for children with life-limiting illness places unique and at times intense demands on the pediatrician. The ability to care effectively for dying children and their families is not a skill shared by all. Most pediatricians have had little, if any, formal palliative care education and limited clinical experience in how to care for a dying child. In addition, there are situations and times in the professional's own life when the demands of end-of-life care for their patients may be especially difficult (e.g., at times of the physician's own personal losses). At such times the availability of supportive colleagues is invaluable, and it may be appropriate and in the patient's best interest to refer to others. However, for most physicians, the duty to care for their patients through the illness spectrum including the terminal phase is a commitment that reaches to the core of their professional identity. Most physicians have had training that emphasized their role as conquerors of disease. This notion, coupled with limited training in psychosocial care, in communication skills, and in pain and symptom management may promote a feeling of personal and professional failure when facing the death of a patient. Like many aspects of medical practice, palliative medicine requires that physicians evolve their own knowledge, skills, and attitudes about healing and their unique role in caring even when death is the unavoidable outcome for their patients. Pediatricians caring for dying children and their families may require supervision from other trained professionals in examining their personal feelings, values, and attitudes about the meaning and goals of their work.

American Academy of Pediatrics: Palliative care for children. *Pediatrics* 2000;106(2):351–7.

Armstrong-Dailey D, Zarbock S (editors): *Hospice Care for Children*, 2nd ed. Oxford, Oxford University Press, 2001.

Goldman A (editor): *Care of the Dying Child*, 2nd printing. Oxford, Oxford University Press, 1998.

National Hospice Organization: *The Compendium of Pediatric Palliative Care*. Virginia, National Hospice Organization, 2000. www.nhpco.org.

Sourkes BM: *Armfuls of Time: The Psychological Experience of the Child with Life-Threatening Illness*. Pittsburgh, University of Pittsburgh Press, 1995.

Wolfe J, Grier HE, Klar N, et al: Symptoms and suffering at the end of life in children with cancer. *N Engl J Med* 2000;342(5):326–33.

Wolfe J, Klar N, Grier HE, et al: Understanding of prognosis among parents of children who died of cancer. *JAMA* 2000;284(19):2469–75.

World Health Organization: *Cancer Pain Relief and Palliative Care in Children*. Geneva, WHO, 1998.

Chapter 39
Children at Special Risk

Richard E. Behrman

In this chapter, the health issues faced by some of the most socioculturally and economically disadvantaged children in the United States are discussed: Native Americans, migrants, immigrants, homeless children, and runaways. Children in foster care are discussed in Chapter 31. The role of poverty in the lives of these and other children has a special significance. The biologic causes of special risk are covered elsewhere. The nonbiologic and biologic causes of special risk often overlap and may confound the risks.

Most children in the United States today grow up loved and supported, although many have problems that disturb their parents and blight their future. However, for a small but significant number of children, their circumstances are so dismal that one wonders how they survive with hope for any quality of future life. Examples of children with even more dismal futures than these also exist elsewhere in the world, such as children growing up in the midst of the Israel-Palestine conflict or in Northern Ireland, Bosnia, Rwanda, or Afghanistan. Many of the children growing up in these environments will be damaged and their futures will be compromised, unless effective interventions are mounted. However, in all of these situations, a few children are so resilient that they survive and actually thrive. Werner has characterized these children as "vulnerable but invincible." The fact that a few defy the odds does not absolve society from attempting to help the majority of those who do not, although these resilient ones can teach us what it takes to survive.

The majority of children at special risk need a nurturing environment but have had their futures compromised by actions or policies arising from their families, schools, communities, and nation. The challenge is to improve the environment of these children so that most can achieve their full potential. Many of their problems are due to several causes, and many of these causes are similar, whether the end result is homeless children, runaways, children in foster care, or other disadvantaged groups. From a preventive point of view, the most effective approach involves alleviation of poverty, poor housing, and lack of jobs. From a treatment point of view, optimal care of these children requires specially organized programs, multidiscipline teams, and special financing.

CHILDREN IN POVERTY

Poverty and economic loss diminish the capacity of parents to be supportive, consistent, and involved with their children. Clinicians need to be especially alert to the development and behavior of children whose parents have lost their jobs or who live in permanent poverty. Fathers who become unemployed frequently develop psychosomatic symptoms, and their children often develop similar symptoms. Young children who grew up in the Great Depression and whose parents were subject to acute poverty suffered more than older children, especially if the older ones were able to take on responsibilities for helping the family economically. Such responsibilities during adolescence seem to give purpose and direction to an adolescent's life. But the younger children, faced with parental depression and unable to do anything to help, suffered a higher frequency of illness and a diminished capacity to lead productive lives even as adults. Children who are poor have higher than average rates of death and illness from almost all causes (exceptions being suicide and motor vehicle accidents, which are most common among white, nonpoor children) (Table 39–1). Also see Chapter 1.

TABLE 39–1. Relative Frequency of Health Problems in Low-Income Children Compared with Other Children

Health Problem	Relative Frequency in Low-Income Children
Low birthweight	Double
Delayed immunization	Triple
Asthma	Higher
Bacterial meningitis	Double
Rheumatic fever	Double to triple
Lead poisoning	Triple
Neonatal death	1.5 times
Postneonatal death	Double to triple
Child deaths due to accidents	Double to triple
Child deaths due to disease	Triple to quadruple
Complications of appendicitis	Double to triple
Diabetic ketoacidosis	Double
Complications of bacterial meningitis	Double to triple
Per cent with conditions limiting school activity	Double to triple
Lost school days	40% more
Severely impaired vision	Double to triple
Severe iron-deficiency anemia	Double

From Starfield B: Effectiveness of Medical Care: Validating Clinical Wisdom. Baltimore, Johns Hopkins University Press, 1985. In Starfield B: Child and adolescent health status measures. Future Child 1992;2:25.

Although physicians cannot cure poverty, they have a responsibility to ask parents about their economic resources, adverse changes in their financial situation, and the family's attempts to cope. Encouraging concrete methods of coping, suggesting ways to reduce stressful social circumstances while increasing social networks that are supportive, and referring patients and their families to appropriate welfare, job training, and family agencies can significantly improve the health and functioning of children at risk when their families live in poverty. In many cases, special services, especially social services, need to be added to the traditional medical services, and outreach is required to find and encourage parents to use health services and bring their children into the health care system.

Poverty among children in the United States was 16.2% in 2000, a rate among the highest of developed countries. The rates are higher for children than adults and are highest for infants and toddlers. The rates also vary substantially among ethnic groups (Chapter 1). Many factors associated with poverty are responsible for the illnesses seen in these children—crowding, poor hygiene and health care, poor diet, environmental pollution, poor education, and stress.

NATIVE AMERICANS, INCLUDING ALASKAN ESKIMOS AND ALEUTS

Children of Native Americans have higher than average rates of many physical and psychologic disorders. They are one group in the United States for whom a separately organized health service has long been in place, the Indian Health Service. There are approximately 2.5 million Native Americans, with a much higher proportion of children than for the remainder of the U.S. population. More than 50% of Native Americans live in urban areas, not on or near native lands. The unemployment and poverty levels of Native Americans are, respectively, three- and fourfold that of the white population and far fewer Native Americans graduate from high school or go on to college.

The rate of low birthweight is more than the white rate and less than the black rate. The neonatal mortality rate and the postneonatal mortality rate are higher for Native Americans living in urban areas than for urban white Americans. Deaths during the 1st yr of life due to sudden infant death syndrome and pneumonia and influenza are higher than the average in the United States, whereas deaths due to congenital anomalies, respiratory distress syndrome, and disorders relating to short gestation and low birthweight are similar.

Accidental death among Native Americans occurs at twice the rate for other U.S. populations, whereas deaths due to malignant neoplasms are lower. During adolescence and young adulthood, suicide and homicide are the second and third causes of death in this population and occur at about twice the rates of the rest of the population. There may be significant underreporting of deaths of Native American children.

Recurrent otitis media is an especially frequent problem among Native American children. As many as three quarters of these children have recurrent otitis media and high rates of hearing loss. This results in learning problems for many children. Other infectious disorders, such as tuberculosis and gastroenteritis, which were so much more common among Native Americans in the past, now occur at about the national average. The asthma-related hospitalization patterns of Native American children are similar to those in white children despite having socioeconomic characteristics more similar to those of black children.

Psychosocial problems are more prevalent in these populations than in the general population: depression, alcoholism, drug abuse, out-of-wedlock teenage pregnancy, school failure and dropout, and child abuse and neglect. The reasons for these differences are not clear, but the cultural disruption of Native American populations is probably, in part, responsible.

Indian Health Service. Since 1954, the Indian Health Service has been the responsibility of the Public Health Service but the 1975 Indian Self-Determination Act gave tribes the option of managing Native American health services in their communities. Thus, today, the Indian Health Service is managed through local administrative units, and some tribes contract outside of the Indian Health Service for health care. A great deal of the emphasis is on adult services: treatment for alcoholism, nutrition and dietetic counseling, and public health nursing services. In addition to programs on Native American reservations, there are currently more than 40 urban programs for Native Americans, with an emphasis on increasing access of this population to existing health services, providing special social services, and developing self-help groups. In an effort to accommodate traditional Western medical, psychologic, and social services to the Native American cultures, such programs increasingly include the "Talking Circle," the "Sweat Lodge," and other interventions based on Native American culture (see Chapter 3). The efficacy of any of these programs, especially those to prevent and treat the sociopsychologic problems particular to Native Americans, has not been assessed.

CHILDREN OF MIGRANT FARM WORKERS

There are estimated to be 3–5 million migrant and seasonal farm workers and their families in the United States. The eastern stream of workers winters primarily in Florida, whereas the western stream comes from Texas and the border states, as well as from Mexico. Many children travel with their parents in the migrant streams. The circumstances of migrants often include poor housing, frequent moves, and a socioeconomic system controlled by a crew boss who arranges the jobs, provides transportation, and often, together with the farm owners, provides food, alcohol, and drugs under a "company store" system that leaves migrant families with little money or even in debt at the end of the year. Children often go without schooling because of the moves, and medical care is usually limited.

The medical problems of children of migrant farm workers are similar to those of children of homeless families: increased frequency of infections (including human immunodeficiency virus [HIV] and AIDS), trauma, poor nutrition, poor dental care, low immunization rates, exposures to toxic chemicals, anemia, and developmental delays.

In 1964, the Public Health Service initiated a special program to provide funds for local groups to organize medical care for migrant families. This program has continued to grow. In addition, many migrant health projects, which were staffed initially by part-time providers and were open for only part of the year, have been transformed into community health care centers that provide services not only for migrants but also for other residents in the area. However, health services for migrant farm workers often need to be organized separately from existing primary care programs because the families are migratory. Special record-keeping systems that link the health care provided during winter months in the south with the care provided during the migratory season in the north are difficult to maintain in ordinary group practices or individual physicians' offices. Outreach programs that take medical care to the often remote farm sites are necessary, and specially organized Head Start, early education, and remedial education programs should also be provided. Similar to other groups discussed in this section, children of migrant farm workers require health care that is more extensive than physicians' services, and this sort of health care often requires separate organizations to deliver it.

CHILDREN OF IMMIGRANTS

The United States has always been a country of immigrants, and it is in the midst of a wave of immigration larger than that experienced in the early 1900s. There has been a marked increase in immigration from Southeast Asia, South America, and the Soviet Union. About 240,000 children legally immigrate each year, and an estimated 50,000/yr enter the country illegally. During the past decade, about 9 million immigrants attained permanent residency status. There may be 850,000 to 1 million illegal immigrant children currently in residence. Families of different origins obviously bring different health problems and different cultural backgrounds, which influence health practices and use of medical care and need to be understood to provide appropriate services (see Chapter 3). Children from Southeast Asia and South America have growth patterns that are generally below the norms established for children of Western European origin, and high rates of hepatitis, parasitic diseases, and nutritional deficiencies are prevalent, as well as high degrees of psychosocial stress. The high prevalence of hepatitis among women from Southeast Asia makes use of hepatitis B vaccine essential for newborns in this group.

Refugee children who escape from war or political violence and whose families have been subjected to extreme stress are a subset of immigrant children. They have a particularly high incidence of mental and behavioral problems. Also see Chapter 22 for discussion of traumatic stress disorder.

Although special health care programs have been developed for many of these children (e.g., children of immigrant migrant workers), children of legal immigrant families have usually been more readily incorporated into traditional medical practice in the United States than some of the other groups of children at special risk. However, "linguistically isolated households," in which no one older than 14 yr of age speaks English, often present significant obstacles to providing quality health care to children because of difficulties in understanding and communicating basic concerns and instructions and in avoiding compromising privacy and confidentiality interests and obtaining informed consent when using translators.

HOMELESS CHILDREN

Families with children are the fastest growing segment of the homeless population (about 40%). Children make up about 25% of the homeless population, with an estimated 100,000 children living in shelters on a given night and about 500,000 homeless each year. Many homeless are not in shelters, and thus, these figures are low estimates. In addition, an unknown number of thrown-away and runaway children and adolescents are homeless, living in shelters, on the streets, and elsewhere (see later). The population of homeless children has been increasing as a consequence of more families with children living in poverty or near poverty, fewer available affordable dwellings for these families, decreasing public assistance programs for the non-elderly poor, and the rising prevalence of substance abuse.

Homeless children have an increased frequency of illness, including intestinal infections, anemia, neurologic disorders, seizures, behavioral disorders, mental illness, and dental problems, as well as increased frequency of trauma and substance abuse. Homeless children are admitted to hospitals at a much higher rate than the national average. They have higher school failure rates, and the likelihood of their being victims of abuse and neglect is much higher. In one study, 50% of such children were found to have psychosocial problems, such as developmental delays, severe depression, or learning disorders. The increased frequency of maternal psychosocial problems, especially depression, in homeless households has a significant untoward impact on the mental and physical health of these children.

Because families tend to break apart under the strain of poverty and homelessness, many homeless children end up in foster care. And even if their families remain intact, frequent moves make it very difficult for them to receive continuity of medical care. Homeless persons rarely have a family physician, and therefore special programs generally need to be developed to provide health services for this population. Mobile vans, with a team consisting of a physician, nurse, social worker, and welfare worker, have been shown to provide effective comprehensive care, ensure delivery of immunizations, link the children to school health services, and bring the children and their families into a stable relation with the traditional medical system. A special record-keeping system is necessary to enhance continuity and to provide a record of care once the family has moved to a permanent location. Because of the high frequency of developmental delays in this group, linkage of preschool homeless children to Head Start programs is an especially important service. Medical and social services for the parents of homeless children are also essential for preservation of these families.

The basic problem of homeless families cannot be solved by physicians. Provision of adequate housing, job retraining for the parents, and mental health and social services are necessary to prevent homelessness from occurring. Physicians can have an important role in motivating society to adopt the social policies that will prevent homelessness from occurring by pointing out the likelihood that these homeless children will become burdens both to themselves and to society if their special health needs are not met.

RUNAWAY AND THROWN-AWAY CHILDREN

The number of runaway and thrown-away children and youths are estimated at about half a million, and several hundred thousand of these children have no secure and safe place to stay. Teenagers make up most of both groups. The usual definition of a runaway is a youth younger than 18 yr who is gone for at least one night from his or her home without parental permission. Most runaways leave home only once, stay overnight with friends, and have no contact with the police or other agencies. This group is no different from their "healthy" peers in psychologic status. A smaller but unknown number become multiple or permanent "runners" and are significantly different from the one-time runners. Thrown-aways include children directly told to leave the household, children who have been away from home and are not allowed to return, abandoned or deserted children, and children who run away but whose caretaker makes no effort to recover them or does not care if they return.

The same constellation of causes common to many of the other special-risk groups is characteristic of permanent runaways. These causes include environmental problems (family dysfunction, abuse, poverty), as well as personal problems of the young person (poor impulse control, psychopathology, substance abuse, or school failure). Thrown-aways experienced more violence and conflicts within their families. The reason why one child enters the group of runaways while another child enters foster care, the juvenile justice system, or mental health systems is not clear.

The minority of runaway youths who become homeless street people have a high frequency of problem behaviors. Three quarters engage in some type of criminal activity and half engage in prostitution as a means of support. A majority of permanent runaways have serious mental problems; more than one third are the product of families who engage in repeated physical and sexual abuse. These children also have a high frequency of medical problems, including traditional infections, hepatitis, sexually transmitted diseases, and drug abuse. Although runaways usually distrust most social agencies, they will come to and use medical services. Thus, medical care may become the point of re-entry into mainstream society and the path to needed services.

Services for permanent runaways and thrown-aways need to be comprehensive and should include social, psychiatric, foster home, drug detoxification, and more traditional medical services. The only approach that has been successful has been long-term team efforts by people who develop the trust of runaway youths and then can help them to work out a better solution to their problems than by running away, drug use, and prostitution.

Although legal considerations involved in the treatment of homeless minor adolescents may be significant, most states, through their "Good Samaritan" laws and definitions of emancipated minors, authorize treatment of homeless youths. Physician liability is based on the usual malpractice standards. Legal barriers should not be used as an excuse to refuse medical care to runaway or thrown-away youths.

The Runaway Youth Act, Title III of the Juvenile Justice and Delinquency Prevention Act of 1974 (Public Law 93-414) and its amended version (Public Law 95-509) have supported shelters and provide a toll-free 24-hr telephone number (1-800-621-4000) for youths who wish to contact their parents or request help after having run away.

Parents who seek a physician's advice about a runaway child should be asked about the child's history of running away, the presence of family dysfunction, and personal aspects of the child's development. If the youth contacts the physician, he or she should be examined and the youth's health status should be assessed, as well as his or her willingness to return home. If it is not feasible for the youth to return home, foster care, a group home, or an independent living arrangement should be sought by referral to a social worker or a social agency.

INHERENT STRENGTHS IN VULNERABLE CHILDREN AND INTERVENTIONS

By age 20–30 yr, many children who were at special risk will have made moderate successes of their lives. Furstenberg's study of teenage mothers and Werner's study of children in Kauai, most of whom were born prematurely or in poverty, demonstrate that by this age, the majority in each study had defied the odds and made the transition to stable marriages and jobs and were accepted by their communities as responsible citizens.

Certain biologic characteristics are associated with success over the long term, such as being born with an accepting temperament. Avoidance of additional social risks is even more important. Premature infants or preadolescent boys with conduct disorders and poor reading skills, who must also face a broken family, poverty, frequent moves, and family violence, are at much greater risk than children with only one of these handicaps. Perhaps most important are the protective buffers that have been found to enhance children's resilience because these can be aided by an effective health care system and community. Children generally do better if they can gain social support, either from family members or from a nonjudgmental adult outside the family, especially an older mentor or peer. Providers of medical services should develop ways to "prescribe" supportive "other" persons for children who are at risk and isolated. Promotion of self-esteem and self-efficacy seems to be a very central factor in protecting against risks. It is essen-

tial to promote competence in some area of these children's lives.

Providers of medical services need the patience to work over a long time frame and the willingness to accept limited improvement. In addition, prediction of the consequences of risk is never 100% accurate. Health professionals as well as families should have hope. However, the confidence that, even without aid, many such children will achieve a good outcome by age 30 yr does not justify ignoring or withholding services from them in early life. It should teach us how to focus our resources on those most in need and provide a basis for hope in individual cases.

Programs that seem to work for high-risk children have a similar group of characteristics. A team is needed, because it is rare for one individual to be able to provide the multiple services needed for high-risk children. At the same time, successful programs are characterized by at least one caring person who can make personal contact with these children and their families. Most successful programs are relatively small (or are large programs divided up into small units) and nonbureaucratic but are intensive, comprehensive, and flexible. They work not only with the individual but also with the family, school, community, and even at broader societal levels. In addition, generally the earlier the programs are started, in terms of the age of the children involved, the better is the chance of success. It is also important for services to be continued over a long period.

General

Dalaker J: *Poverty in the United States: 2000 Current Population Reports: Consumer income, P60-214.* Washington, DC, U.S. Census Bureau, September 2001.

Moore KA, Vandivere S: *Stressful Family Lives: Child and Parent Well-Being.* Child Trends 2000, Series B, No 3-17.

Newacheck PW, Hughes DC, Hung Y, et al: The unmet health needs of America's children. *Pediatrics* 2000;105:989–99.

Scott S, Knapp M, Harrison J, et al: Financial costs of social exclusion: Follow-up study of antisocial children into adulthood. *BMJ* 2001;323:1–5.

Starfield B: Child and adolescent health status measures. *Future Child* 1992; 2:25.

Werner EE: *Vulnerable but Invincible: A Longitudinal Study of Resilient Children and Youth.* New York, McGraw-Hill, 1982.

Native American, Alaskan Eskimo, and Aleut Children

Grossman DC, Krieger JW, Sugarman JR, et al: Health status of urban American Indians and Alaska Natives. *JAMA* 1994;271:845.

Potthoff SJ, Bearinger LH, Skay CL, et al: Dimensions of risk behaviors among American Indian youth. *Arch Pediatr Adolesc Med* 1998;152:157.

The State of Native American Youth Health. University of Minnesota Health Center, 1994.

Homeless Children

Bassuk EL, Weinreb LF, Buckner JC, et al: The characteristics and needs of sheltered homeless and low-income housed mothers. *JAMA* 1996;276: 640.

Ensign J, Santelli J: Health status and service use: Comparison of adolescents at a school-based health clinic with homeless adolescents. *Arch Pediatr Adolesc Med* 1998;152:20.

Ringwalt CL, Greene JM, Robertson M, et al: The prevalence of homelessness among adolescents in the United States. *Am J Public Health* 1998;88: 1325–9.

Wood DL, Valdez RB, Hayashi T, et al: Health of homeless children and housed, poor children. *Pediatrics* 86:858, 1990.

Zima BT, Bussing R, Forness SR, et al: Sheltered homeless children: Their eligibility and unmet need for special education evaluations. *Am J Public Health* 1997;87:236.

Children of Migrant Farm Workers and Immigrants

American Academy of Pediatrics: Health care for children of immigrant families. *Pediatrics* 1997;100:153.

Centers for Disease Control and Prevention: Pregnancy-related behaviors among migrant farm workers—four states, 1989–1993. *MMWR* 1997;46:283.

Dever GEA: *Migrant Health Status: Profile of a Population with Complex Health Problems.* Monograph Series. Migrant Clinicians Network. National Migrant Resource Program, 1991.

Hjern A, Angel B: Organized violence and mental health of refugee children in exile: A six year follow-up. *Acta Paediatr* 2000;89:722–7.

National Commission to Prevent Infant Mortality: *HIV/AIDS: A Growing Crisis Among Migrant and Seasonal Farmworker Families,* 1993.

Runaway and Thrown-Away Children

Finkelhor D, Hotaling G, Sedlak A: *Missing, Abducted, Runaway, and Thrown-away Children in America*. Washington, DC, Office of Justice Programs. Attorney General U.S., 1990.

Greene JM, Ennett ST, Ringwalt CL: Substance use among runaway and homeless youth in three national samples. *Am J Public Health* 1997;87:229

Greene JM, Ringwalt CL: Youth and family substance use associated with suicide attempts among runaway and homeless youth. *Subst Use Misuse* 1996;31:1058.

Chapter 40
Nutritional Requirements
William C. Heird

The dramatic growth of infants during the 1st yr of life (e.g., a three-fold increase in weight and a two-fold increase in length) and continued growth, albeit at lower rates, from 1 yr of age through adolescence impose unique nutritional needs (see Chapters 7–16). Moreover, these needs for growth are superimposed on relatively high maintenance needs incident to the higher metabolic and nutrient turnover rates of infants and children vs. adults. Furthermore, because the rapid rates of growth are accompanied by marked developmental changes in organ function and composition, failure to provide adequate nutrients during this time is likely to have adverse effects on development as well as growth. Unfortunately, provision of these special nutrient needs, particularly during early life, is complicated by the young infant's lack of teeth and immature digestive and metabolic processes.

Recommended (or reference) intakes of most nutrients have been established, and these appear to fulfill the unique nutritional needs of the infant and young child. The most recent recommendations of the Food and Nutrition Board, National Academy of Sciences (1–5), for the 0–6 mo old infant, the 6–12 mo old infant, the 1–3 yr old child, and the 4–8 yr old child are summarized in Table 40–1. Some of these recommendations are discussed briefly in this chapter. Other aspects of nutrition relevant to each age group, including how to provide the recommended or reference intakes, are discussed in Chapter 41.

Requirement vs. Recommended Intake. The Estimated Average Requirement (EAR) of a specific nutrient is the amount of that nutrient that results in some predetermined physiologic endpoint. In infants, this end-point is usually maintenance of satisfactory rates of growth and development and/or prevention of specific nutritional deficiencies. The EAR is usually defined experimentally, often over a relatively short period and in a relatively small study population. Thus, the EAR, by definition,

TABLE 40–1. Daily Reference Intakes of Nutrients for Normal Infants

Nutrient	Reference Intake Per Day			
	0–6 Mo (6 kg)	*7–12 Mo (9 kg)*	*1–3 Yr (13 kg)*	*4–8 Yr (22 kg)*
Energy (kcal (kJ)/24 hr)*	550 (2310)	720 (3013)	1074 (4494)	—
Fat (g/24 hr)	31 (AI)	30 (AI)	—	—
Linoleic Acid (g/24 hr)	4.4 (AI)	4.6 (AI)	7 (AI)	10 (AI)
α-Linolenic Acid (g/24 hr)	0.5 (AI)	0.5 (AI)	0.7 (AI)	0.9 (AI)
Carbohydrate (g/24 hr)	60 (EAR)	95 (EAR)	130 (RDA)	130 (RDA)
Protein (g/24 hr)*	9.3 (EAR)	11 (RDA)	—	21 (RDA)
Electrolytes and Minerals:				
Calcium (mg/24 hr)	210[†]	270[†]	500[†]	800[†]
Phosphorus (mg/24 hr)	100[†]	275[†]	460*	500*
Magnesium (mg/24 hr)	30[†]	75[†]	80*	130*
Sodium (mg/24 hr)*	120	200	225	300
Chloride (mg/24 hr)*	180	300	350	500
Potassium (mg/24 hr)*	500	700	1000 (1 yr)	1400
Iron (mg/24 hr)	0.27[†]	11*	7*	10*
Zinc (mg/24 hr)	2[†]	3*	3*	5*
Copper (µg/24 hr)	200[†]	220[†]	340*	440*
Iodine (µg/24 hr)	110[†]	130[†]	90*	90*
Selenium (µg/24 hr)	15[†]	20[†]	20*	30*
Manganese (mg/24 hr)	0.003[†]	0.6[†]	102[†]	1.5[†]
Fluoride (mg/24 hr)	0.01[†]	0.5[†]	0.7[†]	1.0[†]
Chromium (µg/24 hr)	0.2[†]	5.5[†]	11[†]	15[†]
Molybdenum (µg/24 hr)	2[†]	3[†]	17	22
Vitamins:				
Vitamin A (µg/24 hr)	400[†]	500[†]	300*	400*
Vitamin D (µg/24 hr)	5[†]	5[†]	5[†]	5[†]
Vitamin E (mg α-TE/24 hr)	4[†]	6[†]	6*	7*
Vitamin K (µg/24 hr)	2.0[†]	2.5[†]	30[†]	55[†]
Vitamin C (mg/24 hr)	40[†]	50[†]	15*	25*
Thiamine (mg/24 hr)	0.2[†]	0.3[†]	0.5*	0.6*
Riboflavin (mg/24 hr)	0.3[†]	0.4[†]	0.5*	0.6*
Niacin (mg NE/24 hr)	2[†]	4[†]	6*	8*
Vitamin B$_6$ (µg/24 hr)	0.1[†]	0.3[†]	0.5*	0.6*
Folate (µg)	65[†]	80[†]	150*	200*
Vitamin B$_{12}$ (µg/24 hr)	0.4[†]	0.5[†]	0.9*	1.2*
Biotin (µg/24 hr)	5[†]	6[†]	8[†]	12[†]
Pantothenic acid (mg/24 hr)	1.7[†]	1.8[†]	2[†]	3[†]
Choline (mg/24 hr)	125[†]	150[†]	200[†]	250[†]

*RDA.
[†]Adequate intake (e.g., for infants <1 yr of age; this is the mean intake of normal breast-fed infants).
Estimated minimum requirement (for sodium, chloride, and potassium) from Recommended Dietary Allowances, 10th edition.

meets the needs of roughly half of the population in which it was established but not the needs of the other half. For some, it may be excessive, whereas, for others, it may be inadequate.

The recommended daily allowance (RDA) of a specific nutrient, on the other hand, is the intake of that nutrient deemed to meet the "requirement" for that nutrient by most healthy members of a population. If the EAR of a specific nutrient is known and is normally distributed within the population in which it was established, the RDA for that nutrient is the mean requirement (i.e., the EAR) plus 2 standard deviations. Because the requirements of many nutrients are not normally distributed, other considerations of population variability frequently are necessary. For example, if the "requirement" appears to be adequate for most of the study population, the RDA may be less than the requirement plus 2 standard deviations. RDAs are useful for assessing the nutrient intakes of individuals or groups but not for ascertaining the adequacy, inadequacy, or excess of an individual subject's intake of a specific nutrient.

Because the mean requirement of many nutrients is not known with certainty, it is often difficult to establish a valid RDA. This is particularly true for infants. In recognition of the lack of a valid EAR for most nutrients and the uncertainty of an RDA based on limited information, the latest recommendations of the Food and Nutrition Board, National Academy of Sciences, are Dietary Reference Intakes (DRIs). These include RDAs for those nutrients for which an EAR has been established; and a RDA, therefore, can reliably be established as well as other "reference intakes." The other reference intakes include Adequate Intake (AI) and Tolerable Upper Intake Level (UL).

The AI of a specific nutrient is a recommended daily intake based on the observed or approximated intake of that nutrient by a group of healthy individuals. It is used when an RDA cannot be established, but it is not synonymous with an RDA. The content of a specific nutrient in the average volume of milk consumed by healthy, normally growing, breast-feeding infants is considered an adequate intake of that nutrient for infants younger than 6 mo of age. This definition is consistent with national and international recommendations for exclusive breast-feeding for the first 4–6 mo of life. For the 6–12 mo old infant, the AI of most nutrients is set at the amount of the nutrient in the average volume of human milk plus the average amount of complementary foods consumed by healthy, normally growing 6–12 mo old infants. The EAR of a few nutrients has been established for older children. These were determined directly or by extrapolation from data obtained in adults or older children. For these, an RDA can be established. However, this is impossible for most nutrients and, for these, an AI based on the mean intake of apparently "normal" infants and/or children has been established.

The Tolerable Upper Intake Level (UL) is the highest daily intake of a specific nutrient that is likely to pose no risk. It is not a recommended level of intake but, rather, an aid for avoiding excessive intake and adverse effects secondary to such intake. ULs of those nutrients for which one has been or can be established are summarized in Table 40–2.

THE 0–6 MO OLD INFANT

Energy. Expressed per unit of body weight, the normal infant requires approximately three times more energy than the adult. This reflects primarily the higher metabolic rate of the infant vs. the adult and the infant's special needs for growth and development. The inefficient intestinal absorption of the infant vs. the adult contributes only minimally to the higher energy needs of the infant fed human milk or modern infant formulas.

The currently recommended energy intakes are based on total energy expenditure measured by the doubly labeled water technique plus a reasonable allowance for growth based on changes in body composition. These are about 15% lower than the previous RDA or established requirements.

There is no evidence that either carbohydrate or fat is a superior source of energy. Sufficient carbohydrate to prevent ketosis and/or hypoglycemia is required (~5.0 g/kg/24 hr), as is enough fat to provide essential fatty acid requirements (0.5–1.0 g/kg/24 hr of linoleic acid plus a smaller amount of α-linolenic acid). Currently, there is concern that infants also require long-chain, polyunsaturated fatty acids (LC-PUFA). These fatty acids are more than 18 carbons in length and have two or more double bonds. Those that are most relevant to infant nutrition are arachidonic acid (20:4ω6) and docosahexaenoic (22:6ω3) acid. (By convention, the first number indicates the length of the carbon chain, the number after the colon indicates the number of double bonds, and ω6 and ω3 indicate the site of the first double bond from the noncarboxyl [ω] end of the molecule.) These two fatty acids are the most prevalent ω6 and ω3 fatty acids, respectively, in the central nervous system, and the latter comprises up to 40% of the fatty acid content of retinal photoreceptor membranes. Both are synthesized by the same series of desaturation and elongation reactions from the essential fatty acids linoleic (18:2ω6) and α-linolenic (18:3ω3) acid.

Although infants can convert linoleic and α-linolenic acid, respectively, to arachidonic acid and docosahexaenoic acid, the content of arachidonic and docosahexaenoic acid in plasma and erythrocyte lipids is lower in formula-fed vs. breast-fed infants, and autopsy studies show that the low erythrocyte lipid content of docosahexaenoic acid, but not arachidonic acid, is accompanied by a lower concentration in brain. These differences are assumed to reflect the presence of LC-PUFA in human milk but not formula, suggesting that the synthetic pathway, while intact, does not synthesize enough LC-PUFA. The generally better visual and cognitive development of breast-fed vs. formula-fed infants also has been attributed to the presence of LC-PUFA in human milk but not formula.

Because human milk contains a number of factors other than LC-PUFA that might be important for development, the specific role of LC-PUFA in visual and cognitive development of infants cannot be determined by studies of formula-fed vs. breast-fed infants. Moreover, there are major psychosocial and socioeconomic differences between mothers who choose breast-feeding vs. formula feeding. Thus, over the past decade, many studies have addressed differences in visual function and/or neurodevelopmental status of infants fed LC-PUFA–supplemented vs. unsupplemented formulas. Some of these have shown distinct advantages of LC-PUFA supplementation, but others have not; and the reasons for the different findings are not clear. A meta-analysis of the available data concerning the effect of LC-PUFA supplementation on visual function of term infants shows that supplementation confers advantages at some, but not all, ages. When detected, the magnitude of the advantage equates to approximately one line on a Snellen chart. No such analysis of data concerning neurodevelopmental outcomes, some positive and some negative, is available.

Although a report prepared to advise the U.S. Food and Drug Administration concerning desirable nutrient contents of term infant formulas marketed in the United States did not recommend inclusion of LC-PUFA, similar groups in other countries have advised supplementation. Formulas containing arachidonic and docosahexaenoic acid have been available for some time in many parts of the world and are now available in the United States. These appear to be safe and, in theory, may confer developmental advantages.

In total, the specific needs for carbohydrate and fat, including LC-PUFA, amount to no more than 30 kcal (125.5 kJ)/kg/24 hr, or only about a third of the 0–6 mo old infant's total energy need. Whether the remainder should be comprised predominantly of carbohydrate, fat, or equicaloric amounts of each is not known. Human milk and most currently available formulas contain roughly equicaloric amounts of each. Because a higher percentage of energy as carbohydrate will increase osmolality

TABLE 40–2. Tolerable Upper Intake Levels of Nutrients for Infants and Young Children

Nutrient	Intake Per Day			
	0–6 Mo (6 kg)	7–12 Mo (9 kg)	1–3 Yr (13 kg)	4–8 Yr (22 kg)
Energy (kcal (kJ)/24 hr)	ND	ND	ND	ND
Fat (g)	ND	ND	ND	ND
Carbohydrate	ND	ND	ND	ND
Protein (g/24 hr)	ND	ND	ND	ND
Electrolytes and Minerals:				
Calcium (mg/24 hr)	ND	ND	2500	2500
Phosphorus (g/24 hr)	ND	ND	3	3
Magnesium (mg/24 hr)	ND	ND	65	110
Sodium (mg/24 hr)	NA			
Chloride (mg/24 hr)	NA			
Potassium (mg/24 hr)	NA			
Iron (mg/24 hr)	40	40	40	40
Zinc (mg/24 hr)	4	5	7	12
Copper (µg/24 hr)	ND	ND	1000	3000
Iodine (µg/24 hr)	ND	ND	200	300
Selenium (µg/24 hr)	45	60	90	150
Manganese (mg/24 hr)	ND	ND	2	3
Fluoride (mg/24 hr)	0.7	0.9	1.3	2.2
Chromium (µg/24 hr)	ND	ND	ND	ND
Molybdenum (µg/24 hr)	ND	ND	300	600
Vitamins:				
Vitamin A (µg/24 hr)	600	600	600	900
Vitamin D (µg/24 hr)	[1000 IU (25µg)/day]		2000 IU (50µg)/day	2000 IU/day
Vitamin E (mg α-TE/24 hr)	ND	ND	200	300
Vitamin K (µg/24 hr)	ND	ND	ND	ND
Vitamin C (mg/24 hr)	ND	ND	ND	650
Thiamine (mg/24 hr)	ND	ND	ND	ND
Riboflavin (mg/24 hr)	ND	ND	ND	ND
Niacin (mg/24 hr)	ND	ND	10	15
Vitamin B_6 (µg/24 hr)	ND	ND	30	40
Folate (µg)	ND	ND	300	400
Vitamin B_{12} (µg/24 hr)	ND	ND	ND	ND
Biotin (µg/24 hr)	ND	ND	ND	ND
Pantothenic acid (mg/24 hr)	ND	ND	ND	ND
Choline (mg/24 hr)	ND	ND	1 g/day	1 g/day

NA = Not available; ND = data insufficient to establish a tolerable upper intake level.

and a higher percentage as fat may exceed the limited ability of the infant to digest and absorb fat, roughly equicaloric amounts of each seems appropriate.

Protein. The protein requirement of the normal infant also is greater per unit of body weight than that of the adult. In addition, it is thought that the infant requires a higher proportion of essential amino acids than the adult. These include the amino acids recognized as essential (or indispensable) for the adult (i.e., leucine, isoleucine, valine, threonine, methionine, phenylalanine, tryptophan, lysine, and histidine) as well as cysteine, tyrosine, and, perhaps, arginine. The need for cysteine is thought to be secondary to delayed development of hepatic cystathionase activity; this key enzyme in conversion of methionine to cysteine does not reach adult levels until at least 4 mo of age. The reason for the infant's apparent need for tyrosine is not clear; the hepatic activity of phenylalanine hydroxylase, the rate-limiting enzyme for conversion of phenylalanine to tyrosine, is at or near adult levels early in gestation. It also appears that even preterm infants can convert phenylalanine to tyrosine.

In general, human milk protein and all proteins currently used in infant formulas contain adequate amounts of all essential amino acids, including cysteine, tyrosine, and arginine. Furthermore, the sum of the highest estimates of the requirement of each amino acid is considerably less than the overall protein requirement. However, the required intake of a specific protein depends on its quality, which is usually defined as how closely its amino acid pattern resembles that of human milk. The overall quality of a specific protein can be improved by supplementing it with the essential amino acid(s) that result(s) in its quality being low, i.e., the limiting amino acid. Native soy protein, for example, has insufficient methionine, but when it is fortified with methionine its quality approaches that of bovine milk protein.

Although the amino acid composition of human milk protein is considered ideal, the total protein content of human milk, though quite variable, averages only approximately 1.0 g/dL. Thus, on average, about 200 mL/kg/24 hr must be ingested to meet the current RDA for protein (i.e., 2.0–2.2 g/kg/24 hr). However, because few, if any, breast-fed infants develop protein deficiency, the high quality and easy digestibility of human milk protein obviously compensate for any quantitative deficiency. Bovine milk protein and modern preparations of soy protein, the protein sources of most infant formulas, also are very high quality proteins. Furthermore, if properly processed, these proteins are utilized nearly as well, perhaps as well, as human milk protein. Thus, the amount of these proteins needed to support normal growth is likely to be only minimally, if at all, higher than the amount of human milk protein needed. This possibility is reflected by the protein intakes recommended recently by an International Dietary Energy Consultative Group (IDECG). The "safe" protein intake recommended by this group is approximately 30% higher than the estimated requirement but considerably less than the most recent RDA, particularly for infants older than 3 mo of age. The new AI for protein, released by the Food and Nutrition Board, National Academy of Sciences, is based on the intake of exclusively breast-fed infants.

Electrolytes, Minerals, and Vitamins. Estimated safe and adequate intakes of sodium, chloride, and potassium have been available for some time (see Table 40–1), and infants who receive these intakes experience few problems. More recently, adequate intakes of most minerals and vitamins have been recommended.

In general, these represent the amount of each nutrient in the average intake of breast milk by a healthy, normally growing, 0–6 mo old breast-fed infant.

Although the normal newborn infant is thought to have sufficient stores of iron to meet requirements for 4–6 mo, iron deficiency is common during infancy (see Chapter 447). This reflects the fact that iron stores at birth as well as the absorption of iron are quite variable. Interestingly, although human milk contains less iron than most formulas, iron deficiency is less common in breast-fed infants. Nonetheless, to prevent iron deficiency, routine iron supplementation of breast-fed infants and use of iron-fortified formulas for formula-fed infants is often recommended. The widespread use of iron-fortified formulas over the past several years is thought to have dramatically reduced the incidence of iron deficiency.

If protein intake is adequate, vitamin deficiencies are rare; if not, deficiencies of nicotinic acid and choline, which are synthesized, respectively, from tryptophan and methionine, may develop. In contrast, if bovine milk and bovine milk formulas were not supplemented with vitamin D, hypovitaminosis D would be endemic among formula-fed infants, particularly those with limited exposure to sunlight. Breast-fed infants may not be as susceptible to development of vitamin D deficiency as formula-fed infants, but routine vitamin D supplementation of breast-fed infants is often recommended. Reports of rickets in both breast-fed and formula-fed, dark-skinned infants and infants chronically protected from sunlight have led some to suggest routine vitamin D supplementation for all infants.

Routine perinatal administration of vitamin K is recommended as prophylaxis against hemorrhagic disease of the newborn (see Chapters 92 and 472). Thereafter, deficiency of this vitamin is uncommon except in infants with conditions associated with fat malabsorption.

Water. The normal infant's absolute requirement for water probably is 75–100 mL/kg/24 hr. However, because of higher obligate renal, pulmonary, and dermal water losses as well as a higher overall metabolic rate, the young infant is more susceptible to development of dehydration, particularly with vomiting and/or diarrhea or if solute intake is high, as it is in bovine milk. Thus, intake of bovine milk before 1 yr of age is discouraged and provision of a fluid intake of 150 mL/kg/24 hr is recommended. Because human milk and common formulas are at least 90% water, the typical breast-fed infant as well as the typical formula-fed infant usually consumes this amount for the first several weeks to months of life and, hence, does not need additional water.

THE 6–12 MO OLD INFANT

The nutritional needs of the infant during the last half of the 1st yr of life are no more firmly based on experimental data than those of the younger infant. The AI for most nutrients cited for this age group by the Food and Nutrition Board, National Academy of Sciences (see Table 40–1), reflects the amount of that nutrient in the average volume of human milk consumed by the 6–12 mo old infant plus the amount in the average intake of complementary foods based on national surveys. The AI for other nutrients relies heavily on extrapolation of data obtained in older children and/or adults. These recommendations reflect the developmental differences between younger and older infants as well as the greater level of activity and somewhat slower rate of growth after 6 mo of age. Despite the lack of experimental data concerning the nutrient needs during the second 6 mo of life, the reference intakes for this age group appear to be appropriate.

The most recent EAR for energy (720 kcal [3,013 kJ]/24 hr) reflects estimates of energy needs based on measurement of energy expenditure by the doubly labeled water method and energy deposition as protein and fat (i.e., ~90 kcal [376.6 kJ]/kg/24 hr), throughout the 1st yr of life.

THE CHILD OLDER THAN 1 YR

After 1 yr of age, the child's rate of growth slows and the nutrient needs for growth consequently decrease. However, the rate of growth remains appreciable. Moreover, activity increases. Thus, on a body weight basis, nutrient needs after the 1st yr of life are only minimally less than those during the 1st yr of life (see Table 40–1).

Although the Food and Nutrition Board, National Academy of Sciences, provides reference intakes for the 1–3 yr old and the 4–8 yr old, the major physiologic reason for differentiating between these two periods is the somewhat greater rate of increase in height between 1–3 vs. 4–8 yr of age. On the other hand, there are many practical reasons for differentiating these two periods. Children begin entering school at about 4 yr of age, and availability of reference intakes for the 4–8 yr old child makes it easier for school systems to design meals. This also makes it easier to assess the intake of individual children. In addition, a reasonable amount of data on which to establish EARs are available in this age group. Ending this period at 8 (or 9) yr of age, of course, circumvents the necessity of considering the effect of endocrine changes associated with puberty on nutrient needs.

After 2 yr of age, most children are eating the same foods as the rest of the family. Thus, after this age a diet based on an appropriate number of servings from the various food groups of the food guide pyramid, as modified for children older than 2 yr of age, will provide adequate amounts of most if not all nutrients. Table 40–3 summarizes the recommended number of servings from each food group as well as the size of a serving for a 4–6 yr old child. Two to 3 yr old children need the same number of servings of each food group as 4–6 yr old children, but the size of each serving should be only about two thirds that recommended for 4–6 yr old children.

USING THE DRIs

The DRIs are useful for assessing the nutrient intake of individuals as well as groups. For the individual, the EAR can be used to examine the possibility that the reported intake of a specific nutrient is adequate or inadequate. For example, a reported intake below the EAR suggests inadequacy. However, because individual requirements vary, such an intake may or may not be inadequate for an individual subject. Similarly, a reported intake of a specific nutrient that is greater than the EAR suggests that the intake is likely to be adequate but, because of individual differences in requirements, it may not be.

TABLE 40–3. Use of Food Pyramid Guidelines

Food Group	Serving Size*	Servings/Day
Grain	1 slice bread ½ cup rice (cooked) ½ cup pasta	6
Vegetables	½ cup raw or cooked 1 cup leafy	3
Fruit	¼ medium melon 1 whole fruit ¾ cup juice ½ cup canned ½ cup berries, grapes	2
Milk	1 cup milk, yogurt 2 oz cheese	2
Meat	2–3 oz cooked, lean ½ cup dried beans† 1 egg† 2 Tbsp peanut butter	2
Fats/sweets		Limit

*These serving sizes are for 4–6 yr old children; serving sizes for 2–3 yr old children, except for milk, should be about two thirds of these.

†These amounts are equal to 1 oz lean meat; two servings are equal to one meat serving.

Assessment of a reported intake against the AI or RDA, if one has been established, is likely to be more useful, particularly for assessing the adequacy of a reported intake. An intake equal to or greater than the AI or RDA is likely to be adequate. However, an intake below the AI or RDA also may be adequate for many individuals.

The EAR can be used to estimate the prevalence of inadequate intakes in a group (e.g., the percentage of the group that has an intake below the EAR). Similarly, mean intakes at the AI imply a low prevalence of inadequate intakes. Individual or mean group intakes above the UL suggest the risk of adverse effects for both the individual and the group.

For planning purposes, either for an individual or for a group, the aim should be to achieve intakes equal to the AI or the RDA and to avoid intakes above the UL. This helps ensure adequate intakes of all nutrients with minimal risk of adverse effects due to excessive intakes.

Using the reference intakes just described requires an accurate assessment of the usual intake. For individuals, this is best obtained from a food diary maintained over a period of several days. Any reasonable, statistically valid estimate of the mean intake of groups can be used.

Heird WC: Nutritional requirements during infancy. In Bowman BA, Russell RM (editors): *Present Knowledge in Nutrition*, 8th ed. Washington, DC, International Life Sciences Institute (ILSI) Press, 2001; 38:416–25.

Heird WC: Nutritional requirements during infancy. In Shils ME, Olson JA, Shike M, et al (editors): *Modern Nutrition in Health and Disease*, 9th ed. Baltimore, Williams & Wilkins, 1999; 51:839–55.

Heird WC: The role of polyunsaturated fatty acids in term and preterm infants and breastfeeding mothers. *Pediatr Clin North Am* 2001;48:173–88.

Panel on Dietary Antioxidants and Related Compounds, Subcommittees on Upper Reference Levels of Nutrients and Interpretation and Uses of Dietary Reference Intakes, and the Standing Committee on the Scientific Evaluation of Dietary Reference Intakes, Food and Nutrition Board, Institute of Medicine: *Dietary Reference Intakes for Vitamin C, Vitamin E, Selenium and Carotenoids*. Washington, DC, National Academy Press, 2000.

Panel on Micronutrients, Subcommittees on Upper Reference Levels of Nutrients and of Interpretation and Use of Dietary Reference Intakes, and the Standing Committee on the Scientific Evaluation of Dietary Reference Intakes, Food and Nutrition Board, Institute of Medicine: *Dietary Reference Intakes for Energy, Carbohydrate, Fiber, Fat, Fatty Acids, Cholesterol, Protein and Amino Acids*. Washington, DC, National Academy Press, 2002.

Panel on Micronutrients, Subcommittees on Upper Reference Levels of Nutrients and of Interpretation and Use of Dietary Reference Intakes, and the Standing Committee on the Scientific Evaluation of Dietary Reference Intakes, Food and Nutrition Board, Institute of Medicine: *Dietary Reference Intakes for Vitamin A, Vitamin K, Arsenic, Boron, Chromium, Copper, Iodine, Iron, Manganese, Molybdenum, Nickel, Silicon, Vanadium, and Zinc*. Washington, DC, National Academy Press, 2001.

Standing Committee on the Scientific Evaluation of Dietary Reference Intakes and Its Panel on Folate, Other B Vitamins and Choline and Subcommittee on Upper Reference Levels of Nutrients, Food and Nutrition Board, Institute of Medicine: *Dietary Reference Intakes for Thiamin, Riboflavin, Niacin, Vitamin B$_6$, Folate, Vitamin B$_{12}$, Pantothenic Acid, Biotin and Choline*. Washington, DC, National Academy Press, 1998.

Standing Committee on the Scientific Evaluation of Dietary Reference Intakes, Food and Nutrition Board, Institute of Medicine: *Dietary Reference Intakes for Calcium, Phosphorus, Magnesium, Vitamin D and Fluoride*. Washington, DC, National Academy Press, 1997.

Subcommittee on the 10th Edition of the RDAs Food and Nutrition Board, Commission on Life Sciences: *Recommended Dietary Allowances*, 10th ed. Washington, DC, National Academy Press, 1989.

Chapter 41
The Feeding of Infants and Children *William C. Heird*

The establishment of feeding practices that are comfortable and satisfying for both the mother and the infant is crucial for the emotional well-being of both and for ensuring adequate nutrient intakes for the infant. Maternal feelings are readily transmit-

ted to the infant and are a major determinant of the emotional setting in which feeding takes place. Thus, mothers who are tense, anxious, irritable, easily upset, or emotionally labile are more likely to experience a difficult feeding relationship. However, appropriate guidance and support from an empathetic and experienced relative, friend, lactation consultant, or physician can increase such a mother's confidence, which, in turn, makes her more relaxed and increases the likelihood of establishing successful feeding practices, not only during infancy but throughout childhood and beyond.

FEEDING DURING THE FIRST 6 MO OF LIFE

Feedings should be initiated as soon after birth as possible, depending on the infant's ability to tolerate enteral nutrition. This not only maintains normal metabolism during the transition from fetal to extrauterine life but also promotes maternal-infant bonding. Most infants can start breast-feeding shortly after birth, almost always within 4–6 hr. Hence, mothers who wish to initiate breast-feeding in the delivery room and continue to do so on a demand basis should be supported in doing so. However, if any question about the infant's tolerance of feeding arises, feedings should be withheld until the infant is carefully evaluated. It if appears that feedings must be withheld for several hours, parenteral fluids should be administered.

The successful feeding of infants requires practical interpretation of specific nutritional needs and the wide variability among normal infants in appetite and behavior regarding food. For example, the time required for an infant's stomach to empty may vary from 1–4 hr or more during a single day. Thus, the infant's desire for food will vary at different times of the day. Ideally, the feeding schedule established should be based on this reasonable "self-regulation" by the infant. However, the establishment of this "self-regulation" is not immediate and considerable variation in the time between feedings and in the amount taken per feeding is to be expected during the first few weeks of life. Most infants will have established a suitable and reasonably regular schedule by 1 mo of age.

By the end of the 1st wk of life, most healthy infants will want 6–9 feedings/24 hr. Some will take enough at one feeding to be satisfied for as long as 4 hr, but others will want to be fed as often as every 2–3 hr. In general, breast-fed infants prefer shorter feeding intervals than formula-fed infants. Most infants will be taking 80–90 mL per feeding by the end of the 1st wk of life. Feeding can be considered to have progressed satisfactorily if the infant is no longer losing weight by the end of the 1st wk of life and is gaining weight by the end of the 2nd wk. Although most infants will awaken for a middle-of-the-night feeding until 3–6 wk of age, some never desire this feeding and others continue to desire it well beyond 3–6 wk of age. Between 4–8 mo of age, many infants will lose interest in the late evening feeding; and by 9–12 mo of age, most will be satisfied with 3 meals/day plus snacks. However, not all infants conform to these general guidelines. Individual feeding needs are quite variable, and not all infants can be expected to fit the same pattern.

It is important to appreciate that infants cry for reasons other than hunger and that they do not need to be fed every time they cry. Those who awaken and cry consistently at short intervals may not be receiving enough milk, or they may have discomfort from some cause other than hunger (e.g., too much clothing; colic; soiled, wet, or uncomfortable diapers; swallowed air ("gas"); an uncomfortably hot or cold environment; illness). Some infants cry to gain sufficient or additional attention, whereas others become indifferent to lack of attention. Some cry because they simply need to be held. Those who stop crying as soon as they are picked up or held usually do not need food. Those who continue to cry when held and when food is offered should be carefully evaluated for other causes of distress. The habit of offering frequent, small feedings or holding and feeding to pacify all crying should not be allowed to develop.

At the same time, satisfying the infant's true hunger as it is expressed has several advantages. This allows physiologic requirements to be met promptly. Moreover, the infant is less likely to associate prolonged crying and discomfort with feeding and, also, is less likely to develop eating practices such as gulping an entire feeding or taking small amounts too frequently. Most infants establish a regular feeding schedule that permits the family to resume normal functioning within a few weeks after the infant's birth. If not, individual feedings or the whole day's schedule can be moved ahead or delayed sufficiently to avoid conflicts with necessary family activities.

Some mothers will not understand the goals of infant "self-regulation," and some will misinterpret the physician's instructions or be unable to adjust to the infant's regimen. These as well as orderly, overanxious, and compulsive parents may do better with more specific instructions for the infant's feeding activities.

The postpartum period is a time of great anxiety and insecurity, particularly for the first-time mother who often is temporarily overwhelmed by the responsibilities of motherhood. Thus, it is important for the physician to set aside sufficient time shortly after birth to address the questions and concerns of inexperienced or uncertain mothers. Ideally, these anticipatory guidance sessions should include fathers and other household members. Knowing the personalities and expectations of both parents is invaluable in helping avert physical and psychologic problems centered on feeding. Also, because parental misconceptions and confusion about the dietary and satiety needs of infants are often the basis for abnormal parent-child relations, appropriate counseling can help avoid or lessen these problems.

Breast-Feeding vs. Formula-Feeding. One of the first decisions a new mother must make—ideally, some time before the infant is born—is whether the infant will be breast-fed or formula-fed. Human milk is uniquely adapted to the infant's needs and, hence, is the most appropriate milk for the human infant. Breast-feeding also has practical and psychologic advantages. Thus, all mothers should be encouraged to at least consider breast-feeding her baby.

ADVANTAGES OF BREAST-FEEDING. Breast milk is the natural food for full-term infants during the first months of life. It is always available at the proper temperature and requires no preparation time. It is fresh and free of contaminating bacteria, thereby reducing the chances of gastrointestinal disturbances. Although there is little if any difference in mortality rates between formula-fed and breast-fed infants receiving good care, the protective effects of breast milk against enteric and other pathogens result in less morbidity. These effects are particularly important in developing countries or any locality without a safe supply of potable water and effective methods for disposal of human waste.

Breast-feeding is associated with fewer feeding difficulties incident to allergy and/or intolerance to bovine milk. These include diarrhea, intestinal bleeding, occult melena, "spitting up," colic, and atopic eczema. Breast-fed infants also appear to have a lower frequency of certain allergic and chronic diseases in later life than formula-fed infants.

Human milk contains bacterial and viral antibodies, including relatively high concentrations of secretory IgA that prevents microorganisms from adhering to the intestinal mucosa. It also contains substances that inhibit growth of many common viruses. Antibodies in human milk are thought to provide local gastrointestinal immunity against organisms entering the body via this route. They probably account, at least partially, for the lower incidence of diarrhea as well as otitis media, pneumonia, bacteremia, and meningitis during the 1st yr of life in infants who are breast-fed exclusively vs. formula-fed for the first 4 mo of life.

Macrophages in human milk may synthesize complement, lysozyme, and lactoferrin. In addition, breast milk contains lactoferrin, an iron-binding whey protein that is normally about one-third saturated with iron and has an inhibitory effect on the growth of *Escherichia coli* in the intestine. The lower pH of the stool of breast-fed infants is thought to contribute to the favorable intestinal flora of infants fed human milk vs. formula (i.e., more bifidobacteria and lactobacilli; fewer *E. coli*), which helps protect against infections caused by some species of *E. coli*. Human milk also contains bile salt–stimulated lipase, which kills *Giardia lamblia* and *Entamoeba histolytica*. Transfer of tuberculin responsiveness by breast milk suggests passive transfer of T-cell immunity.

Milk from the mother whose diet is sufficient and properly balanced will supply all the necessary nutrients except, perhaps, fluoride and, after several months, vitamin D. If the water supply is not adequately fluoridated ($\leq$0.3 ppm), the breast-fed infant should receive at least 10 μg of fluoride daily for the first 6 mo of life; thereafter, the fluoride intake should approximate the adequate intake (see Table 40–1). If the maternal vitamin D intake is inadequate and the infant's exposure to sunlight is limited (e.g., dark-skinned infants and infants who are chronically protected from sunlight), 10 μg/24 hr of vitamin D is recommended. The iron content of human milk is somewhat low. However, most normal infants have sufficient iron stores for the first 6 mo of life. Moreover, human milk iron is well absorbed. Nonetheless, by 4–6 mo of age, the breast-fed infant's diet should be supplemented with iron-fortified complementary foods or a ferrous iron preparation.

The vitamin K content of human milk also is low and may contribute to hemorrhagic disease of the newborn. Parenteral administration of 1 mg of vitamin K_1 at birth is recommended for all infants, and this is especially important for those who will be breast-fed.

The psychologic advantages of breast-feeding for both mother and infant are well recognized. The mother is personally involved in the nurturing of her infant, resulting both in a feeling of being essential and a sense of accomplishment while the infant is provided with a close and comfortable physical relationship with the mother.

The resumption of menstruation should not deter continued breast-feeding. However, temporary behavior changes of the mother and/or the baby may call for reassurance. Pregnancy does not necessitate immediate cessation of nursing, but the combined demands of supplying milk to the infant and nutrients to the developing fetus are formidable, necessitating special attention to maternal nutrition.

Transmission of HIV by breast-feeding is well documented. Thus, if safe alternatives are available, breast-feeding by HIV-infected mothers is not recommended. However, in many developing countries, breast-feeding may be crucial to infant survival; if so, the risk of HIV transmission by breast-feeding may be less than the risks of other feeding methods. The World Health Organization recommends that breast-feeding be continued, even in areas of high endemic rates of HIV infection, unless safe infant formula is readily available. This reflects the belief that the risk of formula-feeding in many developing countries is significantly greater than the risk of HIV infection with breast-feeding.

Cytomegalovirus (CMV), human T-cell lymphotropic virus type 1, rubella virus, hepatitis B virus, and herpes simplex virus also have been demonstrated in breast milk. Of these, the presence of CMV is the most troublesome. About two thirds of seronegative breast-fed infants may become infected with CMV. In term infants, this appears to be without symptoms or sequelae, but the risk of infection in preterm infants may be substantially greater. Thus, the use of fresh donor milk for feeding preterm infants is contraindicated unless the milk is known to be CMV negative.

Evidence of breast milk transmission of other viruses is rare. However, vesicles have been noted in the mouth of infants whose mothers' milk contained herpes simplex virus. Thus, nursing women with active herpes simplex lesions should observe scrupulous handwashing technique and should avoid nursing if there are active lesions on or near the nipple.

Although hepatitis B virus has been isolated from maternal milk, the predominant means of mother-infant transmission of this virus appears to be at delivery. Active immunization of the infant within the first 24 hr of life coupled with administration of specific high-titer hepatitis B immune globulin and a follow-up active vaccination should permit the mother who is infected with hepatitis B to nurse with minimal risk to the infant. If a nursing mother acquires hepatitis B, the infant should receive the accelerated protocol of immunization (see Chapter 282).

PREPARATION OF THE PROSPECTIVE MOTHER FOR BREAST-FEEDING. Most women, if encouraged and protected from discouraging experiences and comments while the secretion of breast milk is becoming established, can successfully breast-feed their infant. The physician interested in helping the prospective mother breast-feed successfully should discuss the advantages of breast-feeding with her as early as the midtrimester of pregnancy or whenever the mother begins planning for her infant. Many mothers who are ambivalent toward breast-feeding are able to nurse successfully if they are reassured and supported. However, if the mother adamantly rejects the suggestion that she nurse her infant, overpersuasion may be detrimental to mother-infant relationships.

Factors that are conducive to successful breast-feeding include good health, a proper balance of rest and exercise, freedom from worry, early and sufficient treatment of any intercurrent disease, and adequate nutrition. Retracted and/or inverted nipples are detractors but not contraindications to breast-feeding. Retracted nipples usually benefit from daily manual breast-pump traction during the latter weeks of pregnancy, and truly inverted nipples may be helped by the use of milk cups, starting as early as the 3rd mo of pregnancy.

If the mother's diet is adequate, she need not gain or lose weight while breast-feeding. Nursing will help the uterus return to its normal size sooner and, also, may help the mother return to her prepregnancy weight sooner. Many women must be reassured that breast tone will be preserved by the use of a properly fitted brassiere to support the breasts, especially before delivery and during the nursing period.

ESTABLISHING AND MAINTAINING THE MILK SUPPLY. The most satisfactory stimulus to the secretion of human milk is regular and complete emptying of the breasts. Thus, efforts should be directed toward the early establishment of normal, vigorous nursing, even during the first few days after birth when there appears to be little, if any, milk. Breast-feeding should begin as soon after delivery as the conditions of the mother and the infant permit, preferably within the 1st hr or so. Infants who cannot be fed on demand should be brought to the mother for feeding about every 3 hr during the day and night. Once lactation is well established, most mothers are capable of producing more milk than their infant needs.

Appropriate care for tender or sore nipples should be instituted before severe pain from abrasions and cracking develops. Exposing the nipples to air; applying pure lanolin; avoiding soap, alcohol, and tincture of benzoin; changing disposable nursing pads lining the brassiere cups frequently; nursing more frequently; manually expressing milk; nursing in different positions; and keeping the breast dry between feedings are recommended. If nipple tenderness is sufficient to make the mother apprehensive, the milk-ejection reflex may be delayed. This leads to frustration of the infant and increasingly vigorous nursing, which further injures the nipple and areolar area. Nipple shields may be helpful in these situations.

The first 2 wk after birth are crucial for establishing breast-feeding. Daily weight gains of the infant, while important for ascertaining the volume of milk produced, should not be overly emphasized during this time. In addition, supplemental bottle feedings to achieve weight gain should be limited because these may compromise attempts at breast-feeding.

Although the difference between breast and bottle nipples may confuse the infant, this is usually not a serious problem. It is perfectly satisfactory to have the mother pump her breasts and feed the infant breast milk via a bottle for the first 1–2 wk. Then, when she is relaxed and less anxious, she can attempt breast-feeding one or two times daily until she and the infant have achieved a successful nursing routine. The additional pumping will usually increase milk production, thereby helping to ensure an adequate supply. Even after nursing is well established, it may be appropriate for the mother to pump extra milk and store it (in a freezer for up to 1 mo or refrigerator for up to 24 hr) for use when she is not available. This allows the mother some freedom and, at the same time, allows the father or other caregivers to be more involved in the infant's feeding and care.

Lactation usually is not well established before the mother is discharged from the hospital, and the excitement of going home may impede an initially successful in-hospital nursing experience. It is wise to anticipate this possibility and discuss it with the mother. Providing her with enough formula for a few complementary feedings may prevent discouragement that might prejudice further nursing.

No factor is more important for successful breast-feeding than a happy, relaxed state of mind. Mothers may worry that their infants are abnormal when they cry, are drowsy, sneeze, or regurgitate milk. They are often upset by any suggestion that their milk may be lacking in quantity or quality, and they may be disturbed by the scanty supply of colostrum, nipple tenderness, and the fullness of the breasts on the fourth or fifth day after delivery. Many mothers do not feel comfortable when trying to nurse in an open ward or, even, with another person in the room. Many also may worry about what is going on at home while they are in the hospital or about what is going to happen when they arrive home. An alert physician recognizes and appreciates these worries, particularly if the infant is a first born, and provides tactful reassurance and explanations that minimize worry and enhance the likelihood of successful breast-feeding. The support plan for individual mothers, of course, must include consideration of social and cultural factors.

HYGIENE. Proper hygiene will help prevent irritation and infection of the nipples caused by prolonged initial nursing, maceration from wetness of the nipple, or rubbing of clothing.

The breasts should be washed at least once a day. If soap appears to dry the nipple and areolar area, a milder, nondrying soap should be substituted or use of soap should be temporarily discontinued. The nipple area should be kept as dry as possible.

Many mothers are more comfortable wearing a properly fitted brassiere day and night. If doing so, plastic liners should be removed and a commercially available absorbent pad or clean cloth should be placed inside the brassiere to absorb any leaked milk.

MATERNAL DIET AND OTHER FACTORS. The breast-feeding mother's diet should contain enough calories and other nutrients to compensate for those secreted in the milk as well as for those required to produce it. A varied diet sufficient to maintain weight and generous in fluid, vitamins, and minerals is important. Weight-reducing diets should be avoided, particularly while the infant is exclusively breast-fed. Milk is an important component of the mother's diet, but it should not replace other essential foods. If the mother is allergic to milk or dislikes it, her diet should be supplemented with 1 g calcium daily. Daily fluid intake should approximate 3 qt.

Ingestion of some foods (e.g., berries, tomatoes, onions, members of the cabbage family, chocolate, spices, and condiments) by the mother may occasionally cause gastric distress or loose stools in the infant. However, no food need be withheld from the mother unless it is known to cause, or is strongly suspected of causing, distress to the infant.

Nursing mothers should not take drugs unless they are absolutely necessary. Many preparations are harmful to the neonate, and many have not been evaluated. Antithyroid medications, lithium, anticancer agents, isoniazid, recreationally abused drugs, and phenindione are contraindicated for the breast-feeding mother. If any of these agents or diagnostic radiopharmaceuticals, chloramphenicol, metronidazole, sulfonamides, and/or anthraquinone-derivative laxatives are required, temporary cessation of breast-feeding should be considered. Nursing mothers should not eat fish from waters contaminated with polychlorinated biphenyls or other substances (e.g., mercury). Smoking cigarettes and drinking alcoholic beverages should be discouraged during breast-feeding. It is important for the breast-feeding mother to avoid fatigue. However, she should exercise sufficiently to promote her sense of physical well-being.

TECHNIQUE OF BREAST-FEEDING. Breast-feeding sometimes becomes impossible simply because the attending physician fails to recognize that the difficulties are in the feeding technique. Hence, it is important to review the technical aspects of breast-feeding with the mother, particularly the mother who has not breast-fed before.

At feeding time, the infant should be hungry, dry, and neither too cold nor too warm. He or she should be held in a comfortable, semi-sitting position to prevent vomiting with eructation. The mother, too, should be comfortable and completely at ease. A moderately low chair with an armrest is preferable, and a low stool for resting her foot and raising her knee on the nursing side is advantageous. The infant should be supported comfortably with the face held close to the mother's breast by one arm and hand while the other hand supports the breast, making the nipple easily accessible to the infant's mouth without obstructing nasal breathing. The infant's lips should engage considerable areola as well as nipple.

Success in breast-feeding depends, in large part, on the adjustments made during the first few days of life. Difficulties often result from attempts to adapt the infant to a nursing procedure rather than designing a procedure that satisfies the infant. Most problems can be avoided by conforming to the infant's spontaneous pattern. If the infant is breast-fed when hungry and his or her appetite is satisfied, the fundamental requirements are met.

Several reflexes or behavior patterns that facilitate breast-feeding are present at birth. These include the rooting, sucking, swallowing, and satiety reflexes. The *rooting reflex* is the first to come into play. When the infant smells milk, he or she moves the head in an attempt to find the source of the smell. If the cheek is touched by a smooth object (e.g., the mother's breast), the infant will turn toward that object and open his or her mouth in anticipation of grasping the nipple (i.e., rooting with the mouth for the nipple).

The infant's rooting reflex brings the entire areolar area into the infant's mouth, and contact of the nipple against the infant's palate and posterior tongue elicits sucking, while the buccal fat pads help keep the nipple in place. This *sucking reflex* is a process of squeezing the sinuses of the areola rather than simply sucking on the nipple, as is required for bottle-feeding. Finally, milk in the infant's mouth triggers the *swallowing reflex.*

The breast-feeding infant's sucking results in afferent impulses to the mother's hypothalamus and, then, to both anterior and posterior pituitary. Prolactin release from the anterior pituitary stimulates milk secretion by the cuboidal cells in the acini or alveoli of the breast while secretion of oxytocin by the posterior pituitary results in contraction of the myoepithelial cells surrounding the alveoli deep in the breast and, in turn, "squeezes" milk into the larger ducts, where it is more easily available to the sucking infant. When this "let down" or *milk ejection reflex* functions well, milk flows from the opposite breast as the infant begins to nurse. The reflex is often absent or erratic

during periods of pain, fatigue, or emotional distress; and this is thought to be a common cause of milk retention in women who are unsuccessful in breast-feeding.

Mothers should know that the infant who is not hungry will not search for the nipple or suck. Most infants are usually sleepy for several days after birth and, hence, are not avid suckers. By the 3rd day of life when there has been some weight loss, many mothers become anxious if the infant seems uninterested in nursing. It reassures them to learn that most healthy infants "wake up" and become good nursers by the 4th or 5th day of life. Infants whose mothers were sedated during labor usually suck at lower rates and pressures and, also, consume less milk than infants of nonsedated mothers.

Some infants will empty a breast in 5 min; others will nurse more leisurely, sometimes for 20 min or longer. Most of the milk is obtained early in the feeding (i.e., 50% in the first 2 min and 80–90% in the first 4 min). Unless the mother has sore nipples, the infant should be allowed to suck until satisfied. If the infant does not "unlatch" from the breast after a reasonable period, a finger can be inserted into the corner of his or her mouth to decrease suction and facilitate removal. The infant should not be pulled from the breast.

At the end of the nursing period, the infant should be held erect over the mother's shoulder or on her lap with or without gently rubbing or patting the back to assist in expelling swallowed air. This "burping" procedure often is necessary one or more times during the feeding as well as 5–10 min after the infant has been returned to the crib. It is an essential procedure during the early months of life but should not be overdone.

ONE OR BOTH BREASTS PER FEEDING. The infant should empty at least one breast at each feeding; otherwise, it will not be stimulated sufficiently to refill. Both breasts should be used at each feeding in the early weeks to encourage maximal milk production. After the milk supply is established, the breasts may be alternated at successive feedings. The infant will usually be satisfied with the amount obtained from one. If milk secretion becomes too great, both breasts may be offered at each feeding but incompletely emptied, thereby decreasing milk production.

DETERMINING ADEQUACY OF MILK SUPPLY. If the infant is satisfied after each nursing period, sleeps 2–4 hr between feedings, and gains weight adequately, the milk supply is sufficient. Infants who are "light sleepers" usually require considerable body contact with the mother during the first months of life; hence, it should not be assumed automatically that mothers of such infants have a poor milk supply. On the other hand, if the infant nurses avidly and completely empties both breasts but appears unsatisfied afterward (e.g., does not go to sleep after nursing or sleeps fitfully and awakens after 1–2 hr) and fails to gain weight satisfactorily, the milk supply is probably inadequate. The La Leche League, which establishes close relationships between successful nursing mothers and mothers needing assistance with nursing, is often helpful in such circumstances.*

In general, weighing the infant before and after every nursing to judge the adequacy of the milk supply is neither necessary nor desirable. The amount of milk that an infant takes at a single feeding ranges from one to several ounces throughout a 24 hr period and, hence, is usually unimportant with respect to daily intake. Small gains may worry the mother and, in turn, may diminish her milk supply. In addition, she may give the infant a bottle to reassure herself that the infant is getting enough to eat and the better result with the "test bottle" may discourage breast-feeding, even if she has an adequate milk supply.

---

*La Leche League International, 9616 Minneapolis Avenue, Franklin Park, IL 60131, has many local affiliates composed of successfully nursing mothers willing to assist other mothers desiring to nurse.

Three possibilities should be excluded before assuming that a mother cannot produce sufficient milk: (1) errors in feeding technique; (2) remediable maternal factors related to diet, rest, or emotional distress; and (3) physical disturbances of the infant that interfere with nursing or with weight gain. Infrequently, infants who seem to be nursing well may not thrive because of inadequate milk supply. In such cases, more frequent feedings may be indicated. Nursing more often than every 2 hr, however, may inhibit prolactin secretion and further decrease milk production. This usually is not a problem with feeding at 2 hr intervals. Other aids include stimulation of prolactin secretion by small doses of chlorpromazine for a few days or by devices such as the LactAid, which supplement the infant's intake.

EXPRESSION OF BREAST MILK. Although manual expression of breast milk is useful to relieve engorgement of the breasts, the cost of battery-operated and electric breast pumps is often prohibitive. Pumping can increase milk production and relieve sore nipples because it does not cause as much nipple irritation as suckling. Breast milk can be safely stored in the freezer or refrigerator and used for feeding the infant at a later time.

SUPPLEMENTAL FEEDINGS. Most mothers who are returning to work plan to pump enough milk while at work to feed her infant while she's at work. However, because of stress and time constraints at work, this often is not possible. These mothers should be reassured that it is acceptable to feed the infant a commercial formula during the day and continue nursing in the evening. Breast milk production will gradually decrease so that the mother is not plagued by engorged, leaking breasts but most will continue to produce enough milk for two or three feedings a day for several months.

If formula or stored breast milk is to be given after the infant has completed a breast-feeding, the warmed bottle should be available so that it can be offered immediately after the infant has been "burped." The holes in the nipples should not be so large that the infant gets this portion of food without effort; if this happens, he or she may quickly abandon any efforts to suck adequately at the mother's breast. Some employers provide childcare at the workplace, thus enabling mothers to continue nursing successfully. Others provide convenient facilities for pumping. Such efforts by employers should be commended and encouraged.

WEANING FROM BREAST-FEEDING. Most infants gradually reduce the volume and the frequency of breast-feedings between 6 and 12 mo of age after they become accustomed to solid foods and liquids by bottle and/or cup. As they demand less milk, the mother's supply gradually diminishes without causing discomfort from engorgement. Weaning can be initiated when mutually desired by the mother and infant by substituting formula or bovine milk by bottle or cup for part and, subsequently, for all of a breast-feeding. The breast-feedings are eventually replaced with formula, usually over several days, and the infant is weaned completely. Occasionally, an infant takes a cup as readily as a bottle. If so, the intermediate transfer from breast to bottle before transferring from bottle to cup can be avoided. These changes should be made gradually and should be a pleasant experience, not a conflict, for both the mother and the infant. Praise, loving attention, and cuddling are vital to successful weaning.

When cessation of nursing is necessary at an earlier age, use of a tight breast binder and application of ice bags may help decrease milk production. Restriction of the mother's fluid intake is also helpful. Small doses of estrogen for 1–2 days also may help decrease milk production at the termination of nursing.

CONTRAINDICATIONS TO BREAST-FEEDING. Provided the mother's milk supply is ample, her diet is adequate, and she is not infected with HIV, there are no disadvantages of breast-feeding for the healthy term infant. Allergens to which the infant is sensitized can be conveyed in the milk, but the presence of such allergens is rarely a valid reason to stop breast-feeding.

Rather, an attempt should be made to identify the allergen and remove it from the mother's diet.

There also are few maternal contraindications to breast-feeding. Markedly inverted nipples may be troublesome, as may fissuring or cracking of the nipples, but the latter can usually be avoided by preventing engorgement. Mastitis also may be alleviated by continued and frequent nursing on the affected breast to keep it from becoming engorged, but local heat applications and antibiotics may occasionally be necessary. Acute maternal infection may contraindicate breast-feeding if the infant does not have the same infection; otherwise, there is no need to stop nursing unless the condition of either the mother or the infant necessitates it. When the infant is unaffected, the breast may be emptied if the mother's condition permits and the milk given to the infant by bottle or cup. Mothers with septicemia, active tuberculosis, typhoid fever, breast cancer, or malaria should not breast-feed. Substance abuse and severe neuroses or psychoses also are contraindications to breast-feeding.

Formula-Feeding. Objective nutritional studies of growing infants younger than 4–6 mo of age (e.g., rate of growth in weight and length, normality of various constituents in blood, performance in metabolic studies, body composition) differ minimally, if at all, between infants fed human milk and infants fed modern infant formulas. Although such techniques may not detect small but important variations and/or differences, these investigations attest to the ability of modern infant formulas to support normal growth and development. Thus, the mother who is unable or does not wish to nurse her infant need have no less sense of accomplishment or of affection for her infant than the nursing mother. Modern infant formulas are excellent substitutes for human milk. Moreover, the quality of attachment and mothering as well as the degree of security and affection provided the infant need not be different with formula-feeding vs. breast-feeding.

TECHNIQUE OF FORMULA-FEEDING. The setting for formula-feeding should be similar to that for breast-feeding, with the mother or caregiver and infant in a comfortable position, unhurried, and free from distractions. The infant should be hungry, fully awake, warm, and dry. He or she should be held as though being breast-fed. The nipple holes should be of a size that allows the milk to drop slowly, and the bottle should be held so that milk, not air, channels through the nipple. Bottle propping, even with a "safe" holder, should be avoided; this not only deprives the infant of the physical contact and security of being held but, also, may be dangerous, particularly for small infants who may aspirate if unattended. Otitis media is more common in infants fed with the propped bottle.

The bottle of milk is customarily warmed to body temperature, but no harmful effects from feeding formula at room or, even, refrigerator temperature have been demonstrated. The temperature may be tested by dropping milk onto the wrist.

Eructation of air swallowed during feeding is important for avoiding regurgitation and abdominal discomfort, especially during the first 6–7 mo of life. The technique of "burping" should be the same as described for the breast-fed infant. A few infants relieve themselves best after being returned to the crib. All infants occasionally will regurgitate or "spit up" a small amount of milk after feeding, a fact that the mother should know. Spitting up seems to occur more often in the formula-fed than in the breast-fed infant.

A feeding may last from 5–25 min, depending on the age and the vigor of the infant. Because the appetite varies from one feeding to another, each bottle should contain more than the average amount taken per feeding. In no case, however, should the infant be urged to take more than desired. Excess milk should be discarded.

COMPOSITION OF INFANT FORMULAS. The nutrient content of infant formulas marketed in the United States is regulated by the Infant Formula Act, and most industrialized and many developing countries have similar regulations. All must contain minimum amounts of all nutrients known or thought to be required by infants, and increasing emphasis is being placed on not exceeding a reasonable maximum content of each. The most recent recommendations for the minimum and maximum nutrient contents of infant formulas marketed in the United States are shown in Table 41–1. Note that the minimum recommended amount of each nutrient is greater than the amount of that nutrient in human milk and, hence, greater than the most recent Dietary Reference Intake for that nutrient (see Table 40–1). This, most likely, reflects the perceived lower bioavailability of formula vs. human milk nutrients.

Manufacturers of infant formulas are responsible for assuring the Food and Drug Administration (FDA) that each formula contains the minimum recommended amount and no more than the maximum recommended amount of each nutrient for the intended shelf life of the formula and, also, that the formula was manufactured safely and hygienically. To this end, each batch of manufactured formula is assayed continually over the shelf life of the product. Manufacturers also are responsible for assuring the FDA that each marketed formula, as the infant's source of nutrition, supports normal growth and development for at least the first 4 mo of life. This is usually done by conducting growth studies during the first 4 mo of life in a sufficient number of infants to detect a 3 g/24 hr difference in rate of weight gain. The efficacy and safety of substituting alternative

TABLE 41–1. Recently Recommended Minimum and Maximum Contents of Various Nutrients for Infant Formula Manufactured in the United States*

	Minimum	Maximum
Energy (kcal/dL):	63	71
Fat (g)	4.4	6.4
Linoleic acid (%)	8	35
α-Linolenic acid (%)	1.75	4
Carbohydrate (g)	9	13
Protein (g)	1.7	3.4
Electrolytes and Minerals:		
Calcium (mg)	50	140
Phosphorus (mg)	20	70
Magnesium (mg)	4	17
Sodium (mg)	25	50
Chloride (mg)	50	160
Potassium (mg)	60	160
Iron (mg)	0.2	1.65
Zinc (mg)	0.4	1.0
Copper (μg)	60	160
Iodine (μg)	8	35
Selenium (μg)	1.5	5
Manganese (μg)	1.0	100
Fluoride (μg)	0	60
Chromium	0	0
Molybdenum	0	0
Vitamins:		
Vitamin A (IU)	200	500
Vitamin D (IU)	40	100
Vitamin E (mg α-TE)	0.5	5.0
Vitamin K (μg)	1	25
Vitamin C (mg)	6	15
Thiamine (μg)	30	200
Riboflavin (μg)	80	300
Niacin (μg)	550	2000
Vitamin B_6 (μg)	30	130
Folate (μg)	11	40
Vitamin B_{12} (μg)	0.08	0.7
Biotin (μg)	1	15
Pantothenic acid (μg)	300	1200
Other ingredients:		
Carnitine (mg)	1.2	2.0
Taurine (mg)	0	12
*Myo*inositol (mg)	4	40
Choline (mg)	7	30

Amounts/100 kcal, unless otherwise indicated.

sources of various nutrients also must be demonstrated by appropriate studies.

Most infant formulas contain a protein source, usually a mixture of bovine milk proteins but also soy protein or a variety of hydrolyzed proteins, lactose and/or other sugars, a mixture of vegetable oils, mineral salts, and vitamins. The composition of selected formulas available in the United States is shown in Table 41–2. Most are available in powder, concentrated liquid (intended to be diluted 1:1 with water), and ready-to-feed forms. Similarities to bovine milk from which they evolved are virtually nonexistent.

NUMBER OF FEEDINGS DAILY. The number of feedings required per day decreases throughout the 1st yr of life from eight or more shortly after birth to only three or four at 1 yr of age. The desired interval between feedings differs considerably among infants but, in general, ranges from 3–5 hr during the 1st yr of life, averaging about 4 hr. For the first 1–2 mo, feedings are taken throughout the 24 hr period; thereafter, as the quantity of milk consumed at each feeding increases and the infant adjusts his or her demand to the family pattern of daytime activities, the infant usually sleeps for longer periods at night. As the infant develops psychologically and the relationship between the parent and infant evolves, demand feeding should gradually be replaced by a feeding regimen that accommodates the needs of the infant as well as the rest of the family.

QUANTITY OF FORMULA. The quantity of formula taken at a feeding varies among infants of the same age and within infants at different feedings. Rarely will an infant want more than 7–8 oz at a single feeding. The desire for formula (or breast milk) is somewhat less during the first 2 wk of life than during the following 5–6 mo. After 6 mo of age, formula (or breast milk) is rarely the sole source of the infant's nutrient intake. However, it remains an important source of many nutrients (e.g., calcium).

It is rarely necessary to use more than 1 qt of formula per day. By the time the infant is taking this amount, other foods should be added to the diet. Ingesting more than this volume has no advantages and may displace intake of other essential foods.

INFANT FORMULA VS. BOVINE MILK. Although current recommendations are to avoid intake of bovine milk, particularly low fat or skimmed milk, before at least 1 yr of age, surveys suggest that a sizable percentage of infants older than 6 mo of age are fed homogenized bovine milk rather than infant formula and almost half of these are fed low-fat or skimmed milk—often on the advice of their physician.

The consequences of these practices are not known with certainty. However, infants fed bovine milk, on average, ingest roughly three times the recommended intake of protein and about 50% more sodium than the upper limit of the "safe range" of intake of this mineral but only about two thirds of the recommended intake of iron and only half of the recommended intake of linoleic acid. Ingestion of bovine milk also increases intestinal blood loss and, hence, further contributes to development of iron-deficiency anemia. The protein and sodium intakes of infants fed skimmed rather than whole bovine milk are even higher, the iron intake is equally low, and the intake of linoleic acid is very low. Ironically, while the most common reason for substituting low-fat or skimmed milk for whole milk or formula is to reduce fat and energy intakes, the total energy intake of infants fed skimmed milk is not necessarily lower than that of infants fed whole milk or formula. It appears that infants compensate for the lower energy density of low-fat or skimmed milk by taking more of it and/or increasing intake of other foods.

Whether the high protein and sodium intakes of infants fed either whole or skimmed milk are undesirable is not known with certainty. The low iron intake, clearly, is undesirable but medicinal iron supplementation should prevent development of deficiency. The low intake of linoleic acid may be more problematic. Whereas signs and/or symptoms of essential fatty acid defi-

TABLE 41–2. Composition of Standard Formulas for Normal Infants*

Component	Similac[†]	Enfamil[‡]	Good Start[§]	Isomil[†]	Prosobee[‡]
Protein (g)	2.07 (cow's milk, whey)	2.1 (cow's milk, whey)	2.4 (whey)	2.45 (soy protein isolate)	2.5 (soy protein isolate)
Fat (g)	5.5 (high-oleic safflower, coconut, and soy oils)	5.3 (soy, coconut, and high-oleic sunflower oils)	5.1 (palmolein, soy, coconut, and high-oleic safflower oils)	5.46 (soy and coconut oils)	5.3 (palmolein, soy, coconut, and high-oleic sunflower oils)
Carbohydrate (g)	10.56 (lactose)	10.9 (lactose)	11.0 (lactose, maltodextrin)	10.3 (corn syrup, sucrose)[∥]	10.6 (corn syrup solids)[∥]
Electrolytes and Minerals:					
Calcium (mg)	78	78	64	105	105
Phosphorus (mg)	42	53	36	75	83
Magnesium (mg)	6	8	6.7	7.5	11
Iron (mg)	1.8	1.8	1.5	1.8	1.8
Zinc (mg)	0.75	1	0.75	0.75	1.2
Manganese (µg)	5	15	7	25	25
Copper (µg)	90	75	90	75	75
Iodine (µg)	6	10	6	15	15
Selenium (µg)		2.8			2.8
Sodium (mg)	24	27	24	44	36
Potassium (mg)	105	108	98	108	120
Chloride (mg)	65	63	59	62	80
Vitamins:					
Vitamin A (IU)	300	300	300	300	300
Vitamin D (IU)	60	60	60	60	60
Vitamin E (IU)	1.5	2	2	3	2
Vitamin K (µg)	8	8	8.2	11	8
Thiamine (µg)	100	80	60	60	80
Riboflavin (µg)	150	140	135	90	90
Vitamin B_6 (µg)	60	60	75	60	60
Vitamin B_{12} (µg)	0.25	0.3	0.22	0.45	0.3
Niacin (µg)	1,050	1,000	750	1,350	1,000
Folic acid (µg)	15	16	15	15	16
Pantothenic acid (µg)	450	500	450	750	500
Biotin (µg)	4.4	3	2.2	4.5	3
Vitamin C (mg)	9	12	8	9	12
Choline (mg)	16	12	12	8	12
Inositol (mg)	4.7	6	18	5	6

*Amount/100 kcal.
[†]Ross Laboratories, Columbus, OH.
[‡]Mead-Johnson Nutritionals, Evansville, IN.
[§]Carnation Nutritional Products, Glendale, CA.
[∥]Isomil-SF (sucrose free) has similar composition except that glucose polymers are substituted for corn syrup and sucrose.

ciency appear to be uncommon in infants fed either whole or skimmed milk, an exhaustive search for such symptoms has not been made. Moreover, biochemical evidence of essential fatty acid deficiency without overt signs and symptoms occurs in both younger and older infants fed formulas with a low content of linoleic acid; thus, it is likely that an exhaustive search, including biochemical indices, would reveal a reasonably high incidence of essential fatty acid deficiency. On the other hand, infants who were breast-fed or fed formulas with a high linoleic acid content earlier in life may have sufficient body stores to limit the consequences of a low intake later. However, because essential fatty acid deficiency in animals is associated with long-term deleterious effects on development, it is not wise to assume that biochemical essential fatty acid deficiency without clinically detectable symptoms is without consequences.

Resolving the issues concerning the use of bovine milk in feeding the infant is important for economic as well as health reasons. Because the cost of bovine milk is considerably less than that of infant formula, replacing formula with homogenized bovine milk obviously has important economic advantages for most families, particularly those with limited income. In addition, if the federal food assistance programs could provide homogenized bovine milk rather than formula to infants, even infants older than 6 mo of age, the program's current funds would permit expansion of benefits to many more needy infants. Clearly, this cannot be considered without further data concerning the consequences of feeding bovine milk.

FEEDING DURING THE SECOND 6 MO OF LIFE

By 6 mo of age, the infant's capacity to digest and absorb a variety of dietary components as well as to metabolize, utilize, and excrete the absorbed products of digestion is near the capacity of the adult. Moreover, teeth are beginning to erupt and the infant is more active and beginning to explore his or her surroundings. With the eruption of teeth, the role of dietary carbohydrate in development of dental caries must be considered. Consideration of the long-term effects of inadequate or excessive intakes during infancy also assumes greater importance, as does consideration of the psychosocial role of foods during development.

These considerations rather than concerns about delivery of adequate amounts of nutrients are the basis for many of the feeding practices advocated during the second 6 mo of life. Although it is clear that all nutrient needs during this period can be met with reasonable amounts of currently available infant formulas, addition of other foods after 4–6 mo of age is recommended. In contrast, the volume of milk produced by many women may not be adequate to meet all nutrient needs of the breast-fed infant beyond about 6 mo of age. This is particularly true for iron. Thus, for breast-fed infants, complementary foods are an important source of nutrients.

Complementary foods (i.e., the additional foods, including formulas, given to the breast-fed infant) or replacement foods (i.e., food other than formula given to formula-fed infants) should be introduced in a stepwise fashion to both breast-fed and formula-fed infants, beginning about the time the infant is able to sit unassisted, usually between 4–6 mo of age. Cereals, a good source of iron, should usually be the first such foods given. Vegetables and fruits are introduced next, followed shortly by meats and, finally, eggs. The order in which these foods are introduced probably is not crucial, but only one new food should be introduced at a time, and additional new foods should be spaced by at least 3–4 days to allow detection of any adverse reactions to each newly introduced food. This is particularly important if there is a family history of food and/or other allergies.

Either home-prepared or manufactured complementary or replacement foods can be used. The latter are convenient and also likely to contain less salt. Many such products also have

supplemental nutrients (e.g., iron). These also are available in different consistencies to match the infant's ability to tolerate larger size particles as he or she matures.

Prepared dinners and soups containing a meat and one or more vegetables are quite popular. However, the protein content of these products is not as high as that of strained meat. Puddings and desserts also are popular items but, aside from their milk and egg content, are poor sources of nutrients other than energy; thus, intakes of these should be limited. Moreover, intake of egg-containing products generally should be delayed, especially if there is a family history of food and/or other allergies, until after the infant has demonstrated tolerance to eggs (either a mashed hard boiled egg yolk or a commercial egg yolk preparation).

Aside from the association of bottle-feeding with dental caries after teeth have erupted, little is known about either the potential hazards or the non-nutritional role of diet during the latter half of the 1st yr of life. Thus, feeding practices during this period vary widely. Nonetheless, most recent surveys indicate that infants fed according to current practices receive adequate intakes of most nutrients.

FEEDING PROBLEMS DURING THE 1ST YR OF LIFE

Underfeeding. Underfeeding is suggested by restlessness and crying as well as by failure to gain weight adequately. It may also result from the infant's failure to take a sufficient quantity of food even when offered. In these cases, the frequency of feedings, the mechanics of feeding, the size of the holes in the nipple, the adequacy of eructation of air, the possibility of abnormal mother-infant "bonding," and possible systemic disease in the infant should be investigated.

The extent and duration of underfeeding determine the *clinical manifestations*. Constipation, failure to sleep, irritability, and excessive crying are to be expected. Weight gain may be slow, or there may be an actual loss of weight. In the latter case, the skin becomes dry and wrinkled, subcutaneous tissue disappears, and the infant assumes the appearance of an "old man." Deficiencies of vitamins A, B, C, and D as well as of iron and protein may be responsible for characteristic clinical manifestations (see Chapters 42 and 44).

Treatment of underfeeding includes increasing nutrient intake, correcting deficiencies of vitamins and/or minerals, and instructing the mother in the art and practice of infant feeding. If some underlying systemic disease, child abuse/neglect, or psychologic problem is responsible, specific management of these disorders is necessary (see Chapters 35 and 36).

Overfeeding. As a rule, postprandial discomfort from excessive intake limits the amount of food an infant voluntarily ingests, but there are exceptions. If so, regurgitation and vomiting are the most frequent symptoms. Diets that are too high in fat delay gastric emptying, cause distention and abdominal discomfort, and may cause excessive weight gain. Diets too high in carbohydrate are likely to cause undue fermentation in the intestine, resulting in distention and flatulence as well as a more rapid weight gain than desirable. Because neither breast milk nor formulas contain either excessive fat or excessive carbohydrate, such diets usually result from supplementation. This practice tends to dilute the protein, vitamin, and mineral contents of formula and, hence, should be avoided (also see Chapter 43).

Regurgitation and Vomiting. Regurgitation refers to the return of small amounts of swallowed food during or shortly after eating. Vomiting, on the other hand, is the more complete emptying of the stomach, often occurring some time after feeding. Within limits, regurgitation is a natural occurrence, especially during the first several months of life. It can be reduced to a negligible amount by adequate eructation of swallowed air during and after eating, by gentle handling, by avoiding emotional conflicts, and by placing the infant on the right side immediately after eating (but not for napping or sleeping). The head should not be lower than the rest of the body to avoid gastroesophageal reflux, which is common during the first 4–6 mo of life.

Vomiting is one of the most common symptoms in infancy and may be associated with a variety of disturbances—some trivial and some serious. Its cause should always be investigated.

Loose or Diarrheal Stools. The stool of the breast-fed infant is naturally softer than that of the formula-fed infant. From about the 4th to the 6th day of life, the stools of the breast-fed infant go through a transitional stage of being loose and greenish yellow and containing mucus to the typical "milk stool." Subsequently, the use of laxatives or the ingestion of certain foods by the mother may be temporarily responsible for a breast-fed infant's loose stools. Excessive intake of breast milk may also increase the frequency and the water content of the stool. Actual diarrhea from overfeeding, however, is unusual; thus, diarrhea should be considered infectious until proved otherwise.

Although the stools of formula-fed infants tend to be firmer than those of breast-fed infants, loose stools also may result from artificial feeding. For example, overfeeding may cause loose, frequent stools, particularly during the first 2 wk or so of life. Later, formulas that are too concentrated or too high in sugar content, especially in lactose, may produce loose, frequent stools. However, as noted earlier, this is unlikely unless sugar has been added to the formula. Many diarrheal disturbances in formula-fed infants result from contaminants that would not disturb an older child. These usually are not serious enough to cause prolonged difficulty for the infant. The ease with which formula-fed infants acquire diarrheal disturbances and their potential seriousness are strong arguments for extreme care in preparation to assure that the formula or food is free of pathogenic bacteria.

Mild diarrheal disturbances caused by overfeeding respond quickly to temporary decrease or cessation of feeding. Withholding all solid food as well as one or several feedings and substituting boiled water or a balanced electrolyte solution are usually all that is required.

Constipation (see Chapters 5 and 287) Constipation is practically unknown in breast-fed infants receiving an adequate amount of milk and is rare in formula-fed infants receiving an adequate intake. The consistency of the stool, not its frequency, is the basis for diagnosis. Most infants have one or more stools daily, but some occasionally have a stool of normal consistency at intervals of up to 36–48 hr.

Whenever constipation or obstipation is present from birth or shortly after birth, a rectal examination should be performed. Tight or spastic anal sphincters may occasionally be responsible for obstipation, and finger dilation is frequently corrective. Anal fissures or cracks may also cause constipation. If irritation is alleviated, healing usually occurs quickly. Aganglionic megacolon may be manifested by constipation in early infancy; the absence of stool in the rectum on digital examination suggests this possibility, but further diagnostic work-up is indicated (see Chapter 313.3).

Constipation may be caused by an insufficient amount of food or fluid. In some cases, it may result from diets that are too high in fat or protein or deficient in bulk. Simply increasing the amount of fluid or sugar in the formula may be corrective during the first few months of life. After this age, better results are obtained by adding or increasing the amounts of cereal, vegetables, and fruits. Prune juice ($1/2$ to 1 oz) may be helpful, but adding foods with some bulk is usually more effective. Enemas and suppositories should never be more than temporary measures. Milk of magnesia may be given in doses of 1–2 tsp but should be reserved for unresponsive or severe constipation.

Colic. Colic is a symptom complex of paroxysmal abdominal pain, presumably of intestinal origin, and severe crying. It usually occurs in infants younger than 3 mo of age. The *clinical manifestations* are characteristic. The attack usually begins suddenly with a loud, more or less continuous cry. The so-called paroxysms may persist for several hours. The face may be flushed, or there may be circumoral pallor. The abdomen is usually distended and tense. The legs may be extended for short periods but are usually drawn up on the abdomen. The feet are often cold, and the hands are usually clenched. The attack may not terminate until the infant is completely exhausted. Sometimes, however, the passage of feces or flatus appears to provide relief.

Some infants seem to be particularly susceptible to colic. The *etiology* usually is not apparent, but, in some infants, the attacks appear to be associated with hunger or with swallowed air that has passed into the intestine. Overfeeding may also cause discomfort and distention; and some foods, especially those of high carbohydrate content, may be responsible for excessive intestinal fermentation. However, a change of diet rarely prevents further colic attacks.

Crying with intestinal discomfort occurs in infants with intestinal allergy, but colic is not limited to this group. Colic may mimic intestinal obstruction or peritoneal infection. Attacks commonly occur late in the afternoon or evening, suggesting that events in the household routine may be involved. Worry, fear, anger, or excitement may cause vomiting in an older child and may cause colic in an infant, but no single factor consistently accounts for colic and no treatment consistently provides satisfactory relief. Careful physical examination is important to eliminate the possibility of intussusception, strangulated hernia, or other disorders that cause abdominal pain.

Holding the infant upright or prone across the lap or on a hot water bottle or heating pad occasionally helps. Passage of flatus or fecal material spontaneously or with expulsion of a suppository or enema sometimes affords relief. Carminatives before feedings are ineffective in preventing the attacks. Sedation is occasionally indicated for a prolonged attack. If other measures fail, both the child and the parent may be sedated for a period of time. Temporary hospitalization of the infant, often with no more than a change in feeding routine and a period of rest for the mother, may help in extreme cases. Prevention of attacks should be sought by improving feeding techniques, including "burping," providing a stable emotional environment, identifying possibly allergenic foods in the infant's or nursing mother's diet, and avoiding underfeeding or overfeeding. Colic rarely persists after 3 mo of age. Although not serious, it can be particularly disturbing for the parents as well as the infant. Thus, a supportive and sympathetic physician can be particularly helpful, even if attacks do not resolve immediately.

FEEDING DURING THE 2ND YR OF LIFE

By the end of the 1st yr of life, most infants have adapted to a schedule of 3 meals a day plus one to two snacks. Although considerable latitude in the diet of each infant should be permitted to allow for personal idiosyncrasies and family habits, the mother should be given an outline of the basic daily dietary needs. Equally important, she should be aware of what to expect in terms of eating behavior as the child matures.

Reduced Food Intake. Toward the end of the 1st yr of life, the rate of growth decreases and the child's intake, accordingly, also decreases or fails to increase as rapidly as it did during the 1st yr of life. It is not unusual for the child to have temporary periods of not being interested in certain foods or, indeed, in any food. Failure to expect and recognize these changes in eating behavior often results in attempts to force feed. The child naturally rebels and feeding problems ensue. Because preventing problems is more effective than correcting them, the changing pattern of food habits during the 2nd yr of life should be explained to the mother before it is apparent. She should be reassured that the lack of interest in food is probably temporary and that attempts to force feed not only are futile but also likely to result in more severe feeding problems.

Self-Selection of Diet. Children's strong likes or dislikes of particular foods become apparent after about 1 yr of age and, if possible and practicable, should be respected. For example, the virtues of some foods (e.g., spinach) that are nonessential have been overemphasized; certainly, conflicts about such foods should not be allowed to occur. Often a food that is refused when it is first offered will be accepted when it is offered again a few days or weeks later. On the other hand, if basic staples such as milk and cereal are consistently rejected, food allergy should be considered. If this is not a problem, alternative forms of these basic staples (e.g., cheese, yogurt, breads) should be offered.

Children tend to select diets that, over several days, are well balanced. Thus, the child may be permitted a wide choice of foods, as long as he or she eats adequately over the longer period. Normally, the child determines the quantity of a given food as well as an entire meal that will be eaten. At this age, eating habits, particularly food likes and dislikes, also may be influenced by older children in the family. Thus, because eating patterns and habits developed in the first 2 yr of life usually persist for several years, such influences should be monitored closely.

Self-Feeding by Infants. Infants should be permitted to participate in feeding themselves as soon as they seem physically able to do so, usually long before 1 yr of age. By approximately 6 mo of age, infants can hold a bottle and, within another 2–3 mo, can hold a cup. Zwieback, graham crackers, or other hand-held foods can be introduced by the age of 7–8 mo. The infant may be allowed to use a spoon as soon as it can be held and directed to the mouth, usually between 10–12 mo of age. Mothers often inhibit this important learning process because of its messiness, but it is an important aspect of the infant's overall development and should be encouraged. By the end of the 2nd yr of life, infants should be largely responsible for feeding themselves. However, because the risk of aspiration is reasonably high until approximately 4 yr of age, infants younger than this should not be given foods that are easily aspirated (e.g., grapes, nuts, chunks of cheese and meat) unless a responsible adult is present.

Basic Daily Diet. Parents should be given a basic daily diet plan for the child from which the family menu can be prepared. Daily selection from each of the food groups (grains, fruits, vegetables, meats, and dairy products) provides a balanced diet with sufficient macronutrients and micronutrients. The quantity of intake after the basic requirements have been met can usually be determined by the healthy growing child. The child's dietary history is essential for evaluating the nutrient intake but, unless an accurate dietary diary is kept for several days, such histories are often unreliable. Correcting the diet can be much more effective if reliable information is available.

The older child should learn the content of a basic well-balanced diet and its importance to proper growth and good health. However, this information should never be presented as a threat to enforce rigid feeding practices.

Eating Habits. Eating habits formed in the 1st and 2nd yr of life distinctly affect those of the subsequent years. Feeding difficulties frequently result from excessive parental insistence on eating and subsequent anxiety of the parents and the child if the child fails to heed this insistence. The child's negative reactions often result from undue mealtime stress, the correction of which requires improvement in parent-child relations. Other factors that disturb eating are too much confusion at mealtime, insufficient time for eating on the part of either the adults and older children of the household or the child, food dislikes of other members of the family, and poorly prepared, unattrac-tively served food. Mealtimes should be happy, with conversation concerning subjects of interest to the entire family. A comfortable chair of proper height with a footrest is important for the smaller child's ease at the table.

The child's appetite should be respected; if his or her desire for food is below average at times, there should be no persuasion to eat more. Adults should realize that eating habits are taught better by example than by formal explanation.

Snacks Between Meals. During the 2nd yr of life and for several years thereafter, orange juice or other fruit juice or fruit, together with a cracker, may be given at either or both of the between-meal periods. Snacks served in childcare facilities should be similarly nutritious.

Vegetarian Diets. All-vegetable diets can supply all necessary nutrients but, to do so, the vegetables and grains comprising the diet must be selected from different classes. Vegetables are high in fiber content, vitamins, and minerals. Because of the higher fiber intake, vegetarians usually have faster gastrointestinal transit time, bulkier stools, and lower serum cholesterol levels; as adults, they may be less likely to develop diverticulitis and appendicitis than meat eaters. Vegetarians who consume eggs (ovovegetarians) and milk (lactovegetarians) obviously have more choices for constructing a well-balanced diet than those who consume neither (vegans). Vegans may develop vitamin B_{12} deficiency and, because of high fiber intake, may develop trace mineral deficiencies. Nursing vegan mothers must be given supplemental vitamin B_{12} to prevent methylmalonic acidemia in their infants. There also is some concern that vegetarian infants may not grow as rapidly as omnivores during the first 2 yr of life.

FEEDING DURING LATER CHILDHOOD

After 2 yr of age, a child's diet should not differ from that of the rest of the family. All known required nutrients are supplied by a varied diet selected according to the Food Pyramid Guidelines (Fig. 41–1). These guidelines with emphasis on grains, fruits, and vegetables are consistent with the recommendations of the National Cholesterol Education Program, including restriction of dietary fat to approximately 30% of the total daily energy intake, saturated fatty acids to less than 10% of energy, and cholesterol to no more than 100 mg/1,000 kcal. Polyunsaturated fatty acids should supply 7–8% of energy and monounsaturated fatty acids should supply 12–13%. This diet, the American Heart Association Step One Diet, is recommended to decrease athero-sclerotic heart disease in adulthood and may also be effective in limiting the development of obesity. There is some argument about the importance of such a diet before adolescence, except for those children with a strong family history of atherosclerotic heart disease. However, such diets support normal growth of children as young as 1 yr of age and implementing it after about 2 yr of age may be easier than doing so at adolescence.

Although initially developed for older children and adults, the Food Guide Pyramid has recently been adapted for 2–6 yr old children. This pyramid is shown in Figure 41–1. The suggested number of servings per day from the various food groups as well as the suggested serving sizes for each group are shown in Table 41–3. These are targeted to meet the recommended daily allowances (RDAs) for energy, protein, vitamins, and minerals established by the Food and Nutritional Board, National Academy of Sciences, in 1989. The more recent Dietary Reference Intakes (see Table 40–1) for some nutrients differ from these but, because most are lower, are not likely to have a major impact on the number of servings needed daily from each food group.

The number of servings from each food group needed for well-balanced 1,600 kcal/24 hr, 2,200 kcal/24 hr, and 2,800 kcal/24 hr diets are shown in Table 41–3. The 1,600 kcal/24 hr diet is appropriate for the moderately active 4–6 yr old child.

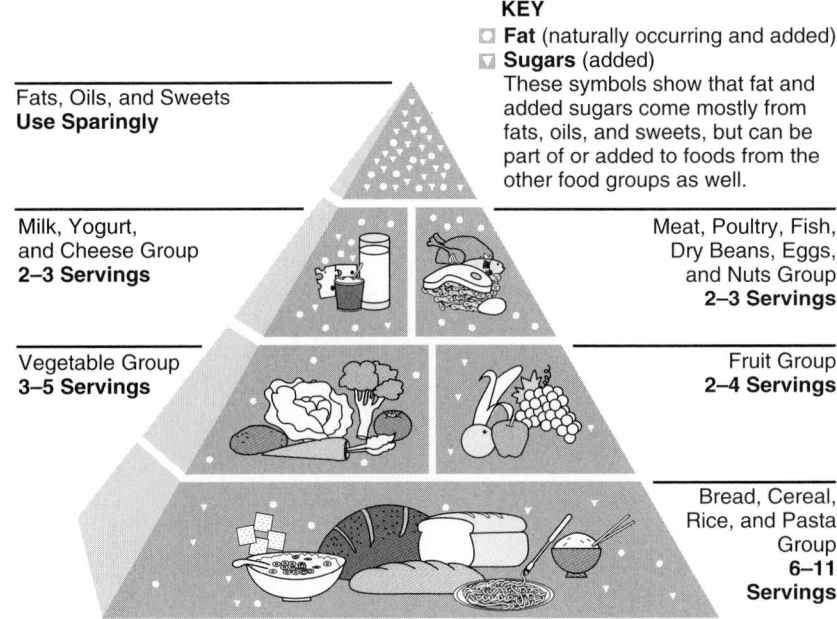

KEY

☐ **Fat** (naturally occurring and added)
☑ **Sugars** (added)

These symbols show that fat and added sugars come mostly from fats, oils, and sweets, but can be part of or added to foods from the other food groups as well.

Fats, Oils, and Sweets
Use Sparingly

Milk, Yogurt, and Cheese Group
2–3 Servings

Meat, Poultry, Fish, Dry Beans, Eggs, and Nuts Group
2–3 Servings

Vegetable Group
3–5 Servings

Fruit Group
2–4 Servings

Bread, Cereal, Rice, and Pasta Group
6–11 Servings

FIGURE 41–1. Food guide pyramid for 2–6 yr old children. (From U.S. Department of Agriculture/USDHHS.)

SOURCE: U.S. Department of Agriculture/U.S. Department of Health and Human Services

However, this energy intake may be excessive for less active children, and it may not be sufficient for the very active child. The goal should be to support normal rates of weight gain without excessive fat deposition. Most children, if not forced to eat more, will adjust intake to achieve this goal.

The 2,200 kcal/24 hr diet is appropriate for most moderately active 6–10 yr old children. Older, very active children of this age group may require somewhat more energy, and younger, less active children may need less. Active teenage boys may require at least 2,800 kcal/24 hr, sometimes more. In general, the energy needs of girls are somewhat less than those of boys.

Note that the increasing requirements with age can be met by increasing the number of servings of each food group rather than the size of the servings. For example, the number of servings suggested for the 2,800 kcal/24 hr diet is the same as suggested for active adults, some of whom need less and some of whom need more than 2,800 kcal/24 hr.

Although these guidelines are useful and can be used to design an appropriate diet for all children older than 2 yr of age, the variation in energy needs among children of the same age is considerable. The level of activity is a major determinant of the amount of energy needed, but this is not the only factor. Variations in energy expenditure among seemingly similar groups of children can vary by as much as 15–20%. Thus, even those children whose diets are based on the Food Guide Pyramid must be observed closely to ensure that growth is adequate but not excessive.

As children become older and more independent, an increasing number of meals are eaten away from home, often at "fast food" restaurants where adherence to the Food Guide Pyramid principles is difficult, if not impossible. An obvious solution is to limit such occasions to once or, at most, twice per week. However, this is often resisted by the child. Moreover, with the increasing number of mothers in the work force, many family meals are either eaten at the same establishment or purchased there for consumption at home. Perhaps the most a pediatrician or nutritionist can hope for is that the parents understand the importance of a well-balanced diet and how best to achieve this without undue hardship for themselves or their children.

Center for Nutrition Policy and Promotion Committee: *Tips for Using the Food Guide Pyramid for Young Children 2 to 6 Years Old*. United States Department of Agriculture, Program Aid 1647, March 1999.

Heird WC: Nutritional requirements during infancy. In Bowman BA, Russell RM (editors): *Present Knowledge in Nutrition*, 8th ed. Washington, DC, International Life Sciences Institute (ILSI) Press, 2001, pp 416–425.

Heird WC: Nutritional requirements during infancy. In Shils ME, Olson JA, Shike M, et al (editors): *Modern Nutrition in Health and Disease*, 9th ed. Baltimore, Williams & Wilkins, 1999, pp 839–855.

La Leche League International: *The Womanly Art of Breast Feeding*. Franklin Park, IL, La Leche League International, 1976.

Lawrence RA: *Breast Feeding, a Guide for the Medical Profession*, 4th ed. St. Louis, CV Mosby, 1994.

National Cholesterol Education Program (NCEP): Reports of the Expert Panel on Blood Cholesterol in Children and Adolescents. *Pediatrics* 1992;89(Suppl):525.

Raiten DJ, Talbot JM, Waters JH: Assessment of nutrient requirements for infant formulas. *J Nutr* 1998;128:2059S–2293S.

Work Group on Breastfeeding, American Academy of Pediatrics: Breastfeeding and the use of human milk. *Pediatrics* 1997;100:1035–39.

Chapter 42

Food Insecurity, Hunger, and Undernutrition *William C. Heird*

Food insecurity, hunger, and undernutrition are often viewed as a continuum, with food insecurity resulting in hunger and, ultimately, if sufficiently severe and/or of sufficient duration, in undernutrition. According to this view, food insecurity indicates inadequate access to food for whatever reason, hunger is the

TABLE 41–3. Servings Needed to Provide Differing Energy Intakes

Food Group	Servings Needed for Daily Energy Intake of:		
	1600 kcal	*2200 kcal*	*2800 kcal*
Bread	6	9	11
Fruit	2	3	4
Vegetable	3	4	5
Meat	5 oz	6 oz	7 oz
Milk	2–3	2–3	2–3
Total fat (g)	53	73	93
Added sugar (tsp)	6	12	18

immediate physiologic manifestation of inadequate intake, and undernutrition describes the biochemical and/or physical consequences of chronically or acutely inadequate intake. However, it is now recognized that this view is incomplete. Although the continuum from food insecurity to hunger and, ultimately, to undernutrition is often true, particularly in developing countries, all food-insecure children do not experience hunger and all undernourished children do not experience food insecurity before becoming undernourished. Each condition, not only undernutrition, has consequences for the individual, the family, and society. Thus, viewing these conditions as an inevitable continuum distorts estimates of the prevalence, causes, and consequences of each condition. It also may lead to inappropriate policy responses as well as to inappropriate treatment and/or failure to recognize and, it is hoped, remedy conditions other than overt undernutrition. It is important to understand the nature of each of these problems and their relationships to each other.

FOOD INSECURITY

Food insecurity can be defined in a number of ways. The broadest definition is "limited or uncertain availability of nutritionally adequate and safe foods in socially acceptable form and by socially acceptable ways." This definition encompasses concepts of the certainty of both short-term and long-term availability of and access to food; concerns about the sufficiency, nutritional quality, and safety of food; and the cultural and social acceptability of accessible food and the means by which this food is acquired.

The concept of food security differs depending on whether it is viewed from a global, a national, a household, or an individual perspective. Globally, food security concerns the overall availability of sufficient food to feed the population of the world. Food security from a national perspective also concerns availability of food. However, the issue is not whether enough food is produced globally to feed the population of the world but whether enough food is produced and/or imported to feed the population of the country. From a household perspective, food security concerns availability of and access to adequate food from household production, local purchase, or some combination of production and purchase. Food security, from an individual perspective, concerns the amount and quality of food available for consumption by the individual. This is a function of the availability of and access to food by the household and the distribution of food within the household.

In some developing countries, food insecurity results from the lack of sufficient food to feed the entire population of the country. This often is a result of war, famine, or some other disaster, but it also can result from a lack of resources to assure adequate production, importation, and/or distribution of food. However, the consequences of food insecurity in such countries as well as in food-rich countries is experienced primarily at the household and individual levels. At the household level, these consequences usually result from a managed process in which inadequate means to obtain food, either because it is not available or because resources are limited, leads to anxiety about the supply of food and this anxiety, in turn, results in a variety of coping tactics (e.g., stretching food money). If these coping tactics are not successful, intake eventually is restricted, resulting not only in nutritional consequences but also emotional consequences for the household as well as individual members of the household. The anxiety over the availability of food usually leads, first, to lower intakes of food or intake of less nutritionally adequate food by women, then a lower quantity and/or quality of the overall household food supply, and, eventually, to a lower quantity and/or quality of children's intakes.

Food insecurity in both developing and developed countries is a form of deprivation, either deprivation per se or the feeling of deprivation. The subjective experience of food insecurity at the individual level is central. Thus, the relevant assessment of food security is that perceived by the household or individual rather than what is decided by researchers or policymakers; if individuals do not believe that food is secure, food insecurity is a problem. Moreover, this problem is a multilevel and multidimensional one, with implications for how food security is assessed and for efforts to improve food security.

Measurement. Estimates of global and national levels of food insecurity are made by estimating the number of people whose intake does not provide enough energy to meet basic energy requirements. This is often equated to the number of undernourished individuals. However, this definition reflects only national food availability, not an individual's ability to access food. Thus, while the number of undernourished individuals is a direct measure of food security at the global or national level, it does not reflect access to and utilization of food by individuals. Hence, it is not a measure of food security at the household or individual level.

How to measure household and individual food security is not clear. Certainly, food insecurity affects intake and, ultimately, nutritional status. Furthermore, measuring intakes of individuals either directly or indirectly by the number of undernourished individuals assesses some aspects of food security (e.g., energy adequacy). However, it does not assess the cognitive and affective components of the uncertainty of food security, nor does it assess the unacceptability and unsustainability of food insecurity. For example, food insecurity exists if there is anxiety that food, although sufficient at the present time, may soon become inadequate. Not only does growth status, per se, not assess many components of food security, it is also an indirect outcome that depends on health and care as well as intake. Thus, in assessing food insecurity, it is important to measure not only the availability and access to food but also the experience of food insecurity, (i.e., how individuals feel about the security of their food supply).

A variety of questionnaires have been used to assess food insecurity in developed countries. These include questions concerning availability of food, concern about availability of food, and whether lack of availability was associated with hunger. These have reliability coefficients ranging from about 0.75 for all households to about 0.8 for households with children. The scores, as expected, are related to income, indicating that food insecurity is more prevalent among families with incomes close to the poverty level. Scores on these questionnaires defining food insecurity also are in agreement with data concerning weekly food expenditures.

Prevalence. Food insecurity is much more prevalent in developing countries than in developed countries. Current estimates of the prevalence of food insecurity in developing countries, based on estimates of undernutrition, indicate that about 18% of all individuals in developing countries are undernourished. Estimates of prevalence vary throughout the world, ranging from about 33% of all individuals in most parts of Africa and about 17% of those in Asia and the Pacific to much lower percentages in most other parts of the world. Because these estimates are based on the number of undernourished individuals, they obviously include only those individuals whose intakes are sufficiently low to result in undernutrition. Hence, the prevalence of food insecurity, as broadly defined, is likely to be considerably greater. On the other hand, these estimates equate food insecurity with undernutrition that results from some combination of inadequate nutrient intake and inadequate care.

Based on questionnaires assessing food security, about 10% of all households in the United States were food insecure in 1999. The prevalence of food insecurity without hunger was 7% of all households, and the prevalence with hunger was 3% of all households. This prevalence equates to 31 million persons in food insecure households. The prevalence of food insecurity is higher in central city and rural areas than in suburban areas. It also is much higher among black and Hispanic households as well as households headed by single women. Estimates of the prevalence of food insecurity without hunger in these households range from 20–30%.

A typical food-insecure household in the United States is not necessarily one in which there is no working member. Rather, at least one member of the household is likely to be employed, albeit in jobs that pay barely enough to enable the family to "get by." In such households, food becomes expendable when the available resources are needed to meet expenses such as rent and/or utilities, transportation in order to continue employment, medical care, and/or other basic needs.

Consequences. Biologic consequences of food insecurity are secondary to inadequate intake. However, the social and behavioral consequences can be secondary to the aspects of food insecurity experienced at the household or individual level as well as the biologic consequences. For example, food insecurity among women of sufficient severity to result in nutrient insufficiency and, hence, undernutrition leads to a higher prevalence of low birthweight infants and may affect breast milk production adversely. These effects, in turn, result in impaired cognitive and neurologic development of the offspring, lower educational achievement, and, hence, a lower likelihood of finding productive work in adulthood. The more severely affected individuals may also have a poor capacity to work, further decreasing their ability to be food secure. This vicious cycle may continue from one generation to the other and perpetuate both the biologic consequences of food insecurity and consequences secondary to the behavioral responses to food insecurity.

Even food insecurity that does not result in overt undernutrition may be associated with a low intake of foods such as fresh fruits and vegetables and, hence, a low intake of several essential nutrients (e.g., vitamins A, E, C, and B_6 as well as magnesium, potassium, and/or fiber [see Table 44–1]). Some studies suggest that women from food-insecure households are more likely to have higher body mass indices and to be obese than women from food-secure households. However, this is not a linear relationship; neither the incidence of obesity nor the body mass indices of women from households with more severe problems (i.e., childhood hunger) differ from those of women from food-secure households.

Clinical Manifestations and Treatment. Unless food insecurity is of sufficient severity to result in food insufficiency and undernutrition, it is not associated with obvious signs and/or symptoms. Thus, it is not likely to be recognized by physicians and other health care workers. Furthermore, even if food insecurity is suspected, a physician can do little except offer understanding and support. Nonetheless, considering the apparent prevalence of food insecurity among poor families, physicians caring for these families are likely to encounter children from food-insecure households. If food insecurity is suspected, further inquiries should be made, both to confirm that the family is food insecure and to assess the severity of the insecurity. These assessments should include information about the child's diet.

A food frequency interview, which provides such information as the number of servings per week of each major food group (see Fig. 41–1), is a reasonable place to start. Should this suggest an imbalanced diet (e.g., low intake of any of the food groups), the next step is to have the mother complete a 3–5 day food diary. If obtained and analyzed appropriately, this can provide quantitative information about dietary intake, including estimates of the intake of specific nutrients. This can be done by the physician, a nutritionist, or a dietitian.

If an intake of any nutrient is less than the Dietary Reference Intake, appropriate dietary advice should be given and/or appropriate supplements prescribed. Many food insecure children are likely to benefit from a multivitamin supplement, but fewer are likely to require macronutrient supplements. If no specific deficiencies are identified, the family may benefit from nutritional counseling, including not only the desired number of servings from each food group but also the most economical source of these foods. The physician should also ensure that the family is aware of the federal, state, and/or local resources available for assistance.

HUNGER

Hunger is the uneasy sensation that results from lack of food. It is a potential, although not inevitable, consequence of food insecurity. However, the concept of hunger differs among individuals, even individuals with similar dietary intakes. Thus, it is even more difficult to define and assess than is food insecurity.

A questionnaire developed by the Community Childhood Hunger Identification Project reliably categorize families as "hungry," "at risk for hunger," or "not hungry" on the basis of answers to eight standarized questions about child and family experiences of food insecurity or insufficiency attributable to constrained resources. Using this measure of food insufficiency as the principal indicator of hunger, this project estimates that 8% of poor children younger than age 12 yr in the United States experience hunger from time to time and that an additional 21% are "at risk for hunger." However, hunger is even more prevalent in children from families with the lowest incomes. Among these families, as many as 21% of children may be hungry and an additional 50% may be "at risk for hunger." This suggests that almost three fourths of the poorest children in the United States may experience food insecurity or insufficiency. It also suggests that hunger is an issue for many of these children and is a serious problem for some. On the other hand, all of these children obviously do not experience food insecurity of sufficient severity to result in undernutrition.

Psychosocial problems, like food insecurity and hunger, also are common among children from low-income families. Estimates of the prevalence of such problems in these children range from 10–30%; estimates of the prevalence of such problems among children from more advantaged families are considerably lower. There also is a relationship between the prevalence of psychosocial problems among low-income families and hunger. In one study, 29% of "hungry" children, 15% of "at risk for hunger" children, and 14% of "not hungry" children were receiving special education services. In the same study, 21% of "hungry" children, 12% of children "at risk for hunger," but only 5% of "not hungry" children had a history of mental health counseling. "Hungry" children also were more likely to have a history of academic failure as well as to demonstrate higher levels of anxious, irritable, aggressive, and oppositional behaviors than their low income, but "not hungry," peers. These findings are similar to the behavioral findings of more severe, chronic undernutrition in developing countries.

The above conclusions are based on correlations that do not necessarily prove a cause-and-effect relationship. Although it is possible that hunger causes the types of behavior problems documented, it also is possible that hunger is a correlate of still another variable rather than the direct cause of the problems. For example, parents who are emotionally drained by chronic illness or the constant struggle to make ends meet are less likely to be able to cope with planning for nutritious and economic food purchases. In other words, hunger may be more prevalent in such families but the other problems of the families may play an equal or a larger role in determining the children's functioning.

Clinical Manifestations and Treatment. The nature of hunger makes it difficult to recognize. Moreover, because the perception of hunger varies considerably both among individuals, even individuals ingesting the same diet, and within the same individual from day to day, asking the child if he or she is ever hungry or questioning the parent may not be helpful.

If hunger is suspected, use of the parental questionnaire developed by the Community Childhood Hunger Identification Project or a similar questionnaire may be useful. Children identified by this instrument as "hungry" or "at risk for hunger" should be evaluated for the possibility of nutrient deficiencies. If present, these should be treated with either supplements or dietary advice. Their parents should be referred to the appropriate agency for assistance.

In some cases, a change in meal patterns without an increase in overall intake may be useful. For example, if entire meals are missed to stretch the available food money, it might help to decrease the quantity of other meals to provide an appropriate number of meals per day.

UNDERNUTRITION

For decades, investigators have searched unsuccessfully for a single cause or a specific set of causes of undernutrition and the appropriate intervention strategies to correct that cause or set of causes. For example, attention has shifted from inadequate protein to inadequate energy to inadequate micronutrients with accompanying shifts of focus concerning appropriate intervention strategies. Problems and causes of undernutrition that are being debated currently include growth faltering, low birthweight, maternal undernutrition, deficiencies of specific nutrients (e.g., iodine, vitamin A, iron, and zinc), diarrhea, HIV infection and other infectious diseases, inadequate infant and child feeding practices, female time constraints, limited household income, limited agricultural production, food insecurity, environmental degradation, and urbanization. A wide array of solutions to these problems also are debated. These include growth monitoring, promotion of more optimal breast-feeding and complementary feeding practices, nutrition education, oral rehydration programs, child spacing, food fortification, supplementation of specific or multiple nutrients (e.g., vitamin A, iron, and/or zinc), income generation, food aid, home gardening, and agricultural intensification. To a great extent, this shifting illustrates the poor understanding of many aspects of the major worldwide problem of undernutrition.

The problem of undernutrition is multifaceted, and solving it at a national level requires understanding, trust, and cooperation among diverse governmental agencies accustomed to dealing solely with health, agriculture, education, or finance issues. The frequent shifting of focus has not generated a coherent and understandable approach to the problem but, rather, has helped create the perception among many national policy makers and planners that the nutrition problem is "too complicated." This, in turn, has delayed coordination of efforts across international and governmental agencies and, equally important, has not generated a consensus within the nutrition community about priority problems and the actions and strategies needed to solve them.

In response to this situation, the United Nations Children Fund (UNICEF) has developed and is promoting an inclusive conceptual framework for organizing scientific knowledge and experience concerning undernutrition (or malnutrition), fostering a common understanding and developing coherent strategies for addressing the problem. A key feature of this framework is the recognition that undernutrition, or malnutrition, is a biologic manifestation of the combined effects of inadequate dietary intake and disease, both of which are closely related to social and economic development. Thus, malnutrition cannot be viewed as distinct from other development problems but, rather, as a reflection of these other problems.

Another feature of this framework is that the assumptions underlying various approaches to malnutrition are stated explicitly so that they can be questioned and debated. This is in contrast to the usual tendency to assume implicitly that malnutrition is due solely to a specific cause (e.g., lack of food, inadequate health care, limited education, poor breast-feeding practices, inadequate agricultural production). Another key feature of the UNICEF framework is that the relative importance of the underlying causes of malnutrition (food, health care) must be recognized widely across households, communities, and countries. This implies that universal causes and solutions do not exist and that constraints in providing adequate food and health care must be assessed and acted on in each setting. A highly decentralized approach to assessment, analysis, and action is required rather than imposed national or global solutions.

Measurement. The traditional approach to nutritional assessment measures only the physical manifestations of the problem (i.e., clinical, anthropometric, and biochemical indicators) and, perhaps, some of the immediate causes related to dietary intake. These indicators may be adequate for estimating the magnitude of the problem, but additional methods and approaches are needed to assess the broader nutrition situation. These approaches include consideration not only of dietary intake but also of health care and control of resources at household, community, and national levels.

Despite the need for additional methods and approaches, a number of anthropometric indices have been used successfully for many years to estimate the prevalence of undernutrition among preschool-aged children. These include height for age, weight for age, and weight for height. The first is an index of the cumulative effects of undernutrition during the life of the child, the second reflects the combined effects of both recent and longer-term levels of nutrition, and the last reflects recent nutritional experiences. Values below 80–90% of expected are considered abnormally low.

These indices are reasonably sensitive indicators of the immediate and underlying general causes of undernutrition, but they are not specific for any particular cause. They do not reveal the relative importance of dietary intake, infectious diseases, food insecurity, inadequate health/environmental services, low birthweight, suboptimal childcare practices, income constraints, or disparities in control of resources. These factors are part of the assessment of the overall nutrition situation and are distinct from the biochemical and/or anthropometric indicators that merely reflect the severity and extent of the problem, its distribution across geographic and social groups, and trends over time.

Prevalence. In 2000, 26.7% of preschoolers in the developing world were estimated to be underweight, as reflected by a low weight for age, and 32.5% were estimated to be stunted based on a low height for age. These estimates are about 11% and about 15% lower, respectively, than estimates in 1980, suggesting considerable improvement, at least in some regions, over these 2 decades. However, the population of the developing world increased during this time; thus, the total number of underweight and stunted children has not changed dramatically since 1980.

Data from the United States and other developed countries indicate that the prevalence of undernutrition as manifested by a low weight for age or height for age is very low. Data from the National Health and Nutrition Examination Survey (NHANES) III (1988–1991) indicate that the prevalence of low height for age (below the 5th percentile) was 4–5% among children from 2 mo to 11 yr of age, about the same prevalence noted by NHANES I (1971–1974) 2 decades earlier. The NHANES III data also show that populations with a high prevalence of poverty do not have a higher prevalence of undernutrition than the general population, emphasizing the importance not only of adequate intake but also of adequate care as defined in the United Nations International Child's Emergency Fund (UNICEF) framework.

In contrast to the low prevalence of undernutrition among the general population of children in the United States and other developed countries, the prevalence among hospitalized children is often as high as in developing countries.

Consequences. The cumulative evidence suggests that undernutrition has pervasive effects on immediate health and survival as well as on subsequent performance. These include not only acute effects on morbidity and mortality but also longer-term effects on cognitive and social development, physical work capacity, productivity, and economic growth. The magnitude of both the acute and longer-term effects are considerable. Prospective studies suggest that severely underweight children (<60% of reference weight for age) have more than an eight-fold greater risk for mortality than normally nourished children, that moderately underweight children (60–69% of reference weight for age) have a four- to five-fold greater risk, and that even mildly underweight children (70–79% of reference weight for age) have a two- to three-fold greater risk. The high prevalence of mortality in those with mild and moderate undernutrition suggests that more than half of child deaths may be caused directly or indirectly by undernutrition. Moreover, 83% of these deaths result from mild to moderate forms of undernutrition. A major factor is the potentiation of infectious diseases by undernutrition.

Survivors of childhood undernutrition frequently have deficits in height and weight that persist beyond adolescence into adulthood. These deficits are often accompanied by deficits in frame size as well as muscle circumference and strength. The implications of these deficits with respect to the work capacity of both men and women and to women's reproductive performance are obvious. Survivors of childhood malnutrition also have deficits in cognitive function and school performance relative to normally nourished children from the same environment. Mean deficits in scores on standard tests of cognition range from 5–15 points. The fact that severely undernourished children, as assessed by low length-for-age, have greater deficits in cognitive performance than children with mild or moderate undernutrition strongly suggests that the intellectual deficits are related to the severity of undernutrition.

The extent to which intellectual deficits can be decreased by dietary intervention alone is not clear. However, these deficits can be decreased by a combination of dietary and behavioral interventions coupled with improvements in the overall quality of the home and/or school environment. Such interventions appear to be much more effective if instituted in early life.

Prevention. Food insecurity and undernutrition are the behavioral or biologic manifestations of problems that are rooted in the social world from the level of individuals and households to the community, national, and international levels. Thus, a wide range of scientific disciplines must be drawn on to maximize the possibility of effective and sustainable solutions. For example, an intervention as simple as supplementing the population with vitamin A requires an understanding of the behavior of households, communities, clinical workers, program managers, and policymakers. Scientific approaches for addressing such problems must include, but go well beyond, the biologic sciences that have formed the core of the discipline of nutrition.

The evolution of thought concerning food security and undernutrition in developed and developing countries has some commonalities with significant policy implications. The major commonality is the recognition that the causes of these problems, while strongly related globally to poverty, are highly contextual and, hence, easily misunderstood. In most developed countries, for example, not all food-insecure individuals live in poverty and all those living in poverty are not food insecure. Similarly, in developing countries, child malnutrition secondary to suboptimal health conditions or caring practices is common even among households with ample food resources. Thus, food insecurity and undernutrition arise from a variety of social, economic, and eco-

logic situations that vary from time to time and from place to place. Therefore, the coping strategies and behaviors of individuals and households as well as communities and nations are highly responsive to a variety of microcontextual factors. Moreover, these coping strategies and behaviors are strongly influenced by the ways in which the food insecure and undernourished experience reality. For example, the risk avoidance and risk management strategies of poor households often discourage their adopting new crop varieties or making other changes in their livelihood strategy despite the fact that such changes appear desirable and rational to outsiders.

Many policies and programs have been ineffective because they do not adequately assess, anticipate, and embrace the coping strategies and likely responses of the population. Some programs that do so have been initiated in communities throughout the developing world and are currently being evaluated. It is hoped that the results of these efforts will suggest strategies to improve the total nutrition situation and reduce high prevalence of childhood undernutrition.

Clinical Manifestations and Treatment. Undernutrition ranges from a lower than desired intake of one or more nutrients with either no symptoms or only vague symptoms to severe malnutrition. The approach to treating mild undernutrition is the same as that suggested for food insecurity of sufficient severity to result in low intake of specific nutrients. Treatment of vitamin deficiencies is discussed in Chapter 44, and treatment of the most severe form of undernutrition is discussed in the following section of this chapter.

PROTEIN/ENERGY MALNUTRITION

Deficiency of a single nutrient is an example of undernutrition or malnutrition. Usually, however, there is deficiency of several nutrients. Protein/energy malnutrition (PEM), for example, is manifested primarily by inadequate dietary intakes of protein and energy, either because the dietary intakes of these two nutrients are less than required for normal growth or because the needs for growth are greater than can be supplied by what, otherwise, would be adequate intakes for growth. However, PEM is almost always accompanied by deficiencies of other nutrients.

The terms *primary* and *secondary* malnutrition refer, respectively, to malnutrition resulting from inadequate food intake and malnutrition resulting from increased nutrient needs, decreased nutrient absorption, and/or increased nutrient losses. Although both primary and secondary malnutrition occur in developing as well as developed countries, primary malnutrition accounts for the major percentage of malnourished children in developing countries, whereas secondary malnutrition accounts for a higher percentage in developed countries.

PEM, whether primary or secondary, is a spectrum ranging from mild undernutrition resulting in some decrease in length and/or weight for age through severe forms of undernutrition resulting in more marked deficits in weight and length for age as well as wasting (i.e., a low weight for length). Historically, the most severe forms of PEM, marasmus, and kwashiorkor, were considered distinct disorders. Marasmus was thought to result primarily from inadequate energy intake, whereas kwashiorkor was thought to result primarily from inadequate protein intake. Currently, a third disorder, marasmic kwashiorkor, which has features of both disorders, also is recognized. The three conditions have distinct clinical and metabolic features, but they also have a number of overlapping features. For example, a low plasma albumin concentration, often thought to be a manifestation of kwashiorkor, is common in children with both clinical marasmus and clinical kwashiorkor. In recognition of the overlapping features of these two clinically distinct conditions, the terms currently preferred are *edematous* (kwashiorkor) and *nonedematous* (marasmus) PEM. The underlying causes of this spectrum of conditions are quite similar. Among these are social and economic factors such as poverty and ignorance, social factors such as food taboos, biologic factors such as maternal malnutrition and inadequate intakes of breast milk and other foods, as well as environmental factors such as overcrowded and unsanitary living conditions.

Clinical Manifestations. In *nonedematous PEM* (marasmus) initially there is failure to gain weight and irritability, followed by weight loss and listlessness until emaciation results. The skin loses turgor and becomes wrinkled and loose as subcutaneous fat disappears. Loss of fat from the sucking pads of the cheeks may occur late, and the infant's face may retain a relatively normal appearance, compared with the rest of the body, eventually becoming shrunken and wizened. The abdomen may be distended or flat with the intestinal pattern readily visible. There is muscle atrophy and resultant hypotonia. The temperature is usually subnormal and the pulse slow. Infants are usually constipated but may develop a starvation diarrhea with frequent small stools containing mucus.

Edematous PEM (kwashiorkor) may initially present as vague manifestations that include lethargy, apathy, or irritability. When well advanced, there is inadequate growth, lack of stamina, loss of muscle tissue, increased susceptibility to infections, vomiting, diarrhea, anorexia, flabby subcutaneous tissues, and edema (Fig. 42–1). The edema usually develops early and may mask the failure to gain weight, but the liver may enlarge early or late. The edema is often present in internal organs before it is recognized in the face and limbs. Dermatitis is common, with darkening of the skin in irritated areas but not in areas exposed to sunlight, in contrast to pellagra (see Chapter 44). Depigmentation may occur after desquamation in these areas, or it may be generalized. The

hair is sparse and thin and, in dark-haired children, may become streaky red or gray. The texture is coarse in chronic disease. Eventually, there is stupor, coma, and death.

Pathophysiology. Many of the manifestations of PEM represent adaptive responses to inadequate energy and/or protein intakes. In the face of inadequate intakes, activity and energy expenditure decrease. However, despite this adaptive response, fat stores are mobilized to meet the ongoing, albeit lower, energy requirement. Once these stores are depleted, protein catabolism must provide the ongoing substrates for maintaining basal metabolism.

Why some children develop edematous PEM and others develop nonedematous PEM is unknown. Although no specific factor has been identified, a number have been suggested. One concerns the variability among infants in nutrient requirements and in body composition at the time the dietary deficit is incurred. In addition, it has been proposed that giving excess carbohydrate to a child with clinical marasmus reverses the adaptive responses to low protein intake, resulting in mobilization of body protein stores. Eventually, albumin synthesis decreases, resulting in hypoalbuminemia with edema. Fatty liver also develops secondary, perhaps, to lipogenesis from the excess carbohydrate. Aflatoxin poisoning as a cause of edematous PEM also has been proposed. Finally, free radical damage has been proposed as an important factor in development of clinical kwashiorkor or edematous PEM. This concept is supported by low plasma concentrations of methionine, a dietary precursor of cysteine, one of the amino acids needed for synthesis of the major antioxidant factor, glutathione. This possibility also is supported by lower rates of glutathione synthesis in children with edematous vs. nonedematous PEM.

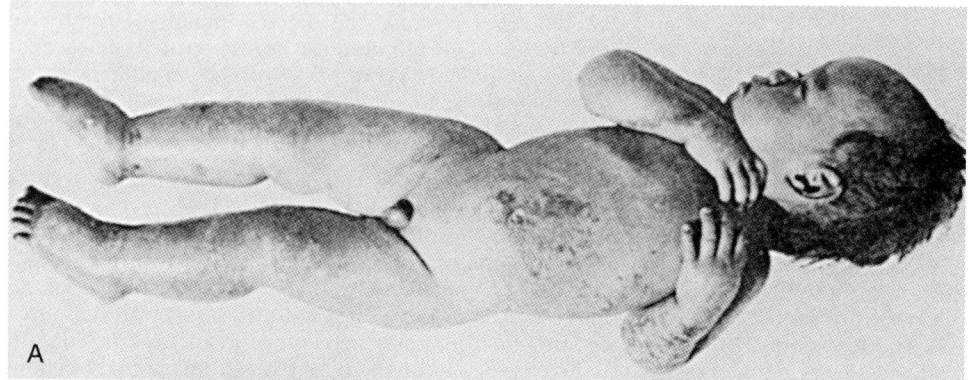

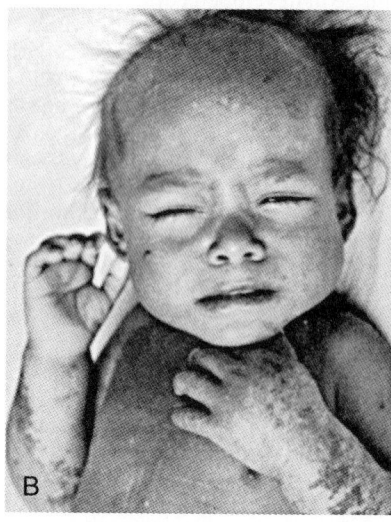

FIGURE 42–1. *A,* Kwashiorkor in a 2 yr old boy. Note the generalized edema, the typical skin lesions, and the state of prostration. *B,* Close-up of the same child showing the hair changes and psychic alterations (apathy and misery); the edema of the face and the skin lesions can be seen more clearly. (Photographs made available by the Institute of Nutrition of Central America and Panama, Guatemala, courtesy of Moises Behar, MD.)

Treatment. The usual approach to treatment of PEM includes three phases. The first relatively brief phase (24–48 hr) is a stabilization phase. During this phase, dehydration, if present, is corrected and antibiotic therapy is initiated to control infection. Because of the difficulty of estimating hydration, oral rehydration therapy is preferred. If intravenous therapy is necessary, estimates of dehydration should be reconsidered frequently, particularly during the first 24 hr of therapy.

The second phase includes continued antibiotic therapy with appropriate changes if the initial combination was not effective and introduction of a diet providing maintenance requirements of energy and protein (~75 cal/kg and ~1 g/kg/24 hr of protein) along with adequate electrolytes, trace minerals, and vitamins. This phase usually lasts for an additional week to 10 days. If the infant is unable to take the feedings from a cup or bottle, administration of feedings by nasogastric tube rather than by the parenteral route is preferred.

By the end of the second phase, any edema that was present has usually been mobilized, infections are under control, the child is becoming more interested in his or her surroundings, and his or her appetite is returning. The child is then ready for the final phase of treatment, which consists primarily of feeding. He or she should be switched gradually to a recovery diet providing up to 150 kcal/kg/24 hr and 4 g/kg/24 hr of protein. After adjustment to this diet, the child can be fed ad libitum. Once ad libitum feedings are allowed, intakes of both energy and protein can be substantial.

In developing countries, this phase is often carried out at home. However, continued hospitalization is much more effective. This allows further focus on maternal education, which is crucial for continued effective treatment as well as prevention of additional episodes.

Iron therapy usually is not started until this final phase of treatment so as to prevent binding of iron to already limited stores of transferrin, which, in turn, may interfere with the protein's host defense mechanisms. There also is concern that free iron during the early phase of treatment may exacerbate oxidant damage, precipitating clinical kwashiorkor or marasmic kwashiorkor in a child with clinical marasmus.

Ashworth A: Treatment of severe malnutrition. *J Pediatr Gastroenterol Nutr* 2001;32:519–20.

Cooper A, Heird WC: Nutritional assessment of the pediatric patient including the low birth weight infant. *Am J Clin Nutr* 1982;35:1132–41.

Karp R: Malnutrition among children in the United States: The impact of poverty. In Shils ME, Olson JA, Shike M, et al (editors): *Modern Nutrition in Health and Disease*, 9th ed. Baltimore, Williams & Wilkins, 1999, pp 989–1001.

Kleinman RE, Murphy M, Little M, et al: Hunger in children in the United States: Potential behavioral and emotional correlates. *Pediatrics* 1998;101(1). www.pediatrics.org/cgi/content/full/101/1/e3; hunger, children, mental health, poverty.

Pelletier DL, Olson CM, Frongillo EA Jr: Food insecurity, hunger, and undernutrition. In Bowman BA, Russell RM (editors): *Present Knowledge in Nutrition*, 8th ed. Washington, DC, ILSI Press, 2001, pp 701–713.

World Health Organization: *Management of Severe Malnutrition: A Manual for Physicians and Other Senior Health Workers*. Geneva, WHO, 1999.

Chapter 43
Obesity *Patricia A. Donohoue*

There has been a significant increase in the prevalence of overweight and obesity in the United States, despite nationwide efforts at reducing fat intake to prevent cardiovascular disease. In pediatrics, the consequences of this epidemic are the occurrence of "adult" diseases in youth, such as type 2 diabetes mellitus, hypertension, and hyperlipidemia.

The definition of obesity may vary depending on the source of the information, but most health care providers agree that individuals whose body mass index (BMI) (weight in kilograms divided by the square of the height in meters; kg/m^2) exceeds the age-gender-specific 95th percentile are obese (see Fig. 15–2A and B). Those whose BMI is between the 85th and 95th percentiles are overweight and are at increased risk for obesity-related co-morbidities (see also Chapter 41). In adults, it is generally considered that an individual whose BMI is more than 30 kg/m^2 is obese. High BMI correlates with excess body fat in all age groups and in both genders, with the exception of persons with very high muscle mass (e.g., "body builders"). Data for age and gender BMI percentiles are derived from the National Health and Nutrition Examination Survey III (NHANES III) and are available from the Centers for Disease Control and Prevention (www.cdc.gov/nchs/about/major/nhanes).

Etiology. The regulation of body fat stores and the etiology of human obesity are multifactorial, reflecting complex interactions between genetic background, environmental stimuli, and developmental processes. During the stage of human evolution when food was obtained through strenuous physical activity (e.g., hunting, digging) and periods of prolonged fasting and famine were constant threats, genotypes developed to favor energy storage. In the environment of plentiful and easily accessible high-calorie food, these so-called thrifty genotypes are highly prevalent and, unfortunately, are now detrimental. This gene-environment interaction must be considered in the prevention and treatment of obesity.

An important factor in maintenance of body weight is the relationship between body weight and total energy expenditure. The trend toward returning to a specific set point for body weight is powerful and results not only from a reduction in total energy expenditure in response to weight loss but also from an increase in energy expenditure with weight gain. There are multiple genetic factors controlling this set point. There is ethnic variability in resting energy expenditure; it is higher in white than in black prepubertal girls and higher in white than in black prepubertal children, independent of percent body fat and sex. Genetic factors may also influence the lower physical activity and resting energy expenditure observed in infants who later become obese children. The genetic control of energy expenditure and heat production may be involved in the etiology of obesity. Energy expenditure and heat production are controlled by interactions with sympathetic neurons and mitochondrial uncoupling proteins, among other systems.

The importance of environmental factors on body size is underscored by the marked increase in obesity over the past 20 yr, a time period whose brevity precludes a significant change in the gene pool. The prevalence of obesity is increasing dramatically not only in adults but also in youth, as demonstrated in the Muscatine Study (Table 43–1). The prevalence is significantly higher, and the trend is even more pronounced in minority groups in the United States, particularly in adult females (Table 43–2). The same minority female preponderance occurs in

TABLE 43–1. Prevalence of Overweight in Muscatine, IA, Schoolchildren*

Year (n)	12–14 yr	15–17 yr	18 yr	Total Percent
Females				
1971 (1,072)	17.5	16.3	25.0	17.4
1981 (906)	18.7	17.9	20.0	18.4
1992 (1,139)	31.4	30.0	22.7	30.5
Males				
1971 (978)	16.8	11.9	26.9	15.4
1981 (921)	19.6	16.5	10.8	17.9
1992 (1,191)	28.5	21.8	33.9	25.9

Age-gender adjusted BMI > 85th percentile.

TABLE 43–2. Prevalence of Obesity (BMI > 30.0 kg/m²) by Race-Ethnic Group: United States, 1988–1994

	Age Group (yr)							Total Age-Adjusted
	20–29	30–39	40–49	50–59	60–69	70–79	80+	20–74 yr
Men								
Non-Hispanic white	12.0	17.1	22.7	30.6	25.3	20.4	7.7	20.0
Non-Hispanic black	19.1	20.3	22.3	21.5	25.6	19.5	11.1	21.3
Mexican-American	13.3	17.9	32.9	37.1	26.6	18.5	4.4	23.1
Women								
Non-Hispanic white	13.1	22.4	22.6	33.5	28.3	23.7	14.3	22.4
Non-Hispanic black	23.4	35.5	44.6	50.1	45.4	38.3	20.5	37.4
Mexican-American	22.4	34.7	44.7	43.0	39.1	24.3	19.1	34.2

youth and is particularly apparent at the onset of puberty and at the time of menarche. The pattern of increasing obesity prevalence has been observed throughout the United States and has accelerated over the past 10 yr. The impact of environment on the epidemic of obesity includes unfavorable trends in food intake and physical activity, as well as barriers to reversing these trends. Other examples of the impact of environment on body size are the development of obesity in patients who have survived leukemia or who have suffered hypothalamic damage, especially patients treated for craniopharyngioma.

The importance of heredity on body size has been demonstrated in multiple studies of dizygotic and monozygotic twins and of adopted individuals and their biologic siblings. Studies of twin pairs have consistently demonstrated higher concordance for body size among monozygotic than dizygotic twins. In adult adoptees and their biologic siblings, both full and half siblings, there is a significant correlation of BMI in biologic siblings across the entire distribution of body sizes.

In large unrelated populations from several ethnic groups, there is statistical evidence for recessive gene effects on body size variables, including BMI, abdominal visceral fat, relative fat pattern, and obesity. Longitudinal studies have demonstrated familial aggregation of obesity and cardiovascular risk. Examples of these include the Muscatine Study, the Bogalusa Heart Study, the San Antonio Family Heart Study, the HERITAGE Study, the Québec Family Study, and studies of American Pima Indians.

Epidemiology. The prediction of risk of adult obesity during childhood is based on several factors. Blood pressure, blood lipid levels, and obesity in childhood track into adulthood. Thus, childhood obesity itself is a predictor of adult obesity and of higher than expected adult morbidity and mortality regardless of the presence of overweight in adulthood. The prevalence of clinically significant obesity-related morbidities in youth is rising and predicts earlier onset of more severe problems in young adults. The increase in type 2 diabetes among children and adolescents is directly related to the obesity epidemic.

Parental obesity, particularly maternal, is predictive of childhood obesity. High birthweight is also a predictor of later obesity, and the most important factor contributing to high birthweight is maternal diabetes and, to a lesser degree, maternal obesity. The relative risk of developing obesity in young adulthood is higher for young children if they have obese parents and higher for older children if they themselves are obese (Table 43–3).

The influence of deficient physical activity on the development of obesity is reflected in the NHANES III data. Lack of physical activity is directly related to television viewing, and hours of television are significantly correlated to weight gain during the growing years. In a study of schoolchildren in California, reduction in television viewing significantly reduced the rate of weight gain in a study of third graders, when compared with third graders with no intervention. Among children

8–16 yr of age, the prevalence of obesity was positively associated with hours of television viewing, even when controlling for age, race, income, caloric intake, and physical activity.

Pathogenesis

ANIMAL MODELS OF SINGLE GENE DEFECTS. In rodents, multiple examples of naturally occurring single gene mutations producing obesity are known and form the basis for a candidate gene approach to identify the genes responsible for human obesity (Table 43–4). Several human counterparts of these rodent obesity syndromes have been identified. The prototypic obese mice with single gene defects are the obese (ob/ob, Lep^ob) and diabetes (db/db, Lepr^db) autosomal recessive mutations. If present on the same genetic background strain, they cause identical phenotypes of severe hyperphagia, obesity, type 2 diabetes, defective thermogenesis, and infertility due to hypogonadotropic hypogonadism. The mutant gene responsible for the phenotype in Lep^ob mice encodes a protein termed *leptin*, which is deficient in these animals. The gene encoding human leptin has been studied extensively, but with the exception of leptin deficiency caused by rare *LEP* gene mutations its importance in altered human satiety and abnormal body size determination has not been clearly demonstrated. Studies of this genetic locus in populations, and in large panels of obese and/or diabetic individuals, have failed to demonstrate linkage or mutations. The cloning of the leptin receptor gene *Lepr* led to characterization of the mutations causing the mouse *db/db* phenotype and its rat homologues, the Zucker fatty (*fa/fa*) and obese Koletsky phenotypes. Thus, mutation of the same gene, *Lepr*, occurred spontaneously in three different strains and produced the same phenotype. Mice that are heterozygous for either the *ob* or the *db* mutation have body composition and leptin homeostasis phenotypes that are intermediate between homozygous wild type and mutant animals. Severe early-onset human obesity caused by a mutant leptin receptor has been identified in three female siblings. These homozygotes had failure of pubertal development and reduced growth hormone and thyroid-stimulating hormone secretion. In

TABLE 43–3. Odds Ratios for Obesity in Young Adulthood According to Obesity Status in Childhood and Parents' Obesity Status

	Obese as Child	Number of Obese Parents	
Age (yr)	Yes vs No	1 vs 0	2 vs 0
1–2	1.3	3.2	13.6
3–5	4.7	3.0	15.3
6–9	8.8	2.6	5.0
10–14	22.3	2.2	2.0
15–17	17.5	2.2	5.6

Data from Whitaker RC, Wright JA, Pepe MS, et al: Predicting obesity in young adulthood from childhood and parental obesity. N Engl J Med 1997; 337:869–73.

TABLE 43–4. Rodent Obesity Mutations, Human Regions of Synteny, and Human Homologues

	Mutation	Gene	Mode of Inheritance (Autosomal)	Rodent Chromosome	Human Syntenic Region	Human Mutation Described	Mutant Protein
Mouse	Agouti	A^y	Dominant	2	20q11	No*	ASP
	Diabetes	db	Recessive	4	1p31	Yes	Lepr
	Fat	fat	Recessive	8	4q21	No†	Carboxypeptidase
	Obese	ob	Recessive	6	7q31	Yes	Leptin
	Tubby	tub	Recessive	7	11p15	No	Phosphodiesterase
Rat	Fatty	fa	Recessive	5	1p31	Yes	Lepr
	Corpulent	fa^K	Recessive	5	1p31	Yes	Lepr

* ASP prevents binding of αMSH to its receptor MC4R. Several MC4R mutations are associated with human obesity.
† CPE is required for normal prohormone processing by prohormone convertase 1 (PC1). PC1 mutations are associated with human obesity.
ASP = agouti signaling protein; Lepr = leptin receptor; CPE = carboxypeptidase E.

linkage studies of large populations, the leptin receptor locus seems more important than the leptin locus in its contribution to variability in body size.

The tubby *(tub)* mutation in mice is an autosomal recessive trait that is associated with less severe obesity and insulin resistance than *ob* or *db*, is not associated with significant hyperphagia, causes variable degrees of hyperlipidemia depending on background strain, and is more severe in males than females. The phenotype also includes retinal degeneration and sensorineural hearing loss similar to the human Usher, Alström, and Bardet-Biedl syndromes, but human *TUB* mutations have not yet been described.

In the fatty *(fat/fat)* mouse, the recessively inherited mutation causes hyperinsulinemia without hyperglycemia and postpubertal obesity that is less severe than that seen in *ob/ob* or *db/db* mice. The "hyperinsulinemia" is caused by hyperproinsulinemia. The molecular defect is in the gene encoding carboxypeptidase E (CPE), an endoprotease required for normal processing of prohormones to active hormones, including proinsulin to insulin and pro-opiomelanocortin (POMC) to adrenocorticotropic hormone (ACTH), melanocyte-stimulating hormone (MSH), β-endorphin, and β-lipoprotein. The role of CPE mutations in human obesity is unknown; however, a possible correlate has been described in which there are mutations of the prohormone convertase 1 (PC1) gene. These patients have obesity along with impaired processing of insulin, leading to diabetes, hyperproinsulinemia, and ACTH deficiency from impaired processing of POMC. Several individuals with mutations of the *POMC* gene have been identified, and they have severe early-onset obesity as well as ACTH deficiency. They also have red hair, whereas their family members do not.

The *yellow* mutation of agouti mice is a dominant trait that causes yellow coat color (rather than the wild-type hairs that are banded black and yellow), obesity, and diabetes. This was the first rodent obesity gene to be cloned, and subsequently dozens of agouti *yellow* alleles have been identified, which vary in their phenotypic expression. The molecular defect in the most dominant form *Ay* is a deletion in the 5′ regulatory region. This results in overproduction of agouti signaling protein (ASP) through ectopic expression of normal agouti mRNA in many tissues, rather than its normal site of expression, which is limited to the skin. ASP and another similar peptide, agouti-related peptide (AgRP), act as antagonists of native ligand binding to melanocortin receptors 1–4 (MC1R through MC4R), each of which is expressed differentially in specific tissues. Although ASP mutations have not yet been described in humans, several MC4R mutations are now known to be associated with obesity. Up to 10% of obese subjects (adults and youth) in Germany and France have MC4R mutations. The prevalence rate appears to be lower in the United States. The dominant nature of these mutations is most likely caused by haploinsufficiency and not a dominant negative effect.

CONTROL OF FEEDING. Energy intake and expenditure is under the control of complex interactions between peripheral signaling and effector systems and neuroendocrine systems. The hormone leptin is an important component of this complex system. Plasma levels of leptin correlate with fat mass and are higher in females than males. As has been demonstrated in animals, human leptin is made almost exclusively in adipose tissue and acts centrally in the hypothalamus by modifying two effector systems. Low plasma concentrations of leptin and insulin (e.g., during fasting and weight loss) increase food intake and decrease energy expenditure by stimulating neuropeptide Y (NPY) synthesis, and perhaps by inhibiting sympathetic activity and other catabolic pathways. High leptin and insulin concentrations (e.g., during feeding and weight gain) decrease food intake and increase energy expenditure through release of melanocortin and corticotropin-releasing hormone (CRH), among others. The list of neuropeptides that are known to alter energy balance is growing rapidly. Many of these are listed in Table 43–5. Among the more important peptides that stimulate feeding are orexins A and B, which are secreted by the hypothalamus, and ghrelin, which is secreted by the stomach.

THE HYPOTHALAMIC-PITUITARY-ADRENAL (HPA) AXIS. It has been demonstrated in multiple animal models that adrenalectomy obliterates or attenuates the obesity syndromes

TABLE 43–5. Central Nervous System Proteins (Neuropeptides) Involved in Energy Homeostasis

Neuropeptide	Regulation by Adiposity Signal (Leptin or Insulin)
Orexigenic (stimulates feeding)	
Neuropeptide Y*	Decreased
Agouti related peptide*	Decreased
Melanin-concentrating hormone	Decreased
Orexin A and B (hypocretin 1 and 2)	Decreased
Galanin	Unknown
Norepinephrine	Unknown
Gherlin	Unknown
Anorexigenic (inhibits feeding)	
α-Melanocyte–stimulating hormone*	Increased
Corticotropin-releasing hormone*	Increased
Thyrotropin-releasing hormone*	Increased
Cocaine- and amphetamine-regulated transcript*	Increased
Interleukin-1β*	Increased
Urocortin*	Unknown
Glucagon-like peptide 1	Unknown
Oxytocin	Unknown
Neurotensin	Unknown
Serotonin	Unknown

*Exerts effects on both energy intake and expenditure that result in a change in energy stores.
Majority of information obtained with permission from Schwartz MW, Woods SC, Porte D Jr, et al: Central nervous system control of food intake. Nature 2000;404:661–71.

expressed in genetically obese rats and mice, in diet-induced obesity, and in hypothalamic obesity. Treatment with only trace quantities of glucocorticoid causes rapid return of the obesity, indicating heightened sensitivity to the steroid. In humans and animals with hypercortisolemia, obesity is prominent. However, in adrenalectomized animals, the effects seen could result from a combination of glucocorticoid deficiency alone or in combination with the secondary elevation of hypothalamic CRH and pituitary ACTH production. In animal studies, CNS administration of CRH as well as a related hormone, urocortin, mimics the events seen in the "stress response," including anorexia. These data suggest that therapeutic manipulations of the HPA axis could alter the phenotype of certain genetically obese individuals.

POLYGENIC MODELS. The polygenic mouse models of obesity have allowed identification of multiple genetic loci within individual strains that modify obesity, plasma cholesterol levels, specific deposition of body fat depots, and propensity toward development of obesity on a high-fat diet. These polygenic models more closely resemble the human obesity phenotypes than single gene models; however, the single gene defects producing recessive traits, dominant traits, promoter alterations, and those subject to parental imprinting must also be considered candidates for genetic effects in human obesity.

GENE-TARGETING AND EFFECTS ON BODY FAT/FEEDING. Gene targeting of a variety of genes has been used to study obesity. These, along with other relevant animal models, are summarized in Table 43–6, and they demonstrate both monogenic and polygenic effects on body size variables.

Clinical Manifestations. Human obesity in rare instances may be associated with defects at a single genetic locus. These include Prader-Willi, Bardet-Biedl, and Alström syndromes, in which the causes of obesity are unknown. The presence of these syndromes can usually be detected by demonstration of the typical dysmorphic features on physical examination. Certain hormonal aberrations, such as hypothyroidism, Cushing syndrome, and generalized hypothalamic dysfunction, can result in excessive weight gain. However, these conditions are rarely identified among the typical patients who present for evaluation of obesity.

In children, obesity is most often associated with tall stature, slightly advanced bone age, and somewhat early puberty. In most patients with obesity, rapid growth in height precludes the diagnosis of hypothyroidism and hypercortisolism. By contrast, hypothyroidism and cortisol excess cause delayed skeletal development, short stature, and delayed puberty. Many obese youth also have **acanthosis nigricans,** a hypertrophic hyperpigmentation of the skin most commonly seen on the posterior neck and in skin creases. This condition is associated with insulin resistance and a higher risk of developing type 2 diabetes.

Laboratory Findings, Diagnosis, and Differential Diagnosis. Obesity can be diagnosed in most cases by simple inspection of the patient. If needed, BMI can be plotted on BMI growth curves (see Fig. 15–2) to identify those who are over the 95th percentile. Early identification of children at risk includes the demonstration of early adiposity rebound. Examination of BMI curves (see Fig. 15–2) shows that BMI reaches a nadir after infancy and then rebounds. If this rebound occurs early, especially if the BMI is already high for age, there is a significantly increased risk of developing obesity.

Hypothyroidism and hypercortisolemia can be ruled out by demonstrating normal free thyroxine and thyroid-stimulating hormone levels and 24 hr urinary free cortisol or diurnal salivary cortisol levels. If patients have severe early-onset obesity, out of proportion to the family history, one of the single gene defects mentioned earlier may need to be considered. Leptin levels can help in the diagnosis of leptin deficiency or resistance, and screening for genetic mutations is possible in several research laboratories.

The most important tests in the evaluation and follow-up of obese patients are those that evaluate cardiovascular disease risk and diabetes risk. These include plasma lipid profiles, fasting glucose and insulin levels, and hemoglobin A1C. It may also be necessary to perform studies to test for sleep apnea.

Complications. The 2001 Surgeon General's Call to Action (www.surgeongeneral.gov/topics/obesity/calltoaction) states that there has been a reversal of gains made in cardiovascular health over the recent past, owing to the huge increase in obesity prevalence. Obesity-associated co-morbidities include significantly increased risks for diabetes, cardiovascular disease, cancer, respiratory disease (asthma, sleep apnea), infertility, degenerative joint disease, proteinuria, depression, anxiety, and discrimination both in social life and in the workplace. Obesity shortens life span through its co-morbidities; and the earlier the onset, the shorter the life. It is a chronic disease that requires chronic therapy.

Prevention. Community-wide efforts need to be directed toward increasing physical activity and changing dietary habits. Increasing the safety of streets and playgrounds may be necessary in some settings, but the resources for this are often absent. Responsibility for promoting and organizing opportunities for nutritional education and for increasing physical activity for all citizens should be shared by schools, community organizations, and places of worship. Enhancement of physical education programs should be a priority of the school systems. School meal programs should provide healthy choices for students; vending machines in schools should not provide high-calorie beverages and snacks. Pediatric health care providers should counsel obese parents about the risk of childhood obesity in their children. Breast-fed infants are less likely to develop adult obesity than bottle-fed infants, and this should be communicated to expectant parents.

Treatment. Reduction of dietary calories and fat and increasing dietary fiber are recommended. Diets that are lower in carbohydrates may be useful in some individuals, but the basic goal should be reduction in energy intake and increase in energy expenditure. Any increase in physical activity is good, with regular aerobic exercise being the goal. This should be accompanied by a decrease in television viewing and computer games.

MEDICATIONS. Medical therapeutic options for treatment of obesity are not very promising. Therapy must be long term and ongoing, as is the case with treatment of hypertension and

TABLE 43–6. Transgenic Models for Altered Body Size or Body Fat

Increased	Decreased	No Change on Normal Diet
MC4R-KO	Dopamine D$_1$ receptor KO	CRH KO
5-HT2c receptor KO	UCP-1 overexpression	NPY KO
CRH overexpression	Tyrosine phosphatase 1B KO	TNF-α KO
BAT ablation	GLUT4 KO	UCP 3 KO
β$_3$-AR KO (+/-)	MCH KO	
GLUT4 overexpressed in fat	LPL overexpression in muscle	
NPY receptor 1 KO	PKA RIIβ KO	
Nhlh2 gene KO	PPAR γ KO heterozygotes	
11β-HSD-1 over-expressed in fat		

MC4R = melanocortin receptor 4; KO = knockout; 5-HT2c = 5-hydroxytryptophan 2c; CRH = corticotropin-releasing hormone; BAT = brown adipose tissue; β$_3$-AR = β$_3$-adrenergic receptor; GLUT4 = glucose transporter 4; NPY = neuropeptide Y; Nhlh2 = one of two helix-loop-helix transcription factors expressed in the developing mouse nervous system; UCP = uncoupling protein; MCH = melanin-concentrating hormone; LPL = lipoprotein lipase; PKA RIIβ = protein kinase A regulatory subunit II β; PPAR = peroxisome proliferator-activated receptor; TNF = tumor necrosis factor; 11β-HSD-1 = 11-β-hydroxysteroid dehydrogenase type 1.

diabetes. Anti-obesity drugs are not approved for prolonged use or for use in youth. They have not been extensively tested for safety over long periods of time, may only benefit a minority of patients, and may be associated with serious cardiovascular side effects. The major classes of drugs are those that reduce food intake (monoamine oxidase inhibitors, sympathomimetic drugs), those that increase energy expenditure (ephedrine, caffeine), and those that inhibit fat absorption (orlistat). The use of agents to induce dietary fat malabsorption has been only minimally successful and is associated with significant intestinal discomfort if not accompanied by a low-fat diet. Metformin, a glucose-sensitizing agent developed for use in type 2 diabetes, has shown promise in helping obese patients adhere to a diet; the diet itself may be nearly equally effective over the long term. Certain neuropeptide agonists and antagonists are being developed as therapeutic agents. The roles of some of these compounds in energy homeostasis are shown in Table 43–5.

The use of recombinant leptin in humans resulted in a modest and highly variable loss of weight (loss of fat mass) that was dose related and occurred in both lean and obese subjects. Leptin treatment in the rare leptin-deficient patients produced a rapid reduction in weight and increase in energy expenditure; antibodies to leptin developed after several months of treatment. The impact of these antibodies on efficacy has not yet been demonstrated.

SURGERY. Surgical therapy to reduce the volume of the stomach may be successful in the long term in some patients. Procedures to bypass the absorptive surfaces of the intestine have been associated with many complications, the most predictable being nutritional deficiencies. Surgery to remove fat (liposuction), if used alone, is not a long-term solution. However, it may be a useful cosmetic adjunct in patients who are successful with diet and exercise, with or without surgical gastroplasty.

GOALS OF TREATMENT. As with adults, it is rarely possible for obese youth to achieve an "ideal body weight" for height. The initial goal should be a 10% reduction in weight for older children; in adults, this modest degree of loss is associated with a decrease in plasma lipids, blood pressure, fasting insulin, and other co-morbidities such as asthma symptoms. For younger children, severe caloric restriction may result in an unacceptable decrement in height velocity. In many younger children, simply preventing further weight gain for a period of time will achieve the same goals. In all age groups, permanent lifestyle changes are required. This is not unlike the lifestyle changes needed for optimal control of diabetes, hyperlipidemia, and hypertension. The most significant impact on the obesity epidemic will have to be achieved through patient education and prevention. At present, there is limited value for genetic counseling, but there may be an increasing role as more genetic defects are described.

Bray GA, Tartaglia L: Medicinal strategies in the treatment of obesity. *Nature* 2000;404:672–77.

Clarke WR, Schrott HG, Leaverton PE, et al: Tracking of blood lipids and blood pressures in school age children: The Muscatine study. *Circulation* 1978;58:626–34.

Crespo CJ, Smit E, Troiano RP, et al: Television watching, energy intake, and obesity in US children: Results from the Third National Health and Nutrition Examination Survey, 1988–1994. *Arch Pediatr Adolesc Med* 2001;155:360–65.

Donohoue PA: Disorders of the body mass. In Rimoin DL, Connor JM, Pyeritz RE, et al (editors): *Emery and Rimoin's Principles and Practice of Medical Genetics*, 4th ed. London, Harcourt, 2002.

Fagot-Campagna A, Pettitt DJ, Engelgau MM, et al: Type 2 diabetes among North American children and adolescents: An epidemiological review and a public health perspective. *J Pediatr* 2000;136:664–72.

He Q, Karlberg J: Prediction of adult overweight during the pediatric years. *Pediatr Res* 1999;46:697–703.

Hill J, Peters J: Environmental contributions to the obesity epidemic. *Science* 1998;280:1371–74.

Kimm SYS, Barton BA, Obarzanek E, et al: Racial divergence in adiposity during adolescence: The NHLBI growth and health study. *Pediatrics* 2001;107:e34.

Leibel RL, Rosenbaum M, Hirsch J: Changes in energy expenditure resulting from altered body weight. *N Engl J Med* 1995;332:621–28.

Mokdad AH, Serdula MK, Dietz WH, et al: The spread of the obesity epidemic in the United States, 1991–1998. *JAMA* 1999;282:1519–22.

Moll PP, Burns TL, Lauer RM: The genetic and environmental sources of body mass index variability: The Muscatine ponderosity family study. *Am J Hum Genet* 1991;49:1243–55.

Ogden CL, Kuczmarski RJ, Flegal KM, et al: Centers for Disease Control and Prevention 2000 growth charts for the United States: Improvements to the 1977 National Center for Health Statistics version. *Pediatrics* 2002;109:45–60.

Robinson TN: Reducing children's television viewing to prevent obesity. *JAMA* 1999;282:1561–67.

Schwartz MW, Woods SC, Porte D Jr, et al: Central nervous system control of food intake. *Nature* 2000;404:661–71.

Seeley RJ, Schwartz MW: Neuroendocrine regulation of food intake. *Acta Paediatr Suppl* 1999;88:58–61.

Von Kries R, Koletzko B, Sauerwald T, et al: Breast feeding and obesity: Cross sectional study. *BMJ* 1999;319:147–50.

Whitaker RC, Pepe MS, Wright JA, et al: Early adiposity rebound and the risk of adult obesity. *Pediatrics* 1998;101:e5.

Whitaker RC, Wright JA, Pepe MS, et al: Predicting obesity in young adulthood from childhood and parental obesity. *N Engl J Med* 1997;337:869–73.

Chapter 44

Vitamin Deficiencies and Excesses *William C. Heird*

Vitamins are essential nutrients that must be supplied exogenously either as part of a well-balanced diet or as supplements. The functions of vitamins are summarized in Table 44–1, and the daily reference intakes for infants and children are summarized in Table 40–1. Deficiency states are uncommon in developed countries except, perhaps, among some food-insecure families (see Chapter 42). In contrast, deficiency states (see Table 44–1) are quite common in many developing countries.

Toxicity results from excessive intakes of the fat-soluble vitamins A and D, but toxicity from excessive intakes of the water-soluble vitamins is rare. The vitamin-dependent states are also summarized in Table 44–1.

VITAMIN A

Vitamin A is a generic term encompassing all β-ionone derivatives other than provitamin A carotenoids. These include retinol, retinyl ester, retinal and retinoic acid, and the vitamin A alcohol, ester, aldehyde, and acid. *Provitamin A carotenoids* is a generic term for all carotenoids that have the biologic activity of β-carotene. They or their derivatives with vitamin A activity are required in the diets of adults as well as of infants and children.

β-Carotene is partially absorbed into the intestinal lymphatics. The remainder is cleaved into two molecules of retinol. Dietary retinyl ester is hydrolyzed to retinol in the intestine, esterified with palmitic acid in the mucosal cells, and stored in the liver as retinyl palmitate, which can be hydrolyzed to free retinol for transport by retinol-binding protein to its site of action. Zinc also is required for this mobilization. Normal plasma values of retinol are 20–50 μg/dL in infants and 30–225 μg/dL in older children and adults.

The liver content of vitamin A is low at birth but is rapidly augmented by the large amounts in colostrum and breast milk as well as infant formulas. Other foods (vegetables, fruits, eggs, butter, liver) or vitamin supplements also provide vitamin A. Cooking, canning, and freezing of foodstuffs results in only small losses of vitamin A, but it is destroyed by oxidizing agents. Thus, risk of vitamin A deficiency is small in healthy children receiving a well-balanced diet. However, vitamin A deficiency can also result from inadequate intestinal absorption secondary to chronic intestinal disorders or fat malabsorption syndromes. Low dietary intake of fat can also result in low vitamin A absorption, and low dietary protein intake can result in deficient

TABLE 44–1. Physical and Metabolic Properties and Food Sources of the Vitamins

Names and Synonyms	Characteristics	Biochemical Action	Effects of Deficiency	Effects of Excess	Sources
Vitamin A: retinol (vitamin A_1) is an alcohol of high molecular weight; 1 μg of retinol = 3.3 IU vitamin A Provitamin A: the plant pigments α-, β-, and γ-carotenes and cryptoxanthin; 1/6 activity of retinol	Fat soluble; heat stable; destroyed by oxidation, drying; bile necessary for absorption; stored in liver; protected by vitamin E	Component of retinal pigments, rhodopsin and iodopsin, for vision in dim light; bone and tooth development; formation and maturation of epithelia	Nyctalopia, photophobia, xerophthalmia, conjunctivitis, keratomalacia leading to blindness; faulty epiphyseal bone formation; defective tooth enamel; keratinization of mucous membranes and skin; retarded growth; impaired resistance to infection	Anorexia, slow growth, drying and cracking of skin, enlargement of liver and spleen, swelling and pain of long bones, bone fragility, increased intracranial pressure, alopecia, carotenemia	Liver, fish liver oils, whole milk, milk fat products, egg yolk, fortified margarines Carotenoids from plants: green vegetables, yellow fruits and vegetables
Vitamin B Complex: thiamine: vitamin B_1; antiberiberi vitamin, aneurin	Water and alcohol soluble; fat insoluble; stable in slightly acid solution; labile to heat, alkali, sulfites	Component of thiamine pyrophosphate carboxylases, which act in various oxidative decarboxylations, including that of pyruvic acid	Beriberi, fatigue, irritability, anorexia, constipation, headache, insomnia, tachycardia, polyneuritis, cardiac failure, edema, elevated pyruvic acid in the blood, aphonia	None from oral intake	Liver, meat, especially pork, milk, whole grain or enriched cereals, wheat germ, legumes, nuts
Riboflavin: vitamin B_2	Sparingly soluble in water; sensitive to light and alkali; stable to heat, oxidation, acid	Constituent of flavoprotein enzymes important in hydrogen transfer reactions; amino acid, fatty acid, and carbohydrate metabolism and cellular respiration. Retinal pigment for light adaptation	Ariboflavinosis; photophobia, blurred vision, burning and itching of eyes, corneal vascularization, poor growth, cheilosis	Not harmful	Milk, cheese, liver and other organs, meat, eggs, fish, green leafy vegetables, whole or enriched grains
Niacin: nicotinamide; nicotinic acid; antipellagra vitamin	Water and alcohol soluble; stable to acid, alkali, light, heat, oxidation	Constituent of coenzymes I and II. NAD, NADP cofactors in a number of dehydrogenase systems	Pellagra, multiple B-vitamin deficiency syndrome, diarrhea, dementia, dermatitis	Nicotinic acid (not the amide) is vasodilator; skin flushing and itching; hepatopathy	Meat, fish, poultry, liver, whole grain and enriched cereals, green vegetables, peanuts
Folacin: group of related compounds containing pteridine ring, para-amino benzoic acid, and glutamic acid. Pteroylglutamic acid (PGA)	Slightly soluble in water: labile to heat, light, acid	Concerned with formation and metabolism of one-carbon units; participates in synthesis of purines, pyrimidines, nucleoproteins, and methyl groups	Megaloblastic anemia (infancy, pregnancy) usually is secondary to malabsorption disease, glossitis, pharyngeal ulcers, impaired immunity	Unknown	Liver, green vegetables, nuts, cereals, cheese, fruits, yeast, beans, peas
Cyanocobalamin: vitamin B_{12}	Slightly soluble in water; stable to heat in neutral solution; labile in acid or alkaline ones; destroyed by light. Castle intrinsic factor of the stomach required for absorption	Transfer of one-carbon units in purine and labile methyl group metabolism; essential for maturation of red blood cells in bone marrow; metabolism of nervous tissue; adenosylcobalamin is the coenzyme for methylmalonyl CoA mutase	Juvenile pernicious anemia, due to defect in absorption rather than to dietary lack; also secondary to gastrectomy, celiac disease, inflammatory lesions of small bowel, long-term drug therapy (PAS, neomycin); methylmalonic aciduria; homocystinuria	Unknown	Muscle and organ meats, fish, eggs, milk, cheese
Biotin	Crystallized from yeast; soluble in water	Coenzyme carboxylases; involved in CO_2 transfer	Dermatitis, seborrhea; inactivated by avidin in raw egg white	None known	Yeast, animal products; synthesized in intestine
Vitamin B_6 active forms: pyridoxine, pyridoxal, pyridoxamine	Water soluble; destroyed by ultraviolet light and by heat	Constituent of coenzymes for decarboxylation, transamination, transsulfuration; fatty acid metabolism	Irritability, convulsions, hypochromic anemia; peripheral neuritis in patients receiving isoniazid; oxaluria	Sensory neuropathy	Meat, liver, kidney, whole grains, soybeans, nuts, fish, poultry, green vegetables

Vitamin	Properties	Function	Deficiency	Toxicity/Tolerance	Sources
Vitamin C: ascorbic acid; vitamin C; antiscorbutic vitamin	Water soluble; easily oxidized, accelerated by heat, light, alkali oxidative enzymes, traces of copper or iron	Integrity and maintenance of intercellular material; facilitates absorption of iron and conversion of folic acid to folinic acid; metabolism of tyrosine and phenylalanine; activity of succinic dehydrogenase and serum phosphatase in infants, not in adults	Scurvy and poor wound healing	Oxaluria	Citrus fruits, tomatoes, berries, cantaloupe, cabbage, green vegetables. Cooking has destructive effect
Vitamin D: group of sterols having similar physiologic activity, D_2-calciferol is activated ergosterol. D_3 is activated 7-dehydrocholesterol in skin. 1 µg = 40 IU vitamin D	Fat soluble, stable to heat, acid alkali, and oxidation; bile necessary for absorption. Prohormone for 25-OH cholecalciferol	Regulates absorption and deposition of calcium and phosphorus by affecting permeability of intestinal membrane; regulates level of serum alkaline phosphatase, which is believed to be concerned with calcium phosphate deposition in bones and teeth	Rickets (high serum phosphatase level appears before bone deformities); infantile tetany; poor growth; osteomalacia	Wide variation in tolerance; over 500 µg/24 hr toxic when continued for weeks; prolonged administration of 45 µg/24 hr may be toxic; nausea, diarrhea, weight loss, polyuria, nocturia, calcification of soft tissues, including heart, renal tubules, blood vessels, bronchi, stomach	Vitamin D–fortified milk and margarine, fish liver oils, exposure to sunlight or other ultraviolet sources
Vitamin E: group of related chemical compounds—tocopherols with similar biologic activities	Fat soluble; unstable to ultraviolet light, alkali; readily oxidized by oxygen, iron, rancid fats Antioxidant; bile necessary for absorption	Minimizes oxidation of carotene, vitamin A, and linoleic acid; stabilizes membranes	Requirements related to polyunsaturated fat intake; red blood cell hemolysis in premature infants; loss of neural integrity	Unknown	Germ oils of various seeds, green leafy vegetables, nuts, legumes
Vitamin K: group of naphthoquinones with similar biologic activities; K_1 is phytoquinone	Natural compounds are fat soluble; stable to heat and reducing agents; labile to oxidizing agents, strong acids, alkali, light; bile salts necessary for intestinal absorption	Prothrombin formation; coagulation factors II, VII, IX, and X and osteocalcin are vitamin K–dependent; proteins C, S, Z	Hemorrhagic manifestations; bone metabolism	Not established; analogues may produce hyperbilirubinemia in premature infants	Green leafy vegetables, pork, liver. Widely distributed

NAD(P) = nicotinamide adenine dinucleotide (phosphate); CoA = coenzyme A; PAS = para-aminosalicylic acid.

retinol-binding protein and, hence, a low plasma concentration of vitamin A.

The major role of vitamin A is in vision. The human retina contains two distinct photoreceptor systems—the rods, which are sensitive to light of low intensity, and the cones, which are sensitive to colors and to light of high intensity. Retinal is the prosthetic group of the photosensitive pigment in both. The major difference between the visual pigments in rods (rhodopsin) and in cones (iodopsin) is the nature of the protein bound to retinal. All-*trans*-retinal isomerizes in the dark to 11 *cis*-retinal, which combines with opsin to form rhodopsin. Energy from light quanta reconverts 11-*cis*-retinal to the all-*trans* form, and this energy exchange is transmitted via the optic nerve to the brain, resulting in visual sensation.

Retinoids, in addition to involvement in vision, are essential for cell differentiation, activation of retinoic acid–responsive genes, and membrane stability. Vitamin A also plays a role in keratinization, cornification, bone metabolism, placental development, growth, spermatogenesis, and mucus formation. Characteristic changes of deficiency in epithelium include proliferation of basal cells, hyperkeratosis, and the formation of stratified, cornified squamous epithelium. Epithelial changes in the respiratory system may result in bronchiolar obstruction. Squamous metaplasia of the renal pelves, ureters, urinary bladder, enamel organs, and pancreatic and salivary ducts may lead to an increase in infections in these areas.

Vitamin A Deficiency

Clinical Manifestations. Ocular lesions of vitamin A deficiency develop insidiously and rarely occur before 2–3 yr of age. The posterior segment of the eye is affected initially with impairment of dark adaptation, resulting in night blindness. Later, drying of the conjunctiva (xerosis conjunctivae) and cornea (xerosis corneae) occur, followed by wrinkling and cloudiness of the cornea or keratomalacia (Fig. 44–1). Dry, silver-gray plaques may appear on the bulbar conjunctiva (Bitot spots), with follicular hyperkeratosis and photophobia.

Vitamin A deficiency also may result in retardation of mental and physical growth and in apathy. Anemia with or without hepatosplenomegaly is usually present. The skin is dry and scaly, and follicular hyperkeratosis may be found on the shoulders, buttocks, and extensor surfaces of the extremities. The vaginal epithelium may become cornified, and epithelial metaplasia of the urinary tract may result in pyuria and hematuria. Increased intracranial pressure with wide separation of cranial bones at the sutures may occur, but hydrocephalus, with or without paralyses of the cranial nerves, is an infrequent manifestation of vitamin A deficiency.

Diagnosis. Dark adaptation tests may be helpful in diagnosing vitamin A deficiency. Xerosis conjunctivae can be detected by biomicroscopic examination of the conjunctiva. Examination of the scrapings from the eye and vagina is recommended as a diagnostic aid. The plasma carotene concentration falls quickly, but that of vitamin A decreases more slowly.

Prevention. Infants should receive at least 500 μg of vitamin A daily, and older children, like adults, should receive 600–1500 μg of vitamin A or carotene. Because maternal vitamin A status is reflected in breast milk vitamin A content, mothers of breast-fed infants living in regions where vitamin A deficiency is common should be given 30,000 μg [100,000 IU]) of vitamin A postpartum.

Low-fat diets should be supplemented with vitamin A. In disorders with poor absorption of fat or increased excretion of vitamin A, water-miscible preparations should be administered in amounts several times the usual reference daily intake. Premature infants, who absorb fats and vitamin A less efficiently than do term infants, should also receive water-miscible preparations.

Epidemiologic public health studies in areas of the world where overt or subclinical vitamin A deficiency is prevalent because of insufficient dietary intake, seasonal variance, or intercurrent illness have shown that restoration of vitamin A sufficiency is associated with a 20% increase in survival of deficient children. Effects are not apparent in infants less than 6 mo of age, but older infants supplemented every 4 mo with water-miscible vitamin A, 30,000 μg (100,000 IU), in those between 6 and 11 mo of age and 60,000 μg (200,000 IU) in those older than 12 mo of age, have a lower mortality associated with severe diarrhea and measles. No consistent effect of vitamin A supplementation on the severity or mortality of respiratory disease has been reported. The effect of vitamin A on mortality from infectious diseases may be related to restoration of epithelial integrity and/or upregulation of immunocompetence.

Treatment. A daily supplement of 1,500 μg of vitamin A is sufficient for treating latent vitamin A deficiency. Xerophthalmia is treated by giving 1,500 μg/kg orally for 5 days followed by daily intramuscular injection of 7,500 μg of vitamin A in oil until recovery occurs. Morbidity and mortality rates from viral infections such as measles may be lower in nondeficient children who are given daily doses of 1,500–3,000 μg of vitamin A.

Hypervitaminosis A

Clinical Manifestations. Acute hypervitaminosis A may occur in infants after ingesting 100,000 μg or more. The symptoms are nausea, vomiting, drowsiness, and, in young infants, bulging of

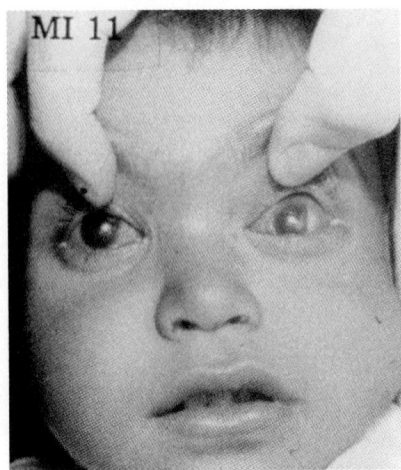
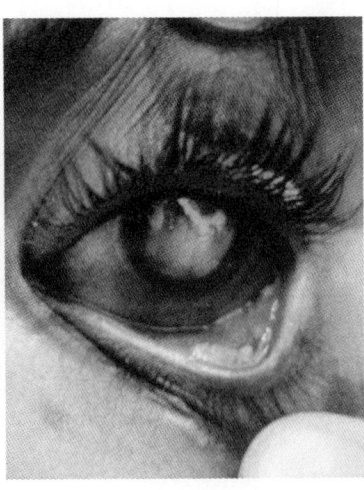

FIGURE 44–1. Recovery from xerophthalmia, showing permanent eye lesion. (From Bloch CE: Blindness and other diseases arising from deficient nutrition [lack of fat-soluble A factor]. *Am J Dis Child* 1924;27:139.)

the fontanel. Diplopia, papilledema, cranial nerve palsies, and other symptoms suggestive of brain tumor (pseudotumor cerebri) may also be present. Toxicity has occurred with supplementation during vaccine administration in developing countries.

Chronic hypervitaminosis A results from ingestion of excessive doses for several weeks or months. An affected child has anorexia, pruritus, and a lack of weight gain. Irritability, limitation of motion, with tender swelling of the bones, alopecia, seborrheic cutaneous lesions, fissuring of the corners of the mouth, increased intracranial pressure, and hepatomegaly also may develop. Craniotabes and desquamation of the palms and soles are common. Radiographs show hyperostosis affecting several long bones; it is most notable at the middle of the shafts (Fig. 44–2). A history of excessive ingestion of vitamin A helps to differentiate vitamin A toxicity from cortical hyperostosis (see Chapter 688). In addition, the serum vitamin A level is elevated. Hypercalcemia and/or liver cirrhosis may occasionally be seen.

Severe congenital malformations may occur in infants of mothers who consume large amounts of oral retinoids for treatment of acne.

Ingested carotenoids, although nontoxic, may result in yellow discoloration of the skin but not of the sclera. This disorder, *carotenemia,* is especially likely to occur in children with liver disease, diabetes mellitus, or hypothyroidism and in those who have congenital absence of enzymes that convert provitamin A carotenoids.

VITAMIN B COMPLEX

Vitamin B complex includes several factors of differing chemical composition and function: thiamine (vitamin B_1), riboflavin, niacin, pyridoxine (vitamin B_6), biotin, folate, and vitamin B_{12}. All are important constituents of enzyme systems that are closely related functionally. Hence, lack of a single factor can interrupt

an entire chain of chemical processes, producing diverse clinical manifestations.

Diets deficient in any one of the B complex vitamins are frequently poor sources of other B vitamins, and manifestations of several vitamin B deficiencies can usually be found in the same person. Because of this, it is generally practical to treat a patient with evidence of deficiency of a specific B vitamin with the entire complex of B vitamins.

Factors such as pantothenic acid, choline, and inositol are important for normal functioning of the human organism, but at present no specific deficiency syndromes can be ascribed to their lack in the diets of children.

Thiamine

Thiamine (vitamin B_1) is water soluble and, as thiamine pyrophosphate or cocarboxylase, functions as a coenzyme in carbohydrate metabolism. It also is required for the synthesis of acetylcholine, and deficiency results in impaired nerve conduction. It is the coenzyme in transketolation and in decarboxylation of α-keto acids and, hence, participates in the hexose monophosphate shunt that generates nicotinamide adenine dinucleotide phosphate and pentose.

Breast milk and bovine milk as well as vegetables, cereals, fruits, and eggs are good sources of thiamine. Thus, most infants and older children whose diets contain these foods do not require thiamine supplements. On the other hand, breast-fed infants of thiamine-deficient mothers are at risk for deficiency. In addition, thiamine is easily destroyed by heat, particularly in neutral or alkaline media; therefore, it is readily extracted from food by cooking water. Furthermore, because the covering of cereal contains most of the vitamin, polishing reduces its availability.

Thiamine absorption from the gastrointestinal tract usually is excellent but may be low in those with gastrointestinal or liver disease. Fever, surgery, and/or stress increase the requirement for thiamine but, because these events are rarely present for very long, they are not likely to result in deficiency.

Thiamine dependence has been described in a child with megaloblastic anemia and in an infant with otherwise typical maple syrup urine disease. In addition, the urine of children with Leigh encephalomyelopathy as well as that of their parents inhibits the formation of thiamine pyrophosphate and large doses of thiamine improve some of the physical abnormalities associated with the disease.

Thiamine Deficiency

Clinical Manifestations. Early manifestations of thiamine deficiency include fatigue, apathy, irritability, depression, drowsiness, poor mental concentration, anorexia, nausea, and abdominal discomfort. Signs of progression include peripheral neuritis with tingling, burning, and paresthesias of the toes and feet, decreased deep tendon reflexes, loss of vibration sense, tenderness and cramping of leg muscles, congestive heart failure, and psychic disturbances. Patients may have ptosis of the eyelids and atrophy of the optic nerve. Hoarseness or aphonia caused by paralysis of the laryngeal nerve is a characteristic sign. Muscle atrophy and tenderness of nerve trunks are followed by ataxia, loss of coordination, and loss of deep sensation. Paralysis occurs in adults but is uncommon in children. Later signs include increased intracranial pressure, meningismus, and coma.

The full-blown deficiency state is called **beriberi**. Two forms of the condition, based primarily on appearance of the patient, are often discussed: wet beriberi and dry beriberi. The child with wet beriberi is undernourished, pale, edematous with dyspnea, vomiting, and tachycardia, and has a waxy skin; the urine often contains albumin and casts. The child with dry beriberi appears plump but is pale, flabby, and listless with dyspnea, tachycardia, and hepatomegaly.

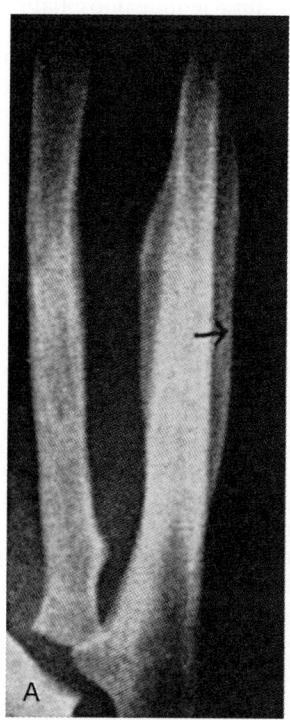
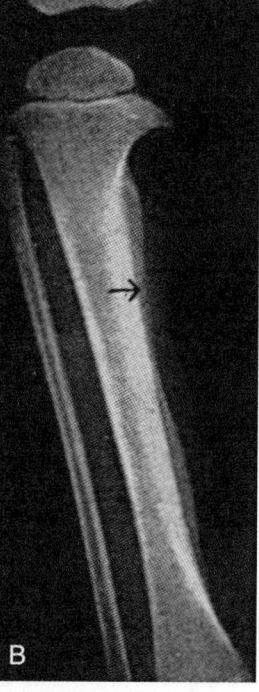

FIGURE 44–2. Hyperostosis of the ulna and the tibia in an infant 21 mo of age, resulting from vitamin A poisoning. *A,* Long, wavy cortical hyperostosis of the ulna. *B,* Long, wavy cortical hyperostosis of the right tibia; striking absence of metaphyseal changes. (From Caffey J: *Pediatric X-ray Diagnosis,* 5th ed. Chicago, Year Book, 1967, p 994.)

Death from thiamine deficiency usually is secondary to cardiac involvement. The initial signs are slight cyanosis and dyspnea, but tachycardia, enlargement of the liver, loss of consciousness, and convulsions may develop rapidly. The heart, especially the right side, is enlarged. The electrocardiogram shows an increased QT interval, inverted T waves, and low voltage. These changes as well as the cardiomegaly rapidly revert to normal with treatment, but, without prompt treatment, cardiac failure can develop rapidly and result in death.

In fatal cases of beriberi, lesions are located principally in the heart, peripheral nerves, subcutaneous tissue, and serous cavities. The heart is dilated, and fatty degeneration of the myocardium is common. Generalized edema or edema of the legs, serous effusions, and venous engorgement are often present. Degeneration of myelin and axon cylinders of peripheral nerves with wallerian degeneration beginning in the distal locations also is common, particularly in the lower extremities. Lesions in the brain include vascular dilatation and hemorrhage.

Diagnosis. The early symptoms of thiamine deficiency are common in many types of nutritional disturbances and, therefore, are not helpful in diagnosing thiamine deficiency. Low red blood cell transketolase and high blood or urinary glyoxylate levels are useful diagnostic indicators. Measurement of urinary thiamine excretion or urinary excretion of its metabolites, thiazole or pyrimidine, after an oral loading dose of thiamine may help to identify the deficiency state. Clinical response to administration of thiamine is the best test for thiamine deficiency.

Prevention. A maternal diet containing sufficient amounts of thiamine prevents thiamine deficiency in breast-fed infants, and infant formulas marketed in all developed countries contain adequate thiamine. A varied diet containing fresh fruits and vegetables as well as whole grain cereals after the period of exclusive breast-feeding or formula feeding will help assure adequate thiamine intake without supplementation. Thiamine requirements are higher if the carbohydrate content of the diet is high, but this is rarely a problem.

Treatment. If a breast-fed infant develops beriberi, both the mother and child should be treated with thiamine. The daily dose for children and adults, respectively, is 10 mg and 50 mg. In the absence of gastrointestinal disturbances, oral administration is effective. However, thiamine should be given intramuscularly or intravenously to children with cardiac failure. Such treatment is usually followed by dramatic improvement, although complete cure requires several weeks of treatment. The heart is not permanently damaged.

Patients with beriberi often have other B complex vitamin deficiencies; therefore, all other vitamins of the B complex also should be administered.

Riboflavin

Riboflavin is a yellow, fluorescent, water-soluble substance that is stable to heat and acid but is destroyed by light and alkali. The coenzymes flavin mononucleotide and flavin adenine dinucleotide (FAD), which form the prosthetic groups of several enzymes important in electron transport, are synthesized from riboflavin. Thus, riboflavin is essential for growth and tissue respiration. It also may play a role in light adaptation, and it is required for conversion of pyridoxine to pyridoxal phosphate. Large amounts are found in liver, kidney, brewer's yeast, milk, cheese, eggs, and leafy vegetables. Cow's milk contains about five times as much riboflavin as human milk.

Riboflavin Deficiency

Riboflavin deficiency, without deficiencies of other members of the vitamin B complex, is rare. It is usually caused by inade-

quate riboflavin intake, but faulty absorption may contribute in patients with biliary atresia or hepatitis as well as in those receiving probenecid, phenothiazines, or oral contraceptives. Phototherapy destroys riboflavin.

Clinical Manifestations. Signs and/or symptoms of riboflavin deficiency include cheilosis (perlèche), glossitis, keratitis, conjunctivitis, photophobia, lacrimation, marked corneal vascularization, and seborrheic dermatitis. Cheilosis begins with pallor at the angles of the mouth and progresses to thinning and maceration of the epithelium. Superficial fissures, often covered by yellow crusts, develop in the angles of the mouth, and extend radially into the skin for distances of 1–2 cm. With glossitis, the tongue is smooth with loss of papillary structure. A normocytic, normochromic anemia with bone marrow hypoplasia is common.

Diagnosis. The signs and symptoms of riboflavin deficiency are too nonspecific to make a definitive diagnosis. Useful diagnostic tests include urinary excretion of riboflavin below 30 μg/24 hr and low levels of erythrocyte glutathionine reductase, a flavoprotein requiring FAD.

Prevention. Reference daily intakes of riboflavin are presented in Table 40–1. Deficiency is usually prevented by a diet that contains adequate amounts of milk, eggs, leafy vegetables, and lean meats.

Treatment. Treatment includes oral administration of 3–10 mg of riboflavin daily. If no response occurs within a few days, intramuscular injections of 2 mg of riboflavin in saline may be given as often as three times daily. The child should also be given a well-balanced diet, including, at least temporarily, generous supplements of other B complex vitamins.

Niacin

Niacin forms part of two cofactors, nicotinamide adenine dinucleotide and nicotinamide adenine dinucleotide phosphate, that are important in electron transfer and glycolysis. Although dietary tryptophan can partially substitute for niacin, other sources of niacin are necessary. Good sources include liver, lean pork, salmon, poultry, and red meat. Most cereals contain only small amounts. Milk and eggs contain little niacin but are good sources of tryptophan from which the active cofactors can be synthesized. Only small losses of niacin occur in cooking.

Niacin Deficiency

Pellagra (*pellis,* "skin"; *agra,* "rough"), a deficiency disease caused by a lack of niacin (nicotinic acid), affects all tissues of the body. It occurs chiefly in countries where corn (maize), a poor source of tryptophan, is a basic foodstuff.

Clinical Manifestations. The early symptoms of pellagra are vague. Anorexia, lassitude, weakness, burning sensations, numbness, and dizziness may be prodromal symptoms. After a long period of deficiency, the classic triad of dermatitis, diarrhea, and dementia appears. Manifestations in children with parasites or chronic disorders may be especially severe.

The dermatitis is the most characteristic manifestation of pellagra. This may develop suddenly or insidiously and may be elicited by irritants, including intense sunlight. The lesions first appear as symmetric areas of erythema on exposed surfaces resembling sunburn. Thus, in mild cases, the dermatitis may not be recognized. The lesions are usually sharply demarcated from the healthy skin around them, and the distribution of the lesions may change frequently. The lesions on the hands often have the appearance of a glove (pellagrous glove). Similar demarcations may also occur on the foot and leg (pellagrous boot) or around the neck (Casal necklace; Fig. 44–3). In some cases, vesicles and bullae develop (wet type); in others, there may be suppuration beneath the scaly, crusted epidermis and, in still others, the

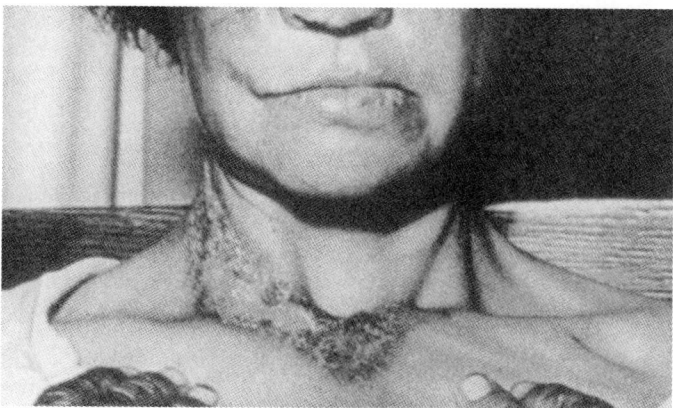

FIGURE 44–3. Pellagra showing an early lesion on the neck (Casal necklace).

swelling may disappear after a short time followed by desquamation. The healed parts of the skin may remain pigmented.

The cutaneous lesions may be preceded by or accompanied by stomatitis, glossitis, vomiting, and/or diarrhea. Swelling and redness of the tip of the tongue and its lateral margins is often followed by intense redness, even ulceration, of the entire tongue and papillae.

Nervous symptoms include depression, disorientation, insomnia, and delirium.

The classic symptoms of pellagra are usually not well developed in infants and young children, but anorexia, irritability, anxiety, and apathy are common. They may also have sore tongues and lips, and their skin is usually dry and scaly. Diarrhea and constipation may alternate, and a moderate secondary anemia may occur. Children who have pellagra often have evidence of other nutritional deficiency diseases.

Pathology. Histologically, there is edema and degeneration of the superficial collagen of the dermis. The papillary vessels are engorged, and there is perivascular lymphocytic infiltration. The epidermis is hyperkeratotic and later becomes atrophic. Changes similar to those in the skin also are present in the tongue, buccal mucous membranes, and vagina. These may be associated with secondary infection and ulceration.

The walls of the colon are thickened and inflamed with patches of pseudomembrane and, usually, mucosal atrophy. Changes in the nervous system occur relatively late in the disease. These include patchy areas of demyelination and degeneration of ganglion cells; demyelination of both the posterior and lateral columns may be seen in the spinal cord.

Diagnosis. Diagnosis is usually made from the physical signs of glossitis, gastrointestinal symptoms, and a symmetric dermatitis. Rapid clinical response to niacin is an important confirming test. N-methylnicotinamide, a normal metabolite of niacin, is almost undetectable in the urine of niacin-deficient individuals.

Prevention. A well-balanced diet containing meat, vegetables, eggs, and milk easily provides adequate intakes of niacin (see Table 40–1). Thus, supplements of niacin are necessary only in breast-fed infants whose mothers have pellagra or in children on very restricted diets.

Treatment. Children usually respond rapidly to antipellagral therapy. A liberal and well-balanced diet should be supplemented with 50–300 mg of niacin daily; in severe cases or in cases of poor intestinal absorption, 100 mg may be given intravenously. Large doses of niacin are often followed by a sensation of heat as well as flushing and burning of the skin. These unpleasant effects, which occur within a half hour of niacin ingestion, are not produced by niacinamide. Large doses of niacin also may cause cholestatic jaundice or hepatotoxicity.

The diet also should be supplemented with other vitamins, especially other B complex vitamins. Sun exposure should be avoided during the active phase of pellagra, and the skin lesions may be covered with soothing applications. Hypochromic anemia, if present, should be treated with iron. Even after successful treatment, the diet should be supervised continuously to prevent recurrence.

Pyridoxine (Vitamin B₆)

Vitamin B_6 includes pyridoxal, pyridoxine, and pyridoxamine. These are converted to pyridoxal-5-phosphate (or pyridoxamine-5-phosphate), which acts as a coenzyme in decarboxylation and transamination of amino acids (e.g., in the decarboxylation of 5-hydroxytryptophan in the formation of serotonin) and in the metabolism of glycogen and fatty acids. Vitamin B_6 also is essential for the breakdown of kynurenine. When this does not occur, xanthurenic acid appears in the urine. In addition, pyridoxine is necessary for adequate functioning of the nervous system. Pyridoxal phosphate is the coenzyme for both glutamic decarboxylase and γ-aminobutyric acid transaminase, each of which is necessary for normal brain metabolism. Other roles of pyridoxine include participation in active transport of amino acids across cell membranes, chelation of metals, and synthesis of arachidonic and docosahexaenoic acids from linoleic and linolenic acids, respectively. If it is lacking, glycine metabolism may lead to oxaluria. Pyridoxine is excreted largely as 4-pyridoxic acid. The pyridoxine content of human milk and infant formulas is adequate. Bovine milk and cereals also are good sources of pyridoxine, but prolonged heat processing of this milk and cereal destroys it. Diseases with fat malabsorption may contribute to vitamin B_6 deficiency.

Pyridoxine antagonists (e.g., isoniazid used in the treatment of tuberculosis), pregnancy, and drugs such as penicillamine, hydralazine, and the oral progesterone-estrogen contraceptives increase the requirements for pyridoxine.

Pyridoxine Deficiency

Clinical Manifestations. There are several types of *vitamin B_6 dependence syndromes.* These include vitamin B_6–dependent convulsions, a vitamin B_6–responsive anemia, xanthurenic aciduria, cystathioninuria, and homocystinuria. They result, presumably, from errors in enzyme structure or function, and patients with these syndromes respond to very large amounts of pyridoxine. *Deficiency symptoms* secondary to one of the vitamin B_6 dependence syndromes or inadequate intake are not as common in children as in adults. Four clinical disturbances caused by vitamin B_6 deficiency have been described in humans: convulsions in infants, peripheral neuritis, dermatitis, and anemia. Pyridoxine and folic acid decrease the frequency of thrombotic events in adults with elevated serum homocysteine levels.

Infants fed a formula deficient in vitamin B_6 for 1 to 6 mo exhibit irritability and generalized seizures. Gastrointestinal distress and an aggravated startle response also are common. Peripheral neuropathy may occur during treatment of tuberculosis with isonicotinic acid hydrazide (INH). The neuropathy responds to administration of pyridoxine or to a decrease in the dose of the drug. Skin lesions include cheilosis, glossitis, and seborrhea around the eyes, nose, and mouth. Microcytic anemia, oxaluria, oxalic acid bladder stones, hyperglycinemia, lymphopenia, decreased antibody formation, and infections also occur.

Convulsions due to vitamin B_6 dependence may occur within several hours to as long as 6 mo after birth. The seizures, typically, are myoclonic with a hypsarrhythmic electroencephalographic (EEG) pattern. In many cases, the mother received large doses of pyridoxine during pregnancy for control of emesis.

In vitamin B_6–dependent anemia, the red blood cells are microcytic and hypochromic. Patients have elevated serum iron concentrations, saturation of iron-binding protein, hemosiderin deposits in bone marrow and liver, and failure of iron utilization for hemoglobin synthesis.

Xanthurenic aciduria after a tryptophan load occurs normally in some families and is apparently benign. Xanthurenic acid excretion decreases after large doses of vitamin B_6. *Cystathioninuria* also is not accompanied by any clear clinical disturbance, although cystathionase is a vitamin B_6–dependent enzyme (see Chapter 73.3).

Cystathionine β-synthase also is a vitamin B_6–dependent enzyme (see Chapter 73.3). In some patients with homocystinuria, serum levels of homocysteine decline after vitamin B_6 administration.

Anemia is not common in infants with pyridoxine deficiency. After administration of 100 mg/kg of tryptophan, large amounts of xanthurenic acid appear in the urine of patients with pyridoxine deficiency; none appears in the urine of normal individuals. Xanthurenic acid excretion also may not increase after a tryptophan load in patients with pyridoxine dependence.

Diagnosis. All infants with seizures should be suspected of having vitamin B_6 deficiency or dependence. If more common causes of infantile seizures (e.g., hypocalcemia, hypoglycemia, infection) are eliminated, 100 mg of pyridoxine should be injected. If the seizure stops, vitamin B_6 deficiency should be suspected and a tryptophan loading test should be performed. In older children, 100 mg of pyridoxine may be injected intramuscularly while the EEG is being recorded; a favorable response of the EEG suggests pyridoxine deficiency.

Erythrocyte glutamic pyruvic transaminase is low in pyridoxine deficiency. Hence, its concentration may be a useful indicator of vitamin B_6 status.

Prevention. Balanced diets usually contain sufficient pyridoxine to prevent deficiency, but children receiving a high-protein diet may require supplemental vitamin B_6. Infants whose mothers have received large doses of pyridoxine during pregnancy are at increased risk of seizures from pyridoxine dependence, and supplements during the first few weeks of life should be considered. Any child receiving a pyridoxine antagonist such as isoniazid should be carefully observed for neurologic manifestations; if these develop, pyridoxine should be administered or the dose of the antagonist should be decreased. A daily intake of 0.3–0.5 mg of pyridoxine in an infant, 0.5–1.5 mg in a child, and 1.5–2.0 mg in an adult prevents deficiency states. However, larger amounts may be necessary in pyridoxine dependency.

Treatment. Convulsions due to pyridoxine deficiency should be treated with 100 mg of the vitamin given intramuscularly. One dose should suffice if the diet is adequate. For pyridoxine-dependent children, daily doses of 2–10 mg intramuscularly or 10–100 mg orally may be necessary.

Pyridoxine Toxicity

Megadoses of pyridoxine have caused neuropathy in adults.

Biotin

Biotin is discussed in Chapter 74.6. Many microorganisms produce biotin. Therefore, biotin deficiency is rare. Deficiency may occur in those consuming the biotin antagonist avidin, found in raw egg white. Deficiency also has been described in infants and children receiving parenteral nutrition exclusively and in infants whose mothers are biotin deficient.

Brawny dermatitis, orofacial lesions, alopecia, somnolence, hallucinations, hypotonia, and hyperesthesia with accumulation of organic acids are common manifestations of deficiency. Other neurologic signs may occur.

Biotin deficiency is suggested by organic aciduria, particularly propionic and dicarboxylic acids. Response of clinical and biochemical abnormalities to biotin administration is confirmatory.

Inclusion of biotin in parenteral nutrition infusates will prevent the most common cause of biotin deficiency in infants. Oral administration of 10 mg is sufficient for treatment of deficiency as well as to confirm the diagnosis of deficiency.

Folic Acid

Folic acid is required primarily for its hematologic effects, which are discussed in Chapter 446.

Folate deficiency before becoming pregnant or during pregnancy results in serious dysmorphologic effects in the fetus. Neurotube defects are among the most common such effects. Consumption of 400 μg of folic acid daily during the periconceptional period markedly decreases the incidence of neurotube and other anatomic defects and may lower the incidence of premature labor. Food may be fortified with folate as a preventive measure to decrease the incidence of neurotube defects. Sufficient fortification to achieve an intake of 100–200 μg/24 hr has been suggested. Cereals and grains are the most commonly fortified food products. It also has been suggested that all women of childbearing age receive a daily folate supplement of 400 μg.

Thrombotic events related to slightly elevated levels of homocystine in adults may be decreased by daily consumption of 1 mg of folic acid together with 5–100 mg of pyridoxine. However, supplements with betaine and vitamin B_{12} may be required to normalize homocystine levels. These doses are considerably less than those given for the inborn error of metabolism homocystinuria (see Chapter 73.3).

Vitamin B_{12}

See Chapters 320 and 446.

VITAMIN C (ASCORBIC ACID)

Ascorbic acid, a potent reducing agent, functions in a number of enzyme systems (see Table 44-1 and Chapter 73.2). For example, transient hypertyrosinemia of the newborn, which is relatively common among low-birthweight infants and to a lesser extent in term infants fed high-protein diets, can be corrected by administering ascorbic acid (see Chapter 73.2). Ascorbic acid also is necessary for conversion of folic acid or other conjugates (see Table 44–1 and Chapters 446 and 320); thus, deficiency may be a factor in some cases of megaloblastic anemia. The major role of ascorbic acid, however, is in the formation of normal collagen. The defects in collagen structure arising from deficiency of the vitamin are due, in part, to failure to incorporate hydroxyproline and proline into collagen, and the resulting alterations in collagen account for the major metabolic and clinical manifestations of vitamin deficiency.

If the mother's intake of vitamin C during pregnancy is adequate, her infant will have adequate stores of vitamin C at birth. The vitamin C content of cord blood plasma is usually two to four times that of maternal plasma. Breast milk produced by a vitamin C–sufficient mother contains adequate vitamin C, as do all infant formulas. However, low maternal vitamin C intake may result in a low breast milk content of the vitamin. Bovine milk contains very little vitamin C; thus, infants fed bovine milk and evaporated milk formulas must receive vitamin C supplements. Fresh fruits, especially citrus fruit, and vegetables are good sources of vitamin C.

The need for vitamin C is increased by febrile illnesses, particularly infectious and diarrheal diseases. Iron deficiency, cold exposure, and protein depletion also increase the need for vitamin C.

Vitamin C Deficiency

Pathophysiology. Vitamin C deficiency results in scurvy, a condition in which formation of collagen and chondroitin sulfate is impaired. This results in a tendency to hemorrhage, defective tooth dentin, and loosening of the teeth. Also, because osteoblasts cannot form osteoid, endochondral bone formation cannot proceed. In addition, the bony trabeculae that have been formed become brittle and fracture easily. The periosteum becomes loosened and subperiosteal hemorrhage occurs, especially at the ends of the femur and tibia. Severe deficiency may result in degeneration of skeletal muscles, cardiac hypertrophy, bone marrow depression, and adrenal atrophy.

Clinical Manifestations. Scurvy can occur at any age but, because clinical manifestations require time to develop, it is unusual in newborn infants. The usual age at onset is between 6 and 24 mo. After variable periods of vitamin C inadequacy, vague symptoms such as irritability, tachypnea, digestive disturbances, and loss of appetite appear. Usually, there is evidence of generalized tenderness. This is particularly noticeable in the legs when the infant is picked up or when the diaper is changed. The pain results in pseudoparalysis; the legs are usually held in a froglike position with the hips and knees semiflexed with the feet rotated outward. Edematous swelling along the shafts of the legs may be present and, in some cases, a subperiosteal hemorrhage can be felt at the end of the femur. The affected child's facial expression is apprehensive. Changes in the gums are most noticeable after teeth have erupted. These include bluish purple, spongy swellings of the mucous membrane, especially over the upper incisors. A "rosary" at the costochondral junctions and depression of the sternum are other typical features (Fig. 44–4). The angulation of scorbutic beads is usually sharper than that of a rachitic rosary.

Petechial hemorrhages are often present in the skin and mucous membranes. Hematuria, melena, and orbital or subdural hemorrhages also may occur. Low-grade fever is usually present. Anemia, if present, may reflect inability to utilize iron or impaired folic acid metabolism (see Chapters 446 and 447). Wound healing is slow, and apparently healed wounds often break down. Swollen joints and follicular hyperkeratosis are additional features, as is the sicca syndrome of Sjögren (xerostomia, keratoconjunctivitis sicca, and enlargement of the salivary glands [see Chapter 152]), which is usually associated with collagen disorders.

Diagnosis. Laboratory tests for scurvy are unsatisfactory. Thus, diagnoses is usually based on the characteristic clinical picture, the radiographic appearance of the long bones, and a history of poor vitamin C intake.

The typical radiographic changes occur at the distal ends of the long bones. These are particularly common in the area of the knee. In the early stages of the condition, the appearance resembles that of simple bone atrophy. The trabeculae of the shaft cannot be discerned and the bone has a ground-glass appearance. The cortex is quite thin, and the epiphyseal ends of the bones are sharply outlined. The white line of Fraenkel, an irregular but thickened white line at the metaphysis, represents the zone of well-calcified cartilage. The epiphyseal centers of ossification also have a ground-glass appearance and are surrounded by a white ring (Fig. 44–5).

Scurvy cannot be diagnosed with certainty from the radiograph until a zone of rarefaction under the white line at the metaphysis becomes apparent. This zone of rarefaction is a linear break in the bone proximal and parallel to the white line. The lateral parts of the zone of rarefaction are seen as a triangular defect (see Fig. 44–5). A spur, or lateral prolongation of the

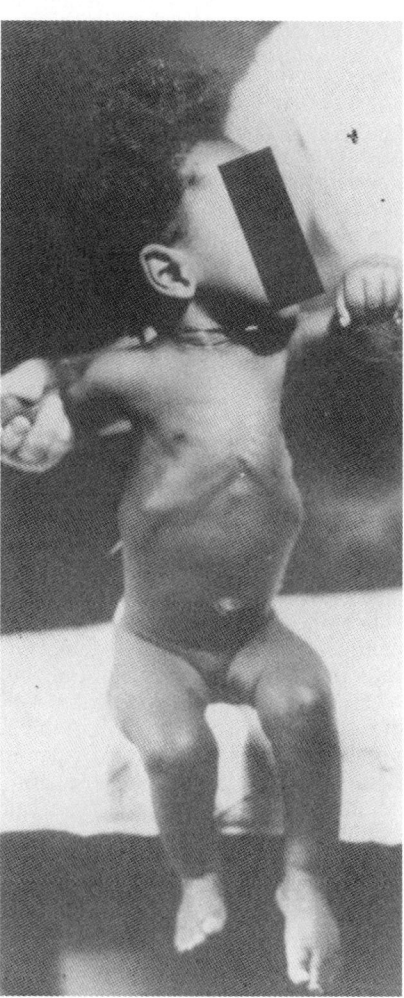

FIGURE 44–4. Scorbutic rosary and depression of sternum.

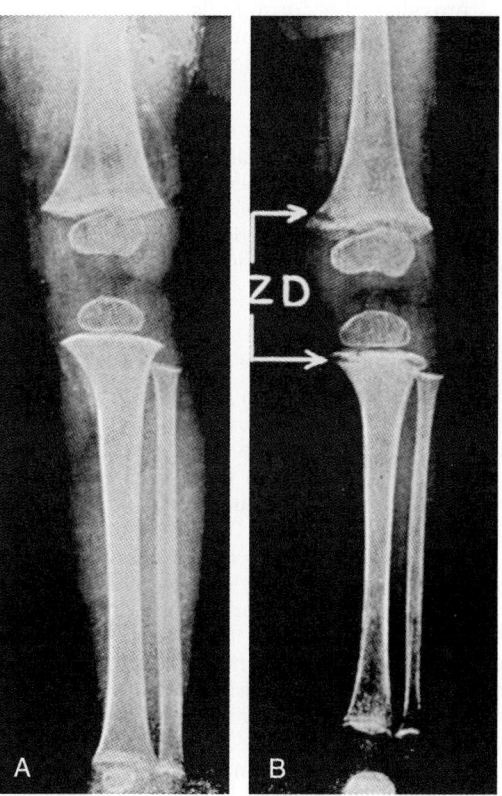

FIGURE 44–5. Radiographs of a leg. *A,* Early scurvy: "white line" is visible on the ends of the shafts of the tibia and fibula; rings are shown around the epiphyses of the femur and tibia. *B,* More advanced scorbutic changes; zones of destruction (ZD) are evident in the femur and tibia.

white line, may be present. Epiphyseal separation may occur along the line of destruction with either linear displacement or compression of the epiphysis against the shaft. Subperiosteal hemorrhages are not visible radiographically during the active phase of scurvy. During healing, however, the elevated periosteum becomes calcified and the affected bone assumes a dumbbell or club shape.

A fasting plasma vitamin C concentration of over 0.6 mg/dL aids in precluding vitamin C deficiency, but an even lower concentration does not necessarily indicate deficiency. The ascorbic acid concentration of the white cell/platelet layer (buffy layer) of centrifuged oxalated blood is a better indicator of vitamin C status. A level of zero in this layer indicates latent scurvy, even in the absence of clinical signs of deficiency. Saturation of the tissues with vitamin C can be estimated from the urinary excretion of the vitamin after a test dose of ascorbic acid. In normal children, 80% of the test dose appears in the urine within 3–5 hr after parenteral administration of the test dose. Generalized, nonspecific aminoaciduria is common in scurvy, but plasma amino acid concentrations remain normal. After a tyrosine load, scorbutic infants excrete metabolites similar to those of premature infants.

Scurvy is often misdiagnosed as arthritis or acrodynia. Copper deficiency also results in a radiographic picture that is very similar to that of scurvy. The pseudoparalysis of scurvy often is confused with that of syphilis; however, the latter usually occurs at an earlier age than does that of scurvy and is usually accompanied by other signs of syphilis. Henoch-Schönlein purpura, thrombocytopenic purpura, leukemia, meningitis, or nephritis may also be suspected.

Prevention. Scurvy can be prevented by an adequate intake of vitamin C. Citrus fruits and juices are excellent sources. Formula-fed infants usually receive adequate amounts of ascorbic acid, provided the formula is not heated excessively. Lactating mothers should consume about 100 mg of vitamin C daily. Older children and adults need somewhat more than infants (see Table 40–1).

Treatment. Daily intake of 3–4 oz of orange juice or tomato juice quickly produces healing in children with scurvy, but ascorbic acid is preferable. The daily therapeutic dose is 100–200 mg, orally or parenterally. Recovery, including resumption of normal growth, is rapid with proper treatment. However, the swelling of subperiosteal hemorrhage may not disappear for months.

VITAMIN D

Two forms of vitamin D, vitamin D_2 and vitamin D_3, are of practical importance. Both are produced synthetically and are available as dietary supplements. Vitamin D_3 also is naturally present in human skin; the provitamin form, 7-dehydrocholesterol, is activated photochemically to vitamin D_3 which is then transferred to the liver. Both vitamin D_2 and vitamin D_3 are hydroxylated in the liver to 25-OH-cholecalciferol and, subsequently, in the renal cortex to 1,25-dihydroxycholecalciferol, which functions as a hormone. Receptors for 1,25-dihydroxycholecalciferol are present in most tissues, but its primary roles are facilitation of intestinal absorption of calcium and phosphorus, renal reabsorption of phosphorus, and possibly a direct effect on bone deposition and reabsorption of calcium and phosphorus. With parathormone and calcitonin, 1,25-dihydroxycholecalciferol plays a major role in calcium and phosphorus homeostasis of both body fluids and body tissues.

The usual diet of infants contains only small amounts of vitamin D. Breast milk content is low, and bovine milk content is even lower. Cereals, vegetables, and fruits contain only negligible amounts. Most marketed cow's milk and infant formulas are fortified with vitamin D. Breast milk vitamin D probably is adequate if the infant is exposed sufficiently to sunlight. Dark-skinned infants who are not exposed adequately to sunlight should receive a supplement.

Children with steatorrhea (e.g., those with disorders such as celiac disease and cystic fibrosis) may become deficient secondary to deficient absorption of vitamin D. Anticonvulsant therapy with the phenytoins or phenobarbital may interfere with metabolism of vitamin D and, hence, increase the requirement. In addition, glucocorticoids appear to be antagonistic to vitamin D in calcium transport.

Vitamin D Deficiency

Vitamin D deficiency results in *rickets,* a term signifying failure to mineralize growing bone or osteoid tissue, or osteomalacia. The early changes of rickets are seen radiographically at the ends of long bones, but evidence of demineralization in the shafts also is present. Subsequently, if healing is not initiated, clinical manifestations appear (see later).

Epidemiology. Formerly, the major cause of rickets in the United States was inadequate intake of vitamin D caused by inadequate direct exposure to sunlight, the rays of which do not pass through ordinary window glass, or inadequate vitamin D intake, or both. These are still important causes in developing countries. However, vitamin D deficiency rickets is now rare among infants and children in industrialized countries. Nevertheless, even in these latter countries, deficiency still occurs in unsupplemented dark-skinned infants, in breast-fed infants of mothers who are not exposed to sunlight, and in breast-fed infants who are not exposed to sunlight. There has been an increase in incidence of rickets in these populations of infants.

In industrialized countries, conditions other than inadequate vitamin D intake account for most of the observed cases of rickets (see Chapters 521.5, 696, 697, and 698). These conditions include clinical entities that interfere with vitamin D absorption or metabolic conversion and activation, such as steatorrhea, hepatic and renal diseases, or conditions that disrupt calcium and phosphorus homeostasis in other ways.

Pathophysiology. New bone formation is initiated by osteoblasts, which are responsible for matrix deposition and subsequent mineralization. Osteoblasts secrete collagen, and changes in polysaccharides, phospholipids, alkaline phosphatase, and pyrophosphatase follow until mineralization occurs. However, mineralization cannot occur unless adequate calcium and phosphorus are present. Resorption of bone occurs when osteoclasts secrete enzymes on the bone surface, which dissolve and remove both matrix and mineral. Osteocytes covered by bone both resorb and redeposit bone. The many factors that affect bone growth are poorly understood, but phosphorus, calcium, fluoride, and growth hormone are known to be involved.

In rickets, defective bone growth results from retardation or suppression of normal epiphyseal cartilage growth and calcification. These changes result from a deficiency of calcium and phosphorus salts in the serum. Cartilage cells fail to complete their normal cycle of proliferation and degeneration, with subsequent failure of capillary penetration, which occurs in a patchy manner. The result is a frayed, irregular epiphyseal line at the end of the shaft. Failure of osseous and cartilaginous matrix to mineralize in the zone of preparatory calcification, followed by deposition of newly formed uncalcified osteoid, results in a wide, irregular, frayed zone of nonrigid tissue (the rachitic metaphysis (Fig. 44–6). This zone is responsible for many of the skeletal deformities of rickets. It becomes compressed and bulges laterally, producing flaring of the ends of the bones and the rachitic rosary (Fig. 44–7). Mineralization is also lacking in subperiosteal bone. Pre-existing cortical bone is resorbed in a normal manner, but it is replaced over the entire shaft by osteoid

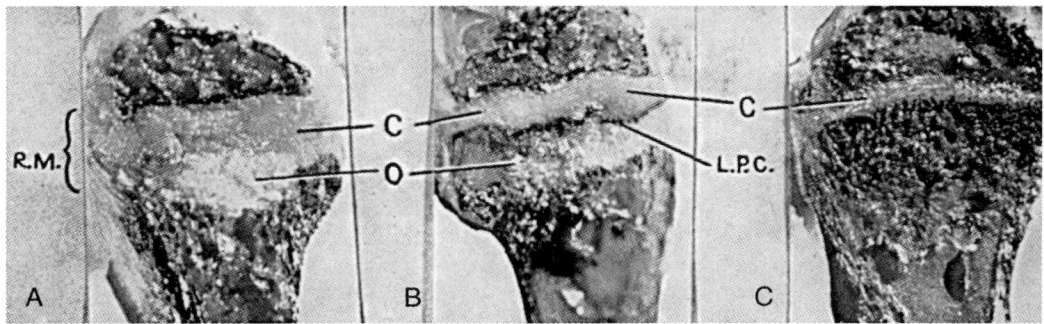

FIGURE 44–6. Line tests in rats (proximal end of the tibia) (calcified tissue stained with silver appears black). *A*, Active rickets. The light broad zone between the epiphysis and the shaft represents the rachitic metaphysis (R.M.) C = cartilage; O = osteoid. *B*, Healing rickets. The line of preparatory calcification (L.P.C.) between the zone of cartilage (C) and the osteoid (O). *C*, Healed rickets. Cartilaginous disc (C) between the epiphysis and the normal shaft.

tissue that fails to mineralize. If this process continues, the shaft loses its rigidity and the softened and rarefied cortical bone is readily distorted by stress, resulting in deformities as well as fractures.

With healing, degeneration of cartilage cells along the metaphyseal-diaphyseal border occurs, capillary penetration of the resultant spaces is resumed, and calcification in the zone of preparatory calcification takes place. This calcification occurs approximately where normal calcification would have occurred had the rachitic process not supervened. It produces a line that is clearly visible on radiographs (Fig. 44–8). As healing progresses, the osteoid tissue between this line of preparatory calcification and the diaphysis also becomes mineralized, as does the osteoid tissue in the cortex and about the trabeculae in the shaft.

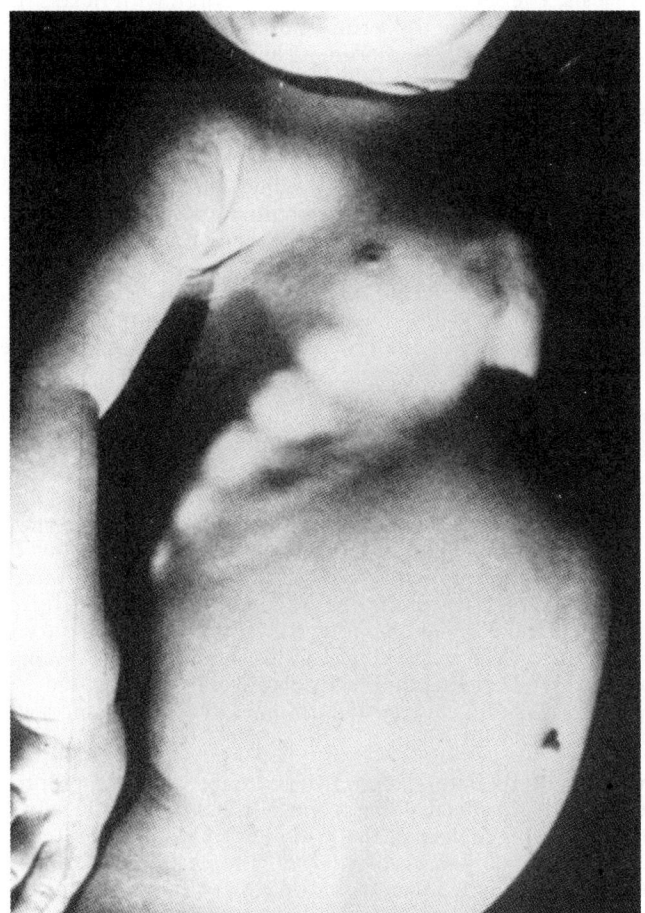

FIGURE 44–7. Rachitic rosary in a young infant.

Vitamin D–deficient rickets can be conceptualized as the body's attempt to maintain normal serum calcium levels. In the absence of vitamin D, less calcium is absorbed from the intestine and, with only a slight decrease in serum calcium concentration, parathormone is secreted. This, in turn, leads to mobilization of calcium and phosphorus from the bone. The serum calcium concentration is, thus, maintained, but secondary effects, including the changes of rickets in bone, a low serum phosphorus concentration (because parathormone decreases phosphorus reabsorption in the kidneys), and elevated serum phosphatase (due to increased osteoblastic activity), take place.

The alkaline phosphatase of serum, less than 200 IU/dL in normal children, increases to more than 500 IU/dL in mild rickets, and much higher levels are not uncommon. However, serum alkaline phosphatase levels may be normal in protein or zinc depleted infants with rickets.

Calcium and phosphorus homeostasis depends on the intestinal absorption of dietary calcium and phosphorus. Maximum calcium absorption occurs when the ratio of calcium to phosphorus in the diet is about 2:1; a lower ratio results in less calcium absorption. Calcium absorption is higher if the intestinal contents are acid and if the dietary sugar is lactose. Chelating agents, including the phytates of cereals, may decrease calcium absorption, and dietary iron may decrease phosphate absorption. High dietary levels of stearic and palmitic acids, which are poorly absorbed, also decrease calcium absorption.

Clinical Manifestations. Craniotabes, one of the early clinical signs of rickets, is caused by thinning of the outer table of the skull. It can be detected by a Ping-Pong ball sensation when pressing firmly over the occiput or posterior parietal bones. Craniotabes near the suture lines is a normal variant. Nonrachitic craniotabes is sometimes present in normal infants during the immediate postnatal period but tends to disappear by the 2nd to 4th mo of life before rachitic softening of the skull would usually become manifest. Craniotabes also occurs in hydrocephalus and osteogenesis imperfecta, but these conditions are easily differentiated from rickets.

Palpable enlargement of the costochondral junctions (the rachitic rosary [see Fig. 44–7]) and thickening of the wrists and ankles (see Fig. 44–8) are other early clinical signs of osseous changes. Enlargement of the costochondral junctions occurs also in scurvy and chondrodystrophy. The enlargements with rickets are rounded knobs, whereas those with scurvy are a ledgelike depression, with the chondral or sternal portion displaced below the osseous ribs. Patients with chondrodystrophy may have irregular, concave outlines of the distal ends of the bones but no radiographic evidence of fraying. Other epiphyseal lesions that may require differentiation from rickets include congenital epiphyseal dysplasia, cytomegalic inclusion disease, syphilis, rubella, and copper deficiency.

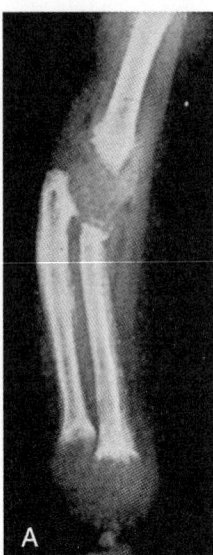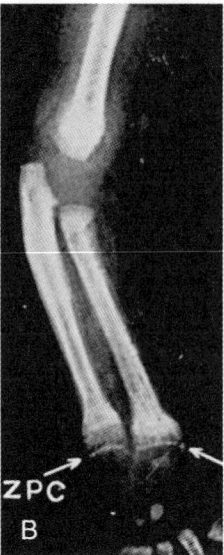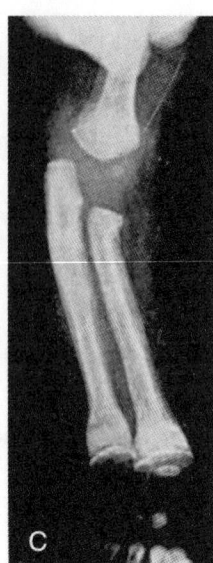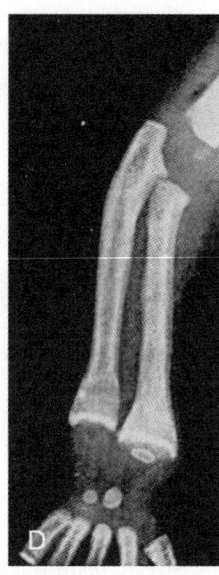

FIGURE 44–8. *A,* Active rickets; cupping and fraying of the distal ends of the radius and ulna; double contour along the lateral outline of the radius (periosteal osteoid). The two dense zones in the shaft of the ulna are calluses of greenstick fractures. *B,* Healing rickets after 12 days of treatment with vitamin D. Zones of preparatory calcification (ZPC); above them in the rachitic metaphyses there is beginning calcification. *C,* Healing rickets after 18 days of treatment. The zones of preparatory calcification are well defined, and the rachitic metaphyses appear well calcified. The epiphysis of the radius has become visible. *D,* Healing rickets after 29 days of treatment. Zones of preparatory calcification, rachitic metaphyses, and shafts have become united.

Enlargement of the costochondral junctions may become prominent; the beading of the ribs is not only palpable but also visible (see Fig. 44–7). The sternum with its adjacent cartilage appears to project forward, the so-called pigeon breast deformity, and a horizontal depression, Harrison groove (Fig. 44–9), develops along the lower border of the chest. These deformities are often difficult to distinguish from congenital deformities.

The softness of the skull may result in flattening and, at times, permanent asymmetry of the head. The anterior fontanel is larger than normal, and its closure may be delayed until after the 2nd yr of life. The central parts of the parietal and frontal bones are often thickened, forming prominences, or bosses, and giving the head a boxlike appearance (caput quadratum). Eruption of the temporary teeth may be delayed, and there may be defects of the enamel and extensive caries. The permanent teeth that are calcifying during the period of vitamin D deficiency may also be affected; the permanent incisors, canines, and first molars almost always have enamel defects.

Children with rickets frequently have a concomitant deformity of the pelvis, which is also retarded in growth. These changes in girls, if they become permanent, add to the hazards of childbirth and may necessitate cesarean section.

As the rachitic process continues, the epiphyseal enlargement at the wrists and ankles becomes more noticeable (see Fig. 44–8), and bending of the softened shafts of the femur, tibia, and fibula results in bowlegs or knock-knees. These are easily distinguishable from familial bow legs.

Greenstick fractures may occur in the long bones, often with no clinical symptoms. Deformities of the spine, pelvis, and legs result in reduced stature or rachitic dwarfism. Relaxation of ligaments contributes to production of the deformities, partly accounting for knock-knees, overextension of the knee joints, weak ankles, kyphosis, and scoliosis. The muscles are poorly developed and lack tone; as a result, children with moderately severe rickets do not stand or walk at the usual ages.

The osseous changes of rickets cannot be recognized radiographically until after several months of vitamin D deficiency. Breast-fed infants of vitamin D–deficient mothers may develop rickets within 2 mo, but rickets usually appears toward the end of the 1st and during the 2nd yr of life. Vitamin D–deficient rickets is rare later in childhood.

Diagnosis. The serum calcium level of children with rickets may be normal or low, but the serum phosphorus level almost always is less than 4 mg/dL. The serum alkaline phosphatase level also is inevitably elevated, and the urinary cyclic AMP level is elevated. Serum 25-hydroxycholecalciferol is low.

Nonspecific findings of vitamin D deficiency include a generalized aminoaciduria, a low bone citrate level with elevated urinary citrate excretion, impaired renal acidification, phosphaturia, and, occasionally, glucosuria. The parathyroid glands hypertrophy in rickets, and urinary cyclic adenosine monophosphate level is increased.

The diagnosis of rickets is based on a history of inadequate intake of vitamin D or inadequate exposure to sunlight and the characteristic clinical signs of the condition. It is confirmed chemically and by radiographic examination.

Prevention. Rickets can be prevented by exposure to ultraviolet light or by oral administration of vitamin D. Formula-fed infants and breast-fed infants of mothers who have adequate exposure to sunlight receive adequate intakes of vitamin D. This remains true after regular bovine milk (but not evaporated milk) replaces breast milk and/or formula.

Breast-fed infants whose mothers are not exposed to adequate sunlight, particularly those who also are protected from sunlight, dark-skinned infants, and infants born during the winter months in temperate climates also should receive a supplement of 400 IU of vitamin D daily, particularly if breast-fed.

Vitamin D should also be administered to pregnant and lactating mothers.

Treatment. Both natural and artificial light of the appropriate wavelength are effective therapeutically, but oral administration of vitamin D is preferred. Daily administration of 50–150 μg of vitamin D$_3$ or 0.5–2 μg of 1,25-dihydroxycholecalciferol produces demonstrable radiographic healing within 2–4 wk, except in cases of vitamin D refractory rickets. Vitamin D$_3$ usually is adequate unless deficiency is secondary to hepatic or renal disease.

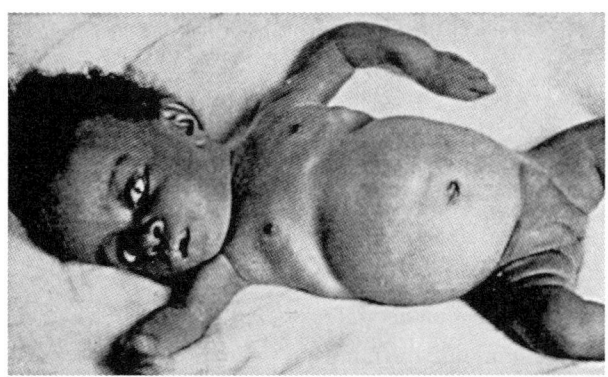

FIGURE 44–9. Deformities in rickets, showing the curvature of the limbs, potbelly, and Harrison groove.

A single dose of 15,000 μg of vitamin D without further therapy for several months may be advantageous. Healing is rapid, possibly allowing earlier differential diagnosis from genetic vitamin D–resistant rickets. If no healing occurs, the rickets is probably resistant to vitamin D (see Chapters 348.1, 521.5, and 696–698).

If sufficient amounts of vitamin D are administered, healing begins within a few days and progresses slowly until the normal bony structure is restored.

Rickets in itself is not a fatal disease, but complications and intercurrent infections are more likely to cause death of rachitic children than normal children.

Tetany of Vitamin D Deficiency (Infantile Tetany)

Tetany due to vitamin D deficiency occasionally accompanies rickets. This type of tetany has virtually disappeared with today's widespread prophylactic use of vitamin D. However, vitamin D deficiency tetany occurs, occasionally, in infants and children with severe steatorrhea, particularly if the serum ionized calcium concentration falls below 3–4 mg/dL. At this level, muscular irritability occurs, apparently due to the loss of the inhibitory control that calcium exerts on the neuromuscular junctions. See also Chapter 48.

Diagnosis is based on the combined presence of rickets, low serum calcium concentration, and symptoms of tetany. The serum phosphorus and alkaline phosphatase levels are similar to those seen in rickets without tetany.

Hypervitaminosis D

Excessive amounts of vitamin D result in signs and symptoms similar to those of idiopathic hypercalcemia (see Chapter 693), which may be due to hypersensitivity to vitamin D. Symptoms, which develop after 1–3 mo of excessive intake, include hypotonia, anorexia, irritability, constipation, polydipsia, polyuria, and pallor. Hypercalcemia and hypercalciuria are notable. Aortic valvular stenosis, vomiting, hypertension, retinopathy, and clouding of the cornea and conjunctiva may occur. Proteinuria may be present and, if excessive intake continues, renal damage and metastatic calcification occur. Radiographs of the long bones reveal metastatic calcification and generalized osteopetrosis.

Metastatic calcification occurs also in chronic nephritis, hyperparathyroidism, and idiopathic hypercalcemia. These conditions, particularly the latter two, also are accompanied by hypercalcemia.

Treatment includes discontinuing vitamin D intake and decreasing calcium intake. For severely affected infants, aluminum hydroxide can be given by mouth. Chelation therapy is rarely necessary.

VITAMIN E

Vitamin E (α-tocopherol) is a fat-soluble antioxidant that may be involved in nucleic acid metabolism, but its precise biochemical action is unclear. It is present in many foods (see Table 44–1).

Deficiency may occur in fat malabsorption states. Diets high in unsaturated fatty acids increase the vitamin E requirement in premature infants who absorb vitamin E poorly. Excess iron administration exaggerates signs of vitamin E deficiency.

Vitamin E Deficiency

Clinical Manifestations. Some vitamin E–deficient individuals have creatinuria, ceroid deposition in smooth muscle, focal necrosis of striated muscle, and muscle weakness. Vitamin E deficiency also has been suggested as a causative factor in the anemia of kwashiorkor. Some premature infants with low serum levels of tocopherol develop hemolytic anemia between 6–10 wk of age that is correctable by administration of vitamin E. Platelet adhesiveness increases in deficiency states, as does the number of platelets. Vitamin E deficiency also has been suggested as a causative factor in retinopathy of prematurity, a possibility that is discussed more fully in Chapters 86 and 621. Patients with malabsorption and vitamin E deficiency secondary to biliary atresia develop a degenerative, potentially reversible, neurologic syndrome consisting of cerebellar ataxia, peripheral neuropathy, and posterior column abnormalities.

Diagnosis. Vitamin E deficiency is best detected by a serum ratio of α-tocopherol to lipid of less than 0.8 mg/g and/or erythrocyte hemolysis in hydrogen peroxide of more than 10%. Three days should elapse before determination of blood levels because orally administered vitamin E may circulate for 1–2 days. Thus, blood levels within 3 days of vitamin E administration may not reliably reflect vitamin E status.

Prevention and Treatment. Minimal daily requirements of vitamin E are not known; 0.7 mg/g of unsaturated fat in the diet appears adequate. Children with deranged fat absorption should receive more. Premature infants may be given up to 15–25 IU per day. Large oral or parenteral doses of vitamin E may prevent permanent neurologic abnormalities in children with biliary atresia or abetalipoproteinemia.

VITAMIN K

Vitamin K is a naphthoquinone that participates in oxidative phosphorylation. Its absence or its failure to be absorbed from the intestinal tract results in hypoprothrombinemia and decreased hepatic synthesis of proconvertin, both of which are important to the second stage of coagulation (see Chapter 467). This stage of coagulation can be assessed by the one-stage prothrombin time (Quick). Administering vitamin K to a newborn infant increases concentrations of prothrombin, proconvertin, plasma thromboplastin component (factor IX), and Stuart-Prower factor (factor X). These four vitamin K–dependent proteins contain γ-carboxyglutamate and require calcium for activity. Other vitamin K–dependent proteins in plasma include proteins C, S, Z, and M. Factors C and S are anticoagulants. Factors Z and M stimulate platelet activity. Vitamin K–dependent calcium-binding proteins such as osteocalcin promote phospholipid interactions in coagulation and in calcium metabolism.

Naturally occurring vitamin K is fat soluble. It is designated vitamin K_1 to distinguish it from vitamin K_2 of bacterial origin and from synthetic naphthoquinones with vitamin K activity. The breast milk content of vitamin K is quite low. That of bovine milk is somewhat higher. The content of infant formulas is adequate. Vitamin K is present in high concentrations in liver, soybeans, and alfalfa and in smaller amounts in vegetables such as spinach, tomatoes, and kale.

Suppression of intestinal bacteria by antibiotics may be responsible for vitamin K deficiency. Irradiated foods have produced vitamin K deficiency in animals.

Vitamin K Deficiency

Clinical Manifestations. Deficiency of vitamin K or hypoprothrombinemia should be considered in all patients with a hemorrhagic disturbance. The incidence of hemorrhagic disease of the newborn (see Chapter 92.4) has dropped sharply since prophylactic administration of vitamin K at birth became common. In childhood, vitamin K deficiency is usually caused by poor fat absorption or factors such as prolonged use of antibiotics that limit synthesis of the vitamin within the intestine. Diarrhea in infants, particularly breast-fed infants, may cause vitamin K deficiency. Diseases of the liver may limit synthesis of prothrombin. Hypoprothrombinemia from this cause usually does not respond to administration of vitamin K.

Hypoprothrombinemia may also result from certain drugs. Dicumarol (or bishydroxycoumarin) is used specifically for the production of hypoprothrombinemia in the prevention and treatment of venous thrombosis. It is thought to prevent the liver from utilizing vitamin K rather than exerting a specific effect on prothrombin. Because blood prothrombin is continually destroyed in the body and dicumarol prevents its replacement, dicumarol treatment results in a decline in prothrombin. If a dangerously low level results, massive doses of vitamin K_1 may be necessary to restore prothrombin levels; whole blood transfusions also may be necessary.

Salicylic acid, a degradation product of dicumarol, produces hypoprothrombinemia by a similar mechanism. The reduction in prothrombin resulting from salicylates, however, is mild compared with that of dicumarol. The hemorrhagic manifestations of acute rheumatic fever may be caused in some cases by large doses of salicylates; this can be reversed by vitamin K adminis-

tration. Thus, its use in children receiving large doses of salicylates appears justified.

Diagnosis. Hypoprothrombinemia that is corrected by vitamin K administration establishes the diagnosis.

Prevention. All infants should receive a prophylactic dose of vitamin K at birth. The breast-fed infant may benefit from additional vitamin K until the diet becomes more varied, but the formula-fed infant receives more than an adequate intake. Infants and children with prolonged diarrhea, as well as those who require prolonged antibiotic treatment or have steatorrhea, should receive supplemental vitamin K.

Treatment. Oral administration of vitamin K may correct mild prothrombin deficiency. For an infant, 1–2 mg every 24 hr usually suffices. If prothrombin deficiency is severe and hemorrhagic manifestations have appeared, 5 mg of vitamin K_1 every 24 hr should be given parenterally. Large doses of synthetic vitamin K analogues, but not vitamin K_1, may result in hyperbilirubinemia and kernicterus in newborns with glucose-6-phosphate dehydrogenase deficiency and in premature infants. Vitamin K can be given for hypoprothrombinemia secondary to liver damage, but whole blood is usually also necessary.

Baxter P, Gardner-Medwin D, Kelly T, et al: Pyridoxine-dependent seizures: Demographic, clinical, MRI and psychometric features, and effect of dose on intelligence quotient. *Dev Med Child Neurol* 1996;38:998.

Bowman BA, Russell RM (editors): *Present Knowledge in Nutrition,* 8th ed. Washington, DC, ILSI Press, 2001, pp 127–270.

DeLuca HF: New concepts of vitamin D functions. *Ann N Y Acad Sci* 1992;669:59.

Hall JG, Solehdin F: Folate and its various ramifications. *Adv Pediatr* 1998;45:1.

Hussey GD, Klein M: A randomized controlled trial of vitamin A in children with severe measles. *N Engl J Med* 1990;323:160.

Leung AKC: Carotenemia. *Adv Pediatr* 1987;34:223.

Neuzil KM, Gruber WC, Chytil F, et al: Serum vitamin A levels in respiratory syncytial virus infection. *J Pediatr* 1994;124:433.

Shils ME, Olson JA, Shike M, et al (editors): *Modern Nutrition in Health and Disease,* 9th ed. Baltimore, Williams & Wilkins 1999, pp 305–483.

Sommer A: Vitamin A prophylaxis. *Arch Dis Child* 1997;77:191.

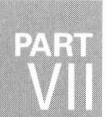

PART VII

Pathophysiology of Body Fluids and Fluid Therapy

Larry A. Greenbaum

Chapter 45

Electrolyte and Acid-Base Disorders

45.1 Composition of Body Fluids

Total Body Water. Water is the most plentiful constituent of the human body. The other components of the body include protein, minerals, fat, and a small amount of carbohydrate. Total body water (TBW) as a percentage of body weight varies with age (Fig. 45–1). The fetus has a very high TBW, which gradually decreases to about 75% of birthweight for a term infant. Premature infants have a higher TBW content than term infants. During the 1st yr of life, TBW decreases to about 60% of body weight and basically remains at this level until puberty. At puberty, the fat content of girls increases more than boys, who acquire more muscle mass than girls. Because fat has very low water content and muscle has high water content, by the end of puberty TBW in boys remains at 60%, but TBW in girls decreases to about 50% of body weight. The high fat content in overweight children causes a decrease in TBW as a percentage of body weight. During dehydration the TBW decreases and, thus, is a smaller percentage of body weight.

Fluid Compartments. TBW is divided between two main compartments: intracellular fluid (ICF) and extracellular fluid (ECF). In the fetus and newborn, the ECF volume is larger than the ICF volume (see Fig. 45–1). The postnatal diuresis causes an immediate decrease in the ECF volume. This is followed by continued expansion of the ICF volume, which results from cellular growth. By 1 yr of age the ratio of the ICF volume to the ECF volume approaches adult levels. The ECF volume is about 20–25% of body weight and the ICF volume is about 30–40% of body weight, close to twice the ECF volume (Fig. 45–2). With puberty, the increased muscle mass of boys causes them to have a higher ICF volume than girls. There is no significant difference in the ECF volume between postpubertal girls and boys.

The ECF is further divided into the plasma water and the interstitial fluid (see Fig. 45–2). The plasma water is normally about 5% of body weight. The blood volume, given a hematocrit of 40%, is usually close to 8% of body weight, although it is higher in newborns and young infants. In premature newborns it is around 10% of body weight. The volume of plasma water can be altered by a variety of pathologic conditions, including dehydration, anemia, polycythemia, heart failure, abnormal

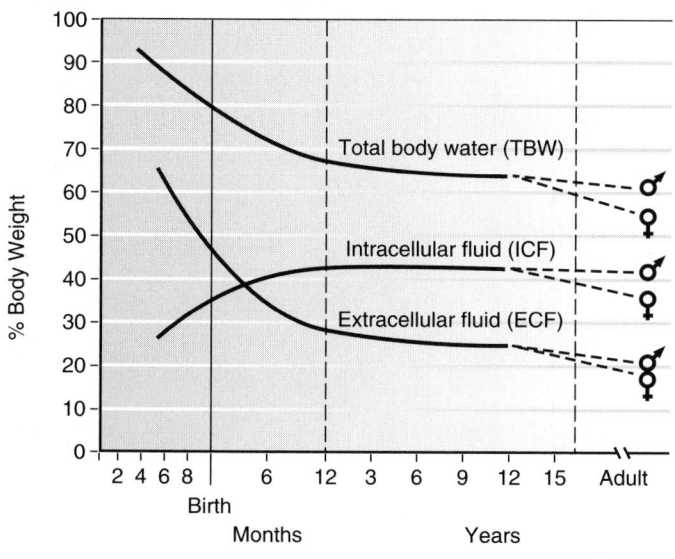

FIGURE 45–1. Total body water, intracellular fluid, and extracellular fluid as a percentage of body weight and a function of age. (From Winters RW: Water and electrolyte regulation. In Winters RW [editor]: *The Body Fluids in Pediatrics.* Boston, Little, Brown & Company, 1973.)

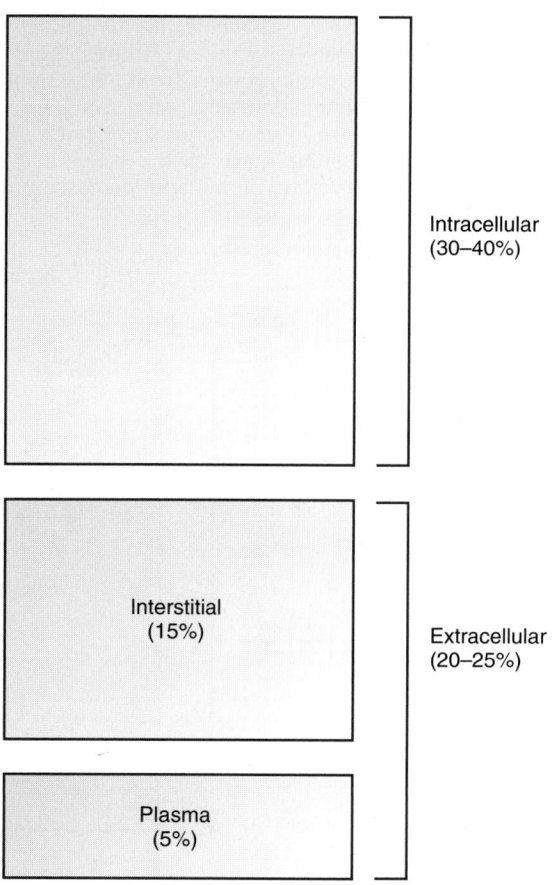

FIGURE 45–2. Compartments of total body water, expressed as a percentage of body weight, in an older child or adult.

plasma osmolality, and hypoalbuminemia. The interstitial fluid, normally about 15% of body weight, can increase dramatically in diseases associated with edema such as heart failure, liver failure, nephrotic syndrome, and other causes of hypoalbuminemia. An increase in interstitial fluid occurs when patients develop ascites or pleural effusions.

There is normally a delicate equilibrium between the intravascular fluid and the interstitial fluid. The balance between hydrostatic and oncotic forces regulates the intravascular volume, which is critical for proper tissue perfusion. The intravascular fluid has a higher concentration of albumin than the interstitial fluid, and the consequent oncotic force draws water into the intravascular space. The maintenance of this gradient depends on the limited permeability of albumin across the capillaries. In contrast, the hydrostatic pressure of the intravascular space, which is due to the pumping action of the heart, drives fluid out of the intravascular space. In the capillaries these forces favor movement into the interstitial space at the arterial end of the capillaries. The decreased hydrostatic forces and increased oncotic forces, which result from the dilutional increase in albumin concentration, cause movement of fluid into the capillaries at the venous end of the capillaries. Overall, there is usually a net movement of fluid out of the intravascular space, but this fluid is returned to the circulation via the lymphatics. An imbalance in these forces may cause expansion of the interstitial volume at the expense of the intravascular volume. In children with hypoalbuminemia, the decreased oncotic pressure of the intravascular fluid contributes to the development of edema. Loss of fluid from the intravascular space may compromise the intravascular volume, placing the child at risk for inadequate blood flow to vital organs. This is especially likely in diseases with capillary leak because the loss of albumin from the intravascular space is associated with an increase in the albumin concentration in the interstitial space, further compromising the oncotic forces that normally maintain intravascular volume. In contrast, with heart failure, there is an increase in venous hydrostatic pressure from expansion of the intravascular volume, which is caused by impaired pumping by the heart, and the increase in venous pressure causes fluid to move from the intravascular space to the interstitial space. Expansion of the intravascular volume and increased intravascular pressure also cause the edema that occurs with acute glomerulonephritis.

Electrolyte Composition. The composition of the solutes in the ICF and ECF are very different (Fig. 45–3). Sodium and chloride are the dominant cations and anions, respectively, in the ECF. The sodium and chloride concentrations in the ICF are much lower. Potassium is the most abundant cation in the ICF, and its concentration within the cells is approximately 30 times higher than in the ECF. Proteins, organic anions, and phosphate are the most plentiful anions in the ICF. The dissimilarity between the anions in the ICF and the ECF is largely determined by the presence of intracellular molecules that do not cross the cell membrane. In contrast, the barrier separating the ECF and the ICF. In contrast, the difference in the distribution of cations—sodium and potassium—is due to the activity of the Na^+,K^+-ATPase, which uses cellular energy to extrude sodium from cells and move potassium into cells. The chemical gradient between the intracellular potassium concentration and extracellular potassium concentration creates the electrical gradient across the cell membrane. Specifically, the concentration-dependent movement of potassium out of the cell makes the intracellular space negative relative to the extracellular space.

The difference in the electrolyte compositions of the ECF and the ICF has important ramifications when evaluating and treating electrolyte disorders. The serum concentration of an electrolyte, which is measured clinically, does not always reflect the body content. This is due to the larger volume of the ICF compared with the ECF and the variation in electrolyte concentrations between these two compartments caused by intracellular processes. For example, the intracellular potassium concentration is much higher than the serum concentration. A shift of potassium from the intracellular potassium pool can maintain a normal or even an elevated serum potassium concentration, despite massive losses of potassium from the intracellular pool. This is dramatically seen in diabetic ketoacidosis, in which a state of significant potassium depletion is often masked because of a shift of potassium from the ICF to the ECF. For potassium and phosphorus, electrolytes with a high intracellular concentration, the serum level may not accurately reflect total body content. This may also be seen with the serum magnesium con-

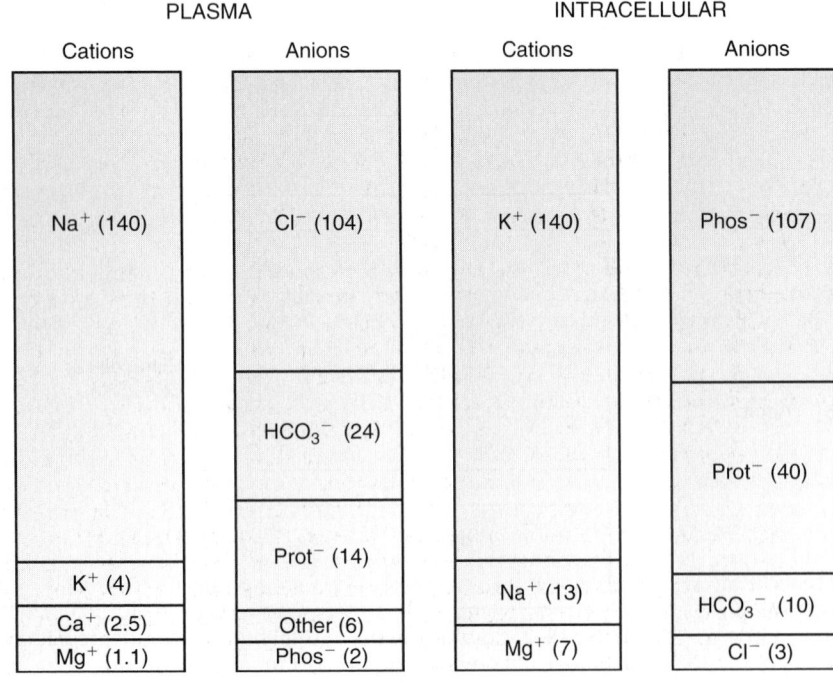

PLASMA		INTRACELLULAR	
Cations	Anions	Cations	Anions
Na⁺ (140)	Cl⁻ (104)	K⁺ (140)	Phos⁻ (107)
	HCO₃⁻ (24)		Prot⁻ (40)
	Prot⁻ (14)		
K⁺ (4)		Na⁺ (13)	HCO₃⁻ (10)
Ca⁺ (2.5)	Other (6)		
Mg⁺ (1.1)	Phos⁻ (2)	Mg⁺ (7)	Cl⁻ (3)

FIGURE 45–3. The concentrations of the major cations and anions in the intracellular space and the plasma, expressed in mEq/L.

centration. Similarly and more dramatically, the serum calcium concentration does not predict the body content of calcium, which is largely in bone.

Osmolality. The ICF and the ECF are in osmotic equilibrium because the cell membrane is freely permeable to water. If the osmolality in one compartment changes, then water movement leads to a rapid equalization of osmolality. This can lead to significant shifts of water between the intracellular space and the extracellular space. Clinically, the primary process is usually a change in the osmolality of the ECF, with a resultant shift of water into the ICF if the ECF osmolality decreases or a shift of water out of the ICF if the ECF osmolality increases. The osmolality of the ECF can be determined, and this equals the ICF osmolality. The plasma osmolality is normally 285–295 mOsm/kg, and it is measured by the degree of freezing point depression. The plasma osmolality can also be calculated based on the following formula:

$$Osmolality = 2 \times [Na] + [Glucose]/18 + [BUN]/2.8$$

Glucose and blood urea nitrogen (BUN) are measured in mg/dL. Division by 18 and 2.8 converts the units into mmol/L. Multiplication of sodium by 2 accounts for its accompanying anions, principally chloride and bicarbonate. The calculated osmolality is usually slightly lower than the measured osmolality.

In most situations, glucose and urea contribute little to the plasma osmolality; multiplication of the sodium by 2 provides a rough approximation of the osmolality. In children with uremia, the urea concentration can have a significant impact on the plasma osmolality. However, urea is not confined to the extracellular space; it readily crosses cell membranes and its intracellular concentration approximately equals its extracellular concentration. Only substances that are confined to the extracellular space are osmotically active. Whereas an elevated sodium concentration causes a shift of water from the intracellular space, with uremia there is no osmolar gradient between the two compartments and consequently no movement of water. Urea is therefore considered an "ineffective osmole," and hyperosmolality from uremia does not cause a fluid shift. The only exception is during hemodialysis, when the decrease in extracellular urea is so rapid that the intracellular urea does not have time to equilibrate. This may lead to the disequilibrium syndrome, in which water shifts into brain cells, potentially causing severe symptoms. Ethanol, because it freely crosses cell membranes, is another ineffective osmole. The effective osmolality can be calculated as follows:

$$Effective \ osmolality = 2 \times [Na] + [Glucose]/18$$

The effective osmolality (also called the tonicity) determines the osmotic force that is mediating the shift of water between the ECF and the ICF.

Hyperglycemia causes an increase in the plasma osmolality and, unlike urea, glucose is an effective osmole because it is not in equilibrium with the intracellular space. During hyperglycemia there is a shift of water from the intracellular space to the extracellular space. This is clinically important in children with hyperglycemia during diabetic ketoacidosis. The shift of water causes dilution of the sodium in the extracellular space, causing hyponatremia despite an elevated plasma osmolality. The magnitude of this effect can be calculated as follows:

$$[Na]_{corrected} = [Na]_{measured} + 1.6 \times ([Glucose] - 100 \ mg/dL)/100$$

where $[Na]_{measured}$ equals the sodium concentration measured by the clinical laboratory and $[Na]_{corrected}$ equals the corrected sodium concentration (the sodium concentration if the glucose concentration were normal and its accompanying water moved back into the cells). The $[Na]_{corrected}$ is the more reliable indicator of the patient's true ratio of total body sodium to TBW, the normal determinant of the sodium concentration.

Normally the measured osmolality and the calculated osmolality are within 10 mOsm/kg. There are some clinical situations in which this does not occur. The presence of "unmeasured osmoles" causes the measured osmolality to be significantly elevated when compared with the calculated osmolality. This difference is the *osmolal gap*, which is present when the measured osmolality is more than 10 mOsm/kg greater than the calculated osmolality. Some examples of unmeasured osmoles include ethanol, ethylene glycol, methanol, and mannitol. These substances increase the measured osmolality, but are not part of the equation for calculating osmolality. The presence of an osmolal gap is a clinical clue to the presence of unmeasured osmoles and may be diagnostically useful when there is clinical suspicion of poisoning with methanol or ethylene glycol. A measured osmolality is necessary when monitoring the effect of mannitol therapy on plasma osmolality.

Pseudohyponatremia is a second situation in which there is discordance between the measured and calculated osmolality. Lipids and proteins are the solids of the serum. In patients with elevated serum lipids or proteins, the water content of the serum decreases because water is displaced by the increased amount of solids. Some clinical laboratories measure sodium concentration by determining the amount of sodium per liter of serum, including the solid component. When the solid component increases, there is a decrease in the sodium concentration per liter of serum, despite a normal concentration of sodium when based on the amount of sodium per liter of serum water. It is the concentration of sodium in serum water that is physiologically relevant. In such situations, the plasma osmolality is normal despite the presence of pseudohyponatremia because the method for measuring osmolality is not appreciably influenced by the percentage of serum that is composed of lipids and proteins. Pseudohyponatremia is diagnosed by finding a normal measured plasma osmolality despite hyponatremia. This laboratory artifact does not occur if the sodium concentration in water is measured directly with an ion-specific electrode, the technique that is increasingly used in clinical laboratories.

When there are no unmeasured osmoles and pseudohyponatremia is not a concern, the calculated osmolality provides an accurate estimate of the plasma osmolality. Measurement of plasma osmolality is useful for detecting or monitoring unmeasured osmoles and confirming the presence of true hyponatremia. Whereas many children with high plasma osmolality are dehydrated—as seen with hypernatremic dehydration or diabetic ketoacidosis—high osmolality does not always equate with dehydration. For example, a child with salt poisoning or uremia has an elevated plasma osmolality, but may be volume overloaded. In many situations it is best to focus on the components of the plasma osmolality and to analyze them individually to reach a correct clinical conclusion. The effective osmolality, which must be calculated, does provide useful information regarding the distribution of water between the ECF and ICF.

45.2 Regulation of Osmolality and Volume

Proper cell functioning requires close regulation of plasma osmolality and intravascular volume. These are controlled by independent systems for water balance, which determines osmolality, and sodium balance, which determines volume status. Maintenance of a normal osmolality depends on control of water balance. Although sodium concentration is the dominant determinant of plasma osmolality, the body does not control osmolality by regulating sodium balance. Normally, control of volume status depends on regulation of sodium balance. However, when volume depletion is present, this takes precedence over regulation of osmolality, and retention of water contributes to maintenance of intravascular volume.

Regulation of Osmolality. The plasma osmolality is tightly regulated to maintain it between 285 and 295 mOsm/kg. Modification of water intake and excretion maintains a normal plasma osmolality. In the steady state, water intake and water produced by the body from oxidation balances water losses from the skin, lungs, urine, and gastrointestinal tract. Only water intake and urinary losses can be regulated.

Osmoreceptors in the hypothalamus sense the plasma osmolality. It is only the effective osmolality that is sensed; this does not include solutes such as urea that readily diffuse across the cell membrane. An elevated effective osmolality leads to secretion of antidiuretic hormone (ADH) by neurons in the supraoptic and paraventricular nuclei in the hypothalamus. The axons of these neurons terminate in the posterior pituitary. Circulating ADH binds to its V_2 receptors in the collecting duct cells of the kidney, and, via the generation of cyclic adenosine monophosphate (cAMP), causes insertion of water channels (aquaporin-2) into the renal collecting ducts. This produces increased permeability to water, permitting reabsorption of water into the hypertonic renal medulla. The end result is that the urine concentration increases and water excretion decreases. Urinary water losses cannot be completely eliminated because there is obligatory excretion of urinary solutes, such as urea and sodium. The regulation of ADH secretion is tightly linked to plasma osmolality, with responses detectable with a 1% change in the osmolality. ADH secretion virtually disappears when the plasma osmolality is low, and this allows excretion of maximally dilute urine. The consequent loss of free water (water without sodium) corrects the plasma osmolality. ADH secretion is not an "all or nothing" response; there is a graded adjustment as the osmolality changes.

Production of concentrated urine under the control of ADH requires a hypertonic renal medulla. The counter current multiplier, produced by the loop of Henle and the vasa recta, generate this hypertonicity. ADH stimulates sodium transport in the loop of Henle, helping to maintain this gradient when water retention is necessary.

Water intake is regulated by hypothalamic osmoreceptors, though these are different from the osmoreceptors that determine ADH secretion. These osmoreceptors, by linking to the cerebral cortex, stimulate thirst when the serum osmolality increases. Thirst occurs with a small increase in the serum osmolality.

Control of osmolality is subordinate to maintenance of an adequate intravascular volume. When volume depletion is present, both ADH secretion and thirst are stimulated, regardless of the plasma osmolality. The sensation of thirst requires moderate volume depletion, but only a 1–2% change in the plasma osmolality. Although all of the mechanisms are not clear, angiotensin II, which is increased during volume depletion, is known to stimulate thirst. Baroreceptors, when sensing volume depletion, may also stimulate thirst.

A number of conditions can limit the kidney's ability to excrete adequate water to correct low plasma osmolality. In the syndrome of inappropriate antidiuretic hormone (SIADH), ADH continues to be produced despite a low plasma osmolality. In the presence of ADH, urinary dilution does not occur, and sufficient water is not excreted. A variety of diseases—mostly central nervous system, but also pulmonary and neoplastic—can cause SIADH (see Chapter 553). Iatrogenic excess of ADH is possible with the use of desmopressin acetate, a synthetic analog of ADH. Other medications, including narcotics, nicotine, cholinergics and barbiturates, stimulate ADH release. Although not as dramatic as SIADH, stress—such as pain, trauma, surgery, or burns—stimulates ADH release, preventing adequate water excretion and potentially causing hyponatremia.

The glomerular filtration rate (GFR) affects the kidney's ability to eliminate water. With a decrease in GFR, less water is delivered to the collecting duct, limiting the amount of water that can be excreted. The impairment in GFR must be quite significant to limit the kidney's ability to respond to an excess of water.

The minimum urine osmolality is approximately 30–50 mOsm/kg. This places an upper limit on the kidney's ability to excrete water; there must be sufficient solute present to permit water loss. Massive water intoxication may exceed this limit, whereas a lesser amount of water is necessary in the child with a diet that has very little solute. This is occasionally seen and can produce severe hyponatremia in children who receive little salt and have little urea production as a result of inadequate protein intake. Volume depletion is an extremely important cause of inadequate water loss by the kidney despite a low plasma osmolality. This "appropriate" secretion of ADH occurs because volume depletion takes precedence over the osmolality in the regulation of ADH.

The normal response to an increased plasma osmolality is conservation of water by the kidney. In central diabetes insipidus this does not occur because of an absence of ADH secretion (see Chapter 552). Ethanol produces a transient decrease in ADH production. Patients with nephrogenic diabetes insipidus (NDI) have an inability to respond to ADH and produce dilute urine despite an increase in plasma osmolality. This is most dramatic in the inherited causes of NDI. X-linked NDI is due to an absence of the ADH receptor. The less common autosomal recessive form is secondary to a deficiency in aquaporin-2, the water channel that is necessary for retention of water by the collecting duct of the kidney. There is an extensive list of secondary causes of NDI, including medications such as lithium and kidney disorders such as renal dysplasia and acute tubular necrosis (see Chapter 522).

The maximum urine osmolality is about 1,200 mOsm/kg. The obligatory solute losses dictate the minimum volume of urine that must be produced, even when maximally concentrated. Obligatory water losses increase in patients with high salt intake or in patients with high urea losses, as may occur after relief of a urinary obstruction or during recovery from acute tubular necrosis. An increase in urinary solute and consequently water losses occurs with an osmotic diuresis, classically seen due to glucosuria in diabetes mellitus, and iatrogenically following mannitol administration. There are developmental changes in the kidney's ability to concentrate the urine. The maximum urine osmolality in a newborn, and especially a premature newborn, is less than in an older infant or child. This limits the ability to conserve water and makes these patients more vulnerable to hypernatremic dehydration. Very high fluid intake, as seen with psychogenic polydipsia, can dilute the high osmolality in the renal medulla, which is necessary for maximal urinary concentration. If fluid intake is restricted in these patients, there may be some impairment in the kidney's ability to concentrate the urine, although this defect corrects after a few days without polydipsia. This may also occur during the initial treatment of central diabetes insipidus with desmopressin acetate; the renal medulla takes time to achieve its normal maximum osmolality. Loop diuretics, such as furosemide, by inhibiting sodium reabsorption in the ascending limb of the loop of Henle, decrease medullary hypertonicity, preventing excretion of maximally concentrated urine.

Regulation of Volume. An appropriate intravascular volume is critical for survival; both volume depletion and volume overload may cause significant morbidity and mortality. Because sodium is the principal extracellular cation and sodium is restricted to the ECF, adequate body sodium is necessary for maintenance of intravascular volume. The principal extracellular anion, chloride, is also necessary, but for simplicity, sodium balance is considered the main regulator of volume status because body content of sodium and chloride usually changes proportionally given the need for equal numbers of cations and anions. In some situations, chloride depletion is considered the dominant derangement causing volume depletion (e.g., metabolic alkalosis with volume depletion). In other situations, such as volume depletion with metabolic acidosis, sodium depletion may exceed chloride depletion.

The kidney determines sodium balance because there is little homeostatic control of sodium intake, even though salt craving does occasionally occur, typically in children with chronic renal salt loss. The kidney regulates sodium balance by altering the percentage of filtered sodium that is reabsorbed along the nephron. Normally, the kidney excretes less than 1% of the sodium filtered at the glomerulus. In the absence of disease, extrarenal losses and urinary output match intake, with the kidney having the capacity to adapt to large variations in sodium intake. When necessary, urinary sodium excretion can be reduced to virtually undetectable levels or increased dramatically.

Urinary sodium excretion is regulated by both intrarenal and extrarenal mechanisms. The most important determinant of renal sodium excretion is the volume status of the child. More precisely, it is the *effective* intravascular volume that influences urinary sodium excretion. The effective intravascular volume is the volume status that is sensed by the body's regulatory mechanisms. For example, congestive heart failure is a state of volume overload, but the effective intravascular volume is low because poor cardiac function prevents adequate perfusion of the kidneys and other organs. This explains the avid renal sodium retention that is often present in such patients.

Sodium reabsorption occurs throughout the nephron (also see Chapter 520). Whereas the majority of filtered sodium is reabsorbed in the proximal tubule and the loop of Henle, the distal tubule and collecting duct are the main sites for precise regulation of sodium balance. Approximately 65% of the filtered sodium is reclaimed in the proximal tubule, which is the major site for reabsorption of bicarbonate, glucose, phosphate, amino acids, and other substances that are filtered by the glomerulus. The transport of all these substances is linked to sodium reabsorption by co-transporters or a sodium-hydrogen exchanger in the case of bicarbonate. This is clinically important for bicarbonate and phosphate because their reabsorption parallels sodium reabsorption. For example, in patients with metabolic alkalosis and volume depletion, correction of the metabolic alkalosis requires urinary loss of bicarbonate, but the volume depletion stimulates sodium and bicarbonate retention, preventing correction of the alkalosis. Similarly, volume expansion causes increased urinary losses of phosphate, even when there is phosphate depletion. In addition, reabsorption of uric acid and urea occurs in the proximal tubule and increases when sodium retention increases. This accounts for the elevated uric acid and BUN measurements that often accompany dehydration, which is a stimulus for sodium retention in the proximal tubule. The cells of the proximal tubule are permeable to water and thus water reabsorption in this segment parallels sodium reabsorption.

The loop of Henle is, in terms of absolute amount, the second most important site of sodium reabsorption along the nephron. The $Na^+,K^+,2Cl^-$ co-transporter on the luminal side of the membrane reclaims filtered sodium and chloride, while most of the potassium is recycled back into the lumen. This is the transporter that is inhibited by furosemide and other loop diuretics, which are highly effective at increasing sodium excretion. The ascending limb of the loop of Henle is not permeable to water, permitting sodium retention without water. ADH stimulates sodium retention in this segment; this helps to create a more hypertonic medulla, which maximizes water conservation when ADH acts in the medullary collecting duct. Because loop diuretics inhibit sodium retention in this segment, their use

causes a less hypertonic medulla, and this prevents excretion of maximally concentrated urine in the presence of ADH.

Sodium retention in the distal tubule is mediated by the thiazide-sensitive Na^+,Cl^- co-transporter. This segment of the nephron is relatively impermeable to water and, along with sodium and chloride retention, the distal tubule is important for delivery of fluid with a low sodium concentration to the collecting duct. This allows for excretion of water without sodium in patients who stop secreting ADH due to low plasma osmolality. Thiazide diuretics, by inhibiting sodium and chloride retention in this segment, prevent the excretion of water without electrolytes. This is a partial explanation for the severe hyponatremia that occasionally develops in patients on chronic thiazide diuretics.

The collecting duct, the final segment of the nephron, is important for regulation of excretion of water, potassium, acid, and sodium. Even though the amount of sodium reabsorbed in this segment is less than in any other segment, this is the critical site for the regulation of sodium balance. Sodium reabsorption occurs via a sodium channel that aldosterone regulates. When these channels are open under the influence of aldosterone, almost all of the sodium can be reabsorbed. The uptake of sodium creates a negative charge in the lumen of the collecting duct, which facilitates the secretion of potassium and hydrogen ions. The potassium-sparing diuretics amiloride and triamterene block these sodium channels, and the inhibition of sodium uptake decreases potassium excretion. In contrast, the potassium-sparing diuretic spironolactone blocks the binding of aldosterone to its receptor, and thus indirectly decreases the activity of the sodium channels. The collecting duct is important for regulation of water balance because it responds to ADH by inserting water channels that increase the permeability to water, and the hypertonicity of the renal medulla allows for maximal concentration of the urine.

Given the importance of sodium balance, it is not surprising that a number of systems are involved in the regulation of renal sodium excretion. The amount of sodium filtered at the glomerulus is directly proportional to the GFR. If sodium reabsorption in the nephron were constant, this would lead to complete reabsorption of sodium with a small decrease in the GFR and significant renal sodium wasting with a small increase. This does not occur, however, because sodium reabsorption in the nephron is proportional to sodium delivery, a principle called *glomerular tubular balance*.

The renin-angiotensin system is an important regulator of renal sodium excretion. The juxtaglomerular apparatus produces renin in response to decreased effective intravascular volume. Specific stimuli for renin release are decreased perfusion pressure in the afferent arteriole, decreased delivery of sodium to the distal nephron, and ß1-adrenergic agonists, which increase during intravascular volume depletion. Renin, a proteolytic enzyme, cleaves angiotensinogen, producing angiotensin I. Angiotensin-converting enzyme (ACE) converts angiotensin I into angiotensin II. The actions of angiotensin II include direct stimulation of the proximal tubule to increase sodium reabsorption and stimulation of the adrenal gland to increase aldosterone secretion. Through its actions in the distal nephron, specifically the late distal convoluted tubule and the collecting duct, aldosterone increases sodium reabsorption. Aldosterone also stimulates potassium excretion, causing increased urinary losses. Along with decreasing urinary loss of sodium, angiotensin II is a vasoconstrictor, which helps to maintain an adequate blood pressure in the presence of volume depletion.

Volume expansion stimulates the synthesis of atrial natriuretic peptide (ANP), which is produced by the atria in response to distention. Along with increasing GFR, ANP inhibits sodium reabsorption in the medullary portion of the collecting duct, facilitating an increase in urinary sodium excretion.

Volume overload occurs when sodium intake exceeds output. In children with kidney failure there is an impaired ability to excrete sodium. This tends to be proportional to the decrease in GFR, although in some kidney diseases, such as renal dysplasia or juvenile nephronophthisis, damaged tubules cause significant sodium loss until the GFR is almost zero. In general, as the GFR decreases, restriction of sodium intake becomes increasingly necessary. The GFR is low at birth, which limits a newborn's ability to excrete a sodium load. In other situations there is a loss of the appropriate regulation of renal sodium excretion. This occurs in patients with excessive aldosterone, as is seen in primary hyperaldosteronism or renal artery stenosis, wherein excess renin production leads to high aldosterone levels. In acute glomerulonephritis, even without a significantly reduced GFR, the normal intrarenal mechanisms that regulate sodium excretion malfunction, causing excessive renal retention of sodium and volume overload.

Renal retention of sodium occurs during volume depletion, but this appropriate response causes the severe excess in total body sodium that is present in congestive heart failure, liver failure, nephrotic syndrome, and other causes of hypoalbuminemia. In these diseases, the effective intravascular volume is decreased, causing the kidney and the various regulatory systems to respond, leading to renal sodium retention and edema formation.

Volume depletion usually occurs when losses of sodium exceed intake. The most common etiology in children is gastroenteritis. Along with the gastrointestinal tract, excessive losses of sodium may occur from the skin in children with burns, in sweat in patients with cystic fibrosis, or after vigorous exercise. Inadequate intake of sodium is uncommon except in neglect, famine, or with an inappropriate choice of liquid diet in a child who cannot take solids. Urinary sodium wasting may occur in a range of renal diseases, from renal dysplasia to tubular disorders such as Bartter syndrome. The neonate, especially if premature, has a mild impairment in the ability to conserve sodium. Iatrogenic renal sodium wasting takes place during diuretic therapy. Renal sodium loss occurs as a result of derangement in the normal regulatory systems. An absence of aldosterone, seen most commonly in children with congenital adrenal hyperplasia due to 21-hydroxylase deficiency, causes sodium wasting. In cerebral salt wasting, there may be a brain natruretic peptide that produces volume depletion secondary to renal sodium loss.

Isolated disorders of water balance can affect volume status and sodium balance. Because the cell membrane is permeable to water, changes in TBW influence both the extracellular volume and the intracellular volume. In isolated water loss, as occurs in diabetes insipidus, the impact is greater on the intracellular space because of its higher volume compared with the extracellular space. This is why, compared with other types of dehydration, hypernatremic dehydration has less impact on plasma volume; most of the fluid loss comes from the intracellular space. Yet, significant water loss does eventually affect intravascular volume and will stimulate renal sodium retention, even if total body sodium content is normal. Similarly with acute water intoxication or SIADH, there is an excess of TBW, but most is in the intracellular space. However, there is some impact on the intravascular volume, and this causes renal excretion of sodium. Children with SIADH or water intoxication have high urine sodium concentrations despite hyponatremia. This reinforces the concept that there are independent control systems for water and sodium, yet the two systems interact when pathophysiologic processes dictate, and control of effective intravascular volume always takes precedence over control of osmolality.

45.3 Sodium

SODIUM METABOLISM

Body Content and Physiologic Function. Sodium is the dominant cation of the ECF (see Fig. 45–3), and it is the principal determi-

nant of extracellular osmolality. Sodium is therefore necessary for the maintenance of intravascular volume. Less than 3% of sodium is intracellular. More than 40% of total body sodium is in bone; the remainder is in the interstitial and intravascular spaces. The low intracellular sodium concentration, about 10 mEq/L, is maintained by Na^+,K^+-ATPase, which exchanges intracellular sodium for extracellular potassium. The chemical gradient created by the high extracellular sodium concentration and the low intracellular sodium concentration provides the energy for the movement of a variety of substances into cells.

Intake. A child's diet determines the amount of sodium ingested—a predominantly cultural determination in older children. An occasional child has salt craving due to an underlying salt-wasting disease. Children in the United States tend to have very high sodium intakes because their diets include a large amount of "junk food" and "fast food." Infants receive sodium from breast milk (about 7 mEq/L) and formula (7–13 mEq/L for 20 calorie/oz formula).

Sodium is absorbed throughout the gastrointestinal tract, with limited regulation. Mineralocorticoids increase sodium transport into the body, although this has limited clinical significance. The presence of glucose enhances sodium absorption due to the presence of a co-transport system. This is the rationale for including sodium and glucose in oral rehydration solutions.

Excretion. Sodium excretion occurs in stool and sweat, but the kidney regulates sodium balance and is normally the principal site of sodium excretion. There is some sodium loss in stool, but this is minimal unless diarrhea is present. Normally, sweat has 5–40 mEq/L of sodium. There is increased sweat sodium concentration in children with cystic fibrosis, aldosterone deficiency, or pseudohypoaldosteronism. The higher sweat losses in these conditions may cause or contribute to sodium depletion.

Sodium is unique among electrolytes because water balance, not sodium balance, usually determines its concentration. Normally, when the sodium concentration increases, the resultant higher plasma osmolality causes increased thirst and increased secretion of ADH, which leads to renal conservation of water. Both of these mechanisms increase the water content of the body, and the sodium concentration returns to normal. During hyponatremia, the decrease in plasma osmolality stops ADH secretion, and consequent renal water excretion leads to an increase in the sodium concentration. Even though water balance is usually regulated by osmolality, volume depletion does stimulate thirst, ADH secretion, and renal conservation of water. In fact, volume depletion takes precedence over osmolality; volume depletion stimulates ADH secretion even if a patient has hyponatremia. This principle is critical for understanding the pathophysiology of many causes of hyponatremia.

The excretion of sodium by the kidney is *not* regulated by the plasma osmolality. The patient's effective plasma volume determines the amount of sodium in the urine. This is mediated by a variety of regulatory systems, including the renin-angiotensin-aldosterone system and intrarenal mechanisms. In hyponatremia or hypernatremia, the underlying pathophysiology determines the amount of urinary sodium, not the serum sodium concentration.

HYPERNATREMIA

Hypernatremia is a sodium concentration greater than 145 mEq/L, although it is sometimes defined as greater than 150 mEq/L. Mild hypernatremia is fairly common in children, especially among infants with gastroenteritis. Hypernatremia in hospitalized patients is frequently iatrogenic, caused by inadequate water administration or excessive sodium administration. Moderate or severe hypernatremia has significant morbidity, the result of underlying disease, the effects of hypernatremia on the brain, and the risks of overly rapid correction.

Etiology and Pathophysiology. There are three basic mechanisms of hypernatremia (Box 45–1). Sodium intoxication is frequently iatrogenic in a hospital setting as a result of correction of metabolic acidosis with sodium bicarbonate. Baking soda, a putative remedy for upset stomach, is another source of sodium bicarbonate; the hypernatremia is accompanied by a profound metabolic alkalosis. In hyperaldosteronism, there is excessive renal retention of sodium.

The classic causes of hypernatremia from a water deficit are nephrogenic and central diabetes insipidus (see Chapters 522 and 552). Hypernatremia in diabetes insipidus only develops if the patient does not have access to water or cannot drink adequately because of neurologic impairment, emesis, or anorexia. Infants are at high risk because of their inability to control their own water intake. Central diabetes insipidus and the genetic forms of nephrogenic diabetes insipidus typically cause massive urinary water losses and very dilute urine. In contrast, the water losses are less dramatic and the urine often has the same osmolality as plasma when nephrogenic diabetes insipidus is secondary to diseases such as obstructive uropathy, renal dysplasia, or sickle cell disease. The other causes of a water deficit are also secondary to an imbalance between losses and intake. Newborns, especially if premature, have high insensible water losses. Losses are further increased under a radiant warmer or if the baby is receiving phototherapy for hyperbilirubinemia. The renal concentrating mechanisms are not optimal at birth, providing an additional source of water loss. Ineffective breast-feeding, often in a primipara, can cause severe hypernatremic dehydration. Adipsia, the absence of thirst, is usually secondary to damage to the hypothalamus, such as from trauma, tumor, hydrocephalus, or histiocytosis. Primary adipsia is rare.

When hypernatremia occurs in conditions with deficits of sodium and water, the water deficit exceeds the sodium deficit. This only occurs if the patient is unable to ingest adequate water. Diarrhea results in both sodium and water depletion. Because diarrhea is hypotonic—typical sodium concentration of 35–65 mEq/L—water losses are in excess of sodium losses, potentially leading to hypernatremia. Most children with gastroenteritis do not develop hypernatremia because they drink enough hypotonic fluid to compensate for stool water losses. Fluids such as water, juice, and formula are more hypotonic than the stool losses, allowing correction of the water deficit, and potentially even causing hyponatremia. Hypernatremia is most likely in the child with diarrhea who has inadequate intake, either due to emesis, lack of access to water, or anorexia.

Osmotic agents, including mannitol or glucose in diabetes mellitus, lead to excessive renal losses of water and sodium. Because the urine is hypotonic—sodium concentration of about 50 mEq/L—during an osmotic diuresis, water loss exceeds sodium loss, and hypernatremia may occur if water intake is inadequate. Certain chronic kidney diseases, such as renal dysplasia and obstructive uropathy, are associated with tubular dysfunction, leading to excessive losses of water and sodium. Many such children have disproportionate water loss and are at risk for hypernatremic dehydration, especially if gastroenteritis supervenes. Similar mechanisms occur during the polyuric phase of acute tubular necrosis and following relief of urinary obstruction (postobstructive diuresis). These patients may have an osmotic diuresis from urinary losses of urea and an inability to conserve water because of tubular dysfunction.

Clinical Manifestations. Most children with hypernatremia are dehydrated and have the typical signs and symptoms of dehydration (see Chapter 47). Children with hypernatremic dehydration tend to have better preservation of intravascular volume because of the shift of water from the intracellular space to the extracellular space. This maintains blood pressure and urine output, and allows hypernatremic infants to be less symptomatic initially and potentially become more dehydrated before seeking medical attention. Breast-fed infants with hypernatremia are often profoundly dehydrated. Probably because of intracellular water loss, the pinched abdominal skin of a dehydrated, hypernatremic infant has a "doughy" feel.

Hypernatremia, even without dehydration, causes central nervous system symptoms that tend to parallel the degree of sodium elevation and the acuity of the increase. Patients are irritable, restless, weak, and lethargic. Some infants have a high-pitched cry and hyperpnea. Alert patients are very thirsty, even though nausea may be present. Hypernatremia causes fever, although many patients have an underlying process that contributes to the fever. Hypernatremia is associated with hyperglycemia and mild hypocalcemia; the mechanisms are unknown. Beyond the sequelae of dehydration, there is no clear direct effect of hypernatremia on other organs or tissues except the brain.

Brain hemorrhage is the most devastating consequence of hypernatremia. As the extracellular osmolality increases, water moves out of brain cells, resulting in a decrease in brain volume. This can result in tearing of intracerebral veins and bridging blood vessels as the brain moves away from the skull and the meninges. Patients may have subarachnoid, subdural, and parenchymal hemorrhage. Seizures and coma are possible sequelae of the hemorrhage, even though seizures are more common during treatment. The cerebral spinal fluid protein is often elevated in infants with significant hypernatremia, probably due to leakage from damaged blood vessels. Neonates, especially if premature, seem especially vulnerable to hypernatremia and excessive sodium intake. There is an association between

---

BOX 45–1. Causes of Hypernatremia

EXCESSIVE SODIUM
Improperly mixed formula
Excess sodium bicarbonate
Ingestion of seawater or sodium chloride
Intentional salt poisoning (child abuse or Münchhausen syndrome by proxy)
Intravenous hypertonic saline
Hyperaldosteronism

WATER DEFICIT
Nephrogenic diabetes insipidus
  Acquired
  X-linked (MIM* 304800)
  Autosomal recessive (MIM 222000)
Central diabetes insipidus
  Acquired
  Autosomal dominant (MIM 125700)
Increased insensible losses
  Premature infants
  Radiant warmers
  Phototherapy
Inadequate intake
  Ineffective breast-feeding
  Child neglect or abuse
  Adipsia (lack of thirst)

WATER AND SODIUM DEFICITS
Gastrointestinal losses
  Diarrhea
  Emesis/Nasogastric suction
  Osmotic cathartics (e.g., lactulose)
Cutaneous losses
  Burns
  Excessive sweating
Renal losses
  Osmotic diuretics (e.g., mannitol)
  Diabetes mellitus
  Chronic kidney disease (e.g., dysplasia and obstructive uropathy)
  Polyuric phase of acute tubular necrosis
  Postobstructive diuresis

---

*MIM refers to the database number from the Mendelian Inheritance in Man (http://www3.ncbi.nlm.nih.gov/Omim/).

rapid or hyperosmolar sodium bicarbonate administration and development of intraventricular hemorrhages in neonates. Even though central pontine myelinolysis (CPM) is classically associated with overly rapid correction of hyponatremia, both CPM and extrapontine myelinolysis can occur in children with hypernatremia. Thrombotic complications occur in severe hypernatremic dehydration and include stroke, dural sinus thrombosis, peripheral thrombosis, and renal vein thrombosis. This is secondary to dehydration and possibly hypercoagulability associated with hypernatremia.

Diagnosis. The etiology of hypernatremia is usually apparent from the history. Hypernatremia resulting from water loss only occurs if the patient does not have access to water or is unable to drink. In the absence of dehydration, it is important to ask about sodium intake. Children with excess sodium intake do not have signs of dehydration, unless another process is present. Severe sodium intoxication causes signs of volume overload such as pulmonary edema. In hyperaldosteronism, hypernatremia is usually mild or absent and is associated with hypertension, hypokalemia, and metabolic alkalosis.

When there is isolated water loss, the signs of volume depletion are usually less severe initially because much of the loss is from the intracellular space. When pure water loss causes signs of dehydration, the hypernatremia and water deficit are usually severe. In the child with renal water loss, either central or nephrogenic diabetes insipidus, the urine is inappropriately dilute and urine volume is not low. The urine is maximally concentrated and urine volume is low if the losses are extrarenal or due to inadequate intake. With extrarenal losses of water, the urine osmolality should be greater than 1,000 mOsm/kg. When diabetes insipidus is suspected, the evaluation may include measurement of ADH and a water deprivation test, including a trial of desmopressin acetate (synthetic ADH analog) to differentiate nephrogenic and central diabetes insipidus (see Chapters 522 and 552). A water deprivation test is unnecessary if the patient has simultaneous documentation of hypernatremia and poorly concentrated urine (osmolality less than plasma). In children with central diabetes insipidus, administration of desmopressin acetate increases the urine osmolality above the plasma osmolality, even though maximum osmolality does not occur immediately because of the decreased osmolality of the renal medulla from the chronic lack of ADH. In children with central diabetes insipidus, urine is concentrated when desmopressin acetate is given, but in children with nephrogenic diabetes insipidus, there is no such response.

With combined sodium and water deficits, analysis of the urine differentiates renal and nonrenal etiologies. When the losses are extrarenal, the kidney responds to volume depletion with low urine volume, a concentrated urine, and sodium retention (urine sodium less than 20 mEq/L). With renal causes, the urine volume is not appropriately low, the urine is not maximally concentrated, and the urine sodium may be inappropriately elevated.

Treatment. As hypernatremia develops, the brain generates idiogenic osmoles to increase the intracellular osmolality and prevent the loss of brain water. This mechanism is not instantaneous and is most prominent when hypernatremia has developed gradually. If the serum sodium concentration is lowered rapidly, there is movement of water from the serum into the brain cells to equalize the osmolality in the two compartments (Fig. 45–4). The resultant brain swelling is clinically similar to the consequences of acute hyponatremia and most commonly manifests as seizures in infants.

Because of the dangers of overly rapid correction, hypernatremia should not be corrected rapidly. The goal is to decrease the serum sodium by less than 12 mEq/L every 24 hr, a rate of 0.5 mEq/L/hr. The most important component of correcting moderate or severe hypernatremia is frequent monitoring of the

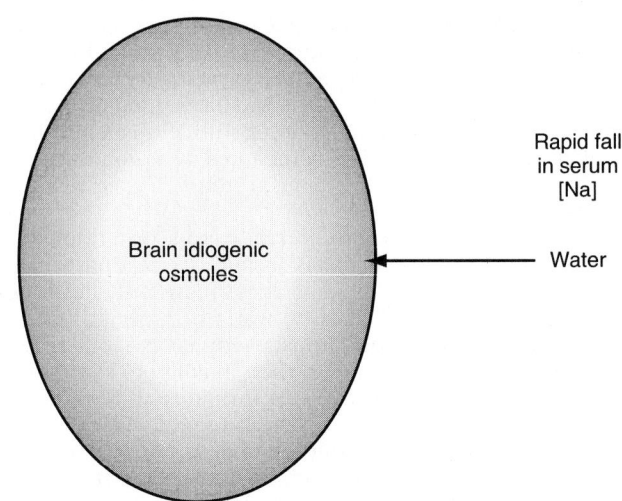

FIGURE 45–4. Mechanism of brain edema during correction of hypernatremia. A rapid decrease of the serum concentration during treatment of hypernatremia causes movement of water into brain cells, leading to cerebral edema. The presence of idiogenic osmoles in brain cells is responsible for the osmotic gradient.

serum sodium so that fluid therapy can be adjusted to provide adequate correction, neither too slow nor too fast. If a child develops seizures from brain edema secondary to overly rapid correction, administration of hypotonic fluid should be stopped and an infusion of 3% saline can acutely increase the serum sodium, reversing the cerebral edema. This is similar to the approach for correcting symptomatic hyponatremia.

In the child with hypernatremic dehydration, as in any child with dehydration, the first priority is restoration of intravascular volume with isotonic fluid (see Chapter 46). Normal saline is preferable to lactated Ringer solution because the lower sodium concentration of the lactated Ringer solution can cause the serum sodium to decrease too rapidly, especially if multiple fluid boluses are given.

The sodium concentration of the fluid, the rate of fluid administration, and the presence of continued water losses determine the rate of decrease of the sodium concentration. The following formula is often cited for calculating the water deficit:

$$\text{Water deficit} = \text{Body weight} \times 0.6 \, (1 - 145/[\text{Current sodium}])$$

This is equivalent to between 3 and 4 mL of water per kilogram for each 1 mEq that the current sodium is greater than 145. The utility of such formulas has never been proven in clinical practice. Most patients with hypernatremic dehydration do well with a fluid sodium concentration between $1/4$ NS and $1/2$ NS, but with a fluid rate that is only 20–50% greater than maintenance. This prevents excessive delivery of free water and too rapid a decrease in the serum sodium. Excessive water and sodium losses may also need to be replaced. If signs or symptoms of volume depletion develop, the patient receives additional boluses of isotonic saline. Monitoring of the rate of decrease of the serum sodium concentration permits adjustment in the rate and sodium concentration of the fluid that the patient is receiving, avoiding overly rapid correction of the hypernatremia.

Acute, severe hypernatremia, usually secondary to sodium administration, can be corrected more rapidly because idiogenic osmoles have not had time to accumulate. This balances the high morbidity and mortality from hypernatremia with the dangers of overly rapid correction. When hypernatremia is due to sodium intoxication and the hypernatremia is severe, it may be impossible to administer enough water to rapidly correct the hypernatremia without worsening volume overload. In this situation, peritoneal dialysis allows for removal of the excess sodium. This requires dialysis fluid with a high glucose concentration and a low sodium concentration. In less severe cases, the addition of a loop diuretic increases removal of excess sodium and water, decreasing the risk of volume overload. With sodium overload, hypernatremia is corrected with sodium-free intravenous fluid (e.g., D5W).

Hyperglycemia from hypernatremia is not usually treated with insulin because the acute decrease in glucose, by lowering plasma osmolality, may precipitate cerebral edema. Rather, the glucose concentration of intravenous fluids should be reduced (e.g., change from D5 to D2.5). The secondary hypocalcemia is treated as needed.

It is important, if possible, to address the underlying cause of the hypernatremia. The child with central diabetes insipidus should receive desmopressin acetate. Since this reduces renal excretion of water, excessive intake of water must consequently be avoided to prevent overly rapid correction of the hypernatremia or the development of hyponatremia. Long term, reduced sodium intake and medications can somewhat ameliorate the water losses in nephrogenic diabetes insipidus (see Chapter 522). The daily water intake of a child who is on tube feeding may need to be increased to compensate for high losses. The patient with significant ongoing losses such as diarrhea may need supplemental water and electrolytes (see Chapter 46). Sodium intake is reduced if this contributed to the hypernatremia.

HYPONATREMIA

Hyponatremia, a very common electrolyte abnormality in hospitalized patients, is a serum sodium level below 135 mEq/L. Both total body sodium and TBW determine the serum sodium concentration. Hyponatremia exists when the ratio of water to sodium is increased. This can occur with low, normal, and high levels of body sodium. Similarly, body water can be low, normal, or high.

Etiology and Pathophysiolgy. The causes of hyponatremia are listed in Box 45–2. Pseudohyponatremia is a laboratory artifact that is present when the plasma contains very high concentrations of protein or lipid. It does not occur if a direct ion-selective electrode determines the sodium concentration, a technique that is increasingly used in clinical laboratories. In true hyponatremia, the measured osmolality is low, whereas it is normal in pseudohyponatremia. Hyperosmolality due to mannitol or glucose causes a low serum sodium concentration because water moves down its osmotic gradient from the intracellular space into the extracellular space, diluting the sodium concentration. However, because the manifestations of hyponatremia are due to the low plasma osmolality, patients with hyponatremia resulting from hyperosmolality do not have symptoms of hyponatremia. When the etiology of the hyperosmolality resolves, such as hyperglycemia in diabetes mellitus, water moves back into the cells and the sodium concentration increases to its "true" value.

The classification of hyponatremia uses the patient's volume status. The hypovolemic child with hyponatremia has lost sodium from the body. Water balance may be positive or negative, but there has been a higher proportion of sodium loss than water loss. The pathogenesis of the hyponatremia is usually due to a combination of sodium loss and water retention to compensate for the volume depletion. The patient has a pathologic increase in fluid loss, and this fluid contains sodium. However, most fluid that is lost has a lower sodium concentration than plasma so would actually cause hypernatremia if the patient only has fluid loss. For example, viral diarrhea has, on average, a sodium concentration of 50 mEq/L. Hypernatremia does not occur because the patient drinks a low sodium–containing fluid such as formula or water. By replacing diarrheal fluid, which has a sodium concentration of 50 mEq/L, with formula, which has

BOX 45–2. Causes of Hyponatremia

PSEUDOHYPONATREMIA
HYPEROSMOLALITY
Hyperglycemia
Mannitol

HYPOVOLEMIC HYPONATREMIA
Extrarenal losses
  Gastrointestinal (emesis, diarrhea)
  Skin (sweating or burns)
  Third space losses
Renal losses
  Thiazide or loop diuretics
  Osmotic diuresis
  Postobstructive diuresis
  Polyuric phase of ATN
  Juvenile nephronophthisis (MIM* 256100/ 602088/ 266900/ 604387)
  Autosomal recessive polycystic kidney disease (MIM 263200)
  Tubulointerstitial nephritis
  Obstructive uropathy
  Cerebral salt wasting
  Proximal (Type II) RTA (MIM 604278†)
  Lack of aldosterone effect (high serum potassium)
    Absent aldosterone (e.g., 21-hydroxylase deficiency [MIM 201910])
    Pseudohypoaldosteronism type I (MIM 264350 and 177735)
    Urinary tract obstruction and/or urinary tract infection

EUVOLEMIC HYPONATREMIA
Syndrome of inappropriate antidiuretic hormone
Desmopressin acetate
Glucocorticoid deficiency
Hypothyroidism
Water intoxication
  Iatrogenic (i.e., excess hypotonic intravenous fluids)
  Swimming lessons
  Tap water enema
  Child abuse
  Psychogenic polydipsia
  Diluted formula
  Beer potomania

HYPERVOLEMIC HYPONATREMIA
Congestive heart failure
Cirrhosis
Nephrotic syndrome
Renal failure
Capillary leak due to sepsis
Hypoalbuminemia due to gastrointestinal disease

*MIM refers to the database number from the Mendelian Inheritance in Man (http://www3.ncbi.nlm.nih.gov/Omim/).
†Most cases of proximal renal tubular acidosis are not due to this primary genetic disorder. Proximal RTA is usually part of Fanconi syndrome, which has multiple etiologies (see Chapter 521).

only about 10 mEq/L of sodium, there is a reduction in the sodium concentration. Intravascular volume depletion interferes with renal water excretion, the body's usual mechanism for preventing hyponatremia. The volume depletion stimulates ADH synthesis, resulting in renal water retention in the collecting duct. In addition, volume depletion decreases the GFR and enhances water reabsorption in the proximal tubule, which reduces water delivery to the collecting duct.

Diarrhea due to gastroenteritis is the most common cause of hypovolemic hyponatremia in children. Emesis causes hyponatremia if the patient takes in hypotonic fluid, either intravenously or enterally, despite the emesis. However, most patients with emesis have either a normal sodium concentration or hypernatremia. Burns may cause massive losses of an isotonic fluid and volume depletion. Hyponatremia develops if the patient receives hypotonic fluid. Losses of sodium from sweat are especially high in children with cystic fibrosis, aldosterone deficiency, or pseudohypoaldosteronism, although high losses can occur simply due to a hot climate. Third space losses are isotonic and can cause significant volume depletion, leading to ADH production and water retention, which can cause hyponatremia if the patient receives hypotonic fluid. In diseases with volume depletion due to extrarenal sodium loss, the urine sodium should be low (<10 mEq/L) as part of the renal response to maintain the intravascular volume. The only exceptions are diseases with both extrarenal sodium losses and renal losses: adrenal insufficiency and pseudohypoaldosteronism.

Renal sodium loss may occur in a variety of situations. In some situations, the urine sodium concentration is higher than 140 mEq/L, and, thus, hyponatremia may occur without any fluid intake. In many cases, the urine sodium is less than the serum concentration, and thus the intake of hypotonic fluid is necessary for hyponatremia to develop. In diseases with urinary sodium loss, the urine sodium is more than 20 mEq/L despite volume depletion. This may not be true if the urinary sodium loss is no longer occurring, as is frequently the case if diuretics are stopped. Because loop diuretics prevent generation of a maximally hypertonic renal medulla, patients can neither maximally dilute nor concentrate the urine. The inability to maximally retain water provides some protection against severe hyponatremia. Patients receiving thiazide diuretics can concentrate the urine and are at higher risk for severe hyponatremia. Osmotic diuretics, such as glucose during diabetic ketoacidosis, cause loss of both water and sodium. Urea accumulates during renal failure and then acts as an osmotic diuretic after relief of urinary tract obstruction and during the polyuric phase of acute tubular necrosis. Transient tubular damage in these conditions further impairs sodium conservation. The serum sodium concentration in these conditions is dependent on the sodium concentration of the fluid used to replace the losses. Hyponatremia develops when the fluid is hypotonic relative to the urinary losses.

Renal salt wasting occurs in hereditary kidney diseases such as juvenile nephronophthisis and autosomal recessive polycystic kidney disease. Obstructive uropathy, most commonly a consequence of posterior urethral valves, produces salt wasting, but these patients may also develop hypernatremia due to impaired urinary concentrating ability and high water loss. Acquired tubulointerstitial nephritis, usually secondary to either medications or infections, may cause salt wasting, along with other evidence of tubular dysfunction. Central nervous system injury may produce cerebral salt wasting, which appears to be mediated by production of a natriuretic peptide that causes renal salt wasting (see Chapter 553.2). In type II renal tubular acidosis (RTA), usually associated with Fanconi syndrome, there is increased excretion of sodium and bicarbonate in the urine. Patients with Fanconi syndrome also have glycosuria, aminoaciduria, and hypophosphatemia due to renal phosphate wasting.

Aldosterone is necessary for renal sodium retention and for excretion of potassium and acid. In congenital adrenal hyperplasia due to 21-hydroxylase deficiency, the absence of aldosterone produces hyponatremia, hyperkalemia, and metabolic acidosis. In pseudohypoaldosteronism, aldosterone levels are elevated, but there is no response because of either a defective sodium channel or a lack of aldosterone receptors. A lack of tubular response to aldosterone may occur in children with urinary tract obstruction, especially during an acute urinary tract infection.

In hypervolemic hyponatremia, there is an excess of TBW and sodium, although the increase in water is greater than the increase in sodium. The pathogenesis of hypervolemic hyponatremia is somewhat similar to hypovolemic hyponatremia. In most of the conditions that cause hypervolemic hyponatremia, there is a decrease in the effective blood volume, due to either third spacing of fluid or poor cardiac function. The regulatory systems of the body sense this decrease and attempt to retain water and sodium in order to correct the problem. ADH causes renal water retention and the kidney, under the influence of aldosterone and other intrarenal mechanisms, retains sodium. The patient's sodium concentration decreases because water intake exceeds sodium intake, and ADH prevents the normal loss of excess water.

In these disorders, there is a low urine sodium concentration (<10 mEq/L) and an excess of both water and sodium. The only exception is the patient with renal failure and hyponatremia. These patients have an expanded intravascular volume, and hyponatremia can therefore appropriately suppress ADH production. Water cannot be excreted because very little urine is being made. Serum sodium is diluted by ingesting water. Because of renal dysfunction, urine sodium concentration may be elevated, but urine volume is so low that patients have not kept up with their sodium intake and therefore are also sodium overloaded. The urine sodium concentration in renal failure varies. In acute glomerulonephritis, because it does not affect the tubules, the urine sodium is usually low, whereas in patients with acute tubular necrosis, the urine sodium is elevated due to tubular dysfunction.

Patients with hyponatremia and no evidence of volume overload or volume depletion have euvolemic hyponatremia. These patients typically have an excess of TBW and a slight decrease in total body sodium. Some of these patients have an increase in weight, implying that they are technically overloaded. Nevertheless, from a clinical standpoint they usually appear normal or have subtle signs of fluid overload.

In SIADH, there is secretion of ADH that is not inhibited by either low serum osmolality or expanded intravascular volume (see Chapter 553.1). The result is that the child with SIADH is unable to excrete water. This results in dilution of the serum sodium and hyponatremia. In addition, the expansion of the extracellular volume due to the retained water causes a mild increase in intravascular volume. The kidney increases sodium excretion in an effort to decrease intravascular volume to normal and, thus, these patients have a mild decrease in body sodium. SIADH most commonly occurs with central nervous system pathology, but lung disease and tumors are other potential causes. In addition, a variety of medications may cause SIADH. The diagnosis of SIADH is one of exclusion, because other causes of hyponatremia must be eliminated (Box 45–3). Because SIADH is a state of intravascular volume expansion, low serum uric acid and BUN levels are supportive of the diagnosis.

Hyponatremia in the hospital frequently occurs in children who inappropriately produce ADH as a result of stress and who receive hypotonic intravenous fluids. The synthetic analog of ADH, desmopressin acetate, causes water retention and may cause hyponatremia if fluid intake is not appropriately limited. The main uses of desmopressin acetate in children are for the management of central diabetes insipidus and nocturnal enuresis.

Excess water ingestion can produce hyponatremia. In these cases, the sodium concentration decreases as a result of dilution. This suppresses ADH secretion and there is a marked water diuresis by the kidney. Hyponatremia only develops because the

---

BOX 45–3. Diagnostic Criteria for Syndrome of Inappropriate Antidiuretic Hormone

Absence of:
Renal, adrenal, or thyroid insufficiency
Congestive heart failure, nephrotic syndrome, or cirrhosis
Diuretic ingestion
Dehydration
Urine osmolality > 100 (usually > plasma)
Serum osmolality < 280 and serum sodium < 135
Urine sodium > 25

intake of water exceeds the kidney's ability to eliminate water. This is more likely to occur in infants because their lower GFR limits their ability to excrete water. In some situations, the water intoxication causes acute hyponatremia and is due to a massive acute water load. Examples include infant swimming lessons, inappropriate hypotonic intravenous fluids, water enemas, and forced water intake as a form of child abuse. Chronic hyponatremia occurs in children who receive water, but limited sodium and protein. The minimum urine osmolality is approximately 50 mOsm/kg so the kidney can only excrete a liter of water if there is enough solute ingested to produce 50 mOsm for urinary excretion. Because sodium and urea—a breakdown product of protein—are the principal urinary solutes, a lack of sodium and protein intake prevents adequate water excretion. This occurs with diluted formula or other inappropriate diets. Subsistence on beer, a poor source of sodium and protein, causes hyponatremia resulting from the inability to excrete the high water load ("beer potomania").

The pathogenesis of the hyponatremia in glucocorticoid deficiency or hypothyroidism is incompletely understood. There is an inappropriate retention of water by the kidney, but the precise mechanisms are not clearly elucidated.

Clinical Manifestations. Hyponatremia causes a decrease in the osmolality of the extracellular space. Because the intracellular space then has a higher osmolality, water inevitably moves from the extracellular space to the intracellular space to maintain osmotic equilibrium. The increase in intracellular water causes cells to swell. Cell swelling is not problematic in most tissues of the body. It is, however, potentially catastrophic in the brain. This is because the brain is contained in a fixed shell, the skull. As brain cells swell, there is an increase in intracranial pressure. Acute, severe hyponatremia can cause brainstem herniation and apnea; respiratory support is often necessary. Brain cell swelling is responsible for most of the symptoms of hyponatremia. Neurologic symptoms of hyponatremia include anorexia, nausea, emesis, malaise, lethargy, confusion, agitation, headache, seizures, coma, and decreased reflexes. Patients may develop hypothermia and Cheyne-Stokes respirations. Hyponatremia can cause muscle cramps and weakness.

The symptoms of hyponatremia are mostly due to the decrease in extracellular osmolality and the resulting movement of water down its osmotic gradient into the intracellular space. However, brain swelling can be significantly obviated if the hyponatremia develops gradually. This is because the brain adapts to the decreased extracellular osmolality by decreasing its internal osmolality. Initially, this is mostly through loss of sodium, potassium, and chloride. More chronically there is loss of intracellular osmoles such as amino acids, which accounts for why the degree of symptoms in hyponatremia is related to both the serum sodium level and its rate of decrease. A patient with chronic hyponatremia may be asymptomatic with a level of 110 mEq/L, but another patient may have seizures due to an acute decline from 140 to 125 mEq/L.

Patients with hyponatremic dehydration have more manifestations of intravascular volume depletion than patients who have equivalent water loss but normal or increased sodium concentrations. During hyponatremia, there is movement of water into the cells, which depletes the water of the extracellular space, including the plasma volume.

Diagnosis. The history usually points to a likely etiology of the hyponatremia. Most patients with hyponatremia have a history of volume depletion. Diarrhea and diuretic use are very common etiologies of hyponatremia in children. A history of polyuria, perhaps with enuresis, and/or salt craving is present in children with primary kidney diseases or absence of aldosterone effect. Children may have signs or symptoms supportive of a diagnosis of hypothyroidism or adrenal insufficiency (see Chapters 559 and 569). Brain injury raises the possibility of SIADH or cerebral

salt wasting. Liver disease, nephrotic syndrome, renal failure, or congestive heart failure may be acute or chronic. The history should include a review of the patient's intake, both intravenous and enteral, with careful attention to water, sodium, and protein amounts.

The traditional first step in the diagnostic process is the determination of the plasma osmolality. This is done because some patients with a low serum sodium value do not have a low osmolality. The clinical effects of hyponatremia are secondary to the associated low osmolality. Without a low osmolality, there is no movement of water into the intracellular space.

A patient with hyponatremia can have a low, normal, or high osmolality. A normal osmolality and hyponatremia occurs in pseudohyponatremia. Children with an elevated serum glucose concentration or another effective osmole (e.g., mannitol) have a high plasma osmolality and hyponatremia. The presence of a low osmolality indicates "true" hyponatremia. These patients are at risk for neurologic symptoms and require further evaluation to determine the etiology of their hyponatremia.

In some situations, true hyponatremia is present despite a normal or elevated plasma osmolality. The presence of an ineffective osmole, most commonly urea, increases the plasma osmolality, but, because it has the same concentration in the intracellular space, does not cause fluid to move into the extracellular space. There is no dilution of the serum sodium by water, and the sodium concentration remains unchanged if the ineffective osmole is eliminated. Most importantly, the ineffective osmole does not protect the brain from edema as a result of hyponatremia. Hence, a patient may develop symptoms from hyponatremia despite a normal or increased osmolality caused by uremia.

The role of determining the plasma osmolality in patients with hyponatremia is open to question. Pseudohyponatremia, a laboratory artifact, does not occur in most clinical laboratories and is simple to ascertain. Even if it is a possibility, hyperlipidemia is apparent by inspection of blood, which is lipemic. High serum protein almost never occurs in children; it is mostly an issue in adult disorders (e.g., multiple myeloma). Measuring a serum glucose level and evaluating for a history of intravenous mannitol easily assesses for hyponatremia secondary to increased effective osmoles. Finally, the presence of ineffective osmoles, such as urea or ethanol, confuses the usual assumption about true hyponatremia only occurring with a low plasma osmolality.

In patients with true hyponatremia, the next step in the diagnostic process is to clinically evaluate the patient's volume status. Patients with hyponatremia can be hypovolemic, hypervolemic, or euvolemic. The diagnosis of volume depletion relies on the usual findings with dehydration (see Chapter 47). Children with hypervolemia are edematous on physical examination. They may have ascites, pulmonary edema, pleural effusion, or hypertension.

Hypovolemic hyponatremia can have renal or nonrenal causes. When the losses are nonrenal and the kidney is working properly, there is renal retention of sodium, a normal homeostatic response to volume depletion. Thus, the urinary sodium concentration is low, typically less than 10 mEq/L, although sodium conservation in neonates is less avid. In contrast, when the kidney is the cause of the sodium loss, the urine will have a sodium concentration of greater than 20 mEq/L, reflecting the defect in renal sodium retention. Therefore, in the child with hypovolemic hyponatremia, the urine sodium is very useful in differentiating between renal and nonrenal causes. The interpretation of the urine sodium is challenging with diuretics because it is high when diuretics are being used but low after the diuretic effect is gone. This becomes an issue only when the diuretic use is surreptitious. The urine sodium is not useful if a metabolic alkalosis is present; the urine chloride must be used instead (see Chapter 45.8).

Differentiating among the nonrenal causes of hypovolemic hyponatremia is usually facilitated by the history. The renal causes are more challenging to distinguish. The serum potassium value is often helpful in this regard. Specifically, a high serum potassium concentration is associated with disorders in which the sodium wasting is due to absent or ineffective aldosterone.

In the patient with hypervolemic hyponatremia, the urine sodium concentration is a helpful parameter. It is usually <10 mEq/L, except in the patient with renal failure. An elevated urine sodium concentration is a useful indication that a child may have acute tubular necrosis superimposed on one of the other causes of hypervolemic hyponatremia.

Treatment. The management of hyponatremia is based on the pathophysiology of the specific etiology. In general, diseases that have a similar pathogenesis are treated similarly. In addition, the management of all causes requires judicious monitoring and avoidance of an overly quick normalization of the serum sodium concentration. Yet, a patient with severe symptoms, no matter the etiology, should be given a bolus of hypertonic saline to produce a small, rapid increase in the serum sodium.

With all causes of hyponatremia, it is important to avoid "overly rapid" correction of the hyponatremia. This is because rapid correction of hyponatremia may cause *central pontine myelinolysis* (CPM). This syndrome produces neurologic symptoms, including confusion, agitation, flaccid or spastic quadriparesis, and death. There are usually characteristic pathologic and radiologic changes in the brain, especially in the pons.

CPM is more common in patients who are treated for chronic hyponatremia than for acute hyponatremia. Presumably this is based on the adaptation of brain cells to the hyponatremia. The reduced intracellular osmolality that is an adaptive mechanism for chronic hyponatremia makes brain cells susceptible to dehydration during rapid correction of the hyponatremia, and this may be the mechanism of CPM. Even though CPM is rare in pediatric patients, it is advisable to avoid correcting the serum sodium by more than 12 mEq/L each day. This guideline does not apply to acute hyponatremia, as may occur with water intoxication, because the hyponatremia is more often symptomatic and there has not been time for the adaptive decrease in brain osmolality. The consequences of brain edema in acute hyponatremia exceed the small risk of CPM.

Patients with hyponatremia can have severe neurologic symptoms such as seizures and coma. The seizures from hyponatremia are generally poorly responsive to anticonvulsants. The child with hyponatremia and severe symptoms needs to receive treatment that will quickly reduce cerebral edema. This is best accomplished by increasing the extracellular osmolality so that water moves down its osmolar gradient from the intracellular space to the extracellular space.

Intravenous hypertonic saline rapidly increases the serum sodium, and the effect on serum osmolality leads to a decrease in brain edema. Each milliliter of 3% sodium chloride increases the serum sodium by approximately 1 mEq/L. A child with active symptoms often improves after receiving 4–6 mL/kg of 3% sodium chloride.

The child with hypovolemic hyponatremia has a deficiency in sodium and may have a deficiency in water. The cornerstone of therapy is to replace the sodium deficit and any water deficit that is present. The first step in any dehydrated patient is to restore the intravascular volume with isotonic saline. This is frequently needed in hyponatremic dehydration because the low serum osmolality causes water to move intracellularly, further depleting the intravascular volume. Ultimately, complete restoration of intravascular volume suppresses ADH production, which permits excretion of the excess water. Chapter 47 discusses the management details of hyponatremic dehydration. Close monitoring of the sodium concentration is essential to avoid overly rapid correction, especially given the water diuresis that may occur with restoration of the intravascular volume.

The management of hypervolemic hyponatremia is difficult. These patients have an excess of both water and sodium. Administration of sodium leads to worsening volume overload and edema. In addition, these patients are retaining water and sodium because of their ineffective intravascular volume or renal insufficiency. The cornerstone of therapy is water and sodium restriction because these patients are overloaded. Diuretics may be helpful by causing excretion of both sodium and water. Patients with low albumin due to nephrotic syndrome have a better response to diuretics after an infusion of albumin. A child with congestive heart failure may have an increase in renal water and sodium excretion if there is an improvement in cardiac output. This will "turn off" the regulatory hormones that are causing renal water (ADH) and sodium (aldosterone) retention. The patient with renal failure cannot respond to any of these therapies except fluid restriction. Insensible fluid losses eventually result in an increase in the sodium concentration as long as insensible and urinary losses are greater than intake. A more definitive approach in children with renal failure is to perform dialysis, which removes water and sodium.

In isovolemic hyponatremia, there is usually an excess of water and a mild sodium deficit. Therapy is directed at eliminating the excess water. The child with excessive water intake loses water in the urine because ADH production is turned off as a result of the low plasma osmolality. It takes time to eliminate the excess water, and limiting water intake allows this process to occur more quickly. For acute, symptomatic hyponatremia due to water intoxication, hypertonic saline may be needed to reverse cerebral edema. For chronic hyponatremia from poor solute intake, the child needs to receive an appropriate formula, and excess water intake should be eliminated.

Hormone replacement is the cornerstone of therapy for the hyponatremia of hypothyroidism or cortisol deficiency. Correction of the underlying defect permits appropriate elimination of the excess water. SIADH is a condition of excess water with a limited ability of the kidney to excrete water. The mainstay of therapy is fluid restriction. The sodium concentration will increase as long as intake of water is less than insensible losses. Fluid restriction obviously requires time and, thus, there is a temptation to treat these patients with normal saline or hypertonic saline. However, therapy with saline can create problems in children with SIADH. Infusions of saline temporarily increase the sodium concentration, but increase the child's blood pressure and this causes the kidneys to eliminate almost all of the sodium, eliminating any benefit from the therapy. In addition, the water contained in the saline is retained and thus the hyponatremia may actually worsen. Saline, by itself, is likely to produce hypertension and minimal long-term therapeutic benefit.

Furosemide is more successful in the patient with SIADH and severe hyponatremia. Even in a patient with SIADH, furosemide causes an increase in water and sodium excretion. The loss of sodium is somewhat counterproductive, but this sodium can be replaced with hypertonic saline. Because the patient has a net loss of water and the urinary losses of sodium have been replaced, there is an increase in the sodium concentration but no significant increase in blood pressure.

Treatment of chronic SIADH is challenging. Fluid restriction in children is difficult for nutritional and behavioral reasons. The mainstays of adult therapy, demeclocycline and lithium, which blunt the effect of ADH, are problematic in children because of their potential toxicity. Another option is chronic furosemide therapy with sodium supplementation.

45.4 Potassium

POTASSIUM METABOLISM

Body Content and Physiologic Function. The intracellular concentration of potassium, approximately 150 mEq/L, is much higher than the plasma concentration (see Fig. 45–3). The majority of body potassium is contained in muscle. As muscle mass increases, there is an increase in body potassium. There is thus an increase in body potassium during puberty, which is more significant in boys. The majority of extracellular potassium is in bone; less than 1% of total body potassium is in plasma.

Because most potassium is intracellular, the plasma concentration does not always reflect the total body potassium content. A variety of conditions alter the distribution of potassium between the intracellular and extracellular compartments. The Na^+,K^+-ATPase maintains the high intracellular potassium concentration by pumping sodium out of the cell and potassium into the cell. This balances the normal leak of potassium out of cells via potassium channels, which is driven by the favorable chemical gradient. Insulin increases potassium movement into cells by activating the Na^+,K^+-ATPase. Because hyperkalemia stimulates insulin secretion, this may have a protective effect during hyperkalemia. Acid-base status affects potassium distribution, probably via potassium channels and the Na^+,K^+-ATPase. A decrease in pH drives potassium extracellularly; an increase in pH has the opposite effect. β-Adrenergic agonists stimulate the Na^+,K^+-ATPase, increasing the cellular uptake of potassium. This may also be protective in that hyperkalemia stimulates adrenal release of catecholamines. α-Adrenergic agonists and exercise cause a net movement of potassium out of the intracellular space. An increase in plasma osmolality, as with mannitol infusion, leads to water movement out of the cells and potassium follows as a result of solvent drag. The serum potassium concentration increases by approximately 0.6 mEq/L with each 10-mOsm increase in the plasma osmolality. This occurs in diabetic ketoacidosis as a result of the increase in osmolality from hyperglycemia. Hyperglycemia in patients without insulin deficiency does not increase the plasma potassium concentration because the secondary insulin production causes potassium to move intracellularly.

The high intracellular concentration of potassium, the principal intracellular cation, is maintained via the Na^+,K^+-ATPase. The resulting chemical gradient is used to produce the resting membrane potential of cells. Potassium is necessary for the electrical responsiveness of nerve and muscle cells, and for the contractility of cardiac, skeletal, and smooth muscle. The changes in membrane polarization that occur during muscle contraction or nerve conduction make these cells susceptible to changes in serum potassium levels. The ratio of intracellular to extracellular potassium determines the threshold for a cell to generate an action potential and the rate of cellular repolarization. The intracellular potassium concentration affects cellular enzymes and the intracellular pH. Low intracellular potassium raises the pH while high intracellular potassium lowers the pH. These acid-base changes modify cell functions. Potassium is necessary for maintaining cell volume because of its important contribution to intracellular osmolality.

Intake. Potassium is plentiful in food. Dietary consumption varies considerably, even though 1–2 mEq/kg is the recommended intake. The intestines normally absorb approximately 90% of ingested potassium. Most absorption occurs in the small intestine, whereas the colon exchanges body potassium for luminal sodium. Regulation of intestinal losses normally has a minimal role in maintaining potassium homeostasis, although renal failure, aldosterone, and glucocorticoids increase colonic secretion of potassium. The increase in intestinal losses in the setting of renal failure and hyperkalemia, which stimulates aldosterone production, is clinically significant, helping to protect against hyperkalemia. Colonic secretion is important following an acute potassium load. Patients with kidney failure who develop constipation or receive an ACE-inhibitor, an indirect inhibitor of aldosterone production, may have less colonic secretion, and therefore develop hyperkalemia. However, colonic secretion is never more than a small part of overall potassium excretion.

Excretion. There is some loss of potassium in sweat, but this is normally minimal. The colon has the ability to eliminate some potassium. In addition, following an acute potassium load, much of the potassium, more than 40%, moves intracellularly, through the actions of epinephrine and insulin, which are produced in response to hyperkalemia. This provides transient protection from hyperkalemia, but most ingested potassium is eventually excreted in the urine. The kidneys are the principal regulator of chronic potassium balance and they alter excretion in response to a variety of signals. Potassium is freely filtered at the glomerulus, but 90% is reabsorbed before the distal tubule and collecting duct, the principal sites of potassium regulation. The distal tubule and the collecting duct have the ability to absorb and secrete potassium. It is the amount of tubular secretion that regulates the amount of potassium that appears in the urine. The plasma potassium concentration directly influences secretion in the distal nephron. As the potassium concentration increases, secretion increases.

The principal hormone regulating potassium secretion is aldosterone, which is released by the adrenal cortex in response to increased plasma potassium. Its main site of action is the cortical collecting duct, where aldosterone stimulates sodium movement from the tubule into the cells. This creates a negative charge in the tubular lumen, facilitating potassium excretion. In addition, the increased intracellular sodium stimulates the basolateral Na^+,K^+-ATPase, causing more potassium to move into the cells lining the cortical collecting duct. Urinary potassium excretion is also increased by glucocorticoids, ADH, high urinary flow rate, and high sodium delivery to the distal nephron. In contrast, potassium excretion is decreased by insulin, catecholamines, and urinary ammonia. Loop and thiazide diuretics increase potassium secretion by increasing sodium delivery to the distal nephron and increasing the urinary flow rate in the distal nephron. Whereas ADH increases potassium secretion, it also causes water reabsorption, decreasing urinary flow. The net effect is that ADH has little overall impact on potassium balance. Alkalosis causes potassium to move into cells, including the cells lining the collecting duct. This increases potassium secretion, and because acidosis has the opposite effect, it decreases potassium secretion.

The kidney can dramatically vary potassium excretion in response to changes in intake. Normally, about 10–15% of the filtered load is excreted. In an adult, excretion of potassium can vary between 5 and 1,000 mEq per day.

HYPERKALEMIA

Hyperkalemia—because of the potential for lethal arrhythmias—is one of the most alarming electrolyte abnormalities.

Etiology and Pathophysiology. There are three basic mechanisms that cause hyperkalemia (Box 45–4). In the individual patient, the etiology is sometimes multifactorial.

Fictitious hyperkalemia is very common in children because of the difficulties in obtaining blood specimens. This is usually due to hemolysis during phlebotomy, but it can be the result of prolonged tourniquet application or fist clinching, which cause local potassium release from muscle.

The serum potassium level is normally 0.4 mEq/L higher than the plasma value, secondary to release from cells during clot formation. This phenomenon is exaggerated with thrombocytosis because of potassium release from platelets. For every $100,000/m^3$ increase in the platelet count, the serum potassium increases by approximately 0.15 mEq/L. This also occurs with the marked white blood cell elevations sometimes seen with leukemia. Elevated white blood cells counts, typically greater than $200,000/m^3$, can cause a dramatic elevation in the serum potassium concentration. Analysis of a plasma sample usually provides an accurate result. It is important to analyze the sample promptly to avoid potassium release from cells. This occurs if the sample is stored in the cold, whereas room temperature

BOX 45–4. Causes of Hyperkalemia

SPURIOUS LABORATORY VALUE
Hemolysis
Tissue ischemia during blood drawing
Thrombocytosis
Leukocytosis

INCREASED INTAKE
Intravenous or oral
Blood transfusions

TRANSCELLULAR SHIFTS
Acidemia
Rhabdomyolysis
Tumor lysis syndrome
Tissue necrosis
Hemolysis/hematomas/GI bleeding
Succinylcholine
Digitalis intoxication
Fluoride intoxication
Beta-adrenergic blockers
Exercise
Hyperosmolality
Insulin deficiency
Malignant hyperthermia (MIM 145600)
Hyperkalemic periodic paralysis (MIM 170500)

DECREASED EXCRETION
Renal failure
Primary adrenal disease
  Acquired Addison disease
  21-hydroxylase deficiency (MIM 201910)
  3β-hydroxysteroid dehydrogenase deficiency (MIM 201810)
  Lipoid congenital adrenal hyperplasia (MIM 201710)
  Adrenal hypoplasia congenita (MIM 300200)
  Aldosterone synthase deficiency (MIM 203400)
  Adrenoleukodystrophy (MIM 300100)
Hyporeninemic hypoaldosteronism
  Urinary tract obstruction
  Sickle cell disease (MIM 603903)
  Kidney transplant
  Lupus nephritis
Renal tubular disease
  Pseudohypoaldosteronism type I (MIM 264350 and 177735)
  Pseudohypoaldosteronism type II (MIM 145260)
  Urinary tract obstruction
  Sickle cell disease
  Kidney transplant
Medications
  Angiotensin-converting enzyme inhibitors
  Angiotensin II blockers
  Potassium-sparing diuretics
  Cyclosporin
  Nonsteroidal anti-inflammatories
  Trimethoprim

---

*MIM refers to the database number from the Mendelian Inheritance in Man (http://www3.ncbi.nlm.nih.gov/Omim/).

---

syndrome, tissue necrosis, or hemolysis, releases potassium into the extracellular milieu. The potassium from red blood cells in internal bleeding, such as hematomas, is resorbed and enters the extracellular space.

Normal doses of succinylcholine or β-blockers and fluoride or digitalis intoxication all cause a shift of potassium out of the intracellular compartment. Succinylcholine should not be used during anesthesia in patients at risk for hyperkalemia. β-blockers prevent the normal cellular uptake of potassium mediated by binding of β-agonists to the $β_2$-adrenergic receptors. Potassium release from muscle cells occurs during exercise, and levels can increase by 1–2 mEq/L with high activity. With an increased plasma osmolality, water moves from the intracellular space and potassium follows as a result of solvent drag. This occurs with hyperglycemia, although in nondiabetic patients the resultant increase in insulin causes potassium to move intracellularly. In diabetic ketoacidosis, the absence of insulin causes potassium to leave the intracellular space, and this is compounded by the hyperosmolality. The effect of hyperosmolality causes a transcellular shift of potassium into the extracellular space after mannitol or hypertonic saline infusions. Malignant hyperthermia, which is triggered by some inhaled anesthetics, causes muscle release of potassium. Hyperkalemic periodic paralysis is an autosomal dominant disorder caused by a mutated sodium channel and results in episodic cellular release of potassium and attacks of paralysis.

The kidneys excrete most of the daily potassium intake so a decrease in kidney function can cause hyperkalemia. The decrease in potassium excretion and the risk of hyperkalemia is proportional to the degree of renal insufficiency. Newborn infants in general, and especially premature infants, have decreased kidney function at birth and thus are at increased risk for hyperkalemia, despite an absence of intrinsic renal disease.

A wide range of primary adrenal disorders, both hereditary and acquired, can cause decreased production of aldosterone, with secondary hyperkalemia (see Chapters 569 and 570). These patients typically have metabolic acidosis and salt wasting with hyponatremia. Children with more subtle adrenal insufficiency may only develop electrolyte problems during acute illnesses. With less severe adrenal insufficiency, hyponatremia may be the only electrolyte abnormality. Causes of acquired adrenal dysfunction include hemorrhage (e.g., Waterhouse-Friderichsen syndrome in meningococcemia), tuberculous, and autoimmune disease. The most common form of congenital adrenal hyperplasia, 21-hydroxylase deficiency, typically presents in infant boys with hyperkalemia, metabolic acidosis, hyponatremia, and volume depletion. Girls with this disorder usually are diagnosed as newborns because of their ambiguous genitalia; treatment prevents the development of electrolyte problems.

Renin, via angiotensin II, stimulates aldosterone production. A deficiency in renin, a result of kidney damage, can lead to decreased aldosterone production. Hyporeninemia occurs in many kidney diseases, with some of the more common pediatric causes listed in Box 45–4. These patients typically have hyperkalemia and a metabolic acidosis, without hyponatremia. Some of these patients have impaired renal function, partially accounting for the hyperkalemia, but the impairment in potassium excretion is more extreme than expected for the degree of renal insufficiency.

A variety of renal tubular disorders impair renal excretion of potassium. Children with pseudohypoaldosteronism type 1 have hyperkalemia, metabolic acidosis, and salt wasting leading to hyponatremia and volume depletion; aldosterone levels are elevated. In the autosomal recessive variant, there is a defect in the renal sodium channel that is normally activated by aldosterone. These patients have severe symptoms, beginning in infancy. In the autosomal dominant form, patients have a defect in the aldosterone receptor, and the disease is milder, often

storage can lead to cellular uptake of potassium and spurious hypokalemia.

Because of the kidney's ability to excrete potassium, it is unusual for excessive intake, by itself, to cause hyperkalemia. This can occur in a patient who is receiving large quantities of intravenous or oral potassium as a result of excessive losses that are no longer present. Frequent or rapid blood transfusions can acutely increase the potassium level because of the potassium content of blood, which is variably elevated. Increased intake may precipitate hyperkalemia if there is an underlying defect in potassium excretion.

The intracellular space has a very high potassium concentration, so a shift of potassium from the intracellular space to the extracellular space can have a significant impact on the plasma potassium. This occurs with metabolic acidosis, but the effect is minimal with an organic acid (e.g., lactic acidosis or ketoacidosis). A respiratory acidosis has less impact than a metabolic acidosis. Cell destruction, as seen with rhabdomyolysis, tumor lysis

remitting in adulthood. Pseudohypoaldosteronism, type 2, also called *Gordon syndrome*, is an autosomal dominant disorder characterized by hypertension due to salt retention and impaired excretion of potassium and acid, leading to hyperkalemia and metabolic acidosis. Activating mutations in either WNK1 or WNK4, both serine-threonine kinases located in the distal nephron, cause Gordon syndrome.

Acquired renal tubular dysfunction, with an impaired ability to excrete potassium, occurs in a number of conditions. These disorders, all characterized by tubulointerstitial disease, are often associated with impaired acid secretion and a secondary metabolic acidosis. In some children, the metabolic acidosis is the dominant feature, although a high potassium intake may unmask the defect in potassium handling. The tubular dysfunction can cause renal salt wasting, potentially leading to hyponatremia. A defect in water handling, secondary nephrogenic diabetes insipidus, takes place in some children. This predisposes to dehydration and may lead to hypernatremia. Among the disorders listed in Box 45–4, the children with obstructive uropathy, primarily posterior urethral valves, are at risk for the most significant tubular dysfunction. Because of the tubulointerstitial damage, these conditions may also cause hyperkalemia as a result of hyporeninemic hypoaldosteronism.

The risk of hyperkalemia resulting from medications is greatest in patients with underlying renal insufficiency. The predominant mechanism of medication-induced hyperkalemia is impaired renal excretion, even though ACE inhibitors may worsen hyperkalemia in anuric patients, probably by inhibiting gastrointestinal potassium loss, which is normally upregulated in renal insufficiency. The hyperkalemia caused by trimethoprim generally only occurs at the very high doses used to treat *Pneumocystis carinii* pneumonia in patients with AIDS. Potassium-sparing diuretics may easily cause hyperkalemia, especially because they are often used in patients who are receiving oral potassium supplements.

Clinical Manifestations. The most import effects of hyperkalemia are due to the role of potassium in membrane polarization. The cardiac conduction system is usually the dominant concern. Electrocardiographic (ECG) changes begin with peaking of the T waves. This is followed, as the potassium level increases, by an increased PR interval, flattening of the P wave, and widening of the QRS complex. This can eventually progress to ventricular fibrillation. Asystole may also occur. Some patients have paresthesias, weakness, and tingling, but cardiac toxicity usually precedes these clinical symptoms, emphasizing the danger of assuming that an absence of symptoms implies an absence of danger.

Diagnosis. The etiology of hyperkalemia is often readily apparent. Spurious hyperkalemia is very common in children, so a repeat potassium level is often appropriate. If there is a significant elevation of the white blood cells or platelets, then the repeat sample should be from plasma that is evaluated promptly. The history should initially focus on potassium intake, risk factors for transcellular shifts of potassium, medications that cause hyperkalemia, and the presence of signs of renal insufficiency such as oliguria or an abnormal urinalysis. Initial laboratory evaluation should include creatinine, BUN, and assessment of acid-base status. Many etiologies of hyperkalemia cause a metabolic acidosis, and a metabolic acidosis worsens hyperkalemia by the transcellular shift of potassium out of cells. Renal insufficiency is a common cause of the combination of metabolic acidosis and hyperkalemia. This association is also seen in diseases with aldosterone insufficiency or aldosterone resistance. Children with absent or ineffective aldosterone often have hyponatremia and volume depletion due to salt wasting. Genetic diseases such as congenital adrenal hyperplasia and pseudohypoaldosteronism usually present in infancy and should be strongly considered in the infant with hyperkalemia

and metabolic acidosis, especially if hyponatremia is present. It is important to consider the various etiologies of a transcellular shift of potassium. In some of these disorders, the potassium continues to increase despite the elimination of all potassium intake, especially when there is concurrent renal insufficiency. This is potentially seen in tumor lysis syndrome, hemolysis, rhabdomyolysis, and other causes of cell death. All of these entities can cause concomitant hyperphosphatemia and hyperuricemia. Rhabdomyolysis produces an elevated creatinine phosphokinase (CPK) and hypocalcemia, whereas children with hemolysis have hemoglobinuria and a decreasing hematocrit. For the child with diabetes, an elevated blood glucose level suggests a transcellular shift of potassium.

When there is no clear etiology of hyperkalemia, the diagnostic approach should focus on differentiating decreased potassium excretion from the other etiologies. Measuring urinary potassium assesses renal excretion of potassium. The transtubular potassium gradient (TTKG) is a useful method to evaluate the renal response to hyperkalemia:

$$TTKG = [K]_{urine}/[K]_{plasma} \times (plasma\ osmolality/urine\ osmolality)$$

where $[K]_{urine}$ is the urine potassium concentration and $[K]_{plasma}$ is the plasma potassium concentration. The urine osmolality must be greater than the serum osmolality for the result to be valid. The TTKG normally varies widely, ranging from 5–15. The TTKG should be greater than 10 in the setting of hyperkalemia, assuming normal renal excretion of potassium. A TTKG of less than 8 during hyperkalemia suggests a defect in renal potassium excretion, which is usually due to lack of aldosterone or an inability to respond to aldosterone. Measurement of aldosterone is useful for differentiating these possible mechanisms. Patients with a lack of aldosterone respond to fludrocortisone, an oral mineralocorticoid, by increasing urinary potassium and decreasing the serum potassium. An appropriate TTKG with normal kidney function argues for a nonrenal cause of hyperkalemia.

Treatment. The plasma potassium level, the ECG, and the risk of the problem worsening determine the aggressiveness of the therapeutic approach. High serum potassium levels and the presence of ECG changes require more vigorous treatment. An additional source of concern is the patient with increasing plasma potassium despite minimal intake. This can happen if there is cellular release of potassium (e.g., tumor lysis syndrome), especially in the setting of diminished excretion (e.g., renal failure).

The first action in a child with a concerning elevation of plasma potassium is to stop all sources of additional potassium (oral and intravenous). Washed red blood cells can be used for patients who require blood transfusions. If the potassium level is greater than 6.0–6.5 mEq/L, an ECG should be obtained to help assess the urgency of the situation. The therapy of the hyperkalemia has two basic goals: (1) to stabilize the heart to prevent life-threatening arrhythmias and (2) to remove potassium from the body. The treatments that acutely prevent arrhythmias all have the advantage of working quickly (i.e., within minutes), but do not remove potassium from the body. Calcium stabilizes the cell membrane of heart cells, preventing arrhythmias. It is given over a few minutes intravenously and its action is almost immediate. Calcium should be given over 30 minutes in a patient receiving digitalis because it may cause arrhythmias. Bicarbonate causes potassium to move intracellularly, lowering the plasma potassium. It is especially efficacious in a patient with a metabolic acidosis. Insulin causes potassium to move intracellularly, but it must be given with glucose to avoid hypoglycemia. The combination of insulin and glucose works within 30 minutes. Nebulized albuterol, by stimulation of β_1-receptors, leads to intracellular movement of potassium. This has the advantage of not requiring an intravenous route of administration, allowing it to be given concurrently with the other measures.

It is important to begin measures that remove potassium from the body. Because none of these work quickly, it is important to start them as soon as possible. In patients who are not anuric, a loop diuretic increases renal excretion of potassium. This may require a high dose in a patient with significant renal insufficiency. Sodium polystyrene sulfonate (Kayexalate) is an exchange resin that is given either rectally or orally. Sodium in the resin is exchanged for body potassium and the potassium-containing resin is then excreted from the body. Some patients require dialysis for acute potassium removal. Dialysis is often necessary if there is severe renal failure or if there is an especially high rate of endogenous potassium release as is sometimes present with tumor lysis syndrome or rhabdomyolysis. Hemodialysis rapidly lowers plasma potassium levels. Peritoneal dialysis is not nearly as quick or reliable, even though it is usually adequate as long as the acute problem can be managed with medications and the endogenous release of potassium is not extremely high.

Chronic management of hyperkalemia includes reducing intake via dietary changes and eliminating or reducing medications that cause hyperkalemia. Some patients require medications to increase potassium excretion. These include sodium polystyrene sulfonate and loop or thiazide diuretics. Some infants with chronic renal failure may need to start dialysis to allow adequate caloric intake without hyperkalemia. It is unusual for an older child to require dialysis principally to control chronic hyperkalemia. The disorders that are due to a deficiency in aldosterone respond to replacement therapy with fludrocortisone.

HYPOKALEMIA

Hypokalemia is common in children, with most cases related to gastroenteritis.

Etiology and Pathophysiology. There are four basic mechanisms of hypokalemia (Box 45–5). Low intake, nonrenal losses, and renal losses are all associated with total body potassium depletion. With a transcellular shift, there is no change in total body potassium, although there may be concomitant potassium depletion resulting from other factors. Spurious hypokalemia occurs in patients with leukemia and very elevated white blood cell counts if plasma for analysis is left at room temperature, permitting the white cells to take up potassium from the plasma. High white counts may cause fictitious hyperkalemia if a serum sample is analyzed or a plasma sample is stored in the cold.

Because the intracellular potassium concentration is much higher than the plasma level, a significant amount of potassium can move into cells without markedly changing the intracellular potassium concentration. Alkalemia is one of the more common causes of a transcellular shift. The effect is much greater with a metabolic alkalosis than with a respiratory alkalosis. The impact of exogenous insulin on potassium movement into cells is substantial in patients with diabetic ketoacidosis. It can be endogenous insulin when a patient is given a bolus of glucose. Both endogenous (e.g., epinephrine in stress) and exogenous (e.g., albuterol) ß-adrenergic agonists stimulate cellular uptake of potassium. Theophylline overdose, barium intoxication, and toluene intoxication from paint or glue sniffing cause a transcellular shift hypokalemia, often with severe clinical manifestations. Children with hypokalemic periodic paralysis, a rare autosomal dominant disorder, have acute cellular uptake of potassium, producing the symptomatology (see Chapter 602).

Inadequate potassium intake occurs in anorexia nervosa; accompanying bulimia and laxative or diuretic abuse exacerbates the potassium deficiency. Sweat losses of potassium can be significant during vigorous exercise in a hot climate. Associated volume

BOX 45–5. Causes of Hypokalemia

SPURIOUS
High white blood cell count

TRANSCELLULAR SHIFTS
Alkalemia
Insulin
β-adrenergic agonists
Drugs/toxins (theophylline, barium, toluene)
Hypokalemic periodic paralysis (MIM* 170400)

DECREASED INTAKE

EXTRARENAL LOSSES
Diarrhea
Laxative abuse
Sweating

RENAL LOSSES
With metabolic acidosis
  Distal renal tubular acidosis (RTA) (MIM 179800/602722)
  Proximal RTA (MIM 604278†)
  Ureterosigmoidostomy
  Diabetic ketoacidosis
Without specific acid-base disturbance
  Tubular toxins: amphotericin, cisplatin, aminoglycosides
  Interstitial nephritis
  Diuretic phase of acute tubular necrosis
  Postobstructive diuresis
  Hypomagnesemia
  High urine anions (e.g., penicillin or penicillin derivatives)
With metabolic alkalosis
  Low urine chloride
    Emesis nasogastric suction
    Chloride losing diarrhea (MIM 214700)
    Cystic fibrosis (MIM 219700)
    Low chloride formula
    Posthypercapnia
    Previous loop or thiazide diuretic use
  High urine chloride and normal blood pressure
    Gitelman syndrome (MIM 263800)
    Bartter syndrome (MIM 602023)
    Loop and thiazide diuretics
  High urine chloride and high blood pressure
    Adrenal adenoma or hyperplasia
    Glucocorticoid-remedial aldosteronism (MIM 103900)
    Renovascular disease
    Renin-secreting tumor
    17α-hydroxylase deficiency (MIM 202110)
    11β-hydroxylase deficiency (MIM 202010)
    Cushing syndrome
    11β-hydroxysteroid dehydrogenase deficiency (MIM 218030)
    Licorice ingestion
    Liddle syndrome (MIM 177200)

*MIM refers to the database number from the Mendelian Inheritance in Man (http://www3.ncbi.nlm.nih.gov/Omim/).
†Most cases of proximal RTA are not due to this primary genetic disorder. Proximal RTA is usually part of Fanconi syndrome, which has multiple etiologies (see Chapter 521).

depletion and hyperaldosteronism increases renal losses of potassium (see later text). Diarrhea has a high concentration of potassium and the resulting hypokalemia is usually associated with a metabolic acidosis resulting from stool losses of bicarbonate. In contrast, a normal acid-base balance or a mild metabolic alkalosis is seen with laxative abuse.

Urinary potassium wasting may be accompanied by a metabolic acidosis (proximal or distal renal tubular acidosis [RTA]). In diabetic ketoacidosis, although often associated with normal plasma potassium caused by transcellular shifts, there is significant total body potassium depletion from urinary losses due to the osmotic diuresis, and the potassium level may dramatically decrease with insulin therapy (see Chapter 583). Both the polyuric phase of acute tubular necrosis and postobstructive diuresis cause transient, highly variable potassium wasting and may be associated with a metabolic acidosis. Tubular damage, either directly from medications or secondary to interstitial nephritis, is often accompanied by other tubular losses, including magnesium, sodium, and water. Such tubular damage may cause a secondary RTA with a metabolic acidosis. Isolated magnesium deficiency causes renal potassium wasting. Penicillin is an anion that is excreted in the urine, resulting in increased potassium excretion because the penicillin anion must be accompanied by a cation. Hypokalemia from penicillin only occurs with the sodium salt of penicillin, not with the potassium salt.

Urinary potassium wasting is often accompanied by a metabolic alkalosis. This is usually associated with increased aldosterone, which increases urinary potassium and acid losses, contributing to the hypokalemia and the metabolic alkalosis. Other mechanisms often contribute to both the potassium losses and the metabolic alkalosis. With emesis or nasogastric suction there is gastric loss of potassium, but this is fairly minimal given the low potassium content of gastric fluid (~10 mEq/L). More important is the gastric loss of HCl, leading to a metabolic alkalosis and a state of volume depletion. The kidney compensates for the metabolic alkalosis by excreting bicarbonate in the urine, but there is obligate loss of potassium and sodium with the bicarbonate. The volume depletion increases aldosterone levels, which prevents correction of the metabolic alkalosis and hypokalemia until the volume depletion is corrected. Urinary chloride is low as a response to the volume depletion. Because the volume depletion is secondary to chloride loss, this is a state of chloride deficiency. There were cases of chloride deficiency resulting from infant formula deficient in chloride, which caused a metabolic alkalosis with hypokalemia and low urine chloride. Current infant formula is not deficient in chloride. A similar mechanism occurs in cystic fibrosis because of a chloride loss in sweat. In congenital chloride-losing diarrhea, an autosomal recessive disorder, there is high stool loss of chloride, leading to metabolic alkalosis, an unusual sequelae of diarrhea. Because of stool potassium losses, chloride deficiency, and metabolic alkalosis, these patients have hypokalemia. During respiratory acidosis, there is renal compensation, with retention of bicarbonate and excretion of chloride. After the respiratory acidosis is corrected, patients have chloride deficiency and post-hypercapnic alkalosis with secondary hypokalemia. Patients with chloride deficiency, metabolic alkalosis, and hypokalemia have urinary chloride of less than 10 mEq/L. Loop and thiazide diuretics lead to hypokalemia, metabolic alkalosis, and chloride deficiency. During treatment, these patients have high urine chloride resulting from the effect of the diuretic. However, after the diuretics are discontinued, there is residual chloride deficiency, the urinary chloride is appropriately low, and neither the hypokalemia nor the alkalosis resolves until the chloride deficiency is corrected.

The combination of metabolic alkalosis, hypokalemia, high urine chloride, and normal blood pressure is characteristic of Bartter syndrome, Gitelman syndrome, and current diuretic use. These patients have high urinary losses of potassium and chloride despite a state of relative volume depletion with secondary hyperaldosteronism. Bartter and Gitelman syndromes are autosomal recessive disorders caused by defects in tubular transporters (see Chapter 523). Bartter syndrome is usually associated with hypercalciuria, often with nephrocalcinosis, whereas children with Gitelman syndrome have low urinary calcium losses, but hypomagnesemia due to urinary magnesium losses.

In the presence of high aldosterone, there is urinary loss of potassium, hypokalemia, metabolic alkalosis, and an elevated urinary chloride. There is also renal retention of sodium, leading to hypertension. Primary hyperaldosteronism from adenoma or hyperplasia is much less common in children than in adults (see Chapter 572). Glucocorticoid-remedial aldosteronism, an auto-somal dominant disorder that leads to high levels of aldosterone, is often diagnosed in childhood.

Increased aldosterone may be secondary to increased renin production. Renal artery stenosis leads to hypertension from increased renin and secondary hyperaldosteronism. The increased aldosterone can cause hypokalemia and metabolic alkalosis, even though most patients have normal electrolytes. Renin-producing tumors, which are extremely rare, can cause hypokalemia.

There are a variety of disorders that cause hypertension and hypokalemia without increased aldosterone. Some are due to increased levels of mineralocorticoids other than aldosterone. This occurs in two forms of congenital adrenal hyperplasia (see Chapter 570). In 11ß-hydroxylase deficiency, which is associated with virilization, 11-deoxycorticosterone is elevated, which causes variable hypertension and hypokalemia. A similar mechanism, increased DOC, occurs in 17α hydroxylase deficiency, but these patients are more uniformly hypertensive and hypokalemic, and have a defect in sex hormone production. Cushing syndrome, frequently associated with hypertension, less commonly causes metabolic alkalosis and hypokalemia. This is secondary to the mineralocorticoid activity of cortisol. In 11ß-hydroxysteroid dehydrogenase deficiency, an autosomal recessive disorder, the enzymatic defect prevents conversion of cortisol to cortisone in the kidney. Because cortisol binds and activates the aldosterone receptor, these children have all the features of excessive mineralocorticoids, including hypertension, hypokalemia, and metabolic alkalosis. Patients with this disorder, which is also called "apparent mineralocorticoid excess," respond to spironolactone therapy, which blocks the mineralocorticoid receptor. An acquired form of 11ß-hydroxysteroid dehydrogenase deficiency occurs from the ingestion of substances that inhibit this enzyme. A classic example is glycyrrhizic acid, which is found in natural licorice. Liddle syndrome is an autosomal dominant disorder that results from an activating mutation of the distal nephron sodium channel that is normally upregulated by aldosterone. Patients have the characteristics of hyperaldosteronism—hypertension, hypokalemia, and alkalosis—but low serum aldosterone levels. These patients respond to the potassium-sparing diuretics (triamterene and amiloride) that inhibit this sodium channel.

Clinical Manifestations. The heart and skeletal muscle are especially vulnerable to hypokalemia. ECG changes include a flattened T wave, depressed ST segment, and appearance of a U wave, which is located between the T wave, if still visible, and P wave. Ventricular fibrillation and torsades de pointes may occur, although usually only in the context of underlying heart disease. Hypokalemia makes the heart especially susceptible to digitalis-induced arrhythmias such as supraventricular tachycardia, ventricular tachycardia, and heart block (also see Chapter 428).

The clinical consequences in skeletal muscle include muscle weakness and cramps. Paralysis is a possible complication, generally only at levels less than 2.5 mEq/L. This usually starts with the legs, followed by the arms. Respiratory paralysis may require mechanical ventilation. Some patients develop rhabdomyolysis; the risk increases with exercise. Hypokalemia slows gastrointestinal motility. This manifests as constipation or, with levels less than 2.5 mEq/L, ileus may occur. Hypokalemia impairs bladder function, potentially leading to urinary retention.

Hypokalemia causes polyuria and polydipsia by two mechanisms: primary polydipsia and impaired urinary concentrating ability, producing a nephrogenic diabetes insipidus. Hypokalemia stimulates renal ammonia production, which is clinically significant if hepatic failure is present because the liver cannot metabolize the ammonia. Hypokalemia may therefore worsen hepatic encephalopathy.

Chronic hypokalemia may cause kidney damage, including interstitial nephritis and renal cysts. In children, chronic hypokalemia, as in Bartter syndrome, leads to poor linear growth.

Diagnosis. Most causes of hypokalemia are readily apparent from the history. It is important to review the child's diet, gastrointestinal losses, and medications. Both emesis and diuretic use can be surreptitious. The presence of hypertension suggests excess mineralocorticoids. Concomitant electrolyte abnormalities are useful clues. The combination of hypokalemia and metabolic acidosis is characteristic of diarrhea and of distal and proximal RTA. A concurrent metabolic alkalosis is characteristic of emesis or nasogastric losses, aldosterone excess, use of diuretics, and Bartter and Gitelman syndromes. Alkalosis is also associated with a transcellular shift of potassium intracellularly and increased urinary losses of potassium.

If a clear etiology is not apparent, the measurement of urinary potassium distinguishes between renal and extrarenal losses. The kidneys should conserve potassium in the presence of extrarenal losses. Urinary potassium losses can be assessed with a 24-hour urine collection, a spot potassium/creatine ratio, a fractional excretion of potassium, or calculation of the TTKG, which is the most widely used approach in children:

$$TTKG = [K]_{urine}/[K]_{plasma} \times (plasma\ osmolality/urine\ osmolality)$$

where $[K]_{urine}$ is the urine potassium concentration and $[K]_{plasma}$ is the plasma potassium concentration.

The urine osmolality must be greater than the serum osmolality for the result to be valid. A TTKG of more than 4 in the presence of hypokalemia suggests excessive urinary losses of potassium. The urinary potassium excretion can be misleading if the stimulus for renal losses, such as a diuretic, is no longer present.

Treatment. Factors that influence the therapy of hypokalemia include the potassium level, clinical symptoms, renal function, presence of transcellular shifts of potassium, ongoing losses, and the patient's ability to tolerate oral potassium. Severe, symptomatic hypokalemia receives more aggressive treatment. Supplementation is more cautious if renal function is decreased because of the kidney's limited ability to excrete excessive potassium. The plasma potassium level does not always provide an accurate estimation of the total body potassium deficit. This is because there may be shifts of potassium from the intracellular space to the plasma. Clinically, this occurs most commonly with metabolic acidosis and the insulin deficiency of diabetic ketoacidosis; the plasma potassium underestimates the degree of total body potassium depletion. As these problems are corrected, potassium moves into the intracellular space so these patients require more potassium supplementation to correct their hypokalemia. Likewise, the presence of a transcellular shift of potassium into cells indicates that the total body potassium depletion is less severe. Patients who have ongoing losses of potassium need correction of their deficit and replacement of the ongoing losses.

Because of the risk of hyperkalemia, intravenous potassium should be used cautiously. Oral potassium is safer, albeit not as rapid in urgent situations. The dose of intravenous potassium is 0.5–1 mEq/kg, usually given over 1 hr. The adult maximum dose is 40 mEq. Conservative dosing is generally preferred. Potassium chloride is the usual choice for supplementation, although the presence of concurrent electrolyte abnormalities may dictate other options. Patients with acidosis and hypokalemia can receive potassium acetate or potassium citrate. If hypophosphatemia is present, then some of the potassium deficit can be replaced with potassium phosphate. It is sometimes possible to decrease ongoing losses of potassium. For patients with excessive urinary losses, potassium-sparing diuretics are effective, but they need to be used cautiously in patients with renal insufficiency. If hypokalemia, metabolic alkalosis, and volume depletions are present (e.g., with gastric losses), then restoration of intravascular volume with adequate chloride will decrease urinary potassium losses. Disease-specific therapy is effective in many of the genetic tubular disorders.

45.5 Calcium

CALCIUM METABOLISM

Body Content and Physiologic Function. Ninety-nine percent of body calcium is in bone, mostly as hydroxyapatite. During growth, bone mass increases faster than body weight, which necessitates a concomitant increase in body calcium. In infants, there is approximately 400 mg/kg of calcium, whereas adults have 950 mg/kg of calcium. Calcium has a number of crucial physiologic functions, including blood coagulation, cellular communication, exocytosis, endocytosis, muscle contraction, and neuromuscular transmission. There are two principal goals of calcium homeostasis. First, there must be adequate net intake of calcium to permit normal skeletal growth and mineralization. Second, there is tight regulation of the serum calcium concentration in order to permit normal physiologic functioning. The second goal takes precedence over the first goal: skeletal mineralization may be sacrificed to maintain a normal serum calcium level.

Measurement of Serum Calcium. Because calcium is a divalent cation, the units mmol/L and mEq/L are not equivalent, and there are three different units used for its measurement (Table 45–1). Most laboratories in the United States use mg/dL when reporting the total calcium concentration. However, the ionized calcium concentration is more physiologically relevant than the total calcium concentration, and its value may be reported in any of the three possible units. It is critical to know whether a calcium value is total or ionized and to know which units are used.

Slightly less than half of the total serum calcium exists in the free or ionized form. Most of the remainder is bound to protein (mostly albumin), whereas a smaller percentage, about 10%, complexes with anions such as phosphate, citrate, or sulfate. The ionized calcium is relevant for cell function, and the body's homeostatic system regulates the ionized calcium concentration. Nevertheless, it is the total calcium that is usually measured.

In general, the total calcium provides a satisfactory assessment of physiologic calcium. However, there are a few clinical situations in which the total calcium is not an adequate surrogate for the ionized calcium concentration. The most common and severe problem is the presence of hypoalbuminemia, such as patients with nephrotic syndrome, liver disease, capillary

TABLE 45–1. Conversion Factors for Calcium, Magnesium, and Phosphorus

	Unit	Conversion Factor	Unit
Calcium	mg/dL	0.25	mmol/L
	mEq/L	0.5	mmol/L
	mg/dL	0.5	mEq/L
Magnesium	mg/dL	0.411	mmol/L
	mEq/L	0.5	mmol/L
	mg/dL	0.822	mEq/L
Phosphorus	mg/dL	0.32	mmol/L

Note: Values in the left unit column are converted into the right unit column via multiplying by the conversion factor (e.g., calcium of 10 mg/dL times 0.25 equals 2.5 mmol/L). Division of the right unit column by the conversion factor converts to the units of the left unit column.

leak, or protein-losing enteropathy. Each 1 g/dL of albumin in the serum binds about 0.8 mg/dL of calcium. A low total calcium concentration may be normal in a patient with significant hypoalbuminemia. The following formula can be used to "correct" the total calcium concentration in the setting of hypoalbuminemia:

$$Ca_c = Ca_m + [0.8 \times (\text{decrease in albumin concentration below normal in g/dL})]$$

where Ca_c is total calcium corrected and Ca_m is total calcium measured.

When using this formula, a total calcium concentration that is in the normal range after correction suggests that the patient has a normal ionized calcium concentration; a high or low value indicates hypercalcemia or hypocalcemia, respectively. Unfortunately, this formula is not universally accurate and an ionized calcium concentration should be obtained when the albumin is low and there is clinical suspicion of an abnormal ionized calcium concentration. This is especially true in sicker patients, because very ill children are more likely to have an abnormal calcium concentration, and they frequently have other disturbances that make the total calcium concentration a less accurate gauge of the ionized calcium concentration.

Some of the limitations of the above formula are due to other factors affecting the relationship between the total calcium and the ionized calcium. Serum globulin binds a small amount of calcium and, therefore, has a small impact on this relationship. The serum pH influences the percentage of calcium that is bound to albumin and other ions such as phosphate. Alkalemia produces more binding of calcium and acidemia causes less binding of calcium. As the pH decreases, less calcium is bound, and the ionized calcium concentration increases. This can be clinically relevant when bicarbonate is administered to correct acidosis; the increasing pH increases the amount of bound calcium and the ionized calcium decreases, possibly producing symptoms.

Regulation of Calcium. A complex hormonal system regulates the serum calcium concentration. Acutely, this system relies on the large reservoir of calcium that is present in bone. Chronically, there must be a balance between calcium intake from the gastrointestinal tract and calcium losses, mostly via the urine. In growing children, a net positive calcium balance is necessary for growth and skeletal mineralization.

Maintenance and accretion of body calcium require gastrointestinal absorption, which occurs predominantly in the duodenum and jejunum. Breast milk (300 mg/L), formula (~530 mg/L), and cow's milk (~1,200 mg/L) are excellent sources of calcium, and children in the United States receive most of their dietary calcium from milk and other dairy products. The recommended intake of calcium varies with age (see Chapter 40). Even though there is some passive calcium absorption when dietary intake is high, an active transport system is responsible for most gastrointestinal absorption, especially when dietary intake is low. Through the production of calcium-binding proteins and activation of a calcium pump on the gastrointestinal epithelial cells, 1,25-dihydroxyvitamin D stimulates the active transport of calcium. Without adequate 1,25-dihydroxyvitamin D, the active form of vitamin D, gastrointestinal absorption of calcium decreases substantially.

The synthesis of vitamin D in the skin occurs when its precursor, 7-dehydrocholesterol, is exposed to ultraviolet light, typically from the sun. The main dietary sources of vitamin D are fortified foods, principally milk or formula, and vitamin supplements. The production of 1,25-dihydroxyvitamin D requires that vitamin D is first hydroxylated in the liver, producing 25-hydroxyvitamin D. In the kidney, the enzyme 1α-hydroxylase converts 25-dihydroxyvitamin D into 1,25-dihydroxyvitamin D.

Modifying synthesis of 1,25-dihydroxyvitamin D is an important mechanism for regulating calcium balance. Parathyroid hormone (PTH), released by the parathyroid gland in response to low serum calcium levels, stimulates the 1α-hydroxylase in the kidney to produce more 1,25-dihydroxyvitamin D, ultimately leading to increased absorption of calcium. A calcium-sensing receptor in the parathyroid gland dictates the release of PTH.

Whereas the actions of 1,25-dihydroxyvitamin D on the intestinal tract control calcium intake, the kidneys control calcium excretion. The calcium in the plasma that is not bound to protein, including the ionized calcium and calcium complexed to anions, is freely filtered by the glomerulus and enters the proximal tubule. About 99% of the filtered calcium is reabsorbed by the tubules, with 50% or more reclaimed in the proximal tubule. The loop of Henle, the distal tubule, and the collecting duct are other sites of calcium reabsorption. In the proximal tubule and the loop of Henle, calcium reabsorption parallels sodium reabsorption. This is very important clinically. In the treatment of hypercalcemia, volume expansion with normal saline, which decreases sodium reabsorption, effectively increases calcium excretion by the kidneys. Similarly, the inhibition of sodium reabsorption in the loop of Henle by loop diuretics such as furosemide increases urinary calcium excretion. The resultant hypercalciuria is helpful in treating hypercalcemia, but chronic use of loop diuretics increases the risk of nephrocalcinosis and nephrolithiasis, especially when used in premature infants.

PTH is the principal regulator of urinary calcium excretion. PTH acts on the ascending limb of the loop of Henle and the distal nephron to increase calcium reabsorption. 1,25-dihydroxyvitamin D also stimulates calcium reabsorption in the distal nephron. Urinary calcium excretion increases in the absence of PTH. Urinary calcium excretion is also increased by growth hormone, metabolic acidosis, thyroid hormone, hyperphosphatemia, glucagon, osmotic diuretics, volume expansion, loop diuretics, and prolonged fasting. Even though urinary excretion of calcium is important, intestinal absorption is the primary site of regulation and, thus, there is usually minimal variation in urinary excretion despite variation in dietary intake.

Acute regulation of serum calcium depends on the large bone reservoir of calcium. PTH stimulates bone osteoclasts to dissolve bone and release calcium; it also increases the number of osteoclasts. In addition, PTH stimulates the 1α-hydroxylase in the kidney to convert 25-hydroxyvitamin D into 1,25-dihydroxyvitamin D. This active form of vitamin D acts on bone to increase calcium mobilization. The hormone calcitonin, produced by the parafollicular cells of the thyroid gland and secreted in response to hypercalcemia, inhibits the release of calcium from bone mediated by osteoclasts. Calcitonin also increases urinary excretion of calcium.

PTH and vitamin D have additional effects that are important for understanding the pathophysiology of calcium disorders. PTH increases urinary excretion of phosphate and bicarbonate. This compensates for the release of phosphate and base that occurs as a result of PTH-mediated bone resorption. Urinary phosphate wasting explains the hypophosphatemia often associated with hyperparathyroidism. 1,25-dihydroxyvitamin D participates in a negative feedback loop whereby PTH increases the synthesis of 1,25-dihydroxyvitamin D, which acts on the parathyroid gland to suppress PTH production. This is an important contributor to the secondary hyperparathyroidism of chronic renal failure. The failing kidneys cannot make adequate 1,25-dihydroxyvitamin D, which results in poor absorption of calcium. This leads to PTH synthesis caused by low serum calcium, and the lack of 1,25-dihydroxyvitamin D prevents its normal negative feedback on synthesis of PTH. 1,25-dihydroxyvitamin D also increases intestinal phosphate absorption, although phosphate absorption is not as dependent on vitamin D as calcium absorption.

HYPOCALCEMIA

Because of potentially severe symptoms such as laryngospasm and seizures, hypocalcemia needs to be identified and treated expeditiously. The ionized calcium concentration is low in true hypocalcemia. The total calcium concentration does not accurately predict the ionized calcium concentration in the patient with hypoalbuminemia. As previously discussed, the formula for correcting the total calcium concentration based on the concurrent albumin concentration is not always accurate, especially in the more critically ill child. Hence, the ionized calcium concentration should be determined in patients with suspected hypocalcemia when the patient is hypoalbuminemic and/or is critically ill.

Etiology and Pathophysiology. There are many causes of hypocalcemia (Box 45–6). Hypocalcemia occurs most commonly in neonates. Hypocalcemia is one of the most common causes of neonatal seizures. This is usually due to early neonatal hypocal-

---

■ BOX 45–6. Causes of Hypocalcemia

SPECIFIC CAUSES IN THE NEONATE
Early neonatal hypocalcemia
Late neonatal hypocalcemia
Maternal hypercalcemia

HYPOPARATHYROIDISM
DiGeorge syndrome (MIM* 188400)
X-linked hypoparathyroidism (MIM 307700)
Parathyroid hormone (PTH) gene mutations (MIM 168450)
Calcium-sensing receptor mutation (MIM 601199)
Autosomal recessive hypoparathyroidism with dysmorphic features (MIM 241410)
HDR (or Barakat) syndrome (MIM 146255)
Autoimmune polyglandular syndrome type I (MIM 240300)
Kearns-Sayre syndrome (MIM 530000)
Hemochromatosis
Wilson disease (MIM 277900)
Postsurgical hypoparathyroidism
Radioactive iodine ablation of the thyroid gland
Hypomagnesemia

LACK OF RESPONSE TO PTH
Pseudohypoparathyroidism type IA (MIM 103580)
Pseudohypoparathyroidism type IB (MIM 603233)
Pseudohypoparathyroidism type II
Hypomagnesemia

VITAMIN D DEFICIENCY
Poor intake
Lack of sunlight
Malabsorption
Increased metabolism (e.g., anticonvulsants)
Failure to form 25-hydroxyvitamin D in the liver
Vitamin D–dependent rickets type 1 (MIM 264700)
Vitamin D–dependent rickets type 2 (MIM 277420)
Renal insufficiency

REDISTRIBUTION OF PLASMA CALCIUM
Hyperphosphatemia
Rhabdomyolysis
Tumor lysis syndrome
Blood transfusions
Hungry bone syndrome
Acute pancreatitis
Osteopetrosis, infantile (MIM 259700)

INADEQUATE CALCIUM INTAKE
Calcium-poor diet or total parenteral nutrition
Dietary calcium chelators
Malabsorption

UNKNOWN
Septic shock
Critical illness

---

*MIM refers to the database number from the Mendelian Inheritance in Man (http://www3.ncbi.nlm.nih.gov/Omim/).

---

cemia, also called transient physiologic hypoparathyroidism. Early neonatal hypocalcemia occurs during the first 72 hr of life, usually before achieving a significant oral intake of milk. Serum calcium values correlate directly with gestational age, and less mature infants have a greater chance of developing hypocalcemia.

There are multiple mechanisms that account for early neonatal hypocalcemia. Even healthy term infants have a decrease in serum calcium concentration after birth, with the nadir occurring at approximately 24 hr. This is presumably due to the sudden disappearance of the transplacental delivery of calcium, an active process that maintains a higher calcium level in the fetus than in the mother. In addition, newborns may have a relative hypoparathyroidism, which has been attributed to the increased serum calcium level of the fetus, causing suppression of the parathyroid gland. Newborns may also have a relative refractoriness of the target cells to parathyroid hormone.

Early hypocalcemia in neonates occurs most commonly in low birthweight infants, especially those with intrauterine growth retardation, in infants born of diabetic mothers, and in infants who have been subjected to prolonged, difficult deliveries (see Chapters 95 and 96). The incidence of hypocalcemia is inversely proportional to gestational age and birthweight. Because of the interruption of calcium transfer across the placenta, the rate of calcium delivery invariably decreases after birth. Calcium intake may be further decreased because the infant's small size or illness prevents normal feeding. Excessive secretion of calcitonin may be a contributing factor in persistent hypocalcemia of premature infants, particularly those stressed by anoxia. The incidence of hypocalcemia in prematurely born infants is extremely high, particularly in those with respiratory distress and those who have received intravenous sodium bicarbonate. Hypocalcemia should be suspected as a possible cause of convulsions in such neonates. Infants born of diabetic mothers have a high incidence of hypocalcemia, with a higher risk if the mothers have had poor metabolic control of their diabetes. Infants of diabetic mothers are more likely to be premature and have birth asphyxia. In addition, diabetes, by causing maternal magnesium depletion, may decrease transfer of magnesium to the fetus. The consequent hypomagnesemia in infants of diabetic mothers causes secondary hypoparathyroidism and hypocalcemia. Early preterm infants are often less symptomatic from hypocalcemia. This may be related to their lower serum albumin and their metabolic acidosis, both leading to an increase in the ionized calcium concentration because of less binding of calcium to albumin. Even though the hypocalcemia in premature or asphyxiated infants usually resolves in a few days, some infants of diabetic mothers have a more prolonged course.

Late hypocalcemia in neonates, much less common than early hypocalcemia, is due to intake of milk with a high content of phosphate. The onset of symptoms occurs most commonly during the first 5–10 days of life; clinical manifestations have occasionally appeared as late as 6 wk of age. The incidence of late neonatal hypocalcemia decreased dramatically when the phosphorus content of formula was reduced. It does not occur in breast-fed infants because of the lower phosphate content of breast milk compared to formula; breast milk has about 140 mg/L of phosphorus and current standard formula has at least twice as much phosphorus. The inappropriate use in a neonate of whole cow's milk, which has 956 mg/L of phosphorus, can cause hyperphosphatemia and secondary hypocalcemia. Late neonatal hypocalcemia most often occurs in otherwise healthy, full-term neonates. The intake of a high-phosphate food in a relatively large volume, combined with decreased renal phosphate excretion, leads to an elevated serum phosphorus level. The decreased renal phosphate excretion is due to the physiologically low GFR of the newborn and relatively high tubular reabsorption of phosphate. The elevated serum phosphorus level depresses the serum calcium level through deposition of calcium phosphate in bone and possibly in other tissues. The normal physiologic response is an increased output of PTH, which stimulates calcium release from bone and urine phosphate excretion. This restores the normal serum levels of calcium and phosphorus. Infants with late neonatal hypocalcemia may have normal or elevated PTH, but the PTH response is relatively inadequate because the serum calcium is low. The immature parathyroid gland, in affected children, may not be able to respond appropriately. Alternatively, some of these infants may have an appropriate PTH response to hypocalcemia, but have end-organ resistance to PTH. This "transient pseudohypoparathyroidism" self-resolves.

Hypocalcemia may occur in infants born to mothers with hypercalcemia, which is commonly due to *hyperparathyroidism from a parathyroid adenoma*. The constant in utero suppression of the parathyroid gland can lead to prolonged hypoparathyroidism in the neonate, sometimes lasting for months. The infants usually develop tetany during the first 3 wk of life, but it may occur later if the infant is breast-fed. Often the mother is asymptomatic and the diagnosis depends on obtaining a maternal serum calcium level.

There are multiple causes of primary hypoparathyroidism (see Chapter 565). Along with hypocalcemia, hypoparathyroidism leads to hyperphosphatemia due to decreased renal excretion of phosphate. PTH levels are either low or undetectable, although inappropriately normal levels in the setting of hypocalcemia may occur in children with some residual PTH production. Because PTH and hypophosphatemia are the normal stimuli for the renal 1α-hydroxylase, 1,25-dihydroxyvitamin D levels are low.

In *DiGeorge syndrome* (also called velocardiofacial syndrome), most patients have a small deletion of chromosome 22 (see Chapter 115.1). It occasionally occurs in patients with a small deletion in chromosome 10. Along with a high incidence of congenital heart disease, these children may have facial anomalies, hypoplasia or aplasia of the parathyroid gland, and, rarely, severe immunodeficiency resulting from aplasia of the thymus. If hypocalcemia occurs in these patients, it is often transitory during the neonatal period, although it may be permanent, recur, or only appear later in life.

X-linked hypoparathyroidism is a rare disorder with unaffected female carriers. Affected boys have an absence of parathyroid tissue and present with hypocalcemia during the first 6 mo of life. Mutations in the PTH gene, with either autosomal recessive or autosomal dominant inheritance, are potential causes of hypoparathyroidism. One form of *autosomal dominant hypoparathyroidism* is secondary to an activating mutation of the calcium-sensing receptor. The parathyroid gland perceives a higher calcium concentration than actually exists; PTH levels are inappropriately normal for the degree of hypocalcemia. *Autosomal recessive hypoparathyroidism* with dysmorphic features is rare, with the only descriptions in Middle Eastern families, usually with consanguinity. **HDR syndrome,** an autosomal dominant disorder, is the combination of **h**ypoparathyroidism, nerve **d**eafness, and **r**enal dysplasia. It is due to a mutation in the GATA3 gene, which produces a zinc finger transcription factor. *Autoimmune polyglandular syndrome type I* is an autosomal recessive disorder, due to mutations in the autoimmune regulator (AIRE) gene, with the combination of hypoparathyroidism, Addison diseases, and mucocutaneous candidiasis, although most patients only have two of these three problems. Candidiasis usually precedes parathyroid gland dysfunction. Hypoparathyroidism, when it occurs, does not usually appear until after 5 yr of age in *Kearns-Sayre syndrome*, a mitochondrially inherited disorder. Copper overload in *Wilson disease* or iron overload in *hemochromatosis* may cause hypoparathyroidism. The iron overload may be secondary to multiple transfusions, as in patients with thalassemia. Accidental removal of the parathyroid gland or disruption of its blood supply may occur after thyroid surgery or after neck sur-

gery for non-thyroid cancer. Radioactive iodine ablation of the thyroid gland for Graves' disease may inadvertently damage the parathyroid gland.

Hypomagnesemia causes secondary hypoparathyroidism because an adequate serum magnesium concentration is necessary for normal release of PTH. In addition, magnesium appears to be important for a normal response to the actions of PTH. Hypomagnesemia causes target-organ resistance to PTH.

In *pseudohypoparathyroidism* there is adequate production of PTH, but a lack of response at the target organs (see Chapter 566). Patients have hypocalcemia, hyperphosphatemia, and low levels of 1,25-dihydroxyvitamin D. Most patients have a defect in the alpha-subunit of the stimulatory G protein that is necessary for signal transduction when PTH binds to its receptor. Administration of PTH to these patients fails to increase renal phosphate excretion or to increase serum calcium. Furthermore, there is no increase in urinary cAMP, as normally occurs as a result of G protein–mediated activation of adenylate cyclase after PTH binds to its receptor. The measurement of urinary cAMP after infusion of synthetic PTH is the diagnostic test of choice for establishing the diagnosis. Children with pseudohypoparathyroidism type 1A have the phenotypic features of Albright hereditary osteodystrophy, including short stature, stocky build, round face, and brachydactyly due to shortened metacarpals and metatarsals. Moderate mental retardation occurs in about 50% of these patients. Pseudohypoparathyroidism type 1B is identical to type 1A, except for the absence of the features of Albright hereditary osteodystrophy. This disease is also secondary to a defect in the stimulatory G protein, and patients have an impaired urinary cAMP response to synthetic cAMP. In pseudohypoparathyroidism type II, a rare and poorly described disorder, there is PTH resistance but a normal urinary cAMP response to PTH infusion.

In *vitamin D deficiency*, hypocalcemia is primarily the result of poor intestinal absorption of calcium. PTH levels are increased as a response to the inadequate calcium, and this initially prevents the development of frank hypocalcemia by causing release of calcium from bone, decreasing urinary losses of calcium, and upregulating the activity of the 1α-hydroxylase that converts 25-hydroxyvitamin D into the active form of vitamin D, 1,25-dihydroxyvitamin D. When these compensatory mechanisms are inadequate, hypocalcemia develops. Most children with inadequate vitamin D receive medical attention for rickets before developing hypocalcemia (see Chapter 44.10). Children with vitamin D deficiency have elevated serum levels of PTH, and, because of increased osteoclast activity, elevated serum levels of alkaline phosphatase. Serum phosphorus is usually low as a result of decreased intestinal absorption and increased urinary excretion secondary to the effect of PTH.

Vitamin D deficiency may be secondary to poor intake combined with inadequate exposure to ultraviolet light from the sun. In the United States, it is most common in African-American children who are breast-fed but do not receive vitamin D supplementation. Malabsorption of fat-soluble vitamins, including vitamin D, occurs with liver disease, gastrointestinal disease, and pancreatic insufficiency. Some patients with liver disease have an inability to convert vitamin D into 25-hydroxyvitamin D. Some medications, including the anticonvulsants phenobarbital and phenytoin, by increasing the activity of the P450 system in the liver, increase the metabolic degradation of vitamin D. Patients with vitamin D deficiency due to nutritional deficiency, malabsorption, or increased degradation have low levels of 25-hydroxyvitamin D. Because of upregulation of 1α-hydroxylase, levels of 1,25-dihydroxyvitamin D may be low, normal, or high. Children with vitamin D–dependent rickets type 1, an autosomal recessive disorder, have an absence of the kidney's 1α-hydroxylase, preventing conversion of 25-hydroxyvitamin into 1,25-dihydroxyvitamin D. These patients have normal levels of 25-hydroxyvitamin D but low levels of

1,25 dihydroxyvitamin D. In vitamin D–dependent rickets type 2, the vitamin D receptor is defective, preventing a normal physiologic response to 1,25-dihydroxyvitamin D. Thus, there is not a true deficiency; 1,25-dihydroxyvitamin D levels are typically elevated. Approximately 50% of children with this autosomal recessive disorder have alopecia. With chronic renal failure, there is a loss of activity of the 1α-hydroxylase in the kidney, leading to inadequate 1,25-dihydroxyvitamin D. In chronic renal failure, unlike the other causes of vitamin D deficiency, the patient has an elevated serum phosphorus as a result of decreased renal excretion.

In a variety of situations, there is a *redistribution of plasma calcium*, with a reduction in the ionized calcium concentration without any net loss of calcium from the body. A high serum phosphorus level produces a decrease in the serum calcium concentration. Calcium-phosphate complexes may deposit in tissues and the high phosphate in the blood leads to increased deposition of calcium and phosphate in bone. In addition, hyperphosphatemia inhibits the synthesis of 1,25-dihydroxyvitamin D, decreasing intestinal absorption of calcium. Hyperphosphatemia may be secondary to excessive intake, especially in the setting of decreased renal excretion due to renal insufficiency. Infants are vulnerable to hyperphosphatemia from excessive intake because of their lower GFR. Some laxatives and enemas contain high amounts of phosphorus, potentially producing severe hyperphosphatemia with secondary life-threatening hypocalcemia. The hyperphosphatemia in tumor lysis syndrome, which is due to release of intracellular phosphate, may cause hypocalcemia. In rhabdomyolysis, hypocalcemia is secondary to the combination of hyperphosphatemia due to release of intracellular phosphate and movement of calcium into the damaged muscle cells.

During *pancreatitis* there is release of pancreatic lipase, leading to breakdown of omental fat. The degraded fat then binds calcium and produces hypocalcemia. **Hungry bone syndrome** classically occurs after parathyroidectomy for hyperparathyroidism. In these patients, the sudden removal of the stimulus for osteoclast release of bone calcium causes calcium to move from the serum into bone because osteoblasts continue to deposit calcium into bone. This produces hypocalcemia and, by the same mechanism, hypophosphatemia and hypomagnesemia.

Citrate in transfused blood products complexes calcium. This causes a decrease in the ionized calcium concentration, potentially producing symptomatic hypocalcemia. The risk is highest with multiple transfusions or with exchange transfusions in neonates for hyperbilirubinemia or older children for sickle cell crises. The total calcium concentration, because it includes calcium-citrate complexes, may be either normal or elevated.

The initial presentation in infants with *osteopetrosis*, characterized by very dense bone on x-ray, may be hypocalcemic seizures. Other manifestations include macrocephaly, hepatosplenomegaly, anemia, blindness, and deafness (see Chapter 687). Prompt diagnosis is essential because bone marrow transplantation, which is potentially curative, is best done before severe sequelae develop.

Patients with septic shock and intensive care unit patients in general are at increased risk for hypocalcemia, even though the mechanisms are unclear. Inadequate dietary calcium is an unusual cause of hypocalcemia in the United States, although it may occur with replacement of breast milk or formula with low-calcium milk substitutes in infants, poor calcium absorption due to high dietary phytate content, or inadequate calcium in total parenteral nutrition. In some intestinal disorders, such as celiac disease or intestinal lymphangiectasia, there may be inadequate absorption of both calcium and vitamin D.

Clinical Manifestations. Symptoms of hypocalcemia are related to the degree of hypocalcemia and tend to be worse if the hypocal-

cemia develops acutely. Mild hypocalcemia is usually asymptomatic. The clinical manifestations of hypocalcemia are mostly due to neuromuscular irritability. Older children may complain of paresthesias, which are typically perioral or of the hands and feet. Tetany is the classic manifestation of hypocalcemia, and symptoms may include carpopedal spasm, laryngospasm, and seizures. Contractions of the muscles of the hands and feet produce carpopedal spasm, which can be quite painful. The wrists are flexed and the fingers extended, with the thumbs adducted over the palms. The feet are extended and adducted; the toes are plantar flexed. Laryngospasm is a spasmodic closure of the vocal cords. This produces inspiratory stridor and may be confused with laryngotracheitis. Severe laryngospasm may require intubation as a result of apnea and cyanosis. Seizures may be the first manifestation of hypocalcemia, especially in infants. The seizures, often brief but recurrent, are usually generalized but are occasionally localized. Patients usually do not lose consciousness between seizures, even though repeated seizures may induce a postictal state. Symptoms of tetany may be provoked in patients with hypocalcemia by hyperventilation, which by raising the pH causes calcium to bind to albumin, thereby lowering the ionized calcium concentration.

Newborn infants with hypocalcemia usually do not have carpopedal spasm. Along with seizures, manifestations in newborns may include irritability, muscular twitching, jitteriness, and tremors. Alternatively, newborns with hypocalcemia may have symptoms suggestive of sepsis, such as poor feeding, vomiting, and lethargy.

The consequences of long-standing hypocalcemia depend on the etiology. In children with inadequate vitamin D, there is concomitant hypophosphatemia and secondary hyperparathyroidism. These patients have inadequate bone mineralization, and consequently develop rickets (see Chapter 44.10). Rickets may also occur with severe dietary calcium deficiency. In hypoparathyroidism or pseudohypoparathyroidism, where hyperphosphatemia accompanies the hypocalcemia, there may be calcifications of the basal ganglia. In addition, calcifications of the lens may cause cataracts.

Chvostek and Trousseau signs may be elicited in patients with hypocalcemia. A positive Chvostek sign occurs if tapping the facial nerve anterior to the external auditory meatus elicits a twitch of the upper lip or entire mouth. This is not a very specific sign because it is positive in about 10% of patients without hypocalcemia. A false positive Chvostek sign is especially common in neonates. Trousseau sign is more specific, but quite uncomfortable to elicit and generally not an appropriate test in a child. A blood pressure cuff is inflated slightly above the systolic blood pressure for more than 3 min; carpopedal spasm occurs if hypocalcemia is present as a result of the ischemia of the motor nerves. The classic ECG change with hypocalcemia is a prolonged corrected QT interval. Other possible findings include a prolonged ST interval, peaked T waves, arrhythmias, and heart block. Hypocalcemia may impair cardiac contractility and decrease blood pressure. This is especially important in children with hypocalcemia due to sepsis.

Diagnosis. The history in the child with hypocalcemia focuses on the dietary intake of calcium, phosphorus, and vitamin D. A family history of endocrine disorders or rickets is relevant because some causes of hypocalcemia are familial. In some patients, such as those with pancreatitis or tumor lysis syndrome, the clinical history provides the explanation for the hypocalcemia and extensive diagnostic testing is unnecessary. This also applies to children with sepsis or with multiorgan failure in an intensive care unit. Because hypocalcemia is so common in these settings, no work-up is usually necessary unless the child has disproportionate difficulties with hypocalcemia.

The history in early neonatal hypocalcemia is usually significant for prematurity, maternal diabetes, intrauterine growth retardation, or a difficult birth. Early neonatal hypocalcemia is quite common, and most of these infants do not require an extensive work-up for unusual causes of hypocalcemia, unless the hypocalcemia is refractory to usual therapy or is prolonged. However, the nonspecific symptoms of neonatal hypocalcemia, including seizures and lethargy, often necessitate investigation for sepsis, intracranial bleeds, and meningitis. Late neonatal hypocalcemia is usually associated with hyperphosphatemia, and monitoring of the serum phosphorus helps guide therapy (see later text). A serum magnesium level is useful in both early and late neonatal hypocalcemia because hypomagnesemia may accompany the hypocalcemia and contribute to its pathogenesis. Treatment of the hypomagnesemia may be necessary for correction of the hypocalcemia. For infants with persistent hypocalcemia, a maternal history of hyperparathyroidism should be investigated, with laboratory testing of the mother for hypercalcemia because many mothers are asymptomatic. In addition, a chest roentgenogram should be obtained; the absence of a thymic shadow or findings suggestive of congenital heart disease may be seen in DiGeorge syndrome.

Except for early neonatal hypocalcemia, most children with hypocalcemia and no clear etiology require a comprehensive evaluation. This includes children with late neonatal hypocalcemia, which is so unusual with current infant formula preparations that a work-up for other causes is necessary unless the history reveals excessive phosphorus intake. Initial laboratory testing includes measurement of the serum levels of phosphorus, alkaline phosphatase, magnesium, PTH, BUN, and creatinine. In addition, 1,25-dihydroxyvitamin D and 25-hydroxyvitamin D levels are helpful in differentiating the various etiologies of vitamin D deficiency. The 25-hydroxyvitamin D level is low in nutritional vitamin D deficiency, whether due to poor intake, lack of sun exposure, malabsorption, or excess metabolism. In vitamin D–dependent rickets type 1, the 25-hydroxyvitamin D level is normal, but the 1,25-dihydroxyvitamin D is low. In vitamin D–dependent rickets type 2, the 1,25-dihydroxyvitamin D level is elevated. In vitamin D deficiency, the serum phosphorus is usually low, unless the deficiency in 1,25-dihydroxyvitamin D is secondary to renal failure. This contrasts with the elevated serum phosphorus in children with hypoparathyroidism or pseudohypoparathyroidism. In addition, the alkaline phosphatase level is high with vitamin D deficiency and normal or low with hypoparathyroidism. A low or inappropriately normal PTH level in the presence of hypocalcemia is characteristic of hypoparathyroidism; the PTH level is elevated with pseudohypoparathyroidism. Children with hypomagnesemia may have an inappropriately low PTH level; a normal serum magnesium level eliminates hypomagnesemia as a cause of hypocalcemia.

Treatment. For symptomatic hypocalcemia in neonates, calcium gluconate is given at a dose of 100–200 mg/kg (1–2 mL/kg of a 10% solution; 9–18 mg of elemental Ca/kg). This dose may be repeated every 6–8 hr until the calcium level stabilizes. Alternatively, calcium gluconate may be given as a constant intravenous infusion, with neonates typically requiring 500–750 mg/kg/24 hr of calcium gluconate. Ionized calcium levels should be monitored closely because of the risk of hypercalcemia. The intravenous calcium is gradually tapered while following serum calcium levels. The hypomagnesemia that sometimes accompanies early neonatal tetany is usually mild and transient; occasionally, it requires treatment before the hypocalcemia responds to therapy. With early neonatal hypocalcemia, the serum calcium level typically normalizes within 1–3 days. When feasible, neonates with previously symptomatic early hypocalcemia may transition to oral calcium supplementation, which is typically needed for about a week. Even though asymptomatic early hypocalcemia in premature infants usually resolves spontaneously, oral calcium supple-

mentation, if possible, may prevent the need for intravenous therapy. For ill neonates who cannot tolerate enteral feedings, intravenous calcium is usually necessary.

Late neonatal hypocalcemia is usually at least partially secondary to concomitant hyperphosphatemia. Therapy attempts to lower the serum phosphorus level by decreasing phosphorus intake. Similac PM 60/40 is an infant formula with a low phosphorus content, but it has low calcium content so oral calcium supplementation is necessary. Alternatively, oral calcium can be added to conventional infant formula; calcium binds phosphorus in the lumen of the intestine, decreasing the amount of phosphorus that can be absorbed.

Liquid calcium preparations are available for oral dosing in neonates. The starting dose of calcium gluconate is 500–750 mg/kg/24 hr, divided into 4–6 doses. Calcium glubionate syrup is begun at a dose of 700–1000 mg/kg/24 hr, divided into 4–6 doses.

Beyond the neonatal period, 100–200 mg/kg of intravenous calcium gluconate over 5–10 min is an effective approach for symptomatic hypocalcemia. The adult dose of intravenous calcium gluconate is 1–3 g. One gram is 10 mL of a 10% solution and this supplies 94 mg of elemental calcium. Additional doses are given as necessary. Some patients require a continuous calcium drip, titrated to maintain the desired serum calcium level.

Once the symptoms of hypocalcemic tetany resolve with intravenous therapy, enteral calcium supplementation is usually appropriate. Liquid preparations of calcium carbonate (400 mg of elemental calcium/g), calcium glubionate (64 mg of elemental calcium/g) and calcium gluconate (90 mg of elemental calcium/g) are available. A typical starting dose of elemental calcium is 50 mg/kg/24 hr, usually divided into 3–4 doses. The adult starting dose is 1–3 g of elemental calcium per day. Chewable calcium carbonate is effective in older children. Titration of the dose of enteral calcium is based on serum calcium levels. For many conditions, vitamin D supplementation is also necessary (see later text). Calcium preparations bind with phosphorus in the intestinal lumen and decrease its absorption. This can be advantageous in hypocalcemic disorders that are associated with hyperphosphatemia, including renal failure, tumor lysis syndrome, and hypoparathyroidism. However, in other patients this may cause hypophosphatemia. Giving calcium supplements between meals reduces the phosphorus binding and may help to prevent hypophosphatemia.

Intravenous calcium should only be given with close monitoring. There is a significant risk of tissue necrosis and calcification if intravenous calcium extravasates; calcium cannot be given intramuscularly. A peripheral intravenous line that is infusing calcium must be observed carefully. Central access is preferred if possible. Patients receiving intravenous calcium should be on a cardiac monitor. High blood concentrations of calcium may inhibit the sinus node. This initially causes bradycardia, but can cause cardiac arrest. A gradual decrease or sudden slowing in the heart rate is an indication for stopping or decreasing the rate of a calcium infusion. ECG monitoring is especially important for patients on digoxin because intravenous calcium increases the risk of digitalis toxicity.

In certain situations, such as pancreatitis and rhabdomyolysis, complete correction of the hypocalcemia should be avoided because with resolution of the primary problem there is release of the complexed calcium and hypercalcemia may ensue. If acidemia is present, the hypocalcemia should, if possible, be corrected first. Acidemia increases the ionized calcium concentration by displacing calcium from albumin. The correction of the acidemia causes the ionized calcium concentration to decrease. In renal failure, dialysis using a high calcium dialysate helps to correct hypocalcemia while also correcting the metabolic acidosis. When hypomagnesemia is the etiology of the hypocalcemia, correction of the hypomagnesemia is necessary. In hungry bone syndrome, some patients may need supplemental phosphorus and magnesium, along with calcium.

Many patients with hypocalcemia require vitamin D supplementation. For children with deficiency secondary to poor intake, malabsorption, or increased metabolism, oral vitamin D is appropriate therapy. Correction of nutritional vitamin D deficiency typically requires about 5,000 IU/24 hr. Alternatively, a 1-day dose of 600,000 IU may be given. Most children with nutritional vitamin D deficiency do not need prolonged calcium supplementation, although they should receive a diet with adequate phosphorus and calcium. Children with malabsorption of vitamin D require much higher daily doses of vitamin D; 25,000 to 50,000 IU of vitamin D per day may be necessary. Severe malabsorption may necessitate intravenous vitamin D in total parenteral nutrition or intramuscular vitamin D. Children with renal failure, vitamin D–dependent rickets type 1, hypoparathyroidism, or pseudohypoparathyroidism do not appropriately convert 25-hydroxyvitamin D into 1,25-dihydroxyvitamin D. These children respond to 1,25-dihydroxyvitamin D (Rocaltrol). Starting doses range from 0.01– 0.08 µg/kg/24 hr. Adults normally require 0.25–1 µg/24 hr.

Long-term treatment of hypoparathyroidism and pseudohypoparathyroidism requires monitoring of serum calcium levels to avoid hypercalcemia. In addition, because there is a significant risk of hypercalciuria with the potential for nephrolithiasis and nephrocalcinosis, it is important to also monitor the urinary calcium. The use of a thiazide diuretic may help to decrease urinary calcium.

HYPERCALCEMIA

Hypercalcemia is frequently discovered incidentally on a routine chemistry profile. This is because hypercalcemia is an uncommon electrolyte disorder, and its clinical manifestations are fairly nonspecific. There are, however, some clinical situations in which hypercalcemia should be suspected.

As previously discussed, the ionized calcium concentration, not the total calcium concentration, is physiologically relevant. Hypercalcemia may go undetected in the patient with hypoalbuminemia and a "normal" total calcium concentration. The ionized calcium concentration is the gold standard for evaluating children with calcium disorders.

Etiology and Pathophysiology. The regulation of serum calcium concentration is dependent on parathyroid hormone, vitamin D, appropriate calcium intake, and renal calcium excretion. Derangements in any of these systems can produce hypercalcemia. In addition, bone is a massive potential source of calcium, which, if inappropriately mobilized, produces hypercalcemia. A variety of different mechanisms may cause hypercalcemia (Box 45–7).

A variety of diseases may cause *primary hyperparathyroidism* (see Chapter 567). The excessive PTH causes hypercalcemia by increasing 1,25-dihydroxyvitamin D synthesis, releasing calcium from bone and decreasing urinary calcium excretion. There is hypophosphatemia due to PTH-mediated renal phosphate wasting. Sporadic adenomas are much more common in adults than in children. Adenomas may be part of a genetic disorder such as familial isolated hyperparathyroidism, multiple endocrine neoplasia type I, multiple endocrine neoplasia type II, or hyperparathyroidism-jaw tumor syndrome.

Neonatal hyperparathyroidism is a severe, life-threatening disorder. Most cases are due to an absence of functional calcium-sensing receptors in the parathyroid gland. Without functional sensors, the parathyroid gland is unable to monitor the extracellular calcium concentration. This leads to continued production of PTH despite increasing serum calcium levels. This is an autosomal recessive disorder, with both parents having one defective calcium sensor. The parents therefore have mild, benign hypercalcemia (see the later description of familial hypocalciuric hypercalcemia). Transient secondary neonatal hyperparathyroidism is a complication in neonates born to mothers with

---

BOX 45–7. Causes of Hypercalcemia

EXCESS PARATHYROID HORMONE
Primary hyperparathyroidism
  Sporadic adenoma
  Familial isolated hyperparathyroidism (MIM* 145000)
  Multiple endocrine neoplasia type I (MIM 131100)
  Multiple endocrine neoplasia type II (MIM 171400)
  Hyperparathyroidism–jaw tumor syndrome (MIM 145001)
  Calcium-sensing receptor mutation (MIM 239200)
Transient secondary neonatal hyperparathyroidism
Tertiary hyperparathyroidism

EXCESS VITAMIN D
Hypervitaminosis D
Subcutaneous fat necrosis
Sarcoidosis
Granulomatous diseases (e.g., tuberculosis and fungal infections)
Lymphomas

EXCESS CALCIUM INTAKE
Calcium supplements
Iatrogenic (e.g., total parenteral nutrition)

EXCESS RENAL REABSORPTION OF CALCIUM
Familial benign hypocalciuric hypercalcemia (MIM 145980)
Thiazide diuretics

RELEASE FROM BONE
Thyrotoxicosis
Hypervitaminosis A
Malignancy associated
  Ectopic parathyroid hormone (PTH)
  PTH-related peptide
  Bone metastasis
  Other factors
Immobilization
Renal osteodystrophy
  Low turnover disease
  Aluminum deposition

MISCELLANEOUS
Williams syndrome (MIM 194050)
Hypophosphatemia
Pheochromocytoma
Adrenal insufficiency
Recovery phase of rhabdomyolysis
Jansen metaphyseal chondrodysplasia (MIM 156400)
Hypophosphatasia (MIM 241500)

---

*MIM refers to the database number from the Mendelian Inheritance in Man (http://www3.ncbi.nlm.nih.gov/Omim/).

---

hypocalcemia, usually due to hypoparathyroidism. The mother's hypocalcemia leads to fetal hypocalcemia and secondary hyperparathyroidism. This can cause poor fetal growth, bone demineralization, and even fractures. Some of these infants have hypercalcemia, which is occasionally the only manifestation. The hypercalcemia resolves over days to weeks as parathyroid gland function returns to normal.

Tertiary hyperparathyroidism occurs when prolonged secondary hyperparathyroidism progresses to either an autonomous parathyroid gland or a parathyroid adenoma. The exact mechanism is unknown, but is dependent on sustained hyperactivity of the parathyroid gland. In children, this most commonly occurs with chronic kidney failure due to inadequate 1,25-dihydroxyvitamin D. Tertiary hyperparathyroidism is also occasionally seen in children with X-linked hypophosphatemic rickets, wherein treatment with dietary phosphate decreases calcium absorption, which causes activation of the parathyroid gland. Parathyroidectomy is often necessary in tertiary hyperparathyroidism.

Extremely *high intake of vitamin D* can produce hypercalcemia. PTH levels are appropriately suppressed while the serum phosphorus level is elevated as a result of vitamin D's effect on intestinal absorption of phosphate and the lack of PTH to stimulate renal phosphate excretion. The hypercalcemia of hypervitaminosis D typically persists for weeks to months because of vitamin D's long half-life. Specific therapy includes discontinuation of vitamin D and a low calcium diet. Glucocorticoids are especially useful because they inhibit the action of vitamin D on both bone and intestines and decrease the levels of 1,25-dihydroxyvitamin D and 25-hydroxyvitamin D in the serum.

Subcutaneous fat necrosis is a disorder of the first few months of life (see Chapter 650). Infants are typically full-term and most have a history of birth asphyxia or trauma. The subcutaneous fat necrosis usually appears 1–2 wk after birth. Infants have hard nodules or plaques with overlying erythematous or purple skin. The most common sites are the cheeks, buttocks, back, and thighs. Skin biopsy shows fat necrosis and granulomatous infiltration with multinucleated giant cells. PTH levels are appropriately low. The hypercalcemia is believed to be due to excessive 1,25-dihydroxyvitamin D, which is probably produced by the macrophages infiltrating the areas of fat necrosis. This is presumably analogous to the situation in granulomatous diseases such as sarcoidosis (see later text).

Up to 40% of patients with *sarcoidosis* develop hypercalciuria, whereas a smaller percentage develop hypercalcemia. The mechanism is production of 1,25-dihydroxyvitamin D by pulmonary macrophages. These macrophages have 1-αhydroxylase, the enzyme that converts 25-hydroxyvitamin D into 1,25-dihydroxyvitamin D. Because the macrophages require 25-hydroxyvitamin D as a precursor to synthesize 1,25-dihydroxyvitamin D, the hypercalcemia may be intermittent, with an increased likelihood during the summer months (due to vitamin D production from sun exposure). Likewise, *oral vitamin D* can precipitate an episode of hypercalcemia. The hypercalciuria may produce nephrocalcinosis and nephrolithiasis. Treatment is restriction of vitamin D and sun exposure and corticosteroids. Hypercalcemia is less commonly caused by a number of other granulomatous diseases, such as tuberculosis and pulmonary fungal infections. Both non-Hodgkin lymphomas and Hodgkin disease have been associated with ectopic 1,25-dihydroxyvitamin D production.

Excessive calcium intake can cause hypercalcemia, especially if kidney impairment prevents renal excretion of calcium. While downregulation of 1,25-dihydroxyvitamin D does decrease calcium absorption, even without active vitamin D, there is passive intestinal absorption that is proportional to intake. With intravenous calcium, such as in total parenteral nutrition, there is no mechanism for downregulating absorption, and so the risk for iatrogenic hypercalcemia is higher.

Familial hypocalciuric hypercalcemia (FHH) is an autosomal dominant disorder caused by a mutation in the calcium-sensing receptor. Half the calcium-sensing receptors in the parathyroid glands are defective and, thus, the parathyroid glands do not receive an adequate signal at normal serum calcium concentrations. This results in increased PTH release at normal calcium concentrations. At the mildly elevated calcium concentrations in these patients, the remaining calcium sensors transmit enough signal that the PTH level decreases into the normal range, even though it is slightly increased in some patients. In addition, the deficiency in calcium-sensing receptors in the kidneys causes the renal tubules to avidly reabsorb calcium as a result of the perception that the serum calcium level is low. Urinary calcium levels are very low, with most patients having a urine calcium/creatinine ratio of less than 0.01 mg/mg. This is lower than in patients with primary hyperparathyroidism due to a parathyroid adenoma and is useful in differentiating these two entities. Other laboratory findings include a normal 1,25-dihydroxyvitamin D level, mild hypermagnesemia, and low-normal or decreased serum phosphorus. Because the serum calcium level is only mildly elevated, FHH is a benign condition; no treatment is necessary. Children who inherit a defective calcium-sensing receptor from each parent have

severe neonatal hyperparathyroidism (see earlier text). Some neonates with FHH have skeletal changes of hyperparathyroidism, an elevated PTH, and mild to moderate hypercalcemia. Unlike those with the homozygous disorder, the hypercalcemia is not severe. The bone changes self-resolve, and parathyroidectomy is not necessary.

Thiazide diuretics decrease renal calcium excretion. In patients without another disorder affecting calcium metabolism, thiazide diuretics may cause a subtle increase in the serum calcium concentration, but they never cause hypercalcemia. Thiazide diuretics may precipitate hypercalcemia if there is a second mechanism present (e.g., hyperparathyroidism or high vitamin D intake).

Thyroid hormone directly stimulates bone resorption. Along with hypercalcemia, patients with hyperthyroidism have a decreased PTH level, increased serum phosphorus, and increased alkaline phosphatase. *Vitamin A intoxication* is another unusual cause of hypercalcemia, probably due to excessive bone resorption. Along with discontinuation of vitamin A and hydration, glucocorticoids are effective for treating the hypercalcemia.

Malignancies cause calcium release from bone via a variety of different mechanisms. Some tumors produce hypercalcemia by direct bone invasion and destruction. Parathyroid hormone related peptide (PTH-RP) has the same actions as PTH, but is normally only produced as a local hormone. Some tumor cells can produce PTH-RP in sufficient quantities that it has a systemic effect. Diagnosis requires analysis of blood for PTH-RP because it will not be detected using the assay for PTH. Patients with PTH-RP–induced hypercalcemia have a low serum phosphorus level, low PTH, and, unlike in patients with hyperparathyroidism, normal levels of 1,25-dihydroxyvitamin D. Rarely, tumors produce PTH. Yet another mechanism for malignancy associated hypercalcemia is the elaboration of factors that increase osteoclast resorption of bone.

Hypercalcemia from immobilization occurs in children with injuries such as leg fractures, burns, or spinal cord paralysis. The hypercalcemia is caused by bone resorption, which also explains the loss of bone mass that is associated with immobilization. The hypercalcemia usually occurs within 1–3 wk after leg fractures requiring traction. Following spinal cord injury the hypercalcemia commonly appears in 4–8 wk, but may appear earlier or months later. It is more common to detect isolated hypercalciuria, which may result in nephrocalcinosis, renal insufficiency, or kidney stones. PTH and 1,25-dihydroxyvitamin D are appropriately suppressed and the serum phosphorus level is often mildly elevated. Because of their higher rate of bone remodeling, children, especially adolescents, are affected more commonly than adults.

Some patients with *renal failure* develop bones that have lost their ability to take up calcium. This can be due to aluminum deposition in bone, although it is now more commonly seen without aluminum deposition and is called adynamic bone disease.

Williams syndrome is due to a deletion of a portion of chromosome 7 (see Chapters 97 and 420.5). This results in a contiguous gene syndrome, with multiple missing genes, and it is usually a new chromosomal deletion so the parents are unaffected. Most children have mild to moderate psychomotor retardation. Older children and adults have an outgoing "cocktail party" personality, but can also seem nervous. Facial features in infancy include periorbital fullness, broad nasal bridge, anteverted nares, long philtrum, open mouth, and full cheeks. Older children and adults have a different appearance, with a more elongated face, thicker lips, and a decrease in both the periorbital fullness and the full cheeks. Supravalvular aortic stenosis is the most common cardiovascular anomaly but it is only present in about one third of patients. Narrowing of the pulmonary arteries, the renal arteries, and the cerebral vasculature is also common. The cardiovascular abnormalities are probably due to the disruption of the gene for elastin. The genetic and pathophysiologic explanation for the hypercalcemia is unknown. The hypercalcemia of Williams syndrome is usually diagnosed during infancy and resolves within a couple of years. It occasionally occurs in older children.

Low serum phosphorus can cause hypercalcemia. This may be due to the fact that hypophosphatemia stimulates the enzyme in the kidney (1 α-hydroxylase) that converts 25-hydroxyvitamin D to 1,25-dihydroxyvitamin D. This active form of vitamin D then stimulates calcium absorption in the gut. In addition, the deficiency of phosphate, which is needed for bone mineralization, prevents normal calcium deposition in the skeleton. This can occur in low-birthweight infants who are fed human milk, which has a low phosphate content. Hypercalcemia is a well described but unusual complication of a pheochromocytoma. Hypercalcemia is rarely associated with Addison disease, but the mechanism is unknown. The hypercalcemia resolves with glucocorticoid therapy.

Acute rhabdomyolysis causes hypocalcemia because of hyperphosphatemia, which leads to complexing of calcium and calcium deposition in injured tissues. This leads to appropriately high levels of PTH and 1,25-dihydroxyvitamin D. During the recovery phase, release of tissue calcium can lead to hypercalcemia. In addition, some patients have elevated levels of 1,25-dihydroxyvitamin D, which may further exacerbate the hypercalcemia. Avoiding overly aggressive treatment of the initial hypocalcemia may potentially prevent or lessen the subsequent hypercalcemia.

In *Jansen metaphyseal chondrodysplasia*, a defective PTH receptor sometimes causes hypercalcemia, along with a variety of other clinical manifestations (see Chapter 684). The PTH receptor is constitutively active and thus sends a signal as if PTH were present, which causes PTH effects in the kidney and bone. Therefore, despite a low PTH, there are similarities to hyperparathyroidism such as low-normal serum phosphorus, elevated 1,25-dihydroxyvitamin D, and elevated alkaline phosphatase.

In the *infantile form of hypophosphatasia*, the patients present during the first 6 mo of life with rickets and/or failure to thrive (see Chapter 694). Hypercalcemia is fairly common, and hypercalciuria can cause nephrocalcinosis. A low serum alkaline phosphatase is characteristic of this disorder. The serum phosphorus is normal.

Clinical Manifestations. The signs and symptoms of hypercalcemia are related to the magnitude of the problem. Hypercalcemia is conventionally classified as mild (<12 mg/dL), moderate (12–15 mg/dL), or severe (>15 mg/dL). Many patients with mild or moderate hypercalcemia are asymptomatic, with the diagnosis resulting from an incidental laboratory test. Hypercalcemia has a number of common manifestations (Box 45–8). Infants often present with poor feeding, emesis, and failure to thrive. Severe hypercalcemia is occasionally fatal; ventricular arrhythmias are a serious concern. Psychiatric symptoms may include confusion, disorientation, depression, psychosis, and/or hallucinations. The polyuria of hypercalcemia is due to secondary nephrogenic diabetes insipidus (see Chapter 522). The high urinary water losses, especially when combined with emesis or decreased oral intake, leads to dehydration in a significant percentage of patients. This exacerbates the hypercalcemia and increases the risk of renal failure or kidney stones. In addition, the nephrogenic diabetes insipidus may cause hypernatremia.

The nephrocalcinosis is typically in the renal medulla, although cortical nephrocalcinosis is also seen. Both ultrasound, with hyperechogenicity, and CT scan may capture the nephrocalcinosis, although neither is sensitive enough to detect less severe cases.

Hypercalcemia can cause pancreatitis, which typically causes hypocalcemia. It is therefore important to monitor the serum

---

BOX 45–8. Clinical Manifestations of Hypercalcemia

GASTROINTESTINAL
Nausea and vomiting
Poor feeding
Failure to thrive
Constipation
Abdominal pain
Pancreatitis
Peptic ulcer

CARDIAC
Hypertension
Decreased QT interval
Arrhythmias

CENTRAL NERVOUS SYSTEM
Lethargy
Hypotonia
Psychiatric disturbances
Coma

KIDNEY
Polyuria and dehydration
Hypernatremia
Renal failure
Nephrolithiasis

---

calcium as the pancreatitis resolves because the hypocalcemic effect of the pancreatitis may mask the true extent of the hypercalcemia.

Certain findings in patients with hypercalcemia are related to the underlying disease. Because PTH stimulates the kidney to excrete base, patients with hypercalcemia due to hyperparathyroidism classically have a mild metabolic acidosis. In contrast, most other patients have a metabolic alkalosis, which seems to be mediated by a combination of alkali release from bone and a direct effect of hypercalcemia that causes the kidney to hold onto base. PTH also causes renal phosphate wasting and hypophosphatemia. Other potential electrolyte complications of hypercalcemia include distal RTA, renal salt wasting, hypomagnesemia, and hypokalemia.

Diagnosis. The history focuses on calcium intake, underlying diseases, renal function, and medications, including vitamins. The age of the patient is helpful. In infants, subcutaneous fat necrosis and Williams syndrome are important considerations; hypercalcemia may be the initial presentation of Williams syndrome. Laboratory evaluation should include electrolytes, BUN, creatinine, phosphorus, PTH, urinary calcium, urinary phosphorus, urinary creatinine (for calculation of the calcium/creatinine ratio and the tubular reabsorption of phosphorus), and a 25-hydroxyvitamin D level. In the setting of possible malignancy, a PTH-related peptide level might be helpful. Williams syndrome can be definitively diagnosed by fluorescent in situ hybridization using a probe for the deleted segment on chromosome 7.

Treatment. The therapeutic approach depends on the severity of the hypercalcemia and the underlying etiology. Many patients with hypercalcemia are dehydrated as a result of polyuria from nephrogenic diabetes insipidus, poor oral intake, and/or vomiting. Rehydration lowers the serum calcium via dilution and corrects prerenal azotemia. The resultant increased urine output increases urinary calcium excretion. Urinary calcium excretion is increased by high urinary sodium excretion. Thus, the mainstay of treating hypercalcemia is aggressive therapy with normal saline, with the caveat that caution is mandatory to avoid fluid overload, especially in the setting of renal impairment or underlying cardiac disease. Urinary calcium excretion is further enhanced by the administration of a loop diuretic, which also helps to maintain adequate urinary volume given the high rate of intravenous saline. The loop diuretic is started once the patient has been rehydrated. The high rates of intravenous fluid and urine output combined with a loop diuretic can lead to a variety of electrolyte disturbances. Therefore, along with serum calcium, it is critical to monitor sodium, potassium, bicarbonate, and magnesium.

Normal saline, with or without a loop diuretic, is often adequate for treating mild or moderate hypercalcemia. More significant hypercalcemia often requires other therapies. Glucocorticoids decrease intestinal absorption of calcium by blocking the action of 1,25-dihydroxyvitamin D. There is also a decrease in levels of 25-hydroxyvitamin D and 1,25-dihydroxyvitamin D. The usual dose of prednisone is 1 mg/kg/24 hr. Glucocorticoids are especially effective when vitamin D is central in the pathogenesis of hypercalcemia, such as subcutaneous fat necrosis and vitamin D intoxication. A decrease in calcium, often dramatic, is frequently apparent within 24–72 hr. The direct tumoricidal effect of glucocorticoids may be useful in certain malignancies. In addition, glucocorticoids may block bone resorption, which is especially useful in some cancers. Glucocorticoids are especially effective in sarcoidosis because they also treat the underlying disease.

Calcitonin lowers calcium by inhibiting bone resorption. It also increases urinary calcium excretion, but this is a less important mechanism. The main advantages of calcitonin are limited side effects and a rapid onset of action, often within 2–4 hr. However, the decrease in calcium is usually less than 3 mg/dL, and patients can become resistant to therapy. Sensitivity to calcitonin may sometimes return by adding glucocorticoids or by changing to a regimen of periodic administration. Bisphosphonates are very effective; they inhibit bone resorption through their effects on osteoclasts. Hemodialysis, using a low or zero dialysate calcium, can rapidly lower serum calcium in patients with severe hypercalcemia. This therapy is especially useful in patients with either acute or chronic renal failure because urinary losses are inherently limited. Management of chronic hypercalcemia often requires a diet with decreased calcium and vitamin D.

Some etiologies of hypercalcemia require disease-specific therapy. Severe neonatal hyperparathyroidism is a surgical emergency, necessitating urgent parathyroidectomy. The hypercalcemia of sarcoidosis responds well to glucocorticoids, which both block intestinal action of vitamin D and treat the disease, decreasing the ectopic production of vitamin D by macrophages (see Chapter 155). Sarcoidosis also responds to ketoconazole or chloroquine. These medications inhibit the P450 system that is necessary to convert 25-hydroxyvitamin D into 1,25-dihydroxyvitamin D. Finally, sarcoidosis has also been treated with cellulose phosphate, which binds intestinal calcium, preventing its absorption. The hypercalcemia of thyrotoxicosis responds to treatment of the thyrotoxicosis. Similarly, treatment of Addison disease corrects the hypercalcemia.

45.6 Magnesium

MAGNESIUM METABOLISM

Body Content and Physiologic Function. Magnesium is the fourth most common cation in the body and the third most common intracellular cation (see Fig. 45–3). Fifty percent to 60% of body magnesium is in bone, where it serves as a reservoir because one third is exchangeable, allowing movement to the extracellular space. Most intracellular magnesium is bound to proteins and other negatively charged molecules such as ATP; only about 25% is exchangeable. Because cells with higher metabolic rates have higher magnesium concentrations, most intracellular magnesium is present in muscle and liver.

The normal plasma magnesium concentration is 1.5–2.3 mg/dL (1.2–1.9 mEq/L; 0.62–0.94 mmol/L), with some varia-

tion between clinical laboratories. In the United States, serum magnesium is reported as mg/dL, but conversion from other units is necessary when reading the world literature or talking with colleagues from outside the United States (see Table 45–1). Infants have slightly higher plasma magnesium concentrations than older children and adults. Only 1% of body magnesium is extracellular (60% ionized; 15% complexed; 25% protein bound).

Magnesium is a necessary cofactor for hundreds of enzymes. It is important for membrane stabilization and nerve conduction. ATP and gaunosine triphosphate (GTP) need associated magnesium when they are used by ATPases, cyclases, and kinases.

Intake. Between 30% and 50% of dietary magnesium is absorbed. Good dietary sources include green vegetables, cereals, nuts, meats, and hard water, although many foods contain magnesium. Human milk contains about 35 mg/L of magnesium; formula contains 40–70 mg/L. The small intestine is the major site of magnesium absorption, although the regulation of magnesium absorption is poorly understood. There is passive absorption, which permits high absorption in the presence of excessive intake. Absorption is diminished in the presence of substances that complex with magnesium (e.g., free fatty acids, fiber, phytate, phosphate, and oxalate); increased intestinal motility and calcium also decrease magnesium absorption. Vitamin D and PTH may enhance absorption, even though this effect is fairly limited. Intestinal absorption does increase when intake is decreased, possibly via a saturable active transport system. However, if there is no oral intake of magnesium, obligatory secretory losses prevent the complete elimination of intestinal losses.

Excretion. Renal excretion is the principal regulator of magnesium balance. There is no defined hormonal regulatory system, even though PTH may increase tubular reabsorption. Approximately 15% of reabsorption occurs in the proximal tubule and 70% in the thick ascending limb (TAL) of the loop of Henle. Proximal reabsorption may be higher in neonates. High serum magnesium inhibits reabsorption in the TAL, suggesting that active transport is involved. Approximately 5–10% of filtered magnesium is reabsorbed in the distal tubule. Hypomagnesemia increases absorption in the TAL and the distal tubule.

HYPOMAGNESEMIA

Hypomagnesemia is relatively common in hospitalized patients, although most cases are asymptomatic. Detection requires a high index of suspicion because magnesium is not measured in most basic metabolic panels.

Etiology and Pathophysiology. Gastrointestinal or renal losses are the major causes of hypomagnesemia (Box 45–9). *Diarrhea* has up to 200 mg/L of magnesium; gastric contents have only about 15 mg/L, but high losses can cause depletion. Steatorrhea causes magnesium loss as a result of the formation of magnesium-lipid salts; restriction of dietary fat can decrease losses.

Primary intestinal hypomagnesemia with secondary hypocalcemia, due to malabsorption of magnesium, is a rare autosomal recessive disorder, mapped to chromosome 9. The patients have seizures, tetany, tremor, or restlessness at 2–8 wk of life due to severe hypomagnesemia (0.2–0.8 mg/dL) and secondary hypocalcemia.

Renal losses may occur due to medications that are direct tubular toxins. Amphotericin frequently causes significant magnesium wasting and is typically associated with other tubular defects (especially potassium wasting). Cisplatin produces dramatic renal magnesium losses. Diuretics affect tubular handling of magnesium. Whereas loop diuretics cause a mild increase in magnesium excretion, thiazide diuretics have even less effect.

GASTROINTESTINAL DISORDERS

Diarrhea
Nasogastric suction or emesis
Inflammatory bowel disease
Celiac disease
Cystic fibrosis
Intestinal lymphangiectasia
Small bowel resection or bypass
Pancreatitis
Protein-calorie malnutrition
Primary intestinal hypomagnesemia with secondary hypocalcemia (MIM* 602014)

RENAL DISORDERS

Medications: amphotericin, cisplatin, cyclosporin, loop diuretics, mannitol, pentamidine, aminoglycosides, thiazide diuretics
Diabetes
Acute tubular necrosis (recovery phase)
Postobstructive nephropathy
Chronic kidney diseases: interstitial nephritis, glomerulonephritis, postrenal transplant
Hypercalcemia
Intravenous fluids
Primary aldosteronism
Genetic diseases
    Gitelman syndrome (MIM 263800)
    Bartter syndrome (MIM 602023)
    Familial hypomagnesemia with hypercalciuria and nephrocalcinosis (MIM 603959)
    Autosomal recessive renal magnesium wasting (MIM 248250)
    Autosomal dominant renal magnesium wasting (MIM 154020)
    Autosomal dominant hypoparathyroidism (MIM 601198/601199)
    Mitochondrial disorders

MISCELLANEOUS CAUSES

Poor intake
Hungry bone syndrome
Insulin administration
Pancreatitis
Intrauterine growth retardation
Infants of diabetic mothers
Exchange transfusion

*MIM refers to the database number from the Mendelian Inheritance in Man (http://www3.ncbi.nlm.nih.gov/Omim/).

Potassium-sparing diuretics decrease magnesium losses. Osmotic agents, such as mannitol, glucose in diabetes mellitus, or urea in the recovery phase of acute tubular necrosis, increase urinary magnesium losses. Intravenous fluid, by expanding the intravascular volume, decreases renal reabsorption of sodium and water, which impairs magnesium reabsorption. Hypercalcemia inhibits magnesium reabsorption in the loop of Henle, although this does not occur in the hypercalcemia due to familial hypercalcemic hypocalciuria or lithium.

There are a number of *rare genetic diseases* that cause renal magnesium loss. Gitelman and Bartter syndromes, autosomal recessive disorders, are the most common entities (see Chapter 523). Gitelman syndrome, which is due to a defect in the thiazide-sensitive Na-Cl co-transporter in the distal tubule, is almost always associated with hypomagnesemia. In Bartter syndrome, which can be caused by mutations in at least three different genes, hypomagnesemia is uncommon; when it does occur, it is usually associated with a defect in the basolateral chloride channel. In both disorders there is hypokalemic metabolic alkalosis, but in Gitelman syndrome there is hypocalciuria, and Bartter syndrome patients frequently have hypercalciuria and secondary nephrocalcinosis. In both disorders the hypomagnesemia is typically not severe and is asymptomatic, although tetany due to hypomagnesemia does occasionally occur.

Familial hypomagnesemia with hypercalciuria and nephrocalcinosis (Michellis-Castrillo syndrome), an autosomal recessive disorder, is due to mutations in the gene for paracellin-1, which is located in the tight junctions of the thick ascending limb of the loop of Henle. Patients have severe renal wasting of magnesium and calcium with secondary hypomagnesemia and nephrocalcinosis; serum calcium levels are normal. Chronic renal failure frequently occurs during childhood. Other features include kidney stones, urinary tract infections, hematuria, increased PTH levels, tetany, seizures, hyperuricemia, ocular abnormalities, polyuria, and polydipsia. Autosomal recessive renal magnesium wasting without hypercalciuria is less commonly described and the genetic basis is unknown.

Autosomal dominant renal magnesium wasting is due to a dominant-negative mutation in the gene encoding the Na$^+$,K$^+$-ATPase gamma-subunit and is associated with hypomagnesemia, increased urinary magnesium losses, hypocalciuria, and normocalcemia. Patients may present with seizures; most are asymptomatic despite serum magnesium levels of 0.8–1.5 mg/dL. Autosomal dominant hypoparathyroidism is caused by an activating mutation in the calcium-sensing receptor, which also senses magnesium levels in the kidney. The mutated receptor inappropriately perceives that magnesium and calcium levels are elevated, leading to urinary wasting. PTH levels are low despite hypocalcemia. Severe hypomagnesemia from renal losses is uncommonly present in mitochondrial disorders.

Poor intake is an unusual cause of hypomagnesemia, although it can be seen in children who are hospitalized and only receive intravenous fluids without magnesium. In **hungry bone syndrome,** which most frequently occurs after parathyroidectomy in patients with hyperparathyroidism, magnesium moves into bone as a result of accelerated bone formation. These patients usually have hypocalcemia and hypophosphatemia via the same mechanism. A similar mechanism can occur during the *refeeding phase of protein-calorie malnutrition* in children, with high magnesium utilization during cell growth depleting the patient's limited reserves. Insulin therapy stimulates uptake of magnesium by cells, and in *diabetic ketoacidosis*, in which total body magnesium is low because of osmotic losses, hypomagnesemia frequently occurs. In *pancreatitis*, there is saponification of magnesium and calcium in necrotic fat, causing both hypomagnesemia and hypocalcemia.

Transient hypomagnesemia in newborns, which is sometimes idiopathic, is more commonly seen in infants of diabetic mothers, presumably due to maternal depletion. Other maternal diseases that cause magnesium losses predispose infants to hypomagnesemia. Hypomagnesemia is more common in infants with intrauterine growth retardation. Hypomagnesemia may develop in newborn infants who require exchange transfusions because of magnesium removal by the citrate in banked blood (see Chapter 95).

Clinical Manifestations. Hypomagnesemia causes secondary hypocalcemia by impairing the release of PTH by the parathyroid gland and through blunting the tissue response to PTH. Thus, hypomagnesemia is part of the differential diagnosis of hypocalcemia (see Box 45–6). This usually occurs only at magnesium levels less than 0.7 mg/dL. The dominant manifestations of hypomagnesemia are due to hypocalcemia: tetany, positive Chvostek and Trousseau signs, and seizures. However, with severe hypomagnesemia, these same signs and symptoms may be present despite normocalcemia. Persistent hypocalcemia due to hypomagnesemia is a rare cause of rickets.

Many causes of hypomagnesemia also result in hypokalemia. However, hypomagnesemia may produce renal potassium wasting and hypokalemia that only corrects with magnesium therapy. ECG changes with hypomagnesemia include flattening of the T wave and lengthening of the ST segment. Arrhythmias may occur, almost always in the setting of underlying heart disease.

Diagnosis. The etiology of hypomagnesemia is often readily apparent from the clinical situation. The child should be assessed for gastrointestinal disease, adequate intake, and kidney disease, with close attention to medications that may cause renal wasting. When the diagnosis is uncertain, an evaluation of urinary magnesium losses distinguishes between renal and nonrenal causes. The fractional excretion of magnesium is calculated via the following formula:

$$FE_{Mg} = (U_{Mg} \times P_{Cr})/([0.7 \times P_{Mg}] \times U_{Cr}) \times 100$$

where FE_{Mg} = fractional excretion of magnesium; U_{Mg} = urinary magnesium concentration; P_{Cr} = plasma creatinine concentration; P_{Mg} = plasma magnesium concentration; U_{Cr} = urinary magnesium concentration. The plasma magnesium concentration is multiplied by 0.7 because approximately 30% is bound to albumin and not filtered at the glomerulus.

The fractional excretion of magnesium does not vary with age, but it does change based on the serum magnesium concentration. The fractional excretion ranges from 1 to 8% in children with normal magnesium levels. In the presence of hypomagnesemia due to extrarenal causes, it should be low due to renal conservation, typically less than 2%. The fractional excretion of magnesium is inappropriately elevated in the setting of renal wasting; values are almost always greater than 4% and frequently are greater than 10%. The measurement should not be evaluated during a magnesium infusion because the acute increase in serum magnesium increases urinary magnesium. Other approaches for evaluating urinary magnesium losses include calculation of 24-hr urinary magnesium losses and the ratio of urine magnesium to urine creatinine, both of which vary with age.

The genetic causes of renal magnesium loss are distinguished based on measurement of other serum and urinary electrolytes. Children with Gitelman syndrome and Bartter syndrome have hypokalemia and metabolic alkalosis.

Treatment. Severe hypomagnesemia is treated with parenteral magnesium. Magnesium sulphate is given at a dose of 25–50 mg/kg (0.05–0.1 mL/kg of a 50% solution; 2.5–5.0 mg/kg of elemental magnesium). This is administered as a slow intravenous infusion, although it is frequently given intramuscularly in neonates. The rate of intravenous infusion should be slowed if patients experience diaphoresis, flushing, or a warm sensation. The dose is often repeated every 6 hr (every 8–12 hr in neonates) for a total of 2–3 doses before rechecking the plasma magnesium concentration. Lower doses are used in children with renal insufficiency.

Long-term therapy is usually given orally. Preparations include magnesium gluconate (5.4 mg elemental magnesium/100 mg), magnesium oxide (60 mg elemental magnesium/100 mg), and magnesium sulfate (10 mg elemental magnesium/100 mg). There are sustained-released preparations such as Slow-Mag (60 mg elemental magnesium/tablet) and Mag-Tab SR (84 mg elemental magnesium/tablet). Oral magnesium dosing should be divided to obviate cathartic side effects. Alternatives to oral magnesium are intramuscular injections and nighttime nasogastric infusion, both designed to minimize diarrhea. Magnesium supplementation must be used cautiously in the context of renal insufficiency (see later text).

HYPERMAGNESEMIA

Clinically significant hypermagnesemia is almost always secondary to excessive intake. It is unusual, except in neonates born to mothers who are receiving intravenous magnesium for preeclampsia or eclampsia (see Chapter 95).

Etiology and Pathophysiology. There is no feedback mechanism to prevent magnesium absorption from the gastrointestinal tract. Magnesium is present in high amounts in certain laxatives, enemas, cathartics used to treat drug overdoses, and antacids. It is also usually present in total parenteral nutrition, and neonates may receive high amounts transplacentally if maternal levels are elevated. Usually the kidneys excrete excessive magnesium, but this ability is diminished in patients with chronic renal failure. In addition, neonates and young infants are vulnerable to excessive magnesium ingestion because of their reduced GFR. Most pediatric cases not related to maternal hypermagnesemia are in infants because of excessive use of antacids or laxatives. Mild hypermagnesemia may occur in chronic renal failure, familial hypocalciuric hypercalcemia, diabetic ketoacidosis, lithium ingestion, milk alkali syndrome, and tumor lysis syndrome. The hypermagnesemia in diabetic ketoacidosis occurs despite significant intracellular magnesium depletion due to urinary losses; hypomagnesemia often occurs following insulin treatment.

Clinical Manifestations. Symptoms usually do not appear until the plasma magnesium is more than 4.5 mg/dL. Hypermagnesemia inhibits acetylcholine release at the neuromuscular junction, producing hypotonia, hyporeflexia, and weakness; paralysis occurs at high concentrations. Direct central nervous system depression causes lethargy and sleepiness; infants have a poor suck. Elevated magnesium is associated with hypotension because of vascular dilation, which also causes flushing. Hypotension can be profound at higher concentrations due to a direct effect on cardiac function. ECG changes include prolonged PR, QRS, and QT intervals. Severe hypermagnesemia (>15 mg/dL) causes complete heart block and cardiac arrest. Other manifestations of hypermagnesemia include nausea, vomiting, and hypocalcemia.

Diagnosis. Except for the case of the neonate with transplacental exposure, a high index of suspicion and a good history are necessary to make the diagnosis. Prevention is essential; magnesium-containing compounds should be used judiciously in children with renal insufficiency.

Treatment. Most patients with normal renal function rapidly clear excessive magnesium. Intravenous hydration and loop diuretics can accelerate this process. In severe cases, especially with underlying renal insufficiency, dialysis may be necessary. Hemodialysis works faster than peritoneal dialysis. Exchange transfusion is another option in newborn infants. Supportive care includes monitoring of cardiorespiratory status, fluids, and, if necessary, pressors for hypotension and electrolyte monitoring. In acute emergencies, especially in the context of severe cardiac manifestations, 100 mg/kg of intravenous calcium gluconate is transiently effective.

45.7 Phosphorus

Approximately two thirds of plasma phosphorus is in phospholipids, but these compounds are insoluble in acid and are not measured by clinical laboratories. It is the phosphorus content of plasma phosphate that is determined. The result is reported as either phosphate or phosphorus, although even when the term *phosphate* is used, it is actually the phosphorus concentration that is measured and reported. The end result is that *phosphate* and *phosphorus* are often used interchangeably. The term *phosphorus* is preferred when referring to the plasma concentration. Conversion from the units used in the United Stages (mg/dL) to mmol/L is straightforward (see Table 45–1).

PHOSPHORUS METABOLISM

Body Content and Physiologic Function. Most phosphorus is in bone or is intracellular, with less than 1% in plasma. At a physiologic pH, there are monovalent and divalent forms of phosphate because the pK of these forms is 6.8. Approximately 80% is divalent and the remainder is monovalent at a pH of 7.4. A small percentage of plasma phosphate, about 15%, is protein bound.

The remainder can be filtered by the glomerulus, with most existing as free phosphate and a small percentage complexed with calcium, magnesium, or sodium. Phosphate is the most plentiful intracellular anion, although the majority is part of a larger compound (e.g., ATP).

The phosphorus concentration varies with age more than any other electrolyte (Table 45–2). The teleologic explanation for the high concentration during childhood is the need for phosphorus to facilitate growth. There is diurnal variation in the plasma phosphorus concentration, with the peak during sleep.

Phosphorus, as a component of ATP and other trinucleotides, is critical for cellular energy metabolism. It is necessary for nucleic acid synthesis and it is a component of cell membranes and other structures. Along with calcium, phosphorus is an essential component of bone, and it is necessary for skeletal mineralization. There is a significant need for a net positive phosphorus balance during growth, with the growing skeleton especially vulnerable to deficiency.

Intake. Phosphorus is readily available in food. Milk and milk products are the best sources of phosphorus, but high concentrations are present in meat and fish. Vegetables have more phosphorus than fruits and grains. Gastrointestinal absorption is fairly proportional to intake, with about two thirds of intake being absorbed, even including a small amount that is secreted. Absorption, almost exclusively in the small intestine, occurs via a paracellular diffusive process and a vitamin D–regulated transcellular pathway. However, the impact of the change in phosphorus absorption caused by vitamin D is relatively small compared to the effect of variations in phosphorus intake.

Excretion. Despite the wide variation in phosphorus absorption dictated by oral intake, excretion matches intake, except for the needs for growth. The kidney is the principal regulator of phosphorus balance, which is mostly determined by intrarenal mechanisms. However, a number of hormones affect phosphorus excretion, although phosphorus homeostasis is not their main function.

About 90% of plasma phosphate is filtered at the glomerulus, although there is some variation based on plasma phosphorus and calcium concentrations. There is no significant secretion of phosphate along the nephron. Reabsorption of phosphate occurs mostly in the proximal tubule, even though a small amount of phosphate can be reabsorbed in the distal tubule. Normally about 85% of the filtered load is reabsorbed. The transport of phosphate from the tubular lumen into the cells of the proximal tubule is coupled with the transport of sodium down its chemical gradient. A sodium/phosphate co-transporter mediates the uptake of phosphate into the cells of the proximal tubule.

The dietary phosphorus determines the amount of phosphate reabsorbed by the nephron. There are both acute and chronic changes in phosphate reabsorption based on intake. Most of these changes appear to be mediated by intrarenal mechanisms that are independent of regulatory hormones. PTH, which is secreted in response to low plasma calcium, decreases reabsorption of phosphate, increasing urinary phosphate. This appears to have a minimal effect during normal physiologic variation in PTH levels. However, this does have an impact in the setting of pathologic changes in PTH synthesis (see later text).

TABLE 45–2. Serum Phosphorus During Childhood

Age	Phosphorus
0–5 days	4.8–8.2 mg/dL
1–3 years	3.8–6.5 mg/dL
4–11 years	3.7–5.6 mg/dL
12–15 years	2.9–5.4 mg/dL
16–19 years	2.7–4.7 mg/dL

Low plasma phosphorus stimulates the 1-αhydroxylase in the kidney that converts 25-vitamin D to 1,25-vitamin D (calcitriol). Calcitriol increases intestinal absorption of phosphorus and is necessary for maximal renal reabsorption of phosphate. The effect of a change in calcitriol on urinary phosphate is only significant when the level of calcitriol was initially low, arguing against a role for calcitriol in nonpathologic conditions.

A humoral mediator called *phosphatonin* inhibits renal reabsorption of phosphorus, causing both phosphaturia and hypophosphatemia in a variety of pathologic conditions. In autosomal dominant hypophosphatemic rickets, fibroblast growth factor type 23 has been identified as the phosphatonin. In X-linked hypophosphatemia rickets there is an absence of an endopeptidase that is believed to cleave a phosphatonin. The role of phosphatonins in normal physiology is not clear.

HYPOPHOSPHATEMIA

Because of the wide variation in normal plasma phosphorus, the definition of hypophosphatemia is age-dependent (see Table 45–2). The range reported on a laboratory report may be based on adult normal values and, therefore, may be misleading in children. For example, a serum phosphorus of 3 mg/dL, a normal value in an adult, is clinically significant hypophosphatemia in an infant.

The plasma phosphorus does not always reflect the total body stores because only 1% of phosphorus is extracellular. Thus, a child may have significant phosphorus deficiency despite a normal plasma phosphorus concentration. This is especially common in conditions in which there is a shift of phosphorus from the intracellular space (see later text).

Etiology and Pathophysiology. A variety of mechanisms cause hypophosphatemia (Box 45–10). A transcellular shift of phosphorus into cells occurs with processes that stimulate cellular utilization of phosphorus (e.g., glycolysis). Usually this only causes a minor, transient decrease in plasma phosphorus, but if intracellular phosphorus deficiency is present, the plasma phosphorus can decrease significantly, producing symptoms of acute hypophosphatemia. Glucose infusion stimulates insulin release, which leads to entry of glucose and phosphorus into cells. Phosphorus is then used during glycolysis and other metabolic processes. A similar phenomenon can occur during the treatment of diabetic ketoacidosis, and these patients are typically phosphorus depleted due to urinary phosphorus losses. Refeeding of patients with protein-calorie malnutrition causes anabolism, which leads to significant cellular demand for phosphorus. The increased phosphorus uptake for incorporation into newly synthesized compounds containing phosphorus leads to hypophosphatemia, which can be severe and symptomatic. Refeeding hypophosphatemia in children occurs frequently during therapy of severe anorexia nervosa. It can occur during treatment of children with malnutrition due to any cause, including cystic fibrosis, Crohn disease, burns, neglect, chronic infection, or famine. Hypophosphatemia usually occurs within the first 5 days of refeeding, and is prevented by a gradual increase in nutrition with appropriate supplementation (see Chapter 42.2). Total parenteral nutrition without adequate phosphorus can cause hypophosphatemia.

Phosphorus moves into the intracellular space during a respiratory alkalosis, which may occur as a result of an anxiety attack or in a variety of ill, hospitalized patients due to pain, sepsis, hepatic coma, or salicylate intoxication. The same transcellular shift of phosphorus takes place during recovery from a respiratory acidosis. An acute decrease in the carbon dioxide concentration, by increasing the intracellular pH, stimulates glycolysis, leading to intracellular utilization of phosphorus and hypophosphatemia. Because a metabolic alkalosis has less effect on the intracellular pH (carbon dioxide diffuses across cell membranes much faster than bicarbonate), there is minimal transcellular phosphorus movement with a metabolic alkalosis.

BOX 45–10. Causes of Hypophosphatemia

TRANSCELLULAR SHIFTS

Glucose infusion
Insulin
Refeeding
Total parenteral nutrition
Respiratory alkalosis
Tumor growth
Bone marrow transplantation
Hungry bone syndrome

DECREASED INTAKE

Nutritional
Premature infants
Low phosphorous formula
Antacids and other phosphate binders

RENAL LOSSES

Hyperparathyroidism
Parathyroid hormone–related peptide
X-linked hypophosphatemic rickets (MIM* 307800)
Tumor-induced osteomalacia
Autosomal dominant hypophosphatemic rickets (MIM 193100)
Fanconi syndrome
Dent disease (MIM 300009)
Hypophosphatemic rickets with hypercalciuria (MIM 241530)
Volume expansion and intravenous fluids
Metabolic acidosis
Diuretics
Glycosuria
Glucocorticoids
Kidney transplantation

MULTIFACTORIAL

Vitamin D deficiency
Vitamin D–dependent rickets type 1 (MIM 264700)
Vitamin D–dependent rickets type 2 (MIM 277440)
Alcoholism
Sepsis
Dialysis

*MIM refers to the database number from the Mendelian Inheritance in Man (http://www3.ncbi.nlm.nih.gov/Omim/).

Tumors that grow rapidly, such as leukemia and lymphoma, can lead to a significant phosphorus utilization and hypophosphatemia. A similar phenomenon may occur during the hematopoietic reconstitution that follows a bone marrow transplantation. In hungry bone syndrome, there is avid bone uptake of phosphorus, along with calcium and magnesium, which can produce plasma deficiency of all three ions. Hungry bone syndrome is most common after parathyroidectomy for hyperparathyroidism because the stimulus for bone dissolution is acutely removed, but bone synthesis continues.

Nutritional phosphorus deficiency is unusual because most foods contain phosphorus. However, infants are especially susceptible because of their high demand for phosphorus to support growth, especially of the skeleton. Premature infants have particularly rapid skeletal growth, and can develop phosphorus deficiency and rickets if fed human milk or standard formula. There is also a relative deficiency of calcium. The provision of additional calcium and phosphorus, using breast milk fortifier or special premature infant formula, prevents this complication. Phosphorus deficiency, sometimes with concomitant calcium and vitamin D deficiency, occurs in infants who are not given enough milk or receive a milk substitute that is nutritionally inadequate.

Antacids containing aluminum hydroxide, such as Maalox and Mylanta, bind dietary phosphorus and secreted phosphorus, preventing absorption. This can cause phosphorus deficiency and rickets in growing children. A similar mechanism causes hypophosphatemia in patients who are overtreated for hyperphosphatemia with phosphorus binders. In children with kidney failure, the addition of dialysis to phosphorus binders increases the risk of iatrogenic hypophosphatemia in these normally hyperphosphatemic patients. This complication, more common in infants, can worsen renal osteodystrophy.

Excessive renal losses of phosphorus occur in a variety of inherited and acquired disorders. Because PTH inhibits the reabsorption of phosphorus in the proximal tubule, hyperparathyroidism causes hypophosphatemia (see Chapter 567). The dominant clinical manifestation, however, is hypercalcemia and the hypophosphatemia is usually asymptomatic. The phosphorus level in hyperparathyroidism is not extremely low and there is no continued loss of phosphorus because a new steady-state is achieved at the lower plasma phosphorus level. Renal excretion, therefore, does not chronically exceed intake. There are occasional malignancies that produce PTH-related peptide, which has the same actions as PTH and causes hypophosphatemia and hypercalcemia.

In X-linked hypophosphatemic rickets, there is urinary wasting of phosphorus and hypophosphatemia (see Chapter 696). Even though transmitted on the X chromosome, the disorder affects both males and female carriers, behaving more like an autosomal dominant disorder. Hypophosphatemia normally stimulates synthesis of 1,25 vitamin D, which should, therefore, be elevated when the serum phosphorus is low, but these patients have either low or inappropriately normal levels, and this defect contributes to the pathogenesis of the disease in that 1,25-vitamin D enhances renal retention and gastrointestinal absorption of phosphorus.

Tumor-induced osteomalacia is a rare disorder that clinically resembles X-linked hypophosphatemic rickets, except it is not hereditary (see Chapter 698). Along with renal phosphorus wasting, the 1,25-vitamin D levels are inappropriately low. This disorder is mediated by a humoral factor or factors, called *phosphatonins*, which are secreted by some mesenchymal tumors. Fibroblast growth factor type 23 is the phosphatonin in some of these tumors. Tumor resection is curative. This condition has occasionally been seen in patients with epidermal nevus syndrome, neurofibromatosis, and fibrous dysplasia.

Autosomal dominant hypophosphatemic rickets is due to a mutation that prevents the degradation of fibroblast growth factor type 23. High levels of this phosphatonin lead to renal phosphorus wasting, hypophosphatemia, inappropriately normal 1,25-vitamin D levels, and rickets. Fanconi syndrome is a generalized defect in the proximal tubule leading to urinary wasting of bicarbonate, phosphorus, amino acids, uric acid, and glucose (see Chapter 521). The clinical sequelae are due to the metabolic acidosis and the hypophosphatemia. In children, an underlying genetic disease, most commonly cystinosis, often causes Fanconi syndrome, but it can be secondary to a variety of toxins and acquired diseases. Some patients have an incomplete Fanconi syndrome, and phosphorus wasting may be one of the manifestations. The hypophosphatemia of Fanconi syndrome is generally associated with rickets and does not usually cause symptomatic acute hypophosphatemia.

Dent disease, an X-linked disorder resulting from a defective chloride channel, can cause renal phosphorus wasting and hypophosphatemia, although this is not present in most cases. Other possible manifestations of Dent disease include tubular proteinuria, hypercalciuria, nephrolithiasis, rickets, and chronic renal failure. Hypophosphatemic rickets with hypercalciuria is a rare disorder, principally described in kindreds from the Middle East.

Metabolic acidosis inhibits reabsorption of phosphorus in the proximal tubule. In addition, metabolic acidosis causes a transcellular shift of phosphorus out of cells because of intracellular catabolism. This released phosphorus is subsequently lost in the urine, leading to significant phosphorus depletion, even though the plasma phosphorus may be normal. This classically occurs in diabetic ketoacidosis in which renal phosphorus loss is further increased by the osmotic diuresis. With correction of the metabolic acidosis and the administration of insulin, both of which cause a transcellular movement of phosphorus into cells, there is a marked decrease in the plasma phosphorus.

Volume expansion from any cause, such as hyperaldosteronism or SIADH, inhibits reabsorption of phosphorus in the proximal tubule. This also occurs with high rates of intravenous fluids. Thiazide and loop diuretics can increase renal phosphorus excretion, but this is seldom clinically significant. Glycosuria and glucocorticoids inhibit renal conservation of phosphorus. Hypophosphatemia is common after kidney transplantation due to urinary phosphorus losses. Possible explanations include pre-existing secondary hyperparathyroidism from chronic renal failure, glucocorticoid therapy, and upregulation of phosphatonins before transplantation. The hypophosphatemia usually resolves in a few months.

Both acquired and genetic causes of vitamin D deficiency are associated with hypophosphatemia (see Chapters 44.10 and 697). The pathogenesis is multifactorial. Vitamin D deficiency, by impairing intestinal calcium absorption, causes secondary hyperparathyroidism that leads to increased urinary phosphorus wasting. An absence of vitamin D decreases intestinal absorption of phosphorus and directly decreases renal reabsorption of phosphorus. The dominant clinical manifestation is rickets, although some patients have muscle weakness that may be related to phosphorus deficiency.

Alcoholism is the most common cause of severe hypophosphatemia in adults. Fortunately, many of the risk factors that predispose adult alcoholics to hypophosphatemia are not usually present in adolescents (e.g., malnutrition, antacid abuse, recurrent episodes of diabetic ketoacidosis). Hypophosphatemia often occurs in sepsis, even though the mechanism is not clear. Aggressive, protracted hemodialysis, as might be used for treatment of methanol or ethylene glycol ingestions, can cause hypophosphatemia.

Clinical Manifestations. There are acute and chronic manifestations of hypophosphatemia. Rickets occurs in children with long-term phosphorus deficiency. The clinical features of rickets are described in Chapter 44.10. With phosphorus deficiency, there is inadequate hydroxyapatite, preventing mineralization of osteoid, the organic matrix of bone. Osteomalacia is the general term for poorly mineralized bone; rickets is osteomalacia of the growth plates and can only occur in growing children. Older children and adults with chronic phosphorus deficiency develop isolated osteomalacia. Isolated phosphorus deficiency can cause rickets, although many children with rickets and hypophosphatemia have other pathogenic mechanisms contributing to the rickets. For example, children with vitamin D–deficiency rickets, who frequently have hypophosphatemia, also have inadequate calcium absorption and secondary hyperparathyroidism. In Fanconi syndrome the concurrent metabolic acidosis may contribute to the development of rickets.

Severe hypophosphatemia, typically levels less than 1–1.5 mg/dL, may affect every organ in the body because phosphorus has a critical role in maintaining adequate cellular energy. Phosphorus is a component of ATP and is necessary for glycolysis. With inadequate phosphorus, red blood cell 2,3-diphosphoglycerate levels decrease, impairing release of oxygen to the tissues. Severe hypophosphatemia can cause hemolysis and dysfunction of white cells and platelets. Chronic hypophosphatemia causes proximal muscle weakness and atrophy. In the intensive care unit, phosphorus deficiency may slow weaning from the ventilator or cause acute respiratory failure. Rhabdomyolysis is the most common complication of acute hypophosphatemia, usually in the setting of an acute transcellular shift of phosphorus into cells in a child with chronic phosphorus depletion (e.g., anorexia nervosa). The rhabdomyolysis is actually somewhat protective in that there is cellular release of phosphorus. Other manifestations of severe hypophosphatemia

include cardiac dysfunction and neurologic symptoms such as tremor, paresthesia, ataxia, seizures, and coma.

Diagnosis. The history and basic laboratory evaluation often suggest the etiology of hypophosphatemia. The history should investigate nutrition, medications, and familial disease. Hypophosphatemia and rickets in an otherwise healthy young child suggests a genetic defect in renal phosphorus conservation, Fanconi syndrome, inappropriate use of antacids, poor nutrition, vitamin D deficiency, or a genetic defect in vitamin D metabolism. In Fanconi syndrome, there is usually a metabolic acidosis, glucosuria, aminoaciduria, and a low plasma uric acid. Measurement of 25-vitamin D and 1,25-vitamin D, calcium, and PTH differentiates the various vitamin D deficiency disorders and X-linked hypophosphatemic rickets. Hyperparathyroidism is easily distinguished by the presence of elevated plasma PTH and calcium levels.

Treatment. The plasma phosphorus level, the presence of symptoms, the likelihood of chronic depletion, and the presence of ongoing losses dictate the approach to therapy. Mild hypophosphatemia does not require treatment unless the clinical situation suggests that chronic phosphorus depletion is present or ongoing losses are occurring. Oral phosphorus can cause diarrhea so the doses should be divided. Intravenous therapy is effective in patients who have severe deficiency or cannot tolerate oral medications. Intravenous phosphorus is available as either sodium phosphorus or potassium phosphorus, with the choice usually based on the patient's plasma potassium level. The oral preparations of phosphorus are available with various ratios of sodium and potassium. This is an important consideration because some patients may not tolerate the potassium load while the supplemental potassium may be helpful in diseases such as Fanconi syndrome or malnutrition.

Increasing dietary phosphorus is the only intervention needed in infants with inadequate intake. Other patients may also benefit from increased dietary phosphorus, usually dairy products. Phosphorus-binding antacids should be discontinued in patients with hypophosphatemia. Certain diseases require specific therapy. For example, vitamin D supplementation, not phosphorus, is the principal therapy in nutritional vitamin D deficiency. X-linked hypophosphatemic rickets is usually treated with a combination of 1,25-vitamin D and oral phosphorus.

HYPERPHOSPHATEMIA

Etiology and Pathophysiology. Renal insufficiency is the most common cause of hyperphosphatemia, with the severity proportional to the degree of kidney impairment. This occurs because the gastrointestinal absorption of the large dietary intake of phosphorus is unregulated, and the kidneys normally excrete this phosphorus. As renal function deteriorates, decreased reabsorption of phosphorus, partially mediated by increased PTH levels, is able to compensate. When kidney function is less than one third of normal, hyperphosphatemia usually develops, even though dietary intake of phosphorus does have a significant modulatory effect. Many of the other causes of hyperphosphatemia are more likely to develop in the setting of renal insufficiency (Box 45–11).

Cellular content of phosphorus is high relative to the plasma phosphorus, and cell lysis can release substantial phosphorus. This is the etiology of hyperphosphatemia in tumor lysis syndrome, rhabdomyolysis, and acute hemolysis. These disorders have concomitant potassium release and the risk of hyperkalemia. Additional features of tumor lysis and rhabdomyolysis are hyperuricemia and hypocalcemia, whereas an indirect hyperbilirubinemia and elevated lactate dehydrogenase (LDH) are often present with hemolysis. An elevated creatinine phosphokinase (CPK) is suggestive of rhabdomyolysis. During lactic

TRANSCELLULAR SHIFTS
Tumor lysis syndrome
Rhabdomyolysis
Acute hemolysis
Diabetic ketoacidosis and lactic acidosis

INCREASED INTAKE
Enemas and laxatives
Cow's milk in infants
Treatment of hypophosphatemia
Vitamin D intoxication

DECREASED EXCRETION
Renal failure
Hypoparathyroidism
Acromegaly
Hyperthyroidism
Tumoral calcinosis with hyperphosphatemia (MIM* 211900)

*MIM refers to the database number from the Mendelian Inheritance in Man (http://www3.ncbi.nlm.nih.gov/Omim/).

acidosis or diabetic ketoacidosis, there is a decreased utilization of phosphorus by cells and phosphorus shifts into the extracellular space. This problem reverses when the underlying problem is corrected, and, especially with diabetic ketoacidosis, patients subsequently become hypophosphatemic as a result of previous renal phosphorus loss.

Excessive intake of phosphorus is especially dangerous in children with renal insufficiency. Neonates are at risk because renal function is normally reduced during the first few months of life. In addition, they may erroneously be given doses of phosphorus that are meant for an older child or adult. Infants fed cow's milk, which has higher phosphorus content than breast milk or formula, may develop hyperphosphatemia. Fleet enemas have a high amount of phosphorus, which can be absorbed, especially if there is an ileus. Infants and children with Hirschsprung disease are especially vulnerable. There is often associated hypernatremia due to sodium absorption and water loss from diarrhea. Sodium phosphorus laxatives may cause hyperphosphatemia if the dose is excessive or renal insufficiency is present. Hyperphosphatemia occurs in children who receive overly aggressive treatment for hypophosphatemia. Vitamin D intoxication causes excessive gastrointestinal absorption of both calcium and phosphorus, and the suppression of PTH by hypercalcemia decreases renal phosphorus excretion.

The absence of PTH in hypoparathyroidism or PTH responsiveness in pseudohypoparathyroidism causes hyperphosphatemia because of increased reabsorption of phosphorus in the proximal tubule of the kidney (see Chapters 565 and 566). The associated hypocalcemia is responsible for the clinical symptoms. The hyperphosphatemia in hyperthyroidism or acromegaly is usually minor. It is secondary to increased reabsorption of phosphorus in the proximal tubule due to the actions of thyroxine or growth hormone. Excessive thyroxine can also cause bone resorption, which may contribute to the hyperphosphatemia and cause hypercalcemia. **Tumoral calcinosis** with hyperphosphatemia is a rare autosomal recessive disorder with heterotopic calcification, predominantly affecting black adolescents.

Clinical Manifestations. The principal clinical consequences of hyperphosphatemia are hypocalcemia and systemic calcification. The hypocalcemia is probably due to tissue deposition of calcium-phosphorus salt, inhibition of 1,25-vitamin D production, and decreased bone resorption. Symptomatic hypocalcemia is most likely to occur when the phosphorus increases rapidly or when diseases predisposing to hypocalcemia are pres-

ent (e.g., chronic renal failure, rhabdomyolysis). Systemic calcification occurs because the solubility of phosphorus and calcium in the plasma is exceeded. This is believed to happen when the plasma calcium × plasma phosphorus, both measured in mg/dL, is more than 70. Clinically, this is often apparent in the conjunctiva, where it manifests as injection. More ominous manifestations are hypoxia from pulmonary calcification and renal failure from nephrocalcinosis.

Diagnosis. The plasma creatinine and BUN should be assessed in any patient with hyperphosphatemia. The history should focus on intake of phosphorus and the presence of chronic diseases that may cause hyperphosphatemia. Measurement of potassium, uric acid, calcium, LDH, bilirubin, and CPK may be indicated if rhabdomyolysis, tumor lysis, or hemolysis is suspected. With mild hyperphosphatemia and significant hypocalcemia, measurement of the serum PTH level distinguishes between hypoparathyroidism and pseudohypoparathyroidism.

Treatment. The treatment of acute hyperphosphatemia depends on the severity and etiology of the hyperphosphatemia. Mild hyperphosphatemia in a patient with reasonable renal function spontaneously resolves; this action can be accelerated by dietary phosphorus restriction. If kidney function is not impaired, then intravenous fluids can enhance renal phosphorus excretion. For more significant hyperphosphatemia or a situation such as tumor lysis or rhabdomyolysis, in which endogenous phosphorus generation is likely to continue, addition of an oral phosphorus binder prevents absorption of dietary phosphorus and can remove phosphorus from the body by binding the phosphorus normally secreted and absorbed by the gastrointestinal tract. Phosphorus binders are most effective when given with food. Binders containing aluminum hydroxide are especially efficient, but calcium carbonate is an effective alternative and may be preferred if there is a need to treat concomitant hypocalcemia. Aluminum hydroxide is not used for chronic conditions because of the risk of aluminum intoxication. Preservation of renal function, for example with alkalinization of urine in rhabdomyolysis or tumor lysis, is an important adjunct because this will permit continued excretion of phosphorus. If the hyperphosphatemia is not responding to conservative management, especially if renal insufficiency is supervening, then dialysis may be necessary to increase phosphorus removal.

Dietary phosphorus restriction is necessary for diseases causing chronic hyperphosphatemia. However, such diets are often difficult to follow given the abundance of phosphorus in a variety of foods. Dietary restriction is often sufficient in conditions such as hypoparathyroidism or mild renal insufficiency. For more problematic hyperphosphatemia, such as with moderate renal insufficiency and end-stage renal disease, phosphorus binders are usually necessary. These include calcium carbonate, calcium acetate, and sevelamer hydrochloride. Aluminum-containing phosphorus binders are no longer used in chronic renal insufficiency because of the risk of aluminum toxicity. The risk is especially high if the patient is also taking oral citrate, which increases gastrointestinal absorption of aluminum. The exclusive reliance in renal insufficiency on calcium-containing binders is diminishing as a result of concerns about systemic calcification. Dialysis directly removes phosphorus from the blood in end-stage renal disease, but it is only an adjunct to dietary restriction and phosphorus binders in that phosphorus elimination by dialysis is not efficient enough to keep up with normal dietary intake.

45.8 Acid-Base Balance

ACID-BASE PHYSIOLOGY

Introduction and Terminology. Close regulation of pH is necessary for cellular enzymes and other metabolic processes that function optimally at a normal pH. Chronic mild derangements in acid-base status may interfere with normal growth and development, whereas acute severe changes in pH can be fatal. Control of acid-base balance depends on the kidneys, the lungs, and intracellular and extracellular buffers.

A normal pH is 7.35–7.45. The pH is the negative log of the hydrogen ion concentration. There is an inverse relationship between the pH and the hydrogen ion concentration. When the hydrogen ion concentration decreases, the pH increases, and when the hydrogen ion concentration increases, the pH decreases. At a pH of 7.40, the hydrogen ion concentration is 40 nanomoles/L. In contrast, a normal serum sodium concentration, 140 mEq/L, is more than 1 million times higher. Maintaining a normal pH is necessary because hydrogen ions are highly reactive and are especially likely to combine with proteins, altering their function. This occurs despite the relatively low concentration of hydrogen ions.

An acid is a substance that releases ("donates") a hydrogen ion (H^+). A base is a substance that accepts a hydrogen ion. An acid (HA) can dissociate into a hydrogen ion and a conjugate base (A^-):

$$HA \longleftrightarrow H^+ + A^-$$

A strong acid is highly dissociated, so in the above reaction there is little HA. A weak acid is poorly dissociated; not all of the hydrogen ions are released from HA. A^- acts as a base when the above reaction moves to the left. These reactions are in equilibrium. When HA is added to the system, there is dissociation of some HA until the concentrations of H^+ and A^- increase enough that a new equilibrium is reached. Addition of hydrogen ions causes a decrease in A^- and an increase in HA. Addition of A^- causes a decrease in hydrogen ions and an increase in HA.

Buffers are substances that attenuate the change in pH that occurs when acids or bases are added to the body. Given the extremely low concentration of hydrogen ions in the body at physiologic pH, without buffers a small amount of hydrogen ions could cause a dramatic decline in the pH. Buffers prevent the decrease in pH by binding the added hydrogen ions:

$$A^- + H^+ \rightarrow HA$$

The increase in hydrogen ion concentration drives this reaction to the right. Similarly, when base is added to the body, buffers prevent the pH from increasing by releasing hydrogen ions:

$$HA \rightarrow A^- + H^+$$

The decrease in the hydrogen ion concentration caused by the addition of base to the body drives this reaction to the right. Buffers work by either accepting or donating hydrogen ions. A buffer functions as a base when acid is added to the body and as an acid when base is added to the body. A strong acid, such as hydrochloric acid (HCl), is an ineffective buffer because the hydrogen ion and chloride remain dissociated at all physiologic hydrogen ion concentrations; chloride never functions as a base by accepting a hydrogen ion. The best buffers are weak acids and bases. This is because a buffer works best when it is 50% dissociated (i.e., half HA and half A^-). The pH at which a buffer is 50% dissociated is the pK of a buffer. The best physiologic buffers have a pK close to 7.40. The concentration of a buffer and the pK determine a buffer's effectiveness (buffering capacity). When the pH is less than the pK of a buffer, there is more HA than A^-. At a pH greater than the pK, there is more A^- than HA.

Physiologic Buffers. There are a variety of buffers that protect the body against major changes in pH. They are divided into the bicarbonate and non-bicarbonate buffers. The bicarbonate buffer system is routinely monitored clinically. The bicarbonate buffer system is based on the relationship between carbon dioxide (CO_2) and bicarbonate (HCO_3^-):

$$CO_2 + H_2O \longleftrightarrow H^+ + HCO_3^-$$

Carbon dioxide acts as an acid, in that, after combining with water, it releases a hydrogen ion; bicarbonate acts as its conjugate base, in that it accepts a hydrogen ion. The pK of this reaction is 6.1. The Henderson-Hasselbalch equation expresses the relationship between pH, pK, and the concentrations of an acid and its conjugate base. This relationship is valid for any buffer. The Henderson-Hasselbalch equation for bicarbonate and carbon dioxide is:

$$pH = 6.1 + \log [HCO_3^-]/[CO_2]$$

The Henderson-Hasselbalch equation for the bicarbonate buffer system has three variables: pH, $[HCO_3^-]$, and $[CO_2]$. Thus, if any two of these variables is known, it is possible to calculate the third. In using the Henderson-Hasselbalch equation, it is important that carbon dioxide and bicarbonate have the same units. Carbon dioxide is reported clinically as mm Hg and must be multiplied by its solubility constant, 0.03 mmol/L/mm Hg, before using the Henderson-Hasselbalch equation. Mathematical manipulation of the Henderson-Hasselbalch equation produces the following relationship:

$$[H^+] = 24 \times P_{CO_2} / [HCO_3^-]$$

At a normal hydrogen ion concentration of 40 nanomoles (pH 7.40), the P_{CO_2}, which is expressed as mm Hg in this equation, is 40 when the bicarbonate concentration is 24 mEq/L. This equation emphasizes that hydrogen ion concentration, and hence pH, can be determined by the ratio of P_{CO_2} and the bicarbonate concentration.

The bicarbonate buffer system is very effective as a result of the high concentration of bicarbonate in the body (24 mEq/L) and the fact that the bicarbonate buffer system is an open system. The remaining body buffers are in a closed system. The bicarbonate buffer system is an open system because the lungs increase carbon dioxide excretion when the blood carbon dioxide concentration increases. When acid is added to the body the following reaction occurs:

$$H^+ + HCO_3^- \rightarrow CO_2 + H_2O$$

In a closed system, the CO_2 would increase. The higher CO_2 concentration would lead to an increase in the reverse reaction:

$$CO_2 + H_2O \rightarrow H^+ + HCO_3^-$$

This would increase the concentration of hydrogen ions, limiting the buffering capacity of bicarbonate. However, because the lungs excrete the excess carbon dioxide, the reverse reaction does not increase; this enhances the buffering capacity of bicarbonate. The same principle holds with the addition of base because the lungs decrease carbon dioxide excretion and prevent the level of carbon dioxide from falling. The lack of change in carbon dioxide concentration dramatically increases the buffering capacity of bicarbonate.

The non-bicarbonate buffers include proteins, phosphate, and bone. Protein buffers consist of extracellular proteins, mostly albumin and intracellular proteins, including hemoglobin. Proteins are effective buffers largely due to the presence of the amino acid histidine, which has a side chain that can bind or release hydrogen ions. The pK of histidine varies slightly depending on its position in the protein molecule, but its average pK is approximately 6.5. This is close enough to a normal pH

(7.4) to make histidine an effective buffer. Hemoglobin and albumin have 34 and 16 histidine molecules, respectively.

Phosphate can bind up to three hydrogen molecules so it can exist as PO_4^{3-}, HPO_4^{2-}, $H_2PO_4^{1-}$, or H_3PO_4. However, at a physiologic pH, most phosphate exists as either HPO_4^{2-} or $H_2PO_4^{1-}$. $H_2PO_4^{1-}$ is an acid and HPO_4^{2-} is its conjugate base:

$$H_2PO_4^{1-} \longleftrightarrow H^+ + HPO_4^{2-}$$

The pK of this reaction is 6.8, making phosphate an effective buffer. The concentration of phosphate in the extracellular space is relatively low, which limits the overall buffer capacity of phosphate; it is less important than albumin. However, phosphate is at a much higher concentration in the urine, where it is an important buffer (see later text). In the intracellular space, most phosphate is covalently bound to organic molecules (e.g., ATP), but it still serves as an effective buffer.

Bone is an important buffer. Bone is basic—it is composed of compounds such as sodium bicarbonate and calcium carbonate—and thus dissolution of bone releases base. This can buffer an acid load, although at the expense of bone density if this occurs over an extended period. In contrast, bone formation, by consuming base, helps to buffer excess base.

Clinically, we measure the extracellular pH, but it is the intracellular pH that affects cell function. Measurement of the intracellular pH is unnecessary because changes in the intracellular pH parallel the changes in the extracellular pH. However, the change in the intracellular pH tends to be less than the change in the extracellular pH because of the increased buffering capacity in the intracellular space.

NORMAL ACID-BASE BALANCE

The lungs and the kidneys maintain a normal acid-base balance. Carbon dioxide generated during normal metabolism is a weak acid. The lungs prevent an increase in the partial pressure of CO_2 (Pco_2) in the blood by excreting the massive quantities of CO_2 that the body produces. CO_2 production varies depending on the body's metabolic needs, increasing, for example, with physical activity. The rapid pulmonary response to changes in CO_2 concentration occurs via central sensing of the Pco_2 and a subsequent increase or decrease in ventilation to maintain a normal Pco_2 (35–45 mm Hg). An increase in ventilation decreases the Pco_2 and a decrease in ventilation increases the Pco_2.

While the lungs excrete CO_2, the kidneys must deal with endogenous acid production. An adult normally produces about 1–2 mEq/kg/24 hr of hydrogen ions. Children normally produce 2–3 mEq/kg/24 hr of hydrogen ions. The three principal sources of hydrogen ions are dietary protein metabolism, incomplete metabolism of carbohydrates and fat, and stool losses of bicarbonate. Because metabolism of protein generates hydrogen ions, endogenous acid production varies with protein intake. The complete oxidation of carbohydrates or fats to carbon dioxide and water does not generate hydrogen ions; the lungs remove the carbon dioxide. However, incomplete metabolism of carbohydrates or fats produces hydrogen ions. For example, incomplete glucose metabolism can produce lactic acid and incomplete triglyceride metabolism can produce ketoacids such as ß-hydroxybutyric acid or acetoacetic acid. There is always some baseline incomplete metabolism that contributes to endogenous acid production. This increases in pathologic conditions such as lactic acidosis or diabetic ketoacidosis. Stool loss of bicarbonate is the third major source of endogenous acid production. The stomach secretes hydrogen ions, but most of the remainder of the gastrointestinal tract secretes bicarbonate and the net effect is a loss of bicarbonate from the body. In order to secrete bicarbonate, the cells of the intestine produce hydrogen ions that are released into the bloodstream. For each bicarbonate molecule lost in the stool the body gains one hydrogen ion.

This source of endogenous acid production is normally minimal, but may increase dramatically in a patient with diarrhea.

The hydrogen ions from endogenous acid production are neutralized by bicarbonate, potentially causing the bicarbonate concentration to decrease. The kidneys regenerate this bicarbonate by secreting hydrogen ions. The lungs cannot regenerate bicarbonate even though loss of carbon dioxide does lower the hydrogen ion concentration:

$$H^+ + HCO_3^- \rightarrow CO_2 + H_2O$$

A decrease in carbon dioxide concentration causes the reaction to move to the right, which decreases the hydrogen ion concentration, but it also lowers the bicarbonate concentration. During a metabolic acidosis, hyperventilation can lower the carbon dioxide concentration, decrease the hydrogen ion concentration, and, thus, increase the pH. However, the underlying metabolic acidosis is still present. Similarly, the kidneys cannot correct an abnormally high carbon dioxide concentration:

$$H^+ + HCO_3^- \rightarrow CO_2 + H_2O$$

An increase in the bicarbonate concentration also causes the reaction to move to the right, which increases the carbon dioxide concentration while simultaneously decreasing the hydrogen ion concentration. During a respiratory acidosis, increased renal generation of bicarbonate can decrease the hydrogen ion concentration and lower the pH, but cannot repair the respiratory acidosis. These examples emphasize the independence and interrelationship of the lungs and kidneys in regulating pH. Both the lungs and the kidneys can affect the hydrogen ion concentration and hence the pH. However, only the lungs can regulate the carbon dioxide concentration and only the kidneys can regulate the bicarbonate concentration.

Renal Mechanisms. The kidneys regulate the serum bicarbonate concentration by modifying acid excretion in the urine. This requires a two-step process. First, the renal tubules reabsorb the bicarbonate that is filtered at the glomerulus. Second, there is tubular secretion of hydrogen ions. The urinary excretion of hydrogen ions generates bicarbonate that neutralizes endogenous acid production. The tubular actions necessary for renal acid excretion occur throughout the nephron (Fig. 45–5).

The reabsorption of filtered bicarbonate is a necessary first step in renal regulation of acid-base balance. A normal adult has a GFR of approximately 180 L/24 hr. This fluid enters Bowman's space with a bicarbonate concentration that is essentially identical to the plasma concentration, normally 24 mEq/L. Multiplying 180 L times 24 mEq/L indicates that more than 4,000 mEq of bicarbonate enter Bowman's space each day. This bicarbonate, if not reclaimed along the nephron, would be lost in the urine. Such massive loss of bicarbonate would cause a profound metabolic acidosis.

The proximal tubule reclaims about 85% of the filtered bicarbonate. The final 15% is reclaimed after the proximal tubule, mostly in the ascending limb of the loop of Henle. Figure 45–6 illustrates the mechanisms responsible for bicarbonate reabsorption in the proximal tubule. The key concept is that bicarbonate molecules are not transported from the tubular fluid into the cells of the proximal tubule. Rather, hydrogen ions are secreted into the tubular fluid, leading to conversion of filtered bicarbonate into carbon dioxide and water. The secretion of hydrogen ions by the cells of the proximal tubule is coupled to generation of intracellular bicarbonate, which is transported across the basolateral membrane of the proximal tubule cell, and enters the capillaries. The bicarbonate produced in the cell replaces the bicarbonate filtered at the glomerulus.

Increased bicarbonate reabsorption by the cells of the proximal tubule—the result of increased hydrogen ion secretion—

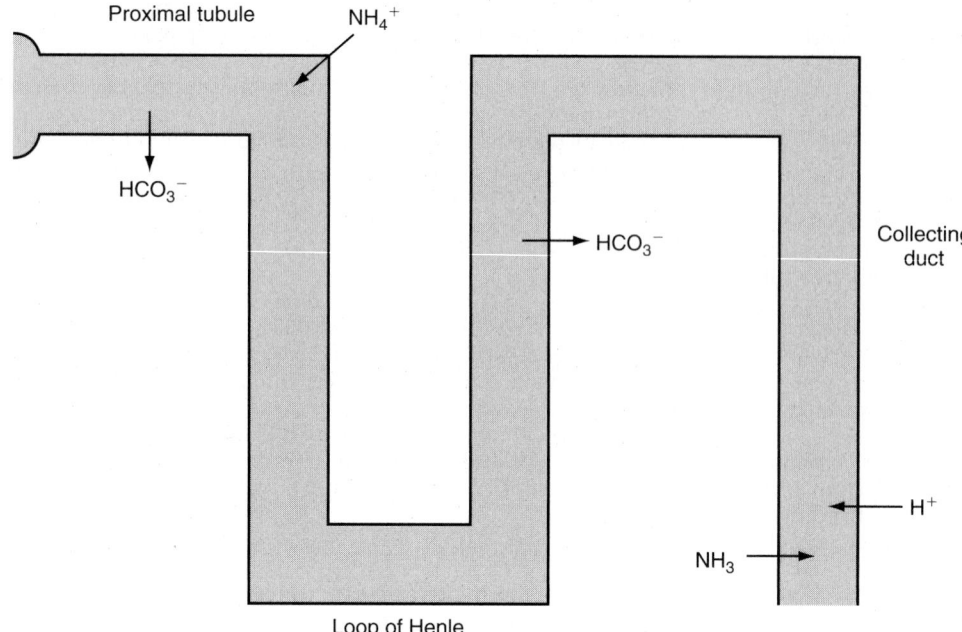

FIGURE 45–5. Tubular sites involved in acid-base balance. The proximal tubule is the site where most filtered bicarbonate is reclaimed, even though other sites along the nephron, especially the thick ascending limb of the loop of Henle, reabsorb some of the filtered bicarbonate. The collecting duct is the principal location for the hydrogen ion secretion that acidifies the urine. The proximal tubule generates the ammonia that serves as a urinary buffer in the collecting duct.

occurs in a variety of clinical situations. Volume depletion increases bicarbonate reabsorption. This is partially mediated by activation of the renin-angiotensin system; angiotensin II increases bicarbonate reabsorption. Increased bicarbonate reabsorption in the proximal tubule is one of the mechanisms that accounts for the metabolic alkalosis that may occur in some patients with volume depletion. Other stimuli that increase bicarbonate reabsorption include hypokalemia and an increased $P{CO_2}$. This partially explains the observations that hypokalemia causes a metabolic alkalosis and that a respiratory acidosis leads to a compensatory increase in serum bicarbonate concentration.

Stimuli that decrease bicarbonate reabsorption in the proximal tubule may cause a decrease in the serum bicarbonate concentration. A decrease in the $P{CO_2}$ (respiratory alkalosis) decreases proximal tubule bicarbonate reabsorption, partially mediating the decrease in the serum bicarbonate concentration that compensates for a respiratory alkalosis. Parathyroid hormone decreases proximal tubule bicarbonate reabsorption; hyperparathyroidism may cause a mild metabolic acidosis. A variety of medications and diseases cause a metabolic acidosis by impairing bicarbonate reabsorption in the proximal tubule. Examples include the medication acetazolamide, which directly inhibits carbonic anhydrase, and the many disorders that cause a proximal RTA (see Chapter 521).

After reclaiming filtered bicarbonate, the kidneys perform the second step in renal acid-base handling, the excretion of endogenous acid production. Excretion of acid occurs mostly in the collecting duct, with a small role for the distal tubule.

Along with secretion of hydrogen ions by the tubular cells lining the collecting duct, adequate excretion of endogenous acid requires the presence of urinary buffers. The hydrogen pumps in the collecting duct cannot lower the urine pH below 4.5. The hydrogen ion concentration at pH 4.5 is less than 0.04 mEq/L; it would require more than 25 L of water with a pH of 4.5 to excrete 1 mEq of hydrogen ions. A 10-kg child, with an endogenous acid production of 20 mEq of hydrogen ions each day, would need to have a daily urinary output of more than 500 L without the presence of urinary buffers. As in the blood, buffers in the urine attenuate the decrease in pH that occurs with the

addition of hydrogen ions. The two principal urinary buffers are phosphate and ammonia.

Urinary phosphate is proportional to dietary intake. Whereas most of the phosphate filtered at the glomerulus is reabsorbed in the proximal tubule, the urinary phosphate concentration is usually much greater than the serum phosphate concentration. This allows phosphate to serve as an effective buffer via the following reaction:

$$H^+ + HPO_4^{2-} \rightarrow H_2PO_4^{1-}$$

The pK of this reaction is 6.8, making phosphate an effective buffer as the urinary pH decreases from 7.0 to 5.0 within the collecting duct. Whereas phosphate is an effective buffer, its buffering capacity is limited by its concentration; there is no mechanism for increasing urinary phosphate excretion in response to changes in acid-base status.

In contrast, ammonia production can be modified, allowing for regulation of acid excretion. The buffering capacity of ammonia is based on the reaction of ammonia with hydrogen ions to form ammonium:

$$NH_3 + H^+ \rightarrow NH_4^+$$

The cells of the proximal tubule are the source of the excreted ammonia, mostly through metabolism of glutamine via the following reactions:

$$Glutamine \rightarrow NH_4^+ + glutamate^-$$

$$Glutamate^- \rightarrow NH_4^+ + \alpha\text{-ketoglutarate}^{2-}$$

The metabolism of glutamine generates two ammonium ions. In addition, the metabolism of α-ketoglutarate generates two bicarbonate molecules. The ammonium ions are secreted into the lumen of the proximal tubule while the bicarbonate molecules exit the proximal tubule cells via the basolateral Na^+, $3HCO_3^-$ co-transporter (see Fig. 45–6). This would seem to accomplish the goal of excreting hydrogen ions (as NH_4^+) and regenerating bicarbonate molecules. However, the ammonium

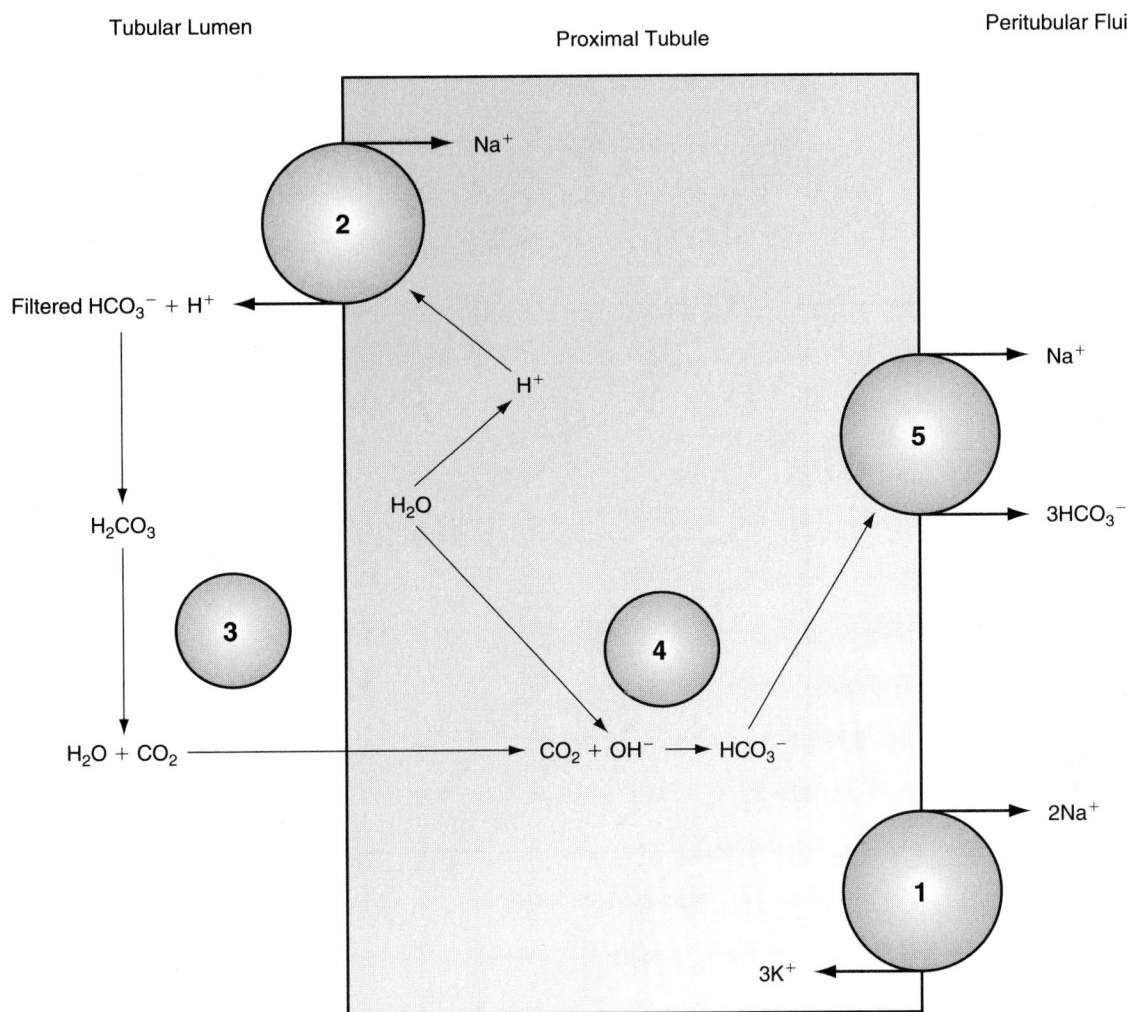

FIGURE 45–6. Reabsorption of filtered bicarbonate in the proximal tubule. The Na+,K+-ATPase (1) excretes sodium across the basolateral cell membrane, maintaining a low intracellular sodium concentration. The low intracellular sodium concentration provides the energy for the Na+,H+ antiporter (2), which exchanges sodium from the tubular lumen for intracellular hydrogen ions. The hydrogen ions that are secreted into the tubular lumen then combine with filtered bicarbonate to generate carbonic acid. Carbon dioxide and water are produced from carbonic acid (H_2CO_3). This reaction is catalyzed by luminal carbonic anhydrase (3). Carbon dioxide diffuses into the cell and combines with OH^- ions to generate bicarbonate. This reaction is catalyzed by an intracellular carbonic anhydrase (4). The dissociation of water generates an OH^- ion and an H+ ion. The Na+,H+ (2) antiporter secretes the hydrogen ions. Bicarbonate ions cross the basolateral membrane and enter the blood via the $3HCO_3^-$/1Na+ co-transporter (5). The energy for the $3HCO3^-$/1Na+ co-transporter comes from the negatively charged cell interior, which makes it electrically favorable to transport a net negative charge (i.e., three bicarbonates and only one sodium) out of the cell.

ions secreted in the proximal tubule do not remain within the tubular lumen. Cells of the thick ascending limb of the loop of Henle reabsorb the ammonium ions. The end result is that there is a high medullary interstitial concentration of ammonia, but the tubular fluid entering the collecting duct does not have significant amounts of ammonium ions. Moreover, the hydrogen ions that were secreted with ammonia, as ammonium ions, in the proximal tubule enter the bloodstream, canceling the effect of the bicarbonate generated in the proximal tubule. The excretion of ammonium ions, and hence hydrogen ions, is dependent on the cells of the collecting duct.

The cells of the collecting duct secrete hydrogen ions and regenerate bicarbonate, which is returned to the bloodstream (Fig. 45–7). This bicarbonate neutralizes endogenous acid production. Phosphate and ammonia buffer the hydrogen ions

secreted by the collecting duct. Ammonia is an effective buffer because of the high concentrations in the medullary interstitium and because the cells of the collecting duct are permeable to ammonia, but not permeable to ammonium. As ammonia diffuses into lumen of the collecting duct, the low urine pH causes almost all of the ammonia to be converted into ammonium. This maintains a low luminal ammonia concentration. Because the luminal pH is lower than the pH in the medullary interstitium, there is a higher concentration of ammonia within the medullary interstitium than in the tubular lumen, favoring movement of ammonia into the tubular lumen. Even though the concentration of ammonium in the tubular lumen is higher than in the interstitium, the cells of the collecting duct are impermeable to ammonium, preventing back diffusion of ammonium out of the tubular lumen. This permits ammonia to be an effective buffer.

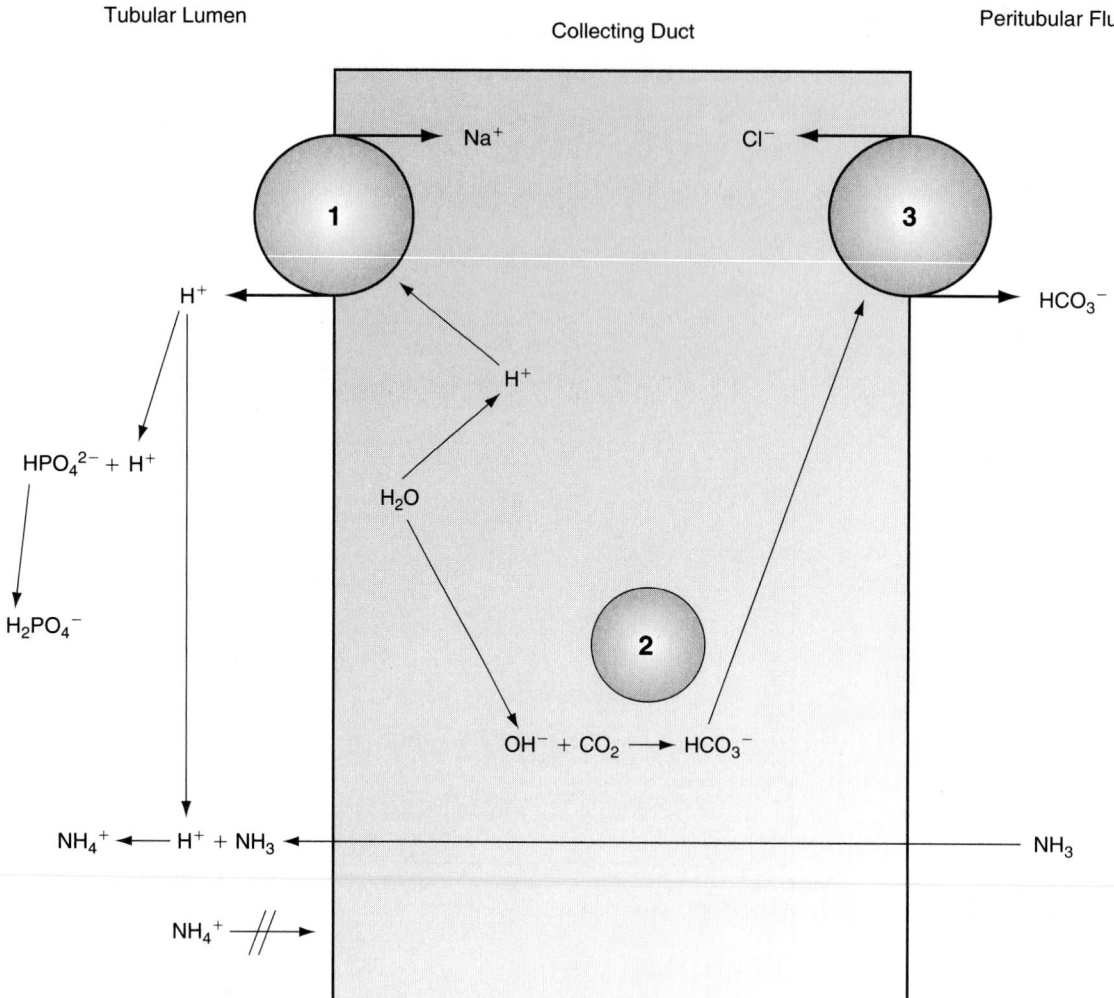

FIGURE 45–7. Secretion of hydrogen ions in the collecting duct. The dissociation of water generates an OH^- ion and an H^+ ion. The H^+ATPase (1) secretes hydrogen ions into the tubular lumen. Bicarbonate is formed when OH^- ion combines with carbon dioxide in a reaction mediated by carbonic anhydrase (2). Bicarbonate ions cross the basolateral membrane and enter the blood via the $HCO3^-$/Cl^- exchanger (3). The hydrogen ions in the tubular lumen are buffered by phosphate and ammonia. Ammonia (NH_3) can diffuse from the peritubular fluid into the tubular lumen, but ammonium ($NH4^+$) cannot pass through the cells of the collecting duct.

The kidneys adjust hydrogen ion excretion based on physiologic needs. There is variation in endogenous acid production, largely due to diet, and pathophysiologic stresses, such as diarrheal losses of bicarbonate, that increase the need for acid excretion. Hydrogen excretion is increased by upregulating hydrogen ion secretion in the collecting duct. This causes the pH of the urine to decrease. This response is fairly prompt, occurring within hours of an acid load, but it is limited by the buffering capacity of the urine; the hydrogen pumps in the collecting duct cannot lower the pH to less than 4.5. A more significant increase in acid excretion requires upregulation of ammonia production by the proximal tubule so that there is more ammonia available to serve as a buffer in the tubular lumen of the collecting duct. This response to a low serum pH reaches its maximum within 5 or 6 days; ammonia excretion can increase approximately 10-fold from baseline.

Acid excretion by the collecting duct increases in a number of different clinical situations. The extracellular pH is the most important regulator of renal acid excretion. A decrease in the extracellular pH from either a respiratory or metabolic acidosis causes an increase in renal acid excretion. Aldosterone stimulates hydrogen ion excretion in the collecting duct, causing an increase

in the serum bicarbonate concentration. This explains the metabolic alkalosis that occurs with primary hyperaldosteronism or secondary hyperaldosteronism due to volume depletion. Hypokalemia increases acid secretion, both by stimulating ammonia production in the proximal tubule and increasing hydrogen ion secretion in the collecting duct. Hypokalemia therefore tends to produce a metabolic alkalosis. Hyperkalemia causes the opposite effects, which may cause a metabolic acidosis.

In patients with an increased pH, the kidney has two principal mechanisms for correcting the problem. First, less bicarbonate is reabsorbed in the proximal tubule, leading to an increase in urinary bicarbonate losses. Second, in a limited number of specialized cells, the process for secretion of hydrogen ions by the collecting duct (see Fig. 45–7) can be reversed, leading to secretion of bicarbonate into the tubular lumen and secretion of hydrogen ions into the peritubular fluid, where they enter the bloodstream.

CLINICAL ASSESSMENT OF ACID-BASE DISORDERS

The following equation, a rearrangement of the Henderson-Hasselbalch equation, emphasizes the relationship between the

P_{CO_2}, the bicarbonate concentration, and the hydrogen ion concentration:

$$[H^+] = 24 \times P_{CO} / [HCO_3^-]$$

An increase in the P_{CO_2} or a decrease in the bicarbonate concentration increases the hydrogen ion concentration; the pH decreases. A decrease in the P_{CO_2} or an increase in the bicarbonate concentration decreases the hydrogen ion concentration; the pH increases.

Terminology. *Acidemia* is a pH below normal (<7.35) and *alkalemia* is a pH above normal (>7.45). An *acidosis* is a pathologic process that causes an increase in the hydrogen ion concentration and an *alkalosis* is a pathologic process that causes a decrease in the hydrogen ion concentration. whereas acidemia is always accompanied by an acidosis, a patient can have an acidosis and a low, normal, or high pH. For example, a patient may have a mild metabolic acidosis, but a simultaneous, severe respiratory alkalosis; the net result may be alkalemia. Acidemia and alkalemia indicate the pH abnormality; acidosis and alkalosis indicate the pathologic process that is taking place.

A *simple acid-base disorder* is a single primary disturbance. During a simple metabolic disorder, there is respiratory compensation. With a metabolic acidosis, the decrease in the pH increases the ventilatory drive, causing a decrease in the P_{CO_2}. The decrease in the carbon dioxide concentration leads to an increase in the pH. This *appropriate respiratory compensation* is expected with a primary metabolic acidosis. Despite the decrease in the carbon dioxide concentration, appropriate respiratory compensation is not a respiratory alkalosis, even though it is sometimes erroneously called a "compensatory respiratory alkalosis." A low P_{CO_2} can be due to a primary respiratory alkalosis or due to appropriate respiratory compensation for a metabolic acidosis. Appropriate respiratory compensation also occurs with a primary metabolic alkalosis, although in this case the carbon dioxide concentration increases to attenuate the increase in the pH. The respiratory compensation for a metabolic process happens quickly and is complete within 12–24 hr.

During a primary respiratory process, there is metabolic compensation, mediated by the kidneys. The kidneys respond to a respiratory acidosis by increasing hydrogen ion excretion, thereby increasing bicarbonate generation and raising the serum bicarbonate concentration. The kidneys increase bicarbonate excretion to compensate for a respiratory alkalosis; the serum bicarbonate concentration decreases. Unlike appropriate respiratory compensation, it takes 3–4 days for the kidneys to complete *appropriate metabolic compensation*. There is, however, a small and rapid compensatory change in the bicarbonate concentration during a primary respiratory process. The expected appropriate metabolic compensation for a respiratory disorder is dependent on whether the process is acute or chronic.

A *mixed acid-base disorder* is present when there is more than one primary acid-base disturbance. For example, an infant with bronchopulmonary dysplasia may have a respiratory acidosis from chronic lung disease and a metabolic alkalosis from the furosemide used to treat the chronic lung disease. More dramatically, a child with pneumonia and sepsis may have severe acidemia due to a combined metabolic acidosis due to lactic acid and respiratory acidosis from ventilatory failure.

There are formulas for calculating the appropriate metabolic or respiratory compensation for the six primary simple acid-base disorders (Table 45–3). The appropriate compensation is expected in a simple disorder; it is not optional. If a patient does not have the appropriate compensation, then a mixed acid-base disorder is present. For example, a patient has a primary metabolic acidosis with a serum bicarbonate concentration of 10 mEq/L. The expected respiratory compensation is a carbon dioxide concentration of 23 mm Hg ± 2 ($1.5 \times 10 + 8 \pm 2 = 23 \pm 2$;

TABLE 45–3. Appropriate Compensation During Simple Acid-Base Disorders

Disorder	Expected Compensation
Metabolic acidosis	$P_{CO_2} = 1.5 \times [HCO_3^-] + 8 \pm 2$
Metabolic alkalosis	P_{CO_2} increases by 7 mm Hg for each 10 mEq/L increase in the serum $[HCO_3^-]$
Respiratory acidosis	
Acute	$[HCO_3^-]$ increases by 1 for each 10 mm Hg increase in the P_{CO_2}
Chronic	$[HCO_3^-]$ increases by 3.5 for each 10 mm Hg increase in the P_{CO_2}
Respiratory alkalosis	
Acute	$[HCO_3^-]$ falls by 2 for each 10 mm Hg decrease in the P_{CO_2}
Chronic	$[HCO_3^-]$ falls by 4 for each 10 mm Hg decrease in the P_{CO_2}

see Table 45–3). If the patient's carbon dioxide concentration is more than 25 mm Hg, then a concurrent respiratory acidosis is present; the carbon dioxide concentration is higher than expected. A patient may have a respiratory acidosis despite a carbon dioxide level below the "normal" value of 35–45 mm Hg. In this example, a carbon dioxide concentration less than 21 mm Hg indicates a concurrent respiratory alkalosis; the carbon dioxide concentration is lower than expected.

Diagnosis. A systematic evaluation of an arterial blood gas, combined with the clinical history, can usually explain the patient's acid-base disturbance. Assessment of an arterial blood gas requires knowledge of normal values (Table 45–4). In most cases this is accomplished via a three-step process (Fig. 45–8):

1. Determine whether acidemia or alkalemia is present.
2. Determine a cause of the acidemia or alkalemia.
3. Determine whether a mixed disorder is present.

The first step in analyzing an acid-base disturbance is usually straightforward. The patient has either acidemia or alkalemia. Most patients with an acid-base disturbance have an abnormal pH, although there are two exceptions. The first exception is in the patient with a mixed disorder, wherein the two processes have opposite effects on the pH (e.g., a metabolic acidosis and a respiratory alkalosis) and cause comparable in magnitude, albeit opposite, changes in the hydrogen ion concentration. The second exception is in the patient with a simple chronic respiratory alkalosis; the appropriate metabolic compensation is, in some instances, enough to normalize the pH. In both of these situations of patients with a normal pH, the presence of an acid-base disturbance is deduced because of the abnormal carbon dioxide and/or bicarbonate levels. Determining the acid-base disturbance in these situations requires proceeding to the third step of this process (see later text).

The second step requires inspection of the serum bicarbonate and carbon dioxide concentrations to determine a cause of the abnormal pH (see Fig. 45–8). In most cases there is only one obvious explanation for the abnormal pH. In some mixed disorders, however, there may be two possibilities (e.g., a high P_{CO_2} and a low $[HCO_3^-]$ in a patient with acidemia). In such cases the patient has two causes of the abnormal pH (a metabolic acidosis and a respiratory acidosis in this instance), and it is unnecessary to proceed to the third step.

TABLE 45–4. Normal Values of an Arterial Blood Gas

pH	7.35–7.45
$[HCO_3^-]$	20–28 mEq/L
P_{CO_2}	35–45 mm Hg

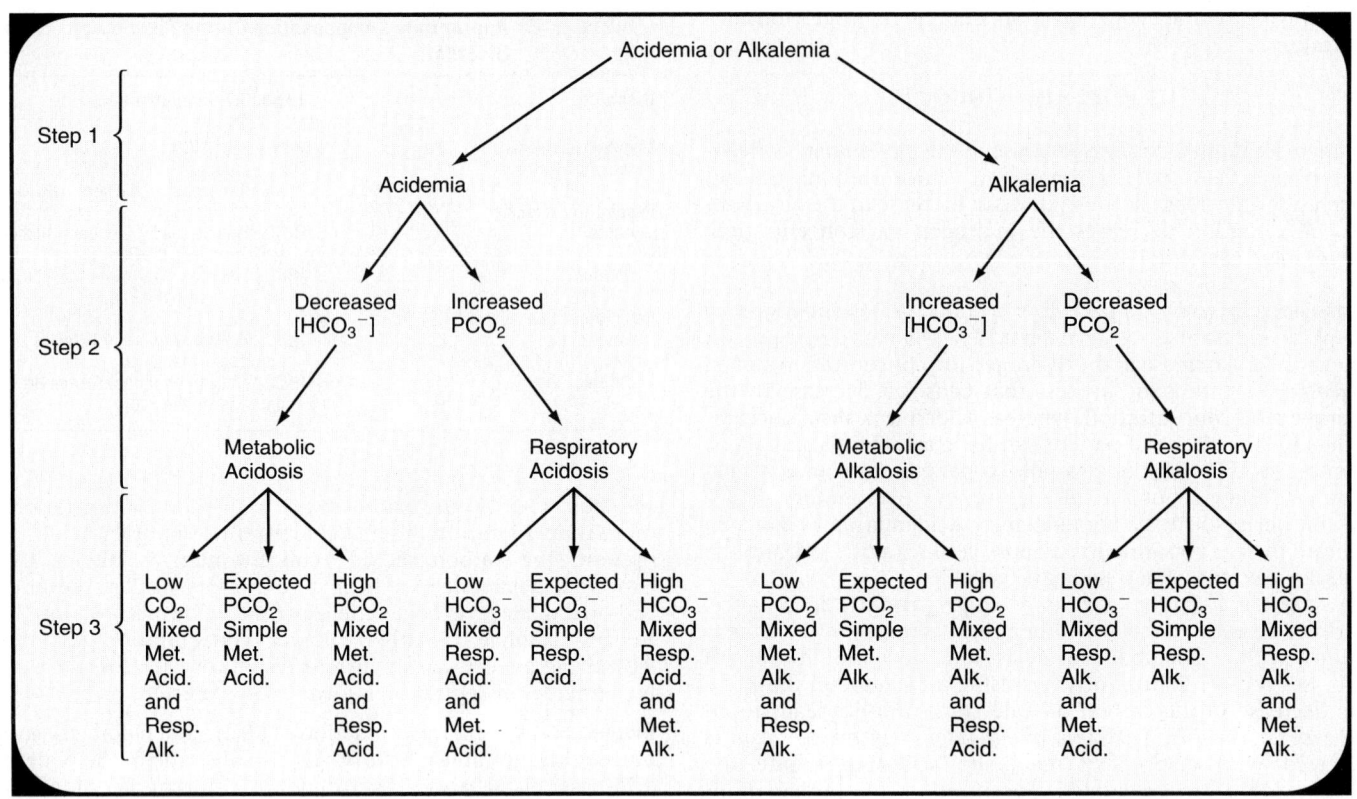

FIGURE 45–8. Three-step process for interpreting acid-base disturbances. In the first step, determine whether the pH is low (acidemia) or high (alkalemia). In the second step, establish an explanation for the acidemia or alkalemia. In the third step, calculate the expected compensation (see Table 45–3) and determine whether a mixed disturbance is present. Met. Alk. = Metabolic alkalosis; Met. Acid. = Metabolic acidosis; Resp. Alk. = Respiratory alkalosis; Resp. Acid. = Respiratory acidosis.

The third step requires determining whether the patient's compensation is appropriate. The patient is assumed to have the primary disorder diagnosed in the second step and the expected compensation is calculated (see Table 45–3). If the compensation is appropriate, then a simple acid-base disorder is present. If the compensation is not appropriate, then a mixed disorder is present. The identity of the second disorder is determined by deciding whether the compensation is too little or too much compared with what was expected (see Fig. 45–8).

The history is always useful in evaluating and diagnosing patients with acid-base disturbances. This is especially true with a respiratory process. The expected metabolic compensation for a respiratory process changes based on whether the process is acute or chronic. This can only be deduced by the history. For example, the metabolic compensation for a patient with an acute respiratory acidosis is less than the compensation for a chronic respiratory acidosis. In a patient with a respiratory acidosis, a small increase in the bicarbonate concentration would be consistent with a simple acute respiratory acidosis or a mixed disorder (a chronic respiratory acidosis and a metabolic acidosis). Only the history can differentiate among these possibilities. Knowledge of the length of the respiratory process and the presence or absence of a risk factor for a metabolic acidosis (e.g., diarrhea) allows the correct conclusion to be reached.

Metabolic Acidosis

Metabolic acidosis occurs frequently in hospitalized children; diarrhea is the most common etiology. For a patient with an unknown medical problem, the presence of a metabolic acidosis is often helpful diagnostically, because it suggests a relatively narrow differential diagnosis.

Patients with a metabolic acidosis have a low serum bicarbonate concentration, although not all patients with a low serum bicarbonate concentration have a metabolic acidosis. The exception is the patient with a respiratory alkalosis, which causes a decrease in the serum bicarbonate as part of appropriate renal compensation. In a patient with an isolated metabolic acidosis, there is a predictable decrease in the blood carbon dioxide concentration:

$$Pco_2 = 1.5 \times [HCO_3^-] + 8 \pm 2$$

A mixed acid-base disturbance is present if the respiratory compensation is not appropriate. If the Pco_2 is greater than predicted, then the patient has a concurrent respiratory acidosis. A lower Pco_2 than predicted indicates a concurrent respiratory alkalosis or, less commonly, an isolated respiratory alkalosis. Because the appropriate respiratory compensation for a metabolic acidosis never normalizes the patient's pH, the presence of a normal pH and a low bicarbonate concentration only occurs if some degree of respiratory alkalosis is present. In this situation, distinguishing an isolated chronic respiratory alkalosis from a mixed metabolic acidosis and acute respiratory alkalosis may only be possible clinically. In contrast, the combination of a low serum pH and a low bicarbonate concentration only occurs if a metabolic acidosis is present.

Etiology and Pathophysiology. There are many causes of a metabolic acidosis (Box 45–12), including the following three basic mechanisms:

BOX 45–12. Causes of Metabolic Acidosis

NORMAL ANION GAP

Diarrhea
Renal tubular acidosis (RTA)
    Distal (type I) (MIM* 179800/602722†)
    Proximal RTA (MIM 604278‡)
    Hyperkalemic (type IV)
Urinary tract diversions
Posthypocapnia
Ammonium chloride intake

INCREASED ANION GAP

Lactic acidosis
    Tissue hypoxia (hypoperfusion, hypoxemia, anemia)
    Liver failure
    Malignancy
    Intestinal bacterial overgrowth
    Inborn errors of metabolism
    Medications (e.g., nucleoside analogues, metformin)
Ketoacidosis
    Diabetic ketoacidosis
    Starvation ketoacidosis
    Alcoholic ketoacidosis
Kidney failure
Poisoning
    Ethylene glycol
    Methanol
    Salicylate
Inborn errors of metabolism

*MIM refers to the database number from the Mendelian Inheritance in Man (http://www3.ncbi.nlm.nih.gov/Omim/)
†Along with these genetic disorders, distal RTA may be secondary to renal disease or medications.
‡Most cases of proximal RTA are not due to this primary genetic disorder. Proximal RTA is usually part of Fanconi syndrome, which has multiple etiologies (see Chapter 521).

- Loss of bicarbonate from the body.
- Impaired ability to excrete acid by the kidney.
- Addition of acid to the body (exogenous or endogenous).

Diarrhea, the most common cause of metabolic acidosis in children, causes a loss of bicarbonate from the body. The amount of bicarbonate lost in the stool depends on the volume of diarrhea and the bicarbonate concentration of the stool, which tends to increase with more severe diarrhea. The kidneys attempt to balance the losses by increasing acid secretion, but metabolic acidosis occurs when this compensation is inadequate. Diarrhea often causes volume depletion as a result of losses of sodium and water, potentially exacerbating the acidosis by causing hypoperfusion and a lactic acidosis. In addition, diarrheal losses of potassium lead to hypokalemia. Moreover, the volume depletion causes increased production of aldosterone. This stimulates renal retention of sodium, helping to maintain intravascular volume, but also leads to increased urinary losses of potassium, exacerbating the hypokalemia.

There are three forms of *renal tubular acidosis* (RTA): distal (type I), proximal (type II), and hyperkalemic (type IV) (see Chapter 521). In distal RTA, children may have accompanying hypokalemia, hypercalciuria, nephrolithiasis, and nephrocalcinosis. Failure to thrive caused by chronic metabolic acidosis is the most common presenting complaint. There are autosomal dominant and autosomal recessive forms of distal RTA. The autosomal dominant form is relatively mild; many patients do not present until adulthood. Autosomal recessively inherited distal RTA is more severe and is often associated with deafness. Patients with distal RTA cannot acidify their urine and, thus, have a urine pH > 5.5 despite a metabolic acidosis.

Proximal RTA is rarely present in isolation. In most patients, proximal RTA is part of Fanconi syndrome, a generalized dysfunction of the proximal tubule. This leads to glycosuria, aminoaciduria, and excessive urinary losses of phosphate and uric acid. The presence of a low serum uric acid level, glycosuria, and aminoaciduria is helpful diagnostically. Chronic hypophosphatemia ultimately leads to rickets in children. Rickets and/or failure to thrive may be the presenting complaint. The ability to acidify the urine is intact in proximal RTA; thus, untreated patients have a urine pH < 5.5. However, bicarbonate therapy increases bicarbonate losses in the urine and the urine pH increases.

In hyperkalemic RTA, renal excretion of acid and potassium is impaired. Hyperkalemic RTA is due to either an absence of aldosterone or an inability of the kidney to respond to aldosterone (see Chapter 521). In severe aldosterone deficiency, as occurs with congenital adrenal hyperplasia due to 21α-hydroxylase deficiency, the hyperkalemia and metabolic acidosis are accompanied by hyponatremia and volume depletion from renal salt wasting. Incomplete aldosterone deficiency causes less severe electrolyte disturbances; children may have isolated hyperkalemic RTA, hyperkalemia without acidosis, or isolated hyponatremia. Patients may have aldosterone deficiency due to decreased renin production by the kidney; renin normally stimulates aldosterone synthesis. Children with hyporeninemic hypoaldosteronism usually have either isolated hyperkalemia or hyperkalemic RTA. The manifestations of aldosterone resistance depend on the severity of the resistance. In the autosomal recessive form of pseudohypoaldosteronism type I, which is due to an absence of the sodium channel that normally responds to aldosterone, there is often severe salt wasting and hyponatremia. In contrast, the aldosterone resistance in kidney transplant patients usually produces either isolated hyperkalemia or hyperkalemic RTA; hyponatremia is unusual. Similarly, the medications that cause hyperkalemic RTA do not cause hyponatremia. Pseudohypoaldosteronism type II, an autosomal recessive disorder called **Gordon syndrome,** is a unique cause of hyperkalemic RTA because the genetic defect causes volume expansion and hypertension.

Children with *abnormal urinary tracts*, usually secondary to congenital malformations, may require diversion of urine through intestinal segments. Ureterosigmoidostomy, anastomosis of a ureter to the sigmoid colon, almost always produces a metabolic acidosis and hypokalemia. Consequently, ileal conduits are now the more commonly used procedure, even though there is still a risk of a metabolic acidosis.

The *appropriate metabolic compensation for a chronic respiratory alkalosis* is a decrease in renal acid excretion. The resultant decrease in the serum bicarbonate concentration lessens the alkalemia caused by the respiratory alkalosis. If the respiratory alkalosis resolves quickly, the patient continues to have a decreased serum bicarbonate concentration, causing acidemia due to a metabolic acidosis. This resolves over 1–2 days via increased acid excretion by the kidneys.

Lactic acidosis most commonly occurs when inadequate oxygen delivery to the tissues leads to anaerobic metabolism and excess production of lactic acid. Lactic acidosis may be secondary to hypoperfusion, severe anemia, or hypoxemia. When the underlying cause of the lactic acidosis is alleviated, the liver is able to metabolize the accumulated lactate into bicarbonate, correcting the metabolic acidosis. There is normally some tissue production of lactate that is metabolized by the liver. In children with severe liver dysfunction, impairment in lactate metabolism may produce a lactic acidosis. Rarely, a metabolically active malignancy grows so fast that its blood supply becomes inadequate, with resultant anaerobic metabolism and lactic acidosis. Patients who have short intestines due to small bowel resection can have bacterial overgrowth. In these patients excessive bacterial metabolism of glucose into lactic acid can cause a lactic acidosis. Lactic acidosis occurs in a variety of inborn errors of metabolism, especially those affecting mitochondrial oxidation. Finally, medications can cause lactic acidosis. Antiretroviral nucleoside analogs that are used to treat HIV infection inhibit mitochondrial replication; lactic acidosis is a rare complication, although elevated serum lactate without acidosis is quite common. Metformin, commonly used for treating type 2 diabetes mellitus, is most likely to cause a lactic acidosis in patients with renal insufficiency.

In *insulin-dependent diabetes mellitus*, inadequate insulin leads to hyperglycemia and diabetic ketoacidosis (see Chapter 583). Production of acetoacetic acid and ß-hydroxybutyric acid causes the metabolic acidosis. Administration of insulin corrects the underlying metabolic problem and permits conversion of acetoacetate and ß-hydroxybutyrate into bicarbonate, which helps to correct the metabolic acidosis. However, in some patients, urinary losses of acetoacetate and ß-hydroxybutyrate may be substantial, preventing rapid regeneration of bicarbonate. In these patients, full correction of the metabolic acidosis requires renal regeneration of bicarbonate, a slower process. The characteristic odor of the breath in diabetic ketoacidosis is from the conversion of some acetoacetic acid into acetone, a volatile ketone that leaves the blood via the lungs. The hyperglycemia causes an osmotic diuresis, usually producing volume depletion, along with substantial losses of potassium, sodium, and phosphate. Despite severe total body potassium depletion, the serum potassium level is initially often normal as a result of a shift of potassium from the intracellular space into the extracellular space because of the lack of insulin and the metabolic acidosis. Hypokalemia develops with insulin therapy unless the patient receives adequate potassium.

In *starvation ketoacidosis*, the lack of glucose leads to ketoacid production. This can produce a metabolic acidosis, although it is usually mild as a result of increased acid secretion by the kidney. In alcoholic ketoacidosis, which is much less common in children than adults, the acidosis usually follows a combination of an alcoholic binge with vomiting and poor intake of food. The acidosis is potentially more severe than with isolated starvation and the blood glucose level may be low, normal, or high.

Renal failure causes a metabolic acidosis because of the need for the kidneys to excrete the acid produced by normal metabolism. With mild or moderate renal insufficiency, the remaining nephrons are usually able to compensate by increasing acid excretion. When the GFR is less than 20–30% of normal, the compensation is inadequate and a metabolic acidosis develops. In some children, especially those with chronic renal failure due to tubular damage, the acidosis develops at a higher GFR because of a concurrent defect in acid secretion by the distal tubule (a distal RTA).

A variety of *toxic ingestions* cause a metabolic acidosis. Salicylate intoxication is much less common since aspirin is no longer recommended for fever control in children. Acute salicylate intoxication occurs after a large overdose. Chronic salicylate intoxication is possible with gradual buildup of the drug. Especially in adults, respiratory alkalosis may be the dominant acid-base disturbance. In children, the metabolic acidosis is usually the more significant finding. Other symptoms of salicylate intoxication include fever, seizures, lethargy, and coma. Hyperventilation may be particularly marked. Tinnitus, vertigo, and hearing impairment are more likely with chronic salicylate intoxication.

Ethylene glycol, a component of antifreeze, is converted in the liver to glyoxylic and oxalic acids, causing a severe metabolic acidosis. Excessive oxalate excretion causes calcium oxalate crystals to appear in the urine, and calcium oxalate precipitation in the kidney tubules can cause renal failure. The toxicity of methanol ingestion is also dependent on liver metabolism; formic acid is the toxic end product that causes the metabolic

acidosis and other sequelae, which include damage to the optic nerve and central nervous system. Symptoms may include nausea, emesis, visual impairment, and altered mental status.

Many *inborn errors of metabolism* cause a metabolic acidosis (see Chapters 74 and 75). The metabolic acidosis may be due to excessive production of ketoacids, lactic acid, and/or other organic anions. Some patients have accompanying hyperammonemia. In most patients, the acidosis only occurs episodically during acute decompensations, which may be precipitated by ingestion of specific dietary substrates, the stress of a mild illness, or poor compliance with dietary or medical therapy. In a few inborn errors of metabolism, patients have a chronic metabolic acidosis.

Clinical Manifestations. The underlying disorder usually produces most of the signs and symptoms in children with a mild or moderate metabolic acidosis. The clinical manifestations of the acidosis are related to the degree of acidemia; patients with appropriate respiratory compensation and less severe acidemia have fewer manifestations than those with a concomitant respiratory acidosis. At a serum pH less than 7.20, there is impaired cardiac contractility and an increased risk of arrhythmias, especially if underlying heart disease or other predisposing electrolyte disorders are present. With acidemia there is a decrease in the cardiovascular response to catecholamines, potentially exacerbating hypotension in children with volume depletion or shock. Acidemia causes vasoconstriction of the pulmonary vasculature, which is especially problematic in newborn infants with persistent pulmonary hypertension (see Chapter 90.7).

The normal respiratory response to metabolic acidosis—compensatory hyperventilation—may be subtle with mild metabolic acidosis, but causes discernible increased respiratory effort with worsening acidemia. The acute metabolic effects of acidemia include insulin resistance, increased protein degradation, and reduced ATP synthesis. Chronic metabolic acidosis causes failure to thrive in children. Acidemia causes potassium to move from the intracellular space to the extracellular space, thereby increasing the serum potassium concentration. This effect is greater with a nonorganic acidosis than with an organic acidosis (e.g., lactic acidosis or ketoacidosis) or a respiratory acidosis. Severe acidemia impairs brain metabolism, eventually resulting in lethargy and coma.

Diagnosis. The etiology of a metabolic acidosis is often apparent from the history and physical examination. Acutely, diarrhea and hypoperfusion are common causes of a metabolic acidosis. Hypoperfusion, which causes a lactic acidosis, is usually apparent on physical examination and can be secondary to dehydration, acute blood loss, shock, or heart disease. Failure to thrive suggests a chronic metabolic acidosis, as happens with renal insufficiency or RTA. New onset of polyuria occurs in children with undiagnosed diabetes mellitus and diabetic ketoacidosis. Metabolic acidosis with seizures and/or a depressed sensorium, especially in an infant, warrants consideration of an inborn error of metabolism. However, meningitis and sepsis with lactic acidosis are a more common explanation for metabolic acidosis with neurologic signs and symptoms. Identification of toxic ingestions, such as ethylene glycol or methanol, is especially important because of the potential excellent response to specific therapy. A variety of medications cause a metabolic acidosis; they may be prescribed or accidentally ingested. Hepatomegaly and metabolic acidosis may occur in children with sepsis, congenital or acquired heart disease, hepatic failure, or inborn errors of metabolism.

Basic laboratory tests in a child with a metabolic acidosis should include BUN, creatinine, serum glucose, urinalysis, and electrolytes. An elevated BUN and creatinine are present in renal insufficiency, whereas an elevated BUN/creatinine ratio (>20:1) supports a diagnosis of prerenal azotemia and the possibility of hypoperfusion with lactic acidosis. Metabolic acidosis, hyperglycemia, glycosuria, and ketonuria support a diagnosis of diabetic ketoacidosis. Less commonly, this combination is secondary to an inborn error of metabolism. Starvation causes ketosis, but the metabolic acidosis, if present, is mild ($HCO_3^- > 18$). A moderate or severe metabolic acidosis with ketosis cannot be explained by starvation. Most children with ketosis due to poor intake and metabolic acidosis have a concomitant disorder such as gastroenteritis with diarrhea as an explanation for the metabolic acidosis. Alternatively, the combination of metabolic acidosis with ketosis occurs in inborn errors of metabolism; these patients may have hyperglycemia, normoglycemia, or hypoglycemia. Adrenal insufficiency may cause metabolic acidosis and hypoglycemia. Metabolic acidosis with hypoglycemia occurs with liver failure. Metabolic acidosis, normoglycemia, and glycosuria occur in children when type II RTA is part of the Fanconi syndrome; the defect in reabsorption of glucose by the proximal tubule of the kidney causes the glycosuria.

The serum potassium level is often abnormal in children with a metabolic acidosis. Even though a metabolic acidosis causes potassium to move from the intracellular space to the extracellular space, many patients with a metabolic acidosis have a low serum potassium level due to excessive body losses of potassium. With diarrhea, there are high stool losses of potassium and often secondary renal losses of potassium, whereas in type I or type II RTA there are increased urinary losses of potassium. In diabetic ketoacidosis, urinary losses of potassium are high, but the shift of potassium out of cells due to lack of insulin and metabolic acidosis is especially significant. Consequently, the initial serum potassium can be low, normal, or high, even though total body potassium is almost always decreased. The serum potassium is usually increased in patients with acidosis due to renal insufficiency; urinary potassium excretion is impaired. The combination of metabolic acidosis, hyperkalemia, and hyponatremia occurs in patients with severe aldosterone deficiency or aldosterone resistance. Patients with less severe type IV RTA often have only hyperkalemia and metabolic acidosis. Very ill children with metabolic acidosis may have an elevated serum potassium level as a result of a combination of renal insufficiency, tissue breakdown, and shift of potassium from the intracellular space to the extracellular space secondary to the metabolic acidosis.

The *plasma anion gap* is useful for evaluating patients with a metabolic acidosis. It divides patients into two diagnostic groups: normal anion gap or increased anion gap. The following formula determines the anion gap:

$$\text{Anion gap} = [\text{Na}^+] - [\text{Cl}^-] - [\text{HCO}_3^-]$$

A normal anion gap is 8–16. Figure 45–9 illustrates the basis for the anion gap. The number of serum anions must equal the number of serum cations in order to maintain electrical neutrality. The anion gap is the difference between the measured cation

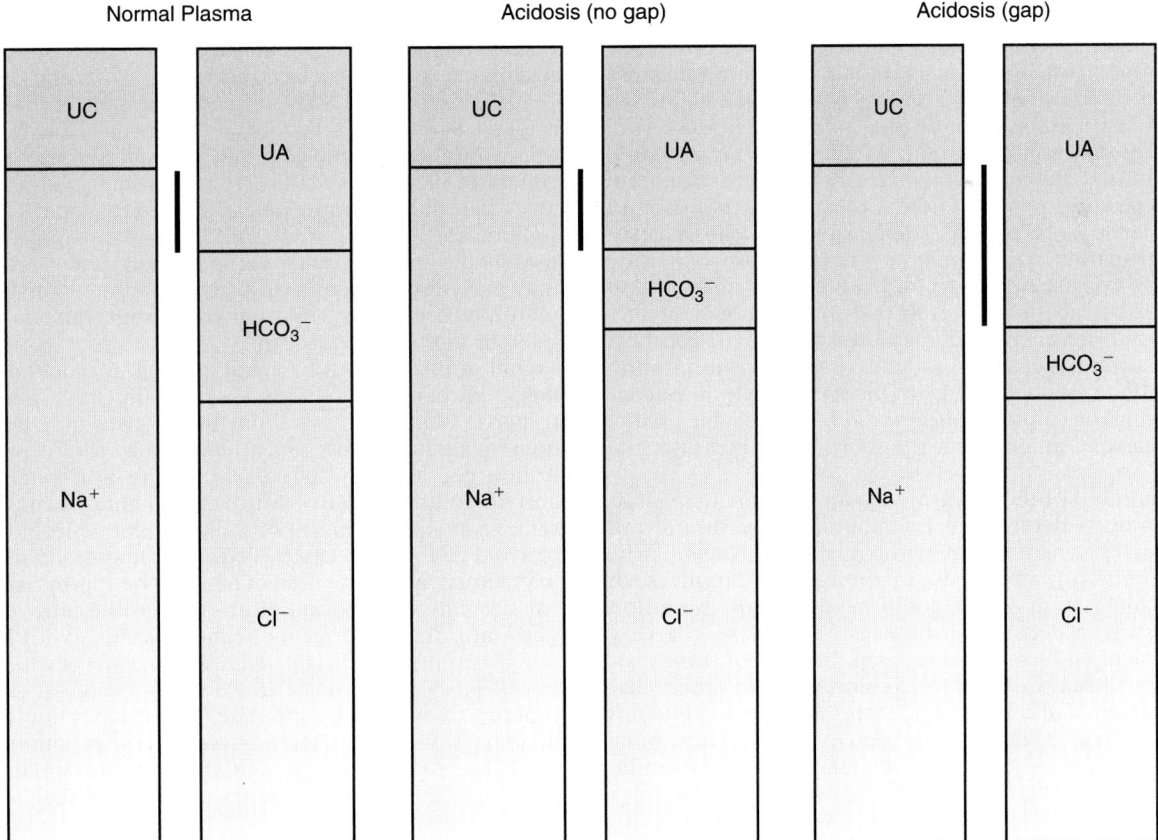

FIGURE 45–9. The anion gap. The anion gap is the difference between the sodium concentration and the combined concentrations of chloride and bicarbonate (*vertical line*). In both a gap and non-gap metabolic acidosis, there is a decrease in the bicarbonate concentration. There is an increase in unmeasured anions (UA) in patients with a gap metabolic acidosis. In a non-gap metabolic acidosis, there is an increase in the serum chloride concentration. UC = unmeasured cations.

(sodium) and the measured anions (chloride + bicarbonate). The anion gap is also the difference between the unmeasured cations (e.g., potassium, magnesium, calcium) and the unmeasured anions (e.g., albumin, phosphate, urate, sulfate). An increased anion gap occurs when there is an increase in unmeasured anions. For example, with a lactic acidosis there is endogenous production of lactic acid, which is composed of positively charged hydrogen ions and negatively charged lactate anions. The hydrogen ions are largely buffered by serum bicarbonate, resulting in a decrease in the bicarbonate concentration. The hydrogen ions that are not buffered by bicarbonate cause the serum pH to decrease. The lactate anions remain, and this causes the increase in the anion gap.

An increase in unmeasured anions, along with hydrogen ion generation, is present in all causes of an increased gap metabolic acidosis (see Box 45–12). In diabetic ketoacidosis, the ketoacids ß-hydroxybutyrate and acetoacetate are the unmeasured anions. In renal failure, there is retention of unmeasured anions, including phosphate, urate, and sulfate. However, the increase in unmeasured anions in renal failure is usually less than the decrease in the bicarbonate concentration. Renal failure is thus a mix of an increased gap and normal gap metabolic acidosis. The normal gap metabolic acidosis is especially prominent in children with renal failure due to tubular damage, as occurs with renal dysplasia or obstructive uropathy, because these patients actually have a concurrent RTA. The unmeasured anions in toxic ingestions vary: formate in methanol intoxication, glycolate in ethylene glycol intoxication, and lactate and ketoacids in salicylate intoxication. In inborn errors of metabolism, the unmeasured anions depend on the specific etiology and may include ketoacids, lactate, and/or other organic anions. In a few inborn errors of metabolism, the acidosis occurs without generation of unmeasured anions and, thus, the anion gap is normal.

A normal anion gap metabolic acidosis occurs when there is a decrease in the bicarbonate concentration without an increase in the unmeasured anions. For example, with diarrhea there is a loss of bicarbonate in the stool, causing a decrease in the serum pH and bicarbonate concentration. As shown in Figure 45–9, the serum chloride concentration increases in order to maintain electrical neutrality. Hyperchloremic metabolic acidosis is an alternative term for a normal anion gap metabolic acidosis. However, calculation of the anion gap is more precise than using the chloride concentration to differentiate a normal and increased gap metabolic acidosis in that the anion gap directly determines the presence of unmeasured anions. In contrast, electrical neutrality dictates that the chloride concentration increases or decreases depending on the serum sodium concentration, making the chloride concentration a less reliable predictor of unmeasured anions than the more direct measure, the anion gap.

Approximately 11 mEq of the anion gap is normally secondary to albumin. A decrease in the albumin concentration of 1 g/dL decreases the anion gap by roughly 4 mEq/L. Similarly, albeit less commonly, an increase in unmeasured cations, such as calcium, potassium, or magnesium, decreases the anion gap. Conversely, a decrease in unmeasured cations is a very unusual cause of an increased anion gap. Because of these variables, the broad range of a normal anion gap and other variables, the presence of a normal or increased anion gap is not always reliable in differentiating the causes of a metabolic acidosis, especially when the metabolic acidosis is mild. Moreover, some patients have more than one explanation for their metabolic acidosis, such as the child with diarrhea and lactic acidosis due to hypoperfusion. The anion gap should not be interpreted in dogmatic isolation; consideration of other laboratory abnormalities and the clinical history improves its diagnostic utility.

Treatment. The most effective therapeutic approach for patients with a metabolic acidosis is repair of the underlying disorder, if possible. For example, the administration of insulin in diabetic ketoacidosis and restoration of adequate perfusion in lactic acidosis eventually result in normalization of acid-base balance. In other diseases, the use of bicarbonate therapy is clearly indicated because the underlying disorder is irreparable. Children with metabolic acidosis due to RTA or chronic renal failure require long-term base therapy. Patients with acute renal failure and metabolic acidosis need base therapy until their kidney's ability to excrete hydrogen normalizes. In other disorders, the cause of the metabolic acidosis eventually resolves, but base therapy is necessary during the acute illness. In salicylate poisoning, for example, alkali administration increases renal clearance of salicylate and decreases the amount of salicylate in brain cells. Short-term base therapy is often necessary in other poisonings (e.g., ethylene glycol or methanol) and inborn errors of metabolism (e.g., pyruvate carboxylase deficiency or propionic acidemia). Some inborn errors of metabolism require chronic base therapy.

The use of base therapy in diabetic ketoacidosis and lactic acidosis is controversial, with little evidence that it improves patient outcome and a variety of potential side effects. The risks of giving sodium bicarbonate include the possibility of causing hypernatremia or volume overload. Furthermore, the patient may have overcorrection of the metabolic acidosis once the underlying disorder resolves because metabolism of lactate or ketoacids generates bicarbonate. The rapid change from acidemia to alkalemia can cause a variety of problems, including hypokalemia and hypophosphatemia. Bicarbonate therapy increases the generation of carbon dioxide, which can accumulate in patients with respiratory failure. Because carbon dioxide readily diffuses into cells, the administration of bicarbonate can lower the intracellular pH, potentially worsening cell function. Despite the potential complications, base therapy is often given to children with severe lactic acidosis and diabetic ketoacidosis.

Oral base therapy is given to children with chronic metabolic acidosis. Sodium bicarbonate tablets are available for older children. Younger children generally take citrate solutions; the liver generates bicarbonate from citrate. Citrate solutions are available as sodium citrate, potassium citrate, and a 1:1 mix of sodium and potassium citrate. The patient's potassium needs usually dictate the choice. Children with type I or type II RTA may have hypokalemia and benefit from potassium supplements, whereas most children with chronic renal failure cannot tolerate additional potassium.

Oral or intravenous base can be used in acute metabolic acidosis; intravenous therapy is generally used when a rapid response is necessary. Sodium bicarbonate may be given as a bolus, usually at a dose of 1 mEq/kg, in an emergency situation. A more gentle approach is to add sodium bicarbonate or sodium acetate to the patient's intravenous fluids, remembering to remove an equal amount of sodium chloride from the solution to avoid giving an excessive sodium load. Careful monitoring is mandatory so that the dose of base can be appropriately titrated. An alternative to sodium bicarbonate is the intravenous agent Carbicarb, which corrects metabolic acidosis with less generation of carbon dioxide, an advantage in patients with respiratory insufficiency. However, Carbicarb has not been shown to be superior to sodium bicarbonate, and it has some of the same potential side effects. Hemodialysis is another option for correcting a metabolic acidosis, and it is an appropriate choice in patients with renal insufficiency, especially if significant uremia or hyperkalemia is also present. Hemodialysis is advantageous for correcting the metabolic acidosis due to methanol or ethylene glycol intoxication because hemodialysis removes the offending toxin. In addition, these patients often have a severe metabolic acidosis that does not respond easily to intravenous bicarbonate therapy. Peritoneal dialysis is another option for correcting the metabolic acidosis due to renal insufficiency, although, because it relies on lactate as the source of base, it may not correct the metabolic acidosis in patients with concomitant renal failure and lactic acidosis.

Many causes of metabolic acidosis require specific therapy. Administration of a glucocorticoid and a mineralocorticoid is necessary in patients with adrenal insufficiency. Patients with diabetic ketoacidosis require insulin therapy, whereas patients with lactic acidosis respond to measures that alleviate tissue hypoxia. Along with correction of acidosis, patients with methanol or ethylene glycol should receive an agent that prevents the breakdown of these agents to their toxic metabolites. Traditionally this has been done with an ethanol infusion, but fomepizole is now an effective alternative with fewer side effects. Both agents work by inhibiting alcohol dehydrogenase, the enzyme that performs the first step in the metabolism of ethylene glycol or methanol. There are a variety of disease-specific therapies for patients with a metabolic acidosis due to an inborn error of metabolism.

Metabolic Alkalosis

Metabolic alkalosis in children is most commonly secondary to emesis or diuretic use. The serum bicarbonate concentration is increased with a metabolic alkalosis, even though a respiratory acidosis also leads to a compensatory elevation of the serum bicarbonate concentration. With a simple metabolic alkalosis, however, the pH is elevated; alkalemia is present. Patients with a respiratory acidosis are acidemic. A metabolic alkalosis, by decreasing ventilation, causes appropriate respiratory compensation. PCO_2 increases by 7 mm Hg for each 10 mEq/L increase in the serum bicarbonate concentration. Appropriate respiratory compensation never exceeds a PCO_2 of 55–60 mm Hg. The patient has a concurrent respiratory alkalosis if the PCO_2 is less than the expected compensation. A greater than expected PCO_2 occurs with a concurrent respiratory acidosis.

Etiology and Pathophysiology. The kidneys normally respond promptly to a metabolic alkalosis by increasing base excretion. Two processes are therefore usually present to produce a metabolic alkalosis. The first process is the generation of the metabolic alkalosis. This requires addition of base to the body. The second process is the maintenance of the metabolic alkalosis. This requires impairment in the kidney's ability to excrete base.

The etiologies of a metabolic alkalosis are divided into two categories based on the urinary chloride (Box 45–13). The alkalosis in patients with a low urinary chloride is maintained by *volume depletion*, and, thus, volume repletion is necessary for correction of the alkalosis. The volume depletion in these patients is due to losses of sodium and potassium, but the loss of chloride is usually greater than that of sodium and potassium combined. Because chloride losses are the dominant cause of the volume depletion, these patients require chloride to correct their volume depletion and their metabolic alkalosis; they are called "chloride responsive." In contrast, the patients with an elevated urinary chloride do not respond to volume repletion; they are called "chloride resistant."

Emesis or nasogastric suction results in *loss of gastric fluid*, which has a high content of HCl. Generation of hydrogen ions by the gastric mucosa causes simultaneous release of bicarbonate into the bloodstream. Normally the hydrogen ions in gastric fluid are reclaimed in the small intestine (by neutralizing secreted bicarbonate). Thus, there is no net loss of acid. With loss of gastric fluid, this does not occur and the patient develops a metabolic alkalosis. This is the generation phase of the metabolic alkalosis.

The maintenance phase of the metabolic alkalosis from gastric losses is due to the volume depletion ("chloride depletion" from gastric loss of HCl). Volume depletion interferes with urinary loss of bicarbonate, the normal renal response to a metabolic alkalosis. During volume depletion, a variety of mechanisms prevent renal bicarbonate loss. First, there is a reduction in the GFR so less bicarbonate is filtered. Second, volume depletion increases reabsorption of sodium and bicarbonate in the proximal tubule, limiting the amount of bicarbonate that can be excreted in the urine. This effect is mediated by angiotensin II and adrenergic stimulation of the kidney, which are both increased in response to volume depletion. Third, the increase in aldosterone during volume depletion increases bicarbonate reabsorption and hydrogen ion secretion in the collecting duct.

In addition to volume depletion, gastric losses are usually associated with hypokalemia as a result of both gastric loss of potassium and, most importantly, increased urinary potassium losses. The increased urinary losses of potassium are mediated by aldosterone, due to volume depletion, and the increase in intracellular potassium secondary to the metabolic alkalosis, which causes potassium to move into the cells of the kidney, causing increased potassium excretion. Hypokalemia contributes to the maintenance of the metabolic alkalosis by decreasing bicarbonate loss. More specifically, hypokalemia increases hydrogen ion secretion in the distal nephron and stimulates ammonia production in the proximal tubule. Ammonia production enhances renal excretion of hydrogen ions.

Many of the effects that maintain the metabolic alkalosis in patients with gastric losses and secondary volume depletion maintain and generate the metabolic alkalosis in the other diseases with chloride responsive metabolic alkalosis. Patients receiving *loop or thiazide diuretics* can develop a metabolic alkalosis. Diuretic use leads to volume depletion, which increases angiotensin II, aldosterone, and adrenergic stimulation of the kidney. Diuretics increase delivery of sodium to the distal nephron, further enhancing acid excretion. Moreover, diuretics cause hypokalemia, which increases acid excretion by the kidney. The increase in renal acid excretion generates the metabolic

---

BOX 45–13. Causes of Metabolic Alkalosis

CHLORIDE RESPONSIVE (urinary chloride <15 mEq/L)

Gastric losses (emesis or nasogastric suction)
Diuretics (loop or thiazide)
Chloride losing diarrhea (MIM* 214700)
Chloride-deficient formula
Cystic fibrosis (MIM 219700)
Post hypercapnia

CHLORIDE RESISTANT (urinary chloride >20 mEq/L)

High blood pressure (BP)
    Adrenal adenoma or hyperplasia
    Glucocorticoid-remedial aldosteronism (MIM 103900)
    Renovascular disease
    Renin-secreting tumor
    17α-hydroxylase deficiency (MIM 202110)
    11β-hydroxylase deficiency (MIM 202010)
    Cushing syndrome
    11β-hydroxysteroid dehydrogenase deficiency (MIM 218030)
    Licorice ingestion
    Liddle syndrome (MIM 177200)
Normal BP
    Gitelman syndrome (MIM 263800)
    Bartter syndrome (MIM 602023)
    Base administration

---

*MIM refers to the database number from the Mendelian Inheritance in Man (http://www3.ncbi.nlm.nih.gov/Omim/).

alkalosis and the decrease in bicarbonate loss maintains the metabolic alkalosis. In addition, patients on diuretics have a "contraction alkalosis." Diuretic use causes fluid loss without bicarbonate, and thus the remaining body bicarbonate is contained in a smaller total body fluid compartment. The bicarbonate concentration increases, helping to generate the metabolic alkalosis.

Diuretics are often used in patients with edema, such as in patients with nephrotic syndrome, heart failure, or liver failure. In many of these patients, metabolic alkalosis resulting from diuretic use develops despite the continued presence of edema. This is because the effective intravascular volume is low, and it is the effective intravascular volume that stimulates the compensatory mechanisms that cause and maintain a metabolic alkalosis. Many of these patients have a decreased effective intravascular volume before beginning diuretic therapy, increasing the likelihood of diuretic-induced metabolic alkalosis.

Diuretic use increases chloride excretion in the urine. Consequently, while a patient is receiving diuretics, the urine chloride is typically high (>20 mEq/L). After the diuretic effect has worn off, the urinary chloride is low (<15 mEq/L) due to appropriate renal chloride retention in response to volume depletion. Thus, categorization of diuretics based on urinary chloride depends on the timing of the measurement. However, the metabolic alkalosis from diuretics is clearly chloride responsive; it only corrects after adequate volume repletion. This is the rationale for including it among the chloride-responsive causes of a metabolic alkalosis.

Most patients with diarrhea develop a metabolic acidosis due to stool losses of bicarbonate. In *chloride-losing diarrhea*, an autosomal recessive disorder, there is a defect in the normal intestinal exchange of bicarbonate for chloride, causing excessive stool losses of chloride (see Chapter 320.12). In addition, stool losses of hydrogen ions and potassium cause metabolic alkalosis and hypokalemia, both of which are exacerbated by increased renal hydrogen and potassium losses due to volume depletion. Treatment is with oral supplements of potassium and sodium chloride. Use of a gastric proton-pump inhibitor, by decreasing gastric HCl production, reduces the volume of diarrhea and decreases the need for electrolyte supplementation.

An *infant formula with an extremely low chloride content* has led to chloride deficiency and volume depletion. The infants fed this formula, which is no longer available, developed a metabolic alkalosis and hypokalemia. *Cystic fibrosis* can cause metabolic alkalosis, hypokalemia, and hyponatremia due to excessive losses of sodium chloride in sweat (see Chapter 393). The volume depletion causes the metabolic alkalosis and hypokalemia through increased urinary losses while the hyponatremia, a less common finding, is secondary to sodium loss combined with renal water conservation in an effort to protect the intravascular volume ("appropriate" ADH production).

A *post-hypercapnic metabolic alkalosis* occurs after the correction of a chronic respiratory acidosis. This is typically seen in patients with chronic lung disease who are placed on a ventilator. During chronic respiratory acidosis, appropriate renal compensation leads to an increase in the serum bicarbonate concentration. This elevated bicarbonate concentration, since it is still present after the acute correction of the respiratory acidosis, causes a metabolic alkalosis. The metabolic alkalosis persists because the patient with a chronic respiratory alkalosis is intravascularly depleted due to chloride loss that occurred during the initial metabolic compensation for the primary respiratory acidosis. In addition, many children with a chronic respiratory acidosis receive diuretics, further decreasing the intravascular volume. The metabolic alkalosis responds to correction of the intravascular volume deficit.

The chloride-resistant causes of metabolic alkalosis can be subdivided based on blood pressure. The *patients with hypertension* have either increased aldosterone or act like they have increased aldosterone. Aldosterone levels are elevated in children with adrenal adenomas or hyperplasia. Aldosterone causes renal retention of sodium, with resultant hypertension. Metabolic alkalosis and hypokalemia result from aldosterone-mediated renal excretion of hydrogen ions and potassium. Urinary chloride is not low in that these patients are volume overloaded, not volume depleted. The volume expansion and hypertension allow normal excretion of sodium and chloride despite the presence of aldosterone. This is known as the "mineralocorticoid escape phenomenon."

In glucocorticoid-remedial aldosteronism, an autosomal dominant disorder, there is excess production of aldosterone due to the presence of an aldosterone synthase gene that is regulated by ACTH (see Chapter 572). Glucocorticoids effectively treat this disorder by inhibiting ACTH production by the pituitary, downregulating the inappropriate aldosterone production. Renovascular disease and renin-secreting tumors both cause excessive renin, leading to an increase in aldosterone, although hypokalemia and metabolic alkalosis are less common findings than hypertension. In two forms of congenital adrenal hyperplasia, 11ß-hydroxylase deficiency and 17α-hydroxylase deficiency, there is excessive production of the mineralocorticoid 11-deoxycorticosterone (see Chapter 570). Hypertension, hypokalemia, and metabolic alkalosis are more likely in 17 α-hydroxylase deficiency than in 11ß-hydroxylase deficiency. These patients respond to glucocorticoids because the excess production of 11-deoxycorticosterone is under the control of ACTH.

Cushing syndrome frequently causes hypertension. Cortisol has some mineralocorticoid activity and high levels can produce hypokalemia and metabolic alkalosis in patients with Cushing syndrome.

Cortisol can bind to the mineralocorticoid receptors in the kidney and function as a mineralocorticoid. This normally does not occur because 11ß-hydroxysteroid dehydrogenase in the kidney converts cortisol to cortisone, which does not bind to the mineralocorticoid receptor. In 11ß-hydroxysteroid dehydrogenase deficiency, cortisol is not converted in the kidney to cortisone. Cortisol is therefore available to bind to the mineralocorticoid receptor in the kidney and act like a mineralocorticoid. These patients, despite low levels of aldosterone, are hypertensive and hypokalemic, and they have a metabolic alkalosis. The same phenomenon can occur with excessive intake of natural licorice because a component of natural licorice, glycyrrhizic acid, inhibits 11ß-hydroxysteroid dehydrogenase. The autosomal dominant disorder **Liddle syndrome** is secondary to an activating mutation of the sodium channel in the distal nephron. Upregulation of this sodium channel is one of the principal actions of aldosterone. Because this sodium channel is continuously open, these children have the features of hyperaldosteronism, including hypertension, hypokalemia, and metabolic alkalosis, but low serum levels of aldosterone.

Bartter syndrome and Gitelman syndrome are autosomal recessive disorders with *normal blood pressure*, elevated urinary chloride, metabolic alkalosis, and hypokalemia (see Chapter 523). In Bartter syndrome, patients have a defect in sodium and chloride reabsorption in the loop of Henle. This leads to excessive urinary losses of sodium and chloride, and, like patients on loop diuretics, there is volume depletion and secondary hyperaldosteronism, causing hypokalemia and metabolic alkalosis. Gitelman syndrome is usually milder than Bartter syndrome. Patients have renal sodium and chloride wasting with volume depletion due to an absence of the thiazide-sensitive sodium-chloride transporter in the distal tubule. Like patients on a thiazide diuretic they develop volume depletion and secondary hyperaldosteronism with hypokalemia and metabolic alkalosis. Children with Gitelman syndrome have hypocalciuria and hypomagnesemia.

Excessive base intake can cause a metabolic alkalosis. These patients do not have a low urine chloride, unless there is associated volume depletion. In the absence of volume depletion, excess base is rapidly corrected via renal excretion of bicarbonate. Rarely, massive base intake can cause a metabolic alkalosis by overwhelming the kidney's ability to excrete bicarbonate. This may occur in infants given baking soda as a "home remedy" for colic or stomach upset. Each teaspoon of baking soda has 42 mEq of sodium bicarbonate. Infants have increased vulnerability due to a lower GFR, limiting the rate of compensatory renal bicarbonate excretion. A metabolic alkalosis may also occur in patients who receive a large amount of sodium bicarbonate during cardiopulmonary resuscitation. Blood products are anticoagulated with citrate, which is converted into bicarbonate by the liver. Patients who receive large amounts of blood products may develop a metabolic alkalosis. Iatrogenic metabolic alkalosis can occur as a result of acetate in total parenteral nutrition. Aggressive use of bicarbonate therapy in a child with a lactic acidosis or diabetic ketoacidosis may cause a metabolic alkalosis. This is especially likely in a patient in whom the underlying cause of the lactic acidosis is successfully corrected (e.g., restoration of intravascular volume in a patient with severe dehydration). Once the cause of the lactic acidosis resolves, lactate can be converted by the liver into bicarbonate, and, when combined with infused bicarbonate, this can create a metabolic alkalosis. A similar phenomenon can occur in a child with diabetic ketoacidosis because the administration of insulin allows ketoacids to be metabolized, producing bicarbonate. However, this rarely occurs because of judicious use of bicarbonate therapy in diabetic ketoacidosis and because there are usually significant pretreatment losses of ketoacids in the urine, preventing massive regeneration of bicarbonate. Base administration is most likely to cause a metabolic alkalosis in patients who have an impaired ability to excrete bicarbonate in the urine. This occurs in patients with concurrent volume depletion or renal insufficiency.

Clinical Manifestations. The symptoms in patients with a metabolic alkalosis are often related to the underlying disease and associated electrolyte disturbances. Children with the chloride-responsive causes of metabolic alkalosis often have symptoms related to volume depletion, such as thirst and lethargy. In contrast, children with chloride unresponsive causes may have symptoms related to hypertension.

Alkalemia causes potassium to shift into the intracellular space, causing a decrease in the extracellular potassium concentration. Moreover, alkalemia leads to increased urinary losses of potassium. Finally, increased potassium losses are present in many of the conditions that cause a metabolic alkalosis. Therefore, most patients with a metabolic alkalosis have hypokalemia, and symptoms may be related to the hypokalemia (see Chapter 45.4).

The symptoms of a metabolic alkalosis are due to the associated alkalemia. The magnitude of the alkalemia is related to the severity of the metabolic alkalosis and the presence of concurrent respiratory acid-base disturbances. During alkalemia, the ionized calcium concentration decreases as a result of increased binding of calcium to albumin. The decrease in the ionized calcium concentration may cause symptoms of tetany (e.g., carpopedal spasm) and seizures.

Arrhythmias are a potential complication of a metabolic alkalosis, and this risk increases if there is concomitant hypokalemia. Alkalemia increases the risk of digoxin toxicity, and antiarrhythmic medications are less effective in the presence of alkalemia. In addition, alkalemia may decrease cardiac output. A metabolic alkalosis causes a compensatory increase in the PCO_2 by decreasing ventilation. In patients with underlying lung disease,

the decrease in ventilatory drive can cause hypoxia. The hypoventilation in patients with severe metabolic alkalosis can cause hypoxia in patients with normal lungs.

Diagnosis. Measurement of the urinary chloride concentration is the most helpful test in differentiating among the causes of a metabolic alkalosis. The urine chloride is low in patients with a metabolic alkalosis resulting from volume depletion, unless there is a defect in renal handling of chloride. Urine chloride is superior to urine sodium in assessing volume status in patients with a metabolic alkalosis because the normal renal response to a metabolic alkalosis is to excrete bicarbonate. Because bicarbonate is negatively charged, it can only be excreted with a cation, usually sodium and potassium. Hence, a patient with a metabolic alkalosis excretes sodium in the urine despite the presence of volume depletion, which normally causes avid sodium retention. Urine sodium cannot be used to assess volume status in the presence of a metabolic alkalosis; urine chloride, in the absence of a defect in renal chloride handling, is a good indicator of volume status and differentiates among the chloride-resistant and chloride-responsive causes of a metabolic alkalosis.

Diuretics and gastric losses are the most common causes of metabolic alkalosis and are usually readily apparent from the patient history. Occasionally, metabolic alkalosis, usually with hypokalemia, may be a clue to the presence of bulimia or surreptitious diuretic use (see Chapter 104). Patients with bulimia have a low urine chloride, indicating that they have volume depletion as a result of an extrarenal etiology, but there is no alternative explanation for their volume depletion. Surreptitious diuretic use may be diagnosed by obtaining a urine toxicology screen for diuretics. The urine chloride is increased while diuretics are being used but is low when the patient stops taking diuretics. Rarely, children with mild Bartter syndrome or Gitelman syndrome are misdiagnosed as having bulimia or abusing diuretics. The urine chloride is always elevated in Bartter syndrome and Gitelman syndrome and the urine toxicology screen for diuretics is negative. Metabolic alkalosis and hypokalemia is occasionally the initial manifestation of cystic fibrosis. An elevated sweat chloride finding is diagnostic.

Patients with a metabolic alkalosis and a high urinary chloride are separated based on blood pressure. Children with a normal blood pressure may have Bartter syndrome or Gitelman syndrome. Excess base administration is another diagnostic possibility, but this is usually apparent from the history. In patients with sodium bicarbonate ingestion (e.g., baking soda), which may be unreported by the parent, the metabolic alkalosis usually occurs with significant hypernatremia. In addition, unless volume depletion is superimposed, the metabolic alkalosis from base ingestion self-resolves once the source of base is eliminated.

Measuring serum concentrations of renin and aldosterone differentiates children with a metabolic alkalosis, a high urinary chloride level, and elevated blood pressure. Both renin and aldosterone are elevated in children with either renovascular disease or a renin-secreting tumor. Aldosterone is high and renin is low in patients with adrenal adenomas or hyperplasia and glucocorticoid-remediable aldosteronism. Renin and aldosterone are low in children with Cushing syndrome, Liddle syndrome, licorice ingestion, 17α-hydroxylase deficiency, 11ß-hydroxylase deficiency, and 11ß-hydroxysteroid dehydrogenase deficiency. An elevated 24-hr urine cortisol level is diagnostic of Cushing syndrome, which is suspected by the presence of the other classic features of this disease (see Chapter 571). 11-Deoxycorticosterone levels are elevated in 17α-hydroxylase deficiency and 11ß-hydroxylase deficiency.

Treatment. The approach to therapy of metabolic alkalosis depends on the severity of the alkalosis and the underlying etiology. In children with a mild metabolic alkalosis ([HCO_3^-] < 32) intervention is often unnecessary, although this depends on the specific circumstances. In a child with congenital heart disease receiving a stable dose of a loop diuretic, a mild alkalosis does not require treatment. In contrast, intervention may be appropriate in a child with a worsening mild metabolic alkalosis due to nasogastric suction. The presence of a concurrent respiratory acid-base disturbance also influences therapeutic decision-making. A patient with a concurrent respiratory acidosis should have some increase in bicarbonate due to metabolic compensation, and thus the severity of the pH elevation is more important than the bicarbonate concentration. In contrast, a patient with a respiratory alkalosis and a metabolic alkalosis is at risk for severe alkalemia; treatment may be indicated, even if the increase in bicarbonate is only mild.

Intervention is usually necessary in children with moderate or severe metabolic alkalosis. The most effective approach is always to address the underlying etiology. In some children, nasogastric suction may be decreased or discontinued. Alternatively, the addition of a gastric proton pump inhibitor reduces gastric secretion and losses of HCl. Diuretics are an important cause of metabolic alkalosis and, if tolerated, they should be eliminated or the dose reduced. Adequate potassium supplementation or the addition of a potassium-sparing diuretic is also helpful in a child with a metabolic alkalosis caused by diuretics. Potassium-sparing diuretics not only decrease renal potassium losses, but, by blocking the action of aldosterone, they decrease hydrogen ion secretion in the distal nephron, increasing urinary bicarbonate excretion. Many children cannot tolerate discontinuation of diuretic therapy, thus potassium supplementation and potassium-sparing diuretics are the principal therapeutic approach. Occasionally, in cases of severe metabolic alkalosis, acetazolamide is an option. Acetazolamide, a carbonic anhydrase inhibitor, decreases reabsorption of bicarbonate in the proximal tubule, causing significant bicarbonate loss in the urine. The patient must be monitored closely because acetazolamide produces major losses of potassium in the urine and increases fluid losses, potentially necessitating a reduction in other diuretics.

Most children with a metabolic alkalosis have one of the chloride-responsive etiologies. In these situations, administration of sufficient sodium chloride and potassium chloride to correct the volume deficit and the potassium deficit is necessary to correct the metabolic alkalosis. This may not be an option in the child who has volume depletion due to diuretics because volume repletion may be contraindicated. Adequate replacement of gastric losses of sodium and potassium in a child with nasogastric tube can minimize or prevent the development of the metabolic alkalosis. With adequate intravascular volume and a normal serum potassium concentration, the kidney is able to excrete the excess bicarbonate within a couple of days.

In children with the chloride resistant causes of a metabolic alkalosis that are associated with hypertension, volume repletion is contraindicated because it exacerbates the hypertension and does not repair the metabolic alkalosis. Ideally, treatment focuses on eliminating the excess aldosterone effect. Adrenal adenomas can be resected, licorice intake can be eliminated, and renovascular disease can be repaired. Glucocorticoid-remediable aldosteronism, 17α-hydroxylase deficiency, and 11ß-hydroxylase deficiency respond to administration of glucocorticoids. The mineralocorticoid effect of cortisol in 11ß-hydroxysteroid dehydrogenase deficiency can be decreased by using spironolactone, which blocks the mineralocorticoid receptor. In contrast, children with Liddle syndrome do not respond to spironolactone; however, either triamterene or amiloride is effective therapy because they block the sodium channel that is constitutively active in Liddle syndrome.

In children with Bartter syndrome and Gitelman syndrome, therapy includes oral potassium supplementation and potassium- sparing diuretics. Children with Gitelman syndrome often require magnesium supplementation, whereas children with severe Bartter syndrome often benefit from indomethacin.

Respiratory Acidosis

A respiratory acidosis is an inappropriate increase in the blood carbon dioxide (PCO_2). Carbon dioxide is a byproduct of metabolism, and it is removed from the body by the lungs. During a respiratory acidosis, there is a decrease in the effectiveness of carbon dioxide removal by lungs. A respiratory acidosis is secondary to either pulmonary diseases, such as severe bronchiolitis, or nonpulmonary disease, such as a narcotic overdose. Even though body production of carbon dioxide can vary, normal lungs are able to accommodate this variation; excess production of carbon dioxide is never an isolated cause of a respiratory acidosis. With impaired alveolar ventilation, the rate of body production of carbon dioxide may affect the severity of the respiratory acidosis, but this is usually not a significant factor.

A respiratory acidosis causes a decrease in the blood pH, but there is normally a metabolic response that partially compensates, minimizing the severity of the acidemia. The acute metabolic response to a respiratory alkalosis occurs within minutes. The metabolic compensation for an acute respiratory acidosis is secondary to titration of acid by non-bicarbonate buffers. This buffering of hydrogen ions causes a predictable increase in the serum bicarbonate concentration: Plasma bicarbonate increases by 1 for each 10 mm Hg increase in the PCO_2 (acute compensation).

With a chronic respiratory acidosis there is more significant metabolic compensation and, thus, less severe acidemia than an acute respiratory acidosis with the same increase in PCO_2. During a chronic respiratory acidosis, the kidneys increase acid excretion. This response occurs over 3–4 days and causes a predictable increase in the serum bicarbonate concentration: Plasma bicarbonate increases by 3.5 for each 10 mm Hg increase in the PCO_2 (chronic compensation).

The increase of serum bicarbonate during a chronic respiratory acidosis is associated with a decrease in body chloride. After acute correction of a chronic respiratory acidosis, the plasma bicarbonate continues to be increased, and the patient has a metabolic alkalosis. Because of the chloride deficit, this is a chloride responsive metabolic alkalosis; it corrects once the patient's chloride deficit is replaced.

A mixed disorder is present if the metabolic compensation is inappropriate. A higher than expected bicarbonate occurs in the setting of a concurrent metabolic alkalosis and a lower than expected bicarbonate occurs in the setting of a concurrent metabolic acidosis. Evaluating whether compensation is appropriate during a respiratory acidosis requires clinical knowledge of the acuity of the process, because the expected compensation is different depending on whether the process is acute or chronic.

The PCO_2 cannot be interpreted in isolation to determine whether a patient has a respiratory acidosis. A respiratory acidosis is always present if a patient has acidemia and an elevated PCO_2. However, an elevated PCO_2 also occurs as appropriate respiratory compensation for a simple metabolic alkalosis. The patient is alkalemic; this is not a respiratory acidosis. During a mixed disturbance a patient can have a respiratory acidosis and a normal or even a low PCO_2. This may occur in a patient with a metabolic acidosis; a respiratory acidosis is present if the patient does not have appropriate respiratory compensation (i.e., the PCO_2 is higher than expected based on the severity of the metabolic acidosis).

Etiology and Pathophysiology. The causes of a respiratory acidosis are either pulmonary or non-pulmonary (Box 45–14). Central nervous system disorders can decrease the activity of the central

BOX 45–14. Causes of Respiratory Acidosis

CENTRAL NERVOUS SYSTEM DEPRESSION
Encephalitis
Head trauma
Brain tumor
Central sleep apnea
Primary pulmonary hypoventilation (Ondine curse)
Stroke
Hypoxic brain damage
Obesity-hypoventilation (Pickwickian syndrome)
Increased intracranial pressure
Medications
  Narcotics
  Barbiturates
  Anesthesia
  Benzodiazepines
  Alcohols

DISORDERS OF THE SPINAL CORD, PERIPHERAL NERVES, OR NEUROMUSCULAR JUNCTION
Diaphragmatic paralysis
Guillain-Barré syndrome
Poliomyelitis
Spinal muscular atrophies
Tick paralysis
Botulism
Myasthenia
Multiple sclerosis
Spinal cord injury
Medications
  Vecuronium
  Aminoglycosides
  Organophosphates (pesticides)

RESPIRATORY MUSCLE WEAKNESS
Muscular dystrophy
Hypothyroidism
Malnutrition
Hypokalemia
Hypophosphatemia
Medications
  Succinylcholine
  Corticosteroids

PULMONARY DISEASE
Pneumonia
Pneumothorax
Asthma
Bronchiolitis
Pulmonary edema
Pulmonary hemorrhage
Adult respiratory distress syndrome
Respiratory distress syndrome, neonatal
Cystic fibrosis
Bronchopulmonary dysplasia
Hypoplastic lungs
Meconium aspiration
Pulmonary thromboembolus
Interstitial fibrosis

UPPER AIRWAY DISEASE
Aspiration
Laryngospasm
Angioedema
Obstructive sleep apnea
Tonsillar hypertrophy
Vocal cord paralysis
Extrinsic tumor
Extrinsic or intrinsic hemangioma

MISCELLANEOUS
Flail chest
Cardiac arrest
Kyphoscoliosis
Decreased diaphragmatic movement due to ascites or peritoneal
  dialysis

respiratory center, reducing ventilatory drive. In addition, a variety of medications and illicit drugs suppress the respiratory center. The signals from the respiratory center need to be trans-mitted to the respiratory muscles via the nervous system. Respiratory muscle failure can be secondary to disruption of the signal from the central nervous system in the spinal cord, the phrenic nerve, or the neuromuscular junction. Disorders directly affecting the muscles of respiration can prevent adequate ventilation, causing a respiratory acidosis.

Mild or moderate lung disease often causes a respiratory alkalosis as a result of hyperventilation secondary to hypoxia or stimulation of lung mechanoreceptors or chemoreceptors. Only more severe lung disease causes a respiratory acidosis. Upper airway diseases, by impairing air entry into the lungs, may decrease ventilation, producing a respiratory acidosis.

Increased production of carbon dioxide is never the sole cause of a respiratory acidosis, but can increase the severity of the disease in a patient with decreased ventilation of carbon dioxide. Increased production of carbon dioxide occurs in patients with fevers, hyperthyroidism, excess caloric intake, and high levels of physical activity. Increased respiratory muscle work also increases carbon dioxide production.

Clinical Manifestations. Patients with a respiratory acidosis are often tachypneic in an effort to correct the inadequate ventilation. Exceptions include patients with a respiratory acidosis resulting from central nervous system depression and patients who are on the verge of complete respiratory failure secondary to fatigue of the respiratory muscles.

The symptoms of respiratory acidosis are related to the severity of the hypercarbia. Acute respiratory acidosis is usually more symptomatic than chronic respiratory acidosis. Symptoms are also increased by concurrent hypoxia or metabolic acidosis. In a patient breathing room air, hypoxia is always present if a respiratory acidosis is present. The potential central nervous system manifestations of respiratory acidosis include anxiety, dizziness, headache, confusion, asterixis, myoclonic jerks, hallucinations, psychosis, coma, and seizures.

Acidemia, no matter the etiology, affects the cardiovascular system. An arterial pH less than 7.20 impairs cardiac contractility and the normal response to catecholamines, both in the heart and the peripheral vasculature. Hypercapnia causes vasodilation, most dramatically in the cerebral vasculature, but hypercapnia produces vasoconstriction of the pulmonary circulation. Respiratory acidosis increases the risk of cardiac arrhythmias, especially in a child with underlying cardiac disease.

Diagnosis. The history and physical often point to a clear etiology. For the obtunded patient with poor respiratory effort, evaluation of the central nervous system is often indicated. This may include imaging studies (e.g., CT or MRI) and potentially a lumbar puncture. A toxicology screen for illicit drugs may also be appropriate. A response to naloxone is both diagnostic and therapeutic. In many of the diseases affecting the respiratory muscles, there is evidence of weakness in other muscles. Stridor is a clue that the child may have upper airway disease. Along with a physical examination, a chest radiograph is often helpful in diagnosing pulmonary disease.

In many patients, respiratory acidosis may be multifactorial. For example, a child with bronchopulmonary dysplasia, an intrinsic lung disease, may worsen due to respiratory muscle dysfunction from severe hypokalemia due to chronic diuretic therapy. Conversely, a child with muscular dystrophy, a muscle disease, may worsen because of an aspiration pneumonia.

For a patient with respiratory acidosis, calculation of the gradient between the alveolar oxygen concentration and the arterial oxygen concentration, the A-a gradient, is useful for distinguishing between poor respiratory effort and intrinsic lung disease. The A-a gradient is increased if the hypoxemia is due to intrinsic lung disease (see Chapters 356 and 357).

Treatment. Respiratory acidosis is best managed by treating the underlying etiology. In some instances, the response is very rapid, such as after the administration of naloxone to a patient with a narcotic overdose. In contrast, the child with pneumonia may require a number of days of antibiotic therapy before the respiratory status improves. In many children with a chronic respiratory acidosis, there is no curative therapy, although an acute respiratory illness superimposed on a chronic respiratory condition is usually reversible.

All patients with an acute respiratory acidosis are hypoxic and therefore need to receive supplemental oxygen. Mechanical ventilation is necessary in some children with a respiratory acidosis. Children with a significant respiratory acidosis due to a central nervous system disease usually require mechanical ventilation because these disorders are unlikely to respond quickly to therapy. In addition, hypercarbia causes cerebral vasodilation, and the increase in intracranial pressure can be dangerous in a child with an underlying central nervous system disease. Readily reversible central nervous system depression, such as from a narcotic overdose, may not require mechanical ventilation. Decisions on mechanical ventilation for other patients depend on a number of factors. Patients with severe hypercarbia—P_{CO_2} greater than 75—usually require mechanical ventilation (see Chapters 57.3, 57.4, and 359). The threshold for intubation is lower if there is concomitant metabolic acidosis, a slowly responsive underlying disease, hypoxia that responds poorly to oxygen, or if the patient appears to be tiring and respiratory arrest seems likely.

In patients with a chronic respiratory acidosis, the respiratory drive is often less responsive to hypercarbia and more responsive to hypoxia. Hence, with chronic respiratory acidosis, excessive use of oxygen can blunt the respiratory drive and, therefore, increase the P_{CO_2}. In these patients, oxygen must be used cautiously.

When possible, it is best to avoid mechanical ventilation in a patient with a chronic respiratory acidosis because extubation is often difficult. However, an acute illness may necessitate mechanical ventilation in a child with a chronic respiratory acidosis. When intubation is necessary, the P_{CO_2} should only be lowered to the patient's normal baseline, which should be done gradually. These patients normally have an elevated serum bicarbonate level as a result of metabolic compensation for their respiratory acidosis. A rapid lowering of the P_{CO_2} can cause a severe metabolic alkalosis, potentially leading to complications, including cardiac arrhythmias, decreased cardiac output, and decreased cerebral blood flow. In addition, prolonged mechanical ventilation at a normal P_{CO_2} causes the metabolic compensation to resolve. When the patient is subsequently extubated, the patient will no longer benefit from metabolic compensation, causing a more severe acidemia due to the respiratory acidosis.

Respiratory Alkalosis

A respiratory alkalosis is an inappropriate reduction in the blood carbon dioxide concentration. This is usually secondary to hyperventilation, initially causing removal of carbon dioxide to surpass production. Eventually, a new steady state is achieved, with removal equaling production, albeit at a lower carbon dioxide tension (P_{CO_2}). A respiratory alkalosis not due to hyperventilation may occur in children receiving extracorporeal membrane oxygenation (ECMO) or hemodialysis, with carbon dioxide lost directly from the blood in the extracorporeal circuit.

With a simple respiratory alkalosis, the pH increases, but there is a normal metabolic response that attenuates some of the change in the blood pH. A metabolic response to an acute respiratory alkalosis occurs within minutes, mediated by hydrogen ion release from non-bicarbonate buffers. The metabolic response to an acute respiratory alkalosis is predictable: Plasma bicarbonate falls by 2 for each 10 mm Hg decrease in the P_{CO_2} (acute compensation).

A chronic respiratory alkalosis leads to more significant metabolic compensation due to the actions of the kidneys, which decrease acid secretion, producing a decrease in the serum bicarbonate concentration. Both the proximal tubule and distal tubule decrease acid secretion. Metabolic compensation for a respiratory alkalosis develops gradually and takes 2–3 days to produce the full effect: Plasma bicarbonate falls by 4 for each 10 mm Hg decrease in the P_{CO_2} (chronic compensation).

A chronic respiratory alkalosis is the only acid-base disturbance wherein appropriate compensation may normalize the pH, albeit above 7.40.

A mixed disorder is present if the metabolic compensation is inappropriate. A higher than expected bicarbonate occurs in the setting of a concurrent metabolic alkalosis and a lower than expected bicarbonate occurs in the setting of a concurrent metabolic acidosis. Evaluating whether compensation is appropriate during a respiratory alkalosis requires clinical knowledge of the acuity of the process, because the expected compensation is different depending on whether the process is acute or chronic.

A low P_{CO_2} does not always indicate a respiratory alkalosis. The P_{CO_2} also decreases as part of the appropriate respiratory compensation for a metabolic acidosis; this is not a respiratory alkalosis. A metabolic acidosis is the dominant acid-base disturbance in a patient with acidemia and a low P_{CO_2}, even though there could still be a concurrent respiratory alkalosis. In contrast, a respiratory alkalosis is always present in a patient with alkalemia and a low P_{CO_2}. Even a normal PCO_2 may be consistent with a respiratory alkalosis in a patient with a metabolic alkalosis because an elevated P_{CO_2} is expected as part of appropriate respiratory compensation for the metabolic alkalosis.

Etiology and Pathophysiology. A variety of stimuli can increase the ventilatory drive and cause a respiratory alkalosis (Box 45–15). Arterial hypoxemia or tissue hypoxia stimulates peripheral chemoreceptors to signal the central respiratory center in the medulla to increase ventilation. The resultant increased respiratory effort increases the oxygen content of the blood, but depresses the P_{CO_2}. The effect of hypoxemia on ventilation begins when the oxygen saturation decreases to about 90% (P_{O_2} = 60 mm Hg), and the hyperventilation increases as hypoxemia worsens. Acute hypoxia is a more potent stimulus for hyperventilation than chronic hypoxia and thus chronic hypoxia, as occurs in cyanotic heart disease, causes a much less severe respiratory alkalosis than an equivalent degree of acute hypoxia. There are many causes of hypoxemia or tissue hypoxia, including primary lung disease, severe anemia, and carbon monoxide poisoning.

The lungs contain chemoreceptors and mechanoreceptors that respond to irritants and stretching, and send signals to the respiratory center to increase ventilation. For example, aspiration or pneumonia may stimulate the chemoreceptors while pulmonary edema may stimulate the mechanoreceptors. Most of the diseases that activate these receptors may also cause hypoxemia and can, therefore, potentially lead to hyperventilation via two mechanisms. Whereas patients with primary lung disease may initially have a respiratory alkalosis, worsening of the disease, combined with respiratory muscle fatigue, often causes respiratory failure and the development of a respiratory acidosis.

Hyperventilation in the absence of lung disease occurs with direct stimulation of the central respiratory center. This occurs with central nervous system diseases such as meningitis, hemorrhage, and trauma. Central hyperventilation due to lesions, such as infarcts or tumors near the central respiratory center in the midbrain, increases the rate and depth of the respiratory effort. This respiratory pattern portends a poor prognosis because these midbrain lesions are frequently fatal. Systemic processes may cause centrally mediated hyperventilation.

BOX 45–15. Causes of Respiratory Alkalosis

HYPOXEMIA OR TISSUE HYPOXIA
Pneumonia
Pulmonary edema
Cyanotic heart disease
Congestive heart failure
Asthma
Severe anemia
High altitude
Laryngospasm
Aspiration
Carbon monoxide poisoning
Pulmonary embolism
Interstitial lung disease
Hypotension

LUNG RECEPTOR STIMULATION
Pneumonia
Pulmonary edema
Asthma
Pulmonary embolism
Hemothorax
Pneumothorax
Respiratory distress syndrome (adult or infant)

CENTRAL STIMULATION
Central nervous system disease
   Subarachnoid hemorrhage
   Encephalitis or meningitis
   Trauma
   Brain tumor
   Stroke
Fever
Pain
Anxiety
Psychogenic hyperventilation or anxiety
Liver failure
Sepsis
Pregnancy
Medications
   Salicylate intoxication
   Theophylline
   Progesterone
   Exogenous catecholamines
   Caffeine
Mechanical ventilation
Extracorporeal membrane oxygenation or hemodialysis

Although the exact mechanisms are not clear, liver disease causes a respiratory alkalosis that is usually proportional to the degree of liver failure. Pregnancy causes a chronic respiratory alkalosis, probably mediated by progesterone acting on the respiratory centers. Salicylates, although often causing a concurrent metabolic acidosis, directly stimulate the respiratory center to produce a respiratory alkalosis. The respiratory alkalosis during sepsis is probably due to cytokine release.

Hyperventilation may be secondary to an underlying disease that causes pain, stress, or anxiety. In psychogenic hyperventilation, there is no disease process accounting for the hyperventilation. This may occur in a child who has had an emotionally stressful experience. Alternatively, it may be part of a panic disorder, especially if there are repeated episodes of hyperventilation. In these patients, the symptoms of acute alkalemia increase anxiety, potentially perpetuating the hyperventilation.

A respiratory alkalosis is quite common in children receiving mechanical ventilation because the respiratory center is not controlling ventilation. In addition, these children may have a decreased metabolic rate and hence less carbon dioxide production because of sedation and paralytic medications. Normally, decreased carbon dioxide production and resultant hypocapnia decreases ventilation, but this physiologic response cannot occur in a child who cannot reduce his ventilatory effort.

Clinical Manifestations. The disease process that is causing the respiratory alkalosis is usually more concerning than the clinical manifestations of the respiratory alkalosis. Chronic respiratory

alkalosis is usually asymptomatic since metabolic compensation decreases the magnitude of the alkalemia.

Acute respiratory alkalosis may cause chest tightness, palpitations, lightheadedness, circumoral numbness, and paresthesias of the extremities. Less common manifestations include tetany, seizures, muscle cramps, and syncope. The lightheadedness and syncope are probably due to the reduction in cerebral blood flow that is caused by hypocapnia. The reduction in cerebral blood flow is the rationale for using hyperventilation to treat children with increased intracranial pressure. The paresthesias, tetany, and seizures may be partially related to the reduction in ionized calcium that occurs because alkalemia causes more calcium to bind to albumin. A respiratory alkalosis also causes a mild reduction in the serum potassium level. Patients with psychogenic hyperventilation tend to be most symptomatic from their respiratory alkalosis, and these symptoms, along with a sensation of breathlessness, exacerbate the hyperventilation.

Diagnosis. In many patients, the hyperventilation producing a respiratory alkalosis is not clinically detectable, even with careful observation of the patient's respiratory effort. Metabolic compensation for a respiratory alkalosis causes a low serum bicarbonate concentration. When the hyperventilation is not appreciated and only serum electrolytes are evaluated, there is often a presumptive diagnosis of a metabolic acidosis. If a respiratory alkalosis is suspected, only a blood gas determination can make the diagnosis.

Hyperventilation does not always indicate a primary respiratory disorder. In some patients, the hyperventilation is appropriate respiratory compensation for a metabolic acidosis. With a primary metabolic acidosis, acidemia is present and the serum bicarbonate is usually quite low if there is clinically detectable hyperventilation. In contrast, the serum bicarbonate never goes below 17 mEq/L as part of the metabolic compensation for acute respiratory alkalosis and simple acute respiratory alkalosis causes alkalemia.

The etiology of a respiratory alkalosis is often apparent from the physical examination or history, such as lung disease, neurologic disease, or cyanotic heart disease. Hypoxemia is a common cause of hyperventilation, and it is important to diagnose because it suggests a significant underlying disease that requires expeditious treatment. Hypoxemia may be detected on physical examination (cyanosis) or by pulse oximetry. However, normal pulse oximetry does not completely eliminate hypoxemia as the etiology of the hyperventilation. There are two reasons why pulse oximetry is not adequate for eliminating hypoxemia as a cause of a respiratory alkalosis. First, pulse oximetry is not very sensitive at detecting a mildly low pO_2. Second, the hyperventilation during a respiratory alkalosis causes the pO_2 to increase, possibly increasing the pO_2 to a level that is not identified as abnormal by pulse oximetry. Only an arterial blood gas can completely eliminate hypoxia as an explanation for a respiratory alkalosis. Along with hypoxemia, it is important to consider processes that cause tissue hypoxia without necessarily causing hypoxemia. Examples include carbon monoxide poisoning, severe anemia, and congestive heart failure.

Lung disease without hypoxemia may cause hyperventilation. Although often apparent by history or physical examination, a chest radiograph may detect more subtle disease. Patients with a pulmonary embolism may have benign chest x-ray findings, normal pO_2, and isolated respiratory alkalosis, even though hypoxia may eventually occur. Diagnosis of a pulmonary embolism requires a high index of suspicion and should be considered in children without another explanation for respiratory alkalosis, especially if risk factors are present, such as prolonged bed rest or a hypercoagulable state (e.g., nephrotic syndrome or lupus anticoagulant).

Treatment. There is seldom a need for specific therapy of respiratory alkalosis. Rather, treatment focuses on the underlying disease. Mechanical ventilator settings are adjusted to correct iatrogenic respiratory alkalosis, unless the hyperventilation has a therapeutic purpose (e.g., treatment of increased intracranial pressure).

For patients with hyperventilation secondary to anxiety, efforts should be undertaken to reassure the child, usually enlisting the parents. Along with reassurance, patients with psychogenic hyperventilation may benefit from benzodiazepines. During an acute episode of psychogenic hyperventilation, rebreathing into a paper bag increases the patient's P_{CO_2}. Using a paper bag, instead of a plastic bag, allows adequate oxygenation, but permits the carbon dioxide concentration in the bag to increase. The resultant increase in the patient's P_{CO_2} decreases the symptoms of the respiratory alkalosis that tend to perpetuate the hyperventilation. Rebreathing should only be done once other causes of hyperventilation have been eliminated; pulse oximetry during the rebreathing is prudent.

Cadnapaphornchai MA, Schrier RW: Pathogenesis and management of hyponatremia. *Am J Med* 2000;109:688–92.

Khan N, Licata A, Rogers D: Intravenous bisphosphonate for hypercalcemia accompanying subcutaneous fat necrosis: A novel treatment approach. *Clin Pediatr (Phila)* 2001;40:217–9.

Manganaro R, Mami C, Marrone T, et al: Incidence of dehydration and hypernatremia in exclusively breast-fed infants. *J Pediatr* 2001;139:673–5.

Schoen EJ, Bhatia S, Ray GT, et al: Transient pseudohypoaldosteronism with hyponatremia-hyperkalemia in infant urinary tract infection. *J Urol* 2002;167:680–2.

Shimada T, Mizutani S, Muto T, et al: Cloning and characterization of fgf23 as a causative factor of tumor-induced osteomalacia. *Proc Natl Acad Sci U S A* 2001;98:6500–5.

Steiner M, Steiner B, Wilhelm S, et al: Severe hypophosphatemia during hematopoietic reconstitution after allogenic peripheral blood stem cell transplantation. *Bone Marrow Transplant* 2000;25:1015–6.

Subramanian R, Khardori R: Severe hypophosphatemia. Pathophysiologic implications, clinical presentations, and treatment. *Medicine (Baltimore)* 2000;79:1–8.

Sullivan JE, Berman BW: The pediatric forum: Hypermagnesemia with lethargy and hypotonia due to administration of magnesium hydroxide to a 4-week-old infant. *Arch Pediatr Adolesc Med* 2000;154:1272–4.

Walton DM, Thomas DC, Aly HZ, et al: Morbid hypocalcemia associated with phosphate enema in a six-week-old infant. *Pediatrics* 2000;106:E37.

Zelikovic I: Molecular pathophysiology of tubular transport disorders. *Pediatr Nephrol* 2001;16:19–35.

Chapter 46
Maintenance and Replacement Therapy

Maintenance intravenous fluids are used in a child who cannot be fed enterally. Along with maintenance fluids, children may require concurrent *replacement fluids* if they have excessive losses such as may occur with drainage from a nasogastric (NG) tube or high urine output due to nephrogenic diabetes insipidus. In addition, if dehydration is present, the patient needs to receive *deficit* therapy. A child awaiting surgery may only need maintenance fluids, whereas a child with diarrheal dehydration needs maintenance and deficit therapy and may also require replacement fluids if the diarrhea continues. This chapter reviews the principles of maintenance therapy and replacement fluids. Chapter 47 discusses dehydration and the administration of deficit therapy.

Maintenance Therapy. Children normally have large variations in their daily intake of water and electrolytes. The only exceptions are patients who receive fixed dietary regimens orally, via gastric tube, or as intravenous total parenteral nutrition. Healthy children can tolerate significant variations in intake because of the many homeostatic mechanisms that can adjust absorption

and excretion of water and electrolytes (see Chapter 45). The calculated water and electrolyte needs that form the basis of maintenance therapy are not absolute requirements. Rather, these calculations provide reasonable guidelines for intravenous therapy. Children do not need to be placed on intravenous fluids simply because their intake is being monitored in a hospital and they are not taking "maintenance fluids" orally, unless there is a pathologic process present that necessitates high fluid intake (e.g., sickle cell crisis).

Maintenance fluids are most commonly necessary in preoperative and postoperative surgical patients. But, many nonsurgical patients also require maintenance fluids. It is important to recognize when it is necessary to begin maintenance fluids. A normal teenager who is given nothing by mouth (NPO) overnight for a morning procedure does not require maintenance fluids because a healthy, older patient can easily tolerate 12 or 18 hours without oral intake. In contrast, a 6-mo-old waiting for a tetralogy of Fallot repair should begin receiving intravenous fluids within 4–6 hr of his last feeding. Infants become dehydrated faster than older patients. This is especially important in a patient with tetralogy of Fallot because even mild dehydration may precipitate a cyanotic spell. More dramatically, a child with obligatory high urine output from nephrogenic diabetes insipidus should begin receiving intravenous fluids soon after being made NPO.

Maintenance fluids are generally composed of a solution of water, glucose, sodium, and potassium. This solution has the advantages of simplicity, long shelf life, low cost, and compatibility with peripheral intravenous administration. Such a solution accomplishes the major objectives of maintenance fluids (Box 46–1). Patients lose water, sodium, and potassium in their urine and stool; water is also lost from the skin and lungs. Maintenance fluids replace these losses and therefore avoid the development of dehydration and deficiencies of sodium or potassium.

The glucose in maintenance fluids provides approximately 20% of the normal caloric needs of the patient. This is enough to prevent the development of starvation ketoacidosis and diminishes the protein degradation that would occur if the patient received no calories.

The goals of maintenance fluid therapy are relatively modest. Maintenance fluids do not provide adequate calories, protein, fat, minerals, or vitamins. This is typically not problematic for a patient receiving intravenous fluids for a few days. But, it is important to remember that a patient on maintenance intravenous fluids is receiving inadequate calories and will actually lose 0.5–1% of weight each day. Thus, it is imperative that patients not remain on maintenance therapy indefinitely; total parental nutrition should be used for children who cannot be fed enterally for more than a few days. This is especially important in a patient with underlying malnutrition.

Prototypical maintenance fluid therapy does not provide electrolytes such as calcium, phosphorous, magnesium, or bicarbonate. For most patients, this is not problematic for a few days. Nevertheless, there are patients who will not tolerate this omission, usually because of excessive losses. For example a child with renal tubular acidosis wastes bicarbonate in urine. Such a patient will rapidly become acidemic unless bicarbonate is added to the maintenance fluids. It is important to remember the limitations of maintenance fluid therapy.

BOX 46–1. Goals of Maintenance Fluids

Prevent dehydration
Prevent electrolyte disorders
Prevent ketoacidosis
Prevent protein degradation

Maintenance Water. Water is a crucial component of maintenance fluid therapy. This is because of the obligatory water losses that occur during the day. These losses are both measurable (urine and stool) and not measurable (insensible losses from the skin and lungs). Failure to replace these losses leads to having a thirsty, uncomfortable child and, ultimately, a dehydrated child.

The goal of maintenance water is to provide enough water to replace these obligatory losses. Urinary losses are approximately 60% of the total. However, the normal kidney has the ability to markedly modify water losses, with daily urine volume potentially varying by more than a factor of 20. Maintenance water is designed to provide enough water so that the kidney does not need to significantly dilute or concentrate the urine. This also provides a nice cushion so that normal homeostatic mechanisms can adjust urinary water losses to keep the patient euvolemic. This adaptability obviates the need for absolute precision in determining water requirements. This is important given the absence of absolute accuracy in the formulas for calculation of water needs. Table 46–1 provides a system for calculating maintenance water based on the patient's weight. This system emphasizes the high water needs of smaller patients. This approach is quite reliable, although calculations based on weight do overestimate the water needs of overweight patients. It is also important to remember that there is an upper limit of 2–2.5 L/24 hr in adult-sized patients. Intravenous fluids are written as an hourly rate. It is therefore often helpful to use the formulas in Box 46–2 to quickly calculate the rate of maintenance fluids.

Maintenance Electrolytes. Sodium, potassium, and chloride are given in maintenance fluids to replace losses from urine and stool. Whereas most patients can adjust their rate of loss, maintenance electrolytes are designed not to stress the body's homeostatic mechanisms and to minimize the development of electrolyte imbalances. Maintenance requirements for sodium and potassium are shown in Box 46–3. Adequate chloride is provided as long as at least half of the sodium and potassium are given as chloride salts.

Glucose. Maintenance fluids usually contain 5% dextrose (D5), which provides 17 calories per 100 mL and close to 20% of the daily caloric needs. This is enough to prevent ketone production and helps minimize protein degradation. It is a diet, and a child will lose weight on this regimen. This is the principal reason why a patient needs to be started on total parental nutrition after a few days of maintenance fluids if enteral feedings are still not possible. Maintenance fluids are also lacking in such crucial nutrients as protein, fat, vitamins, and minerals.

Intravenous Solutions. In designing fluid management, it is important to know the components of the commonly available solutions (Table 46–2). Normal saline (NS) and Ringer lactate are isotonic solutions; they have approximately the same tonicity as plasma. Isotonic fluids are generally used for the acute correction of intravascular volume depletion (see Chapter 47). Half NS and 1/4 NS are the usual choices for maintenance fluid therapy in children. These solutions are available with 5% dextrose. In addition, these solutions are available with 20 mEq/L of potassium chloride, 10 mEq/L of potassium chloride, or no potassium. These are the commercially available solutions. A hospital pharmacy can prepare custom-made solutions with different concentrations of glucose, sodium, or potassium. In addition, other electrolytes such as calcium, magnesium, phosphate, acetate, and bicarbonate can be added to intravenous solutions. Custom-made solutions take time to prepare and are much more expensive than commercial solutions. The use of custom made solutions is only necessary for patients who have underlying disorders that cause significant electrolyte imbalances. The use of premade solution saves both time and expense.

A normal plasma osmolality is 285–295 mOsm/kg. Infusing an intravenous solution peripherally with a much lower osmolality can cause water to move into red blood cells, causing hemolysis. Thus, intravenous fluids are generally designed to have an osmolality that is either close to 285 or greater (moderately higher osmolality fluids do not cause problems). Thus, $1/4$ NS (osmolality = 77) should not be administered peripherally, but D5 $1/4$ NS (osmolality = 355) or D5 $1/2$ NS + 20 mEq/L KCl (osmolality = 472) can be administered.

Selection of Maintenance Fluids. After calculation of water needs and electrolyte needs, children typically receive either D5 $1/4$ NS + 20 mEq/L KCl or D5 $1/2$ NS + 20 mEq/L KCl. Children weighing less than about 20–25 kg do best with the solution containing 1/4 NS because of their high water needs per kilogram. In contrast, larger children and adults may receive the solution with $1/2$ NS. These guidelines assume that there is no disease process present that would require an adjustment in either the volume or electrolyte composition of maintenance fluids (e.g., children with renal insufficiency may not tolerate 20 mEq/L of potassium). These solutions work well in children who have normal homeostatic mechanisms for adjusting urinary excretion of water, sodium, and potassium. In children with complicated pathophysiologic derangements, it may be necessary to empirically adjust the electrolyte composition and rate of maintenance fluids based on electrolyte measurements and assessment of fluid balance.

Variations in Maintenance Water. The calculation of maintenance water is based on standard assumptions regarding water losses. There are patients, however, for whom these assumptions are incorrect. In order to identify such situations, it is helpful to understand the source and magnitude of normal water losses. Box 46–4 lists the three sources of normal water loss: the com-

---

TABLE 46–1. Body Weight Method for Calculating Maintenance Fluid Volume

Body Weight	Fluid per Day
0–10 kg	100 mL/kg
11–20 kg	1,000 mL + 50 mL/kg for each kg > 10 kg
> 20 kg	1,500 mL + 20 mL/kg for each kg > 10 kg*

*The maximum total fluid per day is normally 2,400 mL.

BOX 46–2. Maintenance Water Rate

0–10 kg: 4 mL/kg/hr
10–20 kg: 40 mL/hr + 2 mL/kg/hr × (wt-10 kg)
>20 kg: 60 mL/hr + 1 mL/kg/hr × (wt-20 kg)*

---

*The maximum fluid rate is normally 100 mL/hr.

BOX 46–3. Maintenance Electrolytes

Sodium: 2–3 mEq/kg/24 hr
Potassium: 1–2 mEq/kg/24 hr

TABLE 46–2. Composition of Intravenous Solutions

Fluid	[Na⁺]	[Cl⁻]	[K⁺]	[Ca²⁺]	[Lactate⁻]
Normal saline (0.9% NaCl)	154	154			
½ Normal saline (0.45% NaCl)	77	77			
¼ Normal saline (0.225% NaCl)	38.5	38.5			
Ringer lactate	130	109	4	3	28

ponents of maintenance water. Urine is the most important contributor to normal water loss. Insensible losses represent approximately one third of total maintenance water. Insensible losses are composed of evaporative losses from the skin and the lungs. These losses cannot be quantitated. The evaporative losses from the skin do not include sweat, which should be considered an additional source of water loss. Stool normally represents a minor source of water loss.

Maintenance water needs may be increased or decreased, depending on the clinical situation. This may be obvious in the case of the infant with profuse diarrhea or subtle in the case of the patient who has decreased insensible losses while in a mist tent. It is helpful to consider the sources of normal water loss and determine whether any of these sources is being modified in a specific patient. It is then necessary to adjust maintenance water and electrolyte calculations.

Table 46–3 lists a variety of clinical situations that modify normal maintenance water losses. The skin can be the source of very significant water loss. This is commonly seen in neonates, especially premature infants, who are under radiant warmers or who are receiving phototherapy. Premature infants can have insensible losses of 100–200 mL/kg/24 hr. Burns can result in massive losses of water and electrolytes and there are specific guidelines for fluid management in children with burns (see Chapter 62). Sweat losses of water and electrolytes, especially in a warm climate, can also be significant. Children with cystic fibrosis have increased sodium losses from the skin. Some children with pseudohypoaldosteronism also have increased cutaneous salt losses.

Fever increases evaporative losses from the skin. These losses are somewhat predictable, leading to a 10–15% increase in maintenance water needs for each 1°C increase in temperature above 38°C. These guidelines are for a patient with a persistent fever; a 1-hr fever spike does not cause an appreciable increase in water needs.

Tachypnea or a tracheostomy increases evaporative losses from the lungs. A humidified ventilator causes a decrease in insensible losses from the lungs and can even lead to water absorption via the lungs. Thus, a ventilated patient has a decrease in maintenance water requirements. A mist tent decreases evaporative losses from both the skin and the lungs. Unfortunately, in all of these situations, it is difficult to quantify the changes that take place in the individual patient.

Replacement Fluids. The gastrointestinal (GI) tract is potentially a source of considerable water loss. GI water losses are accompanied by electrolytes and thus may cause disturbances in hydration and electrolyte concentrations. GI losses are often associated with loss of potassium, leading to hypokalemia. Because of the high bicarbonate concentration in stool, children with diarrhea usually develop a metabolic acidosis, which may be accentuated if volume depletion causes hypoperfusion and a concurrent lactic acidosis. In contrast, emesis or losses from an NG tube cause a metabolic alkalosis.

The general strategy for responding to GI losses is the same for all situations. GI losses of water and electrolytes are usually quite small. Therefore, all GI losses are considered excessive and the increase in the water requirement is equal to the volume of fluid losses. Because GI losses can be precisely measured, it is possible to add the GI losses to the calculated maintenance water to determine the adjusted water requirement. The added electrolyte requirements are equal to the GI electrolyte losses. GI losses are best managed by using an appropriate replacement solution.

It is impossible to predict the losses for the next 24 hr. Thus, it is better to replace excessive GI losses as they happen. The child should receive an appropriate maintenance fluid that does not consider the GI losses. The losses should then be replaced as they occur using a solution with the same approximate electrolyte concentration as the GI fluid. The losses are usually replaced every 1–6 hr depending on the rate of loss, with very rapid losses being replaced more frequently. For example, 200 mL of NG output accumulates over 4 hr. The patient is given 200 mL of replacement solution at a rate of 50 mL/24 hr over the next 4 hr. Any NG output from the 4 hr when the patient is receiving the 200 mL is given over the subsequent 4 hr. If the NG losses increase, it may be necessary to provide the replacement solution more frequently, such as every 1–2 hr, in order to avoid dehydration.

Diarrhea is a common cause of fluid loss in children. It can cause dehydration and electrolyte disorders. In the patient with significant diarrhea and a limited ability to take oral fluid, it is important to have a plan for replacing excessive stool losses. The volume of stool should be measured and an equal volume of replacement solution should be given. The electrolyte composition of a replacement solution is always best determined by measuring the electrolyte content of the fluid that is being replaced. There is, however, data on the average electrolyte composition of diarrhea in children (Box 46–5). Using this information, it is possible to design an appropriate replacement solution. The solution shown in Box 46–5 replaces stool losses of sodium, potassium, chloride, and bicarbonate. Each milliliter of stool should be replaced by 1 mL of this solution. The average electrolyte composition of diarrhea is just an average, and there may be considerable variation. It is therefore advisable to consider measuring the electrolyte composition of a patient's diarrhea, particularly if the amount of diarrhea is especially excessive or the patient's serum electrolytes are problematic.

Loss of gastric fluid, either via emesis or NG suction, is also likely to cause dehydration in that most such patients have impaired oral intake of fluids. Electrolyte disturbances, particularly hypokalemia and metabolic alkalosis, are also common. These

TABLE 46–3. Adjustments in Maintenance Water

Source	Causes of Increased Water Needs	Causes of Decreased Water Needs
Skin	Radiant warmer Fever Sweat Burns	Mist tent
Lungs	Tachypnea Tracheostomy	Humidified ventilator Mist tent
Gastrointestinal tract	Diarrhea Emesis Nasogastric suction	
Renal	Polyuria	Oliguria/anuria
Miscellaneous	Surgical drain Third spacing	Hypothyroidism

complications can be avoided by judicious use of a replacement solution. The electrolyte composition of gastric fluid is variable, with significant fluctuation during the course of the day. Moreover, H_2-receptor antagonists and hydrogen pump inhibitors alter gastric electrolytes. The composition of gastric fluid shown in Box 46–6 serves as a useful starting point for designing a replacement solution. Again, direct measurement of gastric electrolytes provides the most precise approach.

Patients with gastric losses frequently develop hypokalemia, although the potassium concentration of gastric fluid is relatively low. The associated urinary loss of potassium is an important cause of hypokalemia in this situation (see Chapter 45). These patients may need additional potassium either in their maintenance fluids or in their replacement fluids to compensate for prior or ongoing urinary losses. Proper hydration of the patient, by decreasing aldosterone synthesis, lessens the urinary potassium losses.

Urine output is normally the largest cause of water loss. Diseases such as renal failure and the syndrome of inappropriate antidiuretic hormone can lead to a decrease in urine volume. The patient with oliguria or anuria has a decreased need for water and electrolytes; continuation of maintenance fluids produces fluid overload. In contrast, other conditions produce an increase in urine volume. Postobstructive diuresis, the polyuric phase of acute tubular necrosis, diabetes mellitus, and diabetes insipidus are examples. The patient must receive more than standard maintenance fluids when the urine output is excessive, else the patient will become dehydrated. The electrolyte losses in patients with polyuria are variable. In diabetes insipidus, the urine electrolyte concentration is usually low, whereas children with diseases such as juvenile nephronophthisis or obstructive uropathy usually have increased losses of both water and sodium.

The approach to decreased or increased urine output is similar (Box 46–7). The patient receives a maintenance fluid that replaces insensible losses. This is accomplished by running this fluid at one third of the normal maintenance rate. Replacing insensible losses in the anuric child will theoretically maintain an even fluid balance, with the caveat that one third of maintenance fluids is an estimate of insensible losses. In the individual patient, this rate may need to be adjusted based on monitoring of the patient's weight and hydration status. Most children with renal insufficiency receive little or no potassium because the kidneys are the principal site for potassium excretion.

For the oliguric child it is important to add a urine replacement solution to prevent dehydration. This is especially important in the patient with acute renal failure because output may slowly increase, which could lead to dehydration and a worsening of renal failure if the patient is left on insensible fluids. A replacement solution of $1/2$ NS is usually appropriate initially, although its composition may need to be adjusted if urine output increases significantly.

The child with polyuria should also be placed on insensible fluids plus urine replacement. This avoids trying to calculate the volume of urine output that is "normal" so that the patient can be given replacement fluid for the excess. In these patients, the urine output is by definition excessive, and it is important to

measure the sodium and potassium concentration of the urine to help in formulating the urine replacement solution.

Surgical drains and chest tubes can produce measurable fluid output. These losses should be replaced when they are significant. They can be measured and replaced with an appropriate replacement solution as they occur. Third space losses are due to a shift of fluid from the intravascular space into the interstitial space. These losses cannot be easily quantitated. Nonetheless, third space losses can be massive and lead to intravascular volume depletion, despite the patient's weight gain and edema. Replacement of third space fluid is empirical but should be anticipated in patients who are at risk, such as children who have had abdominal surgery. Third space losses and chest tube output are isotonic and, thus, usually require replacement with an isotonic fluid such as normal saline or Ringer lactate. Adjustments in the amount of replacement fluid for third space losses are based on continuing assessment of the patient's intravascular volume status. Protein losses from chest tube drainage can be significant, occasionally necessitating that 5% albumin be used as a replacement solution.

Chapter 47
Deficit Therapy

Dehydration, frequently the result of diarrhea, is a common problem in children. Most cases can be managed with oral rehydration, which is discussed in Chapter 48. This chapter focuses on the child who requires intravenous therapy, even though many of the same principles are used in oral rehydration.

Clinical Manifestations. The first step in caring for the child with dehydration is to assess the degree of dehydration. This dictates both the urgency of the situation and the volume of fluid needed for rehydration. Box 47–1 summarizes the clinical features that are present with varying degrees of dehydration.

BOX 46–6. Adjusting Fluid Therapy for Emesis or Nasogastric Losses

AVERAGE COMPOSITION OF GASTRIC FLUID
Sodium: 60 mEq/L
Potassium: 10 mEq/L
Chloride: 90 mEq/L

APPROACH TO REPLACEMENT OF ONGOING LOSSES
Solution: D5 1/2 NS + 10 mEq/L KCl
Replace output mL/mL every 1–6 hr

BOX 46–7. Adjusting Fluid Therapy for Altered Renal Output

OLIGURIA/ANURIA
Place the patient on insensible fluids (1/3 maintenance)
Replace urine output mL/mL with 1/2 NS

POLYURIA
Place the patient on insensible fluids (1/3 maintenance)
Measure urine electrolytes
Replace urine output mL/mL with a solution that is based on the measured urine electrolytes

---

BOX 47–1. Clinical Evaluation of Dehydration

Mild dehydration (3–5%): normal or increased pulse, decreased urine output, thirsty, normal physical examination
Moderate dehydration (7–10%): tachycardia, little or no urine output, irritable/lethargic, sunken eyes and fontanel, decreased tears, dry mucous membranes, mild tenting of the skin, delayed capillary refill, cool and pale
Severe dehydration (10–15%): rapid and weak pulse, decreased blood pressure, no urine output, very sunken eyes and fontanel, no tears, parched mucous membranes, tenting of the skin, very delayed capillary refill, cold and mottled

The infant with mild dehydration has few clinical signs or symptoms. The infant may be thirsty; the alert parent may notice a decline in urine output. The history is most helpful; there is a narrative describing fluid loss. Such an infant is considered 5% dehydrated. The infant with moderate dehydration has clear physical signs and symptoms. The intravascular space is depleted as evidenced by an increased heart rate and limited urine output. This patient is about 10% dehydrated and needs fairly prompt intervention. The infant with severe dehydration is gravely ill. The decrease in blood pressure indicates that vital organs may be receiving inadequate perfusion. Immediate and aggressive intervention is necessary. This child is approximately 15% dehydrated. If possible, the child with severe dehydration should receive intravenous therapy. For older children and adults, mild, moderate, and severe dehydration represent 3%, 6%, and 9%, respectively, of body weight lost. This difference is because water is a higher percentage of body weight in infants (see Chapter 45). For all patients, clinical assessment of dehydration is only an estimate, and thus the patient must be continually re-evaluated during therapy. Moreover, the degree of dehydration tends to be underestimated in hypernatremic dehydration because the movement of water from the intracellular space to the extracellular space helps to preserve the intravascular volume. The opposite occurs with hyponatremic dehydration; dangerous intravascular volume depletion can occur with less severe fluid deficits.

The history usually points to the etiology of the dehydration and may predict whether the patient will have a normal sodium concentration (isotonic dehydration), hyponatremic dehydration, or hypernatremic dehydration. The neonate with dehydration due to poor intake of breast milk often has hypernatremic dehydration. Hypernatremic dehydration is likely in any child with losses of hypotonic fluid and poor water intake such as may occur with diarrhea and poor oral intake due to anorexia or emesis. In contrast, hyponatremic dehydration occurs in the child with diarrhea who is taking in large quantities of low salt fluid such as water or diluted formula.

Some children with dehydration are appropriately thirsty, but in others the lack of intake is part of the pathophysiology of the dehydration. Similarly, even though decreased urine output is present in most children with dehydration, good urine output may be deceptively present if a child has an underlying renal defect such as diabetes insipidus or a salt-wasting nephropathy, or in infants with hypernatremic dehydration.

Physical examination findings are usually proportional to the degree of dehydration. Parents may be helpful when assessing the child for the presence of sunken eyes because this finding may be subtle. Pinching and gently twisting the skin of the abdominal or thoracic wall detects tenting of the skin. Tented skin remains in a pinched position rather than springing quickly back to normal. It is difficult to properly assess tenting of the skin in premature infants or severely malnourished children. Activation of the sympathetic nervous system causes tachycardia in children with intravascular volume depletion; diaphoresis may also be present. Postural changes in blood pressure are often helpful for evaluating and assessing the response to therapy in children with dehydration. Tachypnea in children with dehydration may be present secondary to a metabolic acidosis from stool losses of bicarbonate or due to lactic acidosis from poor tissue perfusion.

Laboratory Findings. A variety of laboratory findings are useful for evaluating the child with dehydration. The serum sodium concentration determines the type of dehydration. Metabolic acidosis may be due to stool bicarbonate losses in children with diarrhea, secondary renal insufficiency, or lactic acidosis from decreased tissue perfusion. The anion gap is useful for differentiating among the various causes of a metabolic acidosis (see Chapter 45). In contrast, emesis or nasogastric losses usually cause a metabolic alkalosis. The serum potassium concentration may be low as a result of diarrheal losses. In children with dehydration due to emesis, the combination of gastric potassium losses, metabolic alkalosis, and urinary potassium losses all contribute to hypokalemia. In contrast, metabolic acidosis, which causes a shift of potassium into cells, and renal insufficiency may lead to hyperkalemia. There is often a combination of mechanisms present and thus it may be difficult to predict the child's acid-base status or serum potassium by the history alone.

Blood urea nitrogen (BUN) and serum creatinine concentration are useful in assessing the child with dehydration. Volume depletion without renal insufficiency may cause a disproportionate increase in the BUN with little or no change in the creatinine concentration. This is secondary to increased passive reabsorption of urea in the proximal tubule due to appropriate renal conservation of sodium and water. This increase in the BUN with moderate or severe dehydration may be absent or blunted in the child with poor protein intake in that urea production is dependent on protein degradation. Conversely, the BUN may be disproportionally increased in the child with increased urea production, as occurs in the child with a gastrointestinal bleed or the child who is receiving glucocorticoids, which increase catabolism. A significant elevation of the creatinine concentration suggests renal insufficiency, although a false elevation in the creatinine can occur in the presence of ketoacidosis. Acute tubular necrosis due to volume depletion is the most common etiology of renal insufficiency in a child with volume depletion, but occasionally the child may have previously undetected chronic renal insufficiency or an alternative explanation for the acute renal failure. For example, renal vein thrombosis is a well-described sequelae of severe dehydration in infants; possible findings include thrombocytopenia and hematuria (see Chapter 512.3). The baseline normal creatinine concentration increases with age (see Fig. 500–6) and thus a normal adult creatinine concentration of 1 mg/dL may indicate significant renal insufficiency in an infant. The BUN and creatinine concentration are dependent on the timing of the disease process. Urea and creatinine are waste products that build up gradually with decreased renal excretion. A child with acute, severe dehydration may have only a minimal elevation of the serum creatinine concentration despite marked renal insufficiency; the creatinine concentration will increase over time.

Urinalysis is most helpful in the measurement of urine specific gravity, which is usually elevated in cases of significant dehydration but returns to normal after rehydration. Although infants have a reduced ability to concentrate the urine, even those who are a few weeks of age can show a clear elevation in specific gravity with significant dehydration. A specific gravity less than 1.020 indicates mild or no dehydration or indicates a urinary concentrating defect, as in chronic renal disease or primary or secondary diabetes insipidus. With dehydration, urinalysis may show hyaline and granular casts, a few white cells and red cells, and 30–100 mg/dL of proteinuria. These findings are not usually associated with significant renal pathology, and they remit with therapy.

Hemoconcentration causes an increase in the hematocrit, hemoglobin, and serum proteins in dehydration. These values normalize with rehydration. A normal hemoglobin concentration during acute dehydration may mask an underlying anemia. A decreased albumin in a dehydrated patient suggests a chronic disease, such as malnutrition, nephrotic syndrome, or liver disease, or an acute process, such as capillary leak. An acute or chronic protein-losing enteropathy may also cause a low serum albumin concentration.

Calculation of Deficits. The child with dehydration has lost water; there is almost always a concurrent loss of sodium and potassium. Most patients have isotonic dehydration and therefore have normal serum sodium values. The guidelines in Box 47–2 are used for calculating the deficits in isotonic dehydration due to gastroenteritis.

The water deficit is the percent dehydration multiplied by the patient's weight. The sodium and potassium deficits are derived from the water deficit (see Box 47–2).

Approach to Dehydration. The child with dehydration requires acute intervention to ensure that there is adequate tissue perfusion. This requires restoration of the intravascular volume with an isotonic solution such as normal saline (NS) or Ringer lactate. The child is given a fluid bolus, usually 20 mL/kg, over about 20 min. The child with mild dehydration does not usually require a fluid bolus. In contrast, the child with severe dehydration may require multiple fluid boluses and may need to receive the boluses at a faster rate.

Blood, 5% albumin, and plasma are occasionally used for fluid boluses. In general, however, normal saline is satisfactory, with both less infectious risk and lower cost. Blood transfusion is indicated in the child with significant anemia or blood loss. Plasma is useful for children with a coagulopathy. The child with hypoalbuminemia may benefit from 5% albumin, although there is evidence that albumin infusions increase mortality in adults.

The initial rehydration is complete when the child has an adequate intravascular volume. Typically, the child will have some general clinical improvement, including a lower heart rate, a normalization of the blood pressure, improved perfusion, and a more alert affect.

When there is adequate intravascular volume, it is appropriate to plan the fluid therapy for the next 24 hr. The general approach is outlined in Box 47–3. In isotonic dehydration, the entire fluid deficit is corrected over 24 hr. The child receives normal maintenance fluids and the fluid deficit. The total amount of water and electrolytes are added together and then an appropriate fluid is selected. For the patient with isotonic dehydration, D5 $1/2$ normal saline with 20 mEq/L KCl is usually an appropriate fluid. For a child weighing less than 10–20 kg with only mild dehydration, a reduction of the sodium concentration is usually reasonable ($1/4$ NS) because the majority of the administered fluid is maintenance fluid. Children with mild dehydration do not require intravenous therapy unless enteral therapy is not possible (see Chapter 48). As detailed herein, the potassium concentration may need to be decreased or, less commonly, increased depending on the clinical situation. Potassium is not usually included in the intravenous fluids until the patient voids. Half of the total fluid is given over the first 8 hr; previous boluses are subtracted from this volume. The remainder is given over the next 16 hr.

It is important to consider ongoing fluid losses of the patient. For example, the child with copious diarrhea must receive an additional replacement solution, or the rehydration will not be complete (see Chapter 46).

BOX 47–2. Calculation of Deficit Water and Electrolytes

WATER DEFICIT
Percent dehydration × weight

SODIUM DEFICIT
Water deficit × 80 mEq/L

POTASSIUM DEFICIT
Water deficit × 30 mEq/L

BOX 47–3. Fluid Management of Dehydration

Restore intravascular volume
   Normal saline: 20 mL/kg over 20 min
   (Repeat until intravascular volume restored)
Calculate 24-hr water needs
   Calculate maintenance water
   Calculate deficit water
Calculate 24-hr electrolyte needs
   Calculate maintenance sodium and potassium
   Calculate deficit sodium and potassium
Select an appropriate fluid (based on total water and electrolyte needs)
   Administer half the calculated fluid during the first 8 hr, first subtracting any boluses from this amount
   Administer the remainder over the next 16 hr
Replace ongoing losses as they occur

Monitoring and Adjusting Therapy. The formulation of a plan for correcting a child's dehydration is only the beginning of management. All calculations in fluid therapy are only approximations. This is especially true with the assessment of percent dehydration. It is equally important to monitor the patient during treatment and to modify therapy based on the clinical situation. The cornerstones of patient monitoring are listed in Box 47–4. The patient's vital signs are useful indicators of intravascular volume status. The child with a decreased blood pressure and an increased heart rate will probably benefit from a fluid bolus. The central venous pressure is an excellent indicator of fluid status in the critically ill child.

The patient's intake and output are critically important in the dehydrated child. The child who, after 8 hr of therapy, has more output than input due to continuing diarrhea needs to be placed on a replacement solution. See Chapter 46 guidelines for selecting an appropriate replacement solution. The urine output and urine specific gravity are useful for evaluating the success of therapy. The presence of a good urine output indicates that rehydration has been successful. This is supported by a decreasing urine specific gravity. For example, if the urine specific gravity is less than 1.005 and the patient is clinically well hydrated, it may be appropriate to decrease the intravenous fluid rate.

The presence of signs of dehydration on physical examination suggests the need for continued rehydration. In contrast, signs of fluid overload, such as edema or pulmonary congestion, are present in the child who is overhydrated. An accurate daily weight measurement is critical for management of the dehydrated child. There should be a gain in weight during successful therapy.

At least daily electrolyte measurements are appropriate for any child who is receiving intravenous rehydration. These children are at risk for disorders of sodium, potassium, and

---

BOX 47–4. Monitoring Therapy

VITALS
Pulse
Blood pressure

INTAKE AND OUTPUT
Fluid balance
Urine output and specific gravity

PHYSICAL EXAMINATION
Weight
Clinical signs of depletion or overload

ELECTROLYTES

acid-base. It is always important to look at trends. For instance, a sodium value of 144 is normal. Yet, if the sodium concentration was 136 mEq/L 12 hr earlier, then there is a distinct risk that the child will be hypernatremic in 12 or 24 hr. It is advisable to be proactive in adjusting fluid therapy.

Both hypokalemia and hyperkalemia are potentially serious (see Chapter 45). Because dehydration can be associated with acute renal failure and hyperkalemia, potassium is withheld from intravenous fluids until the patient has voided. The potassium concentration in the patient's intravenous fluids is not rigidly prescribed. Rather, the patient's serum potassium and underlying renal function are used to modify the potassium delivery. For example, the patient with an elevated creatinine and a potassium level of 5.0 does not receive any potassium until the serum potassium decreases. Conversely, the patient with a potassium level of 2.5 may require additional potassium.

Metabolic acidosis can be severe in dehydrated children. Even though normal kidneys will eventually correct this problem, it is often reasonable to accelerate this process by replacing a portion of the patient's intravenous sodium chloride with sodium bicarbonate or sodium acetate. Adding sodium bicarbonate or sodium acetate to the patient's calculated rehydration solution, without reducing the sodium chloride concentration, could cause hypernatremia as a result of the high sodium load. Base therapy is indicated in the child with a metabolic acidosis and kidneys that are incapable of excreting acid (i.e., the child with renal insufficiency or renal tubular acidosis). In contrast, in the child with a lactic acidosis from hypoperfusion, restoration of intravascular volume permits metabolism of lactate into bicarbonate and thus excessive administration of base may produce a metabolic alkalosis.

The serum potassium level is modified by the patient's acid base status. Acidosis increases the serum potassium by causing intracellular potassium to move into the extracellular space. Thus, as acidosis is corrected, the potassium concentration decreases. Again, it is best to anticipate this problem and to monitor the serum potassium concentration and adjust potassium administration appropriately.

Hyponatremic Dehydration. The pathogenesis of hyponatremic dehydration is usually due to a combination of sodium and water loss and water retention to compensate for the volume depletion. The patient has a pathologic increase in fluid loss, and this fluid contains sodium. However, most fluid that is lost has a lower sodium concentration, so patients with only fluid loss would have hypernatremia. For example diarrhea has, on average, a sodium concentration of 50 mEq/L.

Hypernatremia does not occur because the patient drinks a low sodium containing fluid such as water or formula. By replacing diarrheal fluid with a sodium concentration of 50 mEq/L with water, which has almost no sodium, there is a reduction in the serum sodium concentration. Furthermore, the volume depletion stimulates synthesis of antidiuretic hormone, resulting in reduced renal water excretion. Hence, the body's usual mechanism for preventing hyponatremia, renal water excretion, is blocked. The risk of hyponatremia is further increased if the volume depletion is due to loss of fluid with a higher sodium concentration, as may occur with renal salt wasting, third space losses, or diarrhea with a high sodium content (e.g., cholera).

Hyponatremic dehydration produces more substantial intravascular volume depletion due to the shift of water from the extracellular space into the intracellular space. In addition, some patients develop symptoms, predominantly neurologic, from the hyponatremia (see Chapter 45).

The initial goal in treating hyponatremia is correction of intravascular volume depletion with isotonic fluid (NS or Ringer lactate). Hyponatremic dehydration requires replacement of sodium and water losses. The following formula can be used to calculate a patient's sodium deficit:

$$\text{Sodium deficit} = 0.6 \times \text{Wt} \times ([\text{Na}^+]_d - [\text{Na}^+]_i)$$

where $[\text{Na}^+]_d$ = desired sodium concentration, $[\text{Na}^+]_i$ = initial sodium concentration, and Wt = weight in kilograms.

When calculating the sodium deficit, it is important to choose an appropriate desired sodium concentration. In general, it is not necessary to increase the sodium beyond 135 mEq/L; "overcorrection" is associated with an increased risk of central pontine myelinolysis (CPM). The risk of CPM also increases with overly rapid correction of the serum sodium concentration, so it is important to avoid increasing the sodium by more than 12 mEq/L each 24 hr. Most patients with hyponatremic dehydration do well with the same basic strategy that is outlined in Box 47–3. Despite the increased sodium deficit in these patients compared with patients with isotonic dehydration, D5 $^1/_2$ NS with 20 mEq/L KCl is usually effective. As with isotonic dehydration, half the fluid can be administered over the first 8 hr. Again, potassium delivery is adjusted based on the initial serum potassium and the patient's renal function. Potassium is not given until the patient voids.

The patient's sodium concentration is monitored to ensure appropriate correction and the sodium concentration of the fluid is adjusted appropriately. Patients with ongoing losses require an appropriate replacement solution (see Chapter 46). Patients with neurologic symptoms (e.g., seizures) from hyponatremia need to receive an acute infusion of hypertonic (3%) saline to rapidly increase the serum sodium concentration (see Chapter 45).

Hypernatremic Dehydration. Hypernatremic dehydration is the most dangerous form of dehydration due to complications of hypernatremia and of therapy. Hypernatremia can cause serious neurologic damage, including hemorrhages and thrombosis. This appears to be secondary to movement of water from the brain cells into the hypertonic extracellular fluid, causing brain cell shrinkage and tearing blood vessels within the brain (see Chapter 45).

The movement of water from the intracellular space to the extracellular space during hypernatremic dehydration protects the intravascular volume. Thus, children with hypernatremia often appear less ill than children with a similar degree of isotonic dehydration. Urine output may be preserved longer and there may be less tachycardia. Unfortunately, the milder manifestations often lead to children with hypernatremic dehydration being brought to medical attention with more profound dehydration.

Children with hypernatremic dehydration are often lethargic, but irritable when touched. Hypernatremia may cause fever, hypertonicity, and hyperreflexia. More severe neurologic symptoms may develop if cerebral bleeding occurs.

The treatment of hypernatremic dehydration may cause significant morbidity and mortality. There is generation of idiogenic osmoles within the brain during the development of hypernatremia. These idiogenic osmoles increase the osmolality within the cells of the brain, providing protection against brain cell shrinkage caused by movement of water out of cells into the hypertonic extracellular fluid. However, these idiogenic osmoles dissipate slowly during correction of hypernatremia. With overly rapid lowering of the extracellular osmolality during correction of hypernatremia, there may be an osmotic gradient created that causes water movement from the extracellular space into the cells of the brain, producing cerebral edema. Symptoms of the resultant cerebral edema can range from seizures to brain herniation and death.

To minimize the risk of cerebral edema during correction of hypernatremic dehydration, the serum sodium concentration should not decrease more than 12 mEq/L every 24 hr. Severe hypernatremic dehydration may need to be corrected over 2–4 days (Box 47–5).

The initial management of hypernatremic dehydration requires restoration of the intravascular volume with normal saline. Ringer lactate should not be used because it is more hypotonic than normal saline and may cause too rapid a decrease in the serum sodium concentration, especially if multiple fluid boluses are necessary.

To avoid cerebral edema when correcting hypernatremic dehydration, the fluid deficit is corrected slowly. The rate of correction depends on the initial sodium concentration (see Box 47–5). Unlike patients with isotonic or hyponatremic dehydration, the fluid is not run at a faster rate during the first 8 hr. There is not general agreement on the choice of fluid or the rate of fluid for correcting hypernatremic dehydration. The choice and rate of fluid administration are not nearly as important as vigilant monitoring of the serum sodium concentration and adjustment of the therapy based on the result (see Box 47–5). The rate of decrease of the serum sodium concentration is roughly related to the "free water" delivery, although there is considerable variation between patients. Free water is water without sodium. For example, NS contains no free water, $^1/_2$ NS is 50% free water, and water is 100% free water. In general, smaller patients, to achieve the same decrease in the sodium concentration, tend to need higher amounts of free water delivery per kilogram because of higher insensible fluid losses. D5 $^1/_4$ NS is probably an appropriate starting solution for a neonate with hypernatremic dehydration whereas D5 $^1/_2$ NS may be a better choice in a 3-year-old. Occasionally, fluid with a lower sodium concentration than D5 $^1/_4$ NS or a higher sodium concentration than D5 $^1/_2$ NS is necessary. A child with dehydration due to pure free water loss, as usually occurs with diabetes insipidus, usually needs a more hypotonic fluid than a child with depletion of both sodium and water due to diarrhea.

Adjustment in the sodium concentration of the intravenous fluid is the most common approach for modifying the rate of decrease in the serum concentration (see Box 47–5). For difficult patients with severe hypernatremia, having two intravenous solutions (e.g., D5 $^1/_4$ NS and D5 $^1/_2$ NS, both with the same concentration of potassium) at the bedside can facilitate this approach by allowing for rapid adjustments of the rates of the two fluids. If the serum sodium concentration decreases too rapidly, the rate of D5 $^1/_2$ NS can be increased and the rate of D5 $^1/_4$ NS can be decreased. Adjustment in the total rate of fluid delivery is another approach for modifying free water delivery. For example, if the serum sodium concentration is decreasing too slowly, the rate of the intravenous fluid can be increased, thereby increasing the delivery of free water. There is limited flexibility in modifying the rate of the intravenous fluid because patients generally should receive between 1.25 and 1.5 times the normal maintenance fluid rate. Nevertheless, in some situations this can be a helpful adjustment.

Because increasing the rate of the intravenous fluids increases the rate of decrease of the sodium concentration, signs of volume depletion are treated with additional fluid boluses. The serum potassium concentration and the level of renal function dictate the potassium concentration of the intravenous fluid; potassium is held until the patient voids. Patients with hypernatremic dehydration need an appropriate replacement solution if they have excessive losses (see Chapter 46).

Seizures are the most common manifestation of cerebral edema and result from an overly rapid decrease of the serum sodium concentration during correction of hypernatremic dehydration. Acutely, increasing the serum concentration via an infusion of 3% sodium chloride can reverse the cerebral edema. Each mL/kg of 3% sodium chloride increases the serum sodium concentration by approximately 1 mEq/L. An infusion of 4–6 mL/kg often results in resolution of the symptoms. This is similar to the strategy used for treating symptomatic hyponatremia (see Chapter 45).

In patients with severe hypernatremia, oral fluids must be used cautiously. For example, infant formula, because of its low sodium concentration, has a very high free water content, and, especially if added to intravenous therapy, may contribute to a rapid decrease in the serum sodium concentration. Less hypotonic fluid, such as an oral rehydration solution, may be more appropriate initially (see Chapter 48). If oral intake is allowed, its contribution to free water delivery must be taken into account and adjustment in the intravenous fluid is usually appropriate. Judicious monitoring of the serum sodium concentration is critical.

BOX 47–5. Treatment of Hypernatremic Dehydration

Restore intravascular volume
Normal saline: 20 mL/kg over 20 min
(Repeat until intravascular volume restored)
Determine the time for correction based on the initial sodium concentration
[Na]: 145–157 mEq/L: 24 hr
[Na]: 158–170 mEq/L: 48 hr
[Na]: 171–183 mEq/L: 72 hr
[Na]: 184–196 mEq/L: 84 hr
Administer fluid at a constant rate over the time for correction
Typical fluids: D5 1/4 NS or D5 1/2 NS (both with 20 mEq/L KCl unless contraindicated)
Typical rate: 1.25–1.5 times maintenance
Follow serum sodium concentration
Adjust fluid based on clinical status and serum sodium concentration
Signs of volume depletion: administer NS (20 mL/kg)
Sodium decreases too rapidly
Increase sodium concentration of intravenous fluid, or
Decrease rate of intravenous fluid
Sodium decreases too slowly
Decrease sodium concentration of intravenous fluid, or
Increase rate of intravenous fluid
Replace ongoing losses as they occur

Chapter 48
Fluid and Electrolyte Treatment of Specific Disorders

48.1 Acute Diarrhea and Oral Rehydration

Also see Chapters 287 and 321.

Diarrhea continues to be a serious problem in many areas of the world and may be especially lethal when superimposed on malnutrition. Diarrhea results in large losses of water and electrolytes, especially sodium and potassium, and frequently is complicated by severe systemic acidosis. In approximately 70–80% of patients, the losses of water and sodium are proportionate, with *isotonic dehydration* developing. *Hyponatremic dehydration* is seen in approximately 10–15% of all patients with diarrhea. It occurs when large amounts of electrolytes, especially sodium, are lost in the stool out of proportion to fluid losses. It occurs more frequently with bacillary dysentery or cholera. Hyponatremia may develop or worsen if during diarrhea there is a considerable oral intake of low-electrolyte or electrolyte-free fluids.

Disproportionately large net losses of water compared with losses of electrolytes result in *hypernatremic dehydration*. It is seen in 10–20% of patients with diarrhea and may occur during the course of diarrhea when oral homemade electrolyte solutions with high concentrations of salt are administered or when infants are fed boiled skim milk, which produces a high renal solute load and increased urinary water losses. The potential for hypernatremia also increases with increased evaporative water loss from fever, high environmental temperatures, and hyperventilation and with decreased availability of free water.

The administration of intravenous fluids for treating profound dehydration from severe diarrhea is discussed in Chapter 47. Mild to moderate dehydration from diarrhea of any cause can be treated effectively in a wide range of age groups using a simple oral glucose-electrolyte solution (Table 48–1). These solutions rely on the coupled transport of sodium and glucose in the intestine. Oral rehydration therapy is used in many countries and has significantly reduced the morbidity and mortality from acute diarrhea and lessened diarrhea-associated malnutrition. Oral rehydration is underused in developed countries, but it should be attempted for most patients with mild to moderate diarrheal dehydration when adequate supervision is available. Oral rehydration therapy is less expensive than intravenous therapy and has a lower complication rate. Intravenous therapy may still be required for patients with severe dehydration; those with uncontrollable vomiting; those unable to drink because of extreme fatigue, stupor, or coma; or those with gastric or intestinal distention.

As a guideline for oral rehydration, 50 mL/kg of the oral rehydration solution (ORS) should be given within 4 hr to patients with mild dehydration and 100 mL/kg over 4 hr to those with moderate dehydration. Supplementary ORS is given to replace ongoing losses from diarrhea or emesis. An additional 10 mL/kg of ORS is given for each stool. Fluid intake should be decreased if the patient appears fully hydrated earlier than expected or if the patient develops periorbital edema. Breast-feeding should be allowed after rehydration in infants who are breast-fed; in other patients, their usual formula, milk, or feeding should be offered after rehydration. Along with its nutritional benefits, early refeeding decreases the duration of diarrhea. Most children can tolerate a lactose-containing formula, although some children benefit from a lactose free formula if malabsorption is present.

Vomiting may occur during the first 2 hr of administration of ORS, but it usually does not prevent successful oral rehydration if the ORS is given in small amounts at short intervals (a teaspoon every 1 to 2 min). Emesis usually lessens over time. The volume of ORS can be slowly increased, with an increasing interval between feedings. If sustained and severe vomiting occurs, intravenous therapy should be instituted. The patient's progress should be assessed frequently and changes in body weight monitored, if possible, to determine the degree of rehydration.

When rehydration is complete, maintenance therapy should be started. Patients with mild diarrhea usually can then be treated at home using 100 mL of ORS/kg/24 hr until the diarrhea stops. Breast-feeding or supplemental water intake should be maintained. Patients with more severe diarrhea require continued supervision. The volume of ORS ingested should equal the volume of stool losses. If stool volume cannot be measured, an intake of 10–15 mL of ORS/kg/hr is appropriate.

There is a significant difference in the sodium concentration between the World Health Organization (WHO) solution and the commercially available solutions that are generally used in the United States (see Table 48–1). Low-sodium solutions were advocated because hypernatremia was seen frequently in the United States when oral electrolyte solutions with sodium concentrations of 50 mEq/L or more were used to treat infantile diarrhea. However, extensive use of ORS in many developing countries has shown hypernatremia to be a rare complication, probably because ORS has been used primarily for rehydration (the major previous role for oral therapy was to prevent dehydration or for maintenance); because large amounts of water are ingested in addition to ORS, often a 2:1 ratio of ORS to H_2O; and because ORS has been administered under close supervision by trained personnel. The WHO ORS has also been effective in treating acute diarrheal illnesses in well-nourished children in developed countries. There is a risk of hypernatremia with the WHO ORS if it is used as a maintenance solution without supplemental water or formula. Several commercially available electrolyte solutions for oral use have been reformulated with a sodium concentration of approximately 50 mEq/L. These solutions are effective in the treatment of mild to moderate dehydration. Reduced osmolality solutions (primarily reduced sodium and glucose) are associated with reduced stool output.

48.2 Diarrhea in Chronically Malnourished Children

Severe malnutrition complicated by diarrheal dehydration is common in tropical and subtropical countries and occurs occasionally in the temperate zones. Therapy should be adapted to meet the specific disturbances in body composition characteristic of the dehydrated *and* malnourished infant, in whom there appears to be an overexpansion of the extracellular space, accompanied by extracellular and presumably intracellular hypo-osmolality. Serum sodium, potassium, and magnesium levels tend to be low, and tetany occasionally may result from a magnesium or calcium deficiency. Serum protein levels are frequently less than 3.6 g/dL. The sodium content of muscle is high; potassium and magnesium contents are low. The

TABLE 48–1. Composition of Oral Rehydration Solutions

Solution	Glucose (mmol/L)	Na (mEq/L)	K (mEq/L)	Cl (mEq/L)	Base (mEq/L)	Osmolality (mOsm/kg)
WHO solution	111	90	20	80	30	311
Rehydralyte	140	75	20	65	30	310
Pedialyte	140	45	20	35	30	250
Pediatric Electrolyte	140	45	20	35	48	250
Infalyte	70*	50	25	45	34	200
Naturalyte	140	45	20	35	48	238

Rice syrup solids are the carbohydrate source.
WHO = World Health Organization.

electrocardiogram (ECG) frequently shows tachycardia, low amplitude, and flat or inverted T waves. Cardiac reserve seems lowered, and heart failure is a common complication.

Despite clinical signs of dehydration and reduced body water, urinary osmolality may be low in the chronically malnourished child. This defect in renal concentration may result from the relative absence of urea to contribute to a hypertonic milieu in the renal papillae, a defect associated with a low dietary protein intake, and resulting in a failure of tubular conservation of water. However, the glomerular filtration rate is low, resulting in a smaller loss of water than would otherwise be expected. Renal concentrating ability returns after several days of high-protein feedings. The renal acidifying ability is also limited in patients with malnutrition.

Survival of the malnourished infant with diarrhea is limited by caloric deficit to a greater extent than by water and electrolyte deficit. Reparative calories can be given by slow drip through an indwelling nasogastric tube in conjunction with oral or, when necessary, intravenous rehydration. If appetite is poor and vomiting and gastric distention are absent, feeding is begun early (30–40 cal/kg/24 hr), given by slow intragastric drip. Increases to 50–100 cal/kg/24 hr and 1–2 g of protein/kg/24 hr are made in a few days. Ad libitum intake should be permitted in the succeeding days and weeks, up to 250–300 cal/kg/24 hr, and the diet should include an adequate supply of iron and copper.

Initial parenteral therapy in profound dehydration is designed to improve the circulation and expand extracellular volume. For patients with edema, the quantity of fluid and rate of administration may need to be readjusted from recommended levels to avoid pulmonary edema. Blood should be given if the patient is in shock and severely anemic. Potassium salts can be given early if the urine output is good. Clinical and ECG improvement may be more rapid with magnesium therapy. Seizures occurring during recovery from diarrhea complicating severe malnutrition may respond to magnesium.

48.3 Pyloric Stenosis

Also see Chapter 310.1.

This condition exemplifies the correction of deficits associated with alkalosis. The therapy differs little from that for other causes of dehydration, except that potassium replacement should begin early, as soon as the child has urinated. These patients have a chloride-responsive metabolic alkalosis (see Chapter 45) and only volume repletion, via administration of sodium chloride and potassium chloride, will allow correction of the metabolic alkalosis. Correction of the hypochloremia and alkalosis by administering ammonium chloride without correcting the potassium deficit is not recommended.

Severe depletion of intracellular potassium results in the increased exchange of hydrogen ion for sodium in the distal nephrons of the kidney. The paradoxical presence of an acid urine with systemic alkalosis should be interpreted as signifying a marked potassium deficit and a need to increase the amount of potassium used for repletion.

It is not uncommon for deficits to be replaced and serum levels of electrolytes returned to normal within 6–12 hr. However, except in the mildly ill infant without signs of dehydration, it is preferable to delay surgery for at least 24–48 hr to achieve optimal readjustment of body functions. During this preparation period, adequate fluid therapy prevents dehydration, and the stomach may be decompressed by gentle suction.

48.4 Perioperative Fluids

Preoperatively, preparing a patient having no pre-existing deficit or in whom the deficit has been repaired consists mainly of supplying adequate carbohydrate for sustenance and protein spar-

ing and the usual maintenance requirements of water and electrolytes. Young infants who are not vomiting should receive carbohydrate and electrolyte mixtures by mouth until 3 hr before the operation. Such fluids are readily absorbed from the gastrointestinal tract. Preparing the newborn involves certain unique hazards. Deficits of water and electrolytes from vomiting or from stasis caused by intestinal obstruction should be replaced before the surgery. In cases of intestinal obstruction, conjugated bilirubin may be deglucuronidated by intestinal enzymes; enterohepatic circulation of unconjugated bilirubin can then lead to high serum levels and kernicterus. Hypoprothrombinemia should be prevented by administering 1 mg of vitamin K.

During surgery, blood, plasma, saline, or other volume expanders may be given if blood loss, tissue trauma, third spacing, or excessive evaporative loss occurs. The magnitude of such losses is best judged by the experienced surgeon in the course of the procedure. *The most common error in administering parenteral fluid during and after surgery is excessive administration*, particularly of dextrose in water, rather than use of isotonic solutions. Under most circumstances, little to no potassium need be administered during this time, because extensive tissue trauma or anoxia may result in the release of large amounts of intracellular potassium, with the potential of causing hyperkalemia. If shock occurs, acute renal failure may ensue, impairing the ability to eliminate through the renal route large amounts of released potassium.

Postoperatively, fluid intake should be limited for 24 hr. Thereafter, the usual maintenance therapy is gradually resumed. The water intake should not exceed 85 mL/100 kcal metabolized, because of antidiuresis resulting from trauma, circulatory readjustment, general anesthesia, or narcotic pain relief, unless renal ability to concentrate the urine is limited, as in patients with sickle cell disease, chronic pyelonephritis, or obstructive uropathy. If the intake of water is not limited, whether given parenterally or orally, water intoxication may occur associated with severe hyponatremia and even fatal cerebral edema. This has been reported in post-tonsillectomy patients. Fluid therapy in the postoperative period largely depends on the complex but anticipated response of the body to trauma through modification of water and sodium excretion and the concomitant occurrence of complications from surgery. The patient's clinical condition dictates the final fluid and electrolyte requirements incurred as a result of these processes.

Postoperatively, some children have elevated blood antidiuretic hormone (ADH) levels due to syndrome of inappropriate ADH (SIADH) or to an appropriate response to fluid restriction and resultant volume contraction. If decreasing urine output after surgery is the result of SIADH, the patient is euvolemic and has a normal circulatory status, stable to slightly increased weight, and an elevated urinary sodium excretion. If a child has oliguria related to third spacing and true depletion of intravascular volume, there is decreased urinary sodium excretion associated with clinical signs of hypovolemia, such as weight loss, tachycardia, changes in skin turgor and peripheral perfusion, and hypotension. Isotonic solutions are indicated in this setting.

American Academy of Pediatrics, Provisional Committee on Quality Improvement, Subcommittee on Acute Gastroenteritis: Practice parameter: The management of acute gastroenteritis in young children. *Pediatrics* 1996;97: 424–35.

Dutta P, Mitra U, Manna B, et al: Double blind, randomised controlled clinical trial of hypo-osmolar oral rehydration salt solution in dehydrating acute diarrhoea in severely malnourished (marasmic) children. *Arch Dis Child* 2001;84:237–40.

Guarino A, Albano F, Guandalini S, et al: Oral rehydration: Toward a real solution. *J Pediatr Gastroenterol Nutr* 2001;33:S2–12.

Hahn S, Kim Y, Garner P: Reduced osmolarity oral rehydration solution for treating dehydration due to diarrhoea in children: Systematic review. *Br Med J* 2001;323:81–5.

Ladinsky M, Duggan A, Santosham M, et al: The World Health Organization oral rehydration solution in US pediatric practice: A randomized trial to evaluate parent satisfaction. *Arch Pediatr Adolesc Med* 2000;154:700–5.

Ozuah PO, Avner JR, Stein RE: Oral rehydration, emergency physicians, and practice parameters: A national survey. Pediatrics 2002;109:259–61.

Ramakrishna BS, Venkataraman S, Srinivasan P, et al: Amylase-resistant starch plus oral rehydration solution for cholera. N Engl J Med 2000;342:308–13.

Sarker SA, Mahalanabis D, Alam NH, et al: Reduced osmolarity oral rehydration solution for persistent diarrhea in infants: A randomized controlled clinical trial. J Pediatr 2001;138:532–8.

Victora CG, Bryce J, Fontaine O, et al: Reducing deaths from diarrhoea through oral rehydration therapy. Bull World Health Org 2000;78:1246–55.

Zaman K, Yunus M, Rahman A, et al: Efficacy of a packaged rice oral rehydration solution among children with cholera and cholera-like illness. Acta Paediatr 2001;90:505–10.

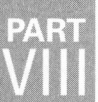

Chapter 49
Evaluation of the Sick Child in the Office and Clinic

Paul L. McCarthy

The approaches to clinical data gathering for the well child evaluation are also useful for the sick child evaluation (see Chapter 6). There are many reasons for a sick child visit, but most are due to acute intercurrent infections, and often the child is febrile.

When evaluating an acutely ill, febrile child, the pediatrician must be aware of categorical statistics about the probable occurrence of serious illness, because one of the major goals of the sick child visit is to identify the seriously ill child who requires specific therapeutic intervention. The risk for and the cause of serious illness in the acutely febrile child vary depending on age. The infant in the first 3 mo of life is more susceptible to sepsis and meningitis caused by group B streptococci and gram-negative organisms. Infants in the first month of life are at highest risk. Urinary tract infections are more frequent in males; infants in this age group more often have an underlying anatomic abnormality of the urinary tract than do older children with urinary tract infections. As the infant matures beyond 3 mo, the bacterial pathogens that usually cause sepsis and meningitis and bacteremia are *Streptococcus pneumoniae, Haemophilus influenzae* type b (if the child is unimmunized or only partially immunized), and *Neisseria meningitidis.* Immunization against some serotypes of *S. pneumoniae* may reduce the occurrence of serious infections caused by that organism as has immunization against *H. influenzae* type b. After infancy, urinary tract infections are seen more often in females. Immunity develops rapidly to the common bacterial pathogens during the first 3–4 yr of life. *N. meningitidis* is the leading cause of bacterial meningitis. In children older than 36 mo, pharyngitis caused by group A streptococci is a common bacterial infection. *Mycoplasma pneumoniae* assumes increasing importance as a cause for pulmonary infiltrates in children older than 5 yr of age. Serious illnesses documented in children in the first 3 yr of life who presented with fever and acute illnesses from a university hospital and private practice are shown in Table 49–1. In other studies, urinary tract infections are the most common serious bacterial infections. Soft tissue infections may include cellulitis, osteomyelitis, and septic arthritis.

The acutely ill child with a serious illness is identified by careful observation, history taking, physical examination, appreciation of age and body temperature as risk factors, and the judicious use of screening laboratory tests. The physician can make informed decisions with the data about the need for more definitive laboratory tests (e.g., urine culture), therapy, and the advisability of hospital admission. Observation, history, and physical examination are integrated into the sick child evaluation; that is, as the child is being observed, historical data are gathered. History taking and observational assessment often continue as the physical examination is performed. If, for example, abdominal tenderness is found on examination, additional

TABLE 49–1. Diagnosis of Serious Illnesses During 996 Episodes of Acute Infectious Illness in Febrile Children Younger Than 36 Mo[*]

	Cases	
Diagnosis	No.	%
Bacterial meningitis	9	0.9
Aseptic meningitis	12	1.2
Pneumonia	30	3.0
Bacteremia	10	1.0
Focal soft tissue infection[†]	10	1.0
Urinary tract infection	8	0.8
Bacterial diarrhea	1	0.1
Abnormal electrolytes, abnormal blood gases	9	0.9
Total	89	8.9

[*]*Nonserious illness includes benign viral diseases such as roseola herpesvirus 6 or 7, enteroviruses, respiratory syncytial virus, influenza, metapneumovirus, parainfluenza, and rotavirus.*
[†]*Includes cellulitis, osteomyelitis, and septic arthritis.*
From McCarthy PL: Acute infectious illness in children. CompTher 1988;14:51.

history about blood in the stool, cramping abdominal pain, and vomiting may be sought.

Observation is important in the evaluation of the acutely ill child. The child should be observed for specific evidence of a serious illness, such as grunting, which might indicate pneumonia or sepsis, or a bulging fontanel, which might indicate bacterial meningitis. *Most observational data that the pediatrician gathers during an acute illness should focus, however, on assessing the child's response to stimuli.* How does the child's crying respond to the parents' comforting? If sleeping, how quickly does the child awaken with a stimulus? Does the child smile when the examiner interacts with him or her? Assessing responses to stimuli, and often providing those stimuli, requires knowledge of normal responses for different age groups, the manner in which those normal responses are elicited, and to what degree a response might be impaired (see Chapter 6).

Sometimes the manner in which the child responds to stimuli is readily apparent. For example, the child may vocalize and smile as the examiner enters the room. At other times, more effort and more stimuli are needed to cause the child to act in a normal manner. Often the fussing, irritable child begins to look around and focus on the examiner when held and walked by the parent. This normal visual behavior is an important indicator of well-being. Thus, during observation, the pediatrician must be both clinically and developmentally oriented.

Six observation items and their scales (the Acute Illness Observation Scales) that have reliably and validly identified serious illness in febrile children are shown in Figure 49–1. A normal finding is scored as 1, a moderate impairment as 3, and severe impairment as 5. The best possible score is 6 items × 1 = 6; the worst score is 6 items × 5 = 30. The chance of serious illness is 1–2% if the total score is 10 or less; if the score is more than 10, the risk of serious illness increases by at least 10-fold. It is not clear whether these scales can be used in the first 2–3 mo of life because infants may not have developed the skills required to score some of these items.

6 OBSERVATION ITEMS AND THEIR SCALES

(PLEASE CHECK BOXES THAT DESCRIBE YOUR CHILD'S APPEARANCE AND BEHAVIOR)

OBSERVATION ITEM	NORMAL	MODERATE IMPAIRMENT	SEVERE IMPAIRMENT
1. **QUALITY OF CRY**	STRONG WITH NORMAL TONE ☐ *OR* CONTENT AND NOT CRYING ☐	WHIMPERING ☐ *OR* SOBBING ☐	WEAK ☐ *OR* MOANING ☐ *OR* HIGH PITCHED ☐
2. **REACTION TO PARENT STIMULATION** (Effect on crying when held, patted on back, jiggled on lap, or carried)	CRIES BRIEFLY, THEN STOPS ☐ *OR* CONTENT AND NOT CRYING ☐	CRIES OFF ☐ AND ON	CONTINUAL CRY ☐ *OR* HARDLY RESPONDS ☐
3. **STATE VARIATION** (Going from awake to asleep or asleep to awake)	IF AWAKE, THEN STAYS AWAKE ☐ *OR* IF ASLEEP AND STIMULATED, THEN WAKES UP QUICKLY ☐	EYES CLOSE BRIEFLY, THEN AWAKENS ☐ *OR* AWAKENS WITH PROLONGED STIMULATION ☐	WILL NOT ROUSE ☐ *OR* FALLS TO SLEEP ☐
4. **COLOR**	PINK ☐	PALE HANDS, FEET ☐ *OR* ACROCYANOSIS (BLUE HANDS AND FEET) ☐	PALE ☐ *OR* BLUE ☐ *OR* ASHEN (GRAY) ☐ *OR* MOTTLED ☐
5. **HYDRATION** (Moisture in skin, eyes, mouth)	SKIN NORMAL *AND* EYES, MOUTH MOIST ☐	SKIN, EYES NORMAL *AND* MOUTH SLIGHTLY DRY ☐	SKIN DOUGHY OR TENTED *AND* EYES MAY BE SUNKEN *AND* DRY EYES AND MOUTH ☐
6. **RESPONSE TO SOCIAL OVERTURES** (Being held, kissed, hugged, touched, talked to, comforted)	SMILES ☐ *OR* ALERTS ☐ (2 months or less)	BRIEF SMILE ☐ *OR* ALERTS BRIEFLY ☐ (2 months or less)	NO SMILE, FACE ANXIOUS ☐ *OR* DULL, EXPRESSIONLESS ☐ *OR* NO ALERTING ☐ (2 months or less)

FIGURE 49–1. Acute Illness Observational Scales for use in clinical evaluation of the well and sick child. (From McCarthy PL, Sharpe MR, Spiesel SZ, et al: Observation scales to identify serious illness in febrile children. *Pediatrics* 1982;70:802, with permission.)

History taking is complex (see Chapters 6 and 17.1). Parents must transmit how a younger child has been "feeling." Parents should also provide information on a specific symptom, such as bloody diarrhea or cyanosis when coughing. The older child's perception of symptoms may reflect a developmentally immature understanding of causation. The examiner pursues the historical information provided by the parents or child to define the symptoms precisely. For example, if the complaint is blood in the stool, additional questions can be asked about other evidence of bowel inflammation, such as watery stools, mucus in the stools, or increased frequency of stooling. If the historical information indicates crying with defecation and streaks of blood on the outer portion of a hard stool, without other changes in the character or frequency of the stool, a diagnosis of a rectal fissure is tenable.

Questions should focus on those entities that are seen most commonly in acute febrile childhood illnesses. The more serious diagnoses are outlined in Table 49–1. Organ-specific questions are helpful, such as fast breathing, cyanosis, retraction, and wheezing with pneumonia, or pain, swelling, and pseudoparalysis with septic arthritis. Because most acute illnesses in children are caused by minor viral infections, specific questions about the epidemiology of the illness can offer important insights. Are

there other children in the family with similar symptoms? Has the child had other illness exposures? Finally, it is important to be aware of any underlying chronic problems that might predispose the child to recurring infections or a serious acute illness; for example, the child with sickle cell anemia or AIDS is at increased risk for recurrent episodes of bacteremia. Benign viral illnesses may produce serious secondary consequences such as dehydration. Additional questions to assess hydration such as wet diapers, tears, or awakeness should be used to assess secondary complications.

The physical examination follows the same sequence for the well child (see Chapter 6). The examiner should be aware of and seek evidence of illnesses that might be present in the acutely ill child. Initially, it is best to seat the child on the parent's lap; the older child may be seated on the examination table. Vital signs are often overlooked but are quite valuable in assessing ill children. The degree of fever, the presence of tachycardia out of proportion to the fever, and the presence of tachypnea and hypotension all suggest a serious infection. In addition to the general level of interaction, color, and hydration, as assessed in the Acute Illness Observation Scales (see Fig. 49–1), the child's respiratory status is evaluated. This evaluation includes determining respiratory rate and noting any evidence of inspiratory stridor, expiratory wheezing, grunting, or coughing. Evidence of increased work of breathing—retractions, nasal flaring, and use of abdominal musculature—is sought. Because acute infections in children are most often caused by viral infections, the presence of nasal discharge is noted. It is possible at this time to assess the skin for rashes. Frequently, viral infections cause an exanthematous eruption, and many of these eruptions are diagnostic (e.g., the reticulated rash and "slapped-cheek" appearance caused by parvovirus infections or the typical appearance of hand-foot-and-mouth disease caused by coxsackieviruses). The skin examination may also yield evidence of more serious infections (e.g., bacterial cellulitis or petechiae associated with bacteremia). Cutaneous perfusion should be assessed by warmth and capillary refill time. When the child is seated and is least perturbed, an assessment of fontanel tension can be completed; it can be determined if the fontanel is depressed, flat, or bulging. It is also important at this time to assess the child's willingness to move and ease of movement. Usually the child with meningitis will hold the neck stiffly and often cry when any attempt is made to move the neck, even during cuddling by the parent. This is termed *paradoxic irritability*. The child with cellulitis, osteomyelitis, or septic arthritis in an extremity will resist movement of that limb. The child with peritoneal inflammation will sit quietly and become irritable during movement. It is reassuring to see the child moving about on the parent's lap with ease and without discomfort.

During this initial portion of the physical examination, when the child is most comfortable, the heart and lungs are auscultated. In the acutely febrile child, because of the relatively frequent occurrence of respiratory illnesses, it is important to assess adequacy of air entry into the lungs, equality of breath sounds, and evidence of adventitial breath sounds, especially wheezes, rales, and rhonchi. The coarse sound of air moving through a congested nasal passage is frequently transmitted to the lungs. The examiner can become attuned to these coarse sounds by placing the stethoscope near the child's nose and then compensating for this sound as the chest is auscultated. The cardiac examination is completed next; findings such as pericardial friction rub, loud murmurs, or distant heart sounds may indicate an infectious process involving the heart. The eyes are examined to identify features that might indicate an infectious process. Often, viral infections result in a watery discharge or redness of the bulbar conjunctivae. Bacterial infection, if superficial, results in purulent drainage; if the infection is more deep-seated, tenderness, swelling, and redness of tissues surrounding the eye are present as well as proptosis, reduced acuity, and altered extraocular movement. The extremities may then be evaluated not only for ease of movement but also for the possibility of swelling, heat, or tenderness; such abnormalities may indicate focal infections.

The components of the physical examination that are more bothersome to the child are completed last. This is best done with the patient on the examination table. Initially, the neck is examined to assess for areas of swelling, redness, or tenderness, as may be seen in cervical adenitis. The neck is then flexed to evaluate suppleness; resistance to flexion is indicative of meningeal irritation. Both Kernig's and Brudzinski's signs may be sought at this time. In children younger than 18 mo, meningeal signs may not always be present with meningitis; if, however, they are present, the diagnostic implications are the same as for the child older than 18 mo. During examination of the abdomen, the diaper is removed. The abdomen is inspected for distention. Auscultation is performed to assess adequacy of bowel sounds, followed by palpation. It is often the case that the child fusses as the abdomen is auscultated and palpated. Every attempt should be made to quiet the child; if this is not possible, increased fussing as the abdomen is palpated may indicate tenderness, especially if this finding is reproducible. In addition to focal tenderness, palpation may elicit involuntary guarding or

rebound; these findings indicate peritoneal irritation, as is seen in appendicitis. The inguinal area and genitals are then sequentially examined. In the febrile child, inguinal adenitis or a strangulated hernia may be the cause of fever. The child is then placed in the prone position, and abnormalities of the back are sought. The spine and costovertebral angle (CVA) areas are percussed to elicit any tenderness; such findings may be indicative of osteomyelitis or diskitis, and pyelonephritis, respectively.

The physical examination is completed by examining the ears and throat. These are usually the most bothersome parts of the examination for the child, and parents frequently can be helpful in minimizing head movement. The oropharyngeal examination is important to document the presence of enanthemas; these may be seen in many infectious processes, such as hand-foot-and-mouth disease caused by coxsackievirus. This portion of the examination is also important in documenting inflammation or exudates on the tonsils, which may be viral or bacterial.

At times, repeating portions of observational assessment and the physical examination is indicated. For example, if the child cried continuously during the initial clinical evaluation, the examiner may not be certain if this was caused by the high fever or stranger anxiety or is indicative of a serious illness. Continual crying also makes portions of the physical examination, such as auscultation of the chest, more difficult. Before a repeat assessment is performed, maneuvers to make the child as comfortable as possible are indicated. Such maneuvers include reducing the fever with antipyretics and allowing the child to take a bottle. Because most children with fever do not have serious illnesses, repeated assessments are more likely to document normal findings. If, on the other hand, the child is persistently irritable, the possibility of serious illness increases.

The sensitivity of the carefully performed clinical assessment, observation, history, and physical examination for the presence of serious illness is approximately 90%. Careful data gathering is necessary in the observation, history, and physical examination, because each component of the evaluation is as effective as the others in identifying serious illness. Other data, however, should be sought to improve this sensitivity level. In the child with an acute febrile illness, the important supplemental data are age, body temperature, and screening laboratory tests. Febrile children in the first 3 mo of life have yet to achieve immunologic maturity and therefore are more susceptible to severe infections and to infections by unusual organisms. Thus, the febrile infant is at greater risk for serious illness than the child beyond 3 mo of age (see Chapter 162). In febrile children, the higher the fever, the greater the risk for serious illness. The risk of bacteremia in infants increases as the degree of fever increases; at 40°C (105°F) or more the risk is 7%. The limit of physiologic thermoregulation is 41.1°C (106°F); fevers in this range and higher indicate not only bacteremia but also possible central nervous system infection, pneumonia, or pathologic hyperthermia.

Screening laboratory tests may be helpful in identifying the febrile child at increased risk for selected serious illnesses. *S. pneumoniae* is currently the most common cause of occult bacteremia not associated with a focal soft tissue infection. A total white blood cell count of 15,000/mm^3 or more and/or absolute neutrophil count of 10,000/mm^3 or more, in addition to age 3–36 mo, higher grades of fever, or a more ill appearance, are indicators of increased risk for occult bacteremia caused by *S. pneumoniae*. A urinalysis and urine culture should be considered when the source of fever is not apparent, especially in females and uncircumcised males younger than 2 yr of age and all boys younger than 1 yr of age—the highest risk groups. The presence of leukocyte esterase, more than 5 white blood cells per high-power field on a spun urine specimen, or bacteria by Gram stain on an unspun urine specimen suggest a urinary tract infection, but the sensitivity of these indicators is, on average, only 75–85% and the urine culture is the definitive test. An elevated

C-reactive protein value may also distinguish bacterial from viral infections.

Diagnostic approach (see also Chapters 98 and 162): If the febrile child is older than 3 mo and appears well, if the history or physical examination does not suggest a serious illness, and if no age or temperature risk factors are present, the child may be followed expectantly. If otitis media is present, it should be treated. This profile applies to most children with acute infectious illnesses. If, on the other hand, the child appears ill or the history or physical examination suggests a serious illness, definitive laboratory tests appropriate for those findings are indicated (e.g., a chest radiograph for a child with grunting). The area of greatest controversy is whether laboratory studies are needed on the febrile child who appears well and has no abnormalities on history and physical examination but who is younger than 3 mo of age or whose temperature is high. Many would agree that a sepsis work-up is indicated in the febrile child younger than age 3 mo (see Chapters 98 and 162). Obtaining blood cultures in children older than 3 mo with higher grades of fever has gained increased acceptance.

If the physician feels comfortable in following as an outpatient the child in whom no specific diagnosis has been established, a follow-up examination often yields a diagnosis. During the initial visit, or from one visit to the next during the acute illness, the change in symptoms or in the physical examination over time may provide important diagnostic clues. For the child in whom a diagnosis has already been established and who does not require hospitalization, follow-up by telephone or an office visit should be used to monitor the course of the illness and to further educate and support the parents.

American Academy of Pediatrics, Committee on Quality Improvement, Subcommittee on Urinary Tract Infection: Practice Parameter: The diagnosis, treatment and evaluation of the initial urinary tract infection in febrile infants and young children. *Pediatrics* 1999;103:843–52.

Baker MD, McCarthy PL: Fever and occult bacteremia in infants and young children. In Jenson HB, Baltimore RS (editors): *Pediatric Infectious Diseases: Principles and Practice.* Philadelphia, WB Saunders, 2002.

Black S, Shinefield H, Fireman B, et al: Efficacy, safety and immunogenicity of heptavalent pneumococcal conjugate vaccine in children. *Pediatr Infect Dis J* 2000; 19:187–95.

Isaacman DJ, Shults J, Gross TK, et al: Predictors of bacteremia in febrile children 3 to 36 months of age. *Pediatrics* 2000;106:977–82.

Kupperman N, Fleisher GR, Jaffe DM: Predictors of occult pneumococcal bacteremia in young, febrile children. *Ann Emerg Med* 1998;31:679–87.

McCarthy P, Freudigman K, Cicchetti D, et al: The mother-child interaction and clinical judgment during acute pediatric illnesses. *J Pediatr* 2000;136:809–17.

McCarthy PL: Fever. *Pediatr Rev* 1998;19:401–7.

Chapter 50
Injury Control

Frederick P. Rivara and David Grossman

Injuries are the most common cause of death during childhood and adolescence beyond the first few months of life and represent one of the most important causes of preventable pediatric morbidity and mortality. Advances have identified the risk factors for injuries and have developed successful programs for prevention and control. Such activities should be applied daily by the pediatrician in the office, emergency department, hospital, or community setting.

Injury Control. The term *accident prevention* has been replaced by *injury control.* The word "accident" implies an event occurring by chance, without pattern or predictability. In fact, most injuries occur under fairly predictable circumstances to high-risk children and families. *Accident* connotes a random event that cannot

be prevented. The use of the term *injury* promotes an awareness of a medical condition with defined risk and protective factors that can be used to define prevention strategies.

The reduction of morbidity and mortality from injuries can be accomplished not only through *primary* prevention (averting the event or injury in the first place) but also through *secondary* and *tertiary* prevention. The latter two approaches include appropriate emergency medical services for injured children; regionalized trauma care for the multiply injured, severely burned, or head-injured child; and specialized pediatric rehabilitation services that attempt to return children to their prior level of functioning. This broadened scope of prevention is more properly described by the term *injury control.*

This expanded definition also encompasses intentional injuries (assaults and self-inflicted injuries). These injuries are important among adolescents and young adults and in some populations rank first or second as causes of death in these age groups. Many of the same principles of injury control can be applied to these problems; for example, limiting access to firearms may reduce both unintentional shootings as well as suicides.

Scope of the Problem

MORTALITY. Injuries cause 45% of the deaths among 1- to 4-yr-old children and three times more deaths than the next leading cause, congenital anomalies. For the rest of childhood and adolescence up to the age of 19 yr, nearly 70% of deaths are due to injuries, more than all other causes combined. In 1999, injuries caused 17,940 deaths among individuals 19 yr and younger in the United States (Table 50–1), resulting in more years of potential life lost than any other cause.

Motor vehicle injuries lead the list of injury deaths at all ages during childhood and adolescence, even in children younger than 1 yr of age. Motor vehicle occupant injuries account for the majority of these deaths during childhood as well as in adults. During adolescence, occupant injuries are the leading cause of injury death, accounting for more than 50% of unintentional trauma mortality in this age group.

Drowning ranks second overall as a cause of unintentional trauma deaths, with peaks in the preschool and later teenage years (see Chapter 61). In some areas of the United States, drowning is the leading cause of death from trauma for preschool-aged children. The causes of drowning deaths vary with age and geographic area. In young children, bathtub and swimming pool drowning predominate, whereas in older children and adolescents, drownings occur predominantly in natural bodies of water while swimming or boating.

Fire and burn deaths account for nearly 6% of all unintentional trauma deaths and 13% in those younger than 5 yr of age (see Chapter 62). The vast majority of these (93%) are due to house fires, with most deaths caused by smoke inhalation and asphyxiation rather than severe burns. Children and the elderly are at greatest risk of these deaths because of difficulty in escaping from burning buildings.

Suffocation accounts for approximately half of all unintentional deaths in children younger than 1 yr of age. The majority of these deaths result from choking on food items such as hot dogs, candies, grapes, and nuts. Nonfood items that can cause choking include undersized infant pacifiers, small balls, and latex balloons.

Homicide is the second leading cause of injury death for infants younger than 1 yr, the second leading cause of injury death for ages 1–4 yr, and the second leading cause of injury death in adolescents (15–19 yr). Homicide in the pediatric age group falls into two patterns: "infantile" and "adolescent." Infantile homicide involves children younger than the age of 5 yr and represents child abuse (see Chapter 35). The perpetrator is usually a caretaker; death is generally the result of blunt trauma to the head and/or abdomen. In contrast, the adolescent pattern of

TABLE 50–1. Injury Deaths in the United States, 1999

Cause of Death	Younger than 1 yr	1–4 yr	5–9 yr	10–14 yr	15–19 yr	0–19 yr
All causes	27,037	5,240	3,474	4,121	13,778	53,650
All injuries	1,231	2,317	1,659	2,158	10,575	17,940
All unintentional	845	1,898	1,459	1,632	6,688	12,522
Motor vehicle occupant	86	203	275	367	2,543	3,474
Pedestrian	13	269	241	210	313	1,046
Other motor vehicle	85	263	286	492	2,342	3,283
Drowning	68	490	192	177	359	1,286
Fire and burn	44	308	171	92	88	703
Poisoning	12	34	12	28	260	346
Bicycle	0	7	74	92	83	256
Firearm	0	12	19	57	126	214
Fall	12	55	25	28	112	232
Suffocation	472	162	54	78	66	832
Other unintentional	53	95	110	11	396	665
All intentional	331	376	188	489	3,728	5,112
Suicide	0	0	2	242	1,615	1,859
Firearm suicide	0	0	0	103	975	1,078
Homicide	331	376	186	247	2,113	2,546
Firearm homicide	8	50	61	164	1,727	2,010
Undetermined intent	55	43	12	37	159	306

From Web-based Injury Statistics Query and Reporting System at http://webapp.cdc.gov/sasweb/ncipc/mortrate.html

homicide involves peers and acquaintances and is due to firearms in more than 80% of cases. The majority of these deaths involve handguns. Children between these two age groups experience homicides of both types.

Suicide is rare in children younger than age 10 yr; only 1% of all suicides occur in children younger than age 15 yr. The suicide rate increases markedly after the age of 10 yr, with the result that suicide is now the third leading cause of death for 15- to 19-yr-olds, accounting for more than 100,000 potential years of life lost. Native American teenagers are at the highest risk, followed by white males; black females have the lowest rate of suicide in this age group. Approximately 60% of teenage suicides involve firearms (see Chapters 24 and 102).

NONFATAL INJURIES. Mortality statistics reflect only a small part of the effects of childhood injuries. Twenty to 25 per cent of children and adolescents receive medical care for an injury each year in hospital emergency departments, and at least an equal number are treated in physicians' offices. Of these, 2.5% require inpatient care and 55% have at least short-term temporary disability from their injuries.

The distribution of these nonfatal injuries is very different from that of fatal trauma (Fig. 50–1). Falls are the leading causes of both emergency department visits and hospitalizations. Bicycle-related trauma is the most common type of sports and recreational injury, accounting for more than 300,000 emergency department visits annually. Nonfatal injuries, such as anoxic encephalopathy from near-drowning, scarring and disfigurement from burns, and persistent neurologic deficits from head injury, may be associated with severe morbidity, leading to substantial changes in the quality of life for victims and families.

TRENDS OVER TIME. The death rate for childhood injuries in the United States and most developed nations has declined throughout the 20th century, with substantial decreases in death rates from unintentional injuries over the past 15 yr. Homicide and suicide are the only leading causes of death in the United States to increase from 1950 to the 1990s. Suicide rates among male teens increased by 50% between 1970 and 1986, largely owing to firearm-related suicides. Since 1986, suicide rates among 15- to 19-yr-olds have decreased; rates in 1998 were 12% lower than in 1986. Homicide rates for 15- to 19-yr-old teens peaked in 1993 and fortunately have decreased by 50% since then. Both the increase and the subsequent drop in homicides were firearm related.

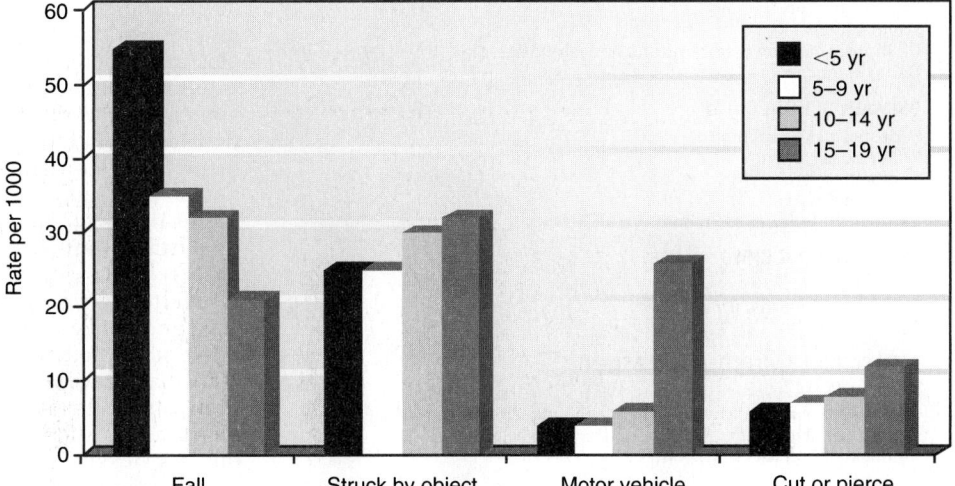

FIGURE 50–1. Emergency department visit rates for leading first-listed causes of injury by age: United States, 1993–1994. (Data from Centers for Disease Control and Prevention, National Center for Health Statistics, and National Hospital Ambulatory Medical Case Survey.)

Principles of Injury Control. For many years, prevention of injuries centered on attempts to pinpoint the innate characteristics of a child that result in greater frequency of injury. Most have discounted the theory of the "accident-prone child." Although longitudinal studies have demonstrated an association between hyperactivity and impulsivity and increased rates of injuries, the sensitivity and specificity of these traits for injury are extremely low. The concept of "accident proneness" is, in fact, counterproductive in that it shifts attention away from potentially more modifiable factors, such as product design or the environment. It is more appropriate to examine the physical and social environment of children with frequent rates of injuries than to try to identify particular personality traits or temperaments, which are difficult to modify. Children at high injury risk are likely to be relatively poorly supervised, have disorganized or stressed families, and live in hazardous environments.

Efforts to control injuries include *education or persuasion, changes in product design,* and *modification of the social and physical environment.* Efforts to persuade individuals, particularly parents, to change their behaviors have constituted the greater part of injury control efforts. Speaking with parents specifically about using child car seat restraints and bicycle helmets, installing smoke detectors, and checking the tap water temperature is likely to be more successful than well-meaning but too-general advice about supervising the child closely, being careful, and "childproofing" the home. This information should be geared to the developmental stage of the child and presented in moderate doses in the form of anticipatory guidance at well-child visits. Important topics to discuss at each developmental stage are shown in Box 50–1.

The most successful injury prevention strategies generally are those involving changes in product design, as shown in Table 50–2. These *passive* interventions protect all individuals in the population, regardless of cooperation or level of skill,

---

BOX 50–1. Injury Prevention Topics for Anticipatory Guidance by the Pediatrician

NEWBORN
Car seats
Tap water temperature
Smoke detectors

INFANT
Car seats
Tap water temperature
Bath safety

TODDLER AND PRESCHOOLER
Car seats
Pedestrian skills training
Water safety
Childproof caps on medicines and household poisons
Syrup of ipecac

PRIMARY SCHOOL CHILD
Pedestrian skills training
Water skills training
Seatbelts
Bicycle helmets
Removal of firearms from home

MIDDLE SCHOOL CHILD
Seatbelts
Removal of firearms from home
Pedestrian skills

HIGH SCHOOL AND OLDER ADOLESCENT
Seatbelts
Alcohol use, especially while driving, boating, and swimming
Occupational injuries
Removal of firearms from home

TABLE 50–2. **Injury Control Interventions**

Product Modification	> Environmental Modification	> Education
Child-resistant caps	Cabinet locks	Anticipatory guidance
Airbags	Roadway design	Public service announcements
Fire-safe cigarettes	Smoke detectors	School safety programs

and are likely to be more successful than *active* measures that require repeated behavior change by the parent or child. However, for some types of injuries, effective passive interventions are not available or feasible; we must rely heavily on attempts to change the behavior of individuals. Turning down the water heater temperature, installing smoke detectors, and using child-resistant caps on medicines and household products are examples of effective product modification. Many interventions require both active and passive measures. For example, smoke detectors provide passive protection when fully functional but behavior change is required to ensure annual battery changes and proper testing.

Modification of the environment often requires greater changes than individual product modification but may be very effective in reducing injuries. Safe roadway design, decreased traffic volume and speed limits in the neighborhood, and elimination of guns from the households are examples of such interventions. Included in this concept are changes in the social environment through legislation such as laws mandating child seat restraint and seatbelt use, bicycle helmet use, and graduated motor vehicle licensing laws.

Prevention campaigns combining two or more of these approaches have been particularly effective in reducing injuries. The classic example is the combination of legislation and education to increase child seat restraint and seatbelt use; other examples are programs to promote bike helmet use among school-aged children and improvements in occupant protection in motor vehicles.

Risk Factors for Childhood Injuries. Major factors that are associated with an increased risk of injuries to children include age, sex, race, socioeconomic status, and the environment.

AGE. Toddlers are at greatest risk for burns, drowning, and falls. As these children acquire mobility and exploratory behavior, poisonings become a risk. Young school-aged children are at greatest risk for pedestrian injuries, bicycle-related injuries (the most serious of which usually involve motor vehicles), motor vehicle occupant injuries, burns, and drowning. During the teenage years, there is a markedly increased risk from motor vehicle occupant trauma, a continued risk from drowning and burns, and the new risk of intentional trauma. Work-related injuries associated with child labor, especially for 14- to 16-yr-olds, are an additional risk.

Injuries occurring at a particular age represent a window of vulnerability during which a child or an adolescent encounters a new task or hazard that he or she may not have the developmental skills to handle successfully. For example, toddlers do not have the judgment to know that medications can be poisonous or that some houseplants are not to be eaten; they do not understand the hazard presented by a swimming pool or an open second-story window. For young children, parents may inadvertently set up this mismatch between the skills of the child and the demands of the task. A walker converts an infant into a mobile toddler and greatly increases contact with hazards. Many parents expect young school-aged children to walk home from school, the playground, or the local candy store, tasks for which most children are not developmentally ready. Likewise, the lack of skills and experience to handle many tasks during the teenage years contributes to an increased risk of injuries, particularly motor vehicle injuries. The high rate of motor vehicle crashes for younger teens is caused in part by inexperience but also appears to reflect their level of development and maturity. Alcohol and other drugs often add to these limitations.

Age also influences the severity of injury as well as the risk of long-term disability. For example, young school-aged children have an incompletely developed pelvis. In a motor vehicle crash, the seatbelt does not anchor onto the pelvis but rides up onto the abdomen, resulting in the risk of serious abdominal injury. Age interacts with the vehicle characteristics in that most children ride in the rear seat, which in the past was equipped only with lap belts and not lap-shoulder harnesses. Proper restraint for 4- to 8-yr-old children requires the use of booster seats. Children younger than the age of 2 yr have much poorer outcomes from closed-head injuries than do older children and adolescents.

SEX. Beginning at 1–2 yr of age and continuing until the 7th decade of life, males have higher rates of injuries than females. During childhood this does not appear to be due to developmental differences between the sexes, differences in coordination, or differences in muscle strength. Variation in exposure to risk may account for the male predominance in some types of injuries. Although boys in all age groups have higher rates of bicycle-related injuries, adjusting for exposure reduces this excess rate. Boys may have higher rates of injuries because they use bicycles more frequently or for more hours. In contrast, sex differences in rates of pedestrian injuries do not appear to be caused by differences in the amount of walking but rather reflect differences in behavior between young girls and boys. Greater risk-taking behavior, combined with greater frequency of alcohol use, may lead to the disproportionately high rate of motor vehicle crashes among teenage males.

RACE. African-Americans have much higher rates of injuries than whites, whereas Asians have lower rates; rates for Hispanics are intermediate between those for African-Americans and whites. Native Americans have the highest death rate from unintentional injuries. These discrepancies are even more pronounced for some injuries. The homicide rate for blacks age 15–19 yr was 63.8 per 100,000 in 1999, compared with 8.84 per 100,000 for whites. The suicide rate for Native American youth is twice the rate for whites and fourfold greater than that for Asians. The rate of fire and burn deaths in black preschool children is more than three times higher than for whites: 5.4 per 100,000 compared with 1.5 per 100,000, respectively.

These racial disparities appear to be primarily related to poverty and educational status of parents, and the presence of hazardous environments, rather than to race. Homicide rates of blacks are nearly equivalent to whites when adjusted for socioeconomic status. It is important to understand racial disparities in injury rates but inappropriate to ascribe the etiology of these differences to race.

SOCIOECONOMIC STATUS. Poverty is one of the most important risk factors for childhood injury. Mortality from fires, motor vehicle crashes, and drowning is two- to fourfold higher in poor children. Death rates for both African-Americans and whites have an inverse relationship with income level: The higher the income level, the lower the death rate. Native Americans have especially high rates. Other factors are single-parent families, teenage mothers, multiple providers, family stress, and multiple siblings; these are primarily a function of poverty rather than independent risk factors.

ENVIRONMENT. Poverty increases the risk of injury to children, at least in part through its effect on the environment. Children who are poor are at increased risk of injury because they are exposed to more hazards in their living environments. For example, they may live in poor housing, which is more likely to be dilapidated and less likely to be protected by smoke detectors. The roads in their neighborhoods are more likely to be major thoroughfares. Their neighborhoods are more likely to

experience higher levels of violence, and they are more likely to be victims of assault than are children and adolescents living in middle-class suburbs. The focus on the environment is also important because it directs attention away from relatively immutable factors, such as family dynamics, poverty, and race, and directs efforts toward factors that can be changed through interventions.

Motor Vehicle Injuries. Motor vehicle injuries are the leading cause of serious and fatal injuries for individuals of all ages. Among adolescents, motor vehicle crashes alone account for 38% of *all* deaths, including deaths from natural causes. Large and sustained reductions in motor vehicle crash injuries can be accomplished by identifiable interventions.

OCCUPANTS. Injuries to passenger vehicle occupants are the predominant cause of motor vehicle deaths among children and adolescents, with the exception of the 5- to 9-yr group, in whom pedestrian injuries make up the largest proportion. The peak injury and death rate for both males and females in the pediatric age group occurs between 15 and 19 yr (see Table 50–1). Proper restraint use in vehicles is the single most effective method for preventing serious or fatal injury.

Much attention has been given to child occupants younger than 4 yr of age. Use of child restraint devices can be expected to reduce fatalities by 71% and the risk of serious injuries by 67% in this age group. All 50 states and the District of Columbia have laws mandating their use. Handouts given to parents by physicians emphasizing the positive benefits of child seat restraints have been successful in improving parent acceptance. Pediatricians should point out to parents that toddlers who normally ride restrained behave better during car trips than children who ride unrestrained.

Excellent films are available that discuss the advantages of child seat restraints; these can be shown to parents in waiting rooms or mothers on postpartum hospital floors. Many hospitals and communities have adopted loan programs, renting restraints at low cost. This is especially important for low-income families, who have the lowest rate of restraint use. A list of acceptable devices is available from the American Academy of Pediatrics. Children weighing less than 20 lb may use an infant seat or be placed in a "convertible" infant-toddler child restraint device. Infants younger than 1 yr or weighing less than 20 lb should be placed in the rear seat facing backward; older toddlers and children can be placed in the rear seat in a forward-facing convertible or toddler seat. Emphasis must be given to correct use of these seats, including placing the seat in the right direction, properly routing the belt, and ensuring that the child is correctly buckled into the seat. Government regulations have made the fit between car seats and the car easier, quicker, and less prone to error. Children younger than age 13 yr should never be placed in the front seat, especially if an airbag is present. Inflating airbags can be lethal to infants in rear-facing seats and to small children in the front passenger seat.

Older children are often not adequately restrained. Many children ride in the rear seat restrained with lap belts only. Unfortunately, the use of lap belts alone has been associated with a marked rise in seatbelt-related injuries, especially fractures of the lumbar spine and hollow-viscus injuries of the abdomen. These flexion-distraction injuries of the spine are usually accompanied by injuries to the abdominal organs; the presence of cutaneous seatbelt contusions in restrained children should alert the clinician to possible abdominal or spine injury. Children should use approved booster seats until large enough to comfortably wear the belt and shoulder harness alone. This occurs when the child is approximately 8 yr old and weighs 80 lb. Shoulder straps placed behind the child or under the arm do not provide adequate crash protection and may increase the risk of serious injury.

Transportation of premature infants presents special problems. The possibility of oxygen desaturation, sometimes associated with bradycardia, among premature infants while in child seat restraints has led the American Academy of Pediatrics to make the following recommendations: monitoring of infants born at less than 37 wk of gestational age in the seat before discharge and the use of oxygen or alternative restraints for infants who experience desaturation or bradycardia, such as seats that can be reclined and used as a car bed. Monitoring in the neonatal intensive care unit should be done for 60–90 min.

Children riding in the back of pickup trucks are at special risk of injury, because of the possibility of ejection from the truck and serious head injury. Children traveling in the back of covered pickup trucks are at risk for carbon monoxide poisoning from faulty exhaust systems.

The rear seat is clearly much safer than the front seat for both children and adults. One study of children younger than the age of 15 yr found that the risk of injury in a crash was 70% lower for children in the rear seat compared with those sitting in the front seat. Frontal airbags appear to offer little protection to children in crashes as well as present a risk of serious or fatal injury from the airbag itself. The implementation of side airbags also poses a risk for children who are in the front seat and are, for example, leaning against the door at the time of a crash. The safest place for children is in the rear seat, properly restrained for their age and size. Educational and legislative interventions to increase the number of children traveling in the rear have been successful.

TEENAGE DRIVERS. Drivers aged 15–17 yr have over twice the rate of collisions than motorists 18 yr of age and older. Formal driver education courses appear to be ineffective as a primary means of decreasing these collisions, and in fact can be counterproductive by allowing younger teens to drive. Risk of serious injury and mortality is directly related to the speed at the time of the crash and inversely related to the size of the vehicle. Small, fast cars greatly increase the risk of a fatal outcome in the event of a crash.

The number of passengers traveling with teen drivers influences the risk of a crash. The risk of death for 17-yr-old drivers is 50% greater driving with one passenger compared with driving alone; this risk is 2.6-fold higher with two passengers and 3-fold higher with three or more passengers. The risk is also increased if the driver is male and if the passengers are younger than age 30 yr.

Teens driving at night are overrepresented in crashes and fatal crashes, with nighttime crashes accounting for over one third of teen motor vehicle fatalities. Almost 50% of the fatal crashes involving drivers younger than age 18 yr occur in the 4 hr before or after midnight. Teens are 5- to 10-fold more likely to be in a fatal crash while driving at night compared with driving during the day. The difficulty of driving at night combined with the inexperience of teen drivers appears to be a deadly combination.

Graduated licensing laws consist of a series of three steps over a period of time before a teen can get full, unrestricted driving privileges. These laws usually place initial restrictions on the number of passengers allowed in the vehicle and limit driving during late night hours. These laws can decrease fatal crashes of 16-yr-old drivers by as much as 50%. Graduated licensing laws have been adopted by many states.

Alcohol use is a major cause of motor vehicle trauma among adolescents. The combination of inexperience in driving and inexperience with alcohol is particularly dangerous. Approximately one fifth of all deaths from motor vehicle crashes in this age group are the result of alcohol intoxication, with impairment of driving seen at blood alcohol concentrations as low as 0.05 g/dL. More than one third of adolescents report riding with a driver who had been drinking. All states have adopted a zero tolerance policy to adolescent drinking while driving. All adolescent motor vehicle injury victims should have their blood alcohol concentration measured in the emergency department and be screened for chronic alcohol use with a standard test (the CAGE or the Short Michigan Alcohol Screening Test) to identify those with alcohol abuse problems. Individuals who have evidence of alcohol abuse should not leave the emergency department or hospital without plans for appropriate alcohol abuse treatment. Interventions for problem drinking can be effective in decreasing the risk of subsequent motor vehicle crashes. Even brief interventions in the emergency department using motivational interviewing can be successful in decreasing adolescent problem drinking.

Bicycle Injuries. Each year in the United States, 250–300 children and adolescents die of injuries incurred while riding bicycles; bicycle-related injuries are one of the most common reasons that children with trauma visit emergency departments. The majority of severe and fatal bicycle injuries involve head trauma. A logical step in the prevention of these head injuries is the use of helmets. Helmets are very effective, reducing the risk of head injury by 85% and brain injury by 88%. Helmets also protect against injuries to the mid and upper face. Pediatricians can be effective advocates for the use of bicycle helmets and should incorporate this advice into their anticipatory guidance schedules for parents and children. Appropriate helmets are those with a firm polystyrene liner that fit properly on the child's head. Parents should avoid buying a larger helmet to give the child "growing room."

Promotion of helmets can and should be extended beyond the office. Community education programs spearheaded by coalitions of physicians, educators, bicycle clubs, and community service organizations have been successful in promoting the use of bicycle helmets, resulting in helmet use rates as high as 60% with concomitant reduction in the number of head injuries. Passage of bicycle helmet laws also leads to increased helmet use.

Consideration should also be given to other types of preventive activities, although the evidence supporting their effectiveness is limited. Bicycle paths are a logical method for separating bicycles and motor vehicles. Safe bicycling training for children can be provided in the school and community.

Pedestrian Injuries. Pedestrian injuries are one of the most common causes of traumatic death for 5- to 9-yr-old children in the United States and most industrialized countries. Although case fatality rates are less than 5%, serious nonfatal injuries constitute a much larger problem. Pedestrian injuries are the most important cause of traumatic coma in children and are a frequent cause of serious lower extremity fractures, particularly in the school-aged child.

Most injuries occur during the day, with a peak in the after-school period. Improved lighting or retroreflective clothing would, therefore, be expected to prevent few injuries. Surprisingly, approximately 30% of pedestrian injuries occur while the individual is in a marked crosswalk, perhaps reflecting a false sense of security and decreased vigilance. The risk of pedestrian injury is greater in neighborhoods with high traffic volumes, speeds greater than approximately 25 mph, absence of play space adjacent to the home, household crowding, and low socioeconomic status.

One important risk factor for childhood pedestrian injuries is the developmental level of the child. Children younger than age 5 yr are at risk of being run over in the driveway. Few children younger than 9 or 10 yr have the developmental skills to successfully negotiate traffic 100% of the time. Young children have poor ability to judge the distance and speed of traffic and are easily distracted by playmates or other factors in the environment. Many parents are not aware of this potential mismatch between the abilities of the young school-aged child and the skills needed to cross streets safely.

Prevention of pedestrian injuries is difficult but should consist of a multifaceted approach. Education of the child in pedestrian safety should be initiated at an early age by the parents and continue into the school-age years. Younger children should be taught never to cross streets when alone; older children should be taught (and practice how) to negotiate quiet streets with little traffic. Major streets should not be crossed alone until the child is 10 yr of age or older.

Pedestrian skills training should constitute part of a more comprehensive pedestrian safety program in a community. Legislation and police enforcement are important components of any campaign to reduce pedestrian injuries. Right-turn-on-red laws increase the hazard to pedestrians. In many cities, few drivers stop for pedestrians in crosswalks, a special hazard for young children. Engineering changes in roadway design are extremely important as passive prevention measures. Most important are measures to slow the speed of traffic and to route traffic away from schools and residential areas. Other modifications include one-way-street networks, proper placement of transit or school bus stops, sidewalks in urban and suburban areas, edge stripping in rural areas to delineate the edge of the road, and curb parking regulations. Comprehensive traffic "calming" schemes employing these strategies have been very successful in reducing child pedestrian injuries in Sweden, the Netherlands, Germany, and increasingly in the United States.

Fire- and Burn-Related Injuries (see Chapter 62). Fire- and burn-related injuries are the fifth most common cause of unintentional injury death in the United States, with about 3,600 fire and burn deaths occurring each year. For both injuries and deaths, the first decade of life is the period of highest risk. The likelihood of burn injury is strongly related to low socioeconomic status, with highest rates among the poor, the less educated, and those living in mobile homes. Burns are much more frequent among males than females. Among children 10–14 yr of age with burns involving flammable substances, males are burned eight times more frequently than females.

One of the first effective interventions involved using non-flammable fabrics. Flame burns resulting from ignition of clothing were a common, serious burn injury, especially in small children. At least one third of those injuries involved infant sleepwear. Such burns averaged 30% of the body surface, requiring hospitalization for an average of 70 days. In 1967, the Federal Flammable Fabrics Act was passed, *requiring children's sleepwear to be flame retardant.* As a result of this and similar state legislation, clothing ignition burns in small children now account for only a small fraction of burns in children. Despite the withdrawal of tromethamine (*TRIS*)-containing clothing because of potential mutagenicity, federal flammability standards still apply to children's sleepwear. Parents should not circumvent these protective regulations by using cotton T-shirts for infant and child sleepwear.

Another hazard modification resulting in substantial reduction of injury involves *scald burns due to tap water.* Scalds account for 40% of the burn injuries in children requiring hospitalization, and a substantial proportion of these scald burns involve tap water. Scalds from hot liquids and foods are the most common reason for a burn admission to the hospital for children younger than age 5 yr. Avoiding the use of electric kettles or frying pans with long cords, not using baby walkers, not drinking hot tea or coffee while holding an infant, and keeping children away from pots cooking on the stove will help to prevent many of these injuries. Unlike those with flame burns, children with scalds generally do not die; however, many children have long hospitalizations, multiple surgical procedures, and severe disfigurement. The risk of full-thickness burns increases geometrically at water temperatures above 125°F. At 150°F, a full-thickness burn will be produced in adult skin in 2 sec. A simple and effective preventive maneuver is to lower the water heater temperature to 125°F (51.6°C). At this setting, dishwashers and washing machines operate effectively, but the risk of serious scald injury is greatly reduced. In many cities, the local power company will turn down the temperature without charge. In 1980, Florida became the first state requiring new water heaters to be preset at a temperature of 125°F.

Fireworks are a seasonal injury, and over 40% of those injured by fireworks are children younger than 15 yr of age. Community restrictions on certain types of fireworks and adult supervision of use of all fireworks have been effective in decreasing burns, amputations, and ocular injuries caused by these devices. Further product modification promises to decrease the hazards associated with certain easy-to-use cigarette lighters commonly found in the home.

Over 80% of all fire deaths in the United States occur in private dwellings. Of these deaths, 60% are caused by smoke asphyxiation and *not* flame burns. *Smoke detectors* are an inexpensive but effective method of preventing the majority of these deaths. Physicians can alter parental behavior and increase smoke detector use by offering information on smoke detectors in their offices.

Cigarettes are estimated to cause 45% of all fires and 22–56% of deaths from house fires. The combination of smoking and alcohol use appears to be particularly lethal. Most cigarettes made in the United States contain additives in both the paper and the tobacco that allow them to burn for as long as 28 min, even if left unattended. If *fire-safe* or *self-extinguishing cigarettes* replaced present types, nearly 2,000 deaths and more than 6,000 burns would be prevented annually.

Some burns result from fire setting by children or adolescents. In young children, this usually represents exploratory play. However, such behavior in older children and adolescents may signify a serious conduct disorder and warrants careful psychiatric and family evaluation. More than half of adolescent fire-setters will be involved in repeat incidents.

Poisoning (see Chapter 704). Deaths by unintentional poisonings among children have decreased dramatically over the past 2 decades, particularly among children younger than 5 yr of age. In 1970, 226 poisoning deaths of children younger than age 5 yr occurred, compared with only 46 in 1999. Poisoning prevention represents the effectiveness of passive strategies—child-resistant packaging and dose limits per container. The Poison Packaging Prevention Act currently includes 28 categories of household products and drugs. This law has been remarkably effective in reducing poisoning deaths and hospitalizations. However, compliance with the law by pharmacists is only 70–75% at present, indicating that physicians should always specify on prescription pads that prescriptions be dispensed in child-resistant containers. In addition, difficulty using child-resistant containers by adults is an important cause of poisoning in young children today. A survey by the Centers for Disease Control and Prevention found that 18.5% of households in which poisoning occurred to children younger than 5 yr of age had replaced the child-resistant closure and 65% of the ones used did not work properly. Nearly 20% of ingestions occur from drugs owned by grandparents, a group that has difficulty using traditional child-resistant containers. There is a need for better child-resistant closures that do not require manual dexterity or strength greater than the capabilities of older adults.

Other poisoning interventions, such as "Mr. Yuk" stickers, are far less effective. They do not deter young children from ingesting labeled medications and may in fact be attractive to children younger than 3 yr of age. The most important feature of the Mr. Yuk sticker is the phone number of the local or regional poison control center. Parents of toddlers should also be given a bottle of syrup of ipecac to store in the medicine chest. In the case of ingestion, they should be instructed to call the regional poison control center or pediatrician before administering ipecac.

Drowning (see Chapter 61). In 1999, 1,286 drownings, primarily associated with recreational activities, occurred in children and adolescents in the United States. In young children, drowning ranks second only to motor vehicle injury as a cause of traumatic death. Although no precise data exist on the number of nonfatal water-related injuries, it is estimated that 140,000 occur annually from swimming activities alone. Diving headfirst into shallow water accounts for the most serious aquatic injuries because of spinal cord damage. Of the estimated 700 spinal cord injuries resulting from aquatic activities each year, the majority result in permanent paralysis.

The proportion of drowning deaths occurring in pools varies by region of the country. In Los Angeles, half of all drowning takes place in residential pools, a rate similar to that in other areas with large numbers of pools. Children younger than the age of 5 yr do not understand the consequences of falling into deep water and usually do not call for help. A majority of child victims drown during lapses in adult supervision. Clearly, the most effective way to prevent childhood pool drowning is through circumferential *fencing*. To give the greatest protection, these barriers should restrict entry to the pool from the yard and residence, use self-closing and self-latching gates, be at least 5 ft high, and have no vertical openings more than 4 inches wide. Ordinances to require appropriate fencing have been demonstrated to be effective. Many people have advocated "water-babies" and other swimming instruction for young children. The efficacy of such techniques is untested. The potential exists for both parent and child to become less vigilant around water, possibly with tragic consequences.

Among adolescents and young adults, alcohol and drug use has been found to be involved in nearly 50% of all drowning deaths. The risk of drowning while boating is increased 10- to 50-fold with alcohol intoxication, both related to the risk of falling overboard and to the increased risk of drowning if drunk while submerged. The *restriction of the sale and consumption of alcoholic beverages* in boating, pool, harbor, marina, and beach areas may combat this dangerous combination of activities. More restrictive licensing of boat owners should also be considered.

Personal flotation devices are thought to be an important device to protect children against drowning. Although the exact protective effect of personal flotation devices (PFDs) is unknown, a study by the U.S. Coast Guard showed that although only 7% of boats involved in mishaps lacked available PFDs, they accounted for 29% of boating fatalities. All children and adolescents should wear a PFD when boating in open water.

The risk of bathtub drowning is markedly increased in children with a seizure disorder, including older children and adolescents. These patients should be instructed to shower instead of using a bathtub.

Firearm Injuries. Injuries to children and adolescents involving firearms occur in three different situations: unintentional injury, suicide attempt, and assault. In each case, the injury induced may be fatal or may result in permanent sequelae.

Unintentional firearm injuries generally occur in a family dwelling; 85% of firearm deaths occur in the home. In gunshot fatalities to children younger than 16 yr of age, poverty is more closely related to shooting deaths than is race or population density. Urban whites have the lowest death rate, rural whites are intermediate, and urban African-American children have the highest fatality rate.

Suicide is the third most common cause of trauma death in teenage males and the fourth for females. During the period from the 1950s to 1970, suicide rates for children and adolescents more than doubled; suicide rates peaked in about 1986 and have decreased since. Rates in 1999 were 13% lower than the peak in 1986. Firearms have played an important role in this increase and are the most common means of suicide in males of all ages. The difference in the rate of suicide between males and females is related less to number of attempts than to the method. Women die less often in suicide attempts because they use less lethal means (mainly drugs) and perhaps have a lower degree of intent. The use of firearms in a suicidal act usually converts an attempt into a fatality.

Homicides are second only to motor vehicle crashes among causes of death in teenagers older than the age of 15 yr. In 1999, 2,546 children and adolescents were homicide victims; nonwhite teenagers accounted for 51.5% of the total, making homicides the most common cause of death among nonwhite teenagers. At present, 85% of homicides among males involve firearms, 75% of which are handguns.

In the United States today, there are an estimated 210 million to 220 million firearms. During the past 2 decades, over 6 million firearms were sold in the United States each year. Handguns account for approximately 20% of the firearms in use today, yet they are involved in 90% of criminal and other firearm misuse. Home ownership of guns increases the risk of adolescent suicide 10-fold and adolescent homicide 4-fold. In homes with guns, the risk to the occupants is far greater than the chance the gun will be used against an intruder; for every death occurring in self-defense, there may be 1.3 unintentional deaths, 4.6 homicides, and 37 suicides.

Handguns pose the greatest risk to children and adolescents of all firearms. Access to handguns by adolescents is surprisingly common and is not restricted to those involved in gang or criminal activity. Stricter regulation of handgun access by youth, rather than all firearms, would appear to be the most appropriate focus of efforts to reduce shooting injuries in children and adolescents.

One approach is information and education campaigns in firearm safety with a particular focus on reducing access by locking and unloading household guns. No data yet exist to support the effectiveness of such programs in decreasing the number of gunshot wounds in children. Safety education alone is also unlikely to have an effect on the use of firearms in homicides and suicides. Most homicides are between relatives or acquaintances and are acts of rage. Elimination of these weapons from the environment of children and adolescents is the key to reduction in firearm fatalities and injuries. Decreasing access to handguns would certainly not eliminate arguments, but it would decrease the likelihood of a fatal conclusion. In an assault, the chance of death is five times greater with a firearm than with a knife.

Physicians have a responsibility to counsel parents and patients about firearm ownership. This should include information informing them of the risks associated with owning a handgun, the risk of gun injury to all members of the household, and the special risks to adolescent males and teens with mental health conditions and alcoholism. Parents should be counseled that the safest approach is to remove the firearm from the household. If the family chooses to keep the gun, parents should be advised to store the gun in a locked container or with a trigger lock, with ammunition stored separately. Further educational information for pediatricians on counseling families and adolescents about guns can be obtained from the American Academy of Pediatrics.

American Academy of Pediatrics Committee on Injury Prevention and Poison Prevention: *Injury Prevention and Control for Children and Youth*, 3rd ed. Elk Grove Village, IL, American Academy of Pediatrics, 1997.

American Academy of Pediatrics Committee on Injury and Poison Prevention: Children in pickup trucks. *Pediatrics* 2000;106:857–9.

Asher KN, Rivara FP, Felix D, et al: Water safety training as a potential means of reducing the risk of young children's drowning. *Injury Prev* 1995;1:228–33.

Baker S, Fowler C, Li G, et al: Head injuries incurred by children and young adults during informal recreation. *Am J Public Health* 1994;84:649–52.

Barrios LC, Davis MK, Kann L, et al: School health guidelines to prevent unintentional injuries and violence. *MMWR Morbid Mortal Wkly Rep* 2001;50(Dec 7):1–73.

Braver ER, Ferguson SA, Greene MA, et al: Reduction in deaths in frontal crashes among right front passengers in vehicles equipped with passenger air bags. *JAMA* 1997;278:1437–9.

Bull MJ, Sheese J: Update for the pediatrician on child passenger safety: Five principles for safer travel. *Pediatrics* 2000;106:1113–16.

Chiavello C, Christoph R, Bond G: Infant walker related injuries: A prospective study of severity and incidence. *Pediatrics* 1994;93:974–76.

Committee on Injury Prevention and Poison Prevention Committee on Community Health Services: Prevention of agricultural injuries among children and adolescents. *Pediatrics* 2001;108:1016–19.

Committee on Sports Medicine and Fitness and Committee on Injury and Poison Prevention, American Academy of Pediatrics: Swimming programs for infants and toddlers. *Pediatrics* 2000;105:868–70.

Coyne-Beasley T, Schoenbach VJ, Johnson RM: "Love our kids, lock your guns": A community-based firearm safety counseling and gun lock distribution program. *Arch Pediatr Adolesc Med* 2001;155:659–64.

Cummings P, Grossman DC, Rivara FP, et al: State gun safe storage laws and child mortality due to firearms. *JAMA* 1997;278:1084–86.

Davidson L, Durkin M, Kuhn L, et al: The impact of the Safe Kids/Healthy Neighborhood Injury Prevention Project in Harlem, 1988 through 1991. *Am J Public Health* 1994;84:580–86.

Foss RD, Feaganes JR, Rodgman EA: Initial effects of graduated driver licensing on 16-year-old driver crashes in North Carolina. *JAMA* 2001;286:1588–92.

Grossman DC, Mang K, Rivara FP: Firearm injury prevention counseling by pediatricians and family physicians: Practices and beliefs. *Arch Pediatr Adolesc Med* 1995;149:973–77.

Harborview Injury Prevention and Research Center: Reviews of child injury prevention strategies. http://www.hiprc.org/childinjury.

Kassirer JP: Guns in the household. *N Engl J Med* 1993;329:1117–19.

Kellermann AL, Somes G, et al: Suicide in the home in relation to gun ownership. *N Engl J Med* 1992;327:467–72.

Kellermann AL, Rivara FP, Rushforth NB, et al: Gun ownership as a risk factor for homicide in the home. *N Engl J Med* 1993;329:1084–91.

Laflamme L, Eilert-Petersson E: Injuries to pre-school children in a home setting: Patterns and related products. *Acta Paediatr* 1998;87:206–11.

Laraque D, Spivak H, Bull M: Serious firearm injury prevention does make sense. *Pediatrics* 2001;107:408–10.

Mallonee S, Istre GR, Rosenberg M: Surveillance and prevention of residential fire injuries. *N Engl J Med* 1996;335:27–31.

Monti PM, Colby SM, Barnett NP, et al: Brief intervention for harm reduction with alcohol-positive older adolescents in a hospital emergency department. *J Consult Clin Psychol* 1999;67:989–94.

Rivara FP, Thompson DC, Patterson MQ, et al: Prevention of bicycle-related injuries: Helmets, education, and legislation. *Ann Rev Public Health* 1998;19:293–318.

Roberts I, Ashton T, Dunn R, Lee-Joe T: Preventing child pedestrian injury: Pedestrian education or traffic calming? *Aust J Public Health* 1994;18:209–12.

Shope JT, Molnar LJ, Elliott MR, et al: Graduated driver licensing in Michigan. *JAMA* 2001;286:1593–98.

Task Force on Community Preventive Services. Motor vehicle occupant injury: Strategies for increasing use of child safety seats, increasing use of safety belts, and reducing alcohol-impaired driving. *MMWR Morbid Mortal Wkly Rep* 2001;50 (May 18).

Thompson DC, Nunn ME, Thompson RS, et al: Effectiveness of bicycle helmets in preventing serious facial injury. *JAMA* 1996;276:1974–75.

Winston FK, Durbin DR, Kallan MJ, et al: The danger of premature graduation to seat belts for young children. *Pediatrics* 2000; 105:1179–83.

Winston FK, Kallan MJ, Elliott MR, et al: Risk injury to child passengers in compact extended-cab pickup trucks. *JAMA* 2002;287:1147–52.

Chapter 51
Emergency Medical Services for Children

M. Denise Dowd and Frederick P. Rivara

Most children who require emergency medical care present to physicians' offices, clinics, and community emergency departments (EDs) and not to specialized pediatric EDs. This requires a community-based approach to emergency care of the child. Emergency medical services for children (EMS-C) is a concept that embodies a continuum of care and encompasses prevention, prehospital care and transport, ED and inpatient care, and necessary follow-up, including rehabilitation (Fig. 51–1).

The Role of the Primary Care Physician. The primary care physician (PCP) has multiple important roles in EMS-C. As *educator*, the PCP's primary goal is prevention. By providing anticipatory guidance, the provider can help shape the attitudes, knowledge, and behaviors of parent and child with the goal of preventing acute medical events such as injury or status asthmaticus and managing them should they occur. As *triage officer*, the PCP receives calls that necessitate directing families to the appropriate site for emergency care. The PCP will frequently serve the role of *emergency care provider* and as such must be prepared (in terms of education, equipment, and policies) to deliver initial emergency care for common problems. Because the majority of children are not treated in a children's hospital ED but are treated in general community hospital EDs or urgent care centers, pediatricians should be *consultants* to these facilities and assist them in planning and delivering high-quality pediatric emergency care. Only 10% of ambulance calls are for pediatric patients; EMS providers may lack training and experience in caring for children; policies or procedures for caring for children may not exist or may be outdated. The pediatrician can be an *advocate* for integrating pediatric emergency care within the existing local EMS system.

Office Preparedness. Providing anticipatory guidance to families regarding injury prevention, prompt recognition and treatment

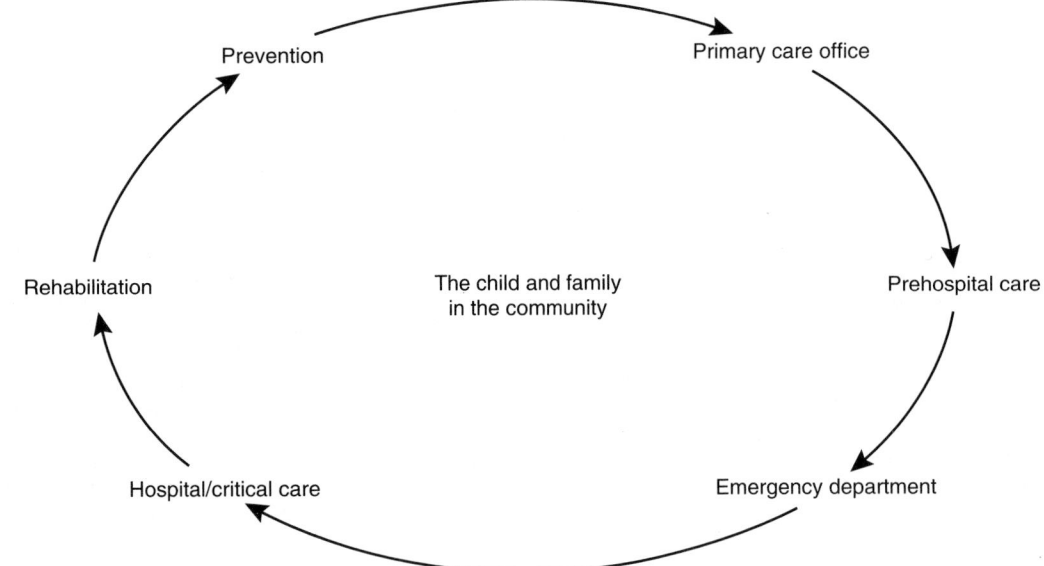

FIGURE 51–1. The EMS-C continuum of care: Seriously ill and injured children interface with a large number of health care personnel as they move through the EMS-C system. The system both begins and ends in the community.

of illness, and accessing emergency care are important roles for the PCP. These may involve providing written materials and developmentally appropriate counseling. Parents and other adult caretakers of medically fragile children should consider learning CPR, and children can be taught to access 911. In addition to teaching the family how to prevent and manage emergencies, the PCP's office should be prepared to handle the medical emergencies that will inevitably present there.

Although the need for full CPR occurs relatively infrequently in an office setting, most practices see children in need of acute intervention or hospitalization on a regular basis. Primary care providers and their staffs may find themselves ill equipped to treat patients with impending shock, respiratory failure, or a seizure in an examination room or for patients whose condition deteriorates while waiting to be seen. Emergency preparedness in the office requires training and continuing education for staff members, policies and procedures for emergency intervention, ready availability of appropriate resuscitation equipment, knowledge of local resources for EMS response and transport, and a working relationship with area EDs to ensure that children are cared for in facilities with expertise in pediatric emergency care.

STAFF TRAINING AND CONTINUING EDUCATION. Initial recognition by an office staff member that a child requires emergency treatment may occur in the course of a telephone call, in the waiting room, or in an examination room. All office personnel, including those seated at the front desk, must be capable of recognizing a child with altered mental status, shock, or respiratory distress/failure and must be aware of an appropriate action plan for rapid intervention.

It is a reasonable expectation that all office staff, including receptionists and medical assistants, be trained in adult and child CPR and first aid and that they maintain their certification on an annual basis. In addition to these requirements, nurses and physicians should have training in a systematic approach to pediatric medical and trauma resuscitation. Core knowledge may be obtained through standardized courses in pediatric advanced life support (ALS) offered by national medical and nursing associations. Frequent recertification is important for maintaining knowledge and skill. Examples of such curricula include the American Heart Association's Pediatric Advanced Life Support (PALS) course, the Advanced Pediatric Life Support (APLS) course sponsored by the American Academy of Pediatrics and the American College of Emergency Physicians, and the Emergency Nurses Pediatric Course (ENPC), the Neonatal Resuscitation Program (NRP), and Pediatric Emergency Nursing self-instruction manual sponsored by the Emergency Nurses Association.

POLICIES AND PROCEDURES. Standardized protocols for telephone triage of seriously ill or injured children are essential, especially if nonphysician personnel take after-hours calls. When a child's status is in question and prehospital care is available, ambulance transport in the care of trained personnel is always preferable to transport by private car. This avoids the potentially serious medical consequences of relying on unskilled and distraught parents without the ability to provide even basic life support (BLS) measures to transport an unstable child to an ED. Written office policies and procedures for the management of status asthmaticus, upper airway obstruction, seizures, ingestions, shock, sepsis/meningitis, trauma, head injury, anaphylaxis, and cardiopulmonary arrest should be generated and made available to all potentially involved staff members.

RESUSCITATION EQUIPMENT. Availability of necessary equipment is a vital part of an emergency response. Every physician's office should have essential resuscitation equipment and medications packaged in a pediatric resuscitation cart or kit (Table 51–1). This kit should be checked on a regular basis and kept in an accessible location known to all office staff. Outdated medications, a laryngoscope with a failed light source, or an

TABLE 51–1. Office Emergency Drugs and Supplies

	Priority
Drugs	
Albuterol for inhalation	E
Epinephrine (1:1000)	E
Activated charcoal	S
Antibiotics	S
Anticonvulsants (diazepam/lorazepam)	S
Corticosteroids (parenteral/oral)	S
Dextrose (25%)	S
Diphenhydramine (parenteral)	S
Epinephrine (1:10,000)	S
Atropine sulfate (0.1 mg/mL)	O
Ipecac	O
Naloxone (0.4 mg/mL)	O
Sodium bicarbonate (4.2%)	O
IV Fluids:	
Normal saline or lactated Ringer's (500-mL bags)	O
5% Dextrose, 0.45 NS (500-mL bags)	O
Airway	
Oxygen and delivery system	E
Bag-valve-mask (450 mL and 1,000 mL)	E
Clear oxygen masks, breather and non-rebreather, with reservoirs	E
Suction device, tonsil tip, bulb syringe	E
Peak flowmeter	E
Nebulizer (or metered-dose inhaler with spacer/mask)	E
Oral airways (sizes 00–5)	E
Nasal airways (sizes 12–30F)	S
Magill forceps (pediatric, adult)	S
Suction catheters (sizes 5–14F)	S
Nasogastric tubes (sizes 6–14F)	S
Pulse oximeter	S
Laryngoscope handle (pediatric, adult) with extra batteries, bulbs	S
Laryngoscope blades (straight 0–4; curved 2–3)	S
Endotracheal tubes (uncuffed 2.5–5.5; cuffed 6.0–8.0)	S
Stylets (pediatric, adult)	S
Fluid Management	
Butterfly needles (19–25 gauge)	S
Catheter-over-needle device (14–24 gauge)	S
Armboards, tape, tourniquet	S
Intraosseous needles (16, 18 gauge)	S
Intravenous tubing, microdrip	S
Miscellaneous Equipment and Supplies	
Color-coded tape or preprinted drug doses	E
Cardiac arrest board/backboard	E
Sphygmomanometer (infant, child, adult, thigh cuffs)	E
Splints, sterile dressings	E
Spot glucose test	S
Stiff neck collars (small/large)	S

E = essential; S = suggested; O = optional.

empty oxygen tank represents a catastrophe in a resuscitation setting; these can be easily avoided if an equipment checklist and maintenance schedule are implemented. Responsible staff should receive routinely scheduled in-service training on equipment location and use, a task that may best be accomplished by a regular schedule of "mock codes" in which all office staff participate. A pediatric kit that includes posters, laminated cards, or resuscitation tapes specifying emergency drug doses and equipment size by age, weight, or height is invaluable in avoiding critical therapeutic errors during resuscitation.

To facilitate emergency response when a child needs rapid intervention in the office, all personnel should have a preassigned role. Organizing a "code team" within the office ensures that necessary equipment is made available to the physician in charge, that an appropriate medical record detailing all interventions and the child's response is generated, and that the call for EMS response or a transport team is made in a timely fashion.

TRANSPORT. A decision must be made on how to transport a child to a facility capable of providing definitive care once the child has been stabilized. If a child has required an artificial airway or cardiovascular support, has altered mental status, continues to have unstable vital signs, or has significant potential to deteriorate en route, it is not appropriate to send the child via private car, regardless of proximity to a hospital. Even when an ambulance is called, it is the primary care provider's responsibility to initiate essential life support measures and attempt to stabilize the child before transport.

In metropolitan centers with numerous public and private ambulance agencies, primary care providers must be knowledgeable about the level of service that is provided by each. The availability of basic life support (BLS) versus advanced life support (ALS) services, transport team configuration, and pediatric expertise vary markedly among agencies. It may be appropriate to consider aeromedical transport when definitive or specialized care is not available within a community or when ground transport times are prolonged. In that case, initial transport via ground to a local hospital for interval stabilization may be undertaken pending arrival of the aeromedical team. When a child is to be transported by air or ground, copies of the child's pertinent medical records as well as any radiologic studies or laboratory results should be sent with the patient (Box 51–1) and a call made to the physicians at the receiving facility to alert them to the referral and any treatments administered. Such prenotification is not merely a courtesy; direct physician-to-physician communication is essential to ensure adequate transmission of patient care information, to allow mobilization of necessary resources in the ED, and to redirect the transport if the emergency physician believes that the child would be better treated at a facility with specialized services. The referring physician is legally responsible for patient safety until the patient's care is taken over by the accepting physician.

Pediatric Prehospital Care. Prehospital care refers to emergency assistance rendered by trained emergency medical personnel before a child reaches a treating medical facility. Although most communities in the United States have a formalized EMS system, the nature of the emergency medical response depends in part on local demographics and population base. EMS may be provided by volunteers or paid professionals. Key points to recognize in considering the interface between the community physician and the local EMS system include access to the system, provider capability, response/transport times, and destination.

ACCESS TO THE EMS SYSTEM. Most metropolitan and many rural communities in the United States have a "911" telephone system that provides direct access to a dispatcher who coordinates police, fire, and EMS response. Some communities have an "enhanced 911" system, in which the location of the caller is automatically provided to the dispatcher, permitting emergency response even if the caller, such as a young child, cannot give an address. The extent of medical training for these dispatchers varies between communities, as do the protocols by which they assign an emergency response. In some smaller communities, no coordinated dispatch exists and emergency medical calls are handled by the local law enforcement agency.

In activating the 911 system, it is important for physicians to make it clear to the dispatcher the nature of the medical emergency and the condition of the child. In many communities, dispatchers are trained to ask a series of questions per protocol, allowing them to send out EMS personnel of an appropriate level of training.

PROVIDER CAPABILITY. There are many levels of training for prehospital EMS providers, ranging from individuals capable of providing only first aid to those trained and licensed to provide ALS in the field. EMS personnel, whether EMT or paramedic, all receive training in pediatric emergencies; however, pediatric cases actually constitute a minority (approximately 10%) of all EMS cases.

First responders may be law enforcement officers, firefighters, or community volunteers who are dispatched to provide emergency medical assistance. They have approximately 40 hr of training in first aid and CPR. Their role is to provide rapid response and stabilization pending the arrival of more highly trained personnel. In some smaller communities, this represents the only prehospital emergency medical response available.

Emergency medical technicians (EMTs) are volunteers or paid professionals who provide the bulk of emergency medical response in the United States. Basic EMTs may staff an ambulance after undergoing an approximately 100-hr training program. They are licensed to provide BLS services but may receive further training to expand their scope of practice to intravenous catheter placement and fluid administration, endotracheal intubation, and use of an automatic external defibrillator, under the direction of a physician advisor.

Paramedics, or EMT-Ps, represent the highest level of EMT response, with medical training and supervised field experience of approximately 1,000 hours. They provide ALS services in the prehospital setting, functioning out of an ambulance equipped as a mobile intensive care unit. Paramedic skills may include endotracheal intubation; the placement of peripheral, central, or intraosseous lines; intravenous administration of drugs; administration of nebulized aerosols; needle thoracotomy; and cardioversion/defibrillation. Paramedics work under the supervision of a physician advisor.

Aeromedical transport team configuration can vary widely and may include physicians, nurses, respiratory therapists, or paramedics. The amount of pediatric training of team members also varies, and it is important to confirm that an appropriate standard of care can be provided during interfacility transport.

The level of training of the prehospital personnel dispatched to the scene of a medical emergency depends on the condition of the patient, available resources, and local protocols. It is important to realize that attention has only recently been focused on *pediatric* prehospital care. Training and equipment for pediatric emergency care have historically been given inadequate attention in national certification curricula and by EMS agencies primarily geared toward adult patients. In some communities, the standard of pediatric prehospital care may not match that offered to adult patients in similar condition. The EMS-C initiative sponsored by the Maternal and Child Health Bureau, U.S. Department of Health and Human Services, has provided program development grants to improve pediatric emergency services in all 50 states. This has led to increased awareness of the special needs of acutely ill and injured children and to the development of many programs and products to enhance their care.

RESPONSE/TRANSPORT TIMES. Depending on the demographics of a community, the location of the incident, and the nature of the EMS available, EMS response times after a call for assistance may range from a few minutes to longer than an hour. Unfortunately, even in communities with relatively rapid response times, individuals may be reluctant to call for help because of a misperception that the 911 system should be activated only for full resuscitations. If a child is physiologically unstable (with marked respiratory distress, cyanosis, signs of early shock, or altered mental status) or has significant potential to deteriorate en route to the ED, or if the parents' ability to comply promptly with recommendations for ED evaluation is in

---

■ **BOX 51–1. Checklist for Patient Transport**

1. Obtain written consent for transfer from the patient's parent or guardian.
2. Call receiving physician and document acceptance of transfer on the appropriate form and patient's medical record, including name of accepting physician and time of acceptance.
3. Call and give report to appropriate transport agency.
4. Copy the medical record, including transport consent forms.
5. Copy all diagnostic tests, including radiograph copies.
6. Document name of transport agency and the time at which the transport occurred.

question, an EMS transport should be initiated. Inherent dangers lie in the attitude that a parent can get to the hospital faster by private car.

DESTINATION. The destination to which a pediatric patient is transported may be defined by parental preference, provider preference, or agency protocol. In communities with an organized trauma system or a system of pediatric designation based on objective capabilities of the area hospitals, seriously ill or injured children may be triaged by protocol to the highest-level center reachable within a reasonable amount of time. The Pediatric Trauma Score (PTS) or Revised Trauma Score (RTS) (see Chapter 57.8) can be used to assess the severity of injury. Children with a PTS less than 8 or an RTS less than 11 should be treated in a designated trauma center. In communities that do not have a hospital with the equipment and personnel resources to provide definitive inpatient care, interfacility transport of a child to a regional center should be undertaken after initial stabilization. The primary care provider may be involved in this decision-making process and must make a critical assessment of the local hospital's capabilities. When interfacility transport is to be undertaken, indications for transfer, parental consent for transfer, and acceptance of the patient by the receiving physician all must be clearly documented in the medical record.

The Emergency Department. The ability of hospital emergency departments to respond to the emergency care of children varies and depends on a number of factors, including available equipment and supplies, training and experience of the staff, and availability of pediatric subspecialties. The majority of children who require emergency care are evaluated in community hospitals by physicians or other health care providers with variable degrees of pediatric training and experience. Children account for 25–30% of all ED visits, but only a fraction of them represent true emergencies. Because the volume of critical pediatric cases is low, emergency physicians and nurses working in community hospitals often have limited opportunities to reinforce their knowledge and skills in pediatric resuscitation. Pediatricians from the community may be consulted when a seriously ill or injured child presents to the ED and should have a structured approach to initial evaluation and treatment in an unstable child of any age, regardless of the underlying diagnosis. Early recognition of life-threatening abnormalities in oxygenation, ventilation, perfusion, and central nervous system (CNS) function and rapid intervention to correct those abnormalities are key to successful pediatric resuscitation.

Because not all EDs are equally capable of treating an ill or injured child, it is the responsibility of the referring physician to be aware of the pediatric capabilities of hospitals in the area. Critically ill and injured patients have an improved outcome when cared for in regional referral centers. This is particularly true for neonatal emergencies, major trauma, burns, head injuries, and specific pediatric surgical problems. Thus, although initial stabilization of these patients may take place in a local community hospital, definitive and long-term care should be delivered in major referral centers especially equipped to provide such care.

Minimal standards must be met by community emergency departments to ensure that children receive the best emergency care possible. Guidelines for care of children in the ED have been published and are endorsed by both the American Academy of Pediatrics (AAP) and the American College of Emergency Physicians (ACEP). These guidelines provide current information on policies, procedures, protocols, quality assurance methods, and equipment and supplies considered essential for managing pediatric emergencies. Specific recommendations on equipment, supplies, and medications for the ED are listed and updates are available on both the AAP and ACEP websites. A list of sample policies and protocols for EDs that care for the ill or injured child are given in Box 51–2.

BOX 51–2. Pediatric Specific Policies and Protocols for the Community Emergency Department

Triage and initial assessment
Child safety
Suspected child abuse or neglect
Family violence
Consent for treatment
Emancipated minors
Sedation and analgesia
Transfer to a higher level of pediatric care
Telephone consultation with pediatric subspecialists
Do not resuscitate (DNR)
Death of a child
Sudden infant death and apparent life-threatening event (ALTE)
Daily verification of location and functioning of pediatric equipment and supplies
Immunizations
Parental presence during procedures
Ground and air transport procedures

Although secondary to an ED staffed by individuals skilled in the emergency care of children, the environment of the ED treating children must be respectful of the needs and expectations of children and their families. A child-safe emergency department is the first priority. Wires and sharps boxes in examination rooms should be out of reach; waste containers should be covered, tall, and stable; and electrical sockets should be covered. Within practical limits the child must be separated from the frightening sights and sounds that are so common in EDs. Examples of ways to meet this goal are (1) a separate ambulance entrance, (2) resuscitation rooms that are private, (3) "quiet rooms" for upset family members, and (4) soundproof procedure rooms. Distraction and entertainment go a long way for the child and the family waiting for or undergoing treatment in an ED. Televisions with VCRs, game boards, interactive toys, and crafts can be considered essential tools of the emergency care of the child. Not only are these techniques comforting to the child and family but also helpful to the practitioner attempting to assess the child. The examination of the calm child is much more reliable than the examination of a frightened, crying child.

The way in which a family supports a child during a crisis is critical in the recovery. Surveys of parents have indicated that the majority of parents want to be with their child during invasive procedures and even resuscitation. This has been shown to reduce parental and patient anxiety and does not interfere with the procedure.

The Community

SCHOOLS. Because children spend a great deal of time in schools, schools must be prepared to attend to emergency needs of normally healthy children as well as children with special health care needs. In 1990, as a result of passage of the Individuals with Disabilities Education Act, more chronically ill and technologically dependent children attend regular school and thus the need for preparation to deal with acute medical problems has increased. Guidelines for emergency medical care in schools have been published by the AAP and include suggested procedures, staff and staff training, documentation, and parental notification.

The range of pediatric emergencies taking place in schools is wide and includes acute emotional/behavioral events (suicide), exacerbation of chronic disease (asthma), injuries, and disclosure of child abuse. School nurses may not be available to assist in the handling of such emergencies, requiring faculty to be prepared to do so. Key factors determining a school's ability to respond to medical emergencies include comprehensive written policies for managing an emergency; basic emergency supplies kit; training of all school personnel required to respond to an emergency in CPR and basic first aid; familiarity and collaborative relationships with local EMS providers and EDs; communication with parents and caretakers concerning the medical needs of their children; and incorporation of injury prevention and basic first aid training activities into the educational curriculum.

DISASTER PREPAREDNESS. Natural and man-made disasters are unfortunate but not uncommon events that affect children and their families. Children's medical and emotional needs should be addressed specifically in any community's disaster plan. Child health specialists can participate in all areas of the EMS-C response to disaster, including planning, acute management, and aftermath activities. Critical elements of a comprehensive disaster plan are guidelines for plan activation; use of space and procurement of extra supplies; security; delineation of responsibilities of key personnel; notification of key personnel; care and transfer of nondisaster patients; care of the deceased; critical incident stress debriefing measures; and plans for disaster drills. Response to threats of bioterrorism is addressed in Chapter 706.

Legal Aspects of EMS-C. The physician treating the child for any emergency condition must be aware of the legal aspects of providing such care. There are numerous federal, state, and local laws with which the physician should become familiar, including issues pertaining to consent, requirements of the Emergency Medical Treatment and Active Labor Act (EMTALA), Good Samaritan laws, and child protection issues.

Written policies that conform to local and state laws regarding consent to treat minors should be developed for all practice settings in which children are treated. Parental consent for medical treatment of a minor is required before treatment, however; physicians may proceed with treatment without consent in the event that a delay would endanger the well-being of the child. The definition of which emergencies fit this category varies among jurisdictions and does not merely include life- or limb-threatening events. If parents or legal guardians are not available to give consent, every attempt must be made to reach them and those attempts documented in the child's chart.

In all 50 states physicians are mandated to report suspected child abuse to the local child protection service (CPS) by state law. Penalties for failure to report vary from state to state but may involve criminal action and substantial fines. Most states provide immunity from civil or criminal litigation if the report was made in good faith. Definitions of abuse and neglect and procedures to report vary from state to state (see Chapter 35).

The Emergency Medical Treatment and Active Labor Act (EMTALA) was enacted by Congress in 1986, and its purpose is to address the concern that hospital EDs were turning away or inappropriately transferring uninsured patients ("patient dumping"). This law applies to hospitals with EDs that participate in Medicare or Medicaid and to individual physicians practicing in those hospitals. There are three requirements of EMTALA:

1. The hospital must provide an appropriate medical screening to assess if the patient has an emergency medical condition.

2. If an emergency condition exists, the patient's condition must be stabilized, or if such measures exceed the hospital's expertise, the patient must be transferred to a hospital capable of stabilization. This aspect of the law applies to any pediatrician who is on call for consultation to the ED.

3. A hospital may transfer an unstable patient only under limited circumstances. Failure to follow EMTALA requirements can result in penalties imposed by the federal authorities.

Good Samaritan laws vary from state to state and are designed to protect individuals rendering emergency assistance at the scene of an emergency. Good Samaritan laws only apply if the physician providing care did not have pre-existing duty to render care. In general these laws will not protect against acts of gross negligence. Some state laws protect only physicians who are licensed in the state where the emergency aid is given. Good Samaritan laws do not apply when giving voluntary medical assistance in air emergencies. Of related importance,

medical kits aboard airplanes are not currently required to carry pediatric equipment.

Psychosocial Aspects of EMS-C. Emergencies involving children are undoubtedly stressful for the child, the parent, and the EMS-C providers. The health care system must be responsive to the emotional and mental health needs of all involved. Parents should be given the opportunity to be with their child in the ED during procedures and even resuscitation and must be involved in decision making. The attitude of the individual communicating with families and the clarity of the information given are crucial to families, especially when the news is bad. Verbal information should be accompanied by written plans and instructions whenever possible.

Staff should be trained in appropriate coping and calming techniques for parents and for children at different developmental levels. Distraction skills, using appropriate level language to explain procedures, and methods to support children and parents should be a priority in continuing education programs for staff.

Screening for and addressing mental health needs should occur in the emergency department. Increasing evidence that post-traumatic stress disorder is both common and impacts on recovery from illness and injury necessitates that patients and families obtain appropriate follow-up services. Attention to substance abuse among adolescents presenting for care, especially with trauma, is as important as dealing with their injuries. Brief interventions in the ED using motivational interviewing can have a significant impact on problem drinking and later risk of injury.

American Academy of Pediatrics, Committee on Pediatric Emergency Medicine: *Childhood Emergencies in the Office, Hospital, and Community: Organizing Systems of Care.* Seidel JS and Knapp JF (editors). Elk Grove Village, IL, AAP, 2000.

American Academy of Pediatrics, Committee on Pediatric Emergency Medicine, and American College of Emergency Physicians, Pediatric Committee Care of Children in the Emergency Department: Guidelines for preparedness. *Pediatrics* 2001;107:777–81.

American Academy of Pediatrics, Committee on Pediatric Emergency Medicine: The pediatrician's role in disaster preparedness. *Pediatrics* 1997;99:130–33.

American Academy of Pediatrics, Committee on School Health: Guidelines for emergency medical care in school. *Pediatrics* 2001;107:435–36.

American Academy of Pediatrics Task Force on Inter-hospital Transport: *Guidelines for Air and Ground Transport of Neonatal and Pediatric Patients.* Elk Grove Village, IL, American Academy of Pediatrics, 1999.

American College of Surgeons, Committee on Trauma: *Advanced Trauma Life Support.* Chicago, American College of Surgeons, 1997.

American Heart Association Emergency Cardiac Care Committee and Subcommittees: Guidelines 2000: Conference on Cardiopulmonary Resuscitation and Emergency Cardiac Care VI: Pediatric advanced life support. *Circulation* 2000;102:I-291–I-342.

Bole ET, Moore GP, Brummett C, et al: Do parents want to be present during invasive procedures performed on their children in the emergency department? A survey of 400 parents. *Ann Emerg Med* 1999;34:70–4.

Chameides L, Hazinski H (editors): *Pediatric Advanced Life Support.* Dallas, American Heart Association, 1997.

Henretig F, Cieslak TJ. Bioterrorism and pediatric emergency medicine. *Clin Pediatr Emerg Med* 2001;2:211–22.

Horowitz L, Kassam-Adams N, Bergstein J: Mental health aspects of emergency medical services for children: Summary of a consensus conference. *Acad Emerg Med* 2001;8:1187–96.

Institute of Medicine Committee on Pediatric Emergency Medical Services: *Emergency Medical Services for Children.* Durch JS and Lohr KN (editors). Washington, DC, National Academy Press, 1993.

Jurkovich GJ, Pierce B, Pananen L, et al: Giving bad news: The family perspective. *J Trauma* 2000;48:865–73.

Monti PM, Colby SM, Barnett NP, et al: Brief intervention for harm reduction with alcohol-positive older adolescents in a hospital emergency department. *J Consult Clin Psychol* 1999;67:989–94.

Seidel J, Tittle S, Hodge D, et al: Guidelines for pediatric equipment and supplies for emergency departments. *Ann Emerg Med* 1998;31:54–7.

Internet Resources for EMS-C

American Academy of Pediatrics, Section of Emergency Medicine (www.aap.org/sections/semed.htm)

American Association of Poison Control Centers (www.aapcc.org)

American College of Emergency Physicians (www.acep.org)

American Heart Association (www.amhrt.org)

Emergency Medical Services for Children (www.ems-c.org)

Chapter 52

Pediatric Critical Care: An Overview *Lorry R. Frankel*

General pediatricians need to understand what constitutes intensive care and should be familiar with the evaluation and stabilization of a child who has an impending life-threatening event or who has recently had a life-threatening event. This knowledge facilitates the management and transfer of the critically ill child to an appropriate facility for care. Pediatric critical care represents a convergence of knowledge, technologies, and approaches to multisystem organ failure from the emergency department, operating room, neonatal intensive care areas, and adult intensive care units (ICUs). Before the development of specialized areas to care for critically ill or injured pediatric patients, most critically ill children were cared for in either adult intensive care or neonatal intensive care units. This resulted in placement of these children alongside geriatric or neonatal patients, whose medical, nursing, and psychosocial needs were significantly different.

Children having acute neurologic deterioration, respiratory distress, cardiovascular compromise, or life-threatening traumatic injuries constitute the most common admissions to a pediatric intensive care unit (PICU). Unlike pediatric patients who require general care, these patients usually have a disease process that affects more than one organ system, commonly referred to as multiple organ system failure (MSOF) or dysfunction (MSOD). Successful PICUs use a multidisciplinary approach to care for these patients. Staff are also trained to manage the psychosocial dynamics encountered among the patients, the parents and other family members, and the various teams of health care professionals including other subspecialists (pediatric cardiology, surgery, pulmonology, neurology) involved in the care of these patients. Communication among the individuals caring for these patients is imperative and involves periodic team conferences with the family, the primary physicians, and the various pediatric subspecialists caring for these complicated and critically ill patients. The pediatric intensivist is a board-eligible or board-certified physician with subspecialty training in the care of critically ill pediatric patients and is usually the team leader. The patient population is diverse in age and disease processes. The most active PICUs admit more than 350 patients per year, with a fairly even mix of medical and surgical diseases; the number and distribution vary with the emphasis on various programs.

Patients are admitted to a PICU because they require a very high level of monitoring of vital signs and other body functions not available in other parts of the hospital (see Chapter 55). These patients may need mechanical ventilation, invasive intravascular monitoring, and frequent attention by both the nursing and the medical staffs (Table 52–1). The children may be admitted directly from physicians' offices, clinics, the emergency department, or the operating rooms. Most PICUs have active transport programs to facilitate the transfer of critically ill children (see Chapter 53). This enables patients to be evaluated and stabilized as well as transported to the appropriate regional PICU. This extension of critical care services to the community and regional areas is essential to provide optimal care to children who have sustained a life-threatening illness or injury.

Unit Organization. PICUs are specially designed and equipped facilities that require nurses, respiratory therapists, pharmacists, and physicians trained to care for critically ill children (see California Children's Services Standards for Pediatric Critical Care Units). The administrative structure for the ICU facilitates the multidisciplinary approach to the care of critically ill patients. It also enables the unit to establish training guidelines for the staff, evaluate equipment, review use of costly resources, and provide objective assessment of the effectiveness of new therapies. A unit director certified in pediatric critical care medicine works closely with nursing leadership and the other physicians to promote integration of critical care and the care provided by other subspecialists who practice in the unit. Assistance from anesthesia is helpful in developing clinical pathways for sedation and pain management and protocols needed to facilitate the transfer of patients from the operating room to the PICU. A surgeon with interests in trauma care is instrumental in developing the appropriate protocols required to care for injured patients. Radiology and laboratory services should be available as emergency "stat" services. Ideally, a pharmacist should be present in the PICU. The creation of a critical care committee is also helpful to formulate policies for the ICU, such as those regarding admission and discharge criteria; the role of the various attending physicians; credential criteria for physicians and physician extenders who practice in the PICU; the role of the house officers in the care of a critically ill child; transfer agreements with other hospitals to accommodate overflow patients during time of high census; and *quality assurance*.

TABLE 52–1. Criteria for PICU and PIICU Admission and Discharge

	Admission Criteria	Discharge Criteria
PICU	Patients who need *invasive monitoring:* arterial and central venous catheters, pulmonary arterial lines, ICP catheters	Patient may be discharged from the PICU once the disease process has reversed itself and care can be provided in a less intense environment:

	Patients with evidence of:
	  Respiratory impairment or failure
	  Cardiovascular compromise: shock, hypotension, hypertensive crisis
	  Acute neurologic deterioration: coma, status epilepticus, increased ICP
	  Acute renal failure requiring dialysis or CVVH
	  Bleeding disorders that necessitate massive transfusions
		Patient no longer requires invasive monitoring
		Patient can protect his/her airway (cough and gag reflexes)
		Patient is hemodynamically stable

PIICU	Patients who do *not* require respiratory assistance for acute respiratory failure but may require continuous noninvasive monitoring of vital signs, BP, Sao$_2$, Tco$_2$, Tcco$_2$ Patients who require chronic respiratory support via tracheostomies or noninvasive ventilation Patients who are in early cardiovascular failure and require monitoring of vital signs (noninvasive monitoring) Patients with acute neurologic injury but with a patent airway that they can protect themselves Patients with MSOD who do not need a PICU, but nursing care is not available elsewhere (e.g., trauma victims, DKA)	Patient may be discharged from the PIICU when it has been determined that care can be provided in general care areas

BP = blood pressure; CVVH = continuous venovenous hemofiltration; DKA = diabetic ketoacidosis; ICP = intracranial pressure; MSOD = multisystem organ dysfunction; PICU = pediatric intensive care unit; PIICU = pediatric intermediate intensive care unit; Sao$_2$ = arterial oxygen saturation; Tco$_2$ = transcutaneous oxygen; Tcco$_2$ = transcutaneous carbon dioxide.

Quality indicators may include mortality, length of ICU stays, adverse neurologic outcomes, reintubation rates for failed extubations, acquired injuries from intubations or other invasive procedures, and unanticipated ICU admissions from various areas within the hospital. Because of the many bioethical issues associated with patients with life-threatening conditions, the hospital should have an ethics committee.

Frankel LR, DiCarlo JV: Pediatric intensive care. In Bernstein D, Shelov SP (editors): *Pediatrics*. Baltimore, Williams & Wilkins, 1996, pp 591–609.

Rabin DS, Wells LA: Admission and discharge criteria and procedures. In Levin DL, Morriss FC (editors): *Essentials of Pediatric Intensive Care*, 2nd ed. New York, 1997, pp 1127–42.

Standards for Pediatric Intensive Care Units; California Children Services: *Manual of Procedures. Department of Health Services*, State of California, Chapter 3.32, revised 2000.

Standards for Pediatric Intensive Care Units; California Children Services: *Manual of Procedures, Department of Health Services, State of California*, Chapter 3.32; April 30, 1992.

Chapter 53
Interfacility Transfer of the Critically Ill Infant and Child

Lorry R. Frankel

Specialized transport programs (interfacility transport) bring patients from community facilities to the regionalized pediatric intensive care unit (PICU). Children are usually taken to the local emergency department by the emergency medical services provider or by their parents where their condition is assessed to determine the extent of injury, severity of illness, and physiologic instability (see Chapter 51). If the local facility does not have the capabilities to provide comprehensive intensive care, the child must be transported to a PICU. If possible, the child should be stabilized in the referring hospital while awaiting the arrival of the pediatric transport team. Regional pediatric centers have a responsibility not only to transport patients as rapidly and safely as possible but also to provide community educational programs that enable the local providers of health care to develop the necessary skills required for physiologic stabilization until the transport team arrives.

The American Academy of Pediatrics, the Association of Air Medical Services, and the Federal Aviation Administration have developed recommendations for pediatric transport programs. The members of the transport team must have the cognitive and technical skills required for the needs of pediatric patients and should be supervised by an attending physician (medical control physician [MCP]) who has expertise in either pediatric emergency medicine or pediatric critical care. All transport teams should have a team leader who is able to interact with the MCP during the transport and who is also able to manage the airway, provide respiratory support, and obtain vascular access and who has basic knowledge of pediatric drug dosing and understands the basic pathophysiology of pediatric disease and the transport environment. The transport program must have a medical director who organizes the overall program and institutes a quality assurance program that reviews transports, the equipment, and the proper use of vehicles.

Dispatch Center/Transfer Center. The regional PICU should provide phone consultation and deploy a team of specialized health care providers to assist in stabilization of patients to transport them in a safe mobile environment to the PICU. Regional centers may develop different protocols for activation of the transport or consultation requests. Some encourage direct access to the unit, some go through the emergency department, and others prefer to use a dispatch center or transfer center to screen the calls and facilitate the coordination of a transport. Once it has been determined that an ill child must be transported to the regional center, the MCP should be consulted to provide further input into the patient's care and to determine the best team composition and vehicle required to transport the patient.

Medical Control Physician. The MCP may have other clinical responsibilities; however, transport requests and consultations should be prioritized so that the necessary clinical information is obtained, appropriate therapeutic interventions can occur, and undue delays are avoided when transferring critically ill patients. The referring hospital provides some of the initial life-sustaining support required for these patients. It is often necessary for the MCP to provide further input into the patient's care while the patient is in the local facility. The MCP may seek additional medical or surgical consultation from other subspecialists if necessary. The MCP has the knowledge required for the stabilization of a critically ill infant or child, the transport requirements needed, the transport environment, the pertinent geography, and the interpersonal skills, which can maintain collegiality during potentially difficult and stressful times for the referring physician and facility. The MCP will assume significant responsibility for a patient who has not yet been seen.

Team Composition. This is based on a number of factors, including the severity of a patient's illness, the distance to the referring facility, the referring facility's insistence that certain team members be present (e.g., a physician), and the ability of the team members to work together in unfamiliar surroundings. The severity of illness is assessed by the MCP from the information provided by the referring hospital. Many transports can be staffed by a nonphysician team leader with phone contact with the MCP. In addition to the team leader, a critical care nurse is helpful for nursing care, monitoring, and administration of medications. If a child requires airway and respiratory support, a respiratory therapist should be included.

Various scoring systems have been developed to predict the need for a physician during the transport. It also appears that the team member's experience and skill in caring for critically ill patients is more important than one's educational degree. These individuals receive this experience through ongoing didactic sessions, skill training in airway management and vascular access, and case review. The use of physicians as team leaders may provide for both cognitive and decision-making capabilities, but the MCP and a nonphysician team leader via phone contact can manage many situations. The evolution of advanced practice nursing has enabled transport programs to utilize these professionals as team leaders. It is mandatory that adequate training in the assessment of the critically ill child includes developing appropriate skills such as airway management and vascular access, understanding the basic pathophysiology of pediatric disease, and having knowledge of the transport environment.

Vehicle Selection. The selection of the vehicle is made by the MCP in coordination with the referring hospital and those who will participate in the transport. Factors to consider are the severity of illness or injury, the distance to the referring hospital, travel time required, weather conditions, vehicle availability, equipment needs, and expense. *Ground ambulance* is used for the majority of transports, which are less than 100 miles. The traffic patterns must be considered in evaluating response time. The major advantages of this mode of transport are the ability to stop en route if the patient's condition worsens and further intervention is required and the ability to take a larger team with more equipment. *Fixed-wing transports* are usually used to reach infants and children who live more than 100–150 miles from the regional PICU. They may be able to fly to areas when the weather or altitude prevents the use of a helicopter. However, the use of fixed-wing aircraft requires several ambulance transfers. In addition, flying at altitude (especially over 5,000 feet) can have serious effects on the partial pressure and volume of gases in various body cavities and closed containers. Thus, patients who have respiratory failure and who require supplemental oxygen or those with a pneumothorax or an ileus require special care to prevent further deterioration. *Helicopters* enable a more rapid response but are expensive; the greatest hazards are poor weather and landing in poorly visualized or nondesignated landing areas. Helicopters are most useful for transports within a 100- to 200-mile radius and for going directly to the site of an injury (e.g., to pick up a trauma victim).

All vehicles must have the capability of radio or telephone contact with the MCP or the base station. In addition, each vehicle must be able to provide on-board oxygen, electrical power, and suction and must have space for adequate supplies and equipment, including oxygen tanks, pharmacy packs, respiratory therapy devices, infusion pumps and solutions, stretchers or Isolettes, and monitors. Additional space may be needed for advanced technologies such as extracorporeal membrane oxygenation and inhaled nitric oxide or helium.

Communication. This is one of the most crucial components of a regional transport system. Dealing with a critically ill or injured infant or child is an uncommon event for community physicians. Therefore, a referring physician needs to know whom, how, and when to call for assistance in the evaluation, stabilization, and transfer of a child. Telephone contact at all levels is required to ensure that physicians talk to physicians and that nurses talk to nurses. A child's condition may change rapidly; the ability to obtain information and provide advice needs to be continuing. Using a dispatch center as the patching system to the MCP and others allows the referring physician or hospital to need only one phone number and to address acute changes that require an immediate response.

The MCP is to determine if more tests should be done at the referring hospital (e.g., various imaging studies) or should various therapeutic interventions be initiated (e.g., elective intubation for progressive respiratory distress or the initiation of inotropic support for cardiovascular failure).

Once the transport team arrives at the referring facility, the team leader should reassess the patient's condition, review all of the pertinent laboratory data and medications, and discuss the situation with the parents and referring physicians. If the patient's condition has changed significantly, the team leader should contact the MCP for additional advice. All medical records including radiographs and scans should be copied to take to the accepting facility. Before departing with the child, the MCP should be consulted again and the PICU contacted to finalize preparations to receive the patient.

The referring physician should provide written documentation of the need to transfer the patient to a higher level of care than can be provided at the referring hospital. This should include a statement that the risks, benefits, and alternatives to care for a critically ill patient have been discussed with the parents and their informed consent has been obtained to have their child transferred to another hospital with PICU capacity. Medicolegal responsibility is probably shared once communication has begun. It is therefore important to document what has been recommended to the referring facility in order to better stabilize the patient.

One problem made by community facilities is transferring a critically ill child either with a team that does not have the expertise or equipment to do so or using some other system that is equally not prepared to care for the unique needs of a pediatric patient. There may be a misconception that the quicker the patient is transported the better the outcome. Unless there is a surgical emergency, it is preferred to stabilize the child and keep the patient in the referring hospital awaiting the arrival of the trained pediatric team. The regional pediatric centers have a responsibility not only to transport a patient in as rapid and safe a process as possible but also to provide educational activities for the community so that personnel can develop the necessary skills required for further stabilization until the transport team arrives.

It is also important that both the referring facility and the regional PICU have realistic expectations about the transport team's capabilities. If it is determined that a physician with significant critical care skills is required for the transport, the PICU has an obligation to provide a team leader with this skill level. The referring hospital should not delay lifesaving interventions while awaiting the arrival of the transport team (i.e., intubation of the trachea, initiation of mechanical ventilation, or pharmacologic support) especially if recommended by the MCP.

Federal legislation prohibits hospitals from refusing, limiting, or terminating patient care for financial reasons. This originates from the Consolidated Omnibus Budget Reconciliation Act (COBRA) passed in 1986 and revised in 1990. This act requires the hospital to evaluate all patients who arrive with emergent conditions and to stabilize patients before transfer. It also requires that the transferring hospital be responsible for the medical capabilities of the receiving hospital. To facilitate the transfer of critically ill pediatric patients, some regional PICUs have developed transfer agreements with referring hospitals. This ensures that the referring hospital has developed a plan as to where and how to transfer a patient. These relationships ensure that the appropriate and safe transfer of the infant or child with a life-threatening illness occurs in as smooth and safe an environment as possible.

As telecommunication systems improve, it will become possible to provide live video viewing of the patient at the referring hospital. The expansion of telemedicine will enable the MCP to work in conjunction with the referring physicians in the evaluation and stabilization of the critically ill child. This will improve outcomes because it provides the necessary critical care expertise at the bedside of the ill patient.

American Academy of Pediatrics, Committee on Pediatric Emergency Medicine, American College of Critical Care Medicine, Society of Critical Care Medicine: Consensus report for regionalization of services for critically ill or injured children. *Pediatrics* 2000;105:152–5.

Linden V, Palmer K, Reinhard J, et al: Inter-hospital transportation of patients with severe acute respiratory failure on extracorporeal membrane oxygenation—national and international experience. *Intensive Care Med* 2001;10:1643–8.

Nieman CT, Merlino JI, Kovach B, et al: Intubated pediatric patients requiring transport: A review of patients, indications, and standards. *Air Med J* 2001;21(1): 22–5.

Woodward GA, Insoft RM, Pearson-Shaver AL, et al: The state of pediatric interfacility transport: Consensus of the second national pediatric and neonatal interfacility transport medicine leadership conference. *Pediatr Emerg Care* 2002; 18:38–43.

Chapter 54

Effective Communication with Families in the PICU

Lawrence H. Mathers and Lorry R. Frankel

The Pediatric Patient in an Unfamiliar Environment. It is difficult to imagine a situation producing more sadness, fright, and anger in families than a child's serious illness that requires admission to a pediatric intensive care unit (PICU). (The terms *family* and *families* are used here to include parents, grandparents, siblings, friends, and others occupying a family-like role in the life of a child.) Young patients and their families may face potentially life-threatening illness or surgery that can result in a permanent disability or death. Families may feel a loss of ability to protect their child from danger, to provide for his or her needs, or to have final determination over which course of treatment should be undertaken. When children are confined to a hospital bed or require restraints to prevent exacerbation of injuries, the child's response is to become more agitated and to reach out to the parents for relief and reassurance. This behavior, limited visitation, and the presence of medical equipment heighten the family's feeling of loss of control and inability to help. Unfamiliar physicians and staff may intensify parental concern and distrust.

Visitation and Presence in the Child's PICU Room. Although patients in a PICU may not be fully alert or able to interact normally with those around them, the goal of care should be to allow the maximum time for families to be with their child and to participate actively in their child's care *(family-centered care)*. Limiting the number of visitors to two at a time has traditionally been considered wise because most PICU patient areas are crowded with equipment, the child may better benefit from contact with one or two individuals rather than a large number of visitors, and large crowds may disturb other patients. Siblings and friends should be allowed to visit but must be screened to ensure that they do not have a communicable illness and are psychologically ready to visit a critically ill child. The patient's appearance and the presence of medical devices may be very frightening to a young sibling. Rules for visitation and access should be tailored to each particular situation and should always respect the principles of patient dignity and confidentiality. Visitors may be asked to leave the room during rounds, during a nursing change of shift, and when invasive procedures are performed. Similar situations applying to another patient sharing the room may require all visitors to leave. The practice of excluding families from patients' rooms during invasive procedures and even emergency resuscitations has been revisited. When families have the option of witnessing such activities, it helps them to understand and adjust to the outcome, even when the resuscitation is unsuccessful. It can be desirable for families to be present during certain procedures to provide comfort to a conscious child.

Families may wish to review their child's medical chart. This should be arranged at a time convenient when both the family and the treating physician can be present together. Such a review may provide an opportunity to answer questions and explain unfamiliar medical terminology, which can provide further family reassurance. All health care professionals caring for a patient should adopt a consistent position on sensitive issues such as witnessing procedures and reviewing the patient's chart.

Identifying Personnel and Their Roles. Large medical centers, especially teaching hospitals, have many physicians, students, nurses, respiratory therapists, social workers, chaplains, and others involved in the care of a patient in a PICU. A single physician (usually the senior attending physician) should assume primary responsibility for communication with the family. If a fellow or other senior trainee is named to temporarily fill this role, the attending physician should reassure the family that he or she will remain fully apprised of the patient's condition and that the fellow is acting as spokesperson with the full support of the attending physician. This person should communicate at least once daily with the family and should have enough experience to place all information in a proper context and avoid hasty and incompletely supported conclusions. Nothing frightens and angers families more than to hear significantly different descriptions of their child's condition from physicians, nurses, and others who are involved in the child's care. It is also extremely helpful if early in a child's PICU course parents receive an explanation of the roles played by the different health care providers. Pamphlets containing this information are useful but cannot

entirely replace a direct discussion with the family. The family should receive reassurance that health care providers in training may act independently in certain situations but are always supervised by an attending physician. Expert consultants must exercise diplomacy when they examine a patient. If significant patient information is sought by the family from a consultant, it may be best to defer providing it until the attending physician can participate in the discussion to ensure that the consultant's observations are put in proper context.

The Role of the Physician. To benefit patients, avoid harm, maintain confidentiality, and respect the dignity of children and their families, an intensivist assumes several roles. The physician may provide information, supporting the family in making difficult decisions about continuation of support, futility of care, withdrawal of support, and organ donation. Families vary widely on the matter of how much they wish to defer painful decisions to the "expert" treating physicians. Most physicians do not simply provide information to families and then ask them to make a decision "on their own," but instead deliver information and follow that with suggestions based on their experience and grasp of the pathophysiology of the illness affecting an individual child. Physicians may assume the role of an important partner supporting the family in making difficult decisions. Physicians can help family members' responses by the manner in which they present the medical information to them. The physician may wish to describe one or two hypothetical situations regarding the future course of an illness and attempt to reach advance agreements about which treatments will be attempted and which will not. As best as possible, the parents and child, if possible, must be asked to articulate their preferences, which, if in the best interest of the patient, must be honored. Each mode of sharing information with families has certain advantages, and an amalgam of these approaches is often used (also see Chapter 2).

Informed Consent. The goal of informed consent is to provide patients or parents or other adults who are responsible for representing the interests of a child with a full understanding of their choices and the benefits and risks of each potential course of action (see Chapter 2). The list of procedures and treatments that require explicit consent grows yearly, and failure to obtain proper consent exposes the caregivers to legal liability. Although informed consent is required only for certain procedures and therapies, the concept should guide all interactions between the physician, the patient, and the patient's family. Caregivers should make efforts to ensure that proper communication occurs despite language barriers or differences in educational or cultural backgrounds (see Chapter 3).

Establishing a Supportive Environment and Rapport. Many children are in the PICU for days, weeks, or even indefinitely before death eventually intervenes. Many children who have sustained very serious injuries evolve into a dependence on mechanical ventilation, assisted feeding and chronic pharmacologic therapies, and transition to the setting of a chronic care facility. Explicit guidelines for palliative care, where the focuses are on doing everything possible to reduce suffering (e.g., pain control), maintain communication wherever possible, protect the patient against fears of abandonment and rejection, protect the patient's dignity, and recognize the difficulty faced by families who must learn to accept the reality of life and death with a severely injured child (see Chapter 38). Each year, in the United States and Canada, approximately 80,000 children die of a wide variety of causes. Although many of these deaths are sudden, many other deaths occur over longer periods of time (chronic diseases, traumatic injuries) and challenge all health care providers to assist patients and their families in facing such tragic events.

Providing Health Information Consistently and Accurately. The goal should be to speak to the family with simple honesty and compassion about the child's condition and prognosis, unless certain circumstances would make such a frank discussion problematic (e.g., psychiatric or other serious illness in a parent). The level of the parents' understanding of medical concepts and terminology should be taken into consideration. Their emotional lability, the need for continued care for other children at home, and career and job responsibilities all guide the physician in choosing the time and circumstances in which to hold a thorough discussion with the parents (see Chapters 38 and 64).

Although informal in-depth discussions among family members and the medical team may be the forum for major decision-making, family members also need discussions to understand the relative significance of monitor readings, laboratory tests, or an examination. A *care conference* with the family and health care providers is used to exchange information and reach a consensus about children with complex problems or those who have extended PICU stays (>7–10 days). A plenary meeting may be held with representation from the various medical and ancillary services involved in a patient's care to reach conclusions and provide information to be shared with the parents and family at another meeting with the attending physician and, if feasible, the child's primary care physician. This also provides an opportunity to evaluate the parent's concerns, emotional response, and understanding. The primary care physician may be particularly helpful in assisting the family with assimilation of the information.

Uncooperative or Hostile Families. The vast majority of families, despite the stress and anxiety provoked by their child's serious illness, want to work with the medical staff toward the goal of improving their child's health. In all but a handful of cases, an appeal to the importance of the cooperation of parents in treating the child will defuse bad feeling and hostility. However, sometimes families feel that the way to express concern and to maintain parental control over what happens to their child is to challenge the recommendations of the medical staff, resist certain suggestions, and refuse to obey visitation and other PICU regulations. The PICU staff should encourage all families to express their concerns and should indicate a willingness to understand and accommodate their positions whenever possible; extensive discussion and counseling of these families may be required.

The frustrations, sadness, and anger associated with the illness of a child can lead some family members to become suspicious, aggressive, and occasionally violent. If there is a threat of intimidation or violence against the medical staff, hospital security and the administration should be alerted that a serious conflict has occurred. In such instances, visitation privileges may be limited, allowed only when a security guard is present, and carried out in the company of an appropriate chaperone. The focus is to care for the child, and any conflicts or animosity between family and hospital must not be allowed to detract from that effort.

Communication Regarding End-of-Life Decisions. When a child's condition irreversibly deteriorates and death is a likely event, health care staff must discuss the possibility of limiting or terminating support. If the possibility of tissue or organ donation exists, then discussions regarding limitation of support must be tailored to that purpose, but in many cases the gravely ill child and his or her family are the sole focus of discussions. Families must be made to feel that their contribution to such a dialogue is valuable and welcome because principles of family-centered care still apply, but at the same time family members should not be made to believe that a decision regarding their child's fate lies solely in their hands. A physician should carefully and thoroughly explain the medical facts and should be prepared to make suggestions about what would be a wise decision. In many cases families badly need to identify a physician whom they can trust, and from whom they will seek not only information but also advice on a very personal level. A family's support network,

including extended family, friends, and faith community, should be recognized as valid participants in end-of-life discussions. Some families may feel poorly informed and excluded from the decision-making process, whereas others may have a positive experience. PICU staff, who are by their nature numerous and frequently moving on and off of the treating team for a given patient, should realize the special need for continuity and consistency in communications with families. Even when death is the tragic outcome of a child's hospitalization, the PICU staff can be a source of strength and compassion and may help families to know that in his or her final days a child will be treated with intelligence, respect, and genuine concern and that the need to recognize and respond to the family's shock and pain was equally important (see also Chapter 38).

Boie E, Moore GP, et al: Do parents want to be present during invasive procedures performed on their children in the emergency department? A survey of 400 parents. *Ann Emerg Med* 1999;34:70–4.

Masri C, Farrell CA, et al: Decision making and end-of-life care in critically ill children. *J Palliat Care* 2000;16:S45–52.

McPherson ML, Sachdeva RC, et al: Development of a survey to measure parent satisfaction in a pediatric intensive care unit. *Crit Care Med* 2000;28:3009–13.

Meyer EC, Burns JP, et al: Parental perspectives on end-of-life care in the pediatric intensive care unit. *Crit Care Med* 2002;30:226–31.

Playfor SD, Thomas DA, et al: Parental perceptions of comfort during mechanical ventilation. *Paediatr Anaesth* 2001;1:99–103.

Powers KS, Rubenstein JS: Family presence during invasive procedures in the pediatric intensive care unit. *Arch Pediatr Adolesc Med* 1999;153:955–58.

Sacchetti A, Carraccio C, et al: Acceptance of family member presence during pediatric resuscitations in the emergency department: Effects of personal experience. *Pediatr Emerg Care* 2000;16:85–87.

Todres ID: Communication between physician, patient and family in the pediatric intensive care unit. *Crit Care Med* 1993;21:S383–86.

Young Seideman R, Watson MA, et al: Parent stress and coping in NICU and PICU. *J Pediatr Nurs* 1977;2:69–77.

Chapter 55

Monitoring Techniques for the Critically Ill Infant and Child *Lorry R. Frankel*

Monitoring critically ill patients obtains biologic-physiologic data by invasive or noninvasive techniques. Noninvasive monitoring can involve continuous evaluation of heart rate and rhythm and respiratory rate, whereas noncontinuous monitoring measures blood pressure and various laboratory values, such as blood gases. Hemodynamic and respiratory monitoring involves the placement of invasive catheters to continuously determine blood pressure and central venous pressure (CVP) and to obtain intermittent arterial blood gas values. Invasive monitoring requires special expertise in the insertion of catheters and nursing care in their maintenance and has potential serious complications (e.g., infections, thrombosis, bleeding). Noninvasive monitoring devices also enable critically ill patients to be monitored on a continuous basis with fewer complications, allowing for greater patient comfort at a reduced expense. Invasive monitoring is widely used particularly in unstable critically ill patients; however, routine bedside monitoring may also incorporate noninvasive devices that allow for continuous and real-time measurements of physiologic data. This combination complements each other and enables the clinician to have a better awareness of minute-to-minute changes.

Monitoring requirements can be divided into hemodynamic, pulmonary, and neurologic; these can be subdivided into invasive and noninvasive (Table 55–1). Both noninvasive and

TABLE 55–1. **Monitoring Devices Commonly Used in the PICU**

Monitoring Devices	Sites	Measured Variables	Limitations/Concerns
Noninvasive Monitoring			
Cardiorespiratory	Chest leads	Heart rate, rhythm, respiratory rate	Only lead II recording, difficulty with dysrhythmia recognition
Pulse oximetry	Digits, palms, ear lobe	Continuous SaO_2	Patient must be well perfused; abnormal hemoglobins and nail polish may affect results
Transcutaneous oxygen and carbon dioxide	Usually chest wall	O_2 and CO_2	Surface electrodes warm skin to 43°C, can cause thermal injury, must be changed every 3–4 hr, useful in young infants
Capnography	End of the endotracheal tube	End-tidal CO_2 using breath-by-breath analysis	Capnographic trace is important to determine actual measurement; it is a true end-tidal representation of alveolar CO_2
Blood pressure	Upper arm, thigh, or calf	Cuff that allows for periodic cycling q 1–15 min	Similar to cuff pressure. Important to have appropriate cuff size
Electroencephalogram	Scalp surface	Provides for continuous monitoring of cranial electrical activity	Requires a specialized technician to place the electrodes and special training in interpreting the waveforms
Invasive Monitoring Techniques			
Arterial	Radial, dorsalis pedis, posterior tibial, femoral, axillary (rarely brachial)	Continuous determination of blood pressure; ability to measure blood gases and other laboratory tests	Expertise in placement and monitoring needed; may require cutdown technique; may lose distal perfusion
Central venous access for pressure measurement (CVP) and infusion	Femoral, subclavian, internal or external jugular, antecubital, or advanced from the saphenous	Allows for CVP determinations and administration of vasoactive agents and hypertonic solutions (TPN)	Requires expertise in placement, especially in very young patients; attempt to use multilumen catheters; need chest x-ray film to determine placement
Pulmonary artery catheter Swan-Ganz (balloon) catheter	Place through a sheath in the internal or external jugular, femoral, or subclavian	Allows for measurements of cardiac output, SvO_2, pulmonary artery pressure; can calculate SVR and PVR	Less commonly used in pediatrics; may assist in titration of inotropic support, vasodilators, adjustment of PEEP
ICP	Skull, either with a subdural bolt, an epidural fiberoptic device, or an IVC	Measures ICP when CNS pathology is associated with cerebral edema (e.g., head injury, Reye's syndrome, or those with unexplained GCS <8)	Requires a neurosurgeon to insert the device; may be done at the bedside; increased risk of infection after 5 days; IVC can be used to remove fluid
Jugular bulb catheter	Internal jugular and threaded to the jugular bulb	Measures SvO_2 at the jugular bulb. Cerebral oxygen extraction can be calculated	Technically difficult to insert; requires training in the utility of the device and the values obtained; may allow modification of therapy

CNS = central nervous system; CVP = central venous pressure; GCS = Glasgow Coma Scale; ICP = intracranial pressure; IVC = intraventricular catheter; PEEP = positive end-expiratory pressure; PVR = pulmonary vascular resistance; SaO_2 = arterial oxygen saturation; SvO_2 = venous oxygen saturation; SVR = systemic vascular resistance; TPN = total parenteral nutrition.

invasive monitors must use age- and disease-specific criteria for setting monitor alarms because normal values for heart rate, blood pressure, and respiratory rate vary with a child's age, whereas acceptable oxygen saturations will vary with different cyanotic congenital heart lesions.

Hemodynamic Monitoring. This is indicated in any patient admitted to the pediatric intensive care unit (PICU) who is in shock, has respiratory failure, or has sustained an acute neurologic insult. Included in hemodynamic monitoring are heart rate and blood pressure as well as CVP and pulmonary capillary wedge pressure (PCWP) and, occasionally in postoperative cardiovascular patients, right atrial and left atrial pressures (RA and LA lines). Heart rate can be measured with conventional electrodes placed on the chest, which can also provide rhythm strips usually in lead II. The lead can be changed if indicated to evaluate for other dysrhythmias, but it should not substitute for a 12-lead electrocardiogram (ECG).

Blood pressure is determined invasively and noninvasively. The choice is determined by the instability of the patient, skill levels of the physicians, and ability of the staff to maintain such devices. Noninvasive blood pressure monitoring provides for manual or automatic repeated but intermittent readings of blood pressure. Whether one chooses a conventional sphygmomanometer or an ultrasonic/Doppler device, appropriate cuff sizes are required to obtain an accurate blood pressure. The cuff should encompass approximately two thirds of the length of the part of the extremity from which it is measuring. The upper

arm, lower leg, and upper leg offer the best sites for obtaining noninvasive blood pressures. Besides the cuff size, factors that affect peripheral blood flow or pulmonary vascular resistance or produce significant peripheral edema may result in abnormal values for noninvasively measured blood pressure.

Because of the technical limitations of noninvasive monitoring, invasive hemodynamic monitoring may be preferred. Sites commonly used to place catheters in an artery for invasive monitoring include the radial, ulnar, posterior tibial, and dorsalis pedis arteries. Less frequently used are the femoral, axillary and brachial arteries and, when available, the umbilical artery. Arterial lines may be inserted either percutaneously or via cutdown if one is unsuccessful with percutaneous attempts. Before attempting to insert an arterial line one should ensure that collateral circulation exists if possible by performing an Allen test (for radial or ulnar lines). Once the catheter is properly inserted, a pressure transducer and pressure tubing are used to connect the catheter to the monitor. A continuous pressure waveform tracing can then be displayed on the monitor screen and should be displayed along with the simultaneous ECG tracing. The arterial waveform may be helpful in diagnosing hypovolemia (very narrowed and blunted dicrotic notch), determining the severity of cardiac dysrhythmias (pulsus alternans), and evaluating the effects of respirations (air trapping) or high pericardial pressure on blood pressure (pulsus paradoxus). Arterial lines also allow for the frequent sampling of blood for various laboratory tests including arterial blood gases, electrolytes, coagulation panels, and others as needed.

Complications from arterial catheterization are rare but may be very serious and require aggressive therapies. Bleeding and infection are relatively rare. Usually, direct pressure to the insertion site will reduce any further bleeding. Cutdowns may require resuturing or placing topical clotting material in the incision. Colonization around the insertion site may produce bacteremia and septicemia. The most serious complication is arterial thrombosis. This is seen in patients with low cardiac output states (shock), in those where heparin was not used in the flush solution, or in those patients who have required prolonged duration of catheter placement. Thrombosis necessitates the immediate removal of the catheter. The use of intravenous heparin or thrombolytic therapy or topical nitroglycerin paste is indicated if the extremity continues to have evidence of poor perfusion. Other complications include vascular spasm, cutaneous mottling, arterial tears, pseudo-aneurysms, peripheral nerve damage, and arteriovenous fistula formation. Temporal artery sites are associated with retrograde flow into the carotid artery resulting in cerebrovascular accidents and therefore should be avoided. Decreased flow distal to an extremity site may result in serious necrosis of an extremity. Excellent nursing care is required to evaluate patients on a frequent and regular basis to monitor for complications. Patients with arterial lines may have excessive blood tests; in small infants this may contribute to the development of anemia.

A *central venous catheter* (CVC) is required to care for many critically ill patients. A CVC provides important information regarding volume status (CVP), but it also permits the safe infusion of hypertonic solutions (parenteral nutrition, bicarbonate, calcium chloride, glucose) and vasoactive agents (epinephrine, norepinephrine, dopamine) that can produce severe peripheral soft tissue damage if they extravasate from peripheral lines into the local tissues. Rapid infusions of large volumes of fluids or blood products are also possible.

CVCs may be inserted from different sites; the catheter is advanced into the thoracic cavity with the tip in the inferior or superior vena cava. Sites include the femoral, subclavian, external jugular, internal jugular, antecubital, and, rarely, saphenous veins. These catheters may be inserted percutaneously or via cutdown and tunneled under the skin to reduce the risk of infection. Catheter sizes vary with the size and age of the patient. Ideally, one should attempt to insert a multilumen catheter because this provides multiple ports for the various infusions required to care for the patient. Before the procedure the patient should have ECG leads placed so that heart rate is monitored during the procedure to detect for any dysrhythmias from inadvertent intracardiac placement. The line should terminate at the atriocaval junction to minimize cardiac perforation and tamponade. An x-ray film ensures that the catheter is in proper position. The catheter is connected via a transducer to the monitor to enable one to evaluate the waveform and obtain a CVP. A true CVP waveform contains characteristic a, c, and v waves. The presence of these waves ensures appropriate placement in the thoracic cavity but not necessarily in the appropriate location, and therefore a chest x-ray film is required. Rarely, an intravenous dye contrast study or fluoroscopy may be needed to confirm placement, because some catheters are not radiopaque. Ultrasonic guided central venous catheterization, via images or sound (Doppler for arteries), is helpful in difficult situations.

Immediate complications of CVC include dysrhythmias, pneumothorax, hydrothorax, hemothorax, air embolism, shearing of the vessel, intravascular loss of the guide wire, bleeding, apnea, oversedation, or airway obstruction. The patient should be monitored for any of these early complications. Infection usually occurs later and is associated with longer duration of catheter placement as well as percutaneous versus tunneled catheters. Thrombosis is a concern because of the duration of the catheters and the potential for associated pulmonary embolic events. The most serious and life-threatening acute or delayed complication is cardiac tamponade. This is usually the result of an intra-atrial catheter. This problem must be immediately recognized and aggressively treated.

Pulmonary artery catheters (PACs) monitor the patient's hemodynamic status when the right- and left-sided circulation's filling pressures may vary. This is common in adults after a myocardial infarction in which the left ventricle is more severely affected than the right, resulting in ventricular discordance. PACs allow one to monitor a number of hemodynamic parameters if a balloon thermodilution catheter is used (Fig. 55–1). One can measure core temperature, CVP as well as pulmonary artery pressures (PAP) and pulmonary artery occlusion pressure (PAOP), cardiac outputs, and mixed venous oxygen saturation and calculate both systemic and pulmonary vascular resistances, oxygen delivery, stroke volume, arteriovenous oxygen content differences, oxygen extraction ratios, and shunt fractions.

PACs are rarely used in pediatric patients. The most common indications are for cardiogenic shock, for severe distributive shock, for the use of very high ventilator pressures to achieve adequate oxygenation, allowing one to modulate therapy in patients with severe pulmonary hypertension, and for the perioperative management of patients who have undergone complex cardiac or other major surgeries. The limitations to the use of these catheters are predominantly patient size and unfamiliarity with these catheters. The smallest thermodilution catheter is 5 Fr, although a single-lumen 4-Fr catheter exists and is useful for measuring PAP or obtaining MvO_2. The single-lumen catheter does not permit one to measure or calculate the data that can be obtained from the larger catheters. The balloon catheters are able to "float" into the pulmonary artery and wedge into a distal position. This provides the pulmonary artery occlusion pressure (PAOP) or pulmonary capillary wedge pressure (PCWP), which is usually reflective of the left ventricle end-diastolic filling pressure. Once this number is determined, the balloon is deflated and allowed to remain in the pulmonary artery. This minimizes potential complications of pulmonary artery erosion or infarction. Other complications include dysrhythmias, damage to the pulmonic valve, coiling in the right ventricle, balloon rupture, and infection. When these complications occur, the PA catheter must be removed.

Pulmonary Monitoring. The monitoring requirements for patients who require significant respiratory support include blood gas determination, either from arterial or, less frequently, capillary and venous blood gases. Arterial blood gas sampling requires special technique similar to inserting an arterial line. Capillary gases usually involve the use of the infant's heel. It must be warmed to "arterialize" the blood. In the laboratory a blood gas analyzer measures the partial pressures of oxygen and carbon dioxide and the pH; the bicarbonate is usually calculated from the pH and P_{CO_2}. The pH and Pa_{CO_2} from a capillary or venous sample should closely resemble the arterial blood gas sample. However, the capillary P_{O_2} does not correlate well with the Pa_{O_2}; and in circumstances in which peripheral blood flow is adversely affected all other parameters obtained from capillary blood gases may not correlate. Capillary and venous blood gas sampling have significant limitations.

Intermittent blood gas sampling is labor intensive and expensive. It does provide the most reliable assessment of acid-base and ventilation-oxygenation status in the critically ill patient. When the patient's clinical status requires both continuous blood pressure monitoring and frequent assessments of respiratory status, an indwelling arterial line is indicated. Devices can provide continuous pH, Pa_{CO_2}, and Pa_{O_2} when the monitoring catheter is placed in an artery; blood flows from the catheter into a closed-loop system passing the blood gas electrodes. The data are obtained in a continuous manner or intermittently. These

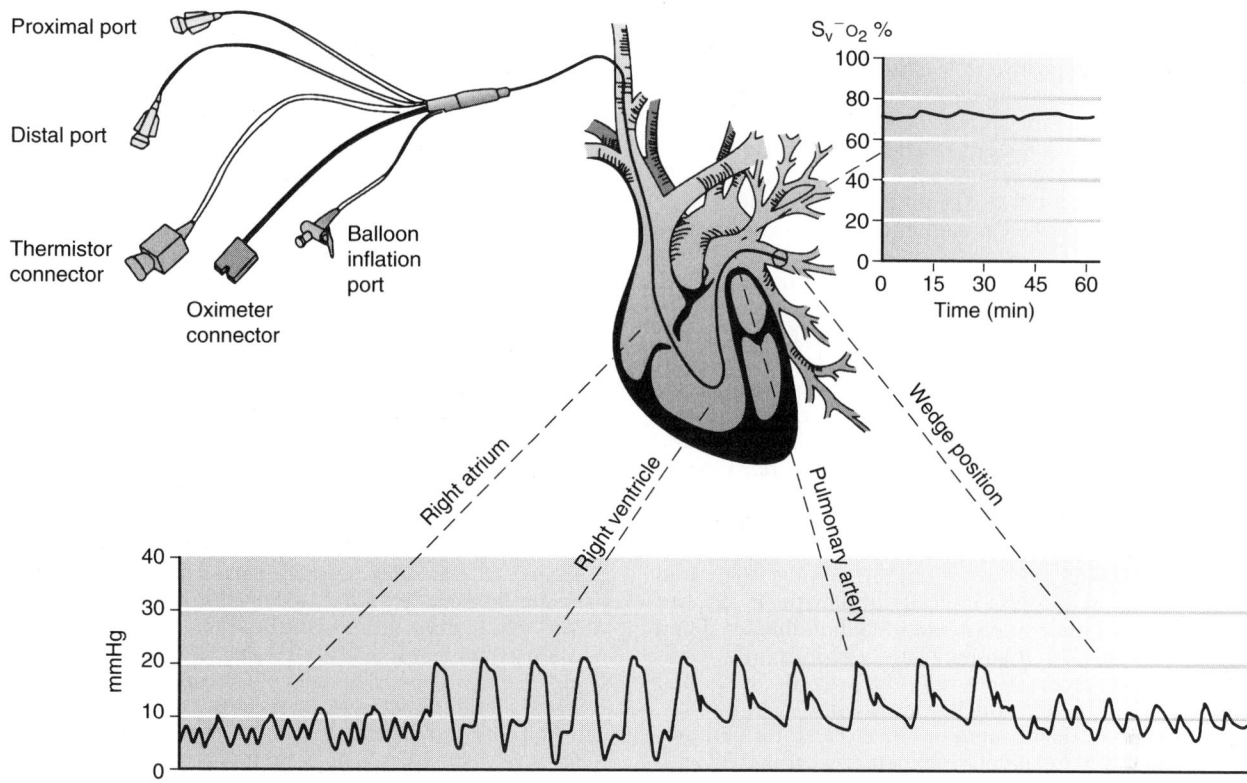

FIGURE 55–1. Components and functional features of a thermodilution flow-directed balloon flotation pulmonary artery catheter (PAC). The flexible multilumen catheter with the balloon at the distal tip inflated is in the wedge position. The proximal ends of the five lumens are labeled. The distal port is connected to a pressure measurement system for catheter insertion and subsequent monitoring. When the distal tip is within the central venous circulation, the balloon is inflated to enhance flow-direction of the tip through the right atrium into the right ventricle and then to the pulmonary artery. Recorded pressures in the lower part of the figure correspond to these locations, confirming the course of the catheter. The last tracing on the right is that corresponding to the "wedge" position, commonly reflecting the pressure transmitted from the left atrium via the pulmonary veins and fiberoptic monitor available on adult-sized catheters. (Redrawn from Daily EK, Tilkian AG: Hemodynamic monitoring. In Tilkian AG, Daily EK [editors]: *Cardiovascular Procedures, Diagnostic Techniques and Therapeutic Procedures.* St. Louis, CV Mosby, 1986.

devices are expensive and require blood vessels of sufficient size to permit the insertion of a large catheter (at least 20 gauge). These devices are useful when placed in central venous lines and used in conjunction with pulse oximetry; this combination demonstrates good correlation of venous pH, with arterial pH and venous Pco_2 with arterial $Paco_2$.

Point of care testing in the PICU and neonatal ICU (NICU) is more expensive yet more expedient and provides valuable information in minutes and at the bedside. Point of care testing may be accomplished with a handheld device that is also useful in the transport environment, in areas where the patient is not in the PICU but must have blood gas analysis performed, such as radiographic imaging suites, or when the patient's condition is so unstable that an instantaneous analysis is required. These simple devices may perform a number of other analyses, such as measuring serum electrolytes, glucose, creatinine, urea, ionized calcium, and hematocrit.

A variety of noninvasive devices and monitors have improved the care of critically ill children. *Transcutaneous instruments* permit the simultaneous determination of transcutaneous carbon dioxide tension ($Tcco_2$) and transcutaneous oxygen tension (Tco_2). Bicarbonate levels or pH cannot be measured by transcutaneous monitoring. Other limitations include skin thickness; transcutaneous monitoring is limited to smaller infants. Transcutaneous electrodes must be warmed to 43°C, which may cause burns; they must be changed every 3–4 hr. The electrodes take 20 min to calibrate; this must be done every 4 hr. Thus,

there may be various delays in obtaining important blood gas information. The major strength of transcutaneous monitoring is the ability to continuously follow $Paco_2$, permitting more rapid ventilator adjustments and facilitating weaning as well as reducing the costs associated with blood gas analysis.

End-tidal CO_2 ($Etco_2$) analysis (capnography) measures the Pco_2 in the exhaled gas. This technique is used in patients who are intubated and have minimal lung disease without significant intrapulmonary shunting. Capnography is based on the principle that the highest concentration of CO_2 sampled in the respiratory circuit represents the alveolar CO_2 concentration, which should also be close to the arterial ($Paco_2$) concentration. Gas is constantly monitored from a side port to the connector from the ventilator to the endotracheal tube. A small amount of gas is diverted from the respiratory circuit and analyzed in a spectrophotometer for Pco_2 determination. The removal of small amounts of respiratory gas must be accounted for when calculating delivered and exhaled tidal volumes.

When interpreting $EtCO_2$ results, one needs to evaluate the graphic picture of the exhalation capnographic image to ensure that the alveolar plateau and peak are achieved. Patients who have significant intrapulmonary shunts or are spontaneously breathing may not produce an acceptable capnographic trace, and thus invalidate end-tidal CO_2 monitoring. This device permits trending and the potential for weaning of patients from mechanical ventilation; it does not replace blood gas analysis.

Capnography can also determine if one has intubated the trachea and is useful in emergent intubations. Using an analyzer that changes color on exposure to levels of CO_2 enables one to differentiate between an esophageal and tracheal intubation. The CO_2 concentration in the stomach is very low, approaching atmospheric levels of close to zero, whereas that in the lungs is markedly higher. With cardiopulmonary arrest and absent pulmonary blood flow, $Etco_2$ will also be undetectable. Indeed, successful reestablishment of the circulation can also be assessed by an elevation of $Etco_2$.

Pulse oximetry is the standard for noninvasive bedside oxygenation monitoring. Pulse oximetry can be used in patients of all ages and does not usually cause tissue damage. Its accuracy is dependent on adequate tissue perfusion; its utility is limited in patients with significant vasoconstriction and poor peripheral perfusion. Pulse oximetry measures oxygen saturation, not the partial pressure of a gas. This is important in interpreting the significance of the value obtained. Normally, arterial oxygen saturation is 95% or more (except in patients with cyanotic congenital heart lesions). Although pulse oximetry does not provide PaO_2, it provides just as good if not better information regarding real-time oxygen saturation. It permits the rapid assessment of oxygenation of a critically ill patient. It requires little, if any, warm-up time and is extremely portable, enabling one to assess oxygenation of patients not only in the PICU but also during transport (see Chapter 53), during procedures that require conscious sedation, and in various non-ICU settings, such as the emergency department or office. The information is extremely reliable and relatively inexpensive compared with blood gas analysis. Pulse oximetry does not provide direct measurements of carbon dioxide tension, acid-base status, or bicarbonate levels.

Neurophysiologic Monitoring. Neurologic monitoring involves careful clinical observation accompanied by highly technical noninvasive devices (e.g., electroencephalography, evoked potentials, near infra-red spectroscopy), or invasive catheters placed to monitor intracranial pressure (ICP).

Acute neurologic deterioration represents a significant number of admissions to a PICU. Trauma, tumors, infections, seizures, vascular malformation, strokes, hypoxia, or various metabolic disorders may produce serious neurologic injury. An experienced PICU nurse should be able to perform careful serial clinical neurologic examinations. These frequent examinations evaluate the cranial nerves, especially the pupillary reflexes, and score a modified Glasgow Coma Scale (GCS) for infants and children. The GCS provides a method to quantitate the patient's level of consciousness and ability to respond to painful stimuli in an easy and standard format (see Chapter 57.1). The scores range from 3–15. Most patients with score less than 12 should be observed in the PICU until they are stable enough to be cared for in less intensely monitored areas.

Advanced techniques in the computerization of electrophysiologic monitoring enable monitoring of the brain's electrical activity through *continuous electroencephalograms (EEGs)*. Managing a child with severe status epilepticus helps determine if anticonvulsant drugs are affecting both the electrical as well as the clinical seizure activity. Patients who have refractory seizures may require a barbiturate coma; monitoring their EEG activity facilitates the suppression of seizure activity. Clinical examinations are not useful in patients requiring paralytic agents or heavy sedation; the ability to monitor seizures through continuous EEGs is essential. When interpreting the data one must be aware that artifacts can be produced from the various monitors, ventilators, or other electrical equipment commonly found in the ICU setting. Video-EEG permits one to record both the electrical changes associated with a seizure and correlate it with a clinical picture.

Evoked potentials enable evaluation of a variety of sensory pathways that include visual evoked responses (VEPs), brainstem auditory evoked potentials (BSAEPs), and somatosensory evoked potentials (SSEPs). These are not affected by the sedative medications, which may produce an isoelectric EEG. The brainstem and somatosensory tests are the most commonly performed evoked potential studies. They may serve as an aid in providing prognostic information. Their utility in diagnosing brain death is not well recognized.

The *Bispectral Index* (BIS) can be used to monitor the neurologic status of both sedated and unsedated critically ill patients. BIS is a statistically derived variable that provides information about the interaction of brain cortical and subcortical regions. The BIS score ranges from 0–100 and is a reliable index of the state of consciousness in normal subjects. Scores more than 95 indicate full consciousness. Of sedated patients, 95% are unconscious if the BIS score is 50. BIS correlates with the depth of sedation of patients who require mechanical ventilation and sedation after surgery or medical illness. BIS has been proposed as a guide to prevent oversedation in the critically ill. Unfortunately, the BIS score may be complicated if the EEG also reflects changes in the neurologic status of the patient that are caused by the illness itself.

Radionuclide imaging is rarely performed in the PICU; it may provide some useful information regarding cerebral blood flow. A portable gamma camera allows tests to be performed at the bedside. Cerebral blood flow studies allow one to confirm brain death if there is equivocation. It also permits one to quantify cerebral blood flow to injured areas of brain. The clinical significance of this is unclear.

Invasive neurologic monitoring involves ICP monitoring and jugular bulb catheterization. The indication for ICP monitoring includes any acute neurologic deterioration where elevated ICP may produce further injury to the patient. Usually, acute traumatic events with a GCS less than 8 will require a monitoring device inserted either in the operating room or at the bedside in the PICU. The type of device and how it is inserted is usually the responsibility of the neurosurgeon placing the device (Fig. 55–2). Ventriculostomy as well as intraparenchymal, subdural, or subarachnoid placement of catheters can be used. All but the intraparenchymal catheters are connected to the transducer via a fluid-filled tubing device. The ventriculostomy and the intraparenchymal fiberoptic devices are the most reliable and most used devices for monitoring ICP. A ventricular catheter allows one to not only measure ICP but also remove fluid if necessary, thereby providing a therapeutic option. The intraparenchymal fiberoptic system provides for a very reliable method of ICP measurements, but does not permit the removal of cerebrospinal fluid (CSF). It is not a fluid-filled system but is easy to use.

The device is connected to a transducer and then to the monitor. A waveform with a numeric value is produced. The ICP should be less than 20 cm H_2O. When monitoring ICP, it is imperative that the systemic arterial blood pressure be determined simultaneously. The difference between the mean arterial pressure and the ICP is the cerebral perfusion pressure. This should be more than 50 in older patients and slightly less in younger children. The complications associated with ICP monitoring include bleeding (check coagulation factors before insertion), infection if left in for more than 5 days, injury to the brain parenchyma (usually only intraventricular catheters), and CSF leak.

Jugular bulb monitoring enables one to obtain continuous oxygen saturation ($JSao_2$) measurements using an indwelling fiberoptic catheter placed in the jugular vein and advanced cephalad to the level of the jugular bulb. The values obtained correlate with the jugular Pao_2 content and do not require blood sampling for actual determination of the oxygen saturations. The jugular bulb is located at the base of the skull and just outside the jugular foramen. It is the point of exit of the blood draining most of the cerebral hemispheres. The clinician is

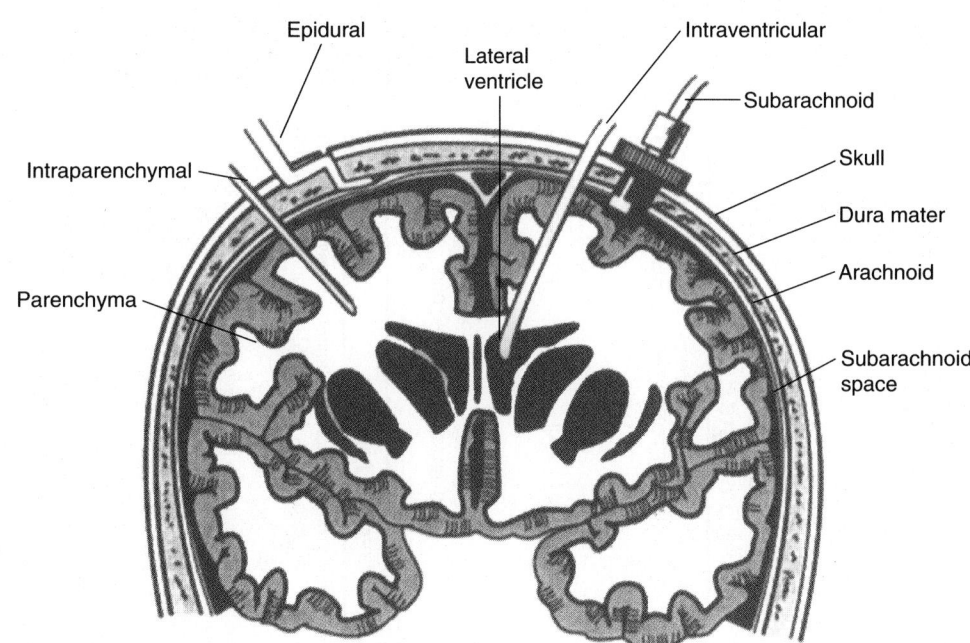

FIGURE 55–2. Sites for monitoring intracranial pressure. A variety of monitor types are shown. Intraventricular catheters are most often fluid-filled tubes connected by pressure tubing to a pressure transducer. CSF can be withdrawn through the catheter. Subarachnoid (also subdural) monitors are fluid-filled, hollow devices that can be bolted to the calvaria connected by pressure tubing to a pressure transducer. CSF cannot be withdrawn. Epidural monitors are waferlike devices of several types, placed in the epidural space. CSF cannot be withdrawn. Intraparenchymal pressure, without the ability to withdraw CSF, can also be monitored. (Redrawn from Lyons MK, Meyer FB: Cerebrospinal fluid physiology and the management of increased intracranial pressure. *Mayo Clin Proc* 1990; 65:684.)

provided with information that enables one to determine how well the injured brain is utilizing oxygen. By knowing the saturations of oxygen in both the systemic arterial and jugular vein, one is able to calculate the arteriojugular difference for oxygen ($AJDo_2$). This is normally 4–9 mg/dL. Levels below this indicate cerebral hyperemia, and the clinician may select therapies designed to decrease cerebral blood flow. Levels greater than 10 mg/dL may indicate ischemia and necessitate further tests to determine the extent of the brain injury. It is hoped that using the values obtained from ICP, $AJDo_2$, and cerebral blood flow, one may alter therapy to improve outcome.

Gilbert TT, Wagner MR, Halukurike V, et al: Use of bispectral electroencephalogram monitoring to assess neurologic status in unsedated, critically ill patients. *Crit Care Med* 2001;29:1996–2000.

Shapiro BA: Bispectral index: Better information for sedation in the intensive care unit? *Crit Care Med* 1999;27:1663–4.

Tobias JD, Connors D, Strauser L, et al: Continuous pH and Pco_2 monitoring during respiratory failure in children with the Paratrend 7 inserted into the peripheral venous system. *J Pediatr* 2000;136:623–7.

Chapter 56
Scoring Systems and Predictors of Mortality

Joseph V. DiCarlo and Lorry R. Frankel

Scoring systems are useful for making triage decisions and assessing the performance of an intensive care unit, but they are of limited use in predicting prognosis in individual cases. Various scoring systems are currently used in the pediatric intensive care unit (PICU): (1) *organ specific*, such as the Glasgow Coma Scale (see Chapter 57.7 and Table 57–3) or the croup score (see Chapter 371), (2) *mechanism of injury*, such as the Pediatric Trauma Score (see Table 57–18) or Injury Severity Score, and (3) *pediatric*, such as the Pediatric Index of Mortality (PIM), the Physiologic Stability Index (PSI), or the Pediatric Risk of Mortality (PRISM).

Pediatric Risk of Mortality. This system, a revision of the PSI, assesses the severity of illness in a population of pediatric patients. The PRISM in its third version (PRISM III) is used to compare and evaluate the performance and resource use among various PICUs. It is based on 17 physiologic variables subdivided into 26 ranges (Fig. 56–1). A patient's past medical history is also taken into account, particularly chronic illness and previous PICU days. The PRISM score has a consistently strong relationship between the number of malfunctioning organ systems at 12 and 24 hr and the mortality risk in a given PICU. Attempts to use PRISM for decision making in a single patient are not valid, owing to less than "adequate certainty." The PRISM is most useful in assessing case mix adjustments between units and the overall outcomes for a population of patients in a PICU. A PICU that performs a periodic self-assessment using PRISM can determine if its performance is on a par with a reference population. If performance is below standard, a chart review may reveal the reasons, such as high secondary infection rates, comorbidity issues, and decisions to withdraw or limit therapy. Changes in the score over time may document improvement or deterioration. PRISM is also useful in research in ensuring that control and experimental groups are similar.

Pediatric Trauma Score (see Table 57–18). This score takes into account a child's size, the accessibility of the airway, the systolic blood pressure, the level of consciousness, and the presence or absence of wounds and fractures. Below a certain cutoff, transfer to a dedicated trauma center is recommended (see Chapter 57).

Other Physiologic Scoring Systems. Other scoring systems are less useful in pediatrics. The Acute Physiology and Chronic Health Evaluation (APACHE) system is used in adult intensive care units. The PRISM III is better suited to the physiology of a child. The PSI is a refinement of APACHE that attempts to make age-related adjustments. The Therapeutic Intervention Scoring System (TISS) relies on the type and amount of therapy given and therefore may indirectly reflect severity of illness and directly reflect resource utilization. A single calculation, the Oxygenation Index [$OI = (Fio_2$ mean airway pressure)/Pao_2] is predictive of survival in many forms of respiratory failure.

Novel Therapies and Refinement of Practice. Intensivists attempt to improve survival by employing new treatments such as

PRISM III

CARDIOVASCULAR/NEUROLOGIC VITAL SIGNS (1–6)

Systolic Blood Pressure (mmHg)

Measurement	Score = 3	Score = 7
Neonate	40–55	<40
Infant	45–65	<45
Child	55–75	<55
Adolescent	65–85	<65

Temperature

Measurement	Score = 3
All ages	<33° C (91.4° F) or >40.0° C (104.0° F)

Mental Status

Measurement	Score = 5
All ages	Stupor/Coma (GCS <8)

Heart Rate (beats per min)

Measurement	Score = 3	Score = 4
Neonate	215–225	>225
Infant	215–225	>225
Child	185–205	>205
Adolescent	145–155	>155

Pupillary Reflexes

Measurement	Score = 7	Score = 11
All ages	One fixed	Both fixed one reactive

ACID-BASE/BLOOD GASES (1, 2, 7, 8)

Acidosis (Total CO$_2$ (mmol/L) or pH)

Measurement	Score = 2	Score = 6
All ages	pH 7.0–7.28 or total CO$_2$ 5–16.9	pH <7.0 or total CO$_2$ <5

pH

Measurement	Score = 2	Score = 3
All ages	7.48–7.55	>7.55

PCO$_2$ (mmHg)

Measurement	Score = 1	Score = 3
All ages	50.0–75.0	>75.0

Total CO$_2$ (mmol/L)

Measurement	Score = 4
All ages	>34.0

PaO$_2$ (mmHg)

Measurement	Score = 3	Score = 6
All ages	42.0–49.9	<42.0

CHEMISTRY TESTS (1, 2, 9)

Glucose

Measurement	Score = 2
All ages	>200 mg/dL or >11.0 mmol/L

Potassium (mmol/L)

Measurement	Score = 3
All ages	>6.9

Creatinine

Measurement	Score = 2
Neonate	>0.85 mg/dL or >75 μmol/L
Infant	>0.90 mg/dL or >80 μmol/L
Child	>0.90 mg/dL or >80 μmol/L
Adolescent	>1.30 mg/dL or >115 μmol/L

Blood Urea Nitrogen (BUN)

Measurement	Score = 3
Neonate	>11.9 mg/dL or >4.3 mmol/L
All other ages	>14.9 mg/dL or >5.4 mmol/L

HEMATOLOGY TESTS (1, 2)

Prothrombin Time (PT) or Partial Thromboplastin Time (PTT) (sec)

Measurement	Score = 3
Neonate	PT >22.0 or PTT >85.0
All other ages	PT >22.0 or PTT >57.0

White Blood Cell Count (cells/mm^3)

Measurement	Score = 4
All ages	<3,000

Platelet Count (cells/mm^3)

Measurement	Score = 2	Score = 4	Score = 5
All ages	100,000–200,000	50,000–99,999	<50,000

TOTAL PRISM III SCORE ____

OTHER FACTORS (10)

☐ Nonoperative CV disease ☐ Chromosomal anomaly ☐ Cancer ☐ Previous PICU admission
☐ Pre-ICU CPR ☐ Post-operative ☐ Acute diabetes (e.g. DKA) ☐ Admission from inpatient
unit (exclude post-operative patients)

Notes:

1. PRISM III mortality risk equations are available for the first 12 hours and the first 24 hours of PICU care.
2. General: Use the highest and/or the lowest values for scoring. When there are both low and high ranges, PRISM III points may be assigned for the low and the high ranges. Readmissions are included as separate patients. Exclude admissions routinely cared for in other hospital locations, staying in the PICU <2 hours; and those admitted in continuous CPR who do not achieve stable vital signs for ≥2 hours. Deaths occurring in the OR are included only if the operation occurred during the PICU stay and was a therapy for the illness requiring PICU care. Terminally ill patients transferred from the PICU for "comfort care" are included as PICU patients for the 24 hours following PICU discharge or, if receiving technologic support, until 24 hours after the technologic support is discontinued. Ages: Neonate = 0–<1 month; Infant = ≥1 month–12 months; Child = ≥12 months–144 months; Adolescent >144 months.
3. Heart Rate: Do not assess during crying or iatrogenic agitation.
4. Temperature: Use rectal, oral, blood, or axillary temperatures.
5. Pupillary Reflexes: Nonreactive pupils must be >3 mm. Do not assess after iatrogenic pupillary dilatation.
6. Mental Status: Include only patients with known or suspected, acute CNS disease. Do not assess within 2 hours of sedation, paralysis, or anesthesia. If there is constant paralysis and/or sedation, use the time period without sedation, paralysis, or anesthesia closest to the PICU admission for scoring. Stupor/coma is defined as GCS score <8 or stupor/coma using other mental status scales.
7. Acid-Base: Use calculated bicarbonate values from blood gases only if total CO$_2$ is not measured routinely. pH and PCO$_2$ may be measured from arterial, capillary, or venous sites.
8. PaO$_2$: Use arterial measurements only.
9. Whole Blood Corrections: Whole blood measurements should be increased as follows: glucose - 10%; sodium - 3 mmol/L; potassium - 0.4 mmol/L. (Pediatric Reference Ranges, Soldin SJ, Hicks JM, AACC Press, Washington, D.C., 1995).
10. Nonoperative CV disease includes acute cardiac and vascular conditions as the primary reasons for admission. Cancer and chromosomal anomalies are acute or chronic. Previous PICU admission and pre-PICU CPR refer to the current hospital admission. Post-operative is the initial 24 hours following an OR surgical procedure. Catheterizations are not post-operative. Acute diabetes includes acute manifestation of diabetes (e.g. DKA) as the primary reason for PICU admission. Admission from routine care area includes all inpatient locations except the operating or recovery rooms.

FIGURE 56–1. The Pediatric Risk of Mortality III (PRISM III) Score. Numbers in parentheses refer to *Notes*. *CV*, cardiovascular; *PICU*, pediatric intensive care unit; *ICU*, intensive care unit; *CPR*, cardiopulmonary resuscitation; *DKA*, diabetic ketoacidosis; *CNS*, central nervous system; *GCS*, Glasgow Coma Scale; *OR*, operating room. (Adapted from Pollack MM, Patel KM, Ruttimann UE: PRISM III: An updated pediatric risk of mortality score. *Crit Care Med* 1996;24:743–52.)

permissive hypercapnia and relative hypoxia in the child with severe respiratory failure; early use of hemofiltration; use of bio-logic modifying products for sepsis; and high-frequency oscilla-tory ventilation, with a concomitant decline in the utilization of jet ventilation and ECMO outside the neonatal period. The hope is for increased survival from septic shock, respiratory failure, and ARDS. Performance deemed acceptable against a predictive score standard developed in 1995 may not be reliable, thus necessitating constant reassessment, reevaluation, and updating of pediatric scores.

Arnold JH, Anas NG, Luckett P, et al: High-frequency oscillatory ventilation in pediatric respiratory failure: A multicenter experience. *Crit Care Med* 2000;28: 3913–19.

Marcin JP, Pollack MM, Patel KM, Ruttimann UE: Decision support issues using a physiology based score. *Intensive Care Med* 1998;24:1299–1304.

Pollack MM, Patel KM, Ruttimann UE: PRISM III: An updated pediatric risk of mortality score. *Crit Care Med* 1996;24:743–52.

Pollack MM, Patel KM, Ruttimann UE: The Pediatric Risk of Mortality III—Acute Physiology Score (PRISM-APS): A method of assessing physiologic instability for pediatric intensive care unit patients. *J Pediatr* 1997;131:575.

Chapter 57
Stabilization of the Critically Ill Child

57.1 Pediatric Emergencies and Resuscitation

Lawrence H. Mathers and Lorry R. Frankel

Each year in the United States there are over 150,000 emergen-cies that threaten the lives of children; approximately 10,000 of these children die, and at least 90,000 survive with permanent disability. These emergencies may need immediate treatment in various settings in the home, community, or hospital. Bystander rescuers, parents, or health care providers may have to provide immediate resuscitation while simultaneously activating the emergency care system and facilitating patient transport to the nearest appropriate facility. The growing number of children with increased vulnerability to serious illness, such as surviving premature infants or children with chronic disease, makes knowledge of how to respond to pediatric emergencies critical (see Chapter 51).

Pediatric emergencies are of various types: respiratory, car-diac, endocrine, traumatic, and infectious. However, most pedi-atric arrests are respiratory, not cardiac. Sudden, unanticipated, nontraumatic cardiac arrests are uncommon in children in con-trast to the primary nature of cardiac arrest in adults from ischemic heart disease and subsequent ventricular fibrillation or ventricular tachycardia. Cardiac arrests in children may develop in the presence of known (preoperative or postoperative con-genital heart disease) or unknown (hypertrophic cardiomyopa-thy, aberrant coronary arteries, prolonged QT syndromes, critical aortic stenosis) lesions during strenuous exercise in ado-lescents (see Chapter 428.6).

Respiratory arrests are more common in children with pre-existing chronic lung disease or those who become acutely ill with shock or airway compromise (Box 57–1). Respiratory fail-ure is a preterminal event following severe asthma, pneumonia, sudden infant death syndrome (SIDS), submersions, trauma, sepsis, and foreign body or gastric content aspiration.

Cardiopulmonary arrests in a hospital setting are usually ini-tially respiratory arrests and are often predictable. Apnea usu-ally precedes bradycardia with poor perfusion; many patients

---

BOX 57–1. Respiratory Emergencies

UPPER AIRWAY OBSTRUCTION

Child usually presents in obvious respiratory distress—with stridor or leaning chin forward and drooling.

Do not put instruments into the airway unless prepared to intubate immediately. This is especially risky in presumed epiglottitis and bacterial tracheitis or foreign body.

Lateral neck radiograph can show enlarged epiglottis at base of tongue or possibly a foreign body.

Major challenge is to avoid irritation of the airway, which can precipitate complete airway obstruction.

SMALL AIRWAYS

Usually this is an exacerbation of a previously existing condition such as asthma, cystic fibrosis, or bronchopulmonary dysplasia. Patients present with wheezing.

Mucus and/or bronchospasm causes air trapping—inspired air more easily enters the alveoli than it leaves them. As a result, the distal airways and alveoli distend with gas and efficient exchange is impaired. Pneumothorax may also occur.

In extreme cases, status asthmaticus or bronchiolitis can be fatal.

Necessary steps for therapy: oxygen, bronchiodilators (aerosols and intravenous), steroids (delayed action), relaxation, and reassurance.

PNEUMONIA

Impaired gas exchange is due to alveolar injury; usually involves surfactant deficiency, plus fluid in alveoli.

Therapy: oxygen, antibiotics, mechanical ventilatory support if serious disease.

Parenchymal disease increases the tendency for intrapulmonary shunts, increasing the hypoxia.

Pneumonia becomes life threatening only when large portions of the lungs are involved.

Sickle cell acute chest syndrome is particularly dangerous.

---

have a pre-existing chronic life-threatening or life-shortening condition. In the hospital, the first recorded electrocardiogram (ECG) is asystole in over 50%; pulseless electrical activity in about 10%; bradycardia with poor perfusion in 25%; and ven-tricular fibrillation or pulseless ventricular tachycardia in about 15%. The older the patient is, the higher the likelihood of ven-tricular fibrillation or ventricular tachycardia.

The proper response to each emergency requires an aware-ness of the mechanisms of disease and the immediate physio-logic threats and their proper treatment. A number of factors contribute to the physiologic instability of infants and young children (Box 57–2). Children with recurring life-threatening illnesses (e.g., seizure disorders, asthma, cardiac dysrhythmias) may be able to take precautions to minimize the risk of such threats. Parental vigilance and anticipation of potential dangers in the home, especially for young children, can prevent many injuries and deaths (see Chapter 50).

Emergency personnel should have an approach that will allow them, in the best interest of the patient, to refrain from initiating or terminating resuscitations when efforts are futile. With many chronically ill children being cared for at home or in care facilities, it is not unusual for emergency personnel to be presented with an advanced directive or other document indi-cating the wish that resuscitation not be performed. It may be difficult to interrupt or not commence a resuscitative effort on the basis of these documents unless a community-wide means of establishing their credibility is developed.

LIFE-THREATENING EMERGENCIES AND PRE-ARREST STATES IN CHILDREN

The most common life-threatening illnesses in children are those involving respiratory (see Chapters 57.3 and 58), cardiac (see Chapters 427–437), or neurologic (see Chapter 57.7) fail-ure. Acute failure of the liver (see Chapter 345), kidneys (see Chapter 527), or adrenals (see Chapter 569) also place pediatric

BOX 57–2. Factors Contributing to Infant Physiologic Instability

TEMPERATURE

Neonates have thin skin (radiating heat) and underdeveloped hypothalamic control. They lack the efficient neural mechanisms for temperature control (e.g., shivering) and are greatly influenced by environmental temperature.

FLUID REQUIREMENTS

Thin skin allows more evaporation; fluid content in an infant's body is higher than in an adult's (75–80% in newborn); kidneys reabsorb electrolytes inefficiently; infants need proportionately more fluid per unit of weight than adults.

AIRWAY

Airway is small and narrow; resistance to gas flow is inversely proportional to the 4th power of the radius, so small mucous obstructions can seriously threaten air movement; laryngeal and tracheal cartilages are softer than in adults and more easily collapse to obstruct the airway.

CARDIAC OUTPUT

Heart rate is the major mechanism for varying cardiac output.

GLUCOSE METABOLISM

Newborn infants, especially, have only marginal glycogen stores and may mobilize fat poorly; hypoglycemia occurs more readily than in adults, because of dependence on exogenous supply of glucose.

patients at risk. Identifying the cause of various organ failures may take considerable time, but treatment of the physiologically unstable child must begin immediately.

Detecting and Assessing Physiologic Instability. A simple and consistent approach is necessary for rapid and efficient evaluation of a pediatric patient who may be in serious distress. *Observation* begins with determination of the alertness of the patient, including response to stimuli, spontaneous vocalization or movement, and muscle tone. In basic life support, this is assessed by asking, "Are you all right?" This is followed by assessment of the *vital signs* (Table 57–1) and other basic indicators of the physiologic state.

Pulse and Heart Rate. The ability to detect a pulse in the compromised patient is unreliable among many lay rescuers. Medical professionals and parents of chronically ill children who were taught to palpate a pulse should do so as part of the initial assessment (Table 57–2). Lay rescuers should check for other physical signs of adequate circulation (breathing, movement, coughing, color) but should not check for a pulse. In children younger than age 8 yr or those with trauma, near-drowning, a drug over-

TABLE 57–2. Chest Compression: Ventilation Relationships

	Neonate	1–8 Yr	>8 Yr
Compression rate	120	At least 100	100
*Compression to ventilation ratio**	3:1	5:1	15:2[†]
Pulse check[‡]	Umbilical artery	Brachial	Carotid

Ventilation should be given without interrupting chest compression. It is asynchronous.
[†]*Once intubated go to 5:1.*
[‡]*For lay rescuers no pulse check is necessary; it actually delays cardiopulmonary resuscitation. Lay rescuers should check for signs of circulation: cyanosis, breathing, coughing, and movement.*

dose, or other obvious respiratory causes of an arrest, the resuscitation should begin before activation of the EMS (the *phone fast protocol*). In children older than age 8 yr or with a history of cardiac disease or with a sudden collapse during exercise, ventricular fibrillation or ventricular tachycardia may be present. This creates a more urgent need to activate EMS to be able to do defibrillation if needed as soon as possible. Therefore, the *phone first protocol* with a lone rescuer involves activating EMS before formal resuscitation. If two rescuers are present, then activation of EMS and resuscitation will be simultaneous. Many community settings (shopping malls, airports, high schools) are equipped with automatic external defibrillators that can be used to rapidly assess the rhythm and to defibrillate (if needed) any child older than 8 yr.

When a child's heart rate lies outside the physiologic parameters, cardiac output may be affected. A rapid heart rate (supraventricular tachycardia or ventricular tachycardia) may be associated with a serious reduction in stroke volume, as reflected in poor perfusion and increased fussiness (see Chapter 428). Cardiac failure may develop with pulmonary edema (see Chapters 57.3 and 394). Bradycardia also may represent a serious pre-arrest condition (see Chapter 428). Alternatively, the heart rate change may reflect an appropriate physiologic response (sinus tachycardia) and may not necessarily constitute significant cardiac pathophysiology. Sinus tachycardia may be distinguished from supraventricular tachycardia (SVT) by the history as well as the presence of upright P waves in sinus tachycardia in leads I and aVF, whereas SVT may demonstrate negative P waves in leads II, III, and aVF. Sinus tachycardia has a rate that is usually less than 220 beats/min in infants and less than 180 beats/min in children. SVT has an abrupt onset and an abrupt termination and can be terminated by vagal maneuvers (Valsalva, ice water bag to face, or gentle carotid massage), intravenous adenosine, or synchronized cardioversion (0.5–1 J/kg).

Blood Pressure (BP). This is most often measured by auscultation, but automated devices such as the Dinamap can be set to measure BP repeatedly and at very short intervals (see Chapter 437). To help define poor perfusion, the lower limit of systolic BP should be less than 60 mm Hg for neonates; less than 70 mm Hg from 1 mo to 1 yr; less than 70 mm Hg + 2 × age from 1–10 yr; and less than 90 mm Hg if older than age 10 yr.

Organ Perfusion. Adequate cardiac output is reflected in good perfusion of the skin (central and of distal extremities). Skin perfusion may be assessed by the temperature of the skin or by capillary refill time (the time required for color to return to the skin after pressure blanching that part of the skin is released). Normal capillary refill time is 2 seconds or less; however, low environmental temperature may cause peripheral vasoconstriction and lengthening of capillary refill. Pulse oximetry is meant to measure hemoglobin oxygen saturation; because it requires

TABLE 57–1. Vital Signs at Various Ages

Age	Heart Rate (beats/min)	Blood Pressure (mm Hg)	Respiratory Rate (breaths/min)
Premature	120–170*	55–75/35–45[†]	40–70[‡]
0–3 mo	100–150*	65–85/45–55	35–55
3–6 mo	90–120	70–90/50–65	30–45
6–12 mo	80–120	80–100/55–65	25–40
1–3 yr	70–110	90–105/55–70	20–30
3–6 yr	65–110	95–110/60–75	20–25
6–12 yr	60–95	100–120/60–75	14–22
12* yr	55–85	110–135/65–85	12–18

In sleep, infant heart rates may drop significantly lower, but if perfusion is maintained, no intervention is required.
[†]*A blood pressure cuff should cover approximately two thirds of the arm; too small a cuff yields spuriously high pressure readings, and too large a cuff yields spuriously low pressure readings.*
[‡]*Many premature infants require mechanical ventilatory support, making their spontaneous respiratory rate less relevant.*

adequate perfusion to produce reliable measurements, the presence of a strong signal indicates good peripheral perfusion.

Core Temperature. The normal temperature range for humans is constant throughout life. Premature infants and small term infants may have difficulty maintaining their appropriate core temperature if they are left uncovered in a cool environment. Infants may not be able to generate an elevated temperature in response to infection (see Chapter 98).

Respiratory Effort and Gas Exchange. Muscle *retractions* in the chest and neck and *flaring* of the nostrils at inspiration are signs of an abnormally high level of effort required to move air into the lungs. *Grunting* is a moaning, crying-like noise at expiration, associated with generation of positive pressure to maintain alveolar patency. A child who is inadequately oxygenated demonstrates *cyanosis* (a blue or dusky color of the skin and mucous membranes) (see Chapters 357 and 359). Although observations of respiratory effort provide useful information about impending respiratory failure, arterial blood gases provide a more accurate assessment of respiratory gas exchange (see Chapters 52 and 359) and evidence of a lactic acidosis due to poor perfusion.

Cardiac Dysrhythmias (see Chapter 428). Disturbances in cardiac rate and rhythm are not rare in children; the majority of these dysrhythmias are transient and not pathologic. Life-threatening cardiac emergencies in children are more likely to be bradycardia or asystole than ventricular fibrillation, which is more common in adolescents and adults. The prevalence of pediatric rhythm disturbances is rising as more children with congenital heart anomalies undergo surgical correction and survive through childhood. Abnormal cardiac rhythms may be manifested as sudden collapse, dyspnea, tachypnea, tachycardia, palpitations (the consciousness of skipped or irregular beats), syncope, dizziness, or angina (rarely). Tachyarrhythmias or bradycardias may not pose any danger to a patient initially; but when they affect the cardiac output, patients become symptomatic.

The diagnosis and the management of specific rhythm disturbances in children are discussed in Chapter 428. *Asystole, symptomatic tachycardias,* and *bradycardia* present distinct resuscitative paradigms that require swift recognition and intervention; personnel in offices, clinics, and inpatient areas need to be prepared to manage these complicated situations (Figs. 57–1 to 57–5). *Electrolyte imbalances* also may produce life-threatening dysrhythmias (see Chapter 45). Children who experience significant fluid

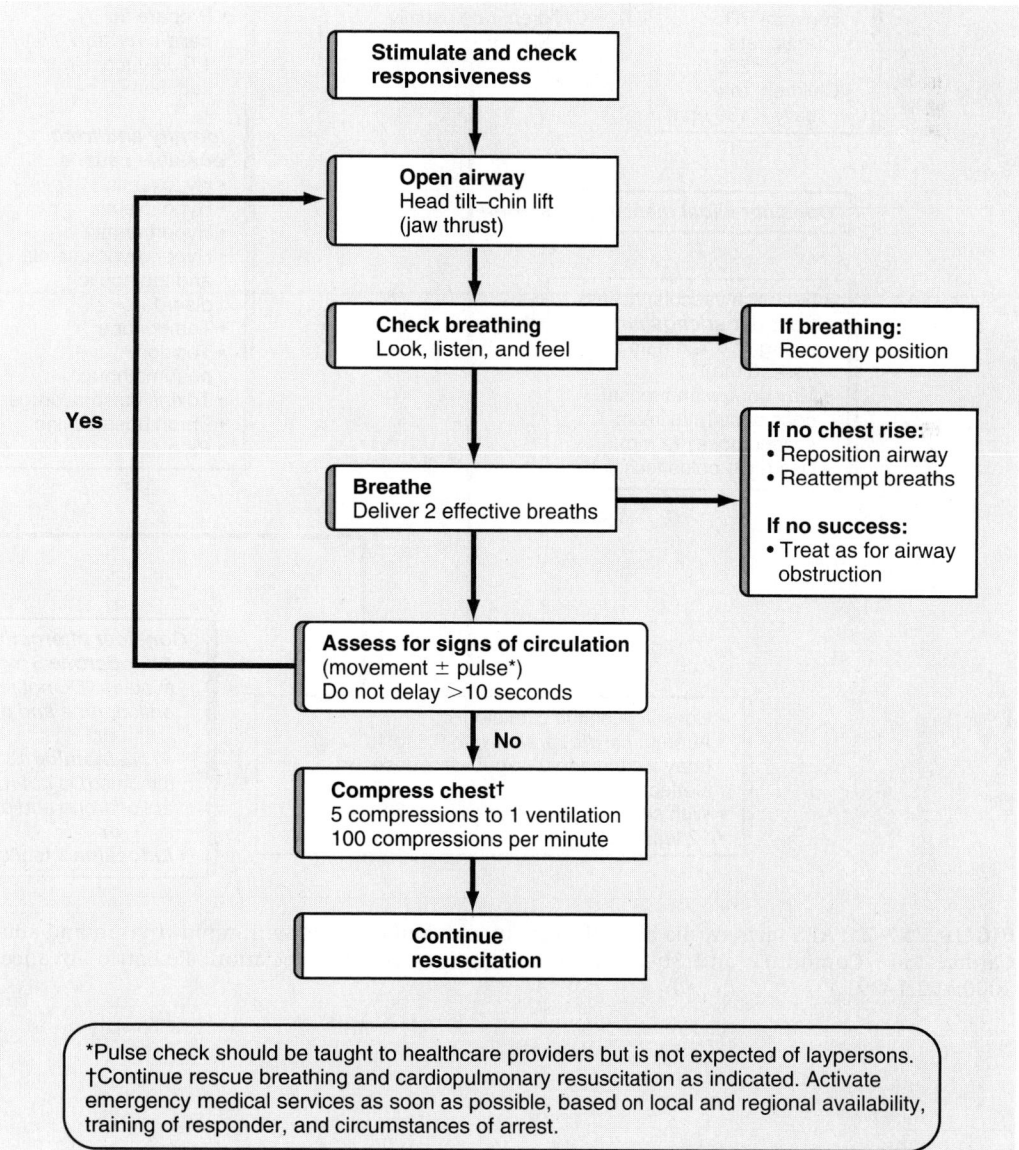

FIGURE 57–1. Pediatric BLS algorithm. (From Emergency Cardiac Care Committee and Subcommittee, American Heart Association: Pediatric basic life support, part 9. *Circulation* 2000; 102:1–253.)

Stimulate and check responsiveness

Open airway
Head tilt–chin lift
(jaw thrust)

Check breathing
Look, listen, and feel

If breathing:
Recovery position

Breathe
Deliver 2 effective breaths

If no chest rise:
• Reposition airway
• Reattempt breaths

If no success:
• Treat as for airway obstruction

Assess for signs of circulation
(movement ± pulse*)
Do not delay >10 seconds

Yes

No

Compress chest†
5 compressions to 1 ventilation
100 compressions per minute

Continue resuscitation

*Pulse check should be taught to healthcare providers but is not expected of laypersons.
†Continue rescue breathing and cardiopulmonary resuscitation as indicated. Activate emergency medical services as soon as possible, based on local and regional availability, training of responder, and circumstances of arrest.

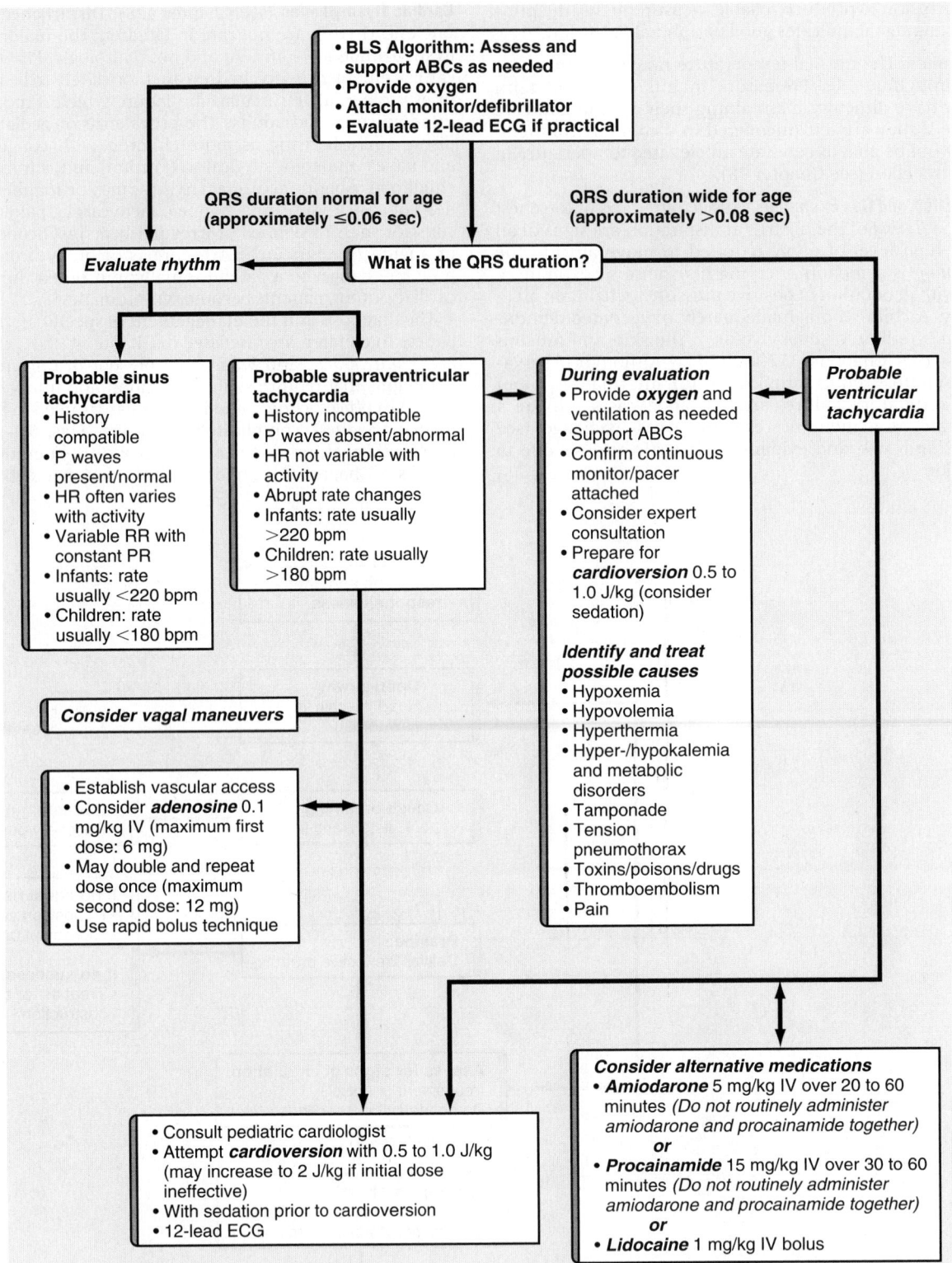

FIGURE 57–2. PALS tachycardia algorithm for infants and children with rapid rhythm and adequate perfusion. (From Emergency Cardiac Care Committee and Subcommittee, American Heart Association: Pediatric advanced life support, part 10. *Circulation* 2000;102:1–291.)

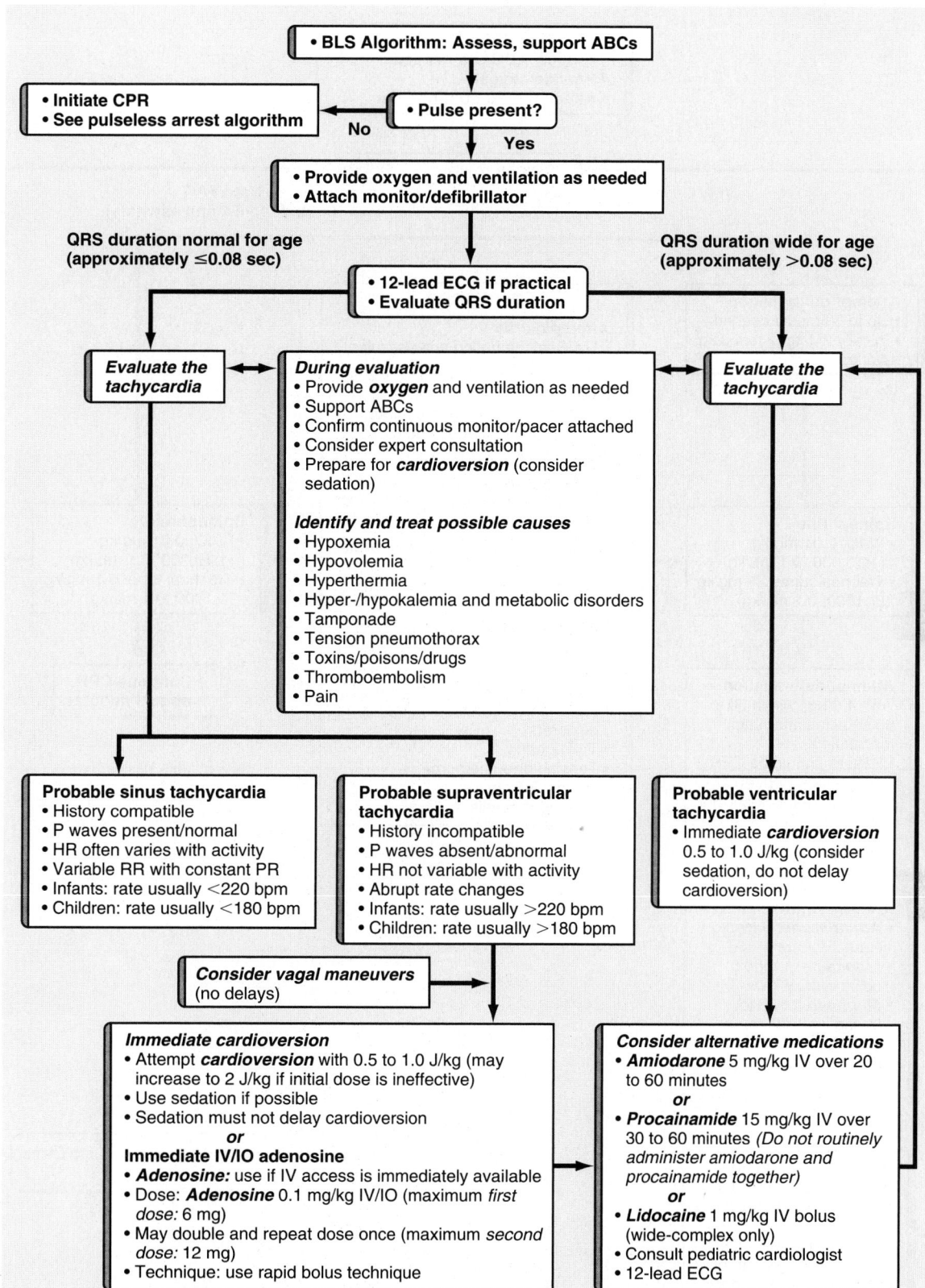

FIGURE 57–3. PALS tachycardia algorithm for infants and children with rapid rhythm and evidence of poor perfusion. (From Emergency Cardiac Care Committee and Subcommittee, American Heart Association: Pediatric advanced life support, part 10. *Circulation* 2000;102:1–291.)

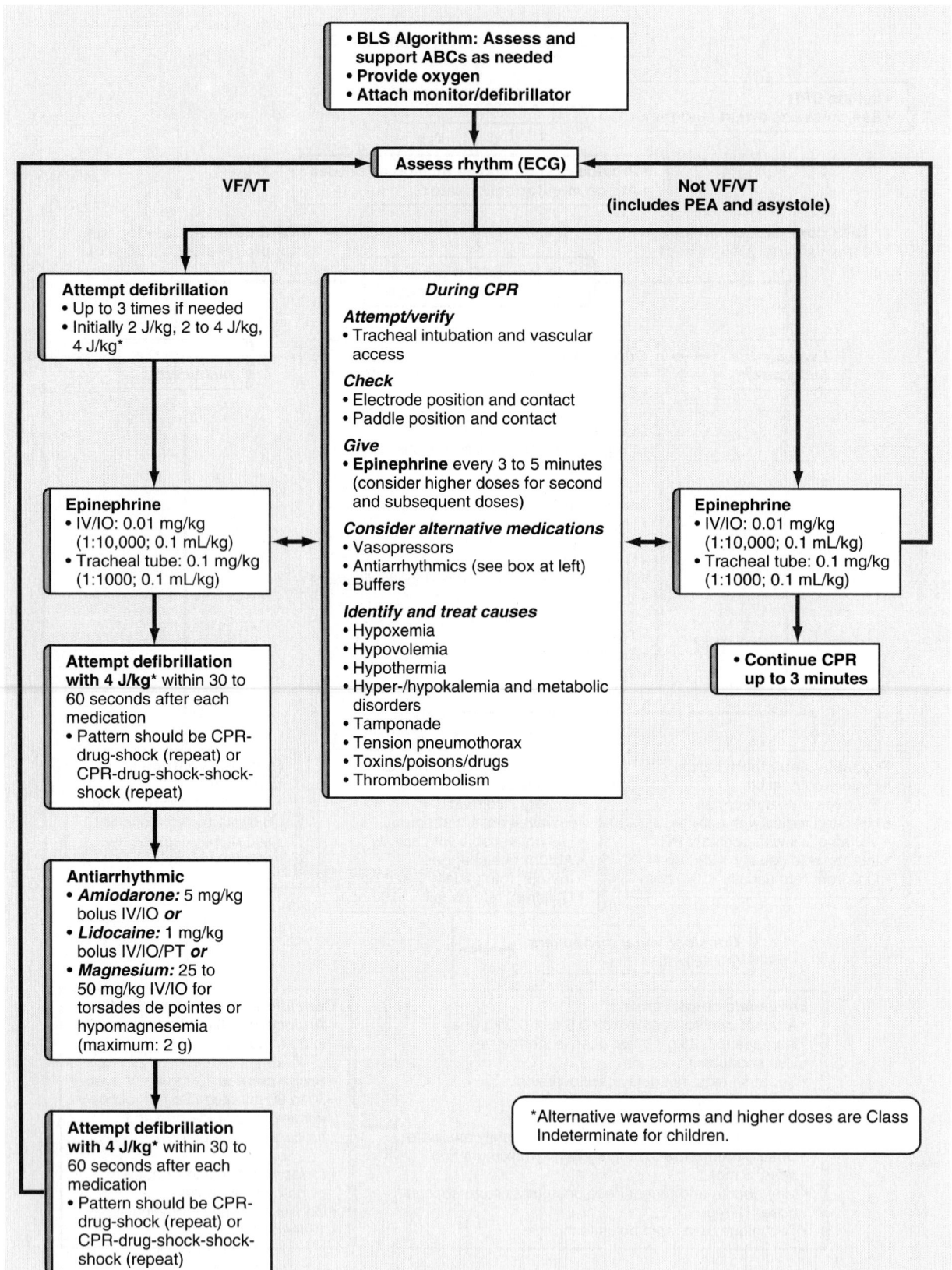

FIGURE 57–4. PALS pulseless arrest algorithm. PEA = pulseless electrical activity; VF = ventricular fibrillation; VT = ventricular tachycardia. (From Emergency Cardiac Care Committee and Subcommittee, American Heart Association: Pediatric advanced life support, part 10. *Circulation* 2000;102:1–291.)

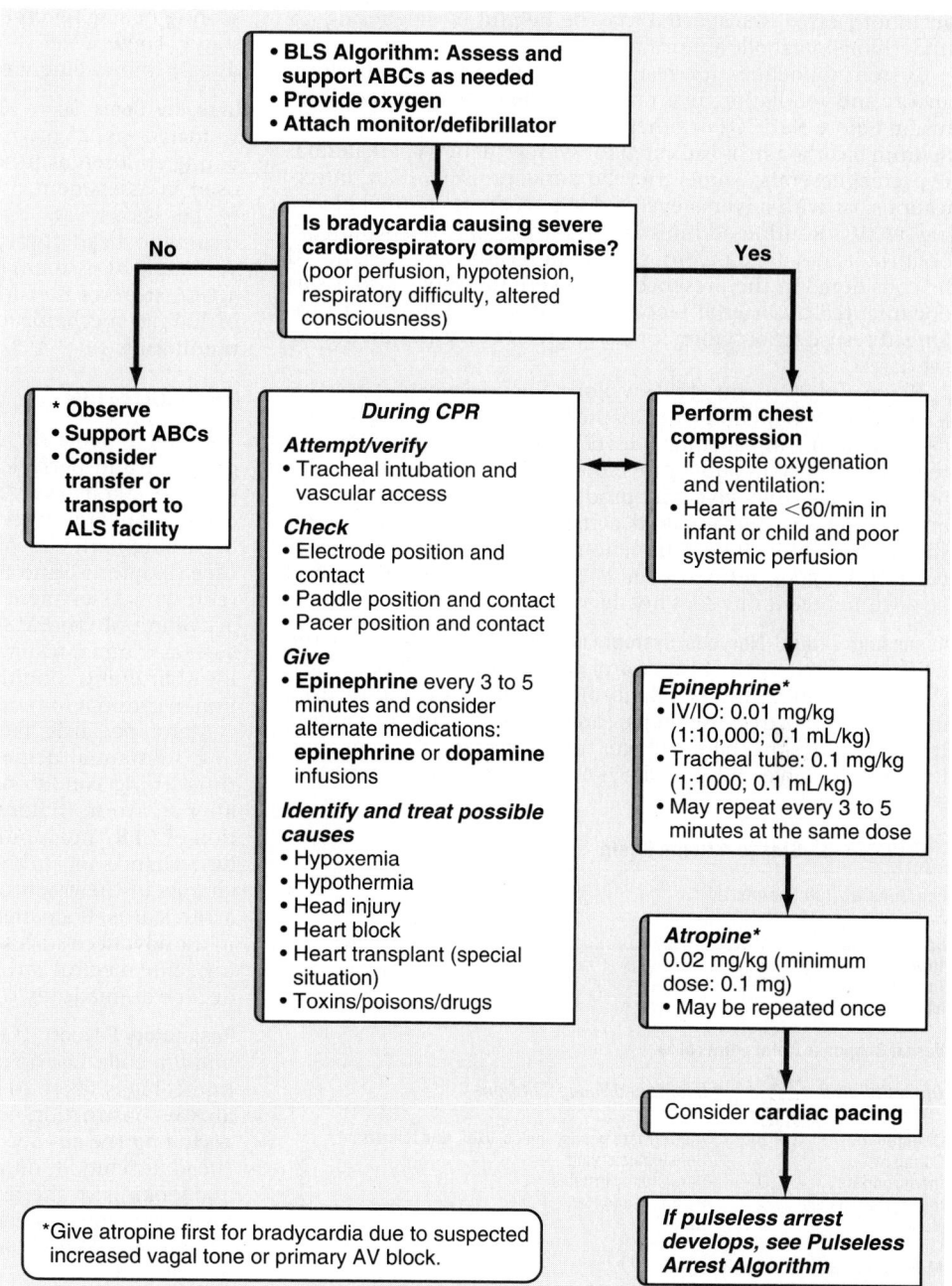

- BLS Algorithm: Assess and support ABCs as needed
- Provide oxygen
- Attach monitor/defibrillator

Is bradycardia causing severe cardiorespiratory compromise? (poor perfusion, hypotension, respiratory difficulty, altered consciousness)

No

Yes

* Observe
- Support ABCs
- Consider transfer or transport to ALS facility

During CPR

Attempt/verify
- Tracheal intubation and vascular access

Check
- Electrode position and contact
- Paddle position and contact
- Pacer position and contact

Give
- **Epinephrine** every 3 to 5 minutes and consider alternate medications: **epinephrine** or **dopamine** infusions

Identify and treat possible causes
- Hypoxemia
- Hypothermia
- Head injury
- Heart block
- Heart transplant (special situation)
- Toxins/poisons/drugs

Perform chest compression if despite oxygenation and ventilation:
- Heart rate <60/min in infant or child and poor systemic perfusion

Epinephrine*
- IV/IO: 0.01 mg/kg (1:10,000; 0.1 mL/kg)
- Tracheal tube: 0.1 mg/kg (1:1000; 0.1 mL/kg)
- May repeat every 3 to 5 minutes at the same dose

Atropine*
0.02 mg/kg (minimum dose: 0.1 mg)
- May be repeated once

Consider **cardiac pacing**

If pulseless arrest develops, see Pulseless Arrest Algorithm

*Give atropine first for bradycardia due to suspected increased vagal tone or primary AV block.

FIGURE 57–5. PALS bradycardia algorithm. (From Emergency Cardiac Care Committee and Subcommittee, American Heart Association: Pediatric advanced life support, part 10. *Circulation* 2000;102:1–291.)

loss or who are receiving diuretics or digoxin are especially at risk.

Alterations of Pulmonary Blood Flow. In various congenital heart conditions and with some physiologic disturbances, blood flow to the lungs meets with resistance, resulting in pulmonary hypertensive crises. These patients are at risk for serious hypoxic/anoxic events (see Chapter 426).

Assessing Metabolic Status. Two important acute destabilizing metabolic disorders are acidosis and hypoglycemia. The causes, consequences, and management of respiratory, metabolic, and mixed *acidosis* are discussed in Chapters 45 and 48. Arterial blood sampling is discussed in Chapter 55. The measurement of the oxygen content of central venous blood (mixed venous oxygen content [Mvo_2]), especially blood from the pulmonary artery (Swan-Ganz) catheter, is helpful in assessing the adequacy of tissue perfusion and increased anaerobic metabolism. Abnormally low oxygen content of venous blood relative to arterial blood suggests that the delivery of blood to tissues is inadequate, resulting in increased extraction of oxygen and metabolic acidosis. If the venous blood oxygen content is abnormally high, either blood is being delivered too rapidly to the tissues (high cardiac output), so that a lower than normal fraction of oxygen is extracted as blood passes through capillary beds, there is abnormal mixing of venous and arterial blood near the heart and great vessels, or the tissue is no longer viable. Assaying a patient's blood and urine for specific organic acids if an inborn error is suspected may be helpful in diagnosing an underlying metabolic abnormality.

Current guidelines for resuscitation emphasize establishing airway and ventilation, heart rate, and adequate peripheral perfusion before NaHCO$_3$ or other buffering agent is administered. Sodium bicarbonate is indicated for symptomatic hyperkalemia, hypermagnesemia, some tricyclic antidepressant drug intoxications, or with adverse events due to sodium channel blocking agents. Routine administration during CPR is discouraged because it may be dangerous. Sodium bicarbonate use should be considered in the presence of a severe metabolic acidosis as documented by arterial blood gas analysis and during a prolonged resuscitation when it may be given every 10 min during the arrest.

Hypoglycemia is defined as low blood glucose level that destabilizes energy production (see Chapters 81 and 96.2). The brain is dependent on an adequate level of circulating glucose and requires a constant supply to support energy-consuming cerebral activities. Hypoglycemia produces weakness and lethargy and can lead to seizures and coma. Emergency resuscitation should usually include intravenous administration of glucose (250–500 mg/kg, infused over 1–2 min; hypoglycemia should be documented if this does not delay treatment).

Assessing Central Nervous System Function. The integrity of the CNS is assessed by the history and physical examination, which should determine the possibility of trauma, toxic and/or drug ingestions, seizures, ischemia, and signs of any expanding intracranial lesion (hemorrhage, tumor, abscess, vascular malformation). Tables 57–3 and 57–4 are examples of important

scoring or staging criteria universally used to assess neurologic status. These scales should be scored serially over time to detect disease improvement or progression.

Glasgow Coma Scale (GCS). Although this scale has not been validated as a prognostic scoring system for infants and young children as it has been in adults, the GCS is commonly used in assessment of pediatric patients with an altered level of consciousness, especially those who have sustained a traumatic head injury (see Table 57–3). The GCS provides very rapid assessment of cerebral cortical function. Patients with a GCS score of 8 or less may require aggressive management, including mechanical ventilation and intracranial pressure monitoring.

RESUSCITATION

The goal in pediatric resuscitation is to maintain adequate oxygenation and perfusion of blood throughout the body while steps are taken to stabilize a child and establish long-term homeostasis. An orderly sequence of events should be instituted, beginning with the ABCs: airway, breathing, and circulation. (See Chapter 51 and Fig. 57–1.) In addition to airway, "A" also represents assessment of responsiveness ("Are you all right?"), activation of the EMS, and anticipation of high-risk situations such as trauma, respiratory distress, or exacerbations of chronic life-shortening conditions. Anticipation is a key to the prevention of cardiopulmonary arrests.

Many pediatric patients undergoing resuscitation recover to a substantial degree. Hospitalized children with acute life-threatening conditions often recover spontaneous circulation after an arrest. Children with a respiratory arrest, a short duration of CPR, and a pulse present at the time of apnea have the best chance of survival. The majority of survivors have no change in their neurologic function compared with their pre-arrest status. If a patient is asystolic on arrival at the hospital or in the advanced stages of a chronic disease process before receiving acute medical care, the chances for a successful resuscitation decline dramatically.

Respiratory Support. If no obstruction by a foreign body is found and if a child has no spontaneous respirations, steps should be immediately taken to breathe for the child. A common cause of airway obstruction in an unresponsive child is the tongue occluding the airway. Assessment includes opening the airway (head tilt/chin lift or jaw thrust if the cervical spine is unstable) and looking for the rise and fall of the chest as well as a foreign body, listening at the nose and mouth for breathing, and feeling air exiting the child's airways (Figs. 57–6 and 57–7). This should be done in less than 10 seconds. If a foreign body is seen, it should be removed; health care workers should perform a tongue/jaw lift if a foreign body is suspected but not initially visualized. If the patient resumes adequate spontaneous ventilation, the patient's body is turned on its side to the recovery position with the head to the side (if in the field).

Rescue breathing should be done by *mouth-to-mouth* or *mouth-to-nose* breathing, a mask over the patient's nose and mouth and *mouth-to-mask* breathing, or *bag-mask* respirations (Figs. 57–8

TABLE 57–3. Glasgow Coma Scale

Eye Opening (total points 4)

Spontaneous	4
To voice	3
To pain	2
None	1

Verbal Response (total points 5)

Older Children		*Infants and Young Children*	
Oriented	5	Appropriate words; smiles, fixes, and follows	5
Confused	4	Consolable crying	4
Inappropriate	3	Persistently irritable	3
Incomprehensible	2	Restless, agitated	2
None	1	None	1

Motor Response (total points 6)

Obeys	6
Localizes pain	5
Withdraws	4
Flexion	3
Extension	2
None	1

Adapted and modified from Teasdale G, Jennett B: Assessment of coma and impaired consciousness: A practical scale. Lancet 1974; 2:81.

TABLE 57–4. Clinical Staging of Encephalopathy

	Clinical Stage			
1	**2**	**3**	**4**	**5**
Lethargic	Combative	Comatose	Comatose	Comatose
Follows commands	Inconsistent following of commands	Occasional response to commands	Responds only to pain	No response to pain
Pupils reactive	Pupils sluggish	Eyes may deviate	Weak pupillary response	No pupillary response
Breathing normal	May hyperventilate	Irregular breathing	Very irregular breathing	Requires mechanical ventilation
Normal muscle tone	Reflexes inconsistent	Decorticate posturing	Decerebrate posturing	Absent tendon reflexes—flaccid

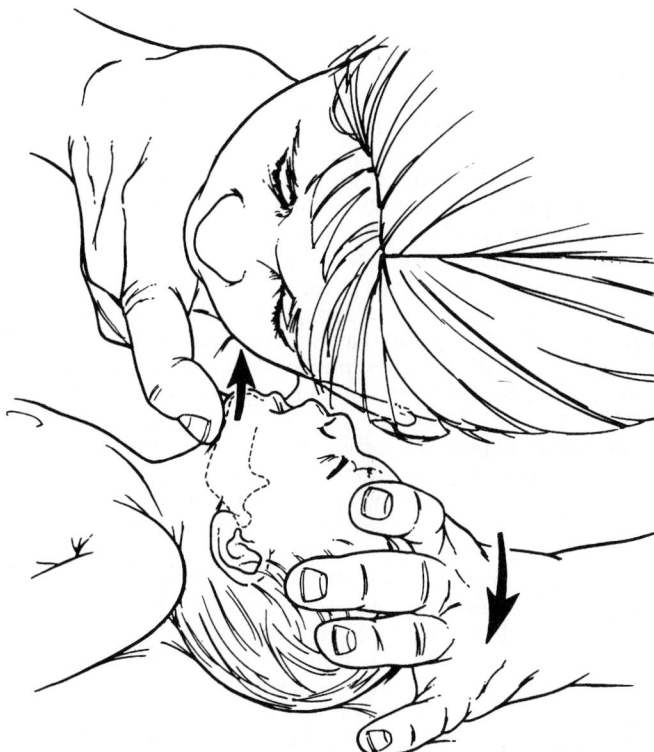

FIGURE 57–6. Opening the airway with the head tilt-chin lift maneuver. One hand is used to tilt the head, extending the neck. The index finger of the rescuer's other hand lifts the mandible outward by lifting on the chin. Head tilt should not be performed if cervical spine injury is suspected. (From Emergency Cardiac Care Committee and Subcommittees, American Heart Association: Pediatric basic life support, part 5. *JAMA* 1992;268:2251.)

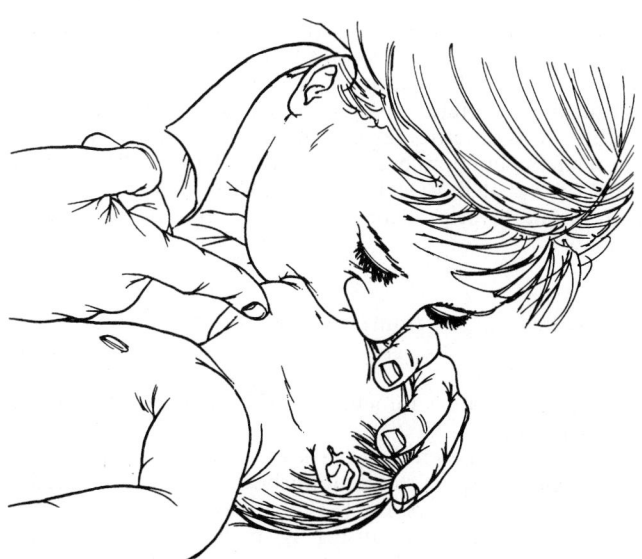

FIGURE 57–8. Rescue breathing in an infant. The rescuer's mouth covers the infant's nose and mouth, creating a seal. One hand performs head tilt while the other hand lifts the infant's jaw. Avoid head tilt if the infant has sustained head or neck trauma. (From Emergency Cardiac Care Committee and Subcommittees, American Heart Association: Pediatric basic life support, part 5. *JAMA* 1992;268:2251.)

entry, recheck that the airway is patent and the seal is tight; if so endotracheal intubation is indicated. Indicators for endotracheal intubation include apnea, loss of CNS control of respirations, airway obstruction unrelieved by airway opening maneuvers, increased work of breathing that may lead to fatigue, the need for positive end-expiratory pressure (PEEP) or

and 57–9). Successful rescue breathing will provide good chest rise and relief of deep cyanosis. Exhaled air is 16–17% oxygen, which corresponds to an alveolar oxygen pressure of 80 mm Hg in the patient. If these measures do not facilitate adequate air

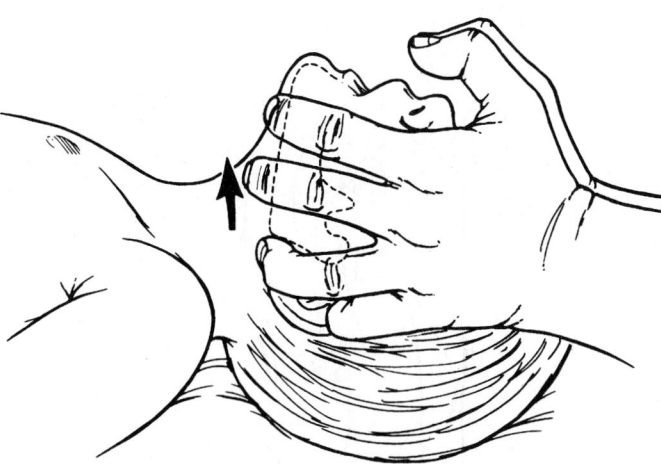

FIGURE 57–7. Combined jaw thrust-spine stabilization maneuver for the pediatric trauma victim. (From Emergency Cardiac Care Committee and Subcommittees, American Heart Association: Pediatric basic life support, part 5. *JAMA* 1992; 268:2251.)

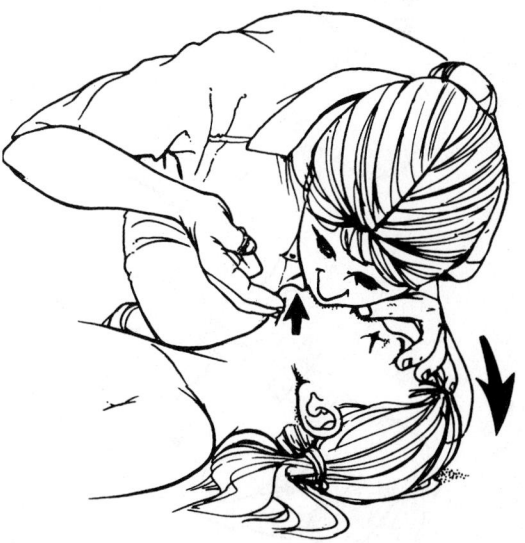

FIGURE 57–9. Rescue breathing in a child. The rescuer's mouth covers the mouth of the child, creating a mouth-to-mouth seal. One hand maintains the head tilt; the thumb and forefinger of the same hand are used to pinch the child's nose. (From Emergency Cardiac Care Committee and Subcommittees, American Heart Association: Pediatric basic life support, part 5. *JAMA* 1992;268:2251.)

a high peak inspiratory pressure (PIP), poor airway protective reflexes, sedation, or the need for paralysis. Once the patient is intubated, proper tube placement is assessed by breath sounds, chest rise, and instantaneous analysis of exhaled carbon dioxide (CO_2) by a colorimetric device placed within the respiratory tubing near the endotracheal tube (ETT). Confirmation of ETT position by exhaled CO_2 is most reliable with a perfusing rhythm. A simple formula for selecting the appropriate size ETT is as follows:

$$\text{Uncuffed ETT size (mm)} = 16 + \frac{\text{Age in yr}}{4}$$

The respiratory rate parameters that should be maintained are indicated in Table 57–2.

In the field, competent bag-mask ventilation may be preferable to repeated attempts at endotracheal intubation by inadequately experienced personnel. The airway in children differs from that of the adult because it is smaller, more anteriorly placed, more difficult to visualize, and more prone to mucosal injuries leading to subglottic stenosis.

Foreign body aspiration always should be suspected if respiratory distress has had a sudden onset (see Chapter 372) or if the chest does not rise when ventilation is first attempted in an unconscious, apneic infant or child. A conscious child suspected of a foreign body partial obstruction should be permitted to cough spontaneously until coughing is not effective (or aphonic), respiratory distress and stridor increase, or the child becomes unconscious. The airway is then opened with the head-tilt/chin-lift maneuver, and ventilation is attempted. If unsuccessful, the airway is repositioned and ventilation again attempted. If there is still no chest rise, attempts to remove a foreign body are indicated. In the infant younger than 1 yr, a com-bination of five back blows and five chest thrusts are administered (Fig. 57–10). The foreign body is removed if it is seen. If no foreign body is visualized, ventilation is again attempted. If this is unsuccessful, the head is repositioned and ventilation attempted again. If there is no chest rise, the series of back blows and chest thrusts are repeated.

A conscious child older than 1 yr is administered a series of five abdominal thrusts (the Heimlich maneuver) with the child standing or sitting (Fig. 57–11). If unconscious, this is done with the child lying down (Fig. 57–12). After the abdominal thrusts, the airway is examined for a foreign body, which should be removed if visualized. If no foreign body is seen, the head is repositioned and ventilation attempted. If unsuccessful, repositioning the head and attempted ventilation are repeated. If unsuccessful, the Heimlich sequence is repeated.

Cardiovascular Support. As resuscitation proceeds and ventilation is started, support of the *circulation* should be provided to sustain adequate blood flow to deliver oxygen to the tissues (Figs. 57–13 to 57–15). Circulation is assessed by lay rescuers without checking for a pulse, while health care workers or trained parents should check for a pulse (see Table 57–2). If there is no pulse or if the pulse is less than 60 beats/min with poor perfusion, chest compressions must be given. Chest compressions are given without interrupting ventilations. The effectiveness of chest compressions is determined by the presence of a palpable pulse. The rate of chest compressions varies with age and size (see Table 57–2). Chest compressions in small infants and newborns may be performed by placing two thumbs on the midsternum with the hands encircling the thorax, or by two fingers over the midsternum and compressing, or by holding the child in the supine posture on one's lap. When feasible, a cardiac resuscitation board should be placed under the child's back to maximize efficiency of compressions. The resuscitation effort should pause

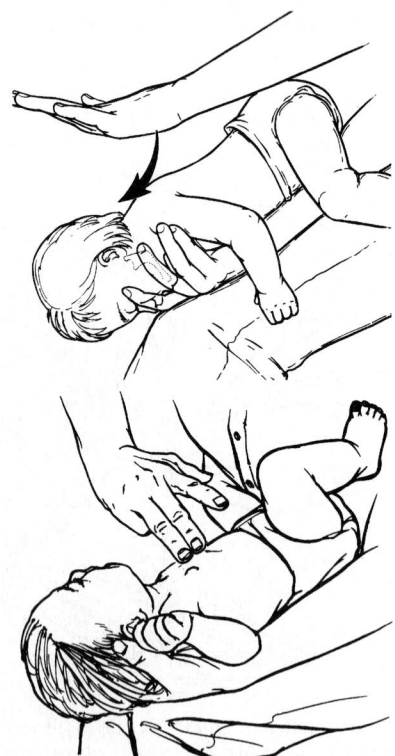

FIGURE 57–10. Back blows *(top)* and chest thrusts *(bottom)* to relieve foreign-body airway obstruction in the infant. (From Emergency Cardiac Care Committee and Subcommittees, American Heart Association. Pediatric basic life support, part 5. *JAMA* 1992;268:2251.)

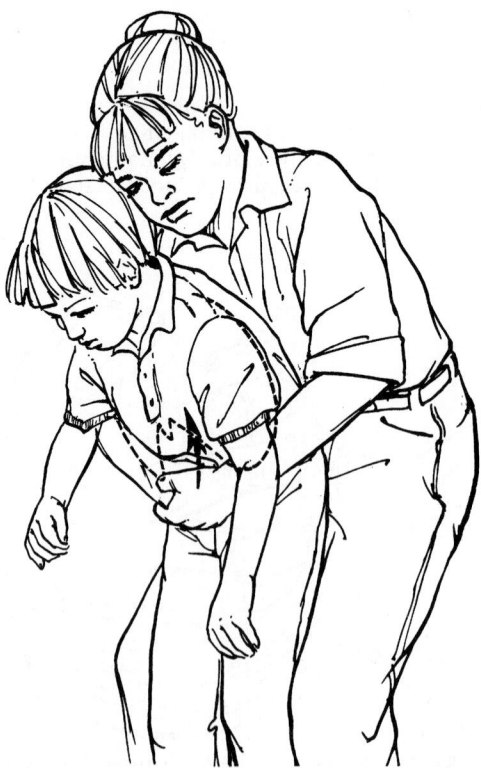

FIGURE 57–11. Abdominal thrusts with victim standing or sitting (conscious). (From Emergency Cardiac Care Committee and Subcommittees, American Heart Association: Pediatric basic life support, part 5. *JAMA* 1992;268:2251.)

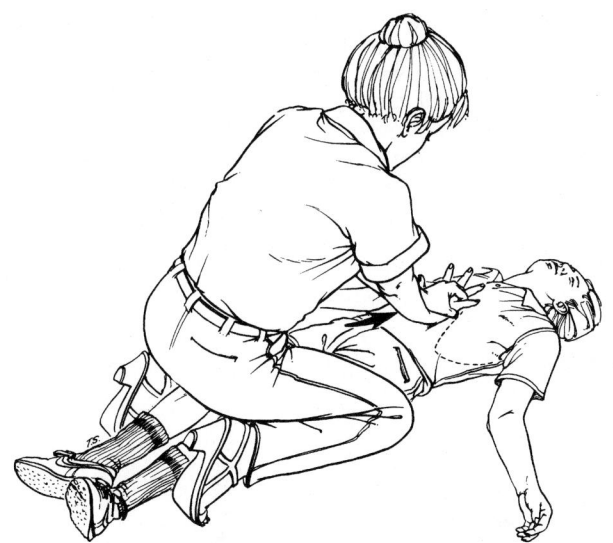

FIGURE 57–12. Abdominal thrusts with victim lying (conscious or unconscious). (From Emergency Cardiac Care Committee and Subcommittees, American Heart Association: Pediatric basic life support, part 5. *JAMA* 1992;268:2251.)

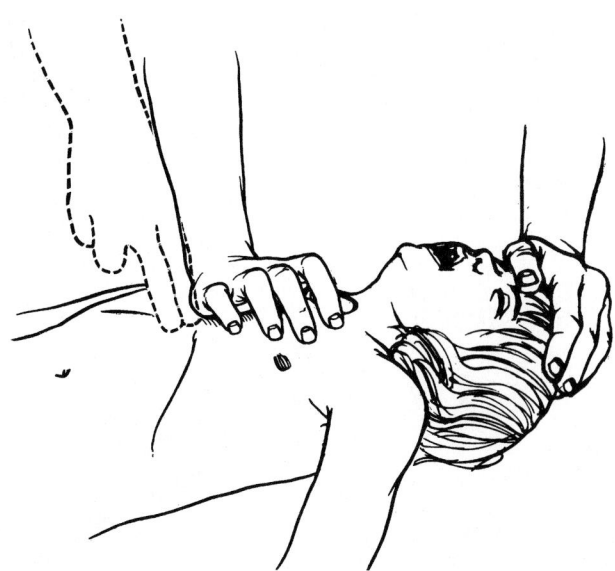

FIGURE 57–14. Locating hand position for chest compression in a child. Note that the rescuer's other hand is used to maintain head position to facilitate ventilation. (From Emergency Cardiac Care Committee and Subcommittees, American Heart Association: Pediatric basic life support, part 5. *JAMA* 1992;268:2251.)

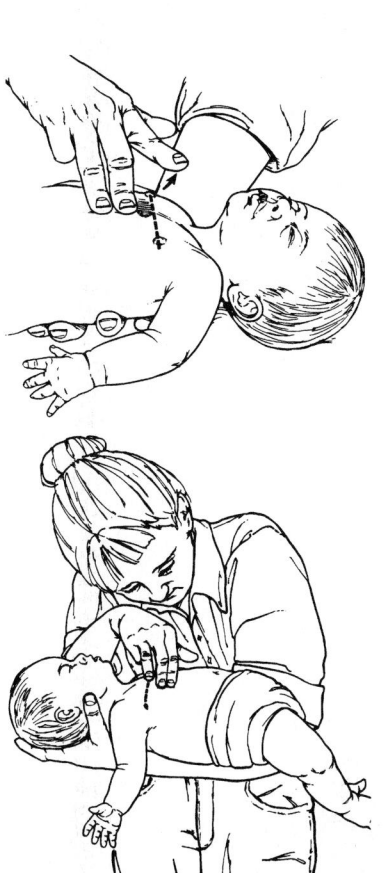

periodically to make an assessment of the possible return of spontaneous heart rate, pulse, and respirations. If the resuscitative efforts do not succeed in re-establishing respiration and heartbeat, the medical team must decide whether continued efforts are warranted or if the resuscitation should be stopped. If resuscitation is to continue and spontaneous heart rate and respirations have not returned, then the patient should be intubated, vascular access established, and administration of resuscitative drugs initiated. In the field with a pulseless child, an automatic external defibrillator may be available and should be used in children older than 8 yr of age if ventricular fibrillation is present.

Intubation and Mechanical Ventilation. Although it is possible to intubate awake infants without sedation, analgesia, or paralysis,

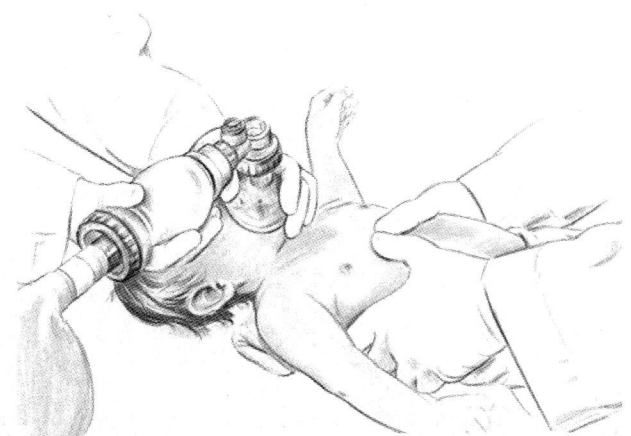

FIGURE 57–13. Cardiac compressions. *Top*, Infant supine on palm of the rescuer's hand. *Bottom*, Performing CPR while carrying the infant or small child. Note that the head is kept level with the torso. (From Emergency Cardiac Care Committee and Subcommittees, American Heart Association: Pediatric basic life support, part 5. *JAMA* 1992;268:2251.)

FIGURE 57–15. Two thumb-encircling hands chest compression technique in infant (2 rescuers). (From Emergency Cardiac Care Committee and Subcommittees, American Heart Association: Pediatric basic life support, part 9. *Circulation* 2000;102:1–253.)

analgesia is recommended to reduce metabolic stress (see Chapter 65). Children 1 mo of age or older should be pretreated with a sedative, an analgesic, and possibly a muscle relaxant unless the situation is an emergency (apnea, asystole, unresponsiveness) and the administration of drugs would cause an unacceptable delay. The intubation technique is shown in Figure 57–16.

In a *controlled intubation*, patients should fast for at least 4 hr or have their stomach emptied by nasogastric tube. The history and physical examination should be reviewed for any allergies or evidence of unusual airway anatomy, or risk for malignant hyperthermia, and informed consent should be obtained. Equipment necessary for intubation and bag-mask ventilation and an emergency cricothyrotomy tray should be available.

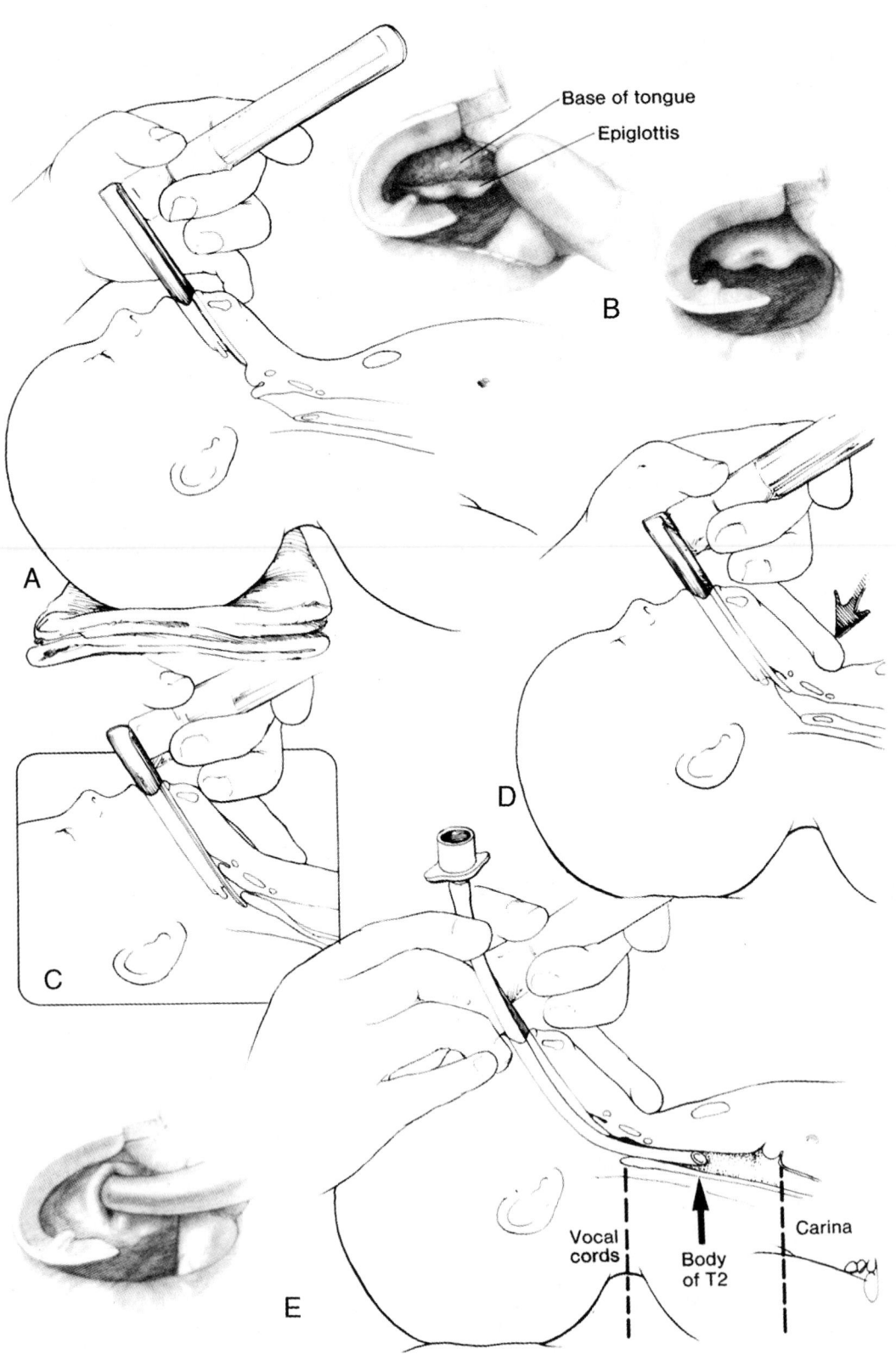

FIGURE 57–16. Intubation technique. (From Fleisher G, Ludwig S: *Textbook of Pediatric Emergency Medicine.* Baltimore, Williams & Wilkins, 1983, p 1250.)

After a period of hyperoxygenation, a benzodiazepine (diazepam, midazolam, lorazepam) should be administered, followed by an opiate (fentanyl, remifentanil, morphine), and a paralytic agent (vecuronium, rocuronium).

Because many intubations in critically ill children are emergent, the foregoing steps often cannot be followed, and procedures for *rapid sequence intubation* (RSI) should be initiated (Table 57–5). The goals of RSI are to induce anesthesia and paralysis and complete intubation rapidly. This minimizes elevations of intracranial and blood pressure that may accompany intubation in awake or lightly sedated patients. Because the stomach generally cannot be emptied before RSI, the **Sellick maneuver** (compression of the cricoid cartilage backward, compressing the esophagus against the vertebral column) should be used to prevent aspiration of gastric contents, which is very likely to occur when the laryngoscope and ETT are inserted into the pharynx and larynx.

Under controlled circumstances, *nasotracheal intubation* may be performed. It is indicated in patients who are going to be lightly sedated or when there is significant oral trauma. A nasotracheal tube causes less noxious sensations than does an *orotracheal tube*, which passes across the tongue and gums, producing a gag reflex in the posterior pharynx. Nasotracheal tubes do, however, obstruct sinus and eustachian tube drainage, and sinus or middle ear infections may result.

Cricothyrotomy. When the airway is obstructed and tracheal intubation has not succeeded, *needle cricothyrotomy* is indicated. The patient should be supine with the face looking directly upward. The midpoint of the cricothyroid membrane is palpated, and a 14-gauge intravenous catheter with stylet is advanced slowly through it, inclined inferiorly at about 45 degrees. Quick aspiration of air through a syringe connected to the catheter indicates entry into the trachea. At this point, the metal stylet is removed and the catheter is pushed farther downward into the trachea. Oxygen should be flushed through the catheter at 10–15 L/min. This supports a child, even one with little or no spontaneous respirations, while plans for a more secure airway are made. *Surgical cricothyrotomy* is rarely necessary in children and should be performed by an experienced surgeon, except in severe emergencies. It involves making a transverse incision in the cricothyroid membrane and advancing a large catheter through the incision downward into the lower trachea. Although similar in principle to a needle cricothyrotomy, the risk of bleeding, upper airway obstruction, and pneumothorax are significantly greater.

Venous Access. Veins suitable for cannulation are numerous, but there is considerable anatomic variation. The *dorsum of the foot* usually has a large vein in the midline, passing across the ankle joint, but a catheter is difficult to maintain in this vein because dorsiflexion tends to dislodge it. A second large vein on the *lateral side of the foot*, running in the horizontal plane, usually 1–2 cm dorsal to the lower margin of the foot, is preferable (Fig. 57–17). The great saphenous vein is accessible in all patients. It is cannulated just anterior to the medial malleolus and may be accessible in the medial leg and thigh in premature infants.

Of the numerous veins on the *dorsum of the hand*, many are suitable for cannulation. The vessels are large and often secured on the flat surface of the dorsum of the hand, and cannulation is well tolerated. There is almost always a large vein lying in the interspace of the 4th and 5th digits, about 1 cm proximal to the metacarpophalangeal joints. The *cephalic vein* is usually cannulated at the wrist, along the forearm, or at the elbow (Fig. 57–18). The *median vein of the forearm* is also suitable because it lies along a flat surface of the forearm. The *basilic vein* is prone to sliding around when attempts are made to cannulate it.

Samples of blood may be obtained from the external and internal *jugular veins* or, in neonates, from various *scalp veins*. The two jugular veins are also potential sites for indwelling catheters (Fig. 57–19). The most notable scalp veins are the superficial temporal (just anterior to the ear) and posterior auricular (just behind the ear).

Deeper and larger veins are very valuable because they provide a reliable access for medications, nutritive solutions, and blood sampling. They may be reached by percutaneous cannulation or by surgical exposure. To cannulate the *femoral vein*, after the skin is cleaned, a needle is inserted about 0.5 cm medial to the pulsing femoral artery (or, if no pulse, about two thirds of the way from the anterior-superior spine to the pubic tubercle

TABLE 57–5. **Rapid Sequence Intubation**

Step	Procedure	Comment/Explanation
1	Brief history and assessment	R/O drug allergies; examine airway anatomy (e.g., micrognathia, cleft palate).
2	Assemble equipment, medications, etc.	See lists below.
3	Preoxygenate patient	With bag/mask, nasal cannula, hood or "blow-by."
4	Premedicate with lidocaine, atropine	Lidocaine minimizes intracranial pressure rise with intubation and can be applied topically to airway mucosa for local anesthesia.
		Atropine helps blunt the bradycardia associated with upper airway manipulation and reduces airway secretions.
5	Sedation and analgesia induced	Sedatives:
		Thiopental (2–5 mg/kg)—very rapid onset; can cause hypotension.
		Diazepam (0.1 mg/kg)—onset 2–5 min; elimination 30–60 min or more.
		Ketamine (2 mg/kg)—onset 1–2 min, elimination 30–40 min. May cause hallucinations if used alone; causes higher ICP, mucous secretions, increased vital signs, and bronchodilation.
		Analgesics:
		Fentanyl: 3–10 µg/kg, may repeat 3–4×. Rapid administration risks "tight chest" response, with no effective ventilation. Effects wear off in 20–30 min.
		Morphine: 0.05–0.1 mg/kg/dose; may last 30–60 min, may lead to hypotension in hypovolemic patients.
6	Pretreat with nondepolarizing paralytic agent	Small dose of nondepolarizing paralytic agent (see below), with intent of diminishing the depolarizing effect of succinylcholine, which is administered next.
7	Administer muscle relaxants	Succinylcholine dose is 1–2 mg/kg; causes initial contraction of muscles, then relaxation. This depolarization can, however, raise ICP and blood pressure. Onset of paralysis in 30–40 sec; duration 5–10 min.
		Increased use of pretreatment with a nondepolarizing muscle relaxant, especially rocuronium (1 mg/kg), which has a very quick onset and short duration. Other nondepolarizing agents include vecuronium and pancuronium, both dosed at 0.1 mg/kg.
8	Sellick maneuver	Pressure on cricoid cartilage, to occlude esophagus and prevent regurgitation or aspiration.
9	Endotracheal intubation	Endotracheal tubes: select proper size for age and weight of child.
		Laryngoscope blades: variety of Miller and Macintosh blades.
		Patient supine: neck extended moderately to "sniffing" position.
10	Secure tube, verify position with roentgenogram	ET tube secured with tape to cheeks and upper lip or to an adhesive patch applied to the skin near the mouth.
11	Begin mechanical ventilation	Verify tube placement before ventilating with positive pressure; if ET in one bronchus, barotrauma may occur.

ICP = intracranial pressure; ET = endotracheal.

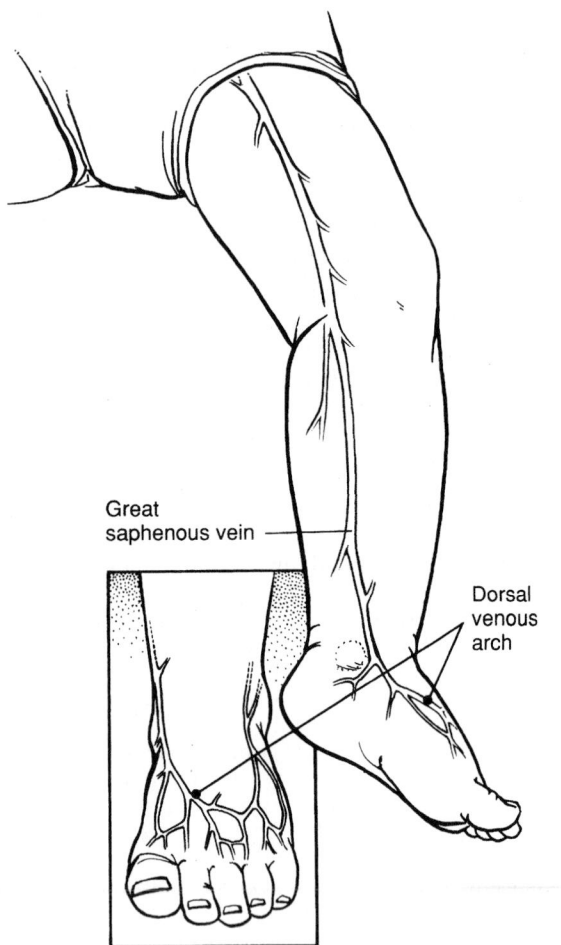

FIGURE 57–17. Veins of the lower extremity. (From American Heart Association: *A Textbook of Pediatric Advanced Life Support.* Dallas, American Heart Association, 1994, with permission. © 1994, American Heart Association.)

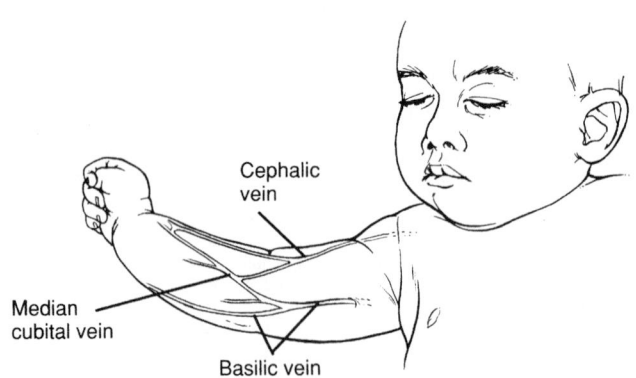

FIGURE 57–18. Veins of the upper extremity. (From American Heart Association: *A Textbook of Pediatric Advanced Life Support.* Dallas, American Heart Association, 1994, with permission. © 1994, American Heart Association.

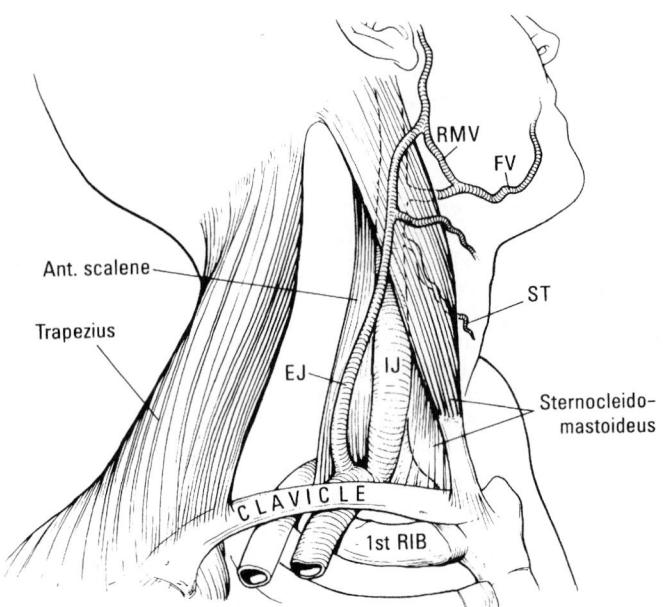

FIGURE 57–19. The internal and external jugular veins. RMV = retromandibular vein; FV = facial vein; ST = superior thyroid vein; IJ = internal jugular vein; EJ = external jugular vein; SCM = sternocleidomastoid muscle. The two heads of the SCM are indicated by the leader lines connecting that word to the diagram. (From Mathers LW, Smim DW, Frankel L: Anatomic considerations in placement of central venous catheters. *Clin Anat* 1992;5:89. Reprinted by permission of Wiley-Liss.)

(Fig. 57–20). Slight backward pressure on the plunger of a connected syringe is maintained so that blood flows easily into the syringe once the vessel is punctured. After the vessel is located, a small wire is advanced through the needle into the lumen of the vessel. The needle is then removed and the catheter is threaded over the wire into the vessel **(Seldinger technique)**. In small infants, the vein is no more than 0.5–1 cm below the surface, so the needle puncture should be at a shallow angle. In large adolescents or very obese patients, the needle may need to be nearly perpendicular to the skin. In either case, once the vein is entered, the needle should be flattened out before advancing it farther into the vein. Similar but distinctive cannulation techniques are used in providing access to the subclavian vein and the internal jugular vein. They involve the risk of pneumothorax in addition to bleeding. Because of its proximity to the median nerve the brachial vein is not often recommended for cannulation.

Current recommendations urge the use of intraosseous cannulation in those patients for whom intravenous access is difficult or unattainable, even in older children. If venous access is not available in an arrest situation within 1 min, an intraosseous line should be placed in the anterior tibia. A wide variety of laboratory tests can be performed and many medications and fluids may be administered through this route, including most involved in emergency resuscitations. Administration of certain drugs is also possible through the ETT. Drugs effective through this route include lidocaine, atropine, naloxone, and epinephrine. Epinephrine should be given at 10 times the intravenous dose.

DRUG THERAPY AND DEFIBRILLATION

If ventilation and chest compressions do not restore the circulation and spontaneous respirations, medications may be needed. If there is ECG evidence of a potentially perfusing rhythm but no pulse is palpated, one should consider the causes of pulseless electrical activity (electrical-mechanical dissociation). These include hypothermia, hypoxia, hypovolemia, hyperkalemia, tension pneumothorax, pericardial tamponade, toxins, and pulmonary thromboembolism (Table 57–6).

If there is bradycardia, asystole, ventricular tachycardia, or ventricular fibrillation, the patient requires drug therapy and, when indicated, defibrillation (Table 57–7; see Figs. 57–1 to 57–5). Epinephrine should initially be used in the standard dose (0.01 mg/kg, which is 0.1 mL/kg of 1:10,000 solution). If the

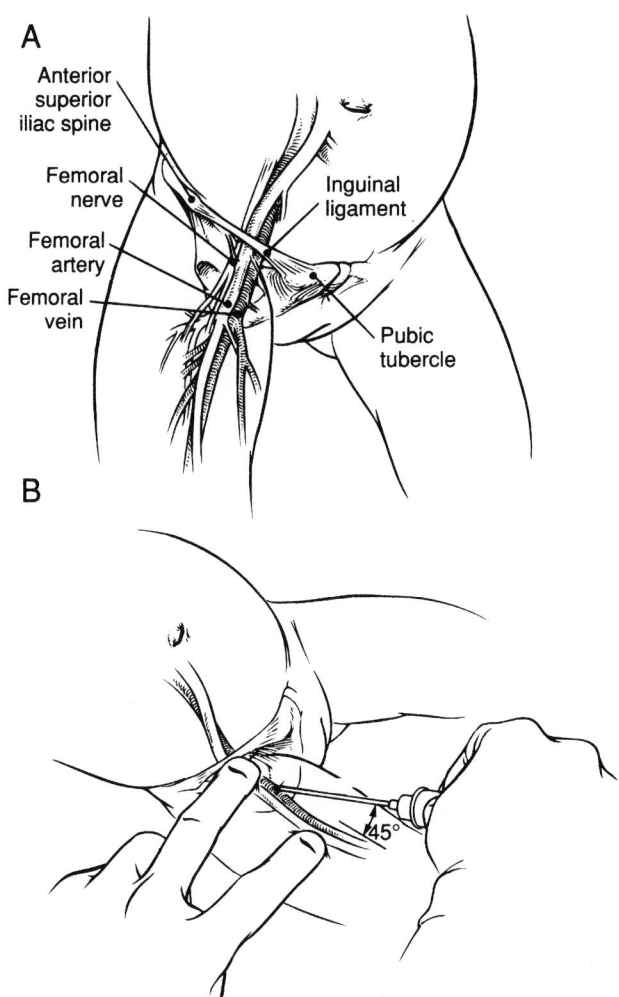

FIGURE 57–20. Femoral vein (A) anatomy and (B) cannulation technique. (From American Heart Association: *Textbook of Pediatric Advanced Life Support.* Dallas, American Heart Association, 1994, with permission. © 1994, American Heart Association.)

first dose is ineffective, it may be repeated every 3 min or increased to 0.1–0.2 mg/kg dose. Vasopressin may also be effective as a one-time dose (40 U in adults) after epinephrine; this is not recommended for children younger than 8 yr of age. Atropine may be effective for pulseless electrical activity, bradycardia, or asystole. Amiodarone is indicated in patients with ventricular fibrillation or pulseless ventricular tachycardia that is shock refractory; lidocaine and procainamide are secondchoice alternate drugs. *Torsades de pointes* may respond to intravenous administration of 25 mg/kg of magnesium sulfate.

Intravenous or intraosseous fluids should be normal saline or lactated Ringer without glucose to support the circulation and to avoid hyperglycemia, which is a poor prognostic factor during an arrest.

Arterial Access. Arterial catheters require special care for insertion and subsequent management because the blood flow to tissue can be compromised and considerable hemorrhage can occur if a catheter is dislodged. In most instances, the child should be in the pediatric intensive care unit (PICU). The adequacy of perfusion distal to the catheter must be monitored (e.g., warmth, capillary filling, edema). Catheters usually need to be heparinized (0.5–1 U/mL) to minimize clotting. The *radial artery* lies on the lateral side of the anterior wrist, just medial to the styloid process of the radius. When cannulating this vessel at

or beyond the crease of the wrist, the superficial branch of the radial artery is being punctured. The *ulnar artery* is used much less often than the radial. At 2–3 cm above the wrist it becomes superficial, lying just lateral to the tendon of flexor carpi ulnaris. Although it is larger than the radial artery, the proximity of the ulnar artery to the ulnar nerve can pose additional risk.

An ulnar or radial artery occasionally may be absent or very small, and cannulation of the normal-sized radial or ulnar vessel may compromise blood flow to the hand. The **Allen test** is used to identify this possibility and consists of simultaneous compression of both the radial and ulnar arteries, instructing patients to clench the fist several times (to blanch the palm of the hand by propelling venous blood upward into the forearm), followed by release of pressure over one of the vessels and observation of how fast and how well the hand regains normal color. The test is then repeated with release of pressure over the other vessel. If, in both cases, the hand quickly becomes pink, it can be adequately perfused with only one of the two main arteries intact, and even if the cannulated artery were to become blocked (a very rare event), the hand would still be adequately perfused.

The *brachial artery* is easily palpable between the brachialis and biceps muscles, on the medial side of the arm, just above the elbow. The median nerve is just medial to the artery and may even lie superficial to the artery. Because cannulating this artery may compromise blood flow distally in the limb, only small catheters should be used (i.e., 22 gauge or smaller) and placed distal to the takeoff of the deep brachial artery. Anatomic landmarks and technique for cannulating or sampling from the *femoral artery* are identical to those for the femoral vein (see Fig. 57–20). The *dorsalis pedis artery* lies on the dorsum of the foot between the tendons of the tibialis anterior and flexor hallucis longus and is usually palpable. However, cannulation requires immobilization of the foot to minimize the risk of dislodging the catheter with flexion and extension of the ankle. Alternatively, cannulation of the *posterior tibial artery* as it passes posterior to the medial malleolus involves risk to the underlying tibial nerve if profuse bleeding occurs.

Intraosseous Line Placement. Intraosseous needles are special rigid large-bore needles that resemble Jamshidi needles for marrow aspiration. There are special flanges on the side of the needle hub and a stylet, which prevents the wedging of bone fragments inside the needle lumen as it passes into the marrow. The most common sites for insertion are the upper tibia (with care taken to avoid traversing the epiphyseal plate), the sternum, and the anterior superior iliac spine. Once positioned in the marrow space, the needle can be used to deliver nearly all intravenous fluids and blood products. Because such needles are often inserted in haste, consideration should be given to empirical antibiotic coverage after the needle is placed and the patient stabilized.

Thoracentesis and Chest Tube Placement (see Chapter 404). *Thoracentesis* is the placement of a needle or catheter (chest tube) into the pleural space to evacuate fluid, blood, or air. Most insertions are performed in an intercostal space between the 4th and 9th ribs, along the midclavicular line in the anterior chest wall (in adolescents and adults), or in the plane of the midaxillary line. After a skin incision is made, dissection through the chest wall is accomplished in layers, using blunt dissection techniques. The needle (and later chest tube) that enters the pleural space should penetrate the intercostal space by passing over the superior edge of the lower rib, because there are larger vessels along the inferior edge of the rib. The chest tube should lie anterior in the pleural space for air and posterior for fluid accumulation. Final penetration of the intercostal membranes, to enter the pleural space, often takes considerable force, and the instrument (usually a hemostat) inserted into the pleural cavity should be grasped in such a way that there is no risk of uncontrolled deep penetration into the mediastinum, with possible contusion of the lung or heart. After the chest tube is inserted, it

TABLE 57–6. Potentially Treatable Conditions Associated with Cardiac Arrest

Condition	Common Clinical Settings	Corrective Actions
Acidosis	Pre-existing acidosis, diabetes, diarrhea, drugs and toxins, prolonged resuscitation, renal disease, and shock	Reassess adequacy of cardiopulmonary resuscitation, oxygenation, and ventilation; reconfirm endotracheal tube placement Hyperventilate Consider intravenous bicarbonate if pH <7.20 after above actions have been taken
Cardiac tamponade	Hemorrhagic diathesis, cancer, pericarditis, trauma, after cardiac surgery, and after myocardial infarction	Administer fluids; obtain bedside echocardiogram, if available Perform pericardiocentesis. Immediate surgical intervention is appropriate if pericardiocentesis is unhelpful but cardiac tamponade is known or highly suspected
Hypothermia	Alcohol abuse, burns, central nervous system disease, debilitated patient, drowning, drugs and toxins, endocrine disease, history of exposure, homelessness, extensive skin disease, spinal cord disease, and trauma	If hypothermia is severe (temperature <30°C), limit initial shocks for ventricular fibrillation or pulseless ventricular tachycardia to three; initiate active internal rewarming and cardiopulmonary support. Hold further resuscitation medications or shocks until core temperature is >30°C If hypothermia is moderate (temperature 30–34°C), proceed with resuscitation (space medications at intervals greater than usual), passively rewarm, and actively rewarm truncal body areas
Hypovolemia, hemorrhage, anemia	Major burns, diabetes, gastrointestinal losses, hemorrhage, hemorrhagic diathesis, cancer, pregnancy, shock, and trauma	Administer fluids Transfuse packed red cells if hemorrhage or profound anemia is present Thoracotomy is appropriate when a patient has cardiac arrest from penetrating trauma and a cardiac rhythm and the duration of cardiopulmonary resuscitation before thoracotomy is <10 min
Hypoxia	Consider in all patients with cardiac arrest	Reassess technical quality of cardiopulmonary resuscitation, oxygenation, and ventilation; reconfirm endotracheal tube placement
Hypomagnesemia	Alcohol abuse, burns, diabetic ketoacidosis, severe diarrhea, diuretics, and drugs (e.g., cisplatin, cyclosporine, pentamidine)	Administer 1–2 g magnesium sulfate intravenously over 2 min
Myocardial infarction	Consider in all patients with cardiac arrest, especially those with a history of coronary artery disease or pre-arrest acute coronary syndrome	Consider definitive care (e.g., thrombolytic therapy, cardiac catheterization or coronary artery reperfusion, circulatory-assist device, emergency cardiopulmonary bypass)
Poisoning	Alcohol abuse, bizarre or puzzling behavioral or metabolic presentation, classic toxicologic syndrome, occupational or industrial exposure, and psychiatric disease	Consult toxicologist for emergency advice on resuscitation and definitive care, including appropriate antidote Prolonged resuscitation efforts may be appropriate; immediate cardiopulmonary bypass should be considered, if available
Hyperkalemia	Metabolic acidosis, excessive administration of potassium, drugs and toxins, vigorous exercise, hemolysis, renal disease, rhabdomyolysis, tumor lysis syndrome, and clinically significant tissue injury	If hyperkalemia is identified or strongly suspected, treat with all of the following: 10% calcium chloride (5–10 mL by slow intravenous push; do not use if hyperkalemia is secondary to digitalis poisoning), glucose and insulin (50 mL of 50% dextrose in water and 10 units of regular insulin intravenously), sodium bicarbonate (50 mmol intravenously; most effective if concomitant metabolic acidosis is present), and albuterol (15–20 mg nebulized or 0.5 mg by intravenous infusion)
Hypokalemia	Alcohol abuse, diabetes, use of diuretics, drugs and toxins, profound gastrointestinal losses, hypomagnesemia	If profound hypokalemia (<2–2.5 mmol of potassium per liter) is accompanied by cardiac arrest, initiate urgent intravenous replacement (2 mmol/min intravenously for 10–15 mmol); then reassess
Pulmonary embolism	Hospitalized patient, recent surgical procedure, peripartum, known risk factors for venous thromboembolism, history of venous thromboembolism, or prearrest presentation consistent with diagnosis of acute pulmonary embolism	Administer fluids; augment with vasopressors as necessary Confirm diagnosis, if possible; consider immediate cardiopulmonary bypass to maintain patient's viability Consider definitive care (e.g., thrombolytic therapy, embolectomy by interventional radiology or surgery)
Tension pneumothorax	Placement of central catheter, mechanical ventilation, pulmonary disease (including asthma, chronic obstructive pulmonary disease, and necrotizing pneumonia), thoracentesis, and trauma	Needle decompression, followed by chest tube insertion

From Eisenberg MS, Mengert TJ: Cardiac resuscitation. N Engl J Med 2001; 344:1304–13.

TABLE 57–7. **Medications for Cardiac Arrest and Symptomatic Arrhythmias**

Drug	Dosage (Pediatric)	Remarks
Adenosine	0.1 mg/kg	Rapid IV/IO bolus
	Repeat dose: 0.2 mg/kg	Rapid flush to central circulation
	Maximum single dose: 12 mg	Monitor ECG during dose.
Amiodarone for pulseless VF/VT	5 mg/kg IV/IO	Rapid IV bolus
Amiodarone for perfusing tachycardias	Loading dose: 5 mg/kg IV/IO	IV over 20–60 min
	Maximum dose: 15 mg/kg/day	Routine use in combination with drugs prolonging QT interval is *not* recommended. Hypotension is most frequent side effect.
Atropine sulfate*	0.02 mg/kg	May give IV, IO, or ET.
	Minimum dose: 0.1 mg	Tachycardia and pupil dilation may occur but *not* fixed dilated pupils.
	Maximum single dose: 0.5 mg in child, 1.0 mg in adolescent. May repeat once.	
Calcium chloride 10% = 100 mg/mL (= 27.2 mg/mL elemental Ca)	20 mg/kg (0.2 mL/kg) IV/IO	Give slow IV push for hypocalcemia, hypermagnesemia, calcium channel blocker toxicity, preferably via central vein. Monitor heart rate; bradycardia may occur.
Calcium gluconate 10% = 100 mg/mL (= 9 mg/mL elemental Ca)	60–100 mg/kg (0.6–1.0 mL/kg) IV/IO	Give slow IV push for hypocalcemia, hypermagnesemia, calcium channel blocker toxicity, preferably via central vein.
Epinephrine for symptomatic bradycardia*	IV/IO: 0.01 mg/kg (1:10,000, 0.1 mL/kg) ET: 0.1 mg/kg (1:1,000, 0.1 mL/kg)	Tachyarrhythmias, hypertension may occur.
Epinephrine for pulseless arrest*	First dose: IV/IO: 0.01 mg/kg (1:10,000, 0.1 mL/kg) ET: 0.1 mg/kg (1:1,000, 0.1 mL/kg) Subsequent doses: Repeat initial dose or may increase up to 10 times (0.1 mg/kg, 1:1,000, 0.1 mL/kg) Administer epinephrine every 3–5 min IV/IO/ET doses as high as 0.2 mg/kg of 1:1,000 may be effective.	
Glucose (10% or 25% or 50%)	IV/IO: 0.5–1.0 g/kg • 1–2 mL/kg 50% • 2–4 mL/kg 25% • 5–10 mL/kg 10%	For suspected hypoglycemia; avoid hyperglycemia.
Lidocaine*	IV/IO/ET: 1 mg/kg	Rapid bolus
Lidocaine infusion (start after a bolus)	IV/IO: 20–50 µg/kg/min	1 to 2.5 mL/kg/h of 120 mg/dL solution or use "rule of 6"
Magnesium sulfate (500 mg/mL)	IV/IO: 25–50 mg/kg, Maximum dose: 2 g per dose	Rapid IV infusion for torsades or suspected hypomagnesemia; 10- to 20-minute infusion for asthma that responds poorly to β-adrenergic agonists.
Naloxone*	≤ 5 years or ≤ 20 kg: 0.1 mg/kg	For total reversal of narcotic effect. Use small repeated doses (0.01–0.03 mg/kg) titrated to desired effect.
	>5 years or > 20 kg: 2.0 mg	
Procainamide for perfusing tachycardias (100 mg/mL and 500 mg/mL)	Loading dose: 15 mg/kg IV/IO	Infusion over 30–60 min; routine use in combination with drugs prolonging QT interval is *not* recommended.
Sodium bicarbonate (1 mEq/mL and 0.5 mEq/mL)	IV/IO: 1 mEq/kg per dose	Infuse slowly and only if ventilation is adequate.

For endotracheal administration use higher doses (2–10 times the IV dose); dilute medication with normal saline to a volume of 3–5 mL and follow with several positive-pressure ventilations.

IV = intravenous; IO = intraosseous; ET = endotracheal; ECG = electrocardiogram; VF = ventricular fibrillation; VT = ventricular tachycardia.
From Emergency Cardiac Care Committee Guidelines on Pediatric Advanced Life Support. Circulation 2000;102: I291–I342.

should be secured firmly to the chest wall and connected to a source of suction (e.g., Pleurovac) at a pressure of 15–20 cm H_2O. A radiograph should be obtained to verify chest tube placement and evacuation of the pleural space.

Pericardiocentesis. When fluid, blood, or gas accumulates in the pericardial sac, a danger is that the heart will be compressed and will not be able to fill and empty with normal volumes of blood, leading to diminution in cardiac output. The cardinal signs of such a restrictive pericardial effusion are tachycardia, hypotension, and decreasing oxygen saturation. Pericardiocentesis is needle aspiration of the sac performed with or without ultrasound verification of needle placement or attachment of a recording electrode. After proper patient positioning, sterile cleansing of the area around the xiphoid process, and sedation/analgesia, pericardiocentesis begins with a short incision in the skin just below the xiphoid process. The needle should be a 22- or 20-gauge spinal needle, 6.25 cm (2.5 inches) in length. The proximal end of the needle is attached to a stopcock and collection syringe. The needle is inserted through the incision and then positioned so that it points toward the space between the left nipple and the medial end of the clavicle. Once the needle is through the skin, its angle should be flattened considerably with respect to the chest wall so that penetration is not too deep (in larger children or adults, the angle must be steeper). During insertion, the syringe attached to the needle is continuously aspirated with gentle pressure so that when the needle enters the pericardial space there will be a rush of gas or fluid. Once the procedure is concluded, a sterile dressing should be placed over the skin incision and a chest radiograph obtained to rule out any complications.

Equipment and Drugs for Resuscitation. An emergency department or intensive care unit should have a full supply of resuscitation equipment that is frequently checked for both presence and functionality (e.g., available catheters and tubes in appropriate sizes and charged batteries). The supplies needed for a pediatric office or clinic emergency are presented in Chapter 51. Those required for a PICU or emergency department are presented in Box 57–3. See Table 57–7 for drugs that may be urgently required for resuscitation. Some resuscitations involve difficulty in establishing vascular access, and a patient whose condition is rapidly deteriorating may die without such access if medications are not administered. In such cases, if an airway has been established, certain drugs may be administered via the endotracheal tube.

BOX 57–3. Supplies Needed for Pediatric Intensive Care/Emergency Department

Storage cart for equipment/materials
Defibrillator/portable ECG monitor
Oxygen cylinder
Airway equipment:
  Laryngoscope handle with batteries
  Assortment of blades—Miller 0, 1, 2, 3 and MacIntosh 2, 3
  Large assortment of endotracheal tubes, cuffed and uncuffed, with stylets
  Nasal and oral airways
  Self-inflating resuscitation bags
  Anesthesia bags with oxygen adapter
Suction equipment, including tongue blades, Yankauer suction tip, several catheters
Various nasogastric tubes
Tapes, sponges, IV adapters, T connectors, stopcocks
Masks for bag-mask ventilation, many sizes
Mapleson system with varied bag sizes
Cardiac equipment:
  Cardiac arrest board for compressions
  IVs, butterflies, intraosseous needles
  Blood pressure measuring equipment
  Several unit doses of epinephrine, bicarbonate, calcium chloride, lidocaine, naloxone $D_{25}W$
IV fluids and medications:
  Various crystalloid and colloid fluids
  Fully equipped IV tray—catheters, alcohol, needles, tape, tourniquets, armboards
  Cutdown tray
  Umbilical catheter tray
  Tracheostomy tray
  Chest tube tray
  Pleurovac pump
  Cardiac surgery open chest tray (if unit cares for postoperative hearts)
  ICP monitor tray
  General minor surgical procedure tray
  Military antishock trousers (MAST) kit
  Warm packs, sandbags, and so on
Monitoring equipment: pulse oximetry, ECG, end-tidal CO_2, blood pressure

ECG = electrocardiogram; IV = intravenous; ICP = intracranial pressure.

POSTRESUSCITATION CARE

When resuscitation is successful, continuous PICU care is usually needed to attend to the potential postischemic multiple organ dysfunction syndrome and continued need for cardiac inotropic support. Most patients do not require hyperventilation. Hyperglycemia and hyperthermia should be avoided. Continuous observation for immediate neurologic deterioration and long-term permanent neurodevelopment sequelae is imperative.

When resuscitation fails and the patient dies, attention is naturally focused on comforting the grieving family. Members of the medical team also need time to adjust to the events and understand how and why their efforts did not succeed. The more senior members of a team should recognize and acknowledge the contributions of those involved in the resuscitation and should convey to the family a detailed description of what took place. Increasingly, families may be present at resuscitations and may need a special kind of "debriefing" to help them accept what they have just witnessed. Where appropriate, families should be reassured that any further data that become available in the days and weeks after a death (autopsy results, etc.) can be shared with them if that should be their wish. Finally, someone on the team must be mindful of the legal and procedural duties involved in a death, such as notification of the coroner and contact with the organ/tissue transplant bank, completion of the death certificate, and arrangements for disposition of the remains of the deceased, depending on local regulations, family wishes, and customs.

Cummins RO, Hazinski MF: The most important changes in the international EED and CPR Guidelines 2000. *Circulation* 2000;102:1371–76.

Eisenberg MS, Mengert TJ: Cardiac resuscitation. *N Engl J Med* 2001;344; 1304–13.

Guidelines 2000 for cardiopulmonary resuscitation and emergency cardiovascular care: Part 9. Pediatric basic life support. American Heart Association in collaboration with the International Liaison Committee on Resuscitation. *Circulation* 2000;102:1–253.

Guidelines 2000 for cardiopulmonary resuscitation and emergency cardiovascular care: Part 10. Pediatric advanced life support. American Heart Association in collaboration with the International Liaison Committee on Resuscitation. *Circulation* 2000;102:1–343.

Guidelines 2000 for cardiopulmonary resuscitation and emergency cardiovascular care: Part 11. Neonatal resuscitation. American Heart Association in collaboration with the International Liaison Committee on Resuscitation. *Circulation* 2000;102:1–343.

Hallstrom A, Cobb L, et al: Cardiopulmonary resuscitation by chest compression alone or with mouth-to-mouth ventilation. *N Engl J Med* 2000;342:1546–53.

Kern K, Halperin HR, et al: New guidelines for cardiopulmonary resuscitation and emergency cardiac care. *JAMA* 2001;285:1267–69.

Kochanek MK, Clark RSB, et al: Cerebral resuscitation after traumatic brain injury and cardiopulmonary arrest in infants and children in the new millennium. *Pediatr Clin North Am* 2001;48:661–81.

Kudenchuk PJ, Cobb LA, Copass MK, et al: Amiodarone for resuscitation after out-of-hospital cardiac arrest due to ventricular fibrillation. *N Engl J Med* 1999; 341:871–78.

Lockey AS, Nolan JP: Cardiopulmonary resuscitation in adults. *BMJ* 2001;323: 819–20.

Mathers LH: Anatomical considerations in obtaining arterial access. *J Intensive Care Med* 1999;5:110.

Mathers LH, Frankel LR, et al: Anatomical considerations in obtaining venous access. *Clin Anat* 1992;4:1.

Morley P: Vasopressin or epinephrine: Which initial vasopressor for cardiac arrests? *Lancet* 2001;358:85–6.

Reis AG, Nadkarni V, Perondi MB, et al: A prospective investigation into the epidemiology of in-hospital pediatric cardiopulmonary resuscitation using the international Utstein reporting style. *Pediatrics* 2002;109:200–9.

Tsai E: Should family members be present during cardiopulmonary resuscitation? *N Engl J Med* 2002;346:1019–21.

57.2 Shock

Lorry R. Frankel and Lawrence H. Mathers

Shock is an acute dramatic syndrome, characterized by inadequate circulatory provision of oxygen, so that the metabolic demands of vital organs and tissues are not met. Insufficient oxygen is delivered to support aerobic cellular metabolism. There is a shift to less efficient anaerobic metabolism, which leads to lactic acidosis (see Chapter 45.8). If inadequate tissue perfusion continues, various endocrine, vascular, inflammatory, metabolic, cellular, and systemic responses occur and the patient becomes more physiologically unstable (see Chapter 163). Shock is a progressive process, owing to the continued presence of the initiating factor plus exaggerated and potentially harmful neurohumoral, inflammatory, and cellular compensatory responses. Initially, shock may be compensated but then may progress to an uncompensated condition, which may still respond to therapy. Untreated shock will lead to irreversible tissue injury (irreversible shock) and death. The specific pattern of response and related pathophysiology, clinical manifestations, and treatments varies with the etiology of shock (Table 57–8). Hypovolemic (hemorrhage, diarrhea-dehydration) and septic shock are the most common causes of shock in children. Cardiogenic shock may be seen in neonates with congenital heart disease and in older patients immediately after repair of congenital heart defects.

Shock often leads to the systemic inflammatory response syndrome and the multiple organ dysfunction syndrome. Sepsis may be present without bacteremia, and bacteremia may be present without sepsis. Sepsis syndrome has more signs of poor tissue perfusion (decreased urine output, restlessness, lactic acidosis, hypoxia), whereas septic shock demonstrates hypotension with blood pressures falling less than the 5th percentile for age. Refractory septic shock is present if despite 1 hr of appropriate therapy shock persists.

TABLE 57–8. Clinical Classification of Shock

Type of Shock	Septic	Cardiogenic	Distributive	Hypovolemic	Obstructive
Characteristics	Infectious organisms release toxins that affect fluid distribution, cardiac output, and so on	Primary pump failure produces inadequate tissue perfusion; resultant metabolic acidosis further impairs cardiac function	Neurologic disturbances may cause uneven distribution of fluids, leading to acidosis. Overdose of drugs can alter fluid distribution	Reduced fluid volume reduces cardiac output; metabolic acidosis can result from low intravascular volume and poor tissue perfusion; serious electrolyte abnormalities may occur	Poor cardiac output, cyanosis, hypotension, narrow pulse pressure
Sample Causes	Bacterial Viral Fungal (all are more likely in immuno-compromised)	Ischemic insult Cardiomyopathy Congenital heart disease	Neurogenic (disturbance of vasomotor tone) Anaphylaxis Toxins Allergic reactions	Enteritis Hemorrhage Extensive burns Diabetes insipidus Adrenal insufficiency	Tension pneumothorax, pericardial tamponade

Epidemiology. Shock occurs in approximately 2% of all hospitalized children and adults in the United States (~400,000 cases/yr). The mortality rate is 20–50%. Most patients do not die in the acute hypotensive phase of shock but rather as a result of one or more complications associated with the shock state. Multiple organ dysfunction syndrome increases the probability of death (one organ system involved, 25%; two organ systems, 60%; three or more organ systems > 85%). The mortality of shock in infected patients increases as one progresses from sepsis to septic shock to refractory sepsis. The mortality rate of shock in pediatric patients has declined as a consequence of educational efforts (pediatric advanced life support [PALS]), which emphasize early recognition and intervention and rapid transfer of critically ill patients to a PICU via a transport service.

Pathophysiology. Shock may result in multiple tissue injury through a number of pathways, which may vary depending on the stage of its development. Production or release of the inflammatory mediators is triggered by the infectious, ischemic, or hypoxic insult, which produces inadequate tissue perfusion. An additional spectrum of injury may occur during the reperfusion stage of shock when blood flow and oxygen delivery are restored to the previously injured tissues. Some of the inflammatory-mediator responses that occur during shock, especially due to infections, are referred to as the systemic inflammatory response syndrome (SIRS). Various inflammatory mediators such as tumor necrosis factor, platelet-activating factor, and proinflammatory interleukins are significant contributing agents to the development of SIRS. SIRS results in capillary fluid loss with edema formation and an unequal distribution of cardiac output further compromising oxygen delivery to the peripheral tissues (Chapter 163).

In the early phases of shock, a number of compensatory physiologic mechanisms act to maintain blood pressure (BP) and preserve tissue perfusion. These responses include increases of heart rate, stroke volume, and vascular smooth muscle tone, regulated through neurohormonal changes in sympathetic nervous system activation and other hormonal responses, to help preserve blood flow to vital organs such as the brain, heart, and kidneys. The respiratory rate is increased to promote the excretion of CO_2 to compensate for increased CO_2 production and the metabolic acidosis. Increased renal excretion of hydrogen ions and retention of bicarbonate occurs in an effort to maintain normal pH (see Chapter 45.8). Maintenance of vascular volume is facilitated by the renin-angiotensin and the atrial natriuretic factor axes (through regulation of sodium), steroid hormone and catecholamine synthesis and release, and secretion of antidiuretic hormone. Despite these compensatory mechanisms, intravascular fluid leaks into the interstitial extracellular space owing to vascular endothelial cell injury.

When the compensatory mechanisms cannot maintain adequate tissue perfusion, further tissue injury, and cell (and eventually patient) death occur (Box 57–4). It is common for more than one of these processes to occur simultaneously. Fluid loss commonly accompanies vomiting and diarrhea, hemorrhagic trauma, and severe burns and can result in an initial increase in vascular resistance as the body attempts to maintain BP and restore circulating intravascular volume. Subsequently, hypotension will develop and produce tissue ischemia. Significant electrolyte alterations may also accompany the fluid loss. When there is a pre-existing *low plasma oncotic pressure*, as occurs with the nephrotic syndrome, malnutrition or hepatic dysfunction, or acute severe burns, there may be excessive capillary leaking; this may result in large fluid loss, which exacerbates shock, produces edema, and potentially worsens the respiratory status. *Abnormal vasodilation* results in vasodilatory shock and is usually caused by sepsis, hypoxia, poisonings (carbon monoxide, cyanide, metformin), anaphylaxis, neurogenic events, and mitochondrial dysfunction (Fig. 57–21). The lower systemic vascular resistance (SVR) is usually accompanied by an increase in cardiac

---

BOX 57–4. Pathophysiology of Shock

EXTRACORPOREAL FLUID LOSS

Hypovolemic shock—may be due to the direct blood loss through hemorrhage or abnormal loss of body fluids (diarrhea, vomiting, burns, diabetes insipidus, nephrosis)

LOWERING PLASMA ONCOTIC FORCES

Hypovolemic shock may also result from hypoproteinemia (liver injury, or as a progressive complication of increased capillary permeability).

ABNORMAL VASODILATION

Distributive shock (neurogenic, anaphylaxis, or septic shock) occurs when intravascular fluid shifts into the extracellular space owing to increase in the rate of blood flow, and blood volume, or hydrostatic pressure in the vascular compartment (sympathetic blockade, local substances affecting permeability, acidosis, drug effects, spinal cord transection, other).

INCREASED VASCULAR PERMEABILITY

Sepsis may change the capillary permeability in the absence of any change in capillary hydrostatic pressure (endotoxins from sepsis, excess histamine release in anaphylaxis, and so on).

CARDIAC DYSFUNCTION

Peripheral hypoperfusion may result from any condition that affects the heart's ability to pump blood efficiently (ischemia, acidosis, drugs, constrictive pericarditis, pancreatitis, sepsis, other).

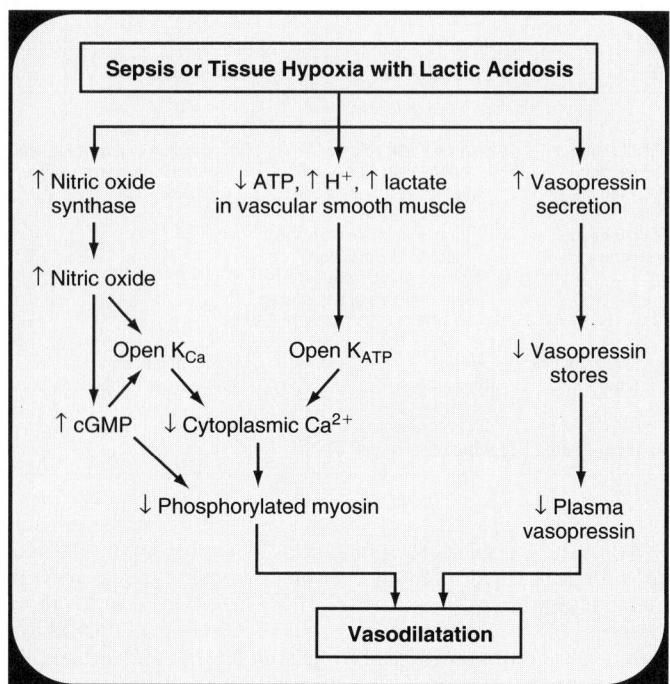

FIGURE 57–21. Mechanisms of vasodilatory shock. Septic shock and states of prolonged shock causing tissue hypoxia with lactic acidosis increase nitric oxide synthesis, activate ATP-sensitive and calcium-regulated potassium channel (K_{ATP} and K_{CA}, respectively) in vascular smooth muscle, and lead to depletion of vasopressin. The abbreviation cGMP denotes cyclic guanosine monophosphate. (From Landry DW, Oliver JA: The pathogenesis of vasodilatory shock. *N Engl J Med* 2001;345: 588–95.)

Figure box contents:

Sepsis or Tissue Hypoxia with Lactic Acidosis

↑ Nitric oxide synthase → ↑ Nitric oxide → Open K_{Ca} → ↑ cGMP / ↓ Cytoplasmic Ca^{2+} → ↓ Phosphorylated myosin

↓ ATP, ↑ H^+, ↑ lactate in vascular smooth muscle → Open K_{ATP} → ↓ Cytoplasmic Ca^{2+}

↑ Vasopressin secretion → ↓ Vasopressin stores → ↓ Plasma vasopressin

→ Vasodilatation

output and a redistribution of blood flow, hence the term *distributive shock.* In addition, prolonged states of intense vasoconstriction due to hemorrhagic or cardiogenic shock may lead to terminal vasodilatory shock. *Increased vascular permeability* is most common with sepsis or anaphylaxis but is also seen in hemorrhagic shock. Bacterial products (endotoxin) and inflammatory mediators (TNF) are implicated and result in significant depletion of intravascular volume. *Cardiogenic shock,* although rare in children, may be associated with a cardiomyopathy, severe congenital heart disease, significant dysrhythmias, or immediately after surgery for congenital heart disease (see Chapter 427). Sepsis, pancreatitis, and SIRS can produce direct myocardial depressant effects, adding a cardiogenic component to patients with septic shock.

A significant misconception is that shock occurs only with low BP (hypotension). Through various compensatory mechanisms, hypotension is often a late finding in shock. It represents an advanced state of *decompensated shock* and has a high mortality rate. Conversely, if blood pressure is low but tissue perfusion is adequate to meet the metabolic demands of the body, shock may not be present. Shock may be present with normal BP if other factors do not permit the patient to maintain adequate tissue oxygen delivery. Anemia and hypoxia will result in reduced oxygen delivery at any given cardiac output. Fever and trauma may increase tissue oxygen requirements. When any of the mechanisms leading to shock progress to the development of hypoxia and lactic acidosis, they pose an immediate risk to cardiac function, lessening the strength of contractions and predisposing to dysrhythmias. Persistent tissue ischemia (hypoxic decreased blood flow) in uncompensated shock results in a cascade of events that, if left uncorrected, result in irreversible shock and death.

The systemic response to an initiating event (infection) may be mediated by genetic polymorphisms of inflammatory genes (e.g., TNF) or its receptor. Patients with a genetic predisposition that causes a more profound inflammatory response are at the greatest risk for shock. Nitric oxide, one central regulator of the control of vascular smooth muscle tone, may soon be joined by locally produced carbon monoxide, for which evidence mounts that it may be a cell-signaling molecule, quite apart from its well-acknowledged role as a toxin. Heat-shock proteins lessen the effects of toxic oxidative molecules during septic shock and other insults to tissues and organs. Their regulation may enhance or modify the circulatory response to shock. Endotoxins involved in sepsis induce production of various inflammatory molecules such as the interleukins; adverse outcomes are associated with high-level inflammatory cytokines. Circulating anti-inflammatory cytokines may modify this response.

Septicemia and septic shock are discussed in Chapters 98 and 163. The associated immune-mediated responses, particularly to endotoxin, leads to the development of SIRS. The vascular endothelium is one of the principal targets of these inflammatory reactions, and changes in the level of nitric oxide and other mediators are a final pathway for both host defense responses and regulation of blood flow to selected tissues (see Fig. 57–21). The production of and the response to these inflammatory mediators varies widely among individuals and may explain why some patients with sepsis who develop shock have a high-mortality and complications such as acute respiratory distress syndrome (ARDS) or hepatic failure.

Clinical Manifestations. A classification of shock is presented in Table 57–8. There is significant overlap in these categories, especially between septic and distributive shock. The clinical presentations of shock depend, in part, on the cause; however, if shock is unrecognized and untreated, a very similar untoward progression of clinical signs and pathophysiologic changes occurs and leads to a common final path (Table 57–9). The clinical features of shock also relate to the stage (duration vs. progression) of the process (early vs late).

Hypovolemic shock usually presents as changes in mental status, tachypnea, tachycardia, hypotension, cool extremities, and oliguria. Table 57–9 outlines the clinical signs of a progressive decrease in perfusion. Supine hypotension and tachycardia are hallmarks of hypovolemia. In adults, postural dizziness and tachycardia (pulse > 30 beats/min over supine value taken 1–2 minutes after standing while counting for 30 seconds) are helpful clues. Dry mucous membranes and a dry axilla and poor skin turgor are variably present. Hypovolemic shock may initially present as normal or only slightly cool distal extremities. *Septic shock* may present initially as compensated or "warm shock" with warm extremities (from peripheral vasodilation secondary to low SVR), bounding pulses and tachycardia (from high stroke volume and widened pulse pressure), tachypnea, adequate urination, and mild metabolic acidosis. In contrast, *cardiogenic shock* presents as cool extremities, delayed (> 2–3 seconds) capillary filling time, hypotension, tachypnea, increasing obtundation, and decreased urination (all caused by peripheral vasoconstriction and decreased cardiac output [see Chapter 427]). Uncompensated or "cool shock" (high vascular resistance, decreased cardiac output, oliguria) occurs late in the progression of shock, regardless of its etiology. Hemodynamic findings in various shock states are noted in Table 57–10.

The transition from warm shock to cool shock is not always easy to identify. At the cellular level, the increase in lactic acid production and very low mixed venous oxygen saturations, indicating inadequate oxygen delivery, are hallmarks of uncompensated shock. Measurement of the oxygen saturation of central mixed venous blood [Mvo_2] from the pulmonary artery, right ventricle, right atrium, and superior or inferior vena cavae

TABLE 57–9. Signs of Decreased Perfusion

Organ System	↓ Perfusion	↓↓ Perfusion	↓↓↓ Perfusion
CNS	—	Restless, apathetic, anxious	Agitated/confused, stuporous, coma
Respiration	—	↑ Ventilation	↑↑ Ventilation
Metabolism	—	Compensated metabolic acidemia	Uncompensated metabolic acidemia
Gut	—	↓ Motility	Ileus
Kidney	↓ Urine volume	Oliguria (<0.5 mL/kg/hr)	Oliguria/anuria
	↑ Urinary specific gravity		
Skin	Delayed capillary refill	Cool extremities	Mottled, cyanotic, cold extremities
CVS	↑ Heart rate	↑↑ Heart rate,	↑↑ Heart rate, ↓ blood pressure, central pulses only
		↓ Peripheral pulses	

CNS = central nervous system; CVS = cardiovascular system; ↑ = increased; ↓ = decreased.
Adapted from Lister G, Apkon M, Fabry JT: Shock. In Emmanouilides GC, Riemenschneider TA, Allen HD, Gutgesell HP (editors): Moss & Adam's Heart Disease in Infants, Children and Adolescents: Including the Fetus and Young Adult, 5th ed. Baltimore, Williams & Wilkins, 1994, pp 1725–46.

TABLE 57–10. Hemodynamic Variables in Different Shock States

	CO	SVR	MAP		Wedge	CVP
Hypovolemic	↓	↑	↔ or	↓	↓↓↓	↓↓↓
Cardiogenic‡						
Systolic	↓↓	↑↑↑	↔ or	↓	↑↑	↑↑
Diastolic	↔	↑↑	↔		↑↑	↑
Obstructive	↓	↑	↔ or	↓	↑↑*	↑↑*
Distributive	↑↑	↓↓↓	↔ or	↓	↔ or ↓	↔ or ↓
Septic						
Early	↑↑↑	↓↓↓	↔ or	↓†	↓	↓
Late	↓↓	↓↓	↓↓		↑	↑ or ↔

Wedge pressure, central venous pressure, and pulmonary artery diastolic pressures are equal.
†*Wide pulse pressure.*
‡*Systolic or diastolic dysfunction.*
From McConnell MS, Perkin RM: Shock states. In Fuhrman BP, Zimmerman JJ (editors): Pediatric Critical Care, 2nd ed. Philadelphia, CV Mosby, 1998.

can determine if overall peripheral oxygen delivery (the true standard for such measurements is the pulmonary artery) is adequate. The Mvo$_2$ should be 20–25% less than the arterial oxygen saturation (normally, the Mvo$_2$ is 75–80%). This can guide caregivers in the use of fluid support and inotropic agents to improve cardiac output in the treatment of shock.

An unusual form of shock is the *hemorrhagic shock encephalopathy syndrome* (HSES). This syndrome initially looks similar to heat stoke. It is usually seen in children younger than 3 yr old and is characterized by encephalopathy, fever, shock, watery diarrhea, severe disseminated intravascular coagulation (DIC), and renal and hepatic dysfunction. In addition to the hemodynamic changes associated with poor perfusion and hypotension, patients with HSES may develop seizures and other severe neurologic findings as a result of cerebral edema. These children have an associated rapid onset of abnormal liver function studies and coagulation tests. These abnormalities persist for 3–4 days. Therapy is directed at fluid resuscitation, maintaining adequate cardiac output, supporting the renal and hepatic failure, and ameliorating acute neurologic abnormalities. Other complications may include myoglobinuria due to rhabdomyolysis. These children have a very high mortality rate, and survivors have a high incidence of neurologic problems.

Treatment

INITIAL MANAGEMENT. In most patients with early shock, a fluid bolus of 20 mL/kg of normal saline or lactated Ringer solution should be given rapidly. If it is not possible to insert an intravenous catheter into a peripheral vein within 90 sec or within three attempts, an intraosseous needle should be inserted to administer fluids (see Chapters 51 and 57.1). After this infusion, the patient is reassessed to determine if more fluid is required or other forms of therapy should be initiated (i.e., antibiotics, vasoactive agents, or other types of fluids). Children in severe hypovolemic shock may require and tolerate fluid boluses totaling 60–80 mL/kg within the first 1–2 hr of presentation. However, the risk of fluid overload must be continually reassessed. If the child's hypovolemia is from loss of blood or protein-rich fluid, replacement with fresh frozen plasma, albumin, whole blood, or packed red blood cells may be appropriate. The use of dextrans (hydroxyethyl starch) or gelatins may be indicated if there is a need to increase plasma oncotic pressure but blood component therapy cannot be administered or is ineffective. There is continuing debate about the relative risks and benefits of choosing crystalloid solutions (normal saline, lactated Ringer solution) versus colloid (e.g., albumin, hetastarch) for fluid resuscitation. The ideal solution is one that remains in the intravascular space (does not produce edema), has a long half-life, and is not toxic. To date, no solution fulfills these criteria. Some hydroxyethyl starches may produce an osmotic renal injury and predisposes the patient to acute renal failure.

If, after what is considered appropriate fluid resuscitation, the patient continues to demonstrate poor perfusion and shock, vasoactive agents are needed. The overall goal is to restore oxygen delivery to vital tissues. This can be accomplished by improving oxygen-carrying capacity (maintain normal hematocrit at 35–40%), improving oxygen saturation (95–99%) and Pao$_2$ (if severely anemic), and enhancing a depressed cardiac output. The latter is influenced by the heart rate, preload (fluid status), afterload (systemic vascular resistance), and state of myocardial contractility. Oxygen delivery need not exceed (supranormal) normal expectations because the "supply-dependency" oxygen relationship is not believed to be a critical factor in managing shock. When achieved, supranormal oxygen delivery does not improve outcome and may increase complications. When oxygen requirements are excessively high (seizures, burns, fever), it may be easier to reduce the metabolic stress with direct therapy (anticonvulsants, antipyretic agents).

CARDIOVASCULAR MANAGEMENT (also see Chapters 427 and 434). Septic, cardiogenic, distributive, and, rarely, hypovolemic shock may require various drugs to stimulate heart rate (*chronotropic*), cardiac contractility (*inotropic*), and enhance peripheral vascular resistance (*blood pressure*). These agents should be infused through a central venous catheter in an intensive care unit. These drugs increase oxygen consumption and the risk of dysrhythmias (Table 57–11). Dopamine is probably the most frequently used initial agent and is preferred for cardiogenic shock. Epinephrine has many of the same properties as dopamine; however, it is more effective in increasing peripheral vascular tone and has a greater effect on the heart. Epinephrine also

TABLE 57–11. Cardiovascular Drug Treatment of Shock

Drug	Effect(s)	Dose Range	Comments
Dopamine	Strengthens contractions (throughout dose range) Increases renal blood flow (low/intermediate doses) Vasoconstriction (high doses)	Low dose = 1–5 µg/kg/min Intermediate dose = 5–15 µg/kg/min High dose = 15–25 µg/kg/min	Increasing risk of dysrhythmias at high dose Should be administered in central vein
Epinephrine	Increases heart rate and strength of contractions Potent vasoconstrictor	0.05–3.0 µg/kg/min	May lessen renal perfusion Causes high O_2 consumption in the heart High risk of dysrhythmias
Dobutamine	Increases strength of heart contraction Little effect on heart rate Peripheral vasodilator, especially in vessels to viscera	1–20 µg/kg/min	Has very weak vasoconstriction (high dose) Good for cardiogenic shock; strengthens heart contraction and produces afterload reduction
Isoproterenol	Strong effect on increasing heart rate A potent bronchodilator Virtually no effect on strength of heart contraction	0.05–2.0 µg/kg/min	Increases O_2 consumption Potential for producing dysrhythmias
Norepinephrine	Strong vasoconstrictor Weak effect on strength of heart contraction	0.05–1.5 µg/kg/min	Produces short-run rise in blood pressure (high SVR) Causes increase in O_2 consumption, tendency for dysrhythmias
Phenylephrine	Strong vasoconstrictor Can be used to slow tachycardia through reflex cardiac slowing	0.5–2.0 µg/kg/min	Can cause sudden hypertension Causes increase in O_2 consumption
Amrinone	Potent inotrope Potent chronotrope Peripheral vasodilator	Load with 1.5–5 mg/kg bolus over 20 min, followed by 5–10 µg/kg/min	Phosphodiesterase inhibitor—slows cyclic AMP breakdown

O_2 = oxygen; SVR = systemic vascular resistance; AMP = adenosine monophosphate.

causes a greater increase in myocardial oxygen consumption and poses a greater risk of dysrhythmias. Dobutamine has a more selective action than either of these agents in cardiogenic shock and provides afterload reduction. Isoproterenol may produce severe tachycardia and decrease coronary perfusion and produce myocardial ischemia. Norepinephrine and phenylephrine are particularly effective in counteracting low systemic vascular resistance. It is not unusual to combine various inotropic agents. Commonly used combinations include low-dose dopamine with epinephrine, dobutamine with norepinephrine, or dopamine with dobutamine. These agents are titrated by continuous intravenous infusions with careful monitoring of BP with an indwelling intra-arterial catheter.

Because of its central role in vasodilatory shock and the demonstration of vasopressin depletion, there is a rationale for using intravenous vasopressin to treat shock that is unresponsive to catecholamines. In addition, in some patients with septic shock and in all patients who are on or who were recently weaned from steroids, intravenous hydrocortisone in stress doses should be started. A significant number of patients with septic shock have secondary adrenal insufficiency; a spot serum cortisol level will confirm the diagnosis, but empirical therapy may need to be started before the laboratory result is known. Afterload reduction is seldom indicated in early shock but may be useful in the recovery phase of cardiogenic shock (Table 57–12). Amrinone and more often milrinone have demonstrated beneficial effects in the advanced treatment of car-

diogenic shock because they increase contractility and promote afterload reduction. Intravenous methylene blue and angiotensin II have also been used in a few patients with unresponsive shock. Methylene blue increases myocardial performance and decreases inotropic drug use and maintains oxygen delivery. Angiotensin II is 40 times more potent as a vasoconstricting agent as norepinephrine.

OTHER MODES OF SUPPORT IN SHOCK. Goal-directed therapy for complications in shock is noted in Table 57–13. Coagulation disorders are frequently found in severe shock; DIC is discussed in Chapter 474. Correction of acidosis and hypocalcemia is discussed in Chapters 48.8 and 48.9, respectively.

Rarely, other invasive techniques may be needed to support children in shock who are not responding to fluid, pharmacologic support, or other modes of treatment when the cause of shock is considered treatable and reversible. Extracorporeal membrane oxygenation (ECMO) may be effective in treating young children with septic shock or severe cardiogenic shock, as a bridge to recovery or transplant in patients who have undergone cardiac surgery, and in those who have difficulty being weaned from bypass. Left ventricular or biventricular assist devices have also been used to manage severe cardiomyopathy and cardiogenic shock as a bridge to transplantation or until the disease process has reversed itself. Dialysis and hemofiltration have been used to manage fluid overload or pulmonary edema and remove inflammatory mediators.

TABLE 57–12. Vasodilators/Afterload Reducers

Nitroprusside	Vasodilator (mainly arterial)	0.5–1.0 µg/kg/min	Rapid effect Prolonged use (>48 hr risks cyanide toxicity)
Nitroglycerin	Vasodilator (mainly venous)	1.0–20 µg/kg/min	Rapid effect Risk of high intracranial pressure
Prostaglandin E₁	Vasodilator Maintains open ductus arteriosus in newborn	0.05–0.2 µg/kg/min	Can lead to hypotension Risk of apnea when given continuously
Hydralazine	Direct arteriolar smooth muscle dilator	0.1–2.0 mg/kg; may start with low dose and repeat with higher doses to effect	Hypotension and reflex tachycardia Lupus-like effect in chronic use

TABLE 57–13. Goal-Directed Therapy of Organ System Dysfunction in Shock

System	Disorders	Goals	Therapies
Respiratory	ARDS Respiratory muscle fatigue Central apnea	Prevent/treat: hypoxia and respiratory acidosis Prevent barotrauma Decrease work of breathing	Oxygen Early endotracheal intubation and mechanical ventilation PEEP Permissive hypercapnia High-frequency ventilation ECMO
Renal	Prerenal failure Renal failure	Prevent/treat: hypovolemia, hypervolemia, hyperkalemia, metabolic acidosis, hyper/ hyponatremia, and hypertension	Judicious fluid resuscitation Monitor serum electrolytes Low-dose dopamine Furosemide (Lasix) Dialysis, ultrafiltration, hemofiltration
Hematologic	Coagulopathy (DIC)	Prevent/treat: bleeding	Vitamin K Fresh frozen plasma Platelets
	Thrombosis	Prevent/treat: abnormal clotting	Heparinization Activated protein C Antithrombin III
Gastrointestinal	Stress ulcers	Prevent/treat: gastric bleeding Avoid aspiration, abdominal distention	H_2 blocking agents or proton pump inhibitors
	Ileus Bacterial translocation	Avoid mucosal atrophy	Nasogastric tube Early enteral feedings
Endocrine	Adrenal insufficiency primary or secondary to chronic steroid therapy	Prevent/treat: adrenal crisis	Stress dose steroids if previously on steroids Physiologic dose for presumed primary insufficiency in sepsis
Metabolic	Metabolic acidosis	Correct etiology Normalize pH	Treat hypovolemia (fluids), poor cardiac function (fluids, inotropic agents) Improve renal acid excretion Low-dose 0.5–2 mEq/kg of sodium bicarbonate if not responding and pH < 7.1 and ventilation (CO_2 elimination) is adequate

ARDS = acute respiratory distress syndrome; PEEP = positive end-expiratory pressure; DIC = disseminated intravascular coagulation; H_2 = histamine₂ receptor; ECMO = extracorporeal membrane oxygenation.

Biologic mediators have shown promise in improving the outcome of septic shock; these include activated protein C and bactericidal permeability increasing protein.

Butt W: Septic shock. *Pediatr Clin North Am* 2001;48:601–26.
Kim KK, Frankel LR: The need for inotropic support in a subgroup of infants with severe life threatening respiratory syncytial virus infection. *J Invest Med* 1997;45:1.
Kirov MY, Evgenov OV, Evgenov NV, et al: Infusion of methylene blue in human septic shock: A pilot, randomized, controlled study. *Crit Care Med* 2001;29:1860–67.
Landry DW, Oliver JA: The pathogenesis of vasodilatory shock. *N Engl J Med* 2001;345:588–95.
Luce JM: Novel molecules and mechanisms in critical care medicine. *Crit Care Med* 2002;30:S1–S95.
McGee S, Abernethy WB, Simel DL: Is this patient hypovolemic? *JAMA* 1999;281:1022–29.
Schortgen F, Lacherade JC, Bruneel F, et al: Effects of hydroxyethylstarch and gelatin on renal function in severe sepsis: A multicentre randomized study. *Lancet* 2001;357:911–16.
Yunge M, Petros A: Angiotensin for septic shock unresponsive to noradrenaline. *Arch Dis Child* 2000;82:388–89.

57.3 Respiratory Distress and Failure

Lorry R. Frankel

Respiratory distress/failure is the primary diagnosis in close to 50% of children admitted to PICUs and is a common cause of cardiopulmonary arrests in children. There is a substantial variability by season, etiology, and severity of illness. Respiratory failure arises from derangements in pulmonary gas exchange. The four principal derangements are hypoventilation, diffusion impairment, intrapulmonary shunting, and ventilation-perfusion ($\dot{V}/\dot{Q}$) mismatch. The causes may be classified by age, anatomic lesions, or abnormalities involving (1) lung and chest wall mechanics, (2) neuromuscular systems, and (3) central nervous system (CNS) control or respiratory drive. The presenting clinical findings usually help to determine the type of problem. Increased respiratory rate and effort (tachypnea and dyspnea) suggest mechanical problems with the lung or chest wall. Neuromuscular disease may result in progressively weaker respiratory efforts and eventually fatigue. CNS pathology may present as other neurologic features (coma, areflexia, weakness) and a variety of respiratory patterns, including bradypnea, apnea, and Cheyne-Stokes respirations. The heterogeneous group of pediatric diseases that can cause respiratory distress and failure requiring mechanical ventilation are discussed in Chapters 357 and 359 and Table 57–14.

Pathogenesis. Respiratory failure is the inability of the respiratory system to provide exchange of oxygen and carbon dioxide between air and blood, resulting in an impaired supply of oxygen and excretion of carbon dioxide to meet the body's metabolic demands. The physiology of respiratory function and gas exchange is discussed in Chapters 356, 357, and 359. The oxygen absorption and carbon dioxide excretion that take place at the respiratory membrane occur because these two gases move along their respective concentration gradients, achieving complete equilibrium of pressure for each gas between the blood phase in the end capillary and the gas phase (air) with the alveolus. Inspired atmospheric room air has a Po_2 of approximately 159 mm Hg, and gas inside the alveoli, the *alveolar air*, normally has a Po_2 of 104 mm Hg. Alveolar air has this lower Po_2 because of humidification and because the oxygen in the alveoli is constantly being absorbed into the pulmonary blood. If the atmospheric air is supplemented with a higher concentration of oxygen, then the alveolar Po_2 (Pao_2) will be higher and the increased oxygen gradient between

TABLE 57–14. Anatomic Classification of Respiratory Failure

Lung	Respiratory Pump
Central Airway Obstruction	**Chest Wall Deformity**
Tracheomalacia	Kyphoscoliosis
Subglottic stenosis	Diaphragmatic hernia
Epiglottitis	Flail chest
Croup	Eventration of diaphragm
Vocal cord paralysis	Prune-belly syndrome
Foreign body aspiration	Asphyxiating thoracic dystrophy
Vascular ring	Pulmonary hypoplasia
Adenotonsillar hypertrophy	
Near-strangulation	**Brainstem**
	Sleep apnea
Peripheral Airway Obstruction	Central hypoventilation
Bronchiolitis	Poisoning
Asthma	Trauma
Aspiration	CNS infection
Cystic fibrosis	
Bronchomalacia	**Spinal Cord**
	Trauma
	Poliomyelitis
Diffuse Alveolar Damage	Werdnig-Hoffmann disease
(Acute Respiratory Distress Syndrome)	
Sepsis	**Neuromuscular**
Pneumonia	Postoperative phrenic nerve injury
Pulmonary edema	Birth trauma
Near-drowning	Infant botulism
Pulmonary embolism	Guillain-Barré syndrome
Lung contusion	Muscular dystrophy
Shock	
SIRS	

CNS = central nervous system; SIRS = systemic inflammatory response syndrome.
Adapted from Helfaer M, Nichols D, Rogers M: Developmental physiology of the respiratory system. In Rogers MC (editor): Textbook of Pediatric Intensive Care, 2nd ed. Baltimore, Williams & Wilkins, 1992, pp 104–33.

alveolar air and pulmonary blood results in increased absorption of oxygen. Carbon dioxide diffuses through the respiratory membrane so quickly that the mixed venous and alveolar Pco_2 are nearly the same. Atmospheric air has a Pco_2 of approximately zero, and a healthy person's alveolar and venous Pco_2 is about 40 mm Hg.

These relationships are described by the alveolar gas equation:

$$Pao_2 = [Fio_2 (Pb - PH_2O)] - (Paco_2/R)$$

Fio_2 is the fraction of inspired oxygen—(e.g., breathing oxygen at room air with a concentration of 21%—an Fio_2 of 0.21). Pb represents the barometric pressure (assumed to be 760 mm Hg at sea level), and PH_2O is the water vapor pressure (which dilutes the dry oxygen content of the atmosphere, about 47 mm Hg). R represents the respiratory quotient, assumed to be 0.8, which can be calculated as follows:

$$R = CO_2 \text{ produced} \div O_2 \text{ consumed}$$

Thus, the Pao_2 of a patient who breathes room air and has a $Paco_2$ of 40 mm Hg would be predicted as:

$$Pao_2 = [0.21 (760 - 47)] - (40/0.8) = 100 \text{ mm Hg}$$

If a patient were breathing a gas mixture with an Fio_2 of 0.5, then the Pao_2 would be 306 mm Hg. The **alveolar-arterial oxygen gradient (A-a gradient)** is the difference between the predicted Pao_2 and the measured arterial Po_2 (Pao_2). This gradi-ent is used to assess the severity of impairment of gas exchange. If a patient is breathing a gas mixture with an Fio_2 of 0.5 and has a Pao_2 of 100 mm Hg and a normal $Paco_2$, the A–a gradient would be 206 (306 – 100). Comparing this with a normal A–a gradient of less than 10 mm Hg (for healthy young subjects breathing air at sea level), it is clear that this child's gas exchange is impaired. An A–a gradient greater than 300 mm Hg while breathing an Fio_2 of 1.0 signifies a serious oxygenation disturbance that may require mechanical ventilation.

Ventilation ($\dot{V}$) is the amount of gas delivered to and exhaled from the lungs, and *perfusion ($\dot{Q}$)* is the amount of mixed venous blood brought to the pulmonary capillary bed. The relationship between these two is referred to the *$\dot{V}/\dot{Q}$ ratio*. This ratio is determined by the amount of pulmonary ventilation and perfusion, and optimal gas exchange occurs if they are distributed in the same proportion to each other throughout the lungs. Therefore, the normal $\dot{V}/\dot{Q}$ ratio = 1. There is a certain amount of nonuniformity in the distribution of ventilation and perfusion of normal lungs (see Chapter 357). Respiratory diseases may cause a spectrum of pathologic derangement from the normal matching of ventilation to perfusion, termed *$\dot{V}/\dot{Q}$ mismatch*. Compensatory mechanisms by which the lungs attempt to restore $\dot{V}/\dot{Q}$ matching may not be adequate, potentially resulting in ventilated but nonperfused alveoli ($\dot{V}/\dot{Q}$ = infinity) and/or perfused but nonventilated alveoli ($\dot{V}/\dot{Q}$ = zero). Supplemental oxygen may improve the Pao_2 in patients with $\dot{V}/\dot{Q}$ mismatch.

Dead space ventilation occurs when the inspired gas is delivered to areas with no perfusion. There is an obligatory amount of normal anatomic dead space because inspired gas must traverse the nose, nasopharynx, trachea, and larger conducting airways. However, alveolar (pulmonary) dead space occurs when alveoli are ventilated but not perfused. This results from a pathophysiologic process that impedes blood flow through the pulmonary capillary bed, such as pulmonary embolism, pulmonary hypotension, and obstructive lung disease.

The volume of gas entering and leaving the mouth or nose per breath is the tidal volume. Alveolar ventilation, the volume of air entering and leaving the alveoli per minute, is defined by the equation

$$\text{Alveolar ventilation} = (\text{tidal volume} - \text{dead space}) \times \text{frequency}$$

Alveolar ventilation determines the rate of carbon dioxide excretion. Diseases that cause increased dead space result in decreased alveolar ventilation, and, unless the tidal volume or frequency of respiration increases enough to compensate, the $Paco_2$ will rise.

When the alveoli are perfused but not ventilated, this portion of lung acts as an *intrapulmonary shunt*, with mixed venous blood being shunted to the systemic arterial circulation without coming into contact with any inspired oxygen. This blood does not participate in gas exchange. The resultant increase in carbon dioxide content of the arterial blood is usually rapidly buffered so the effect on $Paco_2$ is negligible, but the dilution of oxygen content significantly lowers Pao_2. Therefore, diseases that cause increased intrapulmonary shunt cause hypoxemia. The hypoxemia associated with shunt can be severe and is often an indication for mechanical ventilation. Some examples of diseases increasing intrapulmonary shunting are acute respiratory distress syndrome, pneumonia, pulmonary hemorrhage, atelectasis, and pulmonary edema. Supplemental oxygen does not always enhance Pao_2 in patients with shunting.

Respiratory failure may also be classified as due to either lung disease or respiratory pump dysfunction (see Table 57–14). Lung diseases involve the airways, alveoli, or pulmonary circulation alone or in combination and result in hypoxemia. When lung disease leads to respiratory failure, patients have dyspnea, increased respiratory drive, and increased alveolar ventilation, which causes respiratory alkalosis unless the patient develops fatigue leading to failure of the respiratory pump as well. The coordinated activities of the CNS and the respiratory muscles act like a respiratory pump; respiratory failure can result from CNS, neuromuscular, or muscular dysfunction. Failure of the respiratory pump causes hypoventilation, a decrease in alveolar ventilation, and hypercarbia. Hypoxemia may also occur when the respiratory pump fails; it is treated with supplemental oxygen or positive pressure ventilation.

Clinical Manifestations. Children with impending respiratory failure due to lung disease have respiratory distress characterized by rapid breathing or *tachypnea*, exaggerated use of accessory muscles, and intercostal, supraclavicular, and subcostal *retractions*, which may be much more striking in a child than in an adult because of the increased compliance of the chest wall. Impending respiratory failure caused by respiratory pump dysfunction may be more difficult to recognize because these children may not have any signs of respiratory distress. A patient with a neuromuscular disease such as muscular dystrophy or Werdnig-Hoffman disease may be weak, and the degree of retractions may not be obvious. Other causes of respiratory pump failure, such as a narcotic ingestion or a brain tumor, cause decreased ventilatory drive and hypoventilation. An abnormally low respiratory rate or the shallowness of the breathing may identify these children.

Diagnosis. Respiratory distress in children is usually diagnosed by history and physical examination; severe distress may need immediate treatment before performing diagnostic procedures or tests. Some patients may not tolerate procedures such as an arterial puncture for a blood gas determination or a radiologic study; a change into an uncomfortable position may make it more difficult to breathe. It may be best to leave the patient in the position of greatest comfort, provide supplemental oxygen by face mask, and use aerosolized treatments. If these measures are not tolerated and do not result in improvement, then endotracheal intubation is required to secure the airway (see Chapter 57.1).

Laboratory Findings. Although the clinical presentation may require immediate intubation and mechanical ventilation, for the majority of children it is possible and helpful to first obtain an arterial blood sample to analyze blood gas tensions (Pao_2, $Paco_2$, and pH) (see Chapters 48.8 and 359) and initiate noninvasive monitoring by pulse oximetry. Hypoxemic respiratory failure is defined as a Pao_2 less than 60 mm Hg with an Fio_2 greater than 0.6 (in the absence of cyanotic heart disease); hypercarbic respiratory failure is defined as an acute $Paco_2$ greater than 50 mm Hg. In addition to analyzing blood gases, the decision to initiate mechanical ventilation should consider the cause of the respiratory failure, the possibility of reversing the cause of the failure via other interventions, and the overall trend in a patient's clinical status. A patient with respiratory pump failure from narcotic overdose may have an acute $Paco_2$ greater than 50 mm Hg but should respond quickly to administration of a narcotic antagonist and may not require ventilatory support. Conversely, a patient whose lung disease results in hypoxemia and dyspnea that seem adequately treated with supplemental oxygen may have an initially lower than normal $Paco_2$ (respiratory alkalosis). However, if this patient tires, an acute rise in the $Paco_2$ may indicate impending respiratory failure even if the $Paco_2$ is still less than 50 mm Hg.

Treatment. Respiratory arrest or repeated apnea requires immediate respiratory support. Severe shock also may require mechanical ventilation, even if arterial blood gases are within acceptable range, because patients need increased oxygen delivery to vital organs. Patients in shock often have respiratory distress owing to metabolic acidosis; the work of breathing and some lactic acid production may be ameliorated by ventilatory support. Acute neurologic compromise may require venti-

latory support for inadequate or absent ventilation, for loss of protective airway reflexes (cough and gag), or for therapeutic hyperventilation. Intubation and airway management are discussed in Chapters 56 and 57.1. Mechanical ventilation is discussed in Chapter 57.4.

57.4 Mechanical Ventilation

(see also Chapter 357)

Lorry R. Frankel

Underlying Concepts and Terminology. Positive pressure ventilators are the mainstay of providing mechanical ventilation in adult, pediatric, and neonatal ICUs. During positive pressure mechanical ventilation, the flow of gas during inspiration and exhalation is driven by the airway pressure gradient between the airway opening and the alveoli. Pressure may be administered at the airway opening by a tight-fitting mask connected to a ventilator—mask CPAP (continuous positive airway pressure); to a compressible bag attached to a gas source—bag-mask ventilation; or to both—mask BiPAP (bilevel airway pressure). In a PICU setting, ventilator support is most frequently provided by intubation of the trachea, with the placement of an endotracheal tube (ETT) and, on occasion, with a tracheostomy cannula. The ETT adapter, which attaches to the ventilator tubing, is considered the airway opening. During inspiration, the airway opening pressure is greater than alveolar pressure, thereby driving gas into the lungs and inflating them. Exhalation is usually passive and occurs because, at the end of inspiration, alveolar pressure becomes greater than airway pressure.

PRESSURES. *Peak inspiratory pressure* (PIP) occurs during maximal inspiration. *Positive end-expiratory pressure* (PEEP) helps maintain the end-expiratory resting lung volume. Thus, the maximum pressure gradient is the difference between PIP and PEEP. The *mean airway pressure* is a measure of the average pressure to which the lungs are exposed during the respiratory cycle. Mean airway pressure can be increased by increasing PEEP, PIP, the ratio of inspiratory time to expiratory time (I:E ratio), or the inspiratory flow (Fig. 57–22). Adjusting the ventilator to

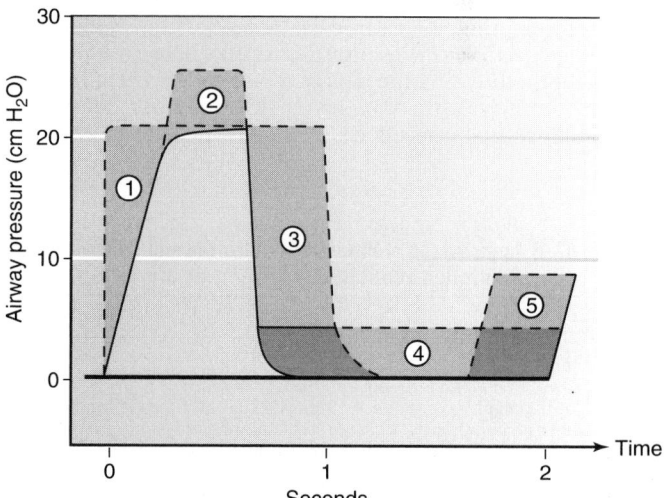

FIGURE 57–22. Five different ways to increase MAP: (1) increase inspiratory flow rate, producing a square-wave inspiratory pattern; (2) increase PIP; (3) reverse the inspiratory-expiratory (I/E) ratio or prolong the inspiratory time without changing the rate; (4) increase PEEP; and (5) increase ventilatory rate by reducing expiratory time without changing the inspiratory time. (From Harris TR, Wood BR: Physiologic principles. In Goldsmith JP, Karotkin EH [editors]: *Assisted Ventilation of the Neonate*, 3rd ed. Philadelphia, WB Saunders, 1996.)

increase mean airway pressure is the therapy for hypoxemia that is not responding to an increasing F_{IO_2}. This probably improves oxygenation by decreasing the number of collapsed alveoli or redistributing lung fluid.

COMPONENTS OF THE VENTILATOR BREATH. Each complete ventilator breath has an allotted time for inspiration (I time) before the ventilator must cycle into exhalation time (E time). The sum of the I time and E time equals the allotted time per breath. The ventilator delivers a set number of breaths per minute, the *ventilator frequency*. The frequency determines the length of each breath. For example, a frequency of 20 would result in 3 sec/breath. Most ventilators allow setting either the I time or the *I:E ratio*. For example, if an I time of 1 sec is ordered and the breath is 3 sec, the I:E ratio will be 1 sec:2 sec. If an I:E ratio of 1:3 is ordered, then the I time would be 0.75 sec, and the E time would be 2.25 sec.

The change in lung volume during the inspiratory period is defined as the *tidal volume* (V_T). It is the volume above the *functional residual capacity* (FRC), that is, the volume above the end-expiratory lung volume. By convention, the gas flow is in units of L/min and the I time is in seconds; in pediatrics the V_T is usually expressed in milliliters rather than as fractions of a liter. From the alveolar gas equation, to adjust $Paco_2$, either the V_T or the ventilator frequency is changed (see Chapter 57.3).

PRESSURE-CONTROLLED VS. VOLUME-CONTROLLED VENTILATION. These are the two primary forms of positive pressure ventilators (Box 57–5). Pressure-controlled ventilators allow a clinician to set the PIP and PEEP. The increase in airway pressure occurs swiftly at the initiation of inspiration to achieve the set PIP. This PIP is then maintained throughout the I time. In pressure-controlled ventilation, the lung volume rises until it reaches its capacity at that PIP or until the ventilator cycles into exhalation. Thus, V_T is not set but rather is determined by both the pressure gradient of the ventilator and the pulmonary mechanics of the patient. In volume-controlled ventilation, the V_T is preset as a product of setting flow and I time. The airway pressure rises throughout inspiration and reaches its peak when the entire V_T has been delivered. Thus, PIP is not set but rather is determined by both the V_T and the pulmonary mechanics of the patient.

VENTILATOR-PATIENT INTERACTIONS. When children are not attempting to breathe spontaneously, the ventilator completely controls the respiratory pattern. For children who can attempt to breathe, the degree to which a ventilator is able to synchronize with the patient's own respiratory efforts may have significant clinical effects. Patients whose lung disease is

improving and who thus are receiving less sedation in an attempt to wean from ventilator support may find that when they need to, they are unable to draw a breath, thereby experiencing dyspnea. Patients also may experience anxiety as gas is pushed into their airway while they are trying to exhale. This dyssynchrony often necessitates pharmacologic interventions with sedation or paralytic agents, which may result in prolonged intubation and ventilation. Patient-ventilator dyssynchrony may also cause barotrauma or pressure injury to the lungs. Advances in mechanical ventilation have attempted to improve patient-ventilator synchronization.

SYNCHRONIZED INTERMITTENT MANDATORY VENTILATION (SIMV). SIMV allows better response by the ventilator to the patient. During SIMV, the ventilator allows the child to trigger a breath by spontaneously attempting to inspire (Fig. 57–23). If the patient takes too long to initiate a spontaneous breath, then inspiration is time triggered by the ventilator: a mandatory breath. Ventilator frequency determines the total time allotted per breath, and some percentage of that time is the window allowed for the patient to initiate inspiration. If the patient does not spontaneously try to breathe during this window of time, then the ventilator initiates inspiration. SIMV may be either volume controlled or pressure controlled. A patient may also breathe spontaneously more often than the set frequency of SIMV inspiring fresh gas from the circuit at the set PEEP, but these breaths are not assisted by a ventilator breath.

SIMV does not allow for complete spontaneous ventilation. Patients trigger inspiration, but they cannot control when inspiration ends and the ventilator cycles to expiration. Patients cannot control the I time of the ventilator-assisted breaths, even though they can control the I time of the nonassisted breaths in between. The *pressure support mode* allows for spontaneous breathing by patients. The ventilator assists every breath a child initiates by applying a predetermined amount of airway pressure above the set PEEP. A child can control the rate of breathing and the duration of inspiration, so the breathing pattern may truly be called spontaneous. Many ventilators allow both

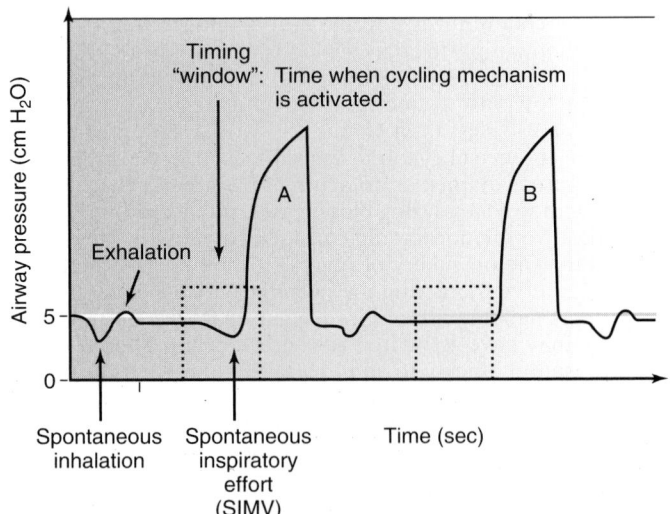

FIGURE 57–23. Synchronized intermittent mandatory ventilation (SIMV). At set intervals, the ventilator's timing circuit becomes activated and a timing "window" appears (*shaded area*). If the patient initiates a breath in the timing "window," then the ventilator delivers a mandatory breath. If no spontaneous effort occurs, then the ventilator delivers a mandatory breath at a fixed time after the timing "window." (From Banner MJ, Gallagher TJ: Respiratory failure in the adult: Ventilatory support. In Kirby RR, Smith RA, Desautels DA [editors]: *Mechanical Ventilation.* New York, Churchill Livingstone, 1985.)

BOX 57–5. Comparison of Pressure-Controlled and Volume-Controlled Ventilation

PRESSURE-CONTROLLED VENTILATION
Constant pressure delivered
Variable volume delivered; reduced risk of barotrauma
Changes in patient's compliance or resistance may lead to alterations in delivered volumes as pressure remains constant
Changes in tidal pressures may result in changes in minute ventilation

VOLUME-CONTROLLED VENTILATION
Constant volume (V_T) delivered; less risk of hypoventilation or hyperventilation
Variable pressure (PIP) delivered
Changes in patient's compliance or resistance leads to potential for dangerously high inflating volume delivered (requires closer monitoring of tidal volume and carbon dioxide, as well as pressure alarms)

V_T = tidal volume; PIP = peak inspiratory pressure.

pressure support and SIMV. The pressure support breaths can occur whenever a child attempts to inspire, unless the patient is breathing within that window of time that results in an SIMV breath.

MONITORING AND ALARMS. What is not controllable is monitored. In pressure-controlled ventilation, the V_T is monitored. In volume-controlled ventilation, the airway pressure is monitored; safety precautions include pop-off limits to the peak airway pressure. An oxygen analyzer allows monitoring of F_{IO_2}.

Alarms can be set for a wide array of events. The common alarms are for high or low airway pressure, absence of flow (apnea), loss of electrical power, high or low exhaled V_T, and high or low minute volume. When alarms occur, they must then be evaluated to determine if there is a malfunction of the ventilator or a change in the patient. The importance of frequent physical examination cannot be overemphasized; it is the fastest means of diagnosing a variety of ventilator problems, such as patient-ventilator dyssynchrony, ETT obstruction, barotrauma pneumothorax, and accidental extubation.

Approach to Mechanical Ventilation. The pressure gradient that inflates the lungs must overcome the pulmonary mechanics of the patient's respiratory system. See Chapter 357 for discussion of compliance, resistance, and time constant of the respiratory system. Respiratory diseases result in decreased lung compliance or increased airway resistance or both. Ventilator strategies are designed to ameliorate physiologic derangements and resulting ventilation-perfusion mismatch.

DISEASES OF DECREASED COMPLIANCE. Compliance is decreased in various diseases that affect the lung parenchyma, such as acute respiratory distress syndrome (ARDS), atelectasis, pneumonia, pulmonary edema, and pulmonary hemorrhage. In all of these diseases, FRC is reduced as terminal air spaces are flooded or collapsed, owing to the presence of abnormal fluid within the alveoli or atelectasis from the decreased amount of surfactant lining the alveoli. These smaller alveoli are more difficult to inflate. Intrapulmonary shunt is increased when blood flows to poorly ventilated lung units. One goal of mechanical ventilation when lung compliance is decreased is to decrease shunting by improving ventilation to the perfused lung units. The ventilator approach to decreased FRC is to increase mean airway pressure in order to recruit atelectatic areas of lung; this increase is usually achieved by higher PEEPs, although higher PIPs also increase mean airway pressure (see Fig. 57–22).

Decreased compliance requires a higher pressure gradient to achieve a given (V_T). This means that with volume-controlled ventilation, the PIP will be higher than it would for a patient with normal lungs. If the ventilator is pressure controlled, then a given PIP may result in a V_T that will be lower than that of a patient with normal lungs. Diseases that decrease compliance also may respond to higher ventilator rates as the lungs empty and fill more quickly. If neither ventilator pressure nor rate is increased sufficiently to compensate for decreased compliance, then hypercarbia develops.

DISEASES OF INCREASED RESISTANCE. Resistance is increased in various diseases that decrease the caliber of the airway lumen by edema, spasm, or obstructing material. Because airways decrease in caliber during exhalation, increased resistance affects expiratory flow more than inspiratory flow. Diseases in which airway resistance is increased include asthma, bronchiolitis, bronchopulmonary dysplasia, smoke inhalation, and cystic fibrosis.

Diseases of increased resistance are often accompanied by both increased intrapulmonary shunt and dead space ventilation. Shunt occurs if the increased resistance greatly impedes gas flow, decreasing ventilation to alveoli that remain perfused. Dead space ventilation occurs if the increased resistance leads to gas trapping in areas of the lung that contain hyperinflated alveoli. These areas of hyperinflated lung units exert pressure on the

surrounding structures, and this results in a reduction of pulmonary capillary blood flow. The increases in both shunt and dead space mean that these diseases produce both significant hypoxemia and hypercarbia. Increased resistance requires that a higher pressure must occur for the flow of gas to reach the terminal air sacs. Therefore, if volume-controlled ventilation is used, an increase in PIP is required to deliver a given V_T. If pressure-controlled ventilation is used, tidal volume is lower than in a normal lung at the same pressure.

Increased resistance may result in significant increases in time constant (see Chapters 355 and 357), unless there is a proportional decrease in compliance, which rarely happens in diseases of increased resistance. A longer time constant (time necessary for gas to fill or empty the alveoli) necessitates long inspiratory and expiratory times. Therefore, these lung diseases may be adversely affected if the ventilator frequency is too high and the expiratory and inspiratory times are too short. This results in a phenomenon known as gas trapping as the ventilator cycles back into inspiration before the lung has had sufficient time to empty. The ventilator breaths stack on each other as more and more gas is trapped, resulting in an increase in the FRC. This eventually leads to lung hyperinflation, a predisposition to pneumothorax and chronic barotrauma, and reduction in compliance.

INITIAL SETTINGS. Mechanical ventilation is initiated to provide support for lungs that function normally or for diseases of decreased compliance, or of increased resistance (Table 57–15). *For supporting normal lungs,* ventilator frequency may be slightly lower than the normal respiratory rate for age because ventilator V_T is usually set higher than a healthy person's V_T of 5–7 mL/kg. The customary range for ventilator V_T has been lowered to 8–10 mL/kg from 10–15 mL/kg. For pressure-controlled ventilation, an initial PIP of 20–25 H_2O is usually sufficient to move an adequate V_T, but this must be immediately assessed by observation of chest expansion and measurement of V_T.

To initiate *support for diseases of decreased compliance,* mean airway pressures need to be higher. A higher PEEP is often used to achieve this. PEEP is titrated upward in an attempt to provide adequate oxygenation at an F_{IO_2} less than 0.6. If volume-controlled ventilation is used, the PIP may be much greater than for normal lungs, and clinicians must pay close attention to pressure alarms. If pressure-controlled ventilation is used, the initial PIP may need to exceed 30 cm H_2O. The V_T has to be closely monitored. Significant hypoxemia results from these diseases, and it is customary to start with an F_{IO_2} of 100% and then reduce it as one attempts to avoid oxygen toxicity. The ventilator frequency may be set higher than normal because a decreased time constant permits a faster rate. A common inspiratory time is 0.8–1 sec.

Diseases of increased resistance often have very high time constants. Ventilator frequency may need to be set as low as 12–16 breaths/min in severe status asthmaticus to allow adequate inspiratory and expiratory times. It is also customary to try to minimize PEEP to 2–3 cm H_2O in these diseases to minimize risk of gas trapping.

COMPLICATIONS. There are many pulmonary and systemic complications of mechanical ventilation. Lung injury may result from positive pressure (*barotrauma*), *oxygen toxicity,* or excessive volume changes in the lung—volutrauma. Volutrauma may be manifested acutely as pulmonary air leak, such as pneumothoraces, pneumomediastinum, pulmonary interstitial emphysema, and bronchopleural fistula. Volutrauma may also be a cause of chronic repetitive lung injury, exacerbating the primary disease. This may result from subjecting alveolar units to repeated overdistention, such as with excessive V_T, or to cyclic collapse and re-expansion, such as with insufficient PEEP to stabilize the resting lung volume. In diseases of decreased compliance, the lung units of higher compliance may receive more of the V_T than the less compliant units, leading to volutrauma of the

TABLE 57–15. Guidelines for Initiating Mechanical Ventilation

	Normal Lungs	Decreased Compliance	Increased Resistance
Tidal Volume (V_T)	8–12 mL/kg (set of volume-controlled and derived if pressure-controlled ventilation)	10–12 mL/kg (may need to use less if the inflating pressures are too high; i.e., risk for volutrauma)	10–12 mL/kg (may need to use less volume if the inflating pressures required are too high; i.e., barotrauma)
Rate (breaths/min)	Physiologic norm for age or lower (depending on the V_T used; e.g., infant rate = 30, toddler rate = 20, adolescent rate = 16)	May require higher rates to maintain adequate minute ventilation	Often requires lower rates to allow adequate emptying time
Peak Inspiratory Pressure PIP (cm H$_2$O)	Initial PIP = 20–25 cm H$_2$O; monitor for adequate chest expansion and V_T	May require higher PIP to obtain acceptable V_T	May require higher PIP to obtain acceptable V_T
Positive End-Expiratory Pressure (PEEP)	2–4 cm H$_2$O to prevent atelectasis	Frequently requires higher PEEP to achieve oxygenation and improved compliance (e.g., 6–10 cm H$_2$O) Anticipate decreased venous return and cardiac output	May need to maintain low PEEP to avoid exacerbation of gas trapping and overinflation
Oxygen Concentration (Fio$_2$)	May not need supplemental oxygen; however, one usually begins with Fio$_2$ of 1.0 and may then quickly wean to an Fio$_2$ ≤0.5	Begin with an Fio$_2$ of 1.0 Attempt to wean to ≤0.6 by adjusting mean airway pressure/PEEP	Begin with an Fio$_2$ of 1, wean to maintain adequate oxygenation and avoid oxygen toxicity
Inspiratory Time (I time)	Normal for age I:E = 1:2, 1:3	Generous I time to allow recruitment of collapsed lung segments (e.g., 1:1.2)	Ensure adequate I time and E time, especially E time, to avoid gas trapping (e.g., I:E of 1:3 or 1:4)

healthier segments of lung. This mechanism may contribute to the chronic lung injury that can develop in ARDS. In diseases of increased resistance, the lung units with higher resistance need more time to fill and empty. This leads to overfilling of the lung units with lower resistance and time constants and to gas trapping and overdistention of the alveoli in the high time constant units with severely obstructed airways.

Positive pressure ventilation also may have effects on the cardiovascular system. Some portion of the mean airway pressure is transmitted through the lungs and raises intrathoracic pressure. This may impede venous return and decrease right ventricular filling. Elevated intrathoracic pressure also may compress the pulmonary circulation and increase the afterload on the right ventricle, which may cause the interventricular septum to shift toward the left ventricle, resulting in a decrease in volume of the left ventricle and a reduction in left ventricular stroke volume. Cardiac output may thus be impeded. Alternatively, elevations in intrathoracic pressure may cause an afterload reduction for the left ventricle. The net result of these many cardiovascular effects may be beneficial or detrimental, depending on the overall cardiovascular status of the child. In general, high mean airway pressures require close observation for possible hemodynamic compromise and may necessitate support with fluids and inotropic drugs (see Chapter 57.2).

An ETT may become obstructed owing to mucus, purulent material, or blood from trauma to the airway or from the child biting on the tube. These are immediately life-threatening complications. An ETT also may cause injury to the tracheal mucosa, resulting in subglottic stenosis, which is usually not symptomatic until the tube is removed. Subglottic stenosis may resolve with time or may ultimately require surgical intervention (see Chapter 373).

Prolonged intubation and mechanical ventilation may predispose the child to nosocomial infections, often by bacteria with resistance to numerous antibiotics. Nosocomial infection, sepsis, and other organ system failures are the leading cause of death of patients with respiratory failure.

Other approaches to the care of the critically ill child with acute respiratory failure include high-frequency modes of ventilation (HFV), the application of permissive hypercapnia, and the use of prone positioning. HFV can be divided into three distinct groups: oscillatory, jet, and flow interruption. All three modes of

ventilation utilize very small tidal volume (<1 mL/kg), very rapid rates (150–1,000 breaths/min), and lower mean airway pressures used to provide a gentler form of mechanical ventilation. *Permissive hypercapnia* allows the patient's Paco$_2$ to rise into the 60–70 mm Hg range as long as the patient is adequately oxygenated (Sao$_2$ > 92%) and the patient is able to tolerate the degree of acidosis. This is used to limit the amount of barotrauma and volutrauma to the patient. Positioning the patient in the prone position has been shown to improve oxygenation and reduce ventilator-induced lung injury in patients with severe lung injury; outcome may not be improved.

Arnold JH, Anas NG, Luckett P, et al: High-frequency oscillatory ventilation in pediatric respiratory failure: A multicenter experience. *Crit Care Med* 2000;28: 3941–42.

Biarent D: New tools in ventilatory support: High frequency ventilation, nitric oxide, tracheal gas insufflation, non-invasive ventilation. *Pediatr Pulmonol Suppl* 1999;18:178–81.

Curley MA: Prone positioning of patients with acute respiratory distress syndrome: A systematic review. *Am J Crit Care* 1999;8:397–405.

Harel Y, Niranjan V, Evans BJ: The current practice patterns of mechanical ventilation for respiratory failure in pediatric patients. *Heart Lung* 1998;27:238–44.

Matthews BD, Noviski N: Management of oxygenation in pediatric acute hypoxemic respiratory failure. *Pediatr Pulmonol* 2001;32:459–70.

Nuckton TJ, Alonso JA, Kallet RH, et al: Pulmonary dead-space fraction as a risk factor for death in the acute respiratory distress syndrome. *N Engl J Med* 2002; 346:1281–86.

57.5 Renal Stabilization

Joseph V. DiCarlo

Etiology and Epidemiology. Renal function is often significantly affected by critical illness that does not involve intrinsic renal disease. Renal dysfunction to some degree is frequently encountered but may be of little consequence or may contribute to the multiple organ dysfunction syndromes. Renal failure in children is most commonly caused by shock, sepsis, hypoxia, or nephrotoxic medications (see Chapter 527). Severe congenital heart disease is a risk factor for life-threatening renal cortical and medullary necrosis resulting from renal ischemia. In infants with renal hypoperfusion and ischemic injury, 50% may have congenital heart disease, 30% may have asphyxial shock or sepsis, whereas only 2% may have gastroenteritis with dehydration. There is usually little association between the renal lesions and the use of radiographic contrast medium. Although renal failure rarely occurs after gastroenteritis and dehydration in children, it can occur as a consequence of hemolytic-uremic syndrome (see Chapter 510) or can be associated with renal vein thrombosis. Renal insufficiency or failure associated with hepatic failure (the hepatorenal syndrome) may also require intensive care. Obstructive uropathy is a potential cause of renal failure necessitating PICU admission. Oliguria may also be caused by excessively high intra-abdominal pressures (abdominal compartment syndrome). Reducing the pressure improves urine output.

Strategies to Improve Renal Function. Although oliguria is common in the PICU and may be associated with poor outcomes, often only additional fluids or low doses of diuretics are needed for correction. In patients with oliguric renal failure, adequate intravascular fluid volumes estimated by the heart rate (within 20% of normal for age) and central venous pressure (at least 4–9 cm H_2O) should be maintained. In addition to treating the underlying cause, loop diuretics may be helpful.

Loop diuretics are commonly used to improve fluid balance in critically ill children. However, tolerance to the effects of the diuretic may require large bolus doses, intravenous drips, a combination of diuretics, or changing drugs. Some children who demonstrate little effect from furosemide respond to bumetanide. Continuous infusion of loop diuretics may decrease dosage requirements, improve response, and minimize adverse effects. Loop diuretics are often used in the hope of decreasing lung water in children with capillary leak syndrome (e.g., ARDS, septic shock), but the effect is often modest. The pairing of a loop diuretic with an infusion of albumin is probably efficacious only in the nephrotic syndrome.

Use of a single loop diuretic may soon lead to drug tolerance owing to hypertrophy of the distal nephron and concomitantly enhanced sodium reabsorption. Resistance can be overcome by the addition of metolazone or thiazides to block distal sodium reabsorption.

In the rare instance that renal failure is caused by (or is impending from) a circulating nephrotoxin or substance that might obstruct the renal tubules (e.g., myoglobin), *forced diuresis* may be beneficial. Crystalloid is infused at up to two times the maintenance rate, followed by mannitol (0.5 g/kg) and/or furosemide (0.5 mg/kg) every 4 hr. However, high infusion rates pose the risk of pulmonary edema, and mannitol may cause osmotic tubular kidney damage if allowed to crystallize in the interstitium.

Vasoactive Medications and Renal Preservation. Although vasopressor agents can theoretically reduce renal blood flow by causing vasoconstriction, renal blood flow and function usually improve when renal perfusion pressure is increased during shock by the infusion of vasopressors. Dopamine at doses of 1–3 µg/kg/min often improves urine output and natriuresis, probably as a result of a direct effect on renal tubules and splanchnic dilatation. However, little evidence shows that dopamine prevents acute renal failure or improves patient outcome. Norepinephrine when used to increase the blood pressure in patients with shock may increase renal blood flow and improve renal function. Early and rapid restoration of the circulating blood volume is probably most efficacious in preserving renal function in shock.

Renal Replacement Therapies (see Chapters 527 and 528). Continuous venovenous hemofiltration (CVVH) is the modality of choice for renal replacement therapy in critically ill children (see Chapter 59). Hemofiltration is usually performed through double-lumen venous catheters, with circulation through the circuit affected by a blood roller-pump fitted with an air trap. CVVH is usually more appropriate than conventional hemodialysis in unstable patients because lower blood flows are needed

(usually 10 mL/kg/min) and the membranes used may be more biocompatible than the standard hemodialysis membrane. The circuit is best anticoagulated by infusing a citrate solution into the filter; the resultant hypocalcemia is counteracted by a calcium infusion for the patient. Reasonably high clearances can be obtained during continuous hemodialysis or hemodiafiltration, even in severely catabolic, septic patients. Countercurrent dialysate flow improves clearance rates, and well-designed replacement solutions can correct acidosis and electrolyte imbalances. CVVH may be beneficial in the management of systemic inflammation (e.g., in septic shock or acute respiratory distress syndrome). The filter removes all substances below a molecular weight of 17,000 daltons that are not protein bound; many pro-inflammatory substances are of this size or smaller. Clearance is best achieved by production of 1 to 4 L of ultrafiltrate per hour.

Australian and New Zealand Intensive Care Society (ANZICS) Clinical Trials Group: Low-dose dopamine in patients with early renal dysfunction: A placebo-controlled randomised trial. *Lancet* 2000;356:2139–43.

Bersten AD: Vasoactive drugs and the importance of renal perfusion pressure. *New Horiz* 1995;3:650–51.

Bhimma R: Post-dysenteric hemolytic uremic syndrome in children during an epidemic of *Shigella* dysentery in Kwazulu, Natal. *Pediatr Nephrol* 1997;11:560–64.

DePriest J: Reversing oliguria in critically ill patients. *Postgrad Med* 1997;102:245.

Eades SK, Christensen ML: The clinical pharmacology of loop diuretics in the pediatric patient. *Pediatr Nephrol* 1998;12:603–16.

O'Leary MJ, Bihari DJ: Preventing renal failure in the critically ill. *BMJ* 2001;322:1437–39.

Stewart CL: Acute renal failure in infants, children and adults. *Crit Care Clin* 1997;13:575–90.

57.6 Nutritional Stabilization

Joseph V. DiCarlo

Critically ill children need nutritional support to ameliorate negative nitrogen balance resulting from excessive catabolism (Tables 57–16 and 57–17, Fig. 57–24) (see Chapter 42). Carbohydrate (glucose infusion of 3–5 mg/kg/min) is given to inhibit the breakdown of endogenous protein. Generally, 70% of calories should be derived from carbohydrates and 30% from lipids. It is often difficult to deliver adequate calories to critically ill children because of enteral intolerance or restrictions in fluid volumes, but the caloric goals should be attainable within the first week of hospitalization.

Amino acids should be provided in reasonable amounts, in any form (1.5 g/kg in older children, 2.0 g/kg in infants). Adequate amounts of glutamine, alanine, and the essential amino acids should be included, but branched-chain amino acids (leucine, cysteine, valine, and lysine) may not confer any special benefit.

Vitamins, particularly water-soluble vitamins B complex and C, are best administered enterally. Vitamin deficiencies, however, can develop even in children receiving parenteral nutrition (e.g., thiamine deficiency leading to Wernicke encephalopathy and riboflavin deficiency).

Essential minerals and trace elements including zinc, magnesium, and selenium should also be provided.

TABLE 57–16. Caloric and Protein Requirements in the Critically III Child

Critical illness	25–30 kcal/kg/24 hr
Mechanical ventilation	20–25 kcal/kg/24 hr
Receiving growth hormone	15–20 kcal/kg/24 hr as carbohydrate
Burn or trauma	40–45 kcal/kg/24 hr
Protein	1.5–2.5 g/kg/24 hr
Protein (burn >20%)	2.0–3.0 g/kg/24 hr

TABLE 57–17. **Relative Effects of Starvation and Hypermetabolism**

Event	Starvation	Hypermetabolism
Energy expenditure	↓	++
Respiratory quotient	0.7	0.8-0.85
Energy source	Glucose/fat	Mixed
Mediator activation	+	+++
Gluconeogenesis	+	+++
Catabolism	+	+++
Protein synthesis relative to catabolism	↓	↓↓
Amino acid oxidation	±	+++
Ureagenesis	±	++
Ketonemia	+++	±
Rate of malnutrition	+	+++

+, Increase; ↓, decrease; ±, minimal change.
From Wesley JR: Nutrient metabolism in relation to systemic stress response. In Pediatric Critical Care. Furhman BP, Zimmerman JJ (editors): CV Mosby, St. Louis 1998. Adapted from Barton R, Cerra FB: Chest 1989;96:1153.

Rarely, growth factors are administered, especially growth hormone. Growth hormone may be beneficial to debilitated children having difficulty in weaning from mechanical ventilation. However, growth hormone aggravates the insulin resis-

tance and hyperglycemia common to critically ill children and produces increased mortality in critically ill adults. Intensive insulin therapy (maintaining blood glucose levels between 80 and 110 mg/dL) has been shown to reduce morbidity and mortality in adults in a surgical ICU. This has not been studied in children.

Enteral Feeding. Early enteral feeding in critically ill children, particularly those with sepsis, may avert ulcerative complications, preserve the indigenous intestinal flora, avoid overgrowth by pathogens, and prevent atrophy of the mucosa. Normal flora also may be restored, in part, by the administration of acidophilus. If the stomach is relatively atonic, early feeding may be accomplished through a weighted tube passed through the pylorus into the jejunum; fluoroscopic guidance or placement via endoscopy may be necessary. However, patients with sepsis often have ileus that precludes enteral nutrition but resolves with time (3–7 days).

Parenteral Nutrition. If the gastrointestinal tract cannot be used, parenteral nutrition is necessary. Conversion of maintenance intravenous fluids to parenteral nutrition is often indicated by the 2nd or 3rd day of hospitalization. There is no need to administer amino acids gradually, although protein restriction may be indicated for renal failure.

Overfeeding. Excessive intake of carbohydrates is manifested as hyperglycemia, which may result in hyperosmolarity, osmotic diuresis, and dehydration. Subsequently, increased carbon dioxide production and an increase in the respiratory quotient may tax an already compromised respiratory system. Excessive administration of lipids can produce hypertriglyceridemia and fatty liver and may increase the risk for infection.

Immunomodulation through Diet. Unfed patients in the PICU, in general, have the highest complication rate. Attempts to enhance immune function through dietary supplementation with glutamine, arginine, omega-3 fatty acids, and nucleotides have failed to demonstrate benefit.

DeBiasse NM, Wilmore DW: What is optimal nutritional support? *New Horiz* 1994; 2:122–30.
Demling R. Growth hormone therapy in critically ill patients. *N Engl J Med* 1999; 341:837–8.
Takala J, Ruokonen E, Webster NR, et al. Increased mortality associated with growth hormone treatment in critically ill adults. *N Engl J Med* 1999;341: 785–92.

57.7 Neurologic Stabilization

Joseph V. DiCarlo and Lorry R. Frankel

Acute neurologic deterioration may be a life-threatening event with numerous causes and a few typical clinical presentations (coma, seizures, weakness, altered mental status). The clinician must act quickly to stabilize the child with an evolving neurologic picture to quickly reverse the process and avoid further permanent injury to the brain. The initial event produces the "primary injury" to the brain that gives rise to the typical signs and symptoms. Failing to recognize the primary events from the clinical manifestations, the child may be at significant risk for further injury referred to as "secondary injury." This is related to systemic hypotension, respiratory failure, and hypoxia as well as progressive cerebral or brainstem herniation resulting from the development of cerebral edema or intracranial bleeding, which if unrecognized and untreated worsen the outcome for the child.

Preservation of global neurologic function, prevention of secondary cerebral edema, and optimizing regeneration are important particular concerns to the intensive care physician. Several disease states can temporarily or permanently profoundly affect

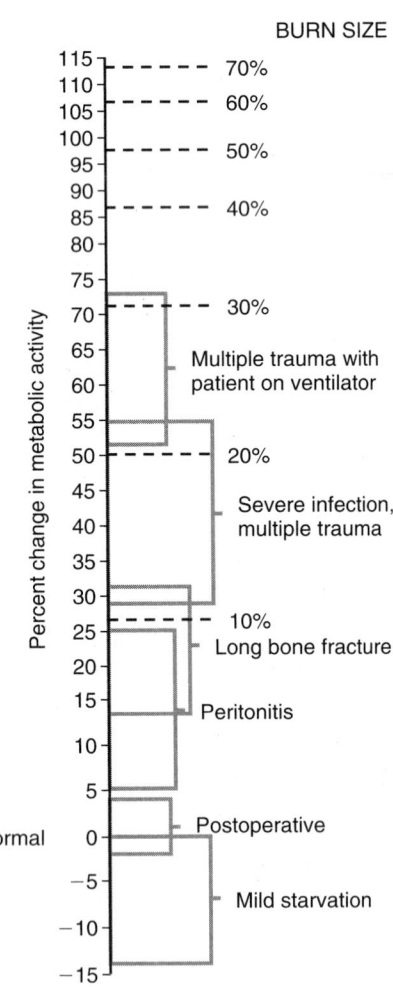

BURN SIZE

FIGURE 57–24. Index of per cent change in metabolic activity caused by various types of stress. (From Wesley JR, et al: *The University of Michigan Hospitals Parenteral and Enteral Nutrition Manual*, 6th ed. Chicago, Abbott Laboratories Hospital Products Division, 1990.)

neurologic function. The intensivist must recognize states that have the potential for permanent dysfunction and support the child in ways that optimize return toward normal. The most common causes of acute global neurologic dysfunction in children are head trauma, hypoxia-ischemia, central nervous system (CNS) infection, and encephalopathies from endogenous metabolites or exogenous toxins. Idiopathic status epilepticus can also cause a moderate or severe encephalopathy. Global neurologic dysfunction coupled with focal signs may be a late presentation of a CNS tumor or abscess.

The manifestations of an acute or evolving neurologic pattern can produce generalized or focal findings. Coma, stupor, and lethargy are more general findings suggestive of an advancing process that has global cerebral implications. Focal findings may reflect a more well-defined process localized to one part of the brain. *Coma* refers to a state in which the patient is unable to arouse or respond to noxious stimuli and is completely unaware of self and surroundings. *Stupor* may be confused with normal sleep, but the patient can be aroused with painful stimuli. *Lethargy* is more subjective and is used to indicate drowsiness or decreased wakefulness. These patients may be more confused but are able to communicate. Because these terms are often used by different physicians with different meaning, it is best to record the physical findings and the Glasgow Coma Scale (GCS) score (see Table 57–3).

Head Trauma. Traumatic brain injury (TBI) is the primary injury that is caused by the direct mechanical disruption of brain tissue and the subsequent secondary injuries that result from the various cerebral and systemic processes worsened by events in the post-traumatic period. TBI in children is different than in adults because of the unique pathophysiology of children associated with the epidemiologic characteristics of pediatric injury. The causes of TBI in children can be separated into injuries associated with child abuse, contact injuries, and inertial injuries.

Nonaccidental trauma, or child abuse, has been thought to produce primary brain injury from repetitive acceleration-deceleration forces, which accompany shaking (therefore the term "shaken baby") (see Chapter 35). The injuries sustained may be more compatible with hypoxic injury secondary to brainstem and spinal injury or the direct effects of the traumatic force. Victims of child abuse may not have signs of external trauma (e.g., bruises, fractures). Instead, they may present with mental status changes (lethargy or irritability), poor feeding, apnea, or seizures. If nonaccidental trauma is suspected, the clinician must obtain a head CT scan to evaluate for acute and subacute injuries such as subdural and epidural hematomas or effusions, punctate intracerebral hemorrhages, skull fractures, cerebral edema, atrophy, and/or hydrocephalus.

Contact injuries occur when an object strikes the head. The force generated by the impact may result in a skull fracture (depressed or linear), cerebral contusion (both coup and contrecoup), or intracranial bleeding (epidural hematoma, subdural hematoma, subarachnoid hemorrhage, or deep intracerebral hematomas). In severe forms of contact injuries, all of aforementioned findings may exist. Those with severe intraparenchymal and intraventricular hemorrhages have a poorer prognosis. In addition, diffuse cerebral edema may develop; this is not always evident on presentation and is not always associated with the severity of the trauma.

Inertial injuries usually occur from rapid acceleration-deceleration forces. This mechanism of injury results from the movement of the intracranial structures within the cranial vault. This may produce severe forms of microscopic injury to the axons resulting in diffuse axonal injury (DAI). Inertial injuries may occur in isolation or in association with contact injuries. The clinical significance of DAI is dependent on the extent and location within the brain. DAI of the brainstem may have more serious consequences than DAI in other parts of the brain.

Secondary brain injuries associated with trauma may occur in the immediate post-traumatic period or develop over the next several days. Secondary injury is associated with systemic hypotension, hypoxia, intracranial hemorrhages, or increased metabolic needs. Cerebral edema is a significant secondary injury that may lead to further neuronal damage, cerebral herniation, and death. TBI may also produce events that may lead to neuronal death via the release of a variety of mediators such as excitatory amino acids (EAAs). This occurs after a generalized depolarization of neurons following the primary brain injury. When this happens, there appears to be cerebrovascular dysfunction (loss of autoregulation), cerebral edema, alterations in the blood-brain barrier, release of free radicals, damage to the mitochondria, apoptosis, and neuronal death.

Children with traumatic head injury may take a long time to recover but often regain significant function during rehabilitation.

Hypoxia-Ischemia. Encephalopathy from poor or absent cerebral perfusion (thus both hypoxia and ischemia) often heralds a poorer outcome than that from trauma; the physician has little to offer to improve the outcome. Often there is diffuse, global brain injury. These children may have experienced a period of asystole and have required cardiopulmonary resuscitation (CPR) such as after near-drowning episodes, acute life-threatening events, smoke inhalation, upper or lower airway obstruction, shock, electrical injuries, and other life-threatening events. The lack of oxygen and perfusion produces primary neuronal damage. Secondary injury occurs from the response of the activation of mediators, which activate a cascade of events that result in cerebral edema and apoptosis and cell death.

Imaging studies may be helpful in evaluating the structural damage seen with hypoxic-ischemic encephalopathy. These changes may not be immediately apparent; they provide an insight into the extent of the cerebral injury. Rapid diffusion weighted imaging MRI demonstrates lesions faster than any other imaging modality. There is often preservation of the brainstem function. Other organ systems may reflect hypoxic-ischemic injury such as the liver, kidneys, intestines, and heart. A poor prognosis is associated with a GCS score of 3, hypotension, cerebral edema, persistent apnea requiring CPR for more than 25 min, persistent loss of cranial nerve reflexes (e.g., corneal), and coma for more than 24 hr. Those patients who have required significant support for these other organ systems have very poor outcomes. Children who have sustained serious hypoxic-ischemic brain injury but have preserved other vital organ function (respiration, blood pressure, pulse) may survive with severe neurologic function and possibly in a persistent vegetative state.

CNS Infection. CNS infections include meningitis, meningoencephalitis, encephalitis, subdural or epidural empyema, and brain abscess. Viruses and bacteria cause meningitis; fungal infections may be noted in patients undergoing transplantation and its inherent requirement for immunosuppression. Important treatable causes for stupor and coma include bacterial meningitis, herpes encephalitis, bacterial abscess, cerebral toxoplasmosis, and tuberculous meningitis. An infectious cause must be considered in any patient with an acute neurologic deterioration associated with fever or leukocytes or in those without a history of trauma. There may or may not be signs of meningeal irritation such as nuchal rigidity or Kernig and Brudzinski signs. Infants may not always have a bulging fontanel. Patients may also present with global encephalopathy such as coma or with status epilepticus.

Early diagnosis and treatment with appropriate antibiotics or antiviral drugs are important. If the patient demonstrates any manifestations of systemic complications (hypotension, apnea) the clinician must address these immediately to prevent secondary neuronal injury and other organ dysfunction. This includes airway management, mechanical ventilation, and cardiovascular support. Complications from acute neurologic infections include cerebrovascular infarcts, cerebritis, cranial nerve compression, development of hydrocephalus, subdural effusion, cerebral edema, and herniation. These findings are detected with imaging studies, which should be performed if the patient is not improving within 24–48 hr or whose condition begins to deteriorate with the development of focal findings or signs of increased intracranial pressure (ICP) (hypertension, bradycardia, irregular respirations, or signs of third or sixth cranial nerve compression). Neurosurgical consultation may be indicated if there is a surgical complication.

Encephalopathies from Endogenous Metabolites or Exogenous Toxins. Profound encephalopathy may result from metabolic defects (inborn errors of metabolism producing hypoglycemia, hyperammonemia, lactic or organic acidosis), from fulminant hepatic failure (hyperammonemia plus other unmeasured neurotoxins), or from the ingestion of certain drugs and substances (ethanol, anticonvulsant drugs). Accidental ingestions are very common in toddlers and young children. Older children may experiment with various chemical substances or ingest wild mushrooms, which may produce acute cerebral signs. Any patient who has an altered level of consciousness without a clear explanation should have a drug toxicology screen.

Other laboratory tests may be helpful in the assessment of the child who presents with obtundation. These tests include routine electrolytes to evaluate for an increased anion gap (acidosis from endogenous acids or exogenous acids such as salicylates), serum osmolarity to detect for differences between calculated and measured osmolarity (alcohol, ethylene glycol ingestion), and arterial blood gas analysis to evaluate respiratory status to determine if there is either a respiratory alkalosis (early salicylate poisoning or hyperammonemia), respiratory acidosis (opiate or barbiturate ingestion producing respiratory depression), or a metabolic acidosis (late salicylate ingestion or endogenous lactic or organic acidosis).

One must always determine if there are alterations in glucose homeostasis because hypoglycemia will produce obtundation, stupor, and coma. Hypoglycemia occurs frequently as a result of various metabolic and endocrine disorders and with intoxication with alcohols. Young infants and children are especially prone to episodes of hypoglycemia because they have limited glycogen stores and can become seriously hypoglycemic as a result of prolonged fasting, inborn errors of metabolism, hyperinsulinism, liver failure, or ingestions. Hypoglycemia is easily reversible and should be aggressively pursued in every comatose child.

Diabetes Mellitus. Severe cerebral edema may occur during treatment of diabetic ketoacidosis (DKA). The cause for such edema is likely due to the action of "idiogenic osmoles," osmotically active particles (e.g., inositol) formed within the cerebral cells during the acute phase to counteract the effects of hyperglycemia. If serum osmolality declines too quickly, these osmolar particles act to attract water into the cell. Cerebral edema in DKA may be associated with significant morbidity and mortality. Coma may also occur in severe DKA or when associated with severe hyperosmolar states before treatment (see Chapter 583). Hyperglycemia and a lactic acidosis (without ketonuria) are common during the hypoxic-ischemic encephalopathy and have a poor prognosis.

Status Epilepticus. Severe status epilepticus will result in stupor or coma and has the potential for permanent cellular damage if the seizures are prolonged or associated with hypoxia, hypercarbia, and hypotension (see Chapter 586). Seizures lasting more than 10 min must be treated aggressively. Intensive therapies are aimed at halting epileptic activity and reducing neurologic cell metabolism in order to limit the extent of the primary neuronal injury. Electrical status may severely affect the brain in the absence of clinically evident seizures; an electroencephalogram will confirm the diagnosis.

Intracranial Hypertension. Acute intracranial hypertension often initially presents first with headache and confusion but may advance at various rates through combativeness, somnolence, and coma. It may be seen as a complication of either global or focal encephalopathies or mass lesions. An increase in the volume of cerebral contents within the rigid cranial cavity (blood, edema, masses, cerebral [ventricular] spinal fluid) produces an increase in ICP. This may result from trauma from hemorrhage or hyperemia; hydrocephalus with cerebrospinal fluid accumulation; tumors or abscesses; severe CNS infections; and metabolic aberrations, including hypoxia-ischemia. As the ICP increases, the effective cerebral perfusion pressure (CPP) decreases (see Chapter 55). CPP is equal to the mean arterial pressure minus the ICP. Autoregulation of the cerebral vasculature provides the initial protection to maintain cerebral perfusion. However, as the ICP increases, autoregulation may be lost and cerebral blood flow decreased. This results in the potential for significant secondary neuronal injury. CPP may be reduced by raised ICP, hypotension, or both. Additional manifestations of increased ICP include papilledema, Cushing triad (bradycardia, hypertension, irregular respirations), bulging fontanel, and signs of third nerve (ptosis, anisocoria) or sixth nerve (lateral rectus weakness) compression. The presence of intracranial hypertension may mimic global encephalopathy with increasing confusion and combativeness progressing to coma and brainstem compression. These are late signs of increased ICP and indicate that herniation of brain structures is occurring; this is life threatening and requires immediate intervention.

Herniation. Coma may precede herniation of intracranial contents. Brainstem herniation proceeds from higher to lower brain centers. Coma is followed by decorticate rigidity, small pupils, and Cheyne-Stokes breathing. As the midbrain and pons become involved, posturing changes to decerebrate, pupils become mid-position and nonreactive, and the breathing pattern is hyperpneic. As the medulla is compromised, the blood pressure and heart rate fluctuate greatly, the patient becomes flaccid, and breathing is irregular and then absent. Unilateral uncal lobe herniation may be heralded by ipsilateral anisocoria, loss of pupillary reflexes, and ptosis caused by compression of the third cranial nerve.

Infratentorial Lesions. Lesions in the infratentorial region can cause coma, cranial nerve palsies, and respiratory abnormalities at an earlier stage in the disease. Obstructive hydrocephalus may result from the compression of the circulatory or cerebrospinal fluid pathways. Such compression is seen with posterior fossa tumors. These may produce brainstem compression without the depth or severity of encephalopathy in more global cortical diseases. The hallmark of infratentorial herniation is early respiratory and autonomic impairment, whereas the pupillary responses may be preserved. Neck pain may be present as well as vocal cord paralysis.

Principles of Support for Global Neurologic Dysfunction
NORMALIZE THE CIRCULATION AND RESPIRATION. The basics of neurologic stabilization include the ABCs of resuscitation (see Chapter 57.1) and maintenance of adequate oxygenation and perfusion. The decision to intubate the trachea and institute mechanical ventilation is determined by the need to control the airway; are protective airway reflexes (i.e., cough and gag) intact to protect the child from aspiration? In some stuporous cases, the patient's respiratory drive may be intact but the gag reflex may be absent or upper airway muscle tone lax. In the case of Guillain-Barré syndrome, one should not wait for respirations to be shallow; the gag reflex may be absent. If the patient can protect the airway, the work of breathing must be maintained to ensure adequate gas exchange and avoid

hypercarbia and hypoxemia. In addition, intubation may be needed to gently hyperventilate the patient to produce mild hypocarbia, thus acutely reducing ICP. The mechanism selected to secure the airway includes the availability of appropriate equipment, medication, and personnel to facilitate the intubation in as rapid and atraumatic manner as possible. The medications and methods used for intubation should not further raise ICP. A form of rapid sequence intubation is used with appropriate positioning and support for the neck (see Chapter 57.1). Once the airway is secured and the patient's oxygenation and ventilation have been stabilized, the clinician can focus on the circulation system.

Circulation should be normalized, with the aim of optimizing perfusion to all tissues. If after appropriate fluid resuscitation the patient still has poor perfusion, one should consider the use of inotropic agents to enhance cardiac output. One must carefully determine if there are ongoing blood or fluid losses that need to be addressed to facilitate fluid resuscitation. Once the patient's cardiac output has been stabilized, modest fluid restriction is beneficial, mainly to avoid fluid overload and attendant hypervolemia. One should not restrict fluids to the point of oliguria. Little benefit has been demonstrated with fluid restriction. The urine output and serum sodium need to be monitored and the fluid restriction considered if hyponatremia from the syndrome of inappropriate antidiuretic hormone secretion (SIADH) begins to develop.

FLUID MANAGEMENT IN THE PRESENCE OF SIADH OR DIABETES INSIPIDUS (DI). *Inappropriate secretion of antidiuretic hormone* is a frequent accompaniment of CNS injury or infection and can occur with many types of brain injury as well as with pulmonary disease. The diagnosis of SIADH is suggested by analyzing urine (higher than expected) and serum (low) osmolalities in the hyponatremic patient. Urine osmolality is often higher than the serum osmolality. The effects of SIADH can be lessened by fluid restriction; SIADH is usually self-limited, although it may persist during mechanical ventilation. Patients with SIADH are normotensive and not edematous in contrast to patients with hyponatremia and heart or hepatic failure (dilutional hyponatremia) or adrenal or renal insufficiency (salt-losing states).

Diabetes insipidus heralds a very poor outcome in the child with significant brain injury. A damaged pituitary or hypothalamus can induce massive unregulated urine output, dehydration, and a rapidly rising serum sodium concentration. The sodium level can rise as much as 30 mEq/L in a few hours. Diabetes insipidus can be managed with vigorous intravenous fluid intake, but it is better controlled with vasopressin or desmopressin.

REDUCTION OF INTRACRANIAL HYPERTENSION. The goal of therapy is to maintain CPP greater than 40 mm Hg in infants and toddlers, greater than 50 mm Hg in young children, and greater than 60–70 mm Hg in adolescents.

Intubation, Ventilation, and Positioning. The initial and most rapid therapeutic intervention for reducing intracranial hypertension requires endotracheal intubation and monitoring of the blood gases to ensure appropriate oxygenation and ventilation to keep the $Paco_2$ at 30–35 mm Hg. Mild hyperventilation is helpful because it reduces cerebral blood flow through vasoconstriction of the cerebral blood vessels. Significant hyperventilation ($Paco_2 < 25$ mm Hg) may possibly cause cerebral ischemia. Proper positioning places the patient's head in the midline and elevated about 30 degrees, to allow optimal venous drainage. Patient movement should be minimized with strong sedation and, if necessary, muscle relaxants (e.g., intermittent or continuous infusions of benzodiazepines, narcotics, and vecuronium).

Ventricular Drainage, Diuretics, Steroids, and Other Therapies. Reduction in cerebrospinal fluid volume may be helpful in managing increased ICP. If a ventriculostomy has been placed, periodic fluid removal will reduce ICP and improve CPP.

Further reduction in circulating blood volume occurs with the use of diuretics. Commonly, diuretic therapy in the form of mannitol or furosemide has been used acutely. Mannitol is commonly useful in the acute treatment of intracranial hypertension. It is an osmotic diuretic and promotes a shift of fluid from the intracellular to the intravascular space. A dose ranging from 0.25–0.5 g/kg is effective. Mannitol is less beneficial with severe disruption of blood-brain barrier because it may enter the CNS and draw fluid into the brain. If mannitol creates a very hyperosmolar circulatory state, renal failure and hemolysis may ensue. Furosemide is a safer but less effective alternative. Usually the combination of both agents is prescribed. Hypertonic saline infusions may also be beneficial. Intravenous corticosteroids are not indicated if there is diffuse cerebral injury, but they have benefit in the localized edema surrounding an intracranial mass (abscess or tumor). Surgical decompression of blood is essential. The use of barbiturate coma with electroencephalographic monitoring has been used with varying success to reduce cerebral metabolic demands and ICP. Unfortunately, barbiturate coma may reduce cardiac output and produce hypotension.

SEIZURES

Benzodiazepines vs. Antiepileptics. Both benzodiazepines and other anticonvulsant drugs reduce cerebral metabolism; the anticonvulsant agents are more effective at suppressing subsequent seizure activity. Seizures lasting longer than 10 min must be treated aggressively. Seizures lasting longer than 30 min are status epilepticus; refractory status epilepticus occurs when despite anticonvulsant therapy, seizures last greater than 60 min. Benzodiazepines (lorazepam or diazepam) are very effective first-line agents for treating seizures in patients with hypoxic-ischemic encephalopathy and other causes of status epilepticus. Both have rapid (3–5 min) onset of action. Because diazepam has a short half-life, it must be followed with another longer-acting agent (phenytoin or phenobarbital). The half-life of phenobarbital is quite long, it has sensitive properties, and at high doses an adequate assessment by the neurologic examination will not be possible. Phenytoin should not cause sedation and should not change the results of neurologic examination; its use is limited by its potential cardiovascular and CNS toxicity (in high doses). The two drugs are often used in combination in refractory status. Fosphenytoin is often used instead of phenytoin. Fosphenytoin and phenobarbital are also used as first-line agents in status epilepticus. Additional agents used in status epilepticus include midazolam and the intravenous form of valproic acid. If seizures are refractory, repeated doses of phenobarbital should be given to achieve high levels (50–100 mg/dL). In addition a continuous intravenous infusion of midazolam may be used. Propofol has also been used with some success in treating refractory seizures.

Barbiturate-Induced Coma. If seizures are refractory to phenobarbital and fosphenytoin, a barbiturate-induced coma may be necessary, using a shorter-acting agent (usually pentobarbital). Therapy may be titrated to a burst suppression pattern of the electroencephalogram; this may not be necessary if seizures cease before this. Monitoring is best conducted with a continuous electroencephalogram. Continuous infusions of midazolam are an alternative approach to treat refractory status. Complications of high-dose barbiturate coma include cardiovascular depression with decreased cardiac output that often requires inotropic drug support.

HYPOTHERMIA. Mild hypothermia (e.g., 32°–34°C) results in a decrease in cerebral metabolism and a reduction of ICP but has the added potential risks of superinfection and dysrhythmias. Hypothermia has not been shown to reliably improve outcome in severe CNS illness. Moderate hypothermia may be beneficial in patients with a GCS score of 5–7 when used for 24 hr. Patients with a GCS score less than 4 may not benefit from hypothermia treatment. Patients with nonpenetrating trauma, age younger than 30 yr, and CPP more than 50 mm Hg and who were hypothermic (<35°C) on admission tend to have a better response to induced hypothermia.

Alves OL, Bullock R: Excitotoxic damage in traumatic brain injury. In Kochanek PM (editor): *Traumatic Brain Injury*. Boston, Kluwer Academic, 2001, pp 1–36.

Berkenbosch JW, et al: The correlation of the bispectral index monitor with clinical sedation scores during mechanical ventilation in the pediatric intensive care unit. *Anesth Analg* 2002;94:506–11.

Butt W: Septic shock. *Pediatr Clin North Am* 2001;48:601–24.

Clifton GL, Miller ER, Choi SC, et al: Lack of effect of induction of hypothermia after acute brain injury. *N Engl J Med* 2001;344:556–63.

Clifton GL, Choi SC, Miller ER, et al: Intercenter variance in clinical trials of head trauma—experience of the National Acute Brain Injury Study: Hypothermia. *J Neurosurg* 2001;95:751–55.

Corbett D, Thornhill J: Temperature modulation (hypothermic and hyperthermic conditions) and its influence on histological and behavioral outcomes following cerebral ischemia. *Brain Pathol* 2000;10:145–52.

Hanhan US, Fiallos MR, Orlowski JP: Status epilepticus. *Pediatr Clin North Am* 2001;48:683–94.

Jacinto SJ, Gieron-Korthals M, Ferreira JA: Predicting outcome in hypoxic-ischemic brain injury. *Pediatr Clin North Am* 2001;48:647–60.

Kochanek PM, Clark RSB, Ruppel RA, Dixon CE: Cerebral resuscitation after traumatic brain injury and cardiopulmonary arrest in infants and children in the new millennium. *Pediatr Clin North Am* 2001;48:661–81.

Verweij BH, Muizelaar JP, Vinas FC, et al: Impaired cerebral mitochondrial function after traumatic brain injury in humans. *J Neurosurg* 2000;93:815–20.

Zipfel GJ, Babcock DJ, Lee JM, Choi DW: Neuronal apoptosis after CNS injury: The roles of glutamate and calcium. *J Neurotrauma* 2000;17:857–69.

57.8 Acute Care of the Multiple Trauma Victim

Peter S. Dayan and Bruce L. Klein

Epidemiology. Injury is the leading cause of death for children aged 1–14 yr in industrialized nations (see Chapter 50). Deaths represent only a small fraction of the total trauma burden. For every child who dies in the Netherlands from home or leisure unintentional injury, there are another 160 hospital admissions and 2,000 emergency department (ED) visits. Many survivors have temporary or permanent functional limitations.

Trauma is classified by the number of significantly injured body parts (one or more), the severity of injury (mild, moderate, or severe), and the mechanism of injury (blunt or penetrating). In childhood blunt trauma predominates, accounting for over 90% of admissions. In adolescence, penetrating trauma increases in frequency and has a higher mortality. This chapter focuses on the emergency management of the child with moderate to severe injury due to blunt trauma.

Regionalization and Trauma Teams. Decreased mortality and morbidity has been noted in geographic regions with comprehensive, coordinated trauma systems. Designated trauma centers, in particular, save lives. At the scene, paramedics should administer necessary advanced life support and do triage (Box 57–6). Generally, it is preferable to bypass local hospitals and rapidly transport a seriously injured child directly to a pediatric trauma center (or trauma center with pediatric commitment).

When the receiving ED is notified before the child's arrival, the trauma team must be mobilized. Each member has defined tasks. A senior surgeon or an emergency physician leads the team. Team compositions vary somewhat from hospital to hospital; the model used at Children's National Medical Center (Washington, DC) is depicted in Figure 57–25. Consultants, especially neurosurgeons and orthopedic surgeons, must be immediately available, and the operating room (OR) staff should be alerted.

Physiologic status, anatomic locations, and/or mechanism of injury are used to determine whether to activate the trauma team. More importance should be placed on physiologic compromise and less on mechanism of injury. Scoring scales using similar parameters have been developed to predict patient outcome (see Chapter 50) (Tables 57–18 and 57–19).

BOX 57–6. Children Requiring Pediatric Trauma Center Care

Patients with serious injury to more than one organ or system
Patients with one-system injury who require critical care or monitoring in an intensive care unit
Patients with signs of shock who require more than one transfusion
Patients with fracture complicated by suspected neurovascular or compartment injury
Patients with fracture of axial skeleton
Patients with two or more long-bone fractures
Patients with potential replantation of an extremity
Patients with suspected or actual spinal cord or column injuries
Patients with head injury with any one of the following:
    Orbital or facial bone fracture
    Cerebrospinal fluid leaks
    Altered state of consciousness
    Changing neural signs
    Open-head injuries
    Depressed skull fracture
    Requiring intracranial pressure monitoring
Patients suspected of requiring ventilator support

From Krug SE: The acutely ill or injured child. In Behrman RE, Kliegman RM (editors): Nelson Essentials of Pediatrics, 4th ed. Philadelphia, WB Saunders, 2002, p 96.

Primary Survey. The American College of Surgeons advocates use of a primary and secondary survey to evaluate trauma victims in the ED. During the primary survey, the physician quickly assesses and treats any life-threatening injuries. The principal causes of death shortly after trauma are airway obstruction, respiratory insufficiency, circulatory collapse from hemorrhage, and central nervous system injury. Therefore, the primary survey addresses the *ABCDE*s: A, Airway; B, Breathing; C, Circulation; D, neurologic Deficit; and E, Exposure of the patient and control of the Environment.

AIRWAY/CERVICAL SPINE. Optimizing oxygenation and ventilation, while protecting the cervical spine from potential further injury, is of paramount importance. Initially, any child sustaining multiple, blunt trauma must be suspected of having a cervical spine injury. Children are at increased risk for such injuries owing to their relatively large heads, which augment flexion-extension forces, and weak neck muscles, which predispose to ligament injuries. Unnecessary movement of the cervical spine can lead to paralysis. The cervical spine should be immobilized in neutral position using a stiff collar, head blocks, and tape or cloth placed across the forehead, torso, and thighs to restrain the child to a rigid backboard.

Airway obstruction presents as snoring, gurgling, hoarseness, stridor, and/or diminished breath sounds despite good respiratory effort. Children are more likely than adults to develop airway obstruction because of their smaller oral cavities, proportionately larger tongues and greater amounts of tonsillar and adenoidal tissue, higher and more anterior glottic openings, and narrower tracheas. Obstruction is common in patients with severe head injuries for several reasons, including decreased muscle tone that allows the tongue to fall posteriorly, occluding the airway. With trauma, obstruction also can result from fractures of the mandible or facial bones, crush injuries of the larynx or trachea, secretions such as blood or vomitus, or foreign body aspiration.

If it is necessary to open the airway, a jaw thrust *without head tilt* is recommended (see Chapter 57.1). This procedure minimizes cervical spine motion. In an unconscious child, an oropharyngeal airway then can be inserted to prevent posterior displacement of the mandibular tissues. A semiconscious child will gag with an oropharyngeal airway but may tolerate a nasopharyngeal airway. If these maneuvers plus suctioning do not clear the airway, oral endotracheal intubation is indicated. Emergent cricothyrotomy is rarely required.

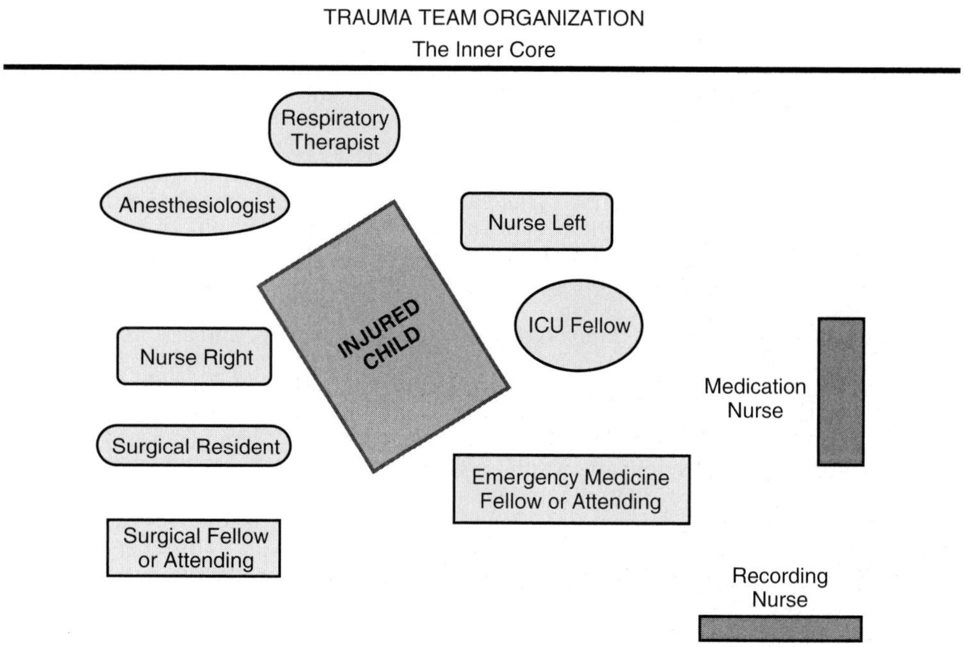

TRAUMA TEAM ORGANIZATION
The Inner Core

FIGURE 57–25. Trauma team inner core members at Children's National Medical Center (Washington, DC). Outer core members include a nursing administrator, social worker, radiology technician, transplant technician, and security officer.

TABLE 57–18. Pediatric Trauma Score

Clinical Category	Score		
	+2	+1	−1
Size	≥ 20 kg	10–20 kg	<10 kg
Airway	Normal	Maintainable	Unmaintainable
Systolic blood pressure*	≥ 90 mm Hg	50–90 mm Hg	<50 mm Hg
Central nervous system	Awake	Obtunded/loss of consciousness	Coma/decerebrate
Open wound	None	Minor	Major/penetrating
Skeletal	None	Closed fracture	Open/multiple fractures

Use this if blood pressure cuff not available: +2 = palpable pulse at wrist; +1 = no palpable pulse in groin; -1 = no palpable pulse. If total score <8, refer to pediatric trauma center.

From Ford EG: Trauma triage. In Ford EG, Andrassy RJ (editors): Pediatric Trauma Initial Assessment and Management. Philadelphia, WB Saunders, 1994, p 112.

BREATHING. Breathing is assessed by counting the respiratory rate; visualizing chest wall motion for symmetry, depth, and accessory muscle use; and auscultating breath sounds in both axillae. In addition to looking for cyanosis, pulse oximetry is standard. If breathing is inadequate, bag-valve-mask ventilation with 100% oxygen must be initiated immediately, followed by endotracheal intubation. End-expiratory CO_2 detectors help verify accurate tube placement.

TABLE 57–19. Revised Trauma Score*

Revised Trauma Score	Glasgow Coma Scale Score	Systolic Blood Pressure (mm Hg)	Respiratory Rate (breaths/min)
4	13–15	>89	10–20
3	9–12	76–89	>29
2	6–8	50–75	6–9
1	4–5	1–49	1–5
0	3	0	0

A score of 0–4 is given for each variable, then added (range, 1–12). A score ≤11 indicates potentially important trauma.

From Fitzmaurice LS: Approach to multiple trauma. In Barkin RM (editor): Pediatric Emergency Medicine, 2nd ed. St. Louis, CV Mosby, 1997, p 224.

Head trauma is the most common cause of respiratory insufficiency. An unconscious child with a severe head injury may develop a variety of breathing abnormalities, including Cheyne-Stokes respirations, slow irregular breaths, or apnea.

Although less common than a pulmonary contusion, tension pneumothorax and massive hemothorax is immediately life threatening (Box 57–7). Tension pneumothorax occurs when air accumulates under pressure in the pleural space. The adjacent lung is compacted, the mediastinum is pushed toward the opposite hemithorax, and the heart, great vessels, and

BOX 57–7. Life-Threatening Chest Injuries

TENSION PNEUMOTHORAX

One-way valve leak from lung parenchyma
Complete collapse with mediastinal and tracheal shift to side opposite the leak
Compromises venous return and decreases ventilation of other lung
Clinically, manifests as respiratory distress, unilateral absent breath sounds, tracheal deviation, distended neck veins, tympany to percussion of involved side, and cyanosis
Relieve first with needle aspiration, then with chest tube drainage

OPEN PNEUMOTHORAX (SUCKING CHEST WOUND)

Effect on ventilation depends on size

MAJOR FLAIL CHEST

Usually caused by blunt injury resulting in multiple rib fractures
Loss of bone stability of thoracic cage
Major disruption of synchronous chest wall motion
Mechanical ventilation and positive end-expiratory pressure required

MASSIVE HEMOTHORAX

Must be drained with large-bore tube
Initiate drainage only with concurrent vascular volume replacement

CARDIAC TAMPONADE

Beck triad:
1. Decreased or muffled heart sounds
2. Distended neck veins from increased venous pressure
3. Hypotension with pulsus paradoxus (decreased pulse pressure during inspiration)
Must be drained

From Krug SE: The acutely ill or injured child. In Behrman RE, Kliegman RM (editors): Nelson Essentials of Pediatrics, 4th ed. Philadelphia, WB Saunders, 2002, p 97.

contralateral lung are compressed. Both ventilation and cardiac output are impaired. Typical findings include cyanosis, tachypnea, retractions, asymmetric chest rise, contralateral tracheal deviation, diminished breath sounds on the ipsilateral side, subcutaneous emphysema, and signs of shock. Needle thoracentesis, followed by thoracostomy tube insertion, is diagnostic and lifesaving.

Hemothorax results from injury to the intercostal vessels, lungs, heart, or great vessels. When ventilation is adequate, fluid resuscitation should begin before evacuation, because a large amount of blood may drain through the chest tube, resulting in shock.

CIRCULATION. The most common type of shock in trauma is hypovolemic shock due to hemorrhage (see Chapter 57.2). Signs of shock include tachycardia, weak peripheral pulses, delayed capillary refill, cool mottled skin, and altered mental status. Early in shock, blood pressure remains normal, because of compensatory increases in heart rate and peripheral vascular resistance. An individual can lose up to 25% of blood volume before the blood pressure declines. It is important to note that 25% of blood volume equals 20 mL/kg, which is only 200 mL in a 10-kg child. With losses greater than 25%, hypotension ensues. Losses greater than 50% cause severe hypotension that, if prolonged, may become irreversible.

Direct pressure should be applied to control external hemorrhage. Blind clamping of bleeding vessels is not advisable because of the risk of damage to adjacent structures.

Cannulating a larger vein, such as an antecubital vein, is usually the quickest way to achieve intravenous access. A short, large-bore catheter offers less resistance to flow, allowing for more rapid administration. Ideally, a second catheter should be placed within the first few minutes of resuscitation in a severely injured child. If intravenous access proves difficult, an intraosseous catheter can be inserted; all medications and fluids can be administered intraosseously. Central venous access using the Seldinger technique (e.g., via the femoral vein) or surgical cutdown (e.g., over the saphenous vein) are other alternatives in experienced hands.

Aggressive, intravenous fluid resuscitation is essential early in shock to prevent further deterioration (20 mL/kg). Isotonic crystalloid solution, such as lactated Ringer or normal saline (20 mL/kg), should be infused rapidly. Currently, no consensus exists supporting routine use of colloid or hypertonic saline solution. When necessary, repeated crystalloid boluses can be given. Many children stabilize with crystalloid solution alone. However, if the patient is still in shock after repeated boluses, 10–15 mL/kg of cross-matched, packed red blood cells should be transfused. Although less desirable, type-specific or O-negative cells can be substituted pending availability of cross-matched blood. When shock persists despite these measures, surgery to stop internal hemorrhage is usually indicated.

NEUROLOGIC DEFICIT. In the primary survey, neurologic status is briefly assessed by evaluating the level of consciousness and determining pupil size and reactivity. Level of consciousness can be classified using the mnemonic *AVPU: A*lert, responsive to *V*erbal commands, responsive to *P*ainful stimuli, or *U*nresponsive.

Head injuries account for approximately 70% of pediatric blunt trauma deaths. Primary direct cerebral injury occurs within seconds of the event and is irreversible. Secondary injury is caused by subsequent anoxia or ischemia. Therefore, the goal is to minimize secondary injury by ensuring adequate oxygenation, ventilation, and perfusion and maintaining normal intracranial pressure (ICP). A child with severe neurologic impairment, such as a Glasgow Coma Scale (GCS) (see Table 57–3) score of 8 or less, should be intubated (see Chapter 57.7).

Signs of increased ICP, including progressive neurologic deterioration or evidence of transtentorial herniation, must be treated immediately. Hyperventilation lowers $Paco_2$, resulting in cerebral vasoconstriction, reduced cerebral blood flow, and decreased ICP. Vigorous, *prolonged* hyperventilation is no longer recommended, because the consequent vasoconstriction may excessively decrease cerebral perfusion. Brief hyperventilation is an option for patients with acute increases in ICP. Mannitol lowers ICP and may improve survival. Because mannitol acts via osmotic diuresis, it can exacerbate hypovolemia and must be used cautiously. Neurosurgical consultation is mandatory. If signs of increased ICP persist, the neurosurgeon must decide whether to obtain a CT scan and/or operate.

EXPOSURE/ENVIRONMENTAL CONTROL. All clothing should be cut away to reveal any injuries. Cutting is quickest and also minimizes unnecessary patient movement.

Children often arrive mildly hypothermic owing to their higher body surface area to mass ratios. They can be warmed using radiant heat as well as heated blankets and intravenous fluids.

Secondary Survey. During the secondary survey, the physician completes a detailed, head-to-toe, physical examination.

HEAD TRAUMA. A GCS or Pediatric GCS score (see Table 57–3) should be assigned to every child with significant head trauma (see Chapter 57.7). This scale assesses eye opening and motor and verbal responses. In the Pediatric GCS, the verbal score is modified for age. The GCS further categorizes neurologic disability, and serial measurements identify improvement or deterioration over time. Patients with low scores 6–24 hr after injury have poorer prognoses.

Head CT scan without contrast medium enhancement has become standard to determine the type of injury. In severely injured children, diffuse cerebral injury with edema is a serious and common finding on CT scan. Focal evacuable hemorrhagic lesions (e.g., epidural hematoma) occur less commonly but may require immediate neurosurgical intervention.

ICP monitoring is used routinely for children with severe brain injuries (e.g., GCS score of 8 or less with an abnormal CT). Although its benefit in improving outcome is uncertain, it has gained wide neurosurgical support. An advantage of an intraventricular catheter, in contrast to an intraparenchymal device, is that cerebrospinal fluid can be drained to treat acute rises in ICP.

A child with a severe brain injury must be treated aggressively in the ED because it can be difficult early in the course to accurately predict long-term neurologic outcome. Compared with adults with similar injuries, children have improved functional outcomes perhaps in part because of the elastic nature of their maturing brains. Nonetheless, diffuse cerebral edema after head trauma has a poor prognosis.

CERVICAL SPINE TRAUMA. Cervical spine injuries occur in less than 2% of children with multisystem trauma but are associated with significant mortality and morbidity. Bony injuries occur mainly from C1-C4 in children younger than 8 yr of age. In older children, they occur equally in the upper and lower cervical spine. The mortality rate, however, is significantly higher in patients with upper cervical spine injuries. *SCIWORA* (cervical spinal cord injury without radiographic [bone] abnormalities on plain films) occurs in approximately 20% of children with cervical spine injuries. Approximately one third of all patients with cervical spine injuries have neurologic deficits.

Evaluation begins with a detailed history and neurologic examination. Identifying the mechanism of injury helps one estimate the likelihood of a cervical spine injury. Both the patient and paramedic should be asked whether there were any neurologic symptoms or signs, such as weakness or abnormal sensation, which resolved before arrival. In a child with transient neurologic complaints and normal x-ray films, SCIWORA still must be considered.

Whenever the history, physical examination, or mechanism of injury suggests a cervical spine injury, radiographs (including lateral, anteroposterior [AP], and odontoid views) should be obtained after initial resuscitation. Cervical spine CT scan can be a valuable adjunct to plain films; some centers use CT as the primary diagnostic tool. Magnetic resonance imaging is especially useful for a child with suspected SCIWORA.

Rapid diagnosis of spinal cord injury is essential. Initiating high-dose intravenous methylprednisolone within 8 hr of spinal cord injury improves motor outcome at 1 year and is standard therapy.

THORACIC TRAUMA. Pulmonary contusions occur frequently in younger children with blunt chest trauma. A child's chest wall is relatively pliable; therefore, less force is absorbed by the rib cage and more is transmitted to the lungs. Respiratory distress may be noted in the ED or develop during the first 24 hr of hospitalization.

Rib fractures result from significant external force and are noted in patients with more severe injuries and are associated with a higher mortality rate. Flail chest, which is caused by multiple rib fractures, is rare in children. The differential diagnosis of life-threatening cardiopulmonary injuries following thoracic trauma is noted in Table 57–20.

ABDOMINAL TRAUMA. Liver and spleen contusions, hematomas, and lacerations account for the majority of intra-abdominal injuries due to blunt trauma. The kidney, pancreas, and duodenum are relatively spared, owing to their retroperitoneal location. Pancreatic and duodenal injuries are more common after a bicycle handlebar impact or a direct blow to the abdomen.

Although a thorough examination for intra-abdominal injuries is essential, this often proves difficult. Misleading findings can result from gastric distention from crying or because a toddler will not cooperate. Calm reassurance and gentle palpation before painful procedures helps with the examination. Important aspects of the examination include looking for distention and bruises, palpating for tenderness, and performing a rectal examination to assess for blood. Specific signs give insight into the mechanism of injury and potential for particular injuries. For example, a lap belt mark across the abdomen suggests the possibility of a bowel or mesentery injury. Pain in the left shoulder may signify splenic trauma.

An abdominal CT scan with intravenous contrast medium enhancement rapidly identifies structural and functional abnormalities and is the preferred study in a stable child. It has excellent sensitivity and specificity for splenic, hepatic, and renal injuries but is less sensitive for intestinal and pancreatic injuries. Administering oral contrast adds little for most injuries. The use of oral contrast in children with possible bowel perforation is controversial, because false-negative scans are common. Ultrasonography may be used to follow injuries.

Nonoperative treatment has become standard for hemodynamically stable children with splenic, hepatic, and renal injuries from blunt trauma. The majority of such children can be treated nonsurgically. In addition to avoiding perioperative complica-

tions, nonoperative treatment also appears to decrease the need for blood transfusions as well as shorten hospital stay. Indications for laparotomy include persistent hemodynamic instability, the need for repeated transfusions (~40 mL/kg/24 hr), and bowel perforation. Splenic repair if possible is preferable to splenectomy in cases of severe splenic injury.

LOWER GENITOURINARY TRAUMA. The perineum should be inspected, pelvic stability assessed, and a rectal examination performed to evaluate for lower genitourinary trauma. Urethral injuries are more common in males. Findings suggestive of a urethral injury include scrotal or labial ecchymoses, blood at the urethral meatus, gross hematuria, and a superiorly positioned prostate (in an adolescent male). Any of these findings represents a contraindication to urethral catheter insertion and warrants consultation with a urologist. A pelvic fracture is also a marker for potential genitourinary injury. Retrograde urethrocystogram and CT scan of the pelvis and abdomen are used to determine the extent of injury.

EXTREMITY TRAUMA. Thorough examination of the extremities is essential because fractures are among the most frequently missed injuries in children with multiple trauma. All limbs should be inspected for deformity, swelling, and bruises; palpated for tenderness; and assessed for active and passive range of motion, sensory function, and perfusion.

Before obtaining x-ray films, suspected fractures and dislocations should be immobilized and an analgesic administered. Splinting a femur fracture helps alleviate pain and may decrease blood loss. An orthopedic surgeon must be consulted immediately to evaluate a child with a compartment syndrome, other causes of neurovascular compromise, or open fracture (Chapter 673).

Radiologic and Laboratory Evaluation. To avoid misdiagnoses, some authorities recommend routinely obtaining a large array of studies in the ED. These include lateral cervical spine, AP chest, and AP pelvis x-ray films; arterial blood gas analysis; complete blood cell count; electrolytes; blood glucose; blood urea nitrogen; creatinine; amylase; liver function tests; prothrombin and partial thromboplastin times; type and cross match; and urinalysis. One benefit of standardizing the evaluation of the major trauma victim is that fewer decisions need to be made on an individual basis, which sometimes expedites ED management.

Research has highlighted some of the advantages and limitations of these studies. The lateral cervical spine x-ray film can miss significant injuries. When it is necessary to assess oxygenation, ventilation, and acid-base status, an arterial blood gas is useful. A large base deficit is associated with a higher mortality rate. Hemoglobin and hematocrit levels provide baseline values in the ED but may not have equilibrated after a hemorrhage at the time of measurement. Abnormal liver function tests or serum amylase levels may be noted in patients with significant abdominal trauma, but most patients with significant blunt trauma to the abdomen have clinical indications for CT scanning or surgery. The vast majority of previously healthy children have normal coagulation profiles; however, these may become abnormal after major head trauma. Although routine urinalysis or dipstick testing for blood has been recommended for children, data from large adult studies suggest this may be unnecessary in patients without gross hematuria or hypotension.

Cardiopulmonary Arrest. Preventing physiologic deterioration is crucial. Children who sustain multiple injuries from blunt trauma have a 0–2% survival rate once pulseless cardiac arrest occurs. Unfortunately, those few who survive resuscitation after pulseless arrest are likely to have severe neurologic impairment.

Psychological and Social Support. Serious multisystem trauma may result in significant long-term psychological and social difficulties for the child and family, particularly when there is a major head injury. Children are at risk of depressive symptoms

TABLE 57–20.	Differential Diagnosis of Immediately Life-Threatening Cardiopulmonary Injuries		
	Tension Pneumothorax	**Massive Hemothorax**	**Cardiac Tamponade**
Breath Sounds	Ipsilaterally decreased	Ipsilaterally decreased	Normal
Percussion Note	Hyperresonant	Dull	Normal
Tracheal Location	Contralaterally shifted	Midline or shifted	Midline
Neck Veins	Distended	Flat	Distended
Heart Tones	Normal	Normal	Muffled

From Cooper A, Foltin GL: Thoracic trauma. In Barkin RM (editor): Pediatric Emergency Medicine, 2nd ed. St. Louis, CV Mosby, 1997, p 325.

and post-traumatic stress disorder. Caregivers face persistent stress and have been noted to have more psychological symptoms. Psychological and social support, therefore, is extremely important.

American College of Surgeons: *Advanced Trauma Life Support for Doctors: Student Course Manual.* Dallas, ACS, 1997.

Dowd MD, McAneney C, Lacher M, et al: Maximizing the sensitivity and specificity of pediatric trauma team activation criteria. *Acad Emerg Med* 2000;7: 1119–25.

Osler TM, Vane DW, Tepas JJ, et al: Do pediatric trauma centers have better survival rates than adult trauma centers? An examination of the National Pediatric Trauma Registry. *J Trauma* 2001;50:95–101.

Povlishock JT (editor): Management and prognosis of severe traumatic brain injury. *J Neurotrauma* 2000;17:449–549.

UNICEF Innocenti Research Centre: A league table of child deaths by injury in rich nations. Innocenti Report Card No. 2, February 2001. (www.unicef-icdc.org/publications/pdf/repcard2e.pdf)

Chapter 58

Acute (Adult) Respiratory Distress Syndrome (ARDS)

Lorry R. Frankel and Joseph V. DiCarlo

Acute respiratory distress syndrome (ARDS) is diagnosed in 2.5–3% of children in the pediatric intensive care unit (PICU); these children account for about 8% of total patient-days and 33% of the deaths. ARDS is more likely to occur in children already compromised by serious illness.

ARDS is an acute process. It may begin with an acute lung injury that progresses rapidly to respiratory failure (Box 58–1). The diagnosis is often delayed in children because pulmonary artery catheters are rarely used in pediatrics and because cardiac function is often abnormal because of hypoxia, shock, or sepsis. The diagnosis can be hastened by a high index of suspicion and an echocardiogram.

Epidemiology and Etiology. Risk factors for ARDS include sepsis, shock, trauma, multiple transfusions, pneumonia, acute chest syndrome (sickle cell anemia), aspiration of gastric contents, pulmonary contusion, fat emboli, near-drowning, inhalation injury, drug overdose, acute pancreatitis, and reperfusion injury after lung transplantation.

Infectious pneumonia and sepsis are the most frequent causes of ARDS. ARDS is associated with viral pneumonia, particularly respiratory syncytial virus, adenovirus, post-measles pneumonia, and, in immunocompromised children, infection with cytomegalovirus or *pneumocystis carinii*.

The mortality of ARDS is 30–40%; risk factors for death include sepsis, shock, multiple organ dysfunction, increased pulmonary dead space, and failure to improve during the first

week of illness. The mortality rate varies from 24% after severe trauma to 88% after bone marrow transplantation. Severe respiratory failure in bone marrow transplant recipients is not always ARDS; diffuse alveolar damage, the histologic hallmark of the ARDS, is present in only 33% of these children.

Pathogenesis. ARDS is a pulmonary manifestation of a systemic inflammatory process triggered by various events. ARDS may progress through 2 or 3 phases. In the *acute exudative phase* there is profound and often refractory hypoxia. The chest x-ray film demonstrates pulmonary edema, whereas CT scans show alveolar fluid, atelectasis, and consolidation in the dependent lung zones (less severe but more generalized findings are noted in the nondependent zones). Inflammation with infiltration by neutrophils and macrophages is caused by an excessive presence of proinflammatory cytokines and an imbalance of the anti-inflammatory cytokines. Diffuse alveolar epithelial damage produces protein-rich edema fluid, hyaline membranes, and inactivation of surfactant. Ventilator management strategies, which result in cyclic recruitment (opening) and de-recruitment (closing) of atelectatic alveolar or which cause alveolar overdistention, cause further cytokine release and exacerbate the original diffuse alveolar injury.

The patient may recover or after 1–2 wk may enter the *fibrosing alveolitis phase*, which manifests as continued hypoxia, increased alveolar dead space, further reductions in compliance, pneumothoraces, and pulmonary hypertension, leading to right ventricular failure (cor pulmonale). Patients who die do so in the exudative or fibrosing phase.

Resolution may take 6–12 mo. Residual effects include airway obstruction, restrictive lung disease, poor carbon monoxide diffusion, and exercise intolerance.

Clinical Manifestations. Acute pulmonary deterioration may not be initially appreciated. During this latent period, patients may exhibit mild respiratory distress with tachypnea, dyspnea, and an increased oxygen requirement. Auscultation of the lungs may reveal clear breath sounds or scattered crackles. Within the next few hours, patients begin to develop more severe hypoxia accompanied by carbon dioxide retention. The onset of ARDS may be quite variable, as seen in patients with infection; very sudden, as with pulmonary gastric fluid aspiration; or insidious, as seen in acute neurologic injury.

Laboratory Findings. Patients are initially monitored with a pulse oximeter. As the oxygen requirements exceed an FIO_2 greater than 0.5% when attempting to maintain the SaO_2 greater than 92%, one must consider the diagnosis of ARDS. An arterial blood gas analysis confirms the increased A-a gradient, and a PaO_2/FIO_2 less than 200 correlates with an intrapulmonary shunt greater than 20%. Radiographic findings are nonspecific; x-ray films are performed to identify other causes of progressive respiratory failure or to determine the presence of cardiomegaly and cardiogenic causes of the pulmonary edema. Over the next few hours the chest films begin to demonstrate interstitial and alveolar pulmonary edema. The use of positive-pressure ventilation may alter the radiographic features of pulmonary edema; based on the alterations in pulmonary function and gas exchange, ARDS is still the most likely diagnosis for the worsening respiratory status. Evidence of barotrauma/volutrauma with alveolar air leak may be seen on serial chest films. CT scans or echocardiography may be occasionally needed to identify other causes of hypoxia and respiratory distress. Although rarely used in pediatrics, a pulmonary artery catheter is helpful in differentiating cardiogenic pulmonary edema from ARDS (see Chapter 55).

Treatment. Once the diagnosis has been made, the patient should be cared for in the intensive care unit by physicians who have the skills and knowledge in the treatment of ARDS. Efforts should be made at treating the underlying disease (e.g., sepsis,

---

BOX 58–1. Criteria for Acute Respiratory Syndromes[*]

Acute onset
Bilateral pulmonary infiltrates on radiography[†]
Absence of left-sided heart failure or elevated left atrial pressure or pulmonary artery wedge pressure $\leq$ 18 mm Hg[‡]
Acute lung injury: $PaO_2:FIO_2 \leq 300$
Acute repiratory distress syndrome: $PaO_2:FIO_2 \leq 200$

---

[*] *Criteria are cause independent.*
[†] *Radiographic features are not specific for ARDS.*
[‡] *Nonhydrostatic pulmonary edema from pulmonary capillary endothelial cell injury.*

aspiration, shock), preventing complications (gastric bleeding), and providing supportive care during this period. Patients with ARDS require invasive monitoring of vital signs and blood gases, as well as the placement of a central venous line used to monitor cardiac filling pressures and to administer fluids. A pulmonary artery catheter may be helpful in titrating various ventilator and pharmacologic therapies.

The mainstay of ventilator therapy is the use of a lung protection strategy that includes positive end-expiratory pressures (PEEP) and a low tidal volume. PEEP improves oxygenation by decreasing intrapulmonary shunting. PEEP is usually titrated in increments of 2–4 cm H_2O with repeated measurement of blood gases. PEEP is adjusted to enable the FIO_2 to be lowered to less than 0.6 and have the PaO_2 in the predetermined range to prevent tissue hypoxia (Pao_2: 55–80 mm Hg; oxygen saturations: 88–95%). If the PEEP exceeds 15 cm H_2O, the patient may experience decreased venous return and reduced cardiac output; additional fluids to improve preload and inotropic agents may be needed to enhance blood pressure and cardiac output.

Permissive hypercapnia (permitting the range of $PaCO_2$ to be 55–70 mm Hg) is the result of low tidal volume (6–7 mL/kg) ventilation used in children with ARDS. Higher ventilator settings, such as tidal volumes of 10–15 mL/kg or peak inspiratory pressures greater than 30 cm Hg, may predispose the child to ventilator-associated lung injury, such as barotrauma or volutrauma (air leak syndromes, i.e., pneumothorax, pneumomediastinum, pneumopericardium, pneumoperitoneum, and the production of inflammatory cytokines).

Fluid balance is also monitored to try to reduce edema formation. Once shock is treated and perfusion established, a moderate fluid restriction may be helpful.

Various rescue therapies are available for patients not responding to a lung protector strategy on a conventional ventilator (see Chapter 57.4). The use of high-frequency ventilation benefits children weighing less than 30 kg by reducing air leak and permitting adequate ventilation to occur with a lower mean airway pressure and less shear forces on the already injured lung. Inhaled nitric oxide and other selective or nonselective pulmonary vasodilator agents have not been consistently beneficial in treating severe ARDS. The value of exogenous surfactant in non-neonatal respiratory failure is suggested from case reports and uncontrolled studies; however, controlled trials have not demonstrated a clear benefit. Extracorporeal membrane oxygenation (ECMO) has been used to rescue patients with refractory ARDS. Earlier intervention (< 7 days) with ECMO demonstrates improvement in survival. During the late fibrosing alveolitis phase, there is some evidence that corticosteroids are beneficial in enhancing recovery. In addition, β-agonists may help clear pulmonary edema fluid.

The physician must also treat the underlying disease, prevent nosocomial infections, provide nutritional support (enteral is preferred to parenteral), maintain an adequate cardiac output, and ensure that the patient remains comfortable. Every effort should be undertaken to elucidate the underlying condition associated with the patient's acute deterioration. All central lines should be placed with respect to the maintenance of sterile technique as well as dressing changes and line care to reduce nosocomial infections. Careful assessments and possibly pharmacologic support of the patient's cardiac output are essential to ensure an adequate cardiac output. Pharmacologic agents, which provide appropriate sedation, analgesia, and amnesia, should be used to facilitate ventilation and reduce the patient's discomfort. Blood transfusions may contribute to endothelial injury and nonhydrostatic pulmonary edema. Although increasing the hemoglobin content potentially increases oxygen delivery at hematocrits greater than 35–40%, there may be an adverse effect on the microcirculation (stasis) and a poor outcome.

Acute Respiratory Distress Syndrome Network: Ventilation with lower tidal volumes as compared with traditional tidal volumes for acute lung injury and the acute respiratory distress syndrome. *N Engl J Med* 2000;342:1301–8.

Arnold JH, Anas NG, Luckett P, et al: High-frequency oscillatory ventilation in pediatric respiratory failure: A multi-center experience. *Crit Care Med* 2000; 28:3913–19.

Dobyns EL, Cornfield DN, Anas NG, et al: Multicenter randomized controlled trial of the effects of inhaled nitric oxide therapy on gas exchange in children with acute hypoxemic respiratory failure. *J Pediatr* 1999;134:406–12.

Masiakos PT, Islam S, Doody DP, et al: Extracorporeal membrane oxygenation for non-neonatal acute respiratory failure. *Arch Surg* 1999;134:375–80.

Matthews BD, Noviski N: Management of oxygenation in pediatric acute hypoxemic respiratory failure. *Pediatr Pulmonol* 2001;32:459–70.

Nuckton TJ, Alonso JA, Kallet RH, et al: Pulmonary dead-space fraction as a risk factor for death in the acute respiratory distress syndrome. *N Engl J Med* 2002; 346:1281–86.

Ranieri VM, Suter PM, Tortorella C, et al: Effect of mechanical ventilation on inflammatory mediators in patients with acute respiratory distress syndrome. *JAMA* 1999;282:54–61.

Ware LB, Matthay MA: The acute respiratory distress syndrome. *N Engl J Med* 2000;342:1334–48.

Chapter 59
Continuous Hemofiltration
Joseph V. DiCarlo

Continuous venovenous hemofiltration (CVVH) was designed as a renal replacement therapy for acute renal failure (see Chapters 57.5 and 527). It is often used instead of hemodialysis for patients with blood pressure instability; it is generally more efficient than peritoneal dialysis and can also remove excessive fluid in overhydrated anuric patients. CVVH is particularly useful in children with multiple organ dysfunction or failure, whose treatment often requires very large amounts of intravenous fluids. A double-lumen dialysis catheter is placed in a large vein and connected to a blood pump and air filter. The hemofilters have an additional port located in the ultrafiltrate compartment that allows for the countercurrent circulation of an added dialysate solution. This converts CVVH into a hemodialysis system (CVVHD), which augments the clearance of solutes of low molecular weight. To avoid increasing blood viscosity, filtration rate is kept below 25–30%, or replacement intravenous fluids are infused at the proximal (inflow) side of the filter, diluting the blood presented to the filter. Predilution reduces sludging within the filter and may increase filter life, but the efficiency of ultrafiltration is compromised, because the ultrafiltrate now contains a portion of the replacement fluid. Overall efficiency may be enhanced, however, if the ultrafiltration rate is increased. The replacement solution should contain dextrose, sodium, and potassium in physiologic concentrations and bicarbonate, calcium, magnesium sulfate, chloride, and phosphate.

Production of large volumes of ultrafiltrate (1 to 4 L/hr) may enhance clearance of the chemical mediators of sepsis and inflammation to a degree that attenuates those disease states. Timely use of hemofiltration may delay the progression of hepatic encephalopathy long enough to allow liver transplantation. Hemofiltration is also quite effective when placed in the extracorporeal membrane oxygenation (ECMO) circuit during prolonged bypass in patients with fluid overload and renal dysfunction.

Gouyon JB, Cochat P, Houzel C, et al: Survey on the practice of extrarenal hemofiltration in pediatrics. *Arch Pediatr* 1996;3:769–74.

Heering P, Morgera S, Schmitz FJ, et al: Cytokine removal and cardiovascular hemodynamics in septic patients with continuous venovenous hemofiltration. *Intensive Care Med* 1997;23:288–96.

Ronco C, Barbacini S, Digito A, et al: Achievements and new directions in continuous renal replacement therapies. *New Horiz* 1995;3:708–16.

Chapter 60

Transplantation Issues in the PICU *Lawrence H. Mathers and*

Lorry R. Frankel

Children in the pediatric intensive care unit (PICU) for pretransplant evaluation or for post-transplant care have unique problems that include sustaining a child with end-organ failure while awaiting a donor; complications after transplant such as sepsis, organ rejection, or multiple organ system dysfunction; and various psychologic, ethical, and social issues. Organ and tissue transplantation is a complex process requiring important decisions involving both the donor and the recipient.

Organ and Tissue Donations. Donors include (1) those who survive the donation (living donor) and (2) those who donate after death (nonliving donor). Living donors include both those who donate a dispensable tissue, such as cartilage, skin, or bone marrow, as well as those who donate a part or all of one of their own vital organs (kidney, partial or split liver, or lung). Acquiring tissue from nonliving donors requires that there be a determination of brain death (see Chapter 64) and that the vital organs remain perfused and oxygenated. In the United States, approximately 20% of nonliving donors are children. Overall the potential to donate is much greater than actual donation, whereas the number of patients on waiting lists exceeds by a factor of 10 the number of needed organs that are donated. Because of this a substantial number of children die while on the waiting list.

Certain medical conditions may preclude donation of organs or tissues: severe organ dysfunction, organ injury from trauma, disseminated malignancy, active infection (including HIV), serious vascular disease, diabetes mellitus, and severe hypertension (Table 60–1). To expand the donor pool, some transplant centers accept organs from patients with bacterial sepsis or meningitis who have been treated with antibiotics for 24–48 hr and have had negative repeat cultures. For some transplants, the size and age of the donor and recipient should be similar.

A potential *recipient* of a transplant is usually identified in advance of the actual transplant, but with potential *donors* there is often little time to discuss the subject of organ donation with the family and secure their support for organ donation. A potential recipient of an organ transplant may be in the same hospital as a potential donor, or they may be separated by many hundreds of miles. The distance over which organs for transplantation can be acquired is limited largely by the readiness of the system to respond to a request and the speed of available transport aircraft. A family whose child or other family member is being considered as a potential donor must comprehend all of the factual information about organ donation and must come to terms with the notion of their loved one being a nonliving donor. The team providing care to the potential donor should introduce the concept of organ donation, beginning with a frank assessment of the degree of injury suffered by the potential donor and the futility of any future care. Accepting the futility of future care and considering the possibility of organ donation, often over a matter of just a few hours, is a difficult emotional hurdle for most families; special sensitivity and compassion on the part of the medical team is mandatory. In many states, the law requires that the local transplant coordination program be contacted when the death of any patient is likely.

Evaluation of potential compatibility between donor and recipient is discussed in Chapter 126 and in chapters addressing specific organ and tissue transplants. *Hyperacute rejection* may occur within minutes of the solid organ transplant in the operating room or in the PICU. It results from the presence of preformed antibodies; blood flow to the transplant is usually compromised by the acute reaction. The organ must be removed immediately or rested as the body is supported (e.g., dialysis, extracorporeal membrane oxygenation [ECMO] in postcardiac transplant recipients). Immune responses, immunosuppression, and *acute* and *chronic rejection* are discussed in Chapters 126 and 128. Admission to a PICU is not required for bone marrow transplantation unless severe complications develop. Solid organ transplants that include heart, heart/lung, liver, or kidney require major surgery and result in admission to a PICU, often before and after the transplantation (kidney transplants in older

TABLE 60–1. Contraindications to Organ Donation

Organ	Relatively Absolute Contraindications	Absolutely Relative Contraindications	Comments
General	Infection: HIV (incl. high-risk groups and hemophiliacs); hepatitis B, antigen-positive; untreated infections	Hepatitis C, CMV, CNS infection, treated infection	Preferably test viral load, p24-antigen; seek to match donor and recipient for CMV
	Malignancies: all except some CNS and nonmelanotic skin tumors	Some CNS tumors	
	SLE and other collagen vascular disease, congenital metabolic disorders, hemoglobinopathies	Hypertension under treatment, diabetes mellitus, sustained hypotension, high-dose inotropes or pressors	
Kidney	Renal disease or trauma amyloidosis, dysproteinemias	Established acute renal failure	Elevated creatinine caused by dehydration is not a contraindication
Liver	Liver disease or trauma, peritonitis	Advanced cardiovascular disease, alcoholism, drug overdose, moderately elevated liver tests	Drug overdose is only a relative contraindication even if paracetamol
Pancreas	Diabetes mellitus, acute or chronic pancreatitis	Previous duodenal or pancreatic surgery	
Heart	Heart disease: valvular, ischemic, cardiomyopathy	Severe chest trauma, prolonged cardiac arrest, varying limits of MAP, CVP, PCWP, ejection fraction, ECG abnormalities	
Lung	History of chronic lung disease, tuberculosis significant acute lung disease, aspiration severe chest trauma or previous surgery	Smoking >20 pack-years, minor opacities on radiography, Pao_2 <300 mm Hg at Fio_2 = 1 and PEEP = 5 mm Hg, positive sputum culture (even yeasts), purulent secretions	Judge both lungs as two separate organs

SLE = systemic lupus erythematosus; CMV = cytomegalovirus; MAP = mean arterial pressure; CVP = central venous pressure; PCWP = pulmonary capillary wedge pressure; PEEP = positive end-expiratory pressure.
From: Lutz-Dettinger N, de Jaeger A, Kerremans I: Care of the potential pediatric organ donor. Pediatr Clin North Am 2001;48:715–49.

children may be an exception). Many children awaiting solid organ transplantation are in a deteriorating state. Pretransplant treatment of the unstable potential recipient is just as important as postoperative care.

Complications of Bone Marrow Transplantation (BMT). Ten to 15 per cent of children having BMT require a PICU because of life-threatening complications, especially those that occur in the first 40 days after transplantation. Complications include significant fluid and electrolyte problems, infections, signs of hemodynamic instability, renal failure, airway obstruction, or progressive respiratory failure. Patients requiring mechanical ventilation after BMT have a very high mortality. Early institution of hemofiltrations may improve outcomes.

Acute *graft versus host disease* (GVHD) may present as cholestasis, erythematous maculopapular rash, and diarrhea requiring PICU management (see Chapter 127). Chronic GVHD often follows acute GVHD.

Veno-occlusive disease, a thrombotic disorder producing clots in the small hepatic venules, is the third most frequent complication of BMT and occurs most often in patients undergoing BMT for malignancy. These patients may have severe hepatic dysfunction, resulting in ascites, respiratory distress, and other evidence of organ failure that may require aggressive treatment, including fluid therapy, anticoagulation, and sometimes thrombolytic agents or procedures.

Infections are of major concern because these children are both immunologically suppressed and neutropenic. Patients should be placed in protective isolation to limit infectious exposures. Opportunistic infections are discussed in Chapter 164. Seizures, encephalopathy, and psychiatric disturbances associated with infections or drug toxicity require aggressive diagnostic and therapeutic interventions.

Thrombocytopenia may result in bleeding from the respiratory and gastrointestinal tract. Efforts are directed at maintaining platelet counts greater than 50,000 when bleeding is present. Children may require nasal packing for severe nosebleeds. Clotting factors may be required if a coagulopathy is present; this is a high risk in children having veno-occlusive disease. Patients also require red blood cell transfusions for a low hematocrit due to bleeding and the inability to produce red blood cells before marrow engraftment.

Oncologists and intensivists need to confer on all BMT recipients in the PICU, to assist the family and the care team in understanding the realistic prospects for success with continued treatment. The PICU staff, in turn, must understand that BMT recipients can become very ill from the immunosuppressive therapy and numerous complications but can still recover. Children with oncologic diseases and their families have typically lived with the disease for months or even years and are prepared for a protracted struggle against complications of their transplants. However, they need to have realistic expectations about the treatment of BMT complications. Frequent care conferences, involving oncologists, intensivists, primary care pediatrician, and family, are often necessary to provide optimal care in these complicated cases.

Heart Transplantation (see Chapter 435.1). Most potential pediatric heart transplant patients are transferred to a PICU before transplant to receive inotropic agents (dobutamine), chronotropic agents (isoproterenol), and afterload-reducing agents (milrinone, dobutamine) aimed at maximizing cardiac output. After transplant, they are admitted to the PICU for close postoperative management and weaning from pressors, intravascular monitors, and respiratory support. Early post-transplant complications include hyperacute rejection, acute rejection, bradycardia, and dysrhythmias. Later, rejection may still occur, along with various infections, accelerated coronary artery atherosclerotic disease (manifest by ischemia, dysrhythmias, heart failure), and lymphoproliferative malignancies secondary to immune sup-

pression. If the transplanted heart begins to fail, vasoreactive agents, extracorporeal membrane oxygenation, or ventricular assist devices may be necessary, and, as a last resort, re-transplantation may be required (most centers place patients with failing recently transplanted organs at the top of their transplant lists). Rejection is confirmed by transcatheter myocardial biopsy.

Lung Transplantation (see Chapter 435.2). Children with cystic fibrosis, primary pulmonary hypertension, and α_1-antitrypsin deficiency are among the primary candidates for pediatric lung transplantation. Recipients about to undergo lung transplantation may need to be placed on cardiopulmonary bypass if they cannot sustain adequate ventilation and oxygenation on only one lung. Hyperacute and acute rejection may occur with lung transplants as with other organs. More than half of all recipients experience some degree of rejection in the first 3 mo after transplant. Transbronchial biopsy may confirm the diagnosis. Bronchial and/or tracheal anastomosis dehiscence is a problem. Infection remains a serious threat, and prophylactic treatment with trimethoprim-sulfamethoxazole (for *Pneumocystis carinii*), fluconazole (for fungus), and ganciclovir (for cytomegalovirus [CMV]) are used by some centers. Bronchiolitis obliterans occurs in 25–50% of survivors and is diagnosed with lung biopsies and treated with pulse steroids and other immunosuppressive agents (see Chapter 378). It may require re-transplant.

Heart-Lung Transplantation (see Chapter 435.2). Postoperatively, these children require mechanical ventilation with the minimum possible intra-airway pressures, because high pressures increase stress on the tracheal suture lines. Fiberoptic bronchoscopies may be needed to clear potential obstructions. For 2–3 wk the denervated lung is sensitive to exogenous fluid overload and is prone to develop pulmonary edema. Rejection of the lung also may occur without evidence of cardiac rejection. This can be assessed with pulmonary function studies that demonstrate alterations in flow patterns, specifically FEF_{25-75}. Bronchoscopy with lavage and biopsies may also be useful in diagnosing rejection. Deaths in the perioperative period are often caused by uncontrollable hemorrhage.

Kidney Transplantation (see Chapter 528). The goal in the immediate postoperative period is to encourage graft organ function; in children, this is achieved by maintaining renal perfusion with high levels of preload fluids producing substantial urine output. Even in the youngest children, the goal is to produce several hundred milliliters of urine per hour. Fluid replacement usually consists of normal saline or another physiologic fluid. This not only encourages sufficient urine production but also helps reduce the risk of thrombi at the vascular suture lines. Urine and insensible losses are replaced, and electrolytes are monitored closely. Blood pressure is tolerated at levels 20–30% higher than normal, particularly if a small child has received a transplanted adult kidney. The large fluid infusions when associated with a capillary leak phenomenon can produce significant pulmonary edema and necessitate meticulous respiratory management.

Ultrasound and Doppler flow studies of the newly transplanted kidney are often performed to confirm proper renal blood flow and to evaluate potential obstructive problems related to the surgery. When oliguria occurs, additional fluid replacement is instituted, assuming that the cause of oliguria is intravascular depletion. If oliguria persists in the presence of adequate intravascular fluid, then a range of problems, from obstruction of the Foley catheter to kinking of the implanted ureter, must be considered. If no fluid or mechanical cause can be found, early rejection or acute tubular necrosis may be the problem. Diuretics may be helpful (a continuous furosemide drip is often effective), but if the problem persists, a graft biopsy may be indicated. Postoperative hypertension should not be treated with angiotensin-converting enzyme inhibitors, because their site of action (at the glomerular arterioles) may jeopardize glomerular perfusion. The treatment of rejection is discussed in Chapter 528.

Liver Transplantation (see Chapter 349). The most common indication for liver transplantation is biliary atresia. Additional indications include other congenital causes of cirrhosis, several inborn errors of metabolism (tyrosinemia, Wilson disease), toxic ingestions (acetaminophen overdose, mushroom poisoning), various forms of acute and chronic hepatitis, certain isolated non-metastatic liver malignancies, and liver trauma. Management of transplantation and immunotherapy are discussed in Chapter 349.

Hepatic failure results in various life-threatening conditions, including acidosis, coagulopathy, hyperammonemia and hepatic coma, hypoalbuminemia and anasarca, and portal hypertension with varices. Hyperammonemic hepatic coma may accelerate the consideration of transplant because it produces unconsciousness and apnea. Children having fulminant hepatic failure should be in a PICU at a liver transplant center for rapid evaluation and transplantation.

The liver graft is subject to an array of potential problems after transplantation. Hyperacute graft rejection is very rare but may occur within minutes of revascularization of a transplanted organ. The organ must be removed and replaced. Acute rejection can occur within the first 5–7 days after transplant and is manifested by rising levels of liver enzymes, worsening coagulopathy, and hepatic encephalopathy. It can be treated with high doses of steroids, increased doses of cyclosporine, or tacrolimus and, if these fail, antithymocyte antibody preparations. Vascular anastomosis breakdown produces hemorrhage and requires surgical re-exploration. Thrombus formation deprives the liver of blood flow and also requires surgery. Hematobilia may require surgical exploration. Intestinal perforations may occur and can be detected by observation of free air in the abdomen. Various abscesses and other fluid accumulations may need surgical exploration. Nonsurgical problems include hypertension (from fluid overload, steroid treatment, cyclosporine); pulmonary edema secondary to fluid overload; effusions; phrenic nerve injury producing basilar atelectasis; seizures; and coagulopathy. Extensive blood product administration may lead to metabolic alkalosis (from the citrate in blood products). Various electrolyte disturbances are possible and require monitoring of electrolytes. The kidney may manifest a mild form of acute tubular necrosis resulting from necessary intraoperative occlusion of the inferior vena cava.

At the time of transplantation, children typically receive corticosteroids and either cyclosporine or tacrolimus. In some cases, small doses of antithymocyte globulin (ATG) or OKT3 are given as well. The early phase of immunosuppression extends for 2–3 wk postoperatively, and most patients continue lifelong small doses of steroids. Patients are also usually treated with antifungal (nystatin, fluconazole), anti-CMV (ganciclovir), and anti-*Pneumocystis* (trimethoprim-sulfamethoxazole, pentamidine) prophylactic medications for a limited time after transplant.

Intestinal Multiorgan Transplantation. Pancreas, small bowel, liver, or various combinations of intestinal viscera transplantation are uncommon. These are experimental procedures for severe, intractable diseases unresponsive to any other form of therapy. In children, the most common reasons for considering intestinal viscera transplantation are short bowel syndrome caused by necrotizing enterocolitis, gastroschisis, volvulus, and intestinal atresias, with complete dependence on total parenteral nutrition.

Many postoperative risks are similar to those in other organ transplant operations. In addition, edema of intestinal tissues, and sometimes the inability to close the abdominal wall, may not allow rapid weaning from mechanical ventilation. Maintaining renal perfusion is critically important. Cleansing bowel preparations before surgery are advisable, as is postoperative treatment

with enteral amphotericin, gentamicin, and polymyxin for several weeks. A short course of ganciclovir (for CMV prophylaxis) is usually also given, and patients may require prophylactic therapy with trimethoprim-sulfamethoxazole for life. Re-introduction of enteral feeding must be done very gradually, while continuing parenteral nutrition. Bowel transplants also should be assessed carefully for the signs and symptoms of bowel dysfunction: obstruction, abdominal tenderness, emesis, diarrhea, and melena. Endoscopic monitoring of the intestinal mucosa and monitoring fluid losses from ileostomy or colostomy sites are essential.

In the postoperative period, usually at the time of reperfusion of the implanted organs, steroids and tacrolimus or acyclovir are administered. Azathioprine may also be added. Prostaglandin E_1 is generally administered for 5–7 days to discourage the formation of clots in the microvasculature of the intestines and to dilate these vascular beds. Graft rejection usually results in fever, pain, distention, emesis, and increased stoma output. Severe rejection can lead to acute ulceration, perforation, and hemorrhage. Any evidence of biliary leakage or obstruction should be pursued vigorously. Vascular problems include microvascular thrombi and breakdown or large clots in vascular anastomoses. The risk of post-transplant infection and lymphoproliferative disease is greater than in other solid organ transplants.

Post-transplant Lymphoproliferative Disorders (PTLD). PTLD involves the unregulated growth of lymphoid tissue, which may occur at sites where lymph nodes are ordinarily found or where nodes do not usually occur. The growing tissue may obstruct nearby structures and produce various symptoms. Stridor or wheezing can result from airway obstruction from the proliferation of mediastinal lymph nodes, adenoidal hypertrophy, or hypertrophy of the glottic structures. Dysphagia can occur when the gastric lymph nodes enlarge around the gastroesophageal junction. A bowel obstruction can occur if mesenteric lymph nodes enlarge and compress the bowel. In addition, PTLD may result in perforation of a hollow viscus, resulting in peritonitis and free air within the abdomen. The diagnosis may require endoscopy or surgical exploration to obtain tissue or relieve an obstruction. Treatment of PTLD involves reduction of immunosuppressive therapy. Adoptive immunotherapy against EBV may have value. Rarely, chemotherapeutic agents used in the treatment of lymphomas unassociated with transplantation are required (see Chapter 488).

Bernstein D, Starnes VA, Baum D: Pediatric heart transplantation. *Adv Pediatr* 1990;37:413–39.

Horak DA, Forman SJ: Critical care of the hematopoietic stem cell patient. *Crit Care Clin* 2001;17:671–76.

Kaufmann SS: Small bowel transplantation: Selection criteria, operative techniques, advances in specific immunosuppression, prognosis. *Curr Opin Pediatr* 2001;13:425–28.

Klingemann HG: Mechanical ventilation for bone marrow transplant patients: When does it become futile? *Crit Care Med* 2000;28:899–900.

Lutz-Dettinger N, de Jaeger A, Kerremans I: Care of the potential pediatric organ donor. *Pediatr Clin North Am* 2001;48:715–49.

Malago M, Rogiers X, Broelsch CE: Liver splitting and liver donor techniques. *Br Med Bull* 1998;53:860–67.

Millan WIT, Sarwal MM, Lemley KV, et al: A 100% 2-year graft survival can be attained in high-risk 15 kg or smaller infant recipients of kidney allografts. *Arch Surg* 2000;135:1063–68; discussion 1068–69.

Neumann M: Evaluation of the pediatric renal transplant recipient. *ANNA J* 1997; 24:515–23.

Patterson GA: Indications: Unilateral, bilateral, heart-lung, and lobar transplant procedures. *Clin Chest Med* 1997;18:225–30.

Salvatierra O Jr: Pediatric renal transplantation. *Transplant Proc* 2000;32: 634–35.

Shah V, Friedman AL, Navarro VJ: Immunology of liver transplantation: Clinical management aspects. *Gastroenterologist* 1997;5:137–47.

Spray TL: Transplantation of the heart and lungs in children. *Annu Rev Med* 1994;45:139–48.

Stokes DC: Pulmonary complications of tissue transplantation in children. *Curr Opin Pediatr* 1994;6:272–79.

Chapter 61
Drowning and Near-Drowning *Harry J. Kallas*

Childhood submersion is a common cause of injury and fatality. After submersion in a liquid medium, suffocation and asphyxia may occur, with or without pulmonary aspiration. Within a few minutes, hypoxia and ischemia can rapidly lead to irreversible multisystem injury and often to death. Treatment in the pediatric intensive care unit (PICU) has reduced mortality from the cardiorespiratory consequences of submersion events; however, neurologic injury from hypoxemia and ischemia is the primary cause of mortality and long-term morbidity.

Death within 24 hr of a submersion is termed *drowning,* which may be immediate or may follow resuscitation. Survival after more than 24 hr is termed *near-drowning,* regardless of whether the victim later dies or recovers. These definitions are somewhat arbitrary but are still widely used; there is no consensus on alternate nomenclature for submersion events.

Epidemiology. Worldwide, it is estimated that 500,000 persons drown each year (approximately 1 person every min); the actual incidence is unknown, because many drowning deaths are not reported. The World Health Organization estimated the 1998 worldwide drowning mortality rate to be 8.4/100,000. As a cause of death globally, drowning ranked 11th for children younger than 5 yr old and 4th for children aged 5–14 yr.

Drowning is a major cause of injury death for children. Children younger than 5 yr old account for nearly 40% of all drowning fatalities. In 1–4 yr old children, drowning is the second leading cause of injury death in the United States and Africa and the leading cause in Australia and several U.S. states (Arizona, California, Florida, and Texas).

Fatality statistics convey only part of the problem, because many submersion victims are resuscitated and survive with neurologic sequelae. There are an estimated 500,000 significant submersions in the United States each year; 50,000 of these will require medical intervention. As many as 50% of all submersion victims are declared dead at the scene and never present to medical facilities for care. Estimates of cumulative risk for males from birth to 19 yr of age indicate that 1/1,098 will drown, 1/301 will be hospitalized for near-drowning, and 1/75 will be treated or observed in an emergency department (ED); comparable risk estimates for females are 1/3,333, 1/913, and 1/228, respectively. Among children younger than 5 yr old, for every pediatric drowning victim there are 14.6 children hospitalized or seen in the ED with near-drowning. For California children (1994), there were 32.8 fatalities for every 100 hospitalized survivors of near-drowning. Of pediatric near-drowning victims treated at a tertiary care facility, 5–12% will survive with profound neurologic damage.

Risk factors for drowning include age, gender, and race. Drowning rates are highest in children younger than 5 yr old and second highest in 15–19 yr olds (predominantly adolescent males). In the United States (1995), 5% of children who drowned were younger than 1 yr old, 37% were 1–4 yr old, 15% were 5–9 yr old, 15% were 10–14 yr old, and 29% were 15–19 yr old. Male drowning victims predominate in all ages, accounting for 74% of drowning deaths; the male:female ratio increases dramatically from 2:1 in toddlers to over 10:1 in teenagers. In the United States, black children have almost double the overall drowning rate of white children. In Cape Town, South Africa, black children have triple the drowning rate of white children. For children older than age 5 yr in the United States, the relative risk of drowning in a swimming pool is 4- to 15-fold greater for black compared with white males and 3- to 10-fold greater for black versus white females.

The proportion of drowning at various sites is greatly influenced by the accessibility to various bodies of water, socioeconomic status, and geographic area. Any body of water can pose a hazard to the child; young children have drowned in a few centimeters of water, owing to their limited developmental abilities. In the United States (1995), 32% of all childhood drowning occurred in artificial pools, 9% occurred at domestic sites (mostly bathtubs), 47% occurred in natural freshwater (mostly rivers and lakes), and 4% occurred in saltwater. Almost 40% of drowning deaths happen during swimming.

The most common site of drowning varies depending on age. In the United States (1995), children younger than 1 yr old who drowned did so mostly in domestic sites (78%), predominantly in the bathtub, and fewer in artificial pools (14%). In drowning victims 1–4 yr old, 55% drowned in artificial pools and 26% died at natural freshwater sites. In most industrialized countries reporting drowning statistics, the swimming pool is the most common drowning site for young children. For U.S. children 5–9 yr old who drowned, 54% died in freshwater and 31% in artificial pools. In young adolescents (10–14 yr old) who drowned, 61% died in freshwater and 21% died in artificial pools. Older teenagers (15–19 yr old) drowned predominantly in freshwater sites (69%) and less commonly in artificial pools (12%) or saltwater (10%).

In warmer climates of the United States, Australia, and South Africa, 50–90% of drowning deaths occur in residential swimming pools; this site accounts for almost 90% of submersion events in children younger than 5 yr old. The U.S. Consumer Product Safety Commission estimated that 3,000 children younger than 5 yr old are seen annually in the ED after submersion in residential pools; up to 80% of these children are hospitalized for at least 1 day. Most pool submersion events occur at the child's own home, and nearly half occur within the first 6 mo of pool exposure. Brief lapses (<5 min) in supervision are associated with most submersion events.

In the United States, more than half of unintentional infant drowning occurs in the bathtub. Of all bathtub drowning, approximately 86% occur in children 7–15 mo old. After the first year of life, bathtub drowning becomes progressively less common (<10%). Often, these infants have inadequate supervision and parents who overestimate their child's abilities or coordination. In Japan, where bathtubs are commonly left filled with water, half of all drowning occurs in the bathtub, and this is the most common drowning site for children younger than 4 yr old.

Hot tubs and spas also pose special hazards, because many have suction devices that can entrap hair, clothing, or body parts, preventing children from surfacing. Brief lapses in supervision are noted in most circumstances; however, drowning from entrapment may occur even when the parents are present and directly supervising the child. Children younger than 2 yr old are the most frequent victims.

Children may also drown in buckets, toilets, washing machines, sinks, and other common house areas containing water. Young children fall headfirst into these water containers and may not be able to extricate themselves because of their relatively cephalad center of gravity and/or insufficient body mass to tip it over. Bucket drowning is common, constituting up to 24% of all toddler drowning in some regions; mortality is high, in part because of cleaning fluids and other caustic substances that buckets may contain.

In older children and teenagers, as much as 70% of drowning occurs in open bodies of water, such as lakes, ponds, streams, ocean beaches, or irrigation ditches, usually where little or no adult supervision exists. The U.S. Lifesaving Association reported 62,747 rescues on U.S. beaches in 1996; there was approximately an 8:1 ratio of near-drowning rescues to drowning deaths. One fifth of open-water drowning events involve boats or other watercraft, and over 50% are associated with alcohol or drug use.

The risk of drowning is increased by the use of alcohol or illicit drugs. Alcohol clouds judgment, increasing the likelihood of injudicious risk-taking behavior, and retards motor coordination. Intoxicated adults are also incapable of providing adequate supervision for younger children near water. In a U.S. survey, 70% of males and 66% of females reported using alcohol during the preceding year while participating in aquatic activities; the largest group of positive respondents was 16–20 yr old. Positive blood alcohol levels are found in 10–50% of adolescent drowning victims.

Concomitant medical conditions may also increase the likelihood of drowning. Children with epilepsy have a 4- to 13-fold increased risk of drowning or near-drowning compared with nonepileptic children. Indeed, drowning is the most likely cause of unintentional injury death in this population. Epilepsy-associated drowning occurs predominately in bathtubs or swimming pools (86%); the majority of cases are in children older than age 5 yr. In nonepileptic children, other mental or motor disabilities may also increase drowning risk.

Child abuse or homicide by submersion does occur and requires a careful history, a high index of suspicion, and an understanding of normal childhood developmental capabilities. Child abuse or neglect may be a factor in 5–19% of submersions in children 1–4 yr of age and in 10–67% of bathtub-related events. Approximately 1 in 30 child homicides is by intentional drowning, mostly in the bathtub; 85% of intentional bathtub drowning involves children 15–30 mo old. Compared with unintentional injuries, victims of abuse are less likely to have resuscitation attempted by bystanders and are more likely to die.

Pathophysiology. It is a common misconception that the submersion victim will signal their distress or call for help. In truth, most pediatric victims drown silently. Studies indicate that young children can only struggle for 10–20 sec before a final submersion event occurs. Indeed, the efforts of a drowning victim to breathe or their splashing may be misconstrued by nearby persons as mere "playing" in the water.

Once submersion occurs, all organs and tissues are at risk for hypoxia. In a short period, hypoxia can lead to cardiac arrest, adding ischemia to the succession of hypoxia-associated injury. The combination of hypoxia and ischemia is a common injury mechanism associated with submersion events, with the severity of injury dependent on the duration. Pulmonary aspiration can further exacerbate hypoxia and subsequent respiratory failure. Some victims may develop hypothermia, which is usually detrimental if not rapidly corrected. In some cases, a fatal catecholamine-induced arrhythmia secondary to one form of the prolonged QT syndrome is responsible for the cardiac arrest and death. In these cases, death does not result from aspiration or suffocation (see Chapter 428.4).

ANOXIC-ISCHEMIC INJURY. After experimental submersion, a conscious animal will initially panic trying to surface. During this stage, small amounts of water enter the hypopharynx, triggering laryngospasm. Most animals struggle violently and swallow copious amounts of water. They soon lose consciousness from hypoxia. Vomiting may ensue, accompanied by involuntary gastric fluid aspiration. In about 10% of animals, the initial laryngospasm persists until death without aspiration into the lungs (aspiration is absent in 10–15% of humans who drown). Profound hypoxia and medullary depression lead to terminal apnea. During these events, cardiovascular changes include an initial tachycardia followed by severe hypertension with reflex bradycardia, presumably from intense catecholamine release; arrhythmias may be seen. By 3–4 min, the circulation abruptly fails as myocardial hypoxia supervenes. The heart may continue to have ineffective contractions or electrical activity for a short time, but there is no effective perfusion. The chance of successful resuscitation quickly becomes impossible as hypoxia and ischemia cause rapid, progressive, and irreversible injury.

The diving reflex may potentially enhance cerebral and myocardial blood flow when the face is submerged in very cold water (<20°C) and is believed by some to contribute to cerebral protection during submersion. Although this reflex is prominent in many sea mammals, it is relatively weak in humans. The extent of neurologic protection afforded humans by the diving reflex is controversial but is probably small.

All organs may be injured from hypoxia and ischemia, but the brain is exquisitely sensitive to hypoxic-ischemic injury. With intensive care, the cardiorespiratory consequences of resuscitated near-drowning are usually manageable and less often the cause of mortality compared with irreversible hypoxic-ischemic central nervous system (CNS) injury. CNS injury is the most frequent cause of mortality and long-term morbidity. Although the duration of anoxia before irreversible CNS injury occurs is uncertain, it is probably on the order of 3–5 min.

Myriad pathophysiologic events occur in the CNS as a result of hypoxemia and ischemia (see Chapter 57.7). The brain has minimal energy stores and requires constant delivery of oxygen and nutrients. After approximately 2 min of anoxia, adenosine triphosphate (ATP) is critically depleted. ATP is necessary to maintain neuronal metabolic functions and ionic gradients; its depletion is a likely trigger for a number of pathogenic cascades.

After cardiopulmonary arrest, cerebral blood flow (CBF) aberrations and impaired autoregulation may persist after resuscitation. After 15 min of global ischemia in dogs followed by the restoration of circulation, there initially is increased CBF (cerebral hyperemia) lasting 15–30 min, followed by delayed hypoperfusion lasting hours to days. This hypoperfusion may or may not be matched to cerebral metabolic demands. The uncoupling of CBF autoregulation to CNS metabolic demands increases the potential of further injury as cerebral metabolic rate of oxygen utilization returns to normal after the ischemic period while CBF remains low.

Secondary CNS injury during reperfusion occurs by various pathways. Injury is exacerbated by the release of glutamate and other "excitatory" amino acids. Glutamate is the predominant excitatory neurotransmitter of the brain and acts through specific receptors: the three principal ionophore-linked receptors are N-methyl-D-aspartate (NMDA), α-amino-3-hydroxy-5-methyl-4-isoxazol-eproprionic acid (AMPA), and kainate receptors. Activation of these receptors on neural cell membranes leads to an influx of calcium and sodium. Glutamate also acts on metabotropic receptors, which trigger secondary messenger systems and lead to release of calcium from intracellular stores. Increased intracellular calcium after hypoxia-ischemia is likely a final pathway toward irreversible cellular injury and death.

Alteration of calcium homeostasis can perpetuate numerous deleterious responses, including activation of phospholipases, proteases, endonucleases, protein kinases, and nitric oxide synthase, and the uncoupling of oxidative phosphorylation. Membrane phospholipid hydrolysis and the release of arachidonic acid metabolites contribute to oxygen free radical generation, the inflammatory response, and cellular damage. The brain is especially vulnerable to injury from free radicals, including superoxide, hydrogen peroxide, peroxynitrite, and nitric acid. Other important contributors to oxygen radical formation include cyclooxygenase, lipoxygenase, purine degradation, the electron transport chain, and inflammatory cells. Oxygen radicals produce cellular injury by various mechanisms, but most importantly lead to lipid peroxidation; the ensuing chain reaction produces more radicals, affects enzymatic function, compromises cell membrane integrity, interrupts DNA synthesis, and disrupts the blood-brain barrier. Additionally, the release of leukotrienes, tumor necrosis factor, metalloproteases, kinins, and other cytokines and mediators also injure the blood-brain barrier. The uncoupling of oxidative phosphorylation and the membrane disruption contribute to mitochondrial and cellular energy failure. A number of triggers for programmed cell death (apoptosis) are also activated, although its contribution to overall CNS injury after hypoxia-ischemia is still not clear.

After cardiopulmonary arrest, cerebral edema may occur. The mechanisms causing cerebral edema are not completely elucidated but are likely mostly due to swelling in astrocyte foot processes and, to a lesser degree, vasogenic edema from disruption of the blood-brain barrier. Astrocyte-mediated uptake of glutamate from the extracellular space appears to be coupled to sodium and water accumulation. Acidosis, potassium, and arachidonic acid also mediate astrocyte swelling. The traditional concept of "cytotoxic" cerebral edema due to cellular energy failure (the pump-leak model) is incomplete, although inability to maintain ionic gradients may still play some role in the production of cerebral edema. Severe cerebral edema can elevate intracranial pressure (ICP), contributing to further ischemia; however, the very presence of ICP is an ominous sign of profound CNS damage.

Hyperglycemia after hypoxia-ischemia may also exacerbate CNS injury. After near-drowning, children with initial serum glucose concentrations of more than 250 mg/dL are more likely to die or survive in a persistent vegetative state compared with normoglycemic victims. Brain-injured hyperglycemic rats have greater CNS damage than injured normoglycemic rats; correction of hyperglycemia with insulin improves CNS outcome to a level equivalent to injured normoglycemic controls. Hyperglycemic rats have significantly lower CNS levels of adenosine and its metabolites compared with normoglycemic animals. Adenosine, proposed to be an endogenous neuroprotecter, causes regional cerebral vasodilatation, inhibits excitotoxin release, decreases calcium conductance, and affects neutrophil-endothelial interactions. Control of hyperglycemia with insulin after near-drowning cannot yet be recommended in humans until clinical trials are performed. It seems prudent to avoid iatrogenic hyperglycemia or hypoglycemia.

Other organs and tissues may also be injured by hypoxia-ischemia. In the lung, damage to pulmonary vascular endothelium, increasing vascular permeability, can lead to acute respiratory distress syndrome (ARDS, see Chapter 58). Aspiration compounds pulmonary injury (see Chapter 380). Myocardial dysfunction, arterial hypotension, decreased cardiac output, arrhythmias, and cardiac infarction may also occur. Acute tubular necrosis or cortical necrosis are common renal complications of major hypoxic-ischemic events (see Chapter 57.5). Vascular endothelial injury can initiate disseminated intravascular coagulation (DIC, see Chapter 474), hemolysis, and thrombocytopenia. Many factors contribute to gastrointestinal damage, including hypoxia-ischemia, hypothermia, catecholamine infusions, and perhaps the diving reflex; a bloody diarrhea with mucosal sloughing may be seen after severe hypoxic-ischemic events and often portends a fatal injury. Levels of hepatic transaminases and serum pancreatic enzymes are often acutely elevated. Violation of normal mucosal protective barriers predisposes the victim to bacteremia and sepsis.

ASPIRATION AND PULMONARY INJURY. Pulmonary aspiration occurs in the great majority of drowning and near-drowning victims, but the amount aspirated is usually small. Nonaspirating victims may acutely succumb from laryngospasm and the consequences of hypoxia. The amount and composition of the aspirated material can affect the patient's clinical course: gastric contents, water salinity, pathogenic organisms, toxic chemicals, and other foreign matter can injure the lung or cause airway obstruction. A few children may have massive aspiration, increasing the likelihood of severe pulmonary dysfunction.

Clinical management is not significantly different in seawater or freshwater aspiration. Seawater is hypertonic (approximately

3% normal saline), establishing an osmotic gradient drawing interstitial and intravascular fluid into the alveoli; furthermore, seawater inactivates surfactant, increasing alveolar surface tension, making the alveolus unstable and prone to atelectasis. On the other hand, hypotonic freshwater aspiration washes out surfactant, also causing alveolar instability and collapse. In either case, hypoxemia and pulmonary insufficiency result from ventilation-perfusion mismatch, increased intrapulmonary shunting, decreased lung compliance, and increased small airway resistance. Profound hypoxia in experimental animals may be seen within 3 min after the aspiration of as little as 2.2 mL/kg. In humans as well, the aspiration of 1–3 mL/kg can lead to marked hypoxemia and a 10–40% reduction in lung compliance.

Pulmonary edema or ARDS may develop from aspiration of liquid or foreign material, hypoxia-ischemia, or marked hypothermia. In some cases, pulmonary edema may be cardiogenic (due to severely impaired myocardial function) or, uncommonly, neurogenic. Pneumonia may result from aspirated contaminated material. Gastric acid or caustic agent aspiration can directly injure the lung without infection being present. Ventilator-associated lung injury (see Chapter 57.4) can also occur with excessive tidal volumes or pressures or prolonged exposure to high concentrations of oxygen.

FLUID AND ELECTROLYTE ALTERATIONS. The great majority of submersion victims do not aspirate large enough volumes of fluid to result in significant electrolyte disturbances. Many do swallow copious amounts of fluid, but even this does not appear to lead to a significant incidence of clinically relevant fluid or electrolyte aberrations. Children who survive long enough to be seen in the ED rarely have electrolyte aberrations requiring therapy.

Rarely, massive seawater ingestion or aspiration can lead to hypernatremia and fluid shifts because of its high sodium concentration and osmolarity. As fluid is osmotically drawn into the lungs or gastrointestinal tract, hemoconcentration may be observed. However, hypernatremia and hemoconcentration due to hyposmolar diuresis also occurs in diabetes insipidus (see Chapter 552), usually a sign of profound CNS injury after hypoxic-ischemic events.

Seldom, water intoxication can occur with massive freshwater aspiration or ingestion, causing hyponatremia and hemodilution. Sudden hyposmolarity can result in red blood cell swelling and hemolysis, hypothetically leading to hemoglobinuria with renal tubular damage and hyperkalemia with subsequent VF. Plasma-free hemoglobin levels in human near-drowning are typically less than 500 mg/dL, usually insufficient to cause renal dysfunction from this mechanism alone. Alternatively, free water overload may be seen with excess antidiuretic hormone (SIADH), which can accompany pulmonary or brain injury (see Chapter 553.1). Excess free water can also increase cerebral edema and ICP.

HYPOTHERMIA (see Chapter 63). Hypothermia (core temperature of less than 35°C) is common after submersion. Children are at increased risk of developing hypothermia owing to their relatively high body surface area to mass ratio, decreased subcutaneous fat, and limited thermogenic capacity. Hypothermia can develop as a result of prolonged surface contact with cold water and potentially after swallowing or aspirating large quantities of very cold fluid. Further drops in body temperature occur after the child is removed from the water as a result of cold air, wet clothes, hypoxia, and hospital transport.

Compensatory mechanisms will usually attempt to restore normothermia at body temperatures above 32°C; below this temperature, thermoregulation fails and spontaneous rewarming will not occur. Moderate hypothermia (core temperature 32–35°C) increases oxygen consumption owing to shivering thermogenesis and increased sympathetic tone. Below 32°C (severe hypothermia), shivering ceases and the cellular metabolic rate decreases approximately 7% per °C in the absence of active thermogenesis.

With moderate to severe hypothermia, progressive bradycardia, impaired myocardial contractility, and loss of vasomotor tone contribute to inadequate perfusion, hypotension, and possible shock. Below 28°C, extreme bradycardia is usually present and the propensity for spontaneous VF or asystole is high. Central respiratory center depression with moderate to severe hypothermia results in hypoventilation and eventual apnea. Deep coma with fixed and dilated pupils and absent reflexes at very low body temperatures (<25–29°C) may give the false appearance of death.

Depending on the duration and severity of the temperature aberration, other systemic adverse consequences of hypothermia may occur acutely and persist even after rewarming. ARDS secondary to hypothermia can be seen in the absence of submersion or aspiration. Depressed hepatorenal metabolism and perfusion reduce drug clearance. Either hypoglycemia from glycogen store exhaustion or hyperglycemia due to catecholamines, altered pancreatic insulin release, and depressed peripheral glucose utilization may be observed. Thrombocytopenia, platelet dysfunction, and DIC also occur. Although hypothermia slows bacterial replication, it also renders the host more susceptible to bacterial and fungal invasion and sepsis by impairing neutrophil and reticuloendothelial function. Hypothermia must be expediently corrected to minimize such adverse consequences.

During initial rewarming efforts, core body temperature may initially decline. This *afterdrop* may occur secondary to the return of colder blood from the extremities to the relatively warmer central core or by the conduction of heat from the warmer core to cooler surface layers. In patients with severe hypothermia, afterdrop may further compromise cardiac, respiratory, or neurologic function or induce arrhythmias. Afterdrop in moderate to severely hypothermic victims may be mitigated if rewarming measures are not applied to the extremities, focusing efforts instead on core rewarming.

Rewarming shock may be observed after rescue. When subjected to the additional metabolic requirements of increasing body temperature and the vasodilatation accompanying surface rewarming, victims with borderline myocardial function may not be able to meet the increased physiologic demands. Hypotension, metabolic acidosis, tissue ischemia, and other consequences of shock (see Chapter 57.2) may therefore be exacerbated during rewarming.

Controversial Issues Related to Hypothermia. The implications and consequences of moderate to severe hypothermia in near-drowning victims are controversial. Misconceptions are fueled by a few case reports of dramatic neurologic recovery after prolonged (10–150 min) icy water submersion. There should be a clear distinction between "cold" and "ice" water. The rare survivor of a prolonged submersion typically has been in freezing water (<5°C) and has a core body temperature less than 30°C (usually much lower). Although hypothermia may confer a degree of cerebral protection from hypoxic-ischemic injury in controlled clinical situations (e.g., the operating room) and in rare individual near-drowning victims, many studies indicate that hypothermia is often a poor prognostic sign.

For hypothermia to be protective, core body temperature must fall extremely rapidly, decreasing cellular metabolic rate before hypoxia-ischemia leads to irreversible injury. Hypothermia has been shown to be effective in protecting the brain and other organs from hypoxia-ischemia for 75–110 min in controlled circumstances in which core body temperature is first cooled to 18°C and then the heart is stopped. However, once processes leading to cell death from hypoxia-ischemia have begun (starting at about 5–6 min), hypothermia does not confer a protective effect or improve recovery.

Surface cooling alone is unlikely to decrease body temperature fast enough to afford neuroprotection. The cooling rate of near-drowning victims is difficult to estimate, because, in addition to surface cooling, victims may swallow or aspirate water. Surface cooling of anesthetized infants with ice packs and ice water decreases rectal temperature by as little as 2.5°C in the first 10 min; it takes a further 32 min for the temperature to fall to 24–26°C. Therefore, hypothermia involving surface cooling would seem to require that prolonged submersion occur in icy water and that the victim continue breathing with the head above water as body temperature gradually cools. This situation is not commonly witnessed.

The hypothesis that the aspiration of icy water accelerates cooling is controversial. Most animals and human submersion victims in warm or cold water drowning aspirate very little. Theoretically, for sufficiently rapid neuroprotective-level hypothermia to develop, a very large quantity of icy water would have to be aspirated or swallowed, or the victim would have to rebreathe a smaller quantity of water for a period of time. In human adults and animals, immersion in icy water results in intense involuntary reflex hyperventilation and a decreased breath-holding ability to less than 10 sec. Thus, it may be that victims of ice-water submersions are more likely to have involuntary respiration and a greater likelihood of aspiration or fluid rebreathing. In such a case, it may be possible for the brain to rapidly cool to a protective level (<30°C) provided that the water aspirated is icy and cardiac output lasts long enough for sufficient heat exchange to occur. Whether this scenario actually occurs is not known.

Hypothermia in non–icy water near-drowning is most commonly an unfavorable prognostic sign. In King County, Washington, where the water is cold but rarely icy, hypothermic protection has not been observed: 92% of survivors with good neurologic outcomes had initial temperatures greater than 34°C, whereas 61% of those who died or had severe neurologic injury had temperatures less than 34°C. Similarly, in Finland where the median water temperature was 16°C, a beneficial effect of hypothermia could not be proved in pediatric submersion victims; submersion duration less than 10 min was most related to good outcome.

Clinical Manifestations and Treatment. A submersion victim's clinical course and outcome are primarily determined by the circumstances of the incident, the duration of submersion, the speed of the rescue, and the effectiveness of resuscitative efforts. Two groups may be identified based on responsiveness at the scene. Children who require minimal amounts of resuscitation at the scene commonly have good outcomes and experience a low incidence of complications. These victims quickly regain spontaneous respiration and typically regain consciousness rapidly. They should be transported to the ED for further evaluation.

Victims in cardiac arrest require aggressive or prolonged resuscitation and have a high risk of multiorgan system complications, major neurologic morbidity, or death. Initial management requires coordinated and experienced prehospital care following the "ABCs" of emergency resuscitation (see Chapter 51). These children often remain comatose and lack brainstem reflexes despite the restoration of oxygenation and circulation. Subsequent ED and PICU care often involves advanced life support strategies and management of multiorgan dysfunction.

INITIAL EVALUATION AND RESUSCITATION (see Chapter 57.1). Once a submersion has occurred, extrication and immediate institution of cardiopulmonary resuscitative efforts at the scene are imperative. Every minute that passes without the re-establishment of adequate breathing and circulation dramatically decreases the possibility of a good outcome. In near-drowning victims with cardiac arrest who receive prehospital CPR, only 7–21% will have neurologically intact survival. Children with good outcomes are almost five times as likely to have had immediate scene resuscitation compared with children with poor outcomes, although this is not demonstrated in all series. Waiting for the arrival of paramedics should not delay bystander resuscitative efforts; even in a model prehospital system, the arrival of paramedics takes longer than 10 min in 91% of submersion cases.

Initial resuscitation must focus on rapidly restoring oxygenation, ventilation, and adequate circulation. The airway should be clear of vomitus or foreign material, which may result in obstruction or aspiration. Abdominal thrusts should not be used for lung fluid removal, as their effectiveness is not established; because many victims have a distended abdomen from swallowed water, abdominal thrusts may increase the risk of regurgitation and aspiration. In cases of suspected airway foreign body, chest compressions or back blows are preferable maneuvers.

The cervical spine should be protected in anyone with potential neck injury (see Chapter 57.8), such as in child abuse, water sport accidents, diving injury, or unknown circumstances surrounding the immersion. The neck should be in a neutral position and protected with a well-fitting cervical collar. Fortunately, neck injuries in submersion victims are uncommon. Approximately 0.5% of submersion victims have cervical-spine injuries. Victims with spine injuries have a history of diving, motorized vehicle crash, fall from height, or submersion in open bodies of water and clinical signs of serious injury. Spinal injuries are exceedingly rare in low-impact submersions.

If the victim has ineffective respiration or apnea, ventilatory support must be initiated immediately (see Chapter 57.1). Mouth-to-mouth or mouth-to-nose breathing by trained bystanders often restores spontaneous ventilation. As soon as it is available, supplemental oxygen should be administered to all victims. Positive pressure bag-mask ventilation with high inspired oxygen concentration should be instituted in patients with respiratory insufficiency.

Gastric distention is often exacerbated by mouth-to-mouth or bag-mask ventilation. Vomiting is seen in 25–75% of victims during resuscitation, and nearly 25% aspirate their gastric contents. Cricoid pressure (the Sellick maneuver) during positive pressure breathing and early nasogastric decompression may decrease the risk of vomiting and aspiration (see Chapter 57.1).

If apnea, cyanosis, hypoventilation, or labored respiration persists, trained personnel should perform endotracheal tube (ETT) intubation as soon as possible. Intubation is also indicated to protect the airway in patients with depressed mental status or hemodynamic instability. Hypoxia must be corrected to optimize the chances of recovery. Oxygen alone may not correct hypoxia in patients with significant pulmonary edema or aspiration; in such cases, the application of positive end-expiratory pressure (PEEP) is necessary to decrease intrapulmonary shunt and improve oxygenation. The routine use of PEEP in near-drowning has made early death from pulmonary insufficiency uncommon. Initial PEEP should be about 5 cm H_2O; it can be increased incrementally up to 10–15 cm H_2O if oxygenation remains inadequate (goal $SaO_2 > 90\%$). During bag-ETT ventilation, PEEP can be maintained by using an adjustable PEEP valve. Tidal volume and breath frequency should initially attempt to achieve normal ventilation without contributing to lung injury. Attempts to acutely or aggressively hyperventilate victims may be harmful.

Concurrent with securing airway control, oxygenation, and ventilation, the child's cardiovascular status must be evaluated. Heart rate and rhythm, blood pressure, temperature, and end-organ perfusion require urgent assessment. CPR should be instituted immediately in pulseless, bradycardic, or severely hypotensive victims (see Chapter 57.1). ECG monitoring assists with the diagnosis and treatment of arrhythmias. Slow capillary refill, cool extremities, or altered mental status are potential indicators of shock (see Chapter 57.2). Core temperature must be evaluated, especially in children, because moderate to severe hypothermia can depress myocardial function and cause arrhythmias.

Often, intravenous fluids and cardioactive medications are required to improve circulation and perfusion (see Chapter 57.1). Venous access should be established as quickly as possible for the administration of fluids or pressors. In many cases, intraosseous catheter placement is a potentially lifesaving vascular access technique that avoids the delay usually associated with multiple attempts to establish intravenous access in critically ill children (see Chapter 57.1). Epinephrine is usually the initial drug of choice in victims with cardiopulmonary arrest (initial IV dose is 0.01 mg/kg of 1:10,000 solution; subsequent IV doses may be as high as 0.1 mg/kg of 1:1000 solution). Epinephrine can be given intratracheally (ETT dose is 0.1–0.2 mg/kg of 1:1,000 concentration) if no intravenous access is available. Bolus intravascular administration of lactated Ringer solution or normal saline is often used to augment preload.

In children with cardiac arrest after submersion, the first recorded rhythm is asystole in 55%, ventricular tachycardia (VT) or VF in 29%, and bradycardia in 16%. Electrical defibrillation or cardioversion is urgently necessary for children with VF or pulseless VT (see Chapter 57.1); other cardioactive medications may be necessary to restore a perfusing rhythm (see Chapter 57.1). Post-resuscitation catecholamine infusions may be required to augment myocardial function and support blood pressure (see Chapters 57.1 and 57.2).

Attention to hypothermia in the field is very important, both to initiate rewarming measures and to prevent the consequences of deeper hypothermia. A low recording thermometer and a high index of suspicion are required to diagnose hypothermia. Core temperature is best measured at the tympanic membrane; rectal temperature determinations are often inadequate, owing to insufficient thermometer insertion depth; oral and axillary temperature readings are unreliable. All hypothermic victims should have damp clothes removed, the skin dried, warm blankets applied, and a warm environmental temperature provided as soon as possible. If available, warmed intravenous fluids (40–43°C) and humidified oxygen (42–46°C) should be used, although their rewarming efficacy is not well established. For victims not in cardiac arrest with core temperatures less than 34°C, external rewarming measures should be applied only to truncal areas, attempting to avoid afterdrop. In poorly perfused hypothermic victims, the application of warm packs and other cutaneous rewarming devices may cause significant burns. Patients with severe hypothermia (core temperature less than 30°C) require active internal warming measures provided as soon as possible (see Chapter 63).

Assessment of blood glucose should be obtained in the field. If a child is hypoglycemic, 0.5–1 g/kg dextrose should be administered as either 10% or 25% solution (maximum: 25 g/dose). In hyperglycemic victims, dextrose-containing solutions initially should be withheld but repeated assessments must be made to avoid unrecognized subsequent hypoglycemia. Although some preliminary data suggest that correction of hyperglycemia may improve outcome, the use of insulin cannot yet be generally recommended for correction of hyperglycemia after submersion injury.

Controversial Issues in the Resuscitation of Severely Hypothermic Victims. The cardiorespiratory management of patients with very severe hypothermia (temperature 28°C) is controversial. Ventricular arrhythmias have been temporally associated with ETT intubation or chest compressions in occasional reports of severely hypothermic patients. Therefore, some authors advocate withholding intubation or chest compressions if any respiratory activity or perfusing rhythm is present to avoid precipitating VF. In a prospective study of severely hypothermic victims, ventricular arrhythmia associated with ETT intubation was not observed. Therefore, gentle ETT placement should be performed in children with hypoxia or insufficient respiration.

No prospective studies are available to guide the clinician regarding chest compressions in severely hypothermic victims who are not in cardiac arrest. Some authors would withhold chest compressions if core temperature is less than 28°C and the electrocardiogram shows a perfusing rhythm with a pulse, regardless of heart rate or hypotension. The logic behind these recommendations follows from observations that effective perfusion often returns with rewarming; rewarming is more effective when any circulation is present; VF or asystole slows rewarming efforts; chest compressions may precipitate VF; cardiopulmonary resuscitation (CPR) is less effective during severe hypothermia. However, given the lack of clinical data, some practitioners would initiate CPR, attempting to thwart life-threatening compromises of cardiac output (see Chapter 63).

Full CPR with chest compressions is indicated for hypothermic victims if (1) narrow-complex QRS activity is absent on ECG or, (2) core temperature is unknown or more than 28°C (82.4°F), no ECG monitor is available, and a pulse cannot be found. When VF is present in severely hypothermic victims, up to three defibrillation attempts should initially be delivered; if defibrillation is unsuccessful, CPR should be reinstituted; some would minimize further defibrillation attempts until the child's temperature is more than 30°C (86°F), at which time successful defibrillation may be possible (see Figure 63-1).

Victims with profound hypothermia may appear clinically dead, but full neurologic recovery is possible, although rare. Attempts at lifesaving resuscitation should not be withheld based on initial clinical presentation unless the victim is obviously dead (e.g., dependent lividity or rigor mortis). Body temperature should be taken into account before resuscitative efforts are terminated. Rewarming efforts, in general, should be continued until temperature is at least 32–34°C (89.6–93.2°F); if the victim then continues to have no effective cardiac rhythm and remains unresponsive to aggressive CPR, resuscitative efforts may be discontinued.

Complete rewarming is not indicated for all arrest victims. Some children with severe hypothermia and the appearance of death are actually dead. In most situations, discontinuing resuscitative efforts in victims of non–icy water submersions who remain asystolic despite 30–45 min of aggressive advanced CPR is probably warranted. Physicians must use their individual clinical judgment when deciding to stop resuscitative efforts, taking into account the unique circumstances of each incident.

HOSPITAL-BASED EVALUATION AND TREATMENT. ED and hospital management of the submersion victim includes and extends the aforementioned resuscitative efforts. Again, patient acuity will determine the extent of further interventions. Some children will present to the ED alert and with minimal symptomatology. More ill children require hospitalization for ongoing evaluation and monitoring. Critically ill victims must be stabilized and admitted to a PICU.

All pediatric submersion victims probably should be hospitalized or observed for at least 8–12 hr, even if they are asymptomatic on presentation to the ED. At a minimum, serial monitoring of vital signs (respiratory rate, heart rate, blood pressure, and temperature); repeated careful pulmonary examination and neurologic assessment; chest radiography; and assessment of oxygenation by arterial blood gas or pulse oximetry should be performed on all submersion victims. Other studies may also be warranted depending on specific circumstances (e.g., possible traumatic injuries or suspected intoxication). Of initially asymptomatic children, almost half may become symptomatic, usually during the first 4–8 hr post-submersion. Mild to rarely severe delayed respiratory symptoms and pulmonary edema can occur even in children with initially normal chest examination and radiography. Among patients who do not require advanced life support in the prehospital setting or during their first 4 hr in the ED and have a Glasgow Coma Scale (GCS) score of 13 or greater on ED presentation, those who develop respiratory deterioration or oxygen desaturation are most likely to do so within 6 hr, if at all. Conversely, most children with minor early respiratory symptoms will become asymptomatic by 18 hr post-submersion. Usually, these children will have the return of normal room air oxygenation and pulmonary examination by 4–6 hr and are unlikely to have subsequent delayed respiratory deterioration. It appears that select low-risk patients who are alert and asymptomatic with normal examination and oxygenation may be considered for discharge after 8–12 hr of observation, as long as appropriate follow-up can be assured.

Respiratory Management. The level of respiratory support should be appropriate to the patient's condition and is a continuation of prehospital management. One must frequently reassess that adequate oxygenation, ventilation, and airway control are maintained. Supplemental oxygen should initially be provided to all victims. Increased inspired oxygen concentration (Fio_2) alone may not resolve hypoxia, and ETT intubation and PEEP are often needed. PEEP increases functional residual capacity, decreases intrapulmonary shunting, improves ventilation-perfusion matching, and may improve pulmonary compliance. The level of PEEP and Fio_2 should restore oxygenation, usually to a goal Sao_2 of more than 90%. Excessive PEEP can impair venous blood return and depress cardiac output. Prolonged use of high Fio_2 (>70–80%) may cause pulmonary oxygen toxicity. An arterial catheter is often required for reliable and frequent arterial blood gas assessment and continuous blood pressure monitoring in critically ill patients.

Unintubated alert children with mild to moderate hypoxemia despite supplemental oxygen who can protect their airway may be candidates for mask continuous positive airway pressure (CPAP) or bilevel positive airway pressure (BiPAP). These noninvasive measures can improve oxygenation and possibly avert ETT intubation. A nasogastric tube may be necessary to prevent gaseous gastric distention. Persistent hypoxemia, impaired ventilation, labored respiration, depressed mental status, or patient intolerance usually requires ETT intubation to secure the airway and breathing.

Hypercapnia should generally be avoided in potentially brain-injured children. Patients with actual or potential hypoventilation or marked elevated work of breathing should have assisted or controlled mechanical ventilation to avoid hypercapnia and decrease the energy expenditures of labored respiration. The usual initial ventilatory goal is a $Paco_2$ of 35–40 mm Hg. Excessive hyperventilation is not indicated; even moderate hyperventilation may potentially contribute to cerebral hypoperfusion.

Children with bronchospasm after near-drowning may benefit from β_2-agonist therapy; however, pulmonary edema or airway foreign body may also cause wheezing and should be considered. Bronchoscopy is indicated if a foreign body is suspected. The routine use of diuretics or corticosteroids for pulmonary edema or lung injury is not recommended. Prophylactic antibiotics are not generally helpful, except in cases where aspirate is known to be grossly contaminated.

ARDS is a serious complication in some submersion victims (see Chapter 58). ARDS can have detrimental effects on oxygenation and pulmonary compliance. Patients administered high airway pressures or tidal volumes during mechanical ventilation are also at increased risk for ventilator-induced lung injury. Studies indicate that the application of peak airway pressures greater than 30–35 cm H_2O may lead to alveolar overdistention and damage, exacerbating lung injury, and promoting pulmonary and systemic inflammatory responses. The use of lower tidal volumes and pressures is associated with decreased ARDS mortality. Patients with ARDS and brain injury pose a difficult challenge because permissive hypercapnia—a strategy commonly employed in ARDS—is normally contraindicated in patients with brain injury or intracranial hypertension. Sedation and, less often, neuromuscular blockade may be necessary to improve thoracic compliance, patient-ventilator synchrony, and gas exchange; these medications can obscure neurologic evaluation, making prognostication and decision-making more difficult.

Various modes of high-frequency ventilation have been successfully used in near-drowning victims failing conventional mechanical ventilation (see Chapter 57.4). In some cases, inhaled nitric oxide may help improve ventilation-perfusion matching and decrease pulmonary hypertension (see Chapter 57.4). Exogenous surfactant after near-drowning has been tried, but indications for its use and guidelines for effective delivery in this population do not exist. Partial liquid ventilation has been performed in individual near-drowning patients with ARDS (see Chapter 58). Extracorporeal life support (ECLS) in near-drowning has been reported; however, the general application of ECLS in submersion victims is controversial and should be limited until better selection criteria and more accurate predictors of neurologic outcome exist.

Cardiovascular Management. Cardiovascular stabilization is a continuation of measures instituted in the prehospital setting. Causes contributing to myocardial insufficiency include hypoxic-ischemic injury, ongoing hypoxia, hypothermia, acidosis, high airway pressures during mechanical ventilation, alterations of intravascular volume, and electrolyte disorders. Heart failure, shock, arrhythmias, or cardiac arrest may occur. Continuous ECG monitoring is mandatory to recognize and treat arrhythmias. Arterial catheterization facilitates continuous blood pressure and laboratory monitoring. Echocardiography, central venous pressure monitoring, or pulmonary artery catheter placement may aid assessment of intravascular volume status and myocardial function.

The provision of adequate oxygenation and ventilation is a prerequisite to improving myocardial function. Fluid resuscitation and inotropic agents are often necessary to improve heart function and restore tissue perfusion. Increasing preload with intravenous fluids may be beneficial by improving stroke volume and cardiac output. Overzealous fluid administration, especially in the presence of poor myocardial function, can worsen pulmonary edema. Epinephrine infusion (dose range: 0.05–1 µg/kg/min) is usually the drug of choice for patients with cardiac dysfunction or hypotension after hypoxic-ischemic events. Others suggest that dobutamine (dose range: 2–20 µg/kg/min) may better improve cardiac output in normotensive patients. Some patients may require other drugs depending on specifics of their cardiovascular dysfunction (see Chapter 57.1). Electrolyte abnormalities, particularly hypocalcemia, and body temperature should be corrected to optimize myocardial performance.

Rewarming Measures (see Chapter 63). Patients with significant hypothermia, if rapidly rewarmed, may have improved stability and decreased morbidity. Adequate circulation greatly facilitates rewarming. Passive rewarming (e.g., warm room, dry blankets) relies on the patient's thermogenic ability and is not sufficient for most significantly hypothermic children. Active external rewarming (e.g., warm blankets, radiant warmers) restores temperature more rapidly ($0.8 \pm 0.4°C/hr$), but decreased surface circulation makes this method less effective. Moderate sources of external heat (e.g., forced-air blanket at about 100 W) may result in skin rewarming and shivering inhibition, but there is little rewarming advantage compared with shivering itself. Placing the subject in a forced warm air box (400 W) produces rates of rewarming double that of shivering (6.1 vs. 3°C/hr).

Active core rewarming more rapidly improves body temperature and is necessary for moderate to severe hypothermia or for victims with impaired shivering thermogenesis. Simple active core rewarming measures include administration of warmed intravenous fluids (36–40°C) and heated humidified inspired oxygen (40–44°C), although the efficacy of these measures is controversial. Gastric, bladder, or peritoneal lavage

with warmed saline may be instituted relatively easily. More aggressive methods include hemodialysis, extracorporeal rewarming (venovenous or arteriovenous), or cardiopulmonary bypass (CPB). Rewarming rates for extracorporeal rewarming ($2.1 \pm 0.7°C/hr$) are significantly faster than external active rewarming methods. For profound hypothermia, especially if circulatory collapse is present, CPB may be required and has a very rapid rewarming rate ($6.9 \pm 1.9°C/hr$). Indications for CPB are not well established; this complex decision requires physician anticipation and rapid transfer to a tertiary care center.

Neurologic Management. Near-drowning victims who present to the hospital awake and alert practically always have normal neurologic outcomes. In comatose victims, the possibility of irreversible CNS injury is a major concern. The primary injury, cell death from hypoxia-ischemia, is not currently treatable. Current therapy emphasizes reducing the duration of the primary insult (i.e., prompt resuscitation) and reducing the potential for secondary CNS injury.

The most effective neurointensive care measures in near-drowning are the rapid restoration of adequate oxygenation, ventilation, and perfusion. Unfortunately, studies of therapies aimed at controlling ICP or maintaining cerebral perfusion pressure have failed to clearly demonstrate improved outcome. Some general measures may be of benefit. Hypoglycemia and iatrogenic hyperglycemia should be avoided. Attempts to control seizures (see Chapter 57.7) and fever are warranted, because they increase cerebral metabolic activity and oxygen utilization. Other neurointensive care measures must be critically scrutinized, given that few have not been shown to improve satisfactory patient outcome after severe global hypoxic-ischemic injuries.

Head CT scans are not generally helpful unless there is a suspicion of associated traumatic injury or to rule out other possible causes of coma. The great majority of near-drowning victims initially have normal scans. An acutely abnormal CT scan is most frequently associated with death. After 24 hr, poor gray-white differentiation and cerebral edema may be seen in children with severe hypoxic-ischemic injuries. Head CT scans cannot adequately distinguish patients with good outcomes versus poor ones. MRI may detect changes associated with hypoxic-ischemic injuries earlier than head CT, but MRI is rarely clinically indicated. There is no advantage to head CT scans or MRI over neurologic examination for prognostication or management of nontraumatic near-drowning.

Many neurointensive care measures have been shown not to benefit the usual near-drowning victim. Although ICP monitoring and therapy to reduce intracranial hypertension would seem likely to preserve cerebral perfusion and prevent herniation, in fact, it does not appear to improve outcome for near-drowning victims. Patients with elevated ICP usually have poor outcomes—either death or persistent vegetative state—regardless of ICP management. Children with normal ICP can also have poor outcomes, although less frequently. Conventional neurointensive care therapies such as osmotic agents, diuretics, fluid restriction, muscle relaxants, hyperventilation, barbiturates, and steroids—measures often used in victims with elevated ICP from different causes—so far have not been shown to benefit the near-drowning victim either individually or in combination. Indeed, there is some evidence that these therapies may decrease overall mortality, but only by increasing the number of survivors in persistent vegetative state: they do not increase the number of neurologically intact survivors or reduce neurologic morbidity.

A number of potential therapies for hypoxic-ischemic brain injury are being studied. Resuscitative or therapeutic cerebral hypothermia in experimental animals may improve neurologic outcome after moderate global hypoxic-ischemic injury; early human studies have shown variable results.

Two randomized controlled trials in a highly selected cohort of adults with out-of-hospital cardiac arrest indicated that early therpeutic hypothermia was associated with decreased mortality and neurologic morbidity. Whether these results are generally applicable to children with hypoxia-induced cardiac arrest (the predominant mechanism of arrest in submersion events) is unknown.

Anti-excitotoxic therapies in humans have not yet proved beneficial; in animals, they must be given within the first 1–2 hr to reduce neurologic injury. Other investigational therapies include oxygen radical scavengers; lipid peroxidation inhibitors; calcium channel antagonists; glutamate pathway antagonists; NMDA-, AMPA-, and GABA-receptor antagonists; glutamate release inhibitors; nitric oxide synthase inhibitors; strategies to improve CBF during delayed hypoperfusion; anti-apoptosis targeted strategies; and a re-investigation of barbiturates.

With optimal management, many initially comatose children can have dramatic neurologic improvement, which usually occurs within the first 24–72 hr. Unfortunately, almost half of deeply comatose children admitted to the PICU will die of their brain injury or survive with severe neurologic damage. Many children become brain dead (see Chapter 64); indeed, submersion injury is the second leading cause of brain death in the PICU. Deeply comatose near-drowning victims who do not substantially improve their neurologic examination by 24–72 hr of aggressive cardiorespiratory support and whose coma cannot be otherwise explained should be seriously considered for limitation of support (see Chapter 64).

Other Management Issues. Some submersion victims may have traumatic injury, especially if they were participating in water sports such as boating, diving, or surfing. A high index of suspicion is required. Spinal precautions should be maintained in victims with altered mental status and suspected traumatic injury. Significant anemia should raise suspicion of trauma and internal hemorrhage.

Hypoxic-ischemic injury can have multiple systemic effects, although protracted organ dysfunction is uncommon in the absence of severe CNS injury. Even after initially severe pulmonary injury, with careful supportive management, lung function returns to normal in most near-drowning victims. Acute renal failure after hypoxic-ischemic injury from acute tubular or cortical injury can result in proteinuria, glucosuria, hemoglobinuria, oliguria, or anuria. Diuretics, fluid restriction, and dialysis are uncommonly needed to treat fluid overload or electrolyte disturbances; renal function usually normalizes in survivors. Rhabdomyolysis after drowning has been reported. Profuse bloody diarrhea and mucosal sloughing usually portend a grim prognosis; conservative management includes bowel rest, nasogastric suction, and gastric pH control. Nutritional support for most near-drowning victims is usually not difficult, because the majority of children either die or recover quickly and resume a normal diet within a few days; enteral tube feeding or parenteral nutrition is occasionally indicated in children who do not quickly recover.

One third to half of near-drowning victims have a fever during the first 48 hr after their submersion. Fever resolves spontaneously without antibiotics in approximately 80% of patients. Prophylactic antibiotics are not recommended. Antimicrobial therapy should be considered in victims with persistent fever, worsening pulmonary or general clinical status, or other evidence of infection. Pulmonary or disseminated infection, either bacterial or fungal, can occur. Reported causes of near-drowning–associated pneumonia include several unusual pathogens, which are frequently specific to the drowning medium and geographic region. Sepsis in critically ill patients can also arise from nonpulmonary sources, requiring careful assessment. Early respiratory and blood cultures should be considered and infectious disease consultation obtained in unusual cases.

Severe anoxic encephalopathy is seen in 10–30% of PICU survivors after near-drowning. Chronic neurologic sequelae include lowered mentation, cerebral dysfunction, spastic quadriplegia, extrapyramidal syndromes, optic and cerebral atrophy, cortical blindness, peripheral neuromuscular damage, or persistent vegetative state.

Psychiatric and psychosocial sequelae are common. Grief, guilt, and anger are frequent. Divorce rates of up to 80% are reported within a few years of severe injury to children, and parents often report difficulties with employment or substance abuse. Friends and family may blame the parents for the event. Professional counseling, pastoral care, or social work referral should be considered for all near-drowning victims and their families.

Prognosis. Overall, about 80% of pediatric submersion victims survive and 92% of survivors have a complete recovery. In those children requiring PICU care, about half survive neurologically intact, but 13–35% die and 7–27% survive with severe brain damage. The outcomes of near-drowning victims are remarkably bimodal: the great majority of victims either have good outcomes (intact or mild neurologic injury) or bad outcomes (persistent vegetative state or death), with very few exhibiting intermediate neurologic injury.

Accurate neurologic prognostication is important for the child, family, physicians, and society. Victims most likely to have good neurologic outcomes should be offered the most aggressive intensive care measures to prevent death from associated injuries; conversely, children with devastating neurologic injuries can be spared the futility of therapies that will not improve their condition. Early and precise prognostication is important to guide triage decisions, counsel families, reduce unnecessary interventions, guide discussions with families regarding limitation of support, and decrease the expenditure of valuable resources on children who will not recover.

Scoring and classification systems as well as individual factors have been used to predict near-drowning outcome. Although many of these systems strongly correlate with outcome, to date, none is accurate enough to completely differentiate good from poor outcomes. In many studies, several factors correlate with outcome, including (1) historical variables, such as submersion duration, interventions at the scene, and patient temperature; (2) treatment variables, such as need for CPR in the ED, apnea and pulselessness, resuscitation duration, GCS and progression, pupillary responsiveness, and brainstem reflexes; and (3) laboratory values, such as pH and glucose.

Prehospital predictors of non–icy water immersion outcomes in King County, Washington, have been comprehensively evaluated (1974–1989). Intact survival or mild neurologic impairment occurred in 91% of children with submersion duration less than 5 min and in 87% who had resuscitation duration less than 10 min. Children at the scene with normal sinus rhythm, reactive pupils, or neurologic responsiveness virtually always had good outcomes (>99%). In cases requiring advanced CPR, death or severe neurologic injury occurred in 93% of patients with submersion duration more than 10 min and in 100% of victims requiring resuscitation for more than 25 min. All victims with submersion duration of more than 25 min died in this study. However, a few authors have rarely noted sporadic intact recovery in non–icy water near-drowning after longer submersion or resuscitation duration, highlighting the difficulty in assigning absolute prognostic classification based on prehospital and ED variables alone.

Other studies of pediatric non–icy water submersions indicate that only a third of victims requiring advanced CPR at the scene survive, but two thirds of survivors have good recoveries. In a study with 89 patients who received CPR in the ED, 41 (46%) survived (8/41 intact and 33/41 with persistent vegetative state). In victims requiring CPR in the ED, functional recovery has been reported in only 0–24% (average 17%). Prolonged CPR after non-icy water submersion almost invariably predicts death or persistent vegetative state. Therefore, the discontinuation of CPR in the hospital is probably warranted for victims of non–icy water submersions who do not respond to aggressive advanced life support within 25–30 min. In any given victim, however, the circumstances surrounding submersion may not be known, especially during the first 25 min of an ongoing resuscitation; therefore, decisions regarding when to discontinue resuscitative efforts must be individualized, understanding that protracted resuscitation efforts generally will not result in survivors with a possibility of a good outcome.

The GCS (see Chapter 57.7) has some utility in predicting recovery. Children with a score of 6 or more on admission to the hospital generally have good outcomes, whereas those with a score of 5 or less have a much higher probability of poor neurologic outcome. However, some children with ED GCS of 3 or 4 uncommonly can have complete recovery. Upward trends in GCS during the first several hours of hospitalization may indicate a better prognosis. Overall, the GCS fails to adequately distinguish children who will survive intact from those with major neurologic injury.

Neurologic examination and progression during the first 24–72 hr are presently the best prognosticators of long-term CNS outcome. Children who regain consciousness within 72 hr, even after prolonged resuscitation, are unlikely to suffer serious neurologic sequelae. In a small series of comatose non–icy water submersion victims, all satisfactory survivors were noted to have spontaneous purposeful movements and normal brainstem function within 24 hr. Good recovery did not occur in any child with abnormal brainstem function and absence of purposeful movements at 24 hr. In another small series of near-drowning victims who remained unconscious more than 24 hr and survived at least 1 yr, 73% remained in a persistent vegetative state and the rest had severe neurologic impairment. These victims continued to have many complications and high mortality: 45% died during the study's post–1-year follow-up period.

The prognostic value of neurologic functional recovery during the first 72 hr of hospitalization was also observed in a larger retrospective series of 274 submersion victims (1985–1994). An initial ED GCS score of 3 was recorded in 100 patients; of these deeply comatose children, only 14% survived intact. There were 185 intact survivors, 95% of whom demonstrated functional recovery (time to first documented purposeful response) within 48 hr. In the 168 patients with a first documented purposeful response within 6 hr, all survived intact. Conversely, only 5.6% of children with poor outcomes (died or survived with persistent vegetative state) had "purposeful" movement within 48 hr. Of note, one child with good outcome and one with an intermediate outcome did not have purposeful movement until 1 and 3 mo, respectively.

Because of inexact prognostication in the prehospital setting and the ED, all near-drowning victims should receive appropriate aggressive support initially. Serial neurologic evaluation should be performed over the ensuing 48–72 hr with consideration of limitation of support in patients failing to demonstrate significant neurologic recovery, even though this may occur before absolute prognostic certainty is achieved.

Laboratory and technologic methods to improve prognostication have not yet proved superior to the neurologic examination. Methods that have received limited investigation include CT scans, MRI, electroencephalography, brainstem auditory evoked responses, somatosensory evoked potentials, visual evoked potentials, cerebrospinal fluid creatine kinase and lactate assays, measurements of CBF and cerebral metabolic rate, positron emission tomography, and magnetic resonance spectroscopy.

Prevention. The best hope for a "cure" of drowning and its serious consequences lies in prevention. These efforts must focus on legislation as well as ongoing education of parents, children, and physicians. Unfortunately, too few physicians are an adequate resource. In a survey of pediatricians in the American Academy of Pediatrics (AAP), 85% of respondents believed that it was the responsibility of pediatricians to become involved in community and legislative efforts to prevent childhood drowning; yet, only 4.1% were involved in such efforts. Despite the fact that drowning is a leading cause of injury death in children, only 50.9% of pediatricians gave any anticipatory guidance to children's parents, and only 33.8% gave any guidance to teenagers. In a study of Los Angeles clinicians, only a third stated they counseled families on drowning prevention. Part of the problem is that only 17.9% of pediatricians noted having received formal drowning prevention education during their residency training.

The residential swimming pool should be a focus of preventive efforts because of the high drowning rate at this site. In one study of pools where children drowned, 75% of pools were inadequately fenced. Only 18% of submersions were witnessed, even though a supervising adult could be identified 84% of the time. Fewer than half of households had any member who knew basic CPR, and 42% of children who died did not receive CPR until paramedics arrived.

Multiple layers of protection are necessary to minimize the risk of pediatric drowning. Education (including basic CPR) in addition to appropriate pool fencing could prevent up to 80% of drowning in young children. Fences should completely isolate the pool from the house and yard (isolation fencing). Isolation fencing is greatly superior to perimeter fencing (three-sided fence that encloses the property and pool) because perimeter fencing allows pool access through the home. Studies indicate that isolated fencing dramatically reduces the risk of drowning. The odds ratio for the risk of drowning or near-drowning in a fenced pool compared with an unfenced pool is 0.27 (95% CI 0.16–0.47). Proper gates are also important and should be self-closing and self-latching, with latches mounted inside and near the top of the fence.

Not all fences are equally effective. The commonly used 4-ft tall, large chain link (2.5-inch mesh) fence can be scaled by 75% of 2-yr olds in an average time of 25.6 sec and by 100% of 4-yr olds in an average 11.5 sec. Obviously, no commonly used barrier is universally insurmountable by young children. However, in one study, the only barrier insurmountable to children age 4 yr and younger was a 5-ft ornamental iron fence (vertical bars 3.25 inches apart; horizontal crossbars 45 inches apart; and no decorative cutouts on the fence). Clever children may still be able to climb any fence using aids such as chairs or boxes, again emphasizing the need for multiple layers of preventative strategies.

Parents need to closely supervise children at every moment during swimming. Toys should be removed from the pool area at the end of swim time. Pool covers should be American Society for Testing Materials approved. However, because pool covers are often cumbersome, they are unlikely to be replaced immediately after swim time and therefore are not likely to be an effective barrier. Lightweight covers should be discouraged, because they do not prevent the child from entering the pool and may obscure visualization of the submerged child. Door alarms and automatically closing and locking doors are untested in efficacy. Swimming pool alarms alone cannot be recommended at this time; in all alarms tested, a significant number of false alarms and failure to alarm were noted.

Infant and toddler swimming programs are popular throughout the United States. Children are not developmentally ready for swimming lessons until they are 4 yr old (AAP recommendations). Aquatic programs for infants and toddlers have not been shown to decrease the risk of drowning, and parents should not feel secure that their child is safe in water or safe from drowning as a consequence of such programs. School-aged children should be taught to swim but nonetheless prevented from swimming in unsupervised circumstances.

Parents must be made aware that any body of water, no matter how innocuous, poses a drowning risk, especially to children 4 yr of age and younger. Educating parents about the risks of common household fixtures, such as bathtubs, buckets, toilets, and washing machines, should be every pediatrician's task. Parents must be taught to remain with children throughout the entire bath time. Buckets containing water should never be left unattended. Toilet covers and bathroom doors should be closed at all times. Children with epilepsy can enjoy swimming as long as close supervision is maintained; these children should be encouraged to shower in a glass-free cubicle rather than in a bathtub.

A National Transportation Safety Board review found that only 15% of boaters who drowned wore a personal flotation device (PFD). In a study of boaters in the northwest United States, only 25% wore a PFD. Use was highest in children younger than age 5 yr (91%) and lowest in those older than age 14 yr (13%). If no adult on a boat wore a PFD, then only 65% of children wore one; if at least one adult wore a PFD, then 95% of children wore one as well. Intensive community boating education efforts have been shown to substantially increase PFD use. Water safety education for children, teenagers, and parents that encourages PFD use and never swimming alone should be reinforced in the school, community, and physician's office. Teenagers should learn CPR and be counseled about alcohol and drug use, which significantly contribute to submersion and drowning.

American Heart Association: International Guidelines 2000 for CPR and ECC. Part 8, Section 3: Advanced challenges in resuscitation, submersion or near-drowning. *Circulation* 2000;102(Suppl):1237.

Biggart MJ, Bohn DJ: Effect of hypothermia and cardiac arrest on outcome of near-drowning accidents in children. *J Pediatr* 1990;117:179–83.

Bratton SL, Jardine DS, Morray JP: Serial neurologic examinations after near-drowning and outcome. *Arch Pediatr Adolesc Med* 1994;148:167–70.

Brenner RA, Trumble AC, Smith GS, et al: Where children drown, United States, 1995. *Pediatrics* 2001;108:85–9.

Christensen DW, Jansen P, Perkin RM: Outcome and acute care hospital costs after warm water near-drowning in children. *Pediatrics* 1997;99:715–21.

Clifton GL, Miller ER, Choi SC, et al: Lack of effect of induction of hypothermia after acute brain injury. *N Engl J Med* 2001;344:556–62.

Griest KJ, Zumwalt RE: Child abuse by drowning. *Pediatrics* 1989;83:41–6.

Hypothermia After Cardiac Arrest Study Group: Mild therapeutic hypothermia to improve the neurologic outcome after cardiac arrest. *N Engl J Med* 2002;346:549–56.

Kyriacou D, Arcinue E, Peek C, et al: Effect of immediate resuscitation on children with submersion injury. *Pediatrics* 1994;94:137–42.

Modell JH: Drowning. *N Engl J Med* 1993;328:253–56.

Quan L, Kinder D: Pediatric submersions: Pre-hospital predictors of outcome. *Pediatrics* 1992;90:909–13.

Rabinovich BA, Lerner ND, Huey RW: Young children's ability to climb fences. *Hum Factors* 1994;36:733–44.

Thompson DC, Rivara FP: Pool fencing for preventing drowning in children. *Cochrane Database Syst Rev 2*, 2000.

Zuckerman GB, Gregory PM, Santos-Damiani SM: Predictors of death and neurologic impairment in pediatric submersion injuries. *Arch Pediatr Adolesc Med* 1998; 152:134–40.

Chapter 62

Burn Injuries

Alia Y. Antoon and Mary K. Donovan

Burns are a leading cause of unintentional death in children, second only to motor vehicle crashes. There has been a decline in the incidence of burn injury requiring medical care over the past decade. This has coincided with an increased focus on burn treatment and prevention, fire and burn prevention education,

availability of regional treatment centers, widespread use of smoke detectors, greater regulation of consumer products and occupational safety, and societal changes such as reduced smoking and alcohol abuse.

Epidemiology. About 1.2 million people in the United States require medical care for burn injuries each year, with 51,000 requiring hospitalization. Thirty to 40 per cent of these patients are younger than 15 yr of age, with an average age of 32 mo. Fires are a major cause of mortality in children, accounting for up to 34% of fatal injuries in those younger than 16 yr. Scald burns account for 85% of total injuries and are most prevalent in children younger than 4 yr of age. Although the incidence of hot water scalding has been reduced by legislation requiring new water heaters to be preset at 120°F, scald injury remains the leading cause of hospitalization for burns. Flame burns account for 13%; the remaining are electrical and chemical burns. Clothing ignition has declined since passage of the Federal Flammable Fabric Act, requiring sleepwear to be flame retardant; however, the Consumer Product Safety Commission voted to relax the existing children's sleepwear flammability standard. Approximately 18% of burns are the result of child abuse, making it important to assess pattern and site of injury and their consistency with history (see Chapter 35). Friction burns from treadmills are also a significant problem. Anoxia and not the actual burn is a major cause of morbidity and mortality in house fires.

Review of the history usually reveals a common pattern: scald burn to the side of face, neck, and arm if liquid is pulled from a table or stove; a pant leg area burn if clothing ignites; splash areas from cooking; and palm of hand contact with a hot stove. However, "glove or stocking" burns of hands and feet, single-area deep burns on the trunk, buttocks, or back, and small-area, full-thickness burns (cigarette burns) in young children should raise the suspicion of child abuse.

Burn care involves a range of activities: prevention, acute care and resuscitation, wound management, pain relief, reconstruction, rehabilitation, and psychosocial adjustment. Children with massive burns require early and appropriate psychologic and social support as well as resuscitation. Surgical débridement, wound closure, and rehabilitative efforts should be instituted concurrently to promote optimal rehabilitation. Aggressive surgical removal of devitalized tissue, infection control, and judicious use of antibiotics as well as early nutrition and cautious use of intubation and mechanical ventilation are necessary to maximize survival. Children who have sustained burn injuries differ in appearance from their peers, necessitating supportive efforts for re-entry to schooling and social and sporting activities.

Prevention. The aim is a continuing reduction in the number of serious burn injuries (Box 62–1). Effective first aid and triage can decrease both the extent (area) and the severity (depth) of injuries. Flame-retardant clothing, smoke detectors, and control of hot water temperature (thermostat settings) within buildings as well as prohibition of cigarette smoking have been partially successful in reducing the incidence of burn injuries. Dedicated burn unit treatment of children with significant burn injuries facilitates medically effective care, improves survival, and leads to greater cost efficiency. Survival of at least 80% of patients with 90% body surface burns is now usual; overall survival of children with burns of all sizes is 99%. Deaths are more likely in children with irreversible anoxic brain injury sustained at the time of the burn.

Pediatricians can play a major role in preventing the most common burns by educating parents and care providers in preventive measures geared to the various stages of child development. Appropriate clothing, smoke detectors, and planned routes for emergency exit from the home are simple, effective, efficient, and cost-effective preventive measures. Child neglect

BOX 62-1. Burn Prophylaxis

PREVENT FIRES

Smoke detectors
Control of hot water thermostat—public buildings (maximum water temperature 120° F)
Learn to use fire-matches-lighter to prevent injury
Prevent cigarette smoking
Flame retardant–treated clothing

PREVENT INJURY

Roll, not run, if clothing catches fire; wrap in blanket
Practice escape procedures
Crawl beneath smoke if indoors
Use of materials for education*

*National Fire Protection Association pamphlets and videos.

and abuse must be seriously considered when the history of the injury and the distribution of the burn do not match.

Acute Care, Resuscitation, and Assessment

INDICATIONS FOR ADMISSION (Box 62–2). Burns covering greater than 10–15% of total body surface area (BSA), burns associated with smoke inhalation, burns resulting from high-tension electrical injuries, and burns associated with suspected child abuse or neglect should be treated as emergencies and the child hospitalized. Small first- and second-degree burns of the hands, feet, face, perineum, and joint surfaces also require admission if close follow-up care is difficult to provide. Children who have been in enclosed-space fires and those who have face and neck burns should be hospitalized for at least 24 hr of observation for signs of central nervous system (CNS) effects of anoxia from carbon monoxide poisoning or pulmonary effects from smoke inhalation.

FIRST AID MEASURES. Acute care should include the following:

1. Extinguish flames by rolling on the ground; cover the child with a blanket, coat, or carpet.

2. After determining that the airway is patent, remove smoldering clothing or clothing saturated with hot liquid. Jewelry, particularly rings and bracelets, should be removed or cut away to prevent constriction and vascular compromise during the edema phase in the first 24–72 hr post burn.

3. In cases of chemical injury, brush off any remaining chemical if powdered or solid; then use copious irrigation or wash the affected area with water. Call Poison Control for the neutralizing agent to treat a chemical ingestion.

4. Cover the burned area with clean, dry sheeting and apply cold (not iced) wet compresses to small injuries. Significant large burn surface area injury (>15–20% BSA) decreases body temperature control and contraindicates the use of cold compress dressings.

5. If the burn is caused by hot tar, use mineral oil to remove the tar.

EMERGENCY CARE (Box 62–3). Life support measures should include the following:

1. Rapidly review the cardiovascular and pulmonary status and document pre-existing or physiologic lesions (e.g., asthma, congenital heart disease, renal or hepatic disease).

2. Ensure and maintain an adequate airway and provide humidified oxygen by mask or endotracheal intubation. The latter may be needed in children who have facial burns or a burn sustained in an enclosed space, before facial or laryngeal edema becomes evident. If hypoxia or carbon monoxide poisoning is suspected, 100% oxygen should be used (see Chapters 57.1 and 57.3).

3. Children with burns greater than 15% of BSA require intravenous fluid resuscitation to maintain adequate perfusion. All inhalation injuries, regardless of the extent of BSA burn, require venous access to control fluid intake. All high-tension and electrical injuries require venous access to ensure forced alkaline diuresis in case of muscle injury to avoid myoglobinuric renal damage. Lactated Ringer solution, 10–20 mL/kg/hr (normal saline may be used if lactated Ringer is not available), is infused until proper fluid replacement can be calculated. Consultation with a specialized burn unit should be made to coordinate fluid therapy, type of fluid, preferred formula for calculation, and preferences for use of colloid agents, particularly if transfer to a burn center is anticipated.

4. Evaluate the child for associated injuries, which are common in patients with a history of high-tension electrical burn, especially if there has been a fall from a height. Injuries to spine, bones, and thoracic or intra-abdominal organs may occur (see Chapter 57.8). The child should be placed on cervical spine precaution until this injury is ruled out. There is a very high risk of cardiac abnormalities, including ventricular tachycardia or ventricular fibrillation, resulting from conductivity of the high electric voltage. Cardiopulmonary resuscitation should be instituted promptly at the scene, and the patient should be placed on a cardiac monitor on arrival at the emergency department (see Chapter 57.1).

5. Children with burns greater than 15% BSA should not receive oral fluids (initially), because they may develop ileus. These children require insertion of a nasogastric tube in the emergency department to prevent aspiration.

6. A Foley catheter should be inserted to monitor urine output in all children who require intravenous fluid resuscitation.

7. All wounds should be wrapped with sterile towels until a decision is made about whether to treat on an outpatient basis or refer the patient to an appropriate facility for treatment.

CLASSIFICATION OF BURNS. Proper triage and treatment of burn injury require assessment of the extent and depth of the injury (Table 62–1). *First-degree burns* involve only the epidermis and are characterized by swelling, erythema, and pain (similar to a mild sunburn). Tissue damage is usually minimal, and there is no blistering. Pain resolves in 48–72 hr; in a small percentage of patients the damaged epithelium will peel off, leaving no residual scars.

A *second-degree burn* involves injury to the entire epidermis and a variable portion of the dermal layer (vesicle and blister formation are characteristic of second-degree burns). A *superficial* second-degree burn is extremely painful because a large

BOX 62-2. Indications for Hospitalization for Burns

Burns greater than 15% body surface area
High-tension wire electrical burns
Inhalation injury regardless of the size of body surface area burn
Inadequate home situation
Suspected child abuse or neglect
Burns to hands, feet, genitals

BOX 62-3. Acute Treatment of Burns

First aid
Fluid resuscitation
Supply energy requirements
Pain control
Prevention of infection—early excision and grafting
Control of bacterial wound flora
Biologic and synthetic dressings to close wound

TABLE 62–1. **Burn Depth Categories**

	First Degree	Second Degree Partial Thickness	Third Degree Full Thickness
Surface Appearance	Dry, no blisters. Minimal or no edema. Erythematous.	Moist blebs, blisters. Underlying tissue is mottled pink and white with good capillary refill.	Dry, leathery eschar. Mixed white, waxy, khaki, mahogany, soot stained.
Pain	Very painful.	Very painful.	Insensate.
Histologic Depth	Epidermal layers only.	Epidermis, papillary, and reticular layers of dermis. May include domes of subcutaneous layers.	Down to and may include fat, subcutaneous tissue, fascia, muscle, and bone.
Healing Time	2–5 days with no scarring.	Superficial: 5–21 days with no grafting. Deep partial: 21–35 days with no infection. If infected, converts to full thickness.	Large areas require grafting. Small areas may heal from the edges after weeks.

number of remaining viable nerve endings are exposed. Superficial second-degree burns heal in 7–14 days as the epithelium regenerates in the absence of infection. *Midlevel* to *deep* second-degree burns also heal spontaneously if wounds are kept clean and infection free. Pain is less than in more superficial burns, because fewer nerve endings remain viable. Fluid losses and metabolic effects of deep dermal (second-degree) burns are essentially the same as those of third-degree burns.

Full-thickness or *third-degree* burns involve destruction of the entire epidermis and dermis, leaving no residual epidermis cells to repopulate the damaged area. The wound cannot epithelialize and can heal only by wound contraction or skin grafting. The absence of painful sensation and capillary filling demonstrates the loss of nerve and capillary elements.

ESTIMATION OF BODY SURFACE AREA OF BURN. Appropriate burn charts for different childhood age groups should be used to accurately estimate the extent of BSA burned. The volume of fluid needed in resuscitation is calculated from the estimation of the extent and depth of burn surface. Mortality and morbidity also depend on the extent and depth of the burn. The variable growth rate of the head and extremities throughout childhood makes it necessary to use surface area charts, such as that modified by Lund and Brower or the chart used at the Shriners Hospital in Boston (Fig. 62–1). The "rule of nines" used in adults may be used only in children older than age 14 yr or as a very rough estimate to institute therapy before transfer to a burn center. In small burns under 10% of BSA, the "rule of palm" may be used, especially in outpatient settings. The area from the wrist crease to finger crease (the palm) in the child equals 1% of the child's BSA.

TREATMENT

OUTPATIENT MANAGEMENT OF MINOR BURNS. First- and second-degree burns less than 10% BSA may be treated on an outpatient basis unless there is inadequate family support or there are issues of child neglect or abuse. These outpatients do not require a tetanus booster or prophylactic penicillin therapy. Children who are not current with immunizations should have their immunizations updated. Blisters should be left intact and dressed with bacitracin or silver sulfadiazine cream (Silvadene). Dressings should be changed once daily, after the wound is washed with lukewarm water to remove any cream left from the previous application. Very small wounds, especially those on the face, may be treated with bacitracin ointment and left open. Débridement of the devitalized skin is indicated when the blisters rupture. Burns to the palm with large blisters usually heal beneath the blisters, with close follow-up on an outpatient basis. The great majority of superficial burns heal in 10–20 days. Deep second-degree burns take longer to heal and may benefit from Polysporin powder placed on the wound and covered with collagenase ointment, which is changed daily. Pain control should be accomplished by using acetaminophen with codeine 1 hour before dressing changes. Wounds that appear deeper than at initial assessment or that have not healed by 21 days may require a short hospital admission for grafting.

The depth of scald injuries is difficult to assess early; conservative treatment is appropriate to allow maturation and declaration of the depth and area involved before closure is attempted. This obviates the risk of anesthesia and unnecessary grafting and diminishes potential scarring in those patients in whom spontaneous healing is likely to occur.

FLUID RESUSCITATION. For most children the Parkland formula is an appropriate starting guideline for fluid resuscitation (4 mL lactated Ringer/kg/% BSA burned). One half of the fluid is given over the first 8 hr calculated from the time of onset of injury. The remaining half is given at an even rate over the next 16 hr. The rate of infusion is adjusted according to the patient's response to therapy. Pulse and blood pressure should return to normal, and an adequate urine output (1 mL/kg/hr) should be accomplished by varying the intravenous infusion rate. Vital signs, acid-base balance, and mental status reflect the adequacy of the resuscitation. Because of interstitial edema and sequestration of fluid in muscle cells, patients may gain up to 20% over baseline pre-burn body weight. Patients with burns of 30% BSA require a large venous access (central venous line) to deliver the fluid required over the critical first 24 hr. Patients with burns greater than 60% BSA may require a multilumen central venous catheter; these patients are best cared for in a specialized burn unit.

During the second 24 hr after the burn, patients will begin to reabsorb edema fluid and to diurese. One half of the first day's fluid requirement is infused as lactated Ringer solution in 5% dextrose. Children younger than age 5 yr may require the addition of 5% dextrose in the first 24 hr of resuscitation. Controversy exists as to whether colloid should be provided in the early period of burn resuscitation. One preference is to use colloid replacement concurrently if the burn is greater than 85% total BSA. Colloid is usually instituted 8–24 hr after the burn injury. In children younger than 12 mo of age, sodium tolerance is limited; volume and sodium concentration of the resuscitation solution should be decreased if urinary sodium is rising. Adequacy of resuscitation should be constantly assessed using vital signs, blood gases, hematocrit, and protein levels. Some patients require arterial and central venous lines, particularly if undergoing multiple excision and grafting procedures as needed, for monitoring and replacement purposes. Central venous pressure monitoring may be indicated to assess circulation and urine output for patients with hemodynamic or cardiopulmonary instability. Femoral vein cannulation is a safe access for fluid resuscitation especially in infants and children. Burn patients who require frequent blood gas monitoring benefit from radial or femoral arterial catheterization.

Oral supplementation may start as early as 48 hr postburn. Milk formula, artificial feedings, homogenized milk, or soy-based products can be given by bolus or constant infusion through a nasogastric or small bowel feeding tube. As oral fluids

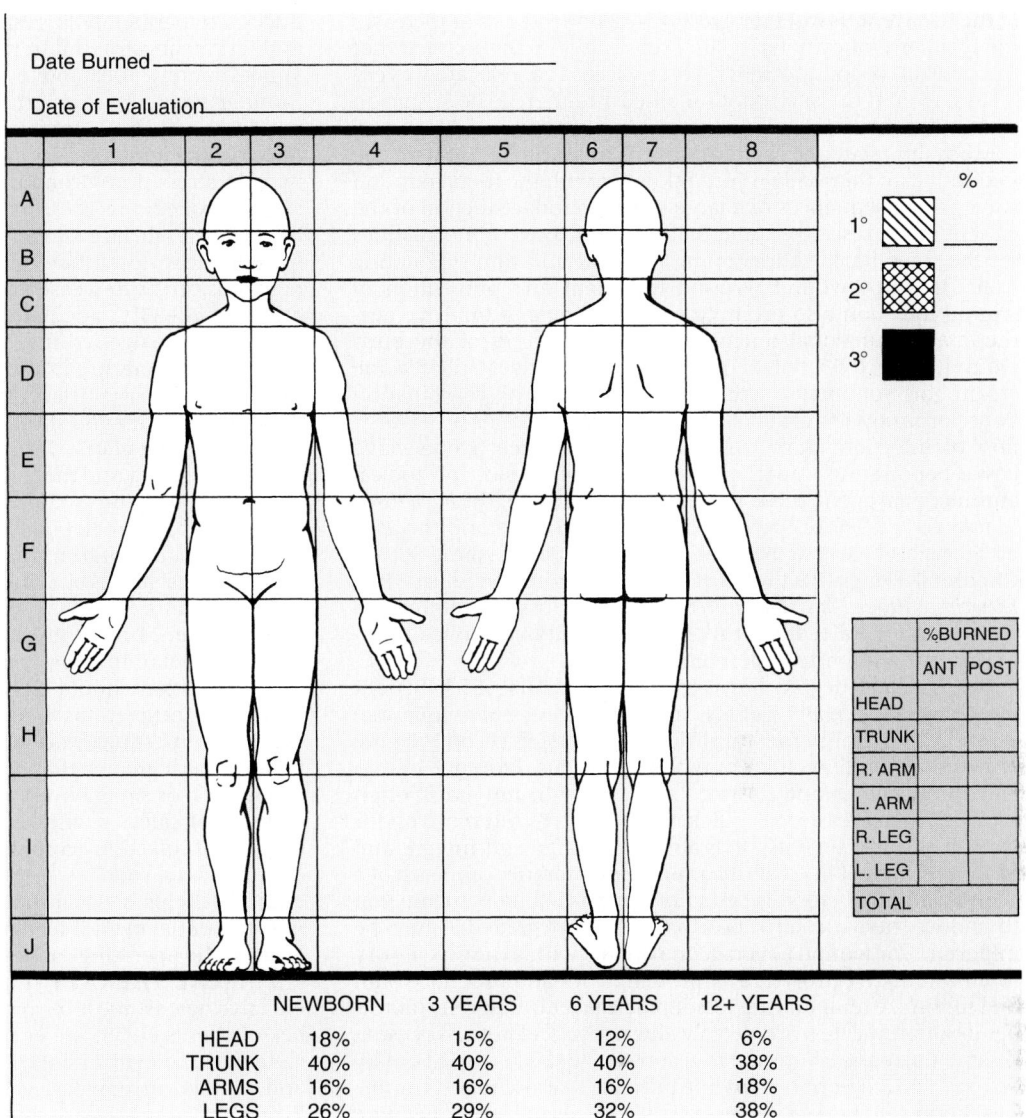

Date Burned_____

Date of Evaluation_____

	1	2	3	4	5	6	7	8
A								
B								
C								
D								
E								
F								
G								
H								
I								
J								

%

1° ▨ ____

2° ▩ ____

3° ■ ____

	%BURNED	
	ANT	POST
HEAD		
TRUNK		
R. ARM		
L. ARM		
R. LEG		
L. LEG		
TOTAL		

	NEWBORN	3 YEARS	6 YEARS	12+ YEARS
HEAD	18%	15%	12%	6%
TRUNK	40%	40%	40%	38%
ARMS	16%	16%	16%	18%
LEGS	26%	29%	32%	38%

FIGURE 62–1. Chart to determine developmentally related per cent body burn surface area. (Courtesy of Shriners Hospital for Crippled Children, Burn Institute, Boston Unit.)

are tolerated, intravenous fluids are decreased proportionately in an effort to keep the total fluid intake constant, particularly if pulmonary dysfunction is present.

Five per cent albumin infusions may be used to maintain the serum albumin levels at a desired 2 g/dL. The following rates are effective: for total BSA burns of 30–50%, 0.3 mL of 5% albumin/kg/% BSA burn is infused over a 24-hr period; for total BSA burns of 50–70%, 0.4 mL/kg/% BSA burn is infused over 24 hr; and for total BSA burns of 70–100%, 0.5 mL/kg/% BSA burn is infused over 24 hr. Packed red cell infusion is recommended if the hematocrit falls below 24% (hemoglobin ≤8 g/dL). Some recommend treating hematocrits below 30% or hemoglobin under 10 g/dL in patients with systemic infections, hemoglobinopathies, cardiopulmonary disease, or anticipated (or ongoing) blood loss when repeated excision and grafting of full-thickness burns is likely to be needed. Fresh frozen plasma is indicated if clinical and laboratory assessment reveals a deficiency of clotting factors, a prothrombin level above 1.5 times control, or a partial thromboplastin time of greater than 1.2 times control in children who are bleeding or are scheduled for an invasive procedure or a grafting procedure that could result in an estimated blood loss of over half the blood volume. Fresh frozen plasma may be used for volume resuscitation within 72 hr of injury in patients younger than 2 yr of age with burns over 20% BSA and associated inhalation injury.

Sodium supplementation may be required for children having burns greater than 20% BSA, if 0.5% silver nitrate solution is used as the topical antibacterial burn dressing. Sodium losses with silver nitrate therapy are regularly as high as 350 mmol sodium/m² burn surface area. Oral sodium chloride supplement of 4 g/m² burn area per 24 hr is usually well tolerated, divided into four to six equal doses to avoid osmotic diarrhea. The aim is to maintain serum sodium levels over 130 mEq/L and urinary sodium concentration over 30 mEq/L. Intravenous potassium supplementation is supplied to maintain serum potassium level over 3 mEq/dL. Potassium losses may be significantly increased when 0.5% silver nitrate solution is used as the topical antibacterial agent or when aminoglycoside, diuretic, or amphotericin therapy is required.

PREVENTION OF INFECTION AND SURGICAL MANAGEMENT OF THE BURN WOUND. Controversy exists over the prophylactic use of penicillin for all acute hospitalized burn patients and the periodic replacement of central venous catheters to prevent infection. In some units a 5-day course of penicillin therapy is used for all acute burns; standard-dose crystalline penicillin is given orally or intravenously in four divided doses. Erythromycin may be used as an alternative in penicillin-allergic children. Other units have discontinued prophylactic use of penicillin therapy without an increase in the infection rate. Similarly, there is conflicting evidence as to whether relocation of the intravenous catheter every 48–72 hr decreases or increases the incidence of catheter-related sepsis. It is recommended that the central venous catheter be replaced and relocated every 7 days, even if the site is not inflamed and there is no suspicion of catheter-related sepsis.

Mortality related to the burn injury is associated not with the toxic effect of thermally injured skin but with the metabolic and bacterial consequences of a large open wound, reduction of the patient's host resistance, and malnutrition. These abnormalities set the stage for life-threatening bacterial infection originating from the burn wound. Wound treatment and prevention of wound infection also promote early healing and improve aesthetic and functional outcomes. *Topical treatment* of the burn wound using 0.5% silver nitrate solution, silver sulfadiazine cream, or Sulfamylon cream, and the use of combination Polysporin powder and collagenase ointment, aims at prevention of infection (Table 62–2). The latter three agents have tissue-penetrating capacity. Regardless of choice of topical antimicrobial agent, it is essential that all third-degree *burn tissue be fully excised* before bacterial colonization occurs and the area be grafted as early as possible to prevent deep wound sepsis. Children having a BSA burn of over 30% should be housed in a *bacteria-controlled nursing unit* to prevent cross contamination and to provide a temperature- and humidity-controlled environment to minimize hypermetabolism.

Deep second-degree burns greater than 10% BSA benefit from early *excision and grafting*. To improve outcome, sequential excision and grafting of third-degree and deep second-degree burns is required in children with large burns. Prompt excision and immediate wound closure is achieved with autografts, often meshed to increase the efficiency of cover. Alternatives for wound closure, such as allografts, xenografts, and Integra and other synthetic skin cover (bilaminate membrane composed of a porous lattice of cross-linked chondroitin-6-sulfate engineered to induce neovascularization as it is biodegraded), may be important for wound coverage in patients with extensive injury to limit fluid, electrolyte, and protein losses and to reduce pain and minimize temperature loss. Epidermal cultured cells (autologous keratinocytes) are a costly alternative and not always successful. Early staged or total excision can be safely carried out by an experienced burn team while burn fluid resuscitation continues. Important keys to success include (1) accurate preoperative and intraoperative determination of burn depth, (2) the choice of excision area and appropriate timing, (3) control of intraoperative blood loss, (4) specific instrumentation, (5) choice and use of perioperative antibiotics, and (6) type of wound coverage chosen. The above process can accomplish early coverage without the use of growth hormone.

NUTRITIONAL SUPPORT. Supporting the increased energy requirements of a burn is a high priority. The burn injury produces a hypermetabolic response characterized by both protein and fat catabolism. Children with a 40% total BSA burn require approximately 50% above predicted basal energy expenditure for their age. Early excision and grafting can decrease the energy requirement. Pain, anxiety, and immobilization increase the physiologic demands. Additional energy expenditure is caused by cold stress if environmental humidity and temperature are not controlled; this is especially true in young infants, in whom the largest surface area:mass ratio allows proportionately greater heat loss than in adolescents and adults. Calorie demands can be decreased by providing environmental temperatures of 28–33°C, adequate covering during transport, and liberal use of analgesics and anxiolytics. Special units to control ambient temperature and humidity may be necessary for children having large surface area burns. Appropriate sleep intervals are necessary and should be part of the regimen.

The objective of caloric supplementation programs is to maintain body weight and meet metabolic demands. This reduces the loss of lean body mass. Calories are provided at one and one half times the basal metabolic rate, 3–4 g/kg of protein per day. Propranolol, in children with more than 40% BSA burns, in sufficient doses to reduce the resting heart rate by 20%, also reduces resting energy expenditure and improves muscle nitrogen balance. Multivitamins, particularly the B vitamin group, vitamin C, vitamin A, and zinc, are also necessary.

Alimentation should be started as soon as is practical, both orally and intravenously, to meet all the caloric needs and keep the gastrointestinal tract active after the resuscitative phase. Patients with greater than 40% total BSA burns need a flexible nasogastric or small bowel feeding tube to facilitate continuous delivery of calories without the risk of aspiration. To decrease the risk of infectious complications, parenteral nutrition is discontinued as soon as is practical after delivery of sufficient enteral calories is established. Continuous gastrointestinal feeding is essential even if feeding is interrupted, owing to frequent visits to the operating room until the full grafting takes place.

TOPICAL THERAPY. Topical therapy is widely used and is effective against most burn pathogens (see Table 62–2). A number of agents (0.5% silver nitrate, sulfacetamide acetate, silver sulfadiazine cream, and the combination of collagenase ointment and Polysporin powder) can be used on small second-degree burns. Preferences vary among burn units. Each topical agent has advantages and disadvantages in application, comfort, and bacteriostatic spectrum. Sulfacetamide acetate is a very effective broad-spectrum agent with the ability to diffuse through the burn eschar and is thus the treatment of choice in injury to cartilaginous surfaces, such as ears. The carbonic anhydrase inhibition activity of sulfacetamide may cause acid-base imbalance if large surface areas are treated, and adverse reactions to the sulfur-containing agents may produce a transient leukopenia.

TABLE 62–2. Topical Agents for Burns

Agent	Effectiveness	Ease of Use
Silver sulfadiazine	Broad spectrum	Closed dressings
Silvadene cream	Good penetration	Changed twice daily
		Residue *must* be washed off with each dressing change
Mafenide acetate	Broad spectrum, including *Pseudomonas*	Closed dressings
		Changed twice daily
	Rapid and deep wound penetration	Residue *must* be washed off with each dressing change
0.5% Silver nitrate solution	Bacteriostatic	Closed bulky dressing soaked every 2 hr and changed once a day
	Broad spectrum, including some fungi Superficial penetration	
Polysporin powder Cover with collagenase ointment	Broad spectrum, enzymatic débridement	Closed dressing; once-a-day change

INHALATIONAL INJURY. This injury is serious in the infant and child, particularly if pre-existing pulmonary conditions are present (see Chapter 57.3). Mortality estimates vary depending on the criteria for diagnosis but are 45–60% in adults; exact figures are not available in children. Evaluation aims at early identification of inhalational airway injuries. These may occur from (1) direct heat (greater problems with steam burns), (2) acute asphyxia, (3) carbon monoxide poisoning, and (4) toxic fumes, including cyanides from combustible plastics. Sulfur and nitrogen oxides and alkalis formed during the combustion of synthetic fabrics produce corrosive chemicals that may erode mucosa and cause significant tissue sloughing. Exposure to smoke may cause degradation of surfactant and decrease its production, resulting in atelectasis. Inhalation injury and burn injury are synergistic, and the combined effect can increase morbidity and mortality.

The pulmonary complications of burns and inhalation can be divided into three syndromes with distinct *clinical manifestations* and temporal patterns:

1. *Early* carbon monoxide poisoning, airway obstruction, and pulmonary edema are major concerns.

2. The acute respiratory distress syndrome usually becomes clinically evident later, at 24–48 hr, although it can occur even later (see Chapter 58).

3. *Late* complications (days to weeks) include pneumonia and pulmonary emboli.

Inhalation injury should be assessed by evidence of obvious injury (swelling or carbonaceous material in nasal passages), wheezing, crackles or poor air entry, and laboratory determination of carboxyhemoglobin (HbCO) and arterial blood gases.

Treatment is initially focused on establishing and maintaining a patent airway through prompt and early nasotracheal intubation and adequate ventilation and oxygenation. Wheezing is common, and β-agonist aerosols or inhaled corticosteroids are useful. Aggressive pulmonary toilet and chest physiotherapy are necessary in prolonged nasotracheal intubation or in the rare patient with a tracheotomy. The availability of less irritating endotracheal tube materials as well as improved tube and cuff design has allowed progressively longer periods of translaryngeal intubation. An endotracheal tube can be maintained for months without the need for tracheostomy. If tracheotomy has to be performed, it should be delayed until burns at and near the site have healed, and then it should be performed electively with the child under anesthesia and using optimal tracheal positioning and hemostasis. In children with inhalation injury or burns of the face and neck, upper airway obstruction can develop rapidly; endotracheal intubation becomes a lifesaving intervention. All should be aware of the potential damage to the columella when both nasotracheal and nasogastric tubes are used for prolonged periods of time. Extubation should be delayed until the patient meets accepted criteria for maintaining the airway.

Signs of CNS injury from hypoxemia due to asphyxia or carbon monoxide poisoning vary from irritability to depression. Carbon monoxide poisoning may be mild (<20% HbCO), with slight dyspnea and decreased visual acuity and higher cerebral functions; moderate (20–40% HbCO), with irritability, nausea, dimness of vision, impaired judgment, and rapid fatigue; or severe (40–60% HbCO), producing confusion, hallucination, ataxia, collapse, acidosis, and coma. Measurement of HbCO is important for diagnosis and treatment. Pao_2 may be normal and the oxyhemoglobin saturation values misleading because HbCO is not detected by the usual tests of oxygen saturation. Carbon monoxide poisoning is assumed until the tests are performed and is treated with 100% oxygen. Significant CO poisoning requires hyperbaric oxygen therapy (see Chapter 704.10).

Patients with severe inhalation injury or with other causes of respiratory deterioration leading to acute respiratory distress syndrome who fail to improve on conventional pressure controlled ventilation (progressive oxygenation failure as manifested by Po_2 below 90% while on Fio_2 between 0.9–1.0 and PEEP of at least 12.5 cm H_2O) may benefit from high-frequency ventilation or nitric oxide inhalation treatment. Nitric oxide usually is administered through the ventilator at 5 parts per minute (ppm) and increased up to 30 ppm. This method of therapy reduces the need of extracorporeal membrane oxygenation.

Pain Relief and Psychologic Adjustment (see also Chapter 66). It is important to provide adequate analgesia, anxiolytics, and psychologic support to reduce early metabolic stress, decrease the potential for post-traumatic stress syndrome (see Chapter 22), and allow future stabilization and rehabilitation. Patients and family require team support to work through a grieving process and accept long-term changes in appearance.

Children having burn injury show frequent and wide fluctuations in pain intensity. Appreciation of pain depends on the depth of the burn, stage of healing, age and stage of emotional development, cognition, experience and efficiency of the treating team, use of analgesics and other drugs, pain threshold, and interpersonal and cultural factors. From the onset of the treatment, preemptive pain control during dressing changes is of paramount importance. The use of a variety of nonpharmacologic interventions as well as pharmacologic agents needs to be reviewed throughout the treatment period. Opiate analgesia prescribed in an adequate dose and timed to cover dressing changes is essential to comfort management. A supportive person who is consistently present and "knows" the patient profile can integrate and encourage patient participation in burn care. The problem of undermedication is most prevalent with adolescents, in whom fear of drug dependency may inappropriately influence treatment. A related problem is that the child's specific pain experience may be misinterpreted; for example, for anxious patients, those who are confused and alone, or those with pre-existing emotional disorders, even small wounds may illicit intense pain. Anxiolytic medication added to the analgesic is usually helpful and has more than a synergistic effect. Equal attention is necessary to decrease stress in the intubated patient. Other modalities of pain and anxiety relief (e.g., relaxation techniques) can decrease the physiologic stress response. Oral morphine sulfate (immediate-release) is recommended on a consistent schedule at a dose of 0.3–0.6 mg/kg q4–6h initially and until wound cover is accomplished. Morphine sulfate intravenous bolus at a dose of 0.05–0.1 mg/kg q2h is administered in older patients using a patient-controlled analgesia (PCA) protocol. Morphine sulfate rectal suppositories may be useful at an added dose of 0.3–0.6 mg/kg q4h. For anxiety, lorazepam (Ativan) is given on a consistent schedule, 0.05–0.1 mg/kg/dose q8h. To control pain during a procedure (dressing changes or débridement), oral morphine at a dose of 0.3–0.6 mg/kg is given 1–2 hr before the procedure, and this is supplemented by a morphine intravenous bolus at a dose of 0.05–0.1 mg/kg given immediately before the procedure. Lorazepam at a dose of 0.04 mg/kg is given orally, or intravenously if necessary, for anxiety before the procedure. Midazolam (Versed) is also very useful for conscious sedation given at a dose of 0.05–0.1 mg/kg/hr as an infusion or a bolus; it may be repeated in 10 min, with a maximum dose of 0.2 mg/kg. During the process of weaning from analgesics, the dose of oral opiates is reduced by 25% over 1–3 days, sometimes with the addition of acetaminophen as opiates are tapered. Antianxiety medications are tapered by reducing the dose of benzodiazepines at 25–50% per dose daily over 1–3 days.

For ventilated patients, pain control is accomplished by using morphine sulfate intermittently as an intravenous bolus at a dose of 0.05–0.1 mg/kg q2h. Doses may need to be increased gradually, and some children may need continuous infusion; a starting dose of 0.05 mg/kg/hr given as an infusion is increased gradually as the need of the child changes. Naloxone is rarely needed but should be immediately available to reverse the effect of morphine, if necessary; if needed for an airway crisis, it should be given in a dose of 0.1 mg/kg up to a total of 2 mg, either intramuscularly or intravenously. For patients on assisted respiration who require treatment of anxiety, midazolam is used as an intermittent intravenous bolus (dose of 0.04 mg/kg given by a slow push q4–6h) or as a continuous infusion. Intubated patients do not require opiates to be discontinued during the process of weaning from the ventilator. Benzodiazepine should be reduced to about half the dose over 24–72 hr before extubation; too rapid weaning from a benzodiazepine can lead to seizures.

Reconstruction and Rehabilitation. To ensure maximum cosmetic and functional outcome, occupational and physical therapy must begin on the day of admission, continue throughout the hospitalization, and, for some patients, continue after discharge. Physical rehabilitation involves body and limb positioning, splinting, exercises (active and passive movement), assistance with activities of daily living, and gradual ambulation. These measures maintain adequate joint and muscle activity with as normal a range of movement as possible after healing or reconstruction. Pressure therapy is necessary to reduce hypertrophic scar formation; a variety of prefabricated and custom-made garments are available for use in different body areas for prevention of hypertrophic scarring. These custom-made garments deliver consistent pressure on scarred areas; they shorten the time of scar maturation and decrease the thickness of the scar as well as the redness and associated itching. Continued adjustments to scarred areas (scar release, grafting, rearrangement) and multiple minor cosmetic surgical procedures are necessary to optimize long-term function and to improve appearance. Replacement of areas of alopecia and scarring has been achieved using tissue expander techniques.

SCHOOL RE-ENTRY AND LONG-TERM OUTCOME. It is best for the child to return to school immediately after discharge. Occasionally, a child may need to attend a few half days (because of rehabilitation needs). However, it is important for the child to return to his or her normal routine of attending school and being with peers. Planning for return to home and school often requires a school re-entry program that is individualized to each child's needs. For a school-aged child, planning for the return to school occurs simultaneously with planning for discharge. The hospital schoolteacher contacts the local school and plans the program with school faculty, nurses, social workers, recreational/child life therapists, and rehabilitation therapists. This team should work with students and staff to ease anxiety, answer questions, and provide information. Burns and scars evoke fears in those who are not familiar with this type of injury and can result in a tendency to withdraw from or reject the burned child. A school re-entry program should be appropriate to a child's development and changing educational needs.

Major advances have made it possible to save lives of children with massive burns; whereas some children have had lingering physical difficulties, most have a satisfactory quality of life. The comprehensive burn care that includes experienced multidisciplinary aftercare plays an important role in recovery.

Special Situations

ELECTRICAL BURNS. There are three types of electrical burns. *Minor electrical burns* usually occur as a result of biting on an extension cord. These injuries produce localized burns to the mouth, which usually involve the upper and lower lip that come in contact with the extension cord. The injury may involve or spare the corners of the mouth. Because these are nonconductive injuries (do not extend beyond the site of injury), hospital admission is not necessary and care is focused on the area of the injury visible in the mouth. Treatment with topical antibiotic creams is sufficient until the patient is seen in a burn unit outpatient department or by a plastic surgeon.

A more serious category of electrical burn is the *high-tension electrical wire burn*, for which children need to be admitted for observation regardless of the extent of the surface area burn. Deep muscle injury is usual and cannot be readily assessed initially. These injuries result from high voltage (>1,000 V) and occur particularly at high-voltage installations, such as electric power stations or railroads; youngsters climb an electric pole and touch an electric box in curiosity or accidentally touch the high-tension electric wire. Such injuries have a mortality rate of 3–15% for children who arrive at the hospital for treatment. Survivors have a high rate of morbidity, including major limb amputations. Points of entry of current through the skin and the exit site show characteristic features consistent with current density and heat. The majority of entrance wounds involve the upper extremity, with small exit wounds in the lower extremity. The electrical path from entrance to exit takes the shortest distance between the two points and may produce injury in any organ or tissue in the path of the current. Multiple exit wounds in some patients attest to the possibility of several electrical pathways in the body, placing virtually any structure in the body at risk (Table 62–3). Damage to abdominal viscera, thoracic structures, and the nervous system in areas remote from obvious extremity injury occurs and must be sought, particularly in multiple current pathway injury or injury in which the victim falls from a high pole. Sometimes arcing occurs and results in a concurrent flame burn and clothing fire. Cardiac abnormalities manifested by ventricular fibrillation or cardiac arrest are common; patients with high-tension electrical injury need cardiac monitoring until they are stable and have been fully assessed. Renal damage from deep muscle necrosis and subsequent myoglobinuria is another complication; such patients need a forced alkaline diuresis to minimize renal damage. Aggressive removal of all dead and devitalized tissue, even with risk of functional loss, remains the key to effective management of the electrically damaged extremity. Early débridement will facilitate early closure of the wound. Damaged major vessels must be isolated and buried in a viable muscle to prevent exposure. Survival depends on the immediate intensive care, whereas a functional result depends on long-term care and delayed reconstructive surgery.

Lightning burns occur when high-voltage current directly strikes a person (most dangerous) or when the current strikes the ground or an adjacent (in-contact) object. A step voltage burn is observed when lightning strikes the ground and travels up one leg and down the other leg (the path of least resistance). Lightning burns are dependent on the current path, the type of clothing, the presence of metal, and cutaneous moisture. Entry, exit, and path lesions are possible; the prognosis is poorest for lesions of the head or legs. Internal organ injury along the path is common and does not relate to the severity of the cutaneous burn. Linear burns are in the locations where sweat is present and are usually first or second degree. Feathering or an arborescent pattern is characteristic of lightning injury. Lightning may ignite clothing or produce serious cutaneous burns from heated metal in the clothing. Internal complications of lightning burns include cardiac arrest caused by asystole, transient hypertension, premature ventricular contractions, ventricular fibrillation, and myocardial ischemia. Most severe cardiac complications resolve if the patient is supported with cardiopulmonary resuscitation (see Chapter 57.1). CNS complications include cerebral edema, hemorrhage, seizures, mood changes, depression, and lower extremity paralysis. Rhabdomyolysis and myoglobinuria (with possible renal failure) also occur.

RENAL FAILURE IN BURN INJURY (also see Chapters 57.5 and 525). Renal failure in burn injury is best classified in relation to the time of onset after the burn injury. Most cases present as a nonoliguric renal failure; careful fluid and electrolyte

TABLE 62–3. **Electrical Injury: Clinical Considerations**

	Clinical Manifestations	Management
General		Extrication; ABCs of resuscitation; immobilize spine History: voltage, type of current CBC with platelets, electrolytes, BUN, creatinine, glucose
Cardiac	Dysrhythmias: asystole, ventricular fibrillation, sinus tachycardia, sinus bradycardia, PVC, PAC, conduction defects, atrial fibrillation, ST-T wave changes	Treat dysrhythmias Cardiac monitor, ECG, and chest x-ray film with suspected thoracic injury CPK with isoenzymes if indicated
Pulmonary	Respiratory arrest, acute respiratory distress, aspiration syndrome	Protect and maintain airway Mechanical ventilation if indicated, chest x-ray film, ABG level
Renal	Acute renal failure, myoglobinuria	Aggressive fluid management unless CNS injury Maintain adequate urine output > 1 mL/kg/hr Consider CVP or pulmonary artery pressure monitoring Urine myoglobin, urinalysis, BUN, creatinine
Neurologic	Immediate: loss of consciousness, motor paralysis, visual disturbances, amnesia, agitation; intracranial hematoma Secondary: pain, paraplegia, brachial plexus injury, SIADH, autonomic disturbances, cerebral edema Delayed: paralysis, seizures, headache, peripheral neuropathy	Treat seizures Fluid restriction if indicated Consider spine x-ray films, especially cervical CT scan of brain if indicated
Cutaneous/oral	Oral commissure burns, tongue and dental injuries; skin burns resulting from ignition of clothes, entrance and exit burns, and arc burns	Search for entrance/exit wound Treat cutaneous burns; tetanus status Plastic surgery or ENT consult if needed
Abdominal	Viscus perforation and solid organ damage; ileus; abdominal injury rare without visible abdominal burns	NG tube if airway compromise or ileus SGOT, SGPT, amylase, BUN, creatinine, CT radiographs as indicated
Musculoskeletal	Compartment syndrome from subcutaneous necrosis limb edema and deep burns Long bone fractures, spine injuries	Follow for compartment syndrome X-ray films and orthopedic/general surgery consultations as indicated
Ocular	Visual changes, optic neuritis, cataracts, extraocular muscle paresis	Ophthalmology consultation as indicated

ABC, Airway, breathing, circulation; CBC, complete blood cell count; BUN, blood urea nitrogen; PVC, premature ventricular contractions; PAC, premature atrial contractions; ECG, electrocardiogram; CPK, creatinine phosphokinase; ABG, arterial blood gas; CNS, central nervous system; CVP, central venous pressure; CT, computed tomography; SIADH, syndrome of inappropriate secretion of antidiuretic hormone; ENT, ear, nose, and throat; NG, nasogastric; SGOT, serum glutamate oxaloacetate transaminase (aspartate aminotransferase); SGPT, serum glutamate pyruvate transaminase (alanine aminotransferase).
From Hall ML, Sills RM: Electrical and lightning injuries. In Barkin RM (editor): Pediatric Emergency Medicine. St. Louis, CV Mosby, 1997, p 484.

monitoring are critical. Special considerations of renal failure in a child with burn injury include the initial phase of capillary leak, making resuscitation difficult; severe catabolic stress with increased risk of hyperkalemia; and rapid development of azotemia. Such children require high caloric and protein intake to prevent catabolic stress and promote wound healing.

Renal failure may occur early or late, after 1–3 wk. *Early* renal failure may occur immediately post burn if late resuscitation with subsequent hypovolemia occurs (acute tubular necrosis) or if severe pigment nephropathy (hemoglobinuria with burn injury in an enclosed space or myoglobinuria secondary to deep muscle injury or post escharotomy) develops. This is associated with early maximal catabolic stress, and frequently dialysis is necessary to sustain the circulation in the presence of marked capillary leak and to provide sufficient calories and protein to minimize the catabolic stress. *Late* renal failure may result from sepsis or drug toxicity. At this time there is less catabolic stress, and standard indications for dialysis apply.

ABLS Advanced Burn Life Support Course Providers Manual. Chicago, American Burn Association, 2000.

Brigham PA, McLoughlin E: Burn incidence and medical care use in the United States: Estimates, trends, and data sources. *J Burn Care Rehabil* 1996;17:95–107.

Carman C, Change B: Treadmill injuries to the upper extremity in pediatric patients. *Ann Plast Surg* 2001;47:15–19.

Goldstein AM, Weber JM, Sheridan RL: Femoral venous access is safe in burned children: An analysis of 224 catheters. *J Pediatr* 1996;130:442–6.

Heimbach D, Luterman A, Burke JF, et al: Artificial dermis for major burns: A multi-center randomized clinical trial. *Ann Surg* 1988;208:313–20.

Herndon DM, Barrow RE, Broemeling LD, et al: Effect of recombinant human growth hormone on the donor site healing in severely burned patients. *Ann Surg* 1990;212:424–9.

Herndon DN, Hart DW, Wolf SE, et al: Reversal of catabolism by beta-blockade after severe burns. *N Engl J Med* 2001;345:1223–9.

Injuries from fireworks in the United States. *Morbid Mortal Wkly Rep MMWR* 2000;49:545–6.

Istre GR, McCoy MA, Osborn L, et al: Deaths and injuries from house fires. *N Engl J Med* 2001;344:1911–16.

Milner S, Hodgetts T, Rylah L: The burns calculator: A simple proposed guide for fluid resuscitation. *Lancet* 1993;342:1089–91.

Monafo W: Initial management of burns. *N Engl J Med* 1996;335:1581–6.

Moore P, Blackeney P, Broemeling L, Portman S: Psychologic adjustment after childhood burn injuries as predicted by personality traits. *J Burn Care Rehabil* 1993;14:80–2.

Musgrave MA, Fingland MD, et al: The use of inhaled nitric oxide as adjuvant therapy in patients with burn injuries and respiratory failure. *J Burn Care Rehabil* 2000;21:551–7.

Remensnyder JP: Acute electrical injuries. In Martyn JAJ (editor): *Acute Management of the Burned Patient.* Philadelphia, WB Saunders, 1990, pp 66–86.

Ryan CM, Schoenfeld DA, Thorpe WP, et al: Objective estimates of probability of death from burn injuries. *N Engl J Med* 1998;338:362–66.

Sheridan RL, Hurford WE, Kacmarek RM, et al: Inhaled nitric oxide in burn patients with respiratory failure. *J Trauma* 1997;42:629–34.

Sheridan RL, Hinson M, et al: Long term outcomes of children surviving massive burns. *JAMA* 2000;283:69–73.

Sheridan RL, Remensnyder JP, et al: Current expectations for survival in pediatric burns. *Arch Pediatr Adolesc Med* 2000;154:245–49.

Sheridan RL, Tompkins RG, Burke JF: Management of burn wounds with prompt excision and immediate closure. *J Intensive Care Med* 1994;9:6–17.

Strongin J, Hales CA: Pulmonary disorders in the burn patient. In Martyn JAJ (editor): *Acute Management of the Burned Patient.* Philadelphia, WB Saunders, 1990, pp 25–45.

Volinsky J, Hanson J, Lustig J: Lightning burns. *Arch Pediatr Adolesc Med* 1994;148:529–30.

Walker A: Emergency department management of house fire burns and carbon monoxide poisoning in children. *Curr Opin Pediatr* 1996;8:239–42.

Weber J: Epidemiology of infections and strategies for control. In Carrougher AJ (editor): *Burn Care and Therapy.* St. Louis, CV Mosby, 1998, pp 185–211.

Chapter 63
Cold Injuries
Alia Y. Antoon and Mary K. Donovan

The involvement of children and youth in snowmobiling, mountain climbing, winter hiking, and skiing places them at risk for cold injury. Cold injury may produce either local tissue damage, with the injury pattern depending on exposure to damp cold (frostnip, immersion foot, or trench foot); dry cold (which leads to local frostbite); or generalized systemic effects (hypothermia).

Pathophysiology. Ice crystals may form between or within cells, interfering with the sodium pump and lead to rupture of cell membranes. Further damage may result from clumping of red blood cells or platelets, causing microembolism or thrombosis. Blood may be shunted away from an affected area by secondary neurovascular responses to the cold injury; this shunting often further damages an injured part while improving perfusion of other tissues. The spectrum of injury ranges from mild to severe and reflects the result of structural and functional disturbance in small blood vessels, nerves, and skin.

Etiology. In general, body heat may be lost by conduction (wet clothing, contact with metal or other solid conducting objects), convection (wind chill), evaporation, and radiation. Susceptibility to cold injury may be increased by dehydration, alcohol or drug use, substance abuse, impaired consciousness, exhaustion, hunger, anemia, impaired circulation due to cardiovascular disease, and sepsis, as well as in very young or aged persons.

Hypothermia occurs when the body can no longer sustain normal core temperature by physiologic mechanisms such as vasoconstriction, shivering, muscle contraction, and nonshivering thermogenesis. When shivering ceases, the body is unable to maintain its core temperature; when the body core temperature falls below 35°C, the syndrome of hypothermia occurs. Wind chill, wet or inadequate clothing, or other factors increase local injury and may cause dangerous hypothermia, even in the presence of an ambient temperature that is not lower than 17–20°C (50–60°F).

Clinical Manifestations

FROSTNIP. This results in the presence of firm, cold white areas on the face, ears, or extremities. Blistering and peeling may occur over the next 24–72 hr, occasionally leaving mild increased hypersensitivity to cold for some days or weeks. Treatment consists of warming the area with an unaffected hand or warm object before the lesion reaches a stage of stinging or aching and before numbness supervenes.

IMMERSION FOOT (TRENCH FOOT). This occurs in cold weather when the feet remain in damp or wet, poorly ventilated boots. The feet become cold, numb, pale, edematous, and clammy. Tissue maceration and infection are likely, and prolonged autonomic disturbance is common. This autonomic disturbance leads to increased sweating, pain, and hypersensitivity to temperature changes, which may persist for years. The treatment is largely prophylactic and consists of using well-fitting, insulated, waterproof, nonconstricting footwear. Once damage has occurred, patients must choose clothing and footwear that are more appropriate, dry, and well fitting. The disturbance in skin integrity is managed by keeping the affected area dry and well ventilated and preventing or treating infection. Only supportive measures are possible for control of autonomic symptoms.

FROSTBITE. With frostbite, initial stinging or aching of the skin progresses to cold, hard, white anesthetic and numb areas.

On rewarming, the area becomes blotchy, itchy, and often red, swollen, and painful. The injury spectrum ranges from complete normality to extensive tissue damage, even gangrene, if early relief is not obtained.

Treatment consists of warming the damaged area. It is important not to cause further damage by attempting to rub the area with ice or snow; initial warming as in frostnip may be tried. The area may be warmed against an unaffected hand, abdomen, or axilla while in transfer to a facility where more rapid warming with a water bath is possible. If the skin becomes painful and swelling occurs, anti-inflammatory agents are helpful, and an analgesic agent is necessary. Freeze and re-thaw cycles are most likely to cause permanent tissue injury, and it may be necessary to delay definitive warming and apply only mild measures if the patient is required to walk on the damaged feet en route to definitive treatment. In the hospital, the affected area should be immersed in warm water (temperature approximately 42°C), being careful not to burn the anesthetized skin. Vasodilating agents, such as prazosin or phenoxybenzamine, may be helpful. Anticoagulants (heparin, dextran) have provided equivocal results; results of chemical and surgical sympathectomy have also been equivocal. Oxygen is of help only at high altitudes. Meticulous local care, prevention of infection, and keeping the rewarmed area dry, open, and sterile provide optimal results. Recovery can be complete, and prolonged observation with conservative therapy is justified before any excision or amputation of tissue is considered. Analgesia and maintenance of good nutrition are necessary throughout the prolonged waiting period.

HYPOTHERMIA. Hypothermia may occur in winter sports when injury, equipment failure, or exhaustion decreases the degree of exertion, particularly if sufficient attention is not paid to wind chill. Immersion in frozen bodies of water and wet wind chill rapidly produce hypothermia. As the core temperature of the body falls, an insidious onset of extreme lethargy, fatigue, incoordination, and apathy follows, followed by mental confusion, clumsiness, irritability, hallucinations, and finally bradycardia. A number of medical conditions, such as cardiac disease, diabetes mellitus, hypoglycemia, sepsis, β-blocking agent overdose, and substance abuse, may need to be considered in a differential diagnosis. The decrease in rectal temperature to less than 34°C (93°F) is the most helpful diagnostic feature. Hypothermia associated with near-drowning is discussed in Chapter 61.

Prevention is a high priority. Of extreme importance for those who participate in winter sports is wearing layers of warm clothing, gloves, socks within insulated boots that do not impede circulation, and a warm head covering, as well as applying adequate waterproofing and protecting against the wind. Thirty per cent of heat loss occurs from the head. Ample food and fluid need to be provided during exercise. Those who participate in sports should be alert to the presence of cold or numbing of body parts, particularly the nose, ears, and extremities, and they should review methods to produce local warming and know to seek shelter if they detect symptoms of local cold injury. Application of petrolatum (Vaseline) to nose and ears give certain protection against frostbite.

Treatment at the scene aims at prevention of further heat loss and early transport to adequate shelter. Dry clothing should be provided as soon as practical, and transport should be undertaken if the victim has a pulse. If no pulse is detected at the initial review, cardiopulmonary resuscitation is indicated (see Chapters 57.1 and 61; Fig. 63–1). During transfer, jarring and sudden motion should be avoided, because these may cause ventricular arrhythmia. It is often difficult to attain a normal sinus rhythm during hypothermia.

If the patient is conscious, mild muscle activity should be encouraged and a warm drink offered. If the patient is unconscious, external warming should be initially undertaken using

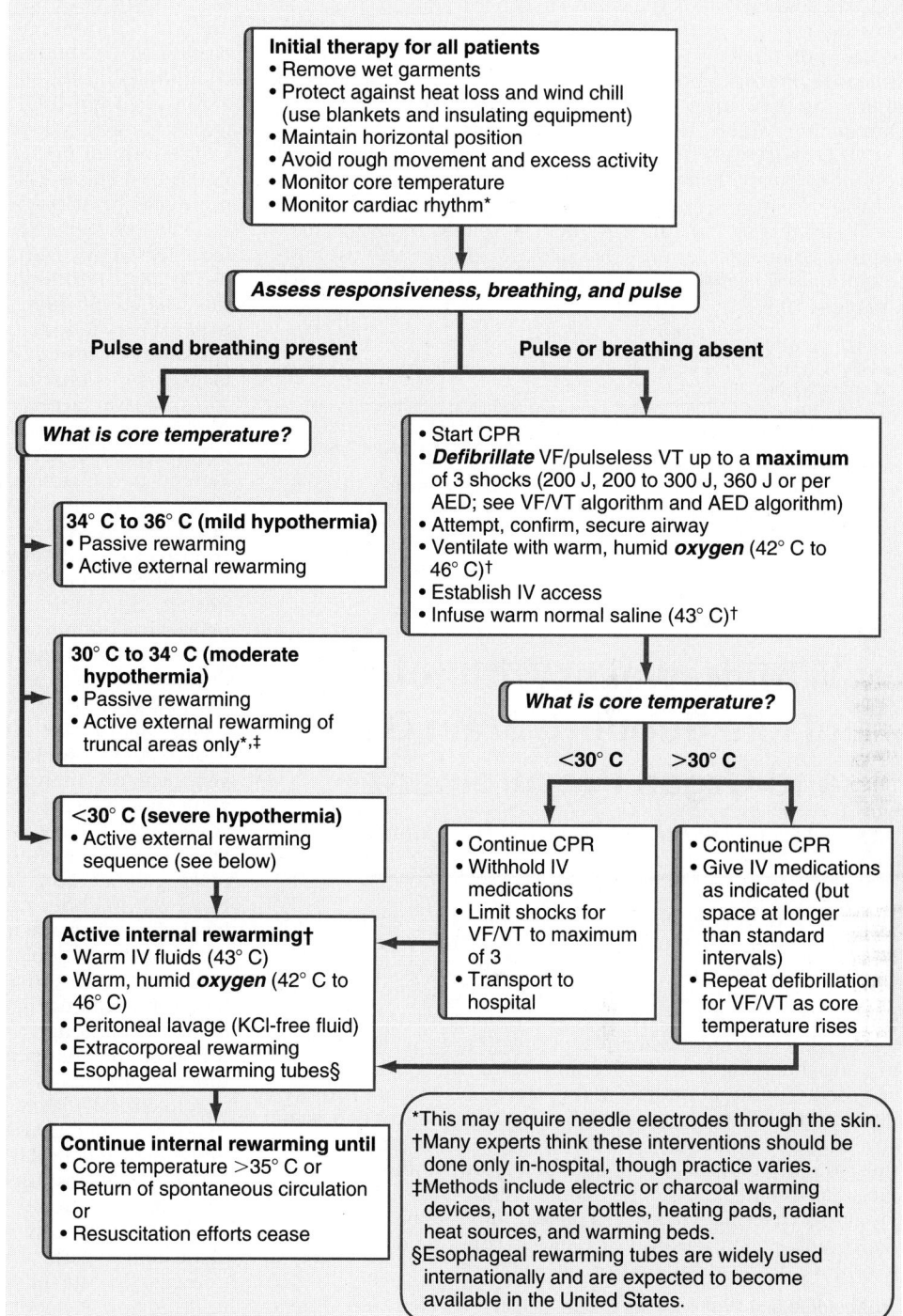

Initial therapy for all patients
- Remove wet garments
- Protect against heat loss and wind chill (use blankets and insulating equipment)
- Maintain horizontal position
- Avoid rough movement and excess activity
- Monitor core temperature
- Monitor cardiac rhythm*

Assess responsiveness, breathing, and pulse

Pulse and breathing present

What is core temperature?

34° C to 36° C (mild hypothermia)
- Passive rewarming
- Active external rewarming

30° C to 34° C (moderate hypothermia)
- Passive rewarming
- Active external rewarming of truncal areas only*,‡

<30° C (severe hypothermia)
- Active external rewarming sequence (see below)

Active internal rewarming†
- Warm IV fluids (43° C)
- Warm, humid *oxygen* (42° C to 46° C)
- Peritoneal lavage (KCl-free fluid)
- Extracorporeal rewarming
- Esophageal rewarming tubes§

Continue internal rewarming until
- Core temperature >35° C or
- Return of spontaneous circulation or
- Resuscitation efforts cease

Pulse or breathing absent

- Start CPR
- *Defibrillate* VF/pulseless VT up to a **maximum** of 3 shocks (200 J, 200 to 300 J, 360 J or per AED; see VF/VT algorithm and AED algorithm)
- Attempt, confirm, secure airway
- Ventilate with warm, humid *oxygen* (42° C to 46° C)†
- Establish IV access
- Infuse warm normal saline (43° C)†

What is core temperature?

<30° C

- Continue CPR
- Withhold IV medications
- Limit shocks for VF/VT to maximum of 3
- Transport to hospital

>30° C

- Continue CPR
- Give IV medications as indicated (but space at longer than standard intervals)
- Repeat defibrillation for VF/VT as core temperature rises

*This may require needle electrodes through the skin.
†Many experts think these interventions should be done only in-hospital, though practice varies.
‡Methods include electric or charcoal warming devices, hot water bottles, heating pads, radiant heat sources, and warming beds.
§Esophageal rewarming tubes are widely used internationally and are expected to become available in the United States.

FIGURE 63–1. Hypothermia treatment algorithm. VF = ventricular fibrillation; VT = ventricular tachycardia. (From American Heart Association: ECC guidelines. Part 8: Advanced challenges in resuscitation. Section 3: Special challenges in ECC. *Circulation* 2002;102:1229.)

blankets and a sleeping bag, often with snuggling with a warm companion to increase the efficiency of warming. On arrival at a treatment center, inhalation of warm, moist air or oxygen, heating pads, or thermal blankets should be used while a warming bath of 45–48°C (113–118°F) is prepared. Monitoring of serum chemistry values and an electrocardiogram are necessary until the core temperature rises above 35°C and can be stabilized. Control of fluid, pH, blood pressure, and oxygen all are necessary in the early phases of the warming period and resuscitation. In severe hypothermia there may be a combined respiratory and metabolic acidosis. Hypothermia may falsely elevate pH; nonetheless most recommend warming the arterial blood gas specimen to 37°C before analysis and considering the result as in a

normothermic patient. In patients with marked abnormalities, warming measures such as gastric or colonic irrigation with warm saline or peritoneal dialysis may be considered, but the effectiveness of these measures to treat hypothermia is unknown. In accidental deep hypothermia (core temperature 28°C) with circulatory arrest, rewarming with cardiopulmonary bypass may be lifesaving for previously healthy young individuals.

CHILBLAIN (PERNIO). Chilblain (pernio) is a form of cold injury in which erythematous, vesicular, or ulcerative lesions occur. The lesions are presumed to be of a vascular or vasoconstrictive origin. They are often itchy and may be painful and result in swelling and scabbing. The lesions are most often found at the ears, tips of fingers, and toes and on exposed areas of the legs. The lesions last for 1–2 wk but may persist longer. *Treatment* consists of prophylaxis—avoiding prolonged chilling and protecting potentially susceptible areas with a cap, gloves, and stockings. Prazosin and phenoxybenzamine may be helpful in improving circulation if this is a recurrent problem. For significant itching, local corticosteroid preparations may be helpful.

COLD-INDUCED FAT NECROSIS (PANNICULITIS). This common, usually benign injury occurs on exposure to cold air, snow, or ice and is manifested in exposed (or, less often, covered) surfaces as red (or, less often, purple to blue) macular, papular, or nodular lesions. *Treatment* is with nonsteroidal anti-inflammatory agents. The lesions may last 10 days to 3 wk. (See Chapter 650.)

Berkow R (editor): Cold injury. In *The Merck Manual of Diagnosis and Therapy*. Rahway, NJ, Merck, Sharp, & Dohme, 1992.
Britt LD, Dascombe WH, Rodriguez A: New horizons in management of hypothermia and frostbite injury. *Surg Clin North Am* 1991;71:345–70.
Shephard RJ: Metabolic adaptations to exercise in the cold: An update. *Sports Med* 1993;16:266–89.
Walpoth BH, Walpoth-Aslan BN, Mattle HP, et al: Outcome of survivors of accidental deep hypothermia and circulatory arrest treated with extracorporeal blood warming. *N Engl J Med* 1997;337:1500–5.

Chapter 64

Withdrawal or Withholding of Life Support, Brain Death, and Organ Procurement

Lorry R. Frankel and Lawrence H. Mathers

The goal of treatment of children with a life-threatening illness is survival with minimal residual injury or cure. When a physician realizes that further treatment is futile in not preventing death and perhaps harmful to a patient, the family should be compassionately informed. It is very important to determine that further treatment will not avoid death and that it may even prolong the dying process. Decisions about such futility should be based on mutual understanding about the prognosis for living, quality of life, and human dignity. The practices of a pediatric intensive care unit (PICU) with patients and families facing these tragic circumstances should be consistent and reflect the most up-to-date knowledge about a disease, its care, and its prognosis (see Chapter 54). If a patient fulfills brain death criteria, compassionate medical care should continue during efforts to remove the dead patient from life support.

Withholding and Withdrawing of Life Support. Two basically different groups of patients die in a PICU: (1) previously healthy children who have recently experienced a catastrophic event (motor vehicle injury, near-drowning, or a serious infection); and (2) children with a severe chronic illness that has become terminal (cystic fibrosis, severe inborn errors of metabolism, major congenital malformations). For these latter children and their families, it may be possible to provide appropriate terminal care in a more comfortable setting than the hospital, such as the home or hospice (see Chapter 38).

The decision to provide palliative care needs to involve the primary and critical care physicians, the child (when appropriate), and parents, social services, and clergy (if appropriate) to come to an understanding that further intervention will not improve the outcome. The management of a dying patient should include consideration of resuscitation measures ("code status"), comfort care, and symptom management (pain, nausea, anxiety, dyspnea). In the majority of cases involving children, families and physicians reach an agreement about limitation of care without involvement of the legal system or ethics committees.

Although not fulfilling the criteria of death, some children may have a very limited quality of continuing life. The most severe form of perpetual debilitation is the *persistent vegetative state* (PVS). This is a state of perpetual unconsciousness in which there may be neurologic responsiveness to some external stimuli. PVS exists when there has been lack of neurologic recovery for at least 6 mo, with preservation of only the autonomic nervous system, resulting in the maintenance of vital signs (heart rate, blood pressure, respirations, and temperature). Such patients may require significant nursing care, including feeding (usually via gastrostomy), bathing, assistance with bowel and bladder function, skin care to prevent pressure ulcers (bed sores), airway access via a tracheotomy, and passive range of motion exercises to minimize joint contractures. These children may be cared for at home or in long-term care nursing facilities. Patients in PVS are susceptible to infections, and death usually occurs as a result of pneumonia, urinary tract infection, or complications of a skin lesion. After months or years of caring for a child in PVS, a family may decide to limit various treatment modalities after careful consideration of the risks and benefits of further interventions for the child. These children may have neocortical but not whole brain death as the brainstem continues to function. Legally they are not brain dead and thus are not dead.

Withdrawal of support represents cessation of medical treatment and support already being provided to patients. This should be the standard in brain dead children. It must be made very clear to a family that as life support is withdrawn from a child who is not brain dead but is dependent on this treatment, the outcome is most likely to be death. In practice, withdrawing therapy or care that has already been instituted is more difficult than making the decision not to institute a therapeutic intervention. However, in either case, the decision not to provide a certain level of care is made in the context in which provision of such care would only prolong an inevitable death, perhaps involving additional pain and suffering. Legally there is no difference between not initiating a therapy (withholding) or withdrawing a therapy. Although there is little moral distinction between the provision of ventilator support (and other highly technical forms of care) and the provision of artificial hydration and nutrition to critically ill patients, most clinicians find it more difficult to advocate withdrawal of the latter than to recommend withdrawing mechanical ventilation or inotropic drugs.

One of the most frightening possibilities is represented by the "locked-in-syndrome," wherein outward signs of responsiveness are lacking, owing to paralysis, muscular dysfunction, or acute neurologic insult, but where consciousness persists, unbeknownst to the observers. This syndrome can occur with injuries to the lower brainstem, sparing the neocortex, and should be suspected and ruled out before any definitive pronouncement of neurologic unresponsiveness is made, especially if this diagnosis likely will lead to withdrawal of support and death of the patient.

Brain Death. Criteria to determine brain death for adult and pediatric patients have been established and are accepted by most states (Table 64–1). Death is defined as irreversible cessation of circulatory and respiratory functions or irreversible cessation of all functions of the entire brain, including the brainstem. Guidelines for assessing brain death in children of different ages also have been established; premature or newborn infants require a longer period of observation than older children or adults (Box 64–1).

The diagnosis of brain death is established once the cause of the coma is determined and the possibility of recovery of any

TABLE 64–1. Diagnosis of Brain Death

Brain Death Criteria	Evaluated by

Prerequisites
1. A recognized cause of coma, sufficient to explain the irreversible cessation of all brain function
2. Potentially reversible causes of coma must be excluded:
  a. Sedatives and neuromuscular blocking drugs
  b. Hypothermia
  c. Metabolic and endocrine disturbances:
    Severe electrolyte disturbances
    Severe hypo- or hyperglycemia
  d. Uncontrolled hypotension
  e. Surgically remediable intracranial conditions
  f. Any other sign that suggests a potentially reversible cause of coma
	History, clinical examination, laboratory, technical investigations

Clinical Evaluation 1. Absence of higher brain function	Lack of consciousness, voluntary movement or responsiveness except for spinal reflexes (stimuli applied to any body region may not elicit motor response within cranial nerve distribution); preferably test in a cranial (trigeminal) dermatome rather than a spinal dermatome; no decorticate or decerebrate posturing, no convulsions

2. Absence of brainstem function
  a. Absence of sympathetic and parasympathetic regulation of the pupils
  b. Disruption of the pathways controlling eye movement in the brainstem
 	
  c. Disruption of afferent trigeminal and efferent facial nerve pathways
  d. Disruption of the afferent and efferent pathways of cranial nerves IX and X in the medulla oblongata
  e. Absence of vagal efferent activity
 	
  f. Disruption of respiratory control centers of the medulla oblongata
	Pupils in midposition or dilated showing neither direct nor indirect reaction to light
	Absence of spontaneous eye movement, absence of reaction to injection of iced water into the ear (vestibulo-ocular reflex), absence of doll's eye phenomenon (oculocephalic reflexes)
	Absence of blink response to (careful) corneal stimulation
	Absence of gag response to stimulation of posterior pharynx, absence of cough on suctioning of the trachea
	No significant increase of heart rate on administration of intravenous atropine or on pressure applied to the eyeballs (oculocardiac reflex)
	No respiratory movement (as assessed by observation ± capnography) at a $Paco_2$ above a set limit during a standardized apnea testing

"Confirmatory" Tests 1. Confirmation of absence of higher brain function 2. Confirmation of complete infarction of the brain and brainstem by confirmation of absence of blood flow	Electrocerebral silence on EEG during at least 30 min Four-vessel contrast angiography or radionuclide imaging
Observation Confirmation of irreversibility	Observation during a set time, ± repeat formal physical examination and confirmatory tests

From Lutz-Dettinger N, de Jaeger A, Kerremans I: Care of the potential pediatric organ donor. Pediatr Clin North Am 2001;48:715–49.

brain function is eliminated. Brain death results from permanent cessation of all brain function in the absence of any factor or agent that could cloud accurate assessment of brain function. Physical examinations by two physicians must demonstrate loss of brainstem responses and include an apnea test, in which the patient is hyperoxygenated and then removed from the ventilator or placed on continuous positive airway pressure. The $Paco_2$ is allowed to rise to a level of 60 mm Hg or greater

---

BOX 64–1. Age-Specific Criteria for Brain Death*

Children 1 wk–2 mo of age: fulfillment of the clinical criteria listed in Table 64–1 in two separate examinations at least 48 hr apart, or one clinical examination followed by an isoelectric EEG at least 48 hr later

Children 2 mo–1 yr: fulfillment of the clinical criteria described in Table 64–1 in two separate examinations, at least 24 hr apart, or one clinical examination followed by an isoelectric EEG or negative results of a cerebral blood flow study at least 24 hr later

Children > 1 yr: fulfillment of the clinical criteria described in Table 64–1 in two separate examinations at least 12 hr apart

---

EEG = electroencephalogram.

*Criteria for brain death in infants younger than 1 wk of age have not been delineated but should be at least as stringent as for those 1 wk–2 mo of age. It is often very difficult to diagnose brain death in premature infants; the wait period should be at least 72 hr. The standard wait period for adults is 6 hr. Some believe the wait period may be shortened if confirmatory testing is employed. Once brain death is determined, that is the medical time of death.

(usually > 10 min) while appropriate oxygenation is maintained. Laboratory tests also are required to establish the cause of the coma and to preclude toxic, metabolic, paralytic, or sedative causes. Electroencephalograms (demonstrating electrical cerebral silence), cerebral perfusion studies (demonstrating absent four-vessel blood flow to the whole brain by contrast angiography), and intracranial pressure monitoring may be helpful in convincing the parents that their child is brain dead and in facilitating the opportunities for organ donation or discontinuation of life support. Additional ancillary tests include radionuclide angiography, Doppler ultrasonography, brainstem evoked potentials, and xenon CT scans. If the prerequisites in Table 64–1 are fulfilled, no confirmatory tests are legally needed.

Brain death is equivalent to cardiorespiratory death, and a child should be considered legally dead at the time brain death criteria are fulfilled. This determination is crucial to the process of organ procurement that requires harvesting heart, lung, liver, or bowel from a donor whose heart is beating. Despite increasing acceptance of organ donation in the United States, fewer than 20% of eligible donors become organ donors. This results in the death of several thousand potential organ recipients each year while awaiting transplantation.

Organ Procurement (see Chapter 60). In the United States there are more than 250 hospitals offering solid organ transplants and at least 75 regional organizations that monitor organ availability and try to match donors with available organs. Every major metropolitan center has its own such organization or network. The number of pediatric transplant centers is considerably smaller. If questions arise about organ transplantation, a 24-hr telephone hotline is maintained at 1-800-355-7427.

When the diagnosis of brain death has been made and the family wishes to pursue organ donation, a transplant donor network should be contacted to assist in the process. A procurement coordinator generally assumes responsibility for the donation process, including family discussions, determining arrangements and logistics, obtaining consent forms, making arrangements for appropriate laboratory tests, contacting various transplant centers to make arrangements for organ retrieval, and checking on recipient lists to match the organs to the patient with the highest priority. The coordinator is able to provide the donor's family long-term follow-up about organ placement; many grieving families find this to be very helpful in dealing with their loss. Most donor organizations assume full financial responsibility for the procurement process and the donated organs.

DuBois J: Non-heart beating organ donation: A defense of the required determination of death. *J Law Med Ethics* 1999;27:126–36.

Flowers WM Jr: Accuracy of clinical evaluation in the determination of brain death. *South Med J* 2000;2:203–6.

Herdman R, Beauchamp TL, Potts JT: The Institute of Medicine's report on non-heart beating organ transplantation. *Kennedy Inst Ethics J* 1998;1:89–90.

Lutz-Dettinger N, de Jaeger A, Kerremans I: Care of the potential pediatric organ donor. *Pediatr Clin North Am* 2001;48:715–49.

Mejia RE, Pollack MM: Variability in brain death determination practices in children. *JAMA* 1995;274:550–53.

Pasquerella R, Smith S, Ladd R: Infants, the dead donor rule, and anencephalic organ donation: Should the rules be changed? *Med Law* 2001;20:417–23.

Staworn D, Lewison L, Marks J, et al: Brain death in pediatric intensive care unit patients: Incidence, primary diagnosis, and the clinical occurrence of Turner's triad. *Crit Care Med* 1994;22:1301–5.

Task Force for the Determination of Brain Death in Children: Guidelines for the determination of brain death in children. *Pediatrics* 1987;80:298–300.

Chapter 65

Anesthesia and Perioperative Care *Randall C. Wetzel*

The perioperative period is a particularly dangerous time for infants and children. Potent drugs are used to blunt physiologic responses to what would be otherwise life-threatening trauma (e.g., surgery). Anesthesia is necessary on humane grounds. In addition, the appropriate application of anesthetic principles decreases mortality from surgery and painful procedures and enhances the child's ability to survive the surgical experience. Intraoperatively, the anesthesiologist is responsible for providing analgesia as well as physiologic and metabolic stability (Box 65–1). These goals are facilitated by a good preanesthesia history (Box 65–2). The increased risk for morbidity and mortality in the perioperative period demands the utmost vigilance. The risk may be increased in certain disease states (Table 65–1). The primary purpose of general anesthesia is to suppress the conscious perception of, and physiologic response to, noxious stimuli and to render the patient unconscious.

GENERAL ANESTHESIA

Analgesia

Providing analgesia perioperatively, and for procedures, is a major responsibility and functions within a spectrum of care (Box 65–3). Techniques exist to provide profound pain relief during operative procedures for even the most critically ill

---

BOX 65–1. The Goals of Anesthesia

1. Analgesia
2. Amnesia and decreased level of consciousness
3. Akinesia
4. Physiologic support and homeostatic management throughout the perioperative process
5. Vigilance

---

infants. Blunting the physiologic responses to painful stimuli inhibits the stress response and its multiple deleterious physiologic and metabolic consequences. The response to painful and stressful stimuli is a potent stimulus of the systemic inflammatory response syndrome (SIRS), which leads to increased catabolism, physiologic instability, and increased mortality. However, appropriate medication use, such as fentanyl anesthesia in neonates, reduces the incidence of postoperative bradycardia, hypotension, acidosis, and hypoglycemia.

Hypnosis and Amnesia

The blunting of consciousness (hypnosis) and conscious recall (amnesia) are crucial aspects of pediatric anesthesia care. Awareness of painful, anxiety-provoking, and stressful conditions for children is just as deleterious, physically and psychologically, as the painful procedures themselves. Management is aimed at blunting the fear and emotional response that surgery, painful procedures (bone marrow aspiration, lumbar punctures), and nonpainful but anxiety-provoking procedures (MRI, CT scans) can invoke. There are many drugs that provide anxiolysis, blunting of recall, and amnesia for such events (Table 65–2). Obtundation of consciousness may accompany the provision of analgesia. Altered consciousness can be induced by hypnotic and sedative agents without producing any analgesia; analgesia and obtunded consciousness are not synonymous. It is also possible to provide analgesia (local analgesia, spinal or epidural analgesia) without obtunding consciousness.

Sedation describes a medically induced state, which is a continuum between awake and general anesthesia (see Box 65–3). General anesthesia obtunds or ablates critical physiologic reflexes; the most important are airway protective reflexes: coughing, gagging, and swallowing. Cardiorespiratory reflexes are also obtunded with general anesthesia, and thus respiratory depression and hemodynamic compromise may occur. As sedation deepens toward general anesthesia, the loss of airway patency, the loss of airway protective reflexes, and the loss of cardiovascular stability occur. Light (minimal) sedation is anxiolysis without loss of these reflexes and airway patency. Deep sedation is when these reflexes are obtunded or lost (see Box 65–3). Adequate sedation in children may be accompanied by the actual or potential loss of vital reflexes. It is mandatory that those providing sedation for children be able to detect the transition into deep sedation and general anesthesia and be prepared to manage the child's airway and provide cardiorespiratory resuscitation if required.

Akinesia

Akinesia is the absence of movement and is necessary to ensure safe and adequate operative conditions and to provide ideal conditions for advanced and meticulous surgery. Akinesia is produced with muscle relaxants (see Table 65–2). These agents facilitate respiratory management in the perioperative period and in critically ill patients. The absence of movement is neither the absence of pain nor the presence of amnesia. Whenever

BOX 65–2. The Preanesthetic History

CHILD'S PREVIOUS ANESTHETIC AND SURGICAL PROCEDURES

Review anesthetic record for information about mask and endotracheal tube size, type and size of laryngoscope used, difficulties with mask ventilation or intubation; history of hyperthermia or acidosis

PERINATAL PROBLEMS (ESPECIALLY FOR INFANTS)

Need for prolonged hospitalization
Need for supplemental oxygen or intubation
History of apnea and bradycardia

OTHER MAJOR ILLNESSES AND HOSPITALIZATIONS

FAMILY HISTORY OF ANESTHETIC COMPLICATIONS, MALIGNANT HYPERTHERMIA, OR PSEUDOCHOLINESTERASE DEFICIENCY

RESPIRATORY PROBLEMS

Chronic exposure to environmental tobacco smoke
Obstructive apnea, breathing irregularities, or cyanosis (especially in infants younger than age 6 mo)
History of snoring or obstructive breathing pattern
Recent upper respiratory tract infection
Recurrent respiratory infections
Previous laryngotracheitis (croup)
Asthma or wheezing during respiratory infections

CARDIAC PROBLEMS

Murmurs
Dysrhythmia
Exercise intolerance
Syncope
Cyanosis

GASTROINTESTINAL PROBLEMS

Reflux and vomiting
Feeding difficulties
Failure to thrive
Liver disease

EXPOSURE TO EXANTHEMS OR POTENTIALLY INFECTIOUS PATHOGENS

NEUROLOGIC PROBLEMS

Seizures
Developmental delay

Neuromuscular diseases
Increased intracranial pressure

HEMATOLOGIC PROBLEMS

Anemia
Bleeding diathesis
Tumor
Immunocompromise
Prior blood transfusions and reactions

RENAL PROBLEMS

Renal insufficiency, oliguria, anuria
Fluid and electrolyte abnormalities

PSYCHOSOCIAL CONSIDERATIONS

Post-traumatic stress
Drug abuse, use of cigarettes or alcohol
Physical or sexual abuse
Family dysfunction
Previous traumatic medical and surgical experiences
Psychosis, anxiety, depression

GYNECOLOGIC CONSIDERATIONS

Sexual history (sexually transmitted diseases)
Possibility of pregnancy

CURRENT MEDICATIONS

Prior administration of corticosteroids

ALLERGIES

Drugs
Iodine
Latex products
Surgical tapes
Food allergies (especially soya and egg albumin)

DENTAL CONDITION (LOOSE OR CRACKED TEETH)

WHEN AND WHAT THE CHILD LAST ATE (ESPECIALLY IN EMERGENCY PROCEDURES)

---

neuromuscular blocking agents are used, analgesia and sedation should be provided.

Physiologic Support

The need for anesthesia increases the need to monitor and support physiologic integrity and homeostasis. Sedation and anesthesia have significant and potentially life-threatening physiologic consequences (see Table 65–2 and Box 65–3). The maintenance of adequate cardiorespiratory function, fluid management, electrolyte control, thermoregulation, and concern for all aspects of the child's health is critical during anesthesia.

Vigilance

Constant, critical attention by physicians who understand the changes in physiologic status and their implications is mandatory to provide safe perioperative care for all children. Careful attention to the child's preoperative condition is mandatory in minimizing the risk in perioperative care (see Box 65–2 and Table 65–1).

INDUCTION OF GENERAL ANESTHESIA

The goal of induction of general anesthesia is to rapidly achieve surgical anesthesia by using intravenous or, more commonly in children, inhalational induction agents. It is routine in children who are too young to tolerate establishing vascular access before the induction of anesthesia to induce anesthesia by inhalation of volatile anesthetics. In the operating room, a child is often accompanied by parents and placed on the operating room table. Before induction of anesthesia, monitors are placed on the child. These include a pulse oximeter, electrocardiogram (ECG) electrodes, and frequently a blood pressure cuff. The child is then cautiously introduced to the face mask, which contains a high gas flow, 5–7 L/min of oxygen, frequently mixed with nitrous oxide. Sixty to 90 sec of inhalation of nitrous oxide and oxygen induces a state of euphoria. The airway responses to inhalational anesthetics are now blunted, and sevoflurane or halothane can be introduced into the inhaled gas mixture. This leads to unconsciousness within 30–60 sec while the child continues to breathe spontaneously.

The child is now "asleep," and the parents can be asked to leave. An intravenous line is then started and comprehensive intraoperative monitoring initiated. Surgical anesthesia can be maintained by spontaneous ventilation with a mask; however, this is safe when the airway is secure and patent, the stomach is empty, and the child is older than 6 mo of age. Procedures over 1 hr are not usually performed with mask inhalational anesthesia. If these conditions are not met or if the surgeon needs to approach the airway (otolaryngologic procedures), securing the airway with an endotracheal intubation is required. Although endotracheal intubation can be performed under

TABLE 65–1. Specific Pediatric Diseases and Their Anesthetic Implications

Disease	Implications
Respiratory System	
Asthma	Intraoperative bronchospasm that may be severe
	Pneumothorax
	Optimal preoperative medical management essential; may require preoperative steroids
Difficult airway	May require special equipment and personnel
	Should be anticipated in children with dysmorphic features or acute airway obstruction as in epiglottitis or laryngotracheobronchitis or with airway foreign body
	Patients with Down syndrome may require evaluation of atlanto-occipital joint
	Patients with storage diseases may be at high risk
Bronchopulmonary dysplasia	Barotrauma with positive pressure ventilation
	Oxygen toxicity, pneumothorax a risk
Cystic fibrosis	Airway reactivity, bronchorrhea
	Risk of pneumothorax, pulmonary hemorrhage
	Atelectasis
	Assess for cor pulmonale
Sleep apnea	Must rule out pulmonary hypertension and cor pulmonale
	Requires careful postoperative observation for obstruction
Cardiac	Need for antibiotic prophylaxis for subacute bacterial endocarditis
	Use of air filters; careful purging of air from intravenous equipment
	Need to understand effects of various anesthetics on the hemodynamics of specific lesions
	Preload optimization and avoidance of hyperviscous states in cyanotic patients
	Possible need for preoperative evaluation of myocardial function and pulmonary vascular resistance
	Provide information about pacemaker function and ventricular device function
Hematologic	
Sickle cell	Possible need for simple or exchange transfusion based on preoperative Hgb and per cent Hgb S
	Importance of avoiding acidosis, hypoxemia, hypothermia, dehydration, and hyperviscosity states
Oncology	Pulmonary evaluation of patients who have received bleomycin, *bis*-chloroethyl-nitrosourea, chloroethyl-cyclohexyl-nitrosourea, methotrexate, or radiation to the chest
	Avoidance of high oxygen concentration
	Cardiac evaluation of patients who have received anthracyclines; risk of severe myocardial depression with volatile agents
	Potential for coagulopathy
Rheumatologic	Limited mobility of temporomandibular joint, cervical spine, arytenoid cartilages
	Requires careful preoperative evaluation
	May be difficult airway
Gastrointestinal	
Esophageal, gastric	Potential for reflux and aspiration
Liver	High overall morbidity and mortality in patients with hepatic dysfunction
	Altered metabolism of some drugs
	Potential for coagulopathy
Renal	Altered electrolyte and acid-base status
	Altered clearance of some drugs
	Need for preoperative dialysis in selected cases
	Succinylcholine to be used with extreme caution and only when serum potassium level is recently shown to be normal
Neurologic	
Seizure disorder	Avoid anesthetics that may lower threshold
	Ensure optimal control preoperatively
	Preoperative anticonvulsant levels
Increased intracranial pressure	Avoid agents that increase cerebral blood flow
	Avoid hypercarbia
Neuromuscular disease	Avoid depolarizing relaxants; at risk for hyperkalemia
	May be at risk for malignant hyperthermia
Developmental delay	May be uncooperative at induction
Psychiatric	Monoamine oxidase inhibitor (or cocaine) may interact with meperidine, resulting in hyperthermia and seizures
	Selective serotonin reuptake inhibitors may induce or inhibit various hepatic enzymes that may alter anesthetic drug clearance
	Illicit drugs may have adverse effects on cardiorespiratory homeostasis and may potentiate the action of anesthetics
Endocrine	
Diabetes	Greatest risk is unrecognized intraoperative hypoglycemia; if insulin is administered, monitor blood glucose level intraoperatively; must provide glucose and insulin with adjustment for fasting condition and surgical stress
Skin	
Burns	Difficult airway
	Risk of rhabdomyolysis and hyperkalemia from succinylcholine
	Fluid shifts
	Bleeding
	Coagulopathy
Immunologic	Retroviral drugs may inhibit benzodiazepine clearance
	Immunodeficiency requires careful infection control practices
	May require cytomegalovirus-negative blood products, irradiation, or leukofiltration
Metabolic	Careful assessment of glucose homeostasis in infants

Hgb = hemoglobin.

BOX 65–3. Definitions of Anesthesia Care

Monitored anesthesia care: Monitored anesthesia care is a specific anesthesia service in which an anesthesiologist has been requested to participate in the care of a patient undergoing a diagnostic or therapeutic procedure.

Monitored anesthesia care includes all aspects of anesthesia care: a preprocedure visit, intraprocedure care, and postprocedure anesthesia management.

During monitored anesthesia care, the anesthesiologist or a member of the anesthesia care team provides a number of specific services, which may include some or all of, but not limited to, the following:

- Monitoring of vital signs, maintenance of the patient's airway, and continual evaluation of vital functions
- Diagnosis and treatment of clinical problems that occur during the procedure
- Administration of sedatives, analgesics, hypnotics, anesthetic agents, or other medications as necessary to ensure patient safety and comfort
- Provision of other medical services as needed to accomplish the safe completion of the procedure
- Anesthesia care often includes the administration of medications for which the loss of normal protective reflexes or loss of consciousness is likely. Monitored anesthesia care refers to those clinical situations in which the patient remains able to protect the airway for the majority of the procedure. If, for an extended period of time, the patient is rendered unconscious and/or loses normal protective reflexes, this will be considered a general anesthetic.

Light sedation: Administration of anxiolysis and/or analgesia that obtunds consciousness but does not obtund normal protective reflexes (cough, gag, swallow, hemodynamic reflexes).

Deep sedation: Sedation that obtunds consciousness and normal protective reflexes or possesses a significant risk of blunting normal protective reflexes (cough, gag, swallow, hemodynamic reflexes).

General anesthesia: Administration of hypnosis, sedation, and analgesia that results in loss of normal protective reflexes.

Regional anesthesia: Induction of neural blockade (either central, neuraxial, epidural, or spinal; or peripheral nerve block, e.g., digital nerve block, brachial plexus block), which provides analgesia and is associated with regional motor blockade. Consciousness is not obtunded by regional anesthesia. Special expertise is required. Frequently, in children, anxiolysis and sedation is also necessary for this technique to be successful. Regional anesthesia (e.g., caudal epidural blockade) is used to supplement general anesthesia and provide postoperative analgesia.

Local anesthesia: Provision of analgesia by local infiltration of an appropriate anesthetic agent. Does not require the presence or involvement of anesthesiology, although an anesthesiologist *may* provide local anesthesia services.

No anesthesiologist: An anesthesiologist will not be involved in the care of the child in any way.

---

deep inhalational anesthesia with respiratory depression and obtunded cough and gag reflexes, the depth of anesthesia required to ablate airway reflexes is very close to that which induces hemodynamic instability. After anesthetic induction, intravenous access is secured and anesthesia is deepened with intravenous agents. Muscle relaxation with intravenous, nondepolarizing muscle relaxants is induced to facilitate endotracheal intubation. Succinylcholine is rarely used. After paralysis is induced, direct laryngoscopy and airway intubation can be performed. The correct endotracheal placement of the endotracheal tube is confirmed by direct laryngoscopy, end-tidal CO_2 measurement, endotracheal tube fogging, and bilateral, equal breath sounds during positive pressure ventilation.

After endotracheal intubation, spontaneous ventilation may be permitted, if muscle relaxants have either not been used or have worn off; however, it is routine to provide controlled mechanical ventilation. When the child is completely anesthetized, positioned for surgery, and hemodynamically stable and maintenance anesthesia is achieved, the surgery can begin.

Inhalational Anesthetics

General anesthesia may be induced and maintained by either inhalation or intravenous routes. Inhalational anesthetics include halothane, enflurane, isoflurane, sevoflurane, and desflurane. Halothane is the prototypical pediatric inhalational anesthetic agent; its use has decreased since the availability of isoflurane and sevoflurane. Enflurane is rarely used in children.

The minimal alveolar concentration (MAC) of an inhalational anesthetic is the alveolar concentration that provides sufficient depth of anesthesia for surgery in 50% of patients. For potent inhalational agents, the alveolar concentration of anesthetic reflects the arterial concentration of anesthetic in the blood perfusing the brain. Thus, the MAC level is an indication of anesthetic potency and is analogous to the ED_{50} of a drug. MAC is age dependent, is lower in premature infants than in full-term infants, and decreases from term through infancy to preadolescence. In adolescence, MAC again increases, falling thereafter. Inhalational anesthetic agents are poorly soluble in blood but rapidly equilibrate between alveolar gas and blood. The less soluble an anesthetic agent is in blood (low blood gas partition coefficient), the more rapid are both the induction and the emergence from inhalational anesthesia. Sevoflurane (0.69) and desflurane (0.42) have lower blood gas partition coefficients (the ratio of anesthetic concentration in the blood compared with the alveolar gas at equilibrium) than halothane (2.4).

Respiratory Effects

The advantages of inhalational anesthesia are rapid onset, rapid offset, convenient route for delivery and excretion (respiratory), and their ability to provide profound analgesia and amnesia. However, inhalational anesthetics are all airway irritants and, in low doses, can cause laryngospasm. All inhalational anesthetics depress ventilation in a dose-dependent manner. One MAC of inhalation anesthesia decreases minute ventilation by approximately 25%, resulting in smaller tidal volumes and decreased respiratory rates. Thus, expired CO_2 and $Paco_2$ increase. One MAC of anesthesia also decreases end-expiratory lung volume (EELV) to below functional residual capacity (FRC) by about 30%. Small lung volumes result in decreased lung compliance, increased total pulmonary resistance, increased work of breathing, and increased intrapulmonary arteriovenous shunting and a restrictive lung defect. Inhalational anesthetics also shift the CO_2 response curve to the right, thus decreasing, but not ablating, the increase in minute ventilation with increasing $Paco_2$.

Inhalational anesthetics may induce apnea and hypoxia in premature infants and newborns and are less frequently used in premature infants and children. General anesthesia always necessitates endotracheal intubation and controlled mechanical ventilation. In older children, spontaneous breathing through a mask, or a laryngeal mask airway (LMA), without controlled ventilation, is possible for shorter operations. The decreased EELV and increased work of breathing always necessitates increased inspired oxygen tension.

Cardiovascular Effects

The cardiovascular effects are depressed cardiac output and peripheral vasodilation; therefore, hypotension is frequent. This is accentuated in hypovolemic patients. This hypotensive effect is more pronounced in neonates than older children and adults. Inhalational anesthetics also decrease baroreceptor and heart rate responses. At one MAC of halothane, cardiac output is depressed approximately 25%. The ejection fraction is

TABLE 65–2. **Selected Drugs Used in Anesthesia**

Drug	Uses and Implications
Muscle Relaxants	Used to facilitate endotracheal intubation and maintain muscle relaxation
Succinylcholine (SDC)	A depolarizing neuromuscular blocking agent with rapid onset and offset properties
	Associated with the development of MH in susceptible patients
	Degraded by plasma cholinesterase, which may be deficient in some individuals and result in prolonged effect
	Fasciculations may be associated with immediate increases in intracranial and intraocular pressure as well as postoperative muscle pain
Pancuronium, vecuronium,	Nondepolarizing neuromuscular blockers
cis-atracurium, D-tubocurarine	Less rapid onset than SDC but longer acting
(curare)	Pancuronium is vagolytic, which may be of benefit in newborns, who have high levels of vagal tone
	Vecuronium and rocuronium are metabolized by the liver and excreted in bile
	Cis-atracurium is metabolized by plasma cholinesterase and therefore may be of benefit in patients with hepatic or renal disease; curare releases histamine and is long acting
Hypnotics	Used to induce a state of unconsciousness
Thiopental	Rapidly acting hypnotic, but not an analgesic
	Offset is by redistribution, not by metabolism
	May cause hypotension because of its myocardial depressant effects and by vasodilation
	Causes respiratory depression
	Releases histamine and may be associated with bronchospasm in susceptible individuals
	Increases seizure threshold
Ketamine	Hypnotic analgesic and amnestic
	Causes sialorrhea and should be co-administered with an antisialogogue such as atropine or glycopyrrolate
	May be associated with laryngospasm
	Causes endogenous catecholamine release, tachycardia, and bronchodilation
	Increases intracranial and intraocular pressure
	Decreases seizure threshold
Etomidate	Cardiovascular stability on induction with no increase in intracranial pressure
	May inhibit corticosteroid synthesis
	Associated with myoclonus, potential difficulty with assisted ventilation, and pain on injection
Propofol	Rapidly acting hypnotic, amnestic but not analgesic
	Like pentothal, may cause hypotension
	Causes respiratory depression
	May increase seizure threshold
	Great utility in titrated doses for sedation and with local anesthetic and short-acting opioid for outpatient procedures
	May suppress nausea
Sedative-Anxiolytics	
Benzodiazepines	May produce sedation, anxiolysis, or hypnosis, depending on dose
	May produce antegrade but not retrograde amnesia
	All raise seizure threshold, are metabolized by the liver, and depress respiration, especially when administered with opioids
	Frequently administered as premedicants
	Diazepam may be painful on injection and has active metabolites
	Midazolam can be administered by various routes and has a short half-life
	Lorazepam has no active metabolites
	Sedation effected by all benzodiazepines may be reversed by flumazenil, but respiratory depression may not be reliably reversed
Analgesic-Sedatives	
Opioids	Gold standard for providing analgesia
	May cause respiratory depression
	Morphine and, to a lesser extent, hydromorphone may cause histamine release
	The synthetic opioids fentanyl, sufentanil, and short-acting alfentanil may have a greater propensity to cause chest wall rigidity when administered rapidly or in high doses and are also associated with the rapid development of tolerance; these three drugs have particular utility in cardiac surgery because of the hemodynamic stability associated with their use
	Remifentanil is an ultra–short-acting synthetic opioid that is metabolized by plasma cholinesterase; it may have particular utility when deep sedation and analgesia are required along with the ability to assess neurologic status intermittently
Inhalational Agents	
Nitrous oxide	Amnesia and mild analgesia at low concentrations
	Danger of hypoxic mixture if oxygen concentration is not monitored and preventive safety mechanisms are not in place
Potent vapors	"Complete anesthetics"—they induce a state of hypnosis, analgesia, and amnesia
	All are myocardial depressants, and some are vasodilators
	All are triggers in MH-susceptible individuals
	Isoflurane and enflurane are fluorinated ethers and isomers
	Enflurane may lower seizure threshold
	Halothane has been the gold standard for performing inhalation induction of anesthesia in children, but sevoflurane, a newer drug, is also well tolerated and has more rapid kinetics (onset and offset) because of its low solubility in blood
	All are bronchodilators at equipotent concentrations
	Isoflurane, enflurane, and especially desflurane are associated with a higher incidence of laryngospasm, when used for anesthetic induction, than either halothane or sevoflurane
	Halothane may be associated with an acute fulminant hepatitis, although this is extremely rare in children.

MH = malignant hyperthermia.

decreased by about 25%. At MAC doses of halothane, heart rate is frequently increased; however, as inhalational anesthetic concentration increases, bradycardia may result, whereas profound bradycardia during anesthesia may indicate an overdose. Halothane and related agents sensitize the heart to catecholamines and may produce arrhythmias. Inhalational anesthesia also blunts the hypoxic pulmonary vasomotor response in the pulmonary circulation, a further factor that contributes to hypoxemia during inhalational anesthesia.

The effect of inhalational anesthesia is decreased oxygen delivery. Perioperatively, catabolism is enhanced and oxygen demands are increased. Therefore, there may be a profound imbalance between oxygen demand and oxygen delivery. Development of a metabolic acidosis perioperatively may reflect this imbalance. Because cardiovascular depressant effects of inhalational anesthesia are greater in premature and newborn infants they are of limited use in these patients. They are widely used for the induction and maintenance of anesthesia in older children.

All inhalational anesthetic agents cause cerebrovasodilation. Halothane is a more potent cerebrovasodilator than sevoflurane or isoflurane. Thus, in children with elevated intracranial pressure, impaired cerebral perfusion, and head trauma, and in premature neonates at risk for intraventricular hemorrhage, halothane and other inhalational agents should be used with extreme caution. Although inhalational anesthetic agents decrease cerebral oxygen consumption, they may disproportionately decrease blood flow, thus worsening oxygen delivery.

Specific Anesthetics

Halothane. Agents that are more pleasant to breathe and induce anesthesia more rapidly have replaced halothane (see earlier and later). Halothane hepatitis is a well-recognized sequelae of halothane and is most likely an idiosyncratic, allergic response. The incidence of hepatitis, which may be mild, leading to elevated levels of liver enzymes and jaundice, or severe, leading to acute hepatic necrosis, occurs at a rate of between 1:6,000 and 1:35,000 cases in adults. This appears to be more rare in children and occurs in between 1:80,000 and 1:200,000 exposures in children. There is no reason to particularly avoid halothane in children with liver disease.

Isoflurane. Isoflurane maintains cardiac output and cerebral perfusion better than halothane. The therapeutic ratio for inducing anesthesia without hemodynamic instability is greater for isoflurane. It is also less of a respiratory depressant than halothane. Isoflurane is pungent and a significant airway irritant with an unacceptably high incidence of complications, such as laryngospasm. Emergence from anesthesia with isoflurane is quite smooth and faster than with halothane. Cerebral blood flow is only minimally affected, and cerebral oxygen delivery is maintained. Isoflurane is not implicated in hepatic disease. Because it is not a suitable induction agent, induction with halothane or sevoflurane, and maintenance with isoflurane, is common pediatric anesthesia practice.

Sevoflurane. Sevoflurane has a low blood gas partition coefficient, predicting rapid alveolar equilibration and a faster rate of induction. Sevoflurane is not a significant airway irritant and leads to a smoother induction than isoflurane and a quicker one than with halothane. Sevoflurane appears to have less hemodynamic effects than halothane; the profile of respiratory effects at one MAC appears similar. Emergence from sevoflurane is quite rapid; however, there is a significant amount of emergence delirium, especially if pain has been inadequately controlled. This can be blunted with pretreatment with midazolam and adequate use of opioid narcotics; however, these delay recovery from anesthesia.

The major use of sevoflurane is induction of inhalational anesthesia in children. Because isoflurane is less expensive and has a similar physiologic profile to sevoflurane, anesthesia is maintained with isoflurane. Metabolism of sevoflurane yields free fluoride, which may cause renal damage and, thus, the U.S. Food and Drug Administration has restricted use of sevoflurane to less than 2 MAC hours, preferably with fresh gas flow rates in excess of 2 L/min.

Desflurane. Desflurane has the lowest blood gas solubility coefficient (0.42) of commonly used anesthetics. It would be predicted that desflurane would provide rapid induction and emergence from anesthesia. Unfortunately, it is a potent airway irritant and causes coughing, breath holding, and laryngospasm during induction and is unsuitable for induction.

Nitrous Oxide (N$_2$O). Nitrous oxide is a tasteless, colorless, odorless gas with potent analgesic properties. It induces a state of euphoria (laughing gas). The MAC of nitrous oxide is greater than 1, and therefore it is not suitable as a sole agent to maintain anesthesia. Nevertheless, nitrous oxide has few complications and little or no hemodynamic or respiratory depression. Commonly, during maintenance of anesthesia the inhalational gas mixture is 70% nitrous oxide and 30% oxygen, with the addition of an inhalational anesthetic or potentiation of analgesia with an opioid or hypnotic agent. It has a remarkably low blood gas partition (0.47), so it rapidly reaches alveolar equilibrium. Induction with and emergence from nitrous oxide–induced anesthesia is quite rapid. The deleterious effects of nitrous oxide are a suspicion of increased postoperative emesis and, in long-term use (days), bone marrow suppression. There is no evidence that there are harmful sequelae of the use of nitrous oxide for routine pediatric anesthesia. Nitrous oxide is a potent analgesic that is safely used in a mixture of 50% nitrous oxide and oxygen (Entonox) in obstetrics and emergency departments to provide analgesia. Although this combination appears to be quite safe, it will potentiate respiratory depressive effects of narcotics and its use, in combination with any other sedative, hypnotic, or narcotic agent requires very close monitoring, because it may produce general anesthesia.

Intravenous Anesthetic Agents

Anesthesia can be both induced and maintained with either boluses or continuous infusions of intravenous anesthetic agents. Intravenous anesthetics include barbiturates, narcotics, benzodiazepines, and miscellaneous drugs, such as ketamine. Intravenous anesthetic agents can induce anesthesia more rapidly than inhalational anesthetics, with fewer complications. On the other hand, an intravenous line needs to be placed and, unless intravenous access is already obtained, inhalation induction may remain the preferred route. For children arriving in the operating room with intravascular access, intravenous induction should be routine, because it rapidly takes the child from awake to anesthetized with less hemodynamic and cardiorespiratory compromise. All intravenous agents affect cardiorespiratory function. The one exception to this may be ketamine, which, in lower doses, releases catecholamines, which maintain cardiac function and blood pressure.

Barbiturates. The most commonly used barbiturate for intravenous induction is sodium thiopental. This drug depresses respiration, induces apnea, and can cause hypotension in the hypovolemic patient. It generally has little impact on myocardial function and in the euvolemic well child is a useful anesthetic induction agent. Induction with 3–5 mg/kg of thiopental usually produces 5 to 10 min of unconsciousness within seconds. Although loss of consciousness can rapidly be induced, barbiturates do not provide analgesia. After intravenous induction with sodium thiopental, maintenance anesthesia can be established using benzodiazepines, intravenous narcotics, or inhalational anesthetics.

Pentobarbital is commonly used for sedation in children. Pentobarbital is an intravenous drug that induces loss of consciousness. It is also a potent respiratory depressant, particularly in conjunction with narcotics and benzodiazepines. It has a very prolonged effect. It is not an analgesic agent, and painful procedures cannot be performed with pentobarbital sedation without supplemental analgesia. Pentobarbital sedation deep enough for anxiolysis and nonpainful procedures generally results in prolonged sleep. Its potency and long duration of action make it difficult to titrate. It is not an ideal drug for sedation for short or painful procedures.

Sodium methohexitone (Brevital) is another intravenous induction agent. It is not dissimilar from sodium thiopental and has a similar spectrum of respiratory depression.

Propofol. Propofol is the most commonly used intravenous induction agent in pediatric anesthesiology and has a rapid onset. In doses between 2–3 mg/kg, propofol induces less respiratory depression than thiopental but does produce hypotension. Propofol can sometimes burn and itch on injection; this frequently leads the child to withdraw or respond after a propofol bolus. After induction of anesthesia, propofol is also a useful agent for maintaining hypnosis and amnesia and can be used as a sole anesthetic agent for nonpainful procedures such as radiotherapy, MRI, and CT scanning. Combined with narcotics, it provides excellent, brief anesthesia for painful procedures such as lumbar punctures and bone marrow aspiration. Propofol is a general anesthetic agent and will obtund airway reflexes, respiration, and hemodynamic function and should not be considered as a "sedation" agent. Although hemodynamic stability, and even spontaneous respirations, can be maintained with propofol sedation, its use in children younger than age 12 yr for prolonged sedation over several hours to days is associated with hemodynamic collapse, metabolic acidosis, cardiac failure, profound shock, and death. Its use for prolonged sedation (>12 hr) in the critical care setting in children is contraindicated.

Ketamine. Ketamine rapidly induces general anesthesia and lasts for 15 to 30 min when given at 2 mg/kg IV. It has few side effects and can maintain adequate blood pressure and cardiac output. Ketamine is also effective given either intramuscularly, subcutaneously, or even orally; however, the dose must be increased for these alternative routes. Ketamine is not only a hypnotic agent, providing obtundation and loss of consciousness, but also an analgesic agent and can act as a sole intravenous agent for the provision of a general anesthesia. In low doses, airway reflexes and spontaneous ventilation may be maintained; in higher doses, loss of airway reflexes, apnea, and respiratory depression occur. It is unwise to rely on ketamine to prevent aspiration of gastric contents during deep sedation. Intravenous ketamine is a useful general anesthetic agent for short procedures.

Ketamine produces disturbing postanesthetic dreams and hallucinations. These can occur during emergence from anesthesia or up to weeks later. In adults, the incidence is 30–50%. In prepubertal children, it may be between 5%–10%. Premedication with a benzodiazepine, such as midazolam, greatly reduces these sequelae, and a benzodiazepine is routinely added in children receiving ketamine anesthesia. The other side effect of ketamine is that it is a potent secretagogue and bronchial secretions are enhanced. A drying agent, such as atropine or glycopyrrolate, is administered before the administration of ketamine.

Ketamine is a bronchial smooth muscle relaxant (bronchodilator) and is a useful agent for sedating asthmatic patients and others in the intensive care unit (ICU). Ketamine has been reported to increase intracranial pressure and is, therefore, not indicated in patients at risk for elevated intracranial pressure. Ketamine can increase myocardial oxygen demand and should be used cautiously in patients with impaired myocardial oxygen delivery or cardiac outflow tract obstruction.

Narcotics. Narcotics are superb analgesic agents providing analgesia for painful procedures and postprocedural pain. Narcotics are well described in Chapter 66. Large doses of morphine, combined with nitrous oxide, provide adequate analgesia for painful procedures and surgery. Narcotic agents suppress the CO_2 response, can induce apnea, and are respiratory depressants. Morphine is frequently associated with hypotension and bronchospasm from histamine release, and its use is cautioned in children with asthma. Morphine is a long-acting agent, and an equivalent dose per kilogram gives much higher blood levels in neonates than in older children, with plasma concentrations approximating three times those in adults. This is caused by a prolonged elimination half-life (14 hr) as compared with adults (2 hr). Because of the prolonged activity and hemodynamic instability induced by morphine, the synthetic fentanyl class of narcotics has largely replaced morphine.

Fentanyl is an effective agent to provide pain relief, analgesia, and sedation for painful procedures with a shorter duration of activity and more stable hemodynamic profile than morphine. In equal analgesic doses, all narcotics are equally potent respiratory depressants. Other anesthetic agents potentiate this respiratory depression, whether they are inhalational anesthetics or intravenous barbiturates or benzodiazepines.

Fentanyl use in a 30–50 µg/kg dosing range provides absence of abnormal hemodynamic response to surgery and provides stable operative conditions. Effective analgesia and anesthesia can be provided with intravenous fentanyl in a 2–3 µg/kg bolus followed by a 1–3 µg/kg/hr continuous infusion. Hemodynamic effects can be blunted and recall totally obtunded using a nitrous anesthetic technique, although muscle tone may remain high and spontaneous movements can occur. Nitrous-narcotic anesthetics usually contain a nondepolarizing muscle relaxant during maintenance anesthesia. If the patient is going to be extubated and resume spontaneous ventilation, reversal of the muscle relaxant is necessary.

Other synthetic narcotics—sufentanil, alfentanil, and remifentanil—have gained some use; fentanyl is the most commonly used. The indications and use for these other synthetic narcotics are guided by their different potencies and altered pharmacokinetics. Both sufentanil and alfentanil have been used for cardiac anesthesia, but they have a different potency than fentanyl. Alfentanil appears to have an increased incidence of muscle rigidity, convulsions, and prolonged respiratory depression compared with fentanyl and is not used in children.

Remifentanil has a very rapid onset and offset of action. In doses of 0.25 µg/kg/min, surgical anesthesia can be maintained. Its short half-life and rapid offset are advantageous for rapid emergence. Unfortunately, the rapid offset of action also leads to postprocedural and postoperative pain and requires analgesic supplementation, frequently with a narcotic, which removes the advantage of a short-acting narcotic anesthesia. Remifentanil may have a place for rapidly deepening anesthesia for particularly painful events or rapidly inducing analgesia. It is a potent respiratory depressant and provides no postprocedural analgesia, which limits its use.

Benzodiazepines. Benzodiazepines induce hypnosis, anxiolysis, sedation, and amnesia and have anticonvulsant activity. In larger doses they cause respiratory depression and apnea; they are synergistic with narcotics and barbiturates in their respiratory depressant effects. Benzodiazepines inhibit neurally mediated γ-aminobutyric acid receptors to induce sedation.

The most commonly used benzodiazepine in pediatric anesthesia is midazolam. It is short acting and water soluble and can be injected intravenously without pain. It is a potent hypnotic-anxiolytic-anticonvulsant and is approximately four times more potent than diazepam. In anxiolytic doses, midazolam (0.15 mg/kg) has no impact on respiratory rate, heart rate, or blood pressure and provides excellent preoperative sedation, frequently accompanied by amnesia. It can be administered orally, nasally, rectally, intravenously, or intramuscularly. Use of *oral* midazolam at a dose between 0.5–1.0 mg/kg, mixed in sweet flavored syrup, induces anxiolysis in approximately 90% of children. Although there are no hemodynamic, oxygenation, or respiratory depressant effects at this dose level, when midazolam is used as a sole agent, children may frequently lose their balance and head control, may have blurred vision, and may, very rarely, become dysphoric. A child sedated with midazolam should not be left unattended and is not safe walking. The vast majority of children rapidly accept an inhalational anesthetic mask after oral midazolam premedication

Complications During Induction of Anesthesia

The period between full wakefulness, with the child in control of airway reflexes, and general anesthesia, with total loss of control, is fraught with difficulty. During induction, laryngospasm, bronchospasm, vomiting, aspiration of gastric contents, and subsequent aspiration pneumonitis are a constant but rare occurrence. Concern for vomiting and aspiration dictates preanesthetic NPO guidelines and the indication for rapid sequence anesthetic induction.

Laryngospasm is the most common complication. During induction of anesthesia, especially with inhalational anesthetics, a period of excitement may occur. This period is associated with heightened airway reflexes, which can lead to coughing, gagging, laryngospasm, and bronchospasm. Laryngospasm is reflex closure of the larynx, which makes it impossible for the child to breathe or to ventilate the child. A child may be witnessed to be making violent respiratory efforts against a closed glottis, generating significantly negative intrathoracic pressure with impact on cardiovascular function and the risk of postobstructive pulmonary edema. Laryngospasm can be prolonged and hypoxia may ensue. Laryngospasm occurs in up to 2% of all anesthetic inductions in children younger than age 9 yr and is half as common in older patients. Laryngospasm occurs twice as frequently in children with active or recent upper respiratory tract infections (URIs). A history of passive smoking from environmental (parental) tobacco smoke increases the likelihood of laryngospasm by 10-fold and even more if the smoker is the child's mother.

Laryngospasm can be relieved during induction of anesthesia by deepening the anesthetic, either intravenously or by inhalational anesthesia (although with the glottis closed, further administration of inhalational anesthesia is not possible). Muscle relaxation will relieve laryngospasm, and this may be, in an acute situation, an indication for succinylcholine. Constant positive airway pressure by someone skilled in airway management to ensure patency of the soft tissues of the oropharynx may be beneficial in alleviating the laryngospasm. Laryngospasm may also occur during emergence as a state of excitement is again traversed between deep anesthesia and wakefulness.

Bronchospasm can occur during induction, either in response to histamine release owing to many of the anesthetic agents or a hyperexcitable stage. Endotracheal intubation may also induce bronchospasm during induction. Bronchospasm during induction is particularly common in children with asthma. Bronchospasm secondary to intubation in a patient with reactive airway disease can be severe, associated with life-threatening hypoxemia and a profound inability to ventilate the child. The use of histamine-releasing anesthetic agents has been associated with total airway obstruction, respiratory failure, and cardiac arrest. Environmental tobacco smoke is a risk factor.

Other pulmonary problems with induction of anesthesia include massive atelectasis with hypoxemia, impaired ventilation and perfusion, blunted hypoxic pulmonary-vasoconstriction, and increased airway secretions with decreased bronchociliary function. Hypersecretion is prevented by the routine use of antisialagogues such as atropine. The newer inhalation agents are less potent secretagogues, and the use of atropine premedication is less common but is probably indicated if ketamine is used.

Hemodynamic complications on induction include hypotension, which in hypovolemic patients can be profound, decreased myocardial function, which in patients with compromised cardiac function can be severe, and tachycardia and cardiac dysrhythmias. Inhalational anesthetics sensitize the myocardium to

circulating catecholamines, and induction and excitement are associated with a hypercatecholaminergic state.

Parental Presence During Induction of Anesthesia

Parents may expect to be with their child during the induction of anesthesia. Removing a terrified child from the comforting arms of a parent is stressful for the child, the parent, and the caregivers. If this parental separation cannot comfortably be achieved with preoperative psychoprophylaxis and behavioral modification, including education and desensitization to the operative environment, or with pharmacologic aids, such as preoperative medications including benzodiazepine and barbiturates, then there may be a need to defer parent-child separation until general anesthesia has been induced. Preoperative oral benzodiazepine premedication more frequently provides calm, smooth induction conditions than parental presence without pharmacologic preparation. Although parental presence in the hands of a confident, competent anesthesia practitioner can replace the need for preoperative medication, it does not reliably predict smooth induction. Parental presence during induction appears neither to decrease emergence phenomena nor the incidence of postoperative behavioral changes and does not appear to add an advantage for the child over that provided by preoperative sedative medication, such as oral midazolam.

MAINTENANCE OF ANESTHESIA

Maintenance of anesthesia is the period between induction and emergence. The child should be asleep, unaware of pain, unresponsive either with motion or hemodynamic responses to painful stimuli, and homeostatically supported. The child is comatose, without protective airway reflexes or suppressed or absent respiration, and has received drugs that suppress hemodynamic maladaptive responses. The child is also exposed to surgical trauma and there may be blood loss and significant fluid shifts (third spacing), decreased intravascular volume, and hypothermia.

Anesthesia is usually maintained with nitrous oxide, an inhalational anesthetic such as isoflurane, and a narcotic for intraoperative analgesia, potentiation and deepening of anesthesia, and postoperative analgesia. A benzodiazepine is added either during premedication or intraoperatively to supplement hypnosis and amnesia. A nondepolarizing muscle relaxant (vecuronium or rocuronium) completes the pharmacologic maintenance of anesthesia. Agents can be given by continuous inhalational anesthesia or by continuous or bolus intravenous infusion.

During maintenance, the child may either breathe spontaneously through an anesthetic mask or endotracheal tube or be mechanically ventilated. All general anesthetic agents lead to decreased end-expiratory lung volume, generally lower than FRC, with an increase in pulmonary closing capacity and increased intrapulmonary shunt. Hypoxia would occur without supplemental oxygenation. These effects are compounded by respiratory depressant effects and the depressed CO_2 response curve. Therefore, it is generally considered that anesthetics that last for more than 1 hr require endotracheal intubation and positive pressure ventilation. For long procedures, spontaneous breathing through a mask is possible; however, in smaller children where the surgical field and the airway may be close together, the need to maintain a patent airway necessitates endotracheal intubation.

Muscle relaxation to facilitate endotracheal intubation was once accomplished with succinylcholine. Succinylcholine has a large risk profile and is associated with postoperative pain (muscle spasms); hyperkalemia; elevated intracranial, intraocular, and intragastric pressures; malignant hyperthermia; and myoglobinuria and renal damage. Succinylcholine is rarely used except to provide rapid relief of laryngospasm. Intubation of the airway is facilitated with a nondepolarizing muscle relaxant of short-acting duration; for procedures that last more than 40 min, vecuronium and alcuronium are adequate. After intubation of the airway, the decision must be made whether to maintain muscle relaxation to facilitate surgery or whether to allow the child to resume spontaneous respiration. Prolonged use of nondepolarizing muscle relaxant is common practice but may contribute to postoperative respiratory compromise.

Thermoregulation is critical during anesthesia. The absence of movements and the inhibition of shivering lead to difficulty in thermogenesis. All factors of heat loss, convection, radiation, evaporation, and conduction, occur during anesthesia. Humidification and warming of inspired air is required. Additional warming devices are quite commonly used, such as the BAIR hugger. General anesthetic agents increase the interthreshold range (the minimal temperature change that will lead to sympathetic response, generally 0.3°C). Although temperature sensing may remain normal, autonomic response to hypothermia is not triggered. Anesthetic agents cause vasoparesis, and this further impairs thermoregulation and causes increased heat loss. In newborns, inhalational anesthetics inhibit nonshivering thermogenesis from brown fat, placing them at higher risk for hypothermia.

Intraoperative Monitoring

Routine monitoring includes electrocardiography, with common chest and limb leads that monitor rate, rhythm, and ST segment depression. Pulse oximetry and monitoring of end-tidal CO_2 are routine. The fraction of inspired oxygen is continuously measured. The fraction of anesthetic vapor in the inspiratory (and expired) gas mixture can be continuously monitored, and the mixture of oxygen, air, and nitrous oxide is continuously visualized, either through the use of rotameters or through direct measurement of the inspiratory gas mixture and digital display. Respiratory rate, tidal volume, and respiratory mechanics may be monitored intraoperatively (compliance and resistance). Blood pressure monitoring, with systolic, diastolic, and mean pressures is also routine. This can be done by Doppler ultrasonic or pneumatic techniques.

Fluid Maintenance During Surgery and Anesthesia

Fluid maintenance differs from the normal resting state owing to the effects of anesthesia and surgery. Patients who are unconscious and immobile have lost venous pump mechanisms and have venous pooling in the periphery. Anesthetic agents cause vasodilation, and patients develop relative hypovolemia. Intravascular volume expansion is frequently required after the induction of anesthesia to maintain adequate perfusion, tissue oxygenation, urine output, and blood pressure. This volume expansion can be an isotonic salt-containing solution (normal saline or lactated Ringer). Surgery may lead to increased autonomic responses as part of the surgical stress response, with vasoconstriction and intravascular volume contraction, diuresis, and intravascular volume loss from hemorrhage and from third space (interstitial space) fluid losses caused by the inflammatory response to stress. Abnormalities in the distribution of renal blood flow and secretion of antidiuretic hormone further complicate the regulation of intravascular volume.

Hypoglycemia due to preoperative fasting was a concern and supported the recommendations that infants and small children receive isotonic solutions with 5% glucose. The occurrence of hyperglycemia and potential neurologic injury during cardiopulmonary bypass, or during neurosurgery and other situations in which CNS injury can occur, and with the recognition that hypoglycemia is rare in non-neonates, has questioned the routine use of glucose-containing solutions. In neonates, glucose monitoring during and after anesthesia is indicated. In older children with normal nutritional status isotonic salt solutions are adequate. In children who are receiving parenteral alimentation with high glucose concentration solution (>10%), continuation of these glucose concentrations should be ensured to avoid hypoglycemia when these high concentration glucose solutions are stopped.

Intraoperative fluid maintenance includes (1) current maintenance fluids and replacement of maintenance deficits while NPO; (2) replacement of third space losses; and (3) replacement of extraordinary losses (hemorrhage). These should be, in infants, glucose-containing, isotonic fluids, such as D_5W with 0.25 normal saline, or isotonic crystalloid solutions. A guideline for determining fluid deficits and maintenance requirement in the operating room is shown in Table 65–3. Replacements of the fluid deficits should be done over the first 2 or 3 hr of the intraoperative management. Deficits are generally calculated as the number of hours that a child was NPO times the hourly maintenance rate for the child. Half of this is replaced during the first hour and one fourth during each of the subsequent 2 hr. If hypotension or tachycardia occur or persist in the early stages of the anesthetic, more rapid replacement of the deficit is indicated. The deficit is replaced with isotonic crystalloid solutions.

Third space losses are replaced with isotonic salt solutions. For large operations, such as abdominal or thoracic operations where there may be a large amount of evaporative loss, as well as a significant amount of third space losses, 8–10 mL/kg/hr of surgery is generally given as intravenous fluid replacement. For smaller operations, such as herniorrhaphy, pyloromyotomy, and minor cases, 3–5 mL/kg/hr of fluid replacement for third space losses is indicated. Even when surgery involves the extremities, and third space losses are minor, it is wise to give an additional 1–2 mL/kg/hr to replace third space losses.

Crystalloid is indicated for blood loss at 3 mL of crystalloid per milliliter of blood loss. This formula could be reduced somewhat if blood is replaced on a milliliter per milliliter basis with packed red blood cells or whole blood equivalent. The use of albumin or other suitable colloid, such as fresh frozen plasma in neonatal surgery, also decreases the amount of crystalloid replacement for blood loss. During maintenance anesthesia, if large volume transfusions are required, warming the blood and crystalloid solutions avoids hypothermia.

Hemodynamic integrity, renal function, cerebral perfusion, thermoregulation, and adequate intraoperative cardiovascular function depend on adequate fluid replacement. With major surgery and the resultant systemic inflammatory response, capillary integrity is lost and losses of interstitial fluid are common. The tissue edema that occurs postoperatively is the result of the surgical stress and occurs whether or not intravascular volume is adequately replaced. Failure to replace this third space loss and restore intravascular volume leads to hypotension, shock, acidemia, and renal failure and further stimulates the systemic inflammatory response and worsens physiologic impairment.

RECOVERING FROM ANESTHESIA

Recovering from anesthesia includes emergence and postoperative recovery from surgery and anesthetics. Emergence describes the period of time and the physiologic response to decreasing depth of anesthesia during return to consciousness. During emergence there is decreased anesthetic effect, increased

---

TABLE 65–3. **Intraoperative Pediatric Fluid Replacement**

4 mL/kg/hr	1 to 10 kg
2 mL/kg/hr	10 to 20 kg
1 mL/kg/hr	per kg over 20 kg

Example: 22 kg child requires: $(4 \times 10) + (2 \times 10) + (1 \times 2) = 62$ mL/hr

stress responses, physiologic and psychologic responses to painful stimuli, excitement, and anxiety. Conscious realization of pain may lead to physiologic responses during emergence. The resumption of normal physiologic functions, such as spontaneous ventilation and improved hemodynamic function, occurs. For routine elective cases, the child should be fully conscious, with intact airway reflexes, the ability to follow simple commands, the effects of muscle relaxants reversed, and airway patency maintained before leaving the operating room. If the child is going to the ICU, or for surgical reasons the decision is made to leave the child intubated, then analgesia and sedation should be maintained along with mechanical ventilation in the postoperative period. Ideally, emergence should be as brief as possible, with maintenance of analgesia and anxiolysis and restoration of cardiorespiratory function. Inhalational anesthetic agents rapidly leave the system during ventilation, and muscle relaxants can be reversed; however, the effects of narcotics, benzodiazepines, and intravenous hypnotic agents may be prolonged.

It is possible to provide perfectly adequate general anesthesia with short-acting narcotics (remifentanil), short-acting muscle relaxants (rocuronium), and inhalational anesthesia. The effects of all of these may entirely dissipate within 5 to 10 min. This is not necessarily ideal because the child may have inadequate analgesia for postoperative pain management and be emerging in an unfamiliar environment.

During emergence, the decision must be made whether to reverse the muscle relaxants. Long-acting, nondepolarizing muscle relaxants (vecuronium and pancuronium) can be reversed using neostigmine, an acetylcholinesterase inhibitor. Atropine, or glycopyrrolate, is frequently administered along with the anticholinesterase drug to prevent bradycardia to which children are particularly sensitive. If the child appears to be weak or have respiratory depression in the postoperative phase, consideration of prolonged neuromuscular blockade is indicated.

PACU

In the post-anesthetic care unit (PACU) the child is observed until there is recovery from anesthesia. Parents should be permitted to comfort their children in the PACU. Achievement of spontaneous breathing, adequate arterial saturations above 95%, and hemodynamic stability are key recovery end-points. The child should be arousable, responsive, and oriented before discharge from the PACU. Duration in the PACU will depend on whether the child is being discharged to an inpatient nursing unit, an ICU, a postrecovery area, or directly home. Discharge from the PACU depends on the child's overall functional status, not merely the physiologic end-points, but also the behavioral end-points, and the adequate provision of analgesia and control of postoperative nausea and vomiting. There are several scoring systems (Table 65-4) for determining whether a child is suitable to be discharged from the ICU.

Complications in the PACU

Respiratory Depression. Prolonged emergence from anesthesia and respiratory depression can be caused by opioids or inadequate antagonism of neuromuscular blocking agents. Pain can cause significant hypoventilation, especially after thoracic or abdominal surgery. Delayed emergence from anesthesia can occur owing to retention of inhaled anesthetic agents worsened by hypoventilation. Hypothermia, especially in neonates, delays metabolism and excretion of anesthetics and also aggravates neuromuscular blockade. If respiratory depression is profound, then maintenance of the airway may require an oral airway. If the patient is severely depressed, endotracheal intubation and mechanical ventilation are indicated.

Only in rare cases, where opioid suppression is suspected, is reversal of the narcotic with naloxone indicated. The reversal of

TABLE 65-4. Recovery Scores

Aldrete Recovery Score	>9 Required for Discharge
Activity–voluntarily or on command	
Moves four extremities	2
Moves two extremities	1
No motion	0
Breathing	
Deep breath, cough, cry	2
Dyspnea or shallow	1
Apnea	0
Blood Pressure	
Within 20% of preanesthetic value	2
Within 20–50% of preanesthetic value	1
Greater than 50% outside preanesthetic value	0
Color	
Pink	2
Pale, blotchy, dusky	1
Cyanotic	0
Consciousness	
Fully aware, responds	2
Arouses to stimulus	1
Unresponsive	0

Steward Recovery Score	6 Required for Discharge
Activity	
Moving limbs purposefully	2
Nonpurposeful movement	1
Still	0
Consciousness	
Awake	2
Responsive	1
Unresponsive	0
Airway	
Coughing on command or crying	2
Maintaining patent airway	1
Requires airway maintenance	0

narcotics with naloxone is not merely reversal of respiratory depression but also reversal of analgesia. A somnolent child with respiratory depression may become excited, agitated in severe pain, uncontrollable, and/or hypertensive after naloxone. Narcotic reversal necessitates bedside attention by the physician to monitor the child's behavioral, hemodynamic, and respiratory status. Naloxone is shorter acting than most narcotic analgesics.

Atelectasis is another respiratory complication occurring in the first 48 hr after anesthesia. Atelectasis raises the suspicion of an inhaled foreign body but is most likely caused by secretions and decreased respiratory effort secondary to pain. Microatelectasis may lead to postoperative infections. Aspiration pneumonia is another postoperative complication.

Postoperative stridor occurs in up to 2% of all pediatric patients. Use of uncuffed, atraumatic, nonirritant endotracheal tubes has decreased the incidence of airway trauma. The use of appropriately sized endotracheal tubes and assurance of a leak below 30 cm H_2O pressure further decreases the risk of airway trauma. A prior history of stridor increases the likelihood of postoperative complications. Stridor may be severe enough post extubation to require re-intubation. Retractions and respiratory distress in the postoperative period should suggest this complication, and stridor or wheezing should confirm the diagnosis. Racemic epinephrine aerosols are effective therapy; however, their use requires prolonged observation owing to the potential of recurrence of the airway obstruction. Stridor in infants should suggest the need for overnight observation.

Hemodynamic instability is much less common in the PACU. Volume expansion may be required to maintain adequate blood pressure, peripheral perfusion, and urine output. Excessive volume replacement (>30 mL/kg) that is required to maintain blood pressure, perfusion, and urine output in the postoperative period is an indication of shock and occult bleeding and requires surgical consultation.

Emergence delirium is noted in less than 3% of children and is more common in ages 3 to 9 yr. In the immediate hours after surgery, the child may become extremely restless, combative, disoriented, screaming, crying, and poorly communicative. These children pose a danger to themselves. This phenomenon is more common when barbiturates are used as part of a premedication or induction and inhalational anesthetics or ketamine form part of the maintenance anesthetic. Although disorientation is common in the postanesthetic stage, erratic, delirious behavior requires attention with gentle restraint and comforting. Potential postoperative complications, such as hypoglycemia and hypoxemia, should be ruled out. Occasionally, it is necessary to sedate the child with benzodiazepines, although these prolong postanesthesia recovery time, and when they wear off emergence delirium may occur.

Postoperative Nausea and Vomiting (PONV). After general anesthesia, as many as 40–50% of children may experience nausea and vomiting. Over 80% of all high-risk children receiving inhalational anesthesia experience postoperative nausea and vomiting. PONV may occur in the immediate postoperative period, within the first 1–2 hr, or can occur several hours after surgery and anesthesia. The etiology may be related to the stress and trauma of surgery, combined with the emetic effects of anesthetic agents. Pain is an important cause of nausea and vomiting. Unfortunately, narcotic analgesics also induce nausea and vomiting. Preoperative fasting does not decrease the incidence of nausea and vomiting. Indeed, hydration and glucose supplementation appear to be important factors in decreasing PONV. The use of analgesic agents other than narcotics (e.g., acetaminophen, ketorolac) and regional or local anesthesia is associated with less nausea and vomiting in the postoperative period.

PONV prolongs recovery room times, requires significant nursing attention, and increases the use of potent antiemetic agents (ondansetron and other serotonin antagonists). Droperidol is beneficial prophylactically and for established vomiting; metoclopramide is useful prophylactically. Droperidol must be used with caution, owing to the rare occurrence of a prolonged QT interval and ventricular arrhythmias. Ondansetron is very efficacious as a prophylactic and a treating agent for PONV. Ondansetron and other serotonin antagonists are recommended for high-risk patients (strabismus surgery) or for actual treatment of PONV.

All inhalational anesthetics are associated with PONV, and their replacement with a nitrous narcotic technique does not decrease PONV. The induction or maintenance of anesthesia with propofol may decrease PONV.

Thermoregulation and Malignant Hyperthermia. In the PACU, thermoregulation remains abnormal for several hours. Shivering is common in the postoperative state, and a feeling of extreme coldness is common. Warm blankets are very comforting and seem to decrease shivering. Hypothermia, especially in neonates, leads to hypotension, bradycardia, acidosis, apnea, and prolongation of the effect of narcotics and neuromuscular blocking agents. Although there are deleterious effects of hypothermia, rewarming must be cautious to avoid burning and cutaneous hyperthermia. Hyperthermia, with temperatures in excess of (39°C), is of concern in the postoperative period. If this occurs within hours of an inhalational anesthetic, especially if succinylcholine was used, malignant hyperthermia must be suspected.

Malignant hyperthermia is an acute hypermetabolic syndrome that is triggered by inhalational anesthetic agents and succinyl-choline. It resembles **neuroleptic malignant syndrome**. The onset of malignant hyperthermia may be acute, and its course may be fulminant and rapidly fatal. This condition, albeit rare (approximately 1:14,000 pediatric anesthetics) is a constant concern. The disease is familial, and hence a family history of death during anesthesia, or the history of a febrile reaction, should alert the anesthesiologist to its potential. Its clinical course is characterized by a rapid onset of fever, acidosis, hypercarbia, and increased expired CO_2. High fever (38.5–46°C, rising 1 degree every 5 min), muscle rigidity, metabolic acidosis, and hemodynamic collapse can occur. Death ensues from shock and cardiac dysrhythmias with unresponsive ventricular fibrillation. The mortality rate for malignant hyperthermia was once in excess of 70%. Aggressive therapy, including discontinuation of all inhalational anesthetic administration, correction of the metabolic acidosis, and treatment with the muscle relaxant sodium dantrolene, has reduced the mortality to less than 5%. Dantrolene and a kit containing supplies necessary to treat malignant hyperthermia should be present at every site where pediatric anesthesia is practiced.

Its exact genetic basis remains elusive owing to the diversity of triggering agents and the range of the response. Malignant hyperthermia is probably genetically heterogeneous, with over ten genes contributing to malignant hyperthermia susceptibility. Genetic mutations in the ryanodine receptor (the calcium channel of the sarcoplasmic reticulum) have been identified in malignant hyperthermia–susceptible swine, and a similar defect has been reported in 20–40% of humans with malignant hyperthermia.

Malignant hyperthermia appears to occur from a massive triggering of excitation-contraction coupling, sarcolemmal calcium release, and propagation of contraction by a complex biochemical process. Phospholipase A_2 activity is primarily triggered, increasing mitochondrial free fatty acids and stimulating calcium release. The prolonged ischemic contraction leads to myolysis with release of myoglobin, very high serum creatine phosphokinase (CPK) levels, and renal failure secondary to myoglobinuria. Malignant hyperthermia generally occurs within the first 2 hr of anesthesia but rarely can occur up to 24 hr later.

Certain phenomena are clues to the risk of developing malignant hyperthermia. The occurrence of masseter spasm during induction, with rigid clenching of the masseter muscles and an inability to open the mouth, may presage full-blown disease. Acute myoglobinuria associated with a malignant hyperthermia–triggering agent is another clue. The child may not be hypermetabolic or febrile but develops dark urine and high serum CPK levels with the risk of myoglobin-induced renal tubular damage. Dark urine after an anesthetic requires investigation for malignant hyperthermia. An elevated CPK value and heme-positive urine in the absence of red blood cells in the urine indicates a need for renal protection with mannitol and alkaline diuresis.

Certain myopathies are associated with the risk for malignant hyperthermia; these include Duchenne muscular dystrophy, Noonan phenotype, and, in children with history of ptosis, squint, scoliosis, and muscle cramping. It is wise to avoid the use of succinylcholine in children with myopathies.

Rapid therapy is essential. All known triggering agents must be stopped. Intravenous administration of dantrolene sodium (2.5 mg/kg IV) as an initial dose is given as soon as possible. Repeated doses are indicated by the persistence of muscle rigidity, acidosis, and tachycardia, up to a maximum dose of 10 mg/kg. After control of the symptoms, the patient should be observed for at least 24 hr after the laboratory values have returned to normal because relapse can occur.

Prevention of malignant hyperthermia in susceptible patients requires the avoidance of triggering agents, which include inhalational anesthetics. Most anesthesiology departments are capable of delivering general anesthetics using anesthesia machines from which all traces of anesthetic vapors have been removed. Intravenous anesthesia and a nitrous-narcotic technique are safe. Dantrolene prophylaxis is not recommended because the disease is rapidly treatable and because the drug has respiratory depressant and muscle weakness. If a child is suspected of having malignant hyperthermia, the malignant hyperthermia hotline, 1-(800)-MHHYPER, should be notified. This will register susceptible patients and provides diagnostic and therapeutic information. Preanesthesia susceptibility testing includes genetic analysis of the ryanodine receptor gene, muscle biopsies, in vitro contraction studies, or possibly measuring muscle CO_2 production in response to intramuscular caffeine.

Postoperative Apnea. Apnea within the first 24–48 hr after surgery and anesthesia in premature infants is common; both central and obstructive apnea (mixed apnea) may occur. The use of respiratory depressants may impair the respiratory control in neonates. Apnea is also a recognized stress response in neonates, and inadequate anesthesia is associated with increased apnea and respiratory complications in neonates.

The risk of developing postoperative apnea in premature neonates is inversely proportional to postconceptual age at the time of surgery. This risk is minimal by the time premature infants have reached the postconceptual age of 60 wk. Apnea is most common within the first 12 hr after surgery; postanesthetic apnea has been reported in premature infants up to 48 hr later. The incidence of apnea in full-term infants is debatable and not clearly demonstrated. It is generally agreed that general anesthesia should be avoided, except for emergent surgery, in full-term children younger than 44 wk postconceptual age. If surgery is required within the first month, overnight observation and monitoring is indicated. Theophyllines decrease the incidence of postoperative apnea; however, they do not ablate it and are, therefore, not routinely used. The safest course is to monitor premature infants younger than 60 wk postconceptual age and full-term infants younger than 1 mo old for at least 24 hr after anesthesia.

PREANESTHETIC EVALUATION

Most previous healthy children require minimal preoperative assessment. The American Society of Anesthesiologists classification system for anesthetic care is the ASA Physical Status classification, which has five levels and an additional classification of "E" for emergency surgery (Box 65–4).

For ASAPS-1 patients, a brief history, notation of medical allergies, and a physical examination, focusing on the airway, lungs, and cardiac function, are sufficient. All children being assessed for anesthesia risk should have a family history obtained for reactions to anesthetics, drug allergies, and for sudden death intraoperatively or hyperthermia after surgery, which may indicate malignant hyperthermia risk. In children who have had a previous anesthetic, questions should be asked

regarding any intraoperative anesthetic complications. In general, the history should focus on determining whether the child is at risk for anesthetic or surgical stress as well as cardiorespiratory disease and airway compromise.

Recent URIs should be noted. A URI is an upper respiratory illness associated with fever, mucopurulent green or yellow nasal discharge, productive cough, injected sclerae, and increased mucus secretions. Clear rhinorrhea is generally not a concern. URIs can increase airway reactivity for up to 6 wk in both normal children and children with a history of reactive airway disease. URIs can also increase the risk of laryngospasm and bronchospasm, cause decreased mucociliary clearance, and increase the risk of intraoperative atelectasis and hypoxemia. It is generally recommended to avoid general anesthesia for elective cases for 4 to 6 wk after a URI. In patients with chronic sinusitis and nasal polyps, infection should be thoroughly treated before elective anesthesia.

Acute, fatal bronchospasm can occur during induction of anesthesia and endotracheal intubation for routine, minor surgery in children with asthma. Those children at particular risk for anesthetic complications with asthma are those who have (1) been admitted to the hospital within the previous year for their asthma, (2) been seen in an emergency department in the past 6 mo, (3) been admitted to an ICU, or (4) been treated with parenteral systemic steroids. The child should be free of wheezing for at least several days before surgery, even if this necessitates an increase in β-agonists and the addition of steroids. Preoperative steroids are indicated for all children with asthma who have received or are receiving asthma therapy within the past year. Prednisone, 1 mg/kg given 24 and 12 hr before surgery, significantly decreases airway reactivity perioperatively. Active wheezing is an indication for canceling elective surgery. If wheezing cannot be controlled while an outpatient with β-agonists, steroids, and other asthma therapy, admission for more aggressive therapy before surgery is indicated.

Bronchopulmonary dysplasia also provides significant intraoperative risks. The same applies to children with cystic fibrosis and other chronic lung diseases where every effort should be made to ensure that these children are in the best possible respiratory status before surgery. Infections should be treated and reactive airways optimally treated without evidence of wheezing.

Airway Evaluation

Because the induction of anesthesia is associated with loss of spontaneous ventilation and airway reflexes, predicting the inability to bag-and-mask ventilate or endotracheally intubate a child before anesthesia is critical. The anesthesiologist must be made aware of children with congenital anomalies that affect the airway (Box 65–5). They include micrognathia syndromes, macroglossia syndromes, and frequently children with thoracic anomalies. Congenital anomalies associated with airway compromise should be diagnosed preoperatively. Conditions that impair mouth opening (temporomandibular joint disease) should be noted. A history of wheezing or stridor may indicate postoperative airway complications and difficult intraoperative airway management.

Mediastinal Masses

Children with anterior mediastinal masses, such as lymphomas and primary mediastinal tumors, are at serious risk from airway compromise, cardiac tamponade, and vascular obstruction. Induction of general anesthesia and even mild sedation can rapidly lead to total loss of the airway with inability to ventilate the child and cardiovascular collapse. These patients often present in a semi-emergent fashion with the need for both a tissue diagnosis before initiating treatment and a surgically placed central line.

BOX 65–4. American Society of Anesthesiology Physical Status Classification

Class 1: Healthy patient, no systemic disease.
Class 2: Mild systemic disease with no functional limitations. (Mild chronic renal failure, iron deficiency anemia, mild asthma)
Class 3: Severe systemic disease with functional limitations. (Hypertension, poorly controlled asthma or diabetes, congenital heart disease, and cystic fibrosis)
Class 4: Severe systemic disease that is a constant threat to life. (Critically and/or acutely ill patients with major systemic disease)
Class 5: Moribund patients not expected to survive 24 hours, either with or without surgery.
Additional classification: "E"; emergency surgery.

BOX 65–5. Syndromes with Difficult Airways

Choanal atresia
Beckwith-Wiedemann
Mucopolysaccharidosis
Pierre Robin
Treacher-Collins
Goldenhar's
DiGeorge
Apert's
Achondroplasia
Turner's
Cornelia de Lange
Smith-Lemli-Opitz
Juvenile rheumatoid arthritis
Fractured mandible
Airway tumors, hemangiomas
Cystic hygroma/teratoma
Trisomy 21

Significant compression of vital structures can occur with seemingly mild symptoms. Tachypnea, orthopnea, wheezing, and sleep disturbances or avoidance of prone or supine positions are significant indications of serious risk. Pericardial tamponade or superior vena cava syndromes are more concerning findings. A CT scan demonstrating greater than 50% compression of the airway at the carina is an indication to prohibit general anesthesia and provide only mild sedation. Echocardiographic or CT evidence of pericardial tamponade, right ventricular compression, or compression of the pulmonary artery suggest severe risk. Biopsy under local anesthesia may be indicated. If anesthesia is required, cardiopulmonary bypass should be considered in the event that it becomes impossible to ventilate the child. In high-risk children, consideration should be given to initiating treatment with steroids, radiotherapy, and chemotherapy before obtaining a tissue diagnosis.

Down Syndrome

Children with Down syndrome are occasionally behaviorally difficult and are especially fearful of medical caregivers. Their cardiac anomalies, macroglossia, and upper airway obstruction can be challenging. Children with Down syndrome have atlantoaxial instability caused by odontoid hypoplasia and joint laxity. In younger Down syndrome children, extension of the neck, routinely used to maintain and intubate the airway, may lead to cervical dislocation and spinal cord trauma. Some anesthesiologists recommend extension and flexion lateral neck films to detect instability before anesthesia. In Down children routine caution to stabilize the cervical spine and avoid flexion and extension is wise.

Cardiovascular System

Because of the depressant effects of anesthetics and the increased demands of surgery, any compromise of myocardial function should be clearly delineated preoperatively. A preoperative ECG, echocardiogram, and cardiology consult are indicated for children with a history of heart disease. The presence of an intracardiac shunt will affect oxygenation status intraoperatively. Because of the significant impact on the oxygen supply and demand relationship caused by general anesthesia and surgical stress, obstructive lesions, such as a valvular stenosis, must also be clearly defined. A past history of cardiac dysrhythmias should be clearly understood, because inhalational anesthetics are dysrhythmogenic.

In neonates, the presence of ductus arteriosus, myocardial compromise, pulmonary edema, or congenital heart disease can significantly complicate oxygen delivery during anesthesia. Accurate diagnosis of cardiac murmurs in neonates is essential. Any cardiovascular compromise preoperatively will be worsened intraoperatively and can catastrophically complicate the perioperative course.

Anemia should be diagnosed and corrected preoperatively if possible. A hematocrit above 30% is generally acceptable for routine elective anesthesia. If there are reasons to expect significant blood loss or prolonged convalescence, anemia should be corrected preoperatively. In the emergent setting, transfusion may be required. Although lower hematocrits can be tolerated in unstressed children, the significant threat to oxygen delivery posed by anesthesia and surgery, especially if blood loss is expected, requires maintaining an adequate hemoglobin concentration perioperatively.

Evidence of coagulopathy should be sought. Easy bruising, the use of aspirin, or familial bleeding disorders should be discussed. Intraoperative hemorrhagic bleeding can be difficult to control; massive blood transfusions in the perioperative period have significant risk for morbidity and mortality. Preoperative correction of coagulopathic disorders is indicated. In neonates, assurance of vitamin K prophylaxis and adequate coagulation status is critical before any significant surgery. In neonates and critically ill children, adequate platelet count and, where indicated, coagulation factors, prothrombin time, and partial thromboplastin time should be assured.

Neurobehavioral Aspects

The child's level of interaction and understanding form a backdrop to providing safe and comfortable anesthesia for the child. The presence of seizures, significant neurologic impairment, altered level of consciousness, respiratory airway compromise secondary to neurologic disease, and neuromuscular disease should be sought and evaluated. Anticonvulsant drug metabolism is often altered perioperatively, and this may alter anticonvulsant drug levels. Anticonvulsants may also complicate the anesthetic management. Maintenance of appropriate anticonvulsant therapy postoperatively is important to avoid new seizures. Cerebrospinal fluid secretion is increased during surgery and general anesthesia. This is significant in patients suspected of elevated intracranial pressure or in children with ventriculoperitoneal shunts. In infants or older children with ventriculoperitoneal shunts, shunt patency and function should be assured before surgery.

Illness and the need for surgery or painful medical procedures are psychologically traumatic events for children and their families. Anxiety results from a host of mechanisms in the child related to loss of control, fear of the unknown, uncertainty, and separation anxiety. Children are also remarkably adept at sensing stressful signals from their parents and caregivers. Many children requiring anesthesia may develop significant levels of fear and anxiety. Most children undergoing surgery develop new-onset negative behavioral changes in the postoperative period, such as maladaptive behavioral responses that include generalized anxiety, enuresis, enhanced separation anxiety, temper tantrums, nighttime crying, and fear of strangers, doctors, and hospitals. Approximately 20% demonstrate these negative behavioral adaptations for 6 mo after surgery. Sleep quality is also altered postoperatively, resulting in further behavioral compromise.

The risk factors for postoperative behavioral changes include preoperative or induction anxiety and behaviors indicating extreme stress, as well as emergence excitation. The type of surgery may be important, with tonsillectomy and genitourinary surgery having a high incidence of postoperative behavioral changes whereas simple procedures (tympanostomy tubes) seem to be associated with fewer changes. Another risk factor is recurrent procedures, such as anesthesia for laser surgery, strabismus surgery, or repeated eye examinations, which lead to difficult behavioral changes and have a significant impact on family dynamics. The type of induction is not a factor.

Preoperative psychologic preparation programs decrease the incidence of postoperative behavioral changes, which last for up to 1 mo. Parental presence during anesthetic induction does not improve postoperative behavior. Oral midazolam (0.5 mg/kg) may decrease negative behavioral changes after surgery. Midazolam has the benefit of providing not only rapid onset anxiolysis in 10 to 20 min but very effective and rapid (10 min) amnesia.

Preoperative Preparation

The child should be in the best nutritional state, and nutritional supplementation, even hyperalimentation in chronically ill children, may be worthwhile. Catabolism is increased after surgery, and the nutritional disorders that accompany major surgery should be prepared for by optimal preoperative nutrition.

Preoperative Fasting. Aspiration of gastric contents is a perioperative disaster and if superimposed on lung disease may be rapidly fatal. Aspiration may lead to laryngospasm and bronchospasm with hypoxemia and hypoxic ischemic encephalopathy. It may also produce intraoperative atelectasis and postoperative pneumonia. It is vital to ensure that the stomach is as empty as possible before the induction of anesthesia. Acid aspiration is less likely with an empty stomach. Preoperative fasting (NPO) guidelines are noted in Table 65–5.

Clear, sweet liquids (Pedialyte, D_5W) facilitate gastric emptying, help avoid hypoglycemia, and can be given up to 2 hr before anesthesia in any child. For older infants and children a fasting period of 4 hr for liquids provides optimal safety and minimal discomfort. Solids must be avoided for *at least* 8 hr before surgery. Because surgery is frequently scheduled in the morning, and for ease and clarity of understanding, the general guideline is NPO for solids after midnight. Many conditions delay gastric emptying, and prolonged periods of fasting may be required in the presence of stress, anxiety, illness, trauma, gross obesity, or biliary atresia or in children with delayed gastric emptying for other reasons.

The Full Stomach. Because of serious complications of gastric contents aspiration, it is desirable to secure the airway as rapidly as possible after obtundation in patients at risk of having a full stomach. Gastric emptying may be delayed for up to 96 hr after an acute episode of trauma or surgical illness. Under these circumstances, induction of general anesthesia and endotracheal intubation are performed in a rapid sequence (rapid sequence induction).

Preparation is of utmost importance. All airway equipment should be available: selection of laryngoscope blades, two laryngoscope handles (in case one fails), and appropriately sized endotracheal tubes with one size above and below the appropriately sized endotracheal tube for age. Two sources of suction with two large-volume suction catheters (Yankauer suction catheters or "tonsil suckers") should be available, because vomiting can be copious. The goal is to place an endotracheal tube through the vocal cords as rapidly as possible after the loss of airway reflexes. Because muscle relaxation with succinylcholine can take 30–45 sec, and nondepolarizing muscle relaxants 45–90 sec, the administration of sedation and muscle relaxation *concurrently* is indicated.

TABLE 65–5. Preoperative Fasting Guidelines*

Time Before Surgery	Oral Intake
2 hours	Clear, sweet liquids
4 hours	Breast milk
6 hours	Infant formula, fruit juices, jello
8 hours	Solid food

*These are general guidelines and may differ among hospitals.

Risks of rapid sequence induction include the possibility that if the airway cannot be intubated, the child is paralyzed without a protected airway and ventilation may be hazardous or impossible. Rapid sequence intubation should be performed by those who will definitely achieve rapid endotracheal intubation. Rapid sequence intubation should be avoided in patients with a history of failed oral endotracheal intubation, or with one of many syndromes (e.g., micrognathia) associated with difficult intubation. Under these circumstances, bronchoscopic awake intubation may be indicated.

Before rapid sequence induction, the child should be preoxygenated by breathing 100% oxygen for 2 min to give an extra margin of safety should intubation be difficult. The child should not be assist-ventilated either before or after the administration of drugs because this may lead to increased gastric air and actually increase the likelihood of vomiting, regurgitation, and aspiration.

A standard regimen for rapid sequence intubation includes the administration of 3–6 mg/kg of sodium thiopental or 1.5–3 mg/kg of propofol concurrently with either 0.9 to 1.2 mg/kg of rocuronium or 1.5 mg/kg of vecuronium. Immediately after the administration of sedation and muscle relaxants, the Sellick maneuver (cricoid pressure) should be performed by applying firm pressure in a posterior direction against the cricoid cartilage. This displaces the cricoid cartilage into the esophagus, forming an artificial sphincter to prevent reflux of gastroesophageal contents. Cricoid pressure should be maintained until it is certain the endotracheal tube is correctly located by direct visualization, fogging of the tube, and, in all circumstances, by positive end-tidal CO_2.

Informed Consent. Consent must be obtained for children undergoing anesthesia. Anesthesia consent (both permission from parents and assent from the child) follows the same guidelines as for other procedures. Whereas the benefits of a surgical procedure are intrinsic to the procedure, the risk of any procedure under anesthesia exposes the child to the additional risks of anesthetic. This particular issue is perhaps unnecessary when discussing surgery with a significant risk (cardiac or complex neurosurgical procedures); when the procedure itself has no intrinsic risks (MRI), the general anesthesia alone may be the only associated risk.

Minor risks include headache, nausea and vomiting, dental or lip trauma, delayed awakening, sore throat, and aspiration. Major risks include hypoxic ischemic encephalopathy, myocardial depression and cardiac arrest, cardiac dysrhythmias, and death (albeit extraordinarily rare). For healthy children undergoing elective surgery, the risks of a serious complication are approximately 1:100,000. In more complex and urgent situations, there is a much higher potential for anesthetic risks.

POSTOPERATIVE PAIN MANAGEMENT

The continuation of analgesia and anxiolysis should follow surgery or painful procedures (see Chapter 66). Incisional and operative pain will persist for hours to days depending on the type and location of the surgery. Complete freedom from pain is not possible. To hold forth the ability of a hospital perioperative service or physician to provide a "pain free" environment is misrepresentation and will disappoint children, families, and caregivers. Every practitioner associated with the care of children should strive to prevent, alleviate, and eradicate pain, fear, and anxiety and maximize comfort.

The combination of narcotic and non-narcotic analgesic agents and an understanding of the benefits and risks is the foundation of pain management. A judicious combination of nonsteroidal anti-inflammatory drugs, cyclooxygenase-2 (COX-2) inhibitors, opioids, and regional analgesia has a role in postoperative pain management. Repeated evaluation is as important as the modality of pain management.

Patient-controlled analgesia (PCA), nurse-controlled analgesia, and parent-controlled analgesia are all used postoperatively (see Chapter 66). PCA provides continuous pain treatment and self-medication (as opposed to intermittent or PRN) as well as control and comfort in an otherwise personally uncontrolled circumstance. PCA provides both a background low dose infusion rate of a continuous narcotic and the opportunity to supplement analgesia with bolus doses as needed. The practitioner can determine the continuous infusion rate, the bolus dose, the bolus frequency, and the number of boluses per unit time that the patient may receive. PCA relies on the theory that patients cannot, or will not, overdose themselves because somnolence will decrease repeated self-administration. In young children, the use of the "pain button" (for pain relief) may be more difficult to ensure; however, children as young as 5 yr have successfully been able to use PCA. In older children and adolescents, PCA should be a standard modality of postoperative pain management.

The concern with nurse-controlled analgesia or parent-controlled analgesia is that an overdose is possible with complications and increased side effects. An overzealous health care provider or parent may continue to medicate the child beyond the point of pain relief and into the dose range associated with complications. Nevertheless, with careful observation and monitoring, as well as intelligent design of the continuous infusion rate, lockout periods, frequency of dosing, and bolus dose, this is a safe modality of therapy.

Regional Anesthesia

Regional anesthesia is the use of anesthetics to block the conduction of afferent neural impulses to the CNS. These can be local analgesic techniques, peripheral nerve blocks, nerve-plexus blocks, or epidural and subarachnoid (spinal) nerve blocks. They may be either by a single injection (single shot) or by continuous infusion, as is common with epidural and occasionally subarachnoid blocks. They may be used for intraoperative anesthesia and postoperative analgesia and have the potential to decrease intraoperative analgesia and anesthetic use, as well as provide postoperative pain management.

Analgesia at the site of need without central cardiorespiratory depressant effects can be valuable. Local anesthesia, with the injection of lidocaine or bupivacaine into the pain area, can provide procedural analgesia, which lasts for several hours. Infiltration of the wound site and edges of an incision decreases postoperative pain in the initial hours after surgery. This can be injected by the surgeon at the conclusion of surgery and may supplement postoperative analgesia.

Epidural analgesia is common in pediatric practice. The epidural space lies below the dura and above the pia and arachnoid membranes, an area through which all nerve roots pass. Bathing these nerve roots in local anesthetics inhibits conduction of pain impulses centrally. A single dose of epidural anesthetic may provide hours of pain relief, and a continuous infusion may provide effective pain relief for hours to days. The epidural injection of opioids can provide analgesia for 12 to 24 hr and is a potential supplement for postoperative analgesia.

A lumbar epidural is placed in the lumbar area to provide analgesia for labor and surgery below the thorax. Caudal epidural analgesia is placed through the sacral hiatus, the distal end of the spinal cord, and is the site most commonly used for anesthesia and analgesia in children and is efficacious for the provision of pelvic and lower limb anesthetic and is beneficial in orthopedic surgery and urologic surgery. A continuous infusion of bupivacaine is the most common means of providing postoperative epidural pain relief; this may be mixed with an opioid (fentanyl or preservative-free morphine). It is also possible to provide epidural PCA with a continuous infusion pump and the ability for the patient to self-medicate with bolus dosing on an as-needed basis. Epidural analgesia can also provide pain relief in patients with chronic pain or pain caused by advanced malignant conditions.

The most *serious* complications of neuraxial anesthesia include cephalad spread of blockade with respiratory depression, paralysis of respiratory muscles and, in extreme cases, brainstem analgesia and depression. The most *common* complications of neuraxial analgesia include mild discomfort; a paresthesia-like feeling of numbness and tingling; pruritus, which, if opioids are used, can occasionally be quite distressing; and occasional nausea and vomiting. Infection and epidural hematoma are extremely rare. Neuraxial opioids, especially administered intrathecally, can cause respiratory depression; their use requires postoperative monitoring. The use of neuraxial opioids often requires treatment with antipruritic as well as antiemetic drugs.

SEDATION

The same drugs that induce general anesthesia are often used to provide sedation. Sedation is the continuum between fully awake and general anesthesia (see Box 65–3). Management of sedated children requires vigilance and knowledge to ensure their safety and is guided by the same guidelines as anesthesia care (Box 65–6). For threatening and nonpainful procedures, anxiolysis or light sedation is frequently sufficient. For painful procedures the combination of sedation with analgesia that is required in children produces deep sedation.

Sedation with chloral hydrate, pentobarbital, or benzodiazepines is often adequate for nonpainful procedures. Nevertheless there can be a high failure rate and complications such as prolonged sedation (hours to overnight), ataxia, nausea and vomiting, desaturation, and occasional need for rapid intervention. The temptation to add narcotics and deepen sedation increases the risk of complications. The most rapid way to ensure safely reversible sedation is with potent anesthetic agents. The ultra–short-acting anesthetics (e.g., methohexital, remifentanil, propofol, thiopental) provide effective procedural sedation, but there is a higher likelihood of inadvertent oversedation and induction of general anesthesia. These anesthetics offer efficient and rapidly reversible procedural sedation, however, with their inherent risks. Therefore, their use requires the presence of an anesthesiologist and/or specially trained physicians.

ANESTHESIA MORTALITY AND MORBIDITY

Anesthetic mortality has decreased to 1:100,000; young age and pre-existing medical conditions present significant risk factors. The overall mortality rate for infants is approximately

---

BOX 65–6. Systematic Approach to Sedation in Children

1. Thorough medical history anticipating underlying medical problems predisposing to sedation problems
2. Careful physical examination focused on the cardiorespiratory system and airway
3. Appropriate fasting
4. Informed consent
5. Pediatric drug dosing (milligrams per kilogram)
6. Appropriate-sized equipment
7. A separate, dedicated observer to monitor sedated patients who may have airway compromise (induced or pre-existing)
8. Documentation of vital signs and condition on a time-based record
9. An emergency backup system, code team, and crash cart
10. A fully equipped and staffed recovery area
11. Discharge criteria documenting recovery from sedation

TABLE 65–6. Risk Control in Anesthesia

	Risk Identification	Risk Modification	Risk Management
The Patient	Underlying medical problems Congenital anomalies Anatomic abnormalities Previous diseases NPO status	Medical interventions Surgical interventions Ensuring NPO status Preoperative physiologic optimization	Fund of knowledge Appropriate, informed consent Parent-child awareness Parental education
The Practitioner	Clinical competence Appropriate training and expertise Impairment Appropriate equipment	Supervision and training Education Equipment maintenance	Credential committees Continuing education Fund of knowledge Drills for rare events Quality improvement monitoring

The Practice	Standards of practice
	Communication among surgeons,
	  neonatologists, and anesthesiologists
		Hospital policies and procedures
		Total quality management programs
		
		Communication skills
		Protocolization
		Combined morbidity and mortality (M&M)
		  conferences with neonatologists,
		  surgeons, and anesthesiologists
			Continuous quality review improvement

Adapted from Holzman RS: Morbidity and mortality in pediatric anesthesia. Pediatr Clin North Am *1994;41:240.*

1:40,000, whereas the risk of a complication in infants is around 4.3:1,000. Severity of illness continues to remain a risk factor, although ASAPS-1 children have a complication risk of 0.4:1,000. This rises to 16.4:1,000 in ASAPS-4–5 and is increased further by an "E" designation.

Anesthesia-related cardiac arrests occur in approximately 1.4:10,000 pediatric anesthetics. Whereas in the past, respiratory events from anesthetic overdose were the common cause of cardiac arrest, the use of pulse oximetry, anesthetic concentration monitoring, and end-tidal CO_2 has greatly reduced this risk. Most cardiac arrests (83%) occur during induction and maintenance of anesthesia, and 21% of all arrests occur during emergency surgery. Infants younger than 1 yr old account for 55% of anesthesia-related cardiac arrests; this is particularly true in the younger than 1 mo age group. Even though these special groups have elevated risk factors, it should be noted that 33% of anesthesia-related cardiac arrests occur in ASAPS-1 and ASAPS-2 patients and are more commonly related to medication-related errors than patient factors. Intraoperative cardiac arrests are commonly stated to have a good likelihood of resuscitation; however, mortality in intraoperative perianesthetic cardiac arrests is 26% in children.

Risk Reduction in Pediatric Anesthesia

Thorough physiologic assessment, attentive intraoperative management, and close perioperative monitoring are essential in minimizing risk to children. Communication among all of the child's caregivers ensures minimizing the risks associated with anesthesia, analgesia, and sedation (Table 65–6).

Betz E: Incidence of PONV not influenced by choice of air or nitrous oxide. *Anesthesiology* 2002;28:2–4.

Bouwmeester NJ, Anand KJ, van Dijk M, et al: Hormonal and metabolic stress responses after major surgery in children aged 0–3 years: A double-blind, randomized trial comparing the effects of continuous versus intermittent morphine. *Br J Anaesth* 2001;87:390–99.

Cote CJ: "Conscious sedation": Time for this oxymoron to go away! *J Pediatr* 2001;139:15–17.

Cote CJ, Notterman DA, Karl HW, et al: Adverse sedation events in pediatrics: A critical incident analysis of contributing factors. *Pediatrics* 2000;105:805–14.

Golianu B, Krane EJ, Galloway KS, et al: Pediatric acute pain management. *Pediatr Clin North Am* 2000;47:559–87.

Hall SC: General pediatric emergencies: Malignant hyperthermia syndrome. *Anesthesiol Clin North Am* 2001;19:367–82.

Hertzog JH, Dalton HJ, Anderson BD, et al: Prospective evaluation of propofol anesthesia in the pediatric intensive care unit for elective oncology procedures in ambulatory and hospitalized children. *Pediatrics* 2000;106:742–7.

Jayabose S, Levendoglu-Tugal O, Giamelli J, et al: Intravenous anesthesia with propofol for painful procedures in children with cancer. *J Pediatr Hematol Oncol* 2001;23:290–93.

Kain ZN: Postoperative behavioral changes in children. *ASA Newsl* 2002;66:14–16.

Krauss B, Green SM: Sedation and analgesia for procedures in children. *N Engl J Med* 2000;342:938–45.

Lowrie L, Weiss AH, Lacombe C: The pediatric sedation unit: A mechanism for pediatric sedation. *Pediatrics* 1998;102:30–37.

Markakis DA: Regional anesthesia in pediatrics. *Anesthesiol Clin North Am* 2000;18:355–81.

Maxwell LG, Yaster M: Perioperative management issues in pediatric patients. *Anesthesiol Clin North Am* 2000;18:601–32.

Melzer W, Dietze B: Malignant hyperthermia and excitation-contraction coupling. *Acta Physiol Scand* 2001;171:367–78.

Monitto CL, Greenberg RS, Kost-Byerly S, et al: The safety and efficacy of parent/nurse-controlled analgesia in patients less than six years of age. *Anesth Analg* 2000;91:573–79.

Morray JP, Geiduschek JM, Ramamoorthy C, et al: Anesthesia-related cardiac arrest in children: Initial findings of the Pediatric Perioperative Cardiac Arrest (POCA) Registry. *Anesthesiology* 2000;93:6–14.

Polaner D, Houck C, Finley G, et al: Sedation, risk, and safety: Do we really have data at last? *Pediatrics* 2001;108:1006–8.

Tobias JD: Therapeutic applications of regional anesthesia in paediatric-aged patients. *Paediatr Anaesth* 2002;12:272–7.

Tobias JD, Martin LD, Wetzel RC: Ketamine by continuous infusion for sedation in the pediatric intensive care unit. *Crit Care Med* 1990;18:19–21.

Urwyler A, Deufel T, McCarthy T, et al: Guidelines for molecular genetic detection of susceptibility to malignant hyperthermia. *Br J Anaesth* 2001;86:283–7.

Wellborn LG, Greenspun JC: Anesthesia and apnea: Perioperative considerations in the former preterm infant. *Pediatr Clin North Am* 1994;41:181–98.

Yaster M: The dose response of fentanyl in neonatal anesthesia. *Anesthesiology* 1987;66:433–35.

Yaster M, Sola JE, Pegoli W Jr, et al: The night after surgery: Postoperative management of the pediatric outpatient—surgical and anesthetic aspects. *Pediatr Clin North Am* 1994;41:199–220.

Chapter 66
Pediatric Pain Management

Brenda Bursch and Lonnie K. Zeltzer

DEVELOPMENT OF PAIN PERCEPTION

Even the smallest neonates respond to noxious stimulation with signs of stress and distress. During the 2nd trimester, afferent pathways in the human peripheral nervous system and spinal cord connect with peripheral targets and rostral projections to the thalamus and cortex develop. Neonates can even be regarded as hypersensitive to painful stimuli since reflex withdrawal is evoked by milder stimuli in neonates than in adults. Noxious stimulation in neonatal animals produces more prolonged discharges in spinal neurons than in older animals. Spinal dorsal horn neurons receive inputs from larger portions of the body surface, with greater overlap of cutaneous receptive fields. Pain inhibitory pathways become active comparatively later in development. Improved medical outcomes have been reported among neonates undergoing intensive care when efforts were undertaken to reduce painful experiences. Related research suggests that younger children may experience higher levels of distress during procedures than older children. Older children tend to display their distress less behaviorally than younger children, reinforcing the need to elicit self-reports of pain when possible.

Short-term benefits of opioid use in newborns receiving ventilatory support have been demonstrated with hemodynamic stability. Surgery in neonates receiving inadequate anesthesia evokes an outpouring of stress hormones with consequences including catabolism, immunosuppression, hemodynamic instability, and marked fluctuations in intracranial pressure.

There may also be long-term consequences of unrelieved pain in infants. More distress is observed in older infants receiving immunizations who were circumcised without anesthesia when compared with an uncircumcised group. Studies of neonatal intensive care unit (NICU) graduates have shown increased sensitivity in the heels of infants who required multiple heelsticks for blood sampling with a wider receptive field of sensitivity than the area in which the heelsticks were made. This work supports studies indicating that early significant pain exposure can sensitize the developing sensory nervous system. Preschoolers demonstrate a relationship between time in the NICU and pain complaints at age 3–4 yr. It is thought that the longer newborns are in the NICU, the more invasive procedures they might experience.

CLINICAL ASSESSMENT OF PAIN

Pain is both a sensory and emotional experience. Whenever feasible, pain is best assessed by directly asking children about the character, location, quality, duration, frequency, and intensity of their pain. Some children may not report pain because of fears such as talking to doctors, disappointing or bothering others, receiving an injection of medication, finding out they are sick, or returning to the hospital. For infants and nonverbal children, parents, pediatricians, nurses, and other caregivers are constantly challenged to interpret whether the distressed behaviors of the children represent pain, fear, hunger, or a range of other perceptions or emotions. Therapeutic trials of comfort measures (cuddling, feeding) and analgesic medications may be helpful in clarifying the situation.

Behavior and physiologic signs are useful but can be misleading. A toddler may scream and grimace during an ear examination because of fear rather than from pain. Conversely, children with inadequately relieved persistent pain from cancer, sickle cell disease, trauma, or surgery may withdraw from their surroundings and appear very quiet, leading observers to conclude falsely that they are comfortable or sedated. In these situations, increased dosing of analgesics may make the child become more, not less, interactive and alert. Similarly, neonates and young infants may close their eyes, furrow their brows, and clench their fists in response to pain. Adequate analgesia is often associated with eye opening and increased involvement in infants' surroundings. A child who is experiencing significant chronic pain may play "normally" as a way to distract attention from pain. This coping behavior is sometimes misinterpreted as evidence of the child "faking" pain at a nondistracted time.

Investigators have devised a range of behavioral distress scales for infants and young children, mostly emphasizing the patient's facial expressions, crying, and body movement. Facial expression measures appear most useful and specific in neonates. Autonomic signs can indicate pain but are nonspecific and may reflect other processes, including fever, hypoxemia, and cardiac or renal dysfunction.

Children ages 3–7 yr become increasingly articulate in describing intensity, location, and quality of pain. Pain is occasionally referred to adjacent areas; referral of hip pain to the leg or knee is not rare in this age range. There are self-report measures for children this age, using drawings, pictures of faces, or graded color intensity (Table 66–1). Children age 8 yr and older can usually use visual analog pain scales accurately. In the United States, regularly documented pain assessments are now required for children who are hospitalized and for children attending outpatient hospital clinics and emergency departments.

The measurement of pain in cognitively impaired children remains a challenge and methods are being studied to determine ways of assessing pain in this group. Understanding pain expression and experience in this population is important because behaviors may be misinterpreted as indicating that cognitively impaired children are more insensitive to pain. Children with Down syndrome may express pain less precisely and more slowly than the general population. Pain in individuals with autism spectrum disorders may be difficult to assess because they may be both hyposensitive and hypersensitive to many different types of sensory stimuli and they may have limited communication abilities.

NONPHARMACOLOGIC APPROACHES TO PAIN MANAGEMENT

There are numerous nonpharmacologic methods that can be used to relieve pain, fear, and anxiety. These approaches have excellent safety and good effectiveness. Studies of childhood chronic headaches provide more robust evidence of effectiveness for cognitive-behavioral treatments than for pharmacologic treatment. Many of these methods are also useful because children can generalize them to new situations and benefit from an increased sense of mastery by managing their symptoms. A child who has cancer and who learns self-hypnosis to reduce distress from lumbar punctures may successfully apply this skill to other stressful situations. Clinical attention to the environment, optimal positioning, physical comforts, and choice/control should be present for every patient and family. Nonpharmacologic techniques alone may not work for some children and should not be used as an excuse for withholding appropriate analgesics.

Information should be given to children (and family members) in a developmentally and situationally appropriate manner as to what to expect with their medical condition, procedures, and treatments. Clinicians should include patients and their families

TABLE 66-1. Pain Measurement Tools

Name	Features	Age Range	Advantages	Limitations
Visual Analog Scale (VAS)	Vertical 10-cm line, subject marks on line between "no pain" (or neutral face) and "worst pain imaginable" (or sad face)	8 yr and older	Good psychometric properties; gold standard	Cannot be used in younger children or those with cognitive limitations
Faces Scale (e.g., Wong-Baker, Oucher, Bieri, McGrath scales)	Subjects compare their pain to line drawings of faces or photos of children	4 yr and older	Can use in younger ages than VAS	Choice of "no pain" face affects responses (neutral vs. smiling)
Color and other analog scales	Horizontal or vertical ruler, on which increasing intensity of red signifies more pain; pain ladder; pain thermometer; blocks	4 yr and older	Can use at younger ages than VAS; converges to VAS at older ages	Cannot be used in toddlers or those with cognitive limitations
Behavioral or combined behavioral-physiological scales (e.g., CHEOPS, OPS, FACS, NIPS)	Scoring of observed behaviors (e.g., facial expression, limb movement) ± heart rate and blood pressure	Some work for any age; some are specific age groups, including preterm infants	Can be used even for infants and nonverbal children	Nonspecific; overrates fear in toddlers and preschool children; underrates persistent pain. Some measures are convenient, others require videotaping and complex processing. Changes can occur unrelated to pain.
Autonomic measures (e.g., heart rate, blood pressure, heart rate spectral analyses)	Scores changes in heart rate, blood pressure, or measures of heart rate variability (e.g., "vagal tone")	All ages	Can be used at all ages Useful for patients receiving mechanical ventilation	Nonspecific; changes can occur unrelated to pain
Hormonal-metabolic measures	Plasma or salivary sampling of hormones (e.g., cortisol, epinephrine)	All ages	Can be used at all ages	Nonspecific; changes can occur unrelated to pain; inconvenient; cannot provide "real-time" information

in the decision-making for pain control to ensure that the pain control option chosen is the most appropriate for the situation and to optimize adherence to treatment protocols.

Relaxation techniques promote muscle relaxation and the reduction of anxiety that often accompanies and increases pain. Controlled breathing and progressive muscle relaxation are commonly used relaxation techniques for children preschool age and older.

Distraction helps a child of any age shift attention away from pain and onto other activities. Common attention-sustainers in the environment include bubbles, music, video games, television, telephone, conversations, school, and play activities.

Hypnotherapy involves helping a child to focus on an imaginative experience that is comforting, safe, fun, or intriguing. Hypnotherapy acts to capture attention, alter sensory experiences, reduce distress, reframe pain experiences, create time distortions, help the child dissociate from the pain, and enhance feelings of mastery and self-control. This intervention is best for children of school-age or older.

Biofeedback involves controlled breathing, relaxation, or hypnotic techniques with a mechanical device that provides visual or auditory "feedback" to the child when the desired action is approximated. Common targets of change include muscle tension, peripheral skin temperature through peripheral vasodilation, or anal control through rectal muscle contraction and relaxation. Biofeedback also enhances the child's sense of mastery and control and is especially useful for the child who needs more "proof" of change than that generated through hypnotherapy alone.

Individual psychotherapy can be used to address the cognitive, behavioral, and psychological contributors to the pain and to pain behaviors. Assessing and treating maladaptive coping, anxiety, depression, learning disorders, social problem-solving deficits, communication problems, relationship issues, unresolved grief or trauma, school avoidance, or other identified problems can reduce acute distress and chronic stress load on the central nervous system, thereby reducing excessive arousal and pain.

Family education and/or psychotherapy may be employed to help family members understand the mechanisms and appropriate treatment of pain, to alter family patterns that may inadver-

tently exacerbate the pain, to help parents better cope with their own and their child's distress, and to develop a plan for the child's optimal self-management of symptoms and independent functioning. Cognitive behavioral family approaches have been shown to be effective for pediatric chronic pain.

Physical therapy can be very useful, especially for children with chronic musculoskeletal pain and/or who have become deconditioned from inactivity. Exercise appears to have both specific benefits related to muscle functioning and posture and more generalized benefits related to improved body image, body mechanics, sleep, and mood.

Transcutaneous electrical nerve stimulation (TENS) is quite safe and can be tried for many forms of localized pain. Children often find TENS helpful and effective; there are no randomized clinical trials of TENS for pain in children.

Acupuncture has been shown in adult studies to be effective in a variety of chronic and postoperative pain states, suggesting usefulness for pediatric myofascial pain, primary dysmenorrhea, sickle cell crisis pain, and sore throat pain. Acupuncture treatment in children can reduce both migraine frequency and intensity and increase panopioid activity that correlates with clinical improvement.

Yoga is another potentially helpful intervention for chronic pain, although studies have been conducted only in adults. Yoga typically involves a series of body poses that promotes a sense of energy, relaxation, strength, balance, and flexibility. Certain types of breathing may also accompany yoga.

Massage therapy can be very useful for children with chronic pain. Reductions in pain in children with juvenile rheumatoid arthritis and cancer and in adolescents with fibromyalgia have been noted using deep tissue massage. In addition to pain reduction and increased function, children were found to have short-term reductions in cortisol levels and improved sleep and mood.

Oral sucrose and pacifiers are effective for procedure-related pain reduction, with the combination being most effective. This approach works best with neonates, but it can be tried in infants up to 3 mo of age. Pacifiers and sucrose should not be used in lieu of analgesic medications when they are necessary and appropriate.

DEVELOPMENTAL PHARMACOLOGY

Because the pharmacokinetics and pharmacodynamics of analgesics vary with age, infants and young children respond to drugs differently from older children and adults. The elimination half-life of most analgesics is prolonged in neonates and young children because of their immature hepatic enzyme systems. Clearance of analgesics also may be variable in young infants and children. Renal blood flow, glomerular filtration, and tubular secretion increase dramatically in the first weeks and approach adult values by 3–5 mo. Renal clearance of analgesics is often greater in toddlers and preschool children than in adults, whereas premature infants tend to have reduced renal clearance of analgesics. There also are age-related differences in body composition and protein binding. Total body water as a fraction of body weight is greater in neonates. Tissues with greater perfusion such as the brain and heart account for a larger proportion of body mass in neonates than do other tissues such as muscle and fat. Because of decreased serum concentrations of albumin and α_1-acid glycoprotein, neonates have reduced protein binding of some drugs, resulting in higher amounts of free, unbound drug. Drug dosing in infants and younger children is often extrapolated from studies in adults and older children using weight-based scaling.

Acetaminophen, Aspirin, and Nonsteroidal Anti-inflammatory Medications. Acetaminophen and nonsteroidal anti-inflammatory drugs (NSAIDs) have replaced aspirin as the most commonly used antipyretics and oral nonopioid analgesics (Table 66–2).

Acetaminophen is generally a safe nonopioid analgesic and antipyretic that has the advantage of rectal, as well as oral, route of administration. In addition, acetaminophen is not associated with the gastrointestinal effects or antiplatelet effects of aspirin and NSAIDs, making it a particularly useful drug in cancer patients. Unlike aspirin and NSAIDs, acetaminophen has little anti-inflammatory action. Toxicity of acetaminophen can occur from either large single doses or excessive cumulative dosing over days (see Chapter 704.2). Acetaminophen overdoses have been associated with fulminant hepatic failure in infants and children.

TABLE 66–2. Commonly Used Nonopioid Medications

Acetaminophen	10–15 mg/kg PO q4h 20–30 mg/kg/PR q4h 35 mg/kg/PR, q6–8h *Maximum daily dosing:* 90 mg/kg/24 hr (children) 60 mg/kg/24 hr (infants) 30–45 mg/kg/24 hr (neonates)	No anti-inflammatory action; no antiplatelet or gastric effects; toxic dosing can produce hepatic failure
Aspirin	10–15 mg/kg PO q4h *Maximum daily dosing:* 120 mg/kg/24 hr (children)	Anti-inflammatory effects; prolonged antiplatelet effects; can cause gastritis; risk of Reye syndrome
Ibuprofen	8–10 mg/kg PO q6h	Anti-inflammatory effects; reversible antiplatelet effects; can cause gastritis; extensive pediatric safety experience
Naprosyn	5–7 mg/kg PO q8–12h	Anti-inflammatory effects; reversible antiplatelet effects; can cause gastritis; more prolonged duration than that of ibuprofen
Ketorolac	Loading dose 0.5 mg/kg then 0.25–0.5 mg/kg IV q6h to a maximum of 5 days; Max. dose 30 mg loading with Max. dosing of 15 mg q6h after that	Anti-inflammatory effects; reversible antiplatelet effects; can cause gastritis; useful for short-term situations when oral dosing is not feasible
Choline magnesium salicylate	10–20 mg/kg PO q8–12h	Weak anti-inflammatory effects; lower risk of bleeding and gastritis than with conventional NSAIDs
Nortriptyline, amitriptyline	Amitriptyline at 0.2–0.5 mg/kg PO qhs, typically with maximum dose at 10–20 mg hs Nortriptyline is typically used at twice the doses described above.	Useful for neuropathic pain; facilitates sleep; can enhance opioid effect; can be useful in sickle cell pain. Rare risk of dysrhythmias; should screen for rhythm disturbances, check for normal QTc before beginning. Side effects include dry mouth, sedation, constipation, urinary retention, orthostatic hypotension, palpitations
Gabapentin (Neurontin)	Start with 100 mg bid or tid and then increase; can use up to 3600 mg/24 h, but no good studies in children to indicate minimum or maximum dosing	Is an anticonvulsant used for neuropathic pain; can be associated with sedation or headache
Thioridazine (Mellaril), resperidone, thorazine, haloperidol	Thioridazine, 5–10 mg tablet or liquid concentrate; start 10 mg PO tid and use prn qh for acute pain exacerbation, especially if nausea accompanies pain (lowest Tab is 10 mg). Resperidone can be especially useful for children with PDD spectrum or tic disorder and chronic pain; dose is 0.25 mg – 1 mg (in 0.25-mg increments) qd or bid. See PDR for other dosing.	Useful when arousal is clearly amplifying pain signaling; often used when first starting SSRI and then weaned off after on therapeutic doses of SSRI for at least 2 wk; check for normal QTc before beginning. Side effects include extrapyramidal reactions and sedation and in high doses can lower the seizure threshold in children with a seizure disorder. Diphenhydramine (Benadryl) can be used to treat or prevent dystonic reactions.
SSRIs (e.g., fluoxetine)	SSRI dosing per psychiatrist recommendation. Fluoxetine can be used in very low doses (e.g., 1 mg) for children with chronic pain and PDD spectrum disorders.	Useful for children with anxiety disorder in which arousal amplifies sensory signaling; useful in PDD spectrum disorders in very low doses; best to use in conjunction with psychiatric evaluation.
Sucrose solution via pacifier or gloved finger	*Preterm Infants (gestational age):* <28 wk: 0.2 mL swabbed into mouth; 28–32 wk: 0.2–2 mL depending on suck/swallow; >32 wk: 2 mL *Term Infants:* 1.5–2 mL PO over 2 min	Wait 2 min before starting procedure. Analgesia may last up to 8 min. The dose may be repeated once.

NSAIDs = nonsteroidal anti-inflammatory drugs; SSRI = selective serotonin reuptake inhibitor; PDD = pervasive developmental disorder.

Fever, alcohol, and dehydration may be risk factors for hepatic injury.

Aspirin is indicated for certain rheumatologic conditions and for inhibition of platelet adhesiveness, as in the treatment of Kawasaki disease. Concerns about Reye hepatic encephalopathy have resulted in a substantial decline in pediatric aspirin use during the past 20 yr (see Chapter 342).

NSAIDs are used widely for the treatment of pain and fever in children. In children with juvenile rheumatoid arthritis, ibuprofen and aspirin are equally effective but ibuprofen is associated with fewer side effects and better compliance. NSAIDs used adjunctively in surgical patients have been found to reduce opioid requirements (and opioid side effects) by as much as 35–40%. Although NSAIDs can be useful postoperatively, they should not be used as an excuse to withhold opioids from patients with unrelieved pain. Ketorolac is useful in treating moderate to severe acute pain when patients are unable to swallow oral medications.

Adverse effects of NSAIDs are rare but include gastrointestinal bleeding, renal dysfunction, and impaired hemostasis. Although the overall incidence of bleeding is very low, NSAIDs should be avoided in children who are at risk for bleeding or when surgical hemostasis is a prominent concern. Renal injury from short-term use of ibuprofen in euvolemic children is quite rare; renal risk is increased by hypovolemia or cardiac dysfunction. The safety of both ibuprofen and acetaminophen for short-term use is well established (see Table 66–2).

NSAIDs and aspirin act by inhibition of cyclooxygenase (COX), which is an enzyme that catalyzes production of prostanoids to form arachidonic acid. Cyclooxygenase has two predominant isoenzymes: a constitutively synthesized form, COX-1, found in platelets, gastric mucosa, liver, and kidneys, and an inducible form, COX-2, found in monocytes, peripheral nerve, and spinal cord and induced by injury and inflammation. Inhibition of COX-1 produces side effects, and inhibition of COX-2 produces analgesia. COX-2 inhibitors may be safer NSAIDs. Clinical trials in adults with several selective COX-2 inhibitors (e.g., rofecoxib [Vioxx] and celecoxib [Celebrex]) suggest that these agents provide analgesia similar to that obtained with NSAIDs but with a dramatic reduction in gastric, hemostatic, hepatic, and renal side effects. Thrombosis and aseptic meningitis are rare complications in adults.

Opioids. Opioids are most frequently administered for moderate and severe pain, such as acute postoperative pain, sickle cell crisis pain, and cancer pain. Opioids can be administered by oral, rectal, oral transmucosal, transdermal, intranasal, intravenous, epidural, intrathecal, subcutaneous, and intramuscular routes. Infants and young children are often underdosed with opioids for fear of significant respiratory side effects. With proper understanding of the pharmacokinetics and pharmacodynamics of opioids, children can receive effective relief of pain and suffering with a good margin of safety (Box 66–1 and Table 66–3).

Opioids act by mimicking actions of endogenous opioid peptides in binding to receptors in the brain, brainstem, spinal cord, and peripheral nervous system. Opioids have dose-dependent respiratory depressant effects and blunt ventilatory responses to hypoxia and hypercarbia. The respiratory depressant effects of opioids can be increased with co-administration of other sedating drugs, such as benzodiazepines or barbiturates. Other common side effects can include constipation, nausea, vomiting, urinary retention, and pruritus. Optimal use of opioids requires proactive and anticipatory management of these side effects. The most common easily treatable side effect is constipation. Stool softeners and stimulant laxatives should be administered to most patients receiving opioids for more than a few days. Constipation often continues to be a problem with long-term opioid adminis-

tration. Specific bowel opiate receptor antagonists may prevent this complication. Nausea sometimes subsides with long-term dosing but often requires treatment with antiemetics, such as phenothiazine, butyrophenones, antihistamines, and the new serotonin receptor antagonists. It is important for pediatricians to understand the phenomena of tolerance, dependence, withdrawal, and addiction (see Box 66–1).

Continuous opioid intravenous infusion is a safe and effective option that permits more constant plasma concentrations and clinical effects than intermittent intravenous opioid bolus dosing. One approach is to permit patients to titrate their own dosing using a patient-controlled analgesia (PCA) device. A basal continuous infusion is often also delivered. Children as young as 5–6 yr can effectively use PCA; parents or nurses can assist younger patients. When compared with children given intermittent intramuscular morphine, children using PCA reported better pain scores and satisfaction. PCA has the advantage of adjusting dosing to account for individual pharmacokinetic and pharmacodynamic variation, as well as changing pain intensity during the day. It also has the psychological advantage of promoting patient control and active coping. There may be lower overall opioid consumption and fewer side effects with use of PCA. Overdoses have been reported when well-meaning, inadequately instructed parents pushed the PCA button in medically complicated situations.

Local Anesthetics. Local anesthetics are widely used in children for topical application, cutaneous infiltration, peripheral nerve block, epidural injection, and intraspinal punctures. Local anesthetics can be used with excellent safety and effectiveness. Excessive systemic concentrations can cause seizures, central nervous system depression, arrhythmia, or cardiac depression. Unlike opioids, there is a strict maximum dosing of local anesthetics. Pediatricians need to be aware of the need to calculate these doses and adhere to the guidelines.

■ **BOX 66–1. Practical Aspects of Prescribing Opioids**

Morphine is typically regarded as a first choice for severe pain.

The right dose is the dose that relieves pain with a good margin of safety.

Dosing should be titrated and individualized. There is no "right" dose for everyone.

Dosing should be more cautious with younger infants, in patients having coexisting diseases that increase risk or impair drug clearance, and with concomitant administration of sedatives.

Anticipate and treat peripheral side effects, including constipation, nausea, and itching.

Give doses at sufficient frequency to prevent return of severe pain before the next dose.

With opioid dosing for more than a week, taper gradually to avoid withdrawal symptoms.

When converting between parenteral and oral opioid doses, use appropriate potency ratios.

Tolerance refers to decreasing effect on continued administration of drug or need for increased dosing to achieve the same effect; patients receiving opioids continually may need increasing doses to achieve analgesia; tolerance to respiratory depression develops parallel with tolerance to analgesic action; thus with the higher doses they do not develop respiratory depression

Dependence refers to the need for continued opioid dosing to prevent withdrawal symptoms (irritability, agitation, autonomic arousal, nasal congestion, piloerection, diarrhea and/or jitteriness; and, in neonates, yawning); produced by regular or high-dose opioids for ≥ 7 days, especially if the opioid is abruptly stopped; slow tapering may be needed

Addiction refers to psychological craving with compulsive drug-seeking behavior. Opioid underdosing does not prevent addiction and may increase drug-seeking behavior for relief of pain; good pain relief allows focus off opioids.

TABLE 66–3. Analgesic Initial Dosage Guidelines

Drug	Equianalgesic Doses Parenteral	Equianalgesic Doses Oral	Usual Starting IV or SC Doses and Intervals Child <50 kg	Usual Starting IV or SC Doses and Intervals Child >50 kg	Parenteral/ Oral Dose Ratio	Usual Starting Oral Doses and Intervals Child <50 kg	Usual Starting Oral Doses and Intervals Child >50 kg	Comments
Codeine	N/R	200 mg	N/R	N/R	1:2	0.5–1 mg/kg q3–4h	30–60 mg q3–4h	Weak opioid; typically given with acetaminophen; doesn't require triplicate
Morphine	10 mg	30 mg	*Bolus:* 0.1 mg/kg q2–4h *Infusion:* 0.01 mg/kg/hr in younger infants to 0.3 mg/kg/hr in older infants and children	*Bolus:* 5–8 mg q2–4h *Infusion:* 1–1.5 mg/hr	1:3	*Immediate release:* 0.3 mg/kg q3–4h *Sustained release:* 20–35 kg: 10–15 mg q8–12h 35–50 kg: 15–30 mg q8–12h	*Immediate release:* 15–20 mg q3–4h *Sustained release:* 30–45 mg q8–12h	Potent opioid for moderate/severe pain; can cause histamine release and wheezing in children with asthma; least expensive opioid. Sustained release must be swallowed whole; cannot be crushed or it becomes immediate acting.
Oxycodone	N/A	30 mg	N/A	N/A	N/A	0.1–0.2 mg q3–4h; available in liquid (1 mg/mL)	5–10 mg q3–4h; available in tablet (5 mg); also comes in long-acting form (q12h) in varying strengths	Weak opioid but more potent than codeine with fewer gastrointestinal side effects; more potent and preferable to hydrocodone, which is always combined with acetaminophen (e.g., Vicodin); available alone without acetaminophen (Percocet is combined form); underutilized because it requires a triplicate.
Methadone	10 mg	20 mg	0.1 mg/kg q4–8h	5–8 mg q4–8h	1:2	0.2 mg/kg q4–8h PO Available in liquid or tablet	10 mg q4–8h	12–24 hr duration; useful in certain types of chronic pain; requires additional vigilance, because it can accumulate and produce delayed sedation. If sedation occurs, doses should be withheld until sedation resolves, then substantially reduced and/or the dosing interval should be extended to 8–12 hr. When patients who are tolerant to morphine or hydromorphone are switched to methadone, they sometimes show incomplete cross tolerance and improved efficacy.
Fentanyl	100 µg (0.1 mg)	N/A	*Bolus:* 0.5–1 µg/kg q1–2h *Infusion:* 0.5–1.5 µg/kg/hr	*Bolus:* 25–50 µg q1–2h *Infusion:* 25–75 µg/hr	N/A	Transdermal patch soon available in 12.5 µg/hr dose	Transdermal patches available; patch reaches steady state at 24 hr and should be changed q72h	Potent analgesic 70–100 times as potent as morphine; rapid onset and shorter duration; with high doses and rapid administration, can cause chest wall rigidity (which can be reversed with naloxone or neuromuscular blockade); useful for short procedures; low gastrointestinal side effect and pruritus profile
Hydromorphone	1.5–2 mg	6–8 mg	*Bolus:* 0.02 mg q2–4h *Infusion:* 0.006 mg/kg/hr	*Bolus:* 1 mg q2–4h *Infusion:* 0.3 mg/hr	1:4	0.04–0.08 mg/kg q3–4h	2–4 mg q3–4h	Similar to morphine except five times as potent; less histamine release than with morphine
Meperidine (pethidine)	75 mg	300 mg	*Bolus:* 0.8–1 mg/kg q2–3h	*Bolus:* 50–75 mg q2–3h	1:4	2–3 mg/kg q3–4h	100–150 mg q3–4h	Avoid if other opioids are available (especially for chronic use) because its metabolite, normeperidine, can cause dysphoria, agitation, and seizures. Primary use in low doses is for treatment of rigors and shivering with amphotericin or blood products.

Topical local anesthetic preparations have diverse uses in reducing pain, such as for suturing lacerations, intravenous catheter placements, lumbar punctures, and accessing indwelling central ports. Application of tetracaine, epinephrine (Adrenalin), and cocaine (TAC) results in good anesthesia for suturing wounds. It should not be used on mucous membranes. Cocaine is not essential; combinations of tetracaine with phenylephrine or lidocaine-epinephrine-tetracaine are equally effective. EMLA is a topical eutectic mixture of lidocaine and prilocaine that is used to anesthetize intact skin and is commonly applied for venipuncture, lumbar puncture, and other needle procedures. EMLA is safe for use in neonates. It is more effective than placebo but probably is less effective than ring block of the penis in providing analgesia for circumcision. EMLA should be used with caution for circumcision, because there was a report of redness and blistering on the penis in a study comparing dorsal penile block to EMLA. A small area should be tested first for hypersensitivity before EMLA is applied more widely.

Lidocaine is the most commonly used local anesthetic for cutaneous infiltration. Maximum safe doses of lidocaine are 5 mg/kg without epinephrine and 6 mg/kg with epinephrine. Concentrated solutions (e.g., 2%) should be avoided, because solutions as dilute as 0.3% are equally effective as 1–2% solutions, and the dilute solutions permit larger doses. For example, a 5-kg infant receiving infiltration for suturing may safely receive up to $5 \times 5 = 25$ mg of lidocaine. This maximum dose would be attained with either 1.25 mL of lidocaine 2%, 2.5 mL of lidocaine 1%, or 5 mL of lidocaine 0.5%.

Regional Anesthesia. Regional anesthesia is widely used for postoperative pain relief in children after many types of surgery, such as abdominal, orthopedic, and thoracic procedures. It also can reduce the need for systemic opioids for patients with severe lung disease. Epidural analgesia and peripheral nerve blocks provide excellent analgesia and are safe even in term and preterm infants. Spinal anesthesia can be used to avoid the need for general anesthesia and for intubated infants with moderate and severe lung disease undergoing herniorrhaphy or lower extremity procedures.

SPECIFIC TYPES OF PAIN

The pharmacologic and nonpharmacologic approaches to pain management should be considered for all pain treatment plans, regardless of the type of pain. Many simple interventions designed to promote relaxation and patient control can be expected to work synergistically with pain medications for optimal relief of pain and related distress. More than one type of pain may be present in the same patient.

Brief Procedural Pain. There is no one way to manage pain and distress for all procedures. The specific approach might vary according to the expected intensity and duration of the pain, the context and meaning of the procedure for the child and family, the coping styles and temperaments of the child and parents, the type of procedure, and the child's pain history (especially during procedures). Interventions that reduce distress for parents and children have been associated with reductions in children's report of pain and in observations of their pain behavior. Therefore, optimal preparation might include education about the procedure, management of procedure-related expectations, development of skills designed to increase active participation and improved coping during the procedure, rehearsal of the procedure to increase mastery, and positive reinforcement for successful coping after the procedure is complete. Imagery, relaxation, and self-regulation and complementary approaches, such as massage or application of cold or heat, may be especially beneficial. Depending on the situation, it may be helpful to have the parents present if they are prepared with specific ways of comforting their child. All pain management strategies will be most effective in a quiet environment (other than entertaining auditory distractors), with calm adults, and with clear and confident instructions.

Procedures may require *analgesia* to make the procedure more comfortable, *anxiolysis* to make the procedure less terrifying, and/or *sedation* to permit a child to lie motionless. Local anesthetics, along with interventions to soothe and minimize distress, should be considered even for simple procedures, such as venipuncture. Newborn circumcisions cause significant pain during the procedure and are associated with irritability and feeding disturbances for several days. For predictably severe procedural pain, such as for bone marrow aspirations, local measures are often insufficient; systemic agents are then required. The use of anxiolytics alone does not provide analgesia and can make a child less able to communicate pain and distress.

Sedation represents a continuum of responses. The term *conscious sedation* refers to a condition in which a patient is sleepy, comfortable, and cooperative but maintains protective airway and ventilatory reflexes. The term *deep sedation* refers to a state of unarousability to voice and greater suppression of reflex responses. A dose of sedative medication that causes minimal sedation in one subject may produce complete unconsciousness and apnea in another. Careful attention to guidelines for appropriate monitoring and managing of sedation in children is imperative. For example, guidelines from the American Academy of Pediatrics recommend that sedation be conducted in a monitored setting with resuscitative drugs and equipment available and that competently trained people administer the sedatives and analgesics. One person should be assigned to monitor the child's condition and another qualified person should be present to respond to medical emergencies (Table 66–4). Most severe adverse events occur during sedations in settings outside the hospital and when these guidelines are not followed.

Operative Pain. Morbidity and mortality can be reduced by good pain treatment. Fortunately, most postoperative pain in children can be well treated in a simple and cost-effective manner without advanced techniques. Education about the surgery and a pain management plan, development of skills designed to decrease anticipatory anxiety, and active participation in treatment planning can be helpful for some children and families. In addition to nonpharmacologic approaches, opioids are indicated to manage moderate to severe postoperative pain. The addition of other analgesics, such as acetaminophen and NSAIDs, can reduce the amount of opioid required. Pain should be controlled as quickly as possible to avoid prolonged pain, escalation of anxiety, and adverse side effects of the analgesic, such as respiratory depression. Consequently, the starting dose should be optimal and subsequent doses should be adjusted depending on patient response. Specifically, attempts should be made to avoid the administration of multiple, small, ineffective doses of analgesic. Oral routes are preferred for mild to moderate pain, and intravenous or regional routes are indicated for moderate to severe pain. Continuous or around-the-clock dosing at fixed intervals is recommended while the pain is moderate to severe. Side effects should be monitored and treated, and the potential synergistic sedative effects of analgesics, anxiolytics, antiemetics, and antihistamines require attention. Treatment of postoperative pain should not stop abruptly at the time of discharge, and a home plan for pain management should be discussed with the family if indicated.

Trauma Pain. The management of trauma pain and distress may be given minimal attention owing to the emphasis on

TABLE 66–4. Drugs Used for Conscious Sedation in Children*

Drug	Suggested Starting Dose(s)	Comments
Midazolam	0.05 mg/kg incremental doses IV q 5–10 min up to 3–5 doses (to a maximum incremental dose of 1 mg) 0.1–0.2 mg/kg IM (maximum dose 10 mg) 0.3–0.6 mg/kg PO (maximum dose 20 mg)	Good anxiolytic Flumazenil is a reversal agent Dose more cautiously when combined with opioids
Fentanyl	0.5 µg/kg increments q 5 min up to 3–5 doses	Rapid infusion of large doses can produce chest wall rigidity Respiratory depression is amplified by co-administration of sedatives
Pentobarbital	1 mg/kg increments IV q 10 min up to 3 doses 2–4 mg/kg IM 4–6 mg/kg PO	Good sedative No analgesia Used often for radiologic procedures Can produce prolonged sedation
Chloral hydrate	25–100 mg/kg PO or PR 30–40 min before the procedure	Higher incidence of failed sedation with 25–50 mg/kg
Ketamine	0.2–0.5 mg/kg increments q 10 min × 3 1–2 mg/kg IM	Co-administration of midazolam or other benzodiazepines can reduce the risk of dysphoria or bad dreams Use should be restricted to cases managed by physicians with deep sedation qualifications
Propofol	Dosing per anesthesiologist	IV anesthetic often referred to as "milk of amnesia" Should be administered by anesthesiologist

*To ensure that patients receive optimal, safe care, it is now required in the United States that hospitals develop conscious sedation guidelines, such as those established by the American Academy of Pediatrics. These guidelines should include recommendations for withholding feeding before procedures, drug dosages, strategies to achieve patient comfort, necessary monitoring, required resuscitation equipment, and a quality improvement program for tracking outcomes and ensuring efficacy and safety. The guidelines also should specify which subgroups of patients are at increased risk and should have sedation performed by pediatric anesthesiologists.

life-supporting, critical care interventions. Pain may be caused by the original trauma, surgical procedures, restricted movement, or underlying disease, and the presence of lines, tubes, and drains. It may be significantly exacerbated by biological and psychological post-traumatic stress responses. The thoughtful choice of analgesics, dosage, timing, and route of administration should be tailored to the individual patient, given the overall context of what is best for the patient and desired by the family. Frequent communication with the family can also serve to optimize appropriate expectations in family members, allowing them to better attend to the needs of their child. When pain is prolonged, dosages should be adjusted to compensate for physical tolerance, and weaning strategies should be used to minimize withdrawal symptoms. Attention should be paid to the child's sleep-wake cycles (because sufficient sleep will enable the child to cope better when awake) and to the child's and family's psychological response to the trauma. Parents can benefit from psychoeducation and/or consultation with a mental health provider to help them monitor their child for signs and symptoms of psychological trauma and to respond to these symptoms in a therapeutically helpful manner.

Cancer Pain. The World Health Organization (WHO) proposed a model for analgesic therapy for cancer pain known as the "analgesic ladder" (Box 66–2). This consists of a hierarchy of oral pharmacologic interventions designed to treat pain of increasing magnitude. It presents a framework for the rational use of oral medication before application of other techniques of drug administration, because of the simplicity and demonstrated efficacy of oral medication. Opioid therapy is the preferred approach for moderate or severe pain. Nonopioid analgesics are used for mild pain, a weak opioid is added for moderate pain, and strong opioids are administered for more severe pain. Adjuvant analgesics can be added, and side effects and co-morbid symptoms are actively managed.

Although the oral route of opioid administration should be encouraged, some children are unable to take oral opioids. Intravenous infusions with a PCA are used next. Small portable infusion pumps are convenient for home use. If venous access is limited, a useful alternative is to administer opioids (especially

---

BOX 66–2. World Health Organization Analgesic Ladder for Cancer Pain

STEP 1:
Patients who present with mild-to-moderate pain should be treated with a nonopioid.

STEP 2:
Patients who present with moderate-to-severe pain or who fail the first-step regimen should be treated with an oral opioid for moderate pain combined with a nonopioid analgesic.

STEP 3:
Patients who present with very severe pain or who fail the second-step regimen should be treated with an opioid used for severe pain with or without a nonopioid analgesic.

Medications for persistent cancer-related pain should be administered on an around-the-clock basis, with additional "as-needed" doses, because regularly scheduled dosing maintains a constant level of drug in the body and helps to prevent a recurrence of pain.

Adjuvant medications can be used to treat opioid side effects and comorbid conditions.

Adjuvant analgesics represent a diverse group of drug classes that have other indications but are analgesic in specific circumstances. Adjuvant medications should be used when indications exist at any step.

Some of the commonly used adjuvant analgesics include anticonvulsants, antidepressants, local anesthetics, corticosteroids, antihistaminics, muscle relaxants, neuroleptics, anticholinergics (for visceral pain caused by bowel obstruction), and psychostimulants (to decrease sedation caused by opioid analgesia).

---

morphine or hydromorphone, not methadone or meperidine) through continuous subcutaneous infusion, with or without a bolus option. A small (e.g., 22-gauge) cannula is placed under the skin and secured on the thorax, abdomen, or thigh. Sites may be changed every 3–7 days as needed. Other alternative routes for opioids include the transdermal and oral transmucosal routes.

Pain Associated with Terminal Illnesses. Patients with terminal illnesses, including cancer, AIDS, neurodegenerative disorders, and cystic fibrosis, need approaches to palliative care that focus on optimal quality of life. Nonpharmacologic and pharmacologic management of pain and other distressing symptoms can be one critical component of comprehensive palliative care. Differences among these conditions related to the progression of underlying illness, associated distressing symptoms, and common emotional responses should shape individual treatment plans (see Chapter 38).

More than 90% of children and adolescents dying of cancer can be made comfortable by standard escalation of opioids according to the WHO protocol. A small subgroup (5%) will have enormous opioid dose escalation to more than 100 times standard morphine infusion rates. In most of these cases, there is spread of solid tumors to the spinal cord, roots, or plexus and signs of neuropathic pain are evident.

The type(s) of pain being experienced by the patient (e.g., neuropathic, myofascial) should determine the need for adjunctive agents. Complementary measures, such as massage, hypnotherapy, or spiritual care, should also be considered in palliative care.

Chronic and Recurrent Nonmalignant Pain. A large proportion of otherwise healthy children experience recurrent episodes or continuous nonspecific headache, chest pain, abdominal pain, or limb pains. These children, who often simply have a neurosensory pain signaling problem, may appear to be growing as expected and may show no signs suggestive of serious disease (see Chapter 158).

A thorough biopsychosocial history, review of systems, and physical examination comprise the cornerstone of diagnosis. It is also important to understand how the pain affects social functioning, school functioning and attendance, and parental behaviors toward the child. Laboratory testing and diagnostic procedures should be sparse and guided by clinical indication. Gastrointestinal barium roentgenographic studies in children with recurrent abdominal pain that appears benign from history and physical examination have a low yield. Recurrent abdominal pain may be one of a variety of functional abdominal symptoms, such as nausea, vomiting, bloating, diarrhea, or constipation, with mechanisms related to neuroenteric dysregulation rather than gastrointestinal structural or inflammatory problems. The absence of findings on radiographic or endoscopic procedures does not indicate that "the problem is fake or is psychological."

Overall, management of chronic benign pain should emphasize nonpharmacologic approaches, rather than excessive reliance on medications in isolation. When it is concluded that a patient's pain is benign, it is very important for the pediatrician to: (1) avoid over medicalization because this can exacerbate the pain and associated disability, (2) maintain an open mind to reassessing the diagnosis if the clinical presentation changes later, and (3) understand and communicate to the family that the pain has a biologic basis (likely related to neural signaling and neurotransmitter dysregulation) and is naturally distressing the child and family. All patients and families should receive a simple explanation of pain physiology that helps them understand the importance of functional rehabilitation to normalize pain signaling, the low risk of causing further injury with systematic increases in normal functioning, and the risks associated with treating the pain as if it were acute. It is counterintuitive for most people to move a part of the body that hurts, and many patients with chronic pain develop atrophy or contractures of a painful extremity because of disuse. Additionally, associated increases in worry and anxiety may exacerbate pain and leave the body even more vulnerable to further illness, injury, and disability.

For a small subgroup of children with chronic pain, school absenteeism is a significant problem. An especially detailed assessment of possible family, cognitive, learning, peer, and anxiety or other emotional problems is indicated to ensure that a successful plan for school re-entry can be developed and implemented. Home schooling for these patients has been shown to predict poor outcome and is, therefore, not recommended as a long-term solution.

Sickle Cell Anemia (see Chapter 454.1). Both recurrent acute severe pain and chronic persistent pain occur in some affected children. There is a marked variation in the frequency and severity of painful episodes; the majority of people with sickle cell disease come to the hospital only rarely and manage most of their symptoms at home. Successful treatment models emphasize (1) self-care and maintenance of normal activities, (2) generous dosing of opioids and NSAIDs at home by the oral route whenever possible, (3) treatment of breakthrough pain in a day-treatment program or clinic rather than in an emergency department or hospital admission, and (4) teaching of biobehavioral techniques and coping strategies before a cycle develops involving negative experiences with health care personnel. Ketorolac may reduce the need for, or the total dose of, opiates and avoid hospitalization. For severe episodes requiring inpatient treatment, intravenous opioid infusions and PCA can be used safely and effectively, although careful dose titration may be needed in many cases. Favorable effects on pain and respiratory function are possible when continuous epidural infusions are used in children at high risk for acute chest syndrome. Other strategies, like acupuncture, should also be considered, as well as amitriptyline for enhanced sleep and opioid efficacy.

Neuropathic Pain. Neuropathic pain is caused by abnormal excitability in the peripheral or central nervous system that may persist after an injury heals or inflammation subsides. The pain, which can be acute or chronic, is often described as burning or stabbing and may be associated with cutaneous hypersensitivity (allodynia). Neuropathic pain conditions may be responsible for more than 35% of referrals to chronic pain clinics and commonly include post-traumatic and postsurgical peripheral nerve injuries, phantom pain after amputation, pain after spinal cord injury, and pain due to metabolic neuropathies. Neuropathic pain frequently responds poorly to opioids. In adults, evidence suggests the efficacy of tricyclic antidepressants (e.g., nortriptyline, amitriptyline) and anticonvulsants (e.g., carbamazepine, gabapentin) for treatment of neuropathic pain. *Complex regional pain syndrome type I* (formerly known as *reflex sympathetic dystrophy*) is the term applied to an affected body part that has become sensitized without any specific nerve injury. Hyperalgesia can occur anywhere on the body, often in no particular neural distribution, including internal organs (e.g., stomach or esophagus). Treatment emphasizes targeted physical therapy and facilitation of functioning.

American Academy of Pediatrics, Committee on Drugs: Guidelines for monitoring and management of pediatric patients during and after sedation for diagnostic and therapeutic procedures. *Pediatrics* 1992;89:1110–15.
American Academy of Pediatrics, Committee on Fetus and Newborn, Committee on Drugs, Section on Anesthesiology, Section on Surgery: Prevention and management of pain and stress in the neonate. *Pediatrics* 2000;105:545–61.
American Academy of Pediatrics, Committee on Psychosocial Aspects of Child and Family Health: The assessment and management of acute pain in infants, children, and adolescents. *Pediatrics* 2000;108:793–97.
American Academy of Pediatrics, Task Force on Circumcision: Circumcision policy statement. *Pediatrics* 1999;103:686–93.
American Pain Society: Pediatric chronic pain: A position statement from the American Pain Society. *Am Pain Soc Bull* 2001;1(11).
American Pain Society: *Guidelines for the Management of Acute and Chronic Pain in Sickle Cell Disease*, 1999.

Berde CB, Sethna NF: Analgesia for the treatment of pain in childhood. *N Engl J Med* 2002;347(14):1094–1103.

Hyman PE (editor): *Pediatric Functional Bowel Disorders.* New York, Academy Professional Information Services, 1999.

Schecter NL, Berde CB, Yaster M (editors): *Pain in Infants, Children, and Adolescents,* 2nd ed. Philadelphia, Lippincott, Williams & Wilkins, 2002.

World Health Organization: *Cancer Pain Relief and Palliative Care in Children,* Geneva, World Health Organization, 1998.

Internet Site

www.pediatric-pain.ca/links.html

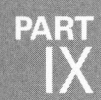

Chapter 67

The Molecular Basis of Genetic Disorders *H. Eugene Hoyme*

THE IMPACT OF GENETICS ON THE CLINICAL PRACTICE OF PEDIATRICS

The etiology of all human disease can be considered a spectrum, from those conditions completely genetically determined to those completely environmentally determined. Most disorders fall somewhere in the middle, with the individual displaying a certain genetic propensity or resistance to a condition, on which the environment acts to determine whether or not an individual is affected.

Despite the perception that individual genetic disorders are rare, taken as a whole they account for a significant proportion of illness and disability in children. The Centers for Disease Control and Prevention has determined that birth defects and genetic disorders represent a major cause of morbidity and mortality in infancy and childhood. Twenty-five per cent to 39% of admissions to children's hospitals involve children with genetically determined or partially genetically determined disorders; 11% of all deaths in childhood are related to an underlying genetic condition.

The Human Genome Project has moved ahead at an advanced pace, and a rough draft of the human genome is now complete, spanning 90% of the sequence, with a high-resolution map anticipated to be available in 2003. The significant and surprising information that the Human Genome Project has already supplied includes the following:

1. The genome is very lumpy—some areas have functional genes packed together; other areas are composed of so-called filler DNA.

2. Humans may have fewer genes than expected, approximately 38,000. Many lower organisms have more genes than humans.

3. Human genes make more proteins per gene (three on average) than many other organisms.

4. Human proteins are more complex than those of many other organisms.

5. Dozens of human genes may be the result of horizontal transfer from bacteria.

6. The repetitive sequences in the human genome provide a fossil record dating back 800 million years.

7. A major component of the filler DNA has an important function.

8. The male mutation rate is approximately twice that of the female mutation rate.

9. Humans (including all different racial and ethnic groups) are 99.9% identical at the functional gene level, implying that there is no genetic basis for precise racial categorization. Nevertheless, various genes and genetic markers are specific for different races.

With the nature of the changes occurring at the level of DNA in genetic disorders becoming more apparent, it is possible to accu-

rately diagnose many genetically determined birth defects and to predict the occurrence of genetic disorders of adult onset by DNA analysis. Modern ability to diagnose genetic conditions exceeds current ability to cure them; however, accurate diagnosis can and does lead to improved treatment of genetic disease such as avoidance of environmental factors that produce or exacerbate disease in the presence of the gene (cigarette smoking and alpha-1 antitrypsin deficiency). In a few instances, gene therapy can cure genetic disorders outright (Chapter 71) and as the altered proteins associated with changed genes are identified, novel methods of treating genetic disorders through replacement of the altered proteins are being developed (Chapter 75).

Pharmacogenomics is an exciting advance in the practice of clinical medicine; the synthesis of new drugs is based on genetic variations in drug response and individualized drug therapy is based on patient genotype of drug metabolizing enzymes or other drug pharmacokinetics or pharmacodynamic principles. What were previously called idiosyncratic drug reactions are now known as variations of alleles in a specific gene or totally different genes that metabolize a drug to a toxic metabolite. Allelic differences of the MDRI (multiple drug resistance gene—multidrug transporter P glycoprotein) or the many drug metabolizing genes of the cytochrome P450 system are two examples of how the same drug dose can have variable clinical effects or achieve different drug levels in patients with different alleles. Drug therapy will become more effective and less likely to be associated with adverse reactions with the application of pharmacogenomics.

THE HUMAN GENOME

The human genome has approximately 38,000 genes, which are the individual units of heredity of all traits. Reproductive or germ line cells contain one copy (N) of this genetic complement and are *haploid*, whereas somatic (non–germ line) cells contain two complete copies (2N) and are *diploid*. The genes are organized into long segments of deoxyribonucleic acid (DNA), which, during cell division, are compacted into intricate structures with proteins to form chromosomes. Each somatic cell has 46 chromosomes (22 pairs of autosomes, or non-sex chromosomes, and 1 pair of sex chromosomes [XY in a male and XX in a female]). Germ cells (eggs, sperm) contain 22 autosomes and 1 sex chromosome, for a total of 23. At fertilization, the full diploid chromosome complement of 46 is again realized in the embryo.

The DNA molecule has three building blocks: a pentose sugar (deoxyribose), a phosphate group, and four types of bases, either purines (adenine and guanine) or pyrimidines (thymine and cytosine) (Fig. 67–1). These four bases form the alphabet of the genetic code. The basic subunit of DNA is the *nucleotide*, composed of one deoxyribose, one phosphate group, and one base. The structure of the DNA molecule is that of a double helix and is a twisted ladder, with the two sides of the ladder formed by the sugar and phosphate components, and the rungs of the ladder composed of the bases (see Fig. 67–1). Each "rung" contains one purine and one pyrimidine, binding with one another in a predictable way: "A" with "T" and "C" with "G." Different long sequences of the nucleotide bases code for different proteins. Individual triplets code for a corresponding transfer RNA, which then corresponds to its specific amino acid. Each haploid set of genes contains about 3 billion nucleotide pairs, the sum of which codes for the complicated array of human proteins.

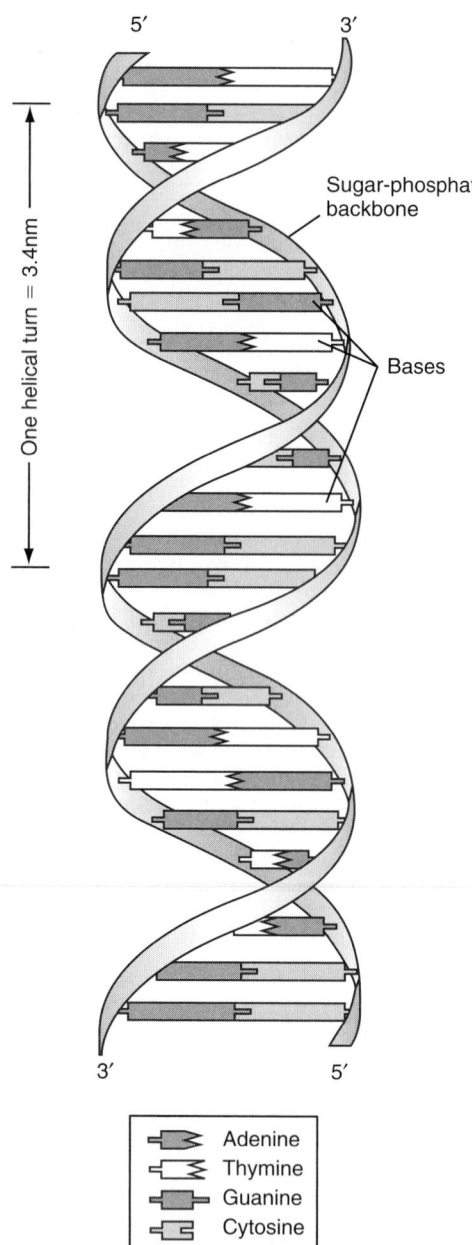

Sugar-phosphate backbone

Bases

One helical turn = 3.4nm

5'   3'

3'   5'

Adenine	
Thymine	
Guanine	
Cytosine	

FIGURE 67–1. The DNA double helix, with sugar-phosphate backbone and nitrogenous bases. (From Jorde LB, Carey JC, Bamshad MJ, et al [editors]: *Medical Genetics*, 2nd ed. St. Louis, Mosby, 1999 p. 8.)

Only a small fraction of the DNA of the cell is functionally working material during the metabolically active portion of the cell cycle; this is estimated to be 10% of the total DNA. Some of the "inactive" genetic material may be important in the regulation of gene expression or in chromosome structure and function.

Most of the genetic material is contained in the cell's nucleus. The mitochondria (the cell's energy-producing organelles) contain their own unique genome. The *mitochondrial chromosome* consists of a double-stranded circular piece of DNA, which contains 16,000 base pairs (bp) of DNA and is completely sequenced. The proteins that comprise the mitochondria may either be produced in the mitochondria (from information contained in the mitochondrial genome) or produced from information contained in the nuclear genome and transported into the organelle. All mitochondria are maternally derived (because sperm do not usually carry mitochondria into fertilized eggs);

different mitochondria within a single cell with a variety of genomes reflect the maternal lines from which they descended.

THE STRUCTURE AND FUNCTION OF GENES

The basic purpose of genes is the production of structural proteins and enzymes. This occurs through a series of events, termed *transcription, processing, and translation*. DNA transmits its information by unwinding into single-stranded DNA, with one strand or the other, or both, acting as a template to be copied. If this occurs during cell replication, each of the DNA strands is copied, forming two new double-stranded daughter DNA molecules during a process termed *replication*. If the process occurs during the metabolically active portion of the cell cycle, only one strand is copied, forming a strand of messenger RNA (*mRNA*) during *transcription*. The complete DNA sequence of each gene is transcribed into mRNA, including the information used to encode amino acids (*exons*) and the noncoding sequences between exons (*introns*) (Fig. 67–2). The resultant mRNA differs from DNA in the substitution of the sugar ribose for deoxyribose and the pyrimidine uracil (U) for thymine (T). This primary transcript of mRNA is processed before leaving the nucleus, by a mechanism in which the noncoding introns are removed from the molecule and the remaining sections are spliced together to form the functional mRNA, which then migrates to the cytoplasm for translation. During *translation*, the mRNA directs the production of proteins on the ribosome by forming base pairs between three of its nucleotides, called *codons*, and three complementary nucleotides on a transfer RNA molecule (tRNA), termed *anticodons*. As the ribosome moves along the RNA sequence, codon by codon, an enzyme joins together the adjacent amino acids associated with the tRNA molecules by forming covalent peptide bonds. The structure of polypeptide chains, and, ultimately, proteins is determined by the mRNA sequence.

MUTATIONS AND THEIR CONSEQUENCES

Medical genetics is concerned with the study of human genetic variation. The basis of that variation is mutation, or change in the DNA sequence. Mutations can and do occur in every cell of the body: When they occur in somatic cells, there is a risk of cancer development; when they occur in the germ line, there is a risk that an offspring may inherit a structural or functional disability. Many mutations are benign or silent; others explain variation in the severity of a genetic disease (polymorphisms), whereas others produce serious consequences.

An awareness of some of the common types of mutations allows for a better understanding of the pathogenesis of many genetic disorders (Fig. 67–3).

If there is a change in a single base pair (a *point mutation*), one of several consequences may result: (1) there may be no change in the amino acid specified, due to the redundancy of the genetic code (a *silent mutation*); (2) a different amino acid may be specified (a *missense mutation*); or (3) a stop codon may be specified, which terminates the polypeptide change prematurely (a *nonsense mutation*). *Deletions* and *insertions* constitute a second major category of mutations; in such changes, one or more base pairs are deleted or inserted into the DNA sequence. If the deletion or insertion of base pairs is not a multiple of three, a *frameshift mutation* results. In such cases, all of the downstream codons are altered, and a markedly changed protein product results. A third common form of mutation affects *tandem repeat DNA sequences*. Some genes contain long series of identical triplet repeats, e.g., CGGCGGCGGCGGCGG, etc. For an unknown reason, in many of these genes, there is a propensity for the number of repeats to expand dramatically during meiosis or early fetal development under certain circumstances (Chapter 70). In such cases, the gene becomes inactivated (through a chemical process, methylation), resulting in marked deficiency or absence of the coded

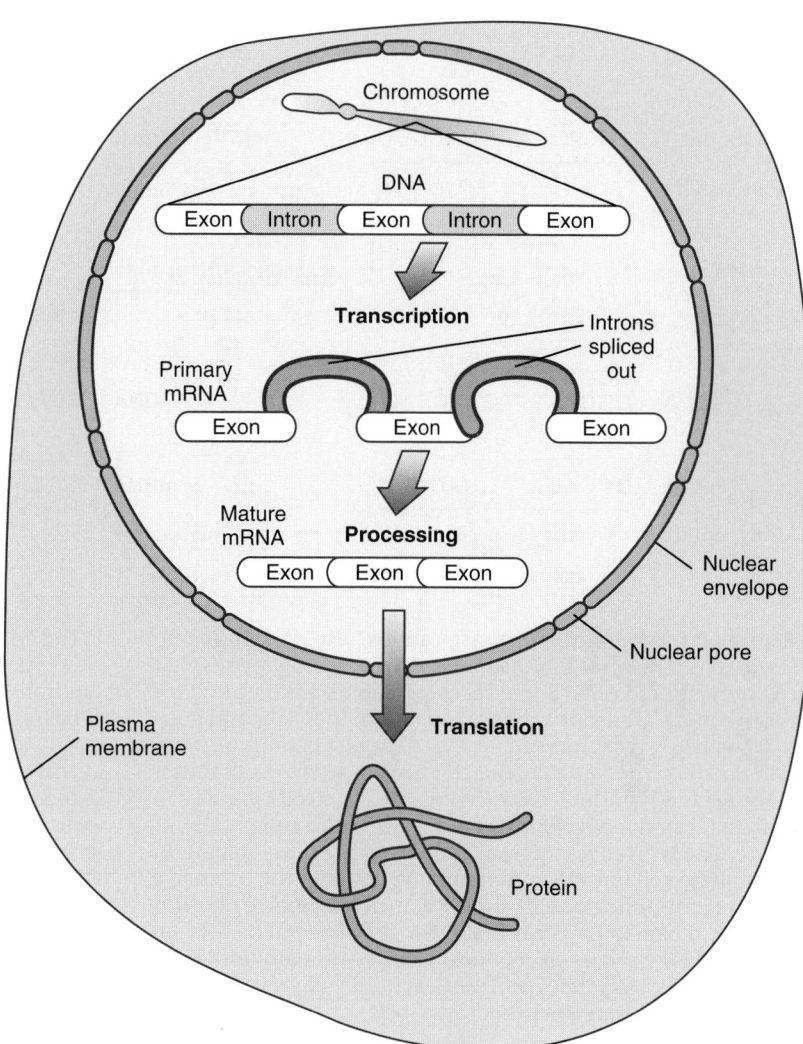

FIGURE 67–2. A summary of the steps leading from DNA to proteins. Replication and transcription occur in the cell nucleus. The mRNA is then transported to the cytoplasm, where translation of the nRNA into amino acid sequences composing a protein occurs. (From Jorde LB, Carey JC, Bamshad MJ, et al [editors]: *Medical Genetics*, 2nd ed. St. Louis, Mosby, 1999, p. 12.)

protein. Many human disorders have been identified that accompany triplet repeat expansions (Table 67–1).

Mutations usually can be classified as causing *gain of function* or *loss of function*. A gain of function mutation can result in an increase in the ability of a protein molecule to perform one or more normal functions, or, more commonly, it can result in overexpression or inappropriate expression of a gene product. Gain of function mutations most frequently produce autosomal dominant disorders (Chapter 69). Charcot-Marie-Tooth disease, type 1A, or *peroneal muscular atrophy*, the most common form of chronic peripheral neuropathy of childhood, results from duplication of the gene for peripheral myelin protein 22, resulting in overexpression of the gene product. The gain of function mutation in achondroplasia, the most common of the short-limbed skeletal dysplasias, exemplifies the enhanced function of a normal protein. Achondroplasia results from a mutation in fibroblast growth receptor 3 (FGFR3), which leads to activation of the receptor, even in the absence of fibroblast growth factor (FGF). Loss of function mutations are frequently observed in autosomal recessive disorders in which loss of 50% enzyme activity in the heterozygote continues to allow for normal function. Alternatively, loss of function mutations can result in conditions in which 50% of the gene product is insufficient for normal function (*haploinsufficiency*). Loss of function mutations can have a *dominant negative effect* when the abnormal protein product actively interferes with the function of the normal protein product.

Another category of mutations may confer a novel property on the protein synthesized, without altering the protein's normal functions. In sickle cell disease an amino acid is substituted into the hemoglobin molecule that has no effect on the ability of the protein to transport oxygen. However, unlike normal hemoglobin, under conditions of deoxygenation, sickle hemoglobin chains aggregate, forming fibers that deform the red cells. A final category of mutations results in abnormal expression of a gene over space and time. Many cancer-causing genes (oncogenes) are normal regulators of cellular proliferation during embryonic development; however, when expressed in adult life, and in cells in which they usually are not expressed, they may result in neoplasia.

Deletions can vary in their extent and, even when not visible at the cytogenetic level, can involve several genes; these are often termed microdeletions. By a variety of rearrangements, conditions referred to as *contiguous gene syndromes* may be generated. The clinician may be alerted to this possibility by an unusually diverse array of clinical features in any individual or the presence of additional features to a known condition. For example, owing to the close physical proximity of a series of genes, different deletions involving the short arm of the X chromosome can produce individuals with various combinations of the following features: ichthyosis, Kallmann syndrome, ocular albinism, mental retardation, chondrodysplasia punctata, and short stature. The individual features in each case depend on the involvement of these genes and the loss of DNA sequences in the underlying rearrangement. Many other contiguous gene syndromes have been described in humans, including Smith-Magenis, Rubinstein-Taybi, DiGeorge, and Prader-Willi syndromes.

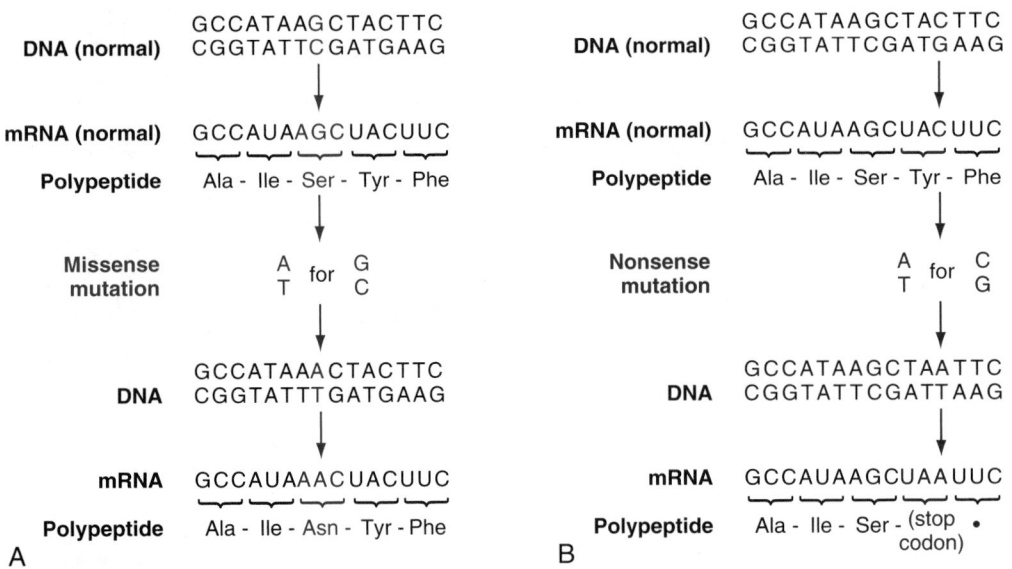

FIGURE 67–3. Missense mutations (*A*) produce a single amino acid change, whereas nonsense mutations (*B*) produce a stop codon in the mRNA. Stop codons terminate translation of polypeptide. (From Jorde LB, Carey JC, Bamshad MJ, et al [editors]: *Medical Genetics*, 2nd ed. St. Louis, Mosby, 1999, p. 30.)

Rearrangements such as translocations also take place in somatic cells. The most understood are the rearrangements that occur in lymphoid cells. Some rearrangements are required for the formation of functional immunoglobulin in B cells and antigen-recognizing receptors on the T cell. Large segments of DNA, which code for the variable and the constant regions of either immunoglobulin or the T-cell receptor, are physically joined at a specific stage in the development of an immunocompetent lymphocyte. The rearrangements take place during development of the lymphoid cell lineage in humans and result in the extensive diversity of immunoglobulin and T-cell receptor molecules. It is as a result of this post–germ line DNA rearrangement that no two individuals, not even identical twins, are really identical, because mature lymphocytes from each will have undergone random DNA rearrangements at these loci.

GENOTYPE-PHENOTYPE CORRELATIONS IN GENETIC DISEASE

Genotype is defined as the genetic constitution of an individual and refers to which particular alternative version (*allele*) of a gene is present at a specific location (*locus*) on a chromosome. Phenotype is defined as the observed structural, biochemical, and physiologic characteristics of an individual, determined by the genotype, and refers to the observed structural and functional effects of a mutant allele at a specific locus. Many mutations result in predictable phenotypes. Therefore, identification of a specific mutation in an individual can often be used to predict clinical outcomes and plan appropriate treatment strategies.

The long QT syndrome exemplifies a disorder with predictable genotype-phenotype correlations (Chapter 428.4). Long QT syndrome (phenotype) can be caused by mutations in several genes (genotypes), which are designated LQT1, LQT2, and LQT3, all encoding cardiac ion channels. The risk for cardiac events (syncope, aborted cardiac arrest, or sudden death) is higher with mutations at the LQT1 locus (63%) or the LQT2 locus (46%) than among subjects with mutations at the LQT3 locus (18%). In addition, those with LQT1 mutations experience most of their episodes during exercise and rarely during rest or sleep; those with LQT2 and LQT3 mutations are more likely to have episodes during sleep or rest, and rarely during exercise.

Mutations in the fibrillin-1 gene associated with the Marfan syndrome represent another example of predictable genotype-phenotype correlations (Chapter 690). Marfan syndrome is characterized by the combination of skeletal, ocular, and aortic manifestations, with the most devastating outcome being aortic root dissection and sudden death. Sixty-five exons comprise the fibrillin-1 gene, and mutations have been found in almost all of these exons. The location of the mutation within the gene (genotype) may play a significant role in determining the severity of the condition (phenotype). Neonatal Marfan syndrome is caused by mutations in exons 24–27 and 31–32, whereas milder forms are caused by mutations in exons 59–65 and in exons 37 and 41.

Genotype-phenotype correlations have also been observed in cystic fibrosis (CF) (Chapter 402). CF is a chronic lung disease caused by mutations in the CF transmembrane conductance

TABLE 67–1. Mutations Showing Triplet Repeat Expansion

Condition	Repeat	Repeat Location	Pathologic Repeat Number
FRAXA	CGG	5′ untranslated	200–1000
FRAXE	CGG		200–1000
FRAXF	CGG		300–500
FRA 16A	CGG		1,000–2,000
Spinal and bulbar muscular atrophy	CAG	Coding region	40–52
Huntington disease	CAG	Coding region	37–86
Spinocerebellar ataxia type I	CAG	Coding region	40–81
Spinocerebellar ataxia type II	CAG	Coding region	35–59
Spinocerebellar ataxia type 6	CAG	Coding region	21–30
Spinocerebellar ataxia type 7	CAG	Coding region	38–130
Dentatorubral-pallidoluysian atrophy	CAG	Coding region	49–75
Myotonic dystrophy	CTG	3′ untranslated	50–2,000
Friedreich ataxia	GAA	1st intron	200–900

Adapted from Willems PJ: Dynamic mutations hit double figures. Nat Genet 1994;8:213.

TABLE 67–2. Useful Internet Genetic Reference Sites

Web Address	Data Base
http://www.ncbi.nlm.nih.gov	General reference maintained by National Library of Medicine
http://www.ncbi.nlm.nih.gov/Omim	Online Mendelian Inheritance in Man (extremely useful for clinicians—over 10,000 entries of genetic traits indexed by gene name, symptoms, and so forth)
http://www.ncbi.nlm.nih.gov/genemap	General reference to current efforts to map the human genome
http://www.ncbi.nlm.nih.gov/Web/Genbank	Searchable repository of all DNA sequence data
http://www.ncbi.nlm.nih.gov/ncicgap	Cancer Genome Anatomy Project (National Cancer Institute)
http://www.nhgri.nih.gov	National Human Genome Research Institute Web Site (useful information about human genetics and ethical issues)
http://www.uwcm.ac.uk/uwcm/mg/hgmd0.html	Human Gene Mutation Database (searchable index of all described mutations in human genes with phenotypes and references)
http://www.geneclinics.org	Links to other genetic databases
	Lists mendelian and nonmendelian diseases
	Genetic testing, diagnosis, and treatment
http://www.genetests.org	Directory of clinics and labs for testing of genetic disorders
	Testing and counseling data
http://www.geneletter.com	Health, clinical, legal, social, and ethical issues
http://www.faseb.org/genetics/ashgmenu.htm	American Society of Human Genetics site
http://www.aap.org/VISIT/cmte18.htm	Committee on Genetics of the American Academy of Pediatrics site. Educational Genetics Compoundium. Health Supervision guidelines for common genetic disorders.

regulator (CFTR) gene. More than 1,000 different mutations have been identified; the most common is the Δ508 mutation, which accounts for 70% of all mutations and is associated with severe disease. Several mutations associated with mild disease have been identified, including 3272-26A>G, 3849+10 kb C>T, IVS8-5T, and 2789+5G>A. Patients with at least one 3272-26A>G allele and a second mutated allele (compound heterozygote) associated with severe disease are more likely to be diagnosed later, have better lung function, have lower incidence of *Pseudomonas aeruginosa* colonization, and have normal pancreatic function. Homozygotes for this mutation are not observed and may not have clinical disease. Conversely, those with 2183AA>G mutations, either homozygous or heterozygous with another CF mutation, are more likely to have early onset, severe disease. Those with this mutation tended to have severe pancreatic involvement, failure to thrive, variable lung involvement, and relatively early death.

With any given mutation, *modifier genes* for a different gene product may attenuate the mutated gene's phenotype. When sickle cell anemia is co-inherited with the gene for hereditary persistence of fetal hemoglobin, the sickle cell phenotypic expression is less severe. Modifier genes in CF may influence the development of congenital meconium ileus, or colonization with *P. aeruginosa*. Modifier genes may also affect the manifestations of Hirschsprung disease, neurofibromatosis type II, craniosynostosis, and congenital adrenal hyperplasia. The combination of genetic mutations producing glucose-6-phosphate dehydrogenase deficiency and Gilbert disease (promoter of glucuronyl transferase) exacerbates neonatal physiologic hyperbilirubinemia.

GENETIC SOURCES

The field of genetics is rapidly expanding and includes molecular basis of disease, rational approaches to disease diagnosis and management, education and counseling of families, and new ethical and social aspects of these newly discovered advances of the genetic basis of disease. To stay current, refer to one of the many constantly updated genetic based websites listed in Table 67–2.

Amaral MD, Pacheco P, Beck S, et al: Cystic fibrosis patients with the 3272-26A>G splicing mutation have milder disease than F508del homozygotes: A large European study. *J Med Genet* 2001;38:777–82.

Beutler E: Discrepancies between genotype and phenotype in hematology: An important frontier. *Blood* 2001;98:2597–2602.

Carnevale A, Hernandez M, Reyes R, et al: The frequency and economic burden of genetic disease in a pediatric hospital in Mexico City. *Am J Med Genet* 1985;20:665–75.

Collins FS, McKusick VA: Implications of the human genome project for medical science. *JAMA* 2001;285:540–4.

Dipple KM, McCabe ER: Modifier genes convert "simple" mendelian disorders to complex traits. *Mol Gen Metabol* 2000;71:43–50.

Dumont-Driscoll M: Genetics and the general pediatrician: Where do we belong in this exploding field of medicine? *Curr Probl Pediatr* 2002;32:1–34.

Harper PS: *Practical Genetic Counseling*, 5th ed. Oxford, Butterworth Heinemann, 2000.

Jorde L, Carey JC, Bamshad MJ, et al: *Medical Genetics*, 2nd ed. St. Louis, Mosby, 1999.

McKusick VA: The anatomy of the human genome. *JAMA* 2001;286:2289–5.

Monaco AP, Bailey AJ: The search for susceptibility genes. *Lancet* 2001;358:83.

Nussbaum RL, McInnes RR, Willard HF: *Thompson & Thompson Genetics in Medicine*, 6th ed. Philadelphia, WB Saunders, 2001.

Palz M, Tiecke F, Booms P, et al: Clustering of mutations associated with mild Marfan-like phenotypes in the 3' region of FBN 1 suggests a potential genotype-phenotype correlation. *Am J Med Genet* 2000;91:212–21.

Preuss N, Brosius U, Biermanns M, et al: PEX1 mutations in complementation group 1 of Zellweger spectrum *patients correlate with severity of disease*. Pediatr Res 2002;51:706–14.

Schwartz PJ, Priori SG, Spazolini C et al: Genotype-phenotype correlation in the long-QT syndrome. *Circulation* 2001;103:89–95.

Telenti A, Aubert V, Spertini F: Individualizing HIV treatment—Pharmacogenetics and immunogenetics. *Lancet* 2002;359:722–3.

Toriello HV: Effect of the human genome project on the practice of adolescent medicine. In Hoyme HE, Greydanus DE (editors): Genetic Disorders in Adolescents. Adolescent Medicine: State of the Art Reviews 2002;13:201–12.

Wolf CR, Smith G, Smith RL: Pharmacogenetics. BMJ 2000;320:987–90.

Yoon PW, Olney RS, Khoury MJ, et al: Contribution of birth defects and genetic diseases to pediatric hospitalizations. *Arch Pediatr Adolesc Med* 1997;151:1096–1103.

Chapter 68

Molecular Diagnosis of Genetic Diseases *H. Eugene Hoyme*

THE APPLICATION OF MOLECULAR GENETIC TECHNOLOGY IN CLINICAL DIAGNOSIS

Because a single gene or short segments of DNA cannot be observed microscopically, molecular genetics techniques are used to detect mutations. Information from the Human Genome Project and other advances in the field of molecular genetics have dramatically improved geneticists' ability to prenatally and postnatally diagnose genetic disorders. These techniques have predictive capabilities for adult-onset disorders that are single-gene conditions or that are multifactorially determined (Chapter 69). Technical capabilities in genetic diagnosis may exceed the ethical framework for decisions about when, or if, such testing should be performed in children and adolescents.

MOLECULAR CYTOGENETIC TECHNIQUES

Chromosomal abnormalities, numerical and structural, are common causes of a variety of cancers and malformation syndromes (Chapter 70). Identification of these chromosomal aberrations is important for counseling families about prognosis and reproductive risks in future pregnancies. Conventional chromosome analysis is the "gold standard" in cytogenetic diagnosis, but it has limited resolution. Fluorescence-tagged assays based on cloning technologies and improved sensitivity of antibody conjugates enable the detection of subtle chromosomal changes beyond the resolution of classic cytogenetics. Such techniques expand the diagnostic capabilities for the investigation of children with mental retardation, malformations, and many other disorders.

FISH TECHNIQUES

FISH (fluorescence in situ hybridization) involves using a unique DNA sequence as a probe, searching for a target DNA sequence on the patient's sample. The locus-specific or gene-specific DNA probe is labeled with a tag (e.g., a fluorochrome), allowing its detection via fluorescence microscopy. The target DNA sequence is a chromosome preparation containing metaphase spreads and interphase (nondividing) nuclei on a microscope slide. Both the probe and target DNA are denatured, resulting in single-stranded DNA. The probe is added to the chromosome preparation and is incubated long enough to allow for the complementary DNA sequences of the probe and target to anneal or hybridize, if the target sequence is present. The DNA will only hybridize to its complementary strands and not to fragments with a different DNA sequence from other parts of the genome. The presence or absence of the bound fluorochrome-labeled probe is ascertained by examination of the sample with a fluorescent microscope. The results are usually unequivocal (Fig. 68–1).

The advantages of FISH include rapid analysis of a large number of cells, high sensitivity and specificity, and the ability to analyze uncultured and nondividing cells. Cells that were once paraffin-embedded can be analyzed. Disadvantages include the inability to provide information regarding the physical state of the DNA or chromosome segment identified. Performing FISH requires knowledge of the loci involved in an aberration as well as the appropriate probes that will detect the aberration. FISH cannot be used as a screening tool; rather it is used to answer specific questions. It is generally used either to complement classic chromosome staining methods, as a substitute for the identification of chromosomes in metaphase or interphase, or to identify specific DNA sequences known to be involved in a recognizable disease (phenotype).

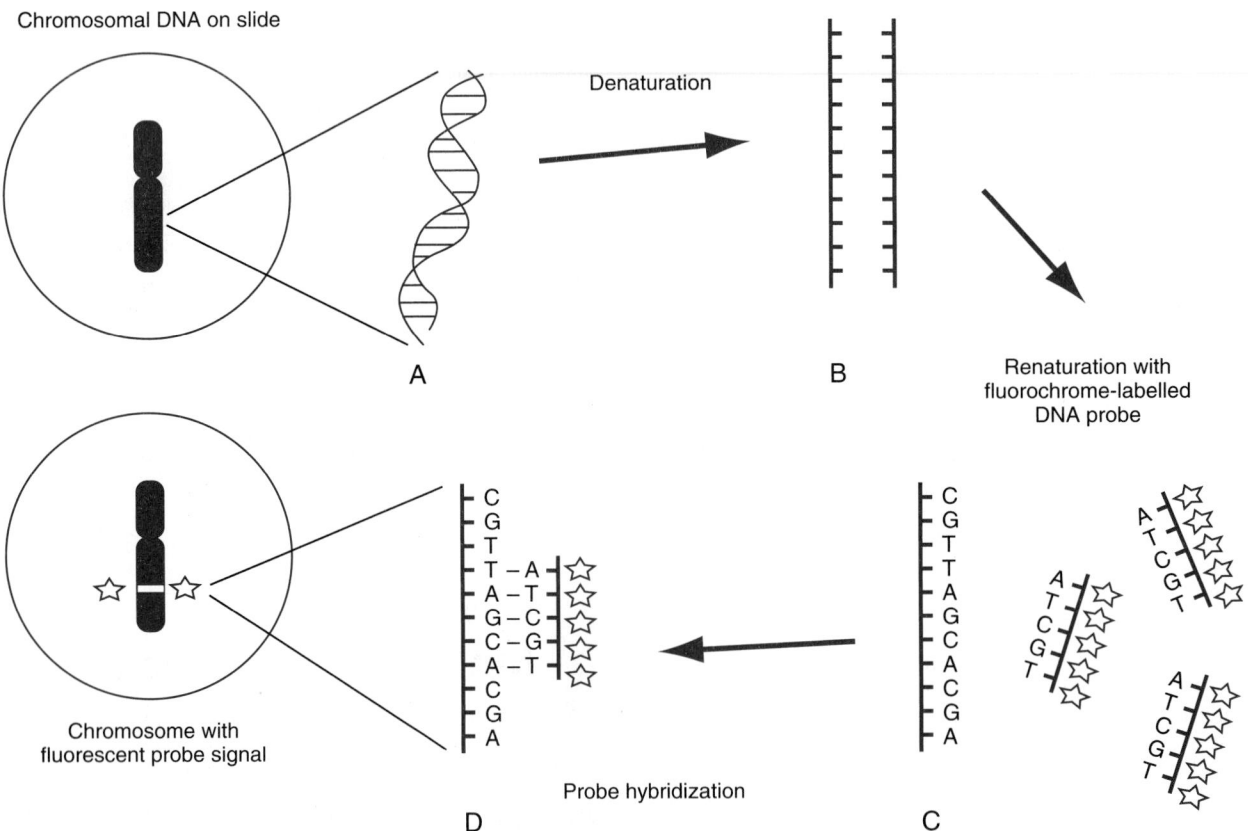

FIGURE 68–1. Fluorescence in situ hybridization (FISH) involves denaturation of double-stranded DNA as present in metaphase chromosomes or interphase nuclei on cytogenetic slide preparations (*A*) into single-stranded DNA (*B*). The slide-bound (in situ) DNA is then renatured or reannealed in the presence of excess copies of a single-stranded, fluorochrome-labeled DNA base pair sequence or probe (*C*). The probe anneals or "hybridizes" to sites of complementary DNA sequence (*D*) within the chromosomal genome. Probe signal is visualized and imaged on the chromosome or nucleus by fluorescent microscopy. (From Lin RL, Cherry AM, Bangs CD, et al: FISHing for answers: The use of molecular cytogenetic techniques in adolescent medicine practice. In Hoyme HE, Greydanus D (editors): *Genetic Disorders in Adolescents. State of the Art Reviews. Adolescent Medicine.* Philadelphia, Hanley and Belfus, 2002, pp. 305–13.)

FISH is used in prenatal diagnosis and in tumor characterization; in pediatric practice, it is usually used to detect submicroscopic chromosome deletions associated with specific malformation syndromes. Microdeletion syndromes are disorders previously thought to be of unknown etiology because the associated chromosomal deletions and rearrangements are usually not visible in conventional chromosome preparations. They are characterized by small deletions in specific chromosomal segments and can be reliably detected by FISH; examples include the Prader-Willi, Angelman, Williams, Miller-Dieker, Smith-Magenis, and velocardiofacial syndromes (Fig. 68–2). FISH has facilitated the diagnosis of these syndromes in atypical cases, especially in infants when all of the diagnostic findings are not present. It is beneficial in adolescents and adults when the typical childhood features have changed.

SUBTELOMERIC REARRANGEMENTS

Most translocations involve the ends of chromosomes (telomeres). A large number of genes for malformation syndromes

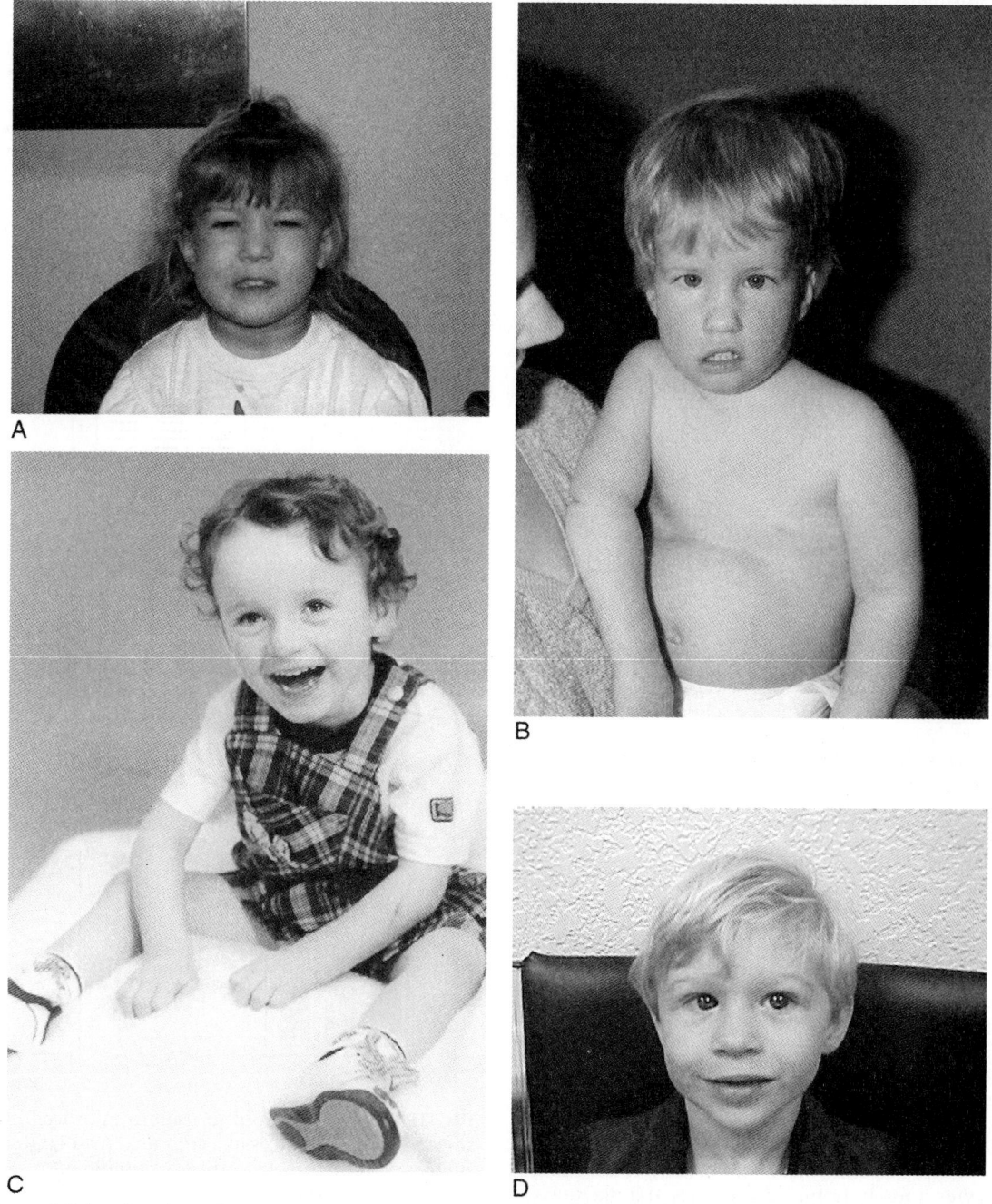

FIGURE 68–2. *A*, Child with velocardiofacial syndrome (deletion 22q11.2). *B*, Child with Prader-Willi syndrome (deletion 15q11-13). *C*, Child with Angelman syndrome (deletion 15q11-13). *D*, Child with Williams syndrome (deletion 7q11.23). (From Lin RL, Cherry AM, Bangs CD, et al: FISHing for answers: The use of molecular cytogenetic techniques in adolescent medicine practice. In Hoyme HE, Greydanus D (editors): *Genetic Disorders in Adolescents. State of the Art Reviews: Adolescent Medicine*. Philadelphia, Hanley and Belfus, 2002, pp. 305–13.)

are located in the regions adjacent to telomeres, the subtelomeric chromosomal regions. Screening telomeres for rearrangements is a useful way to detect submicroscopic chromosome deletions and rearrangements not detected by standard chromosome analysis. FISH screening for submicroscopic chromosome rearrangements in patients with isolated mental retardation has focused on terminal rearrangements; subtelomeric abnormalities are seen in approximately 7.5% of such patients.

COMPARATIVE GENOMIC HYBRIDIZATION

Comparative genomic hybridization (CGH) is a FISH method for genome-wide screening for differences in copy number of any DNA sequence from an individual. CGH was developed for tumor genetics (primarily solid tumors) but is used to identify the location of gains and losses of chromosome material in individuals with potential chromosome abnormalities. The technique involves mixing and hybridizing simultaneously equal amounts of differentially labeled test DNA (e.g., green fluorescence) and normal reference DNA (e.g., red fluorescence) to normal metaphase spreads. A green to red fluorescence ratio profile is produced and areas of amplification of test DNA would be detected as an excess of green fluorescence, losses as red areas reflecting deficiency of test DNA, and equal representation of test and normal DNA as yellow areas. Therefore, CGH produces a map of genome DNA sequence number. Advantages include its applicability to any tissue. The technique is not able to detect balanced chromosomal abnormalities because the DNA copy number remains the same. Chromosome copy changes smaller than 10 Mb are not resolvable, and copy number changes are not detectable if less than half of the analyzed cells contain chromosomal gains or losses.

SPECTRAL KARYOTYPING AND MULTICOLOR FISH

The limitation of CGH in detecting balanced chromosome rearrangements is overcome by multicolor painting of all chromosomes with only one hybridization. *Spectral karyotyping (SKY)* and *multicolor FISH (M-FISH)* are related molecular cytogenetic techniques that can identify balanced rearrangements. In both of these methods, each chromosome of a metaphase spread is labeled with a specific color allowing simultaneous visualization of the entire array of chromosomes. Twenty-four chromosome-painting probes and five fluorochromes are used in combination, resulting in a combinatorial labeling scheme that uniquely labels each of the 22 autosomes, and the X and Y. M-FISH requires the use of specific filter sets for each of the five fluorochromes; SKY uses spectroscopy and an interferometer to evaluate the fluorescence emission patterns. These methods permit the detection of complex rearrangements, small translocations, and marker chromosomes. Disadvantages include the inability to identify small intrachromosomal deletions or duplications and pericentric or paracentric inversions.

METHODS OF DNA ANALYSIS

Molecular cytogenetic techniques have enhanced diagnostic abilities for the detection of chromosomal deletions or duplications (containing tens or hundreds of genes). Other techniques accomplished through DNA analysis allow for detecting changes in single genes. DNA analysis is possible because DNA is a relatively stable molecule that can be isolated from any nucleated cell and stored for future potential diagnostic needs. DNA is most commonly extracted from white blood cells; other tissues include amniocytes and chorionic villi (in prenatal diagnosis), buccal cells (from cheek swabs), and fibroblasts (obtained by skin biopsy). Sampling these tissues usually yields sufficient DNA. DNA amplification techniques, such as the polymerase chain reaction (PCR), allow for amplification of the DNA from as little as one or a few cells.

SOUTHERN/NORTHERN/WESTERN BLOTTING

The *Southern blotting* technique was the first of the molecular diagnostic techniques. PCR-based methods and direct DNA sequencing have largely displaced it. In this procedure, genomic DNA is isolated from the patient and then is cut into small fragments by *restriction enzymes* (bacterial enzymes that cleave DNA at

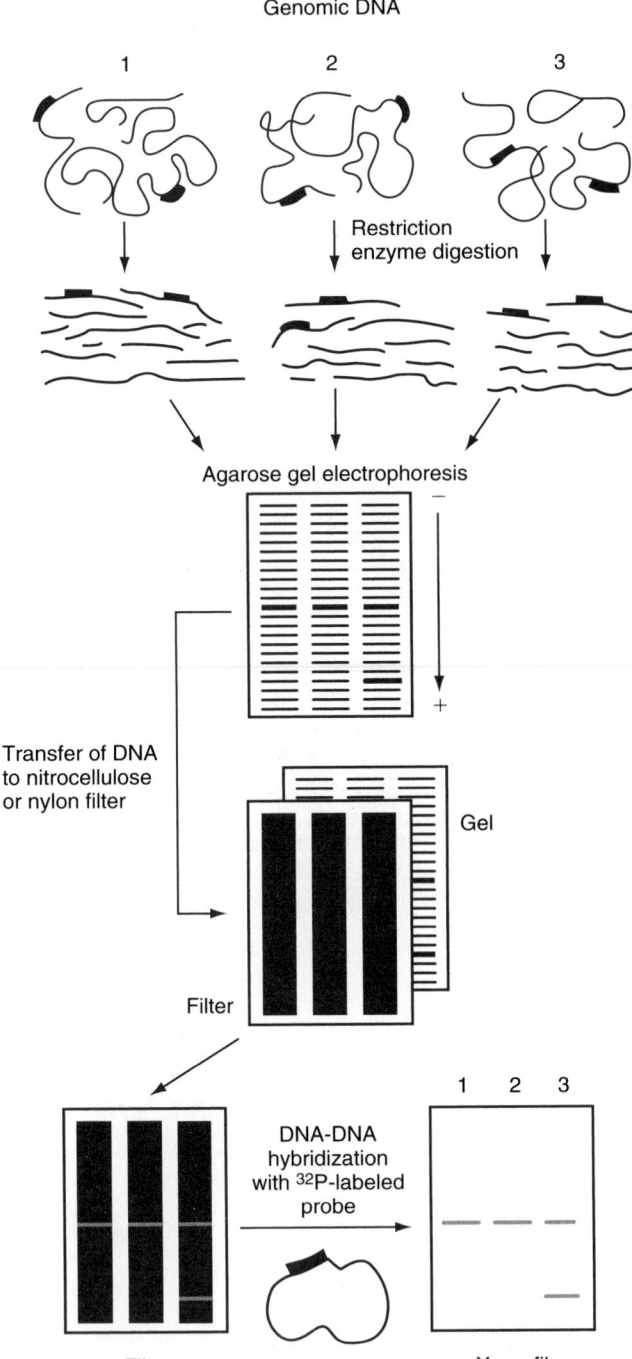

FIGURE 68–3. The Southern blotting procedure for analyzing specific DNA sequences in a complex mix of different sequences, such as genomic DNA. In this example, sample 3 has a different restriction enzyme pattern for the DNA sequence detected by the probe. This variation might be due to a restriction fragment length polymorphism or to a deletion of DNA near the detected sequence. (From Nussbaum RL, McInnes RR, Willard HF: *Thompson & Thompson Genetics in Medicine*, 6th ed. Philadelphia, WB Saunders, 2001.)

very specific sites). The resultant fragments are sorted by size using gel electrophoresis, transferred by "blotting" to a stable nylon filter, fixed to the filter, hybridized against a radiolabeled known gene probe, and displayed by exposure on x-ray film. Mutations can be detected by this method if they alter the length of a DNA fragment (restriction site), which changes the resultant enzyme cleavage banding pattern of the Southern blot. This technique continues to be most useful in detecting "linkage" of a gene to a particular inherited DNA polymorphism within or around the gene in question. The gene can then be tracked through a family, even though the specific molecular defect associated with the genetic disorder cannot be identified (Fig. 68–3).

In *Northern blotting*, the pattern and abundance of messenger RNA produced by a specific gene is analyzed. RNA cannot be cleaved by the restriction enzymes; different RNA transcripts of different lengths are produced depending on the size and number of exons in a gene. Thus, mutations that alter the number and/or lengths of exons can be expected to result in detectable changes in the Northern blot. The laboratory technique is identical to the Southern blot, except that total cellular RNA or purified mRNA, rather than DNA (cleaved by restriction enzymes), is used.

In *Western blotting*, information on the size and amount of mutant protein in cell extracts from patients with specific genetic disorders is analyzed. Proteins from a cell extract are separated according to size by polyacrylamide gel electrophoresis and transferred to a membrane. The membrane is then incubated with specific antibodies to the protein. A second antibody (against the first antibody) tagged with a fluorescent dye or radioactive substance detects the protein-antibody interaction. Western blotting is used to detect the presence or absence and size of the muscle protein dystrophin in patients with X-linked muscular dystrophy.

POLYMERASE CHAIN REACTION

Although in some disorders a high proportion of mutations are the result of large deletions in DNA detectable by Southern blotting, for many conditions, the majority of the gene abnormalities are point mutations. Once a point mutation has been discovered, DNA primers can be constructed that cover the short stretch of sequence affected by the mutation. Obtaining sufficient copies of the altered DNA sequence can be a problem. The PCR technique multiplies the copies of the DNA (gene). PCR uses thermal cycling to amplify the sequence of interest and has revolutionized the detection of mutations by providing a highly sensitive method that can be performed on small samples. The

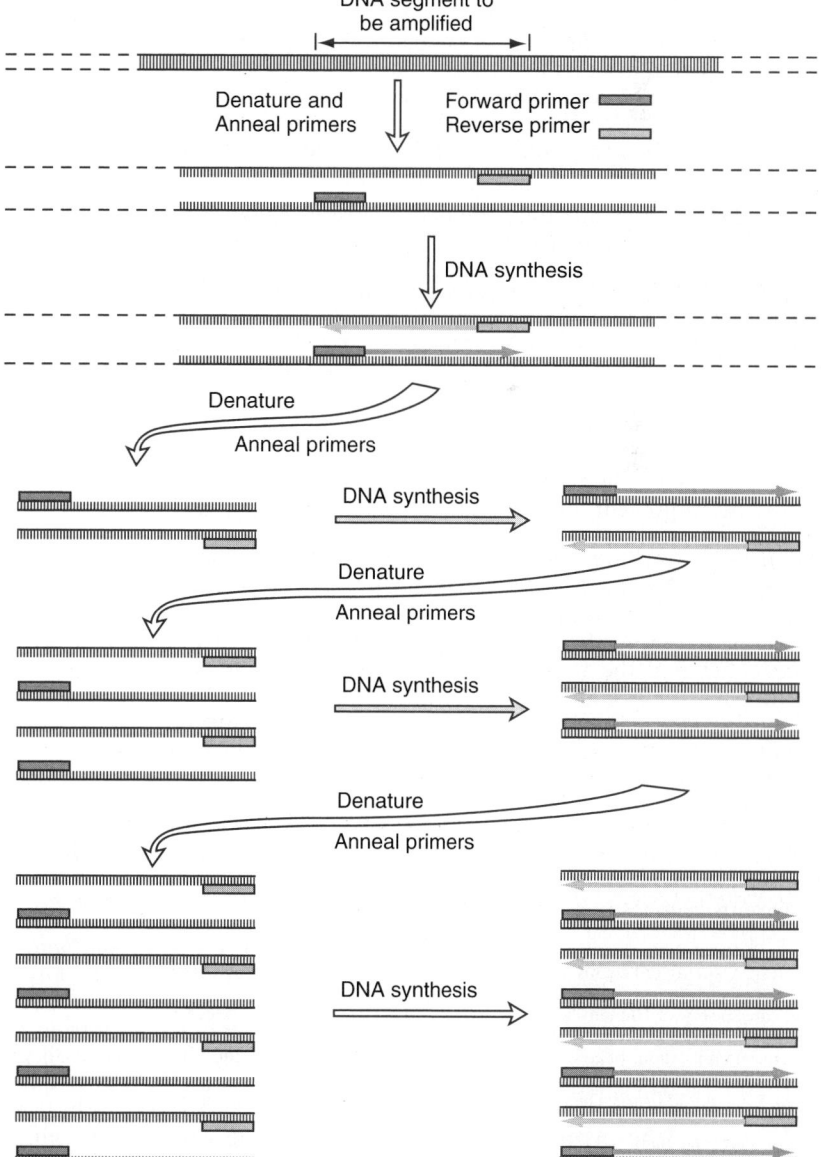

FIGURE 68–4. The polymerase chain reaction. By repeatedly synthesizing a region of DNA located between two DNA primers, this region of DNA is specifically and selectively amplified in an exponential fashion. Three successive rounds of amplification are shown, resulting in a total of eight copies of the targeted sequence. After 30 rounds of amplification, more than a billion copies of the sequence are created. (From Nussbaum RL, McInnes RR, Willard HF: *Thompson & Thompson Genetics in Medicine*, 6th ed. Philadelphia, WB Saunders, 2001.)

technique is standardized and automated. It is relatively inexpensive; billions of copies of a specific DNA sequence can be produced in a few hours (Fig. 68–4).

DIRECT DNA SEQUENCING

Automated DNA sequencing is standard in many clinical molecular genetic laboratories and has permitted the progress of the Human Genome Project. Sequencing is particularly suitable for small genes, and for situations in which the precise mutation in a particular family is not known. All significant findings must be analyzed to determine whether the changes cause disease or are normal polymorphisms.

ETHICAL ISSUES IN GENETIC TESTING IN CHILDREN

Nothing is as personal as one's genetic material. Just because a molecular genetic test can be ordered does not mean that it should. The decision to undergo genetic testing is complicated. The decision of whether or not to perform a genetic test on a child is even more difficult, because the child cannot always participate in discussions about the testing. The ultimate decision hinges on how the results of the test will help or harm the child. The interest of the child is always foremost; thus, open discussion of the pros and cons of testing should always center on the child's interests. Molecular diagnostic tests are often used to diagnose children with malformation syndromes, mental retardation, or other disabilities wherein there is a clear benefit to the child. In other cases, the decision whether to test a child is more difficult.

The American College of Medical Genetics and the American Society of Human Genetics have suggested that the following points be fully discussed with families considering genetic testing for their children:

1. A mature minor and the parents should receive education and counseling about the genetic testing being considered, and consent should be obtained by the physician before genetic testing is done (Chapter 72). Adolescents who are 14 or 15 yr of age or older are usually considered mature minors, and assent/consent should be sought from them (Chapter 2). If a child between the ages of 7 and 14 yr is to be tested, "assent" of the child should be obtained. Assent is the child's affirmative agreement to agree with the decision of the parents.

2. The primary justification for undergoing testing should be timely medical benefit. If the test will not provide medical benefit in terms of prevention or treatment, its necessity should be questioned.

3. If medical benefit is not apparent, one must consider whether substantial psychosocial benefits to the older child or adolescent can justify testing.

4. Genetic testing should be deferred until after age 18 yr if the benefits of the testing will not become apparent until adulthood.

5. In the case of a competent adolescent, if the balance of benefits and harms is unknown, the physician should follow the decision of the adolescent regarding testing, even if it conflicts with the wishes of the parents.

6. The pediatrician should evaluate whether testing is in the best interest of the child, and, if the potential harms of testing outweigh the potential benefits, the physician should dissuade the parents from testing.

American Academy of Pediatrics Committee on Genetics: Molecular genetic testing in pediatric practice: A subject review. *Pediatrics* 2000;106:1494–7.

American Society of Human Genetics Board of Directors, American College of Medical Genetics Board of Directors: Point to consider: Ethical, legal, and psychosocial implications of genetic testing in children and adolescents. *Am J Hum Genet* 1995;57-1233–41.

Harper PS: *Practical Genetic Counseling*, 5th ed. Oxford, Butterworth Heinemann, 2000.

Jorde L, Carey JC, Bamshad MH, et al: *Medical Genetics*, 2nd ed. St. Louis, Mosby, 1999.

Lin RL, Cherry AM, Bangs CD, et al: FISHing for answers: The use of molecular cytogenetic techniques in adolescent medicine practice. In Hoyme HE, Greydanus D (editors): *Genetic Disorders in Adolescents. State of the Art Reviews: Adolescent Medicine*. Philadelphia, Hanley and Belfus, 2002, pp. 305–13.

Nussbaum RL, McInnes RR, Willard HF: *Thompson & Thompson Genetics in Medicine*, 6th ed. Philadelphia, WB Saunders, 2001.

Stevenson DA, Strasburger VC: Advise or consent? Issues in genetic testing of adolescents. In Hoyme HE, Greydanus DE (editors): Genetic disorders in adolescents. State of the art reviews. *Adolesc Med* 2002;13:213–21.

Strom CM, Levin R, Strom S, et al: Neonatal outcomes of preimplantation genetic diagnosis by polar body removal: The first 109 infants. *Pediatrics* 2000;106:650–3.

Chapter 69
Patterns of Inheritance

H. Eugene Hoyme

GENETIC VS FAMILIAL DISORDERS

The diagnosis of a genetic disorder is based on a particular clinical pattern of symptoms and/or signs characteristic of the condition, or by laboratory confirmation of the altered gene or gene products associated with the disorder. The diagnosis is often aided by recognition of the pattern of inheritance within a family. It is important that a distinction be made between diseases that are genetic and those that are familial. A *genetic disorder* is one caused completely or partially by altered genetic material; some genetic disorders occur in multiple family members, others occur sporadically in single individuals in a family with no instances of recurrence. A *familial disorder* is one that is more common in relatives of an affected individual than in the general population; some familial disorders are genetic, and others are caused by environmental exposures (lead poisoning). Recognition of the pattern of inheritance not only assists in clinical diagnosis but also provides essential information for counseling family members about recurrence risks in future pregnancies.

THE PEDIGREE

A *pedigree* is a diagram of a family history and illustrates relationships among family members; it shows which family members are affected with specific medical conditions. Information for a three-generation pedigree should be obtained from a family being evaluated for a genetic disorder. The patient through whom the family is ascertained is called the *proband*. Individuals who share half of their genetic material with the proband are *first-degree relatives* (brothers, sisters, children, parents); those who share one fourth of their genetic material are *second degree relatives* (grandparents, grandchildren, aunts, uncles, nieces, nephews). Third and fourth degree relatives share one eighth and one sixteenth of their genetic material, respectively, with the proband (Fig. 69–1).

AUTOSOMAL DOMINANT INHERITANCE

Autosomal genes are on one of the 22 pairs of non-sex chromosomes. *Autosomal dominant disorders* are those in which a single gene in the heterozygous state is sufficient to cause the phenotype. Autosomal dominant disorders demonstrate certain features that apply in most circumstances: (1) the disorder appears in a vertical pattern in the pedigree, with affected individuals present in every generation; (2) any child of an affected parent has a 50% risk of inheriting the disorder; (3) phenotypically normal family members do not transmit the condition to their offspring; (4) males and females are equally affected; (5) a significant proportion of cases are due to new mutation.

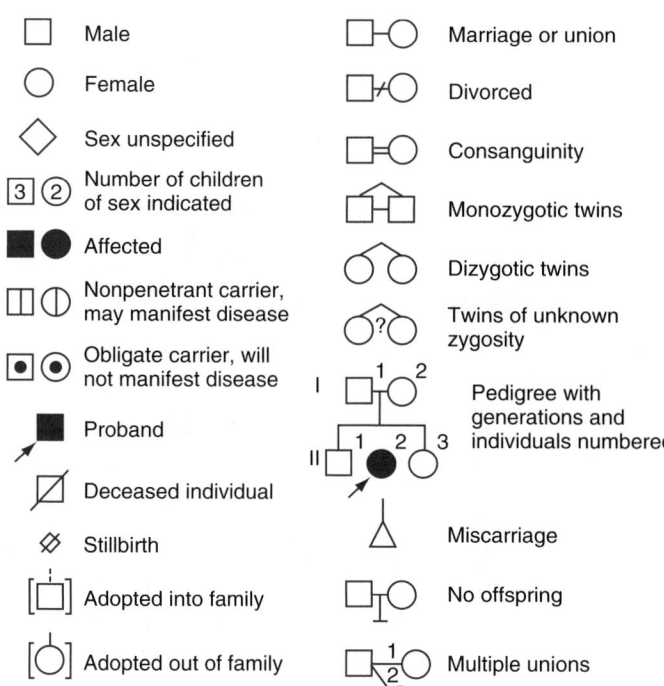

□ Male	□—○ Marriage or union
○ Female	□—/○ Divorced
◇ Sex unspecified	□—○ Consanguinity
③ ② Number of children of sex indicated	Monozygotic twins
■ ● Affected	Dizygotic twins
Nonpenetrant carrier, may manifest disease	Twins of unknown zygosity
Obligate carrier, will not manifest disease	Pedigree with generations and individuals numbered
■ Proband	△ Miscarriage
⊘ Deceased individual	□—○ No offspring
⬦ Stillbirth	
[□] Adopted into family	Multiple unions
[○] Adopted out of family	

FIGURE 69–1. Symbols commonly used in pedigree charts. Although there is no uniform system of pedigree notation, the symbols used here are according to recent recommendations made by the professionals in the field of genetic counseling. (From Bennett RL, Steinhaus KA, Uhrich SB, et al: Recommendations for standardized pedigree nomenclature. *J Genet Counsel* 1995;4: 267–79.)

Autosomal dominant disorders can be distinguished from X-linked conditions by the presence of male-to-male transmission in the former (Fig. 69–2). Because men transmit a Y chromosome, rather than an X chromosome, to their sons, X-linked inheritance is ruled out if a genetic disease is passed from father to son.

Autosomal dominant disorders typically show wide variation in phenotype among affected individuals within a family. This is most commonly due to *variable expressivity* of the mutated gene. The exact cause of variable expressivity is unknown, but it is most likely associated with the effects of modifying genes and the environment on the phenotype. In some families, obligate carriers of an altered gene have no apparent phenotypic manifestations of the condition. This is termed *reduced penetrance* and is an "all or none" phenomenon. In some instances when an individual appears to be nonpenetrant, the patient may actually exhibit either low-grade *somatic mosaicism* or *germ line mosaicism* for the gene. Somatic mosaicism arises in the embryo from a mutation in a somatic cell, leading to an embryo displaying a mixture of genotypes in its cells, some with and others without the mutation. Typically such individuals show fewer or no effects of the altered gene. Germ line mosaicism likewise arises postconception in the embryo and is limited to those cells that are precursors

of eggs or sperm. Germ line mosaicism has been commonly observed in conditions such as osteogenesis imperfecta and the craniosynostosis syndromes: Apert and Crouzon syndromes.

Because only one dose of an altered gene is necessary for phenotypic expression in autosomal dominant disorders, the condition is often the consequence of a new mutation in many affected individuals. The more severe the disorder, the higher the percentage of cases resulting from de novo mutations of the gene; in severe disorders, reduced reproductive capacity limits transmission of the gene from generation to generation. Older paternal age (>40 yr) is observed in some cases of new mutation.

Neurofibromatosis I: A Typical Autosomal Dominant Disorder

Neurofibromatosis is a heterogeneous disorder with two distinct phenotypes: neurofibromatosis 1 (NF1) and neurofibromatosis 2 (NF2). Both conditions are genetically determined, inherited as autosomal dominant traits. NF2 (also known as bilateral acoustic neurofibromatosis) is the less common of the two and is mapped to a locus distinct from NF1.

Neurofibromatosis (NF1) is a common neurocutaneous disorder, with an estimated prevalence of 1 in 3,000 live births (Chapter 589.1). It is due to a mutation in the neurofibromin gene (*NF1*) on the long arm of chromosome 17. Half the patients have NF1 from a new gene mutation, making the mutation rate of the neurofibromin gene among the highest in humans. The offspring of an affected individual have a 50% risk of inheriting the altered *NF1* gene (Fig. 69–3). DNA-based testing for the *NF1* gene is available but is rarely needed for diagnosis or prenatal diagnosis.

Multiple café au lait spots and associated cutaneous findings of neurofibromas, plexiform neurofibromas, and axillary or inguinal freckling characterize NF1. Other manifestations include an increased risk for optic glioma, osseous lesions, and learning disability. As with many autosomal dominant disorders, there is widely variable expressivity in affected patients. The diagnosis of NF1 is based on clinical findings, and consensus diagnostic criteria. The National Institutes of Health diagnostic criteria for NF1 are met in an individual with two or more of the following features:

- Six or more café au lait macules >5 mm in greatest diameter in prepubertal individuals and >15 mm in greatest diameter in postpubertal individuals
- Two or more neurofibromas of any type or one plexiform neurofibroma
- Freckling in the axillary or inguinal regions
- Optic glioma
- Two or more Lisch nodules (iris hamartomas)
- A distinctive osseous lesion such as sphenoid dysplasia or thinning of long bone cortex with or without pseudarthrosis
- A first-degree relative (parent, sibling, or offspring) with NF1 as defined by the above criteria

These criteria are highly specific and sensitive in adults with NF1 but may be inconclusive in young infants. The diagnosis can be confirmed clinically by age 4 yr in nearly all cases. A finding of multiple café au lait spots in a young infant is insufficient to make the diagnosis of NF1 (without a positive family history);

FIGURE 69–2. Pedigree showing typical inheritance of a form of progressive sensorineural deafness (DFNA1) inherited as an autosomal dominant trait. (From Nussbaum RL, McInnes RR, Willard HF: *Thompson & Thompson Genetics in Medicine,* 6th ed. Philadelphia, WB Saunders, 2001.)

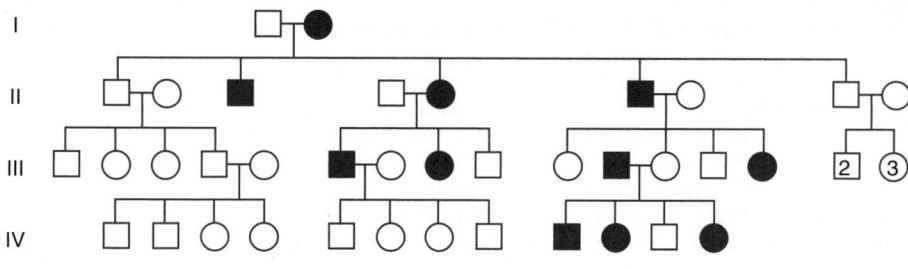

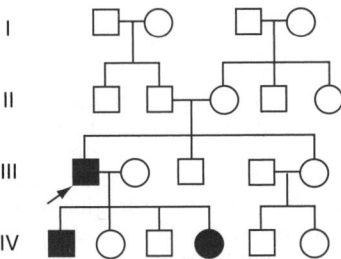

FIGURE 69–3. Pedigree of family with neurofibromatosis, type 1, apparently originating as a new mutation in the proband (*arrow*). (From Nussbaum RL, McInnes RR, Willard HF: *Thompson & Thompson Genetics in Medicine*, 6th ed. Philadelphia, WB Saunders, 2001.)

most will later meet the diagnostic criteria for NF1 and, therefore, should be followed up expectantly. The American Academy of Pediatrics has published guidelines for the health supervision of affected children. These include yearly physical assessment, including blood pressure, scoliosis screening, ophthalmology examination, developmental screening, and neurologic examination. Baseline imaging studies of the cranium are usually not warranted; if there is any suggestion of central nervous system involvement, imaging and referrals should be undertaken immediately.

AUTOSOMAL RECESSIVE INHERITANCE

Autosomal recessive disorders are those in which two copies of the mutant gene in the homozygous state are necessary to cause the phenotype. This implies that both parents of an affected individual are heterozygous carriers of the gene. In general, autosomal recessive disorders are less common than autosomal dominant conditions, although the carrier frequency of many such genes in the heterozygous state may be common in the general population.

The pedigree illustrating this pattern of inheritance (Fig. 69–4) shows the following characteristics: The child of two heterozygous parents has a 25% chance of being homozygous (i.e., a 1 in 2 chance of inheriting the mutant gene from each parent: $1/2 \times 1/2 = 1/4$); males and females are affected with equal frequency; the affected individuals are almost always born in only one generation of the family; the children of the affected (homozygous) person are all heterozygotes; the children of a homozygote can be affected only if the spouse is a heterozygote, which is a rare event because of the low incidence of most adverse recessive genes in the general population.

If the frequency of an autosomal recessive disease is known, the frequency of the heterozygote or carrier state can be calculated from the Hardy Weinberg formula

$$p^2 + 2pq + q^2 = 1$$

in which *p* is the frequency of one of a pair of alleles and *q* is the frequency of the other. For example, if the frequency of cystic fibrosis among white Americans is 1 in 2,500 (p^2), then the frequency of the heterozygote (2 pq) can be calculated; if $p^2 = 1/2,500$, then p = 1/50 and q = 49/50; 2pq = $2 \times 1/50 \times 49/50$, or approximately 1/25 (or 3.92%).

Every human probably has several rare, harmful, recessive genes. Because these mutant genes are frequently not identifiable by laboratory tests, the heterozygous adult usually learns about his or her harmful recessive genes after the birth of a homozygous (and therefore affected) child. Related parents are much more likely to be heterozygous for the same harmful recessive genes because they have a common ancestor.

Autosomal recessive disorders demonstrate certain features that apply in most circumstances: (1) autosomal recessive disor-

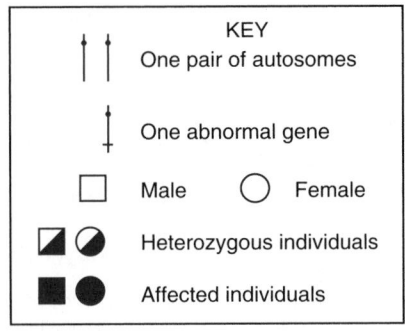

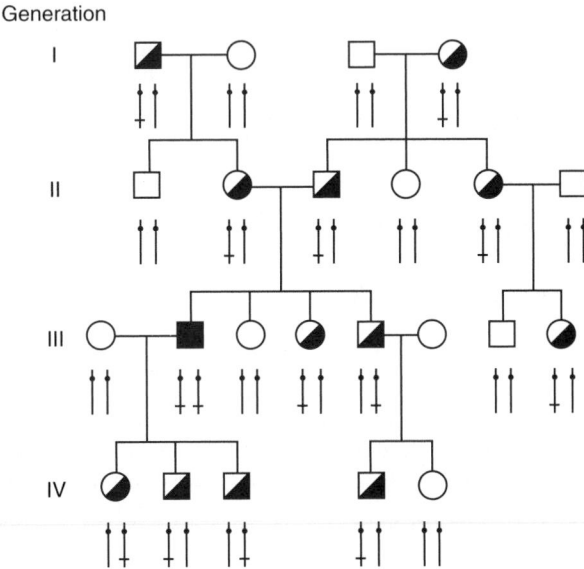

FIGURE 69–4. Autosomal recessive inheritance.

ders display a horizontal pattern in pedigrees (if more than one member of a family is affected, they are typically siblings of the proband, not parents or other relatives); (2) males and females are equally affected; (3) parents of an affected child are asymptomatic heterozygous carriers of the gene; (4) the recurrence risk for siblings of an affected child is 25%.

The chance that any two parents carry an identical mutant allele is increased if the couple is consanguineous (Fig. 69–5). *Consanguinity* is defined as relationship by descent from a common ancestor. Consanguinity between parents of a child with a suspected genetic disorder implies (but does not prove) autosomal recessive inheritance. Although consanguineous unions are uncommon in Western society, in some parts of the world (Southern India, Japan, and the Middle East) they are common. The risk for the offspring of a first cousin marriage (6–8%) is about double the risk in the general population (3–4%). There are some genetic isolates (small populations separated because of geography, religion, culture, or language) in which rare recessive disorders are more common than in the general population. Even though consanguinity may not be increased in these populations, because of limited mate choice, the chance of a couple from an isolated genetic region having a child with an autosomal recessive condition may be as high as that observed in first cousin marriages. Screening programs have been developed in such groups to detect heterozygotes at risk for having affected children. A variety of autosomal recessive conditions are more common among Ashkenazi Jews than in the general population. National practice guidelines recommend screening asymptomatic Ashkenazi Jews for the neurodegenerative disorders Tay Sachs disease (GM_2 gangliosidosis) and Canavan disease (aspartoacylase deficiency); carrier screening for other disorders (Fanconi anemia, Gaucher disease, cystic fibrosis,

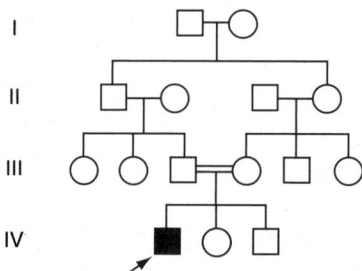

FIGURE 69–5. Pedigree in which parental consanguinity suggests autosomal recessive inheritance. (From Nussbaum RL, McInnes RR, Willard HF: *Thompson & Thompson Genetics in Medicine*, 6th ed. Philadelphia, WB Saunders, 2001.)

familial dysautonomia, nesidioblastosis) is also being considered for inclusion in this population.

The prevalence of carriers of certain autosomal recessive genes in some larger populations is unusually high. In such cases, *heterozygote advantage* is postulated. The carrier frequencies of sickle cell disease in the African population and of cystic fibrosis in the northern European population are much higher than would be expected from new mutations. It is possible that heterozygous carriers have had an advantage in terms of survival and reproduction over noncarriers. In sickle cell disease, the carrier state may confer some resistance to malaria; in cystic fibrosis, the carrier state has been postulated to confer resistance to cholera and enteropathogenic *Escherichia coli* infections. Population-based carrier screening for cystic fibrosis is now recommended for individuals of northern European and Ashkenazi Jewish background; population-based screening for sickle cell disease is recommended for individuals of African background.

X-LINKED INHERITANCE

X-linked disorders are those associated with altered genes on the X chromosome. Most X-linked disorders demonstrate a recessive pattern of inheritance, although a few X-linked dominant conditions have been well described. The characteristics of X-linked conditions differ significantly from autosomal disorders. Because females inherit two copies of the X chromosome, they may be heterozygous or rarely homozygous for any allele at a particular locus; thus, in females, X-linked genes behave like autosomal genes. Because of X-inactivation (a random process occurring early in female embryogenesis), only one X chromosome is active in each cell. Therefore, a female who is heterozygous for a mutant X-linked allele will produce 50% of the normal amount of gene product, similar to a heterozygote for an autosomal recessive condition. This is usually sufficient for a normal phenotype. Because a male inherits only one X chromosome, he is *hemizygous* for all of the genes present at all loci along the chromosome, and all of the genes are expressed. If a male inherits an altered X-linked gene, he will express the condition, because the Y chromosome contains no normal allele to compensate for the mutated gene.

X-LINKED RECESSIVE INHERITANCE

Certain features apply in most circumstances of X-linked recessive inheritance: (1) the incidence of the condition is much higher in males than in females; (2) heterozygous female carriers are usually unaffected; (3) the gene is transferred from an affected man to all of his daughters, and any of his daughters' sons has a 50% chance of inheriting the gene; (4) the gene is never transmitted from father to son; (5) the gene may be transmitted through a series of carrier females, in which case all affected males are related through the carrier females; (6) a significant proportion of sporadic cases are a consequence of new gene mutations (Fig. 69–6).

There are circumstances when females may be affected with X-linked recessive conditions. If both parents carry an X-linked recessive allele, a girl can inherit the altered gene in a homozygous state. However, because most X-linked recessive disorders are rare, this circumstance would be unlikely (except in the case of consanguinity). If a girl has Turner syndrome, accompanying a 45,X chromosome complement, she is hemizygous for all genes on the X chromosome and expresses all genes at all loci, similar to a male. Thus, X-linked recessive disorders are more common in females with Turner syndrome. Finally, because X inactivation is random, it follows a normal distribution in the embryo. Therefore, there will be a few females who by chance have one or the other of their X chromosomes nearly completely inactivated. This *skewed X inactivation pattern* is frequently observed in females who manifest X-linked recessive disorders.

Hemophilia A: A Typical X-Linked Recessive Disorder

Hemophilia A (classic hemophilia) is characterized by a deficiency in coagulation factor VIII, which results in prolonged blood oozing after injuries, tooth extractions, or surgery, renewed bleeding after initial bleeding has stopped, and delayed bleeding (Chapter 468.1). The age of diagnosis and frequency of bleeding episodes are related to the factor VIII clotting activity; mild and severe cases exist. Severe cases are usually diagnosed in infancy; mild cases may not be diagnosed until adolescence or adulthood. Because of skewed X-chromosome inactivation, approximately 10% of carrier females are at risk for mild bleeding.

The diagnosis of hemophilia A is established by documenting low factor VIII clotting activity in the presence of a normal von Willebrand factor (vWF) level. Molecular genetic testing of the factor VIII (*F8*) gene (located on the long arm of the X chromosome, at Xq28) identifies disease-causing mutations in up to 90% of patients with severe hemophilia A and about 80–95% of patients with mild to moderately severe hemophilia A. Such testing is not necessary but is available. Molecular genetic testing is used for genetic counseling of at-risk family members and occasionally in diagnosing mild cases.

Hemophilia A is inherited in an X-linked recessive manner. The risk to siblings of a proband depends on the carrier status of the mother. Carrier females have a 50% chance of transmitting the *F8* mutation in each pregnancy. Sons who inherit the mutation will be affected; daughters who inherit the mutation are carriers. Affected males transmit the mutation to all their daughters and none of their sons. Prenatal testing is possible and is more sensitive if the *F8* disease-causing mutation has been identified in a family member or if informative linked markers are known.

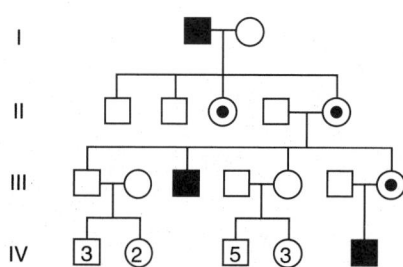

FIGURE 69–6. Pedigree pattern demonstrating an X-linked recessive disorder such as hemophilia A, transmitted from an affected male through females to an affected grandson and great grandson. (From Nussbaum RL, McInnes RR, Willard HF: *Thompson & Thompson Genetics in Medicine*, 6th ed. Philadelphia, WB Saunders, 2001.)

X-LINKED DOMINANT INHERITANCE

An X-linked disorder is described as dominant if the condition is regularly expressed in the heterozygous female carriers. Characteristics of X-linked dominant inheritance include (1) all of the daughters and none of the sons of an affected man have the condition; (2) both male and female offspring of affected females have a 50% risk of inheriting the condition; (3) for rare X-linked dominant conditions, affected females are about twice as common as affected males, but affected females typically have milder (although variable) manifestations of the phenotype (Fig. 69–7).

There are only a few X-linked dominant disorders. One condition is *hypophosphatemic rickets* (vitamin D–resistant rickets); although both males and females express the condition, males are more severely affected than females. Some rare X-linked disorders occur nearly exclusively in women, because the hemizygous state of the condition is lethal in the male embryo. *Incontinentia pigmenti* (IP) is one such disorder that affects the skin, hair, teeth, and nails (Chapter 642). The skin lesions evolve through characteristic stages from blistering in infancy, to a wart-like rash (for several months), and finally, swirling hyperpigmentation and hypopigmentation. Alopecia, hypodontia, abnormal tooth shape, and dystrophic nails are observed. Some patients have retinal vascular abnormalities predisposing to retinal detachment in early childhood, and cognitive delays or mental retardation are occasionally seen (Fig. 69–8). The diagnosis of IP is established by clinical findings and occasionally by corroborative skin biopsy. Molecular genetic testing of the *IKBKG* gene (chromosomal locus Xq28) reveals disease-causing mutation in about 80% of probands. Such testing is available clinically. Females with IP have skewed X-chromosome inactivation; testing for this can be used to support the diagnosis. Affected women have a 50% risk of transmitting the mutant *IKBKG* allele; affected male conceptuses abort. The expected ratio of liveborn children is 33% unaffected females; 33% affected females; 33% unaffected males.

MULTIFACTORIAL INHERITANCE

Most of the common isolated congenital anomalies (e.g., neural tube defects, cleft lip, cleft lip with cleft palate, isolated cleft palate, club feet, and cardiac septal defects) and many of the common disorders of adult life (e.g., diabetes mellitus, hypertension, stroke, coronary artery disease, and schizophrenia) are inherited in a multifactorial manner. *Multifactorially determined disorders* are those that are the product of multiple genetic and environmental factors. The genetic factors predisposing to these disorders are heterogeneous and largely unknown. The *multifactorial model* envisions liability genes predisposing to a particular anomaly or disease as a normal distribution (Fig. 69–9). Theoretically, a point exists on the curve (*threshold of liability*), below which individuals are unaffected and above which the condition is manifest. The threshold can be moved to the left or the right by the environment. For example, in the case of neural

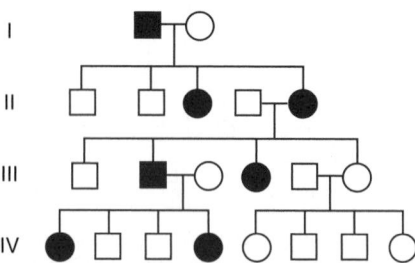

FIGURE 69–7. Pedigree pattern demonstrating X-linked dominant inheritance. (From Nussbaum RL, McInnes RR, Willard HF: *Thompson & Thompson Genetics in Medicine*, 6th ed. Philadelphia, WB Saunders, 2001.)

tube defects, certain teratogens (e.g., valproate) can move the threshold to the left, allowing a child to be affected with a smaller genetic predisposition. Alternatively, the threshold can be moved to the right by maternal folic acid supplementation prior to conception, exerting a protective effect in an embryo with a susceptible genetic background.

Characteristics of multifactorially determined disorders include the following:

1. There is a similar rate of recurrence (typically 3–5%) among all first-degree relatives (parents, siblings, and offspring of the affected child). However, it is unusual to find a substantial increase in risk for relatives related more distantly than second degree to the index case.
2. The risk of recurrence is related to the incidence of the disease.
3. Some disorders have a sex predilection, as indicated by an unequal male:female incidence. Pyloric stenosis is more common in males, whereas congenital dislocation of the hips is more common in females. Where there is an altered sex ratio, the risk is higher for the relatives of an index case in the less commonly affected sex. The risk to the son of an affected female with infantile pyloric stenosis is 18% compared with the 5% risk for the son of an affected male. The female has passed on a greater genetic susceptibility to her offspring.
4. The likelihood that both identical twins will be affected with the same malformation is less than 100% but much greater than the chance that both members of a nonidentical twin pair will be affected. The frequency of concordance for identical twins ranges from 21% to 63%. This distribution contrasts with that of mendelian inheritance, in which identical twins always share a disorder due to a single mutant gene.
5. The risk of recurrence is increased when multiple family members are affected; these instances are often the most problematic for distinguishing a multifactorial from a mendelian etiology. A simple example is that the risk of recurrence for unilateral cleft lip and palate is 4% for a couple with one affected child and increases to 9% with two affected children.
6. The risk of recurrence may be greater when the disorder is more severe. The infant who has long-segment Hirschsprung disease has a greater chance of having an affected sibling than the infant who has short-segment Hirschsprung disease.

NONTRADITIONAL PATTERNS OF INHERITANCE

Genetic disorders are sometimes inherited in ways that do not follow the usual patterns of dominant, recessive, X-linked, or multifactorial inheritance. These atypical patterns of inheritance sometimes involve specific diseases and in other instances may apply to any hereditary disorder.

Certain diseases display an atypical mode of inheritance because they result from mutations in mitochondrial DNA (mtDNA). Mitochondria contain small circular chromosomes that encode 13 proteins that function in the respiratory chain of the organelle. Mutations of the mitochondrial genome (which are often deletions) can produce specific diseases. Abnormalities in these disorders are typically seen in one or more specific organs: the brain, eye, and skeletal muscle. Examples are *Kearns-Sayre syndrome* and *Leber hereditary optic neuropathy*. Because mitochondria are inherited virtually exclusively from the mother, these conditions are passed from mother to offspring, without regard to sex of the latter (thus differing from X-linked recessive inheritance). Because the mitochondria of an individual constitute a heterogeneous mixture of genotypes both within and between cells, the mitochondrial complement passed in the egg is often not representative of the total mitochondrial population of the mother. mtDNA mutations produce disease only in the presence of many mutated mitochondria: 50–60% for single large deletions and 80–90% for point mutations. Mitochondria populations are not equally distributed to all tissues. Some mitochondria demonstrate a replicative

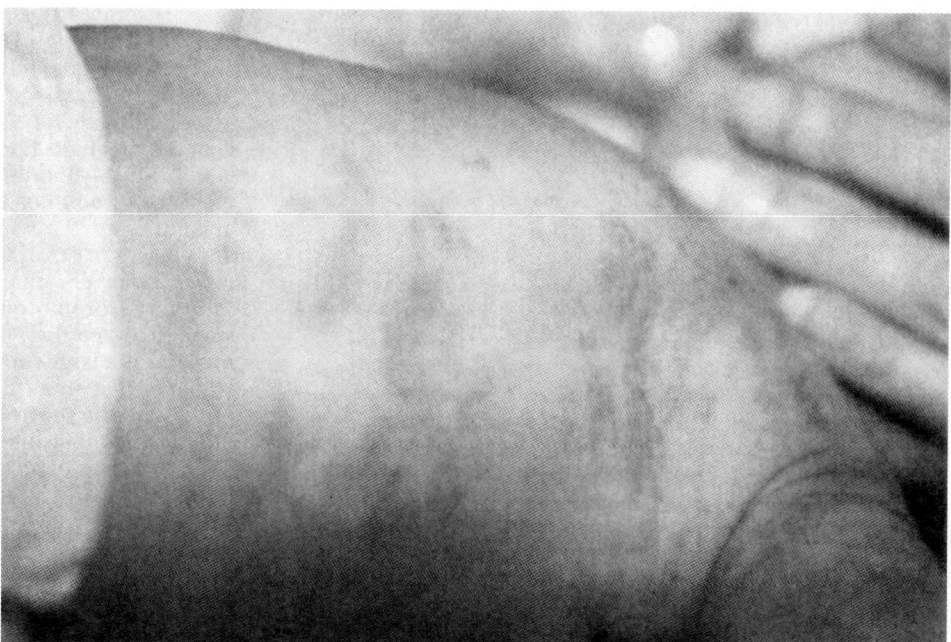

FIGURE 69–8. Typical linear erythema and blistering in a female infant with incontinentia pigmenti. As the child grows older, the skin lesions will become flattened, pigmented streaks. (Photograph courtesy of Virginia Sybert, University of Washington, Seattle, WA. From Nussbaum RL, McInnes RR, Willard HF: *Thompson & Thompson Genetics in Medicine*, 6th ed. Philadelphia, WB Saunders, 2001.)

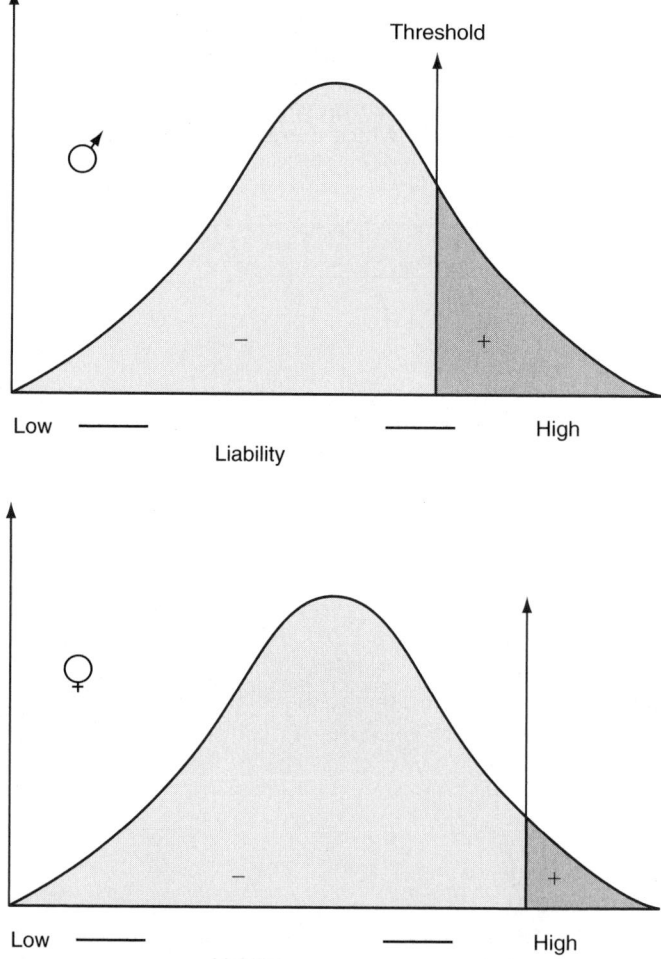

FIGURE 69–9. A liability distribution for a multifactorial disease in a population. To be affected with the disease, an individual must exceed the threshold on the liability distribution. This figure shows two thresholds, a lower one for males and a higher one for females (as in pyloric stenosis).

advantage over other inherited populations of mitochondria. Thus, there is a great variability in symptoms within a family, and the observed inheritance may be more complex than a simple maternal pattern. Although uncommon, mtDNA mutations (deletions) may occur by paternal inheritance. The finding of a myopathy or neurologic disease that seems to come from the mother's side should alert the clinician to the possibility of a mitochondrial etiology. Traditionally, sperm mitochondria undergo destruction by nuclear encoded proteins. For paternal mtDNA inheritance, the father's mitochondria may have a replicative advantage or the destruction of mitochondria may be attenuated.

Another type of nontraditional inheritance is the result of a phenomenon known as *genomic imprinting* (Chapter 70). This takes place in the germ line and results in certain regions of the genome being inherited differently, depending on the parent of origin. Specifically, genes in the relevant region are functionally inactivated (imprinted) during gamete formation and remain inactive in the resulting zygote. The genes imprinted in the two parental germ lines are mutually exclusive sets; otherwise, the offspring would have no active copies of the genes. This imprinting phenomenon leads to clinical consequences in the case of *Prader-Willi syndrome* (PWS). About two thirds of these patients have de novo microdeletions of chromosome 15, and the deletions always occur on the paternally derived chromosome. Similar deletions inherited on the maternal chromosome 15 do not result in PWS and, in fact, give rise to a different disorder, *Angelman syndrome*. In PWS, the relevant gene or genes are silenced on the maternal chromosome 15, so that a deletion on the paternal chromosome leaves the individual with no active alleles (the reverse is true for Angelman patients, in whom silencing of critical paternal genes with deletion of maternal loci results in the absence of active alleles). Most PWS patients who do not have deletions are found to have inherited two copies of their maternal chromosome 15 and are missing the paternal chromosome. Because both maternal chromosomes are silenced in the critical region, these individuals, like the deletion patients, have no active copies of the critical genes. The situation of inheriting both homologous chromosomes from a single parent is called *uniparental disomy*. A number of individuals with abnormal phenotypes have been observed to have uniparental disomy for particular chromosome regions. Thus, at least for certain regions of the genome, it is necessary to have sequences from each parent, so that one can express at least one copy of the relevant genes.

Friedman JM: Neurofibromatosis 1. In Gene Reviews. *http://www.geneclinics.com/*

Harper PS: *Practical Genetic Counseling*, 5th ed. Oxford, Butterworth Heinemann, 2000.

Jones KL: *Smith's Recognizable Patterns of Human Malformation*, 5th ed. Philadelphia, WB Saunders, 1997.

Jorde L, Carey JC, Bamshad MJ, et al (editors): *Medical Genetics*, 2nd ed. St. Louis, Mosby, 1999.

Nussbaum RL, McInnes RR, Willard HF: *Thompson & Thompson Genetics in Medicine*, 6th ed. Philadelphia, WB Saunders, 2001.

Scheuerle AE: Incontinentia pigmenti. In Gene Reviews. *http://www.geneclinics.com/*

Schwartz M, Vissing J: Paternal inheritance of mitochondrial DNA. *N Engl J Med* 2002;347:576–80.

Thompson AR, Johnson M, Fujimura FK: Hemophilia A. In Gene Reviews. *http://www.geneclinics.com*.

Williams RS: Another surprise from the mitochondrial genome. *N Engl J Med* 2002;347:609–11.

Chapter 70

Chromosomal Clinical Abnormalities *Judith G. Hall*

The chromosomes are made up of DNA and other protein complexes and contain most of the genetic information that is passed from one generation to the next. Chromosomes are normally visualized through the microscope only when they are in a contracted state as they go through cell division. Chromosome studies are important because abnormal chromosome number

(e.g., trisomy 13) and abnormal chromosomal arrangements (e.g., microdeletion 15q) may lead to multiple congenital anomalies. Improved culture and staining techniques allow the description of a large number of chromosomal abnormalities associated with specific disorders, and techniques of molecular genetics facilitate the identification of the specific position of genes (FISH—fluorescent in situ hybridization) as well as their presence or absence along the chromosomes (see Chapters 67 and 68).

Cytogeneticists arrange chromosomes by size in pairs—the largest being chromosome 1 and the smallest, chromosome 22 (although chromosome 21 has been found to actually be the smallest)—and then the sex chromosomes X and Y. The X chromosome is a large submetacentric chromosome, and the Y chromosome is a small acrocentric chromosome (Fig. 70–1). The position of the centromere in regard to the chromosome arms is another distinguishing feature of each chromosome (Fig. 70–2). The short arm of a chromosome is referred to as p (for petite) and the long arm as q (for the next letter in the alphabet).

Nomenclature. A karyotype is the designation for the visual display of chromosomes and is obtained after the chromosomes are arrested during cell division in prophase and are photographed and arranged according to size. The visual display can be produced by computer. A description of a karyotype consists of three parts: (1) the number of chromosomes, (2) the sex chromosome constitution, and (3) any abnormalities found. The normal karyotype is 46, XX for females and 46, XY for males. If an abnormality is found, it is noted after the sex chromosome constitution. For example, in the case of a female with cri-du-chat syndrome in which a piece of the short arm of the chromosome 5 is missing, the karyotype would be 46, XX, 5p-. In a male with Down syndrome in which there is an extra chromosome

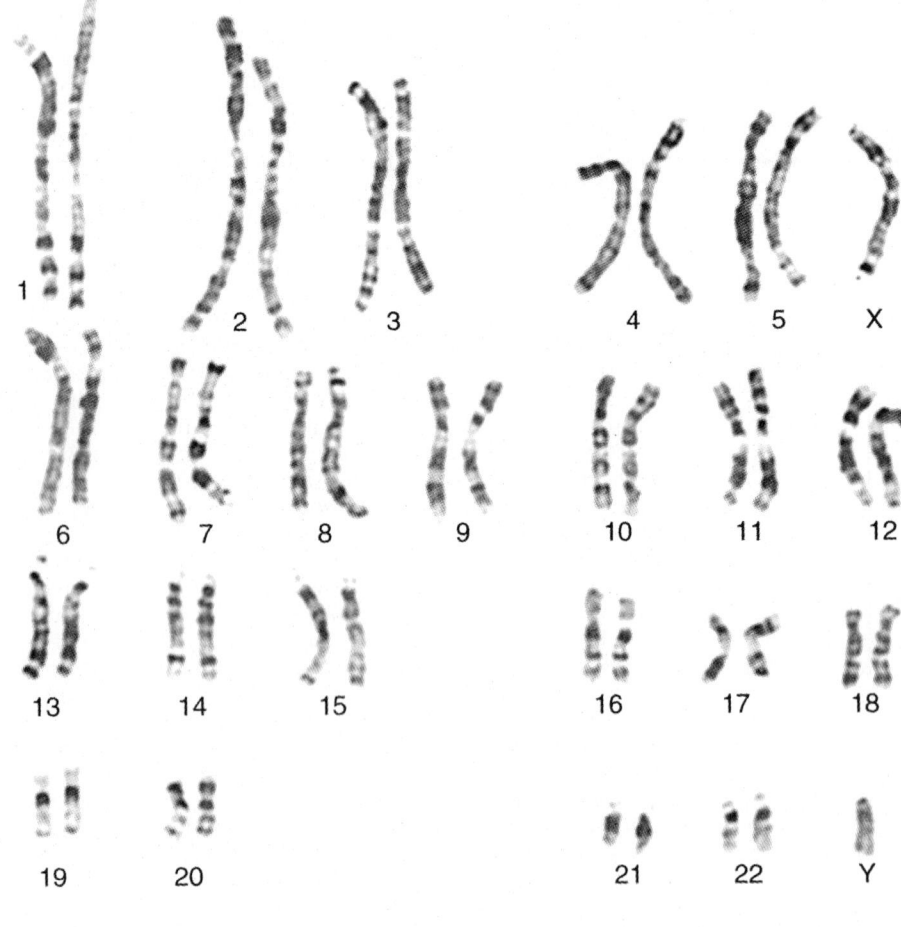

FIGURE 70–1. Karyotype of normal male with chromosomes in late prophase. The chromosomes are longer, and a greater number of bands are seen than when chromosomes are photographed at metaphase.

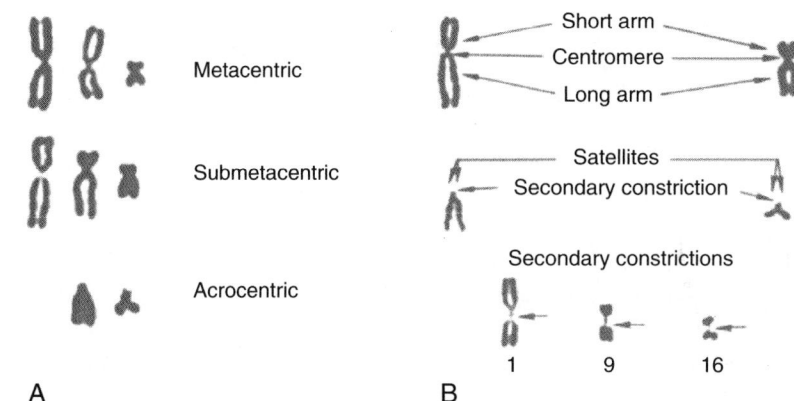

FIGURE 70–2. *A,* Centromere position determining the three types of chromosomes seen in the normal human karyotype—metacentric, submetacentric, and acrocentric. *B,* Morphologic landmarks useful in chromosome identification.

21, the karyotype is 47, XY, +21. In the case of translocations, the chromosomes involved are written in brackets preceded by a "t" as in 45, XX, t(13q14q), indicating a female carrier of a translocation between the long arms of chromosomes 13 and 14. If the chromosome breaks are along an arm of a chromosome, the band position at which the break occurred is also indicated in the brackets, for example, 45, XY, t(13q2.1-14q1.3), indicating a male carrier of a translocation within the long arms of chromosome 13 and 14.

Cell Division. There are two types of cell division: mitosis and meiosis. *Mitosis* is the type of cell division that occurs in most cells of the body. It is during mitosis, specifically the prophase stage of mitosis, that chromosomes are visible and easy to identify for karyotyping. In mitosis, two genetically identical daughter cells are produced from a single parent cell. Before cell division, DNA replication has occurred so that there is a doubled amount of DNA and the chromosomes contain two identical sister chromatids. Mitosis is divided into stages. *Prophase* is characterized by spiraling of the chromosome threads into coils to form microscopically identifiable chromosomes; the nuclear membrane and the nucleolus disappear and the mitotic spindle forms. In *metaphase,* the chromosomes condense and are clearly visible as distinct structures. The centromeres of the chromosomes attach to the microtubules of the mitotic spindle and the chromosomes align at the middle of the cell along the spindle. *Anaphase* is characterized by division of the chromosomes along their longitudinal axis to form two daughter chromatids and migration of each chromatid of the pair to opposite poles of the cell. *Telophase,* which completes mitosis, is characterized by reconstitution of the nuclear membrane and nucleolus, duplication of the centrioles, and cytoplasmic cleavage to form the two daughter cells.

Meiosis is the form of cell division that occurs to produce germ cells or gametes (sperm and egg). A diploid cell (with two sets or 46 chromosomes) divides to form haploid cells (with one set or 23 chromosomes). Meiosis is divided into two parts: meiosis I and meiosis II. DNA replication occurs before meiosis I. In male meiosis, the germ cell begins division with two times the normal cellular amount of DNA. In *meiosis I,* each daughter cell gets one of the duplicated chromosomes of each pair. At the beginning of *meiosis II,* each cell contains 23 chromosomes, each with a duplicated pair of chromatids. In meiosis II, the duplicated pair separate and each daughter cell ends up with one of each of the 23 chromosomes, that is, there are four daughter cells, each with a haploid (half the normal number) set of chromosomes. In female meiosis, rather than going through cell divisions during meiosis I, one diploid set of chromosomes condenses and forms a polar body, and during meiosis II, one of the haploid sets of chromosomes condenses and forms the second polar body, resulting in one egg with a haploid (half the normal number) set of chromosomes and two polar bodies that contain three sets of chromosomes.

There is exchange between chromosomes (crossing over of chromosome segments) during meiosis, leading to new alignment and combination of genes. Two common errors of cell division occur during meiosis that result in abnormal numbers of chromosomes and chromosomal anomalies. The first is *nondisjunction,* in which two chromosomes fail to separate and thus migrate together into one of the new cells, producing one cell with two copies of the chromosome and one cell with no copy. The second is *anaphase lag,* in which a chromatid is lost because it fails to move quickly enough during anaphase to become incorporated into one of the new daughter cells (Fig. 70–3).

Methodology. Chromosome studies can be obtained from any dividing nucleated cell. The techniques for visualization require condensation of chromatin material that occurs at cell division. Cytogenetic studies are usually performed on blood lymphocytes, but cytogenetic studies of fibroblasts must be considered if there is a suspicion of mosaicism. Chromosome studies for prenatal diagnosis are performed with cells obtained from amniotic fluid, chorionic villi tissue, fetal blood, or in preimplantation prenatal diagnosis by analysis of a blastomere.

Karyotyping refers to the systematic arrangement from a photograph or by a computer of previously stained and banded chromosomes of a single cell by pairs (see Fig. 70–1). The cells are cultured, arrested in mitosis during metaphase, and then fixed and stained. If finer details are necessary, prophase chromosomes may be examined. Because prophase chromosomes are longer and less condensed, they show 600–1,200 bands, compared with metaphase chromosomes, in which only 400–600 bands are usually visible. Trypsin-Giemsa staining gives G banding. Quinacrine gives the Q (fluorescent) banding. Special stains are used to demonstrate centromeres.

In situ hybridization is used to identify the presence or absence of specific DNA sequences on a chromosome spread. A molecular probe is used to recognize and attach to homologous DNA sequences on the chromosome spread, identifying a specific chromosome, chromosome segment, or DNA sequence. If fluorescent probes are used, the technique is called FISH (see Chapters 67 and 68).

Comparative *genomic hybridization* is a molecular cytogenetic technique that allows simultaneous enumeration of every chromosome. It involves the isolation of test DNA from a single cell (multiplied by polymerase chain reaction) or multiple cells from the test individual and comparison with DNA from a normal reference individual. The test DNA is labeled in a different way (green fluorochrome) from the reference DNA (red fluorochrome). The test and reference DNA are simultaneously hybridized to normal chromosomes. The fluorescent images reveal ratios of green to red and can be used to identify extra or missing chromosomal material.

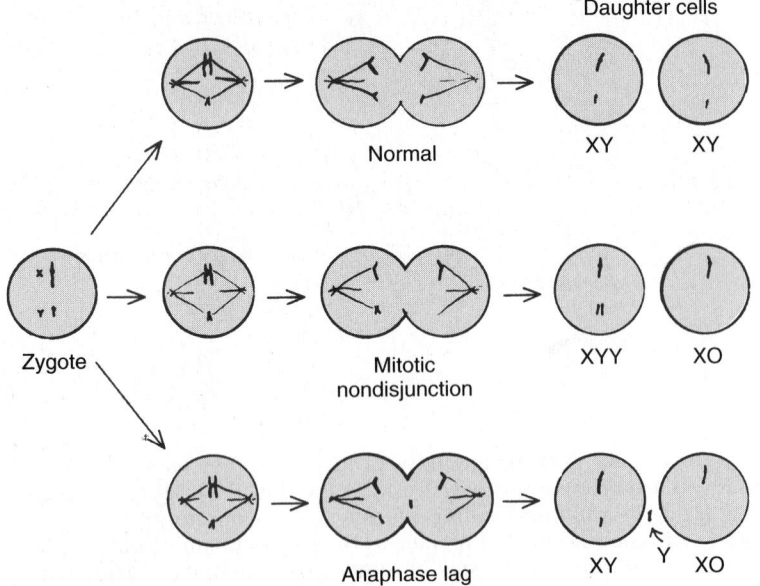

FIGURE 70–3. The formation of mosaicism. The X and Y chromosomes are used to illustrate two common errors leading to chromosomally abnormal cell populations. In normal mitosis *(top)*, duplicated chromosomes separate and become incorporated into daughter cells. If one replicated chromosome fails to separate, mitotic nondisjunction occurs *(middle)*. Occasionally, normal separation occurs, but one member fails to migrate. This is known as anaphase lag *(bottom)*. (From Wisniewski LP, Hirschhorn K: *A Guide to Human Chromosome Defects*, 2nd ed. White Plains, NY, March of Dimes Birth Defects Foundation, Birth Defects:Original Article Series, vol 16, sec 6, 1980, with permission from the copyright holder.)

CHROMOSOMAL ABNORMALITIES

Chromosomal anomalies occur in 0.4% of live births. They are an important cause of mental retardation and congenital anomalies. Chromosomal anomalies are present in much higher frequencies among spontaneous abortions and stillbirths. The phenotypic anomalies that result from chromosomal aberrations are mainly due to imbalance of genetic information. Chromosomal anomalies include abnormalities of chromosome number and structure.

Abnormalities of Chromosome Number

Aneuploidy and Polyploidy. When a human cell has 23 chromosomes, it is referred to as a *haploid cell* (the number of chromosomes in an ova or sperm). Any number of chromosomes that is an exact multiple of the haploid number (e.g., 46, 69, 92 in humans) is referred to as *euploid*. Euploid cells with more than the normal diploid number of 46 chromosomes are called *polyploid cells*. Polyploid conceptions are usually not viable. However, they may be present in mosaic (more than one cell line) forms, which allow survival. Cells with three sets of chromosomes are called triploid and are frequently seen in abortus material and occasionally in viable humans, usually in mosaic form. Cells deviating from the multiples of the haploid number

are called *aneuploid* (i.e., not euploid), indicating a missing or extra chromosome.

Trisomies. The most common abnormalities of chromosome number (aneuploidy) are trisomies. These occur when there are three representatives of a particular chromosome instead of the usual two. Trisomies are usually the result of meiotic nondisjunction (failure of a chromosome pair to separate). Trisomy may be present in all cells or may occur in mosaic form. Most individuals with trisomies exhibit a consistent and specific phenotype depending on the chromosome involved (Table 70–1). The most frequent trisomy in humans is *trisomy 21* or Down syndrome (Fig. 70–4). *Trisomies of chromosome 18* (Fig. 70–5) and *chromosome 13* (Fig. 70–6) are also relatively common and are associated with a characteristic set of congenital anomalies and mental retardation.

The incidence of Down syndrome among conceptions is more than twice as high as it is among live births. More than half the trisomy 21 conceptions spontaneously abort early in pregnancy. The occurrence of trisomy 21 as well as other autosomal trisomies increases with advancing maternal age. The increased risk of trisomy 21 in women older than 35 yr is an indication to offer these women prenatal diagnosis. Amniocentesis, or chorionic villus sampling to examine the fetal chromosomes, is usually offered although maternal serum alpha fetoprotein screening and

TABLE 70–1. Chromosomal Trisomies and Their Clinical Findings

Syndrome	Incidence	Clinical Manifestations
Trisomy 13, Patau syndrome	1/10,000 births	Cleft lip often midline; flexed fingers with polydactyly; ocular hypotelorism, bulbous nose; low-set malformed ears; small abnormal skull; cerebral malformation, especially holoprosencephaly; microphthalmia; cardiac malformations; scalp defects; hypoplastic or absent ribs; visceral and genital anomalies
Trisomy 18, Edwards syndrome	1/6,000 births	Low birthweight, closed fists with index finger overlapping the 3rd digit and the 5th digit overlapping the 4th, narrow hips with limited abduction, short sternum, rocker-bottom feet, microcephaly, prominent occiput, micrognathia, cardiac and renal malformations, and mental retardation; 95% of cases are lethal in the 1st yr
Trisomy 21, Down syndrome	1/600–800 births	Hypotonia, flat face, upward and slanted palpebral fissures and epicanthic folds, speckled irises (Brushfield spots); varying degrees of mental and growth retardation; dysplasia of the pelvis, cardiac malformations, and simian crease; short, broad hands, hypoplasia of middle phalanx of 5th finger, intestinal atresia, and high arched palate; 5% of patients with Down syndrome are the result of a translocation—t(14q21q), t(15q21q), and t(13q21q)—in which the phenotype is the same as trisomy 21 Down syndrome
Trisomy 8, mosaicism	1/20,000 births	Long face, high prominent forehead, wide upturned nose, thick everted lower lip, microretrognathia, low-set ears, high arched, sometimes cleft palate. Osteoarticular anomalies are common; moderate mental retardation.

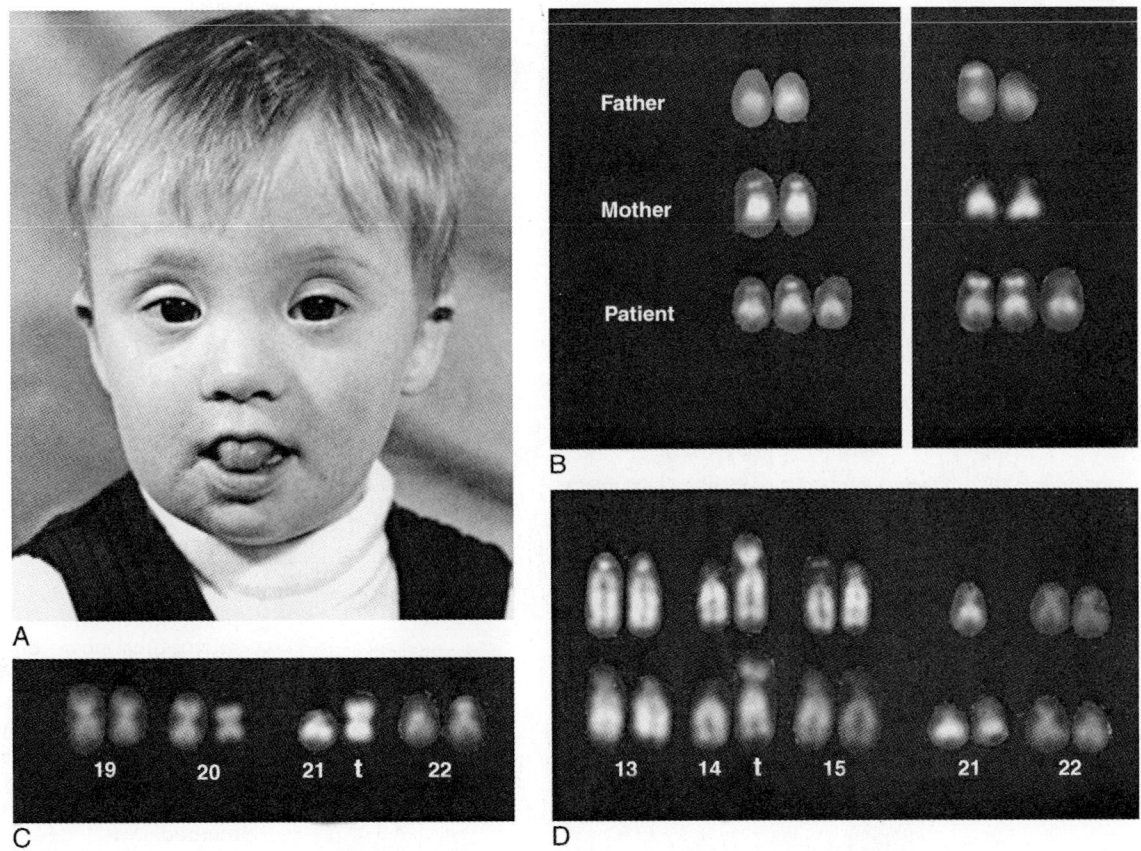

FIGURE 70–4. Partial karyotypes from patients with Down syndrome. *A,* Patient with trisomy 21. *B,* Chromosome 21 from two patients and their parents. *Left:* Two of a patient's chromosomes with brightly fluorescent satellites were transmitted by the mother. *Right:* Another patient's two chromosomes with bright satellites resulted from paternal nondisjunction at second meiotic division. *C,* 21q21q translocation. *D,* 14q21q translocation in a mother *(above)* and her affected child *(below).*

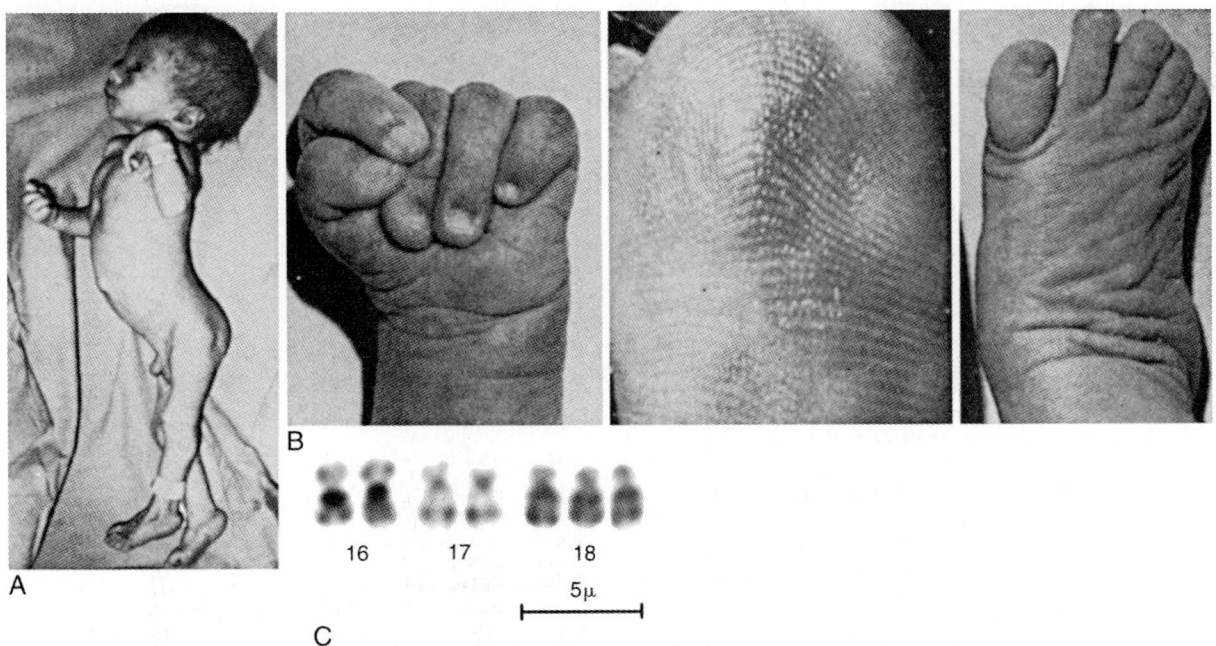

FIGURE 70–5. *A,* Photograph of male infant with trisomy 18, age 4 days. Note prominent occiput, micrognathia, low-set ears, short sternum, narrow pelvis, prominent calcaneus, and flexion abnormalities of the fingers. (Courtesy of Robert E. Carrel.) *B,* Several of the common anomalies in the 18 trisomy syndrome, including the unusual position of the fingers with hypoplasia of fifth fingernail, the simple arch pattern of the finger pads, and the dorsiflexed hallux with hypoplasia of toenails. (From Smith DW: Autosomal abnormalities. *Am J Obstet Gynecol* 1964;90:1055.) *C,* Partial karyotype of trisomy 18 prepared with modified Giemsa stain.

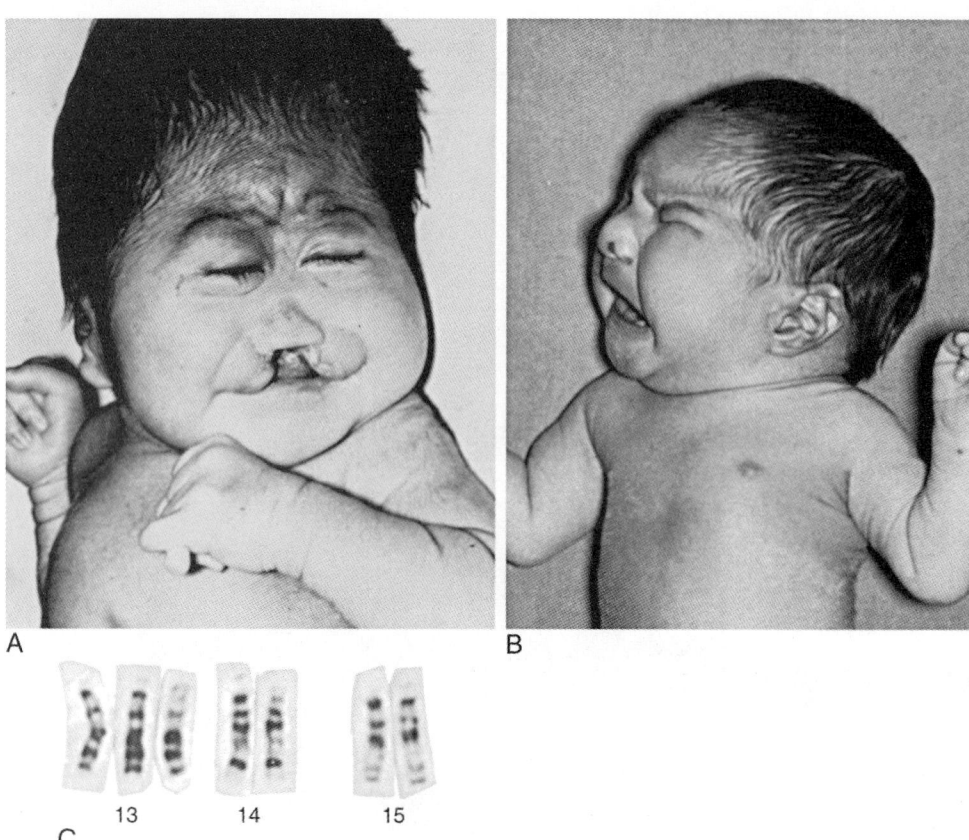

A   B

C   13   14   15

FIGURE 70–6. *A* and *B*, Female infants with trisomy 13 syndrome. Note the midline cleft of the lip and palate, microcephaly, hypotelorism, microphthalmos, bulbous nose, polydactyly, and overlapping of fingers. Scalp defects (not shown) are also present. (Courtesy of Miriam G. Wilson.) *C*, Partial karyotype showing chromosomes 13, 14, and 15 stained with the trypsin-Giemsa method.

recovering fetal DNA or cells from maternal blood are increasingly being used. In women younger than 35 yr of age, maternal serum testing (triple screen) can be efficacious in prenatal screening for Down syndrome. Low maternal serum α-fetoprotein concentration, low unconjugated estriol, and elevated human chorionic gonadotropin are indicators of Down syndrome. Prenatal ultrasonography may detect a thickened nuchal fold, absent nasal bone, a shortened femur, and cardiac or gastrointestinal anomalies associated with trisomy 21 (Chapter 85).

Translocation Down Syndrome. All individuals with Down syndrome have three copies of chromosome 21. About 95% have three freestanding copies of chromosome 21. Approximately 1% of individuals are mosaic with some normal cells. Approximately 4% of Down syndrome individuals have a translocation involving chromosome 21. Translocations account for 9% of the children with Down syndrome born to mothers younger than 30 yr of age. Half the translocations arise de novo in the affected individual, whereas half are inherited from a translocation carrier parent. Parents who are carriers of a translocation involving chromosome 21 produce three types of viable offspring: normal phenotype and karyotype, a phenotypically normal translocation carrier, and the translocation trisomy 21. The majority of translocations that give rise to Down syndrome are fusions at the centromere between chromosomes 13, 14, 15, or 21, for example, t(13q,15q) or t(21q,21q). The phenotype in translocation Down syndrome is not distinguishable from regular trisomy 21 Down syndrome (see Table 70–1). Chromosome studies must be performed on every Down syndrome individual. If a translocation is identified, parental studies must be performed to identify normal individuals who are translocation carriers with a high recurrence risk for a chromosomally abnormal child and who may also have other family members at risk.

Monosomies. Monosomies occur when only one representative of a chromosome is present. They may be complete or partial.

Complete monosomies may be the result of nondisjunction or anaphase lag. In nondisjunction during cell division, the two chromosomes in a replicating pair fail to separate; one cell ends up with only one copy (monosomic) and the other with three copies (trisomic) of the specific chromosome. In anaphase lag, a chromosome fails to move into the new daughter cell and is lost. In humans, all complete autosomal monosomies appear to be lethal early in development and only survive in mosaic forms. Partial monosomies are usually the offspring of a translocation carrier.

Abnormalities of Chromosome Structure

Deletions. Deletions occur when a piece of a chromosome is missing. They may occur as a simple deletion or as a deletion with duplication of another chromosome segment. The latter is usually caused by a crossover in meiosis in a translocation carrier, resulting in an unbalanced reciprocal chromosomal translocation. Deletions may be located at the chromosome ends or in interstitial segments of the chromosome and are usually associated with mental retardation and malformations. Small telomeric deletions may be relatively common in nonspecific mental retardation with minor anomalies. The most commonly observed deletions in humans are 4p-, 5p-, 9p-, 11p-, 13q-, 18p-, and 18q-, which are associated with well-described phenotypes (Table 70–2). Deletions may be observed in routine chromosome preparations, but microdeletions are detectable only under the microscope with prophase chromosome studies. In submicroscopic deletions, the missing piece can be detected only by using molecular probes or DNA studies.

Microdeletions are defined as small chromosome deletions that are detectable only in high-quality (pro)metaphase preparations. These deletions often involve several genes so that the affected individual may be identified by an unusual phenotype associated with an apparent single gene mutation. Williams, Langer-Giedion,

TABLE 70–2. Common Deletions and Their Clinical Manifestations

Deletion	Clinical Abnormalities
4p-	Wolf-Hirschhorn syndrome. The main features are a typical "Greek helmet" facies with ocular hypertelorism, prominent glabella, and frontal bossing; microcephaly, dolichocephaly, hypoplasia of the eye socket, ptosis, strabismus, nystagmus, bilateral epicanthic folds, cleft lip and palate, beaked nose with prominent bridge, hypospadias, cardiac malformations, and mental retardation.
5p-	Cri-du-chat syndrome. The main features are hypotonia, short stature, characteristic cry, microcephaly with protruding metopic suture, moonlike face, hypertelorism, bilateral epicanthic folds, high arched palate, wide and flat nasal bridge, and mental retardation.
9p-	The main features are craniofacial dysmorphology with trigonocephaly, slanted palpebral fissures, discrete exophthalmos, arched eyebrows, flat and wide nasal bridge, short neck with pterygium colli, genital anomalies, long fingers and toes, cardiac malformations, and mental retardation.
13q-	The main features are low birthweight, failure to thrive, and severe mental retardation. Facial features include microcephaly, flat wide nasal bridge, hypertelorism, ptosis, micrognathia. Ocular malformations are common. The hands have hypoplastic or absent thumbs and syndactyly.
18p-	A few patients (15%) are severely affected and have cephalic and ocular malformations, cleft lip and palate, and varying degrees of mental retardation. Most (80%) have only minor malformations and mild mental retardation.
18q-	The main features are hypotonia with "froglike" position with the legs flexed, externally rotated, and in hyperabduction. The face is characteristic with depressed midface and apparent protrusion of the mandible, deep-set eyes, short upper lip, everted lower lip ("carplike" mouth); antihelix of the ears is very prominent; varying degrees of mental retardation and belligerent personality.
21q-	The main features are hypertonia, microcephaly, downward-slanting palpebral fissures, high palate, prominent nasal bridge, large low-set ears, micrognathia, and varying degrees of mental retardation. They may have skeletal malformations.

Prader-Willi, Angelman, Rubinstein-Taybi, Smith-Magenis, Miller-Dieker, Alagille, and velocardiofacial/DiGeorge syndromes have all been found to be associated with microdeletions (Table 70–3). Submicroscopic deletions are not visible by microscopic examination and are detected only with specific probes for a DNA sequence or DNA studies. The deletion is recognized because of the absence of staining or fluorescence.

Translocations. Translocations involve the transfer of chromosomal material from one chromosome to another. Translocations may be Robertsonian or reciprocal. They occur with a frequency of 1/500 liveborn human infants. They may be inherited from a parent or appear de novo, with no other affected family members. *Robertsonian translocations* involve two acrocentric (centromere located at the end) chromosomes that fuse near the centromeric region with subsequent loss of the nonfunctional, very truncated short arms. The translocation chromosome is made up of the long arms of two fused chromosomes, hence the resulting count is only 45 chromosomes. The loss of the short arms of acrocentric chromosomes has no known deleterious effect. Although carriers of a Robertsonian translocation are usually phenotypically normal, they are at increased risk for miscarriages and abnormal offspring. *Reciprocal translocations* are the result of breaks in nonhomologous chromosomes with reciprocal exchange of the broken segments. Carriers of a reciprocal translocation are usually phenotypically normal but also have an increased risk of having chromosomally abnormal offspring and miscarriages because of abnormalities in the segregation of the chromosomes in the germ cells.

Inversions. Inversions require the chromosome to break at two points. The broken piece is then inverted and joined into the same chromosome. Inversions have a frequency of 1/100 liveborns and may be pericentric or paracentric. In *pericentric inversions,* the breaks are in the two opposite arms of the chromosome so that the intervening portion that contains the centromere is reversed. They are usually discovered because they change the position of the centromere. In contrast, *paracentric inversions* involve only chromosomal material from one arm of a chromosome. Carriers of inversions are usually normal, but they may have an increased risk of miscarriages and chromosomally abnormal offspring.

Ring Chromosomes. Ring chromosomes are rare, but they have been found for all human chromosomes. The formation of a ring involves a deletion at each end of the chromosome. The "sticky" ends then join to form the ring. The phenotype of a ring chromosome ranges from mental retardation and multiple congenital anomalies to normal or nearly normal depending on the amount of chromosomal material that is lost. If the ring replaces a normal chromosome, the result is partial monosomy. The phenotype in these cases often overlaps that seen in comparable deletion syndromes of the same chromosome. If there is a ring in addition to the normal chromosomes, the phenotype reflects the partial trisomy for that chromosome.

Duplications. A duplication is the presence of extra genetic material from the same chromosome. Duplications may result from the abnormal segregation in carriers of translocations or inversions.

Insertions. Insertions occur when a piece of chromosome breaks at two points and is incorporated into a break in another part of a chromosome. This requires three breakpoints and may occur between two chromosomes or within one.

Telomere/Subtelomere Deletions. Because chromosomes "cross over" during meiosis, small deletions and duplications of the regions toward the ends of the chromosomes occur relatively frequently. Subtelomeric rearrangements are being found increasingly (5–10%) in children with unexplained moderate to severe mental retardation without very obvious dysmorphic features. Submicroscopic subtelomeric deletions (smaller than 2–3 mb) are the second most common cause of mental retardation after trisomy 21. Clinical features seen in some of these children include prenatal growth retardation (seen in ~40%) and a family history of mental retardation (in 50%). Additional features seen in at least 30% of affected patients include microcephaly, hypertelorism, anomalies of the nose, ear, or hand, cryptorchidism, and short stature. FISH using multiple telomeric probes on metaphase chromosomes should be considered when other causes of developmental delay are excluded.

Sex Chromosome Anomalies

Turner Syndrome. This is one of the most common monosomies in liveborn humans (see Chapter 580.1). The chromosomal finding in Turner syndrome is the loss of part or all of one of the sex chromosomes. Half the affected individuals have 45, X in their lymphocytes. The other half have a variety of abnormalities of one of their sex chromosomes and may be mosaic. The phenotype in Turner syndrome is female and is characterized by short stature and underdeveloped gonads. The frequency at birth is 0.4/1,000 (i.e., 1/4,000 liveborn females or 1/8,000 livebirths), but it occurs much more frequently in spontaneous abortions.

From 5–10% of individuals with Turner syndrome have some Y chromosome material in all or some cells. These individuals may have some masculinization and are at risk for the development of gonadoblastoma. A careful screening for Y chromosome material should be performed on any individual with Turner syndrome in whom no additional X chromosome (in addition to the one normal X) material has been found.

TABLE 70–3. **Microdeletions and Their Clinical Manifestations**

Deletion	Syndrome	Clinical Manifestations
7q11.23	Williams	Round face with full cheeks and lips, stellate pattern in iris, strabismus, supravalvular aortic stenosis and other cardiac malformations, varying degrees of mental retardation, and a very friendly personality
8q24.1-	Langer-Giedion or tricho-rhino-phalangeal, type II	Sparse hair, multiple cone-shaped epiphyses, multiple cartilaginous exostoses, bulbous nasal tip, thickened alar cartilage, upturned nares, prominent philtrum, large protruding ears, and mild mental retardation
11p13-	WAGR	Hypernephroma (Wilms tumor), aniridia, male genital hypoplasia of varying degrees, gonadoblastoma, long face, upward slanting palpebral fissures, ptosis, beaked nose, low-set poorly formed auricles, and mental retardation
15q11-13 (pat)	Prader-Willi	Severe hypotonia at birth, obesity, short stature (responsive to growth hormone), small hands and feet, hypogonadism, and mental retardation
15q11-13 (mat)	Angelman	Hypotonia, fair hair, midface hypoplasia, prognathism, seizures, jerky ataxic movements, uncontrollable bouts of laughter, and severe mental retardation
16p13-	Rubinstein-Taybi	Microcephaly, ptosis, beaked nose with low-lying philtrum, broad thumbs and large toes, and mental retardation
17p11.2	Smith-Magenis	Brachycephaly, midfacial hypoplasia, prognathism, myopia, cleft palate, short stature, behavioral problems, and mental retardation
17p13.3-	Miller-Dieker	Microcephaly, lissencephaly, pachygyria, narrow forehead, hypoplastic male external genitals, growth retardation, seizures, and profound mental retardation
20p12-	Alagille syndrome	Bile duct paucity with cholestasis, heart defects, particularly pulmonary artery stenosis, ocular abnormalities (posterior embryotoxin), skeletal defects such as butterfly vertebrae, long nose with broad midnose
22q11.2	Velocardiofacial-DiGeorge syndrome	Hypoplasia or agenesis of the thymus and parathyroid glands, hypoplasia of auricle and external auditory canal, conotruncal cardiac anomalies, cleft palate, short stature, behavioral problems

Klinefelter Syndrome. These individuals have a male karyotype with an extra X chromosome, 47, XXY, and the phenotype is male (see Chapter 577.1). Individuals with Klinefelter syndrome are usually relatively tall. They may have gynecomastia, and secondary sex development may be delayed. They usually have azoospermia and small testes, and are infertile.

Many other syndromes occur in which there are extra X chromosomes (i.e., 47, XYX, 48, XXY-X, 49, XXXXX, 48, XXXY, and 49, XXXXY). These individuals are often mosaic, having both normal and abnormal cell lines (46, XX/47, YXX). In all these syndromes, the number of abnormalities increases with the number of X chromosomes and is specific to each syndrome. Abnormalities of chromosome Y also exist. The most common abnormality is the XYY male.

47, XYY Male. The frequency of XYY males has been estimated to be 1/1,000 livebirths. Because XYY males do not have any striking phenotypical abnormality, this frequency has been estimated from newborn surveys. XYY males are said to be relatively tall and may have some behavioral problems.

Fragile Sites

Fragile sites are defined as regions of chromosomes that show a tendency to separation, breakage, or attenuation under particular growth conditions. Numerous fragile sites have been identified.

Fragile X Syndrome. The fragile site located on the distal long arm of chromosome X at Xq27.3 is associated with the Fragile X syndrome, which is the most common heritable form of mental retardation in males. This fragile site (FRAXA) becomes visible in chromosome studies only when it is induced under special culture techniques; regular metaphase studies do not demonstrate this fragile site. The fragile site may not always be visible, even with the appropriate chromosome preparation. The diagnosis of fragile X is made by DNA studies, which demonstrate an expanded segment of DNA from the Xq27.3 region. The length of the expanded segment reflects the number of nucleotide triplet repeats. There are two other fragile sites on the X chromosome (FRAXE and FRAXF) also associated with mental retardation and allelic expansion.

The main *clinical manifestations* of Fragile X syndrome in affected males are mental retardation; macroorchidism; large size; characteristic facial features, including long face, prominent jaw, and large prominent ears; stereotyped behavior and speech. Females affected with Fragile X show varying degrees of mental retardation; however, it is a less frequent cause of mental retardation in girls.

The *inheritance of Fragile X* is different from the usual single-gene inheritance patterns. It involves an area of the gene with CGG/CCG repeats (triplet repeats). Three distinct categories of DNA variation occur at the fragile X locus (normal, up to 50 repeats; premutation, 52–200 repeats; symptomatic, 200–2,000 repeats or greater). A person who carries a small increase of trinucleotide repeats without the phenotypic abnormalities is said to be a carrier of a premutation. When inherited, this premutation is unstable and may expand over a few generations, gradually increasing in size when transmitted by females but usually remaining the same size when transmitted by males. When the mutation is transmitted by a female and increases in size, it may become a size (usually an additional 600–3,000 base pairs) that is clinically significant and leads to the typical Fragile X syndrome phenotype with mental retardation. Also see Chapter 68.

Allelic expansion refers to the change of the size of the DNA sequence. Allelic expansion interferes with gene function. The expansion begins as a small increase in the copy number of trinucleotide repeats. The number of repeats is unstable and may lead to different sizes in different cells or tissues. The number of repeats may increase in size from one generation to the next (but occasionally may decrease in size). A change in size of the DNA segment between generations or in tissues means that this type of mutation differs from classic mutations in which the change in DNA sequence usually occurs once and is then passed on from generation to generation. Other disorders associated with allelic expansion include myotonic dystrophy (with CTG repeats), Huntington disease (with CAG repeats), spinobulbar muscular atrophy (with CAG repeats), spinocerebellar ataxia type 1, 2, and 3 (SCA1, SCA2, and SCA3, all with CAG repeats), and dentatorubral-pallidoluysian atrophy (with CAG repeats).

The number of copies seen in disorders associated with allelic expansion seems to determine the age of onset and severity of the disease (Table 70–4). For example, the congenital form of myotonic dystrophy is known to occur with the largest number of repeats but only when the mother transmits it. In Huntington disease, the juvenile onset form of the disease is also associated with the largest number of repeats and occurs primarily when inherited from the father.

Chromosomal Breakage Syndromes

There are a number of recessive disorders that are associated with breakage or rearrangement of chromosomes, or both. The breaks may be spontaneous or they can be induced by a variety of environmental agents and brought out by different laboratory techniques. Chromatid breaks are found in Fanconi anemia, Nijmegen syndrome, Bloom syndrome, and Werner syndrome. Breaks and

TABLE 70–4. Allelic Expansion

Gene	Location	Normal	Premutation	Affected	Parent of Origin Effect
Huntington disease	4p16.3	11–24 repeats	30–38	42–82	Male transmission usually increases repeat
Myotonic dystrophy	19q13.3	5–37 repeats	37–50	>50	Male may decrease repeat
					Female usually increases repeat
Fragile X	Xq23.7	6–54 repeats	52–200	>200	Male constant
					Female may markedly increase repeat

nonrandom rearrangements of chromosomes 7 and 14 have been reported in ataxia-telangiectasia. A special cytogenetic study, sister chromatid exchange, is used in some of these disorders for carrier detection and prenatal diagnosis. These disorders have specific phenotypes, but the growth impairment, malformations, and other dysmorphic features seen in these conditions have not been directly attributed to the chromosome breaks.

Mosaicism

Mosaicism is the term used to describe an individual who has two different cell lines derived from a single zygote (fertilized egg) (see Fig. 70–3). Studies of placental tissue from chorionic villus sampling show that at least 2% of all conceptions are mosaic for chromosomal anomalies at or before 10 wk of pregnancy. Compared with complete trisomies, which are usually nonviable for chromosomes other than 13, 18, and 21, the development of a normal cell line may allow a trisomic conception of the other chromosomes to continue to term and be viable. If a normal cell line develops, the fetus may survive and the original trisomic cell line may even be lost. Normal disomic cells are found in the placenta of infants who are born alive with trisomies 13 and 18.

Germ line mosaicism refers to the presence of mosaicism in the germ cells found in the gonad. This type of mosaicism may be suspected in cases in which there is more than one affected offspring with the same genetic abnormality (usually inherited as a chromosomal or autosomal dominant disorder) with phenotypically normal parents. If germ line mosaicism is present, there is an increased risk for recurrence of an affected child.

Depending on the point at which the new cell line arises during early embryogenesis, an affected individual may have a variety of clinical presentations. Mosaicism may be present in some tissues and not in others, giving the affected individual a patchy or asymmetric distribution of abnormalities. Cytogenetic studies of fibroblasts must be performed if mosaicism is suspected because blood lymphocyte cells may not tolerate some trisomies, deletions, or chromosomal rearrangements, and thus the finding of normal lymphocyte studies will be misleading.

Pallister-Killian Syndrome. This disorder is characterized by coarse facies, pigmentary skin anomalies, localized alopecia, diaphragmatic hernias, cardiovascular anomalies, supernumerary nipples, and profound mental retardation. The syndrome is due to mosaicism for isochromosome 12p. The presence of the isochromosome 12p in cells gives four copies of 12p in the affected cells. The isochromosome 12p is preferentially cultured from fibroblast and is seldom present in lymphocytes. The abnormalities seen in affected individuals probably reflect the presence of abnormal cells during early embryogenesis.

Hypomelanosis of Ito. This entity is characterized by unilateral or bilateral macular hypopigmented whorls, streaks, and patches. Abnormalities of the eyes, musculoskeletal system, and central nervous system may also be present. Patients with hypomelanosis of Ito appear to have two genetically distinct cell lines. The mosaic chromosome anomalies that have been observed involve both autosomes and sex chromosomes and have been demonstrated in about 50% of cases. The mosaicism may not be

visible in chromosome studies carried out on blood but is more likely to be found when the chromosome studies are obtained from skin fibroblasts. Sometimes the distinct cell lines may not be due to observable chromosomal anomalies but to single gene mutations or other mechanisms.

Acquired Cytogenetic Abnormalities

Chromosomal changes are seen in most cancers. It is thought that the chromosomal change affects cancer-promoting and cancer suppressing genes. Loss, gain, and translocations of chromosomes are seen in cancerous tissue, which appear to alter the function of cancer related genes. The particular rearrangements may be useful in predicting prognosis and suggesting the most efficacious therapy.

UNIPARENTAL DISOMY

Uniparental disomy (UPD) is the term used when both chromosomes of a pair of chromosomes in a person with a normal number of chromosomes have been inherited from only one parent. Uniparental isodisomy means that the two chromosomes are identical, whereas uniparental heterodisomy means that the two chromosomes are different members of a pair, both of which were inherited from one parent. The phenotypical result of UPD may vary according to the specific chromosome involved, the parent who contributed the chromosomes, and whether it is isodisomy or heterodisomy. Three types of phenotypic effects are seen in UPD: (1) those related to imprinted genes (see later), that is, the absence of a gene that is expressed only when inherited from a parent of a specific gender, (2) those related to autosomal recessive disorders, and (3) those related to a vestigial aneuploid producing mosaicism. Also see Chapter 69.

In uniparental isodisomy, both chromosomes in the pair are identical; consequently, the genes on both chromosomes are also identical. This becomes particularly important when the parent is a carrier of an autosomal recessive disorder. If the offspring of a carrier parent has uniparental disomy with isodisomy for a chromosome that carries an abnormal gene, the abnormal gene will be present in two copies and the phenotype will be that of the autosomal recessive disorder. In other words, the child has an autosomal recessive disorder when only one parent is actually a carrier of that recessive disorder. It is estimated that all human beings carry five to eight abnormal autosomal recessive genes. The autosomal recessive disorders spinal muscular atrophy, cystic fibrosis, cartilage-hair hypoplasia, α- and β-thalassemias, and Bloom syndrome have occurred because of uniparental disomy. The possibility of uniparental isodisomy should also be kept in mind when an individual is affected with more than one recessive disorder because the abnormal genes for both disorders could be carried on the same isodisomic chromosome. Uniparental isodisomy is a very rare cause of recessively inherited disorders.

Maternal uniparental disomy involving chromosomes 2, 7, 14, and 15 and paternal uniparental disomy involving chromosomes 6, 11, 15, and 20 are associated with phenotypic

PATERNAL

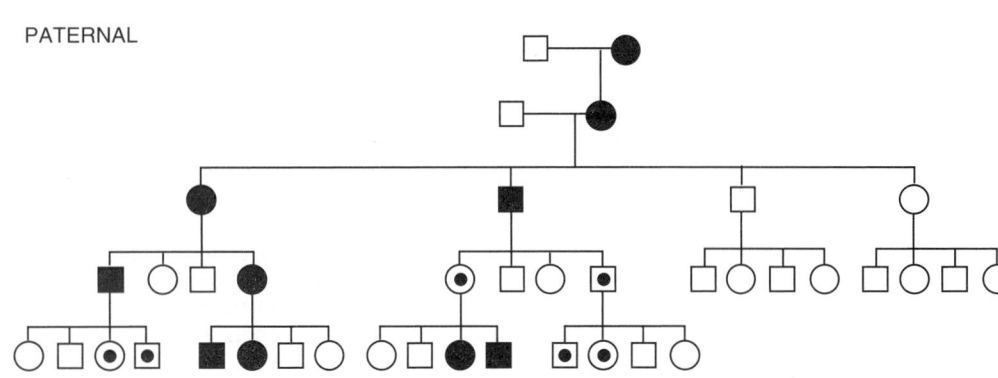

FIGURE 70–7. In pedigrees suggestive of paternal imprinting, phenotypic effects occur only when the gene is transmitted from the mother but not when transmitted from the father. There are equal numbers of males and females affected and nonaffected phenotypically in each generation. A nonmanifesting transmitter gives a clue to the sex of the parent who passes the expressed genetic information; in other words, in paternal imprinting there are "skipped" female nonmanifesting individuals.

abnormalities of growth and behavior. For instance, UPD maternal 7 is associated with a phenotype similar to Russell-Silver syndrome with intrauterine growth retardation. These phenotypic effects may be related to imprinting (see later).

UPD for chromosome 15 is seen in some cases of Prader-Willi syndrome and Angelman syndrome. In *Prader-Willi syndrome*, about 60% of cases have maternal UPD (i.e., missing the paternal chromosome 15). In about 5% of individuals with *Angelman syndrome*, paternal UPD of chromosome 15 is observed (i.e., missing the maternal chromosome 15). The phenotype for both Prader-Willi syndrome and Angelman syndrome in cases of UPD is thought to be due to the lack of the functional contribution from a particular parent of their chromosome 15. These findings suggest there are differences in function of certain regions of chromosome 15, depending on whether it is inherited from the mother or from the father.

Uniparental disomy most likely arises because a pregnancy starts off as a trisomy. Most trisomies are lethal, and the fetus survives only if a cell line loses one of the extra chromosomes and becomes disomic. One third of the time, the disomic cell line is uniparental. Usually, the viable cell line outgrows the trisomic cell line. When mosaic trisomy is found at prenatal diagnosis, care should be taken to determine whether uniparental disomy has resulted and whether the chromosome involved is one of the disomies known to be associated with phenotypic abnormalities. There must always be concern that some residual cells that are trisomic will be present in some tissues, leading to malformations or dysfunction. The presence of aggregates of tri-

somic cells may account for the spectrum of abnormalities seen in individuals with UPD.

IMPRINTING

Genomic imprinting refers to the observation that phenotypic expression depends on the parent of origin for certain genes and chromosome segments. Whether the genetic material is expressed depends on the gender of the parent from whom it was derived. Genomic imprinting is suspected on the basis of a pedigree (Figs. 70–7 and 70–8) with unusual transmission. Imprinting probably occurs in many different parts of the human genome but is thought to be particularly important in gene expression related to development, growth, cancer, evolution, and behavior.

Imprinting in humans is noted by phenotypic differences seen in Prader-Willi and Angelman syndromes, which are associated with deletion and uniparental disomy of the same region of chromosome 15. Thus in uniparental maternal disomy, there is also lack of the paternal segment of chromosome 15, resulting in Prader-Willi syndrome as well. In Prader-Willi syndrome, the deletion, when it occurs, is always of the paternally derived chromosome 15, suggesting that the phenotype of Prader-Willi is due to a lack of paternally derived genetic information carried on that segment of chromosome 15. In contrast, when there is a deleted chromosome 15 in Angelman syndrome, the deleted chromosome is always maternal in origin, and the UPI is always paternal, that is, there is lack of maternal information. There are

MATERNAL

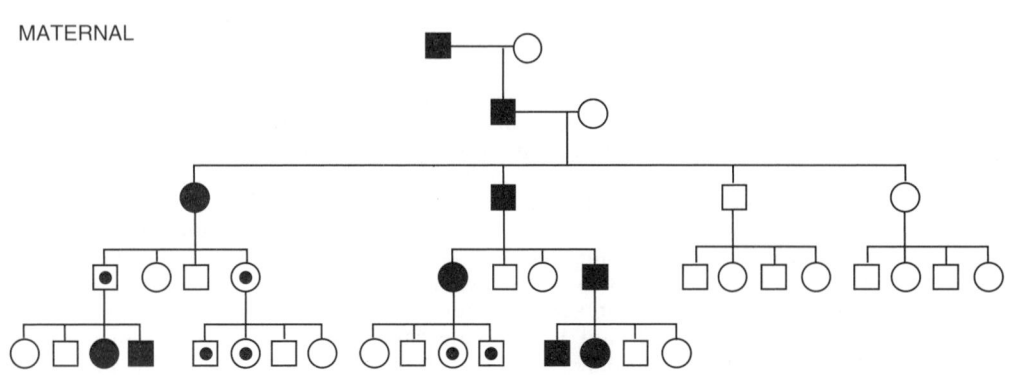

FIGURE 70–8. In pedigrees suggestive of maternal imprinting, phenotypic effects occur only when the gene is transmitted from the father but not when transmitted from the mother. There are equal numbers of males and females affected and nonaffected phenotypically in each generation. A nonmanifesting transmitter gives a clue to the sex of the parent who passes the expressed genetic information; in other words, in maternal imprinting there are "skipped" male nonmanifesting individuals.

likely to be many other disorders with this type of parent of origin effect.

Adinolfi M, Sherlock J: Prenatal detection of chromosome disorders by QF-PCR. *Lancet* 2001;358:1030–1.

Baralle D: Chromosomal aberrations, subtelomeric defects, and mental retardation. *Lancet* 2001;358:7–8.

Cassidy SB, Allanson JE: *Management of Genetic Syndromes.* Wiley-Liss, 2001.

Cassidy SB, Dykens E, Williams CA: Prader-Willi and Angelman syndromes: Sister imprinted disorders. *Am J Med Genet* 2000;97:136–46.

Colleaux L, Rio M, Heuertz S, et al: A novel automated strategy for screening cryptic telomeric rearrangements in children with idiopathic mental retardation. *Eur J Hum Genet* 2001;9:319–27.

Crolla JA: FISH and molecular studies of autosomal supernumerary marker chromosomes excluding those derived from chromosome 15. Review of the literature. *Am J Med Genet* 1998;75:367–81.

Engel E, Antonarakis SE: *Genomic Imprinting and Uniparental Disomy in Medicine: Clinical and Molecular Aspects.* Wiley-Liss, 2002.

Fritz B, Hallermann C, Olert J, et al: Cytogenetic analyses of culture failures by comparative genomic hybridisation (CFH)—Re-evaluation of chromosome aberration rates in early spontaneous abortions. *Eur J Hum Genet* 2001;9:539–47.

International System for Human Cytogenetic Nomenclature (ISCN). Published in collaboration with Cytogenetics and Cell Genetics, 1985.

Kotzot D: Abnormal phenotypes in uniparental disomy (UPD)–fundamental aspects and a critical review with bibliography of UPI other than 15. *Am J Med Genet* 1999;82:265–74.

Langlois S, Lopez-Rangel E, Hall JG: New mechanisms for genetic disease and non-traditional modes of inheritance. *Adv Pediatr* 1995;40:91–111.

Lignon AH, Beaudet AL, Shaffer LG: Simultaneous, multilocus FISH analysis for detection of microdeletions in the diagnostic evaluation of development delay and mental retardation. *Am J Hum Genet* 1997;61:51–9.

Ranke MB, Saenger P: Turner's syndrome. *Lancet* 2001;358:309–14.

Sismani C, Armour JA, Flint J, et al: Screening for subtelomeric chromosome abnormalities in children with idiopathic mental retardation using multiprobe telomeric FISH and the new MAPH telomeric assay. *Eur J Hum Genet* 2001;9:527–32.

Wald NJ, Watt HC, Hackshaw AK: Integrated screening for Down's syndrome based on tests performed during the first and second trimesters. *N Engl J Med* 1999;341:461–7.

Wells D, Sherlock JK, Handyside AH, et al: Detailed chromosomal and molecular genetic analysis of single cells by whole genome amplification and comparative genomic hybridisation. *Nucleic Acids Res* 1999;27:1214–8.

Yang Q, Rasmussen SA, Friedman JM: Mortality associated with Down's syndrome in the USA from 1983 to 1997: A population-based study. *Lancet* 2002;359:1019–25.

Ziauddin J, Sabatini DM: Microarrays of cells expressing defined cDNAs. *Nature* 2001;411:107–10.

Chapter 71

Gene Therapy *Mark A. Kay*

Gene therapy is defined as the introduction of nucleic acids into a tissue to prevent, inhibit, or reverse a pathologic process. Gene therapy was initially considered to treat monogenic disorders; DNA should also be considered to treat both genetic and acquired disorders. Gene therapy is usually restricted for somatic cell therapy. Genetic modification of human germ cells is not currently acceptable. Most of the current clinical trials are performed on adults who are able to give informed consent for experimental procedures. Exceptions may include life-threatening diseases in children for whom no alternative therapy is available. However, as safety and success become demonstrable, gene therapy is likely to impact disease prevention. Currently, there is only one accepted and unequivocal therapeutic benefit in treated patients with X-linked severe combined immunodeficiency (SCID).

GENE TRANSFER STRATEGIES

Most gene therapy involves transferring DNA into target tissues to add expression of the exogenous gene that encodes a protein missing due to a gene mutation or to supply a novel protein with a desired pharmacologic effect. In this situation, the exogenous gene, referred to as the *transgene*, is not localized in the normal chromosomal location in the human genome. Nonetheless, by adding the appropriate promoters or regulatory elements, the added gene can be expressed in the targeted cells (Fig. 71–1). Generic problems include achieving therapeutic levels of gene transfer into the appropriate cell types, control of gene expression, immune reactions to the vector or gene product and the risk of insertional mutagenesis. In some acquired disorders (e.g., cancer or acute infection), short-term transgene expression is desirable; for most genetic diseases, lifelong genetic modification is required.

A second type of gene therapy involves the insertion of nucleic acid in a formulation that instead of randomly inserting itself into a cell's DNA will actually correct a mutation in chromosomal DNA, reverting the inactive gene into a functioning gene or converting an abnormally functioning gene back to normal. Even though there are attractive advantages to correcting a mutation rather than adding exogenous DNA that can in theory have unwanted side effects, it will be very difficult to use gene correction technology to treat diseases where there are hundreds of mutations that cause the same phenotypic disease. This therapy is limited to the treatment of monogenic disorders.

With the clinical efficacy of enzyme replacement for disorders such as Gaucher disease, it may not be obvious why there is an advantage to producing a therapeutic protein within the body compared with exogenous protein therapy. In some cases, it is not possible to target exogenous proteins to the correct tissue or intracellular location required for function. Production of a therapeutic protein within a tissue may achieve a much higher local concentration and may avoid systemic toxicity derived from parenteral protein administration. It is difficult to achieve a constant therapeutic level of most proteins when administered exogenously. Gene transfer produces constitutive and thus steady-state levels of the desired protein.

Gene therapy can be performed ex vivo or in vivo. In ex vivo gene therapy, the target cells are removed, genetically manipulated in the laboratory, and then readministered to the patient. This is not unlike gene therapy with an organ transplant (liver for hyperlipidemia) or a cell transplant (bone marrow for lysosomal diseases) except that it uses autologous cells that are less likely to be immunogenic and lost due to rejection. Even though this approach is easily adaptable to some cell types, including bone marrow derived cells or fibroblasts, it is less feasible to perform in most other tissues. The goal of in vivo gene therapy is to deliver the vector and gene by intravenous infusion or oral or respiratory administration. The vector would then home to the appropriate target organs with minimal dissemination to unnecessary tissues. Further safeguards include using regulatory sequences attached to the gene that only allows for transgene transcription in the targeted tissue.

An important consideration is the risk of humoral immune responses against the corresponding transgene product and/or cellular immune responses directed against the gene-modified cells. This is especially problematic in individuals with genetic disorders who have never been exposed to the normal protein (gene deletions). Polymorphic genetic variances in humans make it likely that responses to gene therapy trials will be much more variable in humans than in inbred animals. Preclinical testing in animals is required before proceeding into human trials, but the limits of animal testing must be considered.

VECTORS–THE VEHICLES OF GENE TRANSFER

Gene transfer vectors are either viral or nonviral (Table 71–1). Viruses are efficient vehicles for transferring genetic information into host cells. The viral shell serves as the physical carrier of the genetic sequences to be transferred into the target cell (see Fig. 71–1). The vector DNA cannot replicate in the absence of viral genes and make new viral particles. The genetic structure of many vectors contains only viral DNA at both ends, which do

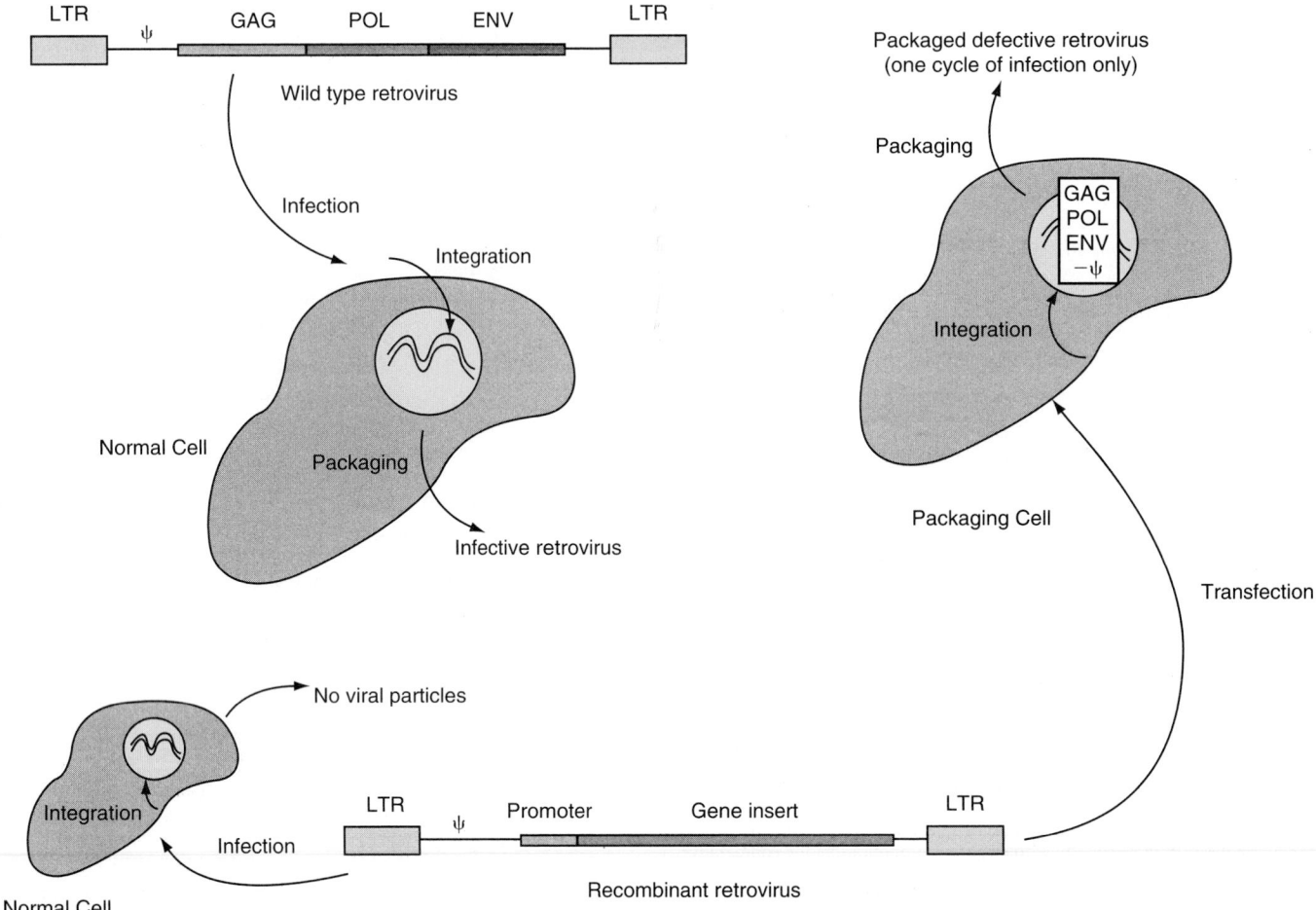

FIGURE 71–1. Life cycle and organization of wild type and recombinant retrovirus genomes. Retroviruses bind to specific cellular receptors on the target cell surface and are internalized by receptor-mediated endocytosis. Following entry, the retroviral RNA genome is removed from its capsid coat and is reverse transcribed by viral reverse transcriptase into DNA that is transported to the nucleus, where integration into the host genome occurs. In wild-type virus, the life cycle is completed by the synthesis of viral proteins and RNA by the host cell, packaging the retroviral particle that is released by budding from the cell surface. Recombinant viruses containing the therapeutic gene or cDNA are replication incompetent, the insert taking the place of the viral genes *GAG, POL,* and *ENV.* "Packaging" lines produce these retroviral gene products in vitro, allowing encapsulation of virus and production of the infectious virions. The "packaged" recombinant virus contains an RNA copy of the therapeutic gene insert that can be used to infect target cells.

not encode viral genes (see Fig. 71–1). The structural ends of the viral vector are recognition signals for packaging the vector DNA into encapsulated virion particles. When a virus is used as a vector, safety concerns related to the inadvertent production of contaminating wild-type (disease causing) virus is important.

There is great effort in developing ways to deliver DNA molecules in the absence of viruses. These include naked DNA and complicated chemical formulations conjugated to the DNA (see Table 71–1). One important limitation is the ability to safely transfer the genes into a specific organ with therapeutic effi-

TABLE 71–1. Properties of Transfection Agents

Transfection Agent	Cell Target	Chromosomal Integration	Immunogenicity	DNA-Carrying Capacity in Kb
Naked DNA	Skeletal muscle, thyroid gland, certain tumor types, liver cells, skin, myocardial cells	No	No	>10
Retrovirus	Dividing cells	Yes	Low	9
Adenovirus	Dividing and nondividing cells	No, episome	High in first generation,	38
				8
			Low in mice	27
Lentivirus	Dividing and nondividing cells	Yes	Low	<8
Adeno-associated virus	Many cells	Rare	Low	<5
Herpes simplex virus	Neurons of sensory ganglia	Extra-chromosomal	Low	25
Liposome	Many cells	Episome	Low	>10
Protein/peptide	Many cells	Episome	Variable	>10

From Balicki D, Beutler E: Gene therapy of human disease. Medicine *2002;81:69–86.*

ciency, resulting in persistent gene expression. In general, viral vectors appear to offer more immediate promise for efficacy, although many future vectors will likely be nonviral.

Retroviral based vectors are the most commonly used vector. The type of retroviral vector used clinically is based on a mouse Moloney retrovirus. These vectors are deleted of all of their viral genes and have a relatively long safety record. To produce the vector, packaging cell lines that are permanently modified with all of the viral genes required for replicating and packaging the vector genome are used (see Fig. 71–1). The vector sequences that contain the therapeutic gene is flanked by structural viral sequence and the packaging signal; a sequence required for packaging the vector DNA into the virion flanks the gene expression cassette. In this approach, only the vector sequences encoding the therapeutic gene of interest are packaged into the viral particle. When exposed to the target cells, the vector genome containing only the therapeutic gene, and no viral genes, is transduced into cells. Retroviral vectors integrate their therapeutic genes into the chromosomes of target cells. This results in stable gene transfer as long as the modified cell or their progenitors survive. This offers an advantage for genetic diseases in which lifelong gene expression is required. Even though these vectors have a long safety record in animal and human trials, the concern with any vector that has the potential to integrate is insertional mutagenesis causing inactivation or overactivation of an unrelated cellular gene that may be involved in carcinogenesis. This vector only transduces cells that are actively dividing. At any one time, most cells in a tissue are not dividing. Unless a stimulus is used to promote cell division, gene transfer efficiencies are low. Most retroviral-based gene transfer clinical protocols are based on ex vivo studies in which the patient's cultured cells (bone marrow) are manipulated in the laboratory to undergo cell cycling. Newer retroviral-based vectors derived from lentiviruses such as HIV have the possible advantage of transducing some cell types that are not actively dividing. Concerns with any viral vector are related to the overlap sequences with wild-type viruses that could result in recombination events leading to the creation of wild-type or rearranged virus. However, with current vector designs, overlap sequences have been eliminated or are very short, making recombination less of a concern.

Recombinant adenoviral vectors do not integrate and can transduce a large proportion of the cells in many different tissues (see Fig. 71–1). The genomic structure of the adenovirus is more complex than that of the retrovirus, and as a result it has been more difficult to remove all of the viral genes from the vectors. The remaining viral genes that are left in the early versions of the vector are transcribed at a very low level, resulting in some level of toxicity and immunogenicity. Whereas adenovirus may offer some advantage in treating diseases such as cancer, the associated vector toxicity resulted in the death of a young man after intravascular infusion. The preclinical studies suggest that vectors without any viral genes have much reduced toxicity.

Recombinant adeno-associated viral vectors are derived from a nonpathogenic human parvovirus. This vector has an outstanding safety record and is efficient at transducing a number of tissues, including the muscle and liver. Clinical trials are ongoing for cystic fibrosis, hemophilia, and muscular dystrophy. The major disadvantage of this vector is that, as a result of its small size, it cannot carry very large genes, which limits its applications for some disorders.

Herpes viruses are probably the least well understood. They are large, have a large DNA capacity, and are efficient at transducing many tissues, including the central nervous system. Preclinical studies are underway and clinical trials are likely to be initiated soon.

Nonviral vectors are made by several different methods and usually consist of DNA complexed with lipids, carbohydrates, proteins, and/or other synthetic chemicals to facilitate delivery or increase vector stability. Gene delivery with naked DNA is also possible; however, the inefficiency of this process probably limits its use. Nonviral vectors are desirable because they eliminate the risk of viral contamination and can be produced under more controlled conditions. Their major disadvantage is low gene transfer rates, at least when compared with most viral vector systems. Novel methods involving coexpression of the vector with protein molecules allow for vector-specific integration into cultured cells or animals. Even though proof-of-concept studies have been demonstrated, additional safety studies are required before clinical implementation will be considered.

For viral vectors, most of these properties are based on the mechanism by which the parent virus is known to infect cells in the wild-type state. Because of these inherent properties, there is great interest in making hybrid vectors that contain desired properties of two different vectors combined into a single vector. Thus future viral vectors may be derived from more than one virus or represent a combination of viral and nonviral components.

Because many of the vectors under development are derived from viruses, similar to what occurs with infection, humoral immunity may prohibit secondary gene transfer with repeated vector administration. Readministration may require a vector derived from a different viral serotype.

TARGETING GENE DELIVERY

An important aspect of gene transfer is expression of the protein in the target or other functional cells. Biologically active factor IX is normally produced in liver, but it can be produced and secreted into the bloodstream via the muscle, endothelium, or fibroblasts. In contrast, globin production for hemoglobinopathies requires regulated gene expression in erythroid-derived cells. It may be possible to deliver the vector into a specific tissue (intramuscular injection for muscle delivery). Retargeting the vector by altering the viral ligand will only allow it to enter the desired cell type. Gene promoter regulatory elements can successfully turn genes on or off in a tissue-specific manner.

Viruses bind to cells based on their outer coat protein and availability of a viral receptor on the host cell. To alter tropism and to get tissue specific uptake of a viral vector, genetic modification of the viral outer proteins is required. Pseudotyping or swapping one coat protein with one derived from a different virus is possible. True tissue-specific engineering of the viral ligand has had technical difficulties. Finally, in some diseases, the ability to turn the gene on or off at desired times, such as with the insulin gene in diabetes (e.g., *on* during high glucose and *off* during low glucose), is required for successful treatment. Regulatory sequences that respond to blood sugar levels have been used. Moreover, drug responsive genes have been constructed such that the gene is either turned on or off with exposure to a specific drug.

DISEASE TARGETS

Even though gene therapy was originally considered for the treatment of monogenic disorders, of the more than 500 clinical trials to date, only about 10% of the proposed or ongoing trials are directed at treating genetic diseases (Table 71–2). Most of the clinical trials are designed to treat cancer. Four major approaches to treat cancer have been considered:

1. *Immune response.* An immune response can result in a robust killing of tumors, thus gene transfer of genes that express potent tumor-specific antigens resulting in a more immunogenic tumor and/or genes for cytokines that stimulate and/or bring more immune-responsive cells to the tumor would be beneficial.

TABLE 71-2. Candidate Diseases for Gene Therapy

Single Gene Defects	Genes Involved	Target Organs/Tissues
Severe combined immunodeficiency	Several	T cells
α_1-Antitrypsin deficiency	α_1-Antitrypsin	Lungs (emphysema), liver (cirrhosis)
Cystic fibrosis	Cystic fibrosis transmembrane regulator	Lungs, pancreas
Hemophilia A and B	Factors VIII and IX	Blood clotting
Gaucher disease	Acid β-glucosidase, glucocerebrosidase	Macrophages; liver, spleen, lungs
β-Hemoglobinopathies	β-Globin	Blood formed elements
Hypercholesterolemia, familial	LDL receptor	Liver; vascular, endothelial; smooth muscle cells
Phenylketonuria	Phenylalanine hydroxylase	Liver

Complex Traits	Genetic Approach	Target Organs/Tissues
Cancer	Cytokine, HLA genes, thymidine kinase, p53 lytic	Various
HIV-1	Antisense constructs, immunoenhancers	Immune system

HIV=human immunodeficiency virus; HLA=human leukocyte antigen; LDL=low-density lipoprotein.

2. *Replacement of tumor suppressor genes.* Administration of genes known to be inactivated in tumors, and at least in part responsible for cellular transformation, can be added to the tumors to revert the cells to a nonmalignant phenotype. It is difficult to envision how this type of approach will be curative because it is unlikely that any vector can truly transduce 100% of malignant cells.

3. *Gene induced toxicity.* The transfer of toxic genes directly to the tumor or neighboring cells is another approach. Transfer of a gene into surrounding tissues that affect tumor vascularization may be effective. Direct targeting of tumor cells with toxic genes or genes that allow prodrug activation into a toxin have been considered. The best example is the thymidine kinase gene (derived from herpes simplex virus), which converts ganciclovir into a DNA analog that interrupts cellular DNA replication resulting in cell death.

4. *Replication lytic viruses.* Some lytic viruses have been engineered to selectively replicate in tumor cells, allowing them to propagate and kill the infected cells.

The demonstration of clinical efficacy as measured by survival has been hampered because most of the clinical trials have been performed in advanced stages of malignancy when all other medical interventions have failed. Gene transfer in the early stages of tumorigenesis greatly enhances the probability of ablation of the tumor. At some point, clinical trials will have to be performed in early onset disease when the therapy has the best chance of being clinically efficacious.

The first effective gene therapy trial was for X-linked SCID due to a deficiency in the interleukin-2 receptor gamma chain gene. These patients have essentially no antigen-specific immunity because of the loss of T cells. Bone marrow–derived cells, which contained a population of "stem" or self-renewing progenitor cells, were removed and transduced with a retroviral vector that expressed the missing protein. Genetically reconstituted cells have a selective advantage and can repopulate the missing T cells. Interestingly, this selective repopulation was sufficient to restore immune function in treated individuals. One patient developed a T cell leukemia like tumor. Insertional mutagenesis is a possible but unproven etiology. Similar positive results were noted when bone marrow or cord blood stem cells were transduced to treat SCID due to adenosine deaminase deficiency. Fanconi anemia is another disease in which a selective advantage has been postulated and a low level of gene transfer may be therapeutic. However, there are at least eight different genes that can cause this disease, requiring a different vector for each. Although bone marrow–derived gene transfer offers hope in treating many diseases, in disorders in which no selective advantage is conferred, higher efficiency gene transfer into stem cells will be required. The rate-limiting step for gene transfer into these cells has not been definitively established.

Gene therapy trials are ongoing for a number of other diseases (see Table 71–2). Gene therapy for cystic fibrosis is complicated by the uncertainty of which cell type is the most critical for gene replacement, the number of cells that need to be genetically modified for clinical efficacy, and the longevity of gene correction in target cells. There are a number of clinical end-points that are possible to measure but the most relevant for establishing success is unclear. Moreover, the lung has evolved efficient barriers to keep viruses out of respiratory epithelium, making it a tough barrier to penetrate. Even though all of the clinical trials have been related to gene addition strategies, because a single mutation (ΔF508) makes up 75% of the mutant alleles, gene correction strategies are viable alternatives.

Hemophilia has been an attractive disease for developing gene transfer strategies. Unlike for cystic fibrosis, the clinical end-points are clear; reconstitution of the plasma with at least 1% of the normal level of coagulation factor VIII or IX in hemophilia A and B, respectively, can convert an individual with severe disease to a much milder phenotype. Even though factor IX is exclusively and factor VIII is primarily made in the liver, not all of the gene therapy attempts for treatment involve the reconstitution of factor production in the liver. Many different approaches include intravenous and/or intramuscular infusions of recombinant retroviral, adenoviral, or adeno-associated viral vectors, ex vivo transplantation of genetically modified fibroblasts, implantation of biochambers containing genetically modified cells, and genetic modification of various endothelial or stem cells.

Vectors derived from adenovirus and adenovirus-associated virus (AAV) are efficient at transferring genes into cells within the central nervous system and skeletal muscle. There is a great interest in attempting to treat neuromuscular and neurodegenerative diseases. Generalized neurodegenerative disorders, especially those that are prenatal in onset are not likely to be treatable with gene therapy in the near future. In contrast, canine models of retinitis pigmentosa have recently been treated.

Expression of a foreign protein from a gene transfer vector can result in a robust humoral or cellular immune response, suggesting that gene transfer can be used in vaccine development. The concept is to express small amounts of the foreign antigen and/or cytokines from antigen presenting cells, resulting in a more robust immune response than for protein-based vaccines. Because transient as well as small amounts of protein synthesis are required in vaccine development, nonviral DNA plasmids have been used for this purpose in early clinical trials. The hope is that this therapy can be developed for current protein vaccines that are not very immunogenic.

Gene transfer approaches for treating acquired infections are being tested. The goal is to interfere with the viral life cycle at different stages of infection, replication, and/or viral assembly. Expression of antiviral proteins (e.g., cytokines, interferon) or protein decoys that interfere with viral proteins critical for viral replication are two current strategies. Therapeutic nucleotides that do not encode proteins but interfere with the viral life cycle also show promise. Molecules known as ribozymes, DNAzymes and antisense and small interfering RNAs are short stretches of nucleotides, which can be delivered directly or expressed from gene transfer vectors. In laboratory studies, these approaches have been shown to either inhibit viral protein synthesis and/or enhance the degradation of the pathogenic viral genome.

Gene transfer strategies for the treatment of juvenile diabetes resulting from autoimmune destruction of beta cells require additional approaches because the target cells are destroyed during the pathogenesis of the disorder. Strategies for therapy include introducing genes into the pancreas or liver progenitor cells that can differentiate into insulin-producing beta cells, or transfecting the insulin gene into hepatocytes containing a glucose-responsive element that regulates gene transcription.

Balicki D, Beutler E: Gene therapy of human disease. *Medicine* 2002;81:69–86.

Baumgartner I, Isner JM: Somatic gene therapy in the cardiovascular system. *Annu Rev Physiol* 2001;63:427–50.

Escolar DM, Scacheri CG: Pharmacologic and genetic therapy for childhood muscular dystrophies. *Curr Neurol Neurosci Rep* 2001;1:168–74.

Ferry N, Heard JM: Liver-directed gene transfer vectors. *Human Gene Ther* 1998;9:1975–81.

Fischer A: Gene therapy of lymphoid primary immunodeficiencies. *Curr Opin Pediatr* 2000;12:557–62.

High KA: Gene transfer as an approach to treating hemophilia. *Circ Res* 2001;88:137.

Kay MA, Glorioso JC, Naldini L: Viral vectors for gene therapy: The art of turning infectious agents into vehicles of therapeutics. *Nat Med* 2001;7:33–40.

Kozarsky KF: Gene therapy for cardiovascular disease. *Curr Opin Pharmacol* 2001;1:197–202.

Kruyt FA, Curiel DT: Toward a new generation of conditionally replicating adenoviruses: Pairing tumor selectivity with maximal oncolysis. *Hum Gene Ther* 2002;13:485–95.

Liu F, Huang L: Development of non-viral vectors for systemic gene delivery. *J Control Release* 2002l8:259–66.

McCormick F: Cancer gene therapy: Fringe or cutting edge? *Nature Rev Cancer* 2001;1:130–41.

Nabel GJ: Immune recognition of malignancies: Relevance to immunotherapy. *Cancer J Sci Am* 1998;4:106–11.

O'Brien KF, Kunkel LM: Dystrophin and muscular dystrophy: Past, present, and future. *Mol Genet Metab* 2001;74:75–88.

Richardson PD, Kren BT, Steer CJ: Gene repair in the new age of gene therapy. *Hepatology* 2002;35:512–18.

Russell DW, Kay MA: Adeno-associated virus vectors and hematology. *Blood* 1999;94:864–74.

Schmidt-Wolf GD, Schmidt-Wolf IG: Immunomodulatory gene therapy for haematological malignancies. *Br J Haematol* 2002;117:23–32.

Yoon JW, Jun HS: Recent advances in insulin gene therapy for type 1 diabetes. *Trends Mol Med* 2002;8:62–68.

Chapter 72
Genetic Counseling *Judith G. Hall*

When a child is born with multiple congenital anomalies or a family is diagnosed with a genetic disorder, talking with the family is not easy. Giving bad news is always difficult, and the information is often somewhat technical. However, it is important to provide the family with as much information as possible so that they can make informed decisions. Genetic counseling has been defined as an educational process that seeks to assist affected and/or at risk individuals to understand the nature of a genetic disorder, its transmission, and the options available to them in management and family planning. There are many indications for genetic counseling. (Box 72–1).

Although the task of providing information about genetic diseases is often done by a team of highly trained medical geneticists and genetic counselors, the information may also be provided by an experienced family physician, pediatrician, or nurse. Genetic counseling must be done based on an under-

---

BOX 72–1. Indications for Genetic Counseling

Advanced parental age
  Maternal age >35 yr
  Paternal age >50 yr
Child with congenital anomalies or dysmorphology
Consanguinity or incest
Family history of heritable disorders or diseases, including:
  Adult onset
  Complex/multifactorial inheritance
  Chromosomal abnormality
  Single gene disorders
Heterozygote screening based on ethnicity, including:
  Sickle cell anemia (West African, Mediterranean, Arab, Indo-Pakistani, Turkish, Southeast Asian)
  Tay-Sachs, Canavan (Ashkenazi-Jewish, French-Canadian)
  Thalassemias (Mediterranean, Arab, Indo-Pakistani)
Pregnancy screening abnormality, including:
  Maternal serum α-fetoprotein
  Maternal serum triple screen
  Prenatal ultrasound examination
Stillborn with congenital anomalies
Teratogen exposure or risk

---

standing of genetic principles, the ability to recognize and diagnose genetic diseases and rare syndromes, and knowledge of the natural history of the disorder and its recurrence risk. Awareness of prenatal diagnosis and screening programs available in a particular region and access to information about advances in genetic disorders and medical techniques are also necessary.

With the sequencing of the human genome, most people think it should be possible to identify the genes responsible for an inherited disorder. However, only about 10% of known or described conditions have had the responsible gene identified. Furthermore, other genes and the environment modify most gene expression so that a wide spectrum of effect can be expected. Developments in molecular genetics provide many options for modification of gene expression, use of alternative pathways, and application of therapeutic approaches once the specific disorder and responsible genes are identified.

TALKING TO FAMILIES

The type of information provided to a family depends on the urgency of the situation, the need to make decisions, and the need to collect additional information. However, there are three general situations in which genetic counseling becomes particularly important.

The first is the prenatal diagnosis of a congenital anomaly or genetic disease. This is a very difficult situation, and the need for information is urgent because a family must often decide whether to continue or to terminate a pregnancy. Risks to the mother must also be considered. The second type of situation occurs when a child is born with a life-threatening congenital anomaly or genetic disease. This also requires urgent information and decisions that must be made immediately with regard to how much support should be provided for the child and whether certain types of therapy should be attempted. The third situation arises later in life when (1) a diagnosis with a genetic implication is made, (2) a couple is planning a family and there is a family history of a genetic problem, including whether one member of a couple carries a translocation or is a carrier of an abnormal gene for an autosomal recessive or X-linked disorder, (3) an adolescent or young adult has a family history of an adult-onset genetic disorder (e.g., Huntington disease or breast cancer), (4) unusual features are present and a diagnosis is wanting or not possible, or (5) there is suspected exposure to a toxic substance or teratogen. It is often necessary to have several meetings with a family in this third category. Urgency is not as much of an issue as being sure that they have as much information and as many options as are available. All of the questions and concerns usually cannot be adequately addressed in one session.

GENETIC COUNSELING

Providing accurate information to families requires (1) taking a careful family history and constructing a pedigree that lists the patient's relatives (including abortions, stillbirths, and deceased individuals) with their sex, age, and state of health up to and including third-degree relatives; (2) gathering information from hospital records about the affected individual (and in some cases, about other family members); (3) documenting prenatal, pregnancy, and delivery histories; (4) reviewing the latest available medical, laboratory, and genetic information concerning the disorder; (5) careful physical examination of the affected individual (with photographs and measurements) and of apparently unaffected individuals in the family; (6) establishing or confirming the diagnosis by the diagnostic tests available; (7) giving the family information about support groups; (8) providing new information to the family as it becomes available (a mechanism for updating needs to be established).

To provide optimal benefits, the counseling session must include certain information:

The Specific Condition or Conditions. If a specific diagnosis is made and confirmed, that should be discussed with the family and information provided in writing. However, often the disorder fits into a spectrum (e.g., 1 of 300 types of arthrogryposis) or the diagnosis is clinically rather than laboratory based. In those situations, the family needs to understand the limits of present knowledge and that additional research will probably lead to better information in the future.

Knowledge of the Diagnosis of the Particular Condition. Although it is not always possible to make an exact diagnosis, having as accurate a diagnosis as possible is important. Estimates of recurrence risk for various family members depend on an accurate diagnosis. When a specific diagnosis cannot be made (as in many cases of multiple congenital anomalies), the various differential diagnoses should be discussed with the family and empirical information provided. If specific diagnostic tests are available, they should be discussed.

Natural History of the Condition. It is very important to discuss the natural history of the specific genetic disorder in the family. Affected individuals and their families will have questions regarding the prognosis and potential therapy that can be answered only with knowledge of the natural history. If there are other possible differential diagnoses, their natural history may also be discussed. If the disorder is associated with a spectrum of clinical outcomes or complications, the worst and best scenario, as well as treatment and referral to the appropriate specialist, should be addressed.

Genetic Aspects of the Condition and Recurrence Risk. This is important information for the family because all family members need to be aware of their reproductive choices. The genetics of the disorder can be explained with visual aids (e.g., figures of chromosomes). It is important to provide accurate occurrence and recurrence risks for various members of the family, including unaffected individuals, cousins, aunts, and so forth. In cases in which a definite diagnosis cannot be made, it is necessary to use empirical recurrence risks. Counseling should give the individuals the necessary information to understand the various options and to make their own informed decisions regarding pregnancies, adoption, artificial insemination, prenatal diagnosis, screening, carrier detection, and termination of pregnancy. To complete this part of the educational process, it may be necessary to have more than one counseling session.

Prenatal Diagnosis and Prevention. Many different methods of prenatal diagnosis are available, depending on the specific genetic disorder. The use of ultrasonography allows prenatal diagnosis of anatomic abnormalities such as congenital heart defects. Amniocentesis and chorionic villus sampling are used to obtain fetal tissue for analysis of chromosomal abnormalities, biochemical disorders, and DNA studies. Maternal blood or serum sampling is used for some types of screening. Fetal cells can be retrieved from the umbilical cord or from maternal blood for testing, although mothers may harbor cells from all previous pregnancies.

Therapies and Referral. A number of genetic disorders require the care of a specialist. For example, individuals with Turner syndrome usually need to be evaluated by an endocrinologist. Prevention of known complications is a priority. The psychologic adjustment of the family may require specific intervention.

Support Groups. A large number of community lay support groups have been formed to provide information and to fund research on specific genetic and nongenetic conditions. An important part of genetic counseling is to give information about these groups to individuals and to suggest a contact person for the families. Many groups have established websites with very helpful information.

Follow-up. Families should be encouraged to continue to ask questions and keep up with new information about the specific disorder. New developments often influence the diagnosis and therapy of specific genetic disorders. Lay support groups are a good source of new information.

Nondirective Counseling. In general, genetic counseling is nondirective. In most developed countries with modern health systems, choices about reproduction are left to the family to decide what is right for them. The role of the counselor (physician, genetic counselor, nurse, medical geneticist) is to provide information in understandable terms and outline the range of options available.

Alliance of Genetic Support Groups: Directory of National Genetic Voluntary Organizations, 35 Wisconsin Circle, Suite 440, Chevy Chase, Maryland 20815-7015.

Bartels DM, LeRoy BS, McCarthy P, et al: Nondirectiveness in genetic counseling: A survey of practitioners. *Am J Med Genet* 1997;72:172–9.

Bowles-Biesecker B, Marteau TM: The future of genetic counseling: An international perspective. *Nat Genet* 1999;22:133–7.

Farrell MH, Certain LK, Farrell PM: Genetic counseling and risk communication services of newborn screening programs. *Arch Pediatr Adolesc Med* 2001;155: 120–6.

Fryer AE: Clinical genetic services: Activity, outcome, effectiveness and quality. Summary of a report of the Clinical Genetics Committee of the Royal College of Physicians. *J Roy Coll Phys Lond* 1997;31:624–7.

Geneclinics: *geneclinics@geneclinics.org*.

Hayflick SJ, Eiff, MP, Carpenter L, et al: Primary care physicians' utilization and perceptions of genetics services. *Genet Med* 1998;1:13–21.

Holtzman NA, Watson MS: Promoting safe and effective genetic testing in the United States: Final report of the task force on genetic testing, Bethesda, Maryland: The Human Genome Research Institute, 1997.

Hubbard R, Lewontin RC: Pitfalls of genetic testing. *N Engl J Med* 1996;334:1192–4.

Press N, Browner CH: Characteristics of women who refuse an offer of prenatal diagnosis: Data from the California maternal serum alpha fetoprotein blood test experience. *Am J Med Genet* 1998;78:433–45.

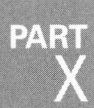

Metabolic Diseases

Chapter 73

An Approach to Inborn Errors of Metabolism *Iraj Rezvani*

Many childhood conditions are caused by gene mutations that encode specific proteins. These mutations can result in the alteration of primary protein structure or the amount of protein synthesized. The functional ability of protein, whether it is an enzyme, receptor, transport vehicle, membrane, or structural element, may be relatively or seriously compromised. These hereditary biochemical disorders are collectively termed *inborn errors of metabolism*.

Most mutations are clinically inconsequential and represent polymorphic differences that set individuals apart *(genetic polymorphism)*. However, some mutations produce disease states that range from very mild to lethal. Most inborn errors of metabolism exhibiting clinical consequences manifest in the newborn period or shortly thereafter.

It is both technologically and economically possible to screen for a large number of metabolic conditions during the first few days of life, before any clinical manifestations of the disease become apparent. Institution of early treatment often prevents the deleterious effects of these conditions, especially on the central nervous system. Intrauterine diagnosis of most genetic conditions is now feasible and is routinely used to detect affected fetuses in the population at risk (see Chapter 85).

Children with inborn errors of metabolism may present with one or more of a large variety of signs and symptoms. These may include high or normal anion gap metabolic acidosis, persistent vomiting, failure to thrive, altered consciousness, seizures, myopathy, developmental delay, hypoglycemia, elevated blood or urinary levels of a particular metabolite (an amino acid, organic acid, or ammonia), a peculiar odor (Table 73–1), or physical changes such as dysmorphology, cardiomegaly, rashes, cataracts, retinitis, optic atrophy, corneal opacity, deafness, skeletal dysplasias, macrocephaly, or hepatomegaly with or without hepatic failure, jaundice, or cirrhosis. Diagnosis is facilitated by considering those disorders presenting in the neonatal period separately from those presenting later in life.

Neonatal Period. Inborn errors of metabolism causing *clinical manifestations* in the neonatal period are usually severe and are often lethal if proper therapy is not promptly initiated. Clinical findings are usually nonspecific and similar to those seen in infants with sepsis. An inborn error of metabolism should be considered in the differential diagnosis of a severely ill neonatal infant, and special studies should be undertaken if the index of suspicion is high (Fig. 73–1).

Infants with metabolic disorders are usually normal at birth; however, signs and symptoms such as lethargy, poor feeding, convulsions, and vomiting may develop as early as a few hours after birth. A history of clinical deterioration in a previously normal neonate should suggest an inborn error of metabolism. This clinical course contrasts to many other genetic disorders or perinatal insults, which cause abnormalities from the time of birth. Occasionally (urea cycle defects, organic acidurias, fatty acid oxidation disorders), vomiting may be severe enough to suggest

the diagnosis of pyloric stenosis, which is usually not present, although it has simultaneously occurred in such infants. Lethargy, poor feeding, convulsions, and coma may also be seen in infants with hypoglycemia (see Chapters 81 and 96) or hypocalcemia (see Chapter 45.5). Measurements of blood concentrations of glucose and calcium and response to intravenous injection of glucose or calcium usually establish these diagnoses. Because most inborn errors of metabolism are inherited as autosomal recessive traits, a history of consanguinity and/or death in the neonatal period should increase suspicion of this diagnosis. Some of these disorders have a high incidence in specific population groups. For instance, tyrosinemia type 1 is more common among French Canadians of Quebec than in the general population. Therefore, knowledge of the ethnic background of the patient may be helpful in diagnosis. *Physical examination* usually reveals nonspecific findings, with most signs related to the central nervous system. Hepatomegaly, however, is a common finding in a variety of inborn errors of metabolism. Occasionally, an unusual odor may offer an invaluable aid to the diagnosis (see Table 73–1). A physician caring for a sick infant should smell the patient and his or her excretions; for example, patients with maple syrup urine disease have the unmistakable odor of maple syrup in their urine and on their bodies.

Diagnosis usually requires a variety of specific *laboratory studies*. Measurements of serum concentrations of glucose, ammonia, bicarbonate, and pH are often very helpful in differentiating major causes of metabolic disorders (see Fig. 73–1). Elevation of blood ammonia levels is usually caused by defects in urea cycle enzymes. Infants with elevated blood ammonia levels commonly have normal serum pH and bicarbonate values; without measurement of blood ammonia they may remain undiagnosed and succumb to their disease. Elevation of serum ammonia levels, however, has also been observed in some infants with certain organic acidemias. These infants are severely acidotic because of accumulation of organic acids in body fluids.

When blood ammonia, pH, and bicarbonate values are normal, other aminoacidopathies (e.g., hyperglycinemia) or galactosemia should be considered; galactosemic infants may also manifest hypoglycemia, cataracts, hepatomegaly, ascites, and jaundice.

Most inborn errors of metabolism presenting in the neonatal period are lethal if specific *treatment* is not initiated immediately. Specific diagnosis, even in an infant in whom death seems inevitable, is of great importance for genetic counseling of the family (see Chapter 72). Therefore, every effort should be made

TABLE 73–1. Inborn Errors of Amino Acid Metabolism Associated with Abnormal Odor

Inborn Error of Metabolism	Urine Odor
Glutaric acidemia (type II)	Sweaty feet, acrid
Hawkinsinuria	Swimming pool
Isovaleric acidemia	Sweaty feet, acrid
Maple syrup urine disease	Maple syrup
Hypermethioninemia	Boiled cabbage
Multiple carboxylase deficiency	Tomcat urine
Oasthouse urine disease	Hops-like
Phenylketonuria	Mousy or musty
Trimethylaminuria	Rotting fish
Tyrosinemia	Boiled cabbage, rancid butter

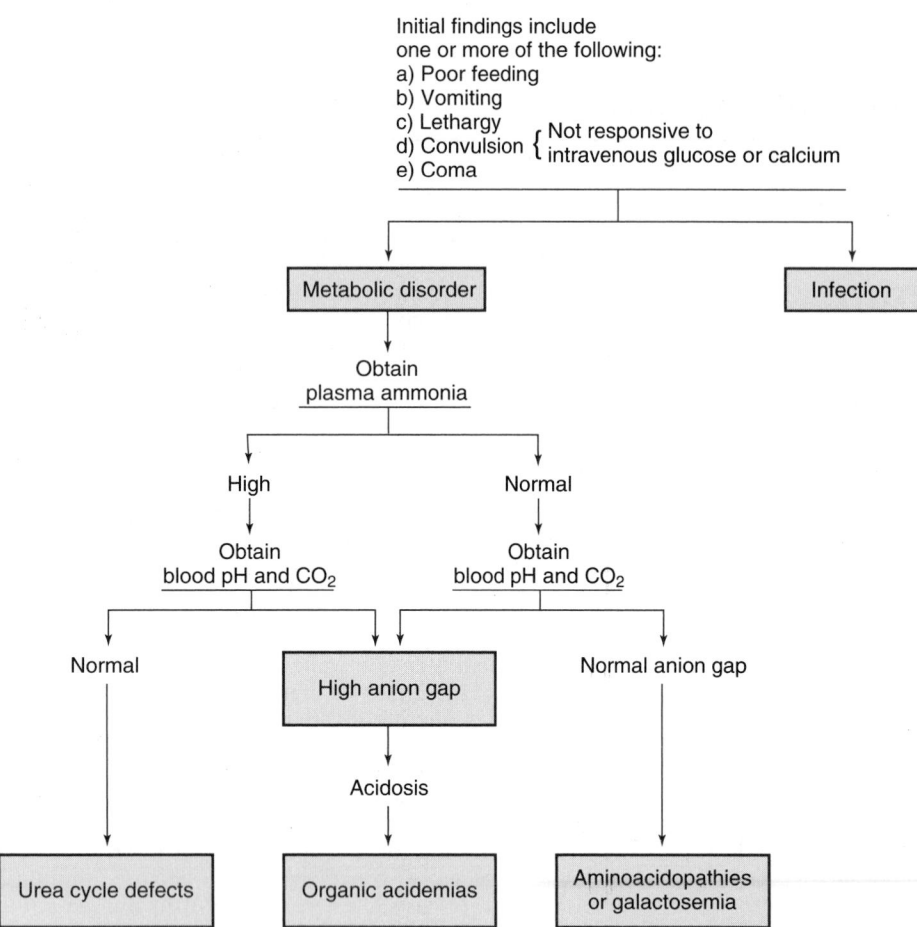

Initial findings include one or more of the following:
a) Poor feeding
b) Vomiting
c) Lethargy
d) Convulsion { Not responsive to intravenous glucose or calcium
e) Coma

Metabolic disorder → Infection

Obtain plasma ammonia

High / Normal

Obtain blood pH and CO_2 / Obtain blood pH and CO_2

Normal / High anion gap / Normal anion gap

Acidosis

Urea cycle defects / Organic acidemias / Aminoacidopathies or galactosemia

FIGURE 73–1. Clinical approach to a newborn infant with a suspected metabolic disorder. This schema is a guide to the elucidation of some of the metabolic disorders in newborn infants. Although some exceptions to this schema exist, it is appropriate for most cases.

to determine the diagnosis while the infant is alive; postmortem examination is usually not helpful. A specific diagnosis is facilitated by direct biochemical assays of metabolites or their metabolic by-products, or of an enzyme's function; by DNA analysis of the gene; by functional tests; by neuroradiology; and with biopsies or postmortem examinations. With tandem mass spectroscopy use in neonatal metabolic screening programs, many disorders are identified in the presymptomatic stage.

Children after the Neonatal Period. Most inborn errors of metabolism that cause symptoms in the first few days of life exhibit milder variant forms that have a more insidious onset. These forms may escape detection during the neonatal period, and the diagnosis may be delayed for months or even years. Early clinical manifestations in children with these forms are commonly nonspecific and may be attributed to unidentified perinatal insults.

Clinical manifestations, such as mental retardation, motor deficits, developmental regression, convulsions, myopathy, recurrent emesis with coma and hepatic dysfunction, and cardiomyopathy are the most constant findings in older children. There may be an episodic or intermittent pattern, with episodes of acute clinical manifestations separated by periods of seemingly disease-free states. The episodes are usually triggered by stress or a nonspecific catabolic insult, such as an infection. The child may die during one of these acute attacks. An inborn error of metabolism should be considered in any child with one or more of the following manifestations: (1) unexplained mental retardation, developmental delay or regression, motor deficits, or convulsions; (2) unusual odor, particularly during an acute illness; (3) intermittent episodes of unexplained vomiting, acidosis, mental deterioration, or coma; (4) hepatomegaly; (5) renal stones; or (6) muscle weakness or cardiomyopathy.

Chapter 74
Defects in Metabolism of Amino Acids

74.1 Phenylalanine

Iraj Rezvani

Phenylalanine is an essential amino acid. Dietary phenylalanine not utilized for protein synthesis is normally degraded by way of the tyrosine pathway (Fig. 74–1). Deficiency of the enzyme phenylalanine hydroxylase or of its cofactor tetrahydrobiopterin causes accumulation of phenylalanine in body fluids and the central nervous system (CNS). The severity of hyperphenylalaninemia depends on the degree of enzyme deficiency and may vary from very high plasma concentrations (>20 mg/dL, or >1200 μM, "classic PKU") to mildly elevated levels (2–6 mg/dL or 120–360 μM). In affected infants with plasma concentrations over 20 mg/dL, excess phenylalanine is metabolized to phenylketones (phenylpyruvate and phenylacetate; see Fig. 74–1) that are excreted in the urine, giving rise to the term *phenylketonuria (PKU)*. These metabolites have no role in pathogenesis of CNS damage in patients with PKU, and their presence in body fluids simply signifies the severity of the condition. The brain is the main organ affected by hyperphenylalaninemia. The CNS damage in affected patients is caused by the elevated concentration of phenylalanine in brain tissue, which interferes with the transport of other

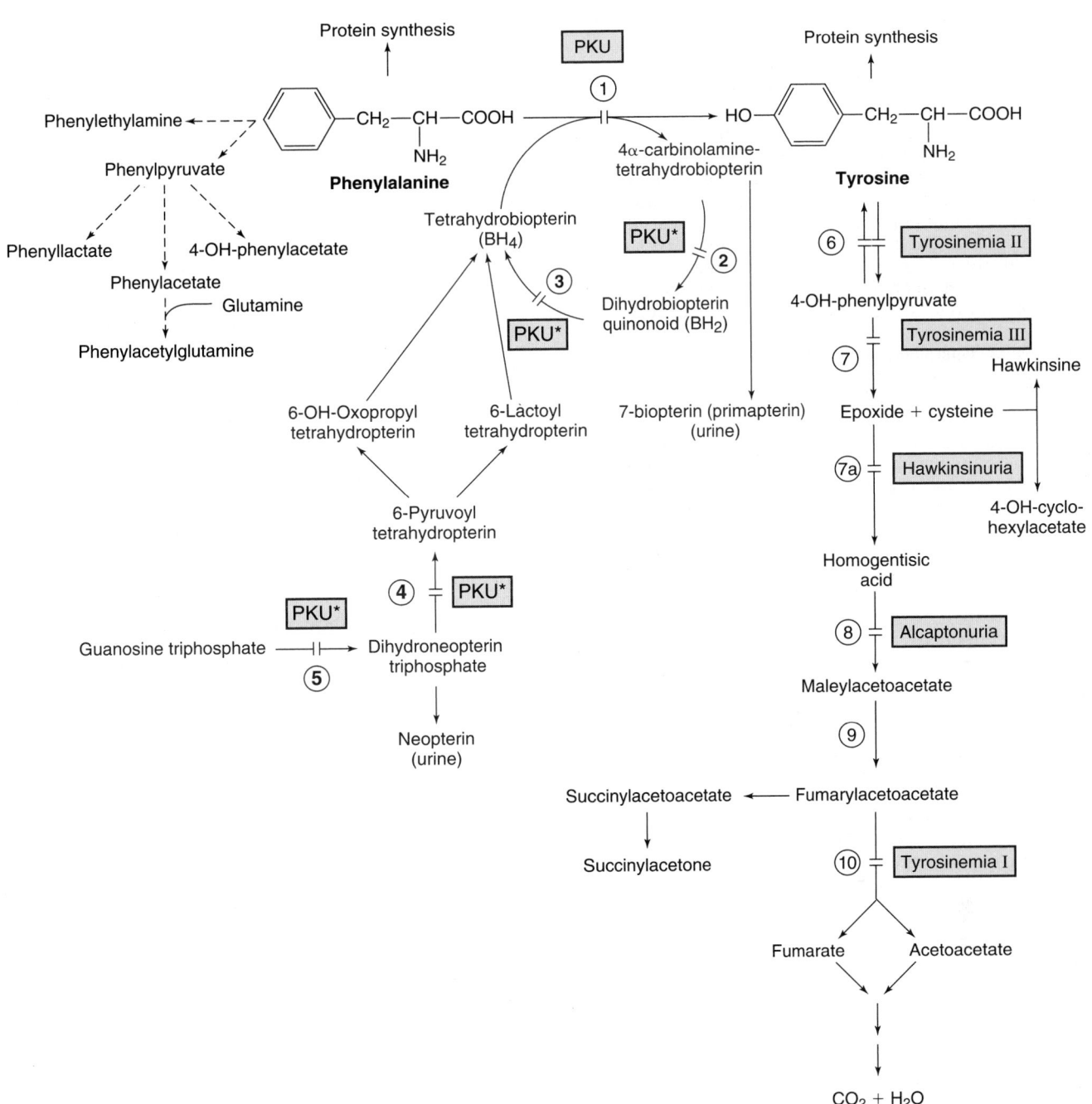

FIGURE 74–1. Pathways of phenylalanine and tyrosine metabolism. Inborn errors are depicted as bars crossing the reaction arrow(s). Pathways for synthesis of cofactor BH_4 are shown in purple. PKU* refers to defects of BH4 metabolism that affect the phenylalanine, tyrosine, and tryptophan hydroxylases. See Figures 74–2 and 74–4. **Enzymes:** (1) phenylalanine hydroxylase; (2) carbinolamine dehydratase; (3) dihydropteridine reductase; (4) 6-pyruvoyltetrahydropterin synthase; (5) guanosine triphosphate (GTP) cyclohydrolase; (6) tyrosine aminotransferase; (7a) intramolecular rearrangement; (7 + 7a) 4-hydroxyphenylpyruvate dioxygenase; (8) Homogentisic acid dioxygenase; (9) maleylacetoacetate isomerase; (10) fumarylacetoacetate hydroxylase.

large neutral amino acids (tyrosine, tryptophan) into the brain. There are a few adults with classic PKU and normal intelligence who have never been treated with a phenylalanine-restricted diet. Phenylalanine content of the brain in these individuals was found to be close to that of normal subjects when studied by magnetic resonance spectroscopy (MRS) and imaging (MRI) techniques.

Classic PKU. Severe hyperphenylalaninemia (plasma phenylalanine levels > 20 mg/dL), if untreated, invariably results in the

development of signs and symptoms of classic PKU, except in rare occasions.

CLINICAL MANIFESTATIONS. The affected infant is normal at birth. Mental retardation may develop gradually and may not be evident for the first few months. It is usually severe, and most patients require institutional care if the condition remains untreated. Vomiting, sometimes severe enough to be misdiagnosed as pyloric stenosis, may be an early symptom. Older untreated children become hyperactive with purposeless movements, rhythmic rocking, and athetosis.

On physical examination these infants are lighter in their complexion than unaffected siblings. Some may have a seborrheic or eczematoid rash, which is usually mild and disappears as the child grows older. These children have an unpleasant odor of phenylacetic acid, which has been described as musty or mousy. There are no consistent findings on neurologic examination. However, most infants are hypertonic with hyperactive deep tendon reflexes. About 25% of children have seizures, and more than 50% have electroencephalographic abnormalities. Microcephaly, prominent maxilla with widely spaced teeth, enamel hypoplasia, and growth retardation are other common findings in untreated children. The clinical manifestations of classic PKU are rarely seen in those countries in which neonatal screening programs for the detection of PKU are in effect.

Milder Forms of Hyperphenylalaninemia, Non-PKU Hyperphenylalaninemias. In any screening program for PKU, a group of infants are identified in whom initial plasma concentrations of phenylalanine are above normal (2 mg/dL, 120 µM) but less than 20 mg/dL (1200 µM). These infants do not excrete phenylketones. Clinically, these infants may remain asymptomatic but progressive brain damage may occur gradually with age. These patients have milder deficiencies of phenylalanine hydroxylase or its cofactor tetrahydrobiopterin (BH$_4$) than those with classic PKU. Attempts have been made to classify these patients in different subgroups depending on the degree of hyperphenylalaninemia, but such a practice seems to have very little clinical or therapeutic advantage. As with classic PKU, deficiency of BH$_4$ should be investigated in all infants with milder forms of hyperphenylalaninemia (see later).

DIAGNOSIS. Because of gradual development of clinical manifestations of hyperphenylalaninemia, early diagnosis can only be achieved by mass screening of all newborn infants (see later). In infants with positive results from the screen for hyperphenylalaninemia, diagnosis should be confirmed by quantitative measurement of plasma phenylalanine. Identification and measurement of phenylketones in the urine has no place in any screening program. However, in countries and places where such programs are not in effect, identification of phenylketones in the urine by ferric chloride may offer a simple test for diagnosis of infants with developmental and neurologic abnormalities. Once the diagnosis of hyperphenylalaninemia is established, deficiency of cofactor (BH$_4$) should be ruled out in all affected infants with proper studies (see later).

NEONATAL SCREENING FOR HYPERPHENYLALANINE-MIA. Effective and relatively inexpensive methods for mass screening of newborn infants have been developed and are being used in the United States and several other countries. The bacterial inhibition assay of Guthrie, which was the first and still the most widely used method for the purpose, is being replaced by more precise and quantitative methods (fluorometric and tandem mass spectrometry). All these methods require a few drops of blood, which are placed on a filter paper and mailed to a central laboratory for assay. Blood phenylalanine in affected infants with PKU may rise to diagnostic levels as early as 4 hr after birth even in the absence of protein feeding. It is recommended, however, that the blood for screening be obtained in the first 24–48 hr of life after feeding protein to reduce the possibility of false-negative results, especially in the milder forms of the condition.

TREATMENT. The goal of therapy is to reduce phenylalanine in the body; formulas low in or free of this amino acid are commercially available. The diet should be started as soon as diagnosis is established. It is generally accepted that infants with persistent plasma levels of phenylalanine over 6 mg/dL (360 µM) should be treated with a phenylalanine-restricted diet similar to that for classic PKU. No dietary restriction is currently recommended for infants whose phenylalanine levels are between 2–6 mg/dL. Plasma concentrations of phenylalanine in treated patients should be maintained as close to normal as possible. Because phenylalanine is not synthesized by the body, "overtreatment" may lead to phenylalanine deficiency manifested by lethargy, failure to thrive, anorexia, anemia, rashes, diarrhea, and even death; moreover, tyrosine becomes an essential amino acid in this disorder and its adequate intake must be ensured. Controversies exist regarding the "allowable" degree of residual hyperphenylalaninemia in treated patients. It is generally believed that plasma phenylalanine levels should be maintained between 2–6 mg/dL (120–360 µM) at least in the first 12 yr of life. The duration of diet therapy is also controversial. Discontinuation of therapy, even in adulthood, may cause deterioration of IQ and cognitive performance. The current recommendation is that all patients be kept on a phenylalanine-restricted diet for life.

Oral administration of the cofactor (BH$_4$) to patients with milder forms of hyperphenylalaninemia from phenylalanine hydroxylase deficiency may produce significant reductions in plasma phenylalanine levels. These children may be able to tolerate a less restricted diet (see later for BH$_4$ therapy). Dietary management of hyperphenylalaninemia requires close monitoring of blood levels of phenylalanine, expert nutritional input, and well-designed educational materials for the patient and the family. Proper management of these patients is best achieved through a regional treatment center.

PREGNANCY IN WOMEN WITH HYPERPHENYLALA-NINEMIA (MATERNAL PKU). Pregnant women with hyperphenylalaninemia who are not receiving a phenylalanine-restricted diet carry a very high risk of having offspring with mental retardation, microcephaly, and congenital heart disease. These complications are related to high levels of maternal plasma phenylalanine during pregnancy. Prospective mothers who have been treated for hyperphenylalaninemia should be maintained on a phenylalanine-restricted diet before and during pregnancy, and every effort should be made to keep blood phenylalanine levels below 6 mg/dL (360 µM) throughout the pregnancy. All women with hyperphenylalaninemia who are of childbearing age should be counseled properly as to the risk of the just described congenital anomalies in their offspring.

Hyperphenylalaninemia from Deficiency of the Cofactor Tetrahydrobiopterin (BH$_4$). In 1–2% of infants with hyperphenylalaninemia, the defect resides in one of the enzymes necessary for production or recycling of the cofactor BH$_4$ (Fig. 74–2). These infants are diagnosed as having PKU, but they deteriorate neurologically despite adequate control of plasma phenylalanine. BH$_4$ is the cofactor for phenylalanine, tyrosine, and tryptophan hydroxylases. The latter two hydroxylases are essential for biosynthesis of the neurotransmitters dopamine (see Fig. 74–2) and serotonin (see Fig. 74–5). BH$_4$ is also a cofactor for nitric oxide synthase, which catalyzes the generation of nitric oxide from arginine. Currently, patients with BH$_4$ deficiency are diagnosed very early in life because all patients with PKU and hyperphenylalaninemia are tested for the possibility of this cofactor deficiency.

BH$_4$ is synthesized from guanosine triphosphate through several enzymatic reactions (see Fig. 74–1). Four enzyme deficiencies leading to defective BH$_4$ formation have been described. More than half of the reported patients have had a deficiency of 6-pyruvoyltetrahydropterin synthase (PTPS).

CLINICAL MANIFESTATIONS. Infants with cofactor deficiency are identified during screening programs for PKU because of evidence of hyperphenylalaninemia. Plasma phenylalanine levels may be as high as those in classic PKU or in the range of milder forms of hyperphenylalaninemia. Neurologic manifestations, such as loss of head control, truncal hypotonia (floppy baby), drooling, swallowing difficulties, and myoclonic seizures, develop after 3 mo of age despite adequate dietary therapy.

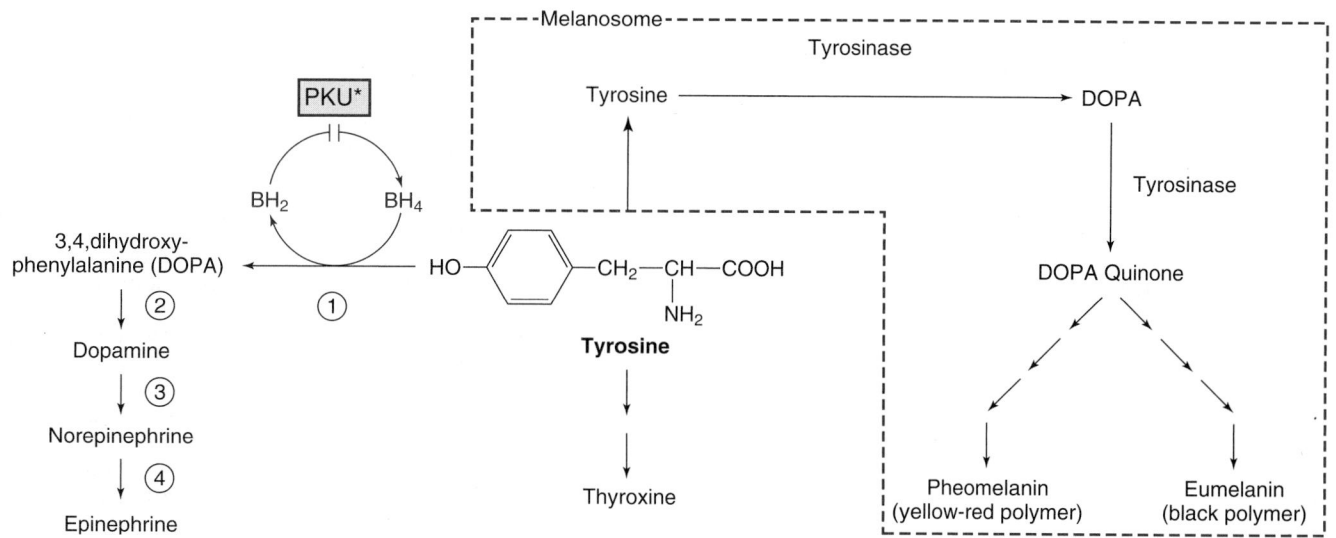

FIGURE 74–2. Other pathways involving tyrosine metabolism. PKU* indicates hyperphenylalaninemia due to tetrahydrobiopterin deficiency (see Fig. 74–1). **Enzymes:** (1) thyrosine hydroxylase; (2) aromatic L-amino acid decarboxylase (AADC); (3) dopamine hydroxylase; (4) phenylethanolamine-*N*-methyltransferase (PNMT).

DIAGNOSIS. BH_4 deficiency and the responsible enzyme defect may be diagnosed by performing any or all of the following tests:

1. Measurement of neopterin (oxidative product of dihydroneopterin triphosphate) and biopterin (oxidative product of dihydrobiopterin and tetrahydrobiopterin) in body fluids, especially urine (see Fig. 74–1). In patients with guanosine triphosphate (GTP) cyclohydrolase deficiency, urinary excretion of both neopterin and biopterin is very low. In patients with 6-pyruvoyltetrahydropterin synthase deficiency, there is a marked elevation of neopterin excretion and a concomitant decrease in biopterin excretion. In patients with dihydropteridine reductase deficiency, the neopterin excretion is normal but that of biopterin is very high. Excretion of biopterin increases in this enzyme deficiency because the quinonoid dihydrobiopterin cannot be recycled into BH_4. Patients with carbinolamine dehydratase deficiency excrete 7-biopterin (an unusual isomer of biopterin) in their urine.

2. BH_4 loading test. An oral dose of BH_4 (20 mg/kg) normalizes plasma phenylalanine in patients with BH_4 deficiency within 4–8 hr. The blood phenylalanine level should be elevated (>400 μM) to be able to interpret the results. This may be achieved by discontinuing diet therapy for 2 days before the test or by administering a loading dose of phenylalanine (100 mg/kg) 3 hr before the BH_4 test.

3. Enzyme assay. The activity of dihydropteridine reductase can be measured in the dry blood spots on the filter paper used for screening purposes. 6-Pyruvoyltetrahydropterin synthase activity can be measured in the liver, kidneys, and erythrocytes. Carbinolamine dehydratase activity can be measured in the liver and kidneys. GTP cyclohydrolase activity can be measured in the liver and in cytokine (interferon γ)-stimulated mononuclear cells or fibroblasts (the enzyme activity is normally very low in unstimulated cells).

TREATMENT. The goals of therapy are to correct hyperphenylalaninemia and to restore neurotransmitter deficiencies in the CNS.

1. The control of hyperphenylalaninemia is important in patients with cofactor deficiency, because high levels of phenylalanine interfere with the transport of neurotransmitter precursors (tyrosine and tryptophan) into the brain tissue. Plasma phenylalanine should be maintained as close to normal as possible (<6 mg/dL). This can be achieved by a combination of a low-phenylalanine diet and oral supplementation of BH_4. Infants with GTP cyclohydrolase or PTPS deficiencies respond more readily to BH_4 therapy (5–10 mg/kg/day) than those with dihydropteridine reductase deficiency. In the latter patients, doses as high as 20 mg/kg/day may be required. BH4 for replacement therapy is commercially available although it remains quite expensive.

2. Administration of deficient neurotransmitters, namely L-dopa and 5-hydroxytryptophan, is recommended even when treatment with BH_4 normalizes plasma levels of phenylalanine. BH_4 does not readily enter the brain tissue to restore local neurotransmitter production. Supplementation with folinic acid is also recommended in patients with dihydropteridine reductase deficiency.

Hyperprolactinemia occurs in patients with BH_4 deficiency and may be due to dopamine deficiency (which is the major prolactin-inhibiting factor) in the hypothalamic region. Measurement of serum prolactin levels may be a convenient method to monitor adequacy of neurotransmitter replacement in affected patients.

Some drugs such as trimethoprim sulfamethoxazole, methotrexate, and other antileukemic agents are known to inhibit dihydropteridine reductase enzyme activity and should be used with great caution in patients with BH_4 deficiency.

GENETICS AND PREVALENCE. All defects causing hyperphenylalaninemia are inherited as autosomal recessive traits. The prevalence of PKU in the United States is estimated at 1:14,000 to 1:20,000 live births. The prevalence of non-PKU hyperphenylalaninemia is estimated at 1:50,000. The condition is more common in whites and Native Americans and less prevalent in blacks, Hispanics, and Asians. The gene for phenylalanine hydroxylase is located on chromosome 12q22-q24.1, and over 400 different disease-causing mutations have been identified in different families. The majority of patients are compound heterozygotes for two different mutant alleles.

Genes for all enzymes involved in biosynthesis of BH_4 have been identified and, as with the phenylalanine hydroxylase gene, many mutations have been identified in different families. The gene for PTP synthase, the most common cause of BH_4 deficiency, resides on chromosome 11q22.3-22.3, the gene for dihydropteridine reductase is located on chromosome 4p15.3, and those of carbinolamine dehydratase and GTP cyclohydrolase are on 10q22 and 17q22.1-22.2, respectively. *Prenatal diagnosis* is possible using specific genetic probes in cells obtained from chorionic villi biopsy.

Tetrahydrobiopterin Defects without Hyperphenylalaninemia

HEREDITARY PROGRESSIVE DYSTONIA, AUTOSOMAL DOMINANT DOPA-RESPONSIVE DYSTONIA, SEGAWA SYNDROME (also see chapter 590.3). This rare form of dystonia, first described in Japan, has been shown to be caused by GTP cyclohydrolase deficiency. It is inherited as an autosomal dominant trait and is more common in females than males (4:1).

Clinical manifestations usually occur around 5–6 yr of age and are heralded by dystonia of the lower limbs, which may spread to all extremities within a few years. Torticollis, dystonia of the arms, and poor coordination may precede dystonia of the lower limbs in some patients. Early development is generally normal. The symptoms usually have an impressive diurnal variation, becoming worse by the end of the day and improving with sleep. Parkinsonian signs may also be present or develop subsequently with advancing age. Patients may be misdiagnosed as having cerebral palsy. Late presentation in adult life has also been reported.

Laboratory findings show no hyperphenylalaninemia, but reduced levels of BH$_4$ and neopterin are found in the spinal fluid. Dopamine and its metabolites (homovanillic acid) may also be reduced in the spinal fluid. It is believed that the enzyme deficiency in this condition is less severe than that of the autosomal recessive form of GTP cyclohydrolase deficiency, which is associated with hyperphenylalaninemia. The existence of asymptomatic carriers indicates that other factors or genes may play a role in pathogenesis of the phenotype.

Diagnosis may be confirmed by reduced levels of BH$_4$ and neopterin in the spinal fluid, by measurement of the enzyme activity (see earlier), and by identification of the gene defect. Clinically, the condition should be differentiated from other causes of dystonias and childhood parkinsonism, especially tyrosine hydroxylase (see Chapter 74.2) and aromatic amino acid decarboxylase deficiencies. The striking diurnal pattern of dystonia is an important clinical finding in favor of GTP cyclohydrolase deficiency.

Treatment with L-dopa in conjunction with a peripheral dopa decarboxylase inhibitor usually produces dramatic improvement.

74.2 Tyrosine

Iraj Rezvani

Tyrosine, obtained from ingested proteins and synthesized endogenously from phenylalanine, is used for protein synthesis and is a precursor of dopamine, norepinephrine, epinephrine, melanin, and thyroxine. Excess tyrosine is metabolized to carbon dioxide and water (see Fig. 74–1). Hypertyrosinemia is observed with deficiencies of tyrosine aminotransferase, 4-hydroxyphenpyruvate dioxygenase (4-HPPD), or fumarylacetoacetate hydrolase (FAH). The causal relationship of high levels of tyrosine with the diseased state has been established only in deficiency of tyrosine aminotransferase (tyrosinemia type II). The significance of hypertyrosinemia in the pathogenesis of the other two enzyme deficiencies is unclear.

Deficiencies of other enzymes involved in tyrosine degradation cause little or no increase in blood levels of tyrosine. *Acquired hypertyrosinemia* may occur in conditions such as severe hepatocellular dysfunction (liver failure), scurvy (vitamin C is the cofactor of 4-HPPD enzyme), and hyperthyroidism.

Tyrosinemia Type I (Tyrosinosis, Hereditary Tyrosinemia, Hepatorenal Tyrosinemia). In this condition, caused by a deficiency of the enzyme fumarylacetoacetate hydrolase, a moderate elevation of serum tyrosine is associated with severe involvement of the liver, kidneys, and central nervous system. These findings are thought to be due to accumulation of intermediate metabolites of tyrosine in the body, especially succinylacetone.

CLINICAL MANIFESTATIONS. The clinical description is based on patients of French-Canadian descent, who have a more severe form of the disease than other ethnic groups.

The affected infant may become symptomatic as early as 2 wk of age or may remain seemingly healthy during the first yr of life. The earlier the presentation, the poorer is the prognosis. The 1-yr mortality, which is about 60% in infants who develop symptoms before 2 mo of age, decreases to 4% in infants who become symptomatic after 6 mo of age.

The major organs affected are the liver, peripheral nerves, and kidneys. An acute *hepatic crisis* commonly heralds the onset of the disease and is usually precipitated by an intercurrent illness that produces a catabolic state. Fever, irritability, vomiting, hemorrhage (melena, hematemesis, hematuria), hepatomegaly, jaundice, elevated levels of serum transaminases, and hypoglycemia are common. An odor resembling boiled cabbage may be present and may be due to increased methionine metabolites. Most hepatic crises resolve spontaneously, but progression to liver failure and death may occur. Between the crises, varying degrees of failure to thrive, hepatomegaly, and coagulation abnormalities often persist. Cirrhosis of the liver and eventually hepatocellular carcinoma occur in children who survive beyond 2 yr. The incidence of hepatic carcinoma may be as high as 37%.

Episodes of acute *peripheral neuropathy* resembling acute porphyria occur in about 40% of affected children. These crises, often triggered by a minor infection, are characterized by severe pain, often in the legs, associated with hypertonia (causing hyperextension of the trunk and neck), vomiting, paralytic ileus, and, occasionally, self-induced injuries. Marked weakness and paralysis occur in about 30% of the episodes, which may lead to respiratory failure and death. These crises may last 1–7 days. Urinary excretion of 5-aminolevulinic acid, which is usually elevated before the crises (see later), is further increased during the episodes. Monitoring the urinary excretion of this compound has little diagnostic or predictive value.

Renal involvement is manifested as a Fanconi-like syndrome with a normal anion gap metabolic acidosis, hyperphosphaturia, hypophosphatemia, and vitamin D–resistant rickets. Nephromegaly and some degree of nephrocalcinosis are often found by ultrasound examination of the kidneys.

Hypertrophic cardiomyopathy is occasionally seen in these infants.

LABORATORY FINDINGS. These include normocytic anemia and marked elevations of serum bilirubin (both conjugated and unconjugated), serum transaminases, and α-fetoprotein. An increase in serum levels of α-fetoprotein is observed in the cord blood of affected infants, indicating intrauterine liver damage. Clotting factors are often markedly decreased. Plasma levels of tyrosine and other amino acids, especially methionine (presumably due to secondary inhibition of methionine adenosyltransferase), are moderately increased. Generalized aminoaciduria occurs. Hyperphosphaturia and hypophosphatemia are common. Urinary excretion of 5-aminolevulinic acid (presumably due to inhibition of 5-aminolevulinic hydratase by succinylacetone) may be increased. The presence of succinylacetoacetate and succinylacetone in serum and urine is diagnostic (see Fig. 74–1). Liver histology is usually compatible with chronic hepatitis and nonspecific cirrhosis. Hyperplasia of pancreatic islet cells is also found.

Diagnosis is established by measurement of fumarylacetoacetate hydroxylase activity in lymphocytes, erythrocytes, and liver biopsy specimens. The degree of residual enzyme activity usually dictates the severity of the disease. This condition should be differentiated from other causes of hepatitis and hepatic failure in infants, including galactosemia, hereditary fructose intolerance, neonatal iron storage disease, biliary atresia, and giant cell hepatitis.

TREATMENT AND OUTCOME. A diet low in phenylalanine and tyrosine may result in some clinical improvement in some patients. However, in most affected infants the progression of the disease cannot be halted by diet alone. Inhibition of the enzyme 4-hydroxyphenylpyruvate dioxygenase by 2-(nitro-4-trifluoromethylbenzoyl)-1,3-cyclohexanedione (NTBC) is a very effective treatment. Acute hepatic and neurologic crises do not occur in patients treated with this agent. Long-term efficacy of NTBC in prevention of hepatic carcinoma, although it seems very promising, awaits further data. It is recommended that patients receive a diet low in phenylalanine and tyrosine in addition to NTBC therapy. Liver transplantation has been considered the most effective therapy for these patients. Whether treatment with NTBC alleviates or delays the need for liver transplantation remains to be determined.

GENETICS AND PREVALENCE. Tyrosinemia type I is an autosomal recessive trait. The *gene* for fumarylacetoacetate hydrolase has been mapped to the long arm of chromosome 15. Over 30 different mutations have been identified in different families. Most reported patients have a French-Canadian or Scandinavian ancestry. The prevalence of the condition is estimated to be 1 in 1,846 live births in the Saguenay-Lac Saint Jean region of the province of Quebec (Canada). The worldwide prevalence is estimated to be 1:100,000 to 1:120,000. *Prenatal diagnosis* has been achieved by measurement of succinylacetone in amniotic fluid and by the enzyme assay in chorionic villi biopsy. Direct gene analysis is possible in some families.

Tyrosinemia Type II (Richner-Hanhart Syndrome, Oculocutaneous Tyrosinemia).

This rare autosomal recessive disorder results in palmar and plantar punctate hyperkeratosis, herpetiform corneal ulcers, and mental retardation. *Clinical manifestations* of excessive tearing, redness, pain, and photophobia may occur before skin lesions. Corneal lesions usually occur during the first few months of life and are presumed to be due to tyrosine deposition. Skin lesions, which may develop later in life, include painful, nonpruritic hyperkeratotic plaques on the soles, palms (especially thenar and hypothenar areas), and fingertips. Mental retardation, which occurs in less than 50% of patients, is usually mild to moderate and may be associated with self-mutilation.

Abnormal *laboratory findings* are limited to significant hypertyrosinemia (20–50 mg/dL) and tyrosinuria. The condition is caused by the deficiency of the cytosolic fraction of hepatic tyrosine aminotransferase. In contrast to tyrosinemia type I, liver and kidney functions, as well as serum concentrations of other amino acids, are normal.

Treatment with a diet low in tyrosine and phenylalanine corrects the chemical abnormalities and results in dramatic healing of the skin and eye lesions. Mental retardation may be prevented by early dietary restriction of tyrosine. The gene for tyrosine aminotransferase is located on the long arm of chromosome 16; about 15 different mutations are identified in different families. About half the reported cases are of Italian descent.

Tyrosinemia Type III (Primary Deficiency of 4-Hydroxyphenylpyruvate Dioxygenase, 4-HPPD).

Only four cases have been reported. All patients have various neurologic findings but no consistent clinical phenotype. There is doubt as to whether this enzyme deficiency causes any clinical abnormalities. Age at onset has been from 1–17 mo. Developmental delay, seizures, intermittent ataxia, and self-destructive behavior have been the main neurologic findings. No liver or renal abnormalities are present.

The *diagnosis* is established by moderate increases in plasma levels of tyrosine (350–700 μM), the presence of 4-hydroxyphenylpyruvic acid and its metabolites (4-hydroxyphenyllactic and 4-hydroxyphenylacetic acids) in urine, and low activity of 4-HPPD enzyme in liver biopsy.

Diets low in tyrosine and phenylalanine in combination with vitamin C cause a dramatic decrease in plasma tyrosine levels. The beneficial effects of the diet on neurologic abnormalities have not been demonstrated. The mode of inheritance is not known.

Transient Tyrosinemia of the Newborn.

In a small number of newborn infants, plasma tyrosine may rise to as high as 60 mg/dL during the first 2 wk of life. Most affected infants are premature and are receiving high-protein diets. The condition is presumably due to delayed maturation of 4-hydroxyphenylpyruvate dioxygenase. Lethargy, poor feeding, and decreased motor activity occur in some of them, but most are asymptomatic and come to medical attention because of a high blood phenylalanine level, from the screening test for PKU. *Laboratory findings* include marked elevation of plasma tyrosine with a moderate increase in plasma phenylalanine. The presence of marked hypertyrosinemia differentiates this condition from phenylketonuria. Four-hydroxyphenylpyruvic acid and its metabolites (4-hydroxyphenyllactic and 4-hydroxyphenylacetic acids) are also present in the urine. Hypertyrosinemia usually resolves spontaneously during the 1st mo of life. The condition is often corrected promptly by reducing the amount of protein in the diet (to 2 g/kg/24 hr) and by administering vitamin C (200–400 mg/24 hr). Mild intellectual deficits have been reported in some full-term infants with this disorder, but the causal relationship to hypertyrosinemia has not been established.

Hawkinsinuria.

This rare condition (named after the first affected family) is caused by a deficiency of one of the components of the 4-hydroxyphenylpyruvate dioxygenase enzyme complex (see Fig. 74–1). A block in the rearrangement step leads to an accumulation of the epoxide intermediate, which either is reduced to form 4-hydroxycyclohexylacetic acid (4-HCAA) or reacts with glutathione to form the unusual organic acid hawkinsin (2-L-cysteine-S-yl-1-4-dihydroxycyclohex-5-en-1-yl-acetic acid); secondary glutathione deficiency may occur.

Individuals with this disorder become symptomatic only during infancy. The symptoms usually appear after weaning from breast-feeding with the introduction of a high-protein diet. Severe metabolic acidosis, ketosis, failure to thrive, mild hepatomegaly, and an unusual odor (of a swimming pool) are common findings. These infants respond well to a diet low in both phenylalanine and tyrosine, and their clinical manifestations resolve spontaneously by 1 yr of age. Adults with this condition are usually asymptomatic despite metabolic abnormalities. Mental development is usually normal.

Affected children and adults excrete 4-hydroxyphenylpyruvic acid and its metabolites (4-hydroxyphenyllactic and 4-hydroxyphenylacetic acids) as well as 5-oxoproline (owing to secondary glutathione deficiency) and the two very unusual organic acids 4-HCAA and hawkinsin in their urine. One patient had mild hypertyrosinemia (196 μM).

Treatment consists of a low-protein diet (such as breast milk) or a diet low in phenylalanine and tyrosine. Large doses of vitamin C (up to 1,000 mg/24 hr) are recommended. No therapy is needed after 1 yr of age. The condition is inherited as an autosomal dominant trait; all patients are presumed to be heterozygous. The gene has not yet been identified.

Alcaptonuria.

This rare (incidence about 1 in 250,000) autosomal recessive disorder is caused by a deficiency of homogentisic acid oxidase, which causes large amounts of homogentisic acid to accumulate in the body and then to be excreted in the urine (see Fig. 74–1). It is most common in the Dominican Republic and Slovakia.

Clinical manifestations consist of ochronosis and arthritis. These findings may not become evident until mid-adult life. The only sign of the disorder in the pediatric age group is a darkening of the urine to almost a black color on standing. This is caused by oxidation and polymerization of the homogentisic acid and is enhanced with an alkaline pH. Therefore, acid urine may not become dark even after many hours of standing. This is one of the reasons why darkening of the urine may never be noted in an affected person, and the diagnosis may be delayed until adulthood, when arthritis or ochronosis occurs. *Ochronosis,* a term used to describe the darkening of tissue, is due to a slow accumulation of the black polymer of homogentisic acid in cartilage and other mesenchymal tissues. It is manifested clinically as dark, blackened spots in the sclera or as diffuse blackish pigmentation of the conjunctiva, cornea, and ear cartilage. *Arthritis* is the only disabling effect, which occurs in almost all affected subjects with advancing age. It involves the large joints (spine, hip, and knee) and is usually more severe in male patients. The arthritis has the clinical characteristics of rheumatoid arthritis, but the radiologic findings are typical of osteoarthritis. Degenerative changes in the lumbar spine are quite characteristic with narrowing of the joint spaces and fusion of the vertebral bodies. The pathogenesis of arthritic changes is unclear. High incidences of heart disease (mitral and aortic valvulitis, calcification of the heart valves, and myocardial infarction) have also been noted.

The *diagnosis* is confirmed by measurement of homogentisic acid in urine. Affected subjects may excrete as much as 4–8 g of this compound daily. Homogentisic acid is a strong reducing agent that produces a positive reaction with Fehling or Benedict reagent (but not with glucose oxidase). The dark urine of phenol poisoning and that associated with melanotic tumors do not have these reducing properties. The enzyme is expressed only in the liver and kidneys. The gene for alcaptonuria has been mapped to the long arm of chromosome 3 and several disease-causing mutations have been identified.

There is no effective *treatment* for this disorder. Nitisinone inhibits homogentisate production; its long term efficacy is unknown.

Tyrosine Hydroxylase Deficiency (Infantile Parkinsonism, Autosomal Recessive Dopa Responsive Dystonia) (see Chapter 590.3) This enzyme catalyzes the formation of L-dopa from tyrosine (see Fig. 74–2). Deficiency of this enzyme is seen in a few children with dystonia and parkinsonism. The clinical picture resembles the autosomal dominant dystonia that is due to GTP cyclohydrolase deficiency (see Chapter 74.1). The spectrum of the condition is not fully appreciated.

Clinical manifestations such as jerky movements of the limbs leading to spasticity and muscle rigidity, expressionless face, ptosis, drooling, oculogyric crises, and parkinsonism may start in early infancy. Psychomotor retardation has been seen in some patients. No diurnal variation of the symptoms has been noted.

Laboratory findings include reduced levels of dopamine and its metabolite HVA (homovanillic acid) and normal concentrations of BH4 and neopterin in the spinal fluid. Serum prolactin levels are usually elevated.

Diagnosis should be considered in any patients with dystonia and parkinsonism. GTP cyclohydroxylase deficiency should be ruled out by proper studies (see earlier). Diagnosis is established by the laboratory findings (see earlier) and gene analysis.

Treatment with L-dopa results in a dramatic response. The condition is inherited as an autosomal recessive trait. The gene for tyrosine hydroxylase is mapped to chromosome 11p.

Albinism. Albinism is caused by defects in the biosynthesis and distribution of melanin. Melanin is synthesized by melanocytes from tyrosine in a membrane-bound intracellular organelle, the melanosome. Melanocytes originate from the embryonic neural crest and migrate to the skin, eyes (choroid and iris), and hair follicles. The melanin in the eye is not secreted into the adjacent tissues, whereas the pigment in skin and hair follicles is secreted into the epidermis and the hair shaft. The rate of melanogenesis is very low in the eye and very high in the skin and hair. The biosynthetic pathway for melanin synthesis is not completely elucidated (see Fig. 74–2). The end products are two pigments *pheomelanin*, which is a yellow-red pigment, and *eumelanin*, a brown-black pigment.

Clinical manifestations common in generalized albinism are hypopigmentation of the skin and hair. Patients with involvement of the eyes may have strabismus, photophobia, decreased visual acuity, and the presence of red reflex. Irides are translucent and pink in infancy and change to light blue or brown with age. Biocular (stereoscopic) vision is absent because of an abnormal decussation and misrouting of the optic fibers at the chiasm. About 90% of optic nerve fibers from one eye cross to the other side at the chiasma in patients with albinism. This defect also causes asymmetric visual evoked potentials. Blindness and skin cancer are major late sequelae of albinism in its severe forms. Melanin is also present in the cochlea. Albino individuals may be more susceptible to ototoxic agents such as gentamicin.

Many clinical forms of albinism have been identified. Some of the seemingly distinct clinical forms are caused by different mutations of the same gene. Several genes (mostly autosomal recessive, rarely autosomal dominant) and at least one on the short arm of the X chromosome have been found to be involved in melanogenesis (Table 74–1). Attempts to differentiate types of albinism based on the mode of inheritance, tyrosinase activity, or the extent of hypopigmentation have failed to yield a comprehensive classification. The following classification is based on the distribution of albinism in the body and the type of mutated gene.

OCULOCUTANEOUS (GENERALIZED) ALBINISM (OCA). Lack of pigment is generalized, affecting skin, hair, and eyes. Three genetically distinct forms exist: OCA_1, OCA_2, and OCA_3. The lack of pigment is usually more severe in patients with OCA_1, however; these types may not be distinguishable clinically because of a great degree of overlap. All are inherited as autosomal recessive traits.

OCA_1 (Tyrosinase-Deficient Albinism). The defect resides in the tyrosinase gene, located on the long arm of chromosome 11. Many mutant alleles have been identified. Most affected individuals are compound heterozygote for two different mutant alleles. The condition can be subdivided to OCA_1A and OCA_1B based on enzyme activity and, to a lesser extent, clinical manifestations.

OCA_1A (Tyrosinase-Negative OCA). A number of mutations in the tyrosinase gene render the enzyme completely inactive. Individuals with this form usually have the most severe case of generalized albinism. Lack of pigment in the skin (milky white), hair (white hair), and eyes (red-gray irides) is evident at birth and remains unchanged throughout life. They do not tan and do not develop pigmented nevi or freckles.

OCA_1B. These mutations in the tyrosinase gene result in enzymes with some residual activities. These individuals, although

TABLE 74–1. Classification of Albinism

Type	Gene	Chromosome
Oculocutaneous Albinism (OCA)		
OCA_1 (tyrosinase deficient)	*TYR*	11_q
OCA_1A (severe deficiency)	*TYR*	11_q
OCA_1B (mild deficiency)*	*TYR*	11_q
OCA_2 (tyrosinase positive)[†]	*p* (pink-eyed dilution)	15_q
Prader-Willi and Angelman syndromes	*p*	15_q
OCA_3 (rufous, red OCA)	*TYRP1*[‡]	9_p
Hermansky-Pudlak syndrome	*HPS1*	10_q
Chédiak-Higashi syndrome	*CHS1*	1_q
Ocular Albinism		
OA_1 (Nettleship-Falls type)	*OA*	x_p
Localized Albinism		
Piebaldism	*KIT*	4_q
Waardenburg syndrome I and III	*PAX3*	2_q
Waardenburg syndrome II	*MITF*	3_p

*This includes Amish, minimal pigment, yellow albinism, platinum, and temperature-sensitive variants.
[†]Includes brown OCA.
[‡]Tyrosinase-related protein 1.

completely depigmented at birth, are capable of developing some pigment with age and become light blond with light blue or hazel eyes. They develop pigmented nevi and freckles and they may tan. These patients, depending on the degree of pigmentation, were once subdivided into different groups and were thought to be genetically different. One interesting form is temperature-sensitive albinism in which the tyrosinase becomes more active in cooler parts of the body such as limbs. These individuals have no pigment in the scalp and trunk but develop some pigment in arms and legs.

OCA$_2$ (Tyrosinase-Positive Albinism). This is the most common form of generalized albinism and is particularly common in African blacks. Patients demonstrate some pigmentation of the skin and eyes at birth and continue to collect pigment throughout their lives. The hair is yellow at birth and may become darker with age. They have pigmented nevi and freckles, but they do not tan. They may be clinically indistinguishable from OCA$_1$B. These individuals have normal tyrosinase activity. The defect is in the *p* (pink-eyed dilution) gene, located on the long arm of chromosome 15. This gene produces the p protein, a melanosome membrane protein the function of which is not completely understood. Patients with *Prader-Willi* and *Angelman* syndromes who have deletion of chromosome 15 have this form of albinism (see Chapter 69).

OCA$_3$ (Rufous Albinism). This form has been identified only in Africans, African-Americans, and natives of New Guinea. Patients have reddish hair with reddish brown skin as an adult. The color of the skin is peculiar to this form. As a youngster the manifestations may be confused with those of OCA$_2$. These patients can make pheomelanin but not eumelanin. The mutation is in the tyrosinase-related protein 1 *(TYRP1)* gene, whose function is not understood.

HERMANSKY-PUDLAK SYNDROME. This tyrosinase-positive oculocutaneous albinism is associated with platelet dysfunction (owing to the absence of platelet-dense bodies) and an accumulation of a ceroid-like material in tissues. The degree of albinism is variable. The condition is most prevalent in Puerto Rico (frequency about 1:2,000). Bleeding tendencies, often manifested as epistaxis and a prolonged bleeding time, are common. The ceroid-like material is histochemically similar to that found in neuronal ceroid-lipofuscinosis. The accumulation of this material in tissues results in restrictive lung disease, inflammatory bowel disease, kidney failure, and cardiomyopathy during the third or fourth decade of life. The condition is caused by mutations in one of the two genes, *HPS1* or *HPS2*. The majority of patients have mutations in *HPS1*, which is located on chromosome 10q. The pathogenesis is not understood.

CHÉDIAK-HIGASHI SYNDROME. Patients with this rare autosomal recessive condition have partial albinism and susceptibility to infection with the presence of giant peroxidase-positive lysosomal granules in granulocytes (see Chapter 120.3). These patients have a reduced number of melanosomes, which are abnormally large (macromelanosomes). Patients who survive early childhood may develop a lymphoproliferative malignancy. Mutations in *CHS1* gene (located on the long arm of chromosome 1) have been identified in these patients.

OCULAR ALBINISM (OA). Albinism is limited to the eyes. All the eye findings of albinism (see earlier) are present. The X-linked recessive form (OA$_1$) has been segregated as a separate entity. Autosomal recessive ocular albinism is a mild variant of OCA$_2$.

Ocular Albinism 1 (OA$_1$ Nettleship-Falls Type). Only the hemizygote male has the complete manifestation while some abnormal retinal pigmentation may be present in heterozygote female carriers. The gene is located on the short arm of the X chromosome. An X-linked ocular albinism with late-onset sensorineural deafness has also been reported.

LOCALIZED ALBINISM. This disorder is characterized by localized hypopigmentation of skin and hair, which may be present at birth or develop with time.

Piebaldism. In this autosomal dominant inherited condition, the individual is usually born with a white forelock. The underlying skin is depigmented. There are usually white macules on the face, trunk, and extremities. The white hair lock and the depigmented underlying skin are devoid of melanocytes. Mutations in the *KIT* gene have been shown in affected patients.

Waardenburg Syndrome. In this syndrome, lateral displacement of inner canthi, broad nasal bridge, heterochromia of irides, and sensorineural deafness are associated with a white forelock. It is inherited as an autosomal dominant trait with four identifiable types. Type I has displacement of inner canthi and is caused by mutations in the *PAX3* gene. Type II has normal inner canthi and mutations in the *MITF* gene in some patients. Type III has all the findings seen in individuals with type I plus hypoplasia and contractures of the upper limbs. The gene abnormality is in *PAX3*. Type IV is associated with Hirschsprung disease and is heterogeneous with mutations in different genes *(EDN3, EDNRB,* or *SOX10)*.

74.3 Methionine

Iraj Rezvani and David S. Rosenblatt

The normal pathway for catabolism of methionine, an essential amino acid, produces *S*-adenosylmethionine (which serves as a methyl group donor for methylation of a variety of compounds in the body), and cysteine, which is formed through a series of reactions called *trans*-sulfuration (Fig. 74–3).

Homocystinuria (Homocystinemia). Most homocysteine, an intermediate compound of methionine degradation, is normally remethylated to methionine. This methionine-sparing reaction is catalyzed by the enzyme methionine synthase, which requires a metabolite of folic acid (5-methyltetrahydrofolate) as a methyl donor and a metabolite of vitamin B$_{12}$ (methylcobalamin) as a cofactor (see Fig. 74–3). Only 20–30% of total homocysteine (and its dimer homocystine) is in free form in the plasma of normal individuals. The rest is bound to protein. Three major forms of homocystinemia and homocystinuria have been identified.

HOMOCYSTINURIA DUE TO CYSTATHIONINE SYNTHASE DEFICIENCY (CLASSIC HOMOCYSTINURIA). This is the most common inborn error of methionine metabolism. About 40% of affected patients respond to high doses of vitamin B$_6$ and usually have milder clinical manifestations than those who are unresponsive to vitamin B$_6$ therapy. These patients possess some residual enzyme activity.

Infants with this disorder are normal at birth. *Clinical manifestations* during infancy are nonspecific and may include failure to thrive and developmental delay. The diagnosis is usually made after 3 yr of age, when subluxation of the ocular lens *(ectopia lentis)* occurs. This causes severe myopia and iridodonesis (quivering of the iris). Astigmatism, glaucoma, staphyloma, cataracts, retinal detachment, and optic atrophy may develop later in life. Progressive *mental retardation* is common. Normal intelligence, however, has been reported. In an international survey of over 600 patients, IQ scores ranged from 10 to 135. The higher IQ scores were noted in vitamin B$_6$ responsive patients. *Psychiatric and behavioral disorders* have been observed in more than 50% of affected patients. Convulsions occur in about 20% of patients. Affected individuals with homocystinuria manifest *skeletal abnormalities* resembling those of Marfan syndrome (see Chapter 690); they are usually tall and thin with elongated limbs and arachnodactyly. Scoliosis, pectus excavatum or carinum, genu valgum, pes cavus, high arched palate, and crowding of the teeth are common. Patients usually have fair complexions, blue eyes, and a peculiar malar flush. Generalized osteoporosis, especially of the spine, is the main radiographic finding. *Thromboembolic episodes* involving both large and small vessels, especially those of the brain, are common and may occur at any age. Optic atrophy, paralysis, cor pulmonale, and

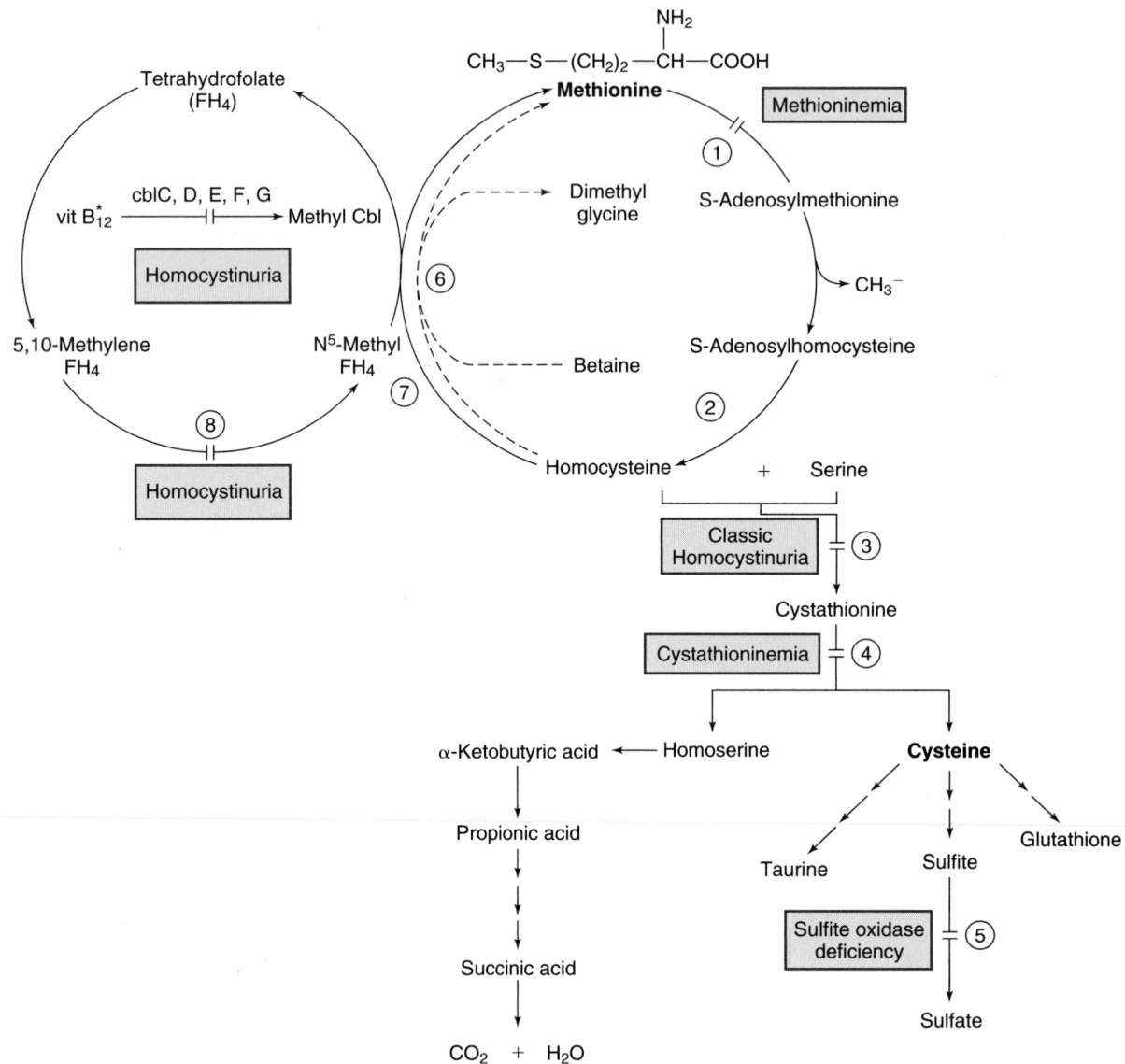

FIGURE 74–3. Pathways in the metabolism of the sulfur-containing amino acids. **Enzymes:** (1) methionine adenosyltransferase; (2) adenosylhomocysteine hydrolase; (3) cystathionine synthase; (4) cystathionase; (5) sulfite oxidase; (6) betaine homocysteine methyltransferase; (7) methionine synthase; (8) methylene tetrahydrofolate reductase.

severe hypertension (from renal infarcts) are among the serious consequences of thromboembolism, which is caused by changes in the vascular walls and by increased platelet adhesiveness secondary to elevated homocystine levels. The risk of thromboembolism increases after surgical procedures.

Elevations of both methionine and homocystine (or total homocysteine) in body fluids are the diagnostic *laboratory findings*. Freshly voided urine should be tested for homocystine, because this compound is unstable and may disappear as the urine is stored. Cystine is low or absent in plasma. The *diagnosis* may be established by assay of the enzyme in liver biopsy specimens, cultured fibroblasts, or phytohemagglutinin-stimulated lymphocytes.

Treatment with high doses of vitamin B₆ (200–1,000 mg/24 hr) causes dramatic improvement in patients who are responsive to this therapy. The degree of response to vitamin B₆ treatment may be different in different families. Some patients may not respond because of folate depletion; a patient should not be considered unresponsive to vitamin B₆ until folic acid (1–5 mg/24 hr) has been added to the treatment regimen. Restriction of methionine intake in conjunction with cysteine supplementation is recom-

mended for patients who are unresponsive to vitamin B₆. The need for dietary restriction and its extent is controversial in patients with vitamin B₆ responsive form. In some patients with this form of the condition, addition of betaine may obviate the need for any dietary restriction. Betaine (trimethylglycine, 6–9 g/24 hr for adults or 200 to 250 mg/kg/day in children) lowers homocysteine levels in body fluids by remethylating homocysteine to methionine (see Fig. 74–3). This treatment has produced clinical improvement (preventing vascular events) in patients who are unresponsive to vitamin B₆ therapy.

More than 100 pregnancies in women with the classic form of homocystinuria have been reported with favorable outcomes for both mothers and infants. The majority of infants were full term and normal. Postpartum thromboembolic events occurred in a few mothers. All but 1 of the 38 affected male patients have had normal offspring.

The *screening* of newborn infants for classic homocystinuria yields a prevalence of 1:200,000 to 1:350,000; most are vitamin B₆ unresponsive. Because almost 40% of patients identified after the newborn period are vitamin B₆ responsive, one must assume that these screening programs miss the majority of infants with the vitamin B_6 responsive form. Newer screening methods (tandem mass spectrometry) may improve the detection process. The condition seems more common in New South Wales, Australia (1:60,000). Early treatment of patients identified by the screening process has produced favorable results. The mean IQ of 16 patients with the vitamin B_6 unresponsive form treated in early infancy is 94. Dislocation of the lens may be preventable.

Homocystinuria is inherited as an autosomal recessive trait. The gene for cystathionine β synthase is located on the long arm of chromosome 21. *Prenatal diagnosis* is feasible by performing an enzyme assay of cultured amniotic cells or chorionic villi. Many disease-causing mutations (over 100) have been identified in different families. The majority of affected patients are compound heterozygotes for two different alleles. Heterozygous carriers are usually asymptomatic, however; thromboembolic events and coronary heart disease are more common than in the normal population.

HOMOCYSTINURIA DUE TO DEFECTS IN METHYL-COBALAMIN FORMATION. Methylcobalamin is the cofactor for the enzyme methionine synthase, which catalyzes remethylation of homocysteine to methionine. There are at least five distinct defects in the intracellular metabolism of cobalamin that may interfere with the formation of methylcobalamin. To better understand the metabolism of cobalamin, see methylmalonic acidemia (see Chapter 74.6 and Figs. 74–3 and 74–5). The five defects are designated as *cbl*C, *cbl*D, *cbl*E (methionine synthase reductase), *cbl*G (methionine synthase), and *cbl*F. Patients with *cbl*C, *cbl*D, and *cbl*F defects have methylmalonic acidemia in addition to homocystinuria because formation of both adenosylcobalamin and methylcobalamin is impaired (see Chapter 74.6).

Patients with *cbl*E and *cbl*G defects are unable to form methylcobalamin and develop homocystinuria without methylmalonic acidemia (see Fig. 74–5); only a few patients with these two defects are known (12 patients with *cbl*E and 24 patients with *cbl*G).

The *clinical manifestations* are similar in patients with all of these defects. Vomiting, poor feeding, lethargy, hypotonia, and developmental delay may occur in the first few months of life. However, one patient with the *cbl*G defect was not symptomatic (except for mild developmental delay) until she was 21 yr old, when she developed difficulty in walking and numbness of the hands. *Laboratory findings* include megaloblastic anemia, homocystinuria, and hypomethioninemia. The presence of megaloblastic anemia differentiates these defects from homocystinuria due to methylenetetrahydrofolate reductase deficiency (see later). The presence of hypomethioninemia differentiates both of these from cystathionine β synthase deficiency (see earlier).

Diagnosis is established by complementation studies performed in cultured fibroblasts. *Prenatal diagnosis* has been accomplished by studies in amniotic cell cultures. The genes for *cbl*E (MTRR) and *cbl*G (MTR) have been identified.

Treatment with vitamin B_{12} in the form of hydroxycobalamin (1–2 mg/24 hr) is used to correct the clinical and biochemical findings. Results vary among both diseases and sibships.

HOMOCYSTINURIA DUE TO DEFICIENCY OF METHYL-ENETETRAHYDROFOLATE REDUCTASE (MTHFR). This enzyme reduces 5–10 methylenetetrahydrofolate to form 5-methyltetrahydrofolate, which provides the methyl group needed for remethylation of homocysteine to methionine (see Fig. 74–3).

The severity of the enzyme defect and of the *clinical manifestations* varies considerably in different families. Complete absence of enzyme activity results in neonatal apneic episodes and myoclonic seizures that may lead rapidly to coma and death. Partial deficiency may result in a more chronic clinical picture, manifested by mental retardation, convulsions, microcephaly, and spasticity. One 15-yr-old patient developed schizophrenia and mental deterioration at 11 yr of age. Premature vascular disease or peripheral neuropathy has been reported as the only

manifestation of this enzyme deficiency in some patients. One affected adult was completely asymptomatic. A common polymorphism (677C→T) causes enzyme thermal lability, mildly elevated total plasma homocysteine levels, and lower levels of plasma folate. Homozygosity for this polymorphism has been implicated as a risk factor for both vascular disease and neural tube defects.

Laboratory findings include moderate homocystinemia and homocystinuria. The methionine concentration is low or low normal. This finding differentiates this condition from classic homocystinuria caused by cystathionine synthase deficiency. Absence of megaloblastic anemia distinguishes this condition from homocystinuria caused by defects in methylcobalamin formation (see earlier). Thromboembolism of vessels has also been observed in these patients. *Diagnosis* may be confirmed by the enzyme assay in cultured fibroblasts and leukocytes.

Treatment with a combination of folic acid, vitamin B_6, vitamin B_{12}, methionine supplementation, and betaine has been tried. Early treatment with betaine seems to have the most beneficial effect.

The gene for this enzyme has been located on the short arm of chromosome 1. The condition is transmitted as an autosomal recessive trait; more than 40 cases have been reported.

Hypermethioninemia. *Secondary hypermethioninemia* occurs in liver disease, tyrosinemia type I, and classic homocystinuria. Hypermethioninemia has also been found in premature and some full-term infants receiving high-protein diets, in whom it may represent delayed maturation of the enzyme methionine adenosyltransferase. Lowering the protein intake usually resolves the abnormality. *Primary hypermethioninemia* caused by the deficiency of hepatic methionine adenosyltransferase (see Fig. 74–3) has been reported in a few patients who have been diagnosed in the neonatal period through screening for homocystinuria. Affected individuals with residual enzyme activity remain asymptomatic throughout life despite persistent hypermethioninemia. Some complain of unusual odor to their breath (boiled cabbage). A few patients with complete enzyme deficiency have had neurologic abnormalities related to demyelination (mental retardation, dystonia, dyspraxia). The gene for methionine adenosyltransferase is located on the long arm of chromosome 10 and several disease-causing mutations have been identified. A novel defect, glycine *N*-methyltransferase deficiency, also causes isolated hypermethioninemia.

Cystathioninemia. Secondary cystathioninuria occurs in patients with vitamin B_6 or B_{12} deficiency, liver disease (particularly with liver damage from galactosemia), thyrotoxicosis, hepatoblastoma, neuroblastoma, ganglioblastoma, or defects in remethylation of homocysteine.

Cystathionase deficiency results in massive cystathioninuria and mild to moderate cystathioninemia; cystathionine is not normally detectable in blood. Deficiency of this enzyme is inherited as an autosomal recessive trait. Affected subjects with a wide variety of clinical manifestations have been reported. Lack of a consistent clinical picture and the presence of cystathioninuria in a number of normal persons suggest that cystathionase deficiency may be of no clinical significance. A majority of reported cases are responsive to oral administration of large doses of vitamin B_6 (100 mg or more/24 hr). When cystathioninuria is discovered in a patient, vitamin B_6 treatment seems indicated, but its beneficial effect has not been established.

74.4 Cysteine/Cystine

Iraj Rezvani

Cysteine is a sulfur-containing nonessential amino acid that is synthesized from methionine (see Fig. 74–3). In the presence of oxygen, two molecules of cysteine are oxidized to form cystine.

The most common disorders of cysteine/cystine metabolism, cystinuria (see Chapter 539) and cystinosis (see Chapter 521.3), are discussed elsewhere.

Sulfite Oxidase Deficiency (Molybdenum Cofactor Deficiency). At the last step in cysteine metabolism, sulfite is oxidized to sulfate by sulfite oxidase, and the sulfate is excreted in the urine (see Fig. 74–3). This enzyme requires a molybdenum-pterin complex named molybdenum cofactor. This cofactor is also necessary for the function of two other enzymes in humans, xanthine dehydrogenase (which oxidizes xanthine and hypoxanthine to uric acid) and aldehyde oxidase. Most patients who were originally diagnosed as having sulfite oxidase deficiency have been proven to have molybdenum cofactor deficiency. Both conditions are inherited as autosomal recessive traits.

Both the enzyme and the cofactor deficiencies produce identical *clinical manifestations*. Refusal to feed, vomiting, severe intractable seizures (tonic, clonic, and myoclonic), and severe developmental delay may develop within a few weeks after birth. Bilateral dislocation of ocular lenses is a common finding in patients who survive the neonatal period.

These children excrete large amounts of sulfite, thiosulfate, S-sulfocysteine, xanthine, and hypoxanthine in their urine. Urinary and serum levels of uric acid and urinary concentration of sulfate are diminished. Fresh urine should be used for screening purposes and for quantitative measurements of sulfite, because oxidation at room temperature may produce false-negative results.

Diagnosis is confirmed by measurement of sulfite oxidase and molybdenum cofactor in fibroblasts and liver biopsies, respectively. *Prenatal diagnosis* is possible by performing an assay of sulfite oxidase activity in cultured amniotic cells or in samples of chorionic villi.

No effective *treatment* is available, and most children die during the first 2 yr of life.

74.5 Tryptophan

Iraj Rezvani

Tryptophan is an essential amino acid and a precursor for nicotinic acid and serotonin (Fig. 74–4). Presumed deficiencies of a variety of enzymes involved in tryptophan catabolism have been reported but no distinct clinical entity has emerged. Hartnup disorder causes disturbance in tryptophan absorption.

Hartnup Disorder. In this autosomal recessive disorder, there is a single defect in the transport of monoamino-monocarboxylic amino acids (neutral amino acids) by the intestinal mucosa and renal tubules. Most children with Hartnup defect remain asymptomatic. The major *clinical manifestation* in the rare symptomatic patient is cutaneous photosensitivity. The skin becomes rough and red after moderate exposure to the sun, and with greater exposure a pellagra-like rash may develop. The rash may be pruritic, and a chronic eczema may appear. The skin changes have been reported in affected infants as young as 10 days of age. Some patients may have intermittent ataxia manifested as an unsteady, wide-based gait. The ataxia may last a few days and usually recovers spontaneously. Mental development is usually normal. However, two individuals in the original kindred were mentally retarded. Episodic psychologic changes, such as irritability, emotional instability, depression and suicidal tendencies, have been observed; these changes are usually associated with bouts of ataxia. Short stature and atrophic glossitis are seen in some patients.

Almost all children who were diagnosed with Hartnup disorder as a result of neonatal screening have remained asymptomatic. This indicates that other factors are also involved in pathogenesis of the clinical condition.

The main *laboratory finding* is aminoaciduria, which is restricted to neutral amino acids (alanine, serine, threonine, valine, leucine, isoleucine, phenylalanine, tyrosine, tryptophan, and histidine). Urinary excretion of proline, hydroxyproline, and arginine remains normal. This important diagnostic finding differentiates Hartnup disorder from other causes of generalized aminoaciduria, such as Fanconi syndrome. Plasma concentrations of neutral amino acids are usually normal. This seemingly unexpected finding is because amino acids are also absorbed as dipeptides; this transport system is intact in Hartnup disorder. The indole derivatives (especially indican) may be found in large amounts in this disorder, owing to bacterial breakdown of unabsorbed tryptophan in the intestines.

Diagnosis is established by the striking intermittent nature of symptoms and the just described urinary findings.

Treatment with nicotinic acid or nicotinamide (50–300 mg/24 hr) and a high-protein diet has resulted in a favorable

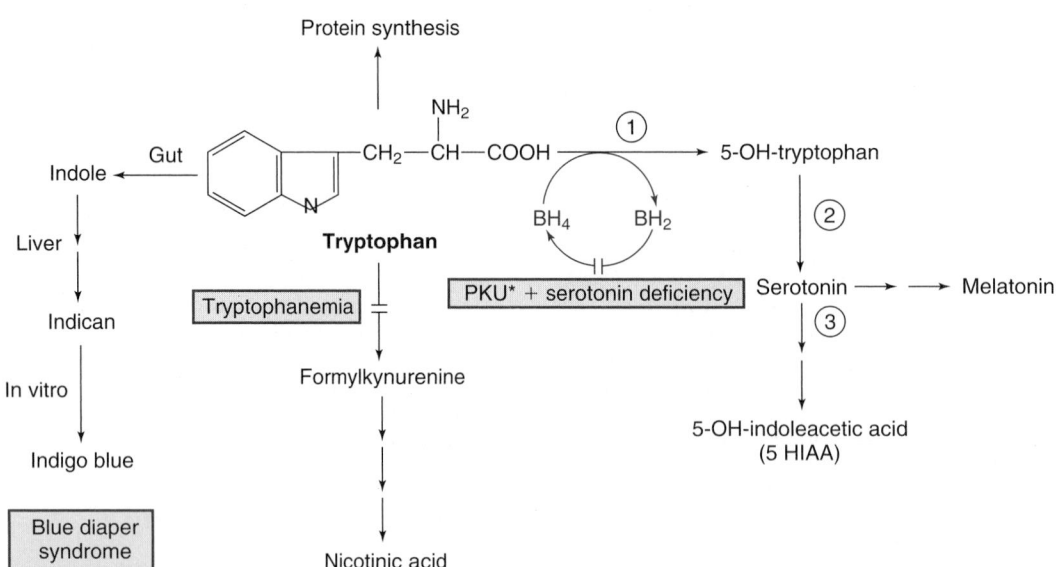

FIGURE 74–4. Pathways in the metabolism of tryptophan. PKU* indicates hyperphenylalaninemia due to tetrahydrobiopterin deficiency (see Fig. 74–1). **Enzymes:** (1) tryptophan hydroxylase; (2) aromatic L-amino acid decarboxylase (AADC); (3) monoamine oxidase (MAO).

response in symptomatic patients. Because of the intermittent nature of the clinical manifestations, the efficacy of these treatments is difficult to evaluate.

74.6 Valine, Leucine, Isoleucine, and Related Organic Acidemias

Iraj Rezvani and David S. Rosenblatt*

The early steps in the degradation of these three essential amino acids, the *branched-chain amino acids*, are similar (Fig. 74–5). The intermediate metabolites are all organic acids, and deficiency of any of the degradative enzymes, except for the transaminases, causes acidosis; in such instances, the organic acids before the enzymatic block accumulate in body fluids and are excreted in the urine. These disorders commonly cause severe metabolic acidosis, which usually occurs during the first few days of life. Although most of the clinical findings are nonspecific, some manifestations may provide important clues to the nature of the enzyme deficiency. An approach to infants suspected of having an organic acidemia is presented in Figure 74–6. Definitive diagnosis is usually established by identifying and measuring specific organic acids in body fluids (blood, urine) and by the enzyme assay.

Organic acidemias are not limited to defects in the catabolic pathways of branched-chain amino acids. Disorders causing accumulation of other organic acids include those derived from lysine (see Chapter 74.13), those associated with lactic acid (see Chapter 76), and dicarboxylic acidemia associated with defective fatty acid degradation (see Chapter 75.1).

Maple Syrup Urine Disease (MSUD). Decarboxylation of leucine, isoleucine, and valine is accomplished by a complex enzyme system (branched-chain α-ketoacid dehydrogenase) using thiamine pyrophosphate (vitamin B_1) as a coenzyme. This mitochondrial enzyme consists of four subunits, $E_{1\alpha}$, $E_{1\beta}$, E_2, and E_3. The E_3 subunit is shared with two other dehydrogenases in the body, namely, pyruvate dehydrogenase and α-ketoglutarate dehydrogenase. Deficiency of this enzyme system causes MSUD (see Fig. 74–5), named after the sweet odor of maple syrup found in body fluids, especially urine. Based on clinical findings and response to thiamine administration, five phenotypes of MSUD have been identified.

CLASSIC MSUD. This form has the most severe *clinical manifestations*. Affected infants are initially normal at birth but develop poor feeding and vomiting during the 1st wk of life; lethargy and coma may ensue within a few days. Physical examination reveals hypertonicity and muscular rigidity with opisthotonos. Periods of hypertonicity may alternate with bouts of flaccidity. Neurologic findings are often mistaken for sepsis and meningitis. Convulsions occur in most infants, and hypoglycemia is common. However, in contrast to most hypoglycemic states, correction of the blood glucose concentration does not improve the clinical condition. Routine *laboratory findings* are usually unremarkable, except for metabolic acidosis, which is not consistently observed. Death usually occurs in untreated patients within the first few weeks or months of life.

Diagnosis is often suspected because of the peculiar odor of maple syrup found in urine, sweat, and cerumen (see Fig. 74–6). It is usually confirmed by amino acid analysis showing marked elevations in plasma levels of leucine, isoleucine, valine, and alloisoleucine (a stereoisomer of isoleucine not normally found in blood) and depression of alanine. Leucine levels are usually higher than those of the other three amino acids. Urine contains high levels of leucine, isoleucine, and valine and their respective

ketoacids. These ketoacids may be detected qualitatively by adding a few drops of 2,4-dinitrophenylhydrazine reagent (0.1% in 0.1 N HCl) to the urine; a yellow precipitate of 2,4-dinitrophenylhydrazone is formed in a positive test. Neuroimaging during the acute state shows cerebral edema, which is most prominent in the cerebellum, dorsal brain stem, cerebral peduncle, and internal capsule. Following the acute state and with advancing age, hypomyelination and cerebral atrophy may develop.

Treatment of the acute state is aimed at rapid removal of the branched-chain amino acids and their metabolites from the tissues and body fluids. Because renal clearance of these compounds is poor, hydration alone may not produce a rapid improvement. Peritoneal dialysis or hemodialysis are the most effective modes of therapy in critically ill infants and should be instituted promptly; significant decreases in plasma levels of leucine, isoleucine, and valine are usually seen within 24 hr of treatment. Providing sufficient calories and nutrients intravenously or orally should reverse the patient's catabolic state.

Treatment after recovery from the acute state requires a low branched-chain amino acid diet with synthetic formulas devoid of leucine, isoleucine, and valine. Because these amino acids cannot be synthesized endogenously, small amounts of them should be added to the diet; the amount should be titrated carefully by performing frequent analyses of the plasma amino acids. A clinical condition resembling *acrodermatitis enteropathica* occurs in affected infants whose plasma isoleucine concentration becomes very low; addition of isoleucine to the diet causes a rapid and complete recovery. Patients with MSUD should remain on the diet for the rest of their lives. Liver transplantation has been performed in a small number of patients with classic MSUD with promising results. These children are able to tolerate a normal diet.

The long-term *prognosis* of affected children remains guarded. Severe ketoacidosis, cerebral edema, and death may occur during any stressful situation, such as infection or surgery, especially in mid childhood. Mental and neurologic deficits are common sequelae.

INTERMITTENT MSUD. In this form, seemingly normal children develop vomiting, odor of maple syrup, ataxia, lethargy, and coma during any stress or catabolic state such as infection or surgery. During these attacks, laboratory findings are indistinguishable from those of the classic form, and death may occur. *Treatment* of the acute attack of intermittent MSUD is similar to that of the classic form. After recovery, although a normal diet is tolerated, a diet low in branched-chain amino acids is recommended. Activity of dehydrogenase in patients with the intermittent form is higher than in the classic form and may reach 5–20% of the normal activity.

MILD (INTERMEDIATE) MSUD. In this form, affected children develop milder disease after the neonatal period. *Clinical manifestations* are insidious and limited to the central nervous system. Patients have mild to moderate mental retardation (usually after 5 mo of age) with or without seizures. They have the odor of maple syrup and excrete moderate amounts of the branched-chain amino acids and their ketoacid derivatives in the urine. Plasma concentrations of leucine, isoleucine, and valine are moderately increased whereas those of lactate and pyruvate are normal. These children are commonly diagnosed during an intercurrent illness when signs and symptoms of classic MSUD may occur. The dehydrogenase activity is 3–30% of normal. Since patients with thiamine-responsive MSUD usually have manifestations similar to those seen in the mild form, a trial of thiamine therapy is recommended. Diet therapy, similar to that of classic MSUD, is needed.

THIAMINE-RESPONSIVE MSUD. Some children with mild or intermediate forms of MSUD who are treated with high doses of thiamine have dramatic clinical and biochemical improvement. Although some responded to treatment with 10 mg/24 hr

---

*David S. Rosenblatt contributed to the section on Methylmalonic Acidemia.

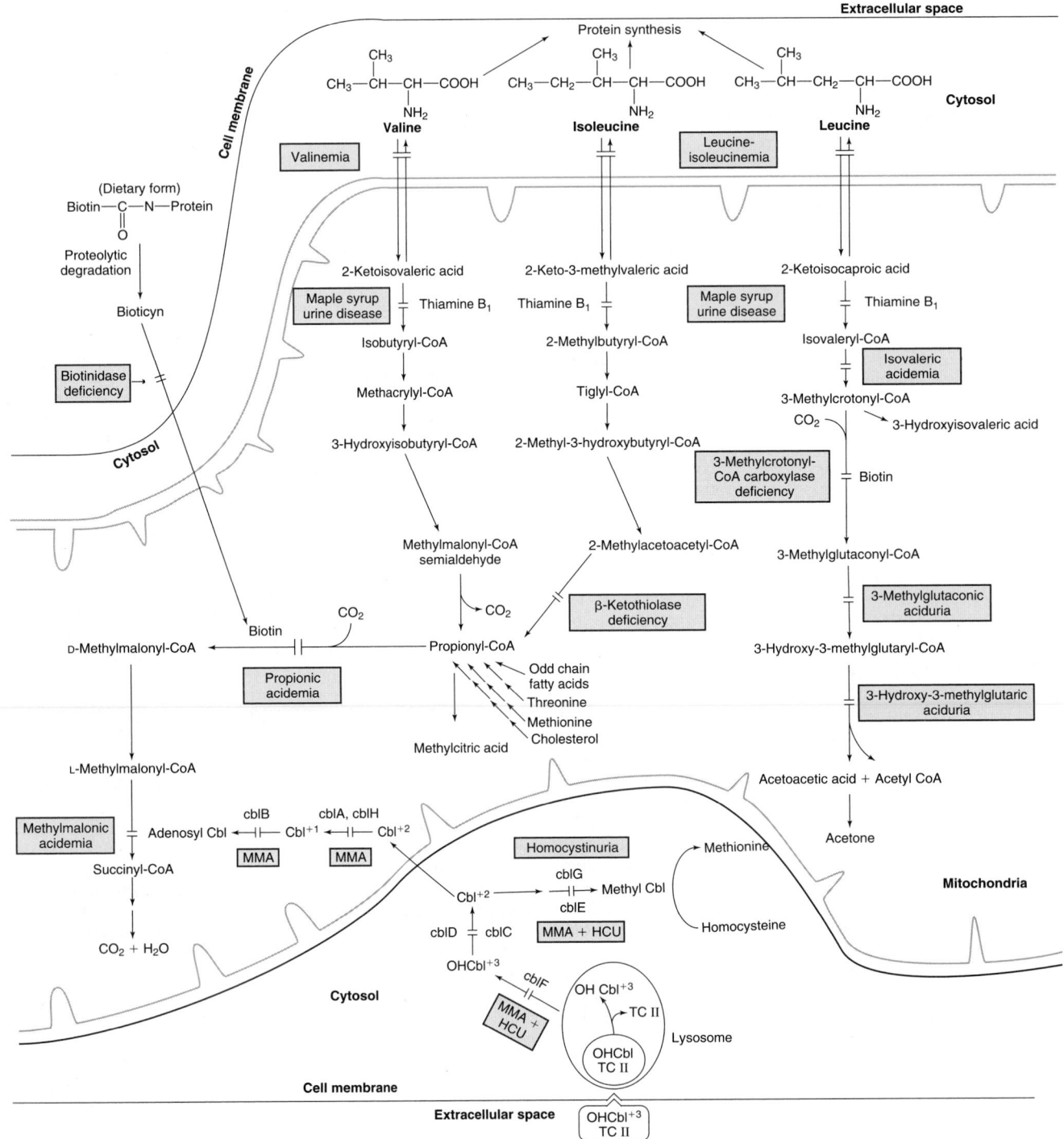

FIGURE 74–5. Pathways in the metabolism of the branched-chain amino acids, biotin, and vitamin B_{12} (cobalamin). MMA = methylmalonic acidemia; HCU = homocystinuria; Cbl = cobalamin; OHCbl = hydroxycobalamin; cbl = defect in metabolism of cobalamin; TC = transcobalamin.

thiamine, others may require as much as 200 mg/24 hr for at least 3 wk before a favorable response is observed. These patients also require diets deficient in branched-chain amino acids. The enzymatic activity in these patients is 2–40% of normal.

MSUD DUE TO A DEFICIENCY OF E3 SUBUNIT (DIHYDROLIPOYL DEHYDROGENASE). This is a very rare disorder. Patients develop lactic acidosis in addition to signs and symptoms similar to those of intermediate MSUD because the E_3 subunit is also a component of pyruvate dehydrogenase and

α-ketoglutarate dehydrogenase. Progressive neurologic impairment manifested by hypotonia and developmental delay occurs after 2 mo of age. Abnormal movements progress to ataxia. Death may occur in early childhood.

Laboratory findings include persistent lactic acidosis with high levels of plasma lactate, pyruvate, and alanine. Plasma concentrations of branched-chain amino acids are moderately increased. Patients excrete large amounts of lactate, pyruvate, α-glutarate, and the three branched-chain ketoacids in their urine.

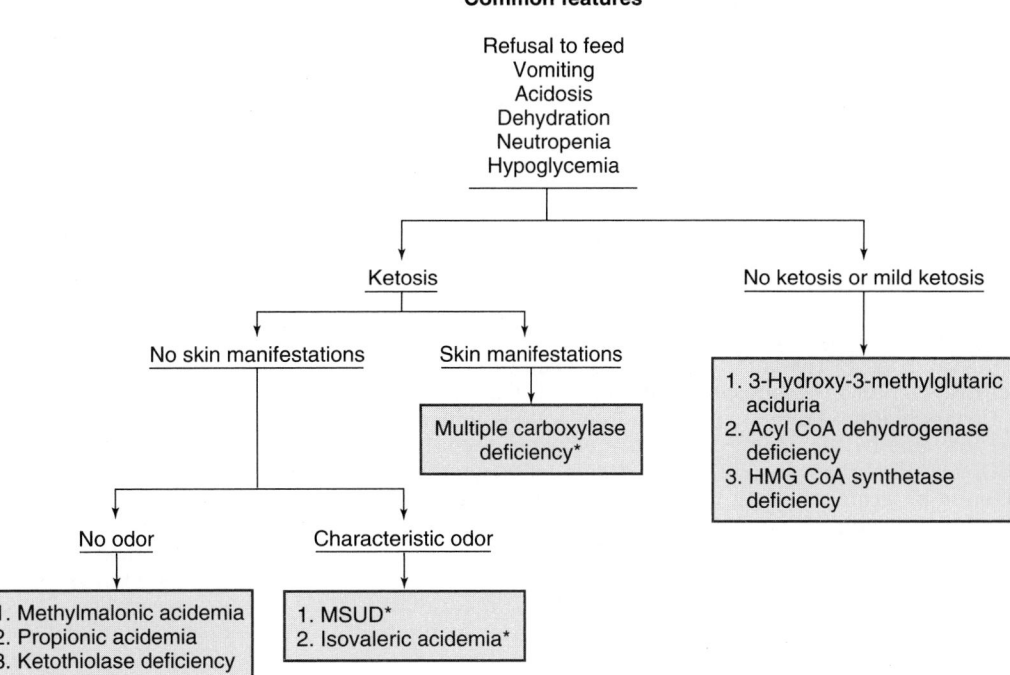

Common features

Refusal to feed
Vomiting
Acidosis
Dehydration
Neutropenia
Hypoglycemia

Ketosis

No ketosis or mild ketosis

No skin manifestations

Skin manifestations

1. 3-Hydroxy-3-methylglutaric aciduria
2. Acyl CoA dehydrogenase deficiency
3. HMG CoA synthetase deficiency

Multiple carboxylase deficiency*

No odor

Characteristic odor

1. Methylmalonic acidemia
2. Propionic acidemia
3. Ketothiolase deficiency

1. MSUD*
2. Isovaleric acidemia*

FIGURE 74–6. Clinical approach to infants with organic acidemia. Asterisks indicate disorders in which patients have a characteristic odor (see text and Table 73–1).

No effective *treatment* is available. Dietary restriction of branched-chain amino acids and treatment with high doses of thiamine, biotin, and lipoic acid has been ineffective.

GENETICS AND PREVALENCE OF MSUD. All forms of MSUD are inherited as an autosomal recessive trait. The enzyme activity can be measured in leukocytes and cultured fibroblasts. The gene for each subunit resides on different chromosomes. The $E_{1\beta}$ gene is on the long arm of chromosome 19; $E_{1\beta}$ is on the short arm of chromosome 6; E_2 is on the short arm of chromosome 1; and E_3 is on the long arm of chromosome 7. Many different disease-causing mutations have been identified in patients with different forms of MSUD. A given phenotype is caused by a variety of genotypes. Patients from different pedigrees with the classic form of MSUD have been shown to have mutations in genes for $E_{1\alpha}$, $E_{1\beta}$, or E_2. Most patients are compound heterozygotes inheriting two different mutant alleles.

The *prevalence* is estimated at 1:185,000. The classic form of MSUD is quite prevalent in the Old Order of Mennonites in the United States and is estimated to be 1:176. Affected patients in this population are homozygous for a specific mutation (Try_{393}-to-Asn) in the $E_{1\alpha}$ subunit gene.

Successful methods for *mass screening* of newborn infants are being used in the United States and other countries. *Prenatal diagnosis* has been accomplished by enzyme assay of the cultured aminocytes, cultured chorionic villi tissue, or direct assay of the chorionic villi samples.

Several successful pregnancies have occurred in women with different forms of MSUD. No ill effects have been observed in the offspring of these patients. Episodes of metabolic decompensations have occurred in the mothers during pregnancy and the postpartum period.

Isovaleric Acidemia. This rare condition is due to the deficiency of isovaleryl CoA dehydrogenase (see Fig. 74–5).

Clinical manifestations in the *acute form* (about 50% of cases) include vomiting and severe acidosis in the first few days of life. Lethargy, convulsions, and coma may ensue, and death may occur if proper therapy is not initiated. The vomiting may be severe enough to suggest pyloric stenosis. The characteristic odor of "sweaty feet" may be present (see Fig. 74–6). Infants

who survive this acute episode will go on to have the chronic intermittent form later on in life. A milder form of the disease *(chronic intermittent form)* also exists in which the first clinical manifestation (vomiting, lethargy, acidosis or coma) may not appear until the infant is a few months or a few years old. In both forms, acute episodes of metabolic decompensations may occur during a catabolic state such as an infection. Both forms of the disease have been observed in the same family.

Laboratory findings during the acute attacks include severe ketoacidosis, neutropenia, thrombocytopenia, and, occasionally, pancytopenia. Hypocalcemia, hyperglycemia, and moderate to severe hyperammonemia may be present in some patients. Increases in plasma ammonia may suggest a defect in the urea cycle. However, in the latter conditions the infant is not acidotic (see Fig. 74–6).

Diagnosis is established by demonstrating marked elevations of isovaleric acid and its metabolites (isovalerylglycine, 3-hydroxyisovaleric acid) in body fluids, especially urine. The main compound in plasma is isovalerylcarnitine, which can be measured even in a few drops of dried blood on a filter paper. Measuring the enzyme in cultured skin fibroblasts confirms the diagnosis.

Treatment of the acute attack is aimed at hydration, reversal of the catabolic state (by providing adequate calories orally or intravenously), correction of metabolic acidosis (by infusing sodium bicarbonate), and removal of the excess isovaleric acid. Because isovalerylglycine has a high urinary clearance, administration of glycine (250 mg/kg/24 hr) is recommended to enhance formation of isovalerylglycine. Carnitine (100 mg/kg/24 hr) also increases removal of isovaleric acid by forming isovalerylcarnitine, which is excreted in the urine. In patients with significant hyperammonemia (blood ammonia > 200 μM), measures that reduce blood ammonia should be employed (see Chapter 74.11). Exchange transfusion and peritoneal dialysis may be needed if the previously mentioned measures fail to induce significant clinical and biochemical improvement. After recovery from the acute attack, the patient should be kept on a low-protein diet (1.0–1.5 g/kg/24 hr) and should be given glycine and carnitine supplements. Pancreatitis (acute or recurrent forms) has been reported in survivors. Normal development can be achieved with early and proper treatment. *Prenatal diagnosis* has been accomplished by measuring isovalerylglycine in amniotic fluid or by enzyme assay in cultured amniocytes. Successful *pregnancy* with favorable outcomes both for the mother and the infant has been reported. Successful methods for *mass screening* of newborn infants are being used in the United States and other countries. Isovaleric acidemia is inherited as an autosomal recessive trait. The gene has been mapped to the long arm of chromosome 15. The gene frequency in the general population is not known.

Multiple Carboxylase Deficiencies (Defects in Utilization of Biotin).

Biotin is a water-soluble vitamin that is a cofactor for all four carboxylase enzymes: pyruvate carboxylase, acetyl CoA carboxylase, propionyl CoA carboxylase, and 3-methylcrotonyl-CoA-carboxylase. The latter two are involved in the metabolic pathways of leucine, isoleucine, and valine (see Fig. 74–5).

Dietary biotin is bound to proteins; free biotin is generated in the intestine by the action of digestive enzymes, by intestinal bacteria and perhaps by biotinidase. The latter enzyme, which is found in serum and most tissues in the body, is also essential for the recycling of biotin in the body by releasing it from the apoenzymes (carboxylases, see Fig. 74–5). Free biotin must form a covalent peptide bond with the apoprotein of the previously mentioned carboxylases to activate them (holocarboxylase). This binding is catalyzed by holocarboxylase synthetase. Deficiencies in this enzyme or in biotinidase result in malfunction of all the carboxylases and in organic acidemia.

HOLOCARBOXYLASE SYNTHETASE DEFICIENCY (MULTIPLE CARBOXYLASE DEFICIENCY—INFANTILE OR EARLY FORM). Infants with this rare autosomal recessive disorder become symptomatic in the first few weeks of life. Symptoms may appear as early as a few hours after birth to 21 mo of age. *Clinically,* the affected infants who seem normal at birth develop breathing difficulties (tachypnea and apnea) shortly after birth. Feeding problems, vomiting, and hypotonia are also commonly present. If the condition remains untreated, a generalized erythematous rash with exfoliation and alopecia (partial or total), failure to thrive, irritability, seizures, lethargy, and even coma may occur. Developmental delay is common. Immune deficiency manifests as susceptibility to infection. The urine may have a peculiar odor, which has been described as similar to tomcat urine. The rash, when present, differentiates this condition from other organic acidemias (see Fig. 74–6).

Laboratory findings include metabolic acidosis, ketosis, hyperammonemia, and the presence of a variety of organic acids, which include lactic acid, propionic acid, 3-methylcrotonic acid, 3-methylcrotonylglycine, methylcitrate, and 3-hydroxyisovaleric acid in body fluids. *Diagnosis* is confirmed by the enzyme assay in lymphocytes or cultured fibroblasts. The mutant enzyme usually has an increased K_m value for biotin. Enzyme activity may be restored by the administration of large doses of biotin.

Treatment with biotin (10 mg/day orally) usually results in an improvement in clinical manifestations and may normalize the biochemical abnormalities. Early diagnosis and treatment are critical to prevent irreversible neurologic damage. In some patients, however, complete resolution may not be achieved even with large doses (up to 80 mg/day) of biotin.

The gene for holocarboxylase synthetase is located on the long arm of chromosome 21, and multiple disease-causing mutations have been identified in different families. All reported cases are compound heterozygotes inheriting two different mutant alleles. Prenatal diagnosis has been accomplished by assaying enzyme activity in cultured amniotic cells and by measurement of intermediate metabolites (3-hydroxyisovalerate and methylcitrate) in amniotic fluid. Two pregnant mothers who had previous offspring with holocarboxylase synthetase deficiency have been treated with biotin late in pregnancy (23 and 34 wk of gestation). Affected infants were normal at birth but the efficacy of the treatment and the outcome remain unclear.

BIOTINIDASE DEFICIENCY (MULTIPLE CARBOXYLASE DEFICIENCY-JUVENILE OR LATE FORM). The absence of biotinidase results in biotin deficiency. The prevalence of this autosomal recessive trait is estimated at 1 in 60,000.

Infants with this deficiency may develop *clinical manifestations* similar to those seen in infants with holocarboxylase synthetase deficiency, but, unlike the latter, symptoms may appear later, when the child is several months or several years old; symptoms may develop as early as 1 wk of age. The term "late form" does not apply to all cases and can be misleading. The delay is presumably because of the presence of sufficient free biotin derived from the mother or the diet. Atopic or seborrheic dermatitis, alopecia, ataxia, myoclonic seizures, hypotonia, developmental delay, sensorineural hearing loss, and immunodeficiency (from T-cell abnormalities) may occur. Children with intractable seborrheic dermatitis may have partial (15–30% activity) deficiency of the enzyme; these children are otherwise asymptomatic, and their dermatitis was resolved with biotin therapy. Asymptomatic children and adults with this enzyme deficiency have been identified in screening programs. Most of these individuals have been shown to have partial deficiency of the enzyme activity.

Laboratory findings and the pattern of organic acids in body fluids resemble those associated with holocarboxylase synthetase deficiency (see earlier). *Diagnosis* can be established by measurement of the enzyme activity in the serum. A simplified method for mass screening of newborn infants is in use in several states in the United States and around the world.

Treatment with free biotin (5–20 mg/24 hr) results in a dramatic clinical and biochemical response. Treatment with biotin is also suggested for individuals with partial biotinidase deficiency.

The gene for biotinidase is located on the short arm of chromosome 3 and several disease-causing mutations have been identified in different families. *Prenatal diagnosis* is possible by the measurement of the enzyme activity in the amniotic cells or by identification of the mutant gene.

MULTIPLE CARBOXYLASE DEFICIENCY DUE TO DIETARY BIOTIN DEFICIENCY. Acquired deficiency of biotin may occur in infants receiving total parenteral nutrition without added biotin, in patients receiving prolonged anticonvulsant drugs (phenytoin, primidone, carbamazepine), or in children with short gut syndrome or chronic diarrhea who are receiving formulas low in biotin. Excessive ingestion of raw eggs may also cause biotin deficiency because the protein avidin in egg white binds biotin and makes it unavailable for absorption. Infants with biotin deficiency develop dermatitis, alopecia, and candidal skin infections.

Isolated 3-Methylcrotonyl-CoA Carboxylase Deficiency.

This enzyme is one of the four carboxylase enzymes in the body that requires biotin as a cofactor (see Fig. 74–5). An isolated deficiency of this enzyme must be differentiated from disorders of biotin metabolism (multiple carboxylase deficiency), which cause diminished activity of all four carboxylases. 3-Methylerotonyl-CoA carboxylase is a heteromeric enzyme consisting of α (biotin-containing) and β subunits. The gene for β subunit *(MCCA)* is located on the long arm of chromosome 3q25-27 and that for the β subunit *(MCCB)* is mapped to the long arm of chromosome 5q12-13. Mutation in either of these genes may result in the deficiency of the enzyme activity. Similar phenotype may be caused by different genotype. Several disease-causing mutations in either gene have been identified in different families.

Clinical manifestations are highly variable, ranging from fatal neonatal onset with acidosis, severe hypotonia and seizures, to asymptomatic adults. Typically, affected infants who have been seemingly normal develop an acute episode of vomiting, hypotonia, lethargy, and convulsions after a minor infection. Death may occur during the acute episode.

Laboratory findings during acute episodes include mild to moderate acidosis, ketosis, severe hypoglycemia, hyperammonemia, and elevated serum levels of liver transaminases. Large amounts of 3-hydroxyisovaleric acid and 3-methylcrotonylglycine are found in the urine. Urinary excretion of 3-methylcrotonic acid is not usually increased in this condition because the accumulated 3-methylcrotonyl CoA is converted to 3-hydroxyisovaleric acid. Severe secondary carnitine deficiency is common. The condition should be differentiated biochemically from multiple carboxylase deficiency (see earlier) in which lactic acid and metabolites of propionic acid are present in body fluids in addition to 3-hydroxyisovaleric acid. *Diagnosis* may be confirmed by measurement of the enzyme activity in cultured fibroblasts. Documentation of normal activities of other carboxylases is necessary for definitive diagnosis.

Aggressive *treatment* of acute episodes with hydration, intravenous infusion of glucose, and alkali is recommended. These patients are unresponsive to biotin therapy. Long-term treatment includes a diet restricted in leucine in conjunction with the oral administration of carnitine (75–100 mg/kg/24 hr) and the prevention of catabolic states. Normal growth and development are expected in these patients. The condition is inherited as an autosomal recessive trait.

Screening programs using tandem mass spectrometry have identified an unexpectedly high number of infants with 3-methylcrotonyl CoA carboxylase deficiencies, suggesting that this condition may be the most common organic acidemia.

3-Methylglutaconic Aciduria. At least three inherited conditions are known to be associated with excessive excretion of 3-methylglutaconic acid in the urine. Deficiency of the enzyme 3-methylglutaconyl CoA hydratase (see Fig. 74–5) is present in type I. In the other two conditions the enzyme activity is normal despite a modest 3-methylglutaconic aciduria.

3-METHYLGLUTACONIC ACIDURIA TYPE I (3-METHYLGLUTACONYL COA HYDRATASE DEFICIENCY) (see Fig. 74–5). This rare autosomal recessive condition is manifested by speech retardation, mild psychomotor delay, and the development of metabolic acidosis during a catabolic state. Patients excrete large amounts of 3-methylglutaconic acid and moderate amounts of 3-hydroxyisovaleric and 3-methylglutaric acids. Deficiency of 3-methylglutaconyl CoA hydratase has been shown in cultured fibroblasts and lymphoblasts. *Treatment* with a low protein diet has been suggested. Beneficial effects of this therapy on the clinical course of the disease are doubtful. Administration of L-carnitine has resulted in clinical improvement in one patient.

3-METHYLGLUTACONIC ACIDURIA TYPE II (X-LINKED CARDIOMYOPATHY, NEUTROPENIA, GROWTH RETARDATION, AND 3-METHYLGLUTACONIC ACIDURIA WITH NORMAL 3-METHYLGLUTACONYL COA HYDRATASE, BARTH SYNDROME). Over 30 male patients with this condition have been reported. *Clinical manifestations*, which usually occur shortly after birth, include dilated cardiomyopathy (manifested as respiratory distress and heart failure), hypotonia, growth retardation, and moderate to severe neutropenia. Mild lactic aciduria and/or hypoglycemia are seen in some patients. If patients survive infancy, relative improvement may occur with advancing age. Cognitive development is usually normal despite delayed motor function.

Laboratory findings include mild to moderate increases in urinary excretion of 3-methylglutaconic, 3-methylglutaric, and 2-ethylhydracrylic acids. Neutropenia is a common finding. Lactic acidosis, hypoglycemia, and abnormal mitochondrial ultrastructure are noted in some patients. Unlike 3-methylglutaconic aciduria type I, urinary excretion of 3-hydroxyisovaleric acid is not elevated.

The condition is inherited as an X-linked recessive trait. The gene has been mapped to the long arm of chromosome X.

The activity of the enzyme 3-methylglutaconyl CoA hydratase is normal. The reason for the increased excretion of the above organic acids is not yet understood. No effective *treatment* is available.

3-METHYLGLUTACONIC ACIDURIA TYPE III (COSTEFF OPTIC ATROPHY SYNDROME). *Clinical manifestations* in these patients include early-onset optic atrophy and later development of choreoathetoid movements, spasticity, ataxia, dysarthria, and mild developmental delay. All reported patients except one were Iraqi Jews living in Israel. These patients excrete moderate amounts of 3-methylglutaconic and 3-methylglutaric acids. The reason for the increased excretion of these organic acids has not been elucidated. Activity of the enzyme 3-methylglutaconyl CoA hydratase has been normal. The condition is inherited as an autosomal recessive trait. The gene for this condition (*OPA3*) is mapped to the long arm of chromosome 19q13.2-13.3. No effective *treatment* is available.

β-Ketothiolase Deficiency (Mitochondrial Acetoacetyl-CoA Thiolase Deficiency). This reversible mitochondrial enzyme cleaves 2-methylacetoacetyl CoA (see Fig. 74–5) or acetoacetyl CoA in one direction and synthesizes these compounds in a reverse action (Fig. 74–7).

Clinical manifestations are quite variable, ranging from an asymptomatic course in an adult to severe episodes of acidosis starting in the 1st yr of life. These children have intermittent episodes of unexplained ketosis and acidosis. These episodes usually occur after an intercurrent infection and respond quickly to intravenous fluids and bicarbonate therapy. Mild to moderate hyperammonemia may also be present during attacks. Both hypoglycemia and hyperglycemia have been reported in isolated cases. The child may be completely asymptomatic between episodes and may tolerate a normal protein diet well. Mental development is normal in most children. The episodes may be misdiagnosed as salicylate poisoning because of the similarity of clinical findings and the interference of elevated blood levels of acetoacetate with the colorimetric assay for salicylate.

Laboratory findings during the acute attack include acidosis, ketosis, and hyperammonemia. The urine contains large amounts of 2-methylacetoacetate and its decarboxylation product, butanone, 2-methyl-3-hydroxybutyrate. Lower concentrations of these urinary metabolites persist during the seemingly well periods. Mild hyperglycinemia may also be present. The clinical and biochemical findings should be differentiated from those seen with propionic and methylmalonic acidemias (see later). *Diagnosis* may be established by assay of the enzyme in cultured fibroblasts.

Treatment of acute episodes includes hydration and infusion of bicarbonate to correct the acidosis; a 10% glucose solution with the appropriate electrolytes and intravenous lipids may be used to minimize the catabolic state. Restriction of protein intake (1–2 g/kg/24 hr) is recommended for long-term therapy. Oral L-carnitine (50–100 mg/kg/24 hr) is also recommended to prevent possible secondary carnitine deficiency. Long-term *prognosis* for achieving normal life seems very favorable. Three patients graduated from high school and one has attended college. All patients continued to have abnormal metabolites in body fluids. Successful pregnancy with normal outcomes for both mother and infant has been reported.

The pathogenesis of ketosis in this condition is not adequately explained because, in this enzyme deficiency, one expects impaired ketone formation (see Fig. 74–7). It is postulated that excess acetoacetyl CoA produced from other sources is used as a substrate for 3-HMG-CoA synthesis in the liver.

This condition is inherited as an autosomal recessive trait and may be more prevalent than has been appreciated. The gene for this enzyme (T$_2$) is located on the long arm of chromosome 11q22.3-23.1.

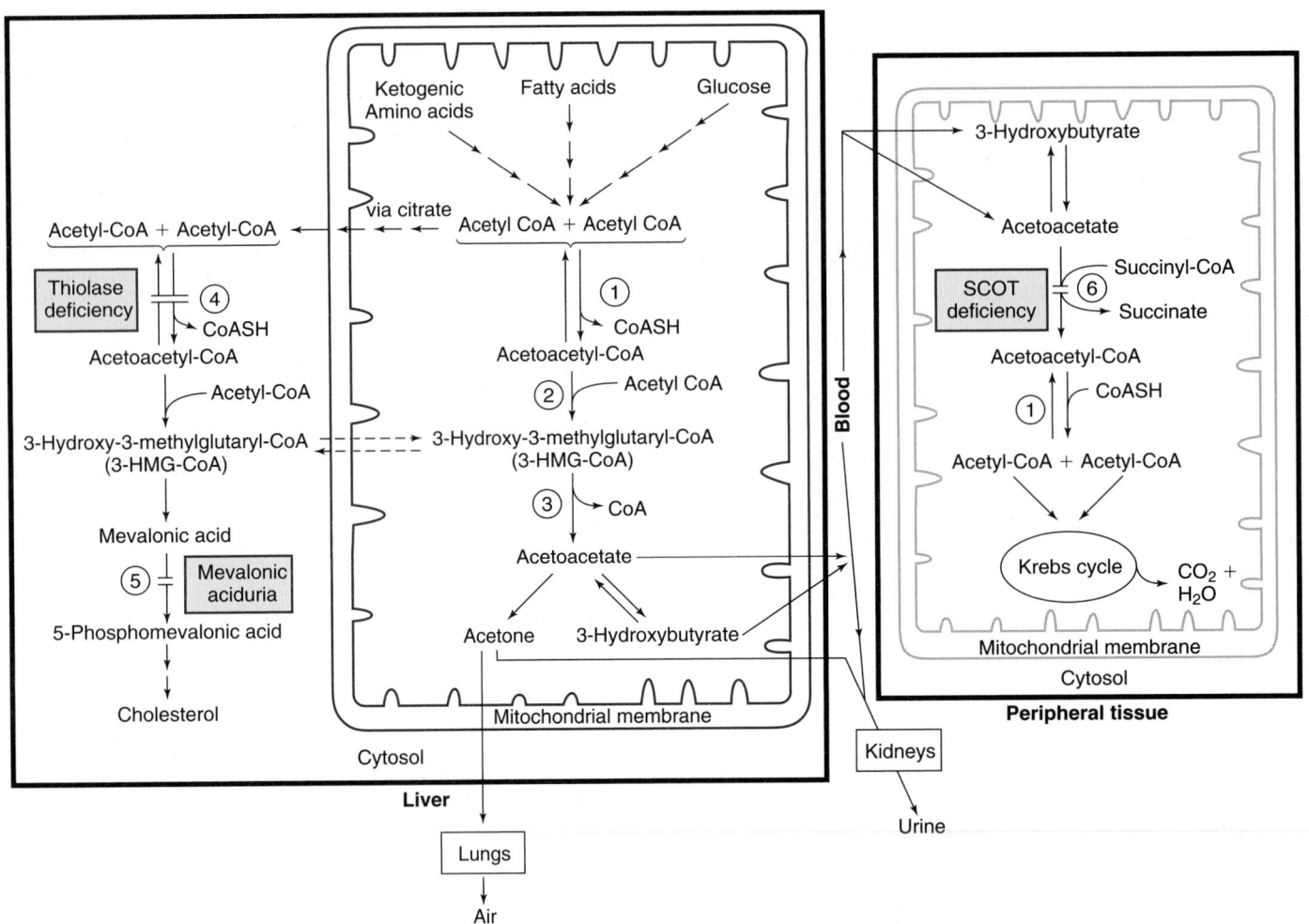

FIGURE 74–7. Formation (liver) and metabolism (peripheral tissues) of ketone bodies and cholesterol synthesis. **Enzymes:** (1) mitochondrial acetoacetyl-CoA thiolase; (2) HMG-CoA synthase; (3) HMG-CoA lyase; (4) cytosolic acetoacetyl-CoA-thiolase; (5) mevalonic kinase; (6) succinyl-CoA; 3-ketoacid CoA transferase (SCOT).

Cystosolic Acetoacetyl CoA Thiolase Deficiency. This enzyme catalyzes the cytosolic production of acetoacetyl CoA from 2 moles of acetyl CoA (see Fig. 74–7). Cytosolic acetoacetyl CoA is the precursor of hepatic cholesterol synthesis. Cytosolic acetoacetyl CoA thiolase is a completely different enzyme from that of mitochondrial thiolase (see earlier and Fig. 74–5). *Clinical manifestations* in patients with this rare enzyme deficiency are similar to those in patients with mevalonic acidemia (see later). Severe progressive developmental delay, hypotonia, and choreoathetoid movements develop in the first few months of life. *Laboratory findings* are nonspecific; elevated levels of lactate, pyruvate, acetoacetate, and 3-hydroxybutyrate may be found in blood and urine. One patient had normal levels of acetoacetate and 3-hydroxybutyrate. *Diagnosis* can be established by demonstrating a deficiency in cytosolic thiolase activity in liver biopsy or in cultured fibroblasts. No effective *treatment* is available. The gene for this condition is mapped to the long arm of chromosome 6q25.3-q26.

Mitochondrial 3-Hydroxy 3-Methylglutaryl-CoA (3-HMG-CoA) Synthase Deficiency. This enzyme catalyzes synthesis of 3-HMG-CoA from acetoacetyl CoA in the mitochondria. This is a critical step in ketone body synthesis in the liver (see Fig. 74–7). Only two unrelated patients with deficiency of this enzyme have been reported. Hypoketotic hypoglycemic episodes occurred in one patient at age 18 mo and in the other at age 6 yr. Both children

were asymptomatic before the episode and are normal afterward except for mild hepatomegaly with fatty infiltration. Laboratory findings were nonspecific; increases in medium-chain and short-chain dicarboxylic acids are found in the urine.

Treatment consisted of provision of adequate calories and avoidance of prolonged periods of fasting. No dietary protein restriction is needed.

The condition is presumably inherited as an autosomal recessive trait. The gene for this condition is located on the short arm of chromosome 1, and different mutations have been identified in the two families. The condition should be considered in any child with fasting hypoglycemia and is perhaps more common than appreciated.

3-Hydroxy-3-Methylglutaric Aciduria. This condition is due to a deficiency of 3-hydroxy-3-methylglutaryl (3-HMG) CoA lyase (see Fig. 74–5). This enzyme catalyzes the conversion of 3-HMG CoA to acetoacetate and is a rate-limiting enzyme for ketogenesis (see Fig. 74–7). *Clinically*, over 60% of patients become symptomatic between 3 and 11 mo of age, whereas about 30% develop symptoms in the first few days of life. One child remained asymptomatic until 15 yr of age. Episodes of vomiting, severe hypoglycemia, hypotonia, acidosis with mild or no ketosis, and dehydration may rapidly lead to lethargy, ataxia, and coma. These episodes often occur during a catabolic state such as fasting or an intercurrent infection. Hepatomegaly is common.

These manifestations may be mistaken for Reye syndrome or medium-chain acyl CoA dehydrogenase (MCAD) deficiency. Patients are usually clinically asymptomatic between the attacks; one patient died of cardiomyopathy at age 7 mo. Development is usually normal, but mental retardation and seizure with MRI abnormalities of white matter have been observed in patients with prolonged episodes of hypoglycemia.

Laboratory findings include hypoglycemia, moderate to severe hyperammonemia, and acidosis. There is mild or no ketosis (see Fig. 74–7 for the explanation). Urinary excretion of 3-hydroxy-3-methylglutaric acid and other proximal intermediate metabolites of leucine catabolism (3-methylglutaconic acid and 3-hydroxy-isovaleric acid) are markedly increased. These organic acids are excreted in the urine as carnitine conjugates resulting in secondary carnitine deficiency. Glutaric and adipic acids may also be increased in urine during acute attacks. *Diagnosis* may be confirmed by enzyme assay in cultured fibroblasts, leukocytes, or liver specimens. *Prenatal diagnosis* is possible with an assay of the enzyme in cultured amniocytes or in a chorionic villi biopsy.

Treatment of acute episodes includes hydration, infusion of glucose to control hypoglycemia, provision of adequate calories, and administration of bicarbonate to correct acidosis. Hyperammonemia should be treated promptly (see Chapter 74.11). Exchange transfusion and peritoneal dialysis may be required in patients with severe hyperammonemia. Restriction of protein and fat intake is recommended for long-term management. Oral administration of L-carnitine (50–100 mg/kg/24 hr, orally) prevents secondary carnitine deficiency. Prolonged fasting should be avoided. One child died after routine immunization. The condition is inherited as an autosomal recessive trait. The gene for 3-HMG-CoA lyase resides on the short arm of chromosome 1 and several disease-causing mutations have been identified in different families. The gene defect appears to be more common in the Arabic population, especially in Saudi Arabia.

Succinyl CoA: 3-Ketoacid CoA Transferase (SCOT) Deficiency.

This enzyme is necessary for the metabolism of ketone bodies (acetoacetate and 3-hydroxybutyrate) in peripheral tissue (see Fig. 74–7). A deficiency of this enzyme results in the underutilization and accumulation of ketone bodies and ketoacidosis. Only a few patients with SCOT deficiency have been reported; the condition may not be rare because many cases are undiagnosed.

The presentation is an acute episode of unexplained severe ketoacidosis in an infant who had been growing and developing normally. About half of the patients present in the 1st wk of life and in all before 2 yr. The acute episode is often precipitated by an intercurrent infection or a catabolic state. Death may occur during these episodes. A chronic subclinical ketosis usually persists between the attacks. Development is usually normal.

Laboratory findings during the acute episode are nonspecific and include metabolic acidosis and ketonuria with high levels of acetoacetate and 3-hydroxybutyrate in blood and urine. No other organic acids are found in the blood or urine. Blood glucose levels are usually normal, but hypoglycemia has been reported in two newborn infants with severe ketoacidosis. Plasma amino acids are usually normal. *Diagnosis* can be established by demonstrating a deficiency of enzyme activity in cultured fibroblasts.

Treatment of acute episodes consists of hydration, correction of acidosis, and the provision of a diet adequate in calories. Long-term treatment with a high carbohydrate diet and avoidance of catabolic states is recommended. *This condition should be considered in any infant with unexplained bouts of ketoacidosis.* The condition is inherited as an autosomal recessive trait. The gene for this enzyme is located on the short arm of chromosome 5, and a limited number of disease-causing mutations have been found in different families.

Mevalonic Aciduria.

Mevalonic acid, an intermediate metabolite of cholesterol synthesis, is converted to 5-phosphomevalonic acid by the action of the enzyme mevalonate kinase (see Fig. 74–7). Based on the severity of clinical manifestations, two forms of this condition have been recognized.

MEVALONIC ACIDURIA, SEVERE FORM. *Clinical manifestations* include mental retardation, failure to thrive, growth retardation, hypotonia, ataxia, hepatosplenomegaly, cataracts, and facial dysmorphism (dolichocephaly, frontal bossing, low-set ears, downward slanting of the eyes, and long eyelashes). Recurrent crises, characterized by fever, vomiting, diarrhea, arthralgia, edema, and morbilliform rash have been observed in all patients. These episodes last 4–5 days and recur up to 25 times per year. Death may occur during these crises.

Laboratory findings include marked elevation of mevalonic acid in urine; the concentration may be as high as 56,000 µmol/mol of creatinine (normal <0.3). Plasma levels of mevalonic acid are also greatly increased (as high as 54 µmol/dL; normal <0.004). This is the only abnormal organic acid found in these patients. The level of mevalonic acid tends to correlate with the severity of the condition and increases during crises. Serum cholesterol concentration is normal or mildly decreased. Serum concentration of creatine kinase (CK) is markedly increased. Sedimentation rate and serum leukotriene-4 are increased during the crises. Serial examination of the brain by MRI reveals progressive atrophy of the cerebellum.

Diagnosis may be confirmed by assay of mevalonate kinase activity in lymphocytes or in cultured fibroblasts. No effective therapy is available. *Treatment* with high doses of prednisone (2 mg/kg/24 hr) causes improvement of the acute crises. The condition is inherited as an autosomal recessive trait. *Prenatal diagnosis* is possible by measurement of mevalonic acid in the amniotic fluid or by assay of the enzyme activity in cultured amniocytes or chorionic villi samples. The gene for mevalonate kinase (MVK) is on the long arm of chromosome 12.

PERIODIC FEVER WITH HYPERGAMMAGLOBULINE-MIA D, MEVALONIC ACIDURIA MILD FORM. Periodic fever with hypergammaglobulinemia D is characterized by periodic bouts of fever associated with abdominal pain, arthralgia, arthritis, lymphadenopathy, and rash. The episodes, which may start in early infancy, occur every 1–2 mo and usually last 2–7 days. Mild to moderate mevalonic aciduria is present during the acute attack and normalizes during the well periods. The serum level of IgD is increased in most patients. The condition is inherited as an autosomal recessive trait with mutations in the gene for mevalonic aciduria (MVK). Although, mutations in most families are different from those with severe forms of mevalonic aciduria, identical mutations have been reported in both types. The discrepancy between genotype and phenotype remains unexplained.

Propionic Acidemia (Propionyl CoA Carboxylase Deficiency).

Propionic acid is an intermediate metabolite of isoleucine, valine, threonine, methionine, odd-chain fatty acids, and cholesterol catabolism. It is normally carboxylated to methylmalonic acid by the mitochondrial enzyme propionyl CoA carboxylase, which requires biotin as a cofactor (see Fig. 74–5). The enzyme is composed of two nonidentical subunits, α and β. Biotin is bound to the α subunit.

Clinical findings are nonspecific. The majority of patients develop symptoms in the first few days or weeks of life. Poor feeding, vomiting, hypotonia, lethargy, dehydration, and clinical signs of severe ketoacidosis progress rapidly to coma and death. Seizures occur in about 30% of affected infants. If an infant survives the first attack, similar episodes may occur during an intercurrent infection or constipation or after ingestion of a high-protein diet. Moderate to severe mental retardation and neurologic abnormalities such as dystonia, choreoathetosis, tremor, and pyramidal signs are common sequelae in the older survivors. Less frequently, the older infant may have mental retardation without acute attacks of ketosis. Some affected children may have episodes of unexplained severe ketoacidosis separated by periods of seemingly normal health. The severity of clinical manifestations may also be variable within a family; in one kindred, a brother was diagnosed at 5 yr of age whereas his 13-yr-old sister, with the same level of enzyme deficiency, was asymptomatic. The reason for this wide variation in the phenotype remains unclear.

Laboratory findings during the acute attack include severe metabolic acidosis with a large anion gap, ketosis, neutropenia, thrombocytopenia, and hypoglycemia. Moderate to severe hyperammonemia is common, and plasma ammonia concentrations usually correlate with the severity. Measurement of plasma ammonia is especially helpful in planning therapeutic strategy during episodes of exacerbation in a patient whose diagnosis has been established. Hyperammonemia is believed to be caused by inhibition of carbamoyl phosphate synthetase (CPS I) by the organic acid. Hyperglycinemia is common in patients with propionic acidemia. Elevations in plasma and urinary levels of glycine have also been observed in patients with methylmalonic acidemia. These disorders were collectively referred to as **ketotic hyperglycinemia** before the specific enzyme deficiencies were elucidated. Concentrations of propionic acid and methylcitric acid (presumably made by the condensation of propionyl CoA with oxaloacetic acid) are markedly elevated in the plasma and urine of infants with propionic acidemia. 3-Hydroxypropionic acid, propionylglycine, and other intermediate metabolites of isoleucine catabolism, such as tiglic acid, tiglyglycine, and 2-methyloacetoacetic acid, are also found in urine. Moderate elevations in blood levels of ammonia, glycine, and the previously mentioned organic acids are usually present between the acute attacks. CT and MRI of the brain may reveal evidence of cerebral atrophy, demyelination, and abnormalities in globus pallidus and basal ganglia. These findings represent infarctions caused by a cerebrovascular accident, which may occur during acute episode of metabolic decompensations. This complication (metabolic stroke) also may occur in patients with other organic acidemias and is a major cause of neurologic sequelae.

The *diagnosis* of propionic acidemia should be differentiated from multiple carboxylase deficiencies (see earlier description and Fig. 74–6). The latter infants may have skin manifestations and excrete large amounts of lactic acid, 3-methylcrotonic acid, and 3-hydroxyisovaleric acid in addition to propionic acid. The presence of hyperammonemia may suggest a genetic defect in the urea cycle enzymes. Infants with defects in the urea cycle are usually not acidotic (see Fig. 73–1). Definitive diagnosis of propionic acidemia can be established by measuring the enzyme activity in leukocytes or cultured fibroblasts.

Treatment of acute attacks includes hydration, correction of acidosis, and prevention of the catabolic state by provision of adequate calories through parenteral hyperalimentation. Minimal amounts of protein (0.25 g/kg/24 hr), preferably a protein deficient in propionate precursors, should be provided in the hyperalimentation fluid very early in the course of treatment. To curtail the possible production of propionic acid by intestinal bacteria, sterilization of the intestinal tract flora by antibiotics (oral neomycin or metronidazole) should be promptly initiated. Constipation should also be treated. Patients with propionic acidemia may develop carnitine deficiency, presumably as a result of urinary loss of propionylcarnitine formed from the accumulated organic acid. Administration of L-carnitine (50–100 mg/kg/24 hr orally or 10 mg/kg/24h intravenously) normalizes fatty acid oxidation and improves acidosis. In patients with concomitant hyperammonemia, measures to reduce blood ammonia should be employed (see Chapter 74.11). Very ill patients with severe acidosis and hyperammonemia require peritoneal dialysis or hemodialysis to remove ammonia and other toxic compounds. Although infants with true propionic acidemia are rarely responsive to biotin, this compound should be administered (10 mg/24 hr orally) to all infants during the first attack and until the diagnosis is established.

Long-term treatment consists of a low-protein diet (1.0–1.5 g/kg/24 hr) and administration of L-carnitine (50–100 mg/kg/24 hr orally). Synthetic proteins deficient in propionate precursors (isoleucine, valine, methionine, and threonine) may be used to increase the amount of dietary protein (to 1.5–2.0 g/kg/24 hr) while causing minimal change in propionate production. However, excessive supplementation with these proteins may cause a deficiency of the essential amino acids. To avoid this problem, natural proteins should comprise most of the dietary protein (50–75%). Some patients require chronic alkaline therapy to correct chronic acidosis. The concentration of ammonia in the blood usually normalizes between attacks, and chronic treatment of hyperammonemia is not usually needed. Catabolic states that may trigger acute attacks (e.g., infections and constipation) should be treated promptly and aggressively. Close monitoring of blood pH, amino acids, urinary content of propionate and its metabolites, and growth parameters is necessary to ensure the proper balance of the diet and the success of therapy.

Long-term *prognosis* is guarded. Death may occur during an acute attack. Normal psychomotor development is possible, but most children manifest some degree of permanent neurodevelopmental deficit such as dystonia, chorea, and pyramidal signs despite adequate therapy. These neurologic findings may be sequelae of a metabolic stroke occurring during an acute decompensation.

Prenatal diagnosis has been accomplished by measuring the enzyme activity in cultured amniotic cells and in samples of uncultured chorionic villi and by measurement of methylcitrate in amniotic fluid. Identification of the mutant gene in the family and in the fetus should provide a more precise method for prenatal DNA diagnosis.

The prevalence of propionic acidemia, inherited as an autosomal recessive trait, is not known. The gene for the α subunit (PCCA gene) is located on chromosome 13 and that of the β subunit (PCCB gene) is mapped to the long arm of chromosome 3. Mutations in either gene have been identified in different patients.

Methylmalonic Acidemia. Methylmalonic acid, a structural isomer of succinic acid, is normally derived from propionic acid as part of the catabolic pathways of isoleucine, valine, threonine, methionine, cholesterol, and odd-chain fatty acids. Two enzymes are involved in the conversion of D-methylmalonic acid to succinic acid, methylmalonyl CoA racemase (which forms the L-isomer) and methylmalonyl CoA mutase (which converts the L-methylmalonic acid to succinic acid) (see Fig. 74–5). The latter enzyme requires adenosylcobalamin, a metabolite of vitamin B_{12}, as a coenzyme. Deficiency of either the mutase or its coenzyme causes the accumulation of methylmalonic acid and its precursors in body fluids. A deficiency of the racemase has not been confirmed.

At least two forms of mutase apoenzyme deficiencies have been identified. These are designated *mut⁰*, meaning no detectable enzyme activity, and *mut⁻*, indicating residual, although abnormal, mutase activity. The majority of reported patients with methylmalonic acidemia have a deficiency of the mutase apoenzyme (*mut⁰* or *mut⁻*). These patients are not responsive to vitamin B_{12} therapy. In the remaining patients with methylmalonic acidemia the defect resides in the formation of adenosylcobalamin.

DEFECTS IN METABOLISM OF VITAMIN B_{12} (COBALAMIN). Dietary vitamin B_{12} requires intrinsic factor, a glycoprotein secreted by the gastric parietal cells, for absorption in the terminal ileum. It is transported in the blood by haptocorrin

(TCI) and transcobalamin II (TCII). The complex of transcobalamin II-cobalamin (TCII-Cbl) is recognized by a specific receptor on the cell membrane and enters the cell by endocytosis. The TCII-Cbl complex is hydrolyzed in the lysosome, and free cobalamin is released into the cytosol (see Fig. 74–5). The cobalt of the molecule is reduced in the cytosol from three valences (cob[III]alamin) to two (cob[II]alamin) before it enters the mitochondria, where further reduction to cob(I)alamin occurs. The latter compound reacts with adenosine to form adenosylcobalamin (coenzyme for methylmalonyl CoA mutase). The free cobalamin in the cytosol may also undergo a series of poorly understood enzymatic steps to form methylcobalamin (coenzyme for methionine synthase; see Fig. 74–3).

At least eight different defects in the intracellular metabolism of cobalamin have been identified. These are designated *cbl* A through H (*cbl* stands for a defect in any step of cobalamin metabolism). *cbl*A, *cbl*H, and *cbl*B cause methylmalonic acidemia only; *cbl*B is caused by a deficiency of adenosylcobalamin transferase. In patients with *cbl*C, *cbl*D, and *cbl*F defects, synthesis of both adenosylcobalamin and methylcobalamin is impaired, causing homocystinuria in addition to methylmalonic acidemia. The *cbl*E defect and the *cbl*G defect involve only the synthesis of methylcobalamin, resulting in homocystinuria without methylmalonic aciduria but usually with megaloblastic anemia.

Clinical manifestations of patients with methylmalonic acidemia due to *mut⁰, mut⁻, cbl*A, *cbl*B, and *cbl*H are similar. There are wide variations in clinical presentation, ranging from very sick newborn infants to asymptomatic adults, regardless of the nature of the enzymatic defect or the biochemical abnormalities. Lethargy, feeding problems, vomiting, tachypnea (due to acidosis), and hypotonia may develop in the first few days of life and may progress to coma and death if untreated. Infants who survive the first attack may go on to develop similar acute metabolic episodes during a catabolic state (such as infection) or after ingestion of a high-protein diet. Between the acute attacks, the patient commonly continues to exhibit hypotonia and feeding problems with failure to thrive. In some patients the condition may present later in life with hypotonia, failure to thrive, and developmental delay. Asymptomatic patients with typical biochemical abnormalities of methylmalonic acidemia have been reported. The reason for this wide variation in clinical presentation remains unclear. It is important to note that mental development and IQ of patients with methylmalonic acidemia remain within the normal range despite repeated acute attacks and regardless of the nature of the enzyme deficiency. In one series with different forms of the condition developmental retardation was noted only in 47%. One adolescent girl with a *mut⁻* deficiency has an IQ of 129.

The episodic nature of the condition and its biochemical abnormalities may be confused with those of ethylene glycol (antifreeze) ingestion. The peak of propionic acid in the assay has been mistaken as that of ethylene glycol.

Laboratory findings include ketosis, acidosis, anemia, neutropenia, thrombocytopenia, hyperglycinemia, hyperammonemia, hypoglycemia, and the presence of large quantities of methylmalonic acid in body fluids (see Fig. 74–6). Propionic acid and its metabolites 3-hydroxypropionate and methylcitrate are also found in the urine. Hyperammonemia may suggest defects in the urea cycle enzymes. Patients with defects in urea cycle enzymes are not acidotic (see Figs. 73–1 and 74–13). The increase in ammonia in patients with methylmalonic acidemia is believed to be caused by inhibition of carbamyl phosphate synthetase I (CPSI) enzyme by the organic acid.

Diagnosis can be confirmed by measuring propionate incorporation or mutase activity and by performing complementation studies in cultured fibroblasts.

Treatment of acute attacks is similar to that of attacks in patients with propionic acidemia (see earlier), except that large doses (1 mg/24 hr) of vitamin B_{12} are used instead of biotin.

Long-term treatment consists of a low-protein diet (1.0–1.5 g/kg/24 hr) and administration of L-carnitine (50–100 mg/kg/24 hr) and vitamin B_{12} (1 mg/24 hr for patients with defects in vitamin B_{12} metabolism; the dose can be decreased depending on the clinical response). The protein composition of the diet is similar to that prescribed for patients with propionic acidemia. Chronic alkaline therapy is usually required to correct chronic acidosis, especially during infancy and early childhood. Blood levels of ammonia usually normalize between the attacks, and chronic treatment of hyperammonemia is rarely needed. Constipation and stressful situations that may trigger acute attacks (such as infection) should be prevented or treated promptly.

Inadequate oral intake secondary to poor appetite is a common and bothersome complication in long-term management of these patients. Consequently, enteral feeding (through a nasogastric tube or gastrostomy) should be considered early in the course of the treatment. Close monitoring of blood pH, amino acid levels, blood and urinary concentrations of methylmalonate, and growth parameters is necessary to ensure proper balance in the diet and the success of therapy. Glutathione deficiency, responsive to high doses of ascorbate, has been described in one patient. Liver and combined liver and kidney transplantations have been attempted with variable success.

Prognosis depends on the severity of symptoms and the occurrence of complications (see later). In general, patients with mutase apoenzyme deficiency *(mut⁰, mut⁻)* have a less favorable prognosis and those with *cbl*A defect have a better outcome than those with *cbl*B.

The main *complication* is chronic renal failure necessitating renal transplant, which has been reported in a number of older patients with the condition and has been observed in all genetic forms of the condition. Tubulointerstitial nephritis has been documented in some of these patients and is thought to be the major cause of renal failure. The pathogenesis remains unclear.

Infarcts of the brain, especially those of the basal ganglia (globus pallidus) and internal capsule, have been reported in a few patients during an acute episode of metabolic decompensation ("metabolic stroke"). These patients have survived with major extrapyramidal (tremor, dystonia) and pyramidal (paraplegia) sequelae. The pathogenesis of this complication also remains unclear.

Acute and recurrent pancreatitis has been reported in the affected patients as young as 13 mo of age. This complication may account for repeated hospitalizations of these children.

The *prevalence* of the condition is estimated at 1:48,000. Diagnosis has been accomplished by the assay of propionate incorporation in cultured amniotic cells. All defects causing methylmalonic acidemia are inherited as autosomal recessive traits. The gene for the mutase has been mapped to the short arm of chromosome 6, and at least 49 different mutations have been identified, including three common mutation (G717V, E117X, and N219Y). The genes for *cbl*A and *cbl*B defects have been cloned, but the gene for the *cbl*H defect has not yet been identified. Neonates with methylmalonic acidemia and severe diabetes caused by the absence of β cells have been reported and have paternal uniparental isodisomy of chromosome 6.

Successful *pregnancy* with normal outcomes for both the mother and the baby has been reported.

Combined Methylmalonic Aciduria and Homocystinuria (*cbl*C, *cbl*D, and *cbl*F Defects).

Almost 200 patients with methylmalonic acidemia and homocystinuria due to *cbl*C, *cbl*D, and *cbl*F defects (see Figs. 74–3 and 74–5) are reported. The majority has the *cbl*C defect; only two brothers with *cbl*D and six patients with *cbl*F defects have been identified.

Neurologic findings are prominent in patients with *cbl*C and *cbl*D defects. Most patients with the *cbl*C defect present in the first few months of life because of failure to thrive, lethargy, poor feeding, mental retardation, and seizures. However, late-onset defects with sudden development of dementia and myelopathy have been reported. Megaloblastic anemia is a common finding in patients with *cbl*C defect. Mild to moderate increases in concentrations of methylmalonic acid and homocysteine are found in body fluids. However, unlike patients with classic homocystinuria, plasma levels of methionine are low to normal in these defects. Neither hyperammonemia nor hyperglycinemia is observed in these patients. The first two patients with *cbl*F defect were females in whom poor feeding, growth and developmental delay, and persistent stomatitis became manifest in the first 3 wk of life. The first patient did not have megaloblastic anemia and homocystinuria, but both these signs were present in the second infant. Moderate methylmalonic acidemia was present in both infants. One patient was not diagnosed until age 10 yr and had findings suggestive of rheumatoid arthritis, a pigmented skin abnormality, and encephalopathy. Vitamin B$_{12}$ malabsorption is noted in patients with *cbl*F defect.

Experience with *treatment* of patients with *cbl*C, *cbl*D, and *cbl*F defects is limited. Large doses of hydroxycobalamin (1–2 mg/24 hr) in conjunction with betaine (6–9 g/24 hr) produce biochemical improvement with little clinical effect. Unexplained severe hemolytic anemia, hydrocephalus, and congestive heart failure are major complications in patients with *cbl*C defect.

Patients with *cbl*E and *cbl*G defects do not have methylmalonic acidemia (see Chapter 74.3).

74.7 Glycine
Iraj Rezvani

Glycine is a nonessential amino acid synthesized mainly from serine and threonine. The main catabolic pathway requires the complex glycine cleavage enzyme to cleave the first carbon of glycine and convert it to carbon dioxide. The glycine cleavage protein, a mitochondrial multienzyme, is composed of four proteins: P protein, H protein, T protein, and L protein.

Hyperglycinemia. Elevated levels of glycine in body fluids occur in propionic acidemia and methylmalonic acidemia that are collectively referred to as *ketotic hyperglycinemia* because episodes of severe acidosis and ketosis occur. The pathogenesis of hyperglycinemia in these disorders is not fully understood, but inhibition of the glycine cleavage enzyme system by the various organic acids has been shown to occur in some patients. The term *nonketotic hyperglycinemia* is reserved for the clinical condition caused by the genetic deficiency of the glycine cleavage enzyme system (Fig. 74–8). In this condition, hyperglycinemia is present without ketosis.

Nonketotic Hyperglycinemia (NKH). Four forms of NKH have been identified: neonatal, infantile, late onset, and transient.

NEONATAL NKH. This is the most common form of NKH. *Clinical manifestations* develop during the first few days of life

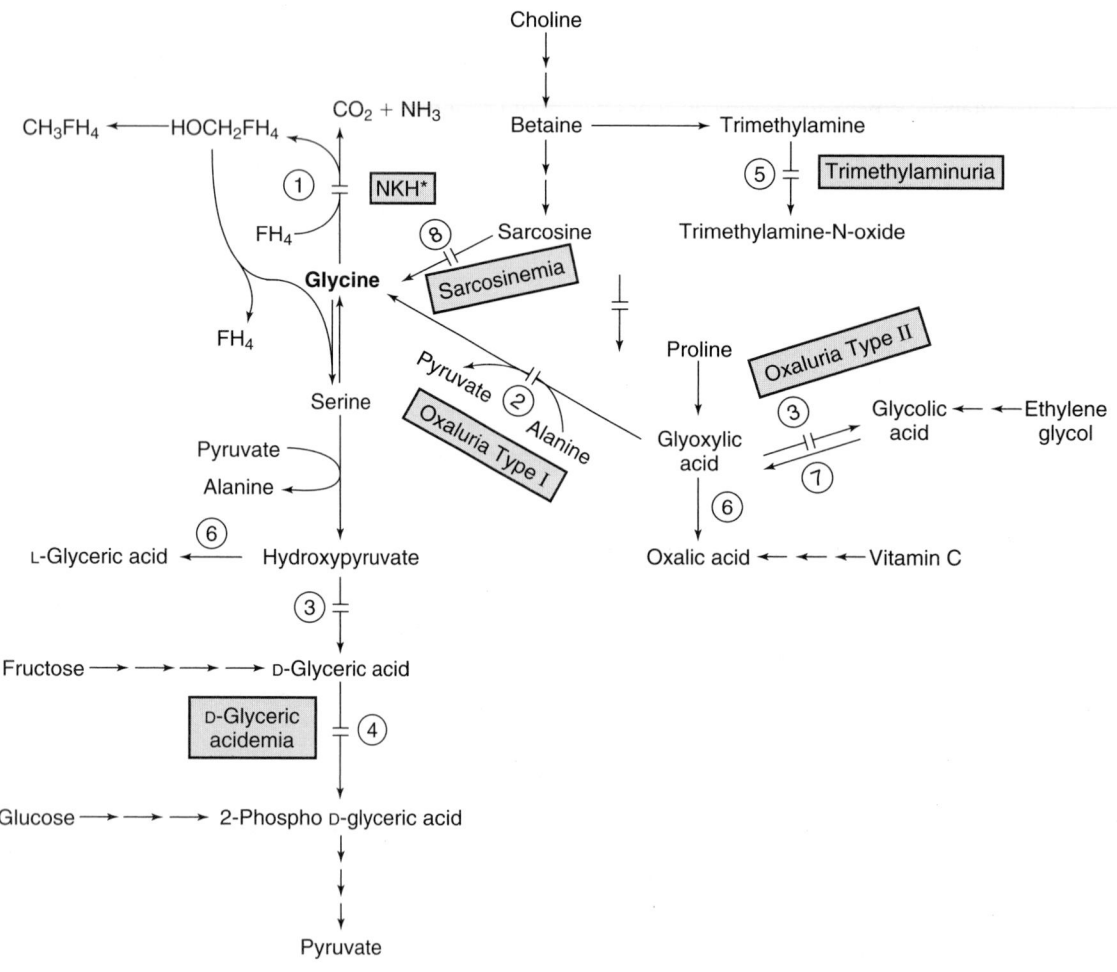

FIGURE 74–8. Pathways in metabolism of glycine and gloxylic acid. **Enzymes:** (1) glycine cleavage enzyme; (2) alanine:glyoxylate aminotransferase; (3) D-glyceric acid dehydrogenase; (4) glycerate kinase; (5) trimethylamine oxidase; (6) lactate dehydrogenase; (7) glycolate oxidase; (8) sarcosine dehydrogenase. NKH* = nonketotic hyperglycinemia; FH$_4$ = tetrahydrofolate.

(between 6 hr to 8 days after birth). Poor feeding, failure to suck, lethargy, and profound hypotonia may progress rapidly to a deep coma, apnea, and death. Convulsions, especially myoclonic seizures and hiccups, are common.

Laboratory findings include moderate to severe hyperglycinemia (as high as eight times normal) and hyperglycinuria. The unequivocal elevation of glycine concentration in the spinal fluid (15–30 times normal) and the high ratio of glycine concentration in spinal fluid to that in plasma (a value greater than 0.08) are diagnostic of NKH. Serum pH is normal; plasma serine levels are usually low.

About 30% of affected infants die despite supportive therapy. Those who survive develop profound psychomotor retardation and intractable seizure disorders (myoclonic and/or grand mal seizures).

INFANTILE NKH. These previously normal infants develop *signs and symptoms* of neonatal NKH (see earlier) after 6 mo of age. Seizures are the common presenting signs. This condition appears to be a milder form; infants usually survive; mental retardation is not as profound as in the neonatal form.

Laboratory findings in these patients are identical to the neonatal form.

LATE-ONSET NKH. This has been reported in a few patients. Progressive spastic paraparesis, optic atrophy, and choreoathetotic movements are the main *clinical manifestations*. Age at onset has been between 2 and 33 yr. Mental development is usually normal, but mild retardation has been reported in three patients. Seizures have occurred in only one patient.

Laboratory findings are similar to, but not as pronounced as in, the neonatal form.

TRANSIENT NKH. This form has been described in six infants. Clinical and laboratory manifestations are indistinguishable from those of the neonatal form. However, by 2 to 8 wk of age, the elevated glycine levels in plasma and cerebrospinal fluid normalize and a complete clinical recovery occurs. Five of these patients had no neurologic abnormalities, but one had severe mental retardation. The etiology of this condition is not known but it is believed to be caused by immaturity of the enzyme system.

All forms of NKH should be differentiated from ketotic hyperglycinemia (see Chapter 74.6), D-glyceric aciduria (see later), and ingestion of valproic acid. The latter compound causes a moderate increase in blood and urinary glycine concentrations. Repeat assays after discontinuation of the drug should establish the diagnosis.

Diagnosis may be established by assay of the enzyme in liver or brain specimens. Enzyme activity in the neonatal form is close to zero, whereas in the other forms some residual activity is present. In over 80% of patients with the neonatal form, the enzyme defect resides in the P protein. The deficit in the remainder of these patients is in the T protein. The enzyme assay in three patients with the infantile and late-onset forms revealed two patients with the defect in the T protein and one in the H protein.

No effective *treatment* is known. Exchange transfusion, dietary restriction of glycine, and administration of sodium benzoate or folate have not altered the neurologic outcome. Drugs that counteract the effect of glycine on neuronal cells, such as strychnine, diazepam, and dextromethorphan have shown some beneficial effects only in patients with the mild forms of the condition.

NKH is inherited as an autosomal recessive trait. The prevalence is not known, but the condition is quite common in northern Finland (1:12,000). The gene for P protein is located on the short arm of chromosome 9. The gene for H and T proteins are mapped to the long arm of chromosome 3. *Prenatal diagnosis* has been accomplished by performing an assay of the enzyme activity in chorionic villi biopsy specimens.

Sarcosinemia. Increased concentrations of sarcosine (*N*-methylglycine) have been observed in both blood and urine, but no consistent clinical picture has been attributed to this metabolic defect. This is a recessively inherited inborn error involving sarcosine dehydrogenase, the enzyme that converts sarcosine to glycine (see Fig. 74–8). The gene for this enzyme is located on the long arm of chromosome 9.

D-Glyceric Aciduria. D-Glyceric acid is an intermediate metabolite of serine and fructose metabolism (see Fig. 74–8). At least two forms of this rare condition have been identified. In one form, clinical manifestations of severe encephalopathy (hypotonia, seizures, and mental and motor deficits) and the laboratory findings of hyperglycinemia and hyperglycinuria were suggestive of nonketotic hyperglycinemia. However, these patients excreted large quantities of D-glyceric acid (this compound is not normally detectable in urine). Enzyme studies indicated a deficiency of glycerate kinase in one patient and decreased activity of D-glyceric dehydrogenase in another.

In the other form, the major findings are persistent metabolic acidosis and developmental delay. This infant excreted large amounts of D-glyceric acid without hyperglycinemia. The enzyme defect in this patient is not known.

No effective therapy is available. Restriction of fructose improved seizures in one patient.

Trimethylaminuria. Trimethylamine is normally produced in the intestine from the breakdown of dietary choline and trimethylamine oxide by bacteria. Eggs and liver are the main sources of choline, and fish is the major source of trimethylamine oxide. Trimethylamine is absorbed and oxidized in the liver by trimethylamine oxidase to trimethylamine oxide, which is odorless, and is excreted in the urine (see Fig. 74–8). Deficiency of this enzyme results in massive excretion of trimethylamine in urine. Several asymptomatic patients with trimethylaminuria have been reported; there is a foul body odor that resembles that of a rotten fish, which may have significant social and psychosocial ramifications. Restriction of fish, eggs, liver, and other sources of choline (such as nuts and grains) in the diet significantly reduces the odor. The gene for trimethylamine oxidase has been mapped to the long arm of chromosome 1.

Hyperoxaluria and Oxalosis. Normally, oxalic acid is derived mostly from oxidation of glyoxylic acid and, to a lesser degree, from oxidation of ascorbic acid (see Fig. 74–8). Glyoxylic acid is formed from the oxidation of glycolic acid in the peroxisomes. The source of glycolic acid remains unclear. Foods containing oxalic acid, such as spinach and rhubarb, are the main exogenous sources of this compound. Oxalic acid cannot be further metabolized in humans and is excreted in the urine as oxalates. Calcium oxalate is relatively insoluble in water and precipitates in tissues (kidneys and joints) if its concentration increases in the body.

Secondary hyperoxaluria has been observed in pyridoxine deficiency (cofactor for alanine-glyoxylate aminotransferase, see Fig. 74–8), after ingestion of ethylene glycol or high doses of vitamin C, after administration of the anesthetic agent methoxyflurane (which oxidizes directly to oxalic acid), and in patients with inflammatory bowel disease or extensive resection of the bowel *(enteric hyperoxaluria)*. Acute, fatal hyperoxaluria may develop after ingestion of plants with a high oxalic acid content, such as sorrel. Precipitation of calcium oxalate in tissues causes hypocalcemia, liver necrosis, renal failure, cardiac arrhythmia, and death. The lethal dose of oxalic acid is estimated to be 5–30 g.

Primary hyperoxaluria is a rare genetic disorder in which large amounts of oxalates accumulate in the body. Two types of primary hyperoxaluria have been identified. The term *oxalosis* refers to deposition of calcium oxalate in parenchymal tissue.

PRIMARY HYPEROXALURIA TYPE I. This rare condition is the most common form of primary hyperoxaluria. It is caused by a deficiency of the peroxisomal enzyme alanine-glyoxylate aminotransferase, which is expressed only in the liver peroxisomes and requires pyridoxine (vitamin B$_6$) as its cofactor. In the absence of this enzyme, glyoxylic acid, which cannot be converted to glycine, is transferred to the cytosol, where it is oxidized to oxalic acid (see Fig. 74–8). It is inherited as an autosomal recessive trait. The gene for this enzyme resides on the long arm of chromosome 2. Several mutations of the gene have been described in patients with this condition. The most common mutation results in the targeting of the enzyme to the mitochondria instead of the peroxisomes. The in vitro enzyme activity in these patients may reach the level found in obligate heterozygotes. However, in vivo function remains defective. About 30% of patients with hyperoxaluria type 1 are estimated to have this defect.

There is a wide variation in the age of presentation. The majority of patients become symptomatic before 5 yr of age. In about 10% of cases symptoms develop before 1 yr of age (neonatal oxaluria). The initial *clinical manifestations* are related to renal stones and nephrocalcinosis. Renal colic and asymptomatic hematuria lead to a gradual deterioration of renal function, manifested by growth retardation and uremia. Most patients die before 20 yr of age from renal failure if the disorder is untreated. Acute arthritis is a rare manifestation and may be misdiagnosed as gout because uric acid is usually elevated in patients with type I hyperoxaluria. Late forms of the disease presenting during adulthood have also been reported.

A marked increase in urinary excretion of oxalate (normal excretion, 10–50 mg/24 hr) is the most important *laboratory finding*. The presence of oxalate crystals in urinary sediment is rarely helpful for diagnosis because such crystals are often seen in normal individuals. Urinary excretion of glycolic acid and glyoxylic acid is increased. *Diagnosis* can be confirmed by performing an assay of the enzyme in liver specimens.

Medical treatment has been largely unsuccessful. In some patients administration of large doses of pyridoxine reduces urinary excretion of oxalate. Renal transplantation in patients with renal failure has not improved the outcome in most cases, because oxalosis has recurred in the transplanted kidney.

Combined liver and kidney transplants have resulted in a significant decrease in plasma and urinary oxalate in a few patients and may be the most effective treatment of this disorder.

Prenatal diagnosis has been achieved by the measurement of fetal hepatic enzyme activity obtained by needle biopsy or by DNA analysis of chorionic villi samples.

PRIMARY HYPEROXALURIA TYPE II (L-GLYCERIC ACIDURIA). This rare condition is due to a deficiency of D-glycerate dehydrogenase/glyoxylate reductase enzyme complex (see Fig. 74–8). A deficiency in the activity of this enzyme results in an accumulation of two intermediate metabolites, hydroxypyruvate (the ketoacid of serine) and glyoxylic acid. Both these compounds are further metabolized by lactate dehydrogenase (LDH) to L-glyceric acid and oxalic acid, respectively. Saulteaux-Ojibway Indians of Manitoba may have a higher risk of this condition.

Clinically, these patients are indistinguishable from those with hyperoxaluria type I. Renal stones presenting as renal colic and hematuria may develop before age 2 yr. Renal failure has not been observed in patients with type II oxaluria; the urine contains large amounts of L-glyceric acid in addition to high levels of oxalate (L-glyceric acid is not normally present in urine). Urinary excretion of glycolic acid and glyoxylic acid is not increased. The presence of L-glyceric acid without increased levels of glycolic and glyoxylic acids in urine differentiate this type from type I hyperoxaluria.

No effective *therapy* is available.

Creatine Deficiency (Guanidinoacetate Methyltransferase Deficiency). Creatine is synthesized in the liver, pancreas, and kidneys from arginine and glycine (Fig. 74–9) and is transported to muscles and the brain, which contain high activities of creatine kinase. Phosphorylation and dephosphorylation of creatine by this enzyme in conjunction with adenosine diphosphate and triphosphate (ADP/ATP) provide high-energy phosphate reactions in these organs. Creatine is nonenzymatically metabolized to creatinine at a constant daily rate and is excreted in the urine. Deficiency of guanidinoacetate methyltransferase causes a severe creatine deficiency state.

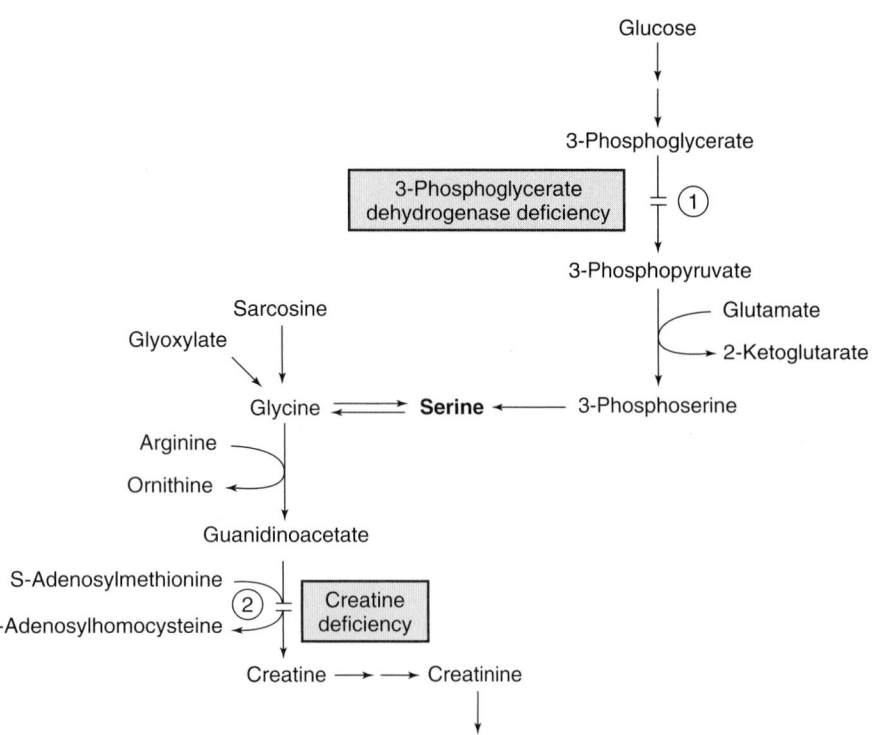

FIGURE 74–9. Pathways for the synthesis of serine and creatine. **Enzymes:** (1) 3-phosphoglycerate dehydrogenase; (2) guanidinoacetate methyltransferase.

Clinical manifestations relate to the brain and muscles and may appear in the first few weeks or months of life. Developmental delay, mental retardation, absence of active speech, autistic behavior with self-mutilation, and profound hypertonia with dyskinetic and dystonic movements are found in most patients. Seizures are a common finding. Somatic growth is normal.

Laboratory findings include decreased creatine and creatinine in blood and urine. Marked elevations of guanidinoacetate in blood, urine, and especially cerebrospinal fluid, are diagnostic. Absence of creatine and creatine phosphate and high levels of guanidinoacetate can be demonstrated in the brain by magnetic resonance spectroscopy (MRS). MRI shows signal hyperintensity of the globus pallidus. *Diagnosis* may be confirmed by measurement of the enzyme in the liver, cultured fibroblasts, stimulated lymphoblasts, or DNA analysis of the gene.

Treatment with creatine monohydrate (350 mg–2 g/kg/day) orally has resulted in a dramatic improvement in muscle tone and mental development and has normalized MRI and electroencephalographic findings. Treatment has no effect on speech development. It is believed that early treatment may ensure normal development.

The condition is inherited as an autosomal recessive trait. The gene for guanidinoacetate methyltransferase has been mapped to the short arm of chromosome 19p13.3, and at least two disease-causing alleles have been identified. This condition must be considered in any patient with brain and muscle disorders, because treatment can produce a dramatic response.

74.8 Serine

Iraj Rezvani

Serine is a nonessential amino acid synthesized from glucose and glycine (see Fig. 74–9).

3-Phosphoglycerate Dehydrogenase Deficiency. A small number of patients with this enzyme deficiency have been reported.

Clinical manifestations usually develop shortly after birth and include severe mental retardation, seizures, hypotonia, and microcephaly. Bilateral cataracts have been reported in at least one patient.

Laboratory findings include low fasting levels of serine and glycine in plasma and very low levels of serine (five times lower than normal) and glycine (two times lower than normal) in cerebrospinal fluid. No abnormal organic acid is found in the urine. MRI of the head shows evidence of cortical atrophy and dysmyelination.

Diagnosis can be confirmed by measurement of the enzyme activity in cultured fibroblasts.

Treatment with serine (200 mg/kg/24 hr, orally) normalizes the serine levels in the blood and in the cerebrospinal fluid. Seizure activity has stopped after 1 wk of treatment. The long-term effectiveness of treatment is unknown. The condition is presumably inherited as an autosomal trait. The gene for 3-phosphoglycerate dehydrogenase enzyme has been mapped to the long arm of chromosome 1. The favorable response of this condition to a simple treatment makes this diagnosis an important consideration in any child with neurologic defects such as psychomotor delay or a seizure disorder.

74.9 Proline and Hydroxyproline

Iraj Rezvani

Proline and hydroxyproline are found in high concentrations in collagen. Neither of these amino acids is normally found in urine in the free form except in early infancy. Excretion of "bound" hydroxyproline (dipeptides and tripeptides containing hydroxyproline) reflects collagen turnover and is increased in disorders of accelerated collagen turnover, such as rickets or hyperparathyroidism.

Hyperprolinemia. Two types of this rare autosomal recessive condition have been described. *Type I hyperprolinemia* is due to a deficiency of proline oxidase (dehydrogenase), and *type II* is due to a defect in Δ′-pyrroline-5-carboxylic acid dehydrogenase enzyme (Fig. 74–10). Neither type causes any specific clinical manifestation. Increased blood concentrations of proline (more pronounced in type II) and prolinuria are found in both types. Hydroxyproline and glycine are also excreted in abnormal amounts in the urine because of the saturation of the common tubular reabsorption mechanism by the massive prolinuria. The presence of Δ′-pyrroline-5-carboxylic acid in plasma and urine differentiates type II from type I. No treatment is recommended for the affected individuals. A 20-mo-old infant with seizures has been found to have prolinuria type II with biochemical evidence of vitamin B$_6$ deficiency. Seizures responded to vitamin B$_6$ therapy. The causal relationships between prolinuria type II, vitamin B$_6$ deficiency, and seizures are unclear.

Hyperhydroxyprolinemia. This rare autosomal recessive condition is presumably caused by a deficiency of hydroxyproline oxidase (see Fig. 74–10). Patients with this disorder are usually asymptomatic. A marked increase in blood concentration of hydroxyproline is diagnostic. These patients also excrete large quantities of proline and glycine in their urine. No treatment is recommended.

Prolidase Deficiency. During collagen degradation imidodipeptides (such as glycylproline) are released and are normally cleaved by tissue prolidase. This enzyme requires manganese for its proper activity. Deficiency of prolidase, which is inherited as an autosomal recessive trait, results in the accumulation of imidodipeptides in body fluids.

The *clinical manifestations* of this rare condition and the age at onset are quite variable (19 mo to 19 yr) and include recurrent, painful skin ulcers, which are typically on hands and legs. Other

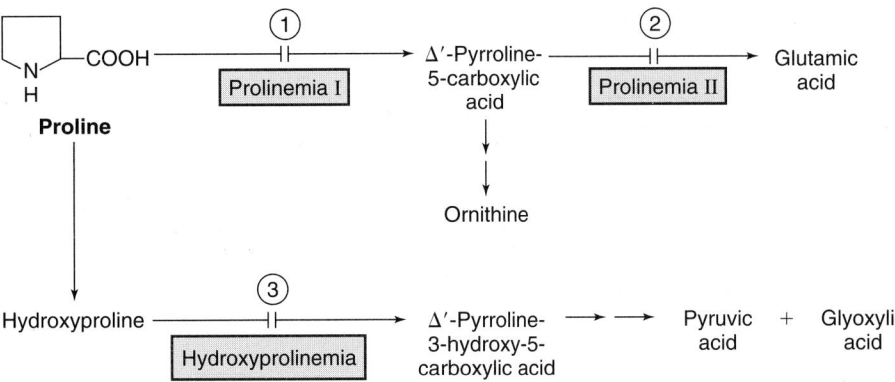

FIGURE 74–10. Pathways in the metabolism of proline. **Enzymes:** (1) proline oxidase; (2) Δ′-pyrroline-5-carboxylic acid dehydrogenase; (3) hydroxyproline oxidase.

skin lesions that may precede ulcers by several years may include scaly erythematous maculopapular rash, purpura, and telangiectasia. Most ulcers become infected. Healing of the ulcers may take 4–7 mo. Mild to severe mental and motor deficits and susceptibility to infections are also present in most patients (recurrent otitis media, sinusitis, respiratory infection, splenomegaly). Infection is the cause of death. Some patients may have some craniofacial abnormalities such as ptosis, ocular proptosis, and prominent cranial sutures. Asymptomatic cases have also been reported. High levels of urinary excretion of imidodipeptides are diagnostic. Enzyme assay may be performed in erythrocytes or cultured skin fibroblasts.

Oral supplementation with proline, ascorbic acid, and manganese and the topical use of proline and glycine result in an improvement in leg ulcers. These treatments are not consistently effective in all patients.

The gene for prolidase enzyme has been mapped to the long arm of chromosome 19q12-13.11, and several disease-causing mutations have been identified in different families

74.10   Glutamic Acid

Iraj Rezvani

Glutathione (γ-glutamylcysteinylglycine) is the major product of glutamic acid in the body. This ubiquitous tripeptide is synthesized and degraded through a complex cycle called the γ-glutamyl cycle (Fig. 74–11). Because of its free sulfhydryl (-SH) group and its abundance in the cell, glutathione protects other sulfhydryl-containing compounds (such as enzymes and coenzyme A) from oxidation. It is also involved in the detoxification of peroxides, including hydrogen peroxide, and in keeping the cell in a reduced state. The common consequence of glutathione deficiency is hemolytic anemia. Glutathione also participates in amino acid transport across the cell membrane through the γ-glutamyl cycle.

Glutathione Synthetase Deficiency (see Part XX, Section 3 and Fig. 74–11). Two forms of this condition have been reported. In the *severe form*, which is due to generalized deficiency of the enzyme, severe acidosis and massive 5-oxoprolinuria are the rule. In the *mild form*, in which the enzyme deficiency causes glutathione deficiency only in the red blood cells, neither 5-oxoprolinuria nor acidosis is observed. In both forms, patients have hemolytic anemia secondary to glutathione deficiency.

GLUTATHIONE SYNTHETASE DEFICIENCY, SEVERE FORM (PYROGLUTAMIC ACIDEMIA, SEVERE 5-OXOPROLINURIA). *Clinical manifestations* of this rare condition occur in the first few days of life and include metabolic acidosis, jaundice, and mild to moderate hemolytic anemia. Chronic acidosis continues after recovery. Similar episodes of life-threatening acidosis may occur during gastroenteritis or infection or after a surgical procedure. In a subgroup of patients, mental retardation and neurologic deficits such as spastic tetraparesis, ataxia, tremor, dysarthria, and seizures are present. Susceptibility to

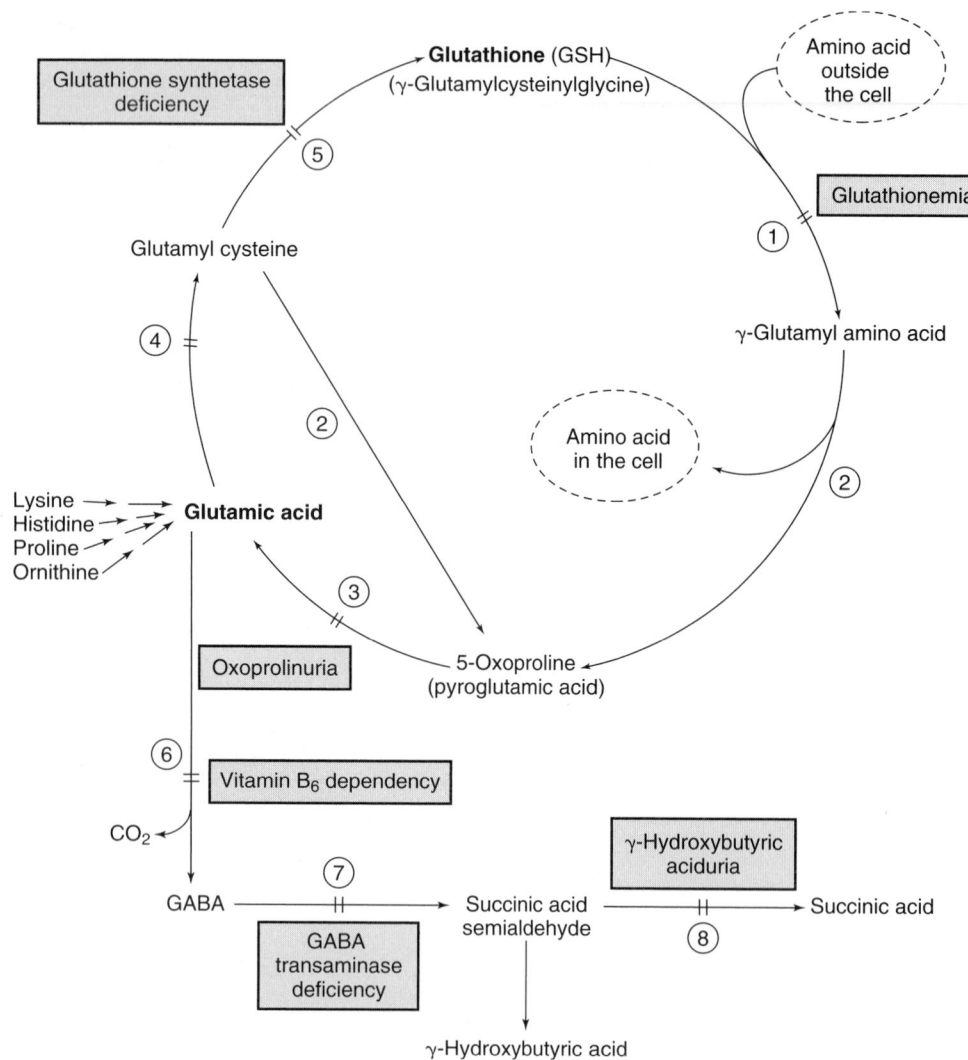

FIGURE 74–11. The γ-glutamyl cycle. Defects of glutathione synthesis and degradation are noted. **Enzymes:** (1) γ-glutamyl transpeptidase; (2) γ-glutamyl cyclotransferase; (3) 5-oxoprolinase; (4) γ-glutamylcysteine synthetase; (5) glutathione synthetase; (6) glutamic acid decarboxylase; (7) GABA transaminase; (8) succinic semialdehyde dehydrogenase.

infection, presumably caused by granulocyte dysfunction, is observed in a few patients.

Laboratory findings include metabolic acidosis, mild to moderate degrees of hemolytic anemia and massive amounts (up to 40 g/24 hr) of 5-oxoprolinuria. High concentrations of this compound are also found in blood. The glutathione content of erythrocytes is markedly decreased. Increased synthesis of 5-oxoproline in this disorder is believed to be caused by the conversion of γ-glutamylcysteine to 5-oxoproline by the enzyme γ-glutamyl cyclotransferase (see Fig. 74–11). γ-Glutamylcysteine production increases greatly because the normal inhibitory effect of glutathione on the γ-glutamylcysteine synthetase enzyme is removed. A deficiency of glutathione synthetase has been demonstrated in a variety of cells including erythrocytes.

Treatment of acute attack includes hydration, correction of acidosis (by infusion of sodium bicarbonate), and measures to correct anemia and hyperbilirubinemia. Chronic administration of alkali is usually needed. Administration of large doses of vitamins C and E is recommended. Drugs and oxidants that are known to cause hemolysis and stressful catabolic states should be avoided. Oral administration of glutathione analogues has had variable success.

Prenatal diagnosis can be achieved by the measurement of 5-oxoproline in amniotic fluid, by enzyme analysis in cultured amniocytes or chorionic villi samples, or by DNA analysis of the gene. Successful pregnancy in affected females with favorable outcomes for both mothers and infants is reported.

The condition is inherited as an autosomal recessive trait. The gene for this enzyme is located on the long arm of chromosome 20q11.2. Several disease-causing mutations have been identified in different families.

GLUTATHIONE SYNTHETASE DEFICIENCY, MILD FORM. This form has been reported only in a few patients. Mild to moderate hemolytic anemia has been the only *clinical finding* in these patients. Splenomegaly has been reported in patients. Mental development is normal; metabolic acidosis and increased concentrations of 5-oxoproline do not occur. This condition is due to mutations in the gene that encodes for glutathione synthetase enzyme. These mutations presumably render the enzyme unstable but with normal catalytic function. The expedited rate of enzyme turnover caused by these mutations is of no consequence for all tissues with normal protein synthesis except for erythrocytes in which the absence of protein synthesis results in a serious deficiency of glutathione. *Treatment* is that of hemolytic anemia and avoidance of drugs and oxidants that can trigger the hemolytic process.

5-Oxoprolinase Deficiency (5-oxoprolinuria). The main cause of massive 5-oxoprolinuria is glutathione synthetase deficiency (see earlier). Moderate 5-oxoprolinuria has been found in a variety of metabolic and acquired conditions, such as in patients with severe burns, Stevens-Johnson syndrome, homocystinuria, urea cycle defects, and tyrosinemia type I.

A few individuals with moderate 5-oxoprolinuria (4–10 g/day) due to 5-oxoprolinase deficiency have been identified. No specific clinical picture has yet emerged. Moderate to severe mental retardation has been reported in two patients. However, asymptomatic individuals with the enzyme deficiency have also been identified. It is, therefore, not clear whether 5-oxoprolinase deficiency is of any clinical consequence. No treatment has been recommended.

γ-Glutamylcysteine Synthase Deficiency. Only a few patients with this enzyme deficiency have been reported. The most consistent *clinical manifestation* has been mild chronic hemolytic anemia. Acute attacks of hemolysis have occurred after exposure to sulfonamides. Peripheral neuropathy and progressive spinocerebellar degeneration have been noted in two siblings in adulthood. *Laboratory findings* of chronic hemolytic anemia were present in all patients. Two patients had generalized

aminoaciduria because the γ-glutamyl cycle is involved in amino acid transport in cells (see Fig. 74–11). *Treatment* is that of hemolytic anemia. The condition is inherited as an autosomal recessive trait.

GLUTATHIONEMIA (γ-GLUTAMYL TRANSPEPTIDASE (GGT) DEFICIENCY). This enzyme is present in any cell that has secretory or absorptive functions. It is especially abundant in the kidneys, pancreas, intestines, and liver. The enzyme is also present in the bile. Measurement of this enzyme in the blood is commonly performed to evaluate liver and bile duct diseases.

Deficiency of this enzyme causes an elevation in glutathione concentrations in body fluids, but cellular levels remain normal. Only a few patients with enzyme deficiency have been reported; therefore, the scope of *clinical manifestations* is not well defined. Mild to moderate mental retardation and severe behavioral problems were observed in three patients. One of the two sisters with this condition had normal intelligence as an adult and the other had Prader-Willi syndrome.

Laboratory findings include marked elevations in urinary concentrations of glutathione (up to 1 g/day), γ-glutamylcysteine, and cysteine. None of the reported patients has had generalized aminoaciduria, a finding that would have been expected to occur in this enzyme deficiency (see Fig. 74–11).

Diagnosis can be confirmed by measurement of the enzyme activity in leukocytes or cultured skin fibroblasts. No effective *treatment* is available.

The condition is inherited as an autosomal recessive trait. The enzyme GGT is a complex protein and is coded by several genes (at least seven). Most of the genes are located on the long arm of chromosome 22.

Inborn Errors of Metabolism of γ-Aminobutyric Acid (GABA). Decarboxylation of glutamic acid by glutamic acid decarboxylate (GAD) is the main biosynthetic pathway for GABA production in the brain and other organs, especially kidneys and the beta cells of the pancreas. This enzyme requires pyridoxine (vitamin B_6) as a cofactor (see Fig. 74–11). Two GAD enzymes (GAD_{65} and GAD_{67}) have been identified. GAD_{67} is the main enzyme in the brain, and GAD_{65} is the major one in the beta cells. Antibodies against GAD_{65} and GAD_{67} are the major markers for type I diabetes and stiff-man syndrome, respectively. The gene for GAD_{65} is mapped to the short arm of chromosome 10p11-23 and that for GAD_{67} to the long arm of chromosome 2q31.

PYRIDOXINE (VITAMIN B_6) DEPENDENCY WITH SEIZURES (also see Chapter 95). This autosomal recessive condition is due to GABA deficiency in the brain, which is presumably caused by decreased activity of glutamic acid decarboxylase (GAD). The main *clinical manifestation* of this condition is seizures, which usually occur in the first few hours of life and are unresponsive to conventional anticonvulsant therapy. Administration of vitamin B_6 in large doses (10–100 mg/kg) usually results in a dramatic improvement of both seizures and electroencephalographic abnormalities. Late-onset forms of the condition (as late as 2 yr of age) have also been reported. A trial with vitamin B_6 therapy has, therefore, been recommended in any infant with intractable seizures. The dependency is usually life long. Other neurologic findings such as delayed speech are noted in some patients.

Laboratory findings include increased glutamate and decreased GABA levels in the brain and in the spinal fluid.

The pathogenesis of this condition remains unclear. Although an increase in the Km of the GAD enzyme for its cofactor (vitamin B_6) in the brain seems a logical explanation, no abnormality in the GAD activity in the brain has been documented. DNA studies of the gene for GAD_{65} and GAD_{67} have also revealed no mutations. Linkage studies have mapped the condition to the long arm of chromosome 5q31.2, a locus completely different from loci of GAD enzymes.

Treatment with high daily doses of vitamin B$_6$ is necessary indefinitely.

GABA TRANSAMINASE DEFICIENCY. This is a very rare autosomal recessive condition that has been reported in three infants from two different families. *Clinical manifestations* include severe psychomotor retardation, hypotonia, hyperreflexia, lethargy, and refractory seizures. Increased linear growth was present in the original report of two siblings. Increased concentrations of GABA and β-alanine are found in the spinal fluid. Evidence of leukodystrophy is noted in the postmortem examination of the brain. GABA transaminase deficiency is demonstrated in the brain and lymphocytes. No effective treatment is available. Treatment with vitamin B$_6$ (natural cofactor of the enzyme) has been ineffective.

γ-HYDROXYBUTYRIC ACIDURIA (SUCCINIC SEMIALDEHYDE DEHYDROGENASE DEFICIENCY). Over 150 patients with this enzyme deficiency (see Fig. 74–11) have been reported. *Clinical manifestations*, which usually begin in early infancy, include mild to moderate mental retardation, delayed speech, marked hypotonia, ataxia, and seizures. Other associated findings are oculomotor apraxia, choreoathetosis, autistic features, and aggressive behavior. Ataxia may improve with advancement of age.

Laboratory findings include marked elevations in γ-hydroxybutyric acid concentrations in the blood (up to 200-fold), spinal fluid (up to 1200-fold), and urine (up to 800-fold). There is no acidosis. Urinary excretion of γ-hydroxybutyric acid decreases with age. Increased concentrations of glycine may also be present in plasma, urine, and spinal fluid.

Diagnosis can be confirmed by measurement of the enzyme activity in lymphocytes. *Prenatal diagnosis* has been achieved by measurement of γ-hydroxybutyric acid in the amniotic fluid and assay of the enzyme activity in the amniocytes or in biopsy specimens of chorionic villi.

Treatment has been largely ineffective; vigabatrin has produced some improvement in ataxia and the mental status in some patients.

The condition is inherited as an autosomal recessive trait. The gene for succinic semialdehyde dehydrogenase has been mapped to the short arm of chromosome 6p22.

The role of γ-hydroxybutyric acid in the pathogenesis of this condition remains unclear and somewhat confusing because administration of this compound to humans and animals has produced some opposite effects. γ-Hydroxybutyrate (GHB) has been used illicitly as a recreational drug with anesthetic effect and is a "date-rape" drug (also see chapter 105).

74.11 Urea Cycle and Hyperammonemia (Arginine, Citrulline, Ornithine)

Iraj Rezvani

Catabolism of amino acids produces free ammonia, which is highly toxic to the central nervous system. Ammonia is detoxified to urea through a series of reactions known as the Krebs-Henseleit or urea cycle (Fig. 74–12). Five enzymes are required for the synthesis of urea: carbamyl phosphate synthetase (CPS), ornithine transcarbamylase (OTC), argininosuccinate synthetase (AS), argininosuccinate lyase (AL), and arginase. A sixth enzyme, *N*-acetylglutamate synthetase, is also required for synthesis of *N*-acetylglutamate, which is an activator of the CPS enzyme. Individual deficiencies of these enzymes have been observed; and, with an overall prevalence of 1 in 30,000 live births, they are the most common genetic causes of hyperammonemia in infants.

Genetic Causes of Hyperammonemia. In addition to defects of the urea cycle enzymes, a marked increase in plasma level of ammonia is also observed in other inborn errors of metabolism (Box 74–1).

Clinical Manifestations of Hyperammonemia. In the *neonatal period*, symptoms and signs are mostly related to brain dysfunction and are similar regardless of the cause of the hyperammonemia. The affected infant is normal at birth but becomes symptomatic within a few days of protein feeding. Refusal to eat, vomiting, tachypnea, and lethargy quickly progress to a deep coma. Convulsions are common. Physical examination may reveal hepatomegaly and neurologic signs of deep coma. In *infants and older children*, acute hyperammonemia is manifested by vomiting and neurologic abnormalities such as ataxia, mental confusion, agitation, irritability, and combativeness. These manifestations may alternate with periods of lethargy and somnolence that may progress to coma.

Routine *laboratory studies* show no specific findings when hyperammonemia is due to defects of the urea cycle enzymes. Blood urea nitrogen is usually low. Serum pH is usually normal or mildly elevated. In infants with organic acidemias, hyperammonemia is commonly associated with severe acidosis. Newborn infants with hyperammonemia are often misdiagnosed as having sepsis; they may succumb without a correct diagnosis. Autopsy is usually unremarkable. It is therefore imperative to measure plasma ammonia levels in any ill infant whose clinical manifestations cannot be explained by an obvious infection.

Diagnosis. The main criterion for diagnosis is hyperammonemia. The plasma ammonia concentration in the ill infant is usually above 200 μM (normal values <35 μM). An approach to the differential diagnosis of hyperammonemia in the newborn infant is illustrated in Figure 74–13. Patients with a deficiency of carbamyl phosphate synthetase or of ornithine transcarbamylase have no specific abnormalities of plasma amino acids except for increased levels of glutamine, aspartic acid, and alanine secondary to hyperammonemia. A marked increase in urinary orotic acid in patients with ornithine transcarbamylase deficiency differentiates this defect from carbamyl phosphate synthetase deficiency. Patients with a deficiency of argininosuccinic acid synthetase, argininosuccinic acid lyase, or arginase have a marked increase in the plasma level of citrulline, argininosuccinic acid, or arginine, respectively. Differentiation between the carbamyl phosphate synthetase deficiency and the *N*-acetylglutamate synthetase deficiency may require an assay of the respective enzymes. Clinical improvement occurring after oral administration of carbamylglutamate, however, may suggest *N*-acetylglutamate synthetase deficiency.

Treatment of Acute Hyperammonemia. Acute hyperammonemia should be treated promptly and vigorously. The goal of therapy

---

BOX 74–1. Inborn Errors of Metabolism Causing Hyperammonemia

Deficiencies of the urea cycle enzymes
  Carbamyl phosphate synthetase (CPS)
  Ornithine transcarbamylase (OTC)
  Argininosuccinate synthetase (AS)
  Argininosuccinate lyase (AL)
  Arginase
  N-Acetylglutamate synthetase
Organic acidemias
  Propionic acidemia
  Methylmalonic acidemia
  Isovaleric acidemia
  β-Ketothiolase deficiency
  Multiple carboxylase deficiencies
  Medium chain fatty acid acyl CoA dehydrogenase deficiency
  Glutaric acidemia type II
  3-Hydroxy-3-methylglutaric aciduria
Lysinuric protein intolerance
Hyperammonemia-hyperornithinemia-homocitrullinemia syndrome
Transient hyperammonemia of the newborn
Congenital hyperinsulinism with hyperammonemia

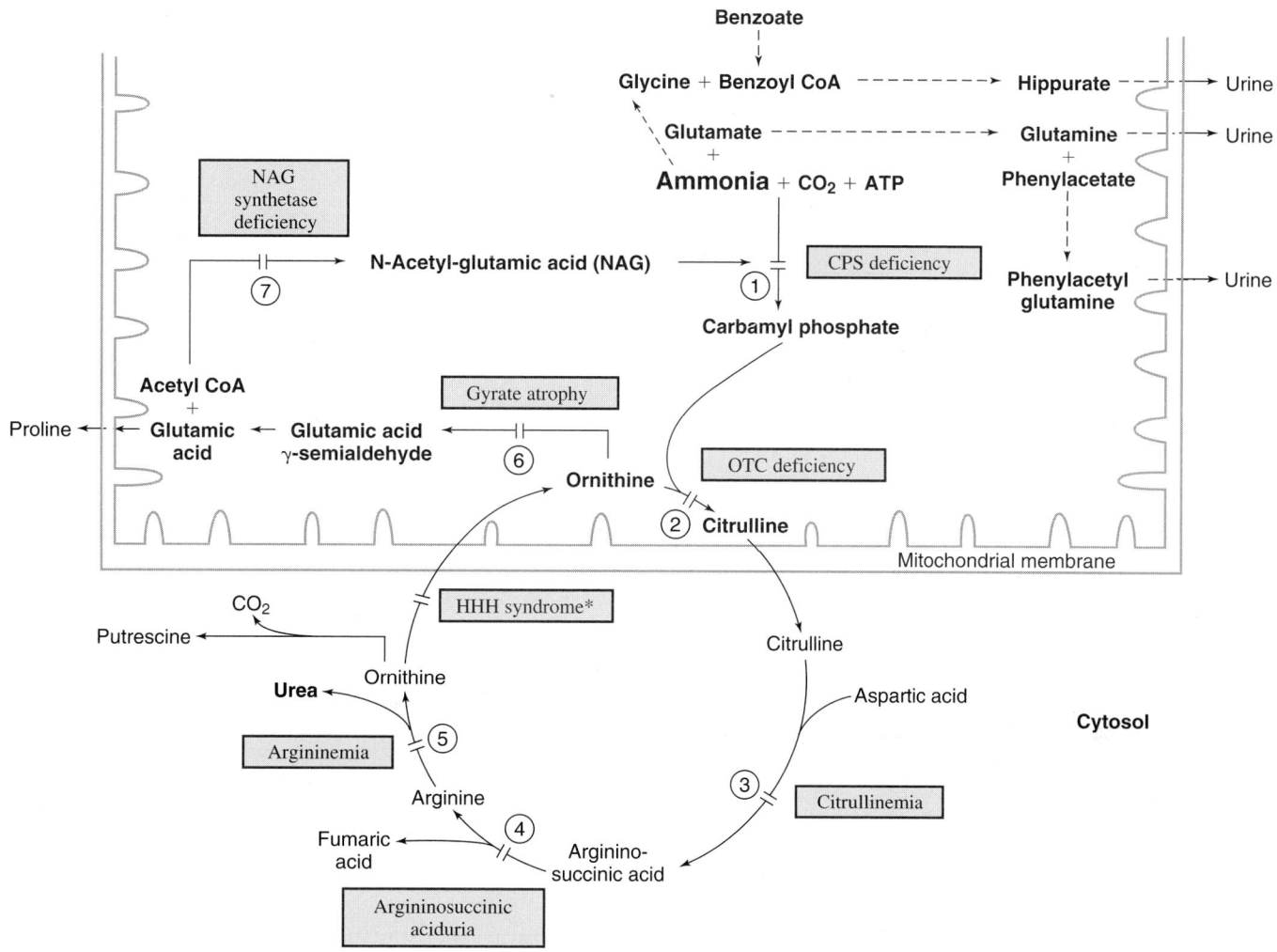

FIGURE 74–12. Urea cycle: pathways for ammonia disposal and ornithine metabolism. Reactions occurring in the mitochondria are depicted in purple. Reactions shown with interrupted arrows are the alternate pathways for the disposal of ammonia. **Enzymes:** (1) carbamylphosphate synthetase (CPS); (2) ornithine transcarbamylase (OCT); (3) argininosuccinic acid synthetase; (4) argininosuccinic acid lyase; (5) arginase; (6) ornithine 5-aminotransferase; (7) *N*-acetylglutamate synthetase. *HHH syndrome: hyperammonemia-hyperornithinemia-homocitrullinemia.

is to remove ammonia from the body and to provide adequate calories and essential amino acids to halt further breakdown of endogenous proteins (Box 74–2). Adequate calories, fluid, and electrolytes should be provided intravenously. Lipids for intravenous use (1 g/kg/24 hr) provide an effective source of calories. Minimal amounts of protein (0.25 g/kg/24 hr), preferably in the form of essential amino acids, should be added to the intravenous fluid to prevent a catabolic state. Oral feeding with a low-protein formula (0.5–1.0 g/kg/24 hr) through a nasogastric tube should be started as soon as sufficient clinical improvement is seen.

Because the kidneys clear ammonia poorly, its removal from the body must be expedited by formation of compounds with a high renal clearance. Sodium benzoate forms hippuric acid with endogenous glycine (see Fig. 74–12). Each mole of benzoate removes 1 mole of ammonia as glycine. Phenylacetate conjugates with glutamine to form phenylacetylglutamine, which is readily excreted in the urine. One mole of phenylacetate removes 2 moles of ammonia as glutamine from the body (see Fig. 74–12).

Arginine administration is effective in the treatment of hyperammonemia that is due to defects of the urea cycle (except in patients with arginase deficiency) because it supplies the urea cycle with ornithine and *N*-acetylglutamate (see Fig. 74–12). In

patients with citrullinemia, 1 mole of arginine reacts with 1 mole of ammonia (as carbamyl phosphate) to form citrulline. In patients with argininosuccinic acidemia, 2 moles of ammonia (as carbamyl phosphate and aspartate) react with arginine to form argininosuccinic acid. Citrulline and argininosuccinic acid are far less toxic and more readily excreted by the kidneys than ammonia. In patients with CPS or ornithine transcarbamylase (OTC) deficiency, arginine administration is indicated because arginine becomes an essential amino acid in these disorders. Patients with OTC deficiency benefit from citrulline supplementation (200 mg/kg/24 hr) because 1 mole of citrulline can accept 1 mole of ammonia (as aspartic acid) to form arginine. Obviously, in patients with arginase deficiency, administration of arginine or citrulline is contraindicated. Arginase deficiency is a rare condition in which acute hyperammonemia rarely occurs as a presenting sign. In patients whose hyperammonemia is secondary to organic acidemias, treatment with arginine is not indicated because no beneficial effect from such therapy can be expected. However, in a newborn infant with a first attack of hyperammonemia, arginine should be used until the diagnosis is established.

Benzoate, phenylacetate, and arginine may be administered together for maximal therapeutic effect. A priming dose of these compounds is followed by continuous infusion until recovery

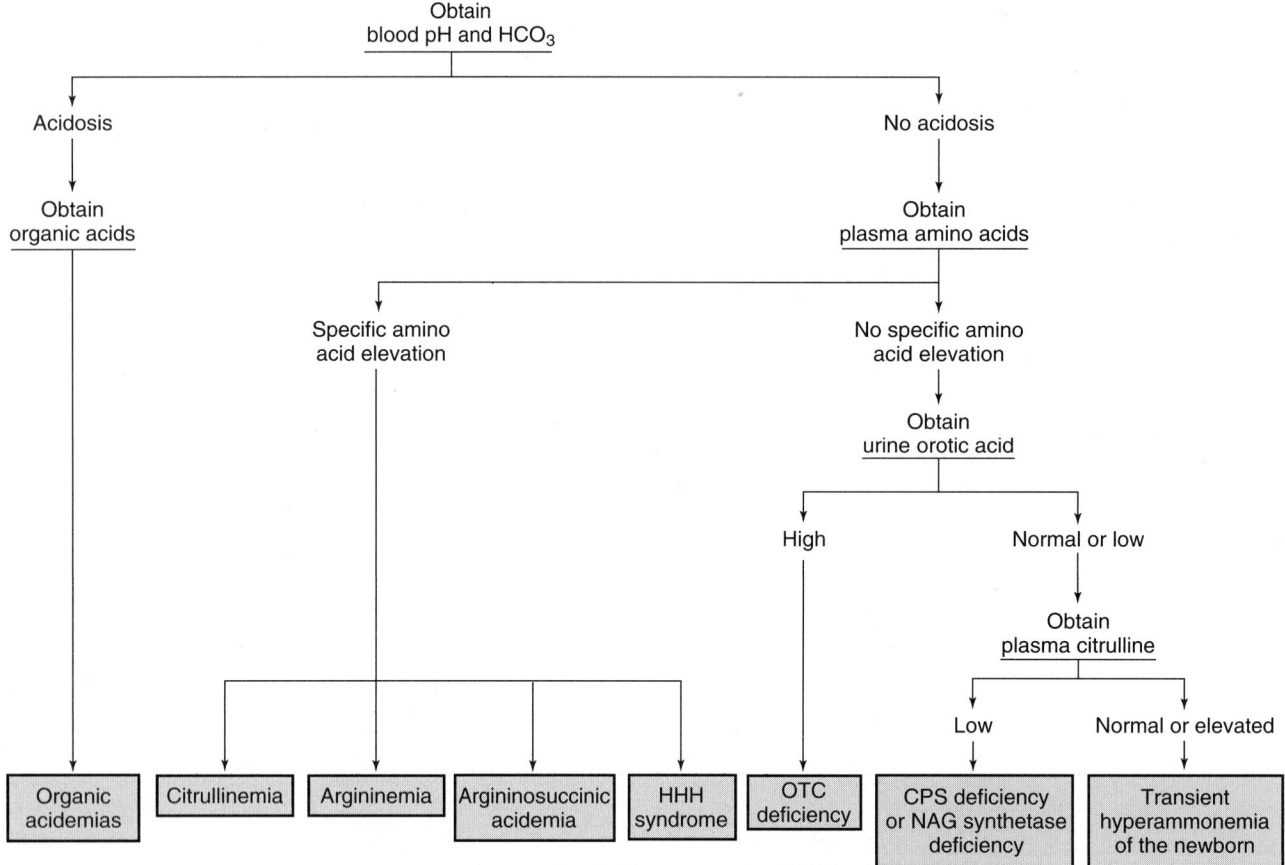

FIGURE 74–13. Clinical approach to a newborn infant with symptomatic hyperammonemia. *HHH syndrome = hyperammonemia-hyperornithinemia-homocitrullinemia.

from the acute state occurs (see Box 74–2). It should be noted that both benzoate and phenylacetate are supplied as concentrated solutions and should be properly diluted (1–2% solution) for intravenous use. The recommended therapeutic doses of both compounds deliver a substantial amount of sodium to the patient that should be calculated as part of the daily sodium requirement. Benzoate and phenylacetate should be used with

caution in newborn infants with hyperbilirubinemia because they may potentiate the risk of indirect hyperbilirubinemia by displacing bilirubin from albumin. In infants at risk, it is advisable to reduce bilirubin to a safe level before administering benzoate or phenylacetate.

If the foregoing therapies fail to produce any appreciable change in the blood ammonia level within a few hours, hemodialysis or peritoneal dialysis should be used. Exchange transfusion has little effect on reducing total body ammonia. It should be used only if dialysis cannot be employed promptly or when the patient is a newborn infant with hyperbilirubinemia (see earlier). Hemodialysis, although the most effective measure for removal of ammonia, is technically difficult to perform and may not be readily available. Peritoneal dialysis, therefore, is the most practical and expeditious method for treatment of patients with severe hyperammonemia; there is usually a dramatic decrease in the plasma ammonia level within a few hours of dialysis, and in most patients the plasma ammonia returns to normal within 48 hr of initiation of peritoneal dialysis. In a patient whose hyperammonemia is due to an organic acidemia, peritoneal dialysis effectively removes both the offending organic acid and ammonia from the body.

To curtail the possible production of ammonia by intestinal bacteria, oral administration of neomycin and lactulose through a nasogastric tube should be initiated very early in the course of therapy. There may be considerable lag between the normalization of ammonia and an improvement in the neurologic status of the patient. Several days may be needed before the infant becomes fully alert.

LONG-TERM THERAPY. Once the infant is alert, therapy should be tailored to the underlying cause of the hyperammonemia. In general, all patients require some degree of protein

---

BOX 74–2. Treatment of Acute Hyperammonemia in an Infant

1. Provide adequate calories, fluid, and electrolytes intravenously (10% glucose and intravenous lipids 1 g/kg/24 hr). Add minimal amounts of protein preferably as a mixture of essential amino acids (0.25 g/kg/24 hr) during the first 24 hr of therapy.
2. Give priming doses of the following compounds:
   To be added to 20 mL/kg of 10% glucose and infused within 1–2 hr
   Sodium benzoate 250 mg/kg (5.5 g/nm²)*
   Sodium phenylacetate 250 mg/kg (5.5 g/nm²)*
   Arginine hydrochloride 200–600 mg/kg (4.0–12.0 g/nm²) as a 10% solution
3. Continue infusion of sodium benzoate* (250–500 mg/kg/24 hr), sodium phenylacetate* (250–500 mg/kg/24 hr), and arginine (200–600 mg/kg/24 hr†) following the above priming doses. These compounds should be added to the daily intravenous fluid.
4. Initiate peritoneal dialysis or hemodialysis if above treatment fails to produce an appreciable decrease in plasma ammonia.

These compounds are usually prepared as a 1–2% solution for intravenous use. Sodium from these drugs should be included as part of the daily sodium requirement.

† The higher dose is recommended in the treatment of patients with citrullinemia and argininosuccinic aciduria. Arginine is not recommended in patients with arginase deficiency and in those whose hyperammonemia is secondary to organic acidemia.

restriction (1–2 g/kg/24 hr) regardless of the enzymatic defect. In patients with defects in the urea cycle, chronic administration of benzoate (250–500 mg/kg/24 hr), phenylacetate (250–500 mg/kg/24 hr), and arginine (200–400 mg/kg/24 hr) or citrulline (in patients with OTC deficiency, 200–400 mg/kg/24 hr) is effective in maintaining blood ammonia levels within the normal range. Phenylbutyrate may be used in place of phenylacetate, because the patient and the family may not accept the latter owing to its offensive odor. Carnitine supplementation has also been recommended for treatment of these patients because benzoate and phenylacetate may cause carnitine depletion, but the clinical benefits of this compound remain to be proved. Catabolic states triggering hyperammonemia should be avoided.

Carbamylphosphate Synthetase (CPS) and N-Acetylglutamate Synthetase Deficiencies

(see Fig. 74–12). Deficiencies of these two enzymes produce similar *clinical and biochemical manifestations*. There is a wide variation in severity of symptoms and in the age of presentation. Most commonly the affected infant becomes symptomatic during the first few days of life with signs and symptoms of hyperammonemia (refusal to eat, vomiting, lethargy, convulsion, and coma). Late forms (as late as 32 yr of age) may present as an acute bout of hyperammonemia in a seemingly normal individual. Coma and death may occur during these episodes. Intermediate forms with mental retardation and chronic subclinical hyperammonemia interspersed with bouts of acute hyperammonemia have also been observed.

Laboratory findings include hyperammonemia without an increase in any specific amino acids in plasma; marked elevations in plasma concentrations of glutamine and alanine seen in these patients are secondary to hyperammonemia. Urinary orotic acid is usually low or may be absent (see Fig. 74–13).

Treatment of patients with CPS deficiency is similar to that outlined earlier for hyperammonemia. Patients with N-acetylglutamate synthetase deficiency were shown to benefit from oral administration of carbamylglutamate. It is therefore important to differentiate between these two enzyme deficiencies by assay of the enzyme activities in biopsy specimens obtained from the liver. Deficiency of this enzyme has rarely been documented in North America.

CPS deficiency is inherited as an autosomal recessive trait; the enzyme is normally present in the liver and intestine. The gene is mapped to the long arm of chromosome 2q35. Several disease-causing mutations have been found in different families.

Ornithine Transcarbamylase (OTC) Deficiency

(see Fig. 74–12). In this X-linked partially dominant disorder the hemizygote males are more severely affected than heterozygote females. The heterozygous females may have a mild form of the disease but the majority (about 75%) are asymptomatic. This is the most common form of the urea cycle disorders.

Clinical manifestations in a male newborn infant are usually those of severe hyperammonemia (see earlier) occurring in the first few days of life. In these patients, the prognosis is poor. Milder forms of the condition are commonly seen in heterozygous females and in some affected males. *Mild* forms characteristically have episodic manifestations, which may occur at any age (usually after infancy). Episodes of hyperammonemia (manifested by vomiting and neurologic abnormalities such as ataxia, mental confusion, agitation, and combativeness) are separated by periods of wellness. These episodes usually occur following a high-protein diet or as a result of a catabolic state such as infection. Hyperammonemic coma and death may occur during one of these attacks. Mental development may proceed normally in mildly affected patients. However, mild to moderate mental retardation is common. Gallstones have been seen in the survivors; the mechanism remains unclear.

The major *laboratory finding* during the acute attack is hyperammonemia without an increase in any specific amino acid in the blood. Elevation of the plasma concentrations of glutamine

and alanine are secondary to hyperammonemia. A marked increase in the urinary excretion of orotic acid differentiates this condition from CPS deficiency (see Fig. 74–13). Orotates may precipitate in urine as gravel or stones. In the mild form, these laboratory abnormalities may revert to normal between attacks. This form should be differentiated from all the episodic conditions of childhood and from poisoning. In particular, lysinuric protein intolerance (see Chapter 74.13) mimics the clinical and biochemical characteristics of OTC deficiency. Increased urinary excretions of lysine, ornithine, and arginine and elevated blood concentrations of citrulline, which are salient features of lysinuric protein intolerance, are not seen in patients with OTC deficiency.

The *diagnosis* may be confirmed by performing an assay of enzyme activity that is normally present only in the liver. *Prenatal diagnosis* has been achieved by means of fetal liver biopsy and by DNA studies of chorionic villi samples. Using an oral protein load, which increases plasma ammonia and urinary orotic acid levels, may identify asymptomatic heterozygous female carriers. A marked increase in urinary excretion of orotidine after an allopurinol-loading test has also been used to detect obligate female carriers. Asymptomatic female carriers usually have mild cerebral dysfunction compared with their unaffected siblings.

Treatment is similar to that described for CPS deficiency except that citrulline may be used in place of arginine. Liver transplantation has been successful as a definite treatment in some patients with OTC deficiency.

The gene for ornithine transcarboxylase has been mapped to the short arm of X chromosome. Many disease-causing mutations (over 150) have been identified in different patients. The degree of enzyme deficiency and the genotype dictate the severity of the phenotype in most cases.

Argininosuccinic Acid Synthetase Deficiency (Citrullinemia)

(see Fig. 74–12). This disorder shows considerable clinical and biochemical heterogeneity. The spectrum of clinical manifestations ranges from severe forms to asymptomatic ones. The signs and symptoms in the neonatal form are identical to those seen in the severe forms of CPS and OTC deficiencies (see earlier). Mild forms may have a gradual onset with failure to thrive, frequent vomiting, developmental delay, and dry, brittle hair or, like mild forms of OTC deficiency, may appear episodically (see earlier). In some patients symptoms may not appear until 20 yr of age.

Laboratory findings are similar to those found in patients with OTC deficiency except that the plasma citrulline concentration is markedly elevated in patients with citrullinemia (see Fig. 74–13). Urinary excretion of orotic acid is moderately increased in patients with citrullinemia, and crystalluria from precipitation of orotates may also occur. Patients with argininosuccinic aciduria also show some increase in the plasma concentration of citrulline in addition to elevated levels of argininosuccinic acid. The *diagnosis* is confirmed by performing an assay of the enzyme activity in cultured fibroblasts. *Prenatal diagnosis* is based on an assay of the enzyme activity in cultured amniotic cells.

Treatment is similar to that for other urea cycle disorders (see earlier). Although *prognosis* is very poor for symptomatic neonates, patients with the mild disease usually do well on a protein-restricted diet. Mild to moderate mental deficiency is a common sequela, even in a well-treated patient.

Citrullinemia is inherited as an autosomal recessive trait. The gene is located on the long arm of chromosome 9q34. Several disease-causing mutations have been identified in different families. The majority of patients are compound heterozygotes for two different alleles.

Argininosuccinate Lyase Deficiency (Argininosuccinic Aciduria)

(see Fig. 74–12). This deficiency is inherited as an autosomal recessive trait with a prevalence of about 1 in 70,000 live births. The gene is located on the long arm of chromosome 7.

The severity of the *clinical and biochemical manifestations* varies considerably. In the neonatal form, severe hyperammonemia develops in the first few days of life and mortality is usually high. In the subacute or late form the major finding is mental retardation, which is associated with failure to thrive and hepatomegaly. Abnormalities of the hair (characterized by dryness and brittleness) are of special diagnostic value. Microscopically, the hair appears similar to that seen in patients with trichorrhexis nodosa. Less severe hair abnormalities are also seen in patients with citrullinemia. Gallstones have been seen in some of the survivors. Acute attacks of severe hyperammonemia commonly occur during a catabolic state.

Laboratory findings include hyperammonemia, moderate elevations in liver enzymes, nonspecific increases in plasma levels of glutamine and alanine, moderate increase in plasma levels of citrulline (less than that seen in citrullinemia), and marked increase in plasma levels of argininosuccinic acid (see Fig. 74–13). In most amino acid analyzers, argininosuccinic acid appears within the isoleucine or methionine region, which may cause confusion in the diagnosis. Argininosuccinic acid can also be found in large amounts in urine and spinal fluid. The levels in the spinal fluid are usually higher than those in plasma. The enzyme is normally present in erythrocytes, the liver, and cultured fibroblasts. *Prenatal diagnosis* is based on measuring the enzyme activity in cultured amniotic cells. Argininosuccinic acid is also elevated in the amniotic fluid of affected fetuses.

Treatment is similar to that described for citrullinemia. Persistent hepatomegaly with mild increases in liver enzymes and bleeding tendencies caused by abnormal clotting factors are common sequelae of the disease.

Arginase Deficiency (Hyperargininemia) (see Fig. 74–12).

This defect is inherited as an autosomal recessive trait. There are two genetically distinct arginases in humans. One is cytosolic and is expressed in the liver and erythrocytes, and the other one is found in the renal mitochondria. The cytosolic enzyme, which is the one deficient in patients with arginase deficiency, is mapped to the long arm of chromosome 6q23. Several disease-causing mutations have been identified in different patients.

The *clinical manifestations* of this rare condition are quite different from those of other urea cycle enzyme defects. The onset is insidious; the infant usually remains asymptomatic in the first few months or, sometimes, years of life. A progressive spastic diplegia with scissoring of the lower extremities, choreoathetoid movements, and loss of developmental milestones in a previously normal infant may suggest a degenerative disease of the central nervous system. Two children were observed for several years with the diagnosis of cerebral palsy before the diagnosis of arginase deficiency was confirmed. Mental retardation is progressive; seizures are common but episodes of severe hyperammonemia are not usually seen in this disorder. Hepatomegaly may be present.

Laboratory findings include marked elevations of arginine in plasma and cerebrospinal fluid (see Fig. 74–13). Urinary orotic acid levels are moderately increased. Plasma ammonia levels may be normal or mildly elevated. Urinary excretions of arginine, lysine, cystine, and ornithine are usually increased, but normal levels have also been noted. Therefore, determination of amino acids in plasma is a critical step in the diagnosis of argininemia. The guanidino compounds (α-keto-guanidinovaleric acid, argininic acid) are markedly increased in urine. The *diagnosis* is confirmed by assaying arginase activity in erythrocytes. Prenatal diagnosis has been achieved.

Treatment consists of a low-protein diet devoid of arginine. Administration of a synthetic protein made of essential amino acids usually results in a dramatic decrease in plasma arginine concentration and an improvement in neurologic abnormalities. The composition of the diet and the daily intake of protein should be monitored by frequent plasma amino acid determina-

tions. Sodium benzoate (250–375 mg/kg/24 hr) is also effective in controlling hyperammonemia. One patient developed type 1 diabetes at age 9 yr while the argininemia was under good control.

Transient Hyperammonemia of the Newborn. Although plasma levels of ammonia in healthy, full-term infants are within normal limits, very low birthweight infants may have a *mild transient hyperammonemia* (40–50 µM), which lasts for 6–8 wk. These infants are asymptomatic, and follow-up studies up to 18 mo of age have not revealed any significant neurologic deficits.

Severe transient hyperammonemia has been observed in newborn infants. The majority of affected infants are premature and have mild respiratory distress syndrome. Hyperammonemic coma may develop within 2–3 days of life, and the infant may succumb to the disease if treatment is not started immediately. Laboratory studies reveal marked hyperammonemia (plasma ammonia value as high as 4,000 µM) with moderate increases in plasma levels of glutamine and alanine. Plasma concentrations of urea cycle intermediate amino acids are usually normal except for that of citrulline, which may be moderately elevated. The cause of the disorder is unknown. Urea cycle enzyme activities are normal. Treatment of hyperammonemia should be initiated promptly and continued vigorously. Recovery without sequelae is common, and hyperammonemia does not recur even with a normal protein diet.

Ornithine. Ornithine is one of the intermediate metabolites of the urea cycle that is not incorporated into natural proteins. Rather, it is generated in the cytosol from arginine and must be transported into the mitochondria where it is used as a substrate for the enzyme OTC to form citrulline. Excess ornithine is catabolized by two enzymes, ornithine 5-aminotransferase, which is a mitochondrial enzyme and converts ornithine to a proline precursor, and ornithine decarboxylase, which resides in the cytosol and converts ornithine to putrescine (see Fig. 74–12). Two genetic disorders result in hyperornithinemia: gyrate atrophy of the retina and hyperammonemia-hyperornithinemia-homocitrullinemia syndrome.

GYRATE ATROPHY OF THE RETINA AND CHOROID. This is a rare autosomal recessively inherited disorder caused by the deficiency of the enzyme ornithine 5-aminotransferase (see Fig. 74–12). About one third of the reported cases are from Finland. *Clinical manifestations* are limited to the eyes and include night blindness, myopia, loss of peripheral vision, and posterior subcapsular cataracts. These eye changes start between 5 and 10 yr of age and progress to complete blindness by the 4th decade of life. Atrophic lesions in the retina resemble cerebral gyri. These patients usually have normal intelligence. There is a 10- to 20-fold increase in plasma levels of ornithine (400 to 1400 µm). There is no occurrence of hyperammonemia and no increases in any other amino acids. In fact, plasma levels of glutamate, glutamine, lysine, creatine, and creatinine are moderately decreased. Some patients respond partially to high doses of pyridoxine (500–1,000 mg/24 hr). Arginine restricted diet in conjunction with supplemental lysine, proline, and creatine has been successful in reducing plasma ornithine concentration and has produced some clinical improvements. The gene for ornithine 5-aminotransferase is mapped to the long arm of chromosome 10q26. Several (at least 60) disease-causing mutations have been identified in different families.

HYPERAMMONEMIA-HYPERORNITHINEMIA-HOMOCITRULLINEMIA SYNDROME (HHH SYNDROME). In this rare autosomal recessively inherited disorder the defect is in the transport system of ornithine from the cytosol into the mitochondria, which causes an accumulation of ornithine in the cytosol and a deficiency of ornithine inside the mitochondria. The former causes hyperornithinemia and the latter results in disruption of the urea cycle and hyperammonemia (see Fig. 74–12). Homocitrulline is presumably formed from the reaction of mitochondrial carbamyl phosphate with lysine, which occurs because of the intramitochondrial deficiency of ornithine. *Clinical manifestations* of hyperammonemia may develop shortly after birth or may be delayed until adulthood. Acute episodes of hyperammonemia manifest as refusal to feed, vomiting, and lethargy; coma may occur during infancy. Progressive neurologic signs, such as lower limb weakness, increased deep tendon reflexes, spasticity, clonus, seizures, and varying degrees of psychomotor retardation may develop if the condition remains undiagnosed. No clinical ocular findings have been observed in these patients.

Laboratory findings reveal marked increases in plasma levels of ornithine and homocitrulline in addition to hyperammonemia. Restriction of protein intake improves hyperammonemia. Ornithine supplementation may produce clinical improvement in some patients. The gene for this disorder *(ORNT1)* is located on the long arm of chromosome 13q14.

74.12 Histidine

Iraj Rezvani

Histidine is an essential amino acid only during infancy. Its synthetic pathway in older children and adults is poorly understood. Histidine is degraded through the urocanic acid pathway to glutamic acid. Several genetic conditions involving the degradative pathway of histidine occur but none has any clinical consequence.

74.13 Lysine

Iraj Rezvani

The major pathway in the catabolism of lysine involves its condensation with α-ketoglutaric acid to form saccharopine. Saccharopine is then broken down to α-aminoadipic acid semialdehyde and glutaric acid. These first two steps are catalyzed by α-aminoadipic semialdehyde synthase, which has two activities, lysine-ketoglutarate reductase and saccharopine dehydrogenase (Fig. 74–14). In a minor pathway for lysine degradation, lysine is transaminated first and then condensed to the cyclic form, pipecolic acid. This is the major pathway for D-lysine in the body and for the L-lysine in the brain (see Fig. 74–14).

Hyperlysinemia, α-aminoadipic acidemia, and α-ketoadipic acidemia are three conditions that are due to inborn errors of metabolism of lysine. Individuals with these conditions are usually asymptomatic.

Glutaric Aciduria Type I. Glutaric acid is an intermediate in the degradation of lysine (see Fig. 74–14), hydroxylysine, and tryptophan. Glutaric aciduria type I, a disorder caused by a deficiency of glutaryl CoA dehydrogenase, should be differentiated from glutaric aciduria type II, a distinct clinical and biochemical disorder caused by defects in the electron transport system (see Chapter 75.1).

CLINICAL MANIFESTATIONS. Affected infants with glutaric aciduria type I may develop normally up to 2 yr of life. Macrocephaly is a common finding in these infants. Symptoms of hypotonia, loss of head control, choreoathetosis, seizures, generalized rigidity, opisthotonos, and dystonia may occur suddenly in a seemingly normal infant after a minor infection. Recovery from the first attack usually occurs slowly, but some residual neurologic abnormalities, especially dystonia and extrapyramidal movements, may persist. Additional acute episodes resembling the first one usually occur during an intercurrent infection. In other patients these signs and symptoms may develop gradually during the first few years of life and hypotonia and choreoathetosis may gradually progress into rigidity and dystonia. Acute episodes of metabolic decompensa-

tion with vomiting, ketosis, seizures, and coma also commonly occur in these patients after infection or other catabolic states. Death usually occurs in the first decade of life during one of these episodes. The intellectual abilities usually remain relatively normal in most patients.

LABORATORY FINDINGS. During acute episodes, mild to moderate metabolic acidosis and ketosis may occur. Hypoglycemia, hyperammonemia, and elevations of serum transaminases have been seen in some patients. High concentrations of glutaric acid are usually found in urine, blood, and cerebrospinal fluid. 3-Hydroxyglutaric acid may also be present in the urine. This finding differentiated glutaric aciduria type I from type II. In glutaric aciduria type II, 2-hydroxyglutaric rather than 3-hydroxyglutaric acid is elevated. Plasma amino acid concentrations are usually within normal limits. Laboratory findings may be unremarkable between attacks. Severely affected children without glutaric aciduria also have been reported. In some of these patients glutaric acid is elevated only in the spinal fluid. Therefore, in any child with progressive dystonia and dyskinesia, activity of the enzyme glutaryl CoA dehydrogenase should be measured in leukocytes or cultured fibroblasts. CT scan and MRI of the brain reveal macrocephaly, dilated lateral ventricles, cortical atrophy, fibrosis, and atrophy of striatum (putamen and caudate).

Prenatal diagnosis has been accomplished by demonstrating increased concentrations of glutaric acid in amniotic fluid or by the enzyme deficiency in amniocytes or chorionic villi samples. The condition is inherited as an autosomal recessive trait. The prevalence is not known. The condition is more prevalent in Sweden and among the Old Order Amish population in the United States.

TREATMENT. A low-protein diet (especially a diet restricted in lysine and tryptophan) and high doses (200–300 mg/24 hr) of riboflavin (the coenzyme for glutaryl CoA dehydrogenase) and carnitine (50–100 mg/kg/24 hr) have resulted in a dramatic decrease in the levels of glutaric acid in body fluids, but the clinical effect has been variable. The addition of a GABA analogue (baclofen) and valproic acid to the therapeutic regimen has produced clinical improvement in some affected children.

The gene is located on the short arm of chromosome 19p13.2.

Lysinuric Protein Intolerance (Familial Protein Intolerance). This rare autosomal recessive disorder is due to a defect in the transport of cationic amino acids, lysine, ornithine, and arginine in both kidneys and intestine. Unlike patients with cystinuria, urinary excretion of cystine is not increased in these patients. About half of the reported cases have been from Finland, where the prevalence has been estimated to be 1 in 60,000.

Clinical manifestations consist of refusal to feed, nausea, aversion to protein, vomiting, and mild diarrhea, which may result in failure to thrive, wasting, and hypotonia. Breast-fed infants usually remain asymptomatic until shortly after weaning. This may be due to the low protein content of breast milk. Episodes of hyperammonemia may occur after ingestion of a high-protein diet. Mild to moderate hepatosplenomegaly, osteoporosis, sparse brittle hair, thin extremities with moderate centripetal adiposity, and growth retardation are common physical findings. Mental development is usually normal, but moderate mental retardation has been observed in 20% of patients. Interstitial pneumonitis manifesting with fever, fatigue, cough, and dyspnea occur as an acute episode or as a chronic progressive process. Some patients have remained undiagnosed until the appearance of pulmonary manifestations. Radiographic evidence of pulmonary fibrosis has been observed in up to 65% of patients without clinical manifestations of pulmonary involvement. Acute attacks of pulmonary proteinosis have occurred in older patients. Renal involvement resembling glomerulonephritis has been observed as part of a multisystem disease that may develop as a terminal event.

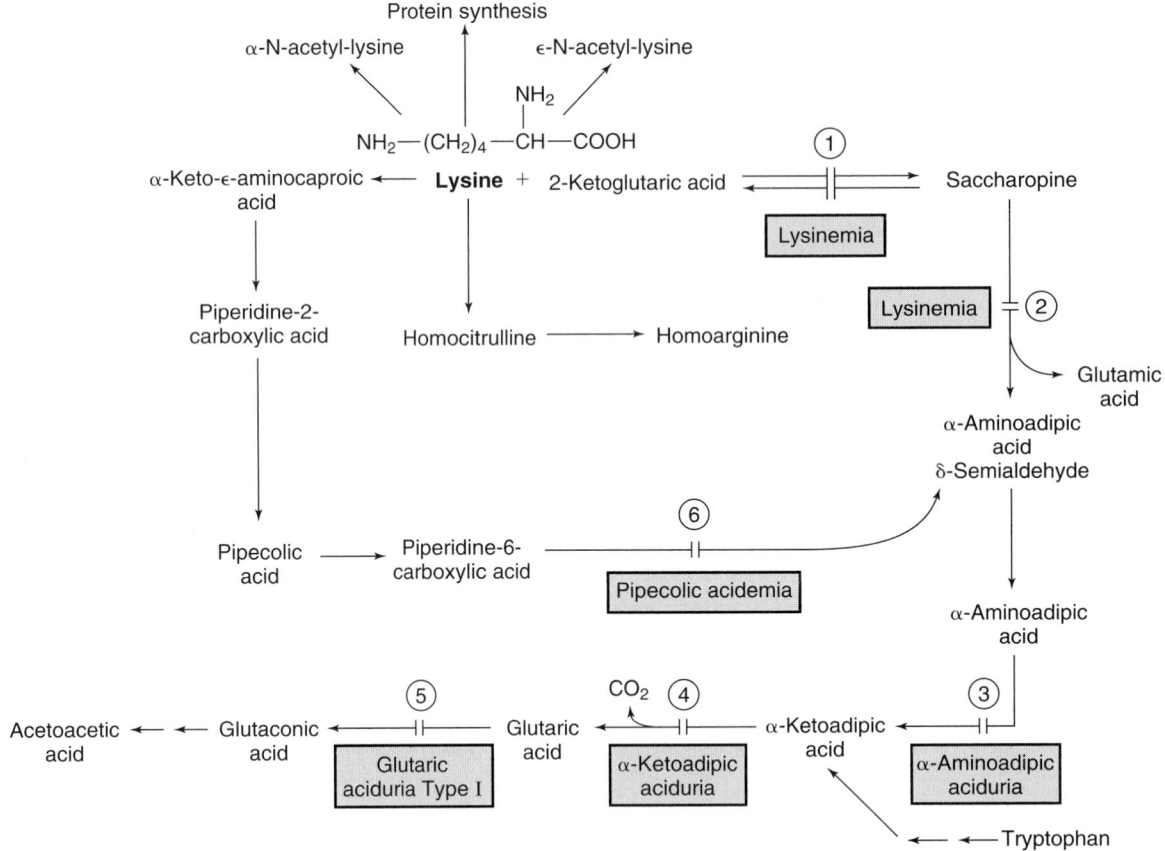

FIGURE 74–14. Pathways in the metabolism of lysine. **Enzymes:** (1) lysine ketoglutarate reductase; (2) saccharopine dehydrogenase; (3) α-aminoadipic acid transferase; (4) α-ketoadipic acid dehydrogenase; (5) glutaryl CoA dehydrogenase; (6) α-aminoadipic semialdehyde oxidase.

Laboratory findings may reveal hyperammonemia and an elevated concentration of urinary orotic acid, which develop only after protein feeding. Fasting blood ammonia and urinary orotic acid excretion are usually normal. Plasma concentrations of lysine, arginine, and ornithine are usually mildly decreased, but urinary levels of these amino acids, especially lysine, are greatly increased. The exact mechanism producing hyperammonemia is not clear. All enzymes of the urea cycle are normal. Hyperammonemia is thought to be related to a disturbance of the urea cycle secondary to a deficiency of arginine and ornithine. However, in patients with cystinuria who also have defects in the transport of lysine, arginine, and ornithine in both intestine and kidneys, hyperammonemia is not observed. Plasma concentrations of alanine, glutamine, serine, glycine, proline, and citrulline are usually increased. These abnormalities may be secondary to hyperammonemia and are not specific to this disorder.

Mild anemia and increased serum levels of ferritin, lactic dehydrogenase (LDH), and thyroxine-binding globulin also have been observed in these patients. This condition should be differentiated from hyperammonemia caused by defects in the urea cycle (see Chapter 74.11), especially in heterozygous females with OTC deficiency. Increased urinary excretion of lysine, ornithine, and arginine and elevated blood levels of citrulline are not seen in patients with OTC deficiency.

The transport defect in this condition resides in the basolateral (antiluminal) membrane of enterocytes and renal tubular epithelia. This explains the observation that cationic amino acids are unable to cross these cells even when administered as dipeptides. Lysine in the form of dipeptide crosses the luminal membrane of the enterocytes but hydrolyzes to free lysine molecules in the cytoplasm. Free lysine, unable to cross the basolateral membrane of the cells, is diffused back into the lumen.

Pregnancies in affected mothers have been complicated by anemia, thrombocytopenia, toxemia, and bleeding, but offspring have been normal.

Treatment with a low-protein diet (1.0–1.5 g/kg/24 hr) supplemented with citrulline (200 mg/kg/24 hr) has produced biochemical and clinical improvements. Episodes of hyperammonemia should be treated promptly (see Chapter 74.11). Supplementation with lysine is not useful because it is poorly absorbed and tends to produce diarrhea and abdominal pain. Treatment with high doses of prednisone and bronchoalveolar lavage has been effective in the management of acute pulmonary complications.

74.14 Aspartic Acid (Canavan Disease)

Reuben K. Matalon

N-Acetylaspartic acid, a derivative of aspartic acid, is synthesized in the brain, where it is found in high concentrations, similar to glutamic acid. Its function is unknown, but excessive amounts of *N*-acetylaspartic acid in urine and a deficiency of the enzyme aspartoacylase that cleaves the *N*-acetyl group from *N*-acetylaspartic acid causes Canavan disease.

Canavan Disease. Canavan disease, an autosomal recessive disorder characterized by spongy degeneration of the white matter of the brain, leads to a severe form of leukodystrophy. It is more prevalent in individuals of Ashkenazi Jewish descent than in other ethnic groups.

ETIOLOGY AND PATHOLOGY. The deficiency of the enzyme aspartoacylase leads to the accumulation of *N*-acetylaspartic acid in the brain, especially in white matter with massive urinary excretion of this compound. Excessive amounts of

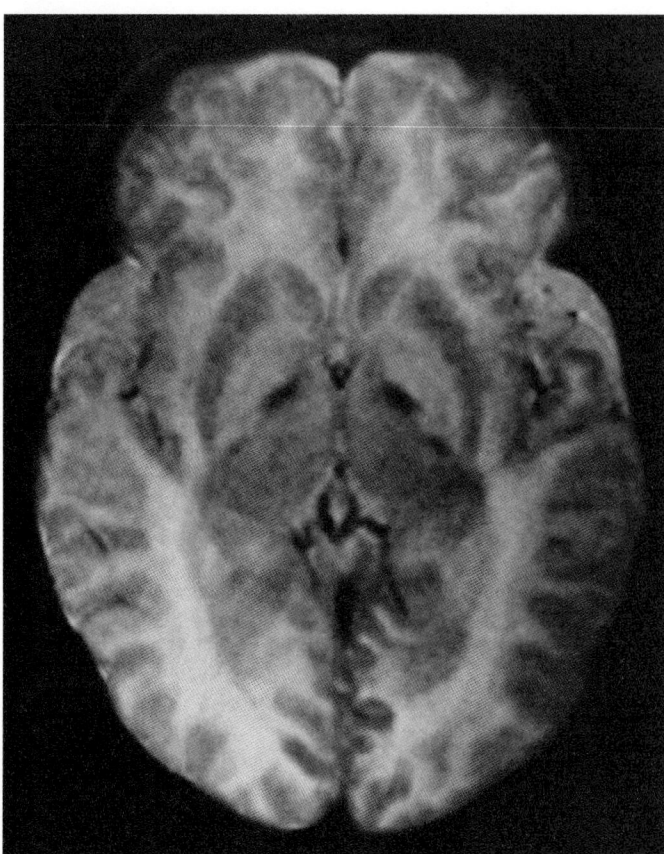

FIGURE 74–15. Axial T-weighted MRI of a 2-yr-old patient with Canavan disease. Extensive thickening of the white matter is seen.

N-acetylaspartic acid are also present in the blood and cerebrospinal fluid. There is striking vacuolization and astrocytic swelling in white matter. Electron microscopy reveals distorted mitochondria. As the disease progresses, the ventricles enlarge from cerebral atrophy.

CLINICAL MANIFESTATIONS. The severity of Canavan disease covers a wide spectrum. Infants usually appear normal at birth and may not manifest symptoms until 3–6 mo of age, when they develop progressive macrocephaly, severe hypotonia, and persistent head lag. As the infant grows older, delayed milestones become evident. These children become hyperreflexic and hypertonic; joint stiffness may be encountered because of disuse. Seizures and optic atrophy develop with time. Feeding difficulties, poor weight gain, and gastroesophageal reflux may occur in the 1st yr of life; swallowing deteriorates during the 2nd and 3rd yr of life, and nasogastric feeding or permanent gastrostomy may be required. Most patients die in the first decade of life; however, with improved nursing care they may survive through the second decade.

DIAGNOSIS. CT scans and MRI reveal diffuse white matter degeneration, primarily in the cerebral hemispheres, with less involvement in the cerebellum and brain stem (Fig. 74–15). Repeated evaluations may be required. Magnetic resonance spectroscopy (MRS) performed at the time MRI is done may show a high peak of *N*-acetylaspartic acid suggesting Canavan disease. The differential diagnosis of Canavan disease should include *Alexander disease*, which is another leukodystrophy with macrocephaly. Progression is usually slow in Alexander disease; hypotonia is not as pronounced as in Canavan disease. Brain biopsy shows spongy degeneration of the myelin fibers, astrocytic swelling, and elongated mitochondria. Definitive diagnosis is established by finding elevated amounts of *N*-acetylaspartic acid in the urine or blood with a deficiency of aspartoacylase in cultured skin fibroblasts. The biochemical method is the preferred choice for diagnosis. Levels of *N*-acetylaspartic acid in normal urine are only trace amounts (24 ± 16 μmol/mmol creatinine), whereas in patients with Canavan disease they are in the range of 1,440 ± 873 μmol/mmol creatinine. High levels of *N*-acetylaspartic acid in plasma, cerebrospinal fluid, and brain tissue can also be detected. The activity of aspartoacylase in the fibroblasts of obligate carriers is about half or less of the activity found in normal individuals.

The gene for aspartoacylase has been cloned, and mutations leading to Canavan disease have been identified. There are two mutations predominant in the Ashkenazi Jewish population. The first is an amino acid substitution (E285A) in which glutamic acid is substituted to alanine. This mutation is the most frequent and encompasses 83% of 100 mutant alleles examined in Ashkenazi Jewish patients. The second common mutation is a change from tyrosine to a nonsense mutation, leading to a stop in the coding sequence (Y231X). This mutation accounts for 13% of the 100 mutant alleles. In the non-Jewish population more diverse mutations have been observed; the two common mutations in Jewish people are rare. A different mutation (A305E), substitution of alanine for glutamic acid, accounts for 40% of 62 mutant alleles in non-Jewish patients. It is important to obtain a molecular diagnosis because this will lead to accurate counseling and prenatal diagnosis for the family. If the mutations are not known, prenatal diagnosis relies on the level of *N*-acetylaspartic acid in the amniotic fluid. In Ashkenazi Jewish patients the carrier frequency may be as high as 1 in 36, which is close to that of Tay-Sachs disease. Ashkenazi Jewish individuals may need to be screened for Canavan disease.

TREATMENT AND PREVENTION. No specific treatment is available. Feeding problems and seizures should be treated on an individual basis. Genetic counseling, carrier testing, and prenatal diagnosis are available. Injection of liposomes with the human aspartoacylase gene was introduced to the ventricles of two children with Canavan disease. The results of this gene therapy have not been encouraging.

General

Leonard JV, Dezateux C: Screening for inherited metabolic disease in newborn infants using tandem mass spectrometry. *BMJ* 2002; 324:4.

Mckusick VA: Online Mendelian Inheritance in Man (OMIM). www.ncbi.nlm.nih.gov/omim.

Scriver CR, Beaudet AL, Valle D, et al (eds): The Metabolic and Molecular Basis of Inherited Disease, 8th ed. New York, McGraw-Hill, 2001.

Phenylalanine

American Academy of Pediatrics: Maternal phenylketonuria. *Pediatrics* 2001;107:427.

Dudesek A, Roschinger W, Muntau AC, et al: Molecular analysis and long term follow up of patients with different forms of 6-pyruvoyltetrahydropterin synthase deficiency. *Eur J Pediatr* 2001;160:267.

Hwu WL, Wan PJ, Hsiao KJ, et al: Dopa-responsive dystonia induced by a recessive GTP cyclohydrolase I mutation. *Hum Genet* 1999;105:226.

Hyland K, Nyggard TG, Trugman JM, et al: Oral phenylalanine loading profiles in symptomatic and asymptomatic gene carriers with dopa-responsive dystonia due to dominantly inherited GTP cyclohydrolase deficiency. *J Inherit Metab Dis* 1999;22:213.

Koch R, Moats R, Guttler F, et al: Blood-brain phenylalanine relationship in persons with phenylketonuria. *Pediatrics* 2000;106:1093.

Leuzzi V, Bianchi MC, Tosetti M, et al: Clinical significance of brain phenylalanine concentration assessed by in-vivo proton magnetic resonance spectroscopy in phenylketonuria. *J Inherit Metab Dis* 2000;23:563.

Levy HL, Guldberg P, Guttler F, et al: Congenital heart disease in maternal phenylketonuria: Report from the maternal PKU collaborative study. *Pediatr Res* 2001;49:636.

Muntau AC, Röschinger W, Habich M, et al: Tetrahydrobiopterin as an alternative treatment for mild phenylketonuria. *N Eng J Med* 2002;347:2122.

Phenylketonuria: Screening and management. Report of the NIH consensus development conference. Bethesda, MD, National Institutes of Health, 2001.

Schweitzer-Krantz S, Burgard P: Survey of national guidelines for the treatment of phenylketonuria. *Eur J Pediatr* 2000;159:S70.

Surtees R, Blau N: The neurochemistry of phenylketonuria. *Eur J Pediatr* 2000; 159:S109.

Waisbren SE, Hanley W, Levy HL, et al: Outcome at age 4 years in offspring of women with maternal phenylketonuria: The maternal PKU collaborative study. *JAMA* 2000;283:756.

Tyrosine

Dionisi-Vivi C, Hoffmann GF, Leuzzi V, et al: Tyrosine hydroxylase deficiency with severe clinical course: Clinical and biochemical investigations and optimization of therapy. *J Pediatr* 2000;136:560.

Grompe M: The pathophysiology and treatment of hereditary tyrosinemia type 1. *Semin Liver Dis* 2001; 4:563.

Macsai MS, Schwartz TL, Hinkle D, et al: Tyrosinemia type II: Nine cases of ocular signs and symptoms. *Am J Ophthalmol* 2001;132:522.

Mohan N, Mekiernan P, Preece MA, et al: Indications and outcome of liver transplantation in tyrosinemia type I. *Eur J Pediatr* 1999;158:S49.

Phornphutkul C, Introne WJ, Perry MB, et al: Natural history of alkaptonuria. *N Eng J. Med* 2002;347:2111.

Pitkanen ST, Salo MK, Heikinheimo M: Hereditary tyrosinemia type I: From basic to progress in treatment. *Ann Med* 2000;32:530.

Russell-Eggitt I: Albinism. *Ophthalmol Clin North Am* 2001;14:533.

Methionine

Kraus JP, Janasik M, Kozich V, et al: Cystathionine beta-synthase mutations in homocystinuria. *Hum Mutat* 1999;13:362.

Schnyder G, Roffi M, Pin R, et al: Decreased rate of coronary restenosis after lowering of plasma homocysteine levels. *N Engl J Med* 2001;345:1593.

Sibani S, Christensen B, O'Ferral E, et al: Characterization of six novel mutations in the methylenetetrahydrofolate reductase (MTHFR) gene in patients with homocystinuria. *Hum Mutat* 2000;15:280.

Topaloglu AK, Sansaricq C, Snyderman SE: Influence of metabolic control on growth in homocystinuria due to cystathionine β-synthase deficiency. *Pediatr Res* 2001;49:796.

Yap S, Rushe H, Howard PM, et al: The intellectual abilities of early treated individuals with pyridoxine-nonresponsive homocystinuria due to cystathionine beta-synthase deficiency. *J Inherit Metab Dis* 2001;24:437.

Valine, Leucine, Isoleucine, and Related Organic Acidemias

Acquaviva C, Benoist JF, Callebaut I, et al: N219Y, a new frequent mutation among mut0 forms of methylmalonic acidemia in Caucasian patients. *Eur J Hum Genet* 2001;9:577.

Bodamer OAF, Rosenblatt DS, Appel SH, et al: Adult-onset combined methylmalonic aciduria and homocystinuria (cblC). *Neurology* 2001;56:1113.

Bodner-Leidecker A, Wendel U, Saudubray JM, et al: Branched-chain L-amino acid metabolism in classical maple syrup urine disease after orthotopic liver transplantation. *J Inherit Metab Dis* 2000;23:805.

Chakrapani A, Sivakumar P, McKiernan PJ, et al: Metabolic stroke in methylmalonic acidemia five years after liver transplantation. *J Pediatr* 2002;140:261.

Chloupkova M, Maclean KN, Alkhateeb A, et al: Propionic acidemia: Analysis of mutant propionyl-CoA carboxylase enzymes expressed in *Escherichia coli*. *Hum Mutat* 2002;19:629.

Cuisset L, Drenth JPH, Simon A, et al: Molecular analysis of MVK mutations and enzymatic activity in hyper IgD and periodic fever syndrome. *Eur J Hum Genet* 2001;9:260.

Danner DJ, Nellis MM: Gene preference in maple syrup urine disease. *Am J Hum Genet* 2001;68:232.

Dobson CM, Wai T, LeClerc D, et al: Identification of the gene responsible for the cblB complementation group of vitamin B$_{12}$-dependent methylmalonic aciduria. *Hum Molec Genet* (in press).

Dobson CM, Wai T, LeClerc D, et al: Identification for the gene responsible for the cblA complementation group of vitamin B$_{12}$-responsive methylmalonic acidemia based on analysis of prokaryotic gene arrangements. *Proc Nat Acad Science* (in press).

Drenth JPH, Van der Meer JWM: Hereditary periodic fever. *N Engl J Med* 2001;345:1748.

Hymes J, Stanley CM, Wolf B: Mutation in BTD causing biotinidase deficiency. *Hum Mutat* 2001;18:375.

Lubrano R, Scopp P, Barsotti P, et al: Kidney transplantation in a girl with methylmalonic acidemia and end stage renal failure. *Pediatr Nephrol* 2001;16:848.

Morton DH, Strauss KA, Robinson DL, et al: Diagnosis and treatment of maple syrup disease: A study of 36 patients. *Pediatrics* 2002;109:999.

Nyhan WL, Rice-Kelts M, Klein J, et al: Treatment of the acute crisis in maple syrup urine disease. *Arch Pediatr Adolesc Med* 1998;152:593.

Sniderman LC, Lambert M, Giguère R, et al: Outcome of individuals with low-moderate methylmalonic aciduria detected through a neonatal screening program. *J Pediatr* 1999;134:675.

Treacy E, Arbour L, Chessex P, et al: Glutathione deficiency as a complication of methylmalonic acidemia: Response to high doses of ascorbate. *J Pediatr* 1996;129:445.

Ugarte M, Perez-Cerda C, Rodriguez-Pombo P, et al: Overview of mutations in PCCA and PCCB genes causing propionic acidemia. *Hum Genet* 1999;14:275.

Varvogli L, Repetto GM, Waisbren SE, et al: High cognitive outcome in an adolescent with mut-methylmalonic acidemia. *Am J Med Genet* 2000;96:192.

Watkins D, Rosenblatt DS: Cobalamin and inborn errors of cobalamin absorption and metabolism. *Endocrinologist* 2001;11:98.

Wilson A, Leclerc D, Rosenblatt DS, et al: Molecular basis for methionine synthase reductase deficiency in patients belonging to the cblE complementation group of disorders in folate/cobalamin. *Hum Mol Genet* 1999;8:2009.

Wilson A, Leclerc D, Saberi F, et al: Functionally null mutations in patients with the cblG-variant form of methionine synthase deficiency. *Am J Hum Genet* 1998;63:409.

Wolf B, Pomponio RJ, Norrgard KJ: Delayed-onset profound biotinidase deficiency. *J Pediatr* 1998;132:362.

Yang X, Aoki Y, Li X, et al: Structure of human holocarboxylase synthetase gene and mutation spectrum of holocarboxylase synthetase deficiency. *Hum Genet* 2001;109:526.

Yorifuji T, Muroi J, Uematsu A, et al: Living related liver transplantation for neonatal-propionic acidemia. *J Pediatr* 2000;137:572.

Glycine

Applegarth DA, Toone JR: Nonketotic hyperglycinemia (glycine encephalopathy): Laboratory diagnosis. *Mol Genet Metab* 2001;74:139.

Cochat P, Nogeeria PCK, Mahmoud MA, et al: Primary hyperoxaluria in infants: Medicoethical and economic issues. *J Pediatr* 1999;135:746.

Glutamic Acid

Beutler E, Gelbart T, Kondo T, et al: The molecular basis of a case of γ-glutamylcysteine synthetase deficiency. *Blood* 1999;94:2890.

Corrons JL, Alvarez R, Pujades A, et al: Hereditary non-spherocytic haemolytic anemia due to red blood cell glutathione synthetase deficiency in four unrelated patients from Spain: Clinical and molecular studies. *Br J Haematol* 2001;112:475.

Medina-Kauwe LK, Tobin AJ, DeMeirleir L, et al: 4-Aminobutyrate aminotransferase (GABA transaminase) deficiency. *J Inherit Metab Dis* 1999;22:414.

Ristoff E, Mayatepek E, Larsson A: Long-term clinical outcome in patients with glutathione synthetase deficiency. *J Pediatr* 2001;139:79.

Urea Cycle

Anadiotis G, Ierardi-Curto L, Kaplan PB, et al: Ornithine transcarbamylase deficiency and pancreatitis. *J Pediatr* 2001;138:123.

Aoshima T, Kajitra M, Sekido Y, et al: Novel mutations (H337 R and 238-362 del) in the CPS I gene cause carbamyl phosphate synthetase I deficiency. *Hum Hered* 2001;52:99.

Arvio P, Arvio M: Progressive nature of aspartylglucosaminuria. *Acta Paediatr* 2002;91:255.

Brusilow SW: Hyperammonemic encephalopathy. *Medicine* 2002;81:240.

Camacho JA, Obie C, Biery B, et al: Hyperornithinemia-hyperammonemia-homocitrullinemia syndrome is caused by mutation in a gene encoding a mitochondrial ornithine transporter. *Nat Genet* 1999;22:151.

Genet S, Cranson T, Middleton-Price HR, et al: Mutation detection in 65 families with a possible diagnosis of ornithine carbamoyltransferase deficiency including 14 novel mutations. *J Inherit Metab Dis* 2000;23:669.

Haberle J, Pauli S, Linnebank M, et al: Structure of human argininosuccinate synthetase gene and an improved system for molecular diagnostics in patients with classical and mild citrullinemia. *Hum Genet* 2002;110:327.

Kaiser-Kupfer MI, Caruso RC, Valle D: Gyrate atrophy of the choroid and retina: Further experience with long-term reduction of ornithine levels in children. *Arch Ophthalmol* 2002;120:146.

Nicolaides P, Liebsch D, Dale N, et al: Neurological outcome of patients with ornithine carbamoyltransferase deficiency. *Arch Dis Child* 2002;86:54.

Scaglia F, O'Brien WE, Henry J, et al: An integrated approach to the diagnosis and prospective management of partial ornithine transcarbamylase deficiency. *Pediatrics* 2002;109:150.

Schultz REH, Salo MK: Under recognition of late onset ornithine transcarbamylase deficiency. *Arch Dis Child* 2000;82:390.

Steiner RD, Cederbaum SD: Laboratory elevation of urea cycle disorders. *J Pediatr* 2001;138:S21.

Summar M: Current strategies for the management of neonatal urea disorders. *J Pediatr* 2001;138:S30.

Summar M, Tuchman M: Proceedings of a consensus conference for the management of patients with urea cycle disorders. *J Pediatr* 2001;138:56.

Tuchman M, Jaleel N, Morizono H, et al: Mutations and polymorphisms in the human ornithine transcarbamylase gene. *Hum Mutat* 2002;19:93.

Weinzimer SA, Stanley CA, Berry GT: A syndrome of congenital hyperinsulinism and hyperammonemia. *J Pediatr* 1997;130:661.

Zammarchi E, Ciani F, Pasquini E, et al: Neonatal onset of hyperornithinemia, hyperammonemia, homocitrullinemia syndrome with favorable outcome. *J Pediatr* 1997;131:440.

Lysine

Bjugstad KB, Goodman SI, Freed CR: Age at symptom onset predicts severity of motor impairment and clinical outcome of glutaric aciduria type I. *J Pediatr* 2000;137:681.

Borsani G, Bassi MT, Spernadeo MP, et al: SLC7A7, encoding a putative permease-related protein, is mutated in patients with lysinuria protein intolerance. *Nat Genet* 1999;21:297.

Kolker S, Ramaekers VT, Zschocke J, et al: Acute encephalopathy despite early therapy in a patient with homozygosity for E365K in the glutamyl coenzyme A dehydrogenase gene. *J Pediatr* 2001;138:277.

Zschocke J, Quak E, Gulberg P, et al: Mutation analysis in glutaric aciduria type I. *J Med Genet* 2000;37:177.

Aspartic Acid

Kaul R, Gao GP, Aloya M, et al: Canavan disease: Mutations among Jewish and non-Jewish patients. *Am J Hum Genet* 1994;55:34.

Leone P, Janson CG, Bilianuk L, et al: Aspartoacylase gene transfer to the mammalian central nervous system with therapeutic implications for Canavan disease. *Ann Neurol* 2000;48:27.

Matalon R, Michals K: Molecular basis of Canavan disease. *Eur J Paediatr Neurol* 1998;2:69.

Matalon R, Michals-Matalon K: Spongy degeneration of the brain, Canavan disease: Biochemical and molecular findings. *Front Biosci* 2000;5:307.

Topcu M, Erdem G, Saatsi I, et al: Clinical and magnetic resonance imaging features of L-2-hydroxyglutaric aciduria: Report of three cases in comparison with Canavan disease. *J Child Neurol* 1996;11:373.

Chapter 75
Defects in Metabolism of Lipids

75.1 Disorders of Mitochondrial Fatty Acid Oxidation

Charles P. Venditti and Charles A. Stanley

Mitochondrial oxidation of fatty acids is an essential energy-producing pathway. It becomes especially important during prolonged periods of starvation when the body switches from using predominantly carbohydrates to predominantly fat as its major fuel. Fatty acids are also important fuels for exercising skeletal muscle and are the preferred substrate for the heart. In these tissues, fatty acids are completely oxidized to carbon dioxide and water. The end products of hepatic fatty acid oxidation are the ketones β-hydroxybutyrate and acetoacetate that cannot be oxidized by the liver but serve as important fuels in peripheral tissues, particularly the brain.

Genetic defects occur in nearly all the steps in the fatty acid oxidation path; all are recessively inherited. *Clinical manifestations* are similar among the disorders. The most common presentation is an acute attack of life-threatening coma and hypoglycemia induced by a period of fasting. Other manifestations frequently may include chronic cardiomyopathy and muscle weakness or, more rarely, acute rhabdomyolysis. These defects can be asymptomatic except during fasting stress and may be misdiagnosed as Reye syndrome or sudden infant death syndrome. Fatty acid oxidation disorders are easily overlooked because the only specific clue to the diagnosis may be the finding of inappropriately low concentrations of urinary ketones in an infant who has hypoglycemia. Genetic defects in ketone utilization may be overlooked because ketosis is an expected finding with fasting hypoglycemia. In some circumstances, clinical manifestations appear to arise from toxic effects of fatty acid metabolites rather than simply inadequate energy production. These include disorders (LCHAD, CPT1, SCAD, see later) in which the presence of an affected fetus has been suggested to increase the risk of a life-threatening illness in the heterozygote mother mimicking acute fatty liver of pregnancy or preeclampsia with HELLP syndrome. Malformations of the brain and kidneys have been described in severe ETF-ETF-DH and CPT-2 deficiency that might reflect in utero toxicity of fatty acid metabolites. Newborn metabolic screening programs that utilize tandem mass spectrometry (MS/MS) can readily detect the abnormal acylcarnitines seen in many of these disorders and permit the presymptomatic diagnosis. Screening programs have shown that fatty acid oxidation disorders are among the most common inborn errors of metabolism.

Figures 75–1 and 75–2 outline the steps involved in mitochondrial oxidation of a typical long-chain fatty acid. In the *carnitine cycle*, fatty acids are carried across the barrier of the inner mitochondrial membrane linked to carnitine. Within the mitochondrial matrix, successive turns of the four-step β-oxidation cycle convert the fatty acid to acetyl-coenzyme A (CoA) units. Two to four chain-length specific isoenzymes are needed for each of these β-oxidation steps to accommodate the different-sized fatty acids. The *electron transfer pathway* carries electrons generated in the first β-oxidation step to the electron transport chain for adenosine triphosphate (ATP) production. Most of the acetyl-CoA generated from hepatic β-oxidation flows through the *ketone synthesis pathway* to β-hydroxybutyrate and acetoacetate.

DEFECTS IN THE β-OXIDATION CYCLE

Medium-Chain Acyl-CoA Dehydrogenase Deficiency

Medium-chain acyl-CoA dehydrogenase (MCAD) deficiency is the most common of the fatty acid oxidation disorders. The disorder shows a strong founder effect: most patients have a northwestern European ancestry, and 85–90% are homozygous for a single common missense mutation: an A→G transition at cDNA position 985.

Clinical Manifestations. Affected patients usually present in the first 2–3 yr of life with episodes of acute illness triggered by prolonged fasting lasting more than 12–16 hr. Signs and symptoms include vomiting and lethargy, which rapidly progress to coma or seizures and cardiorespiratory collapse. The liver may be slightly enlarged with fat deposition. Attacks are rare until the infant is beyond the first few months of life. Affected older infants are at higher risk of illness as they begin to fast through the night or are exposed to fasting stress during an intercurrent childhood illness. Presentation in the first days of life has been reported in newborns who were fasted inadvertently before successful breast-feeding. Diagnosis of MCAD has occasionally been documented in previously healthy teenage and adult individuals, indicating that even patients who are "asymptomatic" are at risk for metabolic decompensation if exposed to sufficient periods of fasting.

Laboratory Findings. During acute episodes, hypoglycemia is usually present. Plasma and urinary ketone concentrations are inappropriately low (hypoketotic hypoglycemia). Because of the absence of ketones, there is little or no acidemia. Tests of liver function are abnormal, with elevations of transaminases, urate, urea, ammonia, and prolonged thrombin and partial thromboplastin times. Liver biopsy results at times of acute illness show increased triglyceride deposition in either a microvesicular or macrovesicular pattern. During fasting stress or at times of acute illness, urinary organic acid profiles by gas chromatography/mass spectrometry show low concentrations of ketones and elevated levels of medium-chain dicarboxylic acids that derive from microsomal and peroxisomal omega oxidation of fatty acids. Plasma and tissue concentrations of total carnitine are reduced to 25–50% of normal, and the fraction of total esterified carnitine is increased. This pattern of *secondary carnitine deficiency* is seen in almost all the fatty acid oxidation defects and reflects competition between increased acylcarnitine levels and free carnitine transport at the plasma membrane. Significant exceptions to this rule are the carnitine transporter, CPT-1, and HMG-CoA synthase deficiencies.

Diagnosis can be made by demonstrating abnormal metabolites in plasma (octanoylcarnitine) or urine (glycine conjugates of hexanoate and phenylpropionate) or by showing deficiency of the enzyme in cultured fibroblasts. Mass spectrometry newborn metabolic screening programs can diagnose presymptomatic infants based on the detection of octanoylcarnitine in filter paper blood spots. In some cases, the diagnosis can be confirmed by finding the common A985G mutation. A rare mutation G583A is associated with severe MCAD deficiency, hypoglycemia, and sudden neonatal death. A second, common

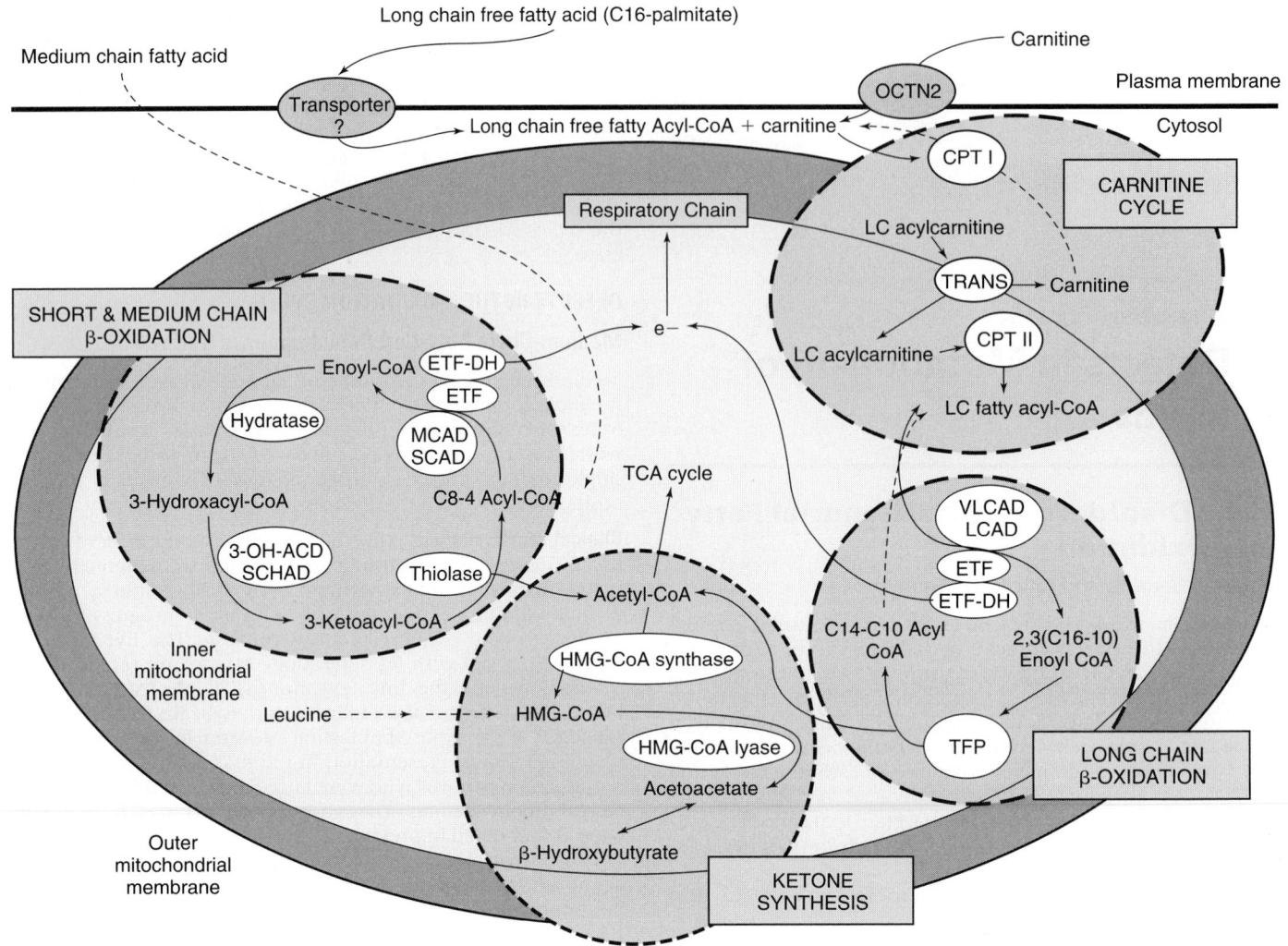

FIGURE 75–1. Mitochondrial fatty acid oxidation. Carnitine enters the cell through the action of the organic cation/carnitine transporter (OCTN2). Palmitate, a typical 16-carbon long-chain fatty acid, is transported across the plasma membrane and can be activated to form a long chain (LC) fatty acyl-CoA. It then enters into the carnitine cycle, where it is transesterified by carnitine palmitoyltransferase-I (CPT-I), translocated across the inner mitochondrial membrane by carnitine/acylcarnitine translocase (TRANS), and then reconverted into a long-chain fatty acyl CoA by carnitine palmitoyltransferase-II (CPT-II) to undergo β-oxidation. Very long chain acyl-CoA dehydrogenase (VLCAD/LCAD) leads to the production of (C16-10) 2,3 enoyl-CoA. Trifunctional protein (TFP) contains the activities of enoyl-CoA hydratase (hydratase), 3-OH-hydroxyacyl CoA dehydrogenase (3-OH-ACD), and β-ketothiolase (thiolase). Acetyl CoA, FADH, and NADH are produced. Medium- and short-chain fatty acids (C8-4) can enter the mitochondrial matrix independent of the carnitine cycle. Medium-chain acyl-CoA dehydrogenase (MCAD), short-chain acyl-CoA dehydrogenase (SCAD), and short-chain hydroxy acyl-CoA dehydrogenase (SCHAD) are required. Acetyl-CoA can then enter the Krebs (TCA) cycle. Electrons are transported from FADH to the respiratory chain via the electron-transfer flavoprotein (ETF) and the electron-transfer flavoprotein dehydrogenase (ETF-DH). NADH enters the electron transport chain through complex I. Acetyl-CoA can be converted into hydroxymethylglutaryl-CoA (HMG-CoA) by β-hydroxy-β-methylglutaryl-CoA synthase (HMG-CoA synthase) and then the ketone body acetoacetate by the action of β-hydroxy-β-methylglutaryl-CoA lyase (HMG-CoA lyase).

mutation, T199C, has been detected in infants with increased octanoylcarnitine in newborn screening tests. This allele has not been seen in symptomatic MCAD patients, however, and may represent a mild mutation that does not cause disease.

Treatment. Acute illnesses should be promptly treated with intravenous fluids containing 10% dextrose to suppress lipolysis as rapidly as possible. Chronic therapy consists of avoiding fasting. This usually requires simply adjusting the diet to ensure that overnight fasting periods are limited to less than 10–12 hr. Restricting dietary fat or treatment with carnitine is controversial.

Prognosis. Up to 25% of patients may die during their first attack of illness. Some patients may have permanent brain injury during an attack. The prognosis for survivors is good because

muscle weakness or cardiomyopathy does not occur in MCAD deficiency. Fasting tolerance improves with age, and the risk of illness decreases. As many as 50% of affected patients never have an episode; therefore, testing of siblings of affected patients is important to detect asymptomatic family members.

Long-Chain/Very Long Chain Acyl-CoA Dehydrogenase Deficiency

Long-chain/very long chain acyl-CoA dehydrogenase (LCAD/VLCAD) deficiency was originally termed *LCAD deficiency* before the existence of an additional VLCAD enzyme specific for longer chain fatty acids was known. All patients previously diagnosed as having LCAD deficiency have VLCAD enzyme deficiency. No patients with isolated LCAD deficiency have been described.

Patients are usually more severely affected than those with MCAD deficiency, presenting earlier in infancy and having more

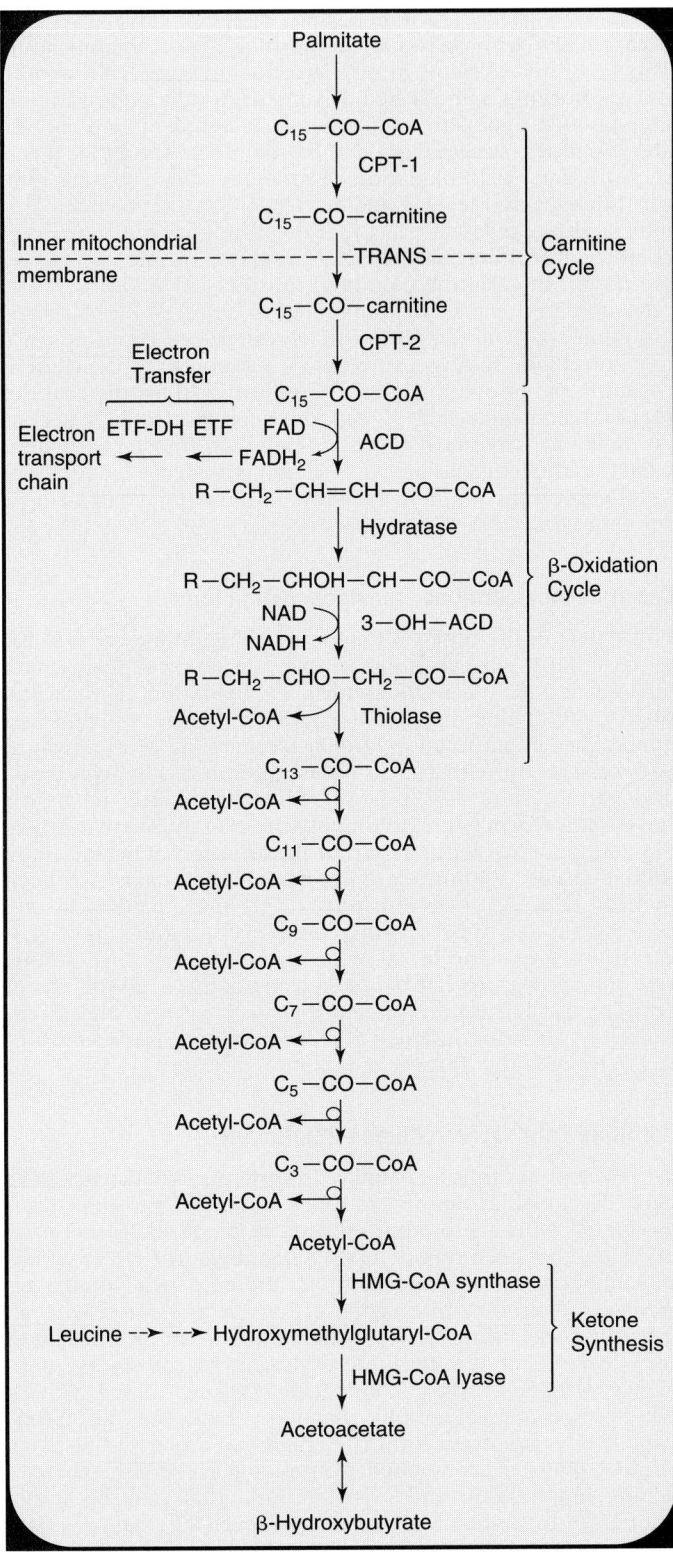

FIGURE 75–2. Pathway of mitochondrial oxidation of palmitate, a typical 16-carbon long-chain fatty acid. Enzyme steps include carnitine palmitoyltransferase (CPT) 1 and 2, carnitine/acylcarnitine translocase (TRANS), electron transfer flavoprotein (ETF), ETF-dehydrogenase (ETF-DH), acyl-CoA dehydrogenase (ACD), enoyl-CoA hydratase (hydratase), 3-hydroxy-acyl-CoA dehydrogenase (3-OH-ACD), β-ketothiolase (thiolase), β-hydroxy-B-methylglutaryl-CoA (HMG-CoA) synthase, and lyase.

chronic problems with muscle weakness or episodes of muscle pain and rhabdomyolysis. Cardiomyopathy may be present during acute attacks associated with fasting. The left ventricle may be hypertrophic or dilated and show poor contractility on echocardiography. Sudden unexpected death has occurred in several patients, but most who survived the initial episode showed improvement, including normalization of cardiac function. Other physical and routine laboratory features are similar to those of MCAD deficiency, including secondary carnitine deficiency. The urinary organic acid profile shows a hypoketotic dicarboxylic aciduria. Increased levels of C_{12-14} dicarboxylic acids may be noted in the urine. *Diagnosis* may be suggested by the demonstration of elevated plasma $C_{14:1}$ fatty acid or acylcarnitine, but the specific diagnosis requires assay of enzyme activities of both LCAD and VLCAD in cultured fibroblasts. The VLCAD gene has been cloned and mutations have been characterized. Inheritance is autosomal recessive. *Treatment* is avoidance of fasts for more than 10–12 hr. Continuous intragastric feeding is useful in some patients.

Short-Chain Acyl-CoA Dehydrogenase Deficiency

A small number of biochemically-verified SCAD patients have been described. Affected individuals do not present with hypoketotic hypoglycemia. Skeletal myopathy seems to predominate in most patients, but a consistent clinical phenotype has not been identified. Some patients have severe metabolic acidosis. Neurologic signs are present in most patients, although mildly affected individuals may be asymptomatic and display only minimal elevations of ethylmalonic acid in the urine. Some of these features suggest a toxicity syndrome, perhaps owing to accumulation of short-chain fatty acid metabolites. One reported patient had normal ketogenesis, implying that there is no impairment of longer chain fatty acid oxidation. Urinary organic acid profile usually shows elevations of short-chain fatty acid metabolites, particularly ethylmalonic acid. Secondary carnitine deficiency is present, and butyrylcarnitine levels may be elevated in the blood.

Diagnosis based solely on the specific metabolite profile in blood and urine may be difficult because some patients do not consistently excrete characteristic metabolites. Confirmation of the diagnosis by enzyme assay in cultured cells and DNA-based testing may be helpful. Mutations have been identified in the SCAD gene in affected patients, and two common SCAD mutations have been associated with ethylmalonic aciduria. *Treatment* is limitation of fasting stress and dietary fat.

Long-Chain 3-Hydroxyacyl-CoA Dehydrogenase Deficiency

Long-chain 3-hydroxyacyl-CoA dehydrogenase (LCHAD) deficiency is the second most common of the fatty acid oxidation disorders. The LCHAD enzyme is part of a trifunctional protein (TFP), which also contains two other steps in β-oxidation, long-chain enoyl-CoA hydratase and β-keto-thiolase. It is a hetero-octameric protein composed of α and β chains that derive from distinct genes. In some patients, only the LCHAD activity of the TFP is affected, whereas others have deficiencies of all three activities. *Clinical manifestations* include attacks of acute hypoketotic hypoglycemia similar to MCAD deficiency; patients often show evidence of more severe disease, including cardiomyopathy, muscle weakness, and abnormal liver function. Toxic effects of fatty acid metabolites may produce retinopathy, progressive liver failure, peripheral neuropathy, and rhabdomyolysis. A life-threatening illness, acute fatty liver of pregnancy (and perhaps HELLP syndrome), has been observed in heterozygotic mothers carrying fetuses affected with LCHAD deficiency. Urinary organic acid profile in patients may show increases in levels of 3-hydroxydicarboxylic acids. Secondary carnitine deficiency is common; plasma 3-hydroxydicarboxylic acid esters of carnitine and 3-hydroxy long-chain fatty acids are increased in blood. A common mutation in the α subunit, E474Q, is seen in more than 80% of LCHAD patients. This mutation in the fetus is significantly associated with **acute fatty liver of pregnancy**.

Treatment is similar to that for MCAD or LCAD/VLCAD deficiency by avoiding a fasting stress. Dietary restriction of long-chain fatty acids with supplementation of medium-chain triglyceride oil may improve hypotonia, hepatomegaly, cardiomyopathy, and lactic acidosis in some patients but does not appear to alter the progressive peripheral neuropathy, pigmentary retinopathy, or myoglobinuria. Liver transplantation does not ameliorate the metabolic abnormalities.

Short-Chain 3-Hydroxyacyl-CoA Dehydrogenase Deficiency

Very few patients with this inborn error have been described. One patient had attacks of fasting hypoglycemia and myoglobinuria associated with deficiency of short-chain 3-hydroxyacyl-CoA dehydrogenase in muscle but not in cultured fibroblasts. The patient died in adolescence with cardiomyopathy and arrhythmias. Another report described two children with recurrent episodes of fasting ketotic hypoglycemia. SCHAD-enzyme activity was reduced in fibroblast mitochondria. Two patients with proven mutations of SCHAD have been reported. One presented with fulminant hepatic failure at age 3 yr and had mutations in the highly conserved NAD binding domain of the SCHAD gene. The other was a 4-mo-old girl with a homozygous missense SCHAD mutation who presented with hypoketotic hypoglycemia but also had evidence of hyperinsulinism and, in contrast to patients with other forms of fatty acid oxidation disorders, required specific therapy for the latter to avoid hypoglycemia.

DEFECTS IN THE CARNITINE CYCLE

Plasma Membrane Carnitine Transport Defect (Primary Carnitine Deficiency)

Primary carnitine deficiency is the only genetic defect in which carnitine deficiency is the cause, rather than the consequence, of impaired fatty acid oxidation. The most common presentation is progressive cardiomyopathy with or without skeletal muscle weakness beginning at 2–4 yr of age. A smaller number of patients may present with fasting hypoketotic hypoglycemia during the 1st yr of life before the cardiomyopathy becomes symptomatic. The underlying defect involves the plasma membrane sodium gradient–dependent carnitine transporter that is present in heart, muscle, and kidney. This transporter is responsible both for maintaining intracellular carnitine concentrations 20- to 50-fold higher than plasma concentrations and for renal conservation of carnitine.

Diagnosis of the carnitine transporter defect is aided by the fact that patients have extremely reduced carnitine levels in plasma and muscle (1–2% of normal). Heterozygote parents have plasma carnitine levels approximately 50% of normal. Fasting ketogenesis may be normal because liver carnitine transport is normal, but it may be impaired if dietary carnitine intake is interrupted. The fasting urinary organic acid profile may show a hypoketotic dicarboxylicaciduria pattern if hepatic fatty acid oxidation is impaired, but it is otherwise unremarkable. The defect in carnitine transport can be demonstrated clinically by severe reduction in renal carnitine threshold or in vitro by assay of carnitine uptake using cultured fibroblasts or lymphoblasts. Mutations in the organic cation/carnitine transporter OCTN2 underlie this disorder. *Treatment* of this disorder with pharmacologic doses of oral carnitine is highly effective in correcting the cardiomyopathy and muscle weakness as well as any impairment in fasting ketogenesis. Muscle total carnitine concentrations remain less than 5% of normal on treatment.

Carnitine Palmitoyltransferase-1 Deficiency

Several infants and children have been described with a deficiency of the liver isozyme of carnitine palmitoyltransferase-1. *Clinical manifestations* include fasting hypoketotic hypoglycemia, occasionally with markedly abnormal liver function tests. The heart and skeletal muscle are not involved because the muscle isozyme is unaffected. Fasting urinary organic acid profile shows a hypoketotic dicarboxylicaciduria but no specific abnormalities. *Diagnosis* is aided by the observation that this is the only fatty acid oxidation disorder in which plasma total carnitine levels are elevated to 150–200% of normal. This may be explained by the fact that the inhibitory effects of long-chain acylcarnitines on the renal tubular carnitine transporter are absent in carnitine palmitoyltransferase-1 deficiency. The enzyme defect can be demonstrated in cultured fibroblasts or lymphoblasts. One patient with elevated free carnitine on a newborn blood spot was subsequently found to be deficient in carnitine palmitoyltransferase-1, indicating that this disorder may be readily detectable by tandom mass spectroscopy neonatal metabolic screening. Carnitine palmitoyltransferase-1 deficiency in the fetus has been associated with acute fatty liver of pregnancy in the mother. *Treatment* with diet to avoid fasting is similar to that for MCAD deficiency.

Carnitine-Acylcarnitine Translocase Deficiency

This defect of the inner mitochondrial membrane carrier protein for fatty acylcarnitines blocks the entry of long-chain fatty acids into the mitochondria for oxidation. The clinical phenotype of this disorder is characterized by a severe and generalized impairment of fatty acid oxidation. Most newborn patients present with attacks of fasting-induced hypoglycemia and cardiorespiratory collapse. All symptomatic newborns have had evidence of cardiomyopathy and muscle weakness. Several patients with a partial translocase deficiency and milder disease without cardiac involvement have also been identified. No distinctive urinary or plasma organic acids are noted, although unusually increased levels of long-chain acylcarnitines are reported. A secondary deficiency of carnitine can occur. *Diagnosis* can be made using cultured fibroblasts or lymphoblasts. The human gene has been cloned, and mutations have been identified in affected patients. *Treatment* is similar to that of other fatty acid oxidation disorders.

Carnitine Palmitoyltransferase-2 Deficiency

Three forms of carnitine palmitoyltransferase-2 deficiency have been described. The antenatal presentation of this disorder is associated with a profound enzyme deficiency, and neonatal death and has been reported in several newborns with dysplastic kidneys, cerebral malformations, and mild facial anomalies. A severe deficiency of enzyme activity is associated with an infantile-onset form. This form shares all the clinical and laboratory features of the carnitine-acylcarnitine translocase deficiency described earlier. A milder defect is associated with an adult presentation of episodic rhabdomyolysis. The first episode usually does not occur until late childhood or early adulthood. Attacks may be precipitated by prolonged exercise. There is aching muscle pain and myoglobinuria that may be severe enough to cause renal failure. Serum levels of creatine kinase are elevated to 5,000–10,000 U/L. Fasting hypoglycemia has not been described, but fasting may contribute to attacks of myoglobinuria; ketogenesis may be impaired. Muscle biopsy shows increased deposition of neutral fat. Diagnosis can be made by demonstrating deficient enzyme activity in muscle or other tissues and in cultured fibroblasts. Mutation analysis can also be performed.

DEFECTS IN ELECTRON TRANSFER PATHWAY

Electron Transfer Flavoprotein and Electron Transfer Flavoprotein Dehydrogenase (ETF-DH) Deficiencies (Glutaric Aciduria Type 2, Multiple Acyl-CoA Dehydrogenation Deficiencies)

Electron transfer flavoprotein (ETF) and electron transfer flavoprotein dehydrogenase (ETF-DH) function to transfer electrons into the mitochondrial electron transport chain from dehydrogenation reactions catalyzed by MCAD, SCAD, LCAD, and VLCAD, as well as glutaryl-CoA dehydrogenase and two enzymes involved in branch-chain amino acid oxidation, isovaleryl-CoA dehydrogenase and branch-chain acyl-CoA dehydrogenase. Deficiencies of ETF or ETF-DH produce illness that combines the features of impaired fatty acid oxidation and impaired oxidation of several of the amino acids, such as leucine and lysine. Complete deficiencies of either enzyme are associated with severe illness in the newborn period, characterized by acidosis, hypoglycemia, coma, hypotonia, and cardiomyopathy. Some affected neonates have had facial dysmorphia and polycystic kidneys, which suggests that toxic effects of accumulated metabolites may occur in utero. *Diagnosis* can be made from the urinary organic acid profile, which shows abnormalities corresponding to blocks in oxidation of fatty acids (ethylmalonate and dicarboxylic acids), lysine (glutarate), and branched-chain amino acids (isovaleryl-, isobutyryl-, and α-methylbutyrylglycine). Most severely affected infants do not survive the neonatal period.

Partial deficiencies of ETF and ETF-DH produce a disorder that may mimic MCAD deficiency or other milder fatty acid oxidation defects. These patients have attacks of fasting hypoketotic coma. The urinary organic acid profile reveals primarily elevations of dicarboxylic acids and ethylmalonate, derived from short-chain fatty acid intermediates. Secondary carnitine deficiency is present. Some patients with mild forms of ETF/ETF-DH deficiency benefit from *treatment* with high doses of riboflavin, the cofactor for these two enzymes as well as for the acyl-CoA dehydrogenases.

DEFECTS IN KETONE SYNTHESIS PATHWAY

β-Hydroxy-β-Methyl Glutaryl-CoA Synthase Deficiency

β-Hydroxy-β-methyl glutaryl-CoA synthase is the rate-limiting step in conversion of acetyl-CoA derived from fatty acid β-oxidation in the liver to ketones. Three patients with this defect have been identified. The presentation is one of fasting hypoketotic hypoglycemia without evidence of impaired cardiac or skeletal muscle function. Urinary organic acid profile showed only a hypoketotic dicarboxylic aciduria. Plasma and tissue carnitine levels were normal, in contrast to all the other disorders of fatty acid oxidation. A separate synthase enzyme, present in cytosol for cholesterol biosynthesis, is not affected. The β-hydroxy-β-methyl glutaryl-CoA synthase defect is expressed only in the liver and cannot be demonstrated in cultured fibroblasts. The gene has been cloned, and mutations in the affected patients have been characterized. Avoiding fasting is usually a successful treatment.

β-Hydroxy-β-Methyl Glutaryl-CoA Lyase Deficiency

See Chapter 74.6.

DEFECTS IN KETONE UTILIZATION

The ketones β-hydroxybutyrate and acetoacetate are the end products of hepatic fatty acid oxidation and are important as metabolic fuels for the brain during fasting. Two defects in utilization of ketones in brain and other peripheral tissues present as episodes of "hyperketotic" with or without hypoglycemia.

Succinyl-CoA Acetoacetyl-CoA Transferase Deficiency

Several patients with succinyl-CoA acetoacetyl-CoA transferase (SCOT) deficiency have been reported. One presented with recurrent episodes of severe ketoacidosis beginning in the newborn period and died at 6 mo of age. Treatment of episodes required infusion of glucose and large amounts of bicarbonate for 3–4 days. All patients exhibit inappropriate hyperketonemia. The enzyme is responsible for activating acetoacetate in peripheral tissues using succinyl-CoA as a donor to form acetoacetyl-CoA. Deficient activity can be demonstrated in brain, muscle, and fibroblasts from affected patients. The gene has been cloned, and mutations have been characterized.

β-Ketothiolase Deficiency

See Chapter 74.6.

Andresen BS, Dobrowolski SF, O'Reilly L, et al: Medium-chain acyl-CoA dehydrogenase (MCAD) mutations identified by MS/MS-based prospective screening of newborns differ from those observed in patients with clinical symptoms: Identification and characterization of a new, prevalent mutation that results in mild MCAD deficiency. *Am J Hum Genet* 2001;68:1408–18.

Bonnefont JP, Demaugre F, Prip-Buus C, et al: Carnitine palmitoyltransferase deficiencies. *Mol Genet Metab* 1999;68:424–40.

Clayton PT, Eaton S, Aynsley-Green A, et al: Hyperinsulinism in short-chain L-3-hydroxyacyl-CoA dehydrogenase deficiency reveals the importance of beta-oxidation in insulin secretion. *J Clin Invest* 2001;108:457–65.

Den Boer MEJ, Wanders RJA, Morris AAM, et al: Long-chain 3-hydroxyacyl-CoA dehydrogenase deficiency: Clinical presentation and follow-up of 50 patients. *Pediatrics* 2002;109:99–104.

Elpeleg ON, Hammerman C, Saada A, et al: Antenatal presentation of carnitine palmitoyltransferase II deficiency. *Am J Med Genet* 2001;102:183–7.

Fukao T, Mitchell GA, Song XQ, et al: Succinyl-CoA:3-ketoacid CoA transferase (SCOT): Cloning of the human SCOT gene, tertiary structural modeling of the human SCOT monomer, and characterization of three pathogenic mutations. *Genomics* 2000; 68:144–51.

Gregersen N, Andresen BS, Corydon MJ, et al: Mutation analysis in mitochondrial fatty acid oxidation defects: Exemplified by acyl-CoA dehydrogenase deficiencies, with special focus on genotype-phenotype relationship. *Hum Mutat* 2001; 18:169–89.

Hsu BY, Iacobazzi V, Wang Z, et al: Aberrant mRNA splicing associated with coding region mutations in children with carnitine-acylcarnitine translocase deficiency. *Mol Genet Metab* 2001;74:248–55.

Ibdah JA, Yang Z, Bennett MJ: Liver disease in pregnancy and fetal fatty acid oxidation defects. *Mol Genet Metab* 2000;71:182–9.

Mathur A, Sims HF, Gopalakrishnan D, et al: Molecular heterogeneity in very-long-chain acyl-CoA dehydrogenase deficiency causing pediatric cardiomyopathy and sudden death. *Circulation* 1999;99:1337–43.

Pourfarzam M, Morris A, Appleton M, et al: Neonatal screening for medium-chain acyl-CoA dehydrogenase deficiency. *Lancet* 2001;251:1063–64.

Saudubray JM, Martin D, de Lonlay P, et al: Recognition and management of fatty acid oxidation defects: A series of 107 patients. *J Inherit Metab Dis* 1999;22:488–502.

Wanders RJ, Vreken P, den Boer ME, et al: Disorders of mitochondrial fatty acyl-CoA beta-oxidation. *J Inherit Metab Dis* 1999;22:442–87.

Yang Z, Yamada J, Zhao Y, et al: Prospective screening for pediatric mitochondrial protein defects in pregnancies complicated by liver disease. *JAMA* 2002;288: 2163–66.

Zschocke J, Schulze A, Lindner M, et al: Molecular and functional characterization of mild MCAD deficiency. *Hum Genet* 2001;108:404–8.

75.2 Disorders of Very Long Chain Fatty Acids

Hugo W. Moser

PEROXISOMAL DISORDERS

The peroxisomal diseases are genetically determined disorders caused by either the failure to form or maintain the peroxisome or a defect in the function of a single enzyme that is normally located in this organelle. These disorders cause serious disability in childhood and occur more frequently and present a wider range of phenotype than has been recognized in the past.

Etiology. Peroxisomal disorders are subdivided into two major categories (Box 75–1).

BOX 75–1. Classification of Peroxisomal Disorders

A: DISORDERS OF PEROXISOME IMPORT

A1: Zellweger syndrome
A2: Neonatal adrenoleukodystrophy
A3: Infantile Refsum disease
A4: Rhizomelic chondrodysplasia punctata

B: DEFECTS OF SINGLE PEROXISOMAL ENZYME

B1: X-linked adrenoleukodystrophy
B2: Acyl-CoA oxidase deficiency
B3: Bifunctional enzyme deficiency
B4: Peroxisomal thiolase deficiency
B5: Classic Refsum disease
B6: 2-Methylacyl-CoA racemase deficiency
B7: DHAP acyltransferase deficiency
B8: Alkyl-DHAP synthase deficiency
B9: Mevalonic aciduria
B10: Glutaric aciduria type III
B11: Hyperoxaluria type I
B12: Acatalasemia

In category A, the peroxisomal biogenesis disorders (PBD), the basic defect is the failure to import one or more proteins into the organelle. In the second category, defects affect a single peroxisomal protein. The peroxisome is present in all cells except mature erythrocytes and is a subcellular organelle surrounded by a single membrane; more than 50 peroxisomal enzymes have been identified. Some enzymes are involved in the production and decomposition of hydrogen peroxide; others are concerned with lipid and amino acid metabolism. Most peroxisomal enzymes are first synthesized in their mature form on free polyribosomes and enter the cytoplasm. Proteins that are destined for the peroxisome contain specific peroxisome targeting sequences (PTS). Most peroxisomal matrix proteins contain PTS1, a 3-amino acid sequence at the carboxyl terminus. PTS2 is an amino-terminal sequence that is critical for the import of enzymes involved in plasmalogen and branched-chain fatty acid metabolism. Import of proteins involves a complex series of reactions that involves at least 23 distinct proteins. These proteins are referred to as peroxins encoded by *PEX* genes. Table 75–1 summarizes the *PEX* genes that are defective in human disease states.

Epidemiology. Except for X-linked adrenoleukodystrophy (X-ALD), all the peroxisomal disorders in Box 75–1 are autosomal recessive traits. X-ALD is the most common peroxisomal disorder, with an estimated incidence of 1:17,000. The combined incidence of the other peroxisomal disorders is estimated to be 1:50,000.

Pathology. Absence or reduction in the number of peroxisomes is pathognomonic for disorders of peroxisome biogenesis. In most disorders there are membranous sacs that contain peroxisomal integral membrane proteins, which lack the normal complement of matrix proteins; these are peroxisome "ghosts." Pathologic changes are observed in many organs and include profound and characteristic defects in neuronal migration; micronodular cirrhosis of the liver; renal cysts; chondrodysplasia punctata; corneal clouding, congenital cataracts, glaucoma, and retinopathy; congenital heart disease; and dysmorphic features.

Pathogenesis. It is likely that all pathologic changes are secondary to the peroxisome defect. Multiple peroxisomal enzymes fail to function in the PBD (Box 75–2). The enzymes that are diminished or absent are synthesized but are degraded abnormally fast because they may be unprotected outside of the peroxisome. It is not clear how defective peroxisome functions lead to the widespread pathologic manifestations.

The PBD are associated with genetically determined import defects. The PBD have been subdivided into 11 complementation groups. The molecular defects have been defined in 10 of these groups (see Table 75–1). The pattern and severity of pathologic features vary with the nature of the import defects and the degree to which import is impaired. These gene defects lead to disorders that were named before their relationship to the peroxisome was recognized, namely, Zellweger syndrome (ZS), neonatal adrenoleukodystrophy (NALD), infantile Refsum disease (IRD), and rhizomelic chondrodysplasia punctata (RCDP). The first three disorders are now considered to form a clinical continuum, with ZS the most severe, IRD the least severe, and NALD intermediate. They can be caused by 10 different gene defects, which involve mainly the import of proteins that contain the PTS1 targeting signal; the gene defects cannot be

TABLE 75–1. Peroxisome Biogenesis Factors (PEX) and Their Alterations in Human PBD Disorders

Peroxin #	Characteristic	Complementation Group			No. Patients Studied at KKI	Phenotype	Chromosome
		KKI	*Japan*	*Ams*	*KKI*		
1	143-kd AAA ATPase	1	E	2	99	ZS, NALD, IRD	7q21-22
2	C$_3$HC$_4$ zinc binding integral peroxisomal membrane protein 35–52 kd	10	F	5	2	ZS	
3	51–52 kd Integral peroxisomal membrane protein						
4	21–24 kd Peroxisomal associated ubiquitin-conjugating enzyme						
5	PTS 1 receptor	2		4	2	ZS, NALD	12p13.3
6	12–127 kd AAA ATPase	4	C	3	16	ZS, NALD	6p21.1
7	PTS 2 receptor	11		1	43	RCDP	6q22-24
8	71–81 kd Peroxisomal associated protein						
9	42-kd Integral peroxisomal membrane protein						
10	C$_3$HC$_4$ zinc-binding integral peroxisomal membrane protein	7	B		5	ZS, NALD	8q21.1
11	27–32 kd Peroxisomal membrane protein involved in peroxisomal proliferation						
12	48-kd C$_3$HC$_4$ zinc binding integral peroxisomal membrane protein	3			6	ZS, NALD, IRD	
13	SH-3 containing 40–43 kd peroxisomal integral peroxisomal membrane protein		H		2	ZS, NALD	
14	41-kd Integral membrane protein						
15	48-kd Cytosolic protein						
16	39-kd Peripheral peroxisomal membrane protein	9	D		1	ZS	
17	27–30 kd Peroxisomal ? intrinsic membrane protein						
18	35–39 kd Peroxisomal membrane protein zinc finger motif						
19	Peroxisomal membrane protein, prenylated		J			ZS	
	Unidentified	8	A		7	ZS, NALD, IRD	
	Unidentified		G			ZS	

KKI = Kennedy Krieger Institute; Ams = Amsterdam
From Moser HW: Genotype-phenotype correlations in disorders of peroxisome biogenesis. Mol Genet Metab 1999; 68:316.

distinguished on the basis of clinical features. The clinical severity varies with the degree to which protein import is impaired. Mutations that abolish import completely often are associated with the ZS phenotype, whereas a missense mutation, in which some degree of import function is retained, leads to the somewhat milder phenotypes. A defect in *PEX7*, which involves the import of proteins that utilize PTS2, is associated with rhizomelic chondrodysplasia punctata (RCDP). *PEX7* defects that leave import partially intact are associated with milder phenotypes, some of which resemble classic Refsum disease.

The genetic disorders that involve single peroxisomal enzymes usually have clinical manifestations that are more restricted and present subsequent to the neonatal period and not infrequently in adolescents or adults. The clinical manifestations may be related to the biochemical defect. For instance, the primary adrenal insufficiency of X-ALD is caused by accumulation of very long chain fatty acids (VLCFA) in the adrenal cortex, and the peripheral neuropathy in Refsum disease is caused by the accumulation of phytanic acid in Schwann cells and myelin.

PBD WITH MILDER OR ATYPICAL PHENOTYPES. Newborn infants with *Zellweger syndrome* show striking and consistent abnormalities that are easily recognized. Of central diagnostic importance are the typical facial appearance (high forehead, unslanting palpebral fissures, hypoplastic supraorbital ridges, and epicanthal folds; Fig. 75–3), severe weakness and hypotonia, neonatal seizures, and eye abnormalities (cataracts, glaucoma, corneal clouding, Brushfield spots, pigmentary retinopathy, and optic nerve dysplasia). Because of the hypotonia and "mongoloid" appearance, Down syndrome may be suspected. Infants with Zellweger syndrome rarely live more than a few months. More than 90% show postnatal growth failure. Table 75–2 lists the main clinical abnormalities.

Patients with *neonatal ALD* show fewer and occasionally no dysmorphic features. Neonatal seizures occur frequently. Some degree of psychomotor development is present; function remains in the severely or profoundly retarded range, and development may regress after 3–5 yr of age, probably from a progressive leukodystrophy. Several patients are now in a stable, albeit disabled, state in their 3rd or 4th decade. Enlarged liver and impaired liver function, pigmentary degeneration of the retina, and severely impaired hearing are invariably present. Adrenocortical function is usually impaired, but overt Addison disease is rare. Chondrodysplasia punctata and renal cysts are absent.

Patients with *infantile Refsum disease* have survived to the 2nd decade or longer. They are able to walk, although gait may be ataxic and broad based. Cognitive function is in the severely retarded range. All have sensorineural hearing loss and pigmentary degeneration of the retina. They have moderately dysmorphic features that may include epicanthal folds, a flat bridge of the nose, and low-set ears. Early hypotonia and enlarged liver with impaired function are common. Levels of plasma cholesterol and high- and low-density lipoprotein are often moderately reduced. Chondrodysplasia punctata and renal cortical

cysts are absent. Postmortem study in infantile Refsum disease reveals micronodular liver cirrhosis and small hypoplastic adrenals. The brain shows no malformations, except for severe hypoplasia of the cerebellar granule layer and ectopic locations of the Purkinje cells in the molecular layer. The mode of inheritance is autosomal recessive.

Some patients with PBD disorders have milder and atypical phenotypes. They may present with peripheral neuropathy or with retinopathy, impaired vision, or cataracts in childhood, adolescence, or adulthood and have been diagnosed to have Charcot-Marie Tooth disease or Usher syndrome. Some patients have survived to the fifth decade.

Rhizomelic Chondrodysplasia Punctata. Rhizomelic chondrodysplasia punctata (RCDP) is characterized by the presence of stippled foci of calcification within the hyaline cartilage and is associated with dwarfing, cataracts (72%), and multiple malformations due to contractures. Vertebral bodies have a coronal cleft filled by cartilage that is a result of an embryonic arrest. Disproportionate short stature affects the proximal parts of the extremities (Fig. 75–4A). Radiologic abnormalities consist of shortening of the proximal limb bones, metaphyseal cupping, and disturbed ossification (see Fig. 75–4B). Height, weight, and head circumference are less than the 3rd percentile, and these children are severely retarded mentally. Skin changes such as those observed in ichthyosiform erythroderma are present in about 25% of patients.

Isolated Defects of Peroxisomal Fatty Acid Oxidation. The disorders labeled B1 through B3 (see Box 75–1) each involve

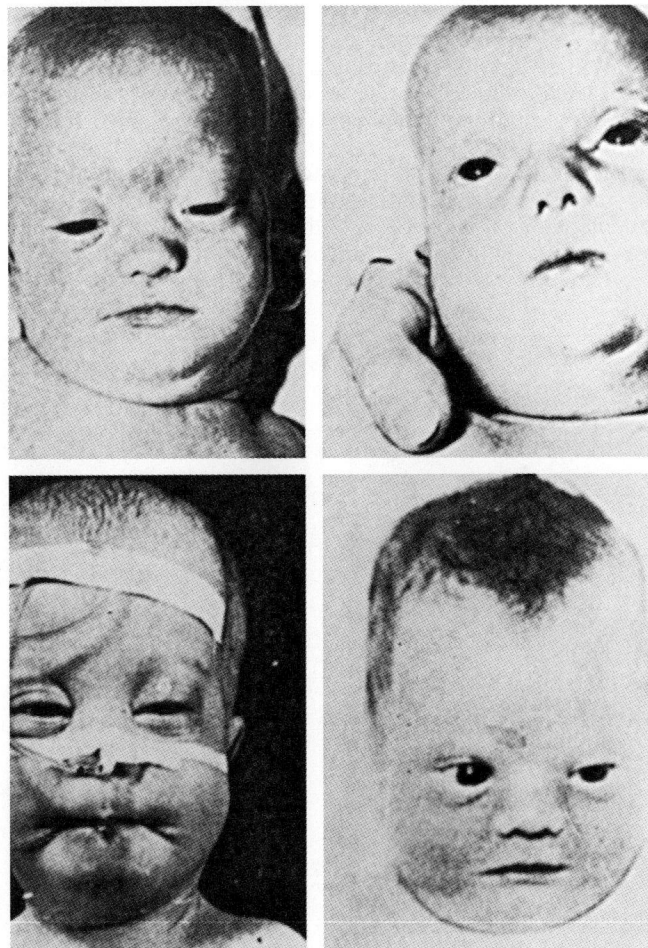

FIGURE 75–3. Four patients with Zellweger cerebrohepatorenal syndrome. Note the high forehead, epicanthal folds, and hypoplasia of supraorbital ridges and midface. (Courtesy of Hans Zellweger, MD.)

TABLE 75–2. Main Clinical Abnormalities in Zellweger Syndrome

Abnormal Feature	Cases in Which Information about the Feature was Available		Cases in Which the Feature was Present	
	No.	*%*	*No.*	*%*
High forehead	60	53	58	97
Flat occiput	16	14	13	81
Large fontanelle(s), wide sutures	57	50	55	96
Shallow orbital ridges	33	29	33	100
Low/broad nasal bridge	23	20	23	100
Epicanthus	36	32	33	92
High arched palate	37	32	35	95
External ear deformity	40	35	39	97
Micrognathia	18	16	18	100
Redundant skinfold of neck	13	11	13	100
Brushfield spots	6	5	5	83
Cataract/cloudy cornea	35	31	30	86
Glaucoma	12	11	7	58
Abnormal retinal pigmentation	15	13	6	40
Optic disc pallor	23	20	17	74
Severe hypotonia	95	83	94	99
Abnormal Moro response	26	23	26	100
Hyporeflexia or areflexia	57	50	56	98
Poor sucking	77	68	74	96
Gavage feeding	26	23	26	100
Epileptic seizures	61	54	56	92
Psychomotor retardation	45	39	45	100
Impaired hearing	21	18	9	40
Nystagmus	37	32	30	81

From Heymans HAS: Cerebro-hepato-renal (Zellweger) syndrome: Clinical and biochemical consequences of peroxisomal dysfunctions. Thesis, University of Amsterdam, 1984.

one of three enzymes involved in peroxisomal fatty acid oxidation. Their clinical manifestations resemble those of the Zellweger syndrome/neonatal ALD/infantile Refsum disease continuum; they can be distinguished from disorders of peroxisome biogenesis by laboratory tests. Defects of bifunctional enzyme are common and are found in approximately 15% of patients with the Zellweger syndrome/neonatal ALD/infantile Refsum disease phenotype. Patients with isolated acyl-coenzyme A (CoA) oxidase deficiency have a somewhat milder phenotype that resembles that of neonatal ALD. Only a single patient with peroxisomal thiolase deficiency has been described. This patient had Zellweger syndrome phenotype.

Isolated Defects of Plasmalogen Synthesis. Plasmalogens are lipids in which the first carbon of glycerol is linked to an alcohol rather than a fatty acid. They are synthesized through a complex series of reactions, the first two steps of which are catalyzed by the peroxisomal enzymes dihydroxyacetone phosphate alkyl transferase and synthase. Deficiency of either of these enzymes (B4 and B5 in Box 75–1) leads to a phenotype that is clinically indistinguishable from the peroxisomal import disorder rhizomelic chondrodysplasia punctata. This latter disorder is caused by a defect in *PEX7*, the receptor for peroxisome targeting sequence 2. It shares the severe deficiency of plasmalogens with disorders B4 and B5, but in addition has defects of phytanic oxidation. The fact that disorders B4 and B5 are associated with the full phenotype of rhizomelic chondrodysplasia punctata suggests that a deficiency of plasmalogens is sufficient to produce it.

Classic Refsum Disease. The defective enzyme (phytanoyl-CoA oxidase) is localized to the peroxisome. The manifestation of classic Refsum disease includes impaired vision from retinitis pigmentosa, ichthyosis, peripheral neuropathy, ataxia, and occasionally cardiac arrhythmias. In contrast to infantile Refsum disease, cognitive function is normal and there are no congenital malformations. Classic Refsum disease often does not manifest until young adulthood, but visual disturbances, such as night blindness, ichthyosis, and peripheral neuropathy may already be present in childhood and adolescence. Early diagnosis is important because institution of a phytanic acid–restricted diet can reverse the peripheral neuropathy and prevent the progression of the visual and central nervous system manifestations.

2-Methylacyl-CoA Racemase Deficiency. This disorder is caused by an enzyme defect that leads to the accumulation of the branched-chain fatty acids (phytanic and pristanic acid) and bile acids. Patients present with adult-type peripheral neuropathy and may also have pigmentary degeneration of the retina.

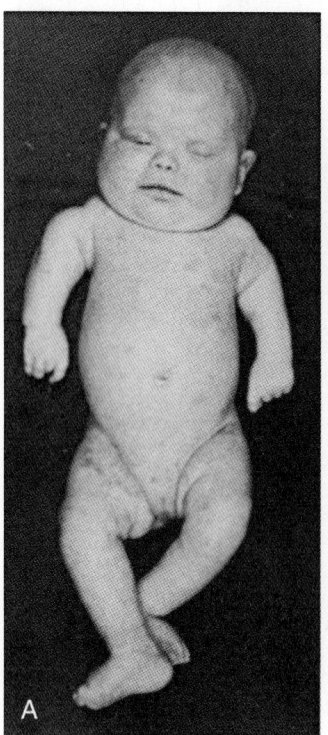
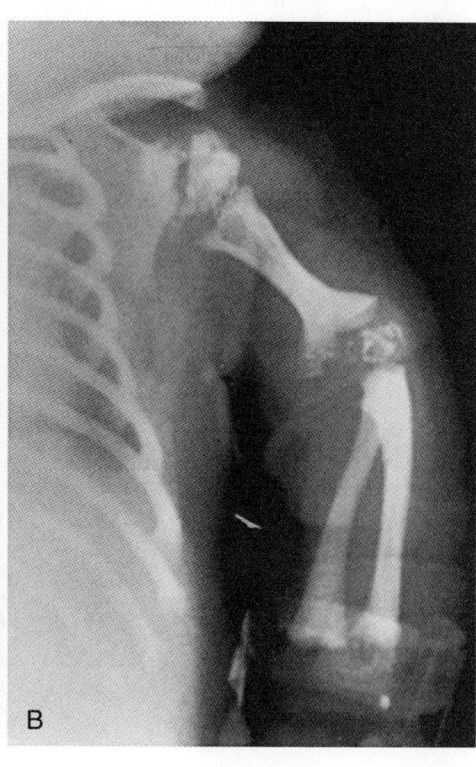

FIGURE 75–4. *A,* A newborn infant with RCDP. Note the severe shortening of the proximal limbs, the depressed bridge of the nose, hypertelorism, and widespread scaling skin lesions. *B,* Note the marked shortening of the humerus and epiphyseal stippling at the shoulder and the elbow joints. (Courtesy of John P. Dorst, MD.)

Laboratory Findings. Laboratory tests for peroxisomal disorders can be viewed at three levels of complexity.

LEVEL 1: DOES THE PATIENT HAVE A PEROXISOMAL DISORDER? This can be resolved by noninvasive tests that are generally available (Table 75–3). Measurement of plasma VLCFA is the most commonly used assay. Whereas plasma VLCFA levels are elevated in many patients with peroxisomal disorders, this is not always the case. The most important exception is RCDP, in which VLCFA levels are normal but plasma phytanic acid levels are increased and red blood cell plasmalogen levels are reduced. In some other peroxisomal disorders the biochemical abnormalities are still more restricted. Therefore, a panel of tests is recommended and includes plasma levels of VLCFA and of phytanic, pristanic, and pipecolic acids and levels of plasmalogens in red blood cells. Tandem mass spectrometry techniques also permit convenient quantitation of bile acids in plasma and urine. This panel of tests can be performed on 2-mL samples of venous blood and permits detection of most peroxisomal disorders, and normal results make the presence of a peroxisomal disorder unlikely.

LEVEL 2: WHAT IS THE PRECISE NATURE OF THE PEROXISOMAL DISORDER? Table 75–3 lists the main biochemical abnormalities in the various peroxisomal disorders. When combined with the clinical presentation the just mentioned panel of tests is often sufficient to identify the precise nature of the defect. Elevated plasma VLCFA levels permit the precise diagnosis of X-ALD in male patients. Marked reduction of erythrocyte plasmalogen levels combined with elevated plasma phytanic acid permits precise diagnosis in a patient with the clinical features of RCDP. Classic Refsum disease can be diagnosed by demonstration of increased plasma phytanic acid combined with normal or reduced levels of pristanic acid levels.

Precise identification of some peroxisomal disorders may require more extensive studies in cultured skin fibroblasts. This may be required for the differentiation of PBD from defects in bifunctional enzyme. In PBD patients peroxisomes are absent and catalase is in the soluble fraction, whereas in bifunctional enzyme defect, peroxisomes are present and catalase is in the particulate fraction. Fibroblast studies are required to identify the nature of the molecular defect in PBD. Whether such specialized studies are clinically warranted depends on individual circumstances. Precise definition of the defect in a proband may improve the precision of prenatal diagnosis in at-risk pregnancies, and it is required for carrier detection. It is also of value in

---

TABLE 75–3. **Peroxisomal Disorders That Involve Fatty Acid Oxidation: Diagnostic Assays**

Disease	Assay		Finding
Zellweger syndrome	Plasma	VLCFA	Increased
Neonatal adrenoleukodystrophy		Phytanic acid	Age-dependent increase
Infantile Refsum disease		Pristanic acid	Age-dependent increase
		Pipecolic acid	Increased
		Bile acid	Increased, abnormal pattern
	RBCs,	Plasmalogen levels	Variably decreased
	Fibroblasts	VLCFA levels	Increased
		VLCFA oxidation	Decreased
		Plasmalogen synthesis	Decreased
		Phytanic, pristanic oxidation	Decreased
		Catalase localization	Cytosolic
		Immunocytochemistry	Peroxisomes absent
		Complementation	See Table 75–1
		DNA	See Table 75–1
Rhizomelic chondrodysplasia punctata	Plasma	Phytanic acid	Increased
		VLCFA	Normal
	RBCs	Plasmalogen levels	Decreased
	Fibroblasts	Plasmalogen synthesis	Decreased
		Phytanic acid oxidation	Decreased
		DNA	*PEX7* defect
X-linked ALD hemizygote	Plasma	VLCFA	Increased
	Fibroblasts	VLCFA levels	Increased
		VLCFA oxidation	Decreased
		ALDP immunoreactivity	Absent 70%
		DNA	*ABCD1* mutation
X-linked ALD heterozygote	Plasma	VLCFA	Variable increase in 85%
	Fibroblasts	VLCFA levels	Variable increase in 90%
		ALDP immunoreactivity	Variable decrease
		DNA	*ABCD1* mutation
Bifunctional enzyme defect	Plasma	VLCFA	Increased
		Phytanic acid	Increased
		Pristanic acid	Increased
		Bile acids	Increased, abnormal pattern
	Fibroblasts	VLCFA levels	Increased
		Pristanic acid oxidation	Decreased
		Catalase localization	Peroxisomal
		Enzyme	D-bifunctional protein deficiency
Acyl-CoA oxidase deficiency	Plasma	VLCFA	Increased
	Fibroblasts	VLCFA levels	Increased
		VLCFA oxidation	Decreased
		Enzyme	Acyl-CoA oxidase defect
2-Methyl acyl-CoA racemase deficiency	Plasma	Pristanic acid	Increased
		Bile acids	Increased, abnormal pattern
	Fibroblasts	Pristanic acid oxidation	Decreased
		Enzyme	2-Methyl acyl CoA oxidase defect
Classic Refsum disease	Plasma	Phytanic acid	Increased
		Pristanic acid	Decreased
	Fibroblasts	Enzyme	Phytanoyl-CoA deficiency

VLCFA = very long chain fatty acids; ALD = adrenoleukodystrophy.

setting prognosis. For example, precise characterization is of prognostic value in patients with *PEX1* defects. This defect is present in about 60% of PBD patients, and about half of the *PEX1* defects have the G843D allele, which is associated with a significantly milder phenotype than is found in other mutations.

LEVEL 3: WHAT IS THE MOLECULAR DEFECT? Table 75–1 shows that the molecular defects in most of the PBD have been defined. Definition of the molecular defect in a proband would speed prenatal diagnosis and is required for carrier detection. Even though mutation analysis of PBD is technically feasible it is not available on a service basis but may become so in the future.

Diagnosis. There are several noninvasive laboratory tests that permit precise and early diagnosis of peroxisomal disorders (see Table 75–3). The challenge in PBD is to differentiate them from the large variety of other conditions that can cause hypotonia, seizures, failure to thrive, or dysmorphic features. Experienced clinicians can readily recognize classic Zellweger syndrome by its clinical manifestations. PBD patients often do not show the full clinical spectrum of disease and may be identifiable only by laboratory assays. Clinical features that may serve as indications for these diagnostic assays include severe psychomotor retardation; weakness and hypotonia; dysmorphic features; neonatal seizures; retinopathy, glaucoma, or cataracts; hearing deficits; enlarged liver and impaired liver function; and chondrodysplasia punctata. The presence of one or more of these abnormalities increases the likelihood of this diagnosis. Atypical milder forms presenting as peripheral neuropathy have also been described.

Some patients with the isolated defects of peroxisomal fatty acid oxidation (group B) resemble those with group A disorders and can be detected by the demonstration of abnormally high levels of VLCFA.

Patients with RCDP must be distinguished from patients with other causes of chondrodysplasia punctata. In addition to warfarin embryopathy and Zellweger syndrome, these disorders include the milder autosomal dominant form of chondrodysplasia punctata *(Conradi-Hunermann syndrome)*, which is characterized by longer survival, absence of severe limb shortening, and usually intact intellect; an X-linked dominant form; and an X-linked recessive form associated with a deletion of the terminal portion of the short arm of the X chromosome. RCDP is suspected clinically because of the shortness of limbs, psychomotor retardation, and ichthyosis. The most decisive laboratory test is the demonstration of abnormally low plasmalogen levels in red blood cells and an impaired capacity to synthesize plasmalogens in cultured skin fibroblasts. These biochemical defects are not present in other types of chondrodysplasia punctata. Chondrodysplasia punctata may also be associated with a defect of 3β-hydroxysteroid-Δ^8,Δ^7-isomerase, an enzyme involved in biosynthesis of cholesterol.

Complications. Patients with Zellweger cerebrohepatorenal syndrome have multiple disabilities involving muscle tone, swallowing, cardiac abnormalities, liver disease, and seizures. These conditions are treated symptomatically, but the prognosis is poor, and most patients succumb during the first few months of life. Patients with rhizomelic chondrodysplasia punctata may develop quadriparesis owing to compression at the base of the brain.

Prevention. See Chapters 72 and 73.

Treatment. The most effective therapy is the dietary treatment of classic Refsum disease with a phytanic acid-restricted diet.

For patients with the somewhat milder variants of the peroxisome import disorders, considerable success has been achieved with multidisciplinary early intervention, including physical and occupational therapy, hearing aids, alternative communication, nutrition, and support for the parents. Although most patients continue to function in the profoundly or severely retarded range, some make significant gains in self-help skills, and several are in stable condition in their teens or even early 20s.

Studies to mitigate some of the secondary biochemical abnormalities include the oral administration of docosahexaenoic acid in a dosage of 50–100 mg/24 hr either as the ethyl ester or in the form of a triglyceride in which one of the fatty acids has been replaced by docosahexaenoic acid. This therapy normalizes the plasma and erythrocyte levels of this substance, which has important physiologic functions in retina and brain, but the levels of which are reduced greatly in patients with disorders of peroxisome biogenesis because the last step of its synthesis takes place in the peroxisome. There are anecdotal reports of clinical improvement. The oral administration of cholic acid and chenodeoxycholic acid in a dosage of 100–250 mg/24 hr, with the aim of reducing the levels of presumably toxic bile acid intermediates, may be effective.

Genetic Counseling. All the peroxisomal disorders can be diagnosed prenatally in the 1st or 2nd trimester, except for hyperoxaluria type 1. The tests are similar to those described for postnatal diagnosis (see Table 75–3) and use chorionic villus sampling or amniocytes. More than 300 pregnancies have been monitored, and more than 60 affected fetuses have been identified without diagnostic error. Because of the 25% recurrence risk, couples, with an affected child, must be advised about the availability of prenatal diagnosis. Heterozygotes can be identified in X-linked adrenoleukodystrophy and in those disorders in which the molecular defect has been identified (see Table 75–1).

Baumgartner MR, Poll-The BT, Verhoeven NM, et al: Clinical approach to inherited peroxisomal disorders: A series of 27 patients. *Ann Neurol* 1998;44:720–30.

Martinez M, Pineda M, Vidal R, et al: Docosahexaenoic acid—a new therapeutic approach to peroxisomal-disorder patients: Experience with two cases. *Neurology* 1993;43:1389–97.

Moser AB, Rasmussen M, Naidu S, et al: Phenotype of patients with peroxisomal disorders subdivided into sixteen complementation groups. *J Pediatr* 1995;127:13–22.

Moser HW: Genotype-phenotype correlations in disorders of peroxisome biogenesis. *Mol Genet Metab* 1999;68:316–27.

Motley AM, Brites P, Gerez L, et al: Mutational spectrum in the *PEX7* gene and functional analysis of mutant alleles in 78 patients with rhizomelic chondrodysplasia punctata type 1. *Am J Hum Genet* 2002;70:612–24.

van Grunsven EG, van Berkel E, Mooijer PA, et al: Peroxisomal bifunctional protein deficiency revisited: Resolution of its true enzymatic and molecular basis. *Am J Hum Genet* 1999;64:99–107.

Walter C, Gootjes J, Mooijer PA: Disorders of peroxisome biogenesis due to mutations in *PEX1*: Phenotypes and PEX1 protein levels. *Am J Hum Genet* 2001;69:35–48.

Wanders RJ, Jansen GA, Skjeldal OH: Refsum disease, peroxisomes and phytanic acid oxidation: A review. *J Neuropathol Exp Neurol* 2001;60:1021–31.

ADRENOLEUKODYSTROPHY (X-LINKED)

X-linked ALD is a genetically determined disorder associated with the accumulation of saturated VLCFA and a progressive dysfunction of the adrenal cortex and nervous system white matter.

Etiology. The key biochemical abnormality is the tissue accumulation of unbranched saturated VLCFA, with a carbon chain length of 24 or more. Excess hexacosanoic acid (C26:0) is the most striking and characteristic feature. This accumulation of fatty acids is caused by genetically deficient peroxisomal degradation of fatty acid. The key biochemical defect involves the impaired function of peroxisomal lignoceroyl-CoA ligase, the enzyme that catalyzes the formation of the CoA derivative of VLCFA. The gene that is defective *(ABCD1)* codes for a peroxisomal membrane (ALDP). More than 400 distinct mutations have been identified, and most families have a mutation that is "private" (unique to that kindred). The gene has been mapped to chromosome Xq28. The mechanism by which the ALDP defect leads to VLCFA accumulation and the pathology of X-ALD is unknown.

Epidemiology. The minimum incidence of X-ALD in males is 1:21,000, and the combined incidence of X-ALD males and heterozygous females in the general population is estimated to be 1:17,000. All races are affected. The various phenotypes often occur in members of the same kindred.

Pathology. Characteristic lamellar cytoplasmic inclusions can be demonstrated with the electron microscope in adrenocortical cells, testicular Leydig cells, and nervous system macrophages. These inclusions probably consist of cholesterol esterified with VLCFA. They are most prominent in cells of the zona fasciculata of the adrenal cortex, which at first are distended with lipid and later atrophy.

The nervous system can display two types of lesions. In the severe childhood cerebral form and in the rapidly progressive adult forms, demyelination is associated with an inflammatory response manifested by the accumulation of perivascular lymphocytes that is most intense in the parieto-occipital region. In the slowly progressive adult form, adrenomyeloneuropathy (AMN), the main finding is a distal axonopathy that affects the long tracts in the spinal cord. The inflammatory response is mild or absent.

Pathogenesis. The adrenal dysfunction is probably a direct consequence of the accumulation of VLCFA. The cells in the zona fasciculata are distended with abnormal lipids. Cholesterol esterified with VLCFA is relatively resistant to adrenocorticotropic hormone (ACTH)-stimulated cholesterol ester hydrolases, and this limits the capacity to convert cholesterol to active steroids. In addition, C26:0 excess increases the viscosity of the plasma membrane and this may interfere with receptor and other cellular functions.

There is no correlation between the neurologic phenotype and the nature of the mutation or the severity of the biochemical defect as assessed by plasma levels of VLCFA or between the degree of adrenal and nervous system involvement. The severity of the illness and rate of progression correlate with the intensity of the inflammatory response. The inflammatory response may be cytokine mediated and may involve an autoimmune response triggered in an unknown way by the excess of VLCFA. A CD1 lipid antigen has been implicated. Approximately half of the patients do not experience the inflammatory response. A modifier gene that sets the "thermostat" for the inflammatory response is postulated.

Clinical Manifestations. There are five relatively distinct phenotypes, three of which present in childhood with symptoms and signs. In all the phenotypes, development is usually normal during the first 3–4 yr.

In the *childhood cerebral* form of ALD, symptoms are first noted most commonly between the ages of 4 and 8 yr (3 yr at the earliest). The most common initial manifestations are hyperactivity, which is often mistaken for an attention deficit disorder, and worsening school performance in a child who had previously been a good student. Auditory discrimination is often impaired, although tone perception is preserved. This may be evidenced by difficulty in using the telephone and greatly impaired performance on intelligence tests in items that are presented verbally. Spatial orientation is often impaired. Other initial symptoms are disturbances of vision, ataxia, poor handwriting, seizures, and strabismus. Visual disturbances often are due to involvement of the cerebral cortex, which leads to variable and seemingly inconsistent visual capacity. Seizures occur in nearly all patients and may represent the first manifestation of the disease. Some patients present with increased intracranial pressure or with unilateral mass lesions. Impaired cortisol response to ACTH stimulation is present in 85% of patients, and mild hyperpigmentation is noted. However, in most patients with this phenotype, adrenal dysfunction is recognized only after the condition is diag-

nosed because of the cerebral symptoms. Cerebral childhood ALD tends to progress rapidly with increasing spasticity and paralysis, visual and hearing loss, and loss of ability to speak or swallow. The mean interval between the first neurologic symptom and an apparently vegetative state is 1.9 yr. Patients may continue in this apparently vegetative state for 10 yr or more.

Adolescent ALD designates patients who experience neurologic symptoms between the ages of 10 and 21 yr. The manifestations resemble those of childhood cerebral ALD except that progression is slower.

About 10% of patients present acutely with status epilepticus, adrenal crisis, acute encephalopathy, or coma.

Adrenomyeloneuropathy first manifests in late adolescence or adulthood as a progressive paraparesis caused by long tract degeneration in the spinal cord. Approximately one half of the patients also have involvement of the cerebral white matter.

The "Addison only" phenotype is an important and underdiagnosed condition. Of male patients with Addison disease, 25% may have the biochemical defect of ALD. Many of these patients have intact neurologic systems, whereas others have subtle neurologic signs. Many acquire adrenomyeloneuropathy in adulthood.

The term *asymptomatic ALD* is applied to persons who have the biochemical defect of ALD but are free of neurologic or endocrine disturbances. Nearly all persons with the gene defect eventually become symptomatic. A few have remained asymptomatic even in the 6th or 7th decade.

Approximately 50% of female heterozygotes acquire a syndrome that resembles adrenomyeloneuropathy but is milder and of later onset. Adrenal insufficiency is rare.

Laboratory and Radiographic Findings. The most specific and important laboratory finding is the demonstration of abnormally high levels of VLCFA in plasma, red blood cells, or cultured skin fibroblasts. The test should be performed in a laboratory that has experience with this specialized procedure. Positive results are obtained in all male patients with X-linked ALD and in approximately 85% of female carriers of X-linked ALD. Mutation analysis is the most reliable method for the identification of carriers.

CT AND MRI. Patients with childhood cerebral or adolescent ALD show cerebral white matter lesions that are characteristic with respect to location and attenuation patterns on MRI. In 80% of patients, the lesions are symmetric and involve the periventricular white matter in the posterior parietal and occipital lobes. About 50% show location of a garland of accumulated contrast material adjacent and anterior to the posterior hypodense lesions (Fig. 75–5A). This zone corresponds to the zones of intense perivascular lymphocytic infiltration where the blood-brain barrier breaks down. In 12% of patients, the initial lesions are frontal. Unilateral lesions that produce a mass effect suggestive of a brain tumor may occur. MRI provides a clearer delineation of normal and abnormal white matter than does CT and may demonstrate abnormalities missed by CT (see Fig. 75–5B).

IMPAIRED ADRENAL FUNCTION. More than 85% of patients with the childhood form of ALD have elevated levels of ACTH in plasma and a subnormal rise of cortisol levels in plasma following intravenous injection of 250 μg of $ACTH_{1B}^{Z}4$ (Cortrosyn).

Diagnosis and Differential Diagnosis. The earliest manifestations of childhood cerebral ALD are difficult to distinguish from the more common attention deficit disorders or learning disabilities. Rapid progression, signs of dementia, or difficulty in auditory discrimination suggest ALD. Even in early stages, CT or MRI may show strikingly abnormal changes. Other leukodystrophies (see Chapters 592.5 and 604.10) or multiple sclerosis (see Chapter 592.5) may mimic these radiographic findings.

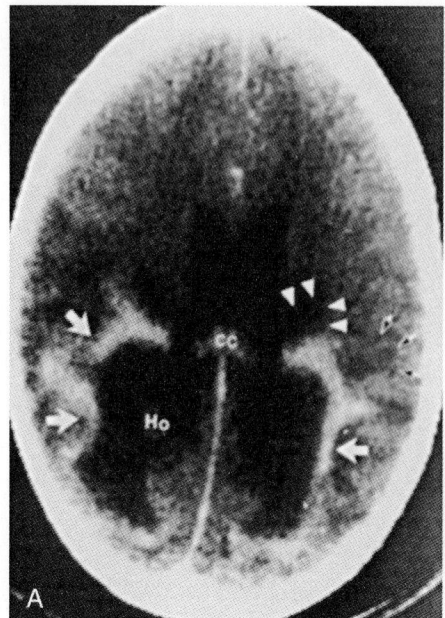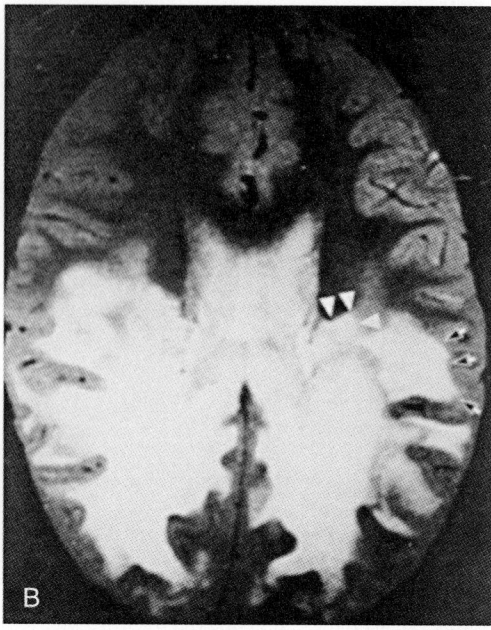

FIGURE 75–5. *A,* Contrast-enhanced CT abnormalities in ALD with typical parieto-occipital location, showing symmetric bilateral hypodense inactive zones (Ho). The enhancing active periphery zone of hypodensity is demarcated by *arrows.* Compare the anterior zone of hypodensity *(arrowheads)* with that on the MRI in *B.* CC = corpus callosum. *B,* MRI of the same patient and area shown by CT. MRI T2-weighted image shows a high-intensity signal of the abnormally bright parieto-occipital white matter. Subcortical involvement is better identified on MRI. Separation of active zones may be better appreciated by CT, because both inactive and active zones are seen at high-signal areas on MRI. However, it is assumed that such major distinctions afforded by CT will also be demonstrable when IV enhancement (paramagnetic enhancement) becomes readily available. Note the hypodense involvement of CT *(arrowheads* and *arrows* in *A)* compared with the well-resolved lesions on MRI in *B.* (From Kumar AJ, Rosenbaum WE, Naidu S, et al: Adrenoleukodystrophy: Correlating MR imaging with CT. *Radiology* 1987;165:697.)

Definitive diagnosis depends on demonstration of VLCFA excess, which occurs only in X-linked ALD and the other peroxisomal disorders. The latter may be distinguished from X-linked ALD by their clinical presentation during the neonatal period.

Cerebral forms of ALD may present as increased intracranial pressure and unilateral mass lesions. These have been misdiagnosed as gliomas, even after brain biopsy, and several patients have received radiotherapy before the correct diagnosis was made. Measurement of VLCFA in plasma or brain biopsy specimens is the most reliable differentiating test.

Adolescent or adult cerebral ALD can be confused with psychiatric disorders, dementing disorders, or epilepsy. The first clue to the diagnosis of ALD may be the demonstration of white matter lesions by CT or MRI; assays of VLCFA are confirmatory.

ALD cannot be distinguished clinically from other forms of Addison disease; it is recommended that assays of VLCFA levels be performed in all male patients with Addison disease. ALD patients usually never have antibodies to adrenal tissue in their plasma.

Complications. An avoidable complication is the occurrence of adrenal insufficiency. The most difficult neurologic problems are those related to bed rest, contracture, coma, and swallowing disturbances. Other complications involve behavioral disturbances and injuries associated with defects of spatial orientation, impaired vision and hearing, and seizures.

Treatment. Corticosteroid replacement for adrenal insufficiency or adrenocortical hypofunction is effective (see Chapter 569). It may be lifesaving and increase general strength and well being, but it does not alter the course of the neurologic disability.

BONE MARROW TRANSPLANTATION. Bone marrow transplantation (BMT) benefits patients who show early evidence of the inflammatory demyelination that is characteristic of the rapidly progressive neurologic disability in boys and adolescents with the cerebral X-ALD phenotype. BMT is a high-risk procedure, and patients must be selected with great care. The mechanism of the beneficial effect is incompletely understood. Bone marrow–derived cells do express ALDP, the protein that is deficient in X-ALD, and approximately 50% of brain microglial cells are bone marrow derived. It is possible that replacement of these cells by cells that contain the normal gene changes the brain milieu sufficiently to correct the brain metabolic disturbance. The favorable effect may also be caused by modification of the brain inflammatory response. Five to 10 yr follow-up of boys and adolescents who had early cerebral involvement has shown stabilization and, in some instances, improvement. On the other hand BMT has not shown favorable effects in patients who had already severe brain involvement and may accelerate disease progression under these circumstances. The nonverbal IQ has been found to be of predictive value, and transplant is not recommended in patients with nonverbal IQ significantly below 80. Unfortunately, in more than half the patients who are diagnosed because of neurologic symptoms, the illness is so advanced that they are not candidates for transplant.

Consideration of BMT is most relevant in neurologically asymptomatic or mildly involved patients. Screening at-risk relatives of symptomatic patients identifies these patients most frequently, and less frequently by measurement of plasma VLCFA levels in patients with Addison disease. Because of its risk (10–20% mortality), and the fact that up to 50% of untreated patients with X-ALD do not develop inflammatory brain demyelination, transplant is not recommended in patients who are free of demonstrable brain involvement. The MRI is also of key importance for the crucial decision of whether transplant should be performed. MRI abnormalities precede clinically evident neurologic or neuropsychologic abnormalities. The brain MRI should be monitored at 6-mo to 1-yr intervals in neurologically asymptomatic boys and adolescents between the ages of

3–15 yr. If the MRI is normal, BMT is not indicated. If brain MRI abnormalities develop, the patient should be evaluated at 3-mo intervals to determine if the abnormality is progressive, in combination with careful neurologic and neuropsychologic evaluation; and if early progressive involvement is confirmed, transplant should be considered. Magnetic resonance spectroscopy improves the capacity to determine whether the brain involvement is progressive. It is not known whether BMT has a favorable effect on the noninflammatory spinal cord involvement in adults with the adrenomyeloneuropathy phenotype.

OTHER THERAPIES. Oral administration of a 4:1 mixture of glyceryl trioleate and glyceryl trierucate (Lorenzo's oil) when combined with a reduced fat intake, normalizes the levels of VLCFA within 4 wk. It has not been found to be effective in patients who are already symptomatic, but it has some preventive effect in asymptomatic boys who are less than 6 yr old. Interferon-β and immunosuppressive therapies have not been found to be effective. Therapies with lovastatin and with 4-phenylbutyrate have been proposed and are being tested in clinical trials. Gene therapy has shown promise in cultured cells and the mouse model of X-ALD but is not yet available for human trial.

SUPPORTIVE THERAPY. The progressive behavioral and neurologic disturbances associated with the childhood form of ALD are extremely difficult for the family. ALD patients require the establishment of a comprehensive management program and partnership among the family, physician, visiting nursing staff, school authorities, and counselors. In addition, parent support groups are often helpful (United Leukodystrophy Foundation, 2304 Highland Drive, Sycamore, IL 60178). Communication with school authorities is important because under the provisions of Public Law 94-142, children with ALD qualify for special services as "other health impaired" or "multi-handicapped." Depending on the rate of progression of the disease, special needs might range from relatively low-level resource services within a regular school program to home and hospital-based teaching programs for children who are not mobile.

Management challenges vary with the stage of the illness. The early stages are characterized by subtle changes in affect, behavior, and attention span. Counseling and communication with school authorities are of prime importance. Changes in the sleep-wake cycle can be benefited by the judicious use at night of sedatives such as chloral hydrate (10–50 mg/kg), pentobarbital (5 mg/kg), or diphenhydramine (2–3 mg/kg).

As the leukodystrophy progresses, the modulation of muscle tone and support of bulbar muscular function are major concerns. Baclofen in gradually increasing doses (5 mg bid to 25 mg qid) is the most effective pharmacologic agent for the treatment of acute episodic painful muscle spasms. Other agents may also be used, with care being taken to monitor the occurrence of side effects and drug interactions. As the leukodystrophy progresses, bulbar muscular control is lost. Although initially this can be managed by changing the diet to soft and pureed foods, most patients eventually require a nasogastric tube or a gastrostomy. At least one third of patients have focal or generalized seizures that usually readily respond to standard anticonvulsant medications.

Genetic Counseling and Prevention. Genetic counseling and primary and secondary prevention of X-ALD are of crucial importance. Extended family screening should be offered to all at-risk relatives of symptomatic patients; one program led to the identification of more than 250 asymptomatic affected males and 1,200 women heterozygous for X-ALD. The plasma assay permits reliable identification of affected males in whom plasma VLCFA levels are increased already on the day of birth. Identification of asymptomatic males permits institution of steroid replacement therapy when appropriate and prevents

the occurrence of adrenal crisis, which may be fatal. Monitoring of brain MRI also permits identification of patients who are candidates for bone marrow transplant at a stage when this procedure has the greatest chance of success. Plasma VLCFA assay is recommended in all male patients with Addison disease. X-ALD has been shown to be the cause of adrenal insufficiency in over 25% of boys with Addison disease of unknown cause. Identification of women heterozygous for X-ALD is more difficult than that of affected males. Plasma VLCFA levels are normal in 15–20% of heterozygous women, and failure to note this has led to serious errors in genetic counseling. If VLCFA levels are normal both in plasma and cultured skin fibroblasts, the risk of false-negative results is reduced but not eliminated. DNA analysis permits accurate identification of carriers provided that the mutation has been defined in a family member. Mutation analysis is available on a service basis.

Prenatal diagnosis of affected male fetuses can be achieved by measurement of VLCFA levels in cultured amniocytes or chorionic villus cells and by mutation analysis. Whenever a new patient with X-linked ALD is identified, a detailed pedigree should be constructed, and efforts should be made to identify all at-risk female carriers and affected males. These investigations should be accompanied by careful and sympathetic attention to social, emotional, and ethical issues during counseling.

Bezman L, Moser AB, Raymond GV, et al: Adrenoleukodystrophy: Incidence, new mutation rate, and results of extended family screening. *Ann Neurol* 2001;49: 512–7.
Boehm CD, Cutting GR, Lachtermacher MB, et al: Accurate DNA-based diagnostic and carrier testing for X-linked adrenoleukodystrophy. *Mol Genet Metab* 1999;66: 128–36.
Kemp S, Pujol A, Waterham HR, et al: X-linked adrenoleukodystrophy mutation database: Role in diagnosis and clinical correlations. *Hum Mutat* 2001;18: 499–515.
Moser AB, Kreiter N, Bezman L, et al: Plasma very long chain fatty acids in 3,000 peroxisome disease patients and 29,000 controls. *Ann Neurol* 1999;45:100–10.
Moser HW, Loes DJ, Melhem ER, et al: X-linked adrenoleukodystrophy: Overview and prognosis as a function of age and brain magnetic resonance imaging abnormality: A study involving 372 patients. *Neuropediatrics* 2000;31:227–39.
Shapiro E, Krivit W, Lockman L, et al: Long-term beneficial effect of bone marrow transplantation for childhood onset cerebral X-linked adrenoleukodystrophy. *Lancet* 2000;356:713–8.
Stephenson DJ, Bezman L, Raymond GV: Acute presentation of childhood adrenoleukodystrophy. *Neuropediatrics* 2000;31:293–7.
Van Geel BM, Assies J, Haverkort EB, et al: Progression of abnormalities in adrenomyeloneuropathy and neurologically asymptomatic X-linked adrenoleukodystrophy despite treatment with "Lorenzo's oil." *J Neurol Neurosurg Psychiatry* 1999; 67:290–9.

75.3 Disorders of Lipoprotein Metabolism and Transport

Andrew M. Tershakovec and Daniel J. Rader

EPIDEMIOLOGY OF BLOOD LIPIDS AND CARDIOVASCULAR DISEASE

There is an association between fat intake and cholesterol levels and adult coronary heart disease (CHD) mortality. Adult cardiovascular disease has its roots in childhood; for example, young American casualties in the Korean and Vietnam wars were found to have a significant prevalence of atherosclerosis. In the Johns Hopkins Precursors Study, cholesterol levels measured in young men in their early 20s were predictive of the risk of CHD developing 3 to 4 decades later. The strongest data linking factors in childhood with adult CHD come from the Bogalusa Heart Study and the Pathobiological Determinants of Atherosclerosis in Youth Research Group. These surveys have found significant correlations between early atherosclerotic changes, identified at autopsy of children and young adults, and both total and low-density lipoprotein (LDL) cholesterol levels.

Although there are no data directly linking cholesterol levels in children with adult heart disease, most of the evidence suggests that such an association exists. Children at risk for the development of premature atherosclerosis in adulthood (those with elevated cholesterol levels) should be identified early in life to try to reduce the associated risk of heart disease. Children, with cholesterol levels greater than the 75th percentile, should be considered hypercholesterolemic and potentially at risk for adult heart disease. Although many experts agree that hypertriglyceridemia is also a risk factor for premature CHD, the risk is less well defined than the risk associated with hypercholesterolemia.

Clinical Trials of Cholesterol Reduction. Multiple trials in adults assessed the impact of cholesterol reduction on a quantitative measure of atherosclerotic disease or on clinical cardiovascular events. A number of trials tested whether treatment to lower cholesterol would influence the course of angiographic coronary disease. These trials have demonstrated that cholesterol reduction resulted in reduced angiographic progression of coronary disease and even modest regression in some cases. The angiographic differences between treated and control groups has generally been small and by themselves of uncertain clinical significance. However, the reductions in clinical cardiovascular events in the treated groups in many of these studies were surprising and disproportionate to the modest differences in measurable atherosclerosis.

Several secondary prevention trials in adults with clinical end points have confirmed that cholesterol reduction in the setting of established coronary disease is highly effective in reducing cardiovascular events and total mortality. These trials have used a wide variety of interventions, including diet, niacin, bile acid sequestrants, partial ileal bypass surgery, and, most effectively, the 3-hydroxy-3-methylglutaryl-coenzyme A (HMG-CoA) reductase inhibitors (statins). Trials with statins that enrolled coronary artery disease patients with average cholesterol levels also demonstrated significant benefit.

Primary prevention of CHD is important, as approximately one fourth to one third of first myocardial infarctions result in death. The Oslo study, which focused on diet intervention and smoking cessation, demonstrated a 47% decrease in fatal and nonfatal myocardial infarction. Three primary prevention trials using different lipid-lowering drugs (clofibrate, cholestyramine, and gemfibrozil) produced mixed results, generally lowering CHD mortality but not overall mortality. The West of Scotland Coronary Prevention Trial demonstrated that treatment with pravastatin resulted in reduced nonfatal myocardial infarctions and CHD mortality, as well as in total mortality, in relatively high-risk men with hypercholesterolemia but no prior history of coronary artery disease. The Air Force/Texas Coronary Artery Prevention Study demonstrated that treatment with lovastatin reduced major coronary events in relatively average-risk men and women with only moderately elevated cholesterol levels, relatively low high-density lipoprotein (HDL) cholesterol levels, and no evidence of baseline vascular disease. These trials have clearly established that drug therapy for hypercholesterolemia is safe and effective in reducing coronary events in adults without prior evidence of CHD.

PLASMA LIPOPROTEIN METABOLISM AND TRANSPORT

Cholesterol and triglycerides are transported in the circulation in macromolecular complexes termed *lipoproteins*; the protein components of the complexes are called *apolipoproteins*. Dietary lipoproteins (chylomicrons) are formed in and secreted by the small intestine; other lipoproteins (very low density lipoproteins, VLDL) are synthesized in the liver; still others (HDL) are secreted as nascent particles by the liver and small intestine and reach their mature form in the circulation only after exchange of components with other circulating lipoproteins or with tissues.

Transport of Exogenous (Dietary) Lipids. After ingestion of a fat-containing meal and hydrolysis of esterified lipids by intestinal and pancreatic lipases, free fatty acids and cholesterol are re-esterified in the intestinal epithelium to form triglycerides and cholesteryl esters, respectively. These lipids are then packaged together with phospholipids, free cholesterol, and the apolipoproteins apoA-I, apo A-IV, and apoB-48 to form chylomicrons (Fig. 75–6). The chylomicrons are then secreted into the intestinal lymph and pass through the thoracic duct into the peripheral circulation. In the circulation, chylomicrons acquire additional apolipoproteins, mainly apoE and several forms of apoC. Triglycerides, which constitute most of the chylomicron mass, are hydrolyzed by lipoprotein lipase at the capillary endothelium; apoC-II is a required cofactor for lipoprotein lipase. The free fatty acid products of this hydrolysis are transferred primarily to adipose tissue for storage as triglycerides or to muscle tissue for β-oxidation. The lipoprotein particles, now smaller and denser because they have lost much of their triglyceride content, are called *chylomicron remnants*. They have retained most of their cholesteryl ester content, have transferred some of their apolipoproteins (apoCs and apoA-I) to HDL, and have become enriched with respect to their apoE content. These remnants are bound and internalized in part via hepatic membrane receptors specific for apoE on the particles. By this mechanism, dietary

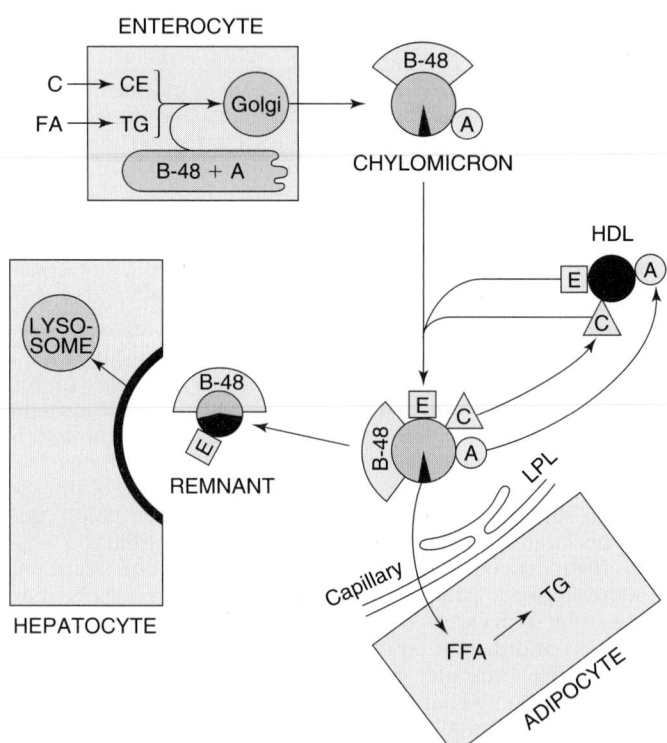

CHYLOMICRON PATHWAY

FIGURE 75–6. Pathway of chylomicron metabolism in human plasma. Fatty acids (FA) and cholesterol (C) are esterified in the intestinal mucosa to form triglycerides (TG) and cholesteryl esters (CE), respectively. They combine with apoA and apoB-48 to form chylomicrons, which are secreted into the circulation: TG *(shaded area)* and CE *(black area)*. Chylomicrons undergo lipolysis in the capillary endothelium near adipose tissue and muscle tissue, losing TG via lipoprotein lipase (LPL), gaining apoE from HDL, and losing apoA and apoC to HDL. The resultant chylomicron remnants are taken up by hepatic apoE receptors for degradation by lysosomes. (Adapted from Havel RJ: Approach to the patient with hyperlipidemia. *Med Clin North Am* 1982;66:319.)

cholesterol is delivered to the liver, where it plays a role in the regulation of hepatic cholesterol metabolism. Under normal circumstances, chylomicrons and their remnants are very short-lived in the circulation; following a 12-hr fast, there are no chylomicrons or chylomicron remnants remaining in the plasma.

Transport of Endogenous Lipids from the Liver. The liver secretes a class of lipoproteins called very low density lipoproteins, which contain free and esterified cholesterol, triglycerides, phospholipids, and several apolipoproteins, notably apoB-100, apoCs, and apoE. Like chylomicrons, VLDL exchange apolipoproteins with other circulating particles and deliver free fatty acids to adipose tissue and muscle after hydrolysis of triglycerides by lipoprotein lipase (Fig. 75–7). In the process, they become smaller and denser and are termed *VLDL remnants* or *intermediate-density lipoproteins* (IDL). Some of these remnant particles are taken up via hepatic receptors specific for apoE, whereas some undergo conversion to LDL. Conversion of LDL particles

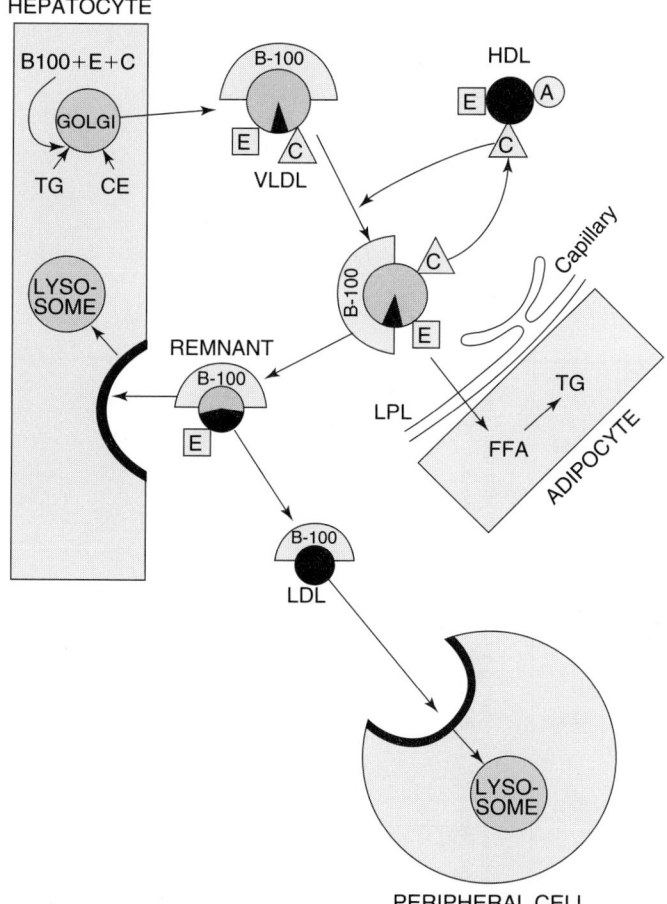

VLDL-LDL PATHWAYS

FIGURE 75–7. Pathways of VLDL and LDL metabolism in human plasma. Triglycerides (TG) and cholesteryl esters (CE) are combined with apoB-100, apoC, and apoE in the liver and then secreted as VLDL, TG *(shaded area)*, and CE *(black area)*. VLDL undergo lipolysis in the capillary endothelium near adipose tissue and muscle tissue, losing TG via lipoprotein lipase (LPL). The resulting VLDL remnants are either converted to low-density lipoproteins (LDL) for transport to peripheral cells via LDL receptor-mediated uptake or are taken up by hepatic receptors. FFA = free fatty acids. (Adapted from Havel RJ: Approach to the patient with hyperlipidemia. *Med Clin North Am* 1982;66:319.)

requires participation of hepatic lipase, which hydrolyzes the remaining triglycerides, as well as some phospholipids. LDL are almost entirely made up of cholesteryl esters and apoB-100. A specific LDL receptor is present on most cell membranes and recognizes, binds, and internalizes LDL. By this mechanism, LDL particles can deliver cholesterol to extrahepatic tissues for use in membrane or steroid hormone synthesis. LDL receptor expression by the liver is a major regulator of plasma LDL cholesterol levels. LDL particles have a half-life of 3–4 days.

High-Density Lipoprotein and Reverse Cholesterol Transport. In contrast to chylomicrons and VLDL, which are secreted into the circulation as mature particles, the liver and small intestine secrete HDL as nascent discoidal particles composed primarily of phospholipids and apolipoproteins. Nascent HDL secreted by the small intestine are rich in apoA-I and apoA-IV, whereas those derived from the liver contain predominantly apoA-I, and apoA-II. Nascent lipid-poor apoA-I accepts unesterified cholesterol from tissues via a process that requires the ATP-binding cassette protein A1 (ABCA1), a cellular protein that facilitates the efflux of unesterified cholesterol and phospholipids from cells to apoA-1. Unesterified cholesterol in nascent HDL is esterified by the enzyme lecithin:cholesterol acyltransferase (LCAT), which is present on HDL, forming cholesteryl esters. HDL cholesteryl esters may be selectively taken up by the liver via a hepatic HDL receptor called scavenger receptor class BI (SR-BI). Alternatively, HDL cholesteryl ester may transfer from HDL to VLDL and LDL by the cholesteryl ester transfer protein (CETP), after which it may be taken up by the liver or redistributed to peripheral tissues. Thus, HDL have two pathways by which they return tissue-derived cholesterol to the liver in a process that has been termed *reverse cholesterol transport*. HDL-derived cholesterol is either converted by the liver to bile acids or directly excreted into the bile.

PLASMA LIPID AND LIPOPROTEIN LEVELS

Table 75–4 presents normal plasma cholesterol and triglyceride levels from birth through the first 2 decades of life. During the first few months of life, cholesterol levels increase largely because of changes in LDL. Over the next 15–20 yr, in both males and females, there is little change in the total cholesterol level; the mean value fluctuates around 150–165 mg/dL. Mean LDL cholesterol levels remain slightly less than 100 mg/dL in both males and females during this period. HDL cholesterol levels are comparable in males and females early in life; they remain essentially constant in females but decline markedly in males during the 2nd decade to a level that is maintained through adulthood. Plasma triglyceride levels, in contrast, rise transiently in both males and females in the 1st year, fall to a mean of 50–60 mg/dL in the ensuing few years, and then rise to a mean of approximately 75 mg/dL by age 20 yr. In early adulthood, there is a rise in plasma cholesterol that is almost exclusively caused by an increase in LDL cholesterol. The rate of increase over the next 30 yr is greater in males than in females. When coupled with their lower HDL cholesterol levels, this puts men at much greater risk than women for atherosclerotic heart disease, at least until women reach the age of menopause. Because of the changes in lipid levels with age, it is more appropriate to use age- and gender-specific percentile figures when comparing levels between individuals and over long periods rather than consider absolute cholesterol levels.

Cholesterol levels track over time. Thus, children with high cholesterol levels tend to have higher levels as young adults, whereas those with low levels as children tend to have lower levels as adults. However, this is not always the case. A significant degree of biologic and laboratory variation in cholesterol measurements contributes to this. Lifestyle changes of participants (weight loss, changes in diet) in longitudinal surveys of cholesterol levels in children and young adults may also have

TABLE 75–4. Plasma Cholesterol and Triglyceride Levels in Childhood and Adolescence: Means and Percentiles

	Total Triglyceride (mg/dL)					Total Cholesterol (mg/dL)					Low-Density Lipoprotein Cholesterol (mg/dL)					High-Density Lipoprotein Cholesterol (mg/dL)*				
	5th	Mean	75th	90th	95th	5th	Mean	75th	90th	95th	5th	Mean	75th	90th	95th	5th	10th	25th	Mean	95th
Cord	14	34	—	—	84	42	68	—	—	103	17	29	—	—	50	13	—	—	35	60
1–4 yr																				
Male	29	56	68	85	99	114	155	170	190	203	—	—	—	—	—	—	—	—	—	—
Female	34	64	74	95	112	112	156	173	188	200	—	—	—	—	—	—	—	—	—	—
5–9 yr																				
Male	28	52	58	70	85	125	155	168	183	189	63	93	103	117	129	38	42	49	56	74
Female	32	64	74	103	126	131	164	176	190	197	68	100	115	125	140	36	38	47	53	73
10–14 yr																				
Male	33	63	74	94	111	124	160	173	188	202	64	97	109	122	132	37	40	46	55	74
Female	39	72	85	104	120	125	160	171	191	205	68	97	110	126	136	37	40	45	52	70
15–19 yr																				
Male	38	78	88	125	143	118	153	168	183	191	62	94	109	123	130	30	34	39	46	63
Female	36	73	85	112	126	118	159	176	198	207	59	96	111	129	137	35	38	43	52	74

*Note that different percentiles are listed for HDL cholesterol.

Data for cord blood from Strong W: Atherosclerosis: Its pediatric roots. In Kaplan N, Stamler J (editors): Prevention of Coronary Heart Disease. Philadelphia, WB Saunders, 1983. Data for children 1–4 yr from Tables 6, 7, 20, and 21, and all other data from Tables 24, 25, 32, 33, 36, and 37 in Lipid Research Clinics Population Studies Data Book, Vol. 1, The Prevalence Study. NIH publication No. 80–1527. Washington, DC, National Institutes of Health, 1980.

contributed to the lower observed degree of tracking. Surveys in adults have described a decline in the prevalence of hypercholesterolemia, presumably related to a decreasing intake of fat in the diet; however, a disturbing increase in the prevalence of obesity is also occurring. This may balance or overwhelm the positive public health effects of lower cholesterol levels.

Children may have moderately raised cholesterol levels for a variety of reasons. Some primary genetic defects may be associated with only mild alterations in blood lipid levels. Furthermore, there are secondary causes of hyperlipoproteinemia (HLP) (other disease states) that need to be considered. Finally, inappropriate dietary habits, by themselves or by interacting with any of the preceding factors, can contribute to moderately raised cholesterol levels. Although some children suffer from well-defined familial hyperlipidemia, the majority of individuals with hyperlipidemia do not have such specific syndromes. In addition, although those with hyperlipidemia are at increased risk for heart disease, not all hyperlipidemic individuals acquire clinical heart disease.

SCREENING FOR HYPERCHOLESTEROLEMIA

The Expert Panel on Blood Cholesterol Levels in Children and Adolescents of the National Cholesterol Education Program and the American Academy of Pediatrics Committee on Nutrition have recommended that children with a parental history of elevated total cholesterol levels (>240 mg/dL) have their total cholesterol level measured. Children with incomplete or unavailable family histories, or those with other risk factors for CHD (obesity, cigarette smoking, hypertension, diabetes, inactivity, low HDL cholesterol), should be screened at the discretion of the pediatric care provider. Cholesterol measurements have been shown to be relatively unreliable when undertaken in settings without adequate quality assurance. To avoid inaccurately labeling children as hypercholesterolemic, screening should be completed using only reliable laboratories and methods.

Children with total cholesterol levels less than 170 mg/dL require no intervention other than that recommended for the general population and should be re-evaluated in 5 yr. Children whose total cholesterol level is greater than 200 mg/dL should have a fasting lipid profile performed. Those with borderline levels (170–199 mg/dL) should have another total cholesterol measurement, and the two values should be averaged; if the average total cholesterol level in these two determinations is greater than 170 mg/dL, a lipid profile is recommended. The expert panel has likewise recommended that children with a family history of premature coronary heart disease (before the age of 55 yr in a parent or grandparent) should have a lipid profile completed. Lipid profiles of parents and other 1st-degree relatives are necessary to establish whether there is a dominantly inherited defect responsible for the hypercholesterolemia.

A lipid profile (total and HDL cholesterol, triglycerides, calculated LDL cholesterol) is obtained after a 12-hr fast. VLDL cholesterol can be estimated by dividing the triglycerides by 5 (in fasting plasma, most triglycerides are in VLDL and the ratio of triglycerides to cholesterol in VLDL is approximately 5:1). LDL cholesterol is calculated using the following equation:

$$\text{LDL cholesterol} = \text{total cholesterol} - [\text{HDL cholesterol} + (\text{triglycerides}/5)]$$

The fasting lipid profile provides more complete information about a child's cholesterol status and helps determine the approach to management (Fig. 75–8). Triglycerides must be less than 400 mg/dL to derive an accurate estimate of LDL cholesterol with this method. The average value from two evaluations is recommended because of the biologic and laboratory variability in lipid values. Children with average LDL cholesterol levels greater than 130 mg/dL are considered to have persistently high

levels, whereas LDL cholesterol levels less than 110 mg/dL are considered acceptable. Levels between 110 and 130 mg/dL are borderline.

These recommendations have been criticized for several reasons. The screening algorithm is complicated to follow for the busy practitioner. Multiple surveys have shown that screening only those with a positive family history misses half or more of the hypercholesterolemic children. This problem is compounded by the fact that many adults do not know their cholesterol levels, as well as the difficulties in obtaining a complete family history. In addition, many parents who may be at risk for CHD are too young to have acquired clinical heart disease while their children are being evaluated; hence their children may not be identified as being at risk.

Those children with *triglyceride* levels greater than the 95th percentile can be a marker of some genetic forms of hyperlipidemia, even if the total cholesterol level is normal. Elevated triglycerides are also sometimes related to secondary hyperlipidemic or to the so-called "metabolic syndrome" (hyperlipidemic, insulin resistance, elevated blood pressure).

TREATMENT OF HYPERLIPIDEMIA

Dietary Management of Hyperlipidemia (see Fig. 75–8). For hypercholesterolemic children (average LDL cholesterol > 110 mg/dL) older than 2 yr, dietary modification is the best initial intervention. Their daily food intake should provide no more than 30% of total calories as fat (approximately equally distributed among saturated, monounsaturated, and polyunsaturated fats), and no more than 100 mg cholesterol/1,000 calories (maximum 300 mg/24 hr) in such a modification program. This has become commonly referred to as the prudent, or Step I American Heart Association, diet. The American Academy of Pediatrics Committee on Nutrition confirms these recommendations and also suggests a lower limit for fat intake of no less than 20% of total calories. It is recommended that all family members older than 2 yr gradually adopt this diet to encourage optimal compliance and health promotion. The minimal goal for dietary intervention is to achieve an LDL cholesterol level less than 130 mg/dL, whereas the ideal goal is to lower it to less than 110 mg/dL. If these goals are not reached even after reinforcing the Step I diet, the Step II diet (< 7% calories as saturated fat and < 66 mg cholesterol/1,000 calories to a maximum of 200 mg/24 hr) should be considered.

When recommending dietary intervention, it is important to explain that the response to dietary management is variable and generally does not lower LDL cholesterol levels by more than 10–15%. Individuals commonly have unrealistic expectations about the cholesterol lowering associated with dietary management, which limits their compliance when the response is modest. Even if the initial response to dietary therapy is limited, the potential for adopting a lifelong healthy style of eating should have long-term benefit.

Dietary modification is safe in the treatment of hyperlipidemia in adults and children older than 2 yr. The Dietary Intervention Study for Children demonstrated the safety and efficacy of a low-fat diet for hypercholesterolemic children. However, it must be emphasized that these recommendations are meant only for children older than 2 yr. Children younger than this placed on a similar or more restrictive diet, and older children placed on more restrictive diets by well-meaning caregivers, have demonstrated poor growth. Children younger than 2 yr require a relatively large amount of calories to maintain their rapid growth. Because of the higher caloric density of high-fat food, it is physically difficult for children younger than 2 yr to eat enough low-fat food to ensure normal growth. Furthermore, the higher fat intake may be necessary to help ensure an adequate supply of appropriate nutrients for the rapidly developing central nervous system. However, despite these concerns, the

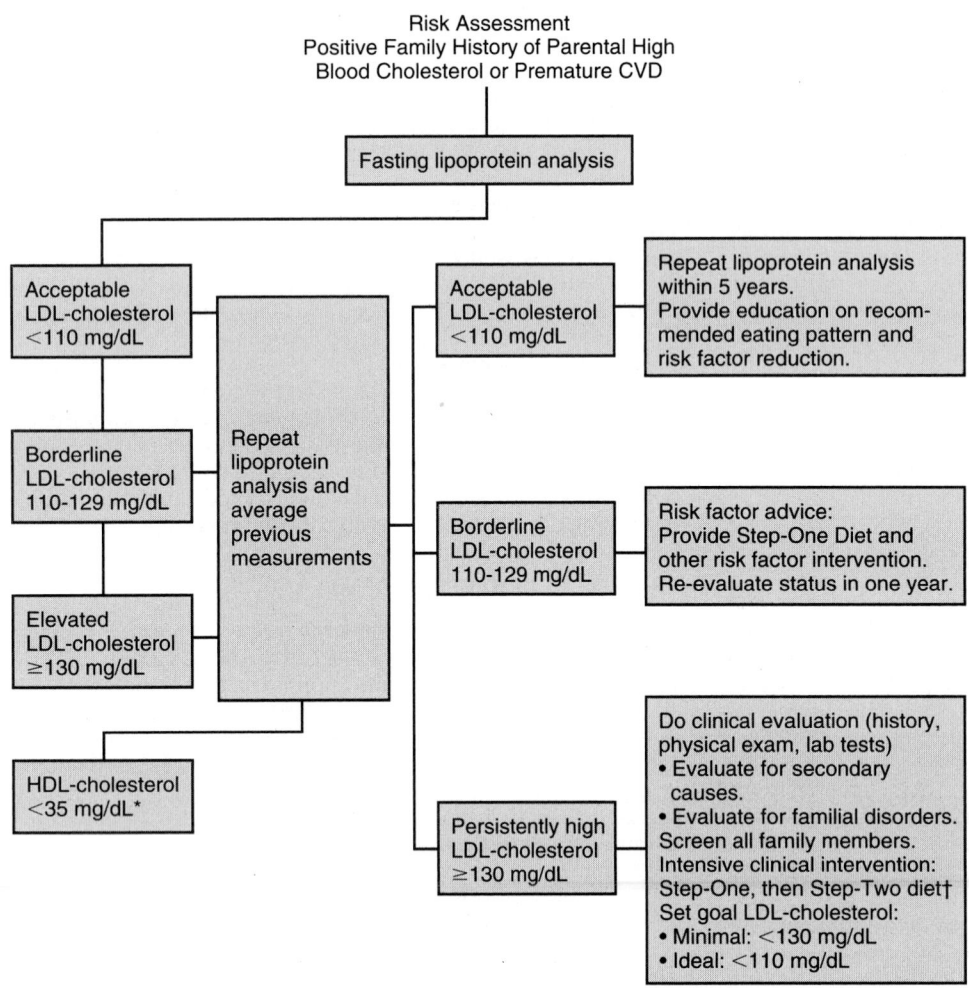

Risk Assessment
Positive Family History of Parental High
Blood Cholesterol or Premature CVD

Fasting lipoprotein analysis

Acceptable
LDL-cholesterol
<110 mg/dL

Borderline
LDL-cholesterol
110-129 mg/dL

Elevated
LDL-cholesterol
≥130 mg/dL

Repeat lipoprotein analysis and average previous measurements

HDL-cholesterol
<35 mg/dL*

Acceptable
LDL-cholesterol
<110 mg/dL

Repeat lipoprotein analysis within 5 years.
Provide education on recommended eating pattern and risk factor reduction.

Borderline
LDL-cholesterol
110-129 mg/dL

Risk factor advice:
Provide Step-One Diet and other risk factor intervention.
Re-evaluate status in one year.

Persistently high
LDL-cholesterol
≥130 mg/dL

Do clinical evaluation (history, physical exam, lab tests)
• Evaluate for secondary causes.
• Evaluate for familial disorders. Screen all family members.
Intensive clinical intervention: Step-One, then Step-Two diet†
Set goal LDL-cholesterol:
• Minimal: <130 mg/dL
• Ideal: <110 mg/dL

*If low HDL-cholesterol is detected, then patients should be counseled regarding cigarette smoking, low saturated fat diet, physical activity, and weight management (if overweight).
†For patients 10 yr old and over and with LDL-C > 190 mg/dL (or > 160 mg/dL with additional risk factors), if diet does not achieve the goal, then pharmacologic intervention should be considered.

FIGURE 75–8. Flow chart of classification, education, and follow-up of children based on LDL cholesterol levels. (From Williams CL, Hayman LL, Daniels SR, et al: Cardiovascular health in childhood. *Circulation* 2002; 106:143–60.)

Special Turhu Coronary Risk Intervention Project has demonstrated that a lower fat diet supports normal growth in children as young as 6 mo old.

There should be proper supervision to ensure the appropriateness of any dietary modification in children, especially for young children. Because most pediatricians are unable to provide detailed guidance for such dietary modifications, referral to a trained pediatric dietitian is indicated. Before undertaking a screening program, the physician should ensure the availability of such referral. The growth and development of any child undergoing dietary intervention should be monitored, and a specific dietary evaluation should be completed if growth or development is altered. It is also important to explain to the child and family that hypercholesterolemia in childhood is only a risk factor and not an illness. Emphasis should be placed on the positive changes the child and the family can make to minimize the risk.

Other Dietary Factors. Dietary fiber, especially soluble fiber, has a modest cholesterol-lowering effect in hypercholesterolemic individuals. However, high-fiber diets must be used with care in children to ensure adequate delivery of calories and nutrients. Monounsaturated fats lower LDL cholesterol levels while maintaining or even raising HDL cholesterol levels, in contrast to the lowering of LDL and HDL cholesterol levels commonly observed with a high polyunsaturated fat diet. *Trans*-fatty acids (partially

hydrogenated vegetable oils), commonly found in processed foods and margarine, seem to raise LDL cholesterol levels. Vegetarian diets have a large and significant cholesterol-lowering effect associated with the substitution of vegetable protein for animal protein and the low fat and cholesterol content of the diet. Although many groups have demonstrated the safety of vegetarian diets for children, care must be taken to ensure the completeness of the diet for the growing child. Plant stanols and sterols have been shown to reduce LDL cholesterol levels modestly in adults if consumed three times per day and are commercially available as functional foods, although their safety and efficacy has not been demonstrated in children. Although fish oil and antioxidants have little, if any, effect on cholesterol levels, they have been reported to be associated with reduced risk of CHD by other mechanisms. (Fish oil is also used as a treatment for severe hypertriglyceridemia.) However, because these compounds are frequently administered in pharmacologic doses, in the absence of additional experience, their use in children should be discouraged. Dietary modification that increases intake of these nutrients can be considered. For example, encouraging appropriate fruit and vegetable intake will help optimize natural sources of antioxidants.

Other Factors Relating to Treatment. Medical management of hypercholesterolemia should be viewed in the context of other lifestyle factors and conditions associated with risk for premature CHD, such as lack of exercise and physical activity and excessive sedentary activity, cigarette smoking, hypertension, obesity, and diabetes. These should be evaluated, controlled, minimized, or eliminated as possible and appropriate. Children already having one risk factor for premature coronary heart disease, such as hyperlipidemia, should be actively treated to minimize any other risk factors. In addition, many of these risk factors are interlinked, and therefore minimizing one may help to ameliorate others (increasing exercise may decrease obesity, which helps to lower blood pressure, LDL cholesterol, and triglyceride levels and, potentially, the risk for type 2 dependent diabetes mellitus, while also helping raise HDL cholesterol levels).

Drug Therapy (see Fig. 75–8). The Expert Panel on Treatment of Hyperlipidemia in Children recommended that drug therapy be considered in children aged 10 yr and older if, after an adequate trial (6 mo–1 yr) of diet therapy:

1. LDL cholesterol remains greater than 190 mg/dL.
2. LDL cholesterol remains greater than 160 mg/dL and (a) there is a positive family history of premature CHD (before 55 yr of age) or (b) two or more other risk factors are present in the child or adolescent after vigorous attempts have been made to control these risk factors (diabetes, hypertension, smoking, low HDL cholesterol, severe obesity, physical inactivity). It should be noted that the Adult Treatment Panel III of the National Cholesterol Education Program recommends an LDL cholesterol level less than 160 mg/dL for adults with one or fewer CHD risk factors. Primary disorders amenable to therapy are noted in Table 75–5.

Bile acid sequestrants or "resins" (cholestyramine, colesevelam, or colestipol) are often the first-line pediatric drugs for the treatment of hypercholesterolemia in children. Bile acid sequestrants primarily reduce LDL cholesterol, and care should be taken in prescribing cholestyramine for patients with triglyceride levels greater than 300 mg/dL because they exacerbate hypertriglyceridemia. These nonabsorbable compounds interrupt the enterohepatic bile acid cycle by the binding of bile acids in the intestine and enhancing their excretion in the stool. This results in shunting of hepatic cholesterol into bile acid synthesis and secondary upregulation of hepatic LDL receptors. As a result, there is increased uptake of LDL from the blood and reduction of LDL cholesterol levels. A 10–32% decrease in LDL cholesterol levels has been reported with cholestyramine therapy in children with familial hypercholesterolemia and familial combined hyperlipidemia (FCHL). However, reported long-term compliance has been poor and related to poor palatability of the medication and gastrointestinal disturbances, including nausea, bloating, and constipation. One packet or scoop contains 4 g of cholestyramine and 5 g of colestipol. The dose is titrated to the severity of hypercholesterolemia and tolerance of the side effects. Generally, resins are started at a dose of one-half packet or scoop twice a day before meals, and the dose is gradually increased over weeks as tolerated and necessary. Doses of three packets or scoops twice a day can be tolerated in some individuals. Colesevelam is available in tablets containing 625 mg. Four to 7 tablets per day is recommended.

The bile acid sequestrants are safe drugs that are not systemically absorbed. However, they are insoluble resins that must be suspended in liquid and are therefore often inconvenient and unpleasant to take. For this reason, some patients may prefer colesevelam tablets. In addition, bile acid sequestrants may bind other drugs and interfere with their absorption, creating the need to take other medications 1 hr before or 4 hr after the bile acid sequestrants. Similarly, these resins may interfere with the absorption of fat-soluble vitamins, suggesting the need for multivitamin supplements (Table 75–6).

HMG-CoA reductase inhibitors (statins) have been used in children with severe hypercholesterolemia who cannot tolerate or have inadequate response to bile acid sequestrants. HMG-CoA reductase is the rate-limiting step in cholesterol biosynthesis, and inhibition of this enzyme decreases cholesterol synthesis and results in upregulation of hepatic LDL receptors. The Canadian Lovastatin in Children Study demonstrated a 21–36% decrease (dose response related) in LDL-cholesterol level in boys with familial hypercholesterolemia treated with 10–40 mg/day lovastatin. No serious side effects were noted over the 8-wk follow-up

TABLE 75–5. Primary Lipoprotein Disorders Amenable to Treatment with Diet and Drug Therapy

Disorder	Mechanisms	Complications	Treatment*
Familial hypertriglyceridemia[†]	Decreased serum triglyceride removal resulting from decreased LPL activity Increased hepatic secretion of triglyceride-rich VLDL	Pancreatitis at triglyceride concentrations >2000 mg/dL (22.6 mmol/L); low risk of CAD	Diet and weight loss Fibrate Nicotinic acid n–3 fatty acids Oxandrolone
Familial combined hyperlipidemia[†]	Increased hepatic secretion of apolipoprotein B–containing VLDL and conversion to LDL Accumulation of VLDL, LDL, or both, depending on efficiency of their removal	CAD, PVD, stroke	Diet and weight loss Statin Nicotinic acid Fibrate[‡]
Remnant removal disease (familial dysbetalipoproteinemia)	Increased secretion of VLDL Impaired removal of remnant lipoproteins resulting from homozygosity ($\varepsilon_2/\varepsilon_2$) or heterozygosity ($\varepsilon_2/\varepsilon_3$ or $\varepsilon_2/\varepsilon_4$) for apolipoprotein E ε_2	PVD, CAD, stroke	Diet, weight loss Fibrate[‡] Nicotinic acid Statin
Familial or polygenic hypercholesterolemia	Diminished LDL-receptor activity Defective apolipoprotein B that is poorly recognized by LDL receptor	CAD, occasionally PVD, stroke	Diet Statin Bile acid–binding resin Nicotinic acid
Familial hypoalphalipoproteinemia (low HDL syndrome)[§]	Diminished apolipoprotein AI formation, increased removal, increased CETP or hepatic lipase activity	CAD, PVD (may be associated with hypertriglyceridemia)	Exercise and weight loss Nicotinic acid Fibrate[‡] Statin

LPL = lipoprotein lipase; VLDL = very-low-density lipoprotein; CAD = coronary artery disease; PVD = peripheral vascular disease; HDL = high-density lipoprotein; CETP = cholesterol-ester transfer protein.
The treatments may be given alone or in combination; the primary treatment is listed first, followed by other treatments in decreasing order of importance.
[†]*Diabetes mellitus can greatly exacerbate the condition. The hyperlipidemia of diabetes is closest mechanistically to familial combined hyperlipidemia.*
[‡]*Combined treatment with a fibrate and a statin can increase the risk of myopathy.*
[§]*This disorder is characterized by low concentrations of HDL cholesterol.*
From Knopp RH: Drug treatment of lipid disorders. N Engl J Med 1999;341:498–512.

TABLE 75–6. Side Effects of Lipid-Lowering Drugs

Drug and Site or Type of Effect	Effect
Statins	
Skin	Rash
Nervous system	Loss of concentration, sleep disturbance, headache, peripheral neuropathy
Liver	Hepatitis, loss of appetite, weight loss, and increases in serum aminotransferases to two to three times the upper limit of the normal range
Gastrointestinal tract	Abdominal pain, nausea, diarrhea
Muscles	Muscle pain or weakness, myositis (usually with serum creatine kinase >1000 U/L), rhabdomyolysis with renal failure
Immune system	Lupus-like syndrome (lovastatin, simvastatin, or fluvastatin)
Protein binding	Diminished binding of warfarin (lovastatin, simvastatin, fluvastatin)
Bile Acid–Binding Resins	
Gastrointestinal tract	Abdominal fullness, nausea, gas, constipation, hemorrhoids, anal fissure, activation of diverticulitis, diminished absorption of vitamin D in children
Liver	Mild serum aminotransferase elevations, which can be exacerbated by concomitant treatment with a statin
Metabolic system	Increases in serum triglycerides of approximately 10% (greater increases in patients with hypertriglyceridemia)
Electrolytes	Hyperchloremic acidosis in children and patients with renal failure (cholestyramine)
Drug interactions	Binding of warfarin, digoxin, thiazide diuretics, thyroxine, statins
Nicotinic Acid	
Skin	Flushing, dry skin, pruritus, ichthyosis, acanthosis nigricans
Eyes	Conjunctivitis, cystoid macular edema, retinal detachment
Respiratory tract	Nasal stuffiness
Heart	Supraventricular arrhythmias
Gastrointestinal tract	Heartburn, loose bowel movements or diarrhea
Liver	Mild increase in serum aminotransferases, hepatitis with nausea and fatigue
Muscles	Myositis
Metabolic system	Hyperglycemia (incidence, approximately 5%; higher in patients with diabetes), increase of 10% in serum uric acid
Fibrates	
Skin	Rash
Gastrointestinal tract	Stomach upset, abdominal pain (mainly gemfibrozil), cholesterol-saturated bile, increase of 1–2% in gallstone incidence
Genitourinary tract	Erectile dysfunction (mainly clofibrate)
Muscles	Myositis with impaired renal function
Plasma proteins	Interference with binding of warfarin, requiring reduction in the dose of warfarin by approximately 30%
Liver	Increased serum aminotransferases

From Knopp RH: Drug treatment of lipid disorders. N Engl J Med 1999;341:498–512.

period. These drugs are metabolized by the cytochrome P450 system, and drugs that inhibit or induce the system will raise or lower the drug level (and effect), respectively.

Potential side effects of statins include gastrointestinal upset, headache, sleep disturbance, fatigue, and muscle or joint pains (see Table 75–6). Severe myopathy and even rhabdomyolysis have been rarely reported with some HMG-CoA reductase inhibitors in adults. The risk of severe myopathy may be increased in patients taking certain other drugs such as erythromycin, antifungal agents, immunosuppressive agents, and fibric acid derivatives such as gemfibrozil and niacin. Liver transaminases should be monitored in patients taking statins, but significant (more than three times normal) elevation in transaminase levels is rare in children. However, because the long-term effects of statins remain uncertain, the risks and benefits of using them in children should be carefully considered. They should be used carefully in girls at risk of pregnancy because of the uncertainty of teratogenic defects.

Nicotinic acid is also frequently used in adults; however, its side effects (flushing, gastrointestinal upset, hepatic toxicity) may preclude its use in children. The practicing pediatrician should consider referral of all children who may be candidates for drug therapy to a specialized pediatric lipid center.

Although drug therapy is used commonly to treat *hypertriglyceridemia* in adults, it is used much less commonly in children (see Table 75–5). The mainstay of therapy in children with hypertriglyceridemia is diet, exercise, and weight loss. In severe cases of hypertriglyceridemia in children with attendant medical complications, a lipid expert should complete a careful risk-benefit analysis considering the use of medication. There are no formal recommendations concerning the treatment of hypertriglyceridemia in children.

SAFETY CONSIDERATIONS. Dietary intervention must be appropriately supervised to ensure that a complete and balanced diet is provided or available. In addition, the potential adverse psychosocial influence of being "labeled" should be considered. Children with heterozygous familial hypercholesterolemia (FH) attending a lipid clinic demonstrated no higher prevalence of psychosocial dysfunction, which could be potentially related to their being labeled "at risk," than control children. Furthermore, in one cholesterol screening program, the parents of hypercholesterolemic children reported better diets and improved perceptions of the children's health 1 yr after cholesterol screening was completed. This may be an effect of the families' active participation in reducing risk and improving health.

There are occasional reports in adults linking low or lowered cholesterol levels with depression, violent tendencies, accidents, and noncardiac illnesses, including some forms of cancer. These reports do not consistently demonstrate the same associations, and other studies present conflicting data (e.g., those reporting an association between high-fat diets and some forms of cancer). In addition, many of the cholesterol-lowering interventions use diet or drugs, or both, and thus negative consequences may be unrelated to the medication. However, the decreased overall mortality reported in well-conducted cholesterol lowering trials using HMG-CoA reductase inhibitors supports the overall safety and efficacy of lowering cholesterol. Data from other countries, in which mean cholesterol levels are lower than those in the United States, do not always support higher overall mortality related to lower cholesterol levels.

Secondary Hyperlipidemias. Most of the hypertriglyceridemia and hypercholesterolemia seen in clinical practice in children is secondary to exogenous factors or underlying clinical disorders. Obesity, for example, is a major cause of elevations of plasma triglycerides, and the hypertriglyceridemia is frequently normalized after a return to desirable weight. Weight loss may also reduce cholesterol levels in overweight individuals.

Pediatric conditions associated with hyperlipidemia include hypothyroidism, diabetes mellitus, nephrotic syndrome, renal failure, storage diseases (glycogen storage disease, Tay-Sachs disease, Niemann-Pick disease), congenital biliary atresia and other causes of cholestasis, hepatitis, anorexia nervosa, and systemic lupus erythematosus. Excessive alcohol intake should be considered in teenagers. Oral contraceptives generally increase triglyceride levels, with varying effects on LDL and HDL cholesterol levels. Other drugs that raise triglyceride levels are 13-*cis*-retinoic acid (isotretinoin or Accutane), thiazide diuretics, steroids, HIV protease inhibitors, immunosuppressants, and some β-adrenergic blocking agents. Treatment of the underlying condition or removal of the offending drug is usually the first approach to management of the patient with secondary hyperlipidemia. If the elevated lipid levels persist, however, consideration must be given to the possibility that the patient has an underlying primary form of HLP, and therapy appropriate to that condition should be initiated.

PRIMARY (GENETIC) DYSLIPIDEMIAS

One third of patients with their first myocardial infarction before the age of 50 yr in men and 60 yr in women have HLP; about one half of cases are due to an inherited disorder of lipoprotein metabolism. The Frederickson and Levy classification is useful as a guide to accurate diagnosis and effective treatment and is based on the type of lipoprotein that is elevated. For example, in type I, chylomicrons are increased; type IIa implies elevation of LDL; type IV, elevation of VLDL; type IIb, elevation of both LDL and VLDL; type III, elevation of chylomicron and VLDL remnants; and type V, elevation of VLDL and chylomicrons. These descriptive classifications do not imply specific genetic etiology; furthermore, as knowledge about the molecular basis of specific genetic defects in lipoprotein metabolism has grown (see Table 75–5), the classification has become less useful and may contribute to misunderstanding. However, because it is still quite prevalent in the literature, physicians need to be aware of the classification.

Disorders Associated with Hypercholesterolemia and Normal Triglycerides (<100 mg/dL)

Elevated cholesterol in the absence of elevated triglycerides generally indicates an elevation in LDL without a concomitant elevation in chylomicrons or VLDL. The LDL receptor plays a major role in regulating the plasma LDL cholesterol levels, and therefore the two major inherited causes of elevated LDL cholesterol both involve the LDL receptor pathway: mutations in the LDL receptor (FH) or in the receptor-binding region of apoB (familial defective apoB).

Familial Hypercholesterolemia. FH is caused by mutations in the LDL receptor, which prevent its synthesis, reduce its appearance on the cell surface, or impair its ability to bind and internalize LDL. Elevated LDL cholesterol levels lead to the major complication of this condition: premature atherosclerotic cardiovascular disease. More than 600 different mutations in the LDL receptor have been described. There are five classes of mutations (null, transport defective, binding defective, internalization defective, and recycling defective) that impair the receptor-mediated uptake of LDL from the circulation (see Fig. 75–7). FH is an autosomal codominant disorder; heterozygotes have hypercholesterolemia, but homozygotes have more severe hypercholesterolemia. One mutant LDL receptor allele results in the production of only about half of the normal number of LDL receptors, whereas two mutant alleles severely reduce or eliminate functional LDL receptors. Heterozygous and homozygous FH differ clinically in a number of important respects.

HETEROZYGOUS FAMILIAL HYPERCHOLESTEROLEMIA. Heterozygous FH occurs in approximately 1/500 people world-wide, making it one of the most common single gene disorders. It is characterized by elevated total and LDL cholesterol levels with normal triglycerides and a family history of hypercholesterolemia or premature cardiovascular disease. The finding of tendon xanthomas is virtually diagnostic of FH, although absence of xanthomas does not exclude the diagnosis, especially in children with heterozygous FH in whom xanthomas are rare. Tendon xanthomas are easily recognized on the Achilles tendons, where they cause thickening and irregularity. Any child with suspected Achilles tendonitis, which may actually be developing Achilles tendon xanthomas, should have cholesterol screening to rule out FH. Another common location for tendon xanthomas is the digit extensor tendons on the dorsum of the hands. Premature corneal arcus is frequently seen in adults with heterozygous FH. There is no widely available definitive diagnostic test for heterozygous FH, which is diagnosed on clinical grounds.

Heterozygous FH is strongly associated with premature atherosclerotic cardiovascular disease, especially CHD. Children with heterozygous FH should be identified and treated to lower the LDL cholesterol and reduce the long-term risk of atherosclerotic CHD. *Treatment* should be initiated with a Step I diet, and followed by the Step II diet if needed. Dietary therapy reduces the LDL cholesterol but rarely normalizes it. Most patients with heterozygous FH require lipid-lowering drug therapy which has proven efficacy and safety in children (see Fig. 75–8).

HOMOZYGOUS FAMILIAL HYPERCHOLESTEROLEMIA. Homozygous FH is caused by the inheritance of two mutant LDL receptor alleles that result in the production of little or no LDL receptors and a severe defect in the catabolism of LDL. Homozygous FH occurs in approximately 1 in 1 million persons worldwide and is a much more severe clinical disorder than heterozygous FH. Patients with homozygous FH are often classified into one of two groups based on the LDL cholesterol level and the amount of LDL receptor activity measured in their skin fibroblasts. "Receptor-negative" patients have less than 2% of normal LDL receptor activity and higher LDL cholesterol levels, whereas "receptor-defective" patients have 2–25% of normal LDL receptor activity and not as high LDL cholesterol levels. Receptor-defective patients have a better prognosis than do receptor-negative patients and sometimes have small responses to drug therapy. The clinical heterogeneity among homozygous FH patients is due to the significant genetic heterogeneity of the LDL receptor gene mutations.

Patients with homozygous FH often present in childhood with cutaneous xanthomas on the hands, wrists, elbows, knees, heels, or buttocks. Some patients with homozygous FH do not have cutaneous xanthomas but acquire tuberous or tendon xanthomas on the elbows, knees, or Achilles tendons as older children or adolescents. The absence of xanthomas in children does not exclude the diagnosis. Arcus cornea may be present to some degree. Total cholesterol levels are usually greater than 500 mg/dL and can be as high as 1200 mg/dL. The major complication of homozygous FH is accelerated atherosclerosis, which can result in clinical sequelae even in childhood. Homozygous FH children often have symptoms of vascular disease before puberty, but symptoms can be atypical or go unreported; sudden death is common. Untreated receptor-negative homozygous FH patients rarely survive beyond the 2nd decade; receptor-defective patients have a better prognosis but invariably experience clinical atherosclerotic vascular disease by age 30 yr and often much sooner.

A child with a total cholesterol level greater than 500 mg/dL and with relatively normal triglycerides, with or without cutaneous or tendon xanthomas, should be suspected of having homozygous FH. The biologic parents and other relatives should be tested for hypercholesterolemia. Obstructive liver disease and nephrotic syndrome should be excluded. The *diagnosis* is made on clinical grounds but can be confirmed in specialized centers by obtaining a skin biopsy specimen and performing an assay of the LDL receptor activity on the skin fibroblasts. Patients with suspected homozygous FH should be referred to a specialized center for confirmation of the diagnosis and recommendations for therapy.

Drug therapy using a statin drug plus a bile acid sequestrant should be attempted. Receptor-defective patients may have a partial response to drug therapy. Liver transplantation is effective in decreasing LDL cholesterol levels but is associated with the substantial risks of surgery and long-term immunosuppression. The current *treatment* of choice for homozygous FH is LDL apheresis, which can promote regression of xanthomas and retard progression of atherosclerosis. The age at which LDL apheresis should be initiated is uncertain. Venous access is often problematic in young children, and central catheters are prone to infections, which are especially risky given the frequent aortic valvular and supravalvular flow disturbances. It is generally recommended that initiation of LDL apheresis be delayed until approximately 5 yr of age except when evidence of atherosclerotic vascular disease is present.

Five patients with homozygous FH were treated in a somatic gene therapy protocol involving ex vivo gene transfer of the LDL receptor gene into autologous hepatocytes with subsequent reimplantation. At 4 mo, all patients had evidence of LDL receptor transgene expression by liver biopsy. LDL cholesterol levels were decreased in two patients by 17% and 22% respectively, but LDL cholesterol levels in the other three patients were essentially unchanged.

Familial Defective Apolipoprotein B-100. Familial defective apoB-100 (FDB) is characterized by elevated LDL cholesterol with normal triglycerides, possible tendon xanthomas, and increased risk of premature atherosclerotic cardiovascular disease. Clinically, it resembles heterozygous FH. In contrast to FH, FDB is caused by mutations in the receptor binding region of apoB-100, the ligand for the LDL receptor, which impairs its binding and delays the clearance of LDL from the blood. The most common mutation causing FDB is a substitution of glutamine for arginine at position 3500 in apoB-100. Other mutations have been reported that have a similar effect on apoB binding to the LDL receptor. FDB is a dominantly inherited disorder and occurs in approximately 1/700 people in Europe and North America. The apoB mutation can be detected in specialized laboratories. There is no compelling reason to make a specific molecular diagnosis because the clinical management of patients with FDB is similar to that of patients with heterozygous FH.

Sitosterolemia. Sitosterolemia is a rare autosomal recessive disease associated with excess intestinal absorption and tissue accumulation of plant-derived sterols such as sitosterol and cholestanol. The molecular etiology of sitosterolemia is related to mutations in one of two different ATP-binding cassette proteins, ABCG5 and ABCG8. These intestinal and hepatic transporters presumably cooperate to limit intestinal absorption and promote biliary excretion of plant sterols and cholesterol.

Sitosterolemia can present with severe hypercholesterolemia, premature atherosclerosis, and tendon xanthomas similar to those seen in patients with homozygous or severe heterozygous FH. Sitosterolemia should be ruled out in patients presenting with these findings. Patients with sitosterolemia often benefit from treatment with bile acid sequestrants but do not benefit from HMG-CoA reductase inhibition. Patients suspected of having sitosterolemia should be referred to specialized centers for further evaluation and management.

Polygenic Hypercholesterolemia. Most forms of hypercholesterolemia are not single gene disorders but rather due to a complex interaction of several genetic and environmental factors. Genetic differences in cholesterol absorption, cholesterol synthesis, or rates of bile acid synthesis may result in very different cholesterol levels in individuals challenged with a fat-rich diet. An elevated cholesterol level with triglyceride levels characterizes polygenic hypercholesterolemia. In polygenic hypercholesterolemia, LDL cholesterol levels usually are not as elevated as they are in heterozygous FH and FDB, and tendon xanthomas are not observed. About half of relatives with FCHL, heterozygous FH, and FDB have dyslipidemia, but fewer first-degree relatives of patients with polygenic hypercholesterolemia are hypercholesteremic. *Treatment* of polygenic hypercholesterolemia follows the same guidelines as the approach to any patient with hypercholesterolemia.

Disorders Associated with Hypercholesterolemia and Moderately Elevated Triglyceride Levels (100–1,000 mg/dL)

Although triglyceride levels more than 1,000 mg/dL are associated with acute pancreatitis (see later) the importance of elevated triglyceride levels in the 100–1,000 mg/dL range is primarily related to their potential association with the risk of the development of atherosclerotic CHD. The major primary causes of elevated triglycerides in the 100–1,000 mg/dL range are FCHL, familial dysbetalipoproteinemia (type III hyperlipidemia), and familial hypertriglyceridemia. It is important to differentiate among them because familial dysbetalipoproteinemia and FCHL are both definitely associated with increased risk of premature atherosclerosis, whereas familial hypertriglyceridemia may not be associated with increased risk.

Familial Combined Hyperlipidemia. FCHL is a common primary lipid disorder, occurring in approximately 1/200 adults. It has been estimated that approximately 20% of patients with CHD younger than 60 yr have a form of FCHL. FCHL is characterized by a mixed dyslipidemia usually associated with moderately reduced HDL-C levels, elevated fasting triglycerides, and/or moderately elevated cholesterol. In this dominantly inherited syndrome, first-degree relatives on one side of the family frequently have hypertriglyceridemia, hypercholesterolemia, or combined elevations of both cholesterol and triglycerides; there is often a family history of premature CHD. The hyperlipidemia tends to be modest, and the lipoprotein abnormalities can change from time to time in the same affected individual. Xanthomas are not generally seen in patients with this disorder. Visceral abdominal obesity, glucose intolerance, hyperinsulinemia, and hypertension are frequently associated with FCHL but are not required for the diagnosis.

FCHL generally presents in adulthood but can be identified in children. In families with FCHL identified through an affected child, half the siblings younger than 20 yr of age have hyperlipidemia, compatible with dominant expression of the trait. A correlation between plasma triglyceride level and age and relative weight in affected children has also been observed, which suggests the gradual expression of hyperlipidemia in some children. It is estimated that at least 0.5% of all children have hyperlipidemia due to FCHL.

The molecular basis of FCHL is not known. Studies of lipoprotein metabolism in carefully selected individuals have indicated that overproduction of VLDL or LDL, or both, is a common metabolic basis of this condition. It has been suggested that a subset of patients with the FCHL phenotype may be heterozygous for lipoprotein lipase (LPL) deficiency, but LPL mutations are probably not a common cause of FCHL. A variant allele at a locus influencing apoB levels predicts FCHL in a large proportion of families ascertained through affected children; however, the function of this gene is unknown. There is evidence that FCHL is not linked to the apoB structural locus. It is likely that more than one genetic cause of the FCHL phenotype exists.

The *diagnosis* of FCHL is suggested by the presence of a mixed hyperlipidemia with fasting triglyceride and cholesterol levels both greater than the 90th percentile, especially if accompanied by decreased HDL cholesterol levels and in the absence of secondary causes of hyperlipidemia. Some affected family members may have only an elevated LDL-C or triglyceride level. The formal diagnosis of FCHL requires the presence of dyslipidemia in at least two first-degree relatives. Familial dysbetalipoproteinemia should be excluded with appropriate testing. The finding of an elevated apoB level (usually greater than the 90th percentile for age) suggests increased levels of "small dense LDL" and supports the diagnosis of FCHL. *Hyperapobetalipoproteinemia* has been used to describe the syndrome of elevated apoB with normal lipid levels and is probably a subset of FCHL.

The risk of premature heart disease for persons with FCHL is increased despite the fact that lipid levels in affected individuals may be only moderately elevated. Children in these families should therefore be identified, and initial dietary *treatment* should be aimed at controlling the hypercholesterolemia and hypertriglyceridemia using the Step I or Step II diet. Dietary modification in children with FCHL has generally demonstrated a 10–15% reduction in the LDL cholesterol level, although fewer than half of the treated children would be expected to have levels less than 130 mg/dL and even fewer would be expected to have levels of less than 110 mg/dL with dietary treatment. When dietary modification alone does not achieve desired results, drug therapy may be considered. Dietary changes resulting in lower LDL-C levels are also commonly associated with some rise in triglyceride levels; within reason, the primary focus remains on lowering LDL-C.

Familial Dysbetalipoproteinemia (Type III Hyperlipoproteinemia). Patients with familial dysbetalipoproteinemia usually present in adulthood with *clinical manifestations* that include distinctive xanthomas, premature atherosclerosis, or asymptomatic hyperlipidemia discovered on routine screening, although children may present with a "strange rash." Two types of xanthomas can be seen in patients with familial dysbetalipoproteinemia. Tuberoeruptive xanthomas begin as clusters of small papules on the elbows, knees, or buttocks and can grow to the size of small grapes. Palmar xanthoma refers to orange-yellow discoloration in the creases of the palms and wrists. The pattern of hyperlipidemia can be a clue to the diagnosis of familial dysbetalipoproteinemia. Patients generally have both hypertriglyceridemia and hypercholesterolemia and, in contrast to most other lipid disorders, the cholesterol and triglyceride are often elevated to a relatively similar degree. In addition, the HDL cholesterol level is often relatively normal, in contrast to most hypertriglyceridemic conditions in which the HDL cholesterol level is usually reduced. The hyperlipidemia can be relatively mild or severe, depending on the presence of other metabolic conditions and unknown factors.

Familial dysbetalipoproteinemia is caused by mutations in the gene for apolipoprotein E (apoE). ApoE is present on chylomicron and VLDL remnants and mediates their removal from the plasma by binding to receptors in the liver. Defective apoE is impaired in its ability to bind to these receptors, resulting in accumulation of chylomicron and VLDL remnants in the plasma. The most common form of familial dysbetalipoproteinemia is related to a common polymorphism of apoE. The "normal" form of apoE is known as apoE3, but another form, apoE2, has an allele frequency of about 7%. The apoE2 protein, which differs from apoE3 by a single amino acid, does not bind to lipoprotein receptors adequately, resulting in defective removal of chylomicron and VLDL remnants. Homozygosity for the E2 allele (the E2/E2 genotype) is the most common cause of familial dysbetalipoproteinemia. However, most individuals with the apoE2/E2 genotype do not have familial dysbetalipoproteinemia; development of this disorder appears to require an additional factor. Some of these factors may include obesity, diabetes mellitus, hypothyroidism, renal disease, and alcohol use; most children with familial dysbetalipoproteine-

mia have one of these conditions in addition to the apoE2/E2 genotype. Many adults with familial dysbetalipoproteinemia do not have an obvious predisposing factor in addition to the E2/E2 genotype. Another common variant of apoE, known as apoE4, has an allele frequency of approximately 14% and is not associated with familial dysbetalipoproteinemia. Other rare mutations in apoE can also cause familial dysbetalipoproteinemia. These mutations generally result in the synthesis of an apoE protein that is severely defective in its ability to bind to lipoprotein receptors and can result in a more severe hyperlipidemia, which may be more likely to present in childhood. Often the inheritance of only one mutant allele is adequate to cause familial dysbetalipoproteinemia, leading to the term *dominant type III HLP*.

The traditional laboratory approach to *diagnosis* is to use lipoprotein electrophoresis, which demonstrates a broad β-band owing to the presence of remnant lipoproteins. A second (and preferred) method is "β quantification" in which plasma is subjected to ultracentrifugation to separate lipoproteins; this is available in specialized laboratories. Because this disorder is associated with increased numbers of VLDL remnants that are enriched in cholesterol relative to triglycerides, an elevated ratio of VLDL cholesterol to triglycerides of greater than 0.3 is confirmatory of the diagnosis. Finally, the apoE2/E2 pattern can be determined by using plasma protein methods (apoE phenotype) or DNA-based methods (apoE genotype). The finding of an apoE2/E2 pattern by phenotyping or genotyping in a patient with suspected familial dysbetalipoproteinemia confirms the diagnosis.

Familial dysbetalipoproteinemia is often sensitive to dietary *treatment*. Weight loss to a level appropriate for height, coupled with institution of the Step I diet, can often cause the lipid levels to return to normal. Discontinuance of alcohol can have a major impact on the dyslipidemia. There is little experience with drug treatment of this disorder in children, but adults with familial dysbetalipoproteinemia have been treated with fibric acid derivatives, nicotinic acid, and HMG-CoA reductase inhibitors, all of which tend to be effective in this disorder, although combination therapy is sometimes required.

Familial Hypertriglyceridemia. Familial hypertriglyceridemia (FHTG) is characterized by moderately elevated triglycerides, usually in the absence of significant hypercholesterolemia. FHTG occurs in approximately 1/500 people and in contrast to FCHL frequently is not associated with premature CHD. Hypertriglyceridemia is often detected by a routine blood test. Triglyceride levels usually range from 250–1,000 mg/dL with normal to mildly increased cholesterol levels and HDL cholesterol levels that are usually decreased. FHTG is inherited as an autosomal dominant trait but is not usually expressed until adulthood. The molecular *etiology* is unknown. The metabolic basis of this disorder is probably heterogeneous but is likely to be related to impaired catabolism of triglyceride-rich lipoproteins. Increased production of VLDL by the liver has been observed in some patients with this phenotype. It is possible that VLDL or chylomicron overproduction, or both, may overload the normal catabolic processes and produce hypertriglyceridemia in some patients. It has been proposed that genetic overproduction of apoC-III could cause this syndrome, but this remains to be proved. Increased dietary fat or simple carbohydrates, a sedentary lifestyle, obesity, insulin resistance, alcohol use, and estrogens can all exacerbate the hypertriglyceridemia.

The *diagnosis* is suggested by elevated triglyceride levels (>90th percentile) with normal or mildly increased cholesterol levels (<90th percentile). Hypertriglyceridemia in at least one first-degree relative is useful in making the diagnosis. It is important to consider and rule out secondary causes of the hypertriglyceridemia. In the differential diagnosis, both familial dysbetalipoproteinemia (type III HLP) and FCHL should be considered. Relative to the triglyceride level, the total cholesterol level is usually lower in FHTG compared with familial dysbetalipoproteinemia and FCHL.

Children older than 2 yr can usually be *treated* adequately with weight control and use of the Step I diet. Occasionally, further modification of the carbohydrate to fat ratio may be required. Alcohol use should be discouraged. Diabetes mellitus should be aggressively controlled. Lipid-lowering drug therapy is generally not indicated in children, except in extreme cases. In such circumstances, fish oils may be an alternative to drug therapy, although the long-term safety in children is not known.

Hepatic Lipase Deficiency. This is a rare autosomal recessive disorder. Hepatic lipase hydrolyzes triglycerides and phospholipids in VLDL remnants and IDL and promotes their conversion to LDL. Genetic deficiency of hepatic lipase impairs the metabolism of VLDL remnants and IDL and is characterized by a mixed hyperlipidemia and the accumulation of lipoprotein remnants in plasma. Hepatic lipase also metabolizes HDL lipids, so levels of HDL cholesterol are often slightly elevated in hepatic lipase deficiency. The *diagnosis* is suggested by a mixed hyperlipidemia with elevation in both triglyceride and cholesterol levels but an HDL cholesterol level that is normal or elevated rather than low. Familial dysbetalipoproteinemia should be excluded by apoE phenotyping or genotyping. Measurements of hepatic lipase can be made in postheparin plasma by specialized laboratories. The association of hepatic lipase deficiency with atherosclerosis is uncertain, but patients should be *treated* for their hyperlipidemia using an approach similar to that used for familial dysbetalipoproteinemia. Acquired (usually partial) defects in hepatic lipase can be seen in hypothyroidism, chronic renal insufficiency, and chronic liver disease.

Disorders Associated with Hypercholesterolemia and Severely Elevated Triglycerides (>1,000 mg/dL)

Fasting triglycerides greater than 1,000 mg/dL in children reflect severe hyperchylomicronemia and indicate an underlying genetic disorder. In some cases, this genetic factor is exacerbated by another medical condition or a hormonal or environmental factor. The major clinical complication of severe hypertriglyceridemia is acute pancreatitis, and initial treatment is focused on decreasing the triglycerides to less than 1,000 mg/dL to prevent this serious complication. Some patients with severe hypertriglyceridemia are at risk for premature atherosclerotic CHD and require more aggressive therapy even when the triglycerides have been decreased to less than the 1,000 mg/dL threshold.

Familial Chylomicronemia Syndrome: Lipoprotein Lipase Deficiency and Apolipoprotein C-II Deficiency. The familial chylomicronemia syndrome is characterized by presentation in childhood with acute pancreatitis in the setting of triglyceride levels greater than 1,000 mg/dL. Recurrent abdominal pain is a common historical feature. Rarely, infants present with recurrent "colic." The massive elevation of plasma triglycerides can be clinically silent and is sometimes discovered incidentally owing to the lipemic appearance of the blood. On physical examination, eruptive xanthomas (small papular lesions that occur in showers on the buttocks and back) may be seen. Lipemia retinalis (a pale appearance to the retinal veins) is a clue to the existence of severe hypertriglyceridemia; hepatosplenomegaly due to ingestion of chylomicrons by the reticuloendothelial system is often found. Premature atherosclerotic cardiovascular disease is not generally a feature of this disease.

Two different genetic defects can cause the familial chylomicronemia syndrome: LPL deficiency and apoC-II deficiency. The hydrolysis of triglycerides in chylomicrons requires the action of LPL in tissue capillary beds, and apoC-II is a required co-factor for the activation of LPL. Mutations in either the LPL gene or the apoC-II gene result in functional inability to hydrolyze triglyc-

erides in chylomicrons and consequent hyperchylomicronemia. The disorder is autosomal recessive, and both alleles of the LPL or apoC-II gene must be affected. Therefore, the parents of children with this disorder generally have normal or near-normal triglyceride levels, and usually there is no family history of severe hyperlipidemia. Both are rare disorders, but of the two, LPL deficiency is more common (approximately 1/1 million persons) than apoC-II deficiency.

The *diagnosis* of the familial hyperchylomicronemia syndrome is usually made based on the clinical presentation and some key laboratory features. The plasma is lactescent and after overnight refrigeration, a cake of chylomicrons forms on the surface. Triglyceride levels are greater than 1,000 mg/dL and may be as high as 10,000 mg/dL or greater. Total cholesterol levels are also elevated because of the presence of cholesterol in chylomicrons. Lipoprotein electrophoresis demonstrates markedly elevated chylomicrons at the origin but is not essential for making the diagnosis. The diagnosis of LPL and apoC-II deficiency can be confirmed at specialized centers by the quantitation of LPL activity in the plasma after intravenous heparin injection (postheparin lipolytic activity). Patients with suspected familial chylomicronemia syndrome should be referred to a specialized lipid center for diagnosis and management.

The mainstay of *treatment* for familial chylomicronemia syndrome is restriction of total dietary fat. Consultation with a registered dietitian familiar with this disorder is essential. Caloric supplementation with medium-chain triglycerides, which are absorbed directly into the portal vein and therefore do not promote chylomicron formation, can be useful. If dietary fat restriction alone is not successful, some patients may respond to a cautious trial of fish oils. For patients with apoC-II deficiency, an attack of acute pancreatitis that fails to resolve can be treated with infusion of fresh frozen plasma to provide an exogenous source of apoC-II in an attempt to clear severe hypertriglyceridemia and promote resolution of the pancreatitis.

Type V Hyperlipoproteinemia (HLP). Type V HLP is common in adults but rare in children. The *diagnosis* of type V HLP is made in a patient with fasting triglyceride levels greater than 1,000 mg/dL (fasting hyperchylomicronemia) who does not have LPL or apoC-II deficiency. Type V HLP is also associated with acute pancreatitis, which can be the initial presentation of this syndrome and is the major rationale for aggressive treatment. Most but not all patients with type V HLP have a family history of hypertriglyceridemia. Type II diabetes mellitus or glucose intolerance frequently accompanies type V hyperlipidemia, but type V hyperlipidemia also occurs in individuals with normal glucose tolerance. Some patients with nephrotic syndrome can acquire severe hypertriglyceridemia. Estrogen-containing therapy can exacerbate moderate hypertriglyceridemia and lead to a more severe type V hyperlipidemia, as can heavy alcohol use. Treatment with isotretinoin or etretinate sometimes causes severe hypertriglyceridemia.

The *treatment* of type V hyperlipidemia is first targeted to decreasing triglycerides to reduce the risk of pancreatitis, followed by further lipid lowering depending on the presence of CHD or other risk factors for cardiovascular disease. Patients taking medications that exacerbate hypertriglyceridemia may need to discontinue them if triglyceride levels are greater than 1,000 mg/dL. Diabetes mellitus should be controlled. Patients should be referred to a registered dietitian for dietary counseling. Dietary management includes restriction of total fat as well as simple sugars in the diet. Alcohol should be avoided. Regular aerobic exercise can have a significant impact on triglyceride levels and should be actively encouraged. If the patient is overweight, weight loss can help to decrease triglyceride levels. When fasting triglyceride levels remain greater than 1,000 mg/dL despite institution of appropriate dietary and lifestyle measures and control of secondary causes, drug therapy should be considered to decrease the risk of acute pancreatitis. None of the agents used in the treatment of hypertriglyceridemia is approved for use in children.

Disorders of High-Density Lipoprotein Metabolism. HDL cholesterol levels are inversely associated with CHD independent of total and LDL cholesterol levels. Although the National Cholesterol Education Program recommends that all adults older than 20 yr should be screened for total cholesterol and HDL cholesterol levels as part of a full fasting lipid profile, it is recommended that only children with a positive family history of premature heart disease have a complete lipid profile including HDL cholesterol. Many causes of low HDL cholesterol are secondary to other factors. Cigarette smoking, obesity, physical inactivity, type II diabetes mellitus, end-stage renal disease, hypertriglyceridemia from any cause, and the use of β-blockers, thiazide diuretics, androgens, progestins, and probucol can all reduce HDL cholesterol levels. A low-fat diet can also result in a low level of HDL cholesterol; the low HDL is not considered to be associated with an increased risk of CHD, because persons who eat low-fat diets are at substantially reduced risk of premature CHD. Several rare genetic disorders can also be associated with low HDL cholesterol levels.

Familial APOA-I Deficiency and Structural APOA-I Mutations. Complete genetic deficiency of apoA-I due to deletions of the apoA-I gene or nonsense mutations that prevent the biosynthesis of apoA-I protein may result in virtually absent plasma HDL. These extremely rare patients acquire corneal opacities and sometimes cutaneous or planar xanthomas. The risk of premature cardiovascular disease in patients with apoA-I deficiency is increased, but onset of CHD symptoms in these kindreds has varied from the 3rd to 7th decades. In contrast, mutations of apoA-1 that permit the secretion of a mutant apoA-1 protein are not generally associated with premature coronary artery disease. Interestingly, a few apoA-I mutations have been described in association with systemic amyloidosis, and the mutant apoA-1 has been found as a component of the amyloid plaque.

Tangier Disease. ABCA1 is a cellular protein that facilitates the efflux of cellular cholesterol to lipid-poor apoA-1. Tangier disease is a rare disorder caused by mutations in *ABCA1*, resulting in a cellular defect in efflux of cholesterol, and particularly affects macrophages and related cells. It is associated with cholesterol accumulation in the reticuloendothelial system, resulting in hepatosplenomegaly, intestinal mucosal abnormalities, and pathognomonic enlarged, orange tonsils. Intermittent peripheral neuropathy can also be seen from cholesterol accumulation in Schwann cells. Tangier disease is frequently diagnosed in childhood because of the finding of enlarged orange-colored tonsils. Patients with Tangier disease have HDL cholesterol levels less than 5 mg/dL and extremely low levels of apoA-I, owing to markedly accelerated HDL catabolism.

Tangier disease is associated with some increased risk of premature atherosclerotic disease, but this risk is not proportional to the markedly decreased HDL cholesterol and apoA-I levels. Tangier disease is an autosomal codominant disease; obligate heterozygotes have moderately reduced HDL cholesterol levels but no evidence of reticuloendothelial cholesterol accumulation. The risk of premature atherosclerosis in obligate heterozygotes is uncertain but may also be increased.

Familial Lecithin:Cholesterol Acyltransferase Deficiency. Unesterified cholesterol effluxed from cells to HDL is esterified by lecithin:cholesterol acyltransferase (LCAT). Two general types of genetic LCAT deficiency have been described in humans: complete deficiency (classic LCAT deficiency) and partial deficiency (fish-eye disease). Both types are extremely rare. Progressive corneal opacification in young adulthood is characteristic of both types; in addition, complete (classic) LCAT deficiency (but not partial deficiency) is characterized by anemia and progressive protein-

uria and renal insufficiency in young adulthood. Both types are characterized by very low plasma levels of HDL cholesterol (usually <10 mg/dL) and variable hypertriglyceridemia. The diagnosis of LCAT deficiency is rarely made in childhood and is suspected when there is corneal opacification, renal insufficiency, or an incidentally discovered very low HDL cholesterol level. The diagnosis can be confirmed in specialized laboratories by quantitation of LCAT and cholesterol esterification activity in the plasma. Remarkably, despite the extremely low levels of HDL cholesterol and apoA-I, there is no apparent increased risk of premature atherosclerotic cardiovascular disease in either complete or partial LCAT deficiency.

Primary Hypoalphalipoproteinemia. The most common inherited form of low HDL is termed *primary* or *familial hypoalphalipoproteinemia*. It is defined as an HDL cholesterol level less than the 10th percentile in the setting of relatively normal cholesterol and triglyceride levels, no apparent secondary causes of low HDL, and no clinical signs of LCAT deficiency or Tangier disease. This syndrome is often referred to as "isolated low HDL." A family history of low HDL cholesterol facilitates the diagnosis of an inherited condition, which usually follows the pattern of an autosomal dominant trait. The genetic etiology of this syndrome is unknown, although the metabolic cause appears to be primarily accelerated catabolism of HDL and its apolipoproteins. The direct relationship of primary hypoalphalipoproteinemia to premature coronary disease is uncertain and may depend on the specific nature of the gene defect or metabolic cause of the low HDL cholesterol level.

CONDITIONS ASSOCIATED WITH LOW CHOLESTEROL LEVELS

Abetalipoproteinemia. This is a rare autosomal recessive disease characterized by fat malabsorption, spinocerebellar degeneration, and pigmented retinopathy. The biochemical hallmark of this disease is the strikingly abnormal plasma lipid and lipoprotein profile. Total cholesterol and triglyceride levels are extremely low; there are no detectable plasma chylomicrons, VLDL, or LDL; and apoB is absent from the plasma. This disease is caused by mutations in the gene for the microsomal triglyceride transfer protein, which mediates the intracellular transport of membrane-associated lipids in the intestine and liver and is necessary for the normal formation of chylomicrons in the enterocyte and VLDL in the hepatocyte.

The most prominent and debilitating *clinical manifestations* of abetalipoproteinemia are neurologic and usually begin in the 2nd decade. The first sign of disease is usually the loss of deep tendon reflexes, followed by decreased distal lower extremity vibratory and proprioceptive senses and cerebellar signs such as dysmetria, ataxia, and spastic gait. The clinical outcome is variable, but the result in untreated patients is often severe ataxia and spasticity by the 3rd or 4th decade. These severe effects on the central nervous system are the ultimate cause of death in most patients and often occur by the 5th decade or earlier. Patients with abetalipoproteinemia also acquire a progressive pigmented retinopathy. The presence of both spinocerebellar degeneration and pigmented retinopathy in this disease may result in a misdiagnosis of Friedreich ataxia. The first ophthalmic symptoms are decreased night and color vision. Daytime visual acuity usually deteriorates inexorably to virtual blindness by the 4th decade.

The majority of the clinical symptoms of abetalipoproteinemia are the result of defects in absorption and transport of fat-soluble vitamins, especially vitamin E. Vitamin E is transported from the intestine to the liver, then "repackaged" in the liver and incorporated into the assembling VLDL particle by a specific protein termed the *tocopherol binding protein*. In the circulation, VLDL is converted to LDL, and vitamin E is transported by LDL to peripheral tissues and delivered to cells via the LDL receptor. Patients with abetalipoproteinemia are markedly deficient in vitamin E. Vitamin E metabolism is greatly altered in patients with abetalipoproteinemia because the plasma transport of vitamin E requires hepatic secretion of apoB-containing lipoproteins. Most of the major clinical symptoms, especially those of the nervous system and retina, are primarily caused by vitamin E deficiency. This concept is supported by the fact that other diseases involving vitamin E deficiency, such as cholestasis and isolated vitamin E deficiency, are characterized by similar symptoms and pathologic changes. Patients with suspected abetalipoproteinemia should be referred to specialized centers for confirmation of the diagnosis and institution of appropriate therapy.

Obligate heterozygotes (parents of patients with abetalipoproteinemia) have no symptoms and no evidence of reduced plasma lipids. Thus, family studies are important in distinguishing abetalipoproteinemia from clinically similar homozygous hypobetalipoproteinemia in which obligate heterozygotes have decreased LDL cholesterol and apoB levels.

Familial Hypobetalipoproteinemia. Familial hypobetalipoproteinemia, in contrast to abetalipoproteinemia, is autosomal codominant. Heterozygotes have levels of LDL cholesterol and apoB that are approximately one half of normal or less, whereas homozygotes have very low or no plasma apoB. Heterozygous familial hypobetalipoproteinemia is not associated with symptoms, whereas some homozygous patients have symptoms that are similar to those in abetalipoproteinemia patients. The gene defect in this disorder resides in most or all cases within the apoB gene itself. Many are nonsense mutations resulting in a truncated apoB protein; at least 25 such mutations have been described to date. One patient who was initially described as having "normotriglyceridemic abetalipoproteinemia" has subsequently been demonstrated to be homozygous for a truncated apoB and therefore has homozygous hypobetalipoproteinemia.

Clinically, heterozygous hypobetalipoproteinemia is associated with LDL cholesterol levels in the 40–80 mg/dL range, is not associated with clinical sequelae, and requires no specific therapy. However, patients with homozygous hypobetalipoproteinemia have markedly reduced to absent LDL cholesterol and apoB levels and may be at risk for many of the sequelae seen in abetalipoproteinemia. Such patients should therefore be referred to specialized centers for confirmation of the diagnosis and institution of appropriate therapy.

Chylomicron Retention Disease. Chylomicron retention disease, or Anderson disease, is associated with the selective inability to secrete apoB from intestinal enterocytes, resulting in fat malabsorption and sometimes neurologic disease similar to that seen in abetalipoproteinemia and homozygous hypobetalipoproteinemia. In contrast to these two disorders, apoB-100 can be detected in the plasma of patients with chylomicron retention disease, because hepatic VLDL secretion is normal. The molecular defect is unknown but appears to be distinct from both the microsomal triglyceride transfer protein and apoB genes.

Smith-Lemli-Opitz Syndrome. This syndrome is a recessive genetic disorder characterized by neurologic developmental defects including microcephaly, hypotonia, and severe mental retardation as well as micrognathia, widespread ears, cataracts, epicanthal folds, blepharoptosis, and syndactyly. Additional features are noted in Boxes 75–3 and 75–4. The prevalence of homozygotes is about 1/20,000 births, and the estimated gene carrier frequency is 1–2%. Smith-Lemli-Opitz syndrome is caused by defects in the gene encoding the enzyme 7-dehydrocholesterol-δ-7-reductase, which is required to convert 7-dehydrocholesterol to cholesterol. Patients have very low plasma cholesterol levels, and the neurologic defects are presumed to be caused by limited cholesterol availability within the central nervous system for neural growth. Cholesterol therapy (50 mg/kg/day) results in improvement in behavioral abnormalities and

improves postnatal growth. Because high concentrations of the cholesterol precursor 7-dehydrocholesterol may be toxic, therapy with simvastatin, an inhibitor of the cholesterol synthetic pathway, may provide additional benefit.

BOX 75–3. Major Clinical Characteristics of Smith-Lemli-Opitz Syndrome: Frequent Anomalies (>50% of Patients)

CRANIOFACIAL
Microcephaly
Blepharoptosis
Anteverted nares
Retromicrognathia
Low-set, posteriorly rotated ears
Midline cleft palate
Broad maxillary alveolar ridges
Cataracts (<50%)

SKELETAL ANOMALIES
Syndactyly of toes II/III
Postaxial polydactyly (<50%)
Equinovarus deformity (<50%)

GENITAL ANOMALIES
Hypospadias
Cryptorchidism
Sexual ambiguity (<50%)

DEVELOPMENT
Pre-and postnatal growth retardation
Feeding problems
Mental retardation
Behavioral abnormalities

From Haas D, Kelley RI, Hoffmann GF: Inherited disorders of cholesterol biosynthesis. *Neuropediatrics* 2001; 32: 113–22.

BOX 75–4. Characteristic Malformations of Internal Organs in Severely Affected Smith-Lemli-Opitz Patients

CENTRAL NERVOUS SYSTEM
Frontal lobe hypoplasia
Enlarged ventricles
Agenesis of corpus callosum
Cerebellar hypoplasia
Holoprosencephaly

CARDIOVASCULAR
Atrioventricular canal
Secundum atrial septal defect
Patent ductus arteriosus
Membranous ventricular septal defect

URINARY TRACT
Renal hypoplasia or aplasia
Renal cortical cysts
Hydronephrosis
Ureteral duplication

GASTROINTESTINAL
Hirschsprung's disease
Pyloric stenosis
Refractory dysmotility
Cholestatic and noncholestatic progressive liver disease

PULMONARY
Pulmonary hypoplasia
Abnormal lobation

ENDOCRINE
Adrenal insufficiency

From Haas D, Kelley RI, Hoffmann GF: Inherited disorders of cholesterol biosynthesis. *Neuropediatrics* 2001; 32: 113–22.

ADDITIONAL DISORDERS OF CHOLESTEROL SYNTHESIS

Mevalonic Aciduria. This malformation syndrome is caused by a deficiency of mevalonate kinase and results in massive excretion of mevalonic acid, an intermediate in cholesterol synthesis (see Chapter 74.6). Patients manifest mental retardation, hypotonia, low-set posteriorly rotated ears, blue sclerae, cataracts, dolichocephaly, hepatosplenomegaly, long eyelashes, and an inflammatory syndrome associated with elevated IgD levels. This periodic fever, hyperimmunoglobulin D syndrome is associated with rash, fever, diarrhea, arthralgias, and an elevated erythrocyte sedimentation rate, which is treated with corticosteroids.

The serum cholesterol level is low or normal.

Conradi-Hünermann Syndrome. These patients have normal or low serum cholesterol levels and malformations consisting of rhizomelic chondrodysplasia. There may be a defect in gene locus for 3β-hydroxysteroid Δ^8, Δ^7 isomerase. The disorder is inherited as an X-linked dominant (affecting only females; lethal to male fetuses) or an autosomal recessive disorder. Patients with the X-linked disease demonstrate rhizomelic limbs, asymmetrically shortened ichthyosis, alopecia, and cataracts (see Chapters 75.2 and 648).

CHILD Syndrome. This X-linked dominant disorder affects females (possibly lethal to male fetuses) and is manifest by a unilateral exfoliative erythematous dermatitis (psoriasis-like) with facial sparing, unilateral hypomelia ipsilateral to the dermatosis, punctate vertebrae, epiphyseal calcification, and airway cartilage calcification. CHILD is an acronym for congenital hemidysplasia, ichthyosiform erythroderma, and limb defects. There may also be unilateral renal aplasia and congenital heart disease.

Desmosterolosis. Deficiency of 3β-hydroxysterol-Δ^{24}-reductase results in this syndrome, manifest by congenital heart defects, ambiguous genitalia in males, rhizomelic limbs, macrocephaly, gingival nodules, and thickened alveolar ridges.

SELECTED GENETIC DISORDERS OF INTRACELLULAR CHOLESTEROL METABOLISM

Cerebrotendinous Xanthomatosis. This is an autosomal recessive disorder caused by mutations in the gene for sterol 27-hydroxylase, a mitochondrial enzyme involved in the normal biosynthesis of bile acids in the liver. As a result of the deficiency in sterol 27-hydroxylase, bile acid intermediates are shunted into the synthesis of cholestanol, which then accumulates in multiple tissues. If untreated, patients acquire cataracts, tendon xanthomas, and progressive disease of the central and peripheral nervous system in the 2nd decade of life. Early diagnosis is crucial, because treatment with chenodeoxycholic acid reduces plasma cholestanol levels and prevents the progression of clinical symptoms.

Cholesterol Ester Storage Disease and Wolman Disease. Cholesterol ester storage disease (CESD) or Wolman disease is an autosomal recessive disorder caused by mutations in the gene for lysosomal acid lipase, a lysosomal enzyme required for hydrolysis of cholesteryl esters and triglycerides in the lysosome. See Chapter 75.4.

Niemann-Pick C Disease. The Niemann-Pick group of diseases includes autosomal recessive diseases characterized by accumulation of cholesterol and sphingomyelin in tissues, especially the liver, reticuloendothelial system, and central nervous system. Niemann-Pick A and B are described in Chapters 75.4 and 592.1. Niemann-Pick C disease is a disorder of intracellular cholesterol transport for which the molecular cause has been established. Niemann-Pick C is characterized by hepatosplenomegaly and progressive neurologic disease, often resulting in severe disability and death by the 2nd decade.

Abramowicz M (editor): Choice of lipid-relating drugs. *Med Lett* 43:2001;43–8.

American Academy of Pediatrics Committee on Nutrition: Cholesterol in childhood. *Pediatrics* 1998;101:141–47.

Clayton PT: Disorders of cholesterol biosynthesis. *Arch Dis Child* 1998;78:185–89.

Defesche JC, Kastelein JJP: Molecular epidemiology of familial hypercholesterolemia. *Lancet* 1998;352:1643–4.

Feoli-Fonseca JC, Levy E, Godard M, et al: Familial lipoprotein lipase deficiency in infancy: Clinical, biochemical, and molecular study. *J Pediatr* 1998;133:417–23.

Haas D, Kelley RI, Hoffmann GF: Inherited Disorders of cholesterol biosynthesis. *Neuropediatrics* 2001;32:113–22.

Hickman TB, Briefel RR, Carroll MD, et al: Distributions and trends of serum lipid levels among United States children and adolescents ages 4–19 years: Data from the Third National Health and Nutrition Survey. *Prev Med* 1998;27:879–90.

Jira PE, Wevers RA, de Jong J, et al: Simvastatin: A new therapeutic approach for Smith-Lemli-Optiz syndrome. *J Lipid Res* 2000;41:1339–46.

Knopp RH: Drug treatment of lipid disorders. *N Engl J Med* 1999;341:498–511.

Lagstrom H, Seppanen R, Jokinen E, et al: Influence of dietary fat on the nutrient intake and growth of children from 1 to 5 yr of age: The Special Turku Coronary Risk Factor Intervention Project. *Am J Clin Nutr* 1999;69:516–23.

National Cholesterol Education Program (NCEP). Executive Summary of the Third Report of the NCEP Expert Panel on Detection, Evaluation and Treatment of High Blood Cholesterol in Adults (Adult Treatment Panel III). *JAMA* 2001;285:2486–97.

Obarzanek EO, Kimm SY, Barton BA, et al: Long-term safety and efficacy of a cholesterol-lowering diet in children with elevated low-density lipoprotein cholesterol: Seven-year results of the Dietary Intervention Study in Children (DISC). *Pediatrics* 2001;107:256–64.

Rask-Nissila L, Jokonen E, Ronnemaa T, et al: Prospective, randomized, infancy-onset trial of the effects of a low-saturated-fat, low cholesterol diet on serum lipids and lipoproteins before school age: The Special Turku Coronary Risk Factor Intervention Project (STRIP). *Circulation* 2000;102:1477–83.

Williams CL, Hayman LL, Daniels SR, et al: Cardiovascular health in childhood: A statement for health professionals from the Committee on Atherosclerosis, Hypertension, and Obesity in the Young (AHOY) of the Council on Cardiovascular Disease in the Young, American Heart Association. *Circulation* 2002;106:143–60.

Winkleby MA, Robinson TN, Sundquist J, et al: Ethnic variation in cardiovascular disease risk factors among children and young adults: Findings from the Third National Health and Nutrition Examination Survey 1998–1994. *JAMA* 281:1006–13.

75.4 Lipidoses

Margaret M. McGovern and Robert J. Desnick

The lysosomal lipid storage diseases are diverse disorders each due to an inherited deficiency of a lysosomal hydrolase leading to the lysosomal accumulation of the enzyme's particular substrate (Table 75–7). With the exception of Wolman disease (cholesterol ester storage disease), the lipid substrates share a common structure that includes a ceramide backbone (2-*N*-acyl-sphingosine) from which the various sphingolipids are derived by substitution of hexoses, phosphorylcholine, or one or more sialic acid residues on the terminal hydroxyl group of the ceramide molecule. The pathway of sphingolipid metabolism in nervous tissue (Fig. 75–9) and in visceral organs (Fig. 75–10) is known; each catabolic step has a genetically determined metabolic defect. Because sphingolipids are essential components of all cell membranes, the inability to degrade these substances and their subsequent accumulation results in the physiologic and morphologic alterations and characteristic clinical manifestations of the lipid storage disorders (see Table 75–7). Progressive lysosomal accumulation of glycosphingolipids in the central nervous system leads to neurodegeneration, whereas storage in visceral cells can lead to organomegaly, skeletal abnormalities, pulmonary infiltration, and other manifestations. The storage of a substrate in a specific tissue is dependent on its normal distribution in the body.

Diagnostic assays for the identification of affected individuals rely on the measurement of the specific enzymatic activity in isolated leukocytes or cultured fibroblasts. For most disorders, carrier identification and prenatal diagnosis are available; a specific diagnosis is essential to permit genetic counseling of the family. The characterization of the genes that encode the specific enzymes required for sphingolipid metabolism permit the development of therapeutic options, such as recombinant enzyme replacement therapy, as well as the potential of gene

Table 75–7. Differential Findings in Lipidoses Lysosomal Storage Diseases

Nomenclature	Enzyme defect	Hydrops fetalis	Coarse facial features / Dysostosis multiplex	Hepatosplenomegaly	Cardiac involvement / Cardiac failure	Mental deterioration	Myoclonus	Spasticity	Peripheral neuropathy	Cherry-red spot	Corneal clouding	Angiokeratomata	Vacuolated lymphocytes	GAG (urine) ↓	Pathologic oligosaccharides ↓
Mucolipidoses															
Mucolipidosis II, I-cell disease	N-Acetylglucosaminylphosphotransferase	(+)	++	+	++	++	–	–	–	–	(+)	–	+	–	–
Mucolipidosis III, Pseudo-Hurler	N-Acetylglucosaminylphosphotransferase	–	+	(+)	–	(+)	–	–	–	–	+	–	+	–	–
Mucolipidosis IV	Unknown	–	–	+	–	(+)	–	–	–	–	+	–	+	–	–
Sphingolipidoses															
Fabry disease	α-Galactosidase	–	–	(+)	+	–	–	–	+	–	+	++	–	–	–
Farber disease	Ceramidase	(+)	–	(+)	++	+	(+)	+	+	(+)	+	–	+	–	–
Galactosialidosis	β-Galactosidase and sialidase	(+)	++	++	+	++	+	+	–	++	+	+	+	–	+
GM1 gangliosidosis	β-Galactosidase	(+)	++	+	(+)	++	+	(+)	–	++	+	+	+	–	+
GM2 gangliosidosis (Tay-Sachs disease, Sandhoff disease)	β-Hexosaminidases A and B	–	–	(+)	–	++	+	+	–	++	–	–	–	–	+
Gaucher type I	Glucocerebrosidase	–	–	+	–	–	–	–	–	–	–	–	–	–	–
Gaucher type II	Glucocerebrosidase	(+)	–	+	–	++	+	+	–	–	–	–	–	–	+
Gaucher type III	Glucocerebrosidase	(+)	–	+	–	+	(+)	(+)	–	–	–	–	+	–	+
Niemann–Pick type I (= A & B)	Sphingomyelinase	–	–	++	–	++	(+)	+	(+)	(+)	(+)	–	+	–	–
Metachromatic leukodystrophy	Arylsulfatase A	–	–	–	–	++	–	+	++	(+)	–	–	+	–	–
Krabbe disease	β-Galactocerebrosidase	–	–	–	–	++	–	+	++	(+)	–	–	+	–	–
Lipid storage disorders															
Niemann–Pick type II (= C & D)	Intracellular cholesterol transport	(+)	–	(+)	(+)	+	–	(+)	–	(+)	–	–	+	–	–
Wolman disease	Acid lipase	–	–	+	–	+	–	–	–	(+)	–	–	+	–	–
Ceroid lipofuscinosis, infantile (Santavuori–Hantia)	Palmitoyl-proteinthioesterase (CLN1)	–	–	–	–	+	+	+	–	–	–	–	+	–	–
Ceroid lipofuscinosis, late infantile (Jansky–Bielschowsky)	Pepstatin-insensitive peptididase (CLN2). Variants in Finland (CLN5), Turkey (CLN7), and Italy (CLN6)	–	–	–	–	+	+	+	+	–	–	–	+	–	–
Ceroid lipofuscinosis, juvenile (Spielmeyer–Vogt)	CLN3, membrane protein	–	–	–	–	+	–	(+)	–	–	–	–	(+)	–	–
Ceroid lipofuscinosis, adult (Kufs, Parry)	CLN4, probably heterogeneous	(+)	–	–	–	+	(+)	–	–	–	–	–	(+)	–	–
Oligosaccharidoses															
Aspartylglucosaminuria	Aspartylglucosaminase	–	+	(+)	(+)	+	+	–	–	–	(+)	(+)	+	–	+
Fucosidosis	α-Fucosidase	–	+	(+)	+	++	–	(+)	–	–	(+)	++	+	–	+
α-Mannosidosis	α-Mannosidase	–	++	+	–	++	–	+	–	–	++	(+)	+	–	+
β-Mannosidosis	β-Mannosidase	–	+	(+)	–	+	–	+	+	–	–	–	–	–	+
Schindler disease	α-N-Acetylgalactosaminidase	–	–	–	+	–	+	+	+	–	–	+	+	–	+
Sialidosis I	Sialidase	(+)	–	–	–	–	++	+	+	++	(+)	–	+	–	+
Sialidosis II	Sialidase	(+)	++	+	+	++	(+)	+	–	++	–	+	+	–	+

++ = prominent; + = often present, (+) = inconstant or occuring later in the disease course; – = not present.
diff, different; GAG, glycosaminoglycans.
Modified from: Hoffmann GF, Nyhan WL, Zschoke J, et al: Storage Disorders in Inherited Metabolic Diseases. Lippincott, Williams & Wilkins, Philadelphia, 2002, pp 346-51.

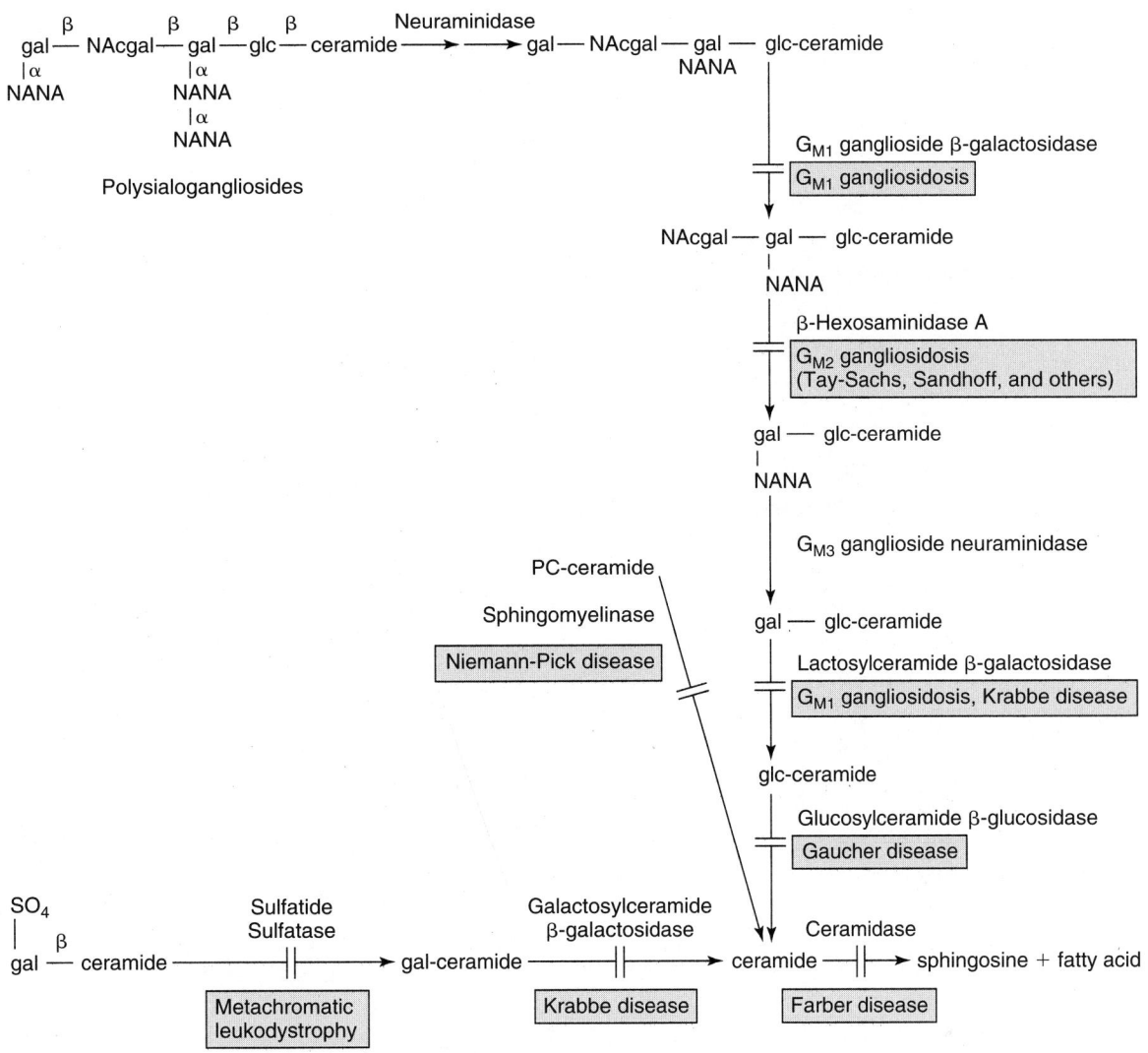

FIGURE 75–9. Pathways in the metabolism of sphingolipids found in nervous tissues. The name of the enzyme catalyzing each reaction is given with the name of the substrate acted on. Inborn errors are depicted as bars crossing the reaction arrows, and the name of the associated defect or defects is given within the nearest box. The gangliosides are named according to the nomenclature of Svennerholm. Anomeric configurations are given only at the largest starting a compound. gal = galactose; glc = glucose; NAcgal = N-acetyl-galactosamine; NANA = N-acetyl-neuraminic acid; PC = phosphorylcholine.

therapy. Identification of specific disease-causing mutations improves diagnosis, prenatal detection, and carrier identification. For some disorders (e.g., Gaucher disease), it has been possible to make genotype-phenotype correlations that predict disease severity and allow more precise genetic counseling. Inheritance is autosomal recessive except for X-linked Fabry disease.

GM1 Gangliosidosis. GM_1 gangliosidosis most frequently presents in early infancy (type 1 disease) but has been described in patients with a juvenile onset (type 2). Both are autosomal recessive traits; each results from the deficient activity of β-galactosidase, a lysosomal enzyme encoded by a gene on chromosome 3 (3p21.33). Although the disorder is characterized by pathologic accumulation of GM_1 gangliosides in the lysosomes of both neural and visceral cells, GM_1 ganglioside accumulation is most marked in the brain. In addition, keratan sulfate, a mucopolysaccharide, accumulates in liver and is excreted in the urine of patients with GM_1 gangliosidosis. The β-galactosidase gene has been isolated and sequenced, and mutations causing either type 1 or type 2 disease have been identified.

The *clinical manifestations* of the infantile form of GM_1 gangliosidosis (type 1 disease) may be evident in the newborn as hepatosplenomegaly, edema, and skin eruptions (angiokeratomata). It most frequently presents within the first 6 mo of life with developmental delay followed by progressive psychomotor retardation and the onset of tonic-clonic seizures. A typical facies characterized by low-set ears, frontal bossing, a depressed nasal bridge, and abnormally long philtrum is also evident. Up to 50% of patients have a macular cherry-red spot. Hepatosplenomegaly and skeletal abnormalities similar to those of the mucopolysaccharidoses, including anterior beaking of the vertebrae, enlargement of the sella turcica, and thickening of the calvarium, are present. By the end of the 1st yr of life, most patients are blind and deaf, with severe neurologic impairment characterized by decerebrate rigidity. Death usually occurs by 3–4 yr of age. The juvenile-onset form of GM_1 gangliosidosis (type 2) is clinically distinct, with a variable age at onset. Affected patients present primarily with neurologic symptoms including ataxia, dysarthria, mental retardation, and spasticity. Deterioration is slow; patients may survive through the 4th decade of life. These patients lack the visceral involvement, facial abnormalities, and

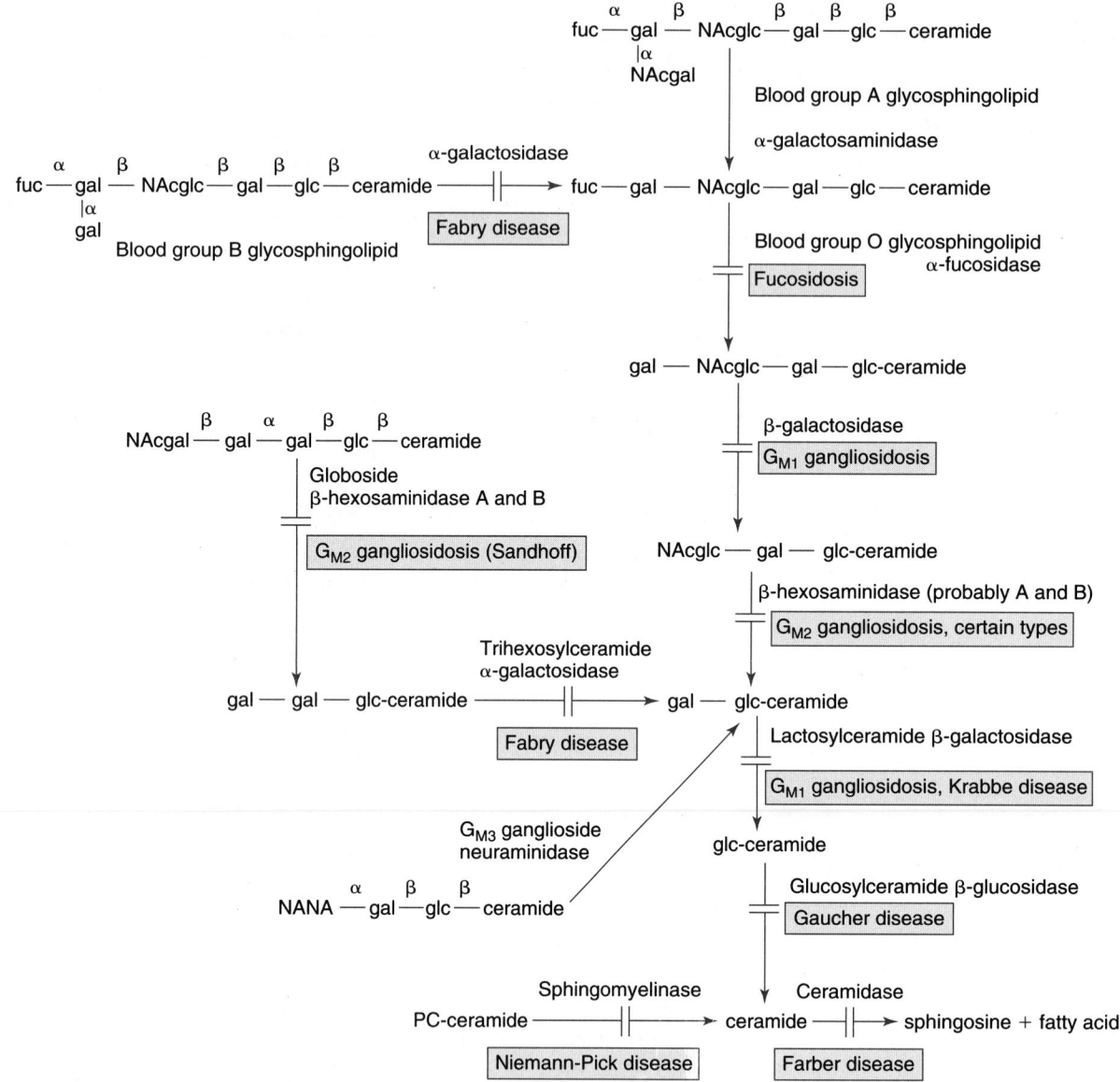

FIGURE 75–10. Pathways in the degradation of sphingolipids found in visceral organs and red or white blood cells. See also the legend for Figure 75–9. fuc = fucose; NAcglc = *N*-acetylglucosamine.

skeletal features seen in type 1 disease. There is no specific *treatment* for either form of GM$_1$ gangliosidosis.

The *diagnosis* of GM$_1$ gangliosidosis should be suspected in infants with typical clinical features and is confirmed by the demonstration of the deficiency of β-galactosidase activity in peripheral leukocytes or cultured skin fibroblasts. Other disorders that share some of the features of the GM$_1$ gangliosidoses include Hurler disease (mucopolysaccharidosis type I), I-cell disease, and Niemann-Pick disease (NPD) type A, which can each be distinguished by the demonstration of their specific enzymatic deficiencies. Carriers of the disorder are detected by the measurement of the enzymatic activity in white blood cells or cultured skin fibroblasts; prenatal diagnosis is accomplished by determination of the enzymatic activity in cultured aminocytes or chorionic villi.

The GM$_2$ Gangliosidoses. The GM$_2$ gangliosidoses include *Tay-Sachs* disease and *Sandhoff disease*; each results from the deficiency of β-hexosaminidase activity and the lysosomal accumulation of GM$_2$ gangliosides, particularly in the central nervous system.

Both disorders have been classified into infantile-, juvenile-, and adult-onset forms based on the age at onset and clinical features. β-Hexosaminidase occurs as two isozymes: β-hexosaminidase A, which is composed of one α and one β subunit, and β-hexosaminidase B, which has two β subunits. β-hexosaminidase deficiency results from mutations in the α subunit and causes Tay-Sachs disease, whereas mutations in the β-subunit gene result in the deficiency of both β-hexosaminidases A and B and cause Sandhoff disease. Both are autosomal recessive traits, with Tay-Sachs disease having a predilection in the Ashkenazi Jewish population, where the carrier frequency is about 1/25.

More than 50 mutations have been identified; most are associated with the infantile forms of disease. Three mutations account for more than 98% of mutant alleles among Ashkenazi Jewish carriers of Tay-Sachs disease, including one allele associated with the adult-onset form. Mutations that cause the subacute or chronic forms result in enzyme proteins with residual enzymatic activities, the levels of which correlate with the severity of the disease.

Patients with the infantile form of Tay-Sachs disease have *clinical manifestations* in infancy of loss of motor skills, increased startle reaction, and macular pallor and retinal cherry-red spots (see Table 75–7). Affected infants usually develop normally until 4–5 mo of age when decreased eye contact and an exaggerated startle response to noise (hyperacusis) are noted. Macrocephaly, not associated with hydrocephalus, may develop. In the 2nd yr of life, seizures requiring anticonvulsant therapy develop. Neurodegeneration is relentless, with death occurring by the age of 4 or 5 yr. The juvenile-onset form initially presents with ataxia and dysarthria and may not be associated with a macular cherry-red spot.

The *clinical manifestations* of Sandhoff disease are similar to those for Tay-Sachs disease. However, infants with Sandhoff disease have hepatosplenomegaly, cardiac involvement, and mild bony abnormalities. The juvenile form of this disorder presents as ataxia, dysarthria, and mental deterioration, but without visceral enlargement or a macular cherry-red spot. There is no *treatment* available for Tay-Sachs disease or Sandhoff disease.

The *diagnosis* of infantile Tay-Sachs disease and Sandhoff disease is usually suspected in an infant with neurologic features and a cherry-red spot. Definitive diagnosis is by determination of the level of β-hexosaminidases A and B in isolated blood leukocytes. The two disorders are distinguished by the enzymatic assay, because in Tay-Sachs disease only the β-hexosaminidase A isozyme is deficient, whereas in Sandhoff disease both the β-hexosaminidase A and B isozymes are deficient. Future at-risk pregnancies for both disorders can be monitored by prenatal diagnosis by amniocentesis or chorionic villus sampling. Identification of carriers within families is also possible by β-hexosaminidases A and B determination. Indeed, for Tay-Sachs disease, carrier screening of all couples in whom at least one member is of Ashkenazi Jewish descent is recommended before the initiation of pregnancy to identify couples at risk. These studies can be conducted by the determination of the level of β-hexosaminidase A activity in peripheral leukocytes or plasma. Molecular studies to identify the exact molecular defect in enzymatically identified carriers should also be performed to permit more specific identification of carriers in the family, and for at-risk couples to allow prenatal diagnosis by both enzymatic and genotype determinations. The incidence of Tay-Sachs disease has been markedly reduced since the introduction of carrier screening programs in the Ashkenazi Jewish population.

Gaucher Disease. This disease is a multisystemic lipidosis characterized by hematologic problems, organomegaly, and skeletal involvement, the latter usually manifested as bone pain and pathologic fractures (see Table 75–7). It is the most common lysosomal storage disease and the most prevalent genetic defect among Ashkenazi Jews. There are three clinical subtypes delineated by the absence or presence and progression of neurologic manifestations: Type 1 or the adult, non-neuronopathic form; type 2, the infantile or acute neuronopathic form; and type 3, the juvenile or Norrbotten form. All are autosomal recessive traits. Type 1, which accounts for 99% of cases, has a striking predilection for Ashkenazi Jews, with an incidence of about 1/1,000 and a carrier frequency of 1/18.

Gaucher disease results from the deficient activity of the lysosomal hydrolase, acid β-glucosidase, which is encoded by a gene located on chromosome 1 q21-q31. The enzymatic defect results in the accumulation of undegraded glycolipid substrates, particularly glucosylceramide, in cells of the reticuloendothelial system. This progressive deposition results in infiltration of the bone marrow, progressive hepatosplenomegaly, and skeletal complications. Four mutations—N370S, L444P, 84insG, and IVS2—account for about 95% of mutant alleles among Ashkenazi Jewish patients, permitting screening for this disorder in this population. Genotype-phenotype correlations have been noted, providing the molecular basis for the clinical het-

erogeneity seen in Gaucher disease type 1, which has a wide range of severity and age at onset. Patients who are homozygous for the N370S mutation tend to have later onset, with a more indolent course than patients with one copy of N370S and another common allele.

Clinical manifestations of type 1 Gaucher disease have a variable age at onset, from early childhood to late adulthood, with most symptomatic patients presenting by adolescence. At presentation, patients may bruise easily owing to thrombocytopenia, chronic fatigue secondary to anemia, hepatomegaly with or without elevated liver function test results, splenomegaly, and bone pain. Occasional patients have pulmonary involvement at the time of presentation. Patients presenting in the 1st decade frequently are not Jewish and have growth retardation and a more malignant course. Other patients may be discovered fortuitously during evaluation for other conditions or as part of routine examinations; these patients may have a milder or even a benign course. In symptomatic patients, splenomegaly is progressive and can become massive. Most patients develop radiologic evidence of skeletal involvement, including an Erlenmeyer flask deformity of the distal femur. Clinically apparent bony involvement, which occurs in more than 20% of patients, can present as bone pain or pathologic fractures. Lytic lesions can develop in the long bones, including the femur, ribs, and pelvis; osteosclerosis may be evident at an early age. Bone crises with severe pain and swelling can occur. Bleeding secondary to thrombocytopenia may manifest as epistaxis or bruising and is frequently overlooked until other symptoms become apparent. With the exception of the severely growth-retarded child, who may experience developmental delay secondary to the effects of chronic disease, development and intelligence are normal.

The pathologic hallmark of Gaucher disease is the Gaucher cell in the reticuloendothelial system, particularly in the bone marrow (Fig. 75–11). These cells, which are 20 to 100 μm in diameter, have a characteristic wrinkled paper appearance resulting from the presence of intracytoplasmic substrate inclusions. The cytoplasm of the Gaucher cell reacts strongly positively with the periodic acid-Schiff stain. The presence of this cell in bone marrow and tissue specimens is highly suggestive of Gaucher disease, although it also may be found in patients with granulocytic leukemia and myeloma.

Gaucher disease type 2 is much less common and does not have an ethnic predilection. It is characterized by a rapid neurodegenerative course with extensive visceral involvement and death within the first 2 yr of life. It presents in infancy with increased tone, strabismus, and organomegaly. Failure to thrive and stridor caused by laryngospasm are typical. After a several-year period of psychomotor regression, death occurs

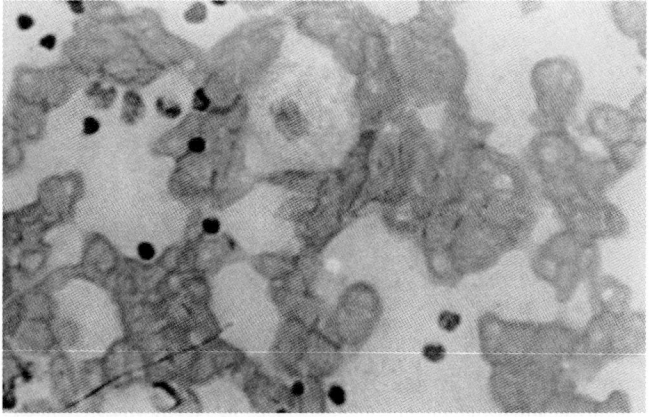

FIGURE 75–11. Cells from a spleen of a patient with Gaucher disease. A characteristic spleen cell is shown engorged with glucocerebroside.

secondary to respiratory compromise. Gaucher disease type 3 presents as clinical manifestations that are intermediate to those seen in types 1 and 2, with presentation in childhood and death by age 10–15 yr. It has a predilection for the Swedish Norrbottnian population, where the incidence is 1/50,000. Neurologic involvement is present but occurs later and with decreased severity compared with type 2 disease. Type 3 disease is further classified as types 3a and 3b based on the extent of neurologic involvement and whether there is progressive myotonia and dementia (type 3a) or isolated supranuclear gaze palsy (type 3b).

Gaucher disease should be considered in the *differential diagnosis* of patients with unexplained organomegaly, who bruise easily, have bone pain, or have a combination of these conditions. Bone marrow examination usually reveals the presence of Gaucher cells. All suspected diagnoses should be confirmed by determination of the acid β-glucosidase activity in isolated leukocytes or cultured fibroblasts. The identification of carriers can be achieved by enzymatic assay, with confirmation of results by molecular testing in most Jewish families. Testing should be offered to all family members, keeping in mind that heterogeneity, even among members of the same kindred, can be so great that nonsymptomatic affected individuals may be diagnosed. Prenatal diagnosis is available by determination of enzyme activity in chorionic villi or cultured amniotic fluid cells.

Treatment of patients with Gaucher disease type 1 includes enzyme replacement therapy, with recombinant acid β-glucosidase (imiglucerase). Most extraskeletal symptoms (organomegaly, hematologic indices) are reversed by an initial debulking dose of enzyme (60 IU/kg) administered by intravenous infusion every other week. Monthly maintenance enzyme replacement improves bone structure, decreases bone pain, and induces compensatory growth in affected children. A small number of patients have undergone bone marrow transplantation, which is curative but results in significant morbidity and mortality from the procedure, making the selection of appropriate candidates limited. Efforts are also under way to develop gene therapy for type 1 disease.

Niemann-Pick Disease (NPD). The original description of NPD was what is now known as type A NPD, a fatal disorder of infancy characterized by failure to thrive, hepatosplenomegaly, and a rapidly progressive neurodegenerative course that leads to death by 2–3 yr of age. Type B is a non-neuronopathic form observed in children and adults. Type C is a neuronopathic form that results from defective cholesterol transport. All the subtypes are inherited as autosomal recessive traits and display variable clinical features (see Table 75–7).

NPD types A and B result from the deficient activity of acid sphingomyelinase, a lysosomal enzyme encoded by a gene on chromosome 11 (11p15.1-p15.4). The enzymatic defect results in the pathologic accumulation of sphingomyelin, a ceramide phospholipid, and other lipids in the monocyte-macrophage system, the primary pathologic site. The progressive deposition of sphingomyelin in the central nervous system results in the neurodegenerative course seen in type A, and in non-neural tissue in the systemic disease manifestations of type B, including progressive lung disease in some patients. The acid sphingomyelinase gene is sequenced, and a variety of mutations that cause types A and B NPD are known.

The *clinical manifestations* and course of type A NPD is uniform and is characterized by a normal appearance at birth (although the newborn period is sometimes complicated by prolonged jaundice). Hepatosplenomegaly, moderate lymphadenopathy, and psychomotor retardation are evident by 6 mo of age, followed by neurodevelopmental regression. With advancing age, the loss of motor function and the deterioration of intellectual capabilities are progressively debilitating; and in later stages, spasticity and rigidity are evident. Affected infants lose contact with their environment. In contrast to the stereotyped type A phenotype, the clinical presentation and course of patients with type B disease are more variable. Most are diagnosed in infancy or childhood when enlargement of the liver or spleen, or both, is detected during a routine physical examination. At diagnosis, type B NPD patients usually have evidence of mild pulmonary involvement, usually detected as a diffuse reticular or finely nodular infiltration on the chest radiograph. Pulmonary symptoms are not usual until adulthood. In most patients, hepatosplenomegaly is particularly prominent in childhood, but with increasing linear growth, the abdominal protuberance decreases and becomes less conspicuous. In mildly affected patients, the splenomegaly may not be noted until adulthood, and there may be minimal disease manifestations.

In some type B patients, decreased pulmonary diffusion caused by alveolar infiltration becomes evident in late childhood or early adulthood and progresses with age. Severely affected individuals may experience significant pulmonary compromise by 15–20 yr of age. Such patients have low P_{O_2} values and dyspnea on exertion. Life-threatening bronchopneumonias may occur, and cor pulmonale has been described. Severely affected patients may have liver involvement leading to life-threatening cirrhosis, portal hypertension, and ascites. Clinically significant pancytopenia due to secondary hypersplenism may require partial or complete splenectomy; this should be avoided if possible because splenectomy frequently causes progression of pulmonary disease, which can be life threatening. In general, type B patients do not have neurologic involvement and have a normal IQ. Some patients with type B disease have cherry red maculae or haloes and subtle neurologic symptoms (peripheral neuropathy).

Type C NPD patients often present with prolonged neonatal jaundice, appear normal for 1–2 yr, and then experience a slowly progressive and variable neurodegenerative course. Their hepatosplenomegaly is less severe than that in patients with types A or B NPD, and they may survive into adulthood. The underlying biochemical defect in type C patients is an abnormality in cholesterol transport, leading to the accumulation of sphingomyelin and cholesterol in their lysosomes and a secondary partial reduction in acid sphingomyelinase activity (see Chapter 75.3).

In type B NPD patients, splenomegaly is usually the first manifestation detected. The splenic enlargement is noted in early childhood; however, in very mild disease, the enlargement may be subtle and detection may be delayed until adolescence or adulthood. The presence of the characteristic NPD cells in the bone marrow aspirates supports the diagnosis of type B NPD. However, patients with type C NPD also have extensive infiltration of NPD cells in the bone marrow and, thus, all suspected cases should be evaluated enzymatically to confirm the clinical diagnosis by measuring the acid sphingomyelinase activity level in peripheral leukocytes, cultured fibroblasts, or lymphoblasts, or a combination of these cells. Patients with types A and B NPD have markedly decreased levels (1–10%), whereas patients with type C NPD have somewhat decreased acid sphingomyelinase activities. The enzymatic identification of NPD carriers is problematic. However, in families in which the specific molecular lesion has been identified, family members can be accurately tested for heterozygote status by DNA analysis. Prenatal diagnosis of types A and B NPD can be made reliably by the measurement of acid sphingomyelinase activity in cultured amniocytes or chorionic villi; molecular analysis of fetal cells can provide the specific diagnosis or serve as a confirmatory test. The clinical diagnosis of type C NPD can be supported by the demonstration of filipin stain positivity in cultured fibroblasts and/or by identifying a specific mutation in the NPC gene.

There is no specific *treatment* for NPD. Orthotopic liver transplantation in an infant with type A disease and amniotic cell transplantation in several type B NPD patients have been attempted with little or no success. Bone marrow transplantation in one type B NPD patient was successful in reducing the spleen and liver volumes, the sphingomyelin content in the liver, the number of NPD cells in the marrow, and the radiologic infiltration of the lungs. However, this patient died 3 mo after transplantation. Lung transplantation has not been performed in any severely compromised type B patient. Future prospects for treatment of type B disease include enzyme replacement and gene therapy. Treatment of types A and C disease is presently precluded by the severe neurologic involvement.

Fabry Disease. This condition is an inborn error of glycosphingolipid metabolism characterized by angiokeratomas (telangiectatic skin lesions), hypohidrosis, corneal and lenticular opacities, acroparesthesias, and vascular disease of the kidney, heart, and/or brain (see Table 75–7). The disease is an X-linked recessive trait that is manifested in affected males and has an estimated prevalence of about 1/50,000 males. Atypical variants with residual α-galactosidase A activity may be asymptomatic or have late-onset, mild disease manifestations primarily limited to the heart. Heterozygous females are usually asymptomatic or exhibit mild manifestations.

The disease results from the deficient activity of α-galactosidase A, a lysosomal enzyme encoded by a gene located on the long arm of the X chromosome (Xq22). The enzymatic defect leads to the systemic accumulation of neutral glycosphingolipids, primarily globotriaosylceramide, particularly in the plasma and lysosomes of vascular endothelial and smooth muscle cells. The progressive vascular glycosphingolipid deposition in affected males results in ischemia and infarction, leading to the major disease manifestations. Affected males who have blood group B or AB have a more severe disease course because the blood group B substances also accumulate, as they are normally degraded by α-galactosidase A. The cDNA and genomic sequences encoding α-galactosidase A have identified over 200 different mutations in the α-galactosidase A gene that are responsible for this lysosomal storage disease, including amino acid substitutions, gene rearrangements, and mRNA splicing defects.

Clinical manifestations include angiokeratomas, which usually occur in childhood and may lead to early diagnosis. They increase in size and number with age and range from barely visible to several millimeters in diameter. The lesions are punctate, dark red to blue-black, and flat or slightly raised. They do not blanch with pressure, and the larger ones may show slight hyperkeratosis. Characteristically, the lesions are most dense between the umbilicus and knees, in the "bathing trunk area," but may occur anywhere, including the oral mucosa. The hips, thighs, buttocks, umbilicus, lower abdomen, scrotum, and glans penis are common sites, and there is a tendency toward symmetry. Variants without skin lesions have been described. Sweating is usually decreased or absent. Corneal opacities and characteristic lenticular lesions, observed under slit lamp examination, are present in affected males as well as in about 70% of asymptomatic heterozygotes. Conjunctival and retinal vascular tortuosity are common and result from the systemic vascular involvement.

Pain is the most debilitating symptom in childhood and adolescence. Fabry crises, lasting from minutes to several days, consist of agonizing, burning pain in the hands and feet and proximal extremities and are usually associated with exercise, fatigue, or fever, or a combination of these factors. These painful acroparesthesias usually become less frequent in the 3rd and 4th decades of life, although in some men they may become more frequent and severe. Attacks of abdominal or flank pain may simulate appendicitis or renal colic.

The major morbid symptoms result from the progressive involvement of the vascular system. Early in the course of the disease, casts, red cells, and lipid inclusions with characteristic birefringent "Maltese crosses" appear in the urinary sediment. Proteinuria, isosthenuria, and gradual deterioration of renal function and development of azotemia occur in the 2nd through 4th decades. Cardiovascular findings may include hypertension, left ventricular hypertrophy, anginal chest pain, myocardial ischemia or infarction, and heart failure. Mitral insufficiency is the most common valvular lesion. Abnormal electrocardiographic and echocardiographic findings are common. Cerebrovascular manifestations result from multifocal small vessel involvement. Other features may include chronic bronchitis and dyspnea, lymphedema of the legs without hypoproteinemia, episodic diarrhea, osteoporosis, retarded growth, and delayed puberty. Death most often results from uremia or vascular disease of the heart or brain. Before hemodialysis or renal transplantation, the mean age at death for affected men was 41 yr. Atypical male variants with residual α-galactosidase A activity who are asymptomatic or mildly affected have been described whose manifestations include late-onset, isolated cardiac disease and proteinuria but normal renal function for age. These patients do not have the early classic manifestations. These "cardiac variants" have cardiomegaly, usually involving the left ventricular wall and interventricular septum, and electrocardiographic abnormalities consistent with cardiomyopathy. Others have had hypertrophic cardiomyopathy and/or myocardial infarction.

The *diagnosis* in classically affected males is most readily made from the history of painful acroparesthesias, hypohidrosis, the presence of characteristic skin lesions, and the observation of the characteristic corneal opacities and lenticular lesions. The disorder is often misdiagnosed as rheumatic fever, erythromelalgia, or neurosis. The skin lesions must be differentiated from the benign angiokeratomas of the scrotum (Fordyce disease) or from angiokeratoma circumscriptum. Angiokeratomas identical to those of Fabry disease have been reported in fucosidosis, aspartylglycosaminuria, late-onset GM_1 gangliosidosis, galactosialidosis, α-N-acetylgalactosaminidase deficiency, and sialidosis. The diagnosis of the mild cardiac variants should be considered in individuals who present with left ventricular hypertrophy or cardiomyopathy, or both. The diagnosis of classic and variant patients is confirmed biochemically by the demonstration of markedly decreased α-galactosidase A activity in plasma, isolated leukocytes, or cultured fibroblasts or lymphoblasts.

Heterozygous females may have corneal opacities, isolated skin lesions, and intermediate activities of α-galactosidase A in plasma or cells. Rare female heterozygotes may have manifestations as severe as those in affected males. However, at-risk females in families affected by Fabry disease who are asymptomatic should be optimally diagnosed by the direct analysis of their family's specific mutation. Prenatal detection of affected males can be accomplished by the demonstration of deficient α-galactosidase A activity or the family's specific gene mutation in chorionic villi obtained in the 1st trimester or in cultured amniocytes obtained by amniocentesis in the 2nd trimester of pregnancy.

Treatment for Fabry disease was once nonspecific and limited to supportive care, which included the use of phenytoin and/or carbamazepine to decrease the frequency and severity of the chronic acroparesthesias and the periodic crises of excruciating pain. Renal transplantation and long-term hemodialysis also have become life-saving procedures for patients with renal failure. Recombinant α-galactosidase is a safe and effective enzyme replacement therapy for Fabry disease. The enzyme is well tolerated. Treatment results in very significant clearance of globotriaosylceramide from the vascular endothelial cells of the kidney, heart, and skin, as well as the cells of the glomerulus.

Fucosidosis. Fucosidosis is a rare, autosomal recessive disorder caused by the deficient activity of α-fucosidase and the accumulation of fucose-containing glycosphingolipids, glycoproteins, and oligosac-charides in the lysosomes of the liver, brain, and other organs (see Table 75–7). The α-fucosidase gene is on chromosome 1 (1p24), and specific mutations are known. Although the disorder is panethnic, most affected patients are from Italy and the United States. There is wide variability in the clinical phenotype, with the most severely affected patients presenting in the 1st yr of life with developmental delay and somatic features similar to those of the mucopolysaccharidoses. These features include frontal bossing, hepatosplenomegaly, coarse facial features, and macroglossia. The central nervous system storage results in a relentless neurodegenerative course with death in childhood. Patients with milder disease have angiokeratomas and longer survival. No specific therapy exists for the disorder, which can be diagnosed by the demonstration of deficient α-fucosidase activity in peripheral leukocytes or cultured fibroblasts. Carrier identification studies and prenatal diagnosis are possible by determination of the enzymatic activity.

Schindler Disease. This disease is an autosomal recessive neurodegenerative disorder that results from the deficient activity of α-*N*-acetylgalactosaminidase and the accumulation of sialylated and asialoglycopeptides and oligosaccharides (see Table 75–7). The gene for the enzyme is mapped to chromosome 22 (22q13.1-13.2). The disease is clinically heterogeneous, and two major phenotypes have been identified. Type 1 disease is an infantile-onset neuroaxonal dystrophy. Affected infants have normal development for the first 9–15 mo of life followed by a rapid neurodegenerative course that results in severe psychomotor retardation, cortical blindness, and frequent myoclonic seizures. Type II disease is characterized by a variable age at onset, mild retardation, and angiokeratomas. There is no specific therapy for either form of the disorder. The diagnosis is by demonstration of the enzymatic deficiency in leukocytes or cultured skin fibroblasts

Metachromatic Leukodystrophy. Metachromatic leukodystrophy (MLD) is an autosomal recessive white matter disease caused by a deficiency of arylsulfatase A (ASA), which is required for the hydrolysis of sulfated glycosphingolipids. An additional form of MLD is caused by a deficiency of a sphingolipid activator protein (SAP1), a protein required for the formation of the substrate-enzyme complex. The deficiency of this enzymatic activity results in the white matter storage of sulfated glycosphingolipids, which leads to demyelination and a neurodegenerative course. The ASA gene is on chromosome 22 (22q13.31qter); specific mutations are known to fall into two groups that correlate with disease severity.

The *clinical manifestations* of the late infantile form of MLD, which is most common, usually presents between 12–18 mo of age as irritability, inability to walk, and hyperextension of the knee, causing genu recurvatum. Deep tendon reflexes are diminished or absent. Gradual muscle wasting, weakness, and hypotonia become evident and lead to a debilitated state. As the disease progresses, nystagmus, myoclonic seizures, optic atrophy, and quadriparesis appear, with death in the 1st decade of life (see Table 75–7). The juvenile form of the disorder has a more indolent course with onset that may occur as late as 20 yr of age. This form of the disease presents as gait disturbances, mental deterioration, urinary incontinence, and emotional difficulties. The adult form, which presents after the 2nd decade, is similar to the juvenile form in its clinical manifestations, although emotional difficulties and psychosis are more prominent features. Dementia, seizures, diminished reflexes, and optic atrophy also occur in both the juvenile and adult forms. The pathologic hallmark of MLD is the deposition of metachromatic bodies, which stain strongly positive with periodic acid–Schiff and alcian blue, in the white matter of the brain. Neuronal inclusions may be seen in the midbrain, pons, medulla, retina, and spinal cord; demyelination occurs in the peripheral nervous system. Attempts to treat patients with MLD

with bone marrow transplantation have resulted in normal enzymatic levels in peripheral blood, but no clear evidence for clinical efficacy in terms of the neurologic course; supportive care remains the primary intervention.

The *diagnosis* of MLD should be suspected in patients with the clinical features of leukodystrophy. Decreased nerve conduction velocities, increased cerebrospinal fluid protein, metachromatic deposits in sampled segments of sural nerve, and metachromatic granules in urinary sediment are all suggestive of MLD. Confirmation of the diagnosis is based on the demonstration of the reduced activity of ASA in leukocytes or cultured skin fibroblasts. Sphingolipid activator protein deficiency is diagnosed by measuring the concentration of SAP1 in cultured fibroblasts using a specific antibody to the protein. Carrier detection and prenatal diagnosis is available for all forms of the disorder.

Multiple Sulfatase Deficiency. This is an autosomal recessive disorder that results from the deficiency of three enzymatic activities: arylsulfatases A, B, and C. Sulfatides, mucopolysaccharides, steroid sulfates, and gangliosides accumulate in the cerebral cortex and visceral tissues, resulting in a clinical phenotype with features of leukodystrophy as well as those of the mucopolysaccharidoses. Severe ichthyosis also may occur. Carrier testing and prenatal diagnosis by measurement of the enzymatic activities can be performed. There is no specific treatment for multiple sulfatase deficiency other than supportive care.

Krabbe Disease. This condition, also called *globoid cell leukodystrophy*, is an autosomal recessive fatal disorder of infancy. It results from the deficiency of the enzymatic activity of galactocerebrosidase and the white matter accumulation of galactosylceramide, which is normally found almost exclusively in the myelin sheath. The galactocerebrosidase gene is on chromosome 14 (14q31), and specific disease-causing mutations are known. The infantile form of Krabbe disease is rapidly progressive and patients present in early infancy with irritability, seizures, and hypertonia (see Table 75–7). Optic atrophy is evident in the 1st yr of life, and mental development is severely impaired. As the disease progresses, optic atrophy and severe developmental delay become apparent; affected children exhibit opisthotonos and die before 3 yr of age. A second, late infantile form of Krabbe disease also exists and patients present after the age of 2 yr. Affected individuals have a disease course similar to that of the early infantile form. Bone marrow transplantation has been attempted in several patients with later-onset disease but without significant results. There is no available therapy. The diagnosis of Krabbe disease relies on the demonstration of the specific enzymatic deficiency in white blood cells or cultured skin fibroblasts. Carrier identification and prenatal diagnosis are available.

Farber Disease. This is an autosomal recessive disorder that results from the deficiency of the lysosomal enzyme, ceramidase, and the accumulation of ceramide in various tissues, especially the joints. Symptoms can begin as early as the 1st yr of life with painful joint swelling and nodule formation (Fig. 75–12), which is sometimes diagnosed as rheumatoid arthritis. As the disease progresses, nodule or granulomatous formation on the vocal cords can lead to hoarseness and breathing difficulties; failure to thrive is common. In some patients, moderate central nervous system dysfunction is present (see Table 75–7). Patients may die of recurrent pneumonias in their teens; there is currently no specific therapy. The diagnosis of this disorder should be suspected in patients who have nodule formation over the joints but no other findings of rheumatoid arthritis. In such patients, ceramidase activity should be determined in cultured skin fibroblasts or white blood cells. Carrier detection and prenatal diagnosis are available.

Wolman Disease and Cholesterol Ester Disease (CESD). Wolman disease and cholesterol ester storage disease are autosomal recessive lysosomal storage diseases that result from the deficiency of

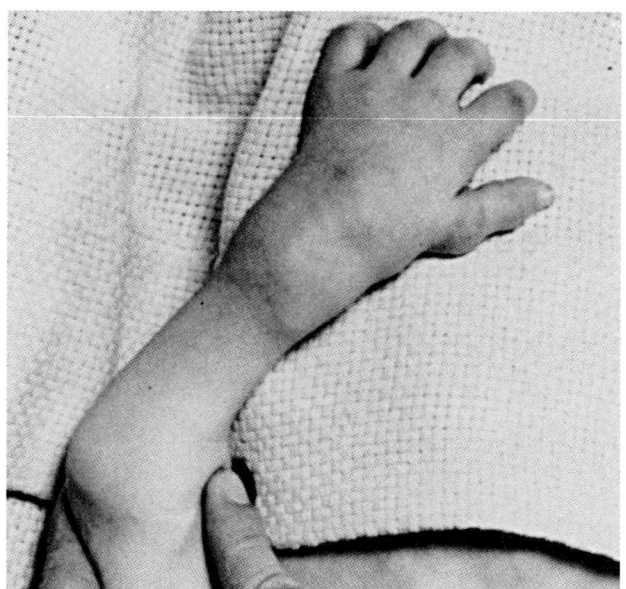

FIGURE 75–12. A forearm of an 18-mo-old girl with Farber disease. Note the painful joint swelling and the nodule formation. The infant was suspected of having rheumatoid arthritis.

acid lipase and the accumulation of cholesterol esters and triglycerides in histiocytic foam cells of most visceral organs. The gene for lysosomal acid lipase is on chromosome 10 (10q24-q25). Wolman disease is the more severe clinical phenotype and is a fatal disorder of infancy. The clinical features of the disease become apparent in the 1st wk of life and include failure to thrive, relentless vomiting, abdominal distention, steatorrhea, and hepatosplenomegaly (see Table 75–7). There usually is hyperlipidemia. Hepatic dysfunction and fibrosis may occur. Calcification of the adrenal glands is pathognomonic for the disorder. Death usually occurs within 6 mo.

Cholesterol ester storage disease is a less severe disorder that may not be diagnosed until adulthood. Hepatomegaly can be the only detectable abnormality, but affected individuals are at significant risk for premature atherosclerosis. Adrenal calcification is not a feature.

Diagnosis and carrier identification are based on measuring acid lipase activity in leukocytes or cultured skin fibroblasts. Prenatal diagnosis depends on measuring decreased enzyme levels in cultured chorionic villi or amniocytes. There is no specific therapy available for either disorder, although the use of pharmacologic agents to suppress cholesterol synthesis in combination with cholestyramine and diet modification has been used in patients with cholesterol ester storage disease (see Chapter 75.3).

Elstein D, Abrahamov A, Hadas-Halpern I, et al: Gaucher's disease. *Lancet* 2001; 358:324–7.
Eng, CM, Banikazemi M, Gordon RE, et al: A phase 1/2 clinical trial of enzyme replacement in Fabry disease: Pharmacokinetic, substrate clearance, and safety studies. *Am J Hum Genet* 2001;68:711–22.
Johnson WG: The clinical spectrum of hexosaminidase deficiency diseases. *Neurology* 1981;31:1453–56.
Mistry PK, Abrahamov A: A practical approach to diagnosis and management of Gaucher's disease. *Baillieres Clin Haematol* 1997;10:817–38.
Schiffmann R, Kopp JB, Austin HA, et al: Enzyme replacement therapy in Fabry disease. *JAMA* 2001;285:2743–49.
Schuchman EH, Desnick RJ: Types A and B Niemann Pick disease. In Scriver CR, Beaudet AL, Sly WS, et al (editors): *The Metabolic and Molecular Bases of Inherited Disease*, 8th ed. New York, McGraw-Hill, 2001.

75.5 Mucolipidoses

Margaret M. McGovern and Robert J. Desnick

I-cell disease (mucolipidosis II, ML-II) and pseudo-Hurler polydystrophy (mucolipidosis III, ML-III) are biochemically related, rare autosomal recessive disorders that share some clinical features with Hurler syndrome. These diseases result from the abnormal transport of newly synthesized lysosomal enzymes that are normally targeted to the lysosome by the presence of mannose-6-phosphate residues and are recognized by specific lysosomal membrane receptors. These mannose-6-phosphate recognition markers are synthesized in a two-step reaction that occurs in the Golgi apparatus and is mediated by two enzymatic activities. The enzyme that catalyzes the first step, UDP-*N*-acetylglucosamine:lysosomal enzymes *N*-acetylglucosamine-1-phosphotransferase, is defective in both ML-II and ML-III. This enzyme deficiency results in abnormal targeting of the lysosomal enzymes that are then secreted into the extracellular matrix. Because the lysosomal enzymes require the acidic medium of the lysosome to function, patients with this defect accumulate a variety of different substrates due to the cellular deficiency of all lysosomal enzymes. The diagnosis of ML-II and ML-III can be made by the determination of the serum lysosomal enzymatic activities, which are elevated, or by the demonstration of reduced enzymatic levels in cultured skin fibroblasts. Direct measurement of the phosphotransferase activity is possible. Prenatal diagnosis and carrier identification studies are available for both disorders by measurement of lysosomal enzymatic activities in cultured cells.

I-Cell Disease. I-cell disease shares many of the clinical manifestations of Hurler syndrome, although there is no mucopolysacchariduria and the presentation is earlier (see Table 75–7). Some patients have clinical features evident at birth, including coarse facial features, craniofacial abnormalities, restricted joint movement, and hypotonia. Nonimmune hydrops may be present in the fetus. The remainder of patients present in the 1st yr with severe psychomotor retardation, coarse facial features, and skeletal manifestations that include kyphoscoliosis and a lumbar gibbus. Patients also may have congenital dislocation of the hips, inguinal hernias, and gingival hypertrophy. Progressive, severe psychomotor retardation leads to death in early childhood. No *treatment* is available.

Pseudo-Hurler Polydystrophy. Pseudo-Hurler polydystrophy is a less severe disorder, with later onset and survival to adulthood reported. Affected children may present around the age of 4 or 5 yr with joint stiffness and short stature. Progressive destruction of the hip joints and moderate dysostosis multiplex are evident. Radiographic evidence of low iliac wings, flattening of the proximal femoral epiphyses with valgus deformity of the femoral head, and hypoplasia of the anterior third of the lumbar vertebrae are characteristic findings. Ophthalmic findings include corneal clouding, retinopathy, and astigmatism; visual complaints are uncommon (see Table 75–7). Some patients have learning disabilities or mental retardation. Treatment, which should include orthopedic care, is symptomatic.

Matsuda I, Arashuma S, Mitsuyama T, et al: Prenatal diagnosis of I-cell disease. *Hum Genet* 1975;30:69.
Scriver CR, Beaudet AL, Sly WS, et al (editors): *The Metabolic Basis of Inherited Disease*, 8th ed. New York, McGraw-Hill, 1995.
Varki A, Reitman ML, Vannier A, et al: Demonstration of the heterozygous state for I-cell disease and pseudo-Hurler polydystrophy by assay of N-acetylglucosaminylphosphotransferase in white blood cells and fibroblasts. *Am J Hum Genet* 1982;34:717–29.

Chapter 76
Defects in Metabolism of Carbohydrates

Carbohydrate synthesis and degradation provide the energy required for most metabolic processes. The important carbohydrates include three monosaccharides—glucose, galactose, and fructose—and a polysaccharide, glycogen. The relevant biochemical pathways of these carbohydrates are shown in Figure 76–1. Glucose is the principal substrate of energy metabolism in humans. A continuous source of glucose from dietary intake, gluconeogenesis, and degradation of glycogen maintains normal blood glucose levels. Metabolism of glucose generates adenosine triphosphate (ATP) via glycolysis (conversion of glu-

cose or glycogen to pyruvate) or mitochondrial oxidative phosphorylation (conversion of pyruvate to carbon dioxide and water), or both. Dietary sources of glucose come from ingesting polysaccharides, primarily starch, and disaccharides, including lactose, maltose, and sucrose. Oral intake of glucose is intermittent and unreliable. Glucose made de novo (gluconeogenesis) contributes to maintaining the euglycemic state, but this process requires time to be active. The breakdown of hepatic glycogen provides the rapid release of glucose, which maintains a constant blood glucose concentration. Glycogen is also the primary stored energy source in muscle, providing glucose for muscle activity during exercise. Galactose and fructose are monosaccharides that provide fuel for cellular metabolism; their role is less significant than that of glucose. Galactose is derived from lactose (galactose + glucose), which is found in milk and milk products. Galactose is an important energy source in infants, but it is first metabolized to glucose. Galactose (exogenous or endogenously synthesized from glucose) is also an important

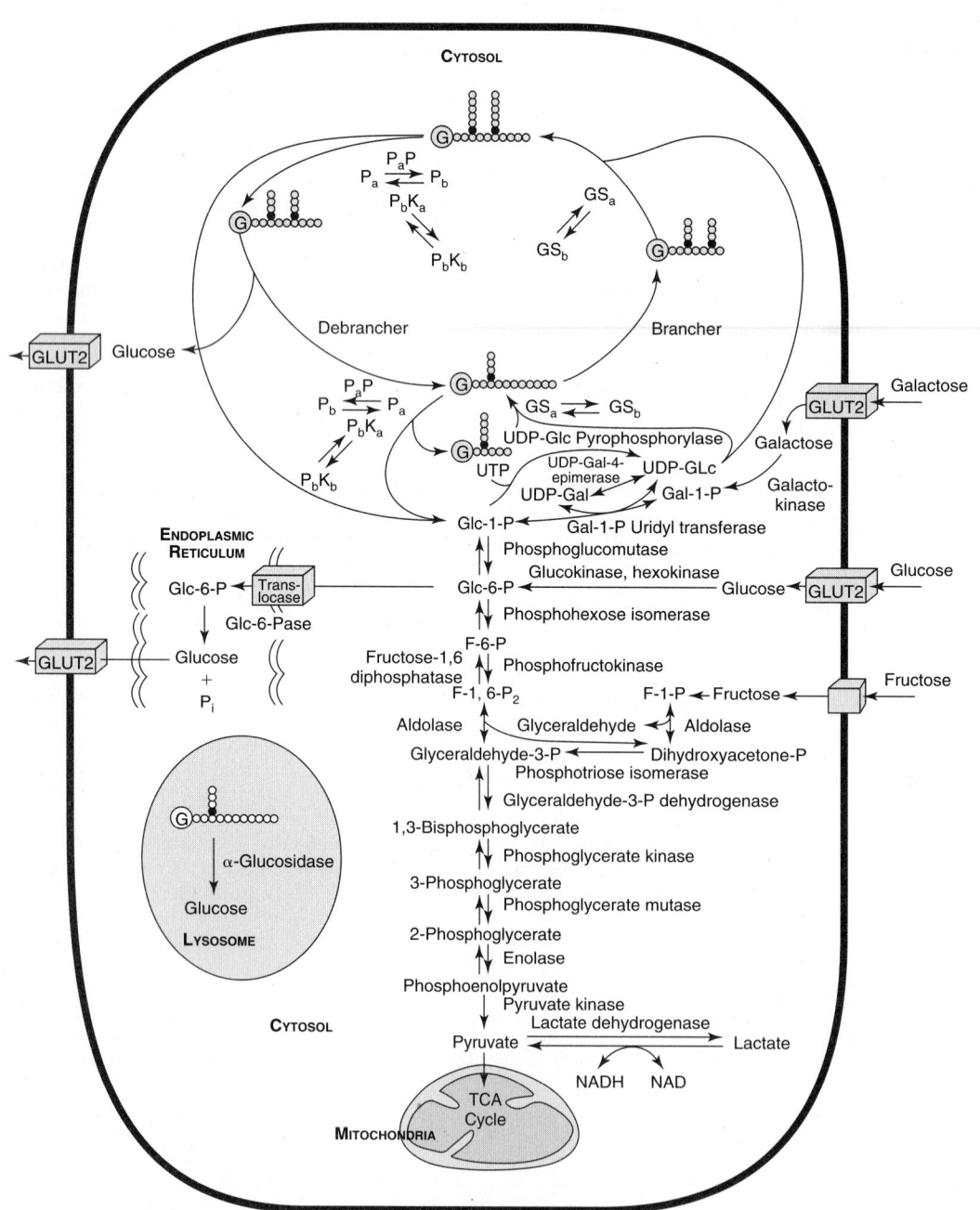

FIGURE 76–1. Pathway related to glycogen storage diseases and galactose and fructose disorders. Nonstandard abbreviations are as follows: GS_a, active glycogen synthetase; GS_b, inactive glycogen synthetase; P_a, active phosphorylase; P_b, inactive phosphorylase; P_aP, phosphorylase a phosphatase; P_bK_a, active phosphorylase b kinase; P_bK_b, inactive phosphorylase b kinase; G, glycogenin, the primer protein for glycogen synthesis. (Modified from AR Beaudet: Glycogen storage disease. In Isselbacher KJ, et al [editors]: *Harrison's Principles of Internal Medicine*, 13th ed. New York, McGraw-Hill, 1994. Reproduced with permission of The McGraw-Hill Companies.)

component for certain glycolipids, glycoproteins, and glycosamino-glycans. The two dietary sources of fructose are sucrose (fructose + glucose) and fructose itself, which is found in fruits, vegetables, and honey.

Defects in glycogen metabolism typically cause an accumulation of glycogen in the tissues, hence the name *glycogen storage disease* (Table 76–1). Defects in gluconeogenesis or the glycolytic pathway, including galactose and fructose metabolism, do not result in an accumulation of glycogen (see Table 76–1). The defects in pyruvate metabolism in the pathway of the conversion of pyruvate to carbon dioxide and water via mitochondrial oxidative phosphorylation are more often associated with lactic acidosis and some tissue glycogen accumulation.

Clinical manifestations of disorders of carbohydrate metabolism differ markedly. The symptoms range from harmless to lethal. Dietary therapy has been effective in many of the carbohydrate disorders. All genes responsible for the inherited defects of carbohydrate metabolism are cloned and mutations identified.

76.1 Glycogen Storage Diseases

Yuan-Tsong Chen

Glycogen storage diseases are inherited disorders affecting glycogen metabolism. Virtually all enzymes involved in the synthesis or degradation of glycogen cause some type of glycogen storage disease (see Fig. 76–1). The glycogen found in these disorders is abnormal in quantity or quality or both. Glycogen storage diseases are categorized by numeric type in accordance with the chronologic order in which these enzymatic defects were identified. This numeric classification is still widely used, at least up to number VII. The glycogen storage diseases can also be classified by organ involvement and clinical manifestations into liver and muscle glycogenoses (see Table 76–1).

There are more than 12 forms of glycogenoses. Glucose-6-phosphatase deficiency (type I), lysosomal acid α-glucosidase deficiency (type II), debrancher deficiency (type III), and liver phosphorylase kinase deficiency (type IX) are the most common that present in early childhood; myophosphorylase deficiency (type V, McArdle disease) is the most common in adults. The frequency of all forms of glycogen storage disease is approximately 1/20,000 live births.

LIVER GLYCOGENOSES

The glycogen storage diseases that principally affect the liver include glucose-6-phosphatase deficiency (type I), debranching enzyme deficiency (type III), branching enzyme deficiency (type IV), liver phosphorylase deficiency (type VI), phosphorylase kinase deficiency (type IX, formerly type VIa), glycogen synthetase deficiency, and glucose transporter-2 defect. Because hepatic carbohydrate metabolism is responsible for plasma glucose homeostasis, this group of disorders typically causes fasting hypoglycemia and hepatomegaly. Some (type III, type IV) are also associated with cirrhosis. Other organs may also be involved and may manifest as renal dysfunction in type I and myopathy in types III and IV as well as in some rare forms of phosphorylase kinase deficiency.

Type I Glycogen Storage Disease (Glucose-6-Phosphatase or Translocase Deficiency, Von Gierke Disease)

Type I glycogen storage disease is caused by the absence or deficiency of glucose-6-phosphatase activity in the liver, kidney, and intestinal mucosa. It can be divided into two subtypes: type Ia, in which the glucose 6-phosphatase enzyme is defective, and type Ib, in which a translocase that transports glucose-6-phosphate across the microsomal membrane is defective. The

defects in both type Ia and type Ib lead to inadequate hepatic conversion of glucose-6-phosphate to glucose and make affected individuals susceptible to fasting hypoglycemia.

Type I glycogen storage disease is an autosomal recessive disorder. The structure gene for glucose-6-phosphatase is on chromosome 17q21 and the gene for translocase is on chromosome 11q23. Common mutations responsible for the disease are known. Carrier detection and prenatal diagnosis are possible with the DNA-based diagnosis.

Clinical Manifestations. Patients with type I glycogen storage disease may present in the neonatal period with hypoglycemia and lactic acidosis; however, they more commonly present at 3–4 mo of age with hepatomegaly or hypoglycemic seizures, or both. These children often have doll-like faces with fat cheeks, relatively thin extremities, short stature, and a protuberant abdomen that is due to massive hepatomegaly; the kidneys are also enlarged, whereas the spleen and heart are normal.

The hallmarks of the disease are hypoglycemia, lactic acidosis, hyperuricemia, and hyperlipidemia. Hypoglycemia and lactic acidosis can develop after a short fast. Hyperuricemia is present in young children; gout rarely develops before puberty. Despite marked hepatomegaly, the liver transaminase levels are usually normal or only slightly elevated. Intermittent diarrhea may occur (the mechanism is unknown). Easy bruising and epistaxis are common and are associated with a prolonged bleeding time as a result of impaired platelet aggregation and adhesion.

The plasma may be "milky" in appearance as a result of a striking elevation of triglyceride levels. Cholesterol and phospholipids are also elevated, but less prominently. The lipid abnormality resembles type IV hyperlipidemia and is characterized by increased levels of very low density lipoprotein, low-density lipoprotein, and a unique apolipoprotein profile consisting of increased levels of apo B, C, and E, with relatively normal or reduced levels of apo A and D. The histologic appearance of the liver is characterized by a universal distention of hepatocytes by glycogen and fat. The lipid vacuoles are particularly large and prominent. There is little associated fibrosis.

All these findings apply to both type Ia and type Ib glycogen storage disease, but type Ib has additional features of recurrent bacterial infections from neutropenia and impaired neutrophil function. Oral and intestinal mucosal ulceration and inflammatory bowel disease are common. Exceptional cases of type Ib without neutropenia and type Ia with neutropenia have been reported.

Although type I glycogen storage disease affects mainly the liver, multiple organ systems are involved. Puberty is often delayed. Virtually all females have ultrasound findings consistent with polycystic ovaries; the other features of polycystic ovary syndrome such as acne and hirsutism are not seen. It remains to be seen whether this ovarian finding actually affects ovulation and fertility. Symptoms of gout usually start around puberty from long-term hyperuricemia. Secondary to the lipid abnormalities, there is an increased risk of pancreatitis. The dyslipidemia together with elevated erythrocyte aggregation predisposes these patients for atherosclerosis. Premature atherosclerosis, however, has not yet been clearly documented except for rare cases. Impaired platelet aggregation and of lipoproteins to oxidation may function as a protective mechanism to help reduce the risk of atherosclerosis. Frequent fractures and radiographic evidence of osteopenia are not uncommon in adult patients, and radial bone mineral content is significantly reduced in the prepubertal patients.

By the 2nd or 3rd decade of life, most patients with type I glycogen storage disease exhibit hepatic adenomas that can hemorrhage and in some cases may become malignant. Other complications include pulmonary hypertension and renal disease.

TABLE 76–1. Features of the Disorders of Carbohydrate Metabolism

Disorders	Basic Defects	Clinical Presentation	Comments
Liver Glycogenoses			
Type/Common Name			
Ia/Von Gierke	Glucose-6-phosphatase	Growth retardation, hepatomegaly, hypoglycemia; elevated blood lactate, cholesterol, triglyceride, and uric acid levels	Common, severe hypoglycemia
Ib	Glucose-6-phosphate translocase	Same as type Ia, with additional findings of neutropenia and impaired neutrophil function	10% of type Ia
II/Pompe Infantile	Acid maltase (acid α-glucosidase)	Cardiomegaly, hypotonia, hepatomegaly; onset: birth–6 mo	Common, cardiorespiratory failure leading to death by age 2 yr
Juvenile	Acid maltase (acid α-glucosidase)	Myopathy, variable cardiomyopathy; onset: childhood	Residual enzyme activity
Adult	Acid maltase (acid α-glucosidase)	Myopathy, respiratory insufficiency; onset: adulthood	Residual enzyme activity
IIIa/Cori or Forbes	Liver and muscle debrancher deficiency (amylo, 1,6 glucosidase)	Childhood: hepatomegaly, growth retardation, muscle weakness, hypoglycemia, hyperlipidemia, elevated transaminase levels; liver symptoms improve with age	Common, intermediate severity of hypoglycemia
IIIb	Liver debrancher deficiency; normal muscle enzyme activity	Liver symptoms same as in type IIIa; no muscle symptoms	15% of type III
IV/Andersen	Branching enzyme	Failure to thrive, hypotonia, hepatomegaly, splenomegaly, progressive cirrhosis (death usually before 5th yr), elevated transaminase levels	Rare neuromuscular variants exist
VI/Hers	Liver phosphorylase	Hepatomegaly, mild hypoglycemia, hyperlipidemia, and ketosis	Rare, benign glycogenosis
Phosphorylase kinase deficiency	Phosphorylase kinase	Hepatomegaly, mild hypoglycemia, hyperlipidemia, and ketosis	Common, benign glycogenosis
Glycogen synthetase deficiency	Glycogen synthetase	Early morning drowsiness and fatigue, fasting hypoglycemia, and ketosis	Decreased liver glycogen store
Fanconi-Bickel syndrome	Glucose transporter-2 (GLUT-2)	Failure to thrive, rickets, hepatorenomegaly, proximal renal tubular dysfunction, impaired glucose and galactose utilization	GLUT-2 expressed in liver, kidney, pancreas, and intestine
Muscle Glycogenoses			
Type/Common Name			
V/McArdle	Myophosphorylase	Exercise intolerance, muscle cramps, increased fatigability	Common, male predominance
VII/Tarui	Phosphofructokinase	Exercise intolerance, muscle cramps, hemolytic anemia, myoglobinuria	Prevalent in Japanese and Ashkenazi Jews
Phosphoglycerate kinase deficiency	Phosphoglycerate kinase	As with type V	Rare, X-linked
Phosphoglycerate mutase deficiency	M subunit of phosphoglycerate mutase	As with type V	Rare, majority of patients are African-American
Lactate dehydrogenase deficiency	M subunit of lactate dehydrogenase	As with type V	Rare
Galactose Disorders:			
Galactosemia with transferase deficiency	Galactose-1-phosphate uridyltransferase	Vomiting, hepatomegaly, cataracts, aminoaciduria, failure to thrive	African-American patients tend to have milder symptoms
Galactokinase deficiency	Galactokinase	Cataracts	Benign
Generalized uridine diphosphate galactose-4-epimerase deficiency	Uridine diphosphate galactose 4-epimerase	Similar to transferase deficiency with additional findings of hypotonia and nerve deafness	A benign variant exists
Fructose Disorders:			
Essential fructosuria	Fructokinase	Urine reducing substance	Benign
Hereditary fructose intolerance	Fructose-1-phosphate aldolase	Acute: vomiting, sweating, lethargy Chronic: failure to thrive, hepatic failure	Prognosis good with fructose restriction
Disorders of Gluconeogenesis:			
Fructose-1,6-diphosphatase deficiency	Fructose-1,6-disphosphatase	Episodic hypoglycemia, apnea, acidosis	Good prognosis, avoid fasting
Phosphoenolpyruvate carboxykinase deficiency	Phosphoenolpyruvate carboxykinase	Hypoglycemia, hepatomegaly, hypotonia, failure to thrive	Rare
Disorders of Pyruvate Metabolism:			
Pyruvate dehydrogenase complex defect	Pyruvate dehydrogenase	Severe fatal neonatal to mild late onset, lactic acidosis, psychomotor retardation, and failure to thrive	Most commonly due to E1 α-subunit defect X-linked
Pyruvate carboxylase deficiency	Pyruvate carboxylase	Same as above	Rare, autosomal recessive
Respiratory chain defects (oxidative phosphorylation disease)	Complex I to V, many mitochondrial DNA mutations	Heterogeneous with multisystem involvement	Mitochondrial inheritance
Other Carbohydrate Disorders:			
Pentosuria	L-Xylulose reductase	Urine reducing substance	Benign

Renal disease is a late complication, and most patients with type I glycogen storage disease older than age 20 yr have proteinuria. Many also have hypertension, renal stones, nephrocalcinosis, and altered creatinine clearance. Glomerular hyperfiltration, increased renal plasma flow, and microalbuminuria are often found in the early stages of renal dysfunction and can occur before the onset of proteinuria. In younger patients, hyperfiltration and hyperperfusion may be the only signs of renal abnormalities. With the advancement of renal disease, focal segmental glomerulosclerosis and interstitial fibrosis become evident. In some patients, renal function has deteriorated and progressed to failure, requiring dialysis and transplantation. Other renal abnormalities include amyloidosis, a Fanconi-like syndrome, hypocitraturia, hypercalciuria, and a distal renal tubular acidification defect.

Diagnosis. The diagnosis of type I glycogen storage disease can be suspected on the basis of clinical presentation and abnormal lactate and lipid values. Administration of glucagon or epinephrine results in little or no rise in blood glucose level, but the lactate level rises significantly. A definitive diagnosis requires a liver biopsy to demonstrate a deficiency of either glucose-6-phosphatase activity or translocase. Identification of the mutations for glucose-6-phosphatase or the translocase gene allows a noninvasive diagnostic method for a majority of patients with type I glycogen storage disease.

Treatment. This is designed to maintain normal blood glucose levels and is achieved by continuous nasogastric infusion of glucose or oral administration of uncooked cornstarch. Nasogastric drip feeding can be introduced in early infancy from the time of diagnosis. It may consist of an elemental enteral formula, or it may contain only glucose or glucose polymer to provide sufficient glucose to maintain normoglycemia during the night. Frequent feedings with high carbohydrate content are given during the day.

Uncooked cornstarch acts as a slow-release form of glucose and can be introduced at a dose of 1.6 g/kg every 4 hr for infants younger than 2 yr of age. The response of young infants is variable. As the child grows older, the cornstarch regimen can be changed to every 6 hr at a dose of 1.75 to 2.5 g/kg of body weight. Because fructose and galactose cannot be converted directly to glucose, their dietary intake should be restricted, and dietary supplements of multivitamins and calcium are required. Dietary therapy improves hyperuricemia, hyperlipidemia, and renal function, slowing the development of renal failure. However, this therapy fails to completely normalize blood uric acid and lipids levels, especially after puberty. The control of hyperuricemia can be further augmented by the use of allopurinol, a xanthine oxidase inhibitor. The hyperlipidemia can be reduced with lipid-lowering drugs such as HMG-CoA reductase inhibitors and fibrate (see Chapter 75.3). Microalbuminuria is an early indicator of renal dysfunction in type I disease and can be treated with angiotensin-converting enzyme (ACE) inhibitors, such as captopril. Citrate supplement may be beneficial in preventing or ameliorating nephrocalcinosis and development of urinary calculi.

In patients with type Ib glycogen storage disease, granulocyte and granulocyte-macrophage colony-stimulating factors are successful in correcting the neutropenia, decreasing the number and severity of bacterial infections, and improving the chronic inflammatory bowel disease.

Orthotopic liver transplantation (OLT) is advocated as a potential cure of type I glycogen storage disease by some groups, but the inherent short- and long-term complications leave this as a treatment of last resort, usually for patients with liver malignancy. A large adenoma may be treated with percutaneous ethanol injection. Before any surgical procedure, the bleeding status should be evaluated, and good metabolic control should be established. Prolonged bleeding times can be normalized by the use of intensive intravenous glucose infusion for 24–48 hr before surgery. Use of 1-deamino-8-D-arginine vasopressin can reduce bleeding complications. Lactated Ringer solution should be avoided because it contains lactate and no glucose. Glucose levels should be maintained in the normal range throughout surgery with the use of 10% dextrose.

Prognosis. Previously, patients with type I glycogen storage disease died, and the prognosis was guarded for those who survived. The long-term complications occur mostly in adults whose disease was not adequately treated during childhood. Early diagnosis and effective treatment have now greatly improved the outcome; however, renal disease and formation of hepatic adenomas remain serious complications.

Type III Glycogen Storage Disease (Debrancher Deficiency, Limit Dextrinosis)

Type III glycogen storage disease is caused by a deficiency of glycogen debranching enzyme activity. Debranching enzymes together with phosphorylase are responsible for complete degradation of glycogen; when debranching enzyme is defective, glycogen breakdown is incomplete and an abnormal glycogen with short outer branch chains and resembling limit dextrin accumulates.

Type III glycogenosis is an autosomal recessive disease that has been reported in many different ethnic groups; the frequency is relatively high in non-Ashkenazic Jews of North African extraction. The gene for debranching enzyme is located on chromosome 1p21. More than 30 different mutations are identified; two exon 3 mutations (17delAG and Q6X) are specifically associated with glycogenosis IIIb, a subtype of glycogenosis III without muscle involvement. Carrier detection and prenatal diagnosis are possible using DNA-based linkage or mutation analysis.

Deficiency of glycogen debranching enzyme causes hepatomegaly, hypoglycemia, short stature, variable skeletal myopathy, and cardiomyopathy. The disorder usually involves both liver and muscle and is termed *type IIIa glycogen storage disease*. However, in about 15% of patients, the disease appears to involve only liver and is classified as type IIIb (Fig. 76–2).

Clinical Manifestations. During infancy and childhood, the disease may be indistinguishable from type I glycogen storage disease, because hepatomegaly, hypoglycemia, hyperlipidemia, and growth retardation are common. Splenomegaly may be present, but the kidney is not enlarged. Remarkably, hepatomegaly and hepatic symptoms in most patients with type III glycogen storage disease improve with age and usually resolve after puberty. Progressive liver cirrhosis and failure may occur and is common in Japanese patients. Hepatic adenomas have been reported; their prevalence may be as high as 25% in French patients. Malignant transformation of adenomas has not been observed, although two patients developed a hepatocellular carcinoma associated with end-stage liver cirrhosis. In patients with muscular involvement (type IIIa), muscle weakness is usually minimal during childhood but can become severe after the 3rd or 4th decade of life, as evidenced by slowly progressive weakness and wasting. Electromyography changes are consistent with a widespread myopathy, and nerve conduction studies may be abnormal. Ventricular hypertrophy is a frequent finding, but overt cardiac dysfunction is rare. Hepatic symptoms in some patients may be so mild that the diagnosis is not made until adulthood, when the patients show symptoms and signs of neuromuscular disease. The initial diagnosis has been confused with Charcot-Marie-Tooth disease. Polycystic ovary appears to be common; the fertility, however, is not reduced.

Hypoglycemia and hyperlipidemia are common. In contrast to type I glycogen storage disease, elevation of liver transaminase levels and fasting ketosis are prominent, but blood lactate

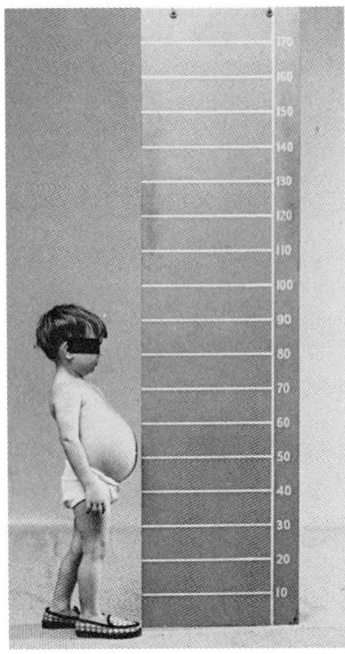
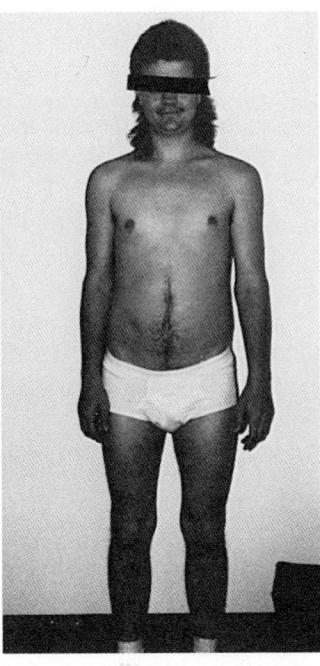

FIGURE 76–2. Growth and development in a patient with type IIIb glycogen storage disease. The patient has debrancher deficiency in liver but normal activity in muscle. As a child he had hepatomegaly, hypoglycemia, and growth retardation. After puberty, he no longer had hepatomegaly or hypoglycemia, and his final adult height is normal. He has no muscle weakness or atrophy; this is in contrast to type IIIa patients, in whom a progressive myopathy is seen in adulthood.

and uric acid concentrations are usually normal. The administration of glucagon 2 hr after a carbohydrate meal provokes a normal increase in blood glucose, but after an overnight fast, glucagon may provoke no change in blood glucose level. Serum creatine kinase levels may be useful to identify patients with muscle involvement; normal levels do not rule out muscle enzyme deficiency.

Diagnosis. The histologic appearance of the liver is characterized by a universal distention of hepatocytes by glycogen and the presence of fibrous septa. The fibrosis and the paucity of fat distinguish type III glycogenosis from type I. The fibrosis, which ranges from minimal periportal fibrosis to micronodular cirrhosis, in most cases appears to be nonprogressive.

Patients with myopathy and liver symptoms have a generalized enzyme defect (type IIIa). The deficient enzyme activity can be demonstrated not only in liver and muscle but also in other tissues such as heart, erythrocytes, and cultured fibroblasts. Patients with hepatic symptoms without clinical or laboratory evidence of myopathy have debranching enzyme deficiency only in the liver, with enzyme activity retained in the muscle (type IIIb). Definite diagnosis requires enzyme assay in liver or muscle, or both. Mutation analysis can provide a noninvasive method for diagnosis and subtype assignment in the majority of patients.

Treatment. Dietary management is less demanding than in type I glycogen storage disease. If hypoglycemia is present, frequent meals high in carbohydrates with cornstarch supplements or nocturnal gastric drip feedings are usually effective. A high-protein diet during the daytime plus overnight protein enteral infusion may also be effective in preventing hypoglycemia, because protein can be used as substrate for gluconeogenesis, a pathway that is intact in type III glycogen storage disease. There is no satisfactory treatment for the progressive myopathy. Patients do not need to restrict dietary intake of fructose and

galactose. Liver transplantation has been performed in patients with end-stage cirrhosis and/or hepatic carcinoma.

Type IV Glycogen Storage Disease (Branching Enzyme Deficiency, Amylopectinosis, or Andersen Disease)

Deficiency of branching enzyme activity results in accumulation of an abnormal glycogen with poor solubility. The disease is referred to as type IV glycogen storage disease or amylopectinosis because the abnormal glycogen has fewer branch points, more α1-4 linked glucose units, and longer outer chains, resulting in a structure resembling amylopectin.

Type IV glycogen storage disease is an autosomal recessive disorder. The glycogen branching enzyme gene is located on chromosome 3p21. Mutations responsible for type IV glycogen storage disease have been identified, and their characterization in individual patients may be useful in predicting the clinical outcome.

Clinical Manifestations. This disorder is clinically variable. The most common and classic form is characterized by progressive cirrhosis of the liver and is manifested in the first 18 mo of life as hepatosplenomegaly and failure to thrive. The cirrhosis progresses to portal hypertension, ascites, esophageal varices, and liver failure that leads to death by 5 yr of age. Rare patients survive without progression of liver disease.

A neuromuscular form of the disease has been reported. These patients may (1) present at birth with severe hypotonia, muscle atrophy, and neuronal involvement with death in the neonatal period; (2) present in late childhood with myopathy or cardiomyopathy; or (3) present as adults with diffuse central and peripheral nervous system dysfunction accompanied by accumulation of polyglucosan body disease in the nervous system (so-called *adult polyglucosan body disease*). For adult polyglucosan disease, leukocyte or nerve biopsy is needed to establish the diagnosis, because the branching enzyme deficiency is limited to those tissues.

Diagnosis. Tissue disposition of amylopectin-like materials can be demonstrated in liver, heart, muscle, skin, intestine, brain, spinal cord, and peripheral nerve. The hepatic histologic findings are characterized by micronodular cirrhosis and faintly stained basophilic inclusions in the hepatocytes. The inclusions consist of coarsely clumped, stored material that is periodic acid–Schiff positive and partially resistant to diastase digestion. Electron microscopy shows, in addition to the conventional α and β glycogen particles, accumulation of the fibrillar aggregations that are typical of amylopectin. The distinct staining properties of the cytoplasmic inclusions, as well as electron microscopic findings, could be diagnostic. However, polysaccharidoses with histologic features reminiscent of type IV disease, but without enzymatic correlation, have been observed. The definitive diagnosis rests on the demonstration of the deficient branching enzyme activity in liver, muscle, cultured skin fibroblasts, or leukocytes. Prenatal diagnosis is possible by measuring the enzyme activity in cultured amniocytes or chorionic villi.

Treatment. There is no specific treatment for type IV glycogen storage disease. For progressive hepatic failure, liver transplantation has been performed, but because it is a multisystem disorder involving many organ systems, the long-term success of liver transplantation is unknown.

Type VI Glycogen Storage Disease (Liver Phosphorylase Deficiency, HERS Disease)

There are few patients with documented liver phosphorylase deficiency. Such patients have a benign course and present with hepatomegaly and growth retardation in early childhood. Hypoglycemia, hyperlipidemia, and hyperketosis are usually mild if present. Lactic acid and uric acid levels are normal. The heart and skeletal muscles are not involved. The hepatomegaly and growth retardation improve with age and usually disappear around puberty. Treatment is symptomatic. A high-carbohydrate diet and frequent feeding are effective in preventing hypoglycemia; most patients require no specific treatment. The liver phosphorylase gene is located on chromosome 14q21-22; mutations responsible for the disease are known.

Type IX Glycogen Storage Disease (Phosphorylase Kinase Deficiency)

This disorder represents a heterogeneous group of glycogenoses. Phosphorylase, the rate-limiting enzyme of glycogenolysis, is activated by a cascade of enzymatic reactions involving adenylate cyclase, cyclic adenosine monophosphate–dependent protein kinase (protein kinase A), and phosphorylase kinase. The latter enzyme has four subunits, each encoded by different genes on different chromosomes and differentially expressed in various tissues. This cascade of reactions is stimulated primarily by glucagon. This glycogenosis could be the result of any enzyme deficiency along this pathway; the most common is the deficiency of phosphorylase kinase.

The numeric classification of phosphorylase kinase deficiency is confusing, ranging from type VIa to VIII to IX. It is advisable to refrain from such a designation and to classify the various disorders according to organ involvement and mode of inheritance.

X-Linked Liver Phosphorylase Kinase Deficiency. This is a common form of liver glycogenoses. Enzyme activity may also be deficient in erythrocytes and leukocytes; it is normal in muscle. Typically a 1–5 yr old presents with growth retardation and an incidental finding of hepatomegaly. Cholesterol, triglycerides, and liver enzymes are mildly elevated. Ketosis may occur after fasting. Lactate and uric acid levels are normal. Hypoglycemia is mild, if present. The response in blood glucose to glucagon is normal. Hepatomegaly and abnormal blood chemistries gradually become normal with age. Most adults achieve a normal final height and are usually asymptomatic despite a persistent phosphorylase kinase deficiency. Liver histologic appearance shows glycogen-distended hepatocytes. The accumulated glycogen (α particles, rosette form) has a frayed or burst appearance and is less compact than the glycogen seen in type I or type III glycogen storage disease. Fibrous septal formation and low-grade inflammatory changes may be present.

The structural gene for the liver isoform of the phosphorylase kinase α subunit is located on chromosome Xp22; mutations of this gene are known.

Autosomal Liver and Muscle Phosphorylase Kinase Deficiency

Several patients have been reported with phosphorylase kinase deficiency in liver and blood cells and an autosomal model of inheritance. As with the X-linked form, hepatomegaly and growth retardation apparent in early childhood are the predominant symptoms. Some also exhibited muscle hypotonia. When measured in a few cases, reduced activity of the enzyme has been demonstrated in muscle. Mutations causing autosomally transmitted liver and muscle phosphorylase kinase deficiency are found in the autosomal gene of the subunit β.

Autosomal Liver Phosphorylase Kinase Deficiency

This form of phosphorylase kinase deficiency is due to mutations in the testis/liver isoform of the γ subunit of the gene (*PHKG2*, γ subunit). In contrast to the benign course of X-linked phosphorylase kinase deficiency, patients with mutations in the *PHKG2* gene have more severe phenotypes and often develop liver cirrhosis

Muscle-Specific Phosphorylase Kinase Deficiency

A few cases of phosphorylase kinase deficiency restricted to muscle are known. Patients, both male and female, present either with muscle cramps and myoglobinuria with exercise or with progressive muscle weakness and atrophy. Phosphorylase kinase activity is decreased in muscle but normal in liver and blood cells. There is no hepatomegaly or cardiomegaly. Mutation in the structure gene of muscle isoform of the α subunit is located on chromosome Xq12; mutation of this gene has been found in male patients with this disorder.

Phosphorylase Kinase Deficiency Limited to Heart

These patients present with cardiomyopathy in infancy and rapidly progress to heart failure and death. Phosphorylase kinase deficiency is demonstrated in heart with normal enzyme activity in skeletal muscle and liver.

Diagnosis. Definitive diagnosis of phosphorylase kinase deficiency requires demonstration of the enzymatic defect in affected tissues. Phosphorylase kinase can be measured in leukocytes and erythrocytes, but because the enzyme has many isozymes, the diagnosis can be missed without studies of liver, muscle, or heart.

Treatment. The treatment for liver phosphorylase kinase deficiency includes high-carbohydrate diet and frequent feedings to prevent hypoglycemia; most patients require no specific treatment. Prognosis is good. There is currently no treatment for the fatal form of isolated cardiac phosphorylase kinase deficiency other than heart transplantation.

Glycogen Synthetase Deficiency

Deficiency of hepatic glycogen synthetase leads to a marked decrease of glycogen stored in the liver. The patients present in infancy with early-morning (before eating breakfast) drowsiness, pallor, emesis, and fatigue and sometimes convulsions associated with hypoglycemia and hyperketonemia. Blood lactate and alanine levels are low, and there is no hyperlipidemia or hepatomegaly. Prolonged hyperglycemia and elevation of lactate with normal insulin levels after administration of glucose suggest a possible diagnosis of deficiency of glycogen synthetase. Definitive *diagnosis* requires a liver biopsy to measure the enzyme activity. *Treatment* consists of frequent meals, rich in protein, and nighttime supplementation with uncooked cornstarch. The disease is due to the mutations in the liver glycogen synthetase gene, located on chromosome 12p12.2.

Hepatic Glycogenosis with Renal Fanconi Syndrome (Fanconi-Bickel Syndrome)

This rare autosomal recessive disorder is caused by defects in the facilitative glucose transporter 2 (GLUT-2), which transports glucose in and out of hepatocytes, pancreatic beta cells, and the basolateral membranes of intestinal and renal epithelial cells. The disease is characterized by proximal renal tubular dysfunction, impaired glucose and galactose utilization, and accumulation of glycogen in liver and kidney.

The affected child presents *clinical manifestations* in the 1st yr of life with failure to thrive, rickets, and a protuberant abdomen from hepatomegaly and renomegaly. Laboratory findings include glucosuria, phosphaturia, generalized aminoaciduria, bicarbonate wasting, hypophosphatemia, increased serum alkaline phosphatase levels, and a radiologic finding of rickets. Mild fasting hypoglycemia and hyperlipidemia may be present. Liver transaminase, plasma lactate, and uric acid levels are usually normal. Oral galactose or glucose tolerance tests show intolerance, which could be explained by the functional loss of GLUT-2 preventing liver uptake of these sugars.

Tissue biopsy results show marked accumulation of glycogen in hepatocytes and proximal renal tubular cells, presumably owing to the altered glucose transport out of these organs.

There is no specific *treatment*. Growth retardation persists through adulthood. Symptomatic replacement of water, electrolytes, and vitamin D; restriction of galactose intake; and a diet similar to that used for diabetes mellitus presented in frequent and small meals with an adequate caloric intake may improve growth.

MUSCLE GLYCOGENOSES

The role of glycogen in muscle is to provide substrates for the generation of ATP for muscle contraction. The muscle glycogen storage diseases are divided into two groups. The first is characterized by progressive skeletal muscle weakness and atrophy or cardiomyopathy, or both, and is represented by a lysosomal glycogen degrading enzyme deficiency of acid α-glucosidase (type II glycogen storage disease). The second is a muscle energy disorder characterized by muscle pain, exercise intolerance, myoglobinuria, and susceptibility to fatigue. This group includes myophosphorylase deficiency (McArdle disease, type V) and deficiencies of phosphofructokinase (type VII), phosphoglycerate kinase, phosphoglycerate mutase, or lactate dehydrogenase. Some of these latter enzyme deficiencies may also be associated with a compensated hemolysis, suggesting a more generalized defect in glucose metabolism.

Type II (Lysosomal Acid α1,4-Glucosidase Deficiency, Pompe Disease)

Type II glycogen storage disease is caused by a deficient activity of lysosomal acid α1,4 glucosidase (acid maltase), an enzyme responsible for the degradation of glycogen in lysosome. The disease is characterized by accumulation of glycogen in lysosomes as opposed to its accumulation in cytoplasm in the other glycogenoses.

Pompe disease is an autosomal recessive disorder with an incidence of 1/40,000 live births with no ethnic predilection. The gene for acid α-glucosidase is on chromosome 17q25.2. A splice site mutation (IVS1-13T→G), commonly seen in adult-onset patients, may be helpful in delineating the phenotypes.

Clinical Manifestations. The disorder encompasses a range of phenotypes, each including myopathy but differing in age at onset, organ involvement, and clinical severity. The most severe is the *infantile-onset disease*, with prominent cardiomegaly, hypotonia, and death before 2 yr of age. Infants appear normal at birth but soon experience generalized muscle weakness with "floppy infant appearance," feeding difficulties, macroglossia, hepatomegaly, and heart failure from a progressively hypertrophic cardiomyopathy. Electrocardiographic findings include a high-voltage QRS complex and a shortened PR interval. Death usually results from cardiorespiratory failure or aspiration pneumonia.

The *juvenile form* presents as delayed motor milestones (if age at onset is early enough) or difficult walking in childhood and is followed by swallowing difficulties, proximal muscle weakness, and respiratory muscle involvement. Death from respiratory failure may occur before the end of the 2nd decade. Cardiomegaly is variable, but overt cardiac failure is not seen.

An *adult form* of type II disease presents as a slowly progressive myopathy without cardiac involvement and has its onset between the 2nd and 7th decades. The clinical picture is dominated by slowly progressive proximal muscle weakness with truncal involvement and greater involvement of the lower limbs than the upper limbs. The pelvic girdle, paraspinal muscle, and diaphragm are the muscle groups most seriously affected. The

initial symptoms in some patients may be respiratory insufficiency manifested by somnolence, morning headache, orthopnea, and exertional dyspnea, which eventually lead to sleep-disordered breathing and respiratory failure.

Laboratory Findings. These include elevated levels of serum creatine kinase, aspartate aminotransferase, and lactate dehydrogenase. Muscle biopsy shows the presence of vacuoles that stain positively for glycogen; acid phosphatase is increased, presumably from a compensatory increase of lysosomal enzymes. Electron microscopy reveals the glycogen accumulation within the membranous sac and in the cytoplasm. Electromyography reveals myopathic features with excessive electrical irritability of muscle fibers and pseudomyotonic discharges. Serum creatine kinase is not always elevated in adult patients; depending on the muscle sampled or tested, the muscle histologic appearance on electromyography may not be abnormal. It is prudent to examine the affected muscle.

Diagnosis. This can be established by demonstration of the absence of or reduced levels of acid α-glucosidase activity in muscle, cultured skin fibroblast, or blood spots. Deficiency is usually more severe in the infantile form than in the juvenile and adult forms. Prenatal diagnosis using amniocytes or chorionic villi is available in the fatal infantile form. A lysosomal glycogen storage disease clinically similar to late-onset type II glycogenosis, but with normal acid α-glucosidase activity, is caused by defects in lysosomal associated membrane protein-2.

Treatment. Definitive therapy is not available; a high-protein diet may be useful for the juvenile and adult forms. Nocturnal ventilatory support in late-onset patients improves the quality of life and is beneficial during a period of respiratory decompensation. Preliminary clinical trials of enzyme replacement therapy have shown that recombinant acid α-glucosidase is capable of improving cardiac and skeletal muscle functions in these patients.

Type V (Muscle Phosphorylase Deficiency, McArdle Disease)

Lack of this enzyme limits muscle ATP generation by glycogenolysis, results in glycogen accumulation, and is the prototype of muscle energy disorder.

Clinical Manifestations. Symptoms usually first develop in late childhood or as an adult and are characterized by exercise intolerance with muscle cramps. Two types of activity tend to cause symptoms: (1) brief exercise of great intensity, such as sprinting or carrying heavy loads, and (2) less intense but sustained activity, such as climbing stairs or walking uphill. Moderate exercise, such as walking on level ground, can be performed by most patients for long periods. Many patients experience a characteristic "second wind" phenomenon. If they slow down or pause briefly at the first appearance of muscle pain, they can resume exercise with more ease.

About half report burgundy-colored urine after exercise, which is the consequence of myoglobinuria secondary to rhabdomyolysis. Intense myoglobinuria after vigorous exercise may cause acute renal failure. In rare cases, electromyographic findings may suggest an inflammatory myopathy and the diagnosis can be confused with polymyositis.

The level of serum creatine kinase is usually elevated at rest and increases more after exercise. Exercise also increases the levels of blood ammonia, inosine, hypoxanthine, and uric acid. The latter abnormalities are attributed to accelerated recycling of muscle purine nucleotides owing to insufficient ATP production.

Clinical heterogeneity is uncommon in type V glycogen storage disease, but late-onset disease with no symptoms as late as the 8th decade and an early-onset, fatal form with hypotonia, generalized muscle weakness, and progressive respiratory insufficiency have been described.

Diagnosis. An ischemic exercise test offers rapid diagnostic screening for metabolic myopathy. Lack of an increase in blood lactate levels and exaggerated blood ammonia elevations indicate muscle glycogenosis and suggest a defect in the conversion of muscle glycogen or glucose to lactate. The abnormal ischemic exercise response is not limited to type V glycogen storage disease. Other muscle defects in glycogenolysis or glycolysis produce similar results (deficiencies of muscle phosphofructokinase, phosphoglycerate kinase, phosphoglycerate mutase, or lactate dehydrogenase).

Phosphorus magnetic resonance imaging (^{31}P MRI) allows for the noninvasive evaluation of muscle metabolism. Patients with type V glycogen storage disease have no decrease in intracellular pH and have excessive reduction in phosphocreatine in response to exercise. The diagnosis should be confirmed by enzymatic evaluation of muscle.

Type V glycogen storage disease is an autosomal recessive disorder. The gene for muscle phosphorylase is located on chromosome 11q13-qter. A nonsense mutation changing arginine to a stop at codon 49 (R49X) and a deletion of a single codon (F708) are prevalent in white and Japanese patients, respectively. This allows DNA-based diagnosis and carrier detection for the two populations.

Treatment. Avoidance of strenuous exercise prevents the symptoms; however, regular and moderate exercise is recommended to improve exercise capacity. Exercise tolerance can also be augmented by oral administration of glucose or fructose or by injection of glucagon. A high-protein diet may increase muscle endurance. Creatine supplement improves muscle function in some patients. Longevity is not generally affected.

Type VII Glycogen Storage Disease (Muscle Phosphofructokinase Deficiency, Tarui Disease)

Type VII glycogen storage disease is caused by a deficiency of muscle phosphofructokinase, which catalyzes the ATP-dependent conversion of fructose-6-phosphate to fructose-1, 6-diphosphate and is a key regulatory enzyme of glycolysis. Phosphofructokinase is composed of three isoenzyme subunits (M [muscle], L [liver], and P [platelet]) that are encoded by different genes and differentially expressed in tissues. Skeletal muscle contains only the M subunit, and red blood cells contain a hybrid of L and M forms. Type VII disease is due to a defective M isoenzyme, which causes a complete enzyme defect in muscle and a partial defect in red blood cells.

Type VII glycogen storage disease is an autosomal recessive disorder and is prevalent among Japanese people and Ashkenazi Jews. The gene for muscle phosphofructokinase is located on chromosome 1cen-1q32. A splicing defect and a nucleotide deletion in the muscle phosphofructokinase gene account for 95% of mutant alleles in Ashkenazi Jews. The molecular diagnosis is possible in this population.

Clinical Manifestations. Five features of type VII are distinctive: (1) Exercise intolerance, usually evident in childhood, is more severe than in type V disease and may be associated with nausea and vomiting. Vigorous exercise causes severe muscle cramps and myoglobinuria. (2) A compensated hemolysis occurs as evidenced by an increased level of serum bilirubin and an elevated reticulocyte count. (3) Hyperuricemia is common and exaggerated by muscle exercise to a more severe degree than that observed in type V or III glycogen storage disease. (4) An abnormal glycogen resembling amylopectin is present in muscle fibers; it is periodic acid–Schiff positive but resistant to diastase digestion. (5) Exercise intolerance is particularly acute after meals that are rich in carbohydrates because glucose cannot be utilized in muscle and because glucose inhibits lipolysis and thus deprives muscle of fatty acid and ketone substrates. In contrast, patients with type V disease can metabolize bloodborne glucose

derived from either liver glycogenolysis or exogenous glucose. Indeed, glucose infusion improves exercise tolerance in type V patients.

Two rare type VII variants occur. One variant presents in infancy with hypotonia and limb weakness and proceeds to a rapidly progressive myopathy that leads to death by 4 yr of age. The other variant presents in adults and is characterized by a slowly progressive, fixed muscle weakness rather than cramps and myoglobinuria.

Diagnosis. To establish a diagnosis, a biochemical or histochemical demonstration of the enzymatic defect in the muscle is required. The absence of the M isoenzyme of phosphofructokinase can also be demonstrated in blood cells and fibroblasts.

Treatment. There is no specific treatment. Avoidance of strenuous exercise is advisable to prevent acute attacks of muscle cramps and myoglobinuria.

Other Muscle Glycogenoses with Muscle Energy Impairment

Six additional enzyme defects—phosphoglycerate kinase, phosphoglycerate mutase, lactate dehydrogenase, fructose-1,6-biphosphate aldolase A, muscle pyruvate kinase, and β-enolase in the pathway of the terminal glycolysis—cause symptoms and signs of muscle energy impairment similar to those of types V. and VII glycogen storage disease. The failure of blood lactate to increase in response to exercise is a useful diagnostic test and can be used to differentiate muscle glycogenoses from disorders of lipid metabolism, such as carnitine palmitoyl transferase II deficiency and very long chain acyl-CoA dehydrogenase deficiency, which also cause muscle cramps and myoglobinuria. Muscle glycogen levels may be normal in the disorders affecting terminal glycolysis; assaying the muscle enzyme activity makes a definite diagnosis. There is no specific treatment. Avoidance of strenuous exercise prevents acute attacks of muscle cramps and myoglobinuria.

76.2 Defects in Galactose Metabolism

Yuan-Tsong Chen

Milk and dairy products contain lactose, the major dietary source of galactose. The metabolism of galactose produces fuel for cellular metabolism through its conversion to glucose-1-phosphate (see Fig. 76–1). Galactose also plays an important role in the formation of galactosides, which include glycoproteins, glycolipids, and glycosaminoglycans. Galactosemia denotes the elevated level of galactose in the blood and is found in three distinct disorders of galactose metabolism defective in one of the following enzymes: galactose-1-phosphate uridyl transferase, galactokinase, and uridine diphosphate galactose-4-epimerase. The term *galactosemia*, although adequate for the deficiencies for any of these three disorders, generally designates the transferase deficiency.

GALACTOSE-1-PHOSPHATE URIDYL TRANSFERASE DEFICIENCY GALACTOSEMIA

"Classic" galactosemia is a serious disease with early onset of symptoms; the incidence is 1/60,000. The newborn infant normally receives up to 20% of caloric intake as lactose, which consists of equal parts of glucose and galactose. Without the transferase enzyme, the infant is unable to metabolize galactose-1-phosphate, the accumulation of which results in injury to kidney, liver, and brain. This injury may begin prenatally in the affected fetus by transplacental galactose derived from the diet of the heterozygous mother or by endogenous production of galactose in the fetus.

Clinical Manifestations. The diagnosis of uridyl transferase deficiency should be considered in newborn or young infants with any of the following features: jaundice, hepatomegaly, vomiting, hypoglycemia, convulsions, lethargy, irritability, feeding difficulties, poor weight gain, aminoaciduria, cataracts, vitreous hemorrhage, hepatic cirrhosis, ascites, splenomegaly, or mental retardation. Patients with galactosemia are at increased risk for *Escherichia coli* neonatal sepsis; the onset of sepsis often precedes the diagnosis of galactosemia. When the diagnosis is not made at birth, damage to the liver (cirrhosis) and brain (mental retardation) becomes increasingly severe and irreversible. Galactosemia should be considered for the newborn or young infant who is not thriving or who has any of the preceding findings.

Diagnosis. Because galactose is injurious to persons with galactosemia, diagnostic challenge tests dependent on administering galactose orally or intravenously should not be used. Galactose administration would result in high concentrations of intracellular galactose-1-phosphate, which can function as a competitive inhibitor of phosphoglucomutase. This inhibition transiently impairs the conversion of glycogen to glucose and produces hypoglycemia. Light and electron microscopy of hepatic tissue reveals fatty infiltration, the formation of pseudoacini, and eventual macronodular cirrhosis. These changes are consistent with a metabolic disease but do not indicate the precise enzymatic defect.

The preliminary diagnosis of galactosemia is made by demonstrating a reducing substance in several urine specimens collected while the patient is receiving human milk, cow's milk, or another formula containing lactose. The reducing substance found in urine by Clinitest can be identified by chromatography or by an enzymatic test specific for galactose. Clinistix or Tes-Tape urine test results are negative because the test materials rely on the action of glucose oxidase, which is specific for glucose and is nonreactive with galactose. Deficient activity of galactose-1-phosphate uridyl transferase is demonstrable in hemolysates of erythrocytes, which also exhibit increased concentrations of galactose-1-phosphate.

Genetics. Transferase deficiency galactosemia is an autosomal recessive trait. There are several enzymatic variants of galactosemia. The Duarte variant, a single amino acid substitution (N314D) has diminished red cell enzyme activity but usually no clinical significance. Some African-American patients have milder symptoms despite the absence of measurable transferase activity in erythrocytes; these patients retain 10% enzyme activity in liver and intestinal mucosa, whereas most white patients have no detectable activity in any of these tissues. In African-Americans, 62% of alleles are represented by the S135L mutation, a mutation that is responsible for the milder disease. In the white population, 70% of alleles are represented by the Q188R and K285N missense mutations and are associated with severe disease. Carrier testing and prenatal diagnosis can be performed by direct enzyme analysis of amniocytes or chorionic villi; testing can also be DNA based.

Treatment and Prognosis. Because of newborn screening for galactosemia, patients are being identified and treated early. Elimination of galactose from diet reverses growth failure and renal and hepatic dysfunction. Cataracts regress, and most patients have no impairment of eyesight. Early diagnosis and treatment have improved the prognosis of galactosemia; however, on long-term follow-up, patients still manifest ovarian failure with primary or secondary amenorrhea, developmental delay, and learning disabilities that increase in severity with age. Most manifest speech disorders, whereas a smaller number demonstrate poor growth and impaired motor function and balance (with or without overt ataxia). The relative control of galactose-1-phosphate levels does not always correlate with long-term outcome, leading to the belief that other factors, such as elevated galactitol, decreased uridine diphos-

phate galactose (UDP-galactose, a donor for galactolipids and proteins), and endogenous galactose production may be responsible.

GALACTOKINASE DEFICIENCY

The deficient enzyme is galactokinase, which normally catalyzes the phosphorylation of galactose. The principal metabolites accumulated are galactose and galactitol. Mutations leading to autosomally inherited galactokinase deficiency are known. The gene coding for galactokinase is located on chromosome 17q24. In contrast to the multiple organs that are affected in transferase deficiency galactosemia, cataracts are usually the sole manifestation of galactokinase deficiency with pseudotumor cerebri as a rare complication. Heterozygotic carriers may have late adult onset cataracts. The affected infant is otherwise asymptomatic. These patients have an increased concentration of blood galactose levels with normal transferase activity and an absence of galactokinase activity in erythrocytes. Treatment is dietary restriction of galactose.

URIDINE DIPHOSPHATE GALACTOSE 4-EPIMERASE DEFICIENCY

The abnormally accumulated metabolites are similar to those in transferase deficiency; however, there is also an increase in cellular UDP-galactose. There are two distinct forms of epimerase deficiency. A benign form has been discovered incidentally through a neonatal screening program. Affected persons are healthy and without problems; the enzyme deficiency is limited to leukocytes and erythrocytes. No treatment is required. The second form of epimerase deficiency is severe, and clinical manifestations resemble transferase deficiency with the additional symptoms of hypotonia and nerve deafness. The enzyme deficiency is generalized, and clinical symptoms respond to restriction of dietary galactose. Although this form of galactosemia is rare, it must be considered in a symptomatic patient who has normal transferase activity.

Patients with epimerase deficiency cannot make galactose. Because it is an essential component of many nervous system structural proteins, patients are placed on a galactose-restricted diet rather than a galactose-free diet.

The gene for UDP-galactose 4-epimerase is located on chromosome 1 at 1p36. Carrier detection is possible by measurement of epimerase activity in the erythrocytes. Prenatal diagnosis for the severe form of epimerase deficiency, using an enzyme assay of cultured amniotic fluid cells is possible.

76.3   Defects in Fructose Metabolism

Yuan-Tsong Chen

DEFICIENCY OF FRUCTOKINASE (BENIGN FRUCTOSURIA)

Deficiency of fructokinase is not associated with any clinical manifestations. It is an accidental finding usually made because the asymptomatic patient's urine contains a reducing substance. No treatment is necessary. Inheritance is autosomal recessive with an incidence of 1/120,000. The gene encoding fructokinase is located on chromosome 2p23.3.

Fructokinase catalyzes the first step of metabolism of dietary fructose: conversion of fructose to fructose 1-phosphate (see Fig. 76–1). Without this enzyme, ingested fructose is not metabolized. Its level is increased in the blood, and it is excreted in urine because there is practically no renal threshold for fructose. Both positive and negative Clinitest results reveal the urinary-reducing substance to be something other than glucose. It can be identified as fructose by chromatography.

DEFICIENCY OF FRUCTOSE-1,6-BISPHOSPHATE ALDOLASE (ALDOLASE B) (HEREDITARY FRUCTOSE INTOLERANCE)

Deficiency of fructose-1,6-bisphosphate aldolase is a severe condition of infants that appears with the ingestion of fructose-containing food and is caused by deficiency of fructose aldolase B activity in the liver, kidney, and intestine. The enzyme catalyzes the hydrolysis of fructose-1,6-bisphosphate into triose phosphate and glyceraldehyde phosphate. The same enzyme also hydrolyzes fructose 1-phosphate. Deficiency of this enzyme activity causes a rapid accumulation of fructose-1-phosphate and initiates severe toxic symptoms when exposed to fructose.

Epidemiology and Genetics. The true incidence of hereditary fructose intolerance is unknown but may be as high as 1/23,000. The gene for aldolase B is on chromosome 9q22.3. Several mutations causing heredity fructose intolerance are known. A single missense mutation, a G→C transversion in exon 5 resulting in the normal alanine at position 149 being replaced by a proline, is the most common mutation identified in northern Europeans. This mutation, plus two other point mutations, account for 80–85% of hereditary fructose intolerance in Europe and the United States. Diagnosis of hereditary fructose intolerance can be made by direct DNA analysis. Prenatal diagnosis should be possible by amniocentesis and chorionic villi, using DNA mutational or linkage analysis.

Clinical Manifestations. Patients with fructose intolerance are perfectly healthy and asymptomatic until fructose or sucrose (table sugar) is ingested (usually from fruit, fruit juice, or sweetened cereal). Symptoms may occur early in life soon after birth if foods or formulas containing these sugars are introduced into the diet. Early clinical manifestations resemble galactosemia and include jaundice, hepatomegaly, vomiting, lethargy, irritability, and convulsions. Laboratory findings include prolonged clotting time, hypoalbuminuria, elevation of bilirubin and transaminase levels, and proximal tubular dysfunction. Acute fructose ingestion produces symptomatic hypoglycemia; chronic ingestion results in failure to thrive and hepatic disease. If the intake of the fructose persists, hypoglycemic episodes recur, and liver and kidney failure progress, eventually leading to death.

Diagnosis. Suspicion of the enzyme deficiency is fostered by the presence of a reducing substance in the urine during an episode. The diagnosis could be supported by an intravenous fructose tolerance test, which will cause a rapid fall, first of serum phosphate and then of blood glucose, and a subsequent increase in uric acid and magnesium. An oral tolerance test should not be performed, because patients may become acutely ill. Definitive diagnosis is made by assay of fructaldolase B activity in the liver.

Treatment. This consists of the complete elimination of all sources of sucrose, fructose, and sorbitol from the diet. This may be difficult because these sugars are widely used additives, found even in most medicinal preparations. With treatment, liver and kidney dysfunction improves, and catch-up in growth is common. Intellectual development is usually unimpaired. As the patient matures, symptoms become milder even after fructose ingestion; the long-term prognosis is good. Because of voluntary dietary avoidance of sucrose, affected patients have few dental caries.

76.4 Defects in Intermediary Carbohydrate Metabolism Associated with Lactic Acidosis

Yuan-Tsong Chen

Lactic acidosis occurs with defects of carbohydrate metabolism that interfere with the conversion of pyruvate to glucose via the pathway of gluconeogenesis or to carbon dioxide and water via the mitochondrial enzymes of the citric acid cycle. Figure 76–3 depicts the relevant metabolic pathways. Type I glycogen storage disease, fructose-1,6-diphosphatase deficiency, and phosphoenolpyruvate carboxylase deficiency are disorders of gluconeogenesis associated with lactic acidosis. Pyruvate dehydrogenase complex deficiency, respiratory chain defects, and pyruvate carboxylase deficiency are disorders in the pathway of pyruvate metabolism causing lactic acidosis. Lactic acidosis can also occur in defects of fatty acid oxidation, organic acidurias (see Chapters 74.6, 74.10, and 75.1), or biotin utilization

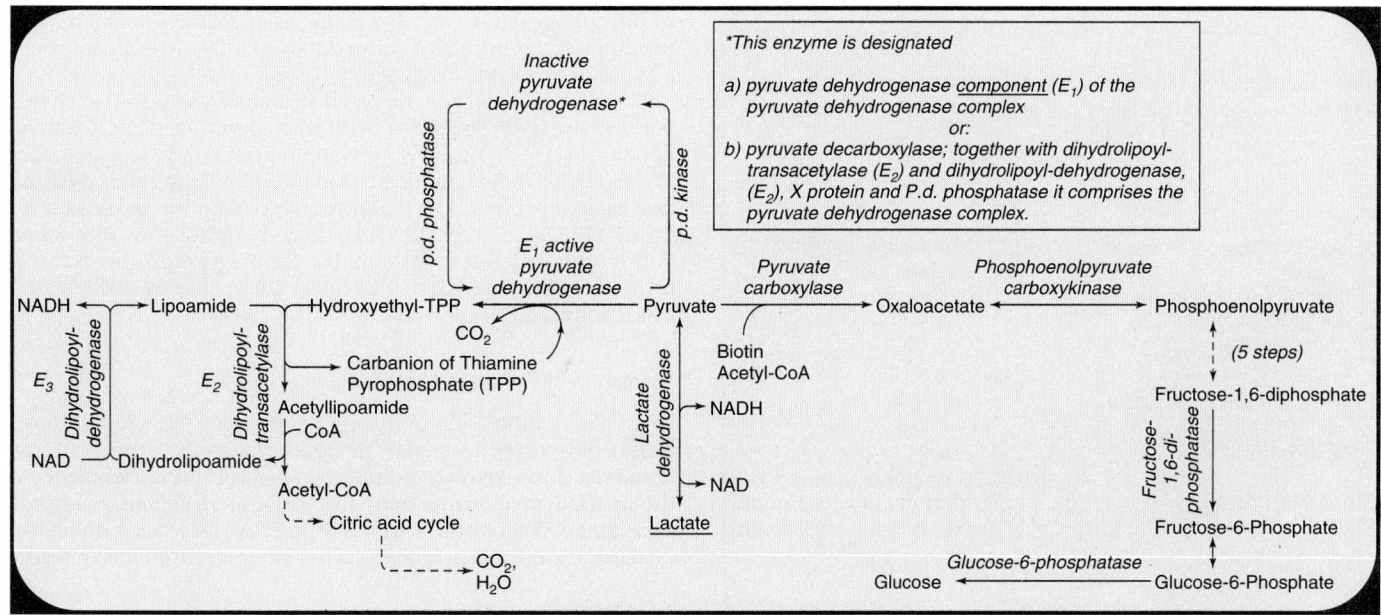

FIGURE 76–3. Enzymatic reactions of carbohydrate metabolism, deficiencies of which may give rise to lactic acidosis, pyruvate elevations, or hypoglycemia. The pyruvate dehydrogenase complex comprises, in addition to E_1, E_2, and E_3, an extra lipoate-containing protein (not shown), called protein X, and pyruvate dehydrogenase phosphatase.

diseases. These disorders are easily distinguishable by the presence of abnormal acylcarnitine profiles in the blood and unusual organic acids in the urine. Therefore, blood lactate and acylcarnitine profiles and the presence of these unusual urine organic acids should be determined in infants and children with unexplained acidosis, especially if there is an increase of anion gap (see Chapter 48).

Lactic acidosis unrelated to an enzymatic defect occurs in hypoxemia. In this case, as well as in defects in the respiratory chain, the serum pyruvate concentration may remain normal (<1.0 mg/dL with an increased lactate:pyruvate ratio), whereas pyruvate is usually increased when lactic acidosis results from an enzymatic defect in gluconeogenesis or pyruvate dehydrogenase complex (both lactate and pyruvate are increased and the ratio is normal). Lactate and pyruvate should be measured in the same blood specimen and on multiple blood specimens obtained when the patient is symptomatic because lactic acidosis may be intermittent. An algorithm for the differential diagnosis of lactic acidosis is shown in Figure 76–4.

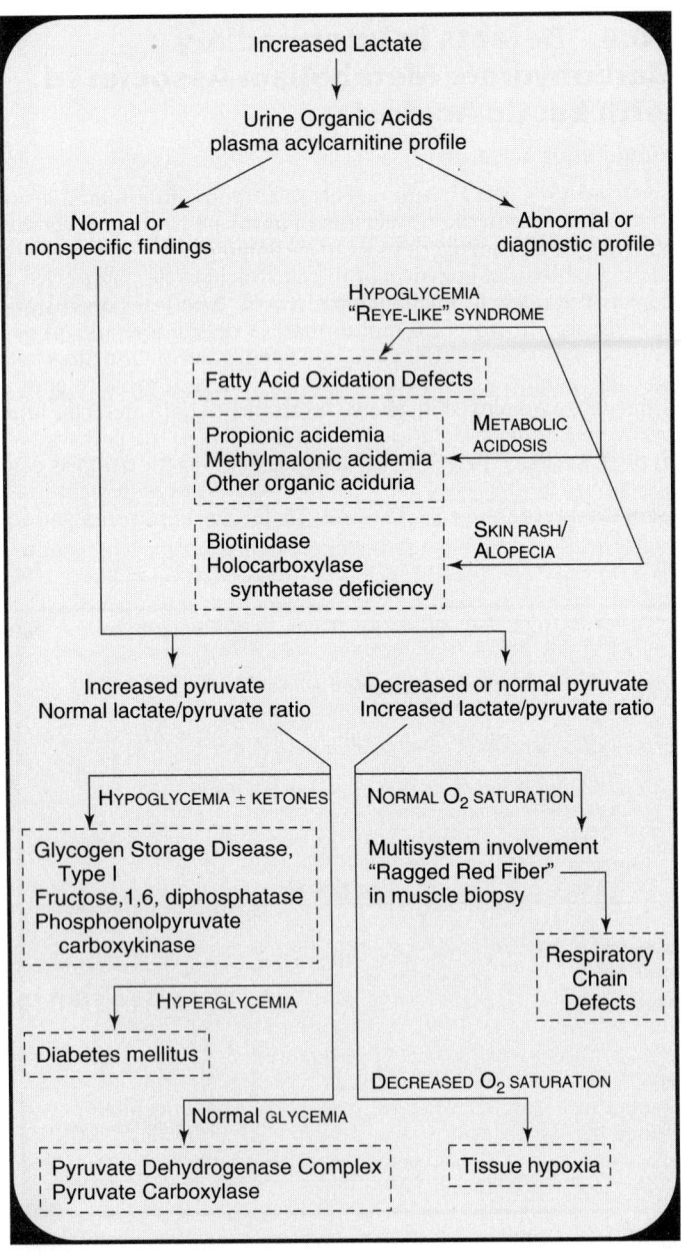

FIGURE 76–4. Algorithm of the differential diagnosis of lactic acidosis.

DISORDERS OF GLUCONEOGENESIS

Deficiency of Glucose-6-Phosphatase (Type I Glycogen Storage Disease)

Type I glycogen storage disease is the only glycogenosis associated with significant lactic acidosis. The chronic metabolic acidosis predisposes these patients to osteopenia, and in an acute setting after prolonged fasting the acidosis associated with hypoglycemia is a life-threatening condition. This disease is discussed further in Chapter 76.1.

Fructose-1,6-Diphosphatase Deficiency

Fructose-1,6-diphosphatase deficiency is not a defect in the fructose pathway; rather, it is a defect involved in gluconeogenesis. The *clinical manifestations* are characterized by life-threatening episodes of acidosis, hypoglycemia, hyperventilation, convulsions, and coma. Half of the patients have an onset in the 1st week of life. In infants and small children, episodes are triggered by febrile infections and gastroenteritis if oral food intake decreases. *Laboratory findings* include low blood glucose and high lactate and uric acid levels and metabolic acidosis. In contrast to hereditary fructose intolerance, there is usually no aversion to sweets; renal tubular and liver functions are normal.

The *diagnosis* is established by demonstrating an enzyme deficiency in either a liver or intestinal biopsy. The enzyme defect may also be demonstrated in leukocytes in some cases. The gene coding for fructose-1,6-diphosphatase is located on chromosome 9q22. Because mutations are being characterized, carrier detection and prenatal diagnosis should be possible using a DNA-based test. *Treatment* of acute attacks consists of correction of hypoglycemia and acidosis by intravenous glucose infusion; the response is usually rapid. Avoidance of fasting and restriction of fructose and sucrose from the diet prevent further episodes. For long-term prevention of hypoglycemia, a slowly released carbohydrate such as cornstarch is useful. Patients who survive childhood develop normally.

Phosphoenolpyruvate Carboxykinase Deficiency

Phosphoenolpyruvate carboxykinase (PEPCK) is a key enzyme in gluconeogenesis. It catalyzes the conversion of oxaloacetate to phosphoenolpyruvate (see Fig. 76–3). PEPCK deficiency has been described both as a mitochondrial enzyme deficiency and as a cytosolic enzyme deficiency.

The disease has been reported in only six cases. The clinical features are heterogeneous, with hypoglycemia, lactic acidemia, hepatomegaly, hypotonia, developmental delay, and failure to thrive as the major manifestations. Hepatic and renal dysfunction may be present. The diagnosis is based on the reduced activity of PEPCK in liver, fibroblasts, or lymphocytes. Fibroblasts and lymphocytes are not suitable for diagnosing the cytosolic form of PEPCK deficiency because these tissues possess only mitochondrial PEPCK.

Disorders of Pyruvate Metabolism

Pyruvate is metabolized through four main enzyme systems: lactate dehydrogenase, alanine aminotransferase, pyruvate carboxylase, and pyruvate dehydrogenase complex. Deficiency of the M subunit of lactate dehydrogenase causes exercise intolerance and myoglobinuria (see Chapter 76.1). Genetic deficiency of alanine aminotransferase has not been reported in humans.

Disorders of Pyruvate Dehydrogenase Complex Deficiency

The pyruvate dehydrogenase complex (PDHC) catalyzes the oxidation of pyruvate to acetyl CoA, which enters the tricarboxylic acid cycle for ATP production. The complex comprises five components: E_1, an α ketoacid decarboxylase; E_2, a dihydrolipoyl transacylase; E_3, a dihydrolipoyl dehydrogenase; protein X, an extra lipoate-containing protein; and pyruvate dehydrogenase phosphatase (see Fig. 76–3).

Deficiency of any of these components is associated with lactic acidosis and central nervous system dysfunction. The central nervous system dysfunction is because the brain obtains its energy primarily from oxidation of glucose.

The E_1 defects are caused by mutations in the gene coding for E_1 α subunit, which is X-linked.

Clinical Manifestations. The disease has a wide spectrum of presentations from the most severe neonatal presentation to a mild late-onset form. The neonatal onset is associated with lethal lactic acidosis, white matter cystic lesions, agenesis of the corpus callosum, and the most severe enzyme deficiency. Infantile onset may be lethal or associated with psychomotor retardation and chronic lactic acidosis, cystic lesions in the brainstem, and basal ganglia pathologic features resembling *Leigh disease*. Older children, usually boys, may have less acidosis, greater enzyme activity, and manifest ataxia with high-carbohydrate diets. Intelligence may be normal. Patients of all ages may have facial dysmorphologic features similar to those of fetal alcohol syndrome.

The E_2 and protein X-lipoate defects are rare and result in severe psychomotor retardation. The E_3 lipoyl dehydrogenase defect leads to deficient activity not only in the pyruvate dehydrogenase complex but also in the α-ketoglutarate and branched-chain ketoacid dehydrogenase complexes. Pyruvate dehydrogenase phosphatase deficiency has also been reported. These other PDHC defects have clinical manifestations within the variable spectrum associated with PDHC deficiency due to E_1 deficiency.

Treatment. The general prognosis is poor except in rare cases in which mutation is associated with altered affinity for thiamine pyrophosphate, which may respond to thiamine supplementation. Because carbohydrates may aggravate lactic acidosis, a ketogenic diet is rational. The diet has lowered the blood lactate level, but limited or no long-term benefit is seen. A potential treatment strategy is to maintain any residual PDHC in its active form by dichloroacetate, an inhibitor of E_1 kinase. Beneficial effects in some patients have been shown. Patients usually respond to a daily dose of 25–100 mg/kg by oral or intravenous (50 mg/kg × 1 may produce a response within 24 hr) routes.

Deficiency of Pyruvate Carboxylase

Pyruvate carboxylase catalyzes the conversion of pyruvate to oxaloacetate as the first step for gluconeogenesis. Clinical manifestations of this deficiency have varied from neonatal severe lactic acidosis accompanied by hyperammonemia, citrullinemia, and hyperlysinemia (type B) to late-onset mild to moderate lactic acidosis and developmental delay (type A). In both types, patients who survived usually had severe psychomotor retardation with seizures, spasticity, and microcephaly. Some patients have pathologic changes in the brainstem and basal ganglia that resemble *Leigh disease*. The clinical severity appears to correlate with the level of the residual enzyme activity. Laboratory findings are characterized by elevated levels of blood lactate, pyruvate, and alanine; in the case of type B, blood ammonia, citrulline, and lysine levels are also elevated, which might suggest a primary defect of the urea cycle. The mechanism is likely caused by depletion of oxaloacetate, which leads to reduced levels of aspartate, which is a substrate for argininosuccinate synthetase in the urea cycle (see Chapter 74.11). Aspartate and citrate supplements restore the metabolic abnormalities; however, whether this treatment can prevent the neurologic deficits is not known. Diagnosis of pyruvate carboxylase deficiency is

made by the measurement of enzyme activity in liver or cultured skin fibroblasts.

Deficiency of Pyruvate Carboxylase Secondary to Deficiency of Holocarboxylase Synthetase or Biotinidase

Deficiency of either holocarboxylase synthetase or biotinidase, which are enzymes of biotin metabolism, results in a secondary deficiency of pyruvate carboxylase (and other biotin-requiring carboxylases and metabolic reactions) and in *clinical manifestations* associated with the respective deficiencies, as well as rash, lactic acidosis, and alopecia (see also Chapter 74.6). The course of holocarboxylase synthetase or biotinidase deficiency can be protracted, with intermittent exacerbation of chronic lactic acidosis, failure to thrive, seizures, and hypotonia leading to spasticity, lethargy, coma, and death. Late-onset milder forms have also been reported. *Laboratory findings* include metabolic acidosis and abnormal organic acids in the urine. *Diagnosis* can be made in skin fibroblasts or lymphocytes by assay for holocarboxylase synthetase activity and in the case of biotinidase in the serum by screening blood spot. *Treatment* consists of biotin supplementation, 5–20 mg/day, and is generally effective if treatment is started before the development of brain damage. Patients identified through newborn screening have been treated with biotin and have remained asymptomatic.

Both enzyme deficiencies are autosomal recessive traits. Holocarboxylase synthetase and biotinidase are located on chromosome 21q22 and 3p25, respectively. Ethnic specific mutations in the holocarboxylase synthetase gene have been identified. Two common mutations (del7/ins3 and R538C) in the biotinidase gene account for 52% of all mutant alleles in symptomatic patients with biotinidase deficiency.

Mitochondrial Respiratory Chain Defects (Oxidative Phosphorylation Disease)

The mitochondrial respiratory chain catalyzes the oxidation of fuel molecules and transfers the electrons to molecular oxygen with concomitant energy transduction into adenosine triphosphate (ATP)—so-called oxidative phosphorylation. The respiratory chain produces ATP from NADH or $FADH_2$ and includes five specific complexes (I: nicotinamide-adenine dinucleotide [NADH]-coenzyme Q reductase; II: succinate-coenzyme Q reductase; III: coenzyme QH_2 cytochrome C reductase; IV: cytochrome C oxidase; V: ATP synthase). Each complex is composed of 9–25 individual proteins and, with the exception of complex II, are encoded by nuclear or mitochondrial DNA (inherited only from the mother by mitochondrial inheritance). Defects in any of these complexes or assembly system produce chronic lactic acidosis presumably due to a change of redox state with increased concentrations of NADH. In contrast to PDHC or pyruvate carboxylase deficiency, skeletal muscle and heart are usually involved in the respiratory chain disorders; and in muscle biopsy, "ragged red fibers" (indicating mitochondrial proliferation) are often seen (see Fig. 76–4). Because of the ubiquitous nature of oxidative phosphorylation, a defect of the mitochondrial respiratory chain accounts for a vast array of clinical manifestations and should be considered in patients in all age groups presenting with multisystem involvement. Some deficiencies resemble Leigh disease, whereas others cause infantile myopathies such as MELAS (mitochondrial encephalopathy, myopathy, lactic acidosis, and strokelike episodes), MERRF (myoclonus epilepsy, with ragged-red fibers), and Kearns-Sayre syndrome (external ophthalmoplegia, acidosis, retinal degeneration, heart block, myopathy, and high cerebrospinal fluid protein) (see also Chapters 591.2 and 602.4). Diagnosis requires measurement of enzyme activities in tissues or analysis of mitochondrial DNA mutation, or both. Treatment remains largely symptomatic and does not significantly alter the outcome of disease. However, some patients appear to respond to cofactor supplements such as coenzyme Q_{10}.

Leigh Disease (Subacute Necrotizing Encephalopathy)

Leigh disease remains a neuropathologic description characterized by demyelination, gliosis, necrosis, relative neuronal sparing, and capillary proliferation in specific brain regions. In decreasing order of severity, the affected areas are the basal ganglia, brain stem cerebellum, and cerebral cortex (see also Chapter 591). Patients with Leigh disease have defects in several enzyme complexes. Dysfunction in cytochrome C oxidase (complex IV) is the most commonly reported defect, followed by NADH-coenzyme Q reductase (complex I), PDHC, and pyruvate carboxylase. Mutations in the nuclear *SURF1* gene, which encodes a factor involved in the biogenesis of cytochrome C oxidase and mitochondrial DNA mutations in the ATPase 6 coding region, are common molecular findings in patients with Leigh disease.

76.5 Deficiency of Xylulose Dehydrogenase (Essential Benign Pentosuria)

Yuan-Tsong Chen

A reducing substance in the urine in an otherwise healthy individual characterizes essential benign pentosuria. Care should be taken not to mistake the reducing substance for glucose. The pentose in the urine reacts with Clinitest but not with glucose oxidase test papers such as Tes-Tape or Clinistix dipsticks.

L-Xylulose dehydrogenase converts L-xylulose (which can arise from D-glucuronate) to xylitol. Xylitol is converted to D-xylulose, which becomes D-xylulose-5-phosphate and enters the pentose phosphate shunt. Deficiency of this enzyme leads to increased concentration of L-xylulose in blood and urine. This rare defect is most common in Jews. No therapy is required.

Pentosuria can be observed in normal individuals if the dietary pentose intake is increased, as with the excessive ingestion of fruit containing pentose. Under these circumstances, there may be urinary excretion of xylose and arabinose up to 200 mg/24 hr in normal individuals.

Amalfitano A, Bengur AR, Morse RP, et al: Recombinant human acid-α-glucosidase enzyme therapy for infantile glycogen storage disease type II: Results of a phase I/II clinical trial. *Genet Med* 2001;3:132–38.

Bandsma RH, Rake JP, Visser G, et al: Increased lipogenesis and resistance of lipoproteins to oxidative modification in two patients with glycogen storage disease type Ia. *J Pediatr* 2002;140:256–60.

Chen YT: Glycogen storage diseases. In Scriver CR, et al (editors): *The Metabolic and Molecular Bases of Inherited Disease,* 8th ed. New York, McGraw-Hill, 2001, pp 1521–51.

Coenen MJ, van Den Heuvel LP, Smeitink JA: Mitochondrial oxidative phosphorylation system assembly in man: Recent achievements. *Curr Opin Neurol* 2001;14:777–81.

Comi GP, et al: β-enolase deficiency: A new metabolic myopathy of distal glycolysis. *Neurology* 2001;56(suppl 13):A231–32.

DiMauro S, Lamperti C: Muscle glycogenoses. *Muscle Nerve* 2001;24:984–99.

Holton JB, et al: Galactosemia. In Scriver CM, et al (editors): *The Metabolic and Molecular Bases of Inherited Disease,* 8th ed. New York, McGraw-Hill, 2001, pp 1553–87.

Shen JJ, Chen YT: Molecular characterization of glycogen storage disease type III. *Curr Molec Med* 2002;2:167–75.

Umapathysivam K, Hopwood JJ, Meikle PJ: Determination of acid alpha-glucosidase activity in blood spots as a diagnostic test for Pompe disease. *Clin Chem* 2001;47:1378–83.

Vorgerd M, Zange J, Kley R, et al: Effect of high-dose creatine therapy on symptoms of exercise intolerance in McArdle disease: Double-blind, placebo-controlled crossover study. *Arch Neurol* 2002;59:97–101.

Weinstein DA, Somers MJ, Wolfsdorf JI: Decreased urinary citrate excretion in type Ia glycogen storage disease. *J Pediatr* 2001;138:378–82.

Yoshikawa M, Fukui K, Kuriyama S, et al: Hepatic adenomas treated with percutaneous ethanol injection in a patient with glycogen storage disease type Ia. *J Gastroenterol* 2001;36:52–61.

76.6 Disorders of Glycoprotein Degradation and Structure

Margaret M. McGovern and Robert J. Desnick

The disorders of glycoprotein degradation and structure include several lysosomal storage diseases that result from defects in glycoprotein degradation and congenital disorders of glycosylation previously called the carbohydrate-deficient glycoprotein syndrome, which is pathophysiologically unrelated. Glycoproteins are macromolecules that are composed of oligosaccharide chains linked to a peptide backbone. They are synthesized by two pathways, the glycosyltransferase pathway, which synthesizes oligosaccharides linked *o*-glycosidically to serine or threonine residues, and the dolichol, lipid-linked pathway, which synthesizes oligosaccharides linked *N*-glycosidically to asparagine.

Glycoprotein lysosomal storage diseases result from the deficiency of the enzymes that normally participate in the degradation of oligosaccharides and include sialidosis, galactosialidosis, aspartylglucosaminuria, and α-mannosidosis (see Box 75–1). In some instances, the abnormality that leads to glycoprotein accumulation also results in abnormal degradation of other classes of macromolecules that contain similar oligosaccharide linkages, such as certain glycolipids and proteoglycans (Table 76–2). In these instances, the underlying enzymatic deficiency results in the accumulation of both glycoproteins and glycolipids. The classification of these types of disorders as lipidoses or glycoproteinoses is dependent on the nature of the predominantly stored substance. Glycoprotein disorders are characterized by autosomal recessive inheritance and a progressive disease course with clinical features that may resemble those seen in the mucopolysaccharidoses.

SIALIDOSIS AND GALACTOSIALIDOSIS

Sialidosis and galactosialidosis are autosomal recessive disorders that result from the isolated deficiency of neuraminidase, and the combined deficiencies of neuraminidase and β-galactosidase, respectively. Neuraminidase cleaves terminal sialyl linkages of several oligosaccharides and glycoproteins. Its deficiency results in the accumulation of oligosaccharides and the urinary excretion of sialic acid terminal oligosaccharides and sialylglycopeptides. Pathologic storage of substrate is seen in many tissues, including liver, bone marrow, and brain. Two different genes may be involved in the expression of the glycoprotein-specific neuraminidase that is deficient in sialidosis patients. The neuraminidase deficiency in one sialidosis patient is a mutation in a structural gene on chromosome 10, whereas the neuraminidase deficiency in a galactosialidosis patient is in a gene located on chromosome 20.

Clinical Manifestations (see Table 75–7). The clinical phenotype of neuraminidase deficiency is variable and includes type I sialidosis, which usually presents in the 2nd decade of life with myoclonus and a cherry-red spot. Patients typically have gait disturbances, myoclonus, or visual complaints. In contrast, type II sialidosis occurs as congenital, infantile, and juvenile forms. The congenital and infantile forms result from isolated neuraminidase deficiency, whereas the juvenile form results from both neuraminidase and β-galactosidase deficiency. Hydrops fetalis, neonatal ascites, hepatosplenomegaly, stippling of the epiphyses, periosteal cloaking, and stillbirth or death characterizes the congenital type II disease during infancy. The type II infantile form presents in the 1st yr of life with dysostosis multiplex, moderate mental retardation, visceromegaly, corneal clouding, cherry-red spot, and seizures. The juvenile type II form of sialidosis, which is sometimes designated galactosialidosis, has a variable age at onset ranging from infancy to adulthood. In infancy, the phenotype is similar to that of GM$_1$ gangliosidosis with edema, ascites, skeletal dysplasia, and a cherry-red spot. Patients with later-onset disease have dysosto-

TABLE 76–2. Characteristics of Congenital Disorders of Glycosylation (CDG)

Name	Defect	Dysmorphology	Neurologic Signs	Gastrointestinal Signs	Other Signs
CDGIa	Phosphomannomutase 2 $M6P \rightarrow M1P$ Incidence 1:80,000	Fat maldistribution: narrow waist, fat in axilla, groin, buttock High nasal bridge Prominal jaw Large ears Inverted nipples	Hypotonia Hyporeflexia Strabismus Ataxia: olivopontocerebellar atrophy or hypoplasia Mental retardation (IQ 40–60) Strokelike episodes Hemorrhagic cerebral infarcts Polyneuropathy Muscle wasting Scoliosis Kyphosis Pigmentary retinal degeneration Contractures Seizures	Poor feeding Failure to thrive Carnitine deficiency Diarrhea Liver failure	Cardiomyopathy Pericardial effusions Nephrotic syndrome Renal tubulopathy Severe infections Hypogonadism Absent puberty TBG deficiency ↓ Levels of: antithrombin III, α_1 acid glycoprotein, α_1-antitrypsin, ferritin, ceruloplasmin, proteins C + S, factor XI, complement-C1, C3a, C4a
CDGIb	Phosphomannose isomerase $F6P \rightarrow M6P$	None	Normal development	Protein-losing enteropathy Failure to thrive Chronic intractable diarrhea Hepatic fibrosis Hyperinsulinemic hypoglycemia Vomiting	Coagulopathy ↓ proteins C, S, antithrombin III
CDGIc	Glucosyltransferase: prevents glucose addition to endoplasmic reticulum lumen	None	Similar to CDGIa but milder Mild cerebellar hypoplasia No neuropathy Pigmentary retinal degeneration Seizures	Failure to thrive	Recurrent eyelid edema Frequent infections Coagulopathy
CDGId	Mannosyltransferase: prevents mannose addition to endoplasmic reticulum lumen	High arched palate Microcephaly	Developmental delay Seizures (severe)	Failure to thrive	
CDGIe	Dolichol-phosphate-mannose synthetase: DPM donates mannose	High arched palate Microcephaly Down slanting palpebral fissures Hemangiomas Short arms Small hands Dysplastic nails	Developmental delay Hypotonia Seizures (severe) Cortical blindness Hyperreflexia Delayed myelination	Failure to thrive	
CDGIIa	N-Acetyl-glucosaminyl-transferase II	Facial dysmorphology	Stereotypic hand movements Developmental delay No neuropathy or cerebellar hypoplasia	Failure to thrive	
CDGIIb	Unknown	Facial dysmorphology	Hypotonia Seizures	Hepatomegaly	
CDGIIc	Unknown	Facial dysmorphology	Developmental delay Hypotonia	Failure to thrive	Recurrent infections with leukocytosis
CDGx or CDGIx	Unknown Unclassified	Like CDGIa Microcephaly	Hypotonia Seizures Cerebellar hypoplasia Developmental delay	Intractable diarrhea Failure to thrive	Nonimmune hydrops Cataracts Thrombocytopenia Renal tubulopathy Distal bone demineralization

M6P = mannose-6-phosphate;
MIP = mannose-1-phosphate;
TBG = thyroid-binding globulin;
FGP = fructose-6-phosphate;
DMP = dolichol-phosphate-mannose.

sis multiplex, visceromegaly, mental retardation, dysmorphism, corneal clouding, progressive neurologic deterioration, and bilateral cherry-red spots.

The *diagnosis* of sialidosis and galactosialidosis is achieved by the demonstration of the specific enzymatic deficiency. Prenatal diagnosis using cultured amniotic cells is possible.

No specific *treatment* exists for any form of the disease.

ASPARTYLGLUCOSAMINURIA

Aspartylglucosaminuria is a rare autosomal recessive lysosomal storage disorder, except in Finland where the carrier frequency is estimated to be 1/36. The disorder results from the deficient activity of aspartylglucosaminidase and the subsequent accumulation of aspartylglucosamine, particularly in the liver, spleen, and thyroid. The gene for the enzyme has been localized to the long arm of chromosome 4. In the Finnish population, a single mutation in the gene (C163S) accounts for most mutant alleles, whereas outside of Finland a large number of private mutations are present. Affected individuals with aspartylglucosaminuria typically present in the 1st yr of life with recurrent infections, diarrhea, and hernias (see Table 75–7). Coarsening of the facies and short stature usually develop later. Other features include joint laxity, macroglossia, hoarse voice, crystal-like lens opacities, hypotonia, and spasticity. Psychomotor development is usually near normal until the age of 5 yr when a decline is noted. Behavioral abnormalities are typical, and the IQ in affected adults is less than 40. Survival to adulthood is common, with most early deaths attributable to pneumonia or other pulmonary causes. Definitive diagnosis requires measurement of the enzyme in peripheral blood leukocytes. Molecular diagnosis by analysis of DNA for the C163S mutation is possible for Finnish patients. Prenatal diagnosis by the determination of the level of aspartylglucosaminidase in cultured amniocytes or chorionic villi is also possible. No specific treatment is available, and care is supportive. Bone marrow transplantation has been attempted in several patients with no improvement in neurologic function.

α-MANNOSIDOSIS

α-Mannosidosis is an autosomal recessive disorder that results from the deficient activity of α-mannosidase and the accumulation of mannose-rich compounds. The gene encoding the enzyme is localized to chromosome 19p13.2-q12. Affected patients with this disorder display clinical heterogeneity. There is a severe infantile form, or type I disease, and a milder juvenile variant, type II disease (see Table 75–7). All patients have psychomotor retardation, facial coarsening, and dysostosis multiplex. However, the infantile form of the disorder is characterized by more rapid mental deterioration, with death occurring between the ages of 3 and 10 yr. Patients with the infantile form also have more severe skeletal involvement and hepatosplenomegaly. The juvenile disorder is characterized by onset of symptoms during early childhood or adolescence with milder somatic features and survival to adulthood. Hearing loss, destructive synovitis, pancytopenia, and spastic paraplegia have all been reported in type II patients. The diagnosis is made by the demonstration of the deficiency of α-mannosidase activity in white blood cells or cultured fibroblasts, and prenatal diagnosis is also possible. No specific therapy exists for the disorder, although bone marrow transplantation has been attempted in several patients.

CONGENITAL DISORDERS OF GLYCOSYLATION

The congenital disorders of glycosylation (CDG), previously known as the carbohydrate-deficient glycoprotein syndrome are autosomal recessive disorders that result from defects in the synthesis and transport (CDG type I) or modification and processing (CGD type II) of the carbohydrate moiety of glycoproteins (see Table 76–2). Because this post-translational modification may affect many proteins in many tissues, the disorders are systemic and heterogeneous. Carbohydrate side glycans are needed for secretion and membrane binding of many proteins. A distinctive biochemical marker of all of these disorders is the presence of carbohydrate-deficient transferrin in serum and cerebrospinal fluid as determined by isoelectric focusing electrophoresis (IEF). Each disorder has its own pattern on IEF. Clinical manifestations are usually both neurologic and multivisceral, involving many different tissues (see Table 76–2).

In patients with CDG type I (type Ia is the most common) the *clinical manifestations* in infancy include hypotonia, weakness, hyperreflexia, strokelike episodes, dysmorphic features, and inverted nipples (see Table 76–2). In childhood, ataxia, muscle atrophy, decreased deep tendon reflexes, toe walking, and continued strokelike episodes are observed. The latter events may be related to reduced factor XI, proteins C and S, and antithrombin III. Strabismus is a consistent finding, and retinitis pigmentosa is common. Growth failure, liver dysfunction, retinal degeneration, and skeletal abnormalities have been described. The skeletal features may include contractures, kyphoscoliosis, and pectus carinatum, all of which may be secondary to the neurologic effects of the disorder. Pericardial effusion in older

patients and hypertrophic obstructive cardiomyopathy in the infant may occur. Transferrin studies have revealed that infantile olivopontocerebellar atrophy is a severe form of some of the CDG. Lipodystrophy with prominent fat pads on the buttocks and suprapubic area is a distinctive feature. Adults with type Ia have hypogonadism and developmental delay and are nonambulatory. These disorders should be considered in patients with failure to thrive, mental retardation, cerebellar hypoplasia, hypotonia, hepatic dysfunction, and episodic strokelike episodes. In contrast, patients with type Ib disease do not have neurologic symptoms and usually present with hypoglycemia, protein-losing enteropathy, vomiting, and diarrhea. The *diagnosis* can be confirmed by analysis of the transferrin pattern by isoelectric focusing. Distinct transferrin patterns are identified in affected patients corresponding to CDG types I and II. *Treatment* is symptomatic. Oral mannose has been effective only in patients with type Ib CDG.

Arvio M, Sauna-Aho O, Peippo M: Bone marrow transplantation for aspartylglucosaminuria: Follow-up study of transplanted and non-transplanted patients. *J Pediatr* 2001;138:288–90.

Grünewald S, Matthijs G, Jaeken J: Congenital disorders of glucosylation; A review. *Pediatr Res* 2002;52:618–24.

Kjaergaard S, Schwartz M, Skovby F: Congenital disorder of glycosylation type Ia (CDG-Ia): Phenotypic spectrum of the R141H/F119L genotype. *Arch Dis Child* 2001;85:236–39.

Leonard J, Grünewald S, Clayton P: Diversity of congenital disorders of glycosylation. *Lancet* 2001;357:1382–83.

Mention K, Michaud L, Dobbelaere D, et al: Neonatal severe intractable diarrhea as the presenting manifestation of an unclassified congenital disorder of glycosylation (CGG-x). *Arch Dis Child Fetal Neonatal Ed* 2001;85:F217–19.

Pearl PL, Krasnewich D: Neurologic course of congenital disorders of glycosylation. *J Child Neurol* 2001;16:409–13.

Chapter 77

Mucopolysaccharidoses

Robert M. Kliegman and Joseph L. Muenzer

Mucopolysaccharidoses (MPSs) are inheritable storage diseases caused by a deficiency of lysosomal enzymes that degrade glycosaminoglycans (GAGs, previously called *mucopolysaccharides*). The MPSs are a heterogeneous group characterized by the intralysosomal accumulation of GAGs, excessive urinary excretion of GAGs, and variable degrees of progressive mental and physical deterioration and, in severe forms, premature death. Each type has a specific lysosomal enzyme deficiency, and many have variable phenotypic expression with characteristic degrees of organ involvement and rates of deterioration (Table 77–1). Depending on the enzyme deficiency, the metabolism of dermatan sulfate, heparan sulfate, or keratan sulfate may be blocked alone or in combination. Lysosomal accumulation of the GAGs eventually results in cell, vascular, tissue, and organ dysfunction. The MPS disorders share many clinical features, although in variable degrees. These include a chronic and progressive course, multisystem involvement, organomegaly, dysostosis multiplex, and abnormal facial features (Tables 77–1 and 77–2). Vision, hearing, airway and cardiovascular function, and joint mobility may be affected. Mental retardation is a common feature of the severe forms. There is clinical similarity among different enzyme deficiencies and, conversely, a wide spectrum of clinical severity within any enzyme deficiency. MPSs are characterized by autosomal recessive traits, except for MPS II, which is an X-linked recessive condition.

Numerous identified mutations are known for each gene in each disorder. Many patients are compound heterozygotes for rare alleles. Mutation analysis is beneficial in establishing genotype-phenotype correlation in Hurler syndrome and the severe

TABLE 77–1. Classification of the Mucopolysaccharidoses

Number	Eponym	Enzyme Deficiency	Stored Glycosaminoglycan	Major Clinical Manifestations
MPS I H	Hurler	α-L-Iduronidase	Dermatan sulfate, heparan sulfate	Mental retardation, heart disease, corneal clouding, coarse facies, dysostosis multiplex, hepatosplenomegaly, cardiac disease, death before 10 yr of age
MPS I S	Scheie	α-L-Iduronidase	Dermatan sulfate, heparan sulfate	Normal intelligence and life span, with corneal clouding, stiff joints, and heart disease
MPS I H/S	Hurler-Scheie	α-L-Iduronidase	Dermatan sulfate, heparan sulfate	Phenotype intermediate between Hurler and Scheie syndromes
MPS II	Hunter*	Iduronate sulfatase	Dermatan sulfate, heparan sulfate	Wide spectrum of severity, mild to severe; dysostosis multiplex, cardiac disease, mental retardation, coarse facies, hepatosplenomegaly, death before 15 yr in severe form; normal intelligence with variable severity of somatic features in the milder form
MPS III A	Sanfilippo A	Heparan-N-sulfatase (sulfamidase)	Heparan sulfate	Hyperactivity, mild somatic features, profound mental deterioration; death usually in 2nd decade
MPS III B	Sanfilippo B	α-N-Acetyl-glucosaminidase	Heparan sulfate	Phenotype similar to Sanfilippo A
MPS III C	Sanfilippo C	Acetyl CoA:α-glucosaminidase acetyltransferase	Heparan sulfate	Phenotype similar to Sanfilippo A and B
MPS III D	Sanfilippo D	N-Acetylglucosamine 6-sulfatase	Heparan sulfate	Phenotype similar to Sanfilippo A and B
MPS IV A	Morquio A	Galactose-6-sulfatase	Keratan sulfate	Unique skeletal abnormalities, odontoid hypoplasia, short trunk and short stature, normal intelligence, nonimmune hydrops fetalis; milder forms exist
MPS IV B	Morquio B	β-Galactosidase	Keratan sulfate	Wild spectrum of clinical severity similar to Morquio A
MPS V	No longer used			
MPS VI	Maroteaux-Lamy	N-Acetylgalactosamine-4-sulfatase	Dermatan sulfate	Normal intelligence, dysostosis multiplex, hepatosplenomegaly, cardiac disease, joint stiffness, corneal clouding; milder forms exist
MPS VII	Sly	β-Glucuronidase	Dermatan sulfate, heparan sulfate	Mental retardation, heart disease, corneal clouding, dysostosis multiplex, hepatosplenomegaly; wide spectrum of clinical severity with fetal (hydrops fetalis) and neonatal form
MPS VIII	No longer used			
MPS IX		Hyaluronidase	Hyaluronan	Periarticular soft tissue masses, short stature

*A mild variant of Hunter syndrome with the same enzyme deficiency and stored glycosaminoglycan has normal intelligence, short stature, and survival into adulthood.

TABLE 77–2. **Management of Mucopolysaccharidosis**

Problem	Disorders	Management
Hydrocephalus	MPS I, II, IV	CT scan
		Ventriculoperitoneal shunting
Corneal clouding	MPS I, IV, VI, VII	Corneal transplant
		Monitor for glaucoma
Retinal degeneration	MPS I, II, III	Night light
Hearing	Many types	Ventilating tubes, hearing aids
Joint stiffness	Most except MPS IV	Range of motion exercises
Carpal tunnel syndrome	Many types	Routine electromyography
		Surgical decompression
Obstructive airways (apnea)	Many types	Tonsillectomy and adenoidectomy
		CPAP at night
		Laser excision of tracheal lesions
		Tracheostomy
Anesthesia	MPS I, II, IV, VI	Avoid atlantoaxial subluxation
		Use small endotracheal tube
		Anticipate prolonged recovery
Mitral regurgitation	MPS I, II	Valve replacement
		Endocarditis prevention
Aortic valve disease	MPS I H/S, IS, IV, VI	As above
Spinal cord compression	MPS IV most common	MRI of cervical spine
	Others except MPS III and IX	Surgical stabilization

CPAP = continuous positive airway pressure.

form of MPS II, but for most mutations the clinical phenotype cannot be predicted.

Clinical Manifestations

MUCOPOLYSACCHARIDOSIS I. Deficiency of iduronidase results in a wide range of clinical involvement from the most severe, Hurler syndrome, to the mild Scheie syndrome, which are ends of a broad clinical spectrum. Hurler syndrome is the prototype for describing MPSs, but this is misleading because it is only representative of the most severe end of a spectrum.

Hurler Syndrome. This form of MPS I is a severe progressive disorder with multiple organ and tissue involvement that results in premature death, usually by 10 yr of age. An infant with Hurler syndrome appears normal at birth. Diagnosis is made between 6–24 mo with evidence of hepatosplenomegaly, skeletal deformity, coarse facial features, corneal clouding, large tongue, prominent forehead, joint stiffness, and short stature. Acute cardiomyopathy may be a feature in some infants younger than 1 yr of age. Most children with Hurler syndrome acquire only limited language skills because of developmental delay, chronic hearing loss, and an enlarged tongue. Hearing loss is common and is caused by a combination of conductive and neurosensory problems. Most patients have recurrent upper respiratory tract and ear infections, noisy breathing, and persistent copious nasal discharge. Progressive ventricular enlargement with increased intracranial pressure caused by communicating hydrocephalus also occurs. Corneal clouding, glaucoma, and retinal degeneration are common. Obstructive airway disease develops in many patients, necessitating tracheostomy. Obstructive airway disease, respiratory infection, and cardiac complications are the common causes of death.

Radiographic changes represent the many skeletal abnormalities in the MPSs and are known as *dysostosis multiplex*. The skull is large, with thickened calvarium, premature closure of lambdoid and sagittal sutures, shallow orbits, enlarged J-shaped sella, and abnormal spacing of teeth with dentigerous cysts. Anterior hypoplasia of the lumbar vertebrae with kyphosis is seen early. The diaphyses of the long bones are enlarged with an irregular appearance of the metaphyses; the epiphyseal centers are not well developed. The pelvis is usually poorly formed with small femoral heads and coxa valga. The clavicles are short, thickened, and irregular. The ribs have been described as oar-shaped—narrowed at the vertebral ends and flat and broad at their sternal ends. The phalanges are short and trapezoid with widening of the diaphyses.

The gene encoding α-iduronidase is on chromosome 4p16.3 and spans 19 kb and includes 14 exons. Mutation analysis has revealed two major alleles, W402X and Q70X, and a minor allele, P533R, that account for more than half the MPS I alleles in the white population. None of these alleles produce functional enzyme (null alleles) and in homozygosity or compound heterozygosity give rise to Hurler syndrome, the severe form of MPS I. There are numerous mutations that occur in only one or a few individuals.

Hurler-Scheie Syndrome. This classification describes a clinical phenotype that is intermediate between Hurler and Scheie syndromes and is characterized by progressive somatic involvement, including dysostosis multiplex with little or no intellectual dysfunction. The onset of symptoms is usually observed between 3–8 yr; survival to adulthood is common. Cardiac involvement and upper airway obstruction contribute to clinical mortality. Patients have micrognathia and spondylolisthesis, which may cause cord compression.

Scheie Syndrome. This mild form of MPS I is characterized by joint stiffness, aortic valve disease, corneal clouding, and few other somatic features. Onset of significant symptoms is usually after the age of 5 yr, with diagnosis made between 10 and 20 yr. Patients with Scheie syndrome have normal intelligence and stature but have significant joint and ocular involvement. Ophthalmic features include severe corneal clouding, glaucoma, and retinal degeneration. Obstructive airway disease, causing sleep apnea, develops in some patients, necessitating tracheostomy. Aortic valve disease is common and has required valve replacement in some patients.

MUCOPOLYSACCHARIDOSIS II. Hunter syndrome (MPS II) comprises two recognized clinical entities, severe and mild, that represents two ends of a wide spectrum. The severe and mild forms of Hunter syndrome are separated on clinical grounds because neither has detectable iduronate sulfatase (IDS) activity. The severe form of Hunter syndrome has features similar to those of Hurler syndrome except for the lack of corneal clouding and the slower progression of somatic and central nervous system (CNS) deterioration. The mild form is somewhat analogous to Scheie syndrome, with a prolonged life span, minimal CNS involvement, and slow progression of somatic deterioration. Coarse facial features, short stature, skeletal deformities, joint stiffness, and mental retardation with onset of disease usually between 2–4 yr of age characterize the severe form of Hunter syndrome. Gastrointestinal storage may produce chronic diarrhea. Communicating hydrocephalus is a common feature of the severe form, which can be difficult to detect because of the concurrent CNS deterioration. Extensive, slowly progressive neurologic involvement similar to the late stages of Sanfilippo syndrome usually precedes death, which usually occurs between 10–15 yr of age.

A milder form of MPS II has been recognized, with preservation of intelligence in adult life but with obvious clinical features of somatic involvement. Somatic features are similar to the severe form of MPS II but occur at a greatly reduced rate of progression. Airway involvement, hearing impairment, carpal tunnel syndrome, and joint stiffness are common and can result in significant loss of function in both the mild and severe forms.

Hunter syndrome is an X-linked disorder. The gene encoding IDS contains nine exons that span 24 kb and is mapped to Xq28. About 20% of patients with the severe form of MPS II have major deletions or rearrangements of the IDS gene. MPS II patients with an unusually severe phenotype have a very large deletion of the IDS locus, including adjoining genes, resulting in a contiguous gene syndrome. Most MPS II mutations are point mutations, small deletions, or insertions, and many occur in only a single family.

MUCOPOLYSACCHARIDOSIS III. Sanfilippo syndrome makes up a biochemically diverse but clinically similar group of four recognized types. Each type is due to a different enzyme deficiency involved in the degradation of heparan sulfate (see Table 77–1). Phenotypical variations exist in MPS III patients but to a lesser degree than other MPS disorders, possibly because a very mild form of MPS III may be difficult to recognize. Patients with Sanfilippo syndrome are characterized by slowly progressive, severe CNS involvement with mild somatic disease. Such disproportionate involvement of the CNS is unique to MPS III. Onset of clinical features usually occurs between 2–6 yr in a child who previously appeared normal. Presenting features can include delayed development, hyperactivity with aggressive behavior, coarse hair, hirsutism, sleep disorders, and mild hepatosplenomegaly. Delays in diagnosis of MPS III are common secondary to the mild physical features, hyperactivity, and slowly progressive neurologic disease. Severe neurologic deterioration occurs in most patients by 6–10 yr, accompanied by rapid deterioration of social and adaptive skills. Severe behavior problems, including sleep disturbance, uncontrolled hyperactivity, temper tantrums, destructive behavior, and physical aggression, are common. Profound mental retardation and behavior problems often occur in patients with normal physical strength, making management particularly difficult.

The gene encoding heparan N-sulfatase (MPS III A [Sanfilipo A]) spans 11 kb and is localized to chromosome 17q25.3. The gene encoding α-N-acetylglucosaminidase (MPS III B [Sanfilipo B]) spans 8.5 kb, comprises six exons, and is localized on chromosome 17q21. Mutations have been found for all the MPS III disorders for which the genes have been isolated. Most MPS III mutations are uncommon, consisting of the missense type, with a few premature terminations and small deletions.

MUCOPOLYSACCHARIDOSIS IV. Morquio syndrome (MPS IV) is caused by defective degradation of keratan sulfate. Two enzyme deficiencies resulting in Morquio syndrome have a wide spectrum of clinical manifestations. Both types of Morquio syndrome are characterized by significant, short-trunk dwarfism, fine corneal deposits, a skeletal dysplasia that is distinct from other mucopolysaccharidoses, and preservation of intelligence. The dominant clinical features of Morquio syndrome are related to the skeleton and its effects on the CNS. Instability of the odontoid process and ligamentous laxity can result in life-threatening atlantoaxial subluxation. Surgery to stabilize the upper cervical spine, usually by posterior spinal fusion, before the development of cervical myelopathy can be lifesaving. The appearance of genu valgus, kyphosis, growth retardation with short trunk and neck, and waddling gait with a tendency to fall are early symptoms of MPS IV. Extraskeletal manifestations may include mild corneal clouding, hepatomegaly, cardiac valvular lesions, and small teeth with abnormally thin enamel and frequent caries formation. Patients with mild forms of MPS IV have been reported with almost normal stature, mild skeletal anomalies with dysplastic hips, corneal clouding, and absent keratosulfaturia.

The gene encoding N-acetylgalactosamine-6-sulfatase (MPS IV A [Morquio A) spans about 50 kb, contains 14 exons, and is on chromosome 16q24.3. About 100 MPS IV A mutations are known, consisting of missense or small deletions. Two mutations are recurring in patients from Northern Ireland and Australia and may explain the relatively high incidence (founder effect) of MPS IV in Northern Ireland. Several missense mutations are described in the β-galactosidase gene that causes MPS IV B, a rare form of Morquio syndrome.

MUCOPOLYSACCHARIDOSIS VI. Maroteaux-Lamy syndrome, caused by deficiency of N-acetylgalactosamine-4-sulfatase, is characterized by preservation of intelligence but with severe to mild somatic involvement, as seen in MPS I. The somatic involvement of the severe form of MPS IV is characterized by corneal clouding, coarse facial features, joint stiffness, valvular heart disease, communicating hydrocephalus, and dysostosis multiplex. In the severe form, growth can be normal for the first few years of life but seems to virtually stop after age 6–8 yr. The mild to intermediate forms of Maroteaux-Lamy syndrome can be easily confused with Scheie syndrome. Spinal cord compression from thickening of the dura in the upper cervical canal with resultant myelopathy is a frequent occurrence in patients with the milder form of MPS VI.

The gene encoding N-acetylgalactosamine-4-sulfatase (arylsulfatase B) is composed of eight exons and has been localized to chromosome 5q13q14. More than 30 mutations are known, most of which are in single families. Mutations found in MPS VI include frameshift, nonsense, and missense mutations.

MUCOPOLYSACCHARIDOSIS VII. Sly syndrome (MPS VII), resulting from a deficiency of β-glucuronidase, is the rarest of all forms of MPS but also has the widest range of clinical involvement from a neonatal form to mild disease in adults. A severe neonatal form is characterized by hydrops fetalis, dysostosis multiplex, and clinical and pathologic findings of a lysosomal storage disease. The severe neonatal form of β-glucuronidase deficiency is one of the few lysosomal storage diseases diagnosable in utero or at birth. The clinical involvement in MPS VII is similar to that seen in MPS I, with coarse facial features, hepatosplenomegaly, umbilical hernias, gibbus, and dysostosis multiplex, with varying degrees of clinical severity and mental retardation. Granulocytes have coarse metachromatic granules.

The gene encoding β-glucuronidase spans 21 kb, contains 12 exons, and is localized to chromosome 7q21.1. More than 35 mutations are known, mostly missense, but also nonsense, frameshift, and splice site.

MUCOPOLYSACCHARIDOSIS IX. Clinical findings in one case are bilateral nodular soft tissue periarticular masses, lysosomal storage of GAGs, mildly dysmorphic craniofacial features, short stature, and normal joint movement and intelligence. The clinical findings may be caused by an inability to degrade the hyaluronan (formerly called hyaluronic acid) that is normally found in cartilage and synovial fluid.

Diagnosis. Analysis of urinary GAGs is an initial diagnostic test. Many methods are available for urinary GAG analysis, ranging from the semiquantitative spot test to more precise qualitative and quantitative analyses. Spot tests are quick, inexpensive, and useful for initial evaluation but are subject to both false-positive and false-negative results, with reliability largely dependent on the testing laboratory. Any individual who is suspected of an MPS disorder based on clinical features, radiographic results, or urinary mucopolysaccharide screening tests should have a definitive diagnosis established by enzyme assay. Serum, leukocytes, or cultured fibroblasts are used as the tissue source for measuring lysosomal enzymes. The choice of tissue used depends on the particular enzyme and the preference of the laboratory. Prenatal diagnosis is available for all MPSs and is carried out on cultured cells from amniotic fluid or chorionic villus biopsy. Measurement of GAGs in amniotic fluid is unreliable. Carrier testing is difficult to perform by enzyme analysis. Carrier testing by enzyme analysis in Hunter syndrome, an X-linked disorder, is problematic and is not recommended. Molecular diagnosis is the preferred method of carrier testing provided that the mutation in the family under consideration is known.

Treatment. Bone marrow transplantation has resulted in significant clinical improvement of somatic disease in MPS I and increased long-term survival. Resolution or improvements have been noted in hepatosplenomegaly, joint stiffness, facial appearance, obstructive sleep apnea, heart disease, communicating hydrocephalus, and hearing loss. However, the skeletal and ocular anomalies are not corrected. Orthopedic procedures, including femoral osteotomies, acetabular reconstruction, and posterior spinal fusion, are necessary for most patients with Hurler syndrome after bone marrow transplantation to maintain function and gait. The neuropsychologic outcomes of MPS vary widely after bone marrow transplantation. Hurler syndrome patients who have undergone transplantation before 24 mo of age and with a baseline mental development index greater than 70 have improved long-term outcome. The microglia cells in the CNS, which are of bone marrow origin, are believed to be the source of the enzyme in the brain after bone marrow transplantation. Preservation of intelligence has not occurred in patients with severe MPS II or MPS III. Bone marrow transplantation is recommended for Hurler syndrome in patients who are younger than 24 mo of age and have no significant neurologic disease at the time of transplantation. Although bone marrow transplantation has significantly modified the natural history of the disease and improved survival in some patients, the procedure is not curative. Somatic disease has generally improved, except for the skeleton and eyes, but neurologic outcomes have varied.

Enzyme replacement using recombinant enzyme is a promising method to treat the somatic features of MPSs. There are ongoing clinical trials of recombinant α-L-iduronidase for MPS I patients. Early results demonstrate normalization of urinary GAG excretion, decreased or normalization of liver and spleen size, improved growth, decreased episodes of sleep apnea, improved joint range of motion, decreased pain, enhanced endurance, and improved activity. Enzyme replacement therapy trials using recombinant enzyme should be initiated in other MPS disorders once adequate quantities of recombinant enzyme are produced. Recombinant enzyme administered peripherally is not expected to cross the blood-brain barrier and improve or stabilize the CNS disease. Complications of enzyme replacement may include antibody formation against the recombinant enzyme and allergic reactions (urticaria).

Because most patients are not candidates for specific therapies at this time, supportive management, with particular attention to respiratory and cardiovascular complications, hearing loss, carpal tunnel syndrome, spinal cord compression, and hydrocephalus, can greatly improve the quality of life for patients and their families (see Table 77–2). The progressive nature of clinical involvement in MPS patients dictates the need for specialized and coordinated evaluation of their clinical status on a regular basis.

Cleary MA, Wraith JE: Management of mucopolysaccharidosis type III. *Arch Dis Child* 1993;69:403–6.

Danos O, Heard JM: Mucopolysaccharidosis. *Mol Cell Biol Hum Dis* 1995;5:350–67.

Guffon N, Souillet G, Maire I, et al: Follow-up of nine patients with Hurler syndrome after bone marrow transplantation. *J Pediatr* 1998;133:119–25.

Hopwood JJ, Bunge S, Morris CP, et al: Molecular basis of mucopolysaccharidosis type II: Mutations in the iduronate-2-sulphatase gene. *Hum Mutat* 1993;2: 435–42.

Hopwood JJ, Morris CP: The mucopolysaccharidoses: Diagnosis, molecular genetics and treatment. *Mol Biol Med* 1990;7:381–404.

Kakkis ED, Muenzer J, Tiller GE, et al: Enzyme-replacement therapy in mucopolysaccharidosis I. *N Engl J Med* 2001;344:182–8.

Mikles M, Stanton RP: A review of Morquio syndrome. *Am J Orthop* 1997;26: 533–40.

Neufeld EF, Muenzer J: The mucopolysaccharidoses. In Scriver CR, Beaudet AL, Sly WS, et al (editors): *The Metabolic Basis of Inherited Disease*, 7th ed, Vol II. New York, McGraw-Hill, 1995, p 2465.

Northover H, Cowie RA, Wraith JE: Mucopolysaccharidosis type IV A (Morquio syndrome): A clinical review. *J Inherit Metab Dis* 1996;19:357–65.

Peters C, Shapiro EG, Anderson J, et al: Hurler syndrome: II. Outcome of HLA-genotypically identical sibling and HLA-haploidentical related donor bone marrow transplantation in fifty-four children. *Blood* 1998;91:2601–8.

Peters C, Shapiro EG, Krivit W: Hurler syndrome: Past, present, and future. *J Pediatr* 1998;133:7–9.

Sands MS, Wolfe JH, Birkenmeier EH, et al: Gene therapy for murine mucopolysaccharidosis type VII. *Neuromuscul Disord* 1997;7:352–60.

Schmidtchen A, Greenberg D, Zhao HG, et al: NAGLU mutations underlying Sanfilippo syndrome type B. *Am J Hum Genet* 1998;62:64–9.

Scott HS, Bunge S, Gal A, et al: Molecular genetics of mucopolysaccharidosis type I: Diagnostic, clinical, and biological implications. *Hum Mutat* 1995;6:288–302.

Shapiro EG, Lockman LA, Balthazor M, et al: Neuropsychological outcomes of several storage diseases with and without bone marrow transplantation. *J Inherit Metab Dis* 1995;18:413–29.

Stone JE: Urine analysis in the diagnosis of mucopolysaccharide disorders. *Ann Clin Biochem* 1998;35:207–25.

Suzuki K, Proia RL, Suzuki K: Mouse models of human lysosomal diseases. *Brain Pathol* 1998;8:195–215.

Tandon V, Williamson JB, Cowie RA, et al: Spinal problems in mucopolysaccharidosis I (Hurler syndrome). *J Bone Joint Surg Am* 1996;78:938–44.

Van Heest AE, House J, Krivit W, et al: Surgical treatment of carpal tunnel syndrome and trigger digits in children with mucopolysaccharide storage disorders. *J Hand Surg [Am]* 1998;23:236–43.

Whitley CB, Belani KG, Chang P, et al: Long-term outcome of Hurler syndrome following bone marrow transplantation. *Am J Hum Genet* 1993;46:209–18.

Wraith JE: The mucopolysaccharidoses: A clinical review and guide to management. *Arch Dis Child* 1995;72:263–67.

Chapter 78

Disorders of Purine and Pyrimidine Metabolism

James C. Harris

Purines provide the primary source of cellular energy through adenosine triphosphate (ATP) and, together with pyrimidines, provide the source for the RNA and DNA that stores, transcribes, and translates genetic information. Purines also provide the basic coenzymes (nicotinamide-adenine dinucleotide [NAD] and its reduced form [NADH]) for metabolic regulation and play a major role in signal transduction and translation (guanosine triphosphate [GTP], cyclic adenosine monophosphate [AMP], cyclic guanosine monophosphate [GMP]). Metabolically active nucleotides are formed from heterocyclic nitrogen-containing purine bases (guanine and adenine) and pyrimidine bases (cytosine, uridine, and thymine). The early steps in the biosynthesis of the purine ring are shown in Figure 78–1. Purines are primarily produced from endogenous sources; dietary purines usually have a small role. The end product of purine metabolism in humans is uric acid (2,6,8-trioxypurine).

The inherited disorders of purine and pyrimidine metabolism cover a broad spectrum of illnesses with various presentations. These include hyperuricemia, acute renal failure, gout, unexplained neurologic deficits (seizures, muscle weakness, choreoathetoid and dystonic movements), developmental disability, mental retardation, compulsive self-injury and aggression, autistic-like behavior, unexplained anemia, failure to thrive, susceptibility to recurrent infection (immune deficiency), and deafness.

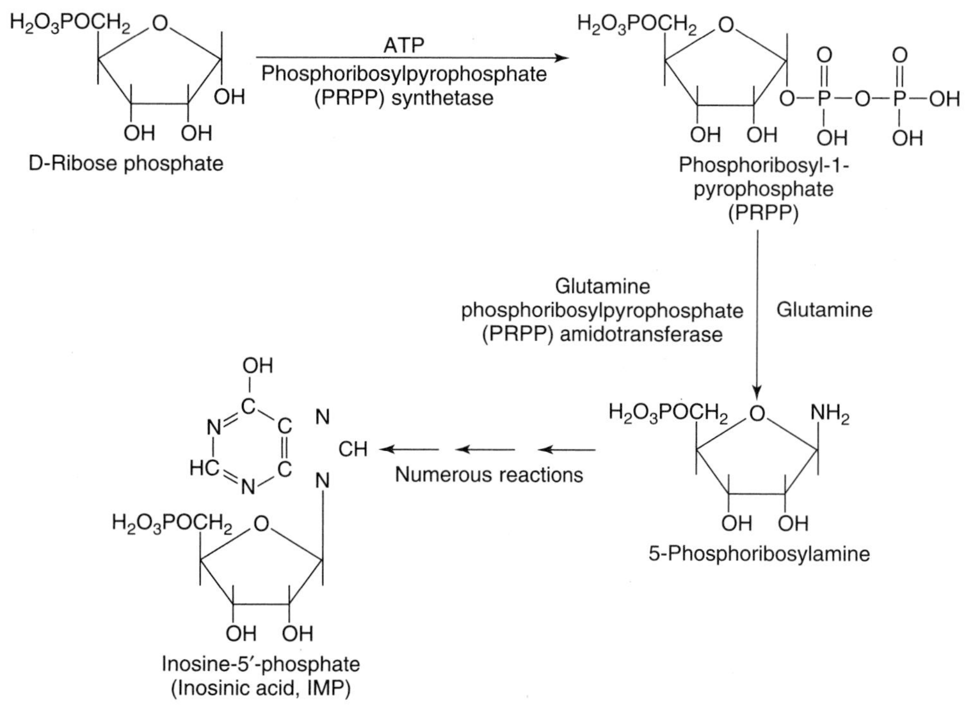

FIGURE 78–1. Early steps in the biosynthesis of the purine ring.

Although uric acid is not a specific disease marker, increased serum levels in children should always lead to the investigation of the cause of its elevation. The level of uric acid present at any time depends on the size of the purine nucleotide pool derived from de novo purine synthesis, catabolism of tissue nucleic acids, and increased turnover of preformed purines. Uric acid is poorly soluble and must be excreted continuously to avoid toxic accumulations in the body. Its renal excretion involves the following components: (1) glomerular filtration, (2) reabsorption in the proximal convoluted tubule, (3) secretion near the terminus of the proximal tubule, and (4) limited reabsorption near these secretory sites. Thus, renal loss of uric acid is a result of renal tube excretion and is a function of serum uric acid concentration and a homeostatic mechanism to avoid hyperuricemia. Serum uric acid levels are a less reliable indicator of uric acid production in children than in adults, and, consequently, measurement of the level in urine may be required to determine excessive production in children. Clearance of a smaller portion of uric acid is via the gastrointestinal tract (biliary and intestinal secretion). Because of the poor solubility of uric acid under normal circumstances, uric acid is near the maximal tolerable limits, and small alterations in production or solubility or changes in secretion may result in high serum levels. In renal insufficiency, urate excretion is increased by residual nephrons and by the gastrointestinal tract. Increased production of uric acid is found in malignancy; Reye syndrome; Down syndrome; psoriasis; sickle cell anemia; cyanotic congenital heart disease; pancreatic enzyme replacement; glycogen storage disease types I, III, IV, and V; hereditary fructose intolerance; acyl-coenzyme A dehydrogenase deficiency; and gout.

The *metabolism* of both purines and pyrimidines can be divided into two biosynthetic pathways and a catabolic pathway. The first involves a multistep biosynthesis from precursors through the de novo pathway that leads to the production of purine and pyrimidine nucleotides from ribose-5-phosphate or carbamyl phosphate, respectively. The second is a single-step salvage pathway that recovers purine and pyrimidine bases derived from either dietary intake or the catabolic pathway (Figs. 78–1, 78–2, and 78–3). In the de novo pathway, the nucleosides guanosine, adenosine, cytidine, uridine, and thymidine

are formed by the addition of ribose-1-phosphate to the purine bases guanine or adenine and to the pyrimidine bases cytosine, uracil, and thymine. The phosphorylation of these nucleosides produces monophosphate, diphosphate, and triphosphate nucleotides. Under usual circumstances, the salvage pathway predominates over the biosynthetic pathway. Synthesis is most active in tissues with high rates of cellular turnover, such as gut epithelium, skin, and bone marrow. The third pathway is catabolism. The end product of the catabolic pathway of the purines is uric acid, whereas catabolism of pyrimidines produces citric acid cycle intermediates. Only a small fraction of the purines turned over each day are degraded and excreted.

Inborn errors in the *synthesis* of purine nucleotides include (1) phosphoribosylpyrophosphate synthetase superactivity and (2) adenylosuccinase deficiency. Disorders resulting from abnormalities in purine *catabolism* include (3) muscle AMP deaminase deficiency, (4) adenosine deaminase deficiency, (5) purine nucleoside phosphorylase deficiency, and (6) xanthine oxidoreductase deficiency. Disorders resulting from the purine *salvage* pathway include (7) hypoxanthine-guanine phosphoribosyltransferase (HPRT) deficiency and (8) adenine phosphoribosyltransferase (APRT) deficiency.

Inborn errors of pyrimidine metabolism include (1) hereditary orotic aciduria (uridine monophosphate synthase deficiency), (2) dihydropyrimidine dehydrogenase deficiency, (3) dihydropyrimidinase deficiency, (4) β-ureidopropionase deficiency, (5) pyrimidine 5'-nucleotidase deficiency, (6) pyrimidine 5'-nucleotidase superactivity, and (7) thymidine phosphorylase deficiency.

GOUT

Gout presents as hyperuricemia, uric acid nephrolithiasis, and acute inflammatory arthritis. Gouty arthritis is due to monosodium urate crystal deposits that result in inflammation in joints and surrounding tissues. The presentation is most commonly monoarticular, typically in the metatarsophalangeal joint of the big toe. Tophi, deposits of monosodium urate crystals, may occur over points of insertion of tendons at the elbows, knees, and feet or over the helix of the ears. *Primary gout,*

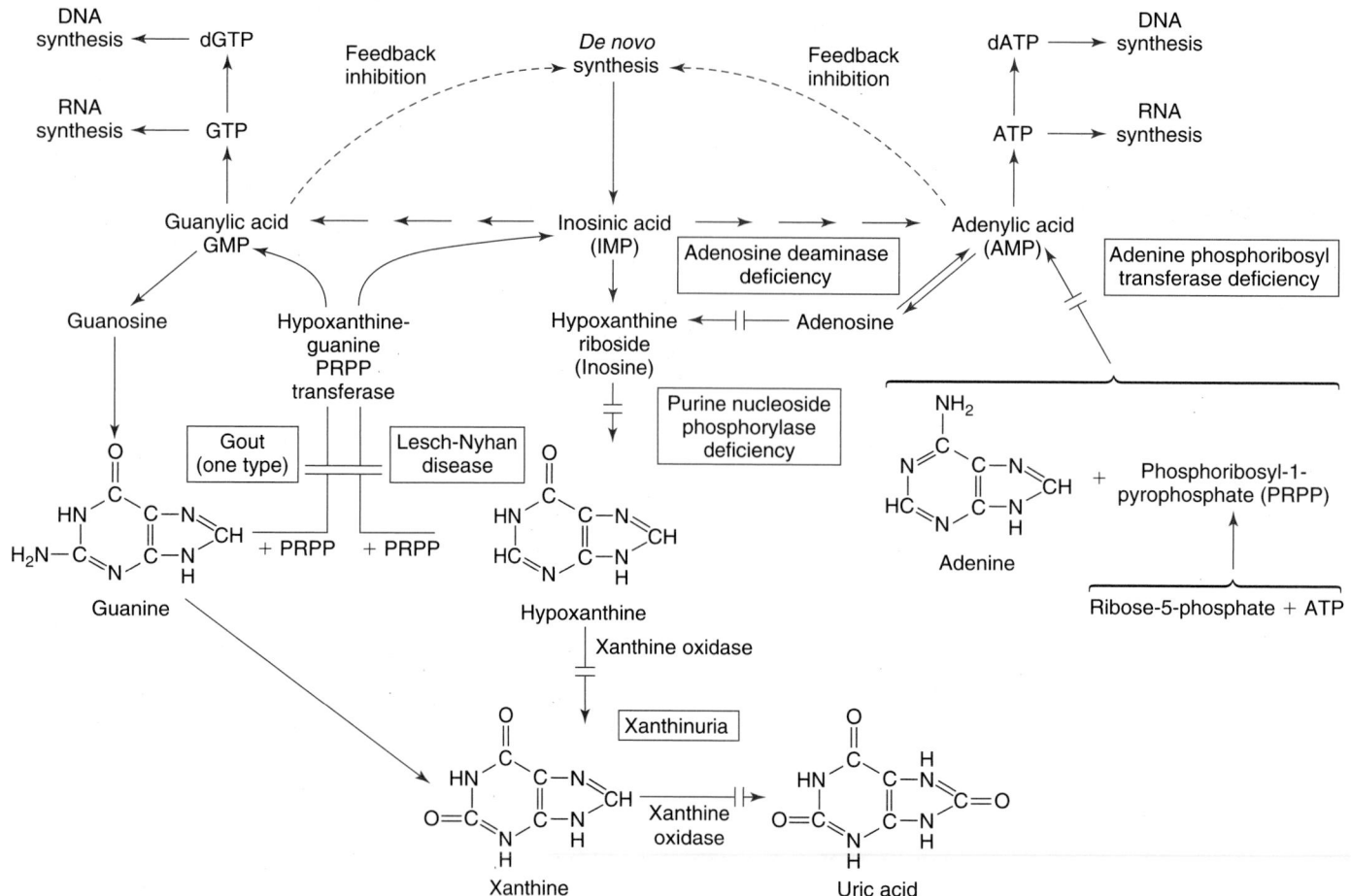

FIGURE 78–2. Pathways in purine metabolism and salvage.

ordinarily occurring in middle-aged men, results from the over-production, decreased renal excretion, or both, of uric acid. Its biochemical etiology is unknown for most of those affected, and it is considered to be a polygenic trait. When hyperuricemia and gout occur in childhood, it is most often *secondary gout*, the result of another disorder in which there is rapid tissue breakdown or cellular turnover leading to increased production or decreased excretion of uric acid. Gout occurs in any condition that leads to reduced clearance of uric acid: during therapy for malignancy or with dehydration, lactic acidosis, ketoacidosis, starvation, diuretic therapy, and renal failure. Excessive purine, alcohol, or carbohydrate ingestion may increase uric acid levels.

Gout is associated with hereditary disorders in three different enzyme disorders that result in hyperuricemia. These include the severe form of HPRT deficiency (Lesch-Nyhan syndrome), partial HPRT deficiency, superactivity of PP-ribose-P synthetase, and glycogen storage disease, type I (glucose-6-phosphatase deficiency) (see Chapter 76.1). In the first two, the basis of hyperuricemia is purine nucleotide and uric acid overproduction, whereas in the third it is both excessive uric acid production and impaired uric acid secretion. Glycogen storage disease types III, V, and VII are associated with exercise-induced hyperuricemia, the consequence of rapid ATP utilization and failure to regenerate it effectively during exercise (see Chapter 76.1).

Familial juvenile gout or familial juvenile hyperuricemic nephropathy (FJHN) is associated with severe renal hypoexcretion of uric acid. Although patients most commonly present from puberty up to the 3rd decade, it has been reported in infancy. It is characterized by hyperuricemia, gout, familial renal disease, and low urate clearance relative to glomerular filtration rate. Familial juvenile hyperuricemic nephropathy is an autosomal dominant disorder, unlike the three inherited purine disorders that are X-linked and the recessively inherited glycogen storage disease. Linkage to 16p12 has been reported in one study of an affected family. It occurs in both males and females and is frequently associated with a rapid decline in renal function that may lead to death unless diagnosed and treated early. Once familial juvenile hyperuricemic nephropathy is recognized, presymptomatic detection is of critical importance to identify asymptomatic family members with hyperuricemia and to begin treatment, when indicated, to prevent nephropathy.

Treatment of hyperuricemia involves the combination of allopurinol (a xanthine oxidase inhibitor) to decrease uric acid production, probenecid to increase uric acid clearance in those with normal renal function, alkalinization of the urine to increase the solubility of uric acid, and increased fluid intake to reduce the concentration of uric acid. A low purine diet, weight reduction, and reduced alcohol intake are recommended.

ABNORMALITIES IN PURINE SALVAGE

Lesch-Nyhan Syndrome

Lesch-Nyhan syndrome (LNS) is a rare X-linked disorder of purine metabolism that results from HPRT deficiency. This enzyme is normally present in each cell in the body, but its highest concentration is in the brain, especially in the basal ganglia. Manifestations include hyperuricemia, mental retardation, cerebral palsy with early choreoathetosis and later spasticity and dystonia, dysarthric speech, and compulsive self-biting, usually beginning with the eruption of teeth.

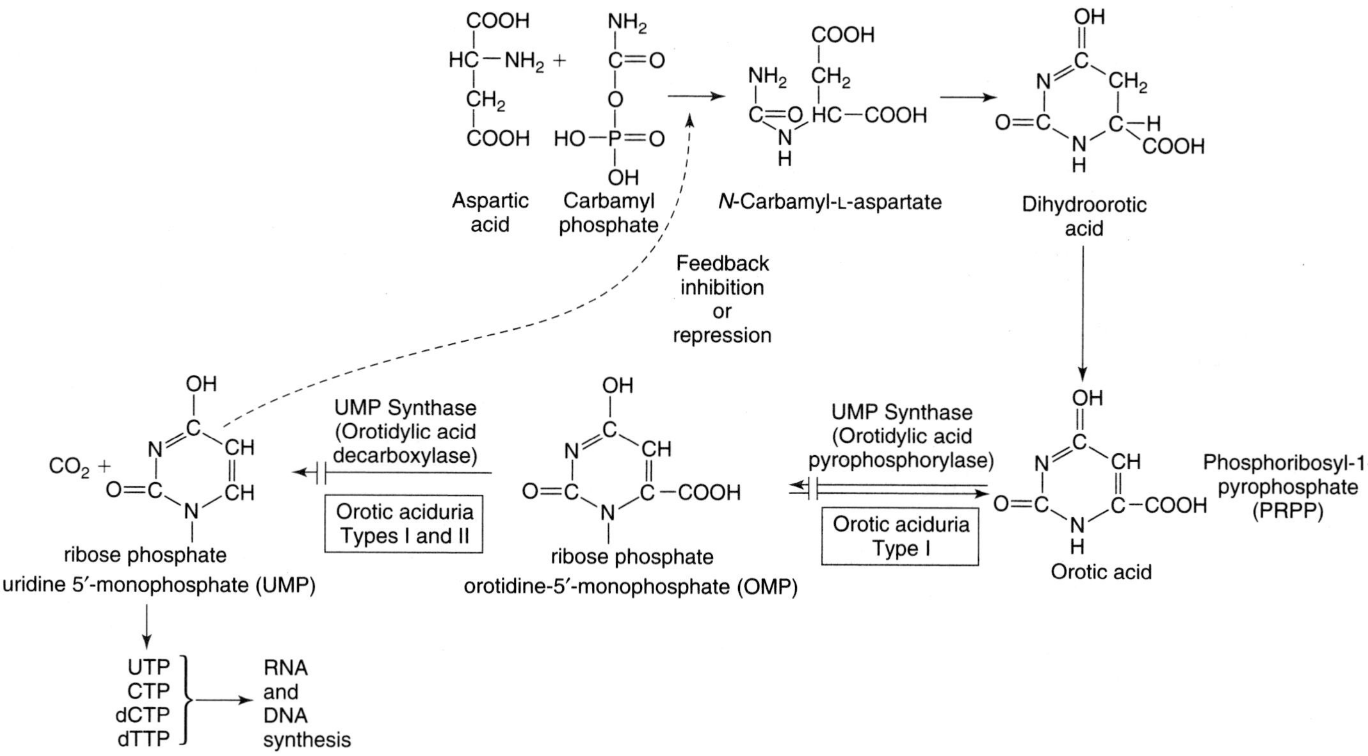

FIGURE 78–3. Pathways in pyrimidine biosynthesis.

There are several clinical presentations of HPRT deficiency. HPRT levels are related to the extent of motor symptoms, to the presence or absence of self-injury, and possibly to the level of cognitive function. The majority of individuals with classic LNS have low or undetectable levels of the HPRT enzyme. Partial deficiency in HPRT (Kelley-Seegmiller syndrome) with more than 1.5–2.0% enzyme is associated with hyperuricemia and variable neurologic dysfunction (neurologic HPRT deficiency). HPRT deficiency with levels over 8% leads to a severe form of gout, with apparently normal cerebral functioning (HPRT-related hyperuricemia), although cognitive deficits may occur. Qualitatively similar cognitive deficit profiles have been reported in both LNS and variant cases. Variants have scores that are intermediate between those of patients with LNS and normal controls on nearly every neuropsychological measure tested.

Genetics. The *HPRT* gene has been localized to the long arm of the X chromosome (q26-q27). The complete amino acid sequence for *HPRT* is known (approximately 44 kb, 9 exons). The disorder appears in males; occurrence in females is extremely rare and ascribed to nonrandom inactivation of the X chromosome. Absence of *HPRT* prevents the normal metabolism of hypoxanthine, resulting in excessive uric acid production and manifestations of gout, necessitating specific drug treatment (allopurinol). Because of the enzyme deficiency, hypoxanthine accumulates in the cerebrospinal fluid, but uric acid does not; uric acid is not produced in the brain and does not cross the blood-brain barrier. The behavior disorder is not caused by hyperuricemia or excess hypoxanthine because patients with partial HPRT deficiency, the variants with hyperuricemia, do not self-injure and infants having isolated hyperuricemia from birth do not develop self-injurious behavior.

The prevalence of classic LNS has been estimated at 1 in 100,000 to 1 in 380,000 based on the number of known cases in the United States. The incidence of partial variants is not known. Those with the classic syndrome rarely survive the 3rd decade because of renal or respiratory compromise. The life span may be normal for patients with partial HPRT deficiency without severe renal involvement.

Pathology. MRI demonstrates reductions in the volume of basal ganglia nuclei. Abnormalities in neurotransmitter metabolism have been identified in three autopsied cases with very low HPRT levels. There was a functional loss of 65–90% of the nigrostriatal and mesolimbic dopamine terminals, although the cells of origin in the substantia nigra did not show dopamine reduction. The brain regions primarily involved were the caudate nucleus, putamen, and nucleus accumbens. The neurochemical changes may be linked to functional abnormalities, possibly resulting from a diminution of arborization or branching of dendrites rather than cell loss. A neurotransmitter abnormality is demonstrated by changes in cerebrospinal fluid neurotransmitters and their metabolites and confirmed by positron emission tomography scans of dopamine function. Reductions in vivo in the presynaptic dopamine transporter have been documented in the caudate and putamen.

The mechanism whereby HPRT leads to the neurologic and behavioral symptoms is unknown. However, both hypoxanthine and guanine metabolism is affected and guanine triphosphate (GTP) and adenosine have substantial effects on neural tissues. There is a functional link between purine nucleotides and the dopamine system that involves guanine, the precursor of GTP. Dopamine binding to its receptor results in either an activation (D_1 receptor) or an inhibition (D_2 receptor) of adenylcyclase. Both receptor effects are mediated by G proteins (GTP-binding proteins) dependent on guanine diphosphate (GDP) in the GDP/GTP exchange for cellular activation. Dopamine and adenosine systems are also linked through the role of adenosine as a neuroprotective agent in preventing neurotoxicity. Adenosine agonists mimic the biochemical and behavioral actions of dopamine antagonists, whereas adenosine receptor antagonists act as functional dopamine agonists. Dopamine reduction in brain is documented in HPRT-deficient strains of mutant mice.

Clinical Manifestations. At birth, infants with LNS have no apparent neurologic dysfunction. After several months, developmental retardation and neurologic signs become apparent. Before the age of 4 mo, hypotonia, recurrent vomiting, and difficulty with secretions may be noted. By 8–12 mo, extrapyramidal signs appear, including chorea and dystonia. By approximately 12 mo, in a significant number of cases, pyramidal tract signs may become evident with hyperreflexia, sustained ankle clonus, positive Babinski sign, and scissoring. Spasticity may become apparent at this time or, in some instances, later in life.

Cognitive function is usually reported to be in the mild-to-moderate range of mental retardation, although some individuals test in the low normal range. Because test scores may be influenced by difficulty in testing the subjects owing to their movement disorder and dysarthric speech, overall intelligence may be underestimated.

The age at onset of self-injury may be as early as 1 yr and occasionally as late as the teens. Self-injury occurs, although all sensory modalities, including pain, are intact. The self-injurious behavior usually begins with self-biting, although other patterns of self-injurious behavior emerge with time. Most characteristically, the fingers, mouth, and buccal mucosa are mutilated. Self-biting is intense and causes tissue damage and may result in the amputation of fingers and substantial loss of tissue around the lips. Extraction of primary teeth may be required. The biting pattern can be asymmetric, with preferential mutilation of the left or right side of the body. The type of behavior is different from that seen in other mental retardation syndromes involving self-injury where self-hitting and head banging are the most common initial presentations. The intensity of the self-injurious behavior generally requires that the patient be restrained. When restraints are removed, the individual with LNS may appear terrified and stereotypically place a finger in the mouth. The patient may ask for restraints to prevent elbow movement; when the restraints are placed or replaced, he may appear relaxed and more good humored. Dysarthric speech may cause interpersonal communication problems; however, the higher-functioning children can express themselves fully and participate in verbal therapy.

The self-mutilation presents as a compulsive behavior that the child tries to control but frequently is unable to resist. Older individuals may enlist the help of others and notify them when they are comfortable enough to have restraints removed. In some instances, the behavior may be followed by deliberate self-harm. The individual with LNS may also show compulsive aggression and inflict injury to others through pinching, grabbing, or hitting or by using verbal forms of aggression. Afterward the person may apologize, stating that this behavior was out of his or her control. Other maladaptive behaviors include head or limb banging, eye poking, and psychogenic vomiting.

Diagnosis. The presence of dystonia along with self-mutilation of the mouth and fingers suggests LNS. With partial HPRT deficiency, recognition is linked to either hyperuricemia alone or hyperuricemia and a dystonic movement disorder, but there is no self-injurous behavior. Serum levels of uric acid that exceed 4–5 mg uric acid/dL and a urine uric acid:creatinine ratio of 3:4 or more are highly suggestive of HPRT deficiency, particularly when associated with neurologic symptoms. The definitive diagnosis requires an analysis of the HPRT enzyme in an erythrocyte lysate. Individuals with classic LNS have near 0% enzyme activity, and those with partial variants show values between 1.5% and 60%. The intact cell HPRT assay in skin fibroblasts offers a good correlation between enzyme activity and the severity of the disease. Molecular techniques are used for gene sequencing and the identification of carriers.

Differential diagnosis includes other causes of infantile hypotonia and dystonia. Children with LNS are often initially incorrectly diagnosed as having athetoid cerebral palsy. When a diagnosis of cerebral palsy is suspected in an infant with a normal prenatal, perinatal, and postnatal course, LNS should be considered. Partial HPRT deficiency may be associated with acute renal failure in infancy; therefore, clinical awareness of partial HPRT deficiency is of particular importance.

An understanding of the molecular disorder has led to effective drug treatment for uric acid accumulation and arthritic tophi, renal stones, and neuropathy. Reduction in uric acid alone does not influence the neurologic and behavioral aspects of LNS. Despite treatment from birth for uric acid elevation, behavioral and neurologic symptoms are unaffected. The most significant complications of LNS are renal failure and self-mutilation.

Treatment. Medical management of this disorder focuses on the prevention of renal failure by pharmacologic treatment of hyperuricemia with allopurinol, efforts to reduce self-mutilation through behavior management and psychosocial support, and the use of restraints or removal of teeth or both. Pharmacologic approaches to decrease anxiety and spasticity with medication have mixed results. Drug therapy focuses on symptomatic management of anticipatory anxiety, mood stabilization, and reduction of self-injurious behavior. Although there is no standard drug treatment, diazepam may be helpful for anxiety symptoms, risperidone for aggressive behavior, and carbamazepine or gabapentin for mood stabilization. Each of these medications may reduce self-injurious behavior by helping to reduce anxiety and/or stabilize mood.

Bone marrow transplantation, which is based on the possibility that the central nervous system damage is produced by a circulating toxin, has been carried out in several patients. Several infant patients have died of complications of bone marrow transplantation. In one adult case in which the transplantation was successful, there was no change in neurologic symptoms or in behavior. In this case, dopamine receptors measured by positron emission tomography before and after the bone marrow transplantation showed no changes in receptor density. There is no evidence that bone marrow transplantation is a beneficial treatment approach. Two patients received partial exchange transfusions every 2 mo for 3–4 years. Erythrocyte hypoxanthine-guanine phosphoribosyltransferase activity was 10–70% of normal during this period, but no reduction of neurologic or behavioral symptoms was apparent. Successful preimplantation genetic diagnosis and in vitro fertilization for LNS has been reported with the birth of an unaffected male infant.

Both the motivation for self-injury and its biologic basis must be addressed in treatment programs. Behavioral techniques alone, using operant conditioning approaches, have not proved to be an adequate general treatment. Although behavioral procedures have had some selective success in reducing self-injury, generalization outside the experimental setting limits this approach and patients under stress may revert to their previous self-injurious behavior. Behavioral approaches may also focus on reducing the self-injurious behavior through the treatment of phobic anxiety associated with being unrestrained. The most common techniques are systematic desensitization, extinction, and differential reinforcement of other (competing) behavior. Stress management has been recommended to assist patients to develop more effective coping mechanisms. Individuals with LNS do not respond to contingent electric shock or similar aversive behavioral measures. An increase in self-injury may be observed when aversive methods are utilized.

Restraint (day and night) and dental procedures are used to prevent self-injury. The time in restraints is linked to the age at onset of self-injury. Children with LNS can participate in making decisions regarding restraints and the type of restraints. The time in restraints may potentially be reduced with systematic behavior treatment programs. Many patients have teeth extracted to prevent self-injury. Others use a protective mouth-guard designed by a dentist. Most parents suggest that stress reduction and awareness of the patient's needs are the most effective in reducing self-injury. Parents reported that they deal with self-injury by attending to physical comfort and adjusting restraints, talking to the child, and finding something more interesting to do. Positive behavioral techniques of reinforcing appropriate behavior are rated effective by almost half of the families. The use of anticonvulsants as mood stabilizers appears promising, but it requires further study.

Adenine Phosphoribosyltransferase Deficiency

Adenine phosphoribosyltransferase (APRT) catalyzes the synthesis of AMP from adenine and 5-phosphoribosyl-1-pyrophosphate (PP-ribose-P). The absence of this enzyme results in the inability to utilize adenine and in the accumulation of 2,8-dihydroxyadenine, which is extremely insoluble. APRT deficiency is present from birth, becoming apparent as early as 5 mo and as late as the 7th decade. *Clinical manifestations* include urinary calculus formation with crystalluria, urinary tract infections, hematuria, renal colic, dysuria, and acute renal failure. The renal calculi, composed of 2,8-dihydroxyadenine, are radiolucent, soft, and easily crushed. These stones are not distinguishable from uric acid stones by routine tests but require confirmation from the ultraviolet (UV) and infrared (IR) spectrums, mass spectroscopy (MS), x-ray crystallography, or capillary electrophoresis for diagnosis. The presence of brownish spots on the infant's diaper or of yellow-brown crystals in the urine is suggestive.

The enzyme deficiency causes suppression of the salvage of adenine from nutritional sources and the polyamine pathway, with adenine being oxidized by xanthine dehydrogenase into 2,8-dihydroxyadenine. Urinary levels of adenine, 8-hydroxyadenine, and 2,8-dihydroxyadenine are elevated, whereas plasma uric acid is normal. The deficiency may be complete (type I) or partial (type II); the partial deficiency is reported in Japan. The diagnosis is made based on the level of residual enzyme in erythrocyte lysates. The disorder is an autosomal recessive trait with considerable clinical heterogeneity. The *APRT* gene is located on chromosome 16q (16q24.3) and encompasses 2.8 kb of genomic DNA. Because identification of 2,8-dihydroxyadenine is complex, the most common diagnostic test is the measurement of APRT activity in erythrocyte lysates.

Treatment includes high fluid intake, dietary purine restriction, and allopurinol, which inhibits the conversion of adenine to its metabolites, further 2,8-dihydroxyadenine excretion, and further stone formation. Alkalinization of the urine is to be avoided, because, unlike that of uric acid, the solubility of 2, 8-dihydroxyadenine does not increase up to pH 9. Shock-wave lithotripsy can be successful. The prognosis depends on renal function at the time of diagnosis. Early treatment is critical in the prevention of stones because severe renal insufficiency may accompany late recognition.

DISORDERS LINKED TO PURINE NUCLEOTIDE SYNTHESIS

Phosphoribosylpyrophosphate Synthetase Superactivity

Phosphoribosylpyrophosphate is a substrate involved in the synthesis of essentially all nucleotides and important in the regulation of the de novo pathways of purine and pyrimidine nucleotide synthesis. Phosphoribosylpyrophosphate synthetase, (PRS) superactivity is inherited as an X-linked trait and presents as two clinical phenotypes with varying degrees of severity. Three distinct PRS cDNAs are known. Two forms are X linked to Xq22-q24 and Xp22.2-p.22.3, respectively, and are widely expressed; the third maps to human chromosome 7 and appears to be transcribed only in the testes. *Clinical manifestations* in the more severe type in affected hemizygous males include signs of uric acid overproduc-

tion that are apparent in infancy or early childhood, neurodevelopmental abnormalities, and sensorineural deafness. Hypotonia, delays in motor milestones, ataxia, and autistic-like behavior occur. Blood uric acid may be two to three times normal values, and the urinary excretion of uric acid is increased. Heterozygous female carriers may also develop gout and hearing impairment. The late juvenile to early adult onset type is found in males who show gout or uric acid urolithiasis but no neurologic signs.

This enzyme produces PRPP from ribose-5-phosphate and ATP, as shown in Figures 78–1 and 78–2. PRPP is the first intermediary compound in the de novo synthesis of purine nucleotides that lead to the formation of inosine monophosphate. Superactivity of the enzyme results in an increased generation of PRPP. Because PRPP amidotransferase, the first enzyme of the de novo pathway, is not physiologically saturated by PRPP, the synthesis of purine nucleotides increases, and, consequently, the production of uric acid is increased. A mechanism for the neurologic symptoms is unknown. The *diagnosis* requires kinetic studies of the enzyme performed in erythrocytes and cultured fibroblasts. This disorder must be differentiated from partial HPRT deficiency involving the salvage pathway, which also results in neurologic HPRT deficiency or hyperuricemia without neurologic features.

Treatment is with allopurinol, which inhibits xanthine oxidase, the last enzyme of the purine catabolic pathway. Uric acid production is reduced and is replaced by hypoxanthine, which is more soluble, and xanthine, which is slightly more soluble than uric acid. The initial dose of allopurinol is 10–20 mg/kg/24 hr in children and is adjusted to maintain normal uric acid levels in plasma. Occasionally, xanthine calculi may form. Consequently, a low purine diet (one free of organ meats, dried beans, and sardines), high fluid intake, and alkalinization of the urine to establish a urinary pH of 6.0–6.5 is necessary. These measures control the hyperuricemia and urate neuropathy but do not affect the neurologic symptoms.

Adenylosuccinate Lyase Deficiency

Adenylosuccinase lyase (ADSL) catalyzes two pathways in de novo synthesis and purine nucleotide recycling. These are the conversion of succinylaminoimidazole carboxamide ribotide (SAICAR) into aminoimidazole carboxamide ribotide (AICAR) in the de novo synthesis of purine nucleotides and the conversion of adenylosuccinate (S-AMP) into adenosine monophosphate (AMP), the second step in the conversion of inosine monophosphate (IMP) into AMP, in the purine nucleotide cycle. ADSL deficiency results in the accumulation in urine, cerebrospinal fluid, and, to a smaller extent, in plasma, of SAICA riboside (SAICAr) and succinyladenosine (S-Ado), dephosphorylated derivatives of SAICAR and S-AMP, respectively. This is an autosomal recessive disorder; the gene is on chromosome 22q13.1-q13.2; about 20 gene mutations are known. *Clinical manifestations* include varying degrees of psychomotor retardation, generally accompanied by a seizure disorder and/or autistic-like behaviors (poor eye contact and repetitive behaviors). Other patients demonstrate moderate to severe mental retardation sometimes associated with growth retardation and muscle hypotonia. One reported case, a girl, tested in the mild range of mental retardation. Type I has profound mental retardation; cases with mild mental retardation are type II. Other patients have an intermediate clinical symptom pattern with moderately delayed psychomotor development, seizures, stereotypes, and agitation. CT and MRI of the brain may show hypotrophy or hypoplasia of the cerebellum, particularly the vermis. Symptoms may be caused by the neurotoxic effects of accumulating succinyl purines. The ratio of S-Ado/SAICAr is linked to phenotype severity, suggesting that SAICAr is the more toxic compound and that S-Ado might be neuroprotective. The *diagnosis* is based on the presence in urine and cerebrospinal fluid of SAICA riboside and S-ADO, both normally undetectable. No successful *treatment* has been demonstrated for this disorder. Prenatal diagnosis is possible. Systematic screening is suggested in infants and children with unexplained psychomotor retardation and/or seizures.

DISORDERS RESULTING FROM ABNORMALITIES IN PURINE CATABOLISM

Myoadenylate Deaminase Deficiency (Muscle Adenosine Monophosphate Deaminase Deficiency)

Myoadenylate deaminase is a muscle-specific isoenzyme of AMP deaminase that is active in skeletal muscle. During exercise, the deamination of AMP leads to increased levels of IMP and ammonia in proportion to the work performed by the muscle. Two forms of myoadenylate deaminase deficiency are known: (1) an inherited (primary) form that may be asymptomatic or associated with cramps or myalgia with exercise and (2) a form that may be associated with other neuromuscular or rheumatologic disorders. *Clinical manifestations* include isolated muscle weakness, fatigue, myalgias following moderate-to-vigorous exercise, or cramps. Myalgias may be associated with an increased serum creatine kinase level and detectable electromyelographic abnormalities. Muscle wasting or histologic changes on biopsy are absent. The age at onset may be as early 8 mo of life, with about 25% of cases recognized between 2 and 12 years of age. The enzyme defect has been identified in asymptomatic family members. Secondary forms of muscle AMP deaminase deficiency have been identified in Werdnig-Hoffmann disease, Kugelberg-Welander syndrome, polyneuropathies, and amyotrophic lateral sclerosis (see Chapter 603.2). The metabolic disorder involves the purine nucleotide cycle (see Fig. 78–2). Muscle dysfunction in AMP deaminase deficiency may result from impaired energy production during muscle contraction. It is unclear how affected individuals can be asymptomatic. A mutation of liver AMP deaminase has been proposed as a cause of primary gout, leading to overproduction of uric acid.

The inherited form of the disorder is an autosomal recessive trait. *AMP-D1*, the gene responsible for encoding muscle AMP deaminase, is located on the short arm of chromosome 1. This mutant allele is found at high frequency in white populations. The disorder may be screened for by performing an exercise test. The elevation of venous plasma ammonia after exercise that is seen in normal subjects is absent in AMP deaminase deficiency. The final diagnosis is made by histochemical or biochemical assays of a muscle biopsy. In the primary form enzyme levels are below 2% with little or no immunoprecipitable enzyme. Affected individuals are advised to exercise with caution to prevent rhabdomyolysis and myoglobinuria. It has been proposed that enhancing the rate of replenishment of the ATP pool might be beneficial. Using this rationale *treatment* with ribose (2–60 g/24 hr orally, in divided doses) or xylitol, which is converted to ribose, improves endurance and muscle strength in some cases but is ineffective in others. Genetic approaches may be feasible in the future for inherited cases whereas treatment of the underlying condition is essential in secondary cases.

Adenosine Deaminase Deficiency

See Chapter 116.1.

Purine Nucleoside Phosphorylase Deficiency

See Chapter 116.2.

Xanthine Oxidoreductase Deficiency

Xanthine oxidoreductase (XOR) is the catalytic enzyme in the final step of the purine catabolic pathway and oxidates hypoxanthine to xanthine and xanthine to uric acid. Because XOR exists in two forms, xanthine dehydrogenase and xanthine oxidase, the deficiency is also referred to as xanthine dehydrogenase/xanthine oxidase (XDH/XO) deficiency. Xanthine, the immediate precursor of uric acid, is less soluble than uric acid in urine, and deficiency of the enzyme results in xanthinuria. Xanthine oxidoreductase deficiency may occur in an isolated form (xanthinuria type 1), in a combined form involving xanthine oxidoreductase deficiency and aldehyde oxidase deficiency (xanthinuria type II), or in a combined form with deficiency of both xanthine oxidoreductase and aldehyde oxidase and sulfite oxidase deficiency (molybdenum co-factor deficiency). The isolated form results in an almost total replacement of uric acid by hypoxanthine and xanthine. Patients with the isolated form are usually asymptomatic or have mild symptoms; renal stones, often not visible on radiography, are a risk for renal damage and may appear at any age. Crystalline xanthine deposits in muscle may result in muscle pain after exertion. Rarely, xanthine stones may develop as a result of allopurinol administration. In type II, the clinical presentation is similar to type 1. Molybdenum co-factor deficiency (failure to synthesize the molybdenum co-factor) involves all three molybdoenzymes and like isolated sulfite oxidase deficiency results in neonatal feeding problems, neonatal seizures, increased or decreased muscle tone, ocular lens dislocation, severe mental retardation, and death in early childhood.

The inheritance of type I and II is autosomal recessive; the human XOR gene is located on chromosome 2p22. In both forms of the deficiency, measuring plasma concentrations of uric acid makes the diagnosis; plasma uric acid is low (<1 mg/dL), and xanthine is elevated in plasma and urine. Urinary uric acid is reduced and is replaced by xanthine and hypoxanthine. In molybdenum co-factor deficiency, there is also an excessive excretion of sulfite and other sulfur-containing metabolites. Enzyme diagnostic measurement requires jejunal or liver biopsy because these are the only human tissues that contain appreciable amounts of xanthine oxoreductase. Sulfite oxidase and the molybdenum co-factor can be measured in liver and fibroblasts. Although the isolated deficiency is generally benign, *treatment* with a low purine diet and increased fluid intake are recommended. Allopurinol has been recommended for those with residual xanthine oxoreductase activity. It completely blocks the conversion of hypoxanthine into the far less soluble xanthine. The prognosis for molybdenum co-factor deficiency is very poor, and drug trials to date have been unsuccessful. This disorder may be a candidate for somatic gene therapy in the future.

DISORDERS OF PYRIMIDINE METABOLISM

The pyrimidines are the building blocks of DNA and RNA and involved in the formation of coenzymes and active intermediates in carbohydrate and phospholipid metabolism. The pyrimidines uracil and thymine are degraded in four steps (see Fig. 78–3). Seven disorders of pyrimidine metabolism are known. The first defect, hereditary orotic aciduria, is in the de novo synthetic pathway, whereas the other disorders involve superactivity (in one syndrome) or defects in the pyrimidine degradation pathway. The first three steps of the degradation pathways for thymine and uracil, respectively, make use of the same enzymes (DPD, DPH, and UP). These three steps result in the conversion into β-alanine from uracil. Pyrimidines may play an important role in the regulation of the nervous system. Reduced production of the neurotransmitter function of β-alanine is hypothesized to produce clinical symptoms. These rare disorders may be overlooked because symptoms are not highly specific; however, they should be considered as possible causes of anemia and neurologic disease and are a contraindication for treatment of cancer patients with certain pyrimidine analogues.

Hereditary Orotic Aciduria (Uridine Monophosphate Synthase Deficiency)

Hereditary orotic aciduria is associated with deficient activity of the last two enzymes of the de novo pyrimidine synthetic pathway (orotate phosphoribosyltransferase and orotidine-5'-monophosphate decarboxylase). The activities of these two enzymes reside in separate domains to a single polypeptide coded by a single gene. This bifunctional protein, uridine 5'-monophosphate (UMP) synthase, catalyzes the two-step conversion of orotic acid to UMP. Hereditary orotic aciduria (UMP synthase deficiency) results in the excessive accumulation of orotic acid. *Clinically*, patients with hereditary orotic aciduria have a macrocytic hypochromic megaloblastic anemia that is unresponsive to the usual forms of therapy (iron, folic acid, and B_{12}) and may have leukopenia. If untreated, this disorder can lead to developmental retardation, failure to thrive, cardiac disease, strabismus, and crystalluria. Renal function is generally normal. Heterozygotes may have mild orotic aciduria but are not affected.

This disorder has autosomal recessive inheritance. The gene for uridine monophosphate synthase is located on the long arm of chromosome 3 (3q13). The clinical features may be related to pyrimidine nucleotide depletion. Metabolites derived from several pharmacologic agents (5-azauridine, allopurinol) produce secondary orotic aciduria and orotidinuria by specifically inhibiting orotidine-5'-monophosphate decarboxylase. Genetic metabolic defects that involve four of the six enzymes associated with the urea cycle may result in orotic aciduria secondary to PP-ribose-P depletion resulting from a substantial increased flux through the de novo pathway. Orotic aciduria may also occur in association with parenteral nutrition, essential amino acid deficiency, and Reye syndrome. The enzymatic defect may be demonstrated in liver, lymphoblasts, erythrocytes, leukocytes, and cultured skin fibroblasts. A carrier detection test is available, as is prenatal diagnosis.

The administration of uridine has been an effective *treatment* in most cases and leads to clinical improvement and reduction in orotic acid excretion. Lifelong treatment is required. Uracil is ineffective because, unlike purines, pyrimidine salvage occurs at the nucleoside level. The long-term *prognosis* in uncomplicated cases is good; congenital malformations and other associated features may adversely affect outcome.

Dihydropyrimidine Dehydrogenase Deficiency

Dihydropyrimidine dehydrogenase (DPD) catalyzes the initial and rate-limiting step in the degradation of the pyrimidine bases uracil and thiamine. DPD has been identified in most tissues, with the highest activity being in lymphocytes. DPD deficiency is characterized by a variable phenotype with accumulation of thiamine and uracil in urine, plasma, and cerebrospinal fluid and no activity in fibroblasts. DPD is the initial and rate-limiting enzyme in the catabolism of the neoplastic drug 5-fluorouracil, being responsible for 80% of its catabolism. Patients with a partial deficiency of this enzyme are at risk for developing a severe 5-fluorouracil–associated toxicity. Several clinical forms are described. The *clinical manifestations* in children may include seizure disorder, mental retardation, and motor delay in half of the patients. Less frequent are growth retardation, microcephaly, autistic-like behavior, and ocular anomalies. Others do not show developmental abnormalities but may have milder neurologic symptoms and language disorder. In most cases, there is an initial period of normal psychomotor development, followed by subsequent developmental delays. Symptoms may link to altered uracil, thymine, and β-alanine homeostasis. In adults, neurotoxicity (headache, somnolence, visual illusions, and memory impairment) is linked to pyrimidinemia after treatment for cancer with 5-fluorouracil.

DPD deficiency is an autosomal recessive disorder mapping to chromosome Ip22 with at least seven known mutations. It is estimated that the frequency of the heterozygote may be as high as 3%. Prenatal *diagnosis* is possible. Diagnostic tests use high-pressure liquid chromatography (HPLC) or gas chromatography/mass spectroscopy (GC/MS). Alternatively, DPD deficiency may be confirmed by measuring the enzyme in cultured fibroblasts and leukoblasts. Uric acid levels are normal. Because β-alanine is a structural analogue of γ-aminobutyric acid and glycine, it may affect inhibitory neurotransmission. There is no established *treatment* for this disorder, however; patients with seizures do respond to anticonvulsant medications. Patients with DPD deficiency should not be given 5-fluorouracil; its deficiency should be suspected when neurologic symptoms emerge after cancer treatment with 5-fluorouracil.

Dihydropyrimidinase Deficiency (Dihydropyrimidinuria)

Dihydropyrimidinase (DPH) is the second enzyme in the three-step degradation pathway of uracil and thiamine leading to increased urinary excretion. Dihydropyrimidinase deficiency is characterized by dihydropyrimidinuria and a variable clinical phenotype. *Clinical manifestations* in three unrelated affected cases include seizures with dysmorphic features and developmental delay in two of these cases. Three unrelated infant and two adult asymptomatic cases were identified in a screening program for pyrimidine-degradation disorders in Japan and were asymptomatic despite the accumulation of pyrimidine degradation products in body fluids.

Inheritance is autosomal recessive with the gene mapped to chromosome 8q22. There may be significant difference in residual activity between mutations observed in symptomatic and asymptomatic individuals. Population prevalence in a Japanese sample is 0.1%. Organic acid screening by GC-MS may identify increased amounts of these compounds in urine. Oral loading tests with uracil, dihydrouracil, thymine, and dihydrothymine have been used to differentiate this disorder from DPD deficiency. In symptomatic cases, *treatment* with β-alanine has been attempted with equivocal results. Increased sensitivity to fluorouracil is expected.

N-Carbamyl-β-Amino Aciduria (Deficiency of β-Ureidopropionase)

The pyrimidine bases uracil and thymine are degraded via the consecutive action of three enzymes to β-alanine and β-aminoisobutyric acid, respectively. The third enzyme in the pathway is β-ureidopropionase (UP), and its deficiency leads to N-carbamyl-β-amino aciduria. Urinary analysis in one case showed elevated levels of N-carbamyl-β-alanine and N-carbamyl-β-aminoisobutyric acid. No activity of β-ureidopropionase could be detected in a liver biopsy. *Clinical manifestations* in one case include muscular hypotonia, dystonic movements, and severe developmental delay. Neuropathology involves both gray and white matter. The human β-ureidopropionase gene is located on chromosome 22q11.2. Ureidopropionase deficiency leads to pathologic accumulation of 3-UPA in body fluids. 3-UPA acts as endogenous neurotoxin via inhibition of mitochondrial energy metabolism, resulting in the initiation of secondary, energy-dependent excitotoxic mechanisms. There is no known *treatment* for ureidopropionase deficiency.

Pyrimidine 5'-Nucleotidase Deficiency (Uridine Monophosphate Hydrolase Deficiency)

Erythrocyte maturation is accompanied by RNA degradation and the release of mononucleotides. Pyrimidine 5'-nucleotidase is the first degradative enzyme of the pyrimidine salvage cycle and catalyzes the hydrolysis of pyrimidine 5'-nucleotides to the corresponding nucleosides. Enzyme deficiency results in the accumulation of high levels of pyrimidine nucleotides in erythrocytes. Homozygous patients with pyrimidine 5'-nucleotidase deficiency present with a nonspherocytic hemolytic anemia with basophilic stippling and splenomegaly, increased indirect bilirubin, and hemoglobinuria. Pyrimidine 5'-nucleotidase deficiency is implicated in the anemia of lead poisoning. This is an autosomal recessive disorder involving a gene on chromosome 7. *Diagnosis* requires demonstration of a complete deficiency of the major isoenzyme, uridine monophosphate hydrolase-1. The enzyme defect should be suspected in patients with nonspherocytic hemolytic anemia with basophilic stippling. The anemia is usually moderate, and transfusions are not usually necessary. There is no specific *treatment*. Splenectomy is not an effective treatment.

Pyrimidine 5'-Nucleotidase Superactivity

Pyrimidine 5'-nucleotidase superactivity may lead to a neurodevelopmental disorder. Four unrelated patients with 6- to 10-fold elevation in the activity of fibroblast pyrimidine 5'-nucleotidase demonstrated normal incorporation of purine bases into nucleotides but decreased incorporation of uridine. *Clinical manifestations* include developmental delay, seizures, ataxia, recurrent infections, severe language deficit, hyperactivity, short attention span, and poor social interaction appearing within the first few years of life. Patients have electroencephalographic abnormalities. Metabolic testing is normal except for persistent hypouricosuria. Increased catabolic activity and decreased pyrimidine salvage may cause a deficiency of pyrimidine nucleotides. *Treatment* is with oral uridine to try to reverse increased nucleotide catabolism. Uridine treatment results in improved speech and behavior, decreased seizure activity, and decreased frequency of infections.

Thymidine Phosphorylase Deficiency

Thymidine phosphorylase catalyzes the conversion of thymidine to thymine. This enzyme is also known as "platelet-derived endothelial cell growth factor," owing to its angiogenic properties, or "gliostatin," indicating its inhibitory effects on glial cell proliferation. It has been implicated in mitochondrial nucleoside metabolism. Loss of function of thymidine phosphorylase causes *mitochondrial neurogastrointestinal encephalomyopathy* (MNGIE), an autosomal recessive disorder with mitochondrial DNA alterations. The gene encoding thymidine phosphorylase is the MNGIE gene and is mapped to chromosome 22q13.32-qter. *Clinical manifestations of MNGIE* include ptosis, progressive external ophthalmoparesis, gastrointestinal dysmotility, cachexia, peripheral neuropathy, and leukoencephalopathy. Muscle biopsies reveal mitochondrial abnormalities. The *diagnosis* is made by assay of thymidine phosphorylase activity in peripheral leukocytes. Plasma thymidine level is increased more than 20-fold in MNGIE. Increased thymidine may cause mitochondrial nucleotide pool imbalance, resulting in mitochondrial DNA alterations through a mitochondria-specific thymidine salvage pathway. Supportive treatment is indicated.

Anderson L, Ernst M: Self-injury in Lesch-Nyhan disease. *J Aut Dev Disord* 1994; 24:67–81.

Augoustides-Savvopoulou P, Papachristou F, Fairbanks LD, et al: Partial hypoxanthine-guanine phosphoribosyltransferase deficiency as the unsuspected cause of renal disease spanning three generations: A cautionary tale. *Pediatrics* 2002;109:E17.

Duran M, Dorland L, Meuleman EEE, et al: Inherited defects of purine and pyrimidine metabolism: Laboratory methods for diagnosis. *J Inherit Metab Dis* 1997;20:227–36.

Jinnah HA, De Gregorio L, Harris JC, et al: The spectrum of inherited mutations causing HPRT deficiency: 75 new cases and a review of 196 previously reported cases. *Mutat Res* 2000;463:309–26.

Marinaki AM, Escuredo E, Duley JA, et al: Genetic basis of hemolytic anemia caused by pyrimidine 5' nucleotidase deficiency. *Blood* 2001;97:3327–32.

McBride MB, Rigden S, Haycock GB, et al: Presymptomatic detection of familial juvenile hyperuricaemic nephropathy in children. *Pediatr Nephrol* 1998;12: 357–64.

Nishino I, Spinazzola A, Hirano M: MNGIE: From nuclear DNA to mitochondrial DNA. *Neuromuscl Disord* 2001;11:7–10.

Nyhan WL: The recognition of Lesch-Nyhan syndrome as an inborn error of metabolism. *J Inherit Metab Dis* 1997;20:171–8.

Page T, Yu A, Fontanes J, et al: Developmental disorder associated with increased cellular nucleotidase activity. *Proc Natl Acad Sci USA* 1997;94:11601–6.

Race V, Marie S, Vincent MF, et al: Clinical, biochemical and molecular genetic correlations in adenylosuccinate lyase deficiency. *Hum Mol Genet* 2000;9:2159–65.

Ray PF, Harper JC, Ao A: Successful preimplantation genetic diagnosis for sex-linked Lesch-Nyhan syndrome using specific diagnosis. *Prenat Diagn* 1999;19: 1237–41.

Schretlen DJ, Harris JC, Park K, et al: Neurocognitive functioning in Lesch-Nyhan disease and partial hypoxanthine-guanine phosphoribosyltransferase deficiency. *J Int Neuropsychol Soc* 2001;7:805–12.

Van Gennip AH, Abeling NGGM, Vrekan P, et al: Inborn errors of pyrimidine degradation: Clinical, biochemical and molecular aspects. *Inherit Metab Dis* 1997;20:203–13.

Van Kuilenburg AB, Vreken P, Abeling NG, et al: Genotype and phenotype in patients with dihydropyrimidine dehydrogenase deficiency. *Hum Genet* 1999;19:1–9.

Van Kuilenburg AB, Van Lenthe H, Assmann B, et al:. Detection of beta-ureidopropionase deficiency with HPLC-electrospray tandem mass spectrometry and confirmation of the defect at the enzyme level. *J Inherit Metab Dis* 2001;24:725–32.

Wilcox WD: Abnormal serum uric acid levels in children. *J Pediatr* 1996;128: 731–41.

Wong DF, Harris JC, Naidu S, et al: Dopamine transporters are markedly reduced in Lesch-Nyham disease in vivo. *Proc Natl Acad Sci* 1996;93:5539.

Chapter 79

Progeria *W. Ted Brown*

Progeria's most striking feature resembles accelerated aging. This rare syndrome, also referred to as the Hutchinson-Gilford syndrome, has a reported incidence of approximately 1:8 million. Affected children do not become sexually mature or reproduce as a result of severe failure to thrive; parent-to-child transmission has not been observed. Although two sets of identical twins have been noted, no examples of recurrence of classic progeria among siblings are documented. Paternal age is significantly increased, but there is no increase in consanguinity or features associated with dominant mutations or autosomal recessive inheritance. Each child with progeria may represent a new sporadic dominant mutation. The molecular basis of such mutations is unknown.

Clinical Manifestations. Children with progeria usually appear normal in early infancy, but manifestations such as midfacial cyanosis, "sculpted nose," and "sclerodema" may suggest the existence of the syndrome at birth. Profound growth failure occurs during the 1st yr of life. The characteristic facies, alopecia, loss of subcutaneous fat, abnormal posture, stiffness of joints, and bone and skin changes usually become apparent during the 2nd yr of life (Fig. 79–1). Motor and mental development is normal. The dominant clinical manifestations include short stature; weight distinctly low for height; diminished subcutaneous fat; head disproportionately large for face; micrognathia; prominent scalp veins; generalized alopecia; prominent eyes; delayed and abnormal dentition; pyriform thorax; short, dystrophic clavicles; "horse-riding" stance; wide-based shuffling gait; coxa valga, thin limbs, and prominent, stiff joints; and failure to complete sexual maturation.

Features frequently present are skin that is thin, taut, dry, wrinkled, and brown spotted in various areas; sclerodermatous skin over the lower abdomen, proximal thighs, and buttocks; prominent superficial veins; loss of eyebrows and eyelashes; persistently patent anterior fontanel; sculpted, beaked nasal tip; faint nasolabial cyanosis; thin lips; protruding ears; absence of ear lobules; thin, high-pitched voice; dystrophic nails; and

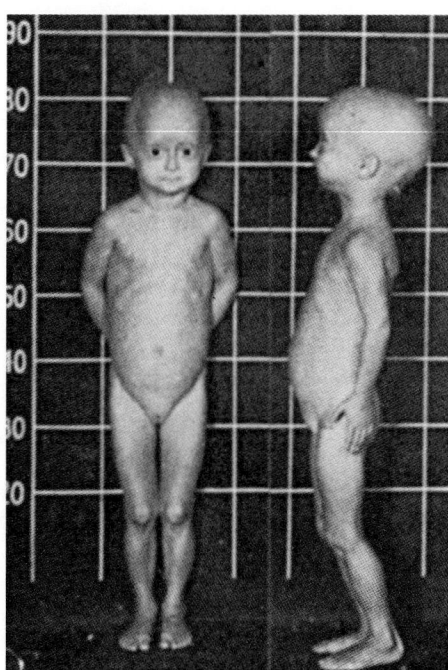

FIGURE 79–1. A 4.5-yr-old girl with height age of 1.75 yr and bone age of 4 yr. (From Wilkins L: *Diagnosis and Treatment of Endocrine Disorders in Childhood and Adolescence*, 3rd ed. Springfield, IL, Charles C Thomas, 1965.)

progressive radiolucency of the terminal phalanges and distal clavicles (acro-osteolysis). A *differential diagnosis* includes neonatal progeroid syndrome, Cockayne syndrome, Hallermann-Streiff syndrome, and mandibular-acral dysplasia. Neonatal progeroid (Weidmann-Rautenstrauch) syndrome is an uncommon autosomal recessive disorder that manifests at birth or thereafter with low birthweight, craniofacial anomalies (pseudohydrocephalus, triangular facies, large fontanel), aged look, lack of subcutaneous fat, natal teeth, developmental delay, and death before the end of the 1st year of life.

Laboratory Findings. Variable degrees of insulin resistance, occasionally insulin-dependent diabetes mellitus, abnormalities of collagen, increased metabolic rate, and inconsistent abnormalities of serum cholesterol and other lipids are found, but there are no demonstrable abnormalities of thyroid, parathyroid, pituitary, or adrenal function. Twenty-four-hour growth hormone levels are normal, but reduced levels of insulin-like growth factor-1 have been noted. Increased levels of hyaluronic acid may occur in the urine of such patients. Variable decrease of DNA repair has also been observed.

Prognosis. Children with progeria usually have severe atherosclerosis, and death occurs as a result of complications of cardiac or cerebrovascular disease generally between age 5–20 yr, with a median life span of approximately 13 yr. Cataracts and tumors have infrequently been noted, but many changes associated with normal aging in adults, such as presbycusis, presbyopia, arcus senilis, osteoarthritis, senile personality changes, or Alzheimer disease, are not found.

Treatment. No specific treatment for this condition exists. There is a progeria family support group. A Progeria Registry exists to help with diagnosis and to define more clearly the incidence and molecular basis of the disorder.

Abdenur JE, Brown WT, Friedman S, et al: Response to nutritional and growth hormone treatment in progeria. *Metabolism* 1997;46:851–6.
Brown WT: Progeria: A human-disease model of accelerated aging. *Am J Clin Nutr* 1992;55:1222S–4.
DeBusk FL: The Hutchinson-Gilford progeria syndrome. *J Pediatr* 1972;80:697–724.
Pivnick EK, Angle B, Kaufman RA, et al: Neonatal progeroid (Wiedemann-Rautenstrauch) syndrome: Report of five new cases and review. *Am J Med Genet* 2000;90:131–40.

Chapter 80
The Porphyrias *Shigeru Sassa*

The porphyrias are inherited and acquired disorders in which the activities of the enzymes of the heme biosynthetic pathway are partially or almost completely deficient. As a result, abnormally elevated levels of porphyrins and/or their precursors are produced, accumulate in tissues, and are excreted in urine and stool. Heme is composed of ferrous iron and protoporphyrin IX (Fig. 80–1) and is an essential molecule for life as the prosthetic group of heme proteins, such as hemoglobin, myoglobin, mitochondrial and microsomal cytochromes, catalase, peroxidases, nitric oxide synthase, and tryptophan pyrrolase. Patients with porphyrias have either cutaneous photosensitivity caused by accumulation of porphyrins in the skin or neurologic disturbances from accumulation of their precursors, or both.

HEME BIOSYNTHETIC PATHWAY

The first step and the last three steps in the heme biosynthetic pathway occur in the mitochondria; the intermediate steps take place in the cytosol (Fig. 80–2). The two major organs that are active in heme synthesis are the liver and the erythroid bone marrow; inherited enzymatic defects in the porphyrias are mainly expressed in these tissues. In erythroid cells, hemoglobin is made in erythroblasts or reticulocytes, which still contain mitochondria; circulating erythrocytes lack the ability to form heme. cDNA and genomic DNA sequences as well as chromosomal assignment have been defined for all heme pathway enzymes (Table 80–1).

Formation of δ-Aminolevulinic Acid (ALA). *δ-Aminolevulinate synthase* (ALAS), the first enzyme of the heme biosynthetic pathway, catalyzes the condensation of glycine and succinyl CoA (see Fig. 80–2, step 1). The enzyme is localized in the inner membrane of mitochondria and requires pyridoxal 5′-phosphate as a cofactor. ALAS activity is very low and rate limiting for heme

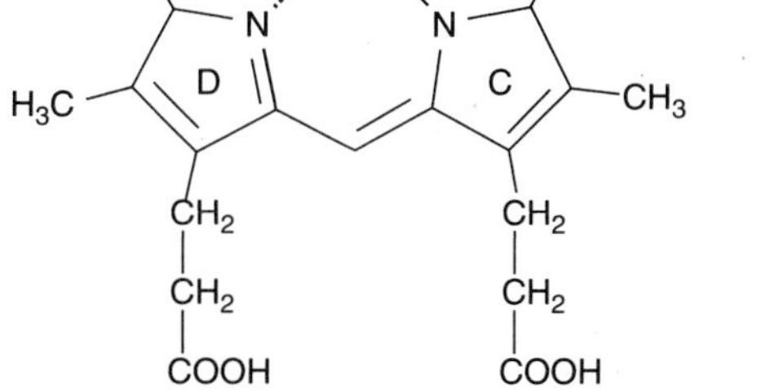

FIGURE 80–1. Structure of heme.

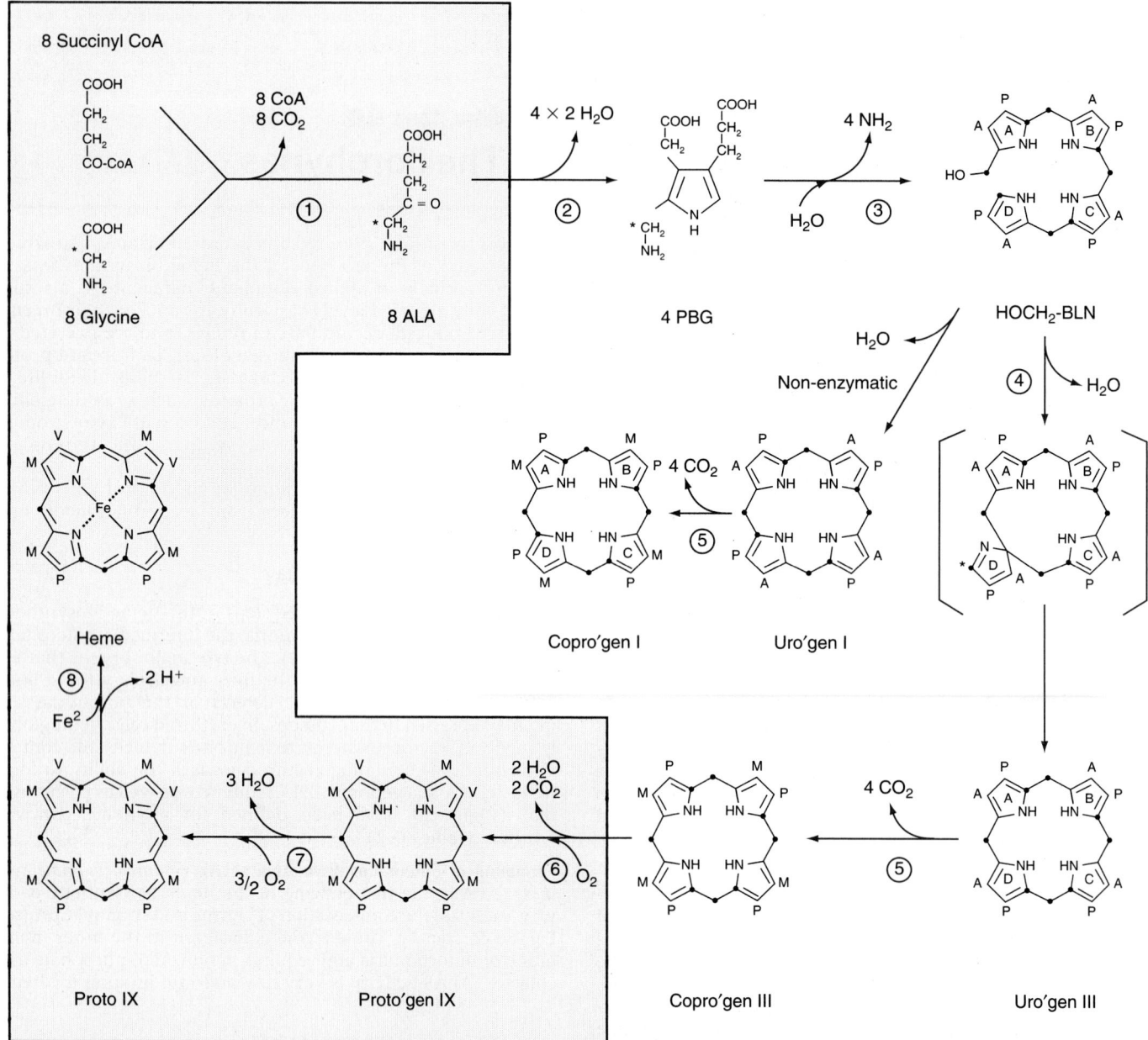

FIGURE 80–2. The heme biosynthetic pathway. A = -CH$_2$- COOH; P = -CH$_2$-CH$_2$-COOH; M = -CH$_3$; V = -CH=CH$_2$; ● = carbon atom derived from the α-carbon of glycine; * = location of the α-carbon atom from glycine in the pyrrole ring that undergoes reversion; [] = a presumed intermediate. (Modified from Hayashi N: The synthesis of heme and its regulation. *Protein Nucl Acid Enzyme (Tokyo)* 1987;32:797.)

formation. Hepatic ALAS (nonspecific, or ALAS-N) and erythroid ALAS (ALAS-E) are isozymes that are encoded by two distinct nuclear genes: *ALAS1* and *ALAS2*. The gene locus for human *ALAS1* is at chromosome 3p21, and that for *ALAS2* is at the Xp11.21. Inherited deficiency of ALAS-E is associated with X-linked sideroblastic anemia.

Formation of Porphobilinogen (PBG) from ALA. Two molecules of ALA are converted by a cytosolic enzyme, *δ-aminolevulinate dehydratase* (ALAD), to a monopyrrole, PBG, with the removal of two molecules of water (see Fig. 80–2, step 2). ALAD deficiency porphyria (ADP) is caused by an almost complete lack of enzyme activity (Fig. 80–3). The human *ALAD* gene is

localized at chromosome 9q34 and contains two promoter regions that generate housekeeping and erythroid-specific transcripts by alternate splicing, analogous to the expression of the human *PBGD* gene. The novel expression of housekeeping and erythroid-specific transcripts apparently evolved to ensure sufficient heme biosynthesis for the high-level tissue-specific production of hemoglobin.

ALAD requires an intact sulfhydryl group and a zinc atom per subunit for full activity. Lead inhibits ALAD by displacing zinc from the enzyme, the essential metal for enzyme activity, and results in neurologic disturbances, some of which resemble those of ADP. The most potent inhibitor of the enzyme is succinylacetone, a structural analogue of ALA, which is found in

TABLE 80–1. Human Enzymes and Genes for Heme Biosynthesis

Enzyme	Gene Symbol	Chromosomal Location	cDNA (bp)	Protein (aa)	Genome Size (kb)	Genome Organization*
δ–Aminolevulinate synthase:						
Housekeeping	ALAS1	3p21.1	2199	640	17	11 exons
Erythroid-specific	ALAS2	Xp11.21	1937	587	22	11 exons
δ–Aminolevulinate dehydratase:	ALAD	9q34				13 exons
Housekeeping			1149	330	15.9	Exons 1A + 2–12
Erythroid-specific			1154	330		Exons 1B+2–12
Porphobilinogen deaminase:	PBGD	11q23.3			11	15 exons
Housekeeping			1086	361		Exons 1+ 3–15
Erythroid-specific			1035	344		Exons 2–15
Uroporphyrinogen III synthase:	UCS	10q25.2-q26.3			34	10 exons
Housekeeping			1296	265		Exon 1+2B–10
Erythroid-specific			1216	265		Exon 2A+2B–10
Uroporphyrinogen decarboxylase	UROD	1p34 ·	1104	367	3	10 exons
Coproporphyrinogen oxidase	CPO	3q12	1062	354	14	7 exons
Protoporphyrinogen oxidase	PPO	1q23	1431	477	5.5	13 exons
Ferrochelatase	FeC	18q21.3	1269	423	45	11 exons

*Number of exons.

urine and blood of patients with hereditary tyrosinemia who often develop a condition similar to ADP.

Formation of Hydroxymethylbilane (HMB) from PBG. *Porphobilinogen deaminase* (PBGD) catalyzes the condensation of four molecules of PBG to yield a linear tetrapyrrole, HMB. In the absence of the subsequent enzyme, uroporphyrinogen III cosynthase (UCS), the bilin is spontaneously cyclized into the first tetrapyrrole, uroporphyrinogen I. In the presence of UCS, uroporphyrinogen III is formed, which has an inverted D-ring pyrrole (see Fig. 80–2, step 3). The gene locus for human *PBGD* is at chromosome 11q23→11qter. The expression of the erythroid-specific mRNA is exclusive to erythroid cells. Two distinct mRNAs are produced through alternative splicing of two primary transcripts arising from two promoters. The upstream promoter is active in all tissues, whereas the other promoter, located 3 kb downstream, is active only in erythroid cells.

Formation of Uroporphyrinogen III from HMB. UCS catalyzes the formation of uroporphyrinogen III from HMB. This involves an intramolecular rearrangement that affects only ring D of the uroporphyrinogen (see Fig. 80–2, step 4). Homozygous deficiency of UCS is associated with congenital erythropoietic porphyria (CEP) (see Fig. 80–3). A single *UCS* gene is at the narrow chromosomal region 10q25.3→q26.3.

Formation of Coproporphyrinogen from Uroporphyrinogen. A cytosolic enzyme, *uroporphyrinogen decarboxylase* (UROD), catalyzes the sequential removal of the four carboxylic groups of the carboxymethyl side chains in uroporphyrinogen to yield coproporphyrinogen (see Fig. 80–2, step 5). The *UROD* gene has been localized to chromosome 1pter→p21. Porphyria cutanea tarda (PCT) is caused by a partial (or heterozygous) deficiency of UROD, whereas hepatoerythropoietic porphyria (HEP) is caused by a homozygous deficiency of the enzyme (see Fig. 80–3). The enzyme functions as a homodimer. The gene locus encoding for *UROD* is on chromosome 1p34.

Formation of Protoporphyrinogen from Coproporphyrinogen. *Coproporphyrinogen oxidase* (CPO) is a mitochondrial enzyme that catalyzes the removal of the carboxyl group and two hydrogens from the propionic groups of pyrrole rings A and B of coproporphyrinogen to form vinyl groups at these positions (see Fig. 80–2, step 6). The *CPO* gene is localized to chromosome 9. Hereditary coproporphyria (HCP) is caused by a partial (or heterozygous) deficiency of CPO (see Fig. 80–3).

Formation of Protoporphyrin from Protoporphyrinogen. The oxidation of protoporphyrinogen to protoporphyrin is mediated by proto-

porphyrinogen *oxidase* (PPO), which catalyzes the removal of six hydrogen atoms from the porphyrinogen nucleus (see Fig. 80–2, step 7). Variegate porphyria (VP) is caused by a partial (or heterozygous) deficiency of PPO (see Fig. 80–3). The human PPO contains noncovalently bound FAD. The *PPO* gene is on chromosome 1q23 or 1q22.

Formation of Heme from Protoporphyrin. The final step of heme biosynthesis is the insertion of iron into protoporphyrin (see Fig. 80–2, step 8). This reaction is catalyzed by the enzyme *ferrochelatase* (FeC). Unlike other steps in the heme biosynthetic pathway, this enzyme uses protoporphyrin IX as a substrate, rather than its reduced form. However, the enzyme specifically requires ferrous, not ferric, iron. The *FeC* gene is on chromosome 18q21.3.

An iron-sulfur cluster, a [2Fe-2S], has been identified in the purified human ferrochelatase at the carboxyl terminus. The putative binding site is a 30-residue region that contains four cysteine residues, which is a fingerprint for a [2Fe-2S] binding motif. The Fe-S cluster is thought to be essential for the mammalian enzyme activity.

REGULATION OF HEME SYNTHESIS

Biosynthesis of heme in the liver is controlled largely by the rate of formation of ALAS, that is, ALAS-N. The enzyme activity in normal liver cells is very low, whereas its level increases dramatically when the liver needs to make more heme and in response to various chemical treatments. The synthesis of the enzyme is also regulated in a feedback fashion by heme, the end product of the biosynthetic pathway. At higher heme concentrations than those that repress the synthesis of ALAS-N, heme induces microsomal heme oxygenase, resulting in enhancement of heme catabolism. Thus, heme concentration is maintained by a balance between the synthesis of ALAS-N and heme oxygenase-1, both of which are under the regulatory influence of heme. In contrast, ALAS-E synthesis in erythroid cells is either refractory to heme treatment or stimulated by such treatment.

PATHOPHYSIOLOGIC CONSEQUENCES OF PORPHYRINS AND THEIR PRECURSORS

Photosensitivity. Free porphyrins occur only in small amounts in normal tissues, but their levels may become markedly elevated in the porphyrias. On illumination at wavelengths of about 400 nm (Soret band) and in the presence of oxygen, porphyrins cause photodynamic damage to tissues, cells, subcellular elements, and biomolecules through the formation of singlet oxygen.

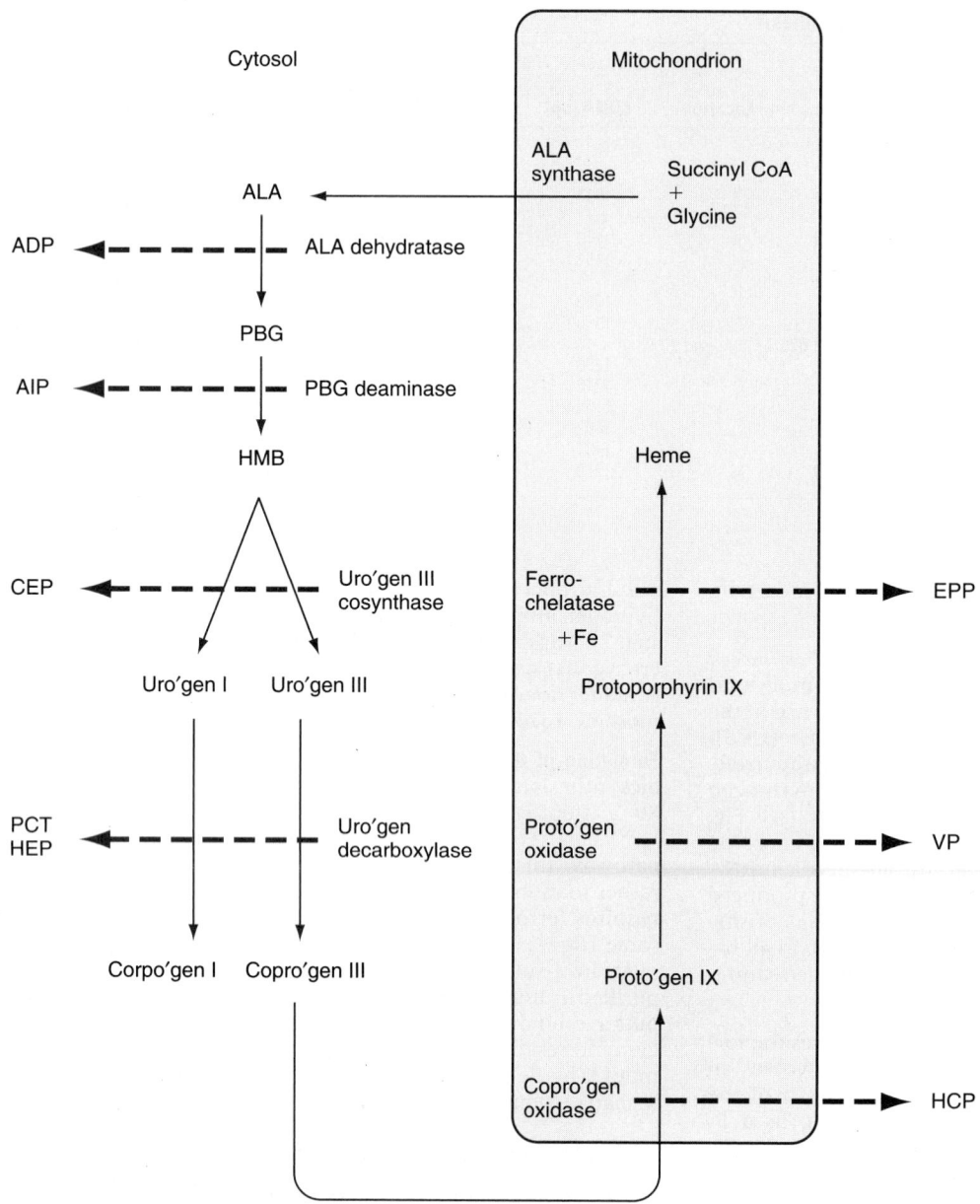

FIGURE 80–3. Enzymatic defects in the porphyrias. The enzymatic defect in each porphyria is shown by a *broken line*. In patients, the substrate for the defective enzymatic step accumulates in the tissue and is excreted in large excess into urine and/or stool. Porphyrin precursors, for example, ALA and PBG, may also be increased in patients with acute hepatic porphyrias as a result of derepression of ALAS-N activity.

Neurologic Disturbances. *Acute hepatic porphyrias*, that is, ADP, AIP, HCP, and VP, are characterized by neurologic disturbances. Most common symptoms are abdominal pain, disturbances in intestinal motility (e.g., diarrhea and constipation), dysesthesia, muscular paralysis, and respiratory failure, which can often be fatal. The exact nature of the neurologic disturbances in the porphyrias remains unclear.

MOLECULAR GENETICS OF THE PORPHYRIAS

Genetic analysis has elucidated the complex nature of molecular defects in the porphyrias and possible consequences of their gene defects on cellular function. It also offers an explanation why hepatic porphyrias do not accompany anemia, or conversely why erythropoietic porphyrias do not exhibit defective drug metabolism, which largely reflects the function of hepatic cytochrome P450. The following general conclusions can be made by molecular genetic studies of the porphyrias.

1. In every porphyria, the molecular defect of the enzyme is heterogeneous. There is more than one mutation resulting clinically in a single porphyria disease. There are more than 100 mutations found in the *PBGD* gene in patients with AIP. There are few founder effect mutations, whereas a pedigree-specific mutation (private mutation) of the enzyme gene is very common.

2. The nature of molecular defects is also highly heterogeneous, including promoter mutations, splicing mutations, consensus sequence mutations, mutations producing nonfunctional mRNAs, and mutations resulting in unstable proteins, gene deletions, and so on.

3. Even among the dominant form of porphyrias, a homozygous form of the disease can be found in a few patients. The homozygous form appears to be caused by mutations with lesser pathophysiologic effects than those found in the heterozygous form. The homozygous disease is clinically more severe than the heterozygous disease due to the combination of two mutant alleles. A subset of homozygous diseases among commonly autosomal dominant diseases has been observed in AIP, HCP, VP, and EPP.

4. Clinically homozygous mutations can be caused by either a *homoallelic* or a *heteroallelic* mutation. However, heteroallelic mutation (*compound heterozygosity*) for two separate mutations is far more common than homoallelic mutation.

5. Tissue-specific regulation of heme pathway enzymes may likely be the basis for the tissue-specific expression of different porphyrias.

6. In the case of *PBGD*, a mutation affecting the splicing of the first intron results in an abnormal enzyme in nonerythroid cells, whereas the same mutation has no effect on the erythroid-specific *PBGD*, because the transcription of the erythroid *PBGD* mRNA utilizes a second AUG that is located approximately 3 kb downstream of the mutated site. Thus, even in a single form of acute hepatic porphyria, there may be distinct tissue-specific expression of the disease, depending on the type of mutation.

7. Most of the acute hepatic porphyrias, such as AIP, HCP, and VP, require an additional factor(s) for their clinical expression. Such a factor can either be genetic or environmental. Thus, porphyrias are not only inborn errors of metabolism but also diseases in which environmental factors have an immense impact on their gene expression.

8. Some hepatic porphyria–like symptoms can be elicited by environmental chemicals, which strongly inhibit heme pathway enzymes. For example, PCT may be caused by UROD inhibition owing to hexachlorobenzene ingestion in normal individuals.

CLASSIFICATION OF PORPHYRIAS

There are eight enzymes involved in the synthesis of heme and, with the exception of the first enzyme, which is ALAS, an enzymatic defect at each step of heme synthesis is associated with each form of porphyria (see Fig. 80–3 and Table 80–2). Porphyrias are classified as either hepatic or erythropoietic, depending on the principal site of expression of the specific enzymatic defect (see Table 80–2). They can also be classified as acute hepatic or cutaneous porphyrias. Acute hepatic porphyrias are characterized clinically by acute episodes of neurologic disturbances and biochemically by an overproduction of porphyrin precursors, whereas cutaneous porphyrias are characterized clinically by cutaneous photosensitivity and biochemically by an excessive production of porphyrins (Table 80–3).

ALAD Deficiency Porphyria (ADP). ADP is an autosomal recessive disorder resulting from a homozygous ALAD deficiency (see Fig. 80–3 and Table 80–2). This is the most rare form of the porphyrias; clinical manifestations have been primarily neuropathic and severity and the age at onset have varied in the four reported cases, including an infant born with the clinical disease. All these cases were unrelated males in Europe.

CLINICAL MANIFESTATIONS. Patients with ADP have vomiting, pain in the arms and legs, and neuropathy, which are exacerbated after stress, alcohol use, or decreased food intake. A rare infant with ADP has been reported who has a clinical course from birth onward that includes general muscle hypotonia and respiratory insufficiency.

LABORATORY FINDINGS. Urinary ALA excretion is markedly elevated, whereas urinary PBG excretion is within the normal range. Urinary and erythrocyte porphyrins are also markedly elevated (100-fold); no satisfactory explanation has yet been advanced to account for this observation. Fecal porphyrin excretion is normal or marginally elevated. Patients with ADP display markedly decreased activities of ALAD in erythrocytes, as well as in nonerythroid cells (2% of normal), and their parents show approximately 50% decreases in enzyme activities.

MOLECULAR PATHOLOGY. One or both alleles probably produce enzyme proteins with decreased activity. The disease is genetically highly heterogeneous, in that nine distinct point mutations in the *ALAD* gene were found in four patients and in an asymptomatic heterozygous carrier. Patients homozygous for the *ALAD* defect are all heteroallelic, having two distinct *ALAD* mutations in each allele.

DIAGNOSIS. Definitive diagnosis depends on the demonstration of impaired ALAD activity and deficiency of enzyme protein in erythrocytes. Supporting evidence includes massive elevations in urinary ALA, substantial elevations of porphyrins in urine and erythrocytes, and perhaps modest elevations in fecal porphyrins. Clinical symptoms of ADP occur only in homozygous patients, whereas heterozygous subjects (parents and certain siblings) of the proband remain clinically unaffected. Because multiple causes of ALAD deficiency have been described, all cases considered to have ADP should be confirmed by molecular studies.

TREATMENT. The similarities in symptoms between ADP and AIP suggest that prudent management of ADP should probably be directed along the same lines as the management of AIP.

Acute Intermittent Porphyria (AIP). AIP, also termed Swedish porphyria, pyrroloporphyria, or intermittent acute porphyria, is an autosomal dominant disorder resulting from a partial PBGD deficiency (see Fig. 80–3 and Table 80–2). The deficient enzyme activity (~50% of normal) is found in all tissues, including erythrocytes, in the majority of patients (~85%). This is consistent with the heterozygous state of affected individuals. However,

TABLE 80–2. The Porphyrias and Their Enzymatic Defects

Enzyme Deficiency	Porphyria	Principal Site of Expression	Mode of Transmission	Remarks
ALAD	ADP	Liver	Recessive	
PBGD	AIP			
	Type I	Liver	Dominant	CRIM (–)
	Type II	Liver	Dominant	Normal erythrocyte PBGD
	Type III	Liver	Dominant	CRIM (+)
UCS	CEP	Bone marrow	Recessive	
UROD	PCT			
	Type I	Liver		Acquired
	Type II	Liver	Dominant	
	Type III	Liver	Dominant	
	HEP	Liver and bone marrow	Recessive	
CPO	HCP	Liver	Dominant	
PPO	VP	Liver	Dominant	
FeC	EPP	Bone marrow	Dominant	

ALAD = δ-aminolevulinate dehydratase; ADP = ALAD deficiency porphyria; PBGD = porphobilinogen deaminase; AIP = acute intermittent porphyria; CRIM = cross-reactive immunologic material; UCS = uroporphyrinogen III cosynthase; CEP = congenital erythropoietic porphyria; UROD = uroporphyrinogen decarboxylase; PCT = porphyria cutanea tarda; HEP = hepatoerythropoietic porphyria; CPO = coproporphyrinogen oxidase; HCP = hereditary coproporphyria; PPO = protoporphyrinogen oxidase; VP = variegate porphyria; FeC = ferrochelatase; EPP = erythropoietic protoporphyria.
From Sassa S, Kappas A: The porphyrias. In Nathan DG, Oski FA (editors): Hematology in Infancy and Childhood, 4th ed. Philadelphia, WB Saunders, 1993, pp 451–71.

TABLE 80–3.　Clinical and Laboratory Features of the Porphyrias

Porphyria	Clinical Features	Laboratory Features			
		Erythrocytes	*Plasma*	*Urine*	*Stool*
ADP	Neurologic (as in AIP)	ZnPP		ALA	
AIP	Neurologic: nausea, vomiting, abdominal pain, diarrhea, constipation, ileus, dysuria, muscle hypotonia, respiratory failure, sensory neuropathy, seizures			ALA, PBG	
CEP	Photosensitivity: bullae, crusts, scar formation, sclerodermoid change, hyper- and hypopigmentation, hypertrichosis, erythrodontia, hemolytic anemia, splenomegaly	Uro, I, Copro I	Uro I, Copro I	Uro I, Copro I	
PCT	Photosensitivity: skin fragility, bullae, crusts, scar formation, sclerodermoid change, hyper- and hypopigmentation, hypertrichosis	Uro I, 7-carboxyl III	Uro I, 7-carboxyl III	Uro, 7-carboxyl, Isocopro	
HEP	Photosensitivity (as in CEP)	ZnPP	Uro I, 7-carboxyl III	Uro I, 7-carboxyl III	Uro, 7-carboxyl, Isocopro
HCP	Neurologic (as in ADP, AIP, and VP) and photosensitive (as in VP)		Copro	Copro, ALA, PBG	Copro
VP	Neurologic (as in ADP, AIP, and HCP) and photosensitive (as in HCP)		Proto	ALA, PBG	Proto
EPP	Photosensitivity: burning sensation, edema, erythema, itching, scarring vesicles	Proto	Proto		Proto

ADP = ALAD deficiency porphyria; AIP = acute intermittent porphyria; ALA = δ-aminolevulinic acid; PBG = porphobilinogen; CEP = congenital erythropoietic porphyria; Uro I = uroporphyrinogen I; PCT = porphyria cutanea tarda; HEP = hepatoerythropoietic porphyria; HCP = hereditary coproporphyria; VP = variegate porphyria; EPP = erythropoietic protoporphyria; Proto = protoporphyrinogen. 7-Carboxyl-7-carboxylporphyrin; Copro-coproporphyrin; Isocopro-isocoproporphyrin; Uro-uroporphyrin; ZnPP-zinc protoporphyrin.

From Sassa S, Kappas A: The porphyrias. In Nathan DG, Oski FA (editors): Hematology in Infancy and Childhood, 4th ed. Philadelphia, WB Saunders, 1993, pp 451–71.

a subset of patients (~15%) show deficient enzyme activity only in nonerythroid cells. The majority (~90%) of individuals with PBGD deficiency remain biochemically and clinically normal. Clinical expression of the disease is usually linked to environmental or acquired factors, for example, nutritional status, drugs, corticosteroids, and other chemicals of endogenous or exogenous origin. The cardinal pathobiology of the disease is a neurologic dysfunction that may affect the peripheral, autonomic, or central nervous systems (see Table 80–3).

EPIDEMIOLOGY. AIP is probably the most common genetic porphyria. The highest incidence occurs in Lapland, Scandinavia, and the United Kingdom, although it has been reported in many population groups. The prevalence of AIP was estimated to be 1–2 in 100,000 in Europe and 2.4 in 100,000 in Finland. The frequency of low PBGD activity, which includes both patients with AIP and latent gene carriers, is as high as 1 in 500 in the general population of Finland. The disorder is expressed clinically after puberty and is more common in women than in men.

CLINICAL MANIFESTATIONS. Abdominal pain, which may be generalized or localized, is the most common symptom and is often the initial sign of an acute attack. Other gastroenterologic features may include nausea, vomiting, constipation or diarrhea, abdominal distention, and ileus. Urinary retention, incontinence, and dysuria may frequently be observed. In severe cases, the urine develops a port-wine color, owing to a high content of porphobilin, an auto-oxidation product of PBG. Tachycardia and hypertension, and, less frequently, fever, sweating, restlessness, and tremor, are also observed. In up to 40% of patients, hypertension may become sustained between acute attacks.

Neuropathy is a common feature of AIP. Muscle weakness often begins proximally in the legs but may involve the arms or the distal extremities. Motor neuropathy may also involve the cranial nerves or lead to bulbar paralysis, respiratory deficiency, and death. Sensory patchy neuropathy may also occur. Seizures, especially in patients with hyponatremia due to vomiting, inappropriate fluid therapy, or the syndrome of inappropriate antidiuretic hormone secretion, may accompany acute attacks of AIP. The course of an acute attack of AIP is highly variable, both in

individuals and among patients, with attacks lasting from a few days to several months. There are no cutaneous manifestations associated with this enzyme deficiency.

Asymptomatic heterozygotes (~90% of subjects with documented PBGD deficiency) may display neither abnormalities in concentrations of porphyrin precursors nor clinical symptoms. Individuals with both latent and previously clinically expressed AIP may be, however, precipitated into an acute attack by endogenous or exogenous environmental factors. There are at least five different classes of *precipitating factors* in this disease:

1. *ALAS-N inducers:* most precipitating factors can be related to an associated increase in the activity of ALAS-N in the liver. An overproduction of ALA then makes the partially deficient PBGD activity rate limiting.

2. *Endocrine factors:* the clinical disease is more common in women, especially at the time of menses. The disease also hardly becomes manifest before puberty.

3. *Calorie intake:* reduced calorie intake often leads to exacerbations of AIP. Additional calories on a diet may reduce PBG excretion and suppress clinical symptoms.

4. *Drugs and foreign chemicals:* many chemicals, for example, barbiturates, sex steroids, and other foreign chemicals that exacerbate porphyria have the potential to induce cytochrome P450. The resultant enhanced demand for heme synthesis may lead to induction of hepatic ALAS-N.

5. *Stress:* stress is known to upregulate the heme oxygenase gene and leads to exacerbations of AIP. Similarly, other forms of stress, including intercurrent illnesses, infections, alcoholic excess, and surgery, are all known to contribute to the genesis of an acute attack of this disorder.

LABORATORY FINDINGS. Patients with clinically expressed AIP, as well as a few individuals with latent AIP, excrete variably increased amounts of ALA and PBG in the urine between attacks. In the majority of cases, the onset of an acute attack is accompanied by further increases in excretion of these precursors. Acute attacks may also be associated with elevations in the serum concentrations of ALA, PBG, and porphyrins, which are normally undetectable. Stool porphyrins are usually normal or only slightly elevated in this disorder. The Watson-Schwartz test is widely used as a screening test for urinary PBG. While this test is highly sensitive, it is neither specific nor quantitative, and its results need to be confirmed and quantified by the column chromatographic. Hemoglobin and bilirubin production are normal.

MOLECULAR PATHOLOGY. Patients with AIP can be classified into three subsets (see Table 80–2). Patients with *type I* mutations are characterized by cross-reactive immunologic material (CRIM)-negative *PBGD* mutation; they exhibit both intermediately reduced enzyme activity and protein content (about 50% of normal). *Type II* mutations are observed in less than 15% of all AIP and are characterized by a decreased PBGD activity in nonerythroid cells, but with normal erythroid PBGD activity. Patients with *type III* mutations are characterized by CRIM-positive mutations, that is, decreased enzyme activity with the presence of structurally abnormal enzyme protein. Various mutations of the human *PBGD* gene have been described in patients with AIP and are summarized in Table 80–3. Mutations found in type I AIP are single base substitutions or deletions that result in a single amino acid change or in truncated proteins. The mutations found in type II AIP are single base substitutions that occur in the exon/intron boundary of exon 1, resulting in a splicing defect that affects only the non-specific form of *PBGD*, but not the erythroid-specific *PBGD*, because the transcription of the gene in erythroid cells starts downstream of the site of mutation. Mutations characterizing type III AIP are observed in the region that is thought to be essential for catalytic activity.

There is marked heterogeneity of the molecular defects in AIP. More than 170 mutations of the *PBGD* gene have been reported in this disorder. The molecular heterogeneity of CRIM-negative forms seems to be more extensive than that of CRIM-positive forms. Most mutations in exons 10 and 12 occur at amino acids in the active site, and several of these are known to be involved in binding the primer, or substrate. The CRIM-positive phenotype of these mutations could be detrimental for activity, but they do not necessarily affect the structure of the enzyme.

DIAGNOSIS. Diagnosis of type I and III AIP can be made by demonstrating decreased PBGD activity in erythrocytes in the majority of patients (about 85%), whereas the distinction between carrier or latent status and clinically expressed AIP requires demonstration of elevated urinary excretion of PBG and ALA. Elevated levels of both ALA and PBG may also be seen in HCP and VP; measurement of urinary and stool porphyrins will usually differentiate these conditions from AIP. The diagnosis of type II AIP requires either the demonstration of PBGD deficiency in nonerythroid cells or DNA hybridization using allele-specific oligonucleotide specific for the mutation.

TREATMENT. The treatment of AIP as well as that of ADP, HCP, and VP is essentially identical. Treatment between attacks consists of adequate nutritional intake, avoidance of drugs known to exacerbate porphyria, and prompt treatment of other intercurrent diseases or infections. Unresponsive severe cases should be treated with intravenous administration of the carbohydrate dextrose to provide a minimum of 300 g of carbohydrate/24 hr. Intravenous hematin (4 mg/kg, q12h) is also effective in reducing ALA and PBG excretion as well as in curtailing acute attacks. Nasal or subcutaneous administration of long-acting agonistic analogues of luteinizing hormone releasing hormone have been shown to inhibit ovulation and greatly reduce the incidence of perimenstrual attacks of AIP in some women with cyclic exacerbations of the disease. Synthetic heme analogues, for example, Sn-mesoporphyrin, which inhibit heme oxygenase activity, have also been shown to diminish the output of ALA, PBG, and/or porphyrins in AIP and VP patients, presumably because of an effective blockade of heme catabolism.

Congenital Erythropoietic Porphyria (CEP). CEP, also referred to as Günther disease, is an autosomal recessive disorder (see Fig. 80–3 and Table 80–2). The primary abnormality is a decreased activity of UCS activity, which results in accumulation and hyperexcretion of predominantly type I porphyrins (see Table 80–3). Clinically, this enzymatic defect is expressed in utero as brownish amniotic fluid caused by excessive amounts of porphyrins and results in cutaneous photosensitivity, hemolysis, and a decreased life expectancy after birth.

EPIDEMIOLOGY. Fewer than 200 cases have been reported, and some of these cases may really have had PCT or HEP. There is no clear racial or sexual predominance.

CLINICAL MANIFESTATIONS. The diagnosis of CEP is suggested at birth by pink to dark brown staining of the diapers in infants, owing to large amounts of porphyrins in urine. Early onset of cutaneous photosensitivity is characteristic and is exacerbated by exposure to sunlight. Subepidermal bullous lesions progress to crusty erosions, which heal with scarring and either hyperpigmentation or, less commonly, hypopigmentation. Hypertrichosis and alopecia are frequent, and erythrodontia (with red fluorescence under ultraviolet light) is virtually pathognomonic of CEP. Patients may display symptoms and signs of hemolytic anemia with splenomegaly and porphyrin-rich gallstones. Bone marrow shows erythroid hyperplasia, which may result in pathologic fractures or vertebral compression-collapse and shortness of stature. Although the onset of symptoms of CEP is most often observed in early infancy, a few patients may first present the syndrome as adults.

PATHOGENESIS. The primary site of expression of the enzymatic defect is the bone marrow; fluorescence secondary to porphyrin accumulation is variably distributed but invariably present. Most marrow normoblasts display fluorescence, principally localized in the nuclei of the cells. Massive elevations of systemic porphyrins in CEP are derived from porphyrin-laden erythrocytes, which accounts for the multiple pathologic processes of the integument.

LABORATORY FINDINGS. Urinary porphyrins are always elevated (20- to 60-fold) above normal levels. Uroporphyrin and coproporphyrin are mostly type I isomers. Occasionally, anemia may be severe and require transfusion.

MOLECULAR PATHOLOGY. A variety of mutations that cause CEP are known. These include missense and nonsense mutations, large and small deletions and insertions, splicing defects, and intronic branch point mutations. Most patients are heteroallelic for the UCS mutations, and they are from diverse racial and demographic groups.

DIAGNOSIS. Pink urine and/or the onset of severe cutaneous photosensitivity in infancy (or rarely in adults) suggest the diagnosis of CEP. Demonstration of elevated urinary, fecal, and erythrocyte porphyrins, with elevated type I isomers of uroporphyrin and coproporphyrin, establishes the diagnosis. Demonstration of a deficiency of UCS activity is definitive.

TREATMENT. The avoidance of sunlight, of trauma to the skin, and of infections is the most important preventive measure in CEP. Topical sunscreens may be of some help, as may oral treatment with β-carotene. Transfusions with packed erythrocytes transiently decrease hemolysis and its attendant drive to increased erythropoiesis and also decrease porphyrin excretion. Splenectomy has been used fairly frequently and has produced short-term reductions in hemolysis, porphyrin excretion, and skin manifestations, but not all cases respond. Treatment with charcoal in a man with CEP was reported to have lowered porphyrin levels and induced complete clinical remission during therapy.

Porphyria Cutanea Tarda (PCT) and Hepatoerythropoietic Porphyria (HEP). PCT is caused by a heterozygous deficiency, and HEP results from a homozygous deficiency of UROD, respectively (see Fig. 80–3 and Table 80–2).

PORPHYRIA CUTANEA TARDA. PCT refers to a heterogeneous group of cutaneous porphyria diseases caused by UROD deficiency, which may be either inherited or, more commonly, acquired. Both forms of the disease display reductions in hepatic UROD activity, but erythrocyte UROD activity may or may not be decreased, depending on their types. *Type I* PCT is an acquired disease that typically presents in adults, with decreased hepatic but not erythrocyte UROD activity. The disease may occur spontaneously but more commonly occurs in conjunction with precipitating environmental factors such as alcohol, estrogen, or drug use, or in association with other disorders. *Type II* PCT is, in contrast, inherited in an autosomal dominant fashion and is associated with decreased UROD activity in all tissues. *Type III* PCT is also inherited, but the defect is confined to the liver and erythrocyte UROD activity and concentrations are normal.

Epidemiology. PCT is probably the most common of all the porphyrias, but its exact incidence is not known. The disease is recognized worldwide and there is no racial predilection except among the Bantus in South Africa, secondary to their high incidence of hemosiderosis. Type I PCT is generally more common than type II PCT in Europe, South Africa, and South America. Previously, PCT was thought to be more common in men than women, perhaps secondary to their higher alcohol intake; the incidence in females has increased to the level seen in males, perhaps owing to increased use of contraceptive steroids, postmenopausal estrogens, and alcohol.

Clinical Manifestations. The pathognomonic clinical feature of PCT is the formation of vesicles on sun-exposed areas of the skin, particularly the dorsa of the hands. Crusting, superficial scar, milia formation, and residual pigmentation supersede the vesicles. Facial hypertrichosis may be present and is conspicuous. Hypopigmented indurated plaques of skin may develop and resemble those seen in scleroderma. Photo-onycholysis is occasionally present. Neurologic dysfunction does not·occur in PCT.

Pathogenesis. Phototoxic porphyrins in the skin may be largely derived from the liver or formed locally in the skin. Activation of the complement system after irradiation has been demonstrated in PCT patients and is presumed to result from the generation of reactive oxygen species. Bullous fluid is known to contain prostaglandin E_2, and photoactivation of uroporphyrin damages lysosomes. Liver from patients with PCT almost invariably displays siderosis with fatty changes, necrosis, chronic inflammatory changes, and granuloma formation. Iron, estrogens, alcohol, and chlorinated hydrocarbons, which are all potential hepatotoxins, may aggravate PCT. Either the homozygous or heterozygous presence of the C282Y and H63D mutations of the hemochromatosis *(HFE)* gene may predispose to the development of PCT. Increased prevalence of the C282Y mutation is increased in both sporadic (type I) and familial (type II) PCT. These associations will be more clearly understood when the function of the *HFE* gene is established and the functional significance of the C282Y and H63D mutations with regard to iron absorption are defined. The incidence of hepatitis B and C infection may also be higher than normal in PCT patients. The incidence of hepatocellular carcinoma in PCT is known to be greater than in the general population. A significant association of HIV-infected patients with PCT has been reported.

Laboratory Findings. Increased concentrations of uroporphyrin (mainly isomer I) and 7-carboxylic porphyrins (isomer III) are found in the urine in PCT, with lesser increases of coproporphyrin and 5- and 6-carboxylic porphyrins. Small quantities of isocoproporphyrin may be detected in serum or in urine, but in feces this is often the dominant porphyrin excreted and represents the most important diagnostic criterion for PCT. Total daily fecal porphyrin excretion exceeds total urinary porphyrin excretion. Skin porphyrins are increased, especially in areas that are protected from photoactivation. Serum iron and ferritin concentrations are frequently elevated.

Molecular Pathology. More than 10 *UROD* mutations responsible for PCT are known. Familial (type II) PCT is associated with heterozygous UROD deficiency. In contrast, HEP is due to homozygous or compound heterozygous state for mutations of the gene encoding this enzyme. Most *UROD* mutations found in HEP have not been found in familial PCT and are associated with residual UROD activity. The heterozygous *UROD* mutations in most cases of familial PCT appear to be more critical to the enzyme activity than those found in HEP. However, a few families with cases of both HEP and PCT have been described.

Diagnosis. The clinical picture in PCT is fairly specific but can be confused with other photosensitive porphyric (VP) and nonporphyric (systemic lupus erythematosus or scleroderma) diseases. Urinary fluorescence under ultraviolet light illumination, quantification of porphyrins and separation and identification of porphyrins by thin-layer chromatography, and high-performance liquid chromatography will assist the diagnosis. Plasma porphyrins are elevated in PCT and in other photosensitizing porphyrias. Fecal porphyrin levels are often elevated; isocoproporphyrin, or an isocoproporphyrin:coproporphyrin ratio of 0.1 or higher, is virtually diagnostic of PCT.

Treatment. In type I PCT, the identification and avoidance of precipitating factors is the first line of treatment. The clinical response to cessation of alcohol ingestion is highly variable; nonetheless, abstinence should be recommended because of the association with a history of heavy alcohol ingestion. Phlebotomy is usually effective in reducing urinary porphyrin concentrations and in induction of clinical remissions. There is strong evidence that the beneficial effects of phlebotomy result from a diminution in the stores of body iron. If phlebotomy is ineffective or contraindicated owing to the presence of other diseases such as anemia, low-dose chloroquine therapy may be considered. Efficacy of chloroquine therapy and phlebotomy is probably similar, and a combined approach may diminish the incidence of side effects. The mechanism of chloroquine therapy may be related to its ability to chelate porphyrins in a water-soluble and, hence, more easily excretable form.

HEPATOERYTHROPOIETIC PORPHYRIA. HEP is a rare form of porphyria probably resulting from a homozygous defect of UROD. Clinically, HEP is characterized by the childhood onset of severe photosensitivity and skin fragility and is indistinguishable from CEP. Some 20 cases are known.

Clinical Manifestations. These findings are very similar to those seen in CEP. Pink urine, severe photosensitivity leading to scarring and mutilation of sun-exposed areas of skin, sclerodermoid changes, hypertrichosis, erythrodontia, anemia (often hemolytic), and hepatosplenomegaly characterize HEP. Onset is usually in early infancy or childhood, but adult onset has also been described. In contrast to PCT, serum iron concentrations are usually normal and phlebotomy has no beneficial effects in HEP patients.

Laboratory Findings. Elevations in urinary porphyrins, predominantly uroporphyrin of isomer type I with lesser quantities of 7-carboxylic porphyrins, mainly type III, are commonly found. Isocoproporphyrin concentrations equal to or greater than coproporphyrin are also found in urine and feces. Elevated erythrocyte Zn-protoporphyrin is commonly observed (see Table 80–3). Anemia and biochemical evidence of impaired hepatic function is highly variable.

Molecular Pathology. In contrast to familial (type II) PCT, which is associated with heterozygous UROD deficiency, HEP is the result of a homozygous, or compound heterozygous, state for mutations of the gene. Although HEP is associated with marked UROD deficiency, there is some residual UROD activity. With a few exceptions, *UROD* mutations found in HEP are unique and not found in familial PCT. *UROD* mutations found in HEP appear to be less severe individually, but in the homozygous or compound heterozygous state they are associated with severe enzyme deficiencies. HEP is genetically heterogeneous. Both CRIM-positive and CRIM-negative mutations have been described.

DIAGNOSIS. The diagnosis must be suspected in patients with severe photosensitivity and especially considered in the differential diagnosis of CEP. Diagnostic criteria include elevated levels of fecal or urinary isocoproporphyrin and erythrocyte Zn-protoporphyrin. Differential diagnosis of HEP includes EPP in which erythrocyte protoporphyrin is also elevated but in which, in contrast to HEP, urinary porphyrins are normal. EPP is also clinically milder than HEP. Measurement of erythrocyte or fibroblast UROD activities typically shows reductions to 2–10% of normal control values with intermediate reductions of UROD activities in family members.

TREATMENT. Avoidance of the sun and the use of topical sunscreens is essentially all that can be offered to these patients. A response to phlebotomy has not been observed, although this is perhaps not surprising because serum iron levels, in contrast to those in PCT patients, are invariably normal.

Hereditary Coproporphyria (HCP). HCP is a disease caused by a heterozygous deficiency of CPO activity, which is inherited in an autosomal dominant manner (see Fig. 80–3 and Table 80–2). Clinically, the disease is similar to ADP or AIP, although it is often milder; additionally, HCP may be associated with photosensitivity. Expression of the disease is variable and influenced by similar precipitating factors responsible for the exacerbation of AIP. Very rarely, homozygous deficiency of this enzyme may occur and is associated with a more severe form of the disease.

EPIDEMIOLOGY. Clinically expressed HCP is much less common than is clinically expressed AIP, but, as with the latter disease, latent HCP or HCP gene carriers are found with greater frequency.

CLINICAL MANIFESTATIONS. Neurovisceral symptomatology is essentially indistinguishable from that of ADP or AIP. Abdominal pain, vomiting, constipation, neuropathies, and psychiatric manifestations are common. Cutaneous photosensitivity is a feature in about 30% of cases. Pregnancy, the menstrual cycle, and contraceptive steroids can precipitate attacks, but the most common precipitating factor is drug administration, most notably phenobarbital.

LABORATORY FINDINGS. The biochemical hallmark of HCP is hyperexcretion of coproporphyrin (predominantly type III) into the urine and feces. Fecal coproporphyrin may be chelated with copper, and fecal protoporphyrin may be modestly elevated. Hyperexcretion of ALA, PBG, and uroporphyrin into the urine may accompany exacerbations of the disease, but, in contrast to AIP, these findings generally normalize between attacks. CPO activity is typically reduced by about 50% in heterozygotes and by about 90–98% in homozygotes.

MOLECULAR PATHOLOGY. The first disease-specific mutation of the CPO gene reported was a C→T transition at position 691, resulting in an Arg→Trp substitution in the protein, in a patient with homozygous HCP. This substitution results in the synthesis of an unstable protein with a residual activity. A G265→A transition, involving the highly conserved glycine residue at the 89th position, was detected in a patient with heterozygous HCP. A transition A→G mutation at position 910 of the coding sequence of the CPO mRNA was found in a variant homozygous form of HCP, *harderoporphyria*; this mutation led to the substitution of a lysine residue by glutamic acid (K304E). Several other mutations in the *CPO* gene are known, but all mutations including two for the homoallelic form of HCP and harderoporphyria, are different.

DIAGNOSIS. The diagnosis of HCP should be suspected in patients with the signs, symptoms, and clinical course characteristic of the acute hepatic porphyrias (ADP, AIP, HCP, and VP) but in whom PBGD activity is normal. Urinary excretion of heme precursors is similar in HCP and VP, but the predominant or exclusive presence of fecal coproporphyrin is highly suggestive of HCP. Fecal or urinary predominance of harderoporphyrin, with greatly reduced CPO activity, was reported in a case of harderoporphyria, a variant form of HCP.

TREATMENT. The identification and avoidance of precipitating factors is essential. Treatment of acute attacks is similar to the treatment of AIP.

Variegate Porphyria (VP). VP, also termed *porphyria variegata*, protocoproporphyria, South African genetic porphyria, or Royal malady, is caused by a heterozygous deficiency in PPO activity and is inherited in an autosomal dominant manner (see Fig. 80–3 and Table 80–2). Patients with this disorder may show neurovisceral symptoms, photosensitivity, or both (Table 80–3). Very rare forms of VP are seen with homozygous deficiencies in PPO activity.

EPIDEMIOLOGY. The incidence of VP of 3 in 1,000 in South Africa is substantially higher than elsewhere. The disease is recognized worldwide, and, with the exception of South Africa, there is no racial or geographic predilection. Outside of South Africa, VP is probably less common than AIP.

CLINICAL MANIFESTATIONS. The neurovisceral symptomatology is identical to that observed in ADP, AIP, and HCP. Photosensitivity is more common, and the resulting lesions tend to be more chronic in VP than in HCP. Cutaneous manifestations comprise vesicles, bullae, hyperpigmentation, milia, hypertrichosis, and increased skin fragility. Lesions are clinically and histologically indistinguishable from PCT. Skin manifestations are less frequently observed in cold climates than in hot climates. The same spectrum of factors that leads to activation of ADP, AIP, and HCP may also exacerbate VP. Barbiturates, dapsone, lead from "moonshine" whiskey, contraceptive steroids, pregnancy, and decreased carbohydrate intake all induce or exacerbate VP.

PATHOGENESIS. PPO activity in most patients with VP is decreased more than 50%. In rare cases of homozygous VP, however, there is a virtual absence of PPO activity. Symptoms include severe photosensitivity, growth and mental retardation, and marked neurologic abnormalities in some cases; onset of homozygous VP starts in childhood.

LABORATORY FINDINGS. The biochemical hallmark of VP is elevated fecal porphyrin, usually with protoporphyrin IX exceeding coproporphyrin (mostly isomer III). Fecal X-porphyrins (ether-acetic acid-insoluble, extracted with urea-Triton), a heterogeneous group of porphyrin-peptide conjugates, are elevated in VP more than in any other type of porphyria. Urinary coproporphyrin (type III), ALA, and PBG are often normal between attacks but may become markedly elevated during acute attacks. Plasma invariably shows a fluorescence emission that probably represents a protoporphyrin-peptide conjugate.

MOLECULAR PATHOLOGY. Various disease-specific PPO mutations have been reported in families with VP from around the world. One of the mutations (R59W) represents the founder gene underlying the high incidence of VP in South Africa. Rare homozygotes for VP have been shown to be mostly *heteroallelic* for defects in the *PPO* gene, with the exception of one who was *homoallelic*.

DIAGNOSIS. VP should be considered in the differential diagnosis of acute porphyria, especially if PBGD activity is normal. Characteristic plasma porphyrin fluorescence, having a different fluorescence emission maximum from PCT, is seen in VP. The differentiation of VP from HCP is usually possible after fecal porphyrin analysis and in patients with only cutaneous manifestations. The demonstration of urinary 8- and 7-carboxylic porphyrins and isocoproporphyrin in PCT is usually sufficient for differentiation from VP. PPO deficiency can be demonstrated in fibroblasts or lymphocytes.

TREATMENT. Identification and avoidance of precipitating factors is essential. Protective clothing can minimize photosensitivity, and canthaxanthin (a β-carotene analogue) may be of some help. The treatment of neurovisceral symptoms is identical to that described for AIP.

Erythropoietic Protoporphyria (EPP). EPP, also referred to as protoporphyria, or erythrohepatic protoporphyria, is associated with a partial deficiency of FeC and is inherited in an autosomal dominant fashion (see Fig. 80–3 and Table 80–2). Biochemically, this defect results in massive accumulations of protoporphyrin in erythrocytes, plasma, and feces. The disease is characterized by the childhood onset of cutaneous photosensitivity in light-exposed areas, but skin lesions are milder and less disfiguring than those seen in CEP.

EPIDEMIOLOGY. EPP is the most common form of erythropoietic porphyria. There is no racial or sexual predilection, and onset is typically in childhood.

CLINICAL MANIFESTATIONS. Cutaneous photosensitivity of EPP is quite different from that seen in CEP or PCT. Stinging or painful burning sensations in the skin occur within 1 hr of exposure to the sun and are followed several hours later by erythema and edema. Some patients experience burning sensations in the absence of such objective signs of cutaneous phototoxicity that result in the erroneous diagnosis of a psychiatric illness. Petechiae, or more rarely, purpura, vesicles, and crusting, may develop and persist for several days after sun exposure. Artificial lights may also cause photosensitivity, especially operating theater lights. Symptoms are usually worse during spring and summer and occur in light-exposed areas, especially on the face and hands. Intense and repeated exposure to the sun may result in onycholysis, leathery hyperkeratotic skin over the dorsa of the hands, and mild scarring. Gallstones, sometimes presenting at an unusually early age, are fairly common, and hepatic disease, although unusual, may be severe and associated with significant morbidity. Anemia is uncommon. There are no known precipitating factors and no neurovisceral manifestations.

PATHOGENESIS. The peak light absorption range for porphyrins corresponds well to the wavelength of light (circa 400 nm) known to trigger photosensitivity reactions in the skin of EPP patients. Light-excited porphyrins generate free radicals and singlet oxygen that may lead to peroxidation of lipids and cross-linking of membrane proteins, which, in erythrocytes, may result in reduced deformability and thus hemolysis. Interestingly, protoporphyrin, but not Zn-protoporphyrin, is released from erythrocytes after irradiation, which may explain why EPP is associated with photosensitivity whereas lead intoxication and iron deficiency are not. Forearm irradiation in EPP patients leads to complement activation and polymorphonuclear chemotaxis. Similar results have been obtained in vitro, and these events may also contribute to the pathogenesis of skin lesions in EPP.

LABORATORY FINDINGS. The biochemical hallmark of EPP is excessive concentrations of free protoporphyrin in erythrocytes, plasma, bile, and feces; this is due to its poor solubility in water, not in urine. The bone marrow and the newly released erythrocytes appear to be the major source of elevated protoporphyrin concentrations, although the liver may contribute in certain cases.

MOLECULAR PATHOLOGY. Molecular analysis of ferrochelatase mutations reveals missense mutations, splicing abnormalities, intragenic deletions, and possible nonsense mutations associated with functional deficiency of ferrochelatase. Exon skipping is the most predominant. Incomplete penetrance and variable clinical expression remain as puzzling features of EPP. There is no strict correlation between the genetic defects

and the erythrocyte protoporphyrin levels or between the abnormal ferrochelatase activity and EPP disease severity.

DIAGNOSIS. Photosensitivity, which is quite distinct from that seen in CEP or PCT, should suggest the diagnosis, which can be confirmed by the demonstration of elevated concentrations of free protoporphyrin in erythrocytes, plasma, and stools with normal urinary porphyrins. The presence of protoporphyrin in both plasma and erythrocytes is specific for EPP. Fluorescent reticulocytes on examination of a peripheral blood smear may also suggest the diagnosis.

TREATMENT. Avoidance of the sun and use of topical sunscreen agents may be helpful. Oral administration of β-carotene may afford systemic photoprotection, resulting in improved, though highly variable, tolerance to the sun. The recommended serum β-carotene level of 600–800 µg/dL is usually achieved with oral doses of 120–180 mg daily, and beneficial effects are typically seen 1–3 mo after the onset of therapy. The mechanism probably involves quenching of activated oxygen radicals.

Bishop TR, Miller MW, Beall J, et al: Genetic regulation of delta-aminolevulinate dehydratase during erythropoiesis. *Nucl Acids Res* 1996;24:2511–18.

Boulechfar S, Da Silva V, Deybach JC, et al: Heterogeneity of mutations in the uroporphyrinogen III synthase gene in congenital erythropoietic porphyria. *Hum Genet* 1992;88:320–24.

Bulaj ZJ, Phillips JD, Ajioka RS, et al: Hemochromatosis genes and other factors contributing to the pathogenesis of porphyria cutanea tarda. *Blood* 2000;95:1565–71.

Cotter PD, Baumann M, Bishop DF: Enzymatic defect in "X-linked" sideroblastic anemia: Molecular evidence for erythroid delta-aminolevulinate synthase deficiency. *Proc Natl Acad Sci USA* 1992;89:4028–32.

Cox TM, Alexander GJ, Sarkany RP: Protoporphyria. *Semin Liver Dis* 1998;18:85–93.

de Verneuil H, Nordmann Y, Phung N, et al: Familial and sporadic porphyria cutanea: Two different diseases. *Int J Biochem* 1978;9:927–31.

Deybach JC, de Verneuil H, Phung N, et al: Congenital erythropoietic porphyria (Gunther's disease): Enzymatic studies on two cases of late onset. *J Lab Clin Med* 1981;97:551–58.

Eales L, Day RS, Blekkenhorst GH: The clinical and biochemical features of variegate porphyria: An analysis of 300 cases studied at Groote Schuur Hospital, Cape Town. *Int J Biochem* 1980;12:837–53.

Elder GH: Porphyria cutanea tarda. *Semin Liver Dis* 1998;18:67–75.

Grandchamp B: Acute intermittent porphyria. *Semin Liver Dis* 1998;18:17–24.

Herrero C, Vicente A, Bruguera M, et al: Is hepatitis C virus infection a trigger of porphyria cutanea tarda? *Lancet* 1993;341:788–9.

Kirsch RE, Meissner PN, Hift RJ: Variegate porphyria. *Semin Liver Dis* 1998;18:33–41.

Martasek P: Hereditary coproporphyria. *Semin Liver Dis* 1998;18:25–32.

Maruno M, Furuyama K, Akagi R, et al: Highly heterogenous nature of δ-aminolevulinate dehydratase (ALAD) deficiencies in ALAD porphyria. *Blood* 2001;97:2972–8.

Mustajoki P: Variegate porphyria. Twelve years experience in Finland. *Q J Med* 1980;194:191–203.

Mustajoki P, Tenhunen R, Tokola O, et al: Haem arginate in the treatment of acute hepatic porphyrias. *BMJ* 1986;293:538–39.

Nakahashi Y, Miyazaki H, Kadota Y, et al: Molecular defect in human erythropoietic protoporphyria with fatal liver failure. *Hum Genet* 1993;91:303–6.

Plewinska M, Thunell S, Holmberg L, et al: δ-Aminolevulinate dehydratase deficient porphyria: Identification of the molecular lesions in a severely affected homozygote. *Am J Hum Genet* 1991;49:167–74.

Rüfenacht U, Gouya L, Schneider-Yin X, et al: Systematic analysis of molecular defects in the ferrochelatase gene from patients with erythropoietic protoporphyria. *Am J Hum Genet* 1998;62:1341–52.

Sassa S: Hematologic aspects of the porphyrias. *Int J Hematol* 2000;71:1–17.

Sassa S, Kappas A: Hereditary tyrosinemia and the heme biosynthetic pathway: Profound inhibition of δ-aminolevulinic acid dehydratase activity by succinylacetone. *J Clin Invest* 1983;71:625–34.

Tenhunen R, Mustajoki P: Acute porphyria: Treatment with heme. *Semin Liver Dis* 1998;18:53–5.

Thunell S, Holmberg L, Lundgren J: Aminolevulinate dehydratase porphyria in infancy: A clinical and biochemical study. *J Clin Chem Clin Biochem* 1987;25:5–14.

Toback AC, Sassa S, Poh Fitzpatrick MB, et al: Hepatoerythropoietic porphyria: Clinical, biochemical, and enzymatic studies in a three-generation family lineage. *N Engl J Med* 1987;316:645–50.

Todd DJ: Clinical implications of the molecular biology of erythropoietic protoporphyria. *J Eur Acad Dermatol Venereol* 1998;11:207–13.

Chapter 81

Hypoglycemia *Mark A. Sperling*

Glucose has a central role in fuel economy and is a source of energy storage in the form of glycogen, fat, and protein (see Chapter 76). Glucose, an immediate source of energy, provides 38 mol of adenosine triphosphate (ATP)/mol of glucose oxidized. It is important for cerebral energy metabolism because it is usually the preferred substrate and its utilization accounts for nearly all the oxygen consumption in brain. Cerebral glucose uptake occurs through a glucose transporter molecule or molecules that are not regulated by insulin. Cerebral transport of glucose is a carrier-mediated, facilitated diffusion process that is dependent on blood glucose concentration. Deficiency of brain glucose transporters can result in seizures because of low cerebral glucose concentrations despite normal blood glucose levels. To maintain the blood glucose concentration and prevent it from precipitously falling to levels that impair brain function, an elaborate regulatory system has evolved.

The defense against hypoglycemia is integrated by the autonomic nervous system and by hormones that act in concert to enhance glucose production through enzymatic modulation of glycogenolysis and gluconeogenesis while simultaneously limiting peripheral glucose utilization. Hypoglycemia represents a defect in one or several of the complex interactions that normally integrate glucose homeostasis during feeding and fasting. This process is particularly important for neonates, in whom there is an abrupt transition from intrauterine life, characterized by dependence on transplacental glucose supply, to extrauterine life, characterized ultimately by the autonomous ability to maintain euglycemia. Because prematurity or placental insufficiency may limit tissue nutrient deposits, and genetic abnormalities in enzymes or hormones may become evident in the neonate, hypoglycemia is common in the neonatal period.

Definition. In neonates, there is not always an obvious correlation between blood glucose concentration and the classic clinical manifestations of hypoglycemia. The absence of symptoms does not indicate that glucose concentration is normal and has not fallen to less than some optimal level for maintaining brain metabolism. There is evidence that hypoxemia and ischemia may potentiate the role of hypoglycemia in causing permanent brain damage. Consequently, the lower limit of accepted normality of the blood glucose level in newborn infants with associated illness that already impairs cerebral metabolism has not been determined (see Chapter 96). Out of concern for possible neurologic, intellectual, or psychologic sequelae in later life, many authorities now urge that any value of blood glucose less than 50 mg/dL in neonates be viewed with suspicion and vigorously treated. This is particularly applicable after the initial 2–3 hr of life, when glucose normally has reached its nadir; subsequently, blood glucose levels begin to rise and achieve values of 50 mg/dL or higher after 12–24 hr. In older infants and children, a whole blood glucose concentration of less than 50 mg/dL (10–15% higher for serum or plasma) represents hypoglycemia.

Significance and Sequelae. Metabolism by the adult brain accounts for the majority of total basal glucose turnover. Most of the endogenous hepatic glucose production in infants and young children can be accounted for by brain metabolism. Furthermore, there is a correlation between glucose production and estimated brain weight at all ages.

Because the brain grows most rapidly during the 1st yr of life and because the larger proportion of glucose turnover is used for brain metabolism, sustained or repetitive hypoglycemia in infants and children can retard brain development and function. In the rapidly growing brain, glucose may also be a source of

membrane lipids and protein synthesis; structural proteins and myelination are important for normal brain maturation. Under conditions of severe and sustained hypoglycemia, these cerebral structural substrates may have to be degraded to energy-usable intermediates such as lactate, pyruvate, amino acids, and ketoacids, which can support brain metabolism at the expense of brain growth. The capacity of the newborn brain to take up and oxidize ketone bodies is about fivefold greater than that of the adult brain. However, the capacity of the liver to produce ketone bodies may be limited in the newborn period, especially in the presence of hyperinsulinemia, which acutely inhibits hepatic glucose output, lipolysis, and ketogenesis, thereby depriving the brain of alternate fuel sources. The deprivation of the brain's major energy source during hypoglycemia and the limited availability of alternate fuel sources during hyperinsulinemia have predictable adverse consequences on brain metabolism and growth: decreased brain oxygen consumption and increased breakdown of endogenous structural components with destruction of functional membrane integrity. Hypoglycemia may thus lead to permanent impairment of brain growth and function. The potentiating effects of hypoxia may exacerbate brain damage or indeed be responsible for it when blood glucose values are not in the classic hypoglycemic range.

The major long-term sequelae of severe, prolonged hypoglycemia are mental retardation or recurrent seizure activity, or both. Subtle effects on personality are also possible but have not been clearly defined. Permanent neurologic sequelae are present in more than half of patients with severe recurrent hypoglycemia who are younger than 6 mo of age, the period of most rapid brain growth. These sequelae may be reflected in pathologic changes characterized by atrophic gyri, reduced myelination in cerebral white matter, and atrophy in the cerebral cortex. Infarcts are absent if hypoxia-ischemia did not contribute to cerebral manifestations, and the cerebellum is spared if hypoglycemia is the sole insult. These sequelae are more likely when alternative fuel sources are limited as occurs with hyperinsulinemia, when the episodes of hypoglycemia are repetitive or prolonged, or when they are compounded by hypoxia. There is no precise knowledge relating the duration or severity of hypoglycemia to subsequent neurologic development of children in a predictable manner. Although less common, hypoglycemia in older children may also produce long-term neurologic defects through neuronal death mediated, in part, by cerebral excitotoxins released during hypoglycemia.

Substrate, Enzyme, and Hormonal Integration of Glucose Homeostasis

IN THE NEWBORN (see also Chapter 96). Under nonstressed conditions, fetal glucose is derived entirely from the mother through placental transfer. Therefore, fetal glucose concentration usually reflects but is slightly lower than maternal glucose levels. Catecholamine release, which occurs with fetal stress such as hypoxia, mobilizes fetal glucose and free fatty acids (FFAs) through β-adrenergic mechanisms, reflecting β-adrenergic activity in fetal liver and adipose tissue. Catecholamines may also inhibit fetal insulin and stimulate glucagon release.

The acute interruption of maternal glucose transfer to the fetus at delivery imposes an immediate need to mobilize endogenous glucose. Three related events facilitate this transition: changes in hormones, changes in their receptors, and changes in key enzyme activity. There is a three- to fivefold abrupt increase in glucagon concentration within minutes to hours of birth. The level of insulin usually falls initially and remains in the basal range for several days without demonstrating the usual brisk response to physiologic stimuli such as glucose. A dramatic surge in spontaneous catecholamine secretion is also characteristic. Epinephrine can also augment growth hormone secretion by α-adrenergic mechanisms; growth hormone levels are elevated at birth. Acting in unison, these hormonal changes at birth mobilize glucose via glycogenolysis and gluco-neogenesis, activate lipolysis, and promote ketogenesis. As a result of these processes, plasma glucose concentration stabilizes after a transient decrease immediately after birth, liver glycogen stores become rapidly depleted within hours of birth, and gluco-neogenesis from alanine, a major gluconeogenic amino acid, can account for approximately 10% of glucose turnover in the human newborn infant by several hours of age. FFA concentrations also increase sharply in concert with the surges in glucagon and epinephrine and are followed by rises in ketone bodies. Glucose is thus spared for brain utilization while FFAs and ketones provide alternative fuel sources for muscle as well as essential gluconeogenic factors such as acetyl-coenzyme A (CoA) and the reduced form of nicotinamide-adenine dinu-cleotide (NADH) from hepatic fatty acid oxidation, which is required for gluconeogenesis.

In the early postnatal period, responses of the endocrine pan-creas favor glucagon secretion so that blood glucose concentra-tion can be maintained. These adaptive changes in hormone secretion are paralleled by similarly striking adaptive changes in hormone receptors. Key enzymes involved in glucose produc-tion also change dramatically in the perinatal period. Thus, there is a rapid fall in glycogen synthase activity and a sharp rise in phosphorylase after delivery. Similarly, the amount of rate-limiting enzyme for gluconeogenesis, phosphoenol-pyruvate carboxykinase, rises dramatically after birth, activated in part by the surge in glucagon and the fall in insulin. This framework can explain several causes of neonatal hypoglycemia based on inap-propriate changes in hormone secretion and unavailability of adequate reserves of substrates in the form of hepatic glycogen, muscle as a source of amino acids for gluconeogenesis, and lipid stores for the release of fatty acids. In addition, appropriate activities of key enzymes governing glucose homeostasis are required (see Fig. 76–1).

IN OLDER INFANTS AND CHILDREN. Hypoglycemia in older infants and children is analogous to that of adults, in whom glucose homeostasis is maintained by glycogenolysis in the immediate postfeeding period and by gluconeogenesis several hours after meals. The liver of a 10-kg child contains 20–25 g of glycogen, which is sufficient to meet normal glucose requirements of 4–6 mg/kg/min for only 6–12 hr. Beyond this period, hepatic gluconeogenesis must be activated. Both glycogenolysis and gluconeogenesis depend on the metabolic pathway summarized in Figure 76–1. Defects in gluconeogene-sis may not be manifested in infants until the frequent feeding of 3- to 4-hr intervals ceases and infants sleep through the night, a situation usually present by 3–6 mo of age. The source of gluco-neogenic precursors is derived primarily from muscle protein. The muscle bulk of infants and small children is substantially smaller relative to body mass than that of adults, whereas glu-cose requirements/unit of body mass are greater in children, so the ability to compensate for glucose deprivation by gluconeo-genesis is more limited in infants and young children, as is the ability to withstand fasting for prolonged periods. The ability of muscle to generate alanine, the principal gluconeogenic amino acid, may also be limited. Thus, in normal young children, the blood glucose level falls after 24 hr of fasting, insulin concentra-tions fall appropriately to levels of less than 5–10 µU/mL, lipoly-sis and ketogenesis are activated, and ketones may appear in the urine.

The switch from glycogen synthesis during and immediately after meals to glycogen breakdown and later gluconeogenesis is governed by hormones, of which insulin is of central impor-tance. Plasma insulin concentrations increase to peak levels of 50–100 µU/mL after meals, which serve to lower the blood glu-cose concentration through the activation of glycogen synthesis, enhancement of peripheral glucose uptake, and inhibition of glucose production. In addition, lipogenesis is stimulated whereas lipolysis and ketogenesis are curtailed. During fasting,

plasma insulin concentrations fall to 5–10 µU/mL or less, and, together with other hormonal changes, this fall results in activation of gluconeogenic pathways (see Fig. 76–1). Fasting glucose concentrations are maintained through the activation of glycogenolysis and gluconeogenesis, inhibition of glycogen synthesis, and activation of lipolysis and ketogenesis. It should be emphasized that a plasma insulin concentration of greater than 5 µU/mL, in association with a blood glucose concentration of 40 mg/dL (2.2 mM) or less, is abnormal, indicating a hyper-insulinemic state and failure of the mechanisms that nor-mally result in suppression of insulin secretion during fasting or hypoglycemia.

The hypoglycemic effects of insulin are opposed by the actions of several hormones whose concentration in plasma increases as blood glucose falls. These counterregulatory hormones, glucagon, growth hormone, cortisol, and epinephrine, act in concert by increasing blood glucose concentrations via activat-ing glycogenolytic enzymes (glucagon, epinephrine); inducing gluconeogenic enzymes (glucagon, cortisol); inhibiting glucose uptake by muscle (epinephrine, growth hormone, cortisol); mobilizing amino acids from muscle for gluconeogenesis (corti-sol); activating lipolysis; providing glycerol for gluconeogenesis and fatty acids for ketogenesis (epinephrine, cortisol, growth hormone, glucagon); and inhibiting insulin release and promo-tion of growth hormone and glucagon secretion (epinephrine).

Congenital or acquired deficiencies in these hormones may rarely result in hypoglycemia, which occurs when endogenous glucose production cannot be mobilized to meet energy needs in the postabsorptive state, that is, 8–12 hr after meals or during fasting. Concurrent deficiency of several hormones (hypopitu-itarism) may result in hypoglycemia that is more severe or appears earlier during fasting than that seen with isolated hor-mone deficiencies. For practical purposes the majority of the causes of hypoglycemia in infancy and childhood reflect inap-propriate adaptation to fasting.

Clinical Manifestations (see also Chapter 96). Clinical features generally fall into two categories. The first includes symptoms associated with the activation of the autonomic nervous system and epinephrine release, usually seen with a rapid decline in blood glucose concentration (Box 81–1). The second category includes symptoms due to decreased cerebral glucose utiliza-tion, usually associated with a slow decline in blood glucose level or prolonged hypoglycemia (see Box 81–1). Although these classic symptoms occur in older children, the symptoms of hypoglycemia in infants may be subtler and include cyanosis, apnea, hypothermia, hypotonia, poor feeding, lethargy, and seizures. Some of these symptoms may be so mild that they are missed. Occasionally, hypoglycemia may be asymptomatic in the immediate newborn period. Newborns with hyperinsu-linemia are often large for gestational age; older infants with hyperinsulinemia may eat excessively because of chronic hypo-glycemia and become obese. In childhood, hypoglycemia may present as behavior problems, inattention, ravenous appetite, or seizures. It may be misdiagnosed as epilepsy, inebriation, per-sonality disorders, hysteria, and retardation. A blood glucose determination should always be performed in sick neonates, who should be vigorously treated if concentrations are less than 50 mg/dL. At any age level, hypoglycemia should be considered a cause of an initial episode of convulsions or a sudden deterio-ration in psychobehavioral functioning.

Classification of Hypoglycemia in Infants and Children. Classification is based on knowledge of the control of glucose homeostasis in infants and children (Box 81–2).

NEONATAL, TRANSIENT, SMALL FOR GESTATIONAL AGE, AND PREMATURE INFANTS (see Chapter 96). The overall incidence of symptomatic hypoglycemia in newborns is 1–3 per 1,000 live births. This incidence is increased severalfold in certain high-risk neonatal groups (see Box 81–2). The prema-

BOX 81–1. Manifestations of Hypoglycemia in Childhood

FEATURES ASSOCIATED WITH ACTIVATION OF AUTONOMIC NERVOUS SYSTEM AND EPINEPHRINE RELEASE*

Anxiety[†]
Perspiration[†]
Palpitation (tachycardia)[†]
Pallor
Tremulousness
Weakness
Hunger
Nausea
Emesis
Angina (with normal coronary arteries)

FEATURES ASSOCIATED WITH CEREBRAL GLUCOPENIA

Headache[†]
Mental confusion[†]
Visual disturbances ($\downarrow$ acuity, diplopia)[†]
Organic personality changes[†]
Inability to concentrate[†]
Dysarthria
Staring
Seizures
Ataxia, incoordination
Somnolence, lethargy
Coma
Stroke, hemiplegia, aphasia
Paresthesias
Dizziness
Amnesia
Decerebrate or decorticate posture

*Some of these features will be attenuated if the patient is receiving β-adrenergic blocking agents.
[†]Common.

ture and small for gestational age (SGA) infants are vulnerable to the development of hypoglycemia. The factors responsible for the high frequency of hypoglycemia in this group, as well as in other groups outlined in Box 81–2, are related to the inadequate stores of liver glycogen, muscle protein, and body fat needed to sustain the substrates required to meet energy needs. These infants are small by virtue of prematurity or impaired placental transfer of nutrients. Their enzyme systems for gluconeogenesis may not be fully developed.

In contrast to deficiency of substrates or enzymes, the hormonal system appears to be functioning normally at birth in most low-risk neonates. Despite hypoglycemia, plasma concentrations of alanine, lactate, and pyruvate are higher, implying their diminished rate of utilization as substrates for gluconeogenesis. Infusion of alanine elicits further glucagon secretion but causes no significant rise in glucose. During the initial 24 hr of life, plasma concentrations of acetoacetate and β-hydroxybutyrate are lower in SGA infants than in full-term infants, implying diminished lipid stores, diminished fatty acid mobilization, or impaired ketogenesis, or a combination of these conditions. Diminished lipid stores are most likely because fat (triglyceride) feeding of newborns results in a rise in the plasma levels of glucose, FFAs, and ketones. In addition, infants with perinatal asphyxia and some SGA newborns may have transient hyperinsulinemia, which promotes hypoglycemia and diminishes FFAs.

The role of FFAs and their oxidation in stimulating neonatal gluconeogenesis is essential. The provision of FFAs as triglyceride feedings from formula or human milk together with gluconeogenic precursors may prevent the hypoglycemia that usually ensues after neonatal fasting. For these and other reasons, milk feedings are introduced early (at birth or within 4–6 hr) after delivery. In the hospital setting, when feeding is precluded by virtue of respiratory distress or when feedings alone cannot maintain blood glucose concentrations at levels greater than 50 mg/dL, intravenous glucose at a rate that supplies 4–8 mg/kg/min should be started. Infants with transient

neonatal hypoglycemia can usually maintain the blood glucose level spontaneously after 2–3 days of life.

INFANTS BORN TO DIABETIC MOTHERS (see Chapter 96). Of the transient hyperinsulinemic states, infants born to diabetic mothers are the most common. Gestational diabetes affects some 2% of pregnant women, and approximately 1/1,000 pregnant women have insulin-dependent diabetes. At birth, infants born to these mothers may be large and plethoric, and their body stores of glycogen, protein, and fat are replete.

Hypoglycemia in infants of diabetic mothers is mostly related to hyperinsulinemia and partly related to diminished glucagon secretion. Hypertrophy and hyperplasia of the islets is present, as is a brisk, biphasic, and typically mature insulin response to glucose; this insulin response is absent in normal infants. Infants born to diabetic mothers also have a subnormal surge in plasma glucagon immediately after birth, subnormal glucagon secretion in response to stimuli and, initially, excessive sympathetic activity that may lead to adrenomedullary exhaustion as reflected by decreased urinary excretion of epinephrine. The normal plasma hormonal pattern of low insulin, high glucagon, and high catecholamines is reversed to a pattern of high insulin, low glucagon, and low epinephrine. As a consequence of this abnormal hormonal profile, the endogenous glucose production is significantly inhibited compared with that in normal infants, thus predisposing them to hypoglycemia.

Infants born with *erythroblastosis fetalis* also may have hyperinsulinemia and share many physical features, such as large body size, with infants born to diabetic mothers. The cause of the hyperinsulinemia in infants with erythroblastosis is not entirely clear.

Mothers whose diabetes has been well controlled during pregnancy, labor, and delivery generally have infants near normal size who are less likely to acquire neonatal hypoglycemia and other complications formerly considered typical of such infants (see Chapter 96). In supplying glucose to hypoglycemic infants, it is important to avoid hyperglycemia that evokes a prompt exuberant insulin release, which may result in rebound hypoglycemia. When needed, glucose should be provided at continuous infusion rates of 4–8 mg/kg/min, but the appropriate dose for each patient should be individually adjusted. During labor and delivery, maternal hyperglycemia should be avoided because it results in fetal hyperglycemia, which predisposes to hypoglycemia when the glucose supply is interrupted at birth. Hypoglycemia persisting or occurring after 1 wk of life requires an evaluation for the causes listed in Box 81–2.

Persistent or Recurrent Hypoglycemia in Infants and Children
HYPERINSULINISM. Most children with hyperinsulinism that causes hypoglycemia present in the neonatal period or in infancy; hyperinsulinism is the most common cause of persistent hypoglycemia in early infancy. Hyperinsulinemic infants may be macrosomic at birth, reflecting the anabolic effects of insulin in utero. There is, however, no history and no biochemical evidence of maternal diabetes. The onset is from birth to 18 mo of age, but occasionally it is first evident in older children. Insulin concentrations are inappropriately elevated at the time of documented hypoglycemia; with non-hyperinsulinemic hypoglycemia, plasma insulin concentrations should be less than 5 µU/mL and no higher than 10 µU/mL. In affected infants, however, plasma insulin concentrations at the time of hypoglycemia are commonly greater than 5–10 µU/mL. Some authorities set more stringent criteria, arguing that any value of insulin higher than 2 µU/mL with hypoglycemia is abnormal. The insulin (µU/mL):glucose (mg/dL) ratio is commonly 0.4 or greater; plasma ketones and FFA levels are low. Macrosomic infants may present with hypoglycemia from the first days of life. Infants with lesser degrees of hyperinsulinemia, however, may manifest hypoglycemia after the first few weeks to months, when the frequency of feedings has been decreased to permit

BOX 81–2. Classification of Hypoglycemia in Infants and Children

NEONATAL TRANSIENT HYPOGLYCEMIA

Associated with inadequate substrate or immature enzyme function
  in otherwise normal neonates
  Prematurity
  Small for gestational age
  Normal newborn
Transient hyperinsulinism
Neonatal hyperinsulinism
  Small for gestational age
  Discordant twin
  Birth asphyxia
  Infant of toxemic mother
  Infant of diabetic mother

NEONATAL, INFANTILE, OR CHILDHOOD PERSISTENT HYPOGLYCEMIAS

Hormonal disorders
  Hyperinsulinism
    Recessive K_{ATP} channel HI
    Focal K_{ATP} channel HI
    Dominant K_{ATP} channel HI
    Dominant glucokinase HI
    Dominant glutamate dehydrogenase HI
      (hyperinsulinism/hyperammonemia syndrome)
    Acquired islet adenoma
    Beckwith-Wiedemann syndrome
    Insulin administration (Munchausen by proxy)
    Oral sulfonylurea drugs
    Congenital disorders of glycosylation
  Counterregulatory hormone deficiency
    Panhypopituitarism
    Isolated growth hormone deficiency
    Adrenocorticotropic hormone deficiency
    Addison's disease
    Epinephrine deficiency
Gluconeogenesis and Glycogenolysis disorders
  Amylo-1,6-glucosidase (debranching enzyme) deficiency (GSD 3)
  Liver phosphorylase deficiency (GSD 6)
  Phosphorylase kinase deficiency (GSD 9)
  Glycogen synthetase deficiency (GSD 0)
  Glucose 6-phosphatase deficiency (GSD 1a)
  Glucose 6-phosphate translocase deficiency (GSD 1b)
  Fructose 1,6-diphosphatase deficiency
  Pyruvate carboxylase deficiency
  Galactosemia
  Hereditary fructose intolerance
Lipolysis disorders
  Propranolol
Fatty acid oxidation disorders
  Carnitine transporter deficiency (primary carnitine deficiency)
  Carnitine palmitoyl-transferase 1 deficiency
  Carnitine translocase deficiency

Carnitine palmitoyl-transferase 2 deficiency
Secondary carnitine deficiencies
Very long – long – medium – short-chain acyl-CoA dehydrogenase
  deficiency

OTHER ETIOLOGIES

Substrate-limited
  Ketotic hypoglycemia
Poisoning—drugs
  Salicylates
  Alcohol
  Oral hypoglycemic agents
  Insulin
  Propranolol
  Pentamidine
  Quinine
  Disopyramide
  Ackee fruit (unripe)—hypoglycin
  Vacor (rat poison)
  Trimethoprim-sulfamethoxazole (with renal failure)
Liver disease
  Reye syndrome
  Hepatitis
  Cirrhosis
  Hepatoma
Amino acid and organic acid disorders
  Maple syrup urine disease
  Propionic acidemia
  Methylmalonic acidemia
  Tyrosinosis
  Glutaric aciduria
  3-Hydroxy-3-methylglutaric aciduria
Systemic disorders
  Sepsis
  Carcinoma/sarcoma (secreting—insulin-like growth factor II)
  Heart failure
  Malnutrition
  Malabsorption
  Anti-insulin receptor antibodies
  Anti-insulin antibodies
  Neonatal hyperviscosity
  Renal failure
  Diarrhea
  Burns
  Shock
  Postsurgical
  Pseudohypoglycemia (leukocytosis, polycythemia)
  Excessive insulin therapy of insulin-dependent diabetes
    mellitus
  Factitious
  Nissen fundoplication (dumping syndrome)
  Falciparum malaria

HI = hyperinsulinemia; GSD = glycogen storage disease; KATP = potassium ATP.

---

the infant to sleep through the night and hyperinsulinemia prevents the mobilization of endogenous glucose. Increasing appetite and demands for feeding, wilting spells, jitteriness, and frank seizures are the most common presenting features. Additional clues include the rapid development of fasting hypoglycemia within 4–8 hr of food deprivation compared with other causes of hypoglycemia (Tables 81–1 and 81–2); the need for high rates of exogenous glucose infusion to prevent hypoglycemia, often at rates greater than 10–15 mg/kg/min; absence of ketonemia or acidosis; and elevated C-peptide or proinsulin levels at the time of hypoglycemia. The latter insulin-related products are absent in factitious hypoglycemia from exogenous administration of insulin. Provocative tests with tolbutamide or leucine are not necessary in infants; hypoglycemia is invariably provoked by withholding feedings for several hours, permitting simultaneous measurement of glucose, insulin, ketones, and FFAs in the same sample at the time of clinically manifested hypoglycemia. The glycemic response to glucagon at the time of

hypoglycemia reveals a brisk rise in glucose of at least 40 mg/dL and implies that glucose mobilization has been restrained by insulin but that glycogenolytic mechanisms are intact (Boxes 81–3, 81–4, and 81–5).

The measurement of serum insulin-like growth factor binding protein-1 (IGFBP-1) concentration may help diagnose hyperinsulinemia. The secretion of IGFBP-1 is acutely inhibited by insulin; IGFBP-1 concentrations are low during hyperinsulinism-induced hypoglycemia. In patients with spontaneous or fasting-induced hypoglycemia with a low insulin level (ketotic hypoglycemia, normal fasting), IGFBP-1 concentrations are significantly higher.

The differential diagnosis of endogenous hyperinsulinism includes *familial and nonfamilial hyperinsulinism of infancy due to diffuse β-cell hyperplasia*, or focal β-cell hyperplasia or adenomas. The plasma levels of insulin alone cannot distinguish these entities. They represent a variety of genetic defects responsible for abnormalities in the endocrine pancreas that is characterized by

BOX 81–3. Analysis of Critical Blood Sample during Hypoglycemia and 30 Minutes After Glucagon[*]

SUBSTRATES

Glucose
Free fatty acids
Ketones
Lactate
Uric acid
Ammonia

HORMONES

Insulin
Cortisol
Growth hormone
Thyroxine, thyroid-stimulating hormone[†]

---

[*]Glucagon 1 mg IV or IM.
[†]Measure once only before or after glucagon administration. Rise in glucose of ≥ 40 mg/dL after glucagon given at the time of hypoglycemia strongly suggests a hyperinsulinemic state with adequate hepatic glycogen stores and intact glycogenolytic enzymes. If ammonia is elevated to 100–200 μM, consider activating mutation of glutamate dehydrogenase.

BOX 81–5. Diagnosis of Acute Hypoglycemia in Infants and Children

ACUTE SYMPTOMS PRESENT

1. Obtain blood sample before and 30 min after glucagon administration.
2. Obtain urine as soon as possible. Examine for ketones; if not present and hypoglycemia confirmed, suspect hyperinsulinemia or fatty acid oxidation defect; if present, suspect ketotic, hormone deficiency, inborn error of glycogen metabolism, or defective gluconeogenesis.
3. Measure glucose in the original blood sample. If hypoglycemia is confirmed, proceed with substrate-hormone measurement as in Box 81–3.
4. If glycemic increment after glucagon exceeds 40 mg/dL above basal, suspect hyperinsulinemia.
5. If insulin level at time of confirmed hypoglycemia is greater than 5 μU/mL, suspect endogenous hyperinsulinemia; if greater than 100 μU/mL, suspect factitious hyperinsulinemia (exogenous insulin injection). Admit to hospital for supervised fast.
6. If cortisol is less than 10 μg/dL or growth hormone is less than 5 ng/mL, or both, suspect adrenal insufficiency or pituitary disease, or both. Admit to hospital for hormonal testing and neuroimaging.

HISTORY SUGGESTIVE: ACUTE SYMPTOMS NOT PRESENT

1. Careful history for relation of symptoms to time and type of food intake, bearing in mind age of patient. Exclude possibility of alcohol or drug ingestion. Assess possibility of insulin injection, salt craving, growth velocity, intracranial pathology.
2. Careful examination for hepatomegaly (glycogen storage disease; defect in gluconeogenesis); pigmentation (adrenal failure); stature and neurologic status (pituitary disease)
3. Admit to hospital for provocative testing:
   a. 24-hr fast under careful observation; when symptoms provoked proceed with steps 1–4 as when acute symptoms present
   b. Pituitary-adrenal function using arginine-insulin stimulation test if indicated
4. Liver biopsy for histologic and enzyme determinations if indicated
5. Oral glucose tolerance test (1.75 g/kg; max 75 g) if reactive hypoglycemia suspected (dumping syndrome, etc.)

---

autonomous insulin secretion and that is not appropriately reduced when blood glucose declines spontaneously or in response to provocative maneuvers such as fasting (see Box 81–5 and Table 81–3). Clinical, biochemical, and molecular genetic approaches now permit classification of congenital hyperinsulinism, formerly termed nesidioblastosis, into distinct entities. One form of persistent hyperinsulinemic hypoglycemia of infancy (PHHI) is inherited in an autosomal recessive pattern, is severe, and is caused by mutations in the regulation of the potassium channel intimately involved in insulin secretion by the pancreatic b cell (Fig. 81–1). Normally, glucose entry into the b cell is enabled by the non–insulin-responsive glucose transporter GLUT-2. On entry, glucose is phosphorylated to glucose-6-phosphate by the enzyme glucokinase, enabling glucose

BOX 81–4. Criteria for Diagnosing Hyperinsulinism Based on "Critical" Samples (Drawn at a Time of Fasting Hypoglycemia: Plasma Glucose <50 mg/dL)

1. Hyperinsulinemia (plasma insulin > 2 μU/mL)[*]
2. Hypofattyacidemia (plasma free fatty acids < 1.5 mmol/L)
3. Hypoketonemia (plasma β-hydroxybutyrate: < 2.0 mmol/L)
4. Inappropriate glycemic response to glucagon, 1 mg IV (delta glucose > 40 mg/dL)

---

[*]Depends on sensitivity of insulin assay.
From: Stanley CA, Thomson PS, Fingold DN, et al: *Hypoglycemia in Neonates and Infants in Pediatric Endocrinology.* 2nd ed, Sperlims M (editor) WB Saunders 2002, pp 135–159.

metabolism to generate ATP. The rise in the molar ratio of ATP relative to adenosine diphosphate (ADP) closes the ATP-sensitive potassium channel in the cell membrane (KATPchannel). This channel is composed of two subunits, the KIR6.2 channel, part of the family of inward-rectifier potassium channels, and a regulatory component in intimate association with KIR6.2 known as the sulfonylurea receptor (SUR). Together, KIR6.2 and SUR constitute the potassium-sensitive ATP channel KATP. Normally, the KATP is open, but with the rise in ATP and closure of the channel, potassium accumulates intracellularly, causing depolarization of the membrane, opening of voltage-gated calcium channels, influx of calcium into the cytoplasm, and secretion of insulin via exocytosis. The genes for both SUR and KIR6.2 are located close together on the short arm of chromosome 11, the site of the insulin gene. Inactivating mutations in the gene for SUR, or, less often, KIR6.2, prevent the potassium channel from opening; it remains essentially closed with constant depolarization and, therefore, constant inward flux

TABLE 81–1. Hypoglycemia in Infants and Children: Clinical and Laboratory Features

Group	Age at Diagnosis (mo)	Glucose (mg/dL)	Insulin (μU/mL)	Fasting Time to Hypoglycemia (hr)
Hyperinsulinemia (n = 12)				
Mean	7.4	23.1	22.4	2.1
SEM	2.0	2.7	3.2	0.6
Nonhyperinsulinemia (n = 16)				
Mean	41.8	36.1	5.8	18.2
SEM	7.3	2.4	0.9	2.9

Adapted from Antunes JD, Geffner ME, Lippe BM, et al: Childhood hypoglycemia: Differentiating hyperinsulinemic from nonhyperinsulinemic causes. J Pediatr 1990; 116:105–8.

TABLE 81–2. Correlation of Clinical Features with Molecular Defects in Persistent Hyperinsulinemic Hypoglycemia in Infancy

Type	Macrosomia	Hypoglycemia/ Hyperinsulinemia	Family History	Molecular Defects	Associated Clinical, Biochemical, or Molecular Features	Response to Medical Management	Recommended Surgical Approach	Prognosis
Sporadic	Present at birth	Moderate/severe in first days to weeks of life	Negative	?SUR1/Kir6.2	Loss of heterozygosity in microadenomatous tissue	Generally poor; may respond to somatostatin better than diazoxide	Partial pancreatectomy if frozen section shows β-cell crowding with small nuclei—microadenoma	Excellent
							Subtotal greater than 95% pancreatectomy if frozen section shows giant nuclei in β-cells—diffuse hyperplasia	Guarded; diabetes mellitus develops in 50% of patients; hypoglycemia persists in 33%
Autosomal recessive	Present at birth	Severe in first days to weeks of life	Positive	SUR/Kir6.2	Consanguinity a feature in some populations	Poor	Subtotal pancreatectomy	Guarded
Autosomal dominant	Unusual	Moderate onset usually post 6 mo of age	Positive	Glucokinase (activating) Some cases gene unknown	None	Very good to excellent	Surgery usually not required Partial pancreatectomy only if medical management fails	Excellent
Autosomal dominant	Unusual	Moderate onset usually post 6 mo of age	Positive	Glutamate dehydrogenase (activating)	Modest hyperammonemia	Very good to excellent	Surgery usually not required	Excellent
Beckwith-Wiedemann syndrome	Present at birth	Moderate, spontaneously resolves after ~6 mo	Negative	Duplicating/imprinting in chromosomal 11p15.1	Macroglossia, omphalocele, hemihypertrophy	Good	Not recommended	Excellent for hypoglycemia; associated with embryonal tumors (Wilms' hepatoblastoma)
Congenital disorders of glycosylation	Not usual	Moderate/onset after 3 mo	Negative	Phosphomannose isomerase deficiency	Hepatomegaly, vomiting, intractable diarrhea	Good with mannose supplement	Not recommended	Fair

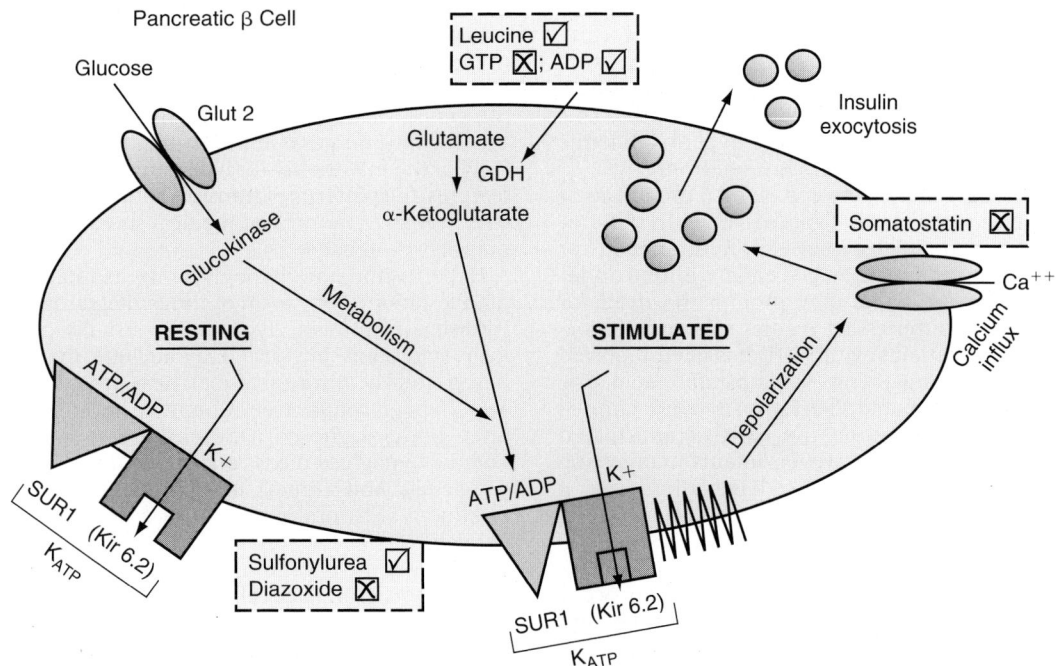

FIGURE 81–1. Schematic representation of the pancreatic cell with some important steps in insulin secretion. The membrane-spanning, adenosine triphosphate (ATP)-sensitive potassium (K$^+$) channel (K$_{ATP}$) consists of two subunits: the sulfonylurea receptor (SUR) and the inward rectifying K channel (K$_{IR}$6.2). In the resting state, the ratio of ATP to adenosine diphosphate (ADP) maintains K$_{ATP}$ in an open state, permitting efflux of intracellular K$^+$. When blood glucose concentration rises, its entry into the β cell is facilitated by the GLUT-2 glucose transporter, a process not regulated by insulin. Within the β cell, glucose is converted to glucose-6-phosphate by the enzyme glucokinase and then undergoes metabolism to generate energy. The resultant increase in ATP relative to ADP closes K$_{ATP}$, preventing efflux of K$^+$, and the rise of intracellular K$^+$ depolarizes the cell membrane and opens a calcium (Ca^{2+}) channel. The intracellular rise in Ca^{2+} triggers insulin secretion via exocytosis. Sulfonylureas trigger insulin secretion by reacting with their receptor (SUR) to close K$_{ATP}$; diazoxide inhibits this process, whereas somatostatin, or its analogue octreotide, inhibits insulin secretion by interfering with calcium influx. Genetic mutations in SUR or K$_{IR}$6.2 that prevent K$_{ATP}$ from being open are responsible for autosomal recessive forms of persistent hyperinsulinemic hypoglycemia of infancy (PHHI). One form of autosomal dominant PHHI is due to an activating mutation in glucokinase. The amino acid leucine also triggers insulin secretion by closure of K$_{ATP}$. Metabolism of leucine is facilitated by the enzyme glutamate dehydrogenase (GDH), and overactivity of this enzyme in the pancreas leads to hyperinsulinemia with hypoglycemia, associated with hyperammonemia from overactivity of GDH in the liver. X = inhibition; 4 = stimulation.

of calcium; hence, insulin secretion is continuous. A milder autosomal dominant form of these defects has also been reported. Likewise, an activating mutation in glucokinase results in closure of the potassium channel through overproduction of ATP and hyperinsulinism. Inactivating mutations of the glucokinase gene are responsible for inadequate insulin secretion and form the basis of type 2 maturity-onset diabetes of youth (see Chapter 583).

The familial forms of PHHI are more common in certain populations, notably Arabic and Ashkenazi Jewish communities, where it may reach an incidence of about 1/2,500, compared with the sporadic rates in the general population of approximately 1/50,000. These *autosomal recessive forms* of PHHI typically present in the immediate newborn period as macrosomic newborns with a weight in excess of 4.0 kg and severe recurrent or persistent hypoglycemia manifesting in the initial hours or days of life. Glucose infusions as high as 15–20 mg/kg/min and frequent feedings fail to maintain euglycemia. Diazoxide, which could function by opening K$_{ATP}$ channels (see Fig. 81–1), fails to control hypoglycemia adequately. Somatostatin, which also opens K$_{ATP}$ and inhibits calcium flux, may be partially effective in about 50% of patients (see Fig. 81–1). Calcium channel blocking agents may have an effect. When affected patients are unresponsive to these measures, pancreatectomy is strongly recommended to avoid the long-term neurologic sequelae of hypoglycemia. If surgery is undertaken, preoperative CT or MRI

rarely reveals an isolated adenoma, permitting local resection. Also, intraoperative ultrasonography may identify a small impalpable adenoma, permitting local resection. Adenomas often present in late infancy or early childhood. Distinguishing between focal and diffuse cases of persistent hyperinsulinism with the use of a combination of transhepatic portal venous catheterization and selective pancreatic venous blood sampling to measure insulin levels as well as intraoperative histologic techniques are possibly helpful. Diffuse hyperinsulinism is characterized by large β cells with abnormally large nuclei, whereas focal adenomatous lesions display small and normal β cell nuclei. Although *SUR1* mutations are present in both types, the focal lesions arise by a random loss of a maternally imprinted growth-inhibitory gene on maternal chromosome 11p in association with paternal transmission of a mutated *SUR1* or K$_{IR}$6.2 paternal chromosome 11p. Local excision of focal adenomatous islet-cell hyperplasia results in a cure with little or no recurrence. If local resection is not possible, near-total resection of 85–90% of the pancreas is recommended. In contrast, the near-total pancreatectomy required for the diffuse hyperplastic lesions is often associated with persistent hypoglycemia and later development of hyperglycemia or frank, insulin-requiring diabetes mellitus.

Further resection of the remaining pancreas may occasionally be necessary if hypoglycemia recurs and cannot be controlled by medical measures, such as the use of somatostatin or diazoxide.

Experienced pediatric surgeons in medical centers equipped to provide the necessary preoperative and postoperative care, diagnostic evaluation, and management should perform surgery. In some patients who have been managed medically, hyperinsulinemia and hypoglycemia regress over months. This is similar to what occurs in children with the hyperinsulinemic hypoglycemia seen in Beckwith-Wiedemann syndrome.

If hypoglycemia first manifests between 3 and 6 mo of age or later, a therapeutic trial using medical approaches with somatostatin, diazoxide, and frequent feedings can be attempted for up to 2–4 wk. Failure to maintain euglycemia without undesirable side effects from the drugs may prompt the need for surgery. Some success in suppressing insulin release and correcting hypoglycemia in patients with PHHI has been reported with the use of the long-acting somatostatin analogue octreotide. Most cases of neonatal PHHI are sporadic; familial forms permit genetic counseling on the basis of anticipated autosomal recessive inheritance. However, infants manifesting hypoglycemia at 3–6 mo of age are likely to have other forms of PHHI.

A second form of familial PHHI suggests *autosomal dominant inheritance*. The clinical features tend to be less severe, and onset of hypoglycemia is most likely, but not exclusively, to occur beyond the immediate newborn period and usually beyond the period of weaning at an average age at onset of about 1 yr. At birth, macrosomia is rarely observed, and response to diazoxide is almost uniform. The initial presentation may be delayed and occur as late as 30 yr, unless provoked by fasting. The genetic basis for this autosomal dominant form has not been delineated; it is not always linked to $K_{IR}6.2$/SUR, and the activating mutation in glucokinase is transmitted in an autosomal dominant manner. If a family history is present, genetic counseling for a 50% recurrence rate can be given for future offspring.

A third form of persistent PHHI is associated with *mild hyperammonemia*, usually as a sporadic occurrence although dominant inheritance occurs. Presentation is more like the autosomal dominant form rather than the autosomal recessive form. Diet and diazoxide control symptoms, but pancreatectomy may be necessary in some cases. The association of hyperinsulinism and hyperammonemia is caused by an inherited or de novo gain-of-function mutation in the enzyme glutamate dehydrogenase. The resulting increase in glutamate oxidation in the pancreatic β cell raises the ATP concentration and, hence, the ratio of ATP:ADP, which closes K_{ATP}, leading to membrane depolarization, calcium influx, and insulin secretion (see Fig. 81–1). In the liver, the excessive oxidation of glutamate to β-ketoglutarate may generate ammonia and divert glutamate from being processed to *N*-acetylglutamate, an essential cofactor for removal of ammonia through the urea cycle via activation of the enzyme carbamoyl phosphate synthetase. The hyperammonemia is mild, with concentrations of 100–200 μM/L, and produces no central nervous system (CNS) symptoms or consequences as seen in other hyperammonemic states. Leucine, a potent amino acid for stimulating insulin secretion and implicated in leucine-sensitive hypoglycemia, acts by allosterically stimulating glutamate dehydrogenase. Thus, *leucine-sensitive hypoglycemia* may be a form of the hyperinsulinemia-hyperammonemia syndrome or a potentiation of mild disorders of the K_{ATP} channel.

Hypoglycemia associated with hyperinsulinemia is also seen in approximately 50% of patients with the *Beckwith-Wiedemann syndrome* (see Chapter 96). This syndrome is characterized by exomphalos, gigantism, macroglossia, microcephaly, and visceromegaly. Distinctive lateral earlobe fissures are present, and hemihypertrophy occurs in many of these infants. Diffuse islet cell hyperplasia occurs in infants with hypoglycemia. The diagnostic and therapeutic approaches are the same as those discussed previously, although microcephaly and retarded brain development may occur independently of hypoglycemia.

Patients with the Beckwith-Wiedemann syndrome may acquire tumors, including Wilms' tumor, hepatoblastoma, adrenal carcinoma, and rhabdomyosarcoma. This overgrowth syndrome is caused by mutations in the chromosome 11p15.5 region close to the genes for insulin, SUR, $K_{IR}6.2$, and IGF-2. Duplications in this region and genetic imprinting from a defective or absent copy of the maternally derived gene are involved in the variable features and patterns of transmission. Hypoglycemia may resolve over weeks to months of medical therapy. Pancreatic resection may also be needed.

Hyperinsulinemic hypoglycemia in infancy is reported as a manifestation of one form of congenital disorder of glycosylation. Disorders of protein glycosylation usually present with neurologic symptoms but also may include liver dysfunction with hepatomegaly, intractable diarrhea, protein-losing enteropathy, and hypoglycemia (see Chapter 76.6). These disorders are often underdiagnosed. One entity associated with hyperinsulinemic hypoglycemia is caused by phosphomannose isomerase deficiency, and clinical improvement followed supplemental treatment with oral mannose at a dose of 0.17 g/kg six times per day.

After the first 12 mo of life, hyperinsulinemic states are uncommon until islet cell adenomas reappear, as a cause after the patient is several years of age. Hyperinsulinemia due to *islet cell adenoma* should be considered in any child 5 yr or older presenting with hypoglycemia. The diagnostic approach is outlined in Table 81–3 and Box 81–5. Fasting for 24–36 hr usually provokes hypoglycemia; coexisting hyperinsulinemia confirms the diagnosis provided that factitious administration of insulin by the parents, a form of *Munchausen syndrome by proxy*, is excluded. Occasionally, provocative tests may be required. Exogenously administered insulin can be distinguished from endogenous insulin by simultaneous measurement of C-peptide concentration. If C-peptide levels are elevated, endogenous insulin secretion is responsible for the hypoglycemia; if C-peptide levels are low but insulin values are high, exogenous insulin has been administered, perhaps as a form of child abuse. Islet cell adenomas at this age are treated by surgical excision; familial multiple endocrine adenomatosis type I (Wermer syndrome) should be considered in the differential diagnosis. Antibodies to insulin or the insulin receptor (insulin mimetic action) are also rarely associated with hypoglycemia. Some tumors produce insulin-like growth factors, thereby provoking hypoglycemia by interacting with the insulin receptor.

A rare form of hyperinsulinemic hypoglycemia has been reported after exercise. Whereas glucose and insulin remain unchanged in most people after moderate, short-term exercise, rare patients manifest severe hypoglycemia with hyperinsulinemia 15–50 min after the same standardized exercise. This form of exercise-induced hyperinsulinism is believed to be caused by an abnormal responsiveness of β-cell insulin release in response to pyruvate generated during exercise.

ENDOCRINE DEFICIENCY. Hypoglycemia associated with endocrine deficiency is usually caused by adrenal insufficiency with or without associated growth hormone deficiency (see Chapters 551 and 569). In panhypopituitarism, isolated adrenocorticotropic hormone (ACTH) or growth hormone deficiency, or combined ACTH deficiency plus growth hormone deficiency, the incidence of hypoglycemia is as high as 20%. In the newborn period, hypoglycemia may be the presenting feature of hypopituitarism; in males, a microphallus may provide a clue to a coexistent deficiency of gonadotropin. Newborns with hypopituitarism often have a form of "hepatitis" and the syndrome of *septo-optic dysplasia*. When adrenal disease is severe, as in congenital adrenal hyperplasia caused by cortisol synthetic enzyme defects, adrenal hemorrhage, or congenital absence of the adrenal glands, disturbances in serum electrolytes with hyponatremia and hyperkalemia or ambiguous genitals may provide diagnostic clues (see Chapter 570). In older children,

TABLE 81–3. Clinical Manifestations and Differential Diagnosis in Childhood Hypoglycemia

Condition	Hypoglycemia	Urinary Ketones (K) or Reducing Sugars	Hepatomegaly	Serum Lipids	Serum Uric Acid	Effect of 24–36-hr Fast on Plasma Glucose	Insulin	Ketones	Alanine	Lactate	Glycemic Response to Glucagon Fed	Fasted	Glycemic Response to Infusion of Alanine	Glycerol
Normal	0	0	0	Normal	Normal	→	→	↑	→	Normal	↑	→	↑	↑
Hyperinsulinemia	Recurrent severe	0	0	Normal or ↑	Normal	↓↓	↑↑	↓↓	Normal	Normal	↑	↑↓	↑	↑
Ketotic hypoglycemia	Severe with missed meals	Ketonuria +++	0	Normal	Normal	↓↓	→	↑↑	↓↓	Normal	↑	↓	↑	↑
Fatty acid oxidation disorder	Severe with missed meals	Absent	0 to + Abnormal liver function test results	Abnormal	↑	Contraindicated					→	↓	Not indicated	
Hypopituitarism	Moderate with missed meals	Ketonuria ++	0	Normal	Normal	↓↓	→	↑↑	↓↓	Normal	↑	↓↓	↑	↑
Adrenal insufficiency	Severe with missed meals	Ketonuria ++	0	Normal	Normal	↓↓	→	↑↑	↓↓	Normal	↑	↓	↑	↑
Enzyme deficiencies Glucose-6-phosphatase	Severe-constant	Ketonuria +++	+++	↑↑	↑↑	↓↓	→	↑↑	↑↑	↑↑	0	0–↓↓	0	0
Debrancher	Moderate with fasting	Ketonuria ++	++	Normal	Normal	↓↓	→	↑↑	↓↓	Normal	↑	0–↓↓	↑	↑
Phosphorylase	Mild-moderate	Ketonuria ++	+	Normal	Normal	→↓↓	→	↑↑	↓↓	Normal	0–↑	0–↓↓	↑↔	→
Fructose-1,6-diphosphatase	Severe with fasting	Ketonuria +++	+++	Normal ↑↑	Normal ↑↑	→↓↓	→	↑↑	↓↓ ↑↑	Normal ↑↑	↑	0–↓↓	↑↔	↓
Galactosemia	After milk or milk products	0 Ketones;(s) +	+++	Normal	Normal	→	→	↑	→	Normal	↑	0–↓↓	↑	↑
Fructose intolerance	After fructose	0 Ketones;(s) +	+++	Normal	Normal	→	→	↑	→	Normal	↑	0–↓↓	↑	↑

0 = absence; ↑ or ↓ indicates respectively small increase or decrease; ↑↑ or ↓↓ indicates respectively large increase or decrease. Details of each condition are discussed in the text.

failure of growth should suggest growth hormone deficiency. Hyperpigmentation may provide the clue to Addison disease with increased ACTH levels or adrenal unresponsiveness to ACTH owing to a defect in the adrenal receptor for ACTH. The frequent association of Addison disease in childhood with hypoparathyroidism (hypocalcemia), chronic mucocutaneous candidiasis, and other endocrinopathies should be considered. Adrenoleukodystrophy should also be considered in the differential diagnosis of primary Addison disease in older children (see Chapter 75.2).

Hypoglycemia in cortisol-growth hormone deficiency may be caused by decreased gluconeogenic enzymes with cortisol deficiency, increased glucose utilization due to a lack of the antagonistic effects of growth hormone on insulin action, or failure to supply endogenous gluconeogenic substrate in the form of alanine and lactate with compensatory breakdown of fat and generation of ketones. Deficiency of these hormones results in reduced gluconeogenic substrate, which resembles the syndrome of ketotic hypoglycemia. Investigation of a child with hypoglycemia, therefore, requires exclusion of ACTH-cortisol or growth hormone deficiency and, if diagnosed, its appropriate replacement with cortisol or growth hormone.

Epinephrine deficiency could theoretically be responsible for hypoglycemia. Urinary excretion of epinephrine has been diminished in some patients with spontaneous or insulin-induced hypoglycemia in whom absence of pallor and tachycardia was also noted, suggesting that failure of catecholamine release, due to a defect anywhere along the hypothalamic-autonomic-adrenomedullary axis, might be responsible for the hypoglycemia. This possibility has been challenged, owing to the rarity of hypoglycemia in patients with bilateral adrenalectomy, provided that they receive adequate glucocorticoid replacement and because diminished epinephrine excretion is found in normal patients with repeated insulin-induced hypoglycemia. Many of the patients described as having hypoglycemia with failure of epinephrine excretion fit the criteria for ketotic hypoglycemia.

Glucagon deficiency in infants or children may rarely be associated with hypoglycemia.

SUBSTRATE LIMITED

Ketotic Hypoglycemia. This is the most common form of childhood hypoglycemia. This condition usually presents between the ages of 18 mo and 5 yr and remits spontaneously by the age of 8–9 yr. Hypoglycemic episodes typically occur during periods of intercurrent illness when food intake is limited. The classic history is of a child who eats poorly or completely avoids the evening meal, is difficult to arouse from sleep the following morning, and may have a seizure or be comatose by midmorning. Another common presentation occurs when parents sleep late and the affected child is unable to eat breakfast, thus prolonging the overnight fast.

At the time of documented hypoglycemia, there is associated ketonuria and ketonemia; plasma insulin concentrations are appropriately low, 5–10 µU/mL or less, thus excluding hyperinsulinemia. A ketogenic provocative diet, formerly used as a diagnostic test, is not essential to establish the diagnosis because fasting alone provokes a hypoglycemic episode with ketonemia and ketonuria within 12–18 hr in susceptible individuals. Normal children of similar age can withstand fasting without hypoglycemia developing during the same period, although even normal children may acquire these features by 36 hr of fasting.

Children with ketotic hypoglycemia have plasma alanine concentrations that are markedly reduced in the basal state after an overnight fast and decline even further with prolonged fasting. Alanine, produced in muscle, is a major gluconeogenic precursor. Alanine is the only amino acid that is significantly lower in these children, and infusions of alanine (250 mg/kg) produce a rapid rise in plasma glucose without causing significant changes in blood lactate or pyruvate levels, indicating that the entire gluconeogenic pathway from the level of pyruvate is intact but that there is a deficiency of substrate. Glycogenolytic pathways are also intact because glucagon induces a normal glycemic response in affected children during the fed state. The levels of hormones that counter hypoglycemia are appropriately elevated, and insulin is appropriately low.

The *etiology* of ketotic hypoglycemia may be a defect in any of the complex steps involved in protein catabolism, oxidative deamination of amino acids, transamination, alanine synthesis, or alanine efflux from muscle. Children with ketotic hypoglycemia are frequently smaller than age-matched controls and often have a history of transient neonatal hypoglycemia. Any decrease in muscle mass may compromise the supply of gluconeogenic substrate at a time when glucose demands per unit of body weight are already relatively high, thus predisposing the patient to the rapid development of hypoglycemia, with ketosis representing the attempt to switch to an alternative fuel supply. Children with ketotic hypoglycemia may represent the low end of the spectrum of children's capacity to tolerate fasting. Similar relative intolerance to fasting is present in normal children, who cannot maintain blood glucose after 30–36 hr of fasting, compared with the adult's capacity for prolonged fasting. Although the defect may be present at birth, it may not be evident until the child is stressed by more prolonged periods of calorie restriction. Moreover, the spontaneous remission observed in children at age 8–9 yr might be explained by the increase in muscle bulk with its resultant increase in supply of endogenous substrate and the relative decrease in glucose requirement per unit of body mass with increasing age. There is also some evidence to support the contention that impaired epinephrine secretion from immaturity of autonomic innervation contributes to ketotic hypoglycemia. Rarely, inborn errors of fatty acid metabolism present as ketotic hypoglycemia, although, typically, fatty acid oxidation defects produce hypoketotic hypoglycemia.

In anticipation of spontaneous resolution of this syndrome, *treatment* of ketotic hypoglycemia consists of frequent feedings of a high-protein, high-carbohydrate diet. During intercurrent illnesses, parents should test the child's urine for the presence of ketones, the appearance of which precedes hypoglycemia by several hours. In the presence of ketonuria, liquids of high carbohydrate content should be offered to the child. If these cannot be tolerated, the child should be offered a short course of corticosteroids or admitted to the hospital for intravenous glucose administration.

Branched-Chain Ketonuria (Maple Syrup Urine Disease) (see Chapter 74.6). The hypoglycemic episodes were once attributed to high levels of leucine, but evidence indicates that interference with the production of alanine and its availability as a gluconeogenic substrate during calorie deprivation is responsible for hypoglycemia.

GLYCOGEN STORAGE DISEASE. See Chapter 76.1.

Glucose-6-Phosphatase Deficiency (Type I Glycogen Storage Disease). Affected children usually display a remarkable tolerance to their chronic hypoglycemia; blood glucose values in the range of 20–50 mg/dL are not associated with the classic symptoms of hypoglycemia, possibly reflecting the adaptation of the CNS to ketone bodies as an alternative fuel.

Affected untreated children manifest growth failure, mental retardation, and a shortened life span unless they are treated. Continuous intragastric feeding improves the metabolic and clinical findings by reducing the frequency and severity of hypoglycemia, thereby avoiding the secondary hormonal changes that appear to be responsible for the metabolic derangements. Continuous intragastric feeding at night, combined with frequent daytime feedings, produces equally effective amelioration of the biochemical disturbances and avoids the inconvenience of 24-hr continuous gastric feeding. The daytime feedings are given every 3–4 hr: 60–70% of the calories as carbohydrate low in fructose and galactose, 12–15% of the calories as protein, and

15–25% of the calories as fat. At night, a small nasogastric tube is passed by the patient (or a parent for younger children), and approximately one third of the daily caloric requirements is continuously infused over 8–12 hr using a small continuous infusion pump. One commercially available formula for nocturnal infusion contains 89% of the calories as glucose and glucose oligosaccharides, 1.8% as safflower oil, and 9.2% as crystalline amino acids (Vivonex, Eaton Laboratories). Nocturnal cornstarch therapy is also beneficial. Transient nocturnal hypoglycemia is not completely prevented, and renal glomerular dysfunction plus formation of hepatic adenoma remain serious complications. Liver transplantation offers promise of long-term cure.

Amylo-1,6-Glucosidase Deficiency (Debrancher Enzyme Deficiency; Type III Glycogen Storage Disease). See Chapter 76.

Liver Phosphorylase Deficiency (Type VI Glycogen Storage Disease) (see also Chapter 76). Low hepatic phosphorylase activity may result from a defect in any of the steps of activation; a variety of defects have been described. Hepatomegaly, excessive deposition of glycogen in liver, growth retardation, and occasional symptomatic hypoglycemia occur. A diet high in protein and reduced in carbohydrate usually prevents hypoglycemia.

Glycogen Synthetase Deficiency (see also Chapter 76). The inability to synthesize glycogen is extremely rare. There is fasting hypoglycemia and hyperketonemia; hyperglycemia with glucosuria occurs after meals. During fasting hypoglycemia, levels of the counterregulatory hormones, including catecholamines, are appropriately elevated or normal, and insulin levels are appropriately low. The liver is not enlarged. Protein-rich feedings at frequent intervals result in dramatic clinical improvement, including growth velocity. This condition mimics the syndrome of ketotic hypoglycemia and should be considered in the differential diagnosis of that syndrome.

DISORDERS OF GLUCONEOGENESIS

Fructose-1,6-Diphosphatase Deficiency (see Chapter 76.3). A deficiency of this enzyme results in a block of gluconeogenesis from all possible precursors below the level of fructose-1,6-diphosphate. Infusion of these gluconeogenic precursors results in lactic acidosis without a rise in glucose; acute hypoglycemia may be provoked by inhibition of glycogenolysis. Glycogenolysis remains intact, and glucagon elicits a normal glycemic response in the fed, but not in the fasted, state. Accordingly, affected individuals have hypoglycemia only during caloric deprivation, as in fasting, or during intercurrent illness. As long as glycogen stores remain normal, hypoglycemia does not develop. In affected families, there may be a history of siblings with known hepatomegaly who died in infancy with unexplained metabolic acidosis.

Clinical features simulate those of type I glycogen storage disease. Hepatomegaly in individuals with fructose-1,6-diphosphatase deficiency is due to lipid storage rather than glycogen storage. Lactic acidosis, ketosis, hyperlipidemia, and hyperuricemia occur; their pathogenesis is related to the severity and duration of hypoglycemia and the resultant low levels of insulin and high levels of counterregulatory hormones. Therapy for these infants, consisting of a diet high in carbohydrates (56%, excluding fructose, which cannot be utilized), low in protein (12%), and normal in fat composition (32%), has permitted normal growth and development. Continuous nocturnal provision of calories through the intragastric infusion system described earlier for type I glycogen storage disease is also applicable to children with fructose-1,6-diphosphatase deficiency. During intercurrent illnesses with vomiting, intravenous glucose infusion is necessary to prevent severe hypoglycemia.

Defects in Fatty Acid Oxidation (see also Chapter 75). The important role of fatty acid oxidation in maintaining gluconeogenesis is underscored by examples of congenital or drug-induced defects in fatty acid metabolism that may be associated with fasting hypoglycemia.

Various congenital enzymatic deficiencies causing defective carnitine or fatty acid metabolism occur. A severe and relatively common form of fasting hypoglycemia with hepatomegaly, cardiomyopathy, and hypotonia occurs with long- and medium-chain fatty acid coenzyme-A dehydrogenase deficiency (LCAD and MCAD). Plasma carnitine levels are low, ketones are not present in urine, but dicarboxylic aciduria is present. Clinically, patients with *acyl CoA dehydrogenase deficiency* present with a Reye-like syndrome, recurrent episodes of severe fasting hypoglycemic coma, and cardiorespiratory arrest (sudden infant death syndrome-like events). Severe hypoglycemia and metabolic acidosis without ketosis also occur in patients with multiple acyl-CoA dehydrogenase disorders. Hypotonia, seizures, and acrid odor are other clinical clues. Survival depends on whether the defects are severe or mild; diagnosis is established from studies of enzyme activity in liver biopsy tissue or in cultured fibroblasts from affected patients. Tandem mass spectrometry can be employed for blood samples, even those on filter paper, for screening of congenital inborn errors. The frequency of this disorder is at least 1/10,000–15,000 births; molecular diagnostic methods are being developed. Avoidance of fasting and supplementation with carnitine may be lifesaving in these patients who generally present in infancy.

Interference with fatty acid metabolism also underlies the fasting hypoglycemia associated with Jamaican vomiting sickness, with atractyloside, and with the drug valproate. In *Jamaican vomiting sickness*, the unripe ackee fruit contains a water-soluble toxin, hypoglycin, which produces vomiting, CNS depression, and severe hypoglycemia. The hypoglycemic activity of hypoglycin derives from its inhibition of gluconeogenesis secondary to its interference with the acyl-CoA and carnitine metabolism essential for the oxidation of long-chain fatty acids. The disease is almost totally confined to Jamaica, where ackee forms a staple of the diet for the poor. The ripe ackee fruit no longer contains this toxin. *Atractyloside* is a reagent that inhibits oxidative phosphorylation in mitochondria by preventing the translocation of adenine nucleotides, such as ATP, across the mitochondrial membrane. Atractyloside is a perhydrophenanthrenic glycoside derived from *Atractylis gummifera*. This plant is found in the Mediterranean basin; ingestion of this "thistle" is associated with hypoglycemia and a syndrome similar to Jamaican vomiting sickness. The anticonvulsant drug *valproate* is associated with side effects, predominantly in young infants, which include a Reye-like syndrome, low serum carnitine levels, and the potential for fasting hypoglycemia. In all these conditions, hypoglycemia *is not associated with ketonuria*.

Acute Alcohol Intoxication. The liver metabolizes alcohol as a preferred fuel, and generation of reducing equivalents during the oxidation of ethanol alters the NADH:NAD ratio, which is essential for certain gluconeogenic steps. As a result, gluconeogenesis is impaired and hypoglycemia may ensue if glycogen stores are depleted by starvation or by pre-existing abnormalities in glycogen metabolism. In toddlers who have been unfed for some time, even the consumption of small quantities of alcohol can precipitate these events. The hypoglycemia promptly responds to intravenous glucose, which should always be considered in a child who presents initially with coma or seizure, after taking a blood sample to determine glucose concentration. The possibility of the child's ingesting alcoholic drinks must also be considered if there was a preceding adult evening party. A careful history allows the diagnosis to be made and may avoid needless and expensive hospitalization and investigation.

Salicylate Intoxication (see also Chapter 704.5). Both hyperglycemia and hypoglycemia occur in children with salicylate intoxication. Accelerated utilization of glucose, resulting from augmentation of insulin secretion by salicylates, and possible interference with gluconeogenesis may contribute to hypoglycemia. Infants are more susceptible than are older children. Monitoring of blood glucose levels with appropriate glucose infusion in the event of hypoglycemia should form part of the therapeutic approach to salicylate intoxication in childhood. Ketosis may occur.

Phosphoenol Pyruvate Carboxykinase Deficiency. Deficiency of this rate-limiting gluconeogenic enzyme is associated with severe fasting hypoglycemia and variable onset after birth. Hypoglycemia may occur within 24 hr after birth, and defective gluconeogenesis from alanine can be documented in vivo. Liver, kidney, and myocardium demonstrate fatty infiltration, and atrophy of the optic nerve and visual cortex may occur. Extensive fatty deposition in liver, kidney, and other tissues also occurs in phosphoenol pyruvate carboxykinase deficiency. Hypoglycemia may be profound. Lactate and pyruvate levels in plasma have been normal, but a mild metabolic acidosis may be present. The fatty infiltration of various organs is caused by increased formation of acetyl-CoA, which becomes available for fatty acid synthesis. Diagnosis of this rare entity can be made with certainty only through appropriate enzymatic determinations in liver biopsy material. Avoidance of periods of fasting through frequent feedings rich in carbohydrate should be helpful because glycogen synthesis and breakdown are intact.

Pyruvate Carboxylase Deficiency (see Chapter 76). This is predominantly a disease of the CNS characterized by a subacute necrotizing encephalomyelopathy and high levels of blood lactate and pyruvate. Hypoglycemia is not a prominent feature of this syndrome, presumably because gluconeogenesis from precursors other than alanine remains intact, and these precursors bypass the pyruvate carboxylase step. The utilization of alanine as well as lactate through pyruvate cannot proceed, however, so these substrates accumulate in blood, and modest hypoglycemia may result during fasting. Affected patients usually die of progressive CNS disease.

OTHER ENZYME DEFECTS

Galactosemia (Galactose-1-Phosphate Uridyl Transferase Deficiency). See Chapter 76.

Fructose Intolerance (Fructose-1-Phosphate Aldolase Deficiency) (see Chapter 76). Acute hypoglycemia is due to the inhibition by fructose-1-phosphate of glycogenolysis via the phosphorylase system and of gluconeogenesis at the level of fructose-1,6-diphosphate aldolase. Affected individuals usually learn to eliminate fructose from their diet spontaneously.

Defects in Glucose Tranporters

GLUT-1 Deficiency. Two infants with a seizure disorder were found to have low cerebrospinal fluid (CSF) glucose concentrations despite normal plasma glucose. Lactate concentrations in CSF were also low, suggesting decreased glycolysis rather than bacterial infection, which causes low CSF glucose with high lactate. The erythrocyte glucose transporter was defective, suggesting a similar defect in the brain glucose transporter responsible for the clinical features. A ketogenic diet reduced the severity of seizures by supplying an alternate source of brain fuel that bypassed the defect in glucose transport.

GLUT-2 Deficiency. Children with hepatomegaly, galactose intolerance, and renal tubular dysfunction (*Fanconi-Bickel syndrome*) have been shown to have a deficiency of the GLUT-2 glucose transporter of plasma membranes. In addition to liver and kidney tubules, GLUT-2 is also expressed in pancreatic β cells. Hence, the clinical manifestations reflect impaired glucose release from liver and defective tubular reabsorption of glucose plus phosphaturia and aminoaciduria resulting from *Fanconi syndrome.*

Systemic Disorders. Several systemic disorders are associated with hypoglycemia in infants and children. Neonatal sepsis is often associated with hypoglycemia, possibly as a result of diminished caloric intake with impaired gluconeogenesis. Similar mechanisms may apply to the hypoglycemia found in severely malnourished infants or those with severe malabsorp-

tion. Hyperviscosity with a central hematocrit of 65% or greater is associated with hypoglycemia in at least 10–15% of affected infants. *Falciparum malaria* has been associated with hyperinsulinemia and hypoglycemia. Heart and renal failure have also been associated with hypoglycemia, but the mechanism is obscure. Infants and children with *Nissen fundoplication*, a relatively common procedure used to ameliorate gastroesophageal reflux, frequently have an associated "dumping" syndrome with hypoglycemia. Characteristic features include significant hyperglycemia of up to 500 mg/dL 30 minutes postprandially and severe hypoglycemia (average 32 mg/dL in one series) 1.5–3 hr later. The early hyperglycemia phase is associated with brisk and excessive insulin release that causes the rebound hypoglycemia. Glucagon responses have been inappropriately low in some. Although the physiologic mechanisms are not always clearly apparent, and attempted treatments not always effective, *acarbose*, an inhibitor of glucose absorption, has been reported to be successful in one small series.

Diagnosis and Differential Diagnosis. Table 81–3 lists the pertinent clinical and biochemical findings in the common childhood disorders associated with hypoglycemia. A careful and detailed history is essential in every suspected or documented case of hypoglycemia (see Box 81–5). Specific points to be noted include age at onset, temporal relation to meals or caloric deprivation, and a family history of prior infants known to have had hypoglycemia or of unexplained infant deaths. In the 1st wk of life, the majority of infants have the transient form of neonatal hypoglycemia either as a result of prematurity/intrauterine growth retardation or by virtue of being born to diabetic mothers. The absence of a history of maternal diabetes, but the presence of macrosomia and the characteristic large plethoric appearance of an "infant of a diabetic mother" should arouse suspicion of hyperinsulinemic hypoglycemia of infancy probably due to a K_{ATP} channel defect that is familial (autosomal recessive) or sporadic; plasma insulin concentrations greater than 10 μU/mL in the presence of documented hypoglycemia confirm this diagnosis. The presence of hepatomegaly should arouse suspicion of an enzyme deficiency; if non–glucose-reducing sugar is present in the urine, galactosemia is most likely. In males, the presence of a microphallus suggests the possibility of hypopituitarism, which also may be associated with jaundice in both sexes.

Past the newborn period, clues to the cause of persistent or recurrent hypoglycemia can be obtained through a careful history, physical examination, and initial laboratory findings. The temporal relation of the hypoglycemia to food intake may suggest that the defect is one of gluconeogenesis, if symptoms occur 6 hr or more after meals. If hypoglycemia occurs shortly after meals, galactosemia or fructose intolerance is most likely, and the presence of reducing substances in the urine rapidly distinguishes these possibilities. The autosomal dominant forms of hyperinsulinemic hypoglycemia need to be considered, with measurement of glucose, insulin, ammonia, and careful history for other affected family members of any age. Measurement of IGFBP-1 may be useful; it is low in hyperinsulinemia states and high in other forms of hypoglycemia. The presence of hepatomegaly suggests one of the enzyme deficiencies in glycogen synthesis or breakdown or in gluconeogenesis, as outlined in Table 81–3. The absence of ketonemia or ketonuria at the time of initial presentation strongly suggests hyperinsulinemia or a defect in fatty acid oxidation. In most other causes of hypoglycemia, with the exception of galactosemia and fructose intolerance, ketonemia and ketonuria are present at the time of fasting hypoglycemia. At the time of the hypoglycemia, serum should be obtained for determination of hormones and substrates, followed by repeated measurement after an intramuscular or intravenous injection of glucagon, as outlined in Box 81–5. Interpretation of the findings is summarized in

Table 81–3. Hypoglycemia with ketonuria in children between ages 18 mo and 5 yr is most likely to be ketotic hypoglycemia, especially if hepatomegaly is absent. The ingestion of a toxin, including alcohol or salicylate, can usually be excluded rapidly by the history.

When the history is suggestive but acute symptoms are not present, a 24–36 hr supervised fast can usually provoke hypoglycemia and resolve the question of hyperinsulinemia or other conditions (see Table 81–3). Such a fast is contraindicated if a fatty acid oxidation defect is suspected; other approaches such as mass tandem spectrometry or molecular diagnosis, or both, should be considered. Because adrenal insufficiency may mimic ketotic hypoglycemia, plasma cortisol levels should be determined at the time of documented hypoglycemia; increased buccal or skin pigmentation may provide the clue to primary adrenal insufficiency with elevated ACTH (melanocyte-stimulating hormone) activity. Short stature or a decrease in the growth rate may provide the clue to pituitary insufficiency involving growth hormone as well as ACTH. Definitive tests of pituitary-adrenal function such as the arginine-insulin stimulation test for growth hormone IGF-1, IGFBP-1, and cortisol release may be necessary.

In the presence of hepatomegaly and hypoglycemia, a presumptive diagnosis of the enzyme defect can often be made through the clinical manifestations, presence of hyperlipidemia, acidosis, hyperuricemia, response to glucagon in the fed and fasted states, and the response to infusion of various appropriate precursors (see Table 81–3 and Box 81–5). These clinical findings and investigative approaches are summarized in Table 81–3. Definitive diagnosis of the glycogen storage disease may require an open liver biopsy (see Chapter 76). Occasional patients with all the manifestations of glycogen storage disease are found to have normal enzyme activity. These definitive studies require special expertise available only in certain institutions.

Treatment. The prevention of hypoglycemia and its resultant effects on CNS development are important in the newborn period. For neonates with hyperinsulinemia not associated with maternal diabetes, subtotal pancreatectomy may be needed, unless hypoglycemia can be readily controlled with long-term somatostatin analogues or diazoxide.

Treatment of acute symptomatic neonatal or infant hypoglycemia includes intravenous administration of 2 mL/kg of $D_{10}W$, followed by a continuous infusion of glucose at 6–8 mg/kg/min, adjusting the rate to maintain blood glucose levels in the normal range.

The management of persistent neonatal or infantile hypoglycemia includes increasing the rate of intravenous glucose infusion to 8–15 mg/kg/min or more, if needed. This may require a central venous or umbilical venous catheter to administer a hypertonic 15–20% glucose solution. If hyperinsulinemia is present, it should be managed with diazoxide, somatostatin analogues, or calcium channel blockers. In addition, intramuscular or intravenous hydrocortisone, 5 mg/kg/24 hr given in divided doses every 8 hr, or oral prednisone, 1–2 mg/kg/24 hr given in divided doses every 6–12 hr, and intramuscular growth hormone, 1 mg/24 hr, may be added temporarily if hypoglycemia is unresponsive to intravenous glucose; if ineffective, these medications should be discontinued after 3–5 days.

Oral diazoxide, 10–25 mg/kg/24 hr given in divided doses q6h, may reverse hyperinsulinemic hypoglycemia but also may produce hirsutism, edema, nausea, hyperuricemia, electrolyte disturbances, advanced bone age, IgG deficiency, and, rarely, hypotension with prolonged use. A long-acting somatostatin analogue (octreotide, formerly SMS 201–995) is effective in controlling hyperinsulinemic hypoglycemia in patients with islet cell disorders not caused by genetic mutations in K_{ATP} channel and islet cell adenoma. Octreotide is administered subcuta-

neously every 6–12 hr in doses of 20–50 μg in neonates and young infants. Potential but unusual complications include poor growth due to inhibition of growth hormone release, pain at the injection site, vomiting, diarrhea, and hepatic dysfunction (hepatitis, cholelithiasis). Octreotide is usually employed as a temporizing agent for various periods before subtotal pancreatectomy for K_{ATP} channel disorders. It may be particularly useful for the treatment of refractory hypoglycemia despite subtotal pancreatectomy. Total pancreatectomy is not optimal therapy, owing to the risks of surgery, permanent diabetes mellitus, and exocrine pancreatic insufficiency. Continued prolonged medical therapy without pancreatic resection if hypoglycemia is controllable is worthwhile because some children have a spontaneous resolution of the hyperinsulinemic hypoglycemia. This should be balanced against the risk of hypoglycemia-induced CNS injury and the toxicity of drugs.

Ahmad A, Kahler SG, Kishnani PS, et al: Treatment of pyruvate carboxylase deficiency with high doses of citrate and aspartate. *Am J Med Genet* 1999;87:331–38.

Amalfitano A, Bengur AR, Morse RP, et al: Recombinant human acid-α-glucosidase enzyme therapy for infantile glycogen storage disease type II: Results of a phase I/II clinical trial. *Genet Med* 2001;3:132–38.

Apak RA, Yurdakok M, Oran O, et al: Preoperative use of octreotide in a newborn with persistent hyperinsulinemic hypoglycemia of infancy. *J Pediatr Endocrinol Metab* 1998;11:143–5.

Bachrach BE, Weinstein DA, Orbo-Melander M, et al: Glycogen synthase deficiency (glycogen storage disease type 0) presenting with hyperglycemia and glucosuria: Report of three new mutations. *J Pediatr* 2002;140:781–83.

Chen YT, Amalfitano A: Towards a molecular therapy for glycogen storage disease, type II (Pompe disease). *Mol Med Today* 2000;6:245–51.

Coenen MJ, van Den Heuvel LP, Smeitink JA: Mitochondrial oxidative phosphorylation system assembly in man: Recent achievements. *Curr Opin Neurol* 2001;14:777–81.

Dacou-Voutetakis C, Psychou F, Maniati-Christidis M: Persistent hyperinsulinemic hypoglycemia of infancy: Long term results. *J Pediatr Endocrinol Metab* 1998;11:131–41.

de Lonlay P, Benelli C, Fouque F, et al. Hyperinsulinism and hyperammonemia syndrome: Report of twelve unrelated patients. *Pediatr Res* 2001;50:353–7.

de Lonlay P, Cuer M, Vuillaumier-Barrot S, et al: Hyperinsulinemic hypoglycemia as a presenting sign in phosphomannose isomerase deficiency: A new manifestation of carbohydrate-deficient glycoprotein syndrome treatable with mannose. *J Pediatr* 1999;135:379–83.

de Lonlay-Debeney P, Poggi-Travert F, Fournet J-C, et al: Clinical features of 52 neonates with hyperinsulinism. *N Engl J Med* 1999;340:1169–75.

DeVivo DC, Trifiletti RR, Jacobson RI, et al: Defective glucose transport across the blood-brain barrier as a cause of persistent hypoglycorrhachia, seizures, and developmental delay. *N Engl J Med* 1991;325:703–9.

DiMauro S, Lamperti C: Muscle glycogenoses. *Muscle Nerve* 2001;24:984–99.

Doctor BA, O'Riordan MA, Kirchner HL, et al: Perinatal correlates and neonatal outcomes of small for gestational age infants born at term gestation. *Am J Obstet Gynecol* 2001;185:652–9.

Dunne MJ, Kane C, Shepherd RM, et al: Familial persistent hyperinsulinemic hypoglycemia of infancy and mutations in the sulfonylurea receptor. *N Engl J Med* 1997;336:703–6.

Elliott M, Maher ER: Beckwith-Wiedemann syndrome. *J Med Genet* 1994;31:560–4.

Elsas LJ II, Lai K: The molecular biology of galactosemia. *Genet Med* 1998;1:40–8.

Freckmann ML, Thorburn DR, Kirby DM, et al: Mitochondrial electron transport chain defect presenting as hypoglycemia. *J Pediatr* 1997;130:431–6.

Glaser B, Kesavan P, Heyman M, et al: Familial hyperinsulinism caused by an activating glucokinase mutation. *N Engl J Med* 1998;338:226–30.

Hatada I, Ohashi H, Fukushima Y, et al: An imprinted gene p57(KIP2) is mutated in Beckwith-Wiedemann syndrome. *Nat Genet* 1996;14:171–3.

Huopio H, Reimann F, Ashfield R, et al: Dominantly inherited hyperinsulinism caused by a mutation in the sulfonylurea receptor type 1. *J Clin Invest* 2000;106:897–906.

Kane C, Lindley KJ, Johnson PRV, et al: Therapy for persistent hyperinsulinemic hypoglycemia of infancy. *J Clin Invest* 1997;100:1888–93.

Katz LE, Ferry RJ Jr, Stanley CA, et al: Suppression of insulin over-secretion by subcutaneous recombinant human insulin-like growth factor 1 in children with congenital hyperinsulinism due to defective beta-cell sulfonylurea receptor. *J Clin Endocrinol Metab* 1999;84:3117–24.

Kelly A, Ng D, Ferry RJ Jr, et al: Acute insulin responses to leucine in children with the hyperinsulinism/hyperammonemia syndrome. *J Clin Endocrinol Metab* 2001;86:3724–8.

Lamberts SWJ, Van Der Lely AJ, De Herder WW, et al: Octreotide. *N Engl J Med* 1996;334:246–54.

Levitt-Katz LE, Satin-Smith MS, Collett-Solberg P, et al: Insulin-like growth factor binding protein-1 levels in the diagnosis of hypoglycemia caused by hyperinsulinism. *J Pediatr* 1997;131:193–9.

Lucas A, Morley R, Cole TJ: Adverse neurodevelopmental outcome of moderate neonatal hypoglycemia. *BMJ* 1988;297:1304–8.

Matern D, Starzl TE, Arnaout W, et al: Liver transplantation for glycogen storage disease types I, III, and IV. *Eur J Pediatr* 1999;158:S43–48.

Mayefsky JH, Sarnaik AP, Postellon DC: Factitious hypoglycemia. *Pediatrics* 1982;69:804–5.

Meissner T, Otonkoski T, Feneberg R, et al: Exercise induced hypoglycaemic hyperinsulinism. *Arch Dis Child* 2001;84:254–7.

Murace M, Gerunda G, Neri D, et al: Hepatocyte transplantation as a treatment for glycogen storage disease type Ia. *Lancet* 2002;359:317–18.

Ng DD, Ferry RJ Jr, Kelly A, et al: Acarbose treatment of postprandial hypoglycemia in children after Nissen fundoplication. *J Pediatr* 2001;139:877–9.

Phillip M, Bashan N, Smith CPA, et al: An algorithmic approach to diagnosis of hypoglycemia. *J Pediatr* 1987;110:387–90.

Plecko B, Stoeckler-Ipsiroglu S, Schober E, et al: Oral β-Hydroxybutyrate supplementation in two patients with hyperinsulinemic hypoglycemia: Monitoring of β-hydroxybutyrate levels in blood and cerebrospinal fluid, and in the brain by *in vivo* magnetic resonance spectroscopy. *Pediatr Res* 2002;52:301–6.

Pollack ES, Pollack CV Jr: Ketotic hypoglycemia: A case report. *J Emerg Med* 1993;11:531–4.

Rivkees SA, Crawford JD: Hypoglycemia pathogenesis in children with dumping syndrome. *Pediatrics* 1987;80:937–42.

Shaiu W, Kishnani P, Shen J, et al: Genotype-phenotype correlation in two frequent mutations and mutation update in Type III glycogen storage disease. *Mol Genet Metab* 2000;69:16–23.

Sperling MA, Menon RK: Hyperinsulinemic hypoglycemia of infancy. *Endocrinol Metab Clin North Am* 1999;28:695–708.

Stanley CA: Dissecting the spectrum of fatty acid oxidation disorders. *J Pediatr* 1998;132:384–6.

Taylor SI, Barbetti F, Accili D, et al: Syndromes of autoimmunity and hypoglycemia: Autoantibodies directed against insulin and its receptor. *Endocrinol Metab Clin North Am* 1989;18:123–43.

Thornton PS, Satin-Smith MS, Herold K, et al: Familial hyperinsulinism with apparent autosomal dominant inheritance: Clinical and genetic differences from the autosomal recessive variant. *J Pediatr* 1998;132:9–14.

Umapathysivam K, Hopwood JJ, Meikle PJ: Determination of acid alpha-glucosidase activity in blood spots as a diagnostic test for Pompe disease. *Clin Chem* 2001;47:1378–83.

Visser G, Rake JP, Fernandes J, et al: Neutropenia, neutrophil dysfunction, and inflammatory bowel disease in glycogen storage disease type Ib: Results of the European study on glycogen storage disease type I. *J Pediatr* 2000;137:187–90.

Vorgerd M, Grehl T, Jager M, et al: Creatine therapy in myophosphorylase deficiency (McArdle disease): A placebo-controlled crossover trial. *Arch Neurol* 2000;57:956–63.

Weber TA, Antognetti MR, Stacpoole PW, et al: Caveats when considering ketogenic diets for the treatment of pyruvate dehydrogenase complex deficiency. *J Pediatr* 2001;138:390–95.

Weinstein DA, Somers MJ, Wolfsdorf JI: Decreased urinary citrate excretion in type Ia glycogen storage disease. *J Pediatr* 2001;138:378–82.

Weston BW, Lin J, Muenzer J, et al: Glucose-6-phosphatase mutation G188R confers an atypical glycogen storage disease type Ib phenotype. *Pediatr Res* 2000; 48:329–34.

White NJ, Marsh K, Turner RC, et al: Hypoglycemia in African children with severe malaria. *Lancet* 1987;1:708–11.

Wolfsdorf JI, Crigler JF Jr: Effect of continuous glucose therapy begun in infancy on the long-term clinical course of patients with type I glycogen storage disease. *J Pediatr Gastroenterol Nutr* 1999;29:136–43.

Wolfsdorf JI, Keller RJ, Landy H, et al: Glucose therapy for glycogenosis type 1 in infants: Comparison of intermittent uncooked cornstarch and continuous overnight glucose feedings. *J Pediatr* 1990;117:384–91.

Yoshikawa M, Fukui K, Kuriyama S, et al: Hepatic adenomas treated with percutaneous ethanol injection in a patient with glycogen storage disease type Ia. *J Gastroenterol* 2001;36:52–61.

Ziadeh R, Hoffman EP, Finegold DN, et al: Medium chain acyl-CoA dehydrogenase deficiency in Pennsylvania: Neonatal screening shows high incidence and unexpected mutation frequencies. *Pediatr Res* 1995;37:675–78.

The Fetus and the Neonatal Infant

SECTION 1 *Noninfectious Disorders*

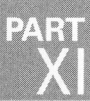

Chapter 82

Overview of Mortality and Morbidity

Barbara J. Stoll and Robert M. Kliegman

Fetal and extrauterine life form a continuum during which human growth and development are affected by genetic, environmental, and social factors. The perinatal period is most often defined as the period from the 28th wk of gestation through the 7th day after birth (additional definitions include the 20th wk of gestation to the 7th day and the 20th wk of gestation to the 28th day). The neonatal period is defined as less than 28 days of life and may be further subdivided into period 1, birth to less than 24 hr; period 2, 24 hr to less than 7 days; and period 3, 7 days to less than 28 days.

Perinatal mortality is influenced by prenatal, maternal, and fetal conditions and by circumstances surrounding delivery. Perinatal deaths are associated with intrauterine growth restriction (IUGR); conditions that predispose the fetus to asphyxia, such as placental insufficiency; severe congenital malformations; and overwhelming early-onset neonatal infections (Table 82–1). Major causes of neonatal mortality are diseases associated with preterm birth and low birthweight (LBW) and lethal congenital anomalies. Neonatal mortality is highest during the first 24 hr of life and overall accounts for 65% of all infant deaths (i.e., deaths before 1 yr of age). Between 1980 and 2000, neonatal mortality rates in the United States declined 46% to 4.6 per 1,000 live births (Fig. 82–1). Factors related to the decline include improved obstetric and neonatal management with a significant reduction in birthweight-specific neonatal mortality (Fig. 82–2). Further reduction in neonatal mortality will depend on prevention of preterm delivery and LBW, prenatal diagnosis and early management of congenital anomalies, and timely effective treatment of diseases that result from factors in gestation and during labor and delivery (see Table 82–1).

In the United States each year, approximately 6 million pregnancies, 4 million live births, 18,000 neonatal deaths, and 28,000 infant deaths occur. Twelve per cent of births are to teenage women between the ages of 15 and 19 yr; 33% are to unmarried women. Births among teenagers (especially first births) declined 22% between 1991 and 2000 (Fig. 82–3). Births to unmarried women remain stable.

Infant mortality rates (deaths occurring from birth to 12 mo of age per 1,000 live births) vary by country; in 1998, rates were lowest in Hong Kong (3.2/1,000 births), moderate in the United States (7.2/1,000), and highest in developing countries (30–150/1,000). Medical, socioeconomic, and cultural factors influence perinatal and neonatal mortality. Preventive variables such as health education, prenatal care, nutrition, social support, risk identification, and obstetric care can effectively reduce perinatal and neonatal mortality. In the United States, 50% of

TABLE 82–1. Major Causes of Perinatal and Neonatal Mortality

Fetal	Preterm	Full Term
Placental insufficiency	Severe immaturity	Congenital anomalies
Intrauterine infection	Respiratory distress syndrome	Birth asphyxia, trauma
Severe congenital malformations (anomalies)	Intraventricular hemorrhage	Infection
Umbilical cord accident	Congenital anomalies	Meconium aspiration pneumonia
Abruptio placentae	Infection	Persistent pulmonary hypertension (PPHN)
Hydrops fetalis	Necrotizing enterocolitis	
	Bronchopulmonary dysplasia (BPD)	

infant deaths in 2000 were due to four causes (classified according to the International Classification of Diseases, 10th edition): congenital malformations, disorders relating to prematurity and unspecified LBW, sudden infant death syndrome (SIDS), and newborns affected by maternal complications of pregnancy.

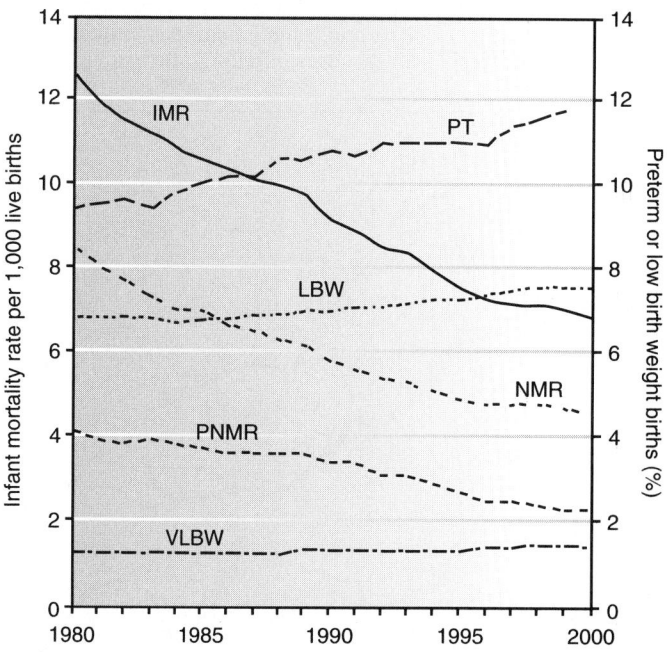

FIGURE 82–1. Infant, neonatal, and postneonatal mortality, LBW and VLBW, and preterm delivery, United States, 1980–2000. IMR = infant deaths per 1,000 live births; NMR = neonatal deaths per 1,000 live births; PNMR = postneonatal deaths per 1,000 live births; LBW = percent low birthweight (<2500 g); VLBW = percent very low birthweight (<1500 g); PT = percent preterm (<37 weeks' gestation). (From Hoyert DL, Freedman MA, Strobino DM, Guyer B: Annual summary of vital statistics: 2000. *Pediatrics* 2001;108:1241.)

519

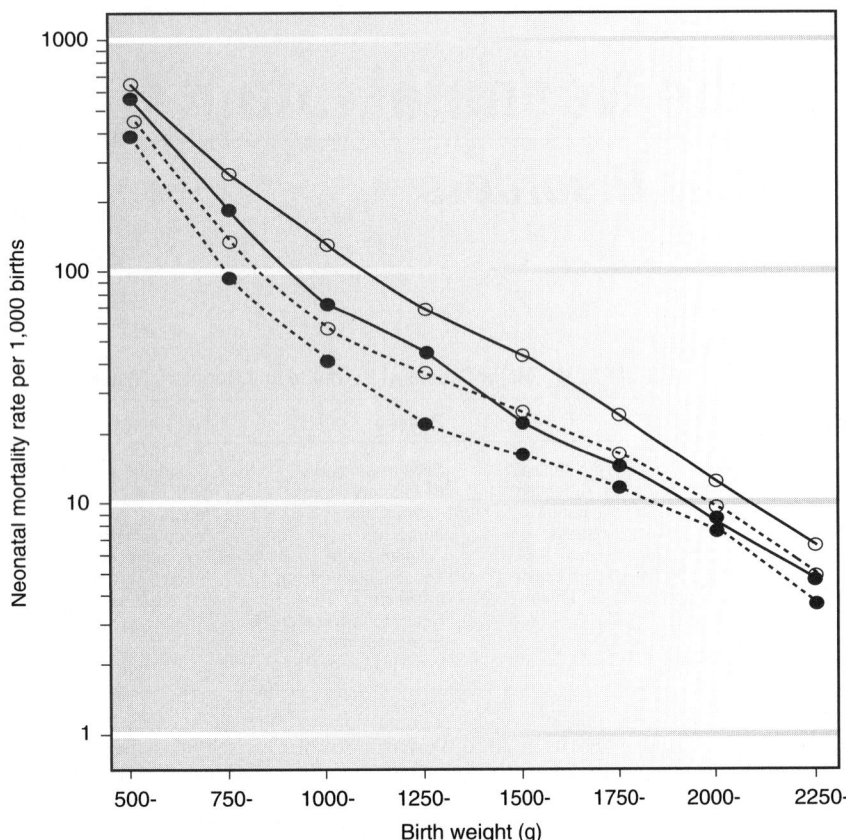

FIGURE 82–2. Neonatal mortality, by birthweight categories, for black *(filled circles)* and for white *(open circles)* infants in the United States. *Solid lines* denote data for 1989; *dashed lines* are for 1997. Data shown are for births of newborn infants weighing less than 2,250 g only. (From Demissie K, Rhoads GG, Ananth CV, et al: Trends in preterm birth and neonatal mortality among Blacks and Whites in the United States from 1989 to 1997. *Am J Epidemiol* 2001;154:307.)

LBW (as a result of preterm delivery and/or IUGR) is a major determinant of both neonatal and infant mortality rates and, together with congenital anomalies (e.g., cardiac, central nervous system, and respiratory), contributes significantly to childhood morbidity. The LBW rate is directly related to the variance of infant mortality rates among different countries.

The *LBW rate* (infants weighing 2,500 g or less at birth each year) in the United States increased from 6.6% to 7.6% between 1981 and 2000, whereas the very low birthweight (VLBW) rate (infants weighing 1,500 g or less at birth) increased from 1.1% to 1.4% of all births. In the past decade, LBW has increased in white infants, mainly because of an increase in multiple births (often associated with assisted reproduction), whereas in blacks, LBW has decreased (Fig. 82–4). Nonetheless, LBW and VLBW rates remain highest among black infants. Reasons for the racial disparity in LBW remain unclear. Despite advances in prenatal and obstetric care, racial disparity in birthweight persists, thus suggesting the need for novel prevention programs. Furthermore, although preterm LBW survival is better among black neonates (see Fig. 82–2), overall neonatal and infant mortality rates remain highest in blacks (Fig. 82–5), even those born to extremely low-risk mothers (married, aged 20–34 yr, ≥13 yr of education, adequate prenatal care, no medical risk factors, no alcohol or tobacco use during pregnancy). A reduction in the racial disparity in mortality is an important public health issue reflected in the U.S. National Health Objectives for the Year 2010.

LBW is caused by preterm birth, IUGR, or both factors. The predominant cause of LBW in the United States is preterm birth, whereas in developing countries, the cause is more often IUGR. Although IUGR does not appear to further increase the risk of mortality in preterm infants, both morbidity and mortality are increased in term growth-restricted infants. VLBW infants are most often premature (<37 wk of gestation), although IUGR may also complicate their early delivery. Even though VLBW occurs in only 1–2% of all infants in the United States, these births represent a large proportion of the neonatal and infant mortality and infants with both short- and long-term complications, including neurodevelopmental handicaps. The etiology of

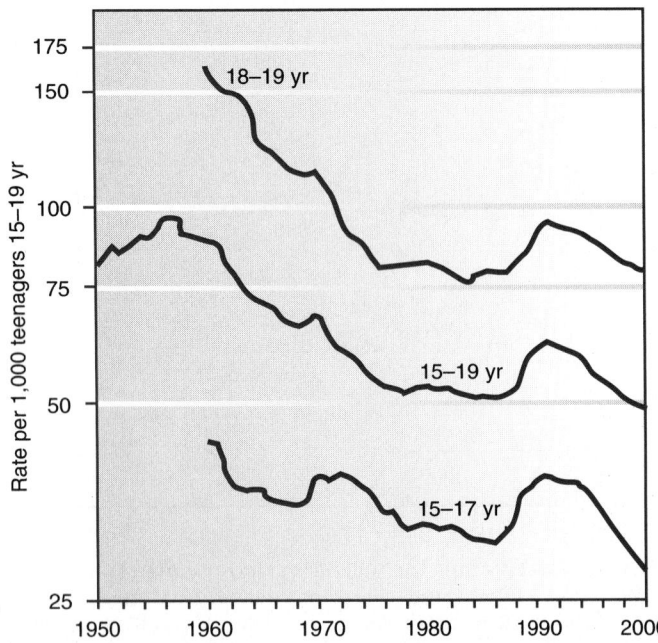

NOTES: Data for 2000 are preliminary. Rates are plotted on a log scale.

FIGURE 82–3. Birthrates for teenagers by age: United States, 1950–2000. (From Ventura SJ, Mathews TJ, Hamilton BE: Births to teenagers in the United States, 1940–2000. *Natl Vital Stat Rep* 2001;49:1.)

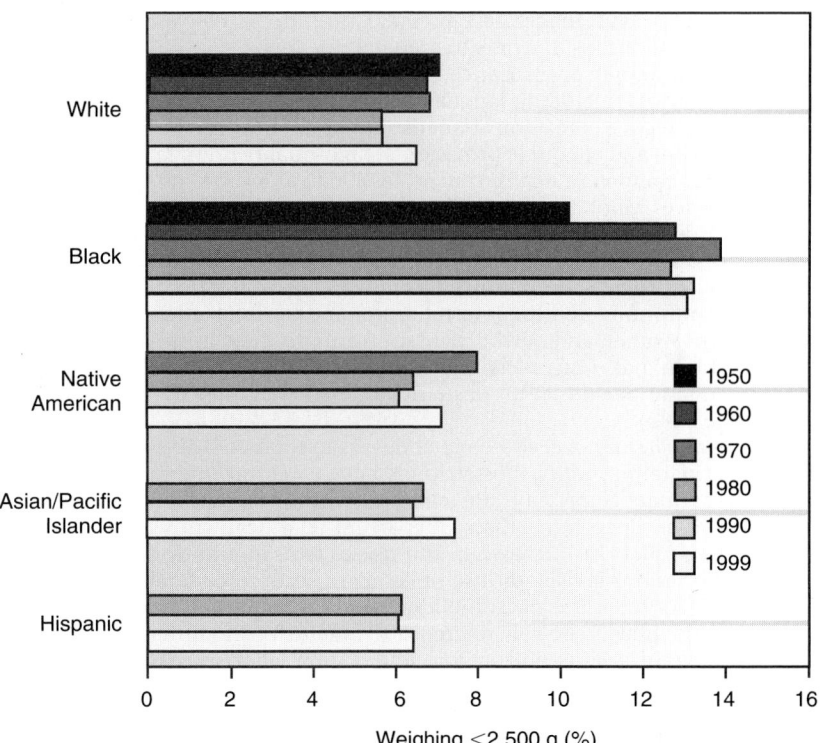

FIGURE 82–4. Percent low birthweight by race and ethnicity, selected years: United States, 1950–1999. (From Guyer B, Freedman MA, Strobino DM, et al: Annual summary of vital statistics: Trends in the health of Americans during the 20th century. *Pediatrics* 2000; 106:1307.)

preterm birth is complex, multifactorial, and not completely understood. Causes include maternal diseases such as severe preeclampsia requiring elective delivery, premature rupture of membranes, uterine abnormalities, placental bleeding (abruptio, previa), multifetus gestation, drug misuse, maternal chronic illnesses, fetal distress, and infection. A complex interaction can be noted between infection, inflammation, and both preterm premature rupture of membranes and preterm birth. Infectious antecedents include maternal urinary tract infection, pyelonephritis, chorioamnionitis, bacterial vaginosis, and upper and lower genitourinary tract infection with a variety of agents (*Chlamydia trachomatis, Ureaplasma urealyticum, Mycoplasma hominis, Gardnerella vaginalis,* and group B streptococcus). In many cases, the cause of preterm delivery is unknown.

Although 99% of births occur in hospitals, only 83% of pregnant women receive *prenatal care* in the 1st trimester. Many

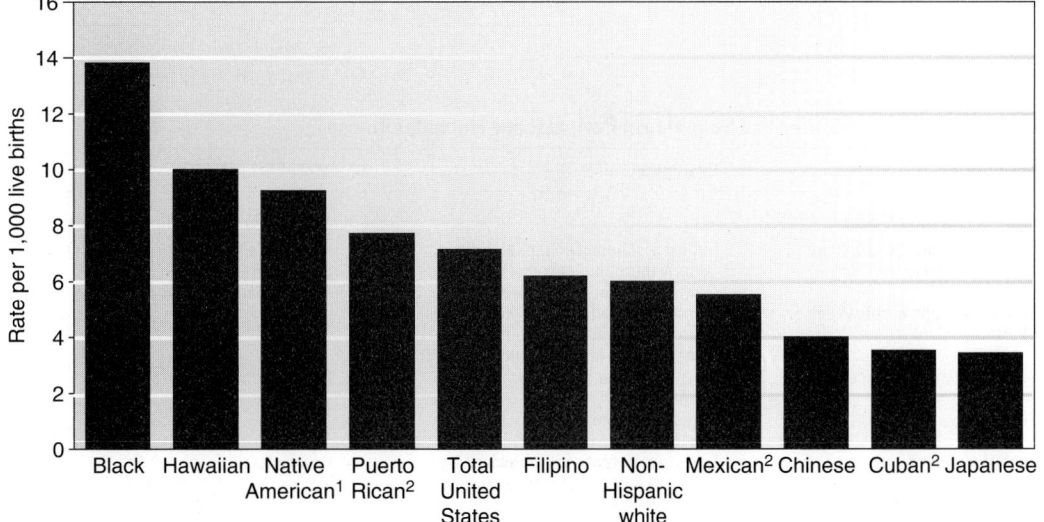

FIGURE 82–5. Infant mortality rates by race and ethnicity, 1998. (From Mathews TJ, Curtin SC, MacDorman MF: Infant mortality statistics from the 1998 period linked birth/infant death data set. *Natl Vital Stat Rep* 2000; 48:1.)

[1]Includes Aleuts and Eskimos.
[2]Persons of Hispanic origin may be of any race.

women who receive inadequate prenatal care are at risk for perinatal complications. Barriers to prenatal care include absent or insufficient money or insurance to pay for care; poor coordination of services, including language and cultural issues; and inadequate effective education about the importance of prenatal care. Successful and adequate provision of high-quality prenatal care requires competent health care professionals and coordination of services among physicians' offices, clinics, community hospitals, special regionalized programs for high-risk mothers and infants, and tertiary care centers. Regional perinatal programs should provide continuing education and consultation in both the community and the referral center and transportation for pregnant women and newborn infants to appropriate hospitals; they should also include a regional hospital with facilities, equipment, and personnel for obstetric and neonatal intensive care (Table 82–2).

Fetal deaths slightly exceed neonatal deaths in their contribution to perinatal mortality. Obstetricians have a central role in reducing perinatal mortality and morbidity. Intrapartum fetal deaths have declined more than antepartum fetal deaths; this decline may reflect an increase in the use of fetal monitoring during labor and more liberal use of cesarean section for fetal distress and other obstetric complications. It is important to emphasize the need to be able to predict the maturity and functional reserve of a fetus both before and during labor so that fetuses and infants at greatest risk can be identified as early as possible. The obstetrician and pediatrician must effectively interact to anticipate perinatal problems and take prompt preventive and therapeutic measures.

Postneonatal mortality refers to deaths between 28 days and 1 yr of life. Historically, these infant deaths were due to causes outside the neonatal period, such as SIDS, infections (respiratory, enteric), and trauma. With the advent of modern neonatal care, many VLBW infants who would have died in the 1st mo of life now survive the neonatal period only to succumb to the sequelae noted in Table 82–3. This delayed neonatal mortality is an important contributor to postneonatal mortality.

For the most immature infants at the limit of viability (22–25 wk gestation), decision-making regarding care is a complex process that involves the physician and other health professionals, the family, and society. The challenge is to not only improve survival but also reduce short-term complications and improve long-term neurodevelopmental outcome.

Adverse neurodevelopmental sequelae include cerebral palsy, seizures, hydrocephalus requiring a shunt, blindness, deafness,

TABLE 82–2. Levels of In-Hospital Perinatal Care

Basic

Maternal	Neonate
Monitor and care for low-risk patients	Resuscitation
	Stabilization
Triage for high risk for transfer	Well neonatal care
Detection and care of unanticipated labor problems	Nursery care
	Visitation
Emergency cesarean delivery within 30 min	General pediatrician staff (capable of neonatal resuscitation)
Blood bank, anesthesia, radiology, ultrasound, and laboratory support	
Care of postpartum problems	
Obstetrician, nurse, midwife staff	

Special Care

Maternal	Neonate
Basic services plus	Basic services plus
Care of high-risk pregnancies	Care of high-risk neonate with short-term problems
Triage, transfer of high-risk pregnancies (<32 wk, IUGR, preeclampsia, severe maternal medical illness)	Stabilization before transfer (<1,500 g, <32 wk, critically ill)
	Accept convalescing back (reverse) transfers

Subspecialty Care

Maternal	Neonate
Basic plus specialty care plus	Basic plus specialty care plus
Experienced perinatologist (24-hr coverage)	Experienced neonatologist (24-hr coverage)
Evaluation of high-risk therapies	Inborn plus transferred patients
Care for severe maternal medical or obstetric illnesses	Evaluation of high-risk therapies
	All pediatric medical, radiologic, and surgical subspecialties
High-risk fetal care (Rh disease, nonimmune hydrops, life-threatening anomalies)	NICU with operating room capabilities
Outcomes research	High-risk follow-up
Community education	Outcomes research
	Community education

IUGR = intrauterine growth retardation; NICU = neonatal intensive care unit.

From American Academy of Pediatrics, American College of Obstetricians and Gynecologists: Guidelines for Perinatal Care, *5th ed. Elk Grove Village, IL, American Academy of Pediatrics, 2002.*

TABLE 82–3. Morbidities and Sequelae of Perinatal and Neonatal Illness

Morbidities	Examples	Morbidities	Examples
Central Nervous System		**Sensation—Peripheral Nerves**	
Spastic diplegic-quadriplegic cerebral palsy	Hypoxic-ischemic encephalopathy, periventricular leukomalacia, undetermined antenatal factors	Reduced visual acuity (blindness)	Retinopathy of prematurity (ROP)
		Strabismus	Undetermined
Choreoathetotic cerebral palsy	Bilirubin encephalopathy (kernicterus)	Hearing impairment (deafness)	Drug toxicity (furosemide, aminoglycosides), bilirubin encephalopathy, hypoxia ± hyperventilation
Microcephaly	Hypoxic-ischemic encephalopathy, intrauterine infection (rubella, CMV)		
Communicating hydrocephalus	Intraventricular hemorrhage, meningitis	Poor speech	Immaturity, chronic illness, hypoxia, prolonged endotracheal intubation, hearing deficit
Seizures	Hypoxic-ischemic encephalopathy, hypoglycemia		
Encephalopathy	Congenital infections (rubella, CMV, human immunodeficiency virus, toxoplasmosis)	Paralysis-paresis	Birth trauma—brachial plexus, phrenic nerve, spinal cord
Educational failure and/or mental retardation	Immaturity, low socioeconomic status, hypoxia, hypoglycemia, cerebral palsy, intraventricular hemorrhage		

TABLE 82–3. Morbidities and Sequelae of Perinatal and Neonatal Illness *Continued*

Morbidities	Examples	Morbidities	Examples
Respiratory		***Gastrointestinal***	Necrotizing enterocolitis, gastroschisis, malrotation-volvulus, cystic fibrosis, intestinal atresia
Bronchopulmonary dysplasia (BPD)	Oxygen toxicity, barotrauma	Short-gut syndrome	
Subglottic stenosis	Endotracheal tube injury		
Sudden infant death syndrome	Prematurity, BPD, infant of illicit drug user	Cholestatic liver disease (cirrhosis, hepatic failure)	Hyperalimentation toxicity, sepsis, short-gut syndrome
Choanal stenosis, nasal septum destruction	Nasotracheal intubation Growth failure	Failure to thrive	Short-gut syndrome, cholestasis, BPD, cerebral palsy, severe congenital heart disease
Cardiovascular			
Cyanosis	Precorrective palliative care of congenital cyanotic heart disease, cor pulmonale from BPD, reactive airway	Poor postnatal weight gain Inguinal hernia	Unknown
		Miscellaneous	
Heart failure	Precorrective palliative care of complex congenital heart disease, BPD, ventricular septal defect	Cutaneous scars	Chest tube or IV placement, hyperalimentation, subcutaneous infiltration, fetal puncture, intrauterine varicella, cutis aplasia
		Absent radial artery pulse	
		Hypertension	Frequent arterial puncture Renal thrombi, repair of coarctation of aorta

CMV = cytomegalovirus; BPD = bronchopulmonary dysplasia; ROP = retinopathy of prematurity

and cognitive impairment. The risk of an adverse outcome increases with decreasing gestational age at birth. Early morbidity and prognostic variables that contribute to adverse neurodevelopmental outcomes include grades 3–4 intraventricular hemorrhage and periventricular leukomalacia, necrotizing enterocolitis requiring extensive bowel resection, bronchopulmonary dysplasia, and postnatal steroid therapy. The association of postnatal steroid use with adverse neurodevelopmental outcome highlights the importance of high-risk infant follow-up after hospital discharge to assess the long-term impact of new and/or frequently used therapies. Many studies have documented the impact of social and family risk factors on outcome. At school age, VLBW infants have poorer physical growth, cognitive function, and school performance. These disadvantages appear to persist into adulthood and therefore have broad implications for society. All VLBW infants must be monitored after discharge to detect neurodevelopmental impairment as early as possible and to ensure that children and families receive any interventions available and adequate support to optimize long-term outcome.

Alexander GR, Kogan MD, Himes JH, et al: Racial differences in birthweight for gestational age and infant mortality in extremely low-risk US populations. *Paediatr Perinat Epidemiol* 1999;13:205.

Barrington KJ: Postnatal steroids and neurodevelopmental outcomes: A problem in the making. *Pediatrics* 2001;107:1425.

Carroli G, Villar J, Piaggio G, et al: WHO systematic review of randomized controlled trials of routine antenatal care. *Lancet* 2001;357:1565.

Centers for Disease Control and Prevention: Infant mortality and low birth weight among black and white infants—United States, 1980–2000. *MMWR Morb Mortal Wkly Rep* 2002;51:589.

Centers for Disease Control and Prevention: Racial and ethnic disparities in infant mortality rates—60 largest U.S. cities, 1995–1998. *MMWR Morb Mortal Wkly Rep* 2002;51:329.

Craig ED, Thompson JMD, Mitchell EA: Socioeconomic status and preterm birth: New Zealand trends, 1980 to 1999. *Arch Dis Child Fetal Neonatal Ed* 2002;86: F142.

Demissie K, Rhoads GG, Ananth CV, et al: Trends in preterm birth and neonatal mortality among Blacks and Whites in the United States from 1989 to 1997. *Am J Epidemiol* 2001;154:307.

Goldenberg RL, Hauth JC, Andrews WW: Mechanisms of disease: Intrauterine infection and preterm delivery. *N Engl J Med* 2000;342:1500.

Goodman DC, Fisher ES, Little GA, et al: The relation between the availability of neonatal intensive care and neonatal mortality. *N Engl J Med* 2002;346:1538.

Gross SJ, Mettelman BB, Dye TD, et al: Impact of family structure and stability on academic outcome in preterm children at 10 years of age. *J Pediatr* 2001;138: 169.

Guyer B, Freedman MA, Strobino DM, et al: Annual summary of vital statistics: Trends in the health of Americans during the 20th century. *Pediatrics* 2000;106: 1307.

Hack M, Flannery DJ, Schluchter M, et al: Outcomes in young adulthood for very-low-birth-weight infants. *N Engl J Med* 2002;346:149.

Healthy People 2010, 2nd ed. Washington, DC, US Government Printing Office. (Conference edition in 2 volumes.) (GPO stock No. 017-001-00547-9.)

Horbar JD, Badger GJ, Carpenter JH, et al: Trends in mortality and morbidity for very low birth weight infants, 1991–1999. *Pediatrics* 2002;110:143.

Hoyert DL, Freedman MA, Strobino DM, et al: Annual summary of vital statistics: 2000. *Pediatrics* 2001;108:1241.

Joseph KS, Marcoux S, Ohlsson A, et al: Changes in stillbirth and infant mortality associated with increases in preterm birth among twins. *Pediatrics* 2001;108:1055.

McIntire DD, Bloom SL, Casey BM, et al: Birth weight in relation to morbidity and mortality among newborn infants. *N Engl J Med* 1999;340:1234.

Saigal S, Hoult LA, Streiner DL, et al: School difficulties at adolescence in a regional cohort of children who were extremely low birth weight. *Pediatrics* 2000;105:325.

Ventura SJ, Mathews TJ, Hamilton BE: Births to teenagers in the United States, 1940–2000. *Natl Vital Stat Rep* 2001;49:1.

Chapter 83

The Newborn Infant (see also Chapter 9)

Barbara J. Stoll and Robert M. Kliegman

The neonatal period is a highly vulnerable time for an infant, who is completing many of the physiologic adjustments required for extrauterine existence. The high neonatal morbidity and mortality rates attest to the fragility of life during this period; in the United States, of all deaths occurring in the 1st yr, two thirds are in the neonatal period. The annual rate of deaths during the 1st yr is unequaled until the 7th decade.

An infant's transition from intrauterine to extrauterine life requires many biochemical and physiologic changes. No longer dependent on maternal circulation via the placenta, a newborn's pulmonary function is activated for self-sufficient respiratory exchange of oxygen and carbon dioxide. Newborn infants also become dependent on gastrointestinal tract function for absorbing food, renal function for excreting waste and maintaining chemical homeostasis, hepatic function for neutralizing and excreting toxic substances, and function of the immunologic system for protecting against infection. The neonatal cardiovascular and endocrine systems also adapt for self-sufficient functioning. Many of a newborn infant's special problems are related to poor adaptation because of asphyxia, premature birth, life-threatening congenital anomalies, or the adverse effects of delivery.

83.1 ■ History in Neonatal Pediatrics

The neonatal history should (1) identify disabling diseases that are amenable to prompt preventive action or treatment (e.g., respiratory distress syndrome), (2) anticipate conditions that may be of later importance (e.g., gonococcal conjunctivitis), and (3) uncover possible causative factors that may explain pathologic conditions regardless of their immediate or future significance (e.g., screening for inborn errors of metabolism). The perinatal history should include demographic and social data (socioeconomic status, age, race); past medical illnesses in the family, including siblings (cardiopulmonary disorders, infectious diseases, genetic disorders, anemia, jaundice, diabetes mellitus); previous maternal reproductive problems (stillbirth, prematurity, blood group sensitization); events occurring in the present pregnancy (vaginal bleeding, medications, acute illness, duration of rupture of membranes); and a description of the labor (duration, fetal presentation, fetal distress, fever) and delivery (cesarean section, anesthesia or sedation, use of forceps, Apgar score, need for resuscitation).

83.2 Physical Examination of the Newborn Infant

Many physical and behavioral characteristics of a normal newborn infant are described in Chapter 9, which should be reviewed.

The initial examination of a newborn infant should be performed as soon as possible after delivery to detect abnormalities and to establish a baseline for subsequent examination. Infants should have temperature, pulse, respiratory rate, color, type of respiration, tone, activity, and level of consciousness monitored every 30 min after birth for 2 hr or until stabilized. For high-risk deliveries, this examination should take place in the delivery room and focus on congenital anomalies and pathophysiologic problems that may interfere with normal cardiopulmonary and metabolic adaptation to extrauterine life. Congenital anomalies may be present in 3–5% of infants. After a stable delivery room course, a 2nd and more detailed examination should be performed within 24 hr of birth. If an infant remains in the hospital longer than 48 hr, a discharge examination should be performed within 24 hr of discharge. With a healthy infant, the mother should be present during this examination; even minor, seemingly insignificant anatomic variations may worry a family and should be explained. The explanation must be careful and skillful so that otherwise unworried families are not unduly alarmed. No infant should be discharged from the hospital without a final examination because certain abnormalities, particularly heart murmurs, often appear or disappear in the immediate neonatal period and, in addition, evidence of disease that has just been acquired may be noted. The pulse (normal, 120–160 beats/min), respiratory rate (normal, 30–60 breaths/min), temperature, weight, length, head circumference, and dimensions of any visible or palpable structural abnormality should be recorded. Blood pressure is determined if a neonate appears ill or has a heart murmur.

Examining a newborn requires patience, gentleness, and procedural flexibility. Thus, if the infant is quiet and relaxed at the beginning of the examination, palpation of the abdomen or auscultation of the heart should be performed first before other, more disturbing manipulations are attempted.

General Appearance. Physical activity may be absent during the relaxation of normal sleep, or it may be decreased by the effects of illness or drugs; an infant may be either lying with the extremities motionless, to conserve energy for the effort of difficult breathing, or be vigorously crying with accompanying activity of the arms and legs. Both active and passive muscle tone and any unusual posture should be recorded. Coarse, tremulous movements with ankle or jaw myoclonus are more common and less significant in newborn infants than at any other age. Such movements tend to occur when an infant is

active, whereas convulsive twitching usually occurs in a quiet state. Edema may produce a superficial appearance of good nutrition. Pitting after applied pressure may or may not be noted, but the skin of the fingers and toes lacks the normal fine wrinkles when filled with fluid. Edema of the eyelids commonly results from irritation caused by the administration of silver nitrate. Generalized edema may occur with prematurity, hypoproteinemia secondary to severe erythroblastosis fetalis, nonimmune hydrops, congenital nephrosis, Hurler syndrome, or unknown cause. Localized edema suggests a congenital malformation of the lymphatic system; when confined to one or more extremities of a female infant, it may be the initial sign of Turner syndrome (Chapters 70 and 580.1).

Skin. Vasomotor instability and peripheral circulatory sluggishness are revealed by deep redness or purple lividity in a crying infant, whose color may darken profoundly with closure of the glottis preceding a vigorous cry, and by harmless cyanosis (acrocyanosis) of the hands and feet, especially when they are cool. Mottling, another example of general circulatory instability, may be associated with serious illness or related to a transient fluctuation in skin temperature. An extraordinary division of the body from the forehead to the pubis into red and pale halves is known as harlequin color change, a transient and harmless condition. Significant *cyanosis* may be masked by the pallor of circulatory failure or anemia; alternatively, the relatively high hemoglobin content of the first few days and the thin skin may combine to produce an appearance of cyanosis at a higher Pao_2 than in older children. Localized cyanosis is differentiated from ecchymosis by the momentary blanching pallor (with cyanosis) that occurs after pressure. The same maneuver also helps in demonstrating *icterus*, possibly significant but unnoticed if the skin is suffused with blood. *Pallor* may represent asphyxia, anemia, shock, or edema. Early recognition of anemia may lead to a diagnosis of erythroblastosis fetalis, subcapsular hematoma of the liver or spleen, subdural hemorrhage, or fetal-maternal or twin-twin transfusion. Without being anemic, postmature infants tend to have paler and thicker skin than term or premature infants do. The ruddy red appearance of *plethora* is seen with polycythemia.

The vernix and common transitory macular capillary hemangiomas of the eyelids and neck are described in Chapter 637. Cavernous hemangiomas are deeper, blue masses that if large, may trap platelets and produce disseminated intravascular coagulation or interfere with local organ function. Scattered petechiae may be seen on the presenting part (usually the scalp or face) after a difficult delivery. Slate blue, well-demarcated areas of pigmentation are seen over the buttocks, back, and sometimes other parts of the body in more than 50% of black, Native American, or Asian infants and occasionally in white ones. These patches have no known anthropologic significance despite their name **mongolian spots**; they tend to disappear within the first year. The vernix, skin, and especially the cord may be stained brownish yellow if the amniotic fluid has been colored by the passage of meconium during or before birth.

The skin of premature infants is thin and delicate and tends to be deep red; in extremely premature infants, the skin appears almost gelatinous and bleeds and bruises easily. Fine, soft, immature hair—**lanugo**—frequently covers the scalp and brow and may also cover the face of premature infants. Lanugo has usually been lost or replaced by vellus hair in term infants. Tufts of hair over the lumbosacral spine suggest an underlying abnormality such as occult spina bifida, a sinus tract, or a tumor. The nails are rudimentary in very premature infants, but they may protrude beyond the fingertips in infants born past term. Postterm infants may have a peeling, parchment-like skin (Fig. 83–1), a severe degree of which suggests ichthyosis congenita (Chapter 637).

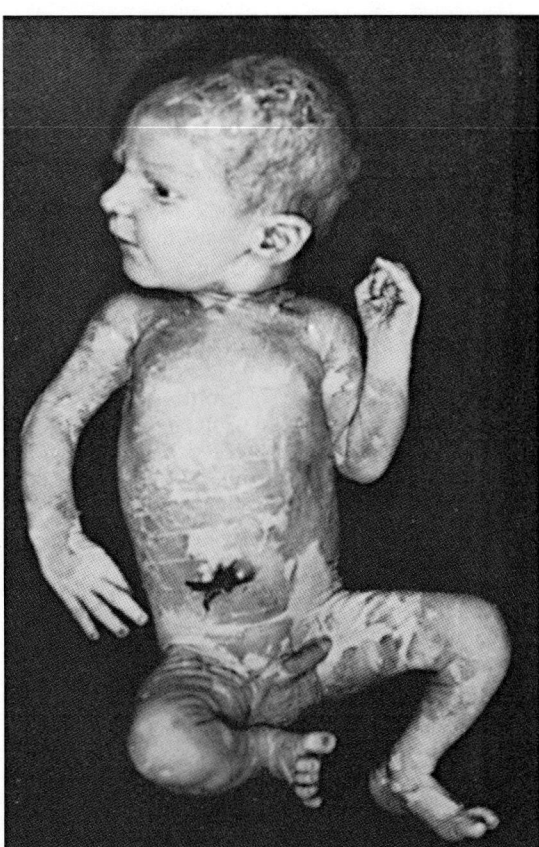

FIGURE 83–1. Infant with intrauterine growth retardation as a result of placental insufficiency. Note the long, thin appearance with peeling, parchment-like dry skin, alert expression, meconium staining of the skin, and long nails. (From Clifford S: *Advances in Pediatrics*, Vol 9. Chicago, Year Book, 1962.)

In many neonates, small, white, occasionally vesiculopustular papules on an erythematous base develop 1–3 days after birth. This benign rash, *erythema toxicum*, persists for as long as 1 wk, contains eosinophils, and is usually distributed on the face, trunk, and extremities (Chapter 637). *Pustular melanosis*, a benign lesion seen predominantly in black neonates, contains neutrophils and is present at birth as a vesiculopustular eruption around the chin, neck, back, extremities, and palms or soles; it lasts 2–3 days. Both lesions need to be distinguished from more dangerous vesicular eruptions such as herpes simplex (Chapter 231) and staphylococcal disease of the skin (Chapter 166.1).

Amniotic bands may disrupt the skin, extremities (amputation, ring constriction, syndactyly), face (clefts), or trunk (abdominal or thoracic wall defects). Their cause is uncertain but may be related to amniotic membrane rupture or vascular compromise with fibrous band formation. Excessive skin fragility and extensibility with joint hypermobility suggest Ehlers-Danlos syndrome, Marfan syndrome, congenital contractural arachnodactyly, or other disorders of collagen synthesis.

Skull. All infants should have their head circumference noted on the chart. The skull may be molded, particularly if the infant is the first-born and if the head has been engaged for a considerable time. The parietal bones tend to override the occipital and frontal bones. The head of an infant born by cesarean section or from a breech presentation is characterized by its roundness. The suture lines and the size and tension of the anterior and posterior fontanels should be determined digitally. Premature fusion of sutures (cranial synostosis) is identified by a hard nonmovable ridge over the suture and an abnormally shaped skull.

Great variation in the size of the fontanels exists at birth; if small, the anterior fontanel usually tends to enlarge during the first few months of life. The persistence of excessively large anterior (normal, 20 ± 10 mm) and posterior fontanels has been associated with several disorders (Box 83–1). Persistently small fontanels suggest microcephaly, craniosynostosis, congenital hyperthyroidism, or wormian bones; a 3rd fontanel suggests trisomy 21 but is seen in preterm infants. Soft areas (craniotabes) are occasionally found in the parietal bones at the vertex near the sagittal suture; they are more common in premature infants and in infants who have been exposed to uterine compression. Though usually insignificant, their possible pathologic cause should be investigated if they persist. Soft areas in the occipital region suggest the irregular calcification and wormian bone formation associated with osteogenesis imperfecta, cleidocranial dysostosis, lacunar skull, cretinism, and occasionally, Down syndrome. Transillumination of an abnormal skull in a dark room or examination by ultrasound or computed tomography rules out hydranencephaly or hydrocephaly (Chapter 585). An excessively large head (megalencephaly) suggests hydrocephaly, storage disease, achondroplasia, cerebral gigantism, neurocutaneous syndromes, or inborn errors of metabolism, or it may be familial. The skull of a premature infant may suggest hydrocephaly because of the relatively larger brain growth in comparison to that of other organs. Depression of the skull (indentation, fracture, Ping-Pong ball deformity) is usually of prenatal onset from prolonged focal pressure by the bony pelvis. Atrophic or alopecic scalp areas may represent *aplasia cutis congenita*, which may be sporadic or autosomal dominant or be associated with trisomy 13, chromosome 4 deletion, or Johanson-Blizzard syndrome. Deformational plagiocephaly may be due to in utero positioning forces on the skull and is manifested as an asymmetric skull and face with ear malalignment. It is associated with torticollis and vertex positioning.

Face. The general appearance should be noted with regard to dysmorphic features, such as epicanthal folds, widely spaced eyes, microphthalmos, asymmetry, long philtrum, and low-set ears, which are often associated with congenital syndromes. The face may be asymmetric as a result of a 7th nerve palsy, hypoplasia of the depressor muscle at the angle of the mouth, or an abnormal fetal posture (Chapter 97); when the jaw has been held against a shoulder or an extremity during the intrauterine period, the mandible may deviate strikingly from the midline. Symmetric facial palsy suggests absence or hypoplasia of the 7th nerve nucleus (Möbius syndrome).

EYES. The eyes often open spontaneously if the infant is held up and tipped gently forward and backward. This maneuver, a result of labyrinthine and neck reflexes, is more successful for inspecting the eyes than forcing the lids apart is. *Conjunctival and retinal hemorrhages* are usually benign. Retinal hemorrhages are more common with vacuum-assisted deliveries (75%) than after cesarean section (7%). They resolve in most infants by 2 wk (85%) and in all infants by 4 wk of age. Pupillary reflexes are present after 28–30 wk of gestation. The iris should be inspected for colobomas and heterochromia. A cornea larger than 1 cm in diameter in a term infant (and photophobia and tearing) suggests

---

BOX 83–1. Disorders Associated with a Large Anterior Fontanel

Achondroplasia	Intrauterine growth retardation
Apert syndrome	Kenny syndrome
Athyrotic hypothyroidism	Osteogenesis imperfecta
Cleidocranial dysostosis	Prematurity
Congenital rubella syndrome	Pyknodysostosis
Hallermann-Streiff syndrome	Russell-Silver syndrome
Hydrocephaly	13-, 18-, 21-trisomies
Hypophosphatasia	Vitamin D deficiency rickets

congenital glaucoma and requires prompt ophthalmologic consultation. The presence of bilateral *red reflexes* suggests the absence of cataracts and intraocular pathology (Chapters 610, 618–624). Leukokoria (white pupillary reflex) suggests cataracts, tumor, chorioretinitis, retinopathy of prematurity, or a persistent hyperplastic primary vitreous and warrants an immediate ophthalmologic consultation.

EARS. Deformities of the pinnae are occasionally seen. Unilateral or bilateral preauricular skin tags occur frequently; if pedunculated, they can be tightly ligated at the base, and dry gangrene and sloughing result. The tympanic membrane, easily seen otoscopically through the short, straight external auditory canal, normally appears dull gray.

NOSE. The nose may be slightly obstructed by mucus accumulated in the narrow nostrils. The nares should be symmetric and patent. Dislocation of the nasal cartilage from the vomerian groove results in asymmetric nares.

MOUTH. A normal mouth may rarely have precocious dentition, with natal (present at birth) or neonatal (eruption after birth) *teeth* in the lower incisor position or aberrantly placed; these teeth are shed before the deciduous ones erupt. Alternatively, such teeth occur in Ellis-van Creveld, Hallermann-Streiff, and other syndromes. Extraction is not usually indicated. Premature eruption of deciduous teeth is even more unusual. The **soft** and **hard palate** should be inspected and palpated for a complete or submucosal cleft and the contour noted if the arch is excessively high or the uvula is bifid. On the hard palate on either side of the raphe may be temporary accumulations of epithelial cells called **Epstein pearls.** Retention cysts of similar appearance may also be seen on the gums. Both disappear spontaneously, usually within a few weeks of birth. Clusters of small white or yellow follicles or ulcers on an erythematous base may be found on the anterior tonsillar pillars, most frequently on the 2nd–3rd day of life. Of unknown cause, they clear without treatment in 2–4 days.

Neonates do not have active salivation. The **tongue** appears relatively large; the **frenulum** may be short, but rarely, if ever is shortness a reason for cutting it. The sublingual mucous membrane occasionally forms a prominent fold. The **cheeks** have a fullness on both the buccal and the external aspects as a result of the accumulation of fat making up the **sucking pads.** These pads, as well as the labial tubercle on the upper lip (sucking callus), disappear when suckling ceases. A marble-sized buccal mass is usually due to benign idiopathic fat necrosis.

The **throat** of a newborn infant is hard to see because of the low arch of the palate; however, it should be clearly viewed because it is easy to miss posterior palatal or uvular clefts. The tonsils are small.

Neck. The neck appears relatively short. Abnormalities are not common but include goiter, cystic hygroma, branchial cleft rests, teratoma, hemangioma, and lesions of the sternocleidomastoid muscle that are presumably traumatic or due to a fixed positioning in utero that produces either a hematoma or fibrosis, respectively. *Congenital torticollis* causes the head to turn toward and the face to turn away from the affected side. Plagiocephaly, facial asymmetry, and hemihypoplasia may develop if it is untreated (see Chapter 670.1). Redundant skin or webbing in a female infant suggests intrauterine lymphedema and Turner syndrome (Chapter 580.1). Both clavicles should be palpated for fractures.

Chest. Breast hypertrophy is common, and milk may be present (but should not be expressed). Asymmetry, erythema, induration, and tenderness should suggest mastitis or a breast abscess. Look for supernumerary nipples, inverted nipples, or widely spaced nipples with a shield-shaped chest; the latter suggests Turner syndrome.

Lungs. Much can be learned by observing breathing. Variations in rate and rhythm are characteristic and fluctuate according to the infant's physical activity, state of wakefulness, or the presence of crying. Because fluctuations are rapid, the respiratory rate should be counted for a full minute with the infant in the resting state, preferably asleep. Under these circumstances, the usual rate for normal term infants is 30–40/min; in premature infants the rate is higher and fluctuates more widely. A rate consistently over 60/min during periods of regular breathing usually indicates pulmonary, cardiac, or metabolic disease. Premature infants may breathe with a Cheyne-Stokes rhythm, known as periodic respiration, or with complete irregularity. Irregular gasping, sometimes accompanied by spasmodic movements of the mouth and chin, strongly indicates serious impairment of the respiratory centers.

The breathing of newborn infants is almost entirely diaphragmatic, so during inspiration the soft front of the thorax is usually drawn inward while the abdomen protrudes. If the baby is quiet, relaxed, and of good color, this "paradoxical movement" does not necessarily signify insufficient ventilation. On the other hand, labored respiration is important evidence of respiratory distress syndrome, pneumonia, anomalies, or mechanical disturbance of the lungs. A weak persistent or intermittent groaning, whining cry or **grunting** during expiration signifies potentially serious cardiopulmonary disease or sepsis and warrants immediate attention. When benign, the grunting resolves between 30 and 60 min after birth. Flaring of the alae nasi and retraction of the intercostal muscles and sternum are common signs of pulmonary pathology.

Normally, the breath sounds are bronchovesicular. Suspicion of pulmonary pathology because of diminished breath sounds, rales, or percussion dullness should always be verified with a chest radiograph.

Heart. Normal variation in the size and shape of the chest makes it difficult to estimate the size of the heart. The location of the heart should be determined to detect dextrocardia. Transitory benign murmurs are common. Congenital heart disease may not initially produce the murmur that will appear later; only a $1/12$ chance exists that a murmur heard at birth represents congenital heart disease. Evaluation of the heart by roentgenography, echocardiography, and electrocardiography is essential when the possibility of a significant lesion exists. The pulse may vary normally from 90/min in relaxed sleep to 180/min during activity. The still higher rate of supraventricular tachycardia (>220) may be determined better on a cardiac monitor or electrocardiogram than by ear. Premature infants, whose resting heart rate is usually 140–150/min, may have a sudden onset of sinus bradycardia. Pulses should be palpated in the upper and lower extremities to detect coarctation of the aorta on both admission and discharge from the nursery.

Blood pressure measurements may be a valuable diagnostic aid in ill infants (Chapter 418). The *oscillometric method* is the easiest and most accurate noninvasive method available. Continuous or intermittent direct measurement of blood pressure with an umbilical artery catheter may be indicated in special circumstances for infants who are under close observation in an intensive care unit (Fig. 83–2).

Abdomen. The liver is usually palpable, sometimes as much as 2 cm below the rib margin. Less commonly, the tip of the spleen may be felt. The approximate size and location of each kidney can usually be determined on deep palpation. At no other period of life does the amount of air in the gastrointestinal tract vary so much, nor is it usually so great under normal circumstances. Gas should normally be present in the rectum on roentgenogram by 24 hr of age. The abdominal wall is normally weak (especially in premature infants), and diastasis recti and umbilical hernias are common, particularly in black infants.

Unusual masses should be investigated immediately by ultrasonography. Renal pathology is the cause of most neonatal abdominal masses. Cystic abdominal masses include hydronephrosis, multicystic-dysplastic kidneys, adrenal hemor-

FIGURE 83-2. Nomogram for mean blood pressure (BP) in neonates with gestational ages of 23–43 wk derived from continuous arterial BP measurements obtained from 103 infants admitted to the neonatal intensive care unit. The graph shows the predicted mean BP of neonates of different gestational age during the first 72 hours of life. Each line represents the lower limit of the 80% confidence interval (two-tail) of the mean BP for each gestational age group; 90% of infants for each gestational age group will be expected to have a mean BP value equal to or above the value indicated by the corresponding line, the lower limit of the confidence interval. (From Nuntnarumit P, Yang W, Bada-Ellzey SB: Blood pressure measurements in the newborn. *Clin Perinatol* 1999;26:981–96.)

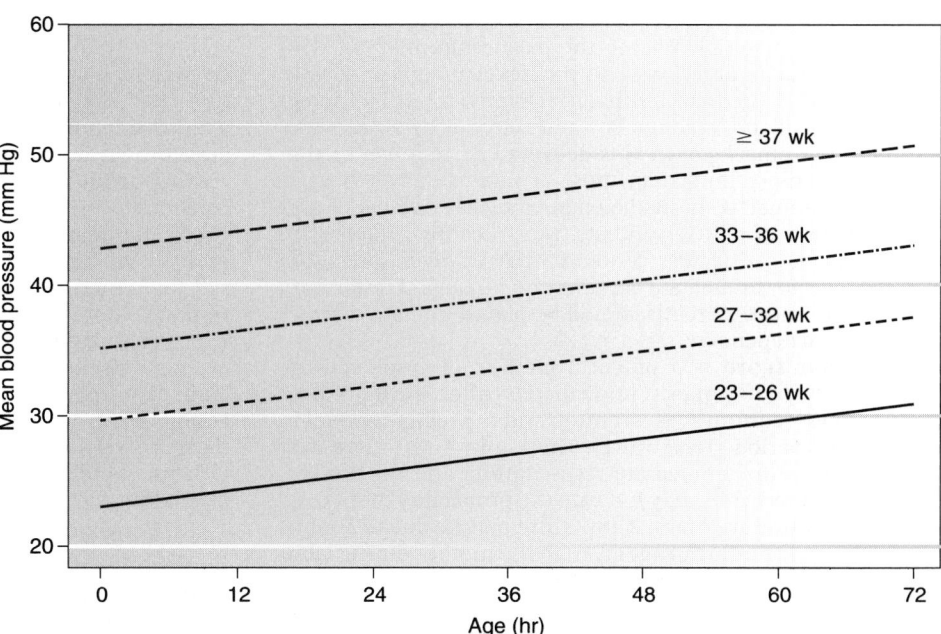

rhage, hydrometrocolpos, intestinal duplication, and choledochal, ovarian, omental, or pancreatic cysts. Solid masses include neuroblastoma, congenital mesoblastic nephroma, hepatoblastoma, and teratoma. A solid flank mass may be caused by renal vein thrombosis, which becomes clinically apparent with hematuria, hypertension, and thrombocytopenia. Renal vein thrombosis in infants is associated with polycythemia, dehydration, diabetic mothers, asphyxia, sepsis, and coagulopathies such as antithrombin III or protein C deficiency.

Abdominal distention at birth or shortly afterward suggests either obstruction or perforation of the gastrointestinal tract, often as a result of meconium ileus; later distention suggests lower bowel obstruction, sepsis, or peritonitis. A scaphoid abdomen in a newborn suggests diaphragmatic hernia. **Abdominal wall defects** produce an omphalocele (Chapter 94) when they occur through the umbilicus and gastroschisis when they occur lateral to the midline. Omphaloceles are associated with other anomalies and syndromes such as Beckwith-Wiedemann, conjoined twins, trisomy 18, meningomyelocele, and imperforate anus. **Omphalitis** is an acute local inflammation of the periumbilical tissue that may extend to the abdominal wall, the peritoneum, the umbilical vein or portal vessels, or the liver and may result in later portal hypertension.

Genitals. The **genitalia** and mammary glands normally respond to transplacentally acquired maternal hormones to produce enlargement and secretion of the breasts in both sexes and prominence of the female genitals, often with considerable nonpurulent discharge. These transitory manifestations require observation but no interference.

An imperforate hymen may result in **hydrometrocolpos** and a lower abdominal mass. A normal scrotum is relatively large; its size may be increased by the trauma of breech delivery or by a **transitory hydrocele,** which is distinguished from a hernia by palpation and transillumination. The testes should be in the scrotum or palpable in the canals. Black male infants usually have dark pigmentation of the scrotum before the rest of the skin assumes its permanent color.

The **prepuce** of a newborn infant is normally tight and adherent. Severe hypospadias or epispadias should always lead one to suspect either that abnormal sex chromosomes are present (Chapter 70) or that the infant is actually a masculinized female with an enlarged clitoris because this finding may be the first evidence of adrenogenital syndrome (Chapter 570). Erection of the penis is common and has no significance. Urine is usually passed during or immediately after birth; a period without voiding may normally follow. However, most void by 12 hr, and about 95% of preterm and term infants void within 24 hr.

Anus. Some passage of meconium usually occurs within the first 12 hr after birth; 99% of term infants and 95% of premature infants pass meconium within 48 hr of birth. Imperforate anus is not always visible and may require evidence obtained by gentle insertion of the little finger or a rectal tube. Roentgenographic study is required. Passage of meconium does not rule out an imperforate anus if a rectal-vaginal fistula is present. The dimple or irregularity in skinfold often normally present in the sacrococcygeal midline may be mistaken for an actual or potential neurocutaneous sinus.

Extremities. In examining the extremities, the effects of fetal posture (Chapter 662) should be noted so that their cause and usual transitory nature can be explained to the mother. Such explanations are particularly important after breech presentations. Observing the extremities in spontaneous or stimulated activity more commonly than by any other means arouses the suspicion of a fracture or nerve injury associated with delivery. The hands and feet should be examined for polydactyly, syndactyly, and abnormal dermatoglyphic patterns such as a simian crease.

The hips of all infants should be examined with specific maneuvers to rule out congenital dislocation (Chapter 668.1).

Neurologic Examination (see Chapters 6 and 584). In utero neuromuscular diseases associated with limited fetal motion produce a constellation of signs and symptoms that are independent of the specific disease. Severe positional deformation and contractures produce arthrogryposis. Other manifestations of fetal neuromuscular disease include breech presentation, polyhydramnios, failure to breathe at birth, pulmonary hypoplasia, dislocated hips, undescended testes, thin ribs, and clubfoot.

83.3 Routine Delivery Room Care

Low-risk infants should be placed head downward immediately after delivery to clear the mouth, pharynx, and nose of fluid, mucus, blood, and amniotic debris by gravity; gentle suction with a bulb syringe or soft rubber catheter may also be helpful in removing this material. Wiping the palate and pharynx with gauze may lead to abrasions and the development of thrush, pterygoid ulcers (Bednar aphthae), or rarely, tooth bud infection with maxillary osteomyelitis and retrobulbar abscess formation. The stomachs of infants delivered by cesarean section may contain more fluid than those of infants delivered vaginally. Their stomachs should be emptied by gastric tube to prevent aspiration of gastric contents. Most healthy infants who appear to be in satisfactory condition may be given directly to their mothers for immediate bonding and nursing. If respiratory distress is a concern, infants should be placed under a warmer with the head dependent.

The **Apgar score** is a practical method of systematically assessing newborn infants immediately after birth to help identify those requiring resuscitation and to predict survival in the neonatal period (Table 83–1). The 1-min Apgar score may signal the need for immediate resuscitation, and the 5-, 10-, 15-, and 20-min scores may indicate the probability of successfully resuscitating an infant. A low score may be due to a number of factors, including drugs given to the mother during labor and immaturity (Table 83–2). The Apgar score was not designed to predict neurologic outcome. Indeed, the score is normal in most patients in whom cerebral palsy subsequently develops, and the incidence of cerebral palsy is low (but higher than in infants with Apgar scores of 7–10) in infants with Apgar scores of 0–3 at 5 min. The Apgar score and umbilical artery blood pH both predict neonatal death. An Apgar score of 0–3 at 5 min is uncommon but is a better predictor of neonatal death (in both term and preterm infants) than an umbilical artery pH of 7.0 or less; combining these two variables increases the relative risk of neonatal mortality in term and preterm infants (Table 83–3).

Infants who fail to initiate respiration should receive prompt resuscitation and close observation (Chapter 89).

Maintenance of Body Heat. Relative to body weight, the body surface of a newborn infant is approximately three times that of an adult, and in low-birthweight infants, the insulating layer of subcutaneous fat is thinner. The estimated rate of heat loss in a newborn is approximately four times that of an adult. Under the usual delivery room conditions (20–25°C), an infant's skin temperature falls approximately 0.3°C/min and deep body temperature decreases approximately 0.1°C/min during the period immediately after delivery; these rates generally result in a cumulative loss of 2–3°C in deep body temperature (corresponding to a heat loss of approximately 200 kcal/kg). The heat loss occurs by *convection* of heat energy to the cooler surrounding air, by *conduction* of heat to the colder materials on which the infant is resting, by heat *radiation* from the infant to other nearby cooler solid objects, and by *evaporation* from moist skin and lungs (a function of alveolar ventilation).

Metabolic acidosis, hypoxemia, hypoglycemia, and increased renal excretion of water and solutes may develop in term infants exposed to cold after birth because of their effort to compensate for heat loss. These conditions augment heat production by increasing the metabolic rate and oxygen consumption and by releasing norepinephrine, which results in nonshivering thermogenesis through oxidation of fat, particularly brown fat. In addition, muscular activity may increase. Hypoglycemic or hypoxic infants cannot increase their oxygen consumption when exposed to a cold environment, and their central temperature decreases. After labor and vaginal delivery, many newborn infants have mild to moderate metabolic acidosis, for which they may compensate by hyperventilating, a response that is more difficult for depressed infants and infants exposed to cold stress in the delivery room. Therefore, it is desirable to ensure that infants are dried and either wrapped in blankets or placed under a warmer while having skin-to-skin contact with the mother. Because carrying out resuscitative measures on a covered infant or one enclosed in an incubator is difficult, a radiant heat source should be used to heat the baby immediately after birth.

Antiseptic Skin and Cord Care. Careful removal of blood from the skin shortly after birth may reduce the risk of infection with blood-borne agents. Once a healthy infant's temperature has stabilized, the entire skin and cord should be cleansed with warm water or a mild non-medicated soap solution and rinsed with water to reduce the incidence of skin and periumbilical colonization with pathogenic bacteria and subsequent infectious complications. To avoid heat loss, infants are then dried and wrapped in sterile blankets. To reduce colonization with *Staphylococcus aureus* and other pathogenic bacteria, the umbilical cord may be treated daily with bactericidal or antimicrobial agents such as triple dye or bacitracin. Alternatively, chlorhexidine washing or, on rare occasion during *S. aureus* epidemics, a single hexachlorophene bath may be used. Routine or repeated total body exposure to hexachlorophene may be neurotoxic, particularly in low-birthweight infants, and is thus contraindicated. Nursery personnel should use chlorhexidine or iodophor-containing antiseptic soaps for routine handwashing before caring for each infant. Rigidly enforcing hand-to-elbow washing for 2 min in the initial wash and 15–30 sec in the 2nd wash is essential for staff and visitors entering the nursery. Equally thorough washes between handling infants are also required.

Other Measures. The eyes of all infants must be protected against gonococcal infection by instilling 1% *silver nitrate* drops, the best-proven therapy; erythromycin (0.5%) and tetracycline (1.0%) sterile ophthalmic ointments are alternative measures. Povidone-iodine (2.5% solution) may also be effective as a one-time prophylactic agent. This procedure may be delayed during the initial short-alert period after birth to promote bonding, but once applied, drops should not be rinsed out. Also see Chapters 177 and 208.3.

Although hemorrhage in newborn infants can be due to factors other than *vitamin K deficiency*, an intramuscular injection of

TABLE 83–1. **Apgar Evaluation of Newborn Infants**

Sign	0	1	2
Heart rate	Absent	Below 100	Over 100
Respiratory effort	Absent	Slow, irregular	Good, crying
Muscle tone	Limp	Some flexion of extremities	Active motion
Response to catheter in nostril (tested after oropharynx is clear)	No response	Grimace	Cough or sneeze
Color	Blue, pale	Body pink, extremities blue	Completely pink

Sixty seconds after complete birth of the infant (disregarding the cord and placenta), the five objective signs above are evaluated, and each is given a score of 0, 1, or 2. A total score of 10 indicates an infant in the best possible condition. An infant with a score of 0–3 requires immediate resuscitation.
Modified from Apgar V: Res Anesth Analg 1953; 32:260.

TABLE 83–2.	Factors Affecting the Apgar Score	

False-Positive (No Fetal Acidosis or Hypoxia; Low Apgar)	False-Negative (Acidosis; Normal Apgar)
Immaturity	Maternal acidosis
Analgesics, narcotics, sedatives	High fetal catecholamine levels
Magnesium sulfate	Some full-term infants
Acute cerebral trauma	
Precipitous delivery	
Congenital myopathy	
Congenital neuropathy	
Spinal cord trauma	
Central nervous system anomaly	
Lung anomaly (diaphragmatic hernia)	
Airway obstruction (choanal atresia)	
Congenital pneumonia and sepsis	
Previous episodes of fetal asphyxia (recovered)	
Hemorrhage-hypovolemia	

Regardless of the etiology, a low Apgar score because of fetal asphyxia, immaturity, central nervous system depression, or airway obstruction identifies an infant needing immediate resuscitation.

1 mg of water-soluble vitamin K_1 (phytonadione) is recommended for all infants immediately after birth to prevent hemorrhagic disease of the newborn (see Chapter 92.4). Higher dose, repeated administration of oral vitamin K may also be useful, but this treatment is not yet established. Larger intravenous doses predispose to the development of hyperbilirubinemia and kernicterus and should be avoided. Administration of vitamin K to the mother during labor is not recommended because of unpredictable placental transfer.

Neonatal screening is available for various genetic, metabolic, hematologic, and endocrine diseases. All states have neonatal screening programs, although the specific tests required vary (Chapter 73). Laboratory tests performed on infant heel puncture blood samples include those for hypothyroidism, phenylketonuria, galactosemia, maple syrup urine disease, homocystinuria, biotinidase deficiency, adrenal hyperplasia, hemoglobinopathy, cystic fibrosis, tyrosinemia, and other organic acid defects or aminoacidopathies. To be effective in the timely identification and prompt management of treatable diseases, screening programs must include not only high-quality laboratory tests but also follow-up of infants with abnormal test results; education, counseling, and psychologic support for families; and prompt referral of the neonate for accurate diagnosis and therapy. Routine screening of the hematocrit or blood glucose is not necessary in the absence of risk factors. *Hearing impairment*, a serious morbidity that affects speech and language development, may be severe in 2/1,000 and overall affects 5/1,000 births. Universal screening of infants is recommended to ensure early detection of hearing loss and appropriate, timely intervention.

TABLE 83–3.	Incidence of Neonatal Death in 132,228 Singleton Infants Born at Term (37 wk of Gestation or Later) in Relation to Apgar Scores at 5 min of Age*

5-min Apgar Score	No. of Live Births	No. Neonatal Deaths (Rate per 1,000 Births)	Relative Risk (95% CI)
0–3	86	21 (244)	1,460 (835–2,555)
4–6	561	5 (9)	53 (20–140)
7–10	131,581	22 (0.2)	1

*Infants with 5-min Apgar scores of 7–10 served as the reference group.
CI = confidence interval.
From Casey BM, McIntire DD, Leveno KJ: The continuing value of the Apgar score for the assessment of newborn infants. N Engl J Med 2001; 344:467–71.*

83.4 Nursery Care

Non–high-risk healthy infants may be taken to the "regular" newborn nursery or be placed in the mother's room if the hospital has rooming-in.

The bassinet, preferably of clear plastic to allow for easy visibility and care, should be cleaned frequently. All professional care should be given in the bassinet, including the physical examination, clothing changes, temperature taking, skin cleansing, and other procedures that if performed elsewhere, would establish a common contact point and possibly provide a channel for cross infection. The clothing and bedding should be minimal, only that needed for an infant's comfort; the nursery temperature should be kept at approximately 24°C (75°F). The infant's temperature should be taken by axillary measurement. Although the interval between temperature taking depends on many circumstances, it need not be shorter than 4 hr during the 1st 2–3 days and 8 hr thereafter. Axillary temperatures of 36.4–37.0°C (97.0–98.5°F) are within normal limits. Weighing at birth and daily thereafter is sufficient. Healthy infants should be placed supine to reduce the risk of sudden infant death syndrome.

Vernix is spontaneously shed within 2–3 days, much of it adhering to the clothing, which should be completely changed daily. The diaper should be checked before and after feeding and when the baby cries; it should be changed when wet or soiled. Meconium or feces should be cleansed from the buttocks with sterile cotton moistened with sterile water. The foreskin of a male infant should not be retracted. Circumcision is an elective procedure.

Early discharge (<48 hr) or very early discharge (<24 hr) may increase the risk of rehospitalization for hyperbilirubinemia, sepsis, failure to thrive, dehydration, and missed congenital anomalies. Early discharge requires careful ambulatory follow-up at home (visiting nurse) or in the office within 48 hr. Additional criteria for the early discharge of term neonates have been developed by the American Academy of Pediatrics and American College of Obstetrics and Gynecology (Box 83–2).

83.5 Parent-Infant Bonding (see also Chapter 9)

Normal infant development depends partly on a series of affectionate responses exchanged between a mother and her newborn infant that binds them together psychologically and physiologically. This bonding is facilitated and reinforced by the emotional support of a loving husband and family. The attachment process may be important in enabling some mothers to provide loving care during the neonatal period and subsequently during childhood. It is initiated before birth with the planning and confirmation of the pregnancy and with the growing acceptance of the fetus as an individual. After delivery and during the ensuing weeks, visual and physical contact between the mother and baby triggers various mutually rewarding and pleasurable interactions such as the mother touching the infant's extremities and face with her fingertips and encompassing and gently massaging the infant's trunk with her hands. Touching an infant's cheek elicits responsive turning toward the mother's face or toward the breast with nuzzling and licking of the nipple, a powerful stimulus for prolactin secretion. An infant's initial quiet alert state provides the opportunity for eye-to-eye contact, which is particularly important in stimulating the loving and possessive feelings of many parents for their babies. An infant's crying elicits the maternal response of touching the infant and speaking in a soft, soothing, higher-toned voice. Initial contact between the mother and infant should take place in the delivery room, and opportunities for extended intimate contact should be provided within the first hours after birth. Delayed or abnormal maternal-infant bonding, as occurs because of prematurity, infant or maternal illness, birth defects,

BOX 83–2. Recommendations for Early Discharge from the Normal Newborn Nursery*

Uncomplicated antepartum, intrapartum, postpartum courses
Vaginal delivery
Singleton at 38–42 wk: appropriate for gestational age
Normal vital signs including respiratory rate <60 breaths/min; axillary temperature 36.1–37°C (97.0–98.6°F) in open crib
Physical examination reveals no abnormalities requiring immediate attention
Urination; stool ×1
At least two uneventful, successful feedings
No excessive bleeding after (2 hr) circumcision
No jaundice within 24 hr of birth
Evidence of parental knowledge, ability, and confidence to care for the baby at home
   Feeding
   Cord, skin, genital care
   Recognition of illness (jaundice, poor feeding, lethargy, fever, etc.)
   Infant safety (car seat, supine sleep position, etc.)
Availability of family and physician support (physician follow-up)
Laboratory evaluation
   Venereal Disease Research Laboratories (VDRL)
   Hepatitis B surface antigen and vaccination or appointment for vaccination
   State screening (e.g., phenylketonuria, thyroid, galactosemia, sickle cell)
   Coombs' test
No social risks
   Substance abuse
   History of child abuse
   Domestic violence
   Mental illness
   Teen mother
   Homeless

*It is not likely that all these criteria will be met before 48 hr of age.
Adapted from American Academy of Pediatrics, American College of Obstetricians and Gynecologists: *Guidelines for Perinatal Care*, 5th ed. Elk Grove Village, IL, American Academy of Pediatrics, 2002.

BOX 83–3. Ten Steps to Successful Breast-Feeding

Every facility providing maternity services and care for newborn infants should accomplish the following:
1. Have a written breast-feeding policy that is routinely communicated to all health care staff.
2. Train all health care staff in the skills necessary to implement this policy.
3. Inform all pregnant women about the benefits and management of breast-feeding.
4. Help mothers initiate breast-feeding within a half hour of birth.
5. Show mothers how to breast-feed and how to maintain lactation even if they should be separated from their infants.
6. Give newborn infants no food or drink other than breast milk unless *medically* indicated.
7. Practice rooming-in (allow mothers and infants to remain together) 24 hr a day.
8. Encourage breast-feeding on demand.
9. Give no artificial teats or pacifiers (also called *dummies* or *soothers*) to breast-feeding infants.
10. Foster the establishment of breast-feeding support groups and refer mothers to them on discharge from the hospital or clinic.

From *Protecting, Promoting and Supporting Breastfeeding: The Special Role of Maternity Services.* A Joint WHO/UNICEF Statement Published by the World Health Organization, 1211 Geneva 27, Switzerland, 1989.

or family stress, may harm infant development and maternal caretaking ability. Hospital routines should be designed to encourage parent-infant contact.

Nurseries and Breast-Feeding. See Chapter 41 for full discussions of breast-feeding and formula feeding. Many hospital practices contribute to difficulties in breast-feeding by enforcing 4-hr feeding schedules, limiting nursing time, using only one breast at a feeding, washing nipples with substances other than water, delaying the 1st feeding, providing formula supplements, and using heavy intrapartum sedation. The Baby-Friendly Hospital Initiative is a global effort (sponsored by the World Health Organization and the United Nations Children's Fund) to promote breast-feeding, which recommends 10 steps to successful breast-feeding (Box 83–3).

Hospital practices that encourage successful breast-feeding include immediate postpartum mother-infant contact with suckling, rooming-in, demand feeding, inclusion of fathers in prenatal breast-feeding education, and support from experienced women. Nursing at least 5 min at each breast is reasonable and allows a baby to obtain most of the available breast contents and provides effective stimulation for increasing the milk supply. Nursing episodes should then be extended according to the comfort and desire of the mother and infant. A confident and relaxed mother, supported by an encouraging home and hospital environment, is likely to nurse well.

Drugs and Breast-Feeding. Maternal medications may affect the production and safety of breast milk (Table 83–4). Although most commonly used medications are safe, the safety of any drug to be used while a woman is breast-feeding must be confirmed before a new drug is initiated and/or breast-feeding is

continued. Maternal sedatives may result in sedation of the infant. Maternal drugs that are weak acids, composed of large molecules, plasma bound, or poorly absorbed from the maternal or neonatal intestine are less likely to affect a neonate. When fresh breast milk is fed by tube or bottle, bacteriologic evaluation of stored milk should be performed within 24 hr.

TABLE 83–4. Drugs and Breast-Feeding

Contraindicated	Avoid or Give with Great Caution	Probably Safe but Give with Caution
Amphetamines	Amiodarone	Acetaminophen
Antineoplastic agents	Anthroquinones	Acyclovir
Bromocriptine	(laxatives)	Aldomet
Chloramphenicol	Aspirin (salicylates)	Anesthetics
Cimetidine	Atropine	Antibiotics (not
Clemastine	Birth control pills	tetracycline)
Cocaine	Bromides	Antiepileptics
Cyclophosphamide	Calciferol	Antihistamines*
Cyclosporine	Cascara	Antihypertensive/
Diethylstilbestrol	Danthron	cardiovascular
Doxorubicin	Dihydrotachysterol	Antithyroid (not
Ergots	Estrogens	methimazole)
Gold salts	Ethanol	Bishydroxycoumarin
Heroin	Metoclopramide	Chlorpromazine*
Immunosuppressants	Metronidazole	Codeine*
Iodides	Narcotics	Digoxin
Lithium	Phenobarbital*	Dilantin (phenytoin)
Meprobamate	Primidone	Diuretics
Methimazole	Psychotropic drugs	Fluoxetine
Methylamphetamine	Reserpine	Furosemide
Nicotine (smoking)	Salicylazosulfapyridine	Haloperidol*
Phencyclidine (PCP)	(sulfasalazine)	Hydralazine
Phenindione		Indomethacin, other
Radiopharmaceuticals		nonsteroidal anti-
Tetracycline		inflammatory drugs
Thiouracil		Methadone*
		Muscle relaxants
		Prednisone
		Propranolol
		Propylthiouracil
		Quinolones
		Sedatives*
		Theophylline
		Vitamins
		Warfarin

*Watch for sedation.

TABLE 83–5. Summary of Infectious Agents Detected in Milk and Newborn Disease

Infectious Agent	Detected in Breast Milk?	Breast Milk Reported Cause of Newborn Disease?	Maternal Infection Contraindication to Breast-Feeding?
Bacteria			
Mastitis/*Staphylococcus aureus*	Yes	No	No, unless breast abscess present
Mycobacterium tuberculosis			
Active disease	Yes	No	Yes, because of aerosol spread
PPD+/CXR–	No	No	No
Escherichia coli, other GNR	Yes, stored	Yes, stored	—
Group B streptococci	Yes	Yes	No*
Listeria monocytogenes	Yes	Yes	No*
Coxiella burnetii	Yes	Yes	No*
Viruses			
HIV	Yes	Yes	Yes, developed countries
Cytomegalovirus			
Term infant	Yes	Yes	No
Preterm infant	Yes	Yes	Evaluate on an individual basis
Hepatitis B virus	Yes, surface antigen	No	No, developed countries
Hepatitis C virus	Yes	No	No†
Hepatitis E virus	Yes	No	No
HTLV-1	Yes	Yes	Yes, developed countries
HTLV-2	Yes	?	Yes, developed countries
Herpes simplex virus	Yes	No/?yes	No, unless breast vesicles present
Rubella			
Wild type	Yes	Yes, rare	No
Vaccine	Yes	No	No
Varicella-zoster virus	Yes	No	No, cover active lesions
Epstein-Barr virus	Yes	No	No
TT virus	Yes	No	No
HHV-6	No	No	No
HHV-7	Yes	No	No
West Nile virus	Possible	Possible	Unknown
Parasites			
Toxoplasmosis	Yes	Yes, one case	No

Provided that the mother and child are taking appropriate antibiotics.
†*Provided that the mother is HIV-seronegative. Mothers should be counseled that breast milk transmission of hepatitis C virus has not been documented, but is theoretically possible.*
PPD = purified protein derivative; CXR = chest x-ray; GNR = gram-negative rods; HTLV = human T-cell leukemia virus; HHV = human herpesvirus.
From Jones CA: Maternal transmission of infectious pathogens in breast milk. J Paediatr Child Health 2001; 37:576–82.

Medical contraindications to breast-feeding in the United States include infection with HIV, human T-cell leukemia virus types 1 and 2, cytomegalovirus (preterm infants), and hepatitis B virus (until an infant receives hepatitis B immune globulin and vaccine) (Table 83–5).

American Academy of Pediatrics, American College of Obstetricians and Gynecologists: *Guidelines for Perinatal Care*, 4th ed. Elk Grove Village, IL, American Academy of Pediatrics, 1997.

American Academy of Pediatrics Committee on Drugs: The transfer of drugs and other chemicals into human milk. *Pediatrics* 2001;108:776–89.

Casey BM, McIntire DD, Leveno KJ: The continuing value of the Apgar score for the assessment of newborn infants. *N Engl J Med* 2001;344:467.

Elliman DAC, Dezateux C, Bedford HE: Newborn and childhood screening programmes: Criteria, evidence, and current policy. *Arch Dis Child* 2002;87:6–9.

Emerson MV, Pieramici DJ, Stoessel KM, et al: Incidence and rate of disappearance of retinal hemorrhage in newborns. *Ophthalmology* 2001;108:36–9.

Iqbal MM, Sobhan T, Ryals T: Effects of commonly used benzodiazepines on the fetus, the neonate, and the nursing infant. *Psychiatric Serv* 2002;53:39–49.

Jones CA: Maternal transmission of infectious pathogens in breast milk. *J Paediatr Child Health* 2001;37:576.

Kennell JH, Klaus MH: Bonding: Recent observations that alter perinatal care. *Pediatr Rev* 1998;19:4.

Lawrence RA: Breastfeeding support benefits very low birth weight infants. *Arch Pediatr Adolesc Med* 2001;155:543–4.

Littlefield TR, Kelly KM, Pomatto JK, et al: Multiple-birth infants at higher risk for development of deformational plagiocephaly: II. Is one twin at greater risk? *Pediatrics* 2002;109:19–25.

Liu LL, Clemens CJ, Shay DK, et al: The safety of newborn early discharge. *JAMA* 1997;278:293.

Maschmann J, Hamprecht K, Dietz K, et al: Cytomegalovirus infection of extremely low birth weight infants via breast milk. *Clin Infect Dis* 2001;33:1998–2003.

Mehl AL, Thomson V: The Colorado newborn hearing screening project, 1992–1999: On the threshold of effective population-based universal newborn hearing screening. *Pediatrics* 2002;109:E7.

Moster D, Lie RT, Irgens LM, et al: The association of Apgar score with subsequent death and cerebral palsy: A population-based study in term infants. *J Pediatr* 2001;138:798–803.

Newborn Screening Task Force: Serving the family from birth to the medical home. A report from the newborn screening task force convened in Washington, DC, May 10–11, 1999. *Pediatrics* 2000;106:386–427.

Nicoll A, Williams A: Breast feeding. *Arch Dis Child* 2002;87:91–2.

Nuntnarumit P, Yang W, Bada-Ellzey SB: Blood pressure measurements in the newborn. *Clin Perinatol* 1999;26:981.

Penny DJ, Shekerdemian LS: Management of the neonate with symptomatic congenital heart disease. *Arch Dis Child* 2001;84:F141–5.

Puckett RM, Offringa M: Prophylactic vitamin K for vitamin K deficiency bleeding in neonates. *Cochrane Database Syst Rev* [computer file] 2000;4:CD002776.

Radford A, Southall DP: Successful application of the baby-friendly hospital initiative contains lessons that must be applied to the control of formula feeding in hospitals in industrialized countries. *Pediatrics* 2001;108:766–8.

Thompson DC, McPhillips H, Davis RL: Universal newborn hearing screening. *JAMA* 2001;286:2000–10.

Wolke D, Dave S, Hayes J, et al: Routine examination of the newborn and maternal satisfaction: A randomized controlled trial. *Arch Dis Child* 2002;86:F155–60.

Yost GC, Young PC, Buchi KF: Significance of grunting respirations in infants admitted to a well-baby nursery. *Arch Pediatr Adolesc* 2001;155:372–5.

Zupan J, Garner P: Topical umbilical cord care at birth. *Cochrane Database of Systematic Reviews* [computer file] 2000;2:CD001057.

Chapter 84
High-Risk Pregnancies

Barbara J. Stoll and Robert M. Kliegman

Pregnancies characterized by factors that increase the likelihood of abortion, fetal death, premature delivery, intrauterine growth restriction, fetal or neonatal disease, congenital malformations, mental retardation, or other handicaps are called high-risk pregnancies (Box 84–1; see also Chapter 85). Some factors, such as ingestion of a teratogenic drug in the 1st trimester, are causally related to the risk; others, such as hydramnios, are associations that alert a physician to determine the etiology and avoid the inherent risks associated with excessive amniotic fluid. Based on their history, 10–20% of pregnant patients can be identified as high risk; nearly half of all perinatal mortality and morbidity is associated with these pregnancies. Although assessing antepartum risk is important in reducing perinatal mortality and morbidity, some women become high risk only during labor and delivery; therefore, careful monitoring is critical throughout the intrapartum course.

Identifying high-risk pregnancies is important not only because it is the 1st step toward prevention but also because therapeutic steps may often be taken to reduce the risks to the fetus or neonate if the physician knows of the potential for difficulty.

BOX 84–1. Factors Associated with High-Risk Pregnancy

ECONOMIC
Poverty
Unemployment
Uninsured, underinsured health insurance
Poor access to prenatal care

CULTURAL-BEHAVIORAL
Low educational status
Poor health care attitudes
No care or inadequate prenatal care
Cigarette, alcohol, drug abuse
Age less than 20 or over 35 yr
Unmarried
Short interpregnancy interval
Lack of support group (husband, family, religion)
Stress (physical, psychologic)
Black race

BIOLOGIC-GENETIC
Previous low-birthweight or preterm infant
Low weight for height
Poor weight gain during pregnancy
Short stature
Poor nutrition
Inbreeding (autosomal recessive?)
Intergenerational effects
Low maternal birthweight
Hereditary diseases (inborn error of metabolism)

REPRODUCTIVE
Previous cesarean section
Previous infertility
Conception by reproductive technology
Prolonged gestation
Prolonged labor
Previous infant with cerebral palsy, mental retardation, birth trauma, congenital anomalies
Abnormal lie (breech)
Multiple gestation
Premature rupture of membranes
Infections (systemic, amniotic, extra-amniotic, cervical)
Preeclampsia or eclampsia
Uterine bleeding (abruptio placentae, placenta previa)
Parity (0 or more than 5)
Uterine or cervical anomalies
Fetal disease
Abnormal fetal growth
Idiopathic premature labor
Iatrogenic prematurity
High or low levels of maternal serum α-fetoprotein

MEDICAL
Diabetes mellitus
Hypertension
Congenital heart disease
Autoimmune disease
Sickle cell anemia
TORCH infection
Intercurrent surgery or trauma
Sexually transmitted diseases
Maternal hypercoagulable states

TORCH = toxoplasmosis, other agents, rubella, cytomegalovirus, herpes simplex.

Genetic Factors. The occurrence of chromosomal abnormalities, congenital anomalies, inborn errors of metabolism, mental retardation, or any familial disease in blood relatives increases the risk of the same condition in the infant. Because many parents recognize only obvious clinical manifestations of genetically determined diseases, specific inquiry should be made about any disease affecting one or more blood relatives.

Maternal Factors. The lowest neonatal mortality rate occurs in infants of mothers who receive adequate prenatal care and who are 20–30 yr of age. Both teenage pregnancies and those in women older than 40 yr, particularly primiparous women, carry an increased risk for intrauterine growth restriction, fetal distress, and intrauterine death. Advanced maternal age increases the risk of both chromosomal and non-chromosomal fetal malformations (Fig. 84–1).

Maternal illness (Table 84–1), multiple pregnancies, particularly those involving monochorionic twinning, infections (Table 84–2), and certain drugs (Chapter 85) increase the risk for the fetus. The use of assisted reproductive technology (in vitro fertilization, intracytoplasmic sperm injection) increases the risk of low birthweight and very low birthweight, as well as major birth defects and multiple-fetus pregnancies. Low birthweight, prematurity, and twinning in these infants also increases the risk of cerebral palsy.

Preterm birth is common in high-risk pregnancies (Chapter 86). Factors associated with prematurity are noted in Box 84–1 and include biologic markers such as cervical shortening, genital infection, fetal fibronectin in cervicovaginal secretions, and preterm premature rupture of membranes (PROM). The latter occurs in 1% of pregnancies but is noted in 30–40% of preterm deliveries, and it is a leading identifiable cause of prematurity. Premature delivery is often difficult to predict. Although women with preterm delivery have more spontaneous uterine contractions before the start of labor, this finding plus the length of the cervix and the presence of fetal fibronectin in cervical secretions has low sensitivity and poor positive predictive value for premature births.

Polyhydramnios and *oligohydramnios* indicate high-risk pregnancies. Although the turnover rate is rapid, during normal pregnancy the amniotic fluid volume gradually increases at a rate of less than 10 mL/day until about the 34th wk of pregnancy, after which it slowly diminishes. Volumes vary widely in normal pregnancy; term volume may be 500–2000 mL. A volume estimated at greater than 2,000 mL in the 3rd trimester constitutes polyhydramnios, and a volume estimated at less than 500 mL indicates oligohydramnios. Polyhydramnios complicates 1–3% and oligohydramnios complicates 1–5% of pregnancies. The ultrasonographic criteria for these diagnoses are based on the *amniotic fluid index,* which is determined by measuring the vertical diameter of amniotic fluid pockets in four quadrants; an index greater than 24 cm suggests polyhydramnios, whereas one less than 5 cm suggests oligohydramnios.

Acute polyhydramnios is rare and is usually associated with premature labor and delivery before 28 wk. Chronic polyhydramnios is diagnosed in the 3rd trimester by the discrepancy between uterine size and gestational age; it is occasionally not diagnosed until the patient has dysfunctional labor or an abnormally large amount of amniotic fluid is noted during delivery. Polyhydramnios is associated with premature labor, abruptio placentae, congenital anomalies, and fetal neuromuscular dysfunction or obstruction of the gastrointestinal tract that interferes with reabsorption of the amniotic fluid swallowed by the fetus (Box 84–2). Increased fetal urination or edema formation is also associated with excessive amniotic fluid volume. Ultrasound demonstrates the increased amniotic fluid surrounding the fetus and detects associated fetal anomalies, hydrops, pleural effusions, and ascites. In 60% of patients, no

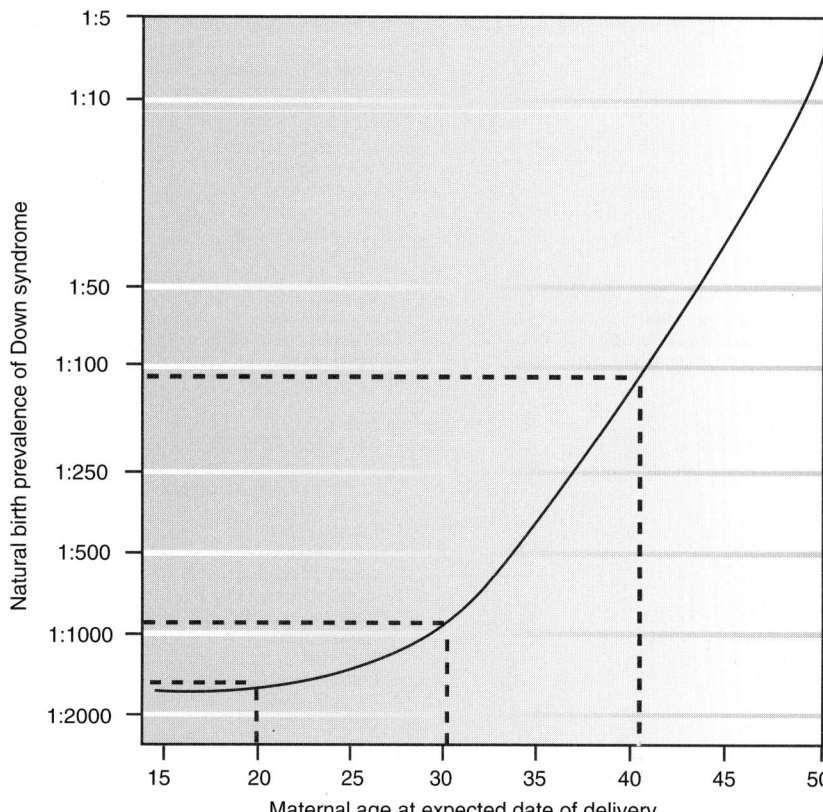

FIGURE 84–1. Natural birth prevalence of Down syndrome according to maternal age. (From Wald NJ, Leck I: *Antenatal and Neonatal Screening,* 2nd ed. Oxford, Oxford University Press, 2000.)

TABLE 84–1. **Maternal Disease Affecting the Fetus or Neonate**

Disorder	Effects	Mechanism
Cholestasis	Preterm delivery	Unknown, possibly hepatitis E
Cyanotic heart disease	Intrauterine growth restriction	Low fetal oxygen delivery
Diabetes mellitus		
Mild	Large for gestational age, hypoglycemia	Fetal hyperglycemia—produces hyperinsulinemia; insulin promotes growth
Severe	Growth restriction	Vascular disease, placental insufficiency
Drug addiction	Intrauterine growth restriction, neonatal withdrawal	Direct drug effect plus poor diet
Endemic goiter	Hypothyroidism	Iodine deficiency
Graves disease	Transient neonatal thyrotoxicosis	Placental immunoglobin passage of thyroid-stimulating antibody
Herpes gestationalis	Bullous rash	Unknown
Hyperparathyroidism	Neonatal hypocalcemia	Maternal calcium crosses to fetus and suppresses fetal parathyroid gland
Hypertension	Intrauterine growth restriction, intrauterine fetal demise	Placental insufficiency, fetal hypoxia
Idiopathic thrombocytopenic purpura	Thrombocytopenia	Nonspecific maternal platelet antibodies cross placenta
Isoimmune neutropenia or thrombocytopenia	Neutropenia or thrombocytopenia	Specific antifetal neutrophil or platelet antibody crosses placenta after sensitization of mother
Malignant melanoma	Placental or fetal tumor	Metastasis
Myasthenia gravis	Transient neonatal myasthenia	Immunoglobin to acetylcholine receptor crosses placenta
Myotonic dystrophy	Neonatal myotonic dystrophy, congenital contractures, respiratory insufficiency	Genetic anticipation
Obesity	Macrosomia, hypoglycemia	Unknown
Phenylketonuria	Microcephaly, retardation	Elevated fetal phenylalanine levels
Preeclampsia, eclampsia	Intrauterine growth restriction, thrombocytopenia, neutropenia, fetal demise	Uteroplacental insufficiency, fetal hypoxia, vasoconstriction
Renal transplant	Intrauterine growth restriction	Uteroplacental insufficiency
Rhesus or other blood group sensitization	Fetal anemia, hypoalbuminemia, hydrops, neonatal jaundice	Antibody crosses placenta directed to fetal cells with antigen
Sickle cell anemia	Preterm birth, intrauterine growth restriction	Maternal sickling producing fetal hypoxia
Systemic lupus erythematosus	Congenital heart block, rash, anemia, thrombocytopenia, neutropenia	Antibody directed to fetal heart, red and white blood cells, and platelets

TABLE 84–2. Maternal Infections Affecting the Fetus or Newborn

Infection	Mode of Transmission	Outcome
Bacteria		
Group B streptococcus	Ascending cervical	Sepsis, pneumonia
Escherichia coli	Ascending cervical	Sepsis, pneumonia
Listeria monocytogenes	Transplacental	Sepsis, pneumonia
Ureaplasma urealyticum	Ascending cervical	Pneumonia, meningitis
Mycoplasma hominis	Ascending cervical	Pneumonia
Chlamydia trachomatis	Vaginal passage	Conjunctivitis, pneumonia
Syphilis	Transplacental, vaginal passage	Congenital syphilis
Borrelia burgdorferi	Transplacental	Prematurity, fetal demise
Neisseria gonorrhoeae	Vaginal passage	Ophthalmia (conjunctivitis), sepsis, meningitis
Mycobacterium tuberculosis	Transplacental	Prematurity, fetal demise, congenital tuberculosis
Granulocytic ehrlichiosis	Transplacental	Sepsis
Virus		
Rubella	Transplacental	Congenital rubella
Cytomegalovirus	Transplacental, breast milk (rare)	Congenital cytomegalovirus or asymptomatic
Human immunodeficiency virus	Transplacental, vaginal passage, breast milk	Congenital acquired immunodeficiency syndrome
Hepatitis B	Vaginal passage, transplacental, breast milk	Neonatal hepatitis, chronic HBsAg carrier
Hepatitis C	Transplacental	Uncommon but neonatal hepatitis, chronic carrier possible
Lymphocytic choriomeningitis	Transplacental	Fetal, neonatal death; hydrocephalus, chorioretinitis
Herpes simplex type 2	Transplacental	Congenital herpes simplex virus
	Vaginal passage, ascending	Neonatal encephalitis, disseminated viremia
Varicella-zoster	Transplacental, early	Congenital anomalies
	Transplacental, late	Neonatal varicella
Parvovirus	Transplacental	Fetal anemia, hydrops
Coxsackie B	Fecal-oral	Myocarditis, meningitis, hepatitis
Poliomyelitis	Transplacental	Congenital poliomyelitis
Epstein-Barr	Transplacental	Anomalies (?)
Rubeola	Transplacental	Abortion, fetal measles
West Nile	Transplacental	Chorioretinitis, focal cerebral necrosis
Parasites		
Toxoplasmosis	Transplacental	Congenital toxoplasmosis or asymptomatic
Malaria	Transplacental	Abortion, prematurty, intrauterine growth restriction
Trypanosomiasis	Transplacental	Congenital Chagas disease
Fungi		
Candida	Ascending, cervical	Sepsis, pneumonia, rash
Prion		
Creutzfeld-Jakob disease	Transplacental, colostrum	Hypothetical route, no long-term data

HBsAg = hepatitis B surface antigen.

cause is identified. Polyhydramnios may be managed by serial amniocentesis or by short-course maternal indomethacin if it is due to excessive fetal urination. Treatment is indicated for acute maternal respiratory distress and threatened preterm labor or to

provide time for the administration of corticosteroids to enhance fetal lung maturity.

Oligohydramnios is associated with congenital anomalies; intrauterine growth restriction; severe renal, bladder, or urethral anomalies; and drugs that interfere with fetal urination (see Box 84–2). The latter becomes most evident after 20 wk of gestation, when fetal urination is the major source of amniotic fluid. Rupture of the membranes must be ruled out when oligohydramnios is suspected, especially if a normal-sized bladder is seen on fetal ultrasonography. Oligohydramnios causes fetal compression abnormalities such as clubfoot, spadelike hands, and a flattened nasal bridge. The most serious complication of chronic oligohydramnios is pulmonary hypoplasia. The risk of umbilical cord compression during labor and delivery is increased in pregnancies complicated by oligohydramnios and may be alleviated by saline amnio-infusion. Ultrasonography may reveal small (1–2 cm) pockets of fluid in addition to the associated growth restriction or anomalies. Oligohydramnios in combination with an elevated α-fetoprotein level, uterine bleeding, or intrauterine growth restriction carries an increased risk of intrauterine fetal demise.

Antenatal screening can be used to detect a number of disorders, including Down syndrome and other chromosomal abnormalities, neural tube defects and other structural anomalies, Tay-Sachs disease and other metabolic genetic diseases, hemoglobinopathies and other blood disorders, and cystic fibrosis. Screening methods include maternal blood tests, fetal ultrasound, and diagnostic tests on cells or fluid obtained by amnio-

---

BOX 84–2. Conditions Associated with Disorders of Amniotic Fluid Volume

OLIGOHYDRAMNIOS

Intrauterine growth restriction
Fetal anomalies
Twin-twin transfusion (donor)
Amniotic fluid leak
Renal agenesis (Potter syndrome)
Urethral atresia
Prune-belly syndrome
Pulmonary hypoplasia
Amnion nodosum
Indomethacin
Angiotensin-converting enzyme inhibitors
Intestinal pseudo-obstruction

POLYHYDRAMNIOS

Congenital anomalies: Anencephaly, hydrocephaly, tracheoesophageal fistula, duodenal atresia, spina bifida, cleft lip or palate, cystic adenomatoid lung malformation, diaphragmatic hernia
Syndromes: Achondroplasia, Klippel-Feil, trisomy 18, trisomy 21, TORCH, hydrops fetalis, multiple congenital anomalad
Other: Diabetes mellitus, twin-twin transfusion (recipient), fetal anemia, fetal heart failure, polyuric renal disease, neuromuscular diseases, nonimmune hydrops, chylothorax, teratoma
Idiopathic

TORCH = toxoplasmosis, other agents, rubella, cytomegalovirus, herpes simplex.

centesis or chorionic villus sampling and by fetal blood or tissue sampling.

Second-trimester screening (15–18 wk) of maternal serum α-fetoprotein (MSAFP) levels is used to screen for open neural tube defects. About 90% of affected pregnancies can be detected by an elevated MSAFP level. Gastroschisis, omphalocele, congenital nephrosis, twins, and other abnormal conditions can also be identified. Low MSAFP is associated with incorrect gestational age estimates, trisomy 18 or 21, and intrauterine growth restriction.

Several effective screening strategies can be used to detect Down syndrome (Fig. 84–2), including a combination of maternal age, nuchal translucency on ultrasound, and a number of serum markers: α-fetoprotein, unconjugated estriol, total human chorionic gonadotropin (HCG), the free β subunit of HCG, inhibin A, and pregnancy-associated plasma protein A. The most effective strategy, the integrated test, combines 1st- and 2nd-trimester screening and can identify 94% of affected pregnancies with a 5% false-positive rate or 85% with a 1% false-positive rate. Absence of the fetal nasal bone is also noted in trisomy 21. Chromosomal analysis of cells obtained by amniocentesis or chorionic villus biopsy makes the diagnosis.

Obstetric conditions are understandably important because fetuses weighing more than 2,500 g make up a very high proportion of total fetal deaths and neonatal mortality is greatest during the 1st 24 hr after delivery. A pregnancy should be considered high risk when the uterus is inappropriately large or small. A uterus large for the estimated stage of gestation suggests the presence of multiple fetuses, hydramnios, or an excessively large infant; an inappropriately small one suggests oligohydramnios or poor intrauterine growth. PROM earlier

than 24 hr before delivery carries a risk of fetal infection; it also increases the risk of premature birth. PROM at term usually results in the onset of labor within 48 hr but poses a risk of chorioamnionitis and umbilical cord compression. PROM before 37 wk has a longer latency until labor starts and has the added risks of cord prolapse, oligohydramnios, abruptio placentae, fetal malposition, and if present for more than 7 days, pulmonary hypoplasia, uterine-induced deformations, and extremity contractures. Prolonged and difficult labor increases the risk for mechanical and hypoxic damage. A tumultuous short labor with a precipitous delivery increases the risk of birth asphyxia and intracranial hemorrhage. Placental separation at any time before delivery and abnormal implantation or compression of the cord increase the possibility of brain damage from fetal anoxia; brown or muddy amniotic fluid suggests that meconium has been passed, possibly during an episode of fetal anoxia.

Although the safety of any type of delivery depends on the skill of the obstetrician, additional hazards accompany particular methods and result from the circumstances that dictated them. The risk of intracranial hemorrhage is greater in infants delivered by vacuum extraction, forceps, or cesarean section with labor than in those with unassisted spontaneous vaginal deliveries. Neonatal deaths after deliveries by mid and high forceps, breech extraction, and version are likely to be related to traumatic intracranial injury.

Infants born by *cesarean section* present problems possibly related to the unfavorable obstetric circumstance that necessitated the operation or to prolonged maternal anesthesia. In normal term pregnancies without any indication of fetal distress, delivery through the abdomen carries a greater risk than

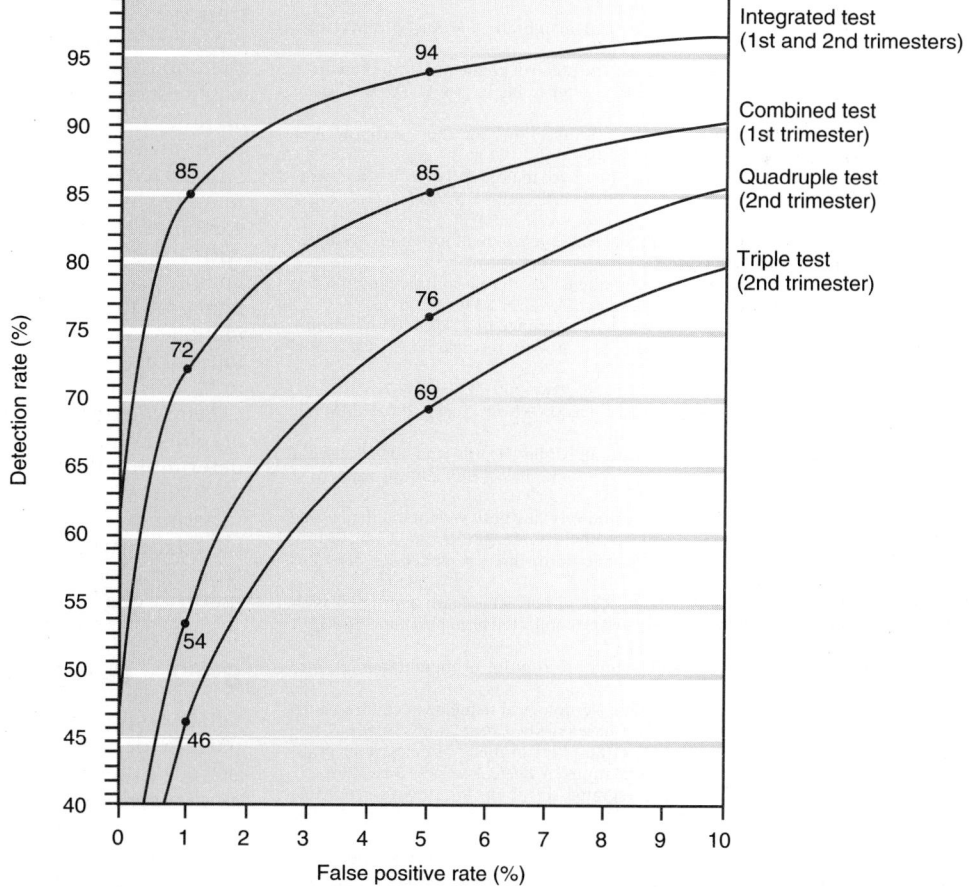

FIGURE 84–2. Rates of detection of Down syndrome and false-positive rates for various screening tests. The triple test includes measurements of serum α-fetoprotein, unconjugated estriol, and human chorionic gonadotropin in the 2nd trimester. The quadruple test includes measurements of serum α-fetoprotein, unconjugated estriol, human chorionic gonadotropin, and inhibin A in the 2nd trimester. The combined test includes measurements of serum pregnancy-associated plasma protein A, free β subunit of human gonadotropin, and nuchal translucency in the 1st trimester. The integrated test includes measurements of serum pregnancy-associated plasma protein A and nuchal translucency in the 1st trimester and measurements of serum α-fetoprotein, unconjugated estriol, human chorionic gonadotropin, and inhibin A in the 2nd trimester. (From Wald NJ, Watt HC, Hackshaw AK: Integrated screening for Down syndrome based on tests performed during the first and second trimester. *N Engl J Med* 1999; 341:461–7.)

delivery through the birth canal does. However, controversy exists regarding the safest type of delivery for a non-distressed, viable immature fetus, especially in a breech presentation; cesarean section may involve less risk than the "stress" of labor and the potentially anoxic effects of uterine contractions during vaginal delivery. Term breech positions (≈3–4% of term births) that do not become vertex after external cephalic version will also benefit from cesarean section. A small percentage of mature infants delivered by cesarean section have some degree of respiratory difficulty for 1–2 days. Although transient tachypnea is the most frequently associated problem, hyaline membrane disease may develop, particularly in infants born to women not in labor, those with uncertain dates or pulmonary maturity, and those born to diabetic mothers or after asphyxia. A trial of labor after a previous cesarean section also increases the risk of perinatal demise.

Anesthesia and analgesia affect the fetus as well as the mother; mild maternal hypoxemia secondary to hypoventilation or hypotension resulting from epidural anesthesia may result in severe fetal hypoxia and shock. Skilled use of medication avoids severe fetal narcosis while securing the benefits of gentle and unhurried delivery. Even skilled administration may result in a mildly depressed infant whose crying and breathing may be delayed 1–2 min and who may be somewhat inactive for several hours. When anesthesia and analgesia are carelessly used or when their milder effects are added to already unfavorable fetal circumstances such as prematurity, anoxia, or trauma, the result may be catastrophic.

ACOG Practice Bulletin. Assessment of risk factors for preterm birth. Clinical management guidelines for obstetrician-gynecologists. Number 31, October 2001. *Obstet Gynecol* 2001;98:709.

Cicero S, Curcio P, Papageorghiou A, et al: Absence of nasal bone in fetuses with trisomy 21 at 11–14 weeks of gestation: An observational study. *Lancet* 2001; 358:1665–7.

Epstein FH: Premature rupture of the fetal membranes. *N Engl J Med* 1998; 338:663.

Goldenberg RL, Iams JD, Mercer BM, et al: The preterm prediction study: Toward a multiple-marker test for spontaneous preterm birth. *Am J Obstet Gynecol* 2001;185:643.

Halliday HL: Elective delivery at "term": Implications for the newborn. *Acta Paediatr* 1999;88:1180.

Hansen M, Kurinczuk JJ, Bower C, et al: The risk of major birth defects after intracytoplasmic sperm injection and in vitro fertilization. *N Engl J Med* 2002; 346:725–30.

Hollier LM, Leveno KJ, Kelly MA, et al: Maternal age and malformations in singleton births. *Obstet Gynecol* 2000;96:701.

Iams JD, Newman RB, Thom EA, et al: Frequency of uterine contractions and the risk of spontaneous preterm delivery. *N Engl J Med* 2002;346:250–5.

Infante-Rivard C, Rivard GE, Yotov WV, et al: Absence of association of thrombophilia polymorphisms with intrauterine growth restriction. *N Engl J Med* 2002;347:19–25.

James D: Caesarean section for fetal distress. *Br Med J* 2001;322:1316–7.

MMWR: Intrauterine West Nile Virus infection—New York, 2002. MMWR 2002;51:1135.

Ross MG, Brace RA: National Institute of Child Health and Development Conference summary: Amniotic fluid biology—basic and clinical aspects. *J Matern Fetal Med* 2001;10:2.

Schieve LA, Meikle SF, Ferre C, et al: Low and very low birth weight in infants conceived with use of assisted reproductive technology. *N Engl J Med* 2002;346:731–6.

Shennan A, Bewley S: How to manage term breech deliveries. *Br Med J* 2001;323:244–5.

Smith GCS, Pell JP, Cameron AD, et al: Risk of perinatal death associated with labor after previous cesarean delivery in uncomplicated term pregnancies. *JAMA* 2002;287:2684–90.

Steer P, Flint C: Preterm labour and premature rupture of membranes. *Br Med J* 1999;318:1059–62.

Stromberg B, Dahlquist G, Ericson A, et al: Neurological sequelae in children born after in vitro fertilization: A population-based study. *Lancet* 2002;359:461–5.

Towner D, Castro MA, Eby-Wilkens E, et al: Effect of mode of delivery in nulliparous women on neonatal intracranial injury. *N Engl J Med* 1999;341:1709.

Wald NJ, Watt HC, Hackshaw AK: Integrated screening for Down's syndrome based on tests performed during the first and second trimesters. *N Engl J Med* 1999;341:461.

Wen SW, Liu S, Kramer MS, et al: Comparison of maternal and infant outcomes between vacuum extraction and forceps deliveries. *Am J Epidemiol* 2001; 153:103.

Chapter 85

The Fetus

Barbara J. Stoll and Robert M. Kliegman

Genetic and environmental influences may affect an embryo and fetus at any time during development; the fetal genome itself has a significant role in development and fetal survival, as does the uterine environment.

The major emphasis in fetal medicine involves (1) assessment of fetal growth and maturity, (2) evaluation of fetal well-being or distress, (3) assessment of the effects of maternal disease on the fetus, (4) evaluation of the effects of drugs administered to the mother on the fetus, and (5) identification and treatment of fetal disease or anomalies. Increasing knowledge of fetal physiology has paved the way for effective fetal therapy, intervention during fetal distress, and improved adaptation of a newborn infant, particularly a premature one, to extrauterine life. Some aspects of human fetal growth and development are summarized in Chapter 8.

85.1 Fetal Growth and Maturity

Ultrasonography of the fetus, a common obstetric procedure, is both safe and accurate. Indications for antenatal ultrasonography include estimation of gestational age (unknown dates, discrepancy between uterine size and dates or suspected growth retardation, multiple gestation, and abnormalities in amniotic fluid volume), location of the placenta, determination of the number and position of fetuses, and identification of congenital anomalies.

Fetal growth can be assessed by ultrasonography as early as 6–8 wk. The most accurate assessment of gestational age is by 1st-trimester ultrasound measurement of crown-rump length. The biparietal diameter is used to assess gestational age beginning in the 2nd trimester. Through 34 wk the biparietal diameter accurately estimates gestation to within ±10 days. Later in gestation, accuracy falls to ±3 wk. Methods used to assess gestational age at term include measurement of abdominal circumference and femoral length. An estimate of gestational age by dating of the last menstrual period should also be obtained. If a single ultrasound examination is performed, the most information can be obtained with a scan at 18 to 20 wk, when both gestational age and fetal anatomy can be evaluated. Serial scans may be useful in assessing fetal growth. Two patterns of fetal growth restriction have been identified: continuous fetal growth 2 SD below the mean for gestational age and a normal fetal growth curve that abruptly slows or flattens later in gestation (Fig. 85–1).

Fetal maturity is usually assessed by accurate ultrasonographic dating of gestational age, but it may also be estimated by determining the surfactant content of amniotic fluid (Chapters 85.5 and 90). Determination of the extent of calcification by ultrasound (placental maturity index), detection of the 1st audible fetal heart tones (16–18 wk), and observation of the initial fetal movements (18–20 wk) may also aid in evaluating the maturity of a fetus.

85.2 Fetal Distress

Fetal compromise may occur during the antepartum or intrapartum periods but may be asymptomatic in the antenatal period. Antepartum fetal surveillance is warranted for women at increased risk for fetal distress, including those with a history of stillbirth, intrauterine growth restriction (IUGR), oligohydramnios or polyhydramnios, multiple gestation, rhesus sensitization, hypertensive disorders, diabetes mellitus or other

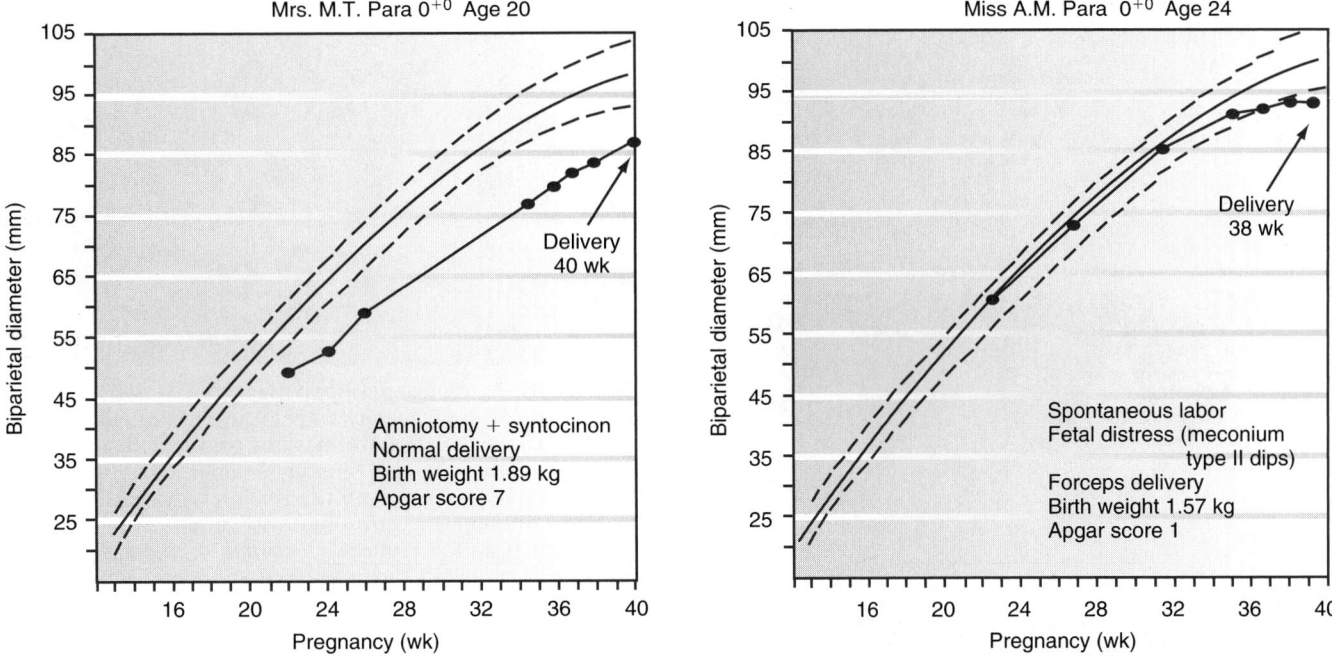

FIGURE 85–1. *A*, Example of a "low-profile" growth retardation pattern in an uneventful pregnancy and labor. The baby cried at 1 min and hypoglycemia did not develop. Birthweight was below the 5th percentile for gestational age. *B*, Example of a "late flattening" growth retardation pattern. The mother had a typical history of preeclampsia, and the infant had intrapartum fetal distress, a low Apgar score, and postnatal hypoglycemia. Birthweight was below the 5th percentile for gestational age. (From Campbell S: *Clin Obstet Gynecol* 1974;1:41.)

chronic maternal disease, decreased fetal movement, and post-term pregnancy. The predominant cause of antepartum fetal distress is uteroplacental insufficiency. Fetal distress may be manifested as IUGR, fetal hypoxia, increased vascular resistance in fetal blood vessels (Figs. 85–2 and 85–3), and when severe, mixed respiratory and metabolic (lactic) acidosis. The goals of antepartum fetal surveillance are to prevent intrauterine fetal demise, prevent hypoxic brain injury, and prolong gestation in women at risk for preterm delivery when such prolongation is safe or deliver a fetus when it is in jeopardy. The most commonly used tests are the *nonstress test* (NST), the *contraction stress test* (CST), and the *biophysical profile* (BPP). Methods for assessing fetal well-being are listed in Table 85–1.

The NST monitors the presence of fetal heart rate accelerations that follow fetal movement. A reactive (normal) NST result demonstrates two fetal heart rate accelerations of at least 15 beats/min lasting 15 sec. A nonreactive NST result suggests fetal compromise and requires further assessment with a CST or the BPP. A CST observes the fetal heart rate response to spontaneous, nipple-, or oxytocin-stimulated uterine contractions. Fetal compromise is suggested when three contractions in 10 min are followed by late decelerations. A CST is contraindicated in women with preterm premature rupture of membranes or a previous uterine scar from a classic cesarean section and in those with multiple gestations, an incompetent cervix, or placenta previa. The goals of fetal monitoring are to prevent intrauterine fetal demise and hypoxic brain injury. Although the CST and NST have low false-negative rates, both have high false-positive rates. The BPP assesses fetal breathing, body movement, tone, heart rate, and amniotic fluid volume, and it is used to improve the accurate and safe identification of fetal compromise (Table 85–2). A score of 2 is given for each observation present. A total score of 8–10 is reassuring; a score of 6 is equivocal, and retesting should be done in 12–24 hr; and a score of 4 or less warrants immediate evaluation and possible delivery. Signs of compromise seen on Doppler ultrasonography include a reduced,

absent, or reversed diastolic waveform velocity in the fetal aorta or umbilical artery (see Fig. 85–3 and Table 85–1). High-risk fetuses often have combinations of abnormalities, such as oligohydramnios, reversed diastolic Doppler umbilical artery blood flow velocity, and a low BPP.

Fetal distress during labor may be detected by monitoring the fetal heart rate, uterine pressure, and fetal scalp blood pH (Fig. 85–4).

Continuous fetal heart rate monitoring detects abnormal cardiac patterns by instruments that compute the beat-to-beat fetal heart rate from a fetal electrocardiographic signal. Signals are derived from an electrode attached to the fetal presenting part, from an ultrasonic transducer placed on the maternal abdominal wall to detect continuous ultrasonic waves reflected from the contractions of the heart, or from a phonotransducer placed on the mother's abdomen. Uterine contractions are simultaneously recorded from an amniotic fluid catheter and pressure transducer or from a tocotransducer applied to the maternal abdominal wall overlying the uterus.

Fetal heart rate patterns show various characteristics, some of which suggest fetal distress. The baseline fetal heart rate is the average rate between uterine contractions, which gradually decreases from about 155 beats/min in early pregnancy to about 135 beats/min at term; the normal range at term is 120–160 beats/min. **Tachycardia** (>160 beats/min) is associated with early fetal hypoxia, maternal fever, maternal hyperthyroidism, maternal β-sympathomimetic or atropine therapy, fetal anemia, infection, and some fetal arrhythmias. The latter do not generally occur with congenital heart disease and may resolve spontaneously at birth. **Fetal bradycardia** (<120 beats/min) occurs with fetal hypoxia, placental transfer of local anesthetic agents and β-adrenergic blocking agents, and occasionally, heart block with or without congenital heart disease.

Normally, the baseline fetal heart rate is variable, with long-term changes of 3–6 cycles/min, as well as short-term beat-to-beat variation. This variability may be decreased or lost with

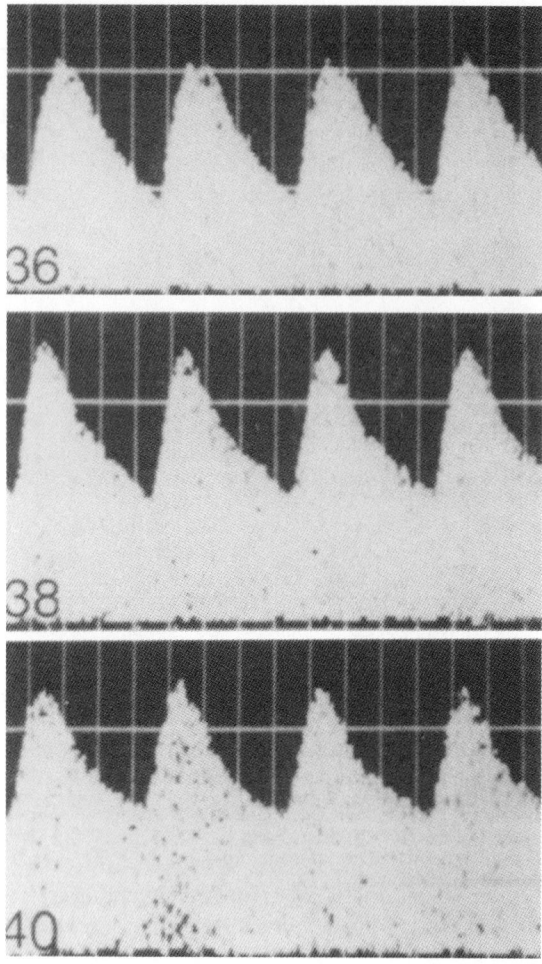

FIGURE 85–2. Normal Doppler velocimetry in sequential studies of fetal umbilical artery flow velocity waveforms from one normal pregnancy. Note the systolic peak flow with lower, but constant flow during diastole. The systolic:diastolic ratio can be determined and, in normal pregnancies, is less than 3 after the 30th wk of gestation. The numbers indicate the week of gestation. (From Trudinger B: Doppler ultrasound assessment of blood flow. In Creasy RK, Resnik R [editors]: *Maternal-Fetal Medicine: Principles and Practice,* 3rd ed. Philadelphia, WB Saunders, 1994.)

Umbilical artery   A/B>6

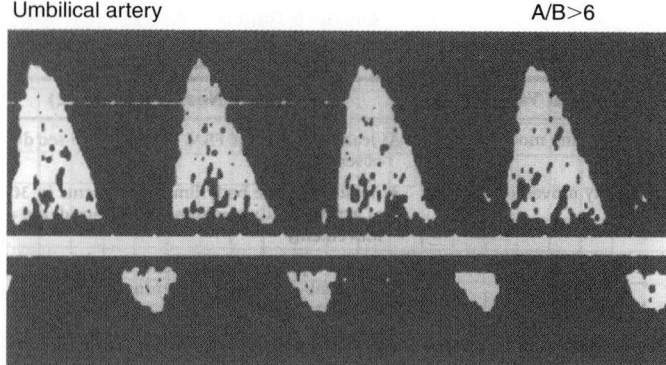

FIGURE 85–3. Abnormal Doppler velocimetry. On an umbilical artery Doppler flow velocity waveform, the umbilical placental impedance is so high that the diastolic component shows flow in a reverse direction. This finding is an indication of severe intrauterine hypoxia and intrauterine growth restriction. (From Trudinger B: Doppler ultrasound assessment of blood flow. In Creasy RK, Resnik R [editors]: *Maternal-Fetal Medicine: Principles and Practice,* 3rd ed. Philadelphia, WB Saunders, 1994.)

fetal hypoxemia or the placental transfer of drugs such as atropine, diazepam, promethazine, magnesium sulfate, and most sedative and narcotic agents. Prematurity, the sleep state, and fetal tachycardia may also diminish beat-to-beat variability.

Periodic accelerations or decelerations of the fetal heart rate in response to uterine contractions may also be monitored (see Fig. 85–4). **Early deceleration** (type I), associated with head compression, is a repetitive pattern of slowing that is synchronous with and proportional to the amplitude of the uterine contraction. **Variable deceleration** (associated with cord compression) is characterized by variable shape, abrupt onset and occurrence with consecutive contractions, and return to baseline at or after the conclusion of the contraction. **Late deceleration** (type II), associated with fetal hypoxemia, occurs repetitively after a uterine contraction is well established, is proportional to its amplitude, and persists into the interval following contractions. The late deceleration pattern is usually associated with maternal hypotension or excessive uterine activity, but it may be a response to any maternal, placental, umbilical cord, or fetal factor that limits effective oxy-

genation of the fetus. Reflex late decelerations with normal beat-to-beat variability are associated with chronic compensated fetal hypoxia, and they occur during uterine contractions that temporarily impede oxygen transport to the heart. Nonreflex late decelerations are more ominous and indicate severe hypoxic depression of myocardial function. The latter, together with decreased beat-to-beat variability or spontaneous decelerations in the absence of uterine contractions, either warrants further assessment by fetal blood sampling or is an indication for delivery.

Fetal scalp blood sampling during labor through a slightly dilated cervix may aid in confirming fetal distress suspected on the basis of variations in fetal heart rate or the presence of meconium in amniotic fluid. The proper use of this technique may result in earlier delivery of depressed infants, who thus have a better chance of successful resuscitation, increased survival, and less morbidity. Alternatively, when continuous fetal heart rate monitoring or general clinical evaluation suggests that a fetus is at risk, a normal fetal scalp blood sample may help avert obstetric intervention.

Fetal scalp blood pH in normal labor decreases from about 7.33 early in labor to approximately 7.25 at the time of vaginal delivery; the base deficit is about 4–6 mEq/L. Changes in the buffer base may be particularly helpful in assessing fetal status because they correspond to the accumulation of fetal lactic acid. A pH less than 7.25 strongly suggests fetal distress, and a pH less than 7.20 is an indication for further assessment and intervention. Determination of the lactate concentration in fetal scalp blood is another tool for monitoring the condition of the fetus.

Complications of fetal scalp sampling and internal monitoring devices are relatively uncommon but include bleeding (usually because of an underlying coagulation defect), puncture of the fontanel, and scalp abscesses with or without adjacent osteomyelitis. Abscesses may be due to *Staphylococcus aureus* or gram-negative rods; more often they are sterile.

Umbilical cord blood samples obtained at the time of delivery are useful to document fetal acid-base status. Although the exact cord blood pH value that defines significant fetal acidemia is unknown, an umbilical artery pH less than 7.0 has been associated with greater need for resuscitation and a higher incidence of respiratory, gastrointestinal, cardiovascular, and neurologic complications. However, when a low pH is detected, many newborn infants will be neurologically normal.

TABLE 85–1. Fetal Diagnosis and Assessment

Method	Comment and Indications
Imaging	
Ultrasound (real-time)	Biometry (growth), anomaly (morphology) detection. Biophysical profile. Amniotic fluid volume, hydrops. Determine gestational age and IUGR
Ultrasound (Doppler)	Velocimetry (blood flow velocity). Detection of increased vascular resistance secondary to fetal hypoxia, IUGR
Embryoscopy	Early diagnosis of limb anomaly
Fetoscopy	Detection of facial, limb, cutaneous anomalies
MRI	Best to define lesions before EXIT procedure
Fluid Analysis	
Amniocentesis	Fetal maturity (L:S ratio), karyotype (cytogenetics), biochemical enzyme analysis, molecular genetic DNA diagnosis, bilirubin, or α-fetoprotein determination. Bacterial culture, pathogen antigen or genome detection
Fetal urine	Prognosis of obstructive uropathy?
Cordocentesis (Percutaneous Umbilical Blood Sampling)	Detection of blood type, anemia, hemoglobinopathies, thrombocytopenia, acidosis, hypoxia, polycythemia, IgM antibody response to infection. Rapid karyotyping and molecular DNA genetic diagnosis. Fetal therapy (see Table 85–5)
Fetal Tissue Analysis	
Chorionic villus biopsy	Karyotype, molecular DNA genetic analysis, enzyme assays
Skin biopsy	Hereditary skin disease*
Liver biopsy	Enzyme assay*
Circulating fetal cells in maternal blood	Molecular DNA genetic analysis
Maternal Serum α-Fetoprotein	
Elevated	Twins, neural tube defects (anencephaly, spina bifida), intestinal atresia, hepatitis, nephrosis, fetal demise, incorrect gestational age
Reduced	Trisomies, aneuploidy
Maternal Cervix	
Fetal fibronectin	Indicates risk of preterm birth
Bacterial culture	Identifies risk of fetal infection (group B streptococcus, *Neisseria gonorrhoeae*)
Fluid	Determination of premature rupture of membranes
Antepartum Biophysical Monitoring	
Nonstress test	Fetal distress; hypoxia
Contraction stress test	Fetal distress; hypoxia
Biophysical profile	Fetal distress; hypoxia
Intrapartum Fetal Heart Rate Monitoring	See Fig. 85–4

DNA genetic analysis on chorionic villus samples, amniocytes from amniocentesis, or fetal cells recovered from the maternal circulation may obviate the need for direct fetal tissue biopsy if the gene or genetic marker is available (e.g., the gene for Duchenne's muscular dystrophy).

IUGR = intrauterine growth restriction; EXIT = ex utero intrapartum treatment (endoscopy, drain placement, surgery); L:S = lecithin:sphingomyelin ratio.

85.3 Maternal Disease and the Fetus

Infectious Diseases (see Table 84–2). Almost any maternal infection with severe systemic manifestations may result in miscarriage, stillbirth, or premature labor. Whether these results are due to infection of the fetus or are secondary to stress is not always clear. Maternal hyperthermia during infections may be associated with an increased incidence of congenital anomalies. Regardless of the severity of the maternal infection, certain agents frequently infect a fetus and result in serious sequelae. Such fetuses are often small for gestational age. Some infections, such as rubella, may also produce congenital malformations if they occur during the period of organogenesis. Intrauterine infection/chorioamnionitis may

be an important risk factor for cerebral white matter injury and subsequent cerebral palsy.

Noninfectious Diseases (see Table 84–1). *Maternal diabetes* may result in organomegaly, hypertrophy and hyperplasia of the β cells of the fetal pancreas, and metabolic derangements in the neonate (Chapter 96.1). A high incidence of intrauterine death occurs after the 36th wk of gestation in unmonitored and poorly controlled mothers. Moreover, maternal diabetes is a risk factor for cardiovascular and other malformations. *Eclampsia-preeclampsia* of pregnancy, chronic hypertension, and chronic renal disease result in small fetal size for gestational age, prematurity, and intrauterine death, all probably caused by diminished uteroplacental perfusion. Uncontrolled maternal *hypothyroidism*

TABLE 85–2. Biophysical Profile Scoring: Technique and Interpretation

Biophysical Variable	Normal Score (2)	Abnormal Score (0)
Fetal breathing movements	At least 1 episode of FBM of at least 30 sec duration in 30 min observation	Absent FBM or no episode of ≥30 sec in 30 min
Gross body movement	At least 3 discrete body/limb movements in 30 min (episodes of active continuous movement considered a single movement)	2 or fewer episodes of body/limb movements in 30 min
Fetal tone	At least 1 episode of active extension with return to flexion of fetal limb(s) or trunk. Opening and closing of hand considered normal tone	Either slow extension with return to partial flexion or movement of limb in full extension or absent fetal movement with fetal hand held in complete or partial deflection
Reactive FHR	At least 2 episodes of FHR acceleration of ≥15 beats/min and at least 15 sec duration associated with fetal movement in 30 min	Less than 2 episodes of acceleration of FHR or acceleration of <15 beats/min in 30 min
Qualitative AFV*	At least 1 pocket of AF that measures at least 2 cm in 2 perpendicular planes	Either no AF pockets or a pocket <2 cm in 2 perpendicular planes

Modification of the criteria for reduced amniotic fluid from less than 1 cm to less than 2 cm would seem reasonable. Ultrasound is used for biophysical assessment of the fetus.

FBM = fetal breathing movement; FHR = fetal heart rate; AFV = amniotic fluid volume; AF = amniotic fluid.

From Creasy RK, Resnik R (editors): Maternal-Fetal Medicine: Principles and Practice, 3rd ed. Philadelphia, WB Saunders, 1994.

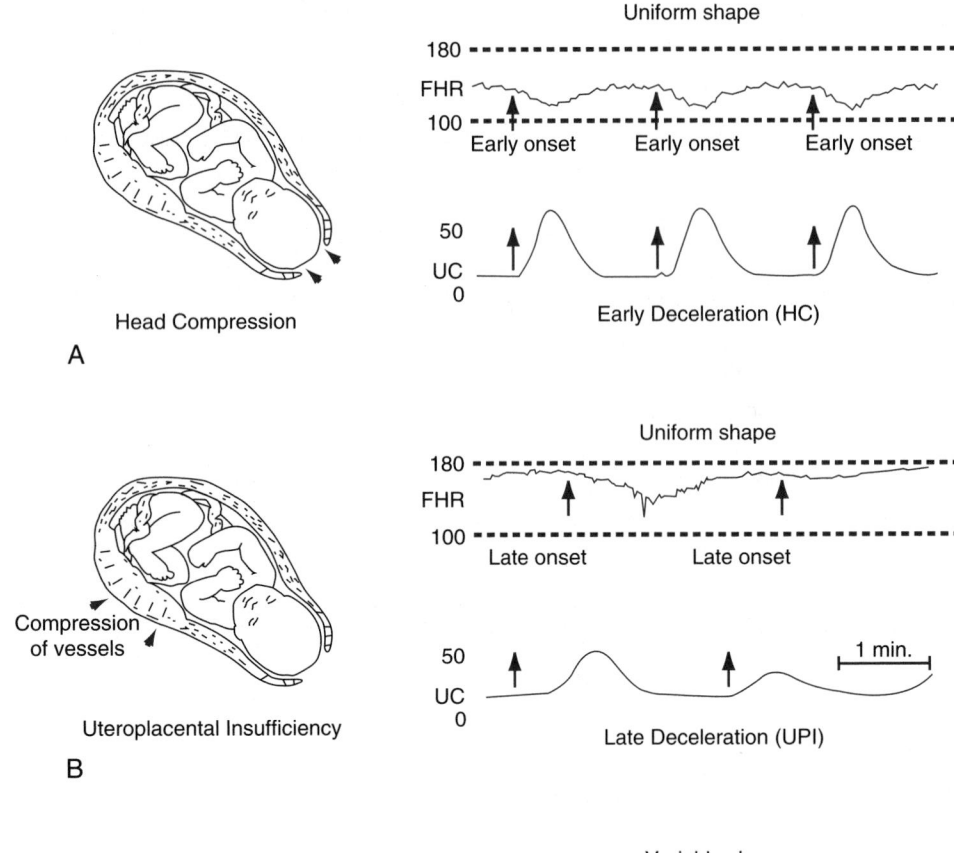

Uniform shape

Early Deceleration (HC)

A Head Compression

Uniform shape

Late Deceleration (UPI)

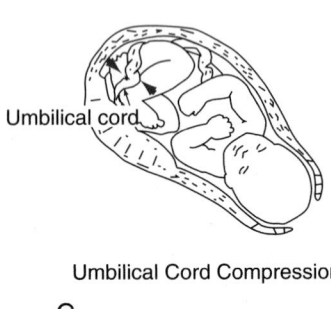

B Compression of vessels — Uteroplacental Insufficiency

Variable shape

Variable Deceleration (CC)

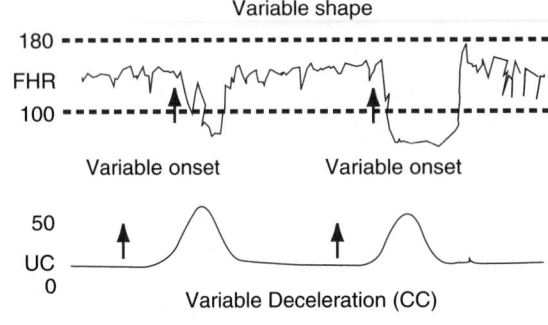

C Umbilical cord — Umbilical Cord Compression

FIGURE 85–4. Patterns of periodic fetal heart rate (FHR) deceleration. The tracing in *A* shows early deceleration occurring during the peak of uterine contractions as a result of pressure on the fetal head. *B,* Late deceleration caused by uteroplacental insufficiency. *C,* Variable deceleration as a result of umbilical cord compression. *Arrows* denote the time relationship between the onset of FHR changes and uterine contractions. (From Hon EH: *An Atlas of Fetal Heart Rate Patterns.* New Haven, CT, Harty Press, 1968.)

or *hyperthyroidism* is responsible for relative infertility, a tendency to abort, premature labor, and fetal death. Hypothyroidism in pregnant women (even if mild or asymptomatic) can adversely affect neurodevelopment of the child. Maternal *immunologic diseases* such as idiopathic thrombocytopenic purpura, systemic lupus erythematosus, myasthenia gravis, and Graves disease, all of which are mediated by IgG autoantibodies that can cross the placenta, frequently result in transient illness in the newborn. Untreated maternal *phenylketonuria* results in miscarriage, congenital cardiac malformations, and injury to the brain of a non-phenylketonuric heterozygotic fetus.

85.4 Maternal Medication and Toxin Exposure and the Fetus

Consumption of medications in pregnancy is frequent; surveys indicate that 90% of pregnant patients have taken at least one drug. The average mother has taken 4 drugs other than vitamins or iron during pregnancy; 4% have taken 10 drugs or more.

Moreover, many women are exposed to potential reproductive toxins, such as occupational, environmental, or household chemicals, including solvents, pesticides, and hair products. The effects of drugs taken by the mother vary considerably, especially in relation to the time in pregnancy when they are taken and perhaps the fetal genotype for drug-metabolizing enzymes. Miscarriage or congenital malformations result from the maternal ingestion of teratogenic drugs during the period of organogenesis. Maternal medications taken later, particularly during the last few weeks of gestation or during labor, tend to affect the function of specific organs or enzyme systems, and they adversely affect the neonate rather than the fetus (Table 85–3 and Box 85–1).

The effects of drugs may be evident immediately in the delivery room or later in the neonatal period, or they may be delayed even longer. The administration of diethylstilbestrol during pregnancy has resulted in vaginal adenosis and vaginal adenocarcinoma in older female children. In addition to in utero carcinogenesis, various reproductive problems have been reported in these women, including cervical anomalies and premature births, ectopic pregnancies, and spontaneous pregnancy loss.

TABLE 85–3. Agents Acting on Pregnant Women That May Adversely Affect the Structure or Function of the Fetus and Newborn

Drug	Effect on Fetus
Accutane (isotretinoin)	Facial-ear anomalies, heart disease
Alcohol	Congenital cardiac, CNS, limb anomalies; IUGR; developmental delay; attention deficits; autism
Aminopterin	Abortion, malformations
Amphetamines	Congenital heart disease, IUGR, withdrawal
Azathioprine	Abortion
Busulfan (Myleran)	Stunted growth; corneal opacities; cleft palate; hypoplasia of ovaries, thyroid, and parathyroids
Carbamazepine	Spina bifida, possible neurodevelopment delay
Carbon monoxide	Cerebral atrophy, microcephaly, seizures
Chloroquine	Deafness
Chorionic villus sampling	Probably no effect, possibly limb reduction
Cigarette smoking	Low birthweight for gestational age
Cocaine/crack	Microcephaly, LBW, IUGR, behavioral disturbances
Cyclophosphamide	Multiple malformations
Danazol	Virilization
17α-Ethinyl testosterone (Progestoral)	Masculinization of female fetus
Hyperthermia	Spina bifida
Lithium	Ebstein's anomaly, macrosomia
6-Mercaptopurine	Abortion
Methyl mercury	Minamata disease, microcephaly, deafness, blindness, mental retardation
Methyltestoserone	Masculinization of female fetus
Misoprostol	Arthrogryposis, cranial neuropathies (Möbius syndrome), equinovarus
Norethindrone	Masculinization of female fetus
Penicillamine	Cutis laxa syndrome
Phenytoin	Congenital anomalies, IUGR, neuroblastoma, bleeding (vitamin K deficiency)
Polychlorinated biphenyls	Skin discoloration—thickening, desquamation, LBW, acne, developmental delay
Prednisone	Oral clefts
Progesterone	Masculinization of female fetus
Quinine	Abortion, thrombocytopenia, deafness
Stilbestrol (diethylstilbestrol [DES])	Vaginal adenocarcinoma in adolescence
Streptomycin	Deafness
Tetracycline	Retarded skeletal growth, pigmentation of teeth, hypoplasia of enamel, cataract, limb malformations
Thalidomide	Phocomelia, deafness, other malformations
Toluene (solvent abuse)	Craniofacial abnormalities, prematurity, withdrawal symptoms, hypertonia
Trimethadione and paramethadione	Abortion, multiple malformations, mental retardation
Valproate	Spina bifida, impaired neurologic function
Vitamin D	Supravalvular aortic stenosis, hypercalcemia
Warfarin (Coumadin)	Fetal bleeding and death, hypoplastic nasal structures

CNS = central nervous system; IUGR = intrauterine growth restriction; LBW = low birthweight.

BOX 85–1. Agents Acting on Pregnant Women That May Adversely Affect the Newborn Infant

Acebutolol—IUGR, hypotension, bradycardia
Acetazolamide—metabolic acidosis
Amiodarone—bradycardia, hypothyroidism
Anesthetic agents (volatile)—CNS depression
Adrenal corticosteroids—adrenocortical failure (rare)
Ammonium chloride—acidosis (clinically inapparent)
Aspirin—neonatal bleeding, prolonged gestation
Atenolol—IUGR, hypoglycemia
Blue cohosh herbal tea—neonatal heart failure
Bromides–rash, CNS depression, IUGR
Captopril, enalapril—transient anuric renal failure, oligohydramnios
Caudal-paracervical anesthesia with mepivacaine (accidental introduction of anesthetic into scalp of baby)—bradypnea, apnea, bradycardia, convulsions
Cholinergic agents (edrophonium, pyridostigmine)—transient muscle weakness
CNS depressants (narcotics, barbiturates, benzodiazepams) during labor—CNS depression, hypotonia
Cephalothin—positive direct Coombs test reaction
Dexamethasone—periventricular leukomalacia
Fluoxetine—possible transient neonatal withdrawal, hypertonicity, minor anomalies
Haloperidol—withdrawal
Hexamethonium bromide—paralytic ileus
Ibuprofen—oligohydramnios, pulmonary hypertension
Imipramine—withdrawal
Indomethacin—oliguria, oligohydramnios, intestinal perforation, pulmonary hypertension

Intravenous fluids during labor (e.g., salt-free solutions)—electrolyte disturbances, hyponatremia, hypoglycemia
Iodide (radioactive)—goiter
Iodides—goiter
Isoxsuprine—ileus, hypocalcemia, hypoglycemia, hypotension
Lead—reduced intellectual function
Magnesium sulfate—respiratory depression, meconium plug, hypotonia
Methimazole—goiter, hypothyroidism
Morphine and its derivatives (addiction)—withdrawal symptoms (poor feeding, vomiting, diarrhea, restlessness, yawning and stretching, dyspnea and cyanosis, fever and sweating, pallor, tremors, convulsions)
Naphthalene—hemolytic anemia (in G6PD-deficient infants)
Nitrofurantoin—hemolytic anemia (in G6PD-deficient infants)
Oxytocin—hyperbilirubinemia, hyponatremia
Phenobarbital—bleeding diathesis (vitamin K deficiency), possible long-term reduction in IQ, sedation
Primaquine—hemolytic anemia (in G6PD-deficient infants)
Propranolol—hypoglycemia, bradycardia, apnea
Propylthiouracil—goiter, hypothyroidism
Pyridoxine—seizures
Reserpine—drowsiness, nasal congestion, poor temperature stability
Sulfonamides—interfere with protein binding of bilirubin; kernicterus at low levels of serum bilirubin, hemolysis with G6PD deficiency
Sulfonylurea—refractory hypoglycemia
Sympathomimetic (tocolytic β-agonist) agents—tachycardia
Thiazides—neonatal thrombocytopenia (rare)

IUGR = intrauterine growth restriction; CNS = central nervous system; G6PD = glucose-6-phosphate dehydrogenase.

Evidence has confirmed an interaction between genetic factors and susceptibility to certain drugs or environmental toxins. For example, phenytoin teratogenesis may be mediated by genetic differences in the enzymatic production of epoxide metabolites, and specific genes may influence the adverse effects of benzene exposure during pregnancy. Polymorphisms of genes encoding enzymes that metabolize the polycyclic aromatic hydrocarbons in cigarette smoke influence the growth-restricting effects of smoking on the fetus.

In view of the limits of current knowledge on the fetal effects of maternal medication, no drugs should be prescribed during pregnancy without weighing maternal need against the risk of fetal damage. All women should be specifically counseled to abstain from the use of alcohol, tobacco, and illicit drugs during pregnancy.

85.5 Teratogens

When an infant or child is malformed or mentally retarded, the parents often wrongly blame themselves and attribute the child's problems to events that occurred during pregnancy. Because infections occur and several drugs are often taken during many pregnancies, the pediatrician must evaluate the presumed viral infections and the drugs ingested to help parents understand their child's birth defect. The causes of approximately 40% of congenital malformations are unknown. Although only a relatively few agents are recognized to be teratogenic in humans (see Tables 84–1, 84–2, 85–3, and Box 85–1), new agents continue to be identified. Overall, only 10% of anomalies are due to recognizable teratogens. The time of exposure is usually at less than 60 days' gestation during organogenesis. Specific agents produce predictable lesions. Some agents have a dose or threshold effect; below the threshold, no alterations in growth, function, or structure occur. The agent's effects may be species specific. Genetic variables such as the presence of specific enzymes may metabolize a benign agent into a more toxic-teratogenic form (phenytoin conversion to its epoxide). In many circumstances, the same agent and dose may not consistently produce the lesion.

Reduced enzyme activity of the folate methylation pathway, particularly the formation of 5-methyltetrahydrofolate, may be responsible for neural tube or other birth defects. The common thermolabile mutation of 5,10-methylene tetrahydrofolate reductase may be one of the enzymes responsible. Folate supplementation for all pregnant women (by direct fortification of cereal grains, mandatory in the United States) during organogenesis may overcome this genetic enzyme defect, thus reducing the incidence of neural tube and perhaps other birth defects.

Mechanisms of teratogenesis include cell death without reparative regeneration; mitotic delay; delayed differentiation; physical or vascular constraining events; reduced histogenesis secondary to cell depletion, necrosis, calcification, or scarring; inhibited cellular migration; and inflammation. Many mechanisms occur secondary to chromosomal or DNA damage and poor molecular repair.

The Food and Drug Administration classifies drugs into five pregnancy risk categories. *Category A* suggests no risk based on evidence from controlled human trials. *Category B* suggests either no risk shown in animal studies but no adequate studies in humans or some risk in animal studies that are not confirmed by human studies. *Category C* is either definite risk shown in animal studies but no adequate human studies or no available data for animals or humans. *Category D* includes drugs with some risk but with a benefit that may exceed that risk for the treated life-threatening condition, such as streptomycin for tuberculosis. *Category X* is for drugs that are contraindicated in pregnancy on the basis of animal and human evidence and whose risk exceeds the benefits.

The specific mechanism of action is known or postulated for very few teratogens. Warfarin, an anticoagulant because it is a vitamin K antagonist, prevents the carboxylation of γ-carboxyglutamic acid, which is a component of osteocalcin and other vitamin K–dependent bone proteins. The teratogenic effect on developing cartilage, especially nasal cartilage, appears to be avoided if the pregnant woman's treatment between weeks 6 and 12 of gestation is switched from warfarin to heparin. Hypothyroidism in the fetus may be caused by the maternal ingestion of an excessive amount of iodides or propylthiouracil; each interferes with the conversion of inorganic to organic iodides. Phenytoin may be teratogenic because of the accumulation of a metabolite as a result of deficiency of epoxide hydrolase.

Recognition of teratogens offers the opportunity for prevention of related birth defects. For example, if a pregnant woman is informed of the potentially harmful effects of alcohol on her unborn infant, she may be motivated to control this problem during pregnancy. A woman with insulin-dependent diabetes mellitus may significantly decrease her risk for having a child with birth defects by achieving good control of her disease *before* conception.

85.6 Radiation (also see Chapter 700)

Accidental exposure of pregnant women to radiation is a common cause for anxiety in women, their families, and their physicians, usually about whether the fetus will have birth defects or genetic abnormalities. It is unlikely that exposure to diagnostic radiation will cause gene mutations; no increase in genetic abnormalities has been identified in the offspring exposed as unborn fetuses to the atomic bomb explosions in Japan in 1945.

A more realistic concern is whether the exposed human fetus will show birth defects or a higher incidence of malignancy. The recommended occupational limit of maternal exposure to radiation from all sources is 500 mrad for the entire 40 wk of a pregnancy. See Chapter 700 for a discussion of gonadal exposure in the mother and whole body exposure of the fetus. The limited data on human fetuses show that large doses of radiation (20,000–50,000 mrad) are harmful to the central nervous system, as evidenced by microcephaly, mental retardation, and IUGR.

Therapeutic abortion is often recommended when exposure exceeds 10,000 mrad. It is more likely that a human fetus will be exposed to 1,000–3,000 mrad, an amount not shown to cause malformations. Whether this level of fetal exposure is associated with an increased risk for childhood cancer or leukemia is controversial.

85.7 Intrauterine Diagnosis of Fetal Disease (see Table 85–1)

See section 85.2 for a discussion of fetal distress.

Diagnostic procedures are used to identify fetal diseases when abortion is being considered, when direct fetal treatment is possible, or when a decision is made to deliver a viable, but premature infant to avoid intrauterine fetal demise. Fetal assessment is also indicated in a broader context when the family, medical, or reproductive history of the mother suggests the presence of a high-risk pregnancy or a high-risk fetus (Chapters 84 and 85.3).

Various methods are used for identifying fetal disease (see Table 85–1). Fetal ultrasonographic imaging may detect fetal growth abnormalities (by biometric measurements of biparietal diameter, femoral length, or head or abdominal circumference) or fetal malformations (Fig. 85–5). Although 95% of fetuses whose biparietal diameter is 9.5 cm or more are at least 37 wk of gestation, the lungs of these fetuses may not be mature. Serial

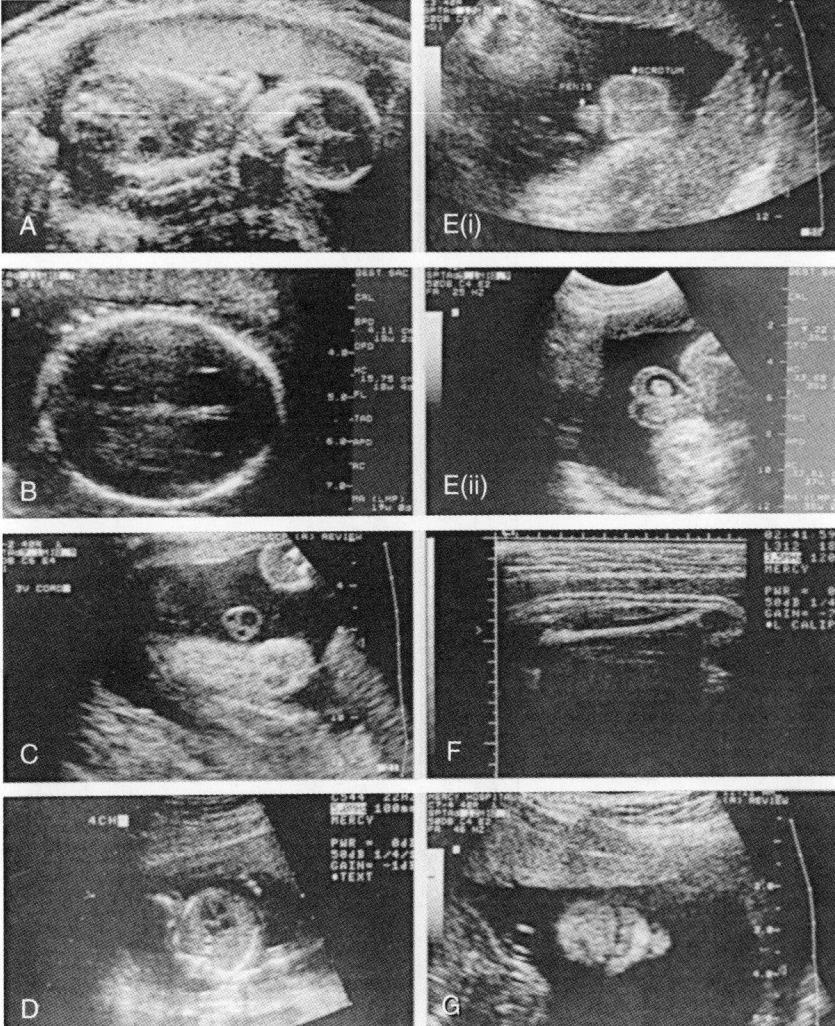

FIGURE 85–5. Assessment of fetal anatomy. *A*, Overall view of the uterus at 24 wk showing a longitudinal section of the fetus and an anterior placenta. *B*, Transverse section at the level of the lateral ventricle at 18 wk showing *(right)* prominent anterior horns of the lateral ventricles on either side of the midline echo of the falx. *C*, Cross section of the umbilical cord showing that the lumen of the umbilical vein is much wider than that of the two umbilical arteries. *D*, Four-chambered view of the heart at 18 wk with equal-sized ventricles shown above equal-sized atria. *E*, *(i)* Normal male genitals near term; *(ii)* hydrocele outlining a testicle within the scrotum projecting into a normal-sized pocket of amniotic fluid at 38 wk. Approximately 2% of male infants after birth have clinical evidence of a hydrocele that is often bilateral, not to be confused with subcutaneous edema occurring during vaginal breech birth. *F*, Section of a thigh near term showing thick subcutaneous tissue (4.6 mm between markers) above the femur of a fetus with macrosomia. *G*, Fetal face viewed from below showing (from right to left) the nose, alveolar margin, and chin at 20 wk. (From Special investigative procedures. In Beischer NA, Mackay EV, Colditz PB (editors): *Obstetrics and the Newborn*, 3rd ed. Philadelphia, WB Saunders, 1997.)

determination of growth velocity and the head-to-abdominal circumference ratio enhances the ability to detect IUGR. Real-time ultrasonography may identify placental abnormalities (abruptio placentae, placenta previa) and fetal anomalies such as hydrocephalus, neural tube defects, duodenal atresia, diaphragmatic hernia, renal agenesis, bladder outlet obstruction, congenital heart disease, limb abnormalities, sacrococcygeal teratoma, cystic hygroma, omphalocele, gastroschisis, and hydrops (Table 85–4).

Real-time ultrasonography also facilitates performance of *cordocentesis* and the BPP by imaging fetal breathing, body movements, tone, and amniotic fluid volume (see Table 85–2). *Doppler velocimetry* assesses fetal arterial blood flow (vascular resistance) (see Figs. 85–2 and 85–3). Roentgenographic examination of the fetus has been replaced by real-time ultrasonography, MRI, and fetoscopy.

Amniocentesis, the transabdominal withdrawal of amniotic fluid during pregnancy for diagnostic purposes (see Table 85–1), is frequently performed to determine the timing of the delivery of fetuses with erythroblastosis fetalis or the need for fetal transfusion. It is also done for genetic indications, usually between the 15th and 16th wk of gestation, with results available within 1–2 wk. The most common indication for genetic amniocentesis is advanced maternal age (the risk for chromosome abnormality at age 21 is 1:526 vs 1:8 at age 49). The amniotic fluid may be directly analyzed for amino acids, enzymes, hormones, and abnormal metabolic products, and amniotic fluid cells may be cultivated to permit detailed cytologic analysis for prenatal detection of chromosomal abnormalities and DNA-gene or enzymatic analysis for the detection of inborn metabolic errors. Analysis of amniotic fluid may also help in identifying neural tube defects (elevation of α-fetoprotein), adrenogenital syndrome (elevation of 17-ketosteroids and pregnanetriol), and thyroid dysfunction. Chorionic villus biopsy (transvaginal or transabdominal) performed in the 1st trimester also provides fetal cells but may pose a slightly increased risk for fetal loss or limb reduction defects. Fetal cells circulating in maternal blood and fetal DNA in maternal plasma are potential noninvasive sources of material for prenatal diagnosis. This new technology may eliminate the need for amniocentesis or chorionic villus sampling.

The best available chemical indices of fetal maturity are provided by determination of amniotic fluid creatinine and lecithin, which reflect the maturity of the fetal kidneys and lungs, respectively. Lecithin is produced in the lungs by type II alveolar cells and eventually reaches the amniotic fluid via the effluent from the trachea. Until the middle of the 3rd trimester, its concentration nearly equals that of sphingomyelin; thereafter, sphingomyelin remains constant in amniotic fluid while lecithin increases. By 35 wk, the lecithin:sphingomyelin (L:S) ratio averages about 2:1, indicative of lung maturity.

Earlier lung maturation may occur in the presence of severe premature separation of the placenta, premature rupture of the fetal membranes, narcotic addiction, or maternal hypertensive

TABLE 85-4. Significance of Fetal Ultrasonographic Anatomic Findings

Prenatal Observation	Definition	Differential Diagnosis	Significance	Postnatal Evaluation
Dilated cerebral ventricles	Ventriculomegaly ≥ 10 mm	Hydrocephalus Hydrancephalus Dandy-Walker cyst Agenesis of corpus callosum	Transient isolated ventriculomegaly common and benign. Persistent or progressive more worrisome. Identify associated cranial and extracranial anomalies	Serial head US or CT. Evaluate for extracranial anomalies
Choroid plexus cysts	1–3% incidence Size ~10 mm: unilateral or bilateral	Abnormal karyotype (trisomy 18, 21) Aneuploidy risk 1:100 if isolated. ↑ Risk (1:3) with other anomalies. Risk ↑ if large, complex, or bilateral cysts or advanced maternal age	Often isolated, benign; resolves by 24–28 wk. Examine for other organ anomalies, then amniocentesis for karyotype	Head US or CT. Examine for extracranial anomalies; karyotype if indicated
Nuchal pad thickening	≥ 6 mm at 15–20 wk; cystic hygroma	Trisomy 21, 18 Turner's syndrome (XO) Nonchromosomal syndromes Normal (~25%)	~50% have chromosome abnormalities Amniocentesis for karyotype	Evaluate for multiple organ malformations; karyotype if indicated
Dilated renal pelvis	Pyelectasis ≥ 5 to 10 mm 0.6–1% incidence	UPJ obstruction Vesicoureteral reflux Posterior ureteral valves Etopic ureterocele Large-volume nonobstruction	Often "physiologic" and transient Reflux is common If >10 mm or with caliectasis, consider pathologic cause. If large bladder, consider posterior urethral valves, megacystic syndrome	Repeat US; VCUG, prophylactic antibiotics
Echogenic bowel	0.6% incidence	CF, meconium peritonitis, trisomy 21 or 18, other chromosomal abnormalities CMV, toxoplasmosis, GI obstruction	Often normal (65%) 10% have CF 1.5% have aneuploidy	Sweat chloride and DNA testing Karyotype Surgery for obstruction TORCH evaluation
Stomach appearance	Small or absent or double bubble	Upper GI obstruction (esophageal atresia) Double bubble signifies duodenal atresia Abnormal karyotype Polyhydramnios Stomach in chest signifies diaphragmatic hernia	Must also consider neurologic disorders that reduce swallowing. Over 30% with double bubble have trisomy 21	Chromosomes, KUB if indicated, upper GI series, neurologic evaluation

US = ultrasonography; UPJ = ureteropelvic junction; VCUG = voiding cystourethrogram; CF = cystic fibrosis; CMV = cytomegalovirus; GI = gastrointestinal; TORCH = toxoplasmosis, other agents, rubella, CMV, herpes simplex; KUB = kidney, ureter, and bladder.

and renal vascular disease. A delay in pulmonary maturation may be associated with hydrops fetalis or maternal diabetes without vascular disease. The likelihood of hyaline membrane disease is greatly reduced with L:S ratios of 2:1 or more, although hypoxia, acidosis, and hypothermia may increase the risk despite this "mature" L:S ratio. Maternal and fetal blood have an L:S ratio of about 1:4; thus, contamination will not alter the significance of a ratio of 2:1 or more. Meconium contamination, storage, and centrifugation all may reduce the reliability of the L:S ratio.

Saturated phosphatidylcholine or phosphatidylglycerol concentrations in amniotic fluid may be more specific and sensitive predictors of pulmonary maturity, especially in high-risk pregnancies such as those occurring in women with diabetes (see Chapters 90 and 96.1).

Although amniocentesis can be carried out with little discomfort to the mother, even in experienced hands the procedure entails some small risk, such as direct damage to the fetus, placental puncture and bleeding with secondary damage to the fetus, stimulation of uterine contraction and premature labor, amnionitis, and maternal sensitization to fetal blood. The earlier in gesta-

tion that amniotic puncture is done, the greater the risk to the fetus. Using ultrasound for placental and fetal localization can reduce the risk. The procedure should be limited to cases in which the potential benefits of the findings will outweigh the risk.

Cordocentesis, or percutaneous umbilical blood sampling, is used to diagnose fetal hematologic abnormalities, genetic disorders, infections, and fetal acidosis (see Table 85–1). Under direct ultrasonographic visualization, a long needle is passed into the umbilical vein at its entrance to the placenta or fetal abdominal wall. Blood may be withdrawn to determine fetal hemoglobin, platelet concentration, lymphocyte DNA, the presence of infection, or Pao_2, pH, Pco_2, and lactate levels. Transfusion or administration of drugs can be given through the umbilical vein (Table 85–5).

85.8 Treatment and Prevention of Fetal Disease

Management of fetal diseases continues to depend on coordinated advances in diagnostic accuracy and knowledge of the dis-

TABLE 85–5. **Fetal Therapy**	
Disorder	**Possible Treatment**
Hematology	
Anemia with hydrops (erythroblastosis fetalis)	Umbilical vein packed red blood cell transfusion
Thalassemia	Fetal stem cell transplantation
Thrombocytopenia	
Isoimmune	Umbilical vein platelet transfusion, maternal intravenous immunoglobulin
Autoimmune (ITP)	Maternal steroids and intravenous immunoglobulin
Chronic granulomatous disease	Fetal stem cell transplantation
Metabolic-Endocrine	
Maternal phenylketonuria (PKU)	Phenylalanine restriction
Fetal galactosemia	Galactose-free diet (?)
Multiple carboxylase deficiency	Biotin if responsive
Methylmalonicacidemia	Vitamin B_{12} if responsive
21-Hydroxylase deficiency	Dexamethasone
Maternal diabetes mellitus	Tight insulin control during pregnancy, labor, and delivery
Fetal goiter	Maternal hyperthyroidism—maternal propylthiouracil
	Fetal hypothyroidism—intra-amniotic thyroxine
Bartter syndrome	Maternal indomethacin may prevent nephrocalcinosis and postnatal sodium losses
Fetal Distress	
Hypoxia	Maternal oxygen, position
Intrauterine growth restriction	Maternal oxygen, position, improve nutrition if deficient
Oligohydramnios, premature rupture of membranes with variable deceleration	Amnioinfusion (antepartum and intrapartum)
Polyhydramnios	Amnioreduction (serial), indomethacin (if due to ↑ urine output) if indicated
Supraventricular tachycardia	Maternal digoxin,* flecainide, procainamide, amiodarone, quinidine
Lupus anticoagulant	Maternal aspirin, prednisone
Meconium-stained fluid	Amnioinfusion
Congenital heart block	Dexamethasone, pacemaker (with hydrops)
Premature labor	Sympathomimetics, magnesium sulfate, antibiotics
Respiratory	
Pulmonary immaturity	Betamethasone
Bilateral chylothorax—pleural effusions	Thoracentesis, pleuroamniotic shunt
Congenital Abnormalities†	
Neural tube defects	Folate, vitamins (prevention); surgery‡
Diaphragmatic hernia	Surgery (correction or plug therapy) (?)‡
Obstructive uropathy (with oligohydramnios but without renal dysplasia)	>24 wk <32 wk, vesicoamniotic shunt plus amnioinfusion
Cystic adenomatoid malformation (with hydrops)	Pleuroamniotic shunt or resection‡
Fetal neck masses	Secure an airway‡
Infectious Disease	
Group B streptococcus	Ampicillin, penicillin (prevention)
Chorioamnionitis	Antibiotics
Toxoplasmosis	Spiramycin, pyrimethamine, sulfadiazine, and folic acid
Syphilis	Penicillin
Tuberculosis	Antituberculosis drugs
Lyme disease	Penicillin, ceftriaxone
Parvovirus	Intrauterine red blood cell transfusion for hydrops, severe anemia
Chlamydia trachomatis	Erythromycin
HIV-AIDS	Zidovudine (AZT) plus protease inhibitors
Cytomegalovirus	Ganciclovir by umbilical vein

Table continued on following page

TABLE 85–5. **Fetal Therapy** *Continued*

Disorder	Possible Treatment
Other	
Nonimmune hydrops (anemia)	Umbilical vein packed red blood cell transfusion
Narcotic abstinence (withdrawal)	Maternal low-dose methadone
Severe combined immunodeficiency disease	Fetal stem cell transplantation
Sacrococcygeal teratoma (with hydrops)	In utero resection or vessel obliteration
Twin-twin transfusion syndrome	Repeated amniocentesis, YAG laser photocoagulation of shared vessels
Twin reversed arterial perfusion syndrome (TRAP)	Digoxin, indomethacin, cord occlusion
Multifetal gestation	Selective reduction

(?) *Denotes possible but not proved efficacy.*
*Drug of choice (may require percutaneous umbilical cord sampling and umbilical vein administration if hydrops is present). Most drug therapy is given to the mother, with subsequent placental passage to the fetus.
†Detailed fetal ultrasonography is needed to detect other anomalies; karyotype is also indicated.
‡Ex utero intrapartum treatment permits surgery and other procedures.

ease's natural history; an understanding of fetal nutrition, pharmacology, immunology, and pathophysiology; the availability of antimicrobial and antiviral drugs; and therapeutic procedures. Progress in providing specific treatments for accurately diagnosed diseases has improved with the advent of real-time ultrasonography and cordocentesis (see Tables 85–1 and 85–5).

The incidence of sensitization of Rh-negative women by Rh-positive fetuses has been reduced by prophylactic administration of Rh(D) immunoglobulin to mothers early in pregnancy and after each delivery or abortion, thus reducing the frequency of hemolytic disease in their subsequent offspring. Fetal erythroblastosis (Chapter 92) may be accurately diagnosed by amniotic fluid analysis and treated with intrauterine intraperitoneal or, more often, intraumbilical vein transfusions of packed Rh-negative blood cells to maintain the fetus until it is mature enough to have a reasonable chance of survival.

Fetal hypoxia or distress may now be diagnosed with moderate success. Treatment, however, remains limited to supplying the mother with high concentrations of oxygen, positioning the uterus to avoid vascular compression, and initiating operative delivery before severe fetal injury occurs.

Pharmacologic approaches to fetal immaturity (e.g., administration of steroids to the mother to accelerate fetal lung maturation and to decrease the incidence of respiratory distress syndrome [Chapter 90] in prematurely delivered infants) are successful. Inhibiting labor with β-sympathomimetic tocolytic agents is unfortunately not successful in most patients with premature labor. Management of definitively diagnosed fetal genetic disease or congenital anomalies consists of parental counseling or abortion; rarely, high-dose vitamin therapy for a responsive inborn error of metabolism (e.g., biotin-dependent disorders) or fetal transfusion (with red blood cells or platelets) may be indicated. Fetal surgery (see Table 85–5) remains an experimental approach to therapy and is available only in a few highly specialized perinatal centers. The nature of the defect and its consequences, as well as ethical implications for the fetus and the parents, must be considered.

Bell EM, Hertz-Picciotto I, Beaumont JJ: A case-control study of pesticides and fetal death due to congenital anomalies. *Epidemiology* 2001;12:148.

Bianchi DW, Lo YM: Fetomaternal cellular and plasma DNA trafficking: The Yin and the Yang. *Ann N Y Acad Sci* 2001;945:119.

Bischoff FZ, Lewis DE, Nguyen DD, et al: Prenatal diagnosis with use of fetal cells isolated from maternal blood: Five-color fluorescent in situ hybridization analysis on flow-sorted cells for chromosomes X, Y, 13, 18, and 21. *Am J Obstet Gynecol* 1998;179:203.

Boyle RJ: Effects of certain prenatal drugs on the fetus and newborn. *Pediatr Rev* 2002;23:17–23.

Castilla EE, Lopez-Camelo JS, Campana H, et al: Epidemiological methods to assess the correlation between industrial contaminants and rates of congenital anomalies. *Mutat Res* 2001;489:123.

Coles CD: Fetal alcohol exposure and attention: Moving beyond ADHD. *Alcohol Res Health* 2001;25:199.

Dudley JA, Haworth JM, McGraw ME, et al: Clinical relevance and implications of antenatal hydronephrosis. *Arch Dis Child* 1997;76:F31.

Electronic fetal heart rate monitoring: Research guidelines for interpretation. National Institute of Child Health and Human Development Research Planning Workshop. *Am J Obstet Gynecol* 1997;177:1385.

Fattibene P, Mazzei F, Nuccetelli, et al: Prenatal exposure to ionizing radiation: Sources, effects and regulatory aspects. *Acta Paediatr* 1999;88:693.

Fetal therapy—ethical considerations. American Academy of Pediatrics. Committee on Bioethics. *Pediatrics* 1999;103:1061.

Flake AW, Zanjani ED: In utero hematopoietic stem cell transplantation. *JAMA* 1997;278:932.

Gonzalez C, Marquez-Dias M, Kim C, et al: Congenital abnormalities in Brazilian children associated with misoprostol misuse in the first trimester of pregnancy. *Lancet* 1998;351:1624.

Graham JM Jr, Edwards MJ, Edwards MJ: Teratogen update: Gestational effects of maternal hyperthermia due to febrile illnesses and resultant patterns of defects in humans. *Teratology* 1998;58:209.

Haddad B, Mercer BM, Livingston JC, et al: Obstetric antecedents to apparent stillbirth (Apgar score zero at 1 minute only). *Obstet Gynecol* 2001;97:961.

Haddow JE, Palomaki GE, Allan WC, et al: Maternal thyroid deficiency during pregnancy and subsequent neuropsychological development of the child. *N Engl J Med* 1999;341:549.

Holmes N, Harrison MR, Baskin LS: Fetal surgery for posterior urethral valves: Long-term postnatal outcomes. *Pediatrics* 2001;108:E7.

Honein MA, Paulozzi LJ, Mathews TJ, et al: Impact of folic acid fortification of the US food supply on the occurrence of neural tube defects. *JAMA* 2001;285:2981–6.

Jones KJ, Lacro RV, Johnson KA, et al: Pattern of malformations in the children of women treated with carbamazepine during pregnancy. *N Engl J Med* 1989;320:1661.

Kaufman RH, Adam E, Hatch EE, et al: Continued follow-up of pregnancy outcomes in diethylstilbestrol-exposed offspring. *Obstet Gynecol* 2000;96:483.

Khattak S, K-Moghtader G, McMartin K, et al: Pregnancy outcome following gestational exposure to organic solvents: A prospective controlled study. *JAMA* 1999;281:1106.

Kimber C, Spitz L, Cuschieri A: Current state of antenatal in utero surgical interventions. *Arch Dis Child* 1997;76:F134.

Koch S, Jäger-Roman E, Lösche G, et al: Antiepileptic drug treatment in pregnancy: Drug side effects in the neonate and neurological outcome. *Acta Paediatr* 1996;84:739.

Koren G, Pastuszak A, Ito S: Drugs in pregnancy. *N Engl J Med* 1998;338:1128.

Kruger K, Hallberg B, Blennow M, et al: Predictive value of fetal scalp blood lactate concentration and pH as markers of neurologic disability. *Am J Obstet Gynecol* 1999;181:1072.

Kulin NA, Pastuszak A, Sage SR, et al: Pregnancy outcome following maternal use of the new selective serotonin reuptake inhibitors. *JAMA* 1998;279:609.

Lammer EJ, Chen CT, Hoar RM, et al: Retinoic acid embryopathy. *N Engl J Med* 1985;313:837.

Lenfant C: Working group report on high blood pressure in pregnancy. *J Clin Hypertens (Greenwich)* 2001;3:75.

Leviton A, Paneth N, Reuss ML, et al: Maternal infection, fetal inflammatory response, and brain damage in very low birth weight infants. *Pediatr Res* 1999;46:566.

Liechty KW, Crombleholme TM, Flake AW, et al: Intrapartum airway management for giant fetal neck masses: The EXIT (ex utero intrapartum treatment) procedure. *Am J Obstet Gynecol* 1997;177:870–4.

Loffredo CA, Wilson PD, Ferencz C: Maternal diabetes: An independent risk factor for major cardiovascular malformations with increased mortality of affected infants. *Teratology* 2001;64:98.

Lumley J, Watson L, Watson M, et al: Periconceptional supplementation with folate and/or multivitamins for preventing neural tube defects (Cochrane Review). *Cochrane Database Syst Rev* 2001;3:CD001056.

Lyerly AD, Gates EA, Cefalo RC: Toward the ethical evaluation and use of maternal-fetal surgery. *Obstet Gynecol* 2001;98:689.

Manning FA, Snijders R, Harman CR, et al: Fetal biophysical profile score. VI. Correlation with antepartum umbilical venous fetal pH. *Am J Obstet Gynecol* 1993;169:755.

McDonnell M, Serra-Serra V, Gaffney G, et al: Neonatal outcome after pregnancy complicated by abnormal velocity waveforms in the umbilical artery. *Arch Dis Child* 1994;70:F84.

Mercer BM, Miodovnik M, Thurnau GR, et al: Antibiotic therapy for reduction of infant morbidity after preterm premature rupture of the membranes. *JAMA* 1997;278:989.

Molloy AM, Daly S, Mills JL, et al: Thermolabile variant of 5,10-methylenetetrahydrofolate reductase associated with low red cell folates: Implications for folate intake recommendations. *Lancet* 1997;349:1591.

Ott WJ: Intrauterine growth restriction and Doppler ultrasonography. *J Ultrasound Med* 2000;19:661.

Park-Wyllie L, Mazzotta P, Pastuszak A, et al: Birth defects after maternal exposure to corticosteroids: Prospective cohort study and meta-analysis of epidemiological studies. *Teratology* 2000;62:385–92.

Pauli RM, Lian JB, Mosher DF, et al: Association of congenital deficiency of multiple vitamin K–dependent coagulation factors and the phenotype of the warfarin embryopathy: Clues to the mechanism of teratogenicity of coumarin derivatives. *Am J Hum Genet* 1987;41:566.

Prontera W, Jaeggi ET, Pfizenmaier M, et al: Ex utero intrapartum treatment (EXIT) of severe fetal hydrothorax. *Arch Dis Child* 2002;86:F58–60.

Stickler SM, Dansky LV, Miller MA, et al: Genetic predisposition to phenytoin-induced birth defects. *Lancet* 1985;2:746.

Sutton L, Sun P, Adzick N: Fetal Neurosurgery. *Neurosurgery* 2001;48:124.

Theion ATA, Soothill P: Antenatal invasive therapy. *Eur J Pediatr* 1998;157:52.

van der Put NM, van den Heuvel LP, Steegers-Theunissen RP, et al: Decreased methylene tetrahydrofolate reductase activity due to the 677C → T mutation in families with spina bifida offspring. *J Mol Med* 1996;74:691.

Wachtel SS, Shulman LP, Sammons D: Fetal cells in maternal blood. *Clin Genet* 2001;59:74.

Wald N, Leck I: *Antenatal & Neonatal Screening*, 2nd ed. Oxford, Oxford University Press, 2000.

Wang X, Chen D, Niu T, et al: Genetic susceptibility to benzene and shortened gestation: Evidence of gene-environment interaction. *Am J Epidemiol* 2000; 152:693.

Wang X, Zuckerman B, Pearson C, et al: Maternal cigarette smoking, metabolic gene polymorphism, and infant birth weight. *JAMA* 2002;287:195–202.

Wu YW, Colford JM Jr: Chorioamnionitis as a risk factor for cerebral palsy. *JAMA* 2000;284:1417.

Chapter 86

The High-Risk Infant

Barbara J. Stoll and Robert M. Kliegman

Infants at risk during the neonatal period should be identified as early as possible to decrease neonatal morbidity and mortality (see also Chapter 82). The term *high-risk infant* designates an infant who should be under close observation by experienced physicians and nurses. Infants in the high-risk category are listed in Box 86–1. Approximately 9% of all births require special or neonatal intensive care. Usually needed for only a few days, such observation may last from a few hours to several months. Some institutions find it advantageous to provide a special or transitional care nursery for high-risk infants, often within the labor and delivery suite. This facility should be equipped and staffed similar to a neonatal intensive care area.

Examination of fresh *placenta, cord,* and *membranes* may alert the physician to newborn infants at high risk and may help confirm a diagnosis in a sick infant. Fetal blood loss may be indicated by placental pallor, **retroplacental hematoma,** and tears in the velamentous cords or chorionic blood vessels supplying the succenturiate lobes. **Placental edema** and subsequent immunoglobulin G deficiency in newborns may be associated with fetofetal transfusion syndrome, hydrops fetalis, congenital nephrosis, or hepatic disease. **Amnion nodosum** (granules on the amnion) and **oligohydramnios** are associated with pulmonary hypoplasia and renal agenesis, whereas small whitish **nodules** on the cord suggest a candidal infection. **Short cords** and non-coiled cords occur with chromosome abnormalities and omphalocele. True umbilical cord **knots** are seen in approximately 1% of births and are associated with a long cord, small fetal size, polyhydramnios, monoamniotic twinning, fetal demise, and low Apgar scores.

Chorioangiomas are associated with prematurity, abruptio, polyhydramnios, and intrauterine growth restriction (IUGR).

Meconium staining suggests in utero stress and increases the risk for pneumonia, and opacity of the fetal placental surface suggests infection. **Single umbilical arteries** are associated with an increased incidence of congenital abnormalities.

Many infants who are born prematurely, are small for gestational age (SGA), have significant perinatal asphyxia, are breech, or are born with life-threatening congenital anomalies do not have previously identified risk factors. For any given duration of gestation, the lower the birthweight, the higher the neonatal mortality; for any given weight, the shorter the gestational duration, the higher the neonatal mortality (Fig. 86–1). The highest risk of neonatal mortality occurs in infants who weigh less than 1,000 g at birth and whose gestation was less than 30 wk. The lowest risk of neonatal mortality occurs in infants with a birth-

---

BOX 86–1. High-Risk Infants

DEMOGRAPHIC SOCIAL FACTORS

Maternal age <16 or >40 yr
Illicit drug, alcohol, cigarette use
Poverty
Unmarried
Emotional or physical stress

PAST MEDICAL HISTORY

Genetic disorders
Diabetes mellitus
Hypertension
Asymptomatic bacteriuria
Rheumatologic illness (SLE)
Long-term medication (see Tables 85–3 and 85–4)

PREVIOUS PREGNANCY

Intrauterine fetal demise
Neonatal death
Prematurity
Intrauterine growth restriction
Congenital malformation
Incompetent cervix
Blood group sensitization, neonatal jaundice
Neonatal thrombocytopenia
Hydrops
Inborn errors of metabolism

PRESENT PREGNANCY

Vaginal bleeding (abruptio placentae, placenta previa)
Sexually transmitted diseases (colonization: herpes simplex, group B streptococcus), chlamydia, syphilis, hepatitis B, HIV
Multiple gestation
Preeclampsia
Premature rupture of membranes
Short interpregnancy time
Poly-oligohydramnios
Acute medical or surgical illness
Inadequate prenatal care
Familial or acquired hypercoagulable states
Treatment of infertility

LABOR AND DELIVERY

Premature labor (<37 wk)
Postdates (>42 wk)
Fetal distress
Immature L:S ratio; absent phosphatidylglycerol
Breech presentation
Meconium-stained fluid
Nuchal cord
Cesarean section
Forceps delivery
Apgar score <4 at 1 min

NEONATE

Birthweight <2,500 or >4,000 g
Birth before 37 or after 42 wk of gestation
SGA, LGA growth status
Tachypnea, cyanosis
Congenital malformation
Pallor, plethora, petechiae

SLE = systemic lupus erythematosus; L:S = lecithin:sphingomyelin ratio; SGA = small for gestational age; LGA = large for gestational age.

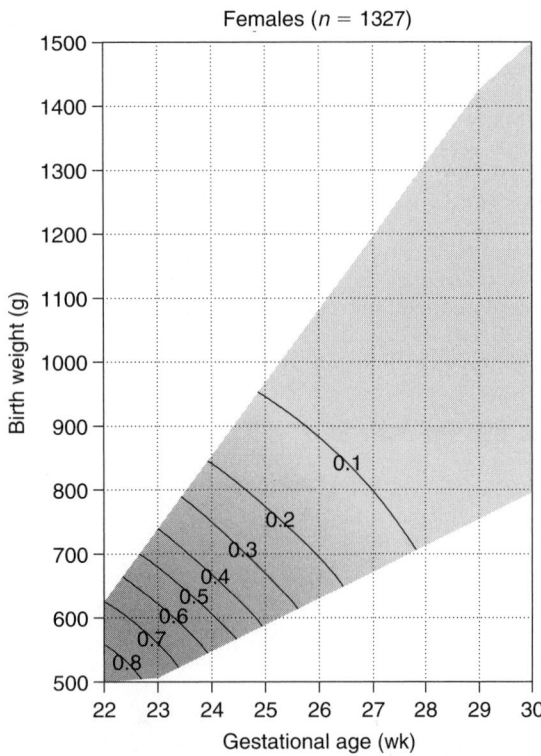
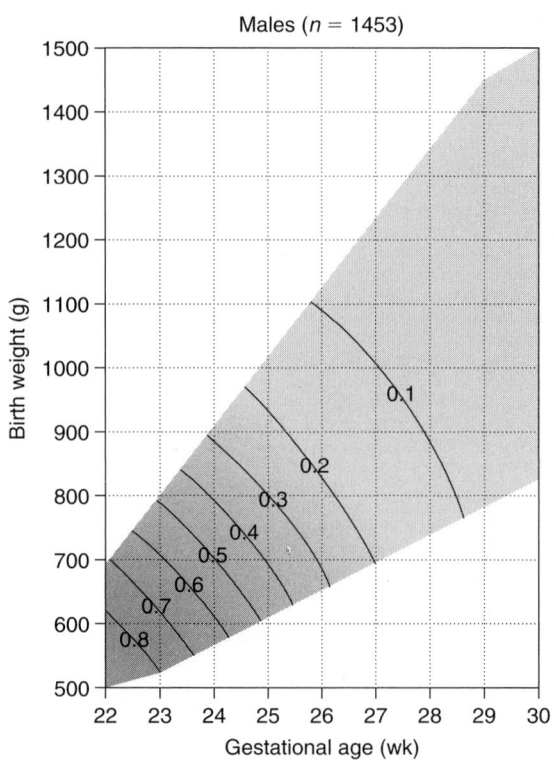

FIGURE 86–1. Estimated mortality risk by birthweight and gestational age based on singleton infants in NICHD Neonatal Research Network Centers between January 1, 1995, and December 31, 1996. (From Lemons JA, Bauers CR, OH W, et al: Very low birthweight outcomes of the National Institute of Child Health and Human Development Neonatal Research Network, January 1995 through December 1996. *Pediatrics* 2001;107. (http://www.pediatrics.org.cgi/content/full/107/1/e1)

weight of 3,000–4,000 g and a gestational age of 38–42 wk. As birthweight increases from 500 to 3,000 g, a logarithmic decrease in neonatal mortality occurs; for every week increase in gestational age from the 25th to the 37th wk, the neonatal mortality rate decreases by approximately half. Nevertheless, approximately 40% of all *perinatal deaths* occur after 37 wk of gestation in infants weighing 2,500 g or more; many of these deaths take place in the period immediately before birth and are more readily preventable than those of smaller and more immature infants. In addition, neonatal mortality rates rise sharply for infants weighing over 4,000 g at birth and for those whose gestational period is 42 wk or longer. Because neonatal mortality largely depends on birthweight and gestational age, Figure 86–1 can be used to help identify high-risk infants quickly. However, this analysis is based on total live births and therefore describes the mortality risk only *at birth*. Because most neonatal mortality occurs within the first hours and days after birth, the outlook improves dramatically with increasing postnatal survival.

Airas U, Heinonen S: Clinical significance of true umbilical knots: A population-based analysis. *Am J Perinatol* 2002;19:127–32.

Amini SB, Catalano PM, Hirsch V, et al: An analysis of birth weight by gestational age using a computerized perinatal data base, 1975–1992. *Obstet Gynecol* 1994;83:342.

Grether JK, Eaton A, Redline R, et al: Reliability of placental histology using archived specimens. *Paediatr Perinat Epidemiol* 1999;13:489.

Hansen AR, Collins MH, Genest D, et al: Very low birthweight infant's placenta and its relation to pregnancy and fetal characteristics. *Pediatr Dev Pathol* 2000;3:419.

Lemons JA, Bauer CR, Oh W, et al: Very low birth weight outcomes of the National Institute of Child Health and Human Development Neonatal Research Network, January 1995 through December 1996. *Pediatrics* 2001;107: http://www.pediatrics.org/cgi/content/full/107/1/e1.

Moster D, Lie RT, Markestad T: Relation between size of delivery unit and neonatal death in low risk deliveries: Population based study. *Arch Dis Child Fetal Neonatal Ed* 1999;80:F221.

Vogler C, Petterchak J, Sotelo-Avila C, et al: Placental pathology for the surgical pathologist. *Adv Anat Pathol* 2000;7:214.

86.1   Multiple Pregnancies

Incidence. The reported incidence of spontaneous twinning is highest among blacks and East Indians, followed by northern European whites, and it is lowest in the Asian races. Specific rates include 1/56 in Belgium, 1/70 in American blacks; 1/86 in Italy; 1/88 in American whites; 1/130 in Greece; 1/150 in Japan; and 1/300 in China. Differences in the incidence of twins mainly involve fraternal (polyovular) dizygotic twins. Triplets are estimated to occur in 1 in 86^2 pregnancies and quadruplets in 1 in 86^3 pregnancies in the United States. The incidence of monozygotic twins is unaffected by racial or familial factors (3–5/1,000). The incidence of twins detected by ultrasonography at 12 wk of gestation (3–5%) is much higher than that occurring later in pregnancy; the vanishing twin syndrome results in a singleton fetus. Although the incidence of spontaneous multifetal gestation is stable, the overall incidence is increasing as a result of treatment of infertility with ovarian stimulants (clomiphene, gonadotropins) and in vitro fertilization. Twins represent about 2.5% of births but 20% of very low birthweight (VLBW) infants.

Etiology. The occurrence of monovular twins appears to be independent of genetic influence. Polyovular pregnancies are more frequent beyond the 2nd pregnancy, in older women, and in families with a history of polyovular twins. They may result from simultaneous maturation of multiple ovarian follicles, but follicles containing two ova have been described as a genetic trait leading to twin pregnancies. Twin-prone women have higher levels of gonadotropin. Polyovular pregnancies occur in many women treated for infertility.

Conjoined twins (Siamese twins—incidence, 1/50,000) probably result from relatively late monovular separation, as does the presence of two separate embryos in one amniotic sac. The latter condition has a high fatality rate that is due to obstruction of the circulation secondary to intertwining of the umbilical cords. The prognosis for conjoined twins depends on the possibility of surgical separation, which in turn depends on the degree that vital organs are shared. The site of connections varies: thoraco-omphalopagus (28% of conjoined twins), thoracopagus (18%), omphalopagus (10%), craniopagus (6%), and incomplete duplication (10%). Most conjoined twins are female.

Superfecundation, or fertilization of an ovum by an insemination that takes place after one ovum has already been fertilized, and *superfetation,* or fertilization and subsequent development of an ovum when a fetus is already present in the uterus, have been proposed as uncommon explanations for differences in size and appearance of certain twins at birth.

A *prenatal diagnosis of pregnancy with twins* is suggested by a uterine size that is greater than that expected for gestational age, auscultation of two fetal hearts, and elevated maternal serum α-fetoprotein or human chorionic gonadotropin levels, and it is confirmed by ultrasound. Ninety per cent of twins are detected before delivery.

Monozygotic vs Dizygotic Twins. Identifying twins as monozygotic or dizygotic (monovular or polyovular) is important because studying monozygotic twins is useful in determining the relative influence of heredity and environment on human development and disease. Twins not of the same sex are dizygotic. In twins of the same sex, zygosity should be determined and recorded at birth through careful examination of the placenta or later through comparison of physical characteristics, detailed blood typing, DNA fingerprinting, or tissue (HLA) typing. Monozygotic twins may have physical and cognitive differences because their in utero environment may be different; differences may exist in the mitochondrial genome, in post-translational gene product modification, and in the expression of nuclear genes in response to environmental factors (nutrition).

EXAMINATION OF THE PLACENTA. If the placentas are separate, they are always dichorionic (present in 75%), but the twins are not necessarily dizygotic because initiation of monovular twinning at the 1st cell division or during the morula stage may result in two amnions, two chorions, and even two placentas. One third of monozygotic twins are dichorionic and diamnionic.

An apparently single placenta may be present with either monovular or polyovular twins, yet inspection of a polyovular placenta usually reveals that each twin has a separate chorion that crosses the placenta between the attachments of the cords and two amnions. Separate or fused dichorionic placentas may be disproportionate in size. The fetus attached to the smaller placenta or the smaller portion of the placenta is usually smaller than its twin or is malformed. Monochorionic twins may be presumed to be monovular. They are usually diamnionic, and almost invariably, the placenta is a single mass.

Problems of twin gestation include polyhydramnios, hyperemesis gravidarum, preeclampsia, premature rupture of membranes, vasa previa, velamentous insertion of the umbilical cord, abnormal presentations (breech), and premature labor. When compared with the first-born twin, the second or B twin is at increased risk for respiratory distress syndrome and asphyxia. Twins are at risk for IUGR, twin-twin transfusion, and congenital anomalies, which occur predominantly in monozygotic twins. Anomalies are due to compression deformation of the uterus from crowding (hip dislocation), vascular communication with embolization (ileal atresia, porencephaly, cutis aplasia) or without embolization (acardiac twin), and unknown factors that cause twinning (conjoined twins, anencephaly, meningomyelocele).

Placental vascular anastomoses occur with high frequency only in monochorionic twins. In monochorionic placentas, the fetal vasculature is usually joined, sometimes in a very complex manner. The vascular anastomoses in monochorionic placentas may be artery to artery, vein to vein, or artery to vein. They are usually well enough balanced so that neither twin suffers. Artery-to-artery communications cross over placental veins, and

when anastomoses are present, blood can readily be stroked from one fetal vascular bed to the other. Vein-to-vein communications are similarly recognized but are less common. A combination of artery-to-artery and vein-to-vein anastomoses is associated with the condition of lethal *acardiac fetus.* This rare lethal anomaly (1/35,000) is secondary to the TRAP sequence—twin reversed arterial perfusion. Nd:YAG laser ablation of the anastomosis or cord occlusion in utero can be used to treat heart failure in the surviving twin. In rare cases, one umbilical cord may arise from the other after leaving the placenta. In such cases, the twin attached to the secondary cord is usually malformed or dies in utero. Table 86–1 lists the more frequent changes associated with a large uncompensated arteriovenous shunt from the placenta of one twin to that of the other; twins of widely discrepant size are usually monochorionic.

In the **fetal transfusion syndrome,** an artery from one twin acutely or chronically delivers blood that is drained into the vein of the other. The latter becomes plethoric and large, and the former is anemic and small. Generally, with chronicity, a 5 g/dL hemoglobin and 20% body weight difference can be noted in this syndrome. Maternal hydramnios in a twin pregnancy suggests fetal transfusion syndrome. Anticipating this possibility by preparing to transfuse the donor twin or bleed the recipient twin may be lifesaving. Death of the donor twin in utero may result in generalized fibrin thrombi in the smaller arterioles of the recipient twin, possibly as the result of transfusion of thromboplastin-rich blood from the macerating donor fetus. Disseminated intravascular coagulation may develop in the surviving twin. Treatment of this highly lethal problem includes maternal digoxin, aggressive amnioreduction for polyhydramnios, selective twin termination, or Nd:YAG laser or fetoscopic ablation of the anastomosis.

POSTNATAL IDENTIFICATION. The following *physical criteria* can be used to determine whether twins are monovular: (1) both must be of the same sex; (2) their features, including ears and teeth, must be obviously alike (but they need not resemble each other more than the lateral halves of one individual); (3) their hair must be identical in color, texture, natural curl, and distribution; (4) their eyes must be of the same color and shade; (5) their skin must be of the same texture and color (nevi may be differently apportioned and distributed); (6) their hands and feet must be of the same conformation and of similar size; and (7) their anthropometric values must show close agreement.

Prognosis. Most twins are born prematurely, and maternal complications of pregnancy are more common than with single pregnancies. Although monochorionic twins have a significant increase in perinatal mortality, there is no significant difference between the neonatal mortality rates of twin and single births in comparable weight groups. Because most twins are premature by weight, their overall mortality is higher than that of single

TABLE 86–1. **Characteristic Changes in Monochorionic Twins with Uncompensated Placental Arteriovenous Shunts**

Twin on	
Arterial Side—Donor	*Venous Side—Recipient*
Prematurity	Prematurity
Oligohydramnios	Polyhydramnios
Small premature	Hydrops
Malnourished	Large premature
Pale	Well nourished
Anemic	Plethoric
Hypovolemia	Polycythemic
Hypoglycemia	Hypervolemic
Microcardia	Cardiac hypertrophy
Glomeruli small or normal	Myocardial dysfunction
Arterioles thin walled	Tricuspid valve regurgitation
	Right ventricular outflow obstruction
	Glomeruli large
	Arterioles thick walled

births. The perinatal mortality of twins is about four times that of singletons. Monoamnionic twins have an increased likelihood of entangling their cords, which may lead to asphyxia. Theoretically, the 2nd twin is more subject to anoxia than the 1st because the placenta may separate after birth of the 1st twin and before birth of the 2nd. In addition, delivery of the 2nd twin may be difficult because it may be in an abnormal presentation (breech, entangled), uterine tone may be decreased, or the cervix may begin to close after the 1st twin's birth. A growth-retarded twin is at high risk for hypoglycemia. Any notable difference in the size of monovular twins at birth usually disappears by the time that the infants are 6 mo of age. The mortality for multiple gestations with four or more fetuses is excessively high for each fetus. Because of this poor prognosis, selective fetal reduction (with transabdominal intrathoracic injection of KCl) to two to three fetuses has been offered as a treatment option. Monozygotic twins have an increased risk of one twin dying in utero. The surviving twin has a greater risk for cerebral palsy and other neurodevelopmental sequelae.

Treatment. Prenatal diagnosis enables the obstetrician and pediatrician to anticipate the birth of infants who are at high risk because of twinning. Close observation is indicated during labor and in the immediate neonatal period so that prompt treatment of asphyxia or fetal transfusion syndrome can be initiated. The decision to perform an immediate blood transfusion in a severely anemic "donor twin" or to perform a partial exchange transfusion of a "recipient twin" must be based on clinical judgment.

Dechaud H, Picot MC, Hedon B, et al: First-trimester multifetal pregnancy reduction: Evaluation of technical aspects and risks from 2,756 cases in the literature. *Fetal Diagn Ther* 1998;13:261.

Donovan EF, Ehrenkranz RA, Shankaran S, et al: Outcomes of very low birth weight twins cared for in the National Institute of Child Health and Human Development Neonatal Research Network's intensive care units. *Am J Obstet Gynecol* 1998;179:742.

Evans MI, Hume RF, Polak S, et al: The geriatric gravida: Multifetal pregnancy reduction, donor eggs, and aggressive infertility treatments. *Am J Obstet Gynecol* 1997;177:875.

Glinianaia S, Pharoah POD, Wright C, et al: Fetal or infant death in twin pregnancy: Neurodevelopmental consequence for the survivor. *Arch Dis Child* 2002;86:F9–15.

Hartley RS, Emanuel I, Hitti J: Perinatal mortality and neonatal morbidity rates among twin pairs at different gestational ages: Optimal delivery timing at 37 to 38 weeks' gestation. *Am J Obstet Gynecol* 2001;184:451.

Kogan MD, Alexander GR, Kotelchuck M, et al: Trends in twin birth outcomes and prenatal care utilization in the United States, 1981–1997. *JAMA* 2000;284:335.

Mari G, Roberts A, Detti L, et al: Perinatal morbidity and mortality rates in severe twin-twin transfusion syndrome: Results of the International Amnioreduction Registry. *Am J Obstet Gynecol* 2001;185:708.

Norwitz ER, Hoyte LPJ, Jenkins KJ, et al: Brief report: Separation of conjoined twins with the twin reversed-arterial-perfusion sequence after prenatal planning with three-dimensional modeling. *N Engl J Med* 2000;343:399.

Pearn J: Bioethical issues in caring for conjoined twins and their parents. *Lancet* 2001;357:1968.

Pharoah POD: Twins and cerebral palsy. *Acta Paediatr Suppl* 2001;436:6–10.

Reynolds MA, Schieve LA, Jeng G, et al: Risk of multiple birth associated with in vitro fertilization using donor eggs. *Am J Epidemiol* 2001;154:1043.

86.2 Prematurity and Intrauterine Growth Retardation

Definitions. Liveborn* infants delivered before 37 wk from the 1st day of the last menstrual period are termed *premature* by the World Health Organization. Low birthweight (LBW; birthweight

---

*Live birth is defined by the World Health Assembly (1950) as "the complete expulsion or extraction from its mother of a product of conception which, after such separation, breathes or shows any other evidence of life such as beating of the heart, pulsation of the umbilical cord, or definite movement of the voluntary muscles, whether or not the umbilical cord has been cut or the placenta is attached." This definition is approved by the American Public Health Association.

of 2500 g or less) is due to prematurity, poor intrauterine growth (IUGR, also referred to as *SGA*), or both. Prematurity and IUGR are associated with increased neonatal morbidity and mortality. Ideally, definitions of LBW for individual populations should be based on data that are as genetically and environmentally homogeneous as possible. Figure 86–1 presents variations in neonatal mortality based on birthweight, gestational age, and gender.

Incidence. In 2000, 7.6% of liveborn neonates in the United States weighed less than 2,500 g; the rate for blacks was almost twice that for whites. Over the past 2 decades, the LBW rate has increased primarily because of an increased number of preterm births. Women whose 1st births are delivered before term are at increased risk for recurrent preterm delivery. Approximately 30% of LBW infants in the United States have IUGR and are born after 37 wk. At LBW rates greater than 10%, the contribution of IUGR increases and that of prematurity decreases. In developing countries, approximately 70% of LBW infants have IUGR. Infants with IUGR have greater morbidity and mortality than do appropriately grown, gestational age–matched infants (see Fig. 86–1).

Very Low Birthweight Infants. VLBW infants weigh less than 1,500 g and are predominantly premature. In the United States in 2000, the VLBW rate was approximately 1.4%, 3.1% in blacks and 1.1% in whites. The VLBW rate is an accurate predictor of the infant mortality rate. VLBW infants account for over 50% of neonatal deaths and 50% of handicapped infants; their survival is directly related to birthweight, with approximately 20% of those between 500 and 600 g and over 90% of those between 1,250 and 1,500 g surviving. The VLBW rate has remained unchanged for black Americans but has increased in whites, perhaps because of a rise in multiple births in whites. Perinatal care has improved the rate of survival of LBW infants. When compared with term infants, VLBW neonates have a higher incidence of rehospitalization during the 1st yr of life for sequelae of prematurity, infections, neurologic complications, and psychosocial disorders (see later discussion in this section on prognosis).

Factors Related to Premature Birth and Low Birthweight. It is difficult to completely separate factors associated with prematurity from those associated with IUGR (see also Chapters 83 and 84). A strong positive correlation exists between both preterm birth and IUGR and low socioeconomic status. Families of low socioeconomic status have higher rates of maternal undernutrition, anemia, and illness; inadequate prenatal care; drug misuse; obstetric complications; and maternal histories of reproductive inefficiency (abortions, stillbirths, premature or LBW infants). Other associated factors such as single-parent families, teenage pregnancies, short inter-pregnancy interval, and mothers who have borne more than four previous children are also encountered more frequently. Systematic differences in fetal growth have also been described in association with maternal size, birth order, sibling weight, social class, maternal smoking, and other factors. The degree to which the variance in birthweight among various populations is due to environmental (extrafetal) rather than genetic differences in growth potential is difficult to determine.

The etiology of preterm birth is multifactorial and involves a complex interaction between fetal, placental, uterine, and maternal factors (Box 86–2).

Premature birth of infants whose LBW is appropriate for their preterm gestational age is associated with medical conditions characterized by an inability of the uterus to retain the fetus, interference with the course of the pregnancy, premature rupture of the amniotic membranes or premature separation of the placenta, or an undetermined stimulus to effective uterine contractions before term.

Overt or asymptomatic bacterial infection (group B streptococci, *Listeria monocytogenes*, *Ureaplasma urealyticum*, *Mycoplasma*

BOX 86–2. Identifiable Causes of Preterm Birth

FETAL
Fetal distress
Multiple gestation
Erythroblastosis
Nonimmune hydrops

PLACENTAL
Placental dysfunction
Placenta previa
Abruptio placentae

UTERINE
Bicornuate uterus
Incompetent cervix (premature dilatation)

MATERNAL
Preeclampsia
Chronic medical illness (e.g., cyanotic heart disease, renal disease)
Infection (e.g., *Listeria monocytogenes*, group B streptococcus, urinary tract infection, bacterial vaginosis, chorioamnionitis)
Drug abuse (e.g., cocaine)

OTHER
Premature rupture of membranes
Polyhydramnios
Iatrogenic
Trauma

BOX 86–3. Factors Often Associated with Intrauterine Growth Restriction

FETAL
Chromosomal disorders (e.g., autosomal trisomies)
Chronic fetal infections (e.g., cytomegalic inclusion disease, congenital rubella, syphilis)
Congenital anomalies—syndrome complexes
Irradiation
Multiple gestation
Pancreatic hypoplasia
Insulin deficiency
Insulin-like growth factor type I deficiency

PLACENTAL
Decreased placental weight or cellularity, or both
Decrease in surface area
Villous placentitis (bacterial, viral, parasitic)
Infarction
Tumor (chorioangioma, hydatidiform mole)
Placental separation
Twin transfusion syndrome

MATERNAL
Toxemia
Hypertension or renal disease, or both
Hypoxemia (high altitude, cyanotic cardiac or pulmonary disease)
Malnutrition or chronic illness
Sickle cell anemia
Drugs (narcotics, alcohol, cigarettes, cocaine, antimetabolites)

hominis, Chlamydia, Trichomonas vaginalis, Gardnerella vaginalis, Bacteroides spp.) of the amniotic fluid and membranes (chorioamnionitis) may initiate preterm labor. Bacterial products may stimulate the production of local inflammatory mediators (interleukin 6, prostaglandins), which may induce premature uterine contractions or a local inflammatory response with focal membrane rupture. Appropriate antibiotic therapy reduces the risk of fetal infection and may prolong gestation. The use of β-sympathomimetic receptor agonists (ritodrine, terbutaline) has not prevented premature birth. Other agents (indomethacin) can lead to significant neonatal complications.

IUGR is associated with medical conditions that interfere with the circulation and efficiency of the placenta, with the development or growth of the fetus, or with the general health and nutrition of the mother (Box 86–3). Many factors are common to both prematurely born and LBW infants with IUGR. IUGR is associated with decreased insulin production or insulin (or insulin-like growth factor [IGF]) action at the receptor level. Infants with IGF-I receptor defects, pancreatic hypoplasia, or transient neonatal diabetes have IUGR. Genetic mutations affecting the glucose-sensing mechanisms of the pancreatic islet cells that result in decreased insulin release (loss of function of the glucose-sensing glucokinase gene) give rise to IUGR.

IUGR may be a normal fetal response to nutritional or oxygen deprivation. Therefore, the issue is not the IUGR but rather the ongoing risk of malnutrition or hypoxia. Similarly, some preterm births signify a need for early delivery from a potentially disadvantageous intrauterine environment. IUGR is often classified as reduced growth that is symmetric (head circumference, length, and weight equally affected) or asymmetric (with relative sparing of head growth) (see Fig. 85–1). Symmetric IUGR often has an earlier onset and is associated with diseases that seriously affect fetal cell number, such as conditions with chromosomal, genetic, malformation, teratogenic, infectious, or severe maternal hypertensive etiologies. Asymmetric IUGR is often of late onset, demonstrates preservation of Doppler waveform velocity to the carotid vessels, and is associated with poor maternal nutrition or with late onset or exacerbation of maternal vascular disease (preeclampsia, chronic hypertension). Problems of infants with IUGR are noted in Table 86–2.

Assessment of Gestational Age at Birth. When compared with a premature infant of appropriate weight, an infant with IUGR has a reduced birthweight and may appear to have a *disproportionately larger head relative to body size*; infants in both groups lack subcutaneous fat. Neurologic maturity (e.g., nerve conduction velocity), in the absence of asphyxia, correlates with gestational age despite reduced fetal weight. Physical signs may be useful in estimating gestational age at birth. Commonly used, the Ballard scoring system is accurate to ±2 wk (Figs. 86–2 to 86–4). An infant should be presumed to be at high risk for mortality or morbidity if a discrepancy exists between the estimation of gestational age by physical examination, the mother's estimated date of her last menstrual period, and fetal ultrasonic evaluation.

Spectrum of Disease in Low-Birthweight Infants. Immaturity tends to increase the severity but reduce the distinctiveness of the clinical manifestations of most neonatal diseases. Immature

TABLE 86–2. Problems of IUGR (SGA) Infants

Problem	Pathogenesis
Intrauterine fetal demise	Hypoxia, acidosis, infection, lethal anomaly
Perinatal asphyxia	↓ Uteroplacental perfusion during labor ± chronic fetal hypoxia-acidosis; meconium aspiration syndrome
Hypoglycemia	↓ Tissue glycogen stores, ↓ gluconeogenesis, hyperinsulinism, ↑ glucose needs of hypoxia, hypothermia, large brain
Polycythemia-hyperviscosity	Fetal hypoxia with ↑ erythropoietin production
Reduced oxygen consumption/ hypothermia	Hypoxia, hypoglycemia, starvation effect, poor subcutaneous fat stores
Dysmorphology	Syndrome anomalads, chromosomal-genetic disorders, oligohydramnios-induced deformations, TORCH infection

Other problems include pulmonary hemorrhage and those common to the gestational age–related risks of prematurity if born at less than 37 wk (see Box 86–4).

IUGR = intrauterine growth restriction; SGA = small for gestational age; TORCH = toxoplasmosis, other agents, rubella, cytomegalovirus, herpes simplex.

Physical maturity	−1	0	1	2	3	4	5
Skin	Sticky, friable, transparent	Gelatinous, red, translucent	Smooth, pink, visible veins	Superficial peeling and/or rash, few veins	Cracking, pale areas, rare veins	Parchment, deep cracking, no vessels	Leathery, cracked, wrinkled
Lanugo	None	Sparse	Abundant	Thinning	Bald areas	Mostly bald	
Plantar surface	Heel–toe 40–50 mm: −1 <40 mm: −2	<50 mm, no crease	Faint red marks	Anterior transverse crease only	Creases on ant. 2/3	Creases over entire sole	
Breast	Impercep-tible	Barely perceptible	Flat areola– no bud	Stripped areola, 1–2 mm bud	Raised areola, 3–4 mm bud	Full areola, 5–10 mm bud	
Eye/ear	Lids fused loosely (−1), tightly (−2)	Lids open, pinna flat, stays folded	Slightly curved pinna; soft; slow recoil	Well-curved pinna, soft but ready recoil	Formed and firm, instant recoil	Thick cartilage, ear stiff	
Genitals, male	Scrotum flat, smooth	Scrotum empty, faint rugae	Testes in upper canal, rare rugae	Testes descending, few rugae	Testes down, good rugae	Testes pendulous, deep rugae	
Genitals, female	Clitoris prominent, labia flat	Prominent clitoris, small labia minora	Prominent clitoris, enlarging minora	Majora and minora equally prominent	Majora large, minora small	Majora cover clitoris and minora	

FIGURE 86–2. Physical criteria for maturity. The expanded New Ballard Score includes extremely premature infants and has been refined to improve accuracy in more mature infants. (From Ballard JL, Khoury JC, Wedig K, et al: New Ballard Score, expanded to include extremely premature infants. *J Pediatr* 1991;119:417.)

organ function, complications of therapy, and the specific disorders that caused the premature onset of labor contribute to neonatal morbidity and mortality associated with premature, LBW infants (Box 86–4). Among VLBW infants, morbidity is inversely related to birthweight. Respiratory distress syndrome is noted in approximately 80% of infants 501–750 g, in 65% of those 751–1,000 g, in 45% between 1,001 and 1,250 g, and in 25% between 1,251 and 1,500 g; severe intraventricular hemorrhage (IVH) is noted in approximately 25% of infants 501–750 g, in 12% between 751 and 1,000 g, in 8% between 1,001 and 1,250 g, and in 3% between 1,251 and 1,500 g. Overall, the risk of late sepsis (24%), bronchopulmonary dysplasia (23%), severe IVH (11%), necrotizing enterocolitis (7%),

and prolonged hospitalization (45–125 days) is high in VLBW infants. Problems associated with IUGR LBW infants are noted in Table 86–2; these added problems are often superimposed on those noted in Box 86–4 if an infant with IUGR is also premature. Poor postnatal growth is an important problem for both preterm and IUGR infants.

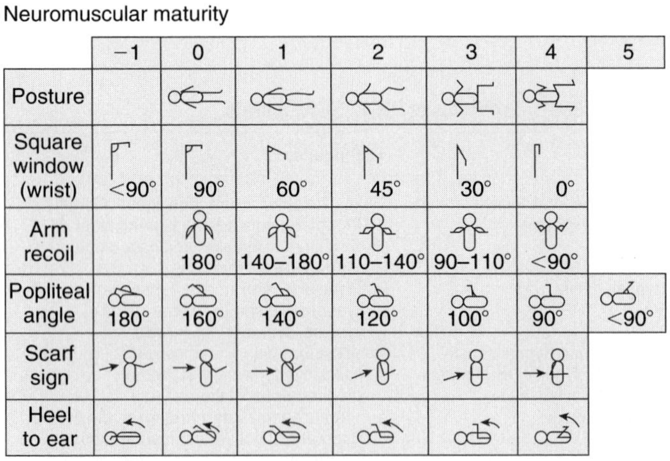

Neuromuscular maturity

	−1	0	1	2	3	4	5
Posture							
Square window (wrist)	<90°	90°	60°	45°	30°	0°	
Arm recoil		180°	140–180°	110–140°	90–110°	<90°	
Popliteal angle	180°	160°	140°	120°	100°	90°	<90°
Scarf sign							
Heel to ear							

FIGURE 86–3. Neuromuscular criteria for maturity. The expanded New Ballard Score includes extremely premature infants and has been refined to improve accuracy in more mature infants. (From Ballard JL, Khoury JC, Wedig K, et al: New Ballard Score, expanded to include extremely premature infants. *J Pediatr* 1991;119:417.)

Maturity Rating

Score	Weeks
−10	20
−5	22
0	24
5	26
10	28
15	30
20	32
25	34
30	36
35	38
40	40
45	42
50	44

FIGURE 86–4. Maturity rating. The physical and neurologic scores are added to calculate gestational age. (From Ballard JL, Khoury JC, Wedig K, et al: New Ballard Score, expanded to include extremely premature infants. *J Pediatr* 1991;119:417.)

BOX 86–4. Neonatal Problems Associated with Premature Infants

RESPIRATORY

Respiratory distress syndrome (hyaline membrane disease)*
Bronchopulmonary dysplasia
Pneumothorax, pneumomediastinum; interstitial emphysema
Congenital pneumonia
Pulmonary hypoplasia
Pulmonary hemorrhage
Apnea*

CARDIOVASCULAR

Patent ductus arteriosus*
Hypotension
Hypertension
Bradycardia (with apnea)*
Congenital malformations

HEMATOLOGIC

Anemia (early or late onset)
Hyperbilirubinemia—indirect*
Subcutaneous, organ (liver, adrenal) hemorrhage*
Disseminated intravascular coagulopathy
Vitamin K deficiency
Hydrops—immune or nonimmune

GASTROINTESTINAL

Poor gastrointestinal function—poor motility*
Necrotizing enterocolitis
Hyperbilirubinemia—direct and indirect
Congenital anomalies producing polyhydramnios
Spontaneous gastrointestinal isolated perforation

METABOLIC-ENDOCRINE

Hypocalcemia*
Hypoglycemia*
Hyperglycemia*
Late metabolic acidosis
Hypothermia*
Euthyroid but low-thyroxin status

CENTRAL NERVOUS SYSTEM

Intraventricular hemorrhage*
Periventricular leukomalacia
Hypoxic-ischemic encephalopathy
Seizures
Retinopathy of prematurity
Deafness
Hypotonia*
Congenital malformations
Kernicterus (bilirubin encephalopathy)
Drug (narcotic) withdrawal

RENAL

Hyponatremia*
Hypernatremia*
Hyperkalemia*
Renal tubular acidosis
Renal glycosuria
Edema

OTHER

Infections* (congenital, perinatal, nosocomial: bacterial, viral, fungal, protozoal)

*Common.

Nursery Care. At birth, the measures needed for clearing the airway, initiating breathing, caring for the cord and eyes, and administering vitamin K are the same in immature infants as in those of normal weight and maturity (Chapter 83). Special care is required to maintain a patent airway and avoid potential aspiration of gastric contents. Additional considerations are the need for (1) thermal control and monitoring of the heart rate and respiration, (2) oxygen therapy, and (3) special attention to the details of feeding. Safeguards against infection can never be relaxed. Everyone involved must be aware that routine procedures that disturb these infants may result in hypoxia. The need for regular and active participation by the parents in the infant's care in the nursery, the need to instruct the mother in at-home care of her infant, and the question of prognosis for later growth and development require special consideration.

THERMAL CONTROL. The survival rate of LBW and sick infants is higher when they are cared for at or near their *neutral thermal environment.* This environment is a set of thermal conditions, including air and radiating surface temperatures, relative humidity, and airflow, at which heat production (measured as oxygen consumption) is minimal and the infant's core temperature is within the normal range. It is a function of the size and postnatal age of an infant; larger, older infants require lower environmental temperatures than smaller, younger infants do. Isolettes (incubators) or radiant warmers can be used to maintain body temperature. Body heat is conserved through provision of a warm environment and standard conditions of humidity. The optimal environmental temperature for minimal heat loss and oxygen consumption for an unclothed infant is one that maintains the infant's core temperature at 36.5–37.0°C. It depends on an infant's size and maturity; the smaller and more immature the infant, the higher the environmental temperature required. An additional Plexiglas heat shield or head cap and body clothing may be required to keep an extremely LBW (ELBW) preterm infant warm. Infant warmth can be maintained by heating the air to a desired temperature or by servo-controlling the infant's body temperature at a desired set point. Continuous monitoring of the infant's temperature is required so that the environmental temperature can be adjusted to maintain optimal body temperature.

Maintaining a relative *humidity* of 40–60% aids in stabilizing body temperature by reducing heat loss at lower environmental temperatures; by preventing drying and irritation of the lining of respiratory passages, especially during the administration of oxygen and after or during endotracheal intubation (usually 100% humidity); and by thinning viscid secretions and reducing insensible water loss from the lungs. An infant should be weaned and then removed from the isolette or radiant warmer only when the gradual change to the atmosphere of the nursery does not result in a significant change in the infant's temperature, color, activity, or vital signs.

Administering *oxygen* to reduce the risk of injury from hypoxia and circulatory insufficiency must be balanced against the risk of hyperoxia to the eyes (retinopathy of prematurity) and oxygen injury to the lungs. Oxygen should be administered via a head hood, nasal cannula, continuous positive airway pressure apparatus, or endotracheal tube to maintain stable and safe inspired oxygen concentrations. Although cyanosis must be treated immediately, oxygen is a drug and its use must be carefully regulated to maximize benefit and minimize potential harm. The concentration of inspired oxygen must be adjusted in accordance with the oxygen tension of arterial blood (Pao_2) or noninvasive methods such as continuous pulse oximetry or transcutaneous oxygen measurements. Capillary blood gases are inadequate for estimating arterial oxygen levels.

FLUID REQUIREMENTS. Fluid needs vary according to gestational age, environmental conditions, and disease states. Assuming minimal water loss in the stool of infants not receiving oral fluids, their water needs are equal to their insensible water loss, excretion of renal solutes, growth, and any unusual ongoing losses. Insensible water loss is indirectly related to gestational age; very immature preterm infants (<1,000 g) may lose as much as 2–3 mL/kg/hr, partly because of immature skin, lack of subcutaneous tissue, and a large exposed surface area. Insensible water loss is increased under radiant warmers, during phototherapy, and in febrile infants. It is diminished when infants are clothed, are covered by a Plexiglas inner heat shield, breathe humidified air, or are of advanced postnatal age. Larger premature infants (2,000–2,500 g) nursed in an incubator may have an insensible water loss of approximately 0.6–0.7 mL/kg/hr.

Adequate fluid intake is essential for excretion of the urinary solute load (e.g., urea, electrolytes, phosphate). The amount varies with dietary intake and the anabolic or catabolic state of nutrition. Formulas with a high solute load, high protein intake, and catabolism increase the end products that require urinary excretion and thus increase the requirement for water. Renal solute loads may vary between 7.5 and 30 mOsm/kg. Newborn infants, especially those with VLBW, are also less able to concentrate urine; thus, their fluid intake required to excrete solutes increases.

Water intake in term infants is usually begun at 60–70 mL/kg on day 1 and increased to 100–120 mL/kg by days 2–3. Smaller, more premature infants may need to start with 70–80 mL/kg on day 1 and advance gradually to 150 mL/kg/day. Fluid volumes should be titrated individually, although it is unusual to exceed 150 mL/kg/24 hr. Infants weighing less than 750 g in the 1st wk of life have immature skin and a large surface area, characteristics that lead to a high rate of transepidermal fluid loss, at times requiring higher rates of intravenous fluids. Daily weights, urine, and serum urea nitrogen with electrolytes should be monitored carefully to determine water balance and fluid needs. Clinical observation and physical examination are poor indicators of the state of hydration of premature infants. Conditions that increase fluid loss, such as glycosuria, the polyuric phase of acute tubular necrosis, and diarrhea, may place additional strain on kidneys that have not yet acquired their maximal capacity to conserve water and electrolytes, the results of which may be severe dehydration. Alternatively, fluid overload may lead to edema, heart failure, patent ductus arteriosus, and bronchopulmonary dysplasia.

TOTAL PARENTERAL NUTRITION. Before enteral feeding has been established or when enteral feeding is impossible for prolonged periods, total intravenous alimentation may provide sufficient fluid, calories, amino acids, electrolytes, and vitamins to sustain the growth of LBW infants. This technique has been lifesaving for ELBW infants and those who have had intractable diarrheal syndromes or extensive bowel resection. Infusions may be administered through a percutaneously or surgically placed indwelling central venous catheter or through a peripheral vein. The umbilical vein may also be used for a short time.

The goal of parenteral alimentation is to deliver sufficient calories from glucose, protein, and lipids to promote optimal growth. The infusate should contain 2.5–3 g/dL of synthetic amino acids and glucose usually in the range of 10–15 g/dL, in addition to appropriate quantities of electrolytes, trace minerals, and vitamins. If a peripheral vein is used, it is advisable to keep the glucose concentration below 12.5 g/dL. If a central vein is used, glucose concentrations as high as 25 g/dL may be used (rarely). Intravenous fat emulsions such as 20% Intralipid (2.2 kcal/mL) may be administered to provide calories without an appreciable osmotic load, thereby decreasing the need for infusion of the higher concentrations of glucose by central or peripheral vein and usually preventing the development of essential fatty acid deficiency. Intralipid may be initiated at 0.5 g/kg/24 hr and advanced to 3 g/kg/24 hr, if triglyceride levels remain normal; 0.5 g/kg/24 hr is sufficient to prevent essential fatty acid deficiency. Electrolytes, trace minerals, and vitamin additives are included in amounts approximating established intravenous maintenance requirements. The content of each day's infusate should be determined after carefully assessing the infant's clinical and biochemical status. Slow and continuous infusion is advisable. A well-trained pharmacist should mix all solutions under a laminar flow hood.

After a caloric intake of greater than 100 kcal/kg/24 hr is established by total parenteral intravenous nutrition, LBW infants can be expected to gain about 15 g/kg/24 hr, with a positive nitrogen balance of 150–200 mg/kg/24 hr, in the absence of episodes of sepsis, surgical procedures, or other severe stress. This goal can usually be achieved (and the catabolic tendency during the 1st wk of life reversed with subsequent weight gain) by peripheral vein infusion of 2.5–3.5 g/kg/24 hr of an amino acid mixture, 10 g/dL of glucose, and 2–3 g/kg/24 hr of Intralipid.

Complications of intravenous alimentation are related to both the catheter and metabolism of the infusate. Sepsis is the most important problem of central vein infusions and can be minimized only by meticulous catheter care and aseptic preparation of the infusate. Coagulase-negative staphylococcus is the most common infecting organism. Treatment includes appropriate antibiotics. If an infection persists (repeatedly positive blood cultures while receiving appropriate antibiotics), the line must be removed. Thrombosis, extravasation of fluid, and accidental dislodgement of catheters have also occurred. Although sepsis is less often attributable to peripheral vein infusion, phlebitis, cutaneous sloughing, and superficial infection may occur. **Metabolic complications** of parenteral nutrition include hyperglycemia from the high glucose concentration of the infusate, which may lead to osmotic diuresis and dehydration; azotemia; a possible increased risk of nephrocalcinosis; hypoglycemia from sudden accidental cessation of the infusate; hyperlipidemia and possibly hypoxemia from intravenous lipid infusions; and hyperammonemia, which may be due to high levels of certain amino acids. Metabolic bone disease and/or cholestatic jaundice and liver disease may develop in infants who require long-term parenteral nutrition. Biochemical and physiologic monitoring of infants receiving intravenous alimentation is indicated because of the frequency and seriousness of complications.

FEEDING. The method of feeding each LBW infant should be individualized. It is important to avoid fatigue and aspiration of food by regurgitation or by the feeding process. No feeding method averts these problems unless the person feeding the infant has been well trained in the method. Oral feeding (nipple) should not be initiated or should be discontinued in infants with respiratory distress, hypoxia, circulatory insufficiency, excessive secretions, gagging, sepsis, central nervous system depression, immaturity, or signs of serious illness. These high-risk infants require parenteral nutrition or gavage feeding to supply calories, fluid, and electrolytes. The process of oral alimentation requires, in addition to a strong sucking effort, coordination of swallowing, epiglottal and uvular closure of the larynx and nasal passages, and normal esophageal motility, a synchronized process that is usually absent before 34 wk gestation.

Preterm infants at 34 wk gestation or more can often be fed by bottle or at the breast. Because the effort of sucking is usually the limiting factor, breast-feeding is less likely to succeed until the infant matures. Bottle-feeding of expressed breast milk may be a temporary alternative. In *bottle-feeding*, effort may be reduced by use of special small, soft nipples with large holes. Smaller or less vigorous infants should be fed by *gavage*: a soft plastic tube with No. 5 French external and approximately 0.05 cm internal diameters and with a rounded atraumatic tip and two holes on alternate sides is preferable. The tube is passed through the nose until approximately 2.5 cm (1 inch) of the lower end is in the stomach. The free end of the tube has an adapter into which the tip of a syringe is fitted, and a measured amount of fluid is given by pump or by gravity. Such tubes may be left in place for 3–7 days before being replaced by a similar tube through the alternate nostril. Infants occasionally have enough local irritation from an indwelling tube that they may gag or troublesome secretions may gather around it in the nasopharynx. In such cases, a catheter may be passed through the mouth by a skilled person and removed at the end of each feeding.

An LBW infant may be fed with intermittent bolus feedings or continuous feeding. In the occasional infant with feeding intolerance, nasojejunal feeding may be successful. However, intestinal perforation is a risk with nasojejunal feeding. A change to breast- or bottle-feeding may be instituted gradually as soon as an infant displays general vigor adequate for oral feeding without fatigue.

Gastrostomy feeding is not usually indicated in premature infants because of an associated increase in mortality, except as an adjunct to surgical management of specific gastrointestinal conditions or in permanently neurologically injured patients unable to suck and swallow normally.

Initiation of Feeding. The optimal time to introduce enteral feeding to a sick LBW infant is controversial. Trophic feeding is the practice of feeding very small amounts of enteral nourishment to VLBW preterm infants to stimulate development of the immature gastrointestinal tract. Many studies have demonstrated benefits of trophic feeding, including enhanced gut motility, improved growth, decreased need for parenteral nutrition, fewer episodes of sepsis, and shortened hospital stay. Once the infant is stable, small-volume feedings are given in addition to intravenous fluids/nutrition. Feeding is gradually advanced and parenteral nutrition decreased. This approach may reduce the incidence of necrotizing enterocolitis. The main principle in feeding premature infants is to proceed cautiously and gradually. Careful early feeding of breast milk or formula tends to reduce the risk of hypoglycemia, dehydration, and hyperbilirubinemia without the additional risk of aspiration, provided that the presence of respiratory distress or other disorders does not present an indication for withholding oral feedings and administering electrolytes, fluids, and calories intravenously.

If an infant is well, is making sucking movements, and is in no distress, oral feeding may be attempted, although most infants weighing less than 1,500 g require tube feeding because they are unable to coordinate breathing, sucking, and swallowing. Intestinal tract readiness for feeding may be determined by active bowel sounds, passage of meconium, and the absence of abdominal distention, bilious gastric aspirates, or emesis. For infants under 1,000 g, the initial feedings are either half- or full-strength breast milk or preterm formula at 10 mL/kg/24 hr as a continuous nasogastric tube drip (or given by intermittent gavage every 2–3 hr). If the initial feeding is tolerated, the volume is increased by 10–15 mL/kg/24 hr. The daily milk volume increment should not exceed 20 mL/kg/24 hr. Once a volume of 150 mL/kg/24 hr

has been achieved, the caloric content may be increased to 24 or 27 kcal/oz. With high caloric density, infants are at risk for dehydration, edema, lactose intolerance, diarrhea, flatus, and delayed gastric emptying with emesis. Intravenous fluids are needed until feedings provide approximately 120 mL/kg/24 hr. The feeding protocol for premature infants weighing over 1,500 g is initiated at a volume of 20–25 mL/kg/24 hr of full-strength breast milk or preterm formula given as a bolus every 3 hr. Thereafter, increments in total daily formula volume should not exceed 20 mL/kg/24 hr. The expected weight increments for premature infants of various birthweights are projected from Figure 86–5. Infants with IUGR may not demonstrate the initial weight loss noted in premature infants.

Regurgitation, vomiting, abdominal distention, or gastric residuals from previous feedings should arouse suspicion of sepsis, necrotizing enterocolitis, or intestinal obstruction; these conditions are indications to drop back in the schedule and increase subsequent feedings slowly or to change to intravenous alimentation and evaluate for more serious problems (Chapter 91.2). Weight gain may not be achieved for 10–12 days, and a daily intake of 130–150 mL/kg or more may be necessary for some infants. Alternatively, in vigorous infants whose feeding schedule is advanced successfully in calories or volume, weight gain may appear within a few days.

When tube feeding is used, the contents of the stomach should be aspirated before each feeding. If only air or small amounts of mucus are obtained, the feeding is given as planned. If all or a substantial part of the previous feeding is aspirated, it is advisable to reduce the amount of the feeding and proceed more gradually with subsequent increases.

The digestive enzyme systems of infants older than 28 wk gestation are mature enough to permit adequate digestion and absorption of protein and carbohydrate. Fat is less well absorbed, primarily because of inadequate amounts of bile salt; unsaturated fats and the fat of human milk are absorbed better than those of cow's milk. The weight gain of infants weighing under 2,000 g at birth should be adequate when human milk or "humanized" milk premature formula (40% casein and 60% whey) with a protein intake of 2.25–2.75 g/kg/24 hr is fed. These two alternatives should provide all amino acids essential

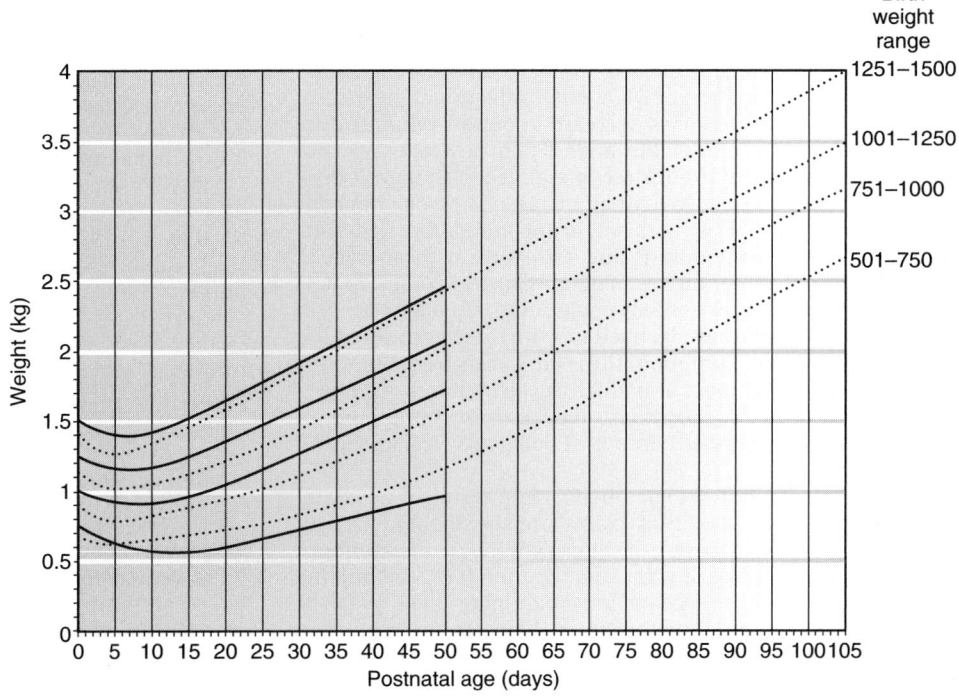

FIGURE 86–5. Average daily weight (grams) vs postnatal age (days) for infants with birthweight ranges of 501–750 g, 751–1,000 g, 1,001–1,250 g, and 1,251–1,500 g (*dotted lines*), plotted with the curves of Dancis and colleagues for infants with birthweights of 750 g, 1,000 g, 1,250 g, and 1,500 g (*solid lines*). (From Wright K, Dawson JP, Fallis D, et al: New postnatal growth grids for very low birth weight infants. *Pediatrics* 1993; 91:922.)

for premature infants, including tyrosine, cystine, and histidine. Higher protein intake may be well tolerated and is generally safe, especially in older, rapidly growing infants. However, protein intake as high as 4–5 g/kg/24 hr may be hazardous: although linear growth may be promoted, high-protein formulas may cause abnormal plasma aminograms; elevations in blood urea nitrogen, ammonia, and sodium concentrations; metabolic acidosis (cow's milk formulas); and untoward effects on neurologic development. Furthermore, the high protein and mineral contents of balanced cow's milk formulas with a high caloric content constitute a large solute load for the kidneys, a fact important in maintaining water balance, especially in infants with diarrhea or fever.

Breast milk from the infant's mother is the preferred milk for all infants, including VLBW infants. In addition to nutritional advantages, the benefits of breast milk include protection against a wide range of infections (through both specific and nonspecific anti-infective factors in breast milk and beneficial effects on intestinal flora), a decreased risk of necrotizing enterocolitis in preterm infants, a lower risk of sudden infant death syndrome, and possible long-term effects, including a lower risk of childhood/adolescent obesity and improved neurodevelopmental outcome. Once a premature infant takes 120 mL/kg/24 hr, breast milk fortifiers are added to supplement breast milk with protein, calcium, and phosphorus. If breast milk is unavailable, special preterm formulas should be used. At approximately 34–36 wk gestation, infants who are not receiving breast milk should be switched to a term formula (unless metabolic bone disease is present—see Chapter 95) because hypercalcemia may develop as a result of the preterm formula's higher calcium and vitamin D levels.

Although formula in amounts necessary for adequate growth probably contains adequate quantities of all vitamins, the volume of milk sufficient to satisfy these requirements may not be ingested for several weeks. Therefore, LBW infants should be given supplemental vitamins. Because requirements for these infants have not been precisely established, the recommended daily allowances for term infants should be given (see Chapter 40.7). Furthermore, these infants may have a special need for certain vitamins. Intermediary metabolism of phenylalanine and tyrosine depends, in part, on vitamin C. Decreased fat absorption with increased fecal fat loss may be associated with decreased absorption of *vitamin D*, other fat-soluble vitamins, and calcium in premature infants. VLBW infants are particularly prone to the development of rickets, but their total intake of vitamin D should not exceed 1,500 IU/24 hr. *Folic acid* is essential for the formation of DNA and production of new cells; serum and erythrocyte levels decrease in preterm infants during the first few weeks of life and remain low for 2–3 mo. Therefore, supplementation is recommended, although it does not result in improved growth or an increased hemoglobin concentration. Deficiency of vitamin E is uncommon but is associated with increased hemolysis and, if severe, with anemia in premature infants. Vitamin E functions as an antioxidant to prevent the peroxidation of excessive polyunsaturated fatty acids in red blood cell membranes; its need may increase because of the increased membrane content of these fatty acids from older formulas with high polyunsaturated fatty acids. Vitamin A supplementation has been shown to reduce bronchopulmonary dysplasia in VLBW infants. Vitamin K deficiency is discussed in Chapter 92.4.

In LBW infants, physiologic anemia as a result of postnatal suppression of erythropoiesis is exacerbated by smaller fetal iron stores and greater expansion of blood volume from the more rapid growth than that of term infants; therefore, the anemia develops earlier and reaches a lower ultimate level. Fetal or neonatal blood loss accentuates this problem. Iron stores, even in VLBW neonates, are usually adequate until an infant's birthweight has doubled or after an infant has been treated with ery-

thropoietin (Chapter 92); iron supplementation (2 mg/kg/24 hr) should then be started.

Properly fed premature infants may have from one to six daily stools of semisolid consistency; a sudden increase in their number, the appearance of occult or gross blood, or change to a watery consistency is more reason for concern than any arbitrarily stated frequency. Premature infants should not vomit or regurgitate. They should be satisfied and relaxed after a feeding but may normally show the activity of hunger shortly before the next feeding.

Prevention of Infection. Premature infants have an increased susceptibility to infection, and thus meticulous attention to infection control is required. Prevention strategies include strict compliance with handwashing and universal precautions, limiting nurse-to-patient ratios and avoiding crowding, minimizing the risk of catheter contamination, meticulous skin care, encouraging early appropriate advancement of enteral feeding, education and feedback to staff, and surveillance of nosocomial infection rates in the nursery. Although no one with an infection should be permitted in the nursery, the risks of infection must be balanced against the disadvantages of limiting the infant's contact with the family. Early and frequent participation by parents in the nursery care of their infant does not significantly increase the risk of infection when preventive precautions are maintained. Routine immunizations should be given on the regular schedule at standard doses (Chapter 282).

Preventing transmission of infection from infant to infant is difficult because often neither term nor premature newborn infants have clear clinical evidence of an infection early in its course. Universal precautions require gloves to be worn with all patient contact. When epidemics occur within a nursery, cohort nursing and isolation rooms should be used.

Immaturity of Drug Metabolism. Renal clearance of almost all substances excreted in the urine is diminished in newborn infants, but more so in premature ones. Intervals between doses may therefore need to be extended when administering drugs excreted chiefly by the kidneys. For instance, highly satisfactory levels of penicillin, gentamicin, and kanamycin are maintained by giving doses at 12 hr intervals. Longer intervals are required for many drugs administered to preterm infants. Drugs detoxified in the liver or requiring chemical conjugation before renal excretion should also be given with caution and in doses smaller than usual.

When possible, blood levels should be determined for potentially toxic drugs, especially if renal or hepatic dysfunction is present. Decisions about the choice and dose of antibacterial agents and the route of administration should be made on an individual basis rather than routinely because of the dangers of (1) development of infections with organisms resistant to antibacterial agents, (2) destruction or inhibition of intestinal bacteria that manufacture significant amounts of essential vitamins (e.g., vitamin K and thiamine), and (3) harmful interference in important metabolic processes.

Many drugs apparently safe for adults on the basis of toxicity studies may be harmful to newborn infants, especially premature ones. Oxygen and a number of drugs have proved toxic to premature infants in amounts not harmful to term infants (Table 86–3). Thus, administering any drug, particularly in large doses, without pharmacologic testing in premature infants should be undertaken carefully after weighing risks against benefits.

Prognosis. Infants born weighing 1,501–2,500 g now have a 95% or greater chance of survival, but those weighing less still have significantly higher mortality (see Fig. 86–1). Intensive care has extended the period during which a VLBW infant is at increased risk of dying of complications of prematurity, such as bronchopulmonary dysplasia, necrotizing enterocolitis, or noso-

TABLE 86–3. Potential Adverse Reactions to Drugs Administered to Premature Infants

Drug	Reaction
Oxygen	Retinopathy of prematurity, bronchopulmonary dysplasia
Sulfisoxazole	Kernicterus
Chloramphenicol	Gray baby—shock, bone marrow suppression
Vitamin K analogs	Jaundice
Novobiocin	Jaundice
Hexachlorophene	Encephalopathy
Benzyl alcohol	Acidosis, collapse, intraventricular bleeding
Intravenous vitamin E	Ascites, shock
Phenolic detergents	Jaundice
NaHCO₃	Intraventricular hemorrhage
Amphotericin	Anuric renal failure, hypokalemia, hypomagnesemia
Reserpine	Nasal stuffiness
Indomethacin	Oliguria, hyponatremia, intestinal perforation
Cisapride	Prolonged Q-Tc interval
Tetracycline	Enamel hypoplasia
Tolazoline	Hypotension, gastrointestinal bleeding
Calcium salts	Subcutaneous necrosis
Aminoglycosides	Deafness, renal toxicity
Enteric gentamicin	Resistant bacteria
Prostaglandins	Seizures, diarrhea, apnea, hyperostosis, pyloric stenosis
Phenobarbital	Altered state, drowsiness
Morphine	Hypotension, urine retention, withdrawal
Pancuronium/ vecuronium	Edema, hypovolemia, hypotension, tachycardia, contractions, prolonged hypotonia
Iodine antiseptics	Hypothyroidism, goiter
Fentanyl	Seizures, chest wall rigidity, withdrawal
Dexamethasone	Gastrointestinal bleeding, hypertension, infection, hyperglycemia, cardiomyopathy, reduced growth
Furosemide	Deafness, hyponatremia, hypokalemia, hypochloremia, nephrocalcinosis, biliary stones
Heparin (not low-dose prophylactic use)	Bleeding, intraventricular hemorrhage, thrombocytopenia
Erythromycin	Pyloric stenosis

BOX 86–5. Sequelae of Low Birthweight

IMMEDIATE	LATE
Hypoxia, ischemia	Mental retardation, spastic diplegia, microcephaly, seizures, poor school performance
Intraventricular hemorrhage	Mental retardation, spasticity, seizures, hydrocephalus
Sensorineural injury	Hearing, visual impairment, retinopathy of prematurity, strabismus, myopia
Respiratory failure	Bronchopulmonary dysplasia, cor pulmonale, bronchospasm, malnutrition, subglottic stenosis, iatrogenic cleft palate, recurrent pneumonia
Necrotizing enterocolitis	Short-bowel syndrome, malabsorption, malnutrition, infectious diarrhea
Cholestatic liver disease	Cirrhosis, hepatic failure, carcinoma, malnutrition
Nutrient deficiency	Osteopenia, fractures, anemia, vitamin E, growth failure
Social stress	Child abuse or neglect, failure to thrive, divorce
Other	Sudden infant death syndrome, infections, inguinal hernia, cutaneous scars (chest tube, patent ductus arteriosus ligation, intravenous infiltration), gastroesophageal reflux, hypertension, craniosynostosis, cholelithiasis, nephrocalcinosis, cutaneous hemangiomas

comial infection (Box 86–5). The post-discharge mortality rate of LBW infants is higher than that of term infants during the 1st 2 yr of life. Because many of these deaths are attributable to infection (e.g., respiratory syncytial virus [RSV]), they are at least theoretically preventable. In addition, premature infants have an increased incidence of failure to thrive, sudden infant death syndrome, child abuse, and inadequate maternal-infant bonding. The biologic risk associated with poor cardiorespiratory regulation because of immaturity or complications of underlying perinatal disease and the social risk associated with poverty also contribute to the high mortality and morbidity of these infants. Congenital anomalies are present in approximately 3–7% of LBW infants.

In the absence of congenital abnormalities, central nervous system injury, VLBW or marked IUGR, the physical growth of LBW infants tends to approximate that of term infants by the 2nd yr; it occurs earlier in premature infants with larger birth size. VLBW infants may not catch up, especially if they have severe chronic sequelae, insufficient nutritional intake, or an inadequate caretaking environment (see Box 86–5). Premature birth in itself may prejudice later development. In general, the greater the immaturity and the lower the birthweight, the greater the likelihood of intellectual and neurologic deficit; as many as 50% of 500–750 g infants have a significant neurodevelopmental handicap (blindness, deafness, mental retardation, cerebral palsy). Small head circumference at birth may be similarly related to a poor neurobehavioral prognosis. Children born after in vitro fertilization have an increased risk of neurologic impairment, especially cerebral palsy. This finding is probably explained by the increased risk associated with prematurity and multiple births, but the long-term safety of the procedure needs to be monitored. Many surviving LBW infants have hypotonia before 8 mo corrected age, which improves by the time that they are 8 mo–1 yr old. This transient hypotonia is not a poor prognostic sign. Thirty to 50% of VLBW children have poor school performance at 7 yr of age (repeat grades, special classes, learn-

ing disorders, poor speech and language), despite a normal IQ. Factors posing a risk for poor academic performance include birthweight below 750 g, severe IVH, periventricular leukomalacia, bronchopulmonary dysplasia, cerebral atrophy, posthemorrhagic hydrocephalus, IUGR, low socioeconomic status, and possibly, low thyroxine levels. Adolescents who were VLBW report satisfactory health; 94% are integrated in regular classes despite neurosensory disabilities (hearing, vision, cerebral palsy, cognition) in 24%.

Predicting Neonatal Mortality. Birthweight and gestational age have traditionally been used as strong indicators for the risk of neonatal death. Indeed, survival at 22 wk of gestation is close to 0%; with increasing gestational age, survival rates increase to approximately 15% at 23 wk, 56% at 24 wk, and 79% at 25 wk. In addition, birthweight-specific neonatal diseases such as grade IV IVH, severe group B streptococcal pneumonia, and pulmonary hypoplasia also contribute to a poor outcome. Scoring systems that have been developed take into consideration physiologic abnormalities (hypotension-hypertension, acidosis, hypoxia, hypercapnia, anemia, neutropenia), as in the Score for Neonatal Acute Physiology (SNAP), or clinical parameters (gestational age, birthweight, anomalies, acidosis, F_{IO_2}), as in the Clinical Risk Index for Babies (CRIB). CRIB includes 6 parameters collected in the first 12 hr after birth, and SNAP has 26 variables collected in the first 24 hr. Although these risk scoring systems may provide prognostic information for mortality, they may not be useful for predicting morbidity in survivors. Furthermore, when compared with the clinical judgment of experienced neonatologists (based on birthweight, illness severity, low Apgar score, IUGR, therapeutic requirements), objective risk scores provide similar predictability. Combining a physician's judgment and an objective score may produce a more accurate assessment of the risk of mortality.

Discharge from the Hospital. Before discharge, a premature infant should be taking all nutrition by nipple, either bottle or breast (Box 86–6). Growth should be occurring at steady increments of approximately 10–30 g/24 hr. Temperature should be stabilized

BOX 86–6. Recommendations for the Discharge of High-Risk Low-Birthweight Infants

Resolution of acute life-threatening illnesses
Ongoing follow-up for chronic but stable problems
    Bronchopulmonary dysplasia
    Intraventricular hemorrhage
    Necrotizing enterocolitis
    Ventricular septal defect, other cardiac lesions
    Anemia
    Retinopathy of prematurity
    Hearing
    Apnea
    Cholestasis
Stable temperature regulation
Gaining weight on oral feedings
    Breast-feeding
    Bottle-feeding
    Gastric tube
Free of significant apnea; home monitoring for apnea if needed
Appropriate immunizations and planning for respiratory syncytial virus prophylaxis if indicated
Hearing screenings
Ophthalmologic examination if <27 wk or <1,250 g at birth
Mother's knowledge, skill, confidence documented in
    Administration of medications (diuretics, methylxanthines, aerosols, etc.)
    Use of oxygen, apnea monitors, oximeters
    Nutritional support
        Timing
        Volume
        Mixing concentrated formulas
    Recognition of illness and deterioration
    Basic cardiopulmonary resuscitation
    Infant safety (see Box 86–1)
Scheduling of referrals
    Primary care provider
    Neonatal follow-up clinic
    Occupational therapy/physical therapy
    Imaging (head ultrasound)
Assessment of and solution to social risks (see Box 86–1)

Adapted from American Academy of Pediatrics, American College of Obstetricians: *Guidelines for Perinatal Care*, 5th ed. Elk Grove Village, IL, American Academy of Pediatrics, 2002.

in an open crib. Infants should have had no recent episodes of apnea or bradycardia, and parenteral drug administration should have been discontinued or converted to oral dosing. Stable infants recovering from bronchopulmonary dysplasia may be discharged on a regimen of oxygen given by nasal cannula as long as careful follow-up is arranged with frequent pulse oximetry monitoring and outpatient visits. All infants with a birthweight under 1500 g and those between 1500 and 2000 g with an unstable clinical course requiring oxygen should have an eye examination to screen for retinopathy of prematurity. All LBW infants should have a hearing test. Those who had indwelling umbilical arterial catheters should have their blood pressure measured to check for renal vascular hypertension. The hemoglobin level or hematocrit should be determined to evaluate for possible anemia. If all major medical problems have resolved and the home setting is adequate, premature infants may then be discharged when their weight approaches 1,800–2,100 g; close follow-up plus easy access to health care providers is essential for early discharge protocols. Alternatively, if the medical or social environment is not ideal, high-risk neonates who have been transported to neonatal intensive care units and whose major illness has resolved may be returned to their hospital of birth for an additional period of hospitalization. Standard vaccinations with full doses should commence after discharge or, if in the hospital, with vaccines that do not contain live viruses. For RSV prophylaxis, see Chapter 239.

Home Care. While the infant is in the hospital, the mother should be instructed in how to care for the baby after discharge. Ideally, this program should include at least one visit to her home by someone capable of evaluating domestic arrangements and advising about any needed improvements.

86.3 Post-Term Infants

Post-term infants are those born after 42 wk of gestation, as calculated from the mother's last menstrual period, regardless of weight at birth. This designation is often used synonymously with the term "postmature" for infants whose gestation exceeds the normal 280 days by 7 or more days. Approximately 25% of all pregnancies end on or after the 287th day of gestation, 12% on or after the 294th day, and 5% on or after the 301st day. The cause of post-term birth or postmaturity is unknown. Large size of the infant correlates poorly with late delivery but does correlate with large size of either parent, multigravidity, or a prediabetic or diabetic state in the mother.

Clinical Manifestations. Post-term infants may be clinically indistinguishable from term infants, but some have received the designation postmature because their appearance and behavior suggest those of an infant 1–3 wk of age. These post-term, postmature infants often have increased birthweight and are characterized by the absence of lanugo, decreased or absent vernix caseosa, long nails, abundant scalp hair, white parchment-like or desquamating skin, and increased alertness. If *placental insufficiency* occurs, the amniotic fluid and fetus may be meconium stained, and abnormal fetal heart rates may be observed; the infant may have growth retardation. Although this syndrome is frequently confused with postmaturity, *only about 20% of infants with placental insufficiency syndrome are post-term.* The majority of those affected are term and preterm infants, particularly those SGA who are infants of toxemic mothers, older primigravidas, and women with chronic hypertension. The placentas are often small or poorly attached. This syndrome has been postulated to result from degenerative changes in the placenta that progressively reduce oxygen and nourishment to the fetus.

Infants born post-term in association with presumed placental insufficiency may have various physical signs. Desquamation, long nails, abundant hair, pale skin, alert faces, and loose skin, especially around the thighs and buttocks, give them the appearance of having recently lost weight; meconium-stained nails, skin, vernix, umbilical cord, and placental membranes may also be noted (see Fig. 83–1).

Prognosis. When delivery is delayed 3 wk or more beyond term, mortality is significantly increased and, in some series, has been approximately three times that of a control group of infants born at term. Mortality has been lowered markedly through improved obstetric management.

Management. Careful obstetric monitoring, including nonstress testing, biophysical profile, or Doppler velocimetry, usually provides a rational basis for choosing a course of nonintervention, induction of labor, or cesarean section. Induction of labor or cesarean section may be indicated in older primigravidas who go more than 2–4 wk beyond term, particularly if evidence of fetal distress is present. Medical problems in the newborn are treated if they arise.

86.4 Large for Gestational Age

See also Chapter 96.

Neonatal mortality rates decrease with increasing birthweight until approximately 4,000 g, after which mortality increases. These oversized infants are usually born at term, but preterm infants with weights high for gestational age also have a significantly higher mortality than do infants of the same size born at term; maternal diabetes and obesity are predisposing factors. Infants who are very large, regardless of their gestational age, have a higher incidence of birth injuries such as cervical and brachial plexus injuries, phrenic nerve damage with paralysis of the diaphragm, fractured clavicles, cephalohematomas, subdural hematomas, and ecchymoses of the head and face.

The incidence of congenital anomalies, particularly congenital heart disease, is also higher than in term infants of normal weight. Intellectual and developmental retardation is statistically more common in high-birthweight term and preterm infants than in babies of appropriate weight for gestational age.

86.5 Infant Transport

With the advent of regionalized care of high-risk neonates, increasing numbers of sick infants are being transported to neonatal intensive care units in hospitals at which they were not born. Ideally, high-risk mothers should be transported to and their babies delivered at centers where these specialized units are located. Neonatal transport should include consultation about the infant's problem and care before transport, ease of access to the transport team, and transport and stabilization by the team before moving the infant. Securing an airway, providing oxygen, assisting with infant ventilation, providing antimicrobial therapy, maintaining the circulation, providing a warmed environment, and placing intravenous or arterial lines or chest tubes should all be initiated, if indicated, before transport. Infant and maternal records, laboratory reports, and a tube of clotted maternal blood should also be provided. Before departing, the mother should be briefly reassured and allowed to see her stabilized infant, if practical; the father should follow the transport vehicle to the unit. The transport officer or nurse should also call ahead to inform the receiving unit about the nature of the patient's illness.

The transport vehicle should be equipped with appropriate medicines, fluids, oxygen tanks, catheters, chest tubes, endotracheal tubes, laryngoscopes, and an infant warming device. It should be well illuminated and have ample room for emergency procedures and monitoring equipment. With efficient transport and appropriately educated nursing and medical staff at the referring hospitals, the mortality of "outborn" neonates should be no higher than that of those born within the tertiary care center.

Akintorin SM, Kamat M, Pildes RS, et al: A prospective randomized trial of feeding methods in very low birth weight infants. *Pediatrics* 1997;100:http://www.pediatrics.org/cgi/content/full/100/4/e4.

American Academy of Pediatrics: *Hospital Care of Newborn Infants.* Evanston, IL, American Academy of Pediatrics, 1997.

Bhutta AT, Cleves MA, Caset PH, et al: Cognitive and behavioral outcomes of school-aged children who were born preterm. *JAMA* 2002;288:728–37.

Blaymore Bier J, Ferguson AE, Morales Y, et al: Breastfeeding infants who were extremely low birth weight. *Pediatrics* 1997;100:http://www.pediatrics.org/cgi/content/full/100/6/e3.

Davey AM, Wagner CL, Cox C, et al: Feeding premature infants while low umbilical artery catheters are in place: A prospective, randomized trial. *J Pediatr* 1994;124:795.

Eckstein Grunau R, Whitfield MF, Davis C: Pattern of learning disabilities in children with extremely low birth weight and broadly average intelligence. *Arch Pediatr Adolesc Med* 2002;156:615–20.

Feldman R, Eidelman AI, Sirota L, et al: Comparison of skin-to-skin (kangaroo) and traditional care: Parenting outcomes and preterm infant development. *Pediatrics* 2002;110:16–26.

Heird WC, Gomez MR: Total parenteral nutrition in necrotizing enterocolitis. *Clin Perinatol* 1994;21:389.

Hollo O, Rautava P, Korhonen T, et al: Academic achievement of small for gestational age children at age 10 years. *Arch Pediatr Adolesc Med* 2002;156:179–87.

Kalhoff H, Diekmann L, Hettrich B, et al: Modified cow's milk formula with reduced renal acid load preventing incipient late metabolic acidosis in premature infants. *J Pediatr* 1997;25:46.

Kliegman RM: Experimental validation of neonatal feeding practices. *Pediatrics* 1999;103:492–3.

Kluckow M, Evans N: Low systemic blood flow and hyperkalemia in preterm infants. *J Pediatr* 2001;139:227–32.

Lau C, Sheena HR, Shulman RJ, et al: Oral feeding in low birth weight infants. *J Pediatr* 1997;130:561.

Lee SK, Zupancic JAF, Pendray M, et al: Transport risk index of physiologic stability: A practical system for assessing infant transport care. *J Pediatr* 2001;139:220–6.

Lemons JA, Bauer CR, Oh W, et al: Very low birth weight outcomes of the National Institute of Child Health and Human Development Neonatal Research Network, January 1995 through December 1996. *Pediatrics* 2001;107:http://www.pediatrics.org/cgi/content/full/107/1/e1.

Lorenz JM, Paneth N, Jetton JR, et al: Comparison of management strategies for extreme prematurity in New Jersey and the Netherlands: Outcomes and resource expenditure. *Pediatrics* 2001;108:1269–74.

Lucas A, Morley R, Cole TJ, et al: A randomised multicentre study of human milk versus formula and later development in preterm infants. *Arch Dis Child* 1994;70:F141.

McCain GC, Gartside PS, Greenberg JM, et al: A feeding protocol for healthy preterm infants that shortens time to oral feeding. *J Pediatr* 2001;139:374–9.

McCormick MC, Richardson DK: Premature infants grow up. *N Engl J Med* 2002;346:197–8.

O'Conner DL, Hall R, Adamkin D, et al: Growth and development in preterm infants fed long-chain polyunsaturated fatty acids: A prospective, randomized controlled trial. *Pediatrics* 2001:108:359–71.

Perlman JM: Neurobehavorial deficits in preterm graduates of intensive care—potential medical and neonatal environmental risk factors. *Pediatrics* 2001;108:1339–48.

Sauer P, Visser M: The neutral temperature of very low birth weight infants. *Pediatrics* 1994;74:788.

Schreuder AM, McDonnell M, Gaffney G, et al: Outcome at school age following antenatal detection of absent or reversed end diastolic flow velocity in the umbilical artery. *Arch Dis Child Fetal Neonatal Ed* 2002;86:F108–14.

Strömberg B, Dahiquist G, Ericson A, et al: Neurological sequelae in children born after in-vitro fertilisation. *Lancet* 2002;359:461.

Tommiska V, Heinonen K, Ikonen S, et al: A national short-term follow-up study of extremely low birth weight infants born in Finland in 1996–1997. *Pediatrics* 2001;107:http://www.pediatrics.org/cgi/content/full/107/1/e2.

Tommiska V, Ostberg M, Fellman V: Parental stress in families of 2 year old extremely low birthweight infants. *Arch Dis Child Fetal Neonatal Ed* 2002;86:F161–4.

Van Wassenaer AG, Kok JH, De Vijlder JJM, et al: Effects of thyroxine supplementation on neurologic development on infants born at less than 30 weeks' gestation. *N Engl J Med* 1997;336:21.

Wariyar U, Tin W, Hey E: Gestational assessment assessed. *Arch Dis Child* 1997;77:F216.

Whitaker AH, Feldman JF, Van Rossem R, et al: Neonatal cranial ultrasound abnormalities in low birth weight infants: Relation to cognitive outcomes at six years of age. *Pediatrics* 1996;98:719.

Wilson DC, Cairns P, Halliday HL, et al: Randomised controlled trial of an aggressive nutritional regimen in sick very low birthweight infants. *Arch Dis Child* 1997;77:F4.

Chapter 87

Clinical Manifestations of Diseases in the Newborn Period *Barbara J. Stoll and Robert M. Kliegman*

The wide variety of disorders that affect the newborn originate in utero, during birth, or in the immediate postnatal period. These disorders may represent genetic mutations, chromosomal aberrations, or acquired diseases and injuries. Recognizing disease in newborn infants depends on knowledge of the disorder and evaluation of a limited number of relatively nonspecific clinical signs and symptoms.

Central cyanosis has respiratory, cardiac, central nervous system (CNS), hematologic, and metabolic causes (Box 87–1). Respiratory insufficiency may be due to pulmonary conditions or may be secondary to CNS depression as a result of drugs, intracranial hemorrhage, or anoxia. If it is caused by the former, respirations tend to be rapid and may be accompanied by retraction of the thoracic cage. If it is due to the latter, respirations tend to be irregular and weak and are often slow. Cyanosis unaccompanied by obvious signs of respiratory difficulty suggests cyanotic congenital heart disease or methemoglobinemia. Cyanosis resulting from congenital heart disease may, however, be difficult to clinically distinguish from cyanosis caused by

BOX 87–1. Differential Diagnosis of Cyanosis in the Newborn

Central or peripheral nervous system hypoventilation
  Birth asphyxia
  Intracranial hypertension, hemorrhage
  Oversedation (direct or through maternal route)
  Diaphragm palsy
  Neuromuscular diseases
  Seizures
Respiratory disease
  Upper airway
    Choanal atresia/stenosis
    Pierre Robin syndrome
    Intrinsic airway obstruction (laryngeal/bronchial/tracheal
      stenosis)
    Extrinsic airway obstruction (bronchogenic cyst, duplication cyst,
      vascular compression)
  Lower airway
    Respiratory distress syndrome
    Transient tachypnea
    Meconium aspiration
    Pneumonia (sepsis)
    Pneumothorax
    Congenital diaphragmatic hernia
    Pulmonary hypoplasia
    Persistent fetal circulation (persistent pulmonary hypertension of
      newborn)
Cardiac right-to-left shunt
  Abnormal connections (pulmonary blood flow normal or increased)
    Transposition of great vessels
    Total anomalous pulmonary venous return
    Truncus arteriosus
    Hypoplastic left heart syndrome
    Single ventricle or tricuspid atresia with large ventricular septal
      defect but without pulmonic stenosis
  Obstructed pulmonary blood flow (pulmonary blood flow
    decreased)
    Pulmonic atresia with intact ventricular septum
    Tetralogy of Fallot
    Critical pulmonic stenosis with patent foramen ovale or atrial
      septal defect
    Tricuspid atresia
    Single ventricle with pulmonic stenosis
    Ebstein malformation of the tricuspid valve
    Persistent fetal circulation (persistent pulmonary hypertension of
      newborn)
Methemoglobinemia
  Congenital (hemoglobin M, methemoglobin reductase deficiency)
  Acquired (e.g., nitrates, nitrites)
Inadequate ambient O_2 or less O_2 delivered than expected (rare)
  Disconnection of O_2 supply to nasal cannula, head hood
  Connection of air, rather than O_2, to a mechanical ventilator
Spurious/artifactual
  Oximeter artifact (poor contact between probe and skin, poor pulse
    searching)
  Arterial blood gas artifact (contamination with venous blood)
Other
  Hypoglycemia
  Adrenogenital syndrome
  Polycythemia
  Blood loss

From Smith F: Cyanosis. In Kliegman: *Practical Strategies in Pediatric Diagnosis and Therapy.* Philadelphia, WB Saunders, 1996.

respiratory disease. Episodes of cyanosis may also be the initial sign of hypoglycemia, bacteremia, meningitis, shock, or pulmonary hypertension. Peripheral acrocyanosis is common and does not usually warrant concern.

Pallor, in addition to anemia or acute hemorrhage, should suggest hypoxia, asphyxia, hypoglycemia, sepsis, shock, or adrenal failure.

Hypotension in term infants suggests shock from hypovolemia (hemorrhage, dehydration), the systemic inflammatory response syndrome (as a result of bacterial sepsis or intrauterine infection), cardiac dysfunction (left heart obstructive lesions—hypoplastic left heart syndrome, myocarditis, asphyxia-induced myocardial stunning, anomalous coronary artery), pneumotho-

rax, pneumopericardium, pericardial effusion, or metabolic disorders (hypoglycemia, adrenal insufficiency–salt-losing adrenogenital syndrome). Hypotension is a common problem in sick preterm infants and may be due to any of the problems noted in a term infant. It may develop in preterm infants with severe respiratory distress syndrome. Strategies used to support blood pressure include volume expansion (normal saline is equally as effective as 5% albumin), pressors (dopamine, epinephrine), and corticosteroids. Some infants weighing less than 1,000 g do not respond to fluids or inotropic agents but may respond to therapy with hydrocortisone (1–2.5mg/kg q4–6h). Sudden onset of hypotension in a very low birthweight infant suggests pneumothorax, intraventricular hemorrhage, or subcapsular hepatic hematoma.

Convulsions (Chapter 586.5) usually point to a disorder of the CNS and suggest hypoxic-ischemic encephalopathy resulting from asphyxia, intracranial hemorrhage, cerebral anomaly, subdural effusion, meningitis, hypocalcemia, hypoglycemia, infarction, benign familial seizures, and rarely, pyridoxine dependence, hyponatremia, hypernatremia, inborn errors of metabolism, or drug withdrawal. Seizures beginning in the delivery room or shortly thereafter may be due to the unintentional injection of maternal local anesthetic into the fetus. Convulsions may also result from hyponatremia and water intoxication in the infant after the administration of large amounts of hypotonic fluid to the mother shortly before and during delivery.

Convulsions should be distinguished from the jitteriness that may be present in normal newborns, in infants of diabetic mothers, in those who experienced birth asphyxia or drug withdrawal, and in polycythemic neonates. Jitteriness resembling simple tremors may be stopped by holding the infant's extremity; it often depends on sensory stimuli and occurs when the infant is active, and it is not associated with abnormal eye movements. Seizures in premature infants are often subtle and associated with abnormal eye (fluttering, deviation, stare) or facial (chewing, tongue thrusting) movements; the motor component is often that of tonic extension of the limbs, neck, and trunk. Term infants may have focal or multifocal, clonic or myoclonic movements, but they may also have more subtle seizure activity. *Apnea* may be the first manifestation of seizure activity, particularly in a premature infant. Seizures may adversely affect the subsequent neurodevelopmental outcome and even predispose to non-neonatal seizures. Seizures should be treated aggressively.

After severe birth asphyxia, infants may have *motor automatisms* characterized by oral-buccal-lingual movements, rotary limb activities (rowing, pedaling, swimming), tonic posturing, or myoclonus. These motor activities are not usually accompanied by time-synchronized electroencephalographic discharges, may not signify cortical epileptic activity, respond poorly to anticonvulsant therapy, but are associated with a poor prognosis. Such automatisms may represent cortical depression that produces a brainstem release phenomenon or subcortical seizures.

Lethargy may be a manifestation of infection, asphyxia, hypoglycemia, hypercapnia, sedation from maternal analgesia or anesthesia, a cerebral defect, and indeed, almost any severe disease, including inborn errors of metabolism. Lethargy appearing after the 2nd day should, in particular, suggest infection. Lethargy with emesis suggests increased intracranial pressure or an inborn error of metabolism.

Irritability may be a sign of discomfort accompanying intraabdominal conditions, meningeal irritation, drug withdrawal, infections, congenital glaucoma, or any condition producing pain. As in later infancy, the eardrums should always be examined as a possible source of pain. *Hyperactivity*, especially in a premature infant, may be a sign of hypoxia, pneumothorax, emphysema, hypoglycemia, hypocalcemia, CNS damage, drug withdrawal, neonatal thyrotoxicosis, bronchospasm, esophageal reflux, or discomfort from a cold environment.

The intensive care of neonates involves a number of painful procedures, including heelstick blood sampling, endotracheal intubation and suctioning, mechanical ventilation, and insertion of intravascular catheters. Pain in neonates results in obvious distress and acute physiologic stress responses, and it may have developmental implications for pain in later life.

Pain and discomfort are potentially avoidable problems during the treatment of sick infants. Pre-emptive relief from painful stimuli should be provided before pain or anxiety develops (Chapter 66). The most frequently used drugs are narcotics (morphine, fentanyl) or benzodiazepines (midazolam, lorazepam). Some minor but painful procedures on well neonates have also been managed with oral concentrated (25–50%) sucrose solutions.

Failure to feed well is seen in most sick newborn infants and should always occasion a careful search for infection, a central or peripheral nervous system disorder, intestinal obstruction, and other abnormal conditions.

Fever may be the result of too high an environmental temperature because of weather, overheated nurseries or isolettes/radiant warmers, or too many clothes. It is also noted in "dehydration fever" of newborn infants. If these causes of fever can be eliminated, serious infection (pneumonia, bacteremia, meningitis, and viral infections, particularly herpes simplex or enteroviruses) must be considered, although such infections often occur without provoking a febrile response in newborn infants (see Chapters 161 and 162). An unexplained *fall in body temperature* may accompany infection or other serious disturbances of the circulation or CNS. A sudden servo-controlled increase in isolette temperature to maintain body temperature is a sign of temperature instability and may be associated with sepsis.

Periods of *apnea*, particularly in premature infants, may be associated with various disturbances (see Chapter 90.2). When apnea recurs or when the intervals are longer than 20 sec or are associated with cyanosis or bradycardia, an immediate diagnostic evaluation is needed.

Jaundice during the 1st 24 hr of life warrants diagnostic evaluation and should be considered to be due to hemolysis until proved otherwise. Septicemia and intrauterine infections such as syphilis, cytomegalovirus, and toxoplasmosis should also be considered, especially in infants with an increase in plasma direct-reacting bilirubin.

Jaundice after the 1st 24 hr may be "physiologic" or may be due to septicemia, hemolytic anemia, galactosemia, hepatitis, congenital atresia of the bile ducts, inspissated bile syndrome after erythroblastosis fetalis, syphilis, herpes simplex, or other congenital infections (see Chapter 91.3).

Vomiting during the 1st day of life suggests obstruction in the upper digestive tract or increased intracranial pressure. Roentgenographic studies are indicated when obstruction is suspected. Vomiting may also be a nonspecific symptom of an illness such as septicemia. It is a common manifestation of overfeeding or inexperienced feeding technique, pyloric stenosis, milk allergy, duodenal ulcer, stress ulcer, or adrenal insufficiency. Vomitus containing dark blood is usually a sign of a serious illness; the benign possibility of swallowed maternal blood should also be considered. Bile-stained vomitus strongly suggests obstruction below the ampulla of Vater and warrants contrast radiography.

Diarrhea may be a symptom of overfeeding (especially high–caloric density formula), acute gastroenteritis, or malabsorption, or it may be a nonspecific symptom of infection. Diarrhea may occur in conditions accompanied by compromised circulation of part of the intestinal or genital tract, such as mesenteric thrombosis, necrotizing enterocolitis, strangulated hernia, intussusception, and torsion of the ovary or testis.

Abdominal distention, usually a sign of intestinal obstruction or an intra-abdominal mass, may also be seen in infants with enteritis, necrotizing enterocolitis, isolated intestinal perforation, ileus accompanying sepsis, respiratory distress, ascites, or hypokalemia.

TABLE 87–1. **Common Life-Threatening Congenital Anomalies**

Name	Manifestations
Choanal atresia	Respiratory distress in delivery room, apnea, unable to pass nasogastric tube through nares. Suspect CHARGE syndrome
Pierre Robin syndrome	Micrognathia, cleft palate, airway obstruction
Diaphragmatic hernia	Scaphoid abdomen, bowel sounds present in chest, respiratory distress
Tracheoesophageal fistula	Polyhydramnios, aspiration pneumonia, excessive salivation, unable to place nasogastric tube in stomach. Suspect VATER syndrome
Intestinal obstruction: volvulus, duodenal atresia, ileal atresia	Polyhydramnios, bile-stained emesis, abdominal distention. Suspect trisomy 21, cystic fibrosis, cocaine
Gastroschisis, omphalocele	Polyhydramnios, intestinal obstruction
Renal agenesis, Potter syndrome	Oligohydramnios, anuria, pulmonary hypoplasia, pneumothorax
Neural tube defects: anencephalus, meningomyelocele	Polyhydramnios, elevated α-fetoprotein, decreased fetal activity
Ductal-dependent congenital heart disease	Cyanosis, hypotension, murmur

CHARGE = Coloboma of the eye, heart anomaly, choanal atresia, retardation, and genital and ear anomalies; VATER = vertebral defects, imperforate anus, tracheoesophageal fistula, and radial and renal dysplasia.

Failure to move an extremity (pseudoparalysis) suggests fracture, dislocation, or nerve injury. It is also seen in osteomyelitis and other infections that cause pain on movement of the affected part.

CONGENITAL ANOMALIES

Congenital anomalies are a major cause of stillbirths and neonatal deaths, but they are perhaps even more important as causes of acute illness, including metabolic disorders, and long-term morbidity. (Anomalies are discussed in general in Chapters 70 and 97 and specifically in the chapters on the various systems of the body.) Early recognition of anomalies is important for planning care; for some, such as tracheoesophageal fistula, diaphragmatic hernia, choanal atresia, and intestinal obstruction, immediate medical and surgical therapy is essential for survival (Table 87–1). Parents are likely to feel anxious and guilty on learning of the existence of a congenital anomaly and require sensitive counseling.

Barker DP, Rutter N: Exposure to invasive procedures in neonatal intensive care unit admissions. *Arch Dis Child Fetal Neonatal Ed* 1995;72:F47.

Brunquell PJ, Glennon CM, DiMario FJ, et al: Prediction of outcome based on clinical seizure type in newborn infants. *J Pediatr* 2002;140:707–12.

Larson BA: Pain management in neonates. *Acta Paediatr* 1999;88:1301.

Levene M: The clinical conundrum of neonatal seizures. *Arch Child Dis Fetal Neonatal Ed* 2002;86:F75–7.

Prevention and management of pain and stress in the neonate. American Academy of Pediatrics. Committee on Fetus and Newborn. Committee on Drugs. Section on Anesthesiology. Section on Surgery. Canadian Paediatric Society. Fetus and Newborn Committee. *Pediatrics* 2000;105:454.

Seri I, Evans J: Controversies in the diagnosis and management of hypotension in the newborn infant. *Curr Opin Pediatr* 2001;13:116.

Chapter 88
Nervous System Disorders
Barbara J. Stoll and Robert M. Kliegman

Central nervous system (CNS) disorders are important causes of neonatal mortality and both short- and long-term morbidity. The etiology is complex and multifactorial and includes developmental abnormalities that may be genetic and/or environmental, acute problems surrounding delivery, and postnatal events. Predisposing factors include chronic or acute maternal illness resulting in uteroplacental dysfunction, intrauterine infection, macrosomia/dystocia, prematurity, intrauterine growth restriction, prolonged labor, breech presentation, and acute and often unavoidable emergencies during delivery that result in mechanical and/or hypoxic-ischemic injury.

88.1 The Cranium

Caput succedaneum is a diffuse, sometimes ecchymotic, edematous swelling of the soft tissues of the scalp involving the portion presenting during vertex delivery. It may extend across the midline and across suture lines. The edema disappears within the first few days of life. Analogous swelling, discoloration, and distortion of the face are seen in face presentations. No specific treatment is needed, but if extensive ecchymoses are present, hyperbilirubinemia may develop. *Molding* of the head and overriding of the parietal bones are frequently associated with caput succedaneum and become more evident after the caput has receded, but they disappear during the first weeks of life. Rarely, a hemorrhagic caput may result in shock and require blood transfusion.

Erythema, abrasions, ecchymoses, and *subcutaneous fat necrosis* of facial or scalp soft tissues may be noted after forceps or vacuum-assisted deliveries. Their location depends on the area of application of the forceps. Ecchymoses may be seen after manipulative deliveries and occasionally in premature infants for no discernible reason.

Subconjunctival and retinal hemorrhages are frequent, and *petechiae* of the skin of the head and neck are common. All are probably secondary to a sudden increase in intrathoracic pressure during passage of the chest through the birth canal. Parents should be assured that these hemorrhages are temporary and the result of *normal* events of delivery.

Cephalohematoma (Fig. 88–1) is a subperiosteal hemorrhage, hence always limited to the surface of one cranial bone. No discoloration of the overlying scalp occurs, and swelling is not usually visible until several hours after birth because subperiosteal bleeding is a slow process. An underlying skull fracture, usually linear and not depressed, is occasionally associated with cephalohematoma. Cranial meningocele may be differentiated from cephalohematoma by pulsation, increased pressure on crying, and roentgenographic evidence of a bony defect. Most cephalohematomas are resorbed within 2 wk–3 mo, depending on their size. They may begin to calcify by the end of the 2nd wk. A sensation of central depression suggesting, but not indicative of an underlying fracture or bony defect is usually encountered on palpation of the organized rim of a cephalohematoma. A few remain for years as bony protuberances and are detectable

roentgenographically as widening of the diploic space; cystlike defects may persist for months or years. Despite these residuals, cephalohematomas require no treatment, although phototherapy may be necessary to ameliorate hyperbilirubinemia. Incision plus drainage is contraindicated because of the risk of introducing infection in a benign condition. A massive cephalohematoma may rarely result in blood loss severe enough to require transfusion. It may also be associated with a skull fracture, coagulopathy, and intracranial hemorrhage.

Fractures of the skull may occur as a result of pressure from forceps or from the maternal symphysis pubis, sacral promontory, or ischial spines. Linear fractures, the most common, cause no symptoms and require no treatment. Depressed fractures are usually indentations of the calvaria similar to a dent in a Ping-Pong ball; they are generally a complication of forceps delivery or fetal compression. Affected infants may be asymptomatic unless they have associated intracranial injury; it is advisable to elevate severe depressions to prevent cortical injury from sustained pressure. Fracture of the occipital bone with separation of the basal and squamous portions almost invariably causes fatal hemorrhage because of disruption of the underlying vascular sinuses. Such fractures may result during breech deliveries from traction on the hyperextended spine of the infant with the head fixed in the maternal pelvis.

88.2 Intracranial-Intraventricular Hemorrhage and Periventricular Leukomalacia

Etiology and Epidemiology. Intracranial hemorrhage may result from trauma or asphyxia and, rarely, from a primary hemorrhagic disturbance or congenital vascular anomaly. Traumatic epidural, subdural, or subarachnoid hemorrhage is especially likely when the fetal head is large in proportion to the size of the mother's pelvic outlet, when for other reasons labor is prolonged, in breech or precipitate deliveries, or as a result of mechanical assistance with delivery. Massive subdural hemorrhage, often associated with tears in the tentorium cerebelli or, less frequently, in the falx cerebri, is rare but is encountered more often in full-term than in premature infants. Primary hemorrhagic disturbances and vascular malformations are rare and usually give rise to subarachnoid or intracerebral hemorrhage. Intracranial bleeding may be associated with disseminated intravascular coagulopathy, isoimmune thrombocytopenia, and neonatal vitamin K deficiency (especially in infants born to mothers receiving phenobarbital or phenytoin). Intracranial hemorrhage often involves the ventricles (**intraventricular hemorrhage** [IVH]) of premature infants delivered spontaneously without apparent trauma.

Pathogenesis. Brain injury is an important problem in very low birthweight (VLBW) preterm infants. The major neuropathologic lesions are IVH and periventricular leukomalacia (PVL). IVH in premature infants occurs in the gelatinous subependymal germinal matrix. This periventricular area is the site of embryonal neurons and fetal glial cells, which migrate outwardly to the cortex. Immature blood vessels in this highly vascular area may be subjected to various forces that, together with poor tissue vascular support, predispose premature infants to IVH. By term, the germinal matrix has become attenuated and the tissue's vascular support has strengthened. *Predisposing factors or events* for IVH include prematurity, respiratory distress syndrome, hypoxic-ischemic or hypotensive injury, reperfusion of damaged vessels, increased or decreased cerebral blood flow, reduced vascular integrity, increased venous pressure, pneumothorax, hypervolemia, and hypertension. These factors result in rupture of the germinal matrix blood vessels. Similar injurious factors (hypoxic-ischemic-hypotensive), venous

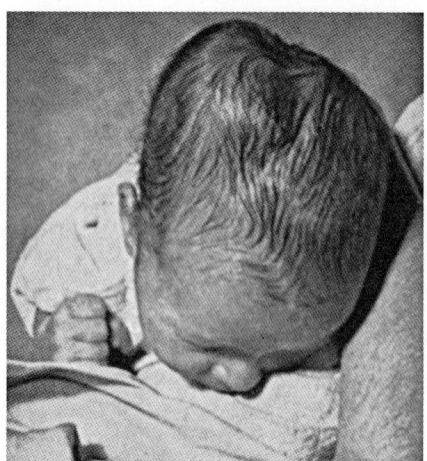

FIGURE 88–1. Cephalohematoma of the right parietal bone.

obstruction from an IVH, or undetected fetal stress may produce periventricular hemorrhage/necrosis (echodensities). PVL is characterized by focal necrotic lesions in the periventricular white matter and/or more diffuse white matter damage. Cranial ultrasound in the first weeks of life can detect focal echodensities and cystic lesions, but more sophisticated imaging techniques are required to detect diffuse injury.

Understanding of the pathogenesis of PVL is evolving, and both intrauterine and postnatal events are involved. A complex interaction exists between the cerebral vasculature and regulation of cerebral blood flow (both gestational age dependent), disturbances in the oligodendrocyte precursors required for myelination, and maternal/fetal infection and/or inflammation. The risk for PVL increases in infants with IVH and/or ventriculomegaly. Cerebral white matter damage/PVL is responsible for a substantial portion of the adverse neurodevelopment of VLBW preterm infants (cerebral palsy). The possible interaction of various factors in the pathogenesis of white matter damage is shown in Figure 88–2.

Clinical Manifestations. The incidence of IVH increases with decreasing birthweight and gestational age: 60–70% of 500–750 g infants and 10–20% of 1,000–1,500 g infants. IVH is rarely present at birth; however, 80–90% of cases occur between birth and the 3rd day of life, 50% occur on the 1st day. Twenty to 40% of cases progress during the 1st wk of life, and delayed hemorrhage may occur in 10–15% of patients after the 1st wk of life. New-onset IVH is rare after the 1st mo of life regardless of birthweight. The most common symptoms are diminished or absent Moro reflex, poor muscle tone, lethargy, apnea, and somnolence. Premature infants with IVH often have a precipitous deterioration on the 2nd or 3rd day of life. Periods of apnea, pallor, or cyanosis; failure to suck well; abnormal eye signs; a high-pitched, shrill cry; muscular twitching, convulsions, decreased muscle tone, or paralysis; metabolic acidosis; shock; and a decreased hematocrit or failure of the hematocrit to increase after transfusion may be the first indications. The fontanel *may* be tense and bulging. Severe neurologic depression progresses to coma after more severe IVH, with associated hemorrhage in the cerebral cortex and ventricular dilatation. A saltatory pattern consists of symptomatic episodes with intervening asymptomatic periods. In some cases (grade I, II) no clinical manifestations may be seen.

PVL is usually asymptomatic until the neurologic sequelae of white matter damage become apparent in later infancy as spastic motor deficits. PVL may be present at birth but usually occurs later as an early echodense phase (3–10 days of life), followed by the typical echolucent (cystic) phase (14–20 days of life).

Diagnosis. Intracranial hemorrhage is diagnosed on the basis of the history, clinical manifestations, transfontanel cranial ultrasonography or CT, and knowledge of the birthweight-specific risks of the type of hemorrhage. The diagnosis of *subdural hemorrhage* in a large for gestational age term infant with cephalopelvic disproportion may be delayed 1 mo until the chronic subdural fluid volume expands and produces megalocephaly, frontal bossing, a bulging fontanel, seizures, and anemia. Late occurrence also warrants suspicion of child abuse. Alternatively, a well neonate with a seizure of short duration may have a benign *subarachnoid hemorrhage*.

Although preterm infants with severe IVH manifest rapid shock, mottling, anemia, coma, or a bulging fontanel, many signs of IVH are nonspecific or absent. Therefore, it is recommended that a premature infant be evaluated with routine real-time *cranial ultrasonography* through the anterior fontanel to detect IVH. Infants weighing under 1,500 g (or <30 wk gestational age) are at high risk for IVH and should be examined within the 1st 7–14 days of life and again at 36–40 wk postmenstrual age. If the 1st scan is abnormal, additional interval examinations are indicated to detect posthemorrhagic hydrocephalus. Ultrasound examination also detects the precystic and cystic symmetric lesions of PVL and the asymmetric intraparenchymal echogenic lesions of cortical hemorrhagic infarction. Furthermore, the delayed development of cortical atrophy, or porencephaly, and the severity, progression, or regression of posthemorrhagic hydrocephalus can be determined by serial ultrasonography. Diffusion-weighted MRI improves the early detection of diffuse PVL/white matter damage and isolated cerebral infarction or stroke.

Three levels of increasing severity of IVH are defined by ultrasound for low-birthweight (LBW) infants: grade I is bleeding confined to the germinal matrix–subependymal region or to less than 10% of the ventricle (≈35% of IVH cases), grade II is intraventricular bleeding with 10–50% filling of the ventricle (≈40% of IVH cases), and grade III is more than 50% involvement with dilated ventricles (Fig. 88–3). Another classification includes a grade IV IVH, which is similar to grade III plus intraparenchymal hemorrhage. Ventriculomegaly is defined as mild (0.5–1 cm), moderate (1.0–1.5 cm) or severe (>1.5 cm).

CT or MRI is indicated for term infants in whom brain injury is suspected because ultrasound may not reveal intraparenchymal hemorrhage or infarction. Lumbar puncture may be indicated in infants with signs of increased intracranial pressure or a deteriorating clinical condition to identify gross subarachnoid hemorrhage or to rule out the possibility of bacterial meningitis; cerebrospinal fluid usually has elevated protein levels with many red blood cells. Not infrequently, hypoglycorrhachia and mild lymphocytosis can be noted. Because a small amount of bleeding into cerebrospinal fluid often occurs in the course of normal and even cesarean deliveries, small numbers of red blood cells or slight xanthochromia in subarachnoid fluid does not necessarily indicate significant intracranial hemorrhage. Conversely, the subarachnoid fluid may be absolutely clear in

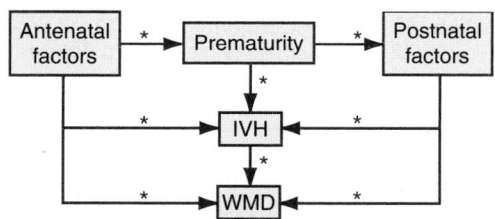

The * represents places in this scheme where factors may diminish or promote the likelihood of developing WMD.

Possible Promoters of WMD Occurrence
Fetal growth restriction
Hypothyroxinemia
Hypocarbia/hypercarbia
Fetal vasculitis
Maternal/placental infection
Other cytokine-promoting factors

Possible Protectors Against WMD Occurrence
Antenatal corticosteroids
Prostaglandin inhibitors
Toxemia/magnesium

FIGURE 88–2. Schematic of possible associations linking prematurity, intraventricular hemorrhage (IVH), and white matter disorders (WMD). Antenatal factors may represent factors that both lead to prematurity and act as an independent marker of risk for IVH and WMD. Factors that occur as a result of or in association with prematurity may in turn modify the likelihood of having IVH or WMD. IVH in its own right may contribute to WMD. (From Kuban K, Sanocka U, Leviton A, et al: White matter disorders of prematurity: Association with intraventricular hemorrhage and ventriculomegaly. *J Pediatr* 1999;134:539.)

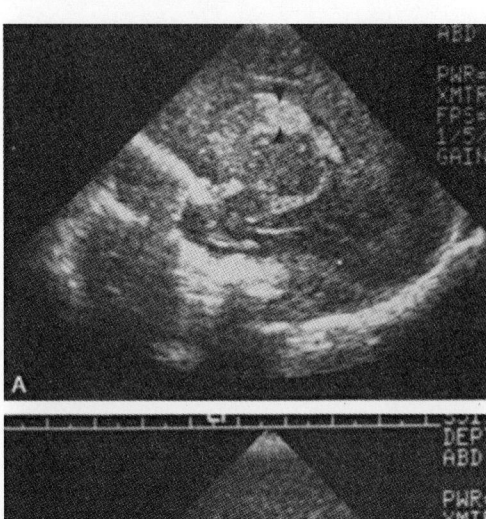

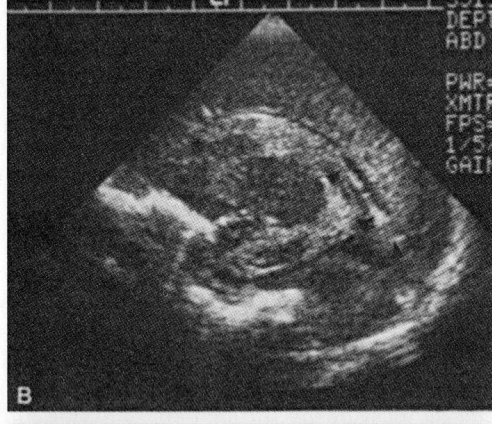

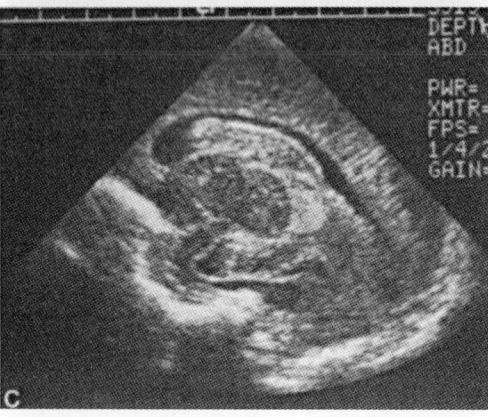

FIGURE 88–3. Grading the severity of germinal matrix intraventricular hemorrhage with parasagittal ultrasound scans. *A,* Grade I. Note the echogenic blood in the germinal matrix *(arrowheads)* just anterior to the anterior tip of the choroid plexus, which (normally) is also echogenic. *B,* Grade II. Note the echogenic blood *(arrowheads)* filling less than 50% of the ventricular area. *C,* Grade III. Note the large blood clot nearly completely filling and distending the entire lateral ventricle. (From Intracranial hemorrhage: Germinal matrix-intraventricular hemorrhage of the premature infant. In Volpe JJ [editor]: *Neurology of the Newborn,* 3rd ed. Philadelphia, WB Saunders, 1995.)

infants with severe subdural or intracerebral hemorrhage and no communication with the subarachnoid space.

Prognosis. Patients with massive hemorrhage caused by tears of the tentorium or falx cerebri rapidly deteriorate and may die after birth. In utero hemorrhage associated with maternal idiopathic or, more often, fetal alloimmune thrombocytopenia may occur as severe cerebral hemorrhage or a porencephalic cyst after resolution of a fetal cortical hemorrhage.

In most infants with IVH and acute ventricular distention, *posthemorrhagic hydrocephalus* does not develop. Ten to 15% of LBW neonates with IVH have hydrocephalus, which may initially be present without clinical signs such as an enlarging head circumference, apnea, bradycardia, lethargy, a bulging fontanel, or widely split sutures. In infants in whom symptomatic hydrocephalus develops, clinical signs may be delayed 2–4 wk despite progressive ventricular distention and compression (thinning) of the cerebral cortex. Posthemorrhagic hydrocephalus is arrested or regresses in 65% of affected infants.

Progressive hydrocephalus requiring ventricular-peritoneal shunting, intraparenchymal hemorrhage, and extensive PVL are associated with a poor prognosis. IVH with intraparenchymal echodensities larger than 1 cm are associated with high mortality and a high incidence of motor and cognitive deficits. Grade I–II IVH may be due to factors other than severe hypoxia-ischemia and has a lower risk of long-term neurologic sequelae if it is not associated with PVL or intraparenchymal hemorrhage.

Prevention. The incidence of traumatic intracranial hemorrhage may be reduced by judicious management of cephalopelvic disproportion and operative (forceps, cesarean section) delivery. Fetal or neonatal hemorrhage caused by maternal idiopathic thrombocytopenic purpura or alloimmune thrombocytopenia may be reduced by maternal treatment with steroids, intravenous immunoglobulin, or fetal platelet transfusion and cesarean section. Vitamin K should be given before delivery to all women receiving phenobarbital or phenytoin during the pregnancy. Wide fluctuations in neonatal blood pressure should be avoided.

A single course of antenatal corticosteroids administered to women in preterm labor reduces both IVH (betamethasone and dexamethasone) and PVL (betamethasone only). The safety plus efficacy of multiple courses of antenatal steroids is unknown. Furthermore, the effect of multiple courses of steroids on brain growth and development has raised concern. The prophylactic administration of low-dose indomethacin to VLBW preterm infants reduces the incidence of severe IVH but does not improve the overall outcome.

Treatment. Although no treatment is available for IVH, it may be associated with other complications that require therapy. Seizures are aggressively treated with anticonvulsant drugs, anemia-shock requires transfusion with packed red blood cells or fresh frozen plasma, and acidosis is treated by the judicious and slow administration of sodium bicarbonate. Neurosurgical placement of an external ventriculostomy catheter may be needed in the early stage of uncontrolled, symptomatic posthemorrhagic hydrocephalus. When a VLBW infant is large enough, a permanent ventricular-peritoneal shunt is placed. Serial lumbar punctures, diuretics, and acetazolamide have no role in the management of posthemorrhagic hydrocephalus.

Symptomatic subdural hemorrhage in large term infants should be treated by removing the subdural fluid collection with a spinal needle placed through the lateral margin of the anterior fontanel. In addition to birth trauma, child abuse should be suspected in all infants with subdural effusions.

88.3 Spine and Spinal Cord

Injury to the spine/spinal cord is rare but can be devastating. Strong traction exerted when the spine is hyperextended or when the direction of pull is lateral, or forceful longitudinal traction on the trunk while the head is still firmly engaged in the pelvis, especially when combined with flexion and torsion of the vertical axis, may produce fracture and separation of the vertebrae. Such injuries, rarely diagnosed clinically, are most likely to occur when difficulty is encountered in delivering the shoulders in cephalic presentations and the head in breech presentations.

The injury occurs most commonly at the level of the 4th cervical vertebra with cephalic presentations and the lower cervical–upper thoracic vertebrae with breech presentations. Transection of the cord may occur with or without vertebral fractures; hemorrhage and edema may produce neurologic signs that are indistinguishable from those of transection except that they may not be permanent. Areflexia, loss of sensation, and complete paralysis of voluntary motion occur below the level of injury, although the persistence of a withdrawal reflex mediated through spinal centers distal to the area of injury is frequently misinterpreted as representing voluntary motion. If the injury is severe, the infant, who from birth may be in poor condition because of respiratory depression, shock, or hypothermia, may deteriorate rapidly to death within several hours before any neurologic signs are obvious. Alternatively, the course may be protracted, with symptoms and signs appearing at birth or later in the 1st wk; immobility, flaccidity, and associated brachial plexus injuries may not be recognized for several days. Constipation may also be present. Some infants survive for prolonged periods, their initial flaccidity, immobility, and areflexia being replaced after several weeks or months by rigid flexion of the extremities, increased muscle tone, and spasms. Apnea on day 1 and poor motor recovery by 3 mo are poor prognostic signs.

The differential diagnosis includes amyotonia congenita and myelodysplasia associated with spina bifida occulta. Ultrasonography or MRI confirms the diagnosis. Treatment of the survivors is supportive, including home ventilation; patients often remain permanently disabled. When a fracture or dislocation is causing compression, the prognosis is related to the time elapsed before the compression is relieved.

88.4 Peripheral Nerve Injuries

Brachial Palsy. Brachial plexus injury is a common problem, with an incidence of 0.6–4.6 per 1,000 live births. Injury to the brachial plexus may cause paralysis of the upper part of the arm with or without paralysis of the forearm or hand or, more commonly, paralysis of the entire arm. These injuries occur in macrosomic infants and when lateral traction is exerted on the head and neck during delivery of the shoulder in a vertex presentation, when the arms are extended over the head in a breech presentation, or when excessive traction is placed on the shoulders. Approximately 45% are associated with shoulder dystocia. In **Erb-Duchenne paralysis**, the injury is limited to the 5th and 6th cervical nerves. The infant loses the power to abduct the arm from the shoulder, rotate the arm externally, and supinate the forearm. The characteristic position consists of adduction and internal rotation of the arm with pronation of the forearm. Power to extend the forearm is retained, but the biceps reflex is absent; the Moro reflex is absent on the affected side (Fig. 88–4). The outer aspect of the arm may have some sensory impairment. Power in the forearm and hand grasp are preserved unless the lower part of the plexus is also injured; the presence of hand grasp is a favorable prognostic sign. When the injury includes the phrenic nerve, alteration in diaphragmatic excursion may be observed fluoroscopically. **Klumpke paralysis** is a rarer form of brachial palsy; injury to the 7th and 8th cervical nerves and the 1st thoracic nerve produces a paralyzed hand and ipsilateral ptosis and miosis (Horner syndrome) if the sympathetic fibers of the 1st thoracic root are also injured. Mild cases may not be detected immediately after birth. Differentiation must be made from cerebral injury; from fracture, dislocation, or epiphyseal separation of the humerus; and from fracture of the clavicle. MRI demonstrates nerve root rupture or avulsion.

Full recovery occurs in most patients, the prognosis depending on whether the nerve was merely injured or was lacerated. If the paralysis was due to edema and hemorrhage about the nerve fibers, function should return within a few months; if due to laceration, permanent damage may result. Involvement of the deltoid is usually the most serious problem and may result in shoulder drop secondary to muscle atrophy. In general, paralysis of the upper part of the arm has a better prognosis than paralysis of the lower part does.

Treatment consists of partial immobilization and appropriate positioning to prevent the development of contractures. In upper arm paralysis, the arm should be abducted 90 degrees with external rotation at the shoulder, full supination of the forearm, and slight extension at the wrist with the palm turned toward the face. This position may be achieved with a brace or splint during the first 1–2 wk. Immobilization should be intermittent through the day while the infant is asleep and between feedings. In lower arm or hand paralysis, the wrist should be splinted in a neutral position and padding placed in the fist. When the entire arm is paralyzed, the same treatment principles should be followed. Gentle massage and range-of-motion exercises may be started by 7–10 days of age. Infants should be closely monitored with active and passive corrective exercises. If the paralysis persists without improvement for 3–6 mo, neuroplasty, neurolysis, end-to-end anastomosis, and nerve grafting offer hope for partial recovery.

The type of treatment and the prognosis depend on the mechanism of injury and the number of nerve roots involved. The mildest injury to a peripheral nerve (neurapraxia) is due to edema and heals spontaneously within a few weeks. Axonotmesis is more severe and is due to nerve fiber disruption with an intact myelin sheath; function usually returns in a few months. Total disruption of nerves (neurotmesis) or root avulsion is the most severe, especially if it involves C5–T1; microsurgical repair may be indicated. Fortunately, most (75%) injuries are at the root level C5–C6 and involve neurapraxia and axonotmesis and should heal spontaneously. Botulism toxin may be used to treat biceps-triceps co-contractions.

Phrenic Nerve Paralysis. Phrenic nerve injury (3rd, 4th, 5th cervical nerves) with diaphragmatic paralysis must be considered

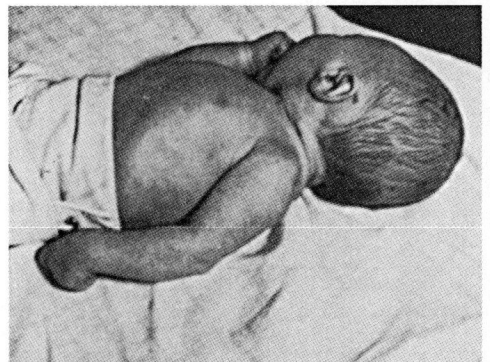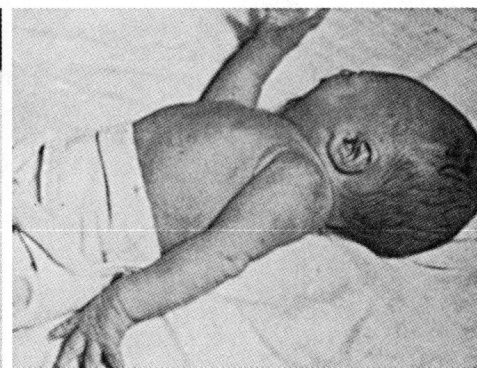

FIGURE 88–4. Brachial palsy of the left arm (asymmetric Moro reflex).

when cyanosis and irregular and labored respirations develop. Such injuries, usually unilateral, are associated with ipsilateral upper brachial palsy. Because breathing is thoracic in type, the abdomen does not bulge with inspiration. Breath sounds are diminished on the affected side. The thrust of the diaphragm, which may often be felt just under the costal margin on the normal side, is absent on the affected side. The *diagnosis* is established by ultrasonography or fluoroscopic examination, which reveals elevation of the diaphragm on the paralyzed side and seesaw movements of the two sides of the diaphragm during respiration.

No specific *treatment* is available; infants should be placed on the involved side and given oxygen if necessary. Initially, intravenous feedings may be needed; later, progressive gavage or oral feeding may be started, depending on the infant's condition. Pulmonary infections are a serious complication. Recovery usually occurs spontaneously by 1–3 mo; rarely, surgical plication of the diaphragm may be indicated.

Facial Nerve Palsy. Facial palsy is usually a peripheral paralysis that results from pressure over the facial nerve in utero, from efforts during labor, or from forceps use during delivery. Rarely, it may result from nuclear agenesis of the facial nerve. Peripheral paralysis is flaccid and, when complete, involves the entire side of the face, including the forehead. When the infant cries, movement occurs only on the nonparalyzed side of the face, and the mouth is drawn to that side. On the affected side the forehead is smooth, the eye cannot be closed, the nasolabial fold is absent, and the corner of the mouth droops. The forehead wrinkles on the affected side with central paralysis because only the lower two thirds of the face is involved. The infant usually also has other manifestations of intracranial injury, most commonly a 6th nerve palsy. The *prognosis* depends on whether the nerve was injured by pressure or whether the nerve fibers were torn. Improvement occurs within a few weeks in the former instance. Care of the exposed eye is essential. Neuroplasty may be indicated when the paralysis is persistent. Facial palsy may be confused with absence of the depressor muscles of the mouth, which is a benign problem.

Other peripheral nerves are seldom injured in utero or at birth except when they are involved in fractures or hemorrhage.

88.5 Hypoxia-Ischemia

Anoxia is a term used to indicate the consequences of complete lack of oxygen as a result of a number of primary causes. *Hypoxia* refers to an arterial concentration of oxygen that is less than normal, and *ischemia* refers to blood flow to cells or organs that is insufficient to maintain their normal function. *Hypoxic-ischemic encephalopathy* is an important cause of permanent damage to CNS cells that may result in neonatal death or be manifested later as cerebral palsy or mental deficiency. Fifteen to 20% of infants with hypoxic-ischemic encephalopathy die in the neonatal period, and 25–30% of survivors are left with permanent neurodevelopmental abnormalities (cerebral palsy, mental retardation). Prevention is critical because no specific therapy can reverse the CNS injury. Death and disability may sometimes be prevented through symptomatic treatment with oxygen or artificial respiration and correction of the associated multiorgan system dysfunction (Table 88–1). *Asphyxia* is considered in infants with fetal acidosis (pH <7.0), a 5-min Apgar score of 0–3, hypoxic-ischemic encephalopathy (altered tone, depressed level of consciousness, seizures), and other multiorgan system signs (see Table 88–1).

Etiology. Fetal hypoxia may be caused by (1) inadequate oxygenation of maternal blood as a result of hypoventilation during anesthesia, cyanotic heart disease, respiratory failure, or carbon monoxide poisoning; (2) low maternal blood pressure as a result

TABLE 88–1. Effects of Asphyxia

System	Effect
Central nervous system	Hypoxic-ischemic encephalopathy, infarction, intracranial hemorrhage, seizures, cerebral edema, hypotonia, hypertonia
Cardiovascular	Myocardial ischemia, poor contractility, cardiac stun, tricuspid insufficiency, hypotension
Pulmonary	Pulmonary hypertension, pulmonary hemorrhage, respiratory distress syndrome
Renal	Acute tubular or cortical necrosis
Adrenal	Adrenal hemorrhage
Gastrointestinal	Perforation, ulceration with hemorrhage, necrosis
Metabolic	Inappropriate secretion of antidiuretic hormone, hyponatremia, hypoglycemia, hypocalcemia, myoglobinuria
Integument	Subcutaneous fat necrosis
Hematology	Disseminated intravascular coagulation

of the hypotension that may complicate spinal anesthesia or that may result from compression of the vena cava and aorta by the gravid uterus; (3) inadequate relaxation of the uterus to permit placental filling as a result of uterine tetany caused by the administration of excessive oxytocin; (4) premature separation of the placenta; (5) impedance to the circulation of blood through the umbilical cord as a result of compression or knotting of the cord; (6) uterine vessel vasoconstriction by cocaine; and (7) placental insufficiency from numerous causes, including toxemia and postmaturity.

Placental insufficiency often remains undetected on clinical assessment. Intrauterine growth restriction may develop in chronically hypoxic fetuses without the traditional signs of fetal distress (e.g., bradycardia). Doppler umbilical waveform velocimetry (demonstrating increased fetal vascular resistance, see Fig. 85–3) and cordocentesis (demonstrating fetal hypoxia and lactic acidosis) identify a chronically hypoxic infant. Uterine contractions further reduce umbilical oxygenation and, as a consequence, depress the fetal cardiovascular system and CNS and thereby result in low Apgar scores and postnatal hypoxia in the delivery room.

After birth, hypoxia may be caused by (1) anemia severe enough to lower the oxygen content of the blood to a critical level, as after severe hemorrhage or hemolytic disease; (2) shock severe enough to interfere with the transport of oxygen to vital organs as a result of overwhelming infection, massive blood loss, and intracranial or adrenal hemorrhage; (3) a deficit in arterial oxygen saturation from failure to breathe adequately postnatally because of a cerebral defect, narcosis, or injury; and (4) failure of oxygenation of an adequate amount of blood as a result of severe forms of cyanotic congenital heart disease or pulmonary disease.

Pathophysiology and Pathology. Within minutes of the onset of total fetal hypoxia, bradycardia, hypotension, decreased cardiac output, and severe metabolic as well as respiratory acidosis occur. The initial circulatory response of the fetus is increased shunting through the ductus venosus, ductus arteriosus, and foramen ovale, with transient maintenance of perfusion of the brain, heart, and adrenals in preference to the lungs (because of pulmonary vasoconstriction), liver, kidneys, and intestine.

The pathology of hypoxia-ischemia is dependent on the affected organ and the severity of the insult. Early congestion, fluid leak from increased capillary permeability, and endothelial cell swelling may then lead to signs of coagulation necrosis and cell death. Congestion and petechiae are seen in the pericardium, pleura, thymus, heart, adrenals, and meninges. Prolonged intrauterine hypoxia may result in PVL and pulmonary arteriole smooth muscle hyperplasia, which predisposes the infant to pulmonary hypertension (Chapter 90.7). If fetal distress produces gasping, the amniotic fluid contents (meconium, squames, lanugo) are aspirated into the trachea or lungs.

The combination of chronic fetal hypoxia and acute hypoxic-ischemic injury after birth results in gestational age–specific neuropathology. Term infants demonstrate neuronal necrosis of the cortex (later, cortical atrophy) and parasagittal ischemic injury. Preterm infants demonstrate PVL (later, spastic diplegia), status marmoratus of the basal ganglia, and IVH. Term more often than preterm infants have focal or multifocal cortical infarcts that produce focal seizures and hemiplegia. Infarctions are best visualized with contrast CT scanning or rapid diffusion MRI. In addition to focal lesions, CT scanning may demonstrate diffuse decreases in tissue attenuation. Cerebral edema with resultant increased intracranial pressure occurs in some infants who have severe hypoxic-ischemic encephalopathy. Excitatory amino acids may have an important role in the pathogenesis of asphyxial brain injury.

Clinical Manifestations. Intrauterine growth restriction with increased vascular resistance may be the first indication of fetal hypoxia. During labor, the fetal heart rate slows, and beat-to-beat variability declines. Continuous heart rate recording may reveal a variable or late (type II dips) deceleration pattern (see Fig. 85–4), and fetal scalp blood analysis may show a pH less than 7.20. The acidosis usually has both metabolic and respiratory components. Particularly in infants near term, these signs should lead to the administration of high concentrations of oxygen to the mother and immediate delivery to avoid fetal death or CNS damage.

At *delivery*, the presence of yellow, meconium-stained amniotic fluid is evidence that fetal distress has occurred. At birth, these infants are frequently depressed and fail to breathe spontaneously. During the ensuing hours, they may remain hypotonic or change from hypotonic to hypertonic, or their tone may appear normal (Table 88–2). Pallor, cyanosis, apnea, a slow heart rate, and unresponsiveness to stimulation are also signs of hypoxic-ischemic encephalopathy. Cerebral edema may develop during the next 24 hr and result in profound brainstem depression. During this time, seizure activity may occur, and it may be severe and refractory to the usual doses of anticonvulsants. Phenobarbital, the drug of choice, is given with an intravenous loading dose (20 mg/kg); additional doses of 10 mg/kg (up to 40–50 mg/kg total) may be needed. Phenytoin (20 mg/kg loading dose) or lorazepam (0.1 mg/kg) may be needed for refractory seizures. Phenobarbital levels should be monitored 24 hr after the loading dose and maintenance therapy (5 mg/kg/24 hr) are begun. Therapeutic phenobarbital levels are 20–40 µg/mL. Though most often a result of the hypoxic-ischemic encephalopathy, seizures in asphyxiated newborns may also be due to hypocalcemia, hypoglycemia, or infection.

In addition to CNS dysfunction, congestive heart failure and cardiogenic shock, persistent pulmonary hypertension (persistent fetal circulation), respiratory distress syndrome, gastrointestinal perforation, hematuria, and acute tubular necrosis are associated with perinatal asphyxia (see Table 88–1).

After delivery, hypoxia is due to respiratory failure and circulatory insufficiency (Chapter 90).

Treatment. Therapy is supportive and directed at the organ system manifestations. Careful attention to ventilatory status and adequate oxygenation, blood volume, hemodynamic status, acid-base balance, and possible infection is important. No established effective treatment is available for the brain tissue injury, although many drugs (phenobarbital, allopurinol, calcium channel blockers) and procedures (total body or local cranial hypothermia) are under study. Aggressive treatment of seizures is critical and may necessitate continuous electroencephalographic monitoring.

Prognosis. The outcome of hypoxic-ischemic encephalopathy ranges from complete recovery to death, the prognosis depending on whether the metabolic and cardiopulmonary complications (hypoxia, hypoglycemia, shock) can be treated, the infant's gestational age (outcome is poorest if the infant is preterm), and the severity of the encephalopathy. Severe encephalopathy (stage 3, see Table 88–2), characterized by flaccid coma, apnea, absent oculocephalic reflexes, and refractory seizures, is associated with a poor prognosis. A low Apgar score at 20 min of age, absence of spontaneous respirations at 20 min of age, and persistence of abnormal neurologic signs at 2 wk of age also predict death or severe cognitive and motor deficits. The combined use of an early electroencephalogram (EEG) and MRI is useful in predicting outcome in term infants with hypoxic-ischemic encephalopathy. Normal MRI and EEG findings are associated with a good recovery, whereas severe MRI and EEG abnormalities predict a poor outcome. All survivors of moderate to severe encephalopathy require comprehensive high-risk medical and developmental follow-up. Early identification of neurodevelopmental problems allows prompt referral for developmental and neurologic care and early intervention services so that the best possible outcome can be achieved.

Brain death after neonatal hypoxic-ischemic encephalopathy is diagnosed by the clinical findings of coma unresponsive to pain, auditory, or visual stimulation; apnea with P_{CO_2} rising from 40 to over 60 mm Hg; and absent brainstem reflexes (pupil, oculocephalic, oculovestibular, corneal, gag, sucking). These findings must occur in the absence of hypothermia, hypotension, and elevated levels of depressant drugs (e.g., phenobarbital). An absence of cerebral blood flow on radionuclide scans and electrical activity on EEG (electrocerebral silence) is inconsistently observed in clinically brain-dead neonatal infants. Persistence of the clinical criteria for 2 days in term and 3 days in preterm infants predicts brain death in most asphyxiated newborns. Nonetheless, no universal agreement has been reached regarding the definition of neonatal brain death. Consideration of withdrawal of life support should include discussions with the family, the health care team, and if there is disagreement, an ethics committee. The best interest of the infant involves judgments about the benefits and harm of continuing therapy or avoiding ongoing futile therapy.

TABLE 88–2. Hypoxic-Ischemic Encephalopathy in Term Infants

Signs	Stage 1	Stage 2	Stage 3
Level of consciousness	Hyperalert	Lethargic	Stuporous, coma
Muscle tone	Normal	Hypotonic	Flaccid
Posture	Normal	Flexion	Decerebrate
Tendon reflexes/clonus	Hyperactive	Hyperactive	Absent
Myoclonus	Present	Present	Absent
Moro reflex	Strong	Weak	Absent
Pupils	Mydriasis	Miosis	Unequal, poor light reflex
Seizures	None	Common	Decerebration
Electroencephalographic	Normal	Low voltage changing to seizure activity	Burst suppression to isoelectric
Duration	<24 hr if progresses; otherwise, may remain normal	24 hr to 14 days	Days to weeks
Outcome	Good	Variable	Death, severe deficits

Modified from Sarnat H, Sarnat M: Neonatal encephalopathy following fetal distress: A clinical and electroencephalographic study. Arch Neurol *1976; 33:696. Copyright 1976, American Medical Association.*

Bager B: Perinatally acquired brachial plexus palsy—a persisting challenge. *Acta Paediatr* 1997;86:1214.

Battin MR, Dezoete A, Gunn TR, et al: Neurodevelopmental outcome of infants treated with head cooling and mild hypothermia after perinatal asphyxia. *Pediatrics* 2001;107:480.

Baud O, Foix-L'Helias L, Kaminski M, et al: Antenatal glucocorticoid treatment and cystic periventricular leukomalacia in very premature infants. *N Engl J Med* 1999;341:1190.

Biagioni E, Mercuri E, Rutherford M, et al: Combined use of electroencephalogram and magnetic resonance imaging in full-term neonates with acute encephalopathy. *Pediatrics* 2001;107:461.

Brown T, Cupido C, Scarfone R, et al: Developmental apraxia arising from neonatal brachial plexus palsy. *Neurology* 2000;55:24.

Cornette LG, Tanner SF, Ramenghi LA, et al: Magnetic resonance imaging of the infant brain: Anatomical characteristics and clinical significance of punctate lesions. *Arch Dis Child* 2002;86:F171–7.

Crowley P: Prophylactic corticosteroids for preterm birth. *Cochrane Database Syst Rev* 2002;Issue 1.

De Felice C, Toti P, Laurini RN, et al: Early neonatal brain injury in histologic chorioamnionitis. *J Pediatr* 2001;138:101.

de Vries LS, Eken P, Groenendaal F, et al: Antenatal onset of haemorrhagic and/or ischaemic lesions in preterm infants: Prevalence and associated obstetric variables. *Arch Dis Child* 1998;78:F51.

Dixon G, Badawi N, Kurinczuk JJ, et al: Early developmental outcomes after newborn encephalopathy. *Pediatrics* 2002;109:26–33.

Ekert P, Perlman M, Steinlin M, et al: Predicting the outcome of postasphyxial hypoxic-ischemic encephalopathy within 4 hours of birth. *J Pediatr* 1997;131:613.

Evans D, Levene M: Neonatal seizures. *Arch Dis Child* 1998;78:F70.

Hall RT, Hall FK, Daily DK: High-dose phenobarbital therapy in term newborn infants with severe perinatal asphyxia: A randomized, prospective study with three-year follow-up. *J Pediatr* 1998;132:345.

Heuchan AM, Evans N, Henderson DJ, et al: Perinatal risk factors for major intraventricular haemorrhage in the Australian and New Zealand neonatal network, 1995–97. *Arch Dis Child* 2002;86:F86–90.

Hoeksma AF, Wolf H, Oei SL: Obstetrical brachial plexus injuries: Incidence, natural course and shoulder contracture. *Clin Rehabil* 2000;14:523.

Inder T, Huppi PS, Zientara GP, et al: Early detection of periventricular leukomalacia by diffusion-weighted magnetic resonance imaging techniques. *J Pediatr* 1999;134:631.

Kennedy CR, Ayers S, Campbell MJ, et al: Randomized, controlled trial of acetazolamide and furosemide in posthemorrhagic ventricular dilation in infancy: Follow-up at 1 year. *Pediatrics* 2001;108:596.

Kuban K, Sanocka U, Leviton A, et al: White matter disorders of prematurity: Association with intraventricular hemorrhage and ventriculomegaly. *J Pediatr* 1999;134:539.

MacKinnon JA, Perlman M, Kirpalani H, et al: Spinal cord injury at birth: Diagnostic and prognostic data in twenty-two patients. *J Pediatr* 1993;122:431.

Ment LR, Bada HS, Barnes P, et al: Practice parameter: Neuroimaging of the neonate. *Neurology* 2002;58:1726–38.

Ment LR, Vohr B, Allan W, et al: The etiology and outcome of cerebral ventriculomegaly at term in very low birth weight preterm infants. *Pediatrics* 1999;104:243.

Mercuri E, Cowan F, Gupte G, et al: Prothrombotic disorders and abnormal neurodevelopmental outcome in infants with neonatal cerebral infarction. *Pediatrics* 2001;107:1400–4.

Mercuri E, Ricci D, Cowan FM, et al: Head growth in infants with hypoxic-ischemic encephalopathy: Correlation with neonatal magnetic resonance imaging. *Pediatrics* 2000;106:235–43.

Mills JF, Dargaville PA, Coleman LT, et al: Upper cervical spinal cord injury in neonates: The use of magnetic resonance imaging. *J Pediatr* 2001;138:105.

Noetzel MJ, Wolpaw JR: Emerging concepts in the pathophysiology of recovery from neonatal brachial plexus injury. *Neurology* 2000;55:5.

Pal BR, Preston PR, Morgan MEI, et al: Frontal horn thin walled cysts in preterm neonates are benign. *Arch Dis Child* 2001;85:F187–93.

Paneth N: Cerebral palsy in term infants—birth or before birth? *J Pediatr* 2001;138:791–2.

Paneth N: Classifying brain damage in preterm infants. *J Pediatr* 1999;134:527.

Pierrat V, Duquennoy C, van Haastert IC, et al: Ultrasound diagnosis and neurodevelopmental outcome of localized and extensive cystic periventricular leukomalacia. *Arch Dis Child* 2002;84:F151–6.

Rollnik JD, Hierner R, Schubert M, et al: Botulinum toxin treatment of co-contractions after birth-related brachial plexus lesions. *Neurology* 2000;55:112.

Schmidt B, Davis P, Moddemann PD, et al: Long-term effects of indomethacin prophylaxis in extremely-low-birth-weight infants. *N Engl J Med* 2001;344:1966.

Strombeck C, Krumlinde-Sundholm L, Forrsberg H: Functional outcome at 5 years in children with obstetrical brachial palsy with and without microsurgical reconstruction. *Dev Med Child Neurol* 2000;42:148.

Vohr B, Allan WC, Scott DT, et al: Early-onset intraventricular hemorrhage in preterm neonates: Incidence of neurodevelopmental handicap. *Semin Perinatol* 1999;23:212.

Volpe JJ: Neurobiology of periventricular leukomalacia in the premature infant. *Pediatr Res* 2001;50:553.

Whitelaw A: Repeated lumbar or ventricular punctures in newborns with intraventricular hemorrhage. *Cochrane Database Syst Rev* 2002;Issue 1.

Whitelaw A, Thoresen, Pople I: Posthaemorrhagic ventricular dilatation. *Arch Dis Child* 2002;86:F72–4.

Wu YW, Colford JM Jr: Chorioamnionitis as a risk factor for cerebral palsy: A meta-analysis. *JAMA* 2000;284:1417.

88.6   Intrauterine Infection (see also Chapter 98)

A variety of agents that infect the mother during pregnancy, labor, and/or delivery can infect the fetus or newborn and cause fetal loss or early neonatal death, multiorgan dysfunction, and/or injury to the developing brain. The most important pathogens are cytomegalovirus (CMV), *Toxoplasma gondii*, herpes simplex virus, *Treponema pallidum*, and rubella virus.

CONGENITAL CYTOMEGALOVIRUS

The greatest risk to the developing fetus is primary CMV infection of the mother during pregnancy. Many women are asymptomatic and the disease may thus go undetected. With primary maternal infection, transmission rates to the fetus range from 24–75%. Like other members of the herpes family, CMV can persist in a latent state after a primary infection. Despite maternal immunity, it can be reactivated during pregnancy and be transmitted to the fetus, or re-infection can occur from a different strain of CMV. The infection is generally less severe in the presence of maternal antibody.

An estimated 0.5–2.5% of all infants are infected with CMV at the time of birth. Approximately 10% of infants with congenital CMV infection in the United States are symptomatic at birth. Less than 10% have generalized *cytomegalic inclusion disease* (CID). CID is characterized by multiorgan involvement, including hepatomegaly, splenomegaly, jaundice, petechiae, microcephaly, chorioretinitis, and fetal growth restriction. About 90% of CMV-infected infants who are symptomatic at birth and 5–15% of those who are asymptomatic will have complications that include sensorineural hearing loss, speech abnormalities, chorioretinitis, optic atrophy, microcephaly, and mental retardation. Prevention efforts have focused on the development of a safe and effective vaccine against CMV. Currently, no treatment has been recommended for maternal infection during pregnancy; however, treatment of symptomatic congenital CMV infection with ganciclovir is being evaluated.

CONGENITAL TOXOPLASMOSIS

Toxoplasmosis during pregnancy can result in fetal infection. The acute signs and symptoms of congenital toxoplasmosis include intrauterine growth restriction, anemia, jaundice, hepatosplenomegaly, intracranial calcifications, hydrocephalus, and microcephaly. Long-term sequelae include visual impairment, blindness, seizures, and mental retardation. The most effective prevention strategy is to avoid risk factors for maternal infection during pregnancy (including contact with infected animals, especially cats, cat feces, or undercooked meat or raw vegetables). Antibiotic treatment during pregnancy (spiramycin for acute maternal infection, pyrimethamine and sulfa for fetal infection) does not appear to reduce the rate of transmission to the fetus, but it does reduce sequelae in infected infants. Postnatal antibiotic treatment of infected infants (pyrimethamine, sulfonamides, and folinic acid) improves the long-term outcome.

HERPES SIMPLEX VIRUS

Both herpes simplex virus types 1 (HSV-1) and 2 (HSV-2) can cause genital infection and can be transmitted from mother to fetus or newborn. HSV infection in the newborn can be acquired in utero (rare), intrapartum (most common), and postnatally. The newborn is at greatest risk for intrapartum transmission if the mother has primary HSV infection at or near the time of delivery (transmission rates of 50% or more with vaginal delivery). Unfortunately, many women are asymptomatic at the time of primary infection. With recurrent maternal infection, intrapartum transmission is reduced to 3–5%, presumably because of pre-existing maternal antibody. Neonatal HSV infection is a life-threatening illness clinically manifested as isolated CNS disease, disseminated disease with CNS involvement, or isolated skin, eye, and/or mouth infection. CNS damage, including microcephaly, hydranencephaly, and/or meningoencephalitis, can result. Therapy with intravenous acyclovir reduces the risk of death (0% for localized skin disease, 5% for encephalitis, 25% for disseminated disease), but morbidity remains high. Whereas 95% of those with skin disease are normal at 2 yr, only 40% of those surviving encephalitis and 60% of those surviving disseminated disease are normal at 2 yr. Long-term neurologic sequelae include microcephaly, porencephalic cysts, chorioretinitis, blindness, spasticity, and mental retardation. A further reduction in morbidity may result from earlier initiation of antiviral therapy.

CONGENITAL SYPHILIS

The risk of congenital syphilis parallels the rates of syphilis in women of childbearing age. Adequate treatment of syphilis during pregnancy prevents the development of congenital syphilis. Untreated or inadequately treated disease can result in fetal and neonatal disease with multisystem involvement, including anemia, thrombocytopenia, hepatosplenomegaly and jaundice, bone abnormalities, and CNS manifestations. Syphilis is an important preventable cause of stillbirth. CNS sequelae include hydrocephalus, cerebral infarction, meningovasculitis, seizures, and mental retardation. Early identification and treatment of infected infants and diagnosis of CNS syphilis are essential to improve both short- and long-term outcomes. Penicillin is the drug of choice for the treatment of congenital syphilis. Between 1997 and 2000, congenital syphilis rates in the United States declined substantially. With adequate screening and treatment of pregnant women, it is believed that elimination of congenital syphilis in the United States is possible.

CONGENITAL RUBELLA SYNDROME

Maternal infection with rubella in early gestation interferes with critical organ development in the fetus. The resulting defects—cataracts, blindness, deafness, cardiovascular anomalies, microcephaly, and mental retardation—are collectively referred to as congenital rubella syndrome (CRS). The prognosis for infants with severe CRS is poor. For those in whom it is diagnosed during the 1st yr, mortality is high, and most survivors are seriously impaired. Vaccination against rubella has made CRS increasingly rare in most developed countries. Rubella remains endemic in many developing countries, however, where it is a major preventable cause of hearing impairment, blindness, and adverse neurodevelopmental outcome. Global immunization programs that include rubella vaccination, as well as efforts to identify and respond to rubella outbreaks, are likely to reduce the global burden of CRS.

Alexander JM, Sheffield JS, Sanchez PJ, et al: Efficacy of treatment for syphilis in pregnancy. *Obstet Gynecol* 1999;93:5.

Bessieres MH, Berrebi A, Rolland M, et al: Neonatal screening for congenital toxoplasmosis in a cohort of 165 women infected during pregnancy and influence of in utero treatment on the results of neonatal tests. *Eur J Obstet Gynecol Reprod Biol* 2001;94:37.

Boppana SB, Fowler KB, Britt WJ, et al: Symptomatic congenital cytomegalovirus infection in infants born to mothers with preexisting immunity to cytomegalovirus. *Pediatrics* 1999;104:55.

Centers for Disease Control and Prevention: Control and prevention of rubella: Evaluation and management of suspected outbreaks, rubella in pregnant women, and surveillance for congenital rubella syndrome. *MMWR Morb Mortal Wkly Rep* 2001;50:1.

Foulon W, Naessens A, Ho-Yen D: Prevention of congenital toxoplasmosis. *J Perinat Med* 2000;28:337.

Kimberlin DW, Lin CW, Jacobs RF, et al: Natural history of neonatal herpes simplex virus infections in the acyclovir era. *Pediatrics* 2001;108:223.

Kimberlin DW, Lin CY, Jacobs RF, et al: Safety and efficacy of high-dose intravenous acyclovir in the management of neonatal herpes simplex virus infections. *Pediatrics* 2001;108:230.

Noyola DE, Demmler GJ, Nelson CT, et al: Early predictors of neurodevelopmental outcome in symptomatic congenital cytomegalovirus infection. *J Pediatr* 2001;138:325.

Plotkin SA: Rubella eradication. *Vaccine* 2001;19:3311.

Sanchez PJ, Wendel GD: Syphilis in pregnancy. *Clin Perinatol* 1997;24:71.

Villena I, Aubert D, Leroux B, et al: Pyrimethamine-sulfadoxine treatment of congenital toxoplasmosis: Follow-up of 78 cases between 1980 and 1997. Reims Toxoplasmosis Group. *Scand J Infect Dis* 1998;30:295.

Whitley RJ, Cloud G, Gruber, et al: Ganciclovir treatment of symptomatic congenital cytomegalovirus infection: Results of a phase II study. National Institute of Allergy and Infectious Diseases Collaborative Antiviral Study Group. *J Infect Dis* 1997;175:1080.

Chapter 89
Delivery Room Emergencies
Barbara J. Stoll and Robert M. Kliegman

The most common and important emergency related to newborn infants in the delivery room is failure to initiate and maintain respirations. Less frequent, but of major importance are shock (Chapter 87), severe anemia (Chapter 92.1), plethora (Chapter 92.3), convulsions (Chapter 586.5), and management of life-threatening congenital malformations (Chapter 87).

Respiratory Distress and Failure. Disorders of respiration in newborn infants can be categorized as either *central nervous system* (CNS) *failure*, representing depression or failure of the respiratory center, or *peripheral respiratory difficulty,* indicating interference with the alveolar exchange of oxygen and carbon dioxide. Cyanosis occurs in both groups (see Table 87–1). Respiratory problems encountered in the delivery room are most frequently those of airway obstruction and depression of the CNS (maternal medications, asphyxia), with an absence of adequate respiratory effort.

Respiratory distress in the presence of good respiratory effort should lead to an immediate consideration of the underlying cause and is an indication for roentgenographic examination of the chest.

If respiratory movements are made with the mouth closed but the infant fails to move air in and out of the lungs, bilateral **choanal atresia** (Chapter 361) or other obstruction of the upper respiratory tract should be suspected. The mouth should be opened and the mouth and posterior of the pharynx cleared of secretions by gentle suction. An oropharyngeal airway should be inserted and the source of the obstruction sought immediately. If effective respiratory flow is not produced by opening the infant's mouth and clearing the airway, laryngoscopy is indicated. With obstructive malformations of the mandible, epiglottis, larynx, or trachea, an endotracheal tube should be inserted; prolonged endotracheal intubation or tracheostomy may be required. Respiratory failure caused by CNS depression or injury may require continuous artificial ventilation with a face mask and bag or through an endotracheal tube.

Hypoplasia of the mandible (Pierre Robin, DiGeorge, and other syndromes) (Chapter 291) with posterior displacement of the tongue may result in symptoms similar to those of choanal atresia and may be temporarily relieved by pulling the tongue forward. A scaphoid abdomen suggests a **diaphragmatic hernia** or **eventration,** as does asymmetry in contour or movement of the chest or a shift of the apical impulse of the heart; these latter manifestations are also compatible with tension pneumothorax. A pneumothorax on the 1st day of life suggests pulmonary hypoplasia, renal malformations, or both.

Pulmonary causes of respiratory difficulty are discussed in Chapter 90.

Failure to Initiate or Sustain Respiration. This problem usually originates in the CNS as a result of asphyxia; immaturity in itself is seldom a causative factor except in infants weighing less than 1,000 g. Intrapulmonary problems, such as the pulmonary hypoplasia associated with Potter syndrome, bilateral pleural effusions (hydrops fetalis), and severe intrauterine pneumonia, may at times result in poorly sustained ventilation. The lungs in these infants are very noncompliant, and standard efforts to begin respirations may be inadequate to initiate sufficient ventilation.

Narcosis results from heavy doses of morphine, meperidine (Demerol), fentanyl, barbiturates, or tranquilizers administered to the mother shortly before delivery or from maternal anesthesia given during the 2nd stage of labor. Infants are cyanotic and hypotonic at birth and slow to cry or breathe; when respiration is established, it is extremely slow.

Narcosis should be avoided by using appropriate analgesic and anesthetic practices. Treatment includes initial physical stimulation and securing of a patent airway. If effective ventilation is not initiated, artificial breathing with a mask and bag must be instituted. At the same time, if the depression is due to morphine or its derivatives, naloxone hydrochloride (Narcan), 0.1 mg/kg, should be given by the intravenous, subcutaneous, intratracheal, or intramuscular routes and repeated two to three times if needed. Narcan is contraindicated for maternal opiate addiction because it precipitates acute neonatal withdrawal with severe seizures. Ventilation is essential before and during administration of this antidote. If depression is due to other anesthetics or analgesics, artificial respiration should be continued until the infant is able to sustain ventilation. CNS stimulant drugs should not be used because they are ineffective and may be harmful.

Prenatal or **perinatal hypoxia** of whatever cause, if sufficiently severe, produces brainstem depression and secondary apnea that is unresponsive to sensory stimulation. Death from apnea may be prevented by resuscitation, provided that the basic cause of the hypoxia can be eliminated within a reasonable time while artificial respiration, if necessary, is being carried out. External cardiac massage, correction of acidosis, and circulatory support with drugs may be important adjuncts to ventilation.

Resuscitation. It is estimated that 5–10% of newborns require some degree of resuscitation at birth. The *goals* of neonatal resuscitation are to prevent the morbidity and mortality associated with hypoxic-ischemic tissue (brain, heart, kidney) injury and to re-establish adequate spontaneous respiration and cardiac output. High-risk situations should be anticipated by the history of the pregnancy, labor, and delivery and by identification of signs of fetal distress. Although the Apgar score is helpful in evaluating patients in need of attention, infants who are born limp, cyanotic, apneic, or pulseless require immediate resuscitation before assignment of the 1-min Apgar score. Rapid and appropriate resuscitative efforts improve the likelihood of preventing brain damage and achieving a successful outcome.

Immediately after birth, an asphyxiated infant should be placed under a radiant heater (to avoid hypothermia), dried, and positioned head down and slightly extended, and the airway should be cleared by suctioning and gentle tactile stimulation provided (slapping the foot, rubbing the back). Simultaneously, the infant's color, heart rate, and respiratory effort should be assessed (Fig. 89–1).

The steps in neonatal resuscitation follow the ABCs: **A,** anticipate and establish a patent *a*irway by suctioning and, if necessary, performing endotracheal intubation; **B,** initiate *b*reathing by using tactile stimulation or positive-pressure ventilation with a bag and mask or through an endotracheal tube; **C,** maintain the *c*irculation with chest compression and medications, if needed. Steps to follow for immediate neonatal evaluation and resuscitation are outlined in Figure 89–1 (also see Chapter 57.1).

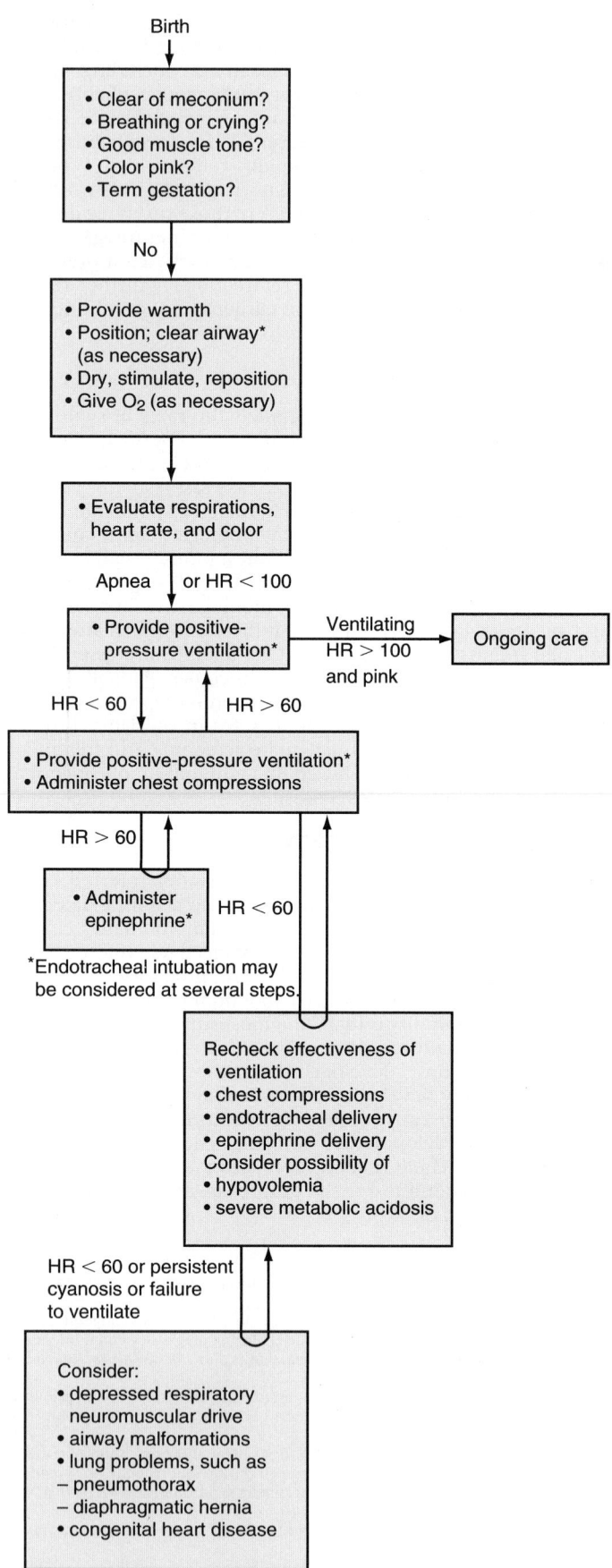

FIGURE 89–1. Neonatal resuscitation: Decision points and sequential steps. HR = heart rate. (From American Heart Association and American Academy of Pediatrics: *Neonatal Resuscitation Textbook,* 4th ed, 2000, with permission.)

If no respirations are noted or if the heart rate is below 100/min, *positive pressure ventilation* is given through a tightly fitted face mask and bag for 15–30 sec. In infants with severe respiratory depression who do not respond to positive pressure ventilation via bag and mask, endotracheal intubation should be performed. Many recommend early intubation for extremely low-birth-weight preterm infants. Guidelines for endotracheal tube size and depth of insertion in infants with different birthweights are shown in Table 89–1. The optimal concentration of oxygen for newborn resuscitation is unknown; most guidelines recommend 100% oxygen. Although the first breath normally requires pressures as low as 15–20 cm H_2O, pressures as high as 30–40 cm H_2O may be needed. Subsequent breaths are given at a rate of 40–60/min with a pressure of 15–20 cm H_2O. Noncompliant stiff lungs secondary to hyaline membrane disease, congenital pneumonia, or meconium aspiration may require higher pressures. Successful ventilation is determined by adequate chest rise, symmetric breath sounds, improved pink color, heart rate greater than 100/min, spontaneous respirations, presence of end-tidal CO_2, and improved tone.

If the mother has a history of analgesic narcotic drug administration, naloxone is given while adequate ventilation is maintained. Breathing in the depressed infant should be maintained until a response to naloxone is noted. Continuous observation of the infant is important because repeated doses of naloxone may be needed even after the infant has been transferred to the nursery.

If the heart rate does not improve after 15–30 sec with bag and mask (or endotracheal) ventilation and remains below 60/min or if the rate is less than 80/min and not rising, ventilation is continued and *chest compression* with two fingers is initiated over the lower third of the sternum at a rate of 120/min. The ratio of compressions to ventilation is 3:1. Bradycardia in neonatal infants is usually due to hypoxia resulting from respiratory arrest and often responds rapidly to effective ventilation alone. Persistent bradycardia despite what appears to be adequate resuscitation suggests more severe cardiac compromise or inadequate ventilation technique. Poor response to ventilation may be due to a loosely fitted mask, poor positioning of the endotracheal tube, intra-esophageal intubation, airway obstruction, insufficient pressure, pleural effusions, pneumothorax, excessive air in the stomach, asystole, hypovolemia, diaphragmatic hernia, or prolonged intrauterine asphyxia.

TABLE 89–1. Guidelines for Tracheal Tube Size and Depth of Insertion

Tube Size (mm ID)	Depth of Insertion from Upper Lip (cm)	Weight (g)	Gestation (wk)
2.5	6.5–7	<1,000	<28
3	7–8	1,000–2,000	28–34
3/3.5	8–9	2,000–3,000	34–38
3.5/4.0	≥9	>3,000	>38

ID = internal diameter.
From Kattwinkel J, Niermeyer S, Nadkarni, et al: Resuscitation of the newly born infant: An advisory statement from the Pediatric Working Group of the International Liaison Committee on Resuscitation. Circulation 1999; 99:1927–38. By permission of the American Heart Association, Inc.

Endotracheal intubation should be performed by an experienced person on any infant who does not respond to initial bag and mask ventilation or who was born apneic, pulseless, cyanotic, and limp.

Medications are rarely required but should be administered when the heart rate is less than 60/min after 30 sec of combined ventilation and chest compressions or during asystole. The umbilical vein can generally be readily cannulated and used for immediate administration of medications during neonatal resuscitation (Fig. 89–2). The endotracheal tube may be used for the administration of epinephrine if intravenous access is not available and/or for naloxone hydrochloride. Epinephrine (0.1–0.3 mL/kg of a 1:10,000 solution, intravenously or intratracheally) is given for asystole or for failure to respond to 30 sec of combined resuscitation. The dose may be repeated every 5 min. If no response is observed, some clinicians recommend using 5 to 10 times the standard dose of epinephrine. Emergency volume expansion is accomplished with 10–20 mL/kg of an isotonic crystalloid solution or O-negative red blood cells (in acute hemorrhage). Sodium bicarbonate (2 mEq/kg, 0.5 mEq/mL of a 4.2% solution) should be given slowly (1 mEq/kg/min) if metabolic acidosis has been documented and the resuscitation is prolonged. Sodium bicarbonate should be given only after effective ventilation has been established because such therapy may increase blood CO_2 and produce respiratory acidosis complicating an existing metabolic acidosis. Restoration of oxygenation

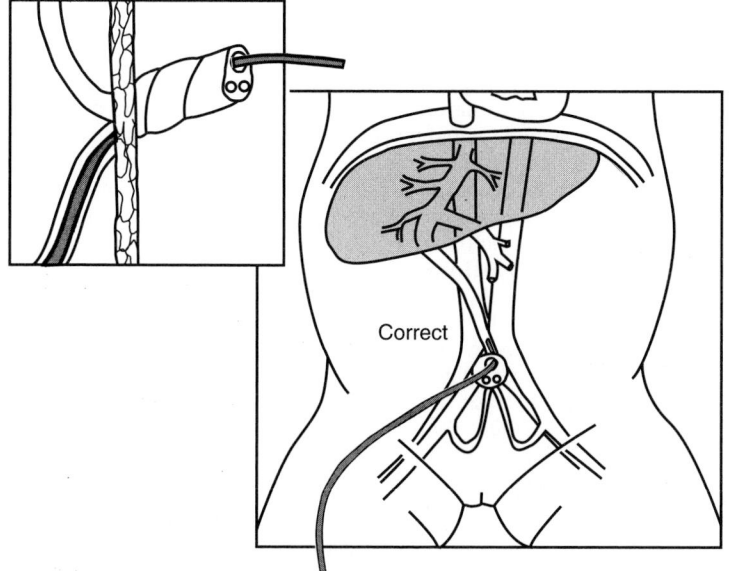
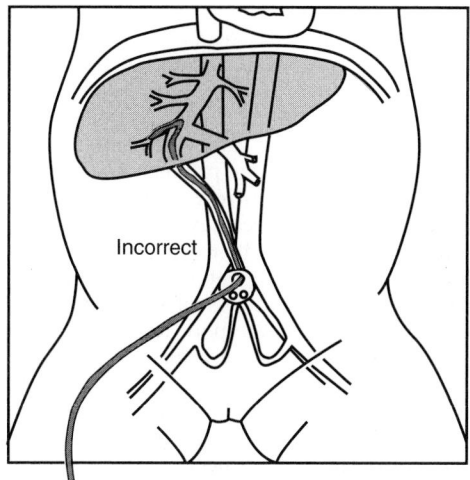

FIGURE 89–2. Use of the umbilical vein for administration of medications during neonatal resuscitation. (From American Heart Association and American Academy of Pediatrics: *Neonatal Resuscitation Textbook,* 4th ed, 2000, with permision.)

and tissue perfusion is the main treatment of metabolic acidosis associated with asphyxia.

Severe asphyxia may also depress myocardial function and cause cardiogenic shock despite the recovery of heart and respiratory rates. Dopamine or dobutamine administered as a continuous infusion (5–20 µg/kg/min) and fluids should be started after the initial resuscitation effort to improve cardiac output in an infant with poor peripheral perfusion, weak pulses, hypotension, tachycardia, and poor urine output. Epinephrine (0.1–1.0 µg/kg/min) may be indicated for infants in severe shock who do not respond to dopamine or dobutamine (Chapter 57.1).

Less severe degrees of asphyxia can usually be managed by brief periods of bag and mask ventilation. Chest compression and medications are not needed for most neonates who have mild to moderate birth depression. Regardless of the severity of asphyxia or the response to resuscitation, asphyxiated infants should be monitored closely for signs of multiorgan hypoxic-ischemic tissue injury (see Table 88–1).

Shock. Circulatory insufficiency may be present at birth as a result of severe asphyxia or hemorrhage during gestation, labor, or delivery. Causes of bleeding include hemolysis; placental abruption, previa or tear; traumatic injury to the umbilical cord or internal organs; and intracranial bleeding. Clinical manifestations include signs of respiratory distress, cyanosis, pallor, flaccidity, cold mottled skin, tachycardia or bradycardia, hepatosplenomegaly, and rarely, convulsions. Edema and hepatosplenomegaly may suggest hydrops fetalis or heart failure without shock. Shock from overwhelming infection may also be present after birth.

Supportive treatment with type O Rh-negative blood or normal saline is indicated for hemorrhage or hypovolemia, respectively. Oxygen should be administered and the metabolic acidosis corrected with sodium bicarbonate. Sympathomimetic agents such as dopamine or dobutamine may be needed to support cardiac output and blood pressure. The diagnosis and treatment of erythroblastosis fetalis are discussed in Chapter 92.2. If infection is present, appropriate antibiotics must be started as soon as possible.

After supportive measures have stabilized the infant's condition, a specific diagnosis should be established and appropriate continuing treatment instituted.

INJURY DURING DELIVERY

Central Nervous System

See Chapter 88.

Viscera

The **liver** is the only internal organ other than the brain that is injured with any frequency during birth. The damage usually results from pressure on the liver during delivery of the head in breech presentations. Large infant size, intrauterine asphyxia, coagulation disorders, extreme prematurity, and hepatomegaly are contributing factors. Incorrect cardiac massage is a less frequent cause. Hepatic rupture may result in the formation of a subcapsular hematoma, but the capsule may tamponade further bleeding. Infants usually appear normal for the 1st 1–3 days. Nonspecific signs related to loss of blood into the hematoma may appear early and include poor feeding, listlessness, pallor, jaundice, tachypnea, and tachycardia. A mass may be palpable in the right upper quadrant, and the abdomen may appear blue. The hematoma may be large enough to cause anemia. Shock and death may occur if the hematoma ruptures into the peritoneal cavity, where the reduced pressure may allow fresh hemorrhage. Early suspicion by means of ultrasonographic diagnosis and prompt supportive therapy can decrease the mortality associated with this disorder. Surgical repair of a laceration

may be required. **Rupture of the spleen** may occur alone or in connection with rupture of the liver. The causes, complications, treatment, and prevention are similar.

Although **adrenal hemorrhage** occurs with some frequency, especially after breech delivery, in infants large for gestational age or infants of diabetic mothers, its cause is undetermined; it may be due to trauma, anoxia, or severe stress, as in overwhelming infection. Ninety per cent are unilateral; 75% are right sided. Calcified central hematomas of the adrenal have been identified roentgenographically or at autopsy in older infants and children, thus suggesting that not all adrenal hemorrhages are immediately fatal. In severe cases, the diagnosis is usually made at postmortem examination. The symptoms are profound shock and cyanosis. A mass may be present in the flank along with overlying skin discoloration; jaundice may also develop. If adrenal hemorrhage is suspected, abdominal ultrasonography may be helpful, and treatment of acute adrenal failure may be indicated (Chapter 569).

Fractures

Clavicle. This bone is fractured during labor and delivery more frequently than any other bone; it is particularly vulnerable with difficult delivery of the shoulder in vertex presentations and the extended arms in breech deliveries. The infant characteristically does not move the arm freely on the affected side; crepitus and bony irregularity may be palpated, and discoloration is occasionally visible over the fracture site. The Moro reflex is absent on the affected side, and spasm of the sternocleidomastoid muscle with obliteration of the supraclavicular depression at the site of the fracture can be noted. Infants with greenstick fractures may not have any limitation of movement, and the Moro reflex may be present. Fracture of the humerus or brachial palsy may also be responsible for limitation of movement of an arm and absence of a Moro reflex on the affected side. The *prognosis* is excellent. *Treatment*, if any, consists of immobilization of the arm and shoulder on the affected side. A remarkable degree of palpable callus develops at the site within a week and may be the initial evidence of the fracture.

Extremities. In fractures of the long bones, spontaneous movement of the extremity is usually absent (pseudoparalysis). The Moro reflex is also absent from the involved extremity. Associated nerve involvement may occur. Satisfactory results of treatment of a fractured humerus are obtained with 2–4 wk of immobilization during which the arm is strapped to the chest, a triangular splint and a Velpeau bandage are applied, or a cast is applied. For fracture of the femur, good results are achieved with traction-suspension of both lower extremities, even if the fracture is unilateral; the legs, immobilized in a spica cast, are attached to an overhead frame. Splints are effective for treatment of fractures of the forearm or leg. Healing is usually accompanied by excess callus formation. The *prognosis* is excellent for fractures of the extremities. Fractures in preterm infants may be related to osteopenia (Chapter 95).

Dislocations and **epiphyseal separations** rarely result from birth trauma. The upper femoral epiphysis may be separated by forcible manipulation of the infant's leg as, for example, in breech extraction or after version. The affected leg shows swelling, slight shortening, limitation of active motion, painful passive motion, and external rotation. The diagnosis is established roentgenographically. The prognosis is good for milder injuries, but coxa vara frequently results from extensive displacement.

Nose. The most prevalent injury to the nose is dislocation of the cartilaginous portion of the septum from the vomerine groove and the columella. The infant may have difficulty nursing and some impairment in nasal respiration. On physical examination, the nares appear asymmetric and the nose flattened. An oral airway rarely is needed, and surgical consultation should be obtained for definitive treatment.

American Heart Association and American Academy of Pediatrics: *Neonatal Resuscitation Textbook,* 4th ed, 2000.

Carrasco M, Martell M, Estol PC: Oronasopharyngeal suction at birth: Effects on arterial oxygen saturation. *J Pediatr* 1997;130:832.

Gunn AJ, Bennet L: Is temperature important in delivery room resuscitation. *Semin Neonatol* 2001;6:241.

Lindner W, Vofsbeck S, Hummler H, et al: Delivery room management of extremely low birth weight infants: Spontaneous breathing or intubation? *Pediatrics* 1999;103:961.

Neonatal Resuscitation Steering Committee of the American Academy of Pediatrics: International guidelines for neonatal resuscitation: An excerpt from the Guidelines 2000 for Cardiopulmonary Resuscitation and Emergency Cardiovascular Care: International consensus on science. *Pediatrics* 2000;106: e29.

Niermeyer S, Van Reempts P, Kattwinkel J, et al: Resuscitation of newborns. *Ann Emerg Med* 2001;37(Suppl):110.

Vento M, Asensi M, Sastre J, et al: Resuscitation with room air instead of 100% oxygen prevents oxidative stress in moderately asphyxiated term neonates. *Pediatrics* 2001;107:642.

Wolkoff LI, Davis JM: Delivery room resuscitation of the newborn. *Clin Perinatol* 1999;26:641.

Chapter 90
Respiratory Tract Disorders

Barbara J. Stoll and Robert M. Kliegman

Respiratory disorders are the most frequent cause of admission for special care in both term and preterm infants. Signs and symptoms include cyanosis, grunting, nasal flaring, retractions, tachypnea, decreased breath sounds with rales and/or rhonchi, pallor, and apnea. A wide variety of pathologic lesions may be responsible for respiratory disturbances (see Table 87–1 and Box 87–1), including hyaline membrane disease (HMD; respiratory distress syndrome [RDS]), aspiration syndrome, pneumonia, sepsis, congenital heart disease, heart failure, pulmonary hypertension, choanal atresia, hypoglycemia, hypoplasia of the mandible with posterior displacement of the tongue, macroglossia, malformation of the epiglottis, malformation or injury of the larynx, cysts or neoplasms of the larynx or chest, pneumothorax, lobar emphysema, pulmonary agenesis or hypoplasia, congenital pulmonary lymphangiectasis, tracheoesophageal fistula, avulsion of the phrenic nerve, hernia or eventration of the diaphragm, intracranial lesions, neuromuscular disorders, and metabolic disturbances.

It is occasionally difficult to distinguish cardiovascular from respiratory causes or sepsis on the basis of clinical signs alone. Any sign of postnatal respiratory distress is an indication for immediate examination and diagnostic evaluation, including a blood gas determination and roentgenogram of the chest. Timely and appropriate therapy is essential to prevent ongoing injury and improve outcome. As a result of important advances in understanding the pathophysiology of respiratory disease, neonatal and infant deaths from early respiratory disease have declined markedly. The challenge is to continue to improve survival, but also to reduce short- and long-term complications related to early lung disease.

90.1 Transition to Pulmonary Respiration

Successful establishment of adequate lung function at birth is dependent on unobstructed anatomy and maturity of respiratory control. Fluid filling the fetal lungs must be removed, gas containing functional residual capacity (FRC) established and

maintained, and a ventilation-perfusion relationship developed that will provide optimal exchange of oxygen and carbon dioxide between alveoli and blood (Chapters 355–357).

The First Breath. During vaginal delivery, intermittent compression of the thorax facilitates removal of lung fluid. Surfactant lining the alveoli enhances the aeration of gas-free lungs by reducing surface tension, thereby lowering the pressure required to open alveoli. Nevertheless, the opening pressures required to inflate the airless lungs are higher than those needed at any other period of life; they range from 10–50 cm (usually 10–20 cm) H_2O vs about 4 cm for normal breathing in term infants and adults. The higher pressures needed to initiate respiration are required to overcome the opposing forces of surface tension (particularly in small airways) and the viscosity of liquid remaining in the airways, as well as to introduce about 50 mL of air into the lungs, 20–30 mL of which remains after the first breath to establish FRC. Most of the liquid in the lungs is removed by the pulmonary circulation, which increases manyfold at birth because all the right ventricular output now perfuses the pulmonary vascular bed. The remainder of the fluid is removed by the pulmonary lymphatics, expelled by the infant, swallowed, or aspirated from the oropharynx; removal may be impaired after cesarean section or as a result of endothelial cell damage, hypoalbuminemia, high pulmonary venous pressure, or neonatal sedation.

Stimuli responsible for the first breath are numerous, and their relative importance is uncertain. These stimuli include a decline in Po_2 and pH and a rise in Pco_2 as a result of interruption of the placental circulation, a redistribution of cardiac output after the umbilical cord is clamped, a decrease in body temperature, and various tactile stimuli.

When compared with term infants, low-birthweight (LBW) infants who have a very compliant chest wall may be at a disadvantage in drawing the first breath. The FRC is least in the most immature infants because of the presence of atelectasis. Abnormalities in the ventilation-perfusion ratio are greater and persist for longer periods, as does gas trapping. LBW infants may have a low Pao_2 (50–60 mm Hg) and an elevated $Paco_2$ as a result of atelectasis, intrapulmonary shunting, and hypoventilation. The smallest immature infants have the most profound disturbances, which may resemble RDS.

Breathing Patterns in Newborns. During sleep in the first months of life, normal full-term infants may have infrequent episodes when regular breathing is interrupted by short pauses. This periodic breathing pattern, which shifts from a regular rhythmicity to cyclic brief episodes of intermittent apnea, is more common in premature infants, who may have apneic pauses of 5–10 sec followed by a burst of rapid respirations at a rate of 50–60/min for 10–15 sec. They rarely have an associated change in color or heart rate, and it often stops without apparent reason. Periodic breathing persists intermittently, usually until premature infants are about 36 wk of gestational age. If an infant is hypoxic, an increase in inspired oxygen concentration often converts periodic to regular breathing. Periodic breathing, a normal characteristic of neonatal respiration, has no prognostic significance.

90.2 Apnea

Apnea is a common problem in preterm infants that may be due to idiopathic apnea of prematurity or an associated illness. In term infants, apnea is always worrisome and demands immediate diagnostic evaluation. Periodic breathing must be distinguished from prolonged apneic pauses because the latter may be associated with serious illnesses. Apnea is a feature of many primary diseases that affect neonates (Table 90–1). These disorders produce apnea by direct depression of the central nervous

TABLE 90–1. Potential Causes of Neonatal Apnea and Bradycardia

Central nervous system	Intraventricular hemorrhage, drugs, seizures, hypoxic injury, herniation, neuromuscular disorders, Leigh syndrome, brainstem infarction or anomalies (e.g., olivopontocerebellar atrophy), after general anesthesia
Respiratory	Pneumonia, obstructive airway lesions, upper airway collapse, atelectasis, extreme prematurity (<1,000 g), laryngeal reflex, phrenic nerve paralysis, severe hyaline membrane disease, pneumothorax, hypoxia
Infectious	Sepsis, necrotizing enterocolitis, meningitis (bacterial, fungal, viral), respiratory syncytial virus
Gastrointestinal	Oral feeding, bowel movement, esophagitis, intestinal perforation
Metabolic	↓ Glucose, ↓ calcium, ↓/↑ sodium, ↑ ammonia, ↑ organic acids, ↑ ambient temperature, hypothermia
Cardiovascular	Hypotension, hypertension, heart failure, anemia, hypovolemia, vagal tone
Other	Immaturity of respiratory center, sleep state

system's control of respiration (e.g., hypoglycemia, meningitis, drugs, hemorrhage, seizures), disturbances in oxygen delivery (shock, sepsis, anemia), or ventilation defects (pneumonia, RDS, persistent pulmonary hypertension of the newborn [PPHN], muscle weakness).

Idiopathic apnea of prematurity occurs in the absence of identifiable predisposing diseases. Apnea is a disorder of respiratory control and may be obstructive, central, or mixed. Obstructive apnea (pharyngeal instability, neck flexion, nasal occlusion) is characterized by absent airflow but persistent chest wall motion. Pharyngeal collapse may follow the negative airway pressures generated during inspiration, or it may result from incoordination of the tongue and other upper airway muscles involved in maintaining airway patency. In central apnea, which is caused by decreased central nervous system (CNS) stimuli to respiratory muscles, airflow and chest wall motion are absent. Gestational age is the most important determinant of respiratory control, with the frequency of apnea being inversely related to gestational age. The immaturity of the brainstem respiratory centers is manifested by an attenuated response to carbon dioxide and a paradoxical response to hypoxia that results in apnea rather than hyperventilation. The most common pattern of idiopathic apnea in preterm neonates has a mixed etiology (50–75%), with obstructive apnea preceding (usually) or following central apnea. Short episodes of apnea are usually central, whereas prolonged ones are often mixed.

Apnea is sleep state dependent; the frequency increases during active (rapid eye movement) sleep. Paradoxical chest wall movement (inspiratory abdominal expansion and inward chest wall movement) is common during active sleep and may cause a fall in Pao_2 because of ventilation-perfusion defects. Furthermore, increased negative pressure during paradoxical breathing and inhibition of pharyngeal muscle tone during active sleep may contribute to upper airway collapse and obstructive apnea.

Clinical Manifestations. The incidence of idiopathic apnea of prematurity varies inversely with gestational age. In preterm infants, it is rare on the 1st day of life; apnea immediately after birth signifies another illness. The onset of idiopathic apnea occurs on the 2nd–7th day of life. The onset of apnea in a previously well premature neonate after the 2nd wk of life or in a term infant at any time is a critical event that warrants immediate investigation. In preterm infants, serious apnea is defined as cessation of breathing for longer than 20 sec, or any duration if accompanied by cyanosis and sinus bradycardia. The incidence of associated bradycardia increases with the length of the preceding apnea and correlates with the severity of hypoxia. Short apnea episodes (10 sec) are rarely associated with bradycardia, whereas longer ones (>20 sec) have a higher incidence of bradycardia. Bradycardia follows the apnea by 1–2 sec in more than

95% of cases; vagal responses and, rarely, heart block are causes of bradycardia without apnea.

Treatment. Infants at risk for apnea should be monitored with apnea monitors. Gentle *cutaneous stimulation* is often adequate therapy for neonatal infants with mild and intermittent episodes. Infants with recurrent and prolonged apnea require immediate *bag and mask ventilation*. *Oxygen* should be administered judiciously to treat hypoxia. Recurrent apnea of prematurity not due to a precipitating identifiable cause may be treated with *theophylline* or *caffeine*. Methylxanthines enhance ventilation through a central mechanism or by improving diaphragmatic strength. Loading doses of 5 mg/kg of theophylline (orally) or aminophylline (intravenously) should be followed by doses of 1–2 mg/kg given every 6–8 hr by the oral or intravenous routes. Loading doses of 10 mg/kg of caffeine are followed 24 hr later by maintenance doses of 2.5 mg/kg/24 hr qd orally. These doses should be monitored by observation of vital signs, clinical response, and serum drug levels (therapeutic levels: theophylline, 6–10 μg/mL; caffeine, 8–20 μg/mL). *Transfusion of packed red blood cells* to reduce the incidence of idiopathic apnea is reserved for severely anemic infants. The role of gastroesophageal reflux in apnea of prematurity is controversial; indeed, there may be no association. Data do not support the use of antireflux medications to reduce the frequency of apnea in preterm infants.

Nasal continuous positive airway pressure (CPAP, 3–5 cm H_2O) and high-flow nasal cannula (1–2.5 L/min) are effective therapies for mixed or obstructive apnea. Continuous positive pressure splints the upper airway and thereby prevents obstruction. When apnea is due to a precipitating illness, airway stability and oxygenation must be maintained in addition to therapy for the underlying disease.

Prognosis. Unless severe, recurrent, and refractory to therapy, apnea of prematurity does not alter an infant's prognosis. Associated problems of intraventricular hemorrhage (IVH), bronchopulmonary dysplasia (BPD), and retinopathy of prematurity are critical in determining the prognosis for apneic infants. Apnea of prematurity usually resolves by 36 wk postconceptional age (gestational age at birth plus postnatal age) and does not predict future episodes of sudden infant death syndrome. Some infants with apnea of prematurity are discharged as long as cardiorespiratory monitoring can be performed at home. In the absence of significant events, home monitoring can be safely discontinued at 44–45 wk postconceptional age.

Arad-Cohen N, Cohen A, Tirosh E: The relationship between gastroesophageal reflux and apnea in infants. *J Pediatr* 2000;137:321.

Darnall RA, Kattwinkel J, Nattie C, et al: Margin of safety for discharge after apnea in preterm infants. *Pediatrics* 1997;100:795.

Eichenwald EC, Aina A, Stark AR: Apnea frequently persists beyond term gestation in infants delivered at 24 to 28 weeks. *Pediatrics* 1997;100:354.

Eichenwald EC, Blackwell M, Lloyd JS, et al: Inter-neonatal intensive care unit variation in discharge timing: Influence of apnea and feeding management. *Pediatrics* 2001;108:928.

Kimball AL, Carlton DP: Gastroesophageal reflux medications in the treatment of apnea in premature infants. *J Pediatr* 2001;138:355.

Martin RJ, Miller MJ, Carlo WA: Pathogenesis of apnea in preterm infants. *J Pediatr* 1986;109:733.

Peter CS, Sprodowski N, Bohnhorst B, et al: Gastroesophageal reflux and apnea prematurity: No temporal relationship. *Pediatrics* 2002;109:8–11.

Ramanathan R, Corwin MJ, Hunt CE, et al: Cardiorespiratory events recorded on home monitors: Comparison of healthy infants with those at increased risk for SIDS. *JAMA* 2001;285:2199.

Ranganathan D, Wall S, Khosnood B, et al: Racial differences in respiratory-related neonatal mortality among very low birth weight infants. *J Pediatr* 2000;136:454.

Sreenan C, Lemke RP, Hudson-Mason A, et al: High-flow nasal cannulae in the management of apnea of prematurity: A comparison with conventional nasal continuous positive airway pressure. *Pediatrics* 2001;107:1081.

Steinhorn DM, Green TP: The treatment of acute respiratory failure in children: A historical examination of landmark advances. *J Pediatr* 2001;139:604.

Sychowski SP, Dodd E, Thomas P, et al: Home apnea monitor use in preterm infants discharged from newborn intensive care units. *J Pediatr* 2001;139:245–8.

Tauman R, Sivan Y: Duration of home monitoring for infants discharged with apnea of prematurity. *Biol Neonate* 2000;78:168.

90.3 Hyaline Membrane Disease (Respiratory Distress Syndrome)

Incidence. HMD occurs primarily in premature infants, and its incidence is inversely proportional to gestational age and birthweight. It occurs in 60–80% of infants less than 28 wk of gestational age, in 15–30% of those between 32 and 36 wk, in about 5% beyond 37 wk, and rarely at term. An increased frequency is associated with infants of diabetic mothers, delivery before 37 wk gestation, multifetal pregnancies, cesarean section delivery, precipitous delivery, asphyxia, cold stress, and a history of previously affected infants. The incidence is highest in preterm male or white infants. The risk of HMD is reduced in pregnancies with chronic or pregnancy-associated hypertension, maternal opiate addiction, prolonged rupture of membranes, and antenatal corticosteroid use.

Etiology and Pathophysiology. Surfactant deficiency (decreased production and secretion) is the primary cause of HMD. The failure of FRC to develop and the tendency of affected lungs to become atelectatic correlate with high surface tension and the absence of pulmonary surfactant. The major constituents of surfactant are dipalmitoyl phosphatidylcholine (lecithin), phosphatidylglycerol, apoproteins (surfactant proteins SP-A, -B, -C, -D), and cholesterol (Fig. 90–1). With advancing gestational age, increasing amounts of phospholipids are synthesized and stored in type II alveolar cells (Fig. 90–2). These surface-active agents are released into the alveoli, where they reduce surface tension and help maintain alveolar stability by preventing the collapse of small air spaces at end-expiration. However, the amounts produced or released may be insufficient to meet postnatal demands because of immaturity. Surfactant is present in high concentrations in fetal lung homogenates by 20 wk of gestation, but it does not reach the surface of the lungs until later. It appears in amniotic fluid between 28 and 32 wk. Mature levels of pulmonary surfactant are usually present after 35 wk. Though rare, genetic disorders may contribute to pulmonary outcome. Abnormalities in surfactant protein genes are associated with severe and/or lethal familial respiratory disease.

Synthesis of surfactant depends in part on normal pH, temperature, and perfusion. Asphyxia, hypoxemia, and pulmonary ischemia, particularly in association with hypovolemia, hypotension, and cold stress, may suppress surfactant synthesis. The epithelial lining of the lungs may also be injured by high oxygen concentrations and the effects of respirator management, thereby resulting in a further reduction in surfactant.

Alveolar atelectasis, hyaline membrane formation, and interstitial edema make the lungs less compliant, so greater pressure is required to expand the small alveoli and airways. In affected infants, the lower part of the chest wall is pulled in as the diaphragm descends, and intrathoracic pressure becomes negative, thus limiting the amount of intrathoracic pressure that can be produced; the result is a tendency for the development of atelectasis. The highly compliant chest wall of preterm infants offers less resistance than that of mature infants to the natural tendency of the lungs to collapse. Thus, at end-expiration, the volume of the thorax and lungs tends to approach residual volume, and atelectasis may develop.

Deficient synthesis or release of surfactant, together with small respiratory units and a compliant chest wall, produces atelectasis and results in perfused, but not ventilated alveoli, which causes hypoxia. Decreased lung compliance, small tidal volumes, increased physiologic dead space, increased work of breathing, and insufficient alveolar ventilation eventually result in hypercapnia. The combination of hypercapnia, hypoxia, and acidosis produces pulmonary arterial vasoconstriction with increased right-to-left shunting through the foramen ovale and ductus arteriosus and within the lung itself. Pulmonary blood flow is reduced, and ischemic injury to the cells producing surfactant and to the vascular bed results in an effusion of proteinaceous material into the alveolar spaces (Fig. 90–3).

Pathology. The lungs appear deep purplish red and are liver-like in consistency. Microscopically, extensive atelectasis with engorgement of the interalveolar capillaries and lymphatics can be observed. A number of the alveolar ducts, alveoli, and respiratory bronchioles are lined with acidophilic, homogeneous, or granular membranes. Amniotic debris, intra-alveolar hemorrhage, and interstitial emphysema are additional, but inconstant findings; interstitial emphysema may be marked when an infant has been ventilated. The characteristic hyaline membranes are rarely seen in infants dying earlier than 6–8 hr after birth.

Clinical Manifestations. Signs of HMD usually appear within minutes of birth, although they may not be recognized for several hours in larger premature infants until rapid, shallow respirations have increased to 60/min or greater. A late onset of tachypnea should suggest other conditions. Some patients require resuscitation at birth because of intrapartum asphyxia or initial severe respiratory distress (especially with a birthweight <1,000 g). Characteristically, tachypnea, prominent (often audible) grunting, intercostal and subcostal retractions, nasal flaring, and duskiness are noted. Cyanosis increases and is often relatively unresponsive to oxygen administration. Breath sounds may be normal or diminished with a harsh tubular quality, and on deep inspiration, fine rales may be heard, especially over the lung bases posteriorly. The natural course of untreated HMD is characterized by progressive worsening of cyanosis and dyspnea. If the condition is inadequately treated, blood pressure may fall; fatigue, cyanosis, and pallor increase, and grunting decreases or disappears as the condition worsens. Apnea and irregular respirations occur as infants tire and are ominous signs requiring immediate intervention. Patients may also have a mixed respiratory-metabolic acidosis, edema, ileus, and oliguria. Respiratory failure may occur in infants with rapid progression of the disease. In most cases, the symptoms and signs reach a peak within 3 days, after which improvement is gradual. Improvement is often heralded by spontaneous diuresis and the ability to oxygenate the infant at lower inspired oxygen levels. Death is rare on the 1st day of illness, usually occurs between days 2 and 7, and is associated with alveolar air leaks (interstitial emphysema, pneumothorax) and pulmonary hemorrhage or

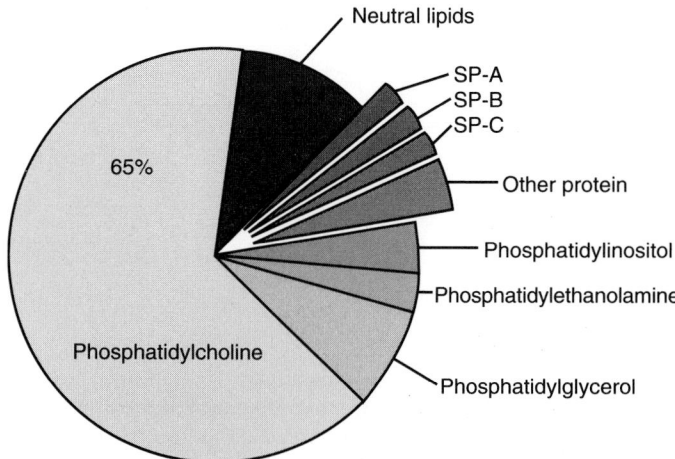

FIGURE 90–1. Composition of surfactant recovered by alveolar wash. The quantities of the different components are similar for surfactant from the mature lungs of mammals. (From Jobe AH: Fetal lung development, tests for maturation, induction of maturation, and treatment. In Creasy RK, Resnik R [editors]: *Maternal-Fetal Medicine: Principles and Practice*, 3rd ed. Philadelphia, WB Saunders, 1994.)

Labels in figure: Neutral lipids; SP-A; SP-B; SP-C; Other protein; Phosphatidylinositol; Phosphatidylethanolamine; Phosphatidylglycerol; Phosphatidylcholine; 65%

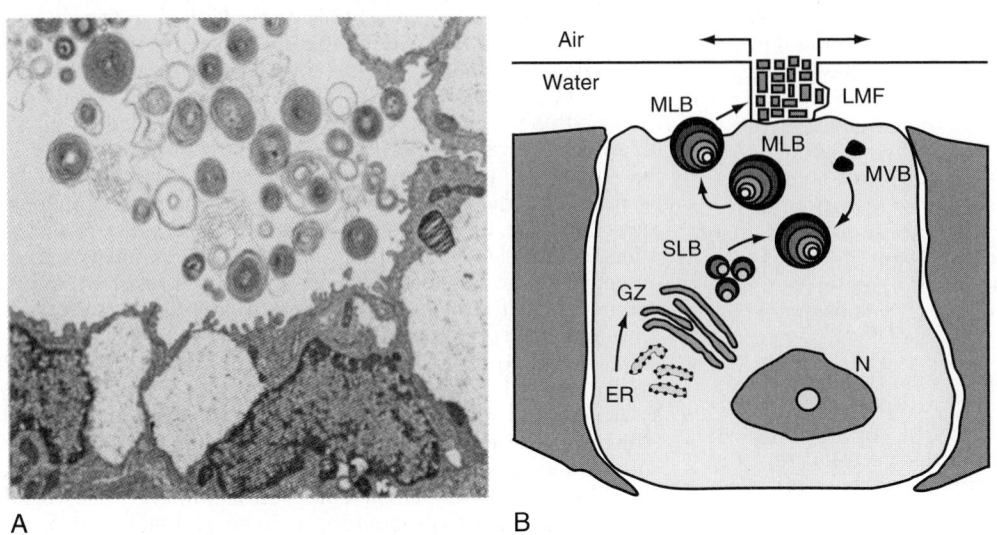

FIGURE 90–2. *A,* Fetal rat lung (low magnification), day 20 (term, day 22), showing developing type II cells, stored glycogen *(pale areas),* secreted lamellar bodies, and tubular myelin. (Courtesy of Mary Williams, M.D., University of California, San Francisco.) *B,* Possible pathway for transport, secretion, and reuptake of surfactant. MLB = mature lamellar body; LMF = lattice (tubular) myelin figure; MVB = multivesicular body; SLB = small lamellar body; GZ = Golgi zone; ER = endoplasmic reticulum; N = nucleus. (From Hansen T, Corbet A: Lung development and function. In Taeusch HW, Ballard RA, Avery MA [editors]: *Schaffer and Avery's Diseases of the Newborn,* 6th ed. Philadelphia, WB Saunders, 1991.)

IVH. Mortality may be delayed weeks or months if BPD develops in mechanically ventilated infants with severe HMD.

Diagnosis. The clinical course, a roentgenogram of the chest, and blood gas and acid-base values help establish the clinical diagnosis. Roentgenographically, the lungs may have a characteristic, but not pathognomonic appearance that includes a fine reticular granularity of the parenchyma and air bronchograms, which are often more prominent early in the left lower lobe because of superimposition of the cardiac shadow (Fig. 90–4). The initial roentgenogram is occasionally normal, with the typical pattern developing at 6–12 hr. Considerable variation in films may be seen, depending on the phase of respiration and the use of CPAP or positive end-expiratory pressure (PEEP); this variation often results in poor correlation between roentgenograms and the clinical course. Laboratory findings are initially characterized by

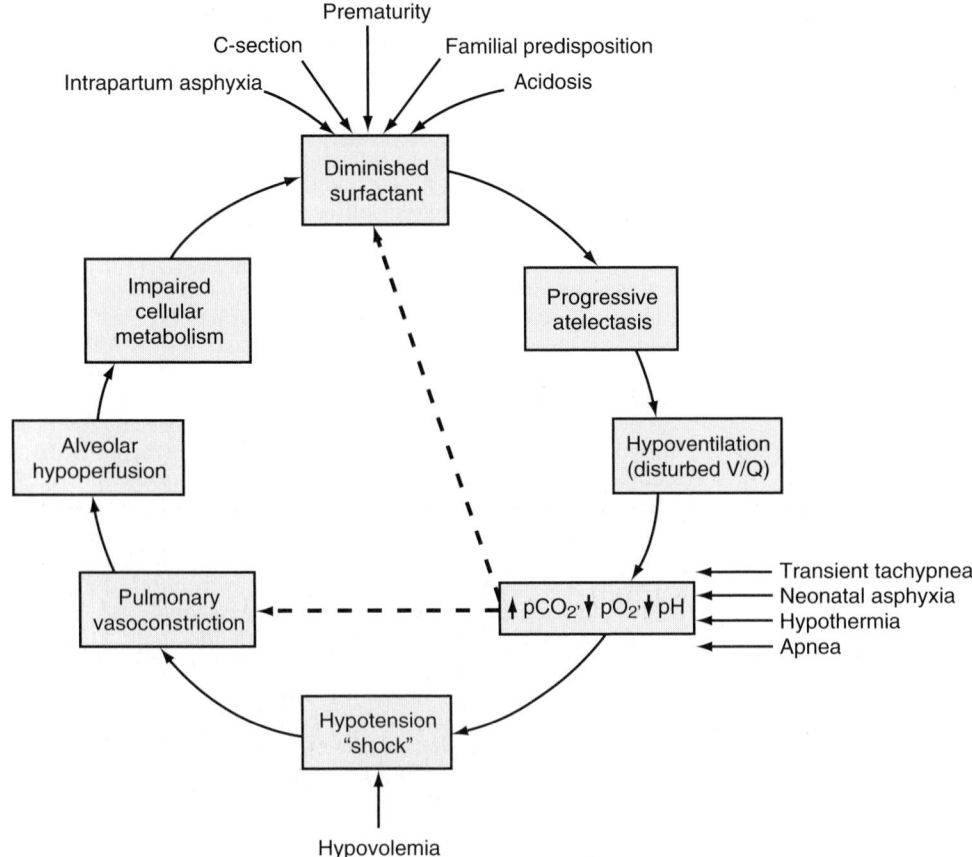

FIGURE 90–3. Contributing factors in the pathogenesis of hyaline membrane disease. The potential "vicious circle" perpetuates hypoxia and pulmonary insufficiency. (From Farrell P, Zachman R: In Quilligan EJ, Kretchmer N [editors]: *Fetal and Maternal Medicine.* New York, John Wiley & Sons, 1980. © 1980. Reprinted by permission of John Wiley & Sons, Inc.)

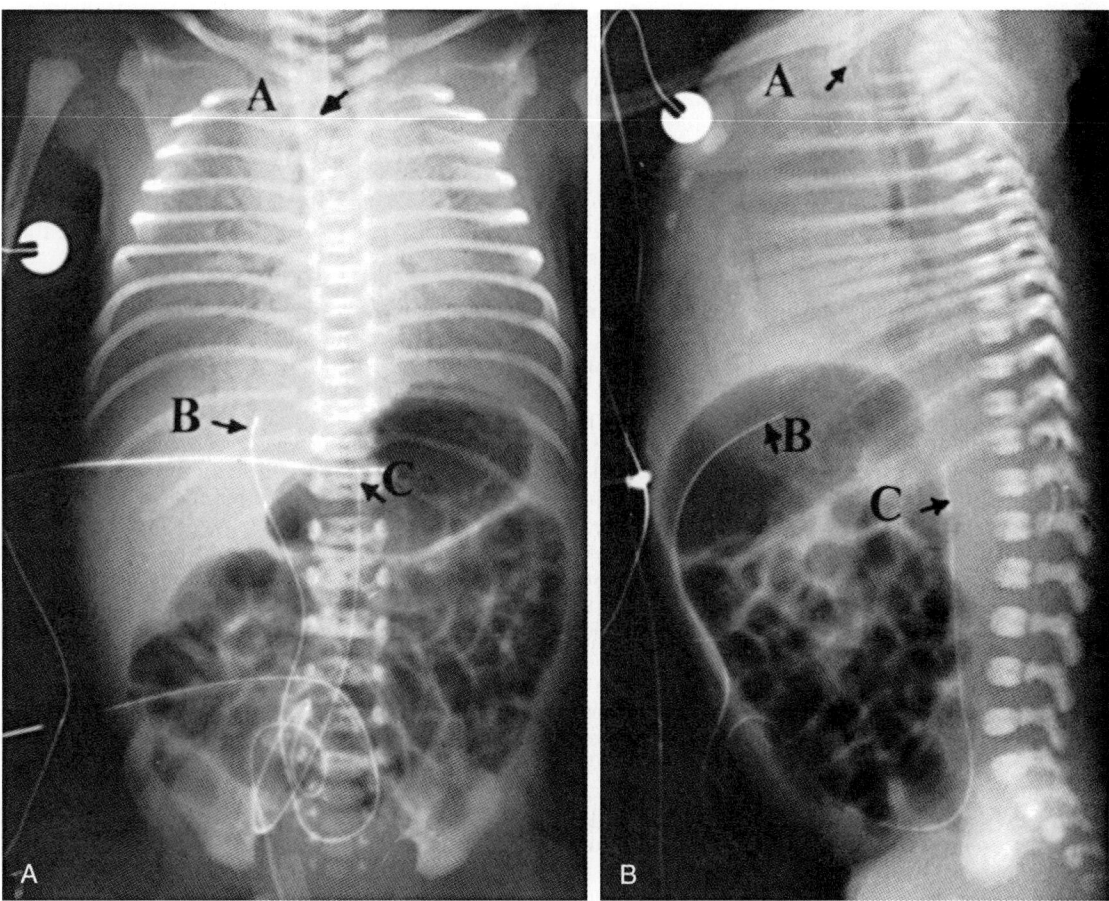

FIGURE 90–4. Infant with hyaline membrane disease. Note the granular lungs, air bronchogram, and air-filled esophagus. Anteroposterior *(A)* and lateral *(B)* roentgenograms are needed to distinguish the umbilical artery from the vein catheter and to determine the appropriate level of insertion. The lateral view clearly shows that the catheter has been inserted into an umbilical vein and is lying in the portal system of the liver. A = endotracheal tube; B = umbilical venous catheter at the junction of the umbilical vein, ductus venosus, and portal vein; C = umbilical artery catheter passed up the aorta to T12. (Courtesy of Walter E. Berdon, Babies Hospital, New York City.)

hypoxemia and later by progressive hypoxemia, hypercapnia, and variable metabolic acidosis.

In the *differential diagnosis,* early-onset sepsis may be indistinguishable from HMD. In pneumonia manifested at birth, the chest roentgenogram may be identical to that for HMD. Maternal group B streptococcal colonization, organisms on Gram stain of gastric or tracheal aspirates or a buffy coat smear, and/or the presence of marked neutropenia may suggest the diagnosis of early-onset sepsis. Cyanotic heart disease (e.g., total anomalous pulmonary venous return), persistent pulmonary hypertension, aspiration syndromes, spontaneous pneumothorax, pleural effusions, and congenital anomalies such as cystic adenomatoid malformation, pulmonary lymphangiectasia, diaphragmatic hernia, and lobar emphysema must be considered and require roentgenographic evaluation. Transient tachypnea may be distinguished by its short and mild clinical course. *Congenital alveolar proteinosis* (e.g., congenital surfactant protein B deficiency) is a rare familial disease that is often manifested as severe and lethal RDS in term and premature infants (see Chapter 389).

Prevention. Most important is prevention of prematurity, including avoidance of unnecessary or poorly timed cesarean section, appropriate management of high-risk pregnancy and labor, and prediction and possible in utero acceleration of pulmonary immaturity (Chapter 85). In timing cesarean section or induction of labor, estimation of fetal head circumference by ultrasonography and determination of the lecithin concentration in

amniotic fluid by the lecithin:sphingomyelin ratio (particularly useful with phosphatidylglycerol in diabetic pregnancies) decrease the likelihood of delivering a premature infant. Intrauterine antenatal and intrapartum monitoring may similarly decrease the risk of fetal asphyxia, which is associated with an increased incidence and severity of HMD.

Administration of *betamethasone* to women 48 hr before the delivery of fetuses between 24 and 34 wk of gestation significantly reduces the incidence and the mortality and morbidity of HMD. It is appropriate to administer corticosteroids intramuscularly to all pregnant women who are likely to deliver a fetus in 1 wk that is between 24 and 34 wk gestation. Only one course of therapy is required even if the infant is not delivered until days to weeks later. Prenatal glucocorticoid therapy decreases the severity of RDS and reduces the incidence of other complications of prematurity, such as IVH, patent ductus arteriosus (PDA), pneumothorax, and necrotizing enterocolitis, without affecting neonatal growth, lung mechanics or growth, or the incidence of infection. Prenatal glucocorticoids may act synergistically with postnatal exogenous surfactant therapy. Prenatal dexamethasone may be associated with a higher incidence of periventricular leukomalacia than is the case with betamethasone.

Administration of a first dose of *surfactant* into the trachea of symptomatic premature infants immediately after birth (prophylactic) or during the first few hours of life (early rescue) reduces air leak and mortality from HMD but does not alter the incidence of BPD.

Treatment. The basic defect requiring treatment is inadequate pulmonary exchange of oxygen and carbon dioxide; metabolic acidosis and circulatory insufficiency are secondary manifestations. Early supportive care of LBW infants, especially in the treatment of acidosis, hypoxia, hypotension (see Chapter 87), and hypothermia, appears to lessen the severity of HMD. Therapy requires careful and frequent monitoring of heart and respiratory rates, Pao_2, $Paco_2$, pH, bicarbonate, electrolytes, blood glucose, hematocrit, blood pressure, and temperature. Arterial catheterization is frequently necessary. Because most cases of HMD are self-limited, the goal of treatment is to minimize abnormal physiologic variations and superimposed iatrogenic problems. Treatment of these infants is best carried out in a specially staffed and equipped hospital unit, the neonatal intensive care unit (NICU).

The general principles for supportive care of any LBW infant should be adhered to, including gentle handling and minimal disturbance consistent with management. To avoid hypothermia and minimize oxygen consumption, infants should be placed in an isolette or radiant warmer and core temperature maintained between 36.5 and 37°C (Chapters 86 and 87). Calories and fluids should be provided intravenously. For the 1st 24 hr, 10% glucose and water should be infused through a peripheral vein at a rate of 65–75 mL/kg/24 hr. Subsequently, electrolytes should be added and fluid volume increased gradually. Excessive fluids contribute to the development of PDA and BPD.

Warm humidified oxygen should be provided at a concentration initially sufficient to keep arterial levels between 55 and 70 mm Hg (>90% saturation) to maintain normal tissue oxygenation while minimizing the risk of oxygen toxicity. If the Pao_2 cannot be maintained above 50 mm Hg at inspired oxygen concentrations of 60% or greater, applying CPAP at a pressure of 6–10 cm H_2O by nasal prongs is indicated and usually produces a sharp rise in Pao_2. CPAP prevents collapse of surfactant-deficient alveoli, improves FRC, and improves ventilation-perfusion matching. The amount of CPAP required usually decreases abruptly at about 72 hr of age, and infants can be weaned from CPAP shortly thereafter. If an infant managed by CPAP cannot maintain an arterial oxygen tension above 50 mm Hg while breathing 70–100% oxygen, assisted ventilation is required.

Infants with severe HMD and those with complications that result in persistent apnea require *assisted mechanical ventilation*. Reasonable indications for its use are (1) arterial blood pH less than 7.20, (2) arterial blood Pco_2 of 60 mm Hg or higher, (3) arterial blood Po_2 of 50 mm Hg or less at oxygen concentrations of 70–100% and CPAP of 8–10 cm H_2O, or (4) persistent apnea. Intermittent positive pressure ventilation delivered by time-cycled, pressure-limited, continuous flow ventilators has been the most common method of conventional ventilation for newborns. Other methods of conventional ventilation include synchronized intermittent mandatory ventilation (the set rate and pressure synchronized with the patient's own breaths), pressure support (the patient triggers each breath and a set pressure is delivered), and volume guarantee (a composite mode in which a specific tidal volume is set and peak pressure is limited). Assisted ventilation for infants with RDS should include PEEP (see Chapter 57.4).

The goals of mechanical ventilation are to improve oxygenation and elimination of carbon dioxide without causing pulmonary barotrauma or oxygen toxicity. Acceptable ranges of blood gas values, after balancing the risks of hypoxia and acidosis against those of mechanical ventilation, are a Pao_2 of 55–70 mm Hg, a Pco_2 of 45–55 mm Hg, and a pH of 7.25–7.35. During mechanical ventilation, oxygenation is improved by increasing the Fio_2 or mean airway pressure. The latter can be increased by increasing the peak inspiratory pressure, gas flow, the inspiratory:expiratory ratio, or PEEP. Excessive PEEP may impede venous return, thereby reducing cardiac output despite improvement in Pao_2 and thus decreasing oxygen delivery. PEEP levels of 4–6 cm H_2O are usually safe and effective. Carbon dioxide elimi-

nation is achieved by increasing the peak inspiratory pressure (tidal volume) or the rate of the ventilator. Many ventilated neonates receive sedation or pain relief with benzodiazepines or opiates (morphine, fentanyl), respectively.

High-frequency ventilation (HFV) was developed to reduce lung injury and/or improve gas exchange in patients with severe respiratory disease. HFV preserves the desired minute ventilation by using smaller tidal volumes and high rates (300–1200 breaths/min or 5–20 Hz). HFV may improve the elimination of carbon dioxide, lower mean airway pressure, and improve oxygenation in patients who do not respond to conventional ventilators and who have severe HMD, interstitial emphysema, many pneumothoraces, or meconium aspiration pneumonia. High-frequency jet ventilation may cause necrotizing tracheal damage, especially in the presence of hypotension or poor humidification, and high-frequency oscillator therapy has been inconsistently associated with an increased risk of air leaks, IVH, and periventricular leukomalacia. Both methods may cause gas trapping. High-frequency oscillation strategies that promote lung recruitment, combined with surfactant therapy, may not reduce the risk for BPD. Complications of endotracheal intubation (plugging of the tube, extubation, subglottic granuloma, and stenosis) and mechanical ventilation (pneumothorax, interstitial emphysema, reduced cardiac output) may be minimized by the interventions of specially trained physicians, nurses, and respiratory therapists in a NICU.

Multidose endotracheal instillation of *exogenous surfactant* to LBW infants requiring 30% oxygen and mechanical ventilation for the treatment (*rescue therapy*) of RDS dramatically improves survival and reduces the incidence of pulmonary air leaks, but it has not consistently reduced the incidence of BPD. Immediate effects include improved alveolar-arterial oxygen gradients, reduced ventilator mean airway pressure, increased pulmonary compliance, and improved appearance of the chest roentgenogram. A number of surfactant preparations have been studied and are widely used, including synthetic surfactants and natural surfactants derived from animal sources. Exosurf is a synthetic surfactant. Natural surfactants include Survanta (bovine), Infasurf (calf), and Curosurf (porcine). Although both synthetic and natural surfactants are effective in the treatment and prevention of RDS, natural surfactants appear to be superior, perhaps because of their surfactant-associated protein content. Natural surfactants have a more rapid onset and are associated with a lower risk of pneumothorax and improved survival. Rapid testing of pulmonary maturity soon after birth by examining tracheal aspirate secretions may reduce the number of unaffected infants treated unnecessarily with surfactant and permit early rescue therapy, usually within the 1st hr of life.

Treatment (rescue) is initiated as soon as possible in the 1st 24 hr of life. Repeated dosing is given via the endotracheal tube every 6–12 hr for a total of two to four doses, depending on the preparation. Exogenous surfactant should be given by a physician who is qualified in neonatal resuscitation and respiratory management and who is able to care for the infant beyond the 1st hr of stabilization. Additional on-site staff support required includes nurses and respiratory therapists experienced in the ventilatory management of LBW infants. Appropriate monitoring equipment must also be available (radiology, blood gas laboratory, and pulse oximetry). Furthermore, each institution should have an approved protocol for the administration of surfactant. Complications of surfactant therapy include transient hypoxia and hypotension, blockage of the endotracheal tube, and pulmonary hemorrhage.

Inhaled nitric oxide (iNO) has acutely improved oxygenation, but it may not improve the overall outcome of infants with HMD.

Weaning from the ventilator varies and is based on the mechanics and special features of the ventilator. Once extubated, many infants are transitioned to nasal CPAP to avoid postextubation atelectasis and hypoxia.

Respiratory acidosis may require short-term or prolonged assisted ventilation. In severe respiratory acidosis and hypoxia, treatment with sodium bicarbonate may exacerbate hypercapnia.

Metabolic acidosis in HMD may be a result of perinatal asphyxia and hypotension and is often encountered when an infant has required resuscitation (Chapter 89). Sodium bicarbonate, 1–2 mEq/kg, may be administered over a 15–20 min period through a peripheral or umbilical vein, with the acid-base determination repeated within 30 min, or it may be administered over a period of several hours. Often, sodium bicarbonate is administered on an emergency basis through an umbilical venous catheter. Alkali therapy may result in skin slough from infiltration, increased serum osmolarity, hypernatremia, hypocalcemia, hypokalemia, and liver injury when concentrated solutions are administered rapidly through an umbilical vein catheter wedged in the liver.

Monitoring of *aortic blood pressure* through an umbilical or peripheral arterial catheter or by oscillometric technique may be useful in managing the shocklike state that may occur during the 1st hr or so after the premature birth of an infant who has been asphyxiated or in whom severe respiratory distress has developed (see Fig. 83–2). Hypotension has been associated with increased CNS morbidity and increased mortality and should be treated with cautious administration of volume (crystalloid) and early use of pressors (usually dopamine). Occasionally, hypotension may be glucocorticoid responsive (see Chapter 87).

Periodic monitoring of Pao_2, $Paco_2$, and pH is an important part of the management; if assisted ventilation is being used, such monitoring is essential. Blood should be obtained from the umbilical or peripheral artery. Tissue Po_2 may also be estimated continuously from transcutaneous electrodes or pulse oximetry (oxygen saturation). Capillary blood samples are of limited value for determining Po_2 but may be useful for evaluating Pco_2 and pH. Radiopaque umbilical catheters should have their position checked roentgenographically after insertion (see Fig. 90–4). The tip of an umbilical artery catheter should lie just above the bifurcation of the aorta (L3–L5) or above the celiac axis (T6–T10). Preferred sites for peripheral catheters are the radial or posterior tibial arteries. Placement and supervision should be carried out by skilled and experienced personnel. Catheters should be removed as soon as patients no longer have any indication for their continued use—usually when the Pao_2 is stable and the Fio_2 is less than 40%.

Because of the difficulty of distinguishing group B streptococcal or other bacterial infections from HMD, empirical antibiotic therapy is indicated until the results of blood cultures are available. Penicillin or ampicillin with kanamycin or gentamicin is suggested; however, the choice of antibiotics is based on the recent pattern of bacterial sensitivity in the hospital where the infant is being treated (Chapter 98).

Complications of HMD and Intensive Care. The most serious complications of **tracheal intubation** are asphyxia from obstruction of the tube, cardiac arrest during intubation or suctioning, and the subsequent development of subglottic stenosis. Other complications include bleeding from trauma during intubation, posterior pharyngeal pseudodiverticula, difficult extubation requiring tracheostomy, ulceration of the nares because of pressure from the tube, permanent narrowing of the nostril as a result of tissue damage and scarring from irritation or infection around the tube, erosion of the palate, avulsion of a vocal cord, laryngeal ulcer, papilloma of a vocal cord, and persistent hoarseness, stridor, or edema of the larynx.

Measures to reduce the incidence of these complications include skillful intubation, adequate securing of the tube, use of

polyvinyl endotracheal tubes, use of the smallest size tube sufficient to reduce local ischemia and pressure necrosis, avoidance of frequent changes and motion of the tube in situ, avoidance of too frequent or vigorous suctioning, and prevention of infection through meticulous cleanliness and frequent sterilization of all apparatus attached to or passed through the tube. The personnel inserting and caring for the endotracheal tube should be experienced and skilled.

Risks associated with **umbilical arterial catheterization** include vascular embolization, thrombosis, spasm, and perforation; ischemic or chemical necrosis of abdominal viscera; infection; accidental hemorrhage; and impaired circulation to a leg with subsequent gangrene. Although the reported incidence of thrombotic complications varies from 1–23% at necropsy, aortography has demonstrated that clots form in or about the tips of 95% of catheters placed in an umbilical artery. Aortic ultrasonography can also be used to investigate the presence of thrombosis. The risk of a serious clinical complication resulting from umbilical catheterization is probably between 2 and 5%.

Transient blanching of the leg may occur during catheterization of the umbilical artery. It is usually due to reflex arterial spasm, the incidence of which is lessened by using the smallest available catheter, particularly in very small infants. The catheter should be removed immediately; catheterization of the other artery may then be attempted. Persistent spasm after removal of the catheter may be relieved by topical nitroglycerin applied over the femoral artery or, rarely, by warming the opposite leg. Blood sampling from a radial artery may similarly result in spasm or thrombosis, and the same treatment is indicated. Intermittent severe spasm or unrelieved spasm may respond to the cautious use of topical nitroglycerin or local infusion of tolazoline (Priscoline), 1–2 mg injected intra-arterially over a 5 min period. Accidentally lodging the catheter in a smaller artery, either blocking it completely or causing unrecognized local vascular spasm, may result in gangrene of the organ or area supplied by the vessel. To prevent this complication, the catheter should be removed promptly if blood cannot be withdrawn from it.

Serious hemorrhage on removal of the catheter is rare. Thrombi may form in the artery or in the catheter, the incidence of which can be lowered by using a smooth-tipped catheter with a hole only at its end, by rinsing the catheter with a small amount of saline solution containing heparin, or by continuously infusing a solution containing 1–5 U/mL of heparin. The risk of thrombus formation with potential vascular occlusion can also be reduced by removing the catheter when early signs of thrombosis are noted, such as narrowing of pulse pressure and disappearance of the dicrotic notch. Some prefer to use the umbilical artery for blood sampling only and leave the catheter filled with heparinized saline between samplings. *Renovascular hypertension* may occur days to weeks after umbilical arterial catheterization in a small number of neonates.

Umbilical vein catheterization is associated with many of the same risks as umbilical artery catheterization. An additional risk is cardiac perforation and pericardial tamponade if the catheter is placed in the right atrium; portal hypertension can subsequently develop from portal vein thrombosis, especially in the presence of omphalitis.

Extrapulmonary extravasation of air is another complication of the management of HMD (Chapter 90.8).

Some neonates with HMD may have clinically significant shunting through a **PDA**, the delayed closure being due to associated hypoxia, acidosis, increased pulmonary pressure secondary to vasoconstriction, systemic hypotension, immaturity, and local release of prostaglandins, which dilate the ductus. There appears to be a link between early adrenal insufficiency, ductal patency, airway inflammation, and the development of BPD. Shunting through the PDA may initially be bidirectional or right to left. As HMD resolves, pulmonary vascular resistance decreases, and left-to-right shunting may occur and lead to left ventricular volume overload and pulmonary edema. Manifestations of PDA may include (1) persistent apnea for unexplained reasons in an infant recovering from HMD; (2) an active heaving precordium, bounding peripheral pulses, wide pulse pressure, and a systolic or to-and-fro murmur; (3) carbon dioxide retention; (4) increasing oxygen dependence; (5) roentgenographic evidence of cardiomegaly and increased pulmonary vascular markings; and (6) hepatomegaly. The diagnosis is confirmed by echocardiographic visualization of a PDA with Doppler flow evidence of left-to-right shunting. Many infants respond to general supportive measures, including diuretics and fluid restriction. In patients in whom spontaneous closure does not occur and deterioration progresses despite supportive and cardiotonic treatment, intravenous indomethacin, 0.2 mg/kg at 12–24 hr intervals for three doses, may induce pharmacologic closure by inhibiting prostaglandin synthesis; repeated courses may be needed. Prophylactic low-dose indomethacin reduces the incidence of both IVH and PDA and improves the rate of permanent ductal closure, but it does not improve the long-term prognosis. Contraindications to indomethacin include thrombocytopenia (<50,000/mm^3), bleeding disorders, oliguria (<1 mL/kg/hr), necrotizing enterocolitis, and an elevated plasma creatinine level (>1.8 mg/dL). Ibuprofen (initial dose of 10 mg/kg, followed at 24 hr intervals by two doses of 5 mg/kg), unlike indomethacin, does not reduce cerebral, mesenteric, or renal blood flow and may be equally effective in closing a PDA. Ibuprofen has rarely been associated with pulmonary hypertension. Indications for surgical closure are failure to close the ductus after one to two courses of drug therapy along with persistent heart failure and ventilator dependence.

BPD is a result of lung injury in infants requiring mechanical ventilation and supplemental oxygen. The BPD described in 1967 by Northway, in an era before the widespread use of antenatal steroids and postnatal surfactant, was a disease of large preterm infants with severe lung injury resulting from mechanical ventilation and oxygen. Today, BPD is a disease primarily of extremely low-birthweight (ELBW) infants, usually under 1,000 g at birth, many of whom have little or no lung disease at birth but in whom progressive disease develops over time.

A consistent pathologic finding in these infants is decreased alveolarization, decreased septation, and minimal airway disease, all of which suggest arrest in lung development. The lung injury is due to an interaction of multiple factors. RDS is a disease of progressive alveolar collapse. Atelectasis (which is affected by

insufficient PEEP), together with ventilator-induced increased lung volume and regional overdistention (volutrauma), promotes injury. Oxygen induces injury by producing free radicals that cannot be metabolized by the immature antioxidant systems of ELBW neonates. Mechanical ventilation and/or oxygen injure the preterm lung by affecting alveolar and vascular development. Moreover, inflammation (measured by circulating neutrophils, neutrophils and macrophages in alveolar fluid, and pro-inflammatory cytokines) contributes to the progression of lung injury. Potential inflammatory or tissue metabolic product markers for BPD have been identified in blood, urine, and tracheal aspirates. Several clinical factors, including immaturity, infection, symptomatic PDA, and malnutrition, contribute to the development of BPD.

BPD is usually defined as a need for supplemental oxygen at 36 wk after conception. Another definition of BPD is based on the severity of disease (Table 90–2). Studies to define BPD based on the physiologic need for oxygen are ongoing. The occurrence of BPD is inversely related to gestational age. Instead of showing improvement on the 3rd–4th day, consistent with the natural course of RDS, some infants who have been maintained by mechanical ventilation with increased concentrations of oxygen show a worsening of their pulmonary condition. The respiratory distress persists and is characterized by hypoxia, hypercapnia, oxygen dependence, and in severe cases, the development of right-sided heart failure. The chest roentgenogram is described as gradually changing from a picture of almost complete opacification with air bronchograms and interstitial emphysema to one of small, round, radiolucent areas alternating with areas of irregular density resembling a sponge (Fig. 90–5). Histologic study at this stage (10–20 days after beginning oxygen therapy) shows less evidence of hyaline membrane formation, progressive alveolar coalescence with atelectasis of the surrounding alveoli, interstitial edema, coarse focal thickening of the basement membrane, and widespread bronchial and bronchiolar mucosal metaplasia and hyperplasia. These findings correspond to a severe maldistribution of ventilation.

Most surviving neonates with persistent roentgenographic changes recover by 6–12 mo, but some require prolonged hospitalization and may have respiratory symptoms persisting through childhood (bronchospasm). Right-sided heart failure and acquired viral necrotizing bronchiolitis (respiratory syncytial virus) are major causes of death in infancy. Pathologic examination reveals cardiac enlargement and pulmonary changes consisting of focal areas of emphysematous alveoli with hypertrophy

TABLE 90–2. Definition of Bronchopulmonary Dysplasia: Diagnostic Criteria

Gestational Age	<32 wk	≥32 wk
Time point of assessment	36 wk PMA or discharge home, whichever comes first	>28 days' but <56 days' postnatal age or discharge home, whichever comes first. Treatment with >21% oxygen for at least 28 days **plus**
	Treatment with >21% oxygen for at least 28 days **plus**	
Mild BPD	Breathing room air at 36 wk PMA or discharge, whichever comes first	Breathing room air by 56 days postnatal age or discharge, whichever comes first
Moderate BPD	Need* for <30% oxygen at 36 wk PMA or discharge, whichever comes first	Need* for <30% oxygen at 56 days' postnatal age or discharge, whichever comes first
Severe BPD	Need* for ≥30% oxygen and/or positive pressure (PPV or NCPAP) at 36 wk PMA or discharge, whichever comes first	Need* for ≥30% oxygen and/or positive pressure (PPV or NCPAP) at 56 days' postnatal age or discharge, whichever comes first

BPD usually develops in neonates being treated with oxygen and PPV for respiratory failure, most commonly respiratory distress syndrome. Persistence of the clinical features of respiratory disease (tachypnea, retractions, crackles) is considered common to the broad description of BPD and has not been included in the diagnostic criteria describing the severity of BPD. Infants treated with greater than 21% oxygen and/or positive pressure for nonrespiratory disease (e.g., central apnea or diaphragmatic paralysis) do not have BPD unless parenchymal lung disease also develops and they have clinical features of respiratory distress. A day of treatment with greater than 21% oxygen means that the infant received greater than 21% oxygen for more than 12 hr on that day. Treatment with greater than 21% oxygen and/or positive pressure at 36 wk PMA or at 56 days' postnatal age or discharge should not reflect an "acute" event, but should rather reflect the infant's usual daily therapy for several days preceding and following 36 wk PMA, 56 days' postnatal age, or discharge.

* A physiologic test confirming that the oxygen requirement at the assessment time point remains to be defined. This assessment may include a pulse oximetry saturation range.

PMA = postmenstrual age; BPD = bronchopulmonary dysplasia; PPV = positive pressure ventilation; NCPAP = nasal continuous positive airway pressure.

From Jobe AH, Bancalari E: Bronchopulmonary dysplasia. Am J Respir Crit Care Med 2001; 163:1723–29.

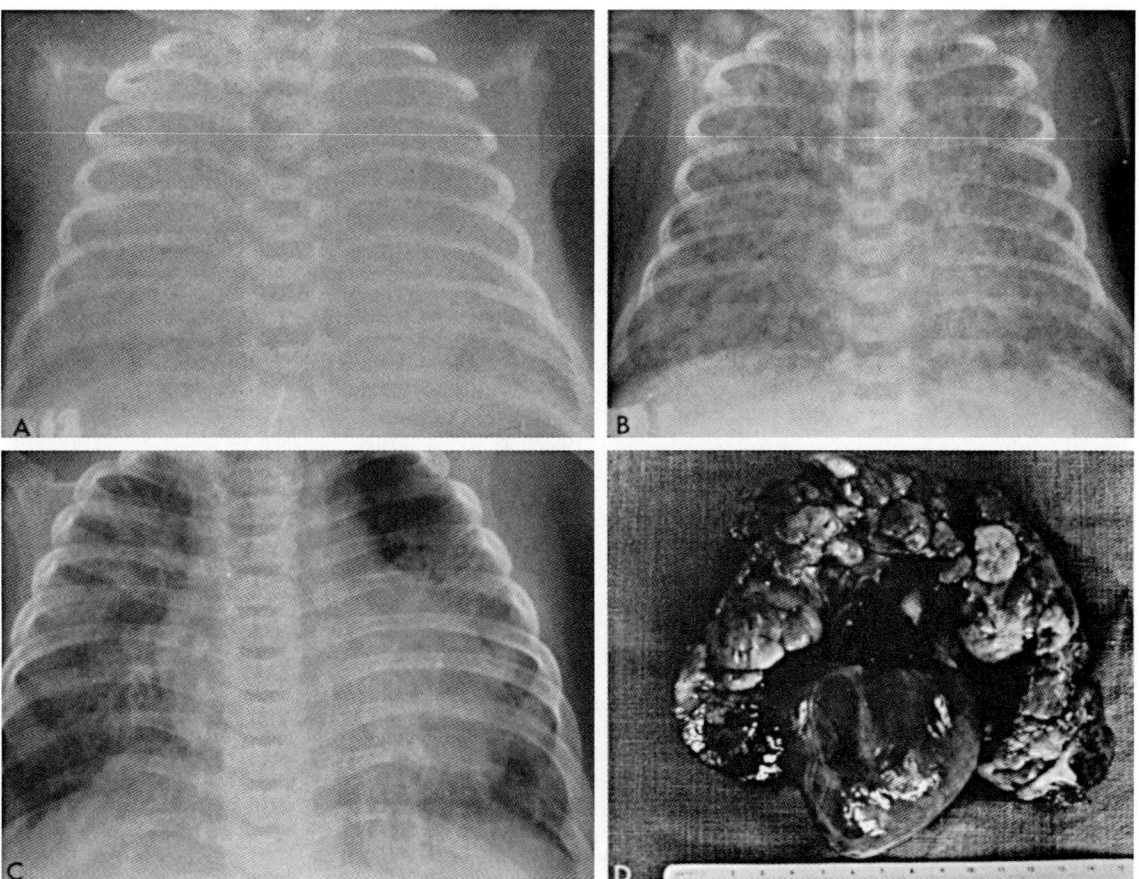

FIGURE 90–5. Pulmonary changes in infants treated with prolonged, intermittent positive pressure breathing with air containing 80–100% oxygen in the immediate postnatal period for the clinical syndrome of hyaline membrane disease. *A*, A 5-day-old infant with nearly complete opacification of the lungs. *B*, A 13-day-old infant with "bubbly lungs" simulating the roentgenographic appearance of the Wilson-Mikity syndrome. *C*, A 7-mo-old infant with irregular, dense strands in both lungs, hyperinflation, and cardiomegaly suggestive of chronic lung disease. *D*, Large right ventricle and a cobbly, irregularly aerated lung of an infant who died at 11 mo of age. This infant also had a patent ductus arteriosus. (From Northway WH Jr, Rosan RC, Porter DY: Pulmonary disease following respirator therapy of hyaline-membrane disease. *N Engl J Med* 1967;276:357.)

of the peribronchial smooth muscle of the tributary bronchioles, some perimucosal fibrosis and widespread metaplasia of the bronchiolar mucosa, thickening of basement membranes, and separation of the capillaries from the alveolar epithelial cells.

Infants at risk for BPD usually have severe respiratory distress requiring prolonged periods of mechanical ventilation and oxygen therapy. Additional associations include the presence of interstitial emphysema, lower gestational age, male sex, low P_{CO_2} during the treatment of HMD, PDA, high peak inspiratory pressure, increased airway resistance in the 1st wk of life, increased pulmonary artery pressure, and possibly a family history of asthma. In some very low birthweight infants without HMD who require mechanical ventilation for apnea or respiratory insufficiency, BPD that does not follow the classic pattern may develop. Vitamin A supplementation (5,000 IU intramuscularly three times per week for 4 wk) in ELBW infants reduces the risk of BPD (1 case prevented for every 14–15 treated).

Severe BPD requires continued mechanical ventilation until weaning from the respirator becomes possible. Acceptable blood gas concentrations for a patient with severe BPD include a P_{CO_2} of 50–70 mm Hg (if pH > 7.30) and a Pa_{O_2} of 55–60 mm Hg with an oxygen saturation of 95% or higher. Lower levels of Pa_{O_2} may exacerbate pulmonary hypertension, produce cor pulmonale, and inhibit growth. Airway obstruction in BPD may be due to mucus and edema production, bronchospasm, and collapse of acquired tracheomalacia. These events may contribute

to "blue spells." Alternatively, blue spells may be due to acute cor pulmonale or myocardial ischemia.

Treatment of BPD includes nutritional support, fluid restriction, drug therapy, maintenance of adequate oxygenation, and prompt treatment of infection. Growth must be monitored because recovery is dependent on the growth of lung tissue and remodeling of the pulmonary vascular bed. Nutritional supplementation to provide added calories (24–30 calories/30 mL formula) and protein (3–3.5 g/kg/24 hr) is needed for growth. Diuretic therapy results in a short-term improvement in lung mechanics and may result in decreased oxygen and ventilatory requirements. Furosemide (1 mg/kg/dose intravenously twice daily [bid] or 2 mg/kg/dose orally bid) given daily or every other day and hydrochlorothiazide alone or in combination with potassium chloride, if needed, or spironolactone are commonly used drugs. Bronchodilators improve lung mechanics by decreasing airway resistance. Both inhaled β_2-adrenergic agents and systemic aminophylline or theophylline (at serum levels of 12–15 mg/L) are used. Adequate oxygenation (pulse oximeter ≥95%) is essential to prevent or treat cor pulmonale and to promote optimal growth and neurodevelopmental outcome. In severe cases, iNO may improve oxygenation. Mortality in infants with BPD ranges from 10–25% and is highest in infants who remain ventilator dependent for over 6 mo. Cardiorespiratory failure (associated with cor pulmonale) and infection (respiratory syncytial virus) are common causes of death.

Postnatal dexamethasone preventive therapy reduces the time to extubation and may decrease the risk of BPD. However, such therapy is associated with substantial short- and long-term risks, including hypertension, hyperglycemia, gastrointestinal bleeding and perforation, hypertrophic cardiomyopathy, sepsis, and poor weight gain and head growth. Survival is not improved, and infants who have been treated with dexamethasone have an apparent increase in neurodevelopmental delay and cerebral palsy. Therefore, the routine use of dexamethasone for the prevention or treatment of BPD is not recommended.

Complications of BPD include growth failure, psychomotor retardation, and parental stress, as well as sequelae of therapy such as nephrolithiasis (from diuretics and total intravenous alimentation), osteopenia, and subglottic stenosis, which may require tracheotomy or an anterior cricoid-split procedure to relieve upper airway obstruction.

Patients with BPD often go home on a regimen of oxygen, diuretics, and bronchodilator therapy. Prevention of sleep-associated hypoxia improves growth, as does hypercaloric formula. The long-term *prognosis* is good for infants who have been weaned from oxygen before discharge from the NICU. Prolonged ventilation, IVH, pulmonary hypertension, cor pulmonale, and oxygen dependence beyond 1 yr of life are poor prognostic signs. Airway obstruction and hyperactivity and hyperinflation may be demonstrated in some adolescents.

Prognosis. Early provision of intensive observation and care of high-risk newborn infants can significantly reduce the morbidity and mortality associated with HMD and other acute neonatal illnesses. Antenatal steroids, postnatal surfactant use, improved modes of ventilation, and supportive NICUs have resulted in low mortality from HMD (≈10%). Mortality increases with decreasing gestational age. Good results depend on the availability of experienced and skilled personnel, specially designed and organized regional hospital units, proper equipment, and lack of complications such as severe asphyxia, intracranial hemorrhage, or irremediable congenital malformation. Surfactant therapy has reduced mortality from HMD approximately 40%; the incidence of BPD has not been measurably affected.

The overall mortality in LBW infants referred to intensive care centers is steadily declining (see Chapter 86.2). Although 85–90% of all infants surviving HMD after requiring ventilatory support with respirators are normal, the outlook is much better for those weighing above 1,500 g. The long-term prognosis for normal pulmonary function in most infants surviving HMD is excellent. However, survivors of severe neonatal respiratory failure may have significant pulmonary and neurodevelopmental impairment.

Ainsworth SB, Beresford MW, Milligan DWA, et al: Pumactant and poractant alfa for treatment of respiratory distress syndrome in neonates born at 25–29 weeks' gestation: A randomized trial. *Lancet* 2000;355:1387.

Aly HZ: Nasal prongs continuous positive airway pressure: A simple yet powerful tool. *Pediatrics* 2001;108:759.

Arlettaz R, Archer N, Wilkinson AR: Closure of the ductus arteriosus and development of pulmonary branch stenosis in babies of less than 32 weeks gestation. *Arch Dis Child* 2001;85:F197–200.

Bancalari E: Changes in the pathogenesis and prevention of chronic lung disease of prematurity. *Am J Perinatol* 2001;18:1.

Bancalari E, del Moral T: Bronchopulmonary dysplasia and surfactant. *Biol Neonate* 2001;80(Suppl 1):7.

Bloom BT, Kattwinkel J, Hall RT, et al: Comparison of Infasurf (calf lung surfactant extract) to Survanta (beractant) in the treatment and prevention of respiratory distress syndrome. *Pediatrics* 1997;100:31.

Bradbury J: Could treatment of neonatal RDS improve further? *Lancet* 2002;360:394.

Cheema IU, Ahluwalia JS: Feasibility of tidal volume–guided ventilation in newborn infants: A randomized, crossover trial using the volume guarantee modality. *Pediatrics* 2001;107:1323.

Clark PL, Ekekezie II, Kafton HA, et al: Safety and efficacy of nitric oxide in chronic lung disease. *Arch Dis Child* 2002;86:F41–5.

Clark RH, Gerstmann DR, Jobe A, et al: Lung injury in neonates: Causes, strategies for prevention, and long-term consequences. *J Pediatr* 2001;139:478.

Clyman RI: Recommendations for the postnatal use of indomethacin: An analysis of four separate treatment strategies. *J Pediatr* 1996;128:601.

Cole FS, Hamvas A, Nogee LM: Genetic disorders of neonatal respiratory function. *Pediatr Res* 2001;50:156.

Gournay V, Savagner C, Thiriez G, et al: Pulmonary hypertension after ibuprofen prophylaxis in very preterm infants. *Lancet* 2002;359:1486.

Greenough A: Update on modalities of mechanical ventilators. *Arch Dis Child* 2002; 87:F3–6.

Greenough A, Milner AD, Dimitriou G: Synchronized mechanical ventilation for respiratory support in newborn infants. *Cochrane Database Syst Rev* 2001;1: CD000456.

Guinn DA, Atkinson MW, Sullivan L, et al: Single vs weekly courses of antenatal corticosteroids for women at risk of preterm delivery. *JAMA* 2001;286:1581.

Halliday HL: Early postnatal dexamethasone and cerebral palsy. *Pediatrics* 2002; 109:1168.

Halliday HL: Elective delivery at "term": Implications for the newborn. *Acta Paediatr* 1999;88:1180.

Halliday HL: Postnatal steroids: A dilemma for the neonatologist. *Acta Paediatr* 2001;90:116–8.

Hamvas A, Nogee LM, Mallory GB Jr, et al: Lung transplantation for treatment of infants with surfactant protein B deficiency. *J Pediatr* 1997;130:231.

Iles R, Edmunds AT: Assessment of pulmonary function in resolving chronic lung disease of prematurity. *Arch Dis Child* 1997;76:F113.

Jobe AH: The new BPD: An arrest of lung development. *Pediatr Res* 1999;46:641.

Jobe AH, Bancalari E: Bronchopulmonary dysplasia: *Am J Respir Crit Care Med* 2001;163:1723.

Kallapur S, Ikegami M: The surfactants. *Am J Perinatol* 2000;17:335.

Kattwinkel J, Bloom BT, Delmore P, et al: High- versus low- threshold surfactant retreatment for neonatal respiratory distress syndrome. *Pediatrics* 2000;106:282.

Klein JM, Thompson MW, Snyder JM, et al: Transient surfactant protein B deficiency in a term infant with severe respiratory failure. *J Pediatr* 1998;132:244.

Kotecha S: Management issues in CLD of prematurity. *Arch Dis Child Fetal Neonatal Ed* 2002;87:F2.

Kotecha S, Allen J: Oxygen therapy for infants with chronic lung disease. *Arch Dis Child Fetal Neonatal Ed* 2002;87:F11-4.

Lago P, Bettiol T, Salvadori S, et al: Safety and efficacy of ibuprofen versus indomethacin in preterm infants treated for patent ductus arteriosus: A randomized controlled trial. *Eur J Pediatr* 2002;161:202–7.

LeFlore JL, Salhab WA, Broyles RS, et al: Association of antenatal and postnatal dexamethasone exposure with outcomes in extremely low birth weight neonates. *Pediatrics* 2002;110:275–9.

McIntosh N: High or low oxygen saturation for the preterm baby. *Arch Dis Child Fetal Neonatal Ed* 2001;84:F149–50.

Nabeel Khalaf M, Brodsky N, Hurley J, et al: A prospective, randomized, controlled trial comparing synchronized nasal intermittent positive pressure ventilation versus nasal continuous positive airway pressure as modes of extubation. *Pediatrics* 2001;108:13.

Nagourney BA, Kramer MS, Klebanoff MA, et al: Recurrent respiratory distress syndrome in successive preterm pregnancies. *J Pediatr* 1996;129:591.

Narayanan M, Cooper B, Weiss H, et al: Prophylactic indomethacin: Factors determining permanent ductus arteriosus closure. *J Pediatr* 2002;136:330.

Nicholl R: Nitric oxide in preterm babies. *Arch Dis Child* 2002;86:59.

Northway WH Jr, Rosan RC, Porter DY: Pulmonary disease following respirator therapy of hyaline-membrane disease. Bronchopulmonary dysplasia. *N Engl J Med* 1976;276:357.

Ogihara T, Hirano K, Morinobu T, et al: KL-6, a mucinous glycoprotein, as an indicator of chronic lung disease of the newborn. *J Pediatr* 2000;137:280.

Overmeire BV, Smets K, Lecoutere D, et al: A comparison of ibuprofen and indomethacin for closure of patent ductus arteriosus. *N Engl J Med* 2000; 343:674.

Postnatal corticosteroids to treat or prevent chronic lung disease in preterm infants. *Pediatrics* 2002;109:330.

Rettwitz-Volk W, Veldman A, Roth B, et al: A prospective, randomized, multicenter trial of high-frequency oscillatory ventilation compared with conventional ventilation in preterm infants with respiratory distress syndrome receiving surfactant. *J Pediatr* 1998;132:249.

Schmidt B, Davis P, Moddemann D, et al: Long-term effects of indomethacin prophylaxis in extremely low birth weight infants. *N Engl J Med* 2001;344:1966.

Seri I, Tan R, Evans J: Cardiovascular effects of hydrocortisone in preterm infants with pressor-resistant hypotension. *Pediatrics* 2001;107:1070.

Singer L, Yamashita T, Lilien L, et al: A longitudinal study of developmental outcome of infants with bronchopulmonary dysplasia and very low birth weight. *Pediatrics* 1997;100:987.

Soll RF, Blanco F: Natural surfactant extract versus synthetic surfactant for neonatal respiratory distress syndrome. *Cochrane Datatabse Syst Rev* 2001;2:CD000144.

Stark AR: High-frequency oscillatory ventilation to prevent bronchopulmonary dysplasia—are we there yet? *N Engl J Med* 2002;347:682.

Stark AR, Carlo WA, Tyson JE, et al: Adverse effects of early dexamethasone treatment in extremely-low-birth-weight infants. *N Engl J Med* 2001;344:95.

Subhedar NV, Hamdan AH, Ryan SW, et al: Pulmonary artery pressure: Early predictor of chronic lung disease in preterm infants. *Arch Dis Child* 1998;78: F20.

Thome UH, Carlo WA: High-frequency ventilation in neonates. *Am J Perinatol* 2000;17:1.

Tyson JE: Does indomethacin prophylaxis benefit extremely low birth weight infants? Results of a placebo-controlled multicenter trial. *Pediatr Res* 2002;51:1.

Tyson JE, Wright LL, Oh W, et al: Vitamin A supplementation for extremely-low-birth-weight infants. *N Engl J Med* 1999;340:1962.

Van Overmeire B, Van de Broek H, Van Laer P, et al: Early versus late indomethacin treatment for patent ductus arteriosus in premature infants with respiratory distress syndrome. *J Pediatr* 2001;138:205.

Watkinson M: Hypertension in the newborn baby. *Arch Dis Child Fetal Neonatal Ed* 2002;86:F78–81.

Watterberg KL: Adrenal insufficiency and cardiac dysfunction in the preterm infant. *Pediatr Res* 2002;51:422.

Watterberg KL, Scott SM, Backstrom C, et al: Links between early adrenal function and respiratory outcome in preterm infants: Airway inflammation and patent ductus arteriosus. *Pediatrics* 2000;105:320.

Yanowitz TD, Yao AC, Werner JC, et al: Effects of prophylactic low-dose indomethacin on hemodynamics in very low birth weight infants. *J Pediatr* 1998;132:28.

90.4 Transient Tachypnea of the Newborn

Transient tachypnea, occasionally called **respiratory distress syndrome type II,** usually follows uneventful normal preterm or term vaginal delivery or cesarean delivery. It may be characterized by the early onset of tachypnea, sometimes with retractions, or expiratory grunting and, occasionally, cyanosis that is relieved by minimal oxygen (<40%). Patients usually recover rapidly within 3 days, although they may rarely appear severely ill and have a more protracted course. The lungs are generally clear without rales or rhonchi, and the chest roentgenogram shows prominent pulmonary vascular markings, fluid lines in the fissures, overaeration, flat diaphragms, and, occasionally, pleural fluid. Hypoxemia, hypercapnia, and acidosis are uncommon. Distinguishing the disease from HMD may be difficult; the distinctive features of transient tachypnea are sudden recovery of the infant and the absence of a roentgenographic reticulogranular pattern or air bronchograms. The syndrome is believed to be secondary to slow absorption of fetal lung fluid resulting in decreased pulmonary compliance and tidal volume and increased dead space.

Avery ME, Gatewood OB, Brumley G: Transient tachypnea of newborn. Possible delayed reabsorption of fluid at birth. *Am J Dis Child* 1966;111:380.

Gross TL, Sokol RJ, Kwong MS, et al: Transient tachypnea of the newborn: The relationship to preterm delivery and significant neonatal morbidity. *Am J Obstet Gynecol* 1983;146:236.

Sundell H, Garrott J, Blankenship WJ, et al: Studies on infants with type II respiratory distress syndrome. *J Pediatr* 1971;78:754.

90.5 Aspiration of Foreign Material (Fetal Aspiration Syndrome, Aspiration Pneumonia)

During prolonged labor and difficult deliveries, infants often initiate vigorous respiratory movements in utero because of interference with the supply of oxygen through the placenta. Under such circumstances, the infant may aspirate amniotic fluid containing vernix caseosa, epithelial cells, meconium, or material from the birth canal, which may block the smallest airways and interfere with alveolar exchange of oxygen and carbon dioxide. Pathogenic bacteria may accompany the aspirated material, and pneumonia may ensue, but even in noninfected cases, respiratory distress accompanied by roentgenographic evidence of aspiration is seen (Fig. 90–6).

Pulmonary aspiration may also occur in newborn infants as a result of tracheoesophageal fistula, esophageal and duodenal obstruction, gastroesophageal reflux, improper feeding practices, and administration of depressant medicines.

The contents of the stomach should be aspirated through a soft catheter just before surgery or other procedures that require anesthesia or significantly disturb an infant. Once aspiration has occurred, treatment consists of general and res-

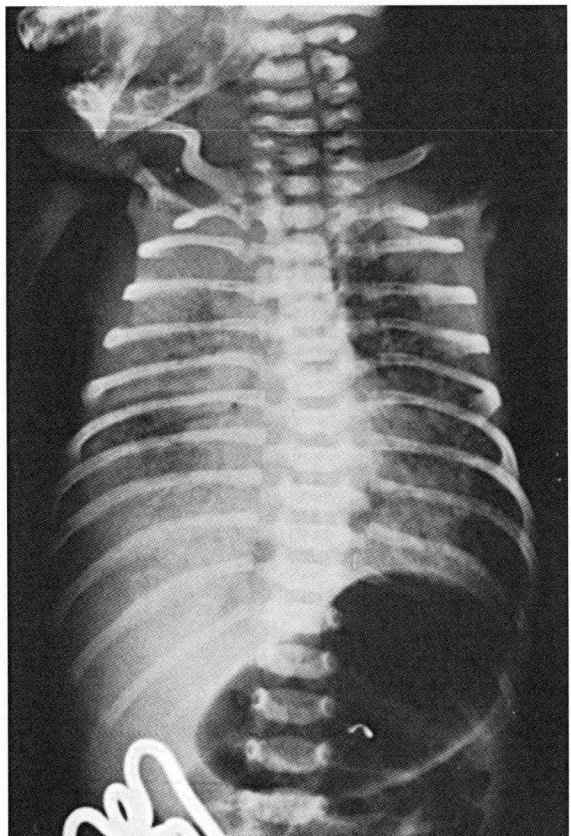

FIGURE 90–6. Fetal aspiration syndrome (aspiration pneumonia). Note the coarsely granular pattern with irregular aeration typical of fetal distress from the aspiration of material contained in amniotic fluid, such as vernix caseosa, epithelial cells, and meconium.

piratory support and treatment of pneumonia (Chapters 90.3 and 380).

Goodwin SR, Graves SA, Haberkern CM: Aspiration in intubated premature infants. *Pediatrics* 1985;75:85.

90.6 Meconium Aspiration

Meconium-stained amniotic fluid is found in 10–15% of births and usually occurs in term or post-term infants. Meconium aspiration pneumonia develops in 5% of such infants; 30% of them require mechanical ventilation, and 3–5% expire. Usually but not invariably, fetal distress and hypoxia occur with passage of meconium into amniotic fluid. These infants are meconium stained and may be depressed and require resuscitation at birth. The pathophysiology is noted in Figure 90–7.

Clinical Manifestations. Either in utero or more often with the first breath, thick, particulate meconium is aspirated into the lungs. The resulting small airway obstruction may produce respiratory distress within the first hours, with tachypnea, retractions, grunting, and cyanosis observed in severely affected infants. Partial obstruction of some airways may lead to pneumothorax or pneumomediastinum, or both. Prompt treatment may delay the onset of respiratory distress, which may consist of only tachypnea without retractions. Overdistention of the chest may be prominent. The condition usually improves within 72 hr, but when its course requires assisted ventilation, it may be severe with a high risk for mortality. Tachypnea may persist for many days or even several weeks. The typical chest roentgenogram is

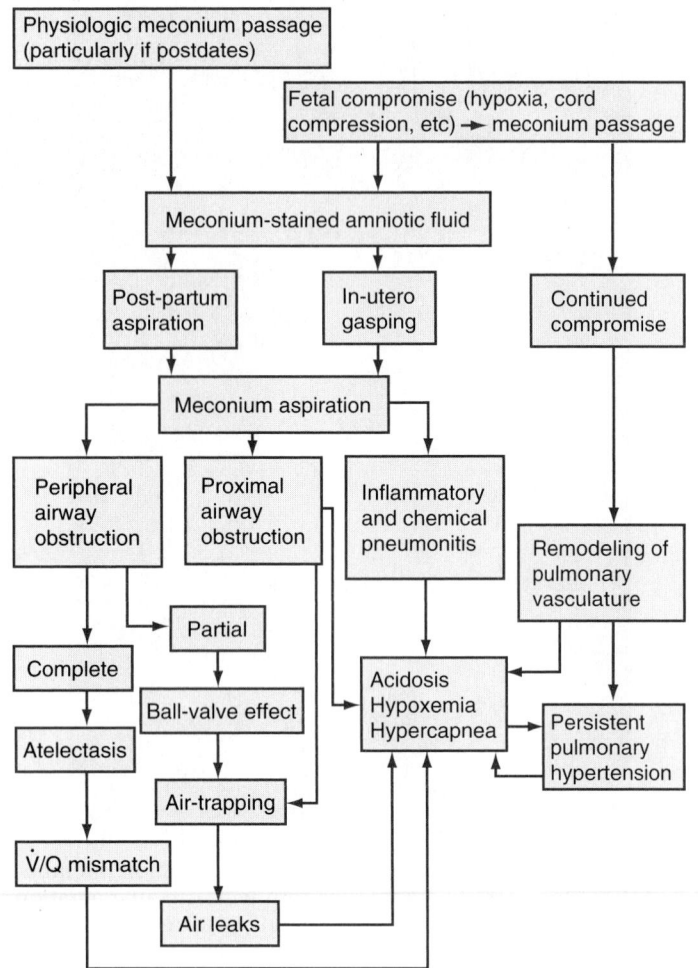

FIGURE 90–7. Pathophysiology of meconium passage and the meconium aspiration syndrome. (From Wiswell TE, Bent RC: Meconium staining and the meconium aspiration syndrome. *Pediatr Clin North Am* 1993;40:955.)

characterized by patchy infiltrates, coarse streaking of both lung fields, increased anteroposterior diameter, and flattening of the diaphragm. A normal chest roentgenogram in an infant with severe hypoxia and no cardiac malformation suggests the diagnosis of pulmonary hypertension (Chapter 90.7). Arterial Po_2 may be low in either disease, and if hypoxia has occurred, metabolic acidosis is usually present.

Prevention. The risk of meconium aspiration may be decreased by paying careful attention to fetal distress and initiating prompt delivery in the presence of fetal acidosis, late decelerations, or poor beat-to-beat variability. Amnio-infusion in cases of meconium-stained fluid lowers the rate of cesarean section and improves neonatal outcome. Immediate DeLee suctioning of the oropharynx after the head is delivered reduces the incidence of meconium aspiration.

Treatment. Routine intubation to aspirate the lungs of vigorous infants born through meconium-stained fluid is not recommended. Depressed infants (those with hypotonia, bradycardia, fetal acidosis, or apnea) should undergo endotracheal intubation, and suction should be applied directly to the endotracheal tube to remove meconium from the airway. The risk associated with laryngoscopy and endotracheal intubation (bradycardia, laryngospasm, hypoxia, posterior pharyngeal laceration with pseudodiverticulum formation) is less than the risk of meconium aspiration syndrome in these severe circumstances.

Treatment of meconium aspiration pneumonia includes supportive care and standard management for respiratory distress. The oxygenation benefit of PEEP must be weighed against the risk of pneumothorax. Severe meconium aspiration may be complicated by persistent pulmonary hypertension and requires similar treatment. Patients who are refractory to conventional mechanical ventilation or HFV may benefit from surfactant therapy (regardless of gestational age), iNO, or extracorporeal membrane oxygenation (ECMO) (see Chapter 90.7).

Prognosis. The mortality rate of meconium-stained infants is considerably higher than that of non-stained infants; meconium aspiration used to account for a significant proportion of neonatal deaths. Residual lung problems are rare but include symptomatic cough, wheezing, and persistent hyperinflation for up to 5–10 yr. The ultimate prognosis depends on the extent of CNS injury from asphyxia and the presence of associated problems such as pulmonary hypertension.

Dargaville PA, South M, McDougall PN: Surfactant and surfactant inhibitors in meconium aspiration syndrome. *J Pediatr* 2001;138:113.
Findlay RD, Taeusch HW, Walther FJ: Surfactant replacement therapy for meconium aspiration syndrome. *Pediatrics* 1996;97:48.
Gregory GA, Gooding CA, Phibbs RH, et al: Meconium aspiration infants; a prospective study. *J Pediatr* 1974;85:848.
Halliday HL: Endotracheal intubation at birth for preventing morbidity and mortality in vigorous, meconium-stained infants born at term. *Cochrane Database Syst Rev* 2001;1:CD000500.
Pierce J, Gaudier FL, Sanchez-Ramos L: Intrapartum amnioinfusion for meconium-stained fluid: Meta-analysis of prospective clinical trials. *Obstet Gynecol* 2000;95:1051.
Ramin KD, Leveno KJ, Kelly MA, et al: Amniotic fluid meconium: A fetal environmental hazard. *Obstet Gynecol* 1996;87:181.
Wiswell TE: Advances in the treatment of the meconium aspiration syndrome. *Acta Paediatr Suppl* 2001;436:28.
Wiswell TE, Gannon CM, Jacob J, et al: Delivery room management of the apparently vigorous meconium-stained neonate: Results of the multicenter, International Collaborative Trial. *Pediatrics* 2000;105:1.
Wiswell TE, Knight GR, Finer NN, et al: A multicenter, randomized, controlled trial comparing Surfaxin (lucinactant) lavage with standard care for treatment of meconium aspiration syndrome. *Pediatrics* 2002;109:1081.

90.7 Persistent Pulmonary Hypertension of the Newborn (Persistent Fetal Circulation)

PPHN occurs in term and post-term infants. Predisposing factors include birth asphyxia, meconium aspiration pneumonia, early-onset sepsis, HMD, hypoglycemia, polycythemia, maternal use of nonsteroidal anti-inflammatory drugs with in utero constriction of the ductus arteriosus, and pulmonary hypoplasia as a result of diaphragmatic hernia, amniotic fluid leak, oligohydramnios, or pleural effusions. PPHN is often idiopathic. Some patients with PPHN have low plasma arginine and nitric oxide metabolite concentrations and polymorphisms of the carbamoyl phosphate synthase gene, findings suggestive of a possible subtle defect in nitric oxide production. The incidence is 1/500–1,500 live births with a wide variation between different clinical centers.

Pathophysiology. Persistence of the fetal circulatory pattern of right-to-left shunting through the PDA and foramen ovale after birth is due to excessively high pulmonary vascular resistance. Fetal pulmonary vascular resistance is usually elevated relative to fetal systemic or postnatal pulmonary pressure. This fetal state permits shunting of oxygenated umbilical venous blood to the left atrium (and brain) through the foramen ovale and bypasses the lungs through the ductus arteriosus to the descending aorta. After birth, pulmonary vascular resistance normally declines rapidly as a consequence of vasodilation secondary to gas filling the lungs, a rise in postnatal Pao_2, a reduction in Pco_2, increased pH, and release of vasoactive substances. Increased neonatal pulmonary vascular resistance may (1) be maladaptive from an acute injury (e.g., not demonstrating normal vasodilation in response to increased oxygen and other changes after birth); (2) be the result of increased pulmonary artery medial muscle thickness and extension of smooth muscle layers into the usually nonmuscular, more peripheral pulmonary arterioles in response to chronic fetal hypoxia; (3) be due to pulmonary hypoplasia (diaphragmatic hernia, Potter syndrome); (4) be obstructive as a result of polycythemia or total anomalous pulmonary venous return; or (5) be due to alveolar capillary dysplasia, a lethal, possibly familial disorder characterized by a thickened alveolar septum and a reduced number of small pulmonary arteries and capillaries. Apart from the etiology, profound hypoxia from right-to-left shunting and normal or elevated Pco_2 are present.

Clinical Manifestations. Infants become ill in the delivery room or within the first 12 hr of life. PPHN related to polycythemia, idiopathic causes, hypoglycemia, or asphyxia may result in severe cyanosis with tachypnea, although initially, signs of respiratory distress may be minimal. Infants who have PPHN associated with meconium aspiration, group B streptococcal pneumonia, diaphragmatic hernia, or pulmonary hypoplasia usually exhibit cyanosis, grunting, flaring, retractions, tachycardia, and shock. Multiorgan involvement may be present (see Table 88–1). Myocardial ischemia, papillary muscle dysfunction with mitral and tricuspid regurgitation, and cardiac stunning produce cardiogenic shock with decreased pulmonary blood flow, tissue perfusion, and oxygen delivery. *The hypoxia is quite labile and often out of proportion to the findings on chest roentgenograms.*

Diagnosis. PPHN should be suspected in all term infants who have cyanosis with or without fetal distress, intrauterine growth restriction, meconium-stained amniotic fluid, hypoglycemia, polycythemia, diaphragmatic hernia, pleural effusions, and birth asphyxia. Hypoxia is universal and is unresponsive to 100% oxygen given by oxygen hood, but it may respond transiently to hyperoxic hyperventilation administered after endotracheal intubation or to the application of a bag and mask. A Pao_2 gradient between a preductal (right radial artery) and a postductal (umbilical artery) site of blood sampling greater than 20 mm Hg suggests right-to-left shunting through the ductus arteriosus. Real-time echocardiography combined with Doppler flow studies demonstrates right-to-left shunting across a patent foramen ovale and a ductus arteriosus. Deviation of the intraatrial septum into the left atrium is seen in severe PPHN. Tricuspid or mitral insufficiency may be noted on auscultation as a holosystolic murmur and can be visualized echocardiographically together with poor contractility when PPHN is associated with myocardial ischemia. The degree of tricuspid regurgitation can be used to estimate pulmonary artery pressure. The 2nd heart sound is accentuated and not split. In asphyxia-associated and idiopathic PPHN, the chest roentgenogram is normal, whereas in PPHN associated with pneumonia and diaphragmatic hernia, it shows the specific lesions of parenchymal opacification and bowel in the chest, respectively. The *differential diagnosis* of PPHN includes cyanotic heart disease (especially obstructed total anomalous pulmonary venous return) and the associated etiologic entities that predispose to PPHN (e.g., hypoglycemia, polycythemia, sepsis).

Treatment. Therapy is directed toward correcting any predisposing disease (hypoglycemia, polycythemia) and improving poor tissue oxygenation. The response to therapy is often unpredictable, transient, and complicated by the adverse effects of drugs or mechanical ventilation. Initial management includes oxygen administration and correction of acidosis, hypotension, and hypercapnia. Persistent hypoxia should be managed with intubation and mechanical ventilation.

The optimal approach to treatment is unclear and variable. One approach to the treatment of severe PPHN consists of insti-

tuting mechanical ventilation with or without pancuronium paralysis; ventilator settings are initially selected to achieve a Pao_2 of 50–70 mm Hg and a Pco_2 of 50–55 mm Hg. Tolazoline (1 mg/kg), a nonselective α-adrenergic antagonist, is sometimes used as an adjunct to nonselectively vasodilate the pulmonary arterial system, but it also results in systemic hypotension, which is treated with volume expansion and dopamine. In another approach to treating severe PPHN, hyperventilation is used to reduce pulmonary vasoconstriction by lowering the Pco_2 (≈25 mm Hg) and increasing the pH (7.50–7.55). Such management requires high peak inspiratory pressures and rapid respiratory rates, often necessitating the use of pancuronium paralysis for control of ventilation to achieve a Pao_2 between 90 and 100 mm Hg. Complications of hyperventilation include hyperinflation with reduced elimination of carbon dioxide, reduced cardiac output, barotrauma, pneumothorax, decreased cerebral blood flow, increased fluid requirements, and edema resulting from paralysis. Alkalinization with sodium bicarbonate also has been used to elevate plasma pH to induce pulmonary arterial vasodilation. Both methods of mechanical ventilation may be successful, and specific indications for one or the other have not been defined. Patients not responding to conventional ventilation may later respond to hyperventilation or HFV. Cardiogenic shock should be treated with inotropic agents such as dopamine and dobutamine.

Exogenous surfactant therapy has been beneficial in some patients. iNO, a potent and selective pulmonary vasodilator (equivalent to endothelium-derived relaxation factor), when given at an initial dose of 1–20 ppm, has improved oxygenation in patients with PPHN and reduced the need for ECMO. Although brief exposure to higher doses (40–80 ppm) appears to be safe, long-term treatment with 80 ppm increases the adverse effects. Responses to iNO include no improvement; initial improvement but not sustained, with ECMO being required; initial and sustained improvement, usually weaned by the 5th day of therapy; and an initial response but prolonged dependency, possibly as a result of pulmonary hypoplasia or alveolar capillary dysplasia. Methemoglobinemia is a rare but possible complication of iNO. The maximal safe duration of iNO therapy is unknown.

EXTRACORPOREAL MEMBRANE OXYGENATION. In 5–10% of patients with PPHN (approximately 1/4,000 births), the response to 100% oxygen, mechanical ventilation, and drugs is poor. In such patients, the alveolar-arterial oxygen gradient (roughly at sea level, [760 - 47] - $Paco_2$ - Pao_2) or the oxygenation index (OI) has been used to predict mortality rates greater than 80%.

$$OI = (Mean\ airway\ pressure \times Fio_2 \times 100) \div Postductal\ Pao_2$$

Alveolar-arterial gradients greater than 620 for 8–12 hr and an OI over 40 that is unresponsive to nitric oxide inhalation predict a high mortality rate and are indications for ECMO. ECMO has also been used to treat carefully selected, severely ill infants with hypoxemic respiratory failure caused by HMD, meconium aspiration pneumonia, congenital diaphragmatic hernia, PPHN, or sepsis.

ECMO is a form of cardiopulmonary bypass that augments systemic perfusion and provides gas exchange. Most experience has been with venoarterial bypass, which requires the placement of large catheters in the right internal jugular vein and carotid artery and, possibly, carotid artery ligation. If the artery is ligated, it should be repaired after stopping ECMO. Venovenous bypass avoids this ligation and provides gas exchange, but it does not support cardiac output. Blood is initially pumped through the ECMO circuit at a rate that approximates 80% of the estimated cardiac output of 150–200 mL/kg/min. Venous return passes through a membrane oxygenator, is warmed, and returns to the aortic arch. Venous oxygen saturation values are used to monitor tissue oxygen delivery and subsequent extraction. The rate of ECMO flow is adjusted to achieve satisfactory venous oxygen saturation (>65%) and cardiovascular stability. When ECMO is started in an infant, the existing ventilator support is weaned to room air at a low rate and pressure to reduce the risk of oxygen toxicity and barotrauma, thus permitting time for the lungs to rest and heal.

Because ECMO requires complete heparinization to prevent clotting in the circuit, patients with or at risk for IVH (weight <2 kg, age <35 wk gestation) are not candidates for this therapy. In addition, infants for whom ECMO is being considered should have reversible lung disease, no signs of systemic bleeding, and an absence of severe asphyxia or lethal malformations, and they should have been ventilated for less than 7–10 days. Complications of ECMO include thromboembolism, air embolization, bleeding, stroke, seizures, atelectasis, cholestatic jaundice, thrombocytopenia, neutropenia, hemolysis, infectious complications of blood transfusions, edema formation, and systemic hypertension.

Prognosis. Survival in patients with PPHN varies with the underlying diagnosis. The long-term outcome for infants with PPHN is related to the associated hypoxic-ischemic encephalopathy and the ability to reduce pulmonary vascular resistance. The long-term prognosis for infants who have PPHN and who survive after treatment with hyperventilation is comparable to that for infants who have underlying illnesses of equivalent severity (e.g., birth asphyxia, hypoglycemia, polycythemia). The outcome for infants who have PPHN treated with ECMO is also favorable; 85–90% survive, and 60–75% of survivors appear normal at 1–3.5 yr of age. Infants who have a diaphragmatic hernia associated with severe PPHN fare poorly if the pre-surgery and post-surgery Pco_2 exceeds 40 mm Hg despite mechanical ventilation. Such patients may respond to ECMO; rarely, it is not possible to wean them from bypass, or they expire after ECMO has been discontinued. Lung transplantation may benefit these infants.

Alano MA, Ngougmna E, Ostrea EM Jr, et al: Analysis of nonsteroidal antiinflammatory drugs in meconium and its relation to persistent pulmonary hypertension of the newborn. *Pediatrics* 2001;107:519.

Bennett CC, Johnson A, Field DJ, et al: UK collaborative randomized trial of neonatal extracorporeal membrane oxygenation: Follow-up to age 4 years. *Lancet* 2001;357:1094.

Clark RH, Kueser TJ, Walker MW, et al: Low-dose nitric oxide therapy for persistent pulmonary hypertension of the newborn. *N Engl J Med* 2000;342:469.

Finer NN, Sun JW, Rich W, et al: Randomized, prospective study of low-dose verus high-dose inhaled nitric oxide in the neonate with hypoxic respiratory failure. *Pediatrics* 2001;108:949.

Gill BS, Neville HL, Khan AM, et al: Delayed institution of extracorporeal membrane oxygenation is associated with increased mortality rate and prolonged hospital stay. *J Pediatr Surg* 2002;37:7.

Hoffman GM, Ross GA, Day SE, et al: Inhaled nitric oxide reduces the utilization of extracorporeal membrane oxygenation in persistent pulmonary hypertension of the newborn. *Crit Care Med* 1997;25:352.

Inhaled nitric oxide in full-term and nearly full-term infants with hypoxic respiratory failure. The Neonatal Inhaled Nitric Oxide Study Group. *N Engl J Med* 1997;336:597.

Inhaled nitric oxide in term and near-term infants: Neurodevelopmental follow-up. The Neonatal Inhaled Nitric Oxide Study Group (NINOS). *J Pediatr* 2000;136:611.

Kinsella JP, Abman SH: Clinical approach to inhaled nitric oxide therapy in the newborn with hypoxemia. *J Pediatr* 2000;136:717.

Lotze A, Mitchell BR, Bulas DI, et al: Multicenter study of surfactant (beractant) use in the treatment of term infants with severe respiratory failure. *Pediatrics* 1998;132:40.

Nakajima W, Ishida A, Arai H, et al: Methaemoglobinaemia after inhalation of nitric oxide in infants with pulmonary hypertension. *Lancet* 1997;350:1002.

Pearson DL, Dawling S, Walsh WF, et al: Neonatal pulmonary hypertension: Urea cycle intermediates, nitric oxide production, and carbamoyl-phosphate synthetase function. *N Engl J Med* 2001;344:1832.

Roy BJ, Rycus P, Conrad SA, et al: The changing demographics of neonatal extracorporeal membrane oxygenation patients reported to the extracorporeal life support organization (ELSO) registry. *Pediatrics* 2000;106:1334.

Walsh-Sukys MC, Tyson JE, Wright LL, et al: Persistent pulmonary hypertension of the newborn in the era before nitric oxide: Practice variation and outcomes. *Pediatrics* 2000;105:14.

90.8 Extrapulmonary Extravasation of Air (Pneumothorax, Pneumomediastinum, Pulmonary Interstitial Emphysema)

Asymptomatic pneumothorax, usually unilateral, is estimated to occur in 1–2% of all newborn infants; symptomatic pneumothorax and pneumomediastinum are less common. Pneumothorax occurs more frequently in males than in females and in term and post-term infants than in premature ones. The incidence is increased in infants with lung disease such as meconium aspiration and HMD; in those who have had vigorous resuscitation or are receiving assisted ventilation, especially if high inspiratory pressure or a continuous elevation of end-expiratory pressure is used; and in infants with urinary tract anomalies.

Etiology and Pathophysiology. The most common cause of pneumothorax is overinflation resulting in alveolar rupture. It may be "spontaneous" and idiopathic or be due to underlying pulmonary disease such as lobar emphysema or rupture of a congenital or pneumonic cyst, to trauma, or to a "ball-valve" type of bronchial or bronchiolar obstruction resulting from aspiration. Air leaks occur during the 1st 24–36 hr in infants with meconium aspiration pneumonia and in infants with HMD when lung compliance is reduced, and later during the recovery phase of HMD if inspiratory pressure and PEEP are not reduced simultaneously with improved respiratory function.

Pneumothorax associated with pulmonary hypoplasia is common, occurs on the 1st day of life, and is due to reduced alveolar surface area and poorly compliant lungs. It is associated with disorders of decreased amniotic fluid volume (Potter syndrome; renal agenesis, renal dysplasia, chronic amniotic fluid leak), decreased fetal breathing movement (oligohydramnios, neuromuscular disease), pulmonary space-occupying lesions (diaphragmatic hernia, pleural effusion, chylothorax), and thoracic abnormalities (asphyxiating thoracic dystrophies).

Air from a ruptured alveolus escapes into the interstitial spaces of the lung, where it may cause *interstitial emphysema* or dissect along the peribronchial and perivascular connective tissue sheaths to the root of the lung. If the volume of escaped air is great enough, it may follow the vascular sheaths and cause mediastinal emphysema or a rupture with subsequent pneumomediastinum, pneumothorax, and subcutaneous emphysema. Rarely, increased mediastinal pressure may compress the pulmonary veins at the hilum and thereby interfere with venous return to the heart and cardiac output. On occasion, air may embolize into the circulation and produce cutaneous blanching, air in intravascular catheters, an air-filled heart on chest roentgenograms, and death.

Tension pneumothorax occurs if an accumulation of air within the pleural space is sufficient to elevate intrapleural pressure above atmospheric pressure. Unilateral tension pneumothorax results in impaired ventilation not only in the collapsed lung but also in the normal lung by a mediastinal shift to the other side. Compression of the vena cava and torsion of the great vessels may interfere with venous return.

Clinical Manifestations. The physical findings of clinically *asymptomatic pneumothorax* are hyperresonance and diminished breath sounds over the involved side of the chest with or without tachypnea.

Symptomatic pneumothorax is characterized by respiratory distress, which varies from only an increased respiratory rate to severe dyspnea, tachypnea, and cyanosis. Irritability and restlessness or apnea may be the earliest signs. The onset is usually sudden but may be gradual; an infant may rapidly become critically ill. The chest may appear asymmetric with an increased anteroposterior diameter and bulging of the intercostal spaces on the affected side, and hyperresonance and diminished or absent breath sounds may be present. The heart is displaced toward the unaffected side, and the diaphragm is displaced downward, as is the liver with right-sided pneumothorax. Because pneumothoraces may be bilateral in approximately 10% of patients, symmetry of findings does not rule out pneumothorax. In tension pneumothorax, signs of shock may be noted, and the apex of the heart is pushed away from the affected side.

Pneumomediastinum occurs in at least 25% of patients with pneumothorax and is usually asymptomatic. The degree of respiratory distress depends on the amount of trapped air. If it is great, bulging of the mid-thoracic area is observed, the neck veins are distended, and blood pressure is low. The last two findings are a result of blockage of the circulation by compression of the systemic and pulmonary veins. Although few clinical signs may exist, subcutaneous emphysema in newborn infants is almost pathognomonic of pneumomediastinum.

Pulmonary interstitial emphysema (PIE) may precede the development of a pneumothorax or may occur independently and result in increasing respiratory distress as a result of decreased compliance, hypercapnia, and hypoxia. The latter is due to an increased alveolar-arterial oxygen gradient and intrapulmonary shunting. Progressive enlargement of blebs or air may result in cystic dilatation and respiratory deterioration resembling pneumothorax. In severe cases, PIE precedes the development of BPD. Avoidance of high inspiratory or mean ventilatory pressure may prevent the development of PIE. Treatment may include bronchoscopy in patients with evidence of mucus plugging, selective intubation and ventilation of the uninvolved bronchus, oxygen, general respiratory care, and HFV.

Diagnosis. Pneumothorax and pneumomediastinum should be suspected in any newborn infant who shows signs of respiratory distress or who is restless or irritable or has a sudden change in condition. The diagnosis of pneumothorax is established roentgenographically, with the edge of the collapsed lung standing out in relief against the pneumothorax (see Fig. 405–1), and pneumomediastinum is diagnosed by hyperlucency around the heart border and between the sternum and the heart border (Fig. 90–8). Transillumination of the thorax is often helpful in the emergency diagnosis of pneumothorax; the affected side transmits excessive light. Associated renal anomalies are identified by ultrasonography. Pulmonary hypoplasia is suggested by signs of uterine compression (extremity contractures), a small thorax on chest roentgenograms, severe hypoxia with hypercapnia, and signs of the primary disease (hypotonia, diaphragmatic hernia, Potter syndrome).

Pneumopericardium may be asymptomatic and require only general supportive treatment, but it is usually manifested as sudden shock with tachycardia, muffled heart sounds, and poor pulses suggesting tamponade, which requires prompt evacuation of entrapped air. **Pneumoperitoneum** from air dissecting through the diaphragmatic apertures during mechanical ventilation may also be confused with intestinal perforation.

Treatment. Without a continued air leak, asymptomatic and mildly symptomatic small pneumothoraces require only close observation. Frequent small feedings may prevent gastric dilatation and minimize crying, which can further compromise ventilation and worsen the pneumothorax. Breathing 100% oxygen accelerates the resorption of free pleural air into blood by reducing the nitrogen tension in blood and producing a resultant nitrogen pressure gradient from the trapped air in the blood, but the benefit must be weighed against the risks of oxygen toxicity. With severe respiratory or circulatory embarrassment, emergency needle aspiration is indicated. Either immediately or after needle aspiration, a chest tube should be inserted and attached to underwater seal drainage. Severe localized interstitial emphysema may respond to selective bronchial intubation. Judicious use of pancuronium (Pavulon) in infants fighting the ventilator may reduce the incidence of pneumothorax. Surfactant therapy for RDS reduces the incidence of pneumothorax.

Primhak RA: Factors associated with pulmonary air leak in premature infants receiving mechanical ventilation. *J Pediatr* 1983;102:764.

Ryan CA, Barrington KJ, Phillips HJ, et al: Contralateral pneumothoraces in the newborn: Incidence and predisposing factors. *Pediatrics* 1987;79:417.

Watkinson M, Tiron I: Events before the diagnosis of a pneumothorax in ventilated neonates. *Arch Dis Child Fetal Neonatal Ed* 2001;85:F201–3.

90.9 Pulmonary Hemorrhage

Pulmonary hemorrhage is a rare, but catastrophic complication with a high risk of morbidity and mortality. Massive pulmonary hemorrhage is present in 15% of neonates who come to autopsy in the 1st 2 wk of life. The reported incidence at autopsy varies

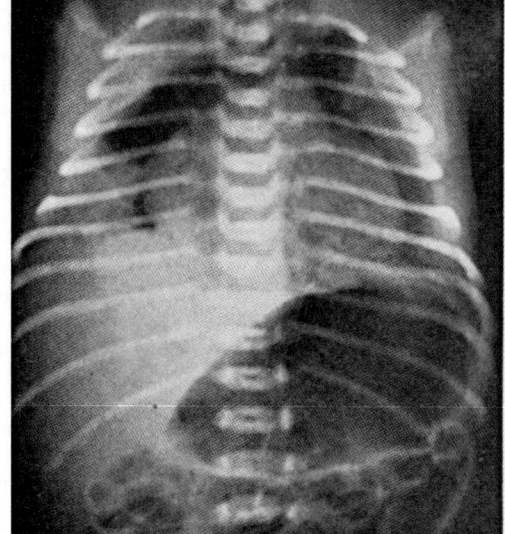
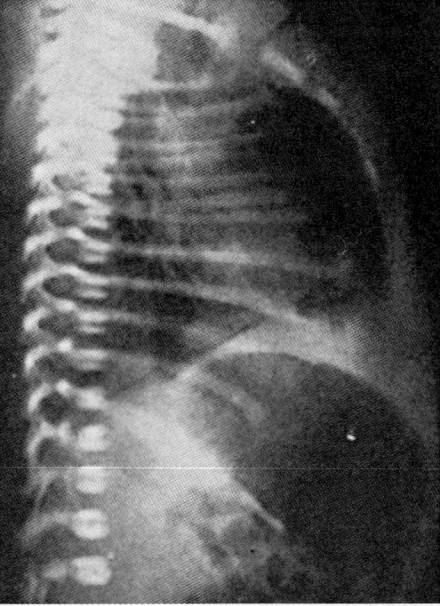

FIGURE 90–8. Pneumomediastinum in a newborn infant. The anteroposterior view demonstrates compression of the lungs, and the lateral view shows bulging of the sternum, each resulting from distention of the mediastinum by trapped air.

from 1 to 4/1,000 live births. About three fourths of patients weigh less than 2,500 g at birth.

Most infants in whom pulmonary hemorrhage is demonstrated at autopsy have had symptoms of respiratory distress that are indistinguishable from those of HMD. The onset may occur at birth or may be delayed several days. Hemorrhagic pulmonary edema is the source of blood in many cases and is associated with significant ductal shunting and high pulmonary blood flow. In severe cases, cardiovascular collapse, poor lung compliance, profound cyanosis, and hypercapnia may be present. Roentgenographic findings are varied and nonspecific and range from minor streaking or patchy infiltrates to massive consolidation.

The incidence of pulmonary hemorrhage is increased in association with acute pulmonary infection, severe asphyxia, HMD, surfactant therapy, assisted ventilation, PDA, congenital heart disease, erythroblastosis fetalis, hemorrhagic disease of the newborn, thrombocytopenia, inborn errors of ammonia metabolism, and cold injury. Although in the majority of instances bleeding into other organs is observed at autopsy, bleeding other than through the nostrils and mouth and intraventricular bleeding are relatively rare during life and should suggest the possibility of an additional bleeding diathesis such as disseminated intravascular coagulation. Bleeding is predominantly alveolar in about two thirds of cases and interstitial in the rest. In some infants, the pulmonary hemorrhage represents hemorrhagic pulmonary edema secondary to severe left-sided heart failure resulting from hypoxia.

The little available information that describes the prognosis of infants who bleed through the mouth or nostrils suggests that it is extremely poor. Death occurs in the 1st 48 hr of life in two thirds of infants who come to autopsy. Treatment includes blood replacement, PEEP, suctioning to clear the airway, intratracheal administration of epinephrine, and in some cases, HFV.

Acute pulmonary hemorrhage may also rarely occur in postneonatal full-term infants. The cause is unknown. These infants have acute respiratory distress with bilateral alveolar infiltrates and usually respond to intensive supportive treatment (see Chapter 388).

Berger TM, Allred EN, Van Marter LJ: Antecedents of clinically significant pulmonary hemorrhage among newborn infants. *J Perinatol* 2000;20:295.

Centers for Disease Control and Prevention: Acute pulmonary hemorrhage among infants—Chicago, April 1992–November 1994. *MMWR Morb Mortal Wkly Rep* 1995;44:67.

Cole VA, Norman ICS, Reynolds EOR, et al: Pathogenesis of hemorrhagic pulmonary edema and massive pulmonary hemorrhage in the newborn. *Pediatrics* 1973;51:175.

Kluckow M, Evans N: Ductal shunting, high pulmonary blood flow, and pulmonary hemorrhage. *J Pediatr* 2000;137:68.

Pappin A, Shenker N, Hack M, et al: Extensive intra-alveolar pulmonary hemorrhage in infants dying after surfactant therapy. *J Pediatr* 1994;124:621.

Chapter 91
Digestive System Disorders

Barbara J. Stoll and Robert M. Kliegman

Vomiting. Vomiting or, more often, regurgitation is a relatively frequent symptom during the neonatal period. In the first few hours after birth, infants may vomit mucus, occasionally blood streaked. This vomiting rarely persists after the first few feedings; it may be due to irritation of the gastric mucosa by material swallowed during delivery. If the vomiting is protracted, gastric lavage with physiologic saline solution may relieve it.

When vomiting occurs shortly after birth and is persistent, the possibilities of intestinal obstruction, metabolic disorders, and increased intracranial pressure must be considered. A history of maternal hydramnios suggests upper gastrointestinal (esophageal, duodenal, ileal) atresia. *Bile-stained emesis* suggests intestinal obstruction beyond the duodenum, but it may also be idiopathic. Abdominal roentgenograms (kidney-ureter-bladder and cross-table lateral views) should be performed in neonates with persistent emesis and in all infants with bile-stained emesis to detect air-fluid levels, distended bowel loops, characteristic patterns of obstruction (double bubble: duodenal atresia), and pneumoperitoneum (intestinal perforation). A barium swallow roentgenogram with small bowel follow-through is indicated in the presence of bilious emesis.

Obstructive lesions of the digestive tract are the most frequent gastrointestinal anomalies (see Chapters 300, 310, 311 and 313). Vomiting from esophageal obstruction occurs with the 1st feeding. The diagnosis of esophageal atresia can be suspected if unusual drooling from the mouth is observed and if resistance is encountered during an attempt to pass a catheter into the stomach. The diagnosis should be made before the infant chokes on oral feedings and is at risk for aspiration pneumonia. Infantile achalasia (cardiospasm), a rare cause of vomiting in newborn infants, is demonstrable roentgenographically by obstruction at the cardiac end of the esophagus without organic stenosis. Regurgitation of feedings because of continuous relaxation of the esophageal-gastric sphincter, or chalasia, is a cause of vomiting. Keeping the infant in a semi-upright position, thickening the feeding, or administering prokinetic drugs can control it.

Vomiting because of *obstruction of the small intestine* usually begins on the 1st day of life and is frequent, persistent, usually non-projectile, copious, and unless the obstruction is above the ampulla of Vater, bile stained; it is associated with abdominal distention, visible deep peristaltic waves, and reduced or absent bowel movements. Malrotation with obstruction from midgut volvulus is an acute emergency that must be considered. Upright roentgenographic films of the abdomen show the distribution of air in the intestine and often aid in locating the site of the obstruction; malrotation will be identified by contrast studies. Normally, air can be demonstrated roentgenographically in the jejunum by 15–60 min, in the ileum by 2–3 hr, and in the colon by 3 hr after birth. Absence of rectal gas at 24 hr is abnormal. Persistent vomiting may occur with congenital diaphragmatic hernia. The vomiting associated with pyloric stenosis may begin any time after birth but does not assume its characteristic pattern before the 2nd–3rd wk. Vomiting with obstipation is a common early sign of Hirschsprung disease. Vomiting may occur with many other disturbances that do not obstruct the digestive tract, such as milk allergy, adrenal hyperplasia of the salt-losing variety, galactosemia, hyperammonemia, organic acidemias, increased intracranial pressure, septicemia, meningitis, and urinary tract infection. In the majority of instances, it is simply regurgitation from overfeeding or from failure to permit the infant to eructate swallowed air. (See Chapter 304 for a discussion of gastric emptying and gastroesophageal reflux.)

Thrush (Oral Candidiasis). Thrush of the mouth occurs in healthy infants. Transmission of fungi from maternal vaginal moniliasis to the infant's oral mucosa is the primary means of infection in healthy newborns. Secondary cases may develop in the hospital nursery as a result of direct or indirect contact with infected infants, caretakers, or contaminated supplies. In an otherwise healthy infant, oral thrush is usually a self-limited infection, but treatment is advised, especially in the presence of candidal diaper rash (Chapter 215.1).

Later in infancy, oral thrush is rare except in debilitated infants, in those receiving antibiotic or immunosuppressive therapy, and in those with AIDS. Infants with AIDS also manifest failure to thrive, psychomotor retardation, hepatosplenomegaly, diarrhea, lymphadenopathy, and hypergammaglobulinemia (see Chapter 254).

Diarrhea. See Chapters 48.1, 48.2, 321, and 322.

Constipation. More than 90% of full-term newborn infants pass meconium within the 1st 24 hr. The possibility of intestinal obstruction should be considered in any infant who does not pass meconium by 24–36 hr. Intestinal atresia, stricture, or stenosis, congenital aganglionic megacolon, milk bolus obstruction, meconium ileus, or meconium plugs may be manifested as constipation. About 20% of very low birthweight (VLBW) infants do not pass meconium within the 1st 24 hr. Constipation not present from birth but appearing during the 1st mo of life suggests short-segment congenital aganglionic megacolon, hypothyroidism, strictures after necrotizing enterocolitis (NEC), or anal stenosis. It must be kept in mind that infrequent bowel movements do not necessarily mean constipation. A breast-fed infant usually has frequent bowel movements, whereas a formula-fed infant may have one to two movements a day or every other day.

Meconium Plugs. Lower colonic or anorectal plugs (Fig. 91–1) with a lower than normal water content may cause intestinal obstruction. Rarely, a firm mass of meconium may form elsewhere in the intestine and cause intrauterine intestinal obstruction and meconium peritonitis unrelated to cystic fibrosis (CF). Anorectal plugs may also cause intestinal ulceration and perforation. Meconium plugs are associated with small left colon syndrome in infants of diabetic mothers and with CF, rectal aganglionosis, maternal drug abuse, and magnesium sulfate therapy for preeclampsia. The plug may be evacuated by irrigating it with isotonic sodium chloride solution. Enemas with the iodinated contrast medium Gastrografin usually induce passage of the plug, presumably because the high osmolarity (1,900 mOsm/L) of the medium draws fluid rapidly into the intestinal lumen and loosens inspissated material. Such rapid loss of fluid into the bowel may result in acute dehydration and shock, so it is advisable to dilute the contrast material with an equal amount of water, correct any existing dehydration, and provide intravenous fluids during and for several hours after the procedure. *After removal of a meconium plug, the infant should be observed closely for the possible presence of congenital aganglionic megacolon.*

91.1 Meconium Ileus in Cystic Fibrosis

In a newborn infant, impaction of meconium causes intestinal obstructions often associated with CF. The absence of fetal pancreatic enzymes limits normal digestive activities in the intestine, and meconium becomes viscid and mucilaginous. It clings to the intestinal wall and moves with difficulty. The inspissated and impacted meconium fills the intestinal canal but is most concentrated in the lower part of the ileum. Clinically, the pattern is that of congenital intestinal obstruction with or without intestinal perforation. Abdominal distention is prominent, and persistent vomiting soon occurs. Infrequently, one or more inspissated meconium stools may be passed shortly after birth.

The *differential diagnosis* involves other causes of intestinal obstruction, including intestinal pseudo-obstruction and pancreatic insufficiency; an exact diagnosis cannot be made except at laparotomy. A presumptive diagnosis can be made on the basis of a history of CF in a sibling, by palpation of doughy or cordlike masses of intestines through the abdominal wall, and by the roentgenographic appearance. Roentgenographically, in contrast to the generally evenly distended intestinal loops above an atresia, the loops may vary in width and are not as evenly filled with gas. At points of heaviest meconium concentration, the infiltrated gas may create a bubbly granular appearance (Figs. 91–2 and 91–3). It is technically difficult to do a sweat test in a neonate. Genetic testing confirms the diagnosis of CF.

Treatment is high Gastrografin enemas as described previously for meconium plugs. If they are unsuccessful or if perforation of the bowel wall is suspected, laparotomy is performed and the ileum opened at the point of greatest diameter of the impaction. Approximately 50% of infants have associated intestinal atresia, stenosis, or volvulus that does not respond to contrast enema and requires surgery. The inspissated meconium is removed by

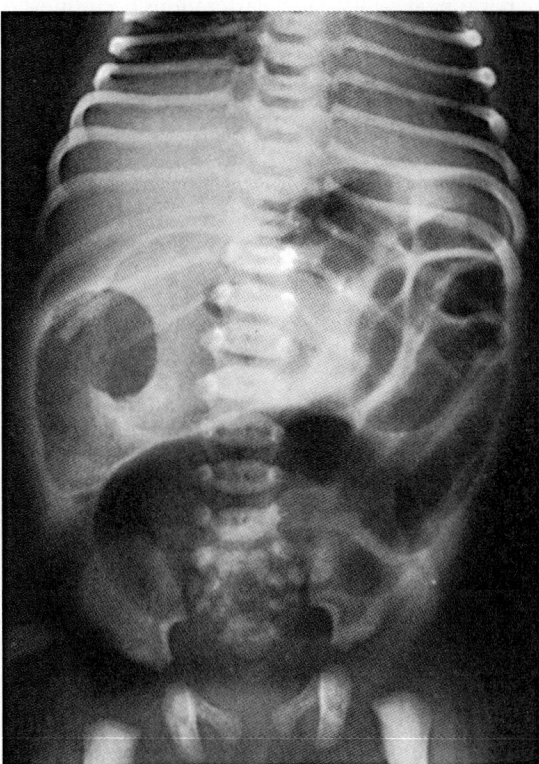

FIGURE 91–2. Meconium ileus. Impacted meconium with small amounts of air interspersed throughout it can be seen in loops of intestine on the right side of the abdomen. The intestinal loops above this impaction are greatly distended.

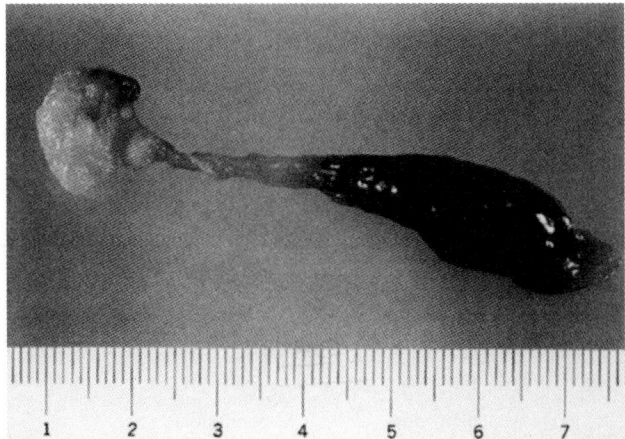

FIGURE 91–1. This plug of meconium and mucus (scale in cm) caused bowel obstruction in a premature infant. A radiograph showed marked gaseous distention and multiple fluid levels at 30 hr of age. Dramatic improvement occurred when the plug was passed after an enema. (From The abnormal fetus. In Beischer NA, Mackay EV, Colditz PB [editors]: *Obstetrics and the Newborn,* 3rd ed. Philadelphia, WB Saunders, 1997.)

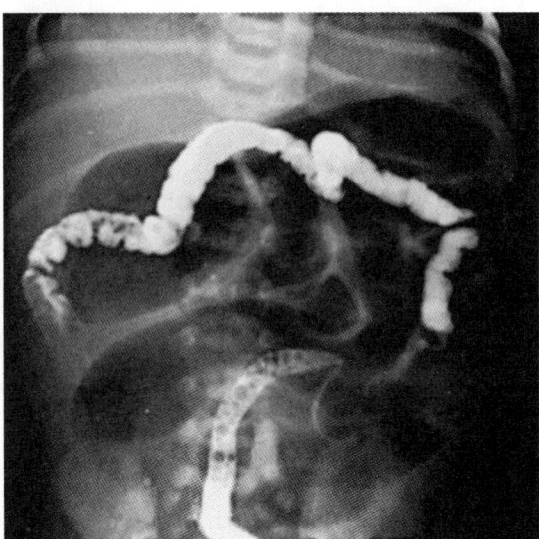

FIGURE 91–3. Meconium ileus. The colon, outlined by contrast material, is small because meconium has not reached it.

gentle and patient irrigation with warm isotonic sodium chloride or acetylcysteine (Mucomyst) solution introduced through a fine catheter, which may be passed between the impaction and the bowel wall. Most infants with meconium ileus survive the neonatal period. If associated with CF, the long-term prognosis depends on the severity of the underlying disease (Chapter 402).

Meconium Peritonitis. Perforation of the intestine may occur in utero or shortly after birth. Either natural processes may seal the tear relatively quickly with only a small amount of meconium escaping, or the meconium contents may largely be emptied into the peritoneal cavity. Such perforations occur most often as a complication of meconium ileus in infants with CF, but the perforation is occasionally due to a meconium plug or intestinal obstruction of another cause.

When an intestinal perforation has spontaneously sealed and only a small amount of meconium has escaped, the event may never be detected, except when meconium becomes calcified and is later fortuitously discovered on roentgenograms of the abdomen. Alternatively, the clinical picture may be dominated by the signs of intestinal obstruction (as in meconium ileus) or peritonitis. Characteristically noted are abdominal distention, vomiting, and absence of stools. Treatment consists primarily of elimination of the intestinal obstruction and drainage of the peritoneal cavity.

91.2 Neonatal Necrotizing Enterocolitis (NEC)

NEC is the most common life-threatening emergency of the gastrointestinal tract in the newborn period. The disease is characterized by various degrees of mucosal or transmural necrosis of the intestine. The cause of NEC remains unclear but is most likely multifactorial. Its incidence is 1–5% of infants in neonatal intensive care units. Both incidence and case fatality rates increase with decreasing birthweight and gestational age. Because very small, ill preterm infants are particularly susceptible to NEC, a rising incidence may reflect improved survival of this high-risk group of patients. The disease is rare in term infants.

Pathology and Pathogenesis. Many factors may contribute to the development of a necrotic segment of intestine, gas accumulation in the submucosa of the bowel wall (pneumatosis intesti-

nalis), and progression of the necrosis to perforation, sepsis, and death. The distal part of the ileum and the proximal segment of colon are involved most frequently; in fatal cases, gangrene may extend from the stomach to the rectum. The concept of "risk factors" for NEC is controversial. The triad of intestinal ischemia, oral feedings (metabolic substrate), and pathogenic organisms has been linked to NEC. The greatest risk factor for NEC is prematurity. Although no proven cause has been established for NEC, the disease probably results from an interaction between mucosal injury caused by a variety of factors (ischemia, infection, inflammation) and the host's response to that injury (circulatory, immunologic, inflammatory). Clustering of cases suggests a primary role for an infectious agent. Various bacterial and viral agents, including *Escherichia coli, Klebsiella, Clostridium perfringens, Staphylococcus epidermidis,* and rotavirus, have been recovered from cultures. Nonetheless, in most situations no pathogen is identified. NEC rarely occurs before the initiation of enteral feeding and is much less common in infants fed human milk. Aggressive enteral feeding may predispose to the development of NEC.

Clinical Manifestations. Infants with NEC have a variety of signs and symptoms and may have either an insidious or sudden catastrophic onset (Box 91–1). The onset of NEC usually occurs in the first 2 wk but can be as late as 3 mo of age in VLBW infants. Age at onset is inversely related to gestational age. The first signs are abdominal distention with gastric retention. Obvious bloody stools are seen in 25% of patients. Because of nonspecific signs, sepsis may be suspected before an intestinal lesion is noted. The spectrum of illness is broad and ranges from mild disease with only guaiac-positive stools to severe illness with bowel perforation, peritonitis, systemic inflammatory response syndrome, shock, and death. Progression may be rapid, but it is unusual for the disease to progress from mild to severe after 72 hr.

Diagnosis. A very high index of suspicion in treating infants at risk is essential. Plain abdominal roentgenograms may demonstrate pneumatosis intestinalis, a finding that is diagnostic of NEC in a newborn infant; 50–75% of patients have pneumatosis when treatment is started (Fig. 91–4). Portal vein gas is a sign of severe disease, and pneumoperitoneum indicates a perforation (Figs. 91–4 and 91–5). Hepatic ultrasonography may detect portal venous gas despite normal abdominal roentgenograms.

The *differential diagnosis* of NEC includes specific infections (systemic or intestinal), obstruction, volvulus, and isolated intestinal perforation. Idiopathic focal intestinal perforation can occur after the early use of postnatal steroids and indomethacin. Pneumoperitoneum develops in such patients, but they are usually less ill than those with NEC.

BOX 91–1. Signs and Symptoms Associated with Necrotizing Enterocolitis

GASTROINTESTINAL	SYSTEMIC
Abdominal distention	Lethargy
Abdominal tenderness	Apnea/respiratory distress
Feeding intolerance	Temperature instability
Delayed gastric emptying	"Not right"
Vomiting	Acidosis (metabolic and/or respiratory)
Occult/gross blood in stool	
Change in stool pattern/diarrhea	Glucose instability
Abdominal mass	Poor perfusion/shock
Erythema of abdominal wall	Disseminated intravascular coagulopathy
	Positive results of blood cultures

From Kanto WP Jr, Hunter JE, Stoll BJ: Recognition and medical management of necrotizing enterocolitis. *Clin Perinatol* 1994; 21:335–46.

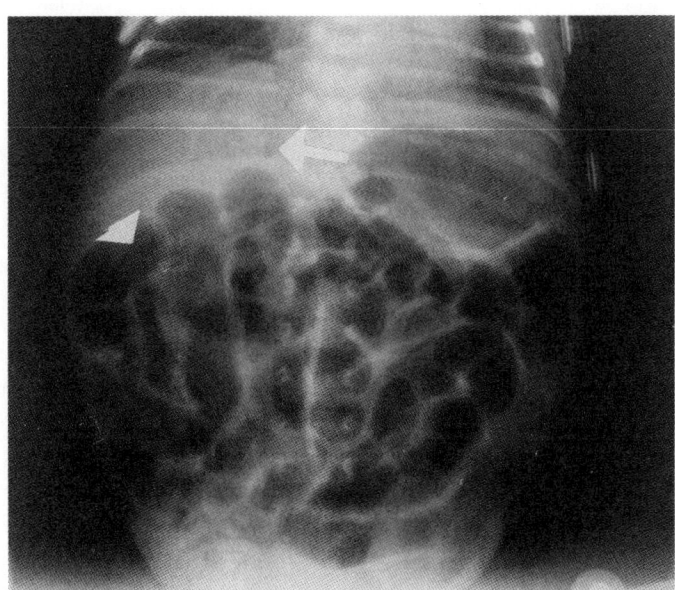

FIGURE 91–4. Necrotizing enterocolitis. A kidney-ureter-bladder film demonstrates abdominal distention, hepatic portal venous gas *(arrow)*, and a bubbly appearance of pneumatosis intestinalis *(arrowhead; right lower quadrant)*. The latter two signs are thought to be pathognomonic for neonatal necrotizing enterocolitis.

Treatment. Intensive therapy is advisable for suspected as well as diagnosed cases. Cessation of feeding, nasogastric decompression, and administration of intravenous fluids with careful attention to respiratory status, coagulation profile, and acid-base and electrolyte balance are very important. Once blood has been drawn for culture, systemic antibiotics (with broad coverage for gram-negative and other organisms) should be started. If present, umbilical catheters should be removed, but with good intravenous access maintained. Ventilation should be assisted if distention is contributing to hypoxia and hypercapnia. If hypotension develops, resuscitation with crystalloid, blood, plasma, and/or dopamine is essential.

The patient's course should be monitored by performing frequent cross-table lateral abdominal roentgenograms to detect perforation and by serial determination of the hematocrit and platelet, electrolyte, and acid-base status. Gown and glove isolation and grouping infants at similar increased risk into cohorts separate from other infants should be instituted to contain an epidemic.

A surgeon should be consulted early in the course of treatment. Evidence of perforation (free air) is an indication for laparotomy and resection of necrotic bowel. Brown paracentesis fluid with organisms on Gram stain suggests perforation. Failure to respond to medical management, a single fixed bowel loop, erythema of the abdominal wall, and a palpable mass are additional indications for exploratory laparotomy, resection of necrotic bowel, and external ostomy diversion. Ideally, surgery should be performed after intestinal necrosis develops, but before perforation and peritonitis occur. Noninvasive diagnosis of intestinal necrosis with abdominal MRI is being studied. The role of peritoneal drainage in lieu of laparotomy in a patient with perforation secondary to NEC is unclear. Peritoneal drainage may be helpful for patients in extremis with peritonitis who are too unstable to withstand surgery. Peritoneal drainage tends to be more successful in patients with isolated intestinal perforation. Such patients tend to have a lower birthweight, are more likely to not be receiving oral feeding, and are prone to perforation at an earlier postnatal age than are patients with perforation related to NEC. In many patients with isolated intestinal perforation treated by drainage, no further surgical procedure is needed; a small subgroup may require later surgery to repair an intestinal stricture or fistula.

Prognosis. Medical management fails in about 20% of patients with pneumatosis intestinalis at diagnosis; of these, 9–25% die. Early postoperative complications include wound infection and dehiscence and stomal problems (prolapse, necrosis). Intestinal strictures develop at the site of the necrotizing lesion in about 10% of surgically or medically managed patients. Resection of the obstructing stricture is curative. Complications of NEC after massive intestinal resection include short-bowel syndrome (malabsorption, growth failure, malnutrition), complications of total parenteral alimentation related to central venous catheters (sepsis, thrombosis), and cholestatic jaundice. No prevention strategy has proved to be effective, although the risk of NEC in preterm infants is significantly lower in infants who are fed only breast milk. Minimal enteric feedings (gut stimulation) prior to bolus feedings may reduce the incidence of NEC; early initiation of aggressive feeding protocols may increase its incidence in VLBW infants.

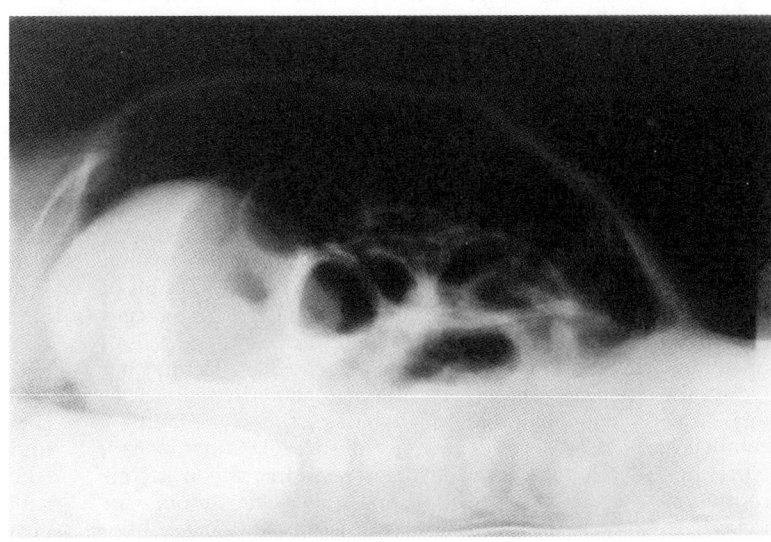

FIGURE 91–5. Intestinal perforation. A cross-table abdominal roentgenogram in a patient with neonatal necrotizing enterocolitis demonstrates marked distention and massive pneumoperitoneum as evidenced by the free air below the anterior abdominal wall.

Amin HJ, Zamora SA, McMillan DD, et al: Arginine supplementation prevents necrotizing enterocolitis in the premature infant. *J Pediatr* 2002;140:425.

Cass DL, Brandt ML, Patel DL, et al: Peritoneal drainage as definitive treatment for neonates with isolated intestinal perforation. *J Pediatr Surg* 2000;35:1531.

Chwals WJ, Blakely ML, Cheng A, et al: Surgery-associated complications in necrotizing enterocolitis: A multiinstitutional study. *J Pediatr Surg* 2001;36:1722.

Grosfeld JL, Molinari F, Chaet M, et al: Gastrointestinal perforation and peritonitis in infants and children: Experience with 179 cases over ten years. *Surgery* 1996;120:650.

Holman R, Stoll B, Clarke M, et al: The epidemiology of necrotizing enterocolitis infant mortality in the United States. *Am J Public Health* 1997;87:2026.

Kanto WP, Hunter JE, Stoll BJ: Recognition and medical management of necrotizing enterocolitis. *Clin Perinatol* 1994;21:335.

Kocoshis S: Evolving concepts and improving prospects for neonates with short bowel syndrome. *J Pediatr* 2001;139:5.

Loh M, Osborn DA, Lui K: Outcome of very premature infants with necrotizing enterocolitis cared for in centres with or without on site surgical facilities. *Arch Dis Child Fetal Neonatal Ed* 2001;85:F114.

Maalouf EF, Fagbemi A, Duggan PJ, et al: Magnetic resonance imaging of intestinal necrosis in preterm infants. *Pediatrics* 2000;105:510.

Moss RL, Dimmitt RA, Henry MC, et al: A meta-analysis of peritoneal drainage versus laparotomy for perforated necrotizing enterocolitis. *J Pediatr Surg* 2001; 36:1210.

Ng SCY: Necrotizing enterocolitis in the full-term neonate. *J Paediatr Child Health* 2001;37:1.

Stoll BJ: Epidemiology of necrotizing enterocolitis. *Clin Perinatol* 1994;21:205.

91.3 Jaundice and Hyperbilirubinemia in the Newborn

Hyperbilirubinemia is a common and, in most cases, benign problem in neonates. Nonetheless, untreated, severe indirect hyperbilirubinemia is potentially neurotoxic, and conjugated-direct hyperbilirubinemia often signifies a serious hepatic or systemic illness. Jaundice is observed during the 1st wk of life in approximately 60% of term infants and 80% of preterm infants. The color usually results from the accumulation in skin of unconjugated, nonpolar, lipid-soluble bilirubin pigment (indirect reacting) formed from hemoglobin by the action of heme oxygenase, biliverdin reductase, and nonenzymatic reducing agents in the reticuloendothelial cells; it may also be due in part to deposition of the pigment after it has been converted in the liver cell microsome by the enzyme uridine diphosphoglucuronic acid (UDP)-glucuronyl transferase to the polar, water-soluble ester glucuronide of bilirubin (direct reacting). The unconjugated form is neurotoxic in infants at certain concentrations and under various conditions. Conjugated bilirubin is not neurotoxic but indicates a potentially serious disorder.

Etiology. A newborn infant's metabolism of bilirubin is in transition from the fetal stage, during which the placenta is the principal route of elimination of the lipid-soluble bilirubin, to the adult stage, during which the water-soluble conjugated form is excreted from hepatic cells into the biliary system and then into the gastrointestinal tract. Unconjugated hyperbilirubinemia may be caused or increased by any factor that (1) increases the load of bilirubin to be metabolized by the liver (hemolytic anemias, polycythemia, shortened red cell life as a result of immaturity or transfused cells, increased enterohepatic circulation, infection), (2) damages or reduces the activity of the transferase enzyme (genetic deficiency, hypoxia, infection, possibly hypothermia and thyroid deficiency), (3) competes for or blocks the transferase enzyme (drugs and other substances requiring glucuronic acid conjugation for excretion), or (4) leads to an absence or decreased amounts of the enzyme or to reduction of bilirubin uptake by liver cells (genetic defect, prematurity). The toxic effects of elevated levels of unconjugated bilirubin in serum are increased by factors that reduce the retention of bilirubin in the circulation (hypoproteinemia, displacement of bilirubin from its binding sites on albumin by competitive binding of drugs such as sulfisoxazole and moxalactam, Chuen-Lin herbal tea, acidosis, increased free fatty acid concentration secondary to hypoglycemia, starvation, or hypothermia) or by factors that increase the permeability of the blood-brain barrier or nerve cell membranes to bilirubin or increase the susceptibility of brain cells to its toxicity, such as asphyxia, prematurity, hyperosmolality, and infection. Early feeding decreases whereas breast-feeding and dehydration increase serum levels of bilirubin. Meconium has 1 mg bilirubin/dL and may contribute to jaundice by the enterohepatic circulation after deconjugation by intestinal glucuronidase (Fig. 91–6). Drugs such as oxytocin and chemicals used in the nursery such as phenolic detergents may also produce unconjugated hyperbilirubinemia. The mnemonic JAUNDICE can be helpful in recalling risk factors for unconjugated hyperbilirubinemia (see Box 91–2).

Clinical Manifestations. Jaundice may be present at birth or may appear at any time during the neonatal period, depending on the cause. Jaundice usually begins on the face and, as serum levels increase, progresses to the abdomen and then the feet. Dermal pressure may reveal the anatomic progression of jaundice (face, ≈5 mg/dL; mid-abdomen, ≈15 mg/dL; soles, ≈20 mg/dL), but clinical examination cannot be depended on to estimate blood levels. Jaundice to the mid-abdomen, signs or symptoms, high-risk factors that suggest nonphysiologic jaundice (Box 91–2), or hemolysis must be evaluated further. Noninvasive techniques for transcutaneous measurement of bilirubin that correlate well with serum levels may be used to screen infants, but determination of a serum bilirubin level is indicated for patients with progressing jaundice, symptoms, or a risk for hemolysis or sepsis. Jaundice resulting from deposition of indirect bilirubin in the skin tends to appear bright yellow or

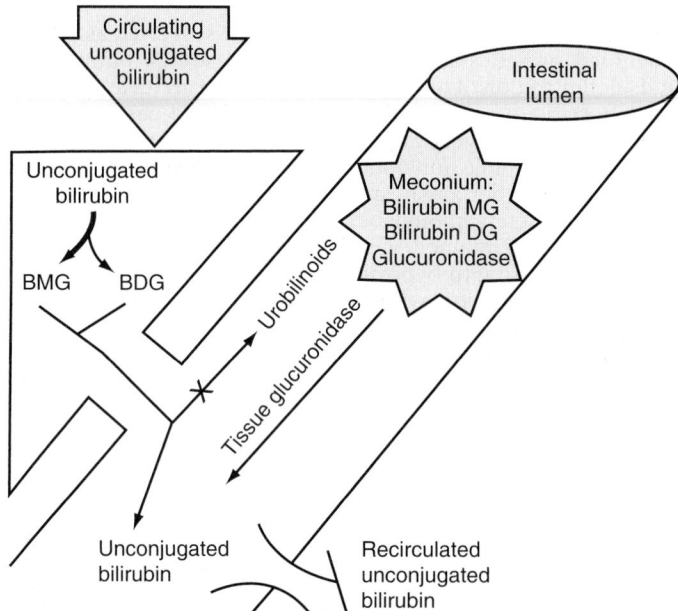

FIGURE 91–6. The neonatal production rate of bilirubin is 6–8 mg/kg/24 hr (in contrast to 3–4 mg/kg/24 hr in adults). Water-insoluble bilirubin is bound to albumin. At the plasma-hepatocyte interface, a liver membrane carrier (bilitranslocase) transports bilirubin to a cytosolic binding protein (ligandin or Y protein, now known to be glutathione *S*-transferase), which prevents back-absorption to plasma. Bilirubin is converted to bilirubin monoglucuronide (BMG) or diglucuronide (BDG) by several classes of the enzyme bilirubin glucuronyl transferase. Neonates excrete more BMG than adults do. In the fetus, conjugated lipid-insoluble BMG and BDG must be deconjugated by tissue β-glucuronidases to facilitate placental transfer of lipid-soluble unconjugated bilirubin across the placental lipid membranes. After birth, intestinal or milk-containing glucuronidases contribute to the enterohepatic recirculation of bilirubin and possibly to the development of hyperbilirubinemia.

orange, and jaundice of the obstructive type (direct bilirubin) has a greenish or muddy yellow cast. This difference is usually apparent only in severe jaundice. Affected infants may be lethargic and may feed poorly. Signs of kernicterus rarely appear on the 1st day of jaundice (Chapter 91.4).

Differential Diagnosis. Jaundice, consisting of either indirect or direct bilirubin, that is present at birth or appears within the 1st 24 hr of life requires immediate attention and may be due to erythroblastosis fetalis, concealed hemorrhage, sepsis, or intrauterine infections, including syphilis, cytomegalic inclusion disease, rubella, and congenital toxoplasmosis. Hemolysis is suggested by a rapid rise in serum bilirubin (>0.5 mg/dL/hr), anemia, pallor, reticulocytosis, hepatosplenomegaly, and a positive family history. An unusually high proportion of direct-reacting bilirubin may characterize jaundice in infants who have received intrauterine transfusions. Jaundice that first appears on the 2nd or 3rd day is usually "physiologic" but may represent a more severe form. Familial nonhemolytic icterus (Crigler-Najjar syndrome) and early-onset breast-feeding jaundice are seen initially on the 2nd or 3rd day. *Jaundice appearing after the 3rd day and within the 1st wk should suggest bacterial sepsis or urinary tract infection;* it may be due to other infections, notably syphilis, toxoplasmosis, cytomegalovirus, or enterovirus. Jaundice secondary to extensive ecchymosis or hematoma may occur during the 1st day or later, especially in premature infants. Polycythemia may lead to early jaundice.

Jaundice that is noted initially after the 1st wk of life suggests breast milk jaundice, septicemia, congenital atresia or paucity of the bile ducts, hepatitis, galactosemia, hypothyroidism, CF, congenital hemolytic anemia (spherocytosis), or possibly the crises of other hemolytic anemias (such as pyruvate kinase and other glycolytic enzyme deficiencies or hereditary nonspherocytic anemia) or hemolytic anemia related to drugs (as in congenital deficiencies of the enzymes glucose-6-phosphate dehydrogenase [G6PD] or glutathione synthetase, reductase, or peroxidase) (Fig. 91–7).

Persistent jaundice during the 1st mo of life suggests inspissated bile syndrome (which may follow hemolytic disease of the newborn), hyperalimentation-associated cholestasis, hepatitis, cytomegalic inclusion disease, syphilis, toxoplasmosis, familial nonhemolytic icterus, congenital atresia of the bile ducts, or

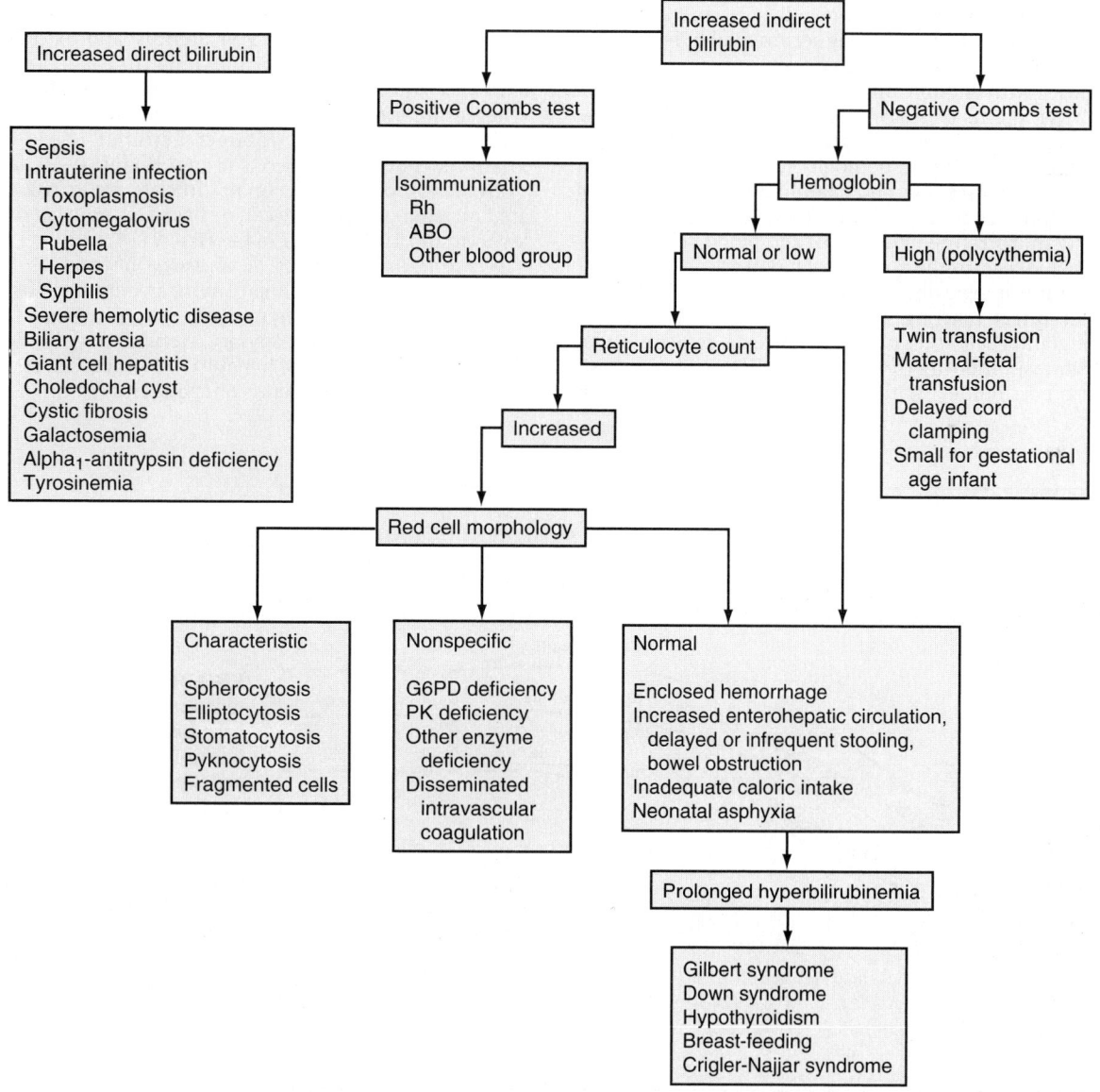

FIGURE 91–7. Schematic approach to the diagnosis of neonatal jaundice. G6PD = glucose-6-phosphate dehydrogenase; PK = pyruvate kinase. (From Oski FA: Differential diagnosis of jaundice. In Taeusch HW, Ballard RA, Avery MA [editors]: *Schaffer and Avery's Diseases of the Newborn,* 6th ed. Philadelphia, WB Saunders, 1991.)

galactosemia. Rarely, physiologic jaundice may be prolonged for several weeks, as in infants with hypothyroidism or pyloric stenosis.

Low-risk jaundiced infants who are full term and asymptomatic may be evaluated by monitoring serum total bilirubin levels. Regardless of the gestational age or time of appearance of jaundice, those with significant hyperbilirubinemia and all patients with symptoms or signs require a complete diagnostic evaluation, which should include determination of the direct and indirect bilirubin fractions, hemoglobin, reticulocyte count, and blood type, a Coombs test, and examination of a peripheral blood smear. Indirect-reacting bilirubinemia, reticulocytosis, and a smear demonstrating evidence of red blood cell destruction suggest hemolysis; in the absence of blood group incompatibility, non-immunologically induced hemolysis should be considered. If direct-reacting hyperbilirubinemia is present, hepatitis, congenital bile duct disorders (atresia, paucity, Byler disease), cholestasis, inborn errors of metabolism, CF, and sepsis are diagnostic possibilities. If the reticulocyte count, Coombs test, and direct bilirubin are normal, physiologic or pathologic indirect hyperbilirubinemia may be present (see Fig. 91–7).

Physiologic Jaundice (Icterus Neonatorum). Under normal circumstances, the level of indirect-reacting bilirubin in umbilical cord serum is 1–3 mg/dL and rises at a rate of less than 5 mg/dL/24 hr; thus, jaundice becomes visible on the 2nd–3rd day, usually peaking between the 2nd and 4th days at 5–6 mg/dL and decreasing to below 2 mg/dL between the 5th and 7th days of life. Jaundice associated with these changes is designated "physiologic" and is believed to be the result of increased bilirubin production after the breakdown of fetal red blood cells combined with transient limitation in the conjugation of bilirubin by the liver.

Overall, 6–7% of full-term infants have indirect bilirubin levels greater than 12.9 mg/dL and less than 3% have levels greater than 15 mg/dL. Risk factors for indirect hyperbilirubinemia include maternal diabetes, race (Chinese, Japanese, Korean, and Native American), prematurity, drugs (vitamin K_3, novobiocin), altitude, polycythemia, male sex, trisomy 21, cutaneous bruising, cephalohematoma, oxytocin induction, breast-feeding, weight loss (dehydration or caloric deprivation), delayed bowel movement, and a sibling who had physiologic jaundice (see Box 91–2). A family history of neonatal jaundice, exclusive breast-feeding, bruising, cephalohematoma, Asian race, and maternal age older than 25 yr identify approximately 60% of cases of extreme hyperbilirubinemia. In infants without these variables, indirect bilirubin levels rarely rise above 12 mg/dL, whereas infants with several risk factors are more likely to have higher bilirubin levels. Indirect bilirubin levels in full-term infants decline to adult levels (1 mg/dL) by 10–14 days of life.

Prediction of which neonatal infants are at risk for exaggerated physiologic jaundice can be based on hour-specific bilirubin levels in the 1st 24–72 hr of life (Fig. 91–8).

Persistent indirect hyperbilirubinemia beyond 2 wk suggests hemolysis, hereditary glucuronyl transferase deficiency, breast milk jaundice, hypothyroidism, or intestinal obstruction. Jaundice associated with pyloric stenosis may be due to caloric deprivation, deficiency of hepatic UDP-glucuronyl transferase, or ileus-induced increased enterohepatic circulation of bilirubin.

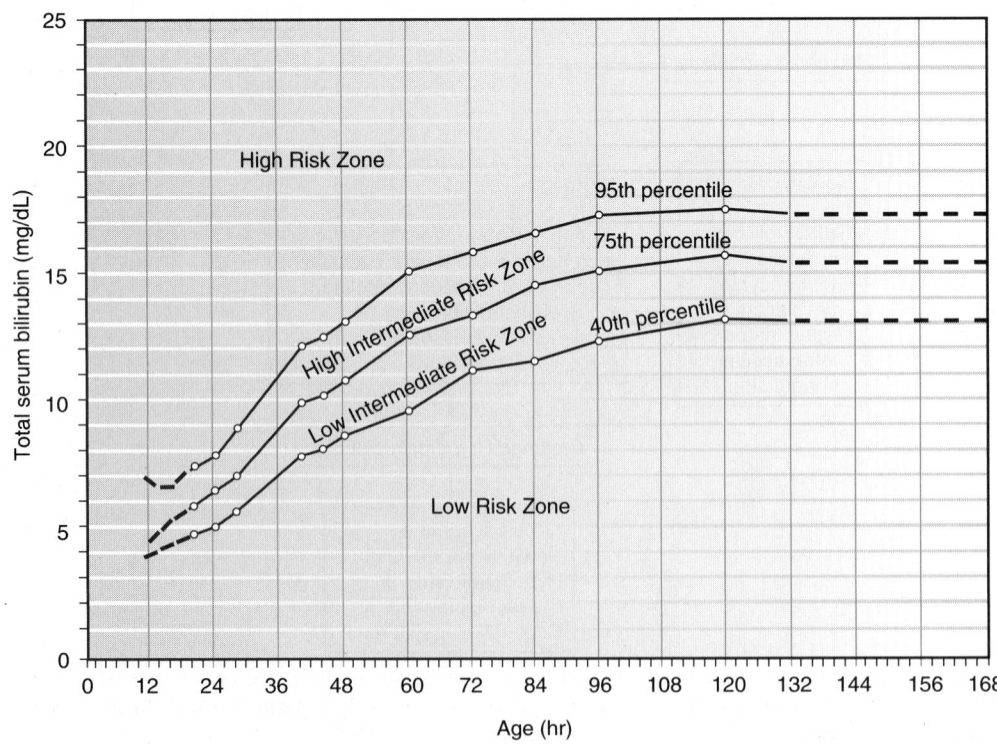

FIGURE 91–8. Risk designation of term and near-term well newborns based on their hour-specific serum bilirubin values. The high-risk zone is designated by the 95th percentile track. The intermediate-risk zone is subdivided into upper and lower risk zones by the 75th percentile track. The low-risk zone has been electively and statistically defined by the 40th percentile track. *(Dotted extensions* are based on less than 300 total serum bilirubin values/epoch.) (From Bhutani VK, Johnson L, Sivieri EM: Predictive ability of a predischarge hour-specific serum bilirubin for subsequent significant hyperbilirubinemia in healthy term and near-term newborns. *Pediatrics* 1999;103:9.)

In premature infants, the rise in serum bilirubin tends to be the same or a little slower than that in term infants, but it is of longer duration, which generally results in higher levels, the peak being reached between the 4th and 7th days; the pattern depends on the time required for the development of mature mechanisms for the metabolism and excretion of bilirubin. Peak levels of 8–12 mg/dL are not usually reached until the 5th–7th day, and jaundice is infrequently observed after the 10th day.

The diagnosis of physiologic jaundice in term or preterm infants can be established only by precluding known causes of jaundice on the basis of the history and clinical and laboratory findings (Table 91–1). In general, a search to determine the cause of jaundice should be made if (1) it appears in the 1st 24–36 hr of life, (2) serum bilirubin is rising at a rate faster than 5 mg/dL/24 hr, (3) serum bilirubin is greater than 12 mg/dL in full-term (especially in the absence of risk factors) or 10–14 mg/dL in preterm infants, (4) jaundice persists after 10–14 days of life, or (5) direct-reacting bilirubin is greater than 2 mg/dL at any time. Among other factors suggesting a nonphysiologic cause of jaundice are a family history of hemolytic disease, pallor, hepatomegaly, splenomegaly, failure of phototherapy to lower bilirubin, vomiting, lethargy, poor feeding, excessive weight loss, apnea, bradycardia, abnormal vital signs (including hypothermia), light-colored stools, dark urine positive for bilirubin, and signs of kernicterus (Chapter 91.4).

Pathologic Hyperbilirubinemia. Jaundice and its underlying hyperbilirubinemia are considered pathologic if their time of appearance, duration, or pattern of serially determined serum bilirubin concentrations varies significantly from that of physiologic jaundice or if the course is compatible with physiologic jaundice but other reasons exist to suspect that the infant is at special risk from the neurotoxicity of unconjugated bilirubin. It may not be possible to precisely determine the cause of an abnormal elevation of unconjugated bilirubin. Many of these infants have an associated risk factor such as Asian race, prematurity, breast-feeding, or weight loss; hence, the terms exaggerated physiologic jaundice and hyperbilirubinemia of the newborn are used for infants whose primary problem is probably a deficiency or inactivity of bilirubin glucuronyl transferase (e.g., Gilbert syndrome) rather than an excessive load of bilirubin for excretion (see Box 91–2). The combination of G6PD deficiency and a mutation of the promoter region of UDP-glucuronyl transferase 1 produces indirect hyperbilirubinemia in the absence of signs of hemolysis. Nonphysiologic hyperbilirubinemia may also be caused by mutations in the gene for bilirubin UDP-glucuronyl transferase.

The greatest risk associated with hyperbilirubinemia is the development of kernicterus (bilirubin encephalopathy) at high indirect serum bilirubin levels (Chapter 91.4). The level of serum bilirubin associated with kernicterus is dependent in part on the cause of the jaundice. Kernicterus develops at lower bilirubin levels in preterm infants and in the presence of asphyxia, intraventricular hemorrhage, hemolysis, or drugs that displace bilirubin from albumin. The exact serum bilirubin level that is harmful for VLBW infants is unclear. Kernicterus does occur in patients with breast milk jaundice but is very uncommon. The duration of exposure to bilirubin and the brain concentration of bilirubin are important factors for neurotoxicity.

Jaundice Associated with Breast-Feeding. Significant elevations in unconjugated bilirubin (breast milk jaundice) develop in an estimated 2% of breast-fed term infants after the 7th day of life, with maximal concentrations as high as 10–30 mg/dL reached during the 2nd–3rd wk. If breast-feeding is continued, the hyperbilirubinemia gradually decreases and may then persist for 3–10 wk at lower levels. If nursing is discontinued, the serum bilirubin level falls rapidly, usually reaching normal levels within a few days. Cessation of breast-feeding for 1–2 days and substitution of formula for breast milk results in a rapid decline in serum bilirubin, after which nursing can be resumed without a return of the hyperbilirubinemia to its previously high levels. If indicated, phototherapy may be of benefit (Chapter 91.4). These infants have no other sign of illness; nonetheless, ker-

TABLE 91–1. Diagnostic Features of the Various Types of Neonatal Jaundice

Diagnosis	Nature of Van den Bergh Reaction	Jaundice Appears	Jaundice Disappears	Peak Bilirubin Concentration mg/dL	Peak Bilirubin Concentration Age in Days	Bilirubin Rate of Accumulation (mg/dL/day)	Remarks
"Physiologic jaundice":							Usually relates to degree of maturity
Full-term	Indirect	2–3 days	4–5 days	10–12	2–3	<5	
Premature	Indirect	3–4 days	7–9 days	15	6–8	<5	
Hyperbilirubinemia due to metabolic factors							Metabolic factors: hypoxia, respiratory distress, lack of carbohydrate
Full-term	Indirect	2–3 days	Variable	>12	1st wk	<5	Hormonal influences: cretinism, hormones, Gilbert syndrome
Premature	Indirect	3–4 days	Variable	>15	1st wk	<5	Genetic factors: Crigler-Najjar syndrome, Gilbert syndrome Drugs: vitamin K, novobiocin
Hemolytic states and hematoma	Indirect	May appear in 1st 24 hr	Variable	Unlimited	Variable	Usually >5	Erythroblastosis: Rh, ABO, Kell Congenital hemolytic states: spherocytic, nonspherocytic Infantile pyknocytosis Drugs: vitamin K Enclosed hemorrhage—hematoma
Mixed hemolytic and hepatotoxic factors	Indirect and direct	May appear in 1st 24 hr	Variable	Unlimited	Variable	Usually >5	Infection: bacterial sepsis, pyelonephritis, hepatitis, toxoplasmosis, cytomegalic inclusion disease, rubella, syphilis Drugs: vitamin K
Hepatocellular damage	Indirect and direct	Usually 2–3 days, may appear by 2nd wk	Variable	Unlimited	Variable	Variable, can be >5	Biliary atresia; paucity of bile ducts, familial cholestasis, galactosemia; hepatitis and infection

From Brown AK: Pediatr Clin North Am 1962;9:589.

nicterus has been reported. The cause is unclear, but in some the milk contains a glucuronidase that may be responsible for jaundice.

This syndrome should be distinguished from an early-onset, accentuated unconjugated hyperbilirubinemia (breast-feeding jaundice) in the 1st wk of life, when breast-fed infants have higher bilirubin levels than formula-fed infants do (Fig. 91–9). Hyperbilirubinemia (>12 mg/dL) develops in 13% of breast-fed infants in the 1st wk of life and may be due to decreased milk intake with dehydration or reduced caloric intake. Giving supplements of glucose water to breast-fed infants is associated with higher bilirubin levels, in part because of reduced intake of the higher caloric density breast milk. Frequent breast-feeding (>10/24 hr), rooming-in with night feeding, and discouraging 5% dextrose or water supplementation may reduce the incidence of early breast-feeding jaundice.

Neonatal Hepatitis. See Chapter 337.1.

Congenital Atresia of the Bile Ducts. See Chapter 337.1. Jaundice persisting for more than 2 wk or associated with acholic stools and dark urine suggests biliary atresia. All such infants should have an immediate diagnostic evaluation, including determination of direct bilirubin.

Inspissated Bile Syndrome. See Late Complications in Chapter 92.

91.4 Kernicterus

Kernicterus, or bilirubin encephalopathy, is a neurologic syndrome resulting from the deposition of unconjugated bilirubin in the basal ganglia and brainstem nuclei. The pathogenesis of kernicterus is multifactorial and involves an interaction between unconjugated bilirubin levels, albumin binding and unbound bilirubin levels, passage across the blood-brain barrier, and neuronal susceptibility to injury. Disruption of the blood-brain barrier by disease, asphyxia, or other factors and maturational changes in blood-brain barrier permeability affect risk.

The precise blood level above which indirect-reacting bilirubin or free bilirubin will be toxic for an individual infant is unpredictable, but kernicterus is rare in healthy term infants and in the absence of hemolysis if the serum level is under 25 mg/dL. In previously healthy, predominantly breast-fed term infants, kernicterus has developed when bilirubin levels exceed 30 mg/dL, although the range is wide (21–50 mg/dL). Its onset is usually in the 1st wk of life, but it may be delayed to the 2nd–3rd wk. The risk in infants with hemolytic disease (erythroblastosis fetalis) is directly related to serum bilirubin levels. The duration of exposure needed to produce toxic effects is also unknown. Little evidence suggests that a level of indirect bilirubin less than 25 mg/dL affects the IQ of healthy term infants without hemolytic disease. *Nonetheless, the less mature the infant, the greater the susceptibility to kernicterus.* Factors that potentiate the movement of bilirubin into brain cells and its adverse effects on them are discussed in Chapter 91.3. In exceptional circumstances, kernicterus in VLBW infants with serum bilirubin concentrations as low as 8–12 mg/dL has been associated with an apparently cumulative effect of a number of these factors.

Clinical Manifestations. Signs and symptoms of kernicterus usually appear 2–5 days after birth in term infants and as late as the 7th day in premature ones, but hyperbilirubinemia may lead to the syndrome at any time during the neonatal period. The early signs may be subtle and indistinguishable from those of sepsis, asphyxia, hypoglycemia, intracranial hemorrhage, and other acute systemic illnesses in a neonatal infant. Lethargy, poor feeding, and loss of the Moro reflex are common initial signs. Subsequently, the infant may appear gravely ill and prostrated, with diminished tendon reflexes and respiratory distress. Opisthotonos with a bulging fontanel, twitching of the face or limbs, and a shrill high-pitched cry may follow. In advanced cases, convulsions and spasm occur, with affected infants stiffly extending their arms in inward rotation with the fists clenched (Box 91–3). Rigidity is rare at this late stage.

Many infants who progress to these severe neurologic signs die; the survivors are usually seriously damaged but may appear to recover and for 2–3 mo show few abnormalities. Later in the 1st yr of life, opisthotonos, muscle rigidity, irregular movements, and convulsions tend to recur. In the 2nd yr, the opisthotonos and seizures abate, but irregular, involuntary movements, muscle rigidity, or in some infants, hypotonia increase steadily. By 3 yr of age, the complete neurologic syndrome is often apparent and consists of bilateral choreoathetosis with involuntary muscle spasms, extrapyramidal signs, seizures, mental deficiency, dysarthric speech, high-frequency hearing loss, squinting, and defective upward movement of the eyes. Pyramidal signs, hypotonia, and ataxia occur in a few infants. In mildly affected infants, the syndrome may be characterized only by mild to moderate neuromuscular incoordination, partial deafness, or "minimal brain dysfunction," occurring singly or in combination; these problems may be inapparent until the child enters school (see Box 91–3).

Pathology. The surface of the brain is usually pale yellow. On cutting, certain regions are characteristically stained yellow by

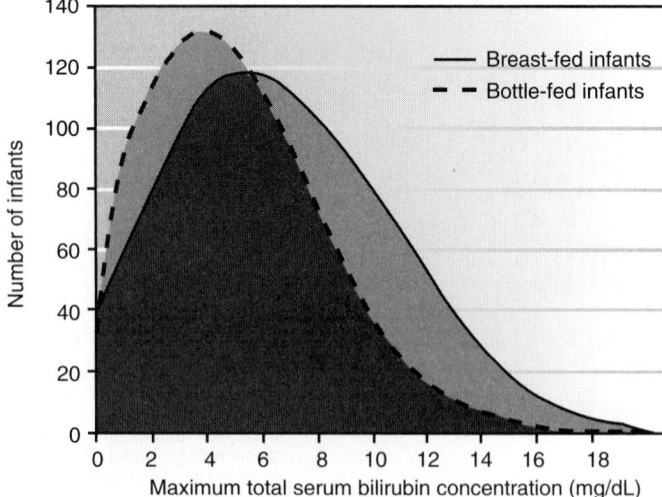

FIGURE 91–9. Distribution of maximal bilirubin levels during the 1st wk of life in breast-fed and formula-fed white infants over 2,500 g. (From Maisels J, Gifford K: Normal serum bilirubin levels in the newborn and the effect of breast-feeding. *Pediatrics* 1986;78:837.)

■ **BOX 91–3. Clinical Features of Kernicterus**

ACUTE FORM

Phase 1 (1st 1–2 days): poor sucking, stupor, hypotonia, seizures
Phase 2 (middle of 1st wk): hypertonia of extensor muscles, opisthotonos, retrocollis, fever
Phase 3 (after the 1st wk): hypertonia

CHRONIC FORM

First year: hypotonia, active deep tendon reflexes, obligatory tonic neck reflexes, delayed motor skills
After 1st yr: movement disorders (choreoathetosis, ballismus, tremor), upward gaze, sensorineural hearing loss

From Dennery PA, Seidman DS, Stevenson DK: Neonatal hyperbilirubinemia. *N Engl J Med* 2001; 344: 581–90.

unconjugated bilirubin, particularly the corpus subthalamicum, hippocampus and adjacent olfactory areas, striate bodies, thalamus, globus pallidus, putamen, inferior clivus, cerebellar nuclei, and cranial nerve nuclei. Nonpigmented areas may also be damaged. Loss of neurons, reactive gliosis, and atrophy of involved fiber systems are found in late disease. The pattern of injury has been related to the development of oxidative enzyme systems in various regions of the brain and overlaps with that found in hypoxic brain damage. Evidence favors the hypothesis that bilirubin interferes with oxygen utilization by cerebral tissue, possibly by injuring the cell membrane; antecedent hypoxic injury increases the susceptibility of brain cells to injury. Gross bilirubin staining without the specific microscopic changes of kernicterus may not be the same entity.

Incidence and Prognosis. By pathologic criteria, kernicterus will develop in one third of infants (all gestational ages) with untreated *hemolytic disease* and bilirubin levels in excess of 25–30 mg/dL. The incidence at autopsy in hyperbilirubinemic premature infants is 2–16% and is related to the risk factors discussed in Chapter 91.3. Reliable estimates of the frequency of the clinical syndrome are not available because of the wide spectrum of manifestations. Overt neurologic signs have a grave prognosis; 75% or more of such infants die, and 80% of affected survivors have bilateral choreoathetosis with involuntary muscle spasms. Mental retardation, deafness, and spastic quadriplegia are common. Infants at risk should have screening hearing tests.

Kernicterus is not a disease of the past; there have been reports of cases associated with high levels of bilirubin and no obvious underlying cause. Some experts recommend universal screening for hyperbilirubinemia in the 1st 24–48 hr of life to detect infants at high risk for severe jaundice and neurotoxicity. The American Academy of Pediatrics (AAP) has identified potentially preventable causes of kernicterus: (1) early discharge (<48 hr) with no early follow-up (within 48 hr of discharge); this problem is particularly important in near-term infants (35–37 wk gestation); (2) failure to check the bilirubin level in an infant noted to be jaundiced in the 1st 24 hr; (3) failure to recognize the presence of risk factors for hyperbilirubinemia; (4) underestimating the severity of jaundice by clinical (i.e., visual) assessment; (5) lack of concern regarding the presence of jaundice; (6) delay in measuring the serum bilirubin level despite marked jaundice or delay in initiating phototherapy in the presence of elevated bilirubin levels; and (7) failure to respond to parental concern regarding jaundice, poor feeding, or lethargy. The AAP recommends the following: (1) any infant who is jaundiced before 24 hr requires measurement of the serum bilirubin level, and if it is elevated, the infant should be evaluated for possible hemolytic disease, and (2) follow-up should be provided within 2–3 days of discharge to all neonates discharged earlier than 48 hr after birth. Early follow-up is particularly important for infants younger than 38 wk gestation. The timing of follow-up depends on the age at discharge and the presence of risk factors. In some cases, follow-up within 24 hr is necessary. Using hour-specific bilirubin levels also helps predict risk (see Fig. 91–8).

Treatment of Hyperbilirubinemia. Regardless of the cause, the goal of therapy is to prevent the concentration of indirect-reacting bilirubin in the blood from reaching levels at which neurotoxicity may occur; it is recommended that phototherapy and, if unsuccessful, exchange transfusion be used to keep the maximal total serum bilirubin below the levels indicated in Tables 91–2 (for preterm) and 91–3 (for healthy term infants without hemolysis). The risk of injury to the central nervous system from bilirubin must be balanced against the risk inherent in the treatment for each infant. Criteria for initiating phototherapy are not generally agreed on. Because phototherapy may require 6–12 hr to have a measurable effect, it must be started at bilirubin levels below those indicated for exchange transfusion.

TABLE 91–2. Suggested Maximal Indirect Serum Bilirubin Concentrations (mg/dL) in Preterm Infants

Birthweight (g)	Uncomplicated	Complicated*
<1,000	12–13	10–12
1,000–1,250	12–14	10–12
1,251–1,499	14–16	12–14
1,500–1,999	16–20	15–17
2,000–2,500	20–22	18–20

Phototherapy is usually started at 50–70% of the maximal indirect level. If values greatly exceed this level, if phototherapy is unsuccessful in reducing the maximal bilirubin level, or if signs of kernicterus are evident, exchange transfusion is indicated.

*Complications include perinatal asphyxia, acidosis, hypoxia, hypothermia, hypoalbuminemia, meningitis, intraventricular hemorrhage, hemolysis, hypoglycemia, or signs of kernicterus.

TABLE 91–3. Approach to Indirect Hyperbilirubinemia in Healthy Term Infants Without Hemolysis*

		Treatment Strategies	
Age (hr)	Phototherapy	Intensive Phototherapy and Preparation for Exchange Transfusion†	Exchange Transfusion if Phototherapy Fails‡
<24	§	§	§
24–48‖	≥15–18	≥25	≥20
49–72	≥18–20	≥30	≥25
>72	≥20	≥30	≥25
>2 wk	¶	¶	¶

*With hemolysis, exchange transfusion is initiated with an indirect bilirubin level of 20 or higher at any age.

The precise level of unconjugated bilirubin in healthy breast-fed term infants that requires therapy is unknown. Treatment options include continued breast-feeding and initiation of phototherapy or interrupted breast-feeding (use formula as a substitute), with or without phototherapy.

If any signs of kernicterus are noted during evaluation or treatment as suggested anywhere in the table or at any level of bilirubin, emergency exchange transfusion must be performed.

†If the initial bilirubin value is high, intense phototherapy should be initiated and preparation made for exchange transfusion. If phototherapy fails to reduce the bilirubin level to the levels noted on the column to the right, initiate exchange transfusion.

‡Intensive phototherapy should be initiated for bilirubin levels in this column and usually reduces serum bilirubin levels 1–2 mg/dL in 4–6 hr. Such treatment is often associated with administration of intravenous fluids at 1–1.5 times maintenance; oral alimentation should also continue.

§Jaundice in the 1st 24 hr of life is not seen in "healthy" infants (see Chapter 91.3).

‖Hyperbilirubinemia of this degree within 48 hr of birth is unusual and should suggest hemolysis, concealed hemorrhage, or causes of conjugated (direct) hyperbilirubinemia.

¶Jaundice suddenly appearing in the 2nd wk of life or continuing beyond the 2nd wk of life with significant hyperbilirubinemia levels to warrant therapy should be investigated in detail because it most probably is due to a serious underlying cause such as biliary atresia, galactosemia, hypothyroidism, or neonatal hepatitis.

When identified, the underlying cause of the icterus should be treated—for example, antibiotics for septicemia. Physiologic factors that increase the risk of neurologic damage should also be treated (e.g., correction of acidosis).

PHOTOTHERAPY. Clinical jaundice and indirect hyperbilirubinemia are reduced on exposure to a high intensity of light in the visible spectrum. Bilirubin absorbs light maximally in the blue range (420–470 nm). Nonetheless, broad-spectrum white, blue, special narrow-spectrum (super) blue, and less often, green lights have been effective in reducing bilirubin levels. Bilirubin in the skin absorbs light energy, which by photo-isomerization converts the toxic native unconjugated 4Z,15Z-bilirubin into the unconjugated configurational isomer 4Z,15E-bilirubin. The latter is the product of a reversible reaction and is excreted in bile without any need for conjugation. Phototherapy also converts native bilirubin, by an irreversible reaction, to the structural isomer lumirubin, which is excreted by the kidneys in the unconjugated state.

The use of phototherapy has decreased the need for exchange transfusion in term and preterm infants with hemolytic and nonhemolytic jaundice. When indications for exchange transfusion are present, phototherapy should not be used as a substitute. However, phototherapy may reduce the need for repeated exchange transfusions in infants with hemolysis.

Phototherapy is indicated only after the presence of pathologic hyperbilirubinemia has been established. The basic cause or causes of the jaundice should be treated concomitantly. Phototherapy may be initiated at the bilirubin levels noted in Tables 91–2 and 91–3. Prophylactic phototherapy in VLBW infants may prevent hyperbilirubinemia and may reduce the incidence of exchange transfusions. VLBW infants receiving phototherapy for 1–3 days have peak serum bilirubin concentrations about half those of untreated infants. In premature infants without significant hemolysis, serum bilirubin usually declines 1–3 mg/dL after 12–24 hr of conventional phototherapy, and peak levels may be decreased by 3–6 mg/dL. The therapeutic effect depends on the light energy emitted in the effective range of wavelengths, the distance between the lights and the infant, and the amount of skin exposed, as well as the rate of hemolysis and in vivo metabolism and excretion of bilirubin. The commercial phototherapy units available vary considerably in spectral output and the intensity of radiation emitted; therefore, the dose can be accurately measured only at the skin surface. Dark skin does not reduce the efficacy of phototherapy.

Maximal intensive phototherapy should be used when indirect bilirubin levels approach those noted in Tables 91–2 and 91–3. Such therapy includes "special blue" fluorescent tubes, placing the lamps within 15–20 cm of the infant, and placing a fiberoptic phototherapy blanket under the infant's back to increase the exposed surface area.

Conventional phototherapy is applied continuously, and the infant is turned frequently for maximal skin exposure. It should be discontinued as soon as the indirect bilirubin concentration has been reduced to levels considered safe in view of the infant's age and condition. Serum bilirubin levels and hematocrit should be monitored every 4–8 hr in infants with hemolytic disease or those with bilirubin levels near the range considered toxic for the individual infant. Others, particularly older infants, may be monitored at 12–24 hr intervals. Monitoring should continue for at least 24 hr after cessation of phototherapy in patients with hemolytic disease because unexpected rises in serum bilirubin sometimes occur and require further treatment. Skin color cannot be relied on for evaluating the effectiveness of phototherapy; the skin of babies exposed to light may appear to be almost without jaundice in the presence of marked hyperbilirubinemia.

The infant's eyes should be closed and adequately covered to prevent exposure to light. Excessive pressure from an eye bandage may injure the closed eyes, or the corneas may be excoriated if the eyes can be opened under the bandage. Body temperature should be monitored, and the infant should be shielded from bulb breakage. If feasible, irradiance should be measured directly and details of the exposure recorded (type and age of the bulbs, duration of exposure, distance from the light source to the infant, and so forth). In infants with hemolytic disease, care must be taken to not overlook developing anemia, which may require transfusion.

Complications of phototherapy include loose stools, erythematous macular rash, a purpuric rash associated with transient porphyrinemia, overheating and dehydration (increased insensible water loss, diarrhea), chilling from exposure of the infant, and bronze baby syndrome. Phototherapy is contraindicated in the presence of porphyria. Eye injury and nasal occlusion from the bandages are uncommon.

The term *bronze baby syndrome* refers to a dark grayish brown discoloration of the skin sometimes noted in infants undergoing phototherapy. Almost all infants observed with this syndrome have had a mixed type of hyperbilirubinemia with significant elevation of direct-reacting bilirubin and often with other evidence of obstructive liver disease. The discoloration may be due to photo-induced modification of porphyrins, which are often present during cholestatic jaundice and may last for many months.

Wide clinical experience suggests that long-term adverse biologic effects of phototherapy are absent, minimal, or unrecognized. However, those using phototherapy should remain alert to these possibilities and avoid any unnecessary use because untoward effects on DNA have been demonstrated in vitro.

EXCHANGE TRANSFUSION. Exchange transfusion is performed if intensive phototherapy has failed to reduce bilirubin levels to a safe range and if the risk of kernicterus exceeds the risk of the procedure or the infant has signs of kernicterus. Potential complications from exchange transfusion are not trivial and include acidosis, electrolyte abnormalities, hypoglycemia, thrombocytopenia, volume overload, arrhythmias, NEC, infection, graft vs host disease, and death. This widely accepted treatment is repeated if necessary to keep indirect bilirubin levels in a safe range (see Tables 91–2 and 91–3). See Exchange Transfusion in Chapter 92.

Various factors may affect the decision to perform an exchange transfusion in an individual patient. The appearance of clinical signs suggesting kernicterus is an indication for exchange transfusion at any level of serum bilirubin. A healthy full-term infant with physiologic or breast milk jaundice may tolerate a concentration slightly higher than 25 mg/dL with no apparent ill effect, whereas kernicterus may develop in a sick premature infant at a significantly lower level. A level approaching that considered critical for the individual infant may be an indication for exchange transfusion during the 1st day or two of life when a further rise is anticipated, but not on the 4th day in term infants or on the 7th day in premature infants, when an imminent fall may be anticipated as the hepatic conjugating mechanism becomes more effective.

OTHER THERAPIES. *Tin (Sn)-protoporphyrin* (or tin-mesoporphyrin) administration has also been proposed for reduction of bilirubin levels. It may inhibit the conversion of biliverdin to bilirubin by heme oxygenase. A single intramuscular dose on the 1st day of life may reduce the need for phototherapy. Such therapy may be beneficial when jaundice is anticipated (G6PD deficiency) or when blood products are discouraged (Jehovah's Witness). In patients with hyperbilirubinemia, bilirubin levels may decline, but the effect is no greater than that achieved with phototherapy. Complications include transient erythema if the infant is receiving phototherapy. More data are needed on efficacy and toxicity before these compounds can be recommended as therapy for hyperbilirubinemia.

Intravenous immunoglobulin (500 mg/kg/dose over a 4 hr period), given q12 hr for 3 doses, is effective in reducing bilirubin levels in patients with Coombs-positive hemolytic anemia, presumably by reducing hemolysis.

Ahlfors CE: Bilirubin-albumin binding and free bilirubin. *J Perinatol* 2001;21 (Suppl):40.

Ahlfors CE: Unbound bilirubin associated with kernicterus: A historical approach. *J Pediatr* 2000;137:540.

Alpay F, Sarici SU, Tosuncuk HD, et al: The value of first-day bilirubin measurement in predicting the development of significant hyperbilirubinemia in healthy term newborns. *Pediatrics* 2000;106 available at http://www.pediatrics.org/cgi/content/full/106/2/e16.

American Academy of Pediatrics, Subcommittee on Neonatal Hyperbilirubinemia: Neonatal jaundice and kernicterus. *Pediatrics* 2001;108: 763.

Bertini G, Dani C, Pezzati M, et al: Prevention of bilirubin encephalopathy. *Biol Neonate* 2001;79:219.

Bhutani V, Johnson L, Sivier E: Predictive ability of a predischarge hour specific serum bilirubin for subsequent significant hyperbilirubinemia in healthy term and near-term newborns. *Pediatrics* 1999;103:6.

Centers for Disease Control and Prevention: Kernicterus in full-term infants—United States, 1994–1998. *MMWR Morb Mortal Wkly Rep* 2001;50:491.

Dennery PA, Seidman DS, Stevenson DK: Neonatal hyperbilirubinemia. *N Engl J Med* 2001;344:581.

Ebbesen F: Recurrence of kernicterus in term and near-term infants in Denmark. *Acta Paediatr* 2000;89:1213.

Hannam S, McDonnell M, Rennie JM: Investigation of prolonged neonatal jaundice. *Acta Paediatr* 2000;89:694.

Hansen TWR: Phototherapy for neonatal jaundice—still in need of fine tuning. *Acta Paediatr* 2000;89:770.

Jackson JC: Adverse events associated with exchange transfusion in healthy and ill newborns. *Pediatrics* 1997;99 http://www.pediatrics.org/cgi/content/full/99/5/e7.

Johnson LH: System-based approach to management of neonatal jaundice and prevention of kernicterus. *J Pediatr* 2002;140:396.

Kappas A, Drummond GS, Valaes T: A single dose of sn-mesoporphyrin prevents development of severe hyperbilirubinemia in glucose-6-phosphate dehydrogenase–deficient newborns. *Pediatrics* 2001;108:25.

Kappas A, Munson DP, Marshall JR: Sn-mesoporphyrin interdiction of severe hyperbilirubinemia in Jehovah's Witness newborns as an alternative to exchange transfusion. *Pediatrics* 2001;108:1374.

Madlon-Kay DJ: Recognition of the presence and severity of newborn jaundice by parents, nurses, physicians, and icterometer. *Pediatrics* 1997;100 www.pediatrics.org/cgi/content/full/100/3/e3.

Maisels MJ, Kring E: Rebound in serum bilirubin level following intensive phototherapy. *Arch Pediatr Adolesc Med* 2002;156:669.

Maisels MJ, Newman TB: Bilirubin and neurological dysfunction—do we need to change what we are doing? *Pediatr Res* 2001;50:677.

Maisels MJ, Newman TB: Kernicterus in otherwise healthy, breast-fed term newborns. *Pediatrics* 1995;96:730.

Maruo Y, Nishizawa K, Sato H, et al: Association of neonatal hyperbilirubinemia with bilirubin UDP-glucuronosyltransferase polymorphism. *Pediatrics* 1999;103: 1224.

Mills JF, Tudehope D: Fibreoptic phototherapy for neonatal jaundice. *Cochrane Database Syst Rev* 2001;1:CD002060.

Monaghan G, Ryan M, Seddon R, et al: Genetic variation in bilirubin UDP-glucuronosyltransferase gene promoter and Gilbert's syndrome. *Lancet* 1996;347: 578.

Newman TB, Xiong B, Gonzales VM, Escobar GJ: Prediction and prevention of extreme neonatal hyperbilirubinemia in a mature health maintenance organization. *Arch Pediatr Adolesc Med* 2000;154:1140.

Rubaltelli FF, Da Riol R, D'Amore ESG, et al: The bronze baby syndrome: Evidence of increased tissue concentration of copper porphyrins. *Acta Paediatr* 1996;85: 381.

Soorani-Lunsing I, Woltil HA, Hadders-Algra M: Are moderate degrees of hyperbilirubinemia in healthy term neonates really safe for the brain? *Pediatr Res* 2001;50:701.

Wennberg RP: The blood-brain barrier and bilirubin encephalopathy. *Cell Mol Neurobiol* 2000;20:97.

Yokochi K: Magnetic resonance imaging in children with kernicterus. *Acta Paediatr* 1995;84:937.

Chapter 92

Blood Disorders *Barbara J. Stoll and Robert M. Kliegman*

92.1 Anemia in the Newborn Infant

Hemoglobin increases with advancing gestational age: at term, cord blood hemoglobin is 16.8 g/dL (14–20 g/dL); hemoglobin levels in very low birthweight (VLBW) infants are 1–2 g/dL below those at term (Fig. 92–1). Less than the normal range of hemoglobin for birthweight and postnatal age is defined as anemia (see Table 438–1). A "physiologic" decrease in hemoglobin content is noticed at 8–12 wk in term infants (hemoglobin, 11 g/dL) and at about 6 wk in premature infants (7–10 g/dL).

Infants born by cesarean section may have a lower hematocrit (Hct) than do those born vaginally. *Anemia at birth* is manifested as pallor, heart failure, or shock (Fig. 92–2). It may be due to acute or chronic blood loss, hemolysis, or underproduction of erythrocytes. It is usually caused by hemolytic disease of the

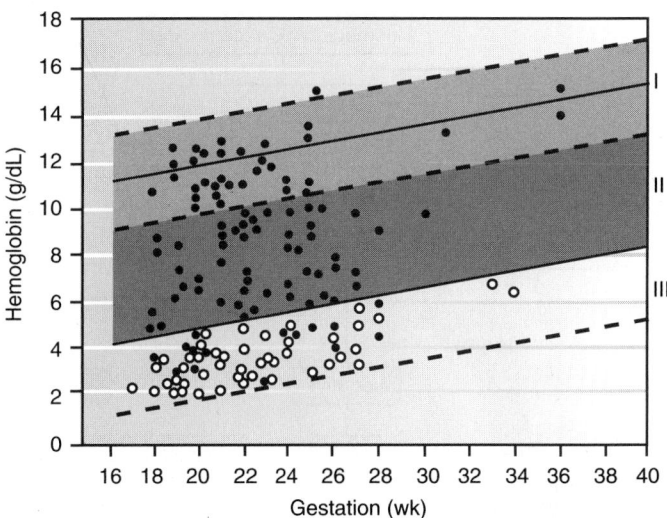

FIGURE 92–1. Range (mean and 95% confidence limits) of hemoglobin concentration from 16 to 40 wk of gestational age from normal (zone I) fetuses obtained by cordocentesis (percutaneous umbilical blood sample). *Solid circles* depict maternal red blood cell isoimmunization; *open circles* indicate hemoglobin levels in fetuses with ultrasonographic evidence of hydrops (zone III). (From Soothill P: Cordocentesis: Role in assessment of fetal condition. *Clin Perinatol* 1989;16:755.)

newborn but may also be a result of tearing or cutting of the umbilical cord during delivery, abnormal cord insertion, communicating placental vessels, placenta previa or abruptio, nuchal cord, incision into the placenta, internal hemorrhage (liver, spleen, or intracranial), α-thalassemia, congenital parvovirus infection or hypoplastic anemia, and twin-twin transfusion in monozygotic twins with arteriovenous placental connections (Chapter 86).

Transplacental hemorrhage with bleeding from the fetal into the maternal circulation has been reported in 5–15% of pregnancies, but unless severe, it is not usually sufficient to cause clinically apparent anemia at birth. The cause of transplacental hemorrhage is not clear, but its occurrence has been proved by demonstrating significant amounts of fetal hemoglobin and red blood cells (RBCs) in maternal blood on the day of delivery by the Kleihauer-Betke test or by flow cytometry methods to detect fetal cells in maternal blood. If the infant has severe anemia with heart failure, emergency exchange transfusion to restore Hct and oxygen-carrying capacity may be needed.

Acute blood loss usually results in severe distress at birth, initially with a normal hemoglobin level, no hepatosplenomegaly, and early onset of shock. In contrast, chronic blood loss in utero produces marked pallor, less distress, a low hemoglobin level with microcytic indices, and if severe, heart failure.

Anemia appearing in the first few days after birth is also most frequently a result of hemolytic disease of the newborn. Other causes are hemorrhagic disease of the newborn, bleeding from an improperly tied or clamped umbilical cord, large cephalohematoma, intracranial hemorrhage, or subcapsular bleeding from rupture of the liver, spleen, adrenals, or kidneys. Rapid decreases in hemoglobin or Hct values during the first few days of life may be the initial clue to these conditions.

Later in the neonatal period, delayed anemia may develop as a result of hemolytic disease of the newborn, with or without exchange transfusion or phototherapy. Congenital hemolytic anemia (spherocytosis) occasionally appears during the 1st mo of life, and hereditary nonspherocytic hemolytic anemia has been described during the neonatal period secondary to deficiency of glucose-6-phosphate dehydrogenase (G6PD) and

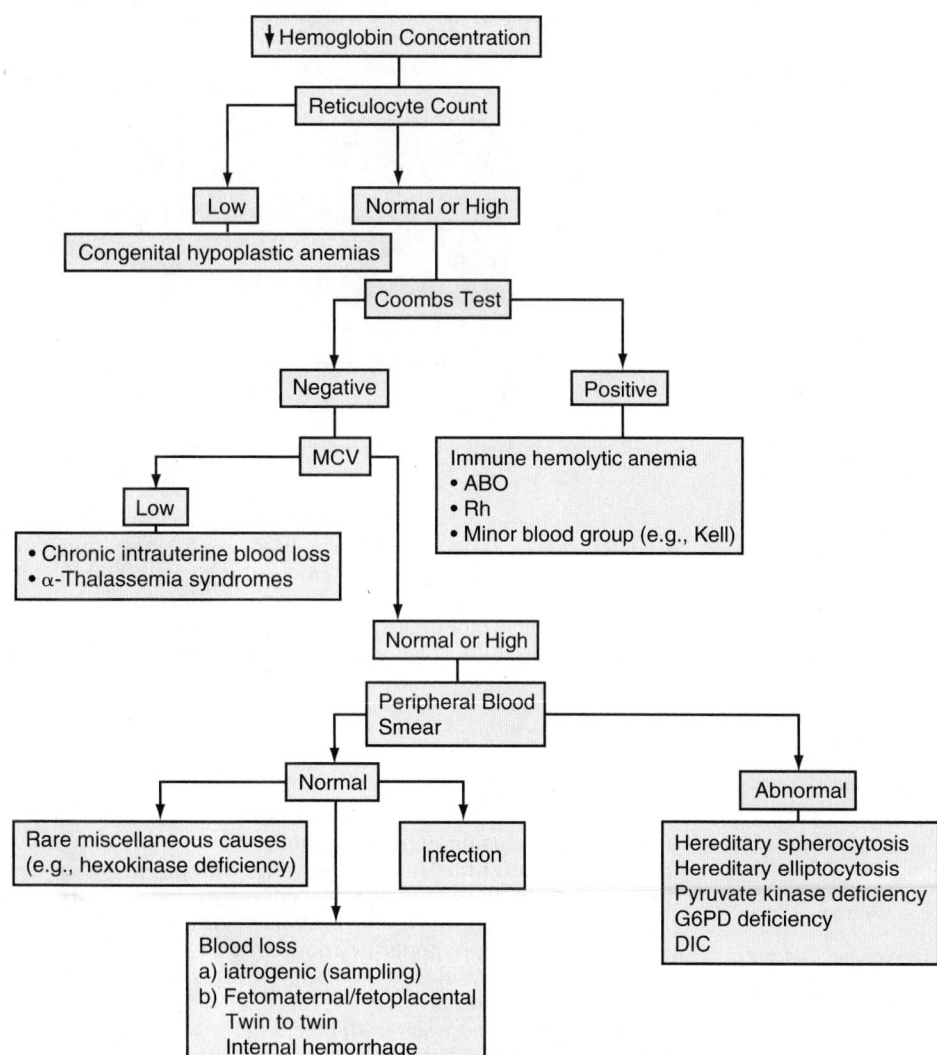

FIGURE 92–2. Diagnostic approach to anemia in newborn infants. MCV = mean corpuscular volume; G6PD = glucose-6-phosphate dehydrogenase. (From Blanchette V, Zipursky A: Assessment of anemia in newborn infants. *Clin Perinatol* 1984;11:489.)

pyruvate kinase. Bleeding from hemangiomas of the upper gastrointestinal tract or from ulcers caused by aberrant gastric mucosa in a Meckel diverticulum or duplication is a rare source of anemia in newborns. Repeated blood sampling of infants requiring frequent monitoring of blood gas and chemistry parameters is a common cause of anemia. Deficiency of minerals such as copper may cause anemia in infants maintained on total parenteral nutrition.

Anemia of prematurity occurs in low-birthweight infants 1–3 mo after birth, is associated with hemoglobin levels below 7–10 g/dL, and is clinically manifested as pallor, apnea, poor weight gain, decreased activity, tachypnea, tachycardia, and feeding problems. Repeated phlebotomy for blood tests, shortened RBC survival, rapid growth, and the physiologic effects of the transition from fetal (low Pao_2 and hemoglobin saturation) to neonatal life (high Pao_2 and hemoglobin saturation) contribute to anemia of prematurity. The oxygen available to neonatal tissue is lower than that in adults, but a neonate's erythropoietin response is attenuated for the degree of anemia, and as a result, hemoglobin and reticulocyte levels are low. In VLBW infants, delayed clamping of the umbilical cord with the infant held below the level of the placenta may enhance placental-infant transfusion and reduce postnatal transfusion needs. This maneuver should not delay any needed resuscitation and may lead to hyperviscosity.

Treatment of neonatal anemia by blood transfusion depends on the severity of symptoms, the hemoglobin level, and the presence of co-morbid diseases (bronchopulmonary dysplasia, cyanotic congenital heart disease, hyaline membrane disease) that interfere with oxygen delivery. The need for treatment with blood should be balanced against the risks of transfusion, including hemolytic transfusion reactions, exposure to blood product preservatives and other potential toxins, volume overload, possible increased risk of retinopathy of prematurity and necrotizing enterocolitis, graft vs host reaction, and transfusion-acquired infection (cytomegalovirus [CMV], HIV, hepatitis B and C). The risk of CMV infection can be almost eliminated by the use of CMV antibody–negative blood and the highly recommended, irradiated white blood cell–poor blood; the risk of acquiring HIV and hepatitis B and C viruses is reduced but not eliminated by antibody screening of donated blood. Blood banking techniques that limit multiple donor exposure should be encouraged. Variations in blood transfusion practices among different neonatal intensive care units have been documented. Although transfusion guidelines for preterm infants have been proposed (Table 92–1), they have not been subjected to rigorous clinical study. Nonetheless, these guidelines have led to a decline in the number of unnecessary transfusions.

Asymptomatic full-term infants with a hemoglobin level of 10 g/dL may be monitored, whereas symptomatic neonates born after abruptio placentae or with severe hemolytic disease of the newborn warrant immediate transfusion. Preterm infants who have repeated episodes of apnea and bradycardia despite

TABLE 92–1. Transfusion Protocol

Hct/Hgb	Respiratory Support and/or Symptoms	Transfusion Volume
Hct ≤35/Hgb ≤11	Infants requiring moderate or significant mechanical ventilation (MAP >8 cm H_2O and F_{IO_2} >0.4)	15 mL/kg PRBC* over period of 2–4 hr
Hct ≤30/Hgb ≤10	Infants requiring minimal respiratory support (any mechanical ventilation or endotracheal/nasal CPAP >6 cm H_2O and F_{IO_2} ≤0.4)	15 mL/kg PRBCs over period of 2–4 hr
Hct ≤25/Hgb ≤8	Infants not requiring mechanical ventilation but who are receiving supplemental O_2 or CPAP with an F_{IO_2} ≤0.4 and in whom 1 or more of the following is present:	20 mL/kg PRBCs over period of 2–4 hr (divide into 2–10 mL/kg volumes if fluid sensitive)
	• ≤24 hr of tachycardia (HR > 180) or tachypnea (RR > 80)	
	• An increased oxygen requirement from the previous 48 hr, defined as a ≥4-fold increase in nasal canula flow (i.e., 0.25 to 1 L/min) or an increase in nasal CPAP ≥20% from the previous 48 hr (i.e., 5 to 6 cm H_2O)	
	• Weight gain <10 g/kg/day over the previous 4 days while receiving ≥100 kcal/kg/day	
	• An increase in episodes of apnea and bradycardia (>9 episodes in a 24-hr period or ≥2 episodes in 24 hr requiring bag and mask ventilation) while receiving therapeutic doses of methylxanthines	
	• Undergoing surgery	
Hct ≤20/Hgb ≤7	Asymptomatic and an absolute reticulocyte count <100 000 cells/μL	20 mL/kg PRBCs over period of 2–4 hr (2–10 mL/kg volumes)

Hct = hematocrit; Hgb = hemoglobin; MAP = mean airway pressure; F_{IO_2} = fractional inspired oxygen; PRBC = packed red blood cells; CPAP = continuous positive airway pressure; HR = heart rate; RR = respiratory rate*. RBC should be irradiated prior to transfusion.

From Ohls RK, Ehrenkranz RA, Wright LL, et al: Effects of early erythropoietin therapy on the transfusion requirements of preterm infants below 1250 grams birth weight: A multicenter, randomized, controlled trial. Pediatrics 2001; 108:934–42.

theophylline therapy and a hemoglobin level of 8 g/dL or lower may benefit from RBC transfusion. In addition, infants with hyaline membrane disease or severe chronic lung disease may need hemoglobin levels of 12–14 g/dL to improve oxygen delivery. No transfusion is needed to replace blood removed for testing or for mild asymptomatic anemia. Asymptomatic neonates with reticulocytopenia and hemoglobin levels of 7 g/dL or lower may require transfusion; if a transfusion is not provided, close observation is essential. Packed RBC transfusion (10–20 mL/kg) is given at a rate of 2–3 mL/kg/hr to raise the hemoglobin concentration; 2 mL/kg raises the hemoglobin level 0.5–1 g/dL. Hemorrhage should be treated with whole blood if available; alternatively, fluid resuscitation is initiated and followed by packed RBC transfusion.

Recombinant human erythropoietin (r-HuEPO) has been used to prevent or treat chronic anemia associated with prematurity, bronchopulmonary dysplasia, and the hyporegenerative anemia of erythroblastosis fetalis. Anemia of prematurity is associated with abnormally low endogenous levels of serum erythropoietin but with r-HuEPO–responsive erythrocyte progenitor cells. Therapy with r-HuEPO may be given by the intravenous or subcutaneous routes and must be supplemented with oral iron and possibly vitamin E. Doses and regimens vary. Treatment with erythropoietin and iron does not have a major impact on transfusion requirements, and therefore routine use of erythropoietin in VLBW infants is not recommended.

92.2 Hemolytic Disease of the Newborn (Erythroblastosis Fetalis)

Erythroblastosis fetalis is caused by the transplacental passage of maternal antibody active against RBC antigens of the infant and is characterized by an increased rate of RBC destruction. It continues to be an important cause of anemia and jaundice in newborn infants despite the development of a method of preventing maternal isoimmunization by Rh antigens. Although more than 60 different RBC antigens capable of eliciting an antibody response in a suitable recipient have been identified, significant disease is associated primarily with the D antigen of the Rh group and with incompatibility of ABO factors. Rarely, hemolytic disease may be caused by C or E antigens or by other RBC antigens such as C^W, C^X, D^U, K (Kell), M, Duffy, S, P, MNS, Xg, Lutheran, Diego, and Kidd. Anti-Lewis antibodies do not cause disease.

HEMOLYTIC DISEASE OF THE NEWBORN CAUSED BY RH INCOMPATIBILITY

The Rh antigenic determinants are genetically transmitted from each parent and determine the Rh type and direct the production of a number of blood group factors (C, c, D, d, E, and e). Each factor can elicit a specific antibody response under suitable conditions; 90% are due to D antigen and the remainder to C or E.

Pathogenesis. Isoimmune hemolytic disease from D antigen is approximately three times more frequent in white persons than blacks. When Rh-positive blood is infused into an Rh-negative woman through error or when small quantities (usually more than 1 mL) of Rh-positive fetal blood containing D antigen inherited from an Rh-positive father enter the maternal circulation during pregnancy, with spontaneous or induced abortion, or at delivery, antibody formation against D antigen may be induced in the unsensitized Rh-negative recipient mother. Once sensitization has taken place, considerably smaller doses of antigen can stimulate an increase in antibody titer. Initially, a rise in IgM antibody occurs, which is later replaced by IgG antibody; the latter readily crosses the placenta and causes hemolytic manifestations.

Hemolytic disease rarely occurs during a first pregnancy because transfusions of Rh-positive fetal blood into an Rh-negative mother tend to occur near the time of delivery, too late for the mother to become sensitized and transmit antibody to her infant before delivery. The fact that 55% of Rh-positive fathers are heterozygous (D/d) and may have Rh-negative offspring and that fetal-to-maternal transfusion occurs in only 50% of pregnancies reduces the chance of sensitization, as does small family size, in which the opportunities for its occurrence are reduced. Finally, the capacity of Rh-negative women to form antibodies is variable, some producing low titers even after adequate antigenic challenge. Thus, the overall incidence of isoimmunization of Rh-negative mothers at risk is low, with antibody to D detected in less than 10% of those studied, even after five or more pregnancies; only about 5% ever have babies with hemolytic disease.

When the mother and fetus are also incompatible with respect to group A or B, the mother is partially protected against sensitization by the rapid removal of Rh-positive cells from her circulation by her pre-existing anti-A or anti-B, which are IgM antibodies and do not cross the placenta. Once a mother has been sensitized, her infant is likely to have hemolytic disease. The severity of Rh illness tends to worsen with successive pregnancies. The possibility that the first affected infant after sensitization may represent the end of the mother's childbearing potential for Rh-positive infants argues urgently for the prevention of sensitization when possible. Such prevention consists of the injection of anti-D gamma globulin (RhoGAM) into the mother immediately after the delivery of each Rh-positive infant (see later).

Clinical Manifestations. A wide spectrum of hemolytic disease occurs in affected infants born to sensitized mothers, depending on the nature of the individual immune response. The severity of the disease may range from only laboratory evidence of mild hemolysis (15% of cases) to severe anemia with compensatory hyperplasia of erythropoietic tissue leading to massive enlargement of the liver and spleen. When the compensatory capacity of the hematopoietic system is exceeded, profound anemia occurs and results in pallor, signs of cardiac decompensation (cardiomegaly, respiratory distress), massive anasarca, and circulatory collapse. This clinical picture of excessive abnormal fluid in two or more fetal compartments (skin, pleura, pericardium, placenta, peritoneum, amniotic fluid), termed *hydrops fetalis,* frequently results in death in utero or shortly after birth. With the use of RhoGAM to prevent Rh sensitization, nonimmune (nonhemolytic) conditions are more frequent causes of hydrops (Table 92–2). The severity of hydrops is related to the level of anemia and the degree of reduction in serum albumin (oncotic pressure), which is due in part to hepatic dysfunction. Alternatively, heart failure may increase right heart pressure, with the subsequent development of edema and ascites. Failure to initiate spontaneous effective ventilation because of pulmonary edema or bilateral pleural effusions results in birth asphyxia; after successful resuscitation, severe respiratory distress may develop. Petechiae, purpura, and thrombocytopenia may also be present in severe cases as a result of decreased platelet production or the presence of concurrent disseminated intravascular coagulation.

Jaundice may be absent at birth because of placental clearance of lipid-soluble unconjugated bilirubin, but in severe cases, bilirubin pigments stain the amniotic fluid, cord, and vernix caseosa yellow. Jaundice is generally evident on the 1st day of life because the infant's bilirubin-conjugating and excretory systems are unable to cope with the load resulting from massive hemolysis. Indirect-reacting bilirubin therefore accumulates postnatally and may rapidly reach extremely high levels and present a significant risk of bilirubin encephalopathy. The risk of kernicterus developing from hemolytic disease is greater than from comparable nonhemolytic hyperbilirubinemia, although the risk in an individual patient may be affected by other complications (e.g., anoxia, acidosis). Hypoglycemia occurs frequently in infants with severe isoimmune hemolytic disease and

TABLE 92–2. Etiology of Hydrops Fetalis*

Category	Disorders	Category	Disorders
Anemia	Immune (Rh, Kell) hemolysis	Teratomas	Choriocarcinoma
	α-Thalassemia		Sacrococcygeal teratoma
	Red blood cell enzyme deficiencies (G6PD)	Tumors and storage diseases	Neuroblastoma
	Fetomaternal hemorrhage		Hepatoblastoma
	Donor in twin-to-twin transfusion		Gaucher disease
Cardiac dysrhythmias	Supraventricular tachycardia		Niemann-Pick disease
	Atrial flutter		Mucolipidosis
	Congenital heart block		GM$_1$ gangliosidosis
Structural heart lesions	Premature closure of foramen ovale		Mucopolysaccharidosis
	Tricuspid insufficiency	Chromosome abnormalities	Trisomy 13, 15, 16, 18, 21
	Hypoplastic left heart		XX/XY, 45XO
	Endocardial cushion defect		Partial duplication of chromosome 11, 15, 17, 18
	Cardiomyopathy		Partial deletion of chromosome 13, 18
	Endocardial fibroelastosis		Triploidy
	Tuberous sclerosis with cardiac rhabdomyoma		Tetraploidy
	Pericardial teratoma	Bone diseases	Osteogenesis imperfecta
Vascular	Chorioangioma of placenta, chorionic vessels, or umbilical vessels		Asphyxiating thoracic dystrophy
			Skeletal dysplasias
	Umbilical artery aneurysm	Congenital infections	Cytomegalovirus
	Angiomyxoma of umbilical cord		Parvovirus
	True knot of umbilical cord		Rubella
	Hepatic hemangioma		Toxoplasmosis
	Cerebral arteriovenous malformation (aneurysm of vein of Galen)		Syphilis
			Leptospirosis
	Angiosteohypertrophy (Klippel-Trénaunay syndrome)		Chagas disease
	Thrombosis of renal or umbilical vein or inferior vena cava	Others	Bowel obstruction with perforation and meconium peritonitis, volvulus
	Recipient in twin-to-twin transfusion		Hepatic fibrosis
Lymphatic	Lymphangiectasia		Beckwith-Wiedemann syndrome
	Cystic hygroma		Prune-belly syndrome
	Chylothorax, chylous ascites		Congenital nephrosis
	Noonan syndrome		Infant of a diabetic mother
	Multiple pterygium syndrome		Myotonic dystrophy
Central nervous system	Absent corpus callosum		Neu-Laxova syndrome
	Encephalocele		Maternal therapy with indomethacin
	Intracranial hemorrhage	Idiopathic	Multiple congenital anomaly syndromes
	Holoprosencephaly		
Thoracic lesions	Cystic adenomatoid malformation of lung		
	Mediastinal teratoma		
	Diaphragmatic hernia		
	Sequestered lung		

The incidence of nonimmune (nonhemolytic) hydrops fetalis is 1/2,000–1/3,500 births.
G6PD = glucose-6-phosphate dehydrogenase.
Modified from Phibbs R: In Polin N, Fox W (editors): Fetal and Neonatal Physiology, 2nd ed. Philadelphia, WB Saunders, 1998.

may be related to hyperinsulinism and hypertrophy of the pancreatic islet cells in these infants.

Infants born after intrauterine transfusion for prenatally diagnosed erythroblastosis may be severely affected because the indications for transfusion are evidence of already severe disease in utero (e.g., hydrops, fetal anemia). Such infants usually have very high (but extremely variable) cord levels of bilirubin, which reflects the severity of the hemolysis and its effects on hepatic function. Infants treated with intra-umbilical vein transfusions in utero may also have a benign postnatal course if the anemia and hydrops resolve before birth. Anemia from continuing hemolysis may be masked by the previous intrauterine transfusion, and the clinical manifestations of erythroblastosis may be superimposed on various degrees of immaturity resulting from spontaneous or induced premature delivery.

Laboratory Data. Before treatment, the direct Coombs test is usually positive, and anemia is generally present. The cord blood hemoglobin content varies and is usually proportional to the severity of the disease; with hydrops fetalis it may be as low as 3–4 g/dL. Alternatively, despite hemolysis, it may be within the normal range because of compensatory bone marrow and extramedullary hematopoiesis. The blood smear typically shows polychromasia and a marked increase in nucleated RBCs. The reticulocyte count is increased. The white blood cell count is usually normal but may be elevated; thrombocytopenia may develop in severe cases. Cord bilirubin is generally between 3 and 5 mg/dL; direct-reacting (conjugated) bilirubin may be substantially elevated. Indirect-reacting bilirubin rises rapidly to high levels in the 1st 6 hr of life.

After intrauterine transfusions, cord blood may show a normal hemoglobin concentration, negative direct Coombs test, predominantly type O Rh-negative adult RBCs, and a relatively normal smear. Marked elevation of both indirect- and direct-reacting bilirubin levels has been reported in these infants.

Diagnosis. Definitive diagnosis of erythroblastosis fetalis requires demonstration of blood group incompatibility and corresponding antibody bound to the infant's RBCs.

ANTENATAL DIAGNOSIS. In Rh-negative women, a history of previous transfusions, abortion, or pregnancy should suggest the possibility of sensitization. Expectant parents' blood types should be tested for potential incompatibility, and the maternal titer of IgG antibodies to D antigen should be assayed at 12–16, 28–32, and 36 wk. Fetal Rh status may be determined by isolating fetal cells or fetal DNA (plasma) from the maternal circulation or by amniocentesis and polymerase chain reaction with primers to the Rh gene. The presence of measurable antibody titer at the beginning of pregnancy, a rapid rise in titer, or a titer of 1:64 or greater suggests significant hemolytic disease, although the exact titer correlates poorly with the severity of disease. If a mother is found to have antibody against D antigen at a titer of 1:16 or greater at any time during a subsequent pregnancy, the severity of fetal disease should be monitored by amniocentesis, percutaneous umbilical blood sampling (PUBS), and ultrasonography. If the mother has a history of a previously affected infant or a stillbirth, an Rh-positive infant is usually equally or more severely affected than the previous infant, and the severity of disease in the fetus should be monitored.

Assessment of the fetus may require information obtained from ultrasonography, amniocentesis, and PUBS. Real-time ultrasonography is used to detect the progression of disease, with hydrops defined as skin or scalp edema, pleural or pericardial effusions, and ascites. Early ultrasonographic signs of hydrops include organomegaly (liver, spleen, heart), the double–bowel wall sign (bowel edema), and placental thickening. Progression to polyhydramnios, ascites, pleural or pericardial effusions, and skin or scalp edema may then follow. If pleural effusions precede ascites and hydrops by a significant length of time, causes other than fetal anemia should be suspected (see Table 92–2). Extramedullary hematopoiesis and, less so, hepatic congestion compress the intrahepatic vessels and produce venous stasis with portal hypertension, hepatocellular dysfunction, and decreased albumin synthesis.

Hydrops is present when fetal hemoglobin is less than 5 g/dL, frequent when under 7 g/dL, and variable between 7 and 9 g/dL. Real-time ultrasonography predicts fetal well-being by the biophysical profile (see Table 85–2), whereas Doppler ultrasonography assesses fetal distress by demonstrating increased vascular resistance. In pregnancies with ultrasonographic evidence of hemolysis (hepatosplenomegaly), early or late hydrops, or fetal distress, amniocentesis or PUBS should be performed.

Amniocentesis is used to assess fetal hemolysis. Hemolysis of fetal RBCs produces hyperbilirubinemia before the onset of severe anemia. Bilirubin is cleared by the placenta, but a significant proportion enters the amniotic fluid and can be measured by spectrophotometry. Amniocentesis is performed if the mother has evidence of sensitization (titer of 1:16), if the father is Rh positive, or if ultrasonographic signs of hemolysis, hydrops, or distress are present. Ultrasonographically guided transabdominal aspiration of amniotic fluid may be performed as early as 18–20 wk of gestation. Spectrophotometric scanning of amniotic fluid wavelengths demonstrates a positive optical density (OD) deviation of absorption for bilirubin from normal at 450 nm (Fig. 92–3). The OD_{450} is a reflection of fetal bilirubin levels and thus hemolysis and indicates the severity of anemia and the risk of intrauterine death. With maturity, the level of amniotic fluid bilirubin normally declines, so fetal risk is assessed during gestation in terms of three relative, but declining zones of OD_{450}, with zone III representing the highest risk. However, some fetuses in zone III do not have life-threatening fetal anemia and thus do not require intrauterine transfusion. If the OD_{450} is in zone III or if hydrops or other signs suggesting fetal anemia are present, PUBS should be performed to determine fetal hemoglobin levels and packed RBCs transfused in those with serious anemia (Hct of 25–30%). Amniocentesis and cordocentesis are invasive procedures with risks to both the fetus and mother, including fetal death, fetal bleeding, fetal bradycardia, worsening of alloimmunization, premature rupture of membranes,

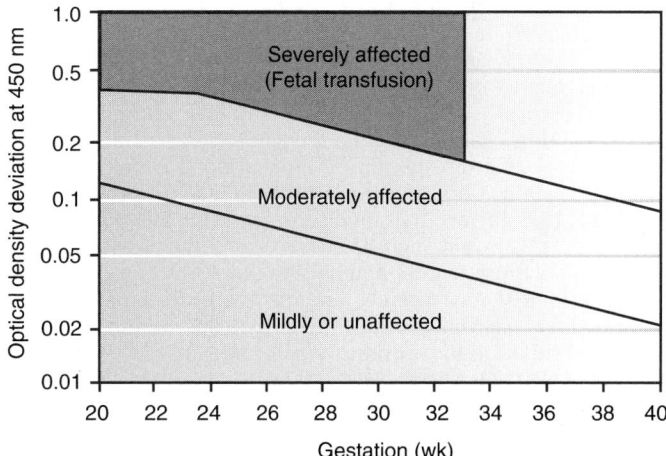

FIGURE 92–3. Optical density of amniotic fluid plotted against weeks of gestation. Severely affected infants are managed by intrauterine transfusion before 32–33 wk and delivery thereafter. A moderately affected fetus warrants repeated amniocentesis, monitoring by cardiotocography, and delivery at 34–37 wk. A mildly affected fetus warrants delivery at 37–40 wk. (From Blood group incompatibility. In Beischer NA, Mackay EV, Colditz PB [editors]: *Obstetrics and the Newborn*, 3rd ed. Philadelphia, WB Saunders, 1997.)

preterm labor, and chorioamnionitis. Noninvasive measurements to detect fetal anemia are desirable. In fetuses without hydrops, moderate to severe anemia can be detected noninvasively by demonstration of an increase in the peak velocity of systolic blood flow in the middle cerebral artery by Doppler ultrasound. This and other noninvasive techniques deserve further study.

POSTNATAL DIAGNOSIS. Immediately after the birth of any infant to an Rh-negative woman, blood from the umbilical cord or from the infant should be examined for ABO blood group, Rh type, Hct and hemoglobin, and reaction of the direct Coombs test. If the Coombs test is positive, a baseline serum bilirubin level should be measured, and a commercially available RBC panel should be used to identify RBC antibodies present in the mother's serum, both tests being performed not only to establish the diagnosis but also to ensure selection of the most compatible blood for exchange transfusion should it be necessary. The direct Coombs test is usually strongly positive in clinically affected infants and may remain so for a few days up to several months.

Treatment. The main goals of therapy are to (1) prevent intrauterine or extrauterine death from severe anemia and hypoxia and (2) avoid neurotoxicity from hyperbilirubinemia.

TREATMENT OF AN UNBORN INFANT. Survival of severely affected fetuses has been improved by the use of ultrasonographic and amniotic fluid analysis to identify the need for in utero transfusion. Intrauterine transfusion into the fetal peritoneal cavity is being replaced by direct intravascular (umbilical vein) transfusion of packed RBCs. Hydrops or fetal anemia (Hct <30%) is an indication for umbilical vein transfusion in infants with pulmonary immaturity (see Fig. 92–1). Intravascular transfusion is facilitated by maternal and hence fetal sedation with diazepam and by fetal paralysis with pancuronium. Packed RBCs are given by slow-push infusion after cross matching with the mother's serum. The cells should be obtained from a CMV-negative donor and irradiated to kill lymphocytes to avoid graft vs host disease. Transfusions should achieve a post-transfusion Hct of 45–55% and can be repeated every 3–5 wk. Indications for delivery include pulmonary maturity, fetal distress, complications of PUBS, or 35–37 wk of gestation.

TREATMENT OF A LIVEBORN INFANT. The birth should be attended by a physician skilled in neonatal resuscitation. Fresh, low-titer, group O, irradiated Rh-negative blood crossmatched against maternal serum should be immediately available. If clinical signs of severe hemolytic anemia (pallor, hepatosplenomegaly, edema, petechiae, or ascites) are evident at birth, immediate resuscitation and supportive therapy, temperature stabilization, and monitoring before proceeding with exchange transfusion may save some severely affected infants. Such therapy should include correction of acidosis with 1–2 mEq/kg of sodium bicarbonate; a small transfusion of compatible packed RBCs to correct anemia; volume expansion for hypotension, especially in those with hydrops; and provision of assisted ventilation for respiratory failure.

EXCHANGE TRANSFUSION. When an infant's clinical condition at birth does not require an immediate full or partial exchange transfusion, the decision to perform one should be based on a judgment that the infant has a high risk of rapid development of a dangerous degree of anemia or hyperbilirubinemia. Cord hemoglobin of 10 g/dL or less and bilirubin of 5 mg/dL or more suggest severe hemolysis but inconsistently predict the need for exchange transfusion. Some physicians consider previous kernicterus or severe erythroblastosis in a sibling, reticulocyte counts greater than 15%, and prematurity to be additional factors supporting a decision for early exchange transfusion. Intrauterine, intravascular transfusions have decreased the need for exchange transfusion.

The hemoglobin concentration, Hct, and serum bilirubin level should be measured at 4–6 hr intervals initially, with extension to longer intervals if and as the rate of change diminishes. The decision to perform an exchange transfusion is based on the likelihood that the trend of bilirubin levels plotted against hours of age indicates that serum bilirubin will reach the levels indicated in Tables 91–2 and 91–3. Term infants with levels of 20 mg/dL or higher have an increased risk of kernicterus. Ordinary transfusions of compatible Rh-negative irradiated RBCs may be necessary to correct anemia at any stage of the disease up to 6–8 wk of age, when the infant's own blood-forming mechanism may be expected to take over. Weekly determinations of hemoglobin or Hct should be done until a spontaneous rise has been demonstrated.

Careful monitoring of the serum bilirubin level is essential until a falling trend has been demonstrated in the absence of phototherapy (Chapter 91.4). Even then, an occasional infant, particularly if premature, may experience an unpredicted significant rise in serum bilirubin as late as the 7th day of life. Attempts to predict the attainment of dangerously high levels of serum bilirubin based on observed levels exceeding 6 mg/dL in the 1st 6 hr or 10 mg/dL in the 2nd 6 hr of life or on rates of rise exceeding 0.5–1.0 mg/dL/hr can be unreliable. Measurement of unbound bilirubin may be a more sensitive predictor of the risk associated with hyperbilirubinemia.

Blood for exchange transfusion should be as fresh as possible. Heparin or citrate-phosphate-dextrose-adenine solution may be used as an anticoagulant. If the blood is obtained before delivery, it should be taken from a type O, Rh-negative donor with a low titer of anti-A and anti-B antibodies and should be compatible with the mother's serum by the indirect Coombs test. After delivery, blood should be obtained from an Rh-negative donor whose cells are compatible with both the infant's and the mother's serum; when possible, type O donor cells are generally used, but cells of the infant's ABO blood type may be used when the mother has the same type. A complete cross match, including an indirect Coombs test, should be performed before the 2nd and subsequent transfusions. Blood should be gradually warmed and maintained at a temperature between 35 and 37°C throughout the exchange transfusion. It should be kept well mixed by gentle squeezing or agitation of the bag to avoid sedimentation; otherwise, the use of supernatant serum with a low RBC count at the end of the exchange will leave the infant anemic. Whole blood or packed irradiated RBCs reconstituted with fresh frozen plasma to an Hct of 40% should be used. The infant's stomach should be emptied before transfusion to prevent aspiration, and body temperature should be maintained and vital signs monitored. A competent assistant should be present to help monitor, tally the volume of blood exchanged, and perform emergency procedures.

With strict aseptic technique, the umbilical vein is cannulated with a polyvinyl catheter to a distance no greater than 7 cm in a full-term infant. When free flow of blood is obtained, the catheter is usually in a large hepatic vein or the inferior vena cava. Alternatively, the exchange may be performed through peripheral arterial (drawn out) and venous (infused in) lines. The exchange should be carried out over a 45–60 min period, with aspiration of 20 mL of infant blood alternating with infusion of 20 mL of donor blood. Smaller aliquots (5–10 mL) may be indicated for sick and premature infants. The goal should be an isovolumetric exchange of approximately two blood volumes of the infant (2×85 mL/kg).

Infants with acidosis and hypoxia from respiratory distress, sepsis, or shock may be further compromised by the significant acute acid load contained in citrated blood, which usually has a pH between 7 and 7.2. The subsequent metabolism of citrate may result in metabolic alkalosis later if citrated blood is used. Fresh heparinized blood avoids this problem. During the exchange, blood pH and Pao_2 should be serially monitored because infants often become acidotic and hypoxic during exchange transfusions. Symptomatic hypoglycemia may occur before or during an exchange transfusion in moderately to severely affected infants; it may also occur 1–3 hr after exchange. Acute complications, noted in 5–10% of infants, include transient bradycardia with or without calcium infusion, cyanosis, transient vasospasm, thrombosis, apnea with bradycardia requiring resuscitation, and death. Infectious risks include CMV, HIV, and hepatitis. Necrotizing enterocolitis is a rare complication of exchange transfusion.

The risk of death from an exchange transfusion performed by an experienced physician is 0.3/100 procedures. However, with the decreasing use of this procedure because of the use of phototherapy and prevention of sensitization, the general level of physician competence is decreasing. Thus, it is best if this procedure is performed in experienced neonatal referral centers.

After exchange transfusion, the bilirubin level must be determined at frequent intervals (every 4–8 hr) because bilirubin may rebound 40–50% within hours. Repeated exchange transfusions should be carried out to keep the indirect fraction from exceeding the levels indicated in Table 91–2 for preterm infants and 20 mg/dL for term infants. Symptoms suggestive of kernicterus are mandatory indications for exchange transfusion at any time.

LATE COMPLICATIONS. Infants who have hemolytic disease or who have had an exchange or an intrauterine transfusion must be observed carefully for the development of anemia and cholestasis. Late anemia may be hemolytic or hyporegenerative. Treatment with supplemental iron, erythropoietin, or blood transfusion may be indicated. A mild graft vs host reaction may be manifested as diarrhea, rash, hepatitis, or eosinophilia.

Inspissated bile syndrome refers to the rare occurrence of persistent icterus in association with significant elevations in direct and indirect bilirubin in infants with hemolytic disease. The cause is unclear, but the jaundice clears spontaneously within a few weeks or months.

Portal vein thrombosis and *portal hypertension* may occur in children who have been subjected to exchange transfusion as newborn infants. It is probably associated with prolonged, traumatic, or septic umbilical vein catheterization.

PREVENTION OF RH SENSITIZATION. The risk of initial sensitization of Rh-negative mothers has been reduced from between 10 and 20% to less than 1% by the intramuscular injection of 300 μg of human anti-D globulin (1 mL of RhoGAM) within 72 hr of delivery of an Rh-positive infant, ectopic pregnancy, abdominal trauma in pregnancy, amniocentesis, chorionic villus biopsy, or abortion. This quantity is sufficient to eliminate approximately 10 mL of potentially antigenic fetal cells from the maternal circulation. Large fetal-to-maternal transfers of blood may require proportionately more RhoGAM. RhoGAM administered at 28–32 wk and again at birth (40 wk) is more effective than a single dose. The use of this technique, combined with improved methods of detecting maternal sensitization and measuring the extent of fetal-to-maternal transfusion, plus the use of fewer obstetric procedures that increase the risk of such fetal-to-maternal bleeding (version, manual separation of the placenta, and so on), should further reduce the incidence of erythroblastosis fetalis.

HEMOLYTIC DISEASE OF THE NEWBORN CAUSED BY A AND B INCOMPATIBILITY

ABO incompatibility is the most common cause of hemolytic disease of the newborn. Approximately 15% of live births are at risk, but manifestations of disease develop in only 0.3–2.2%. Major blood group incompatibility between the mother and fetus generally results in milder disease than Rh incompatibility does. Maternal antibody may be formed against B cells if the mother is type A or against A cells if the mother is type B. However, usually, the mother is type O and the infant is type A or B. Although ABO incompatibility occurs in 20–25% of pregnancies, hemolytic disease develops in only 10% of such offspring, and the infants are generally type A_1, which is more antigenic than A_2. Low antigenicity of the ABO factors in the fetus and newborn infant may account for the low incidence of severe ABO hemolytic disease relative to the incidence of incompatibility between the blood groups of the mother and child. Although antibodies against A and B factors occur without previous immunization ("natural" antibodies), they are ordinarily present in the IgM fraction of gamma globulin, which does not cross the placenta. However, univalent, incomplete (albumin active) antibodies to A antigen may be present in the IgG fraction, which does cross the placenta, so A-O isoimmune hemolytic disease may be found in first-born infants. Mothers who have become immunized against A or B factors from a previous incompatible pregnancy also exhibit IgG antibody. These "immune" antibodies are the primary mediators in ABO isoimmune disease.

Clinical Manifestations. Most cases are mild, with jaundice being the only clinical manifestation. The infant is not generally affected at birth; pallor is not present, and hydrops fetalis is extremely rare. The liver and spleen are not greatly enlarged, if at all. Jaundice usually appears during the 1st 24 hr. Rarely, it may become severe, and symptoms and signs of kernicterus develop rapidly.

Diagnosis. A presumptive diagnosis is based on the presence of ABO incompatibility, a weakly to moderately positive direct Coombs test result, and spherocytes in the blood smear, which may at times suggest the presence of hereditary spherocytosis. Hyperbilirubinemia is often the only other laboratory abnormality. The hemoglobin level is usually normal but may be as low as 10–12 g/dL (100–120 g/L). Reticulocytes may be increased to 10–15%, with extensive polychromasia and increased numbers of nucleated RBCs. In 10–20% of affected infants, the unconjugated serum bilirubin level may reach 20 mg/dL or more unless phototherapy is administered.

Treatment. Phototherapy may be effective in lowering serum bilirubin levels (Chapter 91.4). In rare severe cases, treatment is directed at correcting dangerous degrees of anemia or hyperbilirubinemia by exchange transfusions with type O blood of the same Rh type as the infant. Indications for this procedure are similar to those previously described for hemolytic disease caused by Rh incompatibility. Some infants with ABO hemolytic disease may require transfusion of packed RBCs at several weeks of age because of slowly progressive anemia. Post-discharge monitoring of hemoglobin/Hct is essential in newborns with ABO hemolytic disease.

OTHER FORMS OF HEMOLYTIC DISEASE

Blood group incompatibilities other than Rh or ABO (c, E, K, and so on) account for less than 5% of hemolytic disease of the newborn. The direct Coombs test is invariably positive, and exchange transfusion may be indicated for hyperbilirubinemia and anemia. Hemolytic disease, anemia, and hydrops fetalis as a result of anti-Kell antibodies are not predictable from the previous obstetric history, amniotic fluid OD_{450} bilirubin determinants, or the maternal antibody titer. Erythroid suppression may contribute to the anemia; PUBS is beneficial in actually measuring the fetal Hct.

Congenital infections such as cytomegalic inclusion disease, toxoplasmosis, rubella, and syphilis may be manifested as hemolytic anemia, jaundice, hepatosplenomegaly, and thrombocytopenia, but the direct Coombs test result is negative and these conditions usually have other distinguishing clinical findings. Homozygous α-thalassemia may be associated with severe hemolytic anemia and a clinical picture resembling hydrops fetalis; it can be distinguished by a negative direct Coombs test result and characteristic clinical and laboratory findings (Chapter 454.9). Anemia and jaundice may occur in infancy from hereditary spherocytosis (Chapter 450) and, if untreated, can result in kernicterus. Hemolytic anemia producing jaundice in the 1st wk of life may also be secondary to congenital deficiencies in RBC enzymes, such as pyruvate kinase or G6PD.

92.3 ■ Plethora in the Newborn Infant (Polycythemia) (See Chapters 458 and 459)

Plethora, a ruddy, deep red-purple appearance associated with a high Hct, is often due to polycythemia, defined as a central Hct of 65% or higher. Peripheral (heelstick) Hct values are higher than central values, whereas Coulter counter results are lower than Hct values determined by microcentrifugation. The incidence of neonatal polycythemia is increased at high altitude (5% in Denver vs 1.6% in Texas); in postmature (3%) vs term (1–2%) infants; in small for gestational age (8%) vs large for gestational age (3%) vs average for gestational age (1–2%) infants; during the 1st day of life (peak, 2–3 hr); in the recipient infant of a twin-twin transfusion; after delayed clamping of the umbilical cord; in infants of diabetic mothers; in trisomy 13, 18 or 21; in adrenogenital syndrome; in neonatal Graves disease; in hypothyroidism; and in Beckwith-Wiedemann syndrome. Infants of diabetic mothers and those with growth retardation may have been exposed to chronic fetal hypoxia, which stimulates erythropoietin production and increases RBC production.

Clinical manifestations include anorexia, lethargy, tachypnea, respiratory distress, feeding disturbances, hyperbilirubinemia, hypoglycemia, and thrombocytopenia. Severe complications include seizures, pulmonary hypertension, necrotizing enterocolitis, and renal failure. Many affected infants are asymptomatic. Hyperviscosity is present in most infants with central Hct values of 65% or higher and accounts for the symptoms of polycythemia. Hyperviscosity determined at constant shear rates (e.g., 11.5 sec^{-1}) is present when whole blood viscosity is above 18 cycles/sec. Hyperviscosity is accentuated because neonatal RBCs have decreased deformability and filterability, which predisposes to stasis in the microcirculation.

Treatment of symptomatic polycythemic newborns is partial exchange transfusion (with normal saline). The Hct level (without measurement of viscosity) at which to perform a partial exchange transfusion in an asymptomatic infant is unclear. Partial exchange will lower the Hct and viscosity and improve acute symptoms. The volume to be exchanged is calculated from the following formula:

$$\text{Volume of exchange (mL)} = \text{Blood volume} \times (\text{Observed} - \text{Desired hematocrit})/\text{Observed hematocrit}$$

The long-term *prognosis* of polycythemic infants is unclear. Reported adverse outcomes include speech deficits, abnormal fine motor control, reduced IQ, school problems, and other neurologic abnormalities. It is thought that the underlying etiology (e.g., chronic intrauterine hypoxia) and hyperviscosity contribute to adverse outcomes. It is unclear whether partial exchange transfusion improves the long-term outcome.

92.4 ■ Hemorrhage in the Newborn Infant

Hemorrhagic Disease of the Newborn. A moderate decrease in factors II, VII, IX, and X normally occurs in all newborn infants by 48–72 hr after birth, with a gradual return to birth levels by 7–10 days of age. This transient deficiency of vitamin K–dependent factors is probably due to lack of free vitamin K in the mother and absence of the bacterial intestinal flora normally responsible for the synthesis of vitamin K. Rarely, in term infants and more frequently in premature infants, accentuation and prolongation of this deficiency between the 2nd and 7th days of life result in spontaneous and prolonged bleeding. Breast milk is a poor source of vitamin K, and hemorrhagic complications have appeared more frequently in breast-fed than in formula-fed infants. This classic form of hemorrhagic disease of the newborn, which is responsive to vitamin K therapy, must be distinguished from disseminated intravascular coagulopathy and from the more infrequent congenital deficiencies of one or more of the other factors that are unresponsive to vitamin K (Chapter 474). Early-onset life-threatening vitamin K deficiency–induced bleeding (onset from birth to 24 hr) also occurs if the mother has been treated with drugs (phenobarbital, phenytoin) that interfere with vitamin K function. Late onset (>1 wk) is often associated with vitamin K malabsorption, as noted in neonatal hepatitis or biliary atresia (Table 92–3).

Hemorrhagic disease of the newborn resulting from severe transient deficiencies in vitamin K–dependent factors is characterized by bleeding that tends to be gastrointestinal, nasal, subgaleal, intracranial, or due to circumcision. Prodromal or warning signs (mild bleeding) may occur before serious intracranial hemorrhage. The prothrombin time (PT), blood coagulation time, and partial thromboplastin time are prolonged, and levels of prothrombin (II) and factors VII, IX, and X are significantly decreased. Vitamin K facilitates post-transcriptional carboxylation of factors II, VII, IX, and X. In the absence of carboxylation, such factors form PIVKA (protein induced in vitamin K absence), which is a sensitive marker for vitamin K status. Bleeding time, fibrinogen, factors V and VIII, platelets, capillary fragility, and clot retraction are normal for maturity.

Intramuscular administration of 1 mg of vitamin K at the time of birth prevents the decrease in vitamin K–dependent factors in full-term infants, but it is not uniformly effective in the prophylaxis of hemorrhagic disease of the newborn in premature infants. The disease may be effectively treated with a slow intravenous infusion of 1–5 mg of vitamin K$_1$, with improvement in coagulation defects and cessation of bleeding noted within a few hours. However, serious bleeding, particularly in premature infants or those with liver disease, may require a transfusion of fresh frozen plasma or whole blood. The mortality rate is low in treated patients.

A particularly severe form of deficiency of vitamin K–dependent coagulation factors has been reported in infants born to mothers receiving anticonvulsive medications (phenobarbital and phenytoin) during pregnancy. They may suffer severe bleeding, with onset within the 1st 24 hr of life; the bleeding is usually corrected by vitamin K$_1$, although in some the response is poor or delayed. A PT should be obtained on cord blood and the infant given 1–2 mg of vitamin K intravenously. If the PT is greatly prolonged and fails to improve, 10 mL/kg of fresh frozen plasma should be administered.

The routine use of intramuscular vitamin K for prophylaxis in the United States has been safe and is not associated with an increased risk of childhood cancer or leukemia. Although oral vitamin K (birth, discharge, 3–4 wk: 1–2 mg) has been suggested as an alternative, the effectiveness of oral vitamin K has not been established and it cannot be recommended for routine therapy. The intramuscular route remains the method of choice.

Other forms of bleeding may be clinically indistinguishable from hemorrhagic disease of the newborn responsive to vitamin K, but they are neither prevented nor successfully treated with it. A clinical pattern identical to that of hemorrhagic disease of the newborn may also result from any of the congenital defects in blood coagulation (Chapters 468, 469, and 475). Hematomas, melena, and postcircumcision and umbilical cord bleeding may

TABLE 92–3. **Hemorrhagic Disease of the Newborn**

	Early Onset	Classic Disease	Late Onset
Age	0–24 hr	2–7 days	1–6 mo
Site of hemorrhage	Cephalohematoma	Gastrointestinal	Intracranial
	Subgaleal	Ear-nose-throat–mucosal	Gastrointestinal
	Intracranial	Intracranial	Cutaneous
	Gastrointestinal	Circumcision	Ear-nose-throat–mucosal
	Umbilicus	Cutaneous	Injection sites
	Intra-abdominal	Gastrointestinal	Thoracic
		Injection sites	
Etiology/risks	Maternal drugs (phenobarbital, phenytoin, warfarin, rifampin, isoniazid) that interfere with vitamin K	Vitamin K deficiency Breast-feeding	Cholestasis—malabsorption of vitamin K (biliary atresia, cystic fibrosis, hepatitis)
	Inherited coagulopathy		Abetalipoprotein deficiency
			Idiopathic in Asian breast-fed infants
			Warfarin ingestion
Prevention	Possible vitamin K at birth or to mother (20 mg) before birth	Prevented by parenteral vitamin K at birth. Oral vitamin K regimens require repeated dosing over time	Prevented by parenteral and high-dose oral vitamin K during periods of malabsorption or cholestasis
	Avoid high-risk medications		
Incidence	Very rare	~2% if not given vitamin K	Dependent on primary disease

be present; only 5–35% of cases of factor VIII and IX deficiency become clinically apparent in the newborn period. Treatment of the rare congenital deficiencies of coagulation factors requires fresh frozen plasma or specific factor replacement.

Disseminated intravascular coagulopathy in newborn infants results in consumption of coagulation factors and bleeding. Affected infants are often premature; the clinical course is frequently characterized by hypoxia, acidosis, shock, hemangiomas, or infection. Treatment is directed at correcting the primary clinical problem, such as infection, and interrupting consumption and replacing clotting factors (Chapter 474).

Infants with central nervous system or other bleeding posing an *immediate threat to life* should receive fresh frozen plasma, vitamin K, and blood if needed as soon as possible after blood has been drawn for coagulation studies, which should include a determination of the number of platelets.

The so-called swallowed blood syndrome, in which blood or bloody stools are passed, usually on the 2nd or 3rd day of life, may be confused with hemorrhage from the gastrointestinal tract. The blood may be swallowed during delivery or from a fissure in the mother's nipple. Differentiation from gastrointestinal hemorrhage is based on the fact that the infant's blood contains mostly fetal hemoglobin, which is alkali resistant, whereas swallowed blood from a maternal source contains adult hemoglobin, which is promptly changed to alkaline hematin after the addition of alkali. Apt devised the following test for this differentiation: (1) Rinse a blood-stained diaper or some grossly bloody (red) stool with a suitable amount of water to obtain a distinctly pink supernatant hemoglobin solution. (2) Centrifuge the mixture and decant the supernatant solution. (3) To five parts of the supernatant fluid add one part of 0.25 N (1%) sodium hydroxide. Within 1–2 min a color reaction takes place: a yellow-brown color indicates that the blood is maternal in origin; a persistent pink indicates that it is from the infant. A control test with known adult or infant blood, or both, is advisable.

Widespread subcutaneous ecchymoses in premature infants at or immediately after birth are apparently a result of fragile superficial blood vessels rather than a coagulation defect. Administering vitamin K_1 to the mother during labor has no effect on the incidence of ecchymoses. Occasionally, an infant is born with petechiae or a generalized bluish suffusion limited to the face, head, and neck, probably as a result of venous obstruction by a nuchal cord or sudden increases in intrathoracic pressure during delivery. It may take 2–3 wk for such suffusions to disappear.

Neonatal Thrombocytopenic Purpura. See Chapter 475.

Amin SB, Ahlfors C, Orlando MS, et al: Bilirubin and serial auditory brainstem responses in premature infants. *Pediatrics* 2001;107:664.

Anderson C: Critical haemoglobin thresholds in premature infants. *Arch Dis Child Fetal Neonatal Ed* 2001;84:F146.

Bearer CF, O'Riordan MA, Powers R: Lead exposure from blood transfusion to premature infants. *J Pediatr* 2000;137:549.

Bednarek F, Weisberger S, Richardson DK, et al: Variations in blood transfusions among newborn intensive care units. *J Pediatr* 1998;133:601.

Davis BH, Olsen S, Bigelow NC, et al: Detection of fetal red cells in fetomaternal hemorrhage using a fetal hemoglobin monoclonal antibody by flow cytometry. *Transfusion* 1998;38:749.

de Almeida V, Bowman JM: Massive fetomaternal hemorrhage: Manitoba experience. *Obstet Gynecol* 1994;83:323.

Delaney-Black V, Camp BW, Lubchenco LO, et al: Neonatal hyperviscosity association with lower achievement and IQ scores at school age. *Pediatrics* 1989;83:662.

Franz AR, Pohlandt F: Red blood cell transfusions in very and extremely low birthweight infants under restrictive transfusion guidelines: Is exogenous erythropoietin necessary? *Arch Dis Child Fetal Neonatal Ed* 2001;84:F96.

Hermansen MC: Nucleated red blood cells in the fetus and newborn. *Arch Dis Child* 2001;84:F211.

Janssens HM, de Haan MJJ, van Kamp IL, et al: Outcome for children treated with fetal intravascular transfusions because of severe blood group antagonism. *J Pediatr* 1997;131:373.

Klumper FJ, van Kamp IL, Vandenbussche FP, et al: Benefits and risks of fetal redcell transfusion after 32 weeks gestation. *Eur J Obstet Gynecol Reprod Biol* 2000;92:91.

Kumar D, Greer FR, Super DM, et al: Vitamin K status of premature infants: Implications for current recommendations. *Pediatrics* 2001;108:1117.

Lo D, Hjelm N, Fidler C, et al: Prenatal diagnosis of fetal RhD status by molecular analysis of maternal plasma. *N Engl J Med* 1998;339:1734.

Maier RF, Obladen M, Mueller-Hansen I, et al: Early treatment with erythropoietin β ameliorates anemia and reduces transfusion requirements in infants with birth weights below 1000 g. *J Pediatr* 2002;141:8.

Maier RF, Sonntag J, Walka MM, et al: Changing practices of red blood cell transfusions in infants with birth weights less than 1000 g. *J Pediatr* 2000;136:220.

Mari G, Deter RL, Carpenter RL, et al: Noninvasive diagnosis by Doppler ultrasonography of fetal anemia due to maternal red-cell alloimmunization. Collaborative Group for Doppler Assessment of the Blood Velocity in Anemic Fetuses. *N Engl J Med* 2000;342:9.

Naulaers G, Barten S, Vanhole C, et al: Management of severe neonatal anemia due to fetomaternal transfusion. *Am J Perinatol* 1999;16:193.

Nicaise C, Gire C, Casha P, et al: Erythropoietin as treatment for late hyporegenerative anemia in neonates with Rh hemolytic disease after in utero exchange transfusion. *Fetal Diagn Ther* 2002;17:22.

Ohls RK, Ehrenkranz RA, Wright LL, et al: Effects of early erythropoietin therapy on the transfusion requirements of preterm infants below 1250 grams birth weight: A multicenter, randomized, controlled trial. *Pediatrics* 2001;108:934.

Puckett RM, Offringa M: Prophylactic vitamin K for vitamin K deficiency bleeding in neonates. *Cochrane Database Syst Rev* 2000;CD002776.

Rabe H, Wacker A, Hulskamp G, et al: A randomised controlled trial of delayed cord clamping in very low birth weight preterm infants. *Eur J Pediatr* 2000;159:775.

Robson SC, Lee D, Urbanik S: Anti-D immunoglobulin in RhD prophylaxis. *Br J Obstet Gynaecol* 1998;105:129.

Rothenberg T: Partial plasma exchange transfusion in polycythemic neonates. *Arch Dis Child* 2002;86:60.

Saade GR: Noninvasive testing for fetal anemia. *N Engl J Med* 2000;342:52.

Sekizawa A, Watanabe A, Kimura T, et al: Prenatal diagnosis of the fetal RhD blood type using a single fetal nucleated erythrocyte from maternal blood. *Obstet Gynecol* 1996;87:501.

Stephenson T, Zuccollo J, Mohajer M: Diagnosis and management of nonimmune hydrops in the newborn. *Arch Dis Child* 1994;70:F151.

van Kamp IL, Klumper FJ, Bakkum RS, et al: The severity of immune fetal hydrops is predictive of fetal outcome after intrauterine treatment. *Am J Obstet Gynecol* 2001;185:668.

Vaughan JI, Manning M, Warwick RM, et al: Inhibition of erythroid progenitor cells by anti-Kell antibodies in fetal alloimmune anemia. *N Engl J Med* 1998;338:798.

Waldron P, de Alarcon P: ABO hemolytic disease of the newborn: A unique constellation of findings in siblings and review of protective mechanisms in the fetal-maternal system. *Am J Perinatol* 1999;16:391.

Wong W, Fok TF, Lee CH, et al: Randomized controlled trial: Comparison of colloid or crystalloid for partial exchange transfusion for treatment of neonatal polycythaemia. *Arch Dis Child* 1997;77:F115.

Zipursky A: Prevention of vitamin K deficiency bleeding in newborns. *Br J Haematol* 1999;104:430.

Chapter 93

Genitourinary System

(see also Part XXIII)

Barbara J. Stoll and Robert M. Kliegman

Urinary tract anomalies (hydronephrosis, dysplasia, solitary kidney) are frequently identified by prenatal ultrasonography (see Table 85–5). After birth, the presence/extent of anomalies needs to be confirmed and followed by detailed evaluation and appropriate management. Follow-up of urinary anomalies diagnosed in utero requires renal ultrasonography after birth and again at 2 wk of life. For anomalies such as ureteropelvic junction obstruction and reflux, prenatal diagnosis provides the opportunity for early treatment to minimize functional deterioration and urinary tract infection.

One or both kidneys are often easily palpable in a newborn infant. When both are palpable and similar, infants usually do not have any particular diagnostic problems, but when only one kidney can be felt, a frequent impression is that it is larger than normal or is displaced by an intrinsic or extrinsic mass. Fetal lobulation may contribute to this impression. The problem usually resolves as the kidney becomes progressively less easily palpable during the early months of life. Because palpable enlargement or displacement of a kidney in a newborn may be due to hydronephrosis, neuroblastoma, mesoblastic nephroma, adrenal hemorrhage, or a cystic malformation, ultrasound examination is indicated.

Thrombosis of the Renal Vein. See Chapter 96.

Circumcision (see Chapter 536). Circumcision is the most common elective surgical procedure performed on newborn boys in the United States. The benefits relate to cultural or religious beliefs and to medical benefits and include a reduced incidence of balanitis, penile cancer, sexually transmitted diseases (including HIV), and urinary tract infections (in male infants). The risks are low (local infection, bleeding), but as with any surgical procedure, pain relief must be provided. Analgesia may include concentrated oral sucrose, a dorsal penile nerve block, or topical lidocaine-prilocaine cream.

Circumcision policy statement. American Academy of Pediatrics. Task Force on Circumcision. *Pediatrics* 1999;103:686.

Howard C, Howard F, Garfunkel L, et al: Neonatal circumcision and pain relief: Current training practices. *Pediatrics* 1998;101:423.

Lannon CM, Bailey A, Fleischman A, et al: Circumcision debate. Task Force on Circumcision, 1999–2000. *Pediatrics* 2000;105:641.

Schoen EJ, Colby CJ, Ray GT: Newborn circumcision decreases incidence and costs of urinary tract infections during the first year of life. *Pediatrics* 2000;105:789.

Schoen EJ, Wiswell TE, Moses S: New policy on circumcision—cause for concern. *Pediatrics* 2000;105:620.

Chapter 94

The Umbilicus *Barbara J. Stoll*

and Robert M. Kliegman

Umbilical Cord. The cord contains the two umbilical arteries, the vein, the rudimentary allantois, the remnant of the omphalomesenteric duct, and a gelatinous substance called Wharton jelly. The sheath of the umbilical cord is derived from the amnion. The muscular umbilical arteries contract readily, but the vein does not. The vein retains a fairly large lumen after birth. Abnormally short cords are associated with fetal hypotonia, long cords are at risk for true knots or wrapping around fetal parts (neck, arm), and straight untwisted cords are associated with fetal distress, anomalies, and intrauterine fetal demise.

When the cord sloughs after birth, portions of these structures remain in the base. The blood vessels are functionally closed, but anatomically patent for 10–20 days. The arteries become the lateral umbilical ligaments; the vein, the ligamentum teres; and the ductus venosus, the ligamentum venosum. During this interval, the umbilical vessels are potential portals of entry for infection. The umbilical cord usually sloughs within 2 wk. *Delayed separation of the cord*, after more than 1 mo, has been associated with neutrophil chemotactic defects and overwhelming bacterial infection (Chapter 120.2).

A **single umbilical artery** is present in about 5–10/1,000 births; the frequency is about 35–70/1,000 twin births. Approximately one third of infants with a single umbilical artery have congenital abnormalities, usually more than one, and many such infants are stillborn or die shortly after birth. Trisomy 18 is one of the more frequent abnormalities. Because many abnormalities are not apparent on gross physical examination, it is important that at every delivery the cut cord and the maternal and fetal surfaces of the placenta be inspected. The number of arteries present should be recorded as an aid to the early suspicion and identification of abnormalities in such infants. For infants with a single umbilical artery, some recommend renal ultrasonography.

Patency of the omphalomesenteric (vitelline) *duct* may be responsible for an intestinal fistula, prolapse of the bowel, a polyp (cyst), or a Meckel diverticulum (Chapter 312.2).

A *persistent urachus* (urachal cyst) is due to failure of closure of the allantoic duct and is associated with bladder outlet obstruction. Patency should be suspected if a clear, light yellow, urine-like fluid is being discharged from the umbilicus.

Congenital Omphalocele. An omphalocele is a herniation or protrusion of the abdominal contents into the base of the umbilical cord. In contrast to the more common umbilical hernia, the sac is covered with peritoneum without overlying skin. The size of the sac that lies outside the abdominal cavity depends on its contents. Herniation of intestines into the cord occurs in about 1/5,000 births and herniation of liver and intestines in 1/10,000 births. The abdominal cavity is proportionately small because the impetus to grow and develop is deficient. Immediate surgical repair, before infection has taken place and before the tissues have been damaged by drying (saline-soaked sterile dressings should be applied immediately) or by rupture of the sac, is essential for survival. Mersilene or similar synthetic material may be used to cover the viscera if the sac has ruptured or if excessive mobilization of the skin would be necessary to cover the mass and its intact sac. The risk of associated congenital anomalies/syndromes, including Beckwith-Wiedemann syndrome (omphalocele, macrosomia, hypoglycemia), trisomies 13 and 18, and cardiac anomalies, is increased in patients with omphalocele.

Tumors. Tumors of the umbilicus are rare and include angioma, enteroteratoma, dermoid cyst, myxosarcoma, and cysts of urachal or omphalomesenteric duct remnants.

Hemorrhage. Hemorrhage from the umbilical cord may be due to trauma, inadequate ligation of the cord, or failure of normal thrombus formation. It may also indicate hemorrhagic disease of the newborn or other coagulopathies (factor XIII deficiency), septicemia, or local infection. The infant should be observed frequently during the first few days of life so that if hemorrhage does occur, it will be detected promptly.

Granuloma. The umbilical cord usually dries and separates within 6–8 days after birth. The raw surface becomes covered by a thin layer of skin, scar tissue forms, and the wound is usually healed within 12–15 days. The presence of saprophytic organisms delays separation of the cord and increases the possibility of invasion by pathogenic organisms. Mild infection or incomplete epithelialization may result in a moist granulating area at the base of the cord with a slight mucoid or mucopurulent discharge. Good results are usually obtained by cleansing with alcohol several times daily.

Persistence of granulation tissue at the base of the umbilicus is common. The tissue is soft, vascular and granular, and dull red or pink, and it may have a seropurulent secretion. *Treatment* is cauterization with silver nitrate, repeated at intervals of several days until the base is dry.

Umbilical granuloma must be differentiated from **umbilical polyp,** a rare anomaly resulting from persistence of all or part of the omphalomesenteric duct or the urachus. The tissue of the polyp is firm and resistant, is bright red, and has a mucoid secretion. If the polyp is communicating with the ileum or bladder, small amounts of fecal material or urine may be discharged intermittently. Histologically, the polyp consists of intestinal or urinary tract mucosa. Treatment is surgical excision of the *entire* omphalomesenteric or urachal remnant.

Infections. Although aseptic delivery and routine cord care (daily application of triple dye to the umbilical stump and surrounding skin) decrease the risk of umbilical infection, the necrotic tissue of the umbilical cord is an excellent medium for bacterial growth. Omphalitis may remain localized or may spread to the abdominal wall, the peritoneum, the umbilical or portal vessels, or the liver. Infants with abdominal wall cellulitis or those with necrotizing fasciitis have a high incidence of associated bacteremia. Portal vein phlebitis may develop and result in the later onset of extrahepatic portal hypertension. The general manifestations may be minimal (periumbilical erythema), even when septicemia or hepatitis has resulted. *Treatment* includes prompt antibiotic therapy (effective against *Staphylococcus aureus* and *Escherichia coli)* and, if abscess formation has occurred, surgical incision and drainage.

Umbilical Hernia. Often associated with diastasis recti, an umbilical hernia is due to imperfect closure or weakness of the umbilical ring. Predisposing factors include black race and low birthweight. The hernia appears as a soft swelling covered by skin that protrudes during crying, coughing, or straining and can be reduced easily through the fibrous ring at the umbilicus. The hernia consists of omentum or portions of the small intestine. The size of the defect varies from less than 1 cm in diameter to as much as 5 cm, but large ones are rare.

TREATMENT. Most umbilical hernias that appear before the age of 6 mo disappear spontaneously by 1 yr of age. Even large hernias (5–6 cm in all dimensions) have been known to disappear spontaneously by 5–6 yr of age. Strangulation is extremely rare. It is generally agreed that "strapping" is ineffective. Surgery is not advised unless the hernia persists to the age of 4–5 yr, causes symptoms, becomes strangulated, or becomes progressively larger after the age of 1–2 yr. Defects exceeding 2 cm are less likely to close spontaneously.

Holland AJ, Ford WD, Linke RJ, et al: Influence of antenatal ultrasound on the management of fetal exomphalos. *Fetal Diagn Ther* 1999;14:223.

Lurie S, Sherman D, Bukovsky I: Omphalocele delivery enigma: The best mode of delivery still remains dubious. *Eur J Obstet Gynecol Reprod Biol* 1999;82:19.

O'Donnell KA, Glick PL, Caty MG: Pediatric umbilical problems. *Pediatr Clin North Am* 1998;45:791.

Weber DM, Freeman NV, Elhag KM: Periumbilical necrotizing fasciitis in the newborn. *Eur J Pediatr Surg* 2001;11:86.

Chapter 95
Metabolic Disturbances
Barbara J. Stoll and Robert M. Kliegman

HYPERTHERMIA IN THE NEWBORN (TRANSITORY FEVER OF THE NEWBORN, DEHYDRATION FEVER)

Elevations in temperature (38–39°C or 100–103°F) are occasionally noted on the 2nd–3rd day of life in infants whose clinical course has been otherwise satisfactory. This disturbance is especially likely to occur in breast-fed infants whose intake of fluid has been particularly low or in infants exposed to high environmental temperatures, either in an incubator, in a bassinet near a radiator, or in the sun.

The infant may lose weight. However, a consistent relationship may not be seen between the fever and the extent of weight loss or inadequacy of fluid intake. Urinary output and the frequency of voiding diminish. The fontanel may be depressed. The infant takes fluids avidly, but the apparent vigor of the infant contrasts with the usual appearance of "being sick" in the presence of infection. The rise in temperature may be associated with an increase in serum levels of protein and sodium and with an increase in hematocrit. The possibility of local or systemic infection should be evaluated. Administering oral or parenteral fluids or lowering the environmental temperature leads to prompt reduction of the fever and alleviation of symptoms.

A *more severe form of neonatal hyperthermia* occurs in both newborn and older infants when they are warmly dressed for outdoor low temperatures that do not exist in their immediate indoor environment. The diminished sweating capacity of newborn infants is a contributing factor. Warmly dressed infants left near stoves or radiators, traveling in well-heated automobiles, or left with bright sunlight shining directly on them through the windows of a closed room or automobile are likely to be victims. Excess clothing in hot weather, especially when the infant is left in the sun, is a less common cause. Body temperature is often as high as 41–44°C (106–111°F). The skin is hot and dry, and initially the infant usually appears flushed and apathetic. Tachypnea and irritability may be noted. This stage may be followed by stupor, grayish pallor, coma, and convulsions. Hypernatremia may contribute to the convulsions. Mortality and morbidity rates (brain damage) are high. Hyperthermia has been associated with sudden infant death and with *hemorrhagic shock and encephalopathy syndrome* (Chapter 57.2). The condition is prevented by dressing infants in clothing suitable for the temperature of the *immediate* environment. In newborn infants, exposure of the body to usual room temperature or immersion in tepid water usually suffices to bring the temperature back to normal levels. Older infants may require cooling for a longer time by repeated immersion or by the use of a water-cooled mattress or other apparatus for induction of hypothermia. Attention to possible fluid and electrolyte disturbance is essential.

NEONATAL COLD INJURY

Neonatal cold injury usually occurs in abandoned infants or those in inadequately heated homes during damp cold spells when the outside temperature is in the freezing range (see Chapter 63).

The initial features are apathy, refusal of food, oliguria, and coldness to touch. The body temperature is usually between 29.5 and 35°C (85–95°F), and immobility, edema, and redness of the extremities, especially the hands, feet, and face, are observed. Bradycardia and apnea may also occur. The facial erythema frequently gives a false impression of health and delays recognition that the infant is ill. Local hardening over areas of edema may lead to confusion with scleredema. Rhinitis is common, as are hypoglycemia and acidosis. Hemorrhagic manifestations are frequent; massive pulmonary hemorrhage is a common finding at autopsy. Treatment consists of warming and paying scrupulous attention to recognizing and correcting hypotension and metabolic imbalances, particularly hypoglycemia. Prevention consists of providing adequate environmental heat. The mortality rate is about 10%; about 10% of survivors have evidence of brain damage.

EDEMA

Generalized edema occurs in association with hydrops fetalis and in the offspring of diabetic mothers. In premature infants, edema is often a consequence of a decreased ability to excrete water or sodium, although some have considerable edema without identifiable cause. Infants with hyaline membrane disease may become edematous without heart failure. Edema of the face and scalp may be caused by pressure from the umbilical cord around the neck, and transient localized swelling of the hands or feet may similarly be due to intrauterine pressure. Edema may be associated with heart failure from congenital cardiac lesions; a lag in renal excretion of electrolytes and water may result in edema after a sudden large increase in intake of electrolytes, particularly with feeding of concentrated cow's milk formulas. High-protein formulas may also cause edema as a result of the excessive renal solute load, particularly in premature infants. It is difficult to show a relationship between low serum protein or low hemoglobin levels and the occurrence of edema in older premature infants. Edema also occurs in association with anemia and vitamin E deficiency in premature infants. Rarely, *idiopathic hypoproteinemia* with edema lasting weeks or months is observed in term infants. The cause is unclear, and the disturbance is benign. Persistent edema of one or more extremities may represent congenital lymphedema (Milroy disease) or, in females, *Turner syndrome*. Generalized edema with hypoproteinemia may be seen in the neonatal period with congenital nephrosis and rarely with Hurler syndrome or after feeding hypoallergenic formulas to infants with cystic fibrosis of the pancreas. *Sclerema* is described in Chapter 637.

HYPOCALCEMIA (TETANY) (see Chapters 44.11 and 48.9)

Metabolic Bone Disease. Metabolic bone disease is a common complication in very low birthweight preterm infants. The smallest sickest infants are at greatest risk. Progressive osteopenia with demineralized bones and occasionally pathologic fractures may develop. The major cause is inadequate intake of calcium to meet the demands for growth. Poor intake of phosphorus and vitamin D are additional risk factors. Contributing factors include prolonged parenteral nutrition, vitamin D and calcium malabsorption, intake of unsupplemented human milk, immobilization, and calcium loss from chronic diuretic use. The serum alkaline phosphatase level is used to monitor metabolic bone disease and can be over 1,000 U/L in severe cases. Fortified human milk and formulas designed for preterm infants provide improved intake of calcium, phosphorus, and vitamin D; promote bone mineralization; and may prevent metabolic bone disease. Many extremely low birthweight infants will require additional oral supplements of calcium, phosphorus, and vitamin D. Treatment of fractures requires immobilization and administration of calcium and, if needed, phosphorus (for hypophosphatemia) and vitamin D (not more than 1,000

IU/day unless severe cholestasis or vitamin D resistance is present). See also Chapters 44.10, 44.11, 45.5, 45.7, 48.9, 696, 697.

HYPOMAGNESEMIA

Rarely, hypomagnesemia of unknown cause may occur in newborn infants, usually in association with hypocalcemia. It may also be associated with insufficient stores of skeletal magnesium secondary to deficient placental transfer, decreased intestinal absorption, neonatal hypoparathyroidism, hyperphosphatemia, renal loss (primary or drugs, e.g., amphotericin B), a defect in magnesium and calcium homeostasis, or iatrogenic deficiency caused by loss incurred during exchange transfusion or insufficient replacement during total intravenous alimentation. Infants of diabetic mothers may have serum magnesium levels that are lower than normal. The clinical manifestations of hypomagnesemia are indistinguishable from those of hypocalcemia and tetany and may, in fact, contribute to the accompanying hypocalcemia.

Hypomagnesemia occurs when serum magnesium levels fall below 1.5 mg/dL (0.62 mmol/L), although clinical signs do not usually develop until serum magnesium levels fall below 1.2 mg/dL. During exchange transfusion with citrated blood, which is low in magnesium because of binding by citrate, serum magnesium decreases about 0.5 mg/dL (0.2 mmol/L); approximately 10 days is required for return to normal. In non-iatrogenic hypomagnesemia, the serum magnesium level may be less than 0.5 mg/dL. Serum calcium in either instance is usually at levels noted in hypocalcemic tetany, but the serum phosphorus value is normal or high. Because the hypocalcemia accompanying hypomagnesemia is inadequately corrected by administering calcium alone, hypomagnesemia should also be suspected in any patient with tetany not responding to calcium therapy.

Immediate *treatment* consists of intramuscular injection of magnesium sulfate. For newborn infants, 0.25 mL/kg of a 50% solution daily usually suffices. The accompanying hypocalcemia usually corrects itself as the hypomagnesemia is relieved. The same daily dose can be given for oral maintenance therapy. Four to five times higher doses may be required in malabsorptive states. In most cases, the metabolic defect is transient, and treatment can be discontinued after 1–2 wk. A few patients appear to have a permanent form of the disease that requires continuous oral supplementation with magnesium to prevent recurrence of hypomagnesemia. No residual damage to the central nervous system is evident after prompt treatment.

HYPERMAGNESEMIA

Hypermagnesemia may occur in newborn infants of mothers treated with magnesium sulfate during labor. At high serum levels the central nervous system is depressed, and infants have profound respiratory depression requiring mechanical ventilation. Lower levels may result in hypoventilation, lethargy, flaccidity, hyporeflexia, and poor sucking. Hypermagnesemia may be associated with failure to pass meconium (meconium plug syndrome). The upper limit of normal magnesium is 2.8 mg/dL (1.15 mmol/L), but serious symptoms rarely occur at levels below 5 mg/dL (2.1 mmol/L). In most cases, no specific therapy (beyond supportive care and maintenance of respiratory support) is required. Intravenous calcium and diuresis will reduce magnesium levels. In rare cases, exchange transfusion has been used for rapid removal of magnesium ion from the blood.

OTHER METABOLIC DISEASES

A number of inborn errors of metabolism may be manifested during the neonatal period, including phenylketonuria, galactosemia, the urea cycle defects, methylmalonicacidemia, and maple syrup urine disease (see Chapters 74 to 76). Pyridoxine deficiency and dependence are considered in Chapter 44.6.

SUBSTANCE ABUSE AND NEONATAL ABSTINENCE (WITHDRAWAL)

Substance abuse during pregnancy is a serious problem for both the mother and her newborn. The mother may suffer adverse consequences of her addiction, including episodes of drug withdrawal during pregnancy and illnesses related to high-risk behavior. Effects on the fetus and newborn include chronic or intermittent drug exposure, acute withdrawal shortly after birth, and long-term effects on physical growth and neurodevelopment. Because infants with in utero drug exposure often have social and environmental risk factors and may have been exposed to multiple substances, it may be difficult to evaluate the effects of specific in utero drug exposure on long-term neurodevelopmental outcome.

Pregnancy in women who use illegal drugs or alcohol is, by definition, high risk. Substance misuse in pregnant women is a difficult problem to address from both medical and social aspects. Prenatal care is usually inadequate, and these women have a higher incidence of sexually transmitted diseases, including syphilis, HIV, and hepatitis. In addition, the risk of preterm labor, intrauterine growth restriction, premature rupture of membranes, and perinatal morbidity and mortality is higher. Physiologic addiction to narcotics occurs in most infants born to actively addicted mothers because opiates cross the placenta. Withdrawal may be manifested even before birth by increased activity of the fetus when the mother feels a need for the drug or withdrawal symptoms develop. Heroin and methadone are the drugs most frequently associated with withdrawal syndromes, but such syndromes may also occur with alcohol, phenobarbital, pentazocine, codeine, propoxyphene, hydroxyzine, amphetamines, neuroleptics, antidepressants, and benzodiazepines.

Heroin addiction results in a 50% incidence of low-birthweight infants, half of whom are small for gestational age. Chronic infections, maternal undernutrition, and a direct fetal growth-inhibiting effect are possible causes. The rate of stillbirths is increased, but not the incidence of congenital anomalies. *Clinical manifestations* of withdrawal occur in 50–75% of infants, usually beginning within the 1st 48 hr, depending on the daily maternal dose (<6 mg/24 hr is associated with no or mild symptoms), the duration of addiction (>1 yr has a >70% incidence of withdrawal), and the time of the last maternal dose (the incidence is higher if the last dose was taken within 24 hr of birth). Rarely, symptoms may appear as late as 4–6 wk of age. The incidence of hyaline membrane disease and hyperbilirubinemia may be decreased in preterm infants of heroin users; accelerated production of pulmonary surfactant may explain the former, and enzyme induction of hepatic glucuronyl transferase the latter.

Tremors and hyperirritability are the most prominent symptoms. The tremors may be fine or jittery and indistinguishable from those of hypoglycemia, but they are more often coarse, "flapping," and bilateral; the limbs are frequently rigid, hyperreflexic, and resistant to flexion and extension. Irritability and hyperactivity are generally marked and may lead to skin abrasions. Other signs include wakefulness, hyperacusis, hypertonicity, tachypnea, diarrhea, vomiting, high-pitched cry, fist sucking, poor feeding with weight loss (disorganized sucking), and fever. Sneezing, yawning, hiccups, myoclonic jerks, convulsions, abnormal sleep cycles, nasal stuffiness, apnea, flushing alternating rapidly with pallor, and lacrimation are less common. The risk of sudden infant death syndrome is increased. The *diagnosis* is generally established by the history and clinical findings. Examining the urine for opiates may reveal only low levels during withdrawal, but quinine, which is often mixed with heroin, may be present in higher concentrations. Meconium testing is more accurate than neonatal urine drug testing. Hypoglycemia and hypocalcemia should be excluded.

Methadone addiction is associated with severe withdrawal symptoms, the incidence varying from 20–90%. In general, mothers taking methadone have better prenatal care than those taking heroin; however, these mothers have a high incidence of polysubstance abuse, including alcohol, barbiturates, and tranquilizers, and they are often heavy smokers. The incidence of congenital anomalies is not increased. The average birthweight of infants of mothers taking methadone is higher than that of infants of heroin-addicted mothers; the *clinical manifestations* are similar except that the former group has a higher incidence of seizures (10–20%) and the late onset (2–6 wk of age) of symptoms and signs. Unfortunately, some women continue to abuse heroin, even if they enter a methadone program. Neonates born to these women are more likely to be preterm and/or low birthweight than those born to women who stop using heroin. They are also more likely to suffer withdrawal and have a higher risk of neonatal mortality.

Alcohol withdrawal is uncommon. Infants of women who have been drinking immediately before delivery may have alcohol on their breath for several hours because it rapidly crosses the placenta and blood levels in the infant are similar to those in the mother. Hypoglycemia and acidosis may be present. Infants in whom withdrawal symptoms develop often become agitated and hyperactive, with marked tremors lasting 72 hr, followed by about 48 hr of lethargy before return to normal activity. Seizures may develop.

Phenobarbital withdrawal usually occurs in full-term, appropriate for gestational age infants of addicted mothers. Symptoms begin at a median age of 7 days (range, 2–14 days). Infants may have a brief acute stage consisting of irritability, constant crying, sleeplessness, hiccups, and mouthing movements, followed by a subacute stage consisting of voracious appetite, frequent regurgitation and gagging, episodic irritability, hyperacusis, sweating, and a disturbed sleep pattern, all of which may last 2–4 mo.

Cocaine abuse in pregnant women is common, but withdrawal in their infants is unusual; the pregnancy may be complicated by premature labor, abruptio placentae, and fetal asphyxia. Infants may have intrauterine growth restriction and neurobehavioral deficits characterized by impaired state regulation, impaired auditory information processing, developmental delay, and learning disabilities. At 24 mo of age, they score lower on the mental scale of the Bayley score and are twice as likely to have developmental delay. Family disorganization, polysubstance abuse, sexually transmitted diseases, and child abuse and neglect may also affect these unfortunate families.

Treatment. Infants who are undergoing withdrawal require care in a quiet environment with reduction of external stimuli and swaddling. Not all infants require drug therapy. Therapy is indicated for seizures, for diarrhea, or for such irritability that normal sleep and feeding patterns are disturbed and weight gain is poor. *Treatment* of heroin and methadone withdrawal has been successful with various combinations of narcotics, sedatives, and hypnotics. Methadone withdrawal may require larger amounts of medication for longer periods to control clinical manifestations than are needed for heroin withdrawal. Phenobarbital, 5–10 mg/kg/24 hr in three to four divided doses, can effectively reduce irritability and prevent seizures. Paregoric at a beginning dose of 0.05–0.1 mL/kg is given every 3–4 hr and increased by 0.05 mL every 4 hr if necessary, depending on the size and response of the infant. Paregoric abolishes most withdrawal symptoms, especially diarrhea. Tincture of opium (10 mg/mL) diluted 25-fold results in the same morphine equivalency as paregoric. The recommended dose of diluted tincture of opium is 0.1 mL/kg (≈2 drops/kg) with feedings every 4 hr. The dose may be increased by 2 drops every 4 hr if needed. The dose and duration of therapy may be adjusted according to the clinical response. Parenteral administration of fluids may be necessary to prevent aspiration or dehydration until the symptoms are brought under control.

Current mortality from withdrawal is under 5% and may be negligible with early recognition and treatment. The *prognosis* for normal development is affected by the adverse circumstances of high-risk pregnancy and delivery and by the environment to which the infant is returned after recovery, as well as by the effects of the particular drug on fetal and subsequent neonatal development.

Fetal Alcohol Syndrome. High levels of alcohol ingestion during pregnancy can be damaging to embryonic and fetal development. A specific pattern of malformation identified as the *fetal alcohol syndrome* has been documented, and major and minor components of the syndrome are expressed in 1–2 infants/1,000 live births (Table 95–1). Both moderate and high levels of alcohol intake during early pregnancy may result in alterations in growth and morphogenesis of the fetus; the greater the intake, the more severe the signs. Infants born to heavy drinkers have twice the risk of abnormality as those born to moderate drinkers; 32% of infants born to heavy drinkers had congenital anomalies as compared with 9% in the abstinent and 14% in the moderate group. Additional maternal risk factors associated with fetal alcohol syndrome are advanced maternal age, low socioeconomic status, poor psychologic indicators, and binge drinking.

Characteristics of fetal alcohol syndrome include (1) prenatal onset and persistence of growth deficiency for length, weight, and head circumference; (2) facial abnormalities, including short palpebral fissures, epicanthal folds, maxillary hypoplasia, micrognathia, and a thin upper lip; (3) cardiac defects, primarily septal defects; (4) minor joint and limb abnormalities, including some restriction of movement and altered palmar crease patterns; and (5) delayed development and mental deficiency varying from borderline to severe (see Table 95–1). Fetal alcohol syndrome is a common identifiable cause of mental retardation. The severity of dysmorphogenesis may range from severely affected infants with full manifestations of fetal alcohol syndrome to those mildly affected with only a few manifestations.

The detrimental effects may be due to the alcohol itself or to one of its breakdown products. Some evidence suggests that alcohol may impair placental transfer of essential amino acids and zinc, both necessary for protein synthesis, which may account for the intrauterine growth restriction.

Treatment of these infants is difficult because no specific therapy exists. These infants may remain hypotonic and tremulous despite sedation, and the prognosis is poor. Counseling with regard to recurrence is important. *Prevention* is achieved by eliminating alcohol intake after conception.

Backstrom MC, Kuusela AL, Maki R: Metabolic bone disease of prematurity. *Ann Med* 1996;28:275.

Bandstra ES, Morrow CE, Anthony JC, et al: Intrauterine growth of full-term infants: Impact of prenatal cocaine exposure. *Pediatrics* 2001;108:1309.

Centers for Disease Control and Prevention: Fetal alcohol syndrome—Alaska, Arizona, and New York, 1995–1997. *MMWR Morb Mortal Wkly Rep* 2002;51:433.

Coles CD, Kable JA, Drews-Botsch C, et al: Early identification of risk for effects of prenatal alcohol exposure. *J Stud Alcohol* 2000;61:607.

Coyle MG, Ferguson A, Lagasse L, et al: Diluted tincture of opium (DTO) and phenobarbital versus DTO alone for neonatal opiate withdrawal in term infants. *J Pediatr* 2002;140:561.

Curet LB, Hsi AC: Drug abuse during pregnancy. *Clin Obstet Gynecol* 2002;45:73.

Doberczak TM, Kandall SR, Friedmann P: Relationships between maternal methadone dosage, maternal-neonatal methadone levels, and neonatal withdrawal. *Obstet Gynecol* 1993;81:936.

Fewtrell MS, Cole TJ, et al: Neonatal factors predicting childhood height in preterm infants: Evidence for a persisting effect of early metabolic bone disease? *J Pediatr* 2000;137:668.

Frank DA, Augustyn M, Knight WG, et al: Growth, development, and behavior in early childhood following prenatal cocaine exposure: A systematic review. *JAMA* 2001;285:1613.

Hulse GK, O'Neill G: Methadone and the pregnant user: A matter for careful clinical consideration. *Aust N Z J Obstet Gynaecol* 2001;41:329.

Lester BM, ElSohly M, Wright LL, et al: The maternal lifestyle study: Drug use by meconium toxicology and maternal self-report. *Pediatrics* 2001;107:309.

Mattson SN, Riley EP, Gramling L, et al: Heavy prenatal alcohol exposure with or without physical features of fetal alcohol syndrome leads to IQ deficits. *J Pediatr* 1997;131:718.

Mattson SN, Schoenfeld AM, Riley EP: Teratogenic effects of alcohol on brain and behavior. *Alcohol Res Health* 2001;25:185.

Moore ES, Ward RE, Jamison PL, et al: The subtle facial signs of prenatal exposure to alcohol: An anthropometric approach. *J Pediatr* 2001;139:215.

Neonatal drug withdrawal. American Academy of Pediatrics Committee on Drugs. *Pediatrics* 1998;101:1079.

Ostrea EM Jr, Knapp DK, Tannenbaum L, et al: Estimates of illicit drug use during pregnancy by maternal interview, hair analysis, and meconium analysis. *J Pediatr* 2001;138:344.

Ostrea EM Jr, Ostrea AR, Simpson PM: Mortality within the first 2 years in infants exposed to cocaine, opiate, or cannabinoid during gestation. *Pediatrics* 1997;100:79.

Rantonen T, Kääpa P, Jalonen J, et al: Antenatal magnesium sulphate exposure is associated with prolonged parathyroid hormone suppression in preterm neonate. *Acta Paediatr* 2001;90:278.

Ryan S: Nutritional aspects of metabolic bone disease in the newborn. *Arch Dis Child* 1996;74:F145.

TABLE 95–1. Fetal Alcohol Syndrome Surveillance Network Case Definition Categories

Case Definition Category	Phenotype Positive		
	Face	*Central Nervous System*	*Growth*
Confirmed fetal alcohol syndrome (FAS) phenotype with or without maternal alcohol exposure[*]	Abnormal facial features consistent with FAS as reported by a physician *or* Two of the following: Short palpebral fissures Abnormal philtrum Thin upper lip	Frontal-occipital circumference ≤10th percentile at birth or any age *or* Standardized measure of intellectual function ≤1 SD below the mean *or* Standardized measure of developmental delay ≤1 SD below the mean *or* Developmental delay or mental retardation diagnosed by a qualified examiner (e.g., psychologist or physician) *or* Attention deficit disorder diagnosed by a qualified evaluator	Intrauterine weight or height corrected for gestational age ≤10th percentile *or* Postnatal weight or height ≤10th percentile for age *or* Postnatal weight for height ≤10th percentile
Probable FAS phenotype with or without maternal alcohol exposure[*]	Required; facial features same as above	Must meet either CNS or growth criteria as outlined above	

[*]*Documentation in the records of some level of maternal alcohol use during the index pregnancy.*
From Fetal alcohol syndrome—Alaska, Arizona, and New York, 1995–1997. MMWR Morb Mortal Wkly Rep 2002;51:433.

Singer LT, Arendt R, Minnes S, et al: Cognitive and motor outcomes of cocaine-exposed infants. *JAMA* 2002;287:1952.

Sood B, Delaney-Black V, Covington C, et al: Prenatal alcohol exposure and childhood behavior at age 6 to 7 years: I. dose-response effect. *Pediatrics* 2001;108:http://www.pediatrics.org/cgi/content/full/108/2/e24.

Zuckermann B, Frank DA, Mayes L: Cocaine-exposed infants and developmental outcomes. *JAMA* 2002;287:1990.

Chapter 96

The Endocrine System

Barbara J. Stoll and Robert M. Kliegman

The endocrinopathies are discussed in Part XXV. This chapter focuses on endocrine disturbances that may be identified at birth or during the 1st mo of life.

Pituitary dwarfism is not usually apparent at birth, although panhypopituitary male infants may have neonatal hypoglycemia, hyperbilirubinemia, and micropenis. Conversely, constitutional dwarfs usually have length and weight consistent with prematurity when born after a normal gestational period; otherwise, their physical appearance is normal.

Primary hypothyroidism occurs in approximately 1/4,000 births. Because most of these infants are asymptomatic at birth, all states screen for this serious and treatable disease. *Thyroid deficiency* may also be apparent at birth in genetically determined **cretinism** or in infants of mothers treated with thiouracil or its derivatives during pregnancy. Constipation, prolonged jaundice, goiter, lethargy, or poor peripheral circulation as shown by persistently mottled skin or cold extremities should suggest cretinism. Early diagnosis plus treatment of congenital deficiency of thyroid hormone improves intellectual outcome and is facilitated by screening all newborn infants for this deficiency. Transient hypothyroxinemia of prematurity is most common in ill infants of very low birthweight. These infants are probably chemically euthyroid as suggested by normal levels of serum thyrotropin and other tests of the pituitary-hypothalamic axis. Because the relationship between low thyroid levels and neurodevelopmental outcome is unclear, it remains uncertain whether premature infants with this transient problem should be treated with thyroid hormone.

Temporary *hyperthyroidism* may occur at birth in infants of mothers with hyperthyroidism or in infants whose mothers have been receiving thyroid medication.

Transient *hypoparathyroidism* may be manifested as tetany of the newborn (Chapter 565).

The *adrenal glands* are subject to numerous disturbances, which may become apparent and require lifesaving treatment during the neonatal period. Acute adrenal *hemorrhage* and failure may occur after breech or other traumatic deliveries or in association with overwhelming infection. *Congenital adrenal hyperplasia* is suggested by vomiting, diarrhea, dehydration, hyperkalemia, hyponatremia, shock, ambiguous genitals, or clitoral enlargement. Some infants have ambiguous genitals and hypertension. Because the condition is genetically determined, newborn siblings of patients with the salt-losing variety of adrenocortical hyperplasia should be closely observed for manifestations of adrenal insufficiency. Newborn screening and early diagnosis and therapy for this disorder may prevent severe salt wasting and adverse outcomes.

Congenitally hypoplastic adrenal glands may also give rise to adrenal insufficiency during the first few weeks of life.

Female infants with webbing of the neck, lymphangiectatic edema, hypoplasia of the nipples, cutis laxa, low hairline at the nape of the neck, low-set ears, high-arched palate, deformities of the nails, cubitus valgus, and other anomalies should be suspected of having *gonadal dysgenesis*.

Transient *diabetes mellitus* (Chapter 583) is rare and is encountered only in newborns. It is usually manifested as dehydration, loss of weight, or acidosis in small for gestational age infants.

96.1 Infants of Diabetic Mothers

Control of diabetes mellitus with insulin has led to improved outcomes in diabetic women who bear children. Their infants and the infants of women in whom diabetes later develops share certain distinctive morphologic characteristics, macrosomia, and a high risk of morbidity. Diabetic mothers have a high incidence of polyhydramnios, preeclampsia, pyelonephritis, preterm labor, and chronic hypertension; their fetal mortality rate, which is high at all gestational ages, especially after 32 wk, is greater than that of nondiabetic mothers. Fetal loss throughout pregnancy is associated with poorly controlled maternal diabetes (especially ketoacidosis) and congenital anomalies. Most infants born to diabetic mothers are large for gestational age. If the diabetes is complicated by vascular disease, infants may be growth restricted, especially those born after 37 wk gestation. The neonatal mortality rate is over five times that of infants of nondiabetic mothers and is higher at all gestational ages and in every birthweight for gestational age category.

Pathophysiology. The probable pathogenic sequence is that maternal hyperglycemia causes fetal hyperglycemia, and the fetal pancreatic response leads to fetal hyperinsulinemia; fetal hyperinsulinemia and hyperglycemia then cause increased hepatic glucose uptake and glycogen synthesis, accelerated lipogenesis, and augmented protein synthesis. Related pathologic findings are hypertrophy and hyperplasia of the pancreatic islets with a disproportionate increase in the number of β cells, increased weight of the placenta and infant organs except for the brain, myocardial hypertrophy, increased amount of cytoplasm in liver cells, and extramedullary hematopoiesis. Hyperinsulinism and hyperglycemia produce fetal acidosis, which may result in an increased rate of stillbirth. Separation of the placenta at birth suddenly interrupts glucose infusion into the neonate without a proportional effect on the hyperinsulinism, and hypoglycemia and attenuated lipolysis develop during the first hours after birth.

Hyperinsulinemia has been documented in infants of gestational diabetic mothers and in those of insulin-dependent diabetic mothers without insulin antibodies. The former group also has significantly higher fasting plasma insulin levels than normal newborns do despite similar glucose levels; they respond to glucose with an abnormally prompt elevation in plasma insulin and assimilate a glucose load more rapidly. After arginine administration, they also have an enhanced insulin response and increased disappearance rates of glucose in comparison to normal infants. In contrast, fasting glucose production and utilization rates are diminished. The lower free fatty acid levels in infants of insulin-dependent diabetic mothers probably also reflect their hyperinsulinemia. With good prenatal diabetic control, the incidence of macrosomia and hypoglycemia has decreased.

Although hyperinsulinism is probably the main cause of hypoglycemia, the diminished epinephrine and glucagon responses that occur may be contributing factors. Cortisol and human growth hormone levels are normal. Congenital anomalies correlate with poor metabolic control during the periconception and organogenesis periods and may be due to hyperglycemia-induced teratogenesis.

Clinical Manifestations. Infants of diabetic and gestational diabetic mothers often bear a surprising resemblance to each other (Fig. 96–1). They tend to be large and plump as a result of increased body fat and enlarged viscera, with puffy, plethoric facies resembling that of patients who have been receiving

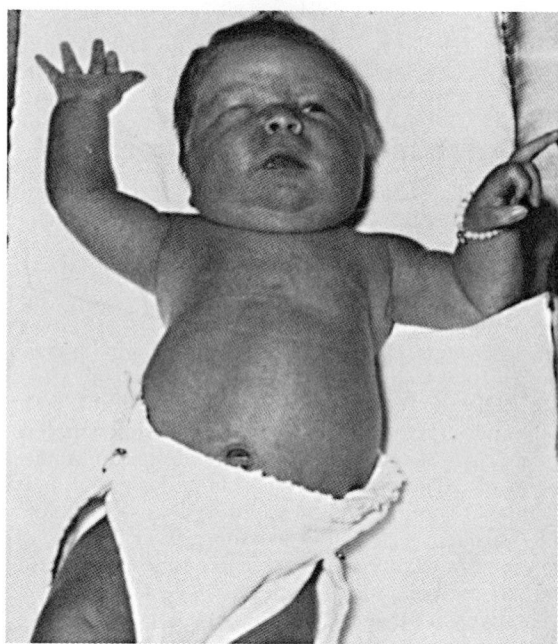

FIGURE 96–1. Large, plump, plethoric infant of a gestational diabetic mother. The baby was born at 38 wk of gestation but weighed 9 lb, 11 oz (4,408 g). Mild respiratory distress was the only symptom other than appearance.

corticosteroids. These infants may, however, also be of normal or low birthweight, particularly if delivered before term or the mother has associated vascular disease.

Hypoglycemia develops in about 25–50% of infants of diabetic mothers and 15–25% of infants of mothers with gestational diabetes, but only a small percentage of these infants become symptomatic. The probability of hypoglycemia developing in the infant increases, and glucose levels are likely to be lower at higher cord or maternal fasting blood glucose levels. The nadir in an infant's blood glucose concentration is usually reached between 1 and 3 hr; spontaneous recovery may begin by 4–6 hr.

The infants tend to be jumpy, tremulous, and hyperexcitable during the 1st 3 days of life, although hypotonia, lethargy, and poor sucking may also occur. They may have any of the diverse manifestations of hypoglycemia. Early appearance of these signs is more likely to be related to hypoglycemia and later appearance related to hypocalcemia; these abnormalities may also occur together. Perinatal asphyxia or hyperbilirubinemia may produce similar signs. Hypomagnesemia may be associated with the hypocalcemia.

Tachypnea develops in many infants of diabetic mothers during the 1st 2 days of life and may be a manifestation of hypoglycemia, hypothermia, polycythemia, cardiac failure, transient tachypnea, or cerebral edema from birth trauma or asphyxia. Infants of diabetic mothers have a higher incidence of respiratory distress syndrome than do infants of nondiabetic mothers born at comparable gestational age; the greater incidence is possibly related to an antagonistic effect of insulin on stimulation of surfactant synthesis by cortisol.

Cardiomegaly is common (30%), and heart failure occurs in 5–10% of infants of diabetic mothers. Asymmetric septal hypertrophy may occur and become manifested similar to idiopathic hypertrophic subaortic stenosis. Inotropic agents worsen the obstruction and are contraindicated. Birth trauma is also a common sequela of fetal macrosomia.

Neurologic development and ossification centers tend to be immature and correlate with brain size (which is not increased) and gestational age rather than total body weight. In addition, these infants have an increased incidence of hyperbilirubinemia, polycythemia, and renal vein thrombosis; the latter should be suspected in infants with a flank mass, hematuria, and thrombocytopenia.

The incidence of congenital anomalies is increased threefold in infants of diabetic mothers; cardiac malformations (ventricular or atrial septal defect, transposition of the great vessels, truncus arteriosus, double-outlet right ventricle, coarctation of the aorta) and lumbosacral agenesis are most common. Additional anomalies include neural tube defects, hydronephrosis, renal agenesis and dysplasia, duodenal or anorectal atresia, situs inversus, double ureter, and holoprosencephaly. These infants may also develop abdominal distention caused by a transient delay in development of the left side of the colon, the *small left colon syndrome*.

Prognosis. The subsequent incidence of diabetes mellitus in infants of diabetic mothers is increased in comparison to that of the general population. Physical development is normal, but oversized infants may be predisposed to childhood obesity that may extend into adult life. Disagreement persists about whether these infants have a slightly increased risk of impaired intellectual development unrelated to hypoglycemia; symptomatic hypoglycemia increases the risk, as does maternal ketonuria.

Treatment. Treatment of infants of diabetic mothers should be initiated before birth by frequent prenatal evaluation of all pregnant women with overt or gestational diabetes, by evaluation of fetal maturity, by biophysical profile, by Doppler velocimetry, and by planning the delivery of these infants in hospitals where expert obstetric and pediatric care is continuously available. Periconception glucose control reduces the risk of anomalies, and glucose control during labor reduces the incidence of neonatal hypoglycemia. Women with type 1 diabetes who have tight glucose control during pregnancy (average daily glucose levels <95 mg/dL) deliver infants with birthweights and anthropomorphic features that are similar to those of infants of nondiabetic mothers. Women with gestational diabetes may be treated successfully with glyburide, which may not cross the placenta. In these mothers, the incidence of macrosomia and neonatal hypoglycemia was similar to that in mothers with insulin-treated gestational diabetes. Regardless of size, all infants of diabetic mothers should initially receive intensive observation and care. Asymptomatic infants should have a blood glucose determination within 1 hr of birth and then every hour for the next 6–8 hr; if clinically well and normoglycemic, oral or gavage feeding with breast milk or formula should be started as soon as possible and continued at 3 hr intervals. If any question arises about an infant's ability to tolerate oral feeding, the feeding should be discontinued and glucose given by peripheral intravenous infusion at a rate of 4–8 mg/kg/min. Hypoglycemia should be treated, even in asymptomatic infants, by frequent feeding and/or intravenous infusion of glucose. Bolus injections of hypertonic glucose should be avoided because they may cause further hyperinsulinemia and potentially produce rebound hypoglycemia. Managing hypoglycemia in sick or symptomatic infants is discussed in the following section. For treatment of *hypocalcemia* and *hypomagnesemia*, see Chapter 95; for *hyaline membrane disease* treatment, see Chapter 90.3; for treatment of *polycythemia*, see Chapter 92.3.

96.2 Hypoglycemia (see also Chapter 88)

Hypoglycemia is present when serum glucose levels are significantly lower than the range in postnatal age-matched normal infants. Although hypoglycemia may also be defined as the presence of neurologic (lethargy, coma, apnea, seizures) or sympathomimetic (pallor, palpitations, diaphoresis) manifestations that respond to glucose, many neonates with low serum glucose levels are asymptomatic, whereas normoglycemic infants may have nonspecific signs of hypoglycemia.

The *incidence of hypoglycemia* varies with the definition, population, method and timing of feeding, and type of glucose assay (serum levels are higher than whole blood values) (Fig. 96–2). Early feeding decreases the incidence, whereas prematurity, hypothermia, hypoxia, maternal diabetes, maternal glucose infusion in labor, and intrauterine growth restriction (IUGR) increase the incidence of hypoglycemia. Serum glucose levels decline after birth until 1–3 hr of age, when levels spontaneously increase in normal infants. In healthy term infants, serum glucose values are rarely less than 35 mg/dL between 1 and 3 hr of life, less than 40 mg/dL from 3 to 24 hr, and less than 45 mg/dL (2.5 mmol/L) after 24 hr. Although previous studies, performed when premature infants were not fed on the 1st day of life, suggested that premature infants have statistically lower glucose levels than term infants do and that preterm infants may be unaffected by low glucose values, evidence does not support these conclusions. Both premature and full-term infants are at risk for serious neurodevelopmental deficits from equally low glucose levels. This risk is related to the depth and duration of the hypoglycemia.

Several pathophysiologic groups of *neonatal infants are at high risk for hypoglycemia*. (1) Hyperinsulinism: Infants of mothers with diabetes mellitus or gestational diabetes and infants with severe erythroblastosis fetalis, insulinomas, leucine sensitivity with hyperammonemia, familial or sporadic hyperinsulinemia, Beckwith syndrome (see later), and panhypopituitarism have hyperinsulinism. *Familial hyperinsulinemic hypoglycemia* (previously called nesidioblastosis) may be an autosomal recessive disease characterized by excessive fetal growth and severe neonatal hypoglycemia, often unresponsive to medical management. This severe form is due to defects in either of the two components of the islet β cell K_{ATP} channel (either the sulfonylurea receptor or the Kir6.2 inward rectifier K^+ channel). A milder autosomal dominant form with delayed onset has an unknown cause. Familial or sporadic hyperammonemic hyperinsulinemia is due to a mutation of the glutamate dehydrogenase gene (increased glutamate oxidation in the β cell releases insulin). (2) IUGR/prematurity: Infants with IUGR or those who are preterm may have experienced intrauterine malnutrition resulting in reduced hepatic glycogen stores and total body fat, especially the smaller of discordant twins (if discordant by 25% or more in weight with a weight <2.0 kg). Other factors in the development of hypoglycemia in this group include impaired gluconeogenesis, diminished free fatty acid oxidation, low cortisol production rates, and possibly increased insulin levels and decreased output of epinephrine in response to hypoglycemia. (3) Increased metabolic demands: Hypoglycemia may develop in very immature or severely ill infants as a result of increased metabolic needs disproportionate to substrate stores and the calories supplied; low-birthweight infants with respiratory distress syndrome, perinatal asphyxia, polycythemia, hypothermia, and systemic infections, as well as infants in heart failure with cyanotic congenital heart disease, are at increased risk. Interruption of intravenous infusions, particularly those with high glucose concentrations, may also result in a precipitous onset of hypoglycemia. (4) Genetic causes: Rare infants with genetic or primary metabolic defects, such as galactosemia, glycogen storage disease, fructose intolerance, propionicacidemia, methylmalonicacidemia, tyrosinemia, maple syrup urine disease, and long- or medium-chain acyl-CoA dehydrogenase deficiency, are also susceptible.

Clinical Manifestations. In contrast to the frequency of chemical hypoglycemia, the incidence of symptomatic hypoglycemia is highest in small for gestational age infants (see Fig. 96–2). These infants usually fall into category 2 or 3 of the earlier pathophysiologic groupings, and some are referred to as having *transient symptomatic idiopathic neonatal hypoglycemia*. Because many of the symptoms also occur together with other conditions such as infections—especially sepsis and meningitis; central nervous system anomalies, hemorrhage, or edema; hypocalcemia and hypomagnesemia; asphyxia; drug withdrawal; apnea of prematurity; congenital heart disease; or polycythemia—and because some may be seen in normoglycemic well infants, the exact incidence of symptomatic hypoglycemia has been difficult to establish. It probably varies between 1 and 3 per 1,000 live births and affects about 5–15% of growth-restricted infants.

The onset of symptoms varies from a few hours to a week after birth. In approximate order of frequency, symptoms include jitteriness or tremors, apathy, episodes of cyanosis, convulsions, intermittent apneic spells or tachypnea, weak or high-pitched cry, limpness or lethargy, difficulty feeding, and eye rolling. Episodes of sweating, sudden pallor, hypothermia, and cardiac arrest and failure also occur. Frequently, a clustering of episodic symptoms may be noted. Because these clinical manifestations may result from various causes, it is critical to measure serum glucose levels and determine whether they disappear with the administration of sufficient glucose to raise the blood sugar to normal levels; if they do not, other diagnoses must be considered.

Treatment. When symptoms other than seizures are present, an intravenous bolus of 200 mg/kg (2 mL/kg) of 10% glucose is effective in elevating the blood glucose concentration. In the presence of convulsions, 4 mL/kg of 10% glucose as a bolus injection is indicated.

After initial therapy, a glucose infusion should be given at 8 mg/kg/min. If hypoglycemia recurs, the infusion rate and concentration should be increased until 15–20% glucose is used. If intravenous infusions of 20% glucose are inadequate to eliminate symptoms and maintain constant normal serum glucose concentrations, hyperinsulinemia is probably present and diazoxide should be administered. If the diazoxide is unsuccessful,

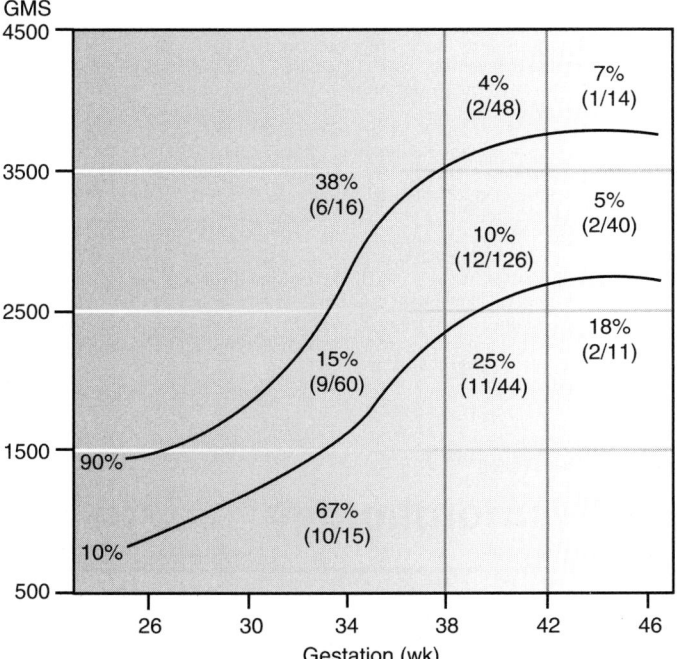

FIGURE 96–2. Incidence of hypoglycemia by birthweight, gestational age, and intrauterine growth. (From Lubchenco LO, Bard H: Incidence of hypoglycemia in newborn infants classified by birth weight and gestational age. *Pediatrics* 1971;47:832.)

octreotide may be useful; many infants with severe persistent hyperinsulinemic hypoglycemia undergo subtotal pancreatectomy. The serum glucose level should be measured every 2 hr after initiating therapy until several determinations are above 40 mg/dL. Subsequently, levels should be measured every 4–6 hr and the treatment gradually reduced and finally discontinued when the serum glucose value has been in the normal range and the baby asymptomatic for 24–48 hr. Treatment is usually necessary for a few days to a week, rarely for several weeks.

Infants at increased risk for hypoglycemia should have their serum glucose measured within 1 hr of birth, every 1–2 hr for the 1st 6–8 hr, and then every 4–6 hr until 24 hr of life. Normoglycemic high-risk infants should receive oral or gavage feeding with human milk or formula started at 1–3 hr of age and continued at 2–3 hr intervals for 24–48 hr. An intravenous infusion of glucose at 4 mg/kg/min should be provided if oral feedings are poorly tolerated or if asymptomatic transient neonatal hypoglycemia develops.

Prognosis. The prognosis is good in asymptomatic patients with hypoglycemia of short duration. Hypoglycemia recurs in 10–15% of infants after adequate treatment. Recurrence is more common if intravenous fluids are extravasated or discontinued too rapidly before oral feedings are well tolerated. Children in whom ketotic hypoglycemia later develops have an increased incidence of neonatal hypoglycemia. The prognosis for normal intellectual function must be guarded because prolonged, recurrent, and severe symptomatic hypoglycemia is associated with neurologic sequelae. Symptomatic infants with hypoglycemia, particularly low-birthweight infants, those with persistent hyperinsulinemic hypoglycemia, and infants of diabetic mothers, have a poorer prognosis for subsequent normal intellectual development than asymptomatic infants do.

HYPOGLYCEMIA WITH MACROGLOSSIA (BECKWITH-WIEDEMANN SYNDROME)

This syndrome includes intractable neonatal hypoglycemia occurring in infants with macroglossia, large size, visceromegaly, mild microcephaly, omphalocele, facial nevus flammeus, a characteristic earlobe crease, an increased risk of tumors (Wilms, hepatoblastoma, gonadoblastoma), and renal medullary dysplasia. The visceromegaly chiefly involves the liver and the kidneys and is due to noncystic hyperplasia. Some infants are also polycythemic, and hyperinsulinemia has been demonstrated. Some infants with Beckwith syndrome have a partial duplication of chromosome 11p, a region that encodes the insulin-like growth factor II gene. Though usually sporadic, familial inheritance has been noted. Treatment is the same as that for hyperinsulinemic hypoglycemia, but in this syndrome, the hypoglycemia may be severe and persist for several months. The prognosis is poor if symptomatic hypoglycemia is severe. Many may be managed medically for the hyperinsulinemic hypoglycemia, but those refractory to such treatment may require subtotal pancreatectomy.

Severe hypoglycemia has also been demonstrated in extremely high birthweight infants who do not have the anomalies present in Beckwith syndrome. These *infant giants* weigh from 3.8 to 5.3 kg, and in some, pancreatic hyperplasia has been described.

Aberg A, Westbom L: Association between maternal pre-existing or gestational diabetes and health problems in children. *Acta Paediatr* 2001;90:746.

Bongers-Schokking JJ, Koot HM, Wiersma D, et al: Influence of timing and dose of thyroid hormone replacement on development in infants with congenital hypothyroidism. *J Pediatr* 2000;136:292.

Briët JM, van Wassenaer AG, Dekker FW, et al: Neonatal thyroxine supplementation in very preterm children: Developmental outcome evaluated at early school age. *Pediatrics* 2001;107:712.

Carrapato MR, Marcelino F: The infant of the diabetic mother: The critical development windows. *Early pregnancy* 2001;5:57.

Clark W, O'Donovan D: Transient hyperinsulinism in an asphyxiated newborn infant with hypoglycemia. *Am J Perinatol* 2001;18:175.

Cordero L, Treuer SH, Landon MB, et al: Management of infants of diabetic mothers. *Arch Pediatr Adolesc Med* 1998;152:249.

Cornblath M, Hawdon JM, Williams AF, et al: Controversies regarding definition of neonatal hypoglycemia: Suggested operational thresholds. *Pediatrics* 2000;105:1141.

Daliva AL, Linder B, DiMartino-Nardi J, et al: Three-year follow-up of borderline congenital hypothyroidism. *J Pediatr* 2000;136:53.

de Lonlay-Debeney P, Poggi-Travert F, Fournet J-C, et al: Clinical features of 52 neonates with hyperinsulinism. *N Engl J Med* 1999;340:1169.

Diwakar KK, Sasidhar MV: Plasma glucose levels in term infants who are appropriate size for gestation and exclusively breast fed. *Arch Dis Child Fetal Neonatal Ed* 2002;87:F46.

Duvanel CB, Fawer C-L, Cotting J, et al: Long-term effects of neonatal hypoglycemia on brain growth and psychomotor development in small-for-gestational-age preterm infants. *J Pediatr* 1999;134:492.

Fisher DA: The importance of early management in optimizing IQ in infants with congenital hypothyroidism. *J Pediatr* 2000;136:273.

Kalhan S, Peter-Wohl S: Hypoglycemia: What is it for the neonate? *Am J Perinatol* 2000;17:11.

Kukuvitis A, Deal C, Arbour L, et al: An autosomal dominant form of familial persistent hyperinsulinemic hypoglycemia of infancy, not linked to the sulfonylurea receptor locus. *J Clin Endocrinol Metab* 1997;82:1192.

Langer O, Conway DL, Berkus MD, et al: A comparison of glyburide and insulin in women with gestational diabetes mellitus. *N Engl J Med* 2000;343:1134.

Langer O, Rodriguez DA, Xenakis EMJ, et al: Intensified versus conventional management of gestational diabetes. *Am J Obstet Gynecol* 1994;170:1036.

Lilien L, Pildes R, Srinivasan G, et al: Treatment of neonatal hypoglycemia with minibolus and intravenous glucose infusion. *J Pediatr* 1980;97:295.

MacNeil S, Dodds L, Hamilton DC, et al: Rates and risk factors for recurrence of gestational diabetes. *Diabetes Care* 2001;24:659.

Marcus C: How to measure and interpret glucose in neonates. *Acta Paediatr* 2001;90:963.

Mello G, Parreti E, Mecacci F, et al: What degree of maternal metabolic control in women with type 1 diabetes is associated with normal body size and proportions in full-term infants? *Diabetes Care* 2000;23:1494.

Menni F, de Lonlay P, Sevin C, et al: Neurologic outcomes of 90 neonates and infants with persistent hyperinsulinemic hypoglycemia. *Pediatrics* 2001;107:476.

Nanchi H, Kulaylat: High incidence of Down's syndrome in infants of diabetic mothers. *Arch Dis Child* 1997;77:242.

Nestorowicz A, Inagaki N, Gonoi T, et al: A nonsense mutation in the inward rectifier potassium channel gene, Kir6.2, is associated with familial hyperinsulinism. *Diabetes* 1997;46:1743.

Osborn DA: Thyroid hormones for preventing neurodevelopmental impairment in preterm infants (Cochrane Review). *Cochrane Database Syst Rev* 2001;4:CD001070.

Rapaport R: Congenital hypothyroidism: Expanding the spectrum. *J Pediatr* 2000;136:10.

Rapaport R, Rose SR, Freemark M: Hypothyroxinemia in the preterm infant: The benefits and risks of thyroxine treatment. *J Pediatr* 2001;139:182.

Simmons D: Persistently poor pregnancy outcomes in women with insulin dependent diabetes. *Br Med J* 1997;315:263.

Stanley CA, Baker L: The causes of neonatal hypoglycemia. *N Engl J Med* 1999;340:1200.

Van der Kamp HJ, Noordam K, Elvers B, et al: Newborn screening for congenital adrenal hyperplasia in the Netherlands. *Pediatrics* 2001;108:1320.

Vela-Huerta MM, Vargas-Origel A, Olvera-López A: Asymmetrical septal hypertrophy in newborn infants of diabetic mothers. *Am J Perinatol* 2000;17:89.

Weinzimer SA, Stanley CA, Berry GT, et al: A syndrome of congenital hyperinsulinism and hyperammonemia. *J Pediatr* 1997;130:661.

Wolfsdorf JI: Hyperinsulinemic hypoglycemia of infancy. *J Pediatr* 1998;132:1.

Xiong X, Saunders LD, Wang FL, et al: Gestational diabetes mellitus: Prevalence, risk factors, maternal and infant outcomes. *Int J Gynaecol Obstet* 2001;75:221.

Zammarchi E, Filippi L, Novembre E, et al: Biochemical evaluation of a patient with a familial form of leucine-sensitive hypoglycemic and concomitant hyperammonemia. *Metabolism* 1996;45:957.

Chapter 97
Dysmorphology *Kenneth Lyons Jones*

The number of recognizable patterns of malformation has more than tripled during the last 25 yr. The potential prenatal effect of various drugs, chemicals, and environmental agents is better appreciated, and the number of genetic and non-genetic defects in which prenatal detection is possible has increased. This chapter provides an approach to children with a prenatal onset of structural defects that is predicated on the concept that the nature of the structural defects represents a clue to the time of onset, mechanism of injury, and possible etiology of the problem, all of which determine the necessary evaluation (Tables 97–1 and 97–2). This approach permits systematic narrowing of the diagnostic possibilities so that other sections of this textbook or one of the basic compendiums on dysmorphology can be used to make a specific diagnosis. The terminology of some malformations is noted in Table 97–3.

Structural defects of prenatal onset can be separated into those that represent a single primary defect in development and those that represent a multiple malformation syndrome. In most cases of a single primary defect, the defect involves only a single structure, the child otherwise being completely normal. The seven most common single primary defects in development are congenital hip dislocation (Chapter 668.1), talipes equinovarus (Chapter 664.3), cleft lip with or without cleft palate (Chapter 291), cleft palate alone (Chapter 291), cardiac septal defects (Chapters 417 and 419), and defects in neural tube closure (Chapter 585). For most, the etiology is unknown, and counseling regarding the risk of recurrence is difficult. However, many of the more common single primary defects are explained on the basis of multifactorial inheritance (Chapter 69), which carries a recurrence risk of between 3% and 5% for the next child of unaffected parents with one affected child. The multifactorial threshold model was developed to explain the empirical 3–5% risk for recurrence in siblings for common single primary defects. Although this figure remains the basis for recurrence risk counseling, the model may not be completely accurate. As the genetic basis for common malformations is elucidated, genetic heterogeneity becomes apparent (Tables 97–4 and 97–5). For some defects, a few major genes rather than many genes may determine genetic susceptibility. For others, a monogenetic etiology may be apparent. For example, a study of the offspring of adults with major heart defects indicates that an atrioventricular septal defect is most likely a single gene defect whereas the tetralogy of Fallot is most likely a polygenic defect with a small number of interacting genes.

Transcription factor mutations are particularly prone to multiple malformations because they regulate gene expression in many different tissues (see Tables 97–4 and 97–5). Rubinstein-Taybi syndrome consists of multiple congenital anomalies and is due to a loss-of-function mutation in CBP (CREB-binding protein), a co-activator of many transcription factors in different tissues. Waardenburg syndrome type I, caused by mutations of the *PAX3* gene, affects neural crest–derived cells. PAX3 is expressed in the developing neural crest and is a tissue-specific transcription factor. Type III Waardenburg syndrome is due to mutations in *MITF* (microphthalmos-associated transcription factor), which is expressed in pigmented cells and may be dependent on transactivation by PAX3. *HOX* (homeotic selector) genes are another class of tissue-specific transcription factors that share a protein motif, the homeodomain, that permits binding to DNA. Homeodomain regions are also present in other transcription factors (e.g., PAX3, PAX6). *HOX* genes are regionalized in the embryo and help select the developmental fate of these cells; HOXA and HOXB act rostral caudally, and HOXA and HOXD act on the axes of the developing limbs. *HOXD13* mutations produce synpolydactyly in humans.

Proteins from one cell can affect the development of a nearby cell in a paracrine-like signal. Morphogens are proteins that affect adjacent cell development along a concentration gradient. The *Sonic hedgehog (SHH)* genes express morphogens involved in cell development of the central nervous system (CNS) and the limb buds. Dominantly inherited *SHH* mutations produce holoprosencephaly; even a 50% reduction in the gene product alters the protein gradient of this morphogen and produces CNS and midfacial anomalies. In some families, a modifier gene or genes may produce variable expressivity of the phenotype despite the

TABLE 97–1. Relative Timing and Developmental Pathology of Certain Malformations

Tissue	Malformation	Defect in	Causes Before	Comment
Central nervous system	Anencephaly	Closure of anterior neural tube	26 days	Subsequent degeneration of forebrain
	Meningomyelocele	Closure in a portion of the posterior neural tube	28 days	80% lumbosacral
Face	Cleft lip	Closure of lip	36 days	42% are associated with cleft palate
	Cleft maxillary palate	Fusion of maxillary palatal shelves	10 wk	
	Branchial sinus and/or cyst	Resolution of branchial cleft	8 wk	Preauricular and along the line anterior to the sternocleidomastoid muscle
Gut	Esophageal atresia plus tracheoesophageal fistula	Lateral septation of foregut into trachea and foregut	30 days	
	Rectal atresia with fistula	Lateral septation of cloaca into rectum and urogenital sinus	6 wk	
	Duodenal atresia	Recanalization of duodenum	7–8 wk	
	Malrotation of gut	Rotation of intestinal loop so that cecum lies to the right	10 wk	Associated incomplete or aberrant mesenteric attachments
	Omphalocele	Return of midgut from yolk sac to abdomen	10 wk	
	Meckel diverticulum	Obliteration of vitelline duct	10 wk	May contain gastric or pancreatic tissue
	Diaphragmatic hernia	Closure of pleuroperitoneal canal	6 wk	
Genitourinary system	Exstrophy of bladder	Migration of infraumbilical mesenchyme	30 days	Associated müllerian and wolffian duct defects
	Bicornuate uterus	Fusion of lower portion of müllerian ducts	10 wk	
	Hypospadias	Fusion of urethral folds (labia minora)	12 wk	
	Cryptorchidism	Descent of testicle into scrotum	7–9 mo	
Heart	Transposition of great vessels	Directional development of bulbus cordis septum	34 days	
	Ventricular septal defect	Closure of ventricular septum	6 wk	
	Patent ductus arteriosus	Closure of ductus arteriosus	9–10 mo	
Limb	Aplasia of radius	Genesis of radial bone	38 days	Often accompanied by other defects of radial side of distal end of limb
	Severe syndactyly	Separation of digital rays	6 wk	
Complex	Cyclopia, holoprosencephaly	Prechordal mesoderm development	23 days	Secondary defects of midface and forebrain

Modified from Jones KL (editor): Smith's Recognizable Patterns of Human Malformation, *5th ed. Philadelphia, WB Saunders, 1997. From Behrman RE, Kliegman (editors):* Nelson's Essentials of Pediatrics, *4th ed. Philadelphia, WB Saunders, 2002.*

TABLE 97–2. Causes of Congenital Malformations

Monogenic (7.5% of Serious Anomalies)
X-linked hydrocephalus
Achondroplasia
Ectodermal dysplasia
Apert disease
Treacher Collins syndrome

Chromosomal (6% of Serious Anomalies)
Trisomies 21, 18, 13
XO, XXY
Deletions 4p–, 5p–, 7q–, 13q–, 18p–, 18q–, 22q–
Prader-Willi syndrome (50% have deletion of chromosome 15)

Maternal Infection (2% of Serious Anomalies)
Intrauterine infections (e.g., herpes simplex, CMV, varicella-zoster, rubella, and toxoplasmosis)

Maternal Illness (3.5% of Serious Anomalies)
Diabetes mellitus
Phenylketonuria
Hyperthermia

Uterine Environment (% Unknown)
Deformation
Uterine pressure, oligohydramnios: clubfoot, torticollis, congenital hip dislocation, pulmonary hypoplasia, 7th nerve palsy

Disruption
Amniotic bands, congenital amputations, gastroschisis, porencephaly, intestinal atresia

Twinning
Conjoined twins, intestinal atresia, porencephaly

Environmental Agents (% Unknown)
Polychlorinated biphenyls
Herbicides
Mercury
Alcohol

Medications (% Unknown)
Thalidomide
Diethylstilbestrol
Phenytoin
Warfarin
Cytotoxic drugs
Isotretinoin (vitamin A)
D-Penicillamine
Valproic acid

Unknown Etiologies
Polygenetic
Anencephaly / spina bifida
Cleft lip / palate
Pyloric stenosis
Congenital heart disease

Sporadic Syndrome Complexes (Anomalads)
CHARGE syndrome
VATER syndrome
Pierre Robin syndrome
Prune-belly syndrome

Nutritional
Low folic acid–neural tube defects

CMV = cytomegalovirus; CHARGE = coloboma, heart defects, atresia choanae, retarded growth, genital anomalies, ear anomalies (deafness); VATER = vertebral defects, anal atresia, tracheoesophageal fistula with esophageal atresia, and radial and renal anomalies.
From Behrman RE, Kliegman RM (editors): Nelson's Essentials of Pediatrics, 4th ed. Philadelphia, WB Saunders, 2002.

same gene mutation. Gene environment interactions may also play a role, such as enzymes that require a higher than normal amount of a cofactor such as folic acid.

The extent to which multifactorial inheritance contributes to the etiology of some of the less common single defects in devel-

opment is unclear. The fact that single primary defects are etiologically heterogeneous implies that some have an environmental etiology and others result from dominantly or recessively inherited single altered genes. Craniosynostosis (Chapter 585.12) secondary to in utero constraint is an example of the

TABLE 97–3. Definitions of Common Clinical Signs

Sign	Definition
Brachycephaly	A condition in which head shape is shortened from front to back along the sagittal plane; the skull is rounder than normal
Brachydactyly	A condition of having short digits
Brushfield spots	Speckled white rings about two thirds of the distance to the periphery of the iris of the eye
Camptodactyly	Permanent flexion of one or more fingers associated with missing inner phalangeal creases indicating lack of finger movement from before 8 wk gestation
Clinodactyly	A medial or lateral curving of the fingers and usually refers to incurving of the 5th finger
Hypoplastic nail	An unusually small nail on a digit
Low-set ears	This designation is made when the helix meets the cranium at a level below a horizontal plane that is an extension of a line through both inner canthi
Melia	A suffix meaning "limb" (e.g., amelia—missing limb; brachymelia—short limb)
Ocular hypertelorism	Increased distance between the pupils of the two eyes
Plagiocephaly	A condition in which head shape is asymmetric in the sagittal or coronal planes; can result from asymmetry in suture closure or from asymmetry of brain growth
Posterior parietal hair whorl	A single whorl occurs to the right or left of midline and within 2 cm anterior to the posterior fontanel in 95% of cases. The whorl represents the focal point from which the posterior scalp skin was under growth tension during brain growth between the 10th and 16th wk of fetal development. Aberrant position of the whorl reflects an early defect in brain development
Preaxial polydactyly	Extra finger or toe present on the medial side of the hand or foot
Postaxial polydactyly	Extra finger or toe present on the lateral side of the hand or foot
Prominent lateral palatine ridges	Relative overgrowth of the lateral palatine ridges secondary to a deficit of tongue thrust into the hard palate
Scaphocephaly	A condition in which the head is elongated from front to back in the sagittal plane; most normal skulls are scaphocephalic
Shawl scrotum	The scrotal skin joins around the superior aspect of the penis and represents a mild deficit in full migration of the labial-scrotal folds
Short palpebral fissures	Decreased horizontal distance of the eye based on measurement from the inner to the outer canthus
Syndactyly	Incomplete separation of the fingers. It most commonly occurs between the 3rd and 4th fingers and between the 2nd and 3rd toes
Synophrys	Eyebrows that meet in the midline
Telecanthus	Lateral displacement of the inner canthi. The inner canthal distance is increased, but the inner pupillary distance is normal
Widow's peak	V-shaped midline, downward projection of the scalp hair in the frontal region. It represents an upper forehead intersection of the bilateral fields of periocular hair growth suppression. It usually occurs because the fields are widely spaced, as in ocular hypertelorism

TABLE 97–4. Examples of Human Developmental Abnormalities According to Primary Cause

Condition	Clinical Findings	Genetics and Pathogenesis
Single Gene		
Aniridia	Reduced or absent iris; frequent retinal, lens, and/or corneal abnormalities	Autosomal semidominant loss-of-function mutations in the paired-like transcription factor *PAX6*; also observed along with Wilms tumor and genitourinary abnormalities as part of the 11p13 WAGR deletion syndrome (Wilms tumor, aniridia, ambiguous genitalia)
Rubenstein-Taybi syndrome	Mental retardation, broad thumbs and toes, down-slanting palpebral fissures, hypoplastic maxilla, prominent nose, congenital heart disease	Heterozygosity for loss-of-function mutations in the autosomal gene encoding CREB-binding protein (CBP), a transcriptional co-activator for many different target genes
Waardenburg syndrome	Deafness, white forelock, pale and/or asymmetric eye pigmentation. Cases caused by *PAX3* mutations have abnormally wide space between the inner eyelids and occasional upper limb defects	Autosomal semidominant loss-of-function mutations in one of two different genes: *PAX3*, which encodes a pairedlike transcription factor expressed in the neural tube and somites, or *MITF*, which encodes a bHLH transcription factor expressed in developing pigment cells
Synpolydactyly	Interphalangeal webbing and extra digits in the hands and feet	Semidominant gain-of-function mutation in *HOXD13*
Holoprosencephaly	Defective morphogenesis with bilateral cleavage of the forebrain and midface causes manifestations ranging from mild (single central incisor) to severe (microcephaly, cyclopia)	Approximately 10% of cases caused by heterozygosity for loss-of-function mutations in *SHH*, which encodes a dosage-sensitive paracrine signaling molecule; other etiologies include single-gene loci, multifactorial causes, and chromosomal imbalance syndromes
Cornelia de Lange syndrome	Growth and mental retardation, upper limb deficiencies, synophrys, depressed nasal bridge, anteverted nares, thin upper lip	Usually sporadic and probably new dominant mutation of unknown gene; rare sibling recurrence may be germline mosaicism
Multifactorial and/or Teratogenic		
Cleft lip with or without cleft palate	Absence of midline tissue from the upper lip; may extend posteriorly to involve the hard and soft palate	Isolated occurrences usually polygenic and associated with recurrence risk of 3–5%; less frequently, associated findings suggest syndromic cause
Fetal alcohol syndrome	Microcephaly, optic nerve hypoplasia, developmental delay, facial abnormalities, hyperactive behavior	Prenatal exposure to ethanol during critical periods of brain development directly causes death of developing neurons
Retinoic acid embryopathy	Microtia (small ears), conotruncal cardiac malformations, posterior fossa malformations, thymus and parathyroid abnormalities	Exposure to isotretinoin causes abnormalities of neural crest– and branchial arch – derived structures
Chromosomal Imbalance		
Trisomy 21	Growth and mental retardation, abnormal facial features, hypotonia, endocardial cushion defect, duodenal atresia	50% increase in dosage for 250 genes on chromosome 21
Velocardiofacial syndrome	Cleft palate, prominent pear-shaped nose, conotruncal heart malformations, learning disabilities	Heterozygous microdeletion in 22q11 that contains 20 genes; individual genes responsible for morphogenetic abnormalities not yet identified

From Nussbaum RL, McInnes RR, Willard HF (editors): Thompson and Thompson Genetics in Medicine, 6th ed. Philadelphia, WB Saunders, 2001.

TABLE 97–5.   **Homologs of *Drosophila* Developmental Control Genes as Causes of Human Abnormalities**

Condition	Gene	Clinical Findings
Nevoid basal cell carcinoma syndrome	*Drosophila patched* gene required for embryonic segmentation; human *PTC* gene is 29% similar	Overgrowth, skeletal abnormalities, increased susceptibility to basal cell carcinoma and medulloblastoma
Greig syndrome; Pallister-Hall syndrome; postaxial polydactyly	*Drosophila cubitus interruptus* gene required for embryonic segmentation; human *GLI3* gene is 22% identical	Extra digits (polydactyly), fusion of bony sutures in skull (craniosynostosis), hypothalamic tumors (in Pallister-Hall syndrome)
Holoprosencephaly (HPE3)	*Drosophila hedgehog* gene required for embryonic segmentation; human *SHH* gene is 38% identical	Reduced or absent development of forebrain and midline facial structures
Saethre-Chotzen syndrome	*Drosophila twist* gene required for mesoderm development; human *TWIST* gene is 32% similar	Craniosynostosis and abnormal facial features
Townes-Brock syndrome	*Drosophila spalt* gene required for specification of head and tail embryonic regions; human *SALL1* gene is 21% identical	Limb deficiency, ear abnormalities, anal atresia or stenosis

From Nussbaum RL, McInnes RR, Willard HF (editors): Thompson and Thompson Genetics in Medicine, *6th ed. Philadelphia, WB Saunders, 2001.*

former, whereas postaxial polydactyly (Chapter 671.7) illustrates the latter. Before multifactorial risk figures are used for counseling when a single primary defect is recognized, references should be consulted to determine whether other risk figures are available.

In contrast to the concept of the single primary defect in development, the designation *multiple malformation syndrome* is used when several observed structural defects all have the same known or presumed etiology. The defects usually include a number of anatomically unrelated errors in morphogenesis. Multiple malformation syndromes are caused by chromosomal abnormalities, by teratogens, and by single-gene defects inherited in mendelian patterns (see Table 97–4). Risks of recurrence range from zero, in cases that represent fresh gene mutations or are caused by teratogens, to 100%, in the case of a child with Down syndrome in which the mother is a balanced 21/21 translocation carrier (Chapter 70).

Single Primary Defects in Development. These defects are subcategorized according to the nature of the error in morphogenesis that has produced the observed structural defect: malformation, deformation, disruption, or dysplasia of a developing structure. A *malformation* is a primary structural defect arising from a localized error in morphogenesis. A *deformation* is an alteration in shape or structure of a part that has differentiated normally. The term *disruption* is used for a structural defect resulting from destruction of a previously normally formed part. The term *dysplasia* refers to an abnormal organization of cells and the structural consequences.

MALFORMATIONS. Most children with a localized malformation, such as cardiac septal defects, are otherwise completely normal. After surgical correction, the prognosis is excellent. When neither dominant nor recessive inheritance is established, multifactorial recurrence risk factors (2–5%) apply to unaffected parents.

DEFORMATIONS. Most deformations involve the musculoskeletal system and are probably caused by intrauterine molding. The pressure producing such molding may be intrinsic, the result of neuromuscular imbalance within the fetus, or extrinsic, secondary to fetal crowding. In either case, the impaired ability of the fetus to kick results in decreased fetal movement, an important factor in development of the normal musculoskeletal system, particularly with respect to normal joint development. In addition, marked positional deformation of any body part can occur when the fetus is unable to change position and thus alter the direction along which potentially deforming forces are being directed.

Intrinsically derived positional deformation of prenatal onset occurs in disorders involving muscle degeneration, such as the Steinert myotonic dystrophy syndrome, and disorders involving motor neurons, such as Werdnig-Hoffmann disease (Chapter 603.2). Early defects in development of the CNS are more common causes of positional deformations and should be seriously considered whenever a structural defect is thought to be intrinsically derived.

Fetal crowding, the most common cause of an extrinsically derived deformation of prenatal onset, is usually due to a decreased volume of amniotic fluid, a situation that occurs normally during the later weeks of gestation when the fetus is undergoing extremely rapid growth, and to the primigravid state. However, it also occurs abnormally with diminished fetal urinary output and chronic leakage of amniotic fluid.

Other extrinsic factors associated with the development of deformations include breech presentation and the shape of the amniotic cavity (Fig. 97–1). When a fetus is in the breech position, the legs may be trapped between the body and the uterine wall. The fetus is unable to kick optimally in this position, and the incidence of deformations is increased 10-fold. The shape of the amniotic cavity, which has a profound effect on the shape of the fetus that lies within it, is influenced by many factors, including uterine shape; volume of amniotic fluid; size and shape of the fetus; presence of more than one fetus; site of placental implantation; presence of uterine tumors; shape of the abdominal cavity, which is influenced by the pelvis, sacral promontory, and neighboring abdominal organs; and tightness of the abdominal musculature.

Various forms of talipes and congenital hip dislocation are the most frequently observed congenital postural deformities. Most children with these deformations are otherwise completely normal, and their prognosis is excellent. Correction usually occurs spontaneously. However, recognizing that a structural defect represents a deformation does not always imply "normal" fetal crowding and should lead to careful consideration of other etiologic possibilities that might have far greater significance to the child. For example, because decreased fetal movement can be secondary to serious neurologic abnormalities, multiple joint contractures should alert the physician to the possibility of a malformation in CNS development. Although congenital hip dislocations and talipes have a 3–5% recurrence risk, most deformations are the result of physiologic crowding and have a lower risk of recurrence. Deformations that are due to pathologic crowding (e.g., uterine tumors or malformation) have a much higher recurrence risk unless the factors leading to crowding are altered before subsequent pregnancies. Deformations that are the result of an underlying malformation (e.g., renal agenesis) have a recurrence risk similar to that of the underlying malformation.

DISRUPTION. Disruption defects occur after destruction of a previously normally formed part. At least two basic mecha-

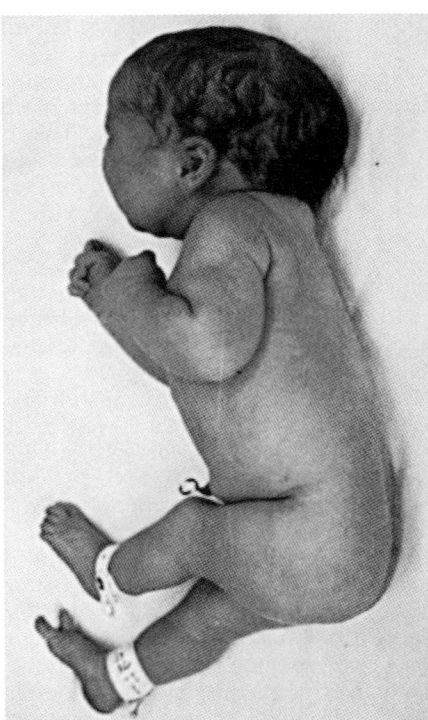

FIGURE 97–1. Breech deformation sequence.

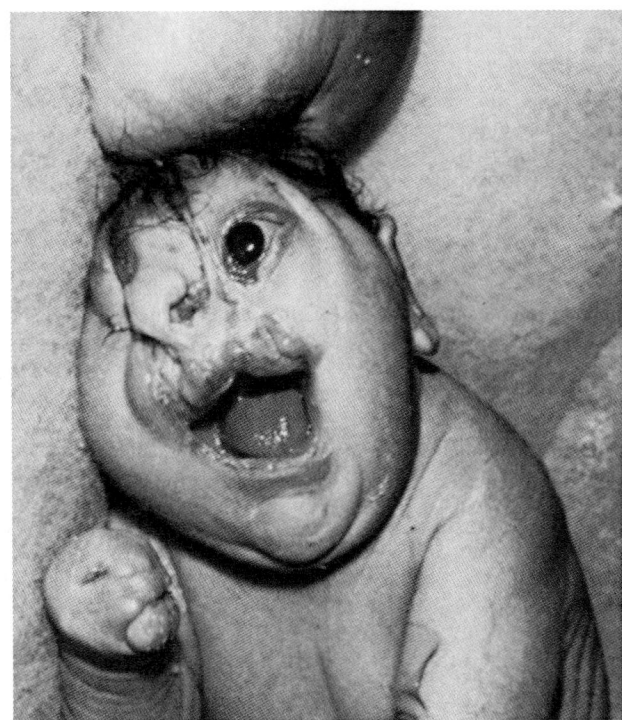

FIGURE 97–2. Amniotic band disruption sequence.

nisms are known to produce disruption. One involves entanglement followed by tearing apart or amputation of a normally developed structure, usually a digit, arm, or leg, by strands of amnion floating within amniotic fluid (i.e., amniotic bands) (Fig. 97–2). The second involves interruption of the blood supply to a developing part, which leads to infarction, necrosis, and/or resorption of structures distal to the insult. If interruption of the blood supply occurs early in gestation, the disruptive defect that is seen at term usually involves atresia or absence of a particular part. If the infarction occurs later, necrosis is more likely to be present. Examples of disruptive single primary defects for which infarctive mechanisms have been implicated include non-duodenal intestinal atresia, gastroschisis (Chapter 83.2), porencephaly (Chapter 585), and terminal transverse limb reduction defects. The extent to which disruption of a developing structure plays a role in dysmorphogenesis is unknown.

Genetic factors play a minor role in the pathogenesis of disruptions; most are sporadic events in otherwise normal families. The prognosis for a disruptive defect is determined entirely by the extent and location of the tissue loss. Thus, a child with a limb amputation has an excellent prognosis for normal function, whereas a child with porencephaly does not.

DYSPLASIA. Dysplasias may be localized or generalized. Localized dysplasias are usually single primary defects in development (e.g., hemangiomas). Localized dysplasia may be due to mosaic expression of a gene mutation occurring in the embryo, or it may be caused by agents (teratogens, viruses) that selectively injure susceptible cells (lens—rubella). However, generalized dysplasias, such as connective tissue disorders, are usually manifested as multiple malformation syndromes with involvement of a wide variety of structures because of the widespread distribution of the dysplastic tissue.

The causes of the vast majority of localized dysplasias are unknown. Because many generalized dysplasias are the result of abnormal genes, it is possible that localized dysplasias will reflect

somatic mutation in specific tissues. The hypothesis is consistent with the observation that the empirical recurrence risk for localized dysplasias is low. The process of dysplasia appears to involve deregulation of growth; hence, most dysplasias change over time. Capillary hemangiomas become involuted, and bathing trunk nevi carry a risk of malignant transformation. Knowledge of the natural history of a lesion is critical in the long-term follow-up of children with localized dysplasias.

SEQUENCE. The pattern of multiple anomalies that occurs when a single primary defect in early morphogenesis produces multiple abnormalities through a cascading process of secondary and tertiary errors in morphogenesis is called a sequence. When evaluating a child with multiple anomalies, the physician must differentiate between multiple anomalies secondary to a single localized error in morphogenesis (a sequence) and a multiple malformation syndrome. In the former, recurrence risk counseling for the multiple anomalies depends entirely on the risk of recurrence for the single localized malformation.

The terms *malformation*, *deformation*, and *disruption sequence* are used to describe only the initiating error in morphogenesis of a sequence if it is known. For example, the Robin malformation sequence (Chapter 292) is a pattern of multiple anomalies, all of which are produced by a single prenatal-onset defect in development—mandibular hypoplasia. Because the tongue is relatively small for the oral cavity, it drops back (glossoptosis), blocks closure of the posterior palatal shelves, and causes a U-shaped cleft palate. Recognizing that all the observed defects are due to a single localized error permits recurrence risk counseling based on the single defect.

The infant shown in Figure 97–1 has bathrocephaly, torticollis, facial asymmetry, a dislocated hip, and valgus anomalies of both feet as a result of compression of developing fetal parts. This pattern is the *breech deformation sequence.* Intrauterine crowding occurred because the large-sized infant was delivered in a breech position from a small, primigravida mother; recurrence risk is therefore negligible. Recognizing the deformational nature of the abnormalities is helpful with respect to prognosis. All the problems should resolve spontaneously or with postural therapy.

In the *amniotic band disruption sequence,* all the craniofacial and limb defects are secondary to constrictions caused by entanglement in multiple fibrous strands of amnion extending from the placental insertion of the umbilical cord to the surface of the amnion-denuded chorion or floating freely within the chorionic sac (see Fig. 97–2). These strands of amnion, which result from disruption of the normally formed membrane, can cause secondary defects through several mechanisms. Malformations occur if a strand of amnion interferes with the normal sequence of development; for example, a strand of amnion may interrupt fusion of the facial processes so that a cleft lip results. Disruptions occur secondary to tearing apart of structures that have previously developed normally; for example, an amniotic band might cleave areas in the developing craniofacies along lines not conforming to the normal planes of facial closure.

Deformations caused by fetal compression occur secondary to *oligohydramnios* or *tethering of a fetal part.* The former may result from rupture of both amnion and chorion and subsequent chronic leakage of amniotic fluid. Tethering occurs when the fetus or one of its parts becomes immobilized by the constraining effect of an amniotic band so that it is unable to change position and thus alter the direction along which potentially deforming forces are being directed. The recurrence risk is based on the recurrence risk for amnion rupture; unaffected parents have not been reported to give birth to more than one child affected with this disorder.

Multiple Malformation Syndromes. This category includes patients in whom one or more developmental anomalies of two or more systems have occurred, all of which are thought to be due to a common etiology. Other than Down syndrome, with an incidence of 1/660, and XXY syndromes (1/500 males), none of these disorders occurs more frequently than 1/3,000 live births.

Multiple malformation syndromes may be caused by chromosomal and genetic abnormalities and by teratogens. A number of them are associated with chromosome abnormalities (Chapter 70).

Disorders that are due to single mutant genes (dominant or X-linked in males) or to pairs of mutant genes (autosomal recessive) also cause a number of recognizable multiple malformation syndromes of prenatal onset. Correct diagnosis depends on clinical recognition because in most cases, no laboratory test is able to confirm the diagnosis. A family history of a similarly affected individual is extremely helpful. However, in many patients with multiple malformation syndromes of genetic etiology, the occurrence is sporadic and thus represents fresh gene mutations. In such situations, all family members are normal, and the diagnosis depends entirely on evaluation of the patient's phenotype. It is important to recognize that variability in expression is the rule in autosomal dominant conditions. The branchio-oto-renal syndrome is an autosomal dominant condition associated with hearing loss, preauricular pits, branchial fistulas or cysts, anomalous pinnae with a malformed middle and/or inner ear, lacrimal duct stenosis/aplasia, and renal dysplasia. In some cases, the parent of a severely affected child could have a preauricular pit as the only manifestation of the altered gene, thus highlighting the importance of a careful physical examination of both parents before providing counseling on the risk of recurrence.

Disorders caused by teratogens include multiple malformation syndromes resulting from the effect of specific infections or pharmacologic or chemical agents with which the embryo or fetus has come in contact during gestation. An example is retinoic acid embryopathy (isotretinoin [Accutane] embryopathy), which is associated with craniofacial anomalies, particularly microtia and/or anotia; cardiovascular defects; CNS

anomalies; thymic abnormalities; and a subnormal range of intelligence. The offspring of women who take isotretinoin between 15 days after conception and the end of the 1st trimester have a 35% risk for this disorder. Such conditions may be prevented before conception, particularly in the case of drugs and chemicals, if the mother is aware that the agent in question can affect her baby. It is difficult, on the other hand, for a pregnant woman to avoid contact with all infectious agents.

A careful history of drug intake (Chapter 85.4) and chemical exposure (Chapter 701) should be obtained from the parents of all children with multiple malformation syndromes, especially when the etiology of the disorder is unknown. *A Catalog of Teratogenic Agents,* by T.H. Shepard, and *Drugs in Pregnancy and Lactation,* by Briggs, Freeman, and Yaffe, as well as on-line references such as REPROTOX and TERIS are excellent references for determining whether the agent that the mother has been exposed to is a known teratogen.

Specific and easily distinguishable phenotypes do not exist for each of the infectious diseases commonly associated with altered fetal development, but intrauterine infection can frequently be suspected in those with an overall pattern of malformation (Chapter 98). An intrauterine infection should be considered if the infant is small for gestational age or developmentally delayed; in addition, the infant may be affected by microcephaly or hydrocephalus; by ocular defects, including microphthalmos, chorioretinitis, cataracts, or glaucoma; and by hepatosplenomegaly and thrombocytopenia. Intrauterine infections have a wide spectrum of clinical manifestations, from a severely affected newborn with multiple malformations to a child with no malformations who has learning disabilities that are first identified at school age.

In addition, some well-recognized multiple malformation syndromes occur in which virtually all cases have been sporadic in otherwise normal families. Examples include the Costello syndrome, a disorder associated with postnatal growth deficiency, mental retardation, macrocephaly, a coarse face, loose skin, hyperkeratotic palms and soles, papillomas in the perioral, nasal, and anal regions, cardiomyopathy, and cerebral atrophy; and the Kabuki syndrome, characterized by postnatal growth deficiency, mental retardation, long palpebral fissures, protuberant ears, preauricular pits, cardiac defects, and prominent fingertip pads. Although the etiology of these two disorders is unknown, it is now possible through molecular techniques to determine the etiology of many of them. For example, studies using fluorescent in situ hybridization indicate that the *Williams syndrome* is due to a deletion of one elastin allele located within chromosome subunit 7q11.23, whereas the *Rubinstein-Taybi syndrome* is due to a microdeletion in 16p13.3 (see Chapter 70). For *Prader-Willi syndrome,* another common sporadic disorder, the presence of the phenotype is dependent on whether the gene has been inherited from the mother or the father, a mechanism known as genetic imprinting. More than 50% of children with Prader-Willi syndrome have a chromosomal deletion involving band q11.2 of the long arm of chromosome 15. In all cases, the deleted chromosome is paternally derived (see Chapters 69 and 70). Although the gene for *Brachmann-de Lange syndrome* has not been localized, most cases are believed to be due to a single gene transmitted in autosomal dominant fashion. The low recurrence risk most likely represents the inability of more severely affected individuals to reproduce. Experience with many children with each of these disorders has provided a vast amount of information that can be extremely helpful to parents in understanding their child's behavior and to educators in planning an appropriate curriculum. For example, a specific behavioral phenotype has been delineated for the de Lange syndrome; the parents' awareness that the child's aberrant behavior is "normal" for the de Lange syndrome rather than being "their fault" can be extremely helpful in relieving their anxiety and guilt. For the *Williams syndrome*, a different, but equally characteristic behavioral phenotype has been documented and includes the following: multiple developmental motor disabilities affecting strength, balance, coordination, and motor planning; sensory integration dysfunction relating primarily to hypersensitivity to sound; hyperactivity; delayed expressive and receptive language skills with simultaneous age-appropriate grammar and articulation; better reading than mathematics ability; and cognitive dysfunction ranging from learning disabilities to mental retardation. This knowledge of a child's particular strengths and weaknesses may allow educators to develop a curriculum that will give affected children a better chance to reach their potential.

In certain nonrandom associations of malformations, it has not been determined whether the pattern is a sequence or a syndrome. Such related malformations are designated **associations**. One important clinical example is the *VATER association*, which includes vertebral defects, anal atresia, tracheoesophageal fistula with atresia, radial upper limb hypoplasia, and renal defects. A single umbilical artery and cardiac and genital anomalies are also seen in this association. These defects are likely to occur together in almost any combination of two or more and usually represent a sporadic occurrence in an otherwise normal family.

The ultimate goal in evaluating a child with structural defects is making a specific overall diagnosis. When such a diagnosis is made, appropriate recurrence risk counseling for the parents, accurate prognostication about the child's future development, and an appropriate plan for achievement of the child's potential are usually possible (see Chapter 37). When an overall diagnosis is lacking, the most that can be expected is a better understanding of the nature and onset of the problem, which may often be helpful to parents and others dealing with the child.

Breuning MH, Dauwerse HG, Fugazza G, et al: Rubinstein-Taybi syndrome caused by submicroscopic deletions within 16p13.3. *Am J Hum Genet* 1993;52:249.

Briggs GG, Freeman RK, Yaffe SJ: *Drugs in Pregnancy and Lactation*, 6th ed. Baltimore, Williams & Wilkins, 2002.

Burn J, Brennan P, Little J, et al: Recurrence risks in offspring of adults with major heart defects: Results from first cohort of British collaborative study. *Lancet* 1998;351:311.

Dilts CV, Morris CA, Leonard CO: Hypothesis for development of a behavioral phenotype in Williams syndrome. *Am J Med Genet* 1990;6:126.

Dunn PM: Congenital postural deformities. *Br Med Bull* 1976;32:71.

Ewart AK, Morris CA, Atkinson D, et al: Hemizygosity at the elastin locus in a developmental disorder, Williams syndrome. *Nat Genet* 1993;5:11.

Gorlin RJ, Cohen MM, Hennekam RCM: *Syndromes of the Head and Neck*, 4th ed. New York, Oxford University Press, 2001.

Higginbottom MC, Jones KL, Hall BD, et al: The amniotic band disruption complex. Timing of amniotic rupture and variable spectra of consequent defects. *J Pediatr* 1979;95:544.

Johnson HG, Ekman P, Frieseu W, et al: A behavioral phenotype in the de Lange syndrome. *Pediatr Res* 1976;10:843.

Jones KL: *Smith's Recognizable Patterns of Human Malformation*, 5th ed. Philadelphia, WB Saunders, 1997.

Kalter H, Warkany J: Congenital malformation, etiologic factors and their role in prevention. *N Engl J Med* 1983;308:424.

Kausseff BG, Newkirk P, Root AW: Brachmann-de Lange syndrome. 1994 update. *Arch Pediatr Adolesc Med* 1994;148:749.

Kazazian HH Jr: The nature of mutation. *Hosp Pract* 1985;20:55.

Lie RT, Wilcox AJ, Skjaerven R: Survival and reproduction among males with birth defects and risk of recurrence in their children. *JAMA* 2001;285:755.

Lie RT, Wilcox AJ, Skjaerven R: A population-based study of the risk of recurrence of birth defects. *N Engl J Med* 1994;331:1.

McKusick VA: *Mendelian Inheritance in Man. Catalog of Autosomal Dominant, Autosomal Recessive and X-linked Phenotypes*, 10th ed. Baltimore, The Johns Hopkins University Press, 1992. www3.ncbi.nlm.nih.gov/omim/REPROTOX: http://reprotox.org/

Shepard TH: *A Catalog of Teratogenic Agents*, 10th ed. Baltimore, The Johns Hopkins University Press, 2001. TERIS:http//depts.washington.edu/~terisweb/

Vrijheid M, Dolk H, Armstrong B, et al: Chromosomal congenital anomalies and residence near hazardous waste landfill sites. *Lancet* 2002;359:320.

Walkowiak J, Wiener JA, Fastabend A, et al: Environmental exposure to polychlorinated biphenyls and quality of the home environment: Effects on psychodevelopment in early childhood. *Lancet* 2001;358:1602.

SECTION 2 *Infections of the Neonatal Infant*

*Barbara. J. Stoll**

Chapter 98

Pathogenesis and Epidemiology

Infections are a frequent and important cause of morbidity and mortality in the neonatal period. As many as 2% of fetuses are infected in utero, and up to 10% of infants have infections in the 1st mo of life. Neonatal infections are unique for several reasons. (1) Infectious agents can be transmitted from the mother to the fetus or newborn infant by diverse modes. (2) Newborn infants are less capable of responding to infection because of one or more immunologic deficiencies. (3) Coexisting conditions often complicate the diagnosis and management of neonatal infections. (4) The clinical manifestations of newborn infections vary and include subclinical infection, mild to severe manifestations of focal or systemic infection, and rarely, congenital malformations resulting from infection in the 1st trimester. The timing of exposure, inoculum size, immune status, and virulence of the etiologic agent influ-

ence the expression of disease in a fetus or newborn infant. (5) Maternal infection that is the source of transplacental fetal infection is often undiagnosed during pregnancy because the mother was either asymptomatic or had nonspecific signs and symptoms at the time of acute infection. (6) A wide variety of etiologic agents infect the newborn, including bacteria, viruses, fungi, protozoa, and mycoplasmas. (7) Finally, with advances in neonatal intensive care, increasingly immature, very low birthweight (VLBW) newborns are surviving and remain in the hospital for a longer time, an environment that puts them at ongoing high risk for infection.

98.1 Modes of Transmission and Pathogenesis

Pathogenesis of Intrauterine Infection. Intrauterine infection is a result of clinical or subclinical maternal infection with a variety of agents (e.g., cytomegalovirus [CMV], *Treponema pallidum, Toxoplasma gondii*, rubella virus, varicella virus, parvovirus B19) and hematogenous transplancental transmission to the fetus. Transplacental infection may occur at any time during gestation, and signs and symptoms may be present at birth or be delayed

---

*Updated and edited from the 16th Edition section by Dr. Sam Gotoff.

for months or years (Fig. 98–1). Infection may result in early spontaneous abortion, congenital malformation, intrauterine growth restriction, premature birth, stillbirth, acute disease in the neonatal period, or asymptomatic persistent infection with sequelae later in life. In some cases, no apparent effects are seen in the newborn infant.

The timing of infection during gestation affects the outcome. First trimester infection may alter embryogenesis, with resulting congenital malformations (congenital rubella). Third trimester infection often results in active infection at the time of delivery (toxoplasmosis, syphilis). Infections that occur late in gestation may lead to a delay in clinical manifestations until some time after birth (syphilis).

Maternal infection is a necessary prerequisite for transplacental infection. For some etiologic agents, maternal immunity is effective and antibody is protective for the fetus (rubella). For other agents, maternal antibody may ameliorate the outcome of infection or have no effect (CMV). Even without maternal antibody, transplacental transmission of infection to a fetus is variable, and the placenta often functions as an effective barrier.

Pathogenesis of Ascending Bacterial Infection. In most cases, the fetus or neonate is not exposed to potentially pathogenic bacteria until the membranes rupture and the infant passes through the birth canal and/or enters the extrauterine environment. The human birth canal is colonized with aerobic and anaerobic organisms that may result in ascending amniotic infection and/or colonization of the neonate at birth. Vertical transmission of bacterial agents that infect the amniotic fluid and/or vaginal canal may occur in utero or more commonly during labor and/or delivery (Fig. 98–2). Chorioamnionitis results from microbial invasion of amniotic fluid, usually as a result of prolonged rupture of the chorioamniotic membrane. On occasion,

amniotic infection occurs with apparently intact membranes or with a relatively brief duration of membrane rupture. Amniotic fluid infection may be asymptomatic or may produce maternal fever, with or without local or systemic signs of chorioamnionitis. The duration of membrane rupture is directly correlated with the development of chorioamnionitis. Previously, longer than 24 hr was considered prolonged rupture of membranes because microscopic evidence of inflammation of the membranes is uniformly present when the duration of rupture exceeds 24 hr. However, at 18 hr of membrane rupture, the incidence of early-onset disease with group B streptococcus (GBS) increases significantly. Therefore, longer than 18 hr is the current cutoff for increased risk of neonatal infection. Difficult or traumatic delivery and premature delivery are also associated with an increased frequency of neonatal infection.

In most cases, bacterial colonization does not result in disease. Factors influencing which colonized infant will develop disease are not well understood but include prematurity, underlying illness, invasive procedures, inoculum size, virulence of the infecting organism, and transplacental maternal antibodies (Fig. 98–3). Aspiration or ingestion of bacteria in amniotic fluid may lead to congenital pneumonia or systemic infection, with manifestations becoming apparent before delivery (fetal distress, tachycardia), at delivery (perinatal asphyxia), or after a latent period of a few hours (respiratory distress, shock). Aspiration or ingestion of bacteria during the birth process may lead to infection after an interval of 1–2 days.

Resuscitation at birth, particularly if it involves endotracheal intubation, insertion of an umbilical vessel catheter, or both, is associated with an increased risk of bacterial infection. Explanations include the presence of infection at the time of birth or acquisition of infection during the invasive procedures associated with resuscitation.

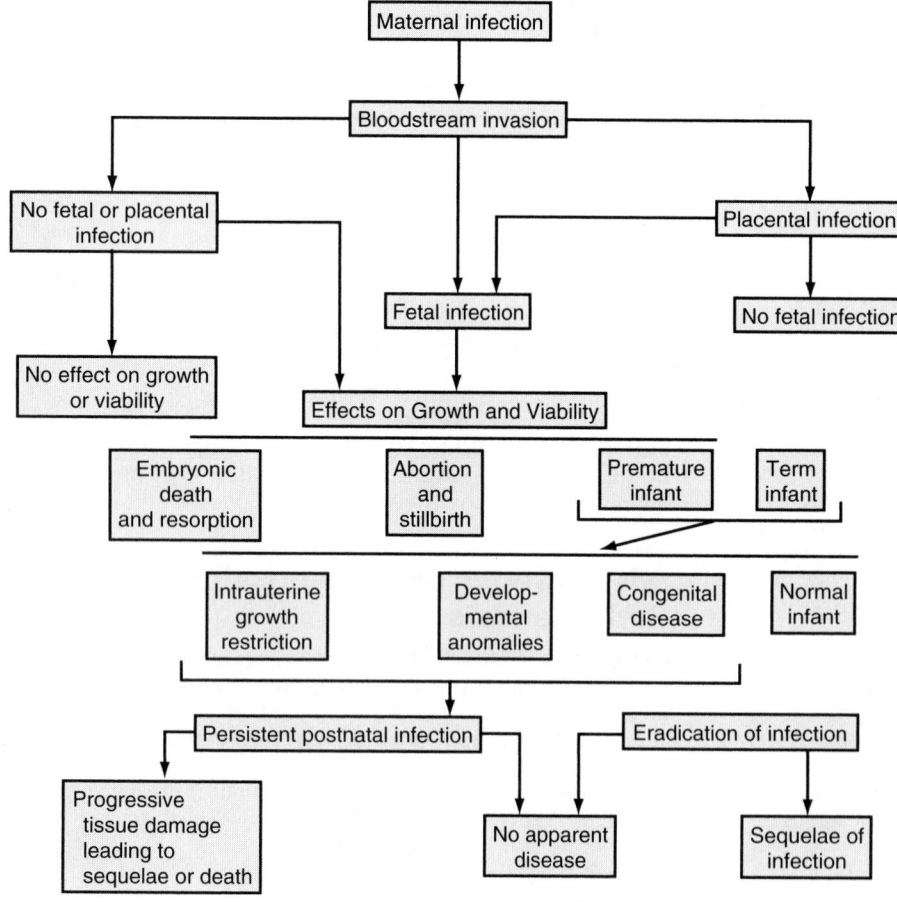

FIGURE 98–1. Pathogenesis of hematogenous transplacental infections. (From Klein JO, Remington JS: Current concepts of infections of the fetus and newborn infant. In Remington JS, Klein JO [editors]: *Infectious Diseases of the Fetus and Newborn Infant,* 5th ed. WB Saunders, Philadelphia, 2002, pp 1–23.)

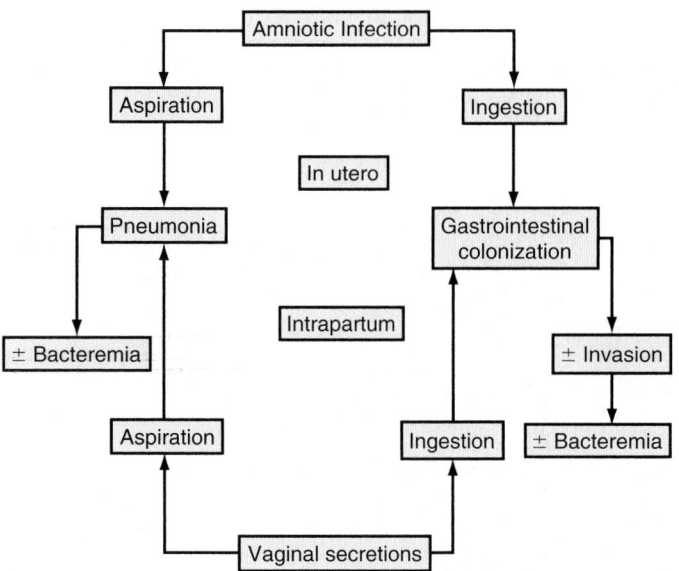

FIGURE 98–2. Pathways of ascending or intrapartum infection.

Pathogenesis of Late-Onset Postnatal Infections. After birth, neonates are exposed to infectious agents in the nursery or in the community. Postnatal infections may be transmitted by direct contact with hospital personnel, the mother, or other family members; from breast milk (HIV, CMV); or from inanimate sources such as contaminated equipment. The most common source of postnatal infections in hospitalized newborns is hand contamination of health care personnel.

Most cases of meningitis result from hematogenous dissemination. Less often, meningitis results from contiguous spread as a result of contamination of open neural tube defects, congenital sinus tracts, or penetrating wounds from fetal scalp sampling or internal fetal electrocardiographic monitors. Abscess forma-

tion, ventriculitis, septic infarcts, hydrocephalus, and subdural effusions are complications of meningitis that occur more often in newborn infants than in older children.

98.2 Immunity

Diminished concentrations of immunoglobulins and other immunologic factors and decreased function of neutrophils and other cells involved in the response to infection have been demonstrated in both term and preterm infants. Despite these alterations in immune function, the rate of systemic infection in newborns is low in the absence of obstetric and neonatal risk factors. All newborns enter an unsterile environment, but infection develops in only a few. The immunologic system is discussed in detail in Part XIII.

Immunoglobulins. IgG is actively transported across the placenta, with concentrations in a full-term infant comparable to those in the mother. The specificity of IgG antibody in cord blood is dependent on the mother's previous antigenic exposure and immunologic response. In premature infants, cord IgG levels are directly proportional to gestational age. Studies of type-specific IgG antibodies to GBS have shown that the ratio of cord to maternal serum concentrations is 1.0, 0.5, and 0.3 at term, 32 wk, and 28 wk of gestation, respectively. Levels of maternally derived IgG fall rapidly after birth. Infants with birthweights less than 1,500 g become significantly hypogammaglobulinemic, with mean plasma IgG concentrations in the range of 200–300 mg/dL in the 1st wk of life. Other classes of immunoglobulins are not transferred across the placenta, although a fetus can synthesize IgA and IgM in response to intrauterine infection.

The presence of passively transferred specific IgG antibody in adequate concentration provides neonates protection against infections to which protection is mediated by antibody (e.g., tetanus, encapsulated bacteria such as GBS). Specific bactericidal and opsonic antibodies against enteric gram-negative bacteria are predominantly in the IgM class. In general, newborn

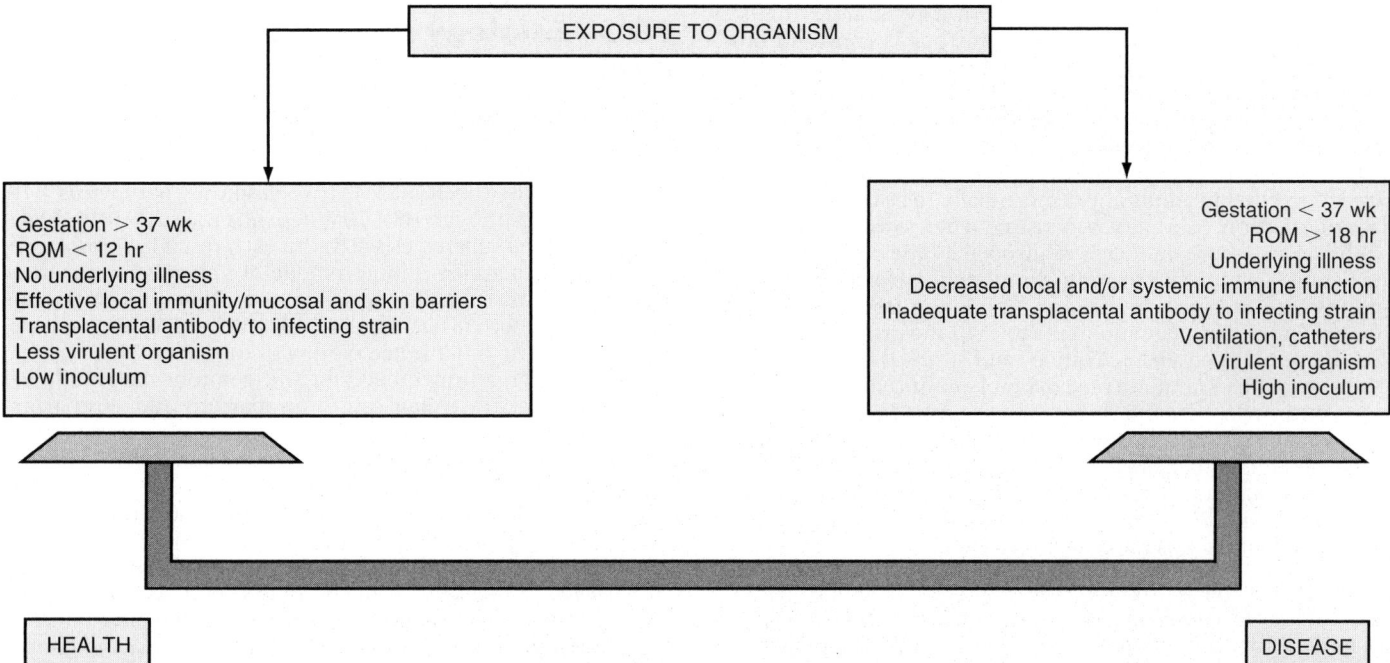

FIGURE 98–3. Factors influencing the balance between health and disease in neonates exposed to a potential pathogen. ROM = rupture of membranes. (Adapted from Baker CJ: Group B streptococcal infections. *Clin Perinatol* 1997;24:59.)

infants lack antibody-mediated protection against *Escherichia coli* and other Enterobacteriaceae.

Complement. The complement system mediates bactericidal activity against certain organisms such as *E. coli* and functions as an opsonin with antibody in the phagocytosis of bacteria such as GBS. Essentially no transplacental passage of complement from the maternal circulation takes place. A fetus begins to synthesize complement components as early as the 1st trimester. Full-term newborn infants have slightly diminished classical pathway complement activity and moderately diminished alternative pathway activity. Considerable variability, however, is seen in both the concentration and activity of complement components. Premature infants have lower levels of complement components and less complement activity than full-term newborns do. These deficiencies contribute to diminished complement-derived chemotactic activity and to a diminished ability to opsonize certain organisms in the absence of antibody. Many studies have been performed with different strains of microorganisms and under different conditions and have examined both the classical and alternative pathways. In general, opsonization of *Staphylococcus aureus* is normal in neonatal sera, but various degrees of impairment have been noted with GBS and *E. coli*.

Neutrophils. Quantitative and qualitative deficiencies of the phagocyte system are important factors contributing to newborns' increased susceptibility to infection. Neutrophil migration (chemotaxis) is abnormal at birth in both term and preterm infants. In addition, neonatal neutrophils have decreased adhesion, aggregation, and deformability, all of which may delay the response to infection. Abnormal expression of cell membrane adhesion molecules (the β_2 integrins and selectins) and abnormalities in the neonatal neutrophil cytoskeleton contribute to abnormal chemotaxis. With adequate opsonization, phagocytosis and killing by neutrophils are comparable in newborn infants and adults. However, in the face of infectious or noninfectious stress (respiratory distress syndrome [RDS]), the ability of neonatal neutrophils to phagocytose gram-negative (but not gram-positive) bacteria appears to be decreased. The oxidative respiratory burst of neonatal neutrophils is impaired and is a factor in the increased risk of sepsis, especially in preterm infants.

The number of circulating neutrophils is elevated after birth in both term and preterm infants, with a peak at 12 hr that returns to normal by 22 hr. Band neutrophils constitute less than 15% in normal newborns and may increase in newborns with infection and other stress responses such as asphyxia.

Neutropenia is frequently observed in preterm infants and those with intrauterine growth restriction, and it increases the risk for sepsis. The neutrophil storage pool in newborn infants is 20–30% of that in adults and is more likely to be depleted in the face of infection. Mortality is increased when sepsis is associated with severe sepsis-induced neutropenia and bone marrow depletion. Granulocyte colony–stimulating factor (G-CSF) and granulocyte-macrophage colony–stimulating factor (GM-CSF) are cytokines that play important roles in the proliferation, differentiation, functional activation, and survival of phagocytes. These cytokines stimulate myeloid progenitor cells, increase the bone marrow neutrophil storage pool, induce peripheral blood neutrophilia, and influence neutrophil function, including enhancement of bactericidal activity. Although these myeloid colony–stimulating factors influence neutrophil number and function, their clinical utility in the treatment and/or prevention of neonatal sepsis remains undetermined.

Monocyte-Macrophage System. The monocyte-macrophage system consists of circulating monocytes and tissue macrophages, particularly in the liver, spleen, and lung. Activated macrophages are involved in antigen presentation, phagocytosis, and immune modulation. The number of circulating monocytes in neonatal blood is normal, but the mass or function of macrophages in the reticuloendothelial system is diminished in newborns, particu-

larly in preterm infants. In both term and preterm infants, chemotaxis of monocytes is impaired; this impairment affects the inflammatory response in tissues and the results of delayed hypersensitivity skin tests. However, monocytes from neonates ingest and kill microorganisms as well as monocytes from adults do.

Natural Killer Cells. Natural killer (NK) cells are a subgroup of lymphocytes that are cytolytic against cells infected with viruses. NK cells also lyse cells coated with antibody in a process called antibody-dependent cell-mediated cytotoxicity (ADCC). NK cells appear early in gestation and are present in cord blood in numbers equivalent to those in adults; however, neonatal NK cells have decreased cytotoxic activity and ADCC in comparison to adult cells. The diminished cytotoxicity against herpes simplex virus (HSV)-infected cells may predispose to disseminated HSV infection in newborns (see Chapter 231).

Cytokines/Inflammatory Mediators. The patient's response to infection and clinical outcome involve a balance between pro-inflammatory and anti-inflammatory cytokines. Several adverse neonatal outcomes, including brain injury, necrotizing enterocolitis, and bronchopulmonary dysplasia (BPD), may be mediated by the cytokine response to infection in the mother, fetus, or newborn. The list of mediators that have been studied in newborns is long and includes tumor necrosis factor-α (TNFα), interleukin 1 (IL-1), IL-4, IL-6, IL-8, IL-10, IL-12, platelet-activating factor, and the leukotrienes. The release of various inflammatory mediators in response to infection offers the potential opportunity to facilitate an early diagnosis of infection. Studies of potential surrogate markers for neonatal infection have focused on the association of bacterial sepsis, pneumonia, and necrotizing enterocolitis with elevated cytokine levels. TNFα, IL-6, and IL-8 are elevated in neonates with sepsis.

Innate immunity involves nonspecific cellular and humoral responses to an infectious agent without previous exposure. Neutrophil granules contain many enzymes; one protein, bactericidal/permeability-increasing protein (BPI), binds to the endotoxin in the cell wall of gram-negative bacteria. It facilitates opsonization and prevents the inflammatory response to endotoxin. BPI activity may also be decreased in neonates.

98.3 Etiology of Fetal and Neonatal Infection

A number of agents may infect newborns in utero, intrapartum, or postpartum (Table 98–1 and Box 98–1). Intrauterine transplacental infections of significance to the fetus and/or newborn include syphilis, rubella, CMV, toxoplasmosis, parvovirus B19, and varicella. Although HSV, HIV, hepatitis B virus (HBV), hepatitis C virus, and tuberculosis (TB) can each result in transplacental infection, the most common mode of transmission for these agents is intrapartum during labor and delivery with passage through an infected birth canal (HIV, HSV, HBV) or postnatal from contact with an infected mother or caretaker (TB).

Any microorganism inhabiting the genitourinary or lower gastrointestinal tract may cause intrapartum and postpartum infection. The most common bacteria are GBS, enteric organisms, gonococci, and chlamydiae. The more common viruses are CMV, HSV, and HIV.

Agents that commonly cause nosocomial infection are coagulase-negative staphylococci, gram-negative bacilli (*E. coli, Klebsiella pneumoniae, Salmonella, Enterobacter, Citrobacter, Pseudomonas aeruginosa, Serratia*), enterococci, *S. aureus*, and *Candida*. Viruses contributing to nosocomial neonatal infection include enteroviruses, CMV, hepatitis A, adenoviruses, influenza, respiratory syncytial virus, rhinovirus, parainfluenza, HSV, and rotavirus. Community-acquired pathogens such as *Streptococcus pneumoniae* may also cause infection in newborn infants after discharge from the hospital.

TABLE 98–1. Bacterial Causes of Systemic Neonatal Infections

Bacteria	Early Onset	Late Onset, Maternal Origin	Late Onset, Nosocomial	Late Onset, Community
Gram Positive				
Clostridia	+		+	*
Enterococci	+		++	
Group B streptococcus	+++	+	+	+
Listeria monocytogenes	+	+		
Other streptococci	++			+
Staphylococcus aureus	+		++	+
Staphylococcus, coagulase negative	+		+++	
Streptococcus pneumoniae	+			++
Viridans streptococcus	+		++	
Gram Negative				
Bacteroides	+		+	
Campylobacter	+			
Citrobacter			+	+
Enterobacter			+	
Escherichia coli	+++		+	++
Haemophilus influenzae	+			+
Klebsiella			+	
Neisseria gonorrhoeae	+			
Neisseria meningitidis	+		+	
Proteus			+	
Pseudomonas			+	
Salmonella		+		+
Serratia			+	
Others				
Treponema pallidum	+	+		
Mycobacterium tuberculosis		+		

*Clostridium tetani *in some developing countries.*
+ = *relative frequency.*

Congenital pneumonia may be caused by CMV, rubella virus, and *T. pallidum* and less commonly by the other agents producing transplacental infection (Table 98–2). Microorganisms causing pneumonia acquired during labor and delivery include GBS, gram-negative enteric aerobes, *Listeria monocytogenes*, genital *Mycoplasma, Chlamydia trachomatis,* CMV, HSV, and *Candida* species.

The bacteria responsible for most cases of nosocomial pneumonia typically include staphylococcal species, gram-negative enteric aerobes, and occasionally, *Pseudomonas*. Fungi are responsible for an increasing number of systemic infections acquired during prolonged hospitalization of neonates. Finally, respiratory viruses cause isolated cases and outbreaks of nosocomial pneumonia. These viruses, usually endemic during the winter months and acquired from infected hospital staff or visitors to the nursery, include respiratory syncytial virus, parainfluenza virus, influenza viruses, and adenovirus. Respiratory viruses are the single most important cause of community-acquired pneumonia and are usually contracted from infected household contacts.

TABLE 98–2. Etiologic Agents of Neonatal Pneumonia According to Timing of Acquisition

Transplacental	Perinatal	Postnatal
Cytomegalovirus	Anaerobic bacteria	Adenovirus
Herpes simplex virus	*Chlamydia*	*Candida species
Mycobacterium tuberculosis	Cytomegalovirus	Coagulase-negative staphylococci
Rubella virus	Enteric bacteria	Cytomegalovirus
Treponema pallidum	Group B streptococci	Echoviruses
Varicella-zoster virus	*Haemophilus influenzae*	*Enteric bacteria
	Herpes simplex virus	Influenza viruses A, B
	Listeria monocytogenes	Parainfluenza
	Mycoplasma	*Pseudomonas
		Respiratory syncytial virus
		Staphylococcus aureus

More likely in infants undergoing mechanical ventilation, with indwelling catheters, or after abdominal surgery.

The most common bacterial causes of neonatal meningitis are GBS, *E. coli*, and *L. monocytogenes. S. pneumoniae*, other streptococci, non-typable *Haemophilus influenzae*, both coagulase-positive and coagulase-negative staphylococci, *Klebsiella, Enterobacter, Pseudomonas, T. pallidum*, and *Mycobacterium tuberculosis* may also produce meningitis. *Citrobacter diversus* is an important cause of brain abscess.

98.4 Epidemiology of Early- and Late-Onset Neonatal Infections

The terms early-onset and late-onset infection refer to the age at onset of infection in the neonatal period (Table 98–3). Originally divided arbitrarily as infections occurring before and after 1 wk of

BOX 98–1. Nonbacterial Causes of Systemic Neonatal Infections

VIRUSES
Adenovirus
Cytomegalovirus
Enteroviruses
Herpes simplex virus
HIV
Parvovirus
Rubella virus
Varicella-zoster virus

MYCOPLASMA
M. hominis
Ureaplasma urealyticum

FUNGI
Candida species
Malassezia species

PROTOZA
Plasmodia
Toxoplasma gondii
Trypanosoma cruzi

TABLE 98–3. Neonatal Infection by Age of Onset

Characteristics	Early Onset	Late Onset	Late, Late Onset
Age at onset	Birth to 7 days usually <72 hr	7 to 30 days	>30 days
Maternal obstetric complications	Common	Uncommon	Varies
Prematurity	Frequent	Varies	Usual
Organism source	Maternal genital tract	Maternal genital tract/environment	Environment/community
Manifestation	Multisystem	Multisystem or focal	Multisystem or focal
Site	Normal nursery, NICU, community	NICU, community	NICU, community

NICU = neonatal intensive care unit.

life, it is more useful to separate early- and late-onset infections according to peripartum pathogenesis. Early-onset infections are acquired before or during delivery. Late-onset infections are acquired after delivery in the normal newborn nursery, neonatal intensive care unit (NICU), or the community. The age at onset depends on the timing of vertical transmission and the virulence of the infecting organism. Pyogenic infections such as GBS are usually clinically apparent within the 1st 24 hr of life. Late, late-onset infections (occurring after 1 mo of life) have been reported, particularly in VLBW preterm infants.

The *incidence of neonatal bacterial sepsis* varies from 1–4 cases per 1,000 live births in developed countries, with considerable fluctuation over time and with geographic location. Term male infants have an approximately twofold higher incidence of sepsis than term females do. This sex difference is less clear in preterm low-birthweight (LBW) infants. Attack rates of neonatal sepsis increase significantly in LBW infants in the presence of maternal chorioamnionitis, congenital immune defects, asple-

nia, galactosemia *(E. coli)*, and malformations leading to high inocula of bacteria (obstructive uropathy).

Intrapartum antibiotics are used to reduce vertical transmission of GBS, as well as lessen neonatal morbidity after preterm rupture of membranes. After the introduction of selective intrapartum antibiotic prophylaxis to prevent perinatal transmission of GBS, rates of early-onset neonatal GBS infection in the United States declined from 1.7 cases per 1,000 live births to 0.6 per 1,000. Intrapartum chemoprophylaxis has had no effect on rates of late-onset GBS disease. Although some studies have reported a decline in non-GBS pathogens, as well as in GBS, others have reported no change in rates of non-GBS pathogens. Of concern are reports of an increase in gram-negative infections (especially *E. coli*) in VLBW infants in the face of a reduction in GBS sepsis.

The *incidence of meningitis* in newborn infants is 0.2–0.4 cases per 1,000 live births and is higher in preterm infants. Bacterial meningitis may be associated with sepsis or may occur as a focal infection. Meningitis currently develops in less than 20% of newborn infants with early-onset invasive bacterial infections.

Prematurity. The most important neonatal factor predisposing to infection is prematurity or LBW. Preterm infants have a 3- to 10-fold higher incidence of infection than full-term, normal-birthweight infants do. A number of possible explanations have been proposed for the increased incidence of infection in preterm infants. (1) Maternal genital tract infection is considered to be an important cause of preterm labor, with an increased risk of vertical transmission to the newborn (Figs. 98–4 and 98–5). (2) The frequency of intra-amniotic infection is inversely related to gestational age. (3) Premature infants have documented immune dysfunction. (4) Premature infants often require prolonged intravenous access, endotracheal intubation, or other invasive procedures that provide a portal of entry or impair clearance mechanisms.

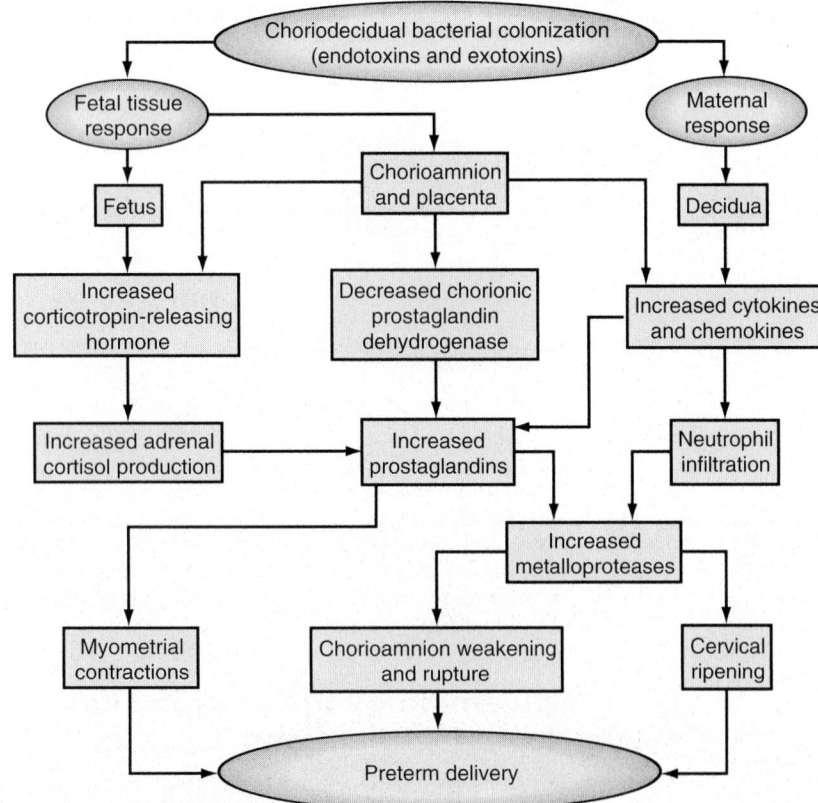

FIGURE 98–4. Potential pathways from choriodecidual bacterial colonization to preterm delivery. (From Goldenberg RL, Hauth JC, Andrews WW: Mechanisms of disease: Intrauterine infection and preterm delivery. *N Engl J Med* 2000;342:1500.)

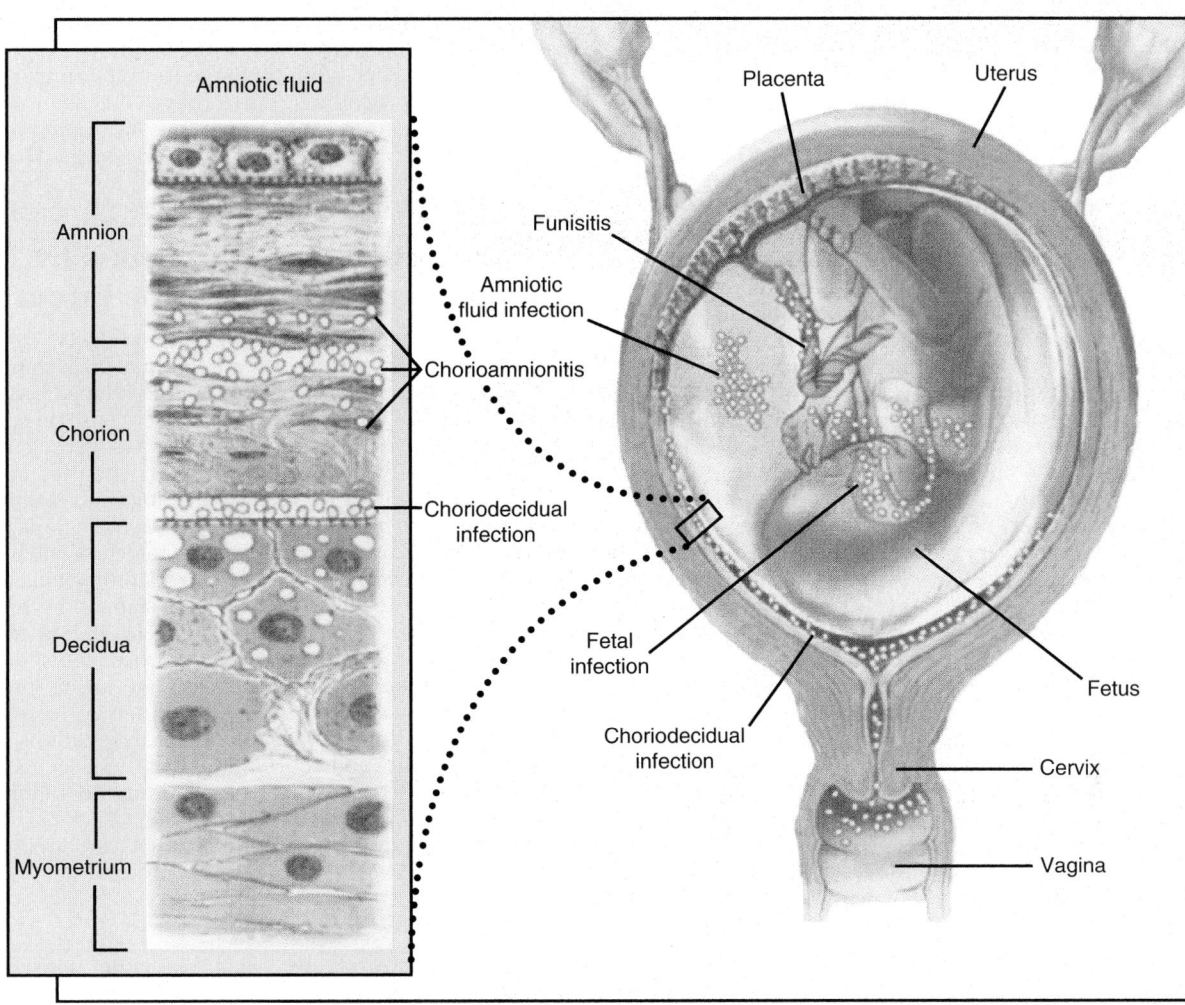

FIGURE 98–5. Potential sites of bacterial infection within the uterus. (From Goldenberg RL, Hauth JC, Andrews WW: Mechanisms of disease: Intrauterine infection and preterm delivery. *N Engl J Med* 2000;342:1500. Copyright 2000 Massachusetts Medical Society.)

Chorioamnionitis. Attack rates of neonatal infection increase significantly in the presence of chorioamnionitis, which is diagnosed by amniotic fluid analysis or histologically. Clinical signs of chorioamnionitis include intrapartum fever (>38°C), maternal leukocytosis (white blood cell [WBC] count >18,000), and uterine tenderness. Rates of histologic chorioamnionitis are inversely related to gestational age and directly related to the duration of membrane rupture.

Nosocomial Infections. Nosocomial, or hospital-acquired, infections are responsible for significant morbidity and late mortality in hospitalized newborns. Neonatal nosocomial infection is not uniformly defined. Many define nosocomial infections as infections occurring after 3 days of life that are not directly acquired from the mother's genital tract. The Centers for Disease Control and Prevention (CDC) defines a nosocomial infection as any infection occurring after admission to the NICU that was not transplacentally acquired. Rates of nosocomial infection in healthy term infants who are either rooming in with their mothers or staying in the well baby nursery are low (less than 1%). The majority of nosocomial infections occur in preterm or term infants who require special care. Risk factors for nosocomial infection in these infants include prematurity, LBW, invasive procedures, indwelling vascular catheters, parenteral nutrition with lipid emulsions, endotracheal tubes, ventricular shunts, alterations in the skin and/or mucous membrane barri-

ers, frequent use of broad-spectrum antibiotics, and prolonged hospital stay. Most nosocomial infections are bloodstream infections associated with an intravascular device. Other serious infections are pneumonia, meningitis, omphalitis, and necrotizing enterocolitis.

Large cohort studies of VLBW infants (under 1500 g birthweight) have reported nosocomial infection rates of 20–25%. Rates increase with decreasing gestational age and birthweight. The National Institute of Child Health and Human Development (NICHD) Neonatal Research Network has reported rates of 43% for infants 401–750 g, 28% for those 751–1000 g, 15% for those 1001–1250 g, and 7% for those 1251–1500 g. The National Nosocomial Infection Surveillance System (NNISS) monitors device-associated nosocomial infection rates. Rates are inversely related to birthweight and range from 11.4 infections/1,000 device days for infants under 1,000 g to 3.8 infections/1,000 device days for those over 2500 g. The widespread differences in practice regarding the inclusion of lumbar puncture in the diagnostic evaluation of an infant with suspected sepsis make it more difficult to determine rates of late-onset meningitis.

Various bacterial and fungal agents colonize hospitalized infants, health care workers, and visitors. Pathogenic agents can be transmitted by direct contact or indirectly via contaminated equipment, intravenous fluids, medications, blood products, or enteral feedings. Colonization of the infant's skin, umbilicus, and respiratory or gastrointestinal tract with pathogenic agents often precedes the development of infection. Antibiotic use interferes with colonization by normal flora, thereby facilitating colonization with more virulent pathogens.

Multiple studies have reported that coagulase-negative staphylococci are the most frequent neonatal nosocomial pathogens. Among a cohort of 6,215 VLBW infants in the NICHD Neonatal Research Network, gram-positive agents were associated with 70%, gram-negative with 18%, and fungi with 12% of cases of late-onset sepsis (Table 98–4). Coagulase-negative staphylococcus, the single most common organism, was isolated in 48% of these infections. The emergence of nosocomial bacterial pathogens resistant to multiple antibiotics is a growing concern. Among NICU patients, methicillin-resistant *S. aureus*, vancomycin-resistant enterococci, and multidrug-resistant gram-negative pathogens are particularly alarming.

Viral organisms may also cause nosocomial infection in the NICU and include respiratory syncytial virus, varicella, influenza, rotavirus, and enteroviruses. For viral as well as bacterial agents, nursery outbreaks may occur in addition to individual cases. Hospital infection control policies are essential to prevent and/or contain nursery outbreaks.

The mean age at onset of the 1st episode of late-onset nosocomial sepsis is 2–3 wk, independent of the infecting pathogen. Nosocomial infections increase the risk of adverse outcomes, including prolonged hospitalization and mortality.

Active surveillance for nosocomial infection is essential to monitor overall rates of infection, rates of infection with specific pathogens, and antibiotic susceptibility patterns and to identify clusters of cases or true infectious outbreaks. Surveillance is based on the ongoing review of nursery infections and data from the microbiology laboratory; routine surveillance to detect colonization is not indicated. Culture results should indicate the bacterial isolate and the antimicrobial sensitivity pattern. Assessment of other microbial markers (biotype, serotype, DNA fingerprint) may be helpful in epidemics. During epidemics, investigation of possible reservoirs of infection, modes of trans-

mission, and risk factors is necessary. Identification of colonized infants and nursery personnel may be helpful.

Infections acquired after discharge from the nursery are usually community acquired. They have the same epidemiologic considerations as other community-acquired infections in infants and children, except for protection provided by maternal antibody.

98.5 Clinical Manifestations of Transplacental Intrauterine Infections

Infection with agents that cross the placenta (CMV, *T. pallidum, T. gondii*, rubella, parvovirus B19, others) may be asymptomatic at birth or may cause a spectrum of disease ranging from relatively mild symptoms to multisystem involvement with severe and life-threatening complications. For some agents, disease is characterized by chronicity, recurrence, or both (in the mother and infant), and the agent may cause ongoing injury. Clinical signs and symptoms do not help make a specific etiologic diagnosis, but rather raise suspicion of an intrauterine infection and help distinguish these infections from acute bacterial infections that occur during labor and delivery. The following signs and symptoms are common to many of these agents (Table 98–5): intrauterine growth restriction, microcephaly or hydrocephalus, intracranial calcifications, chorioretinitis, cataracts, myocarditis, pneumonia, hepatosplenomegaly, direct hyperbilirubinemia, anemia, thrombocytopenia, hydrops fetalis, and skin manifestations, including petechiae, purpura, and vesicles. Many of these agents cause late sequelae, even if the infant is asymptomatic at birth. These adverse outcomes include sensorineural hearing loss, visual disturbances (including blindness), seizures, and neurodevelopmental abnormalities.

BACTERIAL SEPSIS

Neonates with bacterial sepsis may have either nonspecific signs and symptoms or focal signs of infection (Box 98–2, Table 98–6), including temperature instability, hypotension, poor perfusion with pallor and mottled skin, metabolic acidosis, tachycardia or bradycardia, apnea, respiratory distress, grunting, cyanosis, irritability, lethargy, seizures, feeding intolerance, abdominal distention, jaundice, petechiae, purpura, and bleeding. The initial manifestation may involve only limited symptomatology and only one system, such as apnea alone or tachypnea with retractions or tachycardia, or it may be an acute catastrophic manifestation with multiorgan dysfunction. Infants should be re-evaluated over time to determine whether the symptoms have progressed from mild to severe. Later complications of sepsis include respiratory failure, pulmonary hypertension, cardiac failure, shock, renal failure, liver dysfunction, cerebral edema or thrombosis, adrenal hemorrhage and/or insufficiency, bone marrow dysfunction (neutropenia, thrombocytopenia, anemia), and disseminated intravascular coagulopathy (DIC).

A variety of noninfectious conditions can occur together with neonatal infection or can make the diagnosis of infection more difficult. For example, RDS secondary to surfactant deficiency can coexist with bacterial pneumonia. Because bacterial sepsis can be rapidly progressive, the physician must be alert to the signs and symptoms of possible infection and initiate diagnostic evaluation and empirical therapy in a timely manner. The differential diagnosis of many of the signs and symptoms that suggest infection is extensive; these noninfectious disorders must also be considered as the diagnostic evaluation proceeds (Table 98–7).

SYSTEMIC INFLAMMATORY RESPONSE SYNDROME

The clinical manifestations of infection depend on the virulence of the infecting organism and the body's inflammatory

TABLE 98–4. Distribution of Pathogens Associated with the First Episode of Late-Onset Sepsis in VLBW Infants: NICHD Neonatal Research Network, September 1, 1998 Through August 31, 2000

Organism[*]	N	%
Gram-positive organisms	**922**	**70.2**
Staphylococcus—coagulase negative	629	47.9
Staphylococcus aureus	103	7.8
Enterococcus spp.	43	3.3
Group B streptococci	30	2.3
Other	117	8.9
Gram-negative organisms	**231**	**17.6**
Escherichia coli	64	4.9
Klebsiella	52	4.0
Pseudomonas	35	2.7
Enterobacter	33	2.5
Serratia	29	2.2
Other	18	1.4
Fungi	**160**	**12.2**
Candida albicans	76	5.8
Candida parapsilosis	54	4.1
Other	30	2.3
Total	**1,313**	**100**

[*]*Patients with dual infections and patients with presumed coagulase-negative staphylococci (CONS) contaminants excluded. According to the definitions in text, 276 (44%) CONS were definite infections and 353 (56%) were possible infections.*

VLBW = very low birthweight; NICHD = National Institute of Child Health and Human Development.

From Stoll BJ, Hansen N, Fanaroff AA, et al: Late-onset sepsis in very low birthweight neonates: The experience of the NICHD neonatal research network. Pediatrics 2002; 110:285.

TABLE 98–5. Clinical Manifestations of Transplacental Infections

Manifestation	Pathogen
Intrauterine Growth Restriction	CMV, Plasmodium, rubella, toxoplasmosis, Treponema pallidum, Trypanosoma cruzi, VZV
Congenital Anatomic Defects	
Cataracts	Rubella
Heart defects	Rubella
Hydrocephalus	HSV, lymphocytic choriomeningitis virus, rubella, toxoplasmosis
Intracranial calcification	CMV, HIV, toxoplasmosis, T. cruzi
Limb hypoplasia	VZV
Microcephaly	CMV, HSV, rubella, toxoplasmosis
Microphthalmos	CMV, rubella, toxoplasmosis
Neonatal Organ Involvement	
Anemia	CMV, parvovirus, Plasmodium, rubella, toxoplasmosis, T. cruzi, T. pallidum
Carditis	Coxsackieviruses, rubella, T. cruzi
Encephalitis	CMV, enteroviruses, HSV, rubella, toxoplasmosis, T. cruzi, T. pallidum
Hepatitis	CMV, enteroviruses, HSV
Hepatosplenomegaly	CMV, enteroviruses, HIV, HSV, Plasmodium, rubella, T. cruzi, T. pallidum
Hydrops	Parvovirus, T. pallidum, toxoplasmosis
Lymphadenopathy	CMV, HIV, rubella, toxoplasmosis, T. pallidum
Osteitis	Rubella, T. pallidum
Petechiae, purpura	CMV, enteroviruses, rubella, T. cruzi
Pneumonitis	CMV, enteroviruses, HSV, measles, rubella, toxoplasmosis, T. pallidum, VZV
Retinitis	CMV, HSV, lymphocytic choriomeningitis virus, rubella, toxoplasmosis, T. pallidum, West Nile virus
Rhinitis	Enteroviruses, T. pallidum
Skin lesions	Entroviruses, HSV, measles, rubella, T. pallidum, VZV
Thrombocytopenia	CMV, enteroviruses, HIV, HSV, rubella, toxoplasmosis, T. pallidum
Late Sequelae	
Convulsions	CMV, enteroviruses, rubella, toxoplasmosis
Deafness	CMV, rubella, toxoplasmosis
Dental/skeletal	Rubella, T. pallidum
Endocrinopathies	Rubella, toxoplasmosis
Eye pathology	HSV, rubella, toxoplasmosis, T. cruzi, T. pallidum. VZV
Hepatitis	Hepatitis B
Mental retardation	CMV, HIV, HSV, rubella, toxoplasmosis, T. cruzi, VZV
Nephrotic syndrome	Plasmodium, T. pallidum

CMV = cytomegalovirus; VZV = varicella-zoster virus; HSV = herpes simplex virus.

response to that agent. The term *systemic inflammatory response syndrome* (SIRS) is most frequently used to describe this unique process of infection and the subsequent systemic response (Chapters 57.2 and 163). In addition to infection, SIRS may result from trauma, hemorrhagic shock, other causes of ischemia, and pancreatitis.

BOX 98–2. Initial Signs and Symptoms of Infection in Newborn Infants

GENERAL
Fever, temperature
  instability
"Not doing well"
Poor feeding
Edema

GASTROINTESTINAL SYSTEM
Abdominal distention
Vomiting
Diarrhea
Hepatomegaly

RESPIRATORY SYSTEM
Apnea, dyspnea
Tachypnea, retractions
Flaring, grunting
Cyanosis

RENAL SYSTEM
Oliguria

CARDIOVASCULAR SYSTEM
Pallor; mottling; cold, clammy skin
Tachycardia
Hypotension
Bradycardia

CENTRAL NERVOUS SYSTEM
Irritability, lethargy
Tremors, seizures
Hyporeflexia, hypotonia
Abnormal Moro reflex
Irregular respirations
Full fontanel
High-pitched cry

HEMATOLOGIC SYSTEM
Jaundice
Splenomegaly
Pallor
Petechiae, purpura
Bleeding

Patients with SIRS have a spectrum of clinical symptoms that represent progressive stages of the pathologic process. In adults, SIRS is defined by the presence of two or more of the following: (1) fever or hypothermia, (2) tachycardia, (3) tachypnea, and (4) abnormal WBC count or an increase in immature forms. In neonates and pediatric patients, SIRS is manifested as temperature instability, respiratory dysfunction (altered gas exchange, hypoxemia, acute respiratory distress syndrome [ARDS]), cardiac dysfunction (tachycardia, delayed capillary refill, hypotension), and perfusion abnormalities (oliguria, metabolic acidosis, Box 98–3). Increased vascular permeability results in capillary leak into peripheral tissues and the lungs, with resultant pulmonary and peripheral edema. DIC results in the more severely affected cases. The cascade of escalating tissue injury may lead to multisystem organ failure and death.

Fever. Only about 50% of infected newborn infants have a temperature higher than 37.8°C (axillary). Fever in newborn infants does not always signify infection; it may be caused by increased ambient temperature, isolette or radiant warmer malfunction, dehydration, central nervous system (CNS) disorders, hyperthyroidism, familial dysautonomia, or ectodermal dysplasia. A single temperature elevation is infrequently associated with infection; fever sustained over 1 hr is more likely to be due to infection. Most febrile infected infants have additional signs compatible with infection, although a focus of infection may not be apparent. Acute febrile illnesses occurring later in the neonatal period may be caused by urinary tract infection, meningitis, pneumonia, osteomyelitis, or gastroenteritis, in addition to bloodstream infection, thus underscoring the importance of a diagnostic evaluation that includes

TABLE 98–6. Manifestations of Neonatal Bacterial Infections

	Time		Occurrence	
	Early Onset	**Late Onset**	**Common**	**Uncommon**
Abdomen				
Peritonitis	+	+	+	
Hepatitis	+	+		+
Adrenal abscess	+	+		+
Gallbladder hydrops	+	+		+
Brain				
Meningitis	+	+	+	
Abscess		+	+	
Subdural empyema		+	+	
Cerebritis	+	+	+	
Ventriculitis		+	+	
Cardiovascular				
Endovascular infection		+	+	
Endocarditis	+	+		+
Pericarditis	+	+		+
Myocarditis	+	+		+
Ocular				
Conjunctivitis	+	+	+	
Endophthalmitis	+	+		+
Chorioretinitis		+		+
Osteoarticular				
Arthritis	+	+		+
Osteomyelitis		+		+
Dactylitis		+		+
Respiratory Tract				
Pneumonia	+	+	+	
Ethmoiditis	+	+		+
Otitis media		+		+
Mastoiditis		+		+
Salivary glands		+		+
Retropharyngeal cellulitis		+		+
Empyema	+	+	+	
Skin, Soft Tissue				
Breast abscess	+	+	+	
Facial cellulitis	+	+		+
Adenitis		+		+
Fasciitis	+	+		+
Impetigo		+	+	
Purpura fulminans	+	+		+
Omphalitis		+		+
Scalp abscess	+	+		+
Abscess of cystic hygroma		+		+
Urinary tract infection	+	+	+	
No Focus				
Bacteremia	+	+	+	
Sepsis	+	+	+	

TABLE 98–7. Serious Systemic Illness in Newborns: Differential Diagnosis of Neonatal Sepsis

Cardiac
Congenital: Hypoplastic left heart syndrome, other structural disease; PPHN
Acquired: Myocarditis, hypovolemic or cardiogenic shock, PPHN

Gastrointestinal
Necrotizing enterocolitis
Spontaneous GI perforation
Structural abnormalities

Hematologic
Neonatal purpura fulminans
Immune-mediated thrombocytopenia
Immune-mediated neutropenia
Severe anemia
Malignancies (congenital leukemia)
Hereditary clotting disorders

Metabolic
Hypoglycemia
Adrenal disorders: Adrenal hemorrhage, adrenal insufficiency, congenital adrenal hyperplasia
Inborn errors of metabolism: Organic acidurias, lactic acidoses, urea cycle disorders, galactosemia

Neurologic
Intracranial hemorrhage: spontaneous, child abuse
Hypoxic-ischemic encephalopathy
Neonatal seizures
Infant botulism

Respiratory
Respiratory distress syndrome
Aspiration pneumonia: Amniotic fluid, meconium, or gastric contents
Lung hypoplasia
Tracheoesophageal fistula
Transient tachypnea of the newborn

PPHN = persistent pulmonary hypertension of the newborn.

rubella, and parvovirus), congenital neoplastic disease, and Rh hemolytic disease.

Omphalitis. Omphalitis is a unique neonatal infection resulting from inadequate care of the umbilical cord. The umbilical stump is colonized by bacteria from the maternal genital tract and the environment. The necrotic tissue of the umbilical cord is an excellent medium for bacterial growth. Omphalitis may remain a localized infection or may spread to the abdominal wall, the peritoneum, the umbilical or portal vessels, or the liver. Abdominal wall cellulitis or necrotizing fasciitis with associated sepsis and a high mortality rate may develop in infants with omphalitis.

BOX 98–3. Definitions of SIRS and Sepsis: Pediatric Patients

SIRS: The systemic inflammatory response to a variety of clinical insults, manifested by 2 or more of the following conditions:
Temperature instability <35°C or >38.5°C
Respiratory dysfunction
  Tachypnea >2 SD above the mean for age
  Hypoxemia (PaO_2 <70 mm Hg on room air)
Cardiac dysfunction
  Tachycardia >2 SD above the mean for age
  Delayed capillary refill >3 sec
  Hypotension >2 SD below the mean for age
Perfusion abnormalities
  Oliguria (urine output <0.5 mL/kg/hr)
  Lactic acidosis (elevated plasma lactate and/or arterial pH <7.25)
  Altered mental status
Sepsis: The systemic inflammatory response to an infectious process

From Adams-Chapman I, Stoll BJ: Systemic inflammatory response syndrome. *Semin Pediatr Infect Dis* 2001; 12:5–16.

blood culture, urine culture, lumbar puncture, and other studies as indicated (see later). Many agents may cause these late infections, including HSV, enteroviruses, respiratory syncytial virus, and bacterial pathogens. In premature infants, hypothermia or temperature instability is more likely to accompany infection.

Rash. Cutaneous manifestations of infection include impetigo, cellulitis, mastitis, omphalitis, and subcutaneous abscesses. Ecthyma gangrenosum is indicative of infection with *Pseudomonas* species. The presence of small salmon-pink papules suggests *L. monocytogenes* infection. A vesicular rash is consistent with herpesvirus infection. The mucocutaneous lesions of *Candida albicans* are discussed elsewhere (Chapter 215.1). Petechiae and purpura may have an infectious cause. Purple papulonodular lesions are referred to as "blueberry-muffin" rash and represent dermal erythropoiesis. Causes include congenital viral infections (CMV,

Tetanus (see Chapter 194). Neonatal tetanus is an important neonatal infection in several developing countries. It results from unclean delivery and unhygienic management of the umbilical cord in an infant born to a mother who has not been immunized against tetanus. The surveillance case definition of neonatal tetanus requires the ability of a newborn to suck at birth and for the first few days of life, followed by an inability to suck starting between 3 and 10 days of age, difficulty swallowing, spasms, stiffness, seizures, and death. Bronchopneumonia, presumably resulting from aspiration, is a common complication and cause of death. Neonatal tetanus is a preventable disease. It can be prevented by immunizing mothers before or during pregnancy and by ensuring a clean delivery, sterile cutting of the umbilical cord, and proper cord care after birth.

Pneumonia. Early signs and symptoms of pneumonia may be nonspecific, including poor feeding, lethargy, irritability, cyanosis, temperature instability, and the overall impression that the infant is not well. Respiratory symptoms include grunting, tachypnea, retractions, flaring of the alae nasi, cyanosis, apnea, and progressive respiratory failure. If the infant is premature, these signs of progressive respiratory distress may be superimposed on surfactant deficiency (RDS) or BPD. If an infant is being ventilated at the time of infection, the most prominent change may be the need for an increase in ventilatory support.

Signs of pneumonia on physical examination, such as dullness to percussion, change in breath sounds, and the presence of rales or rhonchi, are very difficult to appreciate in a neonate. Roentgenograms of the chest may reveal new infiltrates or an effusion, but if the neonate has underlying RDS or BPD, it is very difficult to determine whether the radiographic changes represent a new process or worsening of the underlying disease.

The progression of neonatal pneumonia can be variable. Fulminant infection is most commonly associated with pyogenic organisms such as GBS (see Chapter 169). Onset may be during the first hours or days of life, with the infant often manifesting rapidly progressive circulatory collapse and respiratory failure. With early-onset pneumonia, the clinical course and radiographs of the chest may be indistinguishable from severe RDS.

In contrast to the rapid progression of pneumonia when caused by pyogenic organisms, older infants with community-acquired infection often have an indolent course. The onset is usually preceded by upper respiratory tract symptoms or conjunctivitis. A nonproductive cough ensues, and the degree of respiratory compromise is variable. Fever is usually absent, and radiographic examination of the chest shows focal or diffuse interstitial pneumonitis. This infection has been called the "afebrile pneumonia syndrome" and is generally caused by *C. trachomatis*, CMV, *Ureaplasma urealyticum*, or one of the respiratory viruses. Although *Pneumocystis carinii* was implicated in the original description of this syndrome, its etiologic role is now in doubt, except in newborns infected with HIV.

98.6 Diagnosis

The maternal history may provide important information about maternal exposure to infection, maternal immunity (natural or acquired), maternal colonization, and obstetric risk factors (prematurity, prolonged ruptured membranes, maternal chorioamnionitis) (Box 98–4).

Sexually transmitted diseases (STDs) that infect a pregnant woman are of particular concern to the fetus and newborn because of the possibility for intrauterine or perinatal transmission. All pregnant women and their partners should be queried about a history of STDs and counseled about the potential adverse effects on the mother and child and the importance of

---

BOX 98–4. Evaluation of a Newborn for Infection or Sepsis

HISTORY (SPECIFIC RISK FACTORS)

Maternal infection during gestation or at parturition (type and duration of antimicrobial therapy)
   Urinary tract infection
   Chorioamnionitis
Maternal colonization with GBS, *Neisseria gonorrhoeae*, herpes simplex
Gestational age/birthweight
Multiple birth
Duration of membrane rupture
Complicated delivery
Fetal tachycardia (distress)
Age at onset (in utero, birth, early postnatal, late)
Location at onset (hospital, community)
Medical intervention
   Vascular access
   Endotracheal intubation
   Parenteral nutrition
   Surgery

EVIDENCE OF OTHER DISEASES*

Congenital malformations (heart disease, neural tube defect)
Respiratory tract disease (RDS, aspiration)
Necrotizing enterocolitis
Metabolic disease, e.g., galactosemia

EVIDENCE OF FOCAL OR SYSTEMIC DISEASE

General appearance, neurologic status
Abnormal vital signs
Organ system disease
Feeding, stools, urine output, extremity movement

LABORATORY STUDIES

Evidence of Infection

Culture from a normally sterile site (blood, CSF, other)
Demonstration of a microorganism in tissue or fluid
Antigen detection (urine, CSF)
Maternal or neonatal serology (syphilis, toxoplasmosis)
Autopsy

Evidence of Inflammation

Leukocytosis, increased immature/total neutrophil count ratio
Acute-phase reactants: CRP, ESR
Cytokines: interleukin 6
Pleocytosis in CSF or synovial or pleural fluid
Disseminated intravascular coagulation: fibrin split proucts

Evidence of Multiorgan System Disease

Metabolic acidosis: pH, Pco_2
Pulmonary function: Po_2, Pco_2
Renal function: BUN, creatinine
Hepatic injury/function: bilirubin, ALT, AST ammonia, PT, PTT
Bone marrow function: neutropenia, anemia, thrombocytopenia

---

*Diseases that increase the risk of infection or may overlap with signs of sepsis.

GBS = group B streptococci; RDS = respiratory distress syndrome; CSF = cerebrospinal fluid; CRP = C-reactive protein; ESR = erythrocyte sedimentation rate; Pco_2 = partial pressure of carbon dioxide; Po_2 = partial pressure of oxygen; BUN = blood urea nitrogen; ALT = alanine aminotransferase; AST = aspartate aminotransferase; PT = prothrombin time; PTT = partial thromboplastin time.

---

avoiding infection during pregnancy. Women should also be counseled about the need for timely diagnosis and therapy for infections during pregnancy. The CDC recommends the following screening tests and appropriate treatment of infected mothers: (1) All pregnant women should be offered voluntary and confidential HIV testing at the 1st prenatal visit. For women at high risk of infection during pregnancy (multiple sexual partners or STDs during pregnancy, intravenous drug use), repeat testing in the 3rd trimester is recommended. (2) A serologic test for syphilis should be performed on all pregnant women at the 1st prenatal visit. Repeat screening early in the 3rd trimester and again at delivery is recommended for women who had positive serology in the 1st trimester and for those at high risk for infection during pregnancy. (3) A serologic test for hepatitis B surface antigen (HBsAg) should be performed at the 1st prenatal visit and repeated late in pregnancy in those who are initially negative but at high risk for infection. (4) A maternal genital culture for *C. trachomatis* should be performed at the 1st prenatal visit. Young women (under 25 yr) and those at increased risk for infection (new or multiple partners during pregnancy) should be retested during the 3rd trimester. (5) A maternal genital culture for *Neisseria gonorrhoeae* should be performed at the 1st prenatal visit for women at risk and for those who live in areas with a high prevalence of gonorrhea. Repeat testing in the 3rd trimester is recommended for those at continued risk. (6) Evaluation for bacterial vaginosis should be considered at the 1st prenatal visit for asymptomatic women at high risk for preterm labor. (7) The CDC has recommended universal screening for rectovaginal GBS col-onization of all pregnant women at 35–37 wk gestation and a screening-based approach to selective intrapartum antibiotic prophylaxis against GBS (Fig. 98–6; also see Chapter 169).

SUSPECTED INTRAUTERINE INFECTION

The acronym *TORCH* refers to *t*oxoplasmosis, *o*ther agents, (syphilis, etc.), *r*ubella, *C*MV, and *H*SV. Although the term may be helpful in remembering some of the etiologic agents of intrauterine infection, the TORCH battery of serologic tests has a poor diagnostic yield, and appropriate diagnostic studies should be selected for each etiologic agent under consideration. CMV and HSV require culture or polymerase chain reaction (PCR) methods, whereas syphilis, toxoplasmosis, and rubella are diagnosed by specific serologic methods (see Box 98–4).

Vaginal and rectal screening cultures at 35–37 wk gestation for ALL pregnant women
(unless patient had GBS bacteriuria during the current pregnancy or a previous infant with invasive GBS disease)

Intrapartum prophylaxis indicated

Patients meeting any of the following criteria **SHOULD** receive intrapartum prophylaxis:

- Previous infant with invasive GBS disease, **OR**
- GBS bacteriuria during **current** pregnancy, **OR**
- Positive GBS screening culture during pregnancy (unless a planned cesarean delivery, in the absence of labor or amniotic membrane rupture, is performed), **OR**
- Unknown GBS status (culture not done, incomplete, or results unknown) **AND**
  - Delivery at < 37 wk gestation,** **OR**
  - Amniotic membrane rupture ≥ 18 hours, **OR**
  - Intrapartum temperature ≥ 100.4°F (≥ 38.0°C)*

Intrapartum prophylaxis NOT indicated

If patient meets none of the stated criteria, intrapartum prophylaxis for GBS is **NOT** indicated. This includes the following circumstances:

- Previous pregnancy with a positive GBS screening culture (unless a culture was ALSO positive during the current pregnancy)

- Planned cesarean delivery performed in the absence of labor or membrane rupture (regardless of maternal GBS culture status)

- Negative vaginal and rectal GBS screening culture during the current pregnancy, regardless of intrapartum risk factors

---

*If amnionitis is suspected, broad-spectrum antibiotic therapy that includes an agent known to be active against GBS should replace GBS prophylaxis.
**If onset of labor or rupture of amniotic membranes occurs at < 37 wk gestation AND there is a significant risk for preterm delivery (as assessed by the clinician), a suggested algorithm for GBS prophylaxis management is outlined below:

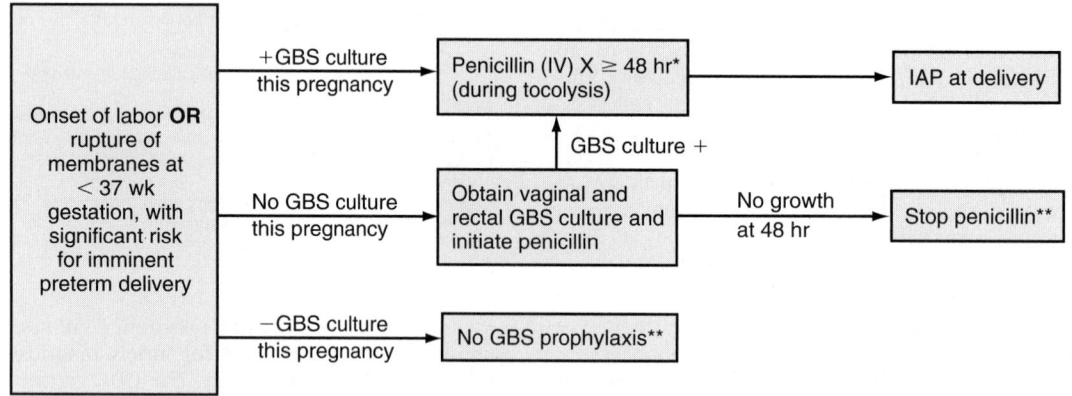

*Penicillin should be continued for a total of at least 48 hr, unless delivery occurs sooner. At the physician's discretion, antibiotic prophylaxis may be continued beyond 48 hr in a GBS culture-positive woman if delivery has not yet occurred. For women who are GBS culture positive, antibiotic prophylaxis should be reinitiated when labor likely to proceed to delivery occurs or recurs.

**If delivery has not occurred within 4 wk, a vaginal and rectal GBS screening culture should be repeated, and the patient should be managed as above, based on the result of the repeat culture.

FIGURE 98–6. Revised perinatal group B streptococcus (GBS) prevention guidelines. IAP = intrapartum antibiotic prophylaxis. (From Schrag S, Gorwitz R, Fultz-Butts K, Schuchat A: Prevention of perinatal group B streptococcal disease: Revised guidelines from CDC MMWR MorbMortalwkly Rep2002;51 [RR-11]:1.)

In most cases of suspected fetal infection, concern is not raised until the pregnant woman has been ill for several weeks or, in retrospect, after delivery. At this time, the maternal immune response to the suspected pathogen may no longer reflect an acute infection—that is, the specific IgM response is no longer detectable and the IgG response has already reached a plateau. Many of the pathogen-specific IgM serologic assays require considerable skill to perform and tend to be less reliable than the more common IgG assays. As a result, IgM assays can be either falsely negative or falsely positive.

Neonatal antibody titers are often difficult to interpret because IgG is acquired from the mother by transplacental passage and determination of neonatal IgM titers to specific pathogens is technically difficult to perform and not universally available. IgM titers to specific pathogens have high specificity but only moderate sensitivity; they should not be used to preclude infection. Paired maternal and fetal-neonatal IgG titers with higher newborn IgG levels or rising IgG titers during infancy may be used to diagnose some congenital infections (e.g., congenital syphilis). Total cord blood IgM or IgA (neither are actively transported across the placenta to the fetus) and the presence of IgM–rheumatoid factor in neonatal serum are nonspecific tests for intrauterine infection.

If the likelihood of maternal infection with a known teratogenic agent is high, fetal ultrasound examination is strongly recommended. If the examination demonstrates either a physical abnormality or delayed growth for gestational age, examination of a fetal blood sample may be warranted. Cordocentesis can provide a sufficient sample for both total and pathogen-specific IgM assays or for PCR or culture. The total IgM value is important because the normal fetal IgM level is less than 5 mg/dL. Any elevation in total IgM may indicate an underlying fetal infection that has stimulated the fetal immune system. Specific IgM antibody tests are available for CMV, *T. pallidum*, parvovirus B19, and toxoplasmosis. However, IgM tests are useful only when the results are strongly positive. A negative pathogen-specific IgM finding does not rule that pathogen out as a cause of fetopathy.

If maternal serologic studies point to a specific pathogen, it is sometimes possible to detect the organism in amniotic fluid (culture, PCR). Amniocentesis can be performed and the fluid sent for analysis. The presence of CMV, *Toxoplasma,* or parvovirus in amniotic fluid indicates that the fetus is infected and at high risk, but it does not always mean that the fetus will have severe sequelae. In contrast, HSV and varicella-zoster virus (VZV) are rarely isolated from amniotic fluid samples. CMV, *Toxoplasma*, and parvovirus can also be identified from cordocentesis sampling.

Parvovirus does not grow in the cell cultures commonly available in the virology laboratory. Furthermore, an IgM response is not always detectable in women with primary infection. When fetal parvovirus infection is suspected, testing of fetal blood or amniotic fluid by PCR is recommended in addition to testing for a specific IgM response in the fetus. PCR may also be used for the diagnosis of toxoplasmosis, CMV, HSV, rubella, and syphilis.

Neonatal infections with CMV, *Toxoplasma,* rubella, HSV, and syphilis present a diagnostic dilemma because (1) their clinical features overlap and may initially be indistinguishable, (2) disease may be inapparent, (3) maternal infection is often asymptomatic, (4) special laboratory studies may be needed, and (5) appropriate treatment of toxoplasmosis, syphilis, and HSV, which may reduce significant long-term morbidity, is predicated on an accurate diagnosis. Common shared features that should suggest the diagnosis of an intrauterine infection include intrauterine growth restriction, hematologic involvement (anemia, neutropenia, thrombocytopenia, petechiae, purpura), ocular signs (chorioretinitis, cataracts, keratoconjunctivitis, glaucoma, microphthalmos), CNS signs (microcephaly, hydrocephaly, intracranial calcifications), other organ system involvement (pneumonia, myocarditis, nephritis, hepa-

titis with hepatosplenomegaly, jaundice), and nonimmune hydrops. Diagnostic studies in newborns with suspected chronic intrauterine infection should specifically test for each diagnostic consideration. Systemic infections with CMV, HSV, and enteroviruses frequently involve the liver; if these infections are suspected, liver function tests should be performed. Neonatal HSV meningitis may be confirmed by isolation of the virus (or by PCR) from cerebrospinal fluid (CSF) or another site (skin, eye, mouth).

SUSPECTED BACTERIAL OR FUNGAL INFECTIONS

Bacterial or fungal infection is diagnosed by isolating the etiologic agent from a normally sterile body site (blood, CSF, urine, joint fluid). Obtaining two blood culture specimens by venipuncture from different sites avoids confusion caused by skin contamination and increases the likelihood of bacterial detection. Samples should be obtained from an umbilical catheter only at the time of initial insertion. A peripheral venous sample should also be obtained when blood is drawn for culture from central venous catheters. Although blood cultures are usually the basis for a diagnosis of bacterial infection, the bacteremic phase of the illness may be missed by poor timing or inadequate blood sample size. Low-level bacteremia (<10 colony-forming units/mL) has been observed in some infants from birth to 2 mo of age with positive cultures. Current automated blood culture systems (BACTEC, Becton Dickinson; BacT/Alert, Organon Teknika), which continuously monitor blood cultures by checking each bottle every few minutes, have led to earlier detection of bacterial growth.

Bacterial antigen detection kits are available for a variety of organisms (GBS, *S. pneumoniae*) but are infrequently used because they are not as sensitive as blood cultures and false-positive results can occur. They may be helpful in the diagnosis of meningitis in the presence of previous antibiotic therapy. DNA probes and PCR technology are available for a number of viral and bacterial agents, but they are more often used in reference or research laboratories than in standard hospital microbiology laboratories. In the future, DNA array technology may permit the near instantaneous detection of pathogens from clinical samples.

Documentation of a positive blood culture is the first diagnostic criterion that must be met for sepsis (see Box 98–4). However, it is important to note that some patients with bacterial infection may have negative blood cultures ("clinical infection"), and other approaches to identification of infection are needed. Although the total WBC count and differential and the ratio of immature to total neutrophils have limitations in sensitivity and specificity, an immature-to-total neutrophil ratio of 0.2 or greater suggests bacterial infection. Neutropenia is more common than neutrophilia in severe neonatal sepsis, but neutropenia also occurs in association with maternal hypertension, preeclampsia, and intrauterine growth restriction. Thrombocytopenia is a nonspecific indicator of infection. Tests to demonstrate an inflammatory response include C-reactive protein, haptoglobin, fibrinogen, and various inflammatory cytokines, including IL-6 and IL-8. It is unclear which surrogate markers for infection are most helpful in determining when infants require a complete course of therapy in the absence of positive culture results.

When the clinical findings suggest an acute infection and the focus is unclear, additional studies should be performed, including, in addition to blood cultures, lumbar puncture, urine examination, and a chest roentgenogram. Urine should be collected by catheterization or suprapubic aspiration; urine culture for bacteria can be omitted in suspected early-onset infections because hematogenous spread to the urinary tract is rare at this point. Examination of the buffy coat with Gram or methylene blue stain may demonstrate intracellular pathogens. Demonstration of bacteria and inflammatory cells in Gram-stained gastric aspirates on the 1st day of life may reflect maternal amnionitis, which is a risk factor for early-onset infection. Stains of endotracheal secretions in infants with early-onset pneumonia may demonstrate intracellular bacteria, and cultures may reveal either pathogens or upper respiratory tract flora. Careful examination of the placenta can be helpful in the diagnosis of both chronic and acute intrauterine infections.

Diagnostic evaluation is indicated for asymptomatic infants born to mothers with chorioamnionitis. The probability of neonatal infection correlates with the degree of prematurity and bacterial contamination of the amniotic fluid. In an asymptomatic term infant whose mother has chorioamnionitis, two blood cultures should be performed and presumptive treatment initiated. Lumbar puncture is not necessary because term infants with bacterial meningitis are almost always symptomatic. If the blood culture result is positive or if the infant becomes symptomatic, lumbar puncture should then be performed. If the mother has been treated with antibiotics for chorioamnionitis, the newborn's blood culture result is usually negative, and the clinician must rely on clinical observation and other laboratory tests.

The diagnosis of pneumonia in a neonate is usually presumptive; microbiologic proof of infection is generally lacking because lung tissue is not easily cultured. Although some rely on the results of bacteriologic culture of material obtained from the trachea as "proof" of cause, interpretation of such cultures has many pitfalls. These cultures often reflect upper respiratory tract commensal organisms and may have no etiologic significance. Even cultures performed on material obtained by bronchoalveolar lavage in a neonate are unreliable because the tiny bronchoscopes used in neonates cannot be protected from contamination as they are introduced into the distal airways. Short of tissue obtained by lung biopsy, the only reliable bacteriologic cultures are those obtained from blood or pleural fluid. Unfortunately, blood culture results are usually negative, and sufficient pleural fluid for culture is rarely present. Interpretation of fungal cultures is associated with the same problems as for bacterial cultures. Cultures of respiratory secretions for *U. urealyticum* and other genital *Mycoplasma* species are of little value because normal neonates are often colonized with these agents as a result of contamination with secretions from the maternal genital tract. Cultures for respiratory viruses and *C. trachomatis* may be valuable; they are never indigenous flora, and isolation of them therefore suggests an etiologic role.

Serologic tests may be helpful in evaluating neonates with suspected pneumonia. Although no serologic tests are useful for bacteria or fungi, reliable tests for respiratory viruses and *C. trachomatis* are available. Serologic tests for *U. urealyticum* are complicated and technically demanding and are therefore not clinically useful at this time. Other tests of potential value in evaluating neonates with possible infectious pneumonitis are discussed under diagnosis of infections (see Chapter 160). The differential diagnosis of pneumonitis in neonates is broad and includes RDS, meconium aspiration syndrome, persistent pulmonary hypertension, diaphragmatic hernia, transient tachypnea of the newborn, congenital heart disease, and BPD.

The diagnosis of meningitis is confirmed by examination of CSF and identification of a bacterium, virus, or fungus by culture, antigen, or the use of PCR. Blood culture and a complete blood count are part of the initial evaluation because 70–85% of neonates with bacterial meningitis have positive results on blood culture. Examination and culture of CSF should be undertaken in infants with bacteremia. Lumbar puncture may be deferred in a severely ill infant if it would further compromise respiratory status. In these situations, blood culture should be performed and treatment initiated for presumed meningitis until lumbar puncture can be safely performed.

Normal, uninfected infants from 0–4 wk of age may have elevated CSF protein levels of 84 ± 45 mg/dL, glucose of 46 ± 10 mg/dL, and elevated CSF leukocyte counts of 11 ± 10 with the 90th percentile being 22. The proportion of polymorphonuclear leukocytes is 2.2 ± 3.8%, with the 90th percentile being 6. Elevated CSF protein levels and leukocyte counts and hypoglycorrhachia may develop in preterm infants after intraventricular hemorrhage. Many nonpyogenic congenital infections can also produce alterations in CSF protein and leukocytes (toxoplasmosis, CMV, HSV, syphilis).

Gram stain of CSF yields a positive result in most patients with bacterial meningitis. The leukocyte count is usually elevated, with a predominance of neutrophils (>70–90%); the number is often greater than 1,000 but may be less than 100 in infants with neutropenia or early in the disease. Microorganisms are recovered from most patients who have not been pretreated with antibiotics. Bacteria have also been isolated from CSF that did not have an abnormal number of cells (<25) or an abnormal protein level (<200 mg/dL), thus underscoring the importance of performing a culture and Gram stain on all CSF specimens. Contamination of CSF by bacteremia after traumatic lumbar puncture may occur rarely. Culture-negative meningitis may be seen with antibiotic pretreatment, a brain abscess, or infection with *Mycobacterium hominis, U. urealyticum, Bacteroides fragilis,* enterovirus, or HSV. Head ultrasonography or CT with contrast enhancement may be helpful in diagnosing ventriculitis and brain abscess.

98.7 Treatment

Treatment of suspected bacterial infection is determined by the pattern of disease and the organisms that are common for the age of the infant and the flora of the nursery. Once appropriate cultures have been obtained, intravenous or intramuscular antibiotic therapy should be instituted immediately. Initial empirical treatment of early-onset bacterial infections should consist of ampicillin and an aminoglycoside (usually gentamicin). Nosocomial infections acquired in a NICU are more likely to be caused by staphylococci, various Enterobacteriaceae, *Pseudomonas* species, or *Candida* species. Thus, an antistaphylococcal drug, methicillin or nafcillin for *S. aureus* or vancomycin for coagulase-negative staphylococci or methicillin-resistant *S. aureus*, should be substituted for ampicillin. A history of recent antimicrobial therapy or the presence of antibiotic-resistant infections in the NICU suggests the need for a different aminoglycoside agent (amikacin). When the history or the presence of necrotic skin lesions suggests *Pseudomonas* infection, initial therapy should be piperacillin, ticarcillin, carbenicillin, or ceftazidime and an aminoglycoside. The use of antifungal therapy should be considered in VLBW infants who have had previous antibiotic therapy, may have mucosal colonization with *C. albicans*, and are at high risk for invasive disease (see Chapter 215.1). Doses of commonly used antibiotics are provided in Table 98–8. Peak and trough levels of gentamicin (peak, 5–10 μg/mL; trough, <2 μg/mL) and vancomycin (peak, 25–40 μg/mL; trough, <10 μg/mL) are useful to ensure therapeutic levels and minimize toxicity if administered for more than 2–3 days.

Once the pathogen has been identified and antibiotic sensitivities determined, the most appropriate drug or drugs should be selected. For most gram-negative enteric bacteria, ampicillin and an aminoglycoside or a third-generation cephalosporin (cefotaxime or ceftazidime) should be used. Enterococci should be treated with both a penicillin (ampicillin or piperacillin) and an aminoglycoside because the synergy of both drugs is needed. Ampicillin alone is adequate for *L. monocytogenes*, and penicillin suffices for GBS. Clindamycin or metronidazole is appropriate for anaerobic infections.

TABLE 98–8. Suggested Dosage Schedules for Antibiotics Used in Newborns

		Dosage (mg/kg) and Interval of Administration				
		Weight <1,200 g*	Weight 1,200–2,000 g		Weight >2,000 g	
Antibiotic	Route	Age 0–4 wk	Age 0–7 Days	Age >7 Days	Age 0–7 Days	Age >7 Days
Amikacin[†]	IV, IM	7.5 q12h	7.5 q12h	7.5 q8h	10 q12h	10 q8h
Ampicillin	IV, IM					
Meningitis		50 q12h	50 q12h	50 q8h	50 q8h	50 q6h
Other infections		25 q12h	25 q12h	25 q8h	25 q8h	25 q6h
Aztreonam	IV, IM	30 q12h	30 q12h	30 q8h	30 q8h	30 q6h
Cefazolin	IV, IM	20 q12h	20 q12h	20 q12h	20 q12h	20 q8h
Cefotaxime	IV, IM	50 q12h	50 q12h	50 q8h	50 q12h	50 q8h
Ceftazidime	IV, IM	50 q12h	50 q12h	50 q8h	50 q8h	50 q8h
Ceftriaxone	IV, IM	50 q24h	50 q24h	50 q24h	50 q24h	75 q24h
Cephalothin	IV	20 q12h	20 q12h	20 q8h	20 q8h	20 q6h
Chloramphenicol[†]	IV, PO	25 q24h	25 q24h	25 q24h	25 q24h	25 q12h
Ciprofloxacin[‡]	IV	—	—	10–20 q24h	—	20–30 q12h
Clindamycin	IV, IM, PO	5 q12h	5 q12h	5 q8h	5 q8h	5 q6h
Erythromycin	PO	10 q12h	10 q12h	10 q8h	10 q12h	10 q8h
Gentamicin[†]	IV, IM	2.5 q18–24h	2.5 q12–18h	2.5 q8h	2.5 q12h	2.5 q8h
Imipenem	IV, IM	—	20 q12h	20 q12h	20 q12h	20 q8h
Methicillin	IV, IM					
Meningitis		50 q12h	50 q12h	50 q8h	50 q8h	50 q6h
Other infections		25 q12h	25 q12h	25 q8h	25 q8h	25 q6h
Metronidazole[§]	IV, PO	7.5 q48h	7.5 q24h	7.5 q12h	7.5 q12h	15 q12h
Mezlocillin	IV, IM	75 q12h	75 q12h	75 q8h	75 q12h	75 q8h
Meropenem[ǁ]	IV, IM	—	20 q12h	20 q12h	20 q12h	20 q8h
Nafcillin	IV	25 q12h	25 q12h	25 q8h	25 q8h	37.5 q6h
Netilmicin[†]	IV, IM	2.5 q18–24h	2.5 q12–18h	2.5 q8–12h	2.5 q12h	2.5 q8h
Oxacillin	IV, IM	25 q12h	25 q12h	25 q8h	25 q8h	37.5 q6h
Penicillin G (U)	IV					
Meningitis		50,000 q12h	50,000 q12h	50,000 q8h	50,000 q8h	50,000 q6h
Other infections		25,000 q12h	25,000 q12h	25,000 q8h	25,000 q8h	25,000 q6h
Penicillin benzathine (U)	IM	—	50,000 (one dose)	50,000 (one dose)	50,000 (one dose)	50,000 (one dose)
Penicillin procaine (U)	IM		50,000 q24h	50,000 q24h	50,000 q24h	50,000 q24h
Piperacillin	IV, IM	—	50–75 q12h	50–75 q8h	50–75 q8h	50–75 q6h
Rifampin	PO, IV	—	10 q24h	10 q24h	10 q24h	10 q24h
Ticarcillin	IV, IM	75 q12h	75 q12h	75 q8h	75 q8h	75 q6h
Tobramycin[†]	IV, IM	2.5 q18–24h	2 q12–18h	2 q8–12h	2 q12h	2 q8h
Vancomycin[†]	IV	15 q24h	10 q12–18h	10 q12h	10 q8h	10 q8h

*Data from Prober CG: The use of antibiotics in neonates weighing less than 1200 grams. Pediatr Infect Dis J 1990; 9:111.

[†]The appropriate dosage schedule should be based on serum concentration measurements; some experts recommend once-daily dosing.

[‡]Suggested doses based on anecdotal clinical experience.

[§]A loading intravenous dose of 15 mg/kg followed 24 hr later (term infants) and 48 hr later (preterm infants) by 7.5 mg/kg every 12 hr has been suggested by other investigators.

[ǁ]Dosages of meropenem suggested are the same as those of imipenem.

IV = intravenous; IM = intramuscular; PO = oral.

Adapted from Sáez-Llorens X, McCracken GH Jr: Clinical pharmacology of antibacterial agents. In Remington JS, Klein JO (editors): Infectious Diseases of the Fetus and Newborn Infant, 5th ed. Philadelphia, WB Saunders, 2001, pp 1419–1466.

Third-generation cephalosporins such as cefotaxime are valuable additions for treating documented neonatal sepsis and meningitis because (1) the minimal inhibitory concentrations needed for treatment of gram-negative enteric bacilli are much lower than those for the aminoglycosides, (2) excellent penetration into CSF occurs in the presence of inflamed meninges, and (3) much higher doses can be given. The end result is much higher bactericidal titers in serum and CSF than achievable with ampicillin-aminoglycoside combinations. However, the routine use of third-generation cephalosporins for suspected sepsis in NICU patients is inappropriate because of the potential for rapid emergence of resistant organisms.

The emergence of antibiotic resistance among pathogens that infect newborns is of great concern. Vancomycin-resistant enterococci and vancomycin-insensitive S. aureus are particularly worrisome. Guidelines to limit the use of vancomycin must be followed. Although vancomycin use cannot be avoided in neonatal units where methicillin-resistant S. aureus is endemic, use can be reduced by limiting empirical therapy to patients with a high suspicion of severe infection with coagulase-negative staphylococci (e.g., severely ill neonate with an indwelling intravascular catheter) and discontinuing therapy after 2–3 days when blood cultures are negative. The rational use of antibiotics in neonates involves using narrow-spectrum drugs when possible, treating infection and not colonization, and limiting the duration of therapy.

Therapy for most bloodstream infections should be continued for a total of 7–10 days or for at least 5–7 days after a clinical response has occurred. A blood culture taken 24–48 hr after initiation of therapy should yield negative results. If the culture results are positive, the possibility of an infected indwelling catheter, endocarditis, an infected thrombus, an occult abscess, subtherapeutic antibiotic levels, or resistant organisms should be considered. A change in antibiotics, longer duration of therapy, or removal of the catheter may be indicated.

Treatment of newborn infants whose mothers received antibiotics during labor should be individualized. If in utero infection is likely, treatment of the infant should be continued until it is shown that no infection has occurred (the infant remains asymptomatic for 24–72 hr) or clinical and laboratory evidence of recovery is apparent.

For pneumonia developing in the 1st 7–10 days of life, a combination of ampicillin and an aminoglycoside or cefotaxime is appropriate. Nosocomial pneumonia, generally manifested after this time, can be treated empirically with methicillin or vancomycin and a third-generation cephalosporin. *Pseudomonas* pneumonia should be treated with an aminoglycoside combined with ticarcillin or ceftazidime. Pneumonia caused by *C. trachomatis* is treated with either erythromycin or trimethoprim-sulfamethoxazole; *U. urealyticum* infection is treated with erythromycin.

Presumptive antimicrobial therapy for bacterial meningitis should include ampicillin in meningitic doses and cefotaxime or gentamicin unless staphylococci are likely, which is an indication for vancomycin. Susceptibility testing of gram-negative enteric organisms is important because resistance to cephalosporins and aminoglycosides has been noted. Most aminoglycosides administered by parenteral routes do not achieve sufficiently high antibiotic levels in the lumbar CSF or ventricles to inhibit the growth of gram-negative bacilli. Therefore, some experts recommend a combination of intravenous ampicillin and a third-generation cephalosporin for the treatment of neonatal gram-negative meningitis. Cephalosporins should not be used as empirical monotherapy because *L. monocytogenes* and enterococcus are resistant to all cephalosporins.

Meningitis caused by GBS usually responds within 24–48 hr and should be treated for 14–21 days. Gram-negative bacilli may continue to grow from repeated CSF samples for 72–96 hr after therapy despite the use of appropriate antibiotics. Treatment of gram-negative meningitis should be continued for 21 days or for at least 14 days after sterilization of the CSF, whichever is longer. *P. aeruginosa* meningitis should be treated with ceftazidime. Metronidazole is the treatment of choice for infection caused by *B. fragilis*. Prolonged antibiotic administration, with or without needle drainage for treatment and diagnosis, is indicated for neonatal cerebral abscesses. CT scans are recommended for patients with suspected ventriculitis, hydrocephalus, or cerebral abscess (initial and follow-up assessments) and for those with an unexpectedly complicated course (prolonged coma, focal neurologic deficits, persistent or recurrent fever). Neonatal herpes meningoencephalitis should be treated with acyclovir, and empirical therapy should be considered in symptomatic infants with a CSF mononuclear pleocytosis. Pleconaril is the treatment of choice for severe enteroviral infections such as meningoencephalitis, carditis, or hepatitis. Treatment of candidal meningitis is discussed in Chapter 215.

Treatment of sepsis and meningitis may be divided into antimicrobial therapy for the suspected or known pathogen and supportive care. Careful attention to respiratory and cardiovascular status is mandatory. Adequate oxygenation of tissues should be maintained; ventilatory support is frequently necessary for respiratory failure caused by sepsis, pneumonia, pulmonary hypertension, or ARDS. Refractory hypoxia and shock may require extracorporeal membrane oxygenation, which has reduced mortality rates in full-term infants with respiratory failure. Shock and metabolic acidosis should be identified and managed with fluid resuscitation and inotropic agents as needed. Corticosteroids should be administered only for adrenal insufficiency. Fluids, electrolytes, and glucose levels should be monitored carefully with correction of hypovolemia, hyponatremia, hypocalcemia, and hypoglycemia and limitation of fluids in those with inappropriate secretion of antidiuretic hormone. Hyperbilirubinemia should be monitored and treated aggressively with phototherapy and/or exchange transfusion because the risk of kernicterus increases in the presence of sepsis and meningitis. Seizures should be treated with anticonvulsants. Parenteral nutrition is needed for any infant who cannot sustain enteral feeding.

DIC may complicate neonatal septicemia. Platelet counts, hemoglobin, and clotting studies should be monitored. DIC is treated by management of the underlying infection, but if bleeding occurs, DIC may require fresh frozen plasma, platelet transfusions, or whole blood.

Because neutrophil storage pool depletion has been associated with a poor prognosis, a number of clinical trials of granulocyte transfusion therapy have been conducted, with variable results. The use of G-CSF or GM-CSF abolishes sepsis-induced neutropenia, but the effect of these cytokines on sepsis-related mortality is unclear. Modern leukapheresis techniques and the use of G-CSF to mobilize polymorphonuclear cells in healthy donors for use in granulocyte transfusion is a promising approach that needs further study. The use of intravenous immunoglobulin (IVIG) has been shown to decrease mortality in patients with sepsis; a meta-analysis of several trials recommended administration of a single dose of 500–750 mg/kg as adjunctive therapy. Selected IVIG preparations containing specific monoclonal antibodies are being studied.

It is important to remember that nonbacterial infectious agents can produce the syndrome of neonatal sepsis. HSV infection requires immediate specific treatment, as does systemic *Candida* infection. Treatment and other aspects of various nonbacterial infections are discussed in detail in other sections: TB (Chapter 197), syphilis (Chapter 200), genital mycoplasmas (Chapter 206), *C. trachomatis* (Chapter 208), *Candida* (Chapter 215), rubella (Chapter 226), enteroviruses (Chapter 229); parvovirus B19 (Chapter 230); HSV (Chapter 231), VZV (Chapter 232), and CMV (Chapter 234).

98.8 Complications and Prognosis

The sequelae of intrauterine infections with specific pathogens are described in their respective chapters. In general, complications of bacterial or fungal infections may be divided into those related to the inflammatory process per se and those that complicate underlying neonatal problems such as respiratory distress and fluid and electrolyte abnormalities.

Complications of bacteremic infections include endocarditis, septic emboli, abscess formation, septic joints with residual disability, and osteomyelitis and bone destruction. Recurrent bacteremia is rare (less than 5% of patients). Candidemia may lead to vasculitis, endocarditis, and endophthalmitis, as well as abscesses in the kidneys, liver, lungs, and brain. Sequelae of sepsis may result from septic shock, DIC, or organ failure.

Mortality rates from the sepsis syndrome depend on the definition of sepsis. In adults, the mortality rate approaches 50%, and the rate in newborn infants is probably at least that high. Reported mortality rates in neonatal sepsis are as low as 10% because all bacteremic infections are included in the definition. Several studies have documented that the sepsis case fatality rate is highest for gram-negative and fungal infections (Table 98–9).

The case fatality rate for neonatal bacterial meningitis is between 20 and 25%. Many of these cases have associated sepsis. Risk factors for death or for moderate or severe disability include a duration of seizures for more than 72 hr, coma, necessity for the use of inotropic agents, and leukopenia. Immediate complications of meningitis include ventriculitis, cerebritis, and brain abscess. Late complications of meningitis occur in 40–50% of survivors and include hearing loss, abnormal behavior, developmental delay, cerebral palsy, focal motor disability, seizure disorders, and hydrocephalus. CT has demonstrated cerebritis, brain abscess, infarct, subdural effusions, cortical atrophy, and diffuse encephalomalacia in newborns surviving meningitis. A number of these sequelae may be encountered in infants with sepsis but without meningitis as a result of cerebritis or septic shock.

98.9 Prevention

A number of intrauterine infections are preventable through maternal immunization, including hepatitis B, rubella, and VZV. CMV vaccines are under study. Toxoplasmosis is preventable with appropriate diet and avoidance of exposure to cat feces.

TABLE 98–9. Infecting Pathogen vs Death Rate, Late-Onset Sepsis Review in VLBW Infants: NICHD Neonatal Research Network, September 1, 1998 through August 31, 2000

Organism*	N	Death n†
All gram-positive organisms	**905**	**101 (11.2%)**
Staphylococcus—coagulase negative	606	55 (9.1%)
Staphylococcus aureus	99	17 (17.2%)
Group B streptococcus	32	7 (21.9%)
All other streptococci	65	7 (10.8%)
All gram-negative organisms	**257**	**93 (36.2%)**
Escherichia coli	53	18 (34.0%)
Klebsiella	62	14 (22.6%)
Pseudomonas	43	32 (74.4%)
Enterobacter	41	11 (26.8%)
Serratia	39	14 (35.9%)
All fungal organisms	**151**	**48 (31.8%)**
Candida albicans	82	36 (43.9%)
Candida parapsilosis	44	7 (15.9%)

*Organisms found on the last positive blood culture before death or discharge. Organism counts differ from those based on the 1st positive blood culture (Table 98–5) because of multiple sepsis episodes. Death rates are not shown for every organism found.

†The odds ratios for death, with control for gestational age, study center, race, and sex, were as follows: gram-positive vs other infections, 0.26 (0.19–0.35), p < .001; gram-negative vs other infections, 3.5 (2.5–4.9), p < .001; and fungi vs other infections, 2.0 (1.3–3.0), p < .01.

VLBW = very low birthweight; NICHD = National Institute of Child Health and Human Development.

From Stoll BJ, Hansen N, Fanaroff AA, et al: Late-onset sepsis in very low birthweight neonates: The experience of the NICHHD neonatal research network. Pediatrics 2002; 110:285.

BOX 98–5. Principles for the Prevention of Nosocomial Infection in the Neonatal Intensive Care Unit

Observe recommendations for universal precautions with all patient contact
  Gloves
  Gowns, mask, and isolation as indicated
Nursery design engineering
  Appropriate nursing:patient ratio
  Avoid overcrowding and excessive workload
  Readily accessible sinks, antiseptic solutions, soap, and paper towels
Handwashing
  Improve handwashing compliance
  Wash hands before and after each patient encounter
  Appropriate use of soap, alcohol-based preparations, or antiseptic solutions
  Alcohol-based antiseptic solution at each patient bedside
  Provide emollients for nursery staff
  Education and feedback for nursery staff
Minimizing risk of CVC contamination
  Maximal sterile barrier precautions during CVC insertion
  Local antisepsis with chlorhexidine gluconate
  Minimize repeated entry into the line for laboratory tests
  Aseptic technique when entering the line
  Minimize CVC days
  Sterile preparation of all fluids to be administered via a CVC
Meticulous skin care
Encourage early and appropriate advancement of enteral feeding
Education and feedback for nursery personnel
Continuous monitoring and surveillance of nosocomial infection rates in the NICU

CVC = central venous catheter; NICU = neonatal intensive care unit.
From Adams-Chapman I, Stoll BJ: Prevention of nosocomial infections in the neonatal intensive care unit. Curr Opin Pediatr 2002; 14:157.

Malaria during pregnancy can be minimized with chemoprophylaxis. Congenital syphilis is preventable by timely diagnosis and appropriate early treatment of infected pregnant women.

Neonatal tetanus can be prevented by maternal tetanus immunization and proper care of the umbilical cord. Aggressive management of suspected maternal chorioamnionitis with antibiotic therapy during labor, along with rapid delivery of the infant, reduces the risk of early-onset neonatal sepsis. Vertical transmission of GBS (Chapter 169) is significantly reduced by selective intrapartum chemoprophylaxis. Neonatal infection with *Chlamydia* can be prevented by identification and treatment of infected pregnant women (Chapter 208). Mother-to-child transmission of HIV is significantly reduced by maternal antiretroviral therapy during pregnancy, labor, and delivery and treatment of the infant after birth (Chapter 254).

PREVENTION OF NOSOCOMIAL INFECTION

Successful strategies to reduce rates of nosocomial infection, especially among VLBW infants in NICUs, are urgently needed. Principles for the prevention of nosocomial infection include adherence to universal precautions with all patient contact, avoiding nursery crowding and limiting nurse-to-patient ratios, strict compliance with handwashing, meticulous neonatal skin care, minimizing the risk of catheter contamination, decreasing the number of venipunctures and heelsticks, reducing the duration of catheter and mechanical ventilation days, providing education and feedback to nursery personnel, and ongoing monitoring and surveillance of nosocomial infection rates in the NICU (Box 98–5).

Most nosocomial infections in the NICU are bloodstream infections associated with an intravascular catheter. Catheters used in neonates include peripheral intravenous catheters, umbilical catheters, peripherally inserted central catheters, and surgically placed central venous catheters (CVCs). Efforts to reduce catheter-related infections include proper antisepsis of the skin before insertion of the catheter, sterile precautions during catheter insertion, aseptic technique when entering the line

and minimizing repeated entry into the line for blood sampling, sterile preparation of fluids to be used with a CVC, and finally, minimizing the number of catheter days.

The skin is an important mechanical barrier to infection. VLBW infants are born with an ineffective epidermal barrier that results in increased transepidermal water loss and an increased risk for infection. Efforts to reduce traumatic injury to this immature skin are important, including a reduction in the number of heelsticks.

Handwashing remains the most important and effective means of reducing nosocomial infections. Several expert groups have established guidelines for effective handwashing. Antimicrobial soaps or alcohol-based preparations are recommended. Proper handwashing is essential before entering the NICU and before each patient contact. Barriers to compliance with handwashing include overcrowding, excessive patient-to-nurse ratios, poorly located sinks and inadequate supplies, lack of easy-to-use alcohol-based products at the bedside, concern about skin irritation, and inadequate knowledge, including the mistaken belief that the use of gloves obviates the need for handwashing.

Ongoing education of staff regarding practices that are likely to reduce nosocomial infections and active surveillance of infection rates are important components of nosocomial infection control.

Adams-Chapman I, Stoll BJ: Prevention of nosocomial infections in the neonatal intensive care unit. *Curr Opin Pediatr* 2002;14:157.

Adams-Chapman I, Stoll BJ: Systemic inflammatory response syndrome. *Semin Pediatr Infect Dis* 2001;12:5.

Ahmed A, Hickey SM, Ehrett S, et al: Cerebrospinal fluid values in the term neonate. *Pediatr Infect Dis J* 1996;15:298.

Baker MD, Bell LM: Unpredictability of serious bacterial illness in febrile infants from birth to 1 month of age. *Arch Pediatr Adolesc Med* 1999;153:508.

Baltimore RS, Huie SM, Meek JI, et al: Early-onset neonatal sepsis in the era of group B streptococcal prevention. *Pediatrics* 2001;108:1094.

Bedford Russell AR, Emmerson AJB, Wilkinson N, et al: A trial of recombinant human granulocyte colony stimulating factor for the treatment of very low birthweight infants with presumed sepsis and neutropenia. *Arch Dis Child Fetal Neonatal Ed* 2001;84:F172.

Benjamin DK, Miller W, Garges H, et al: Bacteremia, central catheters, and neonates: When to pull the line. *Pediatrics* 2001;107:1272.

Bernstein HM, Pollock BH, Calhoun DA, et al: Administration of recombinant granulocyte colony-stimulating factor to neonates with septicemia: A meta-analysis. *J Pediatr* 2001;138:917.

Brodie SB, Sands KE, Gray JE, et al: Occurrence of nosocomial bloodstream infections in six neonatal intensive care units. *Pediatr Infect Dis J* 2000;19:56.

Buttery JP: Blood cultures in newborns and children: Optimizing an everyday test. *Arch Dis Child Fetal Neonatal Ed* 2002;87:F25.

Carr R: Neutrophil production and function in newborn infants. *Br J Haematol* 2000;110:18.

Centers for Disease Control and Prevention: Sexually transmitted diseases treatment guidelines 2002. *MMWR Morb Mortal Wkly Rep* 2002;51(RR-66):1.

Engle WD, Rosenfeld CR, Mouzinho A, et al: Circulating neutrophils in septic preterm neonates: Comparison of two reference ranges. *Pediatrics* 1997;99:10.

Gaynes RP, Edwards JR, Jarvis WR, et al: Nosocomial infections among neonates in high-risk nurseries in the United States. *Pediatrics* 1996;98:357.

Goldenberg RL, Hauth JC, Andrews WW: Mechanisms of disease: Intrauterine infection and preterm delivery. *N Engl J Med* 2000;342:1500.

Hodge D, Puntis JWL: Diagnosis, prevention, and management of catheter related bloodstream infection during long-term parenteral nutrition. *Arch Dis Child Fetal Neonatal Ed* 2002;87:F21.

Hübel K, Dale DC, Liles WC: Granulocyte transfusion therapy: Update on potential clinical applications. *Curr Opin Hematol* 2001;8:161.

Isaacs D: Rationing antibiotic use in neonatal units. *Arch Dis Child Fetal Neonatal Ed* 2000;82:F1.

Jenson HB, Pollock BH: Meta-analyses of the effectiveness of intravenous immune globulin for prevention and treatment of neonatal sepsis. *Pediatrics* http://www.pediatrics.org/cgi/content/full/99/2/e2.

Karlowicz MG, Buescher ES, Surka AE: Fulminant late-onset sepsis in a neonatal intensive care unit, 1988–1997, and the impact of avoiding empiric vancomycin therapy. *Pediatrics* 2000;106:1387.

Kaufman D, Boyle R, Hazen KC, et al: Fluconazole prophylaxis against fungal colonization and infection in preterm infants. *N Engl J Med* 2002;345:1660.

Kellogg JA, Ferrentino FL, Goodstein MH, et al: Frequency of low level bacteremia in infants from birth to two months of age. *Pediatr Infect Dis J* 1997;16:381.

Kenyon SL, Taylor DJ, Tarnow-Mordi W: Broad-spectrum antibiotics for preterm, pre-labour rupture of fetal membranes: The ORACLE I randomised trial. *Lancet* 2001;357:979.

Klein JO, Remington JS: Current concepts of infections of the fetus and newborn infant. In Remington JS, Klein JO (editors): *Infectious Diseases of the Fetus and Newborn Infant*, 5th ed. Philadelphia, WB Saunders, 2001, pp 1–23.

Klinger G, Chin CN, Beyene J, et al: Predicting the outcome of neonatal bacterial meningitis. *Pediatrics* 2000;106:477.

Kumar Y, Qunibi M, Neal TJ, et al: Time to positivity of neonatal blood cultures. *Arch Dis Child Fetal Neonatal Ed* 2001;85:F182.

Levy O: Impaired innate immunity at birth: Deficiency of bactericidal/permeability-increasing protein (BPI) in the neutrophils of newborns. *Pediatr Res* 2002;51:667.

Lewis DB, Wilson CB: Developmental immunology and role of host defenses in neonatal susceptibility to infection. In Remington JS, Klein JO (editors): *Infectious Diseases of the Fetus and Newborn Infant*, 5th ed. Philadelphia, WB Saunders, 2001, pp 25–138.

Lin F-YC, Philips JB III, Azimi PH, et al: Level of maternal antibody required to protect neonates against early-onset disease caused by group B streptococcus type Ia: A multicenter, seroepidemiology study. *J Infect Dis* 2001;184:1022.

Litwin CM, Hill H: Serologic and DNA-based testing for congenital and perinatal infections. *Pediatr Infect Dis J* 1997;16:1166.

MMWR: Intrauterine West Nile virus infection—New York, 2002. *MMWR Morbid Mortal wkly* Rep 2002;51:1135–36.

Mylonakis E, Paliou M, Hohmann EL, et al: Listeriosis during pregnancy. *Medicine (Baltimore)* 2002;81:260.

Oddie S, Embleton ND: Risk factors for early onset neonatal group B streptococcal sepsis: Case-control study. *Br Med J* 2002;325:308.

Sáez-Llorens X, McCracken GH Jr: Clinical pharmacology of antibacterial agents. In Remington JS, Klein JO (editors): *Infectious Diseases of the Fetus and Newborn Infant*, 5th ed. Philadelphia, WB Saunders, 2001, pp 1419–1466.

Saiman L, Ludington E, Pfaller M, et al: Risk factors for candidemia in neonatal intensive care unit patients. *Pediatr Infect Dis J* 2000;19:319.

Schrag S, Gorwitz R, Fultz-Butts K, Schuchat A: Prevention of perinatal group B streptococcal disease: Revised guidelines from CDC. *MMWR Morbid Mortal wkly Rep* 2002;51(RR-11):1.

Schrag SJ, Zell ER, Lynfield R, et al: A population-based comparison of strategies to prevent early onset group B streptococcal disease in neonates. *N Engl J Med* 2002;347:233.

Sohn AH, Garrett DO, Sinkowitz-Cochran RL, et al: Prevalence of nosocomial infections in neonatal intensive care unit patients: Results from the first national point-prevalence survey. *J Pediatr* 2001;139:821.

Stoll BJ, Hansen N, Fanaroff AA, et al: Late-onset sepsis in very low birthweight neonates: The experience of the NICHD Neonatal Research Network. *Pediatrics* 2002;110:285.

Stoll BJ, Hansen N, Fanaroff AA, et al: Changes in pathogens causing sepsis in very low birthweight infants. *N Engl J Med* 2002;347:240.

Weinberg GA, Powell KR: Laboratory aids for diagnosis of neonatal sepsis. In Remington JS, Klein JO (editors): *Infectious Diseases of the Fetus and Newborn Infant*, 5th ed. Philadelphia, WB Saunders, 2001, pp 1327–1344.

Yoon BH, Romero R, Moon JB, et al: Clinical significance of intra-amniotic inflammation in patients with preterm labor and intact membranes. *Am J Obstet Gynecol* 2001;185:1130.

Chapter 99

The Epidemiology of Adolescent Health Problems

Renée R. Jenkins

Behavioral and psychosocial risks, including injuries, account for a substantial proportion of both the utilization of health care services by adolescents and the causes of morbidity and mortality. Adolescents make fewer visits to physicians for ambulatory care than does any other age group, yet school-aged children and adolescents are more likely than younger children to have unmet health needs and delayed medical care. Adolescents and young adults are less likely to be insured than all other age groups, and uninsured adolescents are 5 times as likely to lack a usual source of care, 4 times as likely to have unmet health needs, and twice as likely to go without a physician contact over the course of a year when compared with insured adolescents.

Most ambulatory visits for all age groups occur in physician offices, as compared with outpatient or emergency departments. However, in 1999, 15–24 yr olds received more of their ambulatory care in emergency rooms than did any other age group. In a survey of emergency room visits in the United States, 15–24 yr olds had the highest injury-related visit rate (18.3/100 persons). Although injuries predominated, females presented most often with complaints related to abdominal and chest pain. In the general ambulatory setting, health supervision (10%) and acne led the lists of diagnoses for 10–14 yr olds and 15–19 yr olds, respectively. Acute upper respiratory infections and normal pregnancy completed the list of the most common diag-

noses. Children with disabilities, as a group, access health care services more frequently than do nondisabled children, and adolescents represent the largest proportion of children who are disabled, 84.3 cases/1,000 (ages 12–17 yr) compared with 33.2 cases/1,000 for children younger than 6 yr of age. Overall, impairments of speech, special senses, and intelligence (primarily mental retardation) as well as respiratory disease (primarily asthma) make up the largest categories of disability diagnoses.

The leading causes of hospitalization in adolescents parallel the diagnoses of adolescents seen in the ambulatory setting, with the exception of mental disorders. Hospitalizations for mental disorders composed 17% of the top five discharge diagnoses in 1999 for 10–21 yr olds, with pregnancy and childbirth (55.5%), injuries (10%), diseases of the digestive system (10%), and respiratory tract diseases (7.5%) completing the list. The overall hospitalization rates have declined, with rates for 15–19 yr olds and 20–24 yr olds dropping 29% and 27%, respectively, for the years 1986 to 1996.

The health conditions having the greatest impact on the status of adolescent health are early unintended pregnancy, sexually transmitted diseases (STDs), mental disorders, injuries, and substance use and abuse. The trends in the frequency vary over time relative to prevention programs, legislative actions, and other societal factors. Teen births, at 49 births/1,000 in 2000, have declined steadily since 1991 (see Fig. 109–1) and surpassed the nadir of the early to mid-1980s of 50–53/1,000. Reportable sexually transmitted infections such as gonorrhea and syphilis have the highest prevalence in 15–24 yr olds. Rates for both diseases declined in 1999, compared with 1998 in 15–19 yr olds, but gonorrhea rates for young adults 20–24 yr increased. Chlamydia was the most common STD in adolescents and young adults in 1999, with 1,383/100,000 cases reported in 15–19 yr olds and 1,329/100,000 in 20–24 yr olds, both rates

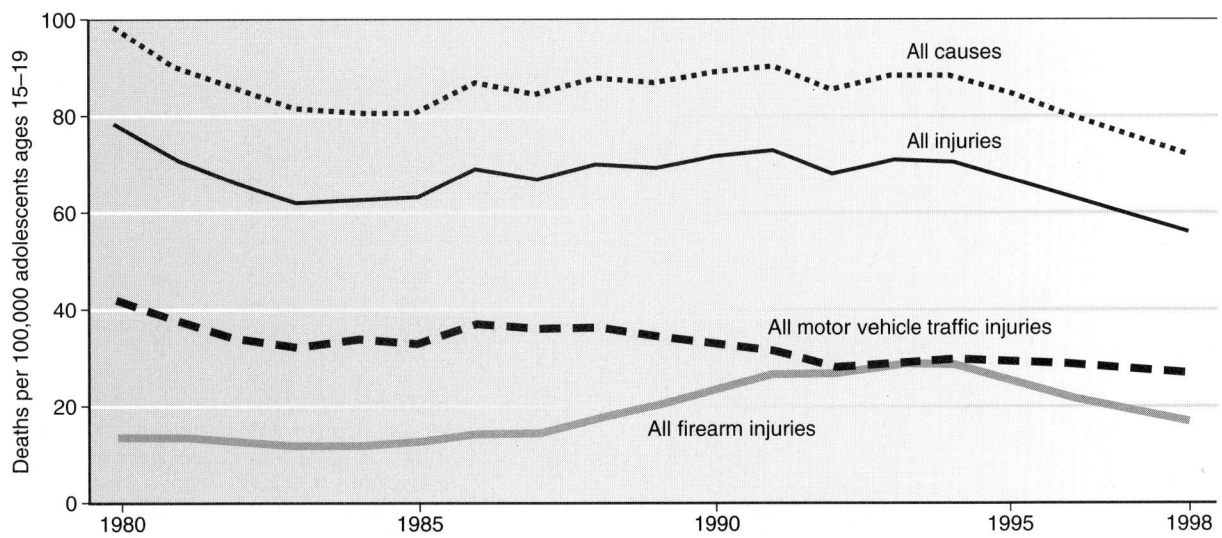

FIGURE 99–1. Death rates among adolescents ages 15 to 19 by cause of death, 1980–98. (From Centers for Disease Control and Prevention, National Center for Health Statistics, National Vital Statistics System.)

reflecting an increase over the previous year. Less comprehensive survey data are available to identify trends for pelvic inflammatory disease, human papillomavirus, and human immunodeficiency virus infection.

Health destructive behavior, such as cigarette and marijuana smoking and the abuse of alcohol and recreational drugs (often in combination with driving), continues to present a serious problem for adolescents. Survey data demonstrate increases in marijuana and alcohol use until 1997, at which time the trend stabilized. See Chapter 105.

Automobile and motorcycle accidents are the leading causes of adolescent morbidity and mortality. Sixteen to 19 yr olds compose 5% of licensed drivers and account for 15% of vehicular fatalities (see Chapter 50). Alcohol is a factor in approximately one third of the fatal accidents involving adolescents. In addition, other factors such as less frequent use of seat belts and the presence of other teen passengers increases the severity of crashes involving teen drivers (Table 99–1). About 100 nonfatal injuries occur for every adolescent killed in a motor vehicle accident. These injuries are the leading cause of disability from head and spinal cord injuries for adolescents. Graduated licensing systems, more vigorously enforced drinking age laws, and nighttime driving restrictions are successful strategies to prevent mortality and morbidity.

Violent deaths and injuries have a significant impact on adolescents (Chapters 1 and 34). Homicides are the second leading cause of death for all adolescents and the most common cause of death for black males. Firearm deaths and injuries are a major contributor to these events. Although reliable national firearm injury data are not available, estimates range as high as 100 nonfatal violent assaults resulting in injury for each firearm death. The trend in the death rate has declined since 1980, reaching its nadir in 1985, then climbing to its height in 1993 (Fig. 99–1). From 1994 to 1998, the firearm homicide rates for black and Hispanic adolescent males declined substantially to 78 and 29 per 100,000, respectively.

International comparisons are becoming more readily available through the World Health Organization and the International Collaborative Effort (ICE) on Injury Statistics. These data are still limited and do not reflect information from Asian and African countries. Health behavior data on smoking

TABLE 99–1. Percentage of Fatal Crashes by Characteristic, 1998

	Driver Age		
	16	**17–19**	**20–49**
Driver error	80	75	62
Speeding	36	31	22
Single vehicle	41	37	30
3+ occupants	33	26	19
Drivers killed with 0.01+ BAC	8	25	47

BAC = blood alcohol concentration.
From Insurance Institute for Highway Safety, Beginning Teenage Drivers, www.iihs.org/safety facts/teens/beginning drivers.htm, accessed 12/27/01.

and drinking in adolescents between ages 11 and 15 years show the United States ranking 24th out of 28 for daily smoking with 12% of 15 yr olds smoking daily. More than 25% of 15 yr olds in Austria, France, Germany, and Hungary smoke daily, leading the nations surveyed. Wales and Greece led the list for teenage drinking; reporting over 50% of 15 yr olds drinking weekly, whereas the United States reported about 23%. Mortality data reveal New Zealand with the highest injury death rate for 15–24 yr olds (Fig. 99–2). The United States leads all nations in the survey for firearm injury deaths.

Certain chronic diseases affecting adults have their origins during adolescence. Heart disease, diabetes, and respiratory conditions related to smoking are most common. Obesity is a major risk factor for cardiovascular diseases in adulthood but is also independently correlated with hypertension, hypercholesterolemia, diabetes mellitus, gallbladder disease, arthritis, and gout. As many as 22% of children aged 6–17 yr are considered overweight with a BMI (body mass index) more than the 85th percentile, whereas 10.9% are obese, with a BMI greater than the 95th percentile (see Chapter 43). Human immunodeficiency virus infection rises in its ranking as a cause of mortality from school-aged children through adulthood; by age 25–34 yr it represents the most common cause of death for black females and ranks among the top six causes of death for whites. According to the natural history of the disease, many of these infections were transmitted during adolescence or young adulthood.

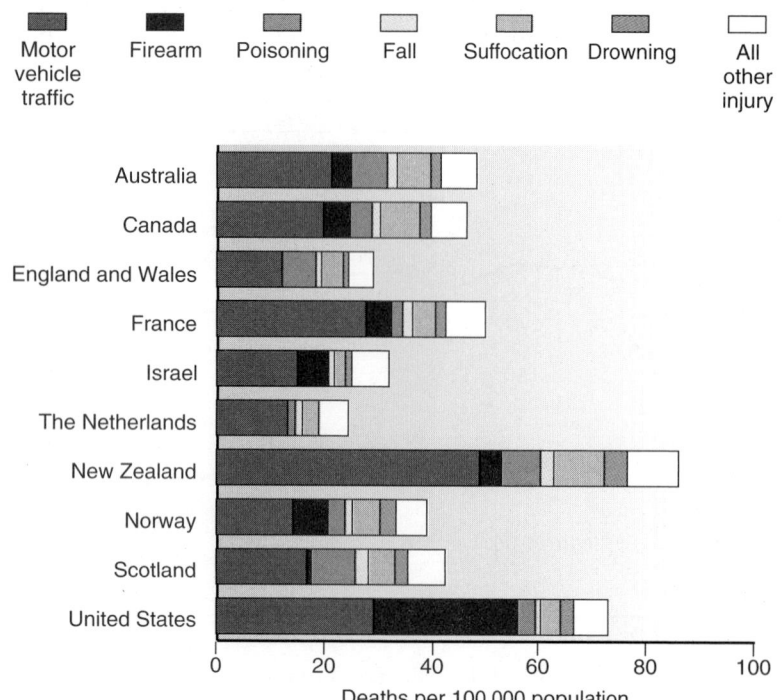

FIGURE 99–2. Average annual injury death rates by mechanism among persons 15–24 years of age: Injury ICE countries, selected recent years. (From Fingerhut LA, Cox CS, Warner M, et al: International comparative analysis of injury mortality: Findings from the ICE on injury statistics. Advance data from vital and health statistics, no. 303. Hyattsville, MD, National Center for Health Statistics, 1998.)

Currie C, Hurrelmann K, Settertobulte W, et al (editors): *Health and Health Behaviour Among Young People.* World Health Organization, Health Policy for Children and Adolescents (HEPCA), Series No. 1, 2000.

Federal Interagency Forum on Child and Family Statistics: America's Children: *Key National Indicators of Well-Being, 2001.* Washington, DC, Federal Interagency Forum on Child and Family Statistics, US Government Printing Office, 2001.

Fingerhut A, Cox CS, Warner M: *International Comparative Analysis of Injury Mortality.* Advance data from vital and health statistics; no. 303. Hyattsville, Maryland, National Center for Health Statistics, 1998.

Maternal and Child Health Bureau: *Child Health USA 2001.* Rockville, MD, US Department of Health and Human Services, HRSA, MCHB.

McCaig LF, Burt CW: National Hospital Ambulatory Medical Care Survey: *1999 Emergency Department Summary.* Advance data from the vital and health statistics: no. 320. Hyattsville, MD, National Center for Health Statistics, 2001.

National Center for Health Statistics: Unpublished data, December 2001.

National Vital Statistics Report, Vol 49, No. 11. October 12, 2001.

Newacheck PW, Brindis CD, Cart CU, et al: Adolescent health insurance coverage: recent changes and access to care. *Pediatrics* 1999:104(2 Pt 1):195–202.

Styne D: Childhood and adolescent obesity: Prevalence and significance. *Pediatr Clin North Am* 2001;48(4):823–54.

Ventura SJ, Mathews MS, Hamilton BE: *Births to Teenagers in the United States, 1940–2000.* National Vital Statistics Report, Vol 49, No. 10, September 25, 2001.

Chapter 100
Delivery of Health Care to Adolescents

Renée R. Jenkins

The leading causes of death and disability among adolescents are preventable, suggesting that society has failed to address the health needs of this age group adequately. Further, teenagers who require medical treatment may not receive the care they need. Although the greatest proportion of health problems in adolescents are behaviorally related and less amenable to prevention and treatment by traditional medical services, there is still much that can be done to improve the effectiveness of adolescent health care. Access, confidentiality, and the delivery of age-appropriate care are the primary issues.

The Society for Adolescent Medicine identified seven criteria critical to adolescents' access to care. *Availability* addresses age-appropriate services at the community level and includes the creation and dissemination of provider education about adolescent preventive health guidelines. The ease of recognition or expectation that an adolescent's needs can be addressed in a setting relates to the *visibility* criterion. The *quality* of care should be kept at a guaranteed standard that is satisfactory to the patient as well. *Confidentiality* and access to care that requires consent by the adolescent should be available, while family involvement should be encouraged. Poor *affordability* is an obvious deterrent to access. Adolescents have the lowest annual rate of visits to office-based physicians compared with all other age groups (Fig. 100–1). For all age groups, including adolescents, individuals without insurance receive less health care, and insurance coverage is worse for adolescents and young adults. In 2000, adolescents (12–17 yr olds) were more likely to be uninsured than children under 12, 12.3% compared with 11.3%. Overall, the percentage of children and adolescents under 18 yr old without health insurance dropped from 12.5% in 1999 to 11.6% in 2000. Older adolescents and young adults (18–24 yr olds) were the least likely to have health insurance coverage, with 72.7% covered for some or all of 2000, more than double the rate of uninsured younger teenagers. Service providers who are *flexible* and adaptable recognize and respond to the cultural, ethnic, and social diversity issues of adolescents. Teens with multiple concerns and a broad range of health-related issues require *coordination* of medical, mental health, social, and other services.

The complexity and interaction of physical, cognitive, and psychosocial developmental processes during adolescence require sensitivity and skill on the part of the pediatrician and a greater number of contacts than is currently appreciated or financed. Health education and promotion as well as disease prevention should be the focus of every visit with a teenager. To ensure that this is carried out comprehensively and systematically, guidelines have been promulgated from several organizations. However, the American Medical Association's Guidelines for Adolescent Preventive Services (GAPS) are the most evidence-based criteria (also see Chapter 5). A comparative analysis of the three sets of guidelines reveals more similarities than differences (Table 100–1). The GAPS guidelines, having been designed exclusively for adolescents, tend to be more specific in stating the criteria for intervention or referral. There is agreement across guidelines for the provision of a comprehensive physical examination (American Academy of Pediatrics [AAP] and Bright Futures [BF], annually; GAPS, three times during adolescence), screening for hypertension and obesity, and obtaining pertinent history for tobacco, alcohol, and drug use. If the teenager is sexually active, all guidelines recommend annual examination and

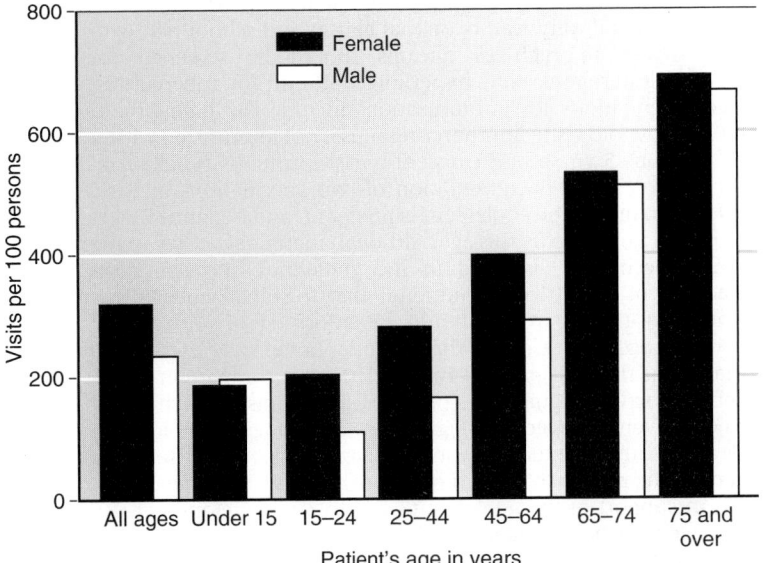

FIGURE 100–1. Annual rate of visits to office-based physicians by patient's age and sex: United States, 1999. (From National Center for Health Statistics, 2001.)

TABLE 100–1. Comparison of Supervision Guidelines

Source	AAP	GAPS	Bright Futures
Periodicity	*Annually*	*Annually*	*Annually*
Anticipatory Guidance			
Parenting	X	X	X
Adolescent development	X	X	X
Safety practices	X	X	X
Diet and fitness	X	X	X
Healthy lifestyles	X	X	X
Oral health	X		X
Screening History			
Tobacco use	X	X	X
Alcohol and drug use	X	X	X
Sexual behavior	X	X	X
School performance	X	X	X
Depression/suicide risk	X	X	X
Eating disorders	X	X	
Learning problems		X	X
Abuse	X	X	X
Physical Assessment with Specific Recommendations			
Hypertension	X*	X	
Obesity	X*	X	X
Breast cancer (self-examination)	X		X
Comprehensive examination	X	X	X
Scoliosis	X		X
Tests			
Hyperlipidemia	X	X	X
Tuberculin	X†	X†	X‡
Vision	X		X
Anemia	X		X
GC, chlamydia, syphilis§	X	X	X
Genital warts (HPV)§		X	
HIV infection	X	X	X
Cervical cancer‖	X	X	X
Immunizations			
MMR	X	X	X
dT	X	X	X
Hepatitis B	X	X	X

*Recommends obtaining and plotting measures only.
†Under specific conditions.
‡At least one during adolescence (14–16 yr old).
§For adolescents who are sexually active.
‖For adolescent girls who are sexually active or ≥ 18 yr old.

testing for sexually transmitted diseases. With varying specificity, recommendations direct physicians to obtain a history of depression; emotional, physical, or sexual abuse; and school performance. Those in high-risk groups should be screened for hypercholesterolemia and hyperlipidemia and for tuberculosis. Recommendations for immunizations include the following at the 11–12 yr old visit: diphtheria-tetanus if not immunized within the previous 5 yr; second trivalent measles-mumps-rubella vaccine if there is no documentation of two vaccinations in early childhood, unless the adolescent is pregnant; and hepatitis B vaccination if not given by this age. Although meningococcal vaccine is not specifically discussed in the guidelines, the American Academy of Pediatrics recommends that freshman college students and their parents should be informed of the risk of meningococcal disease and the potential benefits of the immunization at the visit prior to matriculation. A companion document to the GAPS guidelines provides algorithms for each of the major preventive directives. Figure 100–2 provides a sample using the algorithm for sexuality (also see Chapter 14). A consistent element to the approach of each of the guidelines is the role of parents in support of the adolescent's health and development. BF goes even further in recommending the support and interaction of the community in the adolescent's life.

The time spent on various elements of the screening will vary with the issues that surface during the assessment. For gay and lesbian youth, emotional and psychologic issues related to their experiences, from fear of disclosure to the trauma of homophobia, may direct the clinician to spend more time assessing emotional and psychologic supports in the young person's environment. For youth with chronic illnesses or special needs, the assessment of at-risk behaviors should not be omitted or deemphasized by assuming they do not experience the "normal" adolescent vulnerabilities.

100.1 Legal Issues

In the United States, the right of a minor to *consent* to treatment without parental knowledge is governed by state laws. Some states have age limitations, generally around age 12–15 yr. Usually, the right to self-consent for treatment is granted through public health statutes when there is suspicion of a sexually transmitted disease. Because such diseases are often asymptomatic, this provision is generally interpreted as enabling the physician to perform an examination (including a pelvic examination for a young woman) in any sexually active adolescent solely on his or her own consent. In many states, adolescents may consent to receive care for drug abuse or mental health problems. The minor's right to *contraceptives* has not been

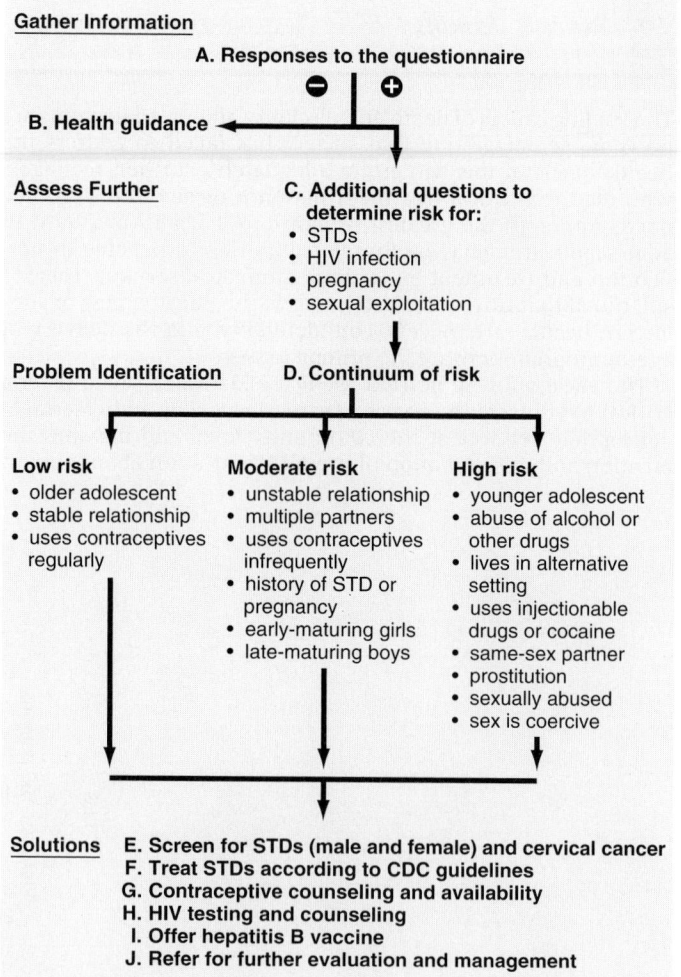

FIGURE 100–2. Sexuality algorithm. (From Levenberg PB, Elster AB: *Guidelines for Adolescent Preventive Services. Clinical Evaluation and Management Handbook.* Chicago, American Medical Association, 1995. © 1995 American Medical Association.)

reviewed by the Supreme Court, although the right to privacy has been upheld (except in a decision allowing searches in schools without due process), and accordingly, most states permit the provision of contraceptives to teenagers on their own consent. Although attempts at restricting Title X–funded programs to provision of contraception only after parents have been informed has not been legislated, the publicity received by the proposal has left many teenagers with the mistaken notion that their parents will be informed if they seek birth control from any physician. The right of an adolescent to obtain an *abortion* without parental consent or over parental objection varies by state.

Minors are also exempt from the requirement of parental consent for medical treatment under the following circumstances:

1. *Emancipated minors.* These are children who live away from home, are no longer subject to parental control, are economically self-supporting, are married, or are members of the military.

2. *Emergencies.* In a medical emergency, a minor may be treated without consent of parents if, in the physician's judgment, the delay resulting from attempts to contact parents would jeopardize the life or health of the minor.

3. *Mature minor rule.* An emerging trend in the law is the recognition that many minors are sufficiently mature to understand the nature of their illness and the potential risks and benefits of proposed therapy and, therefore, should receive such treatment on their own consent. This is particularly the case when the care is low risk, will benefit the minor, and is within established medical practice standards. In these cases, the physician should document that the adolescent has acted in a responsible manner.

Legal policies regarding the confidentiality of information are less consistent than those governing consent. In general, the right to self-consent for health care carries with it the right to confidentiality about that information. Exceptions exist when there are mandatory reporting requirements, as in abuse cases, some legal provision requiring parental disclosure, or a self-imposed danger to the minor. When exceptions exist, this should be divulged to the adolescent and an opportunity for assent or agreement provided.

A chaperone should be present whenever an adolescent female patient is examined by a male physician. The necessity for chaperones in the situation of a female physician examining a male adolescent patient has not yet become an issue.

100.2 Screening Procedures

Interviewing the Adolescent (also see Chapters 5 and 17). The preparation for a successful interview with an adolescent patient varies based on the prior history of the relationship with the patient. Patients, who are going from preadolescence to adolescence while seeing the same provider, and their parents should be guided through the transition. Although the rules for confidentiality are the same for new and continuing patients, the change in the physician-patient relationship, allowing more privacy during the visit and more autonomy in the health process, may be threatening for the parent as well as the adolescent. For new patients, the initial phases of the interview are more challenging given the need to establish rapport rapidly with the patient in order to meet the goals of the encounter. Issues of confidentiality and privacy should be explicitly stated along with the conditions under which that confidentiality may need to be altered, that is, in life- or safety-threatening situations. For new patients, the parents should be interviewed with the adolescent or before the adolescent to ensure that the adolescent does not perceive a breach of confidentiality. The physi-

cian who takes time to listen, avoids judgmental statements and the use of street jargon, and shows respect for the adolescent's emerging maturity will have an easier time communicating with him or her. The use of open-ended questions, rather than closed-ended questions, will further facilitate history-taking (e.g., the close-ended question, "Do you get along with your father?" leading to the answer, "Yes," compared with the question, "What would you like to change in your relationship with your father?" which may lead to an answer such as "I would like to stop him from always putting me down, especially in front of my friends").

The goals of the interview or clinical encounter are to establish an information base, identify problems and issues from the patient's perspective, and identify problems and issues from the perspective of the provider based on knowledge of the health and other issues relevant to the adolescent age group. The adolescent should be given an opportunity to express concerns and the reasons for seeking medical attention. The adolescent as well as the parent should also be given an opportunity to express the strengths and successes of the adolescent, in addition to communicating problems.

Barriers to an effective interview occur when the interviewer is distracted by other events or individuals in the office, when there are extreme time limitations obvious to either party, or when there is expressible discomfort with either the patient or the interviewer. The need for an interpreter when a patient is hearing impaired or if the patient and interviewer are not language-compatible provides a challenge but not necessarily a barrier under most circumstances. Observations during the interview can be useful to the overall assessment of the patient's maturity, presence or absence of depression, and the parent-adolescent relationship. Given the key role of a successful interview in the screening process, adequate training and experience should be sought by physicians wishing to give comprehensive care to adolescent patients.

Psychosocial Assessment. A few questions should be asked to detect the adolescent who is having difficulty with peer relationships (e.g., "Do you have a best friend with whom you can share even the most personal secret?"); self-image (e.g., "Is there anything you would like to change about yourself?" or "What do you consider to be your best features?"); depression (e.g., "What do you see yourself doing 5 yr from now?" or "Are you ever so sad that you think of dying?"); school (e.g., "How are your grades this year compared with last year?" and "How many days have you been absent from school this year compared with last year?"); personal decisions (e.g., "Are you feeling pressured to engage in any behavior for which you do not feel you are ready?" or "Is there anything you would like to change in your relationship with your boyfriend, your father, and so on?"); and an eating disorder (e.g., "Do you ever feel that food controls you rather than vice versa?"). The GAPS material provides questions and algorithms to structure these assessments. Based on those algorithms, appropriate counseling or referrals are recommended for more thorough probing or for in-depth interviewing.

Physical Examination

AUDIOMETRY. Highly amplified music of the kind enjoyed by many adolescents may result in hearing loss (see Chapter 627). Therefore, a hearing screening is recommended by the BF guidelines for adolescents who are exposed to loud noises regularly, have had recurring ear infections, or report problems.

VISION TESTING. The pubertal growth spurt may involve the optic globe, resulting in its elongation and myopia in genetically predisposed individuals. Vision testing should, therefore, be performed in order to detect this problem before it affects school performance.

BLOOD PRESSURE DETERMINATION. Criteria for a diagnosis of hypertension are based on age-specific norms that increase with pubertal maturation (see Chapter 437). An individual whose blood pressure exceeds the 95th percentile for his or her age is suspect for having hypertension, regardless of the absolute reading. Those adolescents with blood pressure between the 90th and 95th percentiles should receive appropriate counseling relative to weight and have a follow-up examination in 6 mo. Those with blood pressure below the 90th percentile should have their blood pressure measured on three separate occasions to determine the stability of the elevation before moving forward with an intervention strategy. The technique is important; false-positive results may be obtained if the cuff covers less than two thirds of the upper arm. The patient should be seated, and an average should be taken of the 2nd and 3rd consecutive readings, using the change rather than the disappearance as the diastolic pressure. Most adolescents with elevations of blood pressure have labile hypertension (see Chapter 437). If the blood pressure is below two standard deviations for age, anorexia nervosa and Addison disease should be considered.

SCOLIOSIS (also see Chapter 669.1). Approximately 5% of male and 10–14% of female adolescents have a mild curvature of the spine. This is two to four times the rate in younger children. Scoliosis is typically manifested during the peak of the height velocity curve, at approximately 12 yr in females and 14 yr in males. Curves measuring greater than 10 degrees should be monitored by an orthopedist until growth is complete.

BREAST EXAMINATION. Examination of the female adolescent's breasts is performed to detect masses (see Chapters 106, 540 and 543), evaluate progression of sexual maturation, provide reassurance about development, and teach the technique of self-examination with the hope that this practice will continue into the higher risk later years. Although self-examination is promoted in two of the three guidelines, there is disagreement on the justification for promoting this routinely, given the rare instances of malignant breast masses in this age group.

SCROTUM EXAMINATION. The peak incidence of germ cell tumors of the testes is in late adolescence and early adulthood. For that reason, palpation of the testes may have an immediate yield and should serve as a model for instruction of self-examination. Because varicoceles often appear during puberty, the examination also provides an opportunity to explain and reassure the patient about this entity (see Chapter 537).

PELVIC EXAMINATION. See Chapter 540.

Laboratory Testing. The increased incidence of iron-deficiency anemia after menarche mandates the performance of a *hematocrit* annually in young women with moderate to heavy menses. The reference standard for this test changes with progression of puberty, as estrogen suppresses erythropoietin (see Chapter 438). Populations with nutritional risk should also have the hematocrit monitored. Androgens have the opposite effect, causing the hematocrit to rise during male puberty; Sex Maturity Rating 1 males have an average hematocrit of 39%, whereas those who have completed puberty (Sexual Maturation Rating 5) have an average value of 43%. *Tuberculosis testing* on an annual basis is important in adolescents with risk factors, such as an adolescent with human immunodeficiency virus (HIV), living in the household with someone with HIV, the incarcerated adolescent, or those with other risk factors, because puberty has been shown to activate this disease in those not previously treated. Sexually active adolescents should undergo screening for *sexually transmitted diseases,* regardless of symptoms (see Chapter 110). During adolescence, a screening *urinalysis* is indicated for the sexually active male and female. Polymorphonuclear leukocytes in the urinary sediment suggest the possibility of either cervicitis, vaginitis, or an asymptomatic infection of the urinary tract in adolescent females and urethritis in adolescent males. *HIV testing* should be included for those at increased risk, e.g., a history of

sexually transmitted diseases, more than one sex partner in the last 6 mo, bisexual and homosexual males, sexual partners of at-risk individuals, and intravenous drug users. *Papanicolaou smears* are also indicated in sexually active females, regardless of age, because 5–35/1,000 have early neoplastic changes. Technique is important; the practice of obtaining two successive cervical scrapes increases the yield by 26% over that obtained by a single cervical specimen. Augmentation or replacement of the traditional Pap smear is occurring with techniques (Thin-Prep, AutoPap, Papnet, cervicography, human papillomavirus [HPV] DNA testing) that increase the sensitivity of the screen and add the ability to identify HPV, a potential cervical cancer risk. Although not included in any of the guidelines, screening tests for *genetic defect carrier states,* such as sickle cell anemia, are commonly performed in affected populations. Age-appropriate counseling should be immediately available to ensure an opportunity to have questions answered and to have unspoken fears allayed. The use of *spirometry* screening for adolescents who smoke may, over time, serve as a deterrent if deterioration of respiratory status can be demonstrated.

100.3 Health Enhancement

The health status of adolescents may be enhanced by application of principles of prevention and anticipatory guidance. Prevention of infectious disease should include immunization and counseling. Prevention of sexually transmitted diseases and pregnancy is an important issue to be addressed in sexually active adolescents of both sexes. Prevention of the use of harmful illicit drugs and alcohol and the potential for related injuries should be reviewed. Prevention of automotive accidents and interpersonal conflicts ending violently, the leading killer of adolescents, and of smoking, the leading killer of adults, should also be discussed. Facilitating an optimal health outcome for the adolescent patient also includes supporting him or her in successfully negotiating adolescence through school, job, and personal and family relations.

American Medical Association: *Guidelines for Adolescent Preventive Services, Recommendations Monograph,* 3rd ed. Chicago, American Medical Association, 1996.

Committee on Infectious Diseases, American Academy of Pediatrics: Meningococcal disease prevention and control strategies for practice-based physicians (Addendum: Recommendations for College Students)(RE0035). *Pediatrics* 2000; 106(6):1500.

Committee on Psychosocial Aspects of Child and Family Health 1995–1996: *Guidelines for Health Supervision III.* Elk Grove Village, IL, American Academy of Pediatrics, 1997.

Elster AB: Comparison of recommendations for adolescent clinical preventive services developed by national organizations. *Arch Pediatr Adolesc Med* 1998;152: 193.

Green M, Palfrey JS (ed): *Bright Futures: Guidelines for Health Supervision of Infants, Children, and Adolescents,* 2nd ed. Arlington, VA, National Center for Education in Maternal and Child Health, 2000.

Kahn JA: An update on human papillomavirus infection and Papanicolaou smears in adolescents. *Curr Opin Pediatr* 2001;13:303.

Society for Adolescent Medicine: Access to health care for adolescents: A position paper of the Society for Adolescent Medicine. *J Adolesc Health* 1992;13:162.

Chapter 101

Depression *Renée R. Jenkins*

(See also Chapter 23.)

Changes in mood are part of the normative developmental "adjustment" to changes in body, roles, and relationships in adolescence (also see Chapter 14). The challenge for a pediatrician is to distinguish between these normative variations and disorders requiring mental health intervention. The widespread belief that major depression in children and adolescents is rare or self-limited has led to underdiagnosis and delayed treatment for approximately two thirds of adolescents with clinical depression.

Epidemiology. The rate of depression in girls and boys changes significantly as a function of puberty. Gender variations are not characteristic of childhood depression, but depression is two to three times higher in postpubertal girls than in postpubertal boys. The lifetime prevalence of major depression is similar to adults and ranges between 15 and 20%. The co-occurrence of depression and another mental health disorder is reported from 40–70% of the time and is common in the adolescent age group. The most frequent co-morbid disorders are anxiety disorders, substance abuse, attention deficit disorder, and disruptive behavior disorders.

Etiology. There appears to be an interactive effect of genetics and environment in major depressive disorders, with studies in adults suggesting individuals with a high genetic risk may be more vulnerable to adverse environmental stressors when compared with those with low genetic risk. A family history of depressed parents increases the adolescent's risk of lifetime major depression threefold. Other parenting factors such as marital conflict, inadequate parenting, or death of a parent are also associated with depression. Controversy exists about the temporal relationship of symptoms such as low self-esteem, high self-criticism, hopelessness, and social skill deficits to their role as risk factors or as a prodrome of depression.

Clinical Manifestations. An adolescent who presents with school failure or another behavioral disorder may have an underlying depressive issue. The *Diagnostic and Statistical Manual for Primary Care, Child and Adolescent Version,* provides the clinical presentation of the range of "sadness" symptoms in young persons from the developmental variation, associated with bereavement or other stressors, through a sadness problem, and on to the full-blown disorder such as major depression. The characteristics of a sadness problem encompass (1) depressed or irritable mood, (2) diminished interest or pleasure, (3) weight loss or gain or failure to make expected weight gains, (4) insomnia or hypersomnia, (5) psychomotor agitation or retardation, (6) fatigue or energy loss, (7) feelings of worthlessness or excessive or inappropriate guilt, and (8) diminished ability to think or concentrate. The quality of these symptoms is less intense with a sadness problem as compared with major depression, and the impact on the adolescent's functioning is mild. When these symptoms occur daily for a period of 2 wk or longer, with or without recurrent thoughts of death and suicidal ideation, the diagnosis falls into the realm of a major depressive disorder. When these symptoms occur within 3 mo of an identifiable stressor, the presentation is considered an adjustment disorder with depressed mood. Persistent but less severe symptoms fall into the category of a dysthymic disorder. The depressed or irritable mood must persist for longer than a year accompanied by additional depressive clinical symptoms to meet the diagnostic criteria. Bipolar affective disorders are associated with child-onset and adolescent-onset depression in up to 30% of cases. The likelihood is increased with a positive family history of bipolar disorder and patients with a history of attention-deficit/hyperactivity disorder occurring with the presentation of depression. Bipolar disorders with depressive and manic features are of specific concern in the spectrum of depression diagnoses because of the potential for more exaggerated manic features being unmasked when these patients are treated with antidepressants.

DIFFERENTIAL DIAGNOSIS. Physical and metabolic disturbances should be ruled out during the assessment of an adolescent with depressive symptoms. Hypothyroidism, nutritional deficiencies, a chronic infection such as mononucleosis, or a chronic systemic disease such as systemic lupus erythematosus

should be considered. Substance abuse can mask the depression symptoms as well as imitate depression. A chronic learning disability leading to low self-esteem can also present with depressive-like symptoms.

OFFICE SCREENING FOR DEPRESSION. Screening for depressive symptoms is recommended as a component of the routine health maintenance assessment for an adolescent. Although the diagnosis of a full depressive disorder is based on interviewing the adolescent and obtaining observational data from parents or primary caretakers, alertness during a medical evaluation can raise suspicion early in the course of the disorder. One strategy recommended in the American Medical Association's Guidelines for Adolescent Preventive Services is to pose a series of screening questions to determine whether depressive symptoms at the level of mild, moderate to severe, or high risk exist. General questions such as, "Have you had fun during the past 2 weeks?" or "In general, are you happy with the way things are going for you these days?" alert the clinician to the need to ask more probing follow-up questions to elicit the presence or absence of diagnostic symptom criteria for depression. Another strategy is to use a depressive screening questionnaire such as the 21-question Beck Depression Inventory to confirm the clinical suspicion of depression. Screening for suicidal ideation must be included as a part of further evaluation in the presence of any depressive symptoms. Referral to a mental health professional for evaluation on an emergent basis is recommended under circumstances in which adolescents have current thoughts about killing themselves.

Treatment. There are several therapeutic modalities for the treatment of depression, including individual and group therapy, family intervention, along with, or independent of, psychopharmacologic treatment (Chapters 28 and 28.2). Antidepressants are generally recommended for moderate to severe cases of major depression and in some cases of dysthymic disorders. The inability to demonstrate efficacy and potential toxicity have limited the use of tricyclic antidepressants in children and adolescents. Selective serotonin reuptake inhibitors are the primary medications used for major depression in children and adolescents. The role of the pediatrician in the timing of a referral to a mental health professional or in prescribing of antidepressants is determined by his or her training and experience in managing mental health problems. The education of parents and patients about depressive disorders is important in successful therapeutic interventions and in removal of the cultural stigma that may be associated with mental health therapy. The significance of timely intervention should be stressed, including the potential for a depressive disorder to disrupt the normal adolescent developmental process. An extended disruption can lead to impaired functioning even after recovery from the depressive episode. The importance of following early identification with prompt treatment cannot be overemphasized. See Chapter 28.2 for discussion of pharmacotherapy.

Prognosis. In one survey of adolescents and young adults, more than one fifth of those with major depression reported ever attempting suicide, the most adverse outcome of a depressive disorder. An untreated major depressive episode can last up to 7–9 mo, with about 40% of cases recurring within 2 yr and 70% within 5 yr. The earlier the onset of depression, the more severe and recurrent the course. Appropriate use of antidepressants can improve depressive symptoms within 1 mo or less in some patients. Outcomes of untreated major depression persist into adulthood and are manifested as impaired psychologic, social, and academic functioning.

Beasley PJ, Beardslee WR: Depression in the adolescent patient. *Adolesc Med* 1998;9:351.

Hagman J: Diagnosis and treatment of depression in adolescence. *Adolescent Health Update* 2001;13(3) (www.aap.org).

Kessler RC, Walters EE: Epidemiology of DSM-III-R major depression and minor depression among adolescents and young adults in the national comorbidity survey. *Depress Anxiety* 1998;7:3.

Levenberg PB, Elster AB: *Guidelines for Adolescent Preventive Services (GAPS), Clinical Evaluation and Management Handbook.* Chicago, American Medical Association, 1995.

Wolraich ML, Felice ME, Drotar D (editors): *The Classification of Child and Adolescent Mental Diagnoses in Primary Care: Diagnostic and Statistical Manual for Primary Care (DSM-PC), Child and Adolescent Version.* Elk Grove Village, IL, American Academy of Pediatrics, 1996.

Chapter 102

Suicide *Renée R. Jenkins*

The recognition of risk factors for suicidal behavior is an important aspect in the prevention efforts directed toward adolescents, particularly those with mood disorders (see also Chapter 24).

Epidemiology. Suicide is the third leading cause of death for all adolescents and young adults 15–24 yr old; it is the second lead-ing cause of death for white males. Higher rates of suicide have also been reported in Alaskan, Asian-American, and Native American youth. From 1981 to 1998, the suicide rate for African-American males aged 10–19 yr doubled (2.9 to 6.1/100,000), further narrowing the gap between the rates for African-American and white males. The chronically ill adolescent is also at increased risk for suicide exacerbated by interpersonal difficulties and increased access to medications that can be used in a suicide attempt. Lithuania, the Russian Federation, and New Zealand lead the international community in reports of youth suicide with rates for males at or above 40/100,000. Although data on the rate of suicide attempts in the United States are not available, estimates range from 50 to 200 attempts per successful suicide. Males more frequently complete suicides, and females attempt suicide more often. Males use more violent methods, such as hanging, shooting, or wrist slashing, than females. Guns and firearms are the most prevalent method used to complete suicide among children and youth.

Etiology. There are at least three proposed models to account for an increased risk of suicidal behavior in adolescents. The traditional psychiatric model of risk factors focuses on interpersonal

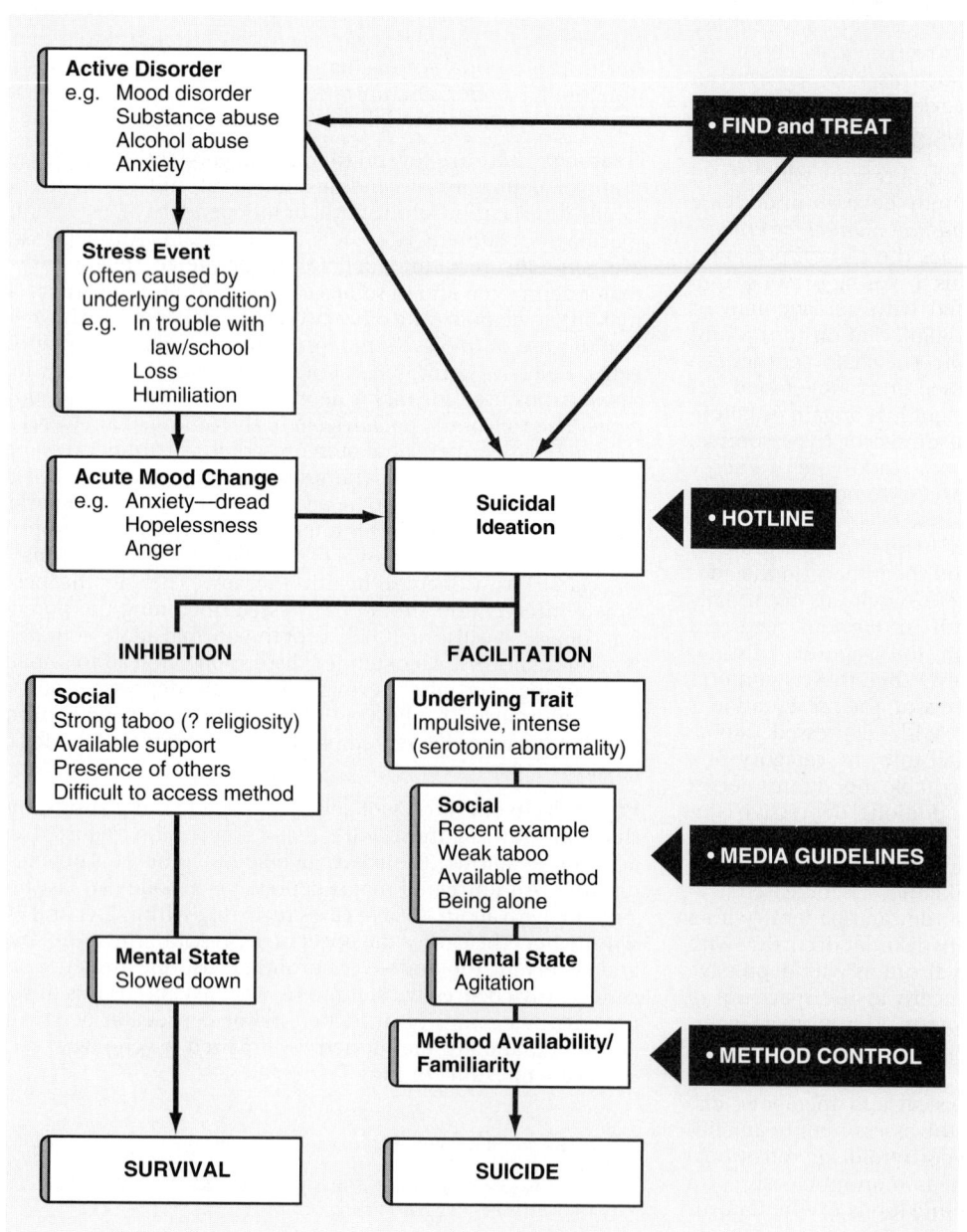

FIGURE 102–1. This model suggests how suicide occurs and highlights types of targeted preventive interventions. (From American Academy of Child and Adolescent Psychiatry: Practice parameter for the assessment and treatment of children and adolescents with suicidal behavior. *J Am Acad Child Adolesc Psychiatry* 2001;40[7 Suppl]: 24S–51S.)

and family factors such as having a psychiatric disorder, family clustering of suicidal behavior, substance use and abuse, sexual and other abuse, and serotonin abnormalities. Low or below average levels of serotonin 5-HT (hydroxytryptamine) or the metabolite 5-HIAA (hydroxy-indoleacetic acid) may be associated with poor impulse control and linked to suicide and violent behavior. Parent-child conflict is more commonly identified as a risk factor in prepubertal adolescents. Gay and bisexual youth may be at greater risk by virtue of gender identity issues, increased use of substances, or the effects of victimization.

The "injury" model for increased suicide risk takes additional community risk factors into account such as local suicide and violence exposure rates, the availability of supportive social networks and suicide prevention programs in the community, and the availability of lethal means such as firearms.

A third approach that is more developmentally driven looks at suicidal risk in the context of other age-related problem behaviors, noting the high correlation between suicide attempts and lack of seatbelt use, carrying a gun in the 30 days prior to the suicide attempt, physical fights in the prior 12 mo, recent tobacco use, and intravenous drug use. Protective factors such as parent-family and school connectedness are emerging as factors modifying the risks for suicide and interpersonal violence. The complex set of factors represented in these approaches has a direct impact on the strategies taken in suicide prevention programs.

Clinical Manifestations. Suicidal ideation alone is not necessarily a risk factor for suicidal behavior. As many as 12–25% of older children and adolescents express some form of suicidal ideation. The risk should be taken much more seriously when the ideation is accompanied by a specific plan. Self-administered suicide scales can be used for screening, but they tend to be oversensitive and underspecific and do not replace the clinical assessment. Psychologic autopsies following successful suicides have also uncovered the frequent occurrence of a stressful event, such as a disciplinary crisis, disappointment, or rejection, immediately preceding the suicide. When a suicide attempt is made, it is often difficult to assess the seriousness of the intent by the actual potency of the method. Beck and associates found medical lethality of methods to correlate poorly with seriousness of intent. There was, however, good correlation between the latter and the patient's expectation of lethality, which was often inaccurate. Although most adolescents who attempt suicide do not become successful, increased risk exists for later morbidity, mortality, depression, behavioral disturbances, and impaired social and academic skills.

Treatment. Consultation with an experienced psychiatrist is essential in the assessment of every teenager who attempts suicide. The evaluation may result in an outpatient referral or hospitalization. When the three most serious risk factors—prior suicide attempt, mood disorder, and substance abuse—are present, there is no proof that hospitalization prevents repeated attempts and the ultimate completion of suicide. However, a hospitalization may assist in resolution of an existing conflict and provide a secure setting in which the patient can have underlying problems addressed. Strategies to improve follow-up outpatient compliance include educating the family about adolescent suicidal behavior and its treatment and the use of a crisis therapist who also serves some case management functions between the family and the treatment provider.

Prevention. The public health approaches to prevention can be targeted to the identification and risk level of the adolescent (Fig. 102–1) and include crisis hotlines, control of access to methods, indirect case finding through identifying "warning signs," direct case finding by primary care providers, providing guidelines to the media, and training professionals to improve skills in recognizing and treating mood disorders. Although considerable attention has been paid to the media impact of conta-

gion and "copy-cat" suicides, clusters involving adolescents and young adults account for 1–5% of suicides in this age group in the United States.

American Academy of Child and Adolescent Psychiatry: Practice parameter for the assessment and treatment of children and adolescents with suicidal behavior. *J Am Acad Child Adolesc Psychiatry* 2001;40(7 Suppl):24S–51S.
Beautrais AL: Risk factors for suicide and attempted suicide among young people. *Aust N Z J Psychiatry* 2000;34:420–36.
Borowsky IW, Ireland M, Resnick MD: Adolescent suicide attempts: Risks and protectors. *Pediatrics* 2001;107(3):485–93.
Greenhill LL, Waslick B: Management of suicidal behavior in children and adolescents. *Psychiatr Clin North Am* 1997;20:641.
United Nations Childrens Fund (UNICEF): *The Progress of Nations, 1996* (www.unicef.org/pon96/insuicid.htm—accessed 4/2/02).

Chapter 103
Violent Behavior *Renée R. Jenkins*

Interpersonal and community violence, physical abuse, and domestic violence lead to significant rates of injury and death for specific age, gender, and racial sectors of the population in the United States (also see Chapter 34). Youth and minority populations are disproportionately affected. Violent behavior permeates the youth culture, whether by media or personal experiences in the family, community, or school. For surveillance and research purposes, the Centers for Disease Control and Prevention has accepted a definition of a violent injury as "a threatened or actual use of physical force against a person or group that either results or is likely to result in injury or death." Youth are perpetrators of violence, victims of violence, or observers of violence with varying severity of impact on the individual. Violent acts may result in, or are contributed to by, mental health problems or disorders. Pediatricians are challenged to screen for these disorders and counsel or refer adolescents with serious disorders to mental health professionals. The public health and educational communities have launched a variety of violence prevention interventions to increase youth prosocial behavior and reduce violence as a societal problem.

Epidemiology. In 1993–1994, the United States led the industrialized world in the number of youth deaths due to firearms, both homicide and unintentional firearm deaths (Fig. 103–1). From 1983–1993, the firearm homicide rate more than tripled from 5 to18/100,000. Since 1993 the rates of fatal and nonfatal firearm injuries have declined. Males are much more likely to be victims than females in fatal and nonfatal injuries; however, 15–24 yr old women have the highest proportion of injuries compared with women in other age groups.

The Youth Risk Behavior Surveillance System reported in 1999 that 17.3% of students (26.6% male and 6% female) carried a weapon such as a gun, knife, or club within the 30 days preceding the survey. However, compared with the baseline survey of 1991, weapon carrying had decreased. Nationally, 36.7% of students also reported being in a fight in the prior year, and this too has declined from 137/100 students/12 mo in 1993 to 106/100 students/12 mo in 1999. Forced sexual intercourse and dating violence were reported at similar rates, 8.8% of students. Females were more likely to report higher rates for both occurrences with the exception of similar rates of dating violence in white males and females (7.3% and 7.4% respectively).

Adolescents are more likely to be victims of violence than are any other age group (Fig. 103–2). In 2000, the victimization rate was 60.1/1,000 for 12–15 yr olds and 64.3/1,000 for 16–19 yr olds, a dramatic decline of almost 50% since 1994. Although adolescents are infrequently the age group that comes to mind when considering child abuse, adolescents make up almost one quarter of the child abuse and neglect cases in the United States

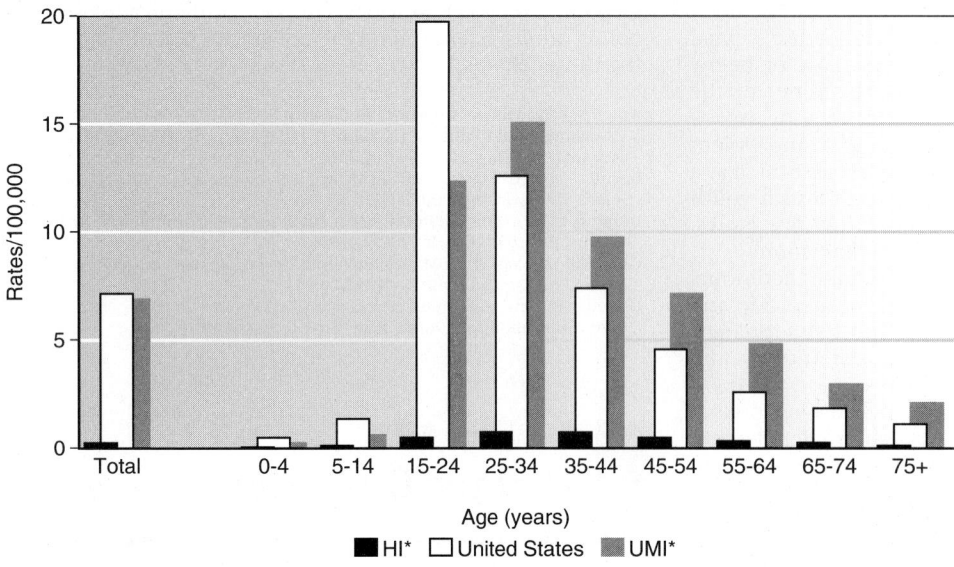

HI* ☐ United States UMI*

* HI indicates high-income countries, and UMI indicates upper-middle-income countries.
NB: Data for 1994 or most recent year available.

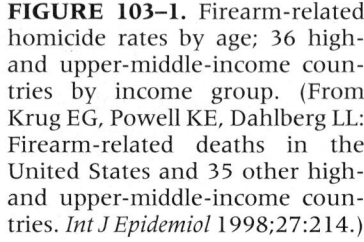

FIGURE 103–1. Firearm-related homicide rates by age; 36 high- and upper-middle-income countries by income group. (From Krug EG, Powell KE, Dahlberg LL: Firearm-related deaths in the United States and 35 other high- and upper-middle-income countries. *Int J Epidemiol* 1998;27:214.)

Violent crime rates by age of victim

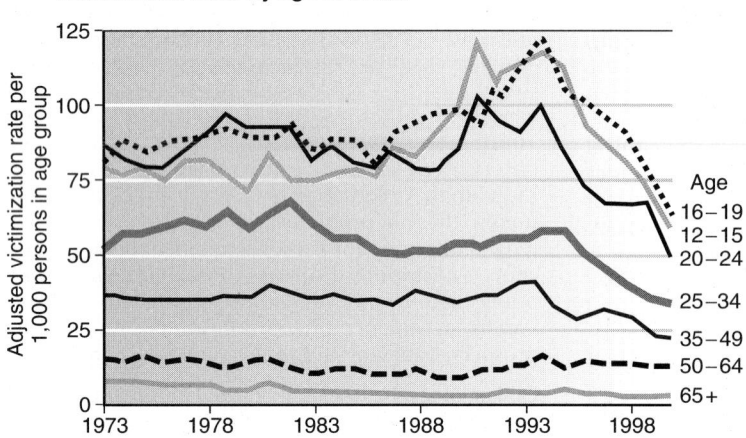

FIGURE 103–2. Violent crimes included are homicide, rape, robbery, and both simple and aggravated assault. The National Crime Victimization Survey redesign was implemented in 1993. The data before 1993 are adjusted to make them comparable with data collected since the redesign. The adjustment methods are described in *Criminal Victimization 1973–95.* Estimates for 1993 and beyond are based on collection year, whereas earlier estimates are based on data year. (From U.S. Department of Justice, Bureau of Justice Statistics, 2001.)

(see Chapter 35). Adolescents and children younger than 5 yr of age are the most likely victims of physical abuse that causes injury.

Etiology. The theories to explain violence come from the perspective of varying disciplines. The development psychopathology model of Mofitt identifies two types of antisocial youth: one that is life course–persistent and one that is life course–limited. Adolescent-limited offenders have no childhood aberrant behaviors and are more likely to commit status offenses such as vandalism, running away, and other behaviors symbolic of their struggle for autonomy from parents. Life course–persistent offenders, in contrast, exhibit aberrant behavior in childhood, such as problems with temperament, behavioral development, and cognition, and as adolescents participate in more victim-oriented crimes. The public health model emphasizes the environment and other external influences. It focuses primarily on preventive strategies that view violence as amenable to systematic, science-based, multidisciplinary, and sustained interventions (Table 103–1). A third theoretical model examines violent behaviors across the spectrum occurring within and outside the family and is referred to as the cycle of violence. This hypothesis

proposes that precursors such as child abuse and neglect, a child witnessing violence, adolescent sexual and physical abuse, and adolescent exposure to violence and violent assaults predispose youth to outcomes of violent behavior, violent crime, delinquency, violent assaults, suicide, or premature death. An additional common paradigm for high-risk violence behavior poses a balance of risk and protective factors at the individual, family, and community level. None of these theories successfully explains violent behavior. Although the media influences violence through a strong effect on aggressive behavior, many questions still remain about the causes of violent behavior.

Clinical Manifestations. There are several clinical entities directly associated with violent behavior that require recognition and intervention. The most common behavioral diagnoses associated with aggressive behavior in adolescents are mental retardation, learning disabilities, moderately severe language disorders, and mental disorders such as attention-deficit/hyperactivity, mood disturbance, anxiety, and personality disorders. Inability to master prosocial skills such as the establishment and maintenance of positive family and peer relations and the resolution of conflict may put adolescents with these disorders at higher risk

TABLE 103–1. Public Health Approach to Youth Violence Prevention Model with Examples

	Victim (Host)	Perpetrator (Vector)	Firearm (Agent)	Social Environment	Physical Environment
Primary prevention	Conflict resolution Violence anticipatory guidance	Substance abuse treatment Home visiting programs for new and single parents	Handgun and assault weapons ban Firearm registration	Job opportunities Adult-supervised activities	Better lighting Zoning-enforced limits in liquor licenses
Secondary prevention	Medical services Psychologic services	Job training Psychosocial rehabilitation	Handgun locks Public education on risks of ownership	School incident debriefing Safe havens	Increased police presence Graffiti removal
Tertiary prevention	Physical rehabilitation Psychosocial services	Incarceration Educational-psychosocial rehabilitation	Firearm surveillance	Foster care Alternative schools	Urban planning, e.g., decrease population density in public housing and mixture of income levels

From Calhoun AD, Clark-Jones F: Theoretical frameworks: Developmental psychopathology, the public health approach to violence, and the cycle of violence. Pediatr Clin North Am *1998; 45:287.*

for physical violence and other risky behaviors. Conduct disorder and oppositional defiant disorder are specific psychiatric diagnoses whose definitions are associated with violent behavior (Table 103–2). They occur co-morbidly with other disorders such as attention-deficit/hyperactivity disorder and increase an adolescent's vulnerability for juvenile delinquency, substance use or abuse, sexual promiscuity, adult criminal behavior, incarceration, and antisocial personality disorder.

In an emergency or urgent care setting, one is very likely to encounter victims of physical and/or sexual assault. Rather than treat the physical injury in isolation, the American Academy of Pediatrics has established a model protocol for physical assault victims and guidelines for caring for sexual assault victims. The guidelines recommend psychologic evaluation and support, social service evaluation of the circumstance surrounding the assault, and a treatment plan on discharge that is designed to protect the adolescent from subsequent injury episodes and minimize the development of psychologic disability. Victims as well as witnesses of violence are at risk for post-traumatic stress disorder (see Chapter 22).

Diagnosis. The assessment of an adolescent at risk for, or with a history of, violent behavior or victimization should be a part of the health maintenance visit of all adolescents. The answers to questions about recent history of involvement in a physical fight, carrying a weapon, or firearms in the household, as well as concerns that the adolescent may have about his or her personal safety may suggest a problem requiring a more in-depth evaluation. The additional factors of physical or sexual abuse, serious problems at school, poor school performance and attendance, multiple incidents of trauma, and symptoms associated with mental disorders are indications for evaluation by a mental

health professional. In a situation of acute trauma, assault victims are not always forthcoming about the circumstances of their injuries for fear of retaliation or police involvement. Stabilization of the injury or the gathering of forensic evidence in sexual assault is the treatment priority; however, once this is achieved, addressing a more comprehensive set of issues surrounding the assault is appropriate.

Treatment. In the instance of acute injury secondary to violent assault, the treatment plan should follow standards established by the American Academy of Pediatrics model protocol, which includes, but is not limited to, the stabilization of the injury, evaluation and treatment of the injury, evaluation of the assault circumstance, psychologic evaluation of the functioning of the victim, rehabilitation of the injury, and outpatient follow-up of the behavioral and physical sequelae. The American College of Emergency Physicians details the required examination and documentation for sexual assault victims in a handbook, *Evaluation and Management of Sexually Assaulted or Sexually Abused Patient.* Specific requirements for forensic evidence, as well as the management of sexually transmitted diseases and pregnancy prevention, are key elements of these recommendations. Specifically, prophylactic treatment of chlamydia and gonorrhea as well as postcoital contraception are recommended (see Chapters 208.2, 177, and 108).

Prevention. Interventions to prevent violence must encompass individual and social factors. Violent behaviors are influenced not only by characteristics of individuals, but also by characteristics of families, such as cohesion and parent practices; characteristics of peers, such as delinquent behaviors; characteristics of schools, such as teacher practices and school atmosphere;

TABLE 103–2. Oppositional Defiant Disorder, Conduct Disorder, and Juvenile Delinquency

Psychiatric Disorder Labels		Legal Label
Oppositional Defiant Disorder	*Conduct Disorder*	*Juvenile Delinquency*
Recurrent pattern of negativistic, defiant, disobedient, and hostile behavior toward authority figures that have a significant adverse effect on functioning (e.g., social, academic, or occupational) Examples: losing temper; arguing with adults; defying or refusing to comply with request or rules of adults; annoying behavior; blaming others; and being irritable, spiteful, resentful	Repetitive and persistent pattern of behavior that violates the basic rights of others or major age-appropriate societal norms or rules Examples: physical fighting, deceitfulness, stealing, destruction of property, threatening or causing physical harm to people or animals, driving without a license, prostitution, rape (even if not adjudicated in the legal system)	Offenses that are illegal because of age; illegal acts Examples: single or multiple instances of being arrested or adjudicated for any of the following: stealing, destruction of property, threatening or causing physical harm to people or animals, driving without a license, prostitution, rape
Diagnosed by a mental health clinician	Diagnosed by a mental health practitioner	Adjudicated in the legal system

From Greydanus DE, Pratt HD, Patel DR, Sloane MA: The rebellious adolescent. Pediatr Clin North Am *1997;44:1460.*

characteristics of community organization, such as the frequency and type of youth activities; and characteristics of the larger society, such as economic opportunity, misuse of firearms, or media exposure. Violence-prevention efforts to date have emphasized individually oriented strategies, directed toward students in school or patients in the clinical setting. These approaches should be continued, but need to be complemented by activities designed to modify exposures at the family, peer, community, and society level.

American Academy of Pediatrics, Committee on Adolescence: Care of the adolescent sexual assault victim. *Pediatrics* 2001;107:1476. (www.aap.org)

American Academy of Pediatrics, Task Force on Adolescent Assault Victim Needs: Adolescent assault victim needs: A review of issues and a model protocol. *Pediatrics* 1996;98:991. (www.aap.org)

American College of Emergency Physicians: *Evaluation and Management of the Sexually Assaulted or Sexually Abused Patient.* Dallas, American College of Emergency Physicians, 1999. (www.acep.org/library/index.cfm/id/2101)

Greydanus DE, Pratt HD, Patel DR, et al: The rebellious adolescent: Evaluation and management of oppositional and conduct disorders. *Pediatr Clin North Am* 1997;44:1457.

Hennes HMA, Calhoun AD (editors): Violence among children and adolescents. *Pediatr Clin North Am* 1998;45:269.

Kann L, Kinchen SA, Williams BI, et al: Youth risk behavior surveillance—U.S., 1999. In: CDC Surveillance Summaries, June 9, 2000. *MMWR* 2000;49(no SS-5):1–94. (www.cdc.gov/YRBSS)

Krug EG, Powell KE, Dahlberg LL: Firearm-related deaths in the United States and 35 other high- and upper-middle-income countries. *Int J Epidemiol* 1998;27:214.

Rennison CM: *Criminal Victimization 2000: Changes 1999–2000 with Trends 1993–2000.* Bureau of Justice Statistics. National Crime Victimization Survey, June 2001. (www.ojp.usdoj.gov/bjs/pub/pdf/cv00.pdf)

Satcher D, Powell KE, Mercy JA, et al: Opening commentary: Violence prevention is as American as apple pie. *Am J Prev Med* 1996;12(Suppl):v.

U.S. Department of Health and Human Services: *Youth Violence: A Report of the Surgeon General.* Rockville, MD, U.S. Department of Health and Human Services, Centers for Disease Control and Prevention, National Center for Injury Prevention and Control; Substance Abuse and Mental Health Services Administration, Center for Mental Health Services; and National Institutes of Health, National Institute of Mental Health, 2001. (www.surgeongeneral.gov/library/youthviolence)

Chapter 104
Anorexia Nervosa and Bulimia *Iris F. Litt*

Epidemiology. The incidence of anorexia nervosa (AN) and bulimia (BN) has increased over the last 2 decades. It is estimated that 1 in every 100 females, 16–18 yr old, has anorexia nervosa. A bimodal distribution occurs, with one peak at 14.5 and the other at 18 yr; 25% may be younger than the age of 13. The increased incidence has been documented in all Western countries, with sporadic reports from other nations. Affected females outnumber males 10:1. Initially reported only in middle and upper socioeconomic groups, AN is now occurring in those from the lower socioeconomic levels and in a variety of ethnic and racial groups. BN is more common than AN. An increased incidence of eating disorders among primary relatives of those with AN and BN suggests a familial basis.

Diagnosis. The *Diagnostic and Statistical Manual of Mental Disorders (DSM-IV)* criteria for the diagnosis of AN include (1) intense fear of becoming obese, which does not diminish as weight loss progresses; (2) disturbance in the way in which one's body weight, size, or shape is experienced (e.g., claiming to "feel fat" even when one is emaciated or believing that one area of the body is "too fat" even when obviously underweight); (3) refusal to maintain body weight over a minimal normal weight for age and height (e.g., weight loss leading to maintenance of body weight 15% below expected, failure to make expected weight gain during period of growth leading to body weight 15% less than that expected); and (4) in females, absence of at least three consecutive menstrual cycles when otherwise expected to occur (primary or secondary amenorrhea).

AN is characterized further by excessive physical activity in the face of apparent inanition; denial of hunger; preoccupation with food preparation, frequently accompanied by bizarre eating behaviors; and often studiousness and academic success. Many are described as having been "model children" before the onset of the illness. Patients who have AN are subdivided into the *restrictor* and *BN* subgroups, according to their method of caloric reduction. Restrictors severely limit their intake of carbohydrate and fat-containing foods, whereas bulimics tend to eat in binges and then to purge themselves of food by self-induced vomiting or the use of cathartics. Excoriations on the dorsum of the hand from self-induced vomiting may suggest the diagnosis.

DSM-IV separates *BN* from AN as a diagnostic entity, defining BN as (1) recurrent episodes of binge eating (rapid consumption of a large amount of food in a discrete period of time, usually less than 2 hr); (2) during the eating binges, a fear of not being able to stop eating; (3) regularly engaging in self-induced vomiting, use of laxatives, or rigorous dieting or fasting in order to counteract the effects of binge eating; (4) a minimum average of two binge eating episodes per week for at least 3 mo; and (5) self-evaluation is unduly influenced by body weight and shape, but the disturbance does not occur exclusively during episodes of AN. The binge-purge pattern may occur in youngsters who have normal weight or are slightly obese.

Etiology and Psychodynamics. Eating disorders commonly begin as innocent dieting behavior, not unlike that seen in many other adolescent women, but those with AN gradually progress to profound weight loss with emaciation. Premorbid psychiatric characteristics of patients with AN may include excessive dependency, developmental immaturity, and isolation. Their families have been described as having difficulty with problem solving and as being intrusive and overprotective. The onset of these conditions at the time of puberty has prompted psychoanalysts to regard them as defenses against emerging sexuality, an opinion that dominated thinking until the 1950s, when Bruch conceptualized AN as a problem in identity development. Others consider that AN may represent a disorder of mood accompanied by manic or depressive symptoms. Patients with AN have also been subcategorized on the basis of psychologic characteristics in order to demonstrate that different subgroups are dynamically and prognostically different. Biogenic amine neurotransmitter abnormalities are found in some patients with AN. Their etiologic significance is unclear.

Clinical Manifestations. AN and BN are associated with disturbances in almost every organ system, although it is uncertain which may be primary and which is the result of severe malnutrition. The death rate in AN is approximately 10% and is usually caused by severe electrolyte disturbance, cardiac arrhythmia, or congestive heart failure in the recovery phase. *Bradycardia* and *postural hypotension* are common, with pulse rates as low as 20 beats/min. Both improve with nutritional therapy. A variety of electrocardiographic abnormalities is common, including low voltage, T-wave inversion and flattening, and ST depression, as well as supraventricular and ventricular dysrhythmias, some preceded by a prolonged QT_c interval. Decreased cardiac output and mitral valve prolapse may result from myofibrillar atrophy. Patients who have abused ipecac may develop myocarditis. Death from congestive heart failure is a late event and may result from unduly rapid rehydration and refeeding. On a regimen achieving a daily weight gain limited to 0.2–0.4 kg, none of our patients has experienced this complication. Other manifestations of the "refeeding syndrome" include hypophosphatemia as a result of insulin-induced shifts of phosphate to intracellular space.

Sleep disturbances occur in some patients with AN and include a short rapid eye movement latency time, similar to that often found in depressed patients. Problems of thermal regulation, particularly hypothermia, are common (15% of our patients had temperatures recorded below 35°C). Hypothermia also occurs in bulimics of normal weight.

Disorders of the hypothalamic-pituitary-ovarian axis are manifested as amenorrhea associated with immature patterns of secretion of luteinizing hormone. These findings may represent a primary hypothalamic defect rather than being secondary to weight loss (which also causes amenorrhea), inasmuch as amenorrhea antedates weight loss in one third to one half of patients with AN, and a similar proportion fail to resume menses when normal weight is restored. One quarter of patients may be amenorrheic for ten or more years, despite weight rehabilitation. Evidence for hypothalamic-pituitary-adrenal axis dysfunction includes increased secretion of cortisol, loss of diurnal variation in its secretion, and failure of dexamethasone to suppress it. The last may also be found in starvation; however, in 44% of our patients with AN, abnormal results of dexamethasone suppression tests have persisted after weight rehabilitation. Growth hormone secretion is abnormally high in these patients, and somatomedin-C is low. Thyroid-stimulating hormone levels are normal, thyroxine and triiodothyronine are low, and reverse triiodothyronine is elevated, presumably in adaptation to a lowered basal metabolic rate as a result of malnutrition and carbohydrate deprivation. In some patients, peripheral edema in the absence of congestive heart failure or hypoproteinemia has been attributed to inappropriate secretion of antidiuretic hormone.

Elevations of blood urea nitrogen level may occur, reflecting dehydration and decreased glomerular filtration rate, but normal levels may be found under these same conditions because of low protein intake even in the dehydrated patient. Mild proteinuria, hematuria, and pyuria, with negative urine cultures, generally resolve with proper rehydration. Pseudoproteinuria is often found because the alkalinity of the urine gives a false-positive reaction to albumin on the dipstick.

Neuropsychologic effects of AN include impairment of concentration and problem solving, as well as attentional-perceptual and motor function. Structural changes occur in the brain, such as deficits in volume of white and gray matter, the latter persisting after weight rehabilitation.

Bone marrow hypoplasia is common in AN, with leukopenia, anemia, and (rarely) thrombocytopenia. Low erythrocyte sedimentation rates are also common, perhaps reflecting low fibrinogen production secondary to malnutrition.

Constipation is a common complication of motility problems in AN, as is esophagitis in those who vomit. Decreased gastrointestinal tract motility may be a cause of perforation following nasogastric tube insertion. Elevations in amylase levels may be associated with bilateral parotid swelling or with pancreatitis.

Electrolyte imbalance (in addition to hypophosphatemia in refeeding) results from vomiting, "waterloading" (a practice of surreptitiously drinking large amounts of water in order to achieve an agreed-upon weight gain), or abuse of diuretics or laxatives. Potassium depletion, associated with a hypochloremic alkalosis, is common. Abnormalities of calcium, magnesium, and phosphorus metabolism may result from laxative abuse, either secondary to malabsorption or resulting from the use of preparations containing phosphate. Paradoxically, cholesterol levels are often elevated in AN. The skin of patients

with AN is dry, and lanugo hair is often seen. Hair loss often occurs in the refeeding phase.

Treatment. Systematic, controlled studies of treatment in these disorders are not available. Most of the regimens in current use combine psychotherapy (individual and family), behavior modification techniques, and nutritional rehabilitation. Pharmacologic therapy (primarily with antidepressant medications) appears to be helpful for that subset of depressed patients with eating disorders. The success rate in short-term follow-up studies is about 70%. The frequent occurrence of medical complications and the possibility of death during the acute or rehabilitation phase require the inclusion of a medically and physiologically oriented physician in the management team.

De Simone G: Cardiac abnormalities in young women with anorexia nervosa. *Br Heart J* 1994;71:287.
Fisher M, Golden NH, Katzman DK, et al: Eating disorders in adolescents: A background paper. *J Adolesc Health* 1995;16:420.
Katzman DK, Zipursky RB, Lambe EK, et al: A longitudinal magnetic resonance imaging study of brain changes in adolescents with anorexia nervosa. *Arch Pediatr Adolesc Med* 1997;151:793.

Chapter 105
Substance Abuse *Renée R. Jenkins*

Cultural and societal norms frame acceptable standards for substance use. These standards also have a historical context. Adolescents are influenced by adult role models and environmental messages related to substances. For example, children of alcoholic parents are 2 to 10 times more likely to develop alcoholism than children of nonalcoholic parents. In the context of the current decade, occasional or situational use of certain substances such as alcohol, marijuana, and cigarettes may be viewed as "normative" given the proportion of youth who report some experience with these substances. Some studies suggest that otherwise normal, healthy, adolescents who "experiment" with drugs may be better adjusted than those who lack that experience. Others view the potential for adverse outcomes even with occasional use in immature adolescents, such as motor vehicle accidents and other injuries, sufficient justification to consider any drug use in younger adolescents a considerable risk.

The developmental considerations are probably most important for this age group. Substance use for most teenagers is not an issue of psychopathology but of the influence on normal functioning. Drug use in younger, less experienced adolescents can act as a substitute for developing age-appropriate coping strategies and enhance vulnerability to poor decision-making. Early adolescent use is also associated with greater vulnerability to adult addictions. When drug use begins to negatively alter functioning in older adolescents at school and in the family, and risk-taking behavior is seen, intervention is warranted. Serious drug use is not an isolated phenomenon. It is a part of a complex set of family and individual issues that should be addressed in a comprehensive fashion. The challenge to the clinician is to determine which type of behavior one is observing and to take the necessary action. The challenge to the community and society is to create norms that decrease the likelihood of adverse health outcomes for adolescents and promote and facilitate opportunities for adolescents to choose healthier and safer options for experimentation.

Etiology. The determinants of adolescent substance use and abuse have been explained using a number of theoretical models. Most of the models include factors at the individual level, the level of significant relationships with others, and the level of the setting, that is, community or other environment. Models have also begun to include a balance of risk and protective or coping factors that tend to account for individual differences among adolescents with similar risk factors who escape adverse outcomes. Duncan and Petrosa also argue for differentiating the risk factors for adolescent use compared with adolescent abuse. Adolescent use is more commonly related to social and peer factors, whereas abuse is more often a function of psychologic and biologic factors. The likelihood that an otherwise normal adolescent would experiment with drugs may be dependent on the availability of the drug to the adolescent, the perceived positive or otherwise functional value to the adolescent, and the presence or absence of restraints as determined by the adolescent's cultural or other important value systems. An abusing adolescent, in contrast, may have genetic or biologic factors coexisting with dependence on a particular drug for coping with day-to-day activities. In addition, such an adolescent may adopt an identification with the addicted role, with a fear of the consequences of withdrawal.

Specific historical questions can assist in determining the severity of the drug problem through a rating system as depicted in Table 105–1. The type of drug used (e.g., marijuana versus heroin), the circumstances of use (e.g., alone or in a group setting), the frequency and timing of use (e.g., daily before school versus rarely on a weekend), the premorbid personality (depressed versus happy), as well as the teenager's general functional status should all be considered in evaluating any youngster found to be abusing a drug. In addition, certain protective factors play a part in buffering the risk factors as well as assisting in anticipating the long-term outcome of experimentation. Emotionally supportive parents with open communication styles, involvement in organized school activities, and recognition of the importance of academic achievement are a few of the important protective factors. Involvement in organized sports activities is usually protective, but it may be a risk factor in regard to the use of anabolic steroids. Any use of a psychoactive drug in the context of the use of machinery or a motor vehicle or in a potentially volatile interpersonal interaction can add an increased health risk, regardless of the extent of any prior use.

Epidemiology. Surveys on adolescent substance use have a variety of limitations due to sampling and questionnaire differences. The National Household Survey on Drug Abuse may reflect refusal to report use within a household. School-based surveys (Monitoring the Future study and Youth Risk Behavior Surveillance) do not capture school dropouts, school absenteeism, and high rates of refusal. The rates of drug use across surveys is not dramatically different and certain observations are consistent across surveys. Alcohol and cigarettes are the most prevalent drugs (Table 105–2). Marijuana tends to be the most commonly reported illicit

TABLE 105–2. Lifetime Use of Cigarettes, Alcohol, Marijuana, MDMA, and Steroids (Anabolic-Androgenic) in 8th, 10th, and 12th Grades, 1997 and 2001

		8th Grade (%)	10th Grade (%)	12th Grade (%)
Cigarettes	1997	47.3	60.2	65.4
	2001	36.6	52.8	61.0
Alcohol	1997	53.8	72.0	81.7
	2001	50.5	70.1	79.7
Marijuana	1997	22.6	42.3	49.6
	2001	20.4	40.1	49.0
MDMA (Ecstasy)	1997	3.2	5.7	6.9
	2001	5.2	8.0	11.7
Steroids (anabolic)	1997	1.8	2.0	2.4
Steroids (anabolic)	2001	2.8	3.5	3.7

From Johnston LD, O'Malley PM, Bachman JG: High School and Youth Trends: 2001 Monitoring the Future Study (MTF), NIDA. U.S. Department of Health and Human Services (www.drugabuse.gov/Infofax/HSYouthtrends.html), accessed 2/24/02.

drug ever used. The prevalence of substance use varies by age, gender, geographic region, race, and other demographic factors. Younger teenagers tend to report less use of most drugs than do older teenagers, with the exception of inhalants (17.1% in 8th grade, 15.2% in 10th grade, and 13.0% in 12th grade, 2001). Males strongly predominate in the lifetime prevalence reports for smokeless tobacco and anabolic steroids compared with females. Marijuana use is reported more frequently in large metropolitan areas, whereas less urbanized areas report more binge drinking and daily cigarette use. In school surveys, Hispanics report more experience with cocaine, whereas white students report high rates of smokeless tobacco and daily cigarette smoking. By 12th grade, blacks report less use of drugs across all categories.

In examining trends in drug use, fewer students reported marijuana, alcohol, and cigarette use over the years since 1997 in 8th, 10th, and 12th grades, with 8th graders showing the greatest declines (see Table 105–2). Alarming trends are seen in MDMA (Ecstasy) and anabolic steroid use, increasing across all grades since 1997.

Pathogenesis. The process of physical growth and development that characterizes puberty may be affected adversely by the use of drugs. For example, one third of adolescent females who use *heroin* have secondary amenorrhea, even in the absence of weight loss. The higher incidence of menstrual abnormalities in the adolescent heroin user probably results from a greater vulnerability of the hypothalamic-pituitary-ovarian axis in the maturing individual. Experiments with naloxone, the opiate antagonist, suggest that endogenous opiates block the release of gonadotropin-releasing hormone. *Amphetamines* interfere with stage 4 sleep and may impair the intimate relationship between sleep and augmentation of secretion of gonadotropin during early adolescence (also see Chapter 20.5). To derive calories mainly from *ethanol* during the peak of the pubertal growth spurt deprives the body of the protein necessary for normal muscle growth.

The metabolism of certain prescribed drugs may be affected by coincident abuse of illicit drugs or alcohol. Induction of hepatic smooth endoplasmic reticulum by barbiturates or alcohol may accelerate the metabolism and enhance the excretion of substances requiring glucuronidation. As a result of this mechanism, estrogen-containing oral contraceptives taken by an abuser of these substances may result in a vulnerability to pregnancy. Conversely, the use of estrogens increases the risk of intoxication from alcohol as a result of decreased ethanol metabolism. The potentiating interaction of alcohol and barbiturates must also be considered when prescribing anticonvulsant medications. Abdominal pain and vomiting occur when metronidazole is ingested by an alcohol-abusing adolescent because of the antagonistic effect of alcohol on acetaldehyde.

TABLE 105–1. Assessing the Seriousness of Adolescent Drug Abuse

Variable	0	+1	+2
Age (yr)	>15 yr	<15 yr	
Sex	Male	Female	
Family history of drug abuse		Yes	
Setting of drug use	In group		Alone
Affect before drug use	Happy	Always poor	Sad
School performance	Good, improving		Recently poor
Use before driving	None		Yes
History of accidents	None		Yes
Time of week	Weekend	Weekdays	
Time of day		After school	Before school
Type of drug	Marijuana, beer, wine	Hallucinogens, amphetamines	Whiskey, opiates, cocaine, barbiturates

Total score: 0–3 less worrisome, 3–8 serious, 8–18 very serious.

Clinical Manifestations. Although manifestations vary by the specific substance of use, adolescents who use drugs often present in an office setting with no obvious physical findings. Drug use is more frequently detected in adolescents who are victims of motor vehicle accidents or intentional injuries. Eliciting appropriate historical information regarding substance use followed by a blood alcohol and a urine drug screen is recommended in emergency settings. In addition, an adolescent presenting to an emergency setting with an impaired sensorium as part of a toxic syndrome should be evaluated for substance use as a part of the differential diagnosis, again accompanied by appropriate screening and physical examination (Box 105–1). Certain psychiatric and behavioral diagnoses are frequently associated with substance use and should be considered once such use is detected. Conversely, screening for substance use is recommended for patients with psychiatric and behavioral diagnoses. Diagnoses that are commonly considered range from conduct disorders, with or without attention deficit disorder, to personality disorders. Other clinical manifestations of substance use are associated with the route of use; intravenous drug use is associated with venous "tracks" and needle marks, and nasal mucosal injuries are associated with nasal insufflation of drugs. Seizures can be a direct effect of drugs such as cocaine and amphetamines or an effect of drug withdrawal in the case of barbiturates or tranquilizers. Additional specific clinical manifestations are described in the following sections on each substance.

Screening for Substance Abuse and Use. The annual health maintenance examination provides an opportunity for identifying adolescents with substance use or abuse issues (see Chapters 17 and 100). The direct questions as well as the assessment of school, family relations, and peer activities may necessitate a more in-depth interview if there are suggestions of difficulties in those areas. Several self-report screening questionnaires are available with varying degrees of standardization, length, and reliability. The classic CAGE mnemonic used for screening adults for alcohol abuse has been modified for use in adolescents and new mnemonics specifically designed for adolescents are in use, e.g., CRAFFT (Box 105–2) and RAFFT. The use of urine screening is recommended in select circumstances, most of which are constructed to provide for the confidentiality and informed choice of the adolescent. Involuntary screening with parental permission is strongly discouraged for older, competent adolescents. Lack of decision-making capacity or very strong medical indications may present a clinical situation in which consent may be waived. Indications for urine screening include (1) psychiatric symptoms, to rule out co-morbidity or dual diagnoses; (2) significant changes in school performance or other daily behaviors; (3) frequently occurring accidents; (4) frequently occurring episodes of respiratory problems; (5) evaluation of serious motor vehicular of other injuries; and (6) as a monitoring procedure for a recovery program. Table 105–3 demonstrates the types of tests commonly used for detection by substance, along with the approximate retention time between the use and the identification of the substance in the urine. Most initial screening uses an immunoassay method such as the enzyme-multiplied immunoassay technique followed by a confirmatory test using the highly sensitive, highly specific gas chromatography-mass spectrometry. The substances that can cause false-positive results should be considered, especially when there is a discrepancy between the physical findings and the urine drug screen result.

Diagnosis. Diagnostic criteria that classify the severity of substance use-abuse range from substance use variation, through the diagnosis of a substance abuse problem, to the definition of a substance abuse disorder. Substance abuse variation refers to the experimentation that commonly occurs in this age group. An adolescent is considered to have a diagnosis of a substance abuse problem if the use occurs more than on a one-time basis and involves impaired memory or other motor function deficits. A substance abuse disorder is diagnosed when there is impaired

---

BOX 105–1. The Most Common Toxic Syndromes

ANTICHOLINERGIC SYNDROMES

Common signs — Delirium with mumbling speech, tachycardia, dry, flushed skin, dilated pupils, myoclonus, slightly elevated temperature, urinary retention, and decreased bowel sounds. Seizures and dysrhythmias may occur in severe cases.

Common causes — Antihistamines, antiparkinsonian medication, atropine, scopolamine, amantadine, antipsychotic agents, antidepressant agents, antispasmodic agents, mydriatic agents, skeletal muscle relaxants, and many plants (notably jimson weed and *Amanita muscaria*).

SYMPATHOMIMETIC SYNDROMES

Common signs — Delusions, paranoia, tachycardia (or bradycardia if the drug is a pure α-adrenergic agonist), hypertension, hyperpyrexia, diaphoresis, piloerection, mydriasis, and hyperreflexia. Seizures, hypotension, and dysrhythmias may occur in severe cases.

Common causes — Cocaine, amphetamine, methamphetamine (and its derivatives 3,4-methylenedioxyamphetamine, 3,4-methylenedioxymethamphetamine, 3,4-methylenedioxyethamphetamine, and 2,5-dimethoxy-4-bromoamphetamine), and over-the-counter decongestants (phenylpropanolamine, ephedrine, and pseudoephedrine). In caffeine and theophylline overdoses, similar findings, except for the organic psychiatric signs, result from catecholamine release.

OPIATE, SEDATIVE, OR ETHANOL INTOXICATION

Common signs — Coma, respiratory depression, miosis, hypotension, bradycardia, hypothermia, pulmonary edema, decreased bowel sounds, hyporeflexia, and needle marks. Seizures may occur after overdoses of some narcotics, notably propoxyphene.

Common causes — Narcotics, barbiturates, benzodiazepines, ethchlorvynol, glutethimide, methyprylon, methaqualone, meprobamate, ethanol, clonidine, and guanabenz.

CHOLINERGIC SYNDROMES

Common signs — Confusion, central nervous system depression, weakness, salivation, lacrimation, urinary and fecal incontinence, gastrointestinal cramping, emesis, diaphoresis, muscle fasciculations, pulmonary edema, miosis, bradycardia or tachycardia, and seizures.

Common causes — Organophosphate and carbamate insecticides, physostigmine, edrophonium, and some mushrooms.

From Kulig K: Initial management of ingestions of toxic substances. *N Engl J Med* 1992; 326:1678.© 1992 Massachusetts Medical Society. All rights reserved.

BOX 105–2. CRAFFT Mnemonic Tool

- Have you ever ridden in a **C**ar driven by someone (including yourself) who was high or had been using alcohol or drugs?
- Do you ever use alcohol or drugs to **R**elax, feel better about yourself or fit in?
- Do you ever use alcohol or drugs while you are by yourself (**A**lone)?
- Do you ever **F**orget things you did while using alcohol or drugs?
- Do your **F**amily or **F**riends ever tell you that you should cut down on your drinking or drug use?
- Have you ever gotten into **T**rouble while you were using alcohol or drugs?

Adapted from Anglin TM: Evaluation by interview and questionnaire. In Schydlower M (editor): *Substance Abuse: A Guide for Health Professionals*, 2nd ed. Elk Grove Village, IL, American Academy of Pediatrics, 2002, p 69.

BOX 105–3. Stages of Adolescent Substance Abuse

STAGE	DESCRIPTION
1	Potential for abuse
	• Decreased impulse control
	• Need for immediate gratification
	• Available drugs, alcohol, inhalants
	• Need for peer acceptance
2	Experimentation: learning the euphoria
	• Use of inhalants, tobacco, marijuana, and alcohol with friends
	• Few, if any, consequences
	• Use may increase to weekends regularly
	• Little change in behavior
3	Regular use: seeking the euphoria
	• Use of other drugs, e.g., stimulants, LSD, sedatives
	• Behavioral changes and some consequences
	• Increased frequency of use; use alone
	• Buying or stealing drugs
4	Regular use: preoccupation with the "high"
	• Daily use of drugs
	• Loss of control
	• Multiple consequences and risk-taking
	• Estrangement from family and "straight" friends
5	Burnout: use of drugs to feel normal
	• Poly substance use/cross-addiction
	• Guilt, withdrawal, shame, remorse, depression
	• Physical and mental deterioration
	• Increased risk-taking, self-destructive, suicidal

From Comerci GD: Recognizing the five stages of substance abuse. *Contemp Pediatr* 1985;2:57–68.

functioning in key settings such as in school, at home, and with peers. The criteria for a disorder encompasses the issues of tolerance, frequency or volume of drug taken, period of time of use, inability to stop the use, and amount of time consumed by drug activities relative to normal activities. Specific diagnostic codes are assigned to substance abuse, substance intoxication, and substance withdrawal. The stages of the progression from substance use to dependence are depicted in Box 105–3. Referral to a specialist in or program for substance abuse treatment should occur by stage 3, unless the primary care physician has additional knowledge or training in addiction medicine.

Complications. Substance use in adolescence has psychologic as well as physical risks. Youth may engage in robbery, burglary, drug dealing, or prostitution for the purpose of acquiring the money necessary to buy drugs or alcohol. Regular use of any drug eventually diminishes judgment and is associated with unprotected sexual activity with its consequences of pregnancy and sexually transmitted diseases, including human immunodeficiency virus (HIV), as well as physical violence and trauma. Drug and alcohol use are closely associated with trauma in the adolescent population. Several studies of adolescent trauma victims have identified cannabinoids and cocaine in blood and urine samples in significant proportions, in addition to the more common identification of alcohol. Any use of injected substances involves the risk of hepatitis and HIV.

Prevention. The model of prevention relevant to the problem of adolescent drug or alcohol use is one that anticipates experimentation with some agent at some point in the normal development of the adolescent and that attempts to delay that event as long as possible, to make its use as limited in amount and setting as possible, and to prevent entirely any use while operating a motor vehicle or any other machinery. The Center for Substance Abuse Prevention has identified 6 program characteristics that have produced statistically significant reduction in 30-day substance use for adolescents: (1) Life Skills Focus—promoting attitudinal and behavioral life skills; (2) Emphasis on Building Connectedness—emphasizing connectedness to positive peers

TABLE 105–3. Urine Screening for Drugs Commonly Abused by Adolescents

Drug	Major Metabolite	Initial	First Confirmation	Second Confirmation	Approximate Retention Time
Alcohol (blood)	Acetaldehyde	GC	IA		7–10 hr
Alcohol (urine)	Acetaldehyde	GC	IA		10–13 hr
Amphetamines		TLC	IA	GC,GC/MS	48 hr
Barbiturates		IA	TLC	GC,GC/MS	Short-acting (24 hr); long-acting (2–3 wk)
Benzodiazepines		IA	TLC	GC,GC/MS	3 days
Cannabinoids	Carboxy- and hydroxymetabolites	IA	TLC	GC/MS	3–10 days (occasional user); 1–2 mo (chronic user)
Cocaine	Benzoyl ecgonine	IA	TLC	GC/MS	2–4 days
Methaqualone	Hydroxylated metabolites	TLC	IA	GC/MS	2 wk
Opiates					
Heroin	Morphine Glucuronide	IA	TLC	GC,GC/MS	2 days
Morphine	Morphine Glucuronide	IA	TLC	GC,GC/MS	2 days
Codeine	Morphine Glucuronide	IA	TLC	GC,GC/MS	2 days
Phencyclidine		TLC	IA	GC,GC/MS	8 days

Modified from Drugs of abuse—Urine screening *[Physician information sheet]. Los Angeles, Pacific Toxicology. From MacKenzie RG, Kipke MD: Substance use and abuse. In Friedman SB, Fisher M, Schonberg SK (eds):* Comprehensive Adolescent Health Care. *St. Louis, Quality Medical Publishing, 1992, p 783.*
GC = gas chromatography; IA = immunoassay; TLC = thin-layer chromatography; MS = mass spectrometry.

and adults; (3) Coherent Program Design and Implementation—linking activities to articulated and coherent prevention theory; (4) Introspective Orientation—encouraging youth to examine their own attitudes and behaviors and their contextual impact; (5) Intensive Contact—4 or more contact hours per week; and (6) After-school Setting—as compared to classroom delivery. Programs that delivered at least 5 of the 6 characteristics demonstrated strong prevention benefits through an 18-month follow-up period.

Treatment. Acute management is discussed in the following sections on specific agents. A variety of chronic treatment programs are available in inpatient and ambulatory settings. Brief interventions, including motivational interviewing, have been used in alcohol and tobacco users with some clinical effectiveness. These interventions are time-limited and patient-centered, with clear advice provided; they are useful in the primary care setting. Important features of successful long-term management of these adolescents include continuing medical evaluation after detoxification and the provision of developmentally appropriate psychosocial support systems.

Prognosis. For adolescent substance abusers who have been referred to a drug treatment program, outcomes are directly related to regular attendance in post-treatment groups. For males with learning problems, these outcomes were worse than were those of their peers without learning problems. Peer use patterns and parental use have a major influence on outcome for males. For females, factors such as self-esteem and anxiety are more important influences on outcomes. The chronicity of a substance abuse disorder makes relapse an issue that must always be kept in mind when managing patients after treatment, and appropriate assistance from a health professional qualified in substance abuse management should be obtained.

105.1   Alcohol

Alcohol use among adolescents has increased during the past decade and poses a threat to the normal functioning of the teenager as well as to the lives of those potentially jeopardized by drunken drivers. The initiation of alcohol use at an early age is associated with an increased risk for alcohol-related problems unless moderate use is deeply rooted in the adolescent's cultural tradition. The usual progression of alcohol use is from beer to wine to hard liquor, although regional differences may alter this pattern. Four ounces of hard liquor (86 proof) consumed on an empty stomach produces a plasma ethanol level of approximately 65 mg/dL in an adult male of average weight and 80 mg/dL in a premenstrual female of adult weight. The legal definition of intoxication in most statutes is a blood ethanol level of 80 or 100 mg/dL (0.08% or 0.10%).

Alcohol is noted as a contributing factor in 8,000 adolescent deaths and 45,000 injuries each year. Approximately 40% of the 10,000 annual nonautomotive accidental deaths, such as drowning and falls, are also associated with alcohol use. The estimates for involvement in suicide and homicide reach about 5,000/diagnosis/year. For a legal drug, alcohol contributes to more deaths in young individuals than all the illicit drugs combined. Therefore, pediatricians should not underestimate the need to recognize alcohol use and abuse in this age group.

Pharmacology and Pathophysiology. Alcohol (ethyl alcohol or ethanol) is rapidly absorbed in the stomach and is transported to the liver and metabolized by two pathways. The primary pathway involves removal of two hydrogen atoms to form acetaldehyde, a reaction catalyzed by alcohol dehydrogenase through reduction of a cofactor nicotinamide-adenine dinucleotide. The removed hydrogen atoms supply energy (7.1 kcal/g of alcohol) and contribute to the excess synthesis of triglycerides, a phenomenon that is responsible for producing a fatty liver, even in those who are well nourished. Engorgement of hepatocytes with fat causes necrosis, triggering an inflammatory process (alcoholic hepatitis), which is followed by fibrosis, the hallmark of cirrhosis. Early hepatic involvement may result in elevation in γ-glutamyl transpeptidase and serum glutamic-pyruvic transaminase. The second metabolic pathway, which is utilized at high serum alcohol levels, involves the microsomal system of the liver, in which the cofactor is reduced nicotinamide-adenine dinucleotide phosphate. The net effect of activation of this pathway is to decrease metabolism of drugs that share this system and to allow for their accumulation, enhanced effect, and possible toxicity (e.g., drinking alcohol and ingesting tranquilizers results in the potentiation of each).

Clinical Manifestations. Alcohol acts primarily as a central nervous system (CNS) depressant. It produces euphoria, grogginess, talkativeness, and impaired short-term memory, and it increases the pain threshold. Alcohol's ability to produce vasodilation and hypothermia is also centrally mediated. At very high serum levels, respiratory depression occurs. Its inhibitory effect on pituitary antidiuretic hormone release is responsible for its diuretic effect. The gastrointestinal complications of alcohol use can occur from a single large ingestion. The most common is acute erosive gastritis, which is manifested by epigastric pain, anorexia, vomiting, and guaiac-positive stools. Less commonly, vomiting and midabdominal pain may be caused by acute alcoholic pancreatitis; diagnosis is confirmed by the finding of elevated serum amylase and lipase activities.

Only a small number of adolescents become young alcoholics; however, problem drinking during adolescence requiring a therapeutic intervention is not uncommon. Adolescents who report having been drunk six or more times in the past year; having problems with school authorities, friends, or the police; having been criticized by dates for drinking habits; or having driven after drinking are considered problem drinkers.

Diagnosis. In addition to the general risk factors noted for substance use, a positive family history of alcohol abuse is significant. The genetic influences for the predisposition to alcoholism are supported by family, twin, and adoption studies. Children of alcoholic parents demonstrate a three- to fourfold increase in the risk for alcoholism. The *alcohol overdose syndrome* should be suspected in any teenager who appears disoriented, lethargic, or comatose (see Box 105–1). Although the distinctive aroma of alcohol may assist in diagnosis, confirmation by analysis of blood is recommended. There is a high correlation between results obtained by serum and breath analyses so that the latter method may be reliably used. At levels greater than 200 mg/dL, the adolescent is at risk of death, and levels greater than 500 mg/dL (median lethal dose) are usually associated with a fatal outcome. When the level of depression appears excessive for the reported blood level, head trauma or ingestion of other drugs should be considered as possible confounding factors.

Treatment. The usual mechanism of death from the alcohol overdose syndrome is respiratory depression, and artificial ventilatory support must be provided until the liver can eliminate sufficient amounts of alcohol from the body. In a patient without alcoholism, it generally takes 20 hr to reduce the blood level of alcohol from 400 mg/dL to zero. Dialysis should be considered when the blood level is higher than 400 mg/dL.

105.2   Marijuana

Marijuana and alcohol, the most popular substances of abuse among adolescents, share a number of psychopharmacologic qualities. Both decrease short-term memory and fine coordination, prolong reaction time, and produce "mental clouding." About 300 mg of cannabis is equivalent to 70 g of alcohol.

Pharmacology. Marijuana (THC, "pot," "weed," "hash," "grass") is synthesized from the resin of the *Cannabis sativa* plant, which flourishes in temperate and hot, dry climates. The tetrahydrocannabinol (THC) fraction of the resin is responsible for its hallucinogenic properties and has been synthesized (δ-9-THC). THC is absorbed rapidly by the nasal or oral routes, producing a peak of subjective effect at 10 min and 1 hr, respectively. Marijuana is generally consumed as a "reefer" or "joint," made by rolling the crushed plant material in paper. Although there is much variation in content, each cigarette contains 8–10% THC. Another popular form that is smoked, a "blunt," is a hollowed-out small cigar refilled with marijuana.

Clinical Manifestations. In addition to the "desired" effects of elation and euphoria, marijuana may cause impairment of short-term memory, poor performance of tasks requiring divided attention (e.g., those involved in driving), loss of critical judgment, and distortion of time perception. Visual hallucinations and perceived body distortions occur rarely, but there may be "flashbacks" or recall of frightening hallucinations experienced under marijuana's influence that usually occur during stress or with fever.

Temperature may be lowered. Tachycardia is apparent within 20 min of smoking marijuana and is followed $\frac{1}{2}$ hr later by transient systolic and diastolic hypertension, which disappears by 3 hr. Heavy users report pharyngitis, sinusitis, bronchitis, and asthma. In placebo-controlled studies of experienced users, smoking marijuana caused hypercapnic ventilation and a decrease in forced expired volume, maximal midexpiratory flow rate, airway conductance, and diffusing capacity. Both δ-9-THC and marijuana (smoking a single joint) cause a significant fall in intraocular pressure, lasting up to 5 hr in normal persons as well as in patients with glaucoma.

Kolodny demonstrated dose-related suppression of plasma testosterone levels and spermatogenesis as a result of smoking marijuana for a minimum of 4 days/wk for 6 mo, prompting concern about the potential deleterious effect of smoking marijuana before completion of pubertal growth and development. There is an antiemetic effect of oral THC or smoked marijuana, often followed by appetite stimulation, which is the basis of the drug's use in patients receiving cancer chemotherapy. Although the possibility of teratogenicity has been raised because of findings in animals, there is no evidence for such effects in humans. An "amotivational" syndrome has been described in chronic marijuana users who lose interest in age-appropriate behavior, yet proof of the causative relationship remains equivocal. The increased THC content of marijuana of almost 5 to 15 times in the 1990s as compared to the 1970s is related to the observation of a withdrawal syndrome, which had not occurred in the past, occurring 24 to 48 hr after discontinuing the drug. Heavy users experience malaise, irritability, agitation, insomnia, drug craving, shakiness, diaphoresis, night sweats, and gastrointestinal disturbance. The symptoms peak by the fourth day and resolve in 10 to 14 days. Certain drugs may interact with marijuana to potentiate sedation (i.e., alcohol, diazepam), potentiate stimulation (i.e., cocaine, amphetamines), or be antagonistic (i.e., propranolol, phenytoin). Long-term heavy cannabis users show memory and attention impairments that last beyond the period of intoxication and worsen with increasing years of regular use.

105.3 Tobacco

CIGARETTES

The average smoker starts at age 12 yr, and most are regular smokers by age 14 yr. Most alarming is the compelling evidence of the addictive nature of cigarette smoking with greater than 90% of adolescent smokers becoming adult smokers. Compared with all other substances and firearms, tobacco kills more individuals in the United States each year than all these other causes combined. The severity of atherosclerosis may be correlated with the duration of smoking, increasing its risk among those who begin smoking during adolescence.

Pharmacology. Human and animal studies confirm the addictive effect of nicotine, the primary active ingredient in cigarettes. It produces a syndrome of dependence as well as withdrawal. Nicotine is absorbed by multiple sites in the body, including lungs, skin, gastrointestinal tract, and buccal and nasal mucosa. The average nicotine content of one cigarette is 10 mg and the average nicotine intake per cigarette ranges from 1.0 mg to 3 mg. Nicotine, as delivered in cigarette smoke, has a half-life of 10–20 min, with an elimination half-life of 2–3 hr. Nicotine's effect on the brain takes less than 20 sec. The action of nicotine is mediated through nicotinic acetylcholine receptors. These receptors are located on noncholinergic presynaptic and postsynaptic sites in the brain. Cotinine is the major metabolite of nicotine via C-oxidation. It has a biologic half-life of 19–24 hr and can be detected in urine, serum, and saliva.

Clinical Manifestations. Adverse health effects of smoking may occur during adolescence. These adverse effects include an increased prevalence of chronic cough, phlegm production, and wheezing. Smoking during pregnancy is associated with an average decrease in fetal weight of 200 g; this, added to the already smaller size of infants born to teenagers, increases perinatal morbidity and mortality. Smoking in combination with the use of estrogen-containing oral contraceptives is associated with an increased risk of myocardial infarction. Tobacco smoke induces hepatic smooth endoplasmic reticulum and, as a result, may also influence metabolism of drugs and of endogenously produced hormones. Phenacetin, theophylline, and imipramine are examples of drugs affected in this manner. In addition, laboratory test results may be affected by smoking, for example, white blood cell count, hemoglobin, hematocrit, mean corpuscular volume, and platelet aggregation are increased and serum creatinine, albumin, globulin (in females), and uric acid (in males) are decreased (see Chapter 710).

Treatment. The approach to smoking cessation in adolescents includes the use of nicotine replacement therapy in addicted teens who are motivated to quit and are not using smokeless tobacco (SLT). The nicotine patch method, available over the counter or by prescription, is the most useful form in this age group; however, gum and spray can also be used. Medications such as bupropion, clonidine, and nortriptyline can be considered if nicotine replacement is ineffective or inappropriate. Additional options may be available through formal smoking cessation programs offered by community agencies. Clinical practice guidelines are available for practical office-based counseling strategies. Health supervision and supportive counseling are necessary components to smoking cessation management in adolescents.

SMOKELESS TOBACCO

Surveys in the late 1980s and 1990s indicating the increased use of smokeless tobacco (SLT) prompted the National Cancer Institute to lead the United States' federal government effort to prevent SLT use, especially in adolescents. Surveys now indicate that since the early to mid-1990s, lifetime prevalence of SLT use has declined in 8th, 10th, and 12th graders. Regular users of SLT risk physical dependence on nicotine. Chewing tobacco may result in lesions, primarily in the mandibular mucobuccal fold. With chronic use, these lesions may become malignant.

105.4 Volatile Substances

The practice of inhalation of a variety of euphoriants has enjoyed popularity among adolescents for centuries. The first well-described documentation of this phenomenon related to an "epidemic" of ether sniffing by Irish teenagers in the 19th century. Young adolescents are attracted to these substances because of their rapid action, easy availability, and low cost. The most popular inhalants among adolescent are glue, gasoline, and volatile nitrites. "Huffing," directly inhaling, or inhaling deeply from a paper bag containing a chemical-soaked cloth is the common method used by teens.

Clinical Manifestations. The major effects of inhalants are psychoactive. Toluene, the main ingredient in airplane glue and some rubber cements, causes relaxation and pleasant hallucinations for up to 2 hr. Tolerance and physical dependence may occur. Gasoline, a popular substance among rural adolescents and Native American youth, contains a complex mixture of organic solvents. Euphoria is followed by violent excitement, and coma may result from prolonged or rapid inhalation. Volatile nitrites, such as amyl nitrite, butyl nitrite, and related compounds marketed as room deodorizers, are used as euphoriants, enhancers of musical appreciation, and aphrodisiacs among older adolescents and young adults. They may result in headaches, syncope, and lightheadedness; profound hypotension and cutaneous flushing followed by vasoconstriction and tachycardia; transiently inverted T waves and depressed ST segments on electrocardiography; methemoglobinemia; increased bronchial irritation; and increased intraocular pressure.

Complications. Airplane glue has been responsible for a wide range of complications, relating to chemical toxicity, to the method of administration (e.g., in plastic bags, with resultant suffocation), and to the often dangerous setting in which the inhalation occurs (e.g., inner-city roof tops). Gasoline toxicity is acute as well as chronic. Death in the acute phase may result from cerebral or pulmonary edema or myocardial involvement. Chronic use may cause pulmonary hypertension, restrictive lung defects or reduced diffusion capacity, peripheral neuropathy, acute rhabdomyolysis, hematuria, tubular acidosis, and possibly cerebral and cerebellar atrophy. Other behavioral disturbances such as inattentiveness, lack of coordination, and general disorientation have been linked to chronic solvent abuse.

Diagnosis. The brief effect of the inhalants makes it unlikely to diagnose unless there is a complication or death from use. Complete blood counts, coagulation studies, and hepatic and renal function studies may identify the complications. In extreme intoxication, a user may manifest symptoms of restlessness, general muscle weakness, dysarthria, nystagmus, disruptive behavior, and occasionally hallucinations, placing inhalant use in the differential diagnosis for acute intoxication of an adolescent. Toluene is excreted rapidly in the urine as hippuric acid, with the residual detectable in the serum by gas chromatography.

Treatment. Treatment is generally supportive and directed toward control of arrhythmia and stabilization of respirations and circulation. Withdrawal symptoms do not usually occur.

105.5 Hallucinogens

Several naturally occurring and synthetic substances have been used by adolescents for their hallucinogenic properties. Lysergic acid diethylamide (LSD) and methylenedioxymethamphetamine (MDMA) or Ecstasy are the most commonly reported hallucinogens in high school. Among high school seniors in 2001, 12.8% reported ever using a hallucinogen, with 10.9% reporting the use of LSD, and 11.7% reporting the use of MDMA. These reports reflect a decreasing trend in use from 1997, with the exception of MDMA, which increased. National household survey rates in 2000 for all hallucinogens report lifetime use for 12–17 yr olds at 5.8%, with use in the prior year at 3.9%. Illicit drugs sold on the street are not labeled and are frequently misrepresented. In one survey, 11% of the confiscated drugs submitted as LSD to the Los Angeles County Street Drug Identification Program contained no identifiable LSD. The reported experiences with these drugs still represent a significant level of experimentation with dangerous chemicals.

LYSERGIC ACID DIETHYLAMIDE

LSD (acid, big "D," blotters) is one of the constituents found in rye fungus. Morning glory seeds contain lysergic acid derivatives, although the commercially packaged varieties have often been treated with toxic chemicals such as insecticides and fungicides. Although the specific mechanisms of action of LSD are still under study, it is proposed to alter neurotransmitters mediated by serotonin. LSD is a very potent hallucinogen with doses as low as 20 μg causing effects in some individuals. Its high potency allows effective doses to be applied to objects as small as postage stamps and paper blotters. It is rapidly absorbed from the gastrointestinal tract. The onset of action can be between 30 and 60 min, and it peaks between 2 and 4 hr. By 10–12 hr, an individual returns to the predrug state.

Clinical Manifestations. The effects of LSD can be divided into three categories: somatic (physical effects), perceptual (altered changes in vision and hearing), and psychic effects (changes in sensorium). The common somatic symptoms are dizziness, dilated pupils, nausea, flushing, elevated temperature, and tachycardia. The sensation of synesthesia or "seeing" smells and "hearing" colors has been reported with LSD use. Delusional ideation, body distortion, and suspiciousness to the point of toxic psychosis are the more serious of the psychic symptoms.

Treatment. An individual is considered to have a "bad trip" when the setting causes the user to become terrified or panicked. These episodes should be treated by removing the individual from the aggravating situation or setting and attempting to reestablish contact with reality through calm verbal interaction. Any physical complications such as hyperthermia, seizure, or hypertension should be treated supportively. "Flashbacks" or LSD-induced states after the drug has worn off and tolerance to the effects of the drug are additional complications of its use.

METHYLENEDIOXYMETHAMPHETAMINE

MDMA ("X," Ecstasy), a phenylisopropylamine hallucinogen, is a synthetic compound similar to mescaline, commonly referred to as a "designer drug." Like other hallucinogens, this drug is proposed to interact with serotoninergic neurons in the CNS. It is the preferential drug at "raves," all night dance parties, and is also known as one of the "club drugs."

Clinical Manifestations. Euphoria, a heightened sensual awareness, and increased psychic and emotional energy are acute effects. Compared with other hallucinogens, MDMA is less likely to produce emotional lability, depersonalization, and disturbances of thought. Adverse effects can be physical as well as psychic. Nausea, jaw clenching, teeth grinding, and blurred vision are somatic symptoms, whereas anxiety, panic attacks, and psychosis are the adverse psychic outcomes. A few deaths have been reported after ingestion of the drug. Hyperthermia in association with vigorous dancing at a "rave" has resulted in severe toxic reactions and death. There are *no specific treatment regimens* recommended for acute toxicity. There is evidence to suggest a link between prenatal MDMA exposure and cardiovascular and musculoskeletal birth defects.

PHENCYCLIDINE

PCP (sternyl, angel dust, "hog," "peace pill," "sheets") is an arylcyclohexalamine whose popularity is related, in part, to its ease of synthesis in home laboratories. One of the by-products of home synthesis causes cramps, diarrhea, and hematemesis. The drug is thought to potentiate adrenergic effects by inhibiting neuronal reuptake of catecholamines. PCP is available as a tablet, liquid, or powder, which may be used alone or sprinkled on cigarettes ("joints"). The powders and tablets generally contain 2–6 mg of PCP, whereas joints average 1 mg for every 150 mg of tobacco leaves, or approximately 30–50 mg per joint.

Clinical Manifestations. The clinical manifestations are dose-related. Euphoria, nystagmus, ataxia, and emotional lability occur within 2–3 min after smoking 1–5 mg and last for hours. Hallucination may involve bizarre distortions of body image that often precipitate panic reactions. With doses of 5–15 mg, a toxic psychosis may occur, with disorientation, hypersalivation, and abusive language lasting for more than 1 hr. Hypotension, generalized seizures, and cardiac arrhythmias commonly occur with plasma concentrations from 40–200 mg/dL. Death has been reported during psychotic delirium, from hypertension, hypotension, hypothermia, seizures, and trauma. The coma of PCP may be distinguished from that of the opiates by the absence of respiratory depression; the presence of muscle rigidity, hyperreflexia, and nystagmus; and lack of response to naloxone. PCP psychosis may be difficult to distinguish from schizophrenia. In the absence of history of use, analysis of urine must be depended on for diagnosis.

Treatment. Management of the PCP-intoxicated patient includes placement in a darkened, quiet room on a floor pad, safe from injury. For recent oral ingestion, gastric absorption is poor and induction of emesis or gastric lavage is useful. Diazepam, in a dose of 5–10 mg orally or 2–5 mg intravenously, may be helpful if the patient is agitated and not comatose. Rapid excretion of the drug is promoted by acidification of the urine. Supportive therapy of the comatose patient is indicated with particular attention to hydration, which may be compromised by PCP-induced diuresis.

105.6 Cocaine

Crack cocaine, the highly addictive smokable form of cocaine, has increased availability and severity of cocaine use in the face of a decrease in use in the overall population. Lifetime or "ever use" in high school seniors dropped from a level of 17.3% in 1985 to 9.4% in 1990. Use in all grades peaked in 1999, and has declined or leveled off by 2001. Use of crack cocaine represents almost half the total cocaine use.

Cocaine, an alkaloid extracted from the leaves of the South American *Erythroxylon coca*, is supplied as the hydrochloride salt in crystalline form. It is rapidly absorbed from the nasal mucosa, detoxified by the liver, and excreted in the urine as benzoyl ecgonine. Its half-life is slightly more than 1 hr. The perceived effect of "snorting" cocaine may be influenced by some of the many diluents now being added to or actually substituted for the drug (heroin, amphetamines, PCP, or fillers such as mannitol or quinine). Smoking the cocaine alkaloid ("freebasing") in pipes or cigarettes, mixed with tobacco, marijuana, parsley, or as a paste, has become a popular method of use. Accidental burns are potential complications of this practice. With crack cocaine, the smoker feels "high" in less than 10 sec. The technique for extracting crack cocaine does not involve ether and is a safer and simpler technique compared with making freebase cocaine. The risk of addiction with this method is higher and more rapidly progressive than from snorting cocaine. Tolerance develops and the user must increase the dose or change the route of administration, or both, to achieve the same effect.

Clinical Manifestations. Cocaine produces euphoria, increased motor activity, decreased fatigability, and occasionally paranoid ideation. Its sympathomimetic properties are responsible for

pupillary dilatation, tachycardia, hypertension, and hyperthermia. Binge patterns of use are common. Neurologic effects such as dizziness, paresthesias, and seizures can occur. Use in group settings has been associated with sexual promiscuity and increased risks of sexually transmitted infections. Lethal effects are possible, especially when cocaine is used in combination with other drugs, such as heroin, in an injectable form known as a "speedball." Although addiction and tolerance develop in the chronic user, withdrawal symptoms on its discontinuation have not been reported, suggesting that physical dependency does not occur. Pregnant adolescents who use cocaine place their fetus at risk for premature delivery, complications of low birthweight, and possibly congenital malformations and developmental disorders.

Treatment. Intensive supportive therapy is directed at the clinical manifestations of acute intoxication.

105.7 Amphetamines

Stimulants, particularly amphetamines, are among the most frequently reported illicit drugs other than marijuana used by high school seniors. Methamphetamine, commonly known as "ice," accounted for more than 25% of stimulant use. Methamphetamine is particularly popular among adolescents and young adults because of its potency and ease of absorption. It can be used by snorting, smoking, ingesting by mouth, or absorption across mucous membranes, such as vaginal mucosa. Its use is especially common in the western and southwestern regions of the United States. Amphetamines have multiple CNS effects, among them the release of neurotramsmitters and an indirect catecholamine agonist effect. In high doses, they may also affect serotonergic receptors.

Clinical Manifestations. The effects of amphetamines can be dose-related. High doses produce slowing of cardiac conduction in the face of ventricular irritability. Hypertensive and hyperpyrexic episodes can occur as can seizures. Binge effects result in the development of psychotic ideation with the potential for sudden violence. Cerebrovascular damage and psychosis can result from chronic use. There is a withdrawal syndrome associated with amphetamine use, with early, intermediate, and late phases. The early phase is characterized as a "crash" phase with depression, agitation, anergia, and desire for more of the drug. Loss of physical and mental energy, limited interest in the environment, and anhedonia mark the intermediate phase. In the final phase, drug craving returns, often triggered by particular situations or objects.

Treatment. Agitation and delusional behaviors can be treated with haloperidol or droperidol. Phenothiazines are contraindicated and may cause a rapid drop in blood pressure or seizure activity. Other supportive treatment consists of a cooling blanket for hyperthermia and treatment of the hypertension and arrhythmias, which may respond to sedation with lorazepam (Ativan) or diazepam (Valium).

105.8 Opiates

Opiate abuse by adolescents decreased considerably during the 1980s, but the magnitude and variety of its medical sequelae warrant continued attention. Although it has been one of the least frequently reported drugs of use since 1991, heroin produces euphoria and analgesia. Heroin is hydrolyzed to morphine, which undergoes hepatic conjugation with glucuronic acid before excretion, usually within 24 hr of administration. It can be detected in urine by thin-layer chromatography up to 48 hr after administration. The route of administration influences the timing of the onset of action. When the drug is inhaled ("snorting"), it requires almost 30 min before the desired effect is achieved. By the subcutaneous route ("skin-popping"), the effect is achieved within minutes; when injected intravenously ("mainlining"), it has an immediate effect. Tolerance develops to the euphoric effect and only rarely to the inhibitory effect on smooth muscle, which causes both constipation and miosis.

Clinical Manifestations. The clinical manifestations are determined by the pharmacologic effects of heroin or its adulterants, combined with the conditions and the route of administration. The cerebral effects include euphoria, diminution in pain, and pinpoint pupils. An effect on the hypothalamus is suggested by the lowering of body temperature. Vasodilation is a major cardiovascular manifestation related to the method of administration of the drug. Respiratory depression is mediated centrally and is characterized by alveolar underventilation. Pulmonary edema is common in death from the overdose syndrome, but it may also be seen as an incidental roentgenologic finding in an otherwise asymptomatic adolescent heroin abuser. The most common dermatologic lesions are the "tracks," the hypertrophic linear scars that follow the course of large veins. Smaller, discrete peripheral scars, resembling healed insect bites, may be easily overlooked. The adolescent who injects heroin subcutaneously may have fat necrosis, lipodystrophy, and atrophy over portions of the extremities. Attempts at concealment of these stigmata may include amateur tattoos in unusual sites. Abscesses secondary to unsterile techniques of drug administration are commonly found. There is a loss of libido; the mechanism is unknown. The female heroin user may resort to prostitution to support the habit, thus increasing the risk of sexually transmitted disease (including HIV), pregnancy, and other hazards. Constipation results from decreased smooth muscle propulsive contractions and increased anal sphincter tone. Hepatic enzyme activities are frequently elevated in heroin users, the majority of whom have serologic evidence suggesting viral infection with hepatitis B. The absence of sterile technique in injection may lead to cerebral microabscesses or endocarditis, usually caused by *Staphylococcus aureus*. Infection with HIV is another complication of needle use. Abnormal serologic reactions are also common, including false-positive Venereal Disease Research Laboratory and latex fixation tests.

WITHDRAWAL. After a period of 8 hr or more without heroin, the addicted individual undergoes, during a period of 24–36 hr, a series of physiologic disturbances referred to collectively as "withdrawal" or the *abstinence syndrome*. The earliest sign is yawning, followed by lacrimation, mydriasis, insomnia, "goose flesh," cramping of the voluntary musculature, hyperactive bowel sounds and diarrhea, tachycardia, and systolic hypertension. The occurrence of grand mal seizures is rare in adolescent addicts. The administration of methadone is the most common method of detoxification. This synthetic opiate is effective by the oral route and is pharmacologically similar to heroin, with the exception of its lack of euphoric effect. A short course of diazepam is also an effective and safe treatment for heroin detoxification.

OVERDOSE SYNDROME. The overdose syndrome is an acute reaction after the administration of an opiate. It is the leading cause of death among drug users. The clinical signs include stupor or coma, seizures, miotic pupils (unless severe anoxia has occurred), respiratory depression, cyanosis, and pulmonary edema. The differential diagnosis includes CNS trauma, diabetic coma, hepatic (and other) encephalopathy, Reye syndrome, as well as overdose of alcohol, barbiturates, PCP, or methadone. Diagnosis of opiate toxicity is facilitated by intravenous administration of the opiate antagonist naloxone, 0.01 mg/kg (2 mg is a common initial dose for an adolescent), which causes dilation of pupils constricted by the opiate. Diagnosis is confirmed by the finding of morphine in the serum.

Treatment. This consists of maintaining adequate oxygenation and continued administration of naloxone every 5 min, when necessary, to improve and maintain adequate ventilation. Naloxone may have to be continued for 24 hr if methadone, rather than shorter-acting heroin, has been taken.

105.9 Anabolic Steroids

The quest for enhanced athletic performance has led to the abuse of anabolic steroids by competitive athletes of both sexes. As with other substances, prevalence data vary across surveys. Reports of anabolic steroids having ever been used range from 0.7–3.7%, usually with male use predominating. However, two of three surveys show significant increases in females who had ever used anabolic steroids in the 1990s. Although the percentages are low, population estimates based on 1995 data suggest that about 375,000 males and 175,000 females of high school age have used anabolic steroids for performance enhancement. Use of anabolic steroids has been associated with a constellation of problem behaviors such as engaging in physical fights with injuries requiring medical attention, weapon carrying, binge drinking, and using other substances of abuse. The evidence for increased muscle mass and strength are controversial but are supported by objective data. The effects appear to be related to the myotrophic action at androgen receptors as well as competitive antagonism at catabolism-mediating corticosteroid receptors. Erythropoietic and psychologic effects may also contribute to their enhancement effects. The most common forms of anabolic steroids used are the oral 17-α-methyl derivatives of testosterone and the injectable esters of testosterone and 19-nortestosterone.

Clinical Manifestations. Some of the adverse side effects of these drugs are reversible; others are not. The most immediate effects for all users is increasing acneform lesions. Other dermatologic manifestations include linear keloids, stria, oily hair, and hirsutism. These findings may be the first recognizable effects. Males can experience gynecomastia, breast pain, testicular atrophy, and azoospermia. Women experience more irreversible side effects such as breast atrophy, clitoral enlargement, and menstrual abnormalities. Serious psychologic effects also have been reported from the use of high doses of these agents (often 100 times the therapeutic doses), including uncontrollable rage, depression, mania, mood fluctuations, and alterations in libido. Users choosing the injectable route increase the risk of HIV if injection equipment is shared with others.

Abnormalities of the liver can be acute, such as hepatitis and hepatomegaly, or more long-term, such as the increased risk of hepatocellular carcinoma, particularly with the 17-α-alkylated forms. Fluid retention is a common side effect that prompts users to take diuretics. In addition to these effects, which occur in individuals of all ages, the early adolescent is at risk for growth retardation because of the possibility of accelerating epiphyseal closure.

Diagnosis and Treatment. The clinical signs noted, coupled with a complete history, provide a diagnosis in most instances. Although urine testing is available and performed at the Olympic and collegiate competitive levels, few laboratories perform these tests and they are very expensive. Therefore, the secondary school approach primarily has been limited to education and prevention. Treatment is supportive.

Center for Substance Abuse Prevention: *The National Cross-site Evaluation of High-Risk Youth Programs, Substance Abuse and Mental Health Services Administration* (www.samhsa.gov/centers), accessed 2/24/02.

Duncan D, Petrosa R: Social and community factors associated with drug use and abuse among adolescents. In Gullotta T, Adams GR (editors): *Substance Misuse in Adolescence.* Thousand Oaks, CA, Sage, 1994.

Hogan MJ: Diagnosis and treatment of teen drug abuse. *Med Clin North Am* 2000;84(4):927–66.

Johnston LD, O'Malley PM, Bachman JG: *High School and Youth Trends: 2001 Monitoring the Future Study* (MTF). NIDA, U.S. Department of Health and Human Services (www.drugabuse.gov/Infofax/HSYouthtrends.html), accessed 2/24/02.

Lieberman DZ: Children of alcoholics: An update. *Curr Opin Pediatr* 2000;12:336.

Lowinson JH, Ruiz P, Millman RB, et al: *Substance Abuse: A Comprehensive Textbook*, 3rd ed. Baltimore, Williams & Wilkins, 1997.

McElhatton PR, Bateman DN, Evans C, et al: Congenital abnormalities after prenatal ecstasy exposure. *Lancet* 1999;354:1441.

Schydlower M (editor): *Substance Abuse: A Guide for Health Professionals*, 2nd ed. Elk Grove Village, IL, American Academy of Pediatrics, 2002.

Solowij N, Stephens RS, Roffman RA, et al: Cognitive functioning of long-term heavy cannabis users seeking treatment. *JAMA* 2002;287:1123–31.

Substance Abuse and Mental Health Services Administration: *Summary of Findings from the 2000 National Household Survey on Drug Abuse*. Office of Applied Studies, NHSDA Series H-13, DHHS Publication No. (SMA) 01-3549. Rockville, MD, 2001. (www.samhsa.gov/oas/NHSDA)

Chapter 106

The Breast *Renée R. Jenkins*

Breast development is one of the first obvious signs of puberty, but it is often the focus of attention and a cause of anxiety in an adolescent, whether the issue is normal progression, some variation in progression, or a definable disorder. Normal breast development during puberty is described using a Sex Maturity Rating scale of 1–5, as the breast becomes more mature (see Chapter 14).

Normal Variants. Minor breast asymmetry is common in adult females and sexually mature adolescent females. Other conditions that rarely occur but should be ruled out include *Poland syndrome* and unilateral breast aplasia, hypoplasia, or hypertrophy. Poland syndrome is marked by a hypoplastic breast nipple and areola with hypoplastic ipsilateral chest wall structures. Unilateral or bilateral juvenile (virginal) hypertrophy occurs with specific histopathologic changes but without any known cause. The enlargement may be mild and cause back pain and postural problems or severe enough to be associated with tissue and skin necrosis. Embarrassment and possible psychologic problems should be addressed in the management of this condition. Reconstructive surgical repair is indicated in severe breast asymmetry but is recommended after sex maturity rating 5 has been reached. Accessory breast tissue (polymastia) can also occur in males and females. This lesion can consist of a supernumerary nipple (polythelia) or breast tissue, or both, and usually occurs along both milk lines of the thorax and the abdomen. Accessory breast tissue beneath the umbilicus, though rare, can be associated with cardiovascular or genitourinary abnormalities.

Female Disorders (also see Chapter 543)

MASSES. The most common adolescent breast disorder is a mass, the majority of which are benign cysts or fibroadenomas. *Cysts* vary in size over the course of a menstrual cycle, so a patient should be re-examined 2 wk after the initial examination. Persistence of the mass or its enlargement over three menstrual cycles is an indication for surgical consultation. Aspiration is usually attempted under local anesthesia, often resulting in curative drainage if it proves to be a cyst. If no fluid is obtained, an excisional biopsy is indicated. When multiple small masses are palpable, associated with pain, a biopsy is rarely indicated. Most fibroadenomas are benign, mobile, well-defined rubbery feeling masses. Multiple fibroadenomas occur in 10–20% of patients. The *fibroadenoma* tends not to vary in size during the menstrual cycle, often distinguishing it from a cyst. *Cystosarcoma phylloides* is a rare variant of a fibroadenoma distinguished by having a more cellular stroma. It is typically larger than a fibroadenoma and can, rarely, be malignant.

In a review of 15 retrospective surgical studies of women younger than age 22 years, the most common lesion was the fibroadenoma (68.3%), followed by fibrocystic changes (18.5%). Malignancies occurred in 0.9% of cases with 5 primary breast cancer patients, and the others having Hodgkin lymphoma, lymphosarcoma, angiosarcomas, and other metastatic tumors. *Carcinoma* of the breast in the adolescent is rare. The efficacy and possible sequelae of mammography in managing adolescent breast masses are unknown. The dense breast tissue of the adolescent obstructs the visualization of a palpable mass; thus mammography is not advised for this age group. Ultrasonography is useful is distinguishing cystic from solid masses.

MASTALGIA. Physiologic swelling and tenderness occur on a cyclic basis, most commonly during the premenstrual phase, and are secondary to hormonal stimulation and resulting proliferative changes. Nodularity, poorly localized tenderness, and a soreness radiating to the axilla and arm are usual accompanying findings. The preferable term for these changes is benign breast changes rather than the classic "fibrocystic disease." Non-cyclic mastalgia is less common in younger women compared with women in their 40s. Treatments recommended for this condition include firm support, heat, analgesics, hormonal therapy, diuretics, and evening primrose oil. Adult doses of evening primrose oil, two 500-mg capsules three times a day, has been associated with an overall response rate of 44%. A 3 mo trial is recommended with a follow-up treatment of 2 mo if the response is positive.

NIPPLE DISCHARGE. Nipple discharge in adolescents is usually due to local stimulation; use of medications, including oral contraceptives; and pregnancy. Rarely, it results from a pituitary or breast neoplasm or infection. Examination of the discharge assists in diagnosis: Benign conditions are associated with a milky, sticky, thick discharge; infection is associated with a purulent discharge; and intraductal papilloma and cancer are associated with a serous, serosanguineous, or bloody discharge. Elevation of the serum prolactin level may occur in the *amenorrhea-galactorrhea syndromes*, associated with the use of certain

---

BOX 106–1. Drugs Associated with Gynecomastia

HORMONES
Estrogens
Aromatizable androgens
Anabolic steroids
Gonadotropins

PSYCHOACTIVE DRUGS
Tricyclic antidepressants
Phenothiazines
Benzodiazepines

CARDIOVASCULAR DRUGS
Calcium channel blockers
Angiotensin-converting enzyme Inhibitors
Digoxin

DIURETICS
Spironolactone
Thiazides

GASTRIC ACID INHIBITORS
Cimetidine
Omeprazole

ANTIBIOTICS
Isoniazid
Ketoconazole
Metronidazole

CYTOTOXIC DRUGS
Cyclophosphamide
Methotrexate
Vincristine

OTHER
Auranofin
Ergotamine
Etretinate
Metoclopramide
Minoxidil
Penicillamine
Sulindac
Theophylline

DRUGS OF ABUSE
Alcohol
Marijuana
Heroin
Methadone
Amphetamines

From Davis AJ, Kulig JW: Adolescent breast disorders. Adolescent Health Update 1996; 9:7.

antihypertensive medications, oral contraceptives, or tranquilizers, or secondary to a pituitary adenoma. The latter is associated with central nervous system signs and is evaluated with a computed tomography scan or magnetic resonance imaging of the head. The possibility of a breast neoplasm is an indication for cytologic examination of the discharge and surgical consultation. Infection in the non–breast-feeding adolescent is rare and may be secondary to a human bite or the initial symptom of diabetes mellitus. Culture of the discharge, followed by appropriate antibiotic therapy (usually directed against *Staphylococcus aureus*) is indicated; surgical drainage is rarely necessary.

MALE DISORDERS. Gynecomastia occurs in approximately one third of normal males during early to midpuberty and often causes concern that may not be openly voiced. The response should be factual information and reassurance of its usually transient nature. Rarely is it of such magnitude or persistence as to warrant surgery. Nonpubertal gynecomastia with hypogonadism is associated with Klinefelter syndrome and places a patient at a higher risk for breast cancer (see Chapter 577). Other conditions associated with nonpubertal gynecomastia are secondary to endocrine disorders, neoplasms, chronic disease, trauma, and medications as well as drugs of abuse (Box 106–1).

Davis AJ, Kulig JW: Adolescent breast disorders. *Adolescent Health Update* 1996;9:1–8.

Neinstein LS: Breast disease in adolescents and young women. *Pediatr Clin North Am* 1999;46(3):607

Chapter 107
Menstrual Problems

Renée R. Jenkins

(See also Chapter 542.)

Some variety of menstrual dysfunction occurs in about 50% of adolescent females. Most of the problems are minor; however, severe dysmenorrhea or prolonged menstrual bleeding can be debilitating to a teenager. Adolescents with mild dysfunction that does not require medical intervention should have their condition explained to them and should be reassured about their reproductive normalcy.

NORMAL MENSTRUATION

The age of normal menarche varies according to the characteristics of the population. In a large office-based study in the United States, 35% of white girls and 62% of African-American girls had initiated menses between ages 12 and 13 yr. The age of menarche in Tanner's English series ranges from ages 9–16 yr, with a mean age of 13.46 yr. The age of menarche is closely related to other parameters of pubertal maturation and correlated closely with bone age. The onset and continuation of normal menstrual cycling depends on the functional and anatomic integrity of (1) the hypothalamus together with higher centers, including possibly the pineal gland; (2) the anterior pituitary; (3) the ovary; and (4) the uterus. The percentage of body fat is also a factor in the onset of menarche, with a minimal fatness of 17% of body weight being necessary for the onset of menstrual cycles and a minimum of 22% fatness necessary to maintain regular ovulatory cycles. Menarche usually occurs about 2.3 yr after the initiation of puberty, with a range of 1–3 yr, and becomes regular after 2–2.5 yr. The length of the menstrual cycle from the first day of menses of one cycle to the first day of the next cycle can range from 21–45 days, although the average is about 28 days. Anovulatory cycles are generally longer. The average blood flow usually results in about 40 mL of blood loss with a range of 25–70 mL. The later the age of menarche, the longer until the establishment of ovulatory cycles.

Menstrual cycle irregularities are described according to variation in frequency of menses, amount, and both frequency and amount (Box 107–1). A complete history for evaluating a patient with menstrual dysfunction should include questions specifically related to puberty and menstrual patterns, a family history of gynecologic problems, and a past medical history noting hospitalizations, chronic illness, medication or substance use, and infections. The related association of weight change, nutrition, exercise, and sports participation can be critically important in considering a differential diagnosis. Regardless of the age of the adolescent, an appropriate history of any type of sexual activity should be elicited, and the pediatrician should be cognizant of the need to rule out sexual abuse as an issue in young adolescents when other findings suggest sexual activity.

In addition to the basic growth parameters of weight, height, blood pressure, heart rate, and body mass index, signs of virilization should be assessed, such as hirsutism and clitoromegaly. A careful external and internal pelvic examination is a key to ruling out anatomic defects and accumulating additional specimens for the evaluation. In the young adolescent, this examination should be performed by someone with expertise in this age group and with the proper-sized equipment.

MENSTRUAL IRREGULARITIES

Etiology. The distinction among menstrual irregularities is somewhat artificial given that the causes of the entities are often similar, e.g., many of the problems of pubertal delay, such as Turner mosaic syndrome, may present as primary amenorrhea or secondary amenorrhea. Thyroid disorders also can be the source of secondary amenorrhea or abnormal vaginal bleeding. The common cause of all of these disorders is a disturbance of the hypothalamic-pituitary-ovarian axis. The amenorrheic disorders are categorized on the basis of follicle-stimulating hormone (FSH) levels into hypergonadotropic hypogonadism (ovarian failure) and hypogonadotropic hypogonadism (hypothalamic or pituitary dysfunction). FSH-luteinizing hormone (LH) patterns in perimenarcheal girls with anovulatory bleeding also suggests the prevalence of a maturational defect for normal negative feedback cyclicity. The rising levels of estrogen do not

---

BOX 107–1. Terms for Menstrual Cycle Irregularities

Variations in frequency
  Polymenorrhea: frequent regular or irregular bleeding at <21-day intervals
  Oligomenorrhea: infrequent irregular bleeding at >45-day intervals
  Primary amenorrhea: no menstrual flow by age 16 yr
  Secondary amenorrhea: absence of vaginal bleeding for > 3 mo
  Irregular menses: bleeding at varying intervals, ≥21-day intervals but <45-day intervals
Variations in amount
  Hypomenorrhea: decreased menstrual flow at regular intervals
  Hypermenorrhea: profuse menstrual flow of normal duration at regular intervals
Variations in amount and duration
  Metrorrhagia: intermenstrual irregular bleeding between regular periods
  Menorrhagia: excessive amount and increased duration of uterine bleeding occurring regularly
  Menometrorrhagia: frequent irregular, excessive, and prolonged episodes of uterine bleeding
  Dysfunctional uterine bleeding: prolonged excessive menstrual bleeding associated with irregular periods: usually due to immaturity of reproductive axis in adolescence if within first 2 yr of menarche

From Blythe MI: Common menstrual problems of adolescence. *Adolesc Med* 1997; 8:87.

cause a fall in FSH and the subsequent suppression of estrogen secretion, and consequently the endometrium becomes thickened, promoting irregular and heavier blood flow with shedding.

Psychogenic factors have been implicated in amenorrhea. It is often difficult to separate psychologic from nutritional factors because weight loss is a common confounding variable in many of these situations, for example, depression, anorexia nervosa, or stress.

Clinical Manifestations. Amenorrhea, or absence of menses, may be primary or secondary. The diagnosis of primary amenorrhea assumes that the patient has passed the age at which menarche normally occurs, from 10–16 yr. Accordingly, the determination of primary amenorrhea should first be based on an assessment of the patient's stage of pubertal development; 10% of girls have menarche at Sex Maturity Rating (SMR) 2, 20% reach menarche at SMR 3, 60% reach it at SMR 4, and 10% reach menarche at SMR 5. If the patient has not entered puberty by the expected time or if pubertal development is completed without the onset of menses, she should be thoroughly evaluated, even if her chronological age is within the normal range. Similarly, the close concordance of the age of menarche between daughters and mothers and among siblings should suggest this diagnosis when the patient is more than 1 yr older than were the mother or sisters when their menarche occurred. The distinguishing characteristic of the clinical presentation of amenorrhea is the presence or absence of virilization. Clinical features such as clitoromegaly, hirsutism, or excessive acne are associated with adrenal or ovarian disease. Other clinical presentations such as slender or obese body habitus or short stature also are characteristic of syndromes associated with amenorrhea.

The first consideration in the adolescent who presents with secondary amenorrhea is pregnancy. This possibility also exists, albeit rarely, as a cause of primary amenorrhea, if fertilization of the first released ovum occurred before menses. A history of sexual intercourse, nausea, and breast tenderness and physical findings of increased pigmentation of nipples and linea alba, cyanosis and softening of the cervix, and an enlarged uterus form the classic picture.

In the clinical presentation of abnormal vaginal bleeding, mild to moderate bleeding may present without any specific clinical findings; however, severe bleeding is accompanied by the abnormal vital signs associated with hypovolemia. Very severe bleeding may progress to syncope and death, making this one of the few gynecologic emergencies of adolescence.

107.1 Amenorrhea

Differential Diagnosis. In *primary amenorrhea,* chromosomal or congenital abnormalities, such as gonadal dysgenesis, the triple X syndrome, isochromosomal abnormalities, testicular feminization syndrome, and, rarely, true hermaphroditism, should be considered in addition to the conditions that cause secondary amenorrhea. Elevated levels of FSH and LH suggest primary gonadal failure, and chromosome analysis elucidates its cause. When primary amenorrhea occurs with advanced pubertal development, a structural anomaly of the müllerian duct system should be suspected. *Imperforate hymen* is most common and is associated with recurrent (monthly) abdominal pain and, after some time has passed, a midline lower abdominal mass, the blood-filled vagina, or *hematocolpos.* Diagnosis is made by inspection of the introitus, revealing a bulging hymen with bluish discoloration. If the obstruction is at the level of the cervix, the blood-filled uterus *(hematometrium)* is apparent on bimanual examination or ultrasonography. Agenesis of the cervix or uterus is rare but occurs in association with sacral agenesis.

Primary or *secondary* amenorrhea may also be caused by chronic illness, particularly that associated with malnutrition or

tissue hypoxia, such as diabetes mellitus, inflammatory bowel disease, cystic fibrosis, or cyanotic congenital heart disease. In most cases, the illness has been diagnosed previously but, occasionally, the amenorrhea is its first manifestation. Polycystic ovarian syndrome is one of the most common endocrine disorders affecting premenopausal women and presents with menstrual abnormalities from amenorrhea to dysfunctional uterine bleeding. A central nervous system (CNS) tumor, most commonly a craniopharyngioma, may present with amenorrhea. Prolactinomas, although rare, are the most common pituitary tumor in adolescence. Abnormalities of the thyroid gland, typically hyperthyroidism, may first be suspected by delayed sexual maturation or amenorrhea, even in the absence of other signs and symptoms. Hypothyroidism may cause precocious puberty but may also be associated with delayed puberty or abnormal uterine bleeding. Anorexia nervosa, which may present with either primary or secondary amenorrhea, is occasionally confused with hyperthyroidism because of weight loss, hyperactivity, and personality changes seen in both entities. Ingestion of drugs, both legal and illegal, may cause amenorrhea and, in the case of phenothiazines, even a false-positive urine pregnancy test. Some drugs, including phenothiazines and certain antihypertensive agents, may cause galactorrhea, further mimicking pregnancy. A thorough drug history is, therefore, necessary.

Laboratory Findings. The approach to the clinical evaluation of delayed menarche (Fig. 107–1) suggests a stepwise progression initiated by the history and physical examination. The pregnancy test, preferably a qualitative serum β-subunit human chorionic gonadotropin (hCG), is the key laboratory test to perform in the evaluation of secondary amenorrhea (Fig. 107–2) regardless of the history or sexual activity given by the patient or signs of virilization. The next step for laboratory determinations follows the scheme and is performed according to the individual's response to an initial progesterone challenge or after the findings of the vaginal smear for estrogen. The direct correlation of bone age to menstrual age enhances the value of a radiograph before proceeding with an extensive work-up. The measurement of FSH is critical in determining whether chromosomal abnormalities (with FSH elevation > 25 mIU/mL) or other endocrinopathies or CNS tumors (with normal or low FSH < 5 mIU/mL) are present.

Prolonged amenorrhea (>6 mo) and persistent oligomenorrhea without an explanation should prompt the measurement of thyroid-stimulating hormone, FSH, LH, and prolactin levels, even in the face of a normal progesterone challenge. Elevated LH and normal FSH levels require the measurement of androgen excess even in the absence of obvious virilization. An LH:FSH ratio greater than 3 and an elevated free testosterone level is common in adolescents with **polycystic ovary syndrome** (PCOS). Hyperinsulinemia is a characteristic feature of PCOS, and there is an increased risk of diabetes mellitus. The criterion for the diagnosis of PCOS is menstrual irregularity in the face of androgen excess with either hirsutism, acne, or increased serum androgens (also see Chapter 544). An elevated prolactin level or other clinical features suggesting a CNS tumor should be followed up with cranial computed tomography scan or, preferably, magnetic resonance imaging.

Endometrial status can be assessed as part of the evaluation when other endocrinologic parameters are normal by a progesterone challenge in which 5 or 10 mg of oral medroxyprogesterone acetate is given for 5 to 10 days. Withdrawal bleeding should occur 2–7 days thereafter when normal endometrium is present. If bleeding does not occur, one must consider insufficient estrogenic priming of the endometrium, an abnormal uterus, or an outflow tract obstruction.

Treatment. Determination of the cause of amenorrhea may permit the initiation of corrective intervention. When the disorder is not amenable to remediation, consideration should be given to establishing regular pseudomenses to allow the adolescent to

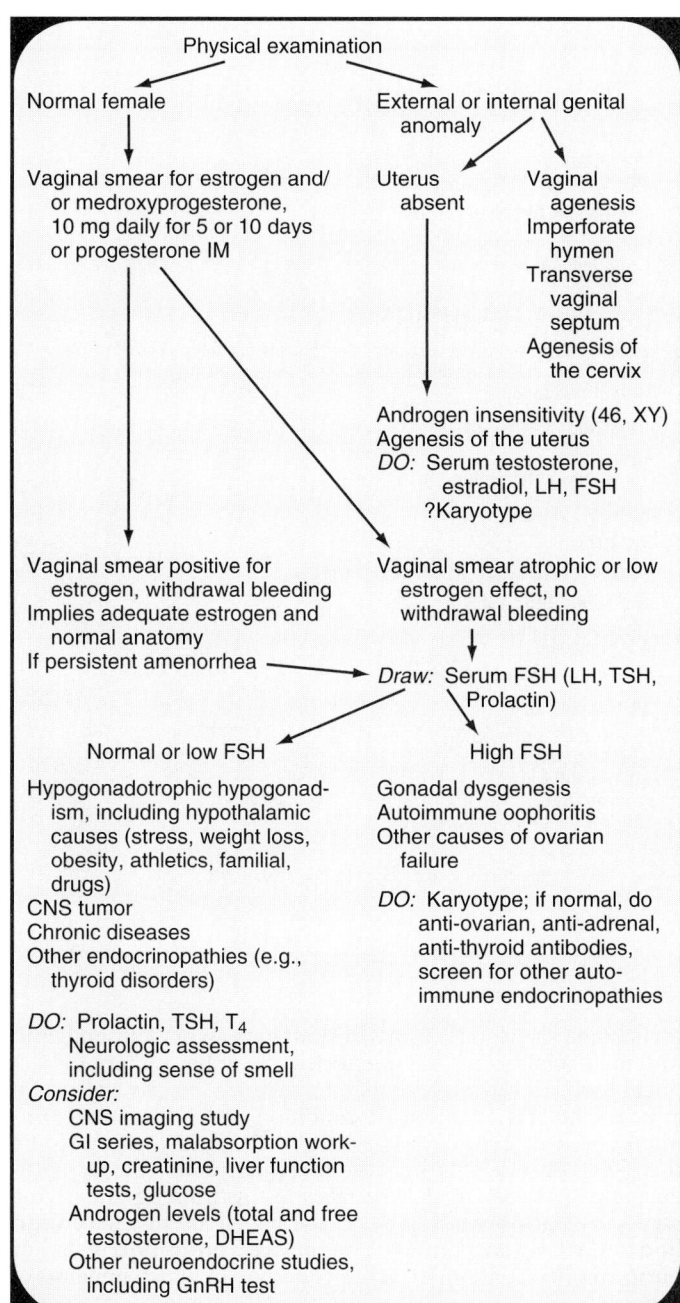

FIGURE 107–1. Delayed menarche. (From Emans SJH, Laufer MR, Goldstein DP [editors]: *Pediatric and Adolescent Gynecology*, 4th ed. Philadelphia, Lippincott-Raven, 1998.)

feel like her peers. If the result of a vaginal smear is positive for estrogen effect, regular cycling can be accomplished using medroxyprogesterone in a dose of 10 mg orally for 10–12 days at least every other month. Combination oral contraceptives can also be used for this purpose in patients with PCOS. In a patient with gonadal dysgenesis, conjugated estrogens must be given first (Premarin in an oral dose of 0.3 mg and increased to 1.25 mg) for feminization to progress. This is followed by medroxyprogesterone, 10 mg orally on days 10–21 of the cycle.

107.2 Abnormal Uterine Bleeding

Differential Diagnosis. Most abnormal vaginal bleeding in adolescents results from anovulatory cycles, normally occurring in the 1st yr of menarche. This is called *dysfunctional uterine bleeding;*

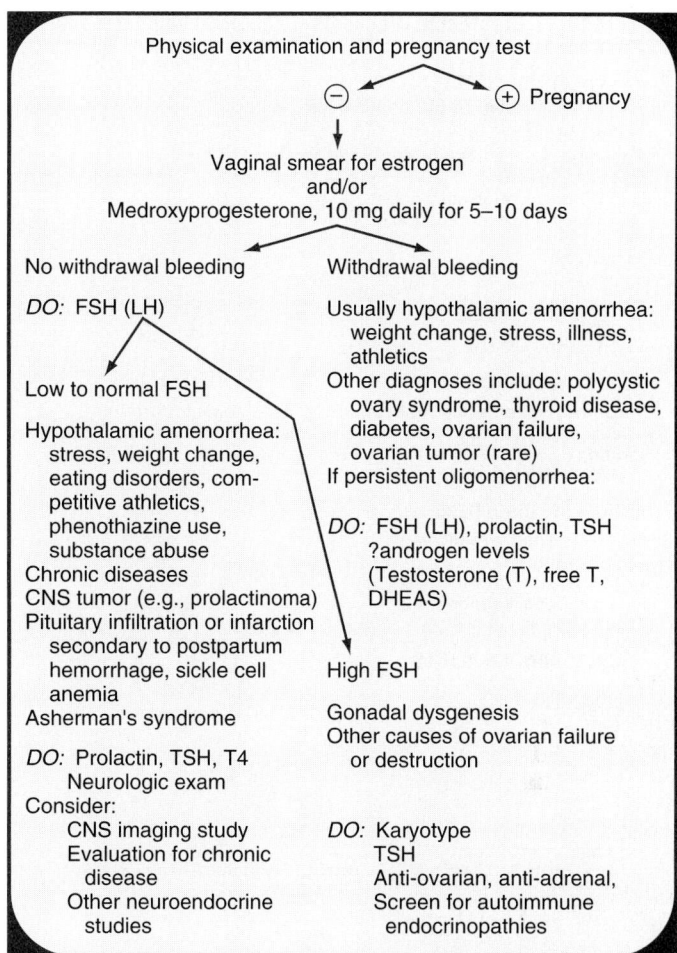

FIGURE 107–2. Evaluation of secondary amenorrhea. (From Emans SJH, Laufer MR, Goldstein DP [editors]: *Pediatric and Adolescent Gynecology*, 4th ed. Philadelphia, Lippincott-Raven, 1998.)

this term is used when no demonstrable organic lesion is identified to account for the abnormal bleeding. Organic lesions are found in about 9% of 10–20 yr old young women; the most common include ectopic pregnancy, threatened abortion, endometritis, and hormonal contraceptives. Box 107–2 lists the full differential diagnosis, which is extensive; however, studies of severe cases that require hospitalization report coagulation disorders (idiopathic thrombocytopenic purpura, von Willebrand disease, leukemia), Glanzmann disease, hypothyroidism, thalassemia major, Fanconi syndrome, and rheumatoid arthritis as the most frequent diagnoses.

Laboratory Findings. The hemoglobin and hematocrit from a complete blood count are the most important elements in the initial evaluation. They establish the severity of the bleeding, with levels less than a hemoglobin of 9 g/dL or a hematocrit of 27% considered severe, 9–11 g/dL and 27–33% considered moderate, and greater than 11 g/dL and greater than 33% considered mild. Hospitalization is generally recommended for adolescents with a hemoglobin less than 7 gm/dL or a hemoglobin less than 10 gm/dL with significant postural blood pressure changes or excessive heavy bleeding. For sexually active teenagers, tests for gonorrhea, chlamydia, and pregnancy are also performed. The secondary evaluation should include liver and thyroid function studies, prothrombin time, partial thromboplastin time, and bleeding time. If these studies are not performed at the first visit, they must be performed before any estrogen therapy is initiated that might interfere with interpreting the results.

BOX 107-2. Differential Diagnosis of Abnormal Vaginal Bleeding in the Adolescent Girl

ANOVULATORY UTERINE BLEEDING
PREGNANCY-RELATED COMPLICATIONS

Threatened abortion
Spontaneous, incomplete, or missed abortion
Ectopic pregnancy
Gestational trophoblastic disease
Complications of termination procedures

INFECTION

Pelvic inflammatory disease
Endometritis
Cervicitis
Vaginitis

BLOOD DYSCRASIAS

Thrombocytopenia (e.g., idiopathic thrombocytopenic purpura,
   leukemia, aplastic anemia, hypersplenism, chemotherapy)
Clotting disorders (e.g., von Willebrand's disease, other disorders of
   platelet function, liver dysfunction)

ENDOCRINE DISORDERS

Hypo- or hyperthyroidism
Adrenal disease
Hyperprolactinemia
Polycystic ovary syndrome
Ovarian failure

VAGINAL ABNORMALITIES

Carcinoma
Laceration

CERVICAL PROBLEMS

Cervicitis
Polyp
Hemangioma
Carcinoma

UTERINE PROBLEMS

Submucous myoma
Congenital anomalies
Polyp
Carcinoma
Use of intrauterine device
Breakthrough bleeding associated with oral contraceptives or other
   hormonal contraceptives
Ovulation bleeding

OVARIAN PROBLEMS

Cyst
Tumor (benign, malignant)

ENDOMETRIOSIS
TRAUMA
FOREIGN BODY (E.G., RETAINED TAMPON)
SYSTEMIC DISEASES

Diabetes mellitus
Renal disease
Systemic lupus erythematosus

MEDICATIONS

Hormonal contraceptives
Anticoagulants
Platelet inhibitors
Androgens
Spironolactone

From Emans SJH, Laufer MR, Goldstein DP (editors): *Pediatric and Adolescent Gynecology*, 4th ed. Philadelphia, Lippincott-Raven, 1998, p 239.

Treatment. In mild cases, iron supplementation is recommended, and the patient should keep a menstrual calendar to follow the subsequent flow patterns. With moderate disturbances, cycling with oral contraceptives, barring any contraindications, should be considered along with monitoring the iron status. Severe bleeding, not requiring hospitalization, can usually be stopped with hormonal therapy, either medroxyprogesterone acetate (Provera) 10 mg/24 hr for 10–14 days or a combination oral contraceptive (OC) using two to four pills per day until the bleeding stops, then one pill per day for the remainder of the cycle. Once a patient is hospitalized, Premarin 20–40 mg every 4 hr up to 24 hr given intravenously is required. At the same time, the combination oral contraceptive regimen or Depo-provera (medroxyprogesterone acetate [DMPA]), 150 mg IM every 12 wk, required for maintenance can be initiated. These estrogen doses are high, but no complications have been reported from short-term use.

In the rare case of a patient whose bleeding cannot be controlled by one of these methods, an endometrial curettage may be indicated. Although this procedure is frequently undertaken in adult women with menometrorrhagia, the rarity of endometrial carcinoma and the usual efficacy of hormonal therapy in adolescence make this procedure unnecessarily invasive in this age group.

107.3 Dysmenorrhea

Painful menstrual cramps are experienced by nearly two thirds of postmenarcheal teenagers in the United States. More than 10% of this group suffer sufficiently to miss school, making dys-

menorrhea the leading cause of short-term school absenteeism in female adolescents. Dysmenorrhea may be primary or secondary. *Primary dysmenorrhea* is characterized by the absence of any specific pelvic pathologic condition and is the more commonly occurring form. Prostaglandins F_2 and E_2, produced by the endometrium, stimulate the myometrium to contract, producing pain. *Secondary dysmenorrhea* results from an underlying **structural abnormality** of the cervix or uterus, a **foreign body** such as an intrauterine device, **endometriosis**, or **endometritis.** Endometriosis, a condition in which implants of endometrial tissue are found at ectopic locations within the peritoneal cavity, is being diagnosed with increasing frequency among adolescents through the use of ultrasonography and laparoscopy. Characteristically, there is severe pain at the time of menses; its specific location depends on the site of the implants.

A pelvic examination must be performed to exclude the causes of secondary dysmenorrhea, and if none is found, a diagnosis of primary dysmenorrhea should be considered. Adolescents suffering from dysmenorrhea have high levels of prostaglandins F_2 and E_2 and experience symptomatic relief when prostaglandin synthetase inhibitors are administered. If given before a menstrual period (or shortly after it begins), administration of a rapidly absorbed prostaglandin synthetase inhibitor, such as naproxen sodium, is effective in destroying the prostaglandins before they produce pain (e.g., two tablets of 275 mg each taken with the onset of menses and one tablet taken every 6–8 hr after that for the 1st 24 hr). Medication is rarely needed beyond the 1st day. For the teenager with dysmenorrhea who requires contraception, oral contraceptive therapy may be indicated. It is not certain whether the beneficial effect of such use derives from the ability of oral contraceptives to inhibit ovulation and thus eliminate progesterone production from the corpus luteum or from their ability to limit endometrial proliferation and therefore the production of prostaglandins.

In adolescent patients with endometriosis, danazol, an anti-gonadotropin, is rarely prescribed because of the unacceptable side effects of weight gain, edema, irregular menses, acne, oily skin, hirsutism, and a deep voice change. The use of gonadotropin-releasing hormone (GnRH) agonists such as nafarelin and leuprolide are more commonly used with the goal of the creation of an acyclic, low-estrogen environment. This prevents bleeding at the site of the implants and further seeding of the pelvis during retrograde menstruation. To reduce the risk of decreased bone density, a long-term side effect of gonadotropin-releasing hormone analog therapy, prescriptions for courses of therapy lasting longer than 6 consecutive mo are not recommended.

107.4 Premenstrual Syndrome

Premenstrual syndrome, or the late luteal phase syndrome, is a complex of physical signs and behavioral symptoms occurring during the second half of the menstrual cycle, which may resolve with the onset of menses. Clinical manifestations may include breast fullness and tenderness; bloating; fatigue; headache; increased appetite, especially for sweets and salty foods; irritability and mood swings; and depression, inability to concentrate, tearfulness, and violent tendencies. About one third of women in the reproductive age group may have premenstrual syndrome, but the absence of objective findings makes this difficult to corroborate. It is not common among adolescents, and it does not relate to the presence of dysmenorrhea, which is much more common in this age group. The popular use of vitamin B_6 and progesterone supplementation is not based on evidence of their effectiveness, nor is there a theoretical basis for their use. Use of a gonadotropin-releasing hormone agonist on a short-term basis is supported by carefully controlled studies, but long-term effects, such as osteoporosis and potential complications, have not yet been evaluated, making its use in adolescents contraindicated.

Bevan JA, Maloney KW, Hillery CA, et al: Bleeding disorders: A common cause of menorrhagia in adolescents. *J Pediatr* 2001;138: 856–61.

Blythe MJ: Common menstrual problems of adolescence. *Adolescent Medicine* 1997;8(1):87–109.

Emans SJH, Laufer MR, Goldstein DP: *Pediatric and Adolescent Gynecology*, 4th ed. Philadelphia, Lippincott-Raven, 1998.

Gordon CM: Menstrual disorders in adolescents: Excess androgens and polycystic ovary syndrome. *Pediatr Clin North Am* 1999; 46(3):519–43.

Neinstein LS: *Adolescent Health Care: A Practical Guide*, 4th ed. Philadelphia, Lippincott, Williams & Wilkins, 2002.

Saenger P: Turner's syndrome. *N Engl J Med* 1996;335(23):1749–59.

Chapter 108

Contraception *Renée R. Jenkins*

Adolescents bear a disproportionate risk for the adverse consequences of sexual activity, sexually transmitted diseases, and early unintended pregnancy. They should be encouraged to postpone sexual activity; however, contraceptive counseling and services should be offered to adolescents who are sexually active.

Epidemiology. The National Survey of Family Growth (1995) reported a decline in sexual activity from 1988–1995, with intercourse in young women aged 15–19 yr dropping from 55–50% and percentages in young men dropping from 60–55%. The Centers for Disease Control and Prevention's Youth Risk

Behavior Survey supports this observation in high school students with "ever had intercourse" rates falling from 54.1% in 1991 to 49.9% in 1999. The survey specifically notes that 64.9% of high school seniors report having ever had intercourse, with 50.6% currently active sexually, which was defined as having had intercourse during the 3 mo preceding the survey. In 9th grade, 38.6% reported ever having had sex, with 26.6% being sexually active. Many factors are associated with early sexual activity, including but not limited to lower expectations for education, poor perception of life options, low school grades, and involvement in other high-risk behaviors.

There is some variability in the reporting of the percentage of teenagers who use contraception depending on the study and the way in which the question was worded. Overall contraceptive use among adolescents aged 15–19 yr, according to the National Survey of Family Growth, increased significantly from 1982–1988 (24.2–32.1%); however, more recent data demonstrate a decline between 1988 and 1995 (29.8%). Contraceptive use at first intercourse, and condom use in general, have increased during this same period. The type of method selected also varies by ethnicity, with nonwhite teens more likely to select pills, and black teens using pills as the first choice, but being two times more likely than whites to use an injectable method (Table 108–1). In a 5-country study of developed nations, United States teens used medical methods at last intercourse less frequently compared to other teens; 52% in U.S. teens, 56% in Swedish 18–19 yr olds, 67% of French 15–19 yr olds, 72% of British 16–19 yr olds, and 73% of Canadian 15–19 yr olds. Sexually active adolescent women in the United States delay going to a clinic or a doctor for a medical contraceptive for an average of 6 mo after initiating intercourse. A higher likelihood of contraceptive use is associated with older age at sexual initiation, aspirations for higher academic achievement, acceptance of one's own sexuality, and a positive attitude toward contraception.

Contraceptive Counseling. The health screening interview during the adolescent preventive visit offers the opportunity both to support the adolescent who is abstinent to continue to be so and to identify the sexually active adolescent who has unsafe sexual

TABLE 108–1. Percentage Distribution of Non-Hispanic White and Non-Hispanic Black Contraceptive Users Aged 15–19 Years by Current Method, 1982–1995

Race-Ethnicity and Method	1982	1988	1995
Non-Hispanic White			
Female sterilization	0	2	0
Male sterilization	0	0	0
Pill	62	56	49
Implant	NA	NA	1
Injectable	NA	NA	8
IUD	0	0	0
Diaphragm	7	1	0
Male condom	23	34	36
Other methods	7	7	7
Non-Hispanic Black			
Female sterilization	0	2	0
Male sterilization	0	0	0
Pill	70	75	32
Implant	NA	NA	5
Injectable	NA	NA	19
IUD	5	0	0
Diaphragm	2	0	0
Male condom	13	21	38
Other methods	10	2	5
TOTAL	100	100	100

IUD = intrauterine device; NA = not available.
Adapted from Piccinino LJ, Mosher WD: Trends in contraceptive use in the United States: 1982–1995. *Fam Plann Perspect* 1998;30:4, 46.

practices (see Chapter 100). Adolescents with chronic diseases are particularly vulnerable to having these issues omitted from the health maintenance visit. There may be particular cautions related to concurrent medication to be noted for these chronically ill teenagers; however, sexuality and contraceptive issues need to be addressed. The goals of a counseling intervention with the adolescent are to understand the adolescent's perceptions and misperceptions about contraceptives, help him or her put the risk of unprotected intercourse in a personal perspective, and educate the adolescent regarding the real risk and contraindications for the various methods available. The likelihood that an adolescent will use a contraceptive method depends on such factors as the developmental level of the adolescent, the reproductive history, the involvement in other high-risk behaviors, and the degree of readiness for using contraception. Readiness to use contraception progresses in stages, from (1) precomtemplative, not thinking about using contraception, (2) contemplative—giving it some thought, but having no immediate plans, (3) preparative, wanting to try a method in the near future, to (4) active—using contraception. The adolescent should also be made aware of the "perfect" use failure rates vs the "typical" failure rates based on patient compliance (Table 108–2). Once an adolescent chooses a method, recognition of the common side effects, with clear plans on management, communication with the provider about the realistic expectation for failure, and a contingency plan for that possibility between the adolescent and the provider give closure to the counseling session and provide strategies for close follow-up. The use of withdrawal as a method is probably underestimated in adolescents and its low efficacy rate should be specifically addressed with young adolescents. The pelvic examination as a requirement to obtain medical contraception creates a barrier for some teenagers; consequently, clinicians have commonly delayed the examination for 3–6 mo for adolescents who might otherwise postpone the acceptance of a contraceptive device. Confidentiality and consent issues related to contraceptive management are discussed in Chapter 100.

108.1 Barrier Methods

Condoms. This method prevents sperm from being deposited in the vagina. There are no major side effects associated with the use of a condom. The AIDS scare appears to have increased the use of condoms among adolescents, with 46.2% of high school students reporting using a condom at last sexual intercourse in 1991 increasing to 58% in 1999. The main advantages of condoms are their low price, availability without prescription, little need for advance planning, and, most important for this age group, their effectiveness in preventing transmission of sexually transmitted diseases, including human immunodeficiency virus (HIV). Condoms are recommended as protection against sexually transmitted diseases (STDs), to be used along with all nonbarrier medical methods for adolescents. A female condom is now available over the counter in single size disposable units. It is a second choice over the male latex condom because of the complexity of properly using the device, its low typical efficacy rate, and the lack of evidence demonstrating its effectiveness against STDs. Most adolescents would require intensive education and hands-on practice to use it effectively.

Diaphragm and Cervical Cap. These methods have few side effects but are much less likely to be used by teenagers. Adolescents tend to object to the messiness of the jelly or to the fact that the insertion of a diaphragm may interrupt the spontaneity of sex, or they may express discomfort about touching their genitals.

108.2 Spermicides

A variety of agents containing the spermicide nonoxynol-9 are available as foams, jellies, creams, films, or effervescent vaginal suppositories. They must be placed in the vaginal cavity shortly before intercourse and reinserted before each subsequent ejaculation in order to be effective. Rare side effects consist of contact vaginitis. There has been some concern regarding the vaginal and cervical mucosal damage observed with nonoxynol-9, and the overall impact on HIV transmission is unknown. Effectiveness is in the range of the barrier methods (approximately 85%), and the finding that nonoxynol-9 is gonococcocidal and spirocheticidal enhances the attractiveness of these agents for adolescents because of their disproportionately high risk for STDs. Spermicides alone probably do not provide protection against STDs, but they should be used in combination with condoms.

108.3 Combination Methods

The conjoint use of the condom by the male and spermicidal foam by the female adolescent is extremely effective; the failure rate is 2% (perfect use), without any of the potential side effects and complications associated with the use of other forms of contraception having comparable efficacy. This combination also prevents STDs, including HIV.

108.4 Hormonal Methods

Hormonal methods currently employ either an estrogenic substance in combination with a progestin or a progestin alone. The action of the estrogen-progestin combination is to prevent the surge of luteinizing hormone and, as a result, to inhibit ovulation. Progestin may prevent ovulation, but it is not reliable. Progestin does, however, affect fallopian tube transport and the composition of cervical mucus in such a way as to make fertilization or implantation less likely.

Combination Oral Contraceptives. Oral contraceptives (OCs) are commonly referred to as "the pill" and currently contain either 50, 35, 30, or 20 μg of estrogenic substance, typically either mestranol or ethinyl estradiol, and a progestin. The pill is one of the most reliable contraceptive methods available, with a perfect-use pregnancy rate in the range of 0.1%/yr. Typical-use failure

---

TABLE 108–2.	First-Year Failure Rates by Contraceptive Method	
	Women Experiencing Pregnancy (%)	
	Typical Use	*Perfect Use*
Implant	0.09	0.09
Injectable	0.3	0.3
IUD		
Copper T380A	0.7	0.6
Progesterone T	2.0	1.5
Oral contraceptive		
Combined	2.5–6.0	0.1
Progestin-only	3.0–10.0	0.5
Male condom	12.0	3.0
Diaphragm with spermicide	16.0–18.0	6.0
Cervical cap	17.4	6.0
Withdrawal	19.0	4.0
Periodic abstinence	20.0	
Calendar "rhythm"		9.0
Cervical mucus		3.0
Symptothermal		2.0
Spermicides	21.0	6.0
Female condom	21.0–26.0	5.0
No method	85.0	85.0

FDA labeled rates noted are adapted from Hatcher RA, Trussell J, Stewart F, et al: Contraceptive Technology, 16th revised ed. New York, Irvington Publishers, 1994; and Jones EF, Forrest JD: Contraceptive failure rates based on 1988 NSFG. Fam Plann Perspect 1992;24:12.

rates in 15–19 yr old women have ranged up to 18.1%. Thrombophlebitis, hepatic adenomas, myocardial infarction, and carbohydrate intolerance are some of the more serious potential complications of exogenous estrogen use. These disorders are, however, exceedingly rare in adolescents. Even though teenage smokers who use OCs have a relative risk of more than 2.0 for myocardial infarction, the likelihood of its occurrence is much smaller, and thus insignificant, than the risk of dying from pregnancy-related complications. Some long-range beneficial effects of estrogen use include decreased risks of benign breast disease, ovarian disease, and anemia.

The short-term adverse effects of OCs, such as nausea and weight gain, often interfere with compliance in adolescent patients. These effects are usually transient and may be overshadowed by the beneficial effects of a shortened menses and the relief of dysmenorrhea. The inhibition of ovulation or the suppressant effect of estrogens on prostaglandin production by the endometrium make OCs effective in preventing dysmenorrhea (see Chapter 107). An initial concern for younger adolescents regarding the potentially untoward effect of estrogens on epiphyseal growth has diminished. This does not occur, either because the amount of estrogen in OCs is small or because they are taken at a time when most growth has been completed. Amenorrhea occurring after cessation of OC use is seen with greater frequency in adolescents than in adults. It may persist for up to 18 mo after the discontinuation of the pill. The increased risk may not be due to age alone but may reflect oligomenorrhea or low body weight (<47 kg) before the initiation of use of the pill. Acne may be worsened by some and improved by other OC preparations. The newer pills with nonandrogenic progestins are particularly effective in reducing acne and hirsutism as side effects. An additional beneficial cardiovascular effect occurs for adolescents taking estrogen-containing OCs; these young women have higher levels of cardioprotective high-density lipoproteins than controls.

Contraindications to the use of estrogen-containing OCs include hepatocellular disease, migraine headaches, breast disease, any condition in which hypercoagulability may be a problem (e.g., replaced cardiac valve, thrombophlebitis, sickle cell anemia) because of the increased levels of factor VIII and decreased production of antithrombin III, and known or suspected pregnancy. The risks of pregnancy must be balanced against the benefits of reliable contraception in patients with chronic diseases such as diabetes, epilepsy, and sickle cell disease. The initial history taken before prescribing OCs should specifically address these risks. Table 108–3 also presents the potential alterations of various laboratory tests that can occur in patients taking OCs.

Other Combination Methods. A *monthly injectable* (estradiol cypionate, 5 μg, and medroxyprogesterone, 25 mg, MPA/E$_2$C, Lunelle) provides the efficacy of the oral contraceptive and the convenience of a monthly injectable. It is administered by a health provider during the first 5 days of the menstrual cycle. The follow-up doses are given every 28 ± 5 days (23–33 days). The mechanism of action and side effect profile are similar to oral contraceptives.

The *transdermal patch* (Evra) contains ethinyl estradiol and norergestromin and is applied to the lower abdomen, buttocks, or upper body. It is worn continuously for 1 wk and changed weekly for a total of 3 wk, then removed to allow menstrual bleeding. It should not be applied to the breast. It appears to be less effective in women who weigh 198 pounds or more, and the common side effects are accidental detachment and skin irritation. Early studies in adults suggest improved compliance with the transdermal patch compared with oral contraceptives.

The *vaginal contraceptive ring* (NuvaRing) is a flexible, transparent, colorless vaginal ring that measures about 2.1 inches in diameter and is inserted into the vagina by the patient. It contains ethinyl estradiol and etonogestrel and remains in place for

TABLE 108–3. Laboratory Tests and Potential Alteration due to Oral Contraceptives

Group	Increased	Decreased
Carbohydrate metabolism	Fasting blood sugar and 2-hr pp Insulin	Glucose tolerance
Hematologic and coagulation	Coagulation factors II, VII, XIII, IX, X, XII Fibrinogen Leukocyte count PTT, PT Plasminogen Platelet count, platelet aggregation, platelet adhesiveness	Antithrombin III Hematocrit PT
Lipid metabolism	Cholesterol, lipoproteins HDL increased by estrogen Triglycerides	HDL decreased by progestins
Liver function and gastrointestinal tests	Alkaline phosphatase Bilirubin, SGOT, SGPT, GGT Protoporphyrin, coproporphyrin excretion (urine)	Haptoglobin Urobilinogen excretion (urine)
Metals	Copper and ceruloplasmin Iron, iron-binding capacity, and transferrin	Magnesium Zinc
Thyroid function	Thyroid-binding globulin Thyroxine	Free thyroxine
Vitamins	Vitamin A	Folate Vitamins B$_6$, B$_{12}$ Vitamin C
Other hormones and enzymes	Aldosterone Angiotensinogen Angiotensin I and II Cortisol Growth hormone Testosterone	Estradiol FSH, LH 17-hydroxycorticosteroids Renin
Miscellaneous	α$_1$-Antitrypsin Antinuclear antibody Lactate Sodium	Albumin Calcium Immunoglobulins A, G, M

FSH = follicle-stimulating hormone; GGT = γ-glutamyltransferase; HDL = high-density lipoprotein; LH = luteinizing hormone; PP = postprandial; PT = prothrombin time; PTT = partial thromboplastin time; SGOT = serum glutamic-oxaloacetic transaminase, SGPT = serum glutamic-pyruvic transaminase.
From Neinstein LS: Adolescent Health Care, 3rd ed. Baltimore, Williams & Wilkins, 1996.

3 wk, during which time these hormones are absorbed. If the ring is accidentally expelled, it should be reinserted; however, if it is out of place for more than 3 hr, a back-up method of contraception should be used.

All of these methods have similar contraindications to oral contraceptives (i.e., smoking, cardiovascular disease, and others).

All-Progestin Contraceptives. Progestin-only contraceptives are available for the adolescent in whom the use of estrogen is potentially deleterious, for example, those with liver disease, replaced cardiac valves, or hypercoagulable states. These agents ("mini-pills") are less reliable in inhibiting ovulation and are associated with a 0.5%/yr pregnancy rate (perfect use). Acceptance by adolescents is limited by the necessity of taking

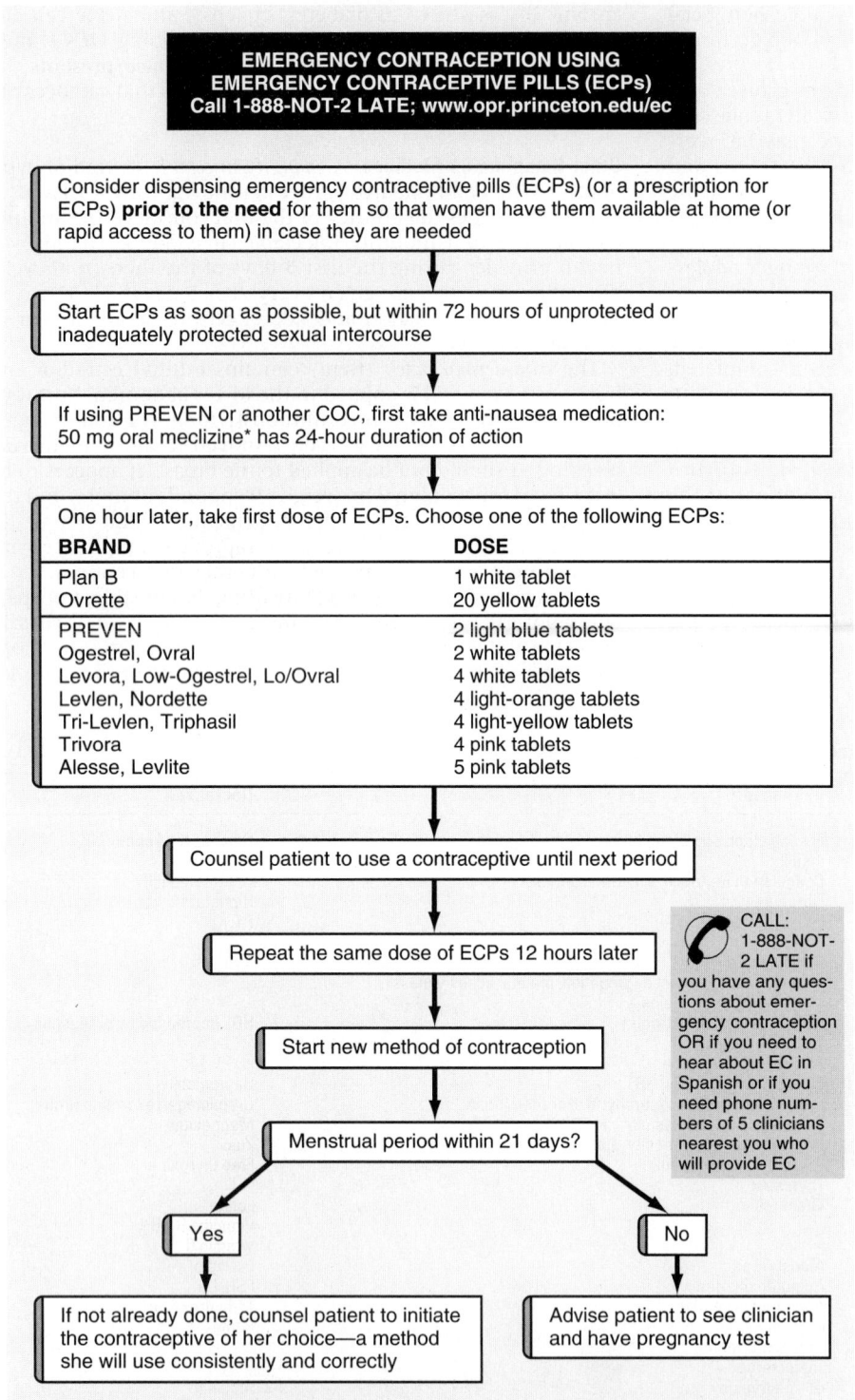

FIGURE 108–1. Emergency contraception using emergency contraceptive pills (ECPs). COC = combination oral contraceptive. (From Hatcher RA, Nelson AL, Zieman M, et al: *A Pocket Guide to Managing Contraception.* Tiger, GA, Bridging the Gap Foundation, 2001.)

the pill daily, the higher incidence of amenorrhea, and increased bleeding.

An *injectable progestin*, medroxyprogesterone (Depo-Provera, DMPA), is highly effective in birth control, with failure rates typically at 0.3–0.4%. This substance needs to be administered only once every 3 mo and is completely reversible in its anovulatory action; furthermore, the cessation of menses is conterminous with its use. The most common side effect of DMPA is menstrual disturbance, either amenorrhea or abnormal vaginal bleeding. Weight gain and lowered bone density have been observed in women taking DMPA; however, the data confirming the agent as the sole cause of these changes are still under study. Issues relative to bone density are of particular concern during adolescence, the developmental period in which the accumulation of bone density is at its greatest. Studies thus far indicate that the effect is reversible on discontinuation of the drug. Until further research is available, one should probably avoid DMPA use in teens at risk for osteoporosis, such as those who have chronic renal disease, who are wheelchair-bound, or who have eating disorders or chronic amenorrhea. In contrast, DMPA is particularly attractive for adolescents who have difficulty with compliance, mentally retarded teenagers, and teenagers with chronic illnesses who have a relative contraindication to estrogen use. Continuation rates are somewhat disappointing and range from 27–45% at 12 months, comparable to adult rates.

A *long-acting progestational agent*, levonorgestrel (Norplant), is contained in six small Silastic tubes that can be implanted subcutaneously. The contraceptive potency remains for 5 yr. This method is the most effective of all reversible birth control methods available, with a typical 1st-yr failure rate for all women at 0.09% and 5-yr failure rates at 0.9–1.1%. Failure rates specifically calculated for adolescent women are not available. Implants have been used primarily in postpartum adolescents with good tolerance and acceptability. When compared with OC use in this population, implant users have better continuation rates and fewer pregnancies over a 1–2 yr period. Requests for early removal of this device have led to its diminished use in adolescent women. Norplant II, with two Silastic rods to be implanted for 3 yr has been approved by the FDA with a similar efficacy and safety profile as Norplant. Another 3-year implant with a single rod containing 3-ketodesogestrol has undergone clinical trials in the United States and Europe. Data on the use of these products in adolescents are not available.

108.5 Emergency Contraception

Unprotected intercourse at midcycle carries a pregnancy risk of 20–30%. At any other time during the cycle, the risk drops to 2–4%. The risk may be reduced or eliminated by intervention within 72 hr after unprotected intercourse. Outside the United States, several agents are used for emergency contraception (EC): oral high-dose estrogens, high-dose combination estrogen-progestins, high-dose progestins, danazol, mifepristone, and the postcoital insertion of a copper intrauterine device (IUD). Strategies are under way to promote more widespread use of EC to reduce unintended pregnancies. One controlled trial with young women documented 2 times as likely use of EC if given in advance as compared to a group who received counseling alone. A protocol for approaching EC is outlined in Figure 108–1. The Yuzpe method is commonly used in the United States, consisting of combination pills totaling 200 µg of ethinyl estradiol and 2.0 mg of norgestrel or 1.0 mg levonorgestrel. Pills that can be utilized for this method appear in Figure 108–1. The high-dose combination OCs disrupt the luteal phase hormone pattern, creating an unstable and unsuitable uterine lining for implantation. If used midcycle, when ovulation is about to occur, the high-dose estrogen and progestin blunt the luteiniz-

ing hormone surge and impair ovulation. This method is effective in reducing the risk of pregnancy by 75%. An emergency contraceptive kit prepackaged for this method (Preven) is FDA approved. The most common side effect is nausea (50%) and vomiting (20%), prompting some clinicians to prescribe or recommend antiemetics along with the OCs. In most health care facilities, a urine pregnancy test is required prior to dispensing the pills to rule out an existing pregnancy. There is some controversy about the need to do this, since there is no evidence to suggest that OCs used in this manner affect early fetal development and the dose as prescribed would not disrupt a previously undetected pregnancy. A progestin-only EC kit was FDA approved in 1999 and contains 2 tablets, each with 0.75 mg of levonorgestrel. Nausea and vomiting are uncommon side effects, and in a recent comparison levonorgestrel proved more effective at preventing pregnancy. Mifepristone (RU-486) is a highly effective EC method with a nearly 0% failure rate; however, it functions as an abortifacient and its use is highly controversial. A 2-wk follow-up appointment is recommended following any of the methods to determine the effectiveness of treatment and to diagnose a possible early pregnancy. The visit also provides an opportunity to counsel the adolescent, explore the situation leading up to the unprotected intercourse, test for STDs, and initiate continuing contraception when appropriate.

108.6 Intrauterine Devices

Intrauterine devices (IUDs) are small, flexible, plastic objects introduced into the uterine cavity through the cervix. They differ in size, shape, and the presence or absence of pharmacologically active substances (e.g., copper or progesterone). The mechanism of action of IUDs is uncertain, although they render the endometrium unsuitable for implantation by inducing a local polymorphonuclear leukocyte response, production of prostaglandins E_2 and F_2, and stimulation of uterine contractility. They are effective in preventing pregnancy in 97–99% of women. Young patients and those with multiple sexual partners are at increased risk of infection, and the prescription of an IUD to teenagers who require passive contraception should be limited to the method of last resort.

Archer DF: New contraceptive options. *Clin Obstet Gynecol* 2001;44(1):122–6.

Audet M, Moreau M, Koltun WD, et al: Evaluation of contraceptive efficacy and cycle control of a transdermal contraceptive patch vs an oral contraceptive. *JAMA* 2001;285(18):2347–54.

Center for Disease Control and Prevention: Youth risk behavior surveillance—United States, 1999, CDC Surveillance Summaries, June 9, 2000. *MMWR* 2000;49 (No. SS- 5).

Darroch JE, Singh SS, Frost JJ, et al: Differences in teenage pregnancy rates among five developed countries: The roles of sexual activity and contraceptive use. *Fam Plann Perspect* 2001;33(6):244. (www.guttmacher.org)

Greydanus DE, Patel DR, Rimsza ME: Contraception in the adolescent: An update. *Pediatrics* 2001;107(3):562–73.

Hatcher RA, Nelson AL, Zieman M, et al: *A Pocket Guide to Managing Contraception.* Tiger, GA, Bridging the Gap Foundation, 2001.

Hewitt G, Cromer B: Update on adolescent contraception. *Obstet Gynecol Clin North Am* 2000;27(1):143–62.

Jenkins RR, Raine T: Helping adolescents prevent unintended pregnancy. *Contemporary Pediatrics* 2000;17(5):75.

Neinstein LS: *Adolescent Health Care: A Practical Guide,* 4th ed. Philadelphia, Lippincott Williams & Wilkins, 2002.

Chapter 109

Pregnancy *Renée R. Jenkins*

Sexual activity at an early age coupled with nonuse or improper use of contraceptives contributes to a disproportionately high rate of teenage pregnancy in the United States when compared with other industrialized nations. By virtue of the trajectory of early sexual activity to early unintended pregnancy, the risk and protective factors are similar. Factors associated with childbearing as the outcome for teenage pregnancy, however, are strongly linked to poverty and the absence of opportunity for other life choices.

Epidemiology. The estimated number of pregnancies in adolescent women fell to approximately 479,067 in 2000. The birthrate of 48.7 births/1,000 for women aged 15–19 yr is the lowest level reported in the United States since 1940 (Fig. 109–1). When considered in the context of the number of sexually active adolescents, the decline is impressive. First births to teens make up the substantial proportion of the reduction, with second births remaining stable since 1996. Most of the pregnancies are unintended, and a significant proportion of young women voluntarily terminate the pregnancy. Forty-one per cent of girls younger than 15 yr of age and 29.1% of 15–19 yr olds elected abortion in 1997, although the overall rates of abortion are also down. Internationally, the United States leads all other industrialized countries in the teen birthrate, and although the birthrate is declining, the drop is less steep than the declines in other developed countries (Fig. 109–2).

Etiology. As with early initiation of intercourse, the factors associated with pregnancy are multifactorial at the individual, family, and environmental levels (Chapter 99). The sexually active female teenager's success in avoiding unintended pregnancy is determined by her ability to use an effective contraceptive method consistently. Young teenagers are likely to be less deliberative and logical about their sexual decisions than are adults, and their sexual activity is likely to be sporadic and coercive, factors contributing to inconsistent contraceptive use and greater risk of pregnancy. Once the pregnancy has occurred, the decision to bear a child, keep or place the child for adoption, or terminate the pregnancy is influenced again by multiple issues. Parents, most often mothers, have a tremendous influence on what the adolescent decides to do. Friends and sexual partners

play a lesser role. Better employment prospects as well as other lifestyle benefits are associated with lowered probability of childbearing. A young woman's attitude toward abortion is the strongest factor associated with that choice. Access to abortion services and individual factors such as high self-esteem and aspirations for further education play a role. Adoption appears to be an option less often considered currently and is associated with younger age, expectations of fewer children and, less often, receiving welfare support prior to pregnancy. Marriage following a first teenager birth is least likely to occur in young teenagers and teenagers with less than a high school education and more likely to occur in some cultural groups, such as Hispanic teens. Overall, adoption and marriage are choices less often selected by pregnant adolescents.

Clinical Manifestations. Adolescents may experience the traditional symptoms of pregnancy, that is, morning sickness, swollen tender breasts, weight gain, and amenorrhea; however, the presentation is often more vague. Headache, fatigue, abdominal pain, and scanty or irregular menses are common presenting symptoms.

Denial of sexual activity and menstrual irregularity should not preclude the diagnosis in face of other clinical or historical information. An unanticipated request for a complete check-up or a visit for contraception may uncover a suspected pregnancy. Pregnancy is still the most common diagnosis when an adolescent presents with secondary amenorrhea.

Diagnosis. On physical examination, the findings of an enlarged uterus, cervical cyanosis (Chadwick sign), a soft uterus (Hegar sign), or a soft cervix (Goodell sign) are highly suggestive of an intrauterine pregnancy. A confirmatory pregnancy test is always recommended. The most commonly used method is a qualitative measurement of the ß-subunit for human chorionic gonadotropin (hCG) by blood or urine. The results are positive in 98% of women within 7 days after implantation. The most sensitive test is a quantitative β-hCG radioimmunoassay, in which results are reliable within 7 days after fertilization. This test is more expensive and less likely to be used under routine circumstances. Evaluation for a possible ectopic pregnancy, a retained placenta following an abortion, or a molar pregnancy are some of its more common uses. Urine pregnancy tests are the enzyme-linked immunosorbent assay type using highly specific monoclonal antibodies to the ß-subunit of hCG. These tests may be positive as early as 3 to 4 days after implantation. One health department study reported 28% of adolescents requesting pregnancy tests had already performed home pregnancy tests prior to the visit. These tests are most often of lower sensitivity and specificity than tests used in the office and should be repeated with more reliable tests before proceeding with clinical management.

Treatment. Confidentiality and privacy are key components of counseling the adolescent in whom pregnancy is suspected. The younger the adolescent, the greater should be the concern that the sexual activity may have been coercive. Special sensitivity is required to explore this issue with the adolescent as is knowledge of proper procedures for enlisting help for the adolescent and reporting suspected abuse. If the adolescent's pregnancy test result is negative, it is prudent to repeat the test in 2 wk. If the repeat test result is negative, the opportunity to counsel the adolescent and provide the appropriate intervention should be seized. If the adolescent is pregnant, the options available to manage the pregnancy should be presented and discussed in the context of her family, and her individual situation. Adolescents should be encouraged to include parents fully in the discussion of their options. When parents are not available or the adolescent is resistant to their initial involvement, the adolescent is urged to involve a trusted adult—for example, a relative or counselor—in the decision-making process. Follow-up is

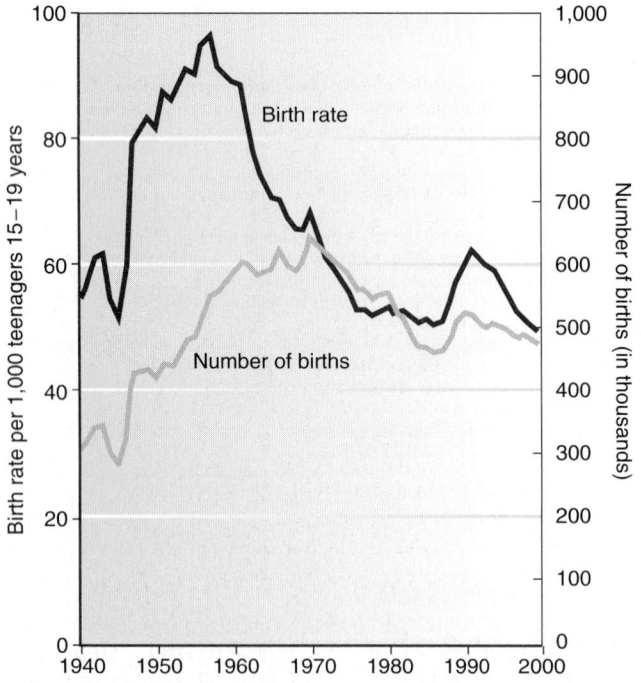

NOTE: Data for 2000 are preliminary.

FIGURE 109–1. Number of births and birthrates for teenagers 15–19 years: United States, 1940–2000. (Adapted from *National Vital Statistics Report*, vol 49, no 19, September 25, 2001.)

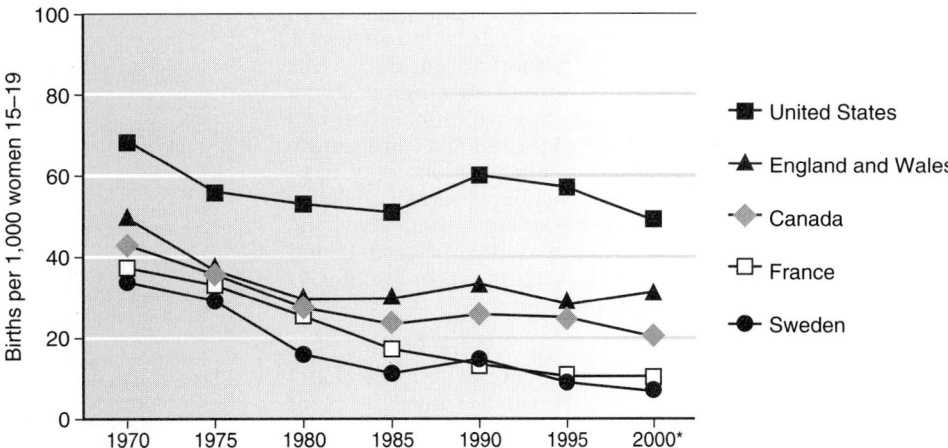

FIGURE 109–2. Teenage birthrates declined less steeply in the United States than in other developed countries between 1970 and 2000. (Adapted from Alan Guttmacher Institute: *Can More Progress Be Made? Teenage Sexual and Reproductive Behavior in Developed Countries.* Executive Summary, 2001, p 2.)

*Data are for 1997 in Canada, 1998 in France, and 1999 in England, Wales and Sweden.

necessary to ensure this involvement, given the possibility that denial, fear, and indecisiveness may delay the adolescent's seeking adult support.

Risks and Consequences of Teenage Childbearing. Adverse outcomes for pregnant teenagers are reduced significantly by early prenatal care. Twenty per cent of teenagers younger than age 15 yr and 12% of all teenagers are likely to receive only third trimester care or no care at all prior to delivery. Adolescent parenting has implications for the adolescent mother, father, and child. When adolescent mothers are compared with their peers, they are less likely to complete high school and have steady employment and are more likely to be on public assistance at some point in their lives and to be in unstable marriages. Infants born to adolescent mothers younger than 15 yr old are at greater risk for low birthweight. The children of adolescents experience more problems in school, showing difficulties with cognitive functioning, and have an increased risk of experiencing an accident within the home and of being hospitalized before 5 yr of age. Men who father the children of adolescent mothers are usually 2–3 yr older than the mother and often not teenagers themselves. However, fathers who are adolescents often suffer the same social and economic risks of the teenage mother, with many fewer resources and programs to assist them. Some controversy exists as to whether the social and economic outcomes are a function of maternal age or maternal and family poverty.

Prevention. The reductions in teenage pregnancy rates, although limited, have been attributed to an increase in contraceptive use at first intercourse and a decrease in sexual activity. Although researchers are still actively seeking successful teenage pregnancy interventions, the multifactorial nature of the issue suggests a multilevel approach. On the individual level, postponing sexual involvement until psychosocial maturity guides a more responsible preventive behavior is the principle underlying a number of successful programs. The pediatrician contributes to this strategy through anticipatory guidance. The next level is to provide birth control counseling to adolescents who are sexually active to protect against pregnancy and sexually transmitted disease. On the community level, there needs to be improved access to protective medical measures, with attention to age-appropriate health care delivery models, and the removal of financial barriers to these services. At a societal level, corroborated by the international experience, improved economic opportunities and the enhancement of life options for young women and young men play a pivotal role in achieving positive outcomes related to teenage sexual behavior and the risk of pregnancy and parenthood.

Alan Guttmacher Institute: *Can More Progress Be Made? Teenage Sexual and Reproductive Behavior in Developed Countries.* Executive Summary, 2001. (www.guttmacher.org)

American Academy of Pediatrics, Committee on Adolescence: Counseling the adolescent about pregnancy options. *Pediatrics* 1998;101:938.

Litt IF: Pregnancy in adolescence [Editorial, Comment. *JAMA* 1996;275:1030.

Moore KA, Miller BC, Sugland BW, et al: *Beginning Too Soon: Adolescent Sexual Behavior, Pregnancy and Parenthood.* Washington, DC, Child Trends, 1995.

Polaneczky M, O'Connor K: Pregnancy in the adolescent patient: Screening, diagnosis and initial management. *Pediatr Clin North Am* 1999;46:649.

Romer D, Stanton B, Galbraith J, et al: Parental influence on adolescent sexual behavior in high-poverty settings. *Arch Pediatr Med* 1999;153:1055–62.

Ventura SJ, Mathews TJ, Hamilton BE: *Births to Teenagers in the United States, 1940–2000.* National vital statistics reports; vol 49, no 10. Hyattsville, MD, National Center for Health Statistics, 2001. (www.cdc.gov/nchs/)

Ventura SJ, Mosher WD, Curtin SC, et al: *Trends in Pregnancy Rates for the United States, 1976–97: An update.* National vital statistics reports; vol 49, no 4. Hyattsville, MD, National Center for Health Statistics, 2001. (www.cdc.gov/nchs/)

Chapter 110

Sexually Transmitted Diseases *Renée R. Jenkins*

The behavioral and physiologic characteristics of adolescence predispose sexually active adolescents to the increased acquisition and adverse consequences of sexually transmitted diseases (STDs). When controlled for sexual activity, age-specific rates of many STDs are highest among sexually experienced adolescents. For STD pathogens, intimate sexual contact is the common mode of transmission; however, the clinical expression can be listed according to STD syndromes based on a constellation of clinical signs and symptoms. Different microorganisms are responsible for similar symptoms. Almost all STD pathogens can also infect an adolescent without manifesting any clinical symptoms. The approach to prevention and control of these diseases lies in education, screening, and early diagnosis and treatment. (See chapters discussing specific microorganisms in Part XVI.)

Etiology. The risk of contracting an STD exists in any adolescent who has had sexual intercourse. The risk is increased for specific STDs when certain factors exist. The younger the adolescent at the time of initiation of sexual activity, the higher the risk. Inadequate time to develop decision-making and cognitive skills as well as biologic status contribute to this susceptibility. The use of drugs and alcohol removes inhibitions and contributes to unplanned and unprotected sexual activity. Intravenous drug use, sex with homosexual or bisexual males, and a history of exchanging sex for food, shelter, money, or drugs are all associated with increasing risk for human immunodeficiency virus (HIV) and other serious STDs. Exposure to uncommon sexual pathogens is increased with anal sex. Sex with more than one partner in 6 mo and failure to use condoms consistently are behaviors for which educational interventions may have some impact. Adolescents who are victims of sexual abuse or rape may not consider themselves "sexually active," given the context of the encounter, and need reassurance, protection, and appropriate intervention when these circumstances are uncovered.

Epidemiology. Adolescents and young adults younger than 25 yr of age have the highest reported prevalence of gonorrheal and chlamydial infection. Rates for gonorrhea in the United States are highest for 15–19 yr old females and 20–24 yr old males. They have dropped from 724.7/100,000 to 715.6/100,000 for females and 373/100,000 to 327/100,000 for males, aged 15–19 yr, for 2000 as compared with 1996. For the 20–24 yr olds, the rates have increased during the same period, 21% higher for females and 10.7% higher for males. Chlamydia is the most common bacterial STD in the United States. The year 2000 is the first year that all 50 states and the District of Columbia reported chlamydial infections to the CDC. The rates show a pattern similar to that of gonococcal infections, with the highest rates in 15–19 yr old females and 20–24 yr old males. After peaking in 1990, the rates for primary and secondary syphilis are declining for all ages. Pelvic inflammatory disease (PID) rates are highest in females aged 15–25 yr when compared with older women. AIDS, but not HIV, is reportable in the United States, giving a somewhat skewed perception of a lower rate of infection in adolescents. In 2000, 342 adolescents with AIDS were reported nationwide, whereas 879 adolescents with HIV were reported from the 34 areas that conduct name-based confidential HIV infection surveillance. The lengthy incubation period coupled with a range of smaller seroprevalence studies underscore the serious risk of HIV disease and the impact of its limited reporting for this population.

Pathogenesis. During puberty, increasing levels of estrogen cause the vaginal epithelium to thicken and cornify and the cellular glycogen content to rise, the latter causing vaginal pH to fall. These changes increase the resistance of the vaginal epithelium to penetration by certain organisms (including *Gonococcus*) and increase the susceptibility to others (e.g., *Candida albicans* and *Trichomonas*). The transformation of the vaginal cells leaves columnar cells on the ectocervix, forming a border of the two cell types on the ectocervix, known as the squamocolumnar junction. The appearance is referred to as *ectopy*. With maturation, this tissue involutes. Prior to involution, it represents a unique vulnerability to infection for adolescent females. A 15 yr old sexually active girl with endocervical colonization has a 1:8 chance of developing PID as compared to the 1:80 chance for a 24 yr old. As a result of these physiologic changes, gonococcal infection becomes primarily cervical and susceptibility to ascending infection is greatest during menses, when the pH is 6.8–7.0. Menstruation in an adolescent with endocervical colonization presents a risk factor for the development of PID.

Clinical Manifestations. STD syndromes are generally characterized by the location of the manifestation (vaginitis) or the type of lesion (genital ulcer). In addition, certain constellations of presenting symptoms suggest the inclusion of a possible STD in the differential diagnosis. The syndromes and the conditions suggestive of STDs are listed in Box 110–1.

URETHRITIS. Urethritis is an inflammation of the urethra classically presenting as a urethral discharge or dysuria, or both. Urgency, frequency of urination, erythema of the urethral meatus, and scrotal pain are less common clinical presenta-

---

BOX 110–1. Sexually Transmitted Disease Clinical Syndromes

SEXUALLY TRANSMITTED DISEASE SYNDROMES
Urethritis
Epididymitis
Vaginitis (vulvitis)
Cervicitis
Pelvic inflammatory disease
Genital ulcer disease
Genital lesions and ectoparasites

CONDITIONS SUGGESTIVE OF SEXUALLY TRANSMITTED DISEASE
Lower abdominal pain (female)
Scrotal swelling and pain
Arthritis
Exanthem, alopecia
Pharyngitis
Conjunctivitis
Hepatitis, perihepatitis
Local and generalized lymphadenitis
Proctitis

From Morse SA, Moreland AA, Holmes KK: *Atlas of Sexually Transmitted Diseases and AIDS*, 2nd ed. London, Mosby-Wolfe, 1996.

---

tions. Asymptomatic or minimally symptomatic presentations are common in males. Adolescent males, in particular, are likely to ignore symptoms that improve spontaneously or sometimes ignore obvious physical signs. Consequently, the genital examination should be thorough, including retraction of the foreskin in uncircumcised males, regardless of the denial of symptoms by the adolescent. Examining a patient prior to a urinary void is an important factor in observing a minimally symptomatic discharge. *C. trachomatis* and *Neisseria gonorrhoeae* are the most common pathogens. *Ureaplasma urealyticum* and *Mycoplasma genitalium* are still considered potential pathogens in nongonococcal urethritis, when *Chlamydia* cannot be confirmed. Diagnostic tests for these pathogens are not readily available. *T. vaginalis* and herpes simplex virus (HSV) are considered in the differential diagnosis when nongonococcal urethritis is resistant to treatment. There are classic descriptions of discharges, associating pathogens with color and consistency, e.g., yellow-green purulent discharge for gonococci and white mucopurulent discharge for chlamydia; however, co-infection and other factors can alter the appearance of discharges. Co-infection with gonococcal and chlamydial urethritis is reported in more than 25% of men with urethritis. Consequently, laboratory evaluation is key to determining the involved pathogens.

EPIDIDYMITIS. The inflammation of the epididymis in adolescent males, unlike that in adult males, is most often associated with an STD. The same pathogens associated with urethritis are prevalent. The presentation of scrotal swelling and tenderness, associated with the history of a spontaneously resolving urethral discharge, constitute the presumptive diagnosis of epididymitis. A urethral discharge may still be present at the time of examination. Males who practice insertive anal intercourse are also vulnerable to *Escherichia coli* infection.

VAGINITIS (VULVITIS). Vaginitis is a superficial infection of the vaginal mucosa frequently presenting as a vaginal discharge, with or without vulvar involvement (see Chapter 541). Pruritus and the presence of an odor help differentiate the cause of the infection. Colonization without infection, as in bacterial vaginosis, can also present as a vaginal discharge. Although bacterial vaginosis is no longer categorized strictly as an STD, sexual activity is associated with increased frequency of vaginosis. Trichomoniasis and candidiasis, together with bacterial vaginosis, are the predominant diseases associated with vaginal discharge. The clinical observations of the color, consistency (frothy, floccular, homogeneous), odor, extent of vulvar involvement, and cervical changes lead one to a presumptive diagnosis. However, laboratory confirmation is recommended in determining the presence of one or more infections that may present in an uncharacteristic manner. The differential diagnosis for vaginitis with the classic presentations is presented in Figure 110–1.

CERVICITIS. The inflammatory process in cervicitis involves the deeper structures in the mucous membrane of the cervix uteri. Vaginal discharge can be a manifestation of cervicitis, if the cervical discharge is profuse. Less subtle clinical manifestations of cervicitis are irregular or postcoital bleeding, mucopurulent discharge from the os, and a friable cervix. The cervical changes associated with cervicitis must be distinguished from cervical ectopy in the younger adolescent to avoid the overdiagnosis of inflammation. The pathogens associated most commonly with cervicitis are *C. trachomatis* and *N. gonorrhoeae*, which are responsible for about 50–60% of cases. HSV is a less common pathogen associated with ulcerative and necrotic lesions on the cervix.

PELVIC INFLAMMATORY DISEASE. A spectrum of inflammatory disorders of the upper genital tract in females is encompassed under the diagnosis of PID. The spectrum includes endometritis, salpingitis, tubo-ovarian abscess, and pelvic peritonitis, usually in combination rather than as separate entities. *N. gonorrhoeae* and *C. trachomatis* predominate as the involved pathogenic organisms in younger adolescents; maturation and recurrent disease increase the appearance of other anaerobic and aerobic bacteria such as *Mycoplasma hominis*, group B streptococci, streptococci, *Peptostreptococcus* spp., *Gardnerella vaginalis*, *E. coli*, and various *Bacteroides* spp.

The clinical diagnosis of PID is based on the minimal criteria of lower abdominal tenderness, adnexal tenderness, and cervical motion tenderness in a sexually active female adolescent with no other causes for illness. Although embarrassment may preclude an adolescent's honest answer regarding prior sexual activity, this history should not preclude gathering of evidence

for this possible diagnosis. The presence of a recent increase in dysmenorrhea, onset of symptoms following menses, fever, urinary symptoms, abnormal vaginal bleeding, and abnormal vaginal discharge add support to the clinical diagnosis.

GENITAL ULCER SYNDROMES. An ulcerative lesion in a mucosal area exposed to sexual contact is the unifying characteristic of diseases associated with these syndromes. These lesions are most commonly seen on the penis and vulva, but also occur on oral and rectal mucosa depending on the sexual practices of the adolescent. HSV, *Treponema pallidum* (syphilis), and *Haemophilus ducreyi* (chancroid) are the organisms associated with genital ulcer syndromes. Although the initial herpetic lesion is a vesicle, by the time the patient presents clinically, the vesicle most often has ruptured spontaneously, leaving a shallow, painful ulcer. Of these syndromes, syphilis and chancroid are less common in adolescents than in adults. HSV-2 predominates as the pathogen in this age group, with an increasing incidence of HSV-1 recovered in genital lesions, especially in women. Clinical characteristics differentiating the lesions are presented in Table 110–1, along with the required laboratory diagnosis to identify the causative agent accurately.

GENITAL LESIONS AND ECTOPARASITES. Lesions that present as outgrowths on the surface of the epithelium and other limited epidermal lesions are included under this categorization of syndromes. Human papillomavirus with its association to cervical cancer causes the most concern for the long-term outcome for individuals infected during adolescence (see Chapter 243). Molluscum contagiosum and condyloma lata associated with secondary syphilis complete this classification of syndromes.

HUMAN IMMUNODEFICIENCY VIRUS DISEASE AND HEPATITIS B. HIV and hepatitis B diseases present as asymptomatic, unexpected occurrences in most infected adolescents. Risk factors identified in the history are much more likely to

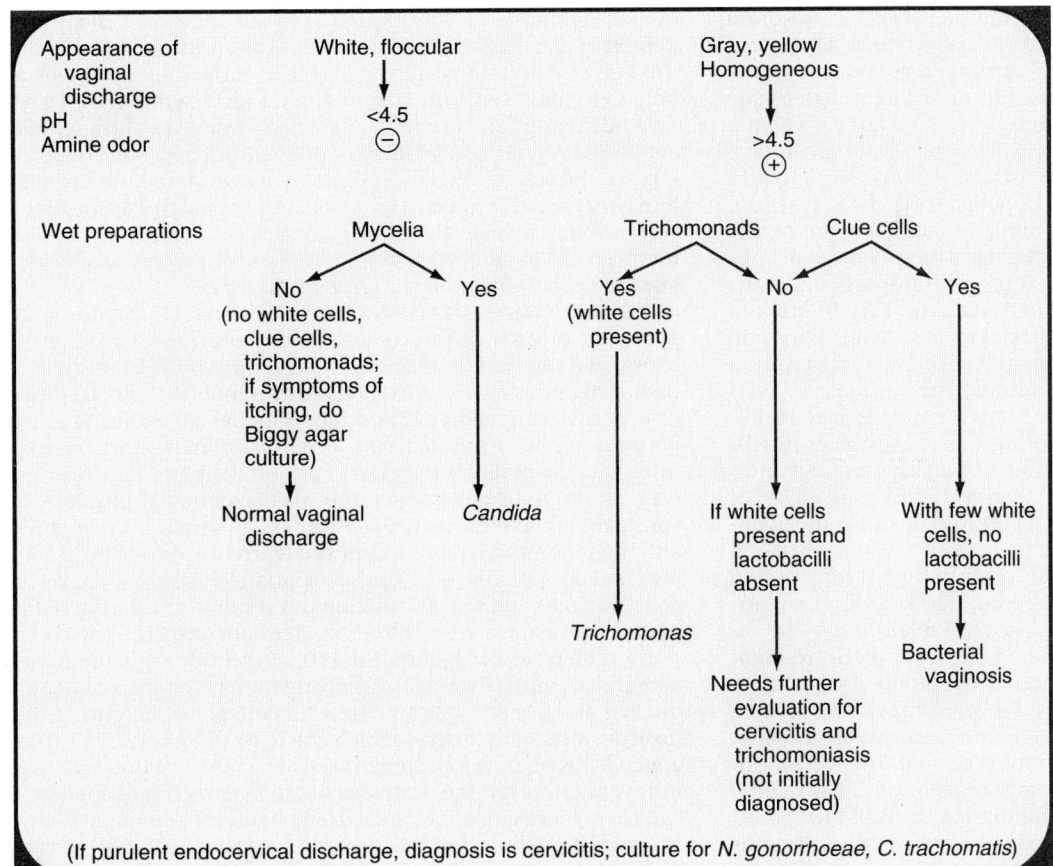

(If purulent endocervical discharge, diagnosis is cervicitis; culture for *N. gonorrhoeae, C. trachomatis*)

FIGURE 110–1. Differential diagnosis of vaginitis. (From Emans SJ, Laufer MR, Goldstein DP [editors]: *Pediatric and Adolescent Gynecology, 4th ed.* Philadelphia, Lippincott-Raven, 1998, p 427.)

TABLE 110–1. Signs, Symptoms, and Presumptive and Definitive Diagnoses of Genital Ulcers

Signs/Symptoms	Herpes Simplex Virus	Syphilis (Primary)	Chancroid
Ulcers	Vesicles rupture to form shallow ulcers	Ulcer with well-demarcated indurated borders and a clean base (chancre)	Unindurated and undermined borders and a purulent base
Painful	Painful	Painless*	Painful
Number of lesions	Usually multiple	Usually single	Multiple
Inguinal lymphadenopathy	First-time infections may cause constitutional symptoms and lymphadenopathy	Usually mild and minimally tender	Unilateral or bilateral painful adenopathy in >50%
			Inguinal bubo formation and rupture may occur
Presumptive diagnosis	Typical lesions plus any of the following: a previously known outbreak, a positive Tzanck smear of lesion scraping, exclusion of other causes of ulcers, or a fourfold increase in acute and convalescent antibody titers (in a first-time infection)	Early syphilis: a typical chancre plus a reactive nontreponemal test (RPR, VDRL) and no history of syphilis or a fourfold increase in a quantitative nontreponemal test in a person with a history of syphilis	Exclusion of other causes of ulcers in the presence of (1) typical ulcers and lymphadenopathy, (2) a typical Gram stain and a history of contact with a high-risk individual (prostitute) or living in an endemic area
Definitive diagnosis	Detection of HSV by culture or nonculture methods (DFA) from ulcer scraping or aspiration of vesicle fluid	Identification T. pallidum, from a chancre or lymph node aspirate, on dark-field microscopy or by DFA	Detection of H. ducreyi by culture

*Primary syphilitic ulcers may be painful if they become co-infected with bacteria or one of the other organisms responsible for genital ulcers.
DFA = direct fluorescent antibody; HSV = herpes simplex virus; RPR = rapid plasma reagin; VDRL = Venereal Disease Research Laboratory.
Data from Centers for Disease Control and Prevention SexuallyTransmitted Disease Clinical Practice Guidelines, May 1991; Centers for Disease Control and Prevention 1993 SexuallyTransmitted DiseaseTreatment Guidelines; and Hoffman I, Schmitz J: Genital ulcers management in the HIV era. Postgrad Med 98:67, 1995.
From Lappa S, Moscicki A:The pediatrician and the sexually active adolescent: A primer for sexually transmitted diseases. Pediatr Clin North Am 44:1430, 1997.

result in suspicion of disease, leading to the appropriate laboratory screening, than are clinical manifestations in this age group.

Diagnosis

ASYMPTOMATIC PATIENTS. Health screening guidelines (see Chapter 100) recommend testing for STDs in asymptomatic patients on an annual basis. Asymptomatic infections with viral pathogens, such as HIV, HSV, and hepatitis B, are the most common presentations for these diseases, whereas asymptomatic infections for chlamydial infection and gonorrhea range from 17–56% and 2–33%, respectively. Adolescent males are more likely to be asymptomatic with chlamydia, whereas adolescent females have a higher rate of asymptomatic gonococcal infections. Urethritis can be documented in an asymptomatic male with a positive leukocyte esterase test on first voided specimen with >10 WBCs per high power field or >5 WBCs per oil immersion field on a Gram stain of urethral secretions. Nucleic acid amplification tests (NAATs) such as polymerase chain reaction, ligase chain reaction, and strand displacement assay are highly recommended for chlamydia screening. Cultures are still preferred for N. gonorrhoeae when holding and transport conditions are adequate to maintain specimen viability. NAATs are not highly recommended for testing rectal swabs. Availability and cost may limit the use of these new tests in some communities. Indirect tests should not be substituted for cultures for STD screening in suspected sexual abuse cases because of the possibility of false-positive results from indirect tests. Advances in HIV testing have also increased opportunities for screening asymptomatic adolescents. Rapid HIV testing with the availability of results in 10–60 min can be useful in settings in which the likelihood of adolescents returning for their results is low, although this does not eliminate the need for confirmatory testing. Based on the preceding observations, the recommendations for screening sexually active adolescents are listed in Table 100–1.

SYMPTOMATIC PATIENTS. Based on the clinical presentation, further evaluations may be needed to identify the causative agent of the syndrome accurately. For urethritis, a Gram stain when a urethral discharge is present confirms the diagnosis of gonorrhea at the time of the presenting symptom. The wet mount is useful in determining the possible pathogen causing a vaginal discharge (see Fig. 110–1). The definitive diagnosis of PID is difficult based on clinical findings alone, and even with an experienced clinician, one third of women are diagnosed incorrectly. In addition to an elevated temperature (>101°F or >38.3°C) and an abnormal cervical or vaginal discharge, the finding of an elevated erythrocyte sedimentation rate or an elevated C-reactive protein level in combination with confirmative laboratory documentation of N. gonorrhoeae or C. trachomatis is recommended to avoid incorrect diagnosis and inappropriate management. Imaging techniques demonstrating thickened fluid-filled fallopian tubes with or without free pelvic fluid or a tubo-ovarian complex are definite criteria. Direct visualization through the laparoscopic technique with cultures from the fallopian tube, while infrequently performed in the United States, is the gold standard for definitive diagnosis. The HSV direct fluorescent antibody test or the herpes culture is readily available in most clinical settings to help determine the pathogen in genital ulcer syndromes. Dark-field microscopy and fluorescent antibody tests to confirm syphilis are less frequently available, with most clinicians relying on serologic confirmation. Tests to confirm the diagnosis of human papillomavirus are discussed in Chapter 243, although Papanicolaou smear often reveals the first evidence of vaginal or cervical involvement in adolescents. Symptomatic or asymptomatic adolescents with STDs should be screened for HIV.

DIFFERENTIAL DIAGNOSES. The differential diagnoses are particular to each of the clinical syndromes. *Reiter's syndrome* is considered an autoimmune response to an STD or enteric pathogen and is characterized by arthritis, nonbacterial urethritis or cervicitis, conjunctivitis, and mucocutaneous lesions. The urinary symptoms associated with urethritis mimic a urinary tract infection, a condition much less common than an STD in adolescent males. Testicular torsion, the main differential diagnosis to consider in scrotal pain, constitutes a surgical emergency, although trauma is a more common occurrence, especially in adolescent males involved in contact sports (see Chapters 538 and 681). Vaginitis and vulvar irritation can result from a foreign body or chemical irritant, for example, bubble bath or spermicide.

The differential diagnosis for PID, presenting as acute lower abdominal pain, is extensive, involving the gastrointestinal, reproductive, and urinary systems. The most emergent differential diagnosis in a sexually active adolescent is to distinguish PID from appendicitis or an ectopic pregnancy, which both require surgical intervention. Given the complexity of the management approach, clinical practice guidelines are extremely useful in moving swiftly and logically to the correct diagnosis (Box 110–2). Most of the conditions in the differential diagnosis of genital ulcerative lesions

BOX 110–2. Uncomplicated Pelvic Inflammatory Disease Clinical Practice Guideline Inclusion Checklist

Patient MUST meet *all* of the following criteria, in the absence of another established cause:
- ☐ lower abdominal pain
- ☐ cervical motion tenderness
- ☐ adnexal tenderness

Patients MUST meet *at least one* of the following criteria:
- ☐ oral temp. > 38.3˚C
- ☐ WBC ≥13,000 K/mm³
- ☐ abnormal cervical or vaginal discharge
- ☐ ESR >20 mm/hr
- ☐ laboratory documentation of cervical infection with *N. gonorrhoeae* or *C. trachomatis*

All patients should have the following as part of the initial evaluation:
- ☐ pelvic examination
- ☐ endocervical culture for *gonorrhoeae*
- ☐ endocervical EIA or culture for chlamydia
- ☐ CBC with differential
- ☐ ESR or C-reactive protein
- ☐ RPR
- ☐ urine βhCG
- ☐ urine dipstick
- ☐ urine culture

The following should be considered:
- ☐ serum βhCG if urine βhCG is negative and suspect ectopic
- ☐ U/S if mass or difficult examination
- ☐ GYN consult immediately if pregnant or if needs U/S
- ☐ surgical consult if suspect appendicitis or other surgical problem

DIFFERENTIAL DIAGNOSIS (partial list):
GI—appendicitis, constipation, diverticulitis, gastroenteritis, IBD, irritable bowel syndrome
GYN—rupture or torsion of ovarian cyst, endometriosis, dysmenorrhea, ectopic pregnancy, mittelschmerz, ruptured follicle, septic or threatened abortion, tubo-ovarian abscess
Urinary tract—cystitis, pyelonephritis, urethritis, nephrolithiasis
- ☐ Check box if patient was placed on the PID clinical practice guideline.

β-hCG = human chorionic gonadotropin; CBC = complete blood count; ESR = erythrocyte sedimentation rate; EIA = enzyme immunoassay; GI = gastrointestinal; GYN = gynecologic; IBD = inflammatory bowel disease; PID = pelvic inflammatory disease; RPR = rapid plasma reagin; U/S = ultrasonography; WBC = white blood cell count.
From Emans SJH, Laufer MR, Goldstein DP (editors): *Pediatric and Adolescent Gynecology*, 4th ed. Philadelphia, Lippincott-Raven, 1998, p 480.

rarely occur in teenagers in the United States (i.e., lymphogranuloma venereum, granuloma inguinale); however, trauma is a common cause that can be detected with a careful history.

Treatment. See Part XVI for chapters on the treatment of specific microorganisms. Treatment regimens using over-the-counter products for *Candida* vaginitis, genital warts, and pediculosis reduce financial and access barriers to rapid treatment for adolescents, but there are potential risks for inappropriate self-treatment and complications from untreated more serious infections that must be considered before using this approach. Minimizing noncompliance with treatment, finding and treating the sexual partner, addressing prevention and contraceptive issues, and making every effort to preserve fertility are additional physician responsibilities. The latter often requires intensive parenteral therapy for PID.

Diagnosis and therapy are often necessarily carried out within the context of a confidential relationship between the physician and the patient. Therefore, the need to report certain sexually transmitted diseases to health department authorities should be clarified at the outset. Most health departments will not violate confidentiality, if assured that treatment and case finding have been accomplished and that the patient can be expected to follow through in a responsible, mature manner.

Prevention. The prevention messages to be communicated to adolescents regarding the avoidance of STDs are in direct contrast to the known risk factors for contracting the disease:

(1) maintaining a healthier sexual behavior, (2) using barrier methods, (3) adopting healthy medical care–seeking behavior, (4) complying with management instruction, and (5) ensuring examination of sexual partners. The elements of maintaining healthier sexual behavior include postponing sexual behavior until *at least* 2–3 yr after menarche, limiting the number of sexual partners, eliciting information about a partner's STD status, inspecting the genitals of sexual partners, and abstaining from sex if STD symptoms develop. The upsurge in sexuality education as a result of the HIV epidemic may have played some role in the increased use of condoms in adolescents (see Chapter 108).

Braverman PK: Sexually transmitted diseases in adolescents. *Med Clin North Am* 2000;84(4):869–89.

Centers for Disease Control and Prevention: Sexually transmitted diseases treatment guidelines 2002. *MMWR* 2002;51(RR-6):1. (www.cdc.gov/nchstp/dstd)

Centers for Disease Control and Prevention: Appendix A: Indications for *Chlamydia trachomatis* testing and test selection specimen type; Appendix B: Indications for *Neisseria gonorrhoeae* testing and test selection specimen type. *MMWR* 2002;51(RR-15):28–33. (www.cdc.gov/mmwr/preview/mmwrhtml/rr5115a3.htm)

Centers for Disease Control and Prevention: *Sexually Transmitted Disease Surveillance, 2000*. Atlanta, GA, U.S. Department of Health and Human Services, Centers for Disease Control and Prevention, September 2001.

Emans SJ, Laufer MR, Goldstein DP (editors): *Pediatric and Adolescent Gynecology*, 4th ed. Philadelphia, Lippincott-Raven, 1998.

Kann L, Kinchen SA, Williams BI, et al: Youth risk behavior surveillance—U.S., 1999. Centers for Disease Control and Prevention. CDC Surveillance Summaries, June 9, 2000. *MMWR* 2000;49(No. SS-5):1.

Neinstein LS: *Adolescent Health Care: A Practical Guide*, 3rd ed. Baltimore, Williams & Wilkins, 1996.

Chapter 111
Chronic Fatigue Syndrome

Hal B. Jenson

Numerous terms (e.g., chronic mononucleosis, chronic Epstein-Barr virus [EBV] infection, and immune dysfunction syndrome) have been applied to the syndrome of easy fatigability associated with mild to debilitating somatic symptoms. This syndrome was formally defined by the Centers for Disease Control and Prevention (CDC) in 1988 as chronic fatigue syndrome because it is fatigue or profound tiredness that is the principal and invariable physical symptom, associated with a variety of physical symptoms and marked and prolonged functional impairment. Chronic fatigue syndrome is neither a new disease nor the result of enhanced appreciation of previously unrecognized clinical illness and is not caused by an identifiable infectious agent, although the differential diagnosis includes many infectious and noninfectious diseases. It is not a single disease with consistent physiologic or pathologic abnormalities but is the subjective experience of symptoms that encompass various clinical conditions of somatic, psychologic, and mixed causes. Current understanding of this condition is largely from studies among adults and adolescents, with limited descriptions of chronic fatigue syndrome in young children.

Epidemiology. Chronic fatigue is a common presenting symptom of adolescents and adults. Approximately 20% of adults in primary care clinics or in surveys complain of chronic fatigue; the incidence in children is unknown. Prevalence rates vary significantly, but chronic fatigue syndrome is encountered in all patient populations. Most patients diagnosed with chronic fatigue syndrome are white, 25–45 yr of age, well educated, high achievers, and in above-average income brackets. These epidemiologic observations may be artifactual because assertive individuals may be less likely to accept being told by their physician that there is nothing physically wrong and are more likely to insist on referral to medical specialists. Women constitute 75% of adult patients. The minimum prevalence in the United States is estimated to be 4–10 cases/100,000 adults 18 yr of age and older. Most cases of chronic fatigue syndrome are sporadic and are not associated with secondary cases. No evidence shows that chronic fatigue syndrome can be transmitted from person to person, in utero to a fetus, or via blood products.

Pathogenesis. The cause of chronic fatigue syndrome is unknown. There is no evidence to support the hypothesis that infection with a known or new virus is the primary cause of the symptoms of chronic fatigue syndrome. Some patients correlate the onset of chronic fatigue syndrome with a history of a virus-like illness such as infectious mononucleosis (EBV) or influenza. In many cases the clinical symptoms of depression, such as fatigue, lack of energy and interest, and inability to concentrate, merge with or are intensified by the weakness often found during convalescence from a systemic infectious disease, resulting in disabling fatigue. Persistent fatigue after an otherwise uncomplicated primary infection is well recognized with many acute infections, especially infectious mononucleosis and influenza. In vulnerable persons, symptoms of fatigue and exhaustion may last for months to a few years and may be accompanied by signs of depression.

Approximately half of adult and adolescent patients fulfill criteria for co-morbid psychiatric disorders, mainly anxiety and depressive disorders. Personality may have special relevance to the predisposition, precipitation, and perpetuation of chronic fatigue. Several studies of convalescence after acute systemic infections support the view that symptomatic recovery is critically dependent on the emotional state and attitude of the individual. Individuals with a propensity to succumb to illness are more likely to respond to acute infection with fatigue and depression-like symptoms than are individuals who do not have such vulnerability.

Up to one half of patients with chronic fatigue syndrome have a concomitant orthostatic intolerance syndrome of circulatory dysfunction including neurally mediated hypotension, instantaneous orthostatic hypotension, and postural tachycardia syndrome. The lightheadedness among patients with chronic fatigue syndrome and orthostatic intolerance appears related to decreased cerebral oxygenated hemoglobin, although factors other than simply reduced cerebral blood flow appear to be operative. Quick control systems of cerebral vasoconstriction such as autonomic reflexes and inhibition of nitric oxide, and increased oxygen consumption by brain tissue have been postulated.

Several diverse and sometimes conflicting in vitro immunologic abnormalities (e.g., hypo- or hypergammaglobulinemia, immunoglobulin subclass deficiencies, elevated levels of circulating immune complexes, mild increased helper/suppressor lymphocyte ratios, natural killer cell dysfunction, monocyte dysfunction) have been reported in patients with chronic fatigue syndrome. A history of food, inhalant, or drug allergy is reported by approximately 67% of patients. No characteristic profile of immune dysfunction has been identified, and the magnitude of the immune abnormalities described is small and does not correlate with the severity of clinical symptoms.

Clinical Manifestations. The symptoms of chronic fatigue syndrome are protean, with a spectrum of gradation from subtle to debilitating. Although the perception of the primary symptom of fatigue is subjective and undoubtedly varies from individual to individual, fatigue as a symptom should not be dismissed as a minor ailment. The syndrome is characterized by numerous somatic complaints of at least 6 mo to several years' duration associated with significant impairment (below 50% of normal) of the work or school schedule, activities of daily living, exercise tolerance, and interpersonal relationships. Fatigue is generally

manifested as lassitude, profound tiredness, weakness, intolerance to exertion with easy fatigability, significant daytime sleeping, and general malaise. Nocturnal sleeping is usually unchanged and does not differ from that of unaffected individuals. Myalgias and low-grade fever in 50–95% of cases characteristically accompany fatigue. Headache and sore throat are common. A multitude of other physical symptoms (e.g., chest palpitations, visual blurring, nausea, dizziness, arthralgias, paresthesias, dry eyes and mouth, diarrhea, cough, night sweats, tender lymphadenopathy, rash) have been reported in 30–60% of cases. Emphasis on one particular physical symptom other than the constitutional symptoms of malaise and fatigability is somewhat uncommon and should prompt further investigation. Weight loss is uncommon in chronic fatigue syndrome. Symptoms of cognitive dysfunction are common and include confusion, difficulty in concentrating, impaired thinking, and forgetfulness. Adult patients often judge these as among the most debilitating symptoms.

Most patients diagnosed with chronic fatigue syndrome relate an abrupt onset to their symptoms, often as part of an initial virus-like illness characterized by low-grade fever accompanied by sore throat and cough. Less frequently, the initial symptoms indicate gastrointestinal tract involvement with nausea and diarrhea. Myalgia is a common symptom.

Symptoms in children appear to be similar to those in adolescents and adults. School absenteeism is a major problem. In a small retrospective study of 23 patients with a median age of 14 yr and a median duration of symptoms of 6 mo, 67% missed 2 wk or more of school and 33% required a home tutor.

Abnormal physical examination findings are conspicuously absent and provide reassurance to both the patient and the physician. Orthostatic intolerance with abnormal heart rate and blood pressure responses to tilt-table testing is common, and impaired cerebral oxygenation measured by near infrared spectroscopy has been documented.

Diagnosis. There are no pathognomonic signs or diagnostic tests for chronic fatigue syndrome; the diagnosis is a clinically defined condition based on inclusionary and exclusionary criteria (Fig. 111–1). Chronic fatigue syndrome in adults is a diagnostic subset of chronic fatigue, a broader category defined as unexplained fatigue of more than 6 mo, which in turn is a subset of prolonged fatigue, which is defined as fatigue lasting more than 1 mo. The diagnostic criteria are applicable to children, with the exception that the required 6 mo duration is too long to be applied to children.

Chronic fatigue syndrome is difficult to diagnose in children, who have trouble describing their symptoms and articulating their concerns. As with any chronic illness in childhood, careful attention must be directed to the family dynamics to identify and resolve family problems or psychopathology that may be contributing to a child's perceptions of his or her symptoms. The diagnosis of chronic fatigue syndrome in a child should be contemplated with caution. Applying the label of chronic fatigue syndrome may delay the diagnosis of a treatable medical illness, avoid the detection of psychologic problems or family dysfunction, and perpetuate inappropriate illness behaviors that may have a profound effect on the child's psychosocial development. Most patients, including children, with chronic fatigue syndrome attribute their symptoms primarily to physical causes and disregard psychologic influences.

The diagnosis of chronic fatigue syndrome can be established only after alternative medical and psychiatric causes of fatigue, many of which are treatable, have been excluded. These include any medical condition that may explain the presence of chronic fatigue, such as untreated hypothyroidism, sleep apnea, narcolepsy, an adverse effect of medication, or severe obesity as defined by a body mass index [body mass index = weight in kg/(height in meters)^2] of 45 or greater. A previously diagnosed

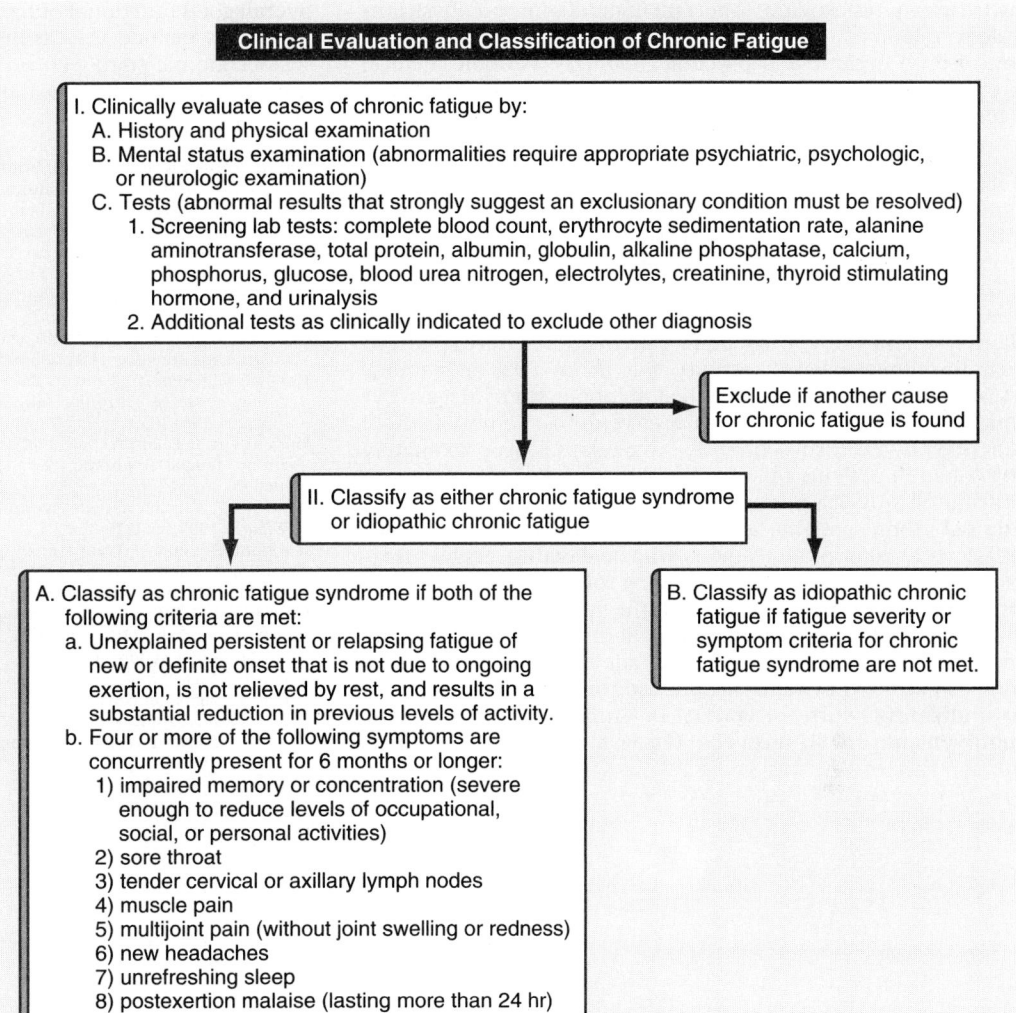

Clinical Evaluation and Classification of Chronic Fatigue

I. Clinically evaluate cases of chronic fatigue by:
   A. History and physical examination
   B. Mental status examination (abnormalities require appropriate psychiatric, psychologic, or neurologic examination)
   C. Tests (abnormal results that strongly suggest an exclusionary condition must be resolved)
      1. Screening lab tests: complete blood count, erythrocyte sedimentation rate, alanine aminotransferase, total protein, albumin, globulin, alkaline phosphatase, calcium, phosphorus, glucose, blood urea nitrogen, electrolytes, creatinine, thyroid stimulating hormone, and urinalysis
      2. Additional tests as clinically indicated to exclude other diagnosis

Exclude if another cause for chronic fatigue is found

II. Classify as either chronic fatigue syndrome or idiopathic chronic fatigue

A. Classify as chronic fatigue syndrome if both of the following criteria are met:
   a. Unexplained persistent or relapsing fatigue of new or definite onset that is not due to ongoing exertion, is not relieved by rest, and results in a substantial reduction in previous levels of activity.
   b. Four or more of the following symptoms are concurrently present for 6 months or longer:
      1) impaired memory or concentration (severe enough to reduce levels of occupational, social, or personal activities)
      2) sore throat
      3) tender cervical or axillary lymph nodes
      4) muscle pain
      5) multijoint pain (without joint swelling or redness)
      6) new headaches
      7) unrefreshing sleep
      8) postexertion malaise (lasting more than 24 hr)

B. Classify as idiopathic chronic fatigue if fatigue severity or symptom criteria for chronic fatigue syndrome are not met.

FIGURE 111–1. The clinical evaluation and classification of unexplained chronic fatigue. The case definition for chronic fatigue syndrome was proposed by the Centers for Disease Control and Prevention in 1988 (Holmes GP, Kaplan JE, Gantz NM, et al: Chronic fatigue syndrome: A working case definition. *Ann Intern Med* 1988;108: 387–9) and refined and simplified by an international working group in 1994 (Fukuda K, Straus SE, Hickie I, et al: The chronic fatigue syndrome: A comprehensive approach to its definition and study. *Ann Intern Med* 1994;121: 953–9).

medical condition with uncertain resolution that may explain chronic fatigue should be clarified, such as unresolved cases of hepatitis B or C virus infection. Chronic fatigue syndrome should not be diagnosed in persons with prior diagnoses of a major depressive disorder with psychotic or melancholic features; bipolar affective disorders; schizophrenia of any subtype; delusional disorders of any subtype; dementias of any subtype; anorexia nervosa; bulimia nervosa; or alcohol or other substance abuse within 2 yr before the onset of the chronic fatigue or at any time afterward.

Fibromyalgia (fibrositis) is a relatively common rheumatic syndrome characterized by symptoms of chronic fatigue syndrome but with widespread musculoskeletal pain in addition to numerous specific tender point sites (see Chapter 158). Fibromyalgia may represent a subset of patients with chronic fatigue syndrome characterized by heightened musculoskeletal symptoms.

Although evaluation of each patient should be individualized, initial laboratory evaluation should be limited to screening laboratory tests to provide reassurance of the lack of significant organic dysfunction (see Fig. 111–1). Further tests should be directed primarily toward excluding treatable diseases that may be suggested by the symptoms or physical findings that are present. Diagnostic evaluation of chronic fatigue should include psychologic evaluation for anxiety and depression disorders, which should precede exhaustive searches for organic causes.

Treatment. Development of definitive treatment for chronic fatigue syndrome awaits delineation of the causes of the symptoms. No specific therapeutic agents are recommended. No data suggest relief of symptoms or cure of chronic fatigue syndrome by dietary or vitamin supplements. Low-dose hydrocortisone is associated with some improvement in symptoms, but the associated adrenal suppression argues against its use. Therapy should be directed toward emotional support for patients and their families, relief of symptoms, and minimizing unnecessary and misleading diagnostic and therapeutic tests. This may include a combination of restoration of a normal sleep pattern, rehabilitation strategies including exercise for fatigue, and optimism. Psychologic or psychiatric intervention is a principal component of treatment if a co-morbid psychiatric disorder is present.

Patients with severe limitation of activity should be started on a schedule of graded remobilization, determined by individual tolerance and, if warranted, physical therapy leading to a regular regimen of moderate exercise. Complete bed rest and lack of exercise only perpetuate immobility and lead to deconditioning; rapid remobilization, for whatever reason, usually exacerbates symptoms and should be avoided. Return to school should also be initiated gradually but systematically to resume normal attendance and socialization. Home tutoring may be an interim alternative. Patients and their families should clearly understand that there is no evidence that activity harms patients with chronic fatigue syndrome. Continued empathy and support by the treating physician are important in maintaining a physician-patient relationship conducive to identification and resolution of both organic and psychologic illness. Periodic medical re-evaluation approximately every 3 mo is warranted for early detection of other identifiable causes of chronic fatigue, especially with interval development of new symptoms.

Prognosis. Chronic fatigue syndrome can persist for years with significant morbidity but no mortality. There are no increased risks of cancer, autoimmune disease, multiple sclerosis, opportunistic infections, or other complications.

The clinical course of chronic fatigue syndrome is highly variable. Patients should be instructed that their symptoms will likely wax and wane. Most adult patients never fully return to their pre-illness level of activity, but about 20% of patients return to their previous state of health for periods of at least 1 yr without any specific medical intervention. Some of these patients, however, subsequently have relapses. Approximately 60% of adult patients report gradual but marked improvement in symptoms over a period of 2–3 yr without specific therapy, although some patients appear to have no improvement or occasionally deteriorate. Patients who deal with stress by somatization and who deny the modulating role of psychosocial factors have a less favorable prognosis. The eventual clinical course is unpredictable, and many adult patients remain functionally impaired for years. Children and adolescents with chronic fatigue appear to have a more optimistic outcome, typically with an undulating course of gradual but substantial symptomatic improvement, or full recovery, 1–4 yr after diagnosis, and an overall good functional outcome in 80% of cases. Poor prognostic factors include increasing time missed from school, lower socioeconomic status, chronic maternal health problems, and untreated co-morbid psychiatric disorder.

Bell DS, Jordan K, Robinson M: Thirteen-year follow-up of children and adolescents with chronic fatigue syndrome. *Pediatrics* 2001;107:994–8.

Carter BD, Edwards JF, Kronenberger WG, et al: Case control study of chronic fatigue in pediatric patients. *Pediatrics* 1995;95:179–86.

Fukuda K, Straus SE, Hickie I, et al: The chronic fatigue syndrome: A comprehensive approach to its definition and study. *Ann Intern Med* 1994;121:953–9.

Gerralda ME, Rangel L: Annotation: Chronic fatigue syndrome in children. *J Child Psychol Psychiatry* 2002;43:169–76.

Krilov LR, Fisher M, Friedman SB, et al: Course and outcome of chronic fatigue in children and adolescents. *Pediatrics* 1998;102:360–6.

Marshall GS: Report of a workshop of the epidemiology, natural history, and pathogenesis of chronic fatigue syndrome in adolescents. *J Pediatr* 1999;134:395–405.

McKenzie R, O'Fallon A, Dale J, et al: Low-dose hydrocortisone for treatment of chronic fatigue syndrome. A randomized controlled trial. *JAMA* 1998;280:1061–6.

Plioplys AV: Chronic fatigue syndrome should not be diagnosed in children. *Pediatrics* 1997;100:270–1.

Schondorf R, Benoit J, Wein T, et al: Orthostatic intolerance in the chronic fatigue syndrome. *J Auton Nerv Syst* 1999;75:192–201.

Smith MS, Mitchell J, Corey L, et al: Chronic fatigue in adolescents. *Pediatrics* 1991;88:195–9.

Stewart JM, Gewitz MH, Weldon A, et al: Orthostatic intolerance in adolescent chronic fatigue syndrome. *Pediatrics* 1999;103:116–21.

Tanaka H, Matsushima R, Tamai H, et al: Impaired postural cerebral hemodynamics in young patients with chronic fatigue with and without orthostatic intolerance. *J Pediatr* 2002;140:412–7.

Wright J, Beverley DW: Chronic fatigue syndrome. *Arch Dis Child* 1998;79:368–74.

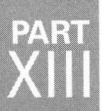

PART XIII

The Immunologic System and Disorders

SECTION 1 *Evaluation of the Immune System*

Rebecca H. Buckley

Chapter 112

Evaluation of Suspected Immunodeficiency

Children with recurrent infections are among the most frequent types of patients seen by primary care physicians. The number of pediatric patients suspected of having primary or secondary immunodeficiency far exceeds the actual number of cases despite the emergence of the human immunodeficiency virus (HIV) epidemic. Most patients with recurrent infections do not have an identifiable immunodeficiency disorder. A major reason for the apparent high rate of recurrent infections is excessive exposure of infants or children to infectious agents in out-of-home child care and other group settings. In addition, excessive use of antibiotics by physicians has masked the classic presentation of many of the primary immunodeficiency diseases.

Primary care physicians must have a high index of suspicion if defects of the immune system are to be diagnosed early enough that appropriate treatment can be instituted before there is irreversible damage. This problem is made more difficult because none of these defects are screened for currently in the perinatal period or later in childhood, and there is widespread use of antibiotics for respiratory infections, which can mask genetic defects in the immune system. Evaluation of immune function should be initiated for children with clinical manifestations of a specific immune disorder or with unusual, chronic, or recurrent infections such as (1) two or more systemic or serious bacterial infections (e.g., sepsis, osteomyelitis, or meningitis); (2) three or more serious respiratory or documented bacterial soft tissue infections (e.g., cellulitis, draining otitis media, or lymphadenitis) within 1 yr; (3) infections occurring at unusual sites (e.g., liver or brain abscess); (4) infections with unusual pathogens (e.g., *Aspergillus, Serratia marcescens, Nocardia,* or *Burkholderia cepacia*); and (5) infections with common childhood pathogens but of unusual severity.

The screening tests selected for immunologic evaluation should be broadly informative, reliable, and cost effective. Familiarity with certain clinical guidelines aids in the initial selection of tests. Patients with deficiencies of antibodies, phagocytic cells, or complement have recurrent infections with encapsulated bacteria. Thus, patients with only repeated viral infections (with the exception of persistent enterovirus infections) are not as likely to have any of these disorders. Children with defects in antibody production, phagocytic cells, or complement proteins may grow and develop normally despite their recurrent infections unless they develop bronchiectasis from repeated lower respiratory tract bacterial infections or have persistent enteroviral infections of the central nervous system. By contrast, patients with deficiencies in T-cell function usually develop opportunistic infections early in life and fail to thrive.

The initial evaluation of immunocompetence includes a thorough history, physical examination, and family history. Most immunologic defects can be excluded at minimal cost with the proper choice of screening tests (Table 112–1). A complete blood count (CBC), manual differential count, and erythrocyte sedimentation rate (ESR) are among the most cost-effective screening tests. If the ESR is normal, chronic bacterial or fungal infection is unlikely. If an infant's neutrophil count is persistently elevated in the absence of any signs of infection, a leukocyte adhesion deficiency should be suspected. If the absolute neutrophil count is normal, congenital and acquired neutropenia and leukocyte adhesion defects are excluded. If the absolute lymphocyte count is normal, the patient is not likely to have a severe T-cell defect. Normal lymphocyte counts are higher in infancy and early childhood than later in life. For example, at 9 mo of age—an age when infants affected with severe T-cell immunodeficiency are likely to present—the lower limit of normal is 4,500 lymphocytes/mm^3 (Chapter 710). Examination of red cells for Howell-Jolly bodies helps exclude congenital asplenia. If the platelet count is normal or platelet size is normal, Wiskott-Aldrich syndrome is excluded. If a CBC and a manual differential were performed on the cord blood of all infants, severe combined immunodeficiency (SCID) could be detected at birth, and lifesaving immunologic reconstitution could then be given to all such infants.

TABLE 112–1. **Initial Immunologic Testing of the Child with Recurrent Infections**

Complete Blood Count, Manual Differential, and Erythrocyte Sedimentation Rate

Absolute lymphocyte count (normal result [Chapter 710] makes T-cell defect unlikely)
Absolute neutrophil count (normal result [Chapter 710] precludes congenital or acquired neutropenia and (usually) both forms of leukocyte adhesion deficiency, in which elevated counts are present even between infections)
Platelet count (normal result excludes Wiskott-Aldrich syndrome)
Howell-Jolly bodies (presence suggests asplenia)
Erythrocyte sedimentation rate (normal result indicates chronic bacterial or fungal infection unlikely)

Screening Tests for B-Cell Defects

IgA measurement; if abnormal, IgG and IgM measurement
Isohemagglutinins
Antibody titers to tetanus, diphtheria, *H. influenzae,* and *S. pneumoniae*

Screening Tests for T-Cell Defects

Absolute lymphocyte count (normal result indicates T-cell defect unlikely)
Candida albicans intradermal skin test: 0.1 mL of a 1:1,000 dilution for patients older than 6 yr, 0.1 mL of a 1:100 dilution for patients younger than 6 yr

Screening Tests for Phagocytic Cell Defects

Absolute neutrophil count
Respiratory burst assay

Screening Test for Complement Deficiency

CH$_{50}$

Patients with abnormalities on any screening tests should be characterized as fully as possible before any type of immunologic treatment is begun unless there is a life-threatening illness. Some "abnormalities" may prove to be laboratory artifacts, and conversely, what may appear to be a straightforward diagnosis may prove to be a much more complex disorder. If results of the initial screening including the CBC and manual differential, immunoglobulin levels, and complement levels are normal, evaluations of T-cell and phagocytic cell functions may be indicated for patients with recurrent or unusual bacterial infections.

B Cells. The presence and titer of antibodies to type A and B red blood cell polysaccharide antigens (isohemagglutinins) is used as a simple screening test. As assayed in most blood banks, this test measures predominantly IgM antibodies. However, isohemagglutinins may be normally absent in the first 2 yr of life and are always absent if the patient is blood type AB. Because most infants and children have received diphtheria-tetanus-pertussis (DTaP), *Haemophilus influenzae* type b (Hib), and conjugate pneumococcal immunizations, it is informative to test for antibodies to diphtheria, tetanus, *H. influenzae* polyribose phosphate, and pneumococcal antigens. If the titers are low, measurement of antibodies to diphtheria or tetanus toxoids before and 2 wk after a pediatric DT booster is helpful in assessing the capacity to form IgG antibodies to protein antigens. To evaluate a patient's ability to respond to polysaccharide antigens, pneumococcal antibodies can be measured before and 3 wk after immunization with the polysaccharide pneumococcal vaccine in patients older than 2 yr. Antibodies detected in these tests are of the IgG isotype. These antibody studies can be performed in many laboratories but it is important to choose a reliable laboratory and to use the same laboratory to test before and after the booster.

Patients with significant or permanent B-cell defects do not produce either IgM or IgG antibodies normally. However, the finding of normal IgM and IgG antibody levels does not preclude IgA deficiency, transient hypogammaglobulinemia of infancy, or protein-losing states. Selective IgA deficiency, the most common B-cell defect, can be excluded by measuring serum IgA. If the IgA concentration is normal, most of the permanent types of hypogammaglobulinemia are also excluded, inasmuch as IgA is usually very low or absent in those conditions as well. If IgA is low, IgG and IgM should also be measured. Patients who are receiving corticosteroids or who have protein-losing states (e.g., nephrosis, protein-losing enteropathy) often have low IgG concentrations but make antibodies normally. Very high serum concentrations of one or more immunoglobulin classes suggest HIV infection or chronic granulomatous disease.

IgG subclass measurements are seldom helpful in assessing immune function in children with recurrent infections. It is difficult to discern the biologic significance of the various mild to moderate deficiencies of IgG subclasses, particularly when completely asymptomatic individuals have been described as totally lacking IgG1, IgG2, IgG4, and/or IgA1 owing to immunoglobulin heavy chain gene deletions. Moreover, a number of healthy children have been described as having low levels of IgG2 but normal responses to polysaccharide antigens when immunized. When children with low IgG2 subclass levels and histories of frequent infections were studied in depth, they were found to have broader immunologic dysfunction, including poor responses to protein antigens as well, suggesting that their condition may have been in the process of developing into common variable immunodeficiency (CVID). Only when antibody deficiencies are detected despite normal levels of immunoglobulins are IgG subclass measurements occasionally helpful. Children who completely lack IgG2 are usually unable to make antibodies to polysaccharide antigens; however, this can be true even in those with normal IgG2 levels. Thus, antibody measurements are far more cost effective than IgG subclass determinations.

Patients found to be agammaglobulinemic should have their blood B cells enumerated by flow cytometry using dye-conjugated monoclonal antibodies to B cell–specific CD antigens, usually CD19 or CD20. Normally, approximately 10% of circulating lymphocytes are B cells. In X-linked agammaglobulinemia (XLA) such cells are missing, whereas in CVID, IgA deficiency, and hyper IgM syndromes, B cells are usually present. This distinction is important because children with hypogammaglobulinemia from XLA and CVID can have different clinical problems, and the two conditions have different inheritance patterns. Patients with XLA have a heightened susceptibility to persistent enteroviral infections, whereas those with CVID have more problems with autoimmune diseases and lymphoid hyperplasia. Specific molecular diagnostic tests for XLA (Chapter 114.1) are necessary in cases without a family history to aid genetic counseling. Molecular testing is also indicated in other defects.

If results of all antibody tests prove to be normal and the immunoglobulins remain low, studies should be performed to confirm that the immunoglobulins are not being lost through the urinary or gastrointestinal tracts, such as occurs in nephrotic syndrome, protein-losing enteropathies, or intestinal lymphangiectasia.

T Cells. The *Candida* skin test is the most cost-effective test of T-cell function. Adults and children older than 6 yr should be tested intradermally with 0.1 mL of a 1:1,000 dilution of a known potent *Candida albicans* extract. If the test result is negative at 24, 48, and 72 hr, a 1:100 dilution should be tested. The latter concentration can be used in the initial testing of children under 6 yr. If the test result is positive, as defined by erythema and induration of greater than 10 mm at 48 hr and the reaction is greater than at 24 hr, virtually all primary T-cell defects are precluded, which obviates the need for more expensive in vitro tests, such as lymphocyte phenotyping or assessments of responses to mitogens.

T cells and T-cell subpopulations can be enumerated by flow cytometry using dye-conjugated monoclonal antibodies recognizing CD antigens present on T cells, such as CD2, CD3, CD4, and CD8. This is a particularly important test to perform on any infant who is lymphopenic, because SCID is a pediatric emergency that can be successfully treated by bone marrow transplantation in more than 95% of cases if diagnosed before untreatable infections develop. CD3 T cells usually constitute 70% of peripheral lymphocytes. Normally there are roughly twice as many CD4 (helper) T cells as there are CD8 (cytotoxic) T cells. Because there are examples of severe immunodeficiency in which phenotypically normal T cells are present, tests of T-cell function are far more informative and cost effective than enumeration of T-cell subpopulations by flow cytometry. T cells are normally stimulated through their T-cell receptors (TCRs) by antigen present in the groove of major histocompatibility complex (MHC) molecules; however, the TCR can also be stimulated directly with mitogens such as phytohemagglutinin (PHA), concanavalin A (Con A), or pokeweed mitogen (PWM). After a 3–5-day period of incubation with the mitogen, the proliferation of T cells is measured by the incorporation of radiolabeled thymidine into DNA. Other stimulants that can be used to assess T-cell function in the same type of assay include antigens (e.g., *Candida* or tetanus toxoid) and allogeneic cells. Additional assays of T-cell function include the measurement of cytokine production by T lymphocytes stimulated with mitogens (see Box 113–1).

Phagocytic Cells. Killing defects of phagocytic cells, which should be suspected if a patient has recurrent staphylococcal abscesses or gram-negative infections, can be evaluated by screening tests measuring the neutrophil respiratory burst after phorbol ester stimulation. The most reliable and useful test of this type is a flow cytometry assessment of the respiratory burst using rhodamine dye; this test has replaced the previously used nitroblue tetrazolium (NBT) dye test, which had technical problems with reproducibility. Leukocyte adhesion deficiencies can be easily diagnosed by flow cytometry assays of blood lymphocytes or neutrophils, using monoclonal antibodies to CD18 or CD11 (LAD1) or to CD15 (LAD2).

Natural killer (NK) cells can be enumerated by flow cytometry using monoclonal antibodies to NK-specific CD antigens, usually CD16 or CD56. NK function is assessed by a radiolabeled chromium-release assay using the K562 human erythroleukemia cell line as target cells, which are readily killed by NK cells.

Phagocytic cell defects can be further defined according to their molecular cause. Mutations in the genes encoding four different components of the electron transport chain have been discovered in various patients with chronic granulomatous disease (CGD). It is important to identify which molecular type of CGD is present as a basis for genetic counseling (one type is X linked, and the other three types are autosomal recessive), prenatal diagnosis, and the eventual prospect of gene therapy. In the case of the leukocyte adhesion deficiencies, early diagnosis is of crucial importance because bone marrow transplantation can be lifesaving. A confirmatory test for LAD1 (if flow cytometry suggests that defect) is NK cell function, because the lack of adhesion molecules prevents the NK cells of such patients from attaching to the target cells.

Complement. The most effective screening test for complement defects is the CH_{50} assay, a bioassay that measures the intactness of the entire complement pathway and yields abnormal results if complement has been consumed from the specimen for any reason. Genetic deficiencies in the complement system are usually characterized by extremely low CH_{50} values. However, the most common cause of an abnormal CH_{50} result is a delay in or improper transport of the specimen to the laboratory. Specific immunoassays for C3 and C4 are commercially available, but further identification of other complement component deficiencies is usually possible only in research laboratories. Nevertheless, it is extremely important to identify which component is missing, because there are different disease susceptibilities depending on whether there are deficiencies of early or late components. Identifying the mode of inheritance is also important for genetic counseling. Properdin deficiency is X linked, but all of the other complement deficiencies are autosomal. Measurement of C4 can be helpful in assessing suspected hereditary angioedema.

Altman PL: Blood leukocyte values: Man. In Dittmer DS (editor): *Blood and Other Body Fluids.* Washington DC, Federation of American Societies for Experimental Biology, 1961.

Fleisher TA: Evaluation of the potentially immunodeficient patient. *Adv Intern Med* 1996;41:1–30.

Heffelfinger JD, Davis TE, Gebrian B, et al: Evaluation of children with recurrent pneumonia diagnosed by World Health Organization criteria. *Pediatr Infect Dis J* 2002;21:108–12.

Holland SM, Gallin JI: Evaluation of the patient with recurrent bacterial infections. *Annu Rev Med* 1998;49:185–99.

Johnston RB: Recurrent bacterial infections in children. *N Engl J Med* 1984;310:1237–43.

Primary immunodeficiency diseases. Report of an IUIS Scientific Committee. International Union of Immunological Societies. *Clin Exp Immunol* 1999;118:1–28.

Shannon DC, Johnson G, Rosen FS: Cellular reactivity to *Candida albicans* antigen. *N Engl J Med* 1966;275:690–3.

SECTION 2 *The T-, B-, and NK-Cell Systems*

Rebecca H. Buckley

Chapter 113

T Lymphocytes, B Lymphocytes, and Natural Killer Cells

Bodily defense against infectious agents is secured through a combination of physical barriers, including the skin, mucous membranes, mucous blanket, and ciliated epithelial cells, and the various components of the immune system. The immune system consists of T lymphocytes, B lymphocytes, natural killer (NK) cells, dendritic and phagocytic cells, and complement proteins. The immune system also serves to protect against autoimmune diseases and malignancy.

LYMPHOPOIESIS IN THE FETUS

Origin of the Lymphoid System. The human immune system arises in the embryo from gut-associated tissue. Pluripotential hematopoietic stem cells first appear in the yolk sac at 2.5–3 wk of gestational age and migrate to the fetal liver at 5 wk of gestation; they later reside in the bone marrow, where they remain throughout life (Fig. 113–1). Lymphoid stem cells develop from such precursor cells and differentiate into T, B, or NK cells, depending on the organs or tissues to which the stem cells traffic. Primary lymphoid organ (thymus and bone marrow) development begins during the middle of the first trimester of gestation and proceeds rapidly; secondary lymphoid organ (spleen, lymph nodes, tonsils, Peyer patches, and lamina propria) development soon follows. These organs continue to serve as sites of differentiation of T, B, and NK lymphocytes from stem cells throughout life. Both the initial organogenesis and the continued cell differentiation occur as a consequence of the interaction of a vast array of lymphocytic and microenvironmental cell surface molecules and proteins secreted by the involved cells. The complexity and number of such cell surface molecules led to the development of an international nomenclature and classification of these differentiation antigens, which are now referred to as **clusters of differentiation (CD)** (Table 113–1).

T and B lymphocytes are the only components of the immune system that have antigen-specific recognition capabilities; they are responsible for adaptive immunity. NK cells are lymphocytes that are also derived from hematopoietic stem cells and are thought to have a role in host defense against viral infections, tumor surveillance, and immune regulation. The proteins synthesized and secreted by T, B, and NK cells, and by the cells with which they interact, are referred to as **cytokines**. Several such

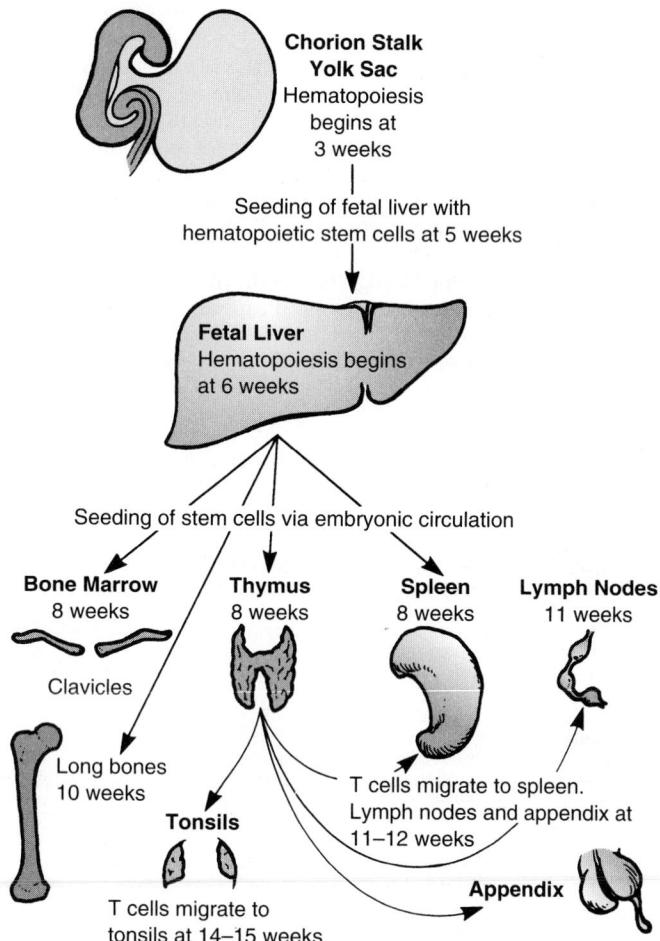

Chorion Stalk Yolk Sac
Hematopoiesis begins at 3 weeks

Seeding of fetal liver with hematopoietic stem cells at 5 weeks

Fetal Liver
Hematopoiesis begins at 6 weeks

Seeding of stem cells via embryonic circulation

Bone Marrow
8 weeks

Clavicles

Long bones
10 weeks

Thymus
8 weeks

Spleen
8 weeks

Lymph Nodes
11 weeks

T cells migrate to spleen.
Lymph nodes and appendix at
11–12 weeks

Tonsils

Appendix

T cells migrate to
tonsils at 14–15 weeks

FIGURE 113–1. Migration patterns of hematopoietic stem cells and mature lymphocytes during human fetal development. (From Haynes BF, Denning SM: Lymphopoiesis. In Stamatoyannopoulis G, Nienhuis A, Majerus P, Varmus H [editors]: *Molecular Basis of Blood Diseases*, 2nd ed. Philadelphia, WB Saunders, 1994.)

proteins have been given an official nomenclature as **interleukins (ILs)** (Box 113–1). Cytokines have the ability to act in an autocrine, paracrine, or endocrine manner to promote and facilitate differentiation and proliferation of the cells of the immune system.

T-Cell Development and Differentiation. The primitive thymic rudiment is formed from the ectoderm of the third branchial cleft and endoderm of the third branchial pouch at 4 wk gestation. Beginning at 7–8 wk, the right and left rudiments move caudally and fuse in the midline. Blood-borne T-cell precursors from the fetal liver then begin to colonize the perithymic mesenchyme at 8 wk gestation. These precursor **pro-T cells** are identified by surface proteins designated as CD7 and CD34. At 8–8.5 wk gestation, CD7 cells are found intrathymically, and some cells also co-express CD4, a protein present on the surfaces of mature T-helper (TH) cells, and CD8, a protein found on both mature cytotoxic cells and NK cells. In addition, some cells bear single T-cell receptor (TCR, Ti) chains (ß, δ, or γ) but none bear complete TCRs.

The mature TCR is a heterodimer of two chains, either α and ß or γ and δ; it is co-expressed on the cell surface with CD3, a complex of five polypeptide chains (γ, δ, ε, ζ, η). TCR gene rearrangement occurs by a process in which large, noncontiguous blocks of DNA are spliced together. These segments, known as **V (variable), D (diversity)**, and **J (joining)**, each have a number of variants. VDJ segments are joined to a constant region of the α gene, and VJ segments are joined to the ß gene to complete the receptor polypeptide genes. Random combinations of the segments account for much of the enormous diversity of TCRs that enables humans to recognize millions of different antigens. TCR gene rearrangement requires the presence of **recombinase activating genes**, referred to as RAG-1 and RAG-2, as well as other recombinase components. This process is flawed in mice with severe combined immunodeficiency (SCID) and in some humans with SCID. Rearrangement of TCR genes signifies commitment of pro-T cells to T-lineage development—that is, to become pre-T cells. TCR gene rearrangement begins shortly after colonization of the thymus with stem cells, and the establishment of the T-cell repertoire begins at 8–10 wk of gestation. By 9.5–10 wk, more than 95% of thymocytes express CD7, CD2, CD4, CD8, and c(cytoplasmic) CD3, and approximately 30% bear the CD1 inner cortical thymocyte antigen. By 10 wk, 25%

TABLE 113–1. **CD Classification of Some Lymphocyte Surface Molecules**

CD Number	Other Names	Tissue/Lineage	Function
CD1	T6	Cortical thymocytes; Langerhans cells	Antigen presentation to TCRγδ cells
CD2	SRBC receptor	T and NK cells	Binds LFA-3 (CD58); alternative pathway of T cell activation
CD3	T3, Leu 4	T cells	TCR-associated; transduces signals from TCR
CD4	T4, Leu3a	Helper T cell subset	Receptor for HLA class II antigens; associated with p56 *lck* tyrosine kinase
CD7	3A1, Leu 9	T and NK cells and their precursors	Co-mitogenic for T lymphocytes
CD8	T8, Leu2a	Cytotoxic T cell subset; also on 30% of NK cells	Receptor for HLA class I antigens; associated with p56 *lck* tyrosine kinase
CD10	cALLA	B cell progenitors	Peptide cleavage
CD11a	LFA-1a α chain	T, B, and NK cells	With CD 18, ligand for ICAMS 1, 2, and 3
CD11b,c	MAC-1,CR3; CR4	NK cells	With CD18, receptors for C3bi
CD16	FcRγIII	NK cells	FcR for IgG
CD19	B4	B cells	Regulates B cell activation
CD20	B1	B cells	Mediates B cell activation
CD21	B2	B cells	C3d and the EBV receptor; CR2
CD34	My10	Precursor cells	Unknown
CD40	CD40	B cells and monocytes	Initiates isotype switching when ligated
CD45	Leukocyte common antigen, T200	All leukocytes	Tyrosine phosphatase that regulates lymphocyte activation; CD45R0 isoform on memory T cells, CD45RA isoform on naive T cells
CD56	N-CAM; NKH-1	NK cells	Mediates NK homotypic adhesion
CD154	CD40 ligand, gp39	Activated CD4 T cells	Ligates CD40 on B cells and initiates isotype switching

CD = clusters of differentiation.

BOX 113–1. Functional Classification of Cytokines*

CYTOKINES INVOLVED IN NATURAL IMMUNE RESPONSES

Type I interferons—IFN-α and IFN-β—inhibit viral replication, inhibit cell proliferation, activate NK cells, upregulate class I MHC molecule expression

TNF-α—mediates host response to gram-negative bacteria and other infectious agents

IL1α and -β—mediate host inflammatory response to infectious agents

IL1Rα—is a natural antagonist of IL1, blocks signals delivered by IL1

IL6—mediates and regulates inflammatory responses

Chemokines (IL8, monocyte chemotactic protein-1 or MCP-1, RANTES, and others)—mediate leukocyte chemotaxis and activation

LYMPHOCYTE REGULATORY CYTOKINES

Immunostimulatory or Growth-Promoting

IL1—co-stimulates activation of T cells

IL2—growth factor for T, B, NK cells; activates effector cells

IL4—T and B cell growth factor; stimulates IgE production; upregulates class I and II MHC molecule and FcRεII expression on macrophages; expansion of T_H2 subset

IL5—B cell growth and activation

IL6—growth factor for B cells

IL7—stromal cell factor; growth factor for precursor B and T cells, T cell homeostatic factor

IL10—growth and differentiation factor for B cells

IL9—growth factor for T cells, B cells, mast cells, eosinophils, neutrophils, endothelial cells

IL12—expansion of T_H1 subset; activates effector cells

IL13—growth and differentiating factor for B cells; stimulates IgE production; upregulates class I and II MHC molecule and FcRεII expression on macrophages

TNF-β—stimulates effector cell function

IL15—growth factor for NK cells

IL18—induces IFN-γ, GM-CSF, TNF-α in immunocompetent cells

IFN-γ—activates macrophages, NK cells; upregulates class I and II MHC molecule expression; inhibits IL4-or IL13-induced IgE production

Immunosuppressive

IL1Rα—regulates IL1 activities

TGF-β—antagonizes lymphocyte responses

IL10—inhibits activities of T_H1 cells

IFNα/β—inhibits production of IFNγ

HEMATOPOIESIS REGULATING CYTOKINES

GM-CSF, G-CSF, M-CSF—colony stimulating factors

Erythropoietin (EPO)—differentiation of erythroid precursors

IL3, SCF, c-kit receptor—regulate stem cell development

IL4—mast cell development

IL5—eosinophil differentiation and proliferation

IL6—differentiation of B cells

IL7—differentiation of B and T cells

IL8—promotes cell survival in response to hematopoietic cytokines

IL11—elevates platelet count in patients given chemotherapy

IL12—expands and activates resting NK cells

IL15—expands and activates resting NK cells

IL21—limits viability of NK cells

PRO-INFLAMMATORY CYTOKINES

IL1, TNF-α, IL6—participate in the acute-phase response and synergize to mediate inflammation, shock, and death

IL12—stimulates INFγ production by T and NK cells

IL17—recruitment and activation of airway neutrophils via chemokines

IL18—induces IFN-γ, GM-CSF, TNFα and upregulates chemokine receptors

ANTI-INFLAMMATORY CYTOKINES

IL4—reduces endotoxin-induced TNF and IL1 production

IL6—inhibits TNF production

IL10—suppresses lymphocyte functions and downregulates production of pro-inflammatory cytokines; anti-atherogenic

IL11—cytoprotective effect on bowel mucosa, skin, and joint inflammation

IL13—downregulates functions of macrophages, suppresses production of proinflammatory cytokines

TGF-β—has immunosuppressive effects, inhibits IL1 and TNF gene expression

IL1Rα—competes with the binding of IL1 to its cell surface receptors and blocks IL1R

TNFsR—soluble TNF receptors, by binding TNF, block interaction of TNF with the target cell

---

IL = interleukin; MHC = major histocompatibility complex; NK = natural killer; SCF = stem cell factor; TNF = tumor necrosis factor.

*This is not an exhaustive list.

Modified from Whiteside TL: Cytokine measurements and interpretation of cytokine assays in human disease. *J Clin Immunol* 1994;14:327–9.

---

of thymocytes bear αβ TCRs. Ti αβ T cells gradually increase in number during embryonic life and represent more than 95% of thymocytes postnatally.

As immature cortical thymocytes begin to express TCRs, the processes of positive and negative selection take place. **Positive selection** occurs through the interaction of immature thymocytes (which express low levels of TCR) with major histocompatibility complex (MHC) antigens present on cortical thymic epithelial cells. As a result, thymocytes with TCR capable of interacting with foreign antigens presented on self MHC antigens are activated and develop to maturity. Mature thymocytes that survive the selection process either express CD4 and are restricted to self class II HLA antigens or express CD8 and are restricted to self class I HLA antigens when they interact with foreign antigens presented by these MHC molecules. **Negative selection** occurs next and is mediated by interaction of the surviving thymocytes, which have much higher levels of TCR expression, with host peptides presented by HLA class I or II antigens present on bone marrow–derived thymic macrophages, dendritic cells, and possibly B cells. This interaction mediates programmed cell death of such autoreactive thymocytes by a process called **apoptosis**. Fetal cortical thymocytes are among the most rapidly dividing cells in the body; they increase in number by 100,000-fold within 2 wk after stem cells enter the thymus. As these cells mature, the previously mentioned selec-

tion process takes place, and as a consequence, 97% of all cortical thymocytes die. The surviving cells are no longer doubly positive for both CD4 and CD8 but are singly positive for either one or the other, and they migrate to the medulla.

T-cell functions are acquired concomitantly with the development of single-positive thymocytes, but they are not fully developed until the cells emigrate from the thymus. It has been estimated that one stem cell gives rise to approximately 3,000 mature medullary thymocytes. Such medullary cells are resistant to the lytic effects of corticosteroids. T cells begin to emigrate from the thymus to the spleen, lymph nodes, and appendix at 11–12 wk of embryonic life and to the tonsils by 14–15 wk. They leave the thymus via the bloodstream and are distributed throughout the body, with heaviest concentrations in the paracortical areas of lymph nodes, the periarteriolar areas of the spleen, and the thoracic duct lymph. Recent thymic emigrants co-express the CD45RA isoforms and CD62L (L-selectin). Rearrangement of the TCR locus during this process leads to the formation of circular episomes as a by-product. These signal joint TCR recombination excision circles (TRECs) can be detected in T cells that are recent thymic emigrants, whereas T cells that develop extrathymically do not contain these episomes. The homing of lymphocytes to peripheral lymphoid organs is directed by the interaction of a lymphocyte surface adhesion molecule, L-selectin, with carbohydrate moieties on specialized regions of lymphoid organ blood vessels, called high endothelial venules. By 12 wk gestation, T cells can proliferate in response to plant lectins, such as phytohemagglutinin (PHA) and concanavalin A (Con A), and to allogeneic cells; antigen-binding T cells have been found by 20 wk gestation. Hassall corpuscles (bodies), which are swirls of terminally differentiated medullary epithelial cells, are first seen in the thymic medulla at 16–18 wk of embryonic life.

B-Cell Development and Differentiation. In parallel with T-cell differentiation, B-cell development begins in the fetal liver before 7 wk gestation. Fetal liver CD34 stem cells are seeded to the bone marrow of the clavicles by 8 wk of embryonic life and to that of the long bones by 10 wk (see Fig. 113–1). **Antigen-independent** stages of B-cell development have been defined according to immunoglobulin gene rearrangement patterns and the surface proteins the cells bear. The **pro–B cell** is the first descendent of the pluripotential stem cell committed to B-lineage development and is detected by the presence of both CD34 and CD10 on its surface; in it the immunoglobulin genes remain germ line (Fig. 113–2). The next stage is the **pre-pre–B cell** stage, during which immunoglobulin genes are rearranged, but there is no cytoplasmic expression of μ heavy chains or surface IgM (sIgM); these cells are further characterized by the co-expression of membrane CD34, CD10, CD19, and CD40, and somewhat later by the additional presence of CD73, CD22, CD24, and CD38. The **pre–B cell** stage is next; these cells are distinguished by the expression of cytoplasmic μ heavy chains but no sIgM, because no immunoglobulin light chains are produced yet. They also continue to express all CD antigens seen at the pre-pre–B cell stage except CD34 and CD10 (which are lost); in addition, they express CD21. Next is the **immature B-cell** stage, during which sIgM is expressed, because light-chain genes have now been rearranged, but not sIgD; CD38 is lost, but all other pre–B-cell CD antigens persist. The last stage of antigen-independent B-cell development is the **mature or virgin B cell**, which co-expresses both sIgM and sIgD; CD23 is also acquired at this stage, and all of the other CD antigens present on immature B cells persist. Pre-B cells can be found in fetal liver at 7 wk gestation, sIgM+ and sIgG+ B cells at between 7 and 11 wk, and sIgD+ and sIgA+ B

cells by 12–13 wk. By 14 wk of embryonic life, the percentage of circulating lymphocytes bearing sIgM and sIgD is the same as in cord blood and slightly higher than in the blood of adults.

Antigen-dependent stages of B-cell development are those that develop after the mature or virgin B cell is stimulated by antigen through its antigen receptor (sIg); the outcome is the differentiation of the cell and its progeny into sIg+ memory (CD27) B cells (for that particular antigen) and plasma cells, which synthesize and secrete antigen-specific immunoglobulin—that is, antibody. Deficiency of activation-induced cytidine deaminase (AID), as seen in one form of autosomal recessive hyper IgM, can result in a failure of isotype switching so that only IgM antibodies are formed. There are five **immunoglobulin isotypes**, which are defined by unique heavy-chain antigens present on each: IgM, IgG, IgA, IgD, and IgE. IgG and IgM, the only complement-fixing isotypes, are the most important immunoglobulins in the blood and other internal body fluids for protection against infectious agents; IgM is confined primarily to the intravascular compartment because of its large size, whereas IgG is present in all internal body fluids. IgA is the major protective immunoglobulin of external secretions—that is, those of the gastrointestinal, respiratory, and urogenital tracts—but it is also present in the circulation. IgE, present in both internal and external body fluids, has a major role in host defense against parasites. However, because of high-affinity IgE receptors on basophils and mast cells, IgE is the principal mediator of allergic reactions of the immediate type. The significance of IgD is still not clear. There are also immunoglobulin subclasses (again defined by unique heavy-chain antigens present on each, in addition to their class-specific heavy-chain antigen), including four subclasses of IgG—IgG1, IgG2, IgG3, and IgG4—and two subclasses of IgA—IgA1 and IgA2. These subclasses each have different biologic roles; for example, antipolysaccharide antibody activity is found predominantly in the IgG2 subclass. Secreted IgM and IgE have been found in abortuses as young as 10 wk, and IgG as early as 11–12 wk. Even though these B-cell developmental stages have been described in the context of B-cell ontogeny, it is important to recognize that the process of B-cell development from pluripotential stem cells goes on throughout postnatal life.

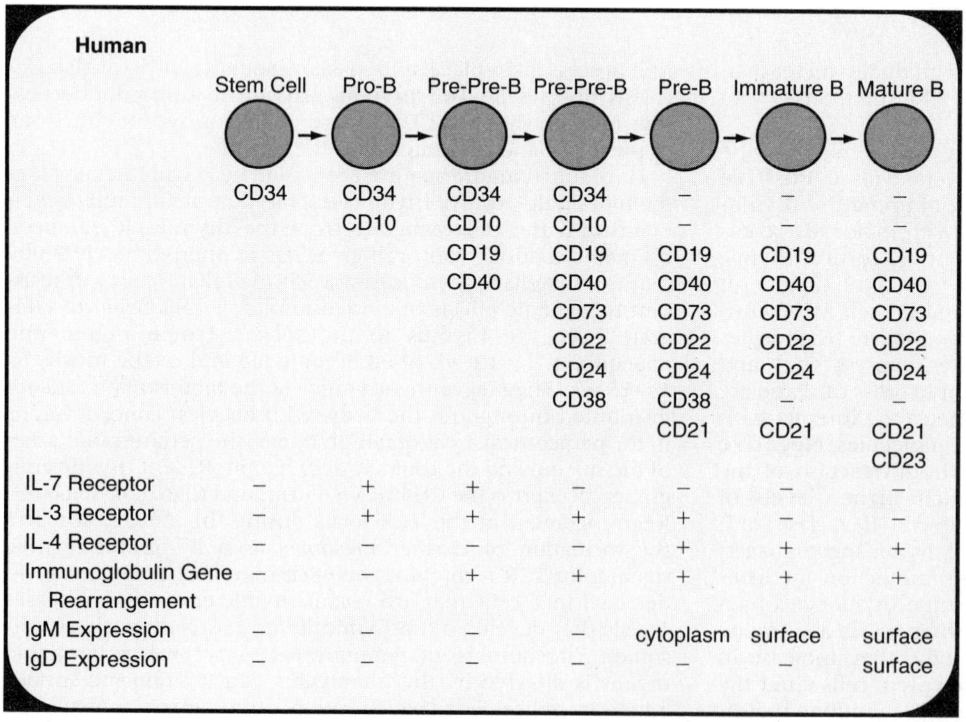

Human	Stem Cell	Pro-B	Pre-Pre-B	Pre-Pre-B	Pre-B	Immature B	Mature B
	CD34	CD34	CD34	CD34	–	–	–
		CD10	CD10	CD10	–	–	–
			CD19	CD19	CD19	CD19	CD19
			CD40	CD40	CD40	CD40	CD40
			CD73	CD73	CD73	CD73	CD73
			CD22	CD22	CD22	CD22	CD22
			CD24	CD24	CD24	CD24	CD24
			CD38	CD38	CD38	–	–
				CD21	CD21	CD21	CD21
							CD23
IL-7 Receptor	–	+	+	–	–	–	–
IL-3 Receptor	–	+	+	+	+	–	–
IL-4 Receptor	–	–	–	–	+	+	+
Immunoglobulin Gene Rearrangement	–	–	+	+	+	+	+
IgM Expression	–	–	–	–	cytoplasm	surface	surface
IgD Expression	–	–	–	–	–	–	surface

FIGURE 113–2. Antigen-independent human B-cell development. (From Haynes BF, Denning SM: Lymphopoiesis. In Stamatoyannopoulis G, Nienhuis A, Majerus P, Varmus H [editors]: *Molecular Basis of Blood Diseases*, 2nd ed. Philadelphia, WB Saunders, 1994.)

Despite the capacity of fetal B lymphocytes to differentiate into immunoglobulin-synthesizing and -secreting cells, plasma cells are not usually found in lymphoid tissues of a fetus until about 20 wk gestation, then only rarely, because of the sterile environment of the uterus. Peyer patches have been found in significant numbers by the 5th intrauterine month, and plasma cells have been seen in the lamina propria by 25 wk gestation. Before birth there may be primary follicles in lymph nodes, but secondary follicles are usually not present.

A human fetus begins to receive significant quantities of maternal IgG transplacentally at around 12 wk gestation, and the quantity steadily increases until at birth cord serum contains a concentration of IgG comparable to or greater than that of maternal serum. IgG is the only class to cross the placenta to any significant degree; all four subclasses do this, but IgG2 does so least well. A small amount of IgM (10% of adult levels) and a few nanograms of IgA, IgD, and IgE are normally found in cord serum; because none of these proteins crosses the placenta, they are presumed to be of fetal origin. These observations raise the possibility that certain antigenic stimuli normally cross the placenta to provoke responses, even in uninfected fetuses. Some atopic infants occasionally have reaginic antibodies to antigens, such as egg white, to which they have had no known exposure during postnatal life, suggesting that synthesis of these IgE antibodies could have been induced in the fetus by antigens ingested by the mother.

Natural Killer (NK)–Cell Development. NK-cell activity has been found in human fetal liver cells at 8–11 wk of gestation. NK lymphocytes are also derived from bone marrow precursors. Thymic processing is not necessary for NK-cell development, although NK cells have been found in the thymus. They are defined by their functional capacity to mediate non–MHC-restricted (classic) cytotoxicity. NK cells also have killer inhibitory receptors (KIRS) that recognize certain MHC antigens and inhibit the killing of normal allogeneic cells in four specific patterns of reactivity. The genetic locus controlling these patterns is different from conventional MHC alloantigenic loci, although it has been mapped to chromosome 6 in the region of the MHC class I genes. Unlike T and B cells, NK cells do not rearrange antigen receptor genes during their development. Virtually all NK cells express CD56, and more than 90% bear CD16 (FcγRIII) molecules on their cell surface. Other CD antigens found on NK cells include CD57 (on 50–60%), CD7 and CD2 (70–90%), and CD8 (30–40%) (see Table 113–1). Because NK cells share surface antigens with T and myeloid cells, the lineage relationship of NK cells to the latter is still unclear. Some humans with SCID and profound deficiencies in T and B cells have abundant NK cells, whereas some humans who have no NK cells may have normal T- and B-cell development. After release from bone marrow, NK cells enter the circulation or migrate to the spleen; there are very few NK cells in lymph nodes. In normal individuals, NK cells represent 10% of lymphocytes; this percentage is often slightly lower in cord blood.

Immune Cell Interactions. Immune cell interaction is of crucial importance to all phases of the adaptive immune response. Unlike the B-cell antigen receptor (Ig), which can recognize native antigen, the TCR can recognize only processed antigenic peptides presented to it by MHC molecules such as **HLA-A,-B, and -C antigens (class I antigens)** and **HLA-DR, -DP, and -DQ (class II antigens)** molecules present on **antigen-presenting cells (APCs).** The MHC molecules have a groove in their protein structure where peptides fit. Class I MHC molecules are found on most nucleated cells in the body. Class II MHC molecules are found on macrophages, dendritic cells, and B cells. The peptides found in the groove of class I HLA molecules come from proteins normally made in the cell that are degraded and inserted into the groove. The peptides include viral peptides if the cell is infected with a virus. The peptides present in the groove of class II molecules come from exogenous native antigens such as vaccine and bacterial proteins. These proteins are taken up by APCs (macrophages, dendritic cells, and B cells), degraded, and expressed on the cell surface in the groove of class II HLA molecules. The TCR then interacts with the peptide-bearing HLA molecule and, through its functional and physical link to the CD3 complex of signal-transducing molecules, sends a signal to the T cell to produce cytokines that ultimately result in T-cell activation and proliferation.

Two of the main functions of T cells are (1) to signal B cells to make antibody by producing cytokines and membrane molecules that can serve as ligands for B-cell surface molecules and (2) to kill virally infected cells or tumor cells. For a T cell to carry out either of these functions, it first must bind to an APC or to a target cell. For high-affinity binding of T cells to APCs or target cells, several molecules on T cells, in addition to TCRs, bind to molecules on APCs or target cells. For example, the CD4 molecule present on TH cells binds directly to MHC class II molecules on APCs. CD8 on killer T cells binds the MHC class I molecule on the target cell. Both CD4 and CD8 molecules are directly involved in the regulation of T-cell activation and are physically linked intracellularly to the p56-lck protein tyrosine kinase. The cytoplasmic tail of CD45 is a tyrosine phosphatase capable of regulating T-cell signal-transduction events by virtue of the fact that p56-lck has been shown to be a substrate for CD45 phosphatase activity. Depending on which isoform of CD45 is present on the T cell (CD45RO on memory T cells, CD45RA on naive T cells), mechanisms by which CD45 could upregulate or downregulate T-cell triggering have been proposed. LFA-1 on the T cell binds a protein called ICAM-1 (intracellular adhesion molecule 1), now designated CD54, on APCs. CD2 on T cells binds LFA-3 (CD58) on the APCs. With the adhesion of T cells to antigen-presenting cells, TH cells are stimulated to make interleukins and upregulate cell surface molecules, such as the CD40 ligand (CD154), that provide help for B cells, and cytotoxic T cells are stimulated to kill their targets.

In the **primary antibody response,** native antigen is carried to a lymph node draining the site, taken up by specialized cells called follicular dendritic cells (FDCs), and expressed on their surfaces. Virgin B cells bearing sIg specific for that antigen then bind to the antigen on the surfaces of the FDCs. If the affinity of the B-cell sIg antibody for the antigen present on the FDCs is high enough, and if other signals are provided by activated T-helper cells, the B cell develops into an antibody-producing plasma cell. If the affinity is not high enough or if T-cell signals are not received, the B cell dies through apoptosis. The signals provided by activated TH cells include those from cytokines they secrete (IL-4, IL-5, IL-6, and IL-13; see Box 113–1) and that from a surface T-cell molecule, CD154, which, on contact of the T cell with the B cell, binds to CD40 on the B-cell surface. CD40 is a type I integral membrane glycoprotein expressed on B cells, monocytes, some carcinomas, and a few other types of cells. It belongs to the tumor necrosis factor (TNF)/nerve growth factor receptor family. Cross linking of CD40 on B cells by allowing CD40 to interact with CD154 in the presence of certain cytokines causes the B cells to undergo proliferation and to initiate immunoglobulin synthesis. In the primary immune response, only IgM antibody is usually made, and most of it is of relatively low affinity. Some B cells become memory B cells during the primary immune response. These cells switch their immunoglobulin genes so that IgG, IgA, and/or IgE antibodies of higher affinity are formed on a secondary exposure to the same antigen. The secondary immune response occurs when these memory B cells again encounter that antigen. Plasma cells form, just as in the primary response; however, many more cells are rapidly generated, and IgG, IgA, and IgE antibodies are made. In addition, genetic changes in immunoglobulin genes (somatic mutation) lead to increased affinity of those antibodies. The exact pattern of isotype response to antigen varies, depending on the type of antigen and the cytokines present in the microenvironment.

For NK-mediated lysis, binding to the target is of crucial importance. This is best exemplified by humans with mutations in CD18, or the β chain of three different adhesion molecules, who also lack NK function. Thus, binding of NK cells to their targets is facilitated by LFA-1-ICAM interactions. CD56 or NCAM (neural cell adhesion molecule) also mediates homotypic adhesion of NK cells. FcγRIII, or the low-affinity IgG receptor, has a higher affinity for IgG when it is present on NK cells than when it is on neutrophils; it permits NK cells also to mediate antibody-dependent cellular cytotoxicity (ADCC). In this reaction, antibody is bound through its Fc region to the FcγRIII. The antibody-combining portion of the IgG attaches to the target. The NK cell, now attached to the target by antibody, kills the target cell.

POSTNATAL LYMPHOPOIESIS

T Cells and T-Cell Subsets. Although the percentage of CD3 T cells in cord blood is somewhat less than in the peripheral blood of children and adults, T cells are actually present in higher number because of a higher absolute lymphocyte count in all normal infants. An additional distinction is that the ratio of CD4 to CD8 T cells is usually higher (3.5–4:1) in cord blood than in blood of children and adults (1.5–2:1). Virtually all T cells in cord blood bear the CD45RA (naive) isoform, and a dominance of CD45RA over CD45RO T cells persists during the first 2–3 yr of life, after which time the numbers of cells bearing these two isoforms gradually equalize. TH cells can be further subdivided according to the cytokines they produce when activated. **TH1 cells** produce IL-2 and IFN-γ, which promote cytotoxic T-cell or delayed hypersensitivity types of responses, whereas **TH2 cells** produce IL-4, IL-5, IL-6, and IL-13 (see Box 113–1), which promote B-cell responses and allergic sensitization. Cord blood T cells have the capacity to respond normally to the two T-cell mitogens, PHA and Con A, and are capable of mounting a normal mixed leukocyte response. Normal newborn infants also have the capacity to develop antigen-specific T cell responses at birth, as evidenced by vigorous tuberculin reactivity a few weeks after BCG vaccination even on day 1 of life. Because patients in the first few months of life may have unrecognized severe T-cell defects, most hospitals now routinely irradiate all blood products given young infants.

B Cells and Immunoglobulins. Newborn infants have increased susceptibility to infections with gram-negative organisms because they have not received IgM antibodies, which are **heat-stable opsonins**, to these organisms from the mother. The level of the **heat-labile opsonin**, C3b, is also lower in newborn serum than in adults. These factors probably account for impaired phagocytosis of some organisms by newborn polymorphonuclear cells. Maternally transmitted IgG antibodies serve quite adequately as heat-stable opsonins for most gram-positive bacteria, and IgG antibodies to viruses afford adequate protection against those agents. However, because there is a relative deficiency of the IgG2 subclass, antibodies to capsular polysaccharide antigens may be deficient. Because premature infants have received less maternal IgG by the time of birth than full-term infants, their serum opsonic activity is low for all types of organisms.

B lymphocytes are present in cord blood in slightly higher percentages but considerably higher numbers than in the blood of children and adults, reflecting the higher absolute lymphocyte counts in all normal infants. However, cord blood B cells do not synthesize the range of immunoglobulin isotypes made by B cells from children and adults when stimulated with pokeweed mitogen (PWM) or anti-CD40 plus IL-4 or IL-10, producing primarily IgM and at a much reduced quantity.

Neonates begin to synthesize antibodies of the IgM class at an increased rate very soon after birth in response to the immense antigenic stimulation of their new environment. Premature infants appear to be as capable of doing this as do full-term infants. At about 6 days after birth, the serum concentration of IgM rises sharply. This rise continues until adult levels are achieved by approximately 1 yr of age. Cord serum from noninfected normal newborns does not contain detectable IgA. Serum IgA is normally first detected at around the 13th day of postnatal life; the level gradually increases during early childhood until adult levels are achieved and preserved between the 6th and 7th yr of life. Cord serum contains an IgG concentration comparable to or greater than that of maternal serum. Maternal IgG gradually disappears during the first 6–8 mo of life, while the rate of infant IgG synthesis increases (IgG1 and IgG3 faster than IgG2 and IgG4 during the 1st year) until adult concentrations of total IgG are reached and maintained by 7–8 yr of age. However, IgG1 and IgG4 reach adult levels first, followed by IgG3 at 10 yr and IgG2 at 12 yr of age. The total immunoglobulin level in infants usually reaches a low point at approximately 3–4 mo of postnatal life. The rate of development of IgE generally follows that of IgA. After adult concentrations of each of the three major immunoglobulins are reached, these levels remain remarkably constant for a normal individual. The capacity to produce specific antibodies to protein antigens is intact at the time of birth. However, normal infants cannot produce antibodies to polysaccharide antigens until usually after age 2 yr unless the polysaccharide is conjugated to a protein carrier, as is the case for the conjugate *Haemophilus influenzae* type b (Hib) and *Streptococcus pneumoniae* vaccines.

NK Cells. The percentage of NK cells in cord blood is usually lower than in the blood of children and adults, but the absolute number of NK cells is approximately the same owing to the higher lymphocyte count. The capacity of cord blood NK cells to mediate target lysis in either NK-cell assays or ADCC assays is roughly two thirds that of adults.

Lymphoid Organ Development. Lymphoid tissue is proportionally small but rather well developed at birth and matures rapidly in the postnatal period. The thymus is largest relative to body size during fetal life and at birth is ordinarily two thirds of its mature weight, which it attains during the 1st year of life. It reaches its peak mass, however, just before puberty, and then gradually involutes thereafter. By 1 yr of age, all lymphoid structures are mature histologically. Absolute lymphocyte counts in the peripheral blood also reach a peak during the 1st yr of life. Peripheral lymphoid tissue increases rapidly in mass during infancy and early childhood. It reaches adult size by approximately 6 yr of age, exceeds those dimensions during the prepubertal years, and then undergoes involution coincident with puberty. The spleen, however, gradually accrues its mass during maturation and does not reach full weight until adulthood. The mean number of Peyer patches at birth is one half the adult number, and gradually increases until the adult mean number is exceeded during adolescent years.

INHERITANCE OF ABNORMALITIES IN T-, B-, AND NK-CELL DEVELOPMENT

More than 100 immunodeficiency syndromes have been described. Until recently, there was little insight into the fundamental problems underlying most of these conditions. However, specific molecular defects have been identified in more than one third of these diseases. Most are recessive traits, several of which are caused by mutations in genes on the X chromosome and others by mutations on autosomal chromosomes. The molecular bases of six X-linked immunodeficiency disorders affecting T, B, and/or NK cells have been reported (Chapters 114–116): X-linked immunodeficiency with hyper IgM, X-linked lymphoproliferative syndrome, X-linked agammaglobulinemia, X-linked SCID, the Wiskott-Aldrich syndrome, and nuclear factor kappa B essential modulator (NEMO). Examples of the autosomal defects include (1) combined immunodeficiencies due to abnormalities of purine salvage pathway enzymes, either adenosine deaminase (ADA, encoded by a gene on chromosome 20q13-ter) or purine nucleoside phosphorylase (PNP, encoded by a gene on chromosome 14q13.1); (2) mutations in the gene encoding ZAP-70 (localized to chromosome 2q12), a non-src family protein tyrosine kinase important in T-cell signaling; and (3) mutations in the gene encoding Janus kinase 3 (Jak3), the primary signal transducer from the common cytokine receptor γ chain (γc). The identification and cloning of the genes for these immunodeficiency diseases have obvious implications for potential future somatic cell gene therapy for these patients.

PRENATAL DIAGNOSIS AND CARRIER DETECTION

Intrauterine diagnosis of ADA and PNP deficiencies can be established by enzyme analyses on amnion cells (fresh or cultured) obtained before 20 wk gestation. Diagnosis of several X-linked defects can be made by direct mutation analysis of the X chromosome of cells obtained by chorionic villus sampling or by amniocentesis from male infants whose mothers have been identified as carriers. Diagnosis of enzyme-normal SCID or other severe T-cell deficiencies, MHC class I and/or II antigen deficiencies, chronic granulomatous disease (CGD), or Wiskott-Aldrich syndrome (by platelet size) can be established by appropriate tests of phenotype or function on small samples of blood obtained by fetoscopy at 18–22 wk of gestation, but this procedure carries significant risk. The same diagnostic procedures can be done on cord blood, but tragically no immunodeficiency disorders are screened for on the cord blood of infants born in the United States or elsewhere. Carriers of ADA and PNP deficiency can be detected by quantitative enzyme analyses of blood samples. Carriers of X-linked agammaglobulinemia, X-linked SCID, or the Wiskott-Aldrich syndrome can be identified by techniques designed to detect nonrandom X-chromosome inactivation in one or more blood cell lineages or by direct mutation analysis if the family's mutation is known.

Buckley RH: Primary immunodeficiency diseases due to defects in lymphocytes. *N Engl J Med* 2000;343:1313–24.

Haynes BF, Denning SM: Lymphopoiesis. In Stamatoyannopoulis G, Nienhuis A, Majerus P, Varmus H (editors): *Molecular Basis of Blood Diseases*, 2nd ed. Philadelphia, WB Saunders, 1994.

Haynes BF, Markert ML, Sempowski GD, et al: The role of the thymus in immune reconstitution in aging, bone marrow transplantation, and HIV-1 infection. *Annu Rev Immunol* 2000;18:529–60.

Primary immunodeficiency diseases. Report of an IUIS Scientific Committee. International Union of Immunological Societies. *Clin Exp Immunol* 1999; 118:1–28.

Schroeder HW, Radbruch A, Berek C: B-cell development and differentiation. In Rich RR, Fleisher TA, Shearer WT, Kotzin BL (editors): *Clinical Immunology: Principles and Practice*. New York, Mosby, 2001.

Chapter 114
Primary Defects of Antibody Production

Of all of the primary immunodeficiency diseases, those affecting antibody production are most frequent. Selective absence of serum and secretory IgA is the most common defect, with rates ranging from 1/333 persons to 1/16,000 among different races. By contrast, it has been estimated that agammaglobulinemia occurs with a frequency of only 1/50,000 persons. Patients with antibody deficiency are usually recognized because they have recurrent infections with encapsulated bacteria or a history of failure of responding to antibiotic treatment, but some individuals with selective IgA deficiency or infants with transient hypogammaglobulinemia may have few or no infections. The defective gene products for many primary antibody deficiency disorders have been identified (Table 114–1). Sometimes the defect is not in the B cell itself but in the T cells that are required for B cell function.

X-LINKED (XLA OR BRUTON) AGAMMAGLOBULINEMIA

Patients with X-linked agammaglobulinemia (XLA) have a profound defect in B lymphocyte development resulting in severe hypogammaglobulinemia, an absence of circulating B cells, small to absent tonsils, and no palpable lymph nodes.

Genetics and Pathogenesis. The abnormal gene in XLA maps to q22 on the long arm of the X chromosome and encodes the B-cell protein tyrosine kinase *Btk* (**Bruton tyrosine kinase**). *Btk* is a member of the *Tec* family of cytoplasmic protein tyrosine kinases that is expressed at high levels in all B-lineage cells, including pre–B cells. This kinase appears to be necessary for pre–B-cell expansion and maturation into surface Ig-expressing B cells, but probably has a role at all stages of B-cell development. It has not

---

TABLE 114–1. Primary Antibody Deficiency Disorders

Chromosome and Region	Gene Product	Disorder	Functional Deficiencies
2p11*	κ chain	κ chain deficiency	Absence of immunoglobulins bearing κ chains
6p21.3	Unknown	Selective IgA deficiency; CVID	Low or absent IgA; low concentrations of all immunoglobulins in CVID
12p13*	Activation-induced cytidine deaminase	Autosomal recessive hyper IgM	Failure to produce IgG, IgA, and IgE antibodies
14q32.3*	Immunoglobulin heavy chains	B cell-negative agammaglobulinemia (μ) or selective deficiencies of other isotypes	Absence of antibody production and lack of B cells in μ chain mutations; subclasses missing but B cells present in others
20*	CD40	Autosomal recessive hyper IgM	Failure to produce IgG, IgA, and IgE antibodies
Xq22*	Bruton tyrosine kinase	X-linked (Bruton) agammaglobulinemia (XLA)	Absence of antibody production, lack of B cells
Xq25*	SLAM-associated protein (SH2D1A)	X-linked lymphoproliferative disease (XLP)	Lack of anti-EBNA and long-lived T-cell immunity; low immunoglobulins
Xq26*	CD154 (CD40 ligand)	X-linked hyper IgM	Failure to produce IgG, IgA, and IgE antibodies
Xq28*	Nuclear factor κB (NF-κB) essential modulator (NEMO)	Anhidrotic ectodermal dysplasia with immunodeficiency	Hyper IgM or IgG subclass and anti-polysaccharide antibodies

Gene cloned and sequenced, gene product known.
CVID = common variable immunodeficiency; EBNA = Epstein-Barr virus nuclear antigen; SLAM = signaling lymphocyte activation molecule.

been detected in any cells of T lineage, but it has been found in cells of the myeloid series. Thus far, all males with known XLA (by family history) have had low or undetectable *Btk* mRNA and kinase activity. Mutations in the *Btk* gene also occur in some agammaglobulinemic boys with no family history of XLA. To date more than 250 different mutations in the human *Btk* gene have been recognized and they encompass most parts of the coding portions of the gene. There is not a clear correlation between the location of the mutation and the clinical phenotype (Fig. 114–1). Carriers are detected by identifying nonrandom X-chromosome inactivation in B cells or by direct mutation analysis. Prenatal diagnosis of affected male fetuses is possible by mutation analysis, if the defect is known in the family.

The expression of *Btk* in cells of myeloid lineage is of interest because boys with XLA often have neutropenia at the height of an acute infection. It is conceivable that *Btk* is only one of the signaling molecules participating in myeloid maturation and that neutropenia is observed in XLA only when rapid production of such cells is needed. Some pre–B cells are found in the bone marrow; however, peripheral blood B lymphocytes are absent or present in very low numbers. In most patients, the percentage of T cells is increased, ratios of T-cell subsets are normal, and T-cell function is intact. The thymus was morphologically normal in patients who underwent autopsy.

Four autosomal recessive defects have also been shown to result in agammaglobulinemia with an absence of circulating B cells, including mutations in the genes encoding (1) the μ heavy chain gene; (2) the Igα signaling molecule; (3) an adaptor protein, B cell linker protein (BLNK); and (4) the surrogate light chain, λ5/14.1 (see Table 114–1).

Clinical Manifestations. Most boys afflicted with XLA remain well during the first 6–9 mo of life by virtue of maternally transmitted IgG antibodies. Thereafter, they acquire infections with extracellular pyogenic organisms, such as *Streptococcus pneumoniae* and *Haemophilus influenzae*, unless given prophylactic antibiotics or immunoglobulin therapy. Infections with *Mycoplasma* are also particularly problematic for these patients. Chronic fungal infections are not usually present, and *Pneumocystis carinii* pneumonia rarely occurs unless there is an associated neutropenia. Viral infections are also usually handled normally, with the exceptions

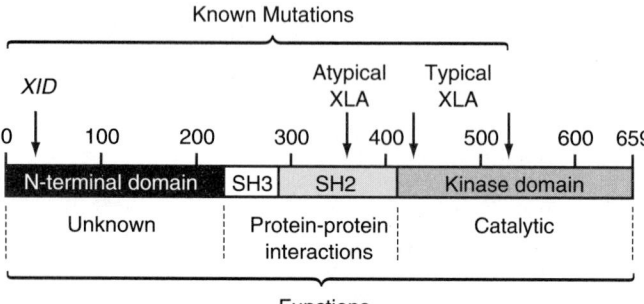

FIGURE 114–1. Location of mutations in the functional domains of the BTK protein. Deletion and point mutations in BTK identified to date in many boys with classic XLA are in the kinase domain, whereas CBA/N xid mice with a less severe B-cell defect have a point mutation causing an amino acid substitution at position 28 in the N-terminal domain. A male with a less severe B-cell defect than in classic XLA has had a point mutation at position 361 in the SH2 domain. However, more recently boys with classic XLA are also reported to have mutations at the xid mutation site and in the SH2 domain. (From Buckley RH: Breakthroughs in the understanding and therapy of primary immunodeficiency. *Pediatr Clin North Am* 1994;41: 665–90.)

of hepatitis viruses and enteroviruses. Several examples of paralysis after live polio vaccine administration have occurred, and chronic, eventually fatal central nervous system infections with various echoviruses have occurred in more than 45 patients. These observations suggest a primary role for antibody, particularly secretory IgA, in host defense against enteroviruses, because normal T-cell function has been present in X-linked agammaglobulinemic patients with such persistent infections. Growth hormone deficiency has also been reported in association with XLA.

The diagnosis of XLA should be suspected if lymphoid hypoplasia is found on physical examination (minimal or no tonsillar tissue and no palpable lymph nodes) and serum concentrations of IgG, IgA, IgM, and IgE are far below the 95% confidence limits for appropriate age- and race-matched controls (Chapter 710), usually <100 mg/dL total immunoglobulin. Tests for natural antibodies to type A and B red blood cell polysaccharide antigens (isohemagglutinins) and for antibodies to antigens given during routine immunizations are abnormal in this disorder, whereas they are normal in transient hypogammaglobulinemia of infancy. Flow cytometry is an important test to demonstrate the absence of circulating B cells, which will distinguish this disorder from common variable immunodeficiency.

COMMON VARIABLE IMMUNODEFICIENCY

Common variable immunodeficiency (CVID) is a syndrome characterized by hypogammaglobulinemia with phenotypically normal B cells. It is also known as **acquired hypogammaglobulinemia** because of a generally later age of onset of infections. CVID patients may appear similar clinically to those with XLA in the kinds of infections experienced and bacterial etiologic agents involved, except that echovirus meningoencephalitis is rare in patients with CVID. In contrast to XLA, the sex distribution in CVID is almost equal, the age of onset is later, and infections are less severe.

Genetics and Pathogenesis. Most patients, if not all, have no identified molecular diagnosis. CVID is a "wastebasket" category of primary immunodeficiency disorders that likely consists of several different genetic defects. As the molecular bases of more and more primary immunodeficiency syndromes are identified, it will be important to consider a variety of genetic mutations that can lead to the hypogammaglobulinemia seen in CVID, including mutations in the *Btk, SH2D1A, CD40L, CD40*, and *AID* genes.

Because CVID occurs in first-degree relatives of patients with selective IgA deficiency, and some patients with IgA deficiency later become panhypogammaglobulinemic, these diseases may have a common genetic basis. The high incidence of abnormal immunoglobulin concentrations, autoantibodies, autoimmune disease, and malignancy in both types of patients and in their families also suggests a shared hereditary influence. This concept is supported by the discovery of a high incidence of C4-A gene deletions and C2 rare gene alleles in the class III major histocompatibility complex (MHC) region in individuals with either IgA deficiency or CVID, suggesting that a common susceptibility gene is in this region on chromosome 6. A small number of HLA haplotypes are shared by individuals affected with IgA deficiency and CVID, with at least one of two particular haplotypes being present in 77% of those affected. In one large family with 13 members, two had IgA deficiency and three had CVID. All of the immunodeficient patients in the family had at least one copy of an MHC haplotype that is abnormally frequent in IgA deficiency and CVID: HLA-DQB1 *0201, HLA-DR3, C4B-Sf, C4A-deleted, G11-15, Bf-0.4, C2a, HSP70-7.5, TNFa-5, HLA-B8, and HLA-A1. However, four immunologically normal members of the pedigree also possessed this haplotype, indicating that its presence is not sufficient for expression of the defects. Environmental factors, particularly drugs such as phenytoin, D-penicillamine, gold, and sulfasalazine are suspected to be triggers for disease expression in individuals with the permissive genetic background.

Despite normal numbers of circulating immunoglobulin-bearing B lymphocytes and the presence of lymphoid cortical follicles, blood B lymphocytes from CVID patients do not differentiate normally into immunoglobulin-producing cells when stimulated with pokeweed mitogen (PWM) in vitro, even when co-cultured with normal T cells. However, studies have shown that CVID B cells can be stimulated both to switch isotype and to synthesize and secrete some immunoglobulin when stimulated with anti-CD40 and IL-4 or IL-10. T cells and T-cell subsets are usually present in normal percentages, although T-cell function is depressed in some patients.

Clinical Manifestations. The serum immunoglobulin and antibody deficiencies in CVID may be as profound as in XLA. Patients with CVID often have autoantibody formation and normal-sized or enlarged tonsils and lymph nodes, and approximately 25% of patients have splenomegaly. CVID has also been associated with a sprue-like syndrome, with or without nodular follicular lymphoid hyperplasia of the intestine; thymoma; alopecia areata; hemolytic anemia; gastric atrophy; achlorhydria; and pernicious anemia. Lymphoid interstitial pneumonia, pseudolymphoma, B-cell lymphomas, amyloidosis, and noncaseating sarcoid-like granulomas of the lungs, spleen, skin, and liver also occur. There is a 438-fold increase in lymphomas among affected women in the 5th and 6th decades of life. CVID is reported to resolve transiently or permanently in patients who acquire human immunodeficiency virus (HIV) infection.

SELECTIVE IgA DEFICIENCY

An isolated absence or near absence (<10 mg/dL) of serum and secretory IgA is the most common well-defined immunodeficiency disorder, with a frequency of 0.33% reported among some apparently healthy blood donors. However, this condition is also commonly associated with ill health.

Genetics and Pathogenesis. As is the case for CVID, the basic defect leading to IgA deficiency is unknown. Phenotypically normal blood B cells are present in both conditions. IgA deficiency occasionally remits spontaneously or after discontinuation of phenytoin (Dilantin) therapy. The occurrence of IgA deficiency in both males and females and in members of successive generations within families suggests autosomal dominant inheritance with variable expressivity. This defect also commonly occurs in pedigrees containing individuals with CVID. Indeed, IgA deficiency has been noted to evolve into CVID, and the finding of rare alleles and deletions of MHC class III genes in both conditions suggests that the susceptibility gene common to these two conditions may reside in the MHC class III region on chromosome 6. IgA deficiency is noted in patients treated with the same drugs associated with producing CVID (phenytoin, D-penicillamine, gold, and sulfasalazine), suggesting that environmental factors may also trigger this disease.

Clinical Manifestations. Infections occur predominantly in the respiratory, gastrointestinal, and urogenital tracts. Bacterial agents responsible are the same as in other antibody deficiency syndromes. Children with IgA deficiency vaccinated with killed poliovirus intranasally produce local IgM and IgG antibodies. Serum concentrations of other immunoglobulins are usually normal in patients with selective IgA deficiency, although IgG2 (and other) subclass deficiency is reported, and IgM (usually elevated) may be monomeric.

Patients with IgA deficiency often have IgG antibodies against cow's milk and ruminant serum proteins. These antiruminant antibodies may cause false-positive results in immunoassays for IgA that use goat (but not rabbit) antisera. A sprue-like syndrome occurs in adults with this defect, which may or may not respond to a gluten-free diet. High incidences of autoantibodies

and autoimmune diseases are noted, and the incidence of malignancy is increased. Serum antibodies to IgA are reported in as many as 44% of patients with selective IgA deficiency. If these antibodies are of the IgE isotype, they can cause severe or fatal anaphylactic reactions after intravenous administration of blood products containing IgA. For this reason, only five-times washed (in 200-mL volumes) normal donor erythrocytes, or blood products from other IgA-deficient individuals, should be administered to these patients. Administration of intravenous immunoglobulin (IVIG), which is greater than 99% IgG, is not indicated because most IgA-deficient patients make IgG antibodies normally. Moreover, many IVIG preparations contain sufficient IgA to cause anaphylactic reactions.

TRANSIENT HYPOGAMMAGLOBULINEMIA OF INFANCY

After birth, the serum level of IgG in an infant diminishes with the decline of maternally derived IgG antibodies, reaching a nadir at 3–4 mo of age, and then rises as an infant's own IgG production gradually increases. Transient hypogammaglobulinemia of infancy (THI) is an extension of this physiologic hypogammaglobulinemia beyond 6 mo of age. B and T lymphocytes are present in normal numbers, and T lymphocyte function is normal. Unlike patients with XLA or CVID, patients with THI synthesize antibodies to type A and B red blood cell polysaccharide antigens (isohemagglutinins) and to diphtheria and tetanus toxoids normally, usually by 6–11 mo of age, and well before total immunoglobulin concentrations become normal. This condition likely represents the extremes of normal variability of the immune system. THI patients may have an increased frequency of otitis media and sinusitis, but infections are not life threatening and respond to appropriate antimicrobial therapy. IVIG therapy is not indicated in this condition.

IgG SUBCLASS DEFICIENCIES

Some patients have deficiencies of one or more of the four subclasses of IgG despite normal or elevated total IgG serum concentration. Most patients with absent or very low concentrations of IgG2 also have IgA deficiency. Other patients with IgG2 deficiency have an evolving pattern of immunodeficiency, such as CVID, suggesting that the presence of IgG subclass deficiency may be a marker for more generalized immune dysfunction. The biologic significance of the numerous moderate deficiencies of IgG subclasses that have been reported is difficult to assess, particularly because commercial laboratory measurement of IgG subclasses is problematic. The more relevant issue is a patient's capacity to make specific antibodies to protein and polysaccharide antigens, because profound deficiencies of antipolysaccharide antibodies have been noted even in the presence of normal concentrations of IgG2. IVIG should not be administered to patients with IgG subclass deficiency unless they are shown to have a deficiency of antibodies to a broad array of antigens.

IMMUNOGLOBULIN HEAVY- AND LIGHT-CHAIN DELETIONS

Some completely asymptomatic individuals have been documented to have a total absence of IgG1, IgG2, IgG4, and/or IgA1 due to gene deletions. These abnormalities were discovered fortuitously in 16 individuals, 15 of whom had no history of undue susceptibility to infection, and all of whom produced antibodies of all other isotypes in normal quantities. These patients illustrate the importance of assessing specific antibody formation before deciding to initiate IVIG therapy in IgG subclass–deficient patients.

HYPER IgM SYNDROME

The hyper IgM syndrome is genetically heterogeneous. Causative mutations have been identified in 2 genes on the X chromosome, the CD40 ligand and NEMO genes, and 2 genes on autosomal chromosomes, the AID gene on chromosome 12 and the CD40 gene on chromosome 20. Distinctive clinical features permit presumptive recognition of the type of mutation in these patients, thereby aiding proper choice of therapy. However, all such patients should undergo molecular analysis to ascertain the affected gene for purposes of genetic counseling, carrier detection, and definitive therapy.

X-Linked Hyper IgM due to Mutations in the CD40 Ligand (CD154) Gene

Boys with this syndrome have very low serum concentrations of IgG and IgA, with a usually normal or sometimes elevated concentration of polyclonal IgM, very small tonsils, no palpable lymph nodes, and often profound neutropenia.

Genetics and Pathogenesis. B cells from boys with the CD40 ligand defect are capable of synthesizing not only IgM but also IgA and IgG when co-cultured with a "switch" T-cell line, indicating that the B cells are actually normal in this condition and that the defect is in the T cells. The abnormal gene is localized to Xq26, and the gene product, CD154, is the ligand for CD40, which is present on B cells and monocytes. CD154 is upregulated on activated T cells. Mutations in CD154 on activated CD4 T cells from males with this defect result in an inability to signal B cells to undergo isotype switching, and thus they produce only IgM. The failure of T cells to interact with B cells through this receptor-ligand pair also causes a failure of upregulation of the B cell and monocyte surface molecules CD80 and CD86 that interact with CD28/CTLA4 on T cells, resulting in failure of "crosstalk" between immune system cells. The failure of interaction of the molecules of those pathways results in a propensity for tolerogenic T cell signaling and defective recognition of tumor cells. More than 73 distinct point mutations or deletions in the gene encoding CD154 have been identified in 87 unrelated families, giving rise to frame shifts, premature stop codons, and single amino acid substitutions, most of which were clustered in the domain with homology to tumor necrosis factor (TNF), located in the carboxy-terminal region.

Clinical Manifestations. Similar to patients with XLA, boys with the CD40 ligand defect have small tonsils and often no palpable lymph nodes, and become symptomatic during the 1st or 2nd year of life with recurrent pyogenic infections, including otitis media, sinusitis, pneumonia, and tonsillitis. Lymph node histology shows only abortive germinal center formation and a severe depletion and phenotypic abnormalities of follicular dendritic cells. However, in contrast to patients with XLA, these patients have normal numbers of circulating B lymphocytes, have a marked susceptibility to *P. carinii* pneumonia, and are often profoundly neutropenic. Circulating T cells are also present in normal number and in vitro responses to mitogens are normal, but there is decreased antigen-specific T-cell function. In a recent retrospective study of 56 patients with the CD40 ligand defect, 13 (23.3%) had died at a mean age at death of 11.7 years. In addition to opportunistic infections such as *P. carinii* pneumonia, there is an increased incidence of extensive verruca vulgaris lesions, *Cryptosporidium* enteritis, subsequent liver disease, and increased risk of malignancy. Because of the poor prognosis, the treatment of choice is an HLA-identical bone marrow transplant at an early age. Alternative treatment for this condition is monthly infusion of IVIG. In some patients with severe neutropenia, the use of G-CSF has been beneficial.

X-Linked Hyper IgM due to Mutations in the Gene Encoding Nuclear Factor κB (NF-κB) Essential Modulator (NEMO or Ikkγ) Deficiency

This is a newly recognized syndrome characterized most often clinically as anhidrotic **ectodermal dysplasia with associ-**

ated immunodeficiency (EDA-ID) in males. The condition results from mutations in the IKBKG gene at position 28q on the X chromosome that encodes **nuclear factor of κB (NF-κB) essential modulator (NEMO)**. Germ line loss-of-function mutations cause the X-linked dominant condition incontinentia pigmenti in females and are lethal in male fetuses. Mutations in the coding region of IKBKG are associated with EDA-ID. The immunodeficiency is variable, with most patients showing impaired antibody responses to polysaccharide antigens. However, some patients with EDA-ID have hyper IgM. Pharmacologic inhibitors of NF-κB activation have been shown to downregulate CD154 mRNA and protein levels, suggesting the mechanism of hyper IgM in this condition. The hyper IgM patients with this defect should be easily recognizable because of the presence of ectodermal dysplasia.

Autosomal Recessive Hyper IgM due to Mutations in the Gene for Activation-Dependent Cytidine Deaminase (AID)

Not all males with hyper IgM have mutations in the gene encoding CD154 or NFKB, and there are many examples in females, indicating that this condition has other causes.

Genetics and Pathogenesis. Patients with autosomal hyper IgM usually have normal numbers of circulating B lymphocytes but, in contrast to patients with the CD40 ligand defect, B cells from these patients are not able to switch from IgM-secreting to IgG-, IgA-, or IgE-secreting cells, even when co-cultured with monoclonal antibodies to CD40 and a variety of cytokines. When their B cells are cultured in vitro, they spontaneously secrete large amounts of IgM, but this is not further augmented by the addition of IL-4 or anti-CD40 with IL-4 or other cytokines. Thus, in these patients, there is truly an intrinsic B-cell abnormality. The defect in many such patients has recently been identified as mutations in a gene on chromosome 12p13 that encodes an activation-dependent cytidine deaminase (AID), an RNA-editing enzyme specifically expressed in germinal center B cells. Deficiency of AID results in impaired terminal differentiation of B cells, a failure of isotype switching, and lack of immunoglobulin gene somatic hypermutation. Unlike patients with X-linked hyper-IgM, who have minimal lymphoid tissue, patients with a mutation of AID have lymphoid hyperplasia because they have enhanced, although defective, germinal center formation.

Clinical Manifestations. As with the X-linked defects, concentrations of serum IgG, IgA, and IgE are very low in the autosomal recessive form of hyper IgM. However, in contrast to the CD40 ligand defect, the serum IgM concentration in patients with autosomal recessive hyper IgM is usually markedly elevated and polyclonal. Patients with AID mutations are generally older at age of onset, do not have susceptibility to *P. carinii* pneumonia, often do have isohemagglutinins, and are much less likely to have neutropenia unless it occurs on an autoimmune basis. With early diagnosis and monthly infusions of IVIG, as well as good management of infections with antibiotics, patients with AID mutations generally have a more benign course than do boys with the CD40 ligand defect.

Autosomal Recessive Hyper IgM due to Mutations in CD40

Patients with autosomal recessive hyper IgM were recently identified who failed to express CD40 on their B-cell surfaces resulting from mutations in the CD40 gene. CD40 is a type I integral membrane glycoprotein encoded by a gene on chromosome 20 and belonging to the TNF and nerve growth factor receptor superfamily. It is expressed on B cells, macrophages, dendritic cells, and a few other types of cells. Mutations in the CD40 gene cause an autosomal recessive form of hyper IgM that is clinically indistinguishable from hyper IgM resulting from the

X-linked CD40 ligand (CD154) defect. However, in contrast to the CD40 ligand defect, the B cells in the autosomal recessive condition are intrinsically abnormal and cannot isotype switch. The T cells are normal except to the extent that they cannot cause upregulation of CD80 and CD86 on B cells and macrophages to interact with CD28/CTLA4 on T cells.

X-LINKED LYMPHOPROLIFERATIVE DISEASE

X-linked lymphoproliferative (XLP) disease, also referred to as **Duncan disease** after the original kindred in which it was described, is an X-linked recessive trait characterized by an inadequate immune response to infection with Epstein-Barr virus (EBV).

Genetics and Pathogenesis. The defective gene in XLP was localized to Xq25, cloned, and initially named SAP (for SLAM Associated Protein) but is now known officially as **SH2D1A**. SLAM (signaling lymphocyte activation molecule) is an adhesion molecule that is upregulated on both T and B cells with infection and other stimulation. SH2D1A is highly expressed in thymocytes and peripheral blood T and NK cells, with a prevalent expression on Th1 cells; its presence in B lymphocytes is unclear. Thus, although antibody deficiency is frequently present, this is really a T and NK cell defect. SH2D1A competes with SHP-2 for binding to SLAM and, as such, is a regulatory molecule. In XLP patients the absence of SH2D1A can lead to an uncontrolled cytotoxic T-cell immune response to EBV. The SH2D1A protein permissively associates with 2B4 on NK cells; thus, selective impairment of 2B4-mediated NK cell activation also contributes to the immunopathology of XLP.

Clinical Manifestations. Affected males are usually healthy until they acquire EBV infection. The mean age of presentation is less than 5 yr. There are 3 major clinical phenotypes: (1) fulminant, often fatal, infectious mononucleosis (50% of cases); (2) lymphomas, predominantly involving B lineage cells (25%); or (3) acquired hypogammaglobulinemia (25%). There is a marked impairment in production of antibodies to the EBV nuclear antigen (EBNA), whereas titers of antibodies to the viral capsid antigen have ranged from absent to markedly elevated. XLP overall has an unfavorable prognosis, inasmuch as 70% of affected boys die by age 10. Only two XLP patients are known to have survived beyond 40 years. Unless there is a family history of XLP, diagnosis prior to the onset of complications is difficult because affected individuals are asymptomatic initially. It is possible to identify affected males of affected kindreds through mutation analysis before they develop primary EBV infection. Approximately half of the limited number of patients with XLP given HLA-identical related or unrelated unfractionated bone marrow transplants are currently surviving without signs of the disease.

Two pedigrees have been reported in which boys in one arm of each pedigree were diagnosed with common variable immunodeficiency (CVID), whereas those in the other arms had fulminant infectious mononucleosis. The family members with CVID never gave a history of infectious mononucleosis. However, all affected members of each pedigree had the same distinct SH2D1A mutation despite the different clinical phenotypes. Because the SH2D1A mutation was the same but the phenotype varied in these families, XLP should be considered in all males with a diagnosis of CVID, particularly if there is more than one male family member with this phenotype.

114.1 Treatment of B-Cell Defects

Except for the CD40 ligand defect and XLP, for which bone marrow transplantation is recommended, judicious use of antibiotics and regular administration of antibodies are the only effective treatments for B-cell disorders. The most common form of replacement therapy is with IVIG. Broad antibody deficiency should be carefully documented before such therapy is initiated. The rationale for the use of these preparations is to provide missing antibodies, not to raise the serum IgG or IgG subclass level. The development of safe and effective IVIG is a major advance in the treatment of patients with severe antibody deficiencies, although it is expensive and there have been frequent national shortages. Almost all commercial preparations are isolated from normal plasma by the Cohn alcohol fractionation method or a modification of this method. Cohn fraction II is then further treated to remove aggregated IgG. Additional stabilizing agents such as sugars, glycine, and albumin are added to prevent re-aggregation and protect the IgG molecule during lyophilization. The ethanol used in preparation of immune serum globulin and IVIG inactivates HIV; an organic solvent/detergent step inactivates hepatitis B and C viruses. Most commercial lots are produced from plasma pooled from more than 60,000 donors and therefore contain a broad spectrum of antibodies. Each pool must contain adequate levels of antibody to antigens in various vaccines, such as tetanus and measles. However, there is no standardization based on titers of antibodies to more clinically relevant organisms, such as *Streptococcus pneumoniae* and *Haemophilus influenzae* type b.

The IVIG preparations available in the United States have similar efficacy and safety. Rare transmission of hepatitis C virus has occurred in the past but the potential transmission of hepatitis C virus has been resolved by additional treatment with an organic solvent/detergent mixture. There has been no documented transmission of HIV by any of these preparations. IVIG (400 mg/kg/mo) achieves trough IgG levels close to the normal range. Systemic reactions to IVIG may occur, but rarely are these true anaphylactic reactions. Anaphylactic reactions caused by a patient's IgE antibodies to IgA in the IVIG preparation may occur, however, in patients with CVID or IgA deficiency. All newly diagnosed patients with CVID should be screened for anti-IgA antibodies through the American Red Cross before undergoing IVIG therapy. If anti-IgA antibodies are detected, IVIG therapy may still be possible by use of carefully screened lots of the one available IVIG preparation containing almost no IgA (Gammagard S/D, Baxter).

Conley ME, Rohrer J, Minegishi Y: X-linked agammaglobulinemia. *Clin Rev Allergy Immunol* 2000;19:183–204.
Conley ME: Autosomal recessive agammaglobulinemia. In Ochs HD, Smith CIE, Puck JM (editors): *Primary Immunodeficiency Diseases: A Molecular and Genetic Approach*. New York, Oxford University Press, 1999.
Cunningham-Rundles C, Bodian C: Common variable immunodeficiency: Clinical and immunological features of 248 patients. *Clin Immunol* 1999;92:34–48.
Morra M, Silander O, Calpe S, et al: Alterations of the X-linked lymphoproliferative disease gene SH2D1A in common variable immunodeficiency syndrome. *Blood* 2001;98:1321–5.
Ochs HD, Smith CIE, Puck JM: *Primary Immunodeficiency Diseases: A Molecular and Genetic Approach*. New York, Oxford University Press, 1999.
Schroeder HW, Zhu Z, March RE, et al: Susceptibility locus for IgA deficiency and common variable immunodeficiency in the HLA-DR3, -B8, -A1 haplotypes. *Mol Med* 1998;4:72–86.

Chapter 115
Primary Defects of Cellular Immunity

In general, patients with defects in T-cell function have infections or other clinical problems that are more severe than in patients with antibody deficiency disorders. These individuals rarely survive beyond infancy or childhood. The defective gene products for some primary T-cell diseases have been identified

(Table 115–1). Transplantation of thymic tissue or of major histocompatibility complex (MHC)–compatible sibling or haploidentical (half-matched) parental bone marrow are currently the treatments of choice for patients with fatal T-cell defects (Chapter 116.3).

THYMIC HYPOPLASIA (DiGEORGE SYNDROME)

Thymic hypoplasia results from dysmorphogenesis of the 3rd and 4th pharyngeal pouches during early embryogenesis, leading to hypoplasia or aplasia of the thymus and parathyroid glands. Other structures forming at the same age are also frequently affected, resulting in anomalies of the great vessels (right-sided aortic arch), esophageal atresia, bifid uvula, congenital heart disease (conotruncal, atrial, and ventricular septal defects), a short philtrum of the upper lip, hypertelorism, an antimongoloid slant to the eyes, mandibular hypoplasia, and low-set, often notched ears. The diagnosis is often first suggested by hypocalcemic seizures during the neonatal period. Similar facial features and conotruncal heart lesions are seen in the fetal alcohol syndrome.

Genetics and Pathogenesis. DiGeorge syndrome occurs in both males and females. Because familial occurrence is rare, the defect was thought unlikely to be heritable. However, microdeletions of specific DNA sequences from chromosome 22q11.2, the DiGeorge chromosomal region (DGCR), are found in more than 95% of cases. Several candidate genes have been identified in this region. There appears to be an excess of 22q11.2 deletions of maternal origin. Polymerase chain reaction (PCR)–based genotyping using microsatellite DNA markers located within the commonly deleted region permits rapid detection of such microdeletions. Similarities are observed between the DiGeorge syndrome, the velocardiofacial syndrome (VCFS), and the conotruncal anomaly face syndrome (CTAFS), inasmuch as all three have conotruncal heart defects and 22q deletions. The **CATCH 22 syndrome** (Cardiac, Abnormal facies, Thymic Hypoplasia, Cleft palate, Hypocalcemia) includes the broad clinical spectrum of conditions with 22q11.2 deletions. Other deletions associated with DiGeorge and velocardiofacial syndromes have been identified on chromosome 10p13 (also see Chapter 70).

Concentrations of serum immunoglobulins are usually normal, but IgA may be diminished and IgE elevated. Absolute lymphocyte counts are usually only moderately low for age. The CD3 T-cell counts are variably decreased in number, corresponding to the degree of thymic hypoplasia, and as a result the percentage of B cells is increased. Lymphocyte responses to mitogen stimulation are absent, reduced, or normal, depending on the degrees of thymic deficiency. Thymic tissue, when found, contains Hassall corpuscles, normal density of thymocytes, and corticomedullary distinction. Lymphoid follicles are usually present, but lymph node paracortical areas and thymus-dependent regions of the spleen show variable degrees of depletion.

Clinical Manifestations. Variable hypoplasia of the thymus and parathyroid glands is more frequent than total aplasia. Children with variable hypoplasia are referred to as having **partial DiGeorge syndrome;** they may have little trouble with infections and grow normally. Patients with **complete DiGeorge syndrome** resemble patients with severe combined immunodeficiency (SCID) in their susceptibility to infections with low-grade or opportunistic pathogens, including fungi, viruses, and *P. carinii*, and to graft versus host disease (GVHD) from nonirradiated blood transfusions.

Treatment. The immune deficiency in the complete DiGeorge syndrome has been corrected by cultured unrelated thymic tissue transplants and by unfractionated HLA-identical sibling bone marrow transplantation (Chapter 116.3).

DEFECTIVE EXPRESSION OF THE T-CELL RECEPTOR–CD3 COMPLEX (TI-CD3)

The first type of this disorder was found in two brothers in a Spanish family. The proband presented with severe infections and died at 31 mo of age with autoimmune hemolytic anemia and viral pneumonia. His lymphocytes had responded poorly to mitogens and to anti-CD3 in vitro and could not be stimulated to develop cytotoxic T cells. However, his antibody responses to protein antigens had been normal, indicating normal T-helper cell function. His 12-yr-old brother was healthy but had almost no CD3-bearing T cells, and had IgG2 deficiency similar to his sibling. The defect in this family is due to mutations in the CD3ε chain.

The second type of this disorder was diagnosed in a 4-yr-old French boy who had recurrent *Haemophilus influenzae* pneumonia and otitis media in early life but is now healthy. He has a partial defect in expression of Ti-CD3, and thus the percentage of CD3 cells is about half-normal but the level of expression is markedly decreased. His T cells do not proliferate in response to anti-CD3 or anti-CD2, nor do they express the IL-2 receptor or have normal calcium influx after these treatments. However, they do respond normally to stimulation with anti-CD28 or antigens, such as tetanus toxoid. The defect was shown to be due to two independent CD3ε gene mutations, leading to defective CD3ε chain synthesis and preventing normal association and membrane expression of the TCR/CD3 complex.

DEFECTIVE CYTOKINE PRODUCTION

Only a few defects of cytokine production are known. One is a selective inability to produce IL-2. In the two reported cases, patients had severe recurrent infections in infancy. The IL-2 gene was present in both, but no IL-2 message or protein was produced. Other T-cell cytokines were produced normally.

TABLE 115–1. Primary Cellular Immunodeficiency Diseases

Chromosome and Region	Gene Product	Disorder	Functional Deficiencies
2q12	ZAP-70*	CD8 lymphocytopenia	Failure of CD4 T cells to respond to usual signals
10p13	Unknown	Thymic hypoplasia (DiGeorge syndrome)/velocardiofacial syndrome	Low number of T cells and impaired T-cell function
11	CD3 γ* or ε*	CD3 deficiency	Poor T-cell responses to mitogens; lack of cytotoxic T cells; IgG subclass deficiency
22q11.22	Unknown	Thymic hypoplasia (DiGeorge syndrome)/velocardiofacial syndrome	Low number of T cells and impaired T-cell function

Gene cloned and sequenced, gene product known.

Another type was found in a single patient who also presented during infancy with severe recurrent infections and failure to thrive. She had defective transcription of several lymphokine genes, including IL-2, IL-3, IL-4, and IL-5, possibly resulting of abnormal binding of nuclear factor of activated T cells (NFAT-1) to response elements in IL-2 and IL-4 enhancers. She was treated with recombinant IL-2 with some clinical improvement.

IL-12, which is produced by activated antigen-presenting cells, promotes the development of Th1 responses and is a powerful inducer of IFN-γ production by T and natural killer (NK) cells. A child with bacille Calmette-Guérin and *Salmonella enteritidis* infections was found to have a large homozygous deletion within the IL-12 p40 subunit gene, precluding expression of functional IL-12 p70 cytokine by activated dendritic cells and phagocytes. As a result, IFN-γ production by the child's lymphocytes was markedly impaired. This suggested that IL-12 is essential for protective immunity to intracellular bacteria such as *Mycobacterium* and *Salmonella*.

T-CELL ACTIVATION DEFECTS

T-cell activation defects are characterized by the presence of normal or elevated numbers of blood T cells that appear phenotypically normal but that fail to proliferate or produce cytokines in response to stimulation with mitogens, antigens, or other signals delivered to the T-cell antigen receptor (TCR), owing to defective signal transduction from the TCR to intracellular metabolic pathways. These patients have problems similar to those of other T-cell–deficient individuals, and some with severe T-cell activation defects may resemble SCID patients clinically.

CD8 LYMPHOCYTOPENIA DUE TO MUTATIONS IN THE GENE ENCODING ZETA-ASSOCIATED PROTEIN 70

Patients with this T-cell activation defect present during infancy with severe, recurrent, and often fatal infections. The majority of cases are reported among Mennonites. These patients have normal or elevated numbers of blood B cells and low to elevated serum immunoglobulin concentrations. Their blood lymphocytes exhibit normal expression of the T-cell surface antigens CD3 and CD4, but CD8 cells are almost totally absent. These cells fail to respond to mitogens or to allogeneic cells in vitro or to generate cytotoxic T lymphocytes. By contrast, NK activity is normal. The thymus of one patient exhibited normal architecture with normal numbers of CD4:CD8 double-positive thymocytes but an absence of CD8 single-positive thymocytes. This condition is due to mutations in the gene encoding **zeta-associated protein 70 (ZAP-70)**, a non-*src* family protein tyrosine kinase important in T-cell signaling, which is localized to chromosome 2q12. The normal number of CD4:CD8 double-positive T cells is because the thymocytes can use the other member of the same tyrosine kinase family, *Syk*, to facilitate positive selection. *Syk* is present at fourfold higher levels in thymocytes than in peripheral T cells, possibly accounting for the lack of normal responses by the CD4 blood T cells.

P56 *ICK* DEFICIENCY

A 2 mo old male infant who presented with bacterial, viral, and fungal infections was found to be lymphopenic and hypogammaglobulinemic. B and NK cells were present, but there was a low number of CD4 T cells. Mitogen responses were variable. The T cells failed to express the activation marker CD69 when stimulated through the T-cell receptor but did when stimulated with phorbol myristate acetate and a calcium ionophore, suggesting a proximal signaling defect. Molecular studies revealed an alternatively spliced transcript for p56 *lck* that lacked the kinase domain.

Buckley RH: Primary immunodeficiency diseases due to defects in lymphocytes. *N Engl J Med* 2000;343:1313–24.

Elder ME, Skoda-Smith S, Kadlecek TA: Distinct T cell developmental consequences in humans and mice expressing identical mutations in the DLAARN motif of ZAP-70. *J Immunol* 2001;166:656–61.

Markert ML, Boeck A, Hale LP, et al: Transplantation of thymus tissue in complete DiGeorge syndrome. *N Engl J Med* 1999;341:1180–9.

Picard C, Fieschi C, Altare F, et al: Inherited interleukin-12 deficiency: IL12B genotype and clinical phenotype of 13 patients from six kindreds. *Am J Hum Genet* 2002;70:336–48.

Primary immunodeficiency diseases. Report of an IUIS Scientific Committee. International Union of Immunological Societies. *Clin Exp Immunol* 1999;118: 1–28.

Sullivan KE. DiGeorge syndrome/chromosome 22q11.2 deletion syndrome. *Curr Allergy Asthma Rep* 2001;1:438–44.

Chapter 116

Primary Combined Antibody and Cellular Immunodeficiencies

Patients with combined antibody and cellular defects have severe, frequently opportunistic infections that lead to death in infancy or childhood unless they are provided bone marrow transplantation early in life. These are thought to be rare defects; however, the true incidences are unknown because there is no screening for any of these defects during infancy. It is possible that many die of infection without being diagnosed. The defective gene products for many combined immunodeficiencies have been identified (Table 116–1).

116.1 Severe Combined Immunodeficiency (SCID)

The syndromes of SCID are caused by diverse genetic mutations that lead to absence of all adaptive immune function and, in some cases, in a lack of natural killer (NK) cells (see Table 116–1). Patients with this group of disorders have the most severe of all of the recognized immunodeficiencies.

Pathogenesis. Typically, patients with SCID have very small thymuses (<1 g) that usually fail to descend from the neck, contain few thymocytes, and lack corticomedullary distinction and Hassall corpuscles. The thymic epithelium appears histologically normal. Both the follicular and paracortical areas of the spleen are depleted of lymphocytes. Lymph nodes, tonsils, adenoids, and Peyer patches are absent or extremely underdeveloped.

Clinical Manifestations. Affected infants present within the first few months of life with diarrhea, pneumonia, otitis media, sepsis, and cutaneous infections. Growth may appear normal initially, but extreme wasting usually ensues after diarrhea and infections begin. Persistent infections with opportunistic organisms such as *Candida albicans*, *P. carinii*, varicella, measles, parainfluenza 3, CMV, Epstein-Barr virus (EBV), adenovirus, and bacillus Calmette-Guérin (BCG) lead to death. Affected infants also lack the ability to reject foreign tissue and are therefore at risk for graft versus host disease (GVHD) from maternal immunocompetent T cells crossing the placenta, or from T lymphocytes in nonirradiated blood products or allogeneic bone marrow.

Infants with SCID have lymphopenia (<2000/mm³) that is present at birth, indicating that the condition could be diagnosed in all affected infants if white blood cell counts with manual differential counts were routinely performed on all cord bloods. These infants also have an absence of lymphocyte

TABLE 116–1. Combined Immunodeficiency Disorders

Chromosome and Region	Gene Product	Disorder	Functional Deficiencies
1q*	RFX5	MHC class II antigen deficiency	Low immunoglobulins, lack of T-cell responses to antigens, CD4 deficiency
5p 13*	IL-7Rα	T–, B+, NK+ SCID	Absence of T and B cell functions
6p21.3*	TAP1, TAP2	MHC class I antigen deficiency	Marked deficiency of CD8 T cells; combined B- and T-cell defects
6q22–q23*	IFN-γR1	Disseminated mycobacterial infections	Failure of macrophages and other cells to produce TNF-α in response to IFN-γ
9p21–p13	Endoribonuclease RNase MRP	Cartilage-hair hypoplasia	Combined B- and T-cell defects of varying severity (including defective antibody-mediated immunity, CID, and SCID)
10p13*	Artemis	T–, B–, NK + SCID	Absence of T and B cell functions
10p14–p15*	IL2Rα	Lymphoproliferative syndrome	Poor T-cell responses; impaired apoptosis; increased bcl-2; autoimmunity
11p13*	RAG1 or RAG2	T–, B–, NK + SCID	Absence of T and B cell functions
11q22.3*	DNA-dependent kinase	Ataxia-telangiectasia	Selective IgA deficiency; T-cell deficiency
13q*	RFXAP	MHC class II antigen deficiency	Low immunoglobulins, lack of T-cell responses to antigens, CD4 deficiency
14q13.1*	Purine nucleosidase	PNP deficiency	Severe T-cell deficiency; may have immunoglobulins
16p13*	CIITA	MHC class II antigen deficiency	Low immunoglobulins, lack of T-cell responses to antigens, CD4 deficiency
19p13.1*	Jak3	T–, B+, NK– SCID	Absence of T-, B- and NK-cell functions
20q13.11*	ADA	T–, B–, NK– SCID	Absence of T- and B-cell functions
Xp11.23*	WASP	Wiskott-Aldrich syndrome	Thrombocytopenia; poor antipolysaccharide antibody production; T-cell deficiency
Xq13.1*	Common γ chain (γc)	T–, B+, NK– SCID	Absence of T-, B- and NK-cell functions

Gene cloned and sequenced, gene product known.
WASP = Wiskott-Aldrich syndrome protein; TH1 = T-helper cell type 1; TH2 = T-helper cell type 2; PNP = purine nucleoside phosphorylase; IL2Rα = interleukin 2 receptor α chain; ADA = adenosine deaminase; Jak3 = Janus kinase 3; IL7Rα = interleukin 7 receptor α chain; RAG1 and RAG2 = recombinase activating genes 1 and 2; IFN-γR1 = interferon γ receptor chain 1; IL-12β1 = interleukin 12 receptor β1 chain; MHC = major histocompatibility complex; SCID = severe combined immunodeficiency; TAP = transporter of antigenic peptide; CIITA = class II transactivator.

proliferative responses to mitogens, antigens, and allogeneic cells in vitro. Patients with adenosine deaminase (ADA) deficiency have the lowest absolute lymphocyte counts, usually <500/mm³. Serum immunoglobulin concentrations are diminished to absent, and no antibodies are formed after immunizations. Analyses of lymphocyte populations and subpopulations demonstrate distinctive phenotypes for the various genetic forms of SCID. T cells are extremely low or absent in all types; when detected, they are in most cases transplacentally derived maternal T cells.

Treatment. This is a true pediatric emergency. Unless immunologic reconstitution is achieved through bone marrow transplantation, death usually occurs in the 1st yr of life and almost invariably before the end of the 2nd yr. If diagnosed at birth or within the first 3 mo of life, more than 95% of cases can be treated successfully with HLA-identical or T-cell–depleted haploidentical (half-matched) related bone marrow stem cells without the need for pretransplant chemoablation or post-transplant GVHD prophylaxis. Recent success in treating X-linked SCID by gene therapy in both Paris and London offers hope that gene therapy will eventually be the treatment of choice for some if not all forms of SCID for which the molecular bases have been identified.

X-LINKED SEVERE COMBINED IMMUNODEFICIENCY (SCIDX1) DUE TO MUTATIONS IN THE GENE ENCODING THE COMMON CYTOKINE RECEPTOR GAMMA CHAIN (γc)

X-linked SCID (SCIDX1) is the most common form of SCID in the United States, accounting for approximately 45% of cases. Clinically, immunologically, and histopathologically, affected individuals appear similar to those with other forms of SCID except for having uniformly low percentages of T and NK cells and an elevated percentage of B cells (T–, B+, NK–), a characteristic feature shared only with Janus kinase 3 (Jak3)–deficient patients with SCID. The abnormal gene in SCIDX1 was mapped to Xq13, cloned, and found to encode the common γ (γc) chain for several cytokine receptors, including IL-2, IL-4, IL-7, IL-9, IL-

15, and IL-21. The shared γc chain functions both to increase the affinity of the receptor for the respective cytokine and to enable the receptors to mediate intracellular signaling. Incapacitation of the receptors for all of these developmentally crucial cytokines by genetic mutations in the common γ chain provides an explanation for the severity of the immunodeficiency in SCIDX1. In the first 136 patients studied, 95 distinct mutations spanning all 8 IL2RG exons were identified, most of them consisting of small changes at the level of one to a few nucleotides. These mutations resulted in abnormal γc chains in two thirds of the cases and absent γc protein in the remainder. Carriers can be detected by demonstrating nonrandom X-chromosome inactivation or the deleterious mutation in their T, B, or NK lymphocytes. Unless donor B or NK cells develop, patients with SCID have very poor B- and NK-cell function after nonablated bone marrow transplantation because of the many cytokine receptor defects, despite excellent reconstitution of T-cell function by donor-derived T cells.

AUTOSOMAL RECESSIVE SEVERE COMBINED IMMUNODEFICIENCY

This pattern of inheritance of SCID is less common in the United States than in Europe. Mutated genes on autosomal chromosomes have been identified in seven forms of SCID: ADA deficiency, Jak3 deficiency, IL-7 receptor α chain (IL-7Rα) deficiency, RAG1 or RAG2 deficiency, Artemis deficiency, and CD45 deficiency.

ADA Deficiency. An absence of the enzyme adenosine deaminase (ADA) is observed in approximately 15% of patients with SCID, resulting from various point and deletional mutations in the ADA gene on chromosome 20q13-ter. Marked accumulations of adenosine, 2′-deoxyadenosine, and 2′-O-methyladenosine lead directly or indirectly to T-cell apoptosis, which causes the immunodeficiency. ADA-deficient patients usually have a much more profound lymphopenia than do infants with other types of SCID, with mean absolute lymphocyte counts of <500/mm³; the absolute numbers of T, B and NK cells are very low. NK function is normal. After T-cell function is conferred by bone marrow transplantation, without pretransplant chemotherapy, there is generally excellent B-cell function. This is because ADA deficiency affects primarily T-cell function. Milder forms of ADA deficiency have led to delayed diagnosis of immunodeficiency, even to adulthood. Other distinguishing features of ADA-deficient SCID include the presence of rib cage abnormalities similar to a rachitic rosary and numerous skeletal abnormalities of chondro-osseous dysplasia, which occur predominantly at the costochondral junctions, at the apophyses of the iliac bones, and in the vertebral bodies where a "bone-in-bone" effect is observed.

As with other types of SCID, ADA deficiency can be cured by HLA-identical or haploidentical T-cell-depleted bone marrow transplantation without the need for pre- or post-transplant chemotherapy; this remains the treatment of choice. Enzyme replacement therapy should not be initiated if bone marrow transplantation is possible because it confers graft-rejection capability. Gene therapy has been attempted several times over the last decade but until very recently had not been successful. A spontaneous in vivo reversion to normal of a mutation in the ADA gene has been reported.

Jak3 Deficiency. Patients with this recently discovered autosomal recessive defect resemble all other types of SCID patients clinically. However, they have a lymphocyte phenotype similar only to that of patients with SCIDX1 with an elevated percentage of B cells and very low or no T and NK cells. Because Jak3 is the only signaling molecule known to be associated with γ_c, it was a candidate gene for mutations leading to autosomal recessive SCID not attributable to ADA deficiency. Jak3 deficiency accounts for approximately 6% of SCID cases. Even after successful T-cell reconstitution by transplantation of haploidentical stem cells, patients with Jak3-deficient SCID fail to develop NK cells or normal B-cell function owing to the defective function of the many types of cytokine receptors that share γ_c.

IL-7Rα Deficiency. Patients with IL-7Rα-deficient SCID have a distinctive lymphocyte phenotype in that, though lacking T cells, they have normal or elevated numbers of both B and NK cells (T-, B+, NK+). This form of SCID represents approximately 10% of SCID cases in the United States. In contrast to patients with γ_c- and Jak3-deficient SCID, the immunologic defect in these patients is completely correctable even by T-cell-depleted haploidentical bone marrow stem cell transplantation.

RAG1 or RAG2 Deficiencies. Infants with these causes of SCID have a different lymphocyte phenotype from those of patients with SCID due to γ_c, Jak3, IL-7Rα, or ADA deficiencies in that they lack both B and T lymphocytes and have primarily NK cells in their circulation (T-, B-, NK+). This suggested a problem with their antigen receptor genes that led to the discovery of mutations in **recombinase activating genes, RAG1 or RAG2.** Such mutations result in a functional inability to form antigen receptors through genetic recombination.

Artemis Deficiency. A very recently discovered cause of human SCID is a deficiency of a novel V(D)J recombination/DNA repair factor that belongs to the metallo-β-lactamase superfamily, which is encoded on chromosome 10p by a gene called Artemis. Deficiency of this factor results in an inability to repair DNA after double-stranded cuts by the RAG1 or RAG2 gene products in rearranging antigen receptor genes from their germline configuration. Similar to RAG1 and RAG2 deficient SCID, this defect results in another form of T-, B-, NK+ SCID, also called **Athabascan SCID.** In addition, there is increased radiation sensitivity of both skin fibroblasts and bone marrow cells of those affected with this type of SCID.

CD45 Deficiency. Another recently discovered molecular defect causing SCID is a mutation in the gene encoding the common leukocyte surface protein CD45. This hematopoietic cell–specific transmembrane protein tyrosine phosphatase functions to regulate *src* kinases required for T- and B-cell antigen receptor signal transduction. A 2-mo-old male infant presented with a clinical picture of SCID and was found to have a very low number of T cells but a normal number of B cells. The T cells failed to respond to mitogens, and serum immunoglobulins diminished with time. He was found to have a large deletion on one CD45 allele and a point mutation causing an alteration of the intervening sequence 13 donor splice site on the other allele. A second case of SCID due to CD45 deficiency has been reported.

RETICULAR DYSGENESIS

Reticular dysgenesis was first described in identical twin boys who exhibited a total lack of both lymphocytes and granulocytes in their peripheral blood and bone marrow. Seven of 8 infants with this defect died between 3 and 119 days of age as a result of overwhelming infections; 7 infants have been cured by bone marrow transplantation. The thymus glands have all weighed <1 g, have no Hassall corpuscles, and few or no thymocytes. Reticular dysgenesis is considered a variant of SCID. The molecular basis of this autosomal recessive disorder is unknown.

116.2 Combined Immunodeficiency (CID)

CID is distinguished from SCID by the presence of low but not absent T-cell function. Like SCID, however, CID is a syndrome of diverse genetic causes. Patients with CID have recurrent or chronic pulmonary infections, failure to thrive, oral or cutaneous candidiasis, chronic diarrhea, recurrent skin infections, gram-negative sepsis, urinary tract infections, and severe varicella in infancy. Although they usually survive longer than infants with SCID, they fail to thrive and die early in life. Neutropenia and eosinophilia are common. Serum immunoglobulins may be normal or elevated for all classes, but selective IgA deficiency, marked elevation of IgE, and elevated IgD levels occur in some cases. Although antibody-forming capacity is impaired in most patients, it is not absent.

Studies of cellular immune function show lymphopenia, profound deficiencies of T cells, and extremely low but not absent lymphocyte proliferative responses to mitogens, antigens, and allogeneic cells in vitro. Peripheral lymphoid tissues demonstrate paracortical lymphocyte depletion. The thymus is very small with a paucity of thymocytes and usually no Hassall corpuscles. An autosomal recessive pattern of inheritance is common.

PURINE NUCLEOSIDE PHOSPHORYLASE DEFICIENCY

More than 40 patients with CID have been found to have purine nucleoside phosphorylase (PNP) deficiency. Point mutations identified in the PNP gene on chromosome 14q13.1 account for these deficiencies. In contrast to ADA deficiency, no characteristic physical or skeletal abnormalities have been noted, and serum and urinary uric acid are usually markedly deficient. Deaths result from generalized vaccinia, varicella, lymphosarcoma, or GVHD mediated by allogeneic T cells in nonirradiated blood or bone marrow. Two thirds of patients have neurologic abnormalities, and one third have autoimmune diseases. Lymphopenia is striking, primarily because of a marked deficiency of T cells; T-cell function is decreased to various degrees. The proportion of circulating NK cells is increased. Prenatal diagnosis is possible. Gene therapy is a possibility for the future, but thus far bone marrow transplantation has been the only successful form of therapy.

INTERLEUKIN 2 RECEPTOR α CHAIN (IL-2R α [CD25]) MUTATION

An infant boy born of a consanguineous union developed cytomegalovirus (CMV) pneumonia, persistent candidiasis, adenoviral gastroenteritis, failure to thrive, lymphadenopathy, hepatosplenomegaly, and chronic inflammation of his lungs and mandible. Biopsy specimens revealed extensive lymphocytic infiltration of his lung, liver, intestines, and bone. Serum IgA level was low. He had T-cell lymphopenia, and the T cells responded poorly to anti-CD3, phytohemagglutinin (PHA) and other mitogens, and IL-2. He was found to have a mutation in the gene encoding the IL-2 receptor α chain (IL-2Rα [CD25]), leading to truncation of the protein. He had no CD1 in his thymus, and an elevation of the anti-apoptotic protein bcl-2. This defect reveals that some components of cytokine receptors normally serve a negative regulatory role. Mutations in those components can result in unchecked lymphoproliferation and autoimmunity in addition to immunodeficiency.

CARTILAGE HAIR HYPOPLASIA

Cartilage hair hypoplasia (CHH) is an unusual form of short-limbed dwarfism with frequent and severe infections. It occurs predominantly among the Pennsylvania Amish, but non-Amish patients have been described.

Genetics and Pathogenesis. CHH is an autosomal recessive condition. Numerous mutations that cosegregate with the CHH phenotype have been identified in the untranslated RNase MRP gene, which has recently been mapped to chromosome 9p21–p13 in Amish and Finnish families (see Table 116–1). The RNase MRP endoribonuclease consists of an RNA molecule bound to several proteins and has at least two functions: cleavage of RNA in mitochondrial DNA synthesis and nucleolar cleaving of pre-RNA. Mutations in RMRP cause CHH by disrupting a function of RNase MRP RNA that affects multiple organ systems. In vitro studies show decreased numbers of T cells and defective T-cell proliferation due to an intrinsic defect related to the G1 phase, resulting in a longer cell cycle for individual cells. However, NK cells are increased in number and function.

Clinical Manifestations. Clinical features include short, pudgy hands; redundant skin; hyperextensible joints of hands and feet but an inability to extend the elbows completely; and fine, sparse, light hair and eyebrows. Severe and often fatal varicella infections, progressive vaccinia, and vaccine-associated poliomyelitis have been observed. Associated conditions include deficient erythrogenesis, Hirschsprung disease, and an increased risk of malignancies. The bones radiographically show scalloping and sclerotic or cystic changes in the metaphyses and flaring of the costochondral junctions of the ribs. Three patterns of immune dysfunction have emerged: defective antibody-mediated immunity, CID (most common), and SCID. The severity of the immunodeficiency varies; in one series, 11 of 77 patients died before age 20 yr but two were still alive at age 76. Bone marrow transplantation has resulted in immunologic reconstitution in some CHH patients with the SCID phenotype.

OMENN SYNDROME

Omenn syndrome is an autosomal recessive, fatal condition characterized by profound susceptibility to infection with T-cell infiltration of skin, intestines, liver, and spleen leading to an exfoliative erythroderma, lymphadenopathy, hepatosplenomegaly, and intractable diarrhea. Mutations in the recombinase activating genes, RAG1 and RAG2, have been found in several patients with this condition. Thus, this is a "leaky" form of SCID. These infants have persistent leukocytosis with marked eosinophilia and lymphocytosis; elevated serum IgE; low IgG, IgA, and IgM; low or absent B cells; and elevated numbers of clonal, likely autoreactive, T cells. There is dominance of TH2-like cells with severely impaired T-cell function due to the restricted heterogeneity of the host T-cell repertoire.

DEFECTIVE EXPRESSION OF MAJOR HISTOCOMPATIBILITY COMPLEX ANTIGENS

The two main forms of immunodeficiency and abnormalities of expression of the major histocopmatibility complex (MHC) are MHC class I (HLA-A, -B, and -C) antigen deficiency and MHC class II (HLA-DR, -DQ, and -DP) antigen deficiency. The associated defects of both B- and T-cell immunity and of HLA expression emphasize the important biologic role for HLA determinants in effective immune cell cooperation.

MHC Class I Antigen Deficiency

Isolated deficiency of MHC class I (HLA-A, -B, and -C) antigens, the **bare lymphocyte syndrome**, is rare. The resulting immunodeficiency is much milder than in SCID, contributing to a later age of presentation. Sera from affected children contain normal quantities of MHC class I antigens and β_2-microglobulin, but MHC class I antigens are not detected on any cells in the body. There is a deficiency of CD8 but not CD4 T cells. Mutations have been found in two genes within the MHC locus on chromosome 6 that encode the peptide transporter proteins, TAP1 and TAP2. TAP functions to transport antigenic peptides from the cytoplasm across the Golgi apparatus membrane to join the α chain of MHC class 1 antigens and β_2-microglobulin. All these are then assembled into a MHC class I complex that can then move to the cell surface. If the assembly of the complex cannot be completed because there is no antigenic peptide, the MHC class I complex is destroyed in the cytoplasm.

MHC Class II Antigen Deficiency

Many affected with MHC class II (HLA-DR, -DQ, and -DP) deficiency are of North African descent. Patients present in early infancy with persistent diarrhea that is often associated with cryptosporidiosis and enteroviral infections (e.g., poliovirus, coxsackievirus). They also have an increased frequency of infections with herpesviruses and other viruses, oral candidiasis, bacterial pneumonia, P. carinii pneumonia, and septicemia. The immunodeficiency is not as severe as in SCID, as evidenced by their failure to develop disseminated infection after BCG vaccination or GVHD from nonirradiated blood transfusions.

Four different molecular defects resulting in impaired expression of MHC class II antigens have been identified (see Table 116–1). One form is a mutation in the gene on chromosome 1q that encodes a protein called RFX5, a subunit of RFX, a multiprotein complex that binds the X box motif of MHC-II promoters. A second form is caused by mutations in a gene on chromosome 13q that encodes a second 36-kD subunit of the RFX complex, called RFX-associated protein (RFXAP). The most recently discovered and most common cause of MHC Class II defects are mutations in RFXANK, the gene encoding a third subunit of RFX. In a fourth type, there is a mutation in the gene on chromosome 16p13 that encodes a novel MHC class II transactivator (CIITA), a non–DNA-binding co-activator that controls the cell-type specificity and inducibility of MHC-II expression. All four of these defects cause impairment in the coordinate expression of MHC class II molecules on the surface of B cells and macrophages.

MHC class II–deficient patients have a very low number of CD4 T cells but normal or elevated numbers of CD8 T cells. Lymphopenia is only moderate. The MHC class II antigens HLA-DP, DQ, and DR are undetectable on blood B cells and monocytes, even though B cells are present in normal number.

Patients are hypogammaglobulinemic owing to impaired antigen-specific responses caused by the absence of these antigen-presenting molecules. In addition, MHC antigen-deficient B cells fail to stimulate allogeneic cells in mixed leukocyte culture. Lymphocyte proliferation studies show normal responses to mitogens but no response to antigens. The thymus and other lymphoid organs are severely hypoplastic, and the lack of class II molecules results in abnormal thymic selection with circulating CD4 T cells that have altered CDR3 profiles.

IMMUNODEFICIENCY WITH THROMBOCYTOPENIA AND ECZEMA (WISKOTT-ALDRICH SYNDROME)

Wiskott-Aldrich syndrome, an X-linked recessive syndrome, is characterized by atopic dermatitis, thrombocytopenic purpura with normal-appearing megakaryocytes but small defective platelets, and undue susceptibility to infection.

Genetics and Pathogenesis. The abnormal gene, on the proximal arm of the X chromosome at Xp11.22–11.23 near the centromere, encodes a 501–amino acid proline-rich cytoplasmic protein restricted in its expression to lymphocytic and megakaryocytic cell lineages. This protein, now referred to as the **Wiskott-Aldrich syndrome protein (WASP),** has been shown to bind CDC42H2 and *rac*, members of the Rho family of guanosine triphosphatases. WASP appears to control the assembly of actin filaments required for microvesicle formation downstream of protein kinase C and tyrosine kinase signaling. Carriers can be detected by nonrandom X-chromosome inactivation in several hematopoietic cell lineages or by demonstration of the deleterious mutation.

Clinical Manifestations. Patients often have prolonged bleeding from the circumcision site or bloody diarrhea during infancy. The thrombocytopenia is not initially due to antiplatelet antibodies. Atopic dermatitis and recurrent infections usually develop during the 1st yr of life. *Streptococcus pneumoniae* and other bacteria having polysaccharide capsules cause otitis media, pneumonia, meningitis, and sepsis. Later, infections with agents such as *P. carinii* and the herpesviruses become more frequent. Survival beyond the teens is rare; infections, bleeding, and EBV-associated malignancies are major causes of death.

Patients with this defect uniformly have an impaired humoral immune response to polysaccharide antigens, as evidenced by absent or markedly diminished isohemagglutinins, and poor or absent antibody responses after immunization with polysaccharide vaccines. IgG2 subclass concentrations, surprisingly, are normal. Anamnestic responses to protein antigens are poor or absent. There is an accelerated rate of synthesis as well as hypercatabolism of albumin, IgG, IgA, and IgM, resulting in highly variable concentrations of different immunoglobulins, even within the same patient. The predominant immunoglobulin pattern is a low serum level of IgM, elevated IgA and IgE, and a normal or slightly low IgG concentration. Percentages of T cells are moderately reduced, and lymphocyte responses to mitogens are variably depressed.

ATAXIA-TELANGIECTASIA

Ataxia-telangiectasia is a complex syndrome with immunologic, neurologic, endocrinologic, hepatic, and cutaneous abnormalities.

Genetics and Pathogenesis. The mutated gene responsible for this defect, **ataxia telangiectasia mutation (ATM)**, was mapped to the long arm of chromosome 11 (11q22–23) and has been cloned. The gene product is a DNA-dependent protein kinase localized predominantly to the nucleus and involved in mitogenic signal transduction, meiotic recombination, and cell cycle control. Cells from patients as well as those of heterozygous carriers have increased sensitivity to ionizing radiation, defective DNA repair, and frequent chromosomal abnormalities.

In vitro tests of lymphocyte function have generally shown moderately depressed proliferative responses to T- and B-cell mitogens. Percentages of CD3 and CD4 T cells are moderately reduced, with normal or increased percentages of CD8 and elevated numbers of Tiγ/δ T cells. Studies of immunoglobulin synthesis have shown both helper T-cell and intrinsic B-cell defects. The thymus is very hypoplastic, exhibits poor organization, and lacks Hassall corpuscles.

Clinical Manifestations. The most prominent clinical features are progressive cerebellar ataxia, oculocutaneous telangiectasias, chronic sinopulmonary disease, a high incidence of malignancy, and variable humoral and cellular immunodeficiency. Ataxia typically becomes evident soon after these children begin to walk and progresses until they are confined to a wheelchair, usually by the age of 10–12 yr. The telangiectasias develop between 3 and 6 yr of age. The most frequent humoral immunologic abnormality is the selective absence of IgA, which is present in 50–80% of these patients. Hypercatabolism of IgA also occurs. IgE concentrations are usually low, and the IgM may be of the low molecular weight variety. IgG2 or total IgG levels may be decreased, and specific antibody titers may be decreased or normal. Recurrent sinopulmonary infections occur in approximately 80% of these patients. Although common viral infections have not usually resulted in untoward sequelae, fatal varicella has occurred. The malignancies associated with ataxia-telangiectasia are usually of the lymphoreticular type, but adenocarcinomas are also found. Unaffected relatives have an increased incidence of malignancy.

INTERFERON-γ RECEPTOR 1 AND 2 AND IL-12 RECEPTOR β1 MUTATIONS

Disseminated BCG infections occur in patients with severe T-cell defects, but no specific host defect is identified in approximately half of such cases. Explanations for this predilection have been discovered. The first was found in a 2.5-mo-old Tunisian girl who had fatal idiopathic disseminated BCG infection and in four children from Malta who had disseminated atypical mycobacterial infections in the absence of a recognized immunodeficiency. There was consanguinity in all, and each had a functional defect in the upregulation of tumor necrosis factor α (TNF-α) production by their blood macrophages in response to stimulation with interferon-γ (IFN-γ). Each was also found to have a mutation in the gene on chromosome 6q22–q23 that encodes the IFN-γ receptor 1 (IFN-γR1). Patients with mutations in the IFN-γR2 have also been identified. A third type of defect was found in other patients who had disseminated mycobacterial infections and who were found to have mutations in the ß1 chain of the IL-12 receptor (IL-12Rβ1). IL-12 is a powerful inducer of IFN-γ production by T and NK cells, and the mutated receptor chain gene resulted in unresponsiveness of these patients' cells to IL-12 and inadequate IFN-γ production. Interestingly, the IFN-γR1, IFN-γR2, and IL-12Rβ1-deficient children appeared not to be susceptible to infection with many agents other than mycobacteria. TH1 responses appeared to be normal in these patients. The susceptibility of these patients to mycobacterial infections thus apparently results from an intrinsic impairment of the IFN-γ pathway response to these particular intracellular pathogens, showing that IFN-γ is obligatory for efficient macrophage antimycobacterial activity.

HYPER IgE SYNDROME

The hyper IgE syndrome is a relatively rare primary immunodeficiency syndrome characterized by recurrent severe staphylococcal abscesses of the skin, lungs, and other viscera and markedly elevated levels of serum IgE. More than 200 patients with hyper IgE syndrome have been reported. The inheritance pattern is as a single locus autosomal dominant trait with variable expression.

Clinical Manifestations. These patients have histories from infancy of recurrent staphylococcal abscesses involving the skin, lungs, joints, and other sites. Persistent pneumatoceles develop as a result of recurrent pneumonias. The pruritic dermatitis that occurs is not typical atopic eczema, and it does not always persist. Allergic respiratory symptoms are usually absent. The first two reported patients were described as having **coarse facial features** including a prominent forehead, deep-set wide-spaced eyes, a broad nasal bridge, a wide fleshy nasal tip, mild prognathism, facial asymmetry, and hemihypertrophy. In older children, delay in shedding primary teeth, recurrent fractures, and scoliosis occur.

These patients demonstrate an exceptionally high serum IgE concentration; an elevated serum IgD concentration; usually normal concentrations of IgG, IgA, and IgM; pronounced blood and sputum eosinophilia; abnormally low anamnestic antibody responses; and poor antibody and cell-mediated responses to neoantigens. In vitro studies show normal percentages of blood T, B, and NK lymphocytes, with the exception of a decreased percentage of T cells with the memory (CD45RO) phenotype. Paradoxically, B cells from these patients demonstrate very low levels of IL-4–stimulated IgE synthesis in vitro, suggesting that they have already been maximally stimulated by a high level of endogenous IL-4. The molecular basis of this disorder remains unknown. Most patients have normal T-lymphocyte proliferative responses to mitogens but very low or absent responses to antigens or allogeneic cells from family members. Blood, sputum, and histologic sections of lymph nodes, spleen, and lung cysts show striking eosinophilia. Hassall corpuscles and thymic architecture are normal. Phagocytic cell ingestion, metabolism and killing, and total hemolytic complement activity are normal in all patients. Results of chemotaxis studies have been mostly normal; thus, defective chemotaxis is not the basic problem in this syndrome.

The most effective therapy is long-term administration of therapeutic doses of a penicillinase-resistant anti-staphylococcal antibiotic, adding other agents as required for specific infections. Intravenous immunoglobulin (IVIG) should be administered to antibody-deficient patients, and appropriate thoracic surgery should be provided for superinfected pneumatoceles or those persisting beyond 6 mo.

116.3 Treatment of Cellular or Combined Immunodeficiency

Transplantation of MHC-compatible sibling or haploidentical (half-matched) parental bone marrow is currently the treatment of choice for patients with fatal T-cell or combined T- and B-cell defects. However, there is considerable optimism that gene therapy will be the treatment of choice for many of these defects in the future. The major risk to the recipient from transplants of bone marrow is that of GVHD. The development of techniques to deplete all post-thymic T cells from donor marrow permits safe and successful use of haploidentical related bone marrow stem cells for the correction of SCID and other fatal immunodeficiency syndromes. Patients with less severe forms of cellular immunodeficiency, including some forms of CID, Wiskott-Aldrich syndrome, cytokine deficiency, and MHC antigen deficiency, reject even HLA-identical marrow grafts unless chemoablative treatment is given before transplantation. Several patients with these conditions have been treated successfully with HLA-identical bone marrow transplantation after conditioning.

From 1968 to 1977, only 14 of 48 infants (29%) with SCID worldwide were long-term survivors after successful HLA class II–compatible bone marrow transplantation. The results of bone marrow transplantation have improved considerably during the past 25 years, possibly because of earlier diagnosis before untreatable opportunistic infections develop. A worldwide survey conducted by the author in 1997 revealed that 224 of 285 (79%) of patients with primary immunodeficiency transplanted with HLA-identical related marrow were surviving. Most encouraging are the results of T-cell–depleted haploidentical related marrow transplants in patients with primary immunodeficiency; 605 patients had had such transplants performed, and of those, 332 (55%) survive. The significance is even more impressive with the realization that most of the 605 recipients would have died had not the T-cell depletion techniques been developed. The greatest success has been in patients with SCID, who do not require pretransplant conditioning or GVHD prophylaxis; 100 of 128 (78%) patients with SCID transplanted by the author during the past 20 years survive, and all but 15 received T-cell–depleted parental marrow. Until somatic cell gene therapy is more fully developed, bone marrow transplantation remains the most important and effective therapy for these inborn errors of the immune system.

Buckley RH: Advances in the understanding and treatment of human severe combined immunodeficiency. *Immunol Res* 2001;22:237–51.

Buckley RH: The hyper-IgE syndrome. *Clin Rev Allergy Immunol* 2001;20:139–54.

Buckley RH: Primary immunodeficiency diseases due to defects in lymphocytes. *N Engl J Med* 2000;343:1313–24.

Buckley RH, Schiff SE, Schiff RI, et al: Hematopoietic stem cell transplantation for the treatment of severe combined immunodeficiency. *N Engl J Med* 1999;340: 508–16.

Casanova JL: Mendelian susceptibility to mycobacterial infection in man. *Swiss Med Wkly* 2001;131:445–54.

Hacein-Bey-Abina S, Le Deist F, Carlier F, et al: Sustained correction of X-linked severe combined immunodeficiency by ex vivo gene therapy. *N Engl J Med* 2002;346:1185–93.

Myers LA, Patel DD, Puck JM: Hematopoietic stem cell transplantation for severe combined immunodeficiency in the neonatal period leads to superior thymic output and improved survival. *Blood* 2002;99:872–78.

Patel DD, Gooding ME, Parrott RE, et al: Thymic function after hematopoietic stem-cell transplantation for the treatment of severe combined immunodeficiency. *N Engl J Med* 2000;342:1325–32.

Reith W, Mach B: The bare lymphocyte syndrome and the regulation of MHC expression. *Annu Rev Immunol* 2001;19:331–73.

Vihinen M, Arredondo-Vega FX, Casanova JL, et al: Primary immunodeficiency mutation databases. *Adv Genet* 2001;43:103–88.

SECTION 3 *The Phagocytic System*

Chapter 117
Neutrophils *Laurence A. Boxer*

The Phagocytic Inflammatory Response. Neutrophils and mononuclear phagocytes share primary functions including the unusual ability to ingest large particles. Neutrophils are of only one type, but there are many varieties of mononuclear phagocytes including the tissue macrophages, and their circulating precursors, monocytes (Chapter 118). Neutrophils develop less rapidly in the bone marrow than monocytes, and remain for only 6 hours in the circulation (Table 117–1).

The hematopoietic progenitor system can be envisioned as a continuum of functional compartments with the most primitive compartment composed of very rare cells known as **pluripotential stem cells**, which have high self-renewal capacity. Pluripotential stem cells give rise to more mature stem cells, including cells that are committed to either lymphoid or myeloid development. Lymphoid stem cells give rise to T- and B-cell precursors and their mature progeny (Chapter 113). Trilineage myeloid stem cells, designated CFU-S for the spleen colony-forming unit described in mice, eventually give rise to committed single-lineage progenitors of the recognizable precursors through a random process of lineage restriction in a stepwise process (Fig. 117–1). The lineage restriction arises from cell-surface expression of lineage-specific growth factor receptors. Single-lineage progenitors, including erythroid burst-forming units (BFU-E), erythroid colony-forming units (CFU-E), megakaryocyte colony-forming units (CFU-Meg), and basophil, granulocyte, monocyte, and eosinophil colony-forming units (CFU-Baso, CFU-G, CFU-M, and CFU-Eo, respectively) proliferate and differentiate into their respective precursors in response to the growth factors that bind to their unique receptors. The capacity of lineage-specific committed progenitors to proliferate and differentiate in response to demand constitutes the most important buffer of the hematopoietic system against increased requirement for mature blood cell production.

Hematopoietic Growth Factors. The proliferation, differentiation, and survival of immature hematopoietic progenitor cells are governed by **hematopoietic growth factors (HGFs),** a family of glycoproteins (Table 117–2). Besides regulating proliferation and differentiation of progenitors, these factors influence the survival and function of mature blood cells. The HGFs include the **interleukins** and the **colony-stimulating factors (CSFs),** which have been named for their ability to stimulate progenitor cells to form colonies of recognizable mature cells in vitro. The majority of lineage-specific progenitors require the presence of additional growth factors such as interleukin 3 (IL-3) or granulocyte-macrophage CSF (GM-CSF) in addition to a lineage-specific HGF to generate the colonies for which they are programmed. Hence, immature committed progenitors bear receptors for IL-3, stem cell factor (SCF), GM-CSF, and IL-6 (Fig. 117–2). These committed progenitors differ from one another with respect to their lineage-specific receptors; this allows the lineage-specific HGF to produce the colonies for which they are programmed. During granulopoiesis and monopoiesis, several cytokines regulate progenitor cells or mature effector cells at each stage of maturation and differentiation from the primitive pluripotent stem cells to nondividing terminally differentiated cells (monocytes, neutrophils, eosinophils, and basophils). The actions of these growth factors are mediated through lineage-specific receptors. As cells mature, they lose receptors for most cytokines, especially those that influence early cell development, such as SCF. Once the cells have matured, however, they express receptors for chemokines, which help direct the cells to sites of inflammation.

Neutrophil Maturation and Kinetics. The bone marrow microenvironment supporting the progenitors and precursors must provide for the normal steady-state rates of renewal of the cellular elements of blood through its ability to provide growth and differentiation factors generated by stromal cells themselves. The growth factors such as granulocyte colony-stimulating factor (G-CSF) and GM-CSF not only stimulate cell division, but also affect the synthesis of many cytoplasmic components of the neutrophil as well as expression of transcription factors that are necessary for myeloid cell differentiation. Transcription factors such as PU.1, Sp-1, C/EBP alpha, and Oct-1 affect myeloid differentiation. For example, the promoter for the myeloblastin gene has a binding site for PU.1, which is engaged following activation of myeloid progenitor cells with G-CSF. Normally, the production rates precisely equal destruction rates. Granulocytes survive intravascularly for only 6–12 hr and therefore daily production of 2×10^4 granulocytes/μL of blood is required to maintain a level of circulating granulocytes of 5×10^3/μL. In contrast, lymphocytes that can exhibit lifetimes measured in months or years require daily renewal of certain lymphocyte progenitors at rates substantially lower than the other hematopoietic progenitors.

The process of intramedullary granulocyte maturation involves changes in nuclear configuration and accumulation of specific intracytoplasmic granules (see Table 117–2). The relatively small peripheral blood pool is compartmentalized into the **circulating pool** and the **marginating pool.** The peripheral blood pool provides entrance into the tissue and is buffered by an immense marrow reserve of identifiable precursors, some of which are undergoing mitosis and some of which are maturing into bands and neutrophils. Proliferation of myeloid cells

TABLE 117–1. Neutrophil and Monocyte Kinetics

Neutrophils

Average time in mitosis (myeloblast to myelocyte)	7–9 day
Average time in postmitosis and storage (metamyelocyte to neutrophil)	3–7 day
Average half-life in the circulation	6 hr
Average total body pool	6.5×10^8 cells/kg
Average circulating pool	3.2×10^8 cells/kg
Average marginating pool	3.3×10^8 cells/kg
Average daily turnover rate	1.8×10^{10} cells/kg

Mononuclear Phagocytes

Average time in mitosis	30–48 hr
Average half-life in the circulation	36–104 hr
Average circulating pool (monocytes)	1.8×10^7 cells/kg
Average daily turnover rate	1.8×10^9 cells/kg
Average survival in tissues (macrophages)	Mo

From Boxer LA: Function of neutrophils and mononuclear phagocytes. In Bennett JC, Plum F (editors): Cecil Textbook of Internal Medicine, 20th ed. Philadelphia, WB Saunders, 1996.

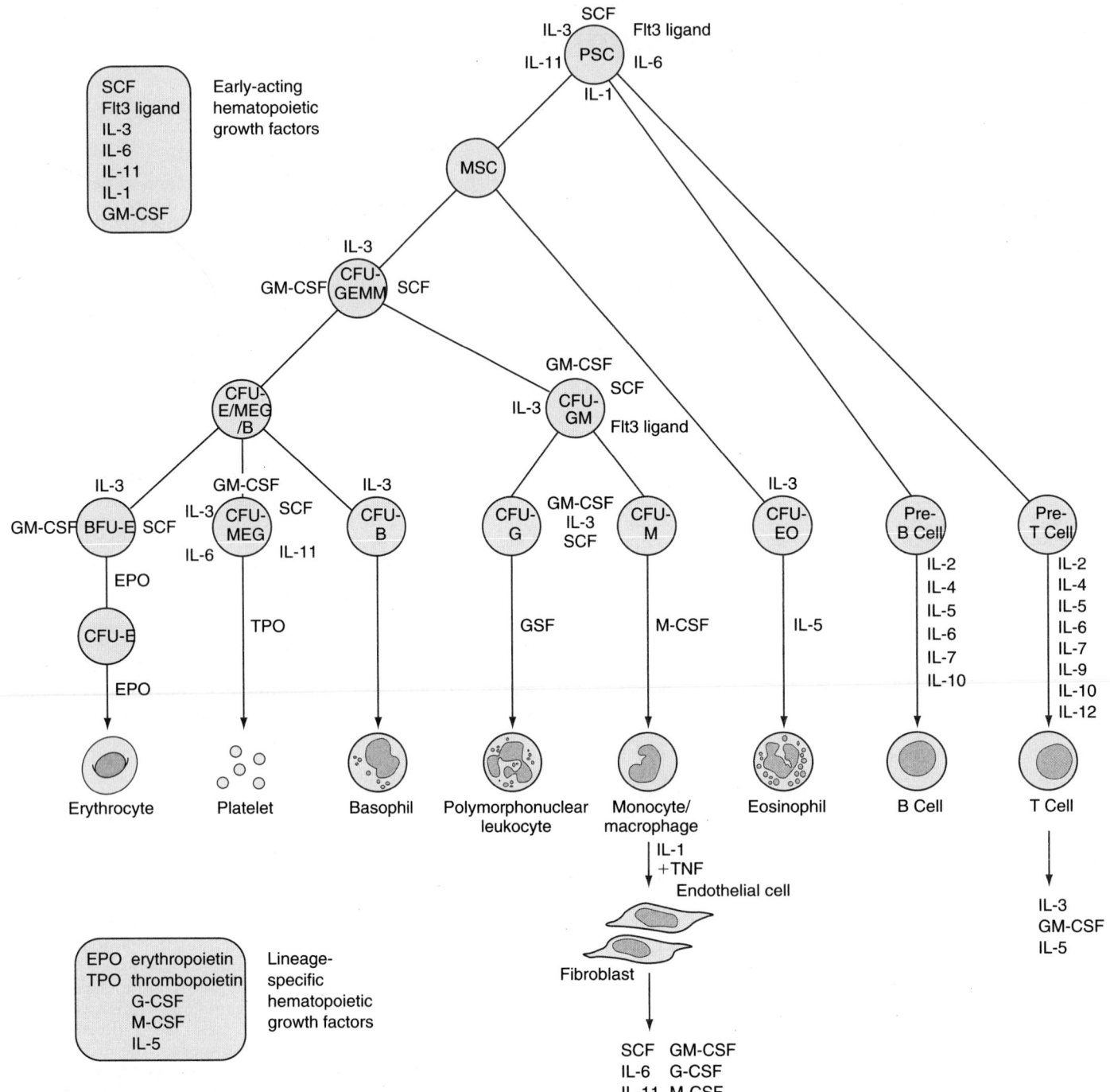

FIGURE 117–1. Major cytokine sources and actions. Cells of the bone marrow microenvironment such as macrophages (ma), endothelial cells (ec), and reticular fibroblastoid cells (fb) produce macrophage colony-stimulating factor (M-CSF), granulocyte-macrophage colony-stimulating factor (GM-CSF), granulocyte colony-stimulating factor (G-CSF), interleukin (IL-6), and probably stem cell factor (SCF; cellular sources not yet precisely determined) after induction with endotoxin (ma) or IL-1/TNF (ec, fb). T cells produce IL-3, GM-CSF, and IL-5 in response to antigenic and IL-1 stimulation. These cytokines have overlapping actions during hematopoietic differentiation, as indicated, and for all lineages optimal development requires a combination of early- and late-acting factors. PSC = pluripotent stem cells; MSC = myeloid stem cells; TNF = tumor necrosis factor. (Modified from Sieff CA, Nathan DG, Clark SC: The anatomy and physiology of hematopoiesis. In Nathan DG and Orkin SH [editors]: *Hematology of Infancy and Childhood,* 5th ed. Philadelphia, WB Saunders, 1997.)

consisting of approximately five divisions takes place only during the first three stages of neutrophil development (myeloblast, promyelocyte, and myelocyte). After the myelocyte stage, the cells terminally differentiate into metamyelocytes, bands, and neutrophils. Neutrophil maturation is associated with changes in the nucleus and with the production of azurophilic primary granules and specific or secondary granules. A myeloblast is a relatively undifferentiated cell with a large oval nucleus, a sizeable nucleolus, and a deficiency of granules. Promyelocytes acquire peroxidase-positive

TABLE 117–2. **Major Human Hematopoietic Growth Factors and Cytokines**

Factor	Synonym	Source	Biologic Activities	
			Progenitors	*Mature Cells*
SCF	Steel factor Stem cell factor Kit ligand	Stromal fibroblasts Vascular endothelium	Synergistic with IL-3, IL-11, IL-6 on blast CFC Synergistic with IL-3, GM-CSF, G-CSF, erythropoietin, thrombopoietin on committed CFC	Mast cell & stem cell growth
Flt, ligand		Spleen Lung	Synergistic with SCF, IL-3, IL-11 on blast CFC Synergistic with IL-3, GM-CSF, G-CSF on committed CFC Synergistic with IL-7, SCF on B-cell progenitors	
IL-3	Multi CSF	T cells Mast cells	All CFC	Eosinophils B cells Monocytes
GM-CSF	CSFα	T cells Endothelium Fibroblasts Monocytes	All CFC	Neutrophils Monocytes Eosinophils
G-CSF	CSFβ	Monocytes Endothelium Fibroblasts	CFU-granulocyte	Neutrophils
IL-5		T cells Mast cells	CFU-eosinophil	Eosinophils
M-CSF	CSF-1	Fibroblasts Endothelial cells	CFU-monocyte	Monocytes
Erythropoietin Thrombopoietin		Kidney Liver Kidney Fibroblasts Endothelium	BFU-erythroid, CFU-erythroid CFU-megakaryocyte	Erythroblasts Megakaryocytes
IL-1α		Monocytes Fibroblasts Endothelium	Synergistic with SCF, IL-3 on blast CFU	Activates cytokine production
IL-1β		Monocytes Fibroblasts Endothelium Kupffer cells Smooth muscle		
IL-2		T cells	T cell growth factor	Activates B cells and NK cells
IL-4		T cells Mast cells	Promotes B cell differentiation and dendritic cell proliferation & differentiation	IgG induction factor
IL-6		Monocytes T cells B cells Fibroblasts Endothelium Kupffer cells	Synergistic: SCF, IL-3, on blast CFU	
IL-7		Stromal cells	Growth factor for B & T cells	
IL-9		TH2 cells	Mast cell growth Synergistic with Epo on BFU	
IL-10		T helper and B cells, keratinocytes, macrophages	Mast cell and B cell proliferation	B cell antibody production suppresser, cytokine production from monocyte and T-helper cells
IL-11		Stromal fibroblasts	Synergistic with SCF, IL-3 on blast CFC Synergistic with IL-3, SCF on CFU-megakaryocyte	Megakaryocytes
IL-12		Macrophages B cells		Induces IFN-γ and cell-mediated immunity from T cells and NK cells
IL-13		T cells	Growth and proliferation of T cells	Promotes IgE production from B cells
IL-14		T cells, some B cell malignancies		Inhibits Ig synthesis
IL-15		Monocytes, neutrophils, fibroblasts	Growth and proliferation of T cells	
IL-16		Activated T helper and T suppressor cells Eosinophils Mast cells		Activates T helper cells
IL-17		T helper and T suppressor		Activates macrophages to secrete cytokines
IL-18		Stromal cells Macrophages		Induces IFNγ secretion from T helper cells & NK cells
IFNα,β		Leukocytes, fibroblasts	Antiproliferative for CFU-GM and BFU-E	Immune modulator of NK cells and monocytes
IFNγ		T cells, NK cells	Antiproliferative like CFU-UM and BFU-E	Immune-modulating and induces cell membrane antigens (MHC class I or II)
TNF α, β		Macrophages, somatic cells, T & B lymphocytes		Immunoenhancing & induces apoptosis of many cells; induces secondary production of cytokines by stromal cells
MIP-1α		T & B cells Neutrophils Macrophages	Inhibits growth of hematopoietic progenitors	

SCF = stem cell factor; CFC = colony-forming cell; CFU = colony-forming unit; BFU-E = erythroid burst-forming unit; IL = interleukin; GM-CSF = granulocyte-macrophage colony-stimulating factor; G-CSF = granulocyte colony-stimulating factor; M-CSF = monocyte colony-stimulating factor; TNF = tumor necrosis factor; IFN = interferon; NK = natural killer.

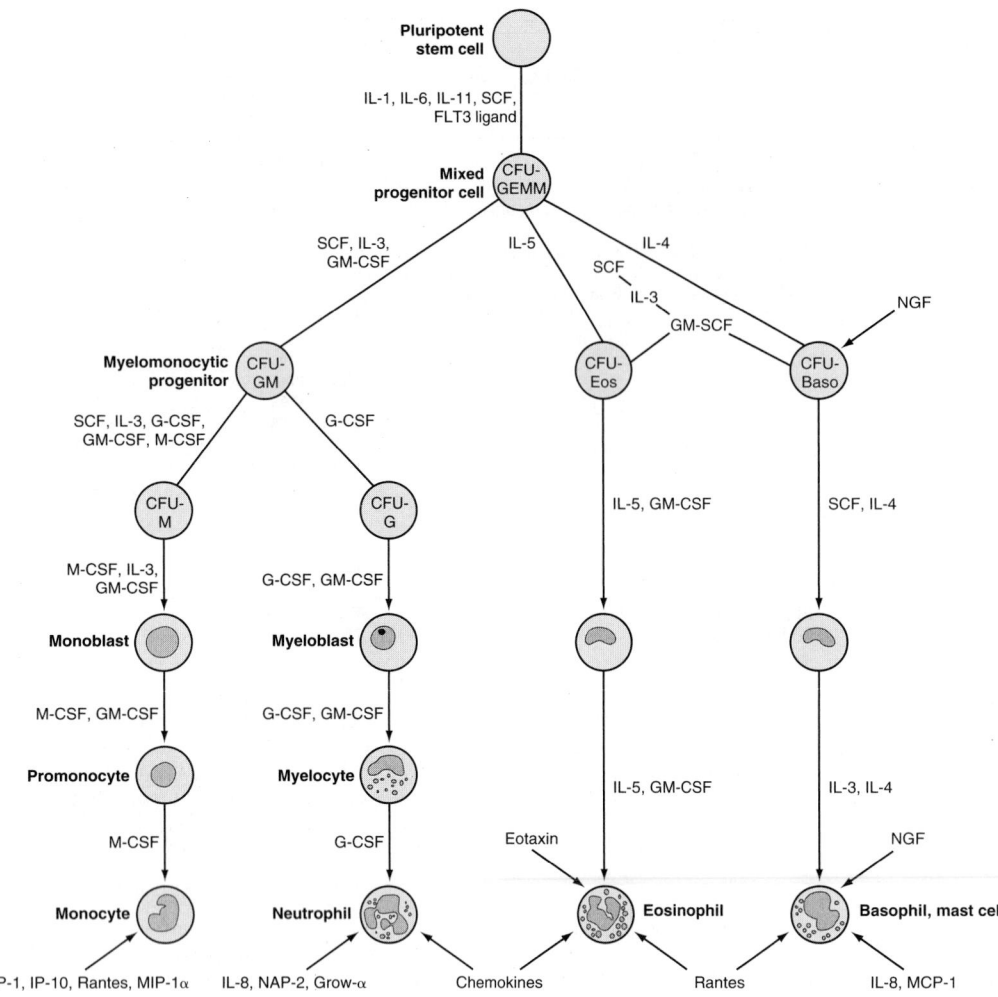

FIGURE 117–2. Various cytokines and chemokines that act at different levels of granulopoiesis and monocytopoiesis. Multiple cytokines regulate progenitor cells or mature effector cells at each stage of maturation/differentiation from the primitive pluripotent stem cell to nondividing terminally differentiated precursors (monocytes, neutrophils, eosinophils, and basophil/mast cells). The cytokines and chemokines also have varying degrees of specificity; some, such as M-CSF and IL-5, act predominantly on the monocytic and eosinophilic pathways, respectively, whereas others, such as CSF-GM, act on multiple granulocytic-monocytic (erythroid not shown) cell types. (Modified from Abboud CN, Liesveld JL: Granulopoiesis and monocytopoiesis. In Hoffman R, Benz EB, Shattil SJ, et al [editors]: *Hematology: Basic Principles and Practice,* 2nd ed. New York, Churchill Livingstone, 1995.)

azurophilic granules, and myelocytes acquire specific granules. Chromatin condensation, loss of nucleoli, and the shape changes of the nucleus result in the morphometric characteristic of the segmented neutrophil.

Neutrophil Function. Neutrophil responses are initiated as circulating neutrophils flowing through the postcapillary venules detect low levels of chemokines and other chemotactic substances released from a site of infection. These soluble effectors of inflammation trigger subtle changes in the array and activity of surface molecules on both endothelial cells and neutrophils. The initial associations are low affinity, reversible, and mediated primarily by cell-selectin-carbohydrate interactions. This leads to the phenomenon known as leukocyte rolling, in which loose adhesions are made and broken, causing neutrophils to move hesitantly along the endothelial surface. The rolling of neutrophils allows more intense exposure of neutrophils to activating factors such as tumor necrosis factor (TNF) or IL-1 (Fig. 117–3). This leads to induction of qualitative and quantitative changes in the family of β2 integrin adhesion receptors on the neutrophils (the CD11/CD18 group of surface molecules). The activated integrin receptors mediate tight heterotypic adhesion between neutrophils and endothelial cells and hemotypic adhesion of neutrophils with each other. The net result of these inter-

dependent intercellular interactions is that neutrophils flatten onto the endothelial cells, while neutrophil/neutrophil and neutrophil/platelet aggregates partially occlude the venule and reduce blood flow.

The next phase involves loosening of the integrin adhesion through the process of mobilizing integrin receptors to the trailing pseudopod of the neutrophil. The neutrophil is able to displace its integrin receptors and undergo conformational changes allowing it to migrate between endothelial cell junctions into the extravascular tissue. Once through the endothelium, the neutrophil senses the gradient of chemokines or other chemoattractants and migrates to sites of infection. Neutrophil migration is a complex process involving rounds of receptor engagement, signal transduction, and remodeling of the actin-microfilaments composing in part the cytoskeleton. Additionally, secretion of specific granules or related secretory vesicular elements containing gelatinase, heparinase, and other enzymes allows the neutrophil to cross the basement membrane and transit through connective tissues. When the neutrophil reaches the site of infection, it recognizes pathogens by means of Fc immunoglobulin and complement receptors, fibronectin receptors, and other adhesion molecules.

The neutrophil ingests microbes that are opsonized (prepared for ingestion) by heat-soluble and heat-labeled factors in human

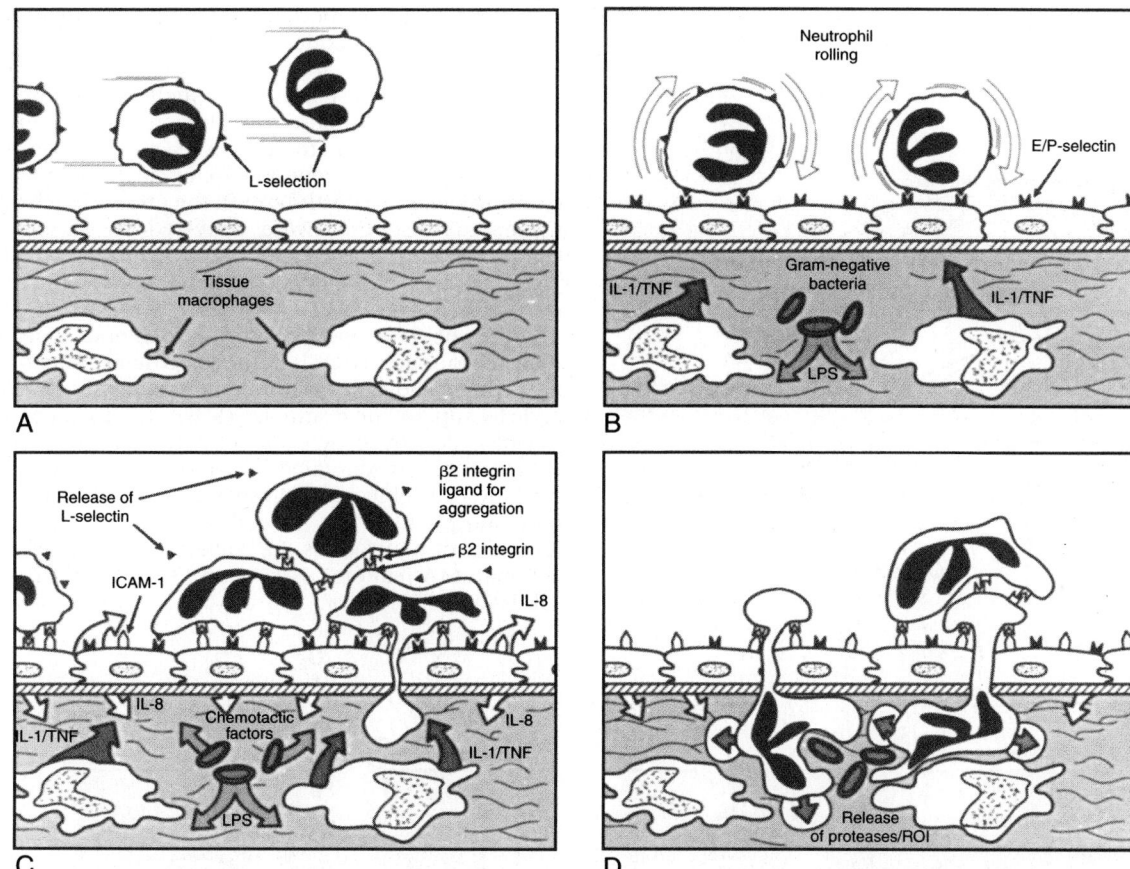

FIGURE 117–3. The neutrophil-mediated inflammatory response. *A,* Unstimulated neutrophils (expressing L-selectin) entering a post capillary venule. *B,* Invasion of gram-negative bacteria with release of lipopolysaccharide stimulates tissue macrophages to secrete inflammatory monokines, IL-1 and TNF, which, in turn, activate endothelial cells to express E- and P-selectins. E- and P-selectins serve as counter receptors for neutrophils sialyl Lewis X and Lewis X to cause low-avidity neutrophil rolling. *C,* Activated endothelial cells express ICAM-1, which serves as a counter-receptor for neutrophil β_2 integrin molecules, leading to high-avidity leukocyte spreading and the start of transendothelial migration. Transendothelial migration of activated neutrophils is stimulated by chemotactic factors such as endothelial cell-derived IL-8 and formylated bacterial factors. Chemoattractants promote neutrophil activation with release of L-selectin and an increase in β_2 integrin affinity for ICAM-1 and for other counter-receptors promoting intravascular and neutrophil aggregation. *D,* Neutrophils invade through the vascular basement membrane with the release of proteases and reactive oxidative intermediates, causing local destruction of surrounding tissue at sites of high concentrations of chemotactic factors. (From Smolen JE, Boxer LA: Functions of neutrophils. In Williams WJ, Beutler E, Erslev AJ, et al [editors]: *Hematology,* 5th ed. New York, McGraw-Hill, 1994, with permission of The McGraw-Hill Companies.)

serum, which include immunoglobulin G (IgG) and C3, respectively. These opsonins facilitate phagocytosis of microbes, in which the pathogens are engulfed into a closed vacuole called a **phagosome** (Fig. 117–4).

As phagocytosis proceeds, two cellular responses essential for optimal microbicidal activity occur concomitantly, **degranulation** and activation of **nicotinamide-adenine dinucleotide phosphate (NADPH)–dependent oxidase**. Fusion of neutrophil granule membranes with the phagosome membrane occurs, resulting in the delivery of potent antimicrobial proteins into the phagosome. In coordinated succession, the contents of the specific granules and then contents of the azurophil granules are secreted into the phagosome. Occurring concomitantly are assembly and activation of NADPH oxidase at the phagosome membrane (Fig. 117–5). This enzyme generates large amounts

of superoxide (O_2^-) from molecular oxygen that in turn decomposes to produce hydrogen peroxide (H_2O_2) and singlet oxygen. H_2O_2 can react with O_2^- to form hydroxyl radicals. In the presence of myeloperoxidase (a major azurophil granule component), a reaction is catalyzed and uses H_2O_2 and ubiquitously present chloride ion to create hypochlorous acid (HOCl) in the phagosome. Although H_2O_2 and HOCl are microbicidal, evidence shows that these agents modulate host defense. First, these oxidants can denature proteins, making them more susceptible to proteolysis. Additionally, some of the neutrophil proteases are activated by the oxidants. These events jointly serve to enhance breakdown or clearance of pathogens from the site of infection. Also, the oxidants can inactivate chemotactic factors and may serve to terminate the process of neutrophil influx, thereby attenuating the inflammatory process.

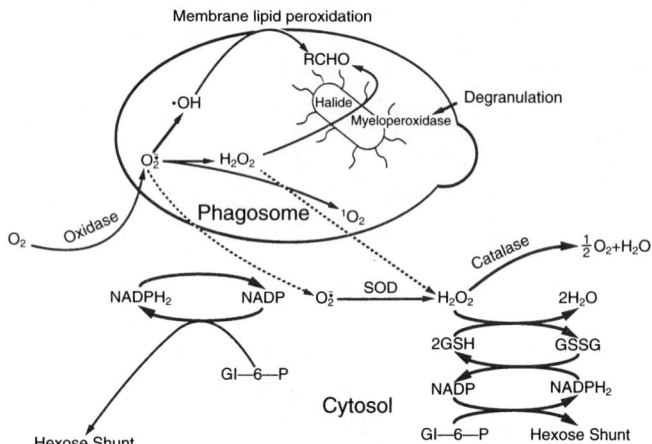

FIGURE 117–4. The mechanisms for the production, action, and detoxification of peroxides in neutrophils. Oxygen is reduced to superoxide (O^-_2) by an oxidase. NADPH is regenerated from NADPH by the hexose monophosphate shunt. Superoxide may spontaneously decompose to hydrogen peroxide in singlet oxygen ($^1O_2$). Hydrogen peroxide can react with superoxide to form hydroxyl radicals and generate bactericidal aldehydes (RCHO) by oxidizing bacterial constituents in the presence of halide ions and myeloperoxidase that were delivered to the phagosome by degranulation. Hydroxyl radicals (●OH) can peroxidize unsaturated fatty acids of the phagosomal membrane and thus yield the potentially bactericidal aldehydes. Hydrogen peroxide in the presence of myeloperoxidase and chloride ion can create hypochlorous acid (HOCl) in the phagosome. Superoxide leaking out of the phagosome may be converted rapidly to hydrogen peroxide by superoxide dismutase (SOD). Hydrogen peroxide in the cytosol is destroyed by catalase or reduced glutathione (GSH). Glutathione is regenerated by coupled reactions that stimulate the flow of glucose-6-phosphate (G-6-P) into the hexose monophosphate shunt. (Modified from Stossel TP, Boxer LA: Functions of neutrophils. In Williams WJ, Beutler E, Erslev AJ, Lichtman MA [editors]: *Hematology*, 3rd ed. New York, McGraw-Hill, 1972, p 751.)

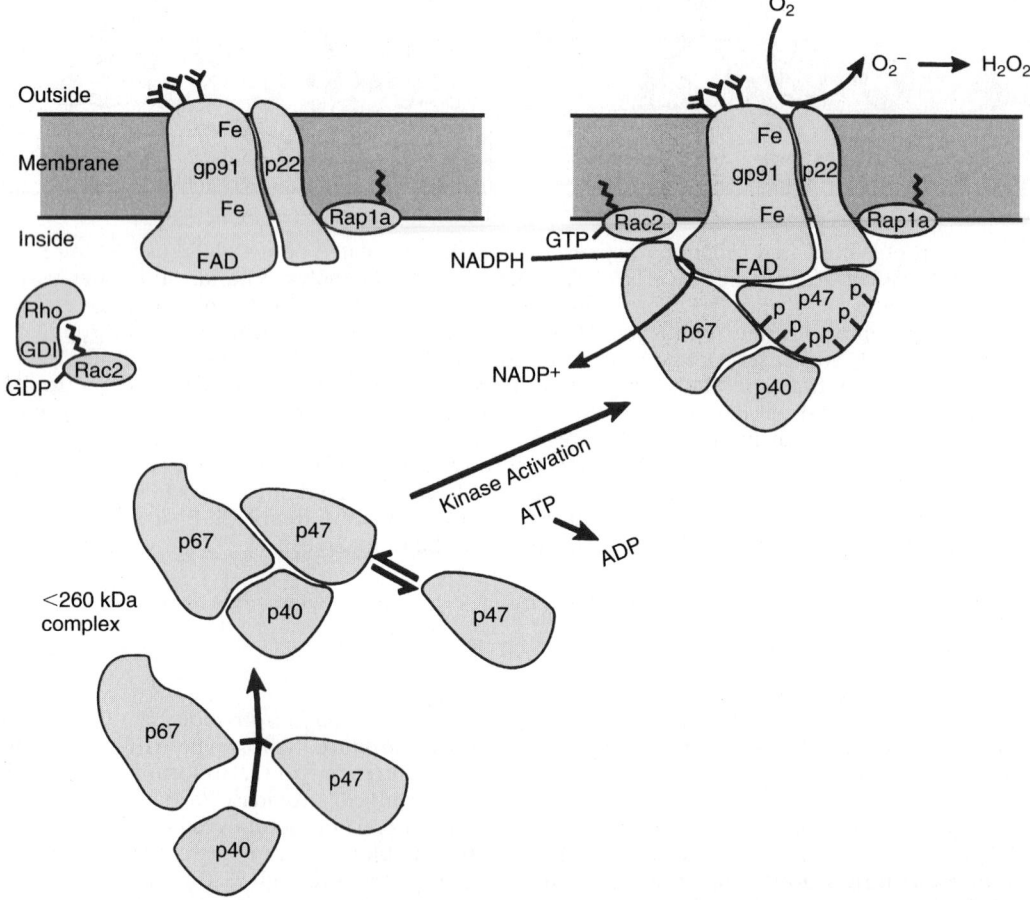

FIGURE 117–5. This is a modification of a hypothetical model of NADPH oxidase activation. Current knowledge suggests that the oxidase in its dormant state *(left)* is composed of both membrane-bound and cytosolic components. The former includes the gp91[phox] and p22[phox] subunits of cytochrome-b (and possibly Rap-1A). The flavin and heme groups (Fe) that mediate the transfer of electrons from NADPH to molecular oxygen are localized in the cytochrome. The cytosolic components p47[phox] and p67[phox] may exist as a preformed complex of 260 kD, which includes a third protein, p40[phox]. The small GTPase Rac2 is present in the cytosol in its inactive guanosine diphosphate-bound state (GDP). Following phagocyte activation, the cytosolic complex translocates to the membrane, which may be under the control of the active guanosine triphosphate (GTP)–bound form of Rac2 and further regulated by phosphorylation of p47[phox]. By a mechanism that is not fully understood, binding of the cytosolic components activates the flavocytochrome to catalyze the transfer of electrons from NADPH to oxygen through the FAD and heme redox centers. (Modified from Curnutte J, Orkin S, Dinauer M: Genetic disorders of phagocyte function. In Stamatopyannopoulous G, Nienhuis AW, Majerus PW, Varmus H [editors]: *The Molecular Basis of Blood Diseases*, 2nd ed. Philadelphia, WB Saunders, 1994, p 522.)

Babior BM: NADPH oxidase: An update. *Blood* 1999;93:1464–76.

Metcalf D: Cellular hematopoiesis in the twentieth century. *Semin Hematol* 1999;36:5–12.

Ward AC, Loeb DM, Soede-Bobok AA, et al: Regulation of granulopoiesis by transcription factors and cytokine signals. *Leukemia* 2000;14:973–90.

Chapter 118
Monocytes and Macrophages *Richard B. Johnston, Jr.*

Mononuclear phagocytes (monocytes and macrophages) have a central and essential role in the immune response, in host defense against infection, and in tissue repair and remodeling. No human has been identified as having congenital absence of this cell line, probably because macrophages are required to remove primitive tissues during fetal development as new tissues develop to replace them. Monocytes and tissue macrophages in their various forms (Box 118–1) constitute the **mononuclear phagocyte system**. These cells are a system because of their common origin, similar morphology, and common functions, particularly efficient phagocytosis.

Development. Monocytes, the circulating precursors of tissue macrophages, develop more rapidly in the bone marrow and remain longer in the circulation than do neutrophils (see Table 117–1). The first recognizable monocyte precursor is the monoblast, followed by the promonocyte, a somewhat larger cell with cytoplasmic granules and an indented nucleus containing finely divided chromatin, and finally the fully developed monocyte. A mature monocyte is larger than a neutrophil and has a cytoplasm filled with granules whose contents include hydrolytic enzymes. The transition from monoblast to mature circulating monocyte requires about 6 days. Monocytes retain a limited capacity to divide, and they undergo considerable further differentiation after entering the tissues, where they may live for weeks to months.

Migration of monocytes into the different tissues appears to occur randomly in the absence of localized inflammation. Once in the tissues, monocytes undergo transformation into tissue macrophages with morphologic and sometimes functional properties that are characteristic for the tissue in which they reside (see Box 118–1). Organ-specific factors influence monocyte differentiation and endow each tissue macrophage with particular metabolic and structural features. Monocytes in the liver become **Kupffer cells** that bridge the sinusoids separating adjacent plates of hepatocytes. Those at the lung airway surface become large ellipsoid **alveolar macrophages**, and those in the bone become **osteoclasts**. All macrophages have at least three major functions in common: presentation of antigens, phagocytosis, and immunomodulation through release of a variety of potent factors broadly termed cytokines. At sites of inflammation, monocytes and macrophages can fuse to form multinucleated giant cells, the terminal stage of development in the mononuclear phagocyte line. Blood monocytes, when exposed to certain cytokines, can differentiate into **dendritic cells**, which are especially effective at presenting antigen to lymphocytes.

Activation. The most important step in the functional maturation of macrophages is the conversion from a resting to an activated macrophage. Activation is driven primarily by certain cytokines, proteins that mediate signaling between cells and thereby influence inflammation or the immune response. **Cytokines** include interferons, interleukins, growth factors, chemokines, and tumor necrosis factors. Cytokines responsible for macrophage activation include interferon-γ (IFN-γ); granulocyte-macrophage colony-stimulating factor (GM-CSF); macrophage-CSF; and tumor necrosis factor–α (TNF-α). Growth hormone and bacterial endotoxin or cell wall proteins also can induce activation. In its most widely accepted sense, the term **activated macrophage** indicates that the cell has an enhanced capacity to kill microorganisms or tumor cells. Activated macrophages are larger, with more pseudopods and pronounced ruffling of the plasma membrane, and they exhibit accelerated activity of many functions (Box 118–2).

Macrophage activation is accomplished during infection through the engagement of CD40 on macrophages with CD40 ligand on antigen-sensitized helper T lymphocytes and through cytokines from these T cells. Activated macrophages and macrophages encountering microorganisms release interleukin (IL)-12, which, in turn, activates the T cells. These interactions constitute the basis of cell-mediated immunity. IFN-γ is an especially important macrophage-activating cytokine that is currently used for preventing infection in patients with chronic granulomatous disease and for treating the decreased bone resorption of congenital osteopetrosis, which is caused by decreased function of osteoclasts.

Macrophages exposed to endotoxin or other inflammatory mediators release TNF-α, which itself can activate other macrophages. As macrophages become activated, they express greater numbers of receptors for TNF-α. Thus, macrophages at sites of inflammation have the potential to activate themselves and thereby achieve enhanced function more rapidly than through the classic cell-mediated immune response, which

---

BOX 118–1. Principal Sites of Macrophages in Tissues

Liver (Kupffer cells)
Lung (interstitial and alveolar macrophages)
Connective tissue
Serous cavities (pleural and peritoneal macrophages)
Bone (osteoclasts)
Brain (reactive microglial cells)
Spleen, lymph nodes, bone marrow
Intestinal wall
Breast milk
Placenta
Granuloma (multinucleated giant cells)

BOX 118–2. Upregulated Functions in Activated Macrophages

Microbicidal activity
Tumoricidal activity
Chemotaxis
Phagocytosis (most particles)
Pinocytosis
Glucose transport and metabolism
Phagocytosis-associated respiratory burst (O_2^-, H_2O_2)
Generation of nitric oxide
Antigen presentation
Secretion
   Complement components
   Lysozyme
   Acid hydrolases
   Collagenase
   Plasminogen activator
   Cytolytic proteinase
   Arginase
   Fibronectin
   Interleukins, including IL-1, -10, -12, and -15
   Tumor necrosis factor-α
   Interferon-α and -β
Angiogenic factors

O_2^- = superoxide anion; H_2O_2 = hydrogen peroxide.

requires accumulation of a population of sensitized T lymphocytes. Conversely, macrophages, as well as helper T cells, secrete IL-10, which inhibits the production of IFN-γ and serves to suppress the potentially damaging effects of uncontrolled macrophage activation.

Functional Activities. Numerous functions are upregulated when the macrophage is activated (see Box 118–2). Obviously important are the ingestion and killing of such intracellular pathogens as *Mycobacterium tuberculosis, Listeria, Leishmania, Toxoplasma,* and some fungi, but macrophages also clear from the bloodstream and eliminate such extracellular pathogens as *Streptococcus pneumoniae.* Killing of the ingested organisms depends heavily on products of the respiratory burst (e.g., hydrogen peroxide) and on nitric oxide; release of these toxic metabolites is enhanced in activated macrophages.

The activity of mononuclear phagocytes against cancers in humans is less well understood. This activity may not involve the phagocytic process. Rather, macrophages may kill tumor cells by means of secreted products including lysosomal enzymes, nitric oxide, oxygen metabolites, cytolytic proteinases, and TNF-α. Proteolytic enzymes and cytocidal factors present on the surface membrane of monocytes may have a role in tumor rejection.

Essential to the monocyte's protective function is its capacity to undergo diapedesis across the endothelial wall of blood vessels and to migrate to sites of microbial invasion in tissues. Chemotactic factors for monocytes include complement products and chemoattractants (chemokines) derived from neutrophils, lymphocytes, and other cell types. Phagocytosis of the invading organisms or cells can then occur, influenced by the presence or absence of opsonins (antibody, complement, mannose-binding and surfactant proteins) for the invader, the inherent surface properties of the microorganism or tumor, and the state of activation of the macrophage.

Other important functions of macrophages are disposal of damaged and dying cells, which helps resolve the immune response, and wound healing. Macrophages lining the sinusoids of the spleen are particularly important in ingesting aged erythrocytes. Macrophages in inflammatory sites can recognize changes in phosphatidylserine on the membrane of lymphocytes and neutrophils undergoing programmed cell death, and these can be removed before they become necrotic and spill their toxic contents into the tissue. Macrophages are phylogenetically primitive and can be identified early in fetal development, where they function to remove debris as one maturing embryonic tissue replaces another. They are also important in removing inorganic particles, such as elements of cigarette smoke or dust that enter the alveoli.

Macrophages are integrally involved in the induction and expression of specific immune responses, including antibody formation and cell-mediated immunity. This involvement depends on their capacity to break down foreign material in phagocytic and pinocytic vesicles and then present individual antigens on their surface as peptides or polysaccharides bound to class II major histocompatibility complex (MHC) molecules. B lymphocytes and, especially, dendritic cells can also present antigen and serve as "accessory cells" for the specific immune response. Expression of MHC class II molecules is increased in activated macrophages, and antigen presentation is more effective.

The heightened capacity of activated macrophages to synthesize and release various hydrolytic enzymes and potentially microbicidal materials (see Box 118–2) probably plays a part in their increased killing capacity, although not every macrophage product is secreted in increased amounts when the cell is activated. The macrophage is an extraordinarily active secretory cell; approximately 100 distinct substances have been identified as being secreted by it, placing this cell in a class with the hepatocyte. Because of the profound effect of some of these secretory

products on other cells, the large number of macrophages, and their widespread distribution, the mononuclear phagocyte system can be viewed as an important endocrine organ. IL-1 illustrates this point well. Microbes and microbial products, burns, ischemia-reperfusion, and other causes of inflammation or tissue damage stimulate the release of IL-1, mainly by monocytes and macrophages. In turn, IL-1 elicits fever, sleep, and release of IL-6, which induces production of acute phase proteins.

Abnormalities of Monocyte-Macrophage Function. Mononuclear phagocytes, as well as neutrophils, from patients with chronic granulomatous disease exhibit a profound defect of phagocytic killing (Chapter 120). The inability of affected macrophages to kill ingested organisms leads to abscess formation and characteristic granulomas at sites of macrophage accumulation in the liver, lungs, spleen, and lymph nodes. Genetic deficiency of the CD11/CD18 complex of membrane adherence glycoproteins (leukocyte adhesion defect), which includes a receptor for opsonic complement component 3, results in impaired phagocytosis by monocytes (Chapter 120).

The monocyte-macrophage system is prominently involved in several lipid storage diseases (sphingolipidoses; Chapter 75.3). In these conditions, the expression in macrophages of a systemic enzymatic defect permits the accumulation of cell debris that is normally cleared by macrophages. Resistance to infection can be impaired, at least partly because of impairment in macrophage function. Gaucher disease is the prototype for these disorders. In this condition, the enzyme glucocerebrosidase functions abnormally, thus allowing accumulation of glucosylceramide (glucocerebroside) from cell membranes in Gaucher cells throughout the body. In all locations, the Gaucher cell is an altered macrophage. These patients can be treated with infusions of the normal enzyme modified to expose mannose residues, which bind to mannose receptors on macrophages.

The cytokine IL-12 is a powerful inducer of IFN-γ production by T cells and natural killer cells. Individuals with inherited deficiency in macrophage receptors for IFN-γ or lymphocyte receptors for IL-12, or in IL-12 itself, suffer a severe, profound, and selective susceptibility to infection by nontuberculous mycobacteria such as *Mycobacterium avium* or bacillus Calmette-Guérin (BCG). About half of these patients have had disseminated *Salmonella* infection. These abnormalities are now grouped under the term **leukocyte mycobactericidal defects**.

Monocyte-macrophage function has been shown to be abnormal in various other clinical conditions. In most of these, however, the abnormality is partial and only a suspected cause of increased infection. For example, cultured mononuclear phagocytes of newborns are more readily infected than adult cells by human immunodeficiency virus (HIV)–1 and measles virus. Macrophages from newborns release less G-CSF and IL-6 in culture, and this deficiency is accentuated in cells from preterm infants. This finding supports the observations that levels of G-CSF are significantly decreased in blood from term and preterm infants, and that the bone marrow granulocyte storage pool is diminished in infants, particularly those born before term. Macrophages from newborns are poorly activated by IFN-γ, which could weaken resistance to infection by intracellular pathogens.

The term **histiocyte** was originally used to describe cells thought to be macrophages in fixed tissue preparations. It is now clear that histiocytosis X represents a malignancy-like overgrowth of Langerhans-type dendritic cells (Chapter 499). Thus, the term **Langerhans cell histiocytoses** better describes these disorders because histiocyte is a histologic term and not cell specific.

Ganz T, Lehrer RI: Production, distribution, and fate of monocytes and macrophages. In Beutler E, Lichtman MA, Coller BS, et al (editors): *Williams Hematology,* 6th ed. New York, McGraw-Hill, 2001, pp 873–6.

Lekstrom-Himes JA, Gallin JI: Immunodeficiency diseases caused by defects in phagocytes. *N Engl J Med* 2000;343:1703–14.

Chapter 119

Eosinophils *Laurence A. Boxer*

Eosinophils are distinguished from other leukocytes by their morphology, constituent products, and association with specific diseases. Eosinophils are nondividing fully differentiated cells with a diameter of approximately 8 μm and a bilobed nucleus. They differentiate from stem cell precursors in the bone marrow under the control of T cell–derived interleukin 3 (IL-3), granulocyte-macrophage colony-stimulating factor (GM-CSF), and especially IL-5. Their characteristic membrane-bound specific granules stain reddish brown with eosin and consist of a crystalline core made up of major basic protein (MBP) surrounded by matrix containing the eosinophil cationic protein (ECP), eosinophil peroxidase (EPO), and eosinophil-derived neurotoxin (EDN). These basic proteins are cytotoxic for the larval stages of helminthic parasites such as *Schistosoma mansoni*, and are also thought to contribute to much of the inflammation associated with asthma, causing sloughing of epithelial cells and contributing to clinical dysfunction (Chapter 134). Both eosinophil MBP and ECP are also present in large quantities in the airways of patients who have died of asthma and are thought to inflict epithelial cell damage that contributes to airway hyperresponsiveness. MBP has the potential to activate other proinflammatory cells including mast cells, basophils, neutrophils, and platelets. Eosinophils have the capacity to generate large amounts of the lipid mediators, platelet-activating factor (PAF) and leukotriene-C4, both of which can cause vasoconstriction and mucus hypersecretion. Eosinophils are a source of a number of proinflammatory cytokines including IL-1, IL-3, IL-5, and GM-CSF. Thus, eosinophils have a potent armory of mediators whose potential to initiate and sustain an inflammatory response is considerable.

Eosinophil migration from the vasculature into the extracellular tissue is mediated by the binding of leukocyte adhesion receptors to their ligands or counterstructures on the postcapillary endothelium. Similar to neutrophils, transmigration begins as the eosinophil selectin receptor binds to the endothelial carbohydrate ligand in loose association, which promotes eosinophils rolling along the endothelial surface until they encounter a priming stimulus such as a chemotactic mediator. Eosinophils then establish a high-affinity bond between integrin receptors and their corresponding immunoglobulin-like ligand. Unlike neutrophils, which become flattened before transmigrating between the tight junctions of the endothelial cells, eosinophils can use unique integrins, known as VLA-4, to bind to vascular cell adhesion molecule (VCAM)–1, which enhances eosinophil adhesion and transmigration through endothelium. Eosinophils are recruited to tissues in inflammatory states by the chemokine, **eotaxin**. These unique pathways account for selective accumulation of eosinophils in allergic and inflammatory disorders. Eosinophils normally dwell primarily in tissues, especially tissues with an epithelial interface with the environment, including the respiratory, gastrointestinal, and lower genitourinary tracts. The life span of eosinophils may extend for weeks within tissues.

In addition to selectively enhancing eosinophil production as well as adhesion to endothelial cells, IL-5 also has a number of important effects on eosinophil function. Considerable evidence shows that IL-5 has a pivotal role in promoting eosinophil accumulation. It is the predominant cytokine in allergen-induced pulmonary late-phase reaction, and antibodies against IL-5 block eosinophil infiltration into the lungs in animal models associated with airway hyperresponsiveness following allergen challenge. Eosinophils also bear unique receptors for several chemokines. These include RANTES, eotaxin, monocyte chemotactic protein (MCP)–3, and MCP-4. These chemokines appear to be key mediators in the induction of tissue eosinophilia.

Blood eosinophil numbers do not always reflect the extent of eosinophil involvement in disease-affected tissues. The **absolute eosinophil count**, calculated as the white blood cell (WBC) count/μL × per cent of eosinophils, is usually less than 450 cells/μL in the blood and varies diurnally, being more abundant in the early morning and diminishing as endogenous glucocorticoid levels rise. Eosinopenia occurs after corticosteroid administration and with some bacterial and viral infections.

DISEASES ASSOCIATED WITH EOSINOPHILIA

Many diseases are associated with eosinophilia (Box 119–1). The genesis of sustained eosinophilia in some patients remains unclear. Patients with sustained blood eosinophilia may develop organ damage, especially cardiac damage as found in the idiopathic hypereosinophilic syndrome, and should be monitored for evidence of cardiac disease.

Allergic Diseases. Allergy is the most common cause of eosinophilia in children in the United States. Acute allergic reactions may cause eosinophilic leukemoid responses with absolute eosinophil counts exceeding 20,000 cells/μL; chronic allergy is rarely associated with absolute eosinophil counts of more than 2,000 cells/μL. Hypersensitivity drug reactions can elicit eosinophilia that is often not accompanied by drug fever or organ dysfunction. Various skin diseases have also been

---

BOX 119–1. Causes of Eosinophilia

Allergic disorders
   Allergic rhinitis
   Asthma
   Acute urticaria
   Hypersensitivity drug reactions
Infectious diseases
   Tissue-invasive helminth infections
      Trichinosis
      Toxocariasis
      Strongyloidosis
      Ascaris
      Filariasis
      Schistosomiasis
      Echinococcosis
   Pneumocystis carinii
   Toxoplasmosis
   Amebiasis
   Malaria
   Bronchopulmonary aspergillosis
   Coccidioidomycosis
   Scabies
Malignant disorders
   Brain tumors
   Hodgkin disease and T-cell lymphomas
   Acute myelogenous leukemia
   Myeloproliferative disorders
Gastrointestinal disorders
   Inflammatory bowel disease
   Peritoneal dialysis
   Eosinophilic gastroenteritis
   Milk precipitin disease
Immunodeficiency disease
   Hyper IgE syndrome
   Wiskott-Aldrich syndrome
   Graft vs host reaction
Pulmonary disease
   Löffler syndrome
   Eosinophilic leukemia
   Hypersensitivity pneumonias
Miscellaneous
   Thrombocytopenia with absent radii
   Vasculitis
   Postirradiation of abdomen
   Histiocytosis with cutaneous involvement

associated with eosinophilia, including atopic dermatitis, eczema, pemphigus, urticaria, and toxic epidermal necrolysis.

Infectious Diseases. Eosinophilia is often associated with infection with multicellular helminthic parasites. The level of eosinophilia tends to parallel the magnitude and extent of tissue invasion, especially by larvae. Eosinophilia often does not occur in established parasitic infections that are well contained within tissues or are solely intraluminal in the gastrointestinal tract, such as *Giardia lamblia* and *Enterobius vermicularis*.

In evaluating patients with unexplained eosinophilia, the dietary history and geographic or travel history may indicate potential exposures to helminthic parasites. It is frequently necessary to examine the stool for ova and larvae at least three times. Additionally, the diagnostic parasite stages of many of the helminthic parasites that cause eosinophilia never appear in feces. Thus, normal results of stool examinations do not absolutely preclude a helminthic cause of eosinophilia, and diagnostic blood tests or tissue biopsy may be needed.

Two fungal diseases may be associated with eosinophilia: aspergillosis in the form of allergic bronchopulmonary aspergillosis (Chapter 218.1) and coccidioidomycosis (Chapter 221) following primary infection, especially in conjunction with erythema nodosum.

Hypereosinophilic Syndrome. The idiopathic hypereosinophilic syndrome is a leukoproliferative disease characterized by sustained overproduction of eosinophils. The three diagnostic criteria for this disorder are (1) eosinophilia of greater than 1,500 cells/μL persisting for longer than 6 mo, (2) lack of another diagnosis to explain the eosinophilia, and (3) signs and symptoms of organ involvement. The clinical signs and symptoms of hypereosinophilic syndrome can be heterogeneous because of the diversity of potential organ involvement. Eosinophilic leukemia may be distinguished from idiopathic hypereosinophilic syndrome by demonstrating probable clonality of X-linked polymorphisms in female patients by using purified populations of eosinophils. One of the most serious and life-threatening complications is cardiac disease due to endomyocardial thrombosis and fibrosis. Other organ systems that can be involved can include the skin, liver, spleen, gastrointestinal tract, brain, and lungs. Therapy is aimed at suppressing eosinophilia and is initiated with corticosteroids. Hydroxyurea or α-interferon may be beneficial in patients unresponsive to corticosteroids. The underlying causes of hypereosinophilic syndrome remain unknown. For patients with prominent organ involvement and those who fail to respond to therapy, the mortality is approximately 75% after 3 years.

Miscellaneous Diseases. Eosinophilia is observed in many patients with primary immunodeficiency syndromes, especially hyper IgE syndrome (Chapter 116) and Wiskott-Aldrich syndrome. Eosinophilia is also frequently present in syndromes of thrombocytopenia with absent radii and in familial reticuloendotheliosis with eosinophilia. Mild eosinophilia is found in 20% of patients with Hodgkin's disease and in gastrointestinal disorders including ulcerative colitis, Crohn's disease during symptomatic phases, gastroenteritis that is associated with milk precipitins, and chronic hepatitis.

Bain BJ: Hypereosinophilia. *Curr Opin Hematol* 2000;7:21–5.
Gompertz S, Stockley RA: Inflammation—role of the neutrophil and the eosinophil. *Semin Respir Infect* 2000;15:14–23.
Leff AR: Regulation of leukotrienes in the management of asthma: Biology and clinical therapy. *Ann Rev Med* 2001;52:1–14.
Lipworth BJ: Eosinophils and airway hyper-responsiveness. *Lancet* 2001;357:1446.
Rankin SM, Conroy DM, Williams TJ: Eotaxin and eosinophil recruitment: Implications for human disease. *Mol Med Today* 2000;6:20–7.
Walsh GM: Eosinophil granule proteins and their role in disease. *Curr Opin Hematol* 2001;8:28–33.
Wardlaw AJ, Brightling C, Green R, et al: Eosinophils in asthma and other allergic diseases. *Br Med Bull* 2000;56:985–1003.

Chapter 120

Disorders of Phagocyte Function *Laurence A. Boxer*

Neutrophils are particularly important in protecting the skin, mucous membranes, and lining of the respiratory and gastrointestinal tracts as part of the first line of defense against microbial invasion. During the critical 2–4-hr period after microbial tissue invasion, phagocytic cells must arrive at the site of inflammation if the infection is to be contained. If not, the resulting infection extends to a larger local lesion and potentially disseminates hematogenously.

Immunologic evaluation of patients with suspected immunodeficiency is formidable (Chapter 112), especially those presenting with recurrent or unusual bacterial infections suggesting disorders of phagocyte function (Table 120–1). The differential diagnosis of diseases can be complicated by similar presentations of neutrophil defects or antibody or complement deficiency. Disorders of phagocyte function should be considered if results of initial screening tests are normal and the patient has had recurrent or unusual bacterial infections (Fig. 120–1). Despite the rarity of the inherited phagocyte disorders, the understanding gleaned from evaluating the molecular mechanisms underlying the inherited disorders has contributed immensely to our knowledge of normal neutrophil function.

Chemotaxis, the direct migration of cells into sites of infection, involves a complex series of events (Chapter 117). Studies of defective in vitro chemotaxis of neutrophils obtained from children having various clinical conditions have not established whether the increased number of infections arises from a chemotactic abnormality or secondary to medical complications of the underlying disorder. The hyper IgE syndrome is characterized by reduced neutrophil motility accompanied by markedly elevated levels of IgE leading to chronic dermatitis and recurrent sinopulmonary infections and is associated with coarse facial features, retention of primary teeth, and a propensity for recurrent bone fractures (Chapter 116).

LEUKOCYTE ADHESION DEFICIENCY

Leukocyte adhesion deficiency–1 (LAD-1) and -2 (LAD-2) are rare autosomal recessive disorders of leukocyte function. LAD-1 affects about 1 per 10 million individuals and is characterized by recurrent bacterial and fungal infections and depressed inflammatory responses despite striking blood neutrophilia.

Genetics and Pathogenesis. LAD-1 results from mutations of the gene on chromosome 21q22.3 encoding CD18, the 95-kD β_2 leukocyte integrin subunit. Normal neutrophils express three heterodimeric adhesion molecules known as LFA-1 (CD11a/CD18), Mac-1 (CD11b/CD18, also known as CR3 or iC3b receptor), and p150, 95 (CD11c/CD18). These three transmembrane adhesion molecules are composed of unique α_1 subunits of 185, 190, and 150 kD, respectively, encoded on chromosome 16 and sharing a common β_2 subunit. This group of leukocyte integrins is responsible for the tight adhesion of neutrophils to the endothelial cell surface, egress from the circulation, and adhesion to iC3b-coated microorganisms, which promotes phagocytosis and particulate activation of the nicotinamide-adenine dinucleotide phosphate (NADPH) oxidase.

Mutations in the CD18 gene either impair or prevent mRNA production or affect the structure of the synthesized CD18 peptide, leading to abnormal post-translational processing and loss of the abnormal CD11/CD18. The CD11α_1 subunits are not stable as polymers, resulting in deficiency of LAD-1 neutrophils in the three CD11α_1 subunits. Some mutations of CD11/CD18

TABLE 120–1. Disorders of Phagocyte Function

Disorder	Etiology	Impaired Function	Clinical Consequence
Degranulation Abnormalities			
Chédiak-Higashi syndrome	Autosomal recessive; disordered coalescence of lysosomal granules. Responsible gene found at 1q42–45. The encoded protein has structural features homologous to a vacuolar sorting protein.	Decreased neutrophil chemotaxis, degranulation and bactericidal activity; platelet storage pool defect; impaired NK function, failure to disperse melanosomes.	Neutropenia; recurrent pyogenic infections, propensity to develop marked hepatosplenomegaly in the accelerated phase; pigment dilution in the skin and fundus.
Specific granule deficiency	Autosomal recessive; abnormal regulation of various myeloid granule genes by a transacting factor.	Impaired chemotaxis and bactericidal activity; bilobed nuclei in neutrophils; reduced content of neutrophil defensins, gelatinase, collagenase, vitamin B_{12}-binding protein, lactoferrin.	Recurrent deep-seated abscesses.
Adhesion Abnormalities			
Leukocyte adhesion deficiency 1	Autosomal recessive; absence of CD11/CD18 surface adhesive glycoprotein (β_2 integrins) on leukocyte membranes most commonly arising from failure to express CD18 mRNA.	Decreased binding of C3bi to neutrophils and impaired adhesion to ICAM1 and ICAM2.	Neutrophilia; recurrent bacterial infection without pus formation.
Leukocyte adhesion deficiency 2	Autosomal recessive; absence of neutrophil sialyl-Lewis X.	Decreased adhesion to activated endothelium expressing ELAM.	Neutrophilia; recurrent bacterial infection without pus formation.
Neutrophil actin dysfunction	Altered polymerization of neutrophil cytoplasmic actin; perhaps arising from the presence of an inhibitor to F-actin formation.	Impaired neutrophil adhesion, chemotaxis, and bacterial killing.	Neutrophilia; recurrent bacterial infections without pus formation.
Disorders of Cell Motility			
Enhanced motile responses: Familial Mediterranean Fever (FMF)	Autosomal recessive gene responsible for FMF on chromosome 16, which encodes for a protein called pyrin that may modify neutrophil activation.	Excessive accumulation of neutrophils at inflamed sites.	Recurrent fever, peritonitis, pleuritis, arthritis, and amyloidosis.
Depressed Motile Responses			
Defects in the generation of chemotactic signals	IgG deficiencies; C3 and properdin deficiency can arise from genetic or acquired abnormalities; mannose binding protein deficiency predominantly in neonates.	Deficiency of serum chemotaxis and opsonic activities.	Recurrent pyogenic infections.
Intrinsic defects of the neutrophil, e.g., leukocyte adhesion deficiency, Chédiak-Higashi syndrome, specific granule deficiency, neutrophil actin dysfunction, neonatal neutrophils	In the neonatal neutrophil there is diminished ability to express β_2-integrins and there is a qualitative impairment in β_2-integrin function.	Diminished chemotaxis.	Propensity to develop pyogenic infections.
Direct inhibition of neutrophil mobility, e.g., drugs	Ethanol, glucocorticoids, cyclic AMP.	Impaired locomotion and ingestion. Impaired adherence.	Possible cause for frequent infections; neutrophilia seen with epinephrine is the result of cyclic AMP release from endothelium.
Immune complexes	Bind to Fc receptors on neutrophils in patients with rheumatoid arthritis, systemic lupus erythematosus, other inflammatory states.	Impaired chemotaxis.	Recurrent pyogenic infections.
Hyperimmunoglobulin E syndrome	Autosomal dominant; variable expression of a soluble inhibitor from mononuclear cells affecting neutrophil chemotaxis; high levels of antistaphylococcal IgE.	Impaired chemotaxis at times; impaired IgG opsonization of *Staphylococcus aureus*.	Recurrent skin and senopulmonary infections.
Defects of Microbicidal Activity			
Chronic granulomatous disease	X-linked and autosomal recessive; failure to express functional gp91^{phox} in the phagocyte membrane in p22^{phox} (autosomal recessive). Other autosomal recessive forms of CGD arise from failure to express protein p47^{phox} or p67^{phox}.	Failure to activate neutrophil respiratory burst leading to failure to kill catalase-positive microbes.	Recurrent pyogenic infections with catalase-positive microorganisms.

Table continued on following page

711

TABLE 120–1. **Disorders of Phagocyte Function** *Continued*

Disorder	Etiology	Impaired Function	Clinical Consequence
G-6-PD deficiency	Less than 5% of normal activity of G-6-PD.	Failure to activate NADPH-dependent oxidase.	Infections with catalase positive microorganisms.
Myeloperoxidase deficiency	Autosomal recessive; failure to process modified precursor protein arising from missense mutation.	H_2O_2-dependent antimicrobial activity not potentiated by myeloperoxidase.	None.
Rac-2 deficiency	Autosomal recessive; dominant negative inhibitor by mutant protein of *Rac-2* mediated functions.	Absent receptor mediated O_2^--generation and chemotaxis. Impaired neutrophil rolling on endothelium.	Neutrophilia; recurrent bacterial infections
Deficiencies of glutathione reductase and glutathione synthetase	Failure to detoxify H_2O_2.	Excessive formation of H_2O_2.	Minimal problems with recurrent pyogenic infections.
Impaired Macrophage Function			
Defects in the interferon γ–interleukin-12 axis	Interferon γ-receptor ligand-binding chain, interferon γ-receptor signalling chain, interleukin-12-receptor β1 chain, interleukin-12p40 deficiency. The interferon γ-receptor abnormalities may be inherited in an autosomal dominant or recessive fashion. The interleukin γ-12 receptor are inherited in an autosomal recessive fashion.	Impaired killing of microorganisms. Fatal BCG infection secondary to inability to either produce interleukin-12 by dendritic cells and macrophages which is necessary to induce secretion of interferon γ by T cells and natural killer cells or secondary to depressed bactercidal activity of macrophages lacking normal function of interferon-γ receptor.	Infection with atypical mycobacteria, *Salmonella*, and *Listeria*.
Impaired Spleen Function			
Splenic absence or splenic dysfunction	Congenital absence of spleen, removal of spleen, vascular occlusion of spleen.	Removal or impaired function of splenic macrophages.	Propensity to infection with encapsulated bacteria.

X = X-linked; AR = autosomal recessive; G-6-PD = glucose-6-phosphate dehydrogenase; CGD = chronic granulomatous disease; ICAM = intracellular adhesion molecule; NK = natural killer; C = complement; m = messenger; H_2O_2 = hydrogen peroxide; NADPH = nicotinamide-adenine dinucleotide phosphate; AMP = adenosine phosphate; BCG = bacille Calmette-Guérin, phox = phagocyte oxidase. Modified from Boxer LA: Quantitative abnormalities of granulocytes. In Beutler E, Lichtman MA, Coller BS, et al (editors): Williams Hematology, 6th ed. New York, McGraw-Hill, 2001, p 836.

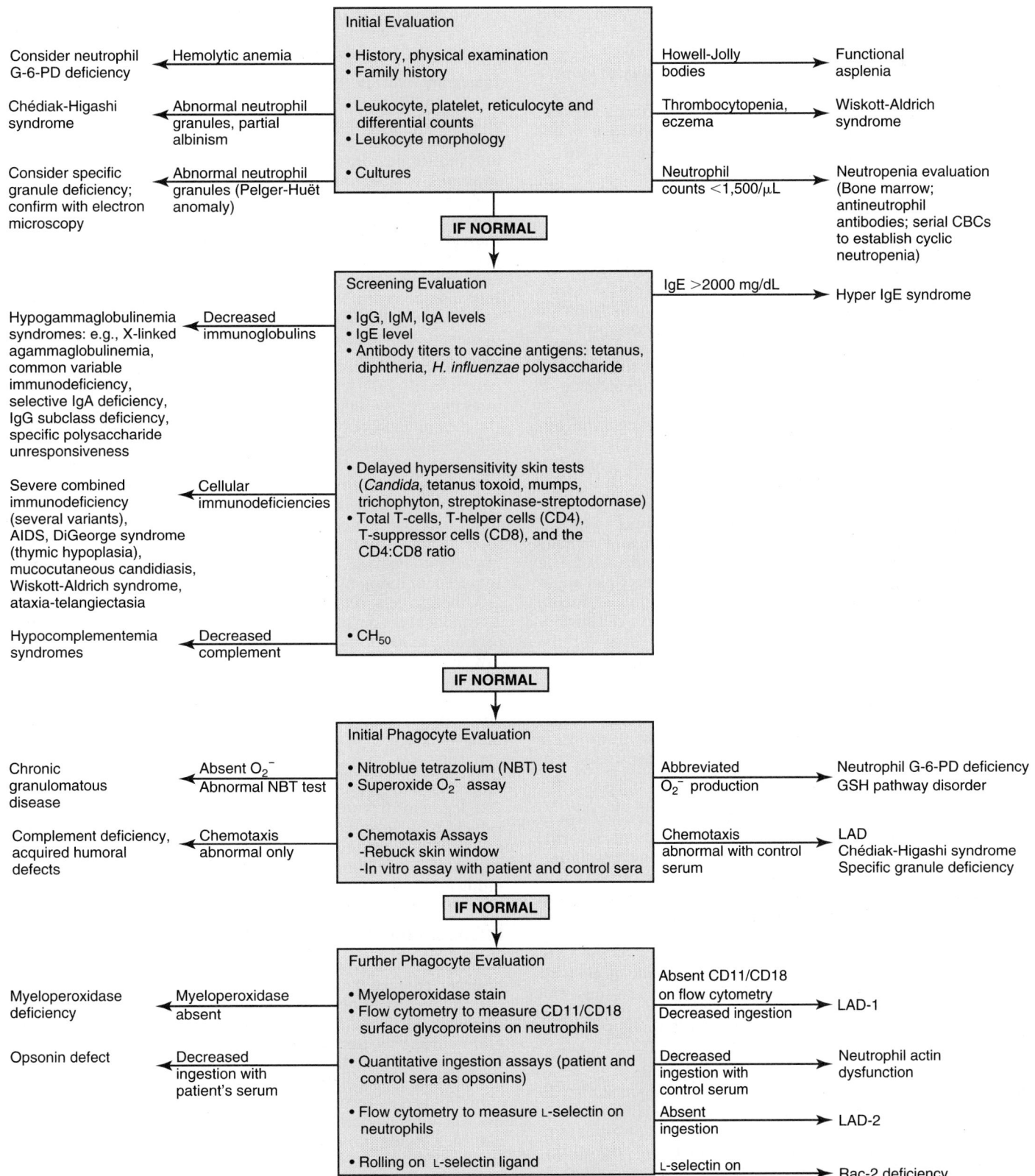

FIGURE 120–1. Algorithm for the evaluation of the patient with recurrent infections suggesting disorders of phagocyte function. CBC = complete blood count; Ig = immunoglobulin; G-6-PD = glucose-6-phosphate dehydrogenase; LAD = leukocyte adhesion deficiency. (Modified from Curnutte JT, Boxer LA: Clinically significant phagocyte cell defects. In Remington JS, Swartz MN [editors]: *Current Clinical Topics in Infectious Diseases,* 6th ed. New York, McGraw-Hill, 1985, p 144.)

allow a low level of assembly and functional active integrin molecules. These children retain some neutrophil integrin adhesion function and have a moderate phenotype. In contrast, failure of neutrophils to bear the β_2 integrins leads to inability to migrate to sites of inflammation outside of the lung because of their inability to adhere firmly to surfaces and undergo transendothelial migration. Failure of the CD11/CD18–deficient neutrophils to undergo transendothelial migration occurs because the β_2 integrins bind to intercellular adhesion molecules–1 and –2 (ICAM-1 and ICAM-2) expressed on inflamed endothelial cells. The neutrophils that do arrive at inflammatory sites in the lungs by CD11/CD18-independent processes fail to recognize microorganisms coated with the opsonin complement fragment iC3b, which is an important stable opsonin formed by the cleavage of C3b by C3b inactivator. Other neutrophil functions such as degranulation and oxidative metabolism normally triggered by iC3b binding are also diminished and markedly compromised in neutrophils from patients with LAD-1 deficiency. Impairment in neutrophil function underlies the propensity for serious and recurrent bacterial infections that is the clinical expression of this disease.

Monocyte function is also impaired, with poor fibrinogen-binding function, an activity promoted by the CD11/CD18 complex; consequently, such cells are unable to participate effectively in wound healing.

Children with LAD-2 share the clinical features of LAD-1 but have normal CD11/CD18 integrins. Features unique to LAD-2 are neurologic defects, cranial facial dysmorphism, and Bombay erythrocyte phenotype. The primary deficiency in LAD-2 is a defect in a specific GDP-L-fucose transporter of the Golgi apparatus. This abnormality prevents the incorporation of fucose into various glycoproteins, which are expressed on cell surface membranes. This provides a biochemical basis both for the abnormalities of erythrocyte carbohydrate blood group markers and the defects in neutrophil adhesion. The neutrophils from patients with LAD-2 are deficient in the carbohydrate structure sialyl-Lewis X, which renders the cells unable to adhere to activated endothelial cells. Thus, the neutrophils from these patients are unable to tether to inflamed venules for subsequent activation and spreading on the endothelium.

Clinical Manifestations. Patients with the severe clinical form of LAD-1 express less than 0.3% of the normal amount of the β_2 integrin molecules, whereas patients with the moderate phenotype may express 2–7%. Children with severe disease present in infancy with recurrent, indolent bacterial infections of the skin, mouth, respiratory tract, lower intestinal tract, and genital mucosa. They may have a history of delayed separation of the umbilical cord, usually with associated infection of the cord stump. Skin infection may progress to large chronic ulcers with polymicrobial infection, including anaerobic organisms. The ulcers heal slowly, require months of antibiotic treatment, and often require plastic surgical grafting. Severe gingivitis similar to what occurs in patients with profound neutropenia is common, with early loss of primary and then secondary teeth.

The pathogens infecting patients with LAD-1 are similar to those affecting patients with severe neutropenia (Chapter 121) and include *Staphylococcus aureus* and enteric gram-negative organisms such as *Escherichia coli*. These patients are also susceptible to fungal infections such as *Candida* and *Aspergillus*. As in profound neutropenia, the typical signs of inflammation, swelling, erythema, and warmth, may be absent. Pus does not form, and few neutrophils may be identified microscopically in biopsy specimens of infected tissues. Despite the paucity of neutrophils within the affected tissue, the circulating neutrophil count during infection may typically exceed 30,000/μL and can surpass 100,000/μL. During intervals between infection, the peripheral blood neutrophil count may chronically exceed 12,000/μL. LAD-1 genotypes, producing small amounts of functional integrins at the surface of the neutrophil, significantly reduce the severity and frequency of infections compared with children with the severe form.

Laboratory Findings. The diagnosis of LAD-1 is established most readily by flow cytometric measurements of surface CD11b in stimulated and unstimulated neutrophils using monoclonal antibodies directed against CD11b. Assessment of neutrophil and monocyte adherence, aggregation, chemotaxis, and iC3b-mediated phagocytosis generally demonstrates striking abnormalities that directly correspond to the molecular deficiency. Delayed-type hypersensitivity reactions are normal, and most individuals have normal specific antibody synthesis. Some patients, however, have impaired T lymphocyte–dependent antibody responses that can be demonstrated by suboptimal responses to repeat vaccination with tetanus toxoid, diphtheria toxoid, and poliovirus. The diagnosis of LAD-2 is established by demonstrating the lack of sialyl-Lewis X on the neutrophil.

Treatment. Treatment of LAD-1 depends on the phenotype as determined by the level of expression of functional CD11/CD18 integrins. Early allogeneic bone marrow transplantation is the treatment of choice for severe LAD-1 associated with complete absence of the CD11/CD18 integrins. Other treatment is largely supportive. Patients can be maintained on prophylactic trimethoprim-sulfamethoxazole and should have close surveillance to identify infections early. Broad-spectrum antibiotics are indicated for empirical therapy when infection occurs. Determination of the etiologic agent by culture and biopsy is important because of the prolonged antibiotic treatment required for indolent infections.

Although gene replacement therapy is not yet available, LAD-1 is an ideal candidate for this approach because the clinical history and mild forms of LAD-1 support the notion that even a low-level correction of neutrophil function attenuates the severity of the disease. One patient but not others responded to fucose supplementation, which induced a rapid reduction in the circulating leukocyte count and appearance of the sialyl-Lewis X molecules accompanied with marked improvement in leukocyte adhesion.

Prognosis. The severity of infectious complication correlates with the degree of β_2 integrin deficiency. Patients with severe deficiency may die in infancy, and those surviving infancy have a susceptibility to severe life-threatening systemic infections. Patients with moderate deficiency have infrequent life-threatening infections and relatively long survival.

CHÉDIAK-HIGASHI SYNDROME

Chédiak-Higashi syndrome (CHS) is a rare autosomal recessive disorder characterized by increased susceptibility to infection owing to defective degranulation of neutrophils, a mild bleeding diathesis, partial oculocutaneous albinism, progressive peripheral neuropathy, and a tendency to develop a life-threatening lymphoma-like syndrome. CHS was initially recognized by giant cytoplasmic granules in neutrophils, monocytes, and lymphocytes but is now recognized as a disorder of generalized cellular dysfunction characterized by increased fusion of cytoplasmic granules. Pigmentary dilution involving the hair, skin, and ocular fundi results from pathologic aggregation of melanosomes and is associated with a failure of decussation of the optic and auditory nerves. Patients exhibit an increased susceptibility to infection that can be explained in part by defects in neutrophil chemotaxis, degranulation, and bactericidal activity. The presence of giant granules in the neutrophils interferes with the cell's ability to traverse the narrow passages between endothelial cells into tissue.

Genetics and Pathogenesis. The mutated gene for CHS, located at chromosome 1q2–q44, has been cloned on the basis of its homology to the murine gene responsible for mouse CHS (beige phenotype). It has structural features homologous to a vacuolar sorting protein termed VPS15 in yeast. The CHS protein is thought to be associated with vesicle transport and to mediate protein-protein interaction and protein-membrane associations.

Almost all cells of patients with CHS show some aspect of the oversized and dysmorphic lysosomes, storage granules, or related vesicular structures. Melanosomes or melanocytes are oversized, and delivery to the keratinocytes and hair follicles is compromised because of the failure to properly disperse the giant melanosomes, resulting in hair shafts devoid of pigment granules. This leads to the macroscopic impression of hair and skin that is lighter than expected from parental coloration. The same abnormality in melanocytes leads to the partial ocular albinism associated with light sensitivity.

Beginning early in neutrophil development there is spontaneous fusion of giant primary granules with each other or with cytoplasmic membrane components, resulting in huge secondary lysosomes that contain reduced content of hydrolytic enzymes including proteinases, elastase, and cathepsin G. In turn, the deficiency of proteolytic enzymes may be responsible for the impaired killing of microorganisms by CHS neutrophils. Because the CHS blood cell membranes are more fluid than cells of normal individuals, it is possible that the altered membrane structure could lead to defective regulation of membrane activation. Changes in membrane fluidity may conceivably affect cell function by altering expression of membrane receptors. This could result in the elevated levels of intracellular cyclic adenosine monophosphate, disordered assembly of microtubules, and defective interaction of microtubules with lysosome membranes, which has been reported.

Clinical Manifestations. Patients with CHS have light skin and silvery hair, and frequently complain of solar sensitivity and photophobia. Other signs and symptoms vary considerably, but frequent infections and neuropathy are common. The infections involve mucous membranes, skin, and respiratory tract. Affected children are susceptible to gram-positive and gram-negative bacteria and fungi, with *S. aureus* being the most common offending organism. The neuropathy may be sensory or motor in type, and ataxia may be a prominent feature. Neuropathy often begins in the teenage years and becomes the most prominent problem.

Patients with CHS have prolonged bleeding times with normal platelet counts, resulting in impaired platelet aggregation associated with a deficiency of the dense granules containing adenosine diphosphate and serotonin. Natural killer cell function is also impaired.

The most life-threatening complication of CHS is the development of an accelerated phase of a lymphoma-like syndrome characterized by pancytopenia, high fever, and lymphohistiocytic infiltration of liver, spleen, and lymph nodes. The accelerated phase may occur at any age. The onset of this accelerated phase may be related to the inability of these patients to contain and control Epstein-Barr virus infection, which leads to features simulating virus-associated hemophagocytic syndrome. The lymphocytic proliferation is associated with recurrent bacterial and viral infections and usually results in death. At autopsy, the lymphohistiocytic infiltrates in the liver, spleen, and lymph nodes are extensive but are not neoplastic by histopathologic criteria.

Laboratory Findings. The diagnosis of CHS is established by finding large inclusions in all nucleated blood cells. These can be seen on Wright-stained blood films but are accentuated by a peroxidase stain.

Treatment. High-dose ascorbic acid (200 mg/24 hr for infants, 2,000 mg/24 hr for adults) improves the clinical status of some children in the stable phase. Although controversy surrounds the efficacy of ascorbic acid, given the safety of the vitamin, it is reasonable to administer ascorbic acid to all patients.

The only curative therapy for the accelerated phase is bone marrow transplantation from an HLA-compatible donor or an unrelated donor compatible at the D locus. Marrow transplantation reconstitutes normal hematopoietic and immunologic function and corrects the natural killer cell deficiency in patients entering the accelerated phase. However, bone marrow transplantation does not correct or prevent the peripheral neuropathy.

MYELOPEROXIDASE DEFICIENCY

Myeloperoxidase (MPO) deficiency is a disorder of oxidative metabolism and is one of the most common inherited disorders of phagocytes, occurring at a frequency approaching 1 per 4,000 individuals. MPO is a green heme protein located in the azurophilic lysosomes of neutrophils and monocytes and is the basis for the greenish tinge to pus accumulated at a site of infection. Most individuals with the trait do not have an increased rate of infection or other clinical manifestations of disease.

Genetics and Pathogenesis. Mutations in the MPO gene causing this defect have been defined and provide insight into the post-translational processing of this granule protein. MPO mRNA is transcribed exclusively during the promyelocytic stage of granulopoiesis. The primary translation product of the MPO gene is a single-chain peptide of 80 kD that undergoes co-translational glycosylation followed by a series of modifications of the oligosaccharides. MPO deficiency is caused by a missense mutation in the MPO gene that replaces an arginine with tryptophan and results in an MPO precursor that does not incorporate heme. Although this mutation is the most common cause of MPO deficiency, many patients are compound heterozygotes with one allele bearing the common mutation and the other being normal or possessing a mutation not yet identified. A partial deficiency results if only one allele is normal.

Partial or complete MPO deficiency leads to diminished production of hypochlorous acid (HOCl) and HOCl-derived chloramines. The deficiency in HOCl leads to early depression of gram-positive and gram-negative bacterial rates of killing in vitro that normalizes after 1 hr incubation. These data indicate that deficient cells use an MPO-independent microbicidal system that is slower to kill pathogens than the MPO-H_2O_2-halide system used by normal neutrophils.

Clinical Manifestations. MPO deficiency usually is clinically silent. Rarely, patients may have disseminated candidiasis, usually in conjunction with diabetes mellitus. Acquired partial MPO deficiency can develop in acute myelogenous leukemia and in myelodysplastic syndromes.

Laboratory Findings. Deficiency of neutrophil and monocyte MPO can be identified by histochemical analysis.

Treatment. There is no specific therapy. Aggressive treatment with antifungal agents should be used in patients with candidal infections. The prognosis is usually excellent.

CHRONIC GRANULOMATOUS DISEASE

Chronic granulomatous disease (CGD) is characterized by the ability of neutrophils and monocytes to ingest but their inability to kill **catalase-positive microorganisms** because of a defect in the generation of microbial oxygen metabolites. CGD is a rare disease with an incidence of 4–5 per million individuals, caused by genes affecting one X-linked and three autosomal recessive chromosomes.

Genetics and Pathogenesis. Activation of NADPH oxidase requires stimulation of the neutrophils and involves assembly from cytoplasmic and integral membrane subunits. Oxidase activation initially arises from phosphorylation of a cationic cytoplasmic protein, p47^phox (47kd "phagocyte oxidase" protein). Phosphorylated p47^phox together with two other cytoplasmic components of the oxidase, p67^phox and a low molecular weight guanine triphosphatase (Rac-2), translocates to the membrane where they interact with the cytoplasmic domains of the transmembrane flavocytochrome b_{558} to form the active oxidase (see Fig. 117–5). The flavocytochrome is a heterodimer of two peptides, p22^phox and highly glycosylated gp91^phox. Current models are consistent with three transmembrane domains within the N-terminus of the flavocytochrome that contain the histidines that coordinate heme binding. The role of p22^phox peptide is required for stability of gp91^phox and for oxidase activity. The role of p40^phox in oxidase activation remains unclear. The gp91^phox peptide is required for electron transport through use of an NADPH-binding domain, a flavin-binding domain, and a heme-binding domain. In turn, the gp91^phox is stabilized by p22^phox. Furthermore, p22^phox provides a docking site for the cytoplasmic subunits. The cytoplasmic p47^phox, p67^phox, and Rac-2 appear to serve as regulatory elements for activation of cytochrome b_{558}.

Approximately two thirds of patients with CGD are males who inherit their disorder as a result of mutations in the X-chromosome gene encoding gp91^phox. About one third of patients inherit CGD in an autosomal recessive fashion resulting from mutations in the gene encoding p47^phox on chromosome 7. Defects in the genes encoding p67^phox (chromosome 1) or p22^phox (chromosome 16) also occur; these are inherited in an autosomal recessive manner and account for about 5% of cases of CGD.

Effective neutrophil phagocytosis requires activation of NADPH-dependent oxidase (Chapter 117). After activation of neutrophils, electrons are passed from NADPH to flavin and then to the heme prosthetic group on cytochrome b_{558} and finally to molecular oxygen to form O_2^- mutations in the gene for cytochrome b_{558}. Alternatively, the cytosolic factor renders the electron transport system ineffective in generating O_2^-.

The metabolic deficiency of the CGD neutrophil predisposes the host to infection; the CGD phagocytic vacuoles remain acidic, and the bacteria are not digested properly (Fig. 120–2). Hematoxylin-eosin–stained sections from patients' macrophages may contain a golden pigment that reflects this abnormal accumulation of ingested material and contributes to the diffuse granulomas that give CGD its descriptive name.

Clinical Manifestations. Although the clinical presentation is variable, several features suggest the diagnosis of CGD. Any patient with recurrent or unusual lymphadenitis, hepatic abscesses, osteomyelitis at multiple sites, a family history of recurrent infections, or unusual infections with catalase-positive organisms (e.g., *S. aureus*) require evaluation for this disorder.

The onset of clinical signs and symptoms may occur from early infancy to young adulthood. The attack rate and severity of infections are exceedingly variable. The most common pathogen is *S. aureus,* although any catalase-positive microorganism may be involved. Other organisms frequently causing infections include *Serratia marcescens, Burkholderia cepacia, Aspergillus, Candida albicans,* and *Salmonella.* Pneumonias, lymphadenitis, and skin infections are the most common illnesses encountered. Patients may suffer from the sequelae of chronic infection, including anemia of chronic disease, lymphadenopathy, hepatosplenomegaly, chronic purulent dermatitis, restrictive lung disease, gingivitis, hydronephrosis, and pyloric outlet narrowing. Perirectal abscesses and recurrent skin infections, including folliculitis, cutaneous granulomas, and discoid lupus erythematosus also suggest the possibility of CGD. Granuloma formation and inflammatory processes are a hallmark of CGD and may be the presenting symptoms that prompt testing for CGD if they cause pyloric outlet obstruction, bladder outlet obstruction, or rectal fistulae simulating Crohn disease.

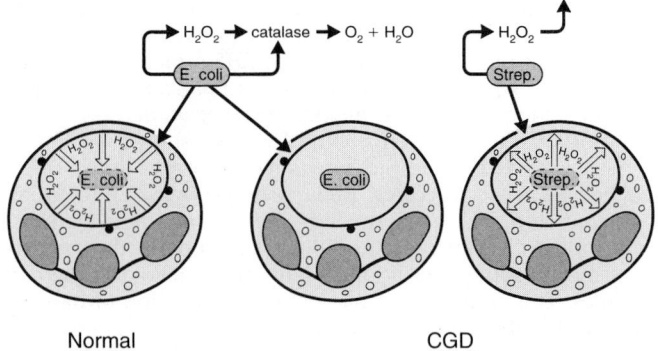

FIGURE 120–2. The pathogenesis of chronic granulomatous disease (CGD). The manner in which the metabolic deficiency of the CGD neutrophil predisposes the host to infection is shown schematically. Normal neutrophils stimulate hydrogen peroxide in the phagosome containing ingested *Escherichia coli*. Myeloperoxidase is delivered to the phagosome by degranulation, as indicated by the closed circles. In this setting, hydrogen peroxide acts as a substrate for myeloperoxidase to oxidize halide to hypochlorous acid and chloramines that kill the microbes. The quantity of hydrogen peroxide produced by the normal neutrophil is sufficient to exceed the capacity of catalase, a hydrogen peroxide–catabolizing enzyme of many aerobic microorganisms, including most gram-negative enteric bacteria, *Staphylococcus aureus, Candida albicans,* and *Aspergillus.* When organisms such as *E. coli* gain entry into CGD neutrophils, they are not exposed to hydrogen peroxide because the neutrophils do not produce it, and the hydrogen peroxide generated by microorganisms themselves is destroyed by their own catalase. When CGD neutrophils ingest streptococci, these organisms, which lack catalase, generate enough hydrogen peroxide to result in a microbicidal effect. As indicated (*middle*), catalase-positive microbes such as *E. coli* can survive within the phagosome of the CGD neutrophil. (Modified from Boxer LA: Quantitative abnormalities of granulocytes. In Beutler E, Lichtman MA, Coller BS, Kipps TJ, Seligsohn V [editors]: *Williams Hematology*, 6th ed. New York, McGraw-Hill, 2001, p 845.)

Laboratory Findings. For screening of CGD, the **nitroblue tetrazolium (NBT) dye test** is still widely used, but it is rapidly being replaced by the more accurate flow cytometry test using **dihydrorhodamine 123 fluorescence (DHR test).** DHR detects oxidant production because it increases fluorescence when oxidized by H_2O_2.

Neutrophils from patients with CGD have normal glucose-6-phosphate dehydrogenase (G6PD) activity. However, a few individuals with apparent CGD have been described as having neutrophils deficient in G6PD activity. The erythrocytes of these patients also lack the enzyme, and the patients have chronic hemolysis. CGD and G6PD deficiency can be distinguished by the hemolytic anemia associated with G6PD deficiency and by the normal erythrocyte G6PD activity in CGD compared with the markedly reduced activity in G6PD deficiency.

Treatment. Bone marrow transplantation is the only known cure for CGD. Vigorous supportive care along with recombinant interferon-γ is used before transplantation. As part of supportive care, patients with CGD should be given daily oral trimethoprim-sulfamethoxazole for prophylaxis of infections. Cultures must be obtained as soon as infection is suspected. Most abscesses require surgical drainage for therapeutic and diagnostic purposes. Prolonged use of antibiotics is often required. If fever occurs without an obvious focus, it is advisable to consider the use of radiographs of the chest and skeleton as well as CT scans of the liver to determine if pneumonia, osteomyelitis, or liver abscesses are present. The cause of fever cannot always be established, and empirical treatment with broad-spectrum parental antibiotics is often required. The erythrocyte sedimentation rate (ESR) may be used to help determine the duration of antibiotic treatment.

Aspergillus infection requires treatment with amphotericin B. Corticosteroids may also be useful for the treatment of children with antral and urethral obstruction. Granulomas may be sensitive to low doses of prednisone (0.5 mg/kg/24 hr); treatment should be tapered over several weeks.

Interferon-γ (50 μg/m², 3 times/wk) can reduce the number of serious infections. The mechanism of action of interferon-γ therapy in CGD is unknown. In the future, somatic gene therapy may be used to correct defective phagocyte oxidase function in selected patients with CGD.

GENETIC COUNSELING. Identifying a patient's specific genetic subgroup is useful primarily for genetic counseling and prenatal diagnosis. In cases of suspected X-linked CGD, further analysis is not necessary if the fetus is initially demonstrated to be a 46,XX female. Fetal blood sampling and NBT slide test analysis of fetal neutrophils can be used for prenatal diagnosis of CGD. DNA analysis of amniotic fluid cells or chorionic villus biopsy is an option for early prenatal diagnosis. Restriction fragment polymorphisms have been identified for gp91^{phox} and p67^{phox} and have proved useful for diagnosis. In families in which the specific mutation is known, prenatal diagnosis is established by analysis of fetal DNA for the presence of mutant alleles using the polymerase chain reaction.

Prognosis. The overall mortality rate for CGD is about 2 patient deaths/year/100 cases, with the highest mortality among young children. The long-term prognosis for patients with CGD has greatly improved during the past 20 yr. This can be attributed to an increased understanding of the biology of CGD, the development of effective infection prophylactic regimens, close surveillance for signs of infections, and aggressive surgical and medical interventions.

Borges WG, Augustine HN, Hill HR: Defective interleukin-12-interferon-γ pathway in patients with hyperimmunoglobulin E syndrome. *J Pediatr* 2000;136:176–80.

Grimbacher B, Holland SM, Gallin JI, et al: Hyper-IgE syndrome with recurrent infections—an autosomal dominant multisystem disorder. *N Engl J Med* 1999;340:692–702.

Lekstrom-Hines JA, Gallin JI: Immunodeficiency diseases caused by defects in phagocytes. *N Engl J Med* 2000;343:1703–14.

Lubke T, Marquardt T, von Figura K, et al: A new type of carbohydrate deficient glycoprotein syndrome due to a decreased import of GDP-fucose into the Golgi. *J Biol Chem* 1999;274:25986–9.

Segal BH, Leto TL, Gallin JI, et al: Genetic, biochemical, and clinical features of chronic granulomatous disease. *Medicine* 2000;79:170–200.

Winkelstein JA, Marino MD, Johnston RB, Jr, et al: Chronic granulomatous disease. Report on a national registry of 368 patients. *Medicine* 2000;79:155–69.

Chapter 121
Leukopenia *Laurence A. Boxer*

Marked developmental changes in normal values for the total white blood cell (WBC) count occur during childhood (Chapter 710). The mean WBC count at birth is high, followed by a rapid fall beginning at 12 hr until the end of the first week. Thereafter, values are stable until 1 yr of age. A slow, steady decline in the WBC count continues throughout childhood until the adult value is reached in adolescence. Leukopenia in adults is defined as a total WBC count less than 4,000/μL. Evaluation of patients with leukopenia, neutropenia, or lymphopenia begins with a through history, physical examination, family history, and screening laboratory tests (Fig. 121–1).

NEUTROPENIA

Neutropenia is an **absolute neutrophil count (ANC)**, calculated as the WBC count/μL × per cent of neutrophils and bands, more than two standard deviations below the normal mean. Normal neutrophil counts must be stratified for age and race. For whites, the lower limit of normal for the neutrophil count is 1,500/μL; for blacks, the lower limit of normal is 1,200/μL. The relatively low counts in blacks probably reflect a relative decrease in neutrophils in the storage compartment of the bone marrow.

Etiology. **Acute neutropenia** evolving over a few days often occurs when neutrophil use is rapid and production is compromised. **Chronic neutropenia** lasting months or years usually arises from reduced production or excessive splenic sequestration of neutrophils. Neutropenia may be classified by whether it arises secondary to factors extrinsic to marrow myeloid cells (Table 121–1), which is common; as an acquired disorder of myeloid and stem cells (Table 121–2), which is less common; or more rarely an intrinsic defect affecting proliferation and maturation of myeloid and stem cells (Table 121–3).

Neutropenia may be characterized as mild, with an ANC of 1,000–1,500/μL; moderate, with an ANC of 500–1,000/μL; or severe, with an ANC <500/μL. This stratification aids in predicting the risk of pyogenic infection because only patients with severe neutropenia have significantly increased susceptibility to life-threatening infections.

INFECTIOUS CAUSES. Transient neutropenia often accompanies viral infections. Neutropenia associated with common childhood viral disease occurs during the first 1–2 days of illness and may persist for 3–8 days. It usually corresponds to a period of acute viremia and is related to virus-induced redistribution of neutrophils from the circulating to the marginating pool. Neutrophil sequestration possibly occurs after virus-induced tissue damage. Moderate to severe neutropenia may also be associated with a wide variety of other infectious causes (Table 121–4). Bacterial sepsis is a particularly serious cause of neutropenia.

Chronic neutropenia often accompanies infection with human immunodeficiency virus (HIV)–1 as a finding associated with AIDS. The neutropenia associated with AIDS probably arises from a combination of impaired neutrophil production and the accelerated destruction of neutrophils mediated by anti-neutrophil antibodies.

DRUG-INDUCED NEUTROPENIA. Drug use remains one of the most common causes of neutropenia (Table 121–5). The incidence of drug-induced neutropenia increases precipitously with age; only 10% of cases occur among children and young adults, with the majority of cases among adults. Drug-induced neutropenia has several underlying mechanisms (i.e., immune-mediated, toxic, idiosyncratic, and hypersensitivity reactions) and should be differentiated from the severe neutropenia that predictably occurs after large doses of cytoreductive cancer drugs or radiotherapy. Cytotoxic chemotherapy preferentially affects myeloid cells and induces neutropenia because of the high proliferative rate of neutrophil precursors and the rapid turnover of blood neutrophils.

Immune-mediated neutropenia usually lasts for about 1 wk and is thought to arise from effects of drugs, such as propylthiouracil or penicillin, that act as haptens to stimulate antibody formation. Other drugs, including the antipsychotic drugs such as the phenothiazines, can cause neutropenia when given in toxic amounts. In contrast, idiosyncratic reactions, such as to chloramphenicol, are unpredictable with regard to dose or duration of use. Hypersensitivity reactions are rare and occasionally may involve arene oxide metabolites of aromatic anticonvulsants.

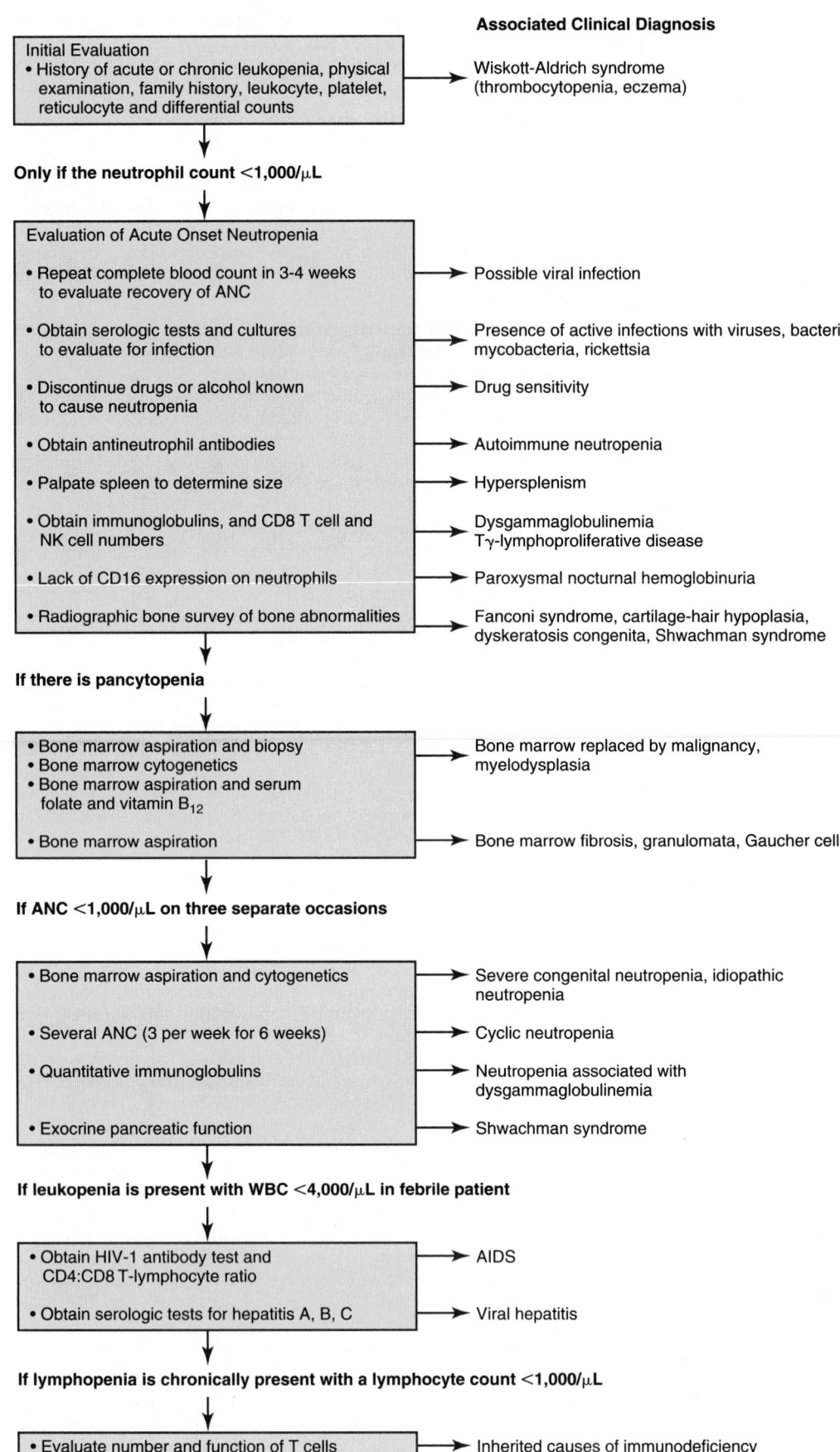

Associated Clinical Diagnosis

Initial Evaluation
- History of acute or chronic leukopenia, physical examination, family history, leukocyte, platelet, reticulocyte and differential counts

→ Wiskott-Aldrich syndrome (thrombocytopenia, eczema)

Only if the neutrophil count <1,000/μL

Evaluation of Acute Onset Neutropenia

- Repeat complete blood count in 3-4 weeks to evaluate recovery of ANC

→ Possible viral infection

- Obtain serologic tests and cultures to evaluate for infection

→ Presence of active infections with viruses, bacteria, mycobacteria, rickettsia

- Discontinue drugs or alcohol known to cause neutropenia

→ Drug sensitivity

- Obtain antineutrophil antibodies

→ Autoimmune neutropenia

- Palpate spleen to determine size

→ Hypersplenism

- Obtain immunoglobulins, and CD8 T cell and NK cell numbers

→ Dysgammaglobulinemia Tγ-lymphoproliferative disease

- Lack of CD16 expression on neutrophils

→ Paroxysmal nocturnal hemoglobinuria

- Radiographic bone survey of bone abnormalities

→ Fanconi syndrome, cartilage-hair hypoplasia, dyskeratosis congenita, Shwachman syndrome

If there is pancytopenia

- Bone marrow aspiration and biopsy
- Bone marrow cytogenetics
- Bone marrow aspiration and serum folate and vitamin B$_{12}$

→ Bone marrow replaced by malignancy, myelodysplasia

- Bone marrow aspiration

→ Bone marrow fibrosis, granulomata, Gaucher cells

If ANC <1,000/μL on three separate occasions

- Bone marrow aspiration and cytogenetics

→ Severe congenital neutropenia, idiopathic neutropenia

- Several ANC (3 per week for 6 weeks)

→ Cyclic neutropenia

- Quantitative immunoglobulins

→ Neutropenia associated with dysgammaglobulinemia

- Exocrine pancreatic function

→ Shwachman syndrome

If leukopenia is present with WBC <4,000/μL in febrile patient

- Obtain HIV-1 antibody test and CD4:CD8 T-lymphocyte ratio

→ AIDS

- Obtain serologic tests for hepatitis A, B, C

→ Viral hepatitis

If lymphopenia is chronically present with a lymphocyte count <1,000/μL

- Evaluate number and function of T cells

→ Inherited causes of immunodeficiency

FIGURE 121–1. Algorithm for the evaluation of a patient with leukopenia. ANC = absolute neutrophil count; NK = natural killer; WBC = white blood cell count. (Modified from Boxer LA: Approach to the patient with leukopenia. In Humes HD [editor]: *Kelley's Textbook of Internal Medicine*, 4th ed. Philadelphia, Lippincott Williams & Wilkins, 2000, p 1578.)

TABLE 121–1. Causes of Neutropenia Extrinsic to Bone Marrow Myeloid Cells

Cause	Etiologic Factors/Agents	Associated Findings
Infection	Viral, bacterial, protozoal, rickettsial, fungal	Redistribution from circulating to marginating pools, impaired production, accelerated destruction
Drug induced	Phenothiazines, sulfonamides, anticonvulsants, penicillins, aminopyrines	Hypersensitivity reaction (fever, lymphadenopathy, rash, hepatitis, nephritis, pneumonitis, aplastic anemia), antineutrophil antibodies
Immune neutropenia	Isoimmune; autoimmune	Variable arrest from metamyelocyte to segmented neutrophils in bone marrow
Reticuloendothelial sequestration	Hypersplenism	Anemia, thrombocytopenia
Bone marrow replacement	Malignancy (leukemia, lymphoma, metastatic solid tumors), Gaucher disease, granuloma, fibrosis	Anemia, thrombocytopenia, presence of immature myeloid and erythroid precursor in peripheral blood
Cancer chemotherapy or radiation therapy to bone marrow	Suppression of myeloid cell production	Bone marrow hypoplasia, anemia, thrombocytopenia
Ineffective myelopoiesis	Malnutrition (marasmus, anorexia nervosa), vitamin B_{12} or folate deficiency	Megaloblastic anemia, hypersegmented neutrophils

Modified from Boxer LA, Blackwood RA: Leukocyte disorders: Quantitative and qualitative disorders of the neutrophil, part I. Pediatr Rev 1996;17:19–28.

TABLE 121–2. Acquired Disorders of Myeloid and Stem Cells

Cause	Associated Findings
Acute myelogenous or acute lymphocytic leukemia	Bone marrow replacement with malignant cells
Myelodysplasias	Bone marrow hypoplasia with megaloblastoid red cell precursors, increased numbers of blasts, increased red cell mean cell volume
Paroxysmal nocturnal hemoglobinuria	Absent expression of CD16 on neutrophils, abnormal Ham test
Aplastic anemia	Marked bone marrow hypoplasia
Vitamin B_{12}/folate deficiency	Megaloblastic anemia
Neutropenia in premature infants	Reduced numbers of bone marrow bands and segmented neutrophils
Chronic idiopathic neutropenia	Bone marrow arrest from promyelocytes through segmented neutrophils may occur

TABLE 121–3. Intrinsic Disorders of Proliferation and Maturation of Myeloid and Stem Cells

Disorder	Mode of Inheritance	Associated Findings	Bone Marrow Findings
Cyclic neutropenia	AD	Periodic oscillation in ANC	Hypoplasia or myeloid maturation arrest, increased number of eosinophils
Severe congenital neutropenia (Kostmann syndrome)	Sporadic occurrence	Profound neutropenia, monocytosis, eosinophilia	Arrest in myeloid maturation at promyelocyte stage
Chronic benign neutropenia	AD, AR, sporadic	Mild neutropenia	Variable pattern, including normal-appearing marrow
Shwachman-Diamond syndrome	AR	Pancreatic insufficiency with fatty replacement and atrophy, anemia, thrombocytopenia, metaphyseal dysostosis	Hypocellularity associated with leukemic transformation
Cartilage-hair hypoplasia	AR	Short-limb dwarfism, fine hair, moderate neutropenia, impaired cellular immunity	Myeloid hypoplasia
Dyskeratosis congenita	X	Nail dystrophy, leukoplakia, reticulated hyperpigmentation of the skin	Marrow hypoplasia
Glycogen storage disease type 1b	AR	Hepatic enlargement, growth retardation, impaired neutrophil motility	Myeloid hypoplasia
Chédiak-Higashi syndrome	AR	Partial albinism, giant granules in myeloid cells, platelet storage pool defect, natural killer cell function impaired, ineffective myelopoiesis	Myeloid hypoplasia
Myelokathexis	AR	Neutrophils have cytoplasmic vacuoles and abnormal nuclei with thin filaments connecting the nuclear lobes	Myeloid hyperplasia
Hyper IgM syndrome	X, AR	Absent IgG, elevated IgM	Maturation arrest at promyelocyte-myelocyte stage

AD = autosomal dominant; AR = autosomal recessive; X = X-linked recessive; ANC = absolute neutrophil count.
Modified from Boxer LA, Blackwood RA: Leukocyte disorders: Quantitative and qualitative disorders of the neutrophil, part I. Pediatr Rev 1996;17:19–28.

TABLE 121–4. Infections Associated with Neutropenia

Viral	Paratyphoid fever
Respiratory syncytial virus	Tuberculosis (disseminated)
Dengue fever	Brucellosis
Colorado tick fever	Tularemia
Mumps	Gram-negative sepsis
Viral hepatitis	Psittacosis
Infectious mononucleosis (EBV)	
Influenza	**Fungal**
Measles	Histoplasmosis (disseminated)
Rubella	
Roseola	**Protozoal**
Varicella	Malaria
Cytomegalovirus	Leishmaniasis (kala-azar)
Human immunodeficiency virus	
Sandfly fever	**Rickettsial**
	Rocky Mountain spotted fever
Bacterial	Typhus fever
Pertussis	Rickettsialpox
Typhoid fever	

From Boxer LA, Blackwood RA: Leukocyte disorders: Quantitative and qualitative disorders of the neutrophil, part 1. Pediatr Rev 1996;17:19–28.

Fever, rash, lymphadenopathy, hepatitis, nephritis, pneumonitis, or aplastic anemia are often associated with hypersensitivity-induced neutropenia. Acute hypersensitivity reactions such as those caused by phenytoin or phenobarbital may last for only a few days if the offending drug is discontinued. Chronic hypersensitivity may last for months to years. Drug-induced neutropenia may occasionally be asymptomatic despite severely reduced numbers of neutrophils and is noted only because of regular monitoring of WBC counts during drug therapy.

Neutropenia complicating the use of anticancer drugs or radiation therapy, especially radiation therapy directed at the pelvis or sternum, is common, secondary to the effects of the cytotoxicity on rapidly replicating cells. A decline in the WBC count typically occurs 7–10 days after administration of the anticancer drug and may persist for 2–3 wk. The neutropenia accompanying both malignancy and following cancer chemotherapy is frequently associated with compromised cellular immunity, thereby predisposing patients to a much greater risk of infection than those disorders associated with isolated neutropenia (Chapter 164).

BONE MARROW REPLACEMENT. Various acquired disorders may lead to neutropenia accompanied by anemia and thrombocytopenia. The most important among these are hematologic malignancies including leukemia and lymphoma, and metastatic solid tumors such as neuroblastoma, rhabdomyosarcoma, and Ewing's sarcoma that infiltrate the bone marrow and lead to suppression of myelopoiesis. Neutropenia may also accompany myelodysplastic disorders or preleukemic syndromes, which typically are characterized by peripheral cytopenias and macrocytic blood cells associated with impaired production of myeloid precursors.

RETICULOENDOTHELIAL SEQUESTRATION. Splenic enlargement resulting from intrinsic splenic disease, portal hypertension, or other causes of splenic hyperplasia can lead to neutropenia. The neutropenia often is mild to moderate and accompanied by a corresponding degree of thrombocytopenia and anemia, and may be corrected by successfully treating the underlying disease. The reduced neutrophil survival corresponds to the size of the spleen, and the extent of the neutropenia is inversely proportional to bone marrow compensatory mechanisms. In selected cases, splenectomy may be necessary to restore the neutrophil count to normal, but this predisposes patients to infections by encapsulated bacterial organisms.

IMMUNE NEUTROPENIA. Immune neutropenias are associated with the presence of circulating antineutrophil antibodies, which may mediate neutrophil destruction by complement-mediated lysis or splenic phagocytosis of opsonized neutrophils.

Alloimmune Neonatal Neutropenia (ANN). This form of neonatal neutropenia occurs after transplacental transfer of maternal alloantibodies directed against antigens on the infant's neutrophils, analogous to Rh hemolytic disease. Prenatal sensitization induces maternal IgG antibodies to neutrophil antigens on fetal cells. The antibodies are usually complement-activating and are frequently directed to neutrophil-specific antigens. The pathogenesis of ANN usually involves phagocytosis of antibody-coated neutrophils by splenic macrophages. Symptomatic infants may present with delayed separation of the umbilical cord, mild skin infections, fever, and pneumonia within the first 2 wk of life; these resolve with antibiotic therapy. The neutropenia is often severe and associated with fever and infections due to the usual microbes that cause neonatal disease. By 7 wk of age, the infant's neutrophil count usually returns to normal, reflecting the duration of survival of maternal antibody in the infant's circulation. Treatment consists of supportive care and appropriate antibiotics for clinical infections.

Autoimmune Neutropenia. Autoimmune neutropenia is analogous to autoimmune hemolytic anemia and thrombocytopenia. Antibodies causing neutropenia have been detected in patients who have no other signs of autoimmune disease, in patients who have additional antibodies against red blood cells and/or platelets, and in patients who have a connective tissue disorder. Autoimmune neutropenia is distinguished from other forms of neutropenia only by the demonstration of antineutrophil antibodies rather than by abnormal bone marrow histology. Autoimmune neutropenia frequently occurs in children with congenital and acquired forms of immune deficiencies, including dysgammaglobulinemia.

Autoimmune Neutropenia of Infancy (ANI). This benign condition has been diagnosed more frequently as reliable techniques for detection of antineutrophil antibodies have become more widely available. The exact incidence of ANI remains unknown, but because of its benign nature, the disorder may be more common than currently appreciated. In one study, ANI occurred with an annual incidence of approximately 1/100,000 among children between infancy and 10 yr. All patients recognized as having ANI have severe neutropenia on presentation, with an ANC usually less than 500/μL, but the total WBC count is always within normal limits. Monocytosis or

TABLE 121–5. Immune-Mediated, Toxic, and Hypersensitivity-Mediated Neutropenia

Characteristic	Immunologic Form	Toxic Form	Hypersensitivity Form
Paradigm drugs	Aminopyrine, propylthiouracil, penicillin	Phenothiazine	Phenytoin, phenobarbital
Time to onset	Days to weeks	Weeks to months	Weeks to months
Clinical appearance	Acute, often explosive symptoms	Often asymptomatic or insidious onset	May be associated with fever, rash, nephritis, pneumonitis, or aplastic anemia
Rechallenge	Prompt recurrence with small test dose	Latent period; high doses required	Latent period; high doses required
Laboratory findings	Antibody test results positive	Evidence of direct toxicity to cells	Evidence of metabolite-mediated damage to cells

From Boxer LA: Approach to the patient with leukopenia. In Humes H (editor): Kelley's Textbook of Internal Medicine, 4th ed. Philadelphia, Lippincott Williams & Wilkins, 2000, p 1579.

eosinophilia may occur but does not seem to affect the rate of infection. The age at diagnosis is between 5 and 15 mo, with a female:male ratio of 6:4. None of the affected children has evidence of other autoimmune diseases. Children with ANI present with minor infections such as otitis media, gingivitis, respiratory tract infections, gastroenteritis, and cellulitis. The diagnosis often is considered only after the blood count reveals neutropenia. Occasionally, children may present with more severe infections including pneumonia, sepsis, or abscesses. Longitudinal studies of infants with ANI demonstrate a median duration of disease of approximately 7 to 24 months. The diagnosis is established by the presence of antineutrophil antibodies in serum. Treatment with recombinant human granulocyte-colony stimulating factor (rhG-CSF) may be useful in providing temporary remission in infants with severe infections or requiring surgical intervention.

Neonatal Autoimmune Neutropenia. Mothers with autoimmune disease may give birth to infants who develop transient neutropenia. The duration of the neutropenia depends on the time required for the infant to clear the maternally transferred circulating IgG antibody. It persists in most cases for a few weeks to a few months. Neonates almost always remain asymptomatic.

INEFFECTIVE MYELOPOIESIS. Ineffective myelopoiesis may be acquired as a result of vitamin B_{12} deficiency, which may result from resection of the distal ileum, or folic acid deficiency. Megaloblastic pancytopenia also can result from extended use of antibiotics such as trimethoprim-sulfamethoxazole, which inhibit folic acid metabolism, and from the use of phenytoin, which may impair folate absorption in the small intestine. Neutropenia also occurs with starvation and marasmus in infants, anorexia nervosa, and occasionally among patients receiving prolonged parenteral feedings.

INTRINSIC DISORDERS OF PROLIFERATION AND MATURATION OF MYELOID STEM CELLS. The isolated disorders of proliferation and maturation of myeloid stem cells are rare. These patients frequently benefit from rhG-CSF therapy. Congenital disorders that have severe neutropenia as a clinical feature include the severe combined immunodeficiencies (Chapter 116), hyper IgM (Chapter 116), and common variable immunodeficiency (Chapter 114).

Cyclic Neutropenia. Cyclic neutropenia, a congenital granulopoietic disorder, is inherited in an autosomal dominant manner in some patients (see Table 121–3). It is characterized by regular, periodic oscillation in the number of peripheral neutrophils from normal to neutropenic values with a mean oscillatory period of 21 ± 3 days. During the neutropenic phase, most patients suffer from oral ulcers, fever, stomatitis, or pharyngitis, occasionally associated with lymph node enlargement. Serious infections occur occasionally and may lead to pneumonia, chronic periodontitis, and recurrent ulcerations of the oral, vaginal, and rectal mucosa. Sepsis, notably with *Clostridium perfringens,* and death may occur. Cyclic neutropenia arises from a regulatory abnormality involving early hematopoietic precursor cells and is associated with mutations in the neutrophil elastase gene. Many patients live for a considerable number of years, with some actually experiencing abatement of symptoms as they age. The cycles tend to become less noticeable in older patients, and the hematologic picture often begins to resemble that of chronic neutropenia.

Severe Congenital Neutropenia. Severe congenital neutropenia, or **Kostmann disease,** is characterized by an arrest in myeloid maturation at the promyelocyte stage of the bone marrow, resulting in an ANC of less than 200/µL (see Table 121–3). This disorder occurs sporadically or as an autosomal dominant or recessive disorder. Patients typically show monocytosis and eosinophilia and suffer from recurrent, severe pyogenic infections, especially of the skin, mouth, and rectum. Anemia associated with chronic inflammatory disease is often present. Approximately 10% of patients develop acute myelogenous

leukemia or myelodysplasia associated with monosomy 7. The neutropenia in the majority of patients is associated with mutations in the neutrophil elastase gene, which in turn leads to accelerated apoptosis of bone marrow myeloid cells. Before the use of rhG-CSF, two thirds of these patients died of fatal infections before reaching adolescence.

Shwachman-Diamond Syndrome. Shwachman-Diamond syndrome is an autosomal recessive disorder characterized by digestive abnormalities and abnormally low WBC counts (see Table 121–3). The initial symptoms are usually diarrhea and failure to thrive because of malabsorption, which develops in almost all infants by 4 mo of age. Growth failure and metaphyseal chondrodysplasia associated with dwarfism are especially prominent during the 1st and 2nd yr of life. Puberty is often delayed. Some patients have respiratory problems with pneumonia and frequent otitis media, as well as eczema. Virtually all patients with Shwachman-Diamond syndrome have neutropenia, with the ANC periodically less than 1,000/µL. Some children have been reported to have a chemotactic defect that may contribute to the increased susceptibility to pyogenic infection. The illness may progress to bone marrow hypoplasia leading to moderate thrombocytopenia and anemia. Myelodysplasia and acute myelogenous leukemia associated with monosomy 7 have also been reported in this syndrome. The neutropenia responds to treatment with rhG-CSF.

Cartilage-Hair Hypoplasia. Cartilage-hair hypoplasia is a multisystem autosomal recessive disorder characterized by short limbs and short stature resulting from abnormal development of long bone cartilage (Chapter 116). The major symptoms include abnormalities of the spine, hyperextensible fingers, and very fine, thin hair, eyebrows, and eyelashes (see Table 121–3). Cartilage-hair hypoplasia is associated with decreased cell-mediated immunity, neutropenia, macrocytic anemia, and increased rates of malignancy. Bone marrow transplantation has restored cellular immunity and corrected the neutropenia.

Glycogen Storage Disease Type Ib. Recurrent infections with neutropenia are a distinctive feature of glycogen storage disease (GSD) type Ib (see Table 121–3). Both classic von Gierke glycogen storage disease (GSDIa) and GSDIb cause massive enlargement of liver and severe growth retardation. In contrast to GSDIa, glucose-6-phosphatase activity is present by in vitro assays but glucose is not liberated from glucose-6-phosphate in vivo with GSDIb. In the liver, glucose-6-phosphatase requires two microsomal membrane components: a specific transfer system, glucose-6-phosphatase translocase, which shuttles glucose-6-phosphate from the cytoplasm to the lumen of the endoplasmic reticulum where it is hydrolyzed by a second enzyme, glucose-6-phosphalase, into glucose and inorganic phosphate. Neutrophils also appear to have a defective transport system resulting in defective neutrophil motility that is associated with the neutropenia. Patients with GSDIb with severe neutropenia are predisposed to recurrent bacterial infections. Treatment with rhG-CSF can correct the neutropenia.

Severe Chronic Neutropenia. Acquired idiopathic chronic symptomatic neutropenia is characterized by onset of neutropenia after 2 yr of age, and more frequently among adults. It is characterized by neutrophil counts that are occasionally less than 500/µL. Patients with an ANC persistently less than 500/µL are afflicted with recurrent pyogenic infections involving the skin, mucous membranes, lungs, and lymph nodes. Bone marrow examination reveals variable patterns of myeloid formation with arrest generally occurring between the myelocyte and band forms (see Table 121–2).

Some forms of chronic neutropenia, such as myelokathexis, arise from an impaired release of neutrophils from the bone marrow into the peripheral blood. Children with myelokathexis have morphologic abnormalities of the neutrophils, with the cells showing cytoplasmic vacuoles of thin strands connecting the nuclear lobes. In some cases, these patients also have cellular immune defects and are predisposed to recurrent bacterial infections (see Table 121–3).

Chronic Benign Neutropenia. In contrast to severe congenital neutropenia, chronic benign neutropenia of childhood represents a common group of disorders characterized by mild to moderate neutropenia that does not lead to an increased risk of pyogenic infections. Spontaneous remissions have often been reported, although these may represent misdiagnosis of autoimmune neutropenia of infancy, in which remissions occur commonly during childhood. Chronic benign neutropenia may be inherited in either a dominant or recessive form. An autosomal recessive form of benign neutropenia is encountered in Yemenite Jews. Because of the relatively low risk of serious infection, patients should be not subjected to the potential toxic effects of prolonged administration of corticosteroids, splenectomy, or cytotoxic therapy (see Table 121–3).

Clinical Manifestations. Individuals with neutrophil counts below 500/μL are at substantial risk for developing infections, primarily from their endogenous flora as well as from nosocomial organisms. Some patients with isolated chronic neutropenia with an ANC below 200/μL may not experience many serious infections, probably because the remainder of the immune system remains intact. In contrast, children whose neutropenia is secondary to acquired disorders of production such as with cytotoxic therapy, immunosuppressive drugs, or radiation therapy, particularly in conjunction with malignancies, are likely to develop serious bacterial infections because many arms of the immune system are markedly compromised.

Leukopenia associated with neutropenia, in addition to monocytopenia and lymphocytopenia, is often more serious than neutropenia alone. The integrity of skin and mucous membranes, the vascular supply to tissues, and the nutritional status of patients influence the risk of infection.

The clinical presentation in most patients with profound neutropenia is fever exceeding 101°F, cellulitis, and furunculosis. Stomatitis, gingivitis, perirectal inflammation, colitis, sinusitis, and otitis media are frequent accompaniments of profound neutropenia in children. Other clinical manifestations of profound neutropenia include hepatic abscesses, recurrent pneumonias, and septicemia. In contrast, isolated neutropenia does not heighten a patient's susceptibility to fungal, parasitic, or viral infections or to bacterial meningitis.

The most common pathogens isolated from neutropenic patients are *Staphylococcus aureus* and gram-negative bacteria. The usual signs and symptoms of local infection and inflammation such as exudate, fluctuance, and regional lymphadenopathy are generally less in the presence of neutropenia because of the inability to form pus. However, neutropenic patients can experience pain at sites of inflammation.

Laboratory Findings. Isolated absolute neutropenia has a limited number of causes (see Tables 121–1, 121–2, and 121–3). The duration and severity of the neutropenia greatly influence the extent of laboratory evaluation. Patients with chronic neutropenia since infancy and a history of recurrent fevers and chronic gingivitis should have WBC counts and differential counts determined three times weekly for 6 wk to evaluate the periodicity suggestive of cyclic neutropenia. Bone marrow aspiration and biopsy should be performed on selected patients to assess cellularity. Additional marrow studies such as cytogenetic analysis and special stains for detecting leukemia and other malignant disorders should be obtained for patients with suspected intrinsic defects in the myeloid cells or the progenitors, and for patients with suspected malignancy. Selection of further laboratory tests is determined by the duration and severity of the neutropenia and the associated findings on physical examination (see Fig. 121–1).

Treatment. The management of acquired transient neutropenia associated with malignancies, myelosuppressive chemotherapy, or immunosuppressive chemotherapy differs from that of congenital or chronic forms of neutropenia. In the former situation, infections sometimes are heralded only by fever, and sepsis is a major cause of death. Early recognition and treatment of infections may be lifesaving (Chapter 164).

Therapy of severe chronic neutropenia is dictated by the clinical manifestations. Patients with benign neutropenia and no evidence of repeated bacterial infections or chronic gingivitis require no specific therapy. Superficial infections in children with mild to moderate neutropenia may be treated with appropriate oral antibiotics. However, in patients who have life-threatening infections, broad-spectrum intravenous antibiotics should be started promptly.

Effective treatment of severe chronic neutropenia including severe congenital neutropenia, chronic symptomatic idiopathic neutropenia, and cyclic neutropenia is now possible. A randomized controlled trial of these patients treated with subcutaneously administered rhG-CSF at doses ranging from 3.4 to 11.50 μg/kg/24 hr led to dramatic increases in neutrophil counts, resulting in marked attenuation of infection and inflammation. rhG-CSF has also been successfully administered to some patients with drug-induced neutropenia whose neutrophil count failed to increase after cessation of the offending drug. The long-term effects of rhG-CSF therapy are unknown but include a propensity for the development of moderate splenomegaly, thrombocytopenia, and, occasionally, vasculitis. Autoimmune neutropenia may be responsive to intermittent corticosteroids, especially if it is part of an underlying disease process such as systemic lupus erythematosus. Although this remains unproved by controlled studies, use of rhG-CSF has benefited some patients who have immune or drug-induced neutropenias.

Those patients with severe congenital neutropenia or Shwachman-Diamond syndrome who develop myelodysplasia or acute myelogenous leukemia respond only to allogeneic bone marrow transplantation. Chemotherapy is ineffective.

LYMPHOPENIA

Lymphocytes account for about 30% of the circulating WBCs in a newborn. The proportion of lymphocytes then increases rapidly within the 1st mo, reaching an average of 60% by 2 yr of age. The normal lymphocyte count in children younger than 2 yr is 3,000–9,500/μL and in adults is 1,000–4,800/μL. At 6 yr of age, the lower limit of normal is 1,500/μL.

Almost 65% of blood T lymphocytes are CD4 (helper) T lymphocytes. Most patients with lymphocytopenia have a reduction in the absolute number of T lymphocytes, particularly in the number of CD4 T lymphocytes. The average number of CD4 T lymphocytes in adult blood is 1,100/μL (range, 300–1,300/μL), and the average number of CD8 (suppressor) T lymphocytes is 600/μL (range, 100–900/μL), with the normal CD4:CD8 ratio of 1.8–2.0.

Lymphocytopenia by itself usually causes no symptoms and is often detected in the evaluation of other illnesses, particularly recurrent viral, fungal, and parasitic infections. Lymphocyte subpopulations can be measured by multiparameter flow cytometry, which uses the pattern of antigen expression to classify and characterize these cells.

INHERITED CAUSES OF LYMPHOCYTOPENIA. Inherited immunodeficiency disorders may have a quantitative or qualitative stem cell abnormality resulting in ineffective lymphocytopoiesis (Box 121–1). Other disorders such as Wiskott-Aldrich syndrome may have associated lymphocytopenia arising from accelerated destruction of T cells. A similar mechanism is present in patients with adenosine deaminase deficiency and purine nucleoside phosphorylase deficiency.

Calderwood S, Kilpatrick L, Douglas SD, et al: Recombinant human granulocyte colony-stimulating factor therapy for patients with neutropenia and/or neutrophil dysfunction secondary to glycogen storage disease type 1b. *Blood* 2001;97:376–82.

Dokal I: Dyskeratosis congenita in all its forms. *Br J Haematol* 2000;110:768–79.

Dror Y, Freedman MD: Shwachman-Diamond syndrome: An inherited preleukemic bone marrow failure disorder with aberrant hematopoietic progenitors and faulty marrow microenvironment. *Blood* 1999;94:3048–54.

Gray PD, Rodwell RL: Neonatal neutropenia associated with maternal hypertension poses a risk for nosocomial infection. *Eur J Pediatr* 1999;158:71–3.

BOX 121–1. Causes of Lymphocytopenia

ACQUIRED CAUSES

Infectious diseases
 AIDS
 Viral hepatitis
 Influenza
 Tuberculosis
 Typhoid fever
 Sepsis
Iatrogenic
 Immunosuppressive therapy
 Corticosteroids
 High-dose PUVA therapy
 Cytotoxic chemotherapy
 Radiation
 Thoracic duct drainage
Systemic and other diseases
 Systemic lupus erythematosus
 Myasthenia gravis
 Hodgkin disease
 Protein-losing enteropathy
 Renal failure
 Sarcoidosis
 Thermal injury
 Aplastic anemia
Dietary deficiency
 Dietary deficiency associated with ethanol abuse

INHERITED CAUSES

Aplasia of lymphopoietic stem cells
Severe combined immunodeficiency associated with defect in IL-2 receptor γ-chain, deficiency of ADA or PNP, or unknown
Ataxia-telangiectasia
Wiskott-Aldrich syndrome
Immunodeficiency with thymoma
Cartilage-hair hypoplasia
Idiopathic CD4T lymphocytopenia

ADA = adenosine deaminase; PNP = purine nucleoside phosphorylase; IL-2 = interleukin-2; PUVA = psoralen and ultraviolet A irradiation.
From Boxer LA: Approach to the patient with leukopenia. In Humes HD (editor): *Kelley's Textbook of Internal Medicine*, 4th ed. Philadelphia, Lippincott Williams & Wilkins, 2000, p 1580.

ACQUIRED LYMPHOCYTOPENIA. Acquired lymphocytopenia is the result of depletion of blood lymphocytes that is not secondary to inherited diseases. AIDS is the most common infectious disease associated with lymphocytopenia, which results from destruction of CD4 T cells infected with HIV-1 or HIV-2. Other viral and bacterial diseases may be associated with lymphocytopenia. In some instances of acute viremia with other viral infections, lymphocytes may undergo accelerated destruction from intracellular viral replication, be trapped in the spleen or nodes, or migrate to the respiratory tract.

Iatrogenic lymphocytopenia is caused by cytotoxic chemotherapy, radiation therapy, and long-term administration of antilymphocyte globulin. Long-term treatment of psoriasis with psoralen and ultraviolet irradiation may destroy T lymphocytes. Corticosteroids can cause lymphopenia through increased cell destruction. Systemic autoimmune diseases such as systemic lupus erythematosus are associated with lymphocytopenia. Other conditions such as protein-losing enteropathy and aberrant or surgical drainage of the thoracic duct are associated with lymphocyte depletion, leading to lymphocytopenia.

Aprikyan AG, Liles WC, Boxer LA, et al: Mutant elastase in pathogenesis of cyclic and severe congenital neutropenia. *J Pediatr Hematol/Oncol* 2002;24:784–6

Aprikyan AG, Liles WC, Parks JR, et al: Myelokathexis, a congenital disorder of severe neutropenia characterized by accelerated apoptosis and defective expression of bcl-x in neutrophil precursors. *Blood* 2000;95:320–7.

Boxer LA: Approach to the patient with leukopenia. In Humes HD (editor): *Kelley's Textbook of Internal Medicine*, 4th ed. Philadelphia, Lippincott-Williams & Wilkins, 2000, pp 1575–82.

Buckley R: Primary immunodeficiency diseases due to defects in lymphocytes. *N Engl J Med* 2000;343:1313–24.

Chapter 122
Leukocytosis *Laurence A. Boxer*

Leukocytosis is an elevation in the total leukocyte, or white blood cell (WBC), count that is two standard deviations above the mean count for a particular age (Chapter 710). The various causes of leukocytosis are categorized by the class of WBCs that is elevated and whether the leukocytosis is acute, chronic, or lifelong.

A WBC count exceeding 50,000/μL is termed a **leukemoid reaction** because of the similarity to features of leukemia. Leukemoid reactions are usually neutrophilic and are most frequently associated with septicemia and severe bacterial infections including shigellosis, salmonellosis, and meningococcemia. Infection in children with leukocyte adhesion deficiency results in WBC counts approaching or exceeding 100,000/μL.

A significant proportion of greater than 5% of immature to mature neutrophil cells is termed a **shift to the left** and indicates rapid release of cells from the bone marrow. This may result in increased circulating band forms, which usually constitute 1–5% of circulating neutrophilic cells, or metamyelocytes and myelocytes, which are not usually found in the peripheral circulation. Higher degrees of shift to the left with more immature neutrophil precursors are indicative of serious bacterial infections but may also be encountered with trauma, burns, surgery, and acute hemolysis or hemorrhage.

Neutrophilia. Neutrophilia is an increase in the total number of blood neutrophils, which for older children and adults is greater than 8,000/μL. During the first day of life, the upper limit of the normal neutrophil count ranges from 7,000 to 12,000/μL. In the 1st mo of life the neutrophil count ranges from 1,800 to 5,400/μL, and by 1 yr of age, the range is 1,500–8,500/μL.

An increase in circulating neutrophils is a result of a disturbance of the normal equilibrium involving bone marrow neutrophil production, movement out of the marrow compartments into the circulation, and neutrophil destruction. Neutrophilia may arise either alone or in combination with enhanced mobilization into the **circulating pool** from either the bone marrow storage compartment or the peripheral blood **marginating pool**, by impaired neutrophil egress into tissues, or after expansion of the circulating neutrophil pool secondary to increased progenitor cell proliferation and terminal differentiation through the myeloid series. Myelocytes are not released to the blood except under extreme circumstances.

ACUTE ACQUIRED NEUTROPHILIA. Neutrophilia is usually an acquired disorder and is a common finding with inflammation, infection, injury, and stress. Acute or chronic bacterial infections, trauma, and surgery are among the most common causes encountered in clinical practice. Neutrophilia is often associated with sickle cell disease, some chronic hemolytic anemias, heatstroke, burns, and diabetic ketoacidosis. Drugs commonly associated with neutrophilia include epinephrine, corticosteroids, and recombinant growth factors such as recombinant human granulocyte colony-stimulating factor (rhG-CSF) and recombinant human granulocyte-macrophage colony stimulating factor (rhGM-CSF). Epinephrine causes release into the circulation of a sequestered pool of neutrophils that normally marginate along the vascular endothelium. Corticosteroids accelerate the release of neutrophils and bands from a large storage pool within the bone marrow and impair the migration of neutrophils from the circulation into tissues. Acute neutrophilia in response to inflammation and infections occurs because of release of neutrophils from the marrow storage pool. The post-mitotic marrow neutrophil pools are approximately 10 times the sizes of the blood neutrophil pool, and about half of these cells are bands and segmented neutrophils. In neutrophil production disorders, such as those associated with malignancies and cancer chemotherapy, the size of this pool may be reduced and the capacity to develop neutrophilia remains impaired. Exposure of blood to foreign substances such as hemodialysis membrane activates the complement system and causes transient neutropenia followed by neutrophilia because of release of bone marrow neutrophils. The colony-stimulating factors, G-CSF and GM-CSF, cause acute and chronic neutrophilia by mobilizing cells from the marrow reserves and by stimulating neutrophil production.

CHRONIC ACQUIRED NEUTROPHILIA. Chronic neutrophilia is usually associated with continued stimulation of neutrophil production resulting from persistent inflammatory reactions or chronic infections such as tuberculosis, vasculitis, postsplenectomy states, Hodgkin disease, chronic myelogenous leukemia, chronic blood loss, and prolonged administration of corticosteroids. Chronic neutrophilia can arise following expansion of cell production secondary to stimulation of cell divisions within the mitotic precursor pool, which consists of promyelocytes and myelocytes (Fig. 122–1). Subsequently, the size of the post-mitotic pool increases. These changes lead to an increase in the marrow reserve pool, which can be readily mobilized for release of neutrophils into the circulation. The neutrophil production rate can increase greatly in response to exogenously administered hemopoietic growth factors such as rhG-CSF, with a maximum response taking at least 1 wk to develop.

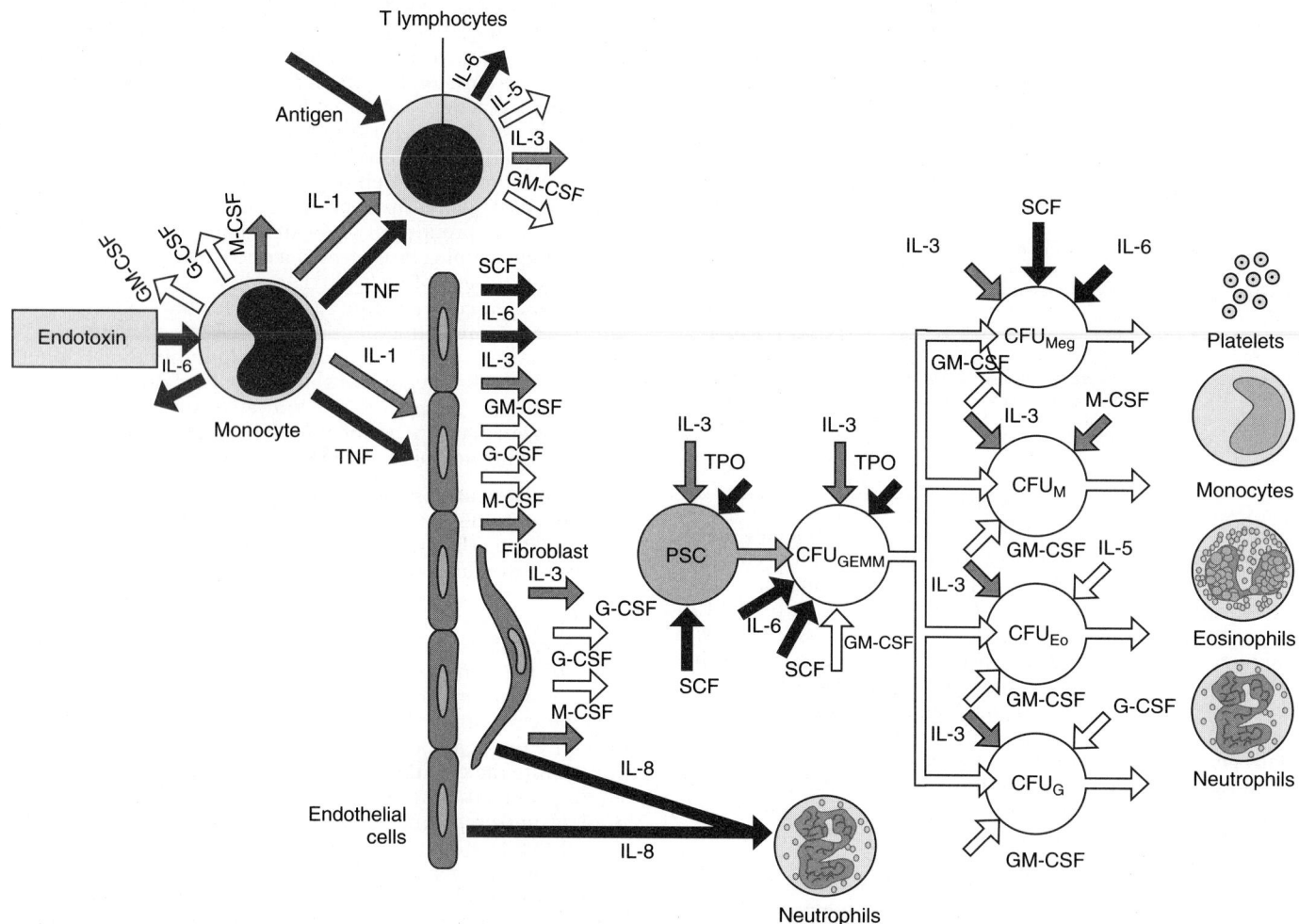

FIGURE 122–1. Cytokine control of the phagocyte production and activation by release of endotoxin during infection. Both endothelial cells and fibroblasts release substantial quantities of both granulocyte macrophage colony-stimulating factor (GM-CSF) and granulocyte colony-stimulating factor (G-CSF) in response to tumor necrosis factor (TNF) and interleukin-1 (IL-1). Both TNF and IL-1 are released from endotoxin-activated monocytes and antigen-activated T-lymphocytes. Stem cell factor (SCF), interleukin-3 (IL-3), GM-CSF, and interleukin-6 (IL-6) each influence the growth and differentiation of multilineage progenitor cells known as colony forming units (CFU)—granulocytes, eosinophils, monocytes, megakaryocytes (CFU_{GEMM})—to the committed colony forming unit macrophage (CFU_M), CFU eosinophil (CFU_{eo}), or CFU granulocyte (CFU_G). Platelet production can also be augmented by expansion of CFU megakaryocyte (CFU_{meg}). Factors that serve as growth and differentiation factors for a specific lineage also act as activation factors for the terminally differentiated forms of the same lineage. Macrophage-colony stimulating factor (M-CSF) enhances antibody-mediated cytotoxicity and phagocyte functions of monocytes. G-CSF promotes neutrophil bactericidal capacity, and interleukin-5 (IL-5) activates eosinophil function. Within hours of an infection, cytokine primed neutrophils move to the invasion site from the circulation under the influence of interleukin-8 (IL-8), which is released from endothelial cells and fibroblasts.

LIFELONG NEUTROPHILIA. Congenital asplenia is associated with lifelong neutrophilia. Uncommon genetic disorders that present with neutrophilia include leukocyte adhesion deficiency, familial myeloproliferative disease, Down syndrome, and Rac-2 mutation. In an autosomal dominant form of hereditary neutrophilia, patients maintain an absolute neutrophil count between 1,400 and 150,000/μL that is associated with hepatosplenomegaly, an increased alkaline phosphatase level, and Gaucher-type histiocytes in the bone marrow.

Evaluation of persistent neutrophilia requires a careful history, physical examination, and laboratory studies to search for infectious, inflammatory, and neoplastic conditions. The leukocyte alkaline phosphatase cytochemical stain of circulating neutrophils is useful to differentiate chronic myelogenous leukemia, in which the level is uniformly near zero, from reactive or secondary neutrophilia, in which normal to elevated levels are found.

Monocytosis. The average absolute blood monocyte count varies with age, which must be considered in the assessment of monocytosis. Given the role of monocytes in antigen presentation and cytokine secretion and as effectors of ingestion of invading organisms, it is not surprising that many clinical disorders give rise to monocytosis (Box 122–1). Most commonly, monocytosis occurs in patients recovering from myelosuppressive chemotherapy and is a harbinger of the return of the neutrophil count to normal. Monocytosis is often a sign of an acute bacterial, viral, protozoal, or rickettsial infection, and also occurs in some forms of chronic neutropenia and postsplenectomy states. Chronic inflammatory conditions can stimulate sustained monocytosis, including preleukemia, chronic myelogenous leukemia, lymphomas, and occasionally Hodgkin disease.

Lymphocytosis. The most common cause of lymphocytosis is an acute viral illness. Lymphocytosis is a normal response to most viral infections because the majority of circulating lymphocytes are T cells. In infectious mononucleosis, the B cells are infected with the Epstein-Barr virus and the T cells react to the viral antigens present in the B cells, resulting in **atypical lymphocytes** with the typical large, vacuolated morphology. Other viral diseases classically associated with lymphocytosis are cytomegalovirus and viral hepatitis. Chronic bacterial infections such as tuberculosis and brucellosis may lead to a sustained lymphocytosis. Pertussis is accompanied by lymphocytosis in approximately 25% of infants infected before 6 mo of age. Thyrotoxicosis and Addison disease are endocrine disorders associated with lymphocytosis. Persistent or profound lymphocytosis suggests acute lymphocytic leukemia.

BOX 122–1. Causes of Monocytosis

INFECTIONS
Bacterial infections
  Tuberculosis
  Brucellosis
  Typhoid fever
  Syphilis
  Infective endocarditis
Nonbacterial infections
  Fungal infections
  Rocky Mountain spotted fever
  Typhus
  Kala-azar
  Malaria

HEMATOLOGIC DISORDERS
Postsplenectomy states
Congenital and acquired neutropenias
Hemolytic anemias

MALIGNANT DISORDERS
Preleukemia
Acute myelogenous leukemia
Chronic myelogenous leukemia
Juvenile chronic myelocytic leukemia
Hodgkin disease
Non-Hodgkin lymphomas

COLLAGEN VASCULAR DISEASES
Systemic lupus erythematosus
Rheumatoid arthritis
Polyarteritis nodosa

GASTROINTESTINAL DISORDERS
Ulcerative colitis
Granulomatous colitis
Cirrhosis

MISCELLANEOUS
Recovery from marrow suppression induced by chemotherapy
Drug reactions
Sarcoidosis

Ward AC, Loeb DM, Soede-Bobok AA, et al: Regulation of granulopoiesis by transcription factors and cytokine signals. *Leukemia* 2000;14:973–90.

Williams DA, Tao W, Yang F, et al: Dominant negative mutation of the hematopoietic-specific Rho GTPase, Rac2, is associated with a human phagocyte immunodeficiency. *Blood* 2000;96:1646–54.

SECTION 4 *The Complement System*

Richard B. Johnston, Jr.

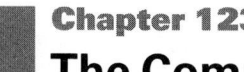

Chapter 123

The Complement System

Complement was originally defined as the nonspecific, heat-labile complementary principle required with specific antibody to lyse bacteria. The first four components were numbered in the order of their discovery and are now termed the classical pathway. Unfortunately for subsequent generations of students and physicians, the components fix to the immune complex in a different order, C1423. Once beyond this regrettable beginning, complement emerges as a logical, exquisitely balanced, and highly influential system that is fundamental to the clinical expression of inflammatory disease.

The complement system can now be broadly conceptualized as the **classical, mannose-binding lectin (MBL), and alternative pathways**, which interact and depend on each other for their full activity; the **membrane attack complex (C5b6789)**, formed from activity of any pathway; the eight serum and four membrane regulatory proteins well defined to date; a serosal regulatory protein; and seven fully defined cell membrane receptors that bind complement components or fragments (Table 123–1). The 24 serum components and regulators together compose about 15% of the globulin fraction of serum. The normal concentrations of serum complement components vary by age (Chapter 710); newborn infants have mild to moderate deficiencies of all plasma components of the complement system.

After C1423, complement nomenclature is logical and consists of only a few rules. Fragments of components resulting from cleavage by other components acting as enzymes are assigned lowercase letters (a, b, c, d, or e); with the exception of C2 fragments, the smaller piece that is released into surrounding fluids is assigned the lowercase letter a, and the major part of the molecule, bound to other components or to some part of the immune complex, is assigned letter b—for example, C3a and C3b. Components of the alternative pathway, B and D, have been assigned uppercase letters, as have the control proteins I and H, which downregulate both pathways. C3, and especially its major fragment C3b, is a component of both the classical and alternative pathways.

Complement is a system of interacting proteins. The biologic functions of the system depend on the interactions of individual components, which occur in sequential, cascade fashion. Activation of each component, except the first, depends on activation of the prior component or components in the sequence. Interaction occurs along three pathways (Fig. 123–1): the classical pathway, in the order antigen–antibody–C142356789; the MBL pathway, in the order microbial mannan–MBL/MBL-associated proteases 1 and 2–C42356789; and the alternative pathway, in the order activator–C3bBD–C356789. Antibody accelerates the rate of activation of the alternative pathway, but activation can occur on appropriate surfaces in the absence of antibody. The classical and the alternative pathways interact with each other through the ability of both to activate C3.

Activation of the early-acting components of complement (C1423) results in the generation of a series of active enzymes, C1, C42, and C423, on the surface of the immune complex or underlying cell. These enzymes cleave and activate the next component in the sequence. In contrast, the interaction among C5b, C6, C7, C8, and C9 is nonenzymatic and depends on changes in molecular configuration.

Classical Pathway. The classical pathway sequence begins with fixation of C1, by way of C1q, to the Fc, non–antigen-binding part of the antibody molecule after antigen-antibody interaction. The C1 tricomplex changes configuration and the C1s subcomponent becomes an active enzyme, C1 esterase.

C-reactive protein (CRP), which reacts with C carbohydrate from microorganisms and is increased in certain inflammatory states, can substitute for antibody in the fixation of C1q and initiate reaction of the entire sequence in the absence of antibody. Other agents that can activate C1 directly, without a requirement for antibody, include certain bacteria, *Mycoplasma*, RNA viruses, uric acid crystals, the lipid A component of bacterial endotoxin, and the products of tissue damage such as apoptotic blebs and mitochondrial membranes.

Mannose-Binding Lectin Pathway. MBL is a member of the collectin family of carbohydrate-binding proteins that are believed to play an important part in innate, nonspecific immunity; its structure is homologous to that of C1q. MBL, in association with two **MBL-associated serine proteases (MASPs),** can bind to mannan on bacterial and fungal surfaces and function like C1s to cleave C4 and C2 and activate the complement cascade. A kinin-like peptide split from C2 can induce vascular permeability and edema through direct action on postcapillary venules. The peptide C4a has weak anaphylatoxin activity; it reacts with mast cells to release the chemical mediators of immediate hypersensitivity, including histamine. C3a and C5a, released later in the sequence, are more potent anaphylatoxins, and C5a is also an important chemotactic factor. Fixation of C4b to the complex permits it to adhere to neutrophils, macrophages, B cells, dendritic cells, and erythrocytes.

Cleavage of C3 and generation of C3b is the next step in the sequence. The C3 concentration is the highest of any component, and its activation is the most crucial step in terms of biologic activity. Cleavage of C3 can be achieved through the **C3 convertase** of the classical pathway, C142, or of the alternative pathway, C3bBb. Once fixed to the complex, C3b permits adherence of the antigen-antibody complex to cells with receptors for C3b **(complement receptor 1 [CR1]),** including B lymphocytes, erythrocytes, and phagocytic cells (neutrophils, monocytes, and macrophages), leading, in the last case, to phagocytosis. Phagocytosis of most microorganisms in vitro, especially by neutrophils, is inefficient without binding of C3 to the microorganism. The severe pyogenic infections that commonly occur in C3-deficient patients indicate that phagocytosis is also inefficient in vivo without C3. The biologic activity of C3b is controlled by cleavage by **factor I (C3b inactivator)** to iC3b, which promotes phagocytosis on binding to the **iC3b receptor (CR3)** on phagocytes. Further degradation of iC3b by I and proteases yields C3dg, then C3d; C3d binds to CR2 on B lymphocytes and thereby serves as a co-stimulator of antigen-induced B-cell activation.

Alternative Pathway. The alternative pathway can be activated by C3b generated through classical pathway activity or through neutrophil or clotting system proteases. It can also be activated by a form of C3 created by low-grade, spontaneous reaction of native C3 with a molecule of water, a "tickover" that occurs constantly in plasma. Once formed, C3b or the hydrolyzed C3 can bind to any nearby cell or to factor B. Factor B attached to C3b in

---

TABLE 123–1. **Constituents of the Complement System**

Serum Components	Membrane Regulatory Proteins
Classical Pathway	CR1
C1q	Membrane cofactor protein (MCP)
C1r	Decay-accelerating factor (DAF)
C1s	CD59 (membrane inhibitor of reactive
C4	lysis)
C2	
C3	*Serosal Regulatory Protein*
	C5a/IL-8 inactivator
Alternative Pathway	
Factor B	*Membrane Receptors*
Factor D	CR1
	CR2 (CD21)
Mannose-Binding Lectin Pathway	CR3 (CD11b/CD18)
Mannose-binding lectin (MBL)	CR4 (CD11c/CD18)
MBL-associated proteases 1 and 2	C3a receptor
	C5a receptor
Membrane Attack Complex	C1q receptor
C5	
C6	
C7	
C8	
C9	
Control Protein, Enhancing	
Properdin	
Control Proteins, Downregulating	
C1 inhibitor (C1 INH)	
C4-binding protein (C4-bp)	
Factor H	
Factor I	
S protein	
Clusterin	
Anaphylatoxin inactivator	

CR = complement receptor; IL = interleukin.
Other downregulating serum factors and membrane receptors have been described but have not been cloned or otherwise fully defined.

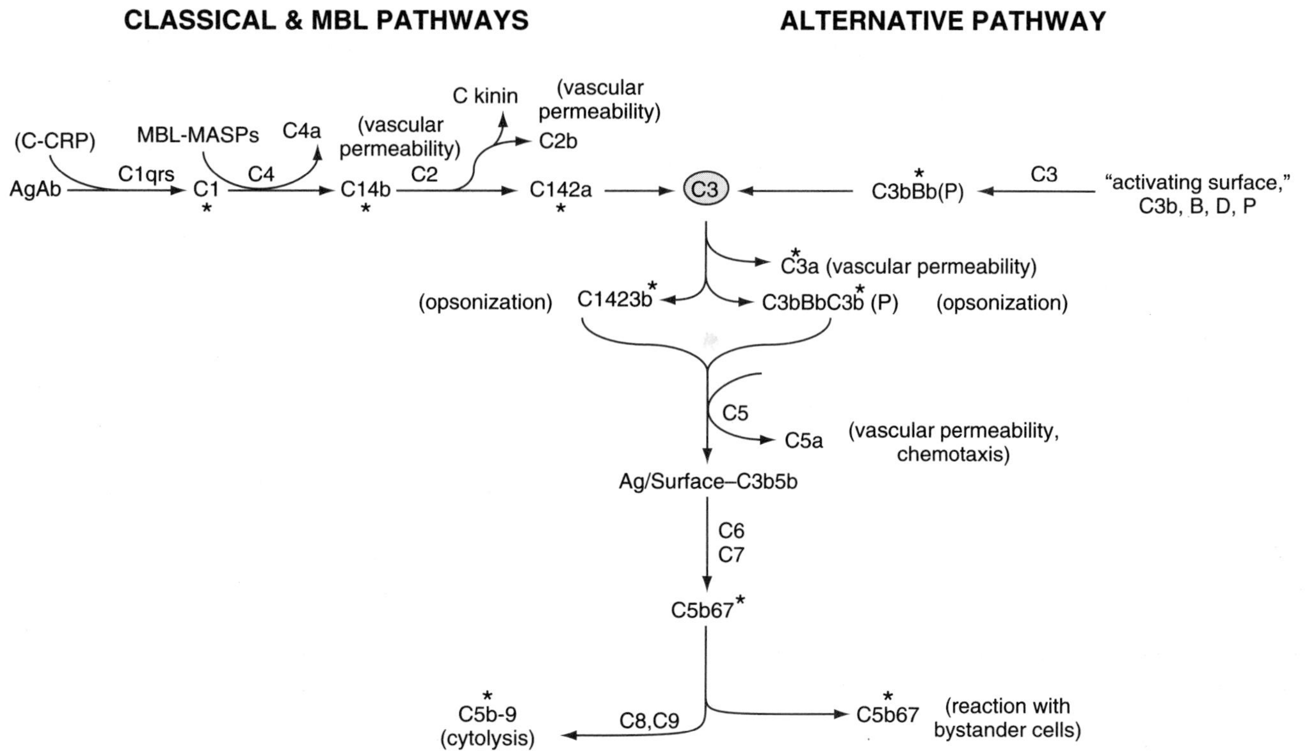

CLASSICAL & MBL PATHWAYS   **ALTERNATIVE PATHWAY**

FIGURE 123–1. Sequence of activation of the components of the classical/MBL pathway of complement and interaction with the alternative pathway. Activation of C3 is the functionally essential target. (Ag = antigen [bacterium, virus, tumor cell, or erythrocyte]; Ab = antibody [IgG or IgM class only]; C-CRP = C carbohydrate–C-reactive protein; B,D,I,H = factors B, D, I, and H; C4-bp = C4-binding protein; MBL = mannose-binding lectin; MASPs = MBL-associated serine proteases.) The multiple sites at which inhibitory regulator proteins act are indicated by asterisks, emphasizing the delicate balance between action and control in this system that is required for host defense yet capable of mediating profound damage to host tissues.

the plasma or on a surface can be cleaved to Bb by D, which exists as an active proteolytic enzyme. The complex C3bBb becomes an efficient C3 convertase, which generates more C3b through an "amplification loop." P can bind to C3bBb, increasing stability of the enzyme and protecting it from inactivation by factors I and H, which modulate the loop and the pathway.

Certain "activating surfaces" promote alternative pathway activation if C3b is fixed to them—for example, bacterial teichoic acid or endotoxin—by protecting the C3bBb enzyme complex from the control otherwise exercised by factors I and H. Rabbit red blood cell membrane is such a surface, which serves as the basis for an assay of serum alternative pathway activity. Endotoxin may alter normally "nonactivating" cell surfaces in vivo so that C3bBb is relatively protected from inactivation, which may partially explain the activation of complement in patients with gram-negative bacteremia. Sialic acid on the surface of microorganisms or cells prevents formation of an effective alternative pathway C3 convertase by promoting activity of I and H. In any case, significant activation of C3 can occur through the alternative pathway, and the resultant biologic activities are qualitatively the same as those achieved through activation by C142 (see Fig. 123–1).

Membrane Attack Complex. The sequence leading to cytolysis begins with the attachment of C5b to the C5-activating enzyme from the classical pathway, C4b2a3b, or from the alternative pathway, C3bBb3b. C6 is bound to C5b without being cleaved, stabilizing the activated C5b fragment. The C5b6 complex then dissociates from C423 and reacts with C7. C5b67 complexes must attach promptly to the membrane of the parent or a bystander cell or they lose their activity. Next, C8 binds, and the C5b678 complex then promotes the addition of multiple C9

molecules. The C9 polymer of at least three to six molecules forms a transmembrane channel, and lysis ensues.

Control Mechanisms. Without control mechanisms, acting at multiple points, there would be no effective complement system, and unbridled consumption of components would generate severe, potentially lethal damage to the host. At the first step, C1 inhibitor (C1 INH) inhibits C1r and C1s enzymatic activity and, thus, the cleavage of C4 and C2. Activated C2 has a short half-life, and this relative instability limits the effective life of C42 and C423. The alternative pathway enzyme that activates C3, C3bBb, also has a short half-life, though it can be prolonged by the binding of **properdin (P)** to the enzyme complex. Serum contains the protein "anaphylatoxin inactivator," an enzyme that cleaves the N-terminus arginine from C4a, C3a, and C5a, thereby markedly reducing their biologic activity. Factor I inactivates C4b and C3b; factor H accelerates inactivation of C3b by I, and an analogous factor, C4-binding protein (C4-bp), accelerates C4b cleavage by I. Three protein constituents of cell membranes, CR1, membrane cofactor protein, and decay-accelerating factor (DAF), promote the disruption of C3 and C5 convertases assembled on those membranes. Other cell membrane–associated proteins (CD59 being the best studied) can bind C8 or both C8 and C9, thereby interfering with insertion of the membrane attack complex (C5b6789). Certain serum proteins (S protein and clusterin being the best studied) can inhibit attachment of the C5b67 complex to cell membranes, bind C8 or C9 in a full membrane attack complex, or otherwise interfere with the formation or insertion of this complex.

Participation in Host Defense. Neutralization of virus by antibody can be enhanced with C1 and C4 and further enhanced by the additional fixation of C3b through the classical or alternative pathway. Complement may, therefore, be particularly important in the early phases of a viral infection when antibody is limited. Antibody and the full complement sequence can also eliminate infectivity of at least some viruses by the production of typical complement "holes," as seen by electron microscopy. Fixation of C1q can opsonize (promote phagocytosis) through binding to the C1q receptor.

C4a, C3a, and C5a can bind to mast cells and thereby trigger release of histamine and other mediators, leading to vasodilatation and the swelling and redness of inflammation. C5a can induce monocytes to release the cytokines tumor necrosis factor and interleukin-1, which amplify the inflammatory response. C5a is a major chemotactic factor for neutrophils, monocytes, and eosinophils, which can efficiently phagocytize microorganisms opsonized with C3b or cleaved C3b (iC3b). Further inactivation of cell-bound C3b by cleavage to C3d removes its opsonizing activity, but it can still bind to B cells. Fixation of C3b to a target cell can enhance its lysis by NK cells or macrophages.

Insoluble immune complexes can be solubilized if they bind C3b, apparently because C3b disrupts the orderly antigen-antibody lattice. Binding C3b to a complex also allows it to adhere to C3 receptors (CR1) on red blood cells, which then transport the complexes to hepatic and splenic macrophages for removal. This phenomenon may at least partially explain the immune complex disease found in patients who lack C1, C4, C2, or C3.

The complement system serves to link the innate and adaptive immune systems. C4b or C3b coupled to immune complexes promotes their binding to antigen-presenting macrophages, dendritic cells, and B cells. Coupling of antigen to C3d allows binding to CR2 on B cells, which reduces the amount of antigen needed to trigger an antibody response by a factor of up to 10,000.

Neutralization of endotoxin in vitro and protection from its lethal effects in experimental animals require later-acting components of complement, at least through C6. Finally, activation of the entire complement sequence can result in lysis of virus-infected cells, tumor cells, and most types of microorganisms. Bactericidal activity of complement has not appeared to be important to host defense, except for the occurrence of *Neisseria* infections in patients lacking later-acting components of complement (Chapter 124).

Berger M, Frank MM: The serum complement system. In Stiehm ER, Ochs HD, Winkelstein JA (editors): *Immunologic Disorders in Infants and Children,* 5th ed. Philadelphia, WB Saunders, 2002.

Holers VM: Complement. In Rich RR, Fleisher TA, Shearer WT, et al (editors): *Clinical Immunology: Principles and Practice,* 2nd ed., vol I. London, Mosby, 2001, pages 21.1–21.18.

Walport MJ: Advances in immunology: Complement. *N Engl J Med* 2001;344: 1058–66, 1140–4.

Chapter 124

Disorders of the Complement System

124.1 Evaluation

Testing for total hemolytic complement activity (CH_{50}) effectively screens for most of the diseases of the complement system. A normal result in this assay depends on the ability of all 11 components of the classical pathway and membrane attack complex to interact and lyse antibody-coated erythrocytes. The dilution of serum that lyses 50% of the cells determines the endpoint. In congenital deficiencies of C1 through C8, the CH_{50}

value is 0 or close to 0; in C9 deficiency, the value is approximately half-normal. Values in the acquired deficiencies vary with the type and severity of the underlying disorder. This assay does not detect deficiencies of the alternative pathway components B or D, or of properdin or mannose-binding lectin (MBL). Deficiency of factor I or H permits consumption of C3, with partial reduction in the CH_{50} value. When clotted blood or serum sits for over about an hour, CH_{50} activity begins to decline, which leads to values that are falsely low, but not zero.

In hereditary angioedema, depression of C4 and C2 during an attack significantly reduces the CH_{50}. Serum concentrations of C4 and C3, and indeed all of the components, can be quantitated using specific antibody. In hereditary angioedema, C4 is characteristically low and C3 normal. Concentrations of C1 inhibitor can be determined with antibody, but a normal result can be anticipated in about 15% of cases. Because C1 acts as an esterase, the specific diagnosis can be made by showing increased capacity of patients' sera to hydrolyze synthetic esters.

Decreased serum concentrations of both C4 and C3 suggest activation of the classical pathway by immune complexes. In contrast, decreased C3 and normal C4 levels suggest activation of the alternative pathway. This difference is particularly useful in distinguishing nephritis secondary to complex deposition from that due to NeF (nephritic factor). In the latter condition and in deficiency of factor I or H, factor B is consumed, and its serum concentration is low. Alternative pathway activity can be measured with a relatively simple and reproducible hemolytic assay that depends on the capacity of rabbit erythrocytes to serve as both an activating (permissive) surface and a target of alternative pathway activity.

A defect of complement function should be considered in any patient with recurrent angioedema, autoimmune disease, chronic nephritis, or partial lipodystrophy, or with recurrent pyogenic infections, disseminated meningococcal or gonococcal infections, or a second episode of bacteremia at any age.

124.2 Primary Deficiencies of Complement Components

Congenital deficiencies of all 11 components of the classical-membrane attack pathway and of factor D of the alternative pathway have been described (Table 124–1).

Most patients with primary **C1q deficiency** have had systemic lupus erythematosus (SLE), an SLE-like syndrome without typical SLE serology, a chronic rash that has shown an underlying vasculitis on biopsy, or membranoproliferative glomerulonephritis (MPGN). Some C1q-deficient children have had serious infections, including septicemia and meningitis.

C1rs deficiency occurs as a complete defect of C1r in association with variable deficiency of C1s, presumably due to the close linkage of the genes for these proteins on chromosome 12. Like individuals with C1q deficiency, patients with **C1r/C1s, C4, C2, or C3 deficiency** have had a high incidence of autoimmune syndromes (see Table 124–1), especially SLE or an SLE-like syndrome in which antinuclear antibody level is not elevated. C4 is encoded by two genes, termed C4A and C4B; complete deficiency of C4A, present in about 1% of the population, also predisposes to SLE though C4 levels are only partially reduced. A few patients with **C5, C6, C7, or C8 deficiency** have had SLE, but recurrent *Neisseria* infections are much more likely to be the major problem in this group. The reason for the concurrence of deficiencies of components of complement and these autoimmune diseases is not entirely clear, but deposition of C3 on autoimmune complexes facilitates their removal from the circulation through binding to complement receptor 1 (CR1) on erythrocytes and transport to the spleen and liver. The early components expedite the clearance of necrotic and apoptotic

TABLE 124–1. Genetic Deficiencies of Plasma Complement Components and Associated Clinical Findings

Deficient Component	Infection*			Autoimmune Disease*		
	Very Common	Common	Occasional	Very Common	Less Common	Occasional
Classical Pathway						
C1q			Pneumococcal B/M, other pyogenic	SLE	GN	DV/DLE
C1rs		Other pyogenic	Pneumococcal B/M, DGI	SLE		GN
C4		Other pyogenic		SLE	Other AD	GN
C2		Other pyogenic, pneumococcal B/M, meningococcal M			SLE, GN, DV/DLE, other AD	
C3	Other pyogenic	Pneumococcal B/M, meningococcal M			GN, DV/DLE	SLE, other AD
C5	Meningococcal M	DGI	Other pyogenic			SLE, GN
C6	Meningococcal M	DGI	Other pyogenic			SLE, GN, other AD
C7	Meningococcal M		DGI, other pyogenic		SLE, other AD	
C8	Meningococcal M	DGI	Other pyogenic			SLE, GN
C9		Meningococcal M				
MBL Pathway						
MBL		Other pyogenic, fungal	HIV			SLE
Alternative Pathway						
Factor D			DGI, meningococcal M			
Factor B	Meningococcal M					
Control Proteins						
C1 INH	Hereditary angioedema†					SLE
Factor I	Other pyogenic, meningococcal M	Pneumococcal B/M				
Factor H		Meningococcal B/M	Other pyogenic	GN		SLE
Properdin		Meningococcal M	Pneumococcal B/M, other pyogenic	DV/DLE		
C4-binding protein						Other AD

*A finding was reported as "very common" if it occurred in 50% or more of reported cases, "common" if reported in about 5–50% of cases, and "occasional" if present in one or two cases or <5% of the more frequent deficiencies.

†Hereditary angioedema is a specific entity not typically associated with infection or autoimmunity.

B/M = Bacteremia or meningitis; DGI = disseminated gonococcal infection; DV/DLE = dermal vasculitis or typical discoid lupus erythematosus; GN = glomerulonephritis in various forms, often membranoproliferative; HIV = human immunodeficiency virus; M = meningitis; MBL = mannose-binding lectin; other AD = other autoimmune diseases (almost all possible diagnoses have been reported); other pyogenic = serious deep or systemic infection due to, or typically caused by, a pyogenic bacterium (abscess, osteomyelitis, pneumonia, bacteremia other than pneumococcal, meningitis other than meningococcal or pneumococcal, cellulitis, myopericarditis, and peritonitis); SLE = typical systemic lupus erythematosus or an SLE-like syndrome without characteristic serologic findings.

Data from Figueroa JE, Densen P: Infectious diseases associated with complement deficiencies. Clin Microbiol Rev 1991;4:359–95; Ross SC, Densen P: Complement deficiency states and infection: Epidemiology, pathogenesis and consequences of neisserial and other infections in an immune deficiency. Medicine 1984;63:243–73, and other case reports and series.

cells, which are sources of autoantigens. Inefficiency of either or both of these processes might explain the particular predisposition to autoimmune disease in individuals with a defect in the classical pathway.

Several patients with **C2 deficiency** have had repeated life-threatening septicemic illnesses, most commonly due to pneumococci. Most have not had problems with increased susceptibility to infection, presumably because of the protective function of the alternative pathway. The genes for C2, factor B, and C4 are situated close to each other on chromosome 6, and a partial depression of factor B levels can occur in conjunction with C2 deficiency. Persons with a deficiency of both proteins may be at particular risk.

Because C3 can be activated by C142 or by the alternative pathway, a defect in the function of either pathway can be compensated for, at least to some extent. Without C3, however, the chemotactic fragment from C5 (C5a) is not generated, and opsonization of bacteria is inefficient. Some organisms must be well opsonized in order to be cleared, and genetic **C3 deficiency** has been associated with recurrent, severe pyogenic infections due to pneumococci and meningococci.

More than half of the individuals reported to have congenital **C5, C6, C7, or C8 deficiency** have had meningococcal meningitis or extragenital gonococcal infection. Patients with **C9 defi-**

ciency retain about half-normal CH_{50} titers; a third of these patients have had *Neisseria* disease. In studies of patients 10 years or older with systemic meningococcal disease, 3–15% have had a genetic deficiency of C5, C6, C7, C8, C9, or properdin. When the infection was caused by an uncommon serogroup (X, Y, Z, W135, 29E, or nongroupable; not A, B, or C), 33–45% of patients had an underlying complement deficiency. It is not clear why patients with a deficiency of one of the late-acting components suffer a particular predisposition to *Neisseria* infections; it may be that serum bacteriolysis is uniquely important in defense against this organism. Some persons with such a deficiency have had no significant illness.

A few individuals have had **factor D deficiency** of the alternative pathway. All have had recurrent infections, often due to *Neisseria*. Hemolytic complement activity in their serum was normal, but alternative pathway activity was markedly deficient or absent.

MBL is an important component of the innate immune system, which protects against infection as the specific immune response emerges. Polymorphisms in the promoter region of the gene encoding MBL and mutations in the structural gene result in pronounced inter-individual variation in the level of circulating MBL. A very low level **(MBL deficiency)** predisposes to recurrent pyogenic and fungal infections, most commonly in infants and young children, but 90% of MBL deficient individuals do not have recurrent infections.

Almost all of the complement components are inherited as autosomal recessive traits of the autosomal co-dominant variety; that is, each parent transmits a gene that codes for synthesis of half the serum level of the component. Deficiency results from inheritance of one null gene from each parent; the hemizygous parents typically have CH_{50} levels that are low normal. Inheritance of deficiency of factors D and B is uncertain but probably also autosomal recessive. Properdin deficiency is transmitted as an X-linked trait.

124.3 Deficiencies of Plasma, Membrane, or Serosal Complement Control Proteins

Congenital deficiencies of 5 plasma complement control proteins have been described (see Table 124–1). **Factor I deficiency** was originally reported as a deficiency of C3 as a result of its hypercatabolism. The first patient described had suffered a series of severe pyogenic infections similar to those seen with agammaglobulinemia or congenital deficiency of C3. Further studies indicated that the primary deficiency was that of factor I, an essential regulator of both pathways. This deficiency permits prolonged existence of C3b in the C3 convertase of the alternative pathway, C3bBb, resulting in constant activation of the alternative pathway and cleavage of more C3 to C3b, in circular fashion. Intravenous infusion of plasma or purified factor I induced a prompt rise in serum C3 concentration in the patient and a return to normal of in vitro C3-dependent functions such as opsonization.

The effects of **factor H deficiency** are like those of factor I deficiency because factor H assists in dismantling the alternative pathway C3 convertase. Levels of C3, factor B, total hemolytic activity, and alternative pathway activity have been low or undetectable in all patients tested. Patients have sustained systemic infections due to pyogenic bacteria, particularly meningococci, and almost half of the cases have had glomerulonephritis. The few patients thus far reported as having **C4-binding protein deficiency** have had about 25% of the normal levels of the protein and no typical disease presentation, although one had angioedema and Behçet's disease.

Persons with **properdin deficiency** have had a striking predisposition to meningococcal meningitis. All reported patients have been male. The predisposition to infection in these patients demonstrates clearly the need for the alternative pathway in host defense against bacterial infection. Serum hemolytic complement activity is normal in these patients, and if the patient has specific antibacterial antibody, the need for the alternative pathway and properdin is greatly reduced. Several patients have had dermal vasculitis or discoid lupus.

Hereditary angioedema occurs in persons born without the ability to synthesize normally functioning C1 inhibitor (C1 INH). In 85% of affected families, the patient has markedly reduced concentrations of inhibitor (5–30% of normal); in the other 15%, normal or elevated concentrations of an immunologically cross-reacting but nonfunctional protein occur. Both forms of the disease are transmitted as an autosomal dominant trait.

In the absence of C1 INH functions, activation of C1 leads to uncontrolled C1 activity, with breakdown of C4 and C2 and release of vasoactive peptides (kinins), which results in episodic, localized, nonpitting edema from the vasodilatory effects of the kinins on the postcapillary venule. The mechanism by which C1 is activated in these patients is not clear.

Swelling of the affected part progresses rapidly, without urticaria, itching, discoloration, or redness, and often without severe pain. Swelling of the intestinal wall, however, can lead to intense abdominal cramping, sometimes with vomiting or diarrhea; concomitant subcutaneous edema is often absent, and patients have undergone abdominal surgery or psychiatric examination before the true diagnosis was established. Laryngeal edema can be fatal. Attacks last 2–3 days and then gradually abate. They may occur at sites of trauma, after vigorous exercise, with menses, or with emotional stress. Attacks can begin in the first 2 years of life but are usually not severe until late childhood or adolescence. **Acquired C1 INH deficiency** can occur in association with B-cell cancer or autoantibody to C1 INH. SLE and glomerulonephritis have been reported in patients with the congenital disease.

Three of the membrane complement control proteins, CR1, membrane cofactor protein, and decay-accelerating factor (DAF), prevent the formation of the full C3-cleaving enzyme, C3bBb, which is triggered by C3b deposition. CD59 (membrane inhibitor of reactive lysis) prevents the full development of the membrane attack complex that creates the "hole." **Paroxysmal nocturnal hemoglobinuria (PNH)** is a hemolytic anemia that occurs when DAF and CD59 are not expressed on the erythrocyte surface. The condition is acquired as a somatic mutation in a hematopoietic stem cell of the *PIG-A* gene on the X chromosome. The product of this gene is required for normal synthesis of a glycosyl-phosphatidylinositol molecule that anchors about 20 proteins to cell membranes, including DAF and CD59. One patient with **genetic isolated CD59 deficiency** had a mild PNH-like disease in spite of normal expression of membrane DAF. In contrast, **genetic isolated DAF deficiency** has not resulted in hemolytic anemia.

Patients with SLE and their asymptomatic family members have a partial **CR1 deficiency**, which is possibly inherited. This deficiency could increase the risk of developing immune complex disease, thereby contributing to the pathogenesis of SLE.

Serosal fluids contain a protease that normally destroys the chemotactic activity of C5a and interleukin 8 (IL-8), important chemotactic factors for neutrophils. A defect in this protease in peritoneal and synovial fluids occurs in **familial Mediterranean fever**. Patients have a missense mutation in a gene encoding a transcription factor termed **pyrin**, which may represent the basic defect. They suffer recurrent episodes of fever in association with painful inflammation of joints and pleural and peritoneal cavities (Chapter 153). Thus, it appears that C5a or IL-8 or both are generated at serosal surfaces under normal conditions and that serosal fluids contain an inhibitor of these chemotactic agents that serves to prevent the inflammatory response that would otherwise ensue.

124.4 Secondary Disorders of Complement

Partial deficiency of C1q has occurred in patients with severe combined immunodeficiency disease or hypogammaglobulinemia, apparently secondary to the deficiency of IgG, which normally binds reversibly to C1q and prevents its rapid catabolism.

Plasma from patients with chronic membranoproliferative glomerulonephritis (MPGN) contains a protein termed **nephritic factor** (NeF) that promotes activation of the alternative pathway. NeF is an IgG antibody to the C3-cleaving enzyme of the alternative pathway, C3bBb, which protects the enzyme from inactivation. The result is increased consumption of C3. Serum C3 concentrations vary widely from patient to patient, however. Pyogenic infections, including meningitis, may occur if the serum C3 level drops below about 10% of normal. This disorder has been found in children and adults with *partial lipodystrophy*. Adipocytes are the main source of factor D and synthesize C3 and factor B; exposure to NeF induces their lysis. An IgG nephritic factor that binds to and protects C42, the classical pathway C3 convertase, has been described in acute postinfectious nephritis and in SLE. The consumption of C3 that characterizes poststreptococcal nephritis and SLE could be due to this factor, to complement activation by immune complexes, or to both. A patient has been described with a circulating inhibitor of factor H and hypocomplementemic MPGN, emphasizing the importance of factor H in restraining the uncontrolled conversion of C3.

Newborn infants have mild to moderate deficiencies of all plasma components of the complement system. Opsonization and generation of chemotactic activity in serum from full-term newborns can be markedly deficient through either the classical or the alternative pathway. Complement activity is even lower in preterm infants. Patients with severe chronic cirrhosis of the liver, hepatic failure, malnutrition, or anorexia nervosa may also have significant depletion of components and functional activity of complement. Although synthesis of components is depressed in these conditions, serum from some patients with malnutrition also appears to contain immune complexes that could accelerate depletion.

Patients with sickle cell disease have normal activity of the classical pathway, but some have defective function of the alternative pathway in opsonization of *Streptococcus pneumoniae*, in bacteriolysis and opsonization of *Salmonella*, and in lysis of rabbit erythrocytes. Deoxygenation of erythrocytes from patients with sickle cell disease alters their membranes to increase exposure of phospholipids that can activate the alternative pathway and consume its components. This activation is accentuated during painful crisis. An alternative pathway defect has been described in about 10% of individuals who have undergone splenectomy and in some patients with β-thalassemia major. The underlying mechanism for this defect in these last two conditions is not known. Children with nephrotic syndrome may have subnormal serum opsonizing activity in association with decreased serum levels of factors B and D.

Immune complexes initiated by microorganisms or their byproducts can induce complement consumption. Activation occurs primarily through fixation of C1 and initiation of the classical pathway. In SLE, immune complexes activate C142, and C3 is deposited at sites of tissue damage, including kidneys and skin; depressed synthesis of C3 is also noted. Formation of immune complexes and consumption of complement have been demonstrated in lepromatous leprosy, bacterial endocarditis, infected ventriculojugular shunts, malaria, infectious mononucleosis, dengue hemorrhagic fever, and acute hepatitis B. Nephritis or arthritis may develop as a result of deposition of immune complexes and activation of complement in these infections. The syndrome of recurrent urticaria, angioedema, eosinophilia, and hypocomplementemia secondary to activation of the classical pathway may be due to circulating immune complexes. Circulating immune complexes and decreased C3 have been reported in some patients with dermatitis herpetiformis, celiac disease, primary biliary cirrhosis, and Reye syndrome.

In patients with bacteremic shock, bacterial products appear to initiate direct activation of the alternative pathway. Intravenous injection of iodinated roentgenographic contrast medium can trigger a rapid and significant activation of the alternative pathway, which may explain at least some of the occasional reactions that occur in patients undergoing this procedure.

Burns can induce massive activation of the complement system, especially the alternative pathway, within a few hours after injury. Generation of C3a and C5a occurs, which stimulates neutrophils and induces their sequestration in the lungs. These events may play an important part in the development of shock lung after burn injury. Cardiopulmonary bypass, plasma exchange, or hemodialysis using cellophane membranes may be associated with a similar syndrome due to activation of plasma complement, with release of C3a and C5a. In patients with erythropoietic protoporphyria or porphyria cutanea tarda, exposure of the skin to light of certain wavelengths activates complement, generating chemotactic activity. Phototoxicity is associated histologically with lysis of capillary endothelial cells, mast cell degranulation, and the appearance of neutrophils in the dermis.

124.5 Treatment of Complement Disorders

No specific therapy is available at present for genetic deficiencies of the complement system except hereditary angioedema, but a great deal can be done to protect patients with any of these disorders from serious complications. Management of hereditary angioedema starts with avoidance of precipitating factors, usually trauma. Infusion of vapor-heated C1 INH concentrate, not yet available in the U.S., aborts acute attacks and is safe and effective in long-term prophylaxis or in preparation for surgery or dental procedures. Adults with hereditary angioedema respond to danazol, a synthetic androgen with weak virilizing and mild anabolic potential. The drug, given orally, increases the level of C1 INH several-fold and prevents attacks. It has not been recommended for use in children.

Effective supportive management is available for other primary diseases of the complement system. Identification of a specific defect in the complement system may have an important impact on management. Concern for the associated complications, such as autoimmune disease and infection, should encourage vigorous diagnostic efforts and earlier institution of therapy. Individuals with SLE and a complement defect generally respond as well to therapy as those without complement deficiency. With the onset of unexplained fever, cultures should be obtained and antibiotic therapy instituted more quickly and with less stringent indications than in a normal child. The parent or patient should be given letters describing any predisposition to systemic bacterial infection associated with the patient's deficiency, along with the recommended approach to management, for possible use by school, camp, or emergency room physicians. The patient and close household contacts should be immunized with vaccines for *Haemophilus influenzae*, *S. pneumoniae*, and *N. meningitidis*. High titers of specific antibody might opsonize effectively without the full complement system, and immunization of household members could reduce the risk of exposing patients to these particularly threatening pathogens.

Eichenfield LF, Johnston RB Jr: Secondary disorders of the complement system. *Am J Dis Child* 1989;143:595–602.

Figueroa JE, Densen P: Infectious disease associated with complement deficiencies. *Clin Microbiol Rev* 1991;4:359–95.

Fijen CAP, Kuijper EJ, te Bulte MT, et al: Assessment of complement deficiency in patients with meningococcal disease in the Netherlands. *Clin Infect Dis* 1999;28:98–105.

Fijen CAP, van den Bogaard R, Schipper M, et al: Properdin deficiency: Molecular basis and disease association. *Mol Immunol* 1999;36:863–7.

Giclas PC: Choosing complement tests: Differentiating between hereditary and acquired deficiency. In Rose NR, Hamilton RG, Detrick B (editors): *Manual of Clinical Laboratory Immunology*, 6th ed. Washington DC, ASM Press, 2002, pp 111–6.

Holers VM: Complement deficiencies. In Rich RR, Fleisher TA, Shearer MT, et al (editors): *Clinical Immunology: Principles and Practice*, 2nd ed, vol II. London, Mosby, 2001, pp 36.1–36.10.

Johnston RB Jr: Complement disorders. In Burg FD, Ingelfinger JR, Wald ER, Polin RA (editors): *Gellis & Kagan's Current Pediatric Therapy 16*. Philadelphia, WB Saunders, 1999, pp 1077–9.

Mold C, Tamerius JD, Phillips G Jr: Complement activation during painful crisis in sickle cell anemia. *Clin Immunol Immunopathol* 1995;76:314–20.

Petersen SV, Thiel S, Jensenius JC: The mannan-binding lectin pathway of complement activation: Biology and disease association. *Mol Immunol* 2001;38:133–49.

Pickering MC, Botto M, Taylor PR, et al: Systemic lupus erythematosus complement deficiency, and apoptosis. *Adv Immunol* 2001;76:227–324.

Ross SC, Densen P: Complement deficiency states and infection: Epidemiology, pathogenesis and consequences of neisserial and other infections in an immune deficiency. *Medicine* (Baltimore) 1984;63:243–73.

Sullivan KE, Winkelstein JA: Complement deficiencies. In Stiehm ER, Ochs HD, Winkelstein JA (editors): *Immunologic Disorders in Infants and Children*, 5th ed. Philadelphia, WB Saunders, 2002.

SECTION 5 *Hematopoietic Stem Cell Transplantation*

Kent A. Robertson

Evolving from clinical trials in the 1970s, bone marrow transplantation for malignant and nonmalignant disorders involved treatment with marrow-ablative chemoradiotherapy followed by an infusion of either the patient's own stored marrow (**autologous transplant**) or marrow from a donor (**allogeneic transplant**). Because only 25% of patients have human leukocyte antigen (HLA)-matched sibling donors, other sources of hematopoietic stem cells have been developed, including mismatched related marrow, unrelated donor marrow, umbilical cord blood, and peripheral blood stem cells (autologous and allogeneic, related and unrelated). The use of multiple hematopoietic stem cells has given rise to the term **hematopoietic stem cell transplantation or**

stem cell transplant (SCT), which is often confused by the general public with the more controversial use of embryonic stem cells. SCT is the treatment of choice for acquired and inherited nonmalignant disorders, such as aplastic anemia and Fanconi anemia, for some malignant diseases, such as chronic myelogenous leukemia, as well as for malignancies that are unresponsive to conventional therapy. The process of SCT also encompasses **gene therapy**, which replaces an absent or defective gene with a normal gene in the patient's own cells. The pediatrician is often called on to participate in the evaluation and consideration of patients for possible transplant and the long-term follow-up of SCT patients.

Chapter 125
Clinical Indications

ACQUIRED DISEASES

Aplastic Anemia. Aplastic anemia, a disorder of unknown cause, results in pancytopenia and bone marrow hypoplasia and, if severe (platelet <20,000/mm^3; absolute neutrophil count <500/mm^3; or reticulocyte count <1% when anemia is present), often results in death within the first 6 mo from infection or bleeding. The marrow dysfunction may result from inherited disorders (e.g., Fanconi anemia or paroxysmal nocturnal hemoglobinuria), autoimmunity, or dysregulated cytokine production, and is occasionally associated with exposure to chemicals (e.g., benzene or chloramphenicol) and non-A, non-B, non-C hepatitis. Blood transfusion should be avoided if possible, because sensitization to blood products increases the likelihood of graft rejection should SCT be needed. SCT is the treatment of choice for patients with severe aplastic anemia who have an HLA-matched family donor; the 2-yr survival rate is 69%, based on data from the International Bone Marrow Transplant Registry. The 15-yr survival rate was 100% among children younger than 6 yr of age (n = 12) and 78% for children 6–19 yr of age (n = 63) receiving HLA-matched sibling SCT in Seattle for aplastic anemia.

Patients transplanted for aplastic anemia exhibit a higher incidence of graft rejection than seen with other kinds of HLA-matched sibling transplants, but the addition of antithymocyte globulin (ATG) to cyclophosphamide for the preparative regimen decreases rejection significantly. Since the institution of this preparative regimen, an actuarial 3-yr survival rate of 92% has been achieved (Fig. 125–1). Transplantation using unrelated donors requires further immunosuppressive therapy, including the addition of irradiation and/or chemotherapy, resulting in a 5-yr survival of 69%. The added therapy has the drawback of an increased incidence of secondary cancers, especially in patients with underlying Fanconi anemia.

Acute Myelogenous Leukemia. Acute myelogenous leukemia (AML) is a heterogeneous group of leukemias derived from myeloid progenitor cells (see Chapter 487–2). SCT is the accepted therapy for AML in first remission. Disease-free survival (DFS) rates range from 55–83% for matched sibling SCT performed during the first complete remission. In a randomized trial in 271 children with AML in first remission following intensive-timed induction therapy, 8-yr DFS rates were 70% for matched sibling SCT, 54% for high-dose chemotherapy alone, and 57% for autologous SCT.

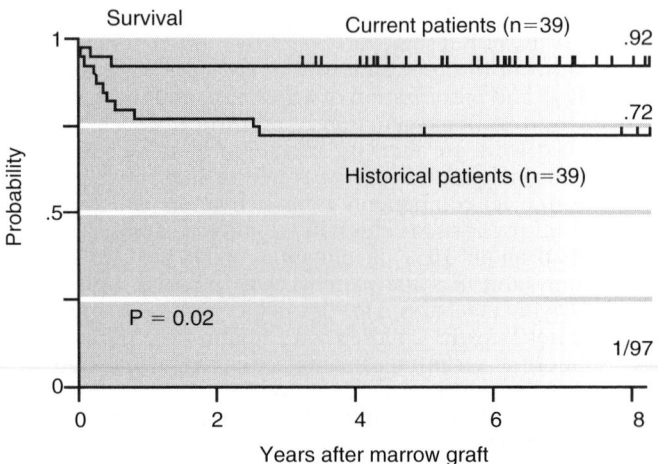

FIGURE 125–1. Marrow grafts for aplastic anemia (AA). Kaplan-Meier estimates of survival in 78 patients with aplastic anemia given HLA-identical marrow transplants. Thirty-nine were conditioned with cyclophosphamide/antithymocyte globulin (current patients), and 39 received cyclophosphamide alone (historical patients). Tick marks indicate surviving patients. (From Storb R, Leisenring W, Anasetti C, et al: Long-term follow-up of allogeneic marrow transplants in patients with aplastic anemia conditioned by cyclophosphamide combined with antithymocyte globulin. *Blood* 1997;89:3890–91.)

SCT also improves survival of children with acute megakaryocytic (M7) leukemia and secondary AML resulting from prior cancer therapy, both of which respond poorly to chemotherapy. SCT is indicated for patients with AML who do not achieve remission, using stem cells from an HLA-identical family donor, mismatched family donor, or unrelated donor. In patients with AML who achieve a first remission, SCT is indicated if they have an HLA-identical family donor. One exception to this strategy is M3 or promyelocytic leukemia, which is quite responsive to all-*trans*-retinoic acid and consolidation chemotherapy. Patients with AML who relapse or are in second remission should be considered for SCT using an HLA-matched family donor, unrelated donor, or previously stored autologous marrow. Patients with numerous relapses, resistant disease, or secondary AML are candidates for higher-risk mismatched SCT.

Acute Lymphoblastic Leukemia. Acute lymphoblastic leukemia (ALL) is the most common malignancy of childhood, and 70–80% of cases are cured by conventional chemotherapy (see Chapter 487–1). A subgroup of these patients are at high risk for relapse with conventional therapy (75–100%) and should be considered for SCT (Box 125–1). DFS rates range from 15–65%, with relapse rates of 30–70%.

Patients with high-risk ALL who have HLA-matched donors may be eligible for allogeneic SCT. Children receiving HLA-matched sibling SCT for high-risk ALL in first complete remission have DFS rates of 70–80% with low relapse rates of 0–10%, although the numbers are small and some high-risk groups such as Philadelphia chromosome–positive ALL have lower survival rates at 50–65%. Patients who do not have high-risk features at the time of diagnosis but who later suffer relapse and have an HLA-identical family donor also benefit from SCT, with DFS rates of 40–60%. Patients have a better outcome if they undergo transplantation in remission, and patients in whom remission occurs earlier have a higher DFS rate. Patients without a family donor may benefit from unrelated donor or cord blood transplant, with DFS rates of 30–40%.

Comparisons of allogeneic and autologous SCT or chemotherapy for ALL relapse support the recommendation that these children should be offered SCT when possible. A review of 376 children receiving HLA-identical sibling SCT compared with 540 children receiving chemotherapy for ALL in second remission revealed DFS rates of 40% and 17%, with relapse rates of 45% and 80%, respectively. Other studies comparing allogeneic and autologous SCT for relapsed ALL have shown DFS rates of 33–61% for allografts and 21–47% for autografts, illustrating the advantage of allogeneic SCT over autologous transplants despite increased toxicity.

The lower incidence of relapse in allogeneic SCT is related to a graft versus host disease (GVHD)/graft versus leukemia (GVL) effect. The probability of relapse was 25 ± 6%, 22 ± 5%, 10 ± 7%, 7 ± 3%, 46 ± 15%, and 41 ± 8% for allogeneic grafts without GVHD, acute GVHD only, chronic GVHD only, acute and chronic GVHD, syngeneic grafts, and allogeneic T cell–depleted grafts, respectively. These results are the same for lymphoblastic and myelogenous leukemia, emphasizing the importance of the immune system in eliminating residual leukemia cells. This concept has been taken a step further with the recent use of low-intensity nonmyeloablative transplant regimens that rely on GVL as a primary therapeutic modality.

Infant leukemia (see Chapter 487.6) occurring within the first 12 mo of life is rare and carries a very poor prognosis, with survival rates of 20–30% after 5 yr with conventional chemotherapy. Cytogenetic abnormalities such as t(4;11)(q21;q23) involving the *MLL* gene (60–70% of cases) and poor response to corticosteroids are recognized as poor prognostic indicators. Infants with a normal 11q23 locus have a very good response to conventional chemotherapy, with a DFS of 80% at a median follow-up of 46 mo, whereas those with a rearranged 11q23 have a very poor response, with a 15% DFS. Studies suggest that SCT is beneficial in these high-risk infants, with DFS rates of 40–50% for patients transplanted in remission compared with 10–20% if SCT is performed after relapse, using various sources of marrow. Children diagnosed within the 1st year of life with acute leukemia with chromosomal rearrangements involving 11q23

are best treated with intense induction chemotherapy followed by bone marrow transplantation if a suitable donor is available.

Myelodysplastic and Myeloproliferative Disorders. Myelodysplastic syndrome (MDS) includes a group of disorders with defects in hematopoietic cell development close to the level of the marrow stem cell, which eventually progresses from a picture of dysplastic ineffective hematopoiesis to aggressive overt myelogenous leukemia. These are classified as refractory anemia, refractory anemia with ringed sideroblasts, refractory anemia with excess blasts, refractory anemia with excess blasts in transformation, and chronic myelomonocytic leukemia (CML). Because of the close relationship to AML, patients with MDS are treated according to AML protocols. The transplant outcome in patients with MDS is similar to that in patients with AML. In one series of 23 pediatric patients, the DFS at 5 yr was 64% using HLA-matched family donors, and for 15 pediatric patients receiving HLA-matched unrelated donor SCT the DFS was 53%. Transplant should be considered early after diagnosis because patients in whom the disease has progressed with increasing blasts have a much poorer outcome and a higher rate of relapse. Conventional chemotherapy and other nontransplant forms of treatment have not made a significant impact of the natural progression of the disease.

These disorders are characterized by a single lineage myeloid proliferation that can progress to an AML-like leukemia and include CML, essential thrombocythemia (ET), polycythemia vera (PV), agnogenic myeloid metaplasia, and juvenile chronic myelogenous leukemia (JCML), also known as juvenile myelomonocytic leukemia. SCT is the treatment of choice for CML (see Chapter 487.5). HLA-identical sibling transplantation results in an 80% long-term DFS compared with 45–74% for matched unrelated SCT. Transplantation is recommended within 1 yr from diagnosis, because delay results in a significant decrease in the DFS to 40–60%. Patients receiving SCT in accelerated phase or blast crisis have DFS rates of 35–40% and 10–20%, respectively, and a 60% chance of relapse compared with a 10–20% chance of relapse in patients receiving SCT in chronic phase.

Successful SCT has also been performed for some of the more uncommon myeloproliferative disorders. SCT should be considered in those patients who fail to respond to conservative management or whose disease progress to an AML-like leukemic condition. SCT is a possible approach for childhood polycythemia vera. SCT has been attempted for ET in a few patients without success. AMM, or idiopathic myelofibrosis, is characterized by splenomegaly and progressive fibrosis of the marrow compartment, resulting in anemia. The mean survival for patients with AMM is 5 yr, and the only known curative therapy is SCT; 7 of 12 patients receiving SCT for AMM survived.

JCML is an aggressive clonal proliferation of immature myeloid precursors associated with neurofibromatosis type 1 and monosomy 7. The clinical course is rapid, with resistance to conventional chemotherapy and death at an average of 9 mo from the time of diagnosis. SCT is curative in these patients and should be pursued aggressively once the diagnosis is confirmed. Multiple studies have yielded DFS rates of 30–40% after receiving SCT from matched sibling donors and 20–30% from mismatched family members/matched unrelated donors. The association of JCML with NF-1 resulting in dysregulation of the *RAS* oncogene and the known response of JCML to retinoic acid has led to current therapy using farnesyl transferase inhibitors, chemotherapy, retinoic acid, and SCT.

Lymphomas. Non-Hodgkin lymphoma (NHL) and Hodgkin disease (HD) are malignant, usually clonal proliferations arising from the lymphoreticular system (see Chapter 488). Childhood lymphomas are quite responsive to conventional chemoradiotherapy, but a subset of these patients have high-risk disease and relapse, requiring more intensive therapy to achieve a cure. SCT

> **BOX 125–1. Risk Factors for Relapse of Acute Lymphoblastic Leukemia (ALL) with Conventional Chemotherapy Alone**
>
> Congenital or infant (<1 yr of age) ALL
> Chromosomal translocations: t(4,11), t(9,22)-Philadelphia, t(8,14)
> FAB L3 morphology (Burkitt)
> White blood cell count ≥100,000/mm³
> More than 1 mo to achieve initial remission
> Failure to achieve a remission
> Relapse while on chemotherapy
> Second and subsequent remissions (when first remission < 30 mo)
> More than one extramedullary site of relapse without a marrow relapse
> Secondary ALL resulting from prior cancer therapy

can cure some patients with NHL and HD and should be offered early after relapse, while the disease is still sensitive to therapy, there is little bulky disease, and there is a greater likelihood of being able to tolerate a transplant regimen. Patients with sensitive disease and little tumor burden have favorable outcomes, with DFS rates of 50–60%, whereas high-risk patients with bulky tumor or refractory disease have a poor outcome with survival rates of 10–20%. Pretransplant salvage chemotherapy including the use of antibodies targeted to specific tumor antigens such as CD20 may be of some benefit to reduce the tumor burden. If an HLA-identical sibling is available, allogeneic transplant should be offered to take advantage of the GVL effect, which has reduced the relapse rate by as much as 25–30% in some series. Use of autologous peripheral blood stem cell transplant (PBSCT) has resulted in earlier engraftment and a decrease in transplant-related morbidity, although the potential for contamination with tumor cells remains. A European Lymphoma Registry study described autologous SCT for children with poor-risk B-cell or Burkitt lymphoma, including those with relapsed or resistant disease. The 5-yr DFS rate was 39.4% in these children with otherwise incurable disease. In a report from six Spanish centers, 46 pediatric patients received SCT for NHL, including lymphoblastic lymphoma, Burkitt, and large cell lymphoma, with a 3-yr DFS rate of 58%. A separate but distinct clinicopathologic entity is the CD30 or Ki-1 positive peripheral T-cell lymphomas including anaplastic large cell lymphomas associated with chromosomal translocation t(2;5). These tumors are aggressive and tend to relapse but have responded well to SCT, with an 80% 5-yr DFS rate.

Hematopoietic SCT has resulted in improved survival for patients with relapsed or refractory Hodgkin's disease, with most series reporting 40–60% DFS rates after 2–5 yr. Using the risk factors of more than one extranodal site of disease, performance status, and progressive disease at the time of transplant, low-risk patients (no risk factors) have a 3-yr DFS rate of 82%, whereas intermediate-risk (one risk factor) and high-risk (two to three risk factors) patients had DFS rates of 56% and 19%, respectively.

Finally, there are several reports of successful SCT performed in children with Langerhans cell histiocytosis, including histiocytosis X (see Chapter 499). Although patients with single-organ involvement histiocytosis fare quite well, patients with multiorgan involvement respond poorly to conventional therapy and should be considered for SCT.

Neuroblastoma. The most common extracranial solid tumor in children is neuroblastoma (see Chapter 490). Although SCT studies show a trend for improvement over those obtained with chemotherapy, randomized trials to compare the two approaches are ongoing. DFS (3 yr) rates for patients receiving SCT after progression of disease are 7–25%, compared with 25–55% for those receiving SCT before progression of disease. Certain high-risk groups have a significant improvement with SCT, including those with *NMYC* amplification, 2 yr of age and older, a partial remission to induction therapy, and bone/bone marrow metastasis. In a Children's Cancer Group study, high-risk patients received chemotherapy, radiation, and surgery and then were randomized to receive autologous SCT and 13-*cis*-retinoic acid (RA), resulting in 3-yr DFS rates for chemotherapy, chemotherapy plus RA, SCT, and SCT plus RA of 18%, 32%, 40%, and 55%, respectively, reflecting the role of biologic agents such as RA as adjuncts to cytotoxic therapy by inducing ganglioneuronal differentiation in neuroblastoma.

Brain Tumors. Tumors of the central nervous system (CNS) are the most common solid tumors in children, accounting for 20% of childhood malignancies (see Chapter 489). For children with disease resistant to conventional chemotherapy and irradiation, the dose-limiting toxicity for intensifying therapy is myelosuppression, thus providing a role for stem cell rescue. Early results

from a multi-institutional study are encouraging in a group of 53 patients with high-risk (19) or average-risk (34) medulloblastoma or supratentorial primitive neuroectodermal tumors (PNET) that were treated sequentially with surgery-topotecan-irradiation followed by four cycles of cyclophosphamide, cisplatin, and vincristine with PBSC support. The 2-yr progression-free survival rates were 93% and 73% in average-risk and high-risk patients, respectively. The Italian group treated 11 children with recurrent medulloblastoma (3), glioblastoma multiforme (2), PNET (2), ependymoma (2), anaplastic astrocytoma (1), and anaplastic oligodendroglioma (1) using a conditioning regimen of etoposide and *bis*-chlorethylnitrosourea (BCNU) or thiotepa followed by autologous marrow infusion; 5 children who had no measurable disease at the time of transplant are alive without evidence of disease after follow-up for a median of 20 mo. A Children's Cancer Group study used carboplatin, thiotepa, and etoposide as a preparative regimen for 23 patients with recurrent medulloblastoma, resulting in a 34% DFS rate after 3 yr. Another study focused on using a similar chemotherapy-only transplant regimen following standard induction therapy (vincristine, cisplatin, cyclophosphamide, and etoposide) for young children with newly diagnosed brain tumors (malignant glioma, 9; ependymoma, 10; brainstem glioma, 6; medulloblastoma, 13; PNET, 14; other, 10) in an effort to avoid the toxicity of cranial radiation; of 62 children enrolled, 37 had no disease progression with induction therapy and went on to autologous marrow transplant with a DFS rate of 41% (27% for all 62 enrolled) after 2 yr.

Solid Tumors. Many solid tumors are quite responsive to conventional chemoradiotherapy; however, a subset of these are associated with a very poor prognosis. These tumors are high risk by virtue of their histology (alveolar rhabdomyosarcomas, anaplastic Wilms tumor), location (pelvic, trunk, or proximal extremity Ewing sarcoma, axial skeletal osteogenic sarcoma), or widespread metastatic presentation. Stem cell rescue allows dose intensification of chemotherapy with or without total body irradiation (TBI). The French Society of Pediatric Oncology reported 28 children who received autologous SCT for refractory or relapsed Wilms tumor (see Chapter 491) using melphalan, etoposide, and carboplatin as a conditioning regimen. Twelve of 28 children remain disease free a median of 48 mo after SCT with a 3-yr DFS rate of 50%. In an update by the European Intergroup Study of high advanced Ewing sarcomas using TBI, melphalan, etoposide, and carboplatin, 9 of 36 patients receiving either autologous or allogeneic SCT survive after 5 yr, with a somewhat poorer DFS for the allogeneic group (20% vs. 25%), owing to toxicity. A more encouraging response was obtained, although with a shorter follow-up, with the use of tandem autologous PBSCT for Ewing sarcoma. After receiving etoposide, carboplatin, and cyclophosphamide followed by stem cell rescue, a second cycle using melphalan and TBI was given 4–6 weeks later with a 3-yr DFS rate of 56%. SCT for high-risk or relapsed rhabdomyosarcoma has been disappointing. In a retrospective review by German/Austrian Transplant Group from multiple centers with eight different conditioning regimens, 9 of 36 patients survive with a median follow-up of 57 mo, showing little difference from salvage chemotherapy regimens. There have been several reports of autologous SCT for retinoblastoma with a 3-yr DFS rate of 67%, with those patients with distant metastasis doing the best and those with CNS extension having a poorer outcome. The most exciting result in SCT for solid tumors comes from studies using less intensive nonmyeloablative PBSCT for refractory renal cell carcinoma. Low-dose therapy (cyclophosphamide and fludarabine) allows engraftment of allogeneic donor T cells to generate a graft versus tumor effect. Nine of 19 patients survive with a median follow-up of 402 days, with 3 patients without evidence of disease. Similar studies are being pursued for other solid tumors.

GENETIC DISEASES

Immunodeficiency Disorders. SCT is the treatment of choice for severe combined immunodeficiency (SCID; see Chapter 116.1). The DFS rate using matched sibling donors is more than 90%, and using T-depleted mismatched family member grafts it is 60–80%. There is less experience with unrelated donor SCT for SCID, but nonetheless it has also been effective. SCT has been performed in other forms of immune deficiency, including Wiskott-Aldrich syndrome, DiGeorge syndrome, Kostmann neutropenia, leukocyte adherence deficiency, chronic granulomatous disease, Chédiak-Higashi syndrome, familial erythrophagocytic lymphohistiocytosis, Duncan syndrome, and neutrophil actin deficiencies. Survival rates are 68% when matched sibling donors are used and 35% when mismatched donors are used. The presentation of DiGeorge syndrome can be variable; however, those patients with initial profoundly depressed T-cell function do not recover over time and are candidates for SCT. If other forms of therapy are available, such as interferon-γ for chronic granulomatous disease or granulocyte colony-stimulating factor (G-CSF) for Kostmann neutropenia, SCT should be reserved for patients who are unresponsive. Other approaches that are promising in these disorders are less toxic nonmyeloablative SCT and gene therapy targeting the specific gene deficiency.

Fanconi Anemia (see Chapter 460). The characteristic sensitivity to DNA cross-linking agents makes children who have Fanconi anemia (FA) quite sensitive to conventional SCT conditioning regimens, requiring dose reduction to avoid excessive toxicity. Transplant-related toxicities include severe oral mucositis, hemorrhagic cystitis, erythroderma, and GVHD. DFS rates are 25–75%, depending on the source of stem cells. Patients receiving reduced conditioning regimens and matched sibling donor SCT have the best outcomes, although mismatched and unrelated donor SCT have been successful. Patients with FA and an HLA-identical family member who has a negative FA screen should be offered SCT at the first sign of pancytopenia. Alternative donor transplants including cord blood should be considered in the absence of a matched family member, given the poor outlook for these patients once leukemic transformation occurs.

Storage Diseases. The metabolic storage diseases are a heterogeneous group of disorders resulting from single gene mutations producing enzyme defects and the subsequent toxic accumulation of metabolites. The end result is progressive neurologic deterioration or visceral infiltration, which is usually fatal. Some disorders, such as adrenoleukodystrophy, respond to dietary measures, whereas others, such as Gaucher disease types I and III, respond to enzyme supplementation; however, in most cases there is no successful supplementation therapy available. SCT provides a source of enzyme through the bone marrow–derived monocyte/phagocytic cell system, which includes the liver (Kupffer cells), brain (microglia), skin (Langerhans cells), marrow (osteoclasts), lung (pulmonary macrophage), and lymph nodes (histiocytes). The results of transplant in several storage disorders are variable, with some patients showing a good response (adrenoleukodystrophy, metachromatic leukodystrophy, globoid cell leukodystrophy, Hurler syndrome), whereas other results have been more dismal (Sanfilippo and Hunter syndromes). The risk of transplant-related mortality is about 10% for matched sibling donors and 37% in mismatched and unrelated donors. Transplant before the disease progresses to extensive end-organ damage is necessary. Efforts should be directed toward early diagnosis and SCT before significant neurologic damage occurs.

Thalassemia (see Chapter 454.9). Three risk factors that influence the outcome of SCT for thalassemia include hepatomegaly, portal fibrosis, and a history of inconsistent iron chelation before transplant. Other factors, such as the number of transfusions, ferritin level, degree of hemosiderosis, hepatic iron concentration, and splenomegaly, have no effect. Patients are classified as class 1, no risk factors; class 2, one to two risk factors; and class 3, all three risk factors. In Italy, more than 500 children age 16 yr or older have received HLA-identical family member SCT (Fig. 125–2). DFS rates of up to 90% are obtained in children undergoing transplants before the development of hepatomegaly or portal fibrosis. Hepatic hemosiderosis and portal fibrosis may improve after transplant if the damage is not too extensive. In the United States, 17/27 children (63%) who received HLA-matched family donor SCT survived disease free; 1 required a second SCT. Another 5 patients survived after graft rejections and lived with recurrent thalassemia for an overall survival of 81%. If an HLA-identical family member is available, SCT should be performed before the patient develops advanced disease. Unrelated donor SCT also have been performed with carefully matched donors, but at a cost of somewhat higher toxicity but a similar DFS.

Sickle Cell Disease (see Chapter 454.1). With supportive care, more than 90% of children with sickle cell disease live into their 3rd and 4th decades, and 60% survive to age 50 yr. Disease severity varies among patients with homozygous hemoglobin S (HbS) disease; 5–20% suffer significant morbidity from vaso-occlusive crises and pulmonary, renal, and CNS damage. New approaches include antisickling agents, gene therapy, and induction of increased hemoglobin F by drugs such as hydroxyurea, but SCT is the only curative treatment for sickle cell disease.

In the United States, 50 patients (ages 3–15 yr) with sickle cell disease have received SCT using HLA-identical sibling donors; two donors had sickle trait. The indications for SCT included history of strokes, recurrent acute chest syndrome, or recurrent vaso-occlusive crises. Forty-seven survive (94%), with 5 patients (10%) experiencing graft rejection or recurrence of sickle cell disease, for a DFS rate of 84% at a median follow-up of 38 mo. Forty-five patients (ages 1–23 yr) received HLA-identical family member SCT for SS disease in Belgium and France. After follow-up of 1–75 mo, 95% survive with a DFS rate of 86%. No vaso-occlusive events have occurred among the 38 patients with successful engraftment, and some have recovered splenic function. Although SCT can cure homozygous HbS disease, selecting appropriate candidates for SCT is difficult.

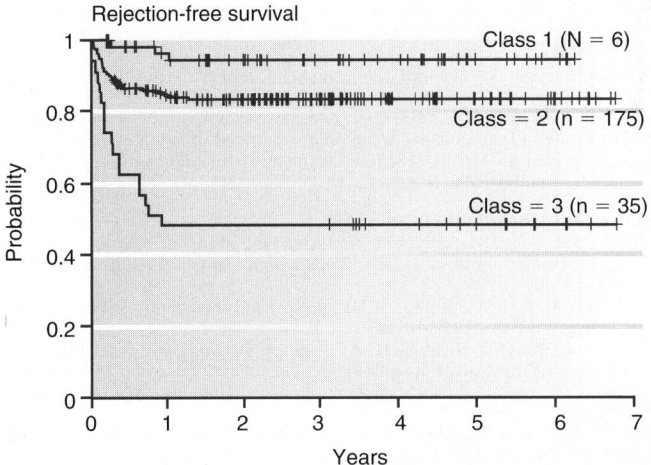

FIGURE 125–2. The probabilities of rejection-free survival for 271 patients younger than 17 yr of age with thalassemia who received marrow transplants from HLA-identical family members after conditioning with busulfan and cyclophosphamide. (From Forman SJ, Blume KG, Thomas ED: *Bone Marrow Transplantation.* Boston, Blackwell, 1994.)

Patients with SS disease may survive for decades, but some patients have a poor quality of life, with repeated hospitalizations for painful vaso-occlusive crises and CNS infarcts. SS patients, such as those with the Central African Republic haplotype, can be predicted to have serious complications. SCT should be considered in young patients who have recurrent severe vaso-occlusive crises, evidence of developing end-organ damage, CNS infarcts, or a history of strokes and have an HLA-identical family member donor.

Other Congenital Anemias. SCT is successful in some other congenital anemias. Diamond-Blackfan syndrome or congenital pure red cell aplasia is characterized by normochromic-macrocytic anemia with a normocellular marrow (see Chapter 440). Patients who fail to respond to initial therapies may benefit from SCT using an HLA-identical sibling donor. Thirty-one of 40 patients who were given SCT for Diamond-Blackfan anemia are alive with a 2-yr DFS rate of 72%. Congenital sideroblastic anemia results from a mitochondrial abnormality in erythroblasts (see Chapter 448). One 34-mo-old child received an SCT from a phenotypically identical cousin and has some persistent liver enlargement after 3 yr but remains transfusion independent with normal serum iron and ferritin levels. There are also reports of curative allogeneic SCT for Shwachman-Diamond syndrome, an autosomal recessive disorder characterized by exocrine pancreatic dysfunction, metaphyseal dysostosis, and marrow dysfunction, including leukemic transformation.

General

Atkinson K (editor): *Clinical Bone Marrow and Blood Stem Cell Transplantation,* 2nd ed. Cambridge, Cambridge University Press, 2000.

Forman SJ, Blume KG, Thomas ED (editors): *Hematopoietic Cell Transplantation,* 2nd ed. Boston, Blackwell Scientific Publications, 1998.

Gross TG, Egeler RM, Smith FO: Pediatric hematopoietic stem cell transplantation. *Hematol Oncol Clin North Am* 2001;15:795–808.

Aplastic Anemia

Doney K, Leisenring W, Storb R, et al: Primary treatment of acquired aplastic anemia: Outcomes with bone marrow transplantation and immunosuppressive therapy. *Ann Intern Med* 1997;126:107–15.

Gillio AP, Boulad F, Small T, et al: Comparison of long-term outcome of children with severe aplastic anemia treated with immunosuppression versus bone marrow transplantation. *Biol Blood Marrow Transplant* 1997;3:18–24.

Kojima S, Matsuyama T, Kato S, et al: Outcome of 154 patients with severe aplastic anemia who received transplants form unrelated donors: the Japan Marrow Donor Program. *Blood* 2002;100:799–803.

Acute Myelogenous Leukemia

Athale UH, Razzouk BI, Raimondi SC, et al: Biology and outcome of childhood acute megakaryoblastic leukemia. *Blood* 2001;97:3727–32.

Hongeng S, Krance RA, Bowman LC, et al: Outcomes of transplantation with matched-sibling and unrelated bone marrow in children with leukemia. *Lancet* 1997;350:767–71.

Langmuir PB, Aplenc R, Lange BJ: Acute myeloid leukaemia in children. *Best Pract Res Clin Haematol* 2001;14:77–93.

Woods WG, Neudorf S, Gold S, et al: A comparison of allogeneic bone marrow transplantation, autologous bone marrow transplantation, and aggressive chemotherapy in children with acute myelogenous leukemia in remission: A report from the Children's Cancer Group. *Blood* 2001;97:56–62.

Acute Lymphoblastic Leukemia

Aricò M, Valsecchi MG, Camitta B, et al: Outcome of treatment in children with Philadelphia chromosome–positive acute lymphoblastic leukemia. *N Engl J Med* 2000;342:998–1006.

Biondi A, Cimino G, Pieters R, et al: Biological and therapeutic aspects of infant leukemia. *Blood* 2000;96:24–33.

Bleakley M, Shaw PJ, Nielsen JM: Allogeneic bone marrow transplantation for childhood relapsed acute lymphoblastic leukemia: Comparison of outcome in patients with and without a matched family donor. *Bone Marrow Transplant* 2002;30:1–7.

Chessells, JM: The role of bone marrow transplantation in first remission of paediatric ALL. *Front Biosci* 2001;6:38–42.

Davies SM, Wagner JE, Shu XO, et al: Unrelated donor bone marrow transplantation for children with acute leukemia. *J Clin Oncol* 1997;15:557–65.

Feig SA, Harris RE, Sather, HN: Bone marrow transplantation versus chemotherapy for maintenance of second remission of childhood acute lymphoblastic leukemia: A study of the Children's Cancer Group (CCG-1884). *Med Pediatr Oncol* 1997;29:534–40.

Saarinen-Pihkala UM, Gustafsson G, Ringdén O, et al: No disadvantage in outcome of using matched unrelated donors as compared with matched sibling donors for

bone marrow transplantation in children with acute lymphoblastic leukemia in second remission. *J Clin Oncol* 2001;19:3406–14.

Weisdorf DJ, Billet AL, Hanan P, et al: Autologous versus unrelated donor allogeneic marrow transplantation for acute lymphoblastic leukemia. *Blood* 1997;90:2962–68.

Myelodysplastic and Myeloproliferative Syndromes

Deeg HJ, Appelbaum FR: Hematopoietic stem cell transplantation in patients with myelodysplastic syndrome. *Leuk Res* 2000;24:653–63.

Dini G, Rondelli R, Miano M, et al: Unrelated-donor bone marrow transplantation for Philadelphia chromosome–positive chronic myelogenous leukemia in children: Experience of eight European countries. *Bone Marrow Transplant* 1996;2:80–85.

Locatelli F, Niemeyer C, Angelucci E, et al: Allogeneic bone marrow transplantation for chronic myelomonocytic leukemia in childhood: A report from the European working group on myelodysplastic syndrome in childhood. *J Clin Oncol* 1997;15:566–73.

Smith FO, King R, Nelson G, et al: Unrelated donor bone marrow transplantation for children with juvenile myelomonocytic leukemia. *Br J Haematol* 2002;116:716–24.

Woods WG, Barnard DR, Alonzo TA, et al: Prospective study of 90 children requiring treatment for juvenile myelomonocytic leukemia or myelodysplastic syndrome: A report from the Children's Cancer Group. *J Clin Oncol* 2002;20:434–40.

Lymphomas

Baker KS, Gordon BG, Gross TG, et al: Autologous hematopoietic stem cell transplantation for relapsed or refractory Hodgkin's disease in children and adolescents. *J Clin Oncol* 1999;17:825–31.

Bureo E, Ortega JJ, Muzoz A, et al: Bone marrow transplantation in 46 pediatric patients with non-Hodgkin's lymphoma. *Bone Marrow Transplant* 1995;15:353–59.

Landenstein R, Pearce R, Hartmann O, et al: High-dose chemotherapy with autologous bone marrow rescue in children with poor-risk Burkitt's lymphoma: A report from the European Lymphoma Bone Marrow Transplantation Registry. *Blood* 1997;90:2921–30.

Schiffman K, Buckner CD, Maziarz R, et al: High-dose busulfan, melphalan, and thiotepa followed by autologous peripheral blood stem cell transplantation in patients with aggressive lymphoma or relapsed Hodgkin's disease. *Biol Blood Marrow Transplant* 1997;3:261–66.

Weisenburger DD, Gordon BG, Vose JM, et al: Occurrence of the t(2;5)(p23;q35) in non-Hodgkin's lymphoma. *Blood* 1996;87:3860–68.

Wheeler C, Eickhoff C, Elias A, et al: High-dose cyclophosphamide, carmustine, and etoposide with autologous transplantation in Hodgkin's disease: A prognostic model for treatment outcomes. *Biol Blood Marrow Transplant* 1997;3:98–106.

Neuroblastoma

Schmidt ML, Lukens JN, Seeger RC, et al: Biologic factors determine prognosis in infants with stage IV neuroblastoma: A prospective Children's Cancer Group Study. *J Clin Oncol* 2000;18:1260–68.

Landenstein R, Philip T, Lasset C, et al: Multivariate analysis of risk factors in stage 4 neuroblastoma patients over the age of one year treated with megatherapy and stem-cell transplantation: A report from the European Bone Marrow Transplantation Solid Tumor Registry. *J Clin Oncol* 1998;16:953–65.

Matthay KK, Villablanca JG, Seeger RC, et al: Treatment of high-risk neuroblastoma with intensive chemotherapy, radiotherapy, autologous bone marrow transplantation, and 13-*cis*-retinoic acid. *N Engl J Med* 1999;341:1165–73.

Brain Tumors

Busca A, Miniero R, Besenzon L, et al: Etoposide-containing regimens with autologous bone marrow transplantation in children with malignant brain tumors. *Childs Nerv Syst* 1997;13:572–77.

Dunkel IJ, Bayett JM, Yates A, et al: High-dose carboplatin, thiotepa, and etoposide with autologous stem-cell rescue for patients with recurrent medulloblastoma. *J Clin Oncol* 1998;16:222–28.

Finlay JL: The role of high-dose chemotherapy and stem cell rescue in the treatment of malignant brain tumors: A reappraisal. *Pediatr Transplant* 1999;1:87–95.

Mason WP, Grovas A, Halpern S, et al: Intensive chemotherapy and bone marrow rescue for young children with newly diagnosed malignant brain tumors. *J Clin Oncol* 1998;16:210–21.

Strother D, Ashley D, Kellie SJ, et al: Feasibility of four consecutive high-dose chemotherapy cycles with stem cell rescue for patients with newly diagnosed medulloblastoma or supratentorial primitive neuroectodermal tumor after craniospinal radiation: Results of a collaborative study. *J Clin Oncol* 2001;19: 2696–704.

Solid Tumors

Burdach S, van Kaick B, Laws HJ, et al: Allogeneic and autologous stem-cell transplantation in advanced Ewing tumors. *Ann Oncol* 2000;11:1451–62.

Childs R, Chernoff A, Contentin N, et al: Regression of metastatic renal cell carcinoma after non-myeloablative allogeneic peripheral blood stem cell transplantation. *N Engl J Med* 2000;343:750–58.

Koscielniak E, Klingebiel TH, Peters C, et al: Do patients with metastatic and recurrent rhabdomyosarcoma benefit from high-dose therapy with hematopoietic rescue? Report of the German/Austrian Pediatric Bone Marrow Transplantation Group. *Bone Marrow Transplant* 1997;19:227–31.

Namouni F, Doz F, Tanguy ML, et al: High-dose chemotherapy with carboplatin, etoposide, and cyclophosphamide followed by a hematopoietic stem cell rescue in patients with high-risk retinoblastoma: a SFOP and SFGM study. *Eur J Cancer* 19979;33:2368–75.

Pein F, Michon J, Valteau-Couanet D, et al: High dose melphalan, etoposide, and carboplatin followed by autologous stem-cell rescue in pediatric high-risk recurrent Wilms' tumor: A French Society of Pediatric Oncology Study. *J Clin Oncol* 1998;16:3295–301.

Immunodeficiency Syndromes

Onodera M, Ariga T, Kawamura N, et al: Successful peripheral T lymphocyte–directed gene transfer for a patient with severe combined immune deficiency caused by adenosine deaminase deficiency. *Blood* 1998;91:30–36.

Dürken M, Finckenstein FG, Janka GE: Bone marrow transplantation in hemophagocytic lymphohistiocytosis. *Leuk Lymphoma* 2001;41:89–95.

Horwitz ME: Stem-cell transplantation for inherited immunodeficiency disorders. *Pediatr Clin North Am* 2000;47:1371–87.

Woolfrey, A, Pulsipher MA, Storb R: Nonmyeloablative hematopoietic cell transplant for treatment of immune deficiency. *Curr Opin Pediatr* 2001;13:539–45.

Fanconi Anemia

Flowers MED, Zanis J, Pasquini R, et al: Marrow transplantation for Fanconi anemia with reduced doses of cyclophosphamide without radiation. *Br J Hematol* 1996;92:699–706.

Guardiola P, Pasquini R, Dokal I, et al: Outcome of 69 allogeneic stem cell transplantations for Fanconi anemia using HLA-matched unrelated donors: A study on behalf of the European Group for Blood and Marrow Transplantation. *Blood* 2000;95:422–29.

Metabolic Storage Diseases

Hoogerbrugge PM, Brouwer OF, Bordigoni P, et al: Allogenic bone marrow transplantation for lysosomal storage diseases. The European Group for Bone Marrow Transplantation. *Lancet* 1995;345:1398–402.

Krivit W, Shapiro EG, Peters C, et al: Hematopoietic stem-cell transplantation for globoid-cell leukodystrophy. *N Engl J Med* 1998;338:1119–26.

Krivit W, Lockman LA, Watkins PA, et al: The future for treatment by bone marrow transplantation for adrenoleukodystrophy, metachromatic leukodystrophy, globoid cell leukodystrophy and Hurler syndrome. *J Inherit Metab Dis* 1995;18:398–412.

Thalassemia

Lucarelli G, Giardini C, Angelucci E: Bone marrow transplantation in thalassemia. *Cancer Treat Res* 1997;77:305–15.

La Nasa G, Giardini, C, Argiolu F, et al: Unrelated donor bone marrow transplantation for thalassemia: The effect of extended haplotypes. *Blood* 2002;99:4350–56.

Walters MC, Sullivan KM, O'Reilly RJ, et al: Bone marrow transplantation for thalassemia: The USA experience. *Am J Pediatr Hematol Oncol* 1994;16:11–7.

Sickle Cell Disease

Vermylen C, Cornu G, Ferster A, et al: Haematopoietic stem cell transplantation for sickle cell anaemia: The first 50 patients transplanted in Belgium. *Bone Marrow Transplant* 1998;221–26.

Walters MC, Storb R, Patience M, et al: Impact of bone marrow transplantation for symptomatic sickle cell disease: An interim report. *Blood* 2000;95:1918–24.

Chapter 126
Matching and Rejection

The long-standing immunologic goal of stem cell transplantation (SCT) has been a graft that can respond to foreign antigens without reacting to the host and that is not rejected; however, current approaches to SCT are now using the immunologic differences between the donor and host tumor antigens as a primary therapeutic modality in nonmyeloablative SCT. These transplants use smaller doses of total body irradiation (TBI) or chemotherapy that supply enough immunosuppression to allow allogeneic donor stem cells to engraft and "reject" the patient's tumor. This technique is also useful in providing a source of donor cells to correct nonmalignant disorders (inborn errors of metabolism, immunodeficiencies, autoimmune disorders, hemoglobinopathies, osteopetrosis) and avoiding the toxic higher doses of TBI and chemotherapy. The tradeoff of this approach is graft versus host disease (GVHD) and risk of rejection.

The most important factor determining tolerance is the histocompatibility between the donor and host. The genes defining histocompatibility are encoded in the **major histocompatibility complex (MHC),** which spans approximately 4,000 kb on the short arm of chromosome 6 and contains the genes for a series of cell surface glycoproteins termed the **human leukocyte antigens (HLA).** The HLA genes are tightly linked and can be divided into class I glycoproteins that dimerize with β_2-microglobulin and class II glycoproteins with α and β peptides that form heterodimers. Although there are more than 35 HLA class I and II genes and more than 1,336 alleles, HLA-A and HLA-B (class I) and HLA-DRB1 (class II) genes are used as the primary determinants for histocompatibility of donors and recipients for SCT. The HLA genes on a single chromosome 6 make up a **haplotype** that, along with the HLA genes on the other copy of chromosome 6, constitute the **genotype.** Class I genes are determined by serotyping, isoelectric focusing gel electrophoresis, and DNA sequence analysis, whereas class II genes are identified primarily by DNA typing. Several potential combinations of donor/recipients may be identified, including syngeneic (twins), genotypically matched siblings (haploidentical), phenotypically matched family members or unrelated donors, and various degrees of mismatch (1, 2, or 3-antigen). Minor mismatches as well as partial matches based on GVHD and rejection vectors may also be identified. Because only 25–30% of patients have an HLA-identical sibling, identification of phenotypically matched unrelated donors is more feasible using large unrelated donor registries (>7 million donors have been typed worldwide). In the United States, the National Marrow Donor Program has typed nearly 5 million volunteer donors and uses 350 network centers to add 40,000 potential new donors each month. The chance of identifying an unrelated donor for a given individual is 20–67%, depending on the ethnic/HLA background. Transplants using one-antigen mismatched, unrelated donors are possible if the mismatch is an allelic mismatch or very closely related HLA antigens.

In an effort to expand the pool of available unrelated donors, umbilical cord blood was found to be an excellent source of hematopoietic stem cells, allowing a greater degree of mismatch (1, 2, or 3 antigen), thus increasing the likelihood of finding a donor and a reduced incidence of GVHD at the cost of a longer time to engraftment. After delivery of an infant and clamping of the cord, 40–200 mL of umbilical cord blood is collected aseptically and stored. Numerous cord blood banks both public and private have been established around the world where cord blood can be donated or stored for potential personal use; more than 30,000 cord units have been made available for transplantation and more than 1,300 umbilical cord blood transplants (CBT) have been performed for nearly every indication for which SCT and peripheral blood stem cell transplantation (PBSCT) has been performed. The overall survival has been 30–65% for both related and unrelated CBT. Immune reconstitution after CBT appears to be complete with normal NK cell function, immunoglobulin production, and B- and T-cell repertoires. Both allogeneic related and unrelated PBSCT have the advantage of earlier engraftment and lower transplant morbidity but at the cost of increased chronic GVHD. Selection of an appropriate stem cell source depends on the patient's clinical status, HLA typing, and availability of adequate numbers of stem cells for engraftment.

Graft failure and graft rejection are influenced by several factors (Box 126–1); HLA disparity is the most important variable. Failure to engraft may occur in autologous as well as allogeneic SCT and may result from an inadequate stem cell dose or from marrow stromal damage by prior therapy in conjunction with the transplant preparative regimen. Graft rejection may occur immediately, without any increase in cell counts, or may follow a brief period of engraftment. Rejection is usually mediated by residual host T cells, cytotoxic antibodies, or lymphokines and is manifested by a fall in donor cell counts with a persistence of host lymphocytes. SCT using marrow from HLA disparate donors increases the risk for graft rejection and failure significantly. For example, the risk of graft failure in an HLA-identical

---

BOX 126–1. Factors Influencing Engraftment and Graft Rejection

HLA disparity
Pretransplant alloimmunization by transfusions
Conditioning regimen
Transplanted stem cell dose
Marrow stroma/microenvironment
Post-transplant/immunosuppression
Donor T cells
Drug toxicity
Viral infections

---

sibling SCT is 1–2%, whereas in haploidentical SCT the risk is 3–15%. Alloimmunization by exposure to multiple transfusions before SCT may sensitize the patient to HLA antigens, increasing the potential for graft rejection; this is observed most often with aplastic anemia. Because adequate immunosuppression of the host before marrow infusion is required to ensure engraftment and prevent rejection, the incidence of rejection depends in part on the conditioning regimen. With matched sibling SCT for aplastic anemia, there is a 24% incidence of graft rejection when cyclophosphamide is used alone as a preparative regimen compared with 3% when antithymocyte globulin is added. Post-transplant immunosuppression is useful to prevent GVHD and to minimize the likelihood of graft rejection. One effective approach to GVHD is to eliminate T cells from the donor marrow before infusion, but elimination of T cells allows the persistence of host lymphocytes, which are capable of mediating graft rejection in about 10% of cases. Graft rejection may be difficult to differentiate from the effects of drugs or viral infections on the graft.

Baker SK, Wagner JE: Novel conditioning regimens and nonmyeloablative stem cell transplants. *Curr Opin Pediatr* 2002;14:17–22.

Petersdorf EW, Hansen JA, Martin PJ, et al: Major histocompatibility-complex class I alleles and antigens in hematopoietic-cell transplantation. *N Engl J Med* 2001;345:1794–800.

Rocha V, Cornish J, Sievers E, et al: Comparison of outcomes of unrelated bone marrow and umbilical cord blood transplants in children with acute leukemia. *Blood* 2001;97:2962–71.

Thomson BG, Robertson KA, Gowan D, et al: Analysis of engraftment, graft-versus-host disease, and immune recovery following unrelated donor cord blood transplantation. *Blood* 2000;96:2703–11.

Vicent MG, Madero L, Ortega JJ, et al: Matched pair analysis comparing allogeneic PBPCT and BMT for HLA-identical relatives in childhood acute lymphoblastic leukemia. *Bone Marrow Transplant* 2002;30:9–13.

GVHD is classified as **acute GVHD,** occurring 100 days or less after stem cell transplantation (SCT), and **chronic GVHD,** occurring more than 100 days after SCT. GVHD can produce a **graft versus leukemia (GVL)** effect resulting in a lower relapse rate in patients transplanted for leukemia. This concept is the driving goal in nonmyeloablative SCT for malignancies by using low-dose or nonmyeloablative conditioning regimens with enough immune suppression to allow engraftment of donor cells, which then effect an antitumor alloreactive response. The process of GVHD represents a loss of "tolerance" normally maintained by thymic elimination of alloreactive lymphocytes; modulation of the T-cell receptor, rendering alloreactive cells anergic; and active suppressor cells that hold activated T cells in check.

Acute GVHD. The acute form of GVHD is set up by release of inflammatory cytokines (e.g., interferons, interleukins, TNF) from damaged cells induced by the conditioning regimen. Host antigen presenting cells (APCs) present MHC-bound host-derived foreign antigens to infused donor T cells in an environment rich in cytokines, resulting in activation and proliferation of donor T cells. Activated donor CD4 and CD8 release additional cytokines, often referred to as a "cytokine storm," to activate effector cytotoxic T cells and NK cells with resultant tissue damage. Clinically, acute GVHD is characterized by erythroderma, cholestatic hepatitis, and enteritis (Table 127–1). Typically, acute GVHD presents as the patient is starting to engraft. It usually starts with a pruritic macular/papular rash on the ears, palms, and soles and may progress to involve the trunk (Fig. 127–1) and extremities, potentially becoming a more confluent erythroderma with bullae formation and exfoliation. Fever may or may not be present. Other diagnostic considerations include toxicity from the preparative regimen, drug rash, and viral or other infectious exanthems. Hepatic manifestations include cholestatic jaundice with elevated liver function tests. The differential diagnosis includes hepatitis, veno-occlusive disease, or drug effect. The intestinal symptoms of acute GVHD include crampy abdominal pain and watery diarrhea, often with blood. The conditioning regimen and infectious agents may produce similar symptoms. Eosinophilia, lymphocytosis, protein-losing enteropathy, bone marrow aplasia (neutropenia, thrombocytopenia, anemia), peripheral edema, and secondary infections may ensue. Factors related to the development of acute GVHD include histocompatibility differences between the

---

Chapter 127
Graft Versus Host Disease (GVHD)

Engraftment by donor lymphocytes in an immunologically compromised host (congenital, irradiation, or chemotherapy-induced immune defects) can result in donor T-cell activation against host major histocompatibility complex (MHC) antigens, with resultant GVHD. Cell death results from cell-mediated cytotoxic activity (e.g., natural killer cells) and a complex cascade of lymphokines released by activated lymphocytes (e.g., tumor necrosis factor [TNF]). For this reaction to occur, the graft must contain immunocompetent cells, the host must be immunocompromised and unable to reject or mount a response to the graft, and there must be histocompatibility differences between the graft and the host.

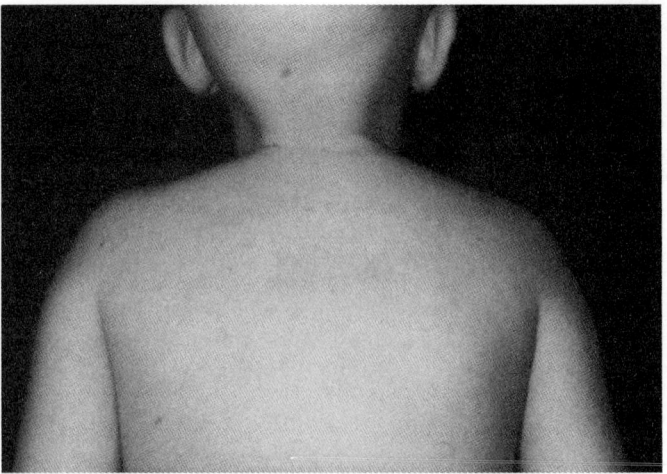

FIGURE 127–1. Acute graft versus host disease of the skin with ear, arm, shoulder, and trunk involvement. (Courtesy of Evan Farmer, MD.) See also color plates.

TABLE 127–1.   **Clinical Staging and Grading of Graft Versus Host Disease**

Stage	Skin	Liver	Intestinal Tract
+	Maculopapular rash <25% of body surface	Bilirubin 2–3 mg/dL	>500 mL diarrhea/day
++	Maculopapular rash <25–50% of body surface	Bilirubin 3–6 mg/dL	>1,000 mL diarrhea/day
+++	Generalized erythroderma	Bilirubin 6–15 mg/dL	>1,500 mL diarrhea/day
++++	Generalized erythroderma with bullous formation and desquamation	Bilirubin >15 mg/dL	Severe abdominal pain with or without ileus

GVHD Grade	Skin Stage	Liver Stage	Intestinal Tract Stage	Decrease in Clinical Performance
I	+ to ++	0	0	None
II	+ to +++	+	+	Mild
III	++ to +++	++ to ++++	++ to +++	Marked
IV	++ to ++++	++ to ++++	++ to ++++	Extreme

Adapted from Thomas ED, Storb R, Clift RA, et al: Bone marrow transplantation. N Engl J Med 1975;292:832–43,895–902.

donor and patient, gender mismatching, donor parity, age, active or relapsed malignancy at the time of BMT, and increasing doses of radiation. The prevention and treatment of GVHD requires various immunosuppressive agents (see Chapter 128). A similar and potentially fatal acute GVHD can occur after transfusion of blood products to individuals who are relatively immunosuppressed, including patients post transplant, those receiving immunosuppressive cancer therapy, those who are HIV positive, those with congenital immunodeficiencies, and preterm infants. All cellular blood products for these patients should be irradiated (2,500–5,000 cGy), but frozen acellular products such as fresh frozen plasma or cryoprecipitate do not need to be irradiated.

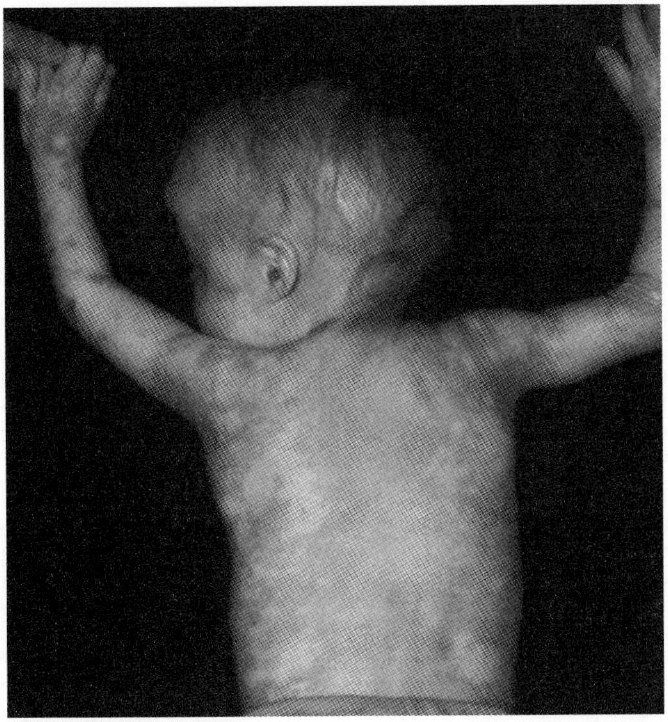

Chronic GVHD. The maturation of the graft may include the development of chronic GVHD, usually after day 100 but as early as day 60. The probability of developing chronic GVHD in children is 24% after HLA-matched sibling SCT and 37% after matched unrelated donor SCT. The pathogenesis of chronic GVHD is poorly understood, but it appears to involve alloreactive donor T cells along with T-cell precursors that have become autoreactive resulting from aberrant thymic processing. Chronic GVHD resembles a multisystem autoimmune process mimicking elements of Sjögren (sicca) syndrome, systemic lupus erythematosus, and scleroderma (Fig. 127–2), lichen planus, bronchiolitis obliterans, and primary biliary cirrhosis. Recurrent infections (e.g., sepsis, sinusitis, pneumonia) with encapsulated bacteria and fungal and viral organisms are common and contribute significantly to transplant-related morbidity and mortality. Prophylaxis with trimethoprim-sulfamethoxazole reduces the incidence of *Pneumocystis carinii* pneumonia. Risks for chronic GVHD include increasing age (donor or host), prior acute GVHD, donor lymphocyte infusions, and a high level of parity of a female donor. Therapy for chronic GVHD consists of additional immunosuppression with agents (prednisone and cyclosporine are front-line drugs) described in Chapter 128, again with the disadvantage of putting the patient at risk for infectious complications. Extensive skin involvement, thrombocytopenia (platelets < 100,000/μL), and progressive onset at diagnosis tend to predict a poor outcome.

FIGURE 127–2. Chronic graft versus host disease of the skin with sclerodermoid changes. (Courtesy of Evan Farmer, MD.) See also color plates.

Goker H, Haznedaroglu IC, Chao NJ: Acute graft-vs-host disease: Pathobiology and management. *Exp Hematol* 2001;29:259–77.

Vogelsang GB: How I treat chronic graft-versus-host disease. *Blood* 2001;97:1196–201.

Zecca M, Prete A, Rondelli R, et al: Chronic graft-versus-host disease in children: Incidence, risk factors, and impact on outcome. *Blood* 2002;100:1192–200.

Chapter 128
Principles of Immunosuppression

Immunosuppressive agents are used to prevent and treat allograft rejection and graft versus host disease (GVHD). Because differences in major or minor histocompatibility antigens induce recipient T-lymphocyte activation and subsequent donor allograft rejection, immunosuppression is needed for all tissue transplantation, except from identical twins and certain instances of stem cell transplantation (SCT) for severe immunodeficiencies. Solid organ transplantation requires lifelong immunosuppression to prevent graft rejection (see Chapters 349, 435, and 528), whereas SCT recipients are treated for 6–12 mo until a state of tolerance is attained. Transplant strategies using selected stem and T cells to enhance engraftment but avoid GVHD and more potent immunosuppressive agents permit successful SCT across greater degrees of mismatched HLA antigens. The ideal immunosuppressive agent inhibits the host lymphocyte subsets that mediate rejection and inhibits donor lymphocytes that mediate GVHD without altering immunity against infection or malignancy (graft versus leukemia [GVL]).

Preparative Regimen. Different preparative regimens are used for SCT for different diseases. Most agents have antineoplastic as well as immunosuppressant activity. Cyclophosphamide (and its isomer ifosfamide) is a nitrogen mustard derivative that requires metabolic activation to generate a bifunctional alkylating metabolite and is the most widely used immunosuppressant in SCT preparative regimens. Total body irradiation (TBI) is also an important therapeutic agent, with excellent antineoplastic activity and immunosuppressive qualities that can effectively treat all parts of the body. Other chemotherapeutic agents that have greater antitumor effects than immunosuppression have been used in combination with TBI and cyclophosphamide and include busulfan, etoposide, melphalan, carmustine (BCNU), cytarabine, thiotepa, and carboplatin. The combinations are designed to achieve adequate immunosuppression, allowing rapid engraftment without excessive toxicity and with the capacity to eliminate a malignant clone. Lower doses of these agents in conjunction with fludarabine have been used in nonmyeloablative SCT to result in a 90–100% engraftment, but GVHD remains a problem; it is still too early to know whether GVL will achieve similar results to conventional high-dose therapy. A nonmyeloablative approach may be most useful in nonmalignant disorders where the presence of normal donor cells (graft) is corrective for the disorder.

T-Cell Depletion. Prevention of graft rejection and GVHD along with treatment of GVHD in the peritransplant period involves several different strategies. Because donor T cells are responsible for GVHD, donor marrows have been depleted of T cells using monoclonal antibodies or physical separation techniques such as soy lectin agglutination. Depletion results in a dramatic reduction in GVHD but can cause graft rejection and relapse. Donor T cells have an important role in eliminating residual host T cells as well as in mediating a GVL effect. Alternatives to T-cell depletion are being explored, including adding back-selected T cells that may help engraftment and retain antitumor activity but without GVHD activity.

Methotrexate. This competitive inhibitor of dihydrofolate reductase is an excellent immunosuppressive agent, in addition to being a cancer chemotherapeutic drug. A regimen of methotrexate given on days 1, 3, 6, and 11 post transplant is effective at preventing GVHD, with additional improvement when used in conjunction with cyclosporine. Methotrexate may aggravate mucositis resulting from the conditioning regimen and may require rescue with leucovorin if a patient has renal impairment or a fluid collection, such as a pleural effusion. Trimetrexate is an antifolate drug with structural similarity to methotrexate, but it is eliminated by the liver and may be an alternative for patients who have significant renal impairment.

Cyclosporine. Cyclosporine is a lipophilic (hydrophobic), cyclic, 11-amino acid peptide that is a potent and specific immunosuppressive agent that blocks T-cell activation by interfering with the T-cell receptor–mediated signal cascade to selectively inhibit the transcription of interleukin (IL)-2. Cyclosporine may also inhibit IL-1, IL-3, and interferon-γ synthesis. Cyclosporine inhibits IL-2 receptor formation at higher doses. Although cyclosporine has no myelosuppressive or anti-inflammatory effects beyond its effects on T cells, it is very useful for preventing graft rejection. Cyclosporine is metabolized by the hepatic cytochrome P450 enzyme system and can be involved in a number of drug interactions. Cyclosporine levels increase in the presence of ketoconazole, erythromycin, warfarin, verapamil, ethanol, imipenem-cilastatin, metoclopramide, itraconazole, and fluconazole. These levels decrease in the presence of phenytoin, phenobarbital, carbamazepine, valproate, nafcillin, octreotide, trimethoprim, and rifampin.

Cyclosporine has significant nonimmunosuppressant adverse effects, including the following: neurotoxicity (tremors, paresthesias, headache, confusion, somnolence, seizures, coma), hypertrichosis, gingival hyperplasia, anorexia, nausea, vomiting, hepatotoxicity (cholestasis, cholelithiasis, hemorrhagic necrosis), endocrinopathies (ketosis, hyperprolactinemia, hypertestosteronism, gynecomastia, impaired spermatogenesis), metabolic disorders (hypomagnesemia, hyperuricemia, hyperglycemia, hyperkalemia, hypocholesterolemia), vascular derangements (hypertension, increased sympathetic nervous system activation, vasculitic-hemolytic uremic syndrome–like illness, atherogenesis), and nephrotoxicity. Renal toxicity is a significant limitation of cyclosporine use and is manifested as an increased creatinine level, oliguria, hypertension, fluid retention, vasoconstriction of the afferent glomerular filtration rate, renal tubular damage, and hemolytic-uremic syndrome–like lesions. Chronic nephrotoxicity (interstitial fibrosis, tubular atrophy) may require a reduction of the cyclosporine dose or a change to other immunosuppressant drugs. Nephrotoxicity may be exacerbated by aminoglycosides, amphotericin B, acyclovir, digoxin, furosemide, indomethacin, or trimethoprim. The renal toxicity may be reduced by adjusting dosing based on blood cyclosporine levels. Levels may also be influenced by clinical conditions affecting absorption, including diarrhea, intestinal disorders (due to GVHD, viral infections, or therapy), or altered hepatic function. Although the drug is lipophilic, obesity does not influence the distribution of the drug and dosing should be based on ideal body weight. Cyclosporine is as effective as methotrexate for post-SCT immunosuppression, and the combination of cyclosporine with methotrexate is better than treatment with either drug alone.

Tacrolimus. Tacrolimus is a macrolide immunosuppressive drug produced by the fungus *Streptomyces tsukubaensis* that is chemically distinct from cyclosporine but with similar effects on the immune system. Although it binds specific proteins, it has the same effects on the expression of IL-2 and the IL-2 receptor as cyclosporine. Tacrolimus has little advantage over cyclosporine, except possibly for the treatment of GVHD of the liver because it is concentrated in the liver. The toxicities and drug interactions are similar to those of cyclosporine. The combination of these drugs causes synergistic toxicity.

Corticosteroids. Prednisone, usually in combination with other immunosuppressive agents, is often used to treat or prevent GVHD and to prevent rejection. Corticosteroids may interfere with T-lymphocyte proliferation by blocking activation of IL-1 and IL-6 through induction of soluble IL-receptor antagonists. Because IL-2 secretion depends in part on IL-1 and IL-6 release, corticosteroids block IL-2 action indirectly. Corticosteroids also produce a more rapid anti-inflammatory response by inducing the production of lipocortin, an inhibitor of phospholipase A_2, which reduces the synthesis of inflammatory prostaglandins. They may also lyse small populations of activated lymphocytes and reduce the migration of monocytes to sites of inflammation. Nonspecific and pronounced immunosuppressant effects of corticosteroids (and other immunosuppressants) place the patient at risk for serious opportunistic infections. Other long-term complications of corticosteroid use include growth failure, cushingoid appearance, hypertension, cataracts, gastrointestinal bleeding, pancreatitis, psychosis, hyperglycemia, osteoporosis, aseptic necrosis of the femoral head, and suppression of the pituitary-adrenal axis.

Antibodies. Antithymocyte globulin (ATG) is a preparation of heterologous antibodies against human thymocytes that have been generated from horses, rabbits, and other sources. These antibody preparations are potent immunosuppressants and have been useful in preparative regimens as well as for treatment of resistant GVHD. Toxicities include fever, hypotension, rash-urticaria, tachycardia, dyspnea, chills, myalgias, serum sickness, and potential anaphylaxis. Diphenhydramine, acetaminophen, and hydrocortisone help to minimize side effects.

Other antibodies such as **anti-CD33 (gemtuzumab ozogamicin)** or **anti-CD20 (rituximab)** alone or conjugated to cytotoxins function to target not only specific immune cellular components but also malignant cells expressing these proteins. These antibody preparations have been used to treat relapsed disease with resultant complete remissions and are now being used in conjunction with conventional preparative regimens. Rituximab is the treatment of choice for post-transplant Epstein-Barr virus–driven lymphoproliferative disease. Anticytokine antibodies (tumor necrosis factor, IL-1, interferon-γ) block the cytokine cascade and have shown promising results in early trials to treat refractory GVHD.

Thalidomide. Initially used as a sedative but found to have immunosuppressive properties, thalidomide has been studied in phase I–II trials for treating patients with high-risk or refractory chronic GVHD; it has shown a 59% response rate with a 76% survival for those with refractory chronic GVHD and 48% for those with high-risk chronic GVHD. Phase III treatment trials have found poor tolerance of higher doses requiring dose modification, whereas prevention trials have demonstrated thalidomide to be ineffective for prevention of chronic GVHD.

Carter P: Improving the efficacy of antibody-based cancer therapies. *Nat Rev Cancer* 2001;1:118–29.

Cohen AD, Luger SM, Sickles C, et al: Gemtuzumab ozogamicin (Mylotarg) monotherapy for relapsed AML after hematopoietic stem cell transplant: Efficacy and incidence of hepatic veno-occlusive disease. *Bone Marrow Transplant* 2002;30:23–28.

Ifthikharuddin JJ, Mieles LA, Rosenblatt JD, et al: CD-20 expression in post-transplant lymphoproliferative disorders: Treatment with rituximab. *Am J Hematol* 2000;65:171–73.

Koc S, Leisenring W, Flowers MED, et al: Thalidomide for treatment patients with chronic graft versus host disease. *Blood* 2000;96:3995–96.

Miniero R, Zecchina G, Nagler A: Non-myeloablative allogeneic stem cell transplantation in children. *Haematologica* 2000;85:12–17.

Sanders JE: Stem-cell transplant preparative regimens. *Pediatr Transplant* 1999;1:23–34.

Chapter 129
Late Effects of Stem Cell Transplantation

As more children are undergoing stem cell transplantation (SCT) for a widening spectrum of indications and an increasing number of these children become long-term survivors, late effects of the transplant process have a lasting impact on the health and well-being of the individual. Possible delayed complications include effects on growth and development, neuroendocrine dysfunction, fertility, second tumors, chronic graft versus host disease (GVHD), cataracts, leukoencephalopathy, and immune dysfunction.

Neurologic Function. Infections, metabolic encephalopathy (resulting from hepatic dysfunction), and drug and irradiation (radiotherapy) all may contribute to neurologic sequelae. Cyclosporine may produce headache, which is usually responsive to propranolol, as well as tremor, confusion, visual disturbance, seizures, and frank encephalopathy. Most of these adverse effects are reversible with discontinuation of the drug.

Leukoencephalopathy is a clinical syndrome characterized by lethargy, slurred speech, ataxia, seizures, confusion, dysphagia, and decerebrate posturing. It may present as minimal symptoms or can result in coma or death in its most severe form. MRI and CT reveal multifocal areas of white matter degeneration with necrosis. Leukoencephalopathy is observed almost exclusively in patients who have received extensive intrathecal chemotherapy or cranial irradiation before transplantation, with an overall incidence of 7% among these patients.

The incidence of cataracts is approximately 80% in patients receiving single-dose total body irradiation (800–1,000 cGy TBI), 20–50% with fractionated TBI, and 20% after regimens with only chemotherapy. A dry eye syndrome, or keratoconjunctivitis sicca, is often related to chronic GVHD and is treated with artificial tears and lubricants.

Secondary Malignancies. The overall risk of developing a secondary form of cancer is six to eight times that in the general population, with the greatest risk being within the 1st yr. Approximately half of the secondary tumors in the 1st year are non-Hodgkin's lymphomas, and two thirds of these are positive for Epstein-Barr virus (EBV). In a study of 3,182 children transplanted for leukemia from 1964–1992, 25 solid tumors developed compared with an expected single case in the general population, with most of the tumors (n = 14) being thyroid and brain tumors. Risk factors that are associated with second malignancies include the diagnosis of immunodeficiency, use of antithymocyte globulin (ATG), T-cell depletion of the donor marrow, younger age at the time of transplant, and TBI in the preparative regimen. EBV-related B-cell lymphomas, which are aggressive and resistant to most therapeutic interventions, have been successfully treated with infusions of donor T cells or anti-CD20 antibody.

Growth. Long-term follow-up studies of patients who have received TBI-containing regimens reveal significant growth depression and growth hormone deficiency, which can diminish adult height. Patients 8 yr after treatment with TBI are 1–2 standard deviations (SD) below the mean height for age, which further decreases to 1.5–3 SD if cranial irradiation was added to TBI. This decrease in growth velocity is similar for boys and girls. Fractionation of irradiation results in less impact (1 SD below the mean height for age) on height compared with single-dose TBI

(2 SD below mean height for age). Children receiving radiation-containing regimens also have no pubertal growth spurt, which depends on the presence of adequate growth hormone and gonadal hormones, both of which may be low after transplantation. A major determinant of adult height is the amount of growth before puberty. A study of 175 children younger than 6 yr of age, 6–12 yr of age, or 12–15 yr of age receiving TBI-based regimens and not treated with growth hormone reported a mean final adult height of 3.49, 1.92, and 0.37 SD below average, respectively. Chronic GVHD and its treatment with corticosteroids may also contribute to growth impairment after transplant. In an attempt to avoid TBI-related growth effects in children, chemotherapy-only regimens such as busulfan/cyclophosphamide have been used. Growth studies indicate that busulfan has much less of an impact on growth but produces the same gonadal failure as TBI-based regimens. Preparative regimens using only cyclophosphamide for aplastic anemia have little effect on normal growth and development. Irradiation of the long bones and vertebral bodies for neuroblastoma also contributes to decreased growth velocity. Therapy with recombinant growth hormone after age 12 yr prevents a further decrease in growth velocity, but little or no catch-up growth is achieved.

Annual growth hormone evaluation is essential for all children after SCT. Current studies are aimed at identifying children with growth hormone deficiencies at an earlier age and administering supplemental growth hormone to achieve a normal pubertal growth spurt. Gonadal hormones are essential for normal pubertal growth as well as development of secondary sexual characteristics. Approximately 75% of patients receiving TBI-containing regimens show delayed development of secondary sexual characteristics, resulting from primary ovarian or testicular failure. Laboratory evaluation reveals elevated follicle-stimulating hormone (FSH) and luteinizing hormone (LH) levels with depressed estradiol and testosterone. These patients require careful follow-up with evaluation of annual Tanner scores and endocrine function. Supplementation of gonadal hormones is useful for primary gonadal failure and is given along with growth hormone to promote pubertal growth.

Thyroid Function. The use of TBI with or without additional conventional irradiation involving the thyroid gland may result in hypothyroidism. Some children who have received single-dose TBI develop compensated (28–56%) or overt (9–13%) hypothyroidism. The use of fractionated TBI has significantly reduced the incidence of both compensated (10–14%) and overt (<5%) hypothyroidism. Risk factors for the development of hypothyroidism appear to be related only to the use of irradiation, with no influence of age, sex, or GVHD. The site of injury by irradiation is at the level of the thyroid gland rather than at the pituitary or hypothalamus. Therapy with thyroxine is very effective for overt hypothyroidism, but treatment of compensated hypothyroidism is more controversial. Despite treatment of hypothyroidism, there remains a risk for thyroid carcinoma. Because the risk of hypothyroidism continues for many years, annual thyroid function studies are important. Chemotherapy-only preparative regimens have far fewer effects on normal thyroid function.

Immune Reconstitution. Chemoradiotherapy for SCT results in complete eradication of host B- and T-cell immunity. After infusion of donor marrow, recovery of the normal immune functions takes many months or years. The ability of newly engrafting B cells to respond to mitogenic stimulation is intact by 2–3 mo. Because the production of antibodies requires B- and T-cell interaction, normal IgM levels are not observed until 4–6 mo after transplant; IgG levels take 7–9 mo to normalize, and it may take 2 yr before normal IgA levels are achieved. T-cell recovery also takes many months. CD8 T cells recover by about 4 mo, but CD4 T cells do not increase until 6–9 mo, resulting in an inverted CD4/CD8 ratio for the first 6–9 mo after transplant. Factors that prolong this interval include T-cell depletion of the marrow, post-transplant immunosuppression, and chronic GVHD. Patients with chronic GVHD have a continued decrease in the number of cytotoxic T lymphocytes and helper T cells, along with increased suppressor T cells.

Live virus vaccines should be avoided in immunocompromised patients. Reimmunization of an individual will be successful only after adequate recovery of immune function. For patients without chronic GVHD, diphtheria and tetanus toxoids, acellular pertussis (in children <7 yr of age), inactivated polio, hepatitis B, *Haemophilus influenzae* type b, and *Streptococcus pneumoniae* immunizations may be given 12 mo after transplant, and measles-mumps-rubella immunizations after 24 mo. Influenza vaccines should be given every fall. If chronic GVHD is present, re-immunization should be postponed and IgG supplemented until it resolves.

Auletta JJ, Fisher VL: Immune reconstitution in pediatric stem-cell transplantation. *Front Biosci* 2001;6:G23–32.

Boulad F, Bromley M, Black P, et al: Thyroid dysfunction following bone marrow transplantation using hyperfractionated radiation. *Bone Marrow Transplant* 1995;15:71–76.

Cohen A: Is endocrinological assessment and follow-up of children after bone marrow transplantation necessary? How, and for how long? *Pediatr Transplant* 1999;3:1–4.

Socié G, Curtis RE, Deeg HJ, et al: New malignant diseases after allogeneic marrow transplantation for childhood acute leukemia. *J Clin Oncol* 2000;18:348–57.

Fisher VL: Long-term follow-up in hematopoietic stem-cell transplant patients. *Pediatr Transplant* 1999;3(Suppl 1):122–29.

Giorgiani G, Bozzola M, Locatelli F, et al: Role of busulfan and total body irradiation on growth of prepubertal children receiving bone marrow transplantation and results of treatment with recombinant human growth hormone. *Blood* 1995;86:825–31.

Sanders JE: Pubertal development of children treated with marrow transplantation before puberty. *J Pediatr* 1997;130:174–75.

Allergic Disorders

Chapter 130

Allergy and the Immunologic Basis of Atopic Disease *Donald Y. M. Leung*

Allergic diseases such as asthma, food allergy, atopic dermatitis, and allergic rhinitis are common illnesses that have been increasing in prevalence during the past 30 years. The term *allergy* was first coined, in 1906, by von Pirquet, who used it to refer to patients who expressed an "altered state of reactivity" to common environmental antigens. With the discovery, in the late 1960s, that most patients with allergy produce IgE antibodies to antigens that trigger their illness, the term *allergy* is often used interchangeably with clinical expression of IgE-mediated allergic disease. This is an oversimplification of the mechanisms involved in allergic disease because a subset of individuals with asthma, atopic dermatitis, and allergic rhinitis have non–Ig E-mediated disease despite manifesting eosinophilia and mast cell activation. Furthermore, certain allergic diseases, such as contact dermatitis, are primarily T cell–mediated without evidence of IgE responses to environmental triggers.

Atopy is derived from the Greek *atopos*, meaning "out of place," and often used to describe patients with IgE-mediated diseases. Such individuals have a familial predisposition to allergic diseases, which are manifest as hyperresponsiveness in their target organs (e.g., the lung, skin, or nose). Importantly, this hyperresponsiveness has both IgE-mediated and non–Ig E-mediated inflammatory components, which lowers the threshold of the target organ to subsequent allergen exposure.

FEATURES OF ALLERGIC DISEASES

Allergens. The term *allergen* refers to an antigen that triggers an IgE response in genetically predisposed individuals. Most allergens are proteins that have molecular weights of 10–70 kd; molecules smaller than 10 kd would not bridge adjacent IgE antibody molecules on the surface of mast cells or basophils, and most molecules larger than 70 kd would not pass through mucosal surfaces needed to reach antigen-presenting cells for stimulation of the immune system. Allergens frequently function in their natural state as proteolytic enzymes, which may contribute to increased mucosal permeability and sensitization. Many major allergens have been identified and cloned, including Der p 1 and Der p 2 from the house-dust mite *(Dermatophagoides pteronyssinus)*, Fel d 1 from cat, and a number of tree, grass, and weed pollens, including Bet v 1 from birch tree, Phl p 1 and Phl p 5 from timothy grass, and Amb a 1, 2, 3, and 5 from giant ragweed.

Type 2 Helper T Cells. All individuals are exposed to potential allergens. Nonatopic subjects respond with the proliferation of T helper type 1 (Th1) cells, which secrete cytokines, including interferon (IFN)-γ, that are involved in the elicitation of allergen-specific IgG antibodies. Th1 cells are generally involved in the eradication of intracellular organisms such as mycobacteria (Fig. 130–1), because of the ability of Th1 cytokines to activate phagocytes and promote the production of opsonizing and complement-fixing antibodies. However, genetically predisposed atopic individuals respond with a brisk expansion of T helper type 2 (Th2) cells that secrete cytokines favoring IgE synthesis and are involved in host defense against extracellular organisms such as parasites.

Atopic responses include the generation of allergen-specific IgE antibodies that are detectable by serum testing or positive immediate reactions to allergen extracts on prick skin testing (see Chapter 131). The Th2 cytokines interleukin (IL)-4 and IL-13 play a key role in immunoglobulin isotype switching to IgE (Fig. 130–2). IL-5 and IL-9 further enhance IgE synthesis and play an important role in the differentiation and development of eosinophils. The combination of IL-3, IL-4, and IL-9 contributes to mast cell development. Thus, Th2 cytokines have been proposed to play an important role in the pathogenesis of asthma and allergic diseases. This is supported by the observation that Th2 cells infiltrate into the affected tissues of acute allergic tissue reactions. Interesting, chronic allergic reactions often are characterized by the infiltration of Th1 and Th2 cells. This is important because Th1-type cytokines such as IFN-γ can potentiate the function of allergic inflammatory effector cells such as eosinophils and thereby contribute to disease severity.

In utero, T cells of the fetus are primarily of the Th2 type, which reduces reactivity of the maternal immune system against the fetal allograft. Postnatally, the nonatopic infant's immune system shifts to a Th1-mediated response to environmental allergens, whereas the atopic infant has a further increase in Th2 cells that were potentially primed in utero by transplacental exposure to allergens. Microbes are the major stimulus for Th1-mediated immunity. Macrophages or dendritic cells stimulated by microbial products, such as endotoxin, secrete IL-12, which is an important inducer of Th1 cells. Because Th1 cells inhibit Th2 cell development, factors that contribute to Th1 cell development reduce allergic responses. High-affinity interactions between T cells and antigen-presenting cells, large amounts of antigen, Th1 cytokines (IL-12 and IL-18), and exposure to microbial DNA containing cytidine-phosphate-guanosine (CpG) repeats are all factors that favor the Th1 phenotype. In contrast, exposure to Th2 cytokines (IL-4), prostaglandin E_2 (PGE_2), nitric oxide, low-affinity interactions between T cells and antigen-presenting cells (APCs), and small amounts of antigen are factors favoring the Th2 phenotype.

Antigen-Presenting Cells. Dendritic cells, Langerhans cells, monocytes, and macrophages play an important role in the induction of allergic inflammation by presenting allergens to T cells and by contributing to the local recruitment of effector cells. APCs are a heterogeneous group of cells with the common property of presenting antigens in the context of the major histocompatibility complex (MHC). Of the various professional APCs, dendritic cells and Langerhans cells are unique in their ability to prime naïve T cells and are thus responsible for the primary immune response, that is, the sensitization phase of allergy. APCs are found primarily in lymphoid organs and the skin. Monocytes and macrophages likely play more of a role in activating memory T-cell responses, the elicitation phase of allergy.

Dendritic cells residing in peripheral sites such as the skin, intestinal lamina propria, and lung are relatively immature. These cells are actively phagocytic but express fewer MHC and

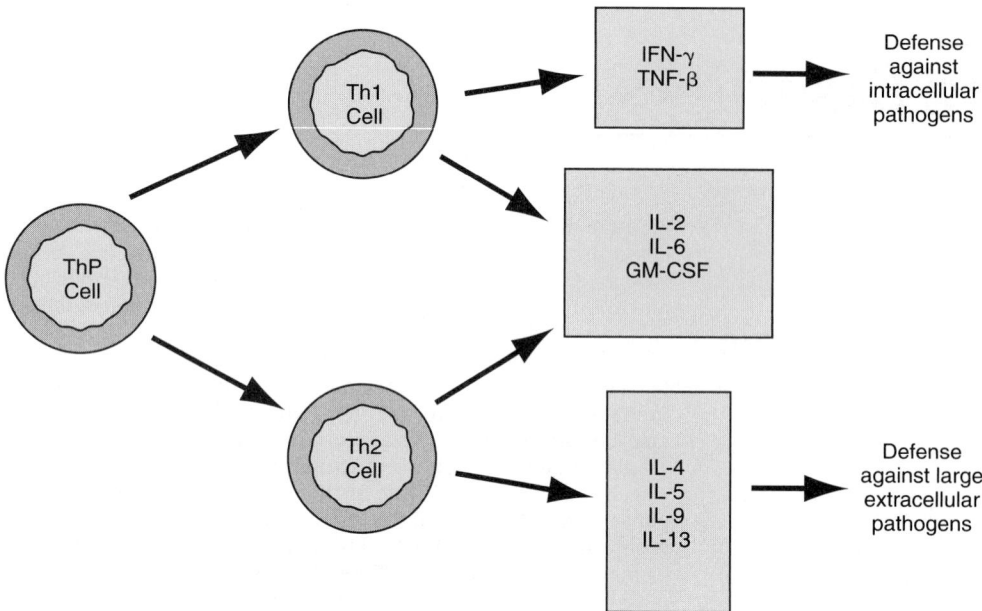

FIGURE 130–1. T-cell differentiation.

co-stimulatory molecules than mature APCs. These immature dendritic cells take up antigens in tissues and then migrate to the T-cell areas in locally draining lymph nodes. During this migration, they undergo phenotypic and functional changes characterized by increased expression of MHC class I, MHC class II, and co-stimulatory molecules that react with CD28 expressed on T cells. In the lymph nodes, they directly present processed antigens to resting T cells to induce their proliferation and differentiation.

Based on their ability to favor Th1 or Th2 differentiation, mature dendritic cells have been called DC1 or DC2, respectively. The critical factor for the polarizing mechanism to Th1

cells is the level of IL-12 produced by DC1 cells. In this regard, a cytokine such as IFN-γ is a potent DC1-promoting factor. Differentiation of T cells in the absence of IL-12 production by DC2 leads to Th2 cells. Histamine and PGE_2 inhibit IL-12 production and contribute to the development of DC2. A unique feature of atopy is the presence of allergen-specific IgE on the cell surface of their APCs. Importantly, the formation of Fc ε receptor I (FcεRI)/IgE/allergen complexes on the APC cell surface markedly facilitates allergen uptake and allergen presentation. The clinical importance of this phenomenon is supported by the observation that FcεRI-positive Langerhans cells bearing IgE molecules is a prerequisite for provocation of eczematous lesions by aeroallergens applied to the skin of patients with atopic dermatitis. The role of the low-affinity IgE receptor Fc ε receptor II (FcεRII, CD23) on monocyte-macrophages is less clear, although it appears that under certain conditions it can also facilitate antigen capture; and cross-linking of this receptor as well as FcεRI on monocyte-macrophages can lead to the release of inflammatory mediators.

IgE and Its Receptors. The acute allergic response is dependent on IgE and its ability to bind selectively to the alpha chain of the high-affinity FcεRI or the low-affinity FcεRII. Cross-linking of receptor-bound IgE molecules by allergen initiates a complex intracellular signaling cascade followed by mast cell or basophil degranulation and the release of various mediators of allergic inflammation. The FcεRI molecule is also found on the surface of antigen-presenting dendritic cells (e.g., Langerhans cells) but differs from the structure found on mast cells/basophils in that the FcεRI molecule found on dendritic cells lacks the β chain. CD23 is found on mononuclear cells, eosinophils, platelets, and follicular dendritic cells.

The induction of IgE synthesis involves two major signals. The initial signal involves activation of germline transcription at the ε immunoglobulin locus by IL-4 or IL-13, and thus dictates isotype specificity. The second signal involves the engagement of CD40 on B cells by CD40 ligand expressed on T cells. This leads to activation of the recombination machinery, resulting in DNA switch recombination. CD40 engagement can be replaced as a second signal by Epstein-Barr virus infection or glucocorticoid treatment. Interactions between several pairs of co-stimulatory molecules (CD28/B7, LFA-1/ICAM-1, and CD2/CD58) can further amplify signal 1 and signal 2 to enhance IgE synthesis. Factors that inhibit IgE synthesis include Th1-type cytokines

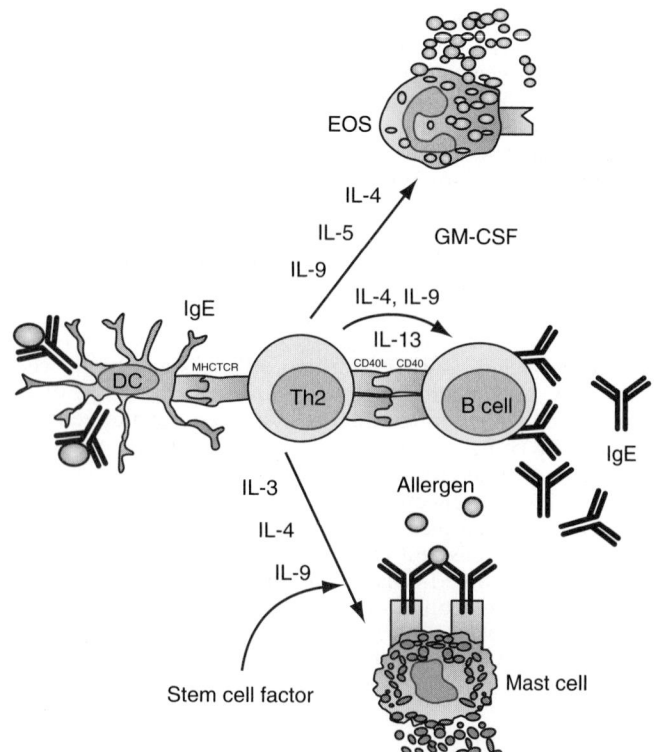

FIGURE 130–2. Role of Th2 cytokines in allergic cascade.

(IL-12, IFN-α and IFN-γ) and microbial DNA containing CpG repeats.

Eosinophils. Allergic diseases are characterized by peripheral blood and tissue eosinophilia. Eosinophils contain dense intracellular granules that are sources of inflammatory proteins. These include major basic protein, eosinophil-derived neurotoxin, peroxidase, and cationic protein. Eosinophil granule proteins have been found to damage epithelial cells, induce airway hyperresponsiveness, and cause degranulation of basophils and mast cells. Major basic protein released from eosinophils can bind to an acidic moiety on the M2 muscarinic receptor and block its function, thereby leading to increased acetylcholine levels and the development of increased airway hyperreactivity. The eosinophil is also a rich source of leukotrienes, particularly cysteinyl leukotriene C4, which contracts airway smooth muscle and increases vascular permeability. Other secretory products of eosinophils include cytokines (IL-4, IL-5, TNF-α), proteolytic enzymes, and reactive oxygen intermediates, all of which can significantly enhance allergic tissue inflammation.

Several cytokines regulate the function of eosinophils in allergic disease. Eosinophils develop and mature in the bone marrow from IL-5–responsive precursor cells. Allergen challenge of clinically allergic patients causes resident bone marrow CD34 cells to express the IL-5 receptor, which stimulates eosinophils to synthesize granule proteins, prolongs their survival, potentiates degranulation of eosinophils, and stimulates the release of eosinophils from the bone marrow. Granulocyte-macrophage colony-stimulating factor (GM-CSF) also enhances proliferation, cell survival, cytokine production, and degranulation of eosinophils. Certain chemokines such as RANTES, macrophage inflammatory protein 1α (MIP-1α), and eotaxins, play an important role in attracting eosinophils into local allergic tissue inflammatory reactions. In particular, eotaxins mobilize IL-5–dependent eosinophil colony-forming progenitor cells from the bone marrow. These progenitors are rapidly cleared from the blood and either return to the bone marrow or are recruited to inflamed tissue sites.

Mast Cells. Mast cells are derived from CD34 hematopoietic progenitor cells that arise in the bone marrow, enter the circulation, and travel to peripheral tissue where they undergo tissue specific maturation. Interactions between the tyrosine kinase receptor c-*kit* expressed on the surface of mast cells and the fibroblast-derived c-*kit* ligand, stem cell factor (SCF), are essential for mast cell development and survival. Unlike mature basophils, mature mast cells do not usually circulate in the blood but are widely distributed throughout connective tissues, where they often lie adjacent to blood vessels and beneath epithelial surfaces that are exposed to the external environment, such as the respiratory tract, gastrointestinal tract, and skin. Thus, mast cells are positioned anatomically to participate in allergic reactions. There are at least two subpopulations of human mast cells: mast cells with tryptase and mast cells with both tryptase and chymase. Mast cells with tryptase are the predominant type found in the lung and small intestinal mucosa, whereas mast cells with both tryptase and chymase are the predominant type found in the skin, gastrointestinal submucosa, and blood vessels.

Mast cells contain or produce on appropriate stimulation a diverse array of mediators that can have different effects on allergic inflammation and organ function. These include preformed granule-associated mediators (e.g., histamine, serine proteases, and proteoglycans) and de novo synthesis and release of membrane-derived lipids, cytokines, and chemokines. The most important mast cell–derived lipid mediators are the cyclo-oxygenase and lipoxygenase metabolites of arachidonic acid, which have potent inflammatory activities. The major cyclo-oxygenase product of mast cells is prostaglandin D_2, and the major lipoxygenase products are the sulfidopeptide leukotrienes: LTC_4 and its peptidolytic derivatives LTD_4 and LTE_4. Mast cells also can produce cytokines, including those that promote Th2-type responses (IL-4, IL-13, GM-CSF) and inflammation (tumor necrosis factor [TNF]-α, IL-6) and regulate tissue remodeling (transforming growth factor, vascular endothelial cell growth factor). Immunologic activation of mast cells and basophils typically begins by cross-linkage of IgE bound to the FcεRI with multivalent allergen. Cell surface FcεRI on mast cells is increased by IL-4 and IgE. Of potential therapeutic interest, surface levels of FcεRI decrease in subjects receiving treatment with anti-IgE antibody that lowers serum IgE. Degranulation of mast cells can also occur via nonimmunologic stimuli such as multivalent lectins (concanavalin A), basic molecules such as compound 48/80, morphine, eosinophil-derived major basic protein, and substance P, and a variety of IgE-dependent and IgE-independent histamine-releasing factors secreted by mononuclear cells.

MECHANISMS OF ALLERGIC TISSUE INFLAMMATION

IgE-mediated immune responses can be classified chronologically according to three patterns of reaction. First, the **early phase response** is the immediate response after introduction of allergen into target organs typically results from mast cell degranulation accompanied by the release of preformed mediators, occurring within 10 min after allergen exposure and resolving within 1–3 hr. Acute reactions are associated with increased local vascular permeability leading to leakage of plasma proteins, tissue swelling, increased blood flow, as well as itching, sneezing, wheezing, and acute abdominal cramps in the skin, nose, lung, and gastrointestinal tract, respectively (depending on the target organ in which the allergen challenge takes place).

Second, a **late phase response** (LPR) can occur within hours of allergen exposure, reaching a maximum at 6–12 hr and resolving by 24 hr. Clinically, cutaneous LPRs are characterized by edema, redness, and induration; in the nose, by sustained nasal blockage; and in the lung, by additional wheezing. LPRs are associated with the early infiltration of neutrophils and eosinophils followed by basophils, monocytes and macrophages, and Th2-type cells. The recruitment of inflammatory cells from the circulation requires the upregulation of adhesion molecules on their cell surface and their ligand on endothelial cells, which are under the control of cytokines. Several hr after allergen exposure, TNF-α, which is released by activated mast cells, induces the endothelial expression of E-selectin and intercellular (ICAM-1) and vascular (VCAM-1) cell adhesion molecules, which leads to the transendothelial migration of various inflammatory cells. Preferential accumulation of eosinophils occurs through the interactions between selective adhesion molecules on the eosinophil (α4β1 integrin or VLA-4) and VCAM-1 that can be further induced by IL-4 and IL-13 on endothelial cells.

Chemokines are chemotactic cytokines that play a central role in the directed migration of inflammatory cells. RANTES, macrophage inflammatory protein 1α, monocyte chemotactic protein (MCP)-3, and MCP-4 are chemoattractants for eosinophils and mononuclear cells, whereas the eotaxins are relatively selective for eosinophils. These chemoattractants have been detected in epithelium, macrophages, lymphocytes, and eosinophils at sites of LPR and allergic tissue inflammation. Blockage of their action leads to significant reduction in tissue-directed migration of allergic effector cells.

Third, in patients with chronic allergic disease, tissue inflammation can persist for days to years. Several factors contribute to persistent tissue inflammation, including recurrent exposure to allergens and microbial agents with repeated stimulation of allergic effector cells such as mast cells, basophils, eosinophils, and Th2 cells. Th2 type cytokines (IL-3, IL-5, and GM-CSF) secreted during allergic reactions can prolong the survival of allergic effector cells because of delayed apoptosis. There is also evidence for local differentiation of tissue-infiltrating eosinophil precursors induced by IL-5 causing self-generation of eosinophils that contributes to continued damage of local tissue. Tissue remodeling leading to irreversible changes in target organs is also a feature of chronic allergic disease. In asthma, remodeling involves thickening of the airway walls, with increased submucosal tissue and smooth muscle and a decline in lung function with age. In atopic dermatitis, lichenification is an obvious manifestation of skin remodeling.

Studies indicate that Th2 cytokines can not only maintain allergic inflammation but also contribute to tissue remodeling by activating resident cells in target organs: IL-4, Il-9, and IL-13 can induce mucus hypersecretion and metaplasia of mucus cells; IL-4 and IL-13 stimulate fibroblast growth and synthesis of extracellular matrix proteins; and IL-5 and IL-9 increase subepithelial fibrosis. Subepithelial fibrosis can result from transforming growth factor-β produced by eosinophils and fibroblasts. IL-11 expressed by eosinophils and epithelial cells also causes subepithelial fibrosis, enhanced deposition of collagen, and the accumulation of myofibroblasts and fibroblasts. Taken together, once the allergic immune response is established it can be self-perpetuating and lead to chronic disease in genetically predisposed individuals.

GENETIC BASIS OF ATOPY

Atopic diseases have a familial predisposition and a genetic basis. However, sorting out the key genes in multifactorial disorders such as asthma, atopic dermatitis, and allergic rhinitis in which environmental and genetic factors are important has been difficult. It is likely that clinical expression of these diseases results from the complex interaction of many genetic loci and that variation in each of these genes contributes to the diversity of phenotypes observed in each atopic disease. The situation is further complicated by the multiple markers that can overlap for various allergic diseases. For example, atopy is frequently defined by positive immediate prick skin tests and elevated serum IgE levels whereas asthma is characterized by airway hyperresponsiveness. Studies suggest that allergic diseases likely have at least two major groups of genes: genes that control systemic expression of atopy (e.g., increased IgE synthesis and eosinophilia) that are commonly expressed among various allergic diseases and genes that control local inflammatory responses in specific target organs (e.g., the skin in atopic dermatitis or the lung in asthma). For example, genome screens for atopic dermatitis have identified linkage on chromosomes 1q21, 3q21, 17q25, and 20p. These regions correspond closely with

known psoriasis loci. The 1q21 locus is known to contain a cluster of genes influencing epidermal differentiation.

The major approaches used for identification of relevant genes in atopic diseases have included the candidate-gene approach, which depends on the identification of polymorphisms that alter the function or expression of genes known to control atopy or inflammation, and positional cloning, which links the inheritance of specific chromosomal regions with the inheritance of a disease. This is followed by physically mapping the target region to identify genes within it. Candidate genes are then screened for mutations and polymorphisms. Several candidate genes associated with atopic diseases have been identified (Table 130–1). Linkage and strong association have been detected particularly to specific alleles on chromosomes 5, 6, 11, 12, and 14.

Chromosome 5. The 5q23-35 region contains several genes implicated in the pathogenesis of allergic diseases. These include the genes coding for Th2 cytokines (IL-3, IL-4, IL-5, IL-9, IL-13, and GM-CSF). IL-4 has been particularly well studied as a potential candidate gene. A cytosine to thymidine exchange at position 589 of the IL-4 promoter region is associated with the formation of a unique binding site for the transcription factor, nuclear factor for activated T cells (NF-AT), increased IL-4 gene transcription, higher NF-AT binding affinity, and increased IgE production. This is consistent with the important role of IL-4 in the development of Th2 cells and immunoglobulin isotype switching to IgE synthesis. Other genes on this chromosome that may alter allergic responses include leukotriene C4 synthase, M-CSF receptor, the glucocorticoid receptor, and β2-adrenergic receptor.

Chromosome 6. This chromosome contains the genes that code for human leukocyte antigen (HLA) class I and class II molecules, which regulate the specificity and intensity of immune responses to specific allergens. It also includes genes that are central to the process of antigen recognition and presentation, including transporters associated with antigen processing (TAP). IgE responses to specific allergens such as ragweed antigen Amb a V and mite allergen Der p I have been linked to specific MHC class II loci. Of note, TNF-α, a key cytokine that contributes to the influx of inflammatory cells, is also located on chromosome 6. TNF-α polymorphisms have been associated with asthma.

Chromosome 11. Several genome-wide searches have linked atopy to chromosome region 11q13. The gene encoding the β subunit of the high-affinity IgE receptor (FcϵR1-β), which amplifies signal transduction through the high-affinity IgE receptor, has been proposed to be the candidate gene in this

TABLE 130–1. Chromosomal Regions and Candidate Genes in Atopic Disease

Chromosome	Candidate Genes	Potential Function
1	IL-10	Anti-inflammatory cytokine
	IL-12 receptor	Induction of IFN-γ
5q23-35	IL-3, IL-4, IL-5, IL-9, IL-13, GM-CSF	IgE synthesis and Th2 response
	Glucocorticoid receptor	Corticosteroid action
	Leukotriene C4 synthase	Leukotriene production
	β_2-Adrenergic receptor	G protein–coupled β_2-agonist receptor
	M-CSF receptor	Inflammatory modulation
6p21-23	MHC, TAP-1, TAP-2; TNF-α	Antigen presentation; inflammatory cytokine
10q	5-Lipoxygenase	Leukotriene production
11q13	FcϵRI β chain	Signal transduction in basophils, mast cells, and dendritic cells.
12q14-24	IFN-γ, STAT-6; SCF	IL-4 inhibition; IL-4 signaling; mast cell development, proinflammatory
	Nitric oxide synthetase	enzyme
14q11-13	TCR α chains	Peptide MHC interaction
16q11-12	IL-4 receptor	IgE class switching, Th2 response
17p12-q11.2	RANTES, eotaxin	Chemokines

IL = interleukin; GM-CSF = granulocyte-macrophage colony-stimulating factor; M-CSF = macrophage colony-stimulating factor; IFN = interferon; SCF = stem cell factor; MHC = major histocompatibility complex; TAP = transporters involved in antigen processing and presentation; STAT = signal transducer and activator of transcription; TCR = T-cell receptor; TNF = tumor necrosis factor.

region. Several genetic variants of FcεRI-β have been associated with asthma, bronchial hyperreactivity, and atopic dermatitis.

Chromosome 12. Linkage of chromosome 12 to asthma and atopy has been observed. Chromosome 12q contains several candidate genes (IFN-γ, nitric oxide synthetase (NOS), stem cell factor (SCF), STAT-6, insulin-like growth factor-1, and the β subunit of nuclear factor-Y (NFYB), which may contribute to the development of asthma. IFN-γ promotes the development of Th1 cells and inhibits Th2 cell function. STAT-6 is activated by IL-4 and is involved in the induction of IgE isotype switching and Th2 cell differentiation. SCF supports the proliferation and differentiation of mast cells.

Other Chromosomes. Chromosome 14 contains the T-cell receptor α chain, which plays an important role in the recognition of allergens. Significant linkage of IgE responses to several allergens and total serum IgE has been found in certain T cell receptor α serotypes, suggesting that a gene in this region modifies specific IgE responses. An association between atopy and a gain-of-function polymorphism in the α subunit of the IL-4R on chromosome 16 has been found. There has also been evidence for linkage between 17p12-q11.2 regions and asthma, which contain genes coding for the C-C chemokines RANTES and eotaxin that play a critical role in eosinophil recruitment into asthmatic airways.

Another means in which genes may influence the course of allergic diseases such as asthma is by altering treatment responses to medications such as corticosteroids, β_2-adrenergic agents, and leukotriene modifiers. Some studies have found that the glutamate-27 β_2-adrenoceptor polymorphism is associated with less reactive airways in asthma. The glycine-16 form of the β_2-adrenergic receptor has been associated with a nocturnal fall in FEV_1. A promoter polymorphism in the 5-lipoxygenase gene has been reported to alter transcription of this leukotriene-generating enzyme. Finally, an IL-4 promoter polymorphism associated with increased IL-4 gene transcription has been found to be associated with corticosteroid resistance and asthma severity, which is of interest because the combination of IL-2 and IL-4 has been found to induce corticosteroid resistance of T cells.

EPIDEMIOLOGIC TRENDS IN ATOPIC DISEASES

The worldwide prevalence of asthma, atopic dermatitis, and allergic rhinitis has been rising, particularly in Westernized metropolitan areas. Several epidemiologic studies suggest that changes in the infectious environment and in the pattern of microbial exposure of children associated with Westernization are important factors underlying the rising prevalence of atopic disorders over the past few decades in developed countries. Proponents of the "hygiene hypothesis" have suggested that the rise in allergy reflects deprivation of the developing immune system to microbial antigens that are needed for stimulation of Th1 cells.

In Western countries, life style has been associated with cleaner living conditions, fewer siblings, and widespread use of antibiotics for minor illnesses. Antibiotic use among young children may alter the microbial flora in the gastrointestinal tract and produce an environment that is less effective in driving a Th1 response. Consistent with this concept are recent studies demonstrating that 1 yr old infants in countries with a low prevalence of atopy have lactobacilli in their gastrointestinal tract whereas infants in countries with a high prevalence of atopy are colonized less often by lactobacilli and have a higher level of aerobic bacteria such as gram-negative bacilli and *Staphylococcus aureus*. This view is further supported by studies demonstrating that exposure of young children to other children at daycare centers protects against the development of asthma, presumably owing to an increased prevalence of viral infections, which are known to stimulate the Th1 response.

These factors, combined with increased exposure to pollutants and indoor allergens, have been proposed to shift the immune system toward a Th2 phenotype and an increased prevalence of allergic disease. These new insights provide new opportunities for the development of novel immunomodulatory therapies directed at restoring the Th1/Th2 imbalance and reducing inflammation in asthma and other allergic diseases.

Adkinson NF, Bochner BS, Busse WW, et al: *Middleton's Allergy: Principles and Practice*, 6th ed. St. Louis, Mosby/Harcourt, 2002.
Busse WW, Lemanske RF Jr: Asthma. *N Engl J Med* 2001;344:350–62.
Kay AB: Allergy and allergic diseases. *N Engl J Med* 2001;344:30–7.
Romagnani S: The role of lymphocytes in allergic disease. *J Allergy Clin Immunol* 2000;105:399–408.
Schleimer RP, Togias AG: Systemic aspects of allergic inflammatory disease. *J Allergy Clin Immunol* 2000;106:S191–310.

Chapter 131
Diagnosis of Allergic Disease *Dan Atkins and*
Donald Y. M. Leung

Allergic diseases arise from the acute or chronic exposure of a sensitized individual to a specific allergen by inhalation, ingestion, contact, or injection. This results in symptoms that most often involve the nose, eyes, lungs, skin, or gastrointestinal tract either individually or in combination. A carefully obtained history, including environmental exposures, and the appropriate laboratory tests or allergen challenges is critical for an accurate diagnosis.

ALLERGY HISTORY

Obtaining a complete history from the allergic patient involves eliciting a description of all symptoms along with their timing and duration, exposure to common allergens, and responses to previous therapies. Because patients often suffer from more that one allergic disease, the presence or absence of other allergic diseases including allergic rhinitis, allergic conjunctivitis, asthma, urticaria, and atopic dermatitis should be determined. A family history of allergic disease is common because this is one of the most important factors predisposing a child to the development of allergies. Prospective studies suggest that the risk of allergic disease in a child approaches 50% when one parent is allergic and 66% when both parents are allergic.

Several characteristic behaviors are often seen in allergic children. Because of nasal pruritus and rhinorrhea, children with allergic rhinitis often perform the **allergic salute** by rubbing their nose upward with the palm of their hand. This maneuver gives rise to the **nasal crease**, a horizontal skinfold over the bridge of the nose. Characteristic vigorous grinding of the eyes with the thumb and side of the fist is frequently observed in children with allergic conjunctivitis. The **allergic cluck** is produced when the tongue is placed against the roof of the mouth to form a seal and withdrawn rapidly in an effort to scratch the palate. Importantly, the presence of other symptoms such as fever, unilateral nasal obstruction, and purulent nasal discharge suggests other diagnoses.

The timing of onset and the progression of symptoms are relevant. For example, the onset of recurrent or persistent nasal symptoms coinciding with placement in a daycare center might suggest recurrent infection rather than allergy. When patients present with a history of episodic acute symptoms it is important to review the setting in which symptoms occur as well as the activities and exposures that immediately precede their onset.

For example, in the patient whose symptoms are associated with lawn mowing, allergy to grass pollen or fungi is suggested, whereas if the symptoms always occur in homes with pets, then animal dander sensitivity is an obvious consideration. Reproducible reactions after the ingestion of a specific food raise the possibility of food allergy. When symptoms wax and wane but evolve gradually and are more chronic in duration, a closer look at whether the timing and progression of symptoms correlates with exposure to a seasonal aeroallergen is warranted.

Aeroallergens such as pollens or fungal spores are prominent causes of allergic disease whose concentration in outdoor air fluctuates seasonally. Correlating symptoms with the seasonal pollination patterns of indigenous plants along with information provided by local pollen counts can aid in identifying the allergen to which the patient is sensitized. Throughout most of the United States, trees pollinate in the early spring. Grasses pollinate in the late spring and early summer, whereas weeds pollinate in late summer through the fall. The presence of fungal spores in the atmosphere follows a seasonal pattern in the northern United States with spore counts increasing with the onset of warmer weather and peaking in the late summer months only to recede again with the onset of colder weather in the late fall through the winter. In warmer regions of the southern United States fungal spores and grass pollens may cause symptoms on a perennial basis.

Rather than experiencing seasonal symptoms, some patients suffer allergic symptoms year round. In these patients sensitization to sources of perennial allergens usually found indoors such as dust mites, animal dander, cockroaches, and fungi warrants consideration. Species of certain fungi such as *Aspergillus* and *Penicillium* are found indoors, whereas *Alternaria* is found in both indoor and outdoor environments. Cockroach allergens are often problematic in urban, inner city environments. Patients sensitive to perennial allergens often also become sensitized to seasonal allergens and experience baseline symptoms year round with worsening during the spring and fall pollen seasons.

The age of the patient is an important consideration in identifying potential allergens. Infants and young children are first sensitized to allergens that are in their environment on a continuous basis, such as dust mites, animal dander, and fungi. Clinically relevant sensitization to seasonal allergens usually takes several seasons of exposure to develop. Food allergies are more common in infants and young children, resulting primarily in cutaneous, gastrointestinal, and, less frequently, respiratory symptoms.

Complete information from all previous evaluations and prior treatments for allergic disease should be reviewed. A list of the medications used and the response to each should be determined. If allergen immunotherapy was previously administered, the duration of the treatment and its success or lack thereof should be noted. Improvement in symptoms during treatment with medications or therapies used to treat allergic disease provides additional evidence that the symptoms are the result of an allergic process.

A thorough environmental survey should be performed with attention to potential sources of allergen and/or irritant exposure. The age and type of the dwelling, how it is heated and cooled, the use of humidifiers or air filtration units (either central or portable), and any history of flooding or water damage should be noted. Forced hot air heating may repeatedly stir up dust mite, fungi, and animal allergens. The irritant effects of wood burning stoves, fireplaces, and kerosene heaters may provoke respiratory symptoms in allergic patients. Increased humidity or water damage in the home is often associated with increased exposure to dust mites and fungi. Carpeting serves as a reservoir for dust mites, fungi, and animal dander. The number of domestic pets and their movements about the house, including where they sleep, should be ascertained. Special attention should be focused on the bedroom because children spend a significant portion of time there. The age and type of bedding, the number of stuffed animals, window treatments, and accessibility of the room to pets should be reviewed. The number of smokers in the home and where they smoke is useful information. Hobbies that might result in exposure to allergens or respiratory irritants such as paint fumes, cleansers, sawdust, or glues should be identified. Similar information should be obtained in regard to other environments where the child spends large portions of time such as a relative's home, the classroom, or daycare center.

PHYSICAL EXAMINATION

In patients with asthma, a peak flow analysis or spirometry should be performed and the results appraised for evidence of airways obstruction. If respiratory distress is observed, pulse oximetry should be performed. The child presenting with a chief complaint of rhinitis or rhinoconjunctivitis should be watched for mouth breathing, paroxysms of sneezing, sniffing, or rubbing of the nose and eyes. Infants taking a bottle or the breast should be observed for nasal obstruction severe enough to interfere with feeding as well as for evidence of aspiration or gastroesophageal reflux. A mental note should be made of the frequency and nature of coughing that occurs during the interview. A positional increase in coughing or wheezing should be noted. Children with asthma should be observed for congested cough, tachypnea at rest, retractions, or audible wheezes. Patients with atopic dermatitis should be monitored for repetitive scratching and the extent of skin involvement.

Because children with severe asthma as well as those receiving oral corticosteroids may suffer growth suppression, an accurate height should be plotted at regular intervals. Poor weight gain in a child with chronic chest symptoms should prompt consideration of cystic fibrosis. The blood pressure should be obtained to evaluate for steroid-induced hypertension. The patient with acute asthma may present with pulsus paradoxus, defined as a drop in systolic blood pressure during inspiration more than 10 mm Hg. Moderate to severe airways obstruction is indicated by a decrease of more than 20 mm Hg. An increased heart rate may be the result of an asthma flare or the use of a β-agonist or decongestant. Fever is not caused by allergy alone and should prompt consideration of an infectious process.

Parents of allergic children are often concerned about a blue-gray to purple discoloration beneath the lower eyelids attributed to venous stasis and referred to as **allergic shiners**. They are found in up to 60% of allergic patients and almost 40% of patients without allergic disease. They are often accompanied by **Dennie lines** (Dennie-Morgan folds), which are prominent symmetric skinfolds that extend in an arc from the inner canthus beneath and parallel to the lower lid margin.

In most patients with allergic conjunctivitis, involvement of the eyes is usually bilateral. Examination of the conjunctiva reveals varying degrees of conjunctival injection and edema. In severe cases, periorbital edema may be observed involving primarily the lower eyelids. The classic discharge associated with allergic conjunctivitis is usually described as "stringy" or "ropy." In children with vernal conjunctivitis, examination of the tarsal conjunctiva may reveal cobblestoning. Children repeatedly receiving large doses of oral corticosteroids for management of severe asthma are at risk for developing posterior subcapsular cataracts. Keratoconus, which is protrusion of the cornea, may occur in patients with atopic dermatitis as a result of repeated trauma produced by persistent rubbing of the eyes.

The external ear should be examined for eczematous changes in patients with atopic dermatitis. Because otitis media with effusion is common in children with allergic rhinitis, pneumatic otoscopic examination of the ear should be performed to evaluate for the presence of fluid in the middle ear and to exclude infection.

Examination of the nose in allergic patients often reveals the presence of a transverse nasal crease on top of the nose at the junction of the cartilaginous and bony portions of the nasal bridge caused by frequent rubbing of the nose. Nasal patency should be assessed and the nose examined for structural abnormalities affecting nasal airflow such as a septal deviation, turbinate hypertrophy, septal spurs, or nasal polyps. A decreased or absent sense of smell should raise concern about the presence of nasal polyps, a feature of cystic fibrosis. The nasal mucosa in allergic rhinitis is classically described as pale to purple in comparison to the beefy red mucosa of patients with nonallergic rhinitis. Allergic nasal secretions are typically thin and clear. Purulent secretions suggest another cause of rhinitis. The frontal and maxillary sinuses should be palpated to identify tenderness to pressure that might be associated with sinusitis.

Examination of the lips may reveal cheilitis caused by drying of the lips from continuous mouth breathing and repeated licking of the lips in an attempt to replenish moisture and relieve discomfort. Tonsillar and adenoidal hypertrophy along with a history of impressive snoring suggests the possibility of obstructive sleep apnea. The posterior pharynx should be examined for the presence of postnasal drip and posterior pharyngeal lymphoid hyperplasia.

Chest findings in asthmatic children vary significantly depending on disease duration, severity, and activity. In a child with mild or well-controlled asthma, the chest may appear entirely normal on examination between asthma exacerbations. However, examination of the same child during an acute episode of asthma may reveal tachypnea, cyanosis, use of accessory muscles, wheezing, and decreased air exchange with a prolonged expiratory time. Tachycardia may be caused by the asthma exacerbation or be accompanied by jitteriness and caused by treatment with β_2-agonists. Decreased airflow or rhonchi and wheezes over the right chest may be noted in children with mucus plugging and right middle lobe atelectasis. Unilateral wheezing after an episode of coughing and choking in a small child without a history of previous respiratory illness suggests aspiration of a foreign body. Wheezing limited to the larynx in association with inspiratory stridor is seen in older children and adolescents with vocal cord dysfunction. In children with chronic asthma an increased anteroposterior diameter of the chest suggests significant air trapping. In infants and younger children with significant asthma a groove along the lower ribs at the site of attachment of the diaphragm may be present. Digital clubbing is rarely seen in patients with uncomplicated asthma and should prompt further evaluation to rule out other potential diagnoses.

The skin of the allergic patient should be examined for evidence of urticaria/angioedema or atopic dermatitis. **Xerosis**, or dry skin, is the most common skin abnormality of allergic children. **Keratosis pilaris**, often found on the extensor surfaces of the upper arms and thighs, is characterized by roughness of the skin caused by keratin plugs lodged in the openings of hair follicles. Examination of the skin of the palms and feet reveals exaggerated palmar and plantar creases in some allergic children.

DIAGNOSTIC TESTING

The laboratory evaluation of the child suspected of having allergic disease should focus on obtaining objective evidence to support the diagnosis, documenting sensitivity to allergens implicated by the history, and ruling out other potential diagnoses.

In Vitro Tests. Allergic diseases are often associated with increased numbers of eosinophils circulating in the peripheral blood and invading the tissues and secretions of target organs. Eosinophilia, generally defined as the presence of more than 450 eosinophils/μL of blood, is the most common abnormality

noted on examination of the blood of allergic patients. Seasonal increases in the number of circulating eosinophils may be observed in sensitized patients after exposure to allergens such as tree, grass, and weed pollens. The number of circulating eosinophils can be suppressed by certain infections and the systemic administration of corticosteroids. In certain pathologic conditions such as drug reactions or eosinophilic pneumonias, significantly increased numbers of eosinophils may be present in the target organ in the absence of peripheral blood eosinophilia. Increased numbers of eosinophils are observed in a wide variety of disorders in addition to allergy (Box 131–1).

Nasal and bronchial secretions are often examined for the presence of eosinophils. The presence of eosinophils in the

---

BOX 131–1. Differential Diagnosis of Childhood Eosinophilia

PHYSIOLOGIC
Prematurity
Infant hyperalimentation
Familial

INFECTIOUS
Parasitic (with tissue-invasive helminths, e.g., trichinosis, strongyloidiasis, pneumocystosis, filariasis, cysticercosis, cutaneous and visceral larva migrans, echinococcosis)
Bacterial (e.g., brucellosis, tularemia, cat-scratch disease, *Chlamydia*)
Fungal (histoplasmosis, blastomycosis, coccidioidomycosis, allergic bronchopulmonary aspergillosis)
Mycobacterial (tuberculosis, leprosy)
Viral (hepatitis A, hepatitis B, hepatitis C, Epstein-Barr virus)

PULMONARY
Allergic (rhinitis, asthma)
Löeffler syndrome
Hypersensitivity pneumonitis
Eosinophilic pneumonia
Pulmonary interstitial eosinophilia

DERMATOLOGIC
Atopic dermatitis
Pemphigus
Dermatitis herpetiformis
Infantile eosinophilic pustular folliculitis
Episodic angioedema and urticaria
Eosinophilic fasciitis (Schulman syndrome)
Eosinophilic cellulitis (Well syndrome)
Kimura disease

ONCOLOGIC
Neoplasm (lung, gastrointestinal, uterine)
Hodgkin disease
Leukemia
Myelofibrosis

IMMUNOLOGIC
T-cell immunodeficiencies
Hyper IgE (Job) syndrome
Wiskott-Aldrich syndrome
Graft versus host disease
Drug hypersensitivity
Post irradiation
Post splenectomy

ENDOCRINE
Post adrenalectomy
Addison disease
Panhypopituitarism

CARDIOVASCULAR
Löeffler disease (fibroplastic endocarditis)
Congenital heart disease
Hypersensitivity vasculitis

GASTROINTESTINAL
Milk protein allergy
Inflammatory bowel disease
Eosinophilic esophagitis
Eosinophilic gastroenteritis

sputum of asthmatic patients is a classic finding. Increased numbers of eosinophils in smears of nasal mucus stained with Hansel stain is a more sensitive indicator of nasal allergies than peripheral blood eosinophilia and aids in distinguishing allergic rhinitis from other causes of rhinitis. In young children, nasal eosinophilia is defined as the presence of more than 4% eosinophils in nasal mucus smears, whereas a finding of more than 10% eosinophils is required in adolescents and adults. Nasal mucus eosinophilia also has therapeutic implications, predicting a higher probability of responsiveness to topical nasal corticosteroid sprays.

An elevated IgE level is often found in the serum of allergic patients, because IgE is the primary antibody associated with allergic reactions. IgE levels are measured in international units (IU), with 1 IU equal to 2.4 ng of IgE. Maternal IgE does not cross the placenta and, although the fetus is capable of producing IgE as early as the 11th week of gestation, infants in developed countries produce little IgE in utero owing to the lack of stimulation by allergens. Serum IgE levels gradually rise over the first years of life to peak in the teen years and decrease steadily thereafter. A variety of factors in addition to age, such as genetic influences, race, gender, certain diseases, and exposure to cigarette smoke and allergens, affect serum IgE levels. Serum IgE levels may increase 2- to 4-fold in allergic patients during and immediately after the pollen season, then gradually decline until the next pollen season. Comparison of total serum IgE levels among patients with allergic disease reveals that those with atopic dermatitis tend to have the highest levels, whereas patients with allergic asthma generally have higher levels than those with allergic rhinitis. Although average total serum IgE levels are higher in populations of allergic patients than in comparable populations without allergic disease, the overlap in levels is such that the diagnostic value of a total serum IgE level is poor. For example, approximately one half of patients with allergic disease have a total serum IgE level in the normal range. However, total serum IgE measurement is indicated when the diagnosis of allergic bronchopulmonary aspergillosis is suspected; total serum IgE concentration greater than 1,000 ng/mL is a criterion for diagnosis of this disorder. Continued monitoring of the total serum IgE in patients with allergic bronchopulmonary aspergillosis is encouraged because serum IgE levels decrease with appropriate therapy and rise again during exacerbations of the disease. The total serum IgE level is also elevated in several nonallergic diseases (Box 131–2).

The presence of IgE specific for a particular allergen can be documented in vivo by skin testing or in vitro by the measurement of allergen-specific IgE levels in the serum (Table 131–1). The most widely employed test for documenting the presence of allergen-specific IgE in the serum is the **radioallergosorbent test (RAST)**. In this test the allergens of an individual allergen extract are bound to a solid phase support. A small amount of the patient's serum is incubated with the allergen-coated support, and any IgE in the patient's serum specific for those allergens binds to them on the support. After rinsing, the allergen-coated support to which the patient's allergen-specific IgE is bound is incubated with radiolabeled antihuman-IgE, which then binds to the patient's allergen-specific IgE. Excess radiolabeled antihuman-IgE is rinsed away and the amount of radioactivity associated with the support to which allergen, the patient's allergen-specific IgE, and radiolabeled antihuman-IgE are attached is measured. Over the years improvements in the assay for allergen-specific IgE have included modification of the solid phase supports to enhance binding of allergen, substituting enzymes for the radiolabels on antihuman-IgE to increase the accuracy of detection while also providing a more stable reagent, and a switch to calibration curves based on known quantities of IgE resulting in quantitative rather than qualitative reporting of results.

The primary advantages of these assays in comparison to allergen skin testing are their safety and that the results are not influenced by skin disease or medications. Overall, the results of these tests correlate well with those obtained by skin testing and provocation challenges; however, the RAST is not as sensitive as the skin test. As a result, in patients with histories of life-threatening reactions to foods, insect stings, drugs, or latex, skin testing is still required because of its higher sensitivity even if the RAST is negative.

In Vivo Tests. Allergen skin testing is the primary in vivo procedure for the diagnosis of allergic disease. Mast cells with allergen-specific IgE antibodies attached to high-affinity receptors on

---

■ BOX 131–2. Nonallergic Diseases Associated with Increased Serum IgE Concentrations

PARASITIC INFESTATIONS
Ascariasis
Capillariasis
Echinococcosis
Fascioliasis
Filariasis
Hookworm
Onchocerciasis
Paragonimiasis
Schistosomiasis
Strongyloidiasis
Trichinosis
Visceral larva migrans

INFECTIONS
Allergic bronchopulmonary aspergillosis
Candidiasis, systemic
Coccidioidomycosis
Cytomegalovirus mononucleosis
Infectious mononucleosis (Epstein-Barr virus)
Leprosy

IMMUNODEFICIENCY
Hyper IgE (Job) syndrome

IgA deficiency, selective
Nezelof syndrome
Thymic hypoplasia (DiGeorge anomaly)
Wiskott-Aldrich syndrome

NEOPLASTIC DISEASES
Hodgkin disease
IgE myeloma

OTHER DISEASES AND DISORDERS
Burns
Cystic fibrosis
Dermatitis, chronic acral
Erythema nodosum, streptococcal
Guillain-Barré syndrome
Hemosiderosis, primary pulmonary
Intestinal nephritis, drug-induced
Kawasaki disease
Liver disease
Pemphigus, bullous
Polyarteritis nodosa, infantile
Rheumatoid arthritis

Ig = immunoglobulin.

TABLE 131–1. Determination of Specific IgE by Radioallergosorbent Test[*] and Skin Testing

Variable	Skin Test	Radioallergosorbent Test
Risk of allergic reaction	Yes	No
Sensitive[†]	Very	Less
Affected by antihistamines	Yes	No
Affected by corticosteroids	Usually not	No
Affected by extensive dermatitis or dermographism	Yes	No
Convenience, less patient anxiety	No	Yes
Broad selection of antigens	Yes	No
Immediate results	Yes	No
Expensive	No	Yes
Semiquantitative	No	Yes
Lability of allergens	Yes	No
Results evident to patient	Yes	No

[*]Radioallergosorbent test as example of other in vitro tests.
[†]Because skin tests are more sensitive, they are more reliable than RAST in confirming life-threatening anaphylactic conditions if maximal sensitivity is required (e.g., penicillin, Hymenoptera hypersensitivity).

their surface reside in the skin of allergic patients. The introduction of minute amounts of an allergen to which the patient is allergic into the skin results in cross-linking by the allergen of allergen-specific IgE antibodies on the mast cell surface, thereby triggering mast cell activation. Once activated, these mast cells release a variety of preformed and newly generated mediators that act on surrounding tissues. Histamine is the mediator most responsible for the immediate wheal and flare reactions observed in skin testing. Examination of the site of a positive skin test reveals a pruritic wheal surrounded by an area of erythema. The time course of these reactions is rapid in onset, reaching a peak within approximately 20 min and usually resolving over the next 20–30 min. However, in some patients a larger area of less distinctly demarcated edema on an erythematous base develops at the skin test site over the next 6–12 hr. This reaction is referred to as a **late-phase response** and usually resolves by 24 hr. Biopsy of the site of a late-phase response reveals the presence of an inflammatory infiltrate consisting of T cells, neutrophils, and eosinophils. These reactions are thought to be similar to the late-phase responses observed in other organs such as the nose and lungs after provocation challenges.

Skin testing in children is usually first performed using the prick/puncture technique. With this technique a small drop of allergen is applied to the skin surface and a tiny amount is introduced into the epidermis by lightly pricking or puncturing the skin through the drop of extract with a small needle. When the prick/puncture skin test is negative and the history is suggestive, selective skin testing using the intradermal technique may be performed. This technique involves using a 26-gauge needle to inject 0.01–0.02 mL of a dilute allergen extract into the dermis of the arm. This technique is more sensitive than the prick/puncture technique and the allergen extracts used are 1,000- to 100-fold less concentrated than extracts used for prick/puncture testing. Intradermal skin tests are not recommended for use with food allergens because of the risk of triggering anaphylaxis. Irritant rather than allergic reactions can occur with intradermal skin testing if higher concentrations of extracts such as 1:100 weight/volume are used. Although less sensitive than intradermal skin tests, positive prick/puncture skin tests tend to correlate better with symptoms on natural exposure to the allergen.

Panels of skin tests are often applied that include the appropriate allergens for a given geographic area in addition to common indoor allergens; however, the number of skin tests performed should be individualized, taking into account the allergens suggested by the history. A positive and negative control skin test, using histamine and saline, respectively, is performed with each set of skin tests. A negative control is necessary to ensure that the patient is not dermatographic and that reactions caused merely by applying pressure to overly sensitive skin are not interpreted as due to allergen sensitivity. A positive control is necessary to establish the presence of a cutaneous response to histamine. Medications with antihistaminic properties in addition to adrenergic agents such as ephedrine and epinephrine have been demonstrated to suppress skin test responses and should be avoided for appropriate intervals before the placement of skin tests. Prolonged courses of systemic corticosteroids may suppress cutaneous reactivity by decreasing the number of tissue mast cells as well as their ability to release mediators.

Under certain circumstances, provocation testing is performed to examine the association between allergen exposure and the development of symptoms. Provocation challenges involving exposure of the skin, conjunctiva, nasal mucosa, oral mucosa, gastrointestinal tract, and lungs to allergens have been performed in a variety of clinical and research settings. Bronchial provocation challenges have been performed by having patients inhale increasingly concentrated solutions of nebulized allergen extracts and monitoring for airways obstruction by clinical observation and the performance of pulmonary function testing. In most studies the results of bronchial provocation challenges have correlated well with other clinical data obtained by skin testing and/or the performance of in vitro testing. Although a large number of bronchial provocation challenges to allergens have been performed safely, the possibility of a severe reaction and the time, expense, and expertise required for the performance of these tests limit their performance to a research setting.

Currently, the bronchial provocation test most frequently performed is to methacholine, which causes potent bronchoconstriction of asthmatic but not of normal airways. **Methacholine challenge testing** is performed to document the presence and degree of bronchial hyperreactivity in a patient suspected of having asthma. After baseline spirometry is obtained, increasing concentrations of nebulized methacholine are inhaled until a specified drop in lung function, such as a 20% decrease in FEV_1, occurs or the patient is able to tolerate the inhalation of a set concentration of methacholine, such as 25 mg/mL, without a significant decrease in lung function.

Oral food challenges are performed to determine if a specific food causes symptoms or if a suspected food can be added to the diet. Food challenges are performed to those foods incriminated by the history and results of skin tests and/or in vitro testing. These challenges may be performed in an open, single-blind, double-blind, or double-blind placebo-controlled fashion and involve the ingestion of gradually increasing amounts of the suspected food at set time intervals until the patient either experiences a reaction or tolerates a normal portion of the food openly. Because of the potential for significant allergic reactions, these challenges should only be performed in an appropriately equipped facility with personnel experienced in the performance of food challenges and the treatment of anaphylaxis, including cardiopulmonary resuscitation.

Beltrani VS: The clinical spectrum of atopic dermatitis. *J Allergy Clin Immunol* 1999; 104:S87–96.
Chusid MJ: Eosinophilia in childhood. *Immunol Allergy Clin North Am* 1999; 19:327–46.
Middleton E, Reed CE, Ellis EF, et al (editors): *Allergy: Principles & Practice*, 5th ed. Philadelphia, WB Saunders, 1998.
Ownby DR: Skin tests in comparison with other diagnostic methods. *Immunol Allergy Clin North Am* 2001;21:355–67.
Tripathi A, Patterson R: Clinical interpretation of skin test results. *Immunol Allergy Clin North Am* 2001;21:291–300.

Chapter 132
Principles of Treatment of Allergic Disease *Dan Atkins and*

Donald Y. M. Leung

The basic principles of the treatment of allergic disease include the avoidance of exposure to allergens and irritants that trigger symptoms and the pharmacologic management of symptoms caused by inadvertent acute and chronic allergen exposures. In selected patients with allergic disease refractory to avoidance measures and optimal pharmacologic management, allergen immunotherapy may be considered.

ENVIRONMENTAL CONTROL MEASURES

Children spend the majority of their time in indoor environments, including their home, a school or daycare center, and the homes of friends and relatives. Over the years in an effort to save energy, houses and buildings have been built tighter and more insulated with fewer air exchanges over a given period. These changes have led to an increase in indoor humidity and higher concentrations of allergens and irritants in indoor air. Examination of indoor environments by epidemiologic studies in a variety of geographic areas suggests that house dust mite, cat, and cockroach allergens are the most common significant triggers of allergic disease in these settings, but exposures to allergens from other pets, pests, fungi, and respiratory irritants such as cigarette smoke can also be a problem.

Over 30,000 species of mites have been identified, but the term **dust mites** usually refers only to the pyroglyphid mites *Dermatophagoides pteronyssinus*, *Dermatophagoides farinae*, and *Euroglyphus maynei*, which are the major sources of allergen in house dust. Respiration and water vapor exchange occurs through the skin of dust mites, rendering them sensitive to decreases in humidity and temperature extremes. The regular use of humidifiers and swamp coolers has been shown to promote dust mite survival. Mites do not survive when the relative humidity drops below 50%. They feed on animal and human skin scales and other debris, which is why they exist in large numbers in mattresses and bedding as well as in carpet and upholstered furniture. They are also found in flour and mixes for baked goods. Several reports have described anaphylaxis following the ingestion of baked goods such as waffles and pancakes prepared with flour infested with dust mites. Dust mite fecal pellets are a major source of allergens. They consist of partially digested food combined with digestive enzymes encased in a permeable membrane, which keeps the fecal pellets intact. These fecal pellets have been likened to pollen grains given their similarities in size (10–40 μm), the amount of allergen they contain, and their ability to rapidly release allergens on contact with moist mucous membranes. Mites can persist in imported furnishings for at least 2 yr, and mite allergens have been shown to remain stable under domestic conditions for periods of at least 4 yr. Most studies have suggested that minimal dust mite allergen becomes airborne during normal household activities and that a vigorous disturbance such as vacuuming without a vacuum bag or shaking a bed sheet is required to launch significant amounts of dust mite allergens into the air. Once airborne, dust mite allergen particles tend to settle out of the air relatively rapidly because of their size and weight. Nonetheless, dust mite allergen exposure likely occurs during sleep on mite-infested pillows and mattresses and during normal household activities when dust mite concentrations in the home are high enough. Studies examining concentrations of dust mite allergens in samples of settled house dust demonstrate that levels as low as 2 μg of dust mite allergen per gram of house dust can lead to sensitization, whereas levels of 10 μg per gram of house dust have been associated with the development of symptoms.

Appropriate environmental control measures can significantly reduce exposure to dust mite allergens. Major emphasis should be placed on reducing exposure to dust mite allergens in the bedroom and the bed because of the large amount of time children spend there. Encasements impermeable to dust mite allergens should be placed on all pillows, the mattress, and the box spring. Dust should be removed from the surface of these covers and the bed frame by vacuuming them weekly. The sheets and mattress pad should be washed weekly in hot water at a temperature hotter than 130°F. Minimizing the number of items in the room that collect dust such as books, drapes, toys, stuffed animals, and any clutter is recommended. Major reservoirs of dust mite allergen often more difficult to deal with include the carpet and upholstered furniture. These should be vacuumed weekly with an efficient double-bagged vacuum cleaner. Although the application of acaricides or denaturing agents to carpets and upholstered furniture has been advised, the actual benefit remains unclear and the amount of effort required may be more than most families are willing to invest. If possible, carpet removal, at least in the bedroom, may prove a better choice for eliminating a large reservoir of dust mite allergen. Other measures for dust mite allergen control include maintaining the indoor relative humidity less than 50% and keeping the air conditioning set at the lowest level during the warmer months.

In many countries more than half of the households have pets, the most common of which are cats and dogs. Cats are considered to be more sensitizing than dogs. With cats, dogs, horses, and cattle the major sources of allergens are hair, dander, and saliva, whereas the major source of rodent allergens is their urine. Studies of airborne cat allergen have shown that a significant portion is found on small particles that behave aerodynamically like spheres of less than 7 μm in diameter. As much as 30% of airborne cat allergen may reside on particles less than 5 μm. Particles this small may not be adequately filtered by the nose and could potentially be deposited in the airways. Their small size enables these particles to remain airborne for longer periods and to be suspended repeatedly by air currents from heating and ventilation systems or just by walking across the carpet or sitting in an upholstered chair. **Fel d 1,** the major cat allergen, is a highly charged protein that readily sticks to a variety of surfaces, including walls, carpeting, and upholstered furniture. Because of this adhesiveness cat allergens bind to their owner's clothing and are routinely transported to public buildings, including schools, where they have been measured in moderately high amounts. From these sites significant amounts of cat allergen can subsequently be carried into homes without cats. Analysis of house dust from homes with cats reveals levels of Fel d 1 ranging from 8 μg–1.5 mg/g of house dust. Levels of Fel d 1 in homes without cats vary from 0.2–80 μg/g of house dust. Sensitization to cat allergen has been associated with levels ranging from 1–8 μg/g of house dust. Carpets, upholstered furniture, and bedding serve as reservoirs of cat allergens, resulting in the persistence of significant amounts in the home for months after a cat has been removed. Complete avoidance of cat allergen is virtually impossible, although significant reduction in exposure to cat allergens is achievable.

Removing the pet from the home is obviously the most effective means of reducing exposure to animal allergens, although it has been demonstrated that without other interventions, such as removing carpeting and upholstered furniture and wiping down walls, it takes 6 mo or more for the levels of cat allergen to drop to a level found in houses without a cat. As a result, cat owners who remove their pets from their homes should be informed not to expect immediate results. Unfortunately, advice to remove a pet from the home or keep it outdoors is often ignored. In contrast to dust mite allergens, cat allergen is light and remains suspended in the air for long periods of time. As a result, HEPA-filtered air cleaners are helpful in reducing the amount of airborne cat allergen. Other suggested methods include washing the cat regularly and maintaining a cat allergen free bedroom from which the cat is excluded and where mattress covers and air-filtering devices are used. The cat should also be restricted from other living areas where the sensitized child spends large amounts of time, such as the family room or other play areas. Regular vacuuming with a HEPA-filtered and double-thickness bag vacuum cleaner is also encouraged. Similar measures are suggested for the control of exposure to other animal allergens, although whether these measures reduce exposure to levels resulting in clinical improvement as demonstrated by decreased symptoms, improved peak flows, or decreases in bronchial hyperreactivity remains to be documented by appropriately controlled studies.

Infestation of the home by insects and other pests such as mice and rats is another potential source of significant allergen exposure in the indoor environment. Studies have identified the importance of exposure to cockroach allergens as a major risk factor for the development of asthma in inner-city children. Once sensitized, inner-city cockroach-sensitive asthmatic children with continued exposure to high levels of cockroach allergens in their bedrooms are at higher risk for urgent care visits and hospitalization than inner-city asthmatic children who are not allergic to cockroaches. Recommended methods to decrease cockroach allergen exposure include reducing access to the home by sealing cracks in the flooring and walls and removing sources of food and water by repairing leaky pipes, putting away food, and frequent cleaning. Regular extermination using baits or chemical treatment of infested areas is also advised.

Efforts to improve indoor air quality should also encompass reducing exposure to respiratory irritants. Passive exposure to environmental tobacco smoke has been shown to worsen asthma and increase nasal symptoms in patients with allergic nasal disease. As a result, smoking cessation should be repeatedly encouraged and smoking indoors should never be permitted. The use of wood-burning stoves and fireplaces and kerosene heaters should be discouraged.

Although exposure to pollens and fungi primarily occurs outdoors, these allergens are detectable indoors during the warmer months when their levels indoors often reflect their prevalence in the outdoor environment. During the winter when the outdoor levels of other fungi are lowest, the indoor fungi *Aspergillus* and *Penicillium* are the most prevalent. Fungi are often found in damp basements and thrive in conditions associated with increased moisture in the home, such as water leaks, flooding, or increased humidity promoted by the excessive use of humidifiers or swamp coolers. As a result, exposure to indoor fungal allergens can be reduced by maintaining the indoor relative humidity less than 50%, removing contaminated carpets, and wiping down washable surfaces prone to fungal growth such as shower stalls, shower curtains, sinks, drip trays, and garbage pails with solutions of detergent and 5% bleach. Dehumidifiers should be placed in damp basements. Standing water at any site in the home should be eliminated and the cause addressed. Removing all items from the home that are prone to fungal contamination and growth is also encouraged. Keeping the windows and doors closed and using air conditioning to filter outdoor air can keep both indoor pollen and fungi levels to a minimum during the warmer months when outdoor levels of these allergens are at their peak. The use of window or attic fans is to be avoided. Laundry should be dried in a dryer rather than on a clothesline. Measures to avoid pollens and fungal spores when out of the house include closing the windows and using the air conditioner when traveling in the car, avoiding moldy vegetation, and wearing a mask when these materials cannot be avoided. Outdoor activities during periods of high pollen counts should be kept to a minimum. Someone other than the sensitized patient should mow the lawn and rake leaves. Frequent hand washing after outdoor play is suggested to avoid transferring pollens from the hands to the eyes and nose. At the end of the day, showering and shampooing is suggested to avoid contamination of the bed with allergens. During the day, the bed should remain covered with a bedspread.

PHARMACOLOGIC THERAPY

Adrenergic Agents. Adrenergic agents exert their effects through the stimulation of cell surface α- and β-adrenergic receptors in a variety of target tissues. These receptors belong to the G protein–coupled superfamily of receptors. In general, α-adrenergic receptor stimulation results in excitatory responses such as vasoconstriction, whereas β-adrenergic stimulation leads to inhibitory responses such as bronchodilation. The α-adrenergic receptors have been classified into α_1- and α_2-adrenergic receptors. Further studies of these receptors in humans have identified three subtypes of α_1-adrenergic receptors and three subtypes of α_2-adrenergic receptors. The β-adrenergic receptors are further divided into three subtypes: β_1, β_2, and β_3. Each of these adrenergic receptors exhibits a distinctive tissue distribution. The physiologic response in a given tissue to the administration of an adrenergic agent depends on the specific receptor binding characteristics of the drug as well as the number and distribution of the various types of adrenergic receptors in the tissue. Epinephrine, the initial adrenergic drug used in Western medicine, remains the drug of choice for the treatment of anaphylaxis because of its combined α- and β-adrenergic effects.

The α-adrenergic agents are effective in the treatment of allergic nasal disease because of their decongestant effects. In the nose, stimulation of α_1-adrenergic receptors on postcapillary venules and α_2-adrenergic receptors on precapillary arterioles leads to vasoconstriction, resulting in a reduction in nasal congestion. The oral decongestants used clinically include pseudoephedrine, phenylephrine, and phenylpropanolamine. They are available individually or in combination with antihistamines in liquid and tablet forms, including sustained-release preparations. Pseudoephedrine and phenylpropanolamine are rapidly and thoroughly absorbed, whereas phenylephrine, the less effective of the three drugs, is incompletely absorbed, resulting in a significantly lower bioavailability of approximately 38%. Peak plasma concentrations of these drugs are reached between 30 min and 2 hr of administration, but the decongestant effect has not been directly correlated to the plasma concentration. Pseudoephedrine and phenylpropanolamine are excreted essentially unchanged by the kidney. The use of oral decongestants should be avoided in patients with hypertension, coronary artery disease, glaucoma, or metabolic disorders such as diabetes or hyperthyroidism. Reported adverse effects of oral decongestants include excitability, headache, nervousness, palpitations, tachycardia, arrhythmias, hypertension, nausea, vomiting, and urinary retention. Decongestants available as topical nasal sprays include phenylephrine, oxymetazoline, naphthazoline, tetrahydrozoline, and xylometazoline. Given their efficacy and rapid onset of action, the potential for excessive use of topical nasal decongestants resulting in rebound nasal congestion is high. When this occurs, refraining from the use of these sprays for 2–3 days is necessary for recovery.

Drugs that stimulate β-adrenergic receptors have been used for years in the treatment of asthma because of their potent bronchodilator effects. The subclassification of β-adrenergic receptors into β_1 and β_2 subtypes led to the development of drugs selective for the β_2-adrenergic receptor that have the advantage of producing significant bronchodilation with less cardiac stimulation. In addition to their bronchodilating effects, β_2-adrenergic agonists have been reported to improve mucociliary clearance, decrease microvascular permeability, inhibit cholinergic nerve transmission, and reduce mediator release in mast cells, basophils, and eosinophils. The β-adrenergic agonists can be delivered orally, by inhalation, or by injection. The inhaled route is generally preferred because of the rapid onset of action and fewer adverse effects. Reported adverse effects of β-adrenergics agents include tremor, palpitations, tachycardia, arrhythmias, central nervous system stimulation, hyperglycemia, hypokalemia, hypomagnesemia, and a transient increase in hypoxia, which is attributed to an increase in perfusion to inadequately ventilated areas of the asthmatic lung.

Anticholinergic Agents. These drugs inhibit vagally mediated reflexes by antagonizing the action of acetylcholine at muscarinic receptors. Of the available anticholinergic agents, ipratropium bromide is the most commonly used. It is a quaternary amine that is poorly absorbed across mucosal surfaces and does not readily cross the blood-brain barrier. As a bronchodilator, it has a slower onset of action than short-acting inhaled β_2-agonists and takes longer to reach maximal effect, which makes it less effective as a rescue medication. Ipratropium is available by prescription as a metered-dose inhaler delivering 18 μg/spray and as a 0.02% nebulized solution (500 μg/2.5 mL). Inhaled anticholinergics have very few adverse effects, although they occasionally trigger coughing.

Ipratropium given as a nasal spray (0.03–0.06%) has been shown to be effective in the reduction of rhinorrhea resulting from perennial nonallergic rhinitis, the common cold, or other triggers such as exposure to irritants or cold air. The use of ipratropium is limited in the treatment of moderate to severe allergic rhinitis because it does not alter other common allergic nasal symptoms, such as sneezing, nasal congestion, or pruritus. Nasal dryness and epistaxis are occasionally encountered with use of the nasal spray.

Antihistamines. The release of histamine and its effects on surrounding tissues is central to the development of the symptoms classically associated with the allergic response. As a result, antihistamines are frequently used medications for the treatment of allergic disease. Histamine exerts its effects through binding with one of its three receptors, referred to as H_1-, H_2-, or H_3-receptors. Histamine effects triggered through H_1-receptor binding are those most relevant to allergic inflammation and include pain, pruritus, vasodilation, increased vascular permeability, smooth muscle contraction, mucus production, and the stimulation of parasympathetic nerve endings and reflexes. The human H_1-receptor gene has been mapped to the distal short arm of chromosome 3. The antimuscarinic effect of some of the early H_1-type antihistamines may be explained by the reported 45% homology of the H_1-receptor with the human muscarinic receptor. The H_1-type antihistamines prevent the effects of H_1-receptor activation through reversible, competitive inhibition of histamine by binding to the H_1-receptor. As a result, antihistamines work best in preventing rather than reversing the actions of histamine and are most effective when given at doses and dosing intervals resulting in the persistent saturation of target organ tissue histamine receptors.

The H_1-type antihistamines are traditionally divided into six classes based on differences in their chemical structures (Table 132–1). These antihistamines are further divided into 1st-generation antihistamines, which, because of their lipophilicity, cross the blood-brain barrier to exert effects on the central nervous system, and 2nd-generation antihistamines, which exert minimal, if any, central nervous system effects because of their inability to cross the blood-brain barrier owing to their size, charge, and lipophobicity. The sedative effects and cognitive impairment associated with the use of 1st-generation antihistamines are well documented. Thus, one of the primary advantages of 2nd-generation antihistamines is that they are nonsedating or much less so than 1st-generation antihista-

TABLE 132–1. Classification of Antihistamines (H1-antagonists)

Class	Examples
Ethylenediamines	
First generation	Antazoline, pyrilamine, tripelennamine
Type II ethanolamines	
First generation	Carbinoxamine, clemastine, diphenhydramine
Type III alkylamines	
First generation	Brompheniramine, chlorpheniramine, triprolidine
Second generation	Acrivastine
Type IV piperazines	
First generation	Cyclizine, hydroxyzine, meclizine
Second generation	Cetirizine
Type V piperidines	
First generation	Azatadine, cyproheptadine
Second generation	Fexofenadine, loratadine
Type VI phenothiazines	
First generation	Methdilazine, promethazine

mines. Both 1st- and 2nd-generation antihistamines are available in oral preparations. A number of 1st-generation antihistamines are available over the counter whereas other 1st-generation and all 2nd-generation antihistamines currently require a prescription. The only antihistamine available as an intranasal spray is azelastine. The benefit of this form of administration is the potential for a rapid onset of action within 15–30 min. Azelastine, which is systemically absorbed and can cross the blood-brain barrier, has been shown to cause central nervous system effects in some patients and is not currently approved for use in children younger than 12 yr of age.

Orally administered antihistamines are well absorbed, reaching peak serum concentrations within approximately 2 hr. High tissue concentrations of antihistamines are usually achieved, which likely accounts for the sustained suppression of wheal and flare reactions even after serum levels have significantly declined. Most antihistamines are metabolized by the hepatic cytochrome P450 enzyme system. As a result, elimination of antihistamines may be reduced in patients with hepatic impairment or by the simultaneous ingestion of inhibitors of this pathway, such as erythromycin and other macrolide antibiotics, ciprofloxacin, ketoconazole, itraconazole, and certain antidepressants such as nefazodone and fluvoxamine. Some antihistamines such as hydroxyzine and loratadine are converted to clinically active metabolites. Clearance of fexofenadine and cetirizine is reduced in patients with impaired renal function. Cetirizine clearance is also reduced in patients with hepatic dysfunction.

The efficacy of antihistamines in the treatment of seasonal and perennial allergic rhinoconjunctivitis is well documented (see Chapter 133). When compared with other medications in regard to the relief of allergic nasal symptoms, antihistamines appear to be more effective than cromolyn sodium but significantly less effective than intranasal corticosteroids. Improvement in symptom relief in patients with allergic rhinitis has been reported when an antihistamine is given in combination with a decongestant or with an intranasal steroid. Numerous formulations combining antihistamines and decongestants are available. Antihistamines have also been shown beneficial in the treatment of acute and chronic urticaria/angioedema. With regard to asthma, a significant clinical effect of antihistamines at conventional doses is difficult to document other than the possible improvement offered by better control of allergic nasal symptoms.

The 2nd-generation antihistamines are often chosen for the treatment of allergic disease in children because of negligible sedative and anticholinergic effects in comparison to 1st-generation antihistamines without a sacrifice in efficacy. In addition, most 2nd-generation antihistamines are effective with once-daily dosing, which, because of the convenience, may improve adherence. However, the widespread availability of 1st-generation antihistamines and their lower cost result in their continued use. The adverse effects most often encountered include the performance impairment and anticholinergic effects noted with the use of 1st-generation antihistamines. The anticholinergic adverse effects encountered may include drying of the mouth and eyes, urinary retention, constipation, excitation, nervousness, palpitations, and tachycardia. Prolongation of the QT interval and ventricular tachycardia (torsades de pointes) was reported in association with the use of two 2nd-generation antihistamines that have since been removed from the market; those currently in use have not been associated with concerning cardiac effects.

Chromones. Cromolyn sodium, the disodium salt of 1,3-*bis* (2-carboxychromon-5-yloxy)-2-hydroxypropane, and nedocromil sodium, a pyranoquinoline dicarboxylic acid, are the two chromones used clinically for the treatment of allergic disorders. Neither cromolyn nor nedocromil is absorbed well orally, with only 1% of the swallowed dose being absorbed. Absorbed drug is not metabolized but is rapidly eliminated in approximately equal amounts by the kidneys and liver. These drugs must be applied topically to the mucosal surface of the target organ to be effective. Both drugs have been demonstrated to inhibit mast cell degranulation and mediator release. They are capable of suppressing the activation of a variety of cells such as eosinophils, neutrophils, macrophages, and epithelial cells and have been shown to inhibit the activity of afferent C-type sensory nerve fibers of the nonadrenergic noncholinergic nervous system. Both drugs inhibit the intracellular increase in free calcium after mast cell activation and have also been shown to phosphorylate a mast cell protein resembling moesin, which is thought to be involved in terminating mediator release. Despite these findings, the molecular mechanism of action of these drugs remains to be completely defined.

Cromolyn and nedocromil prevent both early- and late-phase allergic responses when administered before allergen exposure. They block allergen-induced increases in bronchial hyperresponsiveness as well as seasonal increases in nonspecific bronchial hyperresponsiveness. With prolonged use, both drugs are capable of reducing bronchial hyperresponsiveness. These drugs have no bronchodilator properties but are capable of inhibiting the bronchoconstrictive effects of a variety of stimuli, such as allergen challenge, exercise, hyperventilation with cold air, ultrasonically nebulized distilled water, and exposure to atmospheric and industrial pollutants.

Cromolyn and nedocromil are considered best used for the prophylactic treatment of mild allergic or extrinsic asthma but may also be of benefit in the treatment of nonallergic or intrinsic asthma. Because of their lack of bronchodilator properties, neither drug is useful for the treatment of acute asthma. When their effects are compared, nedocromil is the more potent of the two. Cromolyn is available for the treatment of asthma by prescription as a 1% solution (20 mg/2 mL) for nebulization or by metered-dose inhaler (800 µg/actuation). The suggested dose for the treatment of asthma is 20 mg of cromolyn two to four times/24 hr by nebulization or 1.6 mg two to four times/24 hr by metered-dose inhaler. In numerous studies, cromolyn has been demonstrated to be useful in the treatment of allergic rhinitis and allergic conjunctivitis. Preparations for the nasal and ocular administration of cromolyn are available without a prescription. The suggested dose for the treatment of allergic rhinitis is one spray in each nostril three to four times daily of a nasal spray containing 5.2 mg of cromolyn per spray. For the treatment of allergic conjunctivitis, the suggested dose is 1 drop in each eye four to six times a day of a 4% ophthalmic solution. Nedocromil is not available in a nebulized form but is available by metered-dose inhaler. The recommended dose for the treatment of asthma is 3.5 mg (1.75 mg/puff) two to four times/24 hr. A 2% solution of nedocromil is available by prescription for the treat-

ment of allergic conjunctivitis at a suggested dose of 1–2 drops in each eye twice daily.

The safety of these drugs, even with prolonged administration, has been well documented. Dry throat and transient bronchoconstriction have been the most frequently reported adverse effects of cromolyn use for the treatment of asthma, with only rare reports of patients becoming sensitized to the drug. Some patients using nedocromil complain about its taste. Infrequently reported adverse effects of nedocromil include coughing, sore throat, rhinitis, headache, and nausea.

Glucocorticoids. These are widely used in the treatment of allergic disorders because of their potent anti-inflammatory properties. The diverse anti-inflammatory actions of glucocorticoids are mediated by the regulation of expression of a variety of specific target genes. Glucocorticoids have been shown to inhibit the synthesis of numerous cytokines, including interleukin (IL)-1 through IL-6, tumor necrosis factor-α (TNF-α), and granulocyte-macrophage colony stimulating factor (GM-CSF). They also inhibit the synthesis of the chemokines IL-8, RANTES, eotaxin, macrophage inflammatory protein-1α (MIP-1α), and monocyte chemoattractant protein-1. The expression of enzymes such as nitric oxide synthase, phospholipase A_2, and the inducible form of cyclooxygenase in airway epithelial cells is altered by glucocorticoids. They also regulate the expression of intercellular adhesion molecule-1 (ICAM-1) and vascular cell adhesion molecule-1 (VCAM-1). The administration of glucocorticoids results in (1) alteration in leukocyte number and activity (redistribution, suppression of migration to sites of inflammation, decreased response to mitogens, and suppression of delayed hypersensitivity responses in the skin); (2) suppression of mediator release (decreased histamine synthesis and release, decreased synthesis of prostaglandins, and other products of arachidonic acid metabolism); (3) enhanced response to agents that increase cyclic adenosine monophosphate (prostaglandin E_2 and histamine via the H_2 receptor); and (4) enhanced response to β-adrenergic agonists (increased synthesis of β-adrenergic receptors and increased availability of epinephrine as a result of decreased extraneuronal uptake of catecholamines).

Glucocorticoids are administered topically in ophthalmic preparations, nasal sprays, creams and ointments, and metered-dose inhalers and as a solution for nebulization. Systemic administration is accomplished orally or parenterally. The proper use and efficacy of glucocorticoids in the treatment of allergic disease along with the adverse effects associated with their use are presented in later chapters in this section that include discussions of individual allergic diseases.

Leukotriene-Modifying Agents. Drugs that alter the leukotriene pathway exert their clinical effects either by inhibiting leukotriene production or blocking receptor binding. These agents possess mild anti-inflammatory properties and exhibit bronchodilator effects. In addition to inhibiting the early and late-phase allergic response to inhaled allergen, they diminish bronchoconstriction induced by exercise and exposure to allergen, aspirin, and cold air. These agents are used in the treatment of asthma (see Chapter 134) and are under investigation for treatment of allergic rhinitis.

Theophylline. Because of its bronchodilating effects, theophylline (1,3-dimethyxanthine) has been used for years for the treatment of acute and chronic asthma. Of the molecular mechanisms proposed to explain its mode of action, only nonspecific inhibition of phosphodiesterase isozymes and antagonism of adenosine receptors have been shown to occur at concentrations of the drug of clinical relevance. The bronchodilator effect of theophylline is likely caused by its action as a phosphodiesterase inhibitor, whereas its ability to antagonize adenosine receptors may play a role in other effects, such as the attenuation of diaphragmatic muscle fatigue and diminishing adenosine-enhanced mast cell mediator release. Theophylline has been shown to inhibit the immediate- and late-phase pulmonary response to allergen challenge and to exhibit modest bronchoprotective effects. Selected anti-inflammatory and immunomodulatory effects of this drug have also been reported. Theophylline is available by prescription as both rapidly absorbed and slow-release formulations. It is often administered intravenously when used for the treatment of severe acute asthma. The therapeutic and toxic effects of theophylline are related to the serum concentration, with the incidence of toxic effects significantly increasing as the serum levels approach and exceed 20 µg/mL. A variety of conditions and medications are capable of increasing or decreasing theophylline metabolism. The toxic effects of theophylline range from mild nausea, insomnia, irritability, tremors, and headache to cardiac arrhythmias, seizures, and death. As a result, the routine monitoring of theophylline levels is indicated. Because of the introduction of other effective therapies for the treatment of acute and chronic asthma, the need to monitor theophylline levels routinely and the potential for significant toxicity, the role of theophylline in the treatment of asthma has contracted significantly in recent years (see Chapter 134).

Lodoxamide Tromethamine. This mast cell stabilizer is more effective than topical cromolyn sodium in alleviating signs and symptoms of allergic ocular disease (see Chapter 141). It is used in children older than age 2 yr for vernal keratoconjunctivitis, vernal conjunctivitis, and vernal keratitis. Occasional adverse effects have included transient burning or stinging after instillation.

Olopatadine Hydrocho</ride. This is both a mast cell stabilizer and an H_1-receptor antagonist effective in relieving signs and symptoms of allergic conjunctivitis after topical instillation. It is labeled for use in children at least 3 yr of age. Headaches have occurred in 7% of patients treated; burning and stinging have occurred in fewer than 5%.

New and Future Therapies. An increased understanding of the allergic inflammatory cascade has led to the development and investigation of a variety of new potential therapeutic agents for the treatment of allergic disease. Monoclonal anti-IgE antibodies (anti-IgE) have been developed that bind to circulating IgE at a site that prevents its subsequent attachment to the high affinity receptors for IgE on the mast cell surface. The parenteral administration of anti-IgE has been shown to reduce free serum IgE concentrations, inhibit skin test responses in allergic patients, suppress early- and late-phase responses to allergen, and decrease sputum eosinophilia in asthmatics. Clinical trials have demonstrated a beneficial effect of anti-IgE in the treatment of patients with allergic rhinitis and asthma. Serious adverse effects have not been encountered with this therapy. Anti-IgE may also be of benefit in the treatment of other allergic disorders such as anaphylaxis, atopic dermatitis, and food allergy. The cost of anti-IgE therapy requires careful patient selection with special consideration for those patients with persistent symptoms despite aggressive pharmacotherapy, those suffering from significant adverse effects of their current therapy, and patients with more than one allergic disorder.

Several strategies for inhibiting the actions of proinflammatory cytokines are under investigation. Approaches include the use of recombinant soluble receptors that attach to a specific cytokine and inhibit subsequent binding to cell surface receptors, the development of specific cytokine receptor antagonists and the administration of humanized monoclonal anticytokine antibodies. Recombinant soluble IL-4 receptor antagonists exert their effects by binding to and inactivating IL-4 before it can attach to its cell surface receptor. Initial studies of inhaled

soluble IL-4 receptor in patients with moderate asthma requiring inhaled corticosteroids suggested a beneficial clinical effect, but further investigation is indicated. Humanized monoclonal anti-IL4 antibodies are in development. A soluble receptor antagonist for IL-13, a cytokine with similarities to IL-4, is being developed. Clinical trials of humanized monoclonal anti-IL-5 antibodies administered by injection to asthmatic patients revealed a decrease in circulating eosinophils and sputum eosinophilia, but this effect was unaccompanied by a reduction in methacholine reactivity or a suppression of the early- or late-phase response to allergen.

The use of cytokines with anti-inflammatory effects in the treatment of allergic disorders is under investigation. Unfortunately, initial studies have not demonstrated a beneficial effect of IL-10 or interferons in the treatment of asthma. Although studies have documented that IL-12 administration is associated with a decrease in eosinophil accumulation in response to allergen challenge, inhibition of early- and late-phase responses to allergen or decreases in bronchial hyperreactivity have not been observed. In addition, the high incidence of significant adverse effects encountered with IL-12 administration limits its potential as a viable therapeutic option.

Other therapies under consideration for the treatment of allergic disease include the development of agents to inhibit the actions of chemokines, adhesion receptors, phosphodiesterase-4, and tryptase. Refinement of these potential therapies and continued research examining the molecular and cellular interactions of the allergic inflammatory cascade promises a host of new therapeutic approaches to the treatment and possible cure of allergic disease.

ALLERGEN IMMUNOTHERAPY

Allergen immunotherapy is the process of administering gradually increasing doses of allergens to a person with allergic disease for the purpose of reducing or eliminating the patient's adverse clinical response on subsequent natural exposure to those allergens. When properly administered to an appropriate candidate, allergen immunotherapy is a safe, effective form of therapy capable not only of reducing or preventing symptoms, but of potentially altering the natural history of the disease by minimizing disease duration and preventing disease progression.

Mechanisms. A number of alterations in the immune response to allergen after allergen immunotherapy have been identified. Reciprocal changes in the levels of circulating allergen-specific IgE and IgG have been documented. After an early increase triggered by the onset of allergen administration, serum allergen-specific IgE levels gradually fall below initial levels over the course of treatment. The usual postseasonal rise observed in allergen-specific IgE levels is also blunted. However, clinical improvement often does not correlate well with allergen-specific IgE levels because a reduction in symptoms may occur even while allergen-specific IgE levels are increased or before their decline. In contrast to the reduction in allergen-specific IgE levels, the production of allergen-specific IgG is stimulated by allergen immunotherapy. These allergen-specific IgG antibodies have been called blocking antibodies because their interaction with allergen inhibits its subsequent binding to allergen-specific IgE. In Hymenoptera venom–sensitive patients a rise in venom-specific IgG antibody levels has been shown to correlate with protection over the first few years of treatment. Most studies involving other allergens have demonstrated an association between increasing allergen-specific IgG levels and decreasing symptom-medication scores, although some studies report patients with reduced symptoms in the absence of an allergen-specific IgG response, whereas others describe patients without improvement despite high levels of allergen-specific IgG. Thus, blunting of the allergen-specific IgE response and stimulation of allergen-specific IgG production are not the sole mechanisms responsible for the clinical improvement associated with allergen immunotherapy but represent markers of modulation of the immune response to allergen.

Allergen immunotherapy also leads to changes in cellular elements of the immune response. Not only is the number of mast cells and basophils in target tissues reduced by allergen immunotherapy, but mediator release by these cells after allergen exposure is also diminished. The decline in mast cell and basophil numbers in target tissue combined with a reduction in mediator release by these cells results in decreased numbers of infiltrating inflammatory cells and subsequent suppression of the late-phase allergic response. Regulatory T-cell function is modulated by allergen immunotherapy, as evidenced by documented increases in T-lymphocyte suppressor activity. T-cell cytokine production is shifted with decreases in IL-4 production and increases in the production of interferon-γ, IL-2, and IL-12. In addition, there is a decrease in the production of histamine-releasing factors by a host of other cells, including lymphocytes, alveolar macrophages, platelets, and vascular endothelial cells.

Indications and Contraindications. Allergen immunotherapy is reserved for patients with an allergic disease that has been demonstrated to respond to this form of therapy such as seasonal or perennial allergic rhinoconjunctivitis, asthma triggered by allergen exposures, and insect venom sensitivity. Proof of the efficacy of allergen immunotherapy for the treatment of atopic dermatitis, food allergy, latex allergy, or acute or chronic urticaria is lacking, and therefore allergen immunotherapy is not recommended for the treatment of these disorders. Before considering allergen immunotherapy, sensitivity of the patient to the allergens to be administered should be documented by a positive skin test or an in vitro test revealing an increased serum level of allergen-specific IgE. In addition, the clinical relevance of these allergens should be supported by a history of symptoms on known exposure or a timing of symptoms that correlates well with suspected allergen exposure such as the presence of allergic nasal and ocular symptoms throughout the late summer and fall in a child with a large positive ragweed skin test. The duration and severity of the patient's symptoms should warrant the expense, effort, and risk associated with the administration of allergen immunotherapy. The presence of disabling symptoms in spite of a trial of allergen avoidance and appropriate medications at a suitable dose should be documented. For patients sensitized to seasonal allergens, more than two consecutive seasons of symptoms are usually required before allergen immunotherapy is recommended unless the symptoms are unusually severe or the adverse effects of medication are unacceptable. The obvious exception to this rule is the child with insect sting anaphylaxis who should be started on venom immunotherapy once the sensitivity is correctly diagnosed.

Other factors that may affect the decision to institute allergen immunotherapy include quality of life issues such as the amount of school missed or medical resource utilization, the age of the patient, and other logistical factors. With the exception of venom immunotherapy, few data for the efficacy of allergen immunotherapy in children younger than 5 yr of age are available. Allergen immunotherapy is currently not recommended for children younger than 5 yr because of their increased risk of systemic reactions, the special expertise required to treat anaphylaxis in this age group, their potential inability to communicate clearly with their physician in the event of an allergic reaction, and their age-related potential for emotional distress with frequent injections. Other important logistic factors include the willingness of the patient to comply with a schedule of frequent injections over the course of several years, cost considerations, and the availability of an appropriate setting for the administering allergen immunotherapy.

Allergen immunotherapy is contraindicated in children on β-blocker therapy as well as those with certain immunologic or autoimmune disorders, allergic bronchopulmonary aspergillosis, hypersensitivity pneumonitis, severe psychiatric disturbance, or a medical condition that would impair the ability to survive an allergic reaction. Pregnancy is a contraindication for the initiation of allergen immunotherapy or dosing increases, although pregnant adolescents can continue to receive their usual maintenance dose. Patients with unstable asthma should not be placed on allergen immunotherapy because of their increased risk for fatal anaphylaxis. Allergen immunotherapy is not used for the treatment of allergic bronchopulmonary aspergillosis or hypersensitivity pneumonitis because it has never been proven to be of benefit. Children on β-blockers should be switched to another form of therapy before allergen immunotherapy is considered because of an increased intensity of allergic reactions and a poor response to conventional therapy. Allergen immunotherapy is usually avoided for patients with autoimmune disorders because of the potential for unanticipated stimulation of the immune system, resulting in disease activation.

Allergen Extracts. The potency of the aqueous extracts used in allergen immunotherapy is affected by numerous factors. Allergens from weed and grass pollens are more easily extracted in aqueous solutions and, as a result, are generally more potent than extracts obtained from other sources, such as molds, tree pollens, and dust mites. Allergen extracts from fungal allergens because of their complexity are more variable than extracts of pollen allergens. Refrigeration and appropriate handling of allergen extracts used in allergen immunotherapy are important because degradation of many allergen extracts, such as those from tree, grass, and weed pollens and dust mites, may occur at higher temperatures. Dilute extracts are more susceptible to loss of potency resulting from adherence of allergen to the glass vial than are more concentrated extracts. To combat this effect, human serum albumin is sometimes added to dilute allergen extracts. Some allergen extracts, such as those from cockroaches, dust mites, and fungi, contain proteases capable of degrading other allergens in the extract. As a result it is often recommended that these allergens not be mixed with those from tree, grass, and weed pollens. Insect venoms are never mixed with other allergens. When available, the use of standardized allergen extracts is preferred to ensure consistency in dosing and avoid the variability in allergen content encountered with allergen extracts that are not standardized.

Allergen Extract Administration. The goal of allergen immunotherapy is to gradually increase the dose of allergen extract administered until the injection of an "optimal" maintenance dose containing 4–12 μg of each major allergen in the extract is reached. The mixture of allergen extracts administered during the course of allergen immunotherapy is individually formulated for each patient based on their documented sensitivities. Although various dosing schedules are used, initial injections are most often given at 5–10 day intervals year round. Schedules of allergen administration are selected based on the sensitivity of the patient to the allergens in the extract. The most sensitive patients are advanced to maintenance dose more gradually. Doses of allergen immunotherapy are increased according to a set schedule while taking into account the reaction to the previous injection. Usually 5–6 mo of weekly injections are required to reach the maintenance dose, although it may take longer in patients with marked sensitivity whose dosing schedule must be adjusted because of reactions to the injections. Unique schedules for the administration of insect venoms are used that differ from those for the administration of other allergens. Once the maintenance dose is reached and well tolerated, the time interval between injections is increased to every few weeks to once a month. Because allergen extracts gradually lose potency, the first dose from a fresh replacement vial of maintenance allergen extract is reduced from 25–75% and increased in increments weekly until the usual maintenance dose is reached. The recommended length of a course of allergen immunotherapy is 3–5 yr. Insect venom immunotherapy may be continued longer in patients with histories of life-threatening anaphylaxis. Patients who have not improved after 1 yr of receiving maintenance doses of an appropriate allergen extract are unlikely to benefit and should have their allergen immunotherapy discontinued. Most patients enjoy a sustained improvement after allergen immunotherapy whereas others experience a gradual return of symptoms. Those who experience a relapse may respond to another course of treatment.

Rush immunotherapy involves the administration of multiple injections either in a single day or over several days in an attempt to reach maintenance dose more rapidly. The risk of adverse reactions, including systemic reactions, is higher than that encountered with traditional allergen immunotherapy schedules; and, as a result, these patients are often pretreated with antihistamines and corticosteroids. Because children are at even greater risk for adverse reactions with rush immunotherapy, carefully weighing the benefits versus the risks is warranted before using it.

Although allergen immunotherapy is regarded as safe, the potential for anaphylaxis always exists when patients are injected with extracts containing allergens to which they are sensitized. As a result, allergen immunotherapy should only be offered in medical settings where a physician with access to emergency equipment and medications required for the treatment of anaphylaxis is available. Allergy shots should never be given at home or by untrained personnel. Patients should remain in the office for 20–30 min after the injection because most reactions to allergen immunotherapy begin within this time frame. Fatal anaphylaxis triggered by allergen immunotherapy, although rare, is estimated to occur at an incidence of 1 per 2 million injections. The risk of an adverse reaction is increased by dosage errors and the use of rush immunotherapy schedules. Particular caution is warranted when injections from a new vial are given. Patients with exquisite sensitivity, unstable asthma, or those experiencing exacerbations of allergic rhinitis or asthma are also at increased risk for adverse reactions. Giving allergen immunotherapy to patients on β-blockers is contraindicated. Precautions to reduce significant adverse reactions include using standardized extracts, allowing only trained personnel to administer injections, paying careful attention to detail when giving injections, ensuring that the patient is medically stable beforehand, having appropriate medications and equipment available, and requiring the patient to remain in the office for 20–30 min after each injection. In some asthmatic patients, checking peak flows or spirometry before receiving an injection is also advisable.

Other forms of allergen immunotherapy have been proposed, including local nasal immunotherapy, oral aeroallergen immunotherapy, and the use of alum-precipitated allergen extracts. Local nasal immunotherapy is administered by having the patient spray allergen solutions into the nose at scheduled intervals. Although some studies show encouraging results, adequate long-term data are not available to currently support the routine use of this form of therapy. Although selected studies of oral and sublingual aeroallergen administration have reported favorable results, further studies demonstrating efficacy are required. A desire to decrease the likelihood of allergic reactions induced by the administration of aqueous allergens led to the development of alum-precipitated extracts in which the proteins are precipitated with aluminum hydroxide and alum-precipitated pyridine-extracted extracts. Because of the small number of available extracts and the inability to mix them with other aqueous extracts, their use remains limited. Another method developed to reduce allergenicity while maintaining immunogenicity is the polymerization of allergen extracts with glutaraldehyde. When these extracts are used the maintenance dose can be reached within 2 mo with a markedly reduced incidence of systemic reactions. These extracts have not yet been approved for use in the United States.

Efficacy. The majority of well-designed clinical trials examining the impact of allergen immunotherapy on seasonal or perennial allergic rhinitis or rhinoconjunctivitis recommend it as an effective mode of therapy. In regard to the treatment of allergic rhinitis, birch, mountain cedar, grass, ragweed, and *Cladosporium* are allergens for which the efficacy of allergen immunotherapy has been best documented. Studies examining allergen immunotherapy with other allergens commonly used for the treatment of allergic rhinitis are either lacking or inconclusive. As with allergic rhinitis, most of the controlled trials examining the effects of allergen immunotherapy on seasonal or perennial allergic asthma also report favorable results. A meta-analysis of 20 trials examining the effects of allergen immunotherapy on allergic asthma revealed a significant increase in the odds for improvement after treatment along with fewer symptoms, improved pulmonary functions, less need for medication, and a reduction in bronchial hyperreactivity. The most convincing data for the benefit of allergen immunotherapy in the treatment of allergic asthma are available for birch, mountain cedar, grass, ragweed, and dust mite, with less conclusive, but suggestive data available for *Cladosporium*, *Alternaria*, and cat allergens. As would be expected, studies examining the effects of allergen immunotherapy in the treatment of patients with allergic rhinitis and allergic asthma have usually documented increases in circulating allergen-specific IgG and decreases in allergen-specific IgE after treatment. Reductions in sensitivity to administered allergens have been demonstrated in nasal and bronchial challenges. In addition, these studies have often shown that the late-phase response after allergen challenge is ablated or significantly reduced. The protective benefit as well as the safety of venom immunotherapy in patients with sensitivity to Hymenoptera venoms has also been well documented in several large studies. The efficacy of allergen immunotherapy for the treatment of food allergy, atopic dermatitis, urticaria, and latex allergy has not been documented.

Agosti JM, Sanes-Miller CH: Novel therapeutic approaches for allergic rhinitis. *Immunol Allergy Clin North Am* 2000;20:401–23.

Barnes PJ: Cytokine-directed therapies for asthma. *J Allergy Clin Immunol* 2001; 108:S72–6.

Broide DH: Molecular and cellular mechanisms of allergic disease. *J Allergy Clin Immunol* 2001;108:S65–71.

Bush RK (editor): *Environmental Asthma*. New York, Marcel Dekker, 2001.

Busse WW, Holgate ST (editors): *Asthma & Rhinitis*, 2nd ed. London, Blackwell Science, 2000.

Gentile DA, Friday GA, Skoner PV: Management of allergic rhinitis: Antihistamines and decongestants. *Immunol Allergy Clin North Am* 2000;20: 355–68.

Ledford DK: Efficacy of immunotherapy. *Immunol Allergy Clin North Am* 2000;20: 503–25.

Li JT: Immunotherapy for allergic rhinitis. *Immunol Allergy Clin North Am* 2000;20: 383–400.

Middleton E, Reed CE, Ellis EF, et al (editors): *Allergy: Principles & Practice*, 5th ed. St. Louis, WB Saunders, 1998.

Moss MH, Bush RK: Patient selection and administration of aeroallergen vaccines. *Immunol Allergy Clin North Am* 2000;20:533–52.

Patel NJ, Bush RK: Role of environmental allergens in rhinitis. *Immunol Allergy Clin North Am* 2000;20:323–53.

Peat JK, Dickerson J, Li J: Effect of damp and mould in the home on respiratory health: A review of the literature. *Allergy* 1998;53:120–28.

Platts-Mills TAE, Vervloet D, Thomas WR, et al: Indoor allergens and asthma: Report of Third International Workshop. *J Allergy Clin Immunol* 1997;100: S2–S24.

Williams PV: Treatment of rhinitis: Corticosteroids and cromolyn sodium. *Immunol Allergy Clin North Am* 2000;20:369–81.

Allergic Rhinitis *Henry Milgrom and*

Donald Y. M. Leung

In affluent societies 20–40% of children suffer from allergic rhinitis (AR). Over the past 40 yr there has been a substantial rise in AR in industrialized regions and a smaller increase in undeveloped countries and rural populations. The diagnosis is generally established by 6 yr of age and may be made in infants. The prevalence peaks late in childhood. Risk factors include family history of atopy, serum IgE greater than 100 IU/mL before age 6 yr, and higher socioeconomic group. The risk is increased in children introduced to foods or formula early in infancy, whose mothers smoke heavily especially before the child is 1 yr old, and with heavy exposure to indoor allergens.

Etiology. Two factors required for manifestation of AR are sensitivity to an allergen and its presence in the environment. AR may be seasonal or perennial. Inhalant allergens are the main reason for both. **Seasonal allergic rhinitis** (SAR) follows a well-defined course of cyclical exacerbation, whereas **perennial allergic rhinitis** (PAR) causes year-round symptoms. Approximately 20% of cases are strictly seasonal, 40% perennial, and 40% mixed (perennial with seasonal exacerbations). In temperate climates, airborne pollen responsible for SAR appear in distinct phases: trees pollinate in the spring, grasses in the early summer, and weeds in the late summer. Mold spores are also important aeroallergens that tend to settle in the lower airways. In temperate climates the spores persist outdoors only in the summer, but in warm climates they occur throughout the year. Symptoms of seasonal allergies cease with the appearance of frost. Knowledge of the occurrence of seasonal symptoms, of the regional patterns of pollination and mold sporulation, and of the patient's specific IgE is necessary to establish the cause of SAR. PAR is most often associated with indoor allergens: house dust mites, animal danders, and molds. Cat and dog allergies are of major importance in the United States. The allergens from the saliva and sebaceous secretions can remain airborne for prolonged time. The ubiquitous major cat allergen, Fel d 1, may be found in such "cat-free" settings as schools and hospitals because individuals can carry the allergen in on their clothing.

Pathogenesis. The exposure to an allergen in an atopic host leads to IgE production and the infiltration of the nasal mucosa by inflammatory cells. The clinical reactions on re-exposure to the allergen have been designated as **early-phase responses** and **late-phase allergic responses.** Bridging of the IgE molecules on the surface of mast cells by allergen initiates the early responses, which are characterized by degranulation of mast cells and the release of preformed and newly generated inflammatory mediators, including histamine, prostaglandin E_2, and the cysteinyl leukotrienes. The targets of inflammation in the nasal mucosa are the mucus glands, nerves, blood vessels, and venous sinuses.

Late-phase responses arise 4–8 hr after allergen exposure and are accompanied by the infiltration of cytokine-secreting T cells and eosinophils with secretion of eosinophil-derived mediators—major basic protein, eosinophil cationic protein, and leukotrienes—which cause damage to the epithelium, leading to the clinical and histologic appearance of chronic allergic disease. Repeated intranasal introduction of allergens causes "priming," a brisk response to a reduced provocation dose.

Clinical Manifestations. Symptoms of AR are often ignored or mistakenly attributed to a respiratory infection. Although older children blow their noses, younger ones tend to sniff and snort. Nasal itching brings on grimacing, twitching, and picking of the nose, which may result in epistaxis. Children with AR often perform the **allergic salute,** an upward rubbing of the nose with an open palm or extended fingers. This maneuver gives rise to the **nasal crease,** a horizontal skinfold over the bridge of the nose.

Typical complaints include intermittent nasal congestion, itching, sneezing, clear rhinorrhea, and conjunctival irritation. Symptoms increase with greater exposure to the responsible allergen. The patients may lose their sense of smell and taste. Some experience headaches, wheezing, and coughing. Nasal congestion is often more severe at night, causing mouth breathing and snoring, interfering with sleep and inducing irritability.

Diagnosis. Evaluation of AR should include a patient history, physical examination, and laboratory evaluation. The diagnosis of AR is based on symptoms in absence of an upper respiratory tract infection or structural abnormalities. AR is characterized by symptoms that include sneezing, rhinorrhea, nasal itching, and congestion; and the laboratory findings of elevated IgE, specific IgE antibodies, and positive allergy skin tests. SAR differs from PAR by history and skin test results. Nonallergic rhinitides cause sporadic symptoms and may resemble PAR. Their causes are often unknown. Nonallergic inflammatory rhinitis with eosinophils (NARES) imitates AR in presentation and response to treatment, but the patients do not have elevated IgE antibodies. Vasomotor rhinitis is characterized by excessive responsiveness of the nasal mucosa to physical stimuli. Other nonallergic conditions such as infectious rhinitis, structural problems including nasal polyps and septal deviation, rhinitis medicamentosa (due to the overuse of topical vasoconstrictors), hormonal rhinitis associated with pregnancy or hypothyroidism, neoplasms, vasculitides, and granulomatous disorders may mimic AR.

PHYSICAL EXAMINATION. Signs on physical examination include abnormalities of facial development, dental malocclusion, the **allergic gape** (continuous open-mouth breathing), **allergic shiners** (dark circles under the eyes), and the transverse nasal crease. Conjunctival edema, itching, tearing, and hyperemia are frequent findings. A nasal examination performed with a source of light and a speculum may reveal clear nasal secretions; edematous, boggy, and bluish mucous membranes with little or no erythema; and swollen turbinates that may block the nasal airway. Thick, purulent nasal secretions indicate the presence of infection. Children with AR often have related sinusitis, otitis media, serous otitis, eczema, or asthma.

Laboratory Findings. Epicutaneous skin tests are the best method for detection of allergen-specific IgE. They are inexpensive and sensitive, and the risks and discomfort are minimal. Children younger than 1 yr often do not display any positive reactions to seasonal allergens. Positive skin tests to seasonal respiratory allergens are rare before two seasons of exposure. To avoid false-negative results, montelukast should be withheld for 1 day, most sedating antihistamine preparations for 3–4 days, and nonsedating antihistamines for 5–7 days. Serum immunoassays for IgE to allergens provide a suitable alternative for patients with dermatographism or extensive dermatitis, those taking medications that interfere with mast cell degranulation, those at high risk for anaphylaxis, and those who cannot cooperate with the procedure. Eosinophils in the nasal smear support the diagnosis of AR and neutrophils of infectious rhinitis. Blood eosinophilia and total serum IgE concentrations have relatively low sensitivity.

Treatment. Safe and effective prevention or relief of symptoms is the goal of treatment. The removal or avoidance of offending allergens is advised (see Chapter 132). Sealing the mattress, pillow, and covers in allergen-proof encasings is the most effective strategy for the reduction of mite allergen. Bed linen and blankets should be washed every week in hot water (>130°F).

The only effective measure for evading animal allergens in the home is the removal of the pet. Avoidance of pollen and outdoor molds can be accomplished by staying in a controlled environment. Air conditioning allows for keeping windows and doors closed to lower the pollen exposure. HEPA filters reduce the counts of airborne mold spores.

Oral antihistamines administered as needed are suitable pharmacotherapy for the patient with mild, intermittent symptoms. Antihistamines relieve sneezing and rhinorrhea. The 2nd-generation antihistamines are preferred because they cause less sedation. Four are currently available: cetirizine (2–5 yr: 2.5 mg PO once daily; ≥6 yr: 5–10 mg PO once daily), loratadine (2–5 yr: 5 mg PO once daily; ≥6 yr: 10 mg PO once daily), fexofenadine (6–11 yr: 30 mg PO bid; ≥12 yr: 60 mg PO bid or 180 mg PO qd), and azelastine nasal spray (5–11 yr: 1 spray/nostril bid; ≥12 yr: 2 sprays/nostril bid). Pseudoephedrine (available without prescription; 2–6 yr: 15 mg PO q6h; 6–12 yr: 30 mg PO q6h; >12 yr: 60 mg PO q6h), an oral vasoconstrictor that can be associated with irritability and insomnia, may be used for nasal congestion, and the anticholinergic nasal spray ipratropium bromide (2 sprays/nostril bid or tid, use 0.03% preparation) can be used for serous rhinorrhea. Intranasal decongestants may be used for less than 5 days, not to be repeated more than once a month. Sodium cromoglycate (available without prescription) is effective but requires frequent administration (every 4 hr). Leukotriene-modifying agents have a modest effect on rhinorrhea and nasal blockage.

Patients with more persistent, severe symptoms require treatment with intranasal corticosteroids. These agents are effective for all symptoms of AR with eosinophilic inflammation but not for rhinitis associated with neutrophils or free of inflammation. The older drugs beclomethasone, triamcinolone, and flunisolide are absorbed from the gastrointestinal tract as well as from the respiratory tract. Fluticasone (>4 yr: 1–2 sprays/nostril once daily), mometasone (3–11 yr: 1 spray per nostril once daily; >11 yr: 2 sprays/nostril once daily), and budesonide (>6 yr: 1–2 sprays/nostril once daily) have lower bioavailability and a better safety profile.

A consultation with an allergist is recommended for patients with AR who do not respond to treatment. The allergist may propose more effective avoidance measures and/or immunotherapy. Allergen immunotherapy interferes with IgE production and allergen-induced allergic symptoms and has been found to be effective in the treatment of AR.

Complications. Chronic sinusitis is a frequent complication of AR, most often associated with purulent infection, but a proportion of patients develop marked mucosal thickening, sinus opacification, and nasal polyposis with inflammation but negative cultures. The inflammatory process is characterized by marked eosinophilia. Allergens may be the inciting agents. The sinusitis of **triad asthma** (asthma, sinusitis with nasal polyposis, and aspirin sensitivity) often shows poor response to therapy. Patients who undergo repeated endoscopic surgery derive diminishing benefit with each successive procedure.

Approximately 60% of patients with AR have asthma and even those who do not may manifest bronchial hyperresponsiveness. In patients who have both disorders, the aggravation of AR coincides with exacerbation of asthma and the treatment of nasal inflammation often reduces bronchospasm. Postnasal drip associated with AR commonly causes persistent or recurrent cough. Eustachian tube obstruction and middle ear effusion are frequent complications. Chronic allergic inflammation causes hypertrophy of tonsils and adenoids; the former may be associated with obstructive sleep apnea and the latter with eustachian tube obstruction, serous effusion, and otitis media.

Children with AR experience frustration over their appearance; some have a cognitive impairment. Pediatric Rhinoconjunctivitis Quality of Life measures in these children have documented anxiety and physical, social, and emotional issues that affect learning and the ability to integrate with peers. The disorder contributes to headaches and fatigue, limits daily activities, interferes with sleep, and leads to school absenteeism.

Bousquet J, Van Cauwenberge P, Khaltaev NL: Allergic rhinitis and its impact on asthma. *J Allergy Clin Immunol* 2001;108:S147–334.

Milgrom H: Attainments in atopy: Special aspects of allergy and IgE. *Adv Pediatr* 2002;49:273–97.

New perspectives on pediatric allergic rhinitis. Proceedings of a workshop. Barcelona, Spain. *J Allergy Clin Immunol* 2001;108:S1–64.

Sly RM: Changing prevalence of allergic rhinitis and asthma. *Ann Allergy Asthma Immunol* 1999;82:233–48.

Chapter 134
Childhood Asthma

Andrew H. Liu, Joseph D. Spahn, and Donald Y. M. Leung

Asthma is a chronic inflammatory condition of the lung airways resulting in episodic airflow obstruction. This chronic inflammation heightens the "twitchiness" of the airways—airways hyperresponsiveness—to provocative exposures. Other associated histopathologic abnormalities of the airways characteristic of asthma include epithelial damage, subepithelial collagen deposition with basement membrane thickening, and mucus gland and smooth muscle hypertrophy. These pathologic changes, linked to persistent airways inflammation and hyperresponsiveness, form the chronic basis of this disease.

Clinical manifestations of asthma are intermittent. Dry coughing, expiratory wheezing, chest tightness, and dyspnea are commonly provoked by physical exertion and airways irritants (e.g., cold and dry air, environmental tobacco smoke). Asthma symptoms are usually associated with widespread but variable airflow obstruction that is generally reversible either spontaneously or with treatment. Asthma exacerbations for prolonged periods (i.e., from days to weeks) are induced by common respiratory viral infections and by inhalant allergen exposure in sensitized asthmatics. These exacerbations are characteristically worse at night and can progress to severe airflow obstruction, shortness of breath, and respiratory distress and insufficiency. Rarely, severe sequelae such as hypoxic seizures, respiratory failure, and death can occur.

Current asthma management is aimed at reducing airways inflammation by using daily "controller" anti-inflammatory medications, minimizing proinflammatory environmental exposures, and controlling co-morbid conditions that can worsen asthma. Less inflammation typically leads to better asthma control, including less need for "quick-reliever" asthma medication (i.e., β-agonist bronchodilators) and fewer exacerbations. Exacerbations can, nevertheless, still occur. Early intervention with systemic glucocorticoids can greatly reduce the severity of such episodes. Thus, in contrast to past images of debilitated and frail asthmatic children, recent improvements in asthma management and especially pharmacotherapy enable all but the rare child with severe asthma to live normally. With good asthma management, almost all children with asthma can (1) attend school regularly, (2) participate fully in the sport of their choice, (3) sleep well without disturbance due to asthma, (4) experience little to no adverse effects from asthma pharmacotherapy, and (5) with early intervention, stay safe by keeping asthma exacerbations from becoming severe.

Etiology. Although the cause of childhood asthma has not been pinpointed, contemporary research implicates an interplay between genetic and environmental factors. The strong association of common childhood asthma with concomitant allergies suggests that environmental factors influence immune development toward the asthmatic phenotype in susceptible individuals.

GENETICS. Twin studies have revealed a 0.74 concordance of asthma between monozygotic twins and a 0.35 concordance between dizygotic twins, implicating a genetic contribution to asthma development. More than 22 loci on 15 autosomal chromosomes have been linked to asthma. Although the genetic linkages to asthma have sometimes differed between cohorts, asthma has been consistently linked with loci containing proallergic, proinflammatory genes (e.g., the IL-4 gene cluster on chromosome 5). Genetic variation in receptors for different asthma medications is associated with variation in biologic response to these medications (e.g., polymorphisms in the glucocorticoid, β-adrenergic, and leukotriene receptors). Accordingly, asthma pharmacogenomics should optimize asthma pharmacotherapy in the future by genotyping patients to predict their response to different asthma medication options.

ENVIRONMENT. Common viral infections of the respiratory tract, such as with respiratory syncytial virus (RSV), can induce small airways bronchiolitis. RSV is a common cause of severe bronchiolitis and/or pneumonia in the first 2 yr of life. It is also a common precipitant of asthma exacerbations at any age. Interestingly, whereas nearly all children by age 2 yr have immunologic evidence of previous RSV infection, only 12–40% of those infected report bronchiolitis symptoms. This implies that host features affect the extent of airways injury from viral pathogens. Likewise, injurious viral infections of the airways (i.e., manifesting as pneumonia and/or bronchiolitis requiring hospitalization) are risk factors for persistent asthma in childhood.

Some airways exposures besides viral infections can exacerbate ongoing airways inflammation and increase disease severity. Allergen exposure, in sensitized individuals, can initiate airways inflammation and hypersensitivity to other irritant exposures as well. Indeed, perennial allergen exposure in sensitized asthmatics is a major contributor to disease severity. Consequently, eliminating the offending allergen(s) can lead to resolution of asthma symptoms and can sometimes "cure" asthma. Environmental tobacco smoke, endotoxin, and air pollutants (e.g., ozone, sulfur dioxide) aggravate airways inflammation and increase asthma severity. Cold dry air and strong odors can trigger bronchoconstriction when airways are irritated but do not worsen airways inflammation or hyperresponsiveness.

Epidemiology. Asthma is a common chronic disease, causing considerable morbidity. Based on information collected by the United States National Center for Health Statistics in 1998, 8.65 million children (12.1%) were reported to have physician- or health care professional–diagnosed asthma in their lifetime, and 3.8 million children (5.3%) had experienced an asthma episode in the preceding 12 mo. Childhood asthma in the United States is the most common cause of childhood emergency department visits, hospitalizations, and missed school days, accounting annually for 867,000 emergency department visits, 166,000 hospitalizations, and 10.1 million school days lost. Although death due to asthma is relatively uncommon in children (0.3 deaths per 100,000 population per year), asthma was responsible for 164 deaths of children in the United States in 1998. Many of these asthma deaths could probably have been avoided. Indeed, asthma is generally an underdiagnosed and undertreated condition.

In the United States, asthma morbidity and mortality are particularly high in African-American children. Asthma hospitalization and death rates are more than three times higher in black versus white Americans. A combination of biologic, environmental, economic, and psychosocial risk factors is believed to increase the likelihood of severe asthma exacerbations for ethnic minority asthmatics living in U.S. "inner-city" low-income communities. Although asthma prevalence is slightly higher in black versus white U.S. children (i.e., in 1998, 16.1% vs. 13.2%, respectively), asthma prevalence is not believed to differ significantly with either ethnicity or income status. Therefore, asthma morbidity and mortality is linked with ethnic minority and low-income status whereas asthma prevalence is primarily associated with urban living.

Worldwide, childhood asthma appears to be increasing in prevalence, despite considerable improvements in our management and pharmacopeia to treat asthma. For example, in the United States from 1982 to 1994, childhood asthma prevalence increased 72%. Numerous studies conducted in different countries have reported a similar increase in asthma prevalence of about 50% per decade. Of further interest, childhood asthma prevalence varies widely in different locales. A large international study of childhood asthma prevalence (by report) in 56 countries (International Study of Asthma and Allergies in Childhood) found about a 20-fold variation in asthma prevalence (range, 1.6–36.8%). Furthermore, asthma prevalence correlated well with reported allergic rhinoconjunctivitis and atopic eczema prevalence (R = 0.75 and 0.74, respectively; p <.0001). Childhood asthma seems particularly common in modern metropolitan locales and is strongly linked with other allergic conditions. In contrast, children living in rural areas of developing countries (e.g., rural Africa, China, India) and farming communities (e.g., in Germany, Austria, Switzerland, Finland, Quebec) are less likely to have asthma and allergy. This striking variation in childhood asthma prevalence has led to investigations of potential environmental and lifestyle factors that may explain these differences as well as the recent rise in asthma (see Chapter 130).

Approximately 80% of asthmatics report disease onset before 6 yr of age. However, of all young children who experience recurrent wheezing, only a minority will go on to have persistent asthma in later childhood. Several risk factors for persistent asthma have been identified (Box 134–1). Allergy in these young wheezers has emerged as a major risk factor for persistent childhood asthma and may be evident in the early childhood years as clinical conditions (atopic dermatitis, allergic rhinitis, food allergies).

There are two main types of childhood asthma: (1) recurrent wheezing in early childhood, primarily triggered by common viral infections of the respiratory tract, and (2) chronic asthma associated with allergy that persists into later childhood and often adulthood. A third emerging type of childhood asthma typically occurs in females who develop obesity and early-onset puberty (by 11 years of age). Although asthma mediated by "occupational" exposures is often not considered, some children are raised in settings, on farms or with farm-type animals in the home, where occupational-type exposures can mediate a fourth type of childhood asthma. **Triad asthma,** characteristically

---

BOX 134–1. Early Childhood Risk Factors for Persistent Asthma

Parental asthma
Allergy
    Atopic dermatitis
    Allergic rhinitis
    Food allergy
    Inhalant allergen sensitization
    Food allergen sensitization
Severe lower respiratory tract infection
    Pneumonia
    Bronchiolitis requiring hospitalization
Wheezing apart from colds
Male gender
Low birth weight
Environmental tobacco smoke exposure

associated with hyperplastic sinusitis/nasal polyposis and hypersensitivity to aspirin and nonsteroidal anti-inflammatory medications (e.g., ibuprofen), rarely has its onset in childhood. Current evidence suggests that, of these different types of childhood asthma, the most common form is that associated with allergy. Additionally, allergen sensitization and exposure is associated with more severe asthma.

Pathogenesis. The pathologic changes linked to persistent airways inflammation and hyperresponsiveness underlie the chronic basis of asthma.

AIRWAYS OBSTRUCTION. Airflow obstruction in asthma is the result of numerous pathologic processes. In the small airways, airflow is regulated by smooth muscle encircling the airways lumens; bronchoconstriction of these bronchiolar muscular bands restricts or blocks airflow. A cellular inflammatory infiltrate distinguished by eosinophils, but also including other inflammatory cell types (neutrophils, monocytes, lymphocytes), can fill the airways and induce epithelial damage and desquamation into the airways lumen. Excess production of mucus into the airways and edema of the surrounding tissues also contribute to blockage of airways.

AIRWAYS INFLAMMATION, HYPERRESPONSIVENESS, AND REMODELING. Asthmatic airways tissues have increased numbers of mast cells, activated eosinophils, and activated helper T lymphocytes (see Chapter 130). Helper T lymphocytes that produce proallergic, proinflammatory cytokines (e.g., IL-4, IL-5, IL-13) and chemokines (e.g., RANTES, eotaxin) mediate this inflammatory process. Other immune cells (e.g., cytotoxic T lymphocytes, NK cells, eosinophils, mast cells, basophils) can produce these proallergic, proinflammatory cytokines and chemokines as well. Airways inflammation is strongly linked to hypersensitivity of airways smooth muscle (**airways hyperresponsiveness**) to irritant exposures, such as cold air, dry air, strong odors, and particulate matter in smoke.

Airways inflammation is also linked to less reversible airways changes, such as basement membrane thickening, subepithelial collagen deposition, and smooth muscle and mucus gland hypertrophy and hyperplasia. These airways "remodeling" abnormalities resemble an aberrant tissue repair process in response to persistent tissue injury. Therefore, persistent airways inflammation and remodeling are believed to underlie the chronic functional and pathologic abnormalities as well as the intermittent and episodic clinical manifestations of asthma.

Inhaled allergen challenge studies have revealed two distinct phases of airflow obstructive processes in asthma: (1) an **early phase** (within 15–30 min) consisting of bronchoconstriction and (2) a **late phase** (4–12 hr after allergen exposure) of tissue inflammation and immune cellular infiltration into the airways, in addition to airways edema and excess mucus production. The late phase is also associated with airways hyperresponsiveness that can persist for several weeks. The early phase can be prevented with inhaled β-agonist bronchodilator pretreatment; in contrast, the late phase can be prevented with anti-inflammatory agents (e.g., glucocorticoids) but not β-agonists. Therefore, a quick recovery after an acute allergen-induced exacerbation does not mean that the episode is over; on the contrary, a more serious and sustained late-phase episode can occur hours later.

PROGRESSION OF SEVERE ASTHMA EXACERBATIONS. Airflow obstruction during asthma exacerbations can become extensive, resulting in life-threatening respiratory insufficiency. Often, asthma exacerbations worsen at night (i.e., between midnight and 8 AM), when airways inflammation and hyperresponsiveness are at their peak. Complications that can occur during severe exacerbations include atelectasis and air leaks in the chest (pneumomediastinum or pneumothorax).

Importantly, the first-line pharmacotherapy, β-agonists, can increase pulmonary blood flow through obstructed, unoxygenated areas of the lungs, causing ventilation-perfusion mismatching, and precipitating hypoxemia. Hypoxia perpetuates bronchoconstriction, which further worsens the condition. Severe and progressing asthma exacerbations clearly need to be managed in a medical setting, with administration of supplemental oxygen as first-line therapy.

Clinical Manifestations and Diagnosis. Chronic symptoms are a key aspect of asthma. The medical history typically provides key information in diagnosing asthma. Intermittent dry coughing and/or expiratory wheezing are the most common chronic symptoms of asthma. Older children and adults will report associated shortness of breath and chest tightness; younger children are more likely to report intermittent, nonfocal chest "pain." Respiratory symptoms are characteristically worse at night, especially during prolonged exacerbations triggered by respiratory infections or inhalant allergens. Other asthma symptoms in children can be subtle and include decreased physical activity, general fatigue (possibly due to sleep disturbance), and difficulty keeping up with peers in physical activities. Asking about previous experience with asthma medications (i.e., bronchodilators) may provide a history of symptomatic improvement with treatment that supports the diagnosis of asthma. Lack of improvement with bronchodilator and corticosteroid therapy is inconsistent with underlying asthma and should prompt more vigorous consideration of asthma-masquerading conditions.

Asthma symptoms are typically provoked by numerous common events or exposures: physical exertion and hyperventilation (e.g., laughing), cold or dry air, and airways irritants (Box 134–2). Exposures that induce airways inflammation, such as viral infections and inhaled allergens, also increase airways hyperresponsiveness to irritant exposures. Numerous occupational exposures incite asthma in some adults. Similarly, some children might be chronically exposed to these same airways sensitizers in their home or school environments, leading to "occupational" asthma in children. Accordingly, an environmental history is essential to optimal asthma diagnosis (see Chapter 131) and management.

The presence of risk factors, such as a history of other allergic conditions (allergic rhinitis, allergic conjunctivitis, atopic der-

---

BOX 134–2. Asthma Triggers

Common viral infections of the respiratory tract
Aeroallergens in sensitized asthmatics
  Animal dander
  Indoor allergens:
    Dust mites
    Cockroaches
    Molds
  Seasonal aeroallergens:
    Pollens (trees, grasses, weeds)
    Seasonal molds
Environmental tobacco smoke
Air pollutants
  Ozone
  Sulfur dioxide
  Particulate matter
  Wood- or coal-burning smoke
  Endotoxin, mycotoxins
  Dust
Strong or noxious odors or fumes
  Perfumes, hairsprays
  Cleaning agents
Occupational exposures
  Farm and barn exposures
  Formaldehydes, cedar, paint fumes
Cold air, dry air
Exercise
Crying, laughter, hyperventilation
Co-morbid conditions
  Rhinitis
  Sinusitis
  Gastroesophageal reflux

matitis, and food allergies), parental asthma, and/or asthma symptoms apart from colds, supports the diagnosis of asthma. Because numerous conditions can mimic asthma, the process of excluding common asthma masqueraders such as chronic rhinosinusitis and gastroesophageal reflux should begin in the medical history.

During routine clinic visits, children with asthma commonly present without abnormal signs. Some may exhibit a dry, persistent cough. By auscultation, the chest examination is also often normal. When breath sounds are abnormal, expiratory high-pitched polyphonic wheezing is typically heard by auscultation and is sometimes even audible without a stethoscope. Deeper breaths can sometimes elicit otherwise undetectable wheezing. The physical examination in asthmatics is also helpful in identifying co-morbid conditions (e.g., allergic rhinoconjunctivitis, rhinosinusitis, atopic dermatitis) and abnormalities consistent with other asthma-masquerading conditions (Box 134–3).

During asthma exacerbations, expiratory wheezing and a prolonged expiratory phase can usually be appreciated by auscultation. Decreased breath sounds in some of the lung fields, commonly the right lower posterior, are consistent with regional hypoventilation owing to airways obstruction. Crackles, or rales, and rhonchi can also be heard resulting from excess mucus production and inflammatory exudate in the airways. The combination of segmental crackles and poor breath sounds can indicate lung segmental atelectasis that is difficult to distinguish from bronchial pneumonia and can complicate

---

BOX 134–3. Differential Diagnosis of Childhood Asthma

UPPER RESPIRATORY TRACT CONDITIONS
Allergic rhinitis*
Chronic rhinitis*
Sinusitis*
Adenoidal or tonsillar hypertrophy
Nasal foreign body

MIDDLE RESPIRATORY TRACT CONDITIONS
Laryngotracheobronchomalacia*
Laryngotracheobronchitis (e.g., pertussis)*
Laryngeal web, cyst or stenosis
Vocal cord dysfunction*
Vocal cord paralysis
Tracheoesophageal fistula
Vascular ring, sling, or external mass compressing on the airway (e.g., tumor)
Foreign body aspiration*
Chronic bronchitis from environmental tobacco smoke exposure*
Toxic inhalations

LOWER RESPIRATORY TRACT CONDITIONS
Bronchopulmonary dysplasia or chronic lung disease of preterm infants
Viral bronchiolitis*
Gastroesophageal reflux*
Causes of bronchiectasis:
  Cystic fibrosis
  Immune deficiency
  Allergic bronchopulmonary mycoses (e.g., aspergillosis)
  Chronic aspiration
  Immotile cilia syndrome, primary ciliary dyskinesia
Bronchiolitis obliterans
Interstitial lung diseases
Hypersensitivity pneumonitis
Pulmonary eosinophilia, Churg-Strauss vasculitis
Pulmonary hemosiderosis
Tuberculosis
Pneumonia
Pulmonary edema (e.g., congestive heart failure)
Medications associated with chronic cough
  Acetylcholinesterase inhibitors
  β-Adrenergic antagonists

---

*More common asthma masqueraders.

---

acute asthma management. In severe exacerbations, the greater degree of airways obstruction causes increased work of breathing and respiratory distress manifested as inspiratory and expiratory wheezing, suprasternal and intercostal retractions, nasal flaring, and accessory respiratory muscle use.

DIFFERENTIAL DIAGNOSIS. Many childhood respiratory conditions can present as symptoms and signs similar to asthma (see Box 134–3). Besides asthma, other common causes of chronic, intermittent coughing and/or wheezing include rhinosinusitis and gastroesophageal reflux (GER). Both GER and chronic sinusitis can be challenging to diagnose in children. GER is often clinically silent in children, and children with chronic sinusitis typically do not report sinusitis-specific symptoms such as localized sinus pressure or tenderness. In addition, both GER and rhinosinusitis are often co-morbid conditions with childhood asthma.

In early life, chronic coughing and wheezing can indicate a congenital anatomic abnormality of the airways, foreign body aspiration, recurrent aspiration, cystic fibrosis, or bronchopulmonary dysplasia. In adolescents, vocal cord dysfunction (VCD) can present as intermittent daytime wheezing. In this condition, the vocal cords close inappropriately, during inspiration and sometimes expiration, producing shortness of breath, coughing, throat tightness, and often audible laryngeal wheezing and/or stridor. In most VCD cases, spirometric lung function testing will reveal "truncated" and inconsistent inspiratory and expiratory flow-volume loops, a pattern that differs from the reproducible pattern of airflow limitation in asthma that improves with bronchodilators. However, VCD can also co-exist with asthma. Flexible rhinolaryngoscopy in the symptomatic VCD patient can reveal paradoxical vocal cord movements, with anatomically normal vocal cords. This condition can be well managed with specialized speech therapy training in the relaxation and control of vocal cord movement. Furthermore, treatment of underlying causes of vocal cord irritability (e.g., GER/aspiration, rhinosinusitis, and asthma) can improve VCD. During acute VCD exacerbations, inhalation of heliox (a mixture of 70% helium with 30% oxygen) can relieve vocal cord spasm and VCD symptoms.

In some locales, hypersensitivity pneumonitis (e.g., farming communities, homes of bird owners), pulmonary parasitic infestations (e.g., rural areas of developing countries), or tuberculosis may be common causes of chronic coughing and/or wheezing. Rare asthma-masquerading conditions at any childhood age include bronchiolitis obliterans, interstitial lung diseases, primary ciliary dyskinesias, humoral immune deficiencies, allergic bronchopulmonary mycoses, congestive heart failure, mass lesions in or compressing the larynx, trachea, or bronchi, and medication-induced coughing and/or wheezing as an adverse effect.

Laboratory Findings. Lung or pulmonary function tests including bronchoprovocation challenges are the basis of documenting the presence of asthma and the severity of acute exacerbations.

LUNG FUNCTION TESTING. Measures of expiratory airflow are helpful in diagnosing and monitoring asthma and in assessing efficacy of therapy. Lung function testing is particularly helpful in asthmatics who are poor perceivers of airflow obstruction or when physical signs of asthma do not occur until airflow obstruction has become severe.

Spirometry measures airflow and lung volumes during a forced expiratory maneuver and is considered the gold standard measure of airflow in asthma. Its helpfulness as an objective measure in the initial evaluation and management of asthmatics has led to recommendations for its standard use in the U.S. National Asthma Education and Prevention Program (NAEPP) guidelines sponsored by the U.S. National Institutes of Health. In asthma, airways blockage results in reduced airflow and smaller partial-expiratory lung volumes (Fig. 134–1). Of these measures, normative values for FEV_1 (forced expiratory volume

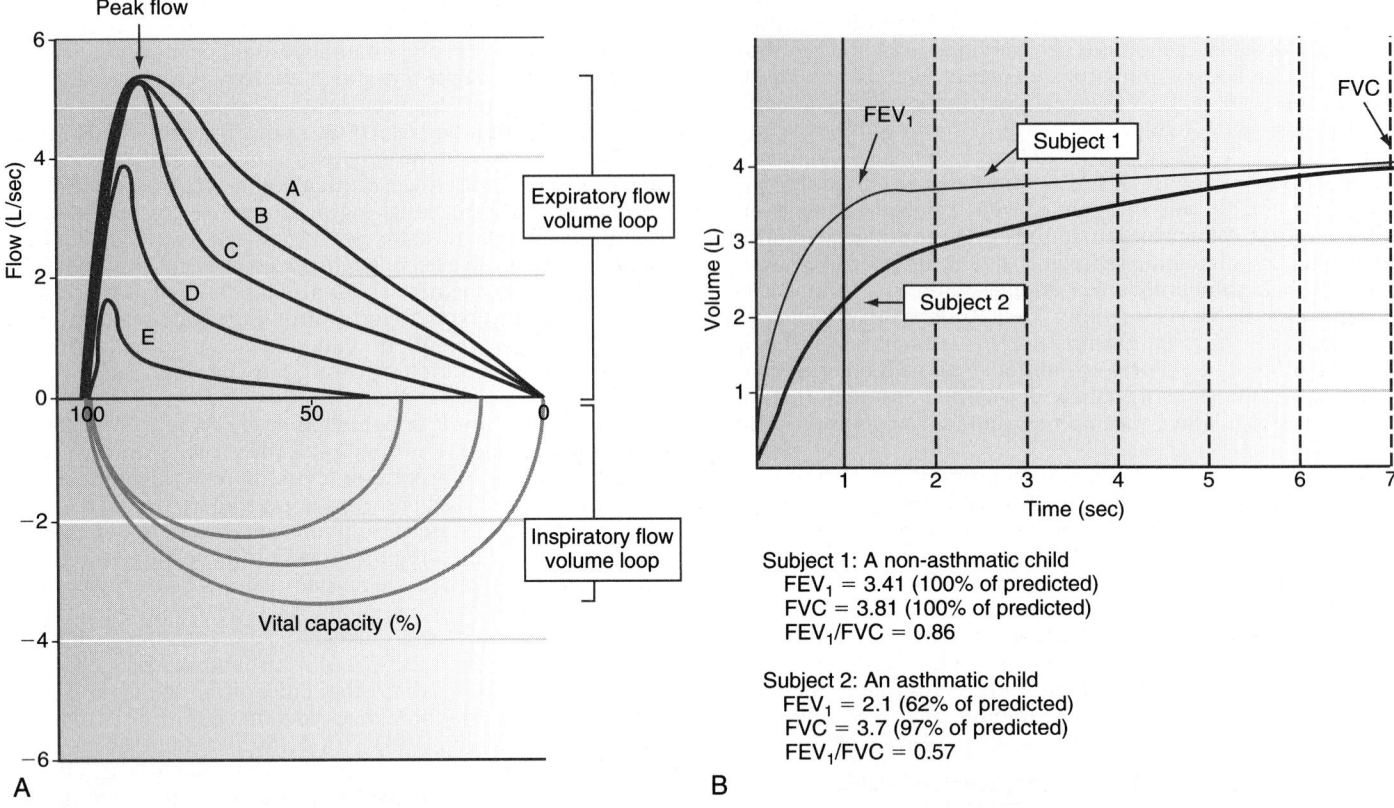

FIGURE 134–1. Spirometry. *A,* Spirometric flow-volume loops. A is an expiratory flow-volume loop of a nonasthmatic, without airflow limitation. B through E are expiratory flow-volume loops in asthmatic patients with increasing degrees of airflow limitation (B is mild; E is severe). Note the "scooped" or concave appearance of the asthmatic expiratory flow-volume loops; with increasing obstruction, there is greater "scooping." *B,* Spirometric volume-time curves. Subject 1 is a nonasthmatic; subject 2 is an asthmatic. Note how the FEV_1 and FVC lung volumes are obtained. The FEV_1 is the volume of air exhaled in the 1st second of a forced expiratory effort. The FVC is the total volume of air exhaled during a forced expiratory effort. Note that subject 2's FEV_1 and FEV_1/FVC ratio are smaller than subject 1's, demonstrating airflow obstruction. Also, subject 2's FVC is very close to what is expected.

in 1 sec) have been standardized for children, based on height, gender, and ethnicity. The reductions in FEV_1 as a percentage of predicted is one of four criteria used to determine asthma severity in the NAEPP guidelines. Because asthmatics are typically hyperinflated, often profoundly, FEV_1 can be simply adjusted for full expiratory lung volume, the forced vital capacity (FVC), with an FEV_1/FVC ratio. Generally, an FEV_1/FVC ratio less than 0.8 indicates significant airflow obstruction (Box 134–4). Such measures of airflow alone, however, are not diagnostic of asthma, because numerous other conditions can cause airflow reduction. Bronchodilator response to inhaled β-agonist medication (i.e., albuterol by nebulizer) is greater in asthmatics vs. nonasthmatics—an improvement in FEV_1 greater than 12% is consistent with asthma. Importantly, valid spirometric measures are dependent on a patient's ability to properly execute a full, forced, and prolonged expiratory maneuver, typically feasible in children older than 6 yr of age (with some younger exceptions). Reproducible spirometric efforts are an indicator of test validity. If, on three consecutive attempts, the FEV_1 is within 5%, then the best FEV_1 effort of the three is used.

Bronchoprovocation challenges can be helpful in diagnosing asthma and optimizing asthma management. Asthmatic airways are hyperresponsive and therefore more sensitive to inhaled methacholine, histamine, and cold or dry air. The degree of airways hyperresponsiveness to these exposures correlates with asthma severity and airways inflammation. Although bronchoprovocation challenges are carefully dosed and monitored in an investigational setting, their use is rarely practical in a general practice setting. **Exercise challenges**

(i.e., aerobic exertion or "running" for 6–8 min) can also help to identify the child with **exercise-induced bronchospasm**. Although the airflow response of nonasthmatics to exercise is to increase functional lung volumes and improve FEV_1 slightly (5–10%), exercise typically induces airflow obstruction in untreated asthmatics. Accordingly, in asthmatics, FEV_1 typically decreases during or after exercise by more than 15% (see Box 134–4). The onset of exercise-induced bronchospasm is usually within 15 min after a vigorous exercise challenge and can spontaneously resolve within 60 min. Studies of U.S. school-age children using such exercise challenges typically identify about 10% with exercise-induced bronchospasm but previously undiagnosed asthma, in addition to the known asthmatics with exercise-induced bronchospasm. Exercise challenges can induce

---

▌BOX 134–4. Lung Function Abnormalities in Asthma

Spirometry
Airflow limitation
  Low FEV_1 (relative to percentage of predicted norms)
  FEV_1/FVC ratio < 0.8
Bronchodilator response (to inhaled β₂-agonist)
  Improvement in FEV_1 ≥12%*
Exercise challenge
  Worsening in FEV_1 ≥15%*
Peak flow morning-to-afternoon variation ≥20%*

---
*Main criteria consistent with asthma.

severe asthma exacerbations in at-risk patients; therefore, careful patient selection for exercise challenges, and preparedness for severe asthma exacerbations, is required.

Peak expiratory flow (PEF) monitoring devices provide a simple and inexpensive home-use tool to measure airflow and can be particularly helpful in many circumstances. PEFs vary in their ability to detect airflow obstruction, and, in some patients, PEF declines only when airflow obstruction is severe. Therefore, PEF monitoring should be started by measuring morning and evening PEFs (best of three consecutive attempts) for several weeks for patients to practice the technique, to determine a "personal best," and to correlate PEF values with symptoms (and ideally spirometry). PEF morning-to-evening variation greater than 20% is consistent with asthma (Fig. 134–2 and see Box 134–4).

RADIOLOGY. Chest radiographs (posteroanterior and lateral views) in children with asthma often appear to be normal, aside from subtle and nonspecific findings of hyperinflation (e.g., flattening of the diaphragms) and peribronchial thickening. Chest radiographs are helpful in identifying abnormalities that are hallmarks of asthma masqueraders (e.g., aspiration pneumonitis, hyperlucent lung fields in bronchiolitis obliterans), and complications during asthma exacerbations (e.g., atelectasis, pneumothorax). Some lung abnormalities can be better appreciated with high-resolution, thin-section chest CT scans. For example, bronchiectasis is sometimes difficult to appreciate on chest radiograph but is clearly seen on CT scan and implicates asthma masqueraders such as cystic fibrosis, allergic bronchopulmonary mycoses (e.g., aspergillosis), ciliary dyskinesias, or immune deficiencies.

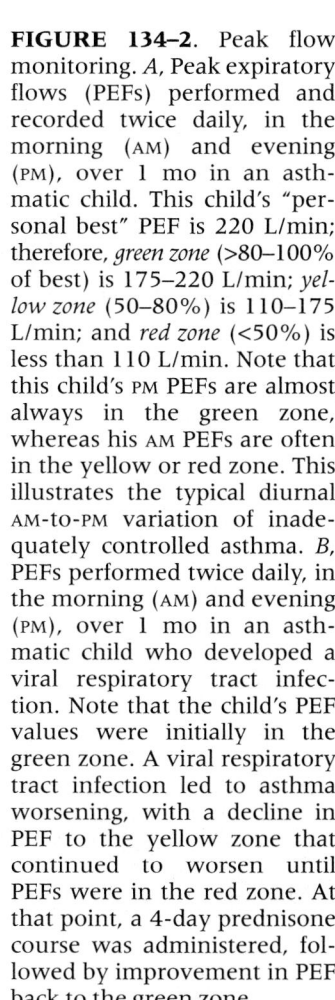

FIGURE 134–2. Peak flow monitoring. *A,* Peak expiratory flows (PEFs) performed and recorded twice daily, in the morning (AM) and evening (PM), over 1 mo in an asthmatic child. This child's "personal best" PEF is 220 L/min; therefore, *green zone* (>80–100% of best) is 175–220 L/min; *yellow zone* (50–80%) is 110–175 L/min; and *red zone* (<50%) is less than 110 L/min. Note that this child's PM PEFs are almost always in the green zone, whereas his AM PEFs are often in the yellow or red zone. This illustrates the typical diurnal AM-to-PM variation of inadequately controlled asthma. *B,* PEFs performed twice daily, in the morning (AM) and evening (PM), over 1 mo in an asthmatic child who developed a viral respiratory tract infection. Note that the child's PEF values were initially in the green zone. A viral respiratory tract infection led to asthma worsening, with a decline in PEF to the yellow zone that continued to worsen until PEFs were in the red zone. At that point, a 4-day prednisone course was administered, followed by improvement in PEF back to the green zone.

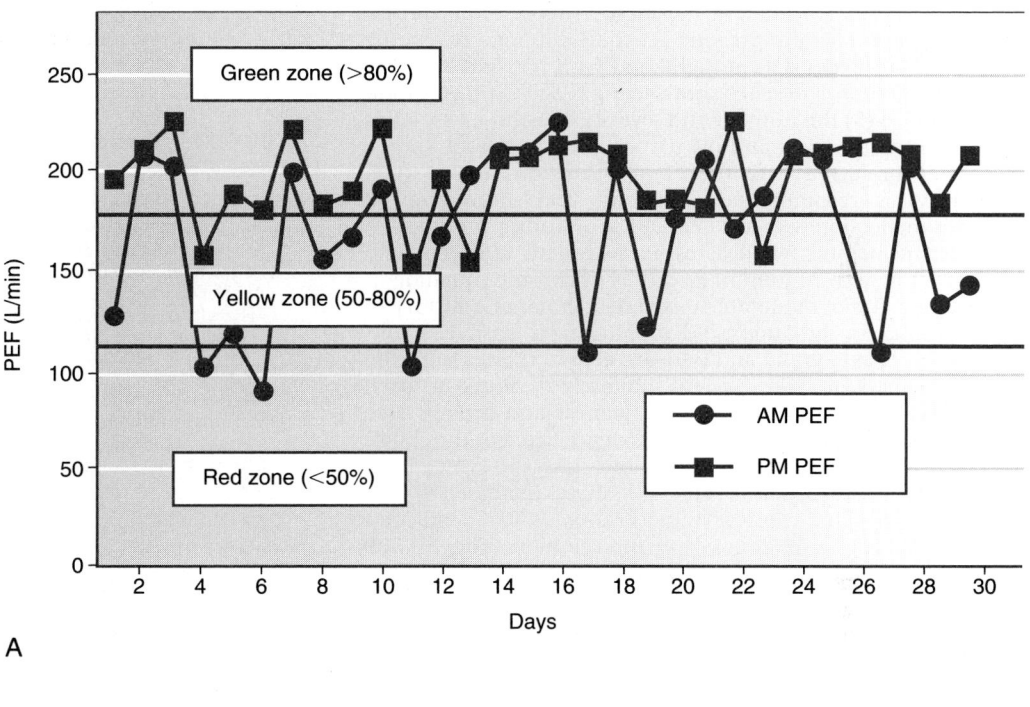

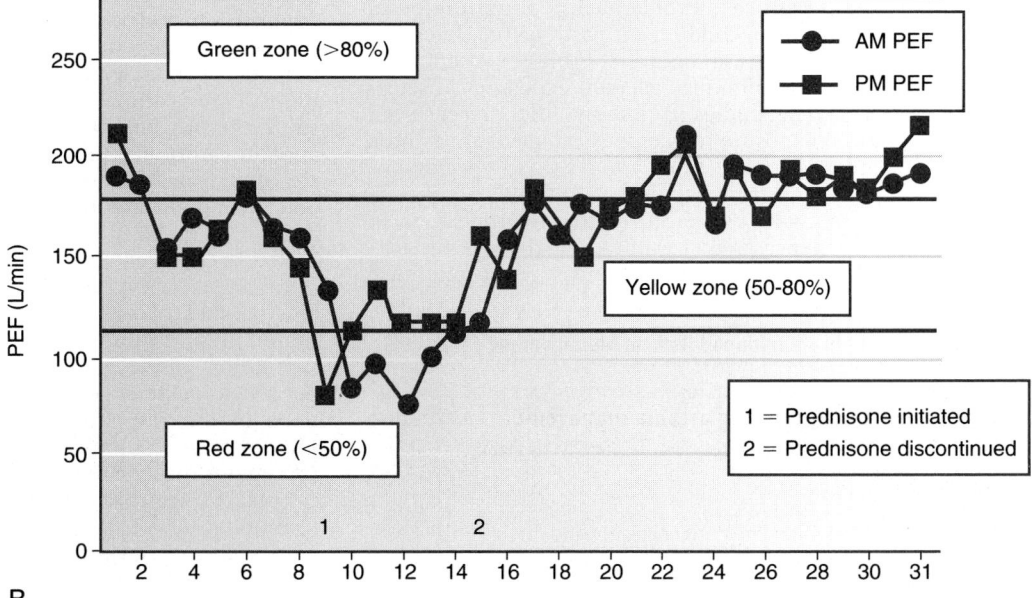

Other tests, such as allergy testing to assess sensitization to inhalant allergens, help with the management and prognosis of asthma. In a comprehensive U.S. study of 5–12 yr old asthmatic children (Childhood Asthma Management Program [CAMP]), 88% had inhalant allergen sensitization by allergy prick skin testing.

Treatment. The goals of childhood asthma management for children can be simply stated (Box 134–5). The NAEPP guidelines have been adapted for childhood asthma in a joint publication of the American Academy of Allergy, Asthma & Immunology and the U.S. National Institutes of Health's National Heart, Lung and Blood Institute and the American Academy of Pediatrics entitled *Pediatric Asthma: Promoting Best Practice*. These guidelines describe four components to optimal asthma management (Box 134–6).

REGULAR ASSESSMENT AND MONITORING. Asthma management can be optimized through regular clinic visits every 2–4 wk until good asthma control is achieved. Two to four regular annual asthma check-ups are recommended to maintain good asthma control. During these visits, asthma control can be assessed by asking about (1) the frequency of asthma symptoms during the day, at night, and with physical exercise; (2) the frequency of "rescue" short-acting β-agonist medication use and refills; (3) the number and severity of asthma exacerbations since the last visit; and (4) participation in school, sports, and other preferred activities. Lung function testing (i.e., spirometry) is recommended annually, and more often if asthma is inadequately controlled. PEF monitoring at home can be especially helpful when assessing asthmatic children with poor symptom perception, other causes of chronic coughing in addition to asthma, moderate-to-severe asthma, or a history of severe asthma exacerbations. PEF monitoring is feasible in children as young as 4 yr old and who are able to master this skill. Use of a "stoplight" zone system, preferably tailored to each child's best PEFs, can optimize effectiveness and interest (see Fig. 134–2): the green zone (80–100% of predicted or the child's best) indicates good control, the yellow zone (50–80%) indicates less than optimal control and necessitates increased awareness and treatment, whereas the red zone (<50%) indicates poor control requiring immediate intervention. The NAEPP guidelines recommend once-daily PEF monitoring, preferably in the morning.

CONTROL OF FACTORS CONTRIBUTING TO ASTHMA SEVERITY. Controllable factors that can significantly worsen asthma can be generally grouped as (1) environmental exposures and (2) co-morbid conditions (Box 134–7).

Eliminate or Reduce Problematic Environmental Exposures. The majority of children with asthma have an allergic component to their disease. Because of this, steps should be taken to investigate and minimize allergen exposures in sensitized asthmatics. Several studies have shown that, in sensitized asthmatics, reduced exposure to allergens can decrease asthma symptoms, the need for medications, and airways hyperresponsiveness.

Asthmatic children who are sensitized to indoor allergens in particular can experience greater asthma severity due to year-round exposure and can benefit from measures to minimize

---

BOX 134–5. Goals of Childhood Asthma Management

Maintain normal activity
  Regular school or daycare attendance
  Full participation in physical exercise, athletics, and other recreational activities
Prevent sleep disturbance
Prevent chronic asthma symptoms
Keep asthma exacerbations from becoming severe
Maintain normal lung function
Experience little to no adverse effects of treatment

BOX 134–6. Four Components of Optimal Asthma Management

REGULAR ASSESSMENT AND MONITORING
Asthma check-ups
  Every 2–4 wk until good control is achieved
  2–4 per year to maintain good control
Lung function monitoring

CONTROL OF FACTORS CONTRIBUTING TO ASTHMA SEVERITY
Eliminate or reduce problematic environmental exposures
Treat co-morbid conditions: rhinitis, sinusitis, gastroesophageal reflux

ASTHMA PHARMACOTHERAPY
Long-term-control versus quick-relief medications
Classification of asthma severity for anti-inflammatory pharmacotherapy
Step-up, step-down approach
Asthma exacerbation management

PATIENT EDUCATION
Provide a two-part care plan
  Daily management
  Action plan for asthma exacerbations

BOX 134–7. Control of Factors Contributing to Asthma Severity

ELIMINATE OR REDUCE PROBLEMATIC ENVIRONMENTAL EXPOSURES
Environmental tobacco smoke elimination or reduction
  In home and automobiles
Allergen exposure elimination or reduction in sensitized asthmatics
  Animal danders
    Pets (cats, dogs, rodents, birds)
    Pests (mice, rats)
  Dust mites
  Cockroaches
  Molds
Other airway irritants
  Wood- or coal-burning smoke
  Strong chemical odors and perfumes (e.g., household cleaners)
  Dusts

TREAT CO-MORBID CONDITIONS
Rhinitis
Sinusitis
Gastroesophageal reflux

GET ANNUAL INFLUENZA VACCINATION (UNLESS EGG-ALLERGIC)

---

allergen exposure in the home. Common perennial allergen exposures include furred or feathered animals as pets or as pests and occult indoor allergens such as dust mites, molds, and cockroaches. Although some sensitized children may report an increase in asthma symptoms on exposure to the allergen source, improvement from allergen avoidance may not become apparent without a sustained period of days to weeks away from the offending exposure. Tobacco, wood, and coal smoke, dusts, and strong or noxious odors and fumes can all aggravate asthma. At the very least, these airways irritants should be eliminated or reduced from the homes and automobiles used by asthmatic children. School classrooms and daycare centers can also be sites of asthma-worsening environmental exposures. Eliminating or minimizing these exposures can reduce asthma symptoms, disease severity, and the amount of medication needed to achieve good asthma control. Common viral infections of the respiratory tract are difficult to avoid; annual influenza vaccination is recommended for all asthmatic children (except for those with egg allergy).

Treat Co-morbid Conditions. Rhinitis, sinusitis, and gastroesophageal reflux commonly accompany asthma and can worsen disease severity. Indeed, these conditions are also common causes of chronic coughing. Effective management of these co-morbid conditions can often improve asthma symptoms and disease severity, so that less medication is needed to achieve good asthma control.

Gastroesophageal reflux (GER) is commonly noted in asthmatics, with a reported incidence of up to 64%. GER may worsen asthma through two postulated mechanisms: (1) aspiration of refluxed gastric contents (micro- or macroaspiration) and (2) reflex bronchospasm. GER should be suspected in all individuals with difficult-to-control asthma, especially patients with prominent symptoms while eating or sleeping (i.e., in a horizontal position). GER can be confirmed by demonstration of reflux of barium into the esophagus during a barium swallow procedure or by esophageal pH monitoring. Because radiographic studies lack sufficient sensitivity and specificity, extended esophageal pH monitoring is the method of choice for diagnosing GER. If significant GER is noted, reflux precautions should be instituted (no food 2 hr before bedtime, head of the bed elevated 6 in) and antacid medications such as H_2-receptor antagonists (e.g., cimetidine, ranitidine) or proton pump inhibitors (e.g., omeprazole, lansoprazole), and possibly prokinetic pharmacotherapy, administered for a 6–8 wk period.

Radiographic evidence for sinus disease is also common in patients with asthma. Several case series have reported significant improvement in asthma control in patients diagnosed and treated for occult sinus disease. A screening CT scan of the sinuses is the current gold standard test for sinus disease. If the patient with asthma has clinical and radiographic evidence for sinusitis, topical therapy to include nasal saline irrigations and intranasal glucocorticoids should be instituted, and a 3 wk course of antibiotics administered.

PRINCIPLES OF ASTHMA PHARMACOTHERAPY. The NAEPP guidelines classify asthma severity before treatment using four parameters: (1) frequency of daytime or (2) nighttime symptoms, (3) degree of airflow obstruction by spirometry, and/or (4) PEF variability (Table 134–1). Asthmatics can be categorized in four disease severity groups, as "mild intermittent" or "persistent" disease that is "mild," "moderate," or "severe." A major objective of this approach is to identify and treat all "persistent" asthma with anti-inflammatory controller medication. The "3 Strikes" rule is a handy memory aid for determining if an asthmatic child should receive controller therapy based on the NAEPP guidelines. Simply put, if an asthmatic child has asthma symptoms or requires quick-relief medication more than three times per week, awakens at night due to asthma more than three times per month, or requires a refill for a quick-relief inhaler prescription more than three times per year, then that patient should receive daily controller therapy. Low-dose inhaled glucocorticoids, leukotriene pathway modifiers, or cromolyn/nedocromil are the recommended controllers for mild persistent asthmatics; sustained-release theophylline is an alternative. The recommended controller medication for moderate persistent asthmatics is medium-dose inhaled glucocorticoids or low-dose inhaled glucocorticoids in combination with a long-acting β-agonist or a leukotriene pathway modifier; sustained release theophylline or long-acting oral β-agonists are alternatives. Severe persistent asthmatics should receive high-dose inhaled glucocorticoids, a long-acting bronchodilator, and routine oral glucocorticoids if needed. "Mild intermittent asthma" is the only level of asthma severity where daily controller therapy

TABLE 134–1. Stepwise Approach for Managing Asthma: Severity Classification and Management*

Asthma Severity	Days with Symptoms	Nights with Symptoms	Lung Function	Long-Term-Control Medication	Quick-Relief Medication	Education
Step 1: Mild Intermittent	<3 per wk	<3 per mo	FEV₁ or PEF ≥80% of predicted; PEF variability <20%	No daily medication needed	**Short-acting β-agonist** as needed and before exercise; Use ≥3 times per wk may indicate need to initiate long-term-control therapy	Asthma facts, MDI and spacer technique, role of medications, action plan, environmental control measures
Step 2: Mild Persistent	≥3 per wk	3–4 per mo	FEV₁ or PEF ≥80% of predicted; PEF variability 20–30%	**Anti-inflammatory:** either low-dose **inhaled glucocorticoid, cromolyn, nedocromil, or leukotriene modifier.** Sustained-release theophylline is an alternative.	**Short-acting β-agonist** as needed and before exercise; daily use or increasing use may indicate need for additional long-term-control therapy	Step 1 actions plus: self-monitoring, group education, review and update self-management plan
Step 3: Moderate Persistent	Daily symptoms, daily use of short-acting β-agonists	>1 time per wk	FEV₁ or PEF >60 and ≤80% predicted; PEF variability >30%	**Anti-inflammatory: inhaled glucocorticoids** (medium-dose) or inhaled glucocorticoids (low-dose) and either **long-acting β-agonist (LABA), leukotriene modifier,** sustained-release theophylline, or LABA tablets.	**Short-acting β-agonist** as needed and before exercise; daily use or increasing use may indicate need for additional long-term-control therapy	Step 1 actions plus: self-monitoring, group education, review and update self-management plan
Step 4: Severe Persistent	Continual symptoms, limited physical activity, frequent exacerbations	Frequent	FEV₁ or PEF ≤60% of predicted; PEF variability >30%	**Anti-inflammatory: inhaled glucocorticoids** (high-dose) and long-acting bronchodilator: either **LABA, leukotriene modifier,** sustained-release theophylline, and/or LABA tablets. Oral glucocorticoid if needed.	**Short-acting β-agonist** as needed and before exercise; daily use or increasing use may indicate need for additional long-term-control therapy	Step 2 and 3 actions plus: referral for individual education/counseling

*Based on clinical features before treatment; classification is determined by the patient's most severe feature; bold print indicates preferred medication; **asthmatics with "persistent" disease of any severity should be treated with a "long-term-control" anti-inflammatory medication.**
Modified from the National Asthma Education & Prevention Program: Expert Panel Report II: Guidelines for the Diagnosis and Management of Asthma. Bethesda, MD, National Institutes of Health, National Heart, Lung, and Blood Institute, 1997.

is not recommended. In these subjects, short-acting inhaled β-agonists are recommended as needed for symptoms and for exercise pre-treatment for those with exercise-induced bronchospasm. Short-acting β-agonists are the recommended reliever medication for all asthma severity levels. They are to be used as needed for acute symptoms.

"Step-Up, Step-Down" Approach. The NAEPP guidelines outline a stepwise approach to asthma therapy that emphasizes initiating higher-level controller therapy at the outset to establish prompt control, with measures to "step-down" therapy once good asthma control is achieved.

Inhalation Technique. Optimal inhalation technique for each puff of metered-dose inhaler (MDI)-delivered medication is a slow (5 sec) inhalation, then a 5–10 sec breath hold. No waiting time between puffs of medication is needed. Spacer devices for the delivery of all medications from MDIs should be used universally in all children with asthma. **Spacer devices** are simple and inexpensive tools that serve three major functions: (1) they decrease the amount of coordination required to use MDIs, especially in young children; (2) they improve the delivery of inhaled drug to the lower airways, which in turn improves medication efficacy; and (3) they minimize the risk of systemic absorption of inhaled glucocorticoids, thus minimizing potential adverse effects of this class of medications. Mouth rinsing is recommended after inhaled glucocorticoid use to rinse out inhaled glucocorticoids deposited on the oral mucosa.

Combination Pharmacotherapy. Most children will have their asthma well controlled on a single controller medication. In children who continue to be symptomatic on low to moderate doses of inhaled glucocorticoid therapy, studies have shown a superior outcome when a long-acting β-agonist or leukotriene pathway modifier is added to the original dose of inhaled glucocorticoids rather than doubling the dose of the inhaled glucocorticoid. Thus, lung function and asthma control can be optimized without increasing the potential for systemic effects from inhaled glucocorticoids.

Adherence. Asthma is a chronic condition that is often best managed with daily controller medication. However, adherence with a daily regimen can be suboptimal. A study that evaluated adherence of asthmatic children to routine inhaled glucocorticoids found that they were underused 60% of the time. In addition, individuals who required an oral glucocorticoid burst due to an asthma exacerbation had used their inhaled glucocorticoids the least (<15% of the time). Other studies have found that adherence is poorer when prescribed frequency of medication administration is greater (i.e., 3–4 times/24 hr). Therefore, treatment strategies should be designed to minimize the frequency with which medications are administered (i.e., once or twice daily).

QUICK-RELIEF OR RELIEVER MEDICATIONS. Asthma medications are used as quick-relief, or "reliever" or "rescue," medications, or long-term-control, or "controller," medications (Table 134–2). Quick-relief medications (inhaled β$_2$-agonists, inhaled anticholinergics, and short-course systemic glucocorticoids) are used in the management of acute episodes of bronchospasm.

Short-Acting β$_2$-Agonists. Given their rapid onset of action, effectiveness, and 4–6 hr duration of action, inhaled short-acting β-agonists (e.g., albuterol, levalbuterol, terbutaline, pirbuterol) are the drugs of choice for acute episodes of bronchospasm (i.e., "rescue" medications) and for preventing exercise-induced bronchospasm. β-Agonists bronchodilate by inducing airway smooth muscle relaxation, reducing vascular permeability airways edema, and improving mucociliary clearance. Studies have reported that overuse of β-agonists is associated with increased death or near-death episodes from asthma. This is a major concern for some patients with asthma who rely on short-acting β-agonists as a "quick fix" for their asthma, rather than using controller medications in a preventive man-

ner. It is helpful to monitor the frequency of inhaled β-agonist use, in that use of >1 canister/mo (200 inhalations/mo) indicates inadequate asthma control and necessitates initiating or intensifying controller therapy.

Anticholinergic Agents. As bronchodilators, the anticholinergic agents (e.g., ipratropium bromide) are much less potent than the β-agonists. Inhaled ipratropium is primarily used in the treatment of acute severe asthma. When used in combination with albuterol, ipratropium has been shown to significantly improve lung function and to reduce the rate of hospitalization in children who present to the emergency department with acute asthma. Ipratropium bromide is the anticholinergic drug of choice because it has few central nervous system adverse effects, and it is available in both MDI and nebulizable formulations. Although widely used in children with asthma exacerbations of all ages, it is approved by the U.S. Food and Drug Administration (FDA) for use in children >12 yr of age.

Systemic Glucocorticoid Therapy. Short-course, systemic glucocorticoid therapy is recommended for use in moderate-to-severe asthma exacerbations, both to hasten recovery and prevent recurrence of symptoms. The efficacy of glucocorticoid therapy for asthma exacerbations in children is firmly established. Studies evaluating single doses of glucocorticoids administered in the emergency department, short courses of oral glucocorticoids in the clinic setting, and both oral and intravenous formulations in hospitalized children have all demonstrated effectiveness. Studies in children hospitalized with acute asthma have found glucocorticoids administered orally to be as effective as intravenous glucocorticoids. Accordingly, oral glucocorticoid therapy can often be used, although children in respiratory distress who require high flow rates of oxygen to adequately treat hypoxemia are obvious candidates for intravenous glucocorticoid therapy. For hospitalized children, the NAEPP guidelines recommend administering methylprednisolone at 1 mg/kg/dose every 6 hr for 48 hr, with a taper to 1–2 mg/kg/24 hr (maximum 60 mg/24 hr) in two divided doses until the patient's PEFs reach 70% of predicted or personal best. For outpatient

TABLE 134–2. Asthma Medications by Category	
Category	**Examples of Medications**
Quick-relief medications ("relievers")	Short-acting inhaled β-agonists:
	Albuterol (Ventolin, Proventil)
	Levalbuterol (Xopenex)
	Terbutaline (Brethaire)
	Pirbuterol (Maxair)
	Metaproterenol (Alupent)
	Inhaled anticholinergics:
	Ipratropium (Atrovent)
	Atropine
	Short-course systemic glucocorticoids:
	Prednisone (Deltasone)
	Methylprednisolone (Medrol)
	Methylprednisolone Sodium Succinate (Solu-Medrol)
Long-term-control medications ("controllers")	Nonsteroidal anti-inflammatory agents:
	Cromolyn (Intal)
	Nedocromil (Tilade)
	Inhaled glucocorticoids:
	Beclomethasone (Vanceril, Beclovent, Qvar)
	Flunisolide (Aerobid)
	Budesonide (Pulmicort)
	Fluticasone (Flovent)
	Triamcinolone (Azmacort)
	Mometasone (Asmanex)
	Sustained-release theophylline (Slobid, Theodur, Uniphyl)
	Long-acting inhaled β-agonists:
	Salmeterol (Serevent)
	Formoterol (Foradil)
	Leukotriene modifiers:
	Montelukast (Singulair)
	Zafirlukast (Accolate)
	Zileuton (Zyflo)
	Oral glucocorticoids (prednisone, methylprednisolone)

management of acute asthma, the NAEPP guidelines suggest 1–2 mg/kg/24 hr (maximum 60 mg/24 hr) of prednisone or methyl-prednisolone in a single or two divided doses for 3–10 days.

LONG-TERM-CONTROL OR CONTROLLER MEDICATIONS. Mild to moderate persistent asthma should be treated with long-term-control medications, which include nonsteroidal anti-inflammatory agents, inhaled glucocorticoids, sustained-release theophylline, long-acting inhaled β-agonists, and leukotriene modifiers.

Nonsteroidal Anti-inflammatory Agents. Cromolyn and nedocromil are "nonsteroidal" anti-inflammatory agents that can inhibit both the early and late phase components of allergen-induced asthmatic responses and can inhibit exercise-induced bronchospasm. Both drugs are indicated for mild to moderate asthma and are considered first-line anti-inflammatory drugs for children with mild persistent asthma according to the NAEPP guidelines. Although largely devoid of adverse effects, these medications must be administered frequently (two to four times/24 hr) and are not nearly as effective as the other two major controller classes of medications, namely, the inhaled glucocorticoids and leukotriene-modifying agents. As a result, they should now be considered alternative agents. Because they inhibit exercise-induced bronchospasm, they can be used in place of short-acting β-agonists, especially in children who develop unwanted adverse effects with β-agonist therapy (e.g., tremor and elevated heart rate). They can also be used in combination with short-acting β-agonists in patients who continue to experience exercise-induced bronchospasm despite short-acting β-agonist pretreatment.

Glucocorticoids. Glucocorticoids are available in inhaled, oral, and parenteral forms. Glucocorticoids are the most potent and effective medications used to treat both the acute (administered systemically) and chronic (administered topically) manifestations of asthma.

Inhaled Glucocorticoid Therapy. The development of inhalation devices, which effectively deliver potent glucocorticoids into the airways, have made inhaled glucocorticoid therapy the treatment of choice for patients with persistent asthma (see Table 134–1). Inhaled glucocorticoid therapy has been shown to reduce asthma symptoms, improve baseline pulmonary function, and reduce bronchial hyperresponsiveness. In addition, inhaled glucocorticoid therapy in children with mild to moderate persistent asthma results in less need for "rescue" short-acting β-agonists use and less need for prednisone and can reduce, by up to 50%, urgent care visits and hospitalizations for acute asthma. Lastly, large epidemiologic studies have now demonstrated low-dose inhaled glucocorticoid therapy to "protect" against asthma death. Inhaled glucocorticoids achieve all of the goals of asthma therapy and as a result have become the gold standard treatment for asthma.

The NAEPP guidelines recommend low-dose inhaled glucocorticoid therapy for all patients with persistent asthma. Whether inhaled glucocorticoids should be first-line therapy in children with mild persistent asthma is controversial. Advocates for inhaled glucocorticoid therapy argue that because this medication reduces airways inflammation, bronchial hyperresponsiveness, and asthma morbidity and mortality, it should be used in all patients with persistent asthma. In contrast, others argue that since inhaled glucocorticoid therapy is not without the potential for adverse effects, its use should be reserved for those with moderate to severe persistent asthma. A few studies have suggested that delay in initiation of inhaled glucocorticoid therapy leads to a diminished therapeutic response. The implication of these studies is that asthma is a progressive condition that requires anti-inflammatory therapy to prevent airway remodeling and subsequent loss of therapeutic response.

There are currently five FDA-approved inhaled glucocorticoids, with a sixth product likely to be approved in 2002 (see Table 134–3). Inhaled glucocorticoids are available for use in MDIs with ozone-friendly propellants, as dry powder inhalers (DPIs), or in suspension for nebulization. All of the available inhaled glucocorticoids are effective in asthma. Fluticasone propionate, mometasone furoate, and, to a lesser extent, budesonide are thought to be "second generation" inhaled glucocorticoids in that they display greater topical to systemic potency compared with other available inhaled glucocorticoids, resulting in a better therapeutic index. Second-generation inhaled glucocorticoids display both increased anti-inflammatory potency and reduced systemic bioavailability, owing to extensive first-pass hepatic metabolism, making these compounds well suited for patients with severe asthma. The NAEPP guidelines recommend starting with higher inhaled glucocorticoid doses and "stepping down" the dose as asthma control improves. Many studies have shown that a fraction of the initial glucocorticoid dose is often sufficient once asthma control is achieved. The ideal inhaled glucocorticoid dose should be large enough to control asthma symptoms yet small enough to avoid the potential for adverse systemic effects (see Table 134–3). Inhaled

TABLE 134–3. Inhaled Glucocorticoids Daily Dosage Guidelines*

Glucocorticoid	Low Dose	Medium Dose	High Dose
Beclomethasone 42, 84 µg/puff (40 µg/puff HFA–propellant)	84–336 µg (2–8 puffs of 42 µg/puff or 1–4 puffs of 84 µg/puff)	336–672 µg (8–16 puffs of 42 µg/puff or 4–8 puffs of 84 µg/puff)	>672 µg (> 16 puffs of 42 µg/puff or > 8 puffs of 84 µg/puff)
Budesonide Turbuhaler (DPI) 200 µg/inhalation Respules (nebulizer) 250, 500 µg/vial	200–400 µg (1–2 inhalations) 500 µg QD	400–800 µg (2–4 inhalations) 1000 µg	> 800 µg (>4 inhalations) 2000 µg
Flunisolide 250 µg/puff (MDI)	500–750 µg (2–3 puffs)	1000–1250 µg (4–5 puffs)	> 1250 µg (>5 puffs)
Fluticasone 44, 110, 220 µg/puff (MDI)	88–176 µg (2–4 puffs of 44 µg/puff)	176–440 µg (4–10 puffs of 44 µg/puff or 2–4 puffs of 110 µg/puff or 1–2 puffs of 220 µg/puff)	> 440 µg (>4 puffs of 110 µg/puff or > 2 puffs of 220 µg/puff)
Triamcinolone 100 µg/puff (MDI with spacer)	400–800 µg (4–8 puffs)	800–1200 µg (8–12 puffs)	>1200 µg (> 12 puffs)

Estimated comparative daily doses for children ≤ 12 yr of age.
Modified from the National Asthma Education & Prevention Program Expert Panel Report: Guidelines for the Diagnosis and Management of Asthma. Update on Selected Topics 2002. Bethesda, MD, National Institutes of Health, National Heart, Lung, and Blood Institute, 2002.

glucocorticoids can be effective when administered once or twice daily.

Although inhaled glucocorticoids have been widely used in adults with persistent asthma, their use in children has been lagging. The reluctance to use inhaled glucocorticoids in childhood asthma has come primarily from their potential for adverse effects with chronic use. Generally, clinically significant adverse effects that occur with chronic systemic glucocorticoid therapy (Box 134–8) have not been seen or have been only rarely reported in children receiving inhaled glucocorticoid therapy in recommended doses. The risk of adverse effects from inhaled glucocorticoid therapy is related to the dose and frequency with which inhaled glucocorticoids are given. High doses (1,000 µg/24 hr in children) administered frequently (e.g., four times/24 hr) have an increased risk for local and systemic adverse effects.

The most commonly encountered adverse effects from inhaled glucocorticoid therapy are local and consist of oral candidiasis (thrush) and dysphonia (hoarse voice). Thrush is thought to occur as a result of local immunosuppression. Dysphonia occurs as a result of vocal cord myopathy. These effects are dose dependent and are most common in individuals on high-dose inhaled and/or oral glucocorticoid therapy. The incidence of these local effects can be greatly minimized by using a holding chamber or "spacer" when using inhaled glucocorticoids delivered via a MDI because these devices effectively reduce the oropharyngeal deposition of the drug. Mouth rinsing using a "swish and spit" technique after inhaled glucocorticoid inhalation is also recommended after administration of any inhaled glucocorticoid.

The potential for growth suppression with long-term inhaled glucocorticoids has long been a concern among health care professionals caring for asthmatic children. Complicating this issue is the long known, but often overlooked observation that asthma, especially poorly controlled asthma, can adversely affect growth. In the long term, prospective Childhood Asthma Management Program (CAMP) study, after a mean of 4.3 yr of therapy, children with mild to moderate asthma randomized to budesonide (400 µg/24 hr) had grown 22.7 cm, whereas those randomized to placebo had grown 23.8 cm—a 1.1 cm difference. Of importance, this 1.1 cm difference occurred primarily in the first year of therapy, indicating that the growth suppression was a transient, not progressive phenomenon. Agertoft and Pedersen, in an open-label, controlled study, found no difference in the measured versus the expected adult heights in a cohort of asthmatics who had received inhaled budesonide (400 µg/24 hr) for longer than 9 yr. They also noted transient growth suppression in the first few years of therapy, with eventual catch-up growth and no adverse effect on final adult height. These two long-term studies support the contention that inhaled glucocorticoid therapy results in a modest and transient effect on growth that is unlikely to have a significant adverse effect on adult height.

Two large pediatric studies that have evaluated the effect of long-term inhaled glucocorticoids on bone mineral density failed to find a relationship between inhaled glucocorticoids use and diminished bone mineral density. Although these studies cannot predict a significant effect of inhaled glucocorticoid therapy on osteoporosis in later adulthood (i.e., after 30 yr of use), improved asthma control may result in less glucocorticoid therapy needed over time. In summary, current evidence suggests that long-term inhaled glucocorticoid therapy has no significant effect on adult attained height or on bone mineral density. These findings were with budesonide at doses of roughly 400 µg/24 hr; higher doses of inhaled glucocorticoids will have a greater potential for adverse effects.

Systemic Glucocorticoid Therapy. Inhaled glucocorticoid therapy has allowed the majority of patients with asthma to maintain good control of their disease. Indeed, inhaled glucocorticoid therapy has allowed many patients with severe asthma to reduce or even discontinue maintenance oral glucocorticoids. Thus, oral glucocorticoid therapy is now used primarily to treat asthma exacerbations and in rare patients with severe disease who remain symptomatic despite optimal use of other asthma medications. In these severe asthmatics, every attempt should be made to exclude any co-morbid conditions and to keep the oral glucocorticoid dose at ≤20 mg administered on alternate days. Doses exceeding this amount are associated with numerous adverse effects (see Box 134–8). To determine the need for continued oral glucocorticoid therapy, a gradual taper of the oral glucocorticoid dose should be considered, with close monitoring of the patient's symptoms and lung function.

When administered orally, prednisone, prednisolone, and methylprednisolone are rapidly and nearly completely absorbed, with peak plasma concentrations occurring within 1–2 hr. Of interest, prednisone is an inactive pro-drug that requires biotransformation via first pass hepatic metabolism to prednisolone, its active form. Glucocorticoids are metabolized in the liver into inactive compounds, with the rate of metabolism influenced by drug interactions and disease states. Anticonvulsants (e.g., phenytoin, phenobarbital, carbamazepine) increase the metabolism of prednisolone, methylprednisolone, and dexamethasone, with methylprednisolone most significantly affected. Rifampin also enhances the clearance of glucocorticoids and can result in diminished therapeutic effect. Other medications

---

BOX 134–8. Adverse Effects Associated with Chronic Systemic Glucocorticoid Use

METABOLIC/ENDOCRINOLOGIC EFFECTS

Hypokalemia
Hyperglycemia
Hyperlipidemia
Adrenal suppression
Growth suppression
Delayed sexual maturation (delayed puberty)
Weight gain
Cushingoid habitus (central obesity with wasting of the extremities)
Diabetes mellitus

MUSCULOSKELETAL EFFECTS

Osteoporosis/vertebral compression fractures
Aseptic necrosis of bone (hips, shoulders, knees)
Myopathy (acute and chronic forms)

DERMATOLOGIC EFFECTS

Dermal thinning and striae
Increased skin fragility
Acne
Hirsutism

OPHTHALMOLOGIC EFFECTS

Cataracts
Glaucoma

IMMUNOLOGIC EFFECTS

Diminished IgG levels
Loss of delayed-type hypersensitivity
Potential for increased risk of opportunistic infection, reactivation of latent tuberculosis, or severe varicella infection

HEMATOLOGIC EFFECTS

Lymphopenia
Neutrophilia

CARDIOVASCULAR EFFECTS

Hypertension
Atherosclerosis

PSYCHOLOGIC/NEUROLOGIC EFFECTS

Mood swings
Steroid withdrawal syndrome
Pseudotumor cerebri
Psychosis

(e.g., ketoconazole, oral contraceptives) can significantly delay glucocorticoid metabolism. Macrolide antibiotics (e.g., erythromycin, clarithromycin) can also delay glucocorticoid clearance; however, this effect is limited to methylprednisolone.

Children who require chronically administered oral glucocorticoids are at risk of developing steroid-induced adverse effects over time (see Box 134–8). Essentially all major organ systems can be adversely affected by chronically administered oral glucocorticoid therapy. These effects can occur immediately (i.e., metabolic effects) or can develop insidiously over several months to years (e.g., growth suppression, osteoporosis, cataracts). Most adverse effects depend on the duration of treatment and occur in a cumulative dose-dependent manner.

Theophylline. Theophylline is rarely used in pediatric asthma because of its potential toxicity. Theophylline, when used chronically, can reduce asthma symptoms and need for supplemental β-agonist use. Because theophylline may have some glucocorticoid-sparing effects in individuals with oral glucocorticoid-dependent asthma, it is still sometimes used in this group of asthmatic children. Theophylline has a narrow therapeutic window; therefore, serum theophylline levels need to be routinely monitored, especially if the patient has a viral illness associated with a fever or is placed on a medication known to delay theophylline clearance, such as macrolide antibiotics, cimetidine, oral antifungals, oral contraceptives, and ciprofloxacin. Elevated theophylline levels have been associated with headaches, vomiting, cardiac arrhythmias, seizures, and death.

Long-Acting Inhaled β-Agonists. Salmeterol and formoterol are long-acting inhaled β-agonists (LABAs), considered as controller medications. Neither is intended for use as a "rescue" medication for acute episodes of bronchospasm or asthma exacerbations, nor recommended as monotherapy for persistent asthma. Salmeterol has a prolonged onset of action, with maximal bronchodilation about 1 hr after administration, whereas formoterol has an onset of action within 5–10 min. Both medications have a prolonged duration of effect of at least 12 hr. Given their long duration of action, they are well suited for patients with nocturnal asthma and for individuals who require frequent use of short-acting β-agonist inhalations during the day to prevent exercise-induced bronchospasm. Their major role is as "add-on" agents in patients who are suboptimally controlled on inhaled glucocorticoid therapy alone. Several studies have found the addition of an LABA to an inhaled glucocorticoid to be superior to doubling the dose of the inhaled glucocorticoid in subjects whose asthma is inadequately controlled on an inhaled glucocorticoid alone. These results suggest that LABAs have some inhaled glucocorticoid-sparing effects. Both LABAs are FDA approved for use in children (salmeterol: > age 4 yr; formoterol: > age 6 yr).

Leukotriene-Modifying Agents. Leukotrienes are potent proinflammatory mediators that can induce bronchospasm, mucus secretion, and airways edema. Two classes of leukotriene modifiers have been developed: inhibitors of leukotriene synthesis and leukotriene receptor antagonists. Zileuton, currently the only leukotriene synthesis inhibitor, is not approved for use in children < 12 yr of age. Because zileuton is administered four times daily, can result in elevated liver function enzymes in 2–4% of patients, and interacts with medications metabolized via the cytochrome-P450 system, it is rarely prescribed for children with asthma.

Leukotriene receptor antagonists (LTRAs) have bronchodilator and targeted anti-inflammatory properties and block exercise-, aspirin-, and allergen-induced bronchoconstriction. Two LTRAs are approved for use in children: zafirlukast and montelukast. Both medications improve asthma symptoms, decrease need for supplemental β-agonist use, and improve pulmonary function in patients with asthma. Montelukast is administered once daily (10 mg for children ≥ 15 yr; 5 mg for children 6–14 yr;

4 mg for children 2–5 yr). Zafirlukast is FDA approved for use in children 7 yr and older and is administered twice daily (10 mg twice daily in children 7–11 yr; 20 mg twice daily in children > 12 yr). Although incompletely studied in children with asthma, LTRAs appear to be less effective than inhaled glucocorticoids in patients with moderate persistent asthma. In general, studies have found inhaled glucocorticoids improve baseline lung function by 10–15%, whereas LTRAs improve baseline lung function by 5–7.5%. These drugs are not thought to have significant adverse effects, although recent case reports described a Churg-Strauss–like syndrome of pulmonary infiltrates, eosinophilia, and cardiomyopathy in adults with glucocorticoid-dependent asthma treated with zafirlukast. It remains to be determined whether these patients had a primary eosinophilic vasculitis masquerading as asthma, which was "unmasked" as their oral glucocorticoid dose was tapered, or whether the disease was a rare adverse effect of the drug.

ASTHMA EXACERBATION MANAGEMENT. Asthma exacerbations are acute or subacute episodes of progressively worsening symptoms associated with expiratory airflow obstruction. It is important to consider asthma severity based on the frequency and severity of previous asthma exacerbations and to identify asthmatics at increased risk for life-threatening exacerbations. Asthma exacerbation severity can be quantified by the number of emergency department visits, hospitalizations, and systemic glucocorticoid courses for asthma exacerbations. Previous severe asthma exacerbations, resulting in respiratory distress, hypoxia, or respiratory failure are probably the best predictors of a future life-threatening exacerbation or fatal asthma episode. Biologic, environmental, economic, and psychosocial risk factors for increased asthma morbidity and mortality have been identified (Box 134–9).

Home Management of Asthma Exacerbations. All asthmatics should have a written action plan that can help guide them in recognizing and assessing their overall asthma control and the severity of acute asthma exacerbations. Recognizing symptoms early and intensifying treatment soon after symptoms worsen

---

BOX 134–9. Risk Factors for Asthma Morbidity and Mortality

BIOLOGIC

Previous severe asthma exacerbation
Severe airflow obstruction
History of rapidly occurring attacks
Severe airways hyperresponsiveness
Increasing and large diurnal variation in peak flows
Decreased chemosensitivity and perception of dyspnea
Poor response to systemic glucocorticoid therapy
Male gender
Low birth weight
Nonwhite (especially black) ethnicity

ENVIRONMENTAL

Allergen exposure
Environmental tobacco smoke exposure
Air pollution exposure
Urban environment

ECONOMIC/PSYCHOSOCIAL

Poverty
Crowding
Mother <20 yr old
Mother with less than high school education
Inadequate medical care
   Inaccessible
   Unaffordable
   No regular medical care (only emergent)
   No care sought for chronic asthma symptoms
   Delay in care of asthma exacerbations
   Inadequate hospital care for asthma exacerbation
Psychopathology in the parent or child
Family problems
Alcohol or substance abuse

can often prevent further worsening and can keep exacerbations from becoming severe. One study found that having a written home action plan was associated with a 70% reduction in the risk of asthma death associated with an acute exacerbation. Clinical signs and symptoms characteristic of an acute episode include cough, shortness of breath, wheezing, chest tightness, use of accessory muscles, and suprasternal retractions. The NAEPP guidelines recommend immediate treatment with "rescue" medication (i.e., inhaled short-acting β-agonist, up to three treatments in 1 hr). A good response is characterized by resolution of symptoms within an hour, no further symptoms over the next 4 hr, and improvement in PEF of 80% predicted or personal best. The child's physician should be contacted for follow-up, especially if bronchodilators are required repeatedly over the next 24–48 hr. If the child has an incomplete response to initial treatment with rescue medication (i.e., persistent symptoms and/or a PEF of 60–80% of predicted or personal best), a short course of oral glucocorticoid therapy (e.g., prednisone 1–2 mg/kg/24 hr for 4 days) in addition to inhaled β-agonist therapy should be instituted. The physician should also be contacted for further instructions. Immediate medical attention should be sought for severe exacerbations, persistent signs of respiratory distress, lack of expected response or sustained improvement after initial treatment, further deterioration, or presence of risk factors for asthma morbidity or mortality. Patients should have medications such as inhaled short-acting β-agonists, oral glucocorticoids, and equipment for treating exacerbations at home.

Emergency Department Management of Asthma Exacerbations. The primary goals of asthma management in the emergency department setting include correction of hypoxemia, rapid improvement of airflow obstruction, and prevention of progression or recurrence of symptoms. Treatment is based on clinical severity on arrival, response to initial therapy, and presence of risk factors that are associated with asthma death. Initial treatment includes close monitoring of clinical status, treatment with supplemental oxygen, inhaled β-agonist every 20 min for 1 hr, and if necessary, systemic glucocorticoids (2 mg/kg/day) given either orally or intravenously. Inhaled ipratropium may be added to the β-agonist treatment if no significant response is seen with the first inhaled β-agonist treatment. A *subcutaneous* injection of epinephrine or other β-agonist may be administered in severe cases. The patient may be discharged to home if there is sustained improvement in symptoms, normal physical findings, PEF greater than 70% of predicted or personal best, and an oxygen saturation greater than 92% on room air for 4 hr. Discharge medications include administration of an inhaled β-agonist up to every 3–4 hr plus a 3–7 day course of oral glucocorticoids.

Hospital Management of Asthma Exacerbations. For patients with a moderate to severe asthma exacerbation that does not significantly improve within 1–2 hr after the initial treatment, associated with PEFs less than 70% or oxygen saturations less than 90–92%, admission to the hospital is warranted. Other indications for hospital admission include prolonged symptoms before the emergency department visit, inadequate access to medical care and medications, difficult psychosocial conditions, or difficulty in obtaining transportation to the hospital in event of further deterioration. Admission to an intensive care unit is indicated for patients with poor response to therapy, persistent severe respiratory distress, or evidence of impending respiratory arrest.

Supplemental oxygen, frequently administered inhaled β-agonists, and systemic glucocorticoid therapy are the treatments of choice for children admitted to the hospital for acute asthma. Supplemental oxygen is administered because many children hospitalized with acute asthma will have hypoxemia, especially at night. Short-acting β-agonists can be delivered frequently and, if needed, continuously. When administered continuously, significant systemic absorption of β-agonist occurs and, as a result, continuous nebulization can obviate the need for intravenous β-agonist therapy. Adverse effects of frequently administered β-agonist therapy include tremor, irritability, tachycardia, and hypokalemia. Patients requiring frequent or continuous nebulized β-agonist therapy should have continuous cardiac monitoring. Because frequent β-agonist therapy can cause ventilation-perfusion mismatch and precipitate hypoxemia, oximetry is indicated with supplemental oxygen. Ipratropium is often added to albuterol every 6 hr, although there is little evidence to support its use in hospitalized children receiving aggressive inhaled β-agonist therapy and systemic glucocorticoids. Patients with persistent severe dyspnea and high-flow oxygen requirements will often require intravenously administered fluids. In this situation, administration of fluids at or slightly below maintenance fluid requirements is recommended, owing to increased antidiuretic hormone (ADH) secretion associated with status asthmaticus.

Despite intensive therapy, some asthmatic children will remain critically ill and at risk for intubation and mechanical ventilation. Complications related to asthma exacerbations increase with intubation and assisted ventilation; therefore, every effort should be made to relieve bronchospasm and prevent respiratory failure. Several therapies, including intravenous β-agonists, intravenous theophylline, heliox, and intravenous magnesium sulfate have some demonstrated benefit as adjunctive therapies in severe status asthmaticus.

Intravenous Theophylline. Although several recent studies have failed to demonstrate the effectiveness of intravenous theophylline in hospitalized children receiving frequent inhaled β-agonist and systemic glucocorticoid therapy, theophylline may still have a role in the treatment of children with severe, life-threatening asthma exacerbations. In a recent study of children with acute severe asthma (mean FEV_1 37% at baseline), intravenous theophylline resulted in a rapid and sustained increase in oxygen saturation and lung function compared with placebo. In addition, fewer patients on intravenous theophylline required intravenous albuterol; in those who did, intravenous albuterol was required for a shorter duration of time. Lastly, all study patients requiring intubation were in the placebo-treated group. This study suggests that intravenous theophylline can be an important adjunctive therapy in acute severe childhood asthma. If a child responds poorly to intensive therapy with nebulized albuterol, ipratropium, and parenteral glucocorticoids, then adding intravenous theophylline should be considered. Because theophylline use is associated with adverse effects, with overdosage resulting in dire consequences, the proper loading and maintenance doses should be used according to the child's age and weight, with serum theophylline level monitoring to ensure values within the therapeutic and nontoxic range.

Heliox. Inhaled heliox (a 70:30 helium:oxygen mixture) has been shown, in several small studies, to be effective in the treatment of acute severe asthma. Because heliox has a density about one-third that of room air, inhalation of this gas mixture can result in decreased airways resistance and clinical improvement within 20 min, even in patients already receiving intensive inhaled β-agonist and intravenous glucocorticoid therapy. Thus, heliox treatment early in the course of status asthmaticus may provide a period with reduced respiratory distress until β-agonist and glucocorticoid therapy can relieve bronchoconstriction and airway narrowing. In severe cases when high-content supplemental oxygen is needed, heliox's 30% oxygen content may limit its use.

Intravenous Magnesium Sulfate. Based on its smooth muscle relaxant properties, many studies have evaluated the effect of magnesium sulfate in acute asthma, but at present it remains controversial whether magnesium is effective in acute asthma. A small controlled study in children who presented to the emergency department with acute asthma found magnesium sulfate (25 mg/kg, maximum dose 2 g) to improve lung function and result in fewer admissions to the hospital when compared with placebo. If magnesium sulfate is to be used, blood pressure should be monitored every 10–15 min during the infusion and for up to 90 min after the infusion, because hypotension is a known adverse effect. Magnesium levels before and 30 min after the infusion should also be obtained.

Mechanical Ventilation. Rarely, a severe asthma exacerbation in children results in respiratory failure, and intubation and mechanical ventilation become necessary. Mechanical ventilation in severe asthma exacerbations requires the careful balance of enough pressure to overcome airways obstruction, while reducing hyperinflation, air trapping, and the likelihood of barotrauma (i.e., pneumothorax, pneumomediastinum). To minimize the likelihood of such complications, mechanical ventilation should be anticipated and asthmatic children at risk for the development of respiratory failure should be managed in a pediatric intensive care setting. Elective tracheal intubation with rapid-induction sedatives and paralytic agents is safer than emergency intubation. Mechanical ventilation aims to achieve adequate oxygenation while tolerating mild to moderate hypercapnia (i.e., PCO_2 40–60 mm Hg) to minimize barotrauma. Volume-cycled ventilators, using short inspiratory and long expiratory times, 10–15 mL/kg tidal volume, 8–15 breaths/min, peak pressures less than 60 cm H_2O, and without positive end-expiratory pressure are starting mechanical ventilation parameters that can achieve these goals. As measures to relieve plugs of mucus in the chest, chest percussion and airways lavage are not recommended because they can induce further bronchospasm. Considering the nature of asthma exacerbations leading to respiratory failure, those of rapid or abrupt onset tend to resolve quickly (i.e., hours to 2 days); in contrast, severe asthma exacerbations that progress gradually to respiratory failure can take days to weeks for airways obstruction to improve enough to allow for cessation of mechanical ventilation. Such prolonged cases are further complicated by muscle atrophy and, when combined with corticosteroid-induced myopathy, profound muscle weakness requiring prolonged rehabilitation.

Management of severe childhood asthma exacerbations in medical centers is usually successful, even when extreme measures are required. Consequently, childhood asthma deaths rarely occur in medical centers; most asthma deaths occur at home or in community settings, before lifesaving medical care can be administered. This highlights the importance of home and community management of asthma exacerbations, emphasizing early intervention measures to keep exacerbations from becoming severe and steps to reduce asthma severity.

MANAGEMENT OF INFANTS AND YOUNG CHILDREN WITH ASTHMA. Not every infant and small child who wheezes in the first few years of life will go on to develop asthma. Nevertheless, young children with recurrent wheezing problems can benefit from conventional reliever and controller asthma medications. As well, with wheezing exacerbations (typically triggered by viral respiratory tract infections), nebulized albuterol, and short courses of oral glucocorticoids mitigate exacerbation progression and can keep them from becoming severe.

There are three FDA-approved controller-class medications for use in young children: nebulized cromolyn, nebulized budesonide, and montelukast. Cromolyn has been widely used in infants and young children because it is available for administration by nebulization and is devoid of serious adverse effects. Unfortunately, it is not a potent medication, and administration four times daily for several weeks is necessary to achieve effective action. Nebulized budesonide is FDA approved for use in children as young as 1 yr of age. It has been extensively studied in infants and young children with recurrent wheezing and is both safe and effective. It is available for use in two concentra-

tions (0.25 mg and 0.50 mg/vial) and can be administered once or twice daily, depending on disease severity. Montelukast is FDA approved for use in children as young as 2 yr of age (recommended dose is 4 mg once daily). Both nebulized budesonide and montelukast appear to be more effective than cromolyn. Nebulized budesonide would be indicated in young children with moderate to severe persistent asthma symptoms and in those who have failed to respond to cromolyn and montelukast. An oral medication such as montelukast that can be administered once daily offers some advantages over nebulized medications in terms of ease of use and convenience.

Treating the infant and young child with asthma with aerosol therapy presents unique challenges. The preferential nasal breathing, small airways, low tidal volume, and high respiratory rate of infants markedly increases the difficulty of drug targeting to the lung airways. Young children are incapable of reliably performing the maneuvers specified for optimal delivery of aerosol therapy delivered via an MDI or DPI. For these reasons, medication delivery devices suitable for young children are limited to those that require minimal cooperation. There are currently two types of delivery systems for inhaled medications for this age group: the nebulizer and the MDI with spacing/holding chamber and face mask. The NAEPP guidelines recommend the nebulizer for the delivery of cromolyn and high-dose short-acting β-agonist. Inhaled glucocorticoid delivered using a MDI with spacing/holding device and face mask is considered acceptable, although perhaps not the preferred means of administering inhaled glucocorticoids to young children and infants, owing to a current paucity of published information or FDA approval.

Nebulizers have been the mainstay of aerosol treatment and remain the first choice of delivery systems for infants and young children. A major advantage of the nebulizer is the simple technique required of relaxed tidal breathing. Multiple studies have demonstrated the effectiveness of both nebulized albuterol in acute episodes and nebulized budesonide in the treatment of recurrent wheezing in infants and young children. Disadvantages of nebulizers include expense, need for a power source, inconvenience in that treatments take about 5 min, and potential for bacterial contamination.

Studies in young children comparing the delivery of short-acting β-agonists via MDI versus nebulizer have shown both devices to be effective in most cases, including the emergency department setting when comparable doses of medication are administered. Studies with radiolabeled albuterol given by MDI with a spacer and face mask to children younger than 5 yr old reveal less than 2% dose delivery to the lower airways. Fluticasone administered via a spacer device and face mask was clinically effective in a European study of infants and young children with recurrent wheezing.

PATIENT EDUCATION. Specific elements in the clinical care of children with asthma, centered around education, are believed to make an important difference in the home management and adherence of families to an optimal plan of care (Box 134–10). With education, the child and family become partners in the asthma management process. In initial patient visits, a basic understanding of the pathogenesis of asthma can help asthmatic children and their parents to understand the importance of recommendations aimed at reducing airways inflammation. Good asthma control in children should be specified so that the expectations of optimal asthma management are made clear (see Box 134–5). Explaining the importance of steps to reduce airways inflammation to achieve good asthma control and addressing concerns about potential adverse effects of asthma pharmacotherapy, and especially their risks relative to their benefits, can be essential to achieve long-term adherence with asthma pharmacotherapy and environmental control measures.

All asthmatic children and their families can benefit from a written asthma management plan with two main components:

(1) a **daily management plan** describing regular asthma medication use and other measures to keep asthma under good control and (2) an **action plan for asthma exacerbations**, describing actions to take when asthma worsens, including what medications to take and when to contact the regular physician and/or obtain emergent or urgent medical care.

Regular follow-up visits can help to maintain optimal asthma control. In addition to the assessment and monitoring of disease severity, follow-up visits should evaluate adherence and concerns with asthma management recommendations, and especially the daily administration of controller medications when prescribed. Reassessment during each visit of the role of different medications in asthma management and the technique used with inhaled medication use can be insightful and lead to important teaching opportunities. Indeed, inhaled medication (and spacer) use and PEF monitoring are important skills for asthmatics to learn and improve with practice and review at each visit. Encouraging open communication of concerns about asthma management recommendations (e.g., daily controller medication use) can be insightful and improve adherence with a management plan that might not have been adequately or properly implemented.

REFERRAL FOR CONSULTATION. NAEPP guidelines recommend referral of asthmatics to an asthma specialist, a board-certified allergist, or pulmonologist for consultation. Asthma specialists can typically provide lung function testing, allergen sensitization assessment and testing, detailed evaluation for asthma masqueraders (e.g., flexible rhinolaryngoscopy or bronchoscopy), bronchoprovocation challenges, environmental assessment and modification recommendations, extensive patient and parent education, and management support of complex or severe asthmatics. Asthmatics with upper airways conditions may require referral to an otolaryngologist. Asthmatics with psychosocial risk factors for asthma morbidity or mortality may benefit from referral to a mental health professional.

Prevention. Currently, asthma prevention strategies are in their infancy. With recent evidence that chronic airways inflammation may result in pathologic remodeling changes, early intervention with anti-inflammatory medications in young children with recurrent wheezing and persistent asthma risk factors may halt disease progression. Investigations into the environmental and lifestyle factors responsible for the lower prevalence of childhood asthma in rural areas and farming communities suggest that early immune modulatory intervention might prevent asthma development. A "hygiene hypothesis" purports that microbial exposures in early life might drive early immune development away from allergen sensitization and allergic inflammation. Accordingly, early life microbial exposures have been associated with a lower likelihood of allergen sensitization and atopic dermatitis in infants and a lower likelihood of asthma and bronchial hyperresponsiveness in later childhood. If these microbial exposures truly have an asthma-protective effect, then these findings may foster new strategies for asthma prevention.

Current evidence also suggests that several other nonpharmacotherapeutic measures with numerous positive health attributes—avoidance of environmental tobacco smoke (beginning prenatally), prolonged breast-feeding (greater than 4 mo), an active lifestyle, and a healthy diet—might reduce the likelihood of asthma development. Immunizations are currently not considered to increase the likelihood of developing asthma; therefore, all standard childhood immunizations are recommended for asthmatic children, including varicella and annual influenza vaccines.

American Academy of Allergy, Asthma & Immunology: *Pediatric Asthma: Promoting Best Practice.* AAAAI, Milwaukee, WI, 1999, pp 1–139. (www.aaaai.org)

Beasley R, Crane J, Lai CK, et al: Prevalence and etiology of asthma. *J Allergy Clin Immunol* 2000;105:S466–72.

Busse WW, Lemanske RF Jr: Asthma. *N Engl J Med* 2001;344:350–62.

Childhood Asthma Management Program Research Group: Long-term effects of budesonide or nedocromil in children with asthma. *N Engl J Med* 2000;343:1054–63.

Martinez FD, Wright AL, Taussig LM, et al: Asthma and wheezing in the first six years of life. The Group Health Medical Associates. *N Engl J Med* 1995;332:133–38.

Milgrom H, Taussig LM: Keeping children with exercise-induced asthma active. *Pediatrics* 1999;104:e38.

National Institutes of Health, National Heart, Lung & Blood Institute. National Asthma Education & Prevention Program: *Expert Panel Report 2: Guidelines for the Diagnosis and Management of Asthma.* Washington DC, 1997, pp 1–86; and *Update on Selected Topics 2002.* Washington, DC, 2002, pp 1–6.. (www.nhlbi.nih.gov/guidelines/asthma)

Szefler SJ, Leung DYM (editors): *Severe Asthma: A Multidisciplinary Approach,* 2nd ed. In Lenfant C (series editor): Lung Biology in Health and Disease Series. New York, Marcel Dekker, 2001, pp 1–635.

Chapter 135

Atopic Dermatitis (Atopic Eczema) *Donald Y. M. Leung*

Atopic dermatitis (AD) is a highly pruritic skin disease that affects more than 10% of children. It is frequently associated with elevated serum IgE levels, and nearly 80% of patients with AD develop allergic rhinitis and/or asthma.

Pathogenesis. Complex interactions between genetic, environmental, and immunologic factors contribute to the pathogenesis of AD. Current therapies in AD have evolved from an understanding of the pathobiology of this disease.

SYSTEMIC IMMUNE RESPONSE. Most patients with AD have peripheral blood eosinophilia and increased serum IgE levels. Peripheral blood T cells from AD patients produce decreased amounts of interferon-gamma (IFN-γ), an inhibitor of T helper type 2 (Th2) cell function. IFN-γ generation ex vivo is inversely correlated with serum IgE concentrations in AD. An increased frequency of allergen-specific T cells producing increased interleukin (IL)-4, IL-5, and IL-13 in the peripheral blood of patients with AD contributes to the eosinophilia and increased IgE levels in AD.

SKIN IMMUNOPATHOLOGY. Clinically *unaffected* skin of AD patients is not normal but reveals mild epidermal hyperplasia and a sparse perivascular T-cell infiltrate. Acute skin lesions are characterized by **spongiosis,** or marked intercellular edema, of the epidermis. The dendritic antigen-presenting cells (APCs) in the skin, Langerhans cells (LCs), in lesional and, to a lesser extent, nonlesional skin of AD exhibit surface-bound IgE molecules. IgE-bearing LCs appear to play an important role in cutaneous allergen presentation to Th2 cells (see Chapter 130). In the acute lesion, there is a marked perivenular T-cell infiltrate with occasional monocyte-macrophages. Mast cells are found in normal numbers in different stages of degranulation.

Chronic lichenified lesions are characterized by a hyperplastic epidermis with elongation of the rete ridges, hyperkeratosis, and minimal spongiosis. There are predominantly IgE-bearing LCs in the epidermis and macrophages in the dermal mononuclear cell infiltrate. The numbers of mast cells and of eosinophils are increased. Eosinophils are thought to contribute to allergic inflammation by the secretion of cytokines and mediators that augment allergic inflammation and induce tissue injury in AD through the production of reactive oxygen intermediates and release of toxic granule proteins.

SKIN IMMUNE RESPONSE. As compared with the skin of normal control subjects, unaffected skin and acute skin lesions of AD have an increased number of cells expressing IL-4 and IL-13. However, acute AD does not contain significant numbers of cells that express IFN-γ or IL-12. Chronic AD skin lesions have significantly fewer cells that express IL-4 and IL-13 but increased numbers of cells that express IL-5, granulocyte-macrophage colony-stimulating factor (GM-CSF), IL-12, and IFN-γ than acute AD. Thus, acute T-cell infiltration in AD is associated with a predominance of IL-4 and IL-13 expression whereas maintenance of chronic inflammation is associated with increased IL-5, GM-CSF, IL-12, and IFN-γ expression and is accompanied by the infiltration of eosinophils and macrophages. The increased expression of IL-12 in chronic AD skin lesions is of interest because cytokine plays a key role in Th1 cell development and its expression in eosinophils and/or macrophages may initiate the switch to Th1 or Th0 cell development in chronic AD.

GENETICS. AD is familially transmitted with a strong maternal influence. Genetic approaches have identified candidate genes, suggesting that AD has a common genetic basis with other allergic diseases. There has been particular interest in the role of chromosome 5q31-33 because it contains a clustered family of cytokine genes, namely, IL-3, IL-4, IL-5, IL-13, and GM-CSF, which are expressed by Th2 cells. A case control comparison has suggested a genotypic association between the T allele of the -590C/T polymorphism of the IL-4 gene promoter region with AD. Because the T allele is associated with increased IL-4 gene promoter activity compared with the C allele, this suggests that genetic differences in transcriptional activity of the IL-4 gene influence AD predisposition. In addition, an association of AD with a gain-of-function mutation in the α subunit of the IL-4 receptor has been reported. A functional mutation in the promoter region of the C-C chemokine RANTES and an IL-13 coding region variant also occurs in AD.

Two genome-wide linkage studies have also identified susceptibility loci for AD. Linkage for AD has been found on chromosome 3q21, a region that encodes the co-stimulatory molecules CD80 and CD86 involved in T-cell activation as well as chromosome 1q21 and 17q25 identifying loci, which closely coincide with regions linked to psoriasis. Thus, AD is also influenced by genes that modulate skin responses independent of allergic mechanisms.

Clinical Manifestations. AD typically begins during infancy. Approximately 50% of patients develop this illness by the first year of life, and an additional 30% are diagnosed between 1–5 yr of age. Intense pruritus and cutaneous reactivity are cardinal features of AD. Pruritus is usually worse at night. Its consequences are scratching that contributes to the induction of eczematous skin lesions. Foods, inhalant allergens, bacterial infection, reduced humidity, excessive sweating, and irritants (e.g., wool, acrylic, soaps, and detergents) can exacerbate pruritus and scratching.

SKIN REACTION PATTERNS. Acute AD skin lesions are intensely pruritic, erythematous papules associated with excoriation and serous exudate. Subacute dermatitis is characterized by erythematous, excoriated, scaling papules. Chronic AD is characterized by lichenification (thickening of the skin with accentuated surface markings) and fibrotic papules (prurigo nodularis). In chronic AD, all three stages of skin reactions can coexist in the same individual. Most AD patients usually also have dry lackluster skin.

The distribution and skin reaction pattern varies with the patient's age and disease activity. During infancy, the AD is generally more acute and involves the face, scalp, and the extensor surfaces of the extremities. The diaper area is usually spared. In older children and in those who have long-standing skin disease, the patient develops chronic AD with lichenification and localization of the rash to the flexural folds of the extremities. AD often goes into remission as the patient grows older, leaving an adolescent or adult with skin that is prone to itching and inflammation when exposed to exogenous irritants.

Diagnosis. Of the major features (Box 135–1), pruritus and chronic remitting eczematous dermatitis with typical morphology and distribution are essential for the diagnosis of AD. Other associated features, including a family history of asthma, hay fever, elevated IgE, and immediate skin test reactivity, are variable.

DIFFERENTIAL DIAGNOSIS. A number of inflammatory skin diseases, immunodeficiencies, skin malignancies, genetic disorders, infectious diseases, and infestations share symptoms and signs with AD and should be considered and excluded before a diagnosis of AD is established. Infants presenting in the 1st year of life with failure to thrive, diarrhea, generalized scaling erythematous rash, and recurrent cutaneous and/or systemic infections should be evaluated for severe combined immunodeficiency syndrome (see Chapter 116.1). In addition, histiocytosis X (see Chapter 499) should be ruled out in any infant with AD and failure to thrive. Wiskott-Aldrich syndrome (see Chapter 116.2) is an X-linked recessive disorder, associated with thrombocytopenia, immune defects, and recurrent severe bacterial infections, characterized by a rash almost indistinguishable from AD. The hyper-IgE syndrome (see Chapter 116.2) is characterized by markedly elevated serum IgE levels, recurrent deep-seated bacterial infections, chronic dermatitis, and recalcitrant dermatophytosis.

Adolescents who present with an eczematous dermatitis with no history of childhood eczema, respiratory allergy, or atopic family history may have allergic contact dermatitis. A contact

---

BOX 135–1. Clinical Features of Atopic Dermatitis

MAJOR FEATURES

Pruritus
Facial and extensor eczema in infants and children
Flexural eczema in adolescents
Chronic or relapsing dermatitis
Personal or family history of atopic disease

ASSOCIATED FEATURES

Xerosis
Cutaneous infections
Nonspecific dermatitis of the hands or feet
Ichthyosis, palmar hyperlinearity, keratosis pilaris
Nipple eczema
White dermatographism and delayed blanch response
Anterior subcapsular cataracts, keratoconus
Elevated serum IgE levels
Positive immediate-type allergy skin tests
Early age at onset
Dennie lines (Dennie-Morgan infraorbital folds)
Facial erythema or pallor
Course influenced by environmental and/or emotional factors

allergen should be considered in any patient whose AD does not respond to appropriate therapy, because chemicals such as parabens and lanolin are commonly used therapeutic topical agents. Topical glucocorticoid contact allergy has been reported increasingly in patients with chronic dermatitis on topical corticosteroid therapy. Eczematous dermatitis has also been reported with HIV infection as well as with a variety of infestations such as scabies. Other conditions that can be confused with AD include psoriasis, ichthyoses, and seborrheic dermatitis.

Treatment. The treatment of AD requires a systematic, multifaceted approach that incorporates skin hydration, topical therapy, identification and elimination of flare factors, and, if necessary, systemic therapy.

TOPICAL THERAPY. Although it is imperative to identify and eliminate the causative factors, topical therapy, especially cutaneous hydration, is usually indicated once symptoms of AD are present.

Cutaneous Hydration. Patients with AD have decreased skin barrier function contributing to the development of **xerosis,** or dry skin, especially during the winter. Lukewarm soaking baths for at least 20 min followed by the application of an occlusive emollient to retain moisture gives patients symptomatic relief. Hydrophilic ointments can be obtained in varying degrees of viscosity according to the patient's preference. Occlusive ointments are sometimes not well tolerated because of interference with the function of the eccrine sweat ducts and may induce the development of folliculitis. In these patients, less-occlusive agents should be used.

Hydration, by baths or wet dressings, promotes transepidermal penetration of topical glucocorticoids. Dressings may also serve as an effective barrier against persistent scratching, which promotes more rapid healing of excoriated lesions. Wet dressings are recommended for use on severely affected or chronically involved areas of dermatitis refractory to skin care. However, they have the potential to promote drying and fissuring of the skin if not followed by topical emollient use. Wet dressing therapy can be complicated by maceration and secondary infection and should be closely monitored by a physician.

Topical Glucocorticoid Treatment. Topical glucocorticoids are frequently the cornerstone of anti-inflammatory treatment for AD. Patients should be carefully instructed on their use of topical glucocorticoids in order to avoid potential adverse effects. There are seven classes of topical glucocorticoids, ranked according to their potency based on vasoconstrictor assays. Because of their potential adverse effects, the ultra-high-potency glucocorticoids should not be used on the face or intertriginous areas and only for very short periods of time on the trunk and extremities. The goal is to use emollients to enhance skin hydration and low-potency glucocorticoids for maintenance therapy. Mid-potency glucocorticoids can be used for longer periods of time to treat chronic AD involving the trunk and extremities.

Compared with creams, ointments have a greater potential to occlude the epidermis, resulting in enhanced systemic absorption. Adverse effects from topical glucocorticoids can be divided into local adverse effects and systemic adverse effects resulting from suppression of the hypothalamic-pituitary-adrenal axis. Local adverse effects include the development of striae and skin atrophy. Systemic adverse effects are related to the potency of the topical glucocorticoid, the site of application, the occlusiveness of the preparation, the percentage of the body surface area covered, and the length of use. The potential for potent topical glucocorticoid to cause adrenal suppression is greatest in infants and young children with severe AD requiring intensive therapy.

Topical Immunomodulators. Topically applied tacrolimus, a calcineurin inhibitor that acts by binding to FK binding protein, has been successfully used in the treatment of AD. Tacrolimus

inhibits the activation of a number of key cells involved in AD, including T cells, Langerhans cells, mast cells, and keratinocytes. AD patients receiving this form of therapy can have markedly diminished pruritus and reduced skin inflammation within several days of initiating therapy. Multicenter, blinded, vehicle-controlled trials have shown tacrolimus ointment to be both safe and effective in children with AD. Local burning sensation has been the only common adverse event. Long-term open-label studies with tacrolimus ointment have demonstrated sustained efficacy and no significant adverse effects. Indeed, *S. aureus* colonization decreases during long-term therapy with tacrolimus ointment. In addition, unlike topical corticosteroids, tacrolimus ointment does not cause cutaneous atrophy and has been used safely for facial and eyelid eczema. Tacrolimus ointment 0.03% has been approved by the U.S. Food and Drug Administration for short-term and intermittent long-term use in AD for children 2–15 yr of age, and 0.03% as well as 0.1% has been approved for patients older than age 16 yr.

Ascomycin compounds, which act by binding to macrophilin 12 to interfere with calcineurin action, have been developed in topical and oral forms, which appear to have preferential drug distribution to the skin. Like tacrolimus, they inhibit Th1 and Th2 cytokine production and have been found to be effective in the treatment of AD.

Tar Preparations. Coal tar preparations have antipruritic and anti-inflammatory effects on the skin. The anti-inflammatory properties of tars, however, are usually not as pronounced as those of topical glucocorticoids or macrolide immunomodulators. Tar preparations are useful in reducing the potency of topical glucocorticoids required in chronic maintenance therapy of AD. Tar shampoos can be particularly beneficial for scalp dermatitis. Adverse effects associated with tar preparations can include skin irritation, folliculitis, and photosensitivity.

Phototherapy. Broad-band ultraviolet B, broad-band ultraviolet A, narrow-band ultraviolet B (311 nm), UVA-1 (340–400 nm), and combined UVA/B phototherapy can be useful adjuncts in the treatment of AD. Investigation of the mechanisms responsible for their therapeutic effectiveness indicate that epidermal Langerhans cells and eosinophils may be targets of ultraviolet A phototherapy with (PUVA) and without psoralen, whereas UVB exerts immunosuppressive effects through blocking of function of antigen-presenting Langerhans cells and altered keratinocyte cytokine production. Photochemotherapy with PUVA may be indicated in patients with severe, widespread AD. Short-term adverse effects with phototherapy include erythema, skin pain, pruritus, and pigmentation. Long-term adverse effects include predisposition to cutaneous malignancies.

IDENTIFICATION AND ELIMINATION OF TRIGGERING FACTORS. It is essential to identify and eliminate triggering factors, both during the period of acute symptoms and on an ongoing basis after symptoms have abated, in an attempt to prevent recurrences.

Irritants. Patients with AD have a low threshold for response to irritants that can trigger their itch-scratch cycle. These include soaps or detergents, contact with chemicals, smoke, abrasive clothing, and exposure to extremes of temperature and humidity. When soaps are used, they should have minimal defatting activity and a neutral pH. New clothing should be laundered before wearing to decrease levels of formaldehyde and other added chemicals. Residual laundry detergent in clothing may be irritating. Using a liquid rather than powder detergent and adding a second rinse cycle will facilitate removal of the detergent.

Every attempt should be made to allow children to be as normally active as possible. Certain sports such as swimming may be better tolerated than other sports involving intense perspiration, physical contact, or heavy clothing and equipment, but chlorine should be rinsed off immediately after swimming and the skin lubricated. Although ultraviolet light may be beneficial to some patients with AD, sunscreens should be used to avoid sunburn.

Foods. Well-controlled studies have demonstrated that food allergens induce rashes in children with AD (see Chapter 142). Based on double-blind, placebo-controlled food challenges, approximately 40% of infants and young children with moderate to severe AD have food allergy. Food allergies in AD patients may induce eczematous dermatitis in some patients, whereas in others urticarial reactions, contact urticaria, wheezing, or nasal congestion is elicited. Increased severity of AD symptoms and younger age of patients correlate directly with the presence of food allergy. Removal of food allergens from the patient's diet can lead to significant clinical improvement but requires a great deal of education because most of the common allergens (e.g., egg, milk, wheat, soy, and peanut) contaminate many foods and are therefore difficult to avoid.

Potential allergens can be identified by taking a careful history and carrying out selective skin prick tests or in vitro blood testing. Negative skin tests or serum tests for allergen-specific IgE have a high predictive value for excluding suspected allergens. Positive skin or in vitro blood tests to foods often do not correlate with clinical symptoms and should be confirmed with controlled food challenges and elimination diets. Extensive elimination diets, which in some cases can be nutritionally deficient, are rarely required because even with multiple positive skin tests the majority of patients will react to fewer than three foods on controlled challenge.

Aeroallergens. In older children, exacerbation of AD can occur after intranasal or epicutaneous exposure to aeroallergens such as fungi, animal dander, grass, or ragweed pollen. In such patients, avoidance of aeroallergens, particularly dust mites, can result in clinical improvement of AD. In dust mite–allergic patients, avoidance measures include use of dust mite–proof encasings on pillows, mattresses, and box springs; washing bedding in hot water weekly; removal of bedroom carpeting; and decreasing indoor humidity levels with air conditioning.

Infections. Patients with AD have an increased tendency to develop bacterial, viral, and fungal skin infections. Antistaphylococcal antibiotics are very helpful in the treatment of patients who are heavily colonized or infected with *S. aureus*. Erythromycin and the newer macrolide antibiotics azithromycin and clarithromycin are usually beneficial for patients who are not colonized with a resistant *S. aureus* strain. However, for macrolide-resistant *S. aureus*, a penicillinase-resistant penicillin (dicloxacillin) or 1st-generation cephalosporin (cephalexin) may be preferred. Topical mupirocin is useful in the treatment of impetiginized lesions; however, in patients with AD and extensive superinfection, a course of systemic antibiotics is most practical. Recent studies demonstrating that IL-4–mediated skin inflammation contributes to skin colonization with *S. aureus* indicate the importance of combining effective anti-inflammatory therapy with antibiotics in the treatment of patients with moderate to severe AD to avoid the need for repeated courses of antibiotics, which can lead to the emergence of antibiotic-resistant strains of *S. aureus*.

Herpes simplex virus (HSV) can provoke recurrent dermatitis and may be misdiagnosed as *S. aureus* infection. The presence of erosive, punched-out erosions, vesicles, and/or infected skin lesions that fail to respond to oral antibiotics should suggest HSV infection. This can be diagnosed by a Giemsa-stained Tzanck smear of cells scraped from the vesicle base or by viral culture. For suspected infection from HSV, topical glucocorticoids are best temporarily discontinued. Antiviral treatment for cutaneous HSV infections is of critical importance in the patient with widespread AD because life-threatening dissemination has been reported.

Dermatophyte infections can contribute to exacerbation of AD disease activity. Patients with dermatophyte infection or IgE antibodies to *Malassezia furfur* (formerly known as *Pityrosporum*

ovale) may benefit from a trial of topical or systemic antifungal therapy.

SYSTEMIC THERAPY. Systemic therapies for AD include antihistamines, glucocorticoids, cyclosporine, and interferons, and are used for more severe cases.

Antihistamines. Systemic antihistamines act primarily by blocking the H_1-receptors in the dermis, thereby reducing histamine-induced pruritus. However, histamine is only one of many mediators that can induce pruritus of the skin and, therefore, patients may derive minimal benefit from antihistaminic therapy. Because pruritus is usually worse at night, the sedating antihistamines (e.g., hydroxyzine or diphenhydramine) may offer an advantage with their soporific adverse effects when used at bedtime. Doxepin hydrochloride has both tricyclic antidepressant and H_1- and H_2-receptor blocking effects. If nocturnal pruritus remains severe, short-term use of a sedative to allow adequate rest may be appropriate. Studies of newer nonsedating antihistamines have shown variable results in the effectiveness of controlling pruritus in AD, although they may be useful in the small subset of AD patients with concomitant urticaria.

Systemic Glucocorticoids. The use of systemic glucocorticoids is rarely indicated in the treatment of chronic AD. The dramatic clinical improvement that may occur with systemic glucocorticoids is frequently associated with a severe rebound flare of AD after discontinuation. Short courses of oral glucocorticoids may be appropriate for an acute exacerbation of AD, whereas other treatment measures are being instituted. If a short course of oral glucocorticoids is given, it is important to taper the dosage and begin intensified skin care, particularly with topical glucocorticoids and frequent bathing followed by application of emollients, to prevent rebound flaring of AD.

Cyclosporine. Cyclosporine is a potent immunosuppressive drug that acts primarily on T cells by suppressing cytokine transcription. The drug binds to an intracellular protein, cyclophilin, and this complex in turn inhibits calcineurin, a molecule required for initiation of cytokine gene transcription. Multiple studies have demonstrated that children with severe AD, refractory to conventional treatment, can benefit from short-term cyclosporine treatment. A dose of 5 mg/kg/24 hr has been utilized with success in short-term and long-term (1 yr) use. Renal impairment and hypertension are specific adverse effects of concern with cyclosporine use.

Interferons. Interferon-gamma (IFN-γ) is known to suppress IgE responses and downregulate TH2 cell proliferation and function. Several studies of patients with AD, including a multicenter, double-blinded, placebo-controlled trial, have demonstrated that treatment with recombinant IFN-γ results in clinical improvement. Reduction in clinical severity of AD correlated with the ability of IFN-γ to decrease total circulating eosinophil counts. Influenza-like symptoms are commonly observed adverse effects early in the treatment course.

Complications. AD is associated with recurrent viral skin infections. The most serious viral infection is **Kaposi varicelliform eruption** or **eczema herpeticum,** which is caused by HSV and affects patients of all ages. After exposure of affected skin to the virus and after an incubation period of 5–12 days, multiple, itchy, vesiculopustular lesions erupt in a disseminated pattern; the vesicular lesions are umbilicated, tend to crop, and often become hemorrhagic and crusted. Patients can also suffer from frequent infection with viruses leading to warts and molluscum contagiosum. Persons with AD are susceptible to **eczema vaccinatum,** a widespread severe viral skin infection caused by variola virus (smallpox), which is similar in appearance to eczema herpeticum and historically follows smallpox vaccination or exposure to individuals vaccinated with smallpox. This form of infection is a potential occurrence in the event of a bioterrorism attack with smallpox (see Chapter 706).

Patients with AD have an increased prevalence of *Trichophyton rubrum* fungal infections compared with nonatopic controls. There has been particular interest in the role of *M. furfur* in AD because it is a lipophilic yeast commonly present in the seborrheic areas of the skin. IgE antibodies against *M. furfur* have been found in patients with head and neck dermatitis. In such patients, a reduction of AD skin severity has been observed after treatment with antifungal agents.

Staphylococcus aureus is found on over 90% of AD skin lesions. Honey-colored crusting, folliculitis, impetigo, and pyoderma are indicators of *S. aureus* skin infection that requires antibiotic therapy. Regional lymphadenopathy is common in such patients. The importance of *S. aureus* in AD is supported by the observation that patients with severe AD, even those without overt infection, can show clinical response to combined treatment with antistaphylococcal antibiotics and topical glucocorticoids.

Patients with extensive skin involvement may develop exfoliative dermatitis. This is associated with generalized redness, scaling, weeping, crusting, systemic toxicity, lymphadenopathy, and fever. It is usually caused by superinfection (e.g., with toxin-producing *S. aureus* or HSV infection) or inappropriate therapy. In some cases, the withdrawal of systemic glucocorticoids used to control severe AD may be a precipitating factor for exfoliative erythroderma.

Eyelid dermatitis and chronic blepharitis may result in visual impairment from corneal scarring. Atopic keratoconjunctivitis is usually bilateral and can have disabling symptoms that include itching, burning, tearing, and copious mucoid discharge. Vernal conjunctivitis is associated with papillary hypertrophy or cobblestoning of the upper eyelid conjunctiva. It usually occurs in younger patients and has a marked seasonal incidence with exacerbation in the spring. Keratoconus is a conical deformity of the cornea believed to result from chronic rubbing of the eyes in patients with AD. Cataracts may be a primary manifestation of AD or from the extensive use of systemic and topical glucocorticoids, particularly around the eyes.

Prognosis. AD generally tends to be more severe and persistent in young children. Periods of remission appear more frequently as the patient grows older. Spontaneous resolution of AD has been reported to occur after age 5 yr in 40–60% of patients affected during infancy, particularly if their disease is mild. Although earlier studies suggested that approximately 84% of children outgrow their AD by adolescence, more recent studies have reported that AD disappears in approximately 20% of children from infancy until adolescence but it had become less severe in 65%. In addition, more than half of those adolescents treated for mild dermatitis may experience a relapse of disease as adults, frequently presenting with hand dermatitis, especially if daily activities require repeated hand wetting. The following predictive factors correlate with a poor prognosis for AD: widespread AD in childhood, concomitant allergic rhinitis and asthma, family history of AD in parents or siblings, early age at onset of AD, being an only child, and very high serum IgE levels.

Prevention. Identification and elimination of triggering factors as part of treatment of AD is also the mainstay of prevention of recurrences.

Bieber T, Leung DYM (editors): *Atopic Dermatitis.* New York, Marcel Dekker, 2002, pp 1–616.

Hoare C, Li Wan Po A, Williams H: Systematic review of treatments for atopic eczema. *Health Technol Assess* 2000;4:1–191.

Leung DYM: Atopic dermatitis: New insights and opportunities for therapeutic intervention. *J Allergy Clin Immunol* 2000;105:860–76.

Luger T, Van Leent EJ, Graeber M, et al: SDZ ASM 981: An emerging safe and effective treatment for atopic dermatitis. *Br J Dermatol* 2001;144:788–94.

Paller A, Eichenfield LF, Leung DYM, et al: A 12-week study of tacrolimus ointment for the treatment of atopic dermatitis in pediatric patients. *J Am Acad Dermatol* 2001;44:S47–57.

Chapter 136
Urticaria and Angioedema (Hives) *Donald Y. M. Leung*

Urticaria and angioedema affects 20% of the population at some point during their life. Urticaria and angioedema is usually classified according to its duration. Skin lesions that last less than 6 wk duration are considered acute, and episodes that persist for more than 6 wk are designated chronic. This distinction is important because the causes and mechanisms of urticaria formation are different in each instance as are the therapeutic approaches.

Etiology and Pathogenesis. Acute urticaria and angioedema is often caused by an allergic (IgE-mediated) reaction (Table 136–1). This form of urticaria is a self-limited process that occurs when an allergen activates mast cells in the skin, which leads to mast cell degranulation and secretion of histamine, leukotrienes, enzymes such as tryptase and chymase, cytokines, and chemokines. Systemically absorbed allergens that can result in generalized urticaria include foods, drugs (particularly antibiotics), and stinging insect venoms. If an allergen can penetrate the skin locally, hives can develop at the site of exposure. Contact urticaria, for example, might occur after exposure to latex gloves if sufficient latex penetrates through the skin. Acute urticaria can also result from non–IgE-mediated stimulation of mast cells, including that from radiocontrast agents, viral agents including hepatitis B and Epstein-Barr virus, opiates, and nonsteroidal anti-inflammatory agents.

Chronic urticaria and angioedema is diagnosed when hives and swelling are present for more than 6 wk, but symptoms commonly exceed 12 wk. Once it has been determined that a protracted episode of urticaria is not physical urticaria or recurrent acute urticaria with repeated exposures to an agent, the diagnosis of chronic urticaria and angioedema can be established.

Urticaria can also be classified according to the rate in which hive formation occurs and the length of time it is evident. One

TABLE 136–1. Diagnostic Testing for Urticaria/Angioedema

Potential Condition	Procedure
Food and drug reactions	Elimination of offending agent, skin testing, and challenge with suspected foods
Inhalant allergens	Skin tests, radioallergosorbent test
Infections	Appropriate cultures or serology
Collagen vascular diseases and cutaneous vasculitis	Skin biopsy, CH_{50}, C4, C3, factor B, immunofluorescence of tissue, antinuclear antibodies, cryoglobulins
Malignancy with angioedema	CH_{50}, C1q, C4, C1 INH determinations
Cold urticaria	Ice cube test
Solar urticaria	Exposure to defined wavelengths of light, red cell protoporphyrin, fecal protoporphyrin, and coproporphyrin
Dermatographism	Stroking with narrow object (e.g., tongue blade, fingernail)
Pressure urticaria	Application of pressure for defined time and intensity
Vibratory angioedema	Vibration for 4 min
Aquagenic urticaria	Challenge with tap water at various temperatures
Urticaria pigmentosa	Skin biopsy, test for dermographism
Hereditary angioedema	C4, C2, CH_{50}, C1 INH by protein and function
Familial cold urticaria	Challenge by cold exposure, measurement of temperature, white blood cell count, erythrocyte sedimentation rate, and skin biopsy
C3b inactivator deficiency	C3, factor B, C3b inactivator determinations
Chronic idiopathic urticaria	Skin biopsy, immunofluorescence (negative result), autologous skin test

form of urticaria has lesions that last 1–2 hr and is typically encountered with physically induced hives with an inciting stimulus that is present only briefly; there is prompt mast cell degranulation, and biopsy of such lesions reveals little or no cellular infiltrate. The second form or urticaria has a prominent cellular infiltrate, and individual lesions can last as long as 36 hr. This can be found with food or drug reactions, delayed pressure urticaria, and chronic urticaria. Serum sickness reactions can be seen as a manifestation of drug reactions and on biopsy reveals a small-vessel cutaneous vasculitis. Urticaria in association with systemic lupus erythematosus or other vasculitides appears similar.

Atypical aspects of the gross appearance of the hives should heighten concern that the urticaria or angioedema may be the manifestation of a more systemic disease process. Lesions that do not blanch or are associated with bleeding into the skin (i.e., purpura) suggest urticarial vasculitis.

PHYSICAL URTICARIAS. Physically induced urticaria and/or angioedema share the common property of being induced by environmental factors, such as a change in temperature or by direct stimulation of the skin with pressure, stroking, vibration, or light (see Table 136–1).

Cold-Dependent Disorders. Cold urticaria is characterized by the rapid onset of pruritus, erythema, and urticaria/angioedema after exposure to a cold stimulus. The location of the swelling is confined to those parts of the body that have been exposed. However, total-body exposure such as occurs with swimming can cause massive release of vasoactive mediators, resulting in hypotension and even death if not promptly treated. The diagnosis is confirmed by challenge testing for an isomorphic cold reaction with an ice cube placed on the patient's skin for 10–15 min. Patients with cold urticaria will have a positive reaction on rewarming of the chilled skin. Cold urticaria can be associated with the presence of **cryoproteins** such as cold agglutinins, cryoglobulins, cryofibrinogen, and the Donath-Landsteiner antibody seen in secondary syphilis (paroxysmal cold hemoglobinuria). In patients with associated cryoglobulins, the isolated proteins appear to transfer cold sensitivity and activate the complement cascade on in vitro incubation with normal plasma. The term **idiopathic cold urticaria** generally applies to patients without abnormal circulating plasma proteins such as cryoglobulins. However, there is evidence that in some patients, chilling initiates an immune reaction mediated by an abnormal IgE bound to mast cells, which, on warming, leads to mediator release into the circulation. Cold urticaria has also been reported after viral infections.

Cholinergic Urticaria. This form of urticaria is characterized by the onset of small punctate wheals surrounded by a prominent erythematous flare associated with exercise, hot showers, and sweating. When the patient cools down, the rash usually subsides in 30–60 min. Also occasionally seen are symptoms of more generalized cholinergic stimulation such as lacrimation, wheezing, salivation, and syncope. These symptoms are mediated by cholinergic nerve fibers that innervate the musculature via parasympathetic neurons and innervate the sweat glands by cholinergic fibers that travel with the sympathetic nerves. Studies of mediator release during attacks of cholinergic urticaria have demonstrated that elevated plasma histamine levels parallel the onset of urticaria triggered by changes in body temperature.

Dermatographism. The ability to write on skin, termed **dermatographism**, can occur as an isolated disorder or accompany chronic urticaria or other physical urticarias, such as cholinergic and cold urticaria. It can be diagnosed by observing the skin after stroking it with a tongue depressor or fingernail. In such patients, a linear response occurs secondary to reflex vasoconstriction, followed by pruritus, erythema, and a linear wheal. In approximately 50% of cases, passive-transfer studies have demonstrated an IgE-dependent mechanism.

Pressure-Induced Urticaria and Angioedema. Pressure-induced urticaria differs from most types of urticaria or angioedema in that symptoms typically occur 4–6 hr after pressure has been applied. The disorder is clinically heterogeneous in that some patients may complain of swelling secondary to pressure with normal-appearing skin (i.e., no urticaria), so that the term **angioedema** is more appropriate. Others are predominantly urticarial and may or may not be associated with significant swelling. When urticaria is present, an infiltrative skin lesion is seen characterized by a perivascular mononuclear cell infiltrate and dermal edema similar to that seen with chronic idiopathic urticaria. Symptoms occur about tight clothing; foot swelling is common after walking; and buttock swelling may be prominent after sitting for a few hours. This condition generally coexists with chronic idiopathic urticaria. The diagnosis is confirmed by challenge testing by pressure applied perpendicular to the skin.

Solar Urticaria. Solar urticaria is a rare disorder in which urticaria develops within 1–3 min of sun exposure. Typically, pruritus occurs first, in about 30 sec, followed by edema confined to the light-exposed area and surrounded by a prominent erythematous zone caused by an axon reflex. The lesions usually disappear within 1–3 hr after sun exposure is avoided. When large areas of the body are exposed, systemic symptoms may occur, including hypotension and wheezing. Solar urticaria has been classified into six types, depending on (1) the wavelength of light that induces skin lesions and (2) the ability or inability to passively transfer the disorder with serum IgE. The rare inborn error of metabolism erythropoietic protoporphyria can be confused with solar urticaria because of the development of itching and burning of exposed skin immediately after sun exposure. In erythropoietic protoporphyria, fluorescence of UV-irradiated red blood cells can be demonstrated.

Aquagenic Urticaria. Patients with aquagenic urticaria develop small wheals after contact with water, regardless of its temperature, and are therefore distinguishable from patients with cold urticaria or cholinergic urticaria. Direct application of a compress of water to the skin is used to test for its presence. The diagnosis should be reserved for those rare cases that test positively for contact with water but negatively for all other forms of physical urticaria.

CHRONIC IDIOPATHIC URTICARIA AND ANGIOEDEMA. This is a common disorder of unknown origin that is often associated with normal routine laboratory studies, including normal white blood cell count and erythrocyte sedimentation rate (ESR), with no evidence of systemic disease. Chronic urticaria does not appear to be an allergic reaction. It differs from allergen-induced skin reactions or from physically induced urticaria in that histologic studies reveal a cellular infiltrate predominantly about small venules. Skin examination reveals infiltrative hives with palpably elevated borders, sometimes varying greatly in size and/or shape but generally being rounded.

Biopsy of the typical lesion consists of a non-necrotizing perivascular mononuclear cell infiltrate. However, many types of histopathologic processes can occur in the skin and manifest as urticaria. For example, patients with hypocomplementemia and cutaneous vasculitis can have urticaria or angioedema and biopsy of patients with urticaria, arthralgias, myalgias, and an elevated ESR as manifestations of necrotizing venulitis can reveal fibrinoid necrosis with a predominant neutrophilic infiltrate. Yet the urticarial lesions may be clinically indistinguishable from those seen in the more typical, nonvasculitis cases.

There is an increased association of chronic urticaria with Hashimoto thyroiditis. Such patients generally have antibodies to thyroglobulin or a microsomal-derived antigen (peroxidase) even if they are euthyroid. The incidence of abnormal thyroid function (either increased or decreased thyroxine [T_4] and/or increased or decreased thyroid stimulating hormone) is approximately 20%. Although some patients show clinical reduction of their urticaria on thyroid replacement therapy, many do not. Therefore, some investigators believe that these are associated, parallel, autoimmune events.

Thirty-five to 40 per cent of patients with chronic urticaria have a positive **autologous skin test:** if serum from the patient is intradermally injected into their skin, a significant wheal and flare reaction is observed. Such patients frequently have an IgG antibody directed to the α subunit of the IgE receptor that could cross link the IgE receptor (α subunit) and degranulate mast cells and basophils. An additional 5–10% of chronic urticaria patients have anti-IgE antibodies rather than anti-IgE receptor antibody. Cutaneous mast cell activation by IgG autoantibodies, however, generally requires the classical complement pathway with involvement of C3a and C5a, which are chemoattractants for inflammatory cells and can activate mast cell degranulation.

Diagnosis. Allergy skin testing can be helpful in sorting out causes of acute urticaria, especially when supported by historical evidence. Drugs and foods are the most common causes of acute urticaria. Dermatographism is frequent in patients with urticaria and can complicate allergy skin testing by causing false-positive reactions. In the absence of any clue suggesting an ingestant cause, elimination diets generally are not useful. The diagnosis is clinical and requires that the physician be aware of the various forms of urticaria.

An exogenous cause of chronic urticaria is rarely identified, reflecting its autoimmune nature. The differential diagnosis of chronic urticaria includes cutaneous or systemic mastocytosis, complement-mediated disorders, malignancies, mixed connective tissue diseases, and cutaneous blistering disorders (e.g., bullous pemphigoid). Only a few screening laboratory tests are useful, including a complete blood cell count with differential, ESR, urinalysis, thyroid autoantibodies, and liver function tests. Further studies are warranted if the patient has fever, arthralgias, or elevated ESR because there is an increased possibility of systemic illness such as malignancy or vasculitis. In such situations, a chest radiograph, skin biopsy, and complement studies may be done (see Table 136–1). C3b inactivator (factor I) deficiency has also been found in some cases of urticaria. Hereditary angioedema, a potentially life-threatening form of angioedema associated with deficient C1 inhibitor activity, is the most important familial form of angioedema (see Chapter 124.3). In patients with eosinophilia, stools for ova and parasites should be obtained because infection with helminthic parasites have been associated with urticaria. A syndrome of episodic angioedema/urticaria and fever with associated eosinophilia has been described in both adults and children. In contrast to other hypereosinophilic syndromes, this entity has a benign course.

Skin biopsy for diagnosis of possible **urticarial vasculitis** is recommended for urticarial lesions that persist at the same location for more than 24 hr or those with pigmented or purpuric components. Additional features suggestive of urticarial vasculitis include painful lesions, poor response to antihistamines, elevated ESR, and features of systemic illness such as fever and arthralgia. Collagen vascular diseases such as systemic lupus may manifest urticarial vasculitis as a presenting feature. The skin biopsy in urticarial vasculitis typically shows endothelial cell swelling of postcapillary venules with necrosis of the vessel wall, perivenular neutrophil infiltrate, diapedesis of red blood cells, and fibrin deposition associated with deposition of immune complexes.

The physical urticarias and clues for their identification should be considered in any patient with chronic urticaria (see Table 136–1). Papular urticaria commonly occurs in small children, generally on the extremities. It presents as grouped or linear highly pruritic wheals or papules mainly on exposed skin at the sites of insect bites. Mastocytosis is characterized by mast cell hyperplasia in the bone marrow, liver, spleen, lymph nodes, and skin. The disease is often associated with clinical effects of mast cell activation, including pruritus, flushing, urtication, abdominal pain, nausea, and vomiting. Urticaria pigmentosa is the most common skin manifestation of mastocytosis and may occur as an isolated skin finding. It appears as small, yellow-tan to reddish-brown macules or raised papules that urticate on scratching **(Darier sign).** The diagnosis is confirmed by a skin biopsy that shows increased numbers of dermal mast cells.

Exercise-induced anaphylaxis presents as varying combinations of pruritus, urticaria, angioedema, wheezing, laryngeal obstruction, or hypotension after exercise (see Chapter 137). Cholinergic urticaria is differentiated by positive results on heat challenge tests and the rare occurrence of anaphylactic shock. The combination of ingestion of various food allergens (shrimp, celery, wheat) and postprandial exercise has been associated with urticaria/angioedema. In such patients, food or exercise alone may not produce this reaction.

Muckle-Wells syndrome is a rare, dominantly inherited condition associated with recurrent urticaria, arthritis, and limb pain that usually appears in adolescence. It is associated with progressive nerve deafness, recurrent fever, elevated ESR, hypergammaglobulinemia, and renal amyloidosis. Eventually these patients develop generalized amyloidosis and die of this complication.

Treatment. Acute urticaria is a self-limited illness requiring little treatment other than antihistamines. Hydroxyzine and diphenhydramine are effective sedating antihistamines commonly used for treatment of urticaria. Loratadine, fexofenadine, and cetirizine are also effective and may be preferable because of reduced frequency of drowsiness. Epinephrine 1:1,000, 0.01 mL/kg, maximum of 0.3 mL, usually provides rapid relief of acute, severe urticaria/angioedema. A short burst of corticosteroids should be given only for very severe episodes of urticaria and angioedema.

Most forms of physical urticaria respond to avoidance of triggering stimuli in combination with oral antihistamines. The exception is delayed pressure urticaria, which often requires oral corticosteroids. Cyproheptadine in divided doses is the drug of choice for cold-induced urticaria. Treatment of dermatographism consists of antihistamines; for severe symptoms, high doses may be needed. The initial objective of therapy is to decrease pruritus so that the stimulation for scratching is diminished. Sunscreens are the only effective treatment for solar urticaria.

The combined use of H_1- and H_2-type antihistamines is sometimes helpful to control chronic urticaria when H_1-type antihistamines alone do not work. Doxepin, an antagonist of both H_1 and H_2 receptors, can be helpful. H_2-type antihistamines alone may exacerbate urticaria. Perpetuation of the inflammatory response by cellular infiltration is critical to disease manifestations and degranulation of mast cells. When maximal H_1-and/or H_2-receptor blockade has been achieved, alternate-day therapy with corticosteroids is the most effective treatment. In general, prednisone, 20 mg orally as a single morning dose on alternate days, is used; the dosage is decreased by 2.5–5.0 mg every 3 wk depending on the patient's response. The goal is a slow gradual decline in dosage toward discontinuing therapy. Antileukotriene agents, in combination with antihistamines, may also be helpful. Treatment with small doses of cyclosporine has been effective in some adults with chronic urticaria, but use of large doses has been limited by nephrotoxicity. Chronic urticaria does not often respond favorably to dietary manipulation. However, in refractory patients, removal of urticarial aggravators, such as salicylates or alcohol, should be considered. Treatment of autoimmune chronic urticaria refractory to medical therapy includes intravenous immunoglobulin or plasmapheresis, or both. Plaquenil has been found to be effective for hypocomplementemic urticarial vasculitis syndrome associated with autoantibodies to C1q.

Grattan C, Powell S, Humphreys F: Management and diagnostic guidelines for urticaria and angio-oedema. *Br J Dermatol* 2001;144:708–14.

Greaves M: Chronic urticaria. *J Allergy Clin Immunol* 2000;105:664–72.

Joint Task Force on Practice Parameters: The diagnosis and management of urticaria: A practice parameter: I. Acute urticaria/angioedema. II. Chronic urticaria/angioedema. *Ann Allergy Asthma Immunol* 2000;85:521–44.

Kozel MM, Mekkes JR, Bossuyt PM, et al: Natural course of physical and chronic urticaria and angioedema in 220 patients. *J Am Acad Dermatol* 2001;45:387–91.

Leung DYM, Cruz P, Kaplan AP: Allergic skin diseases and contact dermatitis. In Rich RR, Fleisher TA, Shearer WT, et al (editors): *Clinical Immunology*, 2nd ed. St. Louis, Mosby–Year Book, 2001, pp 51.1–51.19

Chapter 137

Anaphylaxis *Hugh A. Sampson and Donald Y. M. Leung*

Anaphylaxis is a clinical condition in which there is a sudden release of potent biologically active mediators from mast cells and basophils leading to cutaneous (urticaria, angioedema, flushing), respiratory (bronchospasm, laryngeal edema), cardiovascular (hypotension, dysrhythmias, myocardial ischemia), and gastrointestinal symptoms (nausea, colicky abdominal pain, vomiting, diarrhea). The overall annual incidence of anaphylaxis in the United States is estimated at 30 cases/100,000 persons/year (81,000 cases per year). An Australian parental survey found that 0.59% of children 3–17 yr of age experienced at least one anaphylactic event.

Etiology. The most common causes of anaphylaxis in children differ depending on whether the population surveyed represents in-hospital patients or outpatients. Anaphylaxis occurring in the hospital is primarily the result of allergic reactions to medications and latex, whereas food allergy is the most common cause of anaphylaxis occurring outside the hospital, with about one half of the anaphylactic reactions reported in pediatric surveys from the United States, Italy, and South Australia (Box 137–1). Peanut allergy is becoming the major cause of food-induced anaphylaxis in "Westernized" countries, accounting for the majority of fatal and near-fatal reactions. In the hospital, latex is a particular problem for children undergoing multiple operations, such as patients with spina bifida and urologic disorders, and has prompted many hospitals to switch to latex-free products. Patients with latex allergy also may experience food allergic reactions from homologous proteins in fruits such as bananas, kiwi, avocado, chestnut, and passion fruit.

Pathogenesis. Principal pathologic features in fatal anaphylaxis include acute pulmonary hyperinflation, edema and intra-alveolar hemorrhaging, visceral congestion, laryngeal edema, and urticaria and angioedema. Acute hypotension is attributed to vasomotor dilation and/or cardiac dysrhythmias.

BOX 137–1. Etiology of Anaphylaxis in Children

IN-HOSPITAL
Latex
Antibiotics (especially intravenous)
Intravenous immune globulin
Radiocontrast dye

OUTSIDE OF HOSPITAL
Food (peanut, tree nuts, shellfish, milk, egg)
Insect sting (Hymenoptera, fire ants)
Oral medications (penicillins)
Exercise (including food-associated)
Idiopathic

Most cases of anaphylaxis are the result of activation of mast cells and basophils via cell-bound allergen-specific IgE molecules. As with any IgE-mediated reaction, patients must first be exposed to the responsible allergen to generate allergen-specific antibodies. In many cases the child and the parent are unaware of the initial exposure, which may be passage of food proteins in maternal breast milk. When re-exposed to the sensitizing allergen, mast cells and basophils, and possibly other cells such as macrophages, release a variety of mediators (e.g., histamine, tryptase) and cytokines that can produce allergic symptoms in any or all target organs. Clinical anaphylaxis also may be due to mechanisms other than IgE-mediated reactions, sometimes termed **anaphylactoid reactions**, including direct release of mediators from mast cells by medications and physical factors (e.g., morphine, exercise, cold), disturbances of leukotriene metabolism (aspirin and nonsteroidal anti-inflammatory drugs), immune aggregates and complement activation (blood products), and probable complement activation (e.g., radiocontrast dyes, dialysis membranes).

Clinical Manifestations and Diagnosis. The diagnosis of anaphylaxis is usually apparent owing to the acute and dramatic nature of this disorder. The onset of symptoms may vary somewhat depending on the cause of the reaction; reactions from ingested allergens (foods, medications) are delayed in onset (minutes to 2 hr) compared with injected allergen (insect sting, medications) and tend to have more gastrointestinal symptoms. With the initiation of symptoms, patients may experience pruritus about the mouth and face, a sensation of warmth, weakness, and apprehension. They may develop flushing, urticaria and angioedema, oral pruritus, tightness in the throat, dry staccato cough and hoarseness, periocular pruritus, nasal congestion, sneezing, dyspnea, deep cough, and wheezing. Nausea, abdominal cramping, and vomiting are common with ingested allergens. Uterine contractions, which are manifest as lower back pain, are not uncommon in women, and faintness and loss of consciousness typically occur in severe cases. Some degree of obstructive laryngeal edema is typically encountered with severe reactions. Cutaneous symptoms may be absent, and the acute onset of severe bronchospasm in a previously well asthmatic should suggest the diagnosis of anaphylaxis.

Sudden collapse in the absence of cutaneous symptoms should also raise suspicion of vasovagal collapse, myocardial infarction, aspiration, pulmonary embolism, or seizure disorder. Laryngeal edema, especially with abdominal pain, suggests hereditary angioedema (see Chapter 124.3).

Laboratory Findings. Laboratory studies may indicate the presence of IgE antibodies to a suspected causative agent, but this is not definitive. Plasma histamine is elevated for a brief period but is unstable and difficult to measure in a clinical setting. Plasma β-tryptase is more stable and remains elevated for several hours but is usually not elevated in food-induced anaphylactic reactions.

Treatment. Anaphylactic reaction should be managed aggressively (Box 137–2) with *intramuscular* epinephrine, intramuscular or intravenous H_1 and H_2 antihistamine antagonists, oxygen, intravenous fluids, inhaled β-agonists, and corticosteroids. Patients may experience a biphasic reaction, which occurs when anaphylactic symptoms recur after apparent resolution. The mechanism of this phenomenon is unknown, but it appears to be more common when therapy is initiated late and symptoms at presentation are more severe. It does not appear to be affected by the administration of corticosteroids during the initial therapy. Over 90% of biphasic responses occur within 4 hr, so patients should be observed for at least 4 hr before being discharged from the emergency department.

Prevention. Patients experiencing anaphylactic reactions to foods must be educated in allergen avoidance, including actively

TREATMENT OF REACTION
Dependent on severity of patient's symptoms

Patient
Injectable epinephrine (dependent on history and symptoms)
Oral liquid diphenhydramine (1 mg/kg up to 75 mg)
Transport to emergency facility

Emergency
Supplemental oxygen and airway management

Personnel
Epinephrine IM (IV for severe hypotension)
Intravenous fluid expansion
H_1 antagonist (diphenhydramine)—oral, IM, or IV
Corticosteroids—oral prednisone (1–2 mg/kg up to 75 mg) or intravenous methylprednisolone (1–2 mg/kg up to 125 mg)
Nebulized albuterol
H_2 antagonist (ranitidine)—oral or IV

POST REACTION
H_1 antagonist—cetirizine, fexofenadine, or loratadine for 3 days
Corticosteroids—oral prednisone 1 mg/kg (up to 75 mg) daily for 3 days

PREVENTATIVE TREATMENT
Follow-up evaluation for etiology
Immunotherapy for insect sting allergy
Prescription for EpiPen and antihistamine

PATIENT EDUCATION
Avoidance of causative agent
Recognition of early signs of anaphylaxis
Early treatment of allergic symptoms (anaphylaxis)

reading food labels and knowledge of potential contamination and high-risk situations, as well as in early recognition of anaphylactic symptoms and ready administration of emergency medications. Any child with food allergy and a history of asthma or previous severe anaphylactic reaction should be given an EpiPen, liquid diphenhydramine, and a written emergency plan in case of accidental ingestion. A form can be downloaded from the Food Allergy & Anaphylaxis Network at www.foodallergy.org. Patients with egg allergy should be tested before receiving the influenza or yellow fever vaccines, which contain egg protein. Children experiencing systemic anaphylactic reactions to an insect sting should be evaluated and treated with immunotherapy, which is more than 90% protective. In cases of food-associated exercise-induced anaphylaxis, children must not exercise within 2–3 hr of ingesting the triggering food and, like children with exercise-induced anaphylaxis, they should exercise with a friend, learn to recognize the early signs of anaphylaxis (sensation of warmth and facial pruritus) and stop exercising, and seek help immediately if symptoms develop. Any child who is at risk for anaphylaxis should receive emergency medications, education, and a written emergency plan in case of accidental ingestion.

Reactions to medications can be reduced and minimized by using oral medications in preference to injected forms. New hypo-osmolar radiocontrast dyes can be used in cases where previous reactions are suspected. The use of powder-free, low-allergen gloves and materials should be used in children undergoing multiple surgeries.

American Academy of Allergy, Asthma and Immunology Position Statement: Anaphylaxis in schools and other childcare settings. *J Allergy Clin Immunol* 1998;102:173–6.
American Academy of Pediatrics Position Statement: Guidelines for emergency medical care in school. *Pediatrics* 2001;107:435–6.
Bock SA, Munoz-Furlong A, Sampson HA: Fatalities due to anaphylactic reactions to foods. *J Allergy Clin Immunol* 2001;107:191–3.
Lee JM, Greenes DS: Biphasic anaphylactic reactions in pediatrics. *Pediatrics* 2000;106:762–6.

Novembre E, Cianferoni A, Bernardini R, et al: Anaphylaxis in children: Clinical and allergologic features. *Pediatrics* 1998;101:E8.
Sampson HA, Mendelson L, Rosen JP: Fatal and near-fatal food-induced anaphylaxis in children. *N Engl J Med* 1992;327:380–4.
Sicherer SH, Foreman JA, Noone SA: Use assessment of self-administered epinephrine among food-allergic children and pediatricians. *Pediatrics* 2000;105:359–62

Chapter 138
Serum Sickness *Scott H. Sicherer and Donald Y. M. Leung*

Serum sickness is a systemic, immune complex–mediated hypersensitivity vasculitis classically attributed to the therapeutic administration of foreign serum proteins.

Etiology. In 1905, von Pirquet and Schick gave the first detailed description of the disorder in children treated with horse serum containing diphtheria antitoxin. Animal models later showed that immune complexes involving heterologous serum proteins and complement activation were important pathogenic mechanisms. Reactions described as "serum sickness–like" are now attributed more commonly to drug allergy, triggered in particular by antibiotics (e.g., penicillin, cefaclor) and rarely to other agents such as human gamma globulin and insect venom. For many disorders, the availability of alternative medical therapies, bioengineered antibodies, and biologicals of human origin have supplanted the use of nonhuman antisera. However, antibody therapies derived from the horse are available for treatment of envenomation by the black widow spider and a variety of snakes, botulism in adults, diphtheria infection, and immunosuppression (antithymocyte globulin).

Pathogenesis. Serum sickness is a classic example of a Gell and Coombs type III hypersensitivity reaction caused by antigen-antibody complexes. In the rabbit model using bovine serum albumin as the antigen, symptoms develop with the appearance of antibody against the injected antigen. As free antigen concentration falls and antibody production increases over days, antigen-antibody complexes of various sizes develop in a manner analogous to a precipitin curve. While small complexes usually circulate harmlessly and large ones are cleared by the reticuloendothelial system, intermediate-sized complexes that develop at the point of slight antigen excess may deposit in blood vessel walls and tissues. There the immune microprecipitates induce vascular and tissue damage through activation of complement and granulocytes.

Complement activation (C3a, C5a) promotes chemotaxis and adherence of neutrophils to the site of immune complex deposition. The process of immune complex deposition and of neutrophil accumulation may be facilitated by increased vascular permeability, owing to the release of vasoactive amines from tissue mast cells. Mast cells may be activated by binding of antigen to IgE or through contact with anaphylatoxins (C3a). Tissue injury results from the liberation of proteolytic enzymes and oxygen radicals from the neutrophils.

Clinical Manifestations. The symptoms of serum sickness generally begin 7–12 days after injection of the foreign material but may appear as late as 3 wk afterward. The onset of symptoms may be accelerated if there has been earlier exposure or previous allergic reaction to the same antigen. A few days before the onset of generalized symptoms, the site of injection may become edematous and erythematous. Symptoms usually include fever, malaise, and rashes. Urticaria and morbilliform rashes are the predominant types of skin eruptions, and pruritus is common. In a prospective study of serum sickness induced by administration of equine antithymocyte globulin, an initial rash was noted in most patients that began as a thin serpiginous band of erythema along the sides of the hands, fingers, feet, and toes at the junction of the palmar or plantar skin with the skin of the dorsolateral surface. In most patients, the band of erythema was replaced by petechiae or purpura, presumably because of low platelet counts. Additional symptoms include edema, myalgia, lymphadenopathy, arthralgia or arthritis involving multiple joints, and gastrointestinal complaints including pain, nausea, diarrhea, and melena. The disease generally runs a self-limited course, with recovery in 1–2 wk. Carditis, glomerulonephritis, Guillain-Barré syndrome, and peripheral neuritis are rare complications.

Diagnosis. Circulating immune complexes are usually detectable with peak levels at 10–12 days. Serum complement levels (C3 and C4) are generally decreased and reach a nadir at about day 10. C3a anaphylatoxin may be increased. The erythrocyte sedimentation rate is usually elevated, and thrombocytopenia is often present. Mild proteinuria, hemoglobinuria, and microscopic hematuria may be seen. In serum sickness caused by horse serum proteins, antibodies of the IgG, IgA, IgM, and IgE classes may be found directed against various horse serum proteins. Direct immunofluorescence studies of skin lesions often reveal immune deposits of IgM, IgA, IgE, or C3.

Treatment. Treatment is primarily supportive with antihistamines and analgesics, if needed. When the symptoms are especially severe, systemic corticosteroids can be used. High doses are given and rapidly reduced as the patient improves. The utility of extracorporeal removal of circulating immune complexes via plasmapheresis requires further study.

Prevention. The primary mode of prevention of serum sickness is to seek alternative therapies, if they are available. In some cases, non–equine-derived formulations may be available in limited supply (e.g., human-derived botulinum immune globulin). Other emerging alternatives include partially digested antibodies of animal origin and engineered (humanized) antibodies. However, the potential of these therapies to elicit serum sickness–like disease remains to be determined. When only equine antitoxin/antivenom is available, skin tests should be performed before administration of serum. The results of allergy skin tests reflect primarily the risk of acute anaphylactic reactions to the serum proteins with a positive test indicating an increased likelihood and a negative test indicating a small, but not absent, risk of anaphylaxis. Testing generally begins with prick-puncture using a 1:100 dilution of the serum with positive (histamine) and negative (saline) controls and proceeds through several increasingly higher doses until a positive response is seen or a top dose of 0.02 mL of a 1:100 dilution injected intracutaneously is reached. A negative response to the strongest solution indicates that anaphylactic sensitivity to horse serum is unlikely. Unfortunately, skin tests do not predict the likelihood of development of serum sickness.

For patients who have evidence of anaphylactic sensitivity to horse serum, a risk to benefit assessment must be made to determine the need to proceed with treatment despite an increased risk for anaphylaxis. If needed, the serum can usually be successfully administered by a process of rapid desensitization. The suggested desensitization procedure varies slightly by manufacturer, by estimated degree of sensitivity, and by route (intravenous versus intramuscular/subcutaneous). Starting doses are usually quite small (e.g., 0.1 mL of serum diluted to 1:100,000–1:1,000) and administered in gradually increasing increments such as doubling doses at 15–20 min intervals, as tolerated, until the required cumulative dose is achieved. Generally, the entire amount of antitoxin can be administered safely over a 4–6 hr period. Desensitization is transient, and the patient may regain the previous anaphylactic sensitivity in the

months after treatment. Serum sickness is not prevented by desensitization or pretreatment with methylprednisolone.

Dart RC, Seifert SA, Boyer LV, et al: A randomized multicenter trial of Crotalinae polyvalent immune Fab (Ovine) antivenom for the treatment for crotaline snakebite in the United States. *Arch Intern Med* 2001;161:2030–36.
Kojis FG: Serum sickness and anaphylaxis: Analysis of cases of 6,211 patients treated with horse serum for various infections. *Am J Dis Child* 1942;64:93–143.
Lawley TJ, Bielory L, Gascon P, et al: A prospective clinical and immunological analysis of patients with serum sickness. *New Engl J Med* 1984;311:1407–13.

Chapter 139
Adverse Reactions to Drugs
Mark Boguniewicz

Adverse drug reactions are being increasingly recognized in the pediatric population as the number of drugs approved for use in this population increases. Adverse drug reactions can be divided into predictable and unpredictable reactions. **Predictable reactions** including drug toxicity, drug interactions, and adverse effects are dose dependent, can be related to known pharmacologic actions of the drug, and occur in patients without any unique susceptibility. In contrast, **unpredictable reactions** are dose independent, often not related to the pharmacologic actions of the drug, and occur in susceptible patients. These include idiosyncratic reactions, allergic (hypersensitivity) reactions, and pseudoallergic reactions. **Pseudoallergic reactions** resemble allergic reactions but are distinguished by the fact that an immunologic mechanism is not involved. Allergic reactions require prior sensitization, manifest with signs or symptoms characteristic of an underlying allergic mechanism, such as anaphylaxis or urticaria, and occur in genetically susceptible individuals. They can occur at doses significantly below the therapeutic range.

Epidemiology. The incidence of adverse drug reactions in the general as well as pediatric populations remains unknown, although data from hospitalized patients shows it to be 6.7%, with a 0.32% incidence of fatal adverse drug reactions. Cutaneous reactions are the most common form of adverse drug reactions with ampicillin, amoxicillin, penicillin, and trimethoprim-sulfamethoxazole accounting for the majority of implicated drugs. Although the majority of adverse drug reactions do not appear to be allergic in nature, 6–10% can be attributed to an allergic or immunologic mechanism.

Pathogenesis and Clinical Manifestations. Immunologically mediated adverse drug reactions have been classified according to the **Gell and Coombs classification**: immediate hypersensitivity reactions (type I), cytotoxic antibody reactions (type II), immune complex reactions (type III), and delayed-type hypersensitivity reactions (type IV). Immediate hypersensitivity reactions occur when a drug or drug metabolite interacts with preformed drug-specific IgE antibodies that are bound to the surfaces of tissue mast cells and/or circulating basophils. The cross-linking of adjacent receptor-bound IgE by antigen causes the release of preformed and newly synthesized mediators such as histamine and leukotrienes that contribute to the clinical development of urticaria, bronchospasm, or anaphylaxis. Cytotoxic reactions involve IgG or IgM antibodies that recognize drug antigen on cell membrane. In the presence of serum complement, the antibody coated cell is either cleared by the monocyte-macrophage system or is destroyed. Examples include drug-induced hemolytic anemia or thrombocytopenia. Immune complex reactions are caused by soluble complexes of drug or metabolite in slight antigen excess with IgG or IgM antibodies.

The immune complex is deposited in blood vessel walls and causes injury by activating the complement cascade as seen in serum sickness. Clinical manifestations include fever, urticaria, rash, lymphadenopathy, and arthralgias. Symptoms typically appear 1–3 wk after the last dose of an offending drug and subside when the drug and/or its metabolite are cleared from the body. Delayed-type hypersensitivity reactions are mediated by drug-specific T lymphocytes. Sensitization usually occurs via the topical route of administration, resulting in allergic contact dermatitis. Commonly implicated drugs include neomycin and local anesthetics in topical formulations. Certain adverse drug reactions including drug fever or the morbilliform rash seen with use of ampicillin or amoxicillin in the setting of Epstein-Barr virus infection are not easily classified. Recent studies point to the role of T cells and eosinophils in delayed maculopapular reactions to a number of antibiotics.

DRUG METABOLISM AND ADVERSE REACTIONS. Most drugs and their metabolites are not immunologically detectable until they have become covalently attached to a macromolecule. This multivalent hapten-protein complex forms a new immunogenic epitope that can elicit T and B lymphocyte responses. The penicillins and related β-lactam antibiotics are highly reactive with proteins and can directly haptenate protein carriers, which may account for the frequency of immune-mediated hypersensitivity reactions with this class of antibiotics.

Incomplete or delayed metabolism of some drugs can give rise to toxic metabolites. Hydroxylamine, a reactive metabolite produced by cytochrome P-450 oxidative metabolism, may mediate adverse reactions to sulfonamides. Patients who are slow acetylators appear to be at increased risk. In addition, cutaneous reactions in patients with AIDS treated with trimethoprim-sulfamethoxazole, rifampin, or other drugs may be due to glutathione deficiency resulting in toxic metabolites. Serum sickness–like reactions in which immune complexes have not been documented, which occur most commonly with cefaclor, may result from an inherited propensity for hepatic biotransformation of drugs into toxic or immunogenic metabolites.

RISK FACTORS FOR HYPERSENSITIVITY REACTIONS. Risk factors for adverse drug reactions include previous exposure, previous reaction, age (20–49 yr), route of administration (parenteral or topical), dose (high), and dosing schedule (intermittent), as well as genetic predisposition (slow acetylators). Atopy does not appear to predispose patients to allergic reactions to low molecular weight compounds, but atopic patients who develop an allergic reaction have a significantly increased risk of serious reaction. Atopic patients also appear to be at greater risk for pseudoallergic reactions induced by radiocontrast media. Pharmacogenomics will likely play an increasing role in identifying individuals at risk for certain drug reactions.

Diagnosis. An accurate medical history is an important first step in evaluating a patient with a possible adverse drug reaction. Suspected drugs need to be identified with dosages, route of administration, previous exposures, and dates of administration. In addition, underlying hepatic or renal disease may influence drug metabolism. For past reactions, a detailed description may yield clues to the nature of the adverse drug reaction. The propensity for a particular drug to cause the suspected reaction can be checked with information in the *Physicians' Desk Reference*, the *Drug Eruption Reference Manual*, or directly from the drug manufacturer. However, it is important to remember that the history may be unreliable and many patients are inappropriately labeled as being drug allergic, which can result in inappropriate withholding of a needed drug or class of drugs. In addition, relying solely on the history can lead to overuse of drugs reserved for special indications such as vancomycin in patients suspected of penicillin allergy. In fact, approximately 80% of patients with a history of penicillin allergy will not have evidence of penicillin-specific IgE antibodies on testing.

Skin testing is the most rapid and sensitive method of demonstrating the presence of IgE antibodies to a specific allergen. It can be performed with high molecular weight compounds such as foreign antisera, hormones, enzymes, and toxoids. Reliable skin testing can also be performed with penicillin, but not with most other antibiotics. Most immunologically mediated adverse drug reactions are due to metabolites rather than to parent compounds, and the metabolites for most drugs other than penicillin have not been defined. In addition, many metabolites are unstable or must combine with larger proteins to be useful for diagnosis. Testing with nonstandardized reagents requires caution in interpretation of both positive and negative results because some drugs can induce nonspecific irritant reactions. Whereas a wheal-and-flare reaction is suggestive of drug-specific IgE antibodies, a negative skin test does exclude the presence of such antibodies because the relevant immunogen may not have been used as the testing reagent.

A positive skin test to the major or minor determinants of penicillin has a 60% positive predictive value for an immediate hypersensitivity reaction to penicillin. If skin tests to the major and minor determinants of penicillin are negative, 97–99% of patients (depending on the reagents used) will tolerate the drug without risk of an immediate reaction. The positive and negative predictive values of skin testing to antibiotics other than penicillin are not well established. Nevertheless, positive immediate hypersensitivity skin tests to nonirritant concentrations of nonpenicillin antibiotics may be interpreted as a presumptive risk of an immediate reaction to such agents.

Direct and indirect Coombs tests are often positive in drug-induced hemolytic anemia. Assays for specific IgG and IgM have been shown to correlate with a drug reaction in immune cytopenias, but in most other reactions such assays are not diagnostic. In general, many more patients express humoral or T-cell immune responses to drug determinants than express clinical disease. Serum tryptase is elevated with systemic mast cell degranulation and can be seen with drug associated mast cell activation, although it is not pathognomonic for drug hypersensitivity and nonelevated tryptase levels can be seen in well-defined anaphylaxis.

Treatment. Specific **desensitization,** which involves the progressive administration of an allergen to render effector cells less reactive, is reserved for patients with IgE antibodies to a particular drug for whom an alternative drug is not available or appropriate. Specific protocols for many different drugs have been described. Desensitization should be performed in a hospital setting usually in consultation with an allergist with resuscitation equipment available at all times. While mild complications, such as pruritus or rash, are fairly common and often respond to adjustments in the drug dose or dosing intervals and medications to relieve symptoms, more severe systemic reactions can occur. Oral desensitization may be less likely to induce anaphylaxis than parenteral administration. Pretreatment with antihistamines and/or corticosteroids usually is not recommended.

Graded challenges based on the administration of a drug in an incremental fashion until a therapeutic dose is achieved can be attempted with drugs causing non–IgE-mediated reactions, including trimethoprim-sulfamethoxazole. Graded challenges in aspirin- or nonsteroidal anti-inflammatory drug (NSAID)-intolerant patients, particularly those with respiratory reactions, can also be performed. Gradual introduction of a drug may reveal systemic intolerance early enough to prevent progression to a serious or even life-threatening reaction such as Stevens-Johnson syndrome or toxic epidermal necrolysis.

β-LACTAM HYPERSENSITIVITY. Penicillin is a frequent cause of anaphylaxis and is responsible for the majority of all drug-mediated anaphylactic deaths in the United States. Although IgE-mediated reactions may occur after administration of penicillin by any route, parenteral administration is more likely to cause anaphylaxis. If a patient requires penicillin and has a past history suggestive of penicillin allergy, it is necessary to skin test the patient for the presence of penicillin-specific IgE with both the major and minor determinants of penicillin. Skin tests to both major and minor determinants of penicillin are necessary because about 20% of patients with documented anaphylaxis do not demonstrate skin reactivity to the major determinant. While the major determinant is available commercially (PrePen), minor determinant mixtures are currently not licensed and are synthesized at select centers. Although penicillin G is often used as a substitute for minor determinant mixture, with this approach there is a small but significant risk of false-negative skin test results. Thus, patients should be referred to an allergist capable of performing appropriate testing. If the skin test is positive to either major or minor determinants of penicillin, the patient should receive an alternative non–cross-reacting antibiotic. If administration of penicillin is deemed necessary, desensitization by an allergist in an appropriate medical setting can be performed. Skin testing for penicillin-specific IgE is not predictive for delayed onset cutaneous, bullous, or immune complex reactions. In addition, penicillin skin testing does not appear to resensitize the patient.

Other β-lactam antibiotics including semisynthetic penicillins, cephalosporins, carbacephems, carbapenems, and monobactams share the β-lactam ring structure. Patients with late-onset morbilliform rashes with amoxicillin are not considered to be at risk for IgE-mediated reactions to penicillin and do not require skin testing before penicillin administration. Patients with Epstein-Barr virus infections treated with ampicillin or amoxicillin can develop a nonpruritic rash in up to 100% of cases. Similar reactions occur in patients with elevated uric acid treated with allopurinol or with chronic lymphocytic leukemia. If the rash to ampicillin or amoxicillin is urticarial or systemic, or the history is unclear, the patient should undergo penicillin skin testing if a penicillin is needed. There have been reports of antibodies specific for semisynthetic penicillin side chains in the absence of β-lactam ring-specific antibodies, although the clinical significance of such side chain–specific antibodies is unclear.

Varying degrees of in vitro cross reactivity have been documented between cephalosporins and penicillins. Although the risk of allergic reactions to cephalosporins in patients with positive skin tests to penicillin appears to be low (<2%), anaphylactic reactions have occurred after administration of cephalosporins in patients with a positive history of penicillin anaphylaxis. If a patient has a history of penicillin allergy and requires a cephalosporin, skin testing to major and minor determinants of penicillin should preferably be performed to determine if the patient has penicillin-specific IgE antibodies. If skin tests are negative, the patient can receive a cephalosporin with no greater risk than the general population. If skin tests are positive to penicillin, recommendations may include administration of an alternative antibiotic; cautious graded challenge with appropriate monitoring, recognizing that there may be a 2% chance of inducing an anaphylactic reaction; or desensitization to the required cephalosporin.

Conversely, patients who require penicillin and have a history of an IgE-mediated reaction to a cephalosporin should also undergo penicillin skin testing. If the tests are negative, they can receive penicillin; if positive, they should either receive an alternative medication or undergo desensitization to penicillin. In patients with a history of allergic reaction to one cephalosporin requiring another cephalosporin, skin testing with the required cephalosporin can be performed, recognizing that the negative predictive value is unknown. If the skin test to the cephalosporin is positive, the significance of the test should be checked further in control subjects to determine if the positive response is IgE mediated or an irritant response. The drug can then be administered by graded challenge or desensitization.

Carbapenems (imipenem and meropenem) represent another class of β-lactam antibiotics with a bicyclic nucleus that demonstrate a high degree of cross reactivity with penicillins. In contrast to the other β-lactam antibiotics, monobactams (aztreonam) have a monocyclic ring structure. Aztreonam-specific antibodies have been shown to be predominantly side-chain specific; data suggest that aztreonam can be safely administered to most penicillin-allergic subjects.

SULFONAMIDES. The most common type of reaction to sulfonamides is a maculopapular eruption often associated with fever that occurs after 7–12 days of therapy. Immediate reactions including anaphylaxis as well as other immunologic reactions have also been suggested. For those individuals who develop maculopapular rashes after sulfonamide administration, both graded challenge and desensitization protocols have been shown to be effective. These regimens should not be used in individuals with a history of Stevens-Johnson syndrome or toxic epidermal necrolysis. Hypersensitivity reactions to sulfasalazine, for treatment of inflammatory bowel disease, appear to result from the sulfapyridine moiety. Slow desensitization over approximately 1 mo permits tolerance of the drug in many patients. In addition, oral and enema forms of 5-ASA, thought to be the pharmacologically active agent in sulfasalazine, are effective alternative therapies.

STEVENS-JOHNSON SYNDROME AND TOXIC EPIDERMAL NECROLYSIS. Blistering mucocutaneous disorders induced by drugs encompass a spectrum of reactions, including Stevens-Johnson syndrome and toxic epidermal necrolysis. Epidermal detachment of less than 10% is suggestive of Stevens-Johnson syndrome, detachment of 30% suggests toxic epidermal necrolysis, and 10–30% detachment suggests overlap of the two syndromes. The features of Stevens-Johnson syndrome include confluent purpuric macules on face and trunk and severe, explosive mucosal erosions, usually at more than one mucosal surface, accompanied by fever and constitutional symptoms. Ocular involvement may be particularly severe, and the liver, kidneys, and lungs may also be involved. Toxic epidermal necrolysis, which appears to be related to keratinocyte apoptosis, manifests with widespread areas of confluent erythema followed by epidermal necrosis and detachment with severe mucosal involvement. The risk of infection and mortality are high. Skin biopsy differentiates subepidermal cleavage characteristic of toxic epidermal necrolysis from intraepidermal cleavage characteristic of the scalded skin syndrome induced by staphylococcal toxins. The effectiveness of corticosteroids in the treatment of Stevens-Johnson syndrome is controversial, but, if used, they should be started as early in the course of the disease as possible. Toxic epidermal necrolysis must be treated in a burn unit. Corticosteroids are contraindicated because they can significantly increase the risk of infection. High intravenous doses of immunoglobulin have been shown to be beneficial in patients with toxic epidermal necrolysis likely due to inhibition of Fas-mediated keratinocyte cell death by naturally occurring Fas blocking antibodies in the intravenous immunoglobulin preparation.

PERIOPERATIVE AGENTS. Anaphylactoid reactions occurring during general anesthesia may be caused by induction agents (thiopental) or muscle-relaxing agents (succinylcholine, pancuronium). Quaternary ammonium muscle relaxants (e.g., succinylcholine) can act as bivalent antigens in IgE-mediated reactions. Negative skin tests do not necessarily predict that a drug will be tolerated. Latex allergy should always be considered in the differential diagnosis of a perioperative reaction.

LOCAL ANESTHETICS. Adverse drug reactions associated with local anesthetic agents are primarily toxic reactions resulting from rapid drug absorption, inadvertent intravenous injection, or overdosage. Local anesthetics are classified as esters of benzoic acid (group I) or amides (group II). Group I includes benzocaine and procaine; group II includes lidocaine, bupivacaine, and mepivacaine. In suspected local anesthetic allergy, skin testing followed by a graded challenge can be performed or an anesthetic agent from a different group can be used.

INSULIN. Insulin use has been associated with a spectrum of adverse drug reactions, including local and systemic IgE-mediated reactions, hemolytic anemia, serum sickness reactions, and delayed-type hypersensitivity. In general, human insulin is less allergenic than porcine insulin, which is less allergenic than bovine insulin, but for individual patients porcine or bovine insulin may be the least allergenic. Patients treated with nonhuman insulin have had systemic reactions to recombinant human insulin even on the first exposure. More than 50% of patients who receive insulin develop antibodies against the insulin preparation, although there may not be any clinical manifestations. Local cutaneous reactions usually do not require treatment and resolve with continued insulin administration, possibly owing to IgG blocking antibodies. More severe local reactions can be treated with antihistamines or by splitting the insulin dose between separate administration sites. Local reactions to the protamine component of NPH insulin may be avoided by switching to Lente insulin. Immediate-type reactions to insulin, including urticaria and anaphylactic shock, are unusual and almost always occur after reinstitution of insulin therapy in sensitized patients. Insulin therapy should not be interrupted if a systemic reaction to insulin occurs and continued insulin therapy is essential. Skin testing may identify a less antigenic insulin preparation. The dose following a systemic reaction is usually reduced to one third, and successive doses are increased in 2–5 unit increments until the dose resulting in diabetic control is attained; insulin skin testing and desensitization are required if insulin treatment is subsequently interrupted for more than 24–48 hr. Immunologic resistance usually occurs when a patient develops high titers of predominantly IgG antibodies to insulin. A rare form of insulin resistance caused by circulating antibodies to tissue insulin receptors is associated with acanthosis nigricans and lipodystrophy. Coexisting insulin allergy may be present in up to one third of patients with insulin resistance. Approximately half of affected patients benefit from substitution with a less reactive insulin preparation, based on skin testing.

ANTICONVULSANT HYPERSENSITIVITY SYNDROME. Anticonvulsant hypersensitivity syndrome is a potentially life-threatening syndrome that occurs with exposure of variable lengths to anticonvulsant medications. It appears to result from an inherited deficiency of epoxide hydrolase, an enzyme required for the metabolism of arene oxide intermediates produced during hepatic metabolism of anticonvulsant drugs. It is characterized by fever, maculopapular rash, and generalized lymphadenopathy along with visceral organ involvement. Drug-induced hypersensitivity syndrome has also been described with minocycline, sulfonamides, and dapsone.

RED MAN SYNDROME. This syndrome most commonly described with administration of vancomycin is caused by nonspecific histamine release. It can be prevented by slowing the rate of intravenous infusion and/or preadministration of H_1-blockers.

RADIOCONTRAST MEDIA. Anaphylactoid reactions to radiocontrast media (RCM) or dye can occur after intravascular administration and during myelograms or retrograde pyelograms. No single pathogenic mechanism has been defined, but it is likely that mast cell activation accounts for the majority of these reactions. Complement activation has also been described. There is no evidence that sensitivity to seafood or iodine predisposes to RCM reactions. Although predictive tests are not available, patients with atopic profiles and those using β-blockers appear to be at increased risk for RCM reactions. Patients who have experienced anaphylactoid reactions during the administration of RCM are at increased risk for recurrence with re-exposure. Other diagnostic alternatives should be considered or patients can be given low osmolality RCM with

a pretreatment regimen including oral prednisone, diphenhydramine, and albuterol, with or without cimetidine or ranitidine.

NARCOTIC ANALGESICS. Opiates such as morphine and related narcotics can induce direct mast cell degranulation. Patients may develop generalized pruritus, urticaria, and, occasionally, wheezing. If there is a suggestive history and analgesia is required, a non-narcotic medication should be considered. If this does not control pain, graded challenge with an alternative opiate is an option.

ASPIRIN AND NSAIDS. Aspirin and NSAIDs can cause anaphylactoid reactions or urticaria and/or angioedema in children and rarely asthma with or without rhinoconjunctivitis in adolescents. There is no skin or in vitro test to identify patients who may react to aspirin or other NSAIDs. Once aspirin or NSAIDs intolerance has been established, options include avoidance or pharmacologic desensitization and subsequent continued treatment with aspirin or NSAIDs if indicated. Preliminary studies suggest that cyclo-oxygenase-2 inhibitors are tolerated by patients with aspirin-induced asthma.

Bernstein IL, Gruchalla RS, Lee RE, et al (editors): Disease management of drug hypersensitivity: A practice parameter. *Ann Allergy Asthma Immunol* 1999;83: 678–79.

Carroll MC, Yueng-Yue KA, Esterly NB, et al: Drug-induced hypersensitivity syndrome in pediatric patients. *Pediatrics* 2001;108:485–92.

Gruchalla R: Understanding drug allergies. *J Allergy Clin Immunol* 2000;105: S637–44.

Kelkar PS, Li JT: Cephalosporin allergy. *N Engl J Med* 2001;345:804–9.

Pumphrey RS, Davis S: Under-reporting of antibiotic anaphylaxis may put patients at risk. *Lancet* 1999;353:1157–58.

Reilly TP, Lash LH, Doll MA, et al: A role for bioactivation and covalent binding within epidermal keratinocytes in sulfonamide-induced cutaneous drug reactions. *J Invest Dermatol* 2000;114:1164–73.

Viard I, Wehrli P, Bullani R, et al: Inhibition of toxic epidermal necrolysis by blockade of CD95 with human intravenous immunoglobulin. *Science* 1998;282: 490–3.

Yawalkar N, Egli F, Hari Y, et al: Infiltration of cytotoxic T cells in drug-induced cutaneous eruptions. *Clin Exp Allergy* 2000;30:847–55.

Yawalkar N, Shrikhande M, Hari Y, et al: Evidence for a role for IL-5 and eotaxin in activating and recruiting eosinophils in drug-induced cutaneous eruptions. *J Allergy Clin Immunol* 2000;106:1171–76.

Chapter 140

Insect Allergy *Scott H. Sicherer and Donald Y. M. Leung*

Allergic reactions caused by inhalation of airborne particles of insect origin result in acute and chronic respiratory symptoms. The allergic responses to stinging or, more rarely, biting insects result in reactions that vary from those localized to the skin to systemic anaphylaxis.

Etiology. IgE antibody–mediated allergic responses to airborne particulate matter carrying insect emanations contribute to seasonal and perennial symptoms affecting the upper and lower airway. Seasonal reactions are attributed to exposures to a variety of insects, particularly aquatic insects such as the caddis fly and midge at a time when larvae pupate and adult flies are airborne. The fine wing scales and other emanations from virtually any insect may induce symptoms in select environments; for example, the mayfly is responsible for allergic symptoms in the area around the western end of Lake Erie. In terms of perennial inhalant allergy, cockroach sensitization is associated with increased asthma morbidity for exposed children. The house dust mite plays a similar role as an indoor allergen, but these creatures, unlike the cockroach, have eight rather than six legs and are phylogenetically related to spiders rather than insects.

For insect bite reactions, induced for example by mosquitoes, flies, and fleas, the primary lesion is isolated to the area of the bite and generally does not represent an allergic response. Occasionally, insect bites or stings induce larger local reactions that may be based on immediate or delayed hypersensitivity reactions.

Systemic allergic responses to insects are attributed most typically to IgE antibody-mediated responses, which are caused almost entirely by stings from venomous insects of the order Hymenoptera. Members of this order include apids (honeybee, bumblebee), vespids (yellow jacket, wasp, hornet), and formicids (fire and harvester ants). Among winged stinging insects, yellow jackets are the most notorious for stinging because they are aggressive, are ground dwelling, and linger near human activities involving food. Hornets nest in trees, wasps build honeycomb nests in dark areas such as under porches, and both are aggressive if disturbed. Honeybees are less aggressive, nest in tree hollows, and, unlike the other flying Hymenoptera, almost always leave a barbed stinger with venom sac after an attack. In the United States, red or black fire ants are found in increasing areas of the southeast, living in large mounds of soil. When disturbed, the ants attack in large numbers, anchor themselves to the skin by their mandible and sting multiple times in a semi-circle pattern. Sterile pustules form at the sting sites. Systemic reactions to stinging insects occur in 0.4–0.8% of children and 3% of adults and account for approximately 40 deaths each year in the United States.

Pathogenesis. A variety of proteins derived from insects can become airborne and induce IgE-mediated respiratory responses, causing inhalant allergies. For example, the primary allergenic substance from midge, or lake flies, derives from hemoglobin and the major allergen of caddis fly is a hemocyanin-like protein. Allergens from the cockroach are the best studied and are derived from cockroach saliva, secretions, fecal material, debris from skin casts, and dead cockroaches. Allergenic proteins from the cockroach include proteases, troponin, tropomyosin, and lipocalin.

Localized skin responses to biting insects are likely caused by vasoactive or irritant materials derived from the insect's saliva. There is no evidence for IgE involvement in the local reaction. Systemic IgE-mediated allergic reactions to salivary proteins of biting insects are reported, but uncommon.

Hymenoptera venoms contain numerous components with toxic and pharmacologic activity and with allergenic potential. These constituents include vasoactive materials such as histamine, acetylcholine, and kinins; enzymes such as phospholipase and hyaluronidase; apamin; melittin; and formic acid. The majority of patients who experience systemic reactions after Hymenoptera stings have IgE-mediated sensitivity to antigenic material in the venom. Some venom allergens are homologous among members of the Hymenoptera order; others are family specific. There is substantial cross reactivity among vespid venoms, but these are distinct from honeybee.

Clinical Manifestations. Inhalant allergy caused by insects results in clinical disease that is similar to that induced by other inhalant allergens such as pollens or dust mite. Depending on individual sensitivity and exposure, reactions may result in perennial or seasonal rhinitis, conjunctivitis, and asthma.

Insect bites are usually urticarial but may be papular or vesicular. Papular urticaria affecting the lower extremities in children is usually caused by multiple bites. Occasionally, individuals develop large local reactions. IgE antibody–associated immediate- and late-phase allergic responses to mosquito bites sometimes mimic cellulitis.

Clinical reactions to stinging venomous insects are categorized as local, large local, systemic, toxic, and delayed/late. Simple **local reactions** involve limited swelling, pain and generally last less than a day. **Large local reactions** develop over hours and days, involve swelling of extensive areas that are contiguous with the sting site, and may last for days. **Non–life-threatening systemic reactions** generally progress within minutes and include skin symptoms of urticaria, angioedema, and pruritus distal to the site of the sting. **Life-threatening, immediate systemic reactions** are identical to anaphylaxis from other triggers and include symptoms of laryngeal edema, bronchospasm, and hypotension. Stings from a large number of insects at once may result in **toxic reactions** of fever, malaise, emesis, and nausea owing to the chemical properties of the venom in large doses. Serum sickness, nephrotic syndrome, vasculitis, neuritis, or encephalopathy may occur as **delayed/ late reactions** to stinging insects.

Diagnosis. In the case of inhalant allergy to insects, the diagnosis may be evident by a history of typical symptoms induced seasonally in specific geographic regions (e.g., mayfly induced allergy). A chronic respiratory symptom in the face of chronic exposure, as may occur for cockroach allergy, is a scenario that is less amenable to identification by history. Tests for specific IgE to the insect by skin prick or radioallergosorbent test (RAST) will confirm inhalant insect allergy. In the case of potential cockroach allergy in patients with persistent asthma and known cockroach exposure, allergy tests may be particularly warranted.

The diagnosis of allergy from biting and stinging insects is generally evident from the history of exposure, typical symptoms, and physical examination. The diagnosis of Hymenoptera allergy rests in part on the identification of venom-specific IgE antibody. The primary reasons to pursue testing are to confirm reactivity when venom immunotherapy (VIT) is being considered or when it is clinically necessary to confirm venom hypersensitivity as a cause of a reaction. Venoms of five Hymenoptera (honeybee, yellow jacket, yellow hornet, white-faced hornet, and wasp) and whole-body extracts of fire ant are available for skin testing and treatment. In the context of a convincing clinical history, appropriately performed skin testing is useful in identifying children at risk for systemic anaphylaxis. However, venom skin test negative subjects have been reported to experience anaphylaxis when re-stung. Although the skin tests are considered more sensitive for the detection of venom-specific IgE antibody compared with RAST, if they are negative in the presence of a convincing history it is reasonable to consider additional evaluation with repeat skin tests and RAST. With venom RAST, there is a 20% incidence of both false-positive and false-negative results so it would not be appropriate to exclude venom hypersensitivity based on RAST alone. As many as 40% of skin test–positive subjects may not experience anaphylaxis on sting challenge, so testing without an appropriate history is potentially misleading. Skin tests are usually accurate within 1 wk of a sting reaction, but occasionally a refractory period is observed that warrants re-testing after 4–6 wk if the initial tests were negative.

Treatment and Prevention. Avoidance of the insect is the preferred management of inhalant allergy. This can prove difficult, particularly, for instance, for those living in multiple-dwelling apartments where eradication of cockroaches is problematic. Immunotherapy is occasionally undertaken but beneficial results have not been thoroughly documented.

For cutaneous reactions caused by biting insects and for local reactions to stings, treatment with cold compresses, topical medicaments to relieve itching, and occasionally the use of a systemic antihistamine and oral analgesic are appropriate. Stingers should be removed promptly by scraping with caution not to squeeze the venom sac because this could inject more venom. Sting sites rarely become infected, possibly owing to the antibacterial actions of venom constituents. If the vesicles left by fire ant stings are scratched open, cleansing to prevent secondary infection is appropriate.

Anaphylactic reactions after a Hymenoptera sting are treated in an identical fashion to anaphylaxis from any cause. Therapies may include epinephrine, antihistamines, blood volume expanders, and other treatments (see Chapter 137). Those who have had previous systemic reactions to Hymenoptera stings should have immediate access to self-injectable epinephrine. Adults responsible for allergic children, and older patients who can self-treat, must be carefully taught the indications for and technique of administration of this medication. Particular attention is necessary for children in out-of-home daycare centers, at school, or attending camps to ensure that an emergency action plan is in place. Patients at risk for anaphylaxis from an insect sting should also wear an identification bracelet indicating their allergy. To reduce the risk of stings, they should avoid attractants such as perfumes and bright-colored clothing outdoors, wear gloves when gardening, and wear long pants and shoes when walking in the grass or through fields. Typical insect repellents do not guard against Hymenoptera.

Hymenoptera VIT is highly effective (97%) in decreasing the risk for severe anaphylaxis. The selection of patients for VIT depends on several factors (Table 140–1). Individuals at any age with local reactions are not at increased risk for severe systemic reactions on a subsequent sting and are not candidates for VIT. Those who experience severe systemic reactions (airway involvement or hypotension) and have a positive skin test result should receive immunotherapy. Immunotherapy to winged Hymenoptera is not considered indicated for children younger than age 16 yr in whom stings have caused systemic reactions limited to the skin because their risk for anaphylaxis after a subsequent sting is about 10%, with isolated skin reactions as the most likely event. The risk could be reduced to 1.2% on VIT, so it is an option to consider if multiple future stings are anticipated. Immunotherapy to winged Hymenoptera is indicated in those older than age 17 yr if skin test results are positive to venom and there is a history of systemic reaction, even isolated urticaria, because the risk for future systemic reactions approaches 60%. VIT is usually not indicated if there is no evidence of IgE to venom. The incidence of adverse effects during the course of treatment is not trivial in adults; 50% experience large local reactions and about 7% experience systemic reactions. The incidence of both local and systemic reactions is much lower in children. It is uncertain how long immunotherapy with Hymenoptera venom should continue, but over 85% of adults who have received 5 yr of therapy tolerate challenge stings without systemic reactions for 5–10 yr after completion of treatment.

Less is known about the natural history of fire ant hypersensitivity and efficacy of immunotherapy for this allergy. The criteria for starting immunotherapy are similar to that for other Hymenoptera, but it is controversial as to whether children younger than age 16 yr should receive treatment if they have only experienced systemic reactions confined to the skin. Only whole-body extract is commercially available for diagnosis by allergy skin testing and for treatment by immunotherapy.

Golden DBK, Kagey-Sobotka A, Norman PS, et al: Insect sting allergy with negative venom skin test responses. *J Allergy Clin Immunol* 2001;107:897–901.

Golden DBK, Kagey-Sobotka A, Lichtenstein LM: Survey of patients after discontinuing venom immunotherapy. *J Allergy Clin Immunol* 2000;105:385–90.

Kemp SF, deShazo RD, Moffitt JE, et al: Expanding habitat of the imported fire ant (*Solenopsis invicta*): A public health concern. *J Allergy Clin Immunol* 2000;105: 683–91.

Portnoy JM, Moffitt JE, Golden DBK, et al: Stinging insect hypersensitivity: A practice parameter. *J Allergy Clin Immunol* 1999;103:963–80.

Chapter 141

Ocular Allergies *Mark Boguniewicz*

The eye is a common target of allergic disorders because of its marked vascularity and direct contact with the environment, with the conjunctiva being the most immunologically active tissue of the external eye. Ocular allergies can occur as isolated target organ disease or more commonly in conjunction with nasal allergies. Ocular symptoms can significantly affect quality of life.

Clinical Manifestations

ALLERGIC CONJUNCTIVITIS. Allergic conjunctivitis is the most common hypersensitivity response of the eye, affecting approximately 25% of the general population and 30% of children with atopy. It is caused by direct exposure of the mucosal surfaces of the eye to environmental allergens. Patients complain of itchy eyes, rather than pain. Clinical signs include bilaterally injected conjunctivae with vascular congestion that may progress to **chemosis,** or conjunctival swelling, and a watery discharge. Allergic conjunctivitis occurs in a perennial, or more commonly, seasonal form. Seasonal allergic conjunctivitis is typically associated with allergic rhinitis and most commonly triggered by ragweed or grass pollens. Perennial allergic conjunctivitis is triggered by allergens such as animal danders or dust mites that are present throughout the year. Symptoms are usually not as severe as seen with seasonal allergic conjunctivitis.

VERNAL KERATOCONJUNCTIVITIS. Vernal keratoconjunctivitis is a severe bilateral chronic inflammatory process of the upper tarsal conjunctival surface that occurs in a limbal or palpebral form. It may threaten eyesight if it involves the cornea. Although vernal keratoconjunctivitis is not IgE mediated, it occurs most frequently in children with seasonal allergies, asthma, or atopic dermatitis, with boys being affected twice as often as girls. Vernal keratoconjunctivitis is more common in persons of Asian and African origin. It has a marked seasonal incidence, especially in the springtime. Symptoms include intense pruritus exacerbated by exposure to irritants, light, or perspiration. In addition, patients may complain of photophobia, foreign-body sensation, and lacrimation. Giant papillae occur predominantly on the upper tarsal plate and are typically described as **cobblestoning.** Other signs include a stringy discharge, transient yellow-white points in the limbus **(Trantas dots)** and conjunctiva **(Horner points)** or corneal "shield" ulcers, and **Dennie lines** (Dennie-Morgan folds), which are prominent symmetric skinfolds that extend in an arc from the inner canthus beneath and parallel to the lower lid margin.

ATOPIC KERATOCONJUNCTIVITIS. Atopic keratoconjunctivitis is a chronic inflammatory ocular disorder most commonly involving the lower tarsal conjunctiva. When it involves the cornea, it can lead to blindness. Almost all patients have atopic dermatitis, and a significant number have asthma. Atopic keratoconjunctivitis rarely presents before late adolescence. Symptoms include itching, burning, and tearing that

TABLE 140–1. Indications for Venom Immunotherapy (VIT) to Winged Hymenoptera

Symptoms	Age	Skin test/RAST	Venom Immunotherapy Indicated
Local or large local reaction	All	+ or −	No
Systemic reaction limited to the skin	≤16 yr	+ or −	No
	≥17 yr	+	Yes
		−	No
Systemic reaction beyond the skin	All	+	Yes
		−	No

RAST = radioallergosorbent test.

are much more severe than in allergic conjunctivitis and persist throughout the year. The bulbar conjunctiva is injected and chemotic. Eyelid eczema can extend to the periorbital skin and cheeks with erythema and thick, dry scales. Secondary staphylococcal blepharitis is common because of eyelid induration and maceration.

GIANT PAPILLARY CONJUNCTIVITIS. Giant papillary conjunctivitis has been linked to chronic exposure to foreign bodies, such as contact lenses, both hard and soft, ocular prostheses, and sutures. Symptoms and signs include itching, tearing, and excessive ocular discomfort with mucus production along with white or clear exudate on awakening, which may become thick and stringy. Trantas dots, limbal infiltration, bulbar conjunctival hyperemia, and edema may develop.

CONTACT ALLERGY. Contact allergy typically involves the eyelids but can also involve the conjunctivae. It is being recognized more frequently in association with increased exposure to topical medications, contact lens solutions, and preservatives.

Diagnosis. Nonallergic conjunctivitis can be viral, bacterial, or chlamydial in origin. It can be unilateral or bilateral with stinging or burning rather than itching and often with a foreign body sensation. Ocular discharge can be watery, mucoid, or purulent. Masqueraders of ocular allergy also include nasolacrimal duct obstruction, foreign body, blepharoconjunctivitis, dry eye, uveitis, and trauma.

Treatment. Primary treatment of ocular allergies includes avoidance of allergens, cold compresses, and lubrication. Secondary treatment regimens include the use of oral or topical antihistamines, topical decongestants, mast cell stabilizers, and anti-inflammatory agents (Table 141–1). Children often complain of stinging or burning with use of topical ophthalmic preparations and usually prefer oral antihistamines for allergic conjunctivitis. Using refrigerated medications may decrease some of the discomfort associated with their use. Topical decongestants act as vasoconstrictors, reducing erythema, vascular congestion, and eyelid edema, but do not diminish the allergic response. Adverse effects of topical vasoconstrictors include burning or stinging and rebound hyperemia or conjunctivitis medicamentosa with chronic use. Combined use of an antihistamine and a vasoconstrictive agent is more effective than use of either agent alone. Tertiary treatment of ocular allergy includes topical, or rarely oral, corticosteroids. Local administration of topical corticosteroids may be associated with increased intraocular pressure, viral infections, and cataract formation. Allergen immunotherapy can be very effective in seasonal and perennial allergic conjunctivitis, especially when associated with rhinitis. It can decrease the need for oral or topical medications to control allergy symptoms.

Abelson MB, Spitalny L: Combined analysis of two studies using the conjunctival allergen challenge model to evaluate olopatadine hydrochloride, a new ophthalmic antiallergic agent with dual activity. *Am J Ophthalmol* 1998;125:797–804.
Bielory L: Allergic and immunologic disorders of the eye: II. Ocular allergy. *J Allergy Clin Immunol* 2000;106:1019–32.
Irkec MT, Orhan M, Erdener U: Role of tear inflammatory mediators in contact lens-associated giant papillary conjunctivitis in soft contact lens wearers. *Ocul Immunol Inflamm* 1999;7:35–8.
Leibowitz HM: The red eye. *N Engl J Med* 2000;343:345–51.
New drugs for allergic conjunctivitis. *Med Lett Drugs Ther* 2000;42:39–40.
Verin P: Treating severe eye allergy. *Clin Exp Allergy* 1998;28 Suppl 6:44–48.

Chapter 142
Adverse Reactions to Foods
Hugh A. Sampson and Donald Y. M. Leung

Adverse reactions to foods consist of any untoward reaction after the ingestion of a food or food additive. These reactions are classically divided into **food intolerances,** which are adverse physiologic responses, or **food hypersensitivities,** which are allergies and adverse immunologic responses (Box 142–1). Like other atopic disorders, food allergies have increased over the past 3 decades, primarily in "Westernized" countries, and now affect an estimated 2% of the U.S. population. Up to 6% of infants and young children experience food allergic reactions in the first 3 yr of life; studies from a number of Westernized countries indicate that about 2.5% of infants develop cow's milk allergy, 1.5% develop egg allergy, and 0.6% develop peanut allergy in the first few years of life. Most infants and young children "outgrow" milk and egg allergy, with about one half outgrowing their allergy within 2–3 yr. In contrast, about 80% of those with peanut, nut, or seafood allergy will retain their allergy for life.

Etiology. Adverse food reactions may be the result of intolerances due to functional properties of foods or physiologic responses of the host or of hypersensitivities from adverse immunologic responses of the host (see Box 142–1). Although food represents the largest antigenic load confronting the body, the gut-associated lymphoid tissue (GALT) is able to readily discriminate between "harmless" foods and pathogenic organisms. Ingestion of food leads to **oral tolerance,** or the induction of T-cell anergy and T regulatory cells that enable the systemic immune system to "ignore" the roughly 2% of antigenic protein normally entering the systemic circulation at each meal. In young infants, functional barriers (e.g., stomach acidity, intestinal enzymes, glycocalyx) and immunologic barriers (e.g., secretory IgA) are immature and allow increased penetration of food antigens, and the GALT appears less capable of "tolerizing" compared with the mature system. Consequently, food hypersensitivity reactions most commonly develop during this susceptible age.

Pathogenesis. Food intolerances are the result of a variety of mechanisms, whereas food hypersensitivities are predominantly due to IgE-mediated and/or cell-mediated mechanisms. In susceptible individuals exposed to certain allergens, food-specific IgE antibodies are formed that bind to Fcε receptors on mast cells, basophils, macrophages, and dendritic cells. When food allergens penetrate mucosal barriers and reach cell-bound IgE antibodies, mediators are released that induce vasodilatation, smooth muscle contraction, and mucus secretion, which results in symptoms of immediate hypersensitivity. Activated mast cells and macrophages may release a number of cytokines that attract

TABLE 141–1. Topical Ophthalmic Medications for Allergic Conjunctivitis	
Medications	**Daily Dosing**
Antihistamines	
Levocabastine hydrochloride (Livostin) 0.05%	1 gtt bid-qid
Emedastine difumarate (Emadine) 0.05%	1 gtt qid
Azelastine hydrochloride (Optivar) 0.05%	1 gtt bid
Antihistamine-vasoconstrictor combinations	
Pheniramine maleate 0.3%/naphazoline hydrochloride 0.025% (Naphcon-A)	1–2 gtt qid
Mast cell stabilizers	
Cromolyn sodium (Opticrom) 4%	1–2 gtt q4–6hr
Lodoxamide tromethamine (Alomide) 0.1%	1–2 gtt qid
Nedocromil sodium (Alocril) 2%	1–2 gtt bid
Pemirolast potassium (Alamast) 0.1%	1–2 gtt qid
Antihistamine/mast cell stabilizers	
Olopatadine hydrochloride (Patanol) 0.1%	1 gtt bid (8 hr apart)
Ketotifen fumarate (Zaditor) 0.025%	1 gtt bid q8–12hr
Nonsteroidal anti-inflammatory drugs	
Ketorolac tromethamine (Acular, Acular Preservative-Free) 0.5%	1 gtt qid

BOX 142–1. Adverse Food Reactions

FOOD INTOLERANCE

Host Factors

Enzyme deficiencies—lactase (primary or secondary), fructase (maturational delay)
Gastrointestinal disorders—inflammatory bowel disease, irritable bowel syndrome
Idiosyncratic reactions—caffeine in soft drinks ("hyperactivity")
Psychologic—food phobias
Migraines (rare)

Food Factors

Infectious organisms—*Escherichia coli*, *Staphylococcus aureus*, *Clostridium*
Toxins—histamine (scombroid poisoning), saxitoxin (shellfish)
Pharmacologic agents—caffeine, theobromine (chocolate, tea), tryptamine (tomatoes), tyramine (cheese)
Contaminants—heavy metals, pesticides, antibiotics

FOOD HYPERSENSITIVITIES

IgE Mediated

Cutaneous—urticaria, angioedema, morbilliform rashes and flushing
Gastrointestinal—oral allergy syndrome, gastrointestinal anaphylaxis
Respiratory—acute rhinoconjunctivitis, bronchospasm (wheezing)
Generalized—anaphylactic shock

Mixed IgE and Cell Mediated

Cutaneous—atopic dermatitis
Gastrointestinal—allergic eosinophilic esophagitis and gastroenteritis
Respiratory—asthma

Cell Mediated

Cutaneous—contact dermatitis, dermatitis herpetiformis
Gastrointestinal—food protein–induced enterocolitis, proctocolitis, and enteropathy syndromes, celiac disease
Respiratory—food-induced pulmonary hemosiderosis (Heiner syndrome)

Unclassified

Cow's milk–induced anemia

TABLE 142–1. Major Food Allergens

Class 1		
Food	**Protein**	**Allergen Name**
Cow's milk	Casein	Bos d8
	β-Lactoglobulin	Bos d5
Egg	Ovomucoid	Gal d1
Peanut	Vicilin	Ara h1
	Conglutin	Ara h2
Fish	Paralbumin	Gad c1

Class 2		
Pollen	**Protein**	**Cross-Reacting Food**
Birch	Bet v1	Apple (Mal d1)
		Carrot (Dau c1)
		Potato (Sol t1)
		Cherry (Pru av1)
Ragweed		Watermelon
		Cantaloupe
		Honeydew

highly varied diet. Virtually all milk allergy develops by 12 mo of age and all egg allergy by 18 mo of age, and the median age of first peanut allergic reactions is 14 mo. Class 2 allergens are typically plant or fruit proteins that are partially homologous to pollen proteins (see Table 142–1). With the development of seasonal allergic rhinitis, from birch, grass, or ragweed pollens, ingestion of certain uncooked fruits or vegetables provoke the oral allergy syndrome. Intermittent ingestion of allergenic foods will lead to acute symptoms, whereas prolonged exposure may lead to chronic disorders such as atopic dermatitis and asthma. Cell-mediated sensitivity typically develops to class 1 allergens.

Clinical Manifestations. From a clinical and diagnostic standpoint, it is most useful to subdivide food hypersensitivity disorders by the target organ predominantly affected and immune mechanism (see Box 142–1).

GASTROINTESTINAL MANIFESTATIONS. Gastrointestinal food allergies are often the first form of allergy to affect infants and young children and typically present as irritability, vomiting or "spitting-up," diarrhea, and poor weight gain. Cell-mediated hypersensitivities predominate, making standard allergy tests such as prick skin tests and RAST tests of little diagnostic value.

Food protein–induced enterocolitis syndrome typically presents in the first several months of life with irritability, protracted vomiting, and diarrhea, not infrequently resulting in dehydration. Vomiting generally occurs 1–3 hr after feeding, and continued exposure may result in bloody diarrhea, anemia, abdominal distention, and failure to thrive. Symptoms are most commonly provoked by cow's milk or soy protein–based formulas but occasionally result from food proteins passed in maternal breast milk. A similar enterocolitis syndrome has been reported in older infants and children from egg, wheat, rice, oat, peanut, nuts, chicken, turkey, and fish sensitivity. Hypotension occurs in about 15% of cases after allergen ingestion.

Food protein–induced proctocolitis presents in the first few months of life as blood-streaked stools in otherwise healthy looking infants. About 60% of cases occur in breast-fed infants, with the remainder largely in infants fed cow's milk– or soy protein–based formula. Blood loss is typically modest but occasionally can produce anemia.

Food protein–induced enteropathy often presents in the first several months of life with diarrhea, not infrequently steatorrhea, and poor weight gain. Symptoms include protracted diarrhea, vomiting in up to two thirds of cases, failure to thrive, abdominal distention, early satiety, and malabsorption. Anemia,

and activate other cells, such as eosinophils and lymphocytes, leading to inflammation that is more prolonged. Symptoms elicited during acute IgE-mediated reactions can affect the skin (urticaria, angioedema, and flushing), gastrointestinal tract (oral pruritus and angioedema, nausea, abdominal pain, vomiting, and diarrhea), respiratory tract (nasal congestion, rhinorrhea, pruritus and sneezing, laryngeal edema, and dyspnea, shortness of breath and wheezing), and cardiovascular system (dysrhythmias, hypotension, and loss of consciousness). In the other major form of food hypersensitivities, lymphocytes, primarily food allergen–specific T cells, secrete excessive amounts of various cytokines that lead to a "delayed" inflammatory process affecting the skin (pruritus and erythematous rash), gastrointestinal tract (cachexia, early satiety, abdominal pain, vomiting, and diarrhea) or respiratory tract (food-induced pulmonary hemosiderosis). Mixed IgE and cellular responses to food allergens can also lead to chronic disorders such as atopic dermatitis, asthma, and allergic eosinophilic gastroenteritis.

Children developing IgE-mediated food allergies may be sensitized by food allergens penetrating the gastrointestinal barrier, **class 1 food allergens,** or by partially homologous allergens, such as plant pollens, penetrating the respiratory tract, **class 2 food allergens.** Any food may cause class 1 food allergies, but egg, milk, peanuts, nuts, fish, soy, and wheat account for about 90% of food allergy up to the teenage years. Many of the major allergenic proteins of these foods have been characterized (Table 142–1). Exposure and sensitization to these proteins often occur very early in life, because intact food proteins are passed to the infant through maternal breast milk and, after introduction of solid foods, many parents strive to provide their infant with a

edema, and hypoproteinemia occur occasionally. **Cow's milk sensitivity** is the most frequent cause of this syndrome in young infants, but it also has been associated with sensitivity to soy, egg, wheat, rice, chicken, and fish in older children. **Celiac disease** is the most severe form of enteropathy, characterized by a more extensive loss of absorptive villi and hyperplasia of the crypts leading to malabsorption, chronic diarrhea, steatorrhea, abdominal distention, flatulence, and weight loss or failure to thrive. Oral ulcers and other extraintestinal symptoms secondary to malabsorption are not uncommon. Genetically susceptible individuals (HLA-DQ2 or DQ8) develop a cell-mediated response to tissue transglutaminase (tTGase) deamidated gliadin found in wheat, oat, rye, and barley.

Allergic eosinophilic esophagitis may present from infancy through adolescence. In young children, it is primarily cell-mediated and presents as chronic gastroesophageal reflux (GER), intermittent emesis, food refusal, abdominal pain, dysphagia, irritability, sleep disturbance, and failure to respond to conventional reflux medications. A study of children younger than 1 yr of age presenting with GER found that 40% had cow's milk–induced reflux. **Allergic eosinophilic gastroenteritis** occurs at any age and presents as symptoms similar to esophagitis as well as prominent weight loss or failure to thrive, which are the hallmarks of this disorder. Up to 50% of patients are atopic, and food-induced IgE-mediated reactions have been implicated in a minority of patients. Generalized edema secondary to hypoalbuminemia may occur in some infants with marked protein-losing enteropathy.

Oral allergy syndrome is an IgE-mediated hypersensitivity that occurs in many older children with birch pollen and ragweed-induced allergic rhinitis. Symptoms are usually confined to the oropharynx and consist of the rapid onset of pruritus, tingling, and angioedema of the lips, tongue, palate, and throat, and occasionally a sensation of pruritus in the ears and/or tightness in the throat. Symptoms are generally short-lived and are due to local mast cell activation by fresh fruit and vegetable proteins that cross react with birch pollen (apple, carrot, potato, celery, hazel nuts, and kiwi) and ragweed pollen (banana and melons—watermelon, cantaloupe, etc.).

Gastrointestinal anaphylaxis generally presents as acute abdominal pain and vomiting that accompany other IgE-mediated allergic symptoms.

SKIN MANIFESTATIONS. Cutaneous food allergies are also common in infants and young children.

Atopic dermatitis is a form of eczema that generally begins in early infancy and is characterized by pruritus, chronically relapsing course, and association with asthma and allergic rhinitis (see Chapter 135). Although not often apparent by history, at least one third of children with moderate to severe atopic dermatitis have food allergies. The younger the child and the more severe the eczema, the more likely food allergy is playing a pathogenic role in the disorder.

Acute urticaria and angioedema are among the most common symptoms of food allergic reactions (see Chapter 136). Onset of symptoms may be very rapid, following within minutes of ingesting the responsible allergen. Symptoms are due to activation of IgE-bearing mast cells by circulating food allergens, which are absorbed and circulated rapidly throughout the body. Foods most commonly incriminated in children include egg, milk, peanuts, and nuts, although reactions to various seeds (e.g., sesame, poppy) and fruits (e.g., kiwi) are becoming more common. **Chronic urticaria and angioedema** are rarely due to food allergies.

RESPIRATORY MANIFESTATIONS. Respiratory food allergies are uncommon as isolated symptoms. Although many parents believe that nasal congestion in infants is often due to milk allergy, a number of studies showed this not to be the case. **Food-induced rhinoconjunctivitis** symptoms typically accompany allergic symptoms in other target organs, such as skin, and consist of typical allergic rhinitis symptoms (periocular pruritus and tearing, nasal congestion and pruritus, sneezing, and rhinorrhea). Wheezing occurs in about 25% of IgE-mediated food allergic reactions, but only 5–10% of asthmatic patients have food-induced respiratory symptoms.

Food allergic reactions are the single most common cause of anaphylaxis seen in hospital emergency departments. In addition to the rapid onset of cutaneous, respiratory, and gastrointestinal symptoms, patients may develop cardiovascular symptoms including hypotension, vascular collapse, and cardiac dysrhythmias, presumably caused by massive mast cell mediator release. **Food-associated exercise-induced anaphylaxis** is occurring more frequently among teenage athletes, especially females (see Chapter 137).

Diagnosis. A thorough medical history is necessary to differentiate whether a patient's symptomatology represents an adverse reaction (Box 142–2), if the adverse food reaction is an intolerance or hypersensitivity reaction, and if the latter, whether it is likely to be an IgE-mediated or a cell-mediated response. The following facts should be established: (1) the food suspected of provoking the reaction and the quantity ingested, (2) the time interval between ingestion and the development of symptoms, (3) the type of symptoms elicited by the ingestion, (4) whether ingesting the suspected food produced similar symptoms on other occasions, (5) whether other inciting factors, such as exercise, are necessary, and (6) the time interval from the last reaction to the food. Prick skin tests and radioallergosorbent tests are useful for demonstrating IgE sensitization. Many fruits and vegetables require testing with fresh produce because labile proteins are destroyed during commercial preparation. A negative skin test virtually excludes an IgE-mediated form of food allergy. Conversely, the majority of children with positive skin tests to a food will not react when the food is ingested, so more definitive tests, such as quantitative IgE levels or food elimination and challenge, are often necessary to establish a diagnosis of food allergy. Serum food-specific IgE levels ≥ 15 kU_a/L for milk, $\geq 7\ kU_a/L$ for egg, and $\geq 14\ kU_a/L$ for peanut are associated with a >95% likelihood of clinical reactivity to these foods. In the absence of a clear history of reactivity to a food

---

BOX 142–2. Differential Diagnosis of Adverse Food Reactions

GASTROINTESTINAL DISORDERS (WITH VOMITING AND/OR DIARRHEA)

Structural abnormalities (pyloric stenosis, Hirschsprung disease)
Enzyme deficiencies (primary or secondary)
　Disaccharidase deficiency—lactase, fructase, sucrase-isomaltase
　Galactosemia
Malignancy with obstruction
Other: pancreatic insufficiency (cystic fibrosis), peptic disease

CONTAMINANTS AND ADDITIVES

Flavorings and preservatives—rarely cause symptoms
　Sodium metabisulfite, monosodium glutamate, nitrites
Dyes and colorings—very rarely cause symptoms [urticaria, eczema]
　Tartrazine
Toxins
　Bacterial, fungal (aflatoxin), fish related (scombroid, ciguatera)
Infectious organisms
　Bacteria (*Salmonella, Escherichia coli, Shigella*)
　Virus (rotavirus, enterovirus)
　Parasites (*Giardia, Akis simplex* [in fish])
Accidental contaminants
　Heavy metals, pesticides
Pharmacologic agents
　Caffeine, glycosidal alkaloid solanine (potato spuds), histamine (fish), serotonin (banana, tomato), tryptamine (tomato), tyramine (cheese)

PSYCHOLOGIC REACTIONS

Food phobias

and evidence of food-specific IgE antibodies, definitive studies must be performed before recommending avoidance or the use of highly restrictive diets that may be nutritionally deficient, logistically impractical, and disruptive to the family and the source of future feeding disorders. IgE-mediated food allergic reactions are generally very food specific, so the use of broad exclusionary diets, such as avoidance of all legumes, cereal grains, and animal products, is not warranted. Unfortunately, there are no laboratory studies that help identify foods responsible for cell-mediated reactions. Consequently, elimination diets followed by food challenges are the only way to establish the diagnosis. Allergists experienced in dealing with food allergic reactions and able to treat anaphylaxis should perform **food challenges.** Before initiating a food challenge, the suspected food should be eliminated from the diet for 10–14 days for IgE-mediated food allergy and up to 8 wk for some cell-mediated disorders, such as allergic eosinophilic gastroenteritis. Many children with cell-mediated reactions to cow's milk will not tolerate hydrolysate formulas and must be placed on amino acid–derived products (e.g., ELECARE or Neocate). If symptoms remain unchanged and appropriate elimination diets have been utilized, it is unlikely that food allergy is responsible for the child's disorder.

Treatment. Appropriate identification and elimination of foods responsible for food hypersensitivity reactions are the only validated treatments for food allergies. Complete elimination of common foods (e.g., soy, egg, wheat, rice, chicken, fish, peanut, and nuts) is very difficult, owing to their widespread use in a variety of processed food. The Food Allergy and Anaphylaxis Network (www.foodallergy.org or 800-929-4040) provides excellent information to help parents deal with both the practi-cal and emotional issues surrounding these diets. Children with asthma and IgE-mediated food allergy should be given self-injectable epinephrine and a written emergency plan in case of accidental ingestion (see Chapter 137). Because many food allergies are outgrown, arrangements should be made to have children periodically re-evaluated by an allergist to determine whether they have lost their clinical reactivity. New forms of immunotherapy and use of anti-IgE therapy are under study and may provide definitive means of treating food allergies in future years.

Prevention. There is no consensus as to whether food allergies can be prevented. However, several authorities recommend delaying introduction of major food allergens to infants from atopic families. Recommendations include promotion of breast-feeding with maternal exclusion of peanut and nut products from the mother's diet and delay in introducing major allergenic foods: cow's milk until 1 yr of age; egg until 18–24 mo of age, and peanut, tree nuts, and seafood until 3 yr of age.

American Academy of Pediatrics, Committee on Nutrition: Hypoallergenic infant formulas. *Pediatrics* 2000;106:346–49.
Breiteneder H, Ebner C: Molecular and biochemical classification of plant-derived food allergens. *J Allergy Clin Immunol* 2000;106:27–36.
Sampson HA: Utility of food-specific IgE concentrations in predicting symptomatic food allergy. *J Allergy Clin Immunol* 2001;107:891–96.
Sampson HA, Sicherer SH, Birnbaum AH: AGA technical review on the evaluation of food allergy in gastrointestinal disorders. American Gastroenterological Association. *Gastroenterology* 2001;120:1026–40.
Sampson HA: Food allergy: I. Immunopathogenesis and clinical disorders. *J Allergy Clin Immunol* 1999;103:717–28.
Sampson HA: Food allergy: II. Diagnosis and management. *J Allergy Clin Immunol* 1999;103:981–89.
Sicherer SH: Diagnosis and management of childhood food allergy. *Curr Probl Pediatr* 2001;31:35–57.

Rheumatic Diseases of Childhood (Connective Tissue Diseases, Collagen Vascular Diseases)

PART XV

Chapter 143

Evaluation of Suspected Rheumatic Disease

Michael L. Miller

Rheumatic diseases result from abnormally regulated immune responses that lead to inflammation of target organs. Because many different organs may be affected, rheumatic diseases must be considered for a wide range of presenting complaints. Often, nonrheumatic diseases that can cause similar symptoms need to be excluded during evaluation.

Early diagnosis of rheumatic disease may not always be possible because diagnostic manifestations can take time to develop. Specific diagnostic criteria for rheumatic diseases may not be met for months or, rarely, even years. During that time the clinical evaluation may need to be repeated, and occasionally, a diagnosis will need to be reconsidered. For example, a child meeting diagnostic criteria for juvenile rheumatoid arthritis (JRA) may, after several years, develop anemia, diarrhea, and small bowel biopsy findings more consistent with inflammatory bowel disease. Some patients with JRA, particularly those presenting with high titers of antinuclear antibodies (ANAs), may develop systemic lupus erythematosus (SLE) years after initial presentation. A child with polyarticular arthritis who later develops weakness disproportionate to synovitis may be diagnosed with an inflammatory myositis, such as juvenile dermatomyositis.

Etiology and Pathogenesis. Rheumatic diseases are characterized by autoimmune effects that exaggerate the desired immune response. Normally, the immune system reacts to viruses, bacteria, and other non-self molecules but does not mount a reaction to molecules found in the host's own tissues. This **tolerance** to self is lost in rheumatic diseases. Two possible reasons, which are not mutually exclusive, for self-reactivity are (1) similarity between foreign and self molecules as recognized by immune cells, particularly T lymphocytes, and (2) viral infections with exaggerated immune responses that are otherwise suppressed. The relative contributions of these mechanisms to the pathogenesis of rheumatic diseases are still being investigated. Some genetic factors, such as specific HLA alleles, may influence susceptibility to developing disease, whereas others, such as those that influence levels of baseline immune activities, may affect disease severity.

A series of abnormal cellular and molecular events is present in many rheumatic diseases. T lymphocytes bearing T-cell receptors recognize viruses and other foreign antigens that are bound to surfaces of other cells. After the T-cell receptor binds to antigenic molecules resting in the groove of the HLA molecule, molecular signals are released that activate other cells, such as macrophages. Macrophages produce inflammatory cytokines, including tumor necrosis factor-α (TNFα), interleukin-1 (IL-1), and IL-6. These cytokines can cause tissue damage through direct effects and by attracting additional inflammatory cells to the affected site. Further damage is mediated by B lymphocytes, which are activated by helper T cells to produce excessive antibody, including autoantibodies that bind to self-antigens: The resulting complement fixation can lead to the tissue destruction that is seen with some rheumatic diseases. Normal cells in target organs can be destroyed through cytolysis that is mediated by complement, direct or indirect effects of TNFα, or effects of natural killer or cytolytic T lymphocytes.

In children with rheumatic diseases, products of the immune system may affect function of other organs. For example, IL-6 and other cytokines can bind to neuronal receptors in the central nervous system, causing fever. IL-6 can also interfere with osteoblastic activity, resulting in osteopenia, which is reflected by decreased serum osteocalcin levels. Molecules produced outside the immune system may, in turn, have an effect on immune responses. During a normal immune response, cytokines appear to induce neuroendocrine pathways to produce cortisol, which suppresses cellular and humoral activity. It is possible that defects in these pathways amplify autoimmune responses. The increased incidence of some rheumatic diseases in females may be attributable to the capability of female sex hormones to augment cellular immune responses.

Clinical Manifestations. The history can help distinguish rheumatic conditions from other diseases. For example, parents of children with school phobias are often dubious about the prospect of returning their children to school. In contrast, parents of children with rheumatic diseases, more upset with the school absences themselves, usually are anxious to see their children return to school.

Some symptoms and signs, although not specific, may suggest rheumatic diseases (Table 143–1). Morning stiffness may be reported by children with JRA or postinfectious arthritis. Facial rashes in children with joint complaints or weakness raise the possibility of lupus or dermatomyositis. Raynaud phenomenon can be a presenting complaint of children with scleroderma and overlapping rheumatic syndromes. A history of trauma with monoarticular arthritis near the site of trauma suggests nonrheumatic disease, such as a torn meniscus or osteochondritis. A history of travel, enteric illness in the family, or exposure to sick pets suggests reactive arthritis following an enteric infection. Tick exposure in a child with joint symptoms raises the possibility of Lyme arthritis. Weakness can be present in muscular dystrophies, postviral illnesses, and inflammatory myopathies, of which juvenile dermatomyositis is the most common. Fevers are commonly seen in children with rheumatic diseases; spiking fevers returning to baseline are seen in systemic JRA. However, fever is not specific for rheumatic diseases, and evaluation for infections or malignancies may be necessary. Gait problems are found in children with orthopedic problems, such as Legg-Calvé-Perthes disease, as well as JRA. The inability to walk raises the need for immediate attention to exclude conditions such as osteomyelitis or malignancy.

Physical Examination. The physical examination helps identify the organs involved. Because rheumatic diseases may take time

TABLE 143–1. Symptoms Suggestive of Rheumatic Diseases

Symptom	Rheumatic Diseases	Some Possible Nonrheumatic Diseases Causing Similar Symptoms
Fevers	Systemic juvenile rheumatoid arthritis	Malignancies, infections, inflammatory bowel disease
Arthralgia	Juvenile rheumatoid arthritis, systemic lupus erythematosus, juvenile dermatomyositis, scleroderma	Hypothyroidism, trauma, reactive arthritis, infections
Weakness	Juvenile dermatomyositis	Muscular dystrophies
Malar rash	Systemic lupus erythematosus	Photosensitive dermatitis
Chest pain	Juvenile rheumatoid arthritis, systemic lupus erythematosus (with associated pericarditis or costochondritis)	Costochondritis (isolated), rib fracture, spondylolysis, spondylolisthesis
Back pain	Juvenile rheumatoid arthritis, spondyloarthropathy	Vertebral microfracture, diskitis, intraspinal tumor

to evolve, repeated examinations are often important in detecting new manifestations. The general appearance may suggest certain diagnoses. A depressed or anxious affect may suggest psychiatric disease. Lack of normal movement on the examination table may be a result of muscle weakness, arthritis, central nervous system disease, or skeletal abnormality. Weight loss or decreased weight gain may reflect malnutrition from inflammatory bowel disease. Tachycardia is seen in the child with fevers of any cause or with carditis or pericarditis. **Nailfold capillaroscopy** can detect vasculopathy, reflecting vessel injury in dermatomyositis, scleroderma, and other rheumatic diseases (see Fig. 149–3).

Apparently isolated findings may be clues to target organ involvement in rheumatic diseases. For example, a pericardial friction rub with orthopnea can be seen in pericarditis from lupus or systemic JRA. Persisting oral mucosal lesions are found in lupus; other mucous membrane involvement, such as swollen tongue or lips, raises the possibility of nonrheumatic diseases, including Kawasaki disease, Stevens-Johnson syndrome, and scarlet fever. The eye can be a target in lupus, in which episcleritis may be seen, and in JRA, in which posterior synechiae are a later complication of uveitis. Although persisting joint complaints suggest JRA, other rheumatic diseases, including lupus and dermatomyositis, can also present with arthritis. All children with joint symptoms should be asked about muscle weakness, which is seen in dermatomyositis and mixed connective tissue disease.

The joint examination can detect arthritis, which can be infectious, rheumatic, or secondary to trauma. **Arthritis** is evident by either swelling of the joint or the combination of pain and limited motion. **Arthralgia,** or pain in a joint with full range of motion, can be seen in trauma, psychogenic arthralgia, or early rheumatic disease that cannot yet be specifically diagnosed. The neurologic examination can identify focal deficits resulting from intracranial or intraspinal lesions as well as muscle weakness, which is seen in many diseases including postviral syndromes, inflammatory myositis, other rheumatic diseases, and muscular dystrophies.

Erythema nodosum, a rash characterized by pretibial tender erythematous nodules found in the deep dermis and subcutaneous tissue (Fig. 143–1), is a hypersensitivity reaction resulting from certain infections, inflammatory diseases, or drugs. The finding of erythema nodosum should lead to consideration of possible underlying causes. Common infectious triggers include group A *Streptococcus* pharyngitis, tuberculosis, *Yersinia*, histoplasmosis, and coccidioidomycosis. Erythema nodosum is sometimes the first manifestation of inflammatory bowel disease, sarcoidosis, or spondyloarthropathy. The rash may also develop after exposure to sulfonamides, phenytoin, or oral contraceptive agents. Lesions may evolve from erythematous to bluish, may sometimes be flat, and in severe cases may be found along the entire length of the legs or even involve the arms. New crops

of nodules may develop over several weeks and are sometimes accompanied by fever. Although erythema nodosum is itself a self-limited condition that responds to treatment of the underlying etiology, it must be distinguished from cellulitis, insect bites, thrombophlebitis, and fungal skin infections. When necessary to alleviate pain, supportive treatment includes bed rest, elevation of the legs, and analgesic medication.

Laboratory Findings. The erythrocyte sedimentation rate (ESR) is useful to screen for infectious and rheumatic diseases. However, a normal value does not exclude rheumatic diseases. Although transient infections can increase the ESR, elevated values persisting for more than several weeks require explanation, and extensive evaluation may be necessary. Usually the symptoms, physical findings, or other laboratory abnormalities will guide the focus of further evaluation.

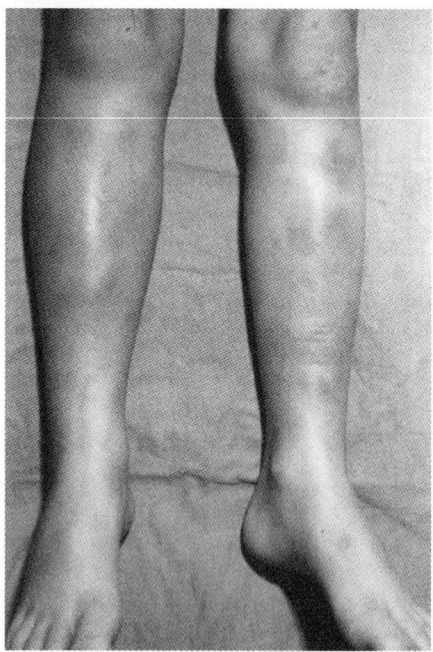

FIGURE 143–1. Erythematous nodules and plaques are present over both shins. The skin overlying the lesions is red, smooth, and shiny. The nodules are usually tender. Erythema nodosum is considered a hypersensitivity reaction and can be associated with a variety of diseases, including sarcoidosis, group A *Streptococcus* infection, tuberculosis, coccidioidomycosis, and ulcerative colitis. See also color plates. (Reprinted from the Clinical Slide Collection on the Rheumatic Diseases; Copyright 1991, 1995, 1997. Used by permission of the American College of Rheumatology.)

The **ANA test** is a screening test for specific antibodies against nuclear constituents, some of which have been characterized (Table 143–2). A positive ANA antibody titer (≥1:80) is a nonspecific reflection of increased lymphocyte activity. Positive ANA tests are found in children with rheumatic diseases and other diseases such as idiopathic thrombocytopenic purpura, Crohn disease, chronic autoimmune hepatitis, Graves disease, and, rarely, leukemia or lymphoma. Children with positive ANA tests who have nonrheumatic diseases may sometimes develop overlapping rheumatic syndromes, such as lupus. In such cases, other laboratory findings typically appear (e.g., antibodies to DNA in lupus patients). Some drugs, such as anticonvulsant medications (e.g., phenytoin, ethosuximide) and antiarrhythmic agents (e.g., procainamide) can cause positive ANA tests, usually without rheumatic disease. Occasionally, lupus develops in such patients. Malaria and some parasitic infections can also cause positive ANA tests.

Some children with positive ANA tests but no persisting symptoms have normal physical examinations and lack other remarkable laboratory findings. Such children rarely develop a rheumatic disease. Other children with positive ANA tests have been found to have arthralgia related to hyperextensible joints; the reason for the association is unknown. These children need to be distinguished from those who develop JRA or other rheumatic disease, which is best detected by periodic re-evaluation to detect changes in physical findings or laboratory abnormalities (e.g., anemia, thrombocytopenia, nephritis).

Other immunologic laboratory tests, although not diagnostic of rheumatic disease, are useful in characterizing the extent of immune activation and in monitoring response to therapy. For example, levels of total hemolytic complement (CH_{50}), C3, and C4 may be decreased in active lupus or vasculitis syndromes. Immune activation may be reflected by elevated levels of immune complexes, serum immunoglobulins, neopterin (a macrophage product), and von Willebrand factor antigen (a molecule found on the surface of vascular endothelium).

Other laboratory results may suggest a nonrheumatic diagnosis. A decrease in two of the three blood cell lines (e.g., leukopenia, anemia, or thrombocytopenia) in a child with limb pain may be seen in acute lymphocytic leukemia. Lactate dehydrogenase levels may be elevated in rheumatic diseases as a result of cell turnover; marked elevations raise the possibility of malignancy. Thyroid function studies can exclude hypothyroidism, which may cause musculoskeletal symptoms. Decreased albumin and serum protein may be seen in nephrosis or inflammatory bowel disease.

Imaging studies also contribute to the evaluation. Bone scans or MRI can detect early osteomyelitis or malignancies. MRI studies with gadolinium for joint evaluation and T2 weighted fat suppression for muscle evaluation can reveal tissue abnormalities seen in such diseases as JRA, dermatomyositis, and sarcoidosis. Findings from MRI studies may also suggest nonrheumatic diseases. Echocardiography can distinguish patients with rheumatic carditis from those with Kawasaki disease or pericarditis resulting from systemic lupus erythematosus or systemic JRA.

Azouz EM, Babyn PS, Mascia AT, et al: MRI of the abnormal pediatric hand and wrist with plain film correlation. *J Comput Assist Tomogr* 1998;22:252–61.
Cabral DA, Tucker LB: Malignancies in children who initially present with rheumatic complaints. *J Pediatr* 1999;134:53–7.
Citera G, Espada G, Maldonado Cocco JA: Sequential development of 2 connective tissue diseases in juvenile patients. *J Rheumatol* 1993;20:2149–52.
Deane PM, Liard G, Siegel DM, et al: The outcome of children referred to a pediatric rheumatology clinic with a positive antinuclear antibody test but without an autoimmune disease. *Pediatrics* 1995;95:892–5.
Malleson PN, Sailer M, Mackinnon MJ: Usefulness of antinuclear antibody testing to screen for rheumatic diseases. *Arch Dis Child* 1997;77:299–304.
ter Meulen DC, Majd M: Bone scintigraphy in the evaluation of children with obscure skeletal pain. *Pediatrics* 1987;79:587–92.
Murray K, Thompson SD, Glass DN: Pathogenesis of juvenile chronic arthritis: Genetic and environmental factors. *Arch Dis Child* 1997;77:530–4.
Passo MH, Fitzgerald JF, Brandt KD: Arthritis associated with inflammatory bowel disease in children. Relationship of joint disease to activity and severity of bowel lesion. *Dig Dis Sci* 1986;31:492–7.
Ramsey SE, Cairns RA, Cabral DA, et al: Knee magnetic resonance imaging in childhood chronic monarthritis. *J Rheumatol* 1999;26:2238–43.
Reed A, Haugen M, Pachman LM, et al: Abnormalities in serum osteocalcin values in children with chronic rheumatic diseases. *J Pediatr* 1990;116:574–80.
Spencer-Green G, Schlesinger M, Bove KE, et al: Nailfold capillary abnormalities in childhood rheumatic diseases. *J Pediatr* 1983;102:341–6.
Wallendal M, Stork L, Hollister JR: The discriminating value of serum lactate dehydrogenase levels in children with malignant neoplasms presenting as joint pain. *Arch Pediatr Adolesc Med* 1996;150:70–3.
Zimmerman SA, Ware RE: Clinical significance of the antinuclear antibody test in selected children with idiopathic thrombocytopenic purpura. *J Pediatr Hematol Oncol* 1997;19:297–303.

Chapter 144
Treatment of Rheumatic Diseases *Daniel J. Lovell,*
Michael L. Miller, and James T. Cassidy

Treatment of children with rheumatic diseases is complex and challenging. The efforts of a team of health care professionals need to be melded into a coordinated system of management that is individualized to meet the needs of each patient and that is sensitive to the capabilities and psychosocial resources of the family. In addition, courses of the rheumatic diseases are not static. For each child, the disease manifestations can vary in severity over time and treatment needs to be adjusted accordingly. The therapeutic program must provide appropriate therapy for currently symptomatic problems, such as arthritis, as well as include appropriate screening methods for often clinically silent problems such as uveitis in patients with juvenile rheumatoid arthritis (JRA) and early nephritis in patients with systemic lupus erythematosus (SLE). The treatment regimen should not focus only on the child with the rheumatic disease. When rheumatic disease occurs in a child, all family members are affected. Indeed, studies have indicated that siblings of a child with a rheumatic disease are often more adversely affected psychosocially than the patient. Furthermore, family dynamics have a significant impact on treatment and outcome. Several studies have documented that the emotional status of the parents at the time of diagnosis of rheumatic disease in their child is one of the strongest predictors of outcome 5–10 yr later. Despite this complex and

TABLE 143–2. Specific Antinuclear Antibodies and Associated Diseases

Antigen	Disease
Histone	Drug-induced lupus
Ribonucleoprotein	Mixed connective tissue disease
Pm-Scl	Scleromatomyositis
Scl	Scleroderma
Sm	Systemic lupus erythematosus
Ro/SSA	Sjögren syndrome, congenital heart block, annular erythema
La/SSB	Sjögren syndrome

The ANA test is a screening test; it does not determine which of various known and unknown nuclear antigens the antinuclear antibody is specific for. Nonspecific elevated ANAs may be detected in healthy children (usually at low titer) and in those with various rheumatic and nonrheumatic diseases. The above specific ANAs are typically found with the corresponding diseases; however, they may sometimes be found in patients without manifestations suggestive of (or diagnostic for) these conditions.

ever-changing therapeutic milieu, current approaches to management supervised by a multidisciplinary team (Table 144–1) experienced in the care of children with rheumatic diseases usually result in acceptable clinical outcomes.

The childhood rheumatic diseases are neither benign nor short-lived in the majority of patients. Optimal treatment for these children requires the coordinated efforts of various health care professionals expert in this highly specialized area. The treatment program includes physical and psychosocial interventions, as well as medications, and requires tailoring to the needs and severity of each particular child's illness that will vary over time. Current therapies are not curative, as evidenced by the chronicity of these diseases.

Pediatric Rheumatology Teams and Primary Care Physicians. The goals for treatment are to maximize the daily functional activities of affected children, relieve discomfort, prevent or reduce organ damage, and avoid or minimize drug toxicity. Although medical therapy is important, nondrug therapy assumes a large role in the treatment of rheumatic diseases. The role of the physician responsible for treating a child with a rheumatic disease includes, in addition to prescribing and monitoring medications, coordinating the efforts of the other team members and educating the child and family about treatments and the nature and expected course of the disease. A key predictor of long-term outcome is early referral to a rheumatology team experienced in the care of children with rheumatic diseases. For example, significant differences in outcome in patients with JRA even 10 yr after disease onset were evident in those patients referred to a pediatric rheumatology center within 6 mo after disease onset compared with those with referral more than 6 mo after disease onset.

The pediatric rheumatology team offers coordinated services for these children and their families. By working closely with the team, the primary care physician helps monitor compliance with treatment plans, check for adverse effects of the medical therapy, evaluate symptoms of intercurrent illnesses, and exclude disease exacerbation or concomitant infections. Communicating with subspecialists and teams at tertiary care centers allows intervention when poor compliance occurs and symptoms flare.

Each member of the pediatric rheumatology team contributes individually and cooperatively to the child's care (Table 144–2). The pediatric rheumatologist establishes the diagnosis, assesses response to treatment, and monitors for changes in disease manifestations. With assistance from other team members, this leader of the team also monitors the child's psychosocial status, including such areas as pain, emotional and behavioral responses to disease, change in roles at home and school, and family response to the child's illness. The nurse provides education about specific chronic illnesses and correct administration of medication. Occupational and physical therapists assess limitations in joint movement and physical function and provide plans for long-term rehabilitation programs. Physical and occupational therapists prescribe and monitor exercise and splinting programs that families perform at home with the child

TABLE 144–1. Multidisciplinary Team for Care of Children with Rheumatic Diseases

Core Team	Consultant Team
Parents and child	Orthopedic surgeon
Pediatric rheumatologist	Psychologist/psychiatrist
Pediatrician or family physician	Dentist
Nurse	School nurse
Social worker	
Physical therapist	
Occupational therapist	
Dietitian	
Ophthalmologist	

TABLE 144–2. Cornerstones of Treatment of Children with Rheumatic Diseases

Accurate diagnosis and education of family	Pediatric rheumatologist Pediatrician Nurse Social Worker
Medications	Nonsteroidal anti-inflammatory drugs (NSAIDs) Methotrexate Hydroxychloroquine Sulfasalazine Intravenous immunoglobulin (IVIG) Cyclophosphamide Cyclosporine Corticosteroids (oral, intravenous, pulse, ophthalmic, intra-articular)
Physical medicine and rehabilitation	Physical therapy Occupational therapy Splints/reconstructive surgery
Physical and psychosocial growth and development	Nutrition School integration Peer group relationships Individual and/or family counseling
Coordination of care	Incorporation of patient/family as critical and active members of team Pediatrician Involvement of school and community resources Nurse, social worker, pediatric rheumatologist

to improve or maintain joint motion in children with arthritis, as well as in patients with myositis to avoid muscle contractures and improve muscle strength. Splints are used to lessen unnecessary mechanical stress on joints that is often associated with routine daily tasks. Splints may also improve muscle or joint contractures and avoid joint deformities, such as subluxation of the wrist. Ophthalmologists should examine children with JRA on a regular basis to screen for uveitis (every 3–12 mo, depending on the type of JRA) and to assess for ocular toxicity from certain medications (every 6–12 mo) such as hydroxychloroquine or glucocorticoids. Social workers are invaluable resources to families by helping them confront the significant social and emotional stresses imposed by the illness, deal with the financial maze of insurance coverage and national and state programs, and identify community resources needed to provide support. Children with rheumatic diseases are often undernourished because of disease- or medication-related anorexia, or they are obese or overnourished as a result of glucocorticoid therapy. Early and ongoing involvement of a nutritionist can significantly improve the health of these patients.

Medications. Medications used for treatment of childhood rheumatic diseases (see Table 144–2) have various mechanisms of action, which is unknown for some, but all share the ability to suppress inflammation. Key to satisfactory short- and long-term outcomes in these children is early induction of a significant and sustained suppression of this inflammation.

NONSTEROIDAL ANTI-INFLAMMATORY DRUGS (NSAIDs). A large number of NSAIDs are approved by the Food and Drug Administration (FDA) for use in adults with rheumatoid arthritis, but a much smaller number are approved for use in children with JRA. NSAIDs can be prescribed to decrease acute and chronic inflammation associated with arthritis, pleuritis, pericarditis, uveitis, and some forms of vasculitis. Lower doses, typically those approved for over-the-counter use, or intermittent dosing can result in analgesia but rarely significant anti-inflammatory effect. To reduce inflammation requires regular administration of adequate doses, on a weight (mg/kg) or body surface area (mg/m^2) basis and for longer periods than for analgesia alone. For example, the mean time to achieve an anti-inflammatory effect in the arthritis associated with JRA was

30 days of consistent administration. NSAIDs work primarily by inhibiting the enzyme **cyclooxygenase (COX),** which is critical in the production of **prostaglandins,** a family of substances that have many physiologic effects, including that of promoting inflammation. Two types of COX receptors have been demonstrated, and several NSAIDs have been approved for use in adults with rheumatoid arthritis that selectively inhibit those receptors responsible for promoting inflammation, which are **selective COX-2 inhibitors.** These selective COX-2 inhibitors have been shown in adults to have similar anti-inflammatory effects with fewer side effects than traditional NSAIDs. Clinical studies of the selective COX-2 inhibitors are in progress in children with JRA.

The most frequent adverse effects with NSAIDs in children are nausea, decreased appetite, and abdominal pain. Gastritis or gastric or duodenal ulceration occurs less frequently in children than in adults. In addition, each of the following side effects occurs in 5% or less of children on long-term NSAID therapy: central nervous system (CNS) symptoms (e.g., mood change, difficulty concentrating that can simulate attention deficit disorder [ADD], sleepiness, irritability, headache, tinnitus), alopecia, anemia, elevated liver enzymes, proteinuria, and hematuria. These NSAID-associated side effects reverse quickly once the medication is stopped. Several NSAID-specific adverse reactions may also occur. Ibuprofen can induce aseptic meningitis in some patients with SLE and rarely in patients with JRA. Naproxen is far more likely in children than other NSAIDs to cause a unique skin reaction called **pseudoporphyria,** which is characterized by small hypopigmented flat scars occurring in areas of even minor skin trauma (skin fragility), such as fingernail scratches, or after small spontaneous blister lesions. Naproxen-induced pseudoporphyria is more likely to occur in fair-skinned individuals and in sun-exposed areas. Confirmation of this skin toxicity should prompt immediate discontinuation of naproxen, because the scars can persist for several years. NSAIDs should be used cautiously in patients with dermatomyositis or systemic vasculitis because there is an increased frequency of gastrointestinal ulceration in these disorders.

The response to NSAIDs varies greatly among individual patients, but overall, approximately 40–60% of children with JRA experience significant improvement in their arthritis. Patients often must try several different NSAIDs before finding the one that demonstrates the most clinical benefit. NSAIDs with longer half-lives or sustained-release formulations have been developed to allow for once- or twice-daily dosing. For patients with JRA or milder cases of SLE, NSAIDs are often a cornerstone of the treatment program. For approximately 20–40% of patients with JRA, NSAIDs are the only drug therapy required to control the arthritis.

METHOTREXATE. Methotrexate has been used and studied in almost all of the rheumatic diseases and in many nonrheumatic conditions, including asthma, inflammatory bowel disease, cystic fibrosis, uveitis, and diabetes. It has a central role in the treatment of arthritis and is used in approximately 60% of patients with polyarticular JRA. Methotrexate given orally in a dose of 10 mg/m^2 once weekly was shown to be significantly better than placebo in a randomized, placebo-controlled trial (63% of methotrexate and 36% of placebo patients responded, p < .001). In a smaller, uncontrolled study in patients with JRA who failed to respond to the 10 mg/m^2/wk dose, methotrexate given intramuscularly in higher doses of 23–29 mg/m^2/wk resulted in prolonged clinical improvement in 70% of the patients. Patients with JRA who demonstrate a clinical response in articular inflammation with methotrexate also have improvement in radiologic evaluation of joint damage, growth rate, and functional ability in daily tasks. Subcutaneous administration of methotrexate has been demonstrated to have similar absorption and pharmacokinetic properties as intramuscular injection, and is much less painful for the children. Methotrexate is commonly

used in treatment of juvenile dermatomyositis that has shown no or inadequate response to glucocorticoids. About 70% of patients with dermatomyositis treated with methotrexate demonstrate improvement in their myositis. It has also been successfully used in a dosage of 10–20 mg/m^2/wk in patients with SLE to treat arthritis, serositis, and, in some cases, nephritis.

Studies in adults have indicated that the mechanism of action of methotrexate, which is an analog of folic acid, in arthritis is not primarily suppression of either folic acid metabolism or bone marrow activity. Methotrexate inhibits dihydrofolate reductase, which is important in purine synthesis, resulting in suppression of inflammation. Methotrexate is well tolerated by children. Because of the lower dose and alternative mechanisms of action, toxicity from methotrexate is much milder and qualitatively different from that observed when methotrexate is used to treat neoplastic diseases. In eight published studies that included 288 patients with JRA on methotrexate therapy, 13% of patients had gastrointestinal toxicity, 3% stomatitis, 15% elevated liver enzymes, 1–2% headache, and <1% leukopenia, interstitial pneumonitis, rash, or alopecia.

Hepatotoxicity observed among adults with rheumatoid arthritis treated with methotrexate has raised concern about similar problems occurring in children. In 46 liver biopsies performed in patients with JRA undergoing long-term methotrexate treatment, 95% of specimens were normal, 5% showed mild fibrosis, but none demonstrated even moderate liver damage. Lymphoproliferative disorders have also been reported in adults, usually after primary Epstein-Barr virus infection, and may not be directly related to the drug per se. However, given the large number of adults on methotrexate, the relative risk of lymphoproliferative disease remains low, at approximately 1.0–1.5%. Thus, methotrexate has become established as one of the cornerstone medications in pediatric rheumatology because of its potential to induce significant improvement in chronic inflammation and to maintain that improvement for long periods because of low toxicity and high patient acceptance.

GLUCOCORTICOIDS. Glucocorticoids are given by various routes for rheumatic diseases, including oral, intravenous, ocular, and intra-articular administration. Oral glucocorticoids are a cornerstone of treatment for moderate to severe SLE, dermatomyositis, and most forms of vasculitis. However, long-term use always leads to adverse effects. Steroid therapy in these chronic diseases must be carefully supervised; a responsible plan requires steroid tapering to acceptable doses for long-term use or the introduction of other anti-inflammatory medications to serve as steroid-sparing agents. Intravenous steroid administration has been used as an alternative to oral administration to treat more severe, acute manifestations of systemic connective tissue diseases such as SLE, dermatomyositis, and vasculitis. The intravenous route allows for much higher therapeutic doses to obtain an immediate, profound anti-inflammatory effect. Methylprednisolone, 10–30 mg/kg/dose up to a maximum of 1 g, has been the intravenous drug of choice. Although generally associated with fewer adverse effects than oral steroids, intravenous administration is not without significant and occasionally life-threatening toxicities, such as cardiac arrhythmias, acute hypertension, hypotension, and shock.

Ocular steroids are prescribed under the supervision of an ophthalmologist either as drops or injections into the soft tissue surrounding the globe (sub-Tenon injection) for the uveitis associated with JRA. Long-term ocular steroid use can lead to cataract formation and glaucoma. However, current ophthalmic management has significantly decreased the frequency of blindness as a complication of JRA-associated uveitis.

Intra-articular steroids are prescribed with increasing frequency for children with JRA in whom one or several joints have not responded to standard parenteral drug therapy or as the initial therapy in patients with arthritis involving only one or two joints. Almost all patients have significant improvement in both symptoms and physical findings within 2–3 days, which persists for at least 6 mo in 60% and for at least 12 mo in 45%. Intraarticular administration may result in subcutaneous atrophy and hypopigmentation of the skin in the area surrounding the injection site, as well as subcutaneous calcifications along the needle tract. These complications are rarely clinically significant.

ETANERCEPT. Etanercept is a genetically engineered fusion protein consisting of two identical chains of the recombinant extracellular tumor necrosis factor (TNF) receptor monomer fused with the Fc domain of human IgG1. Etanercept binds both TNFα and lymphotoxin-α (formerly called TNFβ) and inhibits their activity. A randomized, double-blind, placebo-controlled trial of etanercept (0.4 mg/kg subcutaneously, twice weekly) in children with active polyarticular JRA who had failed methotrexate treatment reported that 74% demonstrated significant clinical improvement after 3 mo of therapy. The children who responded to etanercept were then randomized in a double-blind fashion to either continue treatment with etanercept or begin placebo injections. A significant difference in the frequency of patients who experienced flares (28% versus 81%, p = .003) and the time to demonstrate flare (median of 28 versus >116 days, p > .001) provided evidence in favor of continued treatment with etanercept. The overall frequency and type of adverse events documented in this trial were similar for etanercept and placebo except for injection site reactions and frequency of upper respiratory tract infections, which were both significantly increased among the etanercept-treated subjects. Based on this study, the FDA approved etanercept for the treatment of children with moderate to severe active polyarticular course JRA who have had an inadequate response to one or more second line agents. Etanercept is perhaps helpful in the control of JRA-associated uveitis that is inadequately unresponsive to standard steroid therapy. The role of TNF blockade in the treatment of a variety of rheumatic diseases in both children and adults is still evolving and requires additional longitudinal experience to establish long-term effectiveness and safety. Etanercept is only one of several biologic agents developed to inhibit TNF, but currently it is the only one approved for use in children. TNF is known to have a variety of beneficial functions, and the safety of long-term suppression of TNF function is unknown. TNF blockade is associated with an increased frequency of systemic infections and should not be started in subjects with history of chronic or frequent recurrent infections. Tuberculosis should always be excluded before beginning treatment. TNF blockade has also been shown to be efficacious for treatment of Crohn disease, psoriasis, and psoriatic arthritis, and is being evaluated for treatment of Wegener granulomatosus, spondyloarthropathy, juvenile dermatomyositis, and idiopathic inflammatory myositis in adults.

OTHER DRUGS. Various other medications are used in the treatment of the rheumatic diseases in selected children. **Hydroxychloroquine** sulfate is an antimalarial drug that has an important role in the treatment of SLE and possibly dermatomyositis. Blinded withdrawal of hydroxychloroquine in patients with SLE resulted in a significantly higher frequency of disease worsening compared with placebo. It is especially helpful in the treatment of the cutaneous aspects of SLE and dermatomyositis. It is used infrequently to treat JRA because a prospective trial in patients with JRA failed to demonstrate increased efficacy of hydroxychloroquine compared with placebo. Hydroxychloroquine is given in a dose of 3–6 mg/kg/24 hr; a 3–6 mo trial is necessary to assess therapeutic response. Potential adverse effects include bone marrow suppression, CNS stimulation, gastric irritation, myasthenia-like weakness, and skin rash. The most significant potential side effect is retinal toxicity, which occurs very rarely but may result in blindness or loss of central vision. Complete ophthalmologic examinations including peripheral vision and color fields at baseline every 4–6 mo are mandatory during hydroxy-

chloroquine treatment. The frequency of retinal toxicity is rare (approximately 1/5,000 patients).

Sulfasalazine has been used for many years in the treatment of inflammatory bowel disease. In a randomized, double-blinded, placebo-controlled study of children with JRA, sulfasalazine 50 mg/kg/24 hr (maximum 2,000 mg/24 hr) demonstrated significantly greater improvements in joint inflammation, global assessments, and laboratory parameters when compared with placebo. However, more than 30% of the sulfasalazine-treated patients withdrew from the study because of adverse effects, primarily gastrointestinal irritation and skin rashes. Although none of the adverse effects in this trial was serious, sulfasalazine has been associated with severe systemic hypersensitivity reactions, especially development of the Stevens-Johnson syndrome. These reactions are much more common in patients with active systemic JRA treated with sulfasalazine. The proper role for sulfasalazine in treatment of children with JRA is still evolving. In most centers it is used in polyarticular and pauciarticular JRA and spondyloarthropathy.

Intravenous immunoglobulin (IVIG) is efficacious in various clinical conditions. IVIG has been proven to significantly improve the short- and long-term natural history of Kawasaki disease. Open studies have supported benefit for SLE-associated thrombocytopenia, systemic and polyarticular JRA, and dermatomyositis. A placebo-controlled crossover study demonstrated significant short-term benefit of IVIG in adults with active myositis, although the effect was short-lived after cessation of the therapy. Doses of IVIG generally used in these investigations have been large, 1–2 g/kg/dose, and must be given on a regular basis, usually monthly, to maintain benefit. In addition to being expensive and periodically in short supply, IVIG has been associated with severe systemic allergic reactions and postinfusion aseptic meningitis. IVIG seems to hold promise as a treatment for dermatomyositis, although no controlled trials have involved children.

Cyclophosphamide has been evaluated in controlled trials in both SLE and Wegener granulomatosis. Pulse intravenous cyclophosphamide (500–1,000 mg/m^2) given monthly for 6 mo, then every 3 mo for 12 mo, has been shown to reduce the frequency of renal failure in patients with SLE with diffuse proliferative glomerulonephritis. Open trials also suggest efficacy in severe CNS lupus. Oral cyclophosphamide (2 mg/kg/24 hr) is effective in the treatment of severe Wegener granulomatosis. Cyclophosphamide, an alkylating agent, requires metabolic conversion in the liver to its active metabolites, which alkylate the guanine in DNA, leading to the observed immunosuppression by the inhibition of the S2 phase of mitosis. Decreases in the numbers of T and B lymphocytes result in decreased humoral and cellular immune responses. Cyclophosphamide is a potent cytotoxic drug that is, however, associated with significant short- and long-term toxicities. Potential short-term adverse events include alopecia, nausea, vomiting, anorexia, oral and gastrointestinal tract ulcerations, cystitis, and bone marrow suppression. Long-term complications include an increased risk for sterility and cancer, especially leukemias, lymphomas, and bladder cancer. In adult women with SLE treated with intravenous cyclophosphamide, the overall frequency of permanent sterility has been reported to be 30–40%.

Cyclosporine has been introduced in the treatment of dermatomyositis and active systemic JRA based on uncontrolled clinical studies. Several drugs commonly used in the past are very seldom used currently, including salicylates, gold compounds, azathioprine, and D-penicillamine.

Future Treatments. Rheumatologists have commonly combined several drugs in the treatment of rheumatic diseases to achieve better disease control, often to permit the use of lower dose of steroids. However, only in the last few years have prospective studies been performed to test the efficacy of various combination drug therapies. In adults with rheumatoid arthritis, a combination of methotrexate, hydroxychloroquine, and sulfasalazine has been well tolerated. The combination of these three drugs was more efficacious than any of the drugs taken singly, or any combination of two of the three drugs. In an open study of children with severe systemic JRA, a combination of intravenous methylprednisolone, intravenous cyclophosphamide, and oral methotrexate demonstrated excellent short-term safety and clinical effect. It is anticipated that the development of standardized, sensitive outcome measures and large international consortiums of pediatric rheumatologists will allow various combination therapies to be critically evaluated in clinical trials in children with JRA and other rheumatic diseases.

In addition to inhibitors of TNF, a wide variety of other biologic agents are being studied in adults and many more are in development to modulate individual cell populations or molecular species involved in inflammatory processes. Monoclonal antibodies are being tested that can suppress specific T-cell subpopulations, bind particular cytokines or cytokine receptors, or inhibit anti–double-stranded DNA autoantibodies. These monoclonal antibodies are being widely tested in adults with rheumatic diseases, primarily rheumatoid arthritis and SLE. The potential for these therapies in children with rheumatic diseases is great but largely untested at this time.

Boumpas DT, Austin HA 3rd, Fessler BJ, et al: Systemic lupus erythematosus: Renal, neuropsychiatric, cardiovascular, pulmonary and hematologic disease. *Ann Intern Med* 1995;122:940–50.

Burgos-Vargas R, Vazquez-Mellado J, Pacheco-Tena C, et al: A 26 week randomised, double blind, placebo controlled exploratory study of sulfasalazine in juvenile onset spondyloarthropathies. *Ann Rheum Dis* 2002;61:941–2.

Frank RG, Hagglund KJ, Schopp LH, et al: Disease and family contributors to adaptation in juvenile rheumatoid arthritis and juvenile diabetes. *Arthritis Care Res* 1998;11:166–76.

Giannini EH, Brewer EF, Kuzmina N, et al: Methotrexate in resistant juvenile rheumatoid arthritis. Results of U.S.-U.S.S.R. double-blind, placebo-controlled trial. The Pediatric Rheumatology Collaborative Study Group and the Cooperative Children's Study Group. *N Engl J Med* 1992;326:1043–9.

Giannini EH, Cawkwell GD: Drug treatment in children with juvenile rheumatoid arthritis past, present, and future. *Pediatr Clin North Am* 1995;42:1099–125.

Ilowite NT: Current treatment of juvenile rheumatoid arthritis. *Pediatrics* 2002;109:109–15.

Laxer RM, Gazarian M: Pharmacology and drug therapy. In Cassidy JT, Petty RE (editors): *Textbook of Pediatric Rheumatology*, 4th ed. Philadelphia, WB Saunders, 2001.

Lehman TJ: A practical guide to systemic lupus erythematosus. *Pediatr Clin North Am* 1995;42:1223–38.

Lovell DJ: Juvenile rheumatoid arthritis and juvenile spondyloarthropathy. In Klippel JH (editor): *Primer on the Rheumatic Diseases*, 12th ed. Atlanta, Arthritis Foundation, 2001.

Lovell DJ, Giannini EH, Reiff A, et al: Etanercept in children with polyarticular juvenile rheumatoid arthritis. *N Engl J Med* 2000;342:763–9.

van Rossum MA, Fiselier TJ, Franssen MJ, et al: Sulfasalazine in the treatment of juvenile chronic arthritis: A randomized, double-blind, placebo-controlled, multicenter study. *Arthritis Rheum* 1998;41:808–16.

Wallace CA: The use of methotrexate in childhood rheumatic diseases. *Arthritis Rheum* 1998;41:381–91.

White PH, Shear ES: Transition/job readiness for adolescents with juvenile arthritis and other chronic illness. *J Rheumatol* 1992;19:23–7.

Chapter 145
Juvenile Rheumatoid Arthritis Michael L. Miller
and James T. Cassidy

Juvenile rheumatoid arthritis (JRA) is one of the most common rheumatic diseases of children and a major cause of chronic disability. It is characterized by an idiopathic synovitis of the peripheral joints, associated with soft tissue swelling and effusion. In the classification criteria of the American College of Rheumatology, JRA is regarded not as a single disease but as a category of diseases with three principal types of onset: (1) oligoarthritis, or pauciarticular disease, (2) polyarthritis, and (3) systemic-onset disease (Box 145–1). Nine distinct course subtypes have also been identified. The European League Against Rheumatism (EULAR) has also published classification criteria for a similar constellation of diseases, identified as juvenile chronic arthritis. New international criteria for the classification of seven specific types of onset of peripheral arthritis in children are being developed.

Etiology. The etiology of the diseases classified under JRA is unknown. At least two events are considered necessary: immunogenetic susceptibility and an external, presumably environmental, trigger. Specific HLA subtypes have been identified as rendering children at risk, which may confer varying degrees of susceptibility, or indeed protection, depending on the age of the child. Possible external triggers for JRA include certain viruses (e.g., parvovirus B19, rubella, Epstein-Barr virus), host hyperreactivity to specific self-antigens (type II collagen), and enhanced T-cell reactivity to bacterial or mycobacterial heat shock proteins.

Epidemiology. Although difficult to determine with precision, the incidence of JRA is approximately 13.9/100,000 children/yr among children 15 yr or younger, with an overall prevalence of approximately 113/100,000 children. A report from Australia, however, provided a much higher estimate of prevalence based on examination of school children by a pediatric rheumatologist. This study suggested a need for increased identification and referral of children with arthritis to pediatric rheumatology treatment centers. Different racial and ethnic groups appear to have varying frequencies of the subtypes of JRA. One study reported that black American children with JRA were older at presentation and less likely to have elevated antinuclear antibody (ANA) titers or uveitis.

Pathogenesis. The synovitis of JRA is characterized by villous hypertrophy and hyperplasia with hyperemia and edema of the subsynovial tissues. Vascular endothelial hyperplasia is prominent and characterized by infiltration of mononuclear and plasma cells (Fig. 145–1). Pannus formation occurs in advanced or uncontrolled disease and results in progressive erosion of articular cartilage and contiguous bone (Fig. 145–2).

Although the etiology is unknown, studies suggest exaggerated immune reactivity of several types of cells in predisposed children, suspected but not proved to be in response to exposure to certain viruses. Thus, the onset of JRA may be triggered by a preceding infection. Although trauma may be cited by the

---

BOX 145–1. Criteria for the Classification of Juvenile Rheumatoid Arthritis

Age at onset <16 yr
Arthritis (swelling or effusion, or presence of two or more of the following signs: limitation of range of motion, tenderness or pain on motion, and increased heat) in one or more joints
Duration of disease 6 wk or longer
Onset type defined by type of disease in first 6 mo:
  Polyarthritis: 5 or more inflamed joints
  Oligoarthritis: <5 inflamed joints
  Systemic: arthritis with characteristic fever
Exclusion of other forms of juvenile arthritis

Modified from Cassidy JT, Levison JE, Bass JC, et al: A study of classification criteria for a diagnosis of juvenile rheumatoid arthritis. *Arthritis Rheum* 1986;29;174.

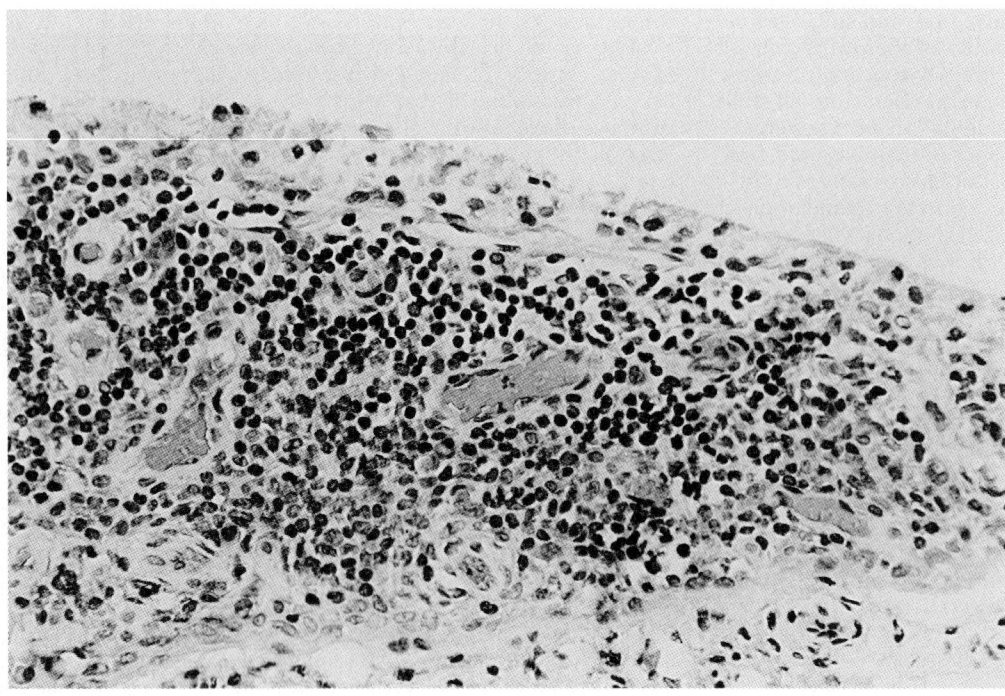

FIGURE 145–1. Synovial biopsy from a 10-yr-old child with pauciarticular juvenile rheumatoid arthritis. There is a dense infiltration of lymphocytes and plasma cells in the synovium.

parents as a trigger, it is more likely the result than the cause of arthritis. Studies of T-cell receptor expression confirm recruitment of T cells specific for antigens, at present uncharacterized, which are present in joint synovium. Specific populations of

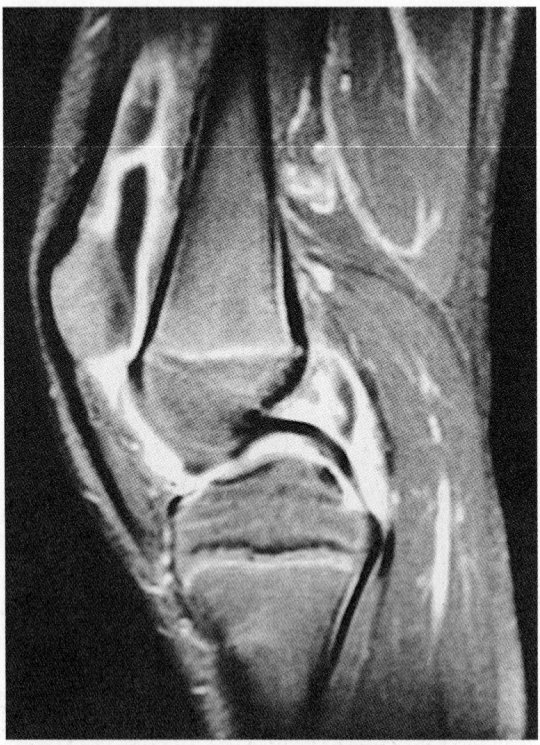

FIGURE 145–2. MRI scan with gadolinium of a 10-yr-old child with juvenile rheumatoid arthritis (same patient as in Fig. 145–1). The dense white signal in the synovium near the distal femur, proximal tibia, and patella reflects inflammation. MRI is useful to exclude ligamentous injury, chondromalacia of the patella, or tumor.

T cells appear to change over time, sometimes with clonal expansion of cells that may be protective (e.g., those reactive toward certain heat shock proteins) and associated with improved responsiveness to medical treatment. However, resistance to treatment may result in part from the migration into synovium of T cells whose surfaces bear molecules permitting chronic activation.

The recruitment of these T cells is made possible by certain HLA types that are found with increased frequency in affected children. HLA-DR4 (particularly the DRB1*0401 allele) is associated with polyarticular disease; pauciarticular JRA has been associated with HLA alleles at the DR8 (particularly DRB1*0801) and DR5 (particularly DRB1*1104) loci.

T-cell activation results in a cascade of events leading to tissue damage in joints and other affected tissues, including B-cell activation, complement consumption, and, in particular, release of interleukin-6 (IL-6), IL-13, tumor necrosis factor-α (TNFα), and other pro-inflammatory cytokines, possibly under the control of specific genetic alleles. Inheritance of certain alleles may predispose to production of greater amounts of these cytokines, resulting in more severe disease.

Clinical Manifestations. Initial symptoms often include morning stiffness and gelling, easy fatigability particularly after school in the early afternoon, joint pain later in the day, and joint swelling. The involved joint is often warm, lacks full range of motion, and is occasionally painful on motion but usually not erythematous.

Oligoarthritis (pauciarticular disease) predominantly affects the joints of the lower extremities, such as the knees and ankles (Fig. 145–3). Involvement of upper extremity large joints, although seen, is not characteristic of this type of onset. Involvement of the hip is almost never a presenting sign of JRA. However, hip disease may occur later, particularly in polyarticular JRA, and is often the first sign of a deteriorating functional course (Fig. 145–4).

Polyarthritis (polyarticular disease) is generally characterized by involvement of both large and small joints (Figs. 145–5 and 145–6). As many as 20–40 separate joints are often affected, although inflammation of only five or more joints is

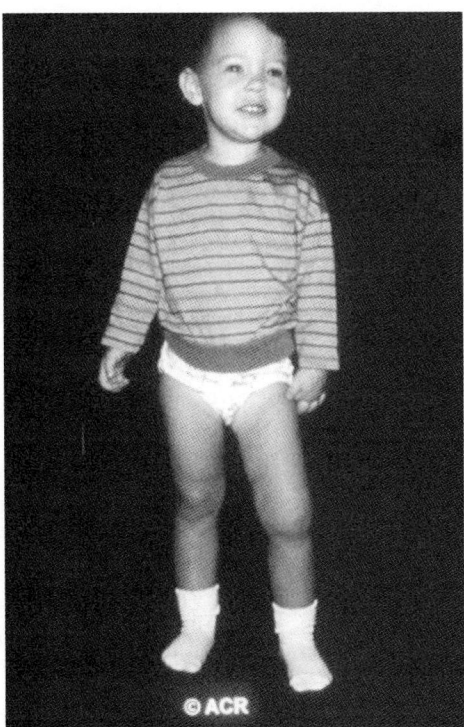

FIGURE 145–3. Pauciarticular juvenile rheumatoid arthritis with involvement of the left knee and hands. (Reprinted from the Clinical Slide Collection on the Rheumatic Diseases; Copyright 1991, 1995, 1997. Used by permission of the American College of Rheumatology.)

required as a criterion for classification of this type of onset or course. Polyarticular disease often resembles the usual presentation of adult rheumatoid arthritis. Rheumatoid nodules found on extensor surfaces of elbows and over the Achilles tendon are associated with a more severe course. Micrognathia reflects chronic temporomandibular joint involvement. Cervical spine involvement of the apophyseal joints (Fig. 145–7) occurs frequently, with risk of atlantoaxial subluxation.

Systemic-onset disease is manifest by arthritis and prominent visceral involvement including hepatosplenomegaly, lymphadenopathy, and serositis, such as a pericardial effusion. It is characterized by a quotidian fever with daily temperature spikes to at least 39°C, sometimes followed by mildly hypothermic temperatures, for a minimum of 2 wk. Each febrile episode is often accompanied by a characteristic faint, erythematous, macular rash; these evanescent **salmon-colored** lesions may be linear or circular, from 2 to 5 mm in size, distributed most commonly over the trunk and proximal extremities (Fig. 145–8). **Koebner phenomenon**, which is cutaneous hypersensitivity to superficial trauma, is elicited by lightly running the edge of the examiner's fingernail along uninvolved skin, is suggestive, but not diagnostic, of systemic-onset disease.

Diagnosis. The diagnosis of JRA is greatly aided by the American College of Rheumatology classification criteria and its subclassification of courses of disease and by the meticulous exclusion of other articular diseases. There is no one pathognomonic finding for these diseases in children. However, the classic intermittent fever in association with the typical rash and objective arthritis is highly suggestive of systemic-onset JRA. The diagnosis is based on a history compatible with inflammatory joint disease and a physical examination that confirms the presence of arthritis, as defined by the classification criteria (see Box 145–1). Laboratory abnormalities characteristic of inflammation include an elevated erythrocyte sedimentation rate (ESR) and C-reactive protein (CRP), leukocytosis, thrombocytosis, and the anemia of chronic disease support the diagnosis.

DIFFERENTIAL DIAGNOSIS. Arthritis can be the presenting manifestation for any of the rheumatic diseases of childhood, including systemic lupus erythematosus (SLE) (see Chapter 148), juvenile dermatomyositis (see Chapter 149), sarcoidosis (see Chapter 155), and the vasculitis syndromes (see Chapter 157). The diagnosis of these diseases will depend on specifically associated manifestations. In scleroderma, the swelling along the digits early in the disease is not confined to the joints, and subsequent loss of motion occurs without articular swelling. Rheumatic fever is characterized by exquisite joint tenderness, high spiking fevers, and polyarthritis that is usually migratory but may also be additive. Autoimmune hepatitis can be associated with arthritis. Lyme disease (see Chapter 204) should be considered in children living in or visiting endemic areas who present with oligoarthritis. Although a history of tick exposure, preceding flulike illness, and subsequent rash should be sought, these are not always present. Joint pain and swelling of a single joint suggests trauma or infection; correlation with history, laboratory, and radiologic findings helps exclude these possibilities.

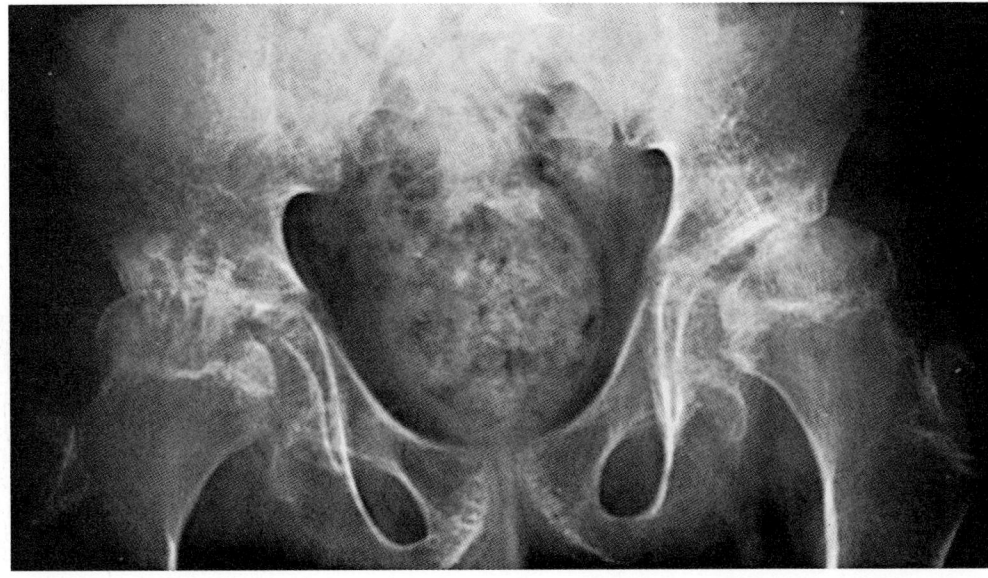

FIGURE 145–4. Severe hip disease in a 13-yr-old boy with active, systemic-onset juvenile rheumatoid arthritis. X-ray shows destruction of the femoral head and acetabula, joint space narrowing, and subluxation of left hip. The patient had received corticosteroids systemically for 9 yr.

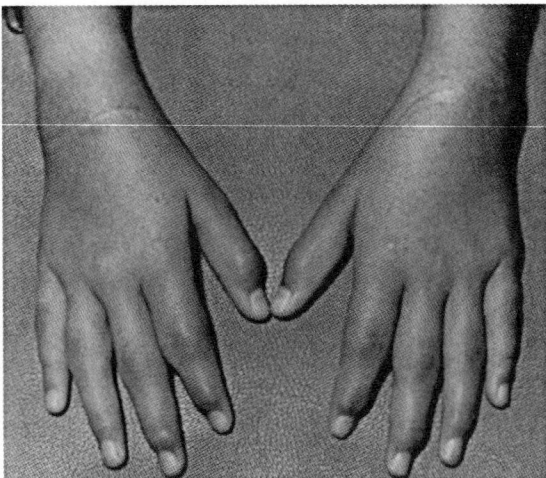

FIGURE 145–5. Hands and wrists of a girl with rheumatoid factor-negative polyarticular juvenile rheumatoid arthritis. Notice the symmetric involvement of the metacarpophalangeal joints, proximal interphalangeal joints, and distal interphalangeal joints. Both wrists are affected.

Monoarticular arthritis unresponsive to anti-inflammatory treatment may be the result of chronic mycobacterial or other infection; the diagnosis is established by synovial biopsy.

Physical findings may suggest other diagnoses. Arthritis and fluid in a single joint suggests bacterial infection, although joint fluid can be significant with JRA, including in the knee joint resulting in a ballotable patella. Chondromalacia of the patella or related femoropatellar syndromes can cause knee pain. Tenderness over insertion of ligaments and tendons raises the possibility of a spondyloarthropathy. Pauciarticular arthritis occurring in an unusual distribution (e.g., small joints of the hand and ankle) can be seen in psoriatic arthritis. However, until psoriasis develops, which may occur years after the arthri-

tis presents, the diagnosis can only be suspected. Isolated hip pain with limited motion raises the possibility of suppurative arthritis, osteomyelitis, Legg-Calvé-Perthes disease, slipped capital femoral epiphysis, and chondrolysis of the hip.

Some children will have persistent arthralgia despite repeated normal physical examination. Although these children do not fulfill the diagnostic criteria for JRA initially, the diagnosis of JRA may sometimes be established as long as 2 yr after initial presentation. Until persisting joint swelling develops, other diagnoses need to be considered. Episodes of joint pain and swelling, usually lasting less than 1 wk with complete resolution between episodes, can be seen in juvenile episodic arthritis, often attributed to hypermobility syndrome. Inflammatory bowel disease may present with pauciarticular arthritis, usually affecting joints in the lower extremities. The presence of diarrhea in a child with arthritis can also follow an enteric infection (see Chapter 147). A fear of returning to school suggests school phobia.

Less commonly, other diseases can produce joint symptoms and abnormal joint examination. Children with leukemia may have joint pain resulting from metaphyseal expansion of malignant bone marrow, sometimes months before demonstrating peripheral blood lymphoblasts. Examination of such a child usually reveals a deeper pain to palpation of the bone; bone marrow aspiration yields the diagnosis. Some diseases, such as cystic fibrosis, diabetes mellitus, and glycogen storage diseases, have associated arthropathies. Swelling that extends beyond the joint can be seen in lymphedema, which may rarely coexist with JRA, and in Henoch-Schönlein purpura. A peripheral arthritis indistinguishable from types of JRA occurs in the presence of humoral immunodeficiency, such as common variable immunodeficiency and X-linked agammaglobulinemia. Some skeletal dysplasias associated with a degenerative arthropathy can be diagnosed by characteristic radiologic abnormalities.

Laboratory Findings. Hematologic abnormalities often reflect the degree of systemic or articular inflammation, with elevated white blood cell and platelet counts and decreased hemoglobin concentration and mean corpuscular volume. The ESR and

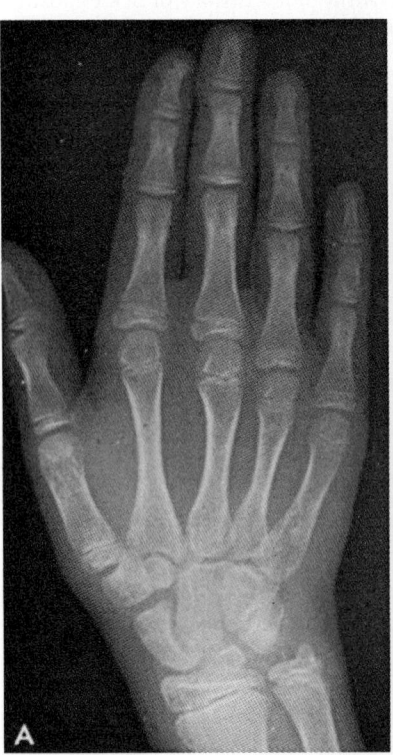

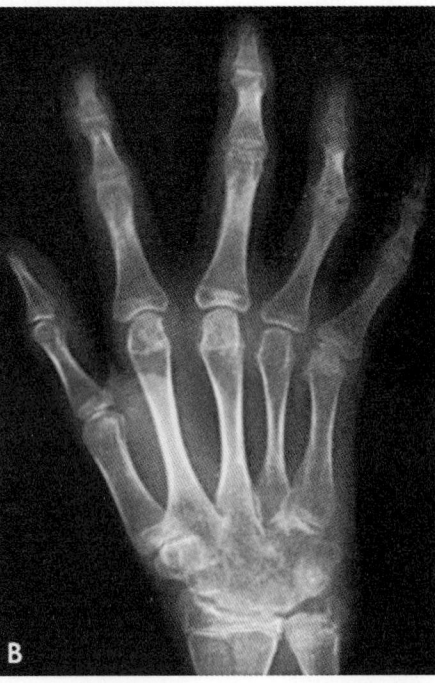

FIGURE 145–6. Progression of joint destruction in a girl with rheumatoid factor-positive juvenile rheumatoid arthritis despite doses of corticosteroids sufficient to suppress symptoms in the interval between *A* and *B*. *A*, Roentgenogram of the hand at onset. *B*, Roentgenogram 4 yr later, showing a loss of articular cartilage and destruction changes in the distal and proximal interphalangeal and metacarpophalangeal joints and destruction and fusion of wrist bones.

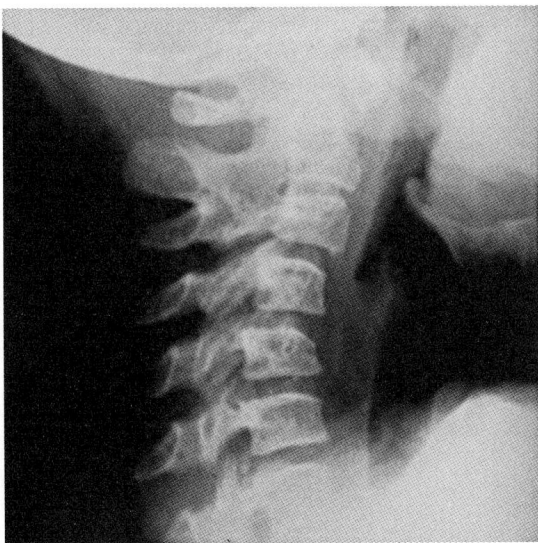

FIGURE 145–7. Radiograph of the cervical spine of a patient with active juvenile rheumatoid arthritis, showing fusion of the neural arch between joints C2-3, narrowing and erosion of the remaining neural arch joints, obliteration of the apophyseal space, and loss of the normal lordosis.

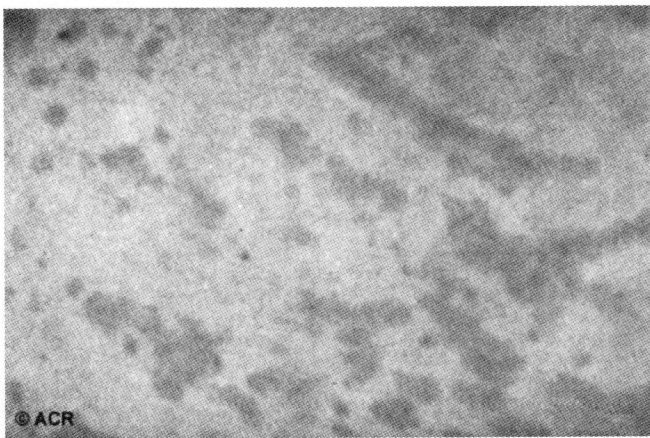

FIGURE 145–8. The rash of systemic-onset juvenile rheumatoid arthritis. The rash is salmon colored, macular, and nonpruritic. Individual lesions are transient and occur in crops over the trunk and extremities. See also color plates. (Reprinted from the Clinical Slide Collection on the Rheumatic Diseases; Copyright 1991, 1995, 1997. Used by permission of the American College of Rheumatology.)

CRP usually mirror these findings, along with elevated serum immunoglobulins. However, it is not unusual for the ESR to be normal in some children with JRA, probably when most activated lymphocytes responsible for disease have shifted from the bloodstream and entered the synovium.

Elevated ANA titers are present in at least 40–85% of all children with pauciarticular or polyarticular JRA but are unusual in children with systemic-onset disease. Detectable ANA, usually with homogeneous or speckled pattern, is associated with increased risk for the development of chronic uveitis but the precise specificities for various ANA patterns have not been determined. A positive rheumatoid factor (RF) may be associated with onset of the disease in an older child with polyarticular involvement (approximately 8%) and the development of rheumatoid nodules, and with a poor overall prognosis and eventual functional disability. Both ANA and RF can occur in association with transient events during childhood, such as viral infections, particularly Epstein-Barr virus; seropositivity must be defined at a specific titer within a laboratory in relation to accepted positive and negative controls and based on consecutive positive tests over a defined period.

Bone mineral metabolism is often abnormal in children with JRA with a history of active synovitis, relatively independent of onset type or course subtype, and predominantly affects appendicular cortical bone, with less effect upon the normal age-related development of trabecular bone. Increased levels of cytokines such as IL-6 may decrease bone formation (reflected by decreased serum levels of osteocalcin and bone-specific alkaline phosphatase) to a greater extent than bone resorption (which may also be decreased, as reflected by decreased levels of tartrate-resistant acid phosphatase). Corresponding abnormalities of skeletal growth become most prominent during the pubertal growth spurt and in postpubertal children (Tanner stages IV–V).

Early radiographic changes include soft tissue swelling, osteoporosis, and periostitis about the affected joints (Fig. 145–9). Regional epiphyseal closure may be accelerated and the local bone growth increased or decreased. Continued disease may lead to subchondral erosions and narrowing of cartilage space, with varying degrees of bony destruction and fusion. Characteristic late radiographic changes of JRA are seen in the hands and cervical spine, most frequently in the neural arch joints at C2-3 (see Fig. 145–7). MRI studies may be helpful to evaluate both joint and soft tissues (see Fig. 145–2).

Treatment. The long-term treatment of children with JRA is initiated and subsequently modified according to disease subtype, severity of the disease, specific manifestations of the illness, and response to therapy. The objectives of treatment are to establish the child in a pattern of adaptation that is as normal as possible

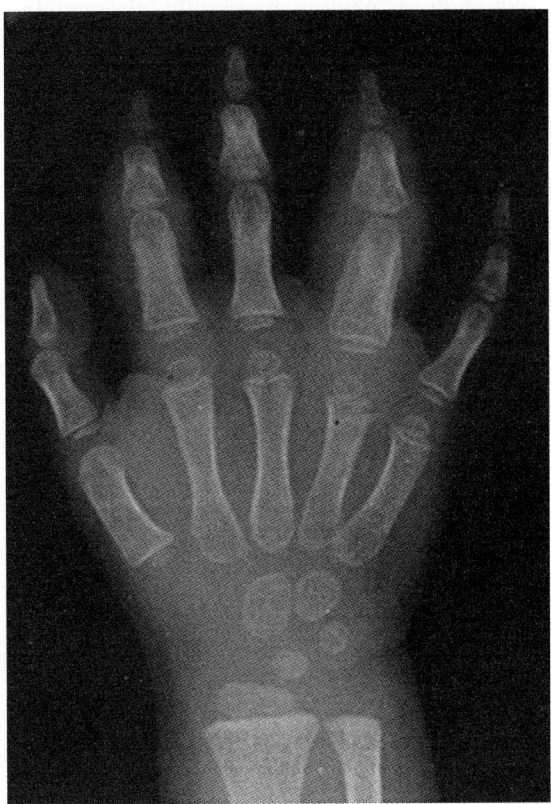

FIGURE 145–9. Early (6-mo duration) radiographic changes of juvenile rheumatoid arthritis, soft tissue swelling, and periosteal new bone formation appear adjacent to the 2nd and 4th proximal interphalangeal joints.

and to accomplish this goal with minimal risk of adverse effects (see Chapter 144).

Most children with oligoarticular JRA respond to nonsteroidal anti-inflammatory drugs (NSAIDs) alone. However, most polyarticular patients, and some oligoarticular patients with aggressive disease, require additional medications. A pyramid therapeutic approach should be considered; combination therapy should begin with the least toxic medications, usually NSAIDs, and proceeding through sulfasalazine, methotrexate, and possibly etanercept or immunosuppressive or experimental drugs (Fig. 145–10). Medications that place the child's present and future health most at risk, such as azathioprine and cyclophosphamide, are reserved for the very few children who do not respond to less aggressive therapy. Newer modes of treatment, such as etanercept, may prove to be more specific for synovial inflammatory disease and potentially less toxic than other current medications.

Glucocorticoids are used for management of overwhelming inflammatory or systemic illness, for **bridge therapy** in lower doses for the child who has not yet responded, in addition to another drug such as methotrexate, and for ocular and intraarticular use. Corticosteroids are very powerful anti-inflammatory drugs, perhaps the most efficacious in current use for systemic disease, but they may be associated with tachyphylaxis and impose upon the child the risk of severe toxicities, including Cushing syndrome, growth retardation, and osteopenia.

Methotrexate is considered the safest, most efficacious, and least toxic of the currently available second-line agents. It may be given either orally or subcutaneously once weekly. Intramuscular gold therapy has been generally supplanted by methotrexate.

Other aspects of management include routine slit-lamp ophthalmologic examination of all patients with JRA to monitor for development of asymptomatic uveitis, dietary evaluation and counseling to ensure appropriate calcium intake, and physical and occupational therapy. Social workers can help families recognize stresses imposed by illness and identify appropriate community resources.

Prognosis. Although the course of JRA in an individual child is unpredictable, some general statements can be made concerning onset type and outcome (Table 145–1). Studies from

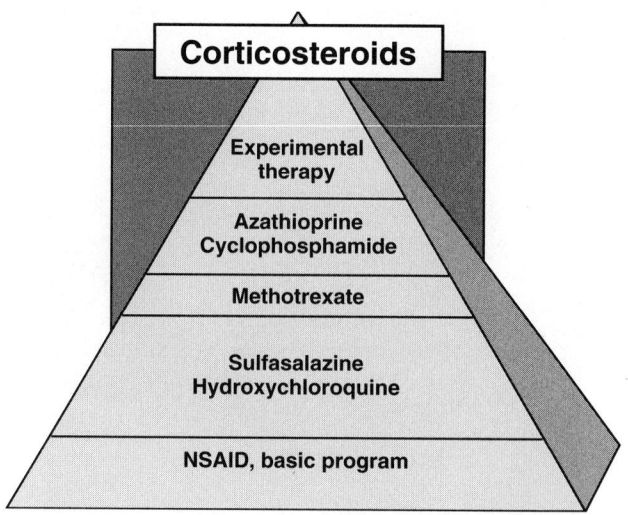

FIGURE 145–10. The "therapeutic pyramid" of juvenile rheumatoid arthritis. (Adapted from Cassidy JT, Petty RE: Juvenile rheumatoid arthritis. In *Textbook of Pediatric Rheumatology*, 3rd ed. Philadelphia, WB Saunders, 1995.)

the United States indicate that, despite current management, approximately 45% of JRA patients have active disease persisting into early adulthood, often with severe limitations of physical function.

Children with oligoarthritis, particularly girls with early onset of arthritis at younger than 6 yr of age, are at risk to develop chronic uveitis. There is usually no association between the course of the arthritis and the chronic uveitis. Anterior uveitis (Fig. 145–11), or iridocyclitis, in children with pauciarticular disease can result in posterior synechiae; untreated or refractory uveitis can result in blindness, which has decreased with more frequent monitoring by slit-lamp examination to exclude asymptomatic uveitis. Many of these children do well, however, with early remission.

The child with polyarticular disease often has a more prolonged course. Functional risk has been associated with older age of onset, the presence of rheumatoid factor seropositivity or

TABLE 145–1. Prognosis of Juvenile Rheumatoid Arthritis by Type of Onset

Onset Type	Course Subtype	Subsequent Clinical Manifestations	Outcome
Polyarthritis	RF-seropositive	Female Older age Hand/wrist Erosions Nodules Unremitting	Poor
	ANA-seropositive	Female Young age	Good
	Seronegative	—	Variable
Oligoarthritis	ANA-seropositive	Female Young age Chronic anterior uveitis (iridocyclitis)	Excellent (except eyes)
	RF-seropositive	Polyarthritis Erosions Unremitting	Poor
	HLA-B27–positive	Male Older age	Good
Systemic disease	Seronegative	—	Good
	Oligoarthritis	—	Good
	Polyarthritis	Erosions	Poor

From Cassidy JT, Petty RE: Juvenile rheumatoid arthritis. In Textbook of Pediatric Rheumatology, *4th ed. Philadelphia, WB Saunders, 2001.*

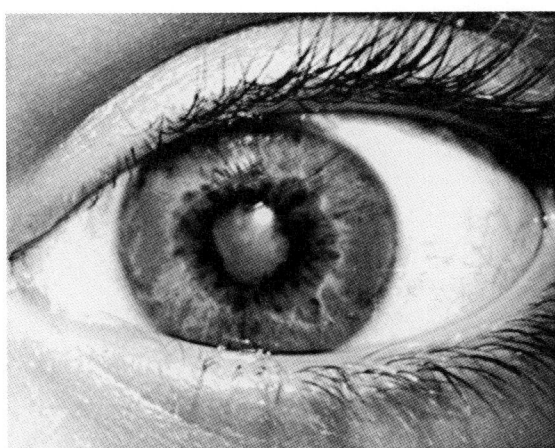

FIGURE 145–11. Chronic anterior uveitis, or iridocyclitis, of juvenile rheumatoid arthritis. Extensive posterior synechiae have resulted in a small, irregular pupil. There is a well-developed cataract and early band keratopathy at the medial and lateral margins of the cornea.

Aasland A, Flato B, Vandvik IH: Psychosocial outcome in juvenile chronic arthritis: A nine-year follow-up. *Clin Exp Rheumatol* 1997;15:561–8.

Cassidy JT, Levinson JE, Bass JC, et al: A study of classification criteria for a diagnosis of juvenile rheumatoid arthritis. *Arthritis Rheum* 1986;29:274–81.

De Benedetti F, Ravelli A, Martini A: Cytokines in juvenile rheumatoid arthritis. *Curr Opin Rheumatol* 1997;9:428–33.

Denardo BA, Tucker LB, Miller LC, et al: Demography of a regional pediatric rheumatology patient population. *J Rheumatol* 1994;21:1553–61.

Feldman BM, Birdi N, Boone JE, et al: Seasonal onset of systemic-onset juvenile rheumatoid arthritis. *J Pediatr* 1996:129:513–8.

Fernandez-Vina M, Fink CW, Stastny P: HLA associations in juvenile arthritis. *Clin Exp Rheumatol* 1994;12:205–14.

Gare BA: Epidemiology of rheumatic disease in children. *Curr Opin Rheumatol* 1996;8:449–54.

Giannini EH, Brewer EJ, Kuzmina N, et al: Methotrexate in resistant juvenile rheumatoid arthritis. Results of the U.S.A.-U.S.S.R. double-blind, placebo-controlled trial. The Pediatric Rheumatology Collaborative Study Group and The Cooperative Children's Study Group. *N Engl J Med* 1992;326:1043–9.

Grom AA, Murray KJ, Luyrink L, et al: Patterns of expression of tumor necrosis factor alpha, tumor necrosis factor beta, and their receptors in synovia of patients with juvenile rheumatoid arthritis and juvenile spondyloarthropathy. *Arthritis Rheum* 1996;39:1703–10.

Lovell DJ, Giannini EH, Reiff A, et al: Etanercept in children with polyarticular juvenile rheumatoid arthritis. Pediatric Rheumatology Collaborative Study Group. *N Engl J Med* 2000;342:763–9.

Manners PJ, Diepeveen DA: Prevalence of juvenile chronic arthritis in a population of 12-year-old children in urban Australia. *Pediatrics* 1996;98:84–90.

Modesto C, Woo P, Garcia-Consuegra J, et al: Systemic onset juvenile chronic arthritis, polyarticular pattern and hip involvement as markers for a bad prognosis. *Clin Exp Rheumatol* 2001;19:211–7.

Mouy R, Stephan JL, Pillet P, et al: Efficacy of cyclosporin A in the treatment of macrophage activation syndrome in juvenile arthritis: Report of five cases. *J Pediatr* 1996;129:750–4.

Pepmueller PH, Cassidy JT, Allen SH, et al: Bone mineralization and bone mineral metabolism in children with juvenile rheumatoid arthritis. *Arthritis Rheum* 1996;39:746–57.

Peterson LS, Mason T, Nelson AM, et al: Juvenile rheumatoid arthritis in Rochester, Minnesota 1960–1993. Is the epidemiology changing? *Arthritis Rheum* 1996;39:1385–90.

Peterson LS, Mason T, Nelson AM, et al: Psychosocial outcomes and health status of adults who have had juvenile rheumatoid arthritis: A controlled, population-based study. *Arthritis Rheum* 1997;40:2235–40.

Prakken AB, van Eden W, Rijkers GT, et al: Autoreactivity to human heat-shock protein 60 predicts disease remission in oligoarticular juvenile rheumatoid arthritis. *Arthritis Rheum* 1996;39:1826–32.

Ragsdale CG, Petty RE, Cassidy JT, et al: The clinical progression of apparent juvenile rheumatoid arthritis to systemic lupus erythematosus. *J Rheumatol* 1980; 7:50–5.

Schwartz MM, Simpson P, Kerr KL, et al: Juvenile rheumatoid arthritis in African Americans. *J Rheumatol* 1997;24:1826–9.

Spiegel LR, Schneider R, Lang BA, et al: Early predictors of poor functional outcome in systemic-onset juvenile rheumatoid arthritis: A multicenter cohort study. *Arthritis Rheum* 2000;43:2402–9.

Thompson SD, Murray KJ, Grom AA, et al: Comparative sequence analysis of the human T cell receptor beta chain in juvenile rheumatoid arthritis and juvenile spondyloarthropathies: Evidence for antigenic selection of T cells in the synovium. *Arthritis Rheum* 1998;41:482–97.

Walco GA, Varni JW, Ilowite NT: Cognitive-behavioral pain management in children with juvenile rheumatoid arthritis. *Pediatrics* 1992;89:1075–9.

Zhang H, Phang D, Laxer RM, et al: Evolution of the T cell receptor beta repertoire from synovial fluid T cells of patients with juvenile onset rheumatoid arthritis. *J Rheumatol* 1997;24:1396–402.

rheumatoid nodules, and the early development of specific articular disease, such as that affecting the cervical spine or hips.

The child with systemic-onset disease is often the most difficult to manage in terms of both articular and systemic manifestations. However, systemic manifestations are usually present only during the first few years after onset. The prognosis after that time is dependent on the number of joints involved and severity of the arthritis.

Anemia, common in active disease or disease of prolonged duration, is usually unresponsive to oral iron administration. Anemia may be exacerbated by gastrointestinal bleeding associated with the use of NSAIDs. Specific complications may occur in subsets of the disease, such as the development of SLE during the course of disease in children with polyarticular JRA, particularly when they develop ANAs with a high titer. Anemia associated with decreases in other blood cell lines raises the possibility of malignancy. Rarely, anemia is a result of hemolytic anemia. Anemia associated with thrombocytopenia or leukopenia with fever, lymphadenopathy, and hepatosplenomegaly suggests **macrophage activation syndrome**, a rare complication of systemic JRA. This diagnosis is confirmed by liver or bone marrow biopsy. Treatment with cyclosporine has been effective in many patients. A rare digital endarteritis threatening autoamputation may respond to parenterally administered prostaglandin E_1. The development of manifestations of other rheumatic diseases suggests that the diagnosis has changed to an overlapping syndrome or another specific disease, such as SLE or dermatomyositis.

Orthopedic complications include leg length discrepancy, which can be treated with a shoe lift on the shorter side to prevent a secondary scoliosis; popliteal cysts, which require no treatment if small; and flexion contractures, particularly of the knees, hips, and wrists. Contractures require medical control of arthritis, appropriate splinting, and a physical therapy program to allow stretching of affected tendons.

Psychosocial adaptation may be affected by JRA. Studies from Scandinavia and the United States indicate that, compared with control subjects, many of these children have problems with lifetime adjustments and obtaining employment. Disability not directly associated with arthritis may continue into young adulthood in as many as 20% of patients, together with continuing chronic pain syndromes in a similar frequency. Psychologic complications, including problems with school attendance and socialization, may respond to counseling by mental health professionals.

Chapter 146

Ankylosing Spondylitis and Other Spondyloarthropathies

Michael L. Miller and Ross E. Petty

The diseases collectively referred to as **spondyloarthropathies** include ankylosing spondylitis, the psoriatic arthritides, arthritis accompanying inflammatory bowel diseases, and chronic reactive arthritis following enteric or genitourinary (GU) tract infections. In the new classification of the International League of

Associations for Rheumatology (ILAR), the term **enthesitis-related arthritis** is used to denote what has traditionally been called juvenile ankylosing spondylitis; psoriatic arthritis is considered distinct.

Epidemiology. Estimates of the prevalence of juvenile ankylosing spondylitis (JAS) range from 11–86/100,000 children, and of psoriatic arthritis from 10–15/100,000 children. JAS occurs most frequently in older boys, adolescents, and young adults. These disorders are frequently familial; the histocompatibility antigen HLA-B27 is strongly associated with JAS (>90%) and is found in increased frequency in persons having spondyloarthropathies with inflammation of the axial skeleton.

Psoriatic arthritis is particularly common in young girls. The arthropathies of inflammatory bowel diseases, reactive arthritis, and Reiter syndrome (a symptom complex consisting of arthritis, urethritis, and conjunctivitis usually associated with HLA-B27) are much less common in childhood; they can affect children of any age and are somewhat more common in boys.

Pathogenesis. The histologic appearance of the synovium in spondyloarthropathies is indistinguishable from that of other idiopathic chronic arthritides. Tenosynovitis may be present, and periostitis may occur. **Enthesitis** (inflammation at the sites of attachments of ligaments, tendons, fascias, and capsules to bone) is characterized by chronic inflammation and, in advanced disease, which is usually found in adults, by calcification of ligaments and fusion of joints.

Chronic reactive arthritis may follow enteric infection with nontyphoidal *Salmonella*, *Shigella*, *Yersinia enterocolitica*, *Campylobacter jejuni*, *Cryptosporidium parvum*, or *Giardia intestinalis*, or GU tract infection with *Chlamydia trachomatis*. The cause of the other spondyloarthropathies is unknown. It is postulated that similarity between self-antigens and bacterial antigens (**molecular mimicry**) permits the development of an autoimmune process in genetically predisposed individuals.

Clinical Manifestations. The spondyloarthropathies are characterized by inflammation of joints of the axial skeleton as well as the limbs, by the presence of enthesitis, and by the absence of rheumatoid factor.

JUVENILE ANKYLOSING SPONDYLITIS. Early JAS is most frequently characterized by oligoarthritis and enthesitis. Joints of the legs are more frequently affected than those of the arms. Abnormalities of the axial skeleton including the sacroiliac joints are usually absent until later in the disease course, although loss of spinal flexibility may eventually be noted (Fig. 146–1). When few joints are affected during the first 6 mo of disease, hip joint arthritis is particularly suggestive of early JAS. Enthesitis, presenting as localized tenderness at characteristic locations around the foot and knee, is particularly common and has led to the description of a syndrome of seronegativity (absence of rheumatoid factor), enthesitis, and arthritis (SEA syndrome), which is probably the most common initial presentation of JAS. The disease course may be characterized by long periods of apparent disease remission. Systemic symptoms such as low-grade fever and weight loss raise the possibility of occult inflammatory bowel disease.

PSORIATIC ARTHRITIS. The most common pattern of psoriatic arthritis is oligoarthritis, which affects large and small joints in an asymmetric pattern. Patients with psoriatic arthritis occasionally have symmetric distal interphalangeal joint disease, or HLA-B27-associated sacroiliitis, although most patients are HLA-B27-negative and do not have arthritis of the sacroiliac joints or lumbosacral spine. The presence of nail pitting (Fig. 146–2), dactylitis, onycholysis, or a family history of psoriasis supports the diagnosis of psoriatic arthritis in a child with oligoarthritis or polyarthritis.

ARTHRITIS WITH INFLAMMATORY BOWEL DISEASE. Two patterns of arthritis complicate Crohn disease and ulcera-

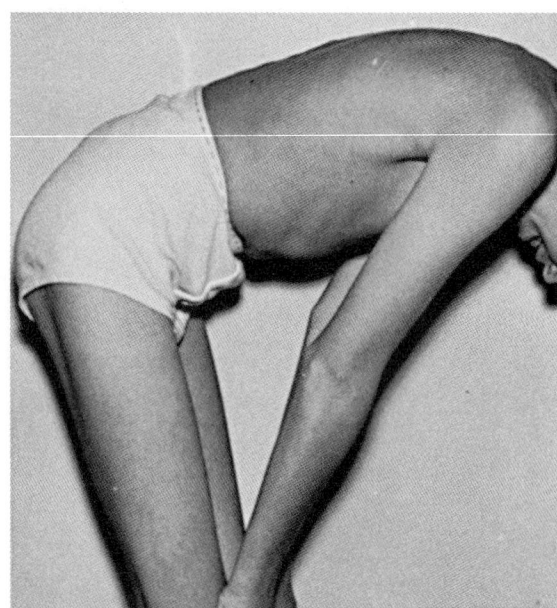

FIGURE 146–1. Loss of lumbodorsal spine mobility in a boy with ankylosing spondylitis: The lower spine remains straight when the patient bends forward.

tive colitis. A polyarthritis affecting large and small joints, which reflects the activity of the intestinal inflammation, is most common and is not truly a spondylarthritis because it does not affect joints of the spine and is not associated with HLA-B27. Less commonly, arthritis of the sacroiliac joints and other peripheral joints occurs in a pattern similar to that in ankylosing spondylitis, which, in most instances, is associated with HLA-B27. Its severity is independent of the activity of the gastrointestinal (GI) inflammation.

REACTIVE ARTHRITIS. Reactive arthritis, including the syndrome of· arthritis, urethritis, and conjunctivitis, is usually preceded by GI or GU infection. The arthritis is usually oligoarticular and may be quite severe, with considerable swelling, pain, and even erythema. Joints of the lower limbs are most commonly affected. Unlike the more common clinical forms of self-limited postinfectious arthritis (see Chapter 147), the arthritis may become chronic, lasting from several weeks to years.

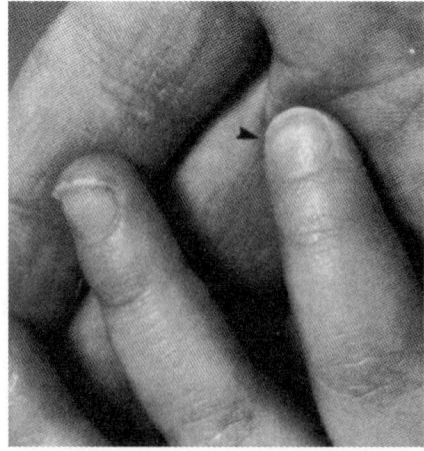

FIGURE 146–2. Nail pitting (*arrow*) and "sausage digit" (dactylitis) of the left index finger of a girl with juvenile psoriatic arthritis. (From Petty RE, Malleson P: Spondyloarthropathies of childhood. *Pediatr Clin North Am* 1986;33:1079.)

Enthesitis may be prominent, and sacroiliitis may eventuate in HLA-B27-positive patients.

Diagnosis. The diagnosis of a spondyloarthropathy is suggested by the onset in an older child, particularly a boy, of oligoarthritis that predominantly affects the hips, knees, ankles, or feet (particularly the intertarsal joints), especially if accompanied by enthesitis. A diagnosis of ankylosing spondylitis is confirmed if there is radiographic evidence of sacroiliitis. Because radiographic changes seldom occur at onset, it may be difficult to differentiate spondylarthritis from oligoarticular juvenile rheumatoid arthritis (JRA) early during the disease course. The presence of synovitis in the upper extremities tends to be more common in patients with JRA than with spondyloarthropathies. In a child with chronic arthritis, the presence of erythema nodosum, pyoderma gangrenosum, significant fever, weight loss, or anorexia suggests inflammatory bowel disease. The acute onset of arthritis, a recent history of diarrhea, and symptoms of urethritis or conjunctivitis may suggest reactive arthritis. Psoriasis, nail changes (see Fig. 146–2), or a family history of psoriasis suggests the diagnosis of psoriatic arthritis in a child (often a young girl) with oligoarthritis or polyarthritis. Early differentiation among the spondyloarthropathies by laboratory or radiographic means is difficult. Sacroiliac joint change or enthesitis may be seen on technetium-99 bone scan, but results of this examination are often difficult to interpret in children and adolescents.

Back pain may occur in children with early ankylosing spondylitis but could also be caused by suppurative arthritis of the sacroiliac joint, osteomyelitis of the pelvis or spine, osteoid osteoma of the posterior elements of the spine, or malignancies such as osteogenic sarcoma, Ewing sarcoma, or leukemia. In addition, mechanical causes such as spondylolysis, spondylolisthesis, and Scheuermann disease should be considered. Back pain secondary to fibromyalgia usually affects the soft tissues of the upper back in a symmetric pattern, as well as other well-localized tender points.

Hip joint arthritis is characterized by pain over the inguinal ligament and loss of internal rotation of the hip joint. Legg-Calvé-Perthes disease, slipped capital femoral epiphysis, and chondrolysis may have presentations similar to spondyloarthropathy.

Laboratory Findings. Laboratory evidence of systemic inflammation is often present at the onset of disease, with elevated erythrocyte sedimentation rate and mild increase in white blood cell count and platelet count. Rheumatoid factor is absent in all children with spondyloarthropathies. Antinuclear antibodies are absent except in children with psoriatic arthritis, in whom antinuclear autoantibodies occur in as many as 50%. HLA-B27 is present in more than 90% of children with JAS but is probably not increased significantly in those with other types of spondylarthritis unless sacroiliitis or acute anterior uveitis is present.

Radiographic changes include periarticular osteoporosis, loss of sharp cortical margins in areas of enthesitis (which may eventually show erosions or bony spurs), indistinct margins and erosions of the sacroiliac joints, with sclerosis on the iliac side of the joint (Fig. 146–3), and, rarely, squaring of the corners of the vertebral bodies. The characteristic **bamboo spine** caused by calcification of ligaments that is so characteristic of advanced ankylosing spondylitis in adults is very rare in childhood.

Treatment. The aims of therapy are to control inflammation, minimize pain, and preserve function. These are accomplished by a combination of anti-inflammatory medications, physical therapy, and psychosocial support. Nonsteroidal anti-inflammatory drugs such as naproxen (15–20 mg/kg/24 hr) may be sufficient. It may be necessary to add sulfasalazine (up to 50 mg/kg/24 hr, no more than 3 g/24 hr in adolescents). Intra-articular triamcinolone hexacetonide is useful for controlling localized joint

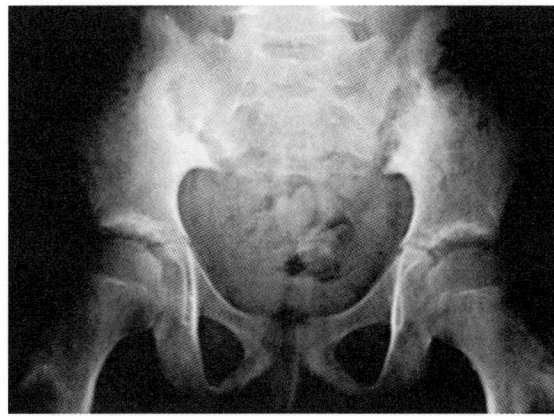

FIGURE 146–3. Well-developed sacroiliitis in a boy with ankylosing spondylitis; both sacroiliac joints show extensive sclerosis, erosion of joint margins, and apparent widening of the joint space.

inflammation. Exercises to maintain range of motion in the back, thorax, and affected joints should be instituted early in the disease course. Custom-fitted insoles are particularly useful in management of painful entheses around the feet.

Complications. Acute iridocyclitis, or anterior uveitis, occurs in as many as 25% of patients with JAS. Chronic iridocyclitis similar to that in JRA occurs in approximately 15% of children with psoriatic arthritis. Aortic valve insufficiency is a rare but important complication of ankylosing spondylitis. Atlantoaxial subluxation has also been reported.

Prognosis. There is little reliable information about long-term outcome of the spondyloarthropathies in childhood. These are chronic diseases with highly variable clinical courses. JAS is often characterized by long periods of active disease followed by long periods of inactivity. Most studies have shown that, over many years, the disease progresses to involve joints of the spine and sacroiliac joints and may cause fusion and significant disability. Psoriatic arthritis tends to be a chronic unremitting disease. Reactive arthritis may be brief (several weeks or months) but may become chronic and progress to ankylosing spondylitis. In children with inflammatory bowel disease, the peripheral arthritis is usually controlled when the GI inflammation is controlled; if the arthritis is associated with HLA-B27, the course tends to be more chronic.

Burgos-Vargas R, Vazquez-Mellado J: The early clinical recognition of juvenile-onset ankylosing spondylitis and its differentiation from juvenile rheumatoid arthritis. *Arthritis Rheum* 1995;38:835–44.

Cabral DA, Oen KG, Petty RE: SEA syndrome revisited: A long-term followup of children with a syndrome of seronegative enthesopathy and arthropathy. *J Rheumatol* 1992;19:1282–5.

Flato B, Aasland A, Vinje O, et al: Outcome and predictive factors in juvenile rheumatoid arthritis and juvenile spondyloarthropathy. *J Rheumatol* 1998;25:366–75.

Foster HE, Cairns RA, Burnell RH, et al: Atlantoaxial subluxation in children with seronegative enthesopathy and arthropathy syndrome: 2 case reports and a review of the literature. *J Rheumatol* 1995;22:548–51.

Jacobs JC, Berdon WE, Johnston AD: HLA-B27-associated spondyloarthritis and enthesopathy in childhood: Clinical, pathologic, and radiographic observations in 58 patients. *J Pediatr* 1982;100:521–8.

Mielants H, Veys EM, Cuvelier C, et al: Gut inflammation in children with late onset pauciarticular juvenile chronic arthritis and evolution to adult spondyloarthropathy—a prospective study. *J Rheumatol* 1993;20:1567–72.

Peh WC, Ho WY, Luk KD: Applications of bone scintigraphy in ankylosing spondylitis. *Clin Imaging* 1997;21:54–62.

Petty RE, Southwood TR, Baum J et al: Revision of the proposed classification for juvenile idiopathic arthritis. Durban, 1997. *J Rheumatol* 1991;25:1991–4.

Roberton DM, Cabral DA, Malleson PN, et al: Juvenile psoriatic arthritis: Followup and evaluation of diagnostic criteria. *J Rheumatol* 1996;23:166–70.

Rosenberg AM, Petty RE: A syndrome of seronegative enthesopathy and arthropathy in children. *Arthritis Rheum* 1982;25:1041–7.

Schaller J, Bitnum S, Wedgwood RJ: Ankylosing spondylitis with childhood onset. *J Pediatr* 1969;74:505–16.

Sheerin KA, Giannini EH, Brewer EJ Jr, et al: HLA-B27-associated arthropathy in childhood: Long-term clinical and diagnostic outcome. *Arthritis Rheum* 1988;31:1165–70.

Shore A, Ansell BM: Juvenile psoriatic arthritis—an analysis of 60 cases. *J Pediatr* 1982;100:529–35.

Southwood TR, Petty RE, Malleson PN, et al: Psoriatic arthritis in children. *Arthritis Rheum* 1989;32:1007–13.

Stamato T, Laxer RM, de Freitas C, et al: Prevalence of cardiac manifestations of juvenile ankylosing spondylitis. *Am J Cardiol* 1995;75:744–6.

Chapter 147
Postinfectious Arthritis and Related Conditions

Michael L. Miller and James T. Cassidy

Infections have been associated with arthritis during their course and as a postinfectious reaction observed several weeks or months afterward. Although certain infectious organisms have been suspected but not proved to trigger juvenile rheumatoid arthritis (JRA), other agents are often associated with a transient arthritis that does not satisfy the classification criteria for JRA. **Reactive arthritis** follows an infection outside the joint, particularly the gastrointestinal or genitourinary tract. The course of reactive arthritis is variable and may progress to chronic spondyloarthropathy (see Chapter 146). **Postinfectious arthritis** implies arthritis that follows infections that are usually viral in origin, with shorter duration than reactive arthritis.

Pathogenesis. Reactive arthritis may follow enteric infection with non-typhoidal *Salmonella, Shigella, Yersinia enterocolitica, Campylobacter jejuni, Cryptosporidium parvum,* or *Giardia intestinalis,* or genitourinary tract infection with *Chlamydia trachomatis.* Reactive arthritis may represent an autoimmune response involving T lymphocytes that cross-react to antigens in joints (**molecular mimicry**). A study of synovial fluid from patients with reactive arthritis suggested that T cells may be more engaged in promoting inflammation than in eliminating bacteria through cytotoxic mechanisms. However, the origin of these abnormal cells may be from outside the joint. Another possible mechanism is lymphocytic reactivity to bacterial DNA found in synovium, perhaps as a by-product of otherwise successfully cleared infection. One study of joint fluid from patients with reactive arthritis, using polymerase chain reaction amplification, demonstrated bacterial DNA. However, a relationship to specific clinical characteristics was not found.

Several viruses (rubella, varicella-zoster, herpes simplex, and cytomegalovirus) have been isolated from the joint space. Antigens from other viruses (hepatitis B, adenovirus 7) have been identified in immune complexes from joint tissue. Postinfectious arthritis following viral infections appears to involve the deposition in joints of immune complexes containing viral antigens.

Certain HLA types may predispose to development of reactive arthritis, possibly by triggering autoreactive T lymphocytes. Adolescents and adults with reactive arthritis following enteric infections have shown persistent gut inflammation even after resolution of gastrointestinal manifestations, particularly in HLA-B27-positive individuals. Uveitis complicating reactive arthritis to *Y. enteritis* has also been associated with HLA-B27. Some children, often HLA-B27 positive, with reactive arthritis eventually develop spondyloarthropathy, further suggesting that HLA type predisposes to reactive arthritis.

Clinical Manifestations. Bacterial enteritis caused by *Shigella, Salmonella, Yersinia,* and *Campylobacter* can be followed within days to several weeks by the development of arthritis and sometimes **enthesitis,** or inflammation of the muscular or tendinous attachment to bone, in a syndrome similar to and overlapping spondyloarthropathy (see Chapter 146). Although the erythrocyte sedimentation rate (ESR) may be elevated, fever and leukocytosis are often absent. Urethritis and conjunctivitis develop occasionally. Postinfectious arthritis following less apparent illness, such as viral upper respiratory tract infections, may precede arthralgia and arthritis by 1–2 mo. Symptoms of arthralgia and joint swelling are transient, usually lasting less than 6 wk.

Certain viruses associated with arthritis (Box 147–1) may result in particular patterns of joint involvement. Rubella and hepatitis B virus typically affect the small joints, and mumps and varicella often involve large joints, especially the knees. The hepatitis B **arthritis-dermatitis syndrome** is characterized by rash and arthritis resembling serum sickness. **Rubella-associated arthropathy** follows natural rubella infection and, infrequently, rubella immunization. It typically occurs in young women, with increased incidence with advancing age, and is uncommon in preadolescent children and in males. Arthralgias of the knees and hands usually begin within 7 days of onset of the rash or 10–28 days after immunization. Parvovirus B19, responsible for erythema infectiosum (fifth disease), can cause arthralgia, symmetric joint swelling, and morning stiffness in adults, particularly women, and less frequently in children. Arthritis occurs occasionally during cytomegalovirus infection and may occur during varicella infections, and is rare after Epstein-Barr virus infection. Varicella may also be complicated by suppurative arthritis, usually due to group A *Streptococcus.*

Arthritis has been reported in children with severe truncal acne, usually in male adolescents. Patients often have fever and superficial infection of skin lesions. Recurrent episodes may be associated with myopathy and may last for several months. Infective endocarditis can be associated with arthralgia, arthritis, or signs suggestive of vasculitis, such as Osler nodes, Janeway lesions, and Roth spots. Arthritis also occurs in children with *Mycoplasma pneumoniae* infections.

Poststreptococcal arthritis may follow infection with either group A or group G *Streptococcus.* Because valvular lesions have been documented by echocardiography after the acute illness in some of these children, some clinicians consider this to be an incomplete form of acute rheumatic fever (see Chapter 168.1). Certain HLA-DRB1 types may predispose children to develop either poststreptococcal arthritis or classic rheumatic fever. Poststreptococcal arthritis is pauciarticular, may affect the small and large joints, and persists for months, compared with the

BOX 147–1. Viruses Associated with Arthritis

Togaviruses	Adenoviruses
Rubivirus	Adenovirus 7
Rubella	Herpesviruses
Alphaviruses	Herpes simplex
Ross River	Cytomegalovirus
Chikungunya	Epstein-Barr
O'nyong-nyong	Varicella-zoster
Mayaro	Paramyxoviruses
Sindbis	Mumps
Ockelbo	Enteroviruses
Pogosta	Echovirus
Parvovirus	Coxsackievirus B
B19	Orthopoxviruses
Hepadnavirus	Variola virus (smallpox)
Hepatitis B	Vaccinia virus

Adapted from Cassidy JT, Petty RE: Arthritis related to infection. In *Textbook of Pediatric Rheumatology.* Philadelphia, WB Saunders, 1995, p 503.

typical course of migratory polyarthritis of rheumatic fever. The symptoms are usually mild and tend to resolve completely.

Transient synovitis (toxic synovitis) typically affects the hip joints, often after an upper respiratory tract infection. Boys from 3–10 yr of age are most commonly affected and have complaints of pain in the hip, thigh, or knee. The ESR and white blood cell count are usually normal. Radiologic or ultrasound examination may reveal widening of the joint space of the hip. Aspiration of the hip may be necessary to exclude suppurative arthritis. The cause of this relatively common syndrome is not known, but it is presumed to be a viral or postinfectious arthritis.

Diagnosis. The diagnosis of reactive postinfectious arthritis is usually established by exclusion only after the arthritis has resolved. Acute arthritis affecting a single joint suggests suppurative arthritis; osteomyelitis may cause joint pain but is associated more often with focal bone pain over the site of infection. Arthritis associated with gastrointestinal symptoms or elevated liver function test results may be caused by infectious or autoimmune hepatitis. Arthritis or spondylarthritis may occur in some children with inflammatory bowel disease, either Crohn disease or chronic ulcerative colitis (see Chapter 317). When two or more blood cell lines show a progressive decrease in a child with arthritis, parvovirus infection, macrophage activation syndrome, and leukemia should be considered. Persistent arthritis suggests the possibility of rheumatic disease, including JRA, spondyloarthropathy, and systemic lupus erythematosus.

Treatment. No specific treatment is necessary for reactive arthritis, except for relief of pain and the functional limitations of arthritis with nonsteroidal anti-inflammatory agents. If swelling or arthralgia recurs, further evaluation may be necessary to preclude active infection or evolving rheumatic disease, such as spondyloarthropathy, JRA, or systemic lupus erythematosus.

Complications and Prognosis. Postinfectious arthritis following viral infections usually resolves without complications unless it is part of a severe viral infection affecting other organs, as with encephalomyelitis. Reactive arthritis, especially after bacterial enteric infection or genitourinary tract infection with *C. trachomatis*, has the potential for evolving to a chronic arthritis and spondyloarthropathy (see Chapter 146). Children with reactive arthritis following enteric infections occasionally develop inflammatory bowel disease months to years after onset. Both uveitis and carditis have been reported in some children diagnosed with reactive arthritis.

Ahmed S, Ayoub EM, Scornik JC, et al: Poststreptococcal reactive arthritis: Clinical characteristics and association with HLA-DR alleles. *Arthritis Rheum* 1998;41: 1096–102.

Birdi N, Allen U, D'Astous J: Poststreptococcal reactive arthritis mimicking acute septic arthritis: A hospital-based study. *J Pediatr Orthop* 1995;15:661–5.

Carroll WL, Balistreri WF, Brilli R, et al: Spectrum of *Salmonella*-associated arthritis. *Pediatrics* 1981;68:717–20.

Chantler JK, Tingle AJ, Petty RE: Persistent rubella virus infection associated with chronic arthritis in children. *N Engl J Med* 1985;313:1117–23.

Cron RQ, Sherry DD: Reiter's syndrome associated with cryptosporidial gastroenteritis. *J Rheumatol* 1995;22:1962–3.

De Cunto CL, Giannini EH, Fink CW, et al: Prognosis of children with poststreptococcal reactive arthritis. *Pediatr Infect Dis J* 1988;7:683–6.

Gerard HC, Wang Z, Wang GF, et al: Chromosomal DNA from a variety of bacterial species is present in synovial tissue from patients with various forms of arthritis. *Arthritis Rheum* 2001;44:1689–97.

Huppertz HI, Sandhage K: Reactive arthritis due to *Salmonella enteritidis* complicated by carditis. *Acta Paediatr* 1994;83:1230–1.

Mertz AK, Ugrinovic S, Lauster R, et al: Characterization of the synovial T cell response to various recombinant *Yersinia* antigens in *Yersinia enterocolitica*-triggered reactive arthritis. Heat-shock protein 60 drives a major immune response. *Arthritis Rheum* 1998;41:315–26.

Meza-Ortiz F. Giardiasis-associated arthralgia in children. *Arch Med Res* 2001;32: 248–50.

Moon RY, Greene MG, Rehe GT, et al: Poststreptococcal reactive arthritis in children: A potential predecessor of rheumatic heart disease. *J Rheumatol* 1995;22: 529–32.

Petty RE, Tingle AJ: Arthritis and viral infection. *J Pediatr* 1988;113:948–9.

Poggio TV, Orlando N, Galanternik L, et al: Microbiology of acute arthropathies among children in Argentina: *Mycoplasma pneumoniae* and *hominis* and *Ureaplasma urealyticum*. *Pediatr Infect Dis J* 1998;17:304–8.

Schaad UB: Reactive arthritis associated with *Campylobacter* enteritis. *Pediatr Infect Dis* 1982;1:328–32.

Tingle AJ, Allen M, Petty RE, et al: Rubella-associated arthritis. I. Comparative study of joint manifestations associated with natural rubella infection and RA 27/3 rubella immunisation. *Ann Rheum Dis* 1986;45:110–4.

Yin Z, Braun J, Neure L, et al: Crucial role of interleukin–10/interleukin–12 balance in the regulation of the type 2 T helper cytokine response in reactive arthritis. *Arthritis Rheum* 1997;40:1788–97.

Chapter 148
Systemic Lupus Erythematosus

Marisa S. Klein-Gitelman and Michael L. Miller

Systemic lupus erythematosus (SLE, or lupus), a rheumatic disease of unknown cause, is characterized by autoantibodies directed against self-antigens and resulting inflammatory damage to target organs including the kidneys, blood-forming cells, and the central nervous system (CNS). The natural history of SLE is unpredictable; patients may present with a history of many years of symptoms or with acute, life-threatening disease. Untreated SLE may be followed by spontaneous remission, years of smoldering disease, or rapid death. Because of its possible manifestations, SLE must be considered in the differential diagnosis of many problems, ranging from fevers of unknown origin to arthralgia, anemia, and nephritis. The initial presentation may be atypical such as parotitis, abdominal pain, transverse myelitis, or dizziness. Lupus should be considered in patients with multiorgan symptoms, usually with an abnormal complete blood count or urinalysis. Early diagnosis and treatment tailored to the particular problems of an individual patient can greatly improve the prognosis for what used to be a fatal disease.

Etiology. The cause and disease mechanisms of SLE remain unknown. Many factors, including genetics, hormones, and the environment, contribute to the immune dysregulation in lupus. The hallmark is autoantibody production against many self-antigens, particularly DNA, as well as other nuclear antigens, ribosomes, platelets, coagulation factors, immunoglobulin, erythrocytes, and leukocytes. Elevated levels of autoantibodies, particularly anti–double-stranded DNA antibodies, are associated with circulating and tissue-bound immune complexes that lead to complement fixation and recruitment of inflammatory cells, and then to tissue injury.

Polyclonal activation of B lymphocytes results in elevated immunoglobulin levels, which may be one cause of elevated autoantibody levels. The mechanism for polyclonal activation is not yet understood. Possible causes include nonspecific response to an antigenic stimulus such as a viral agent or loss of tolerance to self-antigens by loss of suppressor T-lymphocyte function. Investigations have focused on the normal phenomenon of **apoptosis**, or programmed cell death, which is regulated by several proteins including *fas* and *bcl*-2. Dysregulation of apoptosis in SLE may lead to the presence of self-reactive lymphocytes that normally undergo apoptosis before birth.

Other mechanisms may have a role in amplifying the manifestations of SLE. Defects in macrophage phagocytosis and handling of immune complexes have been described. The effects of sex hormones may be responsible for the predominance of females with SLE; one study found higher follicle-stimulating hormone and luteinizing hormone levels and lower free androgen levels in postpubertal boys and girls with SLE. SLE has been associated with complement abnormalities including C1q, C2, and C4 deficiency, a high incidence of C4 null genes, and abnormal complement receptors. Exposure to the ultraviolet rays in sunlight can exacerbate SLE manifestations, perhaps through damage to nuclear material, resulting in release of DNA, which complexes with circulating anti-DNA antibodies.

Genetic associations in SLE are suggested by the frequent findings of antinuclear antibodies (ANAs), hypergammaglobulinemia, and SLE or other autoimmune diseases in family members of patients with SLE. Some HLA types (e.g., HLA-B8, HLA-DR2, and HLA-DR3) may occur with increased frequency among patients with SLE, depending on the racial and ethnic backgrounds of patients studied. **Drug-induced lupus** is a lupus-like disease that occurs after exposure to certain drugs, notably anticonvulsants, sulfonamides, and antiarrhythmic agents. Their similar structure to histone proteins may be one cause, because antihistone antibodies are found in many patients with drug-induced lupus.

Epidemiology. The incidence of SLE is not known but varies by location and ethnicity. Prevalence rates of 4–250/100,000 have been reported, with decreased prevalence in white compared with Native American, Asian, Latin, and black American patients. Although onset before age 8 yr is unusual, SLE has been diagnosed during the 1st year of life. Female predominance varies from less than 4:1 before puberty to 8:1 afterward.

Pathogenesis. Fibrinoid deposits are found in blood vessel walls of affected organs, whose parenchyma may contain hematoxylin bodies, most likely representing degenerated cell nuclei. Rheumatoid nodules and granulomas are also sometimes found in affected tissues.

Clinical Manifestations. Patients can present with various manifestations (Table 148–1). Children most frequently present with fever, fatigue, arthralgia or arthritis, and rash. Symptoms may be intermittent or persistent. A detailed history and physical and laboratory examination can facilitate early diagnosis and treatment.

Cutaneous manifestations are frequently present. The characteristic **malar or butterfly rash** includes the nasal bridge and varies from an erythematous blush to thickened epidermis to scaly patches (Fig. 148–1). Rashes may be photosensitive and extend to all sun-exposed areas. Mucous membrane changes from vasculitic erythema to ulcers occur, particularly on palatal and nasal mucosa (Fig. 148–2). Discoid lesions are unusual in childhood. However, they occur more frequently as a manifestation of SLE than as discoid lupus erythematosis (DLE) alone; 2–3% of all DLE occurs in childhood. Other cutaneous manifestations include vasculitic-appearing erythematous macular eruptions (particularly on fingers, palms, and soles), purpura,

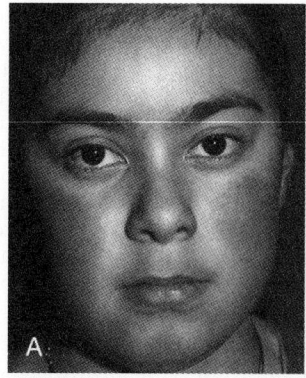
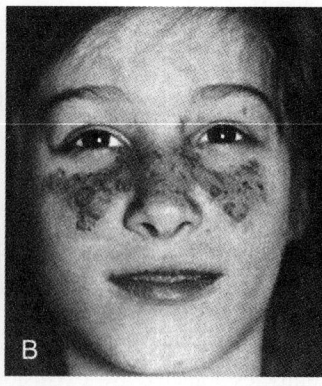

FIGURE 148–1. The butterfly rash of systemic lupus erythematosus. The rash can vary from an erythematous blush (*A*) to thickened epidermis to scaly patches (*B*). See also color plates.

livedo reticularis (Fig. 148–3), and Raynaud phenomenon. Less common findings include subacute psoriasiform or annular skin lesions, bullous lesions, and alopecia.

Musculoskeletal findings include arthralgia, arthritis, tendinitis, and myositis. Deforming arthritis is unusual; hand arthritis can lead to ligament damage and severely lax joints. Osteonecrosis of bone is common and is presumed to be secondary to vasculopathy or corticosteroid treatment.

Serositis can affect pleural, pericardial, and peritoneal surfaces. Hepatosplenomegaly and lymphadenopathy are often found. Other gastrointestinal manifestations, most often resulting from vasculitis, include pain, diarrhea, infarction and melena, inflammatory bowel disease, and hepatitis. Cardiac involvement may affect all cardiac tissues and include valvular thickening and verrucous endocarditis (Libman-Sacks disease), cardiomegaly, myocarditis, conduction abnormalities, heart failure, and coronary artery vasculitis and thrombosis. Pulmonary manifestations include acute pulmonary hemorrhage, pulmonary infiltrates (sometimes with superimposed infection), and chronic fibrosis.

Neurologic manifestations can include the CNS and peripheral nervous system (see Table 148–1). It is likely that many patients with SLE experience memory loss or other cognitive dysfunction during their disease course. Neuropsychiatric manifestations can be severe, and patients may fulfill Diagnostic and

TABLE 148–1. Presenting Manifestations of Systemic Lupus Erythematosus

Target Organ	Manifestations
Constitutional	Fatigue, anorexia, weight loss, prolonged fever, lymphadenopathy
Musculoskeletal	Arthralgias, arthritis
Skin	Malar rash, discoid lesions, livedo reticularis
Renal	Glomerulonephritis, nephrotic syndrome, hypertension, renal failure
Cardiovascular	Pericarditis (cardiac tamponade)
Neurologic	Seizures, psychosis, stroke, cerebral venous thrombosis, pseudotumor cerebri, aseptic meningitis, chorea, global cognitive deficits, mood disorders, transverse myelitis, peripheral neuritis
Pulmonary	Pleuritic pain, pulmonary hemorrhage
Hematologic	Coombs-positive hemolytic anemia, anemia of chronic disease, thrombocytopenia, leukopenia

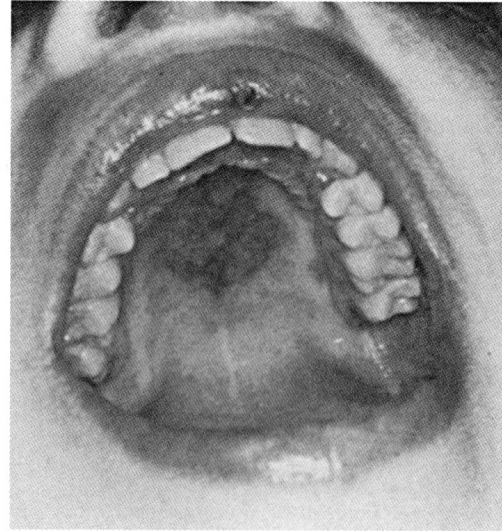

FIGURE 148–2. Erythematous lesion involving the hard palate in a patient with systemic lupus erythematosus. (From Moschella S, Hurley H [editors]: *Dermatology*, 3rd ed. Philadelphia, WB Saunders, 1992.)

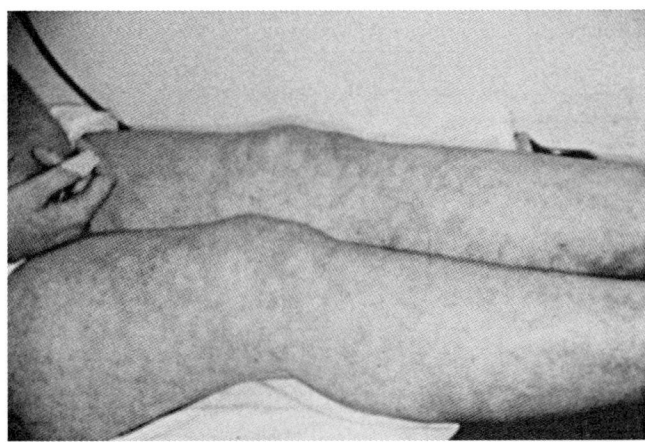

FIGURE 148–3. Livedo reticularis. Lacelike bluish, purplish, or erythematous discoloration of the skin indicating vascular instability. (From Moschella S, Hurley H [editors]: *Dermatology*, 3rd ed. Philadelphia, WB Saunders, 1992.)

Statistical Manual of Mental Disorders (DSM IV) criteria for psychosis. MRI and CT images may be normal although abnormal single-photon emission CT images occur frequently. The occurrence of arterial or venous thrombosis (Fig. 148–4), suggestive of antiphospholipid antibody syndrome, can occur in any organ and can be associated with recurrent fetal loss, livedo reticularis, thrombocytopenia, and Raynaud phenomenon. Thrombotic events can also be associated with the presence of lupus anticoagulant and acquired, activated protein C resistance.

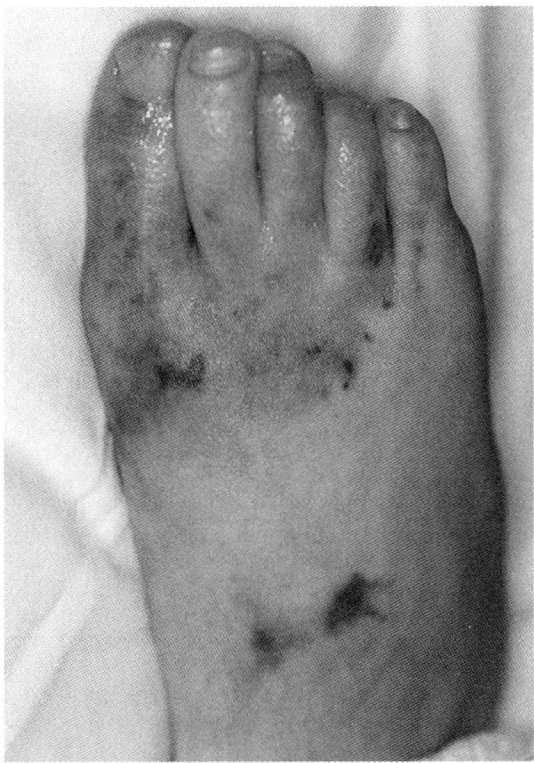

FIGURE 148–4. A 12-yr-old girl with systemic lupus erythematosus and antiphospholipid antibodies with painful cutaneous vasculitis of the right foot. Arterial thrombosis documented by angiography resulted in cyanosis of the large toe. Symptoms resolved with treatment with heparin and corticosteroids. See also clor plates.

Renal disease is manifest by hypertension, peripheral edema, retinal vascular changes, and clinical manifestations associated with electrolyte abnormalities, nephrosis, or acute renal failure (see Chapter 505).

Diagnosis. The diagnosis is confirmed by the combination of clinical and laboratory manifestations revealing multisystem disease. Criteria for the diagnosis of SLE require the presence of 4 of 11 criteria serially or simultaneously (Table 148–2). In 1997, criteria were revised to exclude LE prep and replace it with anti-cardiolipin antibodies or a positive test for lupus anticoagulant; however, this change has not been validated. A positive ANA test result is not required for diagnosis; however, absence of ANA is rare. Patients suspected to have lupus, even if with less than 4 criteria, should receive appropriate medical treatment. Hypocomplementemia is not diagnostic; extremely low levels or absence of total hemolytic complement suggests the possibility of complement component deficiency. Renal biopsy is used to confirm diagnosis of lupus nephritis and to determine treatment.

Laboratory Findings. Elevated ANA titers are often present in children with active SLE. This is an excellent screening tool, although ANA can be found without any disease or can be associated with rheumatic and other conditions (Table 148–3). Levels of anti–double-stranded DNA, which are more specific for lupus, reflect the degree of disease activity. Serum levels of total hemolytic complement (CH_{50}), C3, and C4 are decreased in active disease and provide a second measure of disease activity. Anti-Smith antibody, found specifically in patients with SLE, does not measure disease activity. When present, anti-SSA and anti-SSB antibodies are rarely associated with Sjögren syndrome. Many autoantibodies can be found (Table 148–4). Hypergammaglobulinemia is also frequent.

Treatment. The treatment regimen depends on the affected target organs and disease severity. Patients are treated to support clinical well-being, using serologic markers of disease activity as guidelines, including serum complement levels. Nonsteroidal anti-inflammatory agents, used to treat arthralgia and arthritis, are used with caution because patients with SLE are more susceptible to hepatotoxicity. The antimalarial agent hydroxychloroquine may be used to treat mild manifestations, including skin lesions, fatigue, arthritis, and arthralgia.

Patients with thrombosis and antiphospholipid antibodies or a lupus anticoagulant should receive anticoagulant medication at least until SLE is in remission. The length of therapy is controversial. Low molecular weight heparin is the anticoagulant of choice; however, warfarin can also be used.

Corticosteroids have been demonstrated to control symptoms and autoantibody production in SLE. Treatment with corticosteroids has improved kidney disease and the rate of survival. Corticosteroids, however, can make diagnosis of tuberculosis difficult; all patients should have PPD and control skin tests, when possible, before corticosteroids are initiated. The optimal dose and route of administration of corticosteroids are controversial. Patients with systemic disease are often started on 1–2 mg/kg/24 hr of oral prednisone in divided daily doses. When complement levels increase to within the normal range, the dose is carefully tapered over 2–3 yr to the lowest effective dose. One method is to use alternate-day high-dose corticosteroids to prevent the adverse effects of daily corticosteroid administration. Severely ill patients may require pulse intravenous corticosteroid therapy (30 mg/kg/dose, maximum 1 g, given over 60 min once per day, for 3 days). Intermittent high-dose intravenous therapy in combination with low-dose daily oral corticosteroids has been used as an alternative regimen in some centers. Adverse effects of corticosteroids include hypertension, gastritis, cataracts, osteopenia, and cushingoid body habitus.

TABLE 148–2. **1982 Revised Criteria for Diagnosis of Systemic Lupus Erythematosus**

Criterion*	Definition
Malar rash	Fixed erythema, flat or raised, over the malar eminences, tending to spare the nasolabial folds
Discoid rash	Erythematous raised patches with adherent keratotic scaling and follicular plugging; atrophic scarring may occur in older lesions
Photosensitivity	Rash as a result of unusual reaction to sunlight (elicited by patient history or physician observation)
Oral ulcers	Oral or nasopharyngeal ulceration, usually painless, observed by a physician
Arthritis	Nonerosive arthritis involving two or more peripheral joints, characterized by tenderness, swelling, or effusion
Serositis	Pleuritis—convincing history of pleuritic pain or rub heard by a physician or evidence of pleural effusion or Pericarditis—documented by ECG or rub or evidence of pericardial effusion
Renal disorder	Persistent proteinuria > 0.5 g/day or > 3-plus (+ + +) if quantitation not performed or Cellular casts—may be red blood cell, hemoglobin, granular, tubular, or mixed
Neurologic disorder	Seizures—in the absence of offending drugs or known metabolic derangements (e.g., uremia, ketoacidosis, or electrolyte imbalance) or Psychosis—in the absence of offending drugs or known metabolic derangements (e.g., uremia, ketoacidosis, or electrolyte imbalance)
Hematologic disorder	Hemolytic anemia—with reticulocytosis or Leukopenia—< 4,000/mm^3 total on two or more occasions or Lymphopenia—< 1,500/mm^3 on two or more occasions or Thrombocytopenia—< 100,000/mm^3
Immunologic disorder	Positive LE cell preparation or Anti-DNA antibody to native DNA in abnormal titer or Anti-Sm—presence of antibody to Sm nuclear antigen or False-positive serologic test result for syphilis known to be positive for at least 6 mo and confirmed by *Treponema pallidum* immobilization or fluorescent treponemal antibody absorption test
Antinuclear antibody	An abnormal titer of antinuclear antibody by immunofluorescence or an equivalent assay at any time and in the absence of drugs known to be associated with "drug-induced lupus syndrome"

The proposed classification is based on 11 criteria. For the purpose of identifying patients in clinical studies, a person shall be said to have systemic lupus erythematosus if any 4 or more of the 11 criteria are present, serially or simultaneously, during any interval of observation.
From Tan EM, Cohen AS, Fries JF, et al: The 1982 revised criteria for the classification of systemic lupus erythematosus. Arthritis Rheum 1982;25:1271–7.
A proposed modification deletes the positive LE cell preparation from the immunologic disorder criteria and substitutes the presence of antiphospholipid antibodies for a biologic false-positive test for syphilis (Hochberg MC: Updating the American College of Rheumatology revised criteria for the classification of systemic lupus erythematosus. Arthritis Rheum 1997;40:1725).

Patients with severe disease may require cytotoxic therapy. Pulse intravenous cyclophosphamide has maintained renal function and prevented progression in patients with lupus nephritis, particularly diffuse proliferative glomerulonephritis; however, the optimal length of therapy remains controversial. Cyclophosphamide has been used to treat vasculitis, pulmonary hemorrhage, and CNS disease refractory to corticosteroids. Azathioprine has been used to prevent renal disease progression. Little is known about the long-term sequelae of cytotoxic medications, particularly in children. Adverse effects include secondary infections, gonadal dysfunction, and possibly increased risk of malignancies later in life. Prepubertal children, compared with those who have entered puberty, may be at less risk for subsequent gonadal dysfunction from cytotoxic agents.

Other interventions are being proposed for the treatment of SLE. The role of methotrexate, cyclosporine, and mycophenolate mofetil remains undetermined. Hormonal therapy and autologous and cord stem cell marrow transplantation for patients with severe, persistent disease are undergoing clinical trials in adult patients with SLE. Biologic agents that target cytokine production are also being developed and studied.

The extent of renal involvement may be out of proportion to findings on urinalysis, and renal biopsy for staging can help determine whether an immunosuppressive agent such as cyclophosphamide needs to be added to a corticosteroid regimen (see Chapter 505). Biopsy findings according to the World Health Organization classification correlate with morbidity and mortality. Class I is defined as the absence of abnormalities on light microscopy, immunofluorescence studies, and electron microscopy. Class IIA shows minimal immunoglobulin and complement deposition in mesangium on immunofluorescence and is associated with good prognosis for renal function. Class

TABLE 148–3. **Conditions Associated with Antinuclear Antibodies (ANAs)**

Systemic lupus erythematosus	Scleroderma
Drug-induced lupus	Infectious mononucleosis
Juvenile arthritis	Chronic active hepatitis
Juvenile dermatomyositis	Hyperextensibility
Vasculitis syndromes	

TABLE 148–4. **Autoantibodies Found in Systemic Lupus Erythematosus**

Antibody	Manifestation
Coombs antibodies	Hemolytic anemia
Antiphospholipid antibodies	Antiphospholipid antibody syndrome
Lupus anticoagulant	Coagulopathy
Antithyroid antibodies	Hypothyroidism
Antiribosomal P antibody	Lupus cerebritis

IIB (mesangial glomerulonephritis) shows increased lymphocytic infiltration of the mesangium and has a variable prognosis; it occasionally progresses to more extensive renal involvement. Class III (focal and segmental proliferative glomerulonephritis) is characterized by focal, segmental proliferation of cells near capillaries, with necrosis and lymphocytic infiltration, and is often associated with chronic renal disease. Class IV (diffuse proliferative glomerulonephritis) shows a majority of each glomerulus affected by cellular infiltration, mesangial cellular proliferation, and crescent formation corresponding to scarring and has been correlated with increased risk for developing end-stage renal disease in adulthood; intravenous pulse cyclophosphamide can decrease this risk. Class V disease (membranous glomerulonephritis) shows thickened capillary walls on light microscopy and subepithelial deposits on electron microscopy along the basement membrane. These changes have been associated with proteinuria, which can occur with the other types of lupus nephritis, and variable chronic renal disease, often poorly responsive to treatment.

The most important aspect of management of SLE is meticulous and frequent re-evaluation of patients. This includes clinical and laboratory evaluation, especially for renal and serologic flare of disease. Prompt recognition and treatment of disease flare is essential to patient outcome. Lupus is a lifelong illness, and patients must be monitored indefinitely.

Complications and Prognosis. Childhood SLE was initially viewed as a uniformly fatal disease. With progress in diagnosis and treatment, the 5-yr survival rate is greater than 90%. However, a significant proportion of patients die later of the disease. Major causes of death in patients with SLE currently include infection, nephritis, CNS disease, pulmonary hemorrhage, and myocardial infarction; the latter complication may be a result of chronic corticosteroid administration in the setting of immune complex disease.

148.1 Neonatal Lupus

Lupus in newborns results from maternal transfer of IgG autoantibodies, usually anti-Ro, between the 12th and 16th wk of gestation. Manifestations include congenital heart block, cutaneous lesions, hepatitis, thrombocytopenia, neutropenia, and pulmonary and neurologic disease. Cutaneous lesions occur after ultraviolet exposure at about 6 wk of life and last 3–4 mo. The rash most frequently occurs on the face and scalp; 25% of rashes scar. Treatment is supportive. Most manifestations resolve, although congenital heart block is permanent and often requires cardiac pacing, either after birth or, when detected and severe, antenatally. Even infants of mothers with lupus who are asymptomatic may have slightly prolonged PR intervals. Cardiomyopathy is a rare serious sequela, sometimes requiring heart transplantation.

Neonatal lupus must be distinguished from **infantile multisystem inflammatory disease**, a rare syndrome characterized by fever, rash, arthropathy, chronic meningitis, seizures, uveitis, and lymphadenopathy. This syndrome is difficult to treat and usually requires long-term immunosuppression.

Arisaka O, Obinata K, Sasaki H, et al: Chorea as an initial manifestation of systemic lupus erythematosus. A case report of a 10-year-old girl. *Clin Pediatr* 1984;23: 298–300.

Barron KS, Silverman ED, Gonzales J, et al: Clinical, serologic and immunogenetic studies in childhood-onset systemic lupus erythematosus. *Arthritis Rheum* 1993; 36:348–54.

De Cunto CL, Liberatore DI, San Roman JL, et al: Infantile-onset multisystem inflammatory disease: A differential diagnosis of systemic juvenile rheumatoid arthritis. *J Pediatr* 1997;130:551–6.

Dungan DD, Jay MS: Stroke in an early adolescent with systemic lupus erythematosus and coexistent antiphospholipid antibodies. *Pediatrics* 1992;90:96–9.

Eberhard BA, Laxer RM, Eddy AA, et al: Presence of thyroid abnormalities in children with systemic lupus erythematosus. *J Pediatr* 1991;119:277–9.

Gazarian M, Feldman BM, Benson LN, et al: Assessment of myocardial perfusion and function in childhood systemic lupus erythematosus. *J Pediatr* 1998;132: 109–16.

Hochberg MC: Updating the American College of Rheumatology revised criteria for the classification of systemic lupus erythematosus. *Arthritis Rheum* 1997;40: 1725.

Lane AT, Watson RM: Neonatal lupus. *Am J Dis Child* 1984;138:663–6.

Lehman TJ, Sherry DD, Wagner-Weiner L, et al: Intermittent intravenous cyclophosphamide therapy for lupus nephritis. *J Pediatr* 1989;114:1055–60.

Lehman TJ, McCurdy DK, Bernstein BH, et al: Systemic lupus erythematosus in the first decade of life. *Pediatrics* 1989;83:235–9.

Lehman TJ, Hanson V, Singsen BH, et al: The role of antibodies directed against double-stranded DNA in the manifestations of systemic lupus erythematosus in childhood. *J Pediatr* 1980;96:657–61.

Miller RW, Salcedo JR, Fink RJ, et al: Pulmonary hemorrhage in pediatric patients with systemic lupus erythematosus. *J Pediatr* 1986;108:576–9.

Reed BR, Lee LA, Harmon C, et al: Autoantibodies to SS-A/Ro in infants with congenital heart block. *J Pediatr* 1983;103:889–91.

Seaman DE, Londino AV Jr, Kwoh CK, et al: Antiphospholipid antibodies in pediatric systemic lupus erythematosus. *Pediatrics* 1995;96:1040–5.

Silverman E: What's new in the treatment of pediatric SLE? *J Rheumatol* 1996; 23:1657–60.

Tucker LB, Menon S, Schaller JG, et al: Adult- and childhood-onset systemic lupus erythematosus: A comparison of onset, clinical features, serology and outcome. *Br J Rheumatol* 1995;34:866–72.

Uziel Y, Laxer RM, Blaser S, et al: Cerebral vein thrombosis in childhood systemic lupus erythematosus. *J Pediatr* 1995;126:722–7.

Chapter 149
Juvenile Dermatomyositis
Lauren M. Pachman

Juvenile dermatomyositis (JDM), the most common of the pediatric inflammatory myopathies, is a systemic vasculopathy with characteristic cutaneous findings and focal areas of myositis resulting in progressive proximal muscle weakness that is responsive to the prompt institution of immunosuppressive therapy.

Etiology. The disease appears to be triggered by an antigen driven response in the genetically susceptible child who is positive for the HLA antigen DQA1*0501. The putative agent may be associated with episodic disease, because clusters of new cases of JDM have been observed. Enterovirus (coxsackievirus B) has been implicated in new-onset JDM, both in the United Kingdom by RNA detection and in the United States by elevation in complement-fixing and neutralizing antibody titers. JDM has also followed documented infection with group A *Streptococcus*. Case-control serologic investigations have not substantiated an association of JDM with other potential infectious triggers such as *Toxoplasma gondii*, herpes simplex virus, or hepatitis B. In addition, the gene expression profiles in muscle biopsies from untreated children with JDM (positive for DQA1*0501) show a marked up-regulation of genes induced by interferon (IFN)-α and IFN-β, supporting the concept of an antigen driven immune response.

Epidemiology. The incidence of JDM is 3.2/million children/yr, but there may be some annual variation, which is apparently similar for all racial groups, although 73% of the cases are in whites. The average age of onset is 6.7 yr; children with disease onset before age 7 yr may have a milder course. In the United States, the overall ratio of girls to boys is 2.3:1. Multiple cases of myositis in a kindred are rare, and familial autoimmune disease is not increased in JDM, in contradistinction to juvenile rheumatoid arthritis. Reports of seasonal association have not been verified, although clusters of new cases occur. The prevalence of JDM is difficult to determine because persistent symptoms such as mild skin involvement and loss of range of motion are often disregarded. The long-term consequences of low levels of disease activity have yet to be defined.

Pathogenesis. Disease susceptibility appears to be associated with the class II HLA antigen DQA1*0501, which is found in more than 80% of JDM children in the United States. A chronic disease course appears to be associated with a substitution of an A for a G in the -308 promoter region of the gene for TNF-α. Children who have the TNF-α-308A allele, compared to JDM children without this allele, frequently have increased cellular production of TNF-α, a chronic disease course, requiring immunosuppressive therapy for >36 mo, as well as an increased frequency of pathologic calcifications.

Endothelial cell activation by the putative antigen and/or immune complexes is accompanied by complement activation and release of von Willebrand factor antigen from the damaged endothelium. Occlusion of capillaries and arterioles with local infarction of tissue, perifascicular atrophy, and a mononuclear cellular infiltrate confirm the histologic diagnosis of JDM. New-onset, untreated JDM has four times as many CD56 natural killer (NK) cells in the muscle as in matched peripheral blood, suggesting a role for NK cells. Other T-cell subsets are also represented in diseased muscle; the number of monocytes/macrophages (CD14) correlates with serum levels of neopterin, a macrophage-derived T-cell factor. Extensive fibrosis leads to loss of range of motion. In affected skin, the epidermis thins and the dermis demonstrates edema and vascular inflammation.

Clinical Manifestations. Disease onset is often insidious; constitutional symptoms of fatigue, low-grade fever, weight loss, and irritability are common as are arthralgia and abdominal pain. The characteristic rash appears first in 25% of cases, or at the same time that weakness is recognized in another 50% of children. The rash is prominent in sun-exposed areas, and proximal muscle weakness is usually recognized after a median of 2 mo. Periorbital violaceous (heliotropic) erythema (**heliotrope eyelids**) may cross the nasal bridge (Fig. 149–1). Periorbital edema may be present; edema may be generalized. The rash may involve the upper torso, the extensor surfaces of the arms and legs, the medial malleoli of the ankles, and the buttocks. Facial edema and eyelid telangiectasia occur in 50–90% of cases. Partial baldness is a consequence of chronic scalp inflammation. The skin over the metacarpal and proximal interphalangeal joints may be hypertrophic and reddish pink (**Gottron papules**) during active disease, with a papular, alligator skin–like appearance (Fig. 149–2), which evolves into atrophic colorless bands. Children with an initial amyopathic form of JDM (with the rash only), if not appropriately treated, may develop myositis and subsequent calcinosis later in their disease course. Diffuse vasculopathy (e.g., nailbed telangiectasia, infarction of oral epithelium and skinfolds, digital or gastrointestinal ulceration) is clearly associated with more severe disease; healing may be accompanied by hyperpigmentation or vitiligo.

The onset of proximal muscle weakness is insidious and difficult to recognize. It is often detected by difficulty in climbing stairs, combing hair, or standing from a sitting position. The child cannot rise unassisted from the floor without "climbing up the body" (**Gowers sign**). Neck flexor weakness (inability to raise the head from the bed) or abdominal muscle weakness (inability to perform a sit-up) identifies inflamed muscles that are often tender on compression. Derangement of upper airway function can be detected by hoarseness, a nasal quality to the speech, or difficulty in handling secretions. Dysphagia is a severe prognostic sign and should prompt immediate aggressive therapeutic intervention. Complaints of constipation reflect impaired gastrointestinal (GI) smooth muscle function, and abdominal pain or diarrhea may indicate occult GI bleeding, which can progress and be life threatening. Cardiac involvement with conduction abnormality is frequent at diagnosis; dilated cardiomyopathy has been reported. Lymphadenopathy is not uncommon.

Children with antibody to the polymyositis/scleroderma (Pm/Scl) antigen often have bambooing of the digits with loss of

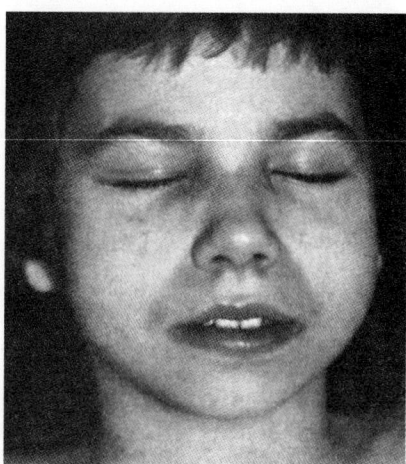

FIGURE 149–1. The facial rash of juvenile dermatomyositis. There is erythema over the bridge of the nose and malar areas, with violaceous (heliotropic) discoloration of the upper eyelids. See also color plates.

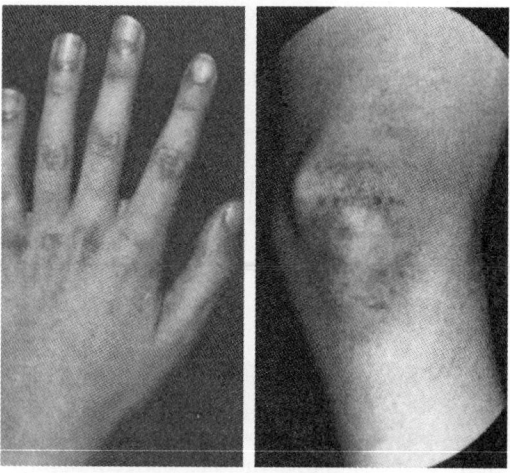

FIGURE 149–2. The rash of juvenile dermatomyositis. The skin over the metacarpal and proximal interphalangeal joints may be hypertrophic and pale red (Gottron papules). See also color plates.

cutaneous elasticity, similar to scleroderma. **Mechanic's hands**, with thickened skin, cuticle overgrowth, and range losses, are indicators of a subset of refractory inflammatory myopathy more common in adults, who may have severe lung involvement and characteristic circulating antibody (Jo–1) to tRNA synthetase.

Less frequent findings include hepatosplenomegaly, retinitis, iritis, central nervous system (CNS) involvement with seizures and depression, and evidence of renal impairment. Association with malignancy at disease onset is observed in adults with dermatomyositis, but not in children.

Diagnosis. The characteristic rash facilitates early diagnosis but should be differentiated from other connective tissue diseases such as systemic lupus erythematosus, scleroderma, or mixed connective tissue disease by both the specific antibody tests and clinical findings associated with each of these disorders. Careful examination of the nailfold capillaries usually documents periungual avascularity with capillary dropout. Those capillaries that remain are usually dilated and have the characteristic terminal bush formation (Fig. 149–3).

If the initial symptom is restricted to weakness, other causes of myopathy should be considered, including acute polymyositis

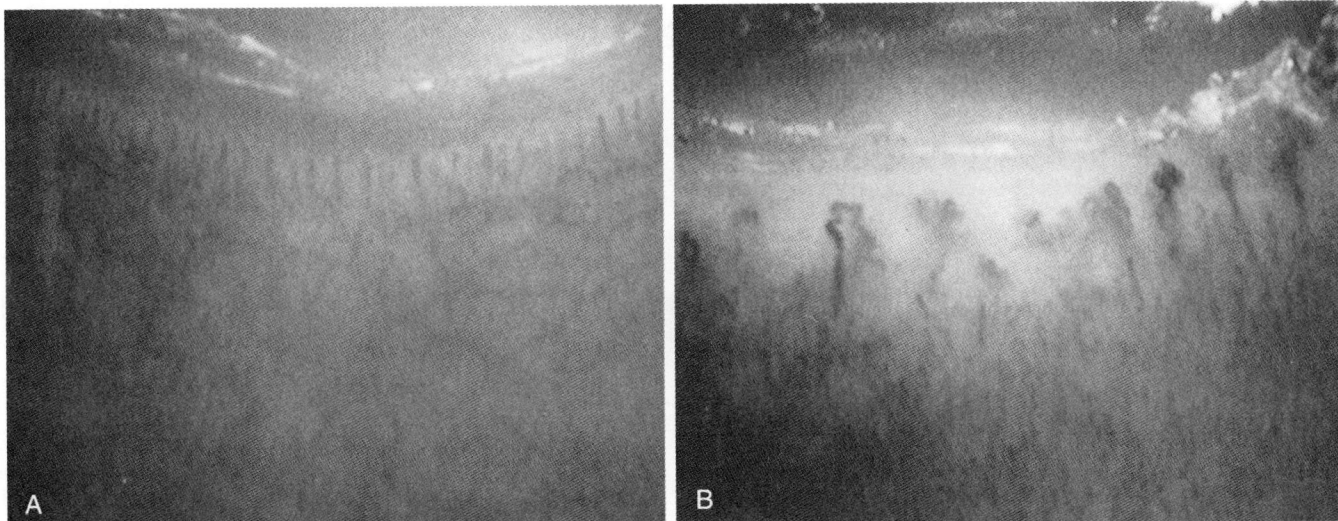

FIGURE 149-3. Nailfold capillary pattern in rheumatic diseases. *A*, Normal nailfold capillary pattern in a healthy child, with a homogeneous distribution and uniform appearance of capillary loops. *B*, The nailfold capillary pattern in a child with juvenile dermatomyositis that shows dropout of capillary end-loops, resulting in a wide band of avascularity. Dilated, tortuous capillaries are also seen, some with terminal bush formation that is found in patients with juvenile dermatomyositis, with scleroderma, and with Raynaud phenomenon that may progress to scleroderma.

associated with influenza B infection, the muscular dystrophies (including Duchenne and Becker muscular dystrophies), myasthenia gravis, Guillain-Barré syndrome, and endocrine or metabolic disorders. Infections associated with muscular symptoms, such as poliomyelitis, trichinosis, or toxoplasmosis, also should be considered. Blunt trauma and crush injuries may lead to transient rhabdomyolysis with myoglobinuria. Other events associated with myositis in children include vaccinations, drugs, growth hormone, and bone marrow transplantation, in which graft versus host myositis occurs as a component of immune activation (see Chapter 127).

Laboratory Findings. Elevated serum levels of muscle-derived enzymes (e.g. creatine kinase, aldolase, serum glutamic-oxaloacetic transaminase, and lactic acid dehydrogenase) reflect the leaky muscle membranes. Antinuclear antibody (ANA) with a speckled pattern (unknown specificity) is present in more than 60% of children, whereas tests for antibodies to SSA, SSB, Sm, RNP, and DNA are negative. Other myositis-specific antibodies, which rarely occur in children, such as to signal recognition particle (SRP), identify children with a protracted disease course, often complicated by pulmonary interstitial fibrosis. Antibodies to Pm/Scl identify a subgroup of myopathies that may not completely resolve and may have cardiac involvement with tachycardia and elevated troponin levels. The erythrocyte sedimentation rate is usually normal, with a Coombs-negative anemia, and the rheumatoid factor is negative.

Indicators of immunologic activation in JDM include increased percentage of peripheral blood CD19 B cells (despite being lymphopenic), and an elevated CD4:CD8 ratio, with decreased CD8 cells, which home to the muscle. In about two thirds of cases there is an increase in levels of von Willebrand factor antigen (vWF:Ag , adjusted for blood group ranges), which is released by damaged endothelial cells, or increased neopterin, which is released by activated macrophages.

MRI using T2 weighted images and fat suppression (Fig. 149-4) can localize the active site of disease for diagnostic muscle biopsy and electromyogram, both of which are nondiagnostic in 20% of instances if not directed by MRI. Extensive rash and abnormal MRI findings are not uncommon despite normal serum levels of muscle-derived enzymes. Muscle biopsy often demonstrates evidence of disease activity and chronicity that is not suspected from the levels of the serum enzymes alone.

A rehabilitation cookie swallow can document significant palatorespiratory dysfunction and an unprotected airway. Pulmonary function testing of the diffusion capacity of the lung for carbon monoxide (DL_{CO}), which can be used for children older than 6 yr, detects decreased respiratory muscle strength as well as alveolar fibrosis associated with other connective tissue diseases. Active disease is frequently associated with decreased bone density with abnormal findings on densitometry and low osteocalcin and vitamin D levels. Calcinosis is detected by plain radiographs.

Treatment. All children with JDM should use a sunscreen (free of *p*-aminobenzoic acid) that provides maximal protection against ultraviolet A and B, even in winter. Vitamin D, at the dose appropriate for weight, with a diet sufficient in calcium, repairs osteopenia and decreases the frequency of bone fracture.

The aid of an experienced pediatric rheumatologist is essential in assessing the need for therapeutic intervention. Children with only mild cutaneous findings, normal immune and serologic markers of disease activity, and a negative family history of color blindness may take hydroxychloroquine (maximum dose of 5 mg/kg/24 hr), with a low daily dose (about 1 mg/kg) of oral corticosteroids. These children should be monitored for the development of muscle involvement by careful physical examination which assesses pediatric muscle strength, as well as the laboratory testing for elevation of immune markers and serum muscle enzymes. If needed, a repeat MRI may identify new areas of muscle involvement.

With minimal muscle damage, oral corticosteroids (prednisone, 1–2 mg/kg/24 hr) may suffice. However, prompt institution of high-dose intermittent intravenous methylprednisolone therapy may rapidly normalize the muscle enzymes, and additional therapy is used if the indicators of inflammation (percentage of CD19 B cells, neopterin, vWf:Ag) remain elevated. Inhibitors of gastric acid secretion are usually also administered to minimize gastric bleeding. Pulse intravenous corticosteroid therapy (30 mg/kg/24 hr of methylprednisolone, not greater than 1 g daily, for 3 days) usually is initially given; thereafter, the frequency of methylprednisolone administration ranges from three times per week to once each week until all the indicators of inflammation normalize. Low-dose oral prednisone

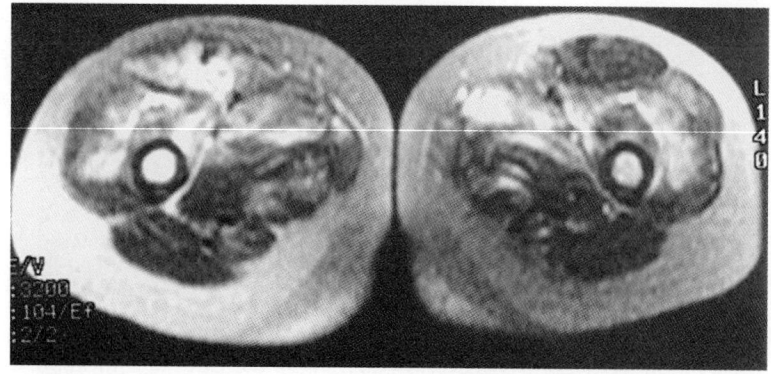

FIGURE 149–4. An MRI scan with T2 weighted image with fat suppression of the proximal muscle of the lower extremities of a child with juvenile dermatomyositis with normal muscle enzymes. There is focal inflammatory myopathy. The white areas reflect the inflammatory response in involved muscle; those areas that are darker are more normal. Identification of the involved areas by MRI aids in directing the location of the muscle biopsy or electromyogram.

(0.5 mg/kg/24 hr) is given on non-intravenous methylprednisolone days. Methotrexate can be added (15–20 mg/m^2) if laboratory values fail to normalize as rapidly as expected, but should be given in conjunction with folic acid (1 mg/24 hr). Cyclophosphamide (500 mg/m^2, given with mesna for bladder protection) is considered for children unresponsive to intravenous methylprednisolone and methotrexate. The associated immunosuppression may result in decreased levels of IgG (<300 mg/dL) and replacement immunoglobulin (0.4 g/kg/mo) may be required to help prevent infections. High-dose intravenous immunoglobulin may initially diminish cutaneous symptoms, but it is not clear that the disease course is altered. Cyclosporine has been successful in some resistant cases and appears to be helpful for primarily cutaneous involvement. Inhibitors of TNF-α have been tried in children with chronic disease with limited success, but may help those with limited range of motion.

Children with dysphagia require a soft diet or nasogastric feedings, if necessary, until treatment restores a functional, protected airway. In rare cases, a respirator and tracheostomy or even extracorporeal membrane oxygenation are required. Absorption of calories and medication may be impaired by extensive GI vasculitis, requiring parenteral hyperalimentation and intravenous administration of drugs. Renal damage secondary to massive creatinine excretion can be averted by appropriate intravenous hydration.

Physical and occupational therapy provide passive stretching early in the disease course and, once active inflammation has resolved, direct reconditioning of muscles to regain strength and range of motion. Bed rest is not indicated; weight bearing improves bone density. Social work services may help facilitate adjustment to the frustration of physical impairment in a previously active child.

Complications. Aspiration pneumonia is a frequent major complication associated with unrecognized impairment in swallowing fluids. Progressive bowel infarction can lead to perforation and death. Depression and mood swings are part of the disease spectrum of CNS involvement and may be accentuated by corticosteroid administration.

Calcinosis is present in about 20% of patients at diagnosis and is associated with increased morbidity and mortality. It is probably a consequence of disease chronicity, fostered by either delay in initiation of therapy or insufficient suppression of inflammation. The calcium deposits form primarily in subcutaneous tissue and fascia; they may drain a white cheesy material and resolve or serve as a nidus for infection (most frequently staphylococcal), which can progress to septicemia and death. Aggressive therapy at the time of diagnosis may be associated with decreased frequency of this unwelcome disease consequence.

Partial lipodystrophy develops in more than 10% of cases of chronic JDM. It is also associated with the TNF-α-308a allele and is characterized by (1) loss of subcutaneous fat on the extremities, giving a hypermuscular appearance; (2) acanthosis nigricans; (3) weakened abdominal muscles resulting in a potbelly appearance; and (4) abnormal glucose and lipid metabolism. Girls may lose their menses, and sterility may result if the onset of JDM is before puberty.

Prognosis. Before the advent of corticosteroids, one third of affected children died and another one third were disabled. The mortality rate is currently about 1%. Although the disease is classified as "chronic," little is known about the consequences of persistent vascular inflammation. The period of active symptoms has decreased from about 3.5 yr to less than 1.5 yr with more aggressive immunosuppressive therapy. Unlike many adults with inflammatory myopathies, children with JDM appear able to repair their vasculature and muscle damage, but follow-up biopsy studies await analysis. The impact of partial lipodystrophy on adult morbidity is not known. Overall, with newer tests to monitor inflammation and disease activity and guide more aggressive therapy, the prognosis for this illness has markedly improved.

Bohan A, Peter JB: Polymyositis and dermatomyositis (parts 1 and 2). *N Engl J Med* 1975;292:344–7,403–7.

Eisenstein DM, O'Gorman MR, Pachman LM: Correlations between change in disease activity and changes in peripheral blood lymphocyte subsets in patients with juvenile dermatomyositis. *J Rheumatol* 1997;24:1830–2.

Feldman BM, Reichlin M, Laxer RM, et al: Clinical significance of specific autoantibodies in juvenile dermatomyositis. *J Rheumatol* 1996;23:1794–7.

Mejlszenkier JD, Safran SE, Healy JJ, et al: The myositis of influenza. *Arch Neurol* 1973;29:441–3.

Mendez EP, Dyer A, Ramsey-Goldman R, et al: U.S. incidence of JDM 1995–1998 from the NIAMS Registry. *Arthritis Care Res* 2003 (in press).

Pachman LM, Hayford JR, Chung A, et al: Juvenile dermatomyositis at diagnosis: Clinical characteristics of 79 children. *J Rheumatol* 1998;25:1198–204.

Pachman LM, Hayford JR, Hochberg MC, et al: New-onset juvenile dermatomyositis: Comparisons with a healthy cohort and children with juvenile rheumatoid arthritis. *Arthritis Rheum* 1997;40:1526–33.

Reed AM, Picornel YJ, Harwood A, et al: Chimerism in children with juvenile dermatomyositis. *Lancet* 2000;356: 2156–7.

Rider LG, Miller FW: Classification and treatment of the juvenile idiopathic inflammatory myopathies. *Rheum Dis Clin North Am* 1997;23:619–21.

Tezak Z, Hoffman EP, Lutz JL, et al: Gene expression profiling in DQA1*0501+ children with untreated dermatomyositis: A novel model of pathogenesis. *J Immunol* 2002;168:4154–63.

Chapter 150

Scleroderma *Michael L. Miller*

Scleroderma, a chronic disease of unknown cause, is characterized by fibrosis affecting the dermis and arteries of the lungs, kidneys, and gastrointestinal (GI) tract. Antinuclear antibodies (ANAs) specific for topoisomerase 1 (SCL70) and the centromere are found in many patients, which suggests that autoimmune processes play a role in pathogenesis. Scleroderma is classified according to the pattern of skin and internal organ involvement (Box 150–1).

SYSTEMIC SCLEROSIS

Diffuse: systemic widespread skin fibrosis, including proximal limbs, trunk, and face; early internal organ involvement
Limited (CREST): systemic distal skin involvement, often face, with late, if any, internal organ involvement
Overlap: sclerodermal skin changes with features of other connective tissue disorders

LOCALIZED SCLERODERMA

Morphea
Generalized morphea
Linear scleroderma
    On face, forehead, or scalp (*coup de sabre*)
    On extremity

EOSINOPHILIC FASCIITIS

SECONDARY FORMS

Drug induced
Chemically induced

PSEUDOSCLERODERMA

From Uzie Y, Miller ML, Laxer RM: Scleroderma in children. *Pediatr Clin North Am* 1995;42:1171.

Epidemiology. Scleroderma is a rare disease. The peak age at onset for systemic sclerosis is 30–50 yr, with a female:male ratio of 3:1. Children represent fewer than 10% of all cases. The cause is unknown but appears to involve injury to vascular endothelium. Rare cases have been reported after exposure to polyvinyl chloride, bleomycin, and pentazocine. Reports of scleroderma in adult women after breast implants may reflect nonrelated conditions, because medical devices (e.g., ventriculoperitoneal shunts) containing silicone have been implanted for many years without reports of similar complications. In children, localized scleroderma is more common than systemic sclerosis. The two forms usually do not overlap.

Pathogenesis. Scleroderma is associated with destruction of vascular endothelium and an increase in the basal lamina. During the initial stages of disease, lymphocytes, macrophages, mast cells, plasma cells, and eosinophils infiltrate the dermis. Factors released from activated platelets may play a role in Raynaud phenomenon and in triggering fibroblast proliferation that increases collagen synthesis, resulting in fibrosis of the dermis, subcutaneous fat, and sometimes muscle.

Studies suggest that a yet unidentified agent, or possibly subclinical graft versus host reaction from persisting cells of maternal origin, injures vascular endothelial cells, resulting in increased expression of adhesion molecules on their surfaces. These molecules entrap platelets and inflammatory cells, resulting in vascular changes of the type associated with such manifestations as Raynaud phenomenon, renovascular hypertension, and pulmonary hypertension. Recruitment of lymphocytes to areas of vascular damage may be the event that leads to specific autoantibody production in many patients. After these events, macrophages and other inflammatory cells appear to leave blood vessels and migrate into tissues affected in scleroderma. These cells secrete interleukin-1 (IL-1), causing platelets to release platelet-derived growth factor (PDGF). These and other molecules induce fibroblasts to reproduce and synthesize excessive amounts of collagen, resulting in fibrosis.

Clinical Manifestations. Raynaud phenomenon, resulting from digital arterial spasm, is often the earliest manifestation and may precede extensive skin and internal organ involvement by months or years. Raynaud phenomenon, which is induced by exposure to cold, affects the fingers, toes, and occasionally the ears and the tip of the nose. It has three stages: pallor, cyanosis, and finally erythema. Two of three stages are considered sufficient for identifying this manifestation. Episodes can vary in duration from minutes to hours.

SYSTEMIC SCLEROSIS. Systemic sclerosis often presents with a preliminary edematous phase that can last several months before chronic fibrosis develops. These early changes include puffiness around the fingers, on the dorsum of the hands, and sometimes on the face. An eventual decrease in edema is associated with tightening of the skin. Skin changes tend to spread proximally from the hands. Loss of subcutaneous tissue in the face can result in a small oral stoma with decreased distance between the upper and lower teeth when the mouth is opened wide (Fig. 150–1). Skin ulceration over pressure points, such as the elbows, may be associated with subcutaneous calcifications. Later, atrophic skin can become shiny and waxy in appearance. Loss of tissue at the fingertips may be associated with ulceration if Raynaud phenomenon is severe (Fig. 150–2). The distal phalanges may exhibit **acro-osteolysis,** or resorption of the distal tufts. The fingers take on a tapered appearance associated with tightened skin (**sclerodactyly**) and eventual development of secondary and often severe flexion contractures and limitation of motion (Fig. 150–3). As lesions spread proximally, flexion contractures in the elbows, hips, and knees may be associated with secondary muscle weakness and atrophy. Other chronic changes include epidermal thinning, hair loss, and decreased sweating. Hyperpigmented postinflammatory changes surrounded by atrophic depigmentation may give a salt-and-pepper appearance to some skin lesions. Over a period of years, remodeling of lesions sometimes results in focal improvement in skin thickening at the same time fibrosis extends elsewhere.

Pulmonary disease includes arterial and interstitial involvement and can vary from minimal disease to a progressive course that eventually results in decreased exercise tolerance, dyspnea at rest, and right-sided heart failure. Chest roentgenograms may appear normal early in the course. Evidence of early involvement may be found only by performing pulmonary function tests, including evaluation of oxygen diffusion by diffusion of carbon monoxide capacity (DLCO). High-resolution CT may also detect changes associated with interstitial disease before they become apparent on chest roentgenograms.

Scleroderma can also affect other organs. Renal arterial disease can cause chronic or severe episodic hypertension. Esophageal dilatation caused by fibrosis can cause dysphagia.

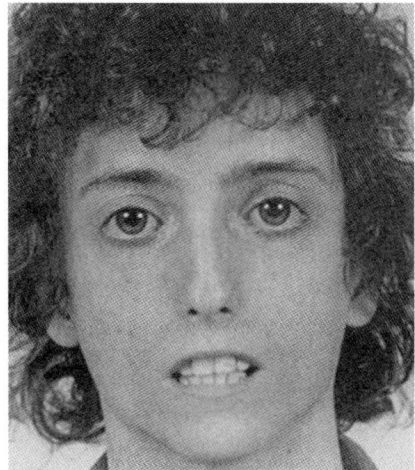

FIGURE 150–1. Facial changes in a 16-yr-old boy with scleroderma. There is a small mouth with puckering of the lips, pinched nose, and hyperpigmentation of the neck. (From Uziel Y, Miller ML, Laxer RM: Scleroderma in children. *Pediatr Clin North Am* 1995;42:1177.)

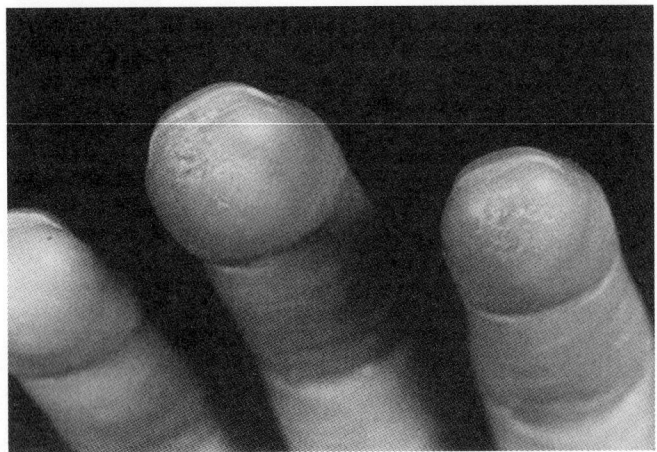

FIGURE 150–2. Tiny digital pitting scars and loss of pulp space resulting from digital ischemia in a 15-yr-old boy with scleroderma. (From Uziel Y, Miller ML, Laxer RM: Scleroderma in children. *Pediatr Clin North Am* 1995;42:1178.)

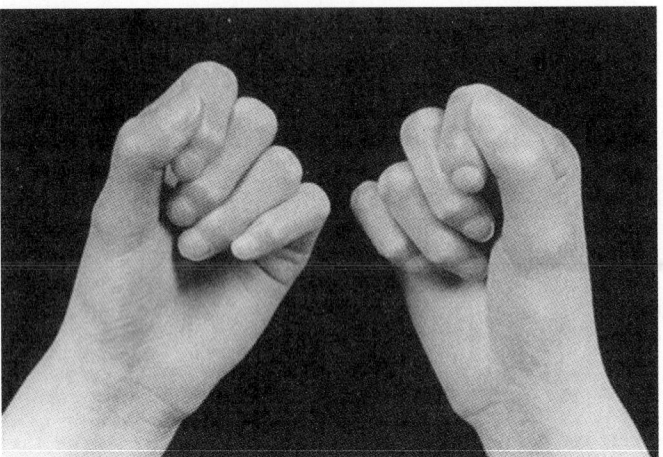

FIGURE 150–3. Inability to make a full fist due to skin and soft tissue tightening in a 10-yr-old girl with scleroderma. (From Uziel Y, Miller ML, Laxer RM: Scleroderma in children. *Pediatr Clin North Am* 1995;42:1176.)

Dilated intestinal loops can result in malabsorption and failure to thrive. Cardiac fibrosis has been associated with arrhythmias, ventricular hypertrophy, and decreased cardiac function.

Scleroderma can present with less extensive involvement. In limited systemic scleroderma, children have less prominent fibrosis that is limited to the distal extremities, face, and neck. Telangiectasias may appear on the fingertips, face, chest wall, and inner surface of lips. The **CREST syndrome** refers to the manifestations of calcinosis, Raynaud phenomenon, esophageal involvement, sclerosis of the skin, and telangiectasias. Severe pulmonary hypertension develops in some patients with CREST syndrome.

MORPHEA AND LINEAR SCLERODERMA. In localized scleroderma, the involvement is restricted to the skin; progression to systemic sclerosis is rare. In children with **morphea**, a form of localized scleroderma, lesions are typically discrete and may occur anywhere on the body but particularly on the face. Early inflammation is followed by indurated, depigmented, atrophic lesions. Children with **linear scleroderma** have lesions affecting the length of extremities; these lesions vary in size from several centimeters to the entire length of the extremity. Fibrosis in the dermis can sometimes extend to muscle, resulting in some instances in total loss of muscle tissue between

the dermis and bone. Resulting leg-length discrepancies, joint flexion contractures (Fig. 150–4), or cosmetic deformities of the face, forehead, or scalp with scarring alopecia (coup de sabre) may require surgical intervention.

Diagnosis. Scleroderma should be suspected in children who develop Raynaud phenomenon followed by skin changes suggestive of sclerodactyly. If Raynaud phenomenon is present for years before classic disease expression, ANA (particularly anti-SCL70) are typically found. Subclinical pulmonary fibrosis, suspected if decreased DLCO is found on pulmonary function testing, may be confirmed by high-resolution CT. Nailfold capillaroscopy of patients with Raynaud phenomenon before progression of disease may reveal a loss of capillaries or abnormal capillary dilatation resulting from vasculopathy (see Fig. 149–3).

According to diagnostic criteria used in adults, the diagnosis of scleroderma requires the presence of the single major criterion (sclerodermatous skin changes proximal to the metacarpophalangeal or metatarsophalangeal joints) or two of the three minor criteria (Box 150–2). The evaluation in these patients should include pulmonary function tests, contrast studies of the upper GI tract to evaluate esophageal motility, and echocardiography to identify pulmonary arterial hypertension.

DIFFERENTIAL DIAGNOSIS. Several conditions present with findings similar to those of scleroderma. Acrocyanosis, in which there is no associated pallor or reflex hyperemia, may be seen following pulmonary arterial hypertension, anorexia nervosa, or frostbite. Diffuse finger swelling extending to the dorsum of the hands can be seen in Henoch-Schönlein purpura and with allergic reactions. Patients with juvenile rheumatoid arthritis usually have swelling in the fingers that is restricted to

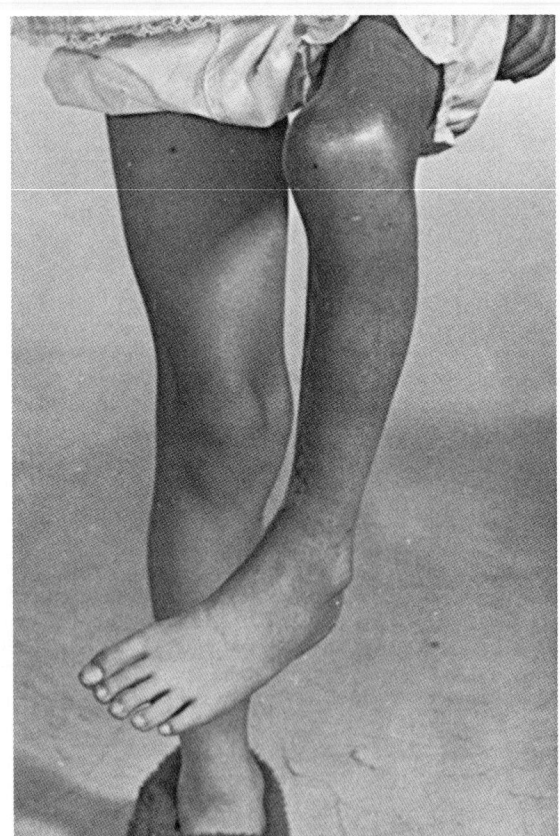

FIGURE 150–4. Extensive morphea involving the entire left leg causing shortening and flexion contractures. The skin has a shiny appearance with patches of hyperpigmentation and vitiligo.

the joints. Flexion contractures in these patients are a result of chronic tendinitis without dermal involvement; therefore, the skin is not tight, compared with that of patients with scleroderma. Manifestations of graft versus host disease after bone marrow transplantation (see Chapter 127) include erythema affecting the face and distal extremities, sclerodermatous skin changes, hepatitis, and diarrhea.

In **Raynaud disease**, Raynaud phenomenon occurs without the subsequent development of skin or internal organ changes of scleroderma. Such patients usually do not have anti-SCL70 or other autoantibodies, and their Raynaud phenomenon does not worsen over time. Weakness, sometimes related to flexion contractures, in patients with skin changes suggestive of early scleroderma raises the possibility of juvenile dermatomyositis or overlap syndromes in which elements of several rheumatic diseases (e.g., systemic lupus erythematosus, dermatomyositis, arthritis, and scleroderma) may be present.

Patients with **eosinophilic fasciitis** develop changes similar to those in localized scleroderma. However, laboratory evaluation shows a striking eosinophilia, elevated erythrocyte sedimentation rate, and occasionally hypergammaglobulinemia. Full-thickness skin biopsy, which extends to and includes muscle fascia, shows a predominately eosinophilic inflammatory infiltration in the dermis and fascial tissues that confirms the diagnosis. Progression to systemic sclerosis is rare. Corticosteroid treatment often ameliorates or prevents progression of lesions. However, some patients develop severe contracting fibrosis involving the entire length of the extremities. Limited experience suggests that it may be possible in some cases to prevent this complication with the use of methotrexate.

Pseudoscleroderma comprises unrelated diseases characterized by patchy or diffuse cutaneous fibrosis without the other manifestations of scleroderma. Patients with phenylketonuria can develop such lesions as well as eczematous changes. **Scleredema of Buschke** is a transient disease of sudden onset often following a febrile illness (especially streptococcal infections) in which patchy sclerodermatous lesions occur on the neck and shoulders, often extending to the face, trunk, and down the arms. These findings usually resolve spontaneously within several months.

Laboratory Findings. Inflammation early in systemic disease may be reflected by anemia and sometimes eosinophilia. Immunoglobulin levels may be nonspecifically elevated. ANAs are often present, with a speckled or nucleolar pattern. If present, anti-SCL70, which is specific for topoisomerase 1, and anticentromere autoantibodies are strongly suggestive of a diagnosis of scleroderma. Autoantibodies usually found in systemic lupus erythematosus (anti-DNA) or mixed connective tissue disease (anti-ribonucleoprotein) suggest the presence of an overlapping

syndrome. In the early phase of the disease, levels of von Willebrand factor antigen, a marker for vascular endothelial damage, may be elevated. In localized scleroderma, laboratory abnormalities are usually restricted to positive ANA (with anti-SCL70 and anticentromere antibodies much less common than in systemic sclerosis) and, on occasion, eosinophilia.

Treatment. Although there is no specific treatment, immunosuppressive agents, including methotrexate and corticosteroids, in the early stages of the disease may be helpful in curbing inflammation. However, corticosteroids later in the course of the disease do not appear to be effective and may exacerbate hypertension. Additional treatment includes physical and occupational therapy to improve flexion contractures and maintain muscle strength, and spring-loaded splints in selected patients.

If Raynaud phenomenon persists despite local measures (e.g., keeping hands warm during cold exposure with Mylar or sheepskin gloves), therapy with calcium channel blockers (e.g., nifedipine, amlodipine besylate), angiotensin-converting enzyme inhibitors (e.g., captopril, enalapril), and topical vasodilators (e.g., nitroglycerin paste) may be successful in preventing or ameliorating fingertip ulcerations. Vascular compromise threatening to lead to gangrene and autoamputation of the distal digits may respond to parenteral administration of prostaglandin E_1 (alprostadil).

Complications. Raynaud phenomenon can become severe enough to lead to early gangrenous changes with the threat of autoamputation of the digits. Arterial disease can also cause esophageal rupture, renovascular hypertensive crises, and pulmonary arterial hypertension with cor pulmonale. Chronic pulmonary insufficiency can result from pulmonary parenchymal disease and pulmonary arterial hypertension. Gastrointestinal involvement can result in malabsorption and failure to thrive. Renal disease and chronic pulmonary arterial hypertension can lead to death.

Prognosis. The course of scleroderma is variable, and findings at presentation are not predictive. Some patients stabilize after several years and have no new skin or visceral involvement. Others show unrelenting progression of disease, with death, either in childhood or later in life, resulting from end-stage pulmonary, cardiac, or renal vascular disease.

Garty BZ, Athreya BH, Wilmott R, et al: Pulmonary functions in children with progressive systemic sclerosis. *Pediatrics* 1991;88:1161–7.
Gerbracht DD, Steen VD, Ziegler GL, et al: Evolution of primary Raynaud phenomenon (Raynaud's disease) to connective tissue disease. *Arthritis Rheum* 1985;28:87–92.
Michels H: Course of mixed connective tissue disease in children. *Ann Med* 1997;29:359–64.
Nelson AM: Localized scleroderma including morphea, linear scleroderma, and eosinophilic fasciitis. *Curr Probl Pediatr* 1996;26:318–24.
Seely JM, Jones LT, Wallace C, et al: Systemic sclerosis: Using high-resolution CT to detect lung disease in children. *AJR Am J Roentgenol* 1998;170:691–7.
Sheiner NM, Small P: Isolated Raynaud's phenomenon—A benign disorder. *Ann Allergy* 1987;58:114–7.

Chapter 151
Behçet Disease *Abraham Gedalia*

Behçet disease, a multisystem disorder originally described as recurrent oral and genital ulceration associated with relapsing iritis or uveitis, is often characterized by cutaneous, arthritic, neurologic, vascular, and gastrointestinal manifestations. Fever, orchitis, myositis, pericarditis, nephritis, splenomegaly, and amyloidosis are rare associated manifestations. The disease is commonly reported in the Mediterranean basin and Asia and is relatively rare in Europe and the United States. The condition is uncommon in children, who account for only an estimated 5% of all cases.

The *etiology* of Behçet disease is unknown, although an association with HLA-B5 and HLA-B51 is clear. A few cases of transient neonatal Behçet disease in offspring of mothers with Behçet disease have been described, suggesting that an antibody-mediated immune process may have a role in the pathogenesis. The basic pathologic lesion is vasculitis of small- and medium-sized arteries with cellular infiltrations leading to fibrinoid necrosis and narrowing and obliteration of the vessel lumens. Necrotizing and granulomatous inflammation of a large vessel such as the aorta or pulmonary artery also may occur.

The *clinical course* is highly variable, with recurrent exacerbations and disease-free intervals of uncertain duration. Painful oral ulcers, usually 2–10 mm in diameter with surrounding erythema, develop over the oronasal cavity and upper airway in all patients, persist for days to weeks, and then heal without scarring. These necrotic ulcers may occur singly or in crops. Genital ulcers occur in most patients and follow a parallel course but may heal with scars. Skin manifestations occur in most patients and include erythema nodosum, pseudofolliculitis, papulopustular lesions, and acneiform nodules. Cutaneous pathergy occurs as an erythematous sterile pustule after 24–48 hr at a needle-prick skin site. Ocular manifestations, including anterior or posterior uveitis and retinal vasculitis, occur less frequently in children than in adults but are more severe in the pediatric population and may progress to blindness. Arthritis is common and is usually acute, recurrent, asymmetric, and polyarticular, involving the large joints. Central nervous system abnormalities such as meningoencephalitis, cranial nerve palsies, and psychosis usually occur later in the course of the disease and indicate a poor prognosis.

Laboratory findings are not diagnostic, although the finding of HLA-B5 or HLA-B51 support the diagnosis.

Treatment is based on anecdotal reports. A wide range of drugs has been used, including systemic corticosteroids, colchicine, chlorambucil, azathioprine, and cyclosporine. Colchicine has been demonstrated to be effective, showing higher efficacy in children than in adults, especially for oral ulcers, skin rash, joint symptoms, and occasionally eye disease. Recently, thalidomide has been reported to be a highly effective and useful therapeutic option for severe oral and genital ulceration that is unresponsive to other therapies. Another potentially important modality is anti–tumor necrosis factor-α therapy, which may also have a role in the management of Behçet disease.

International Study Group for Behçet's Disease: Criteria for diagnosis of Behçet's disease. *Lancet* 1990;335:1078–80.

Kari JA, Shah V, Dillon MJ. Behçet's disease in UK children: Clinical features and treatment including thalidomide. *Rheumatology* 2001;40:933–8.

Kone-Paut I, Yurdakul S, Bahabri SA, et al: Clinical features of Behçet's disease in children: An international collaborative study of 86 cases. *J Pediatr* 1998;132:721–5.

Krause I, Uziel Y, Guedj D, et al: Childhood Behçet's disease: Clinical features and comparison with adult-onset disease. *Rheumatology* 1999;38:457–62.

Lang BA, Laxer RM, Thorner P, et al: Pediatric onset of Behçet's syndrome with myositis: Case report and literature review illustrating unusual features. *Arthritis Rheum* 1990;33:418–25.

Chapter 152
Sjögren Syndrome
Abraham Gedalia

Sjögren syndrome is a chronic inflammatory autoimmune disease characterized by progressive lymphocytic and plasma cell infiltration of the salivary and lacrimal glands leading to xerophthalmia (dry eyes, or keratoconjunctivitis sicca), xerostomia (dry mouth), and associated connective tissue disease features.

Sjögren syndrome typically occurs in women 35–45 yr of age, with a female:male ratio of 9:1. It is uncommon in the pediatric age group, although more than 50 cases in children have been reported. European criteria for the diagnosis of Sjögren syndrome in adult patients have been developed, and recently diagnostic criteria in children have been proposed.

Clinical manifestations are related to exocrine disease of the epithelial surfaces of the eyes, mouth, nose, larynx and trachea, vagina, and skin, leading to the common symptoms of photophobia, burning and itching eyes, and blurred vision; painless unilateral or bilateral enlargement of the parotid glands; decreased sense of taste; dental caries; dysphagia; fissured tongue; and angular cheilitis. Subjective symptoms of xerostomia are less frequent among juvenile cases, indicating that Sjögren syndrome is a slowly progressive disease. Additional manifestations may include a decreased sense of smell and epistaxis; hoarseness; chronic otitis media; and internal organ exocrine disease involving the lungs, hepatobiliary system, pancreas, gastrointestinal tract, and kidneys.

Non-exocrine disease manifestations of Sjögren syndrome may be related to inflammatory vascular disease (in skin, muscle and joints, serosae, peripheral and central nervous system), noninflammatory vascular disease (Raynaud phenomenon), mediator-induced disease (hematologic cytopenias, fatigue, and fever), and autoimmune endocrinopathy (thyroiditis). Because monoclonal B-lymphocyte disease originates chiefly from lymphocytic foci within salivary glands or from parenchymal internal organs, lymphoproliferative forms of Sjögren syndrome occur in adults with potential lymphoid malignancy. Parotitis at onset is much more frequent in children than in adults with Sjögren syndrome. However, positive antinuclear antibodies and articular manifestations are significantly more frequent in adults.

Sjögren syndrome can occur as an isolated disorder, referred to as **primary Sjögren syndrome**, or as a secondary form in association with other rheumatic disorders. Most commonly it accompanies systemic lupus erythematosus or mixed connective tissue disease, and only rarely is it associated with juvenile rheumatoid arthritis. It precedes the associated autoimmune disease by years in half the cases. Maternal Sjögren syndrome can be an antecedent to the neonatal lupus syndrome.

The *diagnosis* is based on clinical features supported by biopsy of the lip or glands demonstrating foci of lymphocytic infiltration, cryoglobulinemia, elevated erythrocyte sedimentation rate, hypergammaglobulinemia, positive rheumatoid factor, and the presence of antibodies to Ro/SSA and La/SSB. A recent study found that anti-α-fodrin autoantibodies are a useful diagnostic marker for juvenile Sjögren syndrome. Ocular tearing may be evaluated by performing **Schirmer test**, which detects abnormal tear production (≤5 mm of wetting of filter paper strip in 5 min). Imaging studies using magnetic resonance, technetium-99 scintigraphy, and sialography are useful in the diagnostic evaluation for Sjögren syndrome.

The *differential diagnosis* of Sjögren syndrome in children includes chronic recurrent parotitis, infectious parotitis, and tumors. In these conditions, sicca complex, rash, arthralgia, and antinuclear antibodies are usually absent.

Treatment is symptomatic, with use of artificial tears, oral lozenges, and fluids to limit the damaging effects of decreased secretions. Corticosteroids with or without immunosuppressive agents may be indicated for severe functional disorders and life-threatening complications.

Anaya JM, Ogawa N, Talal N: Sjögren's syndrome in childhood. *J Rheumatol* 1995;22:1152–8.

Manthrope R, Asmussen K, Oxholm P: Primary Sjögren's syndrome: Diagnostic criteria, clinical features, and disease activity. *J Rheumatol* 1997;24(Suppl 50):8–11.

Bartunkova J, Sediva A, Vencovsky J, et al: Primary Sjögren syndrome in children and adolescents: Proposal for diagnostic criteria. *Clin Exp Rheumatol* 1999;17:381–6.

Maeno N, Takei S, Imanaka H, et al. Anti-alpha-fodrin antibodies in Sjögren's syndrome in children. *J Rheumatol* 2001;28:860–4.

Chapter 153
Familial Mediterranean Fever *Abraham Gedalia*

Familial Mediterranean fever (FMF) is an inherited disorder characterized by brief, acute, self-limited episodes of fever and polyserositis recurring at irregular intervals, as well as development of amyloidosis (see Chapter 154), which, if untreated, leads to end-stage renal failure. FMF appears to be transmitted as an autosomal recessive disease and essentially occurs among ethnic groups of Mediterranean origin, mainly Sephardic Jews, Turks, Armenians, and individuals of Arab descent. In these populations, the carrier frequency is estimated to be as high as one in five persons. Greeks, Hispanics, and Italians are less commonly affected. FMF is rare among Ashkenazi Jews, Germans, and Anglo-Saxons; other ethnic groups report only sporadic cases.

The onset of *clinical manifestations* occurs before age 5 yr in 63–68% of cases and before age 20 yr in 90% of cases. The onset may be as early as 6 mo of age. The typical acute episode lasts 1–4 days and includes fever and one or more symptoms of peritonitis manifested by abdominal pain (90%), arthritis or arthralgia (85%), and pleuritis manifested by chest pain (20%). Other serosal tissues such as the pericardium and tunica vaginalis testis are rarely affected. Erysipelas-like skin rash, myalgia, splenomegaly, scrotal involvement in boys, neurologic involvement, Henoch-Schönlein purpura, and hypothyroidism are other less common clinical manifestations. In about one third to one half of untreated patients with FMF, amyloidosis of AA (amyloid A) type develops and is manifested by proteinuria that progresses to nephrotic syndrome and renal failure over a period of months to several years. Death results from infection, thromboembolism, or uremia. Amyloidosis is common among Sephardic Jews and Turks and less common in Armenians. However, Armenians living in Armenia are reported to have a significantly higher incidence of amyloidosis than do their counterparts in North America, suggesting that environmental factors may also have a role.

The gene responsible for FMF was first mapped to a small interval on the short arm of chromosome 16p13.3, between the gene responsible for adult-onset polycystic kidney disease and the gene linked to Rubinstein-Taybi syndrome. The FMF gene, designated *MEFV*, was then identified and cloned by two independent groups, the international and the French consortia. *MEFV* is a new member of the RoRet gene family; it is approximately 10 kb with 10 exons that express a 3.7-kb transcript encoding a 781 amino acid protein known as **pyrin or marenostrin** that is expressed in myeloid cells. More than 29 mutations, most located in the last exon, were discovered. It is unclear whether all are true disease-related mutations. The five most common mutations (M694V, V726A, M694I, M680I, and E148Q) were found in more than two thirds of tested Mediterranean FMF patients. Haplotypes and mutational analyses showed ancestral relationships among carrier chromosomes that have been separated for centuries. The most common missense mutation is methionine-694-valine (M694V), a mutation occurring in 20–67% of cases and associated with a higher disease severity index and a higher incidence of amyloidosis, followed by the valine-726-alanine (7–35%), which is associated

with milder disease and a lower incidence of amyloidosis. This suggests that phenotypic differences may be related to different mutations. Cloning and identification of the FMF gene now make it possible to establish a diagnosis of FMF, especially in areas where the disease is rare and less familiar to physicians. Genetic screenings using restriction analysis PCR (polymerase chain reaction) systems are now available in some commercial genetic clinical laboratories. However, genetic laboratories usually screen for the 5–10 most common mutations, and rare mutations are missed. Therefore, the diagnosis of FMF is still based on clinical grounds, and genetic screening should be used as a confirmatory test.

The exact *pathogenesis* of the acute episodes of FMF is still not known, although some immunologic abnormalities have been reported. Of special interest is the finding of a C5a inhibitor (inactivating enzyme) deficiency in peritoneal and synovial fluids of patients with FMF. C5a is a fragment of complement, an anaphylatoxin, and a potent chemotactic agent. Normally, small amounts of C5a may be released into serosal cavities and are subsequently neutralized by the inactivating enzyme before they precipitate overt inflammation. One hypothesis is that a deficiency of C5a inhibitor, which is a consequence of pyrin dysfunction in patients with FMF, allows further accumulation of C5a, leading to the acute attack. Better understanding of pyrin function will shed light on its interactions with other proteins involved in the regulation of the inflammatory response.

Attacks of FMF can be *prevented* by prophylactic colchicine therapy at a dose of 0.02–0.03 mg/kg/24 hr (maximum of 2 mg/24 hr) in one or two divided doses. Colchicine therapy not only reduces the frequency of acute attacks but also greatly decreases the probability of development of amyloidosis and may lead to partial regression of existing amyloidosis. Colchicine therapy for FMF during pregnancy has not been reported to harm either the mother or her fetus.

Other conditions of periodic fever syndromes that have been recently recognized need to be considered in the differential diagnosis. There are at least three other separate periodic fever syndromes. **Hyperimmunoglobulin D periodic fever syndrome (HIDS)** is an autosomal recessive condition, reported mostly in families of European descent (Dutch, French), caused by mutations in the mevalonate kinase gene found on chromosome 12q24. Patients with this disorder manifest recurrent short episodes (>14 days) of fever associated with cervical lymphadenopathy, abdominal pain, rash, arthralgia/arthritis, occasional splenomegaly, increased level of acute-phase reactants, and elevated serum level of IgD (>100 U/mL). There is no known therapy for this condition, although glucocorticoids may be of some benefit. **Tumor necrosis factor (TNF)-receptor-associated periodic syndrome (TRAPS)** is a syndrome that was previously known by other names, including familial Hibernian fever, familial periodic fever, and autosomal dominant recurrent fever. This is a rare disorder that has been reported in a few families of Irish or Scottish ancestry and is caused by mutations in the gene encoding for type 1 TNF receptor protein, which has been mapped to chromosome 12p13. Patients with this condition manifest brief (4–6 days) intermittent febrile episodes associated with abdominal pain myalgias, and occasional occurrence of rash, conjunctivitis, and unilateral periorbital edema. Increased level of acute-phase reactants may be seen, but the most specific finding is a low serum level of soluble type 1 TNF receptor. Glucocorticoids may be helpful; using etanercept, a recombinant TNF receptor fusion protein, proved promising in a recent report. A new syndrome referred to as **periodic fever, aphthous stomatitis, pharyngitis, and adenitis (PFAPA)** is associated with arthralgia in some patients. The majority of patients respond to a single dose of oral prednisone (1–2 mg/kg). This syndrome usually develops before age 5 yr, with spontaneous resolution within 4–8 years. The etiology and the pathogenesis are still a puzzle, and it is not clear whether this syndrome represents infectious or immunogenetic dysregulation entities.

Babior BM, Matzner Y: The familial Mediterranean fever gene-cloned at last. *N Engl J Med* 1997;337:1548–9.

Drenth JP, van der Meer JW: Hereditary periodic fever. *N Engl J Med* 2001;348: 1748–57.

Gedalia A, Adar A, Gorodischer R: Familial Mediterranean fever in children. *J Rheumatol Suppl* 1992;19:1–9.

Hull KM, Drewe E, Aksentijevich I, et al: The TNF receptor-associated periodic syndrome (TRAPS): Emerging concept of an autoinflammatory disorder. *Medicine (Baltimore)* 2002;81:349–68.

The International FMF Consortium: Ancient missense mutations in a new member of the RoRet gene family are likely to cause familial Mediterranean fever. *Cell* 1997;90:797–807.

Touitou I: The spectrum of familial Mediterranean fever mutations. *Eur J Hum Genet* 2001;9:473–83.

Chapter 154
Amyloidosis *Abraham Gedalia*

Amyloidosis comprises a group of diseases characterized by extracellular deposition of insoluble fibrous **amyloid proteins** in various body tissues. The deposits are composed of seemingly homogeneous eosinophilic material that stains with Congo red dye and in polarized light demonstrates the pathognomonic apple-green birefringence of amyloid. Amyloid material is composed of microscopic fibrils that are biochemically heterogeneous, with at least 15 different types of protein compositions. However, all amyloid deposits contain an identical nonfibrillar component, **serum amyloid P.** Amyloid fibril deposition may have no apparent consequences, or it may ultimately interfere with organ function. Various disease states result from deposition of different types of amyloid material, and different patterns of tissue deposition result in various patterns of organ dysfunction. Regardless of the cause of amyloidosis, the clinical diagnosis is usually not established until the disease is far advanced.

Classifications of the amyloid proteins and the various amyloid diseases are complex. The **systemic amyloidoses** are multisystem diseases that correspond to clinical patterns of primary, secondary, familial, and dialysis-related amyloidosis. The **localized or organ-limited amyloidoses** are associated with aging and diabetes and occur in isolated organs such as endocrine glands, without evidence of systemic involvement. The most common types of amyloidosis are those related to primary idiopathic amyloidosis and multiple myeloma, with deposition of amyloid composed of pieces of monoclonal light chain of immunoglobulin (AL type). Secondary or reactive amyloidosis occurs in individuals with familial Mediterranean fever (FMF) and chronic inflammatory diseases related to another protein, amyloid A protein (AA type). Finally, a group of amyloid conditions, including those associated with aging (e.g., Alzheimer disease), and several rare familial types of amyloidosis are associated with other amyloid protein precursors.

Primary amyloidosis is extremely rare in children. Only secondary amyloidosis affects children in appreciable numbers, and it occurs in some individuals with FMF and after chronic inflammatory diseases, including juvenile rheumatoid arthritis (JRA), rheumatoid arthritis, ankylosing spondylitis, inflammatory bowel disease, chronic infections such as tuberculosis, and cystic fibrosis. AA protein isolated from amyloid found in these diseases is an N-terminus fragment of serum AA. Because serum AA protein acts as an acute-phase reactant, increased amounts resulting from chronic inflammation may provide an explanation for the occurrence of this form of secondary amyloidosis. Other inflammatory diseases such as lupus erythematosus or dermatomyositis, which are associated with shorter periods of inflammation, are not associated with secondary amyloidosis.

Similar to FMF, secondary amyloidosis affects as many as 10% of children with JRA in some European countries but is rarely seen as a complication of seemingly similar disease in children in the United States and Canada. Reasons for this difference are unknown, although environmental factors may have a role. Secondary amyloidosis usually begins some years after the onset of inflammatory disease and is manifested by anemia, diarrhea, hepatosplenomegaly, proteinuria, and progression to nephrotic syndrome and eventual renal failure.

The *diagnosis* of amyloidosis is established by demonstration of amyloid in affected tissues. Renal biopsies are considered hazardous in the presence of amyloidosis because of potential bleeding. The spleen is often affected but is not a suitable site for biopsy. More accessible biopsy sites include the rectal mucosa and gingival tissue. A method of scintigraphy using serum amyloid P component has been described as a useful diagnostic tool and as a tool for monitoring the status of amyloidosis. Patients with JRA and secondary amyloidosis usually show elevated acute-phase reactants and high levels of immunoglobulins.

Unlike amyloidosis associated with FMF, amyloidosis associated with JRA does not respond to colchicine therapy but instead to chlorambucil, which reverses renal findings and prolongs life. Chlorambucil is associated with chromosome breakage and an unknown risk of subsequent malignancy. There is little experience with other cytotoxic agents and with the therapy for secondary amyloidosis associated with other conditions.

Amyloidosis is the most common serious complication of FMF, leading to end-stage renal disease. There is ethnic variability in the frequency of amyloidosis: among patients with FMF, amyloidosis occurs in up to 60% of Turks, 27% of Sephardic Jews, and 1–2% of Armenians living in the United States. Colchicine has been effective not only in controlling the attacks of FMF, but also in preventing the development of amyloidosis. A recent development is the discovery and cloning of the FMF gene. Phenotype-genotype correlation analysis of children with FMF revealed that patients with M694V homozygous genotype are at higher risk of developing amyloidosis. These children should be given colchicine for life.

Benson MD: Amyloidosis. In Koopman WJ (editor): *Arthritis and Allied Conditions.* Baltimore, Williams & Wilkins, 1997.

David J, Vouyiouka O, Ansell BM, et al: Amyloidosis in juvenile chronic arthritis: A morbidity and mortality study. *Clin Exp Rheumatol* 1993;11:85–90.

Mimouni A, Magal N, Stoffman N, et al: Familial Mediterranean fever: Effect of genotype and ethnicity on inflammatory attacks and amyloidosis. *Pediatrics* 2000;105:E70.

Saatci U, Bakkaloglu A, Ozen S, et al: Familial Mediterranean fever and amyloidosis in children. *Acta Paediatr* 1993;81:705–6.

Woo P: Amyloidosis in children. *Baillieres Clin Rheumatol* 1994;8:691–7.

Chapter 155
Sarcoidosis *Margaret W. Leigh*

Sarcoidosis, a chronic multisystem granulomatous disease of unknown cause, occurs most frequently in young adults but can occur during childhood.

Etiology. The granulomas in sarcoidosis resemble those caused by certain microbial agents, such as mycobacteria and fungi, or by hypersensitivity to organic agents. These similarities have led to speculation that microbes or organic dusts may be inciting agents. However, despite extensive studies, the etiology remains obscure.

Epidemiology. Sarcoidosis has a worldwide distribution involving all ethnic groups. In the southeastern United States, sarcoidosis occurs more frequently in African-Americans than in whites. Familial clustering of this disease has been observed and suggests a genetic predisposition; however, the mode of inheritance is unclear.

Pathology. The noncaseating granulomatous lesions of sarcoidosis may occur in almost any organ of the body. Typically, the granulomas are not necrotic, and they contain epithelioid cells, macrophages, and giant cells in the center surrounded by a mixture of monocytes, lymphocytes, and fibroblasts. Activated lymphocytes and macrophages within the granulomas release various mediators including interleukin-1 (IL-1), IL-2, interferon, and other cytokines that are thought to promote and maintain granulomatous lesions. During active disease, lymphocytes in the granulomas are predominantly helper T (CD4) lymphocytes. These lesions usually heal with complete preservation of the parenchyma; however, in approximately 20% of the lesions, fibroblasts proliferate at the periphery of the granuloma and may produce fibrotic scar tissue. Macrophages within sarcoidosis granulomas produce and secrete $1,25\text{-}(OH)_2\text{-}D_3$, the active form of vitamin D typically produced in the kidneys. Excess vitamin D results in hypercalcemia and hypercalciuria in patients with sarcoidosis.

Clinical Manifestations. The initial clinical presentation is extremely variable, depending on the organ systems involved, but manifestations in children usually include weight loss, cough, fatigue, bone and joint pain, and anemia. In adults and children, the lung is the most frequently affected organ but the pulmonary involvement is variable in its extent and characteristics. Parenchymal infiltrates, miliary nodules, and hilar and paratracheal lymphadenopathy occur (Fig. 155–1). Pulmonary function tests primarily show restrictive changes. Peripheral lymphadenopathy, eye changes consisting of uveitis or iritis, skin lesions, and hepatic involvement occur frequently. Children younger than 4 yr old may have a distinct form of sarcoidosis consisting of a maculopapular erythematous rash, uveitis, and arthritis but minimal to no pulmonary changes. The arthritis, which can be confused with rheumatoid arthritis, produces large, painless, boggy synovial effusions of the tendon sheaths with little limitation of motion.

Diagnosis. There are no specific diagnostic tests. An elevated erythrocyte sedimentation rate, hyperproteinemia, hypercalcemia, hypercalciuria, eosinophilia, and an elevated angiotensin-converting enzyme level are common. The **Kveim test,** consisting of intradermal injection of material from a sarcoid lesion and observation for the formation of a granuloma several weeks later, is used infrequently because of the difficulty in obtaining standardized test material and reports of varying sensitivity and specificity of the test. Definitive diagnosis requires demonstration of the characteristic noncaseating granulomatous lesions in a biopsy of tissue from an affected area. Significant eye disease and renal damage from hypercalciuria can occur without symptoms; therefore, all patients with sarcoidosis should be evaluated at the initial presentation and monitored at regular intervals for evidence of ocular disease and hypercalciuria.

Because of its protean manifestations, the differential diagnosis of sarcoidosis is extremely broad and includes tuberculosis, pulmonary mycoses (histoplasmosis, blastomycosis, and coccidioidomycosis), lymphoma, Crohn disease, and inflammatory ocular lesions such as phlyctenular conjunctivitis.

Treatment. Treatment is symptomatic and supportive. The decision to treat with potentially harmful agents is often difficult because the prognosis and natural history of sarcoidosis in children are uncertain. Spontaneous recovery may occur after a prolonged illness of several months to several years, or the condition may be chronic, with progressive lung disease. Corticosteroids may suppress the acute manifestations, especially the inflammatory ocular lesions, progressive pulmonary disease, and hypercalcemia/hypercalciuria. Methotrexate may be considered in severe cases that are unresponsive to corticosteroid therapy. Eye involvement may lead to blindness; therefore, therapy with topical corticosteroids with careful monitoring is warranted.

Pulmonary function tests are useful in following the progress of lung involvement. Angiotensin-converting enzyme levels have been shown to correlate with disease activity.

Baughman RP, Sharma OP, Lynch JP: Sarcoidosis: Is therapy effective? *Semin Respir Infect* 1998;13:255–73.

Fink CW, Cimaz R: Early onset sarcoidosis: Not a benign disease. *J Rheumatol* 1997;24:174–7.

Newman LS, Rose CS, Maier LA: Sarcoidosis. *N Engl J Med* 1997;336:1224–34.

Pattishall EN, Kendig EL Jr: Sarcoidosis in children. *Pediatr Pulmonol* 1996;22:195–203.

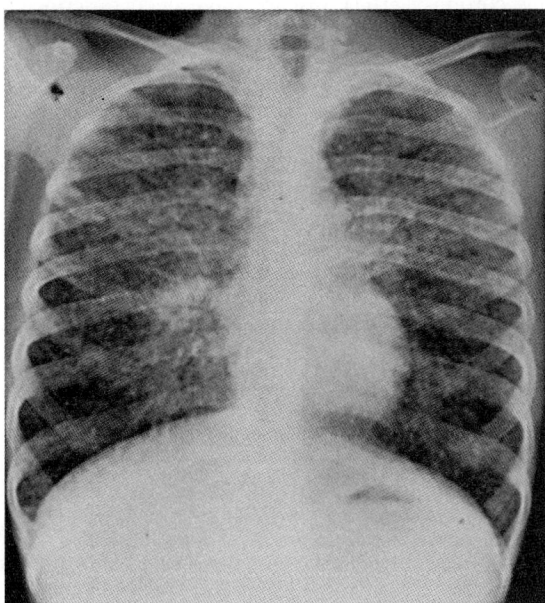

FIGURE 155–1. Sarcoidosis in a white 10-yr-old girl. There are widely disseminated peribronchial infiltrations, multiple small nodular densities, hyperaeration of the lungs, and hilar lymphadenopathy.

Chapter 156

Kawasaki Disease

Anne H. Rowley and Stanford T. Shulman

Kawasaki disease, formerly known as mucocutaneous lymph node syndrome or infantile polyarteritis nodosa, is an acute febrile vasculitis of childhood first described by Dr. Tomisaku Kawasaki in Japan in 1967. The disorder occurs worldwide, with Asians at highest risk. Approximately 20% of untreated patients develop coronary artery abnormalities including aneurysms, with the potential for the development of coronary artery thrombosis or stenosis, myocardial infarction, aneurysm rupture, and sudden death. Kawasaki disease has replaced acute rheumatic fever as the leading cause of acquired heart disease in children in the United States and Japan.

Etiology. The cause of the illness remains unknown, but clinical and epidemiologic features strongly support an infectious origin. These features include the age group affected, the occurrence of periodic epidemics with a wavelike geographic spread of illness during the epidemic, the self-limited nature of the illness, and the clinical features of fever, rash, enanthem, conjunctival injection, and cervical lymphadenopathy. One hypothesis is that a ubiquitous agent causes Kawasaki disease and that symptomatic illness occurs only in genetically predisposed hosts. The infrequent occurrence of the illness in infants younger than 4 mo may be due to passive maternal antibody, and the virtual absence of cases in adults may be due to widespread immunity.

Epidemiology. It is estimated that at least 3,000 cases are diagnosed annually in the United States. The incidence of Kawasaki disease in Asian children is substantially higher than in other racial groups, but the illness occurs worldwide in all ethnic groups. In Japan, more than 170,000 cases have been reported since the 1960s. Kawasaki disease is not a new illness; autopsy reports of infantile periarteritis nodosa before the 1960s appear in retrospect to have represented fatal Kawasaki disease. The disorder bears marked similarities to measles infection and may have been particularly difficult to identify before the development of measles vaccine. The illness occurs predominantly in young children; 80% of patients are younger than 5 yr, and only occasionally are teenagers and adults affected.

Pathogenesis. Kawasaki disease causes a severe vasculitis of all blood vessels but predominantly affecting the medium-sized arteries, with predilection for the coronary arteries. Pathologic examination of fatal cases in the acute or subacute stages reveals edema of endothelial and smooth muscle cells with intense inflammatory infiltration of the vascular wall, initially by polymorphonuclear cells but rapidly changing to macrophages, lymphocytes (which are mostly CD8 T cells), and plasma cells. IgA plasma cells are prominent in the inflammatory infiltrate. In the most severely affected vessels, inflammation involves all three layers of the vascular wall, with destruction of the internal elastic lamina. The vessel loses its structural integrity and weakens, resulting in dilatation or aneurysm formation. Thrombi may form in the lumen and obstruct blood flow. In the healing phase, the lesion becomes progressively fibrotic, with marked intimal proliferation, which may result in stenotic occlusion of the vessel over time.

An inflammatory infiltrate, including IgA plasma cells, is present in selected nonvascular tissues in acute Kawasaki disease, including myocardium, upper respiratory tract, pancreas, kidney, and biliary tract, suggesting that the infectious agent may cause a host immune response in a variety of nonvascular tissues. No significant sequelae appear to occur in any of these nonvascular tissues following the illness.

In the subacute phase of illness, elevated levels of all the serum immunoglobulins are present, suggesting that a vigorous antibody response occurs. It is unclear whether the etiologic agent, the host immune response, or both are the major factors leading to coronary disease.

Clinical Manifestations. Fever is generally high spiking (to 104°F or higher), remittent, and unresponsive to antibiotics. The duration of fever is generally 1–2 wk without treatment but may persist for 3–4 wk. Prolonged fever has been shown to be a risk factor for the development of coronary artery disease. The other characteristic features of the illness are bilateral bulbar conjunctival injection, usually without exudate; erythema of the oral and pharyngeal mucosa with "strawberry" tongue and dry, cracked lips; erythema and swelling of the hands and feet; rash of various forms (maculopapular, erythema multiforme, or scarlatiniform) with accentuation in the groin area; and nonsuppurative cervical lymphadenopathy, usually unilateral, with a node size of 1.5 cm or greater in diameter. Perineal desquamation is common in the acute phase. Periungual desquamation of the fingers and toes begins 1–3 wk after the onset of illness and may progress to involve the entire hand and foot.

Other features include extreme irritability, especially in infants, aseptic meningitis, diarrhea, mild hepatitis, hydrops of the gallbladder, urethritis and meatitis with sterile pyuria, otitis media, and arthritis. Arthritis is more common in girls and may

occur early in the illness with fever and other acute manifestations or may develop during the 2nd–3rd week, generally affecting hands, knees, ankles, or hips.

Cardiac involvement is the most important manifestation of Kawasaki disease. Myocarditis manifested by tachycardia and decreased ventricular function occurs in at least 50% of patients. Pericarditis with a small pericardial effusion is common during the acute illness. Coronary artery aneurysms generally develop in up to 25% of untreated patients during the 2nd–3rd wk of illness and can be detected by two-dimensional echocardiography. Valvular regurgitation and systemic artery aneurysms may occur but are uncommon. Giant coronary artery aneurysms (≥8 mm internal diameter) pose the greatest risk for rupture, thrombosis or stenosis, and myocardial infarction.

Kawasaki disease is generally divided into three clinical phases. The **acute febrile phase**, which usually lasts 1–2 wk, is characterized by fever and the other acute signs of illness. The **subacute phase** begins when fever and other acute signs have abated, but irritability, anorexia, and conjunctival injection may persist. The subacute phase is associated with desquamation, thrombocytosis, the development of coronary aneurysms, and the highest risk of sudden death. This phase generally lasts until about the 4th wk. The **convalescent phase** begins when all clinical signs of illness have disappeared and continues until the erythrocyte sedimentation rate (ESR) returns to normal, approximately 6–8 wk after the onset of illness.

Certain clinical and laboratory findings may predict a more severe outcome. These include male gender, age younger than 1 yr, prolonged fever, recurrent fever after an afebrile period, and the following laboratory values at presentation: low hemoglobin or platelet levels, high neutrophil and band counts, and low albumin and age-adjusted serum IgG levels. However, scoring systems based on these factors have not proven sensitive enough to allow for selective treatment of patients based on risk.

Diagnosis. The diagnosis of Kawasaki disease is based on demonstration of characteristic clinical signs (Box 156–1). The diagnostic criteria require the presence of fever for at least 5 days and at least four of five of the other characteristic clinical features of illness. Atypical or incomplete cases in which a patient has fever with fewer than four other features of the illness and then develops coronary artery disease have been described worldwide. Incomplete cases are most frequent in infants, who unfortunately have the highest likelihood of developing coronary artery disease.

Recognition depends on a high index of suspicion and knowledge of the characteristic clinical features of the illness. Unfortunately, if the diagnosis is not made and treatment not instituted, a patient may suffer sudden death secondary to myocardial infarction or coronary aneurysm rupture, or may

---

BOX 156–1. Diagnostic Criteria for Kawasaki Disease

Fever lasting for at least 5 days[*]
Presence of at least four of the following five signs:
1. Bilateral bulbar conjunctival injection, generally nonpurulent
2. Changes in the mucosa of the oropharynx, including injected pharynx, injected and/or dry fissured lips, strawberry tongue
3. Changes of the peripheral extremities, such as edema and/or erythema of the hands or feet in the acute phase; or periungual desquamation in the subacute phase
4. Rash, primarily truncal; polymorphous but nonvesicular
5. Cervical adenopathy, ≥1.5 cm, usually unilateral lymphadenopathy
Illness not explained by other known disease process

---

[*]Experienced physicians may make the diagnosis of Kawasaki disease (and institute treatment) before the 5th day of fever in patients with classic features of the illness.

develop serious asymptomatic coronary disease that is not diagnosed until symptoms develop in young adulthood.

DIFFERENTIAL DIAGNOSIS. The differential diagnosis of Kawasaki disease includes scarlet fever, toxic shock syndrome, measles, drug hypersensitivity reactions including Stevens-Johnson syndrome, juvenile rheumatoid arthritis, and, more rarely, Rocky Mountain spotted fever and leptospirosis. Some features of uncomplicated measles that help to distinguish it from Kawasaki disease include the presence of exudative conjunctivitis, Koplik spots, rash that begins on the face behind the ears, and a low white blood cell count and ESR. Some features of drug reactions, such as the presence of periorbital edema, oral ulcers, and a low ESR, may help to distinguish these reactions from Kawasaki disease. Toxic shock syndrome may be distinguished by the presence of hypotension, renal involvement, elevated creatine phosphokinase level, and a focus of *Staphylococcus aureus* infection. A common clinical problem is the differentiation of scarlet fever from Kawasaki disease in a child who is a group A streptococcal carrier. Because patients with scarlet fever have a rapid clinical response to penicillin therapy, such treatment for 24–48 hr with clinical reassessment at that time generally clarifies the diagnosis. The presence of lymphadenopathy, hepatosplenomegaly, and an evanescent, salmon-colored rash suggests a diagnosis of juvenile rheumatoid arthritis. Accurate diagnosis of incomplete cases remains a significant challenge for clinicians. Unusual cases should be referred to a center with experience in the diagnosis of Kawasaki disease.

Laboratory Findings. No specific diagnostic test for Kawasaki disease exists, but certain laboratory findings are characteristic. The white blood cell count is normal to elevated, with a predominance of neutrophils and immature forms. Elevated ESR, C-reactive protein, and other acute phase reactants are almost universally present in the acute phase of illness and may persist for 4–6 wk. Normocytic anemia is common. The platelet count is generally normal in the 1st wk of illness and rapidly increases by the 2nd–3rd wk of illness, sometimes exceeding 1,000,000/mm³. Antinuclear antibody and rheumatoid factor are not detectable. Sterile pyuria, mild elevations of the hepatic transaminases, and cerebrospinal fluid pleocytosis may be present.

Two-dimensional echocardiography is the most useful test to monitor the potential development of coronary artery abnormalities and should be performed by a pediatric cardiologist. The test should be performed at diagnosis and again after 2–3 wk of illness. If results of both of these are normal, a repeat study is performed 6–8 wk after onset of illness. If coronary abnormalities are not detected by echocardiography by 6–8 wk after onset of illness, when the ESR has normalized, additional follow-up studies are optional. Some centers routinely perform echocardiography again 1 yr after onset of illness. However, Kawasaki disease is an acute vasculitis; there is no convincing evidence of long-term cardiovascular sequelae in children who do not develop coronary abnormalities within 2 mo after the onset of illness.

For patients who develop coronary artery abnormalities, more frequent echocardiographic studies and potentially angiography may be indicated. Treatment of such patients should be determined in consultation with a pediatric cardiologist.

Treatment. Patients with acute Kawasaki disease should be treated with intravenous immunoglobulin (IVIG) and high-dose aspirin as soon as possible after diagnosis (Box 156–2). The mechanism of action of IVIG in Kawasaki disease is unknown, but treatment results in rapid defervescence and resolution of clinical signs of illness in most patients. IVIG reduces the prevalence of coronary disease from 20–25% in children treated with aspirin alone to 2–4% in those treated with IVIG and aspirin

---

BOX 156–2. Treatment of Kawasaki Disease

ACUTE STAGE
Intravenous immunoglobulin 2 g/kg over 10–12 hr *with* aspirin 80–100 mg/kg/24 hr divided every 6 hr orally until 14th illness day

CONVALESCENT STAGE
Aspirin 3–5 mg/kg once daily orally until 6–8 wk after illness onset

LONG-TERM THERAPY FOR THOSE WITH CORONARY ABNORMALITIES
Aspirin 3–5 mg/kg once daily orally ± dipyridamole 4–6 mg/kg/24 hr divided in two or three doses orally (most experts add warfarin for those patients at particularly high risk of thrombosis)

ACUTE CORONARY THROMBOSIS
Prompt fibrinolytic therapy with tissue plasminogen activator, streptokinase, or urokinase under supervision of a pediatric cardiologist

---

within the first 10 days of illness. In addition, consideration should be given to treatment of patients diagnosed after the 10th illness day if fever has persisted, because the anti-inflammatory effect may be helpful, although the effect of such therapy on the risk of developing coronary aneurysms is unknown. Aspirin is decreased from anti-inflammatory to antithrombotic doses (3–5 mg/kg/24 hr as a single dose) on the 14th illness day or when a patient has been afebrile for at least 3–4 days. Aspirin is continued for its antithrombotic effect until 6–8 wk after onset, when the ESR has normalized, in patients who have not developed abnormalities detected by echocardiography.

Occasional patients do not respond to an initial IVIG infusion or have only a partial response. Strong consideration should be given to re-treatment of these patients with an additional infusion of IVIG, 2 g/kg. The use of corticosteroids in Kawasaki disease remains controversial; if administered, such therapy generally should be reserved for patients with persistent fever following two 2 g/kg infusions of IVIG.

Patients with a small solitary aneurysm should continue aspirin indefinitely. Patients with larger or numerous aneurysms may require the addition of dipyridamole or warfarin therapy; such decisions should be made in consultation with a pediatric cardiologist. Acute thrombosis may occasionally occur in an aneurysmal coronary artery. Thrombolytic therapy may be lifesaving in this circumstance. Abciximab has been used in some patients with Kawasaki disease who develop giant coronary aneurysms or possible thrombosis. Little data regarding efficacy are available, but the drug may reduce thrombotic complications. Long-term follow-up of patients with aneurysms should include echocardiography, stress testing, and possibly angiography. Catheter intervention with percutaneous transluminal coronary rotational ablation, directional coronary atherectomy, and stent implantation are promising therapeutic strategies for the management of coronary stenosis caused by Kawasaki disease.

Patients receiving long-term aspirin therapy are candidates for influenza vaccine to reduce the risk of Reye syndrome. The risk of Reye syndrome in children who take salicylates and who receive varicella vaccine is believed to be much lower than with wild-type varicella. Physicians must weigh the relative risk of vaccine in children on long-term aspirin therapy against the risk of natural varicella infection. Patients treated with 2 g/kg IVIG should have measles-mumps-rubella and varicella vaccines delayed for 11 mo because the presence of specific antiviral antibody in IVIG may interfere with the immune response to parenteral live-virus vaccines.

Complications and Prognosis. Recovery is complete and without apparent long-term effects for patients who do not develop coronary disease. Recurrent illness occurs in only 1–3% of cases.

The prognosis for patients with coronary abnormalities depends on the severity of coronary disease. In Japan, fatality rates are now less than 0.1%. Overall, 50% of coronary artery aneurysms resolve echocardiographically by 1–2 yr after the illness. However, intravascular ultrasonography has demonstrated that resolved aneurysms are associated with marked intimal thickening and abnormal functional behavior of the vessel. Giant aneurysms are unlikely to resolve and are most likely to lead to thrombosis or stenosis. Coronary artery bypass grafting may be required if myocardial perfusion is significantly impaired, and it is best accomplished with the use of arterial grafts, which grow with the child and are more likely to remain patent than venous grafts. Heart transplantation has been required in rare cases in which revascularization is not feasible because of distal coronary stenosis or aneurysms or severe myocardial dysfunction. Whether the presence of coronary artery abnormalities resulting from Kawasaki disease predisposes to the development of atherosclerotic heart disease in young adulthood is unknown.

Akagi T, Ogawa S, Ino T, et al: Catheter interventional treatment in Kawasaki disease: A report from the Japanese Pediatric Interventional Cardiology Investigation Group. *J Pediatr* 2000;137:181–6.

American Heart Association Council on Cardiovascular Disease in the Young, Committee on Rheumatic Fever, Endocarditis, and Kawasaki Disease: Diagnostic guidelines for Kawasaki disease. *Circulation* 2001;103:335–6.

Brown TJ, Crawford SE, Cornwall M, et al: CD8 T cells and macrophages infiltrate coronary artery aneurysms in acute Kawasaki disease. *J Infect Dis* 2001;184:940–3.

Chang RKR: Hospitalizations for Kawasaki disease among children in the United States, 1988–1997. *Pediatrics* 2002;109:e87.

Dajani AS, Taubert KA, Takahashi M, et al: Guidelines for long-term management of patients with Kawasaki disease. *Circulation* 1994;89:916–22.

Han RK, Silverman ED, Newman A, et al: Management and outcome of persistent or recurrent fever after initial intravenous gammaglobulin therapy in acute Kawasaki disease. *Arch Pediatr Adolesc Med* 2000;154:694–9.

Kato H, Sugimura T, Akagi T, et al: Long-term consequences of Kawasaki disease. *Circulation* 1996;94:1379–85.

Newburger JW, Takahashi M, Beiser AS, et al: A single intravenous infusion of gamma globulin as compared with four infusions in the treatment of acute Kawasaki syndrome. *N Engl J Med* 1991;324:1633–9.

Rowley AH, Shulman ST: Kawasaki syndrome. *Pediatr Clin North Am* 1999;46:313–29.

Rowley AH, Shulman ST, Mask CA, et al: IgA plasma cell infiltration of proximal respiratory tract, pancreas, kidney, and coronary artery in acute Kawasaki disease. *J Infect Dis* 2000;182:1183–91.

Stockheim JA, Innocentini N, Shulman ST: Kawasaki disease in older children and adolescents. *J Pediatr* 2000;137:250–2.

Chapter 157
Vasculitis Syndromes

Michael L. Miller and Lauren M. Pachman

Vasculitis in childhood is a result of a spectrum of causes ranging from idiopathic conditions with primary vessel inflammation to syndromes following exposure to known antigens (e.g., infectious agents, drugs causing hypersensitivity reactions). Vasculitis is also a component of many autoimmune diseases. The extent of vessel damage can range from moderate, as in most children with Henoch-Schönlein purpura (HSP), to severe, as in children with polyarteritis nodosa. Most classifications of the vasculitic syndromes are based on the size and location of the blood vessels that are primarily involved, as well as the type of inflammatory infiltrate. The affected target vessels range in size from large afferent vessels, in Takayasu arteritis (TA), to capillary and arteriolar occlusion, characteristic of juvenile dermatomyositis. The inflammatory infiltrate can include various amounts of polymorphonuclear, mononuclear, and eosinophilic cells.

Immune complexes play a key role in the pathophysiology of many vasculitic syndromes. Immune complexes activate complement, releasing chemotactic fragments (C3a, C5a) that attract inflammatory cells. It is speculated in many vasculitic syndromes that immune complexes, after binding to endothelial cells, increase synthesis of adhesion molecules on the cell surfaces. These adhesion molecules bind to other adhesion molecules on circulating polymorphonuclear leukocytes attracted to the vicinity by chemotactic molecules. Subsequent lysosomal release of digestive enzymes from these leukocytes in many vasculitic syndromes destroys the cellular matrix of the blood vessels and surrounding tissues. In the process of degranulation, the polymorphonuclear leukocytes may disintegrate to the "nuclear dust" typical of leukocytoclastic angiitis (Fig. 157–1).

The signs and symptoms of the vasculitic syndromes are nonspecific and tend to overlap, but certain clinical features are useful in distinguishing the type of vasculature that is primarily affected. Palpable purpura suggests small vessel vasculitis located deep in the papillary dermis, whereas a circumscribed tender nodule is more likely a result of involvement of medium-sized vessels.

157.1 Henoch-Schönlein Purpura

HSP, also known as anaphylactoid purpura, is a vasculitis of small vessels. It is the most common cause of nonthrombocytopenic purpura in children.

Epidemiology. The etiology of HSP is unknown, but HSP typically follows an upper respiratory tract infection. The incidence and prevalence of HSP are probably underestimated because cases are not reported to public health agencies. However, of 31,333 new patients seen at 54 pediatric rheumatology centers in the United States, 1,120 had some form of vasculitis and 558 were classified as HSP. Although HSP accounted for 1% of hospital admissions in the past, changes in medical practice have reduced the frequency of admissions; 0.06% of admissions (62/9,083 in 1997) were for HSP at one large Midwestern pediatric center. This illness is more frequent in children than adults, with most cases occurring between 2–8 yr of age, most frequently in the winter months. Males are affected twice as frequently as females. The overall incidence is estimated to be 9/100,000 population.

Pathogenesis. The specific pathogenesis of HSP is not known, although in specific populations, patients with HSP have an significantly higher frequency of HLA-DRB1*07 than geographic controls. Increased serum concentrations of the cytokines tumor necrosis factor-α (TNFα) and interleukin (IL)-6 have been identified in active disease. In one study, almost half of the

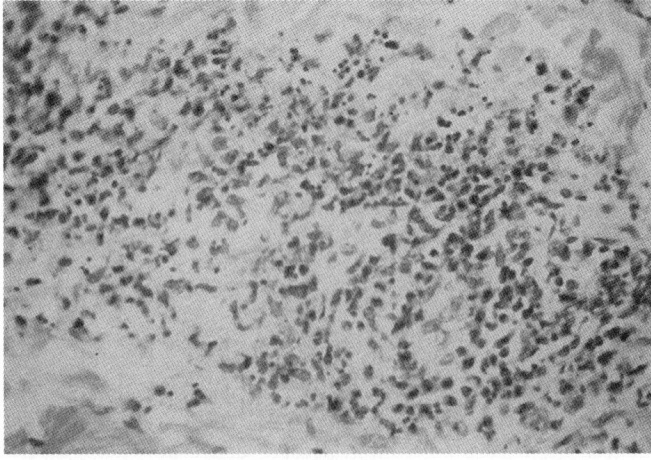

FIGURE 157–1. Histopathology of a skin biopsy from a patient with Henoch-Schönlein purpura showing leukocytoclastic vasculitis with nuclear degeneration ("nuclear dust").

patients had elevated antistreptolysin O (ASO) antibodies, implicating group A *Streptococcus*. This illness is considered by histopathology to be an IgA-mediated vasculitis of small vessels. Immunofluorescence techniques show deposition of IgA and C3 in the small vessels of the skin and the renal glomeruli, but the role of complement activation is controversial.

Clinical Manifestations. The disease onset may be acute, with the appearance of several manifestations simultaneously, or insidious, with sequential occurrence of symptoms over a period of weeks or months. Low-grade fever and fatigue occur in more than half of affected children. The typical rash and the clinical symptoms of HSP are a consequence of the usual location of the acute small vessel damage primarily in the skin, gastrointestinal tract, and kidneys.

The hallmark of the disease is the rash, beginning as pinkish maculopapules that initially blanch on pressure and progress to petechiae or purpura, which are characterized clinically as palpable purpura that evolve from red to purple to rusty brown before they eventually fade (Fig. 157–2). The lesions tend to occur in crops, last from 3–10 days, and may appear at intervals that vary from a few days to as long as 3–4 mo. In fewer than 10% of children, recurrence of the rash may not end until as late as a year, and rarely several years, after the initial episode. Damage to cutaneous vessels also results in local angioedema, which may precede the palpable purpura. Edema occurs primarily in dependent areas—for example, below the waist, over the buttocks (or on the back and posterior scalp in the infant), or in areas of greater tissue distensibility, such as the eyelids, lips, scrotum, or dorsum of the hands and feet.

Arthritis, present in more than two thirds of children with HSP, is usually localized to the knees and ankles and appears to be concomitant with edema. The effusions are serous, not hemorrhagic, in nature and resolve after a few days without residual deformity or articular damage. They may recur during a subsequent reactive phase of the disease.

Edema and damage to the vasculature of the gastrointestinal tract may also lead to intermittent abdominal pain that is often colicky in nature. More than half of patients have occult heme-positive stools, diarrhea (with or without visible blood), or hematemesis. The recognition of peritoneal exudate, enlarged mesenteric lymph nodes, segmental edema, and hemorrhage into the bowel may prevent unnecessary laparotomy for acute abdominal pain. Intussusception may occur, which is suggested by an empty right lower abdominal quadrant on physical examination or by **currant jelly stools**, which may be followed by complete obstruction or infarction with bowel perforation.

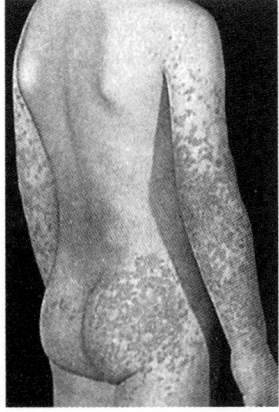

FIGURE 157–2. Henoch-Schönlein purpura. (From Korting GW: *Hautkrankheiten bei Kindern und Jugendlichen*, 3rd ed. Stuttgart, FK SchattauerVerlag, 1982.) See also color plates.

Several other organ systems may be involved during the acute phase of disease. Renal involvement occurs in 25–50% of children, and hepatosplenomegaly and lymphadenopathy may also be present during active disease. A rare but potentially serious outcome of central nervous system (CNS) involvement is the development of seizures, paresis, or coma. Other rare complications include rheumatoid-like nodules, cardiac and eye involvement, mononeuropathies, pancreatitis, and pulmonary or intramuscular hemorrhage.

Diagnosis. The pattern of crops of palpable purpuric lesions of similar hue in dependent areas of the body is characteristic of HSP. Diagnostic uncertainty arises when the symptom complex of edema, rash, arthritis with abdominal complaints, and renal findings occurs for a prolonged period. HSP can occur with other forms of vasculitis or autoimmune disease such as familial Mediterranean fever or inflammatory bowel disease. In polyarteritis nodosa, the cutaneous lesions are different, and peripheral neurologic and cardiac manifestations are more common. Palpable purpura can occur in meningococcemia, if there are pre-existing coagulation abnormalities such as factor V Leiden, protein S, or protein C deficiency. The presentation of unremitting fever, a maculopapular rash that does not reappear in crops but is prominent on the lower extremities, and peripheral arthritis suggests Kawasaki disease. HSP must be distinguished from systemic-onset juvenile rheumatoid arthritis, in which the salmon-pink rash is evanescent and maculopapular, with swelling that does not extend beyond the joint.

Laboratory Findings. Routine laboratory tests are neither specific nor diagnostic. Affected children often have a moderate thrombocytosis and leukocytosis. The erythrocyte sedimentation rate (ESR) may be elevated. Anemia may result from chronic or acute gastrointestinal blood loss. Immune complexes are often present, and 50% of patients have elevated concentrations of IgA as well as IgM but are usually negative for antinuclear antibodies (ANAs), antibodies to nuclear cytoplasmic antigens (ANCAs), and rheumatoid factor (even in the presence of rheumatoid nodules). Anticardiolipin or antiphospholipid antibodies may be present and contribute to the intravascular coagulopathy. Intussusception is usually ileoileal in location; barium enema may be used for both identification and nonsurgical reduction. Renal involvement is manifested by red blood cells, white blood cells, casts, or albumin in the urine.

Definitive diagnosis of vasculitis, confirmed by biopsy of an involved cutaneous site, shows leukocytoclastic angiitis. Renal biopsy may show IgA mesangial deposition and occasionally IgM, C3, and fibrin. Patients with IgA nephropathy may have elevated plasma antibody titers against *H. parainfluenzae*.

Treatment. Symptomatic treatment, including adequate hydration, bland diet, and pain control with acetaminophen, is provided for self-limited complaints of arthritis, edema, fever, and malaise. Avoidance of competitive activities and of maintaining the lower extremities in persistent dependence may decrease local edema. If edema involves the scrotum, elevation of the scrotum and local cooling, as tolerated, may decrease discomfort.

Intestinal complications (e.g., hemorrhage, obstruction, and intussusception) may be life threatening and managed with corticosteroids and, when necessary, reduction (by air or barium) or resection of the intussusception. Therapy with oral or intravenous corticosteroids (1–2 mg/kg/24 hr) is often associated with dramatic improvement of both gastrointestinal and CNS complications, which may recur for as long as 3 yr.

Management of renal involvement is the same as for other forms of acute glomerulonephritis (see Chapter 504). If anticardiolipin or antiphospholipid antibodies are identified and thrombotic events have occurred, aspirin (81 mg; a "baby" aspirin) given once may decrease the risks associated with a hypercoagulable state. Rheumatoid nodules may respond to alternate-day colchicine (0.6 mg/24 hr every other day).

Complications. The major complications of HSP are renal involvement, including nephrotic syndrome, and bowel perforation. An infrequent complication of scrotal edema is testicular torsion, which is quite painful and must be treated promptly.

Prognosis. HSP is a self-limited vasculitic disease with an excellent overall prognosis. Chronic renal disease may result in morbidity: a population-based study indicated that fewer than 1% of patients with HSP develop persistent renal disease and fewer than 0.1% develop serious renal disease. Rarely, death may occur during the acute phase of the disease as a result of bowel infarction, CNS involvement, or renal disease. Occasionally, children who present with an HSP-like syndrome acquire characteristics of other connective tissue diseases.

157.2 Takayasu Arteritis

TA, also known as pulseless disease, is a chronic vasculitis of large vessels.

Epidemiology. TA is infrequently reported in children in the United States but is more common in Asian and Indian populations. Children of all ethnic backgrounds have been affected. After HSP and Kawasaki disease, TA may be the third most common form of childhood vasculitis in the world. There is a 2.5:1 female:male ratio. About one third of cases have onset before age 20 yr, and symptoms usually appear after age 10 yr, although children as young as 8 mo have been affected. The interval from initial presentation to diagnosis in children has been reported to be as long as 19 mo, almost four times the interval reported for adults.

Pathogenesis. TA is a chronic inflammatory and obliterative disease of large vessels, with preference for the aorta and its major branches. Renal lesions include mesangial proliferative, membranoproliferative, and crescentic glomerulonephritis as well as amyloidosis.

Although the antigen responsible for inciting TA has yet to be defined, exposure to tuberculosis has been reported to be associated with the disease in some studies in Asia. Identification of critical amino acid residues of the HLA-B molecule at position 63(Glu) and 67(Ser) suggests a specific antigen-binding site in some cases. Study of non-Asian populations has provided evidence of similarities of sequence. Immune complex formation and complement activation have been frequently identified as well as anti-endothelial antibodies, which up-regulate the expression of endothelial adhesion molecules, but it is uncertain why only large vessels are affected. Cytokines, including IL-6, are increased, and there is a restricted usage of T cell receptors (V and V*), which suggests there is an immune response to an antigen.

Clinical Manifestations. Early disease manifestations, during the prepulseless phase, include night sweats, anorexia, weight loss, fatigue, myalgia, and arthritis, often followed by unexplained hypertension. During the pulseless phase, systemic symptoms are twice as frequent in children compared with adults; splenomegaly may be found. Dermatologic features include erythema nodosum, a malar rash, and erythema induratum. Cardiac involvement includes dilated cardiomyopathy, myocarditis, and pericarditis. Other associated conditions include interstitial lung disease, pneumonic consolidation, ulcerative colitis, rheumatoid arthritis, and polymyositis.

Diagnosis. During the pulseless phase, a characteristic bruit, often over the carotid or subclavian arteries, may be present on auscultation. Children may have diminished or absent radial pulses; limb claudication appears less frequently than in adults.

If these symptoms occur in the 1st yr of life, arterial damage may be accompanied by papular rash, uveitis, symmetric polyarthritis, and granulomatous lesions typical of sarcoid, a condition sometimes termed **juvenile systemic granulomatosis.**

Prompt diagnosis with institution of therapy is essential and may prevent progression of vascular lesions. The presence of intermittent unexplained systemic symptoms of variable duration in conjunction with an elevated ESR should prompt periodic auscultation of large arteries and blood pressure measurements in all four limbs.

This illness must be differentiated from acute rheumatic fever or juvenile arthritis. Because aortitis and aortic regurgitation may develop in TA, other disorders with these findings must also be considered, including Behçet disease, Cogan syndrome (a syndrome of ocular inflammation, vestibuloauditory abnormalities, and systemic vasculitis), relapsing polychondritis, ankylosing spondylitis (enthesitis-related arthritis), and seropositive rheumatoid arthritis. **Juvenile temporal arteritis** is rare, may be associated with a normal ESR, and is not associated with systemic symptoms.

Laboratory Findings. The ESR is significantly elevated, typically 60 mm/hr or greater (Westergren), and a microcytic hypochromic anemia with a leukocytosis is usual. A polyclonal hypergammaglobulinemia is present in one third of cases. Circulating immune complexes may remain elevated when the ESR has normalized, reflecting continued disease activity.

The diagnosis can be confirmed by angiography, which often outlines a massively dilated aortic arch, with aneurysmal dilatation and stenosis of various large vessels—carotids, subclavian, abdominal aorta, or rarely in children, lesions of the coronary artery (Fig. 157–3). Magnetic resonance angiography may be

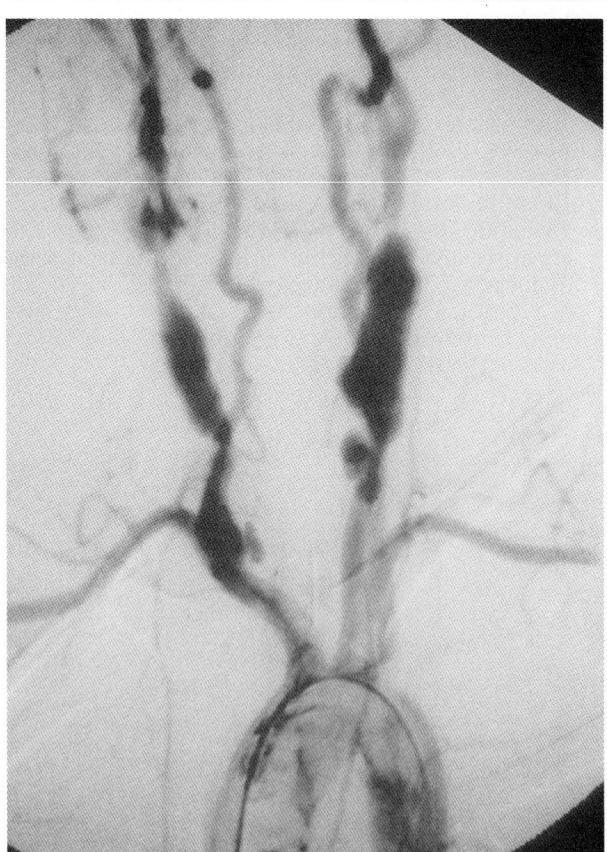

FIGURE 157–3. Angiogram of a child with Takayasu arteritis showing massive bilateral carotid dilatation, stenosis, and poststenotic dilatation.

helpful as a noninvasive test for subsequent monitoring of affected vessels.

Treatment. Early identification and surgical excision of the predominant lesions are essential, in conjunction with institution of appropriate immunosuppressive therapy. Prednisone (orally or intravenously) is administered in conjunction with other agents. Methotrexate has been useful in some situations, but cyclophosphamide (orally or intravenously) may often be needed to control the intense inflammatory response. Cyclophosphamide increases the risk of *Pneumocystis carinii* and therefore prophylactic trimethoprim-sulfamethoxazole is recommended. More than 50% of cases achieve remission after the 1st course of therapy, but about one fourth of cases never achieve remission. The 5-yr mortality has been reported to be as high as 35%. Supportive care includes management of hypertension and psychologic support. There is no indication for genetic counseling.

Complications. The most dreaded complication of this often fatal illness is an aneurysmal rupture. Therefore, the dilated area is often excised and replaced with an ileal vascular graft. Prevention of chronic hypertension and decreased perfusion can sometimes be accomplished by excision of a stenotic area with graft replacement or by insertion of an intraluminal stent to forestall the redevelopment of stenosis.

Prognosis. In the past, the mortality rate has been high. The outlook for these children remains guarded. The best outcome appears to follow early diagnosis and institution of medical and surgical therapy.

157.3 Polyarteritis Nodosa

Polyarteritis nodosa (PAN) is a necrotizing vasculitis affecting small- and medium-sized arteries. Aneurysms and nodules may form at irregular intervals throughout affected arteries.

Epidemiology. PAN occurs rarely during childhood. Boys and girls appear to be equally affected, with a peak at 10 yr of age. The cause is unknown, although the occurrence of PAN after upper respiratory tract infections, group A *Streptococcus* infection, and chronic hepatitis B infection suggests that PAN represents a postinfectious autoimmune response to these agents in susceptible individuals. Other infections, including infectious mononucleosis, tuberculosis, cytomegalovirus, and parvovirus, have also been associated with PAN.

Pathogenesis. Biopsy reveals a necrotizing vasculitis with lymphocytic infiltration affecting all layers of small- and medium-sized muscular arteries (Fig. 157–4). Involvement is usually segmental, including bifurcations of vessels. Different stages of inflammation are found, ranging from mild inflammation to extensive fibrinoid necrosis associated with thrombosis and infarction. Aneurysm formation is common. Vascular occlusion may also occur as a result of postinflammatory fibrosis. Renal arterial involvement is found in the majority of patients; glomerular involvement is variable.

Clinical Manifestations. The clinical presentation is variable but generally reflects the location of vessels that have become inflamed. Children may present with fever of unknown origin before other findings develop. Weight loss and severe abdominal pain suggest mesenteric arterial inflammation and possible thrombosis. Renovascular arteritis can result in hypertension, hematuria, or proteinuria. Vasculitis affecting the skin may be manifested by purpura, edema, and linear erythema with palpable, painful nodules along the course of affected arteries. In cutaneous PAN, the findings are limited to the skin. Arteritis affecting the nervous system may result in cerebrovascular accidents, transient ischemic attacks, psychosis, and ischemic

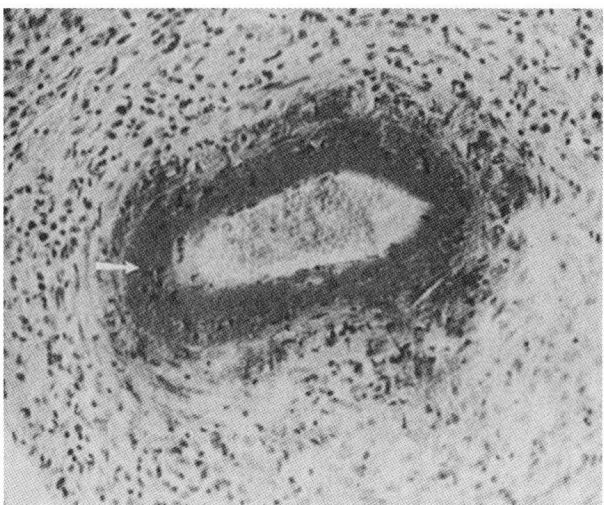

FIGURE 157–4. Biopsy of a medium-sized muscular artery that exhibits marked fibrinoid necrosis of the vessel wall (*arrow*). (From Cassidy JT, Petty RE: Juvenile rheumatoid arthritis. In *Textbook of Pediatric Rheumatology*, 3rd ed. Philadelphia, WB Saunders, 1995.)

peripheral neuropathy, with peripheral paresthesias or weakness. Cardiac involvement characterized by myocarditis may result in myocardial ischemia and heart failure; pericarditis and arrhythmias have also been reported. Less common findings include testicular pain that simulates testicular torsion, bone pain, and retinal arteritis, which may cause blindness. Arthralgia, arthritis, or myalgias may be encountered.

Diagnosis. Diagnosis of PAN requires demonstration of findings characteristic of vasculitis on biopsy or angiography. Biopsy of suggestive cutaneous lesions may reveal vasculitis (see Fig. 157–4). Renal biopsy in patients with renal manifestations may show characteristic necrotizing arteritis. Electromyography in children with peripheral neuropathy may identify affected sites; sural nerve biopsy may show an associated diagnostic vasculitis. Angiography demonstrates areas of aneurysmal dilatation, at branch points of arteries, or segmental stenosis (Fig. 157–5). The renal and mesenteric arteries are often involved. Evidence for previous or active infection should be sought in children with suspected PAN.

DIFFERENTIAL DIAGNOSIS. Early skin lesions may resemble those of HSP; the finding of nodular lesions and systemic findings distinguish PAN. Pulmonary lesions suggest Wegener granulomatosis (WG) or Goodpasture syndrome. Eosinophilia is noted in Churg-Strauss syndrome and eosinophilic fasciitis. Other rheumatic diseases, including systemic lupus erythematosus, dermatomyositis, and scleroderma, have characteristic target organ involvement distinct from PAN. Prolonged fever and weight loss can also characterize inflammatory bowel disease or malignancies.

Laboratory Findings. An elevated ESR is often the earliest finding. Anemia and leukocytosis are usually present eventually. Hypergammaglobulinemia reflects polyclonal B-cell activation. Abnormal urine sediment, proteinuria, and hematuria indicate renal disease. Markers of vasculitis may be useful in monitoring response to therapy. Von Willebrand factor antigen, a molecule found in vascular subendothelium, is released in increased amounts from inflamed vessels. Neopterin is released from macrophages that are activated in some patients with vasculitis. Levels of immune complexes, measured by the Raji cell and C1q assay, may also be elevated. Elevated hepatic enzymes suggest hepatitis B infection, which is more common in adults than in children.

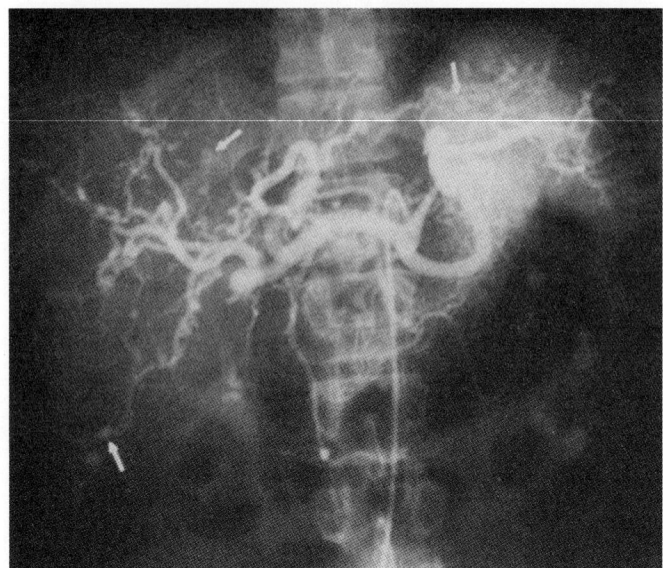

FIGURE 157–5. Celiac angiography of an 18-yr-old boy showing aneurysms in multiple vessels. (From Cassidy JT, Petty RE: Juvenile rheumatoid arthritis. In *Textbook of Pediatric Rheumatology*, 3rd ed. Philadelphia, WB Saunders, 1995.)

Treatment. Oral and intravenous corticosteroids have been used, sometimes in combination with oral or intravenous cyclophosphamide. Iloprost, a prostacyclin analog, may be used for endarteritis that is associated with vascular compromise in the extremities.

Complications. Cutaneous nodules may ulcerate, posing a risk of infection. Hypertension may develop from renal arterial involvement. Cardiac involvement may lead to decreased cardiac function or coronary arterial disease. Hepatic aneurysmal rupture is a rare complication.

Prognosis. The course of PAN varies from mild disease with few complications to a severe, overwhelming, multiorgan disease leading to death. However, aggressive immunosuppressive therapy has resulted in clinical remission. When renal involvement is present, the 1-yr survival rate was 73% and the 5-yr survival rate was 60%.

157.4 Wegener Granulomatosis

WG is a vasculitis affecting the upper and lower respiratory tract and kidneys, characterized by necrotizing granulomas.

Epidemiology. The heterogeneity of clinical presentations suggests that a single causative agent is unlikely. Although most cases occur in adults, children can develop WG, which predominates in whites. The cause is unknown, although proteinase 3 (PR3), normally restricted to neutrophil alpha granules, has been found on the surface of neutrophils of patients with WG. Those ANCAs that bind to PR3 are specific for WG, suggesting an etiologic role for abnormal PR3 expression. Interaction of PR3 with the PiZ variant of α_1-antitrypsin has been found in some studies to increase the risk of developing WG.

Pathogenesis. Necrotizing granulomas are found in affected organs, including the nasal and sinus mucosa, skin, and lower respiratory tract. In the lungs, infiltrates, alveolar hemorrhage, and vasculitis may also be found. Renal involvement can vary from focal proliferative glomerulonephritis to necrotic crescentic glomerulonephritis.

Clinical Manifestations. Children initially often complain of nonspecific constitutional symptoms of fever, malaise, weight loss, myalgia, and arthralgia. Many affected children have seasonal allergies. Later symptoms include cough, congestion, and nasal discharge from chronic sinusitis (often with mucosal ulceration and bone destruction from necrotizing granulomas), and hemoptysis and dyspnea from pulmonary lesions (Fig. 157–6). Ophthalmic involvement includes conjunctival and corneal lesions, uveitis, and an invasive orbital pseudotumor. Cranial and peripheral neuropathies due to intracranial granulomas and peripheral granulomatous lesions have been reported. Hematuria and proteinuria due to glomerulonephritis are often later manifestations. Cutaneous lesions may include palpable purpuric nodules and ulcers.

Diagnosis. The diagnosis of WG should be suspected in children who have severe sinusitis and who develop radiographic pulmonary findings suggestive of granulomas or renal findings consistent with nephritis. High-resolution CT imaging of the chest may reveal interstitial densities consistent with vasculitis or pulmonary hemorrhage. The diagnosis is confirmed by the presence of anti-PR3 ANCAs and the finding of necrotizing granulomatous angiitis on pulmonary, sinus, or renal biopsy.

DIFFERENTIAL DIAGNOSIS. Granulomatous lesions can be found in sarcoidosis, in which antibodies to ANCA are absent. Other granulomatous diseases (e.g., tuberculosis) also lack antibodies to ANCA. **Churg-Strauss syndrome** is a vasculitis that can cause chronic sinus lesions; a history of asthma, circulating eosinophilia, and an eosinophilic cutaneous vasculitis distinguish this syndrome from WG. The lesions in Churg-Strauss syndrome are not usually associated with destructive upper airway disease. Other vasculitic syndromes lack the characteristic granulomas on biopsy of affected organs.

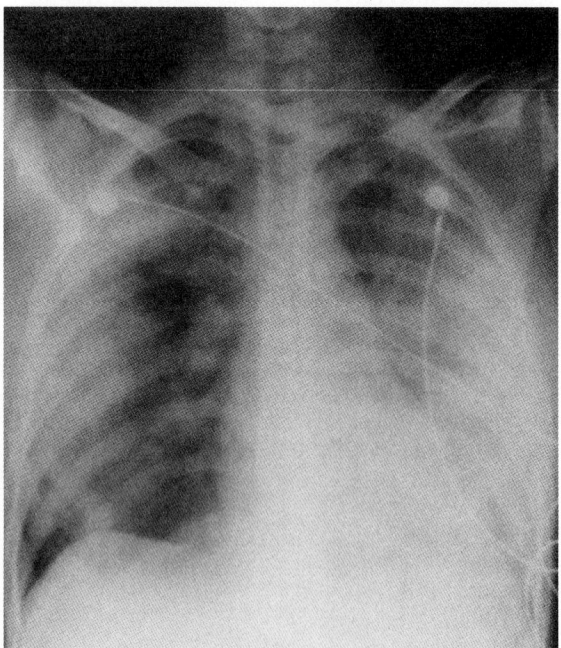

FIGURE 157–6. Chest radiograph of a 14-yr-old girl with Wegener granulomatosis showing widespread infiltrates suggestive of pulmonary hemorrhage. There were considerable day-to-day variability and eventual total resolution of these abnormalities after treatment with prednisone and cyclophosphamide. (From Cassidy JT, Petty RE: Juvenile rheumatoid arthritis. In *Textbook of Pediatric Rheumatology*, 3rd ed. Philadelphia, WB Saunders, 1995.)

Laboratory Findings. Elevated ESR, leukocytosis, thrombocytosis, and anemia may be found. Antibodies to ANCA directed toward PR3 are specific for WG. These antibodies, usually of IgG class, are found on immunofluorescence to be distributed in a diffuse granular staining throughout the cytoplasm (c-ANCA); staining for myeloperoxidase by ANCA in a perinuclear pattern (p-ANCA) is not specific for WG.

Treatment. Oral and intravenous corticosteroids and cyclophosphamide have been effective in many patients. Methotrexate has also been used with success

Complications. Enlarging granulomas may disrupt local anatomy: Intrasinus lesions can invade the orbit; lesions in the ear can result in unilateral deafness. Respiratory complications include pulmonary hemorrhage and upper airway obstruction due to subglottic stenosis. Infectious complications include sinusitis, either as infection of granulomatous lesions or after obstruction, and pneumonia. Chronic glomerulonephritis may result in end-stage renal disease.

Prognosis. The course is variable. Mortality has been reduced with the introduction of cyclophosphamide and other immunosuppressive agents.

157.5 Other Vasculitic Syndromes

Leukocytoclastic vasculitis refers to a spectrum of vasculitic syndromes, including HSP, as well as to specific biopsy findings. It is characterized by cutaneous vessel inflammation affecting both small arteries and postcapillary venules. Purpura and occasionally urticaria are found, particularly on the extremities. The diagnostic term leukocytoclastic vasculitis is sometimes used for cases similar to HSP but with atypical distribution and associated symptoms. **Hypersensitivity angiitis** is cutaneous vasculitis following exposure to drugs, such as sulfonamides. Clinical manifestations include fever, myalgia, and arthralgia but rarely visceral involvement. Subsequent development of systemic findings indicating more extensive vasculitis suggests the likelihood of another diagnosis such as PAN. For both leukocytoclastic vasculitis and hypersensitivity angiitis, biopsy of lesions may reveal fibrinoid necrosis of blood vessels, perivascular polymorphonuclear infiltrate, and nuclear debris or dust.

Merkel PA: Drug induced vasculitis. *Rheum Dis Clin North Am* 2001;27:849–62.
Nadeau SE: Neurologic manifestations of systemic vasculitis. *Neurol Clin* 2002;20: 123–50.
Yalcindag A, Sundel R: Vasculitis in childhood. *Curr Opin Rheumatol* 2001;13: 422–7.

Henoch-Schönlein Purpura
Amoli MM, Thomson W, Hajeer AH, et al: HLA-DRB1*01 association with Henoch-Schönlein purpura in patients from northwest Spain. *J Rheumatol* 2001;28:1266–70.
Rostoker G: Schönlein-Henoch purpura in children and adults: Diagnosis, pathophysiology and management. *BioDrugs* 2001;15:99–138.
Scharer K, Krmar R, Querfeld U, et al: Clinical Outcome of Schönlein-Henoch purpura nephritis in children. *Pediatr Nephrol* 1999;13:816–23.

Takayasu Arteritis
Hoffman GS: Takayasu arteritis: Lessons from the American National Institutes of Health experience. *Int J Cardiol* 1996;54:102–96.
Itazawa T, Noguchi K, Ichida F, et al Magnetic resonance imaging for early detection of Takayasu arteritis. *Pediatr Cardiol* 2001;22:163–4.
Martini A: Behçet's disease and Takayasu disease in children. *Curr Opin Rheumatol* 1995;7:449–54.
Sharma BK, Jain S, Sagar S: Systemic manifestations of Takayasu arteritis: The expanding spectrum. *Int J Cardiol* 1996;54:S149–54.

Polyarteritis Nodosa
Besbas N, Ozen S, Saatci U: Renal involvement in polyarteritis nodosa: Evaluation of 26 Turkish children. *Pediatr Nephrol* 2000;14:325–7.
David J, Ansell BM, Woo P: Polyarteritis nodosa associated with *Streptococcus*. *Arch Dis Child* 1993;69:685–8.

Wegener Granulomatosis
Gottlieb BS, Miller LC, Ilowite NT: Methotrexate treatment of Wegener granulomatosis in children. *J Pediatr* 1996;129:604–7.
Harper L, Savage CO: Leukocyte-endothelial interactions in antineutrophil cytoplasmic antibody-associated systemic vasculitis. *Rheum Dis Clin North Am* 2001;27:887–903.
Rottem M, Fauci AS, Hallahan CW, et al: Wegener granulomatosis in children and adolescents: Clinical presentation and outcome. *J Pediatr* 1993;122:26–31.
Valentini RP, Smoyer WE, Sedman AB, et al: Outcome of antineutrophil cytoplasmic autoantibodies-positive glomerulonephritis and vasculitis in children: A single-center experience. *J Pediatr* 1998;132:325–8.
Wadsworth DT, Siegel MJ, Day DL: Wegener's granulomatosis in children: Chest radiographic manifestations. *Am J Roentgenol* 1994;163:901–4.

Chapter 158
Musculoskeletal Pain Syndromes *Michael L. Miller*

Children with poorly localized pain involving the extremities and with normal findings on physical examination and unremarkable laboratory findings can be considered to have a musculoskeletal pain syndrome (MSPS). MSPS occasionally develops following trauma in children with underlying rheumatic diseases; careful follow up is necessary to distinguish this complication from slowly evolving disease exacerbation. Clinical manifestations of MSPS overlap other conditions, including reflex sympathetic dystrophy (RSD), erythromelalgia, fibromyalgia, and chronic fatigue syndrome (see Chapter 111). Clinical management of these conditions is remarkably similar.

Clinical Manifestations. The history is sometimes related almost entirely by a parent who notes the child to have pain at rest. If symptoms have persisted for years, adolescents may also report chronic pain, often with inconsistent details, when compared with the history offered by the parent. Location of pain can vary from regional, affecting a single extremity, to generalized. Patients often complain of pain refractory to nonsteroidal anti-inflammatory drugs and analgesic agents. Physical therapy programs may have been tried without success.

Other symptoms associated with pain syndromes include fatigue, sleep problems, and poor school attendance. In contrast to many children with pain due to rheumatic diseases, children with MSPS tend to be depressed at the prospect of returning to school instead of staying home from school. Excellent academic performance often precedes prolonged school absences; it is possible that symptoms develop when a child is unable to maintain continuing academic demands. Parents may have a history of organic or functional pain, sometimes in the same anatomic region that is symptomatic in the child.

Results of the physical examination are unremarkable, with normal strength and no joint swelling or limitation of motion. However, exquisite tenderness to light touch is often elicited over various parts of the extremities, which may not be reproducible on repeat examination. Cold, clammy, cyanotic distal extremities occasionally suggest autonomic dysfunction, such as in RSD. These findings may improve after a child has exercised.

Fibromyalgia is distinguished by the presence of **trigger points**, which are localized areas of tenderness to palpation. These are not always reproducible. One study found many children with fibromyalgia to have hypermobile joints.

There are no specific laboratory findings of MSPS. Anemia and hypothyroidism should be excluded. Imaging studies, particularly plain radiographs, may be necessary to exclude fractures or other pathology; MRI studies may be necessary to exclude ligamentous injury. The need for additional tests is individualized, depending on specific symptoms and physical findings.

Diagnosis. The diagnosis of musculoskeletal pain syndromes is one of exclusion if careful, repeated physical examinations and laboratory testing do not reveal an etiology. A history of sleep disturbances and widespread musculoskeletal pain associated with tenderness over trigger points on physical examination suggests fibromyalgia.

DIFFERENTIAL DIAGNOSIS. Because psychiatric disorders can overlap and present with symptoms of MSPS, psychiatric evaluation should be considered for children with these syndromes. Prolonged school absence suggests school phobia (see Chapter 22). When fatigue is more prominent than pain, chronic fatigue syndrome may be considered (see Chapter 111). Physical and sexual abuse may also be manifested by pain syndromes; adolescent girls may have accompanying dizziness. In Munchausen syndrome by proxy (see Chapter 35.3), reports of pain are emphasized with the intent of obtaining unnecessary, often interventional, evaluation.

Repeated physical examinations over time may reveal eventual development of manifestations suggestive of rheumatic or other diseases. Imaging studies, including plain radiographs, MRI, and technetium-99m bone scan, may identify focal pathology resulting from infection, malignancy, or trauma. Weakness may result from thyroid disease, inflammatory myositis, muscular dystrophies, or neurologic disease. Chest pain may be a manifestation of costochondritis, pericarditis, coronary arterial abnormality, or aortic stenosis. Proximal leg pain, often occurring at night, may occur with osteoid osteoma. Back pain may indicate local pathology, including spondylolisthesis, diskitis, and vertebral microfractures. When children with poorly localized pain develop tender entheses, ankylosing spondyloarthropathy should be considered (see Chapter 146).

Treatment. Successful outcome requires that any underlying psychiatric disorder be identified and treated. Therapy should be directed toward emotional support for the patient and family, relief of symptoms, and minimizing unnecessary and misleading diagnostic tests and therapeutic regimens. The approach includes a combination of restoration of a normal sleep pattern, rehabilitation strategies including exercise for fatigue, and optimism. Children have been found to improve when the physician and other health care providers can overcome parental resistance to a vigorous physical therapy program for stretching and joint protection. Increasing physical activity at home to improve the level of physical fitness can also help. Some centers use bedtime doses of antidepressants for MSPS. However, if their use is required for more than several weeks, psychiatric evaluation may be necessary to evaluate for depression. For children with persisting symptoms, a rehabilitation program by a physiatrist or referral to a pain clinic may be indicated.

Complications. Untreated musculoskeletal pain syndromes can result in impaired physical fitness, decreased socialization leading to isolation, prolonged school absences, and lost opportunities for college or vocational training. When families avoid psychologic evaluation or recommendations, children are at risk for developing or exacerbating depression.

158.1 Reflex Sympathetic Dystrophy

Reflex sympathetic (or neurovascular) dystrophy, a condition of unknown cause, is characterized by diffuse limb pain with color and temperature changes thought to result from autonomic nervous system dysfunction. RSD is often a response to physical or emotional distress. A history of physical activities causing repeated impact on the extremities (e.g., ballet dancing) or severe or prolonged emotional trauma (e.g., divorce of the parents, death of a sibling) may be elicited. Children complain of pain worsened by touch or movement, often with dysesthesia

and a sensation of temperature changes and swelling. They tend to maintain the hand or foot in a rigid, unusual position, refusing to allow passive motion. Prolonged disuse of the extremity can cause osteopenia; imaging studies (e.g., Doppler flow studies, technetium-99m bone scan) may show either increased or decreased blood flow. Assurance, physical therapy, and, when indicated, counseling can result in resolution of symptoms and physical findings. Relaxation techniques provided by a psychologist may also be useful. When these measures are unsuccessful, sympathetic blocks may be considered.

158.2 Erythromelalgia

Children with erythromelalgia experience episodes of intense pain, erythema, and heat in the distal portion of their legs (rarely, the hands). Mild heat exposure may trigger symptoms that can last for hours and occasionally for days. Although most cases are sporadic, an autosomal dominant hereditary form has been reported. Erythromelalgia can also be associated with peripheral neuropathy, frostbite, hypertension, and rheumatic disease. Treatment includes avoidance of heat exposure and application of cold during attacks. Propranolol, carbamazepine, or sodium nitroprusside may be effective for some affected children.

Finley WH, Lindsey JR Jr, Fine JD, et al: Autosomal dominant erythromelalgia. *Am J Med Genet* 1992;42:310–5.

Gedalia A, Press J, Klein M, et al: Joint hypermobility and fibromyalgia in school children. *Ann Rheum Dis* 1993;52:494–6.

Gedalia A, Garcia CO, Molina JF, et al: Fibromyalgia syndrome in children: Experience in a pediatric rheumatology clinic. *Clin Exp Rheumatol* 2000;18:415–9.

Mikkelsson M, Sourander A, Phia J, et al: Psychiatric symptoms in preadolescents with musculoskeletal pain and fibromyalgia. *Pediatrics* 1997;100:220–7.

Reid GJ, Lang BA, McGrath PJ: Primary juvenile fibromyalgia: Psychological adjustment, family functioning, coping, and functional disability. *Arthritis Rheum* 1997;40:752–60.

Schanberg LE, Keefe FJ, Lefebvre JC, et al: Pain coping strategies in children with juvenile primary fibromyalgia syndrome: Correlation with pain, physical function, and psychological distress. *Arthritis Care Res* 1996;9:89–96.

Sherry DD: Pain syndromes in children. *Curr Rheumatol Rep* 2000;2:337–42.

Siegel DM, Janeway D, Baum J: Fibromyalgia syndrome in children and adolescents: Clinical features at presentation and status at follow-up. *Pediatrics* 1998;101:377–82.

Stanton RP, Malcolm JR, Wesdock KA, et al: Reflex sympathetic dystrophy in children: An orthopedic perspective. *Orthopedics* 1993;16:773–9.

Wilder RT, Berde CB, Wolohan M, et al: Reflex sympathetic dystrophy in children. Clinical characteristics and follow-up of seventy patients. *J Bone Joint Surg Am* 1992;74:910–9.

Chapter 159

Miscellaneous Conditions Associated with Arthritis

Michael L. Miller

Inflammation of joints or connective tissue may be a manifestation of nonrheumatic conditions. These conditions need to be considered in children with joint complaints whose history, clinical findings, or clinical course are not consistent with rheumatic diseases.

Relapsing Polychondritis. Relapsing polychondritis is characterized by episodic necrotizing inflammation of cartilage in the outer ear, trachea, and nose. Patients may also develop polyarticular arthritis, ocular inflammation, and hearing loss resulting from inflammation near the auditory and vestibular nerves. Children may initially relate only episodes of intense

---

■ **BOX 159–1. Diagnostic Criteria for Relapsing Polychondritis**

Nonerosive seronegative inflammatory polyarthritis
At least three of the following:
    Bilateral auricular chondritis
    Nonerosive seronegative inflammatory polyarthritis
    Nasal chondritis
    Ocular inflammation
    Respiratory tract chondritis
    Audiovestibular chondritis

From McAdam LP, O'Hanlan MA, Bluestone R, et al: Relapsing polychondritis: Prospective study of 23 patients and a review of the literature. *Medicine (Baltimore)* 1976;55:193–215.

---

erythema over the outer ears. Later, inflammation may be so severe that it causes loss of cartilage from the outer ear, nose, or trachea. Diagnostic criteria established for adults are useful guidelines for evaluating children who develop suggestive symptoms (Box 159–1). The differential diagnosis includes Cogan syndrome (characterized by auditory nerve inflammation and keratitis but not chondritis) and Wegener granulomatosis (see Chapter 157.4). The clinical course is variable; although some patients respond to corticosteroids, others experience a relentless, progressive course, culminating in death due to airway obstruction.

Mucha-Habermann Disease. Mucha-Habermann disease, or pityriasis lichenoides et varioliformis acuta (PLEVA), is characterized by recurrent arthritis associated with episodes of vesicular cutaneous lesions, fever, and elevated erythrocyte sedimentation rate. The diagnosis is confirmed by biopsy of skin lesions, which reveals a lymphocytic vasculitis affecting capillaries and venules in the upper dermis.

Sweet Syndrome. Sweet syndrome, or acute febrile neutrophilic dermatosis, occurs most often in young women and is rare in children. It is characterized by recurrent fever and raised, tender erythematous plaques over the face, extremities, and trunk. Some children also have arthritis. The syndrome may be idiopathic or secondary to malignancy, Behçet syndrome (see Chapter 151), or chronic recurrent multifocal osteomyelitis (see Chapter 674). Skin biopsy reveals neutrophilic perivascular infiltrates. The condition is usually responsive to treatment with corticosteroids.

Hypertrophic Osteoarthropathy. Some children with clubbing develop soft tissue swelling over the hands, particularly the distal digits, with arthritis in the distal interphalangeal joints and tender periosteal new bone formation along tubular long bones and bones in the hand. This complication, hypertrophic osteoarthropathy (HOA), can be found in some children with chronic pulmonary disease (e.g., cystic fibrosis), congenital heart disease, gastrointestinal diseases (e.g., malabsorption syndromes, biliary atresia, and inflammatory bowel disease), and malignancies (e.g., nasopharyngeal sarcoma, osteosarcoma, and Hodgkin disease). Although the cause is unknown, some studies suggest that in diseases underlying HOA, platelet fragments escape the pulmonary circulation and interact with peripheral endothelial cells and other tissues. The resulting release of fibroblast and related growth factors causes the clinical manifestations. The symptoms of HOA may improve if the underlying condition can be successfully treated. Evaluation of children presenting with HOA should include a chest radiograph to eliminate pulmonary disease or intrathoracic mass.

Plant Thorn Synovitis. Puncture wounds due to plant thorns or similar foreign objects that penetrate the synovium can cause acute synovitis that may progress to chronic arthritis. The episode of initial trauma often is forgotten. The diagnosis should

be considered in children with chronic monoarticular arthritis unresponsive to anti-inflammatory medication. Diagnosis may require MRI or arthroscopy. Histology often reveals a granulomatous synovitis. Treatment is removal of the foreign body, which may be accomplished by irrigation of the joint during arthroscopy. Chronic synovitis may require synovectomy.

Diabetic Mellitus and Arthropathy. Diabetic cheiroarthropathy (arthropathy of the joints of the hands and fingers) is a complication of juvenile-onset diabetes mellitus, which occurs most often in late childhood or adolescence. The soft tissues of the hands and fingers undergo progressive thickening and tightening, leading to contractures of the small joints in the hand but without the tapering and loss of digital pulp over the fingertips characteristic of sclerodactyly seen in patients with scleroderma (Chapter 161). Occupational therapy can improve loss of motion in affected joints. Diabetic cheiroarthropathy must be distinguished from polyarticular juvenile rheumatoid arthritis, which can coexist with unrelated chronic conditions and in which joint swelling typically precedes flexion contractures.

Cystic Fibrosis and Arthropathy. In addition to hypertrophic osteoarthropathy, some patients with cystic fibrosis experience either episodic or persistent arthritis. The cause is unknown but may reflect synovitis resulting from deposition of immune complexes formed in response to recurrent pulmonary infections. It is also possible that persistent arthritis is a result of expression of coexisting, unrelated juvenile rheumatoid arthritis.

Acute Pancreatitis and Arthritis. Periostitis, nodular skin lesions, and synovial fat necrosis may develop as a result of lipases released during pancreatitis. Affected children may have fever, arthritis, and bone pain for several weeks after blunt abdominal trauma (including child abuse) or other causes of pancreatitis. Elevated serum lipase and amylase levels, periosteal new bone formation, and abnormal findings on bone scintigraphy (revealing fat-induced infarcts) may be found. Drainage of pancreatic pseudocysts may alleviate symptoms of arthritis in some patients.

Immunodeficiency. Some children with B- and T-lymphocyte immunodeficiencies develop rheumatic diseases. There are several potential mechanisms. Defective mucosal immunity in children with B-cell diseases (e.g., IgA deficiency, X-linked agammaglobulinemia, and common variable immunodeficiency) may permit entry from the gut into the circulation of viruses that are either cross-reactive with self antigens or capable of causing infective synovitis. T-cell defects may result in the loss of T-lymphocyte control over autoreactive T lymphocytes. Arthritis, both episodic and chronic, has been described in children with various types of hypogammaglobulinemia, IgA deficiency, and DiGeorge syndrome. IgA deficiency has also been associated with other rheumatic diseases, including lupus, dermatomyositis, scleroderma, and spondyloarthropathy. Patients with Wiskott-Aldrich syndrome have been reported to develop arthritis, vasculitis, and other rheumatic manifestations. The differential diagnosis of arthritis in children with immunodeficiencies includes suppurative arthritis and osteomyelitis.

Akman IO, Ostrov BE, Neudorf S: Autoimmune manifestations of the Wiskott-Aldrich syndrome. *Semin Arthritis Rheum* 1998;27:218–25.

Ansell BM: Hypertrophic osteoarthropathy in the paediatric age. *Clin Exp Rheumatol* 1992;10(Suppl 7):15–8.

Conley ME, Park CL, Douglas SD: Childhood common variable immunodeficiency with autoimmune disease. *J Pediatr* 1986;108:915–22.

Diren HB, Kutluk MT, Karabent A, et al: Primary hypertrophic osteoarthropathy. *Pediatr Radiol* 1986;16:231–4.

Luberti AA, Rabinowitz LG, Ververeli KO: Severe febrile Mucha-Habermann's disease in children: Case report and review of the literature. *Pediatr Dermatol* 1991;8:51–7.

Maillot F, Goupille P, Valat JP: Plant thorn synovitis diagnosed by magnetic resonance imaging. *Scand J Rheumatol* 1994;23:154–5.

Marhaug G, Hvidsten D: Arthritis complicating acute pancreatitis—a rare but important condition to be distinguished from juvenile rheumatoid arthritis. *Scand J Rheumatol* 1988;17:397–9.

McAdam LP, O'Hanlan MA, Bluestone R, et al: Relapsing polychondritis: Prospective study of 23 patients and a review of the literature. *Medicine (Baltimore)* 1976;55:193–215.

Oddone M, Toma P, Taccone A, et al: Relapsing polychondritis in childhood: A rare observation studied by CT and MRI. *Pediatr Radiol* 1992;22:537–8.

Staalman CR, Umans U: Hypertrophic osteoarthropathy in childhood malignancy. *Med Pediatr Oncol* 1993;21:676–9.

Sullivan KE, McDonald-McGinn DM, Driscoll DA, et al: Juvenile rheumatoid arthritis-like polyarthritis in chromosome 22q11.2 deletion syndrome (DiGeorge anomalad/velocardiofacial syndrome/conotruncal anomaly face syndrome). *Arthritis Rheum* 1997;40:430–6.

Wulffraat NM, de Graeff-Meeder ER, Rijkers GT, et al: Prevalence of circulating immune complexes in patients with cystic fibrosis and arthritis. *J Pediatr* 1993;125:374–8.

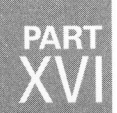

Chapter 160
Diagnostic Microbiology
Anita K. M. Zaidi and Donald A. Goldmann

Laboratory diagnosis of infectious diseases is based on one or more of the following: (1) direct examination of specimens by microscopic or antigenic techniques, (2) isolation of microorganisms in culture, (3) serologic testing for development of antibodies (**serodiagnosis**), and (4) molecular genetic detection. Clinicians must select the appropriate tests and specimens and, when possible, suggest the suspected etiologic agents to the microbiologist, who facilitates selection of the most cost-effective diagnostic approach. Additional roles of the microbiology laboratory include antimicrobial susceptibility testing and assisting the hospital epidemiologist in detecting and clarifying the epidemiology of nosocomial infections.

LABORATORY DIAGNOSIS OF BACTERIAL AND FUNGAL INFECTIONS

Diagnosis of bacterial and fungal infections relies mainly on direct demonstration of the microorganisms by microscopic examination or antigen detection and on growth of microorganisms on nutrient culture media. Molecular diagnostic methods for direct detection of some pathogens have also been developed.

Microscopy. The **Gram stain** remains an extremely useful diagnostic technique because it is a rapid, inexpensive method for demonstrating the presence of bacteria and fungi, as well as inflammatory cells. A preliminary assessment of the etiologic agent can be made by noting the morphology of the microorganisms (e.g., cocci vs rods) and their color (gram-positive microorganisms stain blue, and gram-negative stain red). The presence of inflammatory and epithelial cells can be used to gauge the quality of certain specimens. For example, 10 or more epithelial cells per low-power field in a sputum sample strongly suggests contamination from oral secretions. In many cases, such as in the examination of cerebrospinal fluid (CSF), the Gram stain can provide very rapid and useful results. However, the Gram stain is an insensitive technique, requiring 10^{4-5} microorganisms/mL for detection of organisms. A trained observer may be able to reach a tentative conclusion that there are specific microorganisms in the specimen based on their morphology and Gram reaction (e.g., gram-positive cocci in clusters are likely to be staphylococci), but such preliminary interpretations should be made cautiously and must be confirmed by culture. Many different stains are used in clinical microbiology (Table 160–1).

Rapid Antigen Detection. Several rapid antigen detection tests for bacterial pathogens are commercially available and widely used. These include **latex agglutination** (LA) tests for detection of group A *Streptococcus* in the pharynx, and *Haemophilus influenzae* type b, *Streptococcus pneumoniae*, group B *Streptococcus*, and *Neisseria meningitidis* in CSF. Routinely performing LA tests on CSF is expensive and offers no advantage over a properly performed Gram stain; their use is best limited to patients with CSF pleocytosis who have received prior antimicrobial therapy.

A rapid and sensitive test for the detection of *Streptococcus pneumoniae* (pneumococcus) antigen in the urine of patients with invasive pneumococcal disease (Binax NOW Urinary Antigen Test, Binax Inc., Portland, ME) has recently become available in the United States. Initial data also indicate utility in the detection of pneumococcal antigen in CSF of patients with meningitis. A major limitation of the urinary test is that approximately half of all well children who are merely nasopharyngeal carriers of pneumococci also test positive.

Isolation and Identification. Most medically important bacteria can be cultured on nutrient-rich media such as blood agar and chocolate agar. Specialized agar may be used selectively to grow and differentiate among organisms of different types. For example, MacConkey's agar supports growth of gram-negative rods while suppressing gram-positive organisms; a color change in the media from clear to pink distinguishes lactose-fermenting organisms from other gram-negative rods. Liquid broth media are used for blood cultures and to enhance growth of small numbers of organisms in other clinical specimens. Sabouraud's dextrose agar (with antibiotics to inhibit bacterial growth) is used to culture most fungi. However, many pathogens such as *Bartonella*, *Bordetella pertussis*, *Brucella*, *Francisella*, *Legionella*, anaerobes, mycobacteria, certain fungal pathogens such as *Malassezia furfur*, *Mycoplasma*, and *Chlamydia* require specialized growth media or incubation conditions. Consultation with the laboratory is advised when these pathogens are suspected and cultures are desired.

After isolation in culture, microbial identity can be confirmed by biochemical tests, ability of the organism to grow in the presence of certain substances that inhibit growth of other microorganisms (e.g., selective antibiotics, salt, bile), antigen detection, or molecular probes.

Blood Culture. Several different blood culture systems are available; most use 50–100 mL bottles containing broth that enhances the growth of bacteria and fungi (mainly yeast). Bottles with smaller volumes are also available specifically for pediatric use. Media containing resins are often used to adsorb antibiotics to improve recovery of organisms if the patient has received antibiotics before blood culture. Many laboratories use automated culture systems that greatly reduce the time to microbial detection; more than 80% of all cultures containing pathogens are positive at 24 hours of incubation or sooner.

Proper skin disinfection before blood collection is essential. Povidone-iodine may be used, but this agent must be allowed to dry completely for maximum activity. Alcohol is rapidly bactericidal and is a suitable alternative agent. Iodine is effective but must be

TABLE 160–1. Stains Used for Microscopic Examination

Type of Stain	Clinical Use
Gram stain	Stains bacteria, fungi, leukocytes, and epithelial cells.
Potassium hydroxide (KOH)	A 10% KOH solution dissolves cellular and organic debris and facilitates detection of fungal elements.
Calcofluor white stain	Nonspecific fluorochrome that binds to cellulose and chitin in fungal cell walls. Can be combined with 10% KOH to dissolve cellular material.
Ziehl-Neelson and Kinyoun stains	Acid-fast stains, using basic carbol fuchsin, followed by acid-alcohol decolorization and methylene blue counterstaining. Acid-fast organisms (e.g., *Mycobacterium*, *Cryptosporidium*, and *Cyclospora*) resist decolorization and stain pink or red. A weaker decolorizing agent is used for partially acid-fast organisms (e.g., *Nocardia*).
Acridine orange stain	Fluorescent dye that intercalates into DNA. At acid pH, bacteria and fungi stain orange, and background cellular material stains green.
Auramine-Rhodamine stain	Acid-fast stain using fluorochromes that bind to mycolic acid in mycobacterial cell walls, and resist acid-alcohol decolorization. Acid-fast organisms stain orange-yellow against a black background.
India ink stain	Detects *Cryptococcus neoformans*, an encapsulated yeast, by excluding ink particles from the polysaccharide capsule. (Direct testing for cryptococcal antigen in specimens is much more sensitive than India ink preparations).
Methenamine silver stain	Stains fungal elements, *Pneumocystis* cysts in tissues. Primarily performed in surgical pathology laboratories.
Lugol's iodine stain	Added to wet preparations of fecal specimens for ova and parasites to enhance contrast of the internal structures (nuclei, glycogen vacuoles).
Wright and Giemsa stains	Primarily for detecting blood parasites (*Plasmodium*, *Babesia*, and *Leishmania*), fungi in tissues (yeasts, *Histoplasma*).
Trichrome stain	Stains stool specimens for identification of protozoa.
Direct fluorescent-antibody stain	Used for direct detection of a variety of organisms in clinical specimens by using specific fluorescein-labeled antibodies (e.g., *Bordetella pertussis*, *Legionella*, *Chlamydia trachomatis*, *Pneumocystis carinii*, many viruses).

wiped off with alcohol to avoid skin reactions. The practice of obtaining blood for culture from intravascular catheters without accompanying peripheral venous blood cultures should be discouraged because it is difficult to determine the significance of coagulase-negative staphylococci and other skin flora isolated from blood obtained from "through-the-line" cultures. For patients with suspected bacteremia and fungemia, two or three separate blood cultures are preferred. More than three blood cultures rarely are indicated, even in infective endocarditis. Whenever possible, a minimum of 2 mL of blood should be obtained for culture before administration of antibiotics. Obtaining a larger volume of blood is necessary to maximize yield from blood cultures, because 10–20% of pediatric patients may have low-grade bloodstream infections. For most patients, the most effective approach is to culture the entire volume of blood in a single aerobic bottle because anaerobic bacteremia is rare in children. Blood should also be cultured anaerobically for patients at increased risk for anaerobic sepsis, such as children who are immunocompromised or who have head and neck or abdominal infections. Detection of fungi can be aided by lysis-centrifugation techniques, such as the Isolator 1.5 system (Wampole, Cranbury, NJ). In developing countries with high rates of *Salmonella* bloodstream infections, optimal blood culture practices remain undefined.

CSF CULTURE. CSF should be transported quickly to the laboratory, where it is centrifuged to concentrate organisms for microscopic examination. CSF is routinely plated on blood agar and chocolate agar, which support the growth of the common pathogens that cause meningitis. If tuberculous meningitis is suspected, CSF cultures for mycobacteria should be specifically requested.

URINE CULTURE. Urine for culture and colony count can be obtained by collecting clean-voided midstream specimens, catheterization, or suprapubic aspiration. Urine samples collected by placing bags on the perineum are unacceptable for culture because of frequent contamination, which renders the results uninterpretable. Rapid transport of urine to the laboratory is imperative because gram-negative enteric pathogens have doubling times of 20–30 min, and any delay in transport or plating renders colony counts unreliable. Refrigeration can be used when delay is unavoidable. Culture systems using media-coated "paddles" permit prompt inoculation of the specimen, but confluent growth may be difficult to detect; moreover, accurate antibiotic susceptibility testing requires the presence of individual discrete colonies. Urine obtained by suprapubic puncture should normally be sterile; any bacterial growth is considered significant. Urine colony counts are generally considered significant in urine collected by catheterization if 10^3

organisms/mL or greater, and in urine collected by clean-catch (midstream) void if 10^5 organisms/mL or greater are present. However, lower counts are sometimes found in urinary tract infections in adolescent girls and young women, especially those with bacterial urethritis, or in patients with fungal infections. A Gram stain of unspun urine with at least one bacterium per oil immersion field correlates well with the presence of greater than or equal to 10^5 organisms/mL of urine.

GENITAL TRACT CULTURE. Specimens from the genital tract include urethral, cervical, and anorectal swabs. *Neisseria gonorrhoeae* organisms are fragile, and rapid inoculation at the bedside onto Thayer-Martin medium (warmed to room temperature) or one of its modifications is crucial. Ordinarily, cultures for sexually transmitted pathogens should include specimens obtained from genital, anorectal, and pharyngeal sources to achieve maximum yield. Specimens for *Chlamydia trachomatis* culture are obtained by cotton-tipped, aluminum-shafted urethral swabs. Endocervical specimens, using swabs with aluminum or plastic shafts, should be collected by rubbing the swab vigorously against the endocervical wall to obtain as much cellular material as possible. *C. trachomatis* is cultured by inoculation into cell culture systems, followed by immunofluorescent staining with monoclonal antibody against the organism. However, nonculture methods, such as enzyme immunoassay (EIA) tests, direct immunofluorescent staining by monoclonal antibodies, and DNA amplification methods are widely used and tend to be more cost effective than culture.

THROAT AND RESPIRATORY TRACT CULTURES. Obtaining a throat swab for culture is the most reliable method of diagnosing group A streptococcal pharyngitis and tonsillitis. Vigorous swabbing of the tonsillar area and posterior pharynx is necessary for maximum recovery, but even optimal specimens detect only approximately 90% of infections. The pharynx contains many normal flora; thus, most laboratories screen cultures only for the presence of group A β-hemolytic *Streptococcus*. Some laboratories do not use selective procedures, however, and often report the presence of meningococci, which are usually nontypable and nonpathogenic strains, but occasionally report typable meningococci and other potential pathogens. Most patients harboring such bacteria are carriers, and the culture report serves only to create undue alarm. The laboratory should be alerted when diphtheria, pertussis, gonococcal pharyngitis, or infection with *Arcanobacterium haemolyticum* is clinically suspected. Cultures for *B. pertussis* are obtained by aspiration or a Dacron or flexible wire calcium alginate swab (Calgiswab) of the nasopharynx and inoculation onto special charcoal-blood (Regan-Lowe) or Bordet-Gengou media.

The cause of lower respiratory tract disease in children is not easy to confirm microbiologically because of difficulty in obtaining adequate sputum specimens and lack of correlation between upper respiratory tract flora and organisms causing lower respiratory tract disease. Specimens showing large numbers of epithelial cells or few neutrophils on Gram stain are unsuitable for culture. Patients with cystic fibrosis can usually provide adequate expectorated sputum, and special media should be used to detect important cystic fibrosis pathogens such as *Burkholderia cepacia*.

Endotracheal aspirates from intubated patients may be useful if the Gram stain shows abundant neutrophils and bacteria, although pathogens recovered from such specimens may still reflect only contamination from the endotracheal tube or upper airway. Quantitative cultures of bronchoalveolar lavage fluid or bronchial brush specimens may be valuable for distinguishing upper respiratory tract contamination from lower tract disease in special circumstances.

The diagnosis of pulmonary tuberculosis in young children is best confirmed by culture of early morning gastric aspirates, obtained on 3 successive days, rather than by sputum cultures. Acid-fast stains of gastric aspirates from children with pulmonary tuberculosis are rarely positive. Cultures for *Mycobacterium tuberculosis* should be processed only in laboratories equipped with appropriate biologic safety cabinets and containment facilities.

STOOL CULTURE. Most laboratories in North America routinely culture stool for the presence of *Salmonella, Shigella*, and *Campylobacter* by inoculation onto **selective agar** (to decrease the growth of normal fecal flora) and **differential agar** (to help distinguish pathogenic enteric flora from normal enteric flora). Freshly passed stool is preferred for culture, but rectal swabs may be acceptable. Cultures for *Escherichia coli* O157:H7, *Vibrio cholerae, Yersinia enterocolitica, Aeromonas*, and *Plesiomonas* should be specifically requested when these organisms are suspected. Isolation of enterotoxigenic *E. coli*, the most common cause of traveler's diarrhea, and other pathogenic types of *E. coli*, except for *E. coli* O157:H7, is not routinely attempted. Bacterial stool cultures in the United States rarely yield useful results in patients who have been hospitalized for more than 3 days. Culture for *Clostridium difficile*, the most common bacterial cause of nosocomial diarrhea, has largely been replaced by tests that detect toxin production, such as cell culture assays for cytotoxicity, or EIAs.

CULTURE OF OTHER FLUIDS AND TISSUES. Abscesses, wounds, pleural fluid, peritoneal fluid, joint fluid, and other purulent fluids are cultured onto routine solid agar and broth media. Whenever possible, fluid rather than swabs from infected sites should be sent to the laboratory because culture of a larger volume of fluid may detect organisms present in low concentration. The yield from joint fluid cultures in patients with suppurative arthritis may be increased by inoculation into broth-containing blood culture bottles. Anaerobic organisms are involved in many abdominal and wound abscesses. These specimens should be collected and transported rapidly under anaerobic conditions, preferably in anaerobic transport tubes.

Antimicrobial Susceptibility Testing. Antimicrobial susceptibility tests are generally performed on all organisms of clinical significance except for a few that have predictable antimicrobial susceptibility patterns, such as group A *Streptococcus*, which is currently universally susceptible to penicillin. The most common technique is the **agar disk diffusion method (Bauer-Kirby method)**, in which a standardized inoculum of the organism is seeded onto an agar plate. Antibiotic-impregnated filter paper disks are then placed on the agar surface. After 18–24 hr of incubation, the zone of inhibition of bacterial growth around each disk is measured and compared with nationally determined standards for susceptibility or resistance.

The other widely used technique for susceptibility testing is **dilution testing**, in which a standard concentration of a microorganism is inoculated into serially diluted concentrations of antibiotic, and the **minimum inhibitory concentration (MIC)** in μg/mL, the lowest concentration of antibiotic required to inhibit growth of the microorganism, is determined. Dilution testing also permits determination of the **minimum bactericidal concentration (MBC)**, the lowest concentration of antibiotic required to kill the organism. The MBC is sometimes determined to exclude the possibility of **bacterial tolerance** (MBC > 4 times the MIC). Automated methods that use microtiter wells with pre-made dilutions of antibiotics are now used commonly. However, MICs from automated systems should be interpreted with caution for certain pathogen-antibiotic combinations (e.g., pneumococci resistant to penicillin, enterococci with low-level resistance to vancomycin). Screening agar plate tests, such as oxacillin disk susceptibility to detect penicillin-resistant pneumococci, followed by confirmatory tests, are recommended. The **E-test** is a new method of measuring MICs of individual antibiotics on an agar plate that uses a paper strip impregnated with a known continuous concentration gradient of antibiotic that diffuses across the agar surface, inhibiting microbial growth in an elliptic zone. The MIC is read off the printed strip at the point at which the zone intersects the strip. Major advantages of the E-test are reliable interpretation, reproducibility, and applicability to organisms that require special media or growth conditions, including anaerobic bacteria. However, the cost precludes its use as the principal testing system in clinical laboratories.

Office Bacteriology. Many office practices perform rapid antigen testing for detection of group A streptococcal pharyngitis. The sensitivity depends on the type of kit used and on the concentration of streptococci present in the sample, and as many as 30% of test results may be false-negative. Therefore, all negative results of antigen testing for group A *Streptococcus* should be confirmed by culture.

Other microbiologic tests may be performed in the office setting as long as the site is certified as meeting appropriate quality assurance standards specified by the Clinical Laboratory Improvement Amendments (CLIA) Act of 1988. These include procedures listed under the category of "physician-performed microscopy" including wet mounts, potassium hydroxide (KOH) preparations, pinworm examinations, fecal leukocyte examinations, and urine sediment analysis. Office laboratories licensed for this category are limited to performing these tests but avoid having to undergo periodic inspections and proficiency testing, although they are still subject to CLIA certification requirements specific to these tests. Gram staining, culture inoculation, and isolation of bacteria are considered moderately to highly complex tests under CLIA specifications. Any office laboratory performing Gram stains or cultures must comply with the same requirements and inspections for quality assurance, proficiency testing, and personnel requirements as fully licensed microbiology laboratories.

LABORATORY DIAGNOSIS OF VIRAL INFECTIONS

Specimens for viral diagnosis are selected on the basis of knowledge of the site that is most likely to yield the suspected pathogen. Specimens should be collected early in the course of infection when viral shedding is maximal. Fluids and respiratory secretions should be collected in sterile containers and delivered to the laboratory promptly. Swabs should be rubbed vigorously against mucosal or skin surfaces to obtain as much cellular material as possible, and sent in viral transport media that contain antibiotics to inhibit bacterial growth. Rectal swabs should not be heavily covered with feces because the antibiotics present in viral transport media may be insufficient to kill a large inoculum of bacteria. All specimens for virus culture should be transported on ice. Freezing specimens can result in a significant decrease in culture sensitivity. Consultation with the laboratory is advised for any unusual specimens or suspected pathogens.

Laboratory diagnosis of viral infections may be performed by electron microscopy, antigen detection, virus isolation in culture, serologic testing, or detection of virus genomes by molecular biology techniques. Serologic and molecular tests are the mainstay of diagnosis of viruses such as HIV and Epstein-Barr virus (EBV).

Rapid Antigen Tests. Immunofluorescent-antibody (IFA) techniques or other methods such as EIA that use antibodies to detect viral antigens directly in clinical specimens permit rapid identification of viruses. For example, smears of cellular material from respiratory secretions stained by immunologic reagents can identify the antigens of respiratory syncytial virus (RSV), adenovirus, influenza virus, and parainfluenza virus within 2–3 hr after the specimen is received. In comparison with isolation in cell culture, IFA is approximately 95% sensitive and 98% specific for the diagnosis of RSV and parainfluenza virus type 3 in reference laboratories; the sensitivity of IFA for influenza viruses and adenoviruses is considerably lower. Sensitive IFA staining techniques are also commercially available for identification of varicella-zoster virus (VZV) and herpes simplex virus (HSV). These specific methods have supplanted the Tzanck smear for multinucleated giant cells characteristic of VZV or HSV infections. Several methods for detecting cytomegalovirus (CMV) antigen in blood of high-risk patients also have been developed. IFA is not useful for detecting virus in specimens that do not contain an adequate number of infected cells. When possible, an accompanying specimen for virus isolation usually is advisable.

In addition to providing rapid diagnosis, antigen detection EIA tests are commonly used for the diagnosis of viruses that are difficult or impossible to culture, such as rotavirus, Norwalk virus, and hepatitis B virus.

Isolation and Identification. Viruses require living cells for propagation; the cells used most often are human or animal-derived tissue culture monolayers, such as human embryonic lung fibroblasts or monkey kidney cells. In vivo methods for isolation are sometimes necessary (e.g., suckling mice inoculation for culture of arboviruses and rabies virus). Because viruses require various cell culture systems for isolation, it is important for clinicians to provide relevant clinical information to the laboratory to facilitate inoculation of appropriate cell lines.

Viral growth in susceptible cells can be detected in several ways. Many viruses produce a characteristic **cytopathic effect (CPE)** that is discernible in cell culture by light microscopy under low magnification. For example, RSV and HSV produce multinucleated giant cells and syncytia formation. Other viruses (e.g., influenza virus and mumps virus) can be detected by hemadsorption because hemagglutinins on infected cell membranes facilitate adherence of erythrocytes to infected cells. The most reliable confirmatory method for viral detection in cell culture involves staining cell monolayers with monoclonal antibodies to virus antigens, which are conjugated with a fluorescent or enzyme substrate to permit identification of antigen-antibody binding.

LABORATORY DIAGNOSIS OF PARASITIC INFECTIONS

Most parasites are detected by microscopic examination of clinical specimens. For example, *Plasmodium* and *Babesia* can be detected in stained blood smears, *Leishmania* in bone marrow smears, and helminth eggs, *Entamoeba histolytica* and *Giardia lamblia* cysts, and trophozoites in fecal smears (see Table 160–1). Serologic tests are important in documenting exposure to certain parasites that are difficult to demonstrate in clinical specimens, such as *Trichinella* and *Toxoplasma*. Serologic testing also has a role in the diagnosis of intestinal strongyloidiasis, given the insensitivity of stool examinations.

Fecal specimens should not be contaminated with water or urine because water may contain free-living organisms that can be confused with human parasites, and urine may destroy motile organisms. Mineral oil, barium, and bismuth interfere with the detection of parasites; specimen collection should be delayed for 7–10 days after ingestion of these substances. Because *Giardia* and many worm eggs are shed intermittently into feces, a minimum number of three specimens is required for an adequate examination. The three specimens should be collected on separate days, preferably on alternate days. Because many protozoan parasites are easily destroyed, collection kits with stool preservatives should be used if delay between specimen collection and transport to the laboratory is anticipated.

Ova and parasite examination of fecal specimens includes a wet mount (to detect motile organisms if fresh stool is received), concentration (to improve yield), and permanent staining, such as trichrome, for microscopic examination. These techniques may miss parasites such as *Cryptosporidium*, *Cyclospora*, and microsporidia (*Enterocytozoon bieneusi* and *Septata intestinalis*). *Cryptosporidium* and *Cyclospora* are detected by modified acid-fast stain and microsporidia by a modification of the trichrome stain. The laboratory should be notified if these parasites are suspected. Detection of certain parasites, especially *Giardia* and *Cryptosporidium*, can be simplified by using sensitive EIA antigen detection tests.

SEROLOGIC DIAGNOSIS

Serologic tests are used primarily in the diagnosis of infectious agents that are difficult to culture in vitro or detect by direct examination, such as *Bartonella henselae*, *Legionella*, *Borrelia burgdorferi* (Lyme disease), *Treponema pallidum*, *Mycoplasma pneumoniae*, *Rickettsia*, *Ehrlichia*, some viruses (HIV, EBV, hepatitis viruses), and parasites (*Toxoplasma*, *Trichinella*).

Antibody tests may be specific for immunoglobulin G (IgG) or M (IgM), or may measure antibody response regardless of immunoglobulin class. The IgM response occurs earlier in the illness, generally peaking at 7–10 days after infection, and usually disappears within a few weeks, but for some infections (e.g., hepatitis A) may persist for months. The IgG response peaks at 4–6 weeks and in most cases persists for life. Because the IgM response is transient, the presence of IgM antibody in most cases correlates with recent infection; therefore, a single positive serum specimen is considered diagnostic. Methods for IgM antibody detection are difficult to standardize, however, and false-positive results frequently occur with some tests. The presence of IgG antibody may indicate recent seroconversion or past exposure to the pathogen. To confirm a new infection using IgG testing, it is necessary to demonstrate either **seroconversion**, from seronegative to seropositive, or a significant elevation in IgG titer; a fourfold increase in a **convalescent titer** obtained 2–3 wk after the **acute titer** is considered diagnostic in most situations. However, for some infections (e.g., *Bartonella*, *Legionella*, and rickettsiae) a single positive IgG titer in the appropriate clinical setting is sufficient for diagnosis. The serologic diagnosis of Lyme disease deserves special mention because lack of specificity of the various commercially available enzyme immunoassays remains a problem. To improve specificity, a follow-up confirmatory immunoblot (Western blot) is required for all positive and equivocal results.

MOLECULAR DIAGNOSTIC TECHNIQUES

Molecular diagnostic techniques are most useful for detecting and identifying pathogens for which culture and serologic tests are difficult, slow, or not available. Two of the widely used techniques in clinical microbiology are DNA probes for direct detection and nucleic acid amplification using polymerase chain reaction (PCR).

DNA probes detect or identify organisms by hybridization of the probe to complementary sequences in DNA or ribosomal

RNA. Detection of pathogen nucleic acid directly in clinical specimens requires the presence of relatively large numbers of organisms in the specimen. With the exception of commercially available probes for combined direct detection of *Chlamydia trachomatis* and *Neisseria gonorrhoeae* in the same specimen (e.g., GenProbe PACE2 or Digene Hybrid Capture II CT/GC), the principal use of DNA probe technology remains rapid identification of organisms that already have been isolated in culture but require additional time-consuming or complex confirmation procedures. For example, probes for mycobacterial species can rapidly distinguish *M. tuberculosis* from *M. avium-intracellulare* growing in broth cultures.

The high sensitivity and specificity of PCR amplification make this the method of choice for direct detection of microbial nucleic acid from clinical specimens. The PCR method is based on the ability of thermostable DNA or RNA polymerase to copy targeted gene sequences using complementary nucleotides as primers to amplify a conserved region of the genome. The reaction takes place in a thermal cycler, and, theoretically, each cycle of the reaction doubles the amount of target nucleic acid, resulting in more than a million-fold amplification in 30 cycles of PCR. The number of pathogens that can be detected by PCR is increasing rapidly. PCR tests are available using commercial reagents for HIV, hepatitis C virus, *M. tuberculosis*, and *C. trachomatis*. Additionally, experimental PCR protocols for detection of *Bartonella*, *B. pertussis*, *Legionella*, *M. pneumoniae*, *Chlamydia pneumoniae*, HSV, CMV, and EBV are available in some reference laboratories.

Specimens for PCR should be sent in separate sterile containers and transported rapidly to the laboratory. PCR methods are technically complex and labor intensive. False-positive reactions are a major problem because the extreme sensitivity of the assay can lead to amplification of target nucleic acid from extraneous sources or from crossover contamination from other positive specimens. Clinically relevant diagnostic PCR testing should be performed only in reference laboratories using adequate quality control measures.

Adegbola RA, Obaro SK, Biney E, et al: Evaluation of Binax NOW *Streptococcus pneumoniae* urinary antigen test in children in a community with a high carriage rate of pneumococcus. *Pediatr Infect Dis J* 2001;20:718–9.

American Academy of Pediatrics: Practice parameter: The diagnosis, treatment, and evaluation of the initial UTI in febrile infants and young children. *Pediatrics* 1999;103:843–52.

Dowell SF, Garman RL, Liu G, et al: Evaluation of Binax NOW, an assay for the detection of pneumococcal antigen in urine samples performed among pediatric patients. *Clin Infect Dis* 2001;32:824–5.

Hale YM, Pfyffer GE, Salfinger M: Laboratory diagnosis of mycobacterial infections: New tools and lessons learned. *Clin Infect Dis* 2001;33:834–46.

Isaacman DJ, Karasic RB, Reynolds EA, et al: Effect of number of blood cultures and volume of blood on detection of bacteremia in children. *J Pediatr* 1996;128:190–5.

Kaplan RL, Harper MB, Baskin MN, et al: Time to detection of positive cultures in 28 to 90-day-old febrile infants. *Pediatrics* 2000;106:E74.

Marcos MA, Martinez E, Almela M: New rapid antigen test for diagnosis of pneumococcal meningitis. *Lancet* 2001;357:1499–500.

Maxson S, Lewno MJ, Schutze GE: Clinical usefulness of cerebrospinal fluid bacterial antigen studies. *J Pediatr* 1994;125:235–8.

Mein J, Lum G: CSF bacterial antigen detection tests offer no advantage over gram stain in the diagnosis of bacterial meningitis. *Pathology* 1999;31:67–9.

McGowan KL, Foster JA, Coffin SE: Outpatient pediatric blood cultures: time to positivity. *Pediatrics* 2000;51–5.

Murray PR, Baron EJ, Jorgensen JH, et al (editors): *Manual of Clinical Microbiology*, 8th ed. Washington, DC, American Society for Microbiology, 2003.

Paisley PW, Lauer BA: Pediatric blood cultures. *Clin Lab Med* 1994;14:17–30.

Pfaller MA: Molecular approaches to diagnosing and managing infectious diseases: Practicality and costs. *Emerg Infect Dis* 2001;7:312–8.

Rogers WO, Waites KB, Friedberg RC: Microbiology testing and the pediatrician's office. *Pediatr Infect Dis J* 1997;16:339–45.

Storch GA: Diagnostic virology. *Clin Infect Dis* 2000;31:739–51.

Zaidi AK, Knaut AL, Mirrett S, et al: Value of routine anaerobic blood cultures for pediatric patients. *J Pediatr* 1995;127:263–8.

Zaidi AK, Macone A, Goldmann D: Impact of simple screening criteria on utilization of low-yield bacterial stool cultures in a children's hospital. *Pediatrics* 1999;103:1189–92.

Chapter 161
Fever *Keith R. Powell*

Fever is a controlled increase in body temperature over the normal values for an individual. Body temperature is regulated by **thermosensitive neurons** located in the preoptic or anterior hypothalamus that respond to changes in blood temperature as well as to direct neural connections with cold and warm receptors located in skin and muscle. **Thermoregulatory responses** include redirecting blood to or from cutaneous vascular beds, increased or decreased sweating, extracellular fluid volume regulation (via arginine vasopressin), and behavioral responses, such as seeking a warmer or cooler environmental temperature. Normal body temperature also varies in a regular pattern each day. This circadian temperature rhythm, or **diurnal variation**, results in lower body temperatures in the early morning and temperatures approximately 1°C higher in the late afternoon or early evening.

Pathogenesis. Fever is regulated in the same manner as normal temperature is maintained in a cool environment, the difference being that the body's thermostat has been reset at a higher temperature (Fig. 161–1). Regardless of whether fever is associated with infection, rheumatic disease, or malignancy, the thermostat is reset in response to **endogenous pyrogens** including the cytokines interleukin (IL)-1 and IL-6, tumor necrosis factor-α (TNFα), and interferon (IFN)-ß and -γ. Stimulated leukocytes and other cells produce lipids that also serve as endogenous pyrogens. The best-studied lipid mediator is prostaglandin E_2. Most endogenous pyrogen molecules are too large to cross the blood-brain barrier in an efficient manner. However, circumventricular organs in close proximity to the hypothalamus lack a blood-brain barrier and allow for neuronal contact with circulating factors through fenestrated capillaries.

Microbes, microbial toxins, or other products of microbes are the most common "exogenous pyrogens," which are substances that come from outside of the body, stimulate macrophages and other cells to produce endogenous pyrogens, and result in fever. Some substances produced within the body are not pyrogens but are capable of stimulating endogenous pyrogens. Such substances include antigen-antibody complexes in the presence of complement, complement components, lymphocyte products, bile acids, and androgenic steroid metabolites. Endotoxin is one of the few substances that can directly affect thermoregulation in the hypothalamus as well as stimulate endogenous pyrogen release. Fever may be caused by infection, vaccines, biologic agents (e.g., granulocyte-macrophage colony-stimulating factor, interferons, interleukins), tissue injury (e.g., infarction, pulmonary emboli, trauma, intramuscular injections, burns), malignancy (e.g., leukemia, lymphoma, hepatoma, metastatic disease), drugs (e.g., cocaine, amphotericin B, drug fever), immunologic-rheumatologic disorders (e.g., systemic lupus erythematosus, rheumatoid arthritis), inflammatory diseases (e.g., inflammatory bowel disease), granulomatous diseases (e.g., sarcoidosis), endocrine disorders (e.g., thyrotoxicosis, pheochromocytoma), metabolic disorders (e.g., gout, uremia, Fabry disease, type 1 hyperlipidemia), genetic disorders (e.g., familial Mediterranean fever), and unknown or poorly understood entities. **Factitious fever**, or self-induced fever, may be due to intentional manipulation of the thermometer or injection of pyrogenic material.

Increasing body temperature in response to microbial pathogens is a response observed in reptiles, fish, birds, and mammals. When fish are given an exogenous pyrogen, they swim to warmer water to raise their body temperature. In a similar fashion, lizards given exotoxin lie in the sun until they have raised their body temperature to the febrile range. In humans, increased temperatures

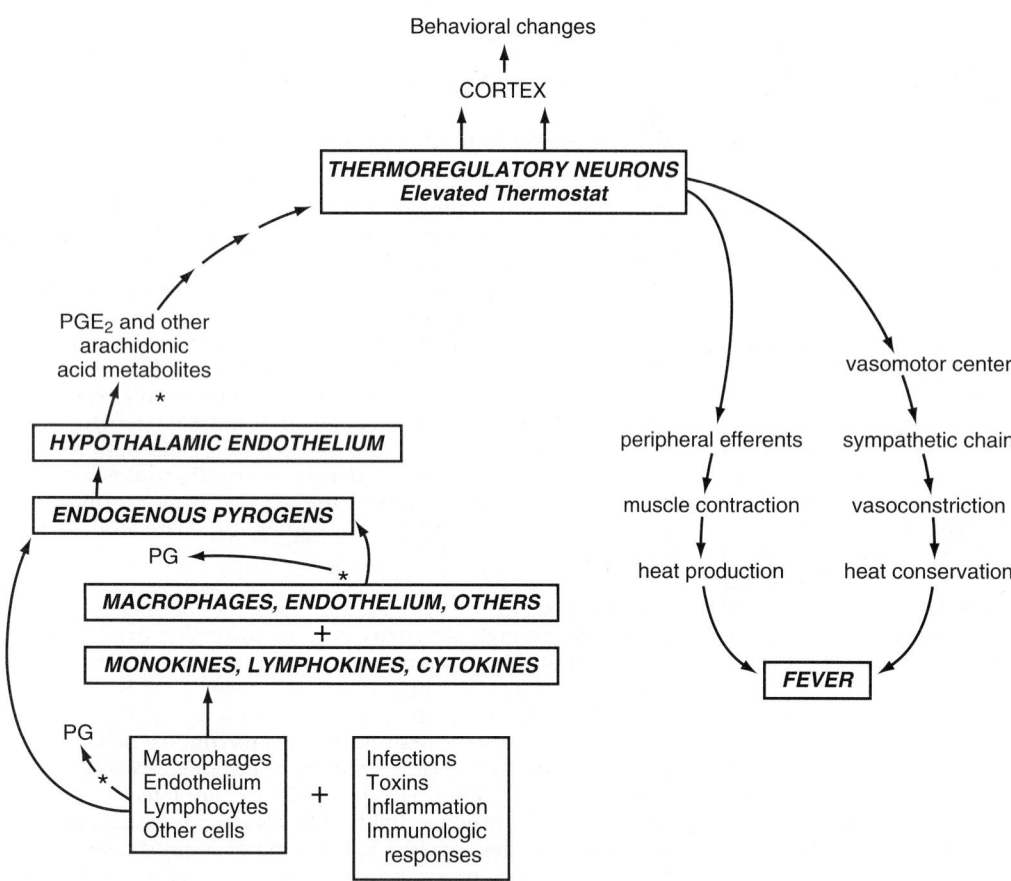

FIGURE 161–1. The pathogenesis of fever. Various infectious toxins and other mediators induce the production of endogenous pyrogens by host inflammatory cells. Endogenous pyrogens include the cytokines interleukin (IL)-1 and IL-6, tumor necrosis factor-α (TNFα), and interferon (IFN)-ß and -γ. Endogenous pyrogenic cytokines directly stimulate the hypothalamus to produce prostaglandin (PG) E_2 (PGE$_2$), which then resets the temperature regulatory set point. Neuronal transmission from the hypothalamus leads to conservation and generation of heat, thus raising core body temperature. (From Dinarello CA, Cannon JG, Wolff SM: New concepts on the pathogenesis of fever. *Rev Infect Dis* 1988;10: 168–89.)

are associated with decreased microbial reproduction and an increased inflammatory response. Thus, most evidence suggests that fever is an adaptive response and should be treated only in selected circumstances. Heat production associated with fever increases oxygen consumption, carbon dioxide production, and cardiac output. Thus, fever may exacerbate cardiac insufficiency in patients with heart disease or chronic anemia (e.g., sickle cell disease), pulmonary insufficiency in those with chronic lung disease, and metabolic instability in children with diabetes mellitus or inborn errors of metabolism. Furthermore, children between the ages of 6 mo and 5 yr are at increased risk of benign febrile seizures, whereas those with idiopathic epilepsy may have an increased frequency of seizures associated with a febrile illness (see Chapter 586.3).

Clinical Manifestations. Although fever patterns per se are not often helpful in determining a specific diagnosis, observing the clinical characteristics of fever can provide useful information. In general, a single isolated fever spike is not associated with an infectious disease. Such a spike can be attributed to the infusion of blood products, some drugs, some procedures, or manipulation of a catheter on a colonized or infected body surface. Similarly, temperatures in excess of 41°C are most often associated with a noninfectious cause. Causes of very high temperatures (>41°C) include **central fever** (resulting from central nervous system dysfunction involving the hypothalamus), malignant hyperthermia, malignant neuroleptic syndrome, drug fever, or heatstroke. Temperatures that are lower than normal (<36°C) can be associated with overwhelming sepsis but are more commonly related to cold exposure, hypothyroidism, or overuse of antipyretics.

Intermittent fever is an exaggerated circadian rhythm that includes a period of normal temperatures on most days; extremely wide fluctuations may be termed **septic or hectic**

fever. Sustained fever is persistent and does not vary by more than 0.5°C/24 hr. **Remittent fever** is persistent and varies by more than 0.5°C/24. **Relapsing fever** is characterized by febrile periods that are separated by intervals of normal temperature; **tertian fever** occurs on the 1st and 3rd days (e.g., malaria caused by *Plasmodium vivax*), and **quartan fever** occurs on the 1st and 4th days (e.g., malaria caused by *Plasmodium malariae*). Diseases characterized by relapsing fevers (Box 161–1) should be distinguished from those infectious diseases that have a tendency to relapse. A **biphasic fever** indicates a single illness with two distinct periods of fever over 1 or more weeks (camelback fever pattern); poliomyelitis is the classic example. A biphasic course is also characteristic of leptospirosis, dengue fever, yellow fever, Colorado tick fever, spirillary rat-bite fever (*Spirillum minus*), and the African hemorrhagic fevers (Marburg, Ebola, and Lassa fever). **Periodic fever** is used narrowly to describe fever syndromes with a regular periodicity (e.g., cyclic neutropenia, and periodic fever, aphthous stomatitis, pharyngitis, and adenopathy [PFAPA]) or more broadly to include disorders characterized by recurrent episodes of fever that do not follow a strictly periodic pattern (e.g., familial Mediterranean fever, Hibernian fever, and hyper IgD syndrome).

The relationship between a patient's pulse rate and temperature can be informative. **Relative tachycardia**, when the pulse rate is elevated out of proportion to the temperature, is usually due to noninfectious diseases or infectious diseases in which a toxin is responsible for the clinical manifestations. **Relative bradycardia (temperature-pulse dissociation)**, when the pulse rate remains low in the presence of fever, suggests typhoid fever, brucellosis, leptospirosis, or drug fever. Bradycardia in the presence of fever also may be a result of a conduction defect resulting from cardiac involvement with acute rheumatic fever, Lyme disease, viral myocarditis, or infective endocarditis.

BOX 161–1. Fevers Prone to Relapse

INFECTIOUS CAUSES

Relapsing fever (*Borrelia recurrentis*)
Trench fever (*Rochalimaea quintana*)
Q Fever (*Coxiella burnetii*)
Typhoid fever (*Salmonella typhi*)
Syphilis (*Treponema pallidum*)
Tuberculosis
Histoplasmosis
Coccidioidomycosis
Blastomycosis
Melioidosis (*Pseudomonas pseudomallei*)
Lymphocytic choriomeningitis (LCM) virus
Dengue fever
Yellow fever
Chronic meningococcemia
Colorado tick fever
Leptospirosis
Brucellosis
Oroya fever (*Bartonella bacilliformis*)
Acute rheumatic fever
Rat-bite fever (*Spirillum minus*)
Visceral leishmaniasis
Lyme disease (*Leptospira burgdorferi*)
Malaria
Babesiosis
Noninfluenza respiratory viruses
Epstein-Barr virus

NONINFECTIOUS CAUSES

Behçet disease
Crohn disease
Weber–Christian disease (panniculitis)
Leukoclastic angiitis
Sweet's syndrome
Systemic lupus erythematosus

PERIODIC FEVER SYNDROMES

Familial Mediterranean fever
Cyclic neutropenia
Periodic fever, aphthous stomatitis, pharyngitis, adenopathy (PFAPA)
Hyper IgD syndrome
Hibernian fever

Modified from Cunha BA: The clinical significance of fever patterns. *Infect Dis Clin North Am* 1996;10:33–44.

Most infections result in some type of injury that induces an inflammatory response and subsequently results in the release of endogenous pyrogens. Administration of antimicrobial agents can result in a very rapid elimination of bacteria, but if tissue injury has been extensive, the inflammatory response and fever can continue for days after all microbes have been eradicated.

Treatment. Fever with temperatures less than 39°C in healthy children generally do not require treatment. As temperatures become higher, patients tend to become more uncomfortable and administration of antipyretics often makes patients feel better. Other than providing symptomatic relief, antipyretic therapy does not change the course of infectious diseases. Antipyretic therapy is beneficial in high-risk patients who have chronic cardiopulmonary diseases, metabolic disorders, or neurologic diseases and in those who are at risk for febrile seizures. Hyperpyrexia (>41°C) indicates greater risk of severe infection, hypothalamic disorders, or central nervous system hemorrhage, and should always be treated with antipyretics. High fever during pregnancy may be teratogenic.

Acetaminophen, aspirin, and ibuprofen are inhibitors of hypothalamic cyclooxygenase, thus inhibiting PGE_2 synthesis. These drugs all are equally effective antipyretic agents. Because aspirin has been associated with Reye syndrome in children and adolescents, its use is not recommended for the treatment of fever. Acetaminophen, 10–15 mg/kg orally every 4 hr, is not associated with significant adverse effects; however, prolonged use may produce renal injury, and massive overdose may produce hepatic failure. Ibuprofen, 5–10 mg/kg orally every 6–8 hr, may cause dyspepsia, gastrointestinal bleeding, reduced renal blood flow, and rarely, aseptic meningitis, hepatic toxicity, or aplastic anemia. Serious injury from ibuprofen overdose is unusual. Tepid sponge bathing in warm water (not alcohol) is another recommended method of reducing hyperpyrexia due to infection or hyperthermia resulting from external causes (e.g., heatstroke). The decline of body temperature after antipyretic therapy does not distinguish serious bacterial from less serious viral diseases.

Crocetti M, Moghbeli N, Serwint J: Fever phobia revisited: Have parental misconceptions about fever changed in 20 years? *Pediatrics* 2001;107:1241–6.
Cunha BA: The clinical significance of fever patterns. *Infect Dis Clin North Am* 1996;10:33–44.
Dinarello CA, Cannon JG, Wolff SM: New concepts on the pathogenesis of fever. *Rev Infect Dis* 1988;10:168–89.
Kluger MJ, Kozak W, Conn C, et al: The adaptive value of fever. *Infect Dis Clin North Am* 1996;10:1–20.
Mackowiak PA, Boulant JA: Fever's glass ceiling. *Clin Infect Dis* 1996;22:525–36.
Saper CB, Breder CD: The neurologic basis of fever. *N Engl J Med* 1994;330:1880–6.
Scholl PR: Periodic fever syndromes. *Curr Opin Pediatr* 2000;12:563–60.

Chapter 162
Fever Without a Focus
Keith R. Powell

Fever is a common manifestation of infectious diseases but is not predictive of severity. Many common viral (e.g., rhinitis, pharyngitis, pneumonia) and bacterial (e.g., otitis media, pharyngitis, impetigo) infections are usually benign in normal hosts and respond well to appropriate antimicrobial or supportive therapy. Other infections (e.g., sepsis, meningitis, pneumonia, osteoarticular infections, pyelonephritis), if untreated, may have significant morbidity or mortality. Most febrile episodes in a normal host can be diagnosed by a careful history and physical examination and require few if any laboratory tests. However, there are well-defined high-risk groups that, on the basis of age, associated diseases, or immunodeficiency status, require a more extensive evaluation and, in certain situations, prompt antimicrobial therapy before a pathogen is identified (Table 162–1).

FEVER WITHOUT LOCALIZING SIGNS

Fever without localizing signs or symptoms, usually of acute onset and present for less than 1 wk, is a common diagnostic dilemma for pediatricians caring for children younger than 36 mo of age. Infants younger than 4 wk of age may acquire community pathogens but are also at risk for late-onset neonatal bacterial diseases and perinatally acquired herpes simplex virus infection. Young infants demonstrate limited signs of infection, often making it difficult to distinguish clinically between serious bacterial infections and self-limited viral illnesses.

Infants Younger than 3 mo of Age. An infectious agent, usually viral, is identified in 70% of infants younger than 3 mo of age with fever; the remainder are presumed to have self-limited but undiagnosed viral infections. However, fever in an infant younger than 3 mo of age should always suggest the possibility of serious bacterial disease. Serious bacterial infections are present in 10–15% of previously healthy term infants presenting with rectal temperatures of 38°C or greater. These infections include sepsis, meningitis, urinary tract infections, enteritis, osteomyelitis, and suppurative arthritis. Bacteremia is present in 5% of febrile infants younger than 3 mo of age; organisms

TABLE 162–1. Febrile Patients at Increased Risk for Serious Bacterial Infections

Risk Group	Diagnostic Considerations
Immunocompetent Patients	
Neonates (<28 days)	Sepsis and meningitis caused by group B *Streptococcus, Escherichia coli, Listeria monocytogenes,* and herpes simplex virus
Infants <3 mo	Serious bacterial disease in 10–15%, including bacteremia in 5%, of febrile infants <3 mo
Infants and children 3–36 mo	Occult bacteremia in 1.5%; increased risk with temperature >39°C and white blood cell count >15,000/μL
Hyperpyrexia (>40°C)	Meningitis, bacteremia, pneumonia, heatstroke, hemorrhagic shock–encephalopathy syndrome
Fever with petechiae	Bacteremia and meningitis caused by *Neisseria meningitidis, Haemophilus influenzae* type b, and *Streptococcus pneumoniae*
Immunocompromised Patients	
Sickle cell disease	Sepsis, pneumonia, and meningitis caused by *S. pneumoniae,* osteomyelitis caused by *Salmonella* (as well as *Staphylococcus*)
Asplenia	Bacteremia and meningitis caused by *N. meningitidis, H. influenzae* type b, and *S. pneumoniae*
Complement/properdin deficiency	Sepsis caused by *N. meningitidis*
Agammaglobulinemia	Bacteremia, sinopulmonary infection
AIDS	*S. pneumoniae, H. influenzae* type b, and *Salmonella* infections
Congenital heart disease	Infective endocarditis; brain abscess with right-to-left shunting
Central venous line	*Staphylococcus aureus,* coagulase-negative staphylococci, *Candida*
Malignancy	Bacteremia with gram-negative enteric bacteria, *S. aureus,* and coagulase-negative staphylococci; fungemia with *Candida* and *Aspergillus*

responsible for bacteremia include group B *Streptococcus* and *Listeria monocytogenes* (late-onset neonatal sepsis and meningitis) and community-acquired pathogens including *Salmonella* (enteritis), *Escherichia coli* (urinary tract infection), *Neisseria meningitidis, Streptococcus pneumoniae,* and *Haemophilus influenzae* type b (sepsis and meningitis), and *Staphylococcus aureus* (osteoarticular infection). Pyelonephritis is more common in uncircumcised infant boys, neonates and infants with urinary tract anomalies, and young girls. Other potential bacterial diseases in this age group include otitis media, pneumonia, omphalitis, mastitis, and other skin and soft tissue infections.

Viral pathogens can be identified in 40–60% of febrile infants younger than 3 mo of age. In contrast to bacterial infections, which have no seasonal pattern, viral diseases have a distinct pattern: respiratory syncytial virus and influenza A virus infections are more common during the winter, whereas enterovirus infections usually occur in the summer and fall.

The approach to febrile patients younger than 3 mo of age includes a careful history and physical examination. Ill-appearing (toxic) febrile infants younger than 3 mo of age require prompt hospitalization and immediate parenteral antimicrobial therapy after cultures of blood, urine, and cerebrospinal fluid (CSF) are obtained. Ceftriaxone (50 mg/kg/dose every 24 hr with normal CSF findings, or 80 mg/kg/dose every 24 hr with CSF pleocytosis) or cefotaxime (50 mg/kg/dose every 6 hr), plus ampicillin (50 mg/kg/dose every 6 hr) to cover for *L. monocytogenes* and *Enterococcus,* is an effective initial antimicrobial regimen for ill-appearing infants without focal findings. This regimen is effective against the usual bacterial pathogens causing sepsis, urinary tract infection, and enteritis in young infants. However, if meningitis is suspected because of CSF abnormalities, vancomycin (15 mg/kg/dose every 6 hr) should be given to cover for possible penicillin-resistant *S. pneumoniae,* in addition to the ceftriaxone/cefotaxime and ampicillin, until the results of culture and susceptibility tests are known.

Infants younger than 3 mo of age with fever who appear generally well; who have been previously healthy; who have no evidence of skin, soft tissue, bone, joint, or ear infection; and who have a total white blood cell (WBC) count of 5,000–15,000 cells/μL, an absolute band count of less than 1,500 cells/μL, and normal urinalysis results are unlikely to have a serious bacterial infection. The negative predictive value with 95% confidence of these criteria for any serious bacterial infection is greater than 98%, and greater than 99% for bacteremia.

Occult Bacteremia in Children 3 Mo–3 Yr of Age. Approximately 30% of febrile children 3 mo–3 yr of age have no localizing signs of infection. Occult bacteremia (bacteremia without an apparent focus of infection) due to *S. pneumoniae, N. meningitidis,* and *Salmonella* occurs in approximately 1.5% of relatively well-appearing children between 3–36 mo of age with fever (rectal temperature ≥38.0°C). The increased incidence of bacteremia among young children may be due in part to a maturational immune deficiency in the production of opsonic IgG antibodies to the polysaccharide antigens present on encapsulated bacteria. *S. pneumoniae* accounts for 90% of cases of occult bacteremia, with *N. meningitidis* and *Salmonella* accounting for most of the remaining positive cultures. *H. influenzae* type b was an important cause of occult bacteremia in young children before the universal use of conjugate *H. influenzae* type b vaccines. Common bacterial infections among children 3–36 mo of age who have localizing signs include otitis media, upper respiratory tract infection, pneumonia, enteritis, urinary tract infection, osteomyelitis, and meningitis. In this age group, bacteremia is present in 11% of febrile children with pneumonia and 1.5% of febrile children with otitis media or pharyngitis.

Risk factors indicating increased probability of occult bacteremia include temperature 39°C or greater, WBC count 15,000/μL or greater, or an elevated absolute neutrophil count, band count, erythrocyte sedimentation rate, or C-reactive protein. The incidence of bacteremia among infants 3–36 mo of age increases as the temperature and WBC count increase. However, no combination of laboratory tests or clinical assessment is completely accurate in predicting the presence of occult bacteremia. Socioeconomic status, race, gender, and age (within the range of 3–36 mo) do not appear to affect the risk for occult bacteremia.

Without therapy, occult bacteremia may resolve spontaneously without sequelae, may persist, or may lead to localized infections, such as meningitis, pneumonia, cellulitis, or suppurative arthritis. The pattern of sequelae may be related to both host factors and the offending organism. In some children, the occult bacteremic illness may represent the early signs of serious localized infection rather than merely a transient disease state. *H. influenzae* type b bacteremia is characteristically of higher grade, as determined by quantitative blood culture techniques, and is associated with a higher risk of localized serious infection than is bacteremia due to *S. pneumoniae.* Hospitalized children with *H. influenzae* type b bacteremia often develop focal infections, such as meningitis, epiglottitis, cellulitis, or osteoarticular infection, whereas fewer than 5% of these bacteremias can be considered transient or occult. In contrast, among all patients with pneumococcal bacteremia (occult, symptomatic, or focal), spontaneous resolution occurs in 30–40%, with a higher rate of spontaneous resolution among well-appearing children with occult pneumococcal bacteremia.

Treatment of toxic-appearing febrile children 3–36 mo of age who do not have focal signs of infection includes hospitalization and prompt institution of antimicrobial therapy after specimens of blood, urine, and CSF are obtained for culture. Meningitis in patients with occult bacteremia that develops after a lumbar puncture does not represent inoculation of bacteria by the puncture but is coincidental and represents meningeal infection that was developing before the lumbar puncture.

A retrospective review of more than 500 well-appearing febrile children discharged from an emergency department since 1987 and subsequently confirmed to be bacteremic with *S. pneumoniae* found 28% of untreated children to have persistent bacteremia or a focal infection (4% had meningitis) compared with only 5% of children who had received oral or parenteral antimicrobials when first seen (1% had meningitis). In addition, children who received antimicrobial therapy were less likely to be febrile upon return. A retrospective study of children with bacterial meningitis showed that children who received antimicrobial therapy before the diagnosis of *S. pneumoniae* meningitis was confirmed had fewer complications attributable to meningitis. These findings argue for empirical antimicrobial therapy for well-appearing children younger than 36 mo of age who have not received *H. influenzae* type b and *S. pneumoniae* conjugate vaccines who have a rectal temperature of 39°C or greater and a WBC count of 15,000/μL or greater.

Consensus practice guidelines published in 1993 recommended that infants 3–36 mo of age who have a temperature less than 39°C and who do not appear toxic can be observed as outpatients without performing diagnostic tests or administering antimicrobial agents. For nontoxic-appearing infants with a rectal temperature of 39°C or greater, two options were suggested: (1) obtain a blood culture and give empirical antimicrobial therapy (ceftriaxone, a single dose of 50 mg/kg, not to exceed 1 g) or (2) if the WBC count is 15,000/μL or greater, obtain a blood culture and give empirical antimicrobial therapy. A third option, not offered in these guidelines, for selected infants is to obtain a blood culture and observe as outpatients without empirical antimicrobial therapy with return for re-evaluation within 24 hr. Regardless of the management option, the family should be instructed to return immediately if the child's condition deteriorates or new symptoms, such as rash, develop.

Studies of febrile infants age 3–36 mo conducted in the United States since the introduction of universal immunization of infants with *H. influenzae* type b conjugate vaccines have demonstrated that this pathogen has been virtually eliminated as a cause of occult bacteremia. In 2000, a heptavalent *S. pneumoniae* conjugate vaccine was introduced and recommended for universal administration during infancy. Based on efficacy trials, it is anticipated that there will be a significant ($\geq$90%) decrease in occult bacteremia caused by *S. pneumoniae* in vaccinated infants. Guidelines for the management of febrile children 3–36 mo of age who have received both *H. influenzae* type b and *S. pneumoniae* conjugate vaccines have yet to be established, but a stronger case for careful observation without the empirical administration of antimicrobial agents can now be made.

If *S. pneumoniae* is isolated from the blood, the child should return to the physician as soon as possible after the culture results are known. If the child appears well, is afebrile, and the physical findings remain normal, a second blood culture should be obtained if the child did not receive antimicrobial treatment at the first visit; all children should receive a total of 7–10 days of oral antimicrobial therapy. If the child appears ill and continues to have fever with no identifiable focus of infection, or if *H. influenzae* or *N. meningitidis* is present in the initial blood culture, the child should have a repeat blood culture, be evaluated for meningitis (including lumbar puncture), and either receive treatment in the hospital with appropriate antimicrobial agents or be given ceftriaxone and be managed as an outpatient. If the child develops a localized infection, therapy is directed toward the specific pathogen and the particular site.

Fever with Petechiae. Independent of age, fever with petechiae with or without localizing signs indicates high risk for life-threatening bacterial infections such as bacteremia, sepsis, and meningitis. From 8–20% of patients with fever and petechiae have a serious bacterial infection, and 7–10% have meningococcal sepsis or meningitis (see Chapter 176). *H. influenzae* type b disease can also present with fever and petechiae (see Chapter 178). Management includes prompt hospitalization, culture of blood and CSF, and administration of appropriate parenteral antimicrobial agents.

Fever in Patients with Sickle Cell Disease. Infection is the most common cause of death among children with sickle cell disease (see Chapter 454.1). The incidence of infection is greatest among children younger than 5 yr of age. The increased risk of infection in these children is due in part to functional asplenia and a defect in the properdin (alternate complement) pathway. Fever without localizing signs in patients with sickle cell disease is a common presentation of infection due to *S. pneumoniae* (sepsis, pneumonia, meningitis), *H. influenzae* type b (meningitis), *Staphylococcus aureus* (osteomyelitis), *Salmonella* (osteomyelitis), and *E. coli* (pyelonephritis).

The management of patients with sickle cell hemoglobinopathies requires culture of blood and, if indicated, CSF, stool, and bone, and administration of antimicrobial agents. Children who appear seriously ill, have temperatures of 40°C or greater, have WBC less than 5,000/μL or greater than 30,000/μL, or who have pulmonary infiltrates or complications of sickle cell disease or severe pain should be hospitalized. Other febrile infants with sickle cell disease can be given intramuscular ceftriaxone and cared for as outpatients after appropriate specimens have been obtained for culture. These children should be re-evaluated within 24 hr, or earlier if their condition deteriorates or new symptoms develop.

Prevention of pneumococcal sepsis is possible by instituting long-term penicillin therapy continued until adolescence (oral penicillin V, 125 mg twice daily for children younger than 5 yr of age and 250 mg orally twice daily for children 5 yr of age and older). Pneumococcal and *H. influenzae* vaccines provide some protection but do not supplant long-term antimicrobial therapy.

Hyperpyrexia. Hyperpyrexia (temperature greater than 41°C) is uncommon and is not associated with higher rates of serious bacterial infections than temperatures of 40.0°C. Infants and children with hyperpyrexia should be carefully evaluated as for all children with fever.

FEVER OF UNKNOWN ORIGIN

The term **fever of unknown origin** (FUO) is best reserved for children with a fever documented by a health care provider and for which the cause could not be identified after 3 wk of evaluation as an outpatient or after 1 wk of evaluation in hospital. Patients with fever not meeting these criteria, and specifically those admitted to the hospital with neither an apparent site of infection nor a noninfectious diagnosis, may be considered to have **fever without localizing signs**. In most of these children, the development of additional clinical manifestations over a relatively short period confirms the infectious nature of the illness.

Etiology. The principal causes of FUO in children, using these rigorous criteria, are infections and rheumatologic (connective tissue or autoimmune) diseases (Box 162–1). Neoplastic disorders should also be seriously considered, although most children with malignancies do not have fever alone. The possibility of drug fever should be considered if the patient is receiving any drug.

■ **BOX 162–1. Diagnostic Considerations of Fever of Unknown Origin in Children**

Abscesses: abdominal, brain, dental, hepatic, pelvic, perinephric, rectal, subphrenic
Diabetes insipidus (non-nephrogenic and nephrogenic)
Infections
  Bacteria
    Caused by specific organism
      Actinomycosis
      Bartonella henselae (cat-scratch disease)
      Brucellosis
      Campylobacter
      Francisella tularensis (Tularemia)
      Listeria monocytogenes (Listeriosis)
      Meningococcemia (chronic)
      Mycoplasma pneumoniae
      Rat-bite fever (*Streptobacillus moniliformis*; streptobacillary
        form of rat-bite fever)
      Salmonella
      Tuberculosis
      Yersiniosis
    Localized infections
      Abscesses: abdominal, brain, dental, hepatic, pelvic,
        perinephric, rectal, subphrenic
      Cholangitis
      Infective endocarditis
      Mastoiditis
      Osteomyelitis
      Pneumonia
      Pyelonephritis
      Sinusitis
  Spirochetes
    Borrelia burgdorferi (Lyme disease)
    Relapsing fever (*Borrelia recurrentis*)
    Leptospirosis
    Rat-bite fever (*Spirillum minus*; spirillary form of rat-bite fever)
    Syphilis
  Fungal diseases
    Blastomycosis (extrapulmonary)
    Coccidioidomycosis (disseminated)
    Histoplasmosis (disseminated)
  Chlamydia
    Lymphogranuloma venereum
    Psittacosis
  Rickettsia
    Ehrlichia canis
    Q fever
    Rocky Mountain spotted fever
    Tick-borne typhus
  Viruses
    Cytomegalovirus
    Hepatitis viruses
    HIV
    Infectious mononucleosis (Epstein-Barr virus)
  Parasitic diseases
    Amebiasis
    Babesiosis
    Giardiasis
    Malaria
    Toxoplasmosis

    Trichinosis
    Trypanosomiasis
    Visceral larva migrans (*Toxocara*)
Rheumatologic diseases
  Behçet's disease
  Juvenile dermatomyositis
  Juvenile rheumatoid arthritis
  Rheumatic fever
  Systemic lupus erythematosus
Hypersensitivity diseases
  Drug fever
  Hypersensitivity pneumonitis
  Pancreatitis
  Serum sickness
  Weber-Christian disease
Neoplasms
  Atrial myxoma
  Cholesterol granuloma
  Hodgkin's disease
  Inflammatory pseudotumor
  Leukemia
  Lymphoma
  Neuroblastoma
  Wilms' tumor
Granulomatous diseases
  Crohn's disease
  Granulomatous hepatitis
  Sarcoidosis
Familial-hereditary diseases
  Anhidrotic ectodermal dysplasia
  Fabry's disease
  Familial dysautonomia
  Familial Mediterranean fever
  Hypertriglyceridemia
  Ichthyosis
  Sickle cell crisis
Miscellaneous
  Chronic active hepatitis
  Diabetes insipidus (non-nephrogenic and nephrogenic)
  Factitious fever
  Hypothalamic-central fever
  Infantile cortical hyperostosis
  Inflammatory bowel disease
  Kawasaki disease
  Kikuchi-Fujimoto disease
  Pancreatitis
  Periodic fever
  Poisoning
  Pulmonary embolism
  Thrombophlebitis
  Thyrotoxicosis
Recurrent or relapsing fever
  See Box 161–1
Undiagnosed fever
  Persistent
  Recurrent
  Resolved

Drug fever is usually sustained and not associated with other symptoms. Discontinuation of the drug is associated with resolution of the fever, generally within 72 hr, although certain drugs, such as iodides, are excreted for a prolonged period with fever that may persist for as long as 1 mo after drug withdrawal.

Most fevers of unknown or unrecognized origin result from atypical presentations of common diseases. In some cases, the presentation as an FUO is characteristic of the disease, such as juvenile rheumatoid arthritis (JRA), but the definitive diagnosis can be established only after prolonged observation because initially there are no associated or specific findings on physical examination and all laboratory results are negative or normal.

In the United States, the systemic infectious diseases most commonly implicated in children with FUO (by the rigorous criteria) are salmonellosis, tuberculosis, rickettsial diseases, syphilis, Lyme disease, cat-scratch disease, atypical prolonged presentations of common viral diseases, infectious mononucleo-

sis, cytomegalovirus (CMV) infection, viral hepatitis, coccidioidomycosis, histoplasmosis, malaria, and toxoplasmosis. Less common infectious causes of FUO include tularemia, brucellosis, leptospirosis, and rat-bite fever. AIDS alone is not usually responsible for FUO, although febrile illnesses frequently occur in patients with AIDS as a result of opportunistic infections.

JRA and systemic lupus erythematosus are the connective tissue diseases associated most frequently with FUO. Inflammatory bowel disease, rheumatic fever, and Kawasaki disease are also commonly reported as causes of FUO. If factitious fever (inoculation of pyogenic material or manipulation of the thermometer by the patient or parent) is suspected, the presence and pattern of fever should be documented in the hospital. Prolonged and continuous observation, which may include electronic surveillance, of patients is imperative. FUO lasting more than 6 mo is uncommon in children and suggests granulomatosis or autoimmune disease. Repeat interval evaluation, including history, physical examination, and roentgenographic studies, is required.

Diagnosis. The evaluation of FUO requires a thorough history and physical examination supplemented by a few screening laboratory tests, and additional laboratory and radiographic tests as indicated by the history or abnormalities found on examination or initial screening.

HISTORY. The *age* of the patient is helpful in evaluating FUO. Children younger than 6 yr of age often have a respiratory or genitourinary tract infection, localized infection (abscess, osteomyelitis), JRA, or, rarely, leukemia. Adolescent patients are more likely to have tuberculosis, inflammatory bowel disease, autoimmune processes, and lymphoma, in addition to the causes of FUO found in younger children.

A history of *exposure to wild or domestic animals* should be solicited. Zoonotic infections in the United States are increasing in frequency and are often acquired from pets that are not overtly ill. Immunization of dogs against specific disorders such as leptospirosis may prevent canine disease but does not always prevent the animal from carrying and shedding leptospires, which may be transmitted to household contacts. A history of ingestion of rabbit or squirrel meat may provide a clue to the diagnosis of oropharyngeal, glandular, or typhoidal tularemia. A history of tick bite or travel to tick- or parasite-infested areas should be obtained.

Any history of *pica* should be elicited. Ingestion of dirt is a particularly important clue to infection with *Toxocara* (visceral larva migrans) or *Toxoplasma gondii* (toxoplasmosis).

A history of unusual dietary habits or travel as early as the birth of the child should be sought. Malaria, histoplasmosis, and coccidioidomycosis may re-emerge years after visiting or living in an endemic area. It is important to identify prophylactic immunizations and precautions taken by the individual against ingestion of contaminated water or food during foreign travel. Rocks, dirt, and artifacts from geographically distant regions that have been collected and brought into the home as souvenirs may serve as vectors of disease.

A *medication history* should be pursued rigorously. This should include over-the-counter preparations and topical agents, including eye drops, which may be associated with atropine-induced fever.

The *genetic background* of a patient also is important. Descendants of the Ulster Scots may have FUO because they are afflicted with nephrogenic diabetes insipidus. Familial dysautonomia (Riley-Day syndrome), a disorder in which hyperthermia is recurrent, is more frequent among Jews than other population groups. Ancestry from the Mediterranean should suggest the possibility of familial Mediterranean fever.

PHYSICAL EXAMINATION. Sweating in a febrile child should be noted. The continuing absence of sweat in the presence of an elevated or changing body temperature suggests dehydration due to vomiting, diarrhea, or central or nephrogenic diabetes insipidus. It also should suggest anhidrotic ectodermal dysplasia, familial dysautonomia, or exposure to atropine.

A careful ophthalmic examination is important. Red, weeping eyes may be a sign of connective tissue disease, particularly polyarteritis nodosa. Palpebral conjunctivitis in a febrile patient may be a clue to measles, coxsackievirus infection, tuberculosis, infectious mononucleosis, lymphogranuloma venereum, and cat-scratch disease. In contrast, bulbar conjunctivitis in a child with FUO suggests Kawasaki disease or leptospirosis. Petechial conjunctival hemorrhages suggest infective endocarditis. Uveitis suggests sarcoidosis, JRA, systemic lupus erythematosus, Kawasaki disease, Behçet's disease, and vasculitis. Chorioretinitis suggests CMV, toxoplasmosis, and syphilis. Proptosis suggests orbital tumor, thyrotoxicosis, metastasis (neuroblastoma), orbital infection, Wegener's granulomatosis, or pseudotumor.

The ophthalmoscope should also be used to examine nailfold capillary abnormalities that are associated with connective tissue diseases such as juvenile dermatomyositis and systemic scleroderma (see Fig. 149–3). Immersion oil or lubricating jelly is placed on the skin adjacent to the nailbed, and the capillary pattern is observed with the ophthalmoscope set on +40.

FUO is sometimes due to hypothalamic dysfunction. A clue to this disorder is failure of pupillary constriction due to absence of the sphincter constrictor muscle of the eye. This muscle develops embryologically when hypothalamic structure and function also are undergoing differentiation.

Fever resulting from familial dysautonomia may be suggested by lack of tears, an absent corneal reflex, or by a smooth tongue with absence of fungiform papillae. Tenderness to tapping over the sinuses or the upper teeth suggests sinusitis. Recurrent oral candidiasis may be a clue to various disorders of the immune system.

Fever blisters are common findings in patients with pneumococcal, streptococcal, malarial, and rickettsial infection. They also are common in children with meningococcal meningitis (which usually does not present as FUO) but rarely are seen in children with meningococcemia. Fever blisters also are rarely seen with *Salmonella* or staphylococcal infections.

Hyperemia of the pharynx, with or without exudate, suggests infectious mononucleosis, CMV infection, toxoplasmosis, salmonellosis, tularemia, Kawasaki disease, or leptospirosis.

The muscles and bones should be palpated carefully. Point tenderness over a bone may suggest occult osteomyelitis or bone marrow invasion from neoplastic disease. Tenderness over the trapezius muscle may be a clue to subdiaphragmatic abscess. Generalized muscle tenderness suggests dermatomyositis, trichinosis, polyarteritis, Kawasaki disease, or mycoplasmal or arboviral infection.

Rectal examination may reveal perirectal lymphadenopathy or tenderness, which suggests a deep pelvic abscess, iliac adenitis, or pelvic osteomyelitis. A guaiac test should be obtained; occult blood loss may suggest granulomatous colitis or ulcerative colitis as the cause of FUO.

Repetitive chills and temperature spikes are common in children with septicemia (regardless of cause), particularly when associated with renal disease, liver or biliary disease, infective endocarditis, malaria, brucellosis, rat-bite fever, or a loculated collection of pus. The general activity of the patient and the presence or absence of rashes should be noted. Hyperactive deep tendon reflexes may suggest thyrotoxicosis as the cause of FUO.

LABORATORY FINDINGS. Ordering a large number of diagnostic tests in every child with FUO according to a predetermined list may waste time and money. Alternatively, prolonged hospitalization for sequential tests may be more costly. The tempo of diagnostic evaluation should be adjusted to the tempo of the illness; haste may be imperative in a critically ill patient, but if the illness is more chronic, the evaluation can proceed more slowly and deliberately and, usually, in an outpatient setting. If there are no clues in the patient's history or on physical examination that suggest a specific infection or area of suspicion, it is unlikely that diagnostic studies will be helpful.

A complete blood cell count with a differential WBC count and a urinalysis should be part of the initial laboratory evaluation. An absolute neutrophil count less than $5,000/\mu L$ is evidence against indolent bacterial infection other than typhoid fever. Conversely, patients with polymorphonuclear leukocytes greater than $10,000/\mu L$ or nonsegmented polymorphonuclear leukocytes greater than $500/\mu L$ have a high likelihood of having a severe bacterial infection. Direct examination of the blood smear with Giemsa or Wright stain may reveal organisms of malaria, trypanosomiasis, babesiosis, or relapsing fever.

An *erythrocyte sedimentation rate* (ESR) greater than 30 mm/hr indicates inflammation and the need for further evaluation for infectious, autoimmune, or malignant diseases. An ESR greater than 100 mm/hr suggests tuberculosis, Kawasaki disease, malignancy, or autoimmune disease. A low ESR does not eliminate the possibility of infection or JRA. C-reactive protein is another acute phase reactant that becomes elevated and returns to normal more rapidly than the ESR. Although experts may prefer use of one over the other, there is no evidence that there is value in measuring both the ESR and C-reactive protein in the same patient.

Blood cultures should be obtained aerobically. Anaerobic blood cultures have an extremely low yield and should be obtained only if there are specific reasons to suspect anaerobic infection. Multiple or repeated blood cultures may be required to detect bacteremia associated with infective endocarditis, osteomyelitis, or deep-seated abscesses. Polymicrobial bacteremia suggests factitious self-induced infection or gastrointestinal (GI) pathology. The isolation of leptospires, *Francisella*, or *Yersinia* may require selective media or specific conditions not routinely used. *Urine culture* should be obtained routinely.

Tuberculin *skin testing* should be performed with intradermal placement of 5 units of purified protein derivative (PPD) that has been kept appropriately refrigerated.

Radiographic examination of the chest, sinuses, mastoids, or GI tract may be indicated by specific historical or physical findings. Radiographic evaluation of the GI tract for inflammatory bowel disease may be helpful in evaluating selected children with FUO and no other localizing signs or symptoms.

Examination of the *bone marrow* may reveal leukemia; metastatic neoplasm; mycobacterial, fungal, or parasitic diseases; and histiocytosis, hemophagocytosis, or storage diseases. If a bone marrow aspirate is performed, cultures for bacteria, mycobacteria, and fungi should be obtained.

Serologic tests may aid in the diagnosis of infectious mononucleosis, CMV infection, toxoplasmosis, salmonellosis, tularemia, brucellosis, leptospirosis, cat-scratch disease, Lyme disease, rickettsial disease, and, on some occasions, JRA. As serologic tests for more diseases become available through commercial laboratories, it is important to ascertain the sensitivity and specificity of each test before relying on these results to make a diagnosis. For example, serologic tests for Lyme disease outside of reference laboratories have been generally unreliable.

Radionuclide scans may be helpful in detecting abdominal abscesses as well as osteomyelitis, especially if the focus cannot be localized to a specific limb or multifocal disease is suspected. Gallium citrate (^{67}Ga) localizes in inflammatory tissues (leukocytes) associated with tumors or abscesses. ^{99m}Tc phosphate is useful for detecting osteomyelitis before plain roentgenograms demonstrate bone lesions. Granulocytes tagged with indium (^{111}In) or iodinated IgG may be useful in detecting localized pyogenic processes. *Echocardiograms* may demonstrate the presence of vegetation on the leaflets of heart valves, suggesting infective endocarditis. *Ultrasonography* may identify intra-abdominal abscesses of the liver, subphrenic space, pelvis, or spleen.

Total body CT or MRI permits detection of neoplasms and collections of purulent material without the use of surgical exploration or radioisotopes. CT and MRI are helpful in identifying lesions of the head, neck, chest, retroperitoneal spaces, liver, spleen, intra-abdominal and intrathoracic lymph nodes, kidneys, pelvis, and mediastinum. CT or ultrasound-guided aspiration or biopsy of suspicious lesions has reduced the need for exploratory laparotomy or thoracotomy. MRI is particularly useful for detecting osteomyelitis if there is concern about a specific limb. Diagnostic imaging can be very helpful in confirming or evaluating a suspected diagnosis but rarely leads to an unsuspected cause.

Biopsy is occasionally helpful in establishing a diagnosis of FUO. Bronchoscopy, laparoscopy, mediastinoscopy, and GI endoscopy may provide direct visualization and biopsy material when organ-specific manifestations are present.

Treatment. Fever and infection in children are not synonymous; antimicrobial agents should not be used as antipyretics, and empirical trials of medication should generally be avoided. An exception may be the use of antituberculous treatment in critically ill children with suspected disseminated tuberculosis. Empirical trials of other antimicrobial agents may be dangerous and can obscure the diagnosis of infective endocarditis, meningitis, parameningeal infection, or osteomyelitis. Hospitalization may be required for laboratory or radiographic studies that are unavailable or impractical in an ambulatory setting, for more careful observation, or for temporary relief of parental anxiety. After a complete evaluation, antipyretics may be indicated to control fever and for symptomatic relief (see Chapter 161).

Prognosis. Children with FUO have a better prognosis than do adults. The outcome in a child is dependent on the primary disease process, which is usually an atypical presentation of a common childhood illness. In many cases, no diagnosis can be established and fever abates spontaneously. In as many as 25% of cases in which fever persists, the cause of the fever remains unclear, even after thorough evaluation.

Bachur R, Harper MB: Reevaluation of outpatients with *Streptococcus pneumoniae* bacteremia. *Pediatrics* 2000;105:502–9.

Baker RC, Seguin JH, Leslie N, et al: Fever and petechiae in children. *Pediatrics* 1989;84:1051–5.

Baraff LJ, Bass JW, Fleisher GR, et al: Practice guidelines for the management of infants and children 0–36 months of age with fever without a source. *Ann Emerg Med* 1993;22:1198–210.

Baroff LJ, Schriger DL, Bass JW, et al: Commentary on pediatric guidelines. *Pediatrics* 1997;100:134–8.

Bauchner H, Pelton SI: Management of the young febrile child: A continuing controversy. *Pediatrics* 1997;100:137–8.

Bonsu BK, Harper MB: Fever interval before diagnosis, prior antibiotic treatment, and clinical outcome for young children with bacterial meningitis. *Clin Infect Dis* 2001;32:566–72.

Dagan R, Hall CB, Powell KR, et al: Epidemiology and laboratory diagnosis of infection with viral and bacterial pathogens in infants hospitalized for suspected sepsis. *J Pediatr* 1989;115:351–6.

Jaskiewicz JA, McCarthy CA, Richardson AC, et al: Febrile infants at low risk for serious bacterial infection—an appraisal of the Rochester criteria and implications for management. *Pediatrics* 1994;94:390–6.

Knockaert DC, Vanneste LJ, Bobbaers HJ: Recurrent or episodic fever of unknown origin. Review of 45 cases and survey of the literature. *Medicine* 1993;72:184–96.

Kramer MS, Shapiro ED: Management of the young febrile child: A commentary on recent pediatric guidelines. *Pediatrics* 1997;100:128–34.

Lee GM, Harper MB: Risk of bacteremia for febrile young children in the post-*Haemophilus influenzae* type b era. *Arch Pediatr Adolesc Med* 1998;152:624–8.

Lohr JA, Hendley JO: Prolonged fever of unknown origin. A record of experiences with 54 childhood patients. *Clin Pediatr* 1977;16:768–73.

McClung HJ: Prolonged fever of unknown origin in children. *Am J Dis Child* 1972;124:544–50.

Miller ML, Szer I, Yogev R, et al: Fever of unknown origin. *Pediatr Clin North Am* 1995;42:999–1015.

Norris AH, Krasinskas AM, Salhany KE, et al: Kikuchi-Fujimoto disease: A benign cause of fever and lymphadenopathy. *Am J Med* 1996;171:401–5.

Pizzo PA, Lovejoy FH Jr, Smith DH: Prolonged fever in children: Review of 100 cases. *Pediatrics* 1975;55:468–73.

Steele RW, Jones SM, Lowe BA, et al: Usefulness of scanning procedures for diagnosis of fever of unknown origin in children. *J Pediatr* 1991;119:526–30.

Wilimas JA, Flynn PM, Harris S, et al: A randomized study of outpatient treatment with ceftriaxone for selected febrile children with sickle cell disease. *N Engl J Med* 1993;329:472–6.

Chapter 163
Sepsis and Shock
Anne Stormorken and Keith R. Powell

The recovery of bacteria in a blood culture, or **bacteremia**, may be a transient phenomenon not associated with disease or may be the serious extension of an invasive bacterial infection originating elsewhere. Local infections, such as meningitis, osteomyelitis, endocarditis, epiglottitis, and facial cellulitis, usually follow or are concomitant with bacteremia. **Transient bacteremia** may follow instrumentation of the respiratory, gastrointestinal, or genitourinary tracts. Bacteremia may be asymptomatic or associated with few symptoms. When bacteria are not effectively cleared by host defense mechanisms, a systemic inflammatory response is set into motion and can progress independently of the original infection. **Sepsis** is the systemic response to infection with bacteria, viruses, fungi, protozoa, or rickettsiae. Sepsis is one of the causes of the **systemic inflammatory response syndrome (SIRS)**, which has noninfectious causes as well. If not recognized and treated early, sepsis can progress to severe sepsis, **septic shock** (sepsis with hypotension), **multiple organ dysfunction syndrome (MODS)**, and death (Fig. 163–1). However, the varied clinical manifestations of sepsis may result in a broad differential diagnosis that includes many noninfectious etiologies (Box 163–1).

Etiology. Sepsis may develop as a complication of localized community-acquired infections (see Box 163–1) or may follow colonization and local mucosal invasion by virulent pathogens (*Neisseria meningitidis, Streptococcus pneumoniae, Haemophilus influenzae* type b, *Salmonella*). Children 3 mo–3 yr of age are at risk for occult bacteremia, which occasionally progresses to sepsis (see Chapter 162).

Nosocomial infections pose a special risk to immunocompromised patients (Chapter 283). Serious gram-negative (*Escherichia coli, Pseudomonas, Acinetobacter, Klebsiella-Enterobacter, Serratia*) sepsis or fungemia occurs in neutropenic patients or intensive care patients who have become colonized with these pathogens. Sepsis caused by *Staphylococcus aureus* or coagulase-negative staphylococci may be associated with intravenous catheters (see Chapter 164) or surgical wounds. Polymicrobial sepsis also occurs in high-risk patients and is associated with central venous catheterization, gastrointestinal disease, neutropenia, and malig-

Infection

Systemic inflammatory response syndrome (SIRS) Response to wide variety of clinical insults • Hyper- or hypothermia • Tachycardia • Tachypnea • Increased or decreased white blood count

Sepsis SIRS with hypotension in response to infection

Severe sepsis Sepsis with organ dysfunction, hypoperfusion or hypotension. May include change in metal status, oliguria, hypoxemia, or lactic acidosis

Septic shock Severe sepsis with persistent hypotension despite adequate fluid resuscitation

Multiple organ dysfunction syndrome (MODS) Presence of altered organ function such that homeostasis cannot be maintained without intervention

Death

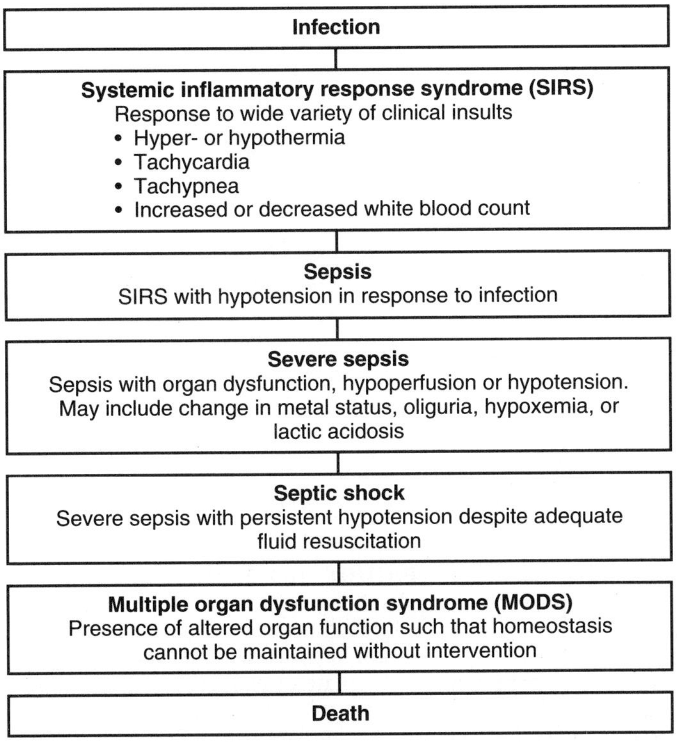

FIGURE 163–1. Progression from infection to sepsis (systemic inflammatory response syndrome [SIRS]) and its complications. (Modified from Sáez-Llorens X, McCracken GH Jr: Sepsis syndrome and septic shock in pediatrics: Current concepts of terminology, pathophysiology, and management. *J Pediatr* 1993;123: 497–508.)

BOX 163–1. Differential Diagnosis of Sepsis

INFECTION
Bacteremia or meningitis (*Streptococcus pneumoniae, Haemophilus influenzae* type b, *Neisseria meningitidis*)
Viral illness (influenza, enteroviruses, hemorrhagic fever group, HSV, RSV, CMV, EBV)
Encephalitis (arboviruses, enteroviruses, HSV)
Rickettsiae (Rocky Mountain spotted fever, *Ehrlichia*, Q fever)
Syphilis
Vaccine reaction (pertussis, influenza, measles)
Toxin-mediated reaction (toxic shock, staphylococcal scalded skin syndrome)

CARDIOPULMONARY
Pneumonia (bacteria, virus, mycobacteria, fungi, allergic reaction)
Pulmonary emboli
Congestive heart failure
Arrhythmia
Pericarditis
Myocarditis

METABOLIC-ENDOCRINE
Adrenal insufficiency (adrenogenital syndrome, corticosteroid withdrawal)
Electrolyte disturbances (hyponatremia or hypernatremia; hypocalcemia or hypercalcemia)
Diabetes insipidus
Diabetes mellitus
Inborn errors of metabolism (organic acidosis, urea cycle, carnitine deficiency)
Hypoglycemia
Reye's syndrome

GASTROINTESTINAL
Gastroenteritis with dehydration
Volvulus
Intussusception
Appendicitis
Peritonitis (spontaneous, associated with perforation or peritoneal dialysis)
Hepatitis
Hemorrhage

HEMATOLOGIC
Anemia (sickle cell disease, blood loss, nutritional)
Methemoglobinemia
Splenic sequestration crisis
Leukemia or lymphoma

NEUROLOGIC
Intoxication (drugs, carbon monoxide, intentional, or accidental overdose)
Intracranial hemorrhage
Infant botulism
Trauma (child abuse, accidental)
Guillain-Barré syndrome
Myasthenia gravis

OTHER
Anaphylaxis (food, drug, insect sting)
Hemolytic-uremic syndrome
Kawasaki disease
Erythema multiforme
Hemorrhagic shock–encephalopathy syndrome

HSV, herpes simplex virus; RSV, respiratory syncytial virus; CMV, cytomegalovirus; EBV, Epstein-Barr virus.

nancy. Unusual pathogens should be considered in patients who have traveled to or been exposed to products from distant lands, or with immunocompromised states such as malignancy, T- or B-lymphocyte defects, and post-splenectomy.

Pseudobacteremia may be associated with contaminated solutions such as heparin flush solutions, intravenous infusates, albumin, cryoprecipitate, and contaminated infusion equipment. Water-associated organisms such as *Burkholderia cepacia, Pseudomonas aeruginosa*, or *Serratia* are often the contaminants.

Pathogenesis. SIRS related to sepsis (see Fig. 163–1) results from tissue damage following the host response to bacterial products such as endotoxin from gram-negative bacteria and the lipoteichoic acid-peptidoglycan complex from gram-positive bacteria. The cardiopulmonary manifestations of gram-negative (e.g., *H. influenzae, N. meningitidis, E. coli, Pseudomonas*) sepsis can be mimicked by injection of endotoxin or tumor necrosis factor (TNF). Inhibition of TNF action by monoclonal anti-TNF antibody greatly attenuates the manifestations of septic shock in experimental models. When bacterial cell wall components are released into the bloodstream, cytokines are activated, and these in turn can lead to further physiologic derangements (Fig. 163–2). Endogenous mediators of sepsis continue to be identified and currently include TNFα; interleukin (IL) –1, –2, –4, –6, and –8; platelet-activating factor (PAF); interferon-γ; eicosanoids (leukotrienes B_4, C_4, D_4, E_4; thromboxane A_2; prostaglandins E_2, I_2); granulocyte-macrophage colony-stimulating factor (GM-CSF); endothelium-derived relaxing factor; endothelin-1; complement fragments C3a and C5a; toxic oxygen radicals and proteolytic enzymes from polymorphonuclear neutrophils; adhesion molecules; platelets; transforming growth factor-ß; vascular permeability factor; macrophage-derived procoagulant and inflammatory cytokine; bradykinin; thrombin; coagulation factors; fibrin; plasminogen activator inhibitors; myocardial depressant substance; ß-endorphin; and heat shock proteins.

Alone or in combination, bacterial products and proinflammatory cytokines trigger physiologic responses to inhibit microbial invaders. These responses include (1) activation of the complement system; (2) activation of Hageman factor (factor XII), which then initiates the coagulation cascade; (3) adrenocorticotropic hormone and ß-endorphin release; (4) stimulation of polymorphonuclear neutrophils; and (5) stimulation of the kallikrein-kinin system (see Fig. 163–2). TNF and other inflammatory mediators increase vascular permeability, producing diffuse capillary leakage, reduced vascular tone, and at the microcirculatory level an imbalance between perfusion and increased tissue metabolic needs (Fig. 163–3).

Shock is a disruption in circulatory function leading to poor perfusion and inadequate delivery of oxygen and other nutrients to tissues (see Chapter 57.2). Shock is not diagnosed by a decrease in blood pressure because compensatory mechanisms work to maintain the blood pressure, initially through an increase in heart rate and then peripheral vasoconstriction as cardiac output decreases further. Hypotension is an ominous indicator that compensatory mechanisms are failing and cardiorespiratory arrest is imminent.

In the early phases of sepsis there is a decrease in systemic vascular resistance and a relative decline in preload, resulting in tachycardia, widened pulse pressure, and increased cardiac output. Cytokine-mediated endothelial damage leads to diffusion of intravascular fluid into tissues, compounding the degree of relative hypovolemia. Clinically, patients in the early phases of sepsis are warm and have bounding pulses with brisk capillary refill. In later phases of septic shock, patients have cool extremities with poor peripheral pulses and decreased blood pressure, reflecting myocardial dysfunction and decreased cardiac output. As tissue oxygen consumption exceeds oxygen delivery, the resultant tissue hypoxia leads to lactic acidosis.

Pulmonary function is often severely impaired. Development of adult respiratory distress syndrome (ARDS) is associated with a poor prognosis (see Chapter 58). Acute renal failure, hepatic dysfunction, pancreatitis, central nervous system dysfunction, and disseminated intravascular coagulation (DIC) can occur alone or in combination in MODS.

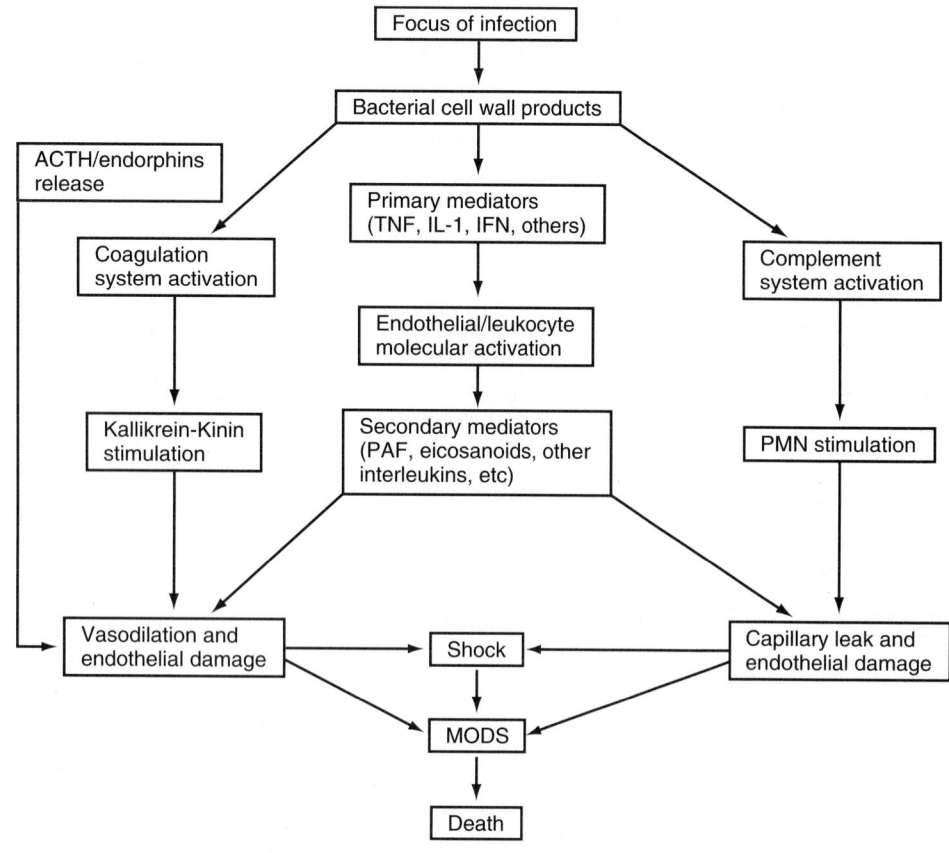

FIGURE 163–2. Hypothetical pathophysiology of the septic process. ACTH, adrenocorticotropic hormone; TNF, tumor necrosis factor; IL-1, interleukin-1; PAF, platelet-activating factor; PMN, polymorphonuclear lymphocytes; IFN, interferon gamma; MODS, multiorgan dysfunction syndrome. (From Sáez-Llorens X, McCracken GH Jr: Sepsis syndrome and septic shock in pediatrics: Current concepts of terminology, pathophysiology, and management. *J Pediatr* 1993;123:497–508.)

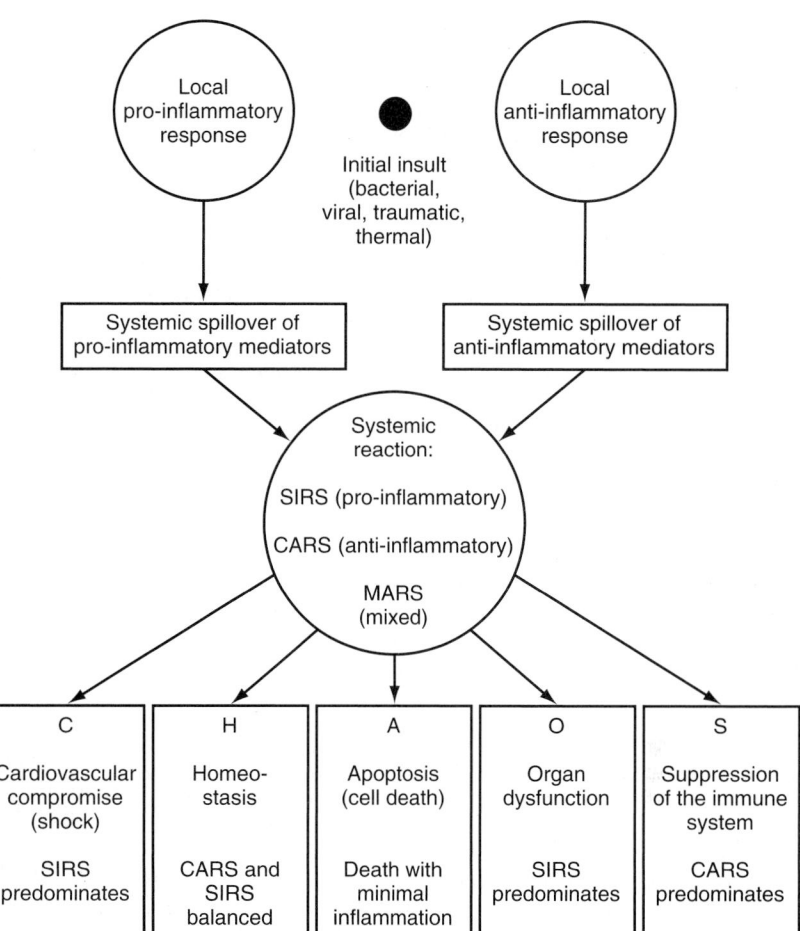

FIGURE 163–3. The hypothetical relationships between pro-inflammatory responses of the systemic inflammatory response syndrome (SIRS), compensatory anti-inflammatory syndrome (CARS), mixed anti-inflammatory syndrome (MARS), and the ensuing "CHAOS" are illustrated. (From Bone RC, Grodzin CJ, Balk RA: Sepsis: A new hypothesis for pathogenesis of the disease process. *Chest* 1997;112: 235–43.)

Clinical Manifestations. The primary signs and symptoms of sepsis and its complications include fever, shaking chills, hyperventilation, tachycardia, hypothermia, cutaneous lesions (e.g., petechiae, ecchymoses, ecthyma gangrenosum, diffuse erythema), and changes in mental status such as confusion, agitation, anxiety, excitation, lethargy, obtundation, or coma. Secondary manifestations include hypotension, cyanosis, symmetric peripheral gangrene (purpura fulminans), oliguria or anuria, jaundice (direct hyperbilirubinemia), and signs of heart failure. There may be evidence of focal infection such as meningitis, pneumonia, arthritis, cellulitis, or pyelonephritis.

Diagnosis. The diagnosis of septic shock includes the clinical diagnosis of shock (Chapter 57.2) with microbiologic confirmation of an infectious etiology such as a positive blood cultures or Gram stain of the serum buffy coat or petechial lesions demonstrating microorganisms. Specimens of blood, urine, and cerebrospinal fluid (CSF) as well as any exudates, abscesses, and cutaneous lesions that are present should be cultured and stained for organisms. A complete blood cell count, platelet count, prothrombin and partial thromboplastin times, fibrinogen level and D-dimer, arterial blood gas, renal and hepatic profiles, and ionized calcium should be obtained. Affected children should be admitted to an intensive care unit where invasive monitoring can be performed and central venous pressure, blood pressure, and cardiac output continuously measured (see Chapter 57).

Laboratory Findings. Laboratory findings often include metabolic acidosis, thrombocytopenia, prolonged prothrombin and partial thromboplastin times, reduced serum fibrinogen levels and elevated fibrin split products, anemia, decreased Pao_2 and increased $Paco_2$,

and alterations in the morphology and number of neutrophils. Elevated neutrophil and band counts (increased immature white blood cells), vacuolation of neutrophils, toxic granulations, and Döhle bodies suggest bacterial infection. Neutropenia is an ominous sign of overwhelming sepsis. Examination of the CSF may reveal neutrophils and bacteria. In the early stages of meningitis, bacteria may be detected in the CSF before development of an inflammatory response.

Treatment. Broad-spectrum bactericidal synergistic antimicrobial agents should be promptly administered to the patient in septic shock. The choice of antimicrobial agents depends on the specific predisposing risk factors. Community-acquired disease (*N. meningitidis, S. pneumoniae, H. influenzae*) can be treated empirically with a third-generation cephalosporin (e.g., ceftriaxone or cefotaxime). Nosocomial sepsis should be treated with a third-generation cephalosporin or an extended gram-negative spectrum penicillin (e.g., mezlocillin, piperacillin-tazobactam), plus an aminoglycoside. Vancomycin should be added to the regimen if the patient has an indwelling medical device (see Chapter 165), to provide coverage for coagulase-negative staphylococci, or if meningitis is suspected to provide coverage for penicillin-resistant *S. pneumoniae*. Empirical use of amphotericin B to treat fungal infections should be considered for selected immunocompromised patients.

Supportive care in an intensive care setting is essential. Supplemental oxygen via a high-flow nonrebreathing system should be administered during initial assessment even if oxygen saturation is normal, because oxygen delivery to the tissues is compromised. Endotracheal intubation and mechanical ventilation may be necessary despite adequate ventilation or oxygenation because of the increased work of breathing. This is especially true in infants and young children who are especially susceptible to developing respiratory failure from the tachypnea secondary to metabolic acidosis. The respiratory status in patients with a deteriorating clinical condition should be maintained and the airway controlled by elective intubation rather than waiting until urgently needed. Initially, 100% oxygen should be administered to maximize oxygen content and oxygen delivery. Positive end-expiratory pressure (PEEP) may be required to improve oxygenation because increased vascular permeability leads to the escape of fluid into the pulmonary interstitium. Hypoxemia refractory to supplemental oxygen suggests severe intrapulmonary shunting; the diagnosis of ARDS is made upon finding diffuse alveolar infiltrates on chest radiograph (see Chapter 58). Sedation and neuromuscular blockade are central to successful ventilator management in ARDS because prolonged inspiratory times and high PEEP are often required. The cardiovascular effects of PEEP should be monitored by central venous pressure and pulmonary capillary wedge pressure measurements.

Concomitant resuscitation of hemodynamic stability is necessary. If possible, two large-bore peripheral intravenous catheters should be placed and prompt administration of crystalloid begun. Although only 25% of crystalloid solutions will remain in the intravascular compartment, clinical studies do not provide evidence of the superiority of colloid to crystalloid for volume expansion. Isotonic solutions such as normal saline and lactated Ringer's solution should be given rapidly in aliquots of 20 mL/kg until perfusion, tachycardia, and hypotension resolve. Successful outcomes depend on the rapidity of infusion and may require drawing fluid into syringes and manually administering the fluid.

If the administration of 60 mL/kg of crystalloid results in no improvement, myocardial dysfunction should be considered. Many of the cytokines released during SIRS are myocardial depressants. Swan-Ganz catheter-derived data may reveal the presence of decreased myocardial contractility, poor diastolic ventricular relaxation, or abnormal systemic vascular resistance (SVR). Inotropic agents such as dopamine or epinephrine improve contractility by stimulating dopaminergic and β-adrenergic receptors, respectively. Pressor agents such as norepinephrine restore SVR through α-adrenergic receptors. However, myocardial hyporesponsiveness to catecholamine administration during septic shock has been documented. Phosphodiesterase inhibitors (milrinone, amrinone) improve contractility, facilitate diastolic relaxation, and decrease SVR. Milrinone has been shown to improve the cardiac index by 20% in pediatric patients with septic shock. Endogenous vasopressin levels decrease during vasodilatory septic shock, and administration of low-dose vasopressin (0.02–0.04 unit/min) restores SVR. The complex etiology of myocardial dysfunction often necessitates a combination of agents.

Correction of metabolic deficiencies can also improve myocardial function. Metabolic acidosis and elevated lactate levels occur secondary to tissue hypoperfusion; however, the administration of sodium bicarbonate has not been shown to decrease morbidity or mortality in these patients. Rather, the base deficit and serum lactate are used to monitor the adequacy of resuscitation. Calcium and potassium ions are integral to the conduction and contractility of the myocardium, and their levels must be monitored and supplemented as needed. Administration of the ions is safest and most expeditious if administered via central venous access; patients must be continuously monitored.

DIC, if present, should resolve as the primary infectious disease is treated. If bleeding occurs or the patient requires an invasive procedure, DIC should be treated with replacement of consumed coagulation factors by transfusion of fresh frozen plasma, cryoprecipitate, and platelets. Decreased serum levels of antithrombin III (AT III) and activated protein C reflect the procoagulant effect of cytokines. At present, patients with documented AT III or protein C deficiency may receive supplementation only as part of a clinical trial or as compassionate use.

Several therapies aimed at modifying overexuberant host responses have met with limited success. Such therapies include intravenous immunoglobulin, monoclonal antiendotoxin antibodies, polyclonal antiendotoxin anticore antibodies, anti-TNFα, IL-1 receptor antagonist, and granulocyte transfusions. Granulocyte transfusions are reserved for patients who have neutropenia prior to the septic episode, do not respond to antimicrobial therapy and remain persistently bacteremic. Corticosteroids are not beneficial in adults with septic shock or early ARDS; however, they may improve the clinical course during the late or fibroproliferative phase of ARDS (see Chapter 58). Stress doses of corticosteroids may be beneficial in patients with adrenal hemorrhage that is part of the Waterhouse-Friderichsen syndrome.

Prognosis. The mortality for septic shock depends on the initial site of infection, the bacterial pathogen, the presence of MODS, and the host immune response. The mortality may be as high as 40–60% for patients with gram-negative enteric sepsis. Urosepsis has a much better prognosis than sepsis without a focus. Poor prognostic signs in meningococcal sepsis include hypotension, coma, leukopenia (<5,000 cells/μL), thrombocytopenia (<100,000/μL), low fibrinogen level (<150 mg/dL), absence of CSF pleocytosis with bacteria noted on Gram stain of the CSF, rapid appearance of petechiae (within 1 hr), and hypothermia. Furthermore, patients who survive septic shock demonstrate an improvement in cardiac indices with therapy as compared with nonsurviving patients.

Prevention. Immunization with the conjugate *H. influenzae* type b and *S. pneumoniae* vaccines is recommended for all infants (see Chapter 282). High-risk patients should also receive the 23-valent pneumococcal vaccine, after priming with the conjugated pneumococcal vaccine, and the quadrivalent (groups A, C, Y, W-135) meningococcal vaccine at age 2 yr. Penicillin prophylaxis to prevent pneumococcal infection is recommended for patients with splenic dysfunction (e.g., sickle cell disease) and those who have had splenectomy. Prophylaxis is recommended for household and other close contacts of patients with invasive *N. meningitidis* or *H. influenzae* type b disease (see Chapters 176 and 178). Prevention of infection and sepsis in immunocompromised patients is discussed in Chapter 164.

Balk RA: Severe sepsis and septic shock: Definitions, epidemiology, and clinical manifestations. *Crit Care Clin* 2000;16:179–92.

Barton P, Garcia J, Giroir B, et al: Hemodynamic effects of IV milrinone lactate in pediatric patients with septic shock. A prospective, double-blinded, randomized, placebo-controlled interventional study. *Chest* 1996;109:1302–12.

Bernard GR, Vincent JL, Laterre PF, et al: Efficacy and safety of recombinant human activated protein C for severe sepsis. *N Engl J Med* 2001;344:699–709.

Bone RC, Grodzin LI, Balk RA: Sepsis: A new hypothesis for pathogenesis of the disease process. *Chest* 1997;112:235–43.

Casey LC, Balk RA, Bone RC: Plasma cytokine and endotoxin levels correlate with survival in patients with sepsis syndrome. *Ann Intern Med* 1993;119:771–8.

Jindal N, Hollenberg SM, Dellinger RP: Pharmacologic issues in the management of septic shock. *Crit Care Clin* 2000;16:233–49.

Landry DW, Oliver JA: The pathogenesis of vasodilatory shock. *N Engl J Med* 2001;345:588–95.

Malay MB, Ashton RC Jr, Landry DW, et al: Low-dose vasopressin in the treatment of vasodilatory septic shock. *J Trauma* 1999;47:699–703.

Saez-Llorens X, McCracken GH Jr: Sepsis syndrome and septic shock in pediatrics: Current concepts of terminology, pathophysiology, and management. *J Pediatr* 1993;123:497–508.

Chapter 164

Infections in Immunocompromised Persons *Marian G. Michaels and*

Michael Green

Microbial agents are encountered throughout life. Infection and disease develop when a host's immune system is insufficient to completely protect against potential pathogens. Infections also occur in individuals with competent immune systems, usually presenting when they are naive to the microbe and have no previous immunity or because the protective barriers of the body such as the skin have been breached. However, the immunocompetent host is able to meet most infectious agents in the world with an immunologic armamentarium capable of preventing significant disease. Once an infection is established, an array of immune responses is set into action to control the disease and prevent it from reappearing. In contrast, children who are immunocompromised may not have this capability and are at increased risk for the balance being tipped in favor of the infectious agent. Depending on the level and type of immune defect, the affected child may not be able to contain the pathogen nor develop an immune response to prevent recurrence.

General practitioners are likely to see children in their practice with abnormal immune systems. Increasing numbers of children survive with primary immunodeficiencies or receive immunosuppressive therapy for treatment of malignancy, autoimmune disorders, or transplantation. For this reason, it is critical that all practitioners be comfortable with recognizing signs and symptoms of infections in these patients.

Primary immunodeficiencies are immunocompromised states that are due to genetic defects affecting one or more arms of the immune system. **Acquired, or secondary, immunodeficiencies** may result from infection, such as with human immunodeficiency virus, malignancy, or as an effect of medications. Perturbations of the mucosal and skin barriers or normal microbial flora can also be characterized as secondary immune deficiencies, leaving the host open to infections if only for a temporary period of time (Box 164–1).

The major pathogenic microbial agents among immunocompetent hosts are also the main pathogens causing infections among children with immunodeficiencies. In addition, organisms that are usually considered to be avirulent in immunocompetent hosts can be pathogenic in hosts with limited immune systems. Normal skin flora, commensal bacteria of the oral pharynx or gastrointestinal tract, environmental fungi, and common community viruses of low-level pathogenicity can cause severe, life-threatening illnesses in immunocompromised patients (Box 164–2). For this reason, close communication with the diagnostic laboratory is critical so that the laboratory does not disregard identifying normal flora and organisms normally considered to be contaminants as being unimportant.

INFECTIONS OCCURRING WITH PRIMARY IMMUNODEFICIENCIES

Abnormalities of the Phagocytic System. Children with abnormalities of the phagocytic and neutrophil system have problems dealing with bacteria as well environmental fungi. Disease manifests as recurrent infections of the skin, mucous membranes, lungs, liver, and bones. Dysfunction of this arm of the immune

BOX 164–1. Major Causes of Increased Risk of Infection in Immunocompromised Hosts

PRIMARY IMMUNODEFICIENCIES
Antibody deficiency (B-cell defects; see Chapter 114)
X-linked agammaglobulinemia
Common variable immunodeficiency
Selective IgA deficiency
IgG subclass deficiencies
Hyper-IgM syndrome

Cell-mediated deficiency (T-cell defects; see Chapter 115)
Thymic dysplasia (DiGeorge's syndrome)
Defective T-cell receptor
Defective cytokine production
T-cell activation defects
CD8 lymphocytopenia

Combined B- and T-cell defects (see Chapter 116)
Severe combined immunodeficiency
Combined immunodeficiency
  Omenn's syndrome
  Thrombocytopenia and eczema (Wiskott-Aldrich syndrome)
  Ataxia telangiectasia
  Hyper-IgE syndrome

Phagocyte defects (see Chapter 120)
  Leukocyte adhesion deficiency
  Chédiak-Higashi syndrome
  Myeloperoxidase deficiency
  Chronic granulomatous disease

Leukopenia (see Chapter 121)
  Congenital neutropenia (Kostmann's syndrome)
  Shwachman-Diamond syndrome

Disorders of the Complement System (see Chapter 124)

SECONDARY IMMUNODEFICIENCIES
HIV
Malignancies (and cancer chemotherapy)
Transplantation
  Bone marrow and stem cell
  Solid organ
Burns
Sickle cell disease
Cystic fibrosis
Diabetes mellitus
Immunosuppressive drugs
Asplenia
Implanted foreign body
Malnutrition

system can be due to inadequate numbers of neutrophils, abnormal movement properties, or aberrant function.

Neutropenia is defined as an absolute neutrophil count less than 1000 cells/mm^3 and can be associated with significant risk of developing severe bacterial and fungal disease, particularly when the absolute count is less than 500 cells/mm^3. Whereas acquired neutropenia secondary to bone marrow suppression from a virus or medication is common, genetic causes of neutropenia also exist. Primary congenital neutropenia (Kostmann syndrome) most often presents during the 1st year of life with cellulitis, perirectal abscesses, or stomatitis from *Staphylococcus aureus* or *Pseudomonas aeruginosa*. Episodes of severe disease, including bacteremia or meningitis, are also possible. Even though the underlying genetic defect causing primary neutropenia remains unknown, bone marrow evaluation shows a failure of maturation of myeloid precursors. Other congenital forms of neutropenia are associated with autosomal recessive mutations, such as some forms of Kostmann syndrome and Shwachman-Diamond syndrome. Patients with Kostmann syndrome appear to have an increased risk of developing myelodysplastic syndrome and acute myelogenous leukemia. Shwachman-Diamond

BOX 164–2. Most Common Causes of Infections in Immunocompromised Children

BACTERIA, AEROBIC

Acinetobacter
Bacillus
Burkholderia cepacia
Citrobacter
Corynebacterium
Enterococcus faecalis
Enterococcus faecium
Escherichia coli
Haemophilus influenzae type b
Klebsiella
Listeria monocytogenes
Mycobacterium
Neisseria meningitidis
Nocardia
Pseudomonas aeruginosa
Staphylococcus aureus
Staphylococcus, coagulase-negative
Streptococcus pneumoniae
Streptococcus, viridans group

BACTERIA, ANAEROBIC

Bacillus
Clostridium
Fusobacterium
Propionibacterium
Peptococcus
Peptostreptococcus
Veillonella

FUNGI

Aspergillus
Candida albicans and other *Candida*
Cryptococcus neoformans
Zygometes (*Absidia, Mucor, Rhizopas, Rhizomucer*)

VIRUSES

Adenoviruses
Cytomegalovirus
Epstein-Barr virus
Herpes simplex virus
Human herpesvirus 6
Respiratory and enteric community-acquired viruses
Varicella-zoster virus

PROTOZOA

Cryptosporidium parvum
Giardia lamblia
Toxoplasma gondii
Pneumocystis carinii

---

syndrome is associated with a variety of other abnormalities including pancreatic insufficiency, skeletal abnormalities, and recurrent infections. Cyclic neutropenia can be an autosomal dominant disorder or sporadic mutation associated with fixed cycles of severe neutropenia between periods of normal counts. The cycles classically occur every 21 days (range, 14–36 days) with neutropenia lasting 3–6 days. Most often the disease is characterized by recurrent aphthous ulcers and stomatitis during the periods of neutropenia. However life-threatening necrotizing cellulitis and systemic disease can occur, especially with *Clostridium perfringens*. Many of the neutropenic syndromes respond to colony-stimulating factor.

Leukocyte adhesion defects are caused by defects in the ß chain of integrin (CD18), which is required for the normal process of neutrophil aggregation and attachment to endothelial surfaces. In the most severe form, there is a total absence of CD18. Children with this defect may have a history of delayed cord separation and recurrent infections of the skin, oral mucosa, and genital tract. Ecthyma gangrenosum and pyoderma gangrenosum also occur. Because the defect is one of transportation and adherence to the affected area, the neutrophil count in the peripheral blood is usually extremely elevated although pus is

not found at the site of infection. Survival is usually less than 10 yr without transplantation.

Chronic granulomatous disease is an inherited neutrophil dysfunction, which can be either X-linked or autosomal recessive. Neutrophils have defects in their NADPH oxidase function, rendering myeloid cells incapable of generating superoxide and thereby impairing intracellular killing. Accordingly, microbes that destroy their own hydrogen peroxide such as *S. aureus, Serratia marcescens, Burkholderia cepacia*, and *Aspergillus* cause recurrent infections in these children, especially involving the lungs, liver, and bone. Prophylaxis with trimethoprim sulfamethoxazole and recombinant human interferon-γ substantially reduces the incidence of severe infections. In addition, many specialists recommend prophylaxis against *Aspergillus* with itraconazole. Patients with life-threatening infections have also been reported to benefit from aggressive treatment with white cell transfusions in addition to antimicrobial agents directed against the specific pathogen.

Defective Opsonization or Complement Deficiency. Children with congenital asplenia, splenic dysfunction due to hemoglobinopathies such as sickle cell disease, or those who have undergone splenectomy are at risk for serious infections from bacteria. Prophylaxis with penicillin should be considered in these patients, particularly in children younger than 5 yr of age. The most common causative organisms are encapsulated bacteria including *Streptococcus pneumoniae, Haemophilus influenzae*, and *Salmonella*. These agents can cause sepsis, pneumonia, meningitis, and osteomyelitis. Defects in the early pathway of complement components, particularly C2 and C3, can be associated with severe infection from these bacteria. Terminal complement defects (C5, C6, C7, C8, C9) are associated with recurrent infections with *Neisseria*. Patients with complement deficiency also have an increased incidence of autoimmune disorders. Vaccines for *S. pneumoniae, H. influenzae* type b, and *N. meningitidis* should be given to all children with abnormalities in opsonization or complement pathways.

B-Cell Defects (Humoral Deficiencies). Antibody deficiencies account for the majority of primary immunodeficiencies found in humans. Patients with defects in the B-cell arm of the immune system fail to produce appropriate antibody responses, with abnormalities that range from complete agammaglobulinemia to failure to produce antibody to a specific antigen or organism. Antibody deficiencies found in children with diseases such as X-linked agammaglobulinemia or common variable immunodeficiency predispose to infections with encapsulated organisms such as *S. pneumoniae* and *H. influenzae* type b. Other bacteria can also be problematic in these children (see Box 164–2). Even though most other classes of microbes (e.g. viruses, fungi) do not cause problems for these patients, some notable exceptions exist. Rotavirus can lead to chronic diarrhea, and enteroviruses can disseminate and cause a chronic meningoencephalitis syndrome. Paralytic polio has developed after immunization with live polio vaccine. In addition, protozoan infections such as giardiasis can be severe and persistent. Children with B-cell defects can develop bronchiectasis over time following chronic or recurrent infections of their lungs.

Children with antibody deficiencies are usually asymptomatic until 5–6 mo of age, when maternal passive antibody wanes. These children then begin to develop recurrent episodes of otitis media, bronchitis, pneumonia, bacteremia, and meningitis. Because many of these infections respond quickly to antibiotics, the diagnosis of antibody deficiency may be delayed. Children, especially boys, who require myringotomy tube placement before 2 yr of age because of recurrent episodes of otitis media (e.g., three or more episodes within 6 mo, or four or more episodes within 12 mo) should be considered for screening measurement of immunoglobulin levels.

The significance and impact of specific IgG subclass deficiencies is less well understood and remains controversial. Deficiencies of specific IgG subclasses were first noted in healthy adult blood donors in whom no increased susceptibility to infections was documented. However, others have identified specific IgG deficiencies to be associated with a predisposition to recurrent bacterial sinopulmonary infection, bacteremia, meningitis, osteomyelitis, and pyoderma. Deficiency of subclass IgG_2 has been associated with poor antibody production after exposure to polysaccharide antigens, either after vaccination or infection with a polysaccharide-encapsulated organism such as *S. pneumoniae* and *H. influenzae* type b.

Selective IgA deficiency leads to a lack of production of secretory antibody at the mucosal membranes. Even though most patients will have no increased risk for infections, some will have mild to moderate disease at sites of mucosal barriers. Accordingly, recurrent sinopulmonary infection and gastrointestinal disease are the major clinical manifestations. These patients also have an increased incidence of allergies and autoimmune disorders compared with the normal population.

Hyper-IgM syndrome is caused by a defect on the CD40 ligand on the T cell and is associated with a deficiency in the production of IgG and IgA antibody. In addition, recurrent neutropenia, hemolytic anemia, or aplastic anemia can be present. Similar to patients with agammaglobulinemia, these individuals are at risk for bacterial sinopulmonary infections, *Pneumocystis carinii* pneumonitis, and *Cryptosporidium* infection.

Replacement of antibody with intravenous immunoglobulin (IVIG) is the mainstay of treatment for most of the primary antibody deficits. The exception to this is IgA deficiency, because these patients can develop antibody against the minute amounts of IgA found in the standard IVIG preparations with an increased risk for anaphylaxis. Prophylaxis with specific antibiotic regimens is controversial and should be individualized for those patients who do not respond to immunoglobulin replacement.

T-Cell Defects (Cell-Mediated Immunity). Children with primary cell-mediated immunodeficiencies, either isolated or more commonly in combination with B-cell defects, present early in life and are susceptible to viral, fungal, and protozoan infections. Clinical manifestations include chronic diarrhea, mucocutaneous candidiasis, pneumonia, rhinitis, and otitis media. In thymic dysplasia (DiGeorge syndrome), hypoplasia or aplasia of the thymus and parathyroid glands occurs during fetal development along with other congenital abnormalities. Hypocalcemia and cardiac anomalies are usually the presenting features of DiGeorge syndrome, which should prompt evaluation of the T-cell system. Chronic mucocutaneous candidiasis is a rare immunodeficiency associated primarily with T-cell dysfunction. These patients may lack delayed hypersensitivity to skin tests to *Candida* antigen despite having chronic infection with yeast, but do not appear to be at increased risk for systemic yeast infections. Endocrinopathies are commonly associated with chronic mucocutaneous candidiasis.

Combined B-Cell and T-Cell Defects. Patients with defects in both the T-cell and B-cell components of the immune system may manifest a variable disease spectrum depending on the extent of the defect. Complete immunodeficiency is found with severe combined immunodeficiency syndrome (SCID), whereas partial defects can be present in such states as ataxia-telangiectasia, Wiskott-Aldrich syndrome, hyper-IgE syndrome, and X-linked immunodeficiency syndrome. Children with SCID present within the first 6 mo of life with recurrent severe infections caused by bacteria, fungi, or viruses. Failure to thrive, chronic diarrhea, mucocutaneous or systemic candidiasis, *P. carinii* pneumonitis, and cytomegalovirus (CMV) infection are common early in life. Passive maternal antibody is relatively protective against the bacterial pathogens during the first few months of life but thereafter patients are susceptible to both gram-positive and gram-negative organisms. Exposure to live virus vaccines can also lead to disseminated disease. Without bone marrow or stem cell transplantation, most children succumb to opportunistic infections within the 1st year of life.

Children with ataxia-telangiectasia develop late onset of recurrent sinopulmonary infections from both bacteria and respiratory viruses. In addition, these children experience an increased incidence of malignancies. Wiskott-Aldrich syndrome is an X-linked recessive disease associated with a reduced number of CD3 lymphocytes, moderately suppressed mitogen responses, and impaired antibody response to polysaccharide antigens. Accordingly, infections with *S. pneumoniae* or *H. influenzae* type b are common, as is *P. carinii* pneumonitis. In addition, affected boys have thrombocytopenia and eczema. Children with hyper-IgE syndrome have markedly elevated levels of IgE and present with recurrent episodes of *S. aureus* abscesses of the skin, lungs, and musculoskeletal system. While the antibody abnormality is notable, these patients also have marked eosinophilia and poor cell-mediated responses to neoantigens, and they are at increased risk for fungal infections.

INFECTIONS OCCURRING WITH ACQUIRED IMMUNODEFICIENCIES

Immunodeficiencies can be secondarily acquired as a result of infections or as a consequence of other underlying disorders such as malignancy, cystic fibrosis, diabetes mellitus, sickle cell disease, or malnutrition. Immunosuppressive medications used to prevent rejection after organ transplantation or graft-versus-host disease (GVHD) after bone marrow transplantation (BMT) leave the host vulnerable to infections. In addition, any process (burns, surgery, or the presence of indwelling catheters) that interrupts or inhibits the normal mucosal and skin barriers can be considered an acquired risk for infection.

Acquired Immunodeficiency from Infectious Agents. Infection with HIV, the causative agent of AIDS, is the most important infectious cause of acquired immunodeficiency (see Chapter 254). If left untreated, the profound effects of HIV infection on the T-cell arm leads to susceptibility to the same types of infections as with primary T-cell immunodeficiencies.

Other viruses can lead to temporary alterations of the immune system. Transient neutropenia associated with many viruses can lead, on rare occasions, to significant disease with bacterial infections. Secondary infections can occur because of impaired immunity or disruption of the normal mucosal immunity, as exemplified by the increased risk of *S. pneumoniae* pneumonia following influenza infection and group A *Streptococcus* cellulitis and fasciitis following chickenpox.

Malignancies. The immune systems of children with malignancies are compromised by the therapies to treat the cancer and, at times, by direct effects of the cancer itself. In addition, the presence of mucous membrane abnormalities, indwelling catheters, malnutrition, prolonged exposure to antibiotics, and frequent hospitalizations all add to the risk for infection in these children. The type, duration, and intensity of anticancer therapy remain the major risk factors for infections in these children and frequently affect more than one arm of the immune system (see Box 164–2).

Even though several arms of the immune system can be affected, the major abnormality associated with infection in children with cancer is neutropenia. The degree and duration of neutropenia have long been relied upon as accurate predictors of the risk of infection in children being treated for cancer. Patients are at particular risk for bacterial infections if the absolute neutrophil count decreases to less than 500 cells/mm^3. Counts greater than 500 cells/mm^3 but less than 1,000 cells/mm^3 still incur some increased risk for infection, but not nearly as great. The lack of neutrophils can lead to a loss of inflammatory response; hence, fever may be the only manifestation of infection. Accordingly, the absence of physical signs and symptoms is not always reliable and the use of empirical antibiotics is required (Fig. 164–1).

Because patients with fever and neutropenia may only have subtle signs and symptoms of infection, the presence of fever warrants thorough physical examination with careful attention to the oropharynx, lungs, perineum and anus, skin, nailbeds, and sites along intravascular catheter sites. In addition, a comprehensive laboratory evaluation including a complete blood cell count, serum creatinine, blood urea nitrogen, and transaminases should be obtained. Blood cultures should be obtained from each port of any central venous catheter, and a peripheral venous sample should be obtained as well. Other microbiologic studies should be done if there are associated clinical symptoms: nasal aspirate for viruses in patients with upper respiratory findings; stool for rotavirus in the appropriate months and *C. difficile* in patients with diarrhea; urine culture in young children, or in older patients with symptoms of urgency, frequency, or dysuria; biopsy and culture of cutaneous lesions. Chest radiographs should be obtained in any individual with respiratory symptoms, although pulmonary infiltrates may be absent in children with severe neutropenia. Sinus films should be obtained if rhinorrhea is prolonged. Abdominal CT scans should also be considered in children with profound neutropenia and abdominal pain to evaluate for the presence of typhlitis. Biopsies for cytology, Gram stain, and culture should be considered if abnormalities are found during endoscopic procedures or if lung nodules are identified radiographically.

Before the routine institution of empirical antimicrobial therapy for fever and neutropenia, 75% of children with fever and neutropenia were ultimately found to have a documented site of infection. Currently, gram-positive cocci are the most common pathogens; however, gram-negative organisms such as *P. aeruginosa*, *E. coli*, and *Klebsiella* can cause life-threatening infection and must be considered in the empirical treatment regimen. Other gram-negative pathogens such as *Enterobacter* and

Acinetobacter are increasing in prevalence as well. While coagulase-negative staphylococci frequently cause infections in these children in association with central venous catheters, these infections are typically indolent and a short delay in treatment will not lead to a detrimental outcome. Other gram-positive bacteria such as *S. aureus* and *S. pneumoniae* cause more fulminant disease and require prompt institution of therapy. *Viridans* streptococci are common pathogens in patients with the oral mucositis that is often associated with the use of cytarabine and selective antibiotics such as quinolones, and can present as an acute septic shock syndrome. Patients with prolonged neutropenia who have received broad antimicrobial therapy are at increased risk for opportunistic fungal infections, especially with *Candida* and *Aspergillus*.

MANAGEMENT. Management of fever and neutropenia includes empirical antimicrobial treatment, which decreases the risks of sepsis and septic shock and the sequelae of ARDS, organ dysfunction, and death. In 2002, the Infectious Diseases Society of America updated their guidelines for the use of antimicrobial agents in neutropenic patients with cancer (see Fig. 164–1). These comprehensive guidelines provide detailed suggestions for management for both children and adults. First-line antimicrobial therapy should take into consideration the types of microbes anticipated and the local resistance patterns encountered at each institution. In addition, antibiotic choices may be limited by specific circumstances, such as the presence of drug allergy and renal or hepatic dysfunction. The empirical use of oral antibiotics has been shown to be safe in some low-risk adults who have no evidence of bacterial focus or signs of significant illness (e.g., rigors, hypotension, mental status changes) and for whom a quick recovery of the bone marrow is anticipated. However, substantive data for this approach is lacking in children and is not currently recommended. The decision to use intravenous monotherapy versus an expanded regimen of antibiotics depends on the severity of illness of the patient, history of

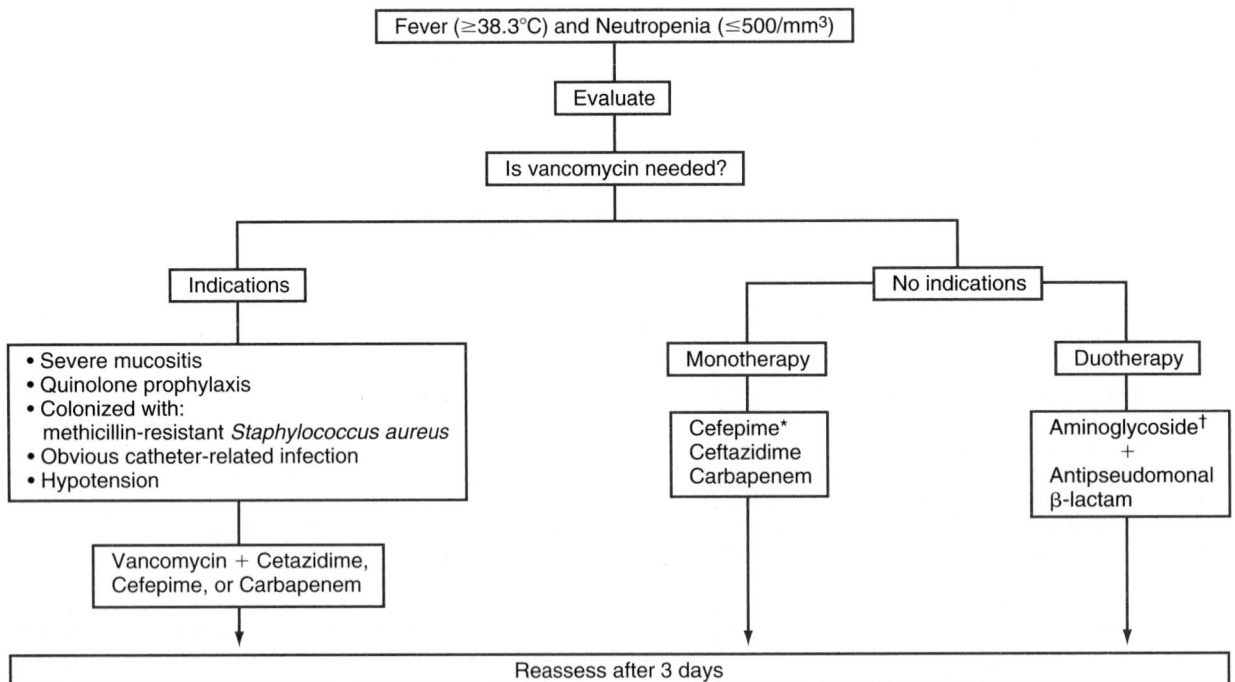

FIGURE 164–1. Guide to the initial management of the febrile neutropenic patient. *Recent studies suggest that cefepime or meropenem may be as effective as ceftazidime or imipenem as monotherapy. †Aminoglycoside antibiotics should be avoided if the patient is also receiving nephrotoxic, ototoxic, or neuromuscular blocking agents; has renal or severe electrolyte dysfunction; or is suspected of having meningitis (because of poor blood-brain perfusion). (Adapted from Hughes WT, Armstrong D, Bodey GP, et al: 2002 Guidelines for the use of antimicrobial agents in neutropenic patients with cancer. *Clin Infect Dis* 2002;34:730–51.)

previous colonization with resistant organisms, and the obvious presence of catheter-related infection (see Fig. 164–1). Vancomycin should be added to empirical initial regimen if the patient has hypotension or other evidence of septic shock, an obvious catheter-related infection, or colonization with methicillin-resistant *S. aureus*, or if the patient is at high risk for viridans streptococci (severe mucositis, prior quinolone prophylaxis). Monotherapy with cefepime, ceftazidime, or a carbapenem (e.g., imipenem/cilastatin, meropenem) has been equally effective. Piperacillin-tazobactam has appropriate coverage and has also been recommended as a potential monotherapy, but it has not been adequately studied.

Regardless of the regimen chosen initially, it is critical to carefully evaluate the patient for response to therapy, development of secondary infections, or adverse effects. Patients without an identified etiology who become afebrile within the first 3–5 days of therapy and who are clinically well with absolute neutrophil counts greater than 100 cells/mm^3 can have antibiotics changed to an oral regimen (e.g., cefixime or amoxicillin/clavulanate) and should receive a minimum of 7 days of therapy. However, if symptoms persist or evolve or if neutrophils remain significantly depressed, the same intravenous regimen should be continued.

Patients without an identified etiology but with persistent fever should be reassessed after 3–5 days. Those remaining clinically well may continue on the same regimen, although consideration should be given to discontinuing vancomycin if it was included initially. Those who remain febrile with clinical progression warrant the addition of vancomycin if not included initially and risk factors exist, as well as consideration for a change of the other antibiotics. In addition, if fever persists for more than 5 days, the addition of an antifungal agent such as fluconazole or amphotericin B is generally warranted. Because not all fevers are due to bacterial or fungal etiologies, patients with persistent fever without an identified cause and without complications may have therapy discontinued 4–5 days after the neutrophil count is greater than 500 cells/mm^3. Clinically stable patients without an identified etiology but with persistent neutropenia after 2 wk of therapy can be considered for discontinuation of antibiotics if continued close observation can be assured.

The use of antiviral agents in fever and neutropenia is not warranted without specific evidence of viral disease. Active herpes simplex or varicella-zoster lesions merit treatment to decrease the time of healing; even if they are not the source of fever they are potential portals of entry for bacteria and fungi. CMV is rarely a cause of fever in children with cancer and neutropenia. If CMV infection is strongly suspected, ganciclovir, foscarnet, or cidofovir may be considered, although ganciclovir can cause bone marrow suppression and foscarnet and cidofovir can be nephrotoxic (see Chapter 234). If influenza is identified, specific treatment with zanamivir, oseltamivir, rimantadine, or amantadine should be administered (see Chapter 237).

The use of hematopoietic growth factors shortens the duration of neutropenia but has not been proven to reduce morbidity or mortality. Accordingly, the 2002 recommendations from the Infectious Diseases Society of America do not endorse the routine use of hematopoietic growth factors in patients with uncomplicated fever and neutropenia.

Infections occur in children with cancer even without neutropenia. Most often these organisms are viral in etiology. However, *P. carinii* can cause pneumonitis regardless of the neutrophil count. Prophylaxis with trimethoprim-sulfamethoxazole against *P. carinii* is an effective preventive strategy and should be provided to all children undergoing active treatment for malignancy (see Chapter 267). Environmental fungi such as *Cryptococcus*, *Histoplasma*, and *Coccidioides* can also cause disease. *Toxoplasma gondii* is an uncommon but occasional pathogen in children with cancer. Infections encountered in healthy children (e.g., *S. pneumoniae*, group A *Streptococcus*) can cause disease in children with cancer regardless of the granulocyte count.

Transplantation. Transplantation of bone marrow, stem cells, and organs including heart, liver, kidney, lungs, pancreas, and intestines is increasingly accepted as therapy for a variety of disorders. Children with transplants are at risk for infections caused by many of the same microbial agents that cause disease in children with primary immunodeficiencies. Although the type and timing of infections after transplantation are in general similar among all recipients of these procedures, some differences exist between patients depending on the type of transplantation performed, the type and amount of immunosuppression given, and the child's previous immunity to specific pathogens.

BONE MARROW AND STEM CELL TRANSPLANTATION. Infections following BMT and stem cell transplantation (SCT) can be classified as occurring during the pretransplantation period, pre-engraftment period (0–30 days after transplantation), postengraftment period (30–100 days), or late post-transplantation (>100 days). Specific defects in host defenses predisposing to infection and their underlying causes vary within each of these time periods (Table 164–1). Neutropenia, abnormalities in cell-mediated immunity, and impaired humoral immune function predictably occur during specific time periods following transplantation, whereas abnormal anatomic barriers, due to the presence of indwelling catheters as well as mucositis secondary to radiation or chemotherapy, create defects in host defenses that may be present during any of the time periods following transplantation.

Pretransplantation Period. Children come to BMT and SCT with a heterogenous history of underlying diseases, chemotherapy exposure, degree of immunosuppression, and previous infections. As many as 12% of all infections among adult BMT recipients are reported to occur during the pretransplantation time period. The majority of infections that occur during the pretransplantation time period are caused by aerobic gram-negative bacilli and are manifest as local infections of the skin, soft tissue, and urinary tract. Importantly, the development of infection during this time period does not either delay engraftment nor alter the success of engraftment.

Pre-engraftment Period. Bacterial infections predominate in the pre-engraftment period (0–30 days). Bacteremia is the most common documented infection and occurs in as many as 50% of all BMT recipients during the first 30 days following transplantation. Bacteremia is typically secondary to either mucositis or the presence of an indwelling catheter but may be associated with pneumonia. Similarly, more than 40% of children undergoing SCT experienced at least one infection in the pre-engraftment period. Gram-positive cocci, gram-negative bacilli, yeast and, less commonly, other fungi all cause infection during this period. *Aspergillus* has been identified in 4–20% of BMT recipients, most often being diagnosed after the 3rd week of neutropenia. Infections with the emerging fungal pathogens *Fusarium* and *Pseudallescheria boydii* are associated with the prolonged neutropenia observed during the pre-engraftment period.

Viral infections also occur during the pre-engraftment period. Among adults, reactivation of herpes simplex virus is the most common viral disease observed but this is a less frequent occurrence among children, which is likely related to absence of the virus in the recipient before BMT or SCT. A history of herpes simplex infection or seropositivity indicates the need for prophylaxis. Nosocomial exposure to community-acquired viral pathogens (e.g., respiratory syncytial virus [RSV], influenza, adenovirus, rotavirus) represents another important source of infection during this time period. There is growing evidence that community-acquired viruses cause both morbidity and mortality for BMT recipients during this time period. Adenovirus is a particularly important viral pathogen that may present early, although it typically presents after engraftment.

Postengraftment Period. The predominant defect in host defenses in the postengraftment period is altered cell-mediated immunity. Accordingly, organisms historically categorized as

TABLE 164–1. Host Defense Defects and Common Pathogens by Time After Bone Marrow Transplantation and Stem Cell Transplantation

Time Period	Host Defense Defects	Causes	Common Pathogens
Pretransplant	Neutropenia Abnormal anatomic barriers	Underlying disease Prior chemotherapy	Aerobic gram-negative bacilli
Pre-engraftment	Neutropenia Abnormal anatomic barriers	Chemotherapy Radiation Indwelling catheters	Aerobic gram-positive cocci Aerobic gram-negative bacilli Candida Aspergillus Herpes simplex virus (in previously infected patients) Community-acquired viral pathogens
Postengraftment	Abnormal cell-mediated immunity Abnormal anatomic barriers	Chemotherapy Immunosuppressive medications Radiation Indwelling catheters Unrelated cord blood donor	Gram-positive cocci Aerobic gram-negative bacilli Cytomegalovirus Adenoviruses Community-acquired viral pathogens Pneumocystis carinii
Late post-transplant	Delayed recovery of immune function (cell-mediated, humoral, and abnormal anatomic barriers)	Time required to develop donor-related immune function Graft-vs-host disease	Varicella-zoster virus Streptococcus pneumoniae

"opportunistic pathogens" predominate during this time period. The risk is especially accentuated 50–100 days after transplant when host immunity is lost and donor immunity is not yet established. *P. carinii* pneumonia presents during this time period if patients are not maintained on appropriate prophylaxis. Reactivation of *T. gondii*, a rare cause of disease in BMT recipients, may also present after engraftment. Hepatosplenic candidiasis frequently presents during the postengraftment period, although seeding likely occurred during the neutropenic phase.

CMV is one of the most important causes of morbidity and mortality among BMT and SCT recipients. Unlike patients undergoing solid organ transplantation, BMT and SCT recipients developing either a primary infection or reactivation of their own latent virus may develop severe CMV disease. Adenovirus is another important viral pathogen, having been recovered from up to 5% of adult BMT and pediatric SCT recipients and causing invasive disease in approximately 20% of cases. Children receiving matched unrelated donors or unrelated cord blood cell transplants have as high as 14% incidence of adenovirus infection during this early postengraftment period. Infections with other community-acquired pathogens have been associated with excess morbidity and mortality during this time period, similar to the pre-engraftment time.

Late Post-transplantation. Infection is unusual after 100 days in the absence of chronic graft-versus-host disease. The presence of chronic graft-versus-host disease significantly affects anatomic barriers and is associated with defects in humoral, splenic, and cell-mediated immune function (see Chapter 127). Viral infections, primarily reactivation of varicella-zoster virus, are responsible for more than 40% of infections during this time period. However, bacterial infections, particularly of the upper and lower respiratory tract, account for approximately one third of infections. These may be associated with deficiencies in immunoglobulin production or synthesis, especially IgG_2. Fungal infections account for less than 20% of confirmed infections during the late post-transplant time period.

SOLID ORGAN TRANSPLANTATION. Factors predisposing to infection after organ transplantation include those that either existed before transplantation or those that are secondary to intraoperative or post-transplant therapies (Box 164–3). Some of these additional risks cannot be prevented, and some risks acquired during or after the operation may be dependent on decisions or actions of members of the transplant team. Currently, the necessity for powerful immunosuppressive agents is the major factor predisposing to infection following transplantation. Despite efforts to develop optimal immunosuppressive regimens to prevent or treat rejection with minimal impairment of immu-

BOX 164–3. Risk Factors for Infections Following Solid Organ Transplantation in Children

PRETRANSPLANT FACTORS
Age of patient
Underlying disease, malnutrition
Specific organ transplanted
Previous exposures to infectious agents
Previous immunizations

INTRAOPERATIVE FACTORS
Duration of transplant surgery
Exposure to blood products
Technical problems
Organisms transmitted with donor organ

POST-TRANSPLANT FACTORS
Immunosuppression
    Induction immunosuppression
    Maintenance immunosuppression
    Augmented treatment for rejection
Indwelling catheters
Nosocomial exposures
Community exposures

nity, all current regimens interfere with the ability of the immune system to fight infection. The majority of these immunosuppressive agents are aimed primarily at controlling cell-mediated immunity; however, regimens may impair many other aspects of the transplant recipient's immune system.

Timing. The timing of specific types of infections is generally predictable, regardless of which organ is transplanted (Table 164–2). Infectious complications typically develop in one of three time intervals: early (0–30 days after transplantation), intermediate (30–180 days, or 1–6 mo), and late (>180 days, or >6 mo); most infections develop in the first 180 days after transplantation. Early infections usually result as either a complication of the transplant surgery itself or the presence of indwelling catheters. Infections during the intermediate time period typically result as a complication of the immunosuppression, which tends to be at its greatest intensity during the first 6 mo following transplantation. This is the time period of greatest risk for infections due to opportunistic pathogens such as CMV and *P. carinii*. Anatomic abnormalities, such as bronchial stenosis and biliary stenosis, developing as a consequence of the transplant surgery can also predispose to recurrent infection that present in this time period. Infections developing late after transplantation typically result as a consequence of uncorrected anatomic abnormalities, chronic rejection or exposure to

TABLE 164–2. Timing of Infectious Complications Following Solid Organ Transplantation

Early Period (0–30 days)	Middle Period (1–6 mo)	Late Period (>6 mo)

Bacterial Infections
  Gram-negative enteric bacilli
    Small bowel, liver, neonatal heart
  Pseudomonas, Burkholderia,
    Stenotrophomonas, Alcaligenes
    Cystic fibrosis lung
  Gram-positive organisms
    All transplant types
Fungal infections
  All transplant types
Viral infections
  Herpes simplex virus
    All transplant types
  Nosocomial respiratory viruses
    All transplant types
	Viral Infections
	  Cytomegalovirus
	    All transplant types
	    Seronegative recipient of seropositive donor
	  Epstein-Barr virus
	    All transplant types (small bowel highest risk group)
	    Seronegative recipient
	  Varicella-zoster virus
	    All transplant types
	Opportunistic infections
	  Pneumocystis carinii
	    All transplant types
	  Toxoplasma gondii
	    Seronegative recipient of cardiac transplant from
	      a seropositive donor
	Bacterial infections
	Pseudomonas, Burkholderia, Stenotrophomonas, Alcaligenes
	  Cystic fibrosis lung
	  Gram-negative enteric bacilli
	    Small bowel
		Viral Infections
		  Epstein-Barr virus
		    All transplant types, but less risk than middle period
		  Varicella-zoster virus
		    All transplant types
		  Community-acquired viral infections
		    All transplant types
		Bacterial Infections
		  Pseudomonas, Burkholderia, Stenotrophomonas, Alcaligenes
		  Cystic fibrosis lung
		  Lung recipients with chronic rejection
		  Gram-negative bacillary bacteremia
		    Small bowel
		Fungal infections
		  Aspergillus
		  Lung transplants with chronic rejection

Adapted from Green M, Michaels MG: Infections in solid organ transplant recipients. In Long SS, Pickering L, Prober C, editors: Principles and Practice of Pediatric Infectious Disease. *New York, Churchill Livingstone, 1997.*

community-acquired pathogens. Acquisition of infection due to community-acquired pathogens, such as RSV, may result in severe infection secondary to the immunocompromised state of the transplant recipient during the early and intermediate periods. Compared to the earlier periods, community-acquired infections in the late period are usually benign because levels of immunosuppression are typically maintained at significantly lower levels. However, certain pathogens, such as varicella-zoster virus (VZV) and Epstein-Barr virus (EBV), may be associated with severe disease even at this late time period.

Bacterial and Fungal Infections. Although there are important graft-specific considerations for bacterial and fungal infections following transplantation, some principles are generally applicable to all transplant recipients. Bacterial and fungal infections following transplantations are usually a direct consequence of the surgery, a breach in an anatomic barrier, presence of foreign body, or an abnormal anatomic narrowing or obstruction. With the exception of infections related to the use of indwelling catheters, sites of bacterial infection tend to occur at or near the transplanted organ. Infections following abdominal transplantation (e.g., liver, intestine, or renal) usually occur in the abdomen or at the surgical wound. The pathogens are typically enteric gram-negative bacteria, *Enterococcus*, and occasionally *Candida*. Infections following thoracic transplantation (e.g., heart, lung) usually occur in the lower respiratory tract or at the surgical wound. Pathogens associated with these infections include *S. aureus* and gram-negative bacteria. Patients undergoing lung transplantation for cystic fibrosis experience a particularly high rate of infectious complications, because they are frequently colonized with *Pseudomonas* or *Aspergillus* before transplantation. Even though the infected cystic lungs are removed, the sinuses and upper airways remain colonized with these same pathogens and subsequent reinfection of the transplanted lungs is not infrequent. Children receiving organ transplants have frequently been hospitalized for long periods and have received many antibiotics, thus recovery of bacteria with multiple antibiotic resistance is common after all types of organ transplantation. Infections due to *Aspergillus* are less common but occur after all types of organ transplantation and are associated with high rates of morbidity and mortality.

Viral Infections. Viral pathogens, especially herpesviruses, are a major source of morbidity and mortality following solid organ transplantation. The patterns of disease associated with individual viral pathogens generally are similar among all organ transplant recipients. However, the frequency, mode of presentation, and severity differ according to type of organ transplanted and pretransplant serologic status of the recipient.

Viral pathogens can be categorized as **donor-associated viruses**, such as CMV and EBV, or as community-acquired viruses. For CMV and EBV, primary infection occurring after transplantation is associated with the greatest degree of morbidity and mortality. The highest risk is in a naive host who receives an organ from a donor who previously was infected with one of these viruses. This "mismatched state" is a frequent cause of severe disease. However, even if the donor is negative for CMV and EBV, these infections can be acquired from a close contact or via blood products. Reactivation of a latent strain within the host, or superinfection with a new strain, tends to result in milder illness unless the patient is greatly immunosuppressed, which may occur in the setting of treatment of significant rejection. CMV is the most commonly recognized transplant viral pathogen and remains a major cause of disease after solid organ transplantation. Disease can range from a syndrome of fatigue and fever to disseminated disease that most often affects the liver, lungs, and gastrointestinal tract. Infection due to EBV is increasingly recognized as another important complication of solid organ transplantation ranging from a mild mononucleosis syndrome to disseminated post-transplant lymphoproliferative disorder (PTLD). PTLD is more common among children than adults because primary EBV infection in the immunosuppressed host is more likely to lead to uncontrolled proliferative disorders, including post-transplant lymphoma. Other donor-associated viral pathogens include hepatitis B virus, hepatitis C virus, HIV, and occasionally adenoviruses.

Community-acquired viruses, including respiratory viruses (e.g., RSV, influenza, and parainfluenza) and enteric viruses (e.g., enteroviruses, rotavirus), may cause important disease in children following organ transplantation. In general, risk factors for more severe infection include young age, acquisition of infection early after transplantation, and augmented immune suppression. Infection in the absence of these risk factors typically results in a clinical illness that is comparable to that seen in immunocompetent children.

Opportunistic Pathogens. Children undergoing solid-organ transplantation are also at risk for symptomatic infections from pathogens that do not usually cause clinical disease in immunocompetent hosts. Even though most frequently recognized in the intermediate time period, these infections can also occur late in patients requiring prolonged and high levels of immunosuppression. *P. carinii* is a well recognized cause of pneumonia following solid organ transplantation, although routine prophylaxis has essentially eliminated this problem. *T. gondii* may complicate cardiac transplantations, because of tropism of the organism for cardiac muscle and risk for donor transmission, and rarely may complicate renal and liver transplants.

PREVENTION OF INFECTION IN IMMUNOCOMPROMISED HOSTS

Infections cannot be completely prevented in children who have defects in one or more arms of their immune system, although some measures can decrease the risks for infection. For example, replacement immunoglobulin is a benefit to children with primary B-cell deficiencies, and IFN-γ and trimethoprim-sulfamethoxazole reduce the number of infections occurring in children with chronic granulomatous disease. Likewise, children with depressed cellular immunity from primary diseases, AIDS, or use of immunosuppressive medications benefit from prophylaxis against *P. carinii*. Immunizations prevent many infections that would be a problem for any host but particularly for children with compromised immune systems. Immunizations should ideally be administered before any treatment that would compromise the child's immune system; however, this is not always possible such as with primary immune defects or in children who require transplants early in life.

While immunodeficient children represent a heterogeneic group, some principles of prevention are generally applicable. Inactivated vaccines do not lead to an increased risk of adverse effects, although their efficacy may be reduced due to an impaired immune response. Live, attenuated virus vaccinations can cause disease in some children with immunologic defects, and therefore alternative immunizations should be used whenever possible, such as the use of inactivated polio vaccine rather than live virus oral polio vaccine. In general, live virus vaccines should not be used in children with primary T-cell abnormalities. However, in some instances in which wild type viral infection can be severe, immunizations, even with live virus vaccine, are warranted. For example, children with HIV infection and CD4 percentage greater than 15% should receive measles vaccination, and they should receive varicella vaccine if CD4 percentage is greater than 25%. Some vaccines should be given to children with immunodeficiencies in addition to routine vaccinations. For example, the meningococcal vaccine and both the polysaccharide pneumococcal vaccine as well as the conjugate pneumococcal vaccine should be given to children with splenic dysfunction or complement deficiency. Influenza vaccination should be strongly considered for immunocompromised children as well as all household contacts, to minimize risk of transmission to the immunocompromised child.

Benjamin Jr DK, Miller WC, Bayliff S, et al: Infections diagnosed in the first year after pediatric stem cell transplantation. *Pediatr Infect Dis J* 2002;21:227–34.

Buckley RH: Primary immunodeficiency disease due to defects in lymphocytes. *N Engl J Med* 2000;343:1313–24.

Burroughs M, Moscona A: Immunization of pediatric solid organ candidates and recipients. *Clin Infect Dis* 2000;30:857–69.

Green M, Michaels MG, Webber SA, et al: The management of Epstein-Barr virus associated post-transplant lymphoproliferative disorders in pediatric solid-organ transplant recipients. *Pediatr Transplant* 1999;3:271–81.

Green M, Wald ER, Fricker FS, et al: Infections in pediatric orthotopic heart transplant recipients. *Pediatr Infect Dis J* 1989;8:87–93.

Hughes WT, Armstrong D, Bodey GP, et al: 2002 Guidelines for the use of antimicrobial agents in neutropenic patients with cancer. *Clin Infect Dis* 2002;34:730–51.

Kusne S, Dummer JS, Singh N, et al: Infection after liver transplantation. An analysis of 101 consecutive cases. *Medicine* 1988;67:132–43.

Mackay IR, Rosen FS: Immunodeficiency diseases caused by defects in phagocytes. Advances in immunology. *N Engl J Med* 2000;343:1703–14.

Palmer SM, Alexander BD, Sanders LL: Significance of bloodstream infection after lung transplantation: analysis in 176 consecutive patients. *Transplantation* 2000;69:2360–6.

Paya C, Fung JJ, Nalesnik MA, et al: Epstein-Barr virus-induced posttransplant lymphoproliferative disorders. *Transplantation* 1999;68:1517–25.

Sable CA, Donowitz GR: Infections in bone marrow transplant recipients. *Clin Infect Dis* 1994;18:273–81.

Their M, Holmberg C, Lautenschlager I, et al: Infections in pediatric kidney and liver patients after perioperative hospitalization. *Transplantation* 2000;69:1617–23.

Chapter 165
Infection Associated with Medical Devices
Patricia M. Flynn and Fred F. Barrett

Despite the therapeutic successes and convenience of the many synthetic devices used in pediatric patients, infectious complications are problematic. The pathogenesis of device-related infection is not completely defined, but many factors are important, including the susceptibility of the host, the composition of the device, the ability of microorganisms to adhere to the device itself or to the biofilm that quickly forms on it, and environmental factors that include the insertion technique and maintenance of the device.

Intravascular Access Devices. Intravascular access devices range from short stainless steel needles to multilumen implantable synthetic plastic catheters that are expected to remain in use for years. Infectious complications include localized infections (exit site infection, tunnel tract infection, suppurative phlebitis) and systemic infections (catheter-related bacteremia and fungemia). The pathogenesis is most often related to local contamination and subsequent colonization of the catheter rather than primary bacteremia or secondary bacteremia from another focus seeding the intravascular device. Infection with the microbial skin flora at the insertion site may extend along the external surface of the catheter. This route of infection is most common in intravascular catheters in place for less than 30 days. Organisms may also gain access to the intraluminal portion of the catheter through improper handling of the catheter hub or contaminated infusate. This route of infection is thought to be more prevalent in catheters in place greater than 30 days. Gram-positive cocci predominate in both categories; more than half are caused by coagulase-negative staphylococci. Gram-negative enteric bacteria are isolated in approximately 20–30% of episodes, and fungi account for 5–10%.

The clinical manifestations of local infection include erythema, tenderness, and purulent discharge at the exit site or along the subcutaneous tunnel tract of the catheter. Catheter-related sepsis may also present as fever without an identifiable focus.

The diagnosis of localized infection is established clinically. A Gram stain and culture of exit site drainage should be performed and may help elucidate the microbiologic cause. The diagnosis of catheter-related bacteremia is confirmed by performing quantitative blood cultures simultaneously from the catheter and the peripheral vein. Evidence of catheter-related bacteremia or fungemia is more than 4–10 times the number of organisms isolated from blood obtained via the catheter as compared to blood obtained via a peripheral vein. If quantitative blood cultures are not available, a catheter blood culture that becomes positive more than 2 hr before a peripheral culture, with equal amounts of blood using a radiometric detection system, may also be used for diagnosis. Catheter-related sepsis can also be diagnosed by isolation of the same organism from the blood and the catheter tip. This method, however, requires catheter removal and is not optimal for patients with long-term devices.

Short-term peripheral catheters are most commonly used in pediatric patients, and infectious complications occur infrequently. The rate of peripheral catheter-related bacteremia is less than 0.15%. Patient age younger than 1 yr, duration of use more than 144 hr, and selected (e.g., total parenteral nutrition, lipid) infusates are associated with increased risk of catheter-related infection.

Central venous catheters (CVCs) are widely used in both adults and pediatric patients and are responsible for the majority of catheter-related infections. They are commonly used in critically ill patients, including neonates, who often have many risk factors for the development of nosocomial infection. Patients who are in an intensive care unit and who have a CVC in place have a fivefold greater risk of developing a nosocomial bloodstream infection than those without a CVC. The means for optimal maintenance of these catheters remains controversial. Although prevalence of infection increases with prolonged duration of catheter use, routine replacement of a CVC results in significant morbidity. Current guidelines suggest placement with full barrier precautions either via a new site or exchange of the catheter over a guide wire, but without a policy for routine replacement.

The use of peripherally inserted central catheters (PICCs), which are inserted into a peripheral vein with the distal end in a central vein, has increased in pediatric patients. Published experience with these devices in children is scanty, but studies in adults document a life span of approximately 3 mo and infection rates of 1.9 episodes/1,000 catheter-days, significantly lower than for CVCs.

When prolonged intravenous access is required, a cuffed silicone rubber (Silastic) catheter may be inserted into the right atrium through the subclavian, cephalic, or jugular vein. The extravascular segment of the catheter passes through a subcutaneous tunnel before exiting the skin, usually on the superior aspect of the chest (Broviac or Hickman catheters). Totally implanted devices consist of a reservoir or port placed in a subcutaneous pocket with a self-sealing silicone septum at the distal end that permits repeated percutaneous needle insertions for administration of drugs. The use of central venous devices has improved the quality of life of high-risk patients but has also increased the risk of various infections. The incidence of local (exit site, tunnel, pocket) infection is 0.2–2.8/1,000 catheter-days. The incidence of Broviac or Hickman catheter-associated sepsis is 0.5–6.8/1,000 catheter days, whereas that for implantable devices is 0.3–1.8/1,000 catheter-days. The risk of catheter infection is increased among premature infants, young children, and those receiving total parenteral nutrition.

If either localized or systemic catheter-related infection is diagnosed in a short-term peripheral catheter or CVC, the device should be removed. Antibiotics should be administered in cases of systemic infection, with the exception of uncomplicated coagulase-negative staphylococcal bacteremia in normal hosts, for which catheter removal is sufficient.

For infections associated with long-term vascular access devices (Hickman, Broviac, totally implantable devices), antibiotic treatment is successful for most systemic bacterial infections without removal of the device. Antibiotic therapy should be directed to the isolated pathogen and given for a total of 10–14 days. Until identification and susceptibility testing are available, empirical therapy with a third-generation cephalosporin or aminoglycoside plus vancomycin is indicated. **"Antibiotic lock" or "dwell" therapy**, with administration of solutions of high concentrations of antibiotics that remain in the catheter for up to 24 hr, may improve outcome. If blood cultures remain positive after 72 hr of appropriate therapy, as confirmed by susceptibility testing, or if a patient deteriorates clinically, the device should be removed. Most experts advocate removal of

the device as well as therapy with systemic antifungals in cases of catheter-related fungemia. Exit-site infections usually respond to local care or systemic antibiotics, but tunnel tract infections require removal of the catheter in approximately two thirds of patients.

PREVENTION OF INFECTION. Prevention of infections of long-term vascular access devices includes placement using meticulous surgical aseptic technique in an operating room–like environment, routine use of antibacterial ointment, avoidance of occlusive or semipermeable dressings, avoidance of bathing or swimming, and careful catheter care. The use of CVCs impregnated with antibiotics may be a future means to prevent catheter-related infection.

Cerebrospinal Fluid Shunts. Cerebrospinal fluid (CSF) shunting is required for the treatment of many children with hydrocephalus. The usual procedure uses a silicone rubber device with a proximal portion inserted into the ventricle, a unidirectional valve, and a distant segment that diverts the CSF from the ventricles to either the peritoneal cavity (ventriculoperitoneal, or VP shunt) or right atrium (ventriculoatrial, or VA shunt). The incidence of shunt infection ranges from 1–20%, with an average of 10%. The highest rates are reported in young infants. Most infections are a result of intraoperative contamination of the surgical wound by skin flora. Accordingly, coagulase-negative staphylococci are isolated in more than half of the cases. *Staphylococcus aureus* is isolated in approximately 20% and gram-negative bacilli in 15%.

Four distinct clinical syndromes have been described: colonization of the shunt, infection associated with wound infection, distal infection with peritonitis, and infection associated with meningitis.

The most common type of infection is "colonization" of the shunt with symptoms that reflect shunt malfunction as opposed to shunt infection per se. Symptoms associated with colonized VP shunts include lethargy, headache, vomiting, and a full fontanel. Low-grade fever is common. Symptoms usually occur within months of the surgical procedure. Colonization of a VA shunt results in more severe systemic symptoms and often without specific symptoms of shunt malfunction. Septic pulmonary emboli, pulmonary hypertension, and infective endocarditis are frequently reported complications of VA shunt colonization. Chronic VA shunt colonization may cause hypocomplementemic glomerulonephritis due to antigen-antibody complex deposition in the glomeruli, which is commonly called **shunt nephritis**; clinical findings include hypertension, microscopic hematuria, elevated blood urea nitrogen (BUN) and serum creatinine levels, and anemia. With shunt colonization, CSF obtained from either lumbar or ventricular puncture is often sterile, and the infecting organism is isolated only from the shunt reservoir. Because of this, it is unusual to observe signs of ventriculitis, and CSF findings are only minimally abnormal. Blood culture results are usually negative in cases of VP colonization but positive in VA shunt colonization.

Wound infection presents with obvious infection or dehiscence along the shunt tract and most often occurs within days to weeks of the surgical procedure. *S. aureus* is the most common isolate. In addition to the physical findings, fever is common, and signs of shunt malfunction eventually ensue in most cases.

Distal infection of VP shunts with peritonitis presents with abdominal symptoms, usually without evidence of shunt malfunction. The pathogenesis is likely related to perforation of bowel at the time of VP shunt placement or translocation of bacteria across the bowel wall. Thus, gram-negative isolates predominate and mixed infection is common. The infecting organisms are often isolated from only the distal portion of the shunt.

The usual meningeal pathogens, *Streptococcus pneumoniae*, *Neisseria meningitidis*, and *Haemophilus influenzae* type b, can also cause bacterial meningitis in patients with shunts in place. The clinical presentation is similar to that for acute bacterial meningitis (see Chapter 594).

Treatment of shunt colonization and distal infection with peritonitis includes the use of antibiotics against the specific organisms isolated and, in most situations, removal of the shunt. Intrashunt antibiotics are indicated because of the poor penetration of most antibiotics into the CNS across uninflamed meninges. If the isolate is susceptible, a parenteral antistaphylococcal penicillin plus intrashunt vancomycin is the treatment of choice. If the organism is resistant to the penicillins, systemic and intrashunt vancomycin is recommended. In cases of gram-negative infections, a combination of a third-generation cephalosporin and intrashunt aminoglycoside is optimal. When using intrashunt antibiotics, monitoring of CSF levels is necessary to avoid toxicity. The best treatment success occurs with initial systemic and intrashunt antibiotics in combination with exteriorization of the distal end of the shunt. After CSF from the reservoir has remained sterile for 48 hr, shunt replacement on the opposite side can be performed. Partial shunt revision with antibiotic therapy or antibiotic therapy alone has been successful in some series, but the relapse rate is higher. When wound infection is diagnosed, the shunt most always needs to be removed. To allow for continued ventricular drainage, a temporary catheter is often placed, with replacement of a new shunt on the opposite side after the wound infection has healed. Only systemic antibiotics are necessary for treatment of bacterial meningitis in patients with a shunt in place; the shunt itself does not need to be removed.

PREVENTION OF INFECTION. Prevention of shunt infection includes meticulous cutaneous preparation and surgical technique. Systemic and intraventricular antibiotics and soaking the shunt tubing in antibiotics have been used to reduce the incidence of infection, with varying success. A meta-analysis of 12 clinical trials using various antimicrobial regimens involving 1,359 randomized patients showed that perioperative use of an antimicrobial agent in CSF shunt placement reduced the risk for infection, although only 1 of the 12 studies individually revealed an effect.

Urethral Catheters. Urinary catheters are a frequent cause of nosocomial infection, with about 14 infections/1,000 admissions. Like other devices, microorganisms adhere to the catheter surface and establish a biofilm that allows proliferation. The physical presence of the catheter reduces the normal host defenses by preventing complete emptying of the bladder, thus providing a medium for growth, distending the urethra, and blocking periurethral glands. Almost all patients catheterized for more than 30 days develop bacteriuria. The urinary tract is considered infected if specimens of urine obtained directly from an indwelling catheter harbor greater than or equal to 100 colony-forming units/mL. Gram-negative bacilli and *Enterococcus* are the predominant organisms isolated in catheter-related urinary tract infection; coagulase-negative staphylococci are implicated in about 15%. Symptomatic urinary tract infections should be treated with antibiotics and catheter removal. Asymptomatic infections can usually be managed with catheter removal alone.

PREVENTION OF INFECTION. All urinary catheters introduce risk for infection, and their casual use should be avoided. When they are in place, their duration of use should be minimized. Technologic advances have led to development of silver- or antibiotic-impregnated urinary catheters that are associated with lower rates of infection. Prophylactic antibiotics do not reduce the infection rates for long-term indwelling urethral catheters.

Peritoneal Dialysis Catheters. During the 1st yr of peritoneal dialysis for end-stage renal disease, 65% of children will have one or more episodes of peritonitis. Bacterial entry comes from luminal or periluminal contamination of the catheter or by translocation across the intestinal wall. Hematogenous infection is rare. Infections can be localized at the exit site, associated with peritonitis, or both. Organisms responsible for peritonitis include coagulase-negative staphylococci (30–40%), *S. aureus* (10–20%), streptococci (10–15%), *Escherichia coli* (5–10%), *Pseudomonas* (5–10%), other gram-negative bacteria (5–15%), *Enterococcus* (3–6%), and fungi (2–10%). *S. aureus* is more common in localized exit or tunnel tract infections (42%). Most infectious episodes are due to a patient's own flora, and carriers of *S. aureus* have been shown to have increased rates of infection as compared with noncarriers.

The clinical manifestations of peritonitis may be subtle and include low-grade fever, mild abdominal pain, and tenderness. Cloudy peritoneal dialysis fluid may be the first and predominant sign. With peritonitis, the peritoneal fluid cell count is usually greater than 100 white blood cells/μL. When peritonitis is suspected, the effluent dialysate should be submitted for cell count, Gram stain (which is positive in up to 40% if peritonitis is present), and culture.

Patients with cloudy fluid and clinical symptoms should receive empirical therapy, preferably guided by results of a Gram stain. If no organisms are visualized, vancomycin and either an aminoglycoside or third-generation cephalosporin with antipseudomonal activity should be given via the intraperitoneal route. Patients without cloudy fluid and with minimal symptoms may have therapy withheld pending culture results. Once the cause is identified by culture, changes in the therapeutic regimen may be needed. Oral rifampin may be added for *S. aureus* infections. Fungal peritonitis should be treated with a combination of oral flucytosine and intraperitoneal or oral fluconazole alone. The duration of therapy is a minimum of 14 days, with longer treatment of 21–28 days for episodes of *S. aureus* and *Pseudomonas*, and 28–42 days for fungi. Repeat episodes of peritonitis within 4 wk of previous therapy represent "apparently relapsing" peritonitis. If the patient responds to reinstitution of antimicrobial therapy, a course of up to 6 wk should be continued. In all cases, if the infection fails to clear on appropriate therapy or if a patient's condition is deteriorating, the catheter should be removed. Exit-site and tunnel infections may occur independently of peritonitis, or may precede it. Appropriate antibiotics should be administered on the basis of Gram stain and culture findings. Some experts recommend that the peritoneal catheter be removed if *Pseudomonas* or fungal organisms are isolated.

Orthopedic Prostheses. Orthopedic prostheses are used infrequently in children although their use is increasing in limb salvage procedures for osteosarcoma. Infection most often follows introduction of microorganisms at surgery or via hematogenous spread. Early postoperative infection occurs within 2–4 wk of surgery with typical manifestations that include fever, pain, and local symptoms of wound infection. Rapid assessment, including isolation of the infecting organism, and antimicrobial treatment may allow salvage of the implant. Late chronic infection occurs more than 1 mo after surgery and is often caused by organisms of low virulence that contaminated the implant at the time of surgery. Typical manifestations include pain and deterioration in function. These infections respond poorly to antibiotic treatment and usually require removal of the implant. Hematogenous infections are most often observed 2 or more yr after surgery. As with other long-term implanted devices, the most common organisms are about equally divided between coagulase-negative staphylococci and *S. aureus*.

The use of systemic antibiotic prophylaxis, antibiotic-containing bone cement, and operating rooms fitted with laminar airflow all have been proposed as beneficial in reducing infection. To date, results from clinical studies are conflicting.

Centers for Disease Control and Prevention: Guidelines for the prevention of intravascular catheter-related infections. *MMWR* 2002;51(RR-10):1–29.
Darouiche RQ: Device-associated infections: A macroproblem that starts with microadherence. *Clin Infect Dis* 2001;33:1567–72.

Mermel LA, Farr BM, Sherertz RH, et al: Guidelines for the management of intravascular catheter-related infections. *Clin Infect Dis* 2001;32:1249–72.

Seifert H, Jansen B, Farr BM (editors): *Catheter-Related Infections.* New York, Marcel Dekker, 1997.

Widmer AF: New developments in diagnosis and treatment of infection in orthopedic implants. *Clin Infect Dis* 2001;33(Suppl 2):S94–106.

SECTION 2 *Gram-Positive Bacterial Infections*

Chapter 166

Staphylococcus James K. Todd

Staphylococci are hardy, aerobic, non–spore-forming, bacteria that are ubiquitous as normal flora of humans and animals and present on fomites in dust. They are resistant to heat and drying and may be recovered from nonbiologic environments weeks to months after contamination. These organisms are gram-positive and grow in clusters as aerobes or facultative anaerobes. Strains are classified as *Staphylococcus aureus* if they are coagulase-positive or as one of the many species of **coagulase-negative staphylococci** (e.g., *S. epidermidis, S. saprophyticus, S. haemolyticus*). Generally, *S. aureus* produces a yellow pigment and β-hemolysis on blood agar and *S. epidermidis* produces a white pigment with variable hemolysis results, although definitive species confirmation requires further testing. *S. aureus* has many virulence factors that mediate various serious diseases, whereas coagulase-negative staphylococci tend to be less pathogenic unless an indwelling foreign body (e.g., intravascular catheter) is present.

166.1 *Staphylococcus aureus*

S. aureus is the most common cause of pyogenic infection of the skin; it also may cause furuncles, carbuncles, osteomyelitis, suppurative arthritis, wound infection, abscesses, pneumonia, empyema, endocarditis, pericarditis, meningitis, and toxin-mediated diseases, including food poisoning, scarlet fever, scalded skin syndrome, and toxic shock syndrome (TSS).

Etiology. Disease may result from tissue invasion or injury caused by various toxins and enzymes. Strains of *S. aureus* can be identified by the virulence factors they produce and classified classically by means of bacteriophage group typing (groups I–IV, miscellaneous) or, more recently, by molecular techniques. Strains within phage groups often have similar pathogenic potential (e.g., phage group I is associated with TSS, phage group II with scalded skin syndrome).

Adhesion of *S. aureus* to mucosal cells is mediated by **teichoic acid** in the cell wall, and exposure to the submucosa or subcutaneous sites increases adhesion to fibrinogen, fibronectin, collagen, and other proteins. Different strains of *S. aureus* produce many virulence factors (Table 166–1), which have one or more of four different roles: protect the organism from host defenses, localize infection, cause local tissue damage, and act as toxins affecting noninfected tissue sites.

TABLE 166–1. Virulence Factors Produced by *Staphylococcus aureus* and Their Role in Disease

Factor	Location	Action	Pathophysiology
Cell Wall Components			
Peptidoglycan	Cell wall		Aggressin, shock
Teichoic acids	Cell wall		Adhesion to epithelium
Slime (coagulase-negative)	Cell wall	Extracellular matrix	Cements and protects
Capsule	Cell wall	Extracellular matrix	Protects from phagocytosis
Protein A	Cell wall	Binds IgG	Protects phagocytosis
Clumping factor	Cell wall	Binds fibrin	Large clumps, blocks phagocytosis
Fibronectin-binding	Cell wall	Attaches to fibronectin	Attachment to cell
PBP2a	Cell wall	Alters penicillin binding	Methicillin resistance
Enzymes			
Catalase	Soluble	Catalyzes H_2O_2	Inhibits PMN killing
Coagulase	Soluble	Clots plasma	Forms abscess wall
Leukocidin	Soluble	Destroys PMNs	Protects from phagocytosis
Hemolysins	Soluble	Cytotoxic	Tissue damage
Lipase	Soluble	Lipolysis	Skin infection
β-Lactamase	Soluble	Penase	Penicillin G resistance
Toxins			
Enterotoxin A, B, C, D, E	Soluble	Vagal stimulator	Food poisoning (TSS)
Exfoliatin A, B	Soluble	Granular layer cleavage	Scalded skin syndrome
TSST-1	Soluble	TNF, IL-1 stimulator	TSS

TSST-1, toxic shock syndrome-1; PMN, polymorphonuclear neutrophil; H_2O_2, hydrogen peroxide; TNF, tumor necrosis factor; IL-1, interleukin 1.

Most strains of *S. aureus* possess factors that protect the organism from host defenses. Many staphylococci produce a loose polysaccharide capsule, or **slime layer**, which may interfere with opsonophagocytosis. Clumping factor interacts with fibrinogen to cause large clumps of organism to form, interfering with effective phagocytosis. Production of **coagulase**, or **clumping factor**, differentiates *S. aureus* from *S. epidermidis* and other coagulase-negative staphylococci. Coagulase causes plasma to clot by interacting with fibrinogen; this may have an important role in localization of infection (i.e., abscess formation). **Protein A**, which is present in most strains of *S. aureus* but not in *S. epidermidis*, reacts specifically with IgG1, IgG2, and IgG4. It is located on the outermost coat of the bacterium and can absorb serum immunoglobulin, preventing antibacterial antibodies from acting as opsonins and thus inhibiting phagocytosis. Other enzymes elaborated by staphylococci include **catalase** (inactivates hydrogen peroxide, promoting intracellular survival), **penicillinase** or **β-lactamase** (inactivates penicillin at the molecular level), and lipase (associated with skin infection). **Leukocidin**, which is produced by most strains of *S. aureus*, combines with the phospholipid of the phagocytic cell membrane, producing increased permeability, leakage of protein, and eventual death of the neutrophil and macrophage.

Many strains of *S. aureus* produce substances that cause local tissue destruction. A number of immunologically distinct hemolysins have been identified: **α-toxin** acts on cell membranes and causes tissue necrosis, injures human leukocytes, and produces aggregation of platelets and spasm of smooth muscle; **β-hemolysin** degrades sphingomyelin, causing hemolysis of red blood cells; **δ-hemolysin** disrupts membranes by a detergent-like action.

Many strains of *S. aureus* release exotoxins. **Exfoliatins A and B** are two serologically distinct proteins that produce localized (e.g., bullous impetigo) or generalized (e.g., scalded skin syndrome, scarlatiniform eruption) dermatologic complications (Chapter 647). Exfoliatins produce skin separation by splitting the desmosome and altering the intracellular matrix in the stratum granulosum.

One or more staphylococcal **enterotoxins (types A, B, C₁, C₂, D, E)** are elaborated by most strains of *S. aureus*. Ingestion of preformed enterotoxin A or B is associated with vomiting and diarrhea and, in some cases, with the development of profound hypotension. By 10 yr of age, almost all individuals have antibodies to at least one enterotoxin.

Toxic shock syndrome toxin-1 (TSST-1) is associated with TSS related to menstruation and focal staphylococcal infection. Enterotoxin A and enterotoxin B also may be associated with nonmenstrual TSS. TSST-1 induces production of interleukin-1 and tumor necrosis factor, resulting in hypotension, fever, and multisystem involvement.

Epidemiology. Most neonates are colonized within the first week of life, and 20–30% of normal individuals carry at least one strain of *S. aureus* in the anterior nares.

The organisms may be transmitted from the nose to the skin, where colonization seems to be more transient. Repeated recovery of *S. aureus* from the skin suggests repeated transfer rather than persistent skin colonization. Persistent umbilical and perianal carriage occurs.

Transmission of *S. aureus* generally occurs by direct contact or by spread of heavy particles over a distance of ≤6 ft. Heavily colonized individual carriers are particularly effective disseminators. Autoinfection is common, and minor infections (e.g., styes, pustules, paronychia) may be the source of disseminated infection. Handwashing between patient contacts decreases the spread of staphylococci from patient to patient. Older children and adults are more resistant than neonates to colonization. Spread via fomites is rare.

Invasive disease may follow colonization. Antibiotic therapy with a drug to which *S. aureus* is resistant favors colonization and the development of infection. Other factors that increase the likelihood of infection include wounds, skin disease, ventriculoperitoneal shunts, intravenous or intrathecal catheterization, corticosteroid treatment, starvation, acidosis, and azotemia. Viral infections of the respiratory tract also may predispose to secondary bacterial infection with staphylococci.

Pathogenesis. The development of staphylococcal disease is related to resistance of the host to infection and to virulence of the organism (Fig. 166–1). The intact skin and mucous membranes serve as barriers to invasion by staphylococci. Defects in the mucocutaneous barriers produced by trauma, surgery, foreign surfaces (e.g., sutures, shunts, intravascular catheters), and burns increase the risk of infection.

Infants may acquire type-specific humoral immunity to staphylococci transplacentally. Older children and adults develop antibodies to staphylococci as a result of intermittent minor infections of the skin and soft tissues. Antibodies acquired after immunization with *S. aureus* capsular material have been shown to temporarily reduce subsequent infection in dialysis patients. Antibody to the various *S. aureus* toxins appears to protect against those specific toxin-mediated diseases but not necessarily focal or disseminated *S. aureus* infection with the same organisms. There is some indication that disseminated *S. aureus* disease in previously healthy children may occur after a viral infection that suppresses neutrophil or respiratory epithelial cell function.

Individuals with congenital or acquired defects in the complement system required for chemotaxis, defective chemotaxis (Job, Chédiak-Higashi, and Wiskott-Aldrich syndromes), defective phagocytosis, and defective humoral immunity (antibodies required for opsonization), as well as those with an impaired intracellular bactericidal capacity, are at increased risk of infection with staphylococci. Patients with chronic granulomatous disease, in which phagocytosis proceeds normally but killing of ingested catalase-positive bacteria is severely impaired, are particularly susceptible to staphylococcal disease. Impaired mobilization of polymorphonuclear leukocytes has been documented in children with diabetic ketoacidosis and in healthy individuals after ingesting alcohol. Patients with HIV infection have neutrophils that are defective in their ability to kill *S. aureus* in vitro.

Clinical Manifestations. The signs and symptoms vary with the location of the infection, which, although most commonly located on the skin, may involve any tissue. Disease states of various degrees of severity are generally a result of local suppuration, systemic dissemination with metastatic infection, or systemic effects of toxin production. Although the nasopharynx and skin of many persons may be colonized with *S. aureus*, disease due to this organism is relatively uncommon. Lesions, especially those of the skin, are considerably more prevalent among persons living in low socioeconomic circumstances and particularly among those in tropical climates.

NEWBORN. *Staphylococcus* is an important cause of neonatal infections (Chapter 98).

SKIN. *Staphylococcus* is an important cause of pyogenic skin infections, including impetigo contagiosa, ecthyma, bullous impetigo, folliculitis, hydradenitis, furuncles, carbuncles, staphylococcal scalded skin syndrome (i.e., Ritter disease), and a syndrome resembling the rash of scarlet fever. Infection may also complicate wounds or occur as superinfection of other noninfectious skin disease (e.g., eczema). Folliculitis, or pyoderma of the hair follicle, may extend to a deep-seated furuncle or carbuncle if more than one hair follicle is involved. Recurrent furunculosis is a disorder of unknown cause and is associated with repeated episodes of pyoderma over months to years. Patients should be evaluated for immune defects associated with recurrent infection, especially those involving neutrophil dysfunction. *Staphylococcus* is also an important cause of nosocomial skin infections (Chapter 283).

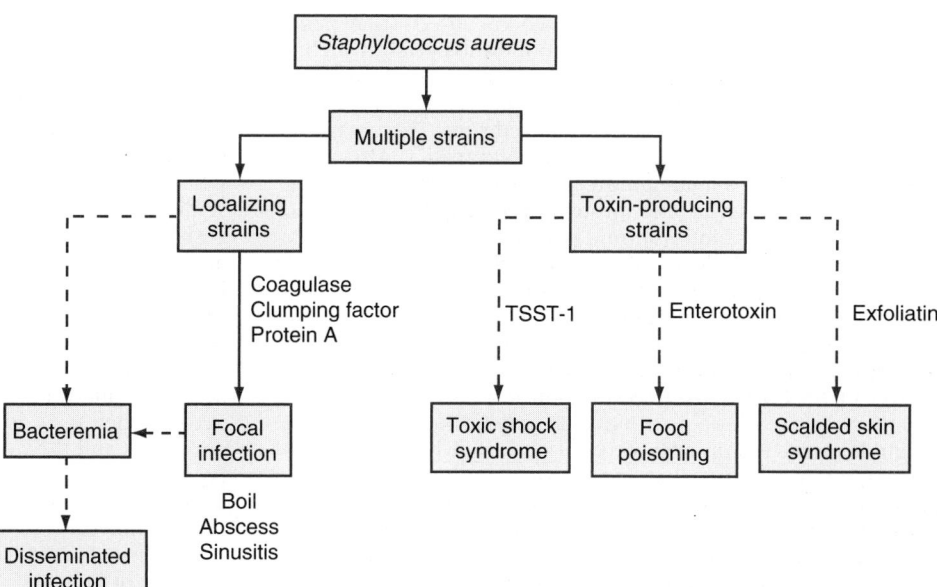

FIGURE 166–1. Relationship of virulence factors to diseases associated with *Staphylococcus aureus*.

RESPIRATORY TRACT. Infections of the upper respiratory tract due to *S. aureus* are rare, considering the frequency with which this area is colonized. Otitis media (Chapter 630) and sinusitis (Chapter 365) due to *S. aureus* may occur rarely. Staphylococcal sinusitis is relatively common in children with cystic fibrosis or defects in white blood cell (WBC) function. Suppurative parotitis is a rare infection, but *S. aureus* is a common cause. Staphylococcal tonsillopharyngitis is rare in otherwise normal children. A membranous tracheitis that complicates viral croup may be infected with *S. aureus* but also by other organisms. Patients typically have high fever, leukocytosis, and evidence of severe upper airway obstruction. Direct laryngoscopy or bronchoscopy shows a normal epiglottis with subglottic narrowing and thick, purulent secretions within the trachea. Treatment requires antibiotics and careful airway management.

Pneumonia (Chapter 389) due to *S. aureus* may be primary (hematogenous) or secondary after a viral infection such as influenza. Hematogenous pneumonia may be secondary to septic emboli, right-sided endocarditis, or the presence of intravascular devices. Inhalation pneumonia is caused by alterations of mucociliary clearance, leukocyte dysfunction, or bacterial adherence initiated by a viral infection. More common are high fever, abdominal pain, tachypnea, dyspnea, and localized or diffuse bronchopneumonia or lobar disease. *S. aureus* causes a necrotizing pneumonitis; empyema, pneumatoceles, pyopneumothorax, and bronchopleural fistulas develop frequently. Staphylococcal pneumonia occasionally produces a diffuse interstitial disease characterized by extreme dyspnea, tachypnea, and cyanosis. Cough may be nonproductive. *S. aureus* is an important pathogen of pneumonia in patients with cystic fibrosis (Chapter 393).

SEPSIS. Staphylococcal bacteremia and sepsis (Chapter 163) may be associated with any localized infection. The onset may be acute and marked by nausea, vomiting, myalgia, fever, and chills. Organisms may localize subsequently at any site but are found especially in the lungs, heart, joints, bones, kidneys, and brain. Even if appropriate antibiotic therapy is provided, patients may remain febrile and blood cultures may remain positive for 24–48 hr.

In some instances, especially in young adolescent males, disseminated staphylococcal disease occurs, characterized by fever, persistent bacteremia despite antibiotics, and focal involvement of two or more separate tissue sites (e.g., skin, bone, joint, kidney, lung, liver, heart). Endocarditis and septic thrombophlebitis must be ruled out.

MUSCLE. Localized staphylococcal abscesses in muscle associated with elevation of muscle enzymes but without septicemia have been called tropical pyomyositis. Although this disorder has been reported most frequently from tropical areas, it also has occurred in the United States in otherwise healthy children. Multiple abscesses occur in 30–40% of cases. Prodromal symptoms may include coryza, pharyngitis, diarrhea, or prior trauma at the site of the abscess. Surgical drainage and appropriate antibiotic therapy are essential.

BONES AND JOINTS. *S. aureus* is the most common cause of osteomyelitis and suppurative arthritis in children (Chapter 674).

CENTRAL NERVOUS SYSTEM. Meningitis (Chapter 594.1) due to *S. aureus* is not common; it is associated with cranial trauma and neurosurgical procedures (e.g., craniotomy, cerebrospinal fluid [CSF] shunt placement) and less frequently with endocarditis, parameningeal foci (e.g., epidural or brain abscess), diabetes mellitus, or malignancy. The CSF profile in *S. aureus* meningitis is indistinguishable from that in other bacterial causes of meningitis.

HEART. Infective endocarditis (Chapter 429) may follow staphylococcal bacteremia. *S. aureus* is a common cause of acute endocarditis on native valves. Perforation of heart valves, myocardial abscesses, heart failure, conduction disturbances, acute hemopericardium, purulent pericarditis, and sudden death may ensue.

KIDNEY. *S. aureus* is a common cause of renal and perinephric abscess (Chapter 530) usually of hematogenous origin. Urinary tract infection due to *S. aureus* is unusual.

TOXIC SHOCK SYNDROME. *S. aureus* is the principal cause of TSS (Chapter 166.2).

INTESTINAL TRACT. Staphylococcal enterocolitis follows overgrowth of normal bowel flora by staphylococci. Although uncommon, this can follow use of broad-spectrum oral antibiotic therapy. Diarrhea is associated with blood and mucus.

Peritonitis associated with *S. aureus* in patients receiving long-term ambulatory peritoneal dialysis usually involves the catheter tunnel. Removal of the catheter is required to achieve a bacteriologic cure.

Food poisoning (Chapter 321) may be caused by ingestion of preformed enterotoxins preformed by staphylococci contaminating foods. Approximately 2–7 hr after ingestion of the toxin, sudden, severe vomiting begins. Watery diarrhea may develop, but fever is absent or low. Symptoms rarely persist longer than 12–24 hr. Rarely, shock and death may occur.

Diagnosis. The diagnosis of staphylococcal infection depends on isolation of the organisms from nonpermissive sites such as skin lesions, abscess cavities, blood, or other sites of infection. Isolation from the nose or skin does not necessarily imply causation because these are normally colonized sites. The organisms can be grown readily in liquid and on solid media. After isolation, identification is made on the basis of Gram stain and coagulase, clumping factor, and protein A reactivity. Patterns of susceptibility to antibiotics should be assessed in serious cases.

Diagnosis of staphylococcal food poisoning generally is made on the basis of epidemiologic and clinical findings. Food suspected of contamination should be examined by Gram stain, cultured, and tested for enterotoxin. Enterotoxin testing can be performed by the Centers for Disease Control and Prevention.

DIFFERENTIAL DIAGNOSIS. Skin lesions due to *S. aureus* and those due to group A streptococci may be indistinguishable. Staphylococcal pneumonia can be suspected on the basis of chest roentgenograms that may reveal pneumatoceles, pyopneumothorax, or lung abscess. These changes, suggesting a necrotizing pneumonitis, are not pathognomonic for staphylococcal infection and may be noted in patients with pneumonia due to other bacteria, including *Klebsiella* and many anaerobes. Fluctuant skin and soft tissue lesions also can be caused by many organisms, including *Mycobacterium tuberculosis*, atypical mycobacteria, *Bartonella henselae* (cat-scratch disease), *Francisella tularensis*, and various fungi.

Treatment. Antibiotic therapy alone is rarely effective in individuals with undrained abscesses or with infected foreign bodies. Loculated collections of purulent material should be relieved by incision and drainage. Foreign bodies should be removed, if possible. Therapy always should be initiated with a penicillinase-resistant antibiotic because more than 90% of all staphylococci isolated, regardless of source, are resistant to penicillin.

For serious infections, parenteral treatment is indicated, at least at the outset, until symptoms are controlled. Serious staphylococcal infections, with or without abscesses, tend to persist and recur, necessitating prolonged therapy.

The antibiotic used as well as the dose, route, and duration of treatment depends on the site of infection, the response of the patient to treatment, and the sensitivity of the organisms recovered from blood or from local sites of infection. For most patients with serious staphylococcal infection, intravenous treatment is recommended until the patient has been afebrile for 72 hr and other signs of infection have disappeared. Oral therapy is continued for a total of 3 wk, longer in selected cases. Treatment of staphylococcal osteomyelitis (see Chapter 674), meningitis (see Chapter 594.1), and endocarditis (see Chapter 429) are discussed in their respective chapters.

In all of these infections, oral treatment may be provided to complete the course of treatment after an initial period of parenteral therapy. Dicloxacillin (50–100 mg/kg/24 hr divided qid PO) and cephalexin (25–100 mg/kg/24 hr divided tid–qid PO) are absorbed well orally and effective. Amoxicillin-clavulanate (40–80 mg amoxicillin/kg/24 hr divided tid PO) also is effective. The duration of oral therapy depends on the response as determined by the clinical, roentgenographic, and laboratory findings.

Skin and soft tissue infection and minor upper respiratory tract infection may be managed by oral therapy alone or by an initial brief course of antibiotics provided parenterally, followed by oral medication.

Individuals with hypersensitivity to penicillin and its derivatives must be treated with other antibiotics or desensitized to the penicillin derivative to be used. About 5% of penicillin-sensitive children are also sensitive to cephalosporins. Clindamycin (30–40 mg/kg/24 hr divided tid–qid PO) has proved effective for the treatment of skin, soft tissue, bone, and joint infections due to *S. aureus* if the organism is susceptible. Clindamycin is bacteriostatic and should *not* be used to treat endocarditis, brain abscess, or meningitis due to *S. aureus*. Vancomycin (40–60 mg/kg/24 hr divided q 6 hr IV) can be used to treat penicillin-sensitive individuals with serious *S. aureus* infections. Serum levels of vancomycin should be monitored, with peak concentrations of 20–40 μg/mL. Vancomycin or teicoplanin (a vancomycin derivative) should be used to treat serious staphylococcal infections when the organism is known or suspected to be resistant to semisynthetic penicillin derivatives, so-called **methicillin-resistant *S. aureus* (MRSA)**. Community acquired MRSA strains are becoming more common throughout the United States even in children without pre-existing risk factors. Rare vancomycin-intermediate strains have also been reported mostly in patients being treated with vancomycin. Despite in vitro susceptibility of *S. aureus* to ciprofloxacin and other quinolone antibiotics, these agents should not be used in serious staphylococcal infections, because their use has not consistently been associated with high cure rates and the quinolones are not recommended for use in patients younger than 18 years of age.

Serious staphylococcal infections (e.g., septicemia, endocarditis, central nervous system infections) can be treated with intravenous nafcillin, oxacillin, or, in penicillin-allergic children, vancomycin or imipenem. Rifampin or gentamicin may be added for synergy.

METHICILLIN-RESISTANT *STAPHYLOCOCCUS AUREUS*. MRSA has emerged as a major nosocomial pathogen. Patients at risk for MRSA infection are those with serious illnesses (e.g., burns, surgical wounds, chronic venous access, lengthy hospitalizations, premature infants) or in contact with other MRSA-infected patients.

Resistance to semisynthetic penicillins is thought to be related to a novel **penicillin-binding protein (PB2A)** that is relatively insensitive to antibiotics containing a β-lactam ring. MRSA strains appear to be as virulent as their methicillin-sensitive counterparts. Vancomycin and its derivative, teicoplanin, are highly effective in the treatment of these infections. Vancomycin is the drug of choice if MRSA is considered a possible cause of serious infection or if MRSA has been isolated. MRSA is also resistant to cephalosporins and imipenem but often remains sensitive to the quinolones. Linezolid and quinupristin-dalfopristin may be useful for serious *S. aureus* infections highly resistant to other antibiotics.

When MRSA is recovered, strict isolation of affected patients has been shown to be the most effective method for preventing nosocomial spread of infection. Thereafter, control measures should be directed toward identification of new isolates and strict isolation of newly colonized or infected patients. It also may be necessary to identify colonized hospital personnel and eradicate carriage in affected individuals.

Strains of *S. aureus* resistant to vancomycin with limited other treatment options have been reported, emphasizing the need for restricting the prescription of unnecessary antibiotics and the importance of isolation of the causative organism and susceptibility testing in serious infections.

Prognosis. Untreated staphylococcal septicemia is associated with a mortality rate of ≥80%. Mortality rates have been reduced significantly by appropriate antibiotic treatment. Staphylococcal pneumonia can be fatal at any age but is more likely to be associated with high morbidity and mortality in young infants or in patients whose therapy has been delayed.

A total WBC count <5,000/mm³ or a polymorphonuclear leukocyte response of <50% is a grave prognostic sign. Prognosis also may be influenced by numerous host factors, including nutrition, immunologic competence, and the presence or absence of other debilitating diseases. In most cases with abscess formation, surgical drainage is necessary.

Prevention. Staphylococcal infection is transmitted primarily by direct contact. Strict attention to handwashing techniques is the most effective measure for preventing the spread of staphylococci from one individual to another (Chapter 283). Use of a detergent containing an iodophor, chlorhexidine, or hexachlorophene is recommended. In hospitals or other institutional settings, all persons with acute staphylococcal infections should be isolated until they have been treated adequately. There should be constant surveillance for nosocomial staphylococcal infections within hospitals.

Patients with recurrent staphylococcal furunculosis may be treated with hexachlorophene washes and dicloxacillin or clindamycin and nasal mupirocin to prevent recurrences.

Food poisoning (Chapter 321) may be prevented by excluding individuals with staphylococcal infections of the skin from the preparation and handling of food. Prepared foods should be eaten immediately or refrigerated appropriately to prevent multiplication of staphylococci with which the food may have been contaminated.

166.2 Toxic Shock Syndrome

TSS is an acute multisystem disease characterized by high fever, hypotension, vomiting, diarrhea, myalgias, nonfocal neurologic abnormalities, conjunctival hyperemia, strawberry tongue, and an erythematous rash with subsequent desquamation on the hands and feet.

Etiology. TSS is caused by TSST-1 producing strains of *S. aureus*, which may colonize the vagina or cause focal sites of staphylococcal infection.

Epidemiology. Many cases occur in menstruating women who are 15–25 yr of age and who use tampons or other vaginal devices (e.g., diaphragm, contraceptive sponge). TSS, however, also occurs in children, nonmenstruating women, and men. Nonmenstrual TSS has occurred with *S. aureus* colonization of nasal packing or infections including wound infections, sinusitis, tracheitis, pneumonia, empyema, abscesses, burns, osteomyelitis, and primary bacteremia. Without antimicrobial therapy, menstrual TSS has a high recurrence rate (30%), with secondary cases being milder and occurring within 3 mo of the original episode; the overall mortality of treated cases is 3%.

Pathogenesis. A majority of *S. aureus* strains isolated from confirmed cases are phage group I and produce a number of extracellular toxins. The primary toxin associated with TSS is TSST-1, which causes massive loss of fluid from the intravascular space directly or after production of interleukin-1 and tumor necrosis factor. However, TSST-1–negative strains have been isolated from patients with TSS, suggesting that other toxins (primarily the enterotoxins) have a role in TSS (especially nonmenstrual). Epidemiologic and in vitro studies suggest that these toxins are selectively produced in a clinical environment consisting of a neutral pH, a high P_{CO_2}, and an "aerobic" P_{O_2}, which are the conditions found in the vagina with tampon use during menstruation. This may explain why 90% of adults have antibody to TSST-1 without a history of clinical TSS—that is, they became colonized with a toxin-producing organism at a site (e.g., anterior nares) where low-grade or inactive toxin exposure resulted in an immune response without disease. The risk factors for symptomatic disease require a nonimmune host colonized with a toxin-producing organism, which is exposed to focal growth conditions (e.g., menstruation plus tampon use or abscess), which induce toxin production.

Clinical Manifestations. The diagnosis of TSS is based on clinical manifestations (Box 166–1). The onset is abrupt, with high fever, vomiting, and diarrhea, and is accompanied by sore throat, headache, and myalgias. A diffuse erythematous macular rash (sunburn-like or scarlatiniform) appears within 24 hr and may be associated with hyperemia of pharyngeal, conjunctival, and vaginal mucous membranes. A strawberry tongue is

BOX 166–1. Diagnostic Criteria of Staphylococcal Toxic Shock Syndrome

MAJOR CRITERIA (ALL REQUIRED)
Acute fever; temperature >38.8°C
Hypotension (orthostatic or shock)
Rash (erythroderma with late desquamation)

MINOR CRITERIA (ANY 3)
Mucous membrane inflammation
Vomiting, diarrhea
Liver abnormalities
Renal abnormalities
Muscle abnormalities
Central nervous system abnormalities
Thrombocytopenia

EXCLUSIONARY CRITERIA
Absence of another explanation
Negative blood cultures (except for *S. aureus*)

common. Symptoms often include alterations in the level of consciousness, oliguria, and hypotension, which in severe cases may progress to shock and disseminated intravascular coagulation. Complications including adult respiratory distress syndrome, myocardial failure, and renal failure are commensurate with the degree of shock. Recovery occurs within 7–10 days and is associated with desquamation, particularly of palms and soles; hair and nail loss have also been observed after 1–2 mo. Many cases of apparent scarlet fever without shock may be caused by TSST-1–producing *S. aureus* strains.

Diagnosis. There is no specific laboratory test; appropriate selective tests reveal involvement of multiple organ systems including the hepatic, renal, muscular, gastrointestinal, cardiopulmonary, and central nervous systems. Bacterial cultures of the associated focus (e.g., vagina, abscess) before administration of antibiotics usually yield *S. aureus*, although this is not a required element of the definition.

DIFFERENTIAL DIAGNOSIS. Group A *Streptococcus* can cause a similar TSS-like illness, termed **streptococcal TSS** (Chapter 168), which is often associated with streptococcal bacteremia or a focal streptococcal infection such as cellulitis or pneumonia.

Kawasaki disease closely resembles TSS clinically but is usually not as severe or rapidly progressive. Both are associated with fever unresponsive to antibiotics, hyperemia of mucous membranes, and an erythematous rash with subsequent desquamation. Many of the clinical features of TSS, however, are absent or rare in Kawasaki disease, including diffuse myalgia, vomiting, abdominal pain, diarrhea, azotemia, hypotension, adult respiratory distress syndrome, and shock (Chapter 156). Kawasaki disease typically occurs in children younger than 5 yr—some cases of "adult Kawasaki disease" may be TSS. Scarlet fever, Rocky Mountain spotted fever, leptospirosis, toxic epidermal necrolysis, sepsis, and measles must also be considered in the differential diagnosis.

Treatment. Parenteral administration of a β-lactamase–resistant antistaphylococcal antibiotic (e.g., nafcillin or a first-generation cephalosporin) is recommended after appropriate cultures have been obtained. The addition of clindamycin in severe or unresponsive cases may terminate toxin production. Drainage of the vagina, by removal of any retained tampons in menstrual TSS, and of focally infected sites in nonmenstrual TSS is important for successful treatment. Antistaphylococcal therapy may also reduce the risk of recurrence in menstrual TSS.

Fluid replacement should be aggressive to prevent or treat hypotension, renal failure, and cardiovascular collapse. Inotropic agents may be needed to treat shock; corticosteroids and intravenous immunoglobulin are reserved for severe cases.

Prevention. The low risk of acquiring TSS (1–2 cases/100,000 menstruating women) may be reduced by not using tampons or by using them intermittently during each menstrual period. If a fever, rash, or dizziness develops during menstruation, any tampon should be removed immediately and medical attention sought.

166.3 Coagulase-Negative Staphylococci

S. epidermidis is just one of many recognized species of coagulase-negative staphylococci (CONS) affecting or colonizing humans. Originally thought to be avirulent commensal bacteria, CONS is now known to produce nosocomial infections in patients with indwelling foreign devices (intravenous catheters—sepsis; hemodialysis shunts and grafts—sepsis; CSF shunts—meningitis; peritoneal dialysis catheters—peritonitis; pacemaker wires and electrodes—pocket infection; prosthetic cardiac valves—endocarditis; urinary catheters—pyelonephritis; prosthetic joints—arthritis), surgical trauma (sternal osteomyelitis, endophthalmitis), immunocompromised states (malignancy, granulocytopenia), and, rarely, community-acquired disease in patients with no underlying disease (urinary tract infection, osteomyelitis). CONS is a common cause of nosocomial neonatal infection. *S. haemolyticus*, another CONS species, is an important cause of invasive infection and may develop resistance to vancomycin and teicoplanin.

Epidemiology. CONS consists of normal inhabitants of the human skin, throat, mouth, vagina, and urethra. *S. epidermidis* is the most common and persistent species, representing 65–90% of staphylococci present on the skin and mucous membranes. Colonization, sometimes with strains acquired from hospital staff, precedes infection; alternatively, direct inoculation during surgery may initiate infection of CSF shunts, prosthetic valves, or indwelling vascular lines. For epidemiologic purposes, CONS can be identified on the basis of phage typing, antibiotic sensitivities, slime layer production, and molecular DNA methods.

Pathogenesis. *S. epidermidis* produces an **exopolysaccharide** protective biofilm, or **slime layer**, that surrounds the organism and may enhance adhesion to foreign surfaces, resist phagocytosis, and impair penetration of antibiotics.

Clinical Manifestations. The low virulence of CONS usually requires the presence of another factor, such as immune compromise or a foreign body, for development of clinical disease.

BACTEREMIA. CONS, specifically *S. epidermidis*, are the most common cause of nosocomial bacteremia. In neonates, CONS bacteremia, with or without a central venous catheter, may be manifested as apnea, bradycardia, temperature instability, abdominal distention, hematochezia, meningitis in the absence of CSF pleocytosis, cutaneous abscesses, and persistence of positive blood cultures for as long as 2 wk despite adequate antimicrobial therapy. CONS bacteremia in patients with bone marrow transplantation and malignancy (e.g., leukemia, lymphoma) is associated with neutropenia, central venous access (Hickman or Broviac catheters), and gastrointestinal colonization. In most circumstances, CONS bacteremia is indolent and is not usually associated with overwhelming septic shock.

ENDOCARDITIS. Infection of native heart valves or the right atrial wall secondary to an infected thrombosis at the end of a central line may produce endocarditis. *S. epidermidis* and other CONS may also produce native valve subacute indolent endocarditis in previously normal patients without a central venous catheter. CONS is a common cause of prosthetic valve endocarditis, presumably due to inoculation at the time of surgery. Infection of the valve sewing ring, with abscess formation and

dissection, produces valve dysfunction, dehiscence, arrhythmias, or valve obstruction. See Chapter 443 for clinical manifestations.

CENTRAL VENOUS CATHETER INFECTION. Central venous catheters become infected through the exit site and subcutaneous tunnel, which provide a direct path to the bloodstream. *S. epidermidis* is the most common CONS, owing in part to its high rate of cutaneous colonization. Line sepsis is manifested as fever, leukocytosis, tenderness, and erythema at the exit site or along the subcutaneous tunnel, and catheter thrombosis.

CEREBROSPINAL FLUID SHUNTS. *S. epidermidis*, introduced at the time of surgery, is the most common pathogen associated with CSF shunt meningitis. Most (70–80%) infections occur within 2 mo of the operation and are manifested by signs of meningeal irritation, fever, increased intracranial pressure (headache), and peritonitis due to the intra-abdominal position of the distal end of the shunt tubing.

URINARY TRACT INFECTION. CONS causes asymptomatic urinary tract infection in hospitalized patients with urinary catheters and after urinary tract surgery or transplantation. *S. saprophyticus* is one of the most common causes of primary urinary tract infections in boys and girls. Manifestations are similar to those characteristic of urinary tract infection due to *Escherichia coli* (Chapter 530).

S. epidermidis is the most common pathogen producing peritonitis in patients on continuous ambulatory peritoneal dialysis. Manifestations of infection include abdominal pain, fever, >100 neutrophils/mm^3, and a positive culture or Gram stain.

Diagnosis. Because *S. epidermidis* is a common skin inhabitant and may contaminate poorly collected blood cultures, differentiating bacteremia from contamination may be difficult. True bacteremia should be suspected when blood cultures grow rapidly (within 24 hr), when two or more blood cultures are positive with the same CONS, when the peripheral venous blood culture has a quantitative colony count comparable to that drawn from a central venous catheter, and when clinical and laboratory signs and symptoms compatible with CONS sepsis are present and subsequently resolve with appropriate therapy. No blood culture that is positive for CONS in a neonate or patient with intravascular catheter should be considered contaminated without careful assessment of the foregoing criteria and examination of the patient. Before initiating presumptive antimicrobial therapy in such patients it is always prudent to draw two separate blood cultures to facilitate subsequent interpretation if CONS is grown.

Treatment. Most CONS strains are resistant to methicillin. Vancomycin is the drug of choice for methicillin-resistant strains. The new quinolones and teicoplanin have some activity against CONS, and the addition of rifampin or gentamicin to vancomycin may increase antimicrobial efficacy. In many cases of CONS infection associated with foreign bodies, the catheter, valve, or shunt must be removed to ensure a cure. Prosthetic heart valves and CSF shunts usually have to be removed to treat the infection adequately.

Antibiotic therapy given through an infected central venous catheter (through each lumen) may effectively cure CONS line sepsis. If the catheter or reservoir is no longer needed, it should be removed. Unfortunately, this is not always possible owing to the therapeutic requirements of the underlying disease (nutrition for short bowel syndrome, chemotherapy for malignancy). A trial of intravenous vancomycin is indicated to attempt to preserve the use of the central line.

Peritonitis due to *S. epidermidis* in patients on continuous ambulatory peritoneal dialysis is another infection that may be treated with intravenous or intraperitoneal antibiotics without removing the dialysis catheter. If the organism is resistant to methicillin, vancomycin adjusted for renal function is appropriate therapy.

Prognosis. Most episodes of CONS bacteremia respond successfully to antibiotics and removal of any foreign body that is present. Poor prognosis is associated with malignancy, neutropenia, and infected prosthetic or native heart valves. CONS increases morbidity, the duration of hospitalization, and mortality rates among patients with underlying complicated illnesses.

Staphylococcus aureus

Centers for Disease Control and Prevention: Four pediatric deaths from community-acquired methicillin-resistant *Staphylococcus aureus*—Minnesota and North Dakota, 1997–1999. *MMWR* 1999;48:707–10.

Farrell AM: Staphylococcal scalded-skin syndrome. *Lancet* 1999;354:880–1.

Gorenstein A, Gross E, Houri S, et al: The pivotal role of deep vein thrombophlebitis in the development of acute disseminated staphylococcal disease in children. *Pediatrics* 2000;106:E87.

Gubbay AJ, Isaacs D: Pyomyositis in children. *Pediatr Infect Dis J* 2000;19:1009–12.

Hussain FM, Boyle-Vavra S, Bethel CD, et al: Current trends in community-acquired methicillin-resistant *Staphylococcus aureus* at a tertiary care pediatric facility. *Pediatr Infect Dis J* 2000;19:1163–6.

Jain A, Daum RS: Staphylococcal infections in children: Part 1. *Pediatr Rev* 1999; 20:183–91.

Luhmann JD, Luhmann SJ: Etiology of septic arthritis in children: An update for the 1990s. *Pediatr Emerg Care* 1999;15:40–2.

Patel JC, Mollitt DL, Tepas JJ 3rd: Infectious complications in critically injured children. *J Pediatr Surg* 2000;35:1174–8.

Shinefield H, Black S, Fattom A, et al: Use of a *Staphylococcus aureus* conjugate vaccine in patients receiving hemodialysis. *N Engl J Med* 2002;346:491–6.

Sugino Y, Iinumab Y, Ichiyama S, et al: In vivo development of decreased susceptibility to vancomycin in clinical isolates of methicillin-resistant *Staphylococcus aureus*. *Diagn Microbiol Infect Dis* 2000;38:159–67.

Winkelstein JA, Marino MC, Johnston RB Jr, et al: Chronic granulomatous disease. Report on a national registry of 368 patients. *Medicine* 2000;79:155–69.

Toxic Shock Syndrome

Todd J, Todd AS: Twenty years of toxic shock syndrome: Evolution of an emerging disease. *Royal Society of Medicine: Int Congress Symp Series* 1998;229:201–204.

Zimbelman J, Palmer A, Todd JK: Improved outcome of clindamycin compared with beta-lactam antibiotics treatment of invasive *Streptococcus pyogenes* infection. *Pediatr Infect Dis J* 1999;18:1096–100.

Coagulase-Negative Staphylococci

Cordero L, Sananes M, Ayers LW: Bloodstream infections in a neonatal intensive-care unit: 12 years' experience with an antibiotic control program. *Infect Control Hosp Epidemiol* 1999;20:242–6.

Karlowicz MG, Furigay PJ, Croitoru DP, et al: Central venous catheter removal versus in situ treatment in neonates with coagulase-negative staphylococcal bacteremia. *Pediatr Infect Dis J* 2002;21:22–7.

Meskin I: *Staphylococcus epidermidis*. *Pediatr Rev* 1998;19:105–6.

Chapter 167

Streptococcus pneumoniae (Pneumococcus)

Jon S. Abramson and Gary D. Overturf

Streptococcus pneumoniae, or pneumococcus, frequently colonizes the upper respiratory tract and may cause upper respiratory tract infection (e.g., otitis media, sinusitis) or invasive disease (e.g., pneumonia, bacteremia, meningitis). *S. pneumoniae* is the most common cause of community-acquired bacterial pneumonia and otitis media. With universal immunization with conjugated *Haemophilus influenzae* type b vaccines, *S. pneumoniae* has become the second most common cause of bacterial meningitis in children and the most common cause of meningitis in adults. The significance of this agent has been emphasized by worldwide emergence of penicillin and multidrug-resistant strains. Introduction of a universal recommendation to give infants the pneumococcal heptavalent conjugate vaccine may have marked effects on the epidemiology of this organism by reducing nasopharyngeal carriage and the burden of pneumococcal disease.

Etiology. *S. pneumoniae* is a gram-positive, lancet-shaped, encapsulated diplococcus, occurring occasionally as individual cocci or in chains. Ninety serotypes have been identified by type-specific capsular polysaccharides. Antisera to some pneumococcal polysaccharides cross react with those of other pneumococcal types and define serogroups (e.g., 6A and 6B), or other bacteria (e.g., *Escherichia coli*, group B *Streptococcus*, and *H. influenzae* type b). Only "smooth," or encapsulated, strains cause serious disease in humans. Capsular material impedes phagocytosis. Virulence is related in part to capsular size, but pneumococcal types with capsules of the same size may vary widely in virulence.

On solid media, *S. pneumoniae* forms unpigmented, umbilicated colonies surrounded by a zone of incomplete (α) hemolysis. *S. pneumoniae* is bile soluble (i.e., 10% deoxycholate) and Optochin-sensitive. Pneumococcal capsules can be microscopically visualized and typed by exposing organisms to type-specific antisera that combine with their unique capsular polysaccharide, rendering the capsule refractile (**Quellung reaction**). Specific antibodies to capsular polysaccharide confer protection on the host, promoting opsonization and phagocytosis. **C substance**, a cell wall antigen that is related to the pneumococcal species rather than a specific serotype, consists of a teichoic acid-containing phosphocholine and galactosamine-6-phosphate. C substance precipitates with a β-globulin, the C-reactive protein, which activates complement, enhancing phagocytosis.

Epidemiology. Most healthy individuals carry *S. pneumoniae* in their upper respiratory tract; >90% of children between 6 mo and 5 yr of age harbor *S. pneumoniae* in the nasopharynx at some time. Serotypes 4, 6B, 9V, 14, 18C, 19F, and 23F constitute the majority of invasive isolates in children and, of these, 6B, 9V, 14, and 19F are frequently not susceptible to penicillin. A single serotype usually is carried for extended periods (45 days–6 mo). Carriage does not consistently induce local or systemic immunity sufficient to prevent later reacquisition of the same serotype. Rates of pneumococcal carriage peak during the first 2 yr of life and decline gradually thereafter. Carriage rates are highest in institutional settings and during the winter, and rates are lowest in summer. Nasopharyngeal carriage of pneumococci is common among young children attending out-of-home care with rates of 21–59% in point prevalence estimates and 65% in longitudinal studies.

S. pneumoniae is the most frequent cause of bacteremia, bacterial pneumonia, and otitis media, and the second most common cause of meningitis in children. The decreased ability in children <2 yr of age to produce antibody against polysaccharide antigens and the high frequency of colonization may explain an increased susceptibility to pneumococcal infection and the decreased effectiveness of polysaccharide vaccines. Males are more commonly affected than females. Native American and African-American children have rates of invasive disease that are 2–10-fold that of other healthy children. Rates of invasive pneumococcal disease in the United States peak at 6–11 mo of age, with attack rates of >540/100,000 in healthy children before the universal use of pneumococcal conjugate immunization.

Pneumococcal disease generally occurs sporadically, but pneumococci can be spread from person to person by respiratory droplet transmission. The frequency and severity of pneumococcal disease are increased in patients with sickle cell disease, asplenia, deficiencies in humoral (B cell) and complement mediated immunity, HIV infection, and certain malignancies (e.g., leukemia, lymphoma); chronic heart, lung, or renal disease (particularly the nephrotic syndrome); and cerebrospinal fluid leak syndromes.

Pathogenesis. Invasion of the host is precipitated by a number of factors. Nonspecific defense mechanisms, including the presence of other bacteria in the nasopharynx, may limit multiplication of pneumococci. Aspiration of secretions containing pneumococci is hindered by epiglottic reflex and by respiratory epithelial cilia, which move infected mucus toward the pharynx. Similarly, normal ciliary flow of fluid from the middle ear through the eustachian tube and sinuses to the nasopharynx usually prevents infection with nasopharyngeal flora, including pneumococci. Interference with these normal clearance mechanisms by allergy, viral infection, or irritants (e.g., smoke) may allow colonization and subsequent infection with these organisms in otherwise normally sterile sites.

Virulent pneumococci are intrinsically resistant to phagocytosis by alveolar macrophages. Pneumococcal disease frequently is facilitated by viral respiratory tract infection, which may produce mucosal injury, diminish epithelial ciliary activity, and depress the function of alveolar macrophages and neutrophils. Phagocytosis may be impeded by respiratory secretions and alveolar exudate. In tissues, pneumococci multiply and spread through the lymphatics or bloodstream (bacteremia) or, less commonly, by direct extension from a local site of infection (e.g., sinuses). The severity of disease is related to the virulence and number of organisms causing bacteremia, and to integrity of specific host defenses. A poor prognosis correlates with very large numbers of pneumococci and high concentrations of capsular polysaccharide in the circulation and cerebrospinal fluid.

Deficiency of many of the complement components is associated with recurrent pyogenic infection, including those caused by *S. pneumoniae*. The increased frequency of pneumococcal disease in asplenic persons is related to both deficient opsonization of pneumococci as well as to absence of the filtering function of the spleen on circulating bacteria. Invasive pneumococcal disease is 30–100-fold more prevalent in children with sickle cell disease and other hemoglobinopathies and in children with congenital or surgical asplenia. This risk is greatest in infants <2 yr of age when antibody production is poor. Children with sickle cell disease have deficits in the antibody-independent properdin (alternative) pathway of complement activation, in addition to functional asplenia. Both pathways contribute to antibody-independent and antibody-dependent opsonophagocytosis of pneumococci. With advancing age (e.g., >5 yr), children with sickle cell disease produce anticapsular antibody, augmenting antibody-dependent opsonophagocytosis and greatly reducing, but not eliminating, the risk of severe pneumococcal disease. The efficacy of phagocytosis also is diminished in patients with B- and T-cell immunodeficiency syndromes (e.g., agammaglobulinemia or severe combined immune deficiency) and is largely caused by a deficiency of opsonic anticapsular antibody. These observations suggest that opsonization of pneumococci depends on the alternative complement pathway in antibody-deficient persons and that recovery from pneumococcal disease depends on the development of anticapsular antibodies that act as opsonins, enhancing phagocytosis and killing of pneumococci. Children with HIV infection also have high rates of invasive pneumococcal infection similar to or greater than that of children with sickle cell disease.

In the lungs and other body tissues, the spread of infection is facilitated by the antiphagocytic properties of the pneumococcal capsule. Surface fluids of the respiratory tract contain only small amounts of IgG and are deficient in complement; both factors promote opsonization of pneumococci. During inflammation, there is an influx of IgG, complement, and neutrophils. Although phagocytosis of bacteria by neutrophils may occur, normal human serum may not opsonize pneumococci and facilitate phagocytosis by alveolar macrophages. The sequence of events evolves over 7–10 days, but can be modified by appropriate antibiotic therapy.

Clinical Manifestations. The signs and symptoms of pneumococcal infection are related to the anatomic site of disease. Common clinical syndromes include pneumonia (Chapter 389), otitis media (Chapter 630), sinusitis (Chapter 365), occult bacteremia in infants and young children (Chapter 162), and sepsis (Chapter 163). Before routine use of the conjugated pneumococcal vaccines, pneumococci caused >80% of bacteremias in infants 2–36 mo of age with fever without an identifiable source. Pneumococcal abscesses of the upper airway (Chapter 367), laryngotracheobronchitis (Chapter 371), and peritonitis (Chapter 352.1) occur, but are rare infections. Local complications of infection may occur, causing empyema, pericarditis, mastoiditis, epidural abscess, or meningitis. Colonizing pneumococci may spread through the eustachian tube, producing otitis media, and aspiration of infected upper respiratory secretions may produce pneumonia. Bacteremia may be followed by meningitis (Chapter 594.1), osteomyelitis and suppurative arthritis (Chapter 674), endocarditis (Chapter 429), and rarely, brain abscess (Chapter 595). Hemolytic-uremic syndrome (Chapter 510) and disseminated intravascular coagulation also occur as rare complications of pneumococcal infections.

Diagnosis. The diagnosis of pneumococcal infection is established by recovery of *S. pneumoniae* from the site of infection or the blood. Although pneumococci may be found in the nose or throat of patients with otitis media, pneumonia, septicemia, or meningitis, they may not be related causally to their disease and therefore throat cultures are not helpful for diagnosis. Blood cultures should be obtained in children with pneumonia, meningitis, arthritis, osteomyelitis, peritonitis, pericarditis, or gangrenous skin lesions. Blood cultures can also be useful in children who are <36 mo of age who have fever without localizing signs of infection, especially those with clinical toxicity or significant leukocytosis (Chapter 162).

Pneumococci can be identified in body fluids as gram-positive, lancet-shaped diplococci. Early in the course of pneumococcal meningitis, many bacteria may be seen in a relatively acellular cerebrospinal fluid. With current methods of continuously monitored blood culture systems, the average time to isolation of pneumococcal organisms is 14–15 hr and rarely >24 hr. Commercially available pneumococcal latex agglutination tests for urine or other sterile body sites suffer from poor sensitivity and add very little to standard cultures and Gram-stained fluids. Leukocytosis often is pronounced, with total white blood cell counts frequently >15,000/mm^3, although severe cases (including meningitis) may have a low white count with a shift to the left.

Before the emergence of penicillin nonsusceptible organisms, penicillin was the treatment of choice for presumed pneumococcal infection. The incidence of intermediate and high-level penicillin resistance and multidrug resistance (e.g., penicillin, tetracycline, chloramphenicol, rifampin, erythromycin, sulfonamides, or clindamycin) have increased during the past decade. In North America, up to 40% of isolates from sterile body sites are nonsusceptible to penicillin G with as many as 50% of these isolates being highly resistant. Multiply resistant strains have been identified in South Africa, Spain, Great Britain, Australia, and the United States. Resistance to antibiotics is most often noted in pneumococcal serogroups 6, 9, 14, 19, and 23, which are the most frequent cause of pneumococcal disease in children.

Problems in treatment may be encountered by organisms that are intermediately resistant to penicillin, defined as minimum inhibitory concentration (MIC) 0.1–1.0 mg/L, or organisms that are highly resistant to penicillin, defined as MIC ≥2.0 mg/L, and organisms that are resistant to several antibiotics. All isolates from children with severe infections should be tested for antibiotic susceptibility. A screening test for susceptibility to penicillin can be performed with a 1-μg oxacillin disk diffusion test, but the use of an E-test or MIC is the preferred method for measuring penicillin susceptibility because of greater specificity, particularly for intermediately resistant strains. Many penicillin-resistant strains are also resistant to the extended spectrum cephalosporins (e.g., ceftriaxone, cefotaxime). Resistance to vancomycin has not been reported.

Empirical treatment of pneumococcal disease should be based on knowledge of susceptibility patterns in specific communities.

Penicillin G is the drug of choice for penicillin-susceptible strains. Oral penicillin V (50–100 mg/kg/24 hr divided q 6–8 hr PO) for minor infections, intravenous penicillin G (200,000–250,000 U/kg/24 hr divided q 4–6 hr IV) for bacteremia or pneumonia, and intravenous penicillin G (300,000 U/kg/24 hr divided q 4–6 hr IV) for meningitis are recommended. For serious infections (e.g., meningitis) with strains that are intermediately resistant to penicillin and for all infections with highly penicillin-resistant strains, vancomycin (60 mg/kg/24 hr divided q6 hr IV) is the treatment of choice until the susceptibilities to other antibiotics are known. Rifampin (20 mg/kg/24 hr divided q 12 hr PO) may be added in severe or unresponsive cases. Resistance to the third-generation cephalosporins, such as cefotaxime and ceftriaxone, is common in penicillin-resistant strains, and treatment failures have been reported when treating meningitis. However, for many intermediately resistant organism, cefotaxime (225–300 mg/kg/24 hr divided q 8 hr IV) or ceftriaxone (100 mg/kg/24 hr divided q 12–14 hr IV) may be added or substituted for vancomycin depending upon the results of susceptibility testing.

For invasive infections outside the central nervous system (e.g., lobar pneumonia with or without bacteremia), high-dose cefotaxime and ceftriaxone are usually effective, even for those infections caused by cephalosporin intermediate or resistant strains (MIC ≥2.0 mg/L). For susceptible strains, clindamycin, erythromycin, cephalosporins, trimethoprim-sulfamethoxazole, and chloramphenicol may provide effective alternative therapy, depending on the site of infection (e.g., clindamycin is often effective for pneumococcal infections other than meningitis), for individuals who are allergic to penicillin. Higher doses of amoxicillin-clavulanate (80–90 mg amoxicillin/kg/day divided tid PO), with modified ratios of amoxicillin and clavulanate to permit higher amoxicillin dosing, have been successful in the treatment of otitis media caused by resistant strains.

Prognosis. Prognosis depends on the integrity of host defenses, virulence and numbers of the infecting organism, the age of the host, the site and extent of the infection, and the adequacy of treatment.

Prevention. Immunologic responsiveness and efficacy following administration of pneumococcal polysaccharide vaccines is unpredictable in children <2 yr of age. Two licensed pneumococcal vaccines contain purified polysaccharide of 23 pneumococcal serotypes responsible for >95% of cases of invasive disease. The clinical efficacy of these vaccines is controversial and studies have yielded conflicting results. Polysaccharide antigens 6A, 14, 19F, and 23F frequently produce childhood disease and are poorly immunogenic in children <5 yr of age.

In contrast, pneumococcal polysaccharide vaccines conjugated to various proteins (e.g., heptavalent pneumococcal polysaccharide conjugated to CRM_{197}) provoke "protective" antibody responses in 90% of infants given these vaccines at 2, 4, and 6 mo of age, and greatly enhanced responses (e.g., immunologic memory) are apparent after "booster" doses given at 12–15 mo of age. In addition, protein conjugate–polysaccharide vaccines reduce nasopharyngeal carriage of vaccine serotypes by up to 60–70%. The currently available heptavalent vaccine contains conjugated capsular polysaccharides of serotypes 4, 6B, 9V, 14, 19F, 23F, and 18C. In efficacy trials in the United States, infant immunization with this vaccine decreased invasive infections by >93% and lobar pneumonias by >73%. Its administration was associated with a 6–7% decrease in otitis media, but greater reduction in complications of otitis media such as tympanostomy tube placement. Adverse events after the administration of heptavalent CRM_{197} conjugate vaccines have included local swelling and redness and slightly increased rates of fever, when used in conjunction with other childhood vaccines. It is likely that vaccines with increased numbers of polysaccharide serotypes, or different protein conjugates, will be licensed in the future.

Immunization with the conjugate polysaccharide vaccine is recommended for all infants in a schedule of four doses administered at 2, 4, 6, and 12–15 mo of age. The number of required immunizations is reduced for children 6–24 mo of age starting immunizations. High-risk children ≥2 yr of age, such as those with asplenia, sickle cell disease, some types of immune deficiency (e.g., antibody deficiencies), HIV infection, or chronic lung, heart, or kidney disease (including nephrotic syndrome), may benefit also from the 23-valent polysaccharide vaccine. After the initial immunization, a single supplemental dose of polysaccharide vaccine may be used 3 yr after the first dose for children <10 yr of age at the time of revaccination, or it may be used at 5 yr after the first dose for children 10 yr of age or older at the time of revaccination.

Immunization with pneumococcal vaccines also may prevent pneumococcal disease caused by nonvaccine serotypes that are serotypically related to a vaccine strain (e.g., 6A and 6B). However, because current vaccines do not eliminate all pneumococcal invasive infections, penicillin prophylaxis is recommended for children at high risk of invasive pneumococcal disease, including children with asplenia or sickle cell disease. Penicillin V potassium (125 mg bid PO for children <3 yr; 250 mg bid PO for children ≥3 yr) substantially decreases the incidence of pneumococcal sepsis in children with sickle cell disease. Once monthly intramuscular benzathine penicillin G (600,000 U q 3–4 wk IM for children <60 lb; 1,200,000 U q 3–4 wk IM for children ≥60 lb) may also provide adequate prophylaxis. Erythromycin may be used in children with penicillin allergy, but its efficacy is unproved. Prophylaxis in sickle cell disease has been safely discontinued after the 5th birthday in children who have received all recommended pneumococcal vaccine doses and who had not experienced invasive pneumococcal disease. Prophylaxis is often administered for at least 2 yr after splenectomy or up to 5 yr of age. Efficacy in children >5 yr of age and adolescents is unproved. If oral antibiotic prophylaxis is used, strict compliance must be encouraged. Given the rapid emergence of penicillin-resistant pneumococci, especially in children receiving long-term, low-dose therapy, prophylaxis cannot be relied on to prevent disease. High-risk children with fever should be promptly evaluated and treated regardless of vaccination history or penicillin prophylaxis.

American Academy of Pediatrics, Committee on Infectious Diseases: Policy statement: Recommendations for the prevention of pneumococcal infections, including the use of pneumococcal conjugate vaccine (Prevnar), pneumococcal polysaccharide vaccine and antibiotic prophylaxis. *Pediatrics* 1000;106:362–6.

Arditi M, Mason EO, Bradley JS, et al: Three-year multicenter surveillance of pneumococcal meningitis in children: Clinical characteristics, and outcome related to penicillin susceptibility and dexamethasone use. *Pediatrics* 1998;102:1087–97.

Black S, Shinefield H, Fireman B, et al: Efficacy, safety, immunogenicity of heptavalent pneumococcal conjugate vaccine in children. *Pediatr Infect Dis J* 2000;19:187–95.

Centers for Disease Control and Prevention: Preventing pneumococcal disease among infants and children: Recommendations of the Advisory Committee on Immunization Practices (ACIP). *MMWR Morb Mortal Wkly Rep* 2000;49(RR-29):1–38.

Eskola J, Kilpi T, Palmu A, et al: Efficacy of a pneumococcal conjugate vaccine against acute otitis media. *N Engl J Med* 2001;344:403–9.

Hausdorff WP, Bryant J, Kloeck C, et al: The contribution of specific pneumococcal serogroups to different disease manifestations: Implications for conjugate vaccine formulation and use, Part II. *Clin Infect Dis* 2000;30:122–40.

Hausdorff WP, Bryant J, Paradiso PR, et al: Which pneumococcal serogroups cause the most invasive disease: Implications for conjugate vaccine formulation and use, Part I. *Clin Infect Dis* 2000;30:100–21.

Kaplan SL, Mason EO, Barson WJ, et al: Three year multicenter surveillance of systemic pneumococcal infections ins children. *Pediatrics* 1998;102:538–45.

Kaplan SL, Mason EO, Barson WJ, et al: Outcome of invasive infections outside the central nervous system caused by *Streptococcus pneumoniae* isolates nonsusceptible to ceftriaxone in children treated with beta-lactam antibiotics. *Pediatr Infect Dis J* 2001;20:392–6.

Overturf GD: Infections and immunizations of children with sickle cell disease. *Adv Pediatr Infect Dis* 1999;14:191–218.

Overturf GD and Committee on Infectious Diseases: Technical report: Prevention of pneumococcal infections, including the use of pneumococcal conjugate

and polysaccharide vaccines and antibiotic prophylaxis. *Pediatrics* 2000;106:
367–75.

Shinefield HR, Black S, Ray P, et al: Safety and immunogenicity of heptavalent pneumococcal CRM₁₉₇ conjugate vaccine in infants and toddlers. *Pediatr Infect Dis J* 1999;18:757–63.

Tan TQ, Mason EO Jr, Wald ER, et al: Clinical characteristics of children with complicated pneumonia caused by *Streptococcus pneumoniae*. *Pediatrics* 2002;110:1–6.

Whitney CG, Farley MM, Hadler J, et al: Increasing prevalence of multidrug-resistant *Streptococcus pneumoniae* in the United States. *N Engl J Med* 2000;343: 1917–24.

Chapter 168

Group A Streptococcus

Michael A. Gerber

Group A streptococcus, also known as *streptococcus pyogenes*, is a common cause of infections of the upper respiratory tract (pharyngotonsillitis) and the skin (impetigo, pyoderma) in children and is a less common cause of perianal cellulitis, vaginitis, septicemia, pneumonia, endocarditis, pericarditis, osteomyelitis, suppurative arthritis, myositis, cellulitis, and omphalitis. These microorganisms are also the cause of two distinct clinical entities, scarlet fever and erysipelas, as well as a toxic shock syndrome and necrotizing fasciitis. Group A streptococcus is also the cause of two potentially serious nonsuppurative complications, rheumatic fever (Chapter 168.1) and acute glomerulonephritis (Chapter 503.1).

Etiology. Group A streptococci are gram-positive coccoid-shaped bacteria that tend to grow in chains. They are broadly classified by their reactions on mammalian red blood cells. The zone of complete hemolysis that surrounds colonies grown on blood agar distinguishes ß-hemolytic (complete hemolysis) from α-hemolytic (green or partial hemolysis) and γ (nonhemolytic) species. The ß-hemolytic streptococci can be divided into groups by a group-specific polysaccharide (Lancefield carbohydrate C) located in the cell wall. More than 20 serologic groups have been identified, designated by the letters A through T. Serologic grouping by the Lancefield method is precise, but group A organisms can be identified more readily by any one of a number of latex agglutination, coagglutination, or enzyme immunoassay procedures. Group A strains can also be distinguished from other groups by differences in sensitivity to bacitracin. A disc containing 0.04 U of bacitracin inhibits the growth of most group A strains, whereas other groups are generally resistant to this antibiotic.

Group A streptococcus can be subdivided into >80 serotypes on the basis of the **M protein** antigen, which is located on the cell surface and in fimbriae (hairlike fuzz) that project from the outer edge of the cell. M typing has relied primarily on the serologic typing of the surface M protein using available polyclonal sera. However, it is frequently difficult to detect M proteins in this way. Recently, a molecular approach to M typing group A streptococcal isolates was developed using the polymerase chain reaction technique and based on sequencing the *emm* gene of group A streptococcus that encodes the M protein. More than 100 distinct M types have been identified using *emm* typing, and there has been a good correlation between the known serotypes and the *emm* types.

M serotyping has been valuable for epidemiologic studies; particular group A streptococcal diseases tend to be associated with certain M types. The M types commonly associated with pharyngitis rarely cause skin infections, and the M types commonly associated with skin infections rarely cause pharyngitis. A few of the "pharyngeal" strains (e.g., M type 12) have been associated with glomerulonephritis, but far more of the "skin" strains (e.g., M types 49, 55, 57, and 60) have been considered nephritogenic. A few of the "pharyngeal" serotypes, but none of the "skin" strains, have been associated with acute rheumatic fever. However, recent evidence suggests that rheumatogenic potential is not solely dependent on the serotype but is a characteristic of specific strains within several serotypes.

Epidemiology. Humans are the natural reservoir for group A streptococcus. These bacteria are highly communicable and can cause disease in normal individuals of all ages who do not have type-specific immunity against the particular serotype involved. Disease in neonates is uncommon, probably because of maternally acquired antibody. The incidence of pharyngeal infections is highest in children >3 yr of age, especially in young school-aged children. These infections are most common in the northern regions of the United States, especially during winter and early spring. Children with untreated acute pharyngitis spread group A streptococcus by airborne salivary droplets and nasal discharge. Transmission is favored by close proximity, and, therefore, the school and the home are important environments for spread. The incubation period for pharyngitis is usually 2–5 days. Recent reports suggest that group A streptococcus has the potential to be an important upper respiratory tract pathogen and to produce outbreaks of disease in the daycare setting. Foods containing group A streptococcus occasionally cause explosive outbreaks of pharyngotonsillitis. Children are usually not infectious 24 hr after appropriate antibiotic therapy has been started. Chronic pharyngeal carriers of group A streptococcus rarely transmit this organism to others.

In contrast to upper respiratory tract infections, streptococcal pyoderma (impetigo) occurs most frequently during the summer in temperate climates, or year round in warmer climates, when the skin is exposed and abrasions and insect bites are more likely to occur. Colonization of healthy skin by group A streptococcus usually precedes the development of impetigo. The impetiguous lesions occur at the site of open lesions (e.g., insect bites, traumatic wounds, or burns) because group A streptococcus cannot penetrate intact skin. Spread is from skin to skin, not via the respiratory tract, although impetigo serotypes may colonize the throat. Fingernails and the perianal region can harbor group A streptococcus and play a role in disseminating impetigo. Multiple cases of impetigo in the same family are common. Both impetigo and pharyngitis are more likely to occur among children living in crowded homes and in poor hygienic circumstances.

The incidence of severe invasive group A streptococcal infections, including bacteremia, streptococcal toxic shock syndrome, and necrotizing fasciitis, has increased in recent years. The incidence appears to be highest in the very young and in older persons. Varicella is the most commonly identified risk factor in children. Other risk factors include diabetes mellitus, human immunodeficiency virus infection, intravenous drug use, and chronic pulmonary or chronic cardiac disease. The portal of entry is unknown in almost 50% of the cases of severe invasive group A streptococcal infection; in most cases, it is believed to be skin or mucous membrane. Severe invasive disease rarely follows group A streptococcal pharyngitis.

Pathogenesis. Apart from its usefulness in typing, M protein has other important properties. Virulence of group A streptococcus depends primarily on the M protein, and strains rich in M protein resist phagocytosis in fresh human blood, whereas M-negative strains do not. Group A streptococcus isolated from chronic pharyngeal carriers contain little or no M protein and are relatively avirulent. The M protein antigen stimulates the production of protective antibodies. These antibodies are type-specific. They protect against infection with a homologous type but confer no immunity against other M types. Therefore, multiple group A streptococcal infections attributable to different types are common during childhood and adolescence. By adult life, individuals are probably immune to many of the common types in the environment, but because of the large number of serotypes it is doubtful that total immunity is ever achieved.

Group A streptococcus produces a large variety of enzymes and toxins, including erythrogenic toxin (known as streptococcal pyrogenic exotoxin). Streptococcal pyrogenic exotoxins A, B, and C are responsible for the rash of scarlet fever and are elaborated by streptococci that are infected with a particular bacteriophage. These exotoxins stimulate the formation of specific antitoxin antibodies that provide immunity against the scarlatiniform rash but not against other streptococcal infections. However, because group A streptococcus can produce three different rash-producing pyrogenic exotoxins (A, B, or C), a second attack of scarlet fever can sometimes occur. Streptococcal pyrogenic exotoxins A, B, and C, as well as several newly discovered exotoxins, appear to be involved in the pathogenesis of invasive group A streptococcal disease, including the streptococcal toxic shock syndrome. In contrast to the streptococcal pyrogenic exotoxins, the roles of most of the streptococcal enzymes and toxins in human disease have yet to be established.

Many of the other extracellular substances are also antigenic and stimulate antibody production after an infection. However, these antibodies bear no relationship to immunity. Their measurement is useful for evidence of a recent streptococcal infection. The test for antibodies against streptolysin O (antistreptolysin O) is well standardized and is the most commonly used antibody determination. Because the immune response to extracellular antigens varies among individuals as well as with the site of infection, it is sometimes necessary to measure other streptococcal antibodies, such as anti-deoxyribonuclease (anti-DNase).

Clinical Manifestations. The most common infections caused by group A streptococcus involve the respiratory tract and the skin and soft tissues.

RESPIRATORY TRACT INFECTIONS. Group A streptococcus is an important cause of acute pharyngitis (Chapter 366) and pneumonia (Chapter 389).

SCARLET FEVER. Scarlet fever is an upper respiratory tract infection associated with a characteristic rash, which is caused by an infection with pyrogenic exotoxin (erythrogenic toxin)-producing group A streptococcus in individuals who do not have antitoxin antibodies. It is now encountered less commonly and is less virulent than in the past, but the incidence is cyclic, depending on the prevalence of toxin-producing strains and the immune status of the population. The modes of transmission, age distribution, and other epidemiologic features are otherwise similar to those for group A streptococcal pharyngitis.

The rash appears within 24–48 hr after onset of symptoms, although it may appear with the first signs of illness. It often begins around the neck and spreads over the trunk and extremities. It is a diffuse, finely papular, erythematous eruption producing a bright red discoloration of the skin, which blanches on pressure. It is often more intense along the creases of the elbows, axillae, and groin. The skin has a goose-pimple appearance and feels rough. The face is usually spared, although the cheeks may be erythematous with pallor around the mouth. After 3–4 days, the rash begins to fade and is followed by desquamation, first on the face, progressing downward, and often resembling that seen subsequent to a mild sunburn. Occasionally, sheetlike desquamation may occur around the free margins of the fingernails, the palms, and the soles. Examination of the pharynx of a patient with scarlet fever reveals essentially the same findings as with group A streptococcal pharyngitis. In addition, the tongue is usually coated and the papillae are swollen. After desquamation, the reddened papillae are prominent, giving the tongue a strawberry appearance.

Typical scarlet fever is not difficult to diagnose; however, the milder form with equivocal pharyngeal findings can be confused with rubella, roseola, Kawasaki disease, and drug eruptions.

Staphylococcal infections are occasionally associated with a scarlatiniform rash. A history of recent exposure to a group A streptococcal infection is helpful. Identification of group A streptococcus in the pharynx confirms the diagnosis, if doubtful.

IMPETIGO. Impetigo has traditionally been classified into two clinical forms: bullous and nonbullous (Chapter 655). Nonbullous impetigo is the more common form and is a superficial infection of the skin that appears first as a discrete papulovesicular lesion surrounded by a localized area of redness. The vesicles rapidly become purulent and covered with a thick, confluent, amber-colored crust that gives the appearance of having been stuck on the skin. The lesions may occur anywhere but are more common on the face and extremities. If untreated, nonbullous impetigo is a mild but chronic illness, often spreading to other parts of the body, but occasionally is self-limited. Regional lymphadenitis is common. Nonbullous impetigo is generally not accompanied by fever or other systemic signs or symptoms. Impetiginized excoriations around the nares are seen with active group A streptococcal infections of the nasopharynx. However, impetigo is not usually associated with an overt streptococcal infection of the upper respiratory tract.

Bullous impetigo is less common and occurs most often in neonates and young infants. It is characterized by flaccid, transparent bullae usually <3 cm in diameter on previously untraumatized skin. The usual distribution involves the face, buttocks, trunk, and perineum. Although S. aureus has traditionally been accepted as the sole pathogen responsible for bullous impetigo, there has been confusion about the organisms responsible for nonbullous impetigo. In most episodes of nonbullous impetigo, either group A streptococcus or S. aureus, or a combination of these two organisms, is isolated. Earlier investigations suggested that group A streptococcus was the causative agent in most cases of nonbullous impetigo and that S. aureus was only a secondary invader. However, studies performed over the past decade have demonstrated the emergence of S. aureus, either alone or in combination with group A streptococcus, as a causative agent in nonbullous impetigo. Culture of the lesions is the only way to distinguish nonbullous impetigo caused by S. aureus from that caused by group A streptococcus.

ERYSIPELAS. Erysipelas is a relatively rare acute group A streptococcal infection involving the deeper layers of the skin and the underlying connective tissue. The skin over the affected area is swollen, red, and very tender. Superficial blebs may be present. The most characteristic finding is the sharply defined, slightly elevated border. At times, reddish streaks of lymphangitis project out from the margins of the lesion. A high fever and other systemic signs and symptoms of infection are present. Cultures obtained by needle aspirate of the inflamed area often reveal the causative agent.

PERIANAL DERMATITIS. Perianal dermatitis, also called **perianal streptococcal disease**, is a distinct clinical entity characterized by well-demarcated, perianal erythema associated with anal pruritus, painful defecation, and blood-streaked stools. Physical examination reveals flat, pink to beefy-red perianal erythema with sharp margins extending as far as 2 cm from the anus. Erythema may involve the vulva and vagina. Lesions may be tender and, particularly when chronic, may fissure and bleed. Systemic symptoms and fever are unusual.

VAGINITIS. Group A streptococcus is a common cause of vaginitis in prepubertal girls (Chapter 541). Patients usually have a serous discharge with marked erythema and irritation of the vulvar area, accompanied by discomfort in walking and in urination.

SEVERE INVASIVE DISEASE. Invasive group A streptococcal infection is defined by isolation of group A streptococcus from a normally sterile body site and includes three overlapping clinical syndromes. The first is group A streptococcal toxic shock syndrome, which is differentiated from other types of invasive group A streptococcal infections by the occurrence of shock and multiorgan system failure early in the course of the infection (Box 168–1). The second is group A streptococcal necrotizing fasciitis characterized by extensive local necrosis of subcutaneous soft tissues and skin. The third is the group of focal and systemic infections that do not meet the criteria for toxic shock syndrome or necrotizing fasciitis and includes bacteremia with no identified focus, meningitis, pneumonia, peritonitis, puerperal sepsis, osteomyelitis, suppurative arthritis, myositis, and surgical wound infections.

The pathogenic mechanisms responsible for severe, invasive group A streptococcal infections, including streptococcal toxic shock syndrome and necrotizing fasciitis, have yet to be defined completely, but an association with streptococcal pyrogenic exotoxins has been suggested. The three original streptococcal pyrogenic exotoxins (A, B, and C), the newly discovered streptococcal pyrogenic exotoxins, and potentially other, as yet unidentified toxins produced by group A streptococcus, act as **superantigens**, which stimulate an intense activation and proliferation of T lymphocytes and macrophages resulting in the production of large quantities of cytokines. These cytokines are capable of producing shock and tissue injury, and are believed to be responsible for many of the clinical manifestations of severe, invasive group A streptococcal infections.

Diagnosis. When attempting to decide whether to perform a microbiological test on a patient presenting with acute pharyngitis, consideration of the clinical and epidemiologic findings should take place before the test is performed. A history of close contact with a well-documented case of group A streptococcal pharyngitis is helpful, as is an awareness of a high prevalence of group A streptococcal infections in the community. Testing usually need not be performed on patients with acute pharyngitis whose clinical and epidemiologic features do not suggest a group A streptococcal etiology. However the signs and symptoms of streptococcal and nonstreptococcal pharyngitis overlap too broadly to allow the requisite diagnostic precision on clinical grounds alone. The clinical diagnosis of group A streptococcal pharyngitis cannot be made with certainty even by the most experienced physicians, and bacteriologic confirmation is required.

Culture of a throat swab on a sheep blood agar plate remains the standard for the documentation of the presence of group A streptococcus in the upper respiratory tract and for the confirmation of the clinical diagnosis of acute streptococcal pharyngitis. If performed correctly, a single throat swab cultured on a blood-agar plate has a sensitivity of 90–95% for detecting the presence of group A streptococcus in the pharynx.

A disadvantage of culturing a throat swab on a blood-agar plate is the delay (overnight or longer) in obtaining the culture result. Rapid antigen detection tests have been developed for the identification of group A streptococcus directly from throat swabs. Although these rapid tests are more expensive than the blood-agar culture, the advantage they offer over the traditional procedure is the speed with which they can provide results.

Rapid identification and treatment of patients with streptococcal pharyngitis can reduce the risk of the spread of group A streptococcus, allowing the patient to return to school or work sooner, and can reduce the acute morbidity of this illness.

The great majority of the rapid antigen detection tests that are currently available have an excellent specificity of >95% when compared with blood-agar plate cultures. False-positive test results are unusual, and, therefore, therapeutic decisions can be made on the basis of a positive test with confidence. Unfortunately, the sensitivity of most of these tests is 80–90%, possibly lower, when compared with the blood-agar plate culture. Newer tests may be more sensitive than other rapid antigen detection tests and perhaps may even be as sensitive as blood-agar plate cultures. However, in view of conflicting data, physicians who elect to use any rapid antigen detection test in children and adolescents without culture backup of negative results should do so only after confirming in their own practice that the rapid test is comparable in sensitivity to the throat culture.

Group A streptococcal infection can also be diagnosed retrospectively on the basis of an elevated or increasing streptococcal antibody titer. The antistreptolysin O assay is the streptococcal antibody test most commonly used. Because streptolysin O also is produced by group C and G streptococcus, the test is not specific for group A infection. The antistreptolysin O response can be feeble in patients with streptococcal impetigo and its usefulness for this condition is limited. In contrast, the anti-DNase B responses are present after both skin and throat infections. A significant antibody increase is usually defined as an increase in titer of two or more dilution increments between the acute phase and convalescent phase specimens, regardless of the actual height of the antibody titer. A single antistreptolysin O titer is generally considered to be elevated if it is at least 240 Todd units in adults and 320 Todd units in children. Anti-DNase B titers of 240 Todd units or greater in school-aged patients, and 120 Todd units or greater in adults, are considered elevated. However, depending on the prevalence of group A streptococcal infections, a varying proportion of the population will show antistreptolysin O or anti-DNase B titers of this magnitude or even greater.

DIFFERENTIAL DIAGNOSIS. Viruses are the most common cause of acute pharyngitis. Adenovirus, influenza virus, parainfluenza virus, rhinovirus, coxsackieviruses, ECHO viruses, herpes simplex virus, and respiratory syncytial virus frequently cause acute pharyngitis. Epstein-Barr virus is a frequent cause of acute pharyngitis that is often accompanied by the other clinical features of infectious mononucleosis (e.g., generalized lymphadenopathy, splenomegaly). Systemic infections with rubeola, cytomegalovirus, rubella, as well as a number of other viral agents may be associated with acute pharyngitis. Other agents such as *Mycoplasma pneumoniae* and *Chlamydia pneumoniae* are uncommon causes of acute pharyngitis.

Although group A streptococcus is the most common cause of bacterial pharyngitis, other bacteria are also capable of producing acute pharyngitis. These include groups C and G β-hemolytic streptococcus (Chapter 170) and *Corynebacterium diphtheriae* (Chapter 172). *Arcanobacterium haemolyticum* is a rare cause of acute pharyngitis that may be associated with a scarlet fever–like rash, particularly in teenagers. *Neisseria gonorrhoeae* can occasionally cause acute pharyngitis in sexually active individuals, and other bacteria such as *Francisella tularensis*, *Yersinia enterocolitica*, and mixed anaerobic infections (i.e., Vincent angina) are rare causes of acute pharyngitis.

Group A streptococcal pharyngitis is the only *commonly occurring* form of acute pharyngitis for which antibiotic therapy is definitely indicated. Therefore, when confronted with a patient with acute pharyngitis, the clinical decision that usually needs to be made is whether the pharyngitis is attributable to group A streptococcus.

BOX 168–1. Definition of Streptococcal Toxic Shock Syndrome

Hypotension plus two or more:
  Renal impairment
  Coagulopathy
  Hepatic involvement
  Adult respiratory distress syndrome
  Generalized erythematous macular rash
  Soft tissue necrosis
Definite case
  Clinical criteria plus group A streptococcus from a normally sterile site
Probable case
  Clinical criteria plus group A streptococcus from a nonsterile site

Treatment. Antibiotic therapy for patients with group A streptococcal pharyngitis can prevent acute rheumatic fever, shorten the clinical course of the illness, reduce transmission of the infection to others, and prevent suppurative complications. For the patient with classic scarlet fever, antibiotic therapy should be started immediately, but for the vast majority of patients who present with much less distinctive findings, treatment should be withheld until there is some form of bacteriologic confirmation either by throat culture or rapid antigen detection test. Rapid antigen detection tests, because of their high degree of specificity, have made it possible to initiate antibiotic therapy immediately for someone with a positive test result.

Group A streptococcus is exquisitely sensitive to penicillin, and resistant strains have never been encountered. Penicillin is, therefore, the drug of choice (except in patients who are allergic to penicillin) for pharyngeal infections as well as for suppurative complications. Treatment with oral penicillin V (250 mg/dose bid–tid PO) for 10 days is recommended but it must be taken for a full 10 days even though there is symptomatic improvement in 3–4 days. Penicillin V (phenoxyethylpenicillin) is preferred over penicillin G because it may be given without regard to mealtime. The major problem with all forms of oral therapy is the risk that the drug will be discontinued before the 10-day course has been completed. Therefore, when oral treatment is prescribed, the necessity of completing a full course of therapy must be emphasized. If the parents seem unlikely to comply because of family disorganization, difficulties in comprehension, or other reasons, parenteral therapy is indicated. A single intramuscular injection of benzathine penicillin G (600,000 IU for ≤60 lb, 1.2 million IU for >60 lb, IM) is the most efficacious and often the most practical method of treatment. Disadvantages include soreness around the site of injection, which may last for several days, and potential for injection into nerves or blood vessels if not administered correctly. The local reaction is diminished when benzathine penicillin G is combined in a single injection with procaine penicillin G, although precautions are necessary to ensure that an adequate amount of benzathine penicillin G is administered.

In some reports, as many as 20% of patients treated with a full course of penicillin continued to harbor group A streptococcus. The reasons for these bacteriologic failures are not clear. For patients who have received oral penicillin, poor compliance always has to be considered a possible explanation. It is likely that many of the failures of penicillin therapy occur in children who are merely group A streptococcal carriers. Therefore, routine follow-up throat cultures of asymptomatic patients who have completed a full course of therapy are not recommended.

Erythromycin (erythromycin estolate 20–40 mg/kg/24 hr divided bid–qid PO, or erythromycin ethylsuccinate 40 mg/kg/24 hr divided bid–qid PO) for 10 days is the drug of choice for patients allergic to penicillin. Although group A streptococcus that is resistant to erythromycin has rarely been encountered in the United States, erythromycin resistance has been a problem in other countries such as Japan and Finland.

A 10-day course of a narrow-spectrum oral cephalosporin is an acceptable alternative for patients allergic to penicillin. However, because up to 15% of penicillin-allergic patients are also cephalosporin-allergic, cephalosporins should not be given to patients with an immediate-type hypersensitivity to penicillin. The additional cost of cephalosporins and their broader spectrum of antibacterial activity compared with penicillin preclude their routine use in patients with group A streptococcal pharyngitis who are not penicillin-allergic. Sulfonamides and the tetracyclines are not indicated for treatment of group A streptococcal infections.

Most oral antibiotics must be administered for the conventional 10 days to achieve maximal pharyngeal eradication rates of group A streptococcus, but certain newer agents have been reported to achieve comparable bacteriologic and clinical cure rates when given for 5 days or less. Definitive results from comprehensive studies, however, are not available to allow final evaluation of these proposed shorter courses of oral antibiotic therapy. Therefore, they cannot be recommended at this time. In addition, these antibiotics have a much broader spectrum than penicillin, and most, even when administered for short courses, are more expensive.

Preliminary investigations have demonstrated that once daily amoxicillin therapy is effective in the treatment of group A streptococcal pharyngitis. If confirmed by additional investigations, once daily amoxicillin therapy, because of its low cost and relatively narrow spectrum, could become an alternative regimen for the treatment of group A streptococcal pharyngitis.

Antibiotic therapy for a patient with nonbullous impetigo can prevent local extension of the lesions, spread to distant infectious foci, and transmission of the infection to others. The ability of antibiotic therapy to prevent poststreptococcal glomerulonephritis, however, has not been clearly demonstrated. Patients with a few superficial, isolated lesions and no systemic signs can be treated with topical antibiotics. Mupirocin is a safe and effective agent that has become the topical treatment of choice. If there are widespread lesions or systemic signs, oral therapy with a β-lactamase–resistant drug (e.g., dicloxacillin, cephalexin) will provide coverage for both group A streptococcus and *S. aureus*. Erythromycin is another alternative, particularly for those allergic to penicillin. However, rapidly emerging resistance to erythromycin among *S. aureus* in many areas suggests that it should not be used as first-line therapy.

Theoretical considerations and experimental data suggest that intravenous clindamycin is a more effective agent for the treatment of severe, invasive group A streptococcal infections than intravenous penicillin. However, because a small proportion of the group A streptococcal isolates in the United States are resistant to clindamycin, clindamycin should be used in combination with penicillin for these infections until susceptibility to clindamycin has been established. If necrotizing fasciitis is suspected, immediate surgical exploration or biopsy is required to identify a deep soft tissue infection that should be debrided immediately. Patients with streptococcal toxic shock syndrome require rapid and aggressive fluid replacement, management of respiratory or cardiac failure, if present, and anticipatory management of multiorgan system failure. Limited data suggest that intravenous gamma globulin is effective in the management of streptococcal toxic shock syndrome, but well-controlled studies have yet to be performed. Currently, intravenous immunoglobulin should be reserved for those patients who do not respond to other therapeutic measures.

Complications. Suppurative complications from the spread of group A streptococcus to adjacent structures were very common before antibiotics became available. Cervical lymphadenitis, peritonsillar abscess, retropharyngeal abscess, otitis media, mastoiditis, and sinusitis still occur in children in whom the primary illness has gone unnoticed or in whom treatment of the pharyngitis has been inadequate. Group A streptococcal pneumonia can rarely occur.

Acute rheumatic fever (Chapter 168.1) and acute poststreptococcal glomerulonephritis (Chapter 503.1) are both nonsuppurative sequelae of infections with group A streptococcus that occur after an asymptomatic latent period. They are both characterized by lesions remote from the site of the group A streptococcal infection. However, acute rheumatic fever and acute glomerulonephritis differ in their clinical manifestations, epidemiology, and potential morbidity. In addition, acute glomerulonephritis can occur after a group A streptococcal infection of either the upper respiratory tract or the skin, but acute rheumatic fever can occur only after an infection of the upper respiratory tract.

POSTSTREPTOCOCCAL REACTIVE ARTHRITIS. Poststreptococcal reactive arthritis has been used to describe a syndrome characterized by the onset of acute arthritis following an episode of group A streptococcal pharyngotonsillitis in a patient whose illness does not otherwise fulfill the Jones criteria for the diagnosis of acute rheumatic fever. There is still considerable debate about whether this entity represents a distinct syndrome or is a manifestation of acute rheumatic fever. Although poststreptococcal reactive arthritis usually involves the large joints, in contrast to the arthritis of acute rheumatic fever, it may involve small peripheral joints as well as the axial skeleton and is typically nonmigratory. The latent period between the antecedent episode of group A streptococcal pharyngitis and the poststreptococcal reactive arthritis is considerably shorter (usually <10 days) than that typically seen with acute rheumatic fever. In contrast to the arthritis of acute rheumatic fever, poststreptococcal reactive arthritis does not respond dramatically to therapy with aspirin or other nonsteroidal inflammatory agents. Even though no more than half of the patients with poststreptococcal reactive arthritis who have a throat culture performed have group A streptococcal isolated, all have serologic evidence of a recent group A streptococcal infection. It has been reported that a small proportion of patients with poststreptococcal reactive arthritis may go on to develop valvular heart disease. Therefore, these patients should be carefully observed for several months for the subsequent development of carditis. Some physicians administer secondary prophylaxis to these patients for a period of up to 1 yr. If carditis is not observed, the prophylaxis can then be discontinued. If carditis is detected, the patient should be classified as having had acute rheumatic fever and should continue to receive secondary prophylaxis.

PEDIATRIC AUTOIMMUNE NEUROPSYCHIATRIC DISORDERS ASSOCIATED WITH *STREPTOCOCCUS PYOGENES* (PANDAS). PANDAS has been used to describe a group of neuropsychiatric disorders (particularly obsessive-compulsive disorders, tic disorders, and Tourette syndrome) for which a possible relationship with group A streptococcal infections has been suggested. It has been demonstrated that patients with Sydenham chorea (a form of acute rheumatic fever) frequently have obsessive-compulsive symptoms and that a subset of patients with obsessive-compulsive and tic disorders will have chorea as well as acute exacerbations following group A streptococcal infections. Therefore, it has been proposed that this subset of patients with obsessive-compulsive and tic disorders produce autoimmune antibodies in response to a group A streptococcal infection that cross-react with brain tissue similar to the autoimmune response believed to be responsible for the manifestations of Sydenham chorea. It has also been suggested that secondary prophylaxis that prevents recurrences of Sydenham chorea might also be effective in preventing recurrences of obsessive-compulsive and tic disorders in these patients. Because of the proposed autoimmune mechanism, it has also been suggested that these patients may benefit from immunoregulatory therapy such as plasma exchange or intravenous immunoglobulin therapy. The possibility that PANDAS could represent an extension of the spectrum of acute rheumatic fever is intriguing but is yet unproven. Until carefully designed and well-controlled studies have established a causal relationship between PANDAS and group A streptococcal infections, secondary prophylaxis to prevent, and immunoregulatory therapy to treat, PANDAS are not recommended.

Prognosis. The prognosis for adequately treated group A streptococcal infections is excellent; most suppurative complications are prevented or readily treated. When therapy is provided promptly, acute rheumatic fever is prevented and complete recovery is the rule. However, there is no evidence that acute poststreptococcal glomerulonephritis can be prevented once pharyngitis or pyoderma with a nephritogenic strain of group A

streptococcus has occurred. In rare instances, particularly in neonates or in children whose response to infection is compromised, fulminant pneumonia, septicemia, and death may occur despite usually adequate therapy.

Prevention. The only specific indication for long-term use of antibiotics to prevent group A streptococcal infections is for patients with a history of acute rheumatic fever or rheumatic heart disease. Mass prophylaxis is generally not feasible except to reduce the number of infections during epidemics of impetigo and to control epidemics of pharyngitis in military populations and in schools.

Because the ability of antimicrobial agents to prevent group A streptococcal infections is limited, a streptococcal vaccine offers the possibility of a more effective approach. Investigators recently have purified and characterized M protein and have succeeded in separating M protein epitopes that evoke protective, type-specific antibodies from M protein epitopes that evoke heart cross-reactive antibodies. Moreover, chemically synthesized subpeptide fragments of M protein, copying known amino acid sequences of different M proteins, also have been found to be effective immunogens without evoking cross-reactive antibodies. Recent evidence suggests that protective antibodies can be produced to conserved, nontype-specific epitopes on the M protein that are shared by many different serologic types. Finally, work on new methods of vaccine delivery, such as intranasal administration, is being performed. An effective group A streptococcal vaccine that could be delivered by way of a mucosal route would have several advantages over parenteral vaccines, including cost, ease of delivery, and the production of protective secretory as well as serum antibodies.

Vaccine candidates have been developed using synthetic or recombinant peptide fragments derived from type-specific sequences of the M protein. Several multivalent, recombinant M protein vaccines have been constructed by placing protective peptide fragments of various M genes in tandem. When tested in rabbits using a parenteral route, a hexavalent M protein vaccine evoked opsonic antibodies with bactericidal activity against all six serotypes and no antibodies reactive with human heart tissue. Studies of this hexavalent vaccine in humans were recently initiated. Another vaccine candidate has been developed using a nonpathogenic commensal organism as a live vector to express a highly conserved region of the M protein that evokes a protective antibody response. Both IgA and IgG antibodies were produced in mice and rabbits following oral and intranasal administration of this vaccine candidate with no evidence of cross-reactive antibodies to human heart tissue. Investigations of this candidate vaccine in humans were recently initiated.

168.1 ■ Rheumatic Fever

Etiology. There is considerable evidence to support the link between group A streptococcus upper respiratory tract infections and acute rheumatic fever and rheumatic heart disease. As many as two thirds of the patients with an acute episode of rheumatic fever have a history of an upper respiratory tract infection several weeks before, and the peak age and seasonal incidence of acute rheumatic fever closely parallel those of group A streptococcal infections. Patients with acute rheumatic fever almost always have serologic evidence of a recent group A streptococcal infection. In addition, their antibody titers are usually considerably higher than those seen in patients with group A streptococcal infections without acute rheumatic fever. Outbreaks of group A streptococcal pharyngitis in closed communities, such as boarding schools or military bases, may be followed by outbreaks of acute rheumatic fever. Finally, antimicrobial therapy that eliminates group A streptococcus from the pharynx also prevents initial episodes of acute rheumatic fever, and long-term, continuous prophylaxis that prevents group A streptococcal pharyngitis also prevents recurrences of acute rheumatic fever.

Not all of the serotypes of group A streptococcus can cause rheumatic fever. When some strains (e.g., M type 4) were present in a very susceptible rheumatic population, no recurrences of rheumatic fever occurred. In contrast, episodes of pharyngitis with other serotypes prevalent in the same population were associated with frequent recurrences. The concept of rheumatogenicity is further supported by the observation that although serotypes of group A streptococcus frequently associated with skin infection are often isolated from the upper respiratory tract, they rarely cause recurrences of rheumatic fever in individuals with a previous history of rheumatic fever. In addition, certain serotypes of group A streptococcus (e.g., M types 1, 3, 5, 6, 18, 24) are more frequently isolated from patients with acute rheumatic fever than are other serotypes.

Epidemiology. In some developing areas of the world, the annual incidence of acute rheumatic fever is currently as high as 282/100,000 population. Worldwide, rheumatic heart disease remains the most common form of acquired heart disease in all age groups, accounting for as much as 50% of all cardiovascular disease and as much as 50% of all cardiac admissions in many developing countries. However, striking differences are evident in the incidence of acute rheumatic fever and rheumatic heart disease among different ethnic groups within the same country; many, but not all, of these differences appear to be related to differences in socioeconomic status.

In the United States, at the beginning of the 20th century, acute rheumatic fever was the leading cause of death among children and adolescents, with annual incidence rates of 100–200/100,000 population. In addition, rheumatic heart disease was the leading cause of heart disease among adults <40 yr of age. At that time, as many as one fourth of the hospital beds in the United States were occupied by patients suffering from acute rheumatic fever or its complications. By the 1940s, the annual incidence of acute rheumatic fever had decreased to 50/100,000, and over the next 4 decades, the decline in incidence accelerated rapidly. By the early 1980s, the annual incidence in some areas of the United States was as low as 0.5/100,000 population. This sharp decline in the incidence of acute rheumatic fever has been observed in other industrialized countries as well.

The explanation for this dramatic decline in the incidence of acute rheumatic fever and rheumatic heart disease in the United States and other industrialized countries is not clear. Historically, acute rheumatic fever has been associated with poverty, particularly in urban areas. Much of the decline in the incidence of acute rheumatic fever in industrialized countries during the preantibiotic era can probably be attributed to improvements in living conditions. A number of studies have suggested that, of the various manifestations of poverty, crowding, which contributes to the spread of group A streptococcal infections, is the one most closely associated with the incidence of acute rheumatic fever. The decline in incidence of acute rheumatic fever in industrialized countries over the past 4 decades has also been attributable in large measure to the greater availability of medical care and to the widespread use of antibiotics. Antibiotic therapy of group A streptococcal pharyngitis has been important in preventing initial attacks and, particularly, recurrences of the disease. In addition, the decline can be attributed, at least in part, to a shift in the prevalent strains of group A streptococcus from rheumatogenic to nonrheumatogenic strains.

A dramatic outbreak of acute rheumatic fever in the Salt Lake City area began in early 1985, and 198 cases were reported by the end of 1989. Other outbreaks were reported between 1984 and 1988 in Columbus and Akron, OH; Pittsburgh, PA; Nashville and Memphis, TN; New York City, NY; Kansas City, MO; Dallas, TX; and among recruits at the San Diego Naval Training Center in California and at the Fort Leonard Wood Army Training Base in Missouri. Evidence suggests that this resurgence of acute rheumatic fever was focal and not nationwide.

Certain rheumatogenic serotypes (e.g., types 1, 3, 5, 6, and 18) that were isolated infrequently during the 1970s and early 1980s dramatically reappeared during these focal outbreaks. The appearance of these rheumatogenic strains in selected communities was probably a major factor in these outbreaks of acute rheumatic fever. Another property of group A streptococcus that has been associated with rheumatogenicity is the formation of highly mucoid colonies. Mucoid strains of group A streptococcus had only rarely been isolated from throat cultures in recent years. However, during these focal outbreaks of acute rheumatic fever, mucoid strains of group A streptococcus were commonly isolated from patients, family members, and members of the surrounding community.

In addition to the specific characteristics of the infecting group A streptococcus, the risk of a particular person developing acute rheumatic fever is also dependent upon various host factors. The incidence of both initial attacks and recurrences of acute rheumatic fever peaks in children aged 5–15 yr, the age of greatest risk for group A streptococcal pharyngitis. Patients who have had one attack of acute rheumatic fever tend to have recurrences, and the clinical features of the recurrences tend to mimic those of the initial attack. In addition, there appears to be a genetic predisposition to acute rheumatic fever. Studies in twins have shown a higher concordance rate of acute rheumatic fever in monozygotic than in dizygotic twin pairs. Recent investigations have also demonstrated an association between the presence of specific HLA markers and a B-cell alloantigen and susceptibility to acute rheumatic fever.

Pathogenesis. The pathogenic link between a group A streptococcal infection of the upper respiratory tract and an attack of acute rheumatic fever, characterized by organ and tissue involvement far removed from the pharynx, is still not clear. One of the major obstacles to understanding the pathogenesis of acute rheumatic fever and rheumatic heart disease has been the inability to establish an animal model. Several theories of the pathogenesis of acute rheumatic fever and rheumatic heart disease have been proposed, but only two are seriously considered: the cytotoxicity theory and the immunologic theory.

The cytotoxicity theory suggests that a group A streptococcal toxin may be involved in the pathogenesis of acute rheumatic fever and rheumatic heart disease. Group A streptococcus produces several enzymes that are cytotoxic for mammalian cardiac cells. For example, streptolysin O has a direct cytotoxic effect on mammalian cells in tissue culture, and most of the proponents of the cytotoxicity theory have focused on this enzyme. However, one of the major problems with the cytotoxicity hypothesis is its inability to explain the latent period between an episode of group A streptococcal pharyngitis and the onset of acute rheumatic fever.

An immune-mediated pathogenesis for acute rheumatic fever and rheumatic heart disease has been suggested by the clinical similarity of acute rheumatic fever to other illnesses produced by immunopathogenic processes and by the latent period between the group A streptococcal infection and the acute rheumatic fever. The antigenicity of a large variety of group A streptococcal products and constituents, as well as the immunologic cross-reactivity between group A streptococcal components and mammalian tissues, also lends support to this hypothesis. Common antigenic determinants are shared between certain components of group A streptococcus (e.g., M protein, protoplast membrane, cell wall group A carbohydrate, capsular hyaluronate) and specific mammalian tissues (e.g., heart, brain, joint). For example, certain M proteins (M1, M5, M6, and M19) share epitopes with human tropomyosin and myosin. Additionally, the involvement of group A streptococcal superantigens such as pyrogenic exotoxins in the pathogenesis of acute rheumatic fever has been proposed.

Clinical Manifestations and Diagnosis. Because no clinical or laboratory finding is pathognomonic for acute rheumatic fever, T. Duckett Jones in 1944 proposed guidelines to aid in diagnosis and to limit overdiagnosis. The Jones criteria, as revised in 1992 by the American Heart Association (Table 168–1), are intended only for the diagnosis of the initial attack of acute rheumatic fever and not for recurrences. There are five major and four minor criteria and an absolute requirement for evidence (microbiologic or serologic) of recent group A streptococcal infection. The diagnosis of acute rheumatic fever can be established by the Jones criteria when a patient fulfills two major criteria or one major and two minor criteria and meets the absolute requirement. Even with strict application of the Jones criteria, overdiagnosis as well as underdiagnosis of acute rheumatic fever may occur. There are three circumstances in which the diagnosis of acute rheumatic fever can be made without strict adherence to the Jones criteria. Chorea may occur as the only manifestation of acute rheumatic fever. Similarly, indolent carditis may be the only manifestation in patients who first come to medical attention months after the onset of acute rheumatic fever. Finally, although most patients with recurrences of acute rheumatic fever fulfill the Jones criteria, some may not.

MAJOR MANIFESTATIONS. There are five major criteria. The presence of two major criteria with evidence (microbiologic or serologic) of recent group A streptococcal infection fulfills the Jones criteria.

Migratory Polyarthritis. Arthritis occurs in about 75% of patients with acute rheumatic fever and typically involves larger joints, particularly the knees, ankles, wrists, and elbows. Involvement of the spine, small joints of the hands and feet, or hips is uncommon. Rheumatic joints are generally hot, red, swollen, and exquisitely tender; even the friction of bedclothes is uncomfortable. The pain can precede and can appear to be disproportionate to the other findings. The joint involvement is characteristically migratory in nature; a severely inflamed joint can become normal within 1–3 days without treatment, as one or more other large joints become involved. Severe arthritis can persist for several weeks in untreated patients. Monoarticular arthritis is unusual unless anti-inflammatory therapy is initiated prematurely, aborting the progression of the migratory polyarthritis. If a child with fever and arthritis is suspected of having acute rheumatic fever, it frequently is useful to withhold salicylates and observe for migratory progression. A dramatic response to even small doses of salicylates is another characteristic feature of the arthritis, and the absence of such a response should suggest an alternative diagnosis. Rheumatic arthritis is typically not deforming. Synovial fluid in acute rheumatic fever usually has 10,000–100,000 white blood cells/mm³ with a predominance of neutrophils, a protein of about 4 g/dL, a normal glucose, and forms a good mucin clot. Frequently, arthritis is the earliest manifestation of acute rheumatic fever and may correlate temporally with peak antistreptococcal antibody titers. There is an apparent inverse relationship between the severity of arthritis and the severity of cardiac involvement.

Carditis. Carditis and resultant chronic rheumatic heart disease are the most serious manifestations of acute rheumatic fever and account for essentially all of the associated morbidity and mortality. Rheumatic carditis is characterized by pancarditis, with active inflammation of myocardium, pericardium, and endocardium. Cardiac involvement during acute rheumatic fever varies in severity from fulminant, potentially fatal exudative pancarditis to mild, transient cardiac involvement. Endocarditis (valvulitis), which is manifest by one or more cardiac murmurs, is a universal finding in rheumatic carditis, whereas the presence of pericarditis or myocarditis is variable. Myocarditis and/or pericarditis without evidence of endocarditis is rarely due to rheumatic heart disease. Most cases consist of either isolated mitral valvular disease or combined aortic and mitral valvular disease. Isolated aortic or right-sided valvular involvement is uncommon. Serious and long-term illness is related entirely to valvular heart disease as a consequence of a single attack or recurrent attacks of acute rheumatic fever. Valvular insufficiency is characteristic of both acute and convalescent stages of acute rheumatic fever, whereas valvular stenosis usually appears several years or even decades after the acute illness. In developing countries, however, where acute rheumatic fever often occurs at a younger age, mitral stenosis and aortic stenosis may develop sooner after acute rheumatic fever than in developed countries, and can occur in young children.

Acute rheumatic carditis usually presents as tachycardia and cardiac murmurs, with or without evidence of myocardial or pericardial involvement. Moderate-to-severe rheumatic carditis can result in cardiomegaly and congestive heart failure with hepatomegaly and peripheral and pulmonary edema. Echocardiographic findings include pericardial effusion, decreased ventricular contractility, and aortic and/or mitral regurgitation. Mitral regurgitation is characterized by a high-pitched apical holosystolic murmur radiating to the axilla. In patients with significant mitral regurgitation, this may be associated with an apical mid-diastolic murmur of relative mitral stenosis. Aortic insufficiency is characterized by a high-pitched decrescendo diastolic murmur at the upper left sternal border. Echocardiographic demonstration of valvular regurgitation without accompanying auscultatory evidence does not satisfy the Jones criteria for carditis.

Carditis occurs in about 50–60% of all cases of acute rheumatic fever. Recurrent attacks of acute rheumatic fever in patients who had carditis with the initial attack are associated with high rates of carditis. The major consequence of acute rheumatic carditis is chronic, progressive valvular disease, par-

---

TABLE 168–1. Guidelines for the Diagnosis of Initial Attack of Rheumatic Fever (Jones Criteria, Updated 1992)

Major Manifestations*	Minor Manifestations	Supporting Evidence of Antecedent Group A Streptococcal Infection

Carditis
Polyarthritis
	Clinical features
	  Arthralgia
	  Fever
		Positive throat culture or rapid streptococcal antigen test
		Elevated or increasing streptococcal antibody titer

Erythema marginatum
Subcutaneous nodules
	Laboratory features
	Elevated acute phase reactants:
	  Erythrocyte sedimentation rate
	  C-reactive protein
	Prolonged PR interval	

*The presence of two major or of one major and two minor manifestations indicates a high probability of acute rheumatic fever if supported by evidence of preceding group A streptococcal infection.
Guidelines for the diagnosis of rheumatic fever: Jones criteria, updated 1992. JAMA 1992;268:2069–73. Copyright American Medical Association.

ticularly valvular stenosis, which can require valve replacement and predispose to infective endocarditis.

Chorea. Sydenham chorea occurs in about 10–15% of patients with acute rheumatic fever and usually presents as an isolated, frequently subtle, neurologic behavior disorder. Emotional lability, incoordination, poor school performance, uncontrollable movements, and facial grimacing, exacerbated by stress and disappearing with sleep, are characteristic. Chorea occasionally is unilateral. The latent period from acute group A streptococcal infection to chorea is usually longer than for arthritis or carditis and can be months. Onset can be insidious, with symptoms being present for several months before recognition. Clinical maneuvers to elicit features of chorea include (1) demonstration of milkmaid's grip (irregular contractions of the muscles of the hands while squeezing the examiner's fingers), (2) spooning and pronation of the hands when the patient's arms are extended, (3) wormian movements of the tongue upon protrusion, and (4) examination of handwriting to evaluate fine motor movements. Diagnosis is based on clinical findings with supportive evidence of group A streptococcal antibodies. However, in patients with a long latent period from the inciting streptococcal infection, antibody levels may have declined to normal. Although the acute illness is distressing, chorea rarely if ever leads to permanent neurologic sequelae.

Erythema Marginatum. Erythema marginatum is a rare (<3% of patients with acute rheumatic fever) but characteristic rash of acute rheumatic fever. It consists of erythematous, serpiginous, macular lesions with pale centers that are not pruritic. It occurs primarily on the trunk and extremities, but not on the face, and it can be accentuated by warming the skin.

Subcutaneous Nodules. Subcutaneous nodules are a rare (≤1% of patients with acute rheumatic fever) and consist of firm nodules approximately 1 cm in diameter along the extensor surfaces of tendons near bony prominences. There is a correlation between the presence of these nodules and significant rheumatic heart disease.

MINOR MANIFESTATIONS. The two clinical minor manifestations are arthralgia (in the absence of polyarthritis as a major criterion) and fever (typically temperature ≥102°F and occurring early in the course of illness). The two laboratory minor manifestations are elevated acute-phase reactants (e.g., C-reactive protein, erythrocyte sedimentation rate) and prolonged PR interval on electrocardiogram (first-degree heart block). However, a prolonged PR interval alone does not constitute evidence of carditis or predict long-term cardiac sequelae.

RECENT GROUP A STREPTOCOCCUS INFECTION. An absolute requirement for the diagnosis of acute rheumatic fever is supporting evidence of a recent group A streptococcal infection. Acute rheumatic fever typically develops 2–4 wk after an acute episode of group A streptococcal pharyngitis at a time when clinical findings of pharyngitis are no longer present and when only 10–20% of the throat culture or rapid streptococcal antigen test results are positive. One third of patients have no history of an antecedent pharyngitis. Therefore, evidence of an antecedent group A streptococcal infection is usually based on elevated or increasing serum antistreptococcal antibody titers. A slide agglutination test (Streptozyme) has been introduced, and it is purported to detect antibodies against five different group A streptococcal antigens. Although this test is rapid, relatively simple to perform, and widely available, it is less standardized and less reproducible than other tests and should not be used as a diagnostic test for evidence of an antecedent group A streptococcal infection. If only a single antibody is measured (usually antistreptolysin O), only 80–85% of patients with acute rheumatic fever have an elevated titer; however, 95–100% have an elevation if three different antibodies (antistreptolysin O, anti-DNase B, antihyaluronidase) are measured. Therefore, when acute rheumatic fever is suspected clinically, multiple antibody tests are performed. Except for patients with chorea,

clinical findings of acute rheumatic fever generally coincide with peak antistreptococcal antibody responses. Most patients with chorea have elevation of antibodies to one or more group A streptococcal antigens, although these antibodies may be waning. The diagnosis of acute rheumatic fever should not be made in patients with elevated or increasing streptococcal antibody titers who do not fulfill the Jones criteria because such titer changes may be coincidental. This is most often true in younger, school-aged children, many of whom have group A streptococcal pyoderma in the summer or unrelated group A streptococcal pharyngitis during the winter and spring months.

DIFFERENTIAL DIAGNOSIS. The differential diagnoses of rheumatic fever include many infectious as well as noninfectious illnesses (Table 168–2). When children present with arthritis, a collagen vascular disease must be considered. Rheumatoid arthritis in particular must be distinguished from acute rheumatic fever. Children with rheumatoid arthritis tend to be younger and usually have less joint pain relative to their other clinical findings than those with acute rheumatic fever. Spiking fevers, lymphadenopathy, and splenomegaly are more suggestive of rheumatoid arthritis than acute rheumatic fever. The response to salicylate therapy is also much less dramatic with rheumatoid arthritis than with acute rheumatic fever. Systemic lupus erythematosus can usually be distinguished from acute rheumatic fever on the basis of the presence of antinuclear antibodies with systemic lupus erythematosus. Other causes of arthritis, such as gonococcal arthritis, malignancies, serum sickness, Lyme disease, sickle cell disease, and reactive arthritis related to gastrointestinal infections (e.g., *Shigella, Salmonella, Yersinia*) should also be considered.

When carditis is the sole major manifestation of suspected acute rheumatic fever, viral myocarditis, viral pericarditis, Kawasaki disease, and infective endocarditis should also be considered. Patients with infective endocarditis may present with both joint and cardiac manifestations. These patients can usually be distinguished from patients with acute rheumatic fever by blood cultures and the presence of associated findings (e.g., hematuria, splenomegaly, splinter hemorrhages). In general, the absence of auscultatory evidence of a significant cardiac murmur excludes the diagnosis of acute rheumatic carditis.

When chorea is the sole major manifestation of suspected acute rheumatic fever, Huntington chorea, Wilson disease, systemic lupus erythematosus, and various encephalitides should also be considered. These other diseases are usually identified by the history, laboratory studies, and clinical findings.

Treatment. All patients with acute rheumatic fever should be placed on bed rest and monitored closely for evidence of carditis. They can be allowed to ambulate as soon as the signs of acute inflammation have subsided. However, patients with carditis require longer periods of bed rest.

ANTIBIOTIC THERAPY. Once the diagnosis of acute rheumatic fever has been established and regardless of the throat

TABLE 168–2. Differential Diagnosis of Acute Rheumatic Fever

Arthritis	Carditis	Chorea
Rheumatoid arthritis	Viral myocarditis	Huntington chorea
Reactive arthritis (e.g., *Shigella, Salmonella, Yersinia*)	Viral pericarditis	Wilson disease
Serum sickness	Infective endocarditis	Systemic lupus erythematosus
Sickle cell disease	Kawasaki disease	Cerebral palsy
Malignancies	Congenital heart disease	Tics
Systemic lupus erythematosus		
	Mitral valve prolapse	Hyperactivity
Lyme disease	Innocent murmurs	
Gonococcal infection		

culture results, the patient should receive 10 days of orally administered penicillin or erythromycin, or a single intramuscular injection of benzathine penicillin to eradicate group A streptococcus from the upper respiratory tract. After this initial course of antibiotic therapy, the patient should be started on long-term antibiotic prophylaxis.

ANTI-INFLAMMATORY THERAPY. Anti-inflammatory agents (e.g., salicylates, corticosteroids) should be withheld if arthralgia or atypical arthritis is the only clinical manifestation of presumed acute rheumatic fever. Premature treatment with one of these agents may interfere with the development of the characteristic migratory polyarthritis and thus obscure the diagnosis of acute rheumatic fever. Agents such as acetaminophen can be used to control pain and fever while the patient is being observed for more definite signs of acute rheumatic fever or for evidence of another disease.

Patients with typical migratory polyarthritis and those with carditis without cardiomegaly or congestive heart failure should be treated with oral salicylates. The usual dose of aspirin is 100 mg/kg/24 hr divided qid PO for 3–5 days, followed by 75 mg/kg/24 hr divided qid PO for 4 wk. Determination of the serum salicylate level is not necessary unless the arthritis does not respond or signs of salicylate toxicity (e.g., tinnitus, hyperventilation) develop. There is no evidence that nonsteroidal anti-inflammatory agents are any more effective than salicylates.

Patients with carditis and cardiomegaly or congestive heart failure should receive corticosteroids. The usual dose of prednisone is 2 mg/kg/24 hr in 4 divided doses for 2–3 wk followed by a tapering of the dose that reduces the dose by 5 mg/24 hr every 2–3 days. At the beginning of the tapering of the prednisone dose, aspirin should be started at 75 mg/kg/24 hr in 4 divided doses for 6 wk. Supportive therapies for patients with moderate-to-severe carditis include digoxin, fluid and salt restriction, diuretics, and oxygen. The cardiac toxicity of digoxin is enhanced with myocarditis.

Termination of the anti-inflammatory therapy may be followed by the reappearance of clinical manifestations or of laboratory abnormalities. These "rebounds" are best left untreated unless the clinical manifestations are severe; salicylates or steroids should be reinstated in such cases.

SYDENHAM CHOREA. Because chorea often occurs as an isolated manifestation after the resolution of the acute phase of the disease, anti-inflammatory agents are usually not indicated. Sedatives may be helpful early in the course of chorea; phenobarbital (16–32 mg q 6–8 hr PO) is the drug of choice. If phenobarbital is ineffective, then haloperidol (0.01–0.03 mg/kg/ 24 hr divided bid PO) or chlorpromazine (0.5 mg/kg q 4–6 hr PO) should be initiated.

Complications. The arthritis and chorea of acute rheumatic fever resolve completely without sequelae. Therefore, the long-term sequelae of rheumatic fever are usually limited to the heart.

Patients with cardiac valvular disease secondary to acute rheumatic fever are at increased risk of developing infective endocarditis during episodes of transient bacteremia. The antibiotic regimens used to prevent recurrences of acute rheumatic fever are inadequate for protection against infective endocarditis. Therefore, these patients require short-term antibiotic prophylaxis before surgical or dental procedures that are associated with transient bacteremia. The current recommendations of the American Heart Association regarding infective endocarditis prophylaxis should be followed (Chapter 429). The importance of good dental hygiene in the prevention of infective endocarditis should also be stressed. Patients who have had rheumatic fever but have no evidence of residual valvular disease do not require endocarditis prophylaxis.

Prognosis. The prognosis for patients with acute rheumatic fever depends on the clinical manifestations present at the time of the initial episode, the severity of the initial episode, and the presence of recurrences. Approximately 70% of the patients with carditis during the initial episode of acute rheumatic fever recover with no residual heart disease; the more severe the initial cardiac involvement, the greater the risk of residual heart disease. Patients without carditis during the initial episode are unlikely to have carditis with recurrences. In contrast, patients with carditis during the initial episode are likely to have carditis with recurrences, and the risk of permanent heart damage increases with each recurrence. Patients who have had acute rheumatic fever are susceptible to recurrent attacks following reinfection of the upper respiratory tract with group A streptococcus. Therefore, these patients require long-term continuous chemoprophylaxis.

Before antibiotic prophylaxis was available, 75% of patients who had an initial episode of acute rheumatic fever had one or more recurrences during their lifetime. These recurrences were a major source of morbidity and mortality. The risk of recurrence is highest immediately after the initial episode and decreases with time.

Approximately 20% of patients who present with "pure" chorea who are not put on secondary prophylaxis develop rheumatic heart disease within 20 yr. Therefore, patients with chorea, even in the absence of other manifestations of rheumatic fever, require long-term antibiotic prophylaxis.

Prevention. Prevention of both initial and recurrent episodes of acute rheumatic fever depends on controlling group A streptococcal infections of the upper respiratory tract. Prevention of initial attacks (primary prevention) depends on identification and eradication of the group A streptococcus that produces episodes of acute pharyngitis. Individuals who have already suffered an attack of acute rheumatic fever are particularly susceptible to recurrences of rheumatic fever with any subsequent group A streptococcus upper respiratory tract infection, whether or not they are symptomatic. Therefore, these patients should receive continuous antibiotic prophylaxis to prevent recurrences (secondary prevention).

PRIMARY PREVENTION. Appropriate antibiotic therapy instituted before the 9th day of symptoms of acute group A streptococcal pharyngitis is highly effective in preventing first attacks of acute rheumatic fever from that episode. However, about one third of patients with acute rheumatic fever do not recall a preceding episode of pharyngitis.

SECONDARY PREVENTION. Secondary prevention is directed at preventing acute group A streptococcal pharyngitis in patients at substantial risk of recurrent acute rheumatic fever. Secondary prevention requires continuous antibiotic prophylaxis, which should begin as soon as the diagnosis of acute rheumatic fever has been made and immediately after a full course of antibiotic therapy has been completed. Because patients who have had carditis with their initial episode of acute rheumatic fever are at a relatively high risk of having carditis with recurrences and of sustaining additional cardiac damage, they should receive antibiotic prophylaxis well into adulthood and perhaps for life.

Patients who did not have carditis with their initial episode of acute rheumatic fever have a relatively low risk of carditis with recurrences. Antibiotic prophylaxis may be discontinued in these patients when they reach their early 20s and after at least 5 yr have elapsed since their last episode of acute rheumatic fever. The decision to discontinue prophylactic antibiotics should be made only after careful consideration of potential risks and benefits and of epidemiologic factors such as the risk of exposure to group A streptococcal infections.

The regimen of choice for secondary prevention is a single intramuscular injection of benzathine penicillin G (1.2 million IU) every 4 wk (Table 168–3). In certain high-risk patients, and in certain areas of the world where the incidence of rheumatic fever is particularly high, use of benzathine penicillin G every 3 wk may be necessary because levels of penicillin may decrease to marginally effective amounts after 3 wk. In compliant patients, continuous oral antimicrobial prophylaxis can be

TABLE 168–3. Secondary Prevention of Rheumatic Fever

Route of Administration	Antibiotic	Dose	Frequency
Intramuscular	Benzathine penicillin G	1,200,000 U	Every 3–4 wk
Oral	Penicillin V	250 mg	Twice daily
	Sulfadiazine	500–1000 mg	Once daily
	Erythromycin	250 mg	Twice daily

used. Penicillin V given twice daily and sulfadiazine given once daily are equally effective when used in such patients. For the exceptional patient who is allergic to both penicillin and sulfonamides, erythromycin given twice daily may be used.

Group A Streptococcus

American Academy of Pediatrics, Committee on Infectious Diseases: Severe invasive group A streptococcal infections: A subject review. *Pediatrics* 1998;101: 136–40.

Bisno AL, Stevens DL: Streptococcal infections of skin and soft tissues. *N Engl J Med* 1996;334:240–5.

Brandt ER, Good MF: Vaccine strategies to prevent rheumatic fever. *Immun Res* 1999;19:89–103.

Cunningham MW: Pathogenesis of group A streptococcal infections. *Clin Microbiol Rev* 2000;13:470–511.

Davis HD, McGeer A, Schwartz B, et al: Invasive group A streptococcal infections in Ontario, Canada. *N Engl J Med* 1996;335:547–54.

Kaul R, McGreer A, Norby-Teglund A, et al: Intravenous immunoglobulin therapy in streptococcal toxic shock syndrome—A comparative observational study. *Clin Infect Dis* 1999;28:800–7.

Mancini AJ: Bacterial skin infections in children; the common and the not so common. *Pediatr Annals* 2000;29:26–35.

Stevens DL: Streptococcal toxic shock syndrome associated with necrotizing fasciitis. *Annu Rev Med* 2000;51:271–88.

Stevens DL, Kaplan EL: *Streptococcal Infections—Clinical Aspects, Microbiology, and Molecular Pathogenesis.* New York, Oxford University Press, 2000.

The Working Group on Prevention of Invasion Group A Streptococcal Infections: Prevention of invasive group A streptococcal disease among household contacts of case-patients. *JAMA* 1998;279:1206–10.

Rheumatic Fever

Ayoub EM, Majeed HA: Poststreptococcal reactive arthritis. *Curr Opin Rheumatol* 2000;12:306–10.

Bisno AL: Group A streptococcal infections and acute rheumatic fever. *N Engl J Med* 1991;325:783–93.

Dajani AS, Ayoub E, Bierman FZ, et al: Guidelines for the diagnosis of rheumatic fever: Jones criteria, 1992 update. *JAMA* 1992;268:2069–73.

Dajani A, Taubert K, Ferrieri P, et al: Treatment of acute streptococcal pharyngitis and prevention of rheumatic fever: A statement for health professionals. *Pediatrics* 1995;96:758–64.

Stollerman GH: Rheumatic fever. *Lancet* 1997;349:935–42.

Stollerman GH: Rheumatogenic GABHS and the return of ARF. *Adv Intern Med* 1990;35:1–25.

Swedo SE, Leonard HL, Garvey M, et al: Pediatric autoimmune neuropsychiatric disorders associated with streptococcal infections: Clinical description of the first 50 cases. *Am J Psychiatry* 1998; 155:264–71.

Taranta A, Markowitz M: *Rheumatic Fever,* 2nd ed. Dordrecht, Kluwer Academic Publishers, 1989.

Veasy LG, Tani LY, Hill HR: Persistence of acute rheumatic fever in the intermountain area of the United States. *J Pediatr* 1994;124:9–16.

Veasy LG, Weidmeier SE, Orsmond GS, et al: Resurgence of acute rheumatic fever in the intermountain area of the United States. *N Engl J Med* 1987;316:421–7.

Chapter 169
Group B Streptococcus

Catherine S. Lachenauer and Michael R. Wessels

Group B streptococcus (GBS), or *Streptococcus agalactiae*, has been recognized as a major cause of neonatal bacterial sepsis in the United States since the 1960s. While advances in prevention strategies have led to a recent decline in the incidence of neonatal disease, GBS remains a major pathogen for neonates, pregnant women, and immunocompromised nonpregnant adults.

Etiology. Group B streptococci are facultative anaerobic gram-positive cocci that form chains or diplococci in broth and small gray-white colonies on solid medium. GBS is definitively identified by demonstration of the Lancefield group B carbohydrate antigen, such as with latex agglutination techniques widely used in clinical laboratories. Presumptive identification can be established on the basis of a narrow zone of β-hemolysis on blood agar, resistance to bacitracin and trimethoprim-sulfamethoxazole, lack of hydrolysis of bile esculin, and elaboration of cAMP factor (cyclic adenosine monophosphate, an extracellular protein that, in the presence of the beta toxin of *Staphylococcus aureus*, produces a zone of enhanced hemolysis on sheep's blood agar). Individual GBS strains are serologically classified according to the presence of one of the structurally distinct capsular polysaccharides (CPS), which are important virulence factors and stimulators of antibody-associated immunity. To date, nine CPS types have been identified: types Ia, Ib, II, III, IV, V, VI, VII, and VIII.

Epidemiology. GBS emerged as a prominent neonatal pathogen in the late 1960s. For the next 2 decades, the incidence of neonatal GBS disease remained fairly constant, affecting 1–5.4/ 1,000 liveborn infants in the United States. Two patterns of disease were seen: early onset disease, which presents <7 days of age, and late-onset disease, which presents at 7 days of age or later. In the 1990s, widespread implementation of maternal chemoprophylaxis led to a striking 65% decrease in the incidence of early onset neonatal GBS disease in the United States, from 1.7/1,000 live births to 0.6/1,000 live births, whereas the incidence of late-onset disease remained essentially stable at approximately 0.4/1,000 (Fig. 169–1). In other developed countries, rates of neonatal GBS disease are similar to those in the United States during the prechemoprophylaxis era. In the developing world, GBS is not a major cause of neonatal sepsis, even though the prevalence of maternal vaginal colonization with GBS (a major risk factor for neonatal disease) among women from developing countries is similar to that reported among women living in the United States. The incidence of neonatal GBS disease is higher in premature and low-birthweight infants, although most cases occur in full-term infants.

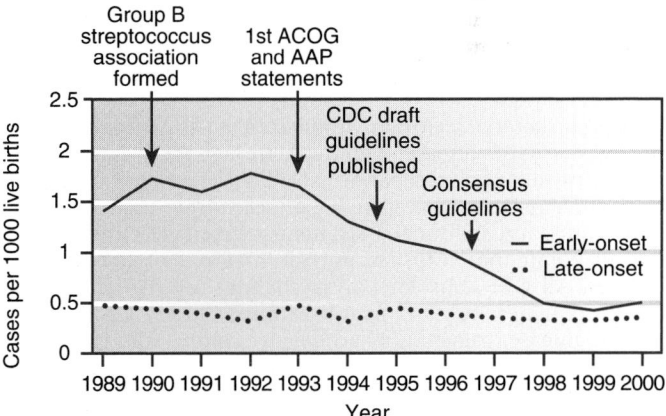

FIGURE 169–1. Incidence of early onset and late-onset invasive group B streptococcus disease in three active surveillance areas (California, Georgia, and Tennessee), 1989 through 2000, and activities for the prevention of group B streptococcus disease. Arrows designate the dates when prevention activities occurred. ACOG, American College of Obstetricians and Gynecologists; AAP, American Academy of Pediatrics. (Adapted from Centers for Disease Control and Prevention: Early-onset group B streptococcal disease—United States, 1998–1999. *MMWR Morb Mortal Wkly Rep* 2000;49:793–6; and Schrag SJ, Zywicki S, Farley MM, et al: Group B streptococcal disease in the era of intrapartum antibiotic prophylaxis. *N Engl J Med* 2000;342:15–20.)

Colonization by GBS in healthy adults is common. Vaginal or rectal colonization occurs in up to approximately 30% of pregnant women and is the usual source for GBS transmission to newborn infants. In the absence of maternal chemoprophylaxis, approximately 50% of infants born to colonized women acquire GBS colonization, and 1–2% of these infants develop invasive disease. Heavy maternal colonization increases the risk of infant colonization and development of early onset disease. Additional risk factors for early onset disease include prolonged rupture of membranes, intrapartum fever, prematurity, maternal bacteriuria during pregnancy, or previous delivery of an infant who developed GBS disease. Risk factors for late onset disease are less well-defined. Whereas late-onset disease may follow vertical transmission, horizontal acquisition from nursery sources also has been described.

GBS is also an important cause of invasive disease in adults. GBS may cause urinary tract infections, bacteremia, endometritis, chorioamnionitis, and wound infection in pregnant and parturient women. In nonpregnant adults with underlying medical conditions such as diabetes mellitus, cirrhosis, or malignancy, GBS may cause serious infections such as bacteremia, skin and soft tissue infections, endocarditis, pneumonia, and meningitis. In the era of maternal chemoprophylaxis, 78% of invasive GBS infections occur in nonpregnant adults.

The serotypes most commonly associated with neonatal GBS disease are types Ia, III, V, Ib, and II. Strains of serotype III are isolated in up to 80–90% of late-onset disease and of meningitis associated with early or late-onset disease. The serotype distribution of colonizing and invasive strains from pregnant women is similar to that from infected newborns. In Japan, serotypes VI and VIII have been reported as common maternal colonizing serotypes, and case reports indicate that type VIII strains may cause neonatal disease indistinguishable from that caused by other serotypes.

Pathogenesis. A major risk factor for the development of early onset neonatal GBS infection is maternal vaginal or rectal colonization by GBS. Infants acquire GBS during passage through the birth canal or, in some cases, via ascending infection. Fetal aspiration of infected amniotic fluid may occur. The incidence of early onset GBS infection increases with the length of rupture of membranes. Infection may also occur through seemingly intact membranes. In cases of late-onset infection, GBS may be vertically transmitted or acquired later from maternal or nonmaternal sources.

Several bacterial factors are implicated in the pathophysiology of invasive GBS disease. Foremost among these is the type-specific capsular polysaccharide. In animals, highly virulent GBS strains elaborate more capsular polysaccharide than do avirulent strains, and, in humans, strains associated with invasive disease elaborate more capsular polysaccharide than do colonizing isolates. All GBS capsular polysaccharides are high molecular weight polymers containing at least three of the following four sugars: glucose, galactose, N-acetylglucosamine, and rhamnose. All contain a short side chain terminating in N-acetylneuraminic acid (sialic acid). Studies in type III GBS show that the sialic acid component of the capsular polysaccharide prevents activation of the alternative complement pathway in the absence of type-specific antibody. Thus, the capsular polysaccharide appears to exert a virulence effect by protecting the organism from opsonophagocytosis in the nonimmune host. In addition, type-specific virulence attributes are suggested by the fact that type III strains are implicated in most cases of late-onset neonatal GBS disease and meningitis. Type III strains are taken up by brain endothelial cells more efficiently in vitro than strains of other serotypes, although studies using acapsular mutant strains demonstrate that it is not the capsule itself that facilitates cellular invasion. Other putative GBS virulence factors include GBS surface proteins, which may play a role in adhesion to host cells;

C5a peptidase, which is postulated to inhibit the recruitment of polymorphonuclear cells into sites of infection; beta hemolysin, which has been associated with cell injury in vitro studies; and hyaluronidase, which has been postulated to act as a spreading factor in host tissues.

Mothers colonized with type III GBS who give birth to healthy infants had higher levels of capsular polysaccharide-specific antibody than women who give birth to infants who developed invasive disease. In addition, there is a high correlation of antibody to type III CPS in mother-infant paired sera. Together, these observations indicate that transplacental transfer of maternal antibody is critically involved in neonatal immunity to GBS. Optimal immunity to GBS also requires an intact complement system. Animal studies using C3- and C4-deficient mice demonstrate that the classic complement pathway is an important component of GBS immunity in the absence of specific antibody, but that antibody-mediated opsonophagocytosis may proceed via the alternative complement pathway. These and other results indicate that anticapsular antibody can overcome the prevention of C3 deposition on the bacterial surface by the sialic acid component of the type III capsule.

The precise steps between GBS colonization and invasive disease remain unclear. In vitro studies showing GBS entry of alveolar epithelium and pulmonary vasculature endothelial cells suggest that GBS may gain access to the bloodstream via invasion from the alveolar space, perhaps following intrapartum aspiration of infected fluid. However, highly encapsulated GBS strains enter eukaryotic cells poorly in vitro compared with capsule-deficient organism, yet they are associated with virulence clinically and in experimental infection models. Additional investigation is needed to define the contribution of GBS entry into host cells in the pathogenesis of GBS infection.

In in vitro and in animal models, GBS induces the release of proinflammatory cytokines. The group B antigen and the peptidoglycan component of the GBS cell wall are potent inducers of tumor necrosis factor (TNF)-α release in vitro, whereas purified type III capsular polysaccharide is not. Wild-type and isogenic unencapsulated mutant GBS strains induced similar amounts of interleukin (IL)-6 or TNF-α in vitro and similar changes in pulmonary vascular resistance and blood gas abnormalities in animals. Thus, it appears that, even though the capsule plays a central role in virulence through avoidance of immune clearance, the capsule does not directly contribute to cytokine release and the resultant inflammatory response.

Clinical Manifestations. Two syndromes of neonatal GBS disease are distinguishable on the basis of age at presentation, epidemiologic characteristics, and clinical features (Table 169–1). **Early onset neonatal GBS disease** presents within the first 7 days of life and is often associated with maternal obstetric complications, including chorioamnionitis, prolonged rupture of membranes, and premature labor. Infants may appear ill at the time of delivery, and most infants become ill within the first 24 hours of birth. In utero infection may result in septic abortion. The most common manifestations of early onset GBS disease are sepsis (50%), pneumonia (30%), and meningitis (15%). Asymptomatic bacteremia is uncommon but can occur. In symptomatic patients, nonspecific signs such as fever, irritability, lethargy, apnea, and bradycardia may be present. Respiratory symptoms are prominent regardless of the presence of pneumonia and include cyanosis, apnea, tachypnea, grunting, flaring, and retractions. A fulminant course with hemodynamic abnormalities including tachycardia, acidosis, and shock may ensue. Persistent fetal circulation may develop. Clinically and radiographically, pneumonia associated with early onset GBS disease is difficult to distinguish from hyaline membrane disease. Patients with meningitis often present with nonspecific findings, with more specific signs of CNS involvement initially being absent.

TABLE 169–1. Characteristics of Early and Late Onset GBS Disease

	Early Onset Disease	Late Onset Disease
Age at onset	0–6 days	7–90 days
Increased risk after obstetric complications	Yes	No
Common clinical manifestations	Sepsis, pneumonia, meningitis	Bacteremia, meningitis, other focal infections
Common serotypes	Ia, III, V, II, Ib	III predominates
Case fatality rate	4.7%	2.8%

Adapted from Schrag SJ, Zywicki S, Farley MM, et al: Group B streptococcal disease in the era of intrapartum antibiotic prophylaxis. N Engl J Med 2000;342:15–20.

Late onset neonatal GBS disease occurs on or after 7 days of life and most commonly manifests as bacteremia (45–60%) and meningitis (25–35%). Focal infections involving bone and joints, skin and soft tissue, the urinary tract, or lungs have been reported in approximately 20% of patients with late-onset disease. Cellulitis and adenitis are often localized to the submandibular or parotid regions. In contrast to early onset disease, maternal obstetric complications are not risk factors for the development of late-onset GBS disease. Infants with late-onset disease are often less severely ill on presentation than infants with early onset disease and the disease is often less fulminant.

Invasive GBS disease in children beyond early infancy is uncommon. In a multistate surveillance study in the 1990s, 2% of all cases of invasive GBS disease were identified in children age 90 days to 14 yr. Two of the more common syndromes associated with childhood GBS disease beyond early infancy are bacteremia and endocarditis. HIV infection should be considered in children with invasive GBS disease beyond the neonatal period.

Diagnosis. A major challenge is distinguishing between hyaline membrane disease and invasive neonatal GBS infection, because the two illnesses share clinical and radiographic features. Severe apnea, early onset of shock, abnormalities in the peripheral leukocyte count, and greater lung compliance may be more likely in infants with GBS disease. Other neonatal pathogens, such as *Escherichia coli* or *Listeria monocytogenes*, may produce illness that is clinically indistinguishable from that due to GBS.

The diagnosis of invasive GBS disease is established by isolation and identification of the organism from a normally sterile site, such as blood, urine, or cerebrospinal fluid (CSF). Isolation of GBS from gastric or tracheal aspirates or from skin or mucous membranes indicates colonization and is not diagnostic of invasive disease. CSF should be examined in all neonates suspected of having sepsis, because specific CNS signs are often absent in the presence of meningitis, especially in early onset disease. Antigen detection methods that use group B polysaccharide-specific antiserum, such as latex particle agglutination, are available for testing of urine, blood, and CSF, but these tests are less sensitive than culture. Moreover, antigen is often detected in urine samples collected by bag from otherwise healthy neonates who are colonized with GBS on the perineum or rectum.

Laboratory Findings. Frequently present are abnormalities in the peripheral white blood cell count, including an increased or decreased absolute neutrophil count, an elevated band count, an elevated ratio of bands to total neutrophils, or leukopenia. Elevations in the C-reactive protein level have been investigated as a potential early marker of GBS sepsis but appear unreliable. Findings on chest radiograph are often indistinguishable from those of hyaline membrane disease and may include reticulogranular patterns, patchy infiltrates, generalized opacification, pleural effusions, or increased interstitial markings.

Treatment. Penicillin G is the treatment of choice of confirmed GBS infection. Initial therapy of neonatal sepsis should include ampicillin and an aminoglycoside, both for the need for broad coverage pending organism identification and for synergistic bactericidal activity. Therapy may be completed with penicillin alone, once GBS has been definitively identified and a good clinical response has occurred. Especially in cases of meningitis, high doses of penicillin (450,000–500,000 U/kg/24 hr) and ampicillin are recommended (300–400 mg/kg/24 hr) because of the relatively high mean inhibitory concentration of penicillin for GBS as well as the potential for a high initial CSF inoculum. Duration of therapy varies according to the site of infection (Table 169–2) and should be guided by clinical circumstances.

In cases of GBS meningitis, some experts recommend that additional CSF be sampled within 24–48 hr to determine whether sterility has been achieved. Persistent GBS growth may indicate an unsuspected intracranial focus or an insufficient antibiotic dose.

Because antibody directed to the capsular polysaccharide has been demonstrated to be protective against GBS infection, administration of intravenous immunoglobulin (IVIG) has been investigated as an adjunctive therapy for neonatal GBS infection. Administration of standard IVIG appears to be safe and well-tolerated, but not clearly of benefit in infants with GBS infection. This may reflect variable and often low concentrations of GBS capsular-specific IgG in normal adults. Attempts have been made at providing large amounts of opsonically active antibody to infants through the use of hyperimmune serum produced by immunizing donors with a GBS vaccine, but to date clinical trials large enough to demonstrate efficacy of hyperimmune IVIG have not been performed.

For recurrent neonatal GBS disease, standard intravenous antibiotic therapy followed by attempted eradication of GBS mucosal colonization has been suggested. This is based on the findings in several studies that invasive isolates from recurrent episodes are often identical to each other and to colonizing strains from the affected infant. Rifampin has most frequently been used for this purpose, but a recent report demonstrates that eradication of GBS colonization in infants is not reliably achieved by rifampin therapy. Optimal management of this uncommon situation remains unclear.

Prognosis. Studies from the 1970s and 1980s showed that up to 30% of infants surviving GBS meningitis had major long-term neurologic sequelae, including developmental delay, spastic quadriplegia, microcephaly, seizure disorder, cortical blindness, or deafness; less severe neurologic complications may be present in other survivors. More contemporary data are not available. Periventricular leukomalacia and severe developmental delay may result from GBS disease and accompanying shock in premature infants, even in the absence of meningitis. The outcome of focal GBS infections outside of the central nervous system, such as bone or soft tissue infections, is generally favorable.

In the 1990s, the case fatality rates associated with early and late-onset neonatal GBS disease were 4.7% and 2.8%, respectively. Mortality is higher in premature infants; one study reported a case fatality rate of 30% in infants whose gestational

TABLE 169–2. Recommended Duration of Therapy for Manifestations of GBS Disease

Treatment	Duration
Bacteremia without a focus	10 days
Meningitis	2–3 wk
Ventriculitis	4 wk
Osteomyelitis	4 wk

Adapted from American Academy of Pediatrics. Group B streptococcal infections. In Pickering, LK, (editor): 2000 Red Book: Report of the Committee on Infectious Diseases, 25th ed, Elk Grove Village, IL, American Academy of Pediatrics, 2000, pp 537–44.

age was <33 wk and 2% in infants whose gestational age was 37 wk or older. The case fatality rate in children aged 3 mo to 14 yr was 9%, and in nonpregnant adults was 11.5%.

Prevention. Persistent morbidity and mortality from perinatal GBS disease despite advances in neonatal care has spurred intense investigation into modes of prevention. Two basic approaches to GBS prevention have been investigated: (1) elimination of colonization from the mother or infant (chemoprophylaxis), and (2) induction of protective immunity (immunoprophylaxis).

CHEMOPROPHYLAXIS. Early studies established that administration of antibiotics to pregnant women before the onset of labor does not reliably eradicate maternal GBS colonization and is not an effective means of preventing neonatal GBS disease. However, interruption of neonatal colonization is achievable through administration of antibiotics to the mother during labor. In a prospective, randomized clinical trial in 1986, infants born to GBS-colonized women with premature labor or prolonged rupture of membranes who were given intrapartum chemoprophylaxis had a substantially lower risk of GBS colonization (9% vs 51%) and of early onset disease (0% vs 6%) than did the infants born to women who were not treated. Maternal postpartum febrile illness was also decreased in the treatment group. This strategy of selective intrapartum chemoprophylaxis, while effective, was not initially widely implemented.

In an effort to enhance prevention practice, specific guidelines for maternal chemoprophylaxis were issued by the Centers for Disease Control and Prevention (CDC) in 1996. These guidelines specified administration of intrapartum antibiotics to women identified as high-risk by either culture-based or risk factor–based criteria. These guidelines were revised in 2002 after epidemiologic data indicated the superior protective effect of the culture-based approach in the prevention of neonatal GBS disease. According to current recommendations, vaginorectal GBS screening cultures should be performed for all pregnant women at 35–37 wk gestation. Any woman with a positive prenatal screening culture, GBS bacteriuria during pregnancy, or a previous infant with invasive GBS disease should receive intrapartum antibiotics. Women whose culture status is unknown (culture not done, incomplete, or results unknown) and who deliver prematurely (<37 wk gestation) or experience prolonged rupture of membranes (≥18 hr) or intrapartum fever (≥38.0°C) should also receive intrapartum chemoprophylaxis. If amnionitis is suspected, broad-spectrum antibiotic therapy that includes an agent active against GBS should replace GBS prophylaxis. Routine intrapartum prophylaxis is not recommended for women with GBS colonization undergoing planned cesarean delivery who have not begun labor or had rupture of membranes.

These guidelines also suggest an approach for the management of infants born to mothers who received intrapartum chemoprophylaxis (Fig. 169–2). Data from a large epidemiologic study indicate that the administration of maternal intrapartum antibiotics does not change the clinical spectrum or delay the onset of clinical signs in infants who developed GBS disease despite maternal prophylaxis. Thus, the CDC guidelines reserve a full diagnostic evaluation for those infants who appear clinically ill or whose mothers are suspected of having chorioamnionitis.

A significant concern with maternal intrapartum prophylaxis has been that large-scale antibiotic use among parturient women might lead to increased rates of antimicrobial resistance or infection in infants with organisms other than GBS. To date, no GBS strains demonstrating resistance to penicillin have been identified, and increases in the incidence of non-GBS early onset neonatal infections have not been demonstrated in most large epidemiologic studies. Continued surveillance is required in this regard. Penicillin remains the preferred agent for chemoprophylaxis, because of its narrow spectrum and the universal penicillin susceptibility of GBS isolates. Because of recent reports indicating

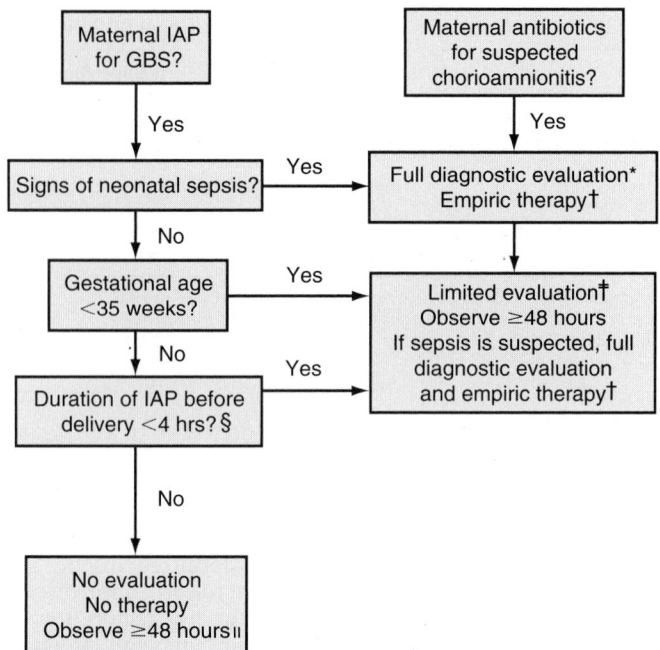

FIGURE 169–2. Empirical management of a newborn whose mother received intrapartum antimicrobial agents for prevention of early onset GBS disease or suspected chorioamnionitis. This algorithm is not an exclusive course of management. Variations that incorporate individual circumstances or institutional preferences may be appropriate. If no maternal intrapartum chemoprophylaxis for GBS was administered despite an indication being present, there are insufficient data available upon which to recommend a single management strategy. *Full diagnostic evaluation includes a complete blood count (CBC) and differential, blood culture, and chest radiograph if respiratory abnormalities are present. When signs of sepsis are present, a lumbar puncture, if feasible, should be performed. †Duration of therapy varies depending on the results of the cultures and laboratory testing and the clinical course of the infant. If laboratory results and clinical course do not indicate bacterial infection, duration may be as short as 48 hr. ‡CBC with differential and blood culture. §Applies only to penicillin, ampicillin, or cefazolin and assumes recommended dosing regimens. ‖A healthy-appearing infant who was ≥38 wk gestational age at delivery and whose mother received ≥4 hr of intrapartum chemoprophylaxis before delivery may be discharged home after 24 hr if other discharge criteria have been met and a person able to comply fully with instructions for home observation will be present. If any of these conditions is not met, the infant should be observed in the hospital for at least 48 hr and until criteria for discharge are achieved. (Adapted from Centers for Disease Control and Prevention: Prevention of perinatal group B streptococcal disease. Revised guidelines from CDC. *MMWR Morb Mortal Wkly Rep* 2002;51[RR-11]:1–22.)

frequent resistance of GBS to erythromycin (up to 25%) and clindamycin (up to 15%), cefazolin should be used in most cases of intrapartum chemoprophylaxis for penicillin-intolerant women. For penicillin-allergic women at high risk for anaphylaxis, clindamycin or erythromycin should be used, if isolates are demonstrated to be susceptible. Vancomycin should be used if isolates are resistant to clindamycin and erythromycin or if susceptibility to these agents is unknown.

A limitation of the maternal chemoprophylaxis strategy is that intrapartum antibiotic use is unlikely to have an impact on late-onset neonatal disease, miscarriages or stillbirths attributed to GBS, or adult GBS disease.

MATERNAL IMMUNIZATION. Another strategy for the prevention of neonatal GBS disease is maternal vaccination. Human studies demonstrate that transplacental transfer of naturally acquired maternal antibody to the GBS capsular polysaccharide protects newborns from invasive GBS infection and that efficient transplacental passage of vaccine-induced GBS antibodies occurs. Conjugate vaccines composed of the GBS capsular polysaccharides coupled to carrier proteins have been produced for human use. In animals, vaccination with these conjugate vaccines induces protective immunity against an otherwise lethal inoculum of GBS in offspring. In early clinical trials, conjugate GBS vaccines were well tolerated and induced levels of functional antibodies well above the range believed to be protective in greater than 90% of recipients. Additional trials are in progress. Administration of a multivalent polysaccharide-protein vaccine before or during pregnancy should lead to transplacental passage of vaccine-induced antibody that protects the fetus and newborn against infection by several GBS serotypes. Such a vaccine would eliminate the need for cumbersome cultures during pregnancy, would circumvent the various risks associated with large-scale antibiotic prophylaxis, and would likely have an impact on both early and late-onset disease. Intrapartum chemoprophylaxis will likely remain an important aspect of prevention, particularly for women in whom opportunities for GBS immunization are missed and for infants born so early that levels of transplacentally acquired antibodies may not be high enough to be protective.

Baker CJ, Kasper DL: Correlation of maternal antibody deficiency with susceptibility to neonatal group B streptococcal infection. *N Engl J Med* 1976;294: 753–6.

Baltimore RS, Huie SM, Meek JI, et al: Early-onset neonatal sepsis in the era of group B streptococcal prevention. *Pediatrics* 2001;108:1094–8.

Boyer KM, Gotoff SP: Prevention of early-onset neonatal group B streptococcal disease with selective intrapartum chemoprophylaxis. *N Engl J Med* 1986;314: 1665–9.

Bromberger P, Lawrence JM, Braun D, et al: The influence of intrapartum antibiotics on the clinical spectrum of early-onset group B streptococcal infection in term infants. *Pediatrics* 2000;106:244–50.

Centers for Disease Control and Prevention: Early-onset group B streptococcal disease—United States, 1998–1999. *MMWR Morb Mortal Wkly Rep* 2000;49: 793–6.

Centers for Disease Control and Prevention: Prevention of perinatal group B streptococcal disease: A public health perspective. *MMWR Morb Mortal Wkly Rep* 1996;45(RR-7):1–24.

Centers for Disease Control and Prevention: Prevention of perinatal group B streptococcal disease. Revised guidelines from CDC. *MMWR Morb Mortal Wkly Rep* 2002;51(RR-11):1–22.

Fernandez M, Rench MA, Albanyan EA, et al: Failure of rifampin to eradicate group B streptococcal colonization in infants. *Pediatr Infect Dis J* 2001;20: 371–6.

Lin F-Y, Azimi P, Weisman LE, et al: Antibiotic susceptibility profiles for group B streptococci isolated from neonates, 1995–1998. *Clin Infect Dis* 2000;31: 76–9.

Lin FYC, Brenner RA, Johnson YR, et al: The effectiveness of risk-based intrapartum chemoprophylaxis for the prevention of early-onset neonatal group B streptococcal disease. *Am J Obstet Gynecol* 2001;184:1204–10.

Lin F-YC, Clemens J, Azimi P, et al: Capsular polysaccharide types of group B streptococcal isolates from neonates with early-onset systemic infection. *J Infect Dis* 1998;177:790–2.

Main E, Slagle T: Prevention of early-onset invasive neonatal group B streptococcal disease in a private hospital setting: The superiority of culture-based protocols. *Am J Obstet Gynecol* 2000;182:1344–54.

Schrag SJ, Zywicki S, Farley MM, et al: Group B streptococcal disease in the era of intrapartum antibiotic prophylaxis. *N Engl J Med* 2000;342:15–20.

Schuchat A: Group B streptococcal disease: From trials and tribulations to triumph and trepidation. *Clin Infect Dis* 2001;33:751–6.

Stoll BJ, Schuchat A: Maternal carriage of group B streptococci in developing countries. *Pediatr Infect Dis J* 1998;17:499–503.

Wessels MR, Butko P, Ma M, et al: Studies of group B streptococcal infection in mice deficient in complement component C3 or C4 demonstrate an essential role for complement in both innate and acquired immunity. *Proc Natl Acad Sci U S A* 1995;92:11490–4.

Yow MD, Mason EO, Leeds LJ, et al: Ampicillin prevents intrapartum transmission of group B streptococcus. *JAMA* 1979;241:1245–7.

Zaleznik DF, Rench MA, Hillier S, et al: Invasive disease due to group B streptococcus in pregnant women and neonates from diverse population groups. *Clin Infect Dis* 2000;30:276–81.

Chapter 170
Non–Group A or B Streptococci *Michael A. Gerber*

The genus *Streptococcus* comprises >30 species. *Streptococcus pneumoniae* (Chapter 167), group A streptococcus (Chapter 168), and group B streptococcus (Chapter 169) are the most common causes of human streptococcal infections. The β-hemolytic streptococci of Lancefield groups C to H and K to O and the nontypable strains that cause α-hemolysis (the **viridans streptococci**) also cause infections in humans (Table 170–1). These organisms commonly colonize intact body surfaces (e.g., the pharynx, skin, gastrointestinal, and genitourinary tracts). Of the non–group A β-hemolytic streptococci, groups C and G streptococcus are the most frequent cause of human disease. Until recently, the enterococci were classified among the group D streptococci but are now a separate genus, *Enterococcus* (Chapter 171).

Group C streptococcus is a much more common cause of infection in animals than in humans. Humans infected with this organism often have had some animal contact. Both group C and group G streptococcus often can be part of the normal human flora of the nasopharynx, skin, and genital tract. Group C streptococcus also can be cultured from the umbilicus of asymptomatic newborns and from routine puerperal vaginal cultures. Group G streptococcus also can be cultured from the gastrointestinal tract. Because of the relatively low virulence of group C and group G streptococci, most humans infected with either of these organisms have some underlying medical disorder (e.g., diabetes mellitus, malignancy, alcohol abuse, immunosuppression).

The clinical features of both group C and group G streptococcal pharyngitis are similar to those of group A streptococcal pharyngitis with fever, mild to moderate sore throat, pharyngeal exudate, and cervical lymphadenitis. Several studies have demonstrated that group C streptococcus is a relatively common cause of acute pharyngitis among college students and among adults who come to an emergency department. In addition to endemic pharyngitis, group C streptococcus can cause epidemic food-borne pharyngitis after ingestion of contaminated products, such as unpasteurized cow's milk. Family and school outbreaks of group C streptococcal pharyngitis have also been described. Group C streptococcus also has been reported as an uncommon cause of a number of other infections, including skin and soft tissue infections, septic arthritis, osteomyelitis, pneumonitis, infective endocarditis, bacteremia and septicemia, meningitis, epiglottitis, pericarditis, urinary tract infections, and sinusitis. These organisms also have been associated with epidemic and nonepidemic cases of puerperal sepsis and endometritis. Recent reports have suggested an association between group C streptococcus and reactive arthritis, as well as a toxic shock–like syndrome.

Even though there have been several well-documented food-borne outbreaks of group G streptococcal pharyngitis, the etiologic role of group G streptococcus in acute, endemic pharyngitis remains unclear. Recently, a community-wide, respiratory outbreak of group G streptococcal pharyngitis in a pediatric population was described in which group G streptococcus was isolated from 56 of 222 (25%) consecutive children with acute pharyngitis seen at a private pediatric office. Results of DNA fingerprinting of the group G streptococcal isolates suggested that 75% of them were the same strain. The patients with group G streptococcal pharyngitis were comparable to those with group A streptococcal pharyngitis with respect to clinical findings, antistreptolysin O titer response, and clinical response to antibiotic therapy. These

TABLE 170–1. Relationship of Streptococci Identified by Lancefield Grouping and Hemolytic Reactions to Sites of Colonization and Disease

	Group A Streptococcus (*S. pyogenes*)	Group B Streptococcus (*S. agalactiae*)	Other β-Hemolytic Streptococci	*Enterococcus*	Viridans Streptococci
Hemolysis	β	β	β	α,β,γ	α
Lancefield group	A	B	C–H, K–V		
Species or strains	M, T types (80)	Serotypes (7)		*E. faecalis* *E. faecium* Many others	*S. bovis* *S. mitis* *S. mutans* *S. sanguis* Many others
Normal flora	Pharynx, skin, anus	Gastrointestinal and genitourinary tracts	Pharynx, skin, gastrointestinal and genitourinary tracts	Gastrointestinal and genitourinary tracts	Pharynx, nose, skin, genitourinary tract
Common human diseases	Pharyngitis, tonsillitis, erysipelas, impetigo, septicemia, wound infections, necrotizing fasciitis, cellulitis, meningitis, pneumonia, scarlet fever, toxic shock–like syndrome, rheumatic fever, acute glomerulonephritis	Puerperal sepsis, chorioamnionitis, endocarditis, neonatal sepsis, meningitis, osteomyelitis, pneumonia	Wound infections, puerperal sepsis, cellulitis, sinusitis, endocarditis, brain abscess, sepsis, nosocomial infections, opportunistic infections	Endocarditis, urinary tract infections, biliary tract infections, peritonitis, wound infections	Endocarditis, human bite infections

α, partial hemolysis; β, complete hemolysis; γ, no hemolysis (nonhemolytic).

findings suggested that antibiotic therapy may have impact on the clinical course of group G streptococcal pharyngitis.

Group G streptococcus has been reported to be an uncommon cause of puerperal sepsis and a neonatal infection that is clinically similar to early onset group B streptococcal disease. Other infections occasionally caused by group G streptococcal include bacteremia, endocarditis, septic arthritis, osteomyelitis, pneumonia, erysipelas and other skin and soft tissue infections, and meningitis. Recently, group G streptococcus has been associated with a toxic shock–like syndrome.

Acute rheumatic fever has not been described as a complication of either group C or group G streptococcal pharyngitis, and, although there have been reports attempting to link acute glomerulonephritis with group G streptococcal pharyngitis, the evidence is anecdotal and a causal relationship has not been established. Acute glomerulonephritis has been reported as a complication of group C streptococcal pharyngitis; however, it is extremely unusual. Therefore, the primary reason to identify either group C or group G streptococcus as the etiologic agent of acute pharyngitis is to initiate antibiotic therapy that may reduce the clinical impact of the illness. However, there is currently no convincing evidence from controlled studies of a clinical response to antibiotic therapy in patients with acute pharyngitis and either group C or group G streptococcus isolated from their upper respiratory tract.

Penicillin is the antibiotic of choice for treating infections due to either group C or group G streptococcus. Pharyngitis usually is treated in a similar manner to group A streptococcal upper respiratory infections, whereas more severe infections require parenteral therapy.

Arditi M, Shulman ST, Davis AT, et al: Group C beta-hemolytic streptococcal infections in children: Nine pediatric cases and review. *Rev Infect Dis* 1989;11: 34–45.

Gerber MA, Randolph MF, Martin NJ, et al: Community-wide outbreak of group C streptococcal pharyngitis. *Pediatrics* 1991;87:598–603.

Meier FA, Centor RM, Graham L Jr, et al: Clinical and microbiological evidence for endemic pharyngitis among adults due to group C streptococci. *Arch Intern Med* 1990;150:825–9.

Turner JC, Hayden FG, Lobo MC, et al: Epidemiologic evidence for Lancefield group C beta-hemolytic streptococci as a cause of exudative pharyngitis in college students. *J Clin Microbiol* 1997;35:1–4.

Chapter 171

Enterococcus David B. Haslam

Enterococcus, long recognized as a pathogen in select populations, in the past 2 decades has become a common and particularly troublesome cause of hospital-acquired infection. These organisms, formerly classified with *Streptococcus bovis* and *Streptococcus equinus* as the Lancefield group D streptococcus, are now placed in a separate genus and are notorious for their frequent resistance to antibiotics.

Etiology. Enterococci are gram-positive, catalase-negative facultative anaerobes that grow in pairs or short chains. Most are nonhemolytic (also called γ-hemolytic) on sheep's blood agar, although some isolates have α- or β-hemolytic activity. Enterococci are distinguished from most Lancefield groupable streptococci by their ability to grow in bile and hydrolyze esculin. Enterococci are able to grow in 6.5% NaCl and hydrolyze L-pyrrolidonyl-β-naphthylamide (the PYR reaction), features used by clinical laboratories to distinguish *Enterococcus* from group D streptococcus. Identification at the species level is enabled by differing patterns of carbohydrate fermentation.

Epidemiology. Enterococci are normal inhabitants of the gastrointestinal tract of humans and animals. Oral secretions and dental plaque, the upper respiratory tract, skin, and vagina may also be colonized by *Enterococcus*. *E. faecalis* is the predominant organism, with colonization commonly occurring in the 1st week of life. By the time of adulthood, *E. faecalis* colonization is nearly ubiquitous. *E. faecium* colonization is less consistent, although approximately 25% of adults harbor this organism.

E. faecalis accounts for 80–90% of enterococcal infections, with almost all of the remaining infections caused by *E. faecium*. Only rarely are other species, such as *E. gallinarium* and *E. cassiliflavus*, associated with invasive infection but these organisms are notable for their intrinsic low-level vancomycin resistance. Typically, the patient's indigenous flora is presumed to be the source of enterococcal infection. However, direct spread from person to person or from contaminated medical devices may occur, particularly within newborn nurseries and intensive care units. Recent studies have demonstrated the importance of nosocomial spread as a source of hospital outbreaks.

Pathogenesis. Enterococci are not aggressively invasive organisms, usually only causing disease in children with damaged mucosal surfaces or impaired immune response. Their dramatic emergence as a cause of nosocomial infection is predominantly due to their resistance to antibiotics commonly used in the hospital setting. Aside from antibiotic resistance genes, few classic virulence factors have been described among enterococci. Adhesion promoting factors likely account for the propensity of these organisms to cause endocarditis and urinary tract infections (UTIs). Many isolates also produce a **cytolysin** that has a broad range of host cells. Released at high bacterial density in a process called quorum sensing, cytolysin contributes to virulence in experimental models of endocarditis, peritonitis, and endophthalmitis. Other proposed virulence factors include aggregation substance, gelatinase, extracellular superoxide, and extracellular surface protein.

ANTIMICROBIAL RESISTANCE. Enterococci are highly resistant to cephalosporins and semisynthetic penicillins such as nafcillin, oxacillin, and methicillin. They are moderately resistant to extended spectrum penicillins such as ticarcillin and carbenicillin. Ampicillin, imipenem, and penicillin are the most active β-lactams against these organisms. Any active drug may be insufficient if used alone for serious infections wherein high bactericidal activity is desired. Some strains of *E. faecalis* produce a plasmid-encoded β-lactamase similar to that found in *Staphylococcus*. These isolates are completely resistant to penicillins, necessitating the combination of a penicillin plus a β-lactamase inhibitor or the use of imipenem or vancomycin.

All enterococci have intrinsic low-level resistance to aminoglycosides because these antibiotics are poorly transported across the *Enterococcus* cell wall (Box 171–1). Concomitant use of a cell wall active agent, such as a β-lactam or glycopeptide antibiotic, improves permeability of the cell wall for the aminoglycosides, resulting in synergistic killing. However, some isolates demonstrate high-level resistance, defined as mean inhibitory concentration (MIC >2,000 μg/mL) due to modification or inactivation of aminoglycoside agents. Strains demonstrating high-level resistance, and even some moderately resistant isolates, are not affected synergistically by aminoglycosides and cell wall–active antibiotics.

Resistance to almost all other antibiotic classes, including tetracyclines, macrolides, and chloramphenicol, has been described among the enterococci, necessitating individual susceptibility testing for these antibiotics when their use is considered. Despite apparent susceptibility in vitro, trimethoprim-sulfamethoxazole has poor activity in vivo, and should not be used as the primary agent against *Enterococcus* infections.

BOX 171–1. Antimicrobial Resistance of *Enterococcus*

INTRINSIC RESISTANCE (CHROMOSOMALLY ENCODED)
Aminoglycosides (low level)
β-lactams (especially semisynthetic penicillins and cephalosporins)
Trimethoprim-sulfamethoxazole
Clindamycin (low level)

ACQUIRED RESISTANCE
Aminoglycosides (high level)
Chloramphenicol
Erythromycin and high-level clindamycin
Quinolones
Penicillins (β-lactamase)
Tetracyclines
Vancomycin
Streptogammins
Oxazolidinones

Vancomycin has traditionally been effective against multiresistant isolates, but resistance to vancomycin and other glycopeptides, including teicoplanin and daptomycin, is increasingly common. Both high- and moderate-level resistance are described in *E. faecalis* and *E. faecium*. High-level resistance (MIC ≥ 64 μg/mL) can be transferred by way of conjugation and is usually due to plasmid-mediated transfer of the *vanA* gene. High-level resistance is most common among *E. fecium* but is increasingly seen among *E. faecalis* isolates. Moderate-level resistance (MIC 8–256 μg/mL) results from a chromosomal homologue of *vanA*, known as *vanB*. Isolates that harbor the *vanB* gene are only moderately resistant to vancomycin and initially demonstrate susceptibility to teicoplanin, although resistance can emerge during therapy.

Clinical Manifestations. Among pediatric patients, *Enterococcus* infections traditionally occurred predominantly in newborn infants. However, infection in older children is increasingly common. Most *Enterococcus* infections occur in patients with breakdown of normal physical barriers such as the gastrointestinal tract, skin, or urinary tract. Other risk factors for *Enterococcus* infection include prolonged hospitalization, indwelling vascular catheters, prior use of antibiotics, and compromised immunity.

NEONATAL INFECTIONS. *Enterococcus* accounts for up to 15% of all neonatal bacteremia and septicemia. Like group B streptococcus infections, *Enterococcus* infections are seen in two distinct settings in neonatal patients. Early onset infection (<7 days of age) may mimic early onset group B streptococcus septicemia, but tends to be milder. Early onset *Enterococcus* sepsis most often occurs in full-term infants who are otherwise healthy. Late-onset infection (≥7 days of age) is associated with risk factors such as extreme prematurity, presence of an intravascular catheter, or necrotizing enterocolitis, or it follows an intra-abdominal surgical procedure. Symptoms in late-onset disease are more severe than those in early onset disease and include apnea, bradycardia, and deteriorating respiratory function. Focal infections such as scalp abscess and catheter infection are commonly associated. Mortality rates range from 6% in early onset septicemia to 15% in late-onset infections associated with necrotizing enterocolitis.

Enterococci are an occasional cause of meningitis. In neonates in particular, meningitis usually occurs as a complication of septicemia. Alternatively, the organism may gain access to the central nervous system by way of contiguous spread, such as through neural tube defect or in association with an intraventricular shunt. *Enterococcus* meningitis can be associated with minimal abnormality of cerebrospinal fluid.

INFECTIONS IN OLDER CHILDREN. *Enterococcus* rarely causes UTI in healthy children, but accounts for approximately 15% of cases of nosocomially acquired UTI, both in children and adults. Presence of an indwelling urinary catheter is the major risk factor for nosocomial UTI. Enterococci are frequently isolated in intra-abdominal infections following intestinal perforation or surgery. Their significance in polymicrobial infections has been questioned, although reported mortality rates are higher when intra-abdominal infections include *Enterococcus*. *Enterococcus* is less commonly associated with bacteremia and endocarditis in children than in adults. Predisposing factors include an indwelling central venous catheter, gastrointestinal surgery, immunodeficiency, and cardiovascular abnormalities.

Treatment. Treatment of invasive *Enterococcus* infections must recognize that these organisms are frequently resistant to antimicrobial agents. In general, in the immunocompetent host, minor localized infections due to *Enterococcus* can be treated with ampicillin alone. Antibiotics containing β-lactamase inhibitors (clavulanate or sulbactam) provide advantage only for the few organisms whose resistance is due to production of β-lactamase. In uncomplicated UTIs, nitrofurantoin is efficacious when the organism is known to be sensitive to this antibiotic.

Invasive infections such as sepsis, meningitis, and endocarditis are usually treated with a combination of penicillin or ampicillin and an aminoglycoside when the isolate is susceptible. Vancomycin can be substituted for the penicillins in allergic patients, but should be used with an aminoglycoside, because vancomycin alone is not bacteriocidal. Endocarditis from strains possessing high-level aminoglycoside resistance may relapse even after prolonged therapy. High-dose or continuous infusion penicillin has been proposed for treatment of these infections in adults, yet ultimately valve replacement may be necessary. In patients with catheter-associated enterococcal bacteremia, the catheter should be removed promptly in almost all cases.

VANCOMYCIN-RESISTANT *ENTEROCOCCUS*. The treatment of serious infections due to multiresistant, vancomycin-resistant strains is particularly challenging. Quinupristin–dalfopristin is a combined streptogammin antibiotic that inhibits bacterial protein synthesis at two different stages. It has activity against most *E. faecium* strains, including those with high-level vancomycin resistance. Approximately 90% of *E. faecium* strains are susceptible to quinupristin–dalfopristin in vitro. Notably, it is inactive against *E. faecalis* and therefore should not be used as the sole agent against gram-positive organisms until culture results exclude the presence of *E. faecalis*. Studies in children suggest that this antibiotic is effective and generally well tolerated. Emergence of resistance to quinupristin–dalfopristin is rare, but has been demonstrated.

Linezolid, an oxazolidinone antibiotic that inhibits protein synthesis, is bacteriostatic against most *E. faecium* and *E. faecalis*, including vancomycin-resistant isolates. Response rates are generally >90%, including cases of bacteremia and sepsis. Anecdotal reports reveal the success of linezolid in treating meningitis due to vancomycin-resistant enterococci. As seen with other antibiotics, however, linezolid resistance is documented and nosocomial spread of these organisms can occur.

Prevention. Strategies for preventing enterococcal infections include early removal of urinary and intravenous catheters and debridement of necrotic tissue. Infection control strategies, including surveillance cultures, patient and staff cohorting, and strict gown and glove isolation are effective at decreasing colonization rates with vancomycin-resistant enterococci. However, these organisms may persist on inanimate objects, such as stethoscopes, complicating efforts to limit their nosocomial spread. To prevent the emergence and spread of vancomycin-resistant organisms, the Centers for Disease Control and Prevention has developed a series of guidelines for prudent vancomycin use.

Bonten MJ, Willems R, Weinstein RA: Vancomycin-resistant enterococci: Why are they here, and where do they come from? *Lancet Infect Dis* 2001;1:314–25.

Centers for Disease Control and Prevention: Recommendations for preventing the spread of vancomycin resistance. Hospital Infection Control Practices Advisory Committee (HICPAC). *MMWR Morbid mortal Wkly Rep* 1995;44(RR-12):1–130.

Gray JW, George RH: Experience of vancomycin-resistant enterococci in a children's hospital. *J Hosp Infect* 2000;45:11–8.

Linden PK: Treatment options for vancomycin-resistant enterococcal infections. *Drugs* 2002;62:425–41.

Malik RK, Montecalvo MA, Reale MR, et al: Epidemiology and control of vancomycin-resistant enterococci in a regional neonatal intensive care unit. *Pediatr Infect Dis J* 1999;18:352–6.

Moellering RC: Quinupristin/dalfopristin: Therapeutic potential for vancomycin-resistant enterococcal infections. *J Antimicrob Chemother* 1999;44:25–30.

Murray BE, Weinstock GM: Enterococci: New aspects of an old organism. *Proc Assoc Am Physicians* 1999;111:328–34.

Ostrowsky BE, Trick WE, Sohn AH, et al: Control of vancomycin-resistant *Enterococcus* in health care facilities in a region. *N Engl J Med* 2001;344:1427–33.

Ray AJ, Hoyen CK, Taub TF, et al: Nosocomial transmission of vancomycin-resistant enterococci from surfaces. *JAMA* 2002;287:1400–1.

Sitges-Serra A, Lopez MJ, Girvent M, et al: Postoperative enterococcal infection after treatment of complicated intra-abdominal sepsis. *Br J Surg* 2002;89:361–76.

Sohn, AH, Garrett DO, Sinkowitz-Cochran RL, et al: Prevalence of nosocomial infections in neonatal intensive care unit patients: Results from the first national point-prevalence survey. *J Pediatr* 2001;139:821–7.

Zachary KC, Bayne PS, Morrison VJ, et al: Contamination of gowns, gloves, and stethoscopes with vancomycin-resistant enterococci. *Infect Control Hosp Epidemiol* 2001;22:560–7.

Zeana C, Kubin CJ, Della-Latta P, et al: Vancomycin-resistant *Enterococcus faecium* meningitis successfully managed with linezolid: Case report and review of the literature. *Clin Infect Dis* 2001;33:477–82.

Chapter 172

Diphtheria (*Corynebacterium diphtheriae*) *Sarah S. Long*

Diphtheria is an acute toxic infection caused by *Corynebacterium diphtheriae*. Diphtheria was the first infectious disease to be conquered on the basis of principles of microbiology, immunology, and public health. Although diphtheria was reduced from a major cause of childhood death in the Western hemisphere in the early 20th century to a medical rarity, modern reminders of the fragility of such success underscore the need to apply those same principles assiduously in an era of vaccine dependence and a single global community.

Etiology. *Corynebacterium* is an aerobic, nonencapsulated, non–spore-forming, mostly nonmotile, pleomorphic, gram-positive bacillus. Not fastidious in growth requirements, its isolation is enhanced by use of a selective medium (i.e., cystine-tellurite blood agar) that inhibits growth of competing organisms and, when reduced by *C. diphtheriae*, renders colonies gray-black. Three biotypes (i.e., *mitis*, *gravis*, and *intermedius*), each capable of causing diphtheria, are differentiated by colonial morphology, hemolysis, and fermentation reactions. A lysogenic bacteriophage carrying the gene that encodes for production of exotoxin confers diphtheria-producing potential to strains of *C. diphtheriae*, but it provides no essential protein to the bacterium. Indigenous nontoxigenic *C. diphtheriae* can be rendered toxigenic and disease-producing after importation of toxigenic *C. diphtheriae*. Diphtheritic toxin can be demonstrated in vitro by the agar immunoprecipitin technique (Elek test), by polymerase chain reaction, or by the in vivo toxin neutralization test in guinea pigs. Toxigenic and nontoxigenic strains are indistinguishable by colony type, microscopy, or biochemical tests.

Epidemiology. Unlike other **diphtheroids (coryneform bacteria)**, which are ubiquitous in nature, *C. diphtheriae* is an exclusive inhabitant of human mucous membranes and skin. Spread is primarily by airborne respiratory droplets, direct contact with respiratory secretions of symptomatic individuals, or exudate from infected skin lesions. Asymptomatic respiratory tract carriers are important in transmission. Where diphtheria is endemic, 3–5% of healthy individuals may harbor toxigenic organisms, but carriage is exceedingly rare if diphtheria is rare. Skin infection and skin carriage are silent reservoirs of diphtheria. Viability in dust and on fomites for up to 6 mo has less epidemiologic significance. Transmission through contaminated milk and an infected food handler has been proved or suspected.

In the 1920s, more than 125,000 cases and 10,000 deaths due to diphtheria were reported annually in the United States, with highest fatality rates among very young and elderly patients. From 1921–1924, diphtheria was the leading cause of death among Canadian children 2–14 yr of age. The incidence then began to decrease, and with the widespread use of diphtheria toxoid in the United States after World War II, it declined steadily, with dramatic reductions in the latter 1970s. Since then, there have been five or fewer cases per year and no epidemics of respiratory tract diphtheria. Similar decreases occurred in Europe.

Although disease incidence has decreased worldwide, diphtheria remains endemic in many developing countries.

When diphtheria was endemic, it primarily affected children <15 yr of age, but epidemiology has shifted to adults who lack natural exposure to toxigenic *C. diphtheriae* in the vaccine era and have low rates of booster vaccinations. In the 27 sporadic cases of respiratory tract diphtheria reported in the United States in the 1980s, 70% occurred in persons >25 yr of age. The largest outbreak of diphtheria in the developed world since the 1960s occurred from 1990–1996 throughout the newly independent countries of the former Soviet Union, causing >150,000 cases in 14 of 15 countries. More than 60% of cases occurred in individuals >14 yr of age. Case fatality rates ranged from 3–23% by state. Factors contributing to the epidemic included a large population of underimmunized adults, decreased childhood immunization, population migration, crowding, and failure to respond aggressively during early phases of the epidemic. Cases of diphtheria among travelers from these endemic areas were transported to many countries in Europe.

Most proven cases of respiratory tract diphtheria in the United States in the 1990s have been associated with importation of toxigenic *C. diphtheriae*, although clonally related, toxigenic *C. diphtheriae* has been demonstrated to persist in the United States and Canada for at least 25 years despite rarity of cases. Protection from serious disease from importation or indigenous exposure depends on immunization.

The estimated minimum protective level of diphtheria antitoxin is 0.01–0.1 IU/mL; the precise protective limit has not been defined. In outbreaks, 90% of individuals with clinical disease have had antibody values <0.01 IU/mL, and 92% of asymptomatic carriers have had values >0.1 IU/mL. In serosurveys in the United States and Western Europe where almost universal immunization during childhood has been achieved, 25% to more than 60% of adults lack protective antitoxin levels, with very low levels especially in the elderly.

Cutaneous diphtheria, a curiosity when diphtheria was common, accounted for >50% of *C. diphtheriae* isolates reported in the United States by 1975. This indolent local infection, compared with mucosal infection, is associated with more prolonged bacterial shedding, increased contamination of the environment, and increased transmission to the pharynx and skin of close contacts. Outbreaks are associated with homelessness, crowding, poverty, alcoholism, poor hygiene, contaminated fomites, underlying dermatosis, and introduction of new strains from exogenous sources. No longer a tropical or subtropical disease, 1,100 *C. diphtheriae* infections were documented in a neighborhood in Seattle, WA, from 1971–1982; 86% were cutaneous, and 40% involved toxigenic strains. Cutaneous diphtheria is an important reservoir for toxigenic *C. diphtheriae* in the United States and is a frequent mode of importation of source cases for subsequent sporadic respiratory tract diphtheria. In an attempt to focus attention on respiratory tract diphtheria, which is much more likely to cause acute obstructive complications and toxic manifestations, skin isolates of *C. diphtheriae* were removed from annual diphtheria statistics reported by the Centers for Disease Control and Prevention (CDC) after 1979.

Pathogenesis. Toxigenic and nontoxigenic *C. diphtheriae* organisms cause skin and mucosal infection and rarely can cause focal infection after bacteremia. The organism usually remains in the superficial layers of skin lesions or respiratory tract mucosa, inducing local inflammatory reaction. The major virulence of the organism lies in its ability to produce the potent 62-kd polypeptide exotoxin, which inhibits protein synthesis and causes local tissue necrosis. Within the first few days of respiratory tract infection, a dense necrotic coagulum of organisms, epithelial cells, fibrin, leukocytes, and erythrocytes forms, advances, and becomes a gray-brown adherent **pseudomem-brane.** Removal is difficult and reveals a bleeding edematous submucosa. Paralysis of the palate and hypopharynx is an early local effect of the toxin. Toxin absorption can lead to necrosis of kidney tubules, thrombocytopenia, cardiomyopathy, and demyelination of nerves. Because the latter two complications can occur 2–10 wk after mucocutaneous infection, the pathophysiologic mechanism in some cases is suspected to be immunologically mediated.

Clinical Manifestations. The manifestations of *C. diphtheriae* infection are influenced by the anatomic site of infection, the immune status of the host, and the production and systemic distribution of toxin.

RESPIRATORY TRACT DIPHTHERIA. In the classic description of 1,400 cases of diphtheria in California in 1954, the primary focus of infection was the tonsils or pharynx in 94%, with the nose and larynx being the next two most common sites. After an average incubation period of 2–4 days, local signs and symptoms of inflammation develop. Infection of the anterior nares, which is more common among infants, causes serosanguineous, purulent, erosive rhinitis with membrane formation. Shallow ulceration of the external nares and upper lip is characteristic. In tonsillar and pharyngeal diphtheria, sore throat is a universal early symptom, but only half of patients have fever, and fewer have dysphagia, hoarseness, malaise, or headache. Mild pharyngeal injection is followed by unilateral or bilateral tonsillar membrane formation, which extends variably to affect the uvula, soft palate, posterior oropharynx, hypopharynx, and glottic areas. Underlying soft tissue edema and enlarged lymph nodes can cause a **bull-neck appearance**. The degree of local extension correlates directly with profound prostration, bull-neck appearance, and fatality due to airway compromise or toxin-mediated complications.

The leather-like adherent membrane, extension beyond the faucial area, relative lack of fever, and dysphagia help differentiate diphtheria from exudative pharyngitis due to group A streptococcus and Epstein-Barr virus. Vincent angina, infective phlebitis and thrombosis of the jugular veins, and mucositis in patients undergoing cancer chemotherapy are usually differentiated by the clinical setting. Infection of the larynx, trachea, and bronchi can be primary or a secondary extension from the pharyngeal infection. Hoarseness, stridor, dyspnea, and croupy cough are clues. Differentiation from bacterial epiglottitis, severe viral laryngotracheobronchitis, and staphylococcal or streptococcal tracheitis hinges partially on the relative paucity of other signs and symptoms in patients with diphtheria and primarily on visualization of the adherent pseudomembrane at the time of laryngoscopy and intubation.

Patients with laryngeal diphtheria are highly prone to suffocation because of edema of soft tissues and the obstructing dense cast of respiratory epithelium and necrotic coagulum. Establishment of an artificial airway and resection of the pseudomembrane are lifesaving, but further obstructive complications are common, and systemic toxic complications are inevitable.

CUTANEOUS DIPHTHERIA. Classic cutaneous diphtheria is an indolent, nonprogressive infection characterized by a superficial, ecthymic, nonhealing ulcer with a gray-brown membrane. Diphtheritic skin infections cannot always be differentiated from streptococcal or staphylococcal impetigo, and they frequently coexist. In most cases, underlying dermatoses, lacerations, burns, bites, or impetigo have become secondarily contaminated. Extremities are more often affected than the trunk or head. Pain, tenderness, erythema, and exudate are typical. Local hyperesthesia or hypesthesia is unusual. Respiratory tract colonization or symptomatic infection and toxic complications occur in the minority of patients with cutaneous diphtheria. Among infected Seattle adults, 3% with cutaneous infections and 21% with symptomatic nasopharyngeal infection, with or without skin involvement, had toxic myocarditis, neuropathy, or obstructive respiratory tract complications. All had received at least 20,000 U of equine antitoxin at the time of hospitalization.

INFECTION AT OTHER SITES. *C. diphtheriae* occasionally causes mucocutaneous infections at other sites, such as the ear (otitis externa), eye (purulent and ulcerative conjunctivitis), and genital tract (purulent and ulcerative vulvovaginitis). The clinical setting, ulceration, membrane formation, and submucosal bleeding help differentiate diphtheria from other bacterial and viral causes. Rare cases of septicemia are described and are universally fatal. Sporadic cases of endocarditis occur, and clusters among intravenous drug users have been reported in several countries; skin was the probable portal of entry, and almost all strains were nontoxigenic. Sporadic cases of pyogenic arthritis, mainly due to nontoxigenic strains, have been reported in adults and children. Diphtheroids isolated from sterile body sites should not be dismissed as contaminants without careful consideration of the clinical setting.

TOXIC CARDIOMYOPATHY. Toxic cardiomyopathy occurs in approximately 10–25% of patients with diphtheria and is responsible for 50–60% of deaths. Subtle signs of myocarditis can be detected in most patients, especially the elderly, but the risk for significant complications correlates directly with the extent and severity of exudative local oropharyngeal disease and delay in administration of antitoxin. The first evidence of cardiac toxicity characteristically occurs in the 2nd–3rd wk of illness as pharyngeal disease improves but can appear acutely as early as the 1st wk, when a fatal outcome is likely, or insidiously as late as the 6th wk of illness. Tachycardia out of proportion to fever is common and may be evidence of cardiac toxicity or autonomic nervous system dysfunction. A prolonged PR interval and changes in the ST-T wave on an electrocardiographic tracing are relatively frequent findings, and dilated and hypertrophic cardiomyopathy detected by echocardiogram have been described. Single or progressive cardiac dysrhythmias can occur, such as first-, second-, and third-degree heart block; atrioventricular dissociation; and ventricular tachycardia. Clinical congestive heart failure may have an insidious or acute onset. Elevation of the serum aspartate aminotransferase concentration closely parallels the severity of myonecrosis. Severe dysrhythmia portends death. Histologic postmortem findings may show little or diffuse myonecrosis with acute inflammatory response. Recovery from toxic myocardiopathy is usually complete, although survivors of more severe dysrhythmias can have permanent conduction defects.

TOXIC NEUROPATHY. Neurologic complications parallel the extent of primary infection and are multiphasic in onset. Acutely or 2–3 wk after onset of oropharyngeal inflammation, hypesthesia and local paralysis of the soft palate occur commonly. Weakness of the posterior pharyngeal, laryngeal, and facial nerves may follow, causing a nasal quality in the voice, difficulty in swallowing, and risk of death due to aspiration. Cranial neuropathies characteristically occur in the 5th wk and lead to oculomotor and ciliary paralysis, which are manifested as strabismus, blurred vision, or difficulty with accommodation. Symmetric polyneuropathy has its onset 10 days–3 mo after oropharyngeal infection and causes principally motor deficits with diminished deep tendon reflexes. Proximal muscle weakness of the extremities progressing distally and, more commonly, distal weakness progressing proximally have been described. Clinical and cerebrospinal fluid findings in the latter are indistinguishable from those of Guillain-Barré syndrome. Paralysis of the diaphragm can ensue. Complete recovery is likely. Rarely, 2–3 wk after onset of illness, dysfunction of the vasomotor centers can cause hypotension or cardiac failure.

Diagnosis. Specimens for culture should be obtained from the nose and throat and any other mucocutaneous lesion. A portion of membrane should be removed and submitted with underlying exudate. The laboratory must be notified to use selective medium. *C. diphtheriae* survives drying. In remote areas, a swab specimen can be placed in a silica gel pack and sent to a reference laboratory. Evaluation of a direct smear using Gram stain or specific fluorescent antibody is unreliable. Culture isolates of coryneform organisms should be identified to the species level, and toxigenicity and antimicrobial susceptibility tests should be performed for *C. diphtheriae* isolates.

Treatment. Specific antitoxin is the mainstay of therapy and should be administered on the basis of clinical diagnosis, because it neutralizes only free toxin. Efficacy diminishes with elapsing time after the onset of mucocutaneous symptoms. Equine diphtheria antitoxin is available in the United States only from the CDC. Physicians treating a case of suspected diphtheria can contact the CDC diphtheria duty officer (404-639-8255, 8 AM–4:30 PM ET; 404-639-2889, all other times). Antitoxin is administered as a single empirical dose of 20,000–120,000 U based on the degree of toxicity, site and size of the membrane, and duration of illness. Antitoxin is probably of no value for local manifestations of cutaneous diphtheria, but its use is prudent because toxic sequelae can occur. Commercially available intravenous immunoglobulin preparations contain low titers of antibodies to diphtheria toxin; their use for therapy of diphtheria is not proved or approved. Antitoxin is not recommended for asymptomatic carriers.

Antimicrobial therapy is indicated to halt toxin production, treat localized infection, and prevent transmission of the organism to contacts. *C. diphtheriae* is usually susceptible to various agents in vitro, including penicillins, erythromycin, clindamycin, rifampin, and tetracycline. Resistance to erythromycin is common in populations if the drug has been used broadly. Only penicillin or erythromycin is recommended; erythromycin is marginally superior to penicillin for eradication of nasopharyngeal carriage. Appropriate therapy is erythromycin (40–50 mg/kg/24 hr divided q 6 hr PO or IV; maximum: 2 g/24 hr), aqueous crystalline penicillin G (100,000–150,000 U/kg/24 hr divided q 5 h IV or IM), or procaine penicillin (25,000–50,000 U/kg/24 hr divided q 12 h IM). Antibiotic therapy is not a substitute for antitoxin therapy. Therapy is given for 14 days. Some patients with cutaneous diphtheria have been treated for 7–10 days. Elimination of the organism should be documented by at least two successive cultures from the nose and throat (or skin) obtained 24 hr apart after completion of therapy. Treatment with erythromycin is repeated if the culture result is positive.

Patients with pharyngeal diphtheria are placed in respiratory isolation, and patients with cutaneous diphtheria are placed in contact isolation until the cultures taken after cessation of therapy are negative. Cutaneous wounds are cleaned thoroughly with soap and water. Bed rest is essential during the acute phase of disease, usually for 2 wk or more until the risk of symptomatic cardiac damage has passed, with a return to physical activity guided by the degree of toxicity and cardiac involvement.

Complications. Respiratory tract obstruction by pseudomembranes may require bronchoscopy or intubation and mechanical ventilation. Recovery from the myocarditis and neuritis is often slow but usually complete. Corticosteroids do not diminish these complications and are not recommended.

Prognosis. The prognosis for patients with diphtheria depends on the virulence of the organism (subspecies *gravis* has the highest fatality), age, immunization status, site of infection, and speed of administration of the antitoxin. Mechanical obstruction from laryngeal diphtheria or bull-neck diphtheria and the complications of myocarditis account for most diphtheria-related deaths.

The case fatality rate of almost 10% for respiratory tract diphtheria has not changed in 50 yr; the rate was 18% in a Swedish outbreak in the 1990s. At recovery, administration of diphtheria toxoid is indicated to complete the primary series or booster doses of immunization, because not all patients develop antibodies after infection.

Prevention. All suspected diphtheria cases should be reported to local and state health departments. Investigation is aimed at preventing secondary cases in exposed individuals and at determining the source and carriers to halt spread to unexposed individuals. Reported rates of carriage in household contacts of case patients are 0–25%. The risk of developing diphtheria after household exposure to a case is approximately 2%, and the risk is 0.3% after similar exposure to a carrier.

ASYMPTOMATIC CASE CONTACTS. All household contacts and those who have had intimate respiratory or habitual physical contact with a patient are closely monitored for illness through the 7-day incubation period. Cultures of the nose, throat, and any cutaneous lesions are performed. Antimicrobial prophylaxis is given, regardless of immunization status, using erythromycin (40–50 mg/kg/24 hr divided qid PO for 7 days; maximum: 2 g/24 hr) or a single injection of benzathine penicillin G (600,000 U IM for <30 kg, 1,200,000 U IM for ≥30 kg). The efficacy of antimicrobial prophylaxis is presumed but not proved. Diphtheria toxoid vaccine, in age-appropriate form, is given to immunized individuals who have not received a booster dose within 5 yr. Children who have not received their fourth dose should be vaccinated. Those who have received fewer than three doses of diphtheria toxoid or who have uncertain immunization status are immunized with age-appropriate preparation on a primary schedule.

ASYMPTOMATIC CARRIERS. When an asymptomatic carrier is identified, antimicrobial prophylaxis is given for 7 days and an age-appropriate preparation of diphtheria toxoid is administered immediately if a booster has not been given within 1 yr. Individuals are placed in respiratory isolation (respiratory tract colonization) or contact isolation (cutaneous colonization only) until at least two subsequent cultures obtained 24 hr apart after cessation of therapy are negative.

Repeat cultures are performed ≥2 wk after completion of therapy for cases and carriers, and, if positive, an additional 10-day course of oral erythromycin should be given and follow-up cultures performed. Susceptibility testing of isolates should be performed as erythromycin resistance is reported. Neither antimicrobial agent eradicates carriage in 100% of individuals. In one report, 21% of carriers had failure of eradication after a single course of therapy. Antitoxin is not recommended for asymptomatic close contacts or carriers, even if inadequately immunized. Transmission of diphtheria in modern hospitals is rare. Only those with an unusual contact with respiratory or oral secretions should be managed as contacts. Investigation of the casual contacts of patients and carriers or persons in the community without known exposure has yielded extremely low carriage rates and is not routinely recommended.

VACCINE. Universal immunization with diphtheria toxoid throughout life to provide constant protective antitoxin levels and to reduce indigenous *C. diphtheriae* is the only effective control measure. Although immunization does not preclude subsequent respiratory or cutaneous carriage of toxigenic *C. diphtheriae*, it decreases local tissue spread, prevents toxic complications, diminishes transmission of the organism, and provides herd immunity when at least 70–80% of a population is immunized.

Diphtheria toxoid is prepared by formaldehyde treatment of toxin, standardized for potency, and adsorbed to aluminum salts, which enhance immunogenicity. Two preparations of diphtheria toxoids are formulated according to the limit of flocculation (Lf) content, a measure of the quantity of toxoid. The pediatric preparation (i.e., DTaP, DT, DTP) contains 6.7–25.0 Lf units of diphtheria toxoid per 0.5-mL dose; the adult preparation (i.e., dT) contains no more than 2 Lf units of toxoid per 0.5-mL dose. The higher-potency (i.e., D) formulation of toxoid is used for primary series and booster doses for children through 6 yr of age because of superior immunogenicity and minimal reactogenicity. For individuals 7 yr of age or older, dT is recommended for the primary series and booster doses because the lower concentration of diphtheria toxoid is adequately immunogenic and because increasing the content of diphtheria toxoid heightens reactogenicity with increasing age.

For children from 6 wk to their 7th birthday, five 0.5-mL doses of diphtheria-containing (D) vaccine are given in a primary series, including three doses at 2, 4, and 6 mo of age, with a fourth dose, an integral part of the primary series, 6–12 mo after the third dose. A booster dose is given at 4–6 yr of age (unless the fourth primary dose was administered after the 4th birthday). For persons 7 yr of age and older, three 0.5-mL doses of diphtheria-containing (d) vaccine are given in a primary series of two doses 4–8 wk apart and a third dose 6–12 mo after the second dose. The only contraindication to tetanus and diphtheria toxoid is a history of neurologic or severe hypersensitivity reaction after a previous dose. For children <7 yr of age in whom pertussis immunization is contraindicated, DT is used. Those begun with DTaP, DTP, or DT before 1 yr of age should have a total of five 0.5-mL doses of diphtheria-containing (D) vaccines by 6 yr of age. For those beginning ≥1 yr of age, the primary series is three 0.5-mL doses of diphtheria-containing (D) vaccine, with a booster given at 4–6 yr, unless the third dose was given after the 4th birthday.

Booster doses of 0.5 mL of dT should be given every 10 yr starting at 11–12 yr of age and no later than by 16 yr of age. Vaccination with diphtheria toxoid should be used whenever tetanus toxoid is indicated, to ensure continuing diphtheria immunity.

There is no known association of DT or dT with increased risk of convulsions. Local side effects alone do not preclude continued use. Persons who experience Arthus-type hypersensitivity reactions or a temperature ≥103°F (39.4°C) after a dose of dT (rare in childhood) usually have high serum tetanus antitoxin levels and should not be given dT more frequently than every 10 yr, even if a significant tetanus-prone injury is sustained. DT or dT preparation can be given concurrently with other vaccines. *Haemophilus influenzae* conjugate vaccines containing diphtheria toxoid (PRP-D) or the variant of diphtheria toxin, CRM_{197} protein (HbOC), are not substitutes for diphtheria toxoid immunization and do not appear to affect reactogenicity.

Bisgard KM, Hardy IR, Popovic T, et al: Respiratory diphtheria in the United States, 1980 through 1995. *Am J Public Health* 1998;88:787–91.

Centers for Disease Control and Prevention: Availability of diphtheria antitoxin through an investigational new drug protocol. *MMWR Morb Mortal Wkly Rep* 1997;46:380.

Gupta RK, Griffin P Jr, Xu J, et al: Diphtheria antitoxin levels in US blood and plasma donors. *J Infect Dis* 1996;173:1493–7.

Kneen R, Giao PN, Solomon T, et al: Penicillin vs. erythromycin in the treatment of diphtheria. *Clin Infect Dis* 1998;27:845–50.

Marston CK, Famieson F, Cahoon F, et al: Persistence of a distinct *Corynebacterium diphtheriae* clonal group within two communities in the United States and Canada where diphtheria is endemic. *J Clin Microbiol* 2001;1586–90.

Scheifele DW, Dobson S, Kallos A, et al: Comparative safety of tetanus-diphtheria toxoids booster immunization in students in grades 6 and 9. *Pediatr Infect Dis J* 1998;17:1121–6.

Vitek CR, Wharton M: Diphtheria in the former Soviet Union: Re-emergence of a pandemic disease. *Emerg Infect Dis* 1998;4:539–50.

Chapter 173

Listeria monocytogenes

Robert S. Baltimore

Listeriosis in humans is caused principally by *Listeria monocytogenes*, one of seven species of the genus *Listeria* that are widely distributed in the environment and throughout the food chain. Human infections can usually be traced to an animal reservoir. Infection occurs most commonly at the extremes of age. In the pediatric population, perinatal infections predominate and usually occur secondary to maternal infection or colonization. Outside the newborn period, disease is most commonly encountered in immunosuppressed children and adults and in the elderly. In the United States, food-borne outbreaks are caused by improperly processed dairy products and contaminated vegetables, and they principally affect the same individuals at risk for sporadic disease.

Etiology. Members of the genus *Listeria* are facultatively anaerobic, non–spore-forming, motile, gram-positive bacilli. The seven *Listeria* species are divided into two genomically distinct groups based on DNA-DNA hybridization studies. One group contains the species *L. murrayi* and *L. grayi*, considered nonpathogenic. The second group contains five species: the nonhemolytic species *L. innocua* and *L. welshimeri* and the hemolytic species *L. monocytogenes*, *L. seeligeri*, and *L. ivanovii*. *L. ivanovii* is pathogenic primarily in animals, and the vast majority of both human and animal disease is due to *L. monocytogenes*.

Subtyping of *L. monocytogenes* isolates for epidemiologic purposes has been attempted using heat-stable somatic O and heat-labile flagellar H antigens, phage typing, ribotyping, and multilocus enzyme electrophoresis. Electrophoretic typing demonstrates the clonal structure of populations of *L. monocytogenes* as well as the sharing of populations between human and animal sources.

Selected biochemical tests together with the demonstration of **tumbling motility, umbrella-type formation** below the surface in semisolid medium, hemolysis, and a typical cyclic adenosine monophosphate (cAMP) test are usually sufficient to establish a presumptive identification of *L. monocytogenes*.

Epidemiology. *L. monocytogenes* is widespread in nature, has been isolated throughout the environment, and is associated with epizootic disease and asymptomatic carriage in more than 42 species of wild and domestic animals and 22 avian species. Epizootic disease in large animals such as sheep and cattle is associated with abortion and "circling disease," a form of basilar meningitis. *L. monocytogenes* is isolated from sewage, silage, and soil, where it survives for more than 295 days. The overall disease rate in the United States is approximately 0.7/100,000; however, in infants it is 10/100,000 and in the elderly it is 1.4/100,000. The rate varies between states. Epidemic human listeriosis has been associated with food-borne transmission in several large outbreaks, especially associated with aged soft cheeses; improperly pasteurized milk and milk products; contaminated raw and ready-to-eat beef, pork, poultry, and packaged meats; and vegetables grown on farms where the ground is contaminated with the feces of colonized animals. The ability of *L. monocytogenes* to grow at temperatures as low as 4°C increases the risk of transmission from aged soft cheeses and stored contaminated food. Small clusters of nosocomial person-to-person transmission have occurred in hospital nurseries and obstetric suites. Sporadic endemic listeriosis is less well characterized. Likely routes include food-borne infection, zoonotic spread, and person-to-person transmission. Zoonotic transmission with cutaneous infections occurs in veterinarians and farmers who handle sick animals.

Reported cases of listeriosis are clustered at the extremes of age. Some studies have shown higher rates in males and a seasonal predominance in the late summer and fall in the northern hemisphere. Outside the newborn period and during pregnancy, disease is usually reported in patients with underlying immunosuppression, with a 100–300 times increased risk in HIV-infected persons and in the elderly (Box 173–1).

The incubation period is defined only for common-source food-borne disease and is 21–30 days. Asymptomatic carriage and fecal excretion are reported in 1% of healthy persons and 5% of abattoir workers, but duration of excretion, when studied, is short (<1 mo).

Pathogenesis. *L. monocytogenes* produces multisystem disease, particularly pyogenic meningitis. Granulomatous reactions and microabscess formation have been reported in many organs, including the liver, lungs, adrenals, kidneys, central nervous system (CNS), and, notably, the placenta. Animal models demonstrate translocation, the transfer of intraluminal organisms across intact intestinal mucosa; whether or not this occurs in humans is not known.

Studies of intracellular and intercellular spread of *L. monocytogenes* have revealed a complex pathogenesis. Four pathogenic steps are described: internalization, escape from the phagocytic vacuole, nucleation of actin filaments, and cell-to-cell spread. Genes involved in each step are known, and isogenic mutants have been shown to have reduced virulence. **Listeriolysin**, a hemolysin and the best-characterized virulence factor, probably mediates lysis of vacuoles and is responsible for the zone of hemolysis when grown on blood-containing solid media. In cell-to-cell spread, locomotion proceeds via cytochalasin-sensitive polymerization of actin filaments, which extrude the bacteria in pseudopods, which are phagocytosed by adjacent cells, necessitating escape from a double-membrane vacuole. This mechanism protects intracellular bacteria from the humoral arm of immunity and is responsible for the well-known requirement of T-cell–mediated activation of monocytes by lymphokines for clearance of infection and establishment of immunity. The role of opsonizing antibody in protecting against infection is unclear.

Clinical Manifestations. The clinical presentation of listeriosis is highly dependent on the age of the patient and the circumstances of the infection.

LISTERIOSIS IN PREGNANCY. Early gestational listeriosis is not well understood. *L. monocytogenes* has been grown from placental and fetal cultures of pregnancies ending in spontaneous abortion. The usual presentation in the 2nd and 3rd trimesters is a flulike illness that may result in bacteremia seeding the uterine contents. Rarely is maternal listeriosis severe, but meningitis in pregnancy has been reported. Recognition and treatment at this stage have been associated with normal pregnancy outcomes, but the fetus may not be infected even if listeriosis in the mother

---

BOX 173–1. Types of *Listeria monocytogenes* Infections

Listeriosis in pregnancy
Neonatal listeriosis
    Early onset
    Late onset
Food-borne outbreaks
Listeriosis in normal children and adults (rare)
Listeriosis in immunocompromised persons
    Lymphohematogenous malignancies
    Collagen vascular diseases
    Diabetes mellitus
    HIV infection
    Transplant recipients
    Renal failure with peritoneal dialysis
Listeriosis in the elderly

is not treated. In other instances, placental listeriosis develops with infection of the fetus that may be associated with stillbirth or premature delivery. Delivery of an infected premature fetus is associated with 50–90% infant mortality. Disseminated disease is apparent at birth, often with a diffuse pustular rash. Infection in the mother usually resolves without specific therapy after delivery, but postpartum fever and infected lochia may occur.

NEONATAL LISTERIOSIS. Two clinical presentations are recognized for neonatal listeriosis: early onset (<5 days, usually within 1–2 days), which is a predominantly septicemic form, and late-onset (>5 days, mean 14 days), which is a predominantly meningitic form (Table 173–1). The principal characteristics of the two presentations resemble the clinical syndromes described for group B streptococcus (Chapter 169).

Early-onset disease occurs from milder transplacental or ascending infections from the female genital tract. There is a strong association with recovery of *L. monocytogenes* from the maternal genital tract, obstetric complications, prematurity, and neonatal sepsis with multiorgan involvement without CNS localization. The mortality rate is approximately 20–30%.

The epidemiology of late-onset disease is poorly understood. Onset is usually after 5 days but before 30 days of age. Affected infants frequently are term, and the mothers are culture negative and asymptomatic. The presenting syndrome is usually of purulent meningitis, which, if adequately treated, has a mortality rate of <20%.

POSTNEONATAL INFECTIONS. Listeriosis beyond the newborn period may rarely occur in otherwise healthy children but is most often encountered in association with underlying malignancies or immunosuppression. The clinical presentation is usually meningitis, less commonly sepsis, and rarely other CNS involvement such as cerebritis, meningoencephalitis, brain abscess, spinal cord abscess, or a focus outside the CNS such as suppurative arthritis, osteomyelitis, endocarditis, peritonitis (associated with peritoneal dialysis), or liver abscess. It is not known whether the frequent gastrointestinal signs and symptoms result from enteric infection, because the mode of acquisition is unknown.

Diagnosis. Listeriosis should be included in the differential diagnosis of infections in pregnancy, neonatal sepsis and meningitis, and of sepsis or meningitis in older children with underlying malignancies, receiving immunosuppressive therapy, or following transplantation. The diagnosis is established by culture of *L. monocytogenes* from blood or cerebrospinal fluid (CSF). Cultures from the maternal cervix, vagina, or lochia and, if possible, placenta should be obtained when intrauterine infections lead to premature delivery or early onset neonatal sepsis. It is helpful to alert the laboratory to suspected cases so that *Listeria* isolates are not discarded as contaminating diphtheroids.

Histologic examination of the placenta is useful. Polymerase chain reaction assays detect *L. monocytogenes,* but commercial assays are not available. Serodiagnostic tests have not proved useful.

DIFFERENTIAL DIAGNOSIS. Listeriosis is indistinguishable clinically from neonatal sepsis and meningitis due to other organisms. The presence of increased peripheral blood monocytes suggests the possibility of listeriosis. Monocytosis or lymphocytosis may be modest or striking. Beyond the neonatal period, *L. monocytogenes* CNS infection is associated with fever, headache, seizures, and signs of meningeal irritation. The brainstem characteristically may be affected. The white blood cell concentration may vary from normal to slightly elevated, and the CSF laboratory findings are variable. Polymorphonuclear leukocytes or mononuclear cells may predominate, with shifts from polymorphonuclear to mononuclear cells in sequential lumbar punctures. A low CSF glucose level that mirrors the severity of disease is usually found. The CSF protein is moderately elevated. *L. monocytogenes* is isolated from the blood in 40–75% of cases of meningitis due to the organism. Deep focal infections, such as endocarditis, osteomyelitis, and liver abscess due to *L. monocytogenes* are also indistinguishable clinically from the more common organisms associated with these sites. Cutaneous infections should be suspected in patients with a history of contact with animals, especially products of conception.

Treatment. The emergence of multiple antibiotic resistance makes routine susceptibility testing of isolates mandatory. Ampicillin alone (100–200 mg/kg/24 hr divided q 6 hr IV; 200–400 mg/kg/24 hr divided q 6 hr IV if meningitis is present) or in combination with an aminoglycoside (5–7.5 mg/kg/24 hr divided q 8 hr IV) is the therapy of choice. Special attention to dosing is required for neonates, who require longer dosing intervals due to the longer half-lives of the antibiotics. Combination therapy is recommended for severe infections. Isolates usually demonstrate tolerance, with the minimum bactericidal concentration ≥32 times the minimum inhibitory concentration, to ampicillin as well as penicillin, erythromycin, and tetracycline. Addition of gentamicin lowers the minimum bactericidal concentration. *L. monocytogenes* is not susceptible to the cephalosporins, including third-generation cephalosporins. If these agents are used for empirical therapy for neonatal sepsis or meningitis in a newborn, it is essential to add ampicillin for possible *L. monocytogenes* infection. Vancomycin, or vancomycin and an aminoglycoside, is an alternative, as are trimethoprim-sulfamethoxazole and erythromycin. The duration of therapy is usually 2–3 wk with 3 wk recommended for immunocompromised persons and meningitis. A longer course is needed for endocarditis brain abscess or osteomyelitis.

Prognosis. Early gestational listeriosis may be associated with abortion or stillbirth, although maternal infection with sparing of the fetus has been reported. No convincing evidence shows that *L. monocytogenes* is associated with repeated spontaneous abortions in humans. The mortality rate is >50% for premature infants infected in utero, 30% for early onset neonatal sepsis, 15% for late-onset neonatal meningitis, and <10% in older children with prompt institution of appropriate antimicrobial therapy. Mental retardation, hydrocephalus, and other CNS sequelae are reported in survivors of *Listeria* meningitis.

Prevention. Listeriosis can be prevented by pasteurization and thorough cooking of foods. Irradiation of meat products may also be beneficial. Consumption of unpasteurized or improperly processed dairy products, especially aged soft cheeses, uncooked and precooked meat products that have been stored at 4°C for extended periods, and unwashed vegetables should be avoided. This is particularly important during pregnancy and for immunocompromised persons. Infected domestic animals should be avoided when possible. Careful handwashing is essential to prevent nosocomial spread within obstetric and neonatal units. Immunocompromised patients given prophylaxis with trimethoprim-sulfamethoxazole are protected from *Listeria* infections.

TABLE 173–1. **Characteristic Features of Early and Late Onset Neonatal Listeriosis**

Early Onset (<5 days)	Late Onset (≥5 days)
Positive maternal *Listeria* culture	Negative maternal *Listeria* culture
Obstetric complications	Uncomplicated pregnancy
Premature delivery	Term delivery
Low birthweight	Normal birthweight
Neonatal sepsis	Neonatal meningitis
Mean age at onset 1.5 days	Mean age at onset 14.2 days
Mortality rate >30%	Mortality rate <10%
	Nosocomial outbreaks

Appleman MD, Cherubin CE, Heseltine PNR, et al: Susceptibility testing of *Listeria monocytogenes*: A reassessment of bactericidal activity as a predictor for clinical outcome. *Diagn Microbiol Infect Dis* 1991;14:311–7.

Lorber B: Listeriosis. *Clin Infect Dis* 1997;24:1–9.

McLauchlin J: Human listeriosis in Britain, 1967–85, a summary of 722 cases: I. Listeriosis during pregnancy and in the newborn. II. Listeriosis in non-pregnant individuals, a changing pattern of infection and seasonal incidence. *Epidemiol Infect* 1990;104:181–9, 191–201.

Michelet C, Avril JL, Cartier F, et al: Inhibition of intracellular growth of *Listeria monocytogenes* by antibiotics. *Antimicrob Agents Chemother* 1994;38:438–46.

Mylonakis E, Hohmann EL, Calderwood SB: Central nervous system infection with *Listeria monocytogenes*: 333 years' experience at a general hospital and review of 776 episodes form the literature. *Medicine* 1998;77:313–36.

Portnoy DA, Chakraborty T, Goebel W, et al: Molecular determinants of *Listeria monocytogenes* pathogenesis. *Infect Immun* 1992;60:1263–7.

Schlech WF III: Foodborne listeriosis. *Clin Infect Dis* 2000;31:770–5.

Schuchat A, Swaminathan B, Broome CV: Epidemiology of human listeriosis. *Clin Microbiol Rev* 1991;4:169–83.

Skogberg K, Syrjanen J, Jahkola M, et al: Clinical presentation and outcome of listeriosis in patients with and without immunosuppressive therapy. *Clin Infect Dis* 1992;14:815–21.

Southwick FS, Purich DL: Intracellular pathogenesis of listeriosis. *N Engl J Med* 1996;334:770–6.

Chapter 174

Actinomyces *Richard F. Jacobs and*
Gordon E. Schutze

Actinomyces are slow-growing, gram-positive bacteria that are part of the normal oral flora in humans. Their filamentous structure gives them a fungus-like appearance. Infection caused by these bacteria is termed **actinomycosis**, which is a chronic, granulomatous, suppurative disease characterized by peripheral spread with extension to contiguous tissue in the formation of numerous draining sinus tracts. These infections usually involve the cervicofacial, thoracic, abdominal, or pelvic regions.

Etiology. *Actinomyces israelii* is the predominant organism causing actinomycoses in humans. Other implicated species, in order of importance, include *Propionibacterium propionicum* (originally described as *A. propionicum*), *A. odontolyticus, A. meyeri, A. naeslundii, A. viscosus, A. europa, A. turicensis,* and *A. radingae*. *Arcanobacterium pyogenes* (previously in the *Actinomyces* genus) also causes human actinomycosis. *Actinobacillus actinomycetemcomitans* is a fastidious, gram-negative rod that frequently complicates actinomycosis caused by *A. israelii*. In addition to being associated with actinomycosis, it is part of the oral flora and has been implicated as a pathogen in periodontal disease. Other bacterial species isolated concomitantly in human actinomycosis are *Eikenella corrodens, Fusobacterium, Bacteroides, Capnocytophaga, Staphylococcus, Streptococcus,* and Enterobacteriaceae.

Actinomyces are non–spore-forming gram-positive, facultative, or strict anaerobes with a variable morphology and are members of the **HACEK group**, which also includes *Haemophilus aphrophilus, Cardiobacterium hominis, Eikenella corrodens,* and *Kingella kingae*. The irregular morphology ranges from diphtheroid to mycelial. *Actinomyces* organisms are found in clinical specimens, such as sputum, purulent exudates, and tissues obtained surgically or at necropsy. Staining of crushed tissue specimens rinsed with sterile saline or purulent exudate stained by Gram or acid-fast procedures can reveal organisms within the classic **sulfur granules**. Cultures on brain-heart infusion agar incubated at 37°C anaerobically (95% nitrogen and 5% carbon dioxide) and a separate set incubated aerobically reveal organisms within the lines of streak at 24–48 hr. *A. israelii* colonies appear as loose masses of delicate branching filaments with a characteristic spider-like growth. Colonies of *A. naeslundii, A. viscosus,* and *P. propionicus* may have similar growth characteristics. Owing to the similarity in growth characteristics from colony morphology, various biochemical tests are performed to identify the specific organism.

Epidemiology. Actinomycosis occurs worldwide without relation to age, sex, race, season, or occupation. In a review of 85 cases of actinomycosis, 27% were in persons <20 yr of age, with 7% of the patients <10 yr of age. The youngest patient in this series was 28 days old. The source of human infection is almost always endogenous flora. Although actinomycosis is usually not an opportunistic infection, disease has been described in patients receiving corticosteroids and those with leukemia, renal failure, congenital immunodeficiency diseases, and HIV infection. In one study, antecedent disease and surgery predisposed 81 of 181 subjects to infection.

Actinomycosis, even in closed infections, is usually part of a polymicrobial infection involving mixed bacteria. In a large study of more than 650 cases, infection with *Actinomyces* was identified in pure culture in only one case and usually was identified with other bacteria, most notably *Actinobacillus actinomycetemcomitans* and *Haemophilus aphrophilus*, as well as other local flora.

Pathogenesis. The organism infects the host after introduction into the tissue by trauma or aspiration into the lung. It spreads locally and, rarely, hematogenously. Actinomycosis is a chronic, suppurative, scarring inflammatory process. Sites of infection show dense cellular infiltrates and suppuration that form many interconnecting abscesses and sinus tracts. This may be followed by cicatricial healing from which the organism then spreads by burrowing along fascial planes. This causes deep communicating scarred sinus tracts. Characteristic **sulfur granules** have an adherent mass of polymorphonuclear neutrophils that are attached to the radially arranged eosinophilic clubs of the granule. A fuzzy outer coat of hairlike fimbriae has been considered to contribute to failure of endodontic therapy due to *A. israelii*.

The three important sites of *Actinomyces* infection in order of frequency are cervicofacial, abdominal, and thoracic. Many less common infections occur, involving every organ in the body. Actinomycosis must be differentiated from several other chronic inflammatory diseases, including tuberculosis, mycotic infections, *Yersinia enterocolitica* "pseudoappendicitis," appendicitis, amebiasis, hepatic abscess, osteomyelitis, nocardiosis, and other chronic bacterial infections. In addition to introduction at wound sites, another route is through use of intrauterine devices (IUDs), which permit the development of pelvic and gastrointestinal actinomycosis. Pulmonary actinomycosis occurs after inhalation or aspiration of organisms, introduction of a colonized foreign body, or spread from an existing cervicofacial or abdominal actinomycotic infection. These masslike lesions may present as a tumor, necessitating invasive approaches for differentiation.

Clinical Manifestations. The three major forms of actinomycosis—cervicofacial, abdominal and pelvic, and pulmonary infections—arise by different routes but may predispose to other forms of the disease. The diagnosis of actinomycosis in children suggests an underlying immunodeficiency disease state, especially chronic granulomatous disease.

CERVICOFACIAL ACTINOMYCOSIS. In cervicofacial actinomycosis, the organisms enter the tissues after trauma that disrupts the mucous membranes of the mouth or pharynx or by way of caries. Patients with this type of actinomycosis often have a history of oral surgery, dental procedures, or trauma to the mouth. Cervicofacial actinomycosis usually presents as a painless, slow growing, hard mass that can produce cutaneous fistulas, a condition commonly known as **lumpy jaw** (Fig. 174–1). Less frequently, cervicofacial actinomycosis can present with findings suggestive of an acute pyogenic infection with an acute, tender, fluctuant mass with trismus, firm swelling, and fistulas with drainage containing the characteristic

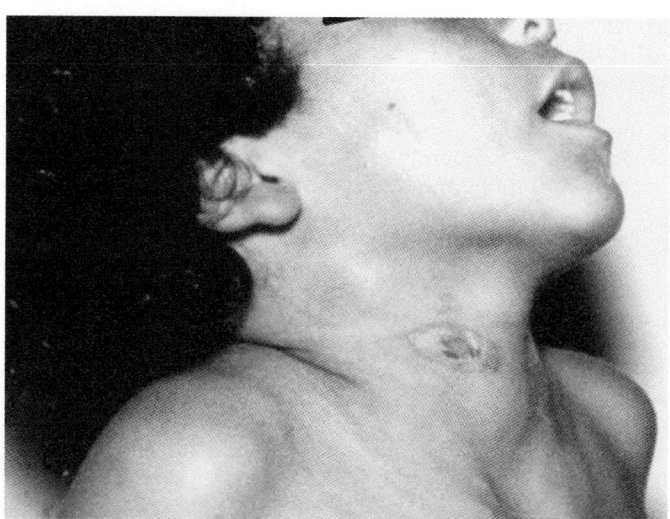

FIGURE 174–1. A 2-yr-old boy with HIV infection who has cervicofacial actinomycosis and a chronic draining fistula.

sulfur granules. Bone is not involved early in the disease, but periostitis, mandibular osteomyelitis, or perimandibular abscess may later develop. Infection may spread by way of sinus tracts to the cranial bones, which may give rise to meningitis. The ability of *Actinomyces* to burrow through tissue planes and even bone is a key differentiating point between actinomycosis and nocardiosis. The cervicofacial type of actinomycosis has the best prognosis, and is usually cured with surgical debridement and excision as an adjunct to appropriate antibiotic therapy.

ABDOMINAL AND PELVIC ACTINOMYCOSIS. Because abdominal actinomycosis also is the result of disruption of the mucosa of the gastrointestinal tract, patients may present with a history of gastrointestinal surgery, diverticulitis, or appendicitis. This disease usually develops as a result of an acute gastrointestinal perforation or after abdominal trauma. Of all the forms of actinomycosis, a delayed diagnosis is typical for abdominal or pelvic disease. Gastrointestinal disease occurs as appendicitis in 25% of cases but can be manifested as various ulcerative diseases. Infection classically appears after appendectomy as a hard, irregular mass in the ileocecal area that softens and then drains to the outside through a fistula. Hepatic involvement has been described in approximately 15% of abdominal actinomycosis cases as solitary or multiple liver abscesses or in a miliary pattern. The clinical course is indolent, with chills, fever, night sweats, and weight loss, and is similar to the presentation of tuberculous peritonitis. Extension from this focus is usually by direct continuity or, rarely, hematogenously to involve any tissue or organ, including muscle, spleen, kidneys, fallopian tubes, ovaries, uterus, testes, bladder, or rectum.

Women wearing IUDs are at risk for developing pelvic actinomycosis. They may present with vaginal discharge, pelvic pain, abdominal pain, menorrhagia, fever, pelvic mass, a history of pelvic inflammatory disease, and/or a history of prolonged IUD use. The risk is more significant if the IUD has been in place for >2–3 yr.

PULMONARY ACTINOMYCOSIS. Neither the clinical nor the radiographic presentation of pulmonary actinomycosis is specific. Pulmonary actinomycosis may present as an endobronchial infection, a tumor-like lesion, diffuse pneumonia, or a pleural effusion. Principal symptoms include fever, productive cough, chest pain, and weight loss. Infection frequently dissects along tissue planes and may extend through the chest wall or diaphragm, producing numerous sinuses. These characteristic sinus tracts contain small abscesses and purulent drainage. Other complications include bony destruction of adjacent ribs,

sternum, and vertebral bodies. Pyogenic mediastinitis has been attributed to *A. odontolyticus* in lung transplant recipients. Multiple lobe involvement is occasionally found in the lung. Associated conditions, such as dental caries, aspiration, inhalation injury, introduction of a colonized foreign body, or pre-existing cervicofacial or abdominal disease, should heighten the index of suspicion. Accurate diagnosis can be more difficult with the propensity of *Actinomyces* to infect pre-existing pulmonary cavities. Diagnosis can be confirmed by examining purulent sinus tract drainage for sulfur granules, and by appropriate cultures. The presence of *Actinomyces* in sputum or bronchoscopy specimens is hampered because these organisms are normal oral flora. The differential diagnosis of pulmonary actinomycosis includes lung abscess and tuberculosis.

OTHER FORMS. Laryngeal actinomycosis rarely has been reported in older teenagers. Colonization of the oropharynx with these organisms may be involved in the development of obstructive tonsillar hypertrophy. *A. pyogenes* only rarely has been implicated as a cause of human infection, but there are reported cases of septicemia, endocarditis, meningitis, arthritis, empyema, pneumonia, otitis media, cystitis, mastoiditis, appendicitis, and cutaneous infection. *A. actinomycetemcomitans* is a pathogen in at least 30% of actinomycotic infections. Failure to recognize this organism and treat it adequately has resulted in clinical relapse and deterioration in infected patients with actinomycosis. Severe forms of periodontitis, particularly localized juvenile periodontitis, are associated with *Actinomyces*, especially in children 10–19 yr of age. Like other HACEK organisms, *Actinomyces* has a propensity for infecting heart valves and results in an insidious presentation of endocarditis, with fever occurring in <50% of cases.

Diagnosis. Microscopic examination with appropriate stains and culture of purulent drainage from fistulas, abscesses, draining sinus tracts, bronchoalveolar lavage, and sputum can reveal *Actinomyces* as an irregular, non–spore-forming, non–acid-fast, non-motile gram-positive bacillus. Inoculation of anaerobic and aerobic cultures enhances the yield on microbiologic cultures. An abdominal CT scan can be helpful in identifying the presence of a contrast-enhancing multicystic lesion that can be approached by CT-guided needle biopsy and culture.

Treatment. The mainstay of treatment for actinomycosis is prolonged antibiotic therapy and an appropriate surgical approach to sinus tracts and abscesses. Prompt use of antibiotics results in a high cure rate. Actinomycosis is treated with penicillin (250,000 U/kg/24 hr divided q 4 hr IV). Other appropriate antibiotics include tetracycline, clindamycin, chloramphenicol, and carbapenems. Although controversy still exists about the dosage and duration of therapy, appropriate therapy usually includes parenteral antibiotics for 2–6 wk followed by oral antibiotics for 3–12 mo. The oral antibiotic of choice is penicillin V (100 mg/kg/24 hr divided q 6 hr PO). Although most *A. israelii* strains are sensitive to penicillin with minimum inhibitory concentrations of 0.03–0.5 mg/mL, some resistant strains have been identified. Antibiotic susceptibility testing should be performed on all isolates from patients with significant disease or who are immunocompromised. Hepatic abscesses or other deep tissue infections should be treated for 6–12 mo. Large abscesses usually require surgical excision. Removal of chronically infected tonsils and treatment of pyorrhea or caries may eliminate possible sources of infection. Generally, the prognosis is excellent with adequate therapy and early diagnosis.

Because co-infection with *A. actinomycetemcomitans* does occur regularly, it is important to consider covering this organism empirically, especially in the critically ill patient. *A. actinomycetemcomitans* is susceptible to newer cephalosporins, rifampin, trimethoprim-sulfamethoxazole, aminoglycosides, ciprofloxacin, tetracycline, and azithromycin. It is susceptible to penicillin and ampicillin in vitro, but test results do not correlate necessarily with clinical outcome. In some patients with periodontitis associated with this organism, a combination of mechanical periodontal treatment with metronidazole plus amoxicillin is effective for subgingival suppression.

Bassiri AG, Girgis RE, Theodore J: *Actinomyces odontolyticus* thoracopulmonary infections: Two cases in lung and heart-lung transplant recipients and a review of the literature. *Chest* 1996;109:1109–11.

Bates M, Cruikshank G: Thoracic actinomycosis. *Thorax* 1952;12:99–124.

Brown JR: Human actinomycosis: A study of 181 subjects. *Hum Pathol* 1973;4: 319–30.

Cintron JR, Del Pino A, Duarte B, et al: Abdominal actinomycosis. *Dis Colon Rectum* 1996;39:105–8.

Feder HM Jr: Actinomycosis manifesting as an acute painless lump of the jaw. *Pediatrics* 1990;85:858–64.

Gahrn-Hansen B, Frederiksen W: Human infections with *Actinomyces pyogenes* (*Corynebacterium pyogenes*). *Diag Microbiol Infect Dis* 1992;15:349–54.

Holm G: Studies on the etiology of human actinomycosis: I. The other microbes of actinomycosis and their importance. *Acta Pathol Microbiol Scand* 1950;27:736–42.

Morris JF, Sewell DL: Necrotizing pneumonia caused by mixed infection with *Actinobacillus actinomycetemcomitans* and *Actinomyces israelii*: Case report and review. *Clin Infect Dis* 1994;18:450–2.

Nelson EG, Tybor AG: Actinomycosis of the larynx. *Ear Nose Throat J* 1992;71: 356–8.

Ramos CP, Falsen E, Alvarez N, et al: *Actinomyces graevenitzii* sp. Nov., isolated from human clinical specimens. *Int J Syst Bacteriol* 1997;47:885–8.

Reddy I, Ferguson DA Jr, Sarubbi FA: Endocarditis due to *Actinomyces pyogenes*. *Clin Infect Dis* 1997;25:1476–7.

Sabbe LJ, Van De Merwe D, Schouls L, et al: Clinical spectrum of infections due to the newly described *Actinomyces* species *A. turicensis*, *A. radingae*, and *A. europaeus*. *J Clin Microbiol* 1999;37:8–13.

Schaal KP, Lee HJ: Actinomycete infections in humans—a review. *Gene* 1992;115: 201–11.

Tyrrell J, Noone P, Prichard JS: Thoracic actinomycosis complicated by *Actinobacillus actinomycetemcomitans*: case report and review of literature. *Respir Med* 1992;86:341–3.

Weisse WC, Smith I: A study of 57 cases of actinomycosis over a 36-year period. *Arch Intern Med* 1975;135:1562–8.

Chapter 175

Nocardia Richard F. Jacobs and

Gordon E. Schutze

Nocardiosis is an acute, subacute, or chronic suppurative infection with a tendency for remissions and exacerbations that cause localized and disseminated disease in children and adults. Recently, larger series of primary cutaneous nocardiosis in children have been reported from the southern United States.

Etiology. *Nocardia* is a member of the order Actinomycetales, which includes gram-positive filamentous bacteria such as *Actinomyces*, *Streptomyces*, and mycobacteria. Soil and decaying vegetable matter are their natural habitat. Numerous taxonomic studies have established the heterogeneity of the species *Nocardia asteroides*, the most common cause of human nocardiosis, and have led to the description of **N. asteroides complex**. *N. brasiliensis* is the second most frequent etiologic agent of human nocardiosis. Current methods of recognition of *N. asteroides* in the clinical laboratory include microscopic and colonial morphology, resistance to lysozyme, and inability to hydrolyze casein, tyrosine, xanthine, and hypoxanthine. *N. asteroides*, *N. farcinica*, *N. otidis-caviarum*, and *N. nova* share similar features and have contributed to the apparent heterogeneity of *N. asteroides*. New identification and rapid diagnostic schemes use molecular typing and identification of preformed enzymes.

In 1988, a susceptibility study of 78 clinical isolates of the *N. asteroides* complex from the United States found that 95% of strains exhibited one of five antibiotic resistance patterns. The most common group, occurring in 35% of isolates, was resistant to ampicillin but susceptible to the broad-spectrum cephalosporins and imipenem. Approximately 20% of isolates, including essentially all isolates in the *N. asteroides* complex, were resistant to cefotaxime, ceftriaxone, and cefamandole, which were subsequently identified as *N. farcinica*. Approximately 20% of the strains were susceptible to ampicillin and erythromycin, which were subsequently identified as *N. nova*. The remaining types had susceptibility patterns that included resistance to broad-spectrum cephalosporins and susceptibility to ampicillin and carbenicillin, but intermediate susceptibility to imipenem. The most active parenteral agents were amikacin (95%), imipenem (88%), ceftriaxone (82%), and cefotaxime (82%). The most active oral agents were sulfonamides (100%), minocycline (100%), and ampicillin (40%).

Systemic nocardiosis is caused most frequently by the bacteria in the *N. asteroides* complex. *N. brasiliensis* is the principal cause of localized nocardial cellulitis and lymphadenitis in immunocompetent children but also causes a form of pulmonary and systemic disease, especially in immunocompromised patients. *Actinomadura madurae* (**Madura foot**), *N. farcinica*, *N. nova*, and *N. transvalensis* are also causes of human disease. *N. asteroides* complex includes the most common agents of systemic nocardiosis in the United States, whereas *N. brasiliensis* is found more commonly in the southern United States, Central America, South America, and Asia. These agents are similar morphologically and can be distinguished only by biochemical and serologic procedures.

Epidemiology. Nocardiosis was once thought to be a rare cause of human disease but is now being recognized more frequently, having been diagnosed in individuals ranging from 4 wk–82 yr of age. Almost all of the patients have one or more severe underlying diseases, usually accompanied by compromised cellular immunity from corticosteroids, primary immunodeficiency (chronic granulomatous disease), organ transplantation, cancer chemotherapy, or HIV infection. HIV-infected patients are at increased risk, although nocardiosis is not considered an AIDS-defining infection. *Nocardia* infections in bone marrow transplant recipients have been associated with a high rate of invasive fungal infection and a lack of protection by trimethoprim-sulfamethoxazole prophylaxis.

Soil is the natural habitat of *Nocardia*, which has been isolated worldwide. The organism is inhaled in aerosolized dust and causes pulmonary infection, with widespread dissemination in susceptible hosts, and it can be transmitted by direct skin inoculation. Cases of nocardiosis following arthropod bite and cat bite have been reported in recent years. Although communicability from human to human has not been proved to be common, a description of human-to-human transmission of *N. farcinica* resulting in sternal wound infections in patients undergoing open heart surgery has raised concern about *Nocardia* as a nosocomial pathogen.

Pathogenesis. *N. asteroides* complex and *N. brasiliensis* organisms are obligate aerobes and grow on ordinary culture media. These organisms are sensitive to various antibiotics; thus, media containing these specific drugs do not support growth. Many isolates of *Nocardia* are thermophilic and can grow at temperatures up to 50°C; however, best growth is achieved at 37°C. At 25°C, the organisms grow very slowly. Colonies appear within 1–2 wk on brain-heart infusion agar and Lowenstein-Jensen media, usually as waxy, folded, or heaped colonies at the edges. With further incubation, these colonies develop aerial hyphae that tend to give them a white, chalky appearance. Classifications of species of *Nocardia* are based on physiologic reactions with various substrates and antibiotic susceptibility testing. An isolated 55-kd protein that has apparent specificity for *N. asteroides* complex is used in an enzyme immunoassay. In biopsy specimens or clinical body fluids using modified Kinyoun acid-fast staining, *Nocardia* demonstrates fragmented bacilli with stain concentrated in a **beaded pattern** along portions of the branching filaments.

Clinical Manifestations. Pulmonary nocardiosis accounts for 75% of cases, which almost all occur in immunocompromised patients or patients with underlying pulmonary disease. Demonstration of tissue invasion is important for identifying active infection because the organism occasionally exists as a respiratory saprophyte (Fig. 175–1). Clinical manifestations include pneumonia and necrotizing pneumonia with single or numerous abscesses. Diagnosis is established in one third of cases in adults by sputum analysis and culture. Bronchoalveolar lavage or lung biopsy may be required to establish the diagnosis in the remaining two thirds of adults and in children. The mortality with nocardiosis is >50% in immunocompromised patients with disseminated disease but may be lower with earlier diagnosis.

Metastatic lesions may occur anywhere in the body, but the brain is the most common secondary site and is affected in 15–40% of cases. Brain lesions may be numerous or single. Brain abscess is the most common presentation, with meningitis the second most common, as manifested by pleocytosis (with a lymphocytic or neutrophilic predominance), elevated cerebrospinal fluid protein, and hypoglycorrhachia. Persistent neutrophilic meningitis with sterile cultures is classic for central nervous system (CNS) infection. The onset of CNS infection may be gradual or sudden and includes manifestations varying from headache to coma. Cranial CT or MRI is recommended in all immunocompromised patients with pulmonary nocardiosis, even when asymptomatic, because of the frequency of CNS involvement, and should be considered in all patients with pulmonary nocardiosis.

The skin is the third most commonly involved organ. Renal nocardiosis is the fourth most common site, presenting with dysuria, hematuria, or pyuria. Lesions may extend from the cortex into the medulla. Gastrointestinal involvement may also be associated, with nausea, vomiting, diarrhea, abdominal distention, and melena. Infection may metastasize to skin, pericardium, myocardium, spleen, liver, or adrenal glands; bone involvement is rare. Almost all of the involved organs have several abscesses, but in contrast to actinomycosis, granules are rarely found. Keratitis due to *N. farcinica* has been associated with the use of semipermeable rigid contact lenses.

Diagnosis. Laboratory diagnosis of nocardiosis requires direct examination of clinical material for characteristic gram-positive, acid-fast organisms and isolation by culture methods. Smears of clinical material are Gram stained or stained by the modified Kinyoun acid-fast stain. *N. asteroides* complex and *N. brasiliensis* appear as delicately branched gram-positive coccoid to bacillary structures that tend to fragment. In properly stained and decolorized acid-fast smears, the organisms may appear as fragmented bacilli with the stain concentrated in a beaded pattern along the portions of the filaments. Antibody titers to the 55-kd *Nocardia* protein of ≥1:256 appear sensitive and specific for diagnosis and have also been used to monitor response to medical treatment.

Treatment. Sulfonamides are the drugs of choice. Sulfisoxazole (120–150 mg/kg/24 hr divided q 6 hr PO), or trisulfapyrimidines, for 3–6 mo is standard therapy. For severe infections, based on susceptibility testing, amikacin (15–30 mg/kg/24 hr divided q 8 hr IV or IM) as a single agent or in combination with a β-lactam antibiotic (e.g., a third-generation cephalosporin or carbapenem) can be used. In addition, and based on in vitro susceptibility testing for specific *N. asteroides* complex isolates, alternative drug combinations may include erythromycin and newer macrolides (azithromycin and clarithromycin), carbapenems, streptomycin, minocycline, quinolones, and third-generation cephalosporins. Clinical trials have shown ampicillin or amoxicillin-clavulanate to be effective in *N. brasiliensis* infections. Antibiotic resistance has become an important issue in many *Nocardia* infections, with resistance to trimethoprim-sulfamethoxazole, streptomycin, and ampicillin reported. Surgical drainage of abscesses is important. Relapses of *Nocardia* have occurred in patients treated for <3 mo. Patients with AIDS probably should be treated indefinitely.

Prognosis. Despite adequate therapy, the overall mortality is >50%, which may be secondary to a delay in diagnosis or to the debilitated state of patients with severely compromised host defenses.

Angeles AM, Sugar AM: Rapid diagnosis of nocardiosis with an enzyme immunoassay. *J Infect Dis* 1987;155:292–6.

Baghdadlian H, Sorger S, Knowles K, et al: *Nocardia transvalensis* pneumonia in a child. *Pediatr Infect Dis J* 1989;8:470–1.

Biehle JR, Cavalieri SJ, Felland T, et al: Novel method for rapid identification of *Nocardia* species by detection of preformed enzymes. *J Clin Microbiol* 1996;34:103–7.

Bottei E, Flaherty JP, Kaplan LJ, et al: Lymphocutaneous *Nocardia brasiliensis* infection transmitted via a cat scratch: A second case. *Clin Infect Dis* 1994;18:649–50.

Burucoa C, Breton I, Ramassamy A, et al: Western blot monitoring of disseminated *Nocardia nova* infection treated with clarithromycin, imipenem, and surgical drainage. *Eur J Clin Microbiol Infect Dis* 1996;15:943–7.

Fergie JE, Purcell K: Nocardiosis in south Texas children. *Pediatr Infect Dis J* 2001;20:711–14.

Lerner PI: Nocardiosis. *Clin Infect Dis* 1996;22:891–903.

McNeil MM, Brown JM, Georghiou PR, et al: Infections due to *Nocardia transvalensis*: Clinical spectrum and antimicrobial therapy. *Clin Infect Dis* 1992;15:453–63.

Paredes BE, Hunger RE, Braathen LR, et al: Cutaneous nocardiosis caused by *Nocardia brasiliensis* after an insect bite. *Dermatology* 1999;198:159–61.

Steingrube VA, Brown BA, Gibson JL, et al: DNA amplification and restriction endonuclease analysis for differentiation of 12 species and taxa of *Nocardia*, including recognition of four new taxa within the *Nocardia asteroides* complex. *J Clin Microbiol* 1995;33:3096–101.

Van Burik JA, Hackman RC, Nadeem SQ, et al: Nocardiosis after bone marrow transplantation: A retrospective study. *Clin Infect Dis* 1997;24:1154–60.

Wallace RJ, Brown BA, Tsukamura M, et al: Clinical and laboratory features of *Nocardia nova. J Clin Microbiol* 1991;29:2407–11.

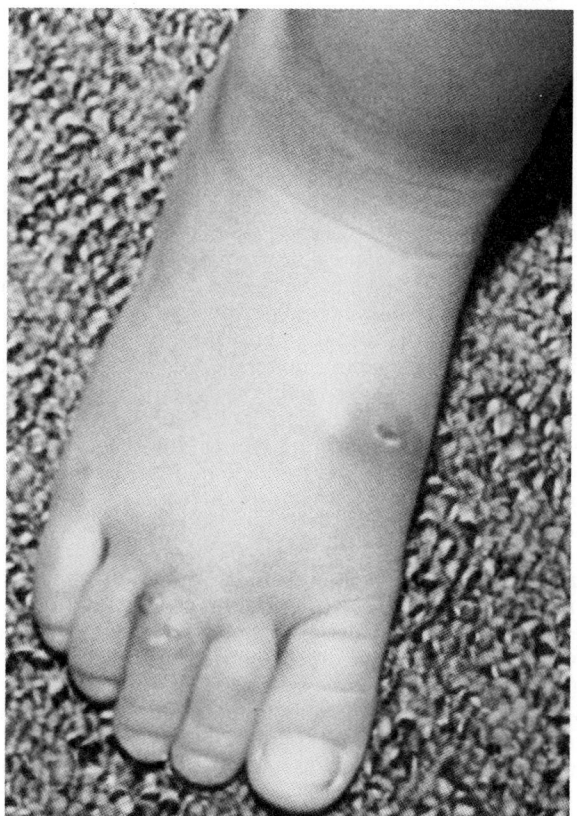

FIGURE 175–1. A 2-yr-old female with multiple pustules on the dorsum of the right foot caused by *Nocardia brasiliensis*. (Photograph courtesy of Jaime E. Fergie, MD.) See also color plates.

Wallace RJ, Septimus EJ, Williams TW, et al: Use of trimethoprim-sulfamethoxazole for treatment of infections due to *Nocardia. Rev Infect Dis* 1982;4:315–25.

Wallace RJ, Steele LC, Sumter G, et al: Antimicrobial susceptibility patterns of *Nocardia asteroides. Antimicrob Agents Chemother* 1988;32:1776–9.

Wallace RJ, Tsukamura M, Brown BA, et al: Cefotaxime-resistant *Nocardia asteroides* strains are isolates of the controversial species *Nocardia farcinica. J Clin Microbiol* 1990;28:2726–32.

SECTION 3 *Gram-Negative Bacterial Infections*

Chapter 176
Neisseria meningitidis (Meningococcus) *Charles R. Woods*

Meningococcal disease, first described by Vieusseaux in 1805 as epidemic cerebrospinal fever, remains a significant health problem worldwide. Most persons with meningococcal infections in developed nations survive, but healthy patients continue to succumb to fulminant disease despite advances in modern critical care medicine. Such cases, especially in the context of community outbreaks of meningococcal infection, create public fear and are not soon forgotten.

Etiology. *Neisseria meningitidis* is a gram-negative diplococcus. In Gram-stained specimens the microbes appear as kidney-shaped pairs with adjacent sides flattened. In most persons, meningococci are commensal colonizers of the nasopharynx. Humans are the only natural reservoir. *N. meningitidis* is fastidious. Growth is facilitated in a moist environment at 35–37°C in a 5–10% carbon dioxide atmosphere. Growth is readily supported by chocolate, blood, and Mueller-Hinton media used routinely in clinical laboratories. On solid media, colonies are transparent, nonpigmented, and nonhemolytic. *N. meningitidis* is identified by its ability to ferment glucose and maltose, but not sucrose or lactose. Indole and hydrogen sulfide are not formed. Meningococci are oxidase-positive due to a cytochrome oxidase in the cell wall and produce superoxide dismutase.

The meningococcal cell wall has lipid A–containing lipooligosaccharides (LOS; i.e., endotoxin) covered by a polysaccharide capsule. Antigenic variation of the capsule has led to recognition of 13 serogroups. The vast majority of meningococcal disease worldwide is caused by serogroups A, B, C, W135, and Y. LOS and several protein families (porin, opacity-associated protein [Opa]) found in the outer membrane complex are used to serotype strains within serogroups.

Epidemiology. Meningococcal infection occurs as endemic disease punctuated by outbreaks of cases that are clustered temporally and geographically. Prevalence of nasopharyngeal carriage typically is 5–10%, but higher rates can be seen among children in daycare centers and in conditions of crowding. Carriage rates can approach 100% in closed populations during epidemics. In the United States, the incidence of reported meningococcal disease ranged from 0.8–1.3/100,000 population during the 1990s, with 2100–3500 cases/yr. Invasive disease is most common among young children, with rates of 9 cases/100,000 population in the 1st year of life and >25 cases/100,000 population during the 1st 4 mo of life.

There is a slight male predominance among cases (55%). Almost 50% of cases occur in children <2 yr of age, with 25% of cases occurring in persons 30 yr of age or older. Recently, higher rates among persons 15–19 yr of age have been observed than occur among younger adolescents and older adults. College students, especially freshmen living in dormitories, are at approximately twofold to eightfold higher risk than noncollegiate peers. Viral infections, especially influenza, smoking and smoke exposure, crowded living conditions, underlying chronic diseases, and low socioeconomic status, are associated with higher risk for meningococcal infection.

Meningitis is present in 58% of cases. *N. meningitidis* is isolated from blood in about two thirds of cases, from cerebrospinal fluid (CSF) in half, and joint fluid in 1%. Serogroups B and C each account for nearly half of cases among young children in developed countries. Cases caused by serogroup Y strains increased during the 1990s, predominantly among adolescents and adults, such that serogroups B, C, and Y now each account for about one third of cases in these age groups.

Endemic disease is caused by heterogeneous meningococcal strains. Analyses with multilocus enzyme electrophoresis and several genotyping methods have shown that outbreaks are caused by single strains (clones). Transcontinental spread of epidemic clones is well documented. In the United States, there were 26 local outbreaks from 1994–1996, compared with six outbreaks from 1980–1989. Outbreaks are defined as three or more cases in a 3-mo period in the same community, such that the attack rate exceeds 10 cases/100,000 persons. Elementary and secondary school outbreaks can occur. The Pacific Northwest recently has experienced increased endemic serogroup B disease, especially among 15–19 year old persons.

Meningococcal disease, particularly group A, remains a major problem in much of the developing world. Many areas, such as in China and Africa, have endemic rates of 10–25/100,000 persons and major periodic epidemics (100–500/100,000). Endemic disease is most common among young children, whereas epidemic disease typically involves older children, adolescents, and young adults. Crowded conditions increase risk of epidemic spread.

Pathogenesis. *N. meningitidis* is acquired primarily by the respiratory route. Nasopharyngeal colonization usually leads to asymptomatic colonization, which can persist for weeks to months. Invasion is rare, tends to occur soon after acquisition of new strains, and sometimes appears facilitated by concurrent viral respiratory tract infection. Meningococci (and gonococci, but not nonpathogenic *Neisseria*) produce an IgA protease that may assist in colonization of mucous membranes by cleaving the proline-rich hinge region of secretory IgA.

Meningococci adhere selectively to nonciliated epithelial cells by way of their type IV pili. Pili attach to CD46 proteins (receptors for C3b, C4b, measles, and other viruses) on the epithelial cell surface. This induces host cytoskeletal rearrangements and microvillus production that lead to endocytosis. Opa extending from the microbial outer membrane interact with the human CD66 family of receptor molecules and facilitate adhesion and endocytosis. Microbes then traverse the cell in membrane-bound vacuoles. Meningococcal porin proteins play roles in endocytosis, intracellular survival, apoptosis of invaded cells, and escape from complement attack through binding of C4b-binding protein.

Once through the epithelium, meningococci may gain entry into the bloodstream. Serum antibody against meningococcal surface antigens, if present, can block this dissemination by initiation of complement-mediated bacterial lysis. Absence of anti-meningococcal antibody is associated with development of meningococcemia. If the bacteremia is not cleared, interaction with phagocytes continues, organisms adhere to endothelial cells (with pili, Opa, and porin proteins again involved), and the complement system is further activated. Endothelial cell expression of surface adhesion molecules is influenced by LOS and capsular polysaccharide, facilitating attachment of white blood cells. Meningococcal survival is enhanced by the polysaccharide capsule, which helps resist phagocytic killing, and an iron scavenging system that can use host transferrin and lactoferrin.

The microbial-phagocyte-endothelial cell-complement interactions lead to production of multiple proinflammatory cytokines, including tumor necrosis factor α (TNFα), interleukin (IL)-1β, IL-6, and IL-8, and activation of both the extrinsic (by way of induction of tissue factor expression on endothelial cell and monocytes) and intrinsic pathways of coagulation. The degree of activation of the complement and clotting cascades, the concentrations of circulating cytokines, and risk of fatality correlate with the concentration of meningococcal LOS in the plasma at presentation. Progression of capillary leak and disseminated intravascular coagulopathy (DIC) can lead to multiple organ system failure, septic shock, and sometimes death. Fatal cases typically have higher concentrations of TNFα and ILs than do survivors, but the causal relationship remains unclear. LOS and TNFα levels decrease rapidly once antibiotics are given, correlating with clearance of viable microbes. Activation of the complement and clotting cascades can continue well beyond this point, especially in fulminant cases.

Non-LOS antigens appear to drive the dendritic cell maturation required for initiation of the adaptive immune response. IL-12 production, driven by meningococcal LOS, creates a Th-1 response environment. Bactericidal antibodies are produced against capsular polysaccharide, outer membrane proteins, and LOS antigens. Natural immunity against *N. meningitidis* develops in most persons after repeated colonization with different serogroups or serotypes and from gastrointestinal colonization with enteric bacteria that express cross-reactive antigens. Infants also have high carriage rates of the unencapsulated, nonpathogenic neisserial strain, *N. lactamica*, which contributes to development of immunity against meningococci. Protective effects of maternally derived IgG wanes during the 1st 3 months of life, with resultant high rates of invasive disease in the 1st year of life.

Invasive meningococcal disease is associated with an acute inflammatory response. Diffuse vasculitis and DIC are common with meningococcemia. Leukocyte-rich fibrin clots are seen in small vessels, including arterioles and capillaries. The resulting focal hemorrhage and necrosis may be seen in any organ system. The heart, central nervous system, skin, mucous and serous membranes, and adrenals are affected in most fatal cases. Myocarditis occurs in >50% of patients who die of meningococcal disease. Diffuse adrenal hemorrhage without vasculitis is common during fulminant meningococcemia (i.e., Waterhouse-Friderichsen syndrome). Meningitis is characterized by acute inflammatory cells in the leptomeninges and perivascular spaces. Focal cerebritis is uncommon.

Persons with primary complement deficiency have an increased risk of developing meningococcal disease, underscoring the important role of complement in host defense against the meningococcus. Among individuals with properdin, factor D, or terminal-component deficiencies, 50–60% will develop serious bacterial infections, caused almost solely by *N. meningitidis*. Some studies suggest disease manifestations with complement deficiencies are less severe than with intact complement function, but this is not certain. Recurrent infection is more common with terminal component deficiencies than with properdin deficiency. Similar increased risk is seen with the acquired complement deficiencies that occur in patients with diseases such as nephrotic syndrome, systemic lupus erythematosus, and hepatic failure. Among persons with meningococcal infections, complement deficiencies are much more prevalent in those >5 yr of age than in younger children.

Host factors that may affect the severity of meningococcal disease include polymorphisms of IL-1, IL-1 receptor antagonist, mannose-binding lectin, and Fc receptor genes (potentially in concert with certain IL-10 alleles) and the promoter regions for the TNFα and plasminogen-activator-inhibitor-1 genes. Presence of factor V Leiden exacerbates purpura fulminans but may not affect mortality.

The group B capsule is a homopolymer of sialic acid, which is poorly immunogenic in humans due in part to its structural homology with mammalian neural cell adhesion molecules. The B capsular antigen also does not activate the alternative complement pathway in humans, which is a key part of the innate immune response essential for protection from infections in the absence of specific antibodies. This may explain in part the higher prevalence of serogroup B meningococcal disease in young children.

Clinical Manifestations. The spectrum of meningococcal disease varies widely from fever and occult bacteremia (Chapter 162) to sepsis and shock (Chapter 163) and death. Recognized patterns of disease include bacteremia without sepsis, meningococcemia (sepsis) without meningitis, and meningitis with or without meningococcemia. At least 80% of cases have overt clinical signs. Occult meningococcal bacteremia often presents as fever with or without associated symptoms that suggest minor viral infections. Resolution may occur without antibiotics, but some cases will develop meningitis.

Acute meningococcemia initially may mimic viral illness with pharyngitis, fever, myalgias, weakness, vomiting, diarrhea, and/or headache. A maculopapular rash can be evident before more serious signs develop. In fulminant cases, the disease progresses rapidly over hours to septic shock characterized by hypotension, DIC, acidosis, adrenal hemorrhage, renal failure, myocardial failure, and coma. Petechiae and purpura may be prominent (purpura fulminans). Meningitis may or may not be present. Concomitant suppurative arthritis, pneumonia, myocarditis, and purulent pericarditis may be present.

The most common clinical manifestation is meningococcal meningitis, which usually responds to appropriate antibiotics and supportive therapy. Headache, photophobia, lethargy, vomiting, and nuchal rigidity and other signs of meningeal irritation typically are present. Seizures and focal neurologic signs occur less frequently than in patients with meningitis caused by pneumococcus or *Haemophilus influenzae* type b. Rarely, meningoencephalitis can occur. This may be more common with serogroup A infection.

In a series of 100 children with invasive meningococcal disease, 71% presented with fever, 42% had hypotension or decreased peripheral perfusion, and 34% had emesis. Petechiae and/or purpura were present in 49%. Purpura fulminans developed in 16%. Maculopapular rashes or pustular or bullous lesions were present in 11%. Additional presenting symptoms and signs were irritability (21%), lethargy (30%), diarrhea (6%), rhinorrhea (10%), seizure (8%), septic arthritis (8%), and non-suppurative arthritis (6%). Radiographic evidence of pneumonia was present initially in 8%.

Uncommon manifestations of meningococcal disease include endocarditis, purulent pericarditis, pneumonia, endophthalmitis, mesenteric lymphadenitis, osteomyelitis, sinusitis, otitis media, and periorbital cellulitis. Primary purulent conjunctivitis can lead to invasive disease. Pleural effusion or empyema occurs in 15% of cases with meningococcal pneumonia. *N. meningitidis* infections of the genitourinary tract are rare, but urethritis, cervicitis, vulvovaginitis, and proctitis can occur.

Chronic meningococcemia occurs rarely and is characterized by fever, nontoxic appearance, arthralgias, headache, and a rash similar to that of disseminated gonococcal infection. Symptoms are intermittent. The mean duration of illness is 6–8 wk. Blood cultures may initially be sterile. Meningitis can develop in untreated cases.

Diagnosis. Definitive diagnosis of meningococcal disease is established by isolation of the organism from a normally sterile body fluid such as blood, CSF, or synovial fluid. Isolation from the nasopharynx is not diagnostic for invasive disease. Blood and CSF are the usual sources of the organism. Cultures often are negative if the patient has received prior antibiotic treatment. Meningococci sometimes can be identified in culture or Gram stain of petechial or papular lesions. Bacteria occasionally are seen on Gram stain of the buffy coat layer of a spun blood sample.

In meningitis, the morphologic and clinical characteristics of CSF are those of acute bacterial meningitis (Chapter 594.1). CSF cultures sometimes are positive in patients with meningococcemia who do not have CSF pleocytosis or clinical evidence of meningitis. Gram stain–positive CSF specimens sometimes are culture-negative. Overdecolorized pneumococci in Gram stains can be mistaken for meningococci (empirical therapy should not be based on Gram stain alone).

Detection of capsular polysaccharide antigens by rapid latex agglutination tests in CSF can support the diagnosis in cases clinically consistent with meningococcal disease. These tests are most useful when results are positive in the setting of partially treated infections with negative cultures. Antigen tests using serum or urine are not helpful. Rapid antigen tests are not reliable for serogroup B strains due to cross-reactions with other bacterial species. Detection of meningococci in blood and CSF using polymerase chain reaction has been used in research laboratories and currently are used clinically in the United Kingdom. These likely will have more widespread use in the future.

Other laboratory findings include leukocytopenia or leukocytosis (often with increased percentages of neutrophils and band forms), thrombocytopenia, proteinuria, and hematuria. Elevated sedimentation rate and C-reactive protein, hypoalbuminemia, hypocalcemia, and metabolic acidosis (often with increased lactate levels) are common. Patients with DIC have decreased serum concentrations of prothrombin and fibrinogen and prolonged coagulation studies.

DIFFERENTIAL DIAGNOSIS. Meningococcal disease can appear similar to sepsis or meningitis caused by many other gram-negative bacteria; *S. pneumoniae*, *S. aureus*, or group A streptococcus; Rocky Mountain spotted fever, ehrlichiosis, or epidemic typhus; and bacterial endocarditis. Viral and other etiologies of encephalitis should be considered in some cases. Autoimmune vasculitides (especially Henoch-Schönlein purpura), serum sickness, hemolytic-uremic syndrome, Kawasaki disease, idiopathic thrombocytopenic purpura, drug eruptions, and ingestion of various poisons can have features that overlap those of meningococcal infection. Infections with echoviruses (particularly types 6, 9, and 16), coxsackieviruses (primarily types A2, A4, A9, and A16), and other viruses also may have severe presentations that initially raise concerns about meningococcal infection.

The petechial or purpuric rash of meningococcemia is similar to that of other generalized vasculitides. Benign petechial rashes are common in viral and group A streptococcal infections. The nonpetechial rashes observed in some meningococcal cases may be confused with a viral exanthem.

Treatment. For hospitalized patients, penicillin G (250,000–400,000 U/kg/24 hr divided q 4–6 hr IV) remains the drug of choice. Cefotaxime (200 mg/kg/24 hr) or ceftriaxone (100 mg/kg/24 hr) are acceptable alternatives and generally are part of initial empiric regimens. Chloramphenicol (75–100 mg/kg/24 hr divided q 6 hr IV) remains effective treatment for patients who are allergic to β-lactam antibiotics. Therapy is continued for 5–7 days.

Early treatment of meningococcal infections may prevent serious sequelae, but timely identification of such patients is difficult in the absence of skin findings. High fever and leukocytosis with increased neutrophil and band counts are common in older children and adolescents with otherwise unsuspected meningococcal infection. Empirical outpatient treatment of selected patients during meningococcal outbreaks and of nontoxic children with petechial rashes can be considered. Most of the latter will not have meningococcal infection. Blood cultures should be obtained before treatment.

Isolates of *N. meningitidis* with relative resistance to penicillin (minimal inhibitory concentration of penicillin of 0.1–1.0 µ/mL) have been reported from Europe, Africa, Canada, and the United States. Decreased susceptibility is caused, at least in part, by altered penicillin-binding protein 2. In 1991 such strains represented ~4% of isolates in the United States. This degree of penicillin resistance does not appear to impact response to therapy. Strains producing β-lactamase remain exceedingly rare. Routine susceptibility testing of meningococcal isolates is not indicated in the United States at this time, but continued surveillance is necessary.

Optimal supportive care is essential (Chapter 57.2). Many adjunctive therapies have been attempted in severe cases. Protein C replacement holds promise for treatment of severe sepsis and DIC and is being evaluated in children. Protein C is an anticoagulant that also downregulates the inflammatory response and is depleted in DIC. Trials of HA-1A human monoclonal antibody to endotoxin and recombinant bactericidal/permeability-increasing protein showed less benefit than expected. Other anticoagulant or fibrinolytic agents and vasodilators have been used with variable success in anecdotal reports. Combinations of such therapies may be useful in selected cases in the future, but have yet to be evaluated.

Children with severe disease who respond poorly to aggressive fluid and inotropic therapies may have adrenal insufficiency and may benefit from hydrocortisone supplementation. Extracorporeal membrane oxygenation has been used with limited success.

Complications. Acute complications are related to the vasculitis, DIC, and hypotension of severe meningococcal disease. Focal skin infarctions often heal but can become secondarily infected (similar to burns), resulting in significant scarring and requiring skin grafting. The gangrene of extremities often seen with purpura fulminans may necessitate amputations. Adrenal hemorrhage, endophthalmitis, arthritis, endocarditis, pericarditis, myocarditis, pneumonia, lung abscess, peritonitis, and renal infarcts can occur during acute infection. Avascular necrosis of epiphyses and epiphyseal-metaphyseal defects can result from the generalized DIC and may lead to growth disturbances and late skeletal deformities.

Deafness is the most frequent neurologic sequela, occurring in 5–10% of children with meningitis in most series. Cerebral arterial or venous thrombosis with resultant cerebral infarction can occur in severe cases. Meningitis rarely is complicated by subdural effusion or empyema or by brain abscess. Other rare neurologic sequelae include ataxia, seizures, blindness, cranial nerve palsies, hemiparesis or quadriparesis, and obstructive hydrocephalus. The latter often presents 3–4 wk after onset of illness.

Nonsuppurative complications of meningococcal disease appear to be immune complex–mediated and become apparent 4–9 days after the onset of illness. Arthritis and cutaneous vasculitis (erythema nodosum) are most common. The arthritis usually is monoarticular or oligoarticular, involves large joints, and has sterile effusions that respond to nonsteroidal anti-inflammatory agents. Long-term sequelae are uncommon. Because most patients with meningococcal meningitis become afebrile by the 7th hospital day, persistence or recrudescence of fever after 5 days of antibiotics warrants evaluation for immune complex–mediated complications.

Reactivation of latent herpes simplex virus infections (primarily herpes labialis) is common during meningococcal infection.

Prognosis. The mortality rate for invasive meningococcal disease remains 8–13% in the United States despite modern interventions. Poor prognostic factors on presentation include hypothermia, hypotension or shock, purpura fulminans, seizures, leukopenia, thrombocytopenia (DIC), acidosis, and high circulating levels of endotoxin and TNFα. The presence of petechiae for <12 hr before admission, the presence of hyperpyrexia, and the absence of meningitis indicate rapid progression and poorer prognosis.

Screening for complement deficiency after resolution of the acute infection can be considered for any person with meningococcal infection and should be performed for older children and adolescents. Recurrent infections also can be severe.

Prevention. Close contacts of patients with meningococcal disease are at increased risk of infection and should be carefully monitored and brought to medical attention if fever develops. Prophylaxis is indicated as soon as possible for household, daycare, and nursery school contacts and for those who have had contact with the patient's oral secretions during the 7 days before onset of illness. Prophylaxis is not routinely recommended for medical personnel except those with intimate exposure, such as with mouth-to-mouth resuscitation, intubation, or suctioning before antibiotic therapy was begun. Children may be given rifampin (10 mg/kg orally q 12 hr for a total of four doses; maximum dose: 600 mg; 5 mg/kg/dose for infants <1 mo of age) or ceftriaxone (125 mg in a single dose IM for children <12 yr; 250 mg in a single dose IM for >12 yr of age). Ciprofloxacin (500 mg orally as a single dose) may be given for persons ≥18 yr. Penicillin does not eradicate nasopharyngeal carriage; patients treated with penicillin should receive prophylaxis before hospital discharge. Hospitalized patients should be placed on droplet precautions for 24 hr after initiation of effective therapy. All confirmed or probable cases of meningococcal infection must be reported to the local public health department.

VACCINE. A quadrivalent vaccine composed of capsular polysaccharide of meningococcal groups A, C, Y, and W135 is licensed in the United States. The vaccine is immunogenic in adults but is unreliable in children younger than 2 yr. No routine immunization use is recommended in the United States at this time. Individuals with anatomic or functional asplenia or complement component deficiencies should be immunized when beyond age 2 yr of age. The vaccine may be beneficial for travelers to countries with a high incidence of meningococcal disease. It is routinely given to American military recruits. It also is used to control sustained local outbreaks of meningococcal disease caused by one of the vaccine serogroups.

College students, especially entering freshmen and those living on campus, and their parents should be informed about the increased risk (both relative and absolute) of meningococcal disease that may be incurred. Vaccine should be made available to those who request it and may be required by some colleges and states before matriculation. Vaccination provides substantial but not absolute protection against the two thirds of meningococcal disease caused by serogroups C and Y in this age group.

Polysaccharide-protein conjugate meningococcal vaccines are immunogenic in infants and are being evaluated in the United States. A group C conjugate vaccine is now being used routinely in the United Kingdom with resulting reduction in the incidence of group C disease. Immune responses to these vaccines are boostable and likely more durable than for nonconjugate vaccines.

Efforts to develop an effective serogroup B vaccine now focus largely on conserved outer membrane proteins. Strain-specific vaccines can be produced if needed for control of serogroup B outbreaks, but such single antigen vaccines are not effective against other strains in the serogroup because of the high frequency of genetic transformation and resultant antigenic variation of *N. meningitidis*.

Alberio L, Lämmle B, Esmon CT: Protein C replacement in severe meningococcemia: Rationale and clinical experience. *Clin Infect Dis* 2001;32:1338–46.

American Academy of Pediatrics, Committee on Infectious Diseases: Meningococcal disease prevention and control strategies for practice-based physicians (Addendum: Recommendation for college students). *Pediatrics* 2000;106:1500–4.

Fijen CAP, Kuijper EJ, te Bulte MT, et al: Assessment of complement deficiency in patients with meningococcal disease in the Netherlands. *Clin Infect Dis* 1999:28:98–105.

Leclerc F, Leteurtre S, Cremer R, et al: Do new strategies in meningococcemia produce better outcomes? *Crit Care Med* 2000;28:S60–3.

Levin M, Quint PA, Goldstein B, et al: Recombinant bactericidal/permeability-increasing protein (rBPI$_{21}$) as adjunctive treatment for children with severe meningococcal sepsis: A randomised trial. *Lancet* 2000;356:961–7.

Pollard AJ, Levin M: Vaccines for prevention of meningococcal disease. *Pediatr Infect Dis J* 2000;9:333–45.

Ramsey ME, Andrews N, Kaczmarski EB, Miller E: Efficacy of meningococcal serogroup C conjugate vaccine in teenagers and toddlers in England. *Lancet* 2001357:195–6

Tzeng Y-L, Stephens DS: Epidemiology and pathogenesis of *Neisseria meningitidis*. *Microbes Infection* 2000;2:687–700.

van Woensel JBM, Biezeveld MH, Alders AMB, et al.: Adrenocorticotropic hormone and cortisol levels in relation to inflammatory response and disease severity in children with meningococcal disease. *J Infect Dis* 2001;184:1532–7.

Wang VJ, Malley R, Fleisher GR, et al: Antibiotic treatment of children with unsuspected meningococcal disease. *Arch Pediatr Adolesc Med* 2000;154:556–60.

Chapter 177
Neisseria gonorrhoeae (Gonococcus) *Toni Darville*

Neisseria gonorrhoeae produces various forms of **gonorrhea**, an infection of the genitourinary tract mucous membranes and rarely of the mucosa of the rectum, oropharynx, and conjunctiva. Gonorrhea transmitted by sexual contact or perinatally is second only to chlamydial infections in the number of cases reported to the Centers for Disease Control and Prevention (CDC) in the United States. This high prevalence and the development of antibiotic-resistant strains have produced significant morbidity in adolescents.

Etiology. *N. gonorrhoeae* is a nonmotile, aerobic, non–spore-forming, gram-negative, intracellular diplococcus with flattened adjacent surfaces. Optimal growth occurs at 35–37°C and at pH 7.2–7.6 in an atmosphere of 3–5% carbon dioxide. The specimen should be inoculated immediately onto fresh, moist modified Thayer-Martin or specialized transport media because gonococci do not tolerate drying. Thayer-Martin medium contains antimicrobial agents that inhibit hardier normal flora present in clinical specimens that may otherwise overgrow gonococci. Presumptive identification may be based on colony appearance, Gram stain, and production of cytochrome oxidase. Gonococci are differentiated from other *Neisseria* species by the fermentation of glucose but not maltose, sucrose, or lactose. Gram-negative diplococci are seen in infected material, often within polymorphonuclear leukocytes.

Like all gram-negative bacteria, *N. gonorrhoeae* possess a cell envelope composed of an inner cytoplasmic membrane, a middle layer of peptidoglycan, and an outer membrane. The outer membrane contains lipo-oligosaccharides (endotoxin), phospholipid, and a variety of proteins that contribute to cell adherence, tissue invasion, and resistance to host defenses. The two systems primarily used to characterize gonococcal strains are auxotyping and serotyping. **Auxotyping** is based on genetically stable requirements of strains for specific nutrients or cofactors as defined by the ability of an isolate to grow on chemically defined media. The most widely used **serotyping** system is based on porin, a trimeric outer membrane protein that makes up a substantial part of the gonococcal envelope structure. Antibodies generated to Por have been used to serotype gonococci (e.g., PorIA-4 and PorIB-12), and changes in porin proteins present in a community are believed to occur, at least in part, as a result of selective immune pressure.

Epidemiology. *N. gonorrhoeae* infection occurs only in humans. The organism is shed in the exudate and secretions of infected mucosal surfaces and is transmitted through intimate contact, such as sexual contact or parturition and, rarely, by contact with fomites. Gonococcal infections in the newborn period generally are acquired during delivery. Gonorrhea is the most common sexually transmitted disease found in sexually abused children. Rarely, *N. gonorrhoeae* may be spread by sexual play among children, but the index patient is likely to be a victim of sexual abuse. Gonococcal infections in children are acquired rarely through household exposure to infected caretakers. In such cases, the possibility of sexual abuse should be seriously considered.

In the United States, the number of reported cases of gonorrhea increased steadily in the United States from 1964–1977, fluctuated through the early 1980s, increased until 1987, and since 1987 have decreased annually. Reported cases have declined from 323 cases/100,000 population in 1987 to 123 cases/100,000 population in 1996. There were 324,901 cases reported to CDC in 1997. The decline in gonorrhea prevalence may be attributed to recommendations by CDC that only highly effective antimicrobial agents be used to treat gonorrhea. The incidence of gonorrhea is highest in high-density urban areas among persons <24 yr of age who have multiple sexual partners and engage in unprotected sexual intercourse. Increases in gonorrhea prevalence have been noted recently among men who have sex with men. Risk factors include nonwhite race, homosexuality, increased number of sexual partners, prostitution, presence of other sexually transmitted diseases (STDs), unmarried status, poverty, and failure to use condoms. Techniques of auxotyping and serotyping, and more recently, molecular typing methods have been used to analyze the spread of individual strains of *N. gonorrhoeae* within a community.

Maintenance and subsequent spread of gonococcal infections in a community require a hyperendemic, high-risk core group such as prostitutes or adolescents with multiple sexual partners. This is because most persons who have gonorrhea cease sexual activity and seek care, unless economic need or other factors (e.g., drug addiction) drive persistent sexual activity. Thus, many core transmitters belong to a subset of infected persons who lack or ignore symptoms and continue to be sexually active. This underscores the importance of seeking out and treating the sexual contacts of infected persons who present for treatment.

Gonococcal infection of neonates usually results from peripartum exposure to infected exudate from the cervix of the mother. An acute infection begins 2–5 days after birth. The incidence of neonatal infection depends on the prevalence of gonococcal infection among pregnant women, prenatal screening for gonorrhea, and neonatal ophthalmic prophylaxis.

Pathogenesis. *N. gonorrhoeae* infect primarily columnar epithelium; stratified squamous epithelium is relatively resistant to invasion. Mucosal invasion by gonococci results in a local inflammatory response that produces a purulent exudate consisting of polymorphonuclear leukocytes, serum, and desquamated epithelium. The gonococcal lipo-oligosaccharide (endotoxin) exhibits direct cytotoxicity, causing ciliastasis and sloughing of ciliated epithelial cells. Once the gonococcus traverses the mucosal barrier, the lipo-oligosaccharide binds bactericidal IgM antibody and serum complement, causing an acute inflammatory response in the subepithelial space. Tumor necrosis factor and other cytokines are thought to mediate the cytotoxicity of gonococcal infections.

Gonococci may ascend the urogenital tract, causing urethritis or epididymitis in postpubertal males, and causing acute endometritis, salpingitis, and peritonitis, which are collectively termed **acute pelvic inflammatory disease (PID),** in postpubertal females. **Perihepatitis (Fitz-Hugh-Curtis syndrome)** follows dissemination through the peritoneum from the fallopian tubes to the liver capsule. Gonococci that invade the lymphatics and blood vessels may lead to inguinal lymphadenopathy; to perineal, perianal, ischiorectal, and periprostatic abscesses; and to **disseminated gonococcal infection (DGI).**

Several gonococcal virulence and host immune factors are involved in the penetration of the mucosal barrier and subsequent manifestations of local and systemic infection. Selective pressure from different mucosal environments probably leads to changes in the outer membrane of the organism, including expression of variants of pili, opacity (Opa) proteins (formerly protein II), and lipo-oligosaccharides. These changes may enhance gonococcal attachment, invasion, replication, and evasion of the host's immune response.

For infection to occur, the gonococcus must first attach to host cells. A gonococcal IgA protease inactivates IgA1 by cleaving the molecule in the hinge region and may be an important factor in colonization or invasion of host mucosal surfaces. Gonococci adhere to the microvilli of nonciliated epithelial cells by hairlike protein structures (pili) that extend from the cell wall. Pili are thought to protect the gonococcus from phagocytosis and complement-mediated killing. Pili undergo high-frequency antigenic variation that may aid in the organism's escape from the host immune response and may provide specific ligands for different cell receptors. Opa proteins, most of which confer an opaque appearance to colonies, are also thought to function as ligands to facilitate binding to human cells. Gonococci that express certain Opa proteins adhere and are phagocytosed by human neutrophils in the absence of serum.

Other phenotypic changes that occur in response to environmental stresses allow gonococci to establish infection. Examples include iron-repressible proteins for binding transferrin or lactoferrin, anaerobically expressed proteins, and synthesis of proteins mediated by contact with epithelial cells. Gonococci may grow in vivo under anaerobic conditions or in an environment with relative lack of iron.

Approximately 24 hr after attachment, the epithelial cell surface invaginates and surrounds the gonococcus in a phagocytic vacuole. This phenomenon is thought to be mediated by the gonococcal outer membrane protein I inserting into the host cell and causing alterations in membrane permeability. Subsequently, phagocytic vacuoles begin releasing gonococci into the subepithelial space by means of exocytosis. Viable organisms may then cause local disease (i.e., salpingitis) or disseminate through the bloodstream or lymphatics.

Serum IgG and IgM directed against gonococcal proteins and lipo-oligosaccharides lead to complement-mediated bacterial lysis. Stable serum resistance to this bactericidal antibody probably results from a particular type of porin protein expressed in gonococci (most contain Por1A), and these strains are often the cause of disseminated disease. *N. gonorrhoeae* differentially subvert the effectiveness of complement and alter the inflammatory responses elicited in human infection. Isolates associated with DGI typically resist killing by normal serum (are serum-resistant), inactivate more C3b, generate less C5a, and result in less inflammation at local sites. PID isolates are serum-sensitive, inactivate less C3b, generate more C5a, and result in more inflammation at local sites. IgG antibody directed against gonococcal reduction modifiable protein (Rmp) blocks complement-mediated killing of *N. gonorrhoeae*. Anti-Rmp blocking antibodies may harbor specificity for outer membrane protein sequences shared with other neisserial species or Enterobacteriaceae or may be directed against unique Rmp upstream cysteine loop specific sequences, or both. Preexisting antibodies directed against Rmp facilitate transmission of gonococcal infection to exposed women; Rmp is highly conserved in *N. gonorrhoeae* and the blocking of mucosal defenses may be one of its functions. Gonococcal adaptation also appears to be important in the evasion of killing by neutrophils. Examples include sialylation of lipo-oligosaccharides, increases in catalase production, and changes in the expression of surface proteins.

Host factors may influence the incidence and manifestations of gonococcal infection. Prepubertal girls are susceptible to vulvovaginitis and, rarely, experience salpingitis. *N. gonorrhoeae* infects noncornified epithelium, and the thin noncornified vaginal epithelium and alkaline pH of the vaginal mucin predispose this age group to infection of the lower genital tract. Estrogen-induced cornification of the vaginal epithelium in neonates and mature females resists infection. Postpubertal females are more susceptible to salpingitis, especially during menses, when diminished bactericidal activity of the cervical mucus and reflux of blood from the uterine cavity into the fallopian tubes facilitate passage of gonococci into the upper reproductive tract.

Populations at risk for DGI include asymptomatic carriers; neonates; menstruating, pregnant, and postpartum women; homosexuals; and immunocompromised hosts. The asymptomatic carrier state implies failure of the host immune system to recognize the gonococcus as a pathogen, the capacity of the gonococcus to avoid being killed, or both. Pharyngeal colonization has been proposed as a risk factor for DGI. The high rate of asymptomatic infection in pharyngeal gonorrhea may account for this phenomenon. Women are at greater risk for developing DGI during menstruation, pregnancy, and postpartum, presumably because of the maximal endocervical shedding and decreased peroxidase bactericidal activity of the cervical mucus during these periods. A lack of neonatal bactericidal IgM antibody is thought to account for a neonate's increased susceptibility to DGI. Persons with terminal complement component deficiencies (C5-C9) are at considerable risk of developing recurrent episodes of DGI.

Clinical Manifestations. Gonorrhea is manifested by a spectrum of clinical presentations, from asymptomatic carriage to the characteristic localized urogenital infections, to disseminated systemic infection.

ASYMPTOMATIC GONORRHEA. The incidence of this form of gonorrhea in children has not been ascertained. Gonococci have been isolated from the oropharynx of young children who have been abused sexually by male contacts; oropharyngeal symptoms are usually absent. Most genital tract infections produce symptoms in children. However, as many as 80% of sexually mature females with urogenital gonorrhea infections are asymptomatic in settings in which most infections are detected through screening or other case-finding efforts; asymptomatic

rectal carriage of *N. gonorrhoeae* has been documented in 40–60% of females with urogenital infection. Most persons with positive rectal cultures are asymptomatic. Most pharyngeal gonococcal infections are asymptomatic. The importance of documenting pharyngeal infection is debated. Most cases resolve spontaneously, transmission from the pharynx to other patients is uncommon, and the pharynx is rarely the only site of infection. On the other hand, pharyngeal infection is sometimes symptomatic and may occasionally be the source of transmission to sexual partners or systemic dissemination.

UNCOMPLICATED GONORRHEA. Genital gonorrhea has an incubation period of 2–5 days in men and 5–10 days in women. Primary infection develops in the urethra of males, the vulva and vagina of prepubertal females, and the cervix of postpubertal females.

Urethritis is usually characterized by a purulent discharge and by dysuria without urgency or frequency. Untreated urethritis in males resolves spontaneously in several weeks or may be complicated by epididymitis, penile edema, lymphangitis, prostatitis, or seminal vesiculitis. Gram-negative intracellular diplococci are found in the discharge.

In prepubertal females, vulvovaginitis usually is characterized by a purulent vaginal discharge with a swollen, erythematous, tender, and excoriated vulva. Dysuria may occur. In postpubertal females, symptomatic gonococcal cervicitis and urethritis are characterized by purulent discharge, suprapubic pain, dysuria, intermenstrual bleeding, and dyspareunia. The cervix may be inflamed and tender. In urogenital gonorrhea limited to the lower genital tract, pain is not enhanced by moving the cervix, and the adnexa are not tender to palpation. Purulent material may be expressed from the urethra or ducts of the Bartholin gland. Rectal gonorrhea, although often asymptomatic, may cause proctitis with symptoms of anal discharge, pruritus, bleeding, pain, tenesmus, and constipation. Asymptomatic rectal gonorrhea may not be due to anal intercourse but may represent colonization from vaginal infection.

Gonococcal ophthalmitis may be unilateral or bilateral. It may occur in any age group after inoculation of the eye with infected secretions. Ophthalmia neonatorum due to *N. gonorrhoeae* usually appears from 1–4 days after birth (Chapter 633). Ocular infection in older patients results from inoculation or autoinoculation from a genital site. The infection begins with mild inflammation and a serosanguineous discharge. Within 24 hr, the discharge becomes thick and purulent, and tense edema of the eyelids with marked chemosis occurs. If the disease is not treated promptly, corneal ulceration, rupture, and blindness may follow.

DISSEMINATED GONOCOCCAL INFECTION. Hematogenous dissemination occurs in 1–3% of all gonococcal infections, more frequently after asymptomatic primary infections than symptomatic infections. Women account for the majority of cases, with symptoms beginning 7–30 days after infection and within 7 days of menstruation. The most common manifestations are asymmetric arthralgia, petechial or pustular acral skin lesions, tenosynovitis, suppurative arthritis, and, rarely, carditis, meningitis, and osteomyelitis. The most common initial symptoms are acute onset of polyarthralgia with fever. Only 25% of patients complain of skin lesions. Most deny genitourinary symptoms; however, primary mucosal infection is documented by genitourinary cultures. Approximately 80–90% of cervical cultures are positive in women with DGI. In males, urethral cultures are positive in 50–60%, pharyngeal cultures are positive in 10–20%, and rectal cultures are positive in 15% of cases.

DGI has been classified into two clinical syndromes that have some overlapping features. The first and more common is the **tenosynovitis-dermatitis syndrome**, which is characterized by fever, chills, skin lesions, and polyarthralgias predominantly involving the wrists, hands, and fingers. Blood culture results are positive in approximately 30–40% of cases, and synovial fluid cultures are almost uniformly negative. The second syndrome is the **suppurative arthritis syndrome**, in which systemic symptoms and signs are less prominent and a monarticular arthritis, often involving the knee, is more common. A polyarthric phase may precede the monarticular infection. In cases of monarticular involvement, synovial fluid culture results are positive in approximately 45–55% and synovial fluid findings are consistent with septic arthritis. Blood culture results are usually negative. DGI in neonates usually occurs as a polyarticular septic arthritis.

Dermatologic lesions usually begin as painful, discrete, 1–20 mm pink or red macules that progress to maculopapular, vesicular, bullous, pustular, or petechial lesions. The typical necrotic pustule on an erythematous base is distributed unevenly over the extremities, including the palmar and plantar surfaces, usually sparing the face and scalp. The lesions number between 5 and 40; 20–30% may contain gonococci. Although immune complexes may be present in DGI, complement levels are normal, and the role of the immune complexes in pathogenesis is uncertain.

Acute endocarditis is an uncommon (1–2%) but often fatal manifestation of DGI that usually leads to rapid destruction of the aortic valve. Acute pericarditis is a rarely described entity in patients with disseminated gonorrhea. Meningitis with *N. gonorrhoeae* has been documented. Signs and symptoms are similar to those of other causes of acute bacterial meningitis.

Diagnosis. It is not possible to distinguish gonococcal from nongonococcal urethritis on the basis of symptoms and signs alone. Gonococcal urethritis and vulvovaginitis must be distinguished from other infections that produce a purulent discharge, including β-hemolytic streptococci, *Chlamydia trachomatis, Mycoplasma hominis, Trichomonas vaginalis,* and *Candida albicans.* Rarely, infection with human herpesvirus type 2 may produce symptoms similar to those of gonorrhea.

In males with symptomatic urethritis, a presumptive diagnosis of gonorrhea can be made by identification of gram-negative intracellular diplococci (within leukocytes) in the urethral discharge. A similar finding in females is not sufficient because *Mima polymorpha* and *Moraxella,* which are normal vaginal flora, have a similar appearance. The sensitivity of the Gram stain for diagnosing gonococcal cervicitis and asymptomatic infections is also low. The presence of commensal *Neisseria* species in the oropharynx prevents the use of the Gram stain for diagnosis of pharyngeal gonorrhea. Nonpathogenic *Neisseria* are not intracellular.

Diagnosis of gonococcal disease depends on isolation of *N. gonorrhoeae.* Antibiotic susceptibility testing necessitates isolation by culture. Male urethral specimens are obtained by placing a small swab 2–3 cm into the urethra. Material for cervical cultures is obtained after wiping the exocervix and placing a swab in the cervical os and rotating it gently for several seconds. Rectal swabs are best obtained by passing a swab 2–4 cm into the anal canal; specimens that are heavily contaminated by feces should be discarded. For optimal culture results, specimens should be obtained with noncotton swabs (e.g., a urethrogenital Calgiswab), inoculated directly onto culture plates, and incubated immediately. The choice of anatomic sites to culture depends on the sites exposed and the clinical manifestations. Samples from the urethra should be cultured for heterosexual men, and samples from the endocervix and rectum should be cultured for all females, regardless of a history of anal intercourse. A pharyngeal culture should be obtained from both men and women if symptoms of pharyngitis are present or in the case of oral exposure to a person known to have genital gonorrhea. In a suspected case of child sexual abuse, rectal, pharyngeal, and urethral (males) or vaginal (females) swabs should be cultured. Culture of the endocervix should not be attempted until after puberty.

Specimens from sites (e.g., cervix, rectum, pharynx) that normally are colonized by other organisms should be inoculated on a selective culture medium, such as modified Thayer-Martin medium (fortified with vancomycin, colistin, nystatin, and trimethoprim to inhibit growth of indigenous flora). Specimens from sites that are normally sterile or minimally contaminated (i.e., synovial fluid, blood, cerebrospinal fluid) should be inoculated on a nonselective chocolate agar medium. If DGI is suspected, blood, pharynx, rectum, urethra, cervix, and synovial fluid (if involved) should be cultured. Cultured specimens should be incubated promptly at 35–37°C in 3–5% carbon dioxide. When specimens must be transported to a central laboratory for culture plating, a reduced, non-nutrient holding medium (i.e., Amies-modified Stuart medium) preserves specimens with minimal loss of viability for up to 6 hr. When transport may delay culture plating by more than 6 hr, it is preferable to inoculate the sample directly onto a culture medium and transport it at an ambient temperature in a candle jar. The Transgrow and JEM-BEC systems of modified Thayer-Martin medium are alternative transport systems.

When microbiology laboratory facilities are not readily available or when patients may be unavailable for follow-up, rapid diagnostic techniques may prove efficacious. Care must be taken in selecting and interpreting results because many rapid tests are less specific than cultures. Nonculture tests include enzyme immunoassay (polyclonal antigonococcal antibodies for detection of gonococcal antigen), enzyme-linked immunosorbent assay (monoclonal antibodies), DNA probes, and nucleic acid amplification tests (polymerase chain reaction or ligase chain reaction). These tests appear to be less reliable than culture in low-risk asymptomatic patients, for nongenital specimens, and for specimens obtained from children. Nucleic acid amplification tests and DNA probes may prove to be comparable to culture in sensitivity and specificity. Nonculture tests cannot replace bacteriologic cultures for definitive diagnosis of *N. gonorrhoeae* or for antimicrobial susceptibility testing and may be more expensive. They may serve as useful adjuvant diagnostic tools in high-prevalence, transient populations (e.g., in adolescent STD clinics), in which a rapid and accurate presumptive diagnosis is required for prompt institution of therapy.

Gonococcal arthritis must be distinguished from other forms of septic arthritis as well as from rheumatic fever, rheumatoid arthritis, inflammatory bowel disease, and arthritis secondary to rubella or rubella immunization. Gonococcal conjunctivitis in the newborn period must be differentiated from chemical conjunctivitis caused by silver nitrate drops as well as from conjunctivitis caused by *C. trachomatis, Staphylococcus aureus,* group A or B streptococcus, *Pseudomonas aeruginosa, Streptococcus pneumoniae,* or human herpesvirus type 2.

Treatment. All patients who are presumed or proven to have gonorrhea should be evaluated for concurrent syphilis, hepatitis B, human immunodeficiency virus, and *C. trachomatis* infection. The incidence of *Chlamydia* co-infection is 15–25% among males and 35–50% among females. Patients beyond the neonatal period should be treated presumptively for *C. trachomatis* infection (Chapter 208.2). Sexual partners exposed in the preceding 60 days should be examined, cultures should be obtained, and presumptive treatment started.

Because of the prevalence of penicillin-resistant *N. gonorrhoeae,* a third-generation cephalosporin, specifically ceftriaxone, is recommended as initial therapy for all ages. Antimicrobial resistance in *N. gonorrhoeae* occurs as plasmid-mediated resistance to penicillin and tetracycline, and chromosomally mediated resistance to penicillins, tetracyclines, spectinomycin, and recently to quinolones.

INFANT AND PEDIATRIC INFECTIONS. Uncomplicated gonococcal infections in children should be treated with ceftriaxone (50 mg/kg in a single dose IM; maximum: 125 mg).

Children who cannot tolerate ceftriaxone may be treated with spectinomycin (40 mg/kg as a single injection IM; maximum: 2 g). Children who have bacteremia or arthritis should be treated with ceftriaxone (50 mg/kg/24 hr; maximum 1 g/day) for a minimum of 7 days if <45 kg and for a minimum of 10–14 days if ≥45 kg. Meningitis should be treated for 10–14 days, and endocarditis for a minimum of 28 days with ceftriaxone (50 mg/kg/dose q 12 hr; maximum: 1–2 g/dose). Neonatal gonococcal ophthalmia is treated effectively with ceftriaxone (50 mg/kg in a single dose IM; maximum: 125 mg); cefotaxime (100 mg/kg in a single dose IM) is an acceptable alternative. The conjunctivae should be irrigated frequently with physiologic saline solution. Infants born to mothers who have gonococcal infection at birth should also receive a single dose of ceftriaxone (50 mg/kg in a single dose IM; maximum: 125 mg). Neonatal sepsis should be treated parenterally for a minimum of 7 days and meningitis for a minimum of 10 days. Cefotaxime is recommended for infants with hyperbilirubinemia. Neonates with gonococcal ophthalmitis must be hospitalized and evaluated for DGI.

ADOLESCENT AND ADULT INFECTIONS. A single dose of ceftriaxone (125 mg IM) eradicates pharyngeal and uncomplicated urogenital gonococcal infections. Ceftriaxone is safe and effective in pregnant women, and it probably aborts incubating syphilis. Alternative regimens include cefixime (400 mg PO), ciprofloxacin (500 mg PO), or ofloxacin (400 mg PO) in a single dose. The efficacy of cefixime against incubating syphilis is uncertain. Ciprofloxacin and ofloxacin should be avoided in pregnant women and are not approved for persons ≤18 yr of age in the United States. These drugs will not abort incubating syphilis. Spectinomycin (40 mg/kg as a single dose IM; maximum: 2 g) remains highly effective for genital and rectal gonorrhea in the United States, but is ineffective for pharyngeal infection and does not inhibit *T. pallidum*. Regardless of the regimen chosen, treatment should be followed by a regimen active against *C. trachomatis*. The recommended regimens are doxycycline (100 mg bid PO for 7 days) or azithromycin (1.0 g in a single dose PO). Most experts recommend a 7–10 day course of erythromycin in pregnant women. Adolescents and adults who are asymptomatic after treatment need not be cultured for a test of cure.

Hospitalization and parenteral administration of ceftriaxone (1 g/24 hr IV) are recommended for initial therapy of DGI. Patients should be examined for clinical evidence of endocarditis and meningitis. Alternatives for adults and older adolescents include intravenous cefotaxime (1 g q 8 hr IV) or ceftizoxime (1 g q 8 hr) or, for patients allergic to β-lactam drugs, ciprofloxacin (500 mg q 12 hr IV), ofloxacin (400 mg q 12 hr IV), or spectinomycin (2 g q 12 hr IM). Treatment may be switched to oral regimens after 24–48 hr when clinical improvement is obvious. Oral regimens include cefixime (400 mg bid PO), ciprofloxacin (500 mg bid PO), or ofloxacin (400 mg bid PO) to complete 7 days of therapy. Gonococcal conjunctivitis should be treated with ceftriaxone (1 g IM in a single dose) with lavage of the infected eye with saline. Meningitis is treated with ceftriaxone (1–2 g q 12 hr IV) for 10–14 days. Endocarditis is treated with ceftriaxone (1–2 g q 12 hr IV) for at least 4 wk. Concurrent therapy for treatment of genital *Chlamydia* infection is important.

PELVIC INFLAMMATORY DISEASE. PID encompasses a spectrum of infectious diseases of the upper genital tract due to *N. gonorrhoeae*, *C. trachomatis*, and endogenous flora (streptococci, anaerobes, gram-negative bacilli). Therapy must cover a broad spectrum and must be given to adolescents as inpatients. A commonly recommended therapeutic regimen is cefoxitin (2 g q 6 hr IV) or cefotetan (2 g q 12 hr IV), plus doxycycline (100 mg bid PO or q 12 hr IV). Therapy is continued for at least 48 hr after a patient shows improvement. Thereafter, oral doxycycline is given for a total of 10–14 days. An alternative recommended regimen is clindamycin (900 mg q 8 hr IV) plus a loading dose of gentamicin (2 mg/kg IV) followed by maintenance gentamicin (1.5 mg/kg q 8 hr IV). Therapy is then continued for

48 hr after improvement and is followed by oral clindamycin (450 mg qid PO) or oral doxycycline (100 mg bid PO) to complete 10–14 days of therapy. If an intrauterine device is present, it must be removed and an alternative form of birth control used. Sexual partners should be examined and treated for uncomplicated gonorrhea. Follow-up culture (test of cure) of cephalosporin-doxycycline therapy of gonococcal STD is not recommended owing to the low treatment failure rate. A follow-up examination and culture are recommended in 1–2 mo to evaluate the possibility of reinfection or, rarely, treatment failure.

Complications. Complications of gonorrhea result from the spread of gonococci from a local site of invasion. The interval between primary infection and development of a complication is usually days to weeks. In postpubertal females, endometritis may occur, especially during menses. This may progress to salpingitis and peritonitis (PID). Manifestations of PID include signs of lower genital tract infection (e.g., vaginal discharge, suprapubic pain, cervical tenderness) and upper genital tract infection (e.g., fever, leukocytosis, elevated erythrocyte sedimentation rate, and adnexal tenderness or mass). The differential diagnosis includes gynecologic (ovarian cyst, ovarian tumor, ectopic pregnancy) and intra-abdominal (appendicitis, urinary tract infection, inflammatory bowel disease) pathology.

Once inside the peritoneum, gonococci may seed the liver capsule, causing a perihepatitis. The resultant right upper quadrant pain, with or without signs of salpingitis, is known as the Fitz-Hugh-Curtis syndrome. Perihepatitis may also be caused by *C. trachomatis*. Progression to PID occurs in about 20% of cases of gonococcal cervicitis. *N. gonorrhoeae* is isolated in approximately 40% of cases of PID in the United States. Untreated cases may lead to hydrosalpinx, pyosalpinx, tubo-ovarian abscess, and eventual sterility. Even with adequate treatment of PID, the risk of sterility caused by bilateral tubal occlusion approaches 20% after one episode of salpingitis and exceeds 60% with three or more episodes. The risk of ectopic pregnancy is increased approximately sevenfold after one or more episodes of salpingitis. Additional sequelae of PID include chronic pain, dyspareunia, and increased risk of recurrent PID.

Urogenital gonococcal infection acquired during the first trimester of pregnancy carries a high risk of septic abortion. After 16 wk, infection causes chorioamnionitis, a major cause of premature rupture of the membranes and premature delivery.

Prognosis. Prompt diagnosis and correct therapy ensure complete recovery from uncomplicated gonococcal disease. Complications and permanent sequelae may be associated with delayed treatment, recurrent infection, metastatic sites of infection (meninges, aortic valve), and delayed or topical therapy of gonococcal ophthalmia.

Prevention. Efforts to develop a gonococcal pilus vaccine have been unsuccessful thus far. The high degree of interstrain and intrastrain antigenic variability of pili poses a formidable deterrent to the development of a single effective pilus vaccine. Other gonococcal surface structures such as the porin protein, stress proteins, and lipo-oligosaccharides may prove more promising as vaccine candidates. In the absence of a vaccine, prevention of gonorrhea can be achieved through education, use of barrier contraceptives (especially condoms), intensive epidemiologic and bacteriologic surveillance (screening sexual contacts), and early identification and treatment of infected contacts.

Gonococcal ophthalmia neonatorum can be prevented by instilling 2 drops of a 1% solution of silver nitrate into each conjunctival sac shortly after birth (Chapter 617). Erythromycin (0.5%) or tetracycline (1%) ophthalmic ointment may also be used.

Centers for Disease Control and Prevention: Sexually transmitted diseases treatment guidelines 2002. *MMWR Morb Mortal Wkly Rep* 2002;51(RR-6):1–80.

Cohen MS, Sparling PF: Mucosal infection with *Neisseria gonorrhoeae*. Bacterial adaptation and mucosal defenses. *J Clin Invest* 1992;89:1699–705.

Fox KK, Knapp JS, Holmes KK, et al: Antimicrobial resistance in *Neisseria gonor-rhoeae* in the United States, 1988–1994: The emergence of decreased susceptibility to the fluoroquinolones. *J Infect Dis* 1997;175:1396–403.

Hobbs MM, Alcorn TM, Davis RH, et al: Molecular typing of *Neisseria gonorrhoeae* causing repeated infections: Evolution of porin during passage within a community. *J Infect Dis* 1999;179:371–81.

Hook EW, Holmes KK: Gonococcal infections. *Ann Intern Med* 1985;102:229–43.

Lind I: Antimicrobial resistance in *Neisseria gonorrhoeae*. *Clin Infect Dis* 1997;24(Suppl 1):S93–7.

O'Brien JP, Goldenberg DL, Rice PA: Disseminated gonococcal infection: A prospective analysis of 49 patients and a review of pathophysiology and immune mechanisms. *Medicine* (Baltimore) 1983;62:395–406.

Plummer FA, Chubb H, Simonsen JN, et al: Antibody to Rmp (outer membrane protein 3) increases susceptibility to gonococcal infection. *J Clin Invest* 1993;91:339–43.

Rice PA, McQuillen DP, Gulati S, et al: Serum resistance of *Neisseria gonorrhoeae*. Does it thwart the inflammatory response and facilitate the transmission of infection? *Ann N Y Acad Sci* 1994;730:7–14.

Chapter 178
Haemophilus influenzae
Robert S. Daum

Approximately 100 yr after the recognition of *Haemophilus influenzae* as the cause of several important syndromes in childhood, an effective vaccine to prevent these illnesses was introduced in the United States, resulting in a dramatic decrease in the prevalence of infections due to this organism. However, mortality and morbidity from *H. influenzae* type b infection remain a problem worldwide, primarily in unimmunized populations.

Etiology. *H. influenzae* is a fastidious, gram-negative, pleomorphic coccobacillus that requires **factor X (hematin)** and **factor V (phosphopyridine nucleotide)** for growth.

Some *H. influenzae* isolates are surrounded by a polysaccharide capsule. Such isolates can be serotyped into six antigenically and biochemically distinct types, designated a–f. The most virulent isolates belong to serotype b.

Epidemiology. Before the advent of effective conjugate vaccine use in 1988, *H. influenzae* was a major cause of certain invasive diseases in children. Serotype b organisms accounted for >95% of these cases. There was a striking age distribution of cases; >90% occurred in children <5 yr of age, and the majority occurred in children <2 yr of age. The annual attack rate of invasive disease was estimated to be 64–129 cases/100,000 children <5 yr of age per year. Invasive disease caused by other capsular serotypes is much less frequent; the incidence of invasive disease has been estimated at about 0.7 cases/100,000 children <5 yr of age per year. The recent descriptions of small clusters of serotype a and f infections may reflect low-level events and important trends for the future. Nonencapsulated (nontypable) *H. influenzae* organisms cause invasive disease in neonates, immunocompromised children, and children in certain developing countries. Nontypable isolates are common etiologic agents in otitis media, in sinusitis, and in chronic bronchitis in adults.

Humans are the only natural hosts for *H. influenzae*. This species is a constituent of the normal respiratory flora in 60–90% of healthy children. Most isolates are nontypable. Colonization by serotype b organisms is infrequent. Before the advent of conjugate vaccine immunization, *H. influenzae* type b could be isolated from the pharynx of 2–5% of healthy preschool and school-aged children; lower rates occurred among infants and adults. Such asymptomatic colonization with *H. influenzae* type b probably occurs at lower rates in immunized populations, although, importantly, the bacterium continues to circulate.

The incidence of *H. influenzae* type b disease has declined by >99% in the vaccine era. From 1989–1997, the incidence of invasive *H. influenzae* type b disease among children <5 yr of age declined 99%, from 34 to 0.4 cases/100,000 children/yr. Because a similar decline in invasive *H. influenzae* disease due to other serotypes or due to nontypable organisms has not occurred, the proportion of cases due to serotype b organisms has also declined and accounted for only 32–41% of reported cases in 1996–1997. Meeting the Centers for Disease Control and Prevention (CDC) objective of eliminating invasive *H. influenzae* type b disease by 2010 will require improved vaccine coverage, standardization of serotyping techniques, complete case ascertainment, and serotype reporting for all cases. The continued circulation of the serotype b organism despite current vaccine coverage levels suggests that meeting this objective may be a formidable task. Also, continued effort will be required to provide currently available conjugate vaccines to children in developing countries where affordability remains an important issue.

The few cases of serotype b invasive disease now occur in both unvaccinated and fully vaccinated children; about half occur in infants <6 mo, too young to have received a three-dose primary series. Among those cases that are age-eligible to have received such a series, about one third had received at least a three-dose primary series, and about one half of these had also received a booster dose.

Certain groups and individuals have been identified to have an increased incidence of invasive disease, including Alaskan Eskimos, Apaches, Navajos, and blacks. In these populations, the proportion of cases of invasive disease in children <12 mo has been relatively high. Persons known to be at an increased risk for invasive disease have also included those with sickle cell disease, asplenia, congenital and acquired immunodeficiencies, and malignancies. Nonvaccinated infants who had previously documented invasive infection are at increased risk for recurrence.

Socioeconomic risk factors for invasive *H. influenzae* type b disease include childcare outside the home, the presence of siblings of elementary school age or younger, short duration of breast-feeding, and parental smoking. Previous hospitalization for invasive *H. influenzae* type b disease and a history of otitis media are associated with an increased risk for invasive disease. Much less is known about the epidemiology of *H. influenzae* infections other than for serotype b.

Among age-susceptible household contacts who have been exposed to a case of invasive *H. influenzae* type b disease, there is increased risk of secondary cases of invasive disease in the first 30 days, especially in susceptible children <24 mo of age.

The mode of transmission is most commonly by direct contact or inhalation of respiratory tract droplets containing *H. influenzae*. The incubation period for invasive disease is variable, and the exact period of communicability is unknown. Most children with invasive *H. influenzae* type b disease are colonized in the nasopharynx before initiation of antimicrobial therapy; 25–40% may remain colonized during the first 24 hr of therapy.

Pathogenesis. The precise mechanisms that facilitate successful colonization of the respiratory epithelium have not been identified. Following bacterial attachment to the respiratory mucosa, the events that result in entry into the intravascular compartment by serotype b organisms are unclear. Once there, however, type b strains resist intravascular clearance mechanisms more readily than do strains of other serotypes and nonencapsulated organisms. Whether it is the type b PRP capsule itself that confers the potential for invasive disease or another closely linked virulence factor is not certain. Once established, the magnitude of *H. influenzae* type b bacteremia and its duration determine the likelihood of dissemination of bacteria into sites such as the meninges or joints.

Noninvasive *H. influenzae* infections such as otitis media, sinusitis, and bronchitis, usually caused by nontypable strains, probably gain access to sites such as the middle ear and sinus cavities by direct extension from the pharynx. The factors facilitating spread from the pharynx include eustachian tube dysfunction and antecedent viral infections of the upper respiratory tract.

ANTIBIOTIC RESISTANCE. Most *H. influenzae* isolates are susceptible to ampicillin or amoxicillin but about one third produce a β-lactamase and are therefore resistant. Rarely, a β-lactamase-negative isolate may be ampicillin-resistant by a different resistance mechanism.

Chloramphenicol is effective against most isolates of *H. influenzae* regardless of β-lactamase production. The disadvantages of chloramphenicol include the need for complex monitoring strategies and the rare occurrence of idiosyncratic aplastic anemia. Isolates of *H. influenzae* type b have been identified as resistant to chloramphenicol, but such resistance has remained relatively rare (about 0.2% of isolates) in the United States and throughout the world, although higher rates have been reported in a few locales. Isolates resistant to both chloramphenicol and ampicillin have been identified rarely (<1% of isolates). Resistance to trimethoprim-sulfamethoxazole (TMP-SMZ) has been infrequent (<10%).

Until recently, amoxicillin-clavulanate was considered uniformly active against *H. influenzae* clinical isolates. However, about 3% of β-lactamase–positive isolates are resistant to amoxicillin-clavulanate. Furthermore, amoxicillin-clavulanate offers no apparent synergy against ampicillin-resistant isolates that do not elaborate β-lactamase. Among the newer macrolides, 99% and 78% of *H. influenzae* isolates were susceptible to azithromycin and clarithromycin, respectively, whereas the activity of erythromycin against *H. influenzae* clinical isolates has been considered to be poor. Resistance to quinolones is believed to be infrequent. Resistance to extended-spectrum cephalosporins, which are commonly used in therapy, has not been documented.

IMMUNITY. The most important element of host defense is antibody directed against the type b capsular polysaccharide, PRP. In the prevaccination era, anti-PRP antibody was acquired in an age-related fashion; its mechanism of action is to facilitate clearance of *H. influenzae* type b from blood. This is related in part to its opsonic activity; other antibodies directed against antigens such as outer membrane proteins or lipopolysaccharides may also have a role in opsonization. Both the classic and alternative complement pathways are important in the opsonization of *H. influenzae* type b. The macrophages of the reticuloendothelial system aid in intravascular clearance of *H. influenzae* type b by affecting intracellular killing after opsonization.

Before the introduction of vaccination and among recipients of unconjugated PRP vaccines, protection from *H. influenzae* type b infection was presumed to correlate with the concentration of circulating anti-PRP antibody at the time of exposure. A serum antibody concentration of 0.15–1.0 μg/mL was considered protective against invasive infection; the higher concentration in vaccines may predict maintenance of a level of >0.15 μg/mL over time. Most infants lack an anti-PRP antibody concentration of this magnitude and are susceptible to disease on encounter with *H. influenzae* type b. This lack of antibody in young infants may reflect a maturational delay in the immunologic response to thymus-independent type 2 (TI-2) antigens such as unconjugated PRP, and it was thought to explain the high incidence of serotype b infections in young infants in the prevaccination era.

Unlike the PRP unconjugated vaccine, the conjugate vaccines—with the exception of PRP-OMP, which also has thymus-independent type 1 (TI-1) properties—act as thymus-dependent (TD) antigens (Table 178–1). They elicit serum antibody responses in young infants, although repeat doses may be required, and prime memory antibody responses on subsequent encounters

TABLE 178–1. *Haemophilus influenzae* Type b Conjugate Vaccines

Abbreviation	Trade Name	Manufacturer	Protein Carrier
HbOC	HibTITER	Wyeth	CRM$_{197}$ (a nontoxic mutant of diphtheria toxin)
PRP-OMP*	PedvaxHIB	Merck	OMP (an outer membrane protein complex of *Neisseria meningitidis*)
PRP-T†	ActHIB	Aventis Pasteur	Tetanus toxoid
	OmniHIB	Aventis Pasteur‡	Tetanus toxoid

*PRP-OMP is also available as a combination vaccine with hepatitis B vaccine (Comvax). This should not be used for hepatitis B immunization at birth.

†PRP-T can be reconstituted with Connaught DTaP vaccine (Tripedia), to produce a combination marketed as TriHIBit, which is acceptable only for the booster (4th) dose in infants ≥15 mo of age.

‡Marketed by GlaxoSmithKline in the United States.

with PRP. The concentration of circulating anti-PRP antibody in a child primed by a conjugate vaccine may not correlate precisely with protection, because a memory response may occur rapidly on exposure to PRP and provide protection.

Less is known about immunity to nontypable *H. influenzae*. Evidence suggests that antibodies directed against one or more outer membrane proteins (OMPs) are bactericidal and protect against experimental challenge. In infant rats, antibody to P6, a major OMP, is bactericidal for encapsulated and nontypable *H. influenzae* and is protective against *H. influenzae* type b disease. Another OMP, P2, has substantial interstrain heterogeneity. Antibody elicited to the nonconserved regions of P2 had complement-dependent bactericidal activity to the homologous strain. Monoclonal antibodies directed against a group of surface-exposed high molecular weight OMPs have provided protection in experimental infection in animals.

Diagnosis. Presumptive identification of *H. influenzae* is established by direct examination of the collected specimen after Gram staining. Because of its small size, pleomorphism, poor uptake of stain by some isolates, and the tendency for fluids, particularly when proteinaceous, to have a red background, *H. influenzae* is sometimes difficult to visualize. Because identification of microorganisms on smear by either technique requires at least 10^5 bacteria/mL, failure to visualize them does not preclude their presence.

Culture of *H. influenzae* requires prompt transport and processing of specimens because the organism is fastidious. Specimens should not be exposed to drying or temperature extremes. Primary isolation of *H. influenzae* can be accomplished on chocolate agar, *Haemophilus* isolation agar, or on blood agar plates using the *Staphylococcus* streak technique.

Serotyping of *H. influenzae* is accomplished by slide agglutination with type-specific antisera. Accurate serotyping is essential to monitor progress toward elimination of serotype b invasive disease. Timely reporting of cases to public health authorities should be ensured.

Clinical Manifestations and Treatment. The clinical manifestations and treatment of all invasive *H. influenzae* disease are similar regardless of serotype. The initial antibiotic therapy of invasive infections possibly due to *H. influenzae* type b should be a parenterally administered antimicrobial agent effective in sterilizing all foci of infection and effective against ampicillin-resistant strains. Extended-spectrum cephalosporins, such as cefotaxime or ceftriaxone, have been used as the initial antimicrobial agent when *H. influenzae* type b is considered a likely pathogen, and they have achieved popularity because of their relative lack of serious adverse effects and ease of administration. Alternatively, chloramphenicol can be used with ampicillin. After the antimicrobial susceptibility of the isolate has been determined, an appropriate agent can be selected to complete the therapy.

Ampicillin remains the drug of choice for the therapy of infections caused by susceptible isolates. If the isolate is resistant to ampicillin, extended-spectrum cephalosporins such as cefotaxime or ceftriaxone are useful; the latter can be administered once daily in selected circumstances for outpatient therapy. Chloramphenicol also has extensive clinical experience.

Oral antimicrobial agents are sometimes used to complete a course of therapy initiated by the parenteral route. If the organism is susceptible to ampicillin, amoxicillin is the drug of choice. An oral third-generation cephalosporin (e.g., cefixime, cefpodoxime) or amoxicillin-clavulanate may be used when the isolate is resistant to ampicillin. Chloramphenicol is another option that continues to enjoy popularity in some countries because of its low cost.

MENINGITIS. Clinically, meningitis due to *H. influenzae* type b cannot be differentiated from that due to *Neisseria meningitidis* or *Streptococcus pneumoniae* and may be complicated by other foci of infection, such as the lungs, joints, bones, or pericardium (Chapter 594.1).

Antimicrobial therapy should be administered parenterally for 7–14 days for uncomplicated cases. Cefotaxime, ceftriaxone, ampicillin, and chloramphenicol all are thought to cross the blood-brain barrier during acute inflammation in concentrations adequate to render them effective for *H. influenzae* meningitis. Chloramphenicol has been administered orally to complete a therapeutic regimen for meningitis.

The prognosis of *H. influenzae* type b meningitis depends on the age at presentation, the duration of illness before appropriate antimicrobial therapy, the CSF capsular polysaccharide concentration, and the rapidity with which it is cleared from CSF, blood, and urine. Low intelligence quotients correlate with clinically manifested inappropriate secretion of antidiuretic hormone and evidence of focal neurologic deficits at presentation. About 6% of patients with *H. influenzae* type b meningitis are left with some hearing impairment, probably because of inflammation of the cochlea and the labyrinth. Dexamethasone (0.6 mg/kg/24 hr divided q 6 hr for 2 days), particularly when given shortly before or concurrent with the initiation of antimicrobial therapy, decreases the incidence of hearing loss. Major neurologic sequelae of *H. influenzae* type b meningitis include behavior problems, language disorders, delayed development of language, impaired vision, mental retardation, motor abnormalities, ataxia, seizures, and hydrocephalus.

CELLULITIS. Children with *H. influenzae* cellulitis often have an antecedent upper respiratory tract infection. They usually have no prior history of trauma, and the infection is thought to represent seeding of the organism to the involved soft tissues during bacteremia. The head and neck, particularly the cheek and preseptal region, are the most common sites of involvement. The involved region generally has indistinct margins and is tender and indurated. Buccal cellulitis is classically erythematous with a violaceous hue, although this sign may be absent. *H. influenzae* may often be recovered directly from an aspirate. The blood culture may reveal the causative organism. Other foci of infection may be present concomitantly, particularly in children <18 mo of age or with fever. A diagnostic lumbar puncture should be considered at the time of diagnosis for these children.

Parenteral antimicrobial therapy is indicated until patients become afebrile, after which an appropriate orally administered antimicrobial agent may be substituted. A 7–10 day course is customary.

PRESEPTAL CELLULITIS. Infection involving the superficial tissue layers anterior to the orbital septum is termed preseptal cellulitis, which may be caused by *H. influenzae*. Uncomplicated preseptal cellulitis does not imply a risk for visual impairment or direct central nervous system extension. However, concurrent bacteremia may be associated with the development of meningitis. *H. influenzae* preseptal cellulitis is characterized by fever, edema, tenderness, warmth of the lid, and, occasionally, purple discoloration. Evidence of interruption of the integument is usually absent. Conjunctival drainage may be associated. *S. pneumoniae*, *Staphylococcus aureus*, and group A streptococcus cause clinically indistinguishable preseptal cellulitis. The latter two pathogens are more likely when fever is absent and with an interruption of the integument (e.g., an insect bite).

Those with preseptal cellulitis in whom *H. influenzae* or *S. pneumoniae* are etiologic considerations (i.e., young age, high fever, intact integument) should have blood submitted for culture, and a diagnostic lumbar puncture should be considered.

Parenteral antibiotics are indicated for preseptal cellulitis. Because *S. aureus*, *S. pneumoniae*, and group A β-hemolytic streptococci are other causes, empirical therapy should include agents active against these pathogens. Patients with preseptal cellulitis without concurrent meningitis should receive parenteral therapy for about 5 days until fever and erythema have abated. In uncomplicated cases, antimicrobial therapy should be given for a total of 10 days.

ORBITAL CELLULITIS. Infections of the orbit are infrequent and usually complicate acute ethmoid and sphenoid sinusitis. Orbital cellulitis may present with lid edema but is distinguished by the presence of proptosis, chemosis, impaired vision, limitation of the extraocular movements, decreased mobility of the globe, or pain on movement of the globe. The distinction between preseptal and orbital cellulitis may be difficult. The extent of the infection is best delineated by CT.

Orbital infections are treated with parenteral therapy for at least 14 days. Underlying sinusitis or orbital abscess may require surgical drainage and more prolonged antimicrobial therapy.

SUPRAGLOTTITIS OR ACUTE EPIGLOTTITIS. Epiglottitis is a cellulitis of the tissues comprising the laryngeal inlet (Chapter 371). It has become exceedingly rare. Direct invasion of the involved tissues by *H. influenzae* type b is probably the initiating pathophysiologic event. This dramatic, potentially lethal condition usually occurs in children 2–7 yr of age. Because of the risk of sudden, unpredictable airway obstruction, supraglottitis is a medical emergency. Pneumonia is detected by chest radiograph in about 25% of cases. Other foci of infection, such as meningitis, are rare. Antimicrobial therapy directed against *H. influenzae* type b should be administered parenterally but only after the airway is secured, and therapy should be continued until patients are able to take fluids by mouth. The duration of antimicrobial therapy typically is 7 days.

PNEUMONIA. The true incidence of *H. influenzae* type b pneumonia in children is unknown because invasive procedures are required to obtain cultures and are seldom performed (Chapter 389). The signs and symptoms of pneumonia due to *H. influenzae* cannot be differentiated from those of pneumonia caused by many other microorganisms. Other foci of infection may be present concomitantly.

Children suspected of having *H. influenzae* type b pneumonia who are <12 mo should receive parenteral antimicrobial therapy initially because of their increased risk for bacteremia and its complications. Older children who do not appear severely ill may be managed with an orally administered antimicrobial. Therapy is continued for 7–10 days of combined parenteral-oral therapy.

Uncomplicated pleural effusion associated with *H. influenzae* pneumonia requires no special intervention. However, if empyema develops, insertion of a chest tube and a more prolonged course of antimicrobial therapy may be necessary.

SUPPURATIVE ARTHRITIS. Large joints, such as the knee, hip, ankle, and elbow, are affected most commonly (Chapter 674). Other foci of infection may be present concomitantly. Although single joint involvement is the rule, multiple joint involvement occurs in about 6% of cases. The signs and symptoms of septic arthritis due to *H. influenzae* are indistinguishable from those of arthritis caused by other bacteria.

Uncomplicated septic arthritis should be treated with an appropriate antimicrobial administered parenterally for at least 5–7 days. If the clinical response is satisfactory the remainder of the course of antimicrobial treatment may be given orally. Therapy is typically given for 3 wk for uncomplicated septic arthritis, but it may be continued beyond 3 wk until the C-reactive protein is normal.

PERICARDITIS. *H. influenzae* is a rare cause of bacterial pericarditis (Chapter 432). Affected children often have had an antecedent upper respiratory tract infection. Fever, respiratory distress, and tachycardia are consistent findings. Other foci of infection may be present concomitantly.

The diagnosis may be established by recovery of the organism from blood or pericardial fluid. Gram stain or detection of PRP in pericardial fluid, blood, or urine (when serotype b organisms are the cause) may aid the diagnosis. Antimicrobials should be provided parenterally in a regimen similar to that used for meningitis (Chapter 594.1). Pericardiectomy is useful for draining the purulent material effectively and preventing tamponade and constrictive pericarditis.

BACTEREMIA WITHOUT AN ASSOCIATED FOCUS. Bacteremia due to *H. influenzae* type b may be associated with fever without any apparent focus of infection (Chapter 162). In this situation, risk factors for "occult" bacteremia include the magnitude of fever (≥39°C) and the presence of leukocytosis (≥15,000 cells/µL). About 25% of children with occult *H. influenzae* type b bacteremia develop meningitis if left untreated. In the vaccine era, this *H. influenzae* type b infection has become exceedingly rare. When it does occur, however, the child should be re-evaluated for a focus of infection and a second blood culture obtained. In general, the child should be hospitalized and given parenteral antimicrobial therapy after a diagnostic lumbar puncture and chest radiograph are obtained.

MISCELLANEOUS INFECTIONS. Urinary tract infection, epididymo-orchitis, cervical adenitis, acute glossitis, infected thyroglossal duct cysts, uvulitis, endocarditis, endophthalmitis, primary peritonitis, osteomyelitis and periappendiceal abscess are rarely caused by *H. influenzae*.

INVASIVE DISEASE IN NEONATES. In neonates with invasive *H. influenzae* infection, nontypable isolates are more common than serotype b isolates, although both are rare. When illness occurs in the first 24 hr of life, especially in association with maternal chorioamnionitis or prolonged rupture of membranes, transmission of the organism to the infant is likely to have occurred through the maternal genital tract, which may be (<1%) colonized with nontypable *H. influenzae*. Manifestations of neonatal invasive infection include bacteremia with sepsis, pneumonia, respiratory distress syndrome with shock, conjunctivitis, scalp abscess or cellulitis, or meningitis. Less commonly, mastoiditis, septic arthritis, or a congenital vesicular eruption may occur.

OTITIS MEDIA. Acute otitis media is one of the most common infectious diseases of childhood (Chapter 630). It is thought to result from the spread of bacteria from the nasopharynx through the eustachian tube into the middle-ear cavity. Usually because of a preceding viral upper respiratory tract infection, the mucosa in the area becomes hyperemic and swollen, resulting in obstruction and an opportunity for bacterial multiplication in the middle ear.

The most common bacterial pathogens are *S. pneumoniae*, *H. influenzae*, and *Moraxella catarrhalis*. Most *H. influenzae* isolates are nontypable. Amoxicillin (80–90 mg/kg/24 hr) is a suitable first-line oral antimicrobial agent; the combined probability of the causative isolate being resistant to amoxicillin and of invasive potential is sufficiently low to continue to justify this approach. Alternatively, a single dose of ceftriaxone may constitute adequate therapy.

In the case of treatment failure or if a β-lactamase–producing isolate is obtained by tympanocentesis or from drainage fluid,

amoxicillin-clavulanate, erythromycin-sulfisoxazole, and cefaclor are among the available alternatives. The latter combination may be useful as first-line agents for patients allergic to β-lactam compounds.

CONJUNCTIVITIS. Acute infection of the conjunctiva is the most common eye infection in childhood (Chapter 617). In neonates, *H. influenzae* is an infrequent cause. However, it is an important pathogen in older children, as are *S. pneumoniae* and *S. aureus*. Most *H. influenzae* isolates associated with conjunctivitis are nontypable, although serotype b isolates and other microorganisms are occasionally found. Empirical treatment of conjunctivitis beyond the neonatal period usually consists of topical antimicrobial therapy with sulfacetamide and erythromycin.

SINUSITIS. *H. influenzae* is an important cause of acute sinusitis in children, second in frequency only to *S. pneumoniae* (Chapter 365). Chronic sinusitis lasting >1 yr or severe sinusitis requiring hospitalization is often caused by *S. aureus* or anaerobes such as *Peptococcus*, *Peptostreptococcus*, or *Bacteroides* species. Nontypable *H. influenzae* and viridans group streptococci are also frequently recovered.

For uncomplicated sinusitis, amoxicillin is acceptable initial therapy. However, if clinical improvement does not occur, a broader-spectrum regimen may be appropriate, such as amoxicillin-clavulanate; hospitalization with parenteral therapy is occasionally required. For uncomplicated sinusitis, a 10-day course is sufficient.

Prevention. Universal immunization with *H. influenzae* type b conjugate vaccine is recommended for all infants. Chemoprophylaxis is indicated if close contacts are unvaccinated.

CHEMOPROPHYLAXIS. Unvaccinated children <48 mo of age in close contact are at increased risk of invasive infection when exposed to an index case with invasive *H. influenzae* type b infection. The risk of secondary disease is inversely related to age (for children >3 mo of age). About half of the cases of secondary disease among susceptible household contacts occur in the 1st wk after hospitalization of the index patient. Because many children are now protected against *H. influenzae* type b by prior immunization, the need for chemoprophylaxis has greatly decreased.

The goal of chemoprophylaxis is to prevent a susceptible child from acquiring *H. influenzae* type b from contacts by eliminating colonization in the close contacts. Rifampin prophylaxis is indicated for all members of the close contact group, including the index patient, if one or more children <48 mo is not fully immunized.

Parents of children hospitalized for invasive *H. influenzae* type b disease should be told that there is an increased risk for secondary infection due to this organism in other young children in the same household if they are partially immunized. Parents of children exposed to a single case of invasive *H. influenzae* type b disease in a child-care center or nursery school should be similarly informed, although there is disagreement about the use of rifampin for these children.

For chemoprophylaxis, children should be given rifampin orally (0–1 mo of age, 10 mg/kg/dose; >1 mo, 20 mg/kg/dose, not to exceed 600 mg/dose), once each a day for 4 consecutive days. The adult dose is 600 mg once daily. It is not recommended for pregnant women, because the effects on a fetus are not established. Because rifampin induces enzymes that metabolize oral contraceptives, other methods of contraception should be implemented during the period of rifampin administration. Rifampin turns body fluids (e.g., urine, saliva, tears) reddish orange and may permanently stain soft contact lenses.

VACCINE. Three *H. influenzae* type b conjugate vaccines are available that differ in the carrier protein used, the saccharide molecular size, and the method of conjugating the saccharide to the protein (see Table 178–1 and Chapter 282). Combination vaccines consisting of a *H. influenzae* type b conjugate vaccine and one or more other vaccines recommended for routine administration in childhood are under development. Currently available combinations are PRP-OMP combined with hepatitis B vaccine (Comvax) and a DtaP vaccine that can be combined with PRP-T for the fourth dose only. Many attempts to combine DTaP (acellular pertussis vaccine) with a *H. influenzae* type b conjugate vaccine have resulted in decreased anti-PRP antibody.

Adderson, EE, Byington CL, Spencer L, et al: Invasive serotype a *Haemophilus influenzae* infections with a virulence genotype resembling *Haemophilus influenzae* type b: Emerging pathogen in the vaccine era? *Pediatrics* 2001;108:18–24.

Barbour ML: Conjugate vaccines and the carriage of *Haemophilus influenzae* type b. *Emerg Infect Dis* 1996;3:176–82.

Bisgard KM, Kao A, Leake J, et al: *Haemophilus influenzae* invasive disease in the United States, 1994–1995: Near disappearance of a vaccine-preventable childhood disease. *Emerg Infect Dis* 1998;4:229–37.

Centers for Disease Control and Prevention: Progress toward elimination of *Haemophilus influenzae* type b invasive disease among infants and children—United States, 1998–2000. *Morb Mortal Wkly Rep* 2002;51:234–6.

Committee on Infectious Diseases, American Academy of Pediatrics: *Haemophilus influenzae* infections. In *Red Book 2000: Report of the Committee on Infectious Diseases*, 25th ed. Elk Grove Village, American Academy of Pediatrics, 2000.

Daum RS, Granoff DM: Lessons from the evaluation of the immunogenicity. In Ellis RW, Granoff DM (editors): *Development and Clinical Uses of Haemophilus b Conjugate Vaccines*. New York, Marcel Dekker, 1994.

McIntyre PB, Berkey CS, King SM, et al: Dexamethoasone as adjunctive therapy in bacterial meningitis. A meta-analysis of randomized clinical trials since 1988. *JAMA* 1997;278:925–31.

Schuchat A, Robinson K, Wenger JD et al: Bacterial meningitis in the United States in 1995. *N Engl J Med* 1997;337:970–6.

Chapter 179
Chancroid (*Haemophilus ducreyi*) *Parvin Azimi*

Chancroid is a sexually transmitted disease characterized by painful genital ulceration and inguinal lymphadenopathy that is caused by *Haemophilus ducreyi*, a fastidious gram-negative bacillus. Chancroid is prevalent in many countries and endemic in some areas of the United States; it is a risk factor for transmission of HIV. Diagnosis of chancroid in infants and children is strong evidence of sexual abuse.

Infection begins with a small inflammatory papule on the preputial orifice or frenulum in men and on the labia, fourchette, or perineal region in women. The lesion becomes pustular, eroded, and ulcerative within 2–3 days. Painful, tender inguinal lymphadenitis (bubo) occurs in >50% of cases. Unlike lymphogranuloma venereum (Chapter 208.4), the ulcer of chancroid is concurrent with lymphadenopathy.

Diagnosis is usually established by the clinical presentation and the exclusion of both *Treponema pallidum* and herpes simplex virus infections. Gram stain of ulcer secretions may show gram-negative coccobacilli in parallel clusters (school of fish). Culture requires special media and is 80% or less sensitive. Indirect immunofluorescence using monoclonal antibodies or polymerase chain reaction may become the best means for diagnosis.

Most *H. ducreyi* organisms are resistant to penicillin and ampicillin because of plasmid-mediated β-lactamase production. Spread of plasmid-mediated resistance among *H. ducreyi* has resulted in lack of efficacy of previously useful drugs such as sulfonamides and tetracyclines as well. The recommended treatment of chancroid is azithromycin (1 g as a single dose PO) or ceftriaxone (250 mg as a single dose IM). Alternative regimens include ciprofloxacin (500 mg bid PO for 3 days, for persons ≥18 yr of age) or erythromycin (500 mg qid PO for 7 days). Fluctuant nodes may require drainage. Symptoms usually resolve within 3–7 days. Relapses can usually be treated successfully with the original treatment regimen. Patients with HIV infection may require longer duration of treatment.

Patients with chancroid should be evaluated for other sexually transmitted diseases; an estimated 10% of patients have concomitant syphilis or genital herpes. Sexual contacts of patients with chancroid should be evaluated and treated.

Mertz KJ, Weiss JB, Webb RM, et al: An investigation of genital ulcers in Jackson, Mississippi, with use of a multiplex polymerase chain reaction assay: High prevalence of chancroid and human immunodeficiency virus infection. *J Infect Dis* 1998;178:1060–6.

Schmid GP: Treatment of chancroid, 1997. *Clin Infect Dis* 1999;28:S14–20.

Trees DL, Morse SA: Chancroid and *Haemophilus ducreyi*: An update. *Clin Microbiol Rev* 1995;8:357–75.

Chapter 180
Pertussis (*Bordetella pertussis* and *B. parapertussis*) *Sarah S. Long*

Pertussis is an acute respiratory tract infection that was well described in the 1500s. Current worldwide prevalence is diminished only by active immunization. Sydenham first used the term *pertussis* (intense cough) in 1670; it is preferable to **whooping cough** because most infected individuals do not "whoop."

Etiology. *Bordetella pertussis* is the sole cause of epidemic pertussis and the usual cause of sporadic pertussis. *B. parapertussis* is an occasional cause of pertussis, accounting for fewer than 5% of isolates of *Bordetella* species in the United States. *B. parapertussis* contributes significantly to total cases of pertussis in other areas such as Scandinavia, the Czech Republic, Slovakia, and the Russian federation. *B. pertussis* and *B. parapertussis* are exclusive pathogens of humans (and some primates). *B. bronchiseptica* is a common animal pathogen; occasional case reports in humans involve any body site and typically occur in immunocompromised patients or young children with unusual exposure to animals. Protracted coughing can be caused by *Mycoplasma*, parainfluenza or influenza viruses, enteroviruses, respiratory syncytial virus, or adenoviruses. None is an important cause of pertussis.

Epidemiology. Sixty million cases of pertussis a year occur worldwide, resulting in more than 500,000 deaths. During the prevaccine era of 1922–1948, pertussis was the leading cause of death due to communicable disease among children <14 yr of age in the United States. Widespread use of pertussis vaccine led to a greater than 99% decline in cases. The pivotal role of vaccine in disease control is reflected in the continued high incidence of pertussis in developing countries, and resurgence in other countries where vaccine coverage is low or where less potent vaccine may have been used. After the lowest number of cases in the United States reported in 1976, lax implementation of policy is partially responsible for the increase in annual pertussis incidence to 1.2 cases/100,000 population from 1980 through 1989 and epidemic pertussis in many states in 1989–1990, 1993, and 1996. The more than 7,500 cases reported to the Centers for Disease Control and Prevention in 1996 are the highest incidence since 1967. During the 1990s in the United States, rates of pertussis during interepidemic years have not returned to baseline, with between 6,000 to 8,000 cases reported annually since 1996. There is good evidence that the diagnosis of pertussis is underconsidered, underproven, and underreported.

Pertussis is endemic, with superimposed epidemic cycles every 3–4 yr after accumulation of a sizable susceptible cohort. The majority of cases occur from July through October. Pertussis is extremely contagious, with attack rates as high as 100% in susceptible individuals exposed to aerosol droplets at close range. *B. pertussis* does not survive for prolonged periods in the environment. Chronic carriage by humans is not documented. After intense exposure as in households, the rate of subclinical infection is as high as 80% in fully immunized and naturally immune individuals. When carefully sought, however, a symptomatic source case can be found for most patients.

Neither natural disease nor vaccination provides complete or lifelong immunity against reinfection or disease. Protection against typical disease begins to wane 3–5 yr after vaccination and is unmeasurable after 12 yr. Subclinical reinfection undoubtedly contributes significantly to immunity against disease ascribed to both vaccine and prior infection. Adults in the United States have inadequate antibody to *B. pertussis*. Despite history of disease or complete immunization, outbreaks of pertussis have occurred in the elderly, in nursing homes, in residential facilities with limited exposures, in highly immunized suburbia, and in adolescents and adults with lapsing time since immunization. Coughing adolescents and adults (usually not recognized as having pertussis) currently are the major reservoir for *B. pertussis* and are the usual sources for "index cases" in infants and children.

In the prevaccine era and in countries such as Germany, Sweden, and Italy where immunization was limited, the peak incidence of pertussis is in children 1–5 yr of age; infants account for <15% of cases. In contrast, in the United States in recent years, approximately one half of cases have occurred in infants younger than 1 yr of age and one fourth in adolescents and adults. Possible explanations for increases in disease incidence and differences in ages affected include decreased vaccine efficacy, waning immunity, increased awareness and diagnosis, and enhanced surveillance. Without natural reinfection with *B. pertussis* or repeated booster vaccinations, adolescents and adults are susceptible to clinical disease if exposed, and mothers provide little if any passive protection to young infants.

Pathogenesis. *Bordetella* organisms are tiny gram-negative coccobacilli that grow aerobically on starch blood agar or completely synthetic media with nicotinamide growth factor, amino acids for energy, and charcoal or cyclodextrin resin to absorb noxious substances. *Bordetella* species share a high degree of DNA homology among virulence genes. Only *B. pertussis* expresses **pertussis toxin** (PT), the major virulence protein. Serotyping is dependent on heat-labile K agglutinogens. Of 14 agglutinogens, six are specific to *B. pertussis*. Serotypes vary geographically and over time.

B. pertussis produces an array of biologically active substances, many of which are postulated to have a role in disease and immunity. After aerosol acquisition, **filamentous hemagglutinin** (FHA), some **agglutinogens** (especially fimbriae [Fim] types 2 and 3), and a 69-kd nonfimbrial surface protein called **pertactin** (Pn) are important for attachment to ciliated respiratory epithelial cells. **Tracheal cytotoxin**, adenylate cyclase, and PT appear to inhibit clearance of organisms. Tracheal cytotoxin, dermonecrotic factor, and adenylate cyclase are postulated to be predominantly responsible for the local epithelial damage that produces respiratory symptoms and facilitates absorption of PT. PT has numerous proven biologic activities (e.g., histamine sensitivity, insulin secretion, leukocyte dysfunction), some of which may account for systemic manifestations of disease. PT causes lymphocytosis immediately in experimental animals by rerouting lymphocytes to remain in the circulating blood pool. PT appears to have a central but not a singular role in pathogenesis.

Clinical Manifestations. Classically, pertussis is a 6-wk disease, divided into catarrhal, paroxysmal, and convalescent stages. The **catarrhal stage** begins after an incubation period ranging from 3–12 days with nondistinctive symptoms of congestion and rhinorrhea variably accompanied by low-grade fever, sneezing, lacrimation, and conjunctival suffusion. As initial symptoms wane, coughing marks the onset of the **paroxysmal stage**. The cough is first as a dry, intermittent, irritative hack and evolves into the inexorable paroxysms that are the hallmark of pertussis. Infants <3 mo do not display classical stages. After the most insignificant startle from a draught, light, sound, sucking, or stretching, a well-appearing young infant begins to choke, gasp, and flail extremities, with face reddened. Cough (expiratory grunt) may not be prominent. **Whoop** (forceful inspiratory gasp) infrequently occurs in infants <3 mo of age who are exhausted or lack muscular strength to create sudden negative intrathoracic pressure. A well-appearing, playful toddler with similarly insignificant provocation suddenly expresses an anxious aura and may clutch a parent or comforting adult before beginning a machine-gun burst of uninterrupted coughs, chin and chest held forward, tongue protruding maximally, eyes bulging and watering, face purple, until coughing ceases and a loud whoop follows as inspired air traverses the still partially closed airway. Adults describe a sudden feeling of strangulation followed by uninterrupted coughs, feeling of suffocation, bursting headache, diminished awareness, and then a gasping breath, usually without a whoop. Post-tussive emesis is common in pertussis at all ages and is a specific clue to the diagnosis in adolescents and adults. Post-tussive exhaustion is universal. The number and severity of paroxysms progress over days to a week (more rapidly in young infants) and remain at that plateau for days to weeks (longer in young infants). At the peak of the paroxysmal stage, patients may have more than one episode hourly. As paroxysmal stage fades into the **convalescent stage**, the number, severity, and duration of episodes diminish. Paradoxically in infants, cough and whoops may become louder and more classic in convalescence.

Immunized children have foreshortening of all stages of pertussis. Adults have no distinct stages. In infants younger than 3 mo, the catarrhal phase is usually a few days or not recognized at all when apnea, choking, or gasping cough herald the onset of disease; convalescence includes intermittent paroxysmal coughing throughout the 1st year of life, including "exacerbations" with subsequent respiratory illnesses; these are not due to recurrent infection or reactivation of *B. pertussis*.

Findings on physical examination generally are uninformative. Signs of lower respiratory tract disease are not expected. Conjunctival hemorrhages and petechiae on the upper body are common.

Diagnosis. Pertussis should be suspected in any individual who has pure or predominant complaint of cough, especially if the following are absent: fever, malaise or myalgia, exanthem or enanthem, sore throat, hoarseness, tachypnea, wheezes, and rales. For sporadic cases, a clinical case definition of cough of ≥14 days' duration with at least one associated symptom of paroxysms, whoop, or post-tussive vomiting has sensitivity of 81% and specificity of 58% for culture confirmation. Approximately 20% of university students who have been studied on many continents, who had no known contact with pertussis and had coughing illness for >7 days, had pertussis. Apnea or cyanosis (before appreciation of cough) is a clue in infants <3 mo of age. *B. pertussis* is an occasional cause of sudden infant death.

Adenoviral infections are usually distinguishable by associated features, such as fever, sore throat, and conjunctivitis. *Mycoplasma* causes protracted episodic coughing, but patients usually have a history of fever, headache, and systemic symptoms at the onset of disease as well as frequent finding of rales on auscultation of the chest. Epidemics of *Mycoplasma* and *B. pertussis* in young adults can be difficult to distinguish on clinical grounds. Although pertussis is often included in the laboratory evaluation of young infants with "afebrile pneumonia," *B. pertussis* is associated uncommonly with staccato cough (breath with every cough), purulent conjunctivitis, tachypnea, rales or wheezes that typify infection due to *Chlamydia trachomatis*, or predominant lower respiratory tract signs that typify infection due to respiratory syncytial virus. Unless an infant with pertussis has secondary pneumonia (and is then ill appearing), the examination findings between paroxysms are entirely normal, including respiratory rate.

Leukocytosis (15,000–100,000 cells/mm^3) due to absolute lymphocytosis is characteristic in the catarrhal stage. Lymphocytes are of T- and B-cell origin and are normal small cells, rather than the large atypical lymphocytes seen with viral infections. Adults and partially immune children have less impressive lymphocytosis. Absolute increase in neutrophils suggests a different diagnosis or secondary bacterial infection. Eosinophilia is not a manifestation of pertussis. A severe course and death are correlated with extreme leukocytosis (median peak white cell count fatal vs nonfatal cases, 94 vs 18 × 10^9 cells/L) and thrombocytosis (median peak platelet count fatal vs nonfatal cases, 782 vs 556 ×10^9/L). Mild hyperinsulinemia and reduced glycemic response to epinephrine have been demonstrated; hypoglycemia is reported only occasionally. The chest radiograph appearance is mildly abnormal in the majority of hospitalized infants, showing perihilar infiltrate or edema (sometimes with a butterfly appearance) and variable atelectasis. Parenchymal consolidation suggests secondary bacterial infection. Pneumothorax, pneumomediastinum, and air in soft tissues can be seen occasionally.

All current methods for confirmation of infection due to *B. pertussis* have limitations in sensitivity, specificity, or practicality. Isolation of *B. pertussis* in culture remains the gold standard for diagnosis. Careful attention must be paid to specimen collection, transport, and isolation technique. The specimen is obtained by deep nasopharyngeal aspiration or by use of a flexible swab, preferably a Dacron or calcium alginate swab, held in the posterior nasopharynx for 15–30 sec (or until coughing). A 1.0% casamino acid liquid is acceptable for holding a specimen up to 2 hr; Stainer-Scholte broth or Regan-Lowe semisolid transport medium is used for longer periods, up to 4 days. Regan-Lowe charcoal agar with 10% horse blood and 5–40 μg/mL cephalexin or Stainer-Scholte media with cyclodextrin resins are the preferred isolation media. Cultures are incubated at 35–37°F in humid environment (with or without 5% carbon dioxide) and examined daily for 7 days for slow-growing, tiny glistening colonies. Direct fluorescent antibody (DFA) testing of potential isolates using specific antibody for *B. pertussis* and *B. parapertussis* maximizes recovery. Direct testing of nasopharyngeal secretions by DFA is a rapid test, especially helpful in patients who have received antibiotics, but is reliable only in laboratories with continuous experience. Polymerase chain reaction (PCR) to test nasopharyngeal specimens has sensitivity similar to culture, averts difficulties of isolation, but is not standardized or available universally. DFA, culture, and PCR are all expected to be positive in unimmunized children during the catarrhal and paroxysmal stage of disease. Less than 10% of any of these tests is positive in partially or remotely immunized individuals tested in the paroxysmal stage. Serologic tests for detection of antibodies to various components of the organism in acute and convalescent samples are the most sensitive tests in immunized individuals and are useful epidemiologically. They are not generally available, are not helpful during acute illness, and are difficult to interpret in immunized individuals. Antibody to pertussis toxin elevated >2 standard deviations above mean of the immunized population is the most reliable result indicating recent infection.

Treatment. Goals of therapy are to limit the number of paroxysms, to observe the severity of the cough, to provide assistance when necessary, and to maximize nutrition, rest, and recovery without sequelae (Box 180–1). Infants <3 mo of age are admit-

---

BOX 180–1. Caveats in Assessment and Care of Infants with Pertussis

- Infants with potentially fatal pertussis may appear well between episodes.
- A paroxysm must be witnessed before deciding between hospital and home care.
- Only analysis of carefully compiled cough record permits assessment of severity and progression of illness.
- Suctioning of nose, oropharynx, or trachea should not be performed on a "preventive" schedule.
- Feeding in the period following a paroxysm may be more successful than following napping.
- Family support begins at the time of hospitalization with empathy for the child's and family's experience to date, transfer of the burden of responsibility for the child's safety to the health care team, and delineation of assessments and treatments to be performed.
- Family education, recruitment as part of the team, and continued support after discharge are essential.

---

ted to hospital almost without exception, as are those between 3–6 mo unless witnessed paroxysms are not severe, and those of any age if significant complications occur. Prematurely born young infants and children with underlying cardiac, pulmonary, muscular, or neurologic disorders have a high risk for severe disease.

The specific, limited goals of hospitalization are to (1) assess progression of disease and likelihood of life-threatening events at peak of disease, (2) prevent or treat complications, and (3) educate parents in the natural history of the disease and in care that will be given at home. Heart rate, respiratory rate, and pulse oximetry are monitored continuously with alarm settings so that paroxysms can be witnessed and recorded by health care personnel. Detailed cough records and documentation of feeding, vomiting, and weight change provide data to assess severity. Typical paroxysms that are not life threatening have the following features: duration <45 sec; red but not blue color change; tachycardia, bradycardia (not <60 beats/min in infants), or oxygen desaturation that spontaneously resolves at the end of the paroxysm; whooping or strength for self-rescue at the end of the paroxysm; self-expectorated mucus plug; and post-tussive exhaustion but not unresponsiveness. Assessing the need to provide oxygen, stimulation, or suctioning requires skilled personnel who can document an infant's ability for self-rescue but who will intervene rapidly and expertly when necessary. Infants whose paroxysms repeatedly lead to life-threatening events despite passive delivery of oxygen or whose fatigue leads to hypercarbia require intubation, paralysis, and ventilation. Subsequent management is complex, with frequent need to suction the airway and intervene when bradycardia or secondary pulmonary processes occur. Mist by tent, specifically avoided by some experts, can be useful in some infants with thick, tenacious secretions and excessively irritable airways. The benefit of a quiet, dimly lighted, undisturbed, comforting environment cannot be overestimated or forfeited in a desire to monitor and intervene. Feeding children with pertussis is challenging. The risk of precipitating cough by nipple feeding does not warrant nasogastric, nasojejunal, or parenteral alimentation in most infants. The composition or thickness of formula does not affect the quality of secretions, cough, or retention. Large-volume feedings are avoided.

Within 48–72 hr, the direction and severity of disease usually are obvious by analysis of recorded information. Many infants have marked improvement upon hospitalization and antibiotic therapy, especially if they are early in the course of disease or have been removed from aggravating environmental smoke, excessive stimulation, or a dry or polluting heat source. Hospital discharge is appropriate if over a 48-hr period disease severity is unchanged or diminished, no intervention is required during paroxysms, nutrition is adequate, no complication has occurred, and parents are adequately prepared for care at home. Apnea and seizures occur in the incremental phase of illness and in those with complicated disease. Portable oxygen, monitoring, or suction apparatus should not be needed at home.

ANTIMICROBIAL AGENTS. An antimicrobial agent is always given when pertussis is suspected or confirmed for potential clinical benefit and to limit the spread of infection. Erythromycin (40–50 mg/kg/24 hr divided qid PO; maximum: 2 g/24 hr) for 14 days is standard treatment. Limited studies of erythromycin salts dosed twice or three times a day for 14 days, erythromycin estolate (40 mg/kg/24 hr divided qid PO; maximum 1 g/24 hr) for 7 days, clarithromycin (15–20 mg/kg/24 hr divided bid PO; maximum 1 g/24hr) for 7 days, and azithromycin (10 mg/kg/24 hr once a day PO) for 5 days have compared favorably with standard treatment for elimination of organisms. Their efficacy is unproved. Erythromycin resistance of *B. pertussis* has been reported rarely. Ampicillin, rifampin, and trimethoprim-sulfamethoxazole are modestly active, but first- and second-generation cephalosporins are not. In clinical studies, erythromycins are superior to amoxicillin for eradication of *B. pertussis* and are the only agents with proven efficacy.

A sevenfold to 10-fold relative risk for infantile hypertrophic pyloric stenosis (IHPS) has been reported in infants <6 wk of age treated with orally administered erythromycin. The highest risk appears to be in the first 2 wk of life in term infants, and with courses of ≥14 days. The risk of IHPS after treatment with azithromycin or clarithromycin is unknown. Physicians should inform families and weigh risks and benefits of prescribing macrolides in this age group. Alternative therapies are not well studied.

OTHER THERAPIES. A handful of small clinical trials and reports suggest a modest reduction of symptoms from the β_2-adrenergic stimulant salbutamol (albuterol). No rigorous clinical trial has demonstrated a beneficial effect; one small study showed no effect. Fussing associated with aerosol treatment triggers paroxysms. No randomized, blinded clinical trial of sufficient size has been performed to evaluate the usefulness of corticosteroids in the management of pertussis; their clinical use is not warranted. Intravenous use of a human hyperimmune pertussis immunoglobulin derived from immunizing adults is under investigation. Standard immunoglobulin for intramuscular or intravenous use is not recommended for treatment of pertussis.

ISOLATION. Patients are placed in respiratory isolation for ≥5 days after initiation of erythromycin therapy. Children and staff with pertussis in child care facilities or schools should be excluded until erythromycin has been taken for 5 days.

CARE OF HOUSEHOLD AND OTHER CLOSE CONTACTS. Erythromycin (40–50 mg/kg/24 hr divided qid PO; maximum 2 g/24 hr) for 14 days should be given promptly to all household contacts and other close contacts, such as those in daycare, regardless of age, history of immunization, or symptoms. Clarithromycin and azithromycin are potential but not proven alternative agents for those who cannot tolerate erythromycin. Visitation and movement of coughing family members in the hospital must be assiduously controlled until erythromycin has been taken for 5 days. Close contacts <7 yr of age who have received less than four doses of pertussis-containing vaccines should have vaccination initiated or continued to complete the recommended series. Children <7 yr of age who received a third dose >6 mo before exposure or a fourth dose ≥3 yr before exposure should receive a booster dose. If infection with *B. pertussis* is proved, the individual should complete the immunization series with at least diphtheria and tetanus toxoids; some experts recommend including the pertussis component as well. Antimicrobial prophylaxis is not routinely recommended for exposed health care workers. Coughing health care workers, with or without known exposure to pertussis, should be promptly evaluated for pertussis. For major hospital outbreaks, multifaceted control procedures have included targeted erythromycin treatment of coughing individuals, mass erythromycin prophylaxis, and immunization of adults.

Complications. Rates of complications are difficult to establish because severe outcomes are preferentially reported, but infants <6 mo of age have excessive mortality and morbidity. Those <2 mo of age have the highest reported rates of pertussis-associated hospitalization (82%), pneumonia (25%), seizures (4%), encephalopathy (1%), and death (1%). Among 23 fatal cases in the United States in 1992–1993, approximately 80% were <6 mo of age. Preterm birth and young maternal age were significantly associated with fatal pertussis, and pneumonia complicated >95% cases.

The principal complications of pertussis are apnea, secondary infections (such as otitis media and pneumonia), and physical sequelae of forceful coughing. The need for intensive care and artificial ventilation is usually limited to infants <3 mo. Apnea, cyanosis, and secondary bacterial pneumonia are events precipitating intubation and ventilation. Bacterial pneumonia or adult respiratory distress syndrome is the usual cause of death at any age; pulmonary hemorrhage has occurred in neonates. Fever, tachypnea or respiratory distress between paroxysms, and absolute neutrophilia are clues to pneumonia. Expected pathogens include *Staphylococcus aureus, S. pneumoniae,* and bacteria of oropharyngeal flora. Bronchiectasis has been reported rarely after pertussis. Children who have pertussis before the age of 2 yr may have abnormal pulmonary function into adulthood.

Increased intrathoracic and intra-abdominal pressure during coughing can result in conjunctival and scleral hemorrhages, petechiae on the upper body, epistaxis, hemorrhage in the central nervous system (CNS) and retina, pneumothorax and subcutaneous emphysema, and umbilical and inguinal hernias. Laceration of the lingual frenulum is not uncommon. Rectal prolapse, once reported as a frequent complication of pertussis, was probably due to pertussis in malnourished children or missed diagnosis of cystic fibrosis. It is distinctly unusual and should elicit evaluation for underlying condition. Especially in infants in developing countries, dehydration and malnutrition following post-tussive vomiting can have a severe impact. Tetany has been associated with profound post-tussive alkalosis.

CNS abnormalities occur at a relatively high frequency and are almost always a result of hypoxemia or hemorrhage associated with coughing or apnea in young infants. Apnea or bradycardia or both may result from apparent laryngospasm or vagal stimulation just before a coughing episode, from obstruction during an episode, or from hypoxemia following an episode. Lack of associated respiratory signs in some young infants with apnea raises the possibility of a primary effect of PT on the CNS. Seizures are usually a result of hypoxemia, but hyponatremia from excessive secretion of antidiuretic hormone during pneumonia can occur. The only neuropathology documented in humans is parenchymal hemorrhage and ischemic necrosis.

Prevention. Universal immunization of children <7 yr of age with pertussis vaccine, beginning in infancy, is central to the control of pertussis (Chapter 282). Despite enormous effort, the critical mechanisms of immunity following disease or vaccination, a serologic correlate of protection, and the cause of vaccine-associated adverse events are not known. The only current standards for vaccine usefulness are clinical efficacy and safety. Current goals of immunization are protection of the individual from a significant coughing illness and control of endemic and epidemic disease.

ACELLULAR VACCINE. Multiple diphtheria and tetanus toxoids combined with acellular pertussis (DTaP) vaccines currently are licensed in the United States and are preferred over those containing whole-cell pertussis (DTP) vaccines because of fewer adverse reactions. Recommendations for use of DTaP are similar to recommendations for use of DTP, which continues to be given to infants and children in many other countries. Acellular pertussis vaccines all contain inactivated PT and may contain one or more other bacterial components (FHA, Pn, Fim 2 and 3). PT is detoxified either chemically or using molecular genetic techniques. Lacking serologic criteria for protection, licensure has been based on clinical efficacy trials conducted in Europe and Africa. Efficacy of licensed products to protect against severe pertussis can be considered similar, with relative protection against milder disease controversial. Mild local and systemic adverse events as well as more serious events (including high fever, persistent crying of ≥3 hr duration, hypotonic hyporesponsive episodes, and seizures) occur significantly less frequently among infants who receive DTaP compared with DTP vaccine. Whether the rare, potentially vaccine-associated events such as encephalopathy or anaphylactic shock will occur less frequently after acellular pertussis vaccine is not known.

DTaP containing vaccines can be administered simultaneously with any other vaccines used in standard schedules for children. Some products are licensed for use for all five doses. Combination of vaccines that include DTaP in place of DTP can affect immunogenicity of products. Combination vaccines should be used only in the dosing series and age group for which each is licensed, and when all components are indicated. When feasible, the same DTaP product is recommended for the first three doses of the vaccination series. Local reactions increase in rate and severity with successive doses of DTaP, although never reaching the magnitude of reactions following similar doses of DTP. Up to 2% of fourth and fifth doses of DTaP can be associated with entire limb swelling, with concurrent pain and erythema in approximately one half of children affected. Swelling subsides spontaneously without sequelae.

The same special considerations, precautions, contraindications, and reporting requirements for serious adverse events that exist for DTP vaccination apply to DTaP as well. Exempting children from pertussis immunization should be considered only in the narrow limits as recommended. Exemptors have been shown to have significantly increased risk for pertussis as well as a role in outbreaks of pertussis in immunized populations. Acellular pertussis vaccines are now licensed for use only among children through 6 yr of age. As studies of impact of pertussis in older individuals and trials of acellular pertussis vaccine in adolescents and adults accumulate, periodic reinforcing doses may be recommended.

American Academy of Pediatrics, Committee on Infectious Diseases: Acellular pertussis vaccine: Recommendations for use as the initial series in infants and children. *Pediatrics* 1997;99:282–8.

Bruss JB, Malley R, Halperin S, et al: Treatment of severe pertussis: A study of the safety and pharmacology of intravenous pertussis immunoglobulin. *Pediatr Infect Dis J* 1999;18:505–11.

Centers for Disease Control and Prevention: Recommendations of the Advisory Committee on Immunization Practices (ACIP): Pertussis vaccination: Use of acellular pertussis vaccines among infants and young children. *MMWR Morb Mortal Wkly Rep* 1997;46(RR-7):1–25.

Deeks S, De Serres G, Boulianne N, et al: Failure of physicians to consider the diagnosis of pertussis in children. *Clin Infect Dis* 1999;28:840–6.

Edwards KM: Is pertussis a frequent cause of cough in adolescents and adults? Should routine pertussis immunization be recommended? *Clin Infect Dis* 2001; 32:1698–9.

Feikin DR, Lezotte DC, Hamman RF, et al: Individual and community risks of measles and pertussis associated with personal exemptions to immunization. *JAMA* 2000;284:3145–50.

Honein MA, Paulozzi LJ, Himelright IM, et al: Infantile hypertrophic pyloric stenosis after pertussis prophylaxis with erythromycin: A case review and cohort study. *Lancet* 1999;354:2101–5.

Mahon BE, Rosenman MB, Kleiman MB: Maternal and infant use of erythromycin and other macrolide antibiotics as risk factors for infantile hypertrophic pyloric stenosis. *J Pediatr* 2001;139:380–4.

Rennels MB, Deloria MA, Pichichero ME, et al: Extensive swelling after booster doses of acellular pertussis-tetanus-diphtheria vaccines. *Pediatrics* 2000;105:1–6.

Strebel P, Nordin J, Edwards K, et al: Population-based incidence of pertussis among adolescents and adults, Minnesota, 1995–1996. *J Infect Dis* 2001;183: 1353–9.

Von König CHW, Rott H, Bogaerts H, et al: A serologic study of organisms possibly associated with pertussis-like coughing. *Pediatr Infect Dis J* 1998;17:645–9.

Wortis N, Strebel PM, Wharton M, et al: Pertussis deaths: Report of 23 cases in the United States, 1992 and 1993. *Pediatrics* 1996;97:607–12.

Chapter 181
Salmonella Thomas G. Cleary

Salmonella infections occur worldwide. Acute enteritis, the most frequent presentation, is usually self-limited, although bacteremia and focal extraintestinal infections may develop, especially in immunocompromised patients. The latter group has become more important and complex because of the increasing number of children who are compromised by AIDS, organ transplantation, or chemotherapy. **Enteric fever**, or **typhoid fever**, is a severe systemic disease that is classically caused by *Salmonella* ser. Typhi (*Salmonella typhi*) and is found mainly in developing countries, but it is encountered worldwide because of international travel.

Molecular technology has enabled classification at the gene level. DNA analysis has proved that all *Salmonella* organisms are closely related genetically as a single species with six subgroups; most isolates causing human or animal disease belong to subgroup 1. The medical slang usage that treated each of the nearly 2,500 serotypes as though it were a separate species has fallen out of favor. The preferred designation currently is the abbreviated version of the formal name by the Centers for Disease Control and Prevention (CDC) (Table 181–1).

181.1 Nontyphoidal Salmonellosis

Etiology. Salmonellae are motile, nonsporulating, nonencapsulated, gram-negative rods. Most strains ferment glucose, mannose, and mannitol to produce acid and gas, but they do not ferment lactose or sucrose. *S.* ser. Typhi does not produce gas. *Salmonella* organisms grow aerobically and are capable of facultative anaerobic growth. They are resistant to many physical agents but can be killed by heating to 130°F (54.4°C) for 1 hr or 140°F (60°C) for 15 min. They remain viable at ambient or reduced temperatures for days and may survive for weeks in sewage, dried foodstuffs, pharmaceutical agents, and fecal material. Like other members of the Enterobacteriaceae, *Salmonella* possesses somatic O antigens and flagellar H antigens. The **O antigens** are the heat-stable lipopolysaccharide components of the outer membrane; the **H antigens** are heat-labile proteins that can be present in phase 1 or 2. The Kauffmann-White scheme commonly used to classify salmonellae serotypes is based on O and H antigens. Serotyping is important clinically because certain serotypes tend to be associated with specific clinical syndromes and because detection of an unusual serotype is sometimes useful in recognizing a common-source outbreak. A virulence capsular polysaccharide (Vi), present on *S.* ser. Typhi, is also found on strains of *S.* ser. Dublin and *S.* ser. Paratyphi C *(S.* ser. Hirschfeldii).

Epidemiology. About 35,000–45,000 cases of culture-proven salmonellosis, approximately 98% of which are caused by nontyphoidal salmonellae, are reported annually in the United States. Because culturing and reporting are incomplete, the actual number of cases has been estimated as 1–5 million/yr. These figures are higher than those of the 1970s and may be related to modern practices of mass food production, which increase the potential for epidemic salmonellosis. About half of reported cases occur in persons <20 yr of age, and one third occur in children ≤4 yr of age; the highest isolation rate is for infants in the first few months of life. The age specific attack rate peaks in the second month of life in the United States at 159 cases/100,000 persons per year; in contrast, the incidence for persons 20–74 yr of age is about 9 cases/100,000 persons per year. Nontyphoidal *Salmonella* infections have a worldwide distribution, with an

TABLE 181-1. *Salmonella* Nomenclature

Traditional Usage	Formal Name	CDC Designation
S. typhi	S. enterica* subsp. enterica ser. Typhi	S. ser. Typhi
S. dublin	S. enterica subsp. enterica ser. Dublin	S. ser. Dublin
S. typhimurium	S. enterica subsp. enterica ser. Typhimurium	S. ser. Typhimurium
S. choleraesuis	S. enterica subsp. enterica ser. Choleraesuis	S. ser. Choleraesuis
S. marina	S. enterica subsp. houtenae ser. Marina	S. ser. Marina

CDC, Centers for Disease Control and Prevention; subsp, subspecies; ser., serotype.
*Some authorities prefer choleraesuis or enteritidis rather than enterica to describe the species.

incidence related to water potability, sewage disposal, and food preparation practices.

In the United States, *Salmonella* infections occur with highest frequency in the warmer months, July through November. Although most reported cases of nontyphoidal salmonellosis occur sporadically, food-borne outbreaks are common. Each year, about 500 food-borne *Salmonella* outbreaks are reported, representing more than 50% of all gastroenteritis outbreaks with a documented bacterial cause. Some of the *Salmonella* outbreaks are widespread—interstate or even international—and affect thousands of individuals. Refinement of outbreak tracing has improved with the development of molecular epidemiology techniques, such as plasmid analysis and endonuclease digestion of chromosomal genes for recognition of small differences in chromosomal structure. These can "fingerprint" a particular clone and are especially useful in tracing outbreaks caused by common serotypes. The *Salmonella* serotypes most often encountered in the United States include *S.* ser. Typhimurium, *S.* ser. Enteritidis, *S.* ser. Heidelberg, and *S.* ser. Newport.

Animals constitute the principal source of human nontyphoidal *Salmonella* disease. Infected animals are often asymptomatic. *Salmonella* has been isolated from many animals, including poultry (i.e., chickens, turkeys, ducks), sheep, cows, pigs, birds, and domestic pets. Specific serotypes are associated with particular animal hosts. For example, children with *S.* ser. Marina typically have exposure to pet iguanas. Pets, especially reptiles, cause about 3% of the outbreaks. Animal-to-animal transmission may occur. Animal feeds containing fishmeal or bone meal contaminated with *Salmonella* are an important source of infection for animals. Moreover, subtherapeutic concentrations of antibiotics are often added to animal feed. Such practices promote the emergence of antibiotic-resistant bacteria, including *Salmonella*, in the gut flora of the animals. During slaughtering, these gut organisms may contaminate the meat, which is subsequently consumed by humans. Data suggest that animal antibiotic exposure may be responsible for antibiotic-resistant *Salmonella* infections in humans.

Poultry and poultry products (mainly eggs) cause about half of the common-source outbreaks. Foods containing raw or undercooked eggs (e.g., Caesar salad, egg-dipped bread, and homemade eggnog) are of special importance. *Salmonella* infections in chickens increase the risk for contamination of eggs. Salmonellae can contaminate the shell surface, penetrate the egg, or be transmitted from an ovarian infection directly to the egg yolk. *Salmonella* serotypes have been isolated in as many as 50% of poultry, 16% of pork, 5% of beef, and 40% of frozen egg products purchased in retail stores. Meats, especially beef and pork, cause about 13% of the outbreaks, and raw or powdered milk and dairy products are the source of about 5% of the outbreaks. Food product–related outbreaks are often caused by contaminated equipment in processing plants or infected food handlers.

The estimated number of bacteria that must be ingested to cause symptomatic disease in healthy adults is 10^6–10^8 *Salmonella* organisms. In infants and in persons with certain underlying conditions, the inoculum size that can produce disease is smaller. Because of the relatively high inoculum size of *Salmonella* infection, ingestion of contaminated food, in which the organisms can multiply, is a major source of human infection. Because of the high infecting dose, person-to-person transmission by direct fecal-oral spread is unusual but can occur, especially in young children. Perinatal transmission during vaginal delivery has been reported. Prior antibiotic therapy during the previous month increases risk of symptomatic infection in children.

Nosocomial infections have been related to contaminated medical instruments (particularly endoscopes) and diagnostic or pharmacologic preparations, particularly those of animal origin (e.g., pancreatic extracts, pituitary extracts, bile salts, pepsin, gelatin, vitamins, carmine dye). Food-borne nosocomial transmission is also possible. Hospitalized patients are at increased risk of severe and complicated *Salmonella* infections. Intravenous transmission by platelet transfusion has been reported.

After infection, nontyphoidal salmonellae are excreted in feces for a median of 5 wk. In young children and in individuals with symptomatic infections, the excretion period is longer. Prolonged carriage of *Salmonella* organisms is rare in healthy children but has been reported in those with underlying immune deficiency. During the period of *Salmonella* excretion, the individual may infect others, directly by the fecal-oral route or indirectly by contaminating foods.

Pathogenesis. Enterocolitis is the typical disorder caused by nontyphoidal *Salmonella* infection. Findings include diffuse mucosal inflammation and edema, sometimes with erosions and microabscesses. Although *Salmonella* organisms are capable of penetrating the intestinal mucosa, neither destruction of epithelial cells nor production of ulcers is usually found. Intestinal inflammation, with polymorphonuclear leukocytes and macrophages, usually involves the lamina propria. Underlying intestinal lymphoid tissue and mesenteric lymph nodes enlarge and may develop small areas of necrosis. Such lymphoid hypertrophy may cause interference with the blood supply to the gut mucosa. Hyperplasia of the reticuloendothelial system is also noted within the liver and spleen. If bacteremia develops, it may lead to localized infection and suppuration in almost any organ.

The development of disease after infection with *Salmonella* depends on the number of infecting organisms, on their virulence traits, and on several host defense factors. Ingested *Salmonella* organisms reach the stomach, where acid is the first protective barrier. The acidity inhibits multiplication of the salmonellae, and most organisms are rapidly killed at gastric pH ≤2.0. Achlorhydria, buffering medications, rapid gastric emptying after gastrectomy or gastroenterostomy, and a large inoculum enable viable organisms to reach the small intestine. Neonates and young infants have hypochlorhydria and rapid gastric emptying, which contribute to their increased vulnerability to symptomatic salmonellosis. Because the transit time through the stomach is faster for drinks than for foods, a lower inoculum may cause disease in water-borne infection.

In the small and large intestines, salmonellae have to compete with normal bacterial flora to multiply and cause disease; prior antibiotic therapy disrupts this competitive relationship. Decreased intestinal motility due to anatomic causes or medications increases the contact time of the ingested salmonellae with the mucosa and the likelihood of symptomatic disease. After multiplication within the lumen, the organisms penetrate through the Peyer patches, typically at the distal part of the ileum and the proximal part of the colon. The penetration process includes specific attachment to the M cells, internalization by receptor-mediated endocytosis, cytoplasmic translocation of the infected endosome to the basal membrane, and release of the salmonellae in the lamina propria. Dendritic cells in the dome of Peyer patches and beneath the gut epithelium begin the processing that leads to stimulation of CD4 T cells, interferon-γ production, and bacterial clearance. Penetration usually occurs without destroying epithelial cells, and ulcers are not produced.

Heat-labile cholera-like enterotoxin is produced by many *Salmonella* isolates. This toxin and the prostaglandins that are produced locally increase cyclic adenosine monophosphate levels within intestinal crypts, causing a net efflux of electrolytes and water into the intestinal lumen.

Genes code for adherence, invasion, a cholera toxin-like enterotoxin, spread beyond the Peyer patches to mesenteric lymph nodes, intracellular growth in the liver and spleen, survival in macrophages, serum resistance, and complement resistance. The genes causing invasion are closely related to the *Shigella* invasion genes. However, *Shigella* lack the genes for spread beyond the intestine and survival in the bloodstream. These genetic differences explain the higher frequency of bacteremia in *Salmonella* infection. Some virulence traits are shared by all salmonellae, but others are serotype restricted. These virulence traits have been defined in tissue culture and murine models; it is likely that clinical features of human *Salmonella* infection will eventually be related to specific DNA sequences.

With most diarrhea-associated nontyphoidal salmonelloses, the infection does not extend beyond the lamina propria and the local lymphatics. *S. ser.* Dublin and *S. ser.* Choleraesuis rapidly invade the bloodstream with little or no intestinal involvement. Specific virulence genes are related to the ability to cause bacteremia. These genes are found significantly more often in strains of *S. ser.* Typhimurium isolated from the blood than the feces of humans. Bacteremia, however, is possible with any *Salmonella* serotype, especially in individuals with reduced host defenses. An impaired reticuloendothelial or cellular immune response is important. Children with chronic granulomatous disease, other white cell disorders, and AIDS are at increased risk. A central role for IL-12 and interferon-γ cell-mediated immunity in clearance of *Salmonella* has been demonstrated by inherited defects in this pathway. These defects (interferon-γ receptor binding chain or signaling chain deficiency, IL-12 receptor beta 1 chain deficiency, IL-12 p40 subunit deletion) cause decreased interferon-γ production. These genetic defects are associated with both *Salmonella* and mycobacterial infections.

Children with sickle cell disease are prone to *Salmonella* septicemia and osteomyelitis. The numerous infarcted areas in the gastrointestinal tract, bones, and reticuloendothelial system may initially permit organisms greater access to the circulation from the intestine and then furnish an optimal environment for localization. The decreased phagocytic and opsonizing capacity of patients with sickle cell disease also contributes to the high infection rate.

Chronic infection is associated with cholelithiasis, *Schistosoma mansoni* infection with hepatosplenic involvement, and *Schistosoma hematobium* infection of the urinary tract. Localized infections are more common in areas with impaired local defenses (e.g., effusions, tumors, hematomas).

Clinical Manifestations. Several distinct clinical syndromes can develop in children infected with nontyphoidal *Salmonella*, depending on host factors and the specific serotype involved.

ACUTE ENTERITIS. The most common clinical presentation of salmonellosis is acute enteritis. After an incubation period of 6–72 hr (mean, 24 hr), there is an abrupt onset of nausea, vomiting, and crampy abdominal pain primarily in the periumbilical area and right lower quadrant, followed by mild to severe watery diarrhea and sometimes by diarrhea containing blood and mucus. Moderate fever (temperature of 101–102°F [38.5–39°C]) affects about 70% of patients. Some children develop severe disease with high fever, headache, drowsiness,

confusion, meningismus, seizures, and abdominal distention. Abdominal examination reveals some tenderness. The stool typically contains a moderate number of polymorphonuclear leukocytes and occult blood. Mild leukocytosis may be detected. Symptoms subside within 2–7 days in healthy children; fatalities are rare.

In certain high-risk groups, the course of *Salmonella* gastroenteritis may be more complicated. Neonates, young infants, and children with primary or secondary immune deficiency may have symptoms persisting for several weeks. In patients with AIDS, the infection may become widespread and overwhelming, causing multisystem involvement, septic shock, and death. In patients with inflammatory bowel disease, especially active ulcerative colitis, *Salmonella* gastroenteritis may cause invasion of the bowel with rapid development of toxic megacolon, systemic toxicity, and death. Patients with schistosomiasis have increased susceptibility to salmonellosis and exhibit persistence of infection unless the schistosomiasis is also treated. *Salmonella* organisms are able to multiply within the schistosomes, where they are protected from antibiotics.

BACTEREMIA. In contrast to adults who usually are immunologically impaired and develop *Salmonella* bacteremia in the absence of diarrhea, the majority of children have no predisposing risk factors and develop bacteremia as a complication of acute enteritis. The older a child is, the more likely he is to have an underlying condition when *Salmonella* bacteremia occurs. Transient bacteremia during nontyphoidal *Salmonella* gastroenteritis is believed to occur in 1–5% of patients. The precise incidence is unclear, because blood cultures often are not obtained from patients with *Salmonella* gastroenteritis, especially those who are not hospitalized, and because most data are from retrospective studies. *Salmonella* bacteremia is associated with fever, chills, and often with a toxic appearance. Bacteremia has been documented, however, in afebrile, well-appearing children, including neonates. Prolonged or intermittent bacteremia is associated with low-grade fever, anorexia, weight loss, diaphoresis, and myalgias. Children with certain underlying conditions and *Salmonella* gastroenteritis are at increased risk of bacteremia (Box 181–1), which may lead to extraintestinal infection. Children who have no underlying disease may be at increased risk of bacteremia if they have been treated with antibiotics in the month before acquisition of *Salmonella* infection. Bacteremic disease after antibiotic treatment is more likely to be due to a resistant *Salmonella*. In patients with AIDS, recurrent septicemia appears despite antibiotic therapy, often with a negative stool culture for *Salmonella* and sometimes with no identifiable focus of infection. In children, persistent bacteremia usually occurs without an intravascular focal infection, although adults with persistent bacteremia may have endocarditis, arteritis, or an infected aortic aneurysm. Prolonged or recurrent bacteremia also occurs in patients with schistosomiasis. Hemolytic anemias, malaria, and bartonellosis are associated with an increased risk

---

BOX 181–1. Conditions That Increase the Risk of *Salmonella* Bacteremia During *Salmonella* Gastroenteritis

Neonates and young infants (≤3 mo of age)
AIDS, chronic granulomatous disease, and other immuno deficiencies
Malignancies, especially leukemia and lymphoma
Immunosuppressive and corticosteroid therapy
Hemolytic anemia, including sickle cell disease, malaria, and bartonellosis
Collagen vascular disease
Inflammatory bowel disease
Gastrectomy or gastroenterostomy
Achlorhydria or antacid medication use
Impaired intestinal motility
Schistosomiasis
Malnutrition

of bacteremia, presumably because of reticuloendothelial system dysfunction. In pregnancy, *Salmonella* septicemia and fetal loss have been reported. *S.* ser. Typhimurium is the most common serotype causing *Salmonella* bacteremia in the United States.

EXTRAINTESTINAL FOCAL INFECTIONS. After salmonellae have entered the bloodstream, they have a unique capability to metastasize and cause a focal suppurative infection of almost any organ. Sites of pre-existing abnormalities are often involved. Extraintestinal infections are most common in the first 3 mo of life, in those with sickle cell disease, and in those who have had prior gastrointestinal surgery. The most common focal infections involve the skeletal system, meninges, and intravascular sites. *Salmonella* is a common cause of osteomyelitis in children with sickle cell disease. *Salmonella* osteomyelitis and suppurative arthritis also occur in sites of previous trauma or skeletal prosthesis. Reactive arthritis may follow *Salmonella* gastroenteritis, usually in adolescents with the HLA-B27 antigen. Meningitis occurs about 100 times less frequently than bacteremia. Although meningitis can occur at any age, the peak incidence is in infancy. Patients may present with little or no fever and minimal symptoms, or rapid deterioration, and neurologic sequelae despite appropriate antibiotic therapy. *Salmonella* meningitis occurs also in patients with AIDS, for whom the mortality rate is more than 50%, and relapse and brain abscesses can occur.

Diagnosis. Definitive diagnosis of the various clinical syndromes is still based on culturing and subsequent identification of *Salmonella* organisms. In children with gastroenteritis, cultures of stools have higher yields than rectal swabs. In patients with sites of local suppuration, aspirated specimens should be Gram stained and cultured. *Salmonella* organisms grow well on nonselective or enriched media, such as blood agar, chocolate agar, or nutrient broth. Normally sterile body fluids (e.g., cerebrospinal fluid, joint fluid, urine) can be cultured on any of these. For specimens normally containing mixed bacterial flora (e.g., stools), selective media, such as MacConkey, XLD, bismuth sulfite (BBL), or *Salmonella-Shigella* (SS) agar, which inhibit the growth of normal flora, should be used.

Several methods are being developed to answer the need for rapid diagnosis. Tests based on latex agglutination and fluorescence are commercially available for the rapid diagnosis of *Salmonella* colonies growing in stool culture enrichment broth or culture plates. Serologic assay for detecting antibodies against *S.* ser. Typhimurium and *S.* ser. Enteritidis has been reported, but clinical usefulness is unclear. The serotype isolated can suggest a source that may be epidemiologically important: *S.* ser. Kentucky and *S.* ser. Heidelberg in broilers; *S.* ser Hadar and *S.* ser. Heidelberg in turkeys; *S.* ser. Derby and *S.* ser. Typhimurium in swine; and *S.* ser. Marina, *S.* ser. Flint, *S.* ser. Kintambo, *S.* ser. Wassenaar, *S.* ser. Ealing, *S.* ser. Carrau, *S.* ser. Stanley, *S.* ser. Java, and *S.* ser. Abaetetuba in reptiles.

DIFFERENTIAL DIAGNOSIS. *Salmonella* gastroenteritis should be differentiated from other bacterial, viral, and parasitic causes of diarrhea. The presentation of inflammatory diarrhea with moderate fever should be particularly differentiated from *Shigella*, enteroinvasive *Escherichia coli*, *Yersinia enterocolitica*, and *Clostridium difficile* infections. Rotavirus infections in infants can mimic *Salmonella* enterocolitis. Etiologic diagnosis on the basis of the clinical picture is seldom possible. Epidemiologic data may be helpful. If abdominal pain and tenderness are severe, appendicitis, perforated viscus, and ulcerative colitis merit consideration in the differential diagnosis.

Treatment. Appropriate therapy depends on the specific clinical presentation of *Salmonella* infection. Assessment of the hydration status, correction of dehydration and electrolyte disturbances, and supportive care (Chapters 46 and 48.1) are the most important aspects of managing *Salmonella* gastroenteritis in children. Antimotility agents prolong intestinal transit time and are thought to increase the risk of invasion; they should not be used when salmonellosis is suspected. In patients with gastroenteritis, antimicrobial agents do not shorten the clinical course, nor do they eliminate fecal excretion of *Salmonella*. By suppressing normal intestinal flora, antimicrobial agents may prolong the excretion of *Salmonella* and increase the risk of creating the chronic carrier state. Antibiotics therefore are not indicated routinely in treating *Salmonella* gastroenteritis. They should be used in infants (≤3 mo of age) and other children who are at increased risk of a disseminated disease (see Box 181–1) and in those with a severe or protracted course. It has been recommended that toxic megacolon should be managed with adequate hydration and insertion of a rectal tube to decompress the dilated colon in an attempt to prevent perforation.

Children with bacteremia or extraintestinal focal *Salmonella* infections should receive antimicrobial therapy. Ampicillin (200 mg/kg/24 hr divided qid) is efficacious and used to be the drug of choice; trimethoprim-sulfamethoxazole (TMP-SMZ; 10 mg/kg/24 hr of the TMP component and 50 mg/kg/24 hr of the SMZ divided bid) is also effective. Because of the increasing worldwide antibiotic resistance of *Salmonella* strains, it is necessary to perform susceptibility tests on all human isolates. About 20% of *Salmonella* isolates in the United States are resistant to ampicillin. Multiresistance to ampicillin, TMP-SMZ, and chloramphenicol has been reported. The third-generation cephalosporins cefotaxime (150–200 mg/kg/24 hr divided q 6–8 hr) or ceftriaxone (100 mg/kg/24 hr in one or two daily doses) are effective if the isolate is susceptible. Ceftriaxone resistant salmonellae are being recognized with increasing frequency in the United States among individuals who have not traveled internationally. Their prevalence has increased from 0.1% in 1996 to 0.5% in 1998. Ceftriaxone resistant organisms have been traced to cattle. Quinolones are also effective, but they are not approved for use in persons ≤18 yr of age because of the potential damage to growing cartilage. Rarely, use of a fluoroquinolone may be appropriate in a child whose organism is resistant to other first-line choices. Unfortunately, *S.* ser. Typhimurium DT104, an organism that has spread from food animals to humans and has caused large outbreaks, is multidrug resistant, sometimes including resistance to quinolones. In children with severe disease, initial treatment with a third-generation cephalosporin is recommended until antibiotic susceptibility is known. Thereafter, antibiotics should be changed on the basis of susceptibility data and clinical syndrome.

The duration of antimicrobial therapy is 10–14 days for children with bacteremia, 4–6 wk for acute osteomyelitis, and 4 wk for meningitis. For children with a focal suppurative process, surgical drainage is necessary in addition to antibiotic treatment. Surgical intervention is often necessary in intravascular *Salmonella* infections and in cases of chronic osteomyelitis.

Prognosis. Complete recovery is the rule in healthy children who develop *Salmonella* gastroenteritis. Young infants and immunocompromised patients often have systemic involvement, a prolonged course, and extraintestinal foci. The prognosis is poor for children with *Salmonella* meningitis or endocarditis.

CHRONIC CARRIER STATE. After clinical recovery from *Salmonella* gastroenteritis, asymptomatic fecal excretion of salmonellae occurs for several months, particularly in younger children or those treated with antibiotics. A chronic carrier state is defined as asymptomatic excretion of *Salmonella* organisms for >1 yr. A prolonged carrier state after nontyphoidal salmonellosis is rare (<1%); it is more common in patients with biliary tract disease (e.g., cholelithiasis). The only significance of asymptomatic fecal excretion of nontyphoidal *Salmonella* is the potential transmission of the infection to other individuals.

Prevention. Chlorinated water, proper sanitary systems, and adequate food hygiene practices are necessary to prevent nontyphoidal salmonellosis in humans. Handwashing is of paramount importance in controlling person-to-person transmission by means of food. In hospitalized patients, enteric precautions should be used for the duration of illness. Individuals with symptomatic or asymptomatic excretion of *Salmonella* strains should be excluded from activities that involve food preparation or child care until repeated stool cultures are negative. Breast-feeding has been shown to reduce infection.

Control of the transmission of *Salmonella* infections to humans requires control of the infection in the animal reservoir, judicious use of antibiotics in dairy and livestock farming, prevention of contamination of foodstuffs prepared from animals, and use of appropriate standards in food processing in commercial and private kitchens. Parents should be advised of the risk of reptiles as pets in households with young infants. Whenever cooking practices prevent food from reaching a temperature greater than 150°F (65.5°C) for >12 min, *Salmonella* may remain viable. Because large outbreaks are often related to mass food production, it should be recognized that contamination of just one piece of machinery used in food processing may cause an outbreak; meticulous cleaning of equipment is essential. No vaccine against nontyphoidal *Salmonella* infections is available. Infections should be reported to public health authorities so that outbreaks can be recognized and investigated.

181.2 Enteric Fever

Etiology. Enteric fever, or **typhoid fever**, is caused by *S.* ser Typhi, *S.* ser. Paratyphi A, *S.* ser. Paratyphi B (Schottmuelleri), and *S.* ser. Paratyphi C (Hirschfeldii). Rarely, other *Salmonella* serotypes can cause a similar prolonged febrile illness.

Epidemiology. The incidence, mode of transmission, and consequences of enteric fever differ significantly in developed and developing countries. The incidence has decreased markedly in developed countries. In the United States, about 400 cases of typhoid fever are reported each year, giving an annual incidence of less than 0.2 cases/100,000 population, which is similar to that in Western Europe and Japan. In Southern Europe, the annual incidence is 4.3–14.5 cases/100,000 population. In developing countries, *S.* ser. Typhi is often the most common *Salmonella* isolate, with an incidence that can reach 500 cases/100,000 population (0.5%) and a high mortality rate. The World Health Organization has estimated that at least 12.5 million cases occur annually worldwide.

Because humans are the only natural reservoir of *S.* ser. Typhi, direct or indirect contact with an infected person (sick or chronic carrier) is necessary for infection. Ingestion of foods or water contaminated with human feces is the most common mode of transmission. Water-borne outbreaks due to poor sanitation and direct fecal-oral spread due to poor personal hygiene are encountered, mainly in developing countries. Oysters and other shellfish cultivated in water contaminated by sewage are also a source of widespread infection. In the United States about 65% of the cases result from international travel. Travel to Asia (especially to India) and Central or South America (especially Mexico) is usually implicated. Domestically acquired enteric fever is most frequent in the southern and western United States and is usually caused by consumption of foods contaminated by individuals who are chronic carriers. Congenital transmission of enteric fever can occur by transplacental infection from a bacteremic mother to her fetus. Intrapartum transmission is also possible, occurring by a fecal-oral route from a carrier mother.

Pathogenesis. In younger children, the morphologic changes of *S.* ser. Typhi infection are less prominent than in older children and adults. Hyperplasia of Peyer patches with necrosis and sloughing of overlying epithelium produces ulcers that may bleed. The mucosa and lymphatic tissue of the intestinal tract are severely inflamed and necrotic. Ulcers heal without scarring.

Strictures and intestinal obstruction virtually never occur after typhoid fever. The inflammatory lesion may occasionally penetrate the muscularis and serosa of the intestine and produce perforation. The mesenteric lymph nodes, liver, and spleen are hyperemic and generally reveal areas of focal necrosis. Hyperplasia of reticuloendothelial tissue with proliferation of mononuclear cells is the predominant finding. A mononuclear response may be seen in the bone marrow in association with areas of focal necrosis. Inflammation of the gallbladder is focal, inconstant, and modest in proportion to the extent of local bacterial multiplication. Bronchitis is common. Inflammation also may be observed in the form of localized abscesses, pneumonia, septic arthritis, osteomyelitis, pyelonephritis, endophthalmitis, and meningitis.

The inoculum size required to cause enteric fever in volunteers is 10^5–10^9 *S.* ser. Typhi organisms. These estimates may be higher than in naturally acquired infection because the volunteers ingested the organisms in milk; stomach acidity is an important determinant of susceptibility to *Salmonella*. The bacteria invade through the Peyer patches. Organisms are transported to intestinal lymph nodes, where multiplication takes place within the mononuclear cells. Monocytes, unable to destroy the bacilli early in the disease process, carry these organisms into the mesenteric lymph nodes. Organisms then reach the bloodstream through the thoracic duct, causing a transient bacteremia. Circulating organisms reach the reticuloendothelial cells in the liver, spleen, and bone marrow and may seed other organs. After proliferation in the reticuloendothelial system, bacteremia recurs. The gallbladder is particularly susceptible to being infected. Local multiplication in the walls of the gallbladder produces large numbers of salmonellae, which reach the intestine through the bile.

Several virulence factors seem to be important. Invasion of Peyer patches is encoded by genes closely related to the invasion genes of *Shigella* and enteroinvasive *E. coli*. However, *S.* ser. Typhi possesses a number of additional genes not found in *Shigella* that are responsible for the features of typhoid fever. The surface Vi capsular antigen found in *S.* ser. Typhi interferes with phagocytosis by preventing the binding of C3 to the surface of the bacterium. The ability of organisms to survive within macrophages after phagocytosis is an important virulence trait encoded by the *phoP* regulon; it may be related to metabolic effects on host cells. Circulating endotoxin, a lipopolysaccharide component of the bacterial cell wall, is thought to cause the prolonged fever and toxic symptoms of enteric fever, although its levels in symptomatic patients are low. Alternatively, endotoxin-induced cytokine production by human macrophages may cause the systemic symptoms. The occasional occurrence of diarrhea may be explained by presence of a toxin related to cholera toxin and *E. coli* heat-labile enterotoxin.

Cell-mediated immunity is important in protecting the human host against typhoid fever. Decreased numbers of T lymphocytes are found in patients who are critically ill with typhoid fever. Carriers show impaired cellular reactivity to *S.* ser. Typhi antigens in the leukocyte migration inhibition test. In carriers, a large number of virulent bacilli pass into the intestine daily and are excreted in the stool, without entering the epithelium of the host.

Clinical Manifestations. The incubation period is usually 7–14 days, but it may range from 3–30 days, depending mainly on the size of the ingested inoculum. The clinical manifestations of enteric fever depend on age.

SCHOOL-AGED CHILDREN AND ADOLESCENTS. The onset of symptoms is insidious. Initial symptoms of fever, malaise, anorexia, myalgia, headache, and abdominal pain develop over 2–3 days. Although diarrhea having a pea soup consistency may be present during the early course of the disease, constipation later becomes a more prominent symptom. Cough and epistaxis may ensue. Severe lethargy may develop in some children. Temperature, which increases in a stepwise fashion, becomes an unremitting and high fever within 1 wk, often reaching 40°C.

During the 2nd week of illness, high fever is sustained, and fatigue, anorexia, cough, and abdominal symptoms increase in severity. Patients appear acutely ill, disoriented, and lethargic. Delirium and stupor may be observed. Physical findings include a relative bradycardia, which is disproportionate to the high fever. Hepatomegaly, splenomegaly, and distended abdomen with diffuse tenderness are very common. In about 50% of patients with enteric fever, a macular or maculopapular rash (**rose spots**) appears on about the 7th–10th day. Lesions are usually discrete, erythematous, and 1–5 mm in diameter; the lesions are slightly raised and blanch on pressure. They appear in crops of 10–15 lesions on the lower chest and abdomen and last 2–3 days. They leave a slight brownish discoloration of the skin on healing. Cultures of the lesions have a 60% yield for *Salmonella* organisms. Rhonchi and scattered rales may be heard on auscultation of the chest. Nausea and vomiting if occurring in the 2nd or 3rd week suggest a complication. If no complications occur, the symptoms and physical findings gradually resolve within 2–4 wk, but malaise and lethargy may persist for an additional 1–2 mo. Patients may be emaciated by the end of the illness. Enteric fever caused by nontyphoidal *Salmonella* is usually milder, with a shorter duration of fever and a lower rate of complications.

INFANTS AND YOUNG CHILDREN (<5 YR). Enteric fever is relatively rare in this age group in endemic areas. Although clinical sepsis can occur, the disease is surprisingly mild at presentation, making the diagnosis difficult. Mild fever and malaise, misinterpreted as a viral syndrome, occur in infants with culture-proven typhoid fever. Diarrhea is more common in young children with typhoid fever than in adults, leading to a diagnosis of acute gastroenteritis.

NEONATES. In addition to its ability to cause abortion and premature delivery, enteric fever during late pregnancy may be transmitted vertically. The neonatal disease usually begins within 3 days of delivery. Vomiting, diarrhea, and abdominal distention are common. Temperature is variable but may be as high as 40.5°C. Seizures may occur. Hepatomegaly, jaundice, anorexia, and weight loss can be marked.

Complications. Severe intestinal hemorrhage and intestinal perforation occur in 1–10% and 0.5–3% of the patients, respectively. These and most other complications usually occur after the 1st week of the disease. Hemorrhage, which usually precedes perforation, is manifested by a decrease in temperature and blood pressure and an increase in the pulse rate. Perforations, which are usually pinpoint size but may be as large as several centimeters, typically occur in the distal ileum and are accompanied by a marked increase in abdominal pain, tenderness, vomiting, and signs of peritonitis. Sepsis with various enteric aerobic gram-negative bacilli and anaerobes may develop. Although disturbed liver function test results are found for many patients with enteric fever, overt hepatitis and cholecystitis are considered complications. An increase in serum amylase levels may sometimes accompany clinically obvious pancreatitis.

Pneumonia caused by superinfection with organisms other than *Salmonella* is more common in children than in adults. In children, pneumonia or bronchitis is common (approximately 10%). Toxic myocarditis with fatty infiltration and necrosis of the myocardium may be manifested by arrhythmias, sinoatrial block, ST-T changes on the electrocardiogram, or cardiogenic shock. Thrombosis and phlebitis occur rarely. Neurologic complications include increased intracranial pressure, cerebral thrombosis, acute cerebellar ataxia, chorea, aphasia, deafness, psychosis, and transverse myelitis. Peripheral and optic neuritis have been reported. Permanent sequelae are rare. Other reported complications include fatal bone marrow necrosis, pyelonephritis,

nephrotic syndrome, meningitis, endocarditis, parotitis, orchitis, and suppurative lymphadenitis. Although osteomyelitis and suppurative arthritis can occur in a normal host, they are more common in children with hemoglobinopathies.

Diagnosis. Culturing the *Salmonella* strain involved is usually the basis for confirming the diagnosis. Results of blood cultures are positive in 40–60% of the patients seen early in the course of the disease, and stool and urine cultures become positive after the 1st week. The stool culture result is also occasionally positive during the incubation period. Because of the intermittent and low-level bacteremia, repeated blood cultures should be obtained in suspect cases. Cultures of bone marrow often yield positive results during later stages of the disease, when blood cultures may be sterile; although seldom obtained, cultures of mesenteric lymph nodes, liver, and spleen may also have positive results at this point. A culture of bone marrow is the single most sensitive method of diagnosis (positive in 85–90%) and is less influenced by prior antimicrobial therapy. Stool and sometimes urine cultures are positive in chronic carriers. In suspected cases with negative results of stool cultures, a culture of aspirated duodenal fluid or of a duodenal string capsule may be helpful in confirming infection. However, the duodenal string culture test cannot be performed on those too young or too ill to cooperate.

Direct detection of *S*. ser. Typhi-specific antigens in the serum or *S*. ser. Typhi Vi antigen in the urine has been attempted by immunologic methods, often using monoclonal antibodies. Polymerase chain reaction has been used to amplify specific genes of *S*. ser. Typhi in the blood of patients, enabling diagnosis within a few hours. This method is specific and more sensitive than blood cultures, given the low level of bacteremia in enteric fever. Serology is of little help in establishing the diagnosis, but it may be useful in epidemiologic studies. The classic **Widal test** measures antibodies against O and H antigens of *S*. ser. Typhi. Because many false-positive and false-negative results occur, diagnosis of typhoid fever by Widal test alone is prone to error.

A normochromic, normocytic anemia often develops after several weeks of illness and is related to intestinal blood loss or bone marrow suppression. Blood leukocyte counts are frequently low in relation to the fever and toxicity, but there is a wide range in counts; leukopenia, usually not less than 2,500 cells/mm^3, is often found after the 1st or 2nd week of illness. When pyogenic abscesses develop, leukocytosis may reach 20,000–25,000/mm^3. Thrombocytopenia may be striking and persist for as long as 1 wk. Liver function test results are often disturbed. Proteinuria is common. Fecal leukocytes and fecal blood are very common.

DIFFERENTIAL DIAGNOSIS. During the initial stage of enteric fever, the clinical diagnosis may mistakenly be gastroenteritis, viral syndrome, bronchitis, or bronchopneumonia. Subsequently, the differential diagnosis includes sepsis with other bacterial pathogens; infections caused by intracellular microorganisms, such as tuberculosis, brucellosis, tularemia, leptospirosis, and rickettsial diseases; viral infections, such as infectious mononucleosis and anicteric hepatitis; and malignancies, such as leukemia and lymphoma.

Treatment. Antimicrobial therapy is essential in treating enteric fever. Because of increasing antibiotic resistance, however, choosing the appropriate empirical therapy is problematic and controversial. Although antibiotic resistance of *S*. ser. Typhi isolates in the United States is relatively low (3–4%), most infections are acquired abroad, where resistance occurs. Increasing rates of plasmid-mediated antibiotic resistance of *S*. ser. Typhi have been reported from Southeast Asia, Mexico, and certain countries in the Middle East. Reports from India describe multiresistance to chloramphenicol, ampicillin, and TMP-SMX in 49–83% of *S*. ser. Typhi isolates. Resistant strains are usually susceptible to third-generation cephalosporins. Quinolones are efficacious but are not approved for children. Most antibiotic regimens are associated with a 5–20% recurrence risk. Chloramphenicol (50 mg/kg/24 hr divided qid PO or 75 mg/kg/24 hr divided q 6 hr IV), ampicillin (200 mg/kg/24 hr divided q 4–6 hr IV), amoxicillin (100 mg/kg/24 hr divided tid PO), and trimethoprim-sulfamethoxazole (10 mg of TMP and 50 mg of SMZ/kg/24 hr divided bid PO) have demonstrated good clinical efficacy. Although chloramphenicol therapy is associated with a more rapid defervescence and sterilization of blood, the rate of relapse is somewhat higher, and this agent can cause potentially serious adverse effects. Most children become afebrile within 7 days; treatment of uncomplicated cases should be continued for at least 14 days, or 5–7 days after defervescence. Data suggest that very short courses of therapy may be adequate with oral cefixime (20 mg/kg/24 hr divided bid for 7 days), ceftriaxone (50 mg/kg/24 hr once daily IM for 5 days) or oral ofloxacin (15 mg/kg/24 hr for 2 days). Chloramphenicol remains the gold standard.

In adults, ciprofloxacin at a dose of 500 mg bid for 7–10 days is effective and associated with a low relapse rate. In children with suspected resistant strains, empirical therapy with ceftriaxone (or cefotaxime) is appropriate until antibiotic susceptibility patterns are available.

In addition to antibiotic therapy, a short course of dexamethasone (3 mg/kg for the initial dose, followed by 1 mg/kg q 6 hr for 48 hr) improves the survival rate of patients with shock, obtundation, stupor, or coma. Supportive treatment and maintenance of appropriate fluid and electrolyte balance are essential. When intestinal hemorrhage is severe, blood transfusion is needed. Surgical intervention and broad-spectrum antibiotics are recommended for intestinal perforation. Surgical resection of 10 cm on each side of the perforation has been reported to improve survival. Platelet transfusions have been suggested for the treatment of thrombocytopenia that is sufficiently severe to cause intestinal hemorrhage in patients for whom surgery is contemplated.

Although attempts to eradicate chronic carriage of *S.* ser. Typhi are recommended for public health considerations, eradication is difficult despite in vitro susceptibility to the usual antibiotics. A course of 4–6 wk of high-dose ampicillin (or amoxicillin) plus probenecid or TMP-SMZ results in an approximately 80% cure rate of carriers if no biliary tract disease is present. Ciprofloxacin has been used successfully in adults. In the presence of cholelithiasis or cholecystitis, antibiotics alone are unlikely to be successful; cholecystectomy within 14 days of antibiotic treatment is recommended.

Prognosis. The prognosis for a patient with enteric fever depends on prompt therapy, the age of the patient, previous state of health, the causative *Salmonella* serotype, and the appearance of complications. In developed countries, with appropriate antimicrobial therapy, the mortality rate is less than 1%. In developing countries, the mortality rate is higher than 10%, usually because of delays in diagnosis, hospitalization, and treatment. Infants and children with underlying debilitating disorders are at higher risk. The appearance of complications, such as gastrointestinal perforation or severe hemorrhage, meningitis, endocarditis, and pneumonia, is associated with high morbidity and mortality rates.

Relapse after the initial clinical response occurs in 4–8% of the patients who are not treated with antibiotics. In patients who have received appropriate antimicrobial therapy, the clinical manifestations of relapse become apparent about 2 wk after stopping antibiotics and resemble the acute illness. The relapse, however, is usually milder and of shorter duration. Numerous relapses may occur. Individuals who excrete *S.* ser. Typhi for ≥3 mo after infection usually become chronic carriers. The risk of becoming a carrier is low in children and increases with age; of all patients with typhoid fever, 1–5% become chronic carriers.

The incidence of biliary tract diseases is higher in chronic carriers than in the general population. Although chronic urinary carriage may also occur, it is rare and found mainly in individuals with schistosomiasis.

Prevention. In endemic areas, improved sanitation and clean running water are essential to control enteric fever. To minimize person-to-person transmission and food contamination, personal hygiene measures, handwashing, and attention to food preparation practices are necessary. Efforts to eradicate *S.* ser. Typhi from carriers are recommended, because humans are the only reservoir of *S.* ser. Typhi. When such efforts are unsuccessful, carriers should be prevented from working in food- or water-processing activities, in kitchens, and in occupations related to patient care. These individuals should be made aware of the potential contagiousness of their condition and of the importance of handwashing and attentive personal hygiene.

VACCINE. Two vaccines against *S.* ser. Typhi are commercially available in the United States. An oral, live-attenuated preparation of the Ty21a strain of *S.* ser. Typhi have been shown to have good efficacy (67–82%). Four enteric-coated capsules are given on alternate days, and the entire series is repeated every 5 yr. Significant adverse effects are rare. The oral vaccine is recommended for persons ≥6 yr of age. Infants and toddlers do not develop immune responses with this preparation. It should not be used in persons with immunodeficiency syndromes. The Vi capsular polysaccharide can be used in persons ≥2 yr of age. It is given as a single intramuscular dose, with a booster every 2 yr.

Typhoid vaccination is recommended to travelers to endemic areas, especially Latin America, Southeast Asia, and Africa. Such travelers need to be cautioned that the vaccine is not a substitute for personal hygiene and careful selection of foods and drinks, because none of the vaccines has efficacy approaching 100%. Vaccination is also recommended to individuals with intimate exposure to a documented carrier and for control of outbreaks.

Nontyphoidal Salmonellosis

Altare F, Lammas D, Revy P, et al: Inherited interleukin 12 deficiency in a child with bacille Calmette-Guerin and Salmonella enteritidis disseminated infection. *J Clin Invest* 1998;102:2035–40.

Chao HC, Chiu CH, Kong MS, et al: Factors associated with intestinal perforation in children's non-typhi *Salmonella* toxic megacolon. *Pediatr Infect Dis J* 2000;19:1158–62.

Cody SH, Abbott SL, Marfin AA, et al: Two outbreaks of multidrug-resistant *Salmonella* serotype Typhimurium DT104 infections linked to raw-milk cheese in Northern California. *JAMA* 1999;281:1805–10.

Cohen JI, Bartlett JA, Corey GP: Extra-intestinal manifestations of *Salmonella* infections. *Medicine* 1987;66:349–88.

de Jong R, Altare F, Haagen IA, et al: Severe mycobacterial and *Salmonella* infections in interleukin-12 receptor-deficient patients. *Science* 1998;280:1435–8.

Delarocque-Astagneau E, Bouillant C, et al: Risk factors for the occurrence of sporadic *Salmonella enterica* serotype Typhimurium infections in children in France: A national case-control study. *Clin Infect Dis* 2000;31:488–92.

Dunne EF, Fey PD, Kludt P, et al: Emergence of domestically acquired ceftriaxone-resistant *Salmonella* infections associated with AmpC beta-lactamase. *JAMA* 2000;284:3151–6.

Fey PD, Safranek TJ, Rupp ME, et al: Ceftriaxone-resistant *Salmonella* infection acquired by a child from cattle. *N Engl J Med* 2000;342:1242–9.

Hedberg CW, David MJ, White KE, et al: Role of egg consumption in sporadic *Salmonella enteritis* and *Salmonella typhimurium* infection in Minnesota. *J Infect Dis* 1993;167:107–11.

Mermin J, Hoar B, Angulo FJ: Iguanas and *Salmonella marina* infection in children: A reflection of the increasing incidence of reptile-associated salmonellosis in the United States. *Pediatrics* 1997 99:399–402.

Molbak K, Baggesen DL, Aarestrup FM, et al: An outbreak of multidrug-resistant, quinolone-resistant *Salmonella enterica* serotype Typhimurium DT104. *N Engl J Med* 1999;341:1420–5.

Olsen SJ, Bishop R, Brenner FW, et al: The changing epidemiology of Salmonella: Trends in serotypes isolated from humans in the United States, 1987–1997. *J Infect Dis* 2001;183:753–61.

Schutze GE, Schutze SE, Kirby RS: Extra-intestinal salmonellosis in a children's hospital. *Pediatr Infect Dis J* 1997;16:482–5.

Shimoni Z, Pitlik S, Leibovici L, et al: Nontyphoid *Salmonella* bacteremia: Age-related differences in clinical presentation, bacteriology, and outcome. *Clin Infect Dis* 1999;28:822–7.

Sirinavin S, Jayanetra P, Thakkinstian A: Clinical and prognostic categorization of extraintestinal nontyphoidal *Salmonella* infections in infants and children. *Clin Infect Dis* 1999;29:1151–6.

Sperber SJ, Schleupner CJ: Salmonellosis during infection with human immuno-deficiency virus. *Rev Infect Dis* 1987;9:925–34.

St. Geme JW, Hodes HL, Marcy SM, et al: Consensus: Management of *Salmonella* infection in the first year of life. *Pediatr Infect Dis J* 1988;7:615–21.

Villar RG, Macek MD, Simons S, et al: Investigation of multidrug-resistant *Salmonella* serotype Typhimurium DT104 infections linked to raw-milk cheese in Washington State. *JAMA* 1999;281:1811–6.

Enteric Fever

Athie CG, Guizar CB, Alcantara AV, et al: Twenty-five years of experience in the surgical treatment of perforation of the ileum caused by *Salmonella typhi* at the General Hospital of Mexico City, Mexico. *Surgery* 1998;123:632–6.

Bhutta ZA, Khan IA, Molla AM: Therapy of multiply resistant typhoid fever with oral cefixime vs intravenous ceftriaxone. *Pediatr Infect Dis J* 1994;13:990–4.

Butler T, Islam A, Kabir I, et al: Patterns of morbidity and mortality in typhoid fever dependent on age and gender: A review of 552 patients hospitalized with diarrhea. *Rev Infect Dis* 1991;13:85–90.

Girgis NI, Sultan Y, Hammad O, et al: Comparison of the efficacy, safety and cost of cefixime, ceftriaxone and aztreonam in the treatment of multidrug-resistant *Salmonella typhi* septicemia in children. *Pediatr Infect Dis J* 1995;14:603–5.

Mahle WT, Levine MM: *Salmonella typhi* infection in children younger than five years of age. *Pediatr Infect Dis J* 1993;12:627–31.

Mermin JH, Townes JM, Gerber M, et al: Typhoid fever in the United States, 1985–1994. Changing risks of international travel and increasing antimicrobial resistance. *Arch Intern Med* 1998;158:633–8.

Misra S, Diaz PS, Rowley AH: Characteristics of typhoid fever in children and adolescents in a major metropolitan area in the United States. *Clin Infect Dis* 1997;24:998–1000.

Mosley JG, Chaudhuri AK: Surgery and *Salmonella*: Complications require prompt diagnosis and treatment. *Br Med J* 1990;300:552–3.

Chapter 182

Shigella Thomas G. Cleary

Although dysenteric syndromes have long been recognized as a scourge of humans, it is only in the past century that the bacteriology of the most common form of epidemic dysentery, shigellosis, has been appreciated.

Etiology. Four species of *Shigella* are responsible for shigellosis: *S. dysenteriae* (serogroup A), *S. flexneri* (serogroup B), *S. boydii* (serogroup C), and *S. sonnei* (serogroup D). There are 13 serotypes in group A, six serotypes and 15 subserotypes in group B, 18 serotypes in group C, and one serotype in group D.

Epidemiology. Infection with shigellae occurs most often during the warm months in temperate climates and during the rainy season in tropical climates. Both sexes are affected equally. Although infection can occur at any age, it is most common in the 2nd and 3rd year of life. Infection in the first 6 mo of life is rare for reasons that are not clear. Breast milk, which in endemic areas contains antibodies to both virulence plasmid-coded antigens and lipopolysaccharides, may partially explain the age-related incidence. Asymptomatic infection of children and adults occurs commonly in endemic areas.

In industrialized societies, *S. sonnei* is the most common cause of bacillary dysentery, with *S. flexneri* second in frequency; in pre-industrial societies, *S. flexneri* is most common, with *S. sonnei* second in frequency. *S. dysenteriae* serotype 1 tends to occur in massive epidemics, although it is also endemic in Asia and Africa.

TRANSMISSION. Contaminated food (often a salad or other item requiring extensive handling of the ingredients) and water are important vectors. However, person-to-person transmission is probably the major mechanism of infection in most areas of the world. Spread within families, custodial institutions, and child-care centers demonstrates the ability of low numbers of organisms to cause disease on a person-to-person basis.

Shigellae require very low inocula to cause illness. Ingestion of as few as 10 *S. dysenteriae* serotype 1 organisms can cause dysentery in some susceptible individuals. This is in contrast to organisms such as *Vibrio cholerae*, which require ingestion of 10^8–10^{10} organisms to cause illness. The inoculum effect explains the ease of person-to-person transmission of shigellae in contrast to *V. cholerae*.

Pathogenesis. The basic virulence trait shared by all shigellae is the ability to invade intestine. This characteristic is encoded on a large (120–140 megadalton) plasmid that is responsible for synthesis of a group of polypeptides involved in cell invasion and killing. Shigellae that lose the virulence plasmid are no longer pathogenic. *Escherichia coli* that harbor this plasmid (enteroinvasive *E. coli*) behave clinically like shigellae. In addition to the major plasmid-encoded virulence traits, chromosomally encoded factors are also required for full virulence; some of these chromosomal traits are important for all shigellae (e.g., lipopolysaccharide synthesis), whereas others are important in some serotypes (e.g., Shiga toxin synthesis by *S. dysenteriae* serotype 1 and ShET-1 by *S. flexneri* 2a). **Shiga toxin**, a potent protein synthesis-inhibiting exotoxin, is produced in significant amounts by *S. dysenteriae* serotype 1, by certain *E. coli*, which are known as Shiga toxin–producing *E. coli* (STEC), and rarely by other organisms. The watery diarrhea phase of shigellosis may be caused by enterotoxins.

The pathologic changes of shigellosis take place primarily in the colon, the target organ for shigellae. The changes are most intense in the distal colon, although pancolitis may occur. Grossly, localized or diffuse mucosal edema, ulcerations, friable mucosa, bleeding, and exudate may be seen. Microscopically, ulcerations, pseudomembranes, epithelial cell death, infiltration extending from the mucosa to the muscularis mucosae by polymorphonuclear and mononuclear cells, and submucosal edema occur.

IMMUNITY. Secretory IgA and serum antibodies develop within days to weeks after infection with *Shigella*. Both antilipopolysaccharide and antivirulence plasmid polypeptide antibodies have been described; protection is serotype specific. Induction of multiple cytokines and brisk inflammatory responses is followed by healing. Interferon-γ produced by NK cells is critically important to resistance.

Clinical Manifestations. Bacillary dysentery is clinically similar regardless of whether the disease is caused by any of the four species of *Shigella* or an enteroinvasive *E. coli* (Chapter 183); however, there are some clinical differences, particularly relating to the greater severity and risk of complications with *S. dysenteriae* serotype 1 infection.

Ingestion of shigellae is followed by an incubation period of 12 hr to several days before symptoms ensue. Severe abdominal pain, high fever, emesis, anorexia, generalized toxicity, urgency, and painful defecation characteristically occur. Physical examination at this point may show abdominal distention and tenderness, hyperactive bowel sounds, and a tender rectum on digital examination.

The diarrhea may be watery and of large volume initially, evolving into frequent small-volume, bloody mucoid stools; however, some children never progress to the stage of bloody diarrhea, whereas in others the first stools are bloody. Significant dehydration related to the fluid and electrolyte losses in both feces and emesis can occur. Untreated diarrhea may last 1–2 wk; only about 10% of patients have diarrhea persisting for more than 10 days. Persistent diarrhea occurs in malnourished infants, those with AIDS, and occasionally previously normal children. Even nondysenteric disease can be complicated by persistent illness.

Neurologic findings are among the most common extraintestinal manifestations of bacillary dysentery, occurring in as many as 40% of hospitalized infected children. Enteroinvasive *E. coli* can cause similar neurologic toxicity. Convulsions, headache, lethargy, confusion, nuchal rigidity, or hallucinations may be present before or after the onset of diarrhea. The cause of these neurologic findings is not understood. In the past, these symptoms were attributed to the neurotoxicity of Shiga toxin, but it is now clear that that explanation is wrong. Seizures sometimes occur when little fever is present, suggesting that simple febrile convulsions do not explain their appearance. Hypocalcemia or hyponatremia may be associated with seizures in a small number of patients. Although symptoms often suggest central nervous system infection, and cerebrospinal fluid pleocytosis with minimally elevated protein levels can occur, meningitis due to shigellae is rare.

The most common complication of shigellosis is dehydration. Inappropriate secretion of antidiuretic hormone with profound hyponatremia may complicate dysentery, particularly when *S. dysenteriae* is the etiologic agent. Hypoglycemia and protein-loosing enteropathy are common. Other major complications, particularly in very young, malnourished children, include sepsis and disseminated intravascular coagulation. Given that shigellae penetrate the intestinal mucosal barrier, these events are surprisingly uncommon. Shigellae and sometimes other gram-negative enteric bacilli are recovered from blood cultures in 1–5% of patients in whom blood cultures are taken; because patients selected for blood cultures represent a biased sample, the risk of bacteremia in unselected cases of shigellosis is presumably lower. Bacteremia is more common with *S. dysenteriae* serotype 1 than with other shigellae. The mortality rate is high (~20%) when sepsis occurs.

S. dysenteriae serotype 1 infection is commonly complicated by hemolysis, anemia, and hemolytic-uremic syndrome. This syndrome is caused by Shiga toxin–mediated endothelial injury; *E. coli* that produce Shiga toxin (e.g., *E. coli* 0157:H7, *E. coli* 0111:NM, *E. coli* 026:H11) also cause hemolytic-uremic syndrome (Chapter 510).

Rectal prolapse, toxic megacolon or pseudomembranous colitis (usually associated with *S. dysenteriae*), cholestatic hepatitis, conjunctivitis, iritis, corneal ulcers, pneumonia, arthritis (usually 2–5 wk after enteritis), Reiter syndrome, cystitis, myocarditis, and vaginitis (typically with a blood-tinged discharge associated with *S. flexneri*) are uncommon events. Death is a rare outcome in well-nourished older children; malnutrition, illness in the 1st year of life, hypothermia, severe dehydration, thrombocytopenia, hyponatremia, renal failure, and bacteremia are common in children who die during bacillary dysentery. The rare syndrome of extreme toxicity, convulsions, extreme hyperpyrexia, and headache followed by brain edema and a rapidly fatal outcome without sepsis or significant dehydration (Ekiri syndrome or "lethal toxic encephalopathy") is not well understood.

Diagnosis. Although clinical features suggest shigellosis, they are insufficiently specific to allow confident diagnosis. Infection by *Campylobacter jejuni, Salmonella,* enteroinvasive *E. coli,* Shiga toxin–producing *E. coli* such as *E. coli* 0157:H7, *Yersinia enterocolitica, Clostridium difficile,* and *Entamoeba histolytica* as well as inflammatory bowel disease may cause confusion. Presumptive data supporting a diagnosis of bacillary dysentery include the finding of fecal leukocytes (confirming the presence of colitis), fecal blood, and demonstration in peripheral blood of leukocytosis with a dramatic left shift (often with more bands than segmented neutrophils). The total peripheral white blood cell count is usually 5,000–15,000 cells/mm³, although leukopenia and leukemoid reactions occur.

Culture of both stool and rectal swab specimens optimizes the chance of diagnosing *Shigella* infection. Culture media should include MacConkey agar as well as selective media such as xylose-lysine deoxycholate (XLD) and SS agar. Transport media should be used if specimens cannot be cultured promptly. Appropriate media should be used to exclude *Campylobacter* and other agents. Studies of outbreaks and illness in volunteers show that the laboratory is often not able to confirm the clinical suspicion of shigellosis even when the pathogen is present. Although additional tools to improve diagnosis (e.g., gene probes) are being developed, the diagnostic inadequacy of cultures makes it incumbent on the clinician to use judgment in the management of clinical syndromes consistent with shigellosis. In children who appear to be toxic, blood cultures should be obtained; this is particularly important in very young or malnourished infants because of their increased risk of bacteremia.

Treatment. As with gastroenteritis of other causes, the first concern about a child with suspected shigellosis should be for fluid and electrolyte correction and maintenance (Chapters 46 and 48.1). Nutrition is a key concern in areas where malnutrition is common. A high protein diet during convalescence enhances growth in the following 6 mo. A single large dose of vitamin A (200,000 IU) lessens severity of shigellosis in settings where vitamin A deficiency is common. Drugs that retard intestinal motility (e.g., diphenoxylate hydrochloride with atropine [Lomotil] or loperamide [Imodium]) should not be used because of the risk of prolonging the illness.

The next concern is a decision about the use of antibiotics. Although some authorities recommend withholding antibacterial therapy because of the self-limited nature of the infection, the cost of drugs, and the risk of emergence of resistant organisms, there is a persuasive logic in favor of empirical treatment of all children in whom shigellosis is strongly suspected. Even if not fatal, the untreated illness may cause a child to be quite ill for 2 wk or more; chronic or recurrent diarrhea may ensue. Malnutrition may develop or worsen during prolonged illness, particularly in children in developing countries. The risk of continued excretion and subsequent infection of family contacts further argues against the strategy of withholding antibiotics.

There are major geographic variations in antibiotic susceptibility of shigellae. In the United States, shigellae are so frequently resistant to ampicillin that it is not appropriate for empirical therapy. However, oral ampicillin (100 mg/kg/24 hr divided qid PO) may be used if the strain is known to be susceptible. Amoxicillin, because of better gastrointestinal absorption, is less effective than ampicillin for treatment of ampicillin-sensitive strains. Many regions of the United States now harbor strains that are also resistant to trimethoprim-sulfamethoxazole (TMP-SMZ). Cefixime (8 mg/kg/24 hr divided bid PO) or ceftriaxone (50 mg/kg/24 hr as a single daily dose IV or IM) can be used for empirical therapy. Nalidixic acid (55 mg/kg/24 hr divided qid PO) is also an acceptable alternative drug. Quinolones such as ciprofloxacin, norfloxacin, or ofloxacin, which have been recommended for use in persons ≥18 yr of age, are not routinely used for children because of the putative risk of arthropathy. Use of these agents is reserved for seriously ill children with bacillary dysentery due to an organism that is suspected or known to be resistant to other agents. Treatment is typically for a 5-day course. Oral first- and second-generation cephalosporins are inadequate as alternative drugs despite in vitro susceptibility.

Treatment of patients suspected on clinical grounds of having *Shigella* infection should be initiated when first examined. Stool culture is obtained to exclude other pathogens and to assist in antibiotic changes should a child fail to respond to empirical therapy. A child who has typical dysentery and who responds to initial empirical antibiotic treatment should be continued on that drug for a full 5-day course even if the stool culture is negative. The logic of this recommendation is based on the difficulty of culturing *Shigella* from stools. In a child who fails to respond to therapy of a dysenteric syndrome in the presence of initially negative stool culture results, cultures should be retaken and the child re-evaluated for other possible diagnoses.

Prevention. Two simple measures decrease the risk of shigellosis in children. The first is to encourage prolonged breast-feeding of infants. Breast-feeding decreases the risk of symptomatic shigellosis and lessens its severity in those infants who acquire infection despite breast-feeding. The second measure is to educate families and child-care center personnel in handwashing techniques, especially after defecation and before food preparation and consumption.

Ashkenazi S, Amir J, Waisman Y, et al: A randomized, double-blind study comparing cefixime and trimethoprim sulfamethoxazole in the treatment of childhood shigellosis. *J Pediatr* 1993;123:817–21.

Bennish ML: Potentially lethal complications of shigellosis. *Rev Infect Dis* 1991;13: S319–24.

Munoz C, Baqar S, van de Verg L, et al: Characteristics of *Shigella sonnei* infection of volunteers: Signs, symptoms, immune responses, changes in selected cytokines and acute-phase substances. *Am J Trop Med Hyg* 1995;53:47–54.

Replogle ML, Fleming DW, Cieslak PR: Emergence of antimicrobial-resistant shigellosis in Oregon. *Clin Infect Dis* 2000;30:515–9.

Salam MA, Bennish ML: Therapy for shigellosis: I. Randomized, double-blind trial of nalidixic acid in childhood shigellosis. *J Pediatr* 1988;113:901–7.

Varsano I, Eidlitz-Marcus T, Nussinovitch M, et al: Comparative efficacy of ceftriaxone and ampicillin for treatment of severe shigellosis in children. *J Pediatr* 1991;118:627–32.

Chapter 183

Escherichia coli Theresa J. Ochoa and

Thomas G. Cleary

Escherichia coli are important causes of enteric infections as well as urinary tract infections (Chapter 530), sepsis and meningitis in the newborn (Chapter 98), and bacteremia and sepsis in immunocompromised patients (Chapter 164) and in patients with intravascular devices (Chapter 165).

Etiology. *E. coli* species are members of the Enterobacteriaceae family. They are oxidase-positive, facultatively anaerobic, gram-negative bacilli. Fermentation of lactose is variable. Five groups of diarrheagenic *E. coli* have been characterized on the basis of clinical, biochemical, and molecular-genetic criteria (Table 183–1): (1) **enterotoxigenic *E. coli* (ETEC)** produce secretory enterotoxins; (2) **enteroinvasive *E. coli* (EIEC)** are capable of invading intestinal epithelial cells and causing a dysenteric illness; (3) **enteropathogenic *E. coli* (EPEC)** are defined by their pattern of adherence to tissue culture cells and their ability to produce a characteristic alteration in the microvillus membrane, the "attaching and effacing" lesion; (4) **shigatoxin-producing *E. coli* (STEC)**, also known as enterohemorrhagic *E. coli* (EHEC), *Shiga*-like toxin-producing *E. coli* (SLT-EC) and verotoxin-producing *E. coli* (VTEC) produce Shiga toxins (Stx) and cause diarrhea, hemorrhagic colitis, and hemolytic-uremic syndrome (HUS); (5) **enteroaggregative *E. coli* (EAggEC)** adhere in vitro to HEp-2 cells in a characteristic aggregative manner and are associated with persistent diarrhea in children.

Epidemiology. In the developing world, the various diarrheogenic serogroups of *E. coli* cause frequent infections in the first few years of life. They occur with increased frequency during the warm months in temperate climates and during rainy season months in tropical climates. Most *E. coli* strains (except STEC and perhaps some EPEC) require a large inoculum of organisms to induce disease; person-to-person spread is atypical, but food-borne or water-borne illness is common. Infection is most likely when food-handling or sewage-disposal practices are suboptimal.

ETEC are a major cause of infantile diarrhea in the developing countries, as well as important etiologic agents of traveler's diarrhea. They account for approximately 20–30% of diarrhea episodes in the developing world.

EIEC are mostly described in outbreaks; however, endemic disease occurs in developing countries where these bacteria can be isolated with relatively high frequency. In the developing world as many as 5% of sporadic diarrhea episodes and 20% of bloody diarrhea cases may be caused by EIEC strains.

EPEC are a major cause of infant diarrhea and mortality in developing countries, primarily in children <2 yr of age. In developed countries EPEC are responsible for occasional outbreaks in daycare centers and pediatric wards. Several studies have shown that breast-feeding is protective against diarrhea due to EPEC.

STEC infections may be asymptomatic. Very young children are not a target group of STEC; rather, severe and complicated illness occurs most often among children from 6 mo to 10 yr of age. The elderly may also be severely affected. STEC are transmitted person to person as well as by food and water, because ingestion of a low number of these organisms is sufficient to cause disease. Poorly cooked hamburger is a common cause of food-borne outbreaks, although many other foods including apple cider, lettuce, mayonnaise, salami, dry fermented sausage and unpasteurized dairy products have also been incriminated. Although most outbreaks of STEC-associated diarrhea in the Northern hemisphere have been attributed to strains of serotype 0157:H7, many other serotypes have been associated with outbreaks and sporadic cases of severe disease.

EAggEC asymptomatic excretion rates can be high. EAggEC are associated with persistent (lasting >14 days) pediatric diarrhea in developing countries, most prominently in children >12 mo of age. EAggEC are etiologic agents in AIDS-associated chronic diarrhea and traveler's diarrhea.

TABLE 183–1. Clinical Characteristics and Pathogenesis of Diarrheogenic *Escherichia coli*

| | | Characteristics of Diarrhea | | | Main Virulence Factors | |
	Populations at Risk	Watery	Bloody	Duration	Adherence Factors	Toxins
ETEC	>1 yr old and travelers	+++	—	Acute	Colonization factor antigens (CFA I, II, IV)	Heat-labile enterotoxin (LT) Heat-stable enterotoxin (ST)
EIEC	>1 yr old	+	++ Dysentery with fever	Acute	Invasion plasmid antigen (IpaABCD)	Sen (?)
EPEC	<2 yr old, especially infants <6 mo	+++	—	Acute or persistent	A/E lesion, intimin/Tir, EspABD BFP	EspF (?)
STEC	6 mo–10 yr and the elderly	+	+++ Afebrile hemorrhagic colitis; hemolytic uremic syndrome	Acute	A/E lesion, intimin/Tir, EspABD	Shiga toxins (Stx1, Stx2, and variants of Stx2)
EAggEC	<1 yr old and travelers	+++		Acute or persistent	Aggregative adherence fimbriae (AAF I-II)	Enteroaggregative heat stable toxin (EAST 1)

ETEC, enterotoxigenic E. coli; EIEC, enteroinvasive E. coli; EPEC, enteropathogenic E. coli; STEC, shigatoxin-producing E. coli; EAggEC, enteroaggregative E. coli; Tir, translocated intimin receptor; EspABD, E. coli secreted proteins A, B, and D; BFP, bundle forming pilus; Sen, Shigella enterotoxin.

Pathogenesis. Because *E. coli* organisms are normal fecal flora, demonstration of virulence characteristics is the usual way by which the diarrheogenic *E. coli* are defined. The mechanism by which *E. coli* produces diarrhea typically involves adherence of organisms to a glycoprotein or glycolipid receptor, followed by production of some noxious substance that injures gut cells or disturbs their function. The genes for virulence properties and for antibiotic resistance are often carried on transferable plasmids, pathogenicity islands, or bacteriophages.

ETEC cause few or no structural alterations in the gut mucosa. Diarrhea is caused by colonization of the small intestine and subsequent elaboration of enterotoxins. ETEC secrete a **heat-labile enterotoxin (LT)** or a **heat-stable enterotoxin (ST)**, or both. LT, a large molecule consisting of five receptor-binding subunits and one enzymatically active subunit, is structurally, functionally, and immunologically related to cholera toxin produced by *Vibrio cholerae*. LT stimulates adenylate cyclase, resulting in increased cyclic adenosine monophosphate. ST is a small molecule not related to LT or cholera toxin. ST stimulates guanylate cyclase, resulting in increased cyclic guanosine monophosphate. A large proportion of ETEC strains also produce EAST1, a heat-stable toxin similar to ST, which was originally identified in EAggEC strains

Colonization of the intestine requires fimbrial colonization factor antigens (CFAs), which promote adhesion to the intestinal epithelium. The most prevalent colonization factors are CFA/I, CFA/II and CFA/IV. CFAs are composed of distinct *E. coli* surface antigens (CS), expressed in different combinations. A large proportion of ETEC strains produce a type IV pilus called longus, which functions as a colonization factor and is found among several gram-negative bacterial pathogens. The binding of enterotoxigenic invasion protein A (Tia), a 25-kd outer membrane protein, to host epithelial cells is mediated at least in part through heparan sulfate proteoglycans; ETEC belong on the growing list of pathogens that use these ubiquitous cell surface molecules as receptors.

Of the >180 *E. coli* serogroups, only a relatively small number typically are ETEC; these serogroups (06, 08, 015, 020, 025, 027, 063, 078, 080, 085, 0115, 0128ac [but not subgroups 0128ab or 0128ad], 0139, 0148, 0153, 0159, and 0167) are generally different from those found in the other diarrhea-associated *E. coli*.

EIEC cause colonic lesions with ulcerations, hemorrhage, and infiltration of polymorphonuclear leukocytes and mucosal and submucosal edema. EIEC strains behave like shigellae in their capacity to invade gut epithelium and produce a dysentery-like illness. The invasive process involves (1) initial entry into cells, (2) intracellular multiplication, (3) intracellular and intercellular spread, and (4) host-cell killing. All bacterial genes necessary for entry into the host cell are clustered within a 30-kb region of a large virulence plasmid, also found in *Shigella*. This region carries the *ipa* and *ipg* genes encoding the entry-mediating proteins and their individual intrabacterial chaperones, and the *mxi* and *spa* genes, which code for proteins forming a type III secretion apparatus required for secretion of the invasins (IpaA-D and IpgD). IpaB and IpaC have been identified as the primary effector proteins of epithelial cell invasion. The type III secretion apparatus is found in many other pathogenic gram-negative bacteria. Its major function is to transport proteins from the bacteria cytoplasm into the host cell plasma membrane and cytoplasm upon contact with host cells.

EIEC encompass a small number of serogroups (028ac, 029, 0124, 0136, 0143, 0144, 0152, 0164, 0167, and some untypable strains). These serogroups have lipopolysaccharide (LPS) antigens related to *Shigella* LPS, and, like shigellae, the organisms are nonmotile (they lack H or flagellar antigens) and are usually nonlactose fermenting.

EPEC are associated with blunting of villi, inflammatory changes, and sloughing of superficial mucosal cells; these lesions are found from the duodenum through the colon. EPEC induce a characteristic **attaching and effacing** (A/E) histopathologic lesion, which is defined by the intimate attachment of bacteria to the epithelial surface and effacement of host cell microvilli. Factors responsible for the A/E lesion formation are encoded by the locus of enterocyte effacement (LEE) which is a pathogenicity island that contains the genes for (1) the type III secretion system, (2) the translocated intimin receptor (Tir) and intimin, and (3) the *E. coli*–secreted proteins (EspA-B-D).

EPEC pathogenesis involves three distinct stages. The first stage is the initial adherence of the bacteria to the host's intestinal epithelium in a pattern known as localized adherence, mediated in part by the type IV bundle forming pilus (BFP) encoded in the EAF plasmid. The second stage involves the production and translocations of bacterial proteins through a "needle complex" or type III secretion system. Filamentous appendages made of EspA form a physical bridge between the bacteria and the host cell for the translocations of bacterial effectors (EspB, EspD, Tir). EspB and EspD form pores in the host's cell membrane. The third stage is characterized by intimate bacterial attachment to the host cell, enterocyte effacement, and pedestal formation. Tir is injected into host cells by way of this conduit. Tir moves to the surface of host cells where it is bound by a bacterial outer membrane protein intimin (encoded by the *eae* gene). Intimin-Tir binding triggers polymerization of actin and other cytoskeletal components at the site of attachment. Other bacterial effectors include a mitochondrial-associated protein (Map) with membrane-potential disrupting activity and EspF, a protein that disrupts the intestinal barrier function and induces host cell death.

Some serogroups are associated with localized adherence and are EAF probe positive (055, 086, 0111, 0119, 0125, 0126, 0127, 0128ab, and 0142), whereas others are nonadherent or diffusely adherent to HEp-2 cells and are usually EAF probe negative (018, 044, 0112, and 0114). There is more evidence that EPEC with localized adherence are true enteropathogens than there is for those with diffuse adherence.

STEC affect the colon most severely. These organisms cause edema, fibrin deposits, hemorrhage in the submucosa, mucosal ulceration, neutrophil infiltration, and microvascular thrombi. Pseudomembranous colitis may be seen. **Shiga toxins** are considered to be the cardinal virulence factor of STEC. There are two major toxin types, Stx1 and Stx2. Some STEC produce only Stx1 and others only Stx2, but most STEC produce both toxins. Stx1 (or SLT-I or VT-1) is essentially identical to Shiga toxin, the protein synthesis-inhibiting exotoxin of *Shigella dysenteriae* serotype 1, whereas Stx2 (or SLT-II or VT-2) and variants of Stx2 are more distantly related. Each toxin is composed of a single A subunit noncovalently associated with a pentamer composed of identical B subunits. The B subunits bind to globotriaosylceramide (Gb_3), a glycosphingolipid receptor on host cells. The A subunit is taken up by endocytosis. The toxin target is the 28S rRNA, which is depurinated by the toxin at a specific adenine residue, causing protein synthesis to cease and affected cells to die. Stx enters the systemic circulation after translocation across the intestinal epithelium and damages endothelial cells. This causes activation of the coagulation cascade, formation of microthrombi, intravascular hemolysis, and ischemia. STEC induce proinflammatory cytokines. Clinical outcome of STEC infection depends on the *stx* genotype of the infecting strain. Stx2 genotype is associated with a more severe disease.

STEC adhere to intestinal cells and produce attaching-effacing lesions like those seen with EPEC. Most pathogenic strains of STEC contain the locus for enterocyte effacement. Most STEC strains also carry a large plasmid encoding proteins such as the enterohemolysin (EhyA), an extracellular serine protease (EspP) and a STEC autoagglutinating adhesin (Saa), which may be accessory virulence factors.

The most common serotypes are *E. coli* O157:H7, *E. coli* 0111:NM, and *E. coli* 026:H11, although a number of other STEC serotypes have also been described. Some *E. coli* 026:H11 and *E. coli* 0111:NM strains produce Shiga toxin, but others do not.

EAggEC form a characteristic mucous biofilm on the intestinal mucosa and induce shortening of the villi, hemorrhagic necrosis, and inflammatory responses. The proposed model of pathogenesis of EAggEC involves three phases: adherence to the intestinal mucosa by way of the aggregative adherence fimbriae (AAF); enhanced mucous production; and production of toxins and inflammation that results in damage of the mucosa and intestinal secretion. Diarrhea caused by EAggEC is predominantly secretory. The intestinal inflammatory response (elevated fecal lactoferrin, IL-8 and IL-1β) may be related to growth impairment and malnutrition.

Putative EAggEC virulence factors include aggregative adherence fimbriae (AAF/I and AAF/II), a 108-kd plasmid-encoded cytotoxin (Pet), hemolysins, various outer membranes proteins, and an enterotoxin designated as enteroaggregative *E. coli* heat stable toxin 1 (EAST 1). The EAST 1 gene, *astA*, is also present in other diarrheogenic *E. coli* and some other human enteric pathogens.

Strains of *E. coli* categorized as EAggEC belong to a diverse range and combination of O and H serotypes. Some EAggEC, however, do not express O antigens, are nonmotile or untypable.

Clinical Manifestations. The clinical features of *E. coli*-associated diarrhea vary in relation to the different mechanisms of disease production.

ETEC are a major cause of dehydrating infantile diarrhea in the developing world. The typical signs and symptoms include explosive watery, nonmucoid, nonbloody diarrhea, abdominal pain, nausea, vomiting, and little or no fever. The illness is usually self-limited in 3–5 days, but occasionally lasts >1 wk.

EIEC infections present most commonly as watery diarrhea, which can be indistinguishable from the secretory diarrhea seen with ETEC. A minority of patients experience a dysentery syndrome, manifested as blood, mucus, and leukocytes in the stools, with fever, systemic toxicity, crampy abdominal pain, tenesmus, and urgency.

EPEC generally cause acute diarrhea, but severe cases can lead to protracted disease. In addition to profuse watery, nonbloody diarrhea with mucus, vomiting and low-grade fever are common symptoms. Chronic diarrhea and malnutrition can occur in infants in the developing world.

STEC have been shown to cause a wide spectrum of diseases. Patients develop intestinal symptoms ranging from mild diarrhea to severe hemorrhagic colitis. The gastrointestinal illness is characterized by abdominal pain with diarrhea that is initially watery but within a few days becomes blood-streaked or grossly bloody. Although this pattern resembles that of shigellosis or EIEC disease, it differs in that fever is an uncommon manifestation. Most individuals infected with STEC recover from the infection without further complication. However, 5–10% of children go on to develop systemic complications such as hemolytic-uremic syndrome, characterized by acute renal failure, thrombocytopenia, and hemolytic anemia. The elderly may also develop HUS or thrombotic thrombocytopenic purpura.

EAggEC typical illness is manifested by watery, mucoid, secretory diarrhea with low-grade fever and little or no vomiting. One third of patients have grossly bloody stools. The watery diarrhea may persist ≥14 days. EAggEC is associated with growth retardation in infants and malnutrition.

Diagnosis. The clinical features of illness are seldom distinctive enough to allow confident diagnosis, and routine laboratory studies are of very limited value. Diagnosis currently depends heavily on laboratory studies that are not readily available to practitioners.

The diagnosis of diarrheogenic *E. coli* infection can be made based on (1) initial isolation of the bacteria from stool cultures,

(2) biochemical criteria (e.g., fermentation patterns), (3) detection of the bacteria serogroup/serotype, (4) animal models (e.g., Sereny test for invasiveness in EIEC), (5) tissue culture (e.g., HEp2-cells assays for EPEC and EAggEC), (6) detection of antibodies against specific virulence factors (e.g., intimin, EspA, EspB), and (7) identification of specific virulence factors of the bacteria by phenotypic (e.g., toxins) or genotypic (e.g. *ipa*, *eae*, *ehyA* genes) detection assays.

DNA probes for genes encoding the various virulence traits are the best diagnostic tests, but are currently available only as a research tool. Therefore, suspected organisms should be forwarded to reference or research laboratories for definitive evaluation. Such efforts are seldom necessary, but they may be important for correct diagnosis when a child has severe or life-threatening complications or for outbreak investigation. DNA probes for genes encoding the various virulence factors are now available for all the diarrheogenic *E. coli*. However, because of the emergence of different combinations of virulence gene sequences (genetic profiles) found in the *E. coli* strains (that might have been transferred horizontally in the intestine and/or environment), multiple phenotypic and genotypic characteristics need to be tested in each strain.

Practical, non-DNA–dependent, methods for routine diagnosis of diarrheogenic *E. coli* have been developed primarily for the STEC. Serotype O157:H7 is suggested by failure to ferment sorbitol on MacConkey sorbitol medium; latex agglutination confirms that the organism contains O157 LPS. Other STEC can be detected in routine hospital laboratories using commercially available enzyme immunoassay or latex agglutination to detect Shiga toxins.

Other laboratory data are at best nonspecific indicators of etiology. Fecal leukocyte examination of the stool is frequently positive with the EIEC but negative with all other diarrheogenic *E. coli*. With EIEC and STEC there may be an elevated leukocyte count with a left shift. Fecal lactoferrin, IL-8 and IL-1β can be used as inflammatory markers. Electrolyte changes are nonspecific, reflecting only fluid loss.

Treatment. The cornerstone of proper management is related to fluid and electrolyte therapy. In general, this therapy should include oral replacement and maintenance with rehydration solutions such as those specified by the World Health Organization. Early refeeding (within 8–12 hr of initiation of rehydration) with breast milk or infant formula should be encouraged. Prolonged withholding of feeding frequently leads to chronic diarrhea and malnutrition.

Specific antimicrobial therapy of diarrheogenic *E. coli* is problematic because of the difficulty of making an accurate diagnosis of these pathogens and the unpredictability of antibiotic susceptibilities. ETEC respond to antimicrobial agents such as trimethoprim-sulfamethoxazole (TMP-SMZ) when the *E. coli* strains are susceptible. However, other than for a child recently returning from travel in the developing world, empirical treatment of severe watery diarrhea with antibiotics is seldom appropriate. EIEC infections are usually treated before the availability of culture results because the clinician typically suspects shigellosis and begins empirical therapy. If the organisms are susceptible, TMP-SMZ is an appropriate choice. Although treatment of EPEC infection with TMP-SMZ intravenously or orally for 5 days is effective in speeding resolution, the lack of a rapid diagnostic test makes treatment decisions difficult. The STEC represent a particularly difficult therapeutic dilemma. The data suggest that antibiotic treatment may increase the risk of hemolytic-uremic syndrome (Chapter 510). Some data suggest that ciprofloxacin, which is seldom used in children, is useful for EAggEC traveler's diarrhea.

Antibiotic resistance is often encoded on the same plasmids that carry virulence proteins and continues to make rational decisions about antibiotic therapy difficult. Because emergence of resistance to widely used regimens is typical, new antimicrobial agents must continue to be evaluated.

Complications. The major complications of diarrheal illness are related to dehydration and electrolyte loss. Some complications are related to specific pathogens. EPEC and EAggEC are likely to cause persistent diarrhea and malnutrition. Infection with STEC can be associated with the hemolytic-uremic syndrome or thrombotic thrombocytopenic purpura (Chapter 510).

Prevention. In the developing world, prevention of disease caused by diarrheogenic *E. coli* is probably best done by maintaining prolonged breast-feeding, paying careful attention to personal hygiene, and following proper food- and water-handling procedures. People traveling to these places can be best protected by consuming only processed water, bottled beverages, breads, fruit juices, fruits that can be peeled, or foods that are served steaming hot.

Prophylactic antibiotic therapy, although effective in adult travelers, has not been studied in children and is not recommended. Public health measures, including sewage disposal and food-handling practices, have made pathogens that require large inocula to produce illness relatively uncommon in industrialized countries. Food-borne outbreaks of STEC are a problem for which no adequate solution has been found. During the occasional hospital outbreak of EPEC disease, attention to enteric isolation precautions and cohorting may be critical.

The nature of protective immunity is not fully understood and no vaccines are available for clinical use. There are several vaccine candidates based on bacterial toxins or colonization factors that are being studied in animals.

Donnenberg MS, Whittam TS: Pathogenesis and evolution of virulence in enteropathogenic and enterohemorrhagic *Escherichia coli. J Clin Invest* 2001;107: 539–548.

Nataro JP, Kaper JB: Diarrheagenic *Escherichia coli. Clin Micro Rev* 1998;11:142–201.

Robins-Browne RM, Hartland EL: *Escherichia coli* as a cause of diarrhea. *J Gastroenterol Hepatol* 2002;17:467–75.

Sekiya K, Ohishi M, Ogino T, et al: Supermolecular structure of the enteropathogenic *Escherichia coli* type III secretion system and its direct interaction with the EspA-sheath-like structure. *Proc Natl Acad Sci U S A* 2001;98:11638–43.

Uzzau S, Fasano A: Cross-talk between enteric pathogens and the intestine. *Cellular Micro* 2000;2:83–9.

Vallance BA; Finlay BB: Exploitation of host cells by enteropathogenic *Escherichia coli. Proc Natl Acad Sci U S A* 2000;97:8799–806.

Chapter 184
Cholera (*Vibrio cholerae*)

Gloria P. Heresi and James R. Murphy

Cholera remains an important public health problem for many poorer communities and an episodic problem for richer communities; the disease is responsible for significant morbidity and mortality worldwide with an estimated 5–7 million cases and >100,000 deaths/yr. The disease can cause the death of a previously healthy individual in hours and must be addressed as an emergency.

The 1990s witnessed the reintroduction of epidemic cholera into the Americas, the emergence of a new epidemic strain, and an outbreak with an extraordinary death rate (12,000 deaths among 70,000 cases). The genome of a representative *V. cholerae* was published in 2000. The long history of studies of cholera is marked with numerous significant medical findings, including Snows' 1850s seminal studies of epidemiology and the studies that led to modern rehydration practices that have saved countless lives. Yet unknown facets of the biology of the organism continue to be discovered and *V. cholerae* continues to cause substantial suffering.

Etiology. The cause of cholera is *V. cholerae*, a gram-negative, non–spore-forming, motile, slightly curved rod (1.5–3.0 × 0.5 μm), with a polar flagellum. *V. cholerae* includes pathogenic and non-pathogenic strains; *V. cholera* O1 and O139 are responsible for causing disease. The two **biogroups (or biotypes)** of *V. cholerae* O1 are differentiated as **classic** and **El Tor** based on hemolysin, hemagglutination, susceptibility to polymyxin B, and susceptibility to bacteriophages. They are also subdivided into **serogroups (or serovars)** based on O antigens. *V. cholerae* O1 has two major O antigenic types (**Ogawa** and **Inaba**) and an unstable intermediate type (**Hikojima**). *V. cholerae* O139 is closely related to the El Tor biotype. Recently, the genome of *V. cholerae* O1 biotype El Tor was published. The genome comprises two circular chromosomes: a larger chromosome of 3 million bp and a smaller chromosome of 1.07 million bp.

Epidemiology. Cholera exists in sporadic, endemic, epidemic, and pandemic forms. The transition from epidemic to endemic may relate to a population acquiring immune resistance. During epidemics, high rates of intrafamilial spread occur (up to 50%). Transmission is usually by fecal-oral spread with contaminated water as the main vehicle but contaminated food and utensils may also play important roles as may houseflies. Water also serves as an environmental reservoir of *V. cholerae*.

Humans are the only known vertebrate reservoirs of *V. cholerae*. However, evidence is scarce that persistent carriers are responsible for intraepidemic maintenance. Other possible explanations for intraepidemic maintenance include the existence of nonculturable but viable strains in water and the existence of O antigen–deficient organisms that may gain O antigen by a variety of means.

A notable feature of cholera is the occurrence of global epidemics or pandemics. In pandemics, an O1 vibrio emerges from an Asian site and spreads globally over ensuing years or decades and then wanes. This pattern was first identified in 1831 when the second pandemic of cholera reached England. In 1961 *V. cholerae* O1 biotype El Tor began spreading from a focus in Indonesia. This marked the start of the still ongoing seventh pandemic. In January 1991, this pandemic strain was found in Peru, marking the first time in >100 yr that epidemic cholera existed in the Americas. At least 20 countries in Latin America have reported cholera cases resulting from this pandemic; Latin American cases exceed 1,000,000 and deaths exceed 10,000. In 1973, a focus of *V. cholerae* O1 biotype El Tor was identified in the Gulf of Mexico. This strain is not the El Tor responsible for the seventh pandemic; it differs by ribotype and restriction fragment length polymorphisms, for example.

In 1992, an epidemic cholera-like disease occurred in southern India. The agent was a *V. cholera* that received the designation *V. cholerae* O139, Bengal. This *V. cholera* was the first non–O1 vibrio with demonstrated epidemic-causing capability. It rapidly spread through the Indian subcontinent raising fears that an eighth pandemic was starting that might run concomitantly with the seventh. For unknown reasons, O139 has not continued its epidemic spread. O139 Bengal is derived genetically from the O1 El Tor strain responsible for the seventh pandemic but has changed its antigenic structure in a way that immunity acquired by exposure to O1 vibrios is ineffective. Thus, many populations and all age groups, even in cholera endemic regions, are susceptible to O139 disease.

In 1994, over 20,000 people died in a 4-wk period from an outbreak of cholera during a Rwandan refugee crisis. The magnitude of this disaster, which recapitulates historical cholera, establishes the continued virulence of the vibrios and what happens if medical interventions are unavailable, delayed, or denied.

Pathogenesis. Severe cholera results from the voluminous loss by diarrhea of fluid isotonic with plasma and with high concentrations of bicarbonate and potassium; these outcomes result from the actions of toxins produced by *V. cholerae* that have colonized the upper small bowel. Colonization usually requires the ingestion of a large number of viable vibrios (>~10^8 viable units), in part, because the organisms are killed by acid environments including the normal stomach. Under conditions in which gastric acidity is neutralized or absent (i.e., hypochlorhydria) the infectious dose is about 10,000-fold less. Once in the upper small intestine, the organisms must associate with the mucosa and produce toxin if disease is to follow. Association with the mucosa is facilitated by bacterial motility, chemotaxis, and the production of a protease that facilitates penetration of the mucus overlying the epithelium.

The primary mechanism of fluid loss is activation of adenylyl cyclase at the cytoplasmic surface of the basolateral membrane by the enterotoxin, **cholera toxin** (CT). To accomplish this, CT must enter the intestinal epithelial cell at the apical end and transit to the basolateral membrane. This is effected by CT co-opting the machinery for membrane traffic endogenous to the epithelial cell. CT traffics as an intact protein through two unique pathways: transcytosis and retrograde movement through the Golgi cisternae to the endoplasmic reticulum. CT comprises an enzymatically active A subunit and five cell-binding B subunits. The structural genes for CT are encoded within a lysogenic phage (CTxv) that is integrated into the large chromosome. Induction of expression of CT production follows an interaction of *V. cholerae* with the intestinal microenvironment. The receptor for subunit B is the ganglioside GM_1. The A1 portion of A subunit is an adenosine diphosphate-ribosyltransferase that activates the α-subunit of the stimulatory G protein to bind and activate adenylate cyclase, resulting in prolonged elevation of cyclic adenosine monophosphate (cAMP) levels. The high cAMP level causes a decrease in active absorption of sodium and chloride by villous cells and an increase in active secretion of chloride by crypt cells. *V. cholerae* produces additional enterotoxins (zonula occludens toxin [*zot*], accessory cholera enterotoxin [*ace*]) that are of lesser clinical importance.

It was recently established that the propagation of the bacteriophage that bears the CT gene is influenced by environmental factors such as temperature, sunlight, and salinity. Knowledge of the switching on of these and similar genes may provide resolution to the long-standing issue of how cholera re-emerges from environmental sources to cause epidemics.

Clinical Manifestations. Toxigenic strains of *V. cholera* O1 and O139 cause a broad spectrum of disease. Most infected people are asymptomatic, about one fourth present with mild to moderate disease, and 2–5% developed severe cholera. The hallmark of cholera is massive loss of fluids and electrolytes. Watery diarrhea and vomiting develop after an incubation period of 6 hr–5 days (average, 2–3 days). Low-grade fever occurs in some children. In severe cases, patients have profuse, painless, watery diarrhea with a rice-water consistency and a fishy odor, sometimes with flecks of mucus but no blood. The fluid and electrolyte losses lead to thirst and tachycardia, followed by tachypnea, irritability, a sunken anterior fontanel, poor skin turgor, and progress to circulatory collapse, stupor, and renal failure if untreated. Diarrhea may be so massive that vascular collapse occurs <24 hr after onset. Fluid losses may continue for as long as 1 wk.

Laboratory Findings. Changes related to dehydration and electrolyte loss are common. Hemoconcentration is manifested with increased serum protein, elevated hematocrit, and increased serum specific gravity. Hyponatremia, hypokalemia, and acidosis are often present in moderate and severe cases. Fecal leukocytes are not present because *V. cholera* does not invade the mucosa.

Diagnosis. In individual cases, diagnosis of cholera remains primarily clinical. In epidemiologic investigations, laboratory confirmation is required. In endemic areas, a child with severe watery diarrhea should be considered to have a possible case of cholera pending laboratory investigations, and treatment should be started. In the United States, the diagnosis should be suspected in any child with severe watery diarrhea and a history of recent travel to an endemic area.

Two selective media are used for culturing *V. cholerae*: thiosulfate-citrate-bile-sucrose (TCBS) and tellurite-taurocholate-gelatin agar (TTGA). The gold standard for cholera diagnosis remains stool culture on TCBS medium. On TCBS, *V. cholerae* appears as large smooth yellow colonies against the bluish-green background of the medium. On TTGA, the colonies are small and opaque, with a zone of cloudiness around them. Colonies of O139 strains grown on TTGA are grayish opaque with dark centers. Biotyping of *V. cholerae* into classic or El Tor is made on the basis of direct hemagglutination with chicken or sheep red blood cells (i.e., El Tor strains agglutinate), sensitivity to polymyxin B (i.e., classic strains are sensitive), or susceptibility to cholera-phage group IV (i.e., classic strains are susceptible). Recently, rapid diagnosis techniques using DNA-based methods have been developed; polymerase chain reaction (PCR) using primers with high sensitivity and specificity for the ctxA gene and an outer membrane protein, OmpW gene, are described. Use of PCR seems a promising method to improve detection of *V. cholerae* in environmental sources. Immunoassays as rapid diagnostics are under evaluation.

Treatment. The mainstay of treatment for cholera is fluid and electrolyte replacement. Oral or parenteral rehydration therapy should be initiated as soon as the diagnosis is suspected. The World Health Organization Oral Rehydration Solution (WHO-ORS) contains per liter 90 mmol of Na$^+$, 20 mmol of K$^+$, 80 mmol of Cl$^-$, 111 mmol of glucose, and 30 mmol of bicarbonate (citrate can be substituted for bicarbonate). Oral rehydration given ad libitum is the treatment of choice, unless the child is obtunded, has an ileus, or is in shock; in these cases, intravenous saline or lactated Ringer solution rather than oral rehydration is appropriate. Vomiting is not a contraindication to oral rehydration. Although all patients with cholera should be carefully monitored, attention to intake and output is especially important for infants. Food should be restarted as soon as deficits are replaced to minimize the nutritional impact of the illness; refeeding does not affect purging rates or the duration of diarrhea. The success of oral rehydration was well demonstrated when epidemic cholera arrived in Peru in 1991; the mortality rate was <1%.

Rehydration is the most important treatment. However, antibiotics are useful in shortening the duration of illness, reducing the period of excretion of the organisms, and decreasing the requirements for fluid replacement. Antimicrobial therapy should be considered for patients with moderate or severe disease. Oral tetracycline (50 mg/kg/24 hr divided qid PO for 3 days; maximum: 2 g/24 hr) or doxycycline (5 mg/kg PO as a single dose, maximum: 200 mg/24 hr) are the drugs of choice for cholera due to *V. cholera* O1 and O139. For children <9 years of age, the use of tetracycline is not recommended. In resistant strains or children <9 years old, trimethoprim-sulfamethoxazole (8–10 mg/kg/24 hr of trimethoprin and 40 mg/kg/24 hr of sulfamethoxazole, divided bid PO), erythromycin (40 mg/kg/24 hr; maximum: 2 g/24 hr), or furazolidone (5–8 mg/kg/24 hr, maximum: 400 mg) may be used. Resistance to tetracycline and other antimicrobials is increasing. Studies show a lower prevalence of antimicrobial resistance in O139 serotypes compared with O1 serotypes. Some African isolates (i.e., from Uganda) are resistant to TMP-SMZ, tetracycline, chloramphenicol, ampicillin, and streptomycin. Quinolones are effective for infection due to *V. cholera* O1 and O139 but they are not recommended in patients <18 years. Recent data show increased resistance to norfloxacin of *V. cholera* O1 El Tor. Antibiotic resistance evaluations should be performed of isolates from sporadic cases and representative cases from an epidemic.

Complications. Lethargy, seizures, altered consciousness, fever, hypoglycemia, hyperglycemia, and death occur more frequently in children than in adults. Inadequate fluid and electrolyte replacement may lead to acute tubular necrosis. In severely ill children with potassium depletion and acidosis, hypokalemic arrhythmia can cause sudden death. Children with low potassium levels can develop paralytic ileus and abdominal distention that can make oral rehydration impossible. In as many as 10% of small children, prolonged drowsiness, coma, or seizures occur. When the seizures are associated with hypoglycemia, they are often followed by coma and death; in one study, 14.3% of children with cholera complicated by hypoglycemia died, compared with 0.7% of children without hypoglycemia. After dehydration, hypoglycemia is the most common life-threatening consequence of cholera in children. Hyperglycemia can be caused by secretion of epinephrine, norepinephrine, cortisol, glucagon, and C peptide in response to the stress of hypovolemia. Pulmonary edema occurs in some children, probably because of fluid overload during rehydration. Transient tetany may occur during correction of electrolyte imbalances. In children treated with excessive sugar and salt, hypernatremia can be observed. Despite its high sodium content, WHO-ORS is not associated with hypernatremia if used properly; it can be used to treat children with hypernatremic dehydration.

Prevention. The most practical method of preventing life-threatening cholera in infants is prolonged breast-feeding. Safe food and water and proper handling of sewage are long-term solutions. Cost, ignorance, and politics have kept these basic needs from being met. The development of an improved vaccine is a high priority.

VACCINE. The only currently approved cholera vaccine in the United States is made of phenol-killed organisms administered parenterally as a two-dose primary series followed by boosters every 6 mo to maintain immunity. This vaccine has about 50% efficacy by 3–6 mo after vaccination, does not protect against O139 vibrios, and is highly reactogenic (i.e., pain, erythema, local induration, fever, headaches). This vaccine should be used only in very high-risk persons (e.g., those with achlorhydria) with a very high probability of exposure. It is not recommended for children <6 mo of age. Travelers to areas endemic for cholera should take appropriate food precautions. Visitors to countries reporting cholera who follow common tourist itineraries and who use standard accommodations are at low risk of infection. Outside of the United States, two additional vaccines may be readily available: an oral killed whole cell cholera toxin recombinant B subunit vaccine, with 80–85% protection through 6 mo, and an oral live attenuated *V. cholerae* (CVD 103 HgR) vaccine, with 62–100% efficacy through 6 mo. Both products have markedly reduced reactogenicity compared with the product available in the United States but neither protects against O139 vibrios.

Dromigny JA, Rakoto-Alson O, Rajaonatahina D, et al: Emergence and rapid spread of tetracycline-resistant *Vibrio cholerae* strains, Madagascar. *Emerg Infect Dis* 2002;8:336–8.

Gunnlaugsson G, Angulo FJ, Einarsdottir J, et al: Epidemic cholera in Guinea-Bissau; the challenge of preventing deaths in rural West Africa. *Int J Infect Dis* 2000;4:8–13.

Heidelberg JF, Eisen JA, Nelson WC, et al: DNA sequence of both chromosomes of the cholera pathogen *Vibrio cholerae*. *Nature* 2000;406:477–83.

Nandi B, Nandi RK, Mukhopadhyay S, et al: Rapid method for species-specific identification of *Vibrio cholerae* using primers targeted to the gene of outer membrane protein Omp W. *J Clin Microbiol* 2000;38:4145–51.

Reidl J, Klose KE: *Vibrio cholerae* and cholera: Out of the water and into the host. *FEMS Microbiol Rev* 2002;26:125–39.

Ryan ET, Calderwood SB: Cholera vaccines. *Clin Infect Dis* 2000;31:561–5.

Shears P: Recent developments in cholera. *Curr Opin Infect Dis* 1001;14:553–8.

Chapter 185
Campylobacter Gloria P. Heresi and
James R. Murphy

The genus *Campylobacter* includes more than 12 species. Those known or considered pathogenic for humans include *C. jejuni*, *C. fetus*, *C. coli*, *C. hyointestinalis*, *C. lari*, *C. upsaliensis*, *C. concisus*, *C. sputorum*, *C. rectus*, *C. mucosalis*, *C. jejuni* subspecies *doylei*, *C. curvus*, *C. gracilis*, and *C. cryaerophila*. Additional *Campylobacter* species have been isolated from clinical specimens, but their roles as pathogens have not been proved. *C. jejuni* and *C. coli* are the most important pathogens of the genus. More than 90 serotypes of *C. jejuni* have been identified. *C. jejuni* infection is one of the most frequent bacterial causes of human enteritis in the United States and may be the most commonly identified bacterial cause of acute gastroenteritis worldwide.

Etiology. *Campylobacter* organisms are thin, curved, gram-negative, non–spore-forming rods that usually have tapered ends; they can be short and S-shaped or long, multispiraled, and filamentous. In older cultures, coccal forms may be seen. The organisms are motile, with a flagellum at one or both poles and form small (0.5–1 mm), slightly raised, smooth colonies on solid media. Visible growth in blood culture is often not apparent until 5–14 days after inoculation. Most *Campylobacter* organisms are microaerophilic. They neither oxidize nor ferment carbohydrates. Selective culture media developed to enhance isolation of *C. jejuni* may not support, and could even inhibit, the growth of other *Campylobacter* species. *C. jejuni* has a circular chromosome of 1.64 million base pairs (30.6% G + C). This is predicted to encode 1,654 proteins and 54 stable RNA species. The genome is unusual in that there are virtually no insertion sequences of phage-associated sequences and very few repeat sequences.

Clinical presentations associated with *Campylobacter* differ, in part, by species (Table 185–1). Intestinal disease is usually associated with *C. jejuni* and *C. coli*, and extraintestinal and systemic infections are usually associated with *C. fetus*. However, *C. jejuni* septicemia is increasingly recognized; this at times occurs without signs. Less frequently, enteritis is recognized in association with isolation of *C. lari*, *C. fetus*, and other species.

Epidemiology. Human campylobacterioses most commonly result from ingestion of contaminated food or water, from direct contact with environmental sources (i.e., a pet), or from person-to-person transmission.

Campylobacter organisms are global in distribution and are ubiquitous in the environment. Although chickens are the classic source of *Campylobacter*, essentially all animal sources of food for humans have been shown to harbor or can harbor *Campylobacter*. Oysters and mussels have recently been shown to harbor these organisms. Additionally, many animals kept as human pets can carry *Campylobacter*. Puppies with diarrhea have been associated with human illness. Beetles and flies that frequent chicken farms may harbor *C. jejuni*. Direct or indirect exposure to this plethora of environmental sources is the primary route by which humans get infection.

Direct transmission of *Campylobacter* between humans is possible. *C. jejuni* and *C. coli* may spread person-to-person, perinatally, and where diapered toddlers are present. Individuals infected with *C. jejuni* usually shed the organism for weeks but may shed for months. The minimum human infectious dose for *C. jejuni* is a few hundred colony-forming units in some volunteers; however, very large inocula fail to make some individuals sick. The infectious dose for other species is unknown.

TABLE 185–1. *Campylobacter* Species Associated with Human Disease

Species	Clinical Illnesses in Humans	Common Sources
C. jejuni	Gastroenteritis, bacteremia	Poultry, raw milk, cats, dogs, cattle, swine, monkeys, water
C. coli	Gastroenteritis, bacteremia	Poultry, raw milk, cats, dogs, cattle, swine, monkeys, oysters, water
C. fetus	Bacteremia, meningitis, endocarditis, mycotic aneurysm, diarrhea, relapsing fevers, abortions	Sheep, cattle, birds
C. hyointestinalis	Diarrhea, bacteremia, proctitis	Swine, cattle, deer, raw milk, oysters
C. lari	Diarrhea, colitis, appendicitis, bacteremia, urinary tract infection	Seagulls, water, poultry, cattle, oysters, mussels
C. upsaliensis	Diarrhea, bacteremia, abscesses, enteritis, colitis, hemolyticuremic syndrome, abortion	Cats, other domestic pets
C. concisus	Diarrhea, gastritis, enteritis, periodontitis	
C. sputorum	Diarrhea, bedsores, abscesses, periodontitis	Swine
C. rectus	Periodontitis	
C. mucosalis	Enteritis	Swine
C. jejuni subspecies doylei	Diarrhea, colitis, appendicitis, bacteremia, urinary tract infection	
C. curvus	Gingivitis	Poultry, raw milk, cats, dogs, cattle, swine, monkeys, water
C. gracilis	Abscesses (head and neck, abdominal, empyema)	
C. cryaerophila	Diarrhea	Swine

Pathogenesis. Widely disparate pathology results from infections with *Campylobacter*. Evidence from the well-studied species *C. jejuni* suggests that most infections do not cause symptoms. The frequency of asymptomatic infections with other *Campylobacter* species is less well known.

When disease follows *Campylobacter* colonization, the pathology generally reflects the site at which the bacteria localize, whether or not septicemia occurs, and whether immunoreactive complications are triggered. Species of *Campylobacter* differ markedly in preferred sites of colonization and propensity to cause bacteremia.

Some studies suggest that in vitro invasion of cultured cells corresponds to isolates from patients with colitis, but others have failed to show relationships between in vitro invasion and clinical disease. A cholera-like enterotoxin that causes fluid accumulation in intestinal loop assays and fluid secretion into intestines in an animal model has been described. This enterotoxin can be detected with ganglioside GM_1-based enzyme-linked immunosorbent assay. *Campylobacter* exhibits various cytotoxic activities (including cytolethal distending toxin, Shiga-like toxin, and hemolysin). Because the inflammatory pathology in some *Campylobacter* infections is consistent with cytotoxins, a role for these in human disease is postulated. As with the enterotoxin, direct evidence of a role for cytotoxins in human disease is not available.

C. fetus possesses a high molecular weight S-layer protein that endows this species with high-level resistance to serum-mediated killing and phagocytosis and is thus thought to be responsible for its propensity to bacteremia. *C. jejuni* and *C. coli* isolates are mostly sensitive to serum-mediated killing, but variants of greater resistance exist. It has been suggested that these serum-killing–resistant variants may be more capable of systemic dissemination.

There is a strong association between Guillain-Barré syndrome and preceding infection with some serotypes of *C. jejuni*. The core oligosaccharides of the lipopolysaccharide of the neuropathic serotypes contain tetrasaccharides or pentasaccharides identical with those of several gangliosides including GM_1, GD_{1a}, and GQ_{1b}. Molecular mimicry between nerve tissue and this group of infectious agents may be the triggering factor in *Campylobacter*-associated Guillain-Barré syndrome and Miller-Fisher syndrome, a variant of Guillain-Barré syndrome characterized by ataxia, areflexia, and ophthalmoplegia.

Clinical Manifestations. There are several clinical presentations of *Campylobacter* infections that link to the species involved and host factors, such as age, immunocompetence, and underlying conditions. The most common presentation is acute enteritis.

ACUTE GASTROENTERITIS. Diarrhea is usually caused by *C. jejuni* (90–95%) or *C. coli* and rarely by *C. lari*, *C. hyointestinalis*, or *C. upsaliensis*. The incubation period is 1–7 days. Patients may have loose, watery stools or bloody and mucus-containing stools (dysentery). Blood appears in the stools 2–4 days after the onset of symptoms. Fever, vomiting, malaise, and myalgia are common. Fever may be the only initial manifestation, but 60–90% of older children also complain of abdominal pain. The abdominal pain is periumbilical; cramping may precede other symptoms or persist after the stools return to normal. Abdominal pain may mimic appendicitis or intussusception.

Mild infection lasts only 1–2 days and resembles viral gastroenteritis. Most patients recover in less than 1 wk, although 20–30% remain ill for 2 wk and 5–10% longer. Persistent or recurrent *Campylobacter* gastroenteritis and emergence of erythromycin resistance during therapy have been reported in immunocompetent persons, patients with hypogammaglobulinemia (congenital or acquired), and patients with AIDS. Persistent infection may mimic chronic inflammatory bowel disease. Fecal shedding of the organisms in untreated patients usually lasts for 2–3 wk. The range may be from a few days to several months. Young children tend to shed the organisms for longer periods. Acute appendicitis, mesenteric lymphadenitis, and ileocolitis have been reported in patients who have had appendectomies during *C. jejuni* infection.

BACTEREMIA. *Campylobacter* bacteremia most often occurs in malnourished children, in patients with chronic illnesses, in those with immunodeficiency, and at the extremes of age. *C. fetus* may cause bacteremia in adults with or without identifiable focal infection. Most have underlying conditions such as malignancy or diabetes mellitus. Bacteremia, when symptomatic, is associated with fever, headache, and malaise. Relapsing or intermittent fever is associated with night sweats, chills, and weight loss when the illness is prolonged. Lethargy and confusion can occur, but focal neurologic signs are unusual without cerebrovascular disease or meningitis. Abdominal pain is frequent; diarrhea, jaundice, and hepatomegaly are less common. A cough may occur, but pulmonary parenchymal involvement is unusual. Results of the physical examination are unimpressive except for the ill appearance of the patient. Moderate leukocytosis may be found. Both transient asymptomatic bacteremia and rapidly fatal septicemia have been described. A prolonged bacteremia of 8–13 wk has been described, with spontaneous remissions and relapses, especially in immunocompromised hosts. In HIV-infected patients, bacteremia is more frequent with increased morbidity and mortality. Occasional reports describe bacteremia with *C. upsaliensis*.

FOCAL EXTRAINTESTINAL INFECTIONS. Focal infections caused by *C. jejuni* occur mainly in neonates or immunocompromised patients. These include meningitis, pancreatitis, cholecystitis, ileocecitis with right lower quadrant pain mimicking appendicitis, urinary tract infection, arthritis, and peritonitis. *C. fetus* shows a predilection for vascular endothelium, causing endocarditis, pericarditis, thrombophlebitis, and mycotic aneurysms; focal infections include meningitis, septic arthritis, osteomyelitis, urinary tract infections, lung abscess, and cholangitis. *C. hyointestinalis* has been associated with proctitis, *C. upsaliensis* with breast abscesses, and *C. rectus* with periodontitis.

PERINATAL INFECTIONS. Severe perinatal infections, although uncommon, are usually caused by *C. fetus* and, rarely, by *C. jejuni*. Maternal *C. fetus* and *C. jejuni* infections, which may be asymptomatic, may result in abortion, stillbirth, premature delivery, or neonatal infection with sepsis and meningitis. Newborn infection with *C. jejuni* is associated with diarrhea that may be bloody; *C. fetus* rarely causes diarrhea.

Diagnosis. The clinical presentation of *Campylobacter* enteritis is similar to that of enteritis caused by other bacterial enteropathogens. The differential diagnosis should include *Shigella*, *Salmonella*, invasive *Escherichia coli*, *E. coli* O157:H7, *Yersinia enterocolitica*, *Aeromonas*, *Vibrio parahaemolyticus*, and amebiasis. Fecal leukocytes are found in as many as 75% of cases and fecal blood in 50%.

The diagnosis of *Campylobacter* is usually confirmed by identification of the organism in culture. Selective media, such as Skirrow or Butzler media, and microaerophilic conditions (5–10% oxygen) are commonly used. Some *C. jejuni* grow best at 42°C. Filtration methods are available and can preferentially enrich for *Campylobacter* by selecting for their smaller size. These methods allow for subsequent culture of the enriched sample on antibiotic free media. This enhances rates of isolation of those *Campylobacter* inhibited by the antibiotics included in standard selective media.

For rapid diagnosis of *Campylobacter* enteritis, direct carbolfuchsin stain of fecal smear, indirect fluorescence antibody test, dark-field microscopy, or latex agglutination can be used. Antigen detection by enzyme immunoassay is nearly as sensitive and specific as culture. Species-specific DNA probes and specific gene amplification by polymerase chain reaction have been described, although clinical experience is limited. Serologic diagnoses may be made with enzyme-linked immunoassays to measure the antibody (IgG, IgM, IgA) levels to *C. jejuni* for epidemiologic investigations.

Treatment. Fluid replacement, correction of electrolyte imbalance, and supportive care are the mainstays of treatment of children with *Campylobacter* gastroenteritis. Antimotility agents may cause prolonged or fatal disease and should not be used.

The need for antibiotic therapy in patients with uncomplicated gastroenteritis is controversial. Some data suggest a shortened duration of symptoms and intestinal shedding if erythromycin ethylsuccinate suspension is initiated early in the disease in patients with the dysenteric form of *Campylobacter* enteritis.

Most *Campylobacter* are susceptible to macrolides, aminoglycosides, chloramphenicol, imipenem, and clindamycin and are resistant to cephalosporins, tetracyclines, rifampin, penicillins, trimethoprim, and vancomycin. Quinolone resistance has developed recently and has been related to the use of quinolones in veterinary medicine. Erythromycin-resistant *Campylobacter* isolates remain uncommon and erythromycin is still the drug of choice if therapy is required. Clarithromycin and azithromycin show good in vitro activity, but clinical evaluation is limited. Antibiotics are recommended for patients with the dysenteric form of the disease, high fever, or a severe course and for children who are immunosuppressed or have underlying diseases.

Extraintestinal infection caused by *Campylobacter* requires parenteral antibiotic therapy with an aminoglycoside, imipenem, or both. In patients with *C. fetus* bacteremia, prolonged therapy

is advised. *C. fetus* isolates resistant to erythromycin have been reported.

Complications. Severe, prolonged *C. jejuni* infection can occur in patients with immunodeficiencies including hypogammaglobulinemia and malnutrition. In patients with AIDS, an increased frequency and severity of *C. jejuni* infection have been reported; severity correlates inversely with CD4 count.

REACTIVE ARTHRITIS. Reactive arthritis may accompany *Campylobacter* enteritis in adolescents and adults, especially those who are positive for HLA-B27. It appears 5–40 days after the onset of diarrhea, involves mainly large joints, and resolves without any sequelae. The arthritis typically is migratory, but the child is afebrile. Synovial fluid is always sterile. Reiter syndrome (i.e., reactive arthritis with conjunctivitis, urethritis, and rash) and erythema nodosum are less common. IgA nephropathy and immune complex glomerulonephritis with *C. jejuni* antigens in the kidneys have been reported. Other complications are hemolytic anemia and rectal bleeding.

GUILLAIN-BARRÉ SYNDROME. Guillain-Barré syndrome is an acute demyelinating disease of the peripheral nervous system characterized clinically by acute flaccid paralysis. *C. jejuni* is an important causal factor for GBS. GBS has been reported 1–12 wk after culture-proven *C. jejuni* gastroenteritis. Stool cultures obtained from patients with Guillain-Barré syndrome at the onset of neurologic symptoms have yielded *C. jejuni* in more than 25% of the cases. Serologic studies suggest that 20–45% of patients with Guillain-Barré syndrome have evidence of recent *C. jejuni* infection. The management of Guillain-Barré syndrome includes supportive care, plasma exchange, and intravenous immunoglobulin (Chapter 607).

Prognosis. Although *Campylobacter* gastroenteritis is usually self-limited, immunosuppressed children, including those with AIDS, may experience a protracted or a severe course. Septicemia in newborns and immunocompromised hosts has a poor prognosis, with an estimated mortality rate of 30–40%.

Prevention. Most human campylobacterioses are acquired indirectly or directly from infected animals. Interventions to minimize transmission include preparing food under conditions that kill *Campylobacter* and that prevent recontamination after cooking (not using the same surfaces, utensils, or containers for both uncooked and cooked food), ensuring that water sources are not contaminated and that water is kept in clean containers, and taking steps to prevent direct transmission from infected persons or infected domestic pets. Breast-feeding appears to decrease symptomatic *Campylobacter* disease but does not reduce colonization.

Several approaches at immunization are being studied, including the use of live-attenuated organisms, subunit vaccines, and killed whole cell vaccines. A candidate whole cell vaccine in combination with an oral adjuvant is in clinical trials.

Allos BM: *Campylobacter jejuni* infections: Update on emerging issues and trends. *Clin Infect Dis* 2001;32:1201–6.

Coker AO, Isokpehi RD, Thomas BN, et al: Human campylobacteriosis in developing countries. *Emerg Infect Dis* 2002;8:237–44.

Engberg J, Aarestrup FM, Taylor DE, et al: I. Quinolone and macrolide resistance in *Campylobacter jejuni* and *C. coli*: Resistance mechanisms and trends in human isolates. *Emerg Infect Dis* 2001;7:24–34.

Hill SL, Cheney JM, Taton-Allen GF, et al: Prevalence of enteric zoonotic organisms in cats. *J Am Vet Med Assoc* 2000;216:687–92.

Hooper DC: Emerging mechanisms of fluoroquinolone resistance. *Emerg Infect Dis* 2001;7:337–41.

Ketley JM: Pathogenesis of enteric infection by *Campylobacter*. *Microbiology* 1997;143(Pt 1):5–21.

McCarthy N, Giesecke J: Incidence of Guillain-Barré syndrome following infection with *Campylobacter jejuni*. *Am J Epidemiol* 2001;153:610–4.

Parkhill J, Wren, BW, Mungall K, et al: The genome sequence of the food-borne pathogen *Campylobacter jejuni* reveals hypervariable sequences. *Nature* 2000;403:665–8.

Saenz Y, Zarazaga M, Lantero M, et al: Antibiotic resistance in *Campylobacter* strains isolated from animals, foods, and humans in Spain in 1997–1998. *Antimicrob Agents Chemother* 2000;44:267–71.

Tsang RS: The relationship of *Campylobacter jejuni* infection and the development of Guillain-Barré syndrome. *Curr Opin Infect Dis* 2002;15:221–8.

Chapter 186

Yersinia *James R. Murphy and*

Gloria P. Heresi

The genus *Yersinia* comprises more than 10 named species, three of which are clearly pathogens of humans. *Yersinia enterocolitica*, by far the most frequent *Yersinia* causing human disease, produces fever, abdominal pain, and diarrhea that may mimic appendicitis. *Yersinia pseudotuberculosis* may cause a similar clinical presentation. *Yersinia pestis*, the agent of plague, most commonly causes an acute febrile lymphadenitis (bubonic plague) and less frequently presents as septicemic, pneumonic, or meningeal plague. Untreated plague carries a significant mortality rate. Other *Yersinia* are infrequent causes of infections of humans and their identification is often an indicator of immune deficit. *Yersinia* is a zoonotic and can be found in most areas of the world. The organisms can colonize domestic pets. Infection of humans most often results from contact with infected animals or their tissues, ingestion of contaminated water, milk, or meat or, for *Y. pestis*, the bite of infected fleas.

186.1 *Yersinia enterocolitica*

Etiology. *Y. enterocolitica* is a large, gram-negative coccobacillus that exhibits little or no bipolarity when stained with methylene blue and carbolfuchsin. These facultative anaerobes grow well on commonly available culture media and are motile at 22°C but not at 37°C. *Y. enterocolitica* comprises pathogenic and nonpathogenic members.

Epidemiology. *Y. enterocolitica* is transmitted to humans through food, water, animal contact, and contaminated blood products. Transmission can occur from mother to newborn. *Y. enterocolitica* appears to have a global distribution but is seldom a cause of tropical diarrhea. There is approximately one culture-proved *Y. enterocolitica* infection per 100,000 population/yr in the United States, but infection may be more frequent in northern Europe. Cases are more frequent in colder months, younger individuals, and males. Most infections in children are in patients <7 yr of age, with the majority of infections in children <1 yr of age.

Natural reservoirs of *Y. enterocolitica* include rodents, rabbits, pigs, sheep, cattle, horses, dogs, and cats. Contact with feral animals or colonized pets is the common source of human infections. Culture and molecular techniques have found the organism in a variety of foods and in water. A major contamination source of sporadic *Y. enterocolitica* infections is edible pig offal (chitterlings). In one study, 71% of human isolates were indistinguishable from the strains isolated from tongues, livers, kidneys, and hearts of pigs, confirming that contaminated pig offal is an important vehicle in the transmission of *Y. enterocolitica* from slaughterhouses to humans. *Y. enterocolitica* has been demonstrated as an occupational threat to butchers.

Over recent decades, *Y. enterocolitica* infections have increased while *Y. pseudotuberculosis* infections have declined, leading to the suggestion that the former organism is replacing the latter in an ecologic niche. In part, the mass production of animals, development of meat factories based on sophisticated chains of cold storage, and international trade of meat products and animals are believed to be the reasons for the increasing prevalence

of yersiniosis in humans. *Y. enterocolitica* can proliferate at refrigerator temperatures.

Pathogenesis. The organisms most often enter by the alimentary tract and cause mucosal ulcerations in the ileum. Necrotic lesions of Peyer patches and mesenteric lymphadenitis occur. If septicemia develops, suppurative lesions can be found in infected organs. Infection may trigger reactive arthritis and erythema nodosum.

Adherence, invasion, and toxin production are established as essential mechanisms of pathogenesis. Recently, it was demonstrated that bacterial components, some associated with the bacterial type III secretion apparatus, can actively suppress immunologic capacities, suggesting that immunosuppression may contribute to pathogenesis. Motility appears to be required for *Y. enterocolitica* pathogenesis. Serogroups that predominate in human illness are 0:3, 0:8, 0:9, and 0:5,27. Virulence traits are both chromosomal and plasmid encoded. Possibly because pathogenic strains require iron, individuals with iron overload like hemochromatosis, thalassemia, and sickle cell disease are at high risk of infection.

Clinical Manifestations. Disease presents most often as enterocolitis with diarrhea, fever, and abdominal pain. Acute enteritis is more common among younger children, and mesenteric lymphadenitis that may mimic appendicitis may be found in older children and adolescents. *Y. enterocolitica* septicemia is less common and most often found in very young children (<3 mo of age) and in individuals with underlying immune-compromising conditions. Systemic infection has been associated with splenic and hepatic abscesses, osteomyelitis, meningitis, endocarditis, and mycotic aneurysms. Exudative pharyngitis, pneumonia, empyema, lung abscess, and acute respiratory distress syndrome may infrequently occur.

Reactive complications include erythema nodosum and polyarthritis. These may be more frequent in selected populations (northern Europeans) and in association with HLA-B27 and are more frequent in females.

Stools may be watery or contain leukocytes and less frequently frank blood and mucus. *Y. enterocolitica* is excreted in stool for 1–4 wk. Family contacts of a case may frequently be found to be asymptomatically colonized with *Y. enterocolitica*.

Diagnosis. Culture of *Y. enterocolitica* is the primary method of diagnosis. The organism is easily cultured from normally sterile sites but requires special procedures for isolation from stool where other bacteria may outgrow *Y. enterocolitica*. Many laboratories do not routinely perform the procedures required to isolate *Y. enterocolitica* and cultures targeted to this organism must be specifically requested. A history indicating contact with environmental sources of *Yersinia* and detection of fecal leukocytes are helpful indicators of a need to culture for *Y. enterocolitica*. The culture isolation of a *Yersinia* from stool should be followed by tests to confirm that the isolate is a pathogen.

DIFFERENTIAL DIAGNOSIS. Clinical presentation is similar to other bacterial causes of enterocolitis. The most common differential is among *Shigella*, *Salmonella*, *Campylobacter*, *Clostridium difficile*, enteroinvasive *Escherichia coli*, and inflammatory bowel disease.

Treatment. Enterocolitis occurring in an immunocompetent individual is a self-limiting disease and no benefit to antibiotic therapy is established. Patients with systemic infection and very young children in whom septicemia is common should be treated. Many *Yersinia* strains are sensitive to trimethoprim-sulfamethoxazole (TMP-SMZ), aminoglycosides, third-generation cephalosporins, and quinolones. TMP-SMZ is recommended as empirical treatment in children because most strains are sensitive and it is well tolerated by children. In more severe infection such as bacteremia, third-generation cephalosporins with or without aminoglycosides have been shown effective. *Y. enterocolitica* produces β-lactamases a and b responsible for resistance to penicillins and cephalosporins. Patients on deferoxamine should discontinue iron chelation therapy during treatment for *Y. enterocolitica*, especially if they have complicated gastrointestinal infection or extraintestinal infection.

Complications. Reactive arthritis, erythema nodosum, erythema multiforme, hemolytic anemia, thrombocytopenia, and systemic dissemination of bacteria have been reported in association with *Y. enterocolitica* infection. Septicemia is more frequent in younger children and reactive arthritis in older patients. Arthritis seems mediated by immune complexes and viable organisms are not present in involved joints.

Prevention. Prevention centers on reducing contact with environmental sources of *Yersinia*. Breaking or sterilization of the chain from animal reservoirs to humans holds the greatest potential to reduce infections and the techniques applied must be tailored to the reservoirs in each area. There is no vaccine available.

186.2 *Yersinia pseudotuberculosis*

Y. pseudotuberculosis is so named because it causes tuberculosis-like lesions in guinea pigs. The agent has a worldwide distribution but *Y. pseudotuberculosis* disease is less frequent than *Y. enterocolitica* disease. The most common form of disease is a mesenteric lymphadenitis that produces an appendicitis-like syndrome. *Y. pseudotuberculosis* also causes a Kawasaki syndrome–like illness.

Etiology. *Y. pseudotuberculosis* is differentiated biochemically from *Y. enterocolitica* on the basis of ornithine decarboxylase activity, fermentation of sucrose, sorbitol, cellobiose, and other tests, although some overlap between species may be noted. Antisera to somatic O antigens and sensitivity to *Yersinia* phages may also be used to differentiate the two species. Subspecies-specific DNA sequences that allow direct probe- and primer-specific differentiation of *Y. pestis*, *Y. pseudotuberculosis*, and *Y. enterocolitica* have been described. *Y. pseudotuberculosis* is more closely related to *Y. pestis* than to *Y. enterocolitica*.

Epidemiology. Yersinioses are zoonotic infections with reservoirs in wild rodents, rabbits, deer, farm animals, various birds, and domestic animals including cats and canaries. Transmission to humans is by consumption of contaminated animals, contact with these animals, or contact with an environmental source, often water, contaminated by these animals. Infections are more commonly reported from Europe, in males, and in the winter.

Pathogenesis. Ileal and colonic mucosal ulceration and mesenteric lymphadenitis are hallmarks of the infection. Necrotizing epithelioid granulomas may be seen in the mesenteric lymph nodes, but the appendix is frequently grossly and microscopically normal. The mesenteric nodes are often the only source of isolation of the organisms. *Y. pseudotuberculosis* antigens bind directly to HLA class II molecules and may function as superantigens, which may account for the clinical illness resembling Kawasaki syndrome caused by this organism.

Clinical Manifestations. Pseudoappendicitis with abdominal pain, right lower quadrant tenderness, fever, and leukocytosis is the most common clinical presentation. Enterocolitis and extraintestinal spread are uncommon. Age, iron overload, diabetes mellitus, and chronic liver disease are often found concomitantly with extraintestinal *Y. pseudotuberculosis* infection. Renal involvement with tubulointerstitial nephritis, azotemia, pyuria, and glucosuria may occur.

Diagnosis. *Y. pseudotuberculosis* is rarely recovered from stool. Involved mesenteric lymph nodes removed at appendectomy may yield the organism by culture. Ultrasound examination of children with unexplained fever and abdominal pain may reveal a characteristic picture of enlarged mesenteric lymph nodes, thickening of the terminal ileum, and no image of the appendix.

DIFFERENTIAL DIAGNOSIS. Appendicitis (most commonly), inflammatory bowel disease, and other intra-abdominal infections should be considered. Kawasaki syndrome, staphylococcal or streptococcal disease, leptospirosis, Stevens-Johnson syndrome, and collagen vascular diseases including acute-onset juvenile rheumatoid arthritis can mimic the syndrome with prolonged fever and rash.

Treatment. Uncomplicated mesenteric lymphadenitis due to *Y. pseudotuberculosis* is a self-limited disease, and antimicrobial therapy is not required. Culture-confirmed bacteremia should be treated with an aminoglycoside, ampicillin, chloramphenicol, or a third-generation cephalosporin.

Complications. An illness with presentation similar to Kawasaki disease may occur. There may be fever of 1–2 days' duration, strawberry tongue, pharyngeal erythema, a scarlatiniform rash, cracked red swollen lips, conjunctivitis, sterile pyuria, periungual desquamation, and thrombocytosis. Coronary aneurysm has been described. Erythema nodosum and arthritis may follow infection.

Prevention. The sporadic nature of the disease makes application of targeted prevention measures difficult. Avoiding exposure to potentially infected animals and good food handling practices could prevent infection.

186.3 Plague (*Yersinia pestis*)

Etiology. *Y. pestis* is a gram-negative coccobacillus belonging to the Enterobacteriaceae. The bacterium has several chromosomal and plasmid-associated factors that are essential to its virulence and survival in mammalian hosts and fleas. The nonmotile bacterium was first isolated by Yersin in 1894 and shares bipolar staining appearance with *Y. pseudotuberculosis*. *Y. pestis* can be differentiated from *Y. pseudotuberculosis* by biochemical reactions, serology, selected *Yersinia* phage sensitivity, and selected molecular techniques. The genome of *Y. pestis* is published.

Epidemiology. Plague is endemic in at least 24 countries. In the United States, plague is most common west of a line from east Texas to east Montana. The epidemic form of disease killed about one fourth of the population of Europe in the Middle Ages. Plague is infrequent in the United States (0–40 reported cases per year) with 80% of cases in the southwestern states of New Mexico, Arizona, and Colorado. Transmission to humans is most commonly from wild animal sources, although most cases of inhalation plague reported recently to the Centers for Disease Control and Prevention (CDC) were associated with exposure to infected free-roaming domestic cats.

The most common mode of transmission of *Y. pestis* to humans is by the bite of infected fleas, and historically most human infections are thought to have resulted from bites of fleas that acquired infection from feeding on infected urban rats. Less frequently, infection is caused by contact with infectious body fluids or tissues or inhaling infectious droplets. Sylvatic plague may exist as a stable enzootic infection or as an epizootic disease with high host mortality. Ground squirrels, rock squirrels, prairie dogs, rats, mice, bobcats, cats, rabbits, and chipmunks may be infected. Transmission among animals is usually by flea bite or by ingestion of contaminated tissue.

The lack of nucleotide diversity in the *Y. pestis* genome supports the view that *Y. pestis* has emerged relatively recently in evolutionary history from the closely related gastrointestinal pathogen *Y. pseudotuberculosis* (probably serotype 0:1b).

Pathogenesis. Infected fleas regurgitate organisms into a patient's skin during feeding attempts. The bacteria appear to migrate via cutaneous lymphatics to the regional lymph nodes where *Y. pestis* replicates, resulting in **bubonic plague**. In the absence of specific therapy, bacteremia may occur, resulting in purulent, necrotic, and hemorrhagic lesions in many organs. Both plasmid and chromosomal genes are required for full virulence.

Pneumonic plague occurs when infected material is inhaled. The organism is highly transmissible from persons with pneumonic plague and from domestic cats with pneumonic infection. This high transmissibility and high morbidity and mortality have provided an impetus for attempts to use *Y. pestis* as a biological weapon (Chapter 706).

Clinical Manifestations. *Y. pestis* infection can present as several clinical syndromes and infection may be subclinical. The three principal clinical presentations of plague are bubonic, septicemic, and pneumonic. Bubonic plague is the most frequent form (80–90% of cases in the United States). From 2–8 days after a flea bite, a 1–10 cm lymph nodes, or **bubo**, which is remarkable for its tenderness, develops in a draining lymph node located in the inguinal (most common), axillary, or cervical region depending on the inoculation site. Fever, chills, weakness, prostration, headache, and the development of septicemia are common. The skin may show insect bites or scratch marks. Purpura and gangrene of the extremities may develop as a result of disseminated intravascular coagulation. These lesions may be the origin of the name **Black Death**. Untreated plague can kill up to 50% of symptomatic individuals and death may occur within 2–4 days after onset of symptoms.

Occasionally, *Y. pestis* may establish systemic infection and induce the systemic symptoms seen with bubonic plague without causing a bubo (**primary septicemic plague**). Because of the delay in diagnosis linked to the lack of the bubo, septicemic plague carries a higher case fatality rate than bubonic plague. In some regions, bubo-free septicemic plague may comprise one fourth of cases.

Pneumonic plague is the least common but most dangerous and fatal form of the disease. Pneumonic plague may result from hematogenous dissemination, or rarely as **primary pneumonic plague** after inhalation of the organism from a human or animal with plague pneumonia or potentially from a biologic attack. Signs of pneumonic plague include severe pneumonia with high fever, dyspnea, and hemoptysis.

Plague meningitis, tonsillitis, or gastroenteritis may occur. Meningitis tends toward a late complication following inadequate treatment. Tonsillitis and gastroenteritis may occur with or without apparent bubo formation or lymphadenopathy.

Diagnosis. A febrile patient who has been exposed to small animals in endemic areas should be suspected of having plague. Thus, bubonic plague is suspected in a patient with a painful swollen lymph node, fever, and prostration who has been exposed to fleas or rodents in the western United States. A history of camping or the presence of flea bites should increase the index of suspicion. Laboratory diagnosis is based on bacteriologic culture or direct visualization using Gram, Giemsa, or Wayson stains of lymph node aspirates, blood, sputum, or exudates. *Y. pestis* grows well under routine culture conditions. Suspected isolates of *Y. pestis* should be forwarded using special containment precautions to a reference laboratory for confirmation. Cases of plague should be reported immediately to local and state health departments and the CDC.

DIFFERENTIAL DIAGNOSIS. Gram stain of *Y. pestis* may be confused with that of *Enterobacter agglomerans*. Mild and subacute forms of bubonic plague may be confused with other disorders causing localized lymphadenitis and lymphadenopathy. Septicemic plague may be indistinguishable from other forms of overwhelming bacterial sepsis.

Treatment. Patients suspected of having bubonic plague should be placed on isolation until 2 days after starting antibiotic treatment to prevent the potential spread of the disease if the patient develops pneumonia. The treatment of choice for bubonic plague has been streptomycin (30 mg/kg/24 hr divided q 12 hr IM for 10 days). However, intramuscular streptomycin is inappropriate for septicemia because absorption from muscles may be erratic when perfusion is poor. The poor central nervous system penetration of streptomycin makes this an inappropriate drug for meningitis. Septicemia and meningitis are usually treated with chloramphenicol (60–100 mg/kg/24 hr divided q 6 hr IV). Resistance to these agents and relapses are rare. *Y. pestis* is susceptible to penicillin in vitro but this is ineffective in treatment of human disease. Mild disease may be treated with oral chloramphenicol or tetracycline in children >9 yr of age. Prophylaxis or expectant treatment should be given to close contacts of patients with pneumonic plague. Recommended regimens include a 7-day course of tetracycline, doxycycline, or trimethoprim-sulfamethoxazole. Contacts of cases of uncomplicated bubonic plague do not require prophylaxis.

Prevention. Avoidance of exposure to infected animals and fleas is the best method of prevention of infection. Patients with plague should be isolated if they have pulmonary symptoms, and infected materials should be handled with extreme care. A vaccine is available for individuals at high risk of infection.

Yersinia enterocolitica
Abdel-Haq NM, Asmar BI, Abuhammour WM, et al: *Yersinia enterocolitica* infection in children. *Pediatr Infect Dis J* 2000;19:954–8.
Bottone EJ: *Yersinia enterocolitica*: Overview and epidemiologic correlates. *Microbes Infect* 1999;1:323–33.
Haller JC, Carlson S, Pederson KJ, et al: A chromosomally encoded type III secretion pathway in *Yersinia enterocolitica* is important in virulence. *Mol Microbiol* 2000;36:1436–46.
Revell PA, Miller VL: *Yersinia* virulence: More than a plasmid. *FEMS Microbiol Lett* 2001;205:159–64.
Satterthwaite P, Pritchard K, Floyd D, et al: A case-control study of *Yersinia enterocolitica* infections in Auckland. *Aust N Z J Public Health* 1999;23:482–5.
Sing A, Roggenkamp A, Geiger AM, et al: *Yersinia enterocolitica* evasion of the host innate immune response by V antigen-induced IL-10 production of macrophages is abrogated in IL-10-deficient mice. *J Immunol* 2002;168: 1315–21.
Uchiyama T, Kato H: The pathogenesis of Kawasaki disease and superantigens. *Jpn J Infect Dis* 1999;52:141–5.

Yersinia pseudotuberculosis
Carnoy C, Mullet C, Muller-Alouf H, et al: Superantigen YPMa exacerbates the virulence of *Yersinia pseudotuberculosis* in mice. *Infect Immunol* 2000;68:2553–9.
Fukushima H, Matsuda Y, Seki R, et al: Geographical heterogeneity between Far Eastern and Western countries in prevalence of the virulence plasmid, the superantigen *Yersinia pseudotuberculosis*-derived mitogen, and the high-pathogenicity island among *Yersinia pseudotuberculosis* strains. *J Clin Microbiol* 2001;39: 3541–7.
Nowgesic E, Fyfe M, Hockin J, et al: Outbreak of *Yersinia pseudotuberculosis* in British Columbia—November 1998. *Can Commun Dis Rep* 1999;25:97–100.
Press N, Fyfe M, Bowie W, et al: Clinical and microbiological follow-up of an outbreak of *Yersinia pseudotuberculosis* serotype Ib. *Scand J Infect Dis* 2001;33:523–6.

Plague (*Yersinia pestis*)
Centers for Disease Control and Prevention: Fatal human plague—Arizona and Colorado, 1996. *MMWR Morb Mortal Wkly Rep* 1997;46:617–20.
Cole ST, Buchrieser C: Bacterial genomics. A plague o' both your hosts. *Nature* 2001;413:467, 469–70.
Drancourt M, Raoult D: Molecular insights into the history of plague. *Microbes Infect* 2002;4:105–9.
Keeling MJ, Gilligan CA: Bubonic plague: A metapopulation model of a zoonosis. *Proc R Soc Lond B Biol Sci* 2000;267:2219–30.
Klevytska AM, Price LB, Schupp JM, et al: Identification and characterization of variable-number tandem repeats in the *Yersinia pestis* genome. *J Clin Microbiol* 2001;39:3179–85.

Chapter 187

Aeromonas and *Plesiomonas* James R. Murphy and

Gloria P. Heresi

Aeromonas and *Plesiomonas* organisms cause enteritis and less frequently skin and soft tissue infections and septicemia. These organisms are common in fresh and brackish water and in and on animals and plants in contact with water.

187.1 *Aeromonas*

Etiology. *Aeromonas* are members of the Vibrionaceae family. They are oxidase-positive, facultatively anaerobic, gram-negative bacilli. The species most often associated with human infection are *A. hydrophila*, *A. veronii* biotype *sobria*, and *A. caviae*.

Aeromonas infect a wide variety of warm- and cold-blooded animals. In humans, infection with *Aeromonas* is associated with three distinct syndromes: gastroenteritis, skin and soft tissue infections, and septicemia. *Aeromonas* strains are divided into two major groups: the nonmotile psychrophilic organisms that infect cold-blooded animals and the motile mesophilic organisms that infect humans and other warm-blooded animals.

Epidemiology. *Aeromonas* organisms are ubiquitous. They are present in numerous environmental fresh and brackish aquatic sources including rivers and streams, well water, and sewage. They are most often cultivated from aquatic sources during warm weather months. However, prevalence of human infection may or may not exhibit seasonality, apparently depending on local conditions. *Aeromonas* organisms have been isolated from meats, milk, and vegetables consumed as human food. Most human infections are associated with exposure to contaminated water. Asymptomatic colonization with *Aeromonas* occurs in humans and is more common in inhabitants of tropical regions.

Pathogenesis. Clinical and epidemiologic data demonstrate that many *Aeromonas* are enteric pathogens. However, adult volunteers fed 10^4–10^{10} colony-forming units of *Aeromonas* did not develop diarrhea or become colonized. *Aeromonas* possesses various potential virulence factors including α- and β-hemolysin, adherence fimbriae, enterotoxin, protease, and chitinase. The β-hemolysin has been shown to be cytotoxic to various cell lines. Enterotoxin causes fluid accumulation in rabbit ileal loops, increases intracellular cyclic adenosine monophosphate in rabbit intestinal epithelium, and cross reacts immunologically with cholera toxin. The protease may have a role in extraintestinal manifestations of *Aeromonas* infections. A few strains produce shiga toxin. It is not clear which of the potential virulence traits define strains that cause illness. Normal human serum generally promotes phagocytosis and intracellular killing of *Aeromonas* and the lack of this serum action has been linked to poor prognosis.

Clinical Manifestations. Colonization with *Aeromonas* may be asymptomatic or cause illness, including gastroenteritis, focal invasive infection, and septicemia. Apparently immunologically normal individuals may present with each manifestation, but invasive disease is more commonly seen in immunologically compromised individuals.

ENTERITIS. The most common clinical manifestation of infection with *Aeromonas* is enteritis. This occurs primarily in children <3 yr old. Studies suggest that, in some locations, it is the third or fourth most common cause of childhood bacterial

diarrhea. *Aeromonas* have been isolated from 2–10% of patients with diarrhea and 1–5% of asymptomatic control subjects in various studies. The diarrheal illness is often watery and self-limited, although a dysentery-like syndrome with blood and mucus in the stool has also been described. Fever and vomiting are common in children. Gastroenteritis caused by *A. hydrophila* and *A. sobria* tends to be acute and self-limited, whereas one third of the patients with *A. caviae* gastroenteritis have chronic or intermittent diarrhea that may last 4–6 wk. Complications of *Aeromonas* gastroenteritis include intussusception, failure to thrive, hemolytic-uremic syndrome, bacteremia, and strangulated intestinal hernia.

SKIN AND SOFT TISSUE INFECTION. *A. hydrophila* is the predominant species associated with skin and soft tissue infections, with peak incidence during the summer months. Skin and soft tissue infection is the second most common presentation of *Aeromonas* infection. Predisposing factors include local trauma and exposure to contaminated fresh water. *Aeromonas* soft tissue infections have been reported to result from alligator bites, water-sport injuries, tick bites, and the use of medicinal leech therapy. The spectrum of skin and soft tissue infections is broad, ranging from a localized skin nodule to life-threatening necrotizing fasciitis and myonecrosis. *Aeromonas* cellulitis is indistinguishable from that due to other bacterial pathogens that cause cellulitis but should be suspected in wounds in contact with a water source, especially during the summer.

SEPTICEMIA. *Aeromonas* septicemia, the third most frequent presentation of infection with *Aeromonas*, is associated with a high mortality rate (reported range 27–73%). *Aeromonas* septicemia usually occurs in patients with underlying conditions such as hepatobiliary disease or malignancy but may occur in an immunocompetent host. *Aeromonas* may be the only organism isolated or may be part of a polymicrobial bacteremic syndrome. *A. hydrophila* septicemia tends to occur in patients with less serious underlying disease. *A. caviae* tends to associate with polymicrobial septicemia and is isolated more often from patients with underlying illnesses.

OTHER INFECTIONS. *Aeromonas* is a rare cause of necrotizing gastroenteritis, endocarditis, meningitis, osteomyelitis, pyogenic arthritis, endophthalmitis, urinary tract infection, peritonitis, myositis, cellulitis, necrotizing fasciitis, cholecystitis, lung abscess, and pneumonia. *Aeromonas* can be associated with aspiration pneumonia after a near-drowning event.

Diagnosis. Diagnosis is by culture isolation of *Aeromonas*. The organism is easily grown on standard media when the source material is normally sterile. However, isolation of the organism from samples containing numerous bacteria is more difficult, presumably because competing bacteria outgrow *Aeromonas*. Use of selective media such as a blood agar supplemented with ampicillin or MacConkey agar containing Tween 80 and ampicillin enhances isolation. Most (~90%) strains produce β-hemolysis on blood agar. Lactose-fermenting strains of *Aeromonas* may be overlooked in stool specimens if the clinical laboratory does not routinely perform oxidase tests on lactose fermenters isolated on MacConkey or does not routinely use selective media for the isolation of *Aeromonas*.

Treatment. *Aeromonas* gastroenteritis is usually self-limited, and antimicrobial therapy may not be indicated. No controlled trials have been carried out; however, data from uncontrolled trials suggest that antimicrobial therapy shortens the course of the illness. Antimicrobial therapy is reasonable to consider in patients with protracted diarrhea, a dysentery-like illness, or underlying conditions such as hepatobiliary disease or immunocompromise. Most isolates are resistant to ampicillin. Septicemia should be treated with an aminoglycoside or a third-generation cephalosporin. Other options include aztreonam, imipenem, chloramphenicol, and trimethoprim-sulfamethoxazole (TMP-SMZ).

187.2 *Plesiomonas shigelloides*

Etiology. *Plesiomonas shigelloides,* the only species in the genera, is a fermentative bacilli that is not an Enterobacteriaceae. The organism has been associated with acute gastroenteritis and very rarely extraintestinal infections. *P. shigelloides* is a member of the family Vibrionaceae, although some authorities believe they are related more closely to Enterobacteriaceae. The bacilli are oxidase-positive, facultatively anaerobic, motile, and gram-negative. Analysis of the sequence of 5S rRNA, 16S rRNA, and 16S rDNA suggests that *P. shigelloides* is closely related to Enterobacteriaceae.

Epidemiology. *P. shigelloides* is ubiquitous in fresh water and historically has been most often found in warmer and tropical waters. There are increasing reports of isolations in colder regions. *P. shigelloides* colonizes numerous warm- and cold-blooded animals and may cause disease in cats. Infection of humans is thought to be the result of consumption of contaminated water or food and possibly through contact with colonized animals. The role that colonized animals play in the ecology of human infection is poorly understood. Asymptomatic colonization with *S. shigelloides* is common in some tropical and subtropical regions and more infrequent in colder climates. A majority of symptomatic patients seen in North America have either traveled abroad or report exposure to potentially contaminated water or food. Clinical disease in humans begins 24 hr to about 4 days after contact with the organism.

Pathogenesis. Epidemiologic evidence indicates that *P. shigelloides* is an enteropathogen. However, diarrhea did not develop in volunteers fed *P. shigelloides.* The mechanism of gastroenteritis is not known, but it appears that the species can cause both secretory and invasive disease.

Clinical Manifestations. *Plesiomonas* gastroenteritis is usually secretory but occasionally may be dysenteric, with blood and mucus. The frequency of secretory vs dysenteric diarrhea clusters by outbreak report, suggesting that either human populations or bacterial populations associate with type of presentation. Symptoms include fever, headache, abdominal cramping, nausea, vomiting, and diarrhea. Blood, mucus, or both may be passed with stool, and white blood cells may be visualized in stained preparations of stool. The illness usually resolves in about 2 wk, but reports describe diarrhea lasting ≥4 wk.

Extraintestinal infections are rare and usually occur in patients with underlying conditions such as immunodeficiency, malignancy, sickle cell disease, or cirrhosis. Rarely, bacteremia accompanying gastroenteritis has been documented in apparently otherwise normal children. Extraintestinal disease includes septicemia, meningitis, osteomyelitis, septic arthritis, reactive arthritis, cellulitis, endophthalmitis, pseudoappendicitis, pseudomembranous colitis, proctitis, and cholecystitis. Early onset neonatal sepsis and meningitis are rare but comprise most of reported cases of *P. shigelloides* meningitis; it has a very high mortality rate (80%). Septicemia has a high mortality rate in adults.

Diagnosis. A history of foreign travel, ingestion of raw seafood, or exposure to contaminated water should raise a suspicion of *P. shigelloides* when clinical presentation matches those described above. Isolation of the organism from stool or sterile body fluids is essential for diagnosis. *P. shigelloides* grows well on traditional enteric media. However, selective techniques may be required to isolate the organism from mixed cultures. It may be underrecognized by clinical laboratories that do not routinely perform an oxidase test. Molecular methodology is under development for diagnostic purposes but is not yet in routine use.

Treatment. Gastroenteritis due to *P. shigelloides* is usually self-limited. Antimicrobial therapy is reserved for those patients with prolonged or bloody diarrhea. Data from uncontrolled trials suggest that antimicrobial therapy decreases the duration of symptoms. *P. shigelloides* is susceptible to TMP-SMZ, cephalosporins, carbapenems, and quinolones (not approved for use in the United States in children <18 yr of age). *P shigelloides* is commonly resistant to penicillin, streptomycin, and azithromycin.

Antibiotics are essential for therapy of extraintestinal disease. Empirical therapy with a third-generation cephalosporin is reasonable, because most isolates are susceptible in vitro. Definitive therapy should be guided by the susceptibility of the individual isolate.

Aeromonas
Essers B, Burnens AP, Lanfranchini FM, et al: Acute community-acquired diarrhea requiring hospital admission in Swiss children. *Clin Infect Dis* 2000;31:192–6.

Lau SM, Peng MY, Chang FY: Outcomes of *Aeromonas* bacteremia in patients with different types of underlying disease. *J Microbiol Immunol Infect* 2000;33:241–7.

Lehane L, Rawlin GT: Topically acquired bacterial zoonoses from fish: A review. *Med J Aust* 2000;173:256–9.

Nayduch D, Honko A, Noblet GP, et al: Detection of *Aeromonas caviae* in the common housefly *Musca domestica* by culture and polymerase chain reaction. *Epidemiol Infect* 2001;127:561–6.

Svenungsson B, Lagergren A, Ekwall E, et al: Enteropathogens in adult patients with diarrhea and healthy control subjects: a 1-year prospective study in a Swedish clinic for infectious diseases. *Clin Infect Dis* 2000;30:770–8.

Vila J, Marco F, Soler L, et al: In vitro antimicrobial susceptibility of clinical isolates of *Aeromonas caviae, Aeromonas hydrophila* and *Aeromonas veronii* biotype *sobria. J Antimicrob Chemother* 2002;49:701–2.

Plesiomonas shigelloides
Aldova E, Shimada T: New O and H antigens of the international antigenic scheme for *Plesiomonas shigelloides.* *Folia Microbiol* (Praha) 2000;45:301–4.

Ampofo K, Graham P, Ratner A, et al: *Plesiomonas shigelloides* sepsis and splenic abscess in an adolescent with sickle-cell disease. *Pediatr Infect Dis J* 2001;20:1178–9.

Chida T, Okamura N, Ohtani K, et al: The complete DNA sequence of the O antigen gene region of *Plesiomonas shigelloides* serotype O17 which is identical to *Shigella sonnei* form I antigen. *Microbiol Immunol* 2000;44:161–72.

Gonzalez-Rey C, Svenson SB, Bravo L, et al: Specific detection of *Plesiomonas shigelloides* isolated from aquatic environments, animals and human diarrhoeal cases by PCR based on 23S rRNA gene. *FEMS Immunol Med Microbiol* 2000;29:107–13.

Jagger T, Keane S, Robertson S: *Plesiomonas shigelloides*—an uncommon cause of diarrhoea in cats? *Vet Rec* 2000;146:296.

Janda JM, Abbott SL: Unusual food-borne pathogens. *Listeria monocytogenes, Aeromonas, Plesiomonas,* and *Edwardsiella* species. *Clin Lab Med* 1999;19:553–82.

Chapter 188

Pseudomonas, Burkholderia, and *Stenotrophomonas*

Robert S. Baltimore

Pseudomonas and *Burkholderia* live abundantly in soil and water and on plants, and are widespread throughout nature. Most human infections due to these species are opportunistic and occur among low-birthweight infants and in older infants and children with impaired host defenses, such as those with traumatic wounds, cystic fibrosis, malignancies, extensive burns, malnutrition (especially in impoverished populations), and primary immunodeficiencies as well as those receiving immunosuppressive therapy. *Pseudomonas aeruginosa* is an important cause of nosocomial infections including postsurgical infections.

A number of species formerly considered under the genus *Pseudomonas* were reclassified on the basis of rRNA homology. Species formerly classified as *P. cepacia, P. mallei,* and *P. pseudomallei* are now *Burkholderia cepacia, B. mallei,* and *B. pseudomallei. P. maltophilia* is now *Stenotrophomonas maltophilia.*

A large number of *Pseudomonas, Burkholderia,* and related organisms have been identified, but only a few are pathogenic for humans; of these, *P. aeruginosa* is by far the most common. Other species occasionally recognized as human pathogens include *B. cepacia, S. maltophilia, P. fluorescens, B. putrefaciens, B. pseudomallei,* and *B. mallei.*

188.1 *Pseudomonas aeruginosa*

P. aeruginosa is a gram-negative rod and is a strict aerobe. It can multiply in most moist environments that contain minimal amounts of organic compounds because it can use any source of carbon. Strains from clinical specimens may produce β-hemolysis on blood agar; >90% of strains produce a bluish-green phenazine pigment (blue pus) as well as fluorescein, which is yellow-green and fluoresces. These pigments diffuse into and color the medium surrounding the colonies. Strains of *Pseudomonas* can be differentiated for epidemiologic purposes by serologic, phage, and pyocin typing and by genome restriction fragment length polymorphisms using pulsed-field gel electrophoresis.

Epidemiology. In a study from Israel the rate of *P. aeruginosa* bacteremia in children was 3.8/1000 patients over 10 yr with a 20% mortality rate, but rates varied according to the prevalent underlying diseases. *P. aeruginosa* and other pseudomonads frequently enter the hospital environment on the clothes, skin, or shoes of patients or hospital personnel, with plants or vegetables brought into the hospital, and in the gastrointestinal tracts of patients. Colonization of any moist or liquid substance may ensue; for example, the organisms may be found growing in distilled water, hospital kitchens and laundries, some antiseptic solutions, and equipment used for respiratory therapy. Colonization of patients' skin, throat, stool, and nasal mucosa is low at admission to the hospital but increases to as high as 50–70% with prolonged hospitalization and the use of broad-spectrum antibiotics, chemotherapy, mechanical ventilation, and urinary catheters. Patients' intestinal microbial flora may be altered by the use of broad-spectrum antibiotics, which reduces resistance to colonization and permits *P. aeruginosa* in the environment to populate the GI tract. Intestinal mucosal breakdown associated with medications, especially cytotoxic agents, and nosocomial enteritis may provide a pathway by which *P. aeruginosa* spreads to the lymphatics or bloodstream.

Pathogenesis. The requirement of oxygen for growth may account for the lack of invasiveness of *Pseudomonas* after it has colonized or even infected the skin. Invasiveness of *P. aeruginosa* is mediated by a host of virulence factors. It produces endotoxin that is weak compared with that of other gram-negative bacilli.

It also produces numerous exotoxins, including exotoxin A, which causes local necrosis and facilitates systemic bacterial invasion, and exoenzyme S, which acts as both an adhesin and a cellular toxin. *Pseudomonas* produces disease in three stages. Bacterial colonization and attachment are facilitated by pili or fimbriae and by opportunistic adhesion to epithelium damaged by prior injury or infection. A mucopolysaccharide may inhibit phagocytosis, whereas extracellular proteins, proteases, elastases, and cytotoxin (formerly leukocidin) digest cell membranes, and antibodies produce capillary vascular permeability and inhibit leukocyte function. Dissemination and bloodstream invasion follow extension of local tissue damage and are facilitated by the antiphagocytic properties of endotoxin, the **mucoid exopolysaccharide**, and protease cleavage of IgG. The host responds to infection by producing antibodies to *Pseudomonas* exotoxin (**exotoxin A**) and lipopolysaccharide. Compromised host defense mechanisms (owing to trauma, neutropenia, mucositis, immunosuppression, impaired mucociliary transport) explain the predominant role of this organism in producing opportunistic infections.

Clinical Manifestations. Most clinical patterns (Table 188–1) are related to opportunistic infections (Chapter 164) or are associated with shunts and indwelling catheters (Chapter 165). *P. aeruginosa* may be introduced into a minor wound of a healthy person as a secondary invader, and cellulitis and a localized abscess that exudes green or blue pus may follow. The characteristic skin lesions of *Pseudomonas*, **ecthyma gangrenosum**, whether caused by direct inoculation or secondary to septicemia, begin as pink macules and progress to hemorrhagic nodules and eventually to ulcers with ecchymotic and gangrenous centers with eschar formation, surrounded by an intense red areola.

Outbreaks of dermatitis and urinary tract infections caused by *P. aeruginosa* have been reported in healthy persons after use of community swimming pools, wading pools, recreational whirlpools, or family-owned hot tubs. Skin lesions of folliculitis develop several hours to 2 days after contact with these water sources. Skin lesions may be erythematous, macular, papular, or pustular. Illness may vary from a few scattered lesions to extensive truncal involvement. In some children, malaise, fever, vomiting, sore throat, conjunctivitis, rhinitis, and swollen breasts may be associated with dermal lesions.

Pseudomonads other than *P. aeruginosa* rarely cause disease in healthy children, but pneumonia and abscesses due to *B. cepacia*, otitis media due to *P. putrefaciens* or *P. stutzeri*, abscesses due to

TABLE 188–1. *Pseudomonas aeruginosa* Infections

Infection	Common Clinical Characteristics
Endocarditis	Native right-sided (tricuspid) valve disease with intravenous drug abuse
Pneumonia	Compromised local (lung) or systemic host defense mechanisms. Nosocomial (respiratory), bacteremic (malignancy), or abnormal mucociliary clearance (cystic fibrosis) may be pathogenetic. Cystic fibrosis is associated with mucoid *Pseudomonas aeruginosa* organisms producing capsular slime.
Central nervous system infection	Meningitis, brain abscess; contiguous spread (mastoiditis, dermal sinus tracts, sinusitis); bacteremia or direct inoculation (trauma, surgery)
External otitis	Swimmer's ear; humid warm climates, swimming pool contamination
Malignant otitis externa	Invasive, indolent, febrile toxic, destructive necrotizing lesion in young infants, immunosuppressed neutropenic patients, or diabetic patients; associated with 17th nerve palsy and mastoiditis
Chronic mastoiditis	Ear drainage, swelling, erythema; perforated tympanic membrane
Keratitis	Corneal ulceration; contact lens keratitis
Endophthalmitis	Penetrating trauma, surgery, penetrating corneal ulceration; fulminant progression
Osteomyelitis/septic arthritis	Puncture wounds of foot and osteochondritis; intravenous drug abuse; fibrocartilaginous joints, sternum, vertebrae, pelvis; open fracture osteomyelitis; indolent; pyelonephritis and vertebral osteomyelitis
Urinary tract infection	Iatrogenic, nosocomial; recurrent urinary tract infections in children, instrumented patients, and those with obstruction or stones
Intestinal tract infection	Immunocompromise, neutropenia, typhlitis, rectal abscess, ulceration, rarely diarrhea; peritonitis in peritoneal dialysis
Ecthyma gangrenosum	Metastatic dissemination; hemorrhage, necrosis, erythema, eschar, discrete lesions with bacterial invasion of blood vessels; also subcutaneous nodules, cellulitis, pustules, deep abscesses
Primary and secondary skin infections	Local infection; burns, trauma, decubitus ulcers, toe web infection, green nail (paronychia); whirlpool dermatitis: diffuse, pruritic, folliculitis, vesiculopustular or maculopapular, erythematous lesions

P. fluorescens, and cellulitis and septicemia and osteomyelitis due to *S. maltophilia* have been reported. Septicemia and endocarditis due to *S. maltophilia* have also been associated with intravenous abuse of drugs.

BURNS AND WOUND INFECTION. The surfaces of burns or wounds are frequently populated by *Pseudomonas* and other gram-negative organisms; this initial colonization with a low number of adherent organisms is a necessary prerequisite to invasive disease. Administration of antibiotics may diminish the susceptible microbiologic flora, permitting strains of relatively resistant *Pseudomonas* to flourish. Multiplication of organisms in devitalized tissues or associated with prolonged use of intravenous or urinary catheters increases the risk of septicemia with *P. aeruginosa,* a major problem in burned patients (Chapter 62).

CYSTIC FIBROSIS. *P. aeruginosa* is common in children with cystic fibrosis; prevalence increases with increasing age and severity of pulmonary disease (Chapter 393). Mucoid strains of *P. aeruginosa* predominate in patients with cystic fibrosis but are rarely encountered in other conditions. The infection begins insidiously or even asymptomatically, and the progression has a highly variable pace. In children with cystic fibrosis, antibody does not eradicate the organism and antibiotics are only partially effective, thus, infection becomes chronic. After repeated courses of antibiotic treatment the *P. aeruginosa* strains may be highly antibiotic-resistant.

IMMUNOCOMPROMISED PERSONS. Children with leukemia or other debilitating malignancies, particularly those who are receiving immunosuppressive therapy and who are neutropenic, are extremely susceptible to septicemia due to invasion of the bloodstream by *Pseudomonas* with which the patient is already colonized, usually in the respiratory or gastrointestinal tract. Signs of sepsis are often accompanied by a generalized vasculitis, and hemorrhagic necrotic lesions may be found in all organs, including the skin, where they appear as purple nodules or ecchymotic areas that become gangrenous (ecthyma gangrenosum). Hemorrhagic or gangrenous perirectal cellulitis or abscesses may occur, associated with ileus and profound hypotension.

NOSOCOMIAL PNEUMONIA. Although not a significant cause of community-acquired pneumonia in children, *P. aeruginosa* is an important cause of nosocomial pneumonia, especially ventilator-associated pneumonia. *P. aeruginosa* has historically been found to contaminate ventilators, tubing, and humidifiers, but this is uncommon today with appropriate disinfection and routine changing of equipment. Nevertheless, colonization of the upper respiratory tract and the gastrointestinal tract may be followed by aspiration of *P. aeruginosa*-contaminated secretions, resulting in severe pneumonia. One of the most challenging situations is distinguishing between colonization and pneumonia in intubated patients. This can often only be resolved by using invasive culture techniques such as bronchoscopy with bronchial brushing.

INFANTS. *P. aeruginosa* is an occasional cause of nosocomial bacteremia in newborns and accounts for 2–5% of positive blood culture results in neonatal intensive care units. A frequent focus preceding bacteremia is conjunctivitis. *P. aeruginosa* has been isolated increasingly from peritoneal fluid in infants with necrotizing enterocolitis. Older infants may occasionally present with community-acquired sepsis due to *P. aeruginosa,* but this is uncommon. In the few reports describing this sepsis, preceding conditions included ecthyma-like skin lesions, virus-associated transient neutropenia, and prolonged contact with contaminated bath water.

Diagnosis. *P. aeruginosa* infection is rarely clinically distinctive. Diagnosis depends on recovery of the organism from the blood, cerebrospinal fluid, urine, or needle aspirate of the lung or from purulent material obtained by aspiration of subcutaneous abscesses or areas of cellulitis. An exception is ecthyma gan-

grenosum, which is characteristic of *Pseudomonas* infection of the skin. Rarely, similar skin lesions may follow septicemia due to *Aeromonas hydrophila,* other gram-negative bacilli, and *Aspergillus.*

Treatment. Systemic infections with *Pseudomonas* should be treated promptly with an antibiotic to which the organism is susceptible in vitro. Response to treatment may be limited, and prolonged treatment may be necessary for systemic infection in immunocompromised hosts.

Septicemia and other aggressive infections should be treated with either one or two bactericidal agents. Little evidence shows that more than one agent is needed for individuals with normal immunity or when treating urinary tract infections, but dual therapy is often used for a synergistic effect in immunocompromised patients or when the susceptibility of the organism is in doubt. Appropriate single agents include ceftazidime, cefoperazone, ticarcillin-clavulanate, and piperacillin-tazobactam. Gentamicin or another aminoglycosides may be used concomitantly for synergistic effect. Carbenicillin, ticarcillin, and mezlocillin alone are not recommended because strains of the organism rapidly become resistant to these agents.

Ceftazidime has proved to be extremely effective in patients with cystic fibrosis (150–250 mg/kg/24 hr divided q 6–8 hr IV). Azlocillin, mezlocillin, or piperacillin-tazobactam (300–450 mg/kg/24 hr divided q 6–8 hr IV) also have proved to be effective therapy for susceptible strains of *P. aeruginosa* when combined with an aminoglycoside. Additional effective antibiotics include imipenem-cilastatin, meropenem, and aztreonam. Ciprofloxacin, is effective but not approved in the United States for persons <18 yr of age. It is important to base continued treatment on the results of susceptibility tests because antibiotic resistance of *P. aeruginosa* to one or more antibiotics is increasing.

Meningitis is best treated with ceftazidime in combination with gentamicin, given intravenously. Concomitant intraventricular or intrathecal treatment with gentamicin (1–2 mg once daily, independent of body weight, until the cerebrospinal fluid is sterile) may be required when intravenous therapy fails but is not recommended for routine use.

Prognosis. The prognosis is dependent in large part on the nature of the underlying disease. In severely immunocompromised patients, the prognosis for patients with *P. aeruginosa* sepsis is poor, unless susceptibility factors such as neutropenia or hypogammaglobulinemia can be reversed. The outcome is improved by combined antimicrobial therapy, a urinary tract portal of entry, absence of neutropenia or recovery from neutropenia, and drainage of local sites of infection. *Pseudomonas* is recovered from the lungs of most children who die of cystic fibrosis and may be responsible for the slow deterioration of these patients; *B. cepacia,* which is frequently resistant to standard antimicrobial agents, has been associated with a more rapid decline in pulmonary function and lower survival rate. The prognosis for normal development is poor in the few infants who survive *Pseudomonas* meningitis.

Prevention. Prevention of infections due to *P. aeruginosa* is not a concern for healthy individuals outside of the hospital but is dependent on limiting contamination of the health care environment and preventing transmission to patients. Effective hospital infection control programs are necessary to identify and eradicate sources of the organism as quickly as possible. *Pseudomonas* may grow in distilled water, some disinfectants, parenteral alimentation solutions, and medications. In newborn nurseries, infection generally has been transmitted to the infants by the hands of personnel, from washbasin surfaces, from catheters, and from solutions used to rinse suction catheters.

Strict attention to handwashing, particularly with an iodophor-containing solution or alcohol-based hand rubs, before and between contacts with neonates, may prevent or interdict epidemic disease. Meticulous care and sterile procedures in suctioning of endotracheal tubes, insertion and care of indwelling catheters, preparation of intravenous solutions, especially those for total parenteral alimentation, and regular replacement of intravenous administration tubing greatly reduce the hazard of extrinsic contamination by *Pseudomonas* and other gram-negative organisms.

Prevention of follicular dermatitis caused by *Pseudomonas* contamination of whirlpools or hot tubs is possible by maintaining pool water at a pH of 7.2–7.8 and free chlorine concentration at 70.5 mg/L.

Infections in burned patients may be minimized by protective isolation, debridement of devitalized tissue, and topical application of sulfadiazine or 10% mafenide acetate cream. Administration of intravenous immunoglobulin may be used. Approaches under investigation to prevent infection include development of *Pseudomonas* vaccine and development of hyperimmune globulin.

Pseudomonas infection of dermal sinuses communicating with the cerebrospinal space can be prevented by early identification and surgical repair. *Pseudomonas* infection of the urinary tract may be minimized or prevented by early identification and corrective surgery of obstructive lesions.

188.2 *Burkholderia*

B. cepacia. *B. cepacia* is a filamentous gram-negative rod. It may be difficult to isolate from respiratory specimens in the laboratory, requiring an enriched, selective media (OFPBL) and as long as 3 days of incubation.

B. cepacia is a classic opportunist that rarely infects normal tissue but can be a pathogen for individuals with pre-existing damage to respiratory epithelium, especially persons with cystic fibrosis. Resistance to many antibiotics appears to be a factor in its emergence as a nosocomial pathogen. Although it is found throughout the environment, human-to-human spread among patients with cystic fibrosis occurs either directly by inhalation of aerosols or indirectly from contaminated equipment or surfaces. This has led to cohorting of patients with cystic fibrosis in some clinics, hospital wards, and social gatherings on the basis of *B. cepacia* colonization. *B. cepacia* in persons with cystic fibrosis may only represent colonization in many patients but in some it is associated with an acute respiratory syndrome of fever, leukocytosis, and progressive respiratory failure. This is in contradistinction to *P. aeruginosa* in cystic fibrosis, which is insidious and less communicable.

Treatment in hospitals should include standard precautions and avoidance of placing colonized and uncolonized patients in the same room. Persons who have cystic fibrosis and who visit or provide care and are not infected or colonized with *B. cepacia* may elect to wear a mask when within 3 ft of a colonized patient. The use of antibiotics is guided by susceptibility studies of a patient's isolates because the susceptibility pattern of this species is quite variable. Ureidopenicillins (e.g., mezlocillin, piperacillin), aminoglycosides, ceftazidime, ciprofloxacin, and trimethoprim-sulfamethoxazole frequently show good activity. Resistance to aminoglycosides is the rule and presence of inducible β-lactamase in many strains is probably the cause of clinical failures reported with ureidopenicillins and ceftazidime. Treatment with two or three agents may be necessary to control the infection and avoid the development of resistance.

B. mallei (Glanders). Glanders is a severe infectious disease of horses and other domestic and farm animals due to *B. mallei*, a nonmotile gram-negative bacillus that is occasionally transmitted to humans. It is acquired by inoculation into the skin, usually at the site of a previous abrasion, or by inhalation of aerosols. Laboratory workers may acquire it from clinical specimens. The disease is relatively common in Asia, Africa, and the

Middle East. The clinical manifestations include septicemia, acute or chronic pneumonitis, and hemorrhagic necrotic lesions of the skin, nasal mucous membranes, and lymph nodes. Glanders is treated with sulfadiazine, tetracycline, or chloramphenicol and streptomycin over a period of many months. Interest in this organism has increased due to the possibility of its use as a bioterrorism agent (Chapter 706).

B. pseudomallei (Melioidosis). This important disease of Southeast Asia and northern Australia occurs in the United States mainly in persons returning from endemic areas. The causative agent is *B. pseudomallei*, an inhabitant of soil and water in the tropics. It is ubiquitous in endemic areas; infection follows inhalation of dust or direct contamination of abrasions or wounds. Human-to-human transmission has only rarely been reported. Serologic surveys demonstrate that asymptomatic infection occurs in endemic areas. The disease may remain latent and appear when host resistance is reduced, sometimes years after the initial exposure.

Melioidosis may present as a single primary skin lesion (vesicle, bulla, or urticaria). Pulmonary infection may be subacute and mimic tuberculosis or it may present as an acute necrotizing pneumonia. Occasionally, septicemia occurs and numerous abscesses are noted in various organs of the body. Myocarditis, pericarditis, endocarditis, intestinal abscess, cholecystitis, acute gastroenteritis, urinary tract infections, septic arthritis, paraspinal abscess, osteomyelitis, and generalized lymphadenopathy all have been observed. Melioidosis may also present as an encephalitic illness with fever and seizures.

Diagnosis is based on visualization of characteristic small gram-negative rods in exudates or growth on laboratory media such as eosin-methylene blue or MacConkey agar. Serologic tests are available, and diagnosis can be established by a fourfold or greater increase in antibody titer in an individual with an appropriate syndrome.

B. pseudomallei is susceptible to many antimicrobial agents, including third-generation cephalosporins, aminoglycosides, tetracycline, cotrimoxazole, sulfisoxazole, chloramphenicol, and amoxicillin-clavulanate. Therapy should be guided by antimicrobial susceptibility tests; two or three agents such as ceftazidime or chloramphenicol plus either trimethoprim-sulfamethoxazole, sulfisoxazole, or an aminoglycoside are usually chosen for severe or septicemic disease. For severe disease, prolonged treatment of 2–6 mo is recommended to prevent relapses. Appropriate antibiotic therapy generally results in recovery.

188.3 *Stenotrophomonas*

S. maltophilia (formerly *Xanthomonas maltophilia* or *Pseudomonas maltophilia*) is a short to medium-sized straight gram-negative bacillus. It is ubiquitous in nature and can be found in the hospital environment. Strains isolated in the laboratory may be contaminants, may be a commensal from the colonized surface of a patient, or may represent an invasive pathogen. The species is an opportunist; serious infections usually afflict those requiring intensive care, typically patients with ventilator-associated pneumonia or catheter-associated infections. Prolonged antibiotic exposure appears to be a frequent factor in nosocomial *S. maltophilia* infections, probably due to its endogenous antibiotic resistance pattern. Common types of infection include pneumonia, urinary tract infection, endocarditis, and osteomyelitis. Strains vary as to antibiotic susceptibility. Treatment should be based on the results of susceptibility testing. Trimethoprim-sulfamethoxazole, minocycline, doxycycline, ticarcillin-clavulanate, and chloramphenicol frequently show good activity. Trimethoprim-sulfamethoxazole is usually the drug combination of choice. Aminoglycosides, cephalosporins, and carbapenems are usually inactive. Among the quinolone antibiotics, ciprofloxacin often has good activity and has been used clinically, and the newer agents sparfloxacin and levofloxacin usually show good activity in vitro.

Baltimore RS, Christie CD, Smith GJ: Immunohistopathologic localization of *Pseudomonas aeruginosa* in lungs from patients with cystic fibrosis. Implications for the pathogenesis of progressive lung deterioration. *Am Rev Respir Dis* 1989;140:1650–61.

Chaowagul W, White NJ, Dance DA, et al: Melioidosis: A major cause of community-acquired septicemia in northeastern Thailand. *J Infect Dis* 1989;159:890–9.

Chen JS, Witzmann KA, Spilker T, et al: Endemnicity and inter-city spread *of Burkholderia cepacia* genomovar III in cystic fibrosis. *J Pediatr* 2001;139:643–9.

Chusid MJ, Hillmann SM: Community-acquired *Pseudomonas* sepsis in previously healthy infants. *Pediatr Infect Dis J* 1987;6:681–4.

Feder HM Jr, Grant-Kels JM, Tilton RG: *Pseudomonas* whirlpool dermatitis. *Clin Pediatr* 1983;22:638–42.

Gales AC, Jones RN, Turnidge J, et al: Characterization of *Pseudomonas aeruginosa* isolates: Occurrence rates, antimicrobial susceptibility patterns and molecular typing in the SENTRY antimicrobial surveillance program, 1997–1999. *Clin Infect Dis* 2001;32(Suppl 2):146–55.

Grisaru-Soen G, Lerner-Geva L, Keller N, et al: *Pseudomonas aeruginosa* bacteremia in children: Analysis of trends in prevalence, antibiotic resistance and prognostic factors. *Pediatr Infect Dis J* 2000;19:959–63.

Hilf M, Yu VL, Sharp JS, et al: Antibiotic therapy for *Pseudomonas aeruginosa* bacteremia: Outcome correlations in a prospective study of 200 patients. *Am J Med* 1989;87:540–6.

Kerem E, Corey M, Gold R, et al: Pulmonary function and clinical course in patients with cystic fibrosis after pulmonary colonization with *Pseudomonas aeruginosa. J Pediatr* 1990;116:714–9.

McManus AT, Mason AD, McManus WF, et al: Twenty-five year review of *Pseudomonas aeruginosa* bacteremia in a burn center. *Eur J Clin Microbiol* 1985;4:219–23.

Rodriguez WJ, Khan WN, Cocchetto DM, et al: Treatment of *Pseudomonas* meningitis with ceftazidime with or without concurrent therapy. *Pediatr Infect Dis J* 1990;9:83–7.

Salmen P, Dwyer DM, Vorse H, et al: Whirlpool associated *Pseudomonas aeruginosa* urinary tract infections. *JAMA* 1983;15:2025–6,.

Srinivasan A, Kraus CN, DeShazer D, et al: Glanders in a military research microbiologist. *N Engl J Med* 2001;345:256–8.

Chapter 189
Tularemia (*Francisella tularensis*) *Gordon E. Schutze and Richard F. Jacobs*

Tularemia is a zoonotic infection caused by the gram-negative bacterium *Francisella tularensis*. Tularemia is primarily a disease of wild animals; human disease is incidental and usually results from contact with blood-sucking insects or wild animals. The illness caused by *F. tularensis* is manifested by different clinical syndromes, the most common of which consists of an ulcerative lesion at the site of inoculation with regional lymphadenopathy or lymphadenitis.

Etiology. *F. tularensis*, the causative agent of tularemia, is a small, nonmotile, pleomorphic, gram-negative coccobacillus. The two main biovars are *F. tularensis* biovar *tularensis* (Jellison type A) and *F. tularensis* biovar *palearctica* (Jellison type B). Type A produces more serious disease in humans and is most commonly found in North America; type B may be found in North America, Europe, and Asia and produces a less virulent disease. Type A is associated with ticks and lagomorphs (i.e., rabbits, hares); type B can be associated with mosquitoes, rodents, and water and marine animals.

Epidemiology. During 1990–2000, a total of 1,368 cases of tularemia were reported in the United States from 44 states, averaging 124 cases (range: 86–193) per year (Fig. 189–1). Four states accounted for 56% of all reported tularemia cases: Arkansas, 315 cases (23%); Missouri, 265 cases, (19%); South Dakota, 96 cases (7%); Oklahoma, 90 cases, (7%).

TRANSMISSION. Of all the zoonotic diseases, tularemia is unusual because of the different modes of transmission of disease. A large number of animals serve as a reservoir for this organism, which can penetrate both intact skin and mucous membranes. Transmission can occur through the bite of infected ticks or other biting insects, by contact with infected animals or their carcasses, by consumption of contaminated foods or water, or through inhalation, as might occur in a laboratory setting. This organism is not, however, transmitted from person to person. In the United States, rabbits and ticks are the principal reservoirs. Most disease due to rabbit exposure occurs in the winter, and disease due to tick exposure occurs in the warmer months (April–September). *Amblyomma americanum* (Lone Star tick), *Dermacentor variabilis* (dog tick), and *Dermacentor andersoni* (wood tick) are the most common tick vectors. These ticks usually feed on infected small rodents and later feed on humans. Taking that blood meal through a fecally contaminated field transmits the infection.

Pathogenesis. The most common portal of entry for human infection is through the skin or mucous membrane. This may occur through the bite of an infected insect or by way of inapparent abrasions. Inhalation or ingestion of *F. tularensis* can also result in infection. More than 10^8 organisms are usually required to produce infection if they are ingested, but as few as 10 organisms may cause disease if they are inhaled or injected into the skin. Within 48–72 hr after injection into the skin, an erythematous, tender, or pruritic papule may appear at the portal of entry. This papule may enlarge and form an ulcer with a black base, followed by regional lymphadenopathy. Once *F. tularensis* reaches the lymph nodes, the organism may multiply and form granulomas. Bacteremia may also be present, and although any organ of the body may be involved, the reticuloendothelial system is the most commonly affected.

Conjunctival inoculation may result in infection of the eye with preauricular lymphadenopathy (**Parinaud oculoglandular syndrome**). Inhalation, aerosolization, or hematogenous spread of the organisms can result in pneumonia. Chest roentgenograms of such patients may reveal patchy infiltrates rather than areas of consolidation. Pleural effusions may also be present and may contain blood. In pulmonary infections, mediastinal adenopathy may be present; in oropharyngeal disease, patients may develop cervical lymphadenopathy. Typhoidal tularemia may be used to describe severe bacteremic disease, regardless of the mode of transmission or portal of entry.

Infection with tularemia stimulates the host to produce antibodies. This antibody response, however, has only a minor role in fighting this infection. The body is dependent on cell-mediated immunity to contain and eradicate this infection. Infection is usually followed by specific protection; thus, chronic infection or reinfection is unlikely.

Clinical Manifestations. Although it may vary, the average incubation period from infection until clinical symptoms appear is 3 days (range, 1–21 days). A sudden onset of fever with other associated symptoms is common (Table 189–1). Physical examination may include lymphadenopathy, hepatosplenomegaly, or skin lesions. Various skin lesions have been described, including erythema multiforme and erythema nodosum. Approximately 20% of patients may develop a generalized maculopapular rash that occasionally becomes pustular. These clinical manifestations of tularemia have been divided into various syndromes (Table 189–2).

Ulceroglandular and glandular disease are the two most common forms of tularemia diagnosed in children. The most common glands involved are usually the cervical or posterior auricular nodes owing to a tick bite on the head or neck. If an ulcer is present, it is erythematous and painful and may last from 1–3 wk. The ulcer is located at the portal of entry. After the ulcer develops, regional lymphadenopathy ensues. These nodes

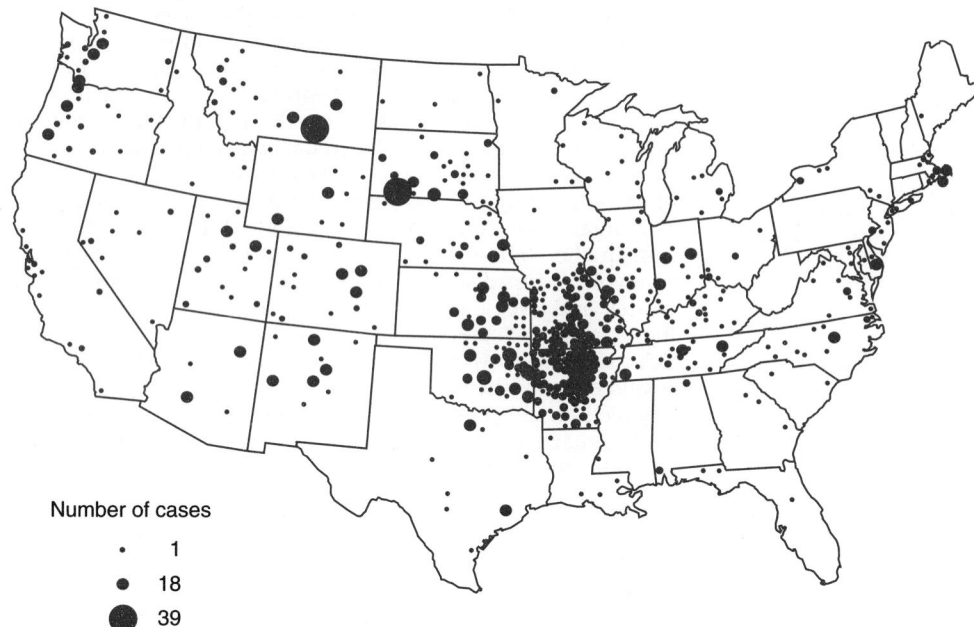

FIGURE 189–1. Reported cases of tularemia in the United States from 1990–2000, based on 1,347 patients reporting county of residence in the lower continental Unites States. Alaska reported ten cases in four counties during 1990–2000. The circle size is proportional to the number of cases, ranging from 1–39 cases. (From Centers for Disease Control and Prevention: Tularemia—United States, 1990–2000. *MMWR* 2002;51:181–4.)

Number of cases

· 1
● 18
● 39

TABLE 189–1.   Common Clinical Manifestations of Tularemia in Children

Sign or Symptom	Frequency (%)
Lymphadenopathy	96
Fever (>38.3°C)	87
Ulcer/eschar/papule	45
Pharyngitis	43
Myalgias/arthralgias	39
Nausea/vomiting	35
Hepatosplenomegaly	35

TABLE 189–2.   Clinical Syndromes of Tularemia in Children

Clinical Syndrome	Frequency (%)
Ulceroglandular	45
Glandular	25
Pneumonia	14
Oropharyngeal	4
Oculoglandular	2
Typhoidal	2
Other*	6

Includes meningitis, pericarditis, hepatitis, peritonitis, endocarditis, osteomyelitis.

may vary in size from 0.5–10 cm and may appear singly or in clusters. These affected nodes may become fluctuant and drain spontaneously, but most usually resolve with treatment. Late suppuration of the involved nodes has been described in 25–30% of patients despite effective therapy. Examination of this material from such lymph nodes usually reveals sterile necrotic material.

Pneumonia due to *F. tularensis* usually presents as variable parenchymal infiltrates that are unresponsive to β-lactam antimicrobial agents. Inhalation-related infection has been described in laboratory workers who are working with the organism; it results in a relatively high mortality rate. Aerosols from farming activities involving rodent contamination (e.g., haying, threshing)

or carcass destruction with lawnmowers have been reported to cause pneumonia as well. Patchy parenchymal infiltrates can also be demonstrated in other forms of tularemia. Patchy segmental infiltrates, hilar adenopathy, and pleural effusions are the most common abnormalities demonstrated on chest roentgenograms. Patients may also complain of a nonproductive cough, dyspnea, or pleuritic chest pain.

Oropharyngeal tularemia results from consumption of poorly cooked meats or contaminated water. This syndrome is characterized by acute pharyngitis, with or without tonsillitis, and cervical adenitis. Infected tonsils may become large and develop a yellowish-white membrane that may resemble the membranes associated with diphtheria. Gastrointestinal disease may also occur and usually presents with mild, unexplained diarrhea but may progress to rapidly fulminant and fatal disease.

Oculoglandular tularemia is uncommon, but when it does occur, the portal of entry is the conjunctiva. Contact with contaminated fingers or debris from crushed insects is the most common way of applying the organisms to the conjunctiva. The conjunctiva is painful and inflamed, with yellowish nodules and pinpoint ulcerations. This purulent conjunctivitis with regional lymphadenopathy (ipsilateral preauricular or submandibular nodes) is referred to as Parinaud oculoglandular syndrome.

Typhoidal tularemia is usually associated with a large inoculum of organisms and usually presents with fever, headaches, and signs or symptoms of endotoxemia. Patients typically are critically ill, and symptoms mimic those with other forms of sepsis. Clinicians practicing in tularemia-endemic regions must always consider this diagnosis in critically ill children.

Diagnosis. The history and physical examination of the patient may suggest the diagnosis of tularemia, especially if the patient lives in or has visited an endemic region. A history of animal or tick exposure may be especially helpful. Hematologic blood tests are nondiagnostic. Results of routine cultures and smears are positive in only approximately 10% of cases. *F. tularensis* can be cultured in the microbiology laboratory on cysteine-glucose-blood agar, but care should be taken to alert the personnel in the laboratory if this is attempted so they can take the proper precautions to protect themselves from acquiring infection.

The diagnosis of tularemia is most commonly established through the use of a standard and highly reliable serum agglutination test. In the standard tube agglutination test, a single titer of ≥1:160 in a patient with a compatible history and physical findings can establish the diagnosis. A fourfold increase in titer from paired serum samples collected 2–3 wk apart is also diagnostic. False-negative serologic responses can be obtained early in the infection, and as many as 30% of individuals require longer than 3 wk before testing positive. Once infected, patients may have a positive agglutination test result (1:20–1:80) that may persist for a lifetime.

Other testing techniques available include a microagglutination test, an enzyme-linked immunosorbent assay, an analysis of urine for tularemia antigen, and polymerase chain reaction. These techniques may become more popular in the future but at this time have a limited role in establishing the diagnosis of tularemia.

DIFFERENTIAL DIAGNOSIS. The differential diagnosis of ulceroglandular or glandular tularemia includes cat-scratch disease *(Bartonella henselae)*; infectious mononucleosis; Kawasaki syndrome; lymphadenopathy due to *Staphylococcus aureus*, group A streptococcus, *Mycobacterium tuberculosis*, *Toxoplasma gondii*, and the nontuberculous mycobacteria, along with *Sporothrix schenckii*; plague; anthrax; melioidosis; and rat-bite fever. Oculoglandular disease may also occur with other infectious agents, such as *B. henselae*, *Treponema pallidum*, *Coccidioides immitis*, herpes simplex virus, adenovirus, and the bacterial agents responsible for purulent conjunctivitis. Oropharyngeal tularemia must be differentiated from the same diseases that cause ulceroglandular/glandular disease and from cytomegalovirus, herpes simplex, adenovirus, and other viral or bacterial etiologies. Pneumonic tularemia must be differentiated from the other non–β-lactam-responsive organisms such as *Mycoplasma*, *Chlamydia*, mycobacteria, fungi, and rickettsia. Typhoidal tularemia must be differentiated from other forms of sepsis as well as from enteric fever (typhoid and paratyphoid fever) and brucellosis.

Treatment. All strains of *F. tularensis* are susceptible to gentamicin and streptomycin. Gentamicin (5 m/kg/24 hr divided bid or tid IV or IM) has become the drug of choice for the treatment of tularemia in children because of the limited availability of streptomycin (30–40 mg/kg/24 hr divided bid IM) and the fewer adverse effects of gentamicin. Therapy is typically continued for 7–10 days, but in mild cases, 5–7 days may be sufficient. Chloramphenicol and tetracyclines have been used in the past, but the high relapse rate has limited their use in children. Early data suggested that *F. tularensis* would be susceptible to the third-generation cephalosporins (e.g., cefotaxime, ceftriaxone), but clinical case reports demonstrate a nearly universal failure rate with these agents. Quinolones are active against *F. tularemia* and have been used for treatment of the milder form of tularemia due to the European biovar *F. tularensis* biovar *palearctica*. Further data are required before quinolone therapy can be recommended for the most common biovar encountered in North America, *F. tularensis* biovar *tularensis*.

Patients typically have defervescence within 24–48 hr after starting therapy, and relapses are uncommon if gentamicin or streptomycin is used. Patients who have not started on appropriate therapy early may respond more slowly to antimicrobial therapy. Late suppuration of involved lymph nodes may occur despite adequate therapy but usually contains sterile material.

Prognosis. Poor outcomes are associated with a delay in recognition and treatment, but with rapid recognition and treatment fatalities are exceedingly rare. The mortality rate for severe untreated disease (e.g., pneumonia, typhoidal disease) can be as high as 30% in these situations, but in general, the overall mortality rate is <1%.

Prevention. Prevention of tularemia is based on avoiding exposure. Children living in tick-endemic regions should be taught to avoid tick-infested areas, and families should have a tick control plan for their immediate environment and for their pets. Protective clothing should be worn when entering a tick-infested area, but more importantly, children should undergo frequent tick checks during and after their time in these areas. Skin repellents such as *N-N*-diethyl-M-toluamide (DEET) can be used but have been described to cause systemic reactions if used incorrectly on small infants. Avoiding taking young infants into tick-endemic regions is the most prudent approach. If DEET-containing compounds are used, they should be used sparingly on the exposed skin, avoiding the hands and face. The repellent should be washed off completely after leaving the high-risk region. Clothing repellents that use permethrin have been demonstrated to be an effective addition to the use of protective clothing. If ticks are found on the child, forceps should be used to pull the tick straight out. The skin should be cleansed before and after this procedure.

Children should also be taught to avoid sick and dead animals. Dogs and cats are most likely to bring these animals to a child's attention. Children should be encouraged to wear gloves while cleaning wild game. A vaccine is available for adults with high-risk vocations (e.g., veterinarians), but there are no recommendations for use in children. Prophylactic antimicrobial agents are not effective in preventing tularemia and should not be used after exposure.

Centers for Disease Control and Prevention: Tularemia—United States, 1990–2000. *MMWR* 2002;51:181–4.

Cross JT, Schutze GE, Jacobs RF: Treatment of tularemia with gentamicin in pediatric patients. *Pediatr Infect Dis J* 1995;14:151–2.

Enderlin G, Morales L, Jacobs RF, et al: Streptomycin and alternative agents for the treatment of tularemia: Review of the literature. *Clin Infect Dis* 1994;19:42–7.

Jacobs RF, Narain JP: Tularemia in children. *Pediatr Infect Dis J* 1983;2:487–91.

Johansson A, Berglund L, Gothefors L, et al: Ciprofloxacin for treatment of tularemia in children. *Pediatr Infect Dis J* 2000;19:449–53.

Sotiropoulos SV: Tularemia. *Semin Pediatr Infect Dis* 1994;5:102–7.

Chapter 190

Brucella Gordon E. Schutze and Richard F. Jacobs

Human brucellosis, caused by organisms of the genus *Brucella*, continues to be a major public health problem worldwide. Humans are accidental hosts and acquire this zoonotic disease from direct contact with an infected animal or consumption of products of an infected animal. Although brucellosis is widely recognized as an occupational risk among adults working with livestock, much of the brucellosis in children is food-borne and is associated with consumption of unpasteurized milk products.

Etiology. *Brucella abortus* (cattle), *B. melitensis* (goat/sheep), *B. suis* (swine), and *B. canis* (dog) are the most common organisms responsible for human disease. These organisms are small, aerobic, non–spore-forming, nonmotile, gram-negative coccobacillary bacteria that are fastidious in their growth but can be grown on various laboratory media including blood and chocolate agars. When brucellosis is suspected, however, the clinical laboratory should be alerted so the cultures can be maintained for ≥21 days to ensure growth if the organism is present.

Epidemiology. Brucellosis exists worldwide but is especially prevalent in the Mediterranean basin, Arabian Gulf, the Indian subcontinent, and parts of Mexico and Central and South America. In industrialized countries, recreational or occupational exposure to infected animals is a major risk factor for the development of disease. Among children, however, geographic locations that are endemic for *B. melitensis* remain areas of increased risk for the development of infection. In such locations, unpasteurized milk from goats or camels may be used to feed children, thus leading to the development of brucellosis. Consequently, a history of travel to endemic regions or consumption of exotic food or unpasteurized dairy or dairy products may be an important clue to the diagnosis of human brucellosis.

Pathogenesis. Routes of infection for these organisms include inoculation through cuts or abrasions in the skin, inoculation of the conjunctival sac of the eye, inhalation of infectious aerosols, or ingestion of contaminated meat or dairy products. The risk of infection depends on the nutritional and immune status of the host, the route of inoculum, and the species of *Brucella*. For reasons that remain unclear, *B. melitensis* and *B. suis* tend to be more virulent than *B. abortus* or *B. canis*.

The major virulence factor for *Brucella* appears to be its cell wall lipopolysaccharide. Strains containing smooth lipopolysaccharide have been demonstrated to have greater virulence and are more resistant to killing by polymorphonuclear leukocytes. These organisms are facultative intracellular pathogens that can survive and replicate within the mononuclear phagocytic cells (monocytes, macrophages) of the reticuloendothelial system. Even though *Brucella* are chemotactic for leukocytes entry into the body, the leukocytes are less efficient in killing these organisms than other bacteria despite the assistance of serum factors such as complement.

Organisms that are not phagocytosed by the leukocytes are ingested by the macrophages and become localized within the reticuloendothelial system. Specifically, they reside within the liver, spleen, lymph nodes, and bone marrow and result in granuloma formation. Antibodies are produced against the lipopolysaccharide and other cell wall antigens. This provides a means of diagnosis and probably has a role in long-term immunity. The major factor in recovery from infection appears to be development of a cell-mediated response resulting in macrophage activation and enhanced intracellular killing. Specifically, sensitized T lymphocytes release cytokines (e.g., interferon-γ and tumor necrosis factor α), which activate the macrophages and enhance their intracellular killing capacity.

Clinical Manifestations. Brucellosis is a systemic illness that can be very difficult to diagnose in children without a history of animal or food exposure. Symptoms can be acute or insidious in nature and are usually nonspecific, beginning 2–4 wk after inoculation. Although the clinical manifestations do vary, the classic triad of fever, arthralgia/arthritis, and hepatosplenomegaly can be demonstrated in most patients. Other associated symptoms include abdominal pain, headache, diarrhea, rash, night sweats, weakness/fatigue, vomiting, cough, and pharyngitis. A common constellation of symptoms in children is refusal to eat, lassitude, refusal to bear weight, and failure to thrive. Besides hepatosplenomegaly, the physical findings on examination are usually few, with the exception of arthritis. The fever pattern can vary widely, and virtually any organ or tissue can be involved.

If abnormalities are demonstrated on physical examination, the bones and joint frequently are involved, with the sacroiliac joint as well as the hips, knees, and ankles being the most common. Although headache, mental inattention, and depression may be demonstrated in patients with brucellosis, invasion of the nervous system occurs in only about 1% of cases. Neonatal and congenital infections with these organisms have also been described. These have been transmitted transplacentally, from breast milk, and through blood transfusions. The signs and symptoms associated with this infection are very vague and nonpathognomonic.

Diagnosis. Routine laboratory examinations of the blood are not helpful, with the exception of the white blood cell count, which may be low or normal. A history of exposure to animals or ingestion of unpasteurized dairy products may be more helpful. A definitive diagnosis is established by recovering the organisms in the blood, bone marrow, or other tissues. Although automated culture systems and the use of the lysis-centrifugation method have shortened the isolation time from weeks to days, it is prudent to alert the clinical microbiology laboratory that brucellosis is suspected. Isolation of the organism still may require as long as 4 wk from a blood culture sample. Caution is also advised when using automated bacterial identification systems, because isolates have been misidentified as other gram-negative organisms (e.g., *Haemophilus influenzae* type b).

In the absence of positive culture results, various serologic tests have been applied to the diagnosis of brucellosis. The serum agglutination test (SAT) is the most widely used and detects antibodies against *B. abortus*, *B. melitensis*, and *B. suis*. This method does not detect antibodies against *B. canis* because this organism lacks the smooth lipopolysaccharide. No single titer is ever diagnostic, but most patients with acute infections have titers of ≥1:160. Low titers may be found early in the course of the illness, requiring the use of acute and convalescent sera testing to confirm the diagnosis. Because patients with active infection have both an IgM and an IgG response and the SAT measures the total quantity of agglutinating antibodies, the total quantity of IgG is measured by treatment of the serum with 2-mercaptoethanol. This fractionation is important in determining the significance of the antibody titer because low levels of IgM can remain in the serum for weeks to months after the infection has been treated. It is important to remember that all titers must be interpreted in light of a patient's history and physical examination. False-positive results due to cross-reacting antibodies to other gram-negative organisms such as *Yersinia enterocolitica*, *Francisella tularensis*, and *Vibrio cholerae* can occur. In addition, the prozone effect can give false-negative results in the presence of high titers of antibody. To avoid this issue, serum that is being tested should be diluted to ≥1:320.

Among newer tests, the enzyme immunoassay appears to be the most sensitive method for detecting *Brucella* antibodies. Polymerase chain reaction assays are also becoming available but at this time are mostly limited to research facilities.

DIFFERENTIAL DIAGNOSIS. Brucellosis may be confused with other infections such as tularemia, cat-scratch disease, typhoid fever, and fungal infections due to histoplasmosis, blastomycosis, or coccidioidomycosis. Infections due to *Mycobacterium tuberculosis*, atypical mycobacteria, rickettsiae, and *Yersinia* can present in a similar fashion to brucellosis.

Treatment. Many antimicrobial agents are active in vitro against the *Brucella* species, but the clinical effectiveness does not always correlate with these results. Doxycycline is the most useful antimicrobial agent and, when combined with an aminoglycoside, is associated with the fewest relapses (Table 190–1). Treatment failures with β-lactam antimicrobial agents, including the third-generation cephalosporins, may be due to the intracellular nature of the organism. Agents that provide intracellular killing are required for eradication of this infection. Similarly, it is apparent that prolonged treatment is the key to preventing disease relapse. Relapse is confirmed by isolation of *Brucella* within weeks to months after therapy has ended and is usually not associated with antimicrobial resistance.

The onset of initial antimicrobial therapy may precipitate a Jarisch-Herxheimer–like reaction presumably due to a large antigen load. It is rarely severe enough to require corticosteroid therapy.

Prognosis. Before the use of antimicrobial agents, the course of brucellosis was often prolonged and may have led to death. Since the institution of specific therapy, most deaths are due to specific organ system involvement (e.g., endocarditis) in complicated cases. The prognosis after specific therapy is excellent if patients are compliant with the prolonged therapy.

TABLE 190–1. Recommended Therapy for the Treatment of Brucellosis

Age and Condition	Antimicrobial Agent	Dose	Route	Duration
≥ 9 yr	Doxycycline +	200 mg/24 hr	PO	6 wk
	Streptomycin or	1 g/24 hr	IM	1–2 wk
	Gentamicin *Alternative:*	3–5 mg/kg/24 hr	IM/IV	1–2 wk
	Doxycycline +	200 mg/24 hr	PO	6 wk
< 9 yr	Rifampin TMP-SMZ	600–900 mg/24 hr Trimethoprim (10 mg/kg/24 hr; maximum: 480 mg/24 hr) and sulfamethoxazole (50 mg/kg/24 hr; maximum: 2.4 gr/24 hr)	PO PO	6 wk 45 days
	+ Rifampin	+ 15–20 mg/kg/24 hr	PO	45 days
Meningitis, osteomyelitis, endocarditis	Doxycycline +	200 mg/24 hr	PO	4–6 mo
	Gentamicin +/–	3–5 mg/kg/24 hr	IV	4–6 mo
	Rifampin	Same as above	PO	4–6 mo

Prevention. Prevention of brucellosis is dependent on effective eradication of the organism from cattle, goats, and swineherds as well as from other animals. Pasteurization of milk and dairy products for human consumption remains an important aspect of prevention. No vaccine currently exists for use in children; therefore, education of the public continues to have a prominent role in prevention of this disease.

Al-Kharfy TM: Neonatal brucellosis and blood transfusion: Case report and review of the literature. *Ann Trop Pediatr* 2001;21:349–52.

Araj GF. Human brucellosis: A classical infectious disease with persistent diagnostic challenges. *Clin Lab Science* 1999;12:207–12.

Ariza J, Corredoira J, Pallares R, et al: Characteristics of and risk factors for relapse of brucellosis in humans. *Clin Infect Dis* 1995;20:1241–9.

Gottesman G, Vanunu D, Maayan MC, et al: Childhood brucellosis in Israel. *Pediatr Infect Dis J* 1996;15:610–5.

Khuri-Bulos NA, Daoud AH, Azab SM: Treatment of childhood brucellosis: Results of a prospective trial on 113 children. *Pediatr Infect Dis J* 1993;12:377–81.

Lubani MM, Dudin KI, Sharda DC, et al: A multicenter therapeutic study of 1100 children with brucellosis. *Pediatr Infect Dis J* 1989;8:75–8.

Young EJ: An overview of human brucellosis. *Clin Infect Dis* 1995;21:283–90.

Young EJ: Serologic diagnosis of human brucellosis: Analysis of 214 cases by agglutination tests and review of the literature. *Rev Infect Dis* 1991;13:359–72.

Chapter 191
Legionella Lucy Tompkins

Legionellosis comprises **legionnaires' disease** (pneumonia), other invasive extrapulmonary infections, and an acute flulike illness known as **Pontiac fever**. In contrast to the syndromes associated with invasive disease, Pontiac fever is a self-limiting illness that develops after aerosol exposure and may represent a toxic or hypersensitivity response to *Legionella*.

Etiology. Legionellaceae are aerobic, non–spore-forming unencapsulated gram-negative bacilli that stain poorly with Gram stain when performed on smears from clinical specimens. Microorganisms in tissue can be better visualized with the Gimenez or silver stains (Dieterle or Warthin-Starry). Stained smears of *Legionella pneumophila* taken from colonial growth resemble *Pseudomonas*. Unlike other *Legionella* species, *L. micdadei* stains acid fast. Although more than 30 species of the genus have now been identified, the majority (90%) of clinical infections are caused by *L. pneumophila*, and most of the remainder are caused by *L. micdadei, L. bozemanii, L. dumoffii,* and *L. longbeachae*.

The organisms are fastidious and require L-cysteine, ferric ion, and α-keto acids for growth. Colonies develop within 3–5 days on buffered charcoal yeast extract agar, which may contain selected antibiotics to inhibit overgrowth by other microorganisms; *Legionella* rarely grows on routine laboratory media.

Epidemiology. Fresh water (e.g., lakes, streams, thermally polluted waters, potable water) is the environmental reservoir of *Legionella* in nature, and invasive pneumonia (legionnaires' disease) is related to exposure to potable water or to aerosols containing the bacteria. Growth of *Legionella* occurs more readily in hot water, and exposure to warm water sources is an important risk factor for disease. *Legionella* organisms are facultative intracellular parasites and grow inside protozoans present in biofilms consisting of organic and inorganic material found in plumbing and water storage tanks and various other bacterial species. Sporadic cases of community-acquired legionnaires' disease can be attributed to potable water in the local environment of the patient. Risk factors for acquisition of sporadic community-acquired pneumonia include nonmunicipal water supply, residential plumbing repairs, and lower water heater temperatures, which facilitate growth of bacteria or lead to release of a bolus of biofilm containing *Legionella* into potable water. The mode of transmission may be by way of inhalation of aerosols or by aspiration. Outbreaks of legionnaires' disease have been associated with protozoans in the implicated water source; replication within these eukaryotic cells presumably amplifies and maintains *Legionella* within the potable water distribution system. Outbreaks of community-acquired pneumonia and some nosocomial outbreaks have been linked to common sources, including potable hot water heaters, evaporative condensers cooling towers, whirlpool baths, humidifiers, and nebulizers.

Hospital-acquired infections are most often linked to potable water. Exposure may occur through two general mechanisms: (1) aspiration of ingested microorganisms, including those in gastric feedings, that are mixed with contaminated tap water; and (2) aerosols from showers and sinks. Extrapulmonary legionellosis may occur through topical application of contaminated tap water into surgical or traumatic wounds. In contrast to legionnaires' disease, Pontiac fever outbreaks have occurred through exposure to aerosols from whirlpool baths, ultrasonic humidifiers, and ventilation systems.

The incidence of community-acquired legionnaires' disease caused by *L. pneumophila* occurring sporadically in adults is estimated at 7–20 cases/100,000 per year and demonstrates geographic differences. *Legionella* infections have no seasonal pattern. Approximately 0.5–5.0% of those exposed to a common source develop pneumonia, whereas the attack rate in Pontiac fever outbreaks is very high (85–100%). In one large community-based study of adults, *Legionella* was associated with 3% of pneumonia cases. Taken together, *Mycoplasma pneumoniae*, *Chlamydia pneumoniae*, and *L. pneumophila* accounted for 10–38% of all community-acquired pneumonia. Therefore, current clinical guidelines for community-acquired pneumonia recommend empirical therapy with macrolides or quinolones.

As estimated by seroconversion to *L. pneumophila* among children hospitalized with pneumonia, the legionnaires' disease rate was found to be quite low. Community-acquired pneumonia occurs most often in children >4 yr of age. Most nosocomial infections have been reported as case reports; therefore, the true incidence of disease in children is unknown. Nosocomial infection rates in adults are difficult to determine because many hospital laboratories do not attempt to isolate *Legionella* by culture. Hospital-acquired legionellosis in children is associated with clinical risk factors and with environmental exposure. Acquisition of antibodies to *L. pneumophila* in healthy children occurs progressively over time, although this presumably reflects subclinical infection or mild respiratory disease or antibodies that cross react with other bacterial species.

Pathogenesis. *Legionella* organisms are facultative intracellular parasites of eukaryotic cells. In humans, the target cell is the alveolar macrophage, although other cell types may also be invaded. Although *Legionella* can be grown on artificial media, the intracellular environment provides the definitive site of growth. Growth in macrophages occurs to the point of cell death, followed by reinfection of new cells, until these cells are activated and can subsequently kill intracellular microorganisms. Acute, severe infection of the lung provokes an acute inflammatory response and necrosis; early on, more bacteria are found in extracellular spaces. Subsequently, macrophage activation and other immune responses produce intense infiltration of tissue by macrophages that contain intracellular bacteria. Corticosteroid therapy poses a high risk of infection by interfering with T cell and macrophage function. Legionnaires' disease rarely occurs in healthy immunocompetent patients with no evidence of respiratory tract disease or dysfunction.

Although certain bacterial factors have been postulated to have a role in virulence, the contribution of each of these to overall pathogenesis is unclear. As in other diseases caused by facultative intracellular microorganisms, the outcome is critically dependent on the specific and nonspecific immune responses of the host, in particular, macrophage and T-cell responses.

Clinical Manifestations. Legionnaires' disease was originally believed to cause a clinical syndrome called atypical pneumonia and was associated with extrapulmonary signs and symptoms, including diarrhea, hyponatremia, hypophosphatemia, abnormal results of liver function tests, confusion, and renal dysfunction. Although a subset of patients may exhibit "classic" manifestations, *Legionella* infection typically causes pneumonia that is indistinguishable from disease produced by other infectious agents. Fever, cough, and chest pain are common presenting symptoms; the cough may be productive of purulent sputum or may be nonproductive. Although the classic chest radiographic appearance showed rapidly progressive alveolar filling infiltrates, in usual cases of pneumonia the chest radiographic appearance is widely variable, appearing as tumor-like shadows, evidence of nodular infiltrates, unilateral or bilateral infiltrates, or cavitation, although cavitation is rarely seen in non-immunocompromised patients. This picture overlaps substantially with disease caused by *Streptococcus pneumoniae*. Although pleural effusion is less commonly associated with legionnaires' disease, its frequency varies so widely that neither the presence or absence of effusion is helpful in differential diagnosis. If present, pleural fluid should be obtained for culture.

A few clinical features may help to differentiate *Legionella* pneumonia from other causes. *Legionella* pneumonia produces an acute-onset febrile illness, the radiograph shows alveolar filling infiltrates, and there is no clinical response to broad-spectrum β-lactam (penicillins and cephalosporins) or aminoglycoside antibiotics.

Concomitant infection with other pathogens occurs in 5–10% of cases of legionnaires' disease; therefore, culture of another potential pulmonary pathogen does not preclude the diagnosis of legionellosis.

Reports of nosocomial *Legionella* pneumonia in children demonstrate that rapid onset, temperature greater than 38.5°C, cough, pleuritic chest pain, and dyspnea are present in most. Abdominal pain, headache, and diarrhea are also common. Chest radiographs reveal lobar consolidations or diffuse bilateral infiltrates, and pleural effusions are noted. Symptoms do not respond to treatment with β-lactam antibiotics or aminoglycosides.

Risk factors for legionnaires' disease in adults include chronic diseases of the lung (e.g., smoking, bronchitis), older age, diabetes and renal failure, immunosuppression associated with organ transplantation, corticosteroid therapy, and episodes of aspiration. The number of reported cases of community-acquired legionnaires' disease in children is small. Among these, immunocompromised status, especially corticosteroid treatment, coupled with exposure to contaminated potable water, are the major risk factors. Infection in a few children with chronic pulmonary disease without immune deficiency has also been reported but infection in children lacking any risk factors is very uncommon. The modes of transmission of community-acquired disease in children include exposure to mists, water coolers, and other aerosol-generating apparatuses. Nosocomial *Legionella* infection occurs more frequently than community-acquired disease in children, and the modes of acquisition include microaspiration, frequently associated with nasogastric tubes, and aerosol inhalation. Bronchopulmonary *Legionella* infections occur in patients with cystic fibrosis and have been associated with aerosol therapy or mist tents. Legionnaires' disease is also reported in pediatric patients with asthma and tracheal stenosis. Chronic steroid therapy for asthma is a reported risk factor for *Legionella* infections in children.

Pontiac fever in adults and children is characterized by high fever, myalgia, headache, and extreme debilitation, lasting for a few days. Cough, breathlessness, diarrhea, confusion, and chest pain may occur, but there is no evidence for invasive infection. The disease is self-limited without sequelae. Virtually all exposed individuals seroconvert to *Legionella* antigens. A very large outbreak in Scotland that affected 35 children was attributed to *L. micdadei*, which was isolated from a whirlpool spa. The onset of illness was 1–7 days (median, 3 days), and all exposed children developed significant titers of specific antibodies to *L. micdadei*. The pathogenesis of Pontiac fever is not known. In the absence of evidence of true infection, the most likely hypothesis is that this syndrome is caused by a toxic or hypersensitivity reaction to microbial, or protozoan, antigens.

Diagnosis. Culture of *Legionella* from sputum, other respiratory tract specimens, blood, or tissue is the gold standard against which indirect methods of detection should be compared. Specimens obtained from the respiratory tract that are contaminated with oral flora must be treated and processed to reduce contaminants and plated onto selective media. Because these are costly and time-consuming methods, many laboratories do not process specimens for culture. The urinary antigen assay that detects *L. pneumophila* serogroup I has 80% sensitivity and

99% specificity. Thus, the assay is a useful method in the prompt diagnosis of legionnaires' disease caused by this serogroup, which accounts for the majority of symptomatic infections. In the United States, this test is frequently used because it is widely available in reference laboratories. The microorganisms can also be identified presumptively by direct immunofluorescence antibody screening, although the sensitivity of the test is generally low in most laboratories, in part because of the lack of antisera directed against other *Legionella* serogroups and species. This method failed to detect the infection in several well-documented pediatric cases. Retrospective diagnosis can be made serologically using the indirect immunofluorescence assay to detect specific antibody production. Seroconversion may not occur for several weeks after onset of infection, and the available serologic assays do not detect all strains of *L. pneumophila* or all species. In view of the low sensitivity of direct detection and the slow growth of the microorganism in culture, the diagnosis of legionellosis should be pursued actively when there is suggestive clinical evidence, including the lack of response to "usual" antibiotics, even when results of other laboratory studies are negative.

Treatment. Erythromycin (40 mg/kg/24 hr PO or IV), with or without rifampin (15 mg/kg/24 hr), has been empirically established as effective therapy. The newer macrolides including azithromycin (10 mg/kg on day 1, not to exceed 500 mg/day then 5 mg/kg daily for 4 days, PO) and clarithromycin (15 mg/kg/24 hr PO) and the quinolones (ciprofloxacin, levofloxacin, trovafloxacin, and sparfloxacin) have excellent activity in vitro, although quinolones are not approved for children <18 yr of age. In serious infections or in high-risk patients, parenteral therapy is recommended initially; a switch to oral therapy can be made when a patient has had a clinical response. Acute hearing loss, which is reversible, is associated with high-dose parenteral erythromycin therapy. The duration of therapy for legionnaires' disease is 2–3 wk for erythromycin. Duration of therapy in immunocompetent patients with newer macrolides is 7–10 days. Treatment of extrapulmonary infections, including prosthetic valve endocarditis and sternal wound infections, may require prolonged therapy. Trimethoprim-sulfamethoxazole (TMP-SMZ; 15 mg TMP/kg/24 hr and 75 mg SMZ/kg/24 hr) has been used as an alternative. β-lactams and aminoglycosides and other antibiotics that do not penetrate mammalian cells are not clinically effective. Relapse (recrudescence) may occur after cessation of erythromycin therapy.

Prognosis. The mortality rate of community-acquired legionnaires' disease in adults who are hospitalized is approximately 15%. The prognosis depends on underlying host factors and possibly on the duration of the illness before appropriate therapy is begun. Despite appropriate antibiotic therapy, patients may succumb to respiratory complications, such as acute respiratory distress syndrome, associated with artificial ventilation and intubation. A high mortality rate is noted in case reports of premature infants and children, virtually all of whom have been immunocompromised.

Abernathy-Carver KJ, Fan LL, Boguniewicz M, et al: *Legionella* and *Pneumocystis* pneumonias in asthmatic children on high doses of systemic steroids. *Pediatr Pulmonol* 1994;18:135–8.

Campins M, Ferrer A, Callis L, et al: Nosocomial legionnaire's disease in a children's hospital. *Pediatr Infect Dis J* 2000;19:228–34.

Famiglietti RF, Bakerman PR, Saubolle MA, et al: Cavitary legionellosis in two immunocompetent infants. *Pediatrics* 1997;99:899–903.

Gervaix A, Beghetti M, Rimensberger P, et al: Bullous emphysema after *Legionella* pneumonia in a two-year-old. *Pediatr Infect Dis J* 2000;19:86–7.

Goldberg DJ, Emslie JA, Fallon RJ, et al: Pontiac fever in children. *Pediatr Infect Dis J* 1992;11:240–1.

Green M, Wald ER, Dashefsky B, et al: Field inversion gel electrophoretic analysis of *Legionella pneumophila* strains associated with nosocomial legionellosis in children. *J Clin Microbiol* 1996;34:175–6.

Holmberg RE Jr, Pavia AT, Montgomery D, et al: Nosocomial *Legionella* pneumonia in the neonate. *Pediatrics* 1993;92:450–3.

Levy I, Rubin LG: *Legionella* pneumonia in neonates: A literature review. *J Perinatol* 1998;18:287–90.

Luck PC, Dinger E, Helbig JH, et al: Analysis of *Legionella pneumophila* strains associated with nosocomial pneumonia in a neonatal intensive care unit. *Eur J Clin Microbiol Infect Dis* 1994;13:565–71.

Luttichau HR, Vinther C, Uldum SA, et al: An outbreak of Pontiac fever among children following use of a whirlpool. *Clin Infect Dis* 1998;26:1374–8.

Chapter 192

Bartonella Barbara W. Stechenberg

The spectrum of disease resulting from human infection with *Bartonella* species has expanded rapidly in the past 2 decades, including the association of bacillary angiomatosis with AIDS and cat-scratch disease (CSD) with the fastidious gram-negative rod initially identified as *Rochalimaea henselae*. However, like *Bartonella bacilliformis*, which has been identified for many years, *Rochalimaea* species grow on the surface of eukaryotic host cells and on blood agar. On the basis of these findings, 16S ribosomal RNA gene sequencing, and other molecular genetic homologies, the *Rochalimaea* genus was transferred to the genus *Bartonella*, as part of the alpha subdivision of proteobacteria. Five major *Bartonella* species have been found to be pathogenic for humans: *B. bacilliformis*, *B. henselae*, *B. quintana*, *B. elizabethae*, and most recently *B. clarridgeiae*. Several other *Bartonella* species have been found in animals, particularly rodents and moles (Table 192–1).

Members of the genus *Bartonella* are gram-negative, oxidase-negative, fastidious aerobic rods that ferment no carbohydrates. Only one species, *B. bacilliformis*, is motile by means of polar flagella. Optimal growth is obtained on fresh media containing 5% or more sheep or horse blood in the presence of 5% carbon dioxide. The use of lysis-centrifugation for specimens from blood on chocolate agar for extended periods (2–6 wk) enhances recovery.

192.1 Bartonellosis (*Bartonella bacilliformis*)

The first human *Bartonella* infection described was bartonellosis, a geographically distinct disease caused by *B. bacilliformis*, which causes two predominant forms of illness: **Oroya fever**, a severe, febrile hemolytic anemia; and **verruca peruana (verruga peruana)**, an eruption of hemangioma-like lesions. The organism also causes asymptomatic infection. Bartonellosis is also called **Carrión disease** in honor of the Peruvian medical student who inoculated himself with blood from a verruca and 21 days later developed Oroya fever. He died 39 days after inoculation, thus proving the unitary etiology of the two clinical illnesses.

Etiology. *B. bacilliformis* is a small, motile gram-negative organism with a brush of 10 or more unipolar flagella, which appear to be important components for invasiveness. An obligate aerobe, it grows best at 28°C in semisolid nutrient agar containing rabbit serum and hemoglobin.

Epidemiology. Bartonellosis is a zoonosis found only in mountain valleys of the Andes Mountains in Peru, Ecuador, Colombia, Chile, and Bolivia at altitudes and environmental conditions favorable for the vector, which is the sandfly, *Lutzomyia verrucarum*.

Pathogenesis. After the bite, *Bartonella* organisms enter the endothelial cells of blood vessels, where they proliferate. Found throughout the reticuloendothelial system, they then re-enter the bloodstream and parasitize the erythrocytes. They bind on the cells, deform the membranes, and then enter intracellular

TABLE 192–1. *Bartonella* Causing Human Disease

Disease	Organism	Vector	Primary Risk Factor
Angiomatosis	*B. bacilli formis*	Human body louse	Immunocompromised
Bartonellosis	*B. bacilliformis*	Sandfly (*Lutzomyia verrucarum*)	Living in endemic area (Andes Mountains)
Cat-scratch disease	*B. henselae*	Cat	Cat scratch or bite
	B. clarridgeiae (1 case)		
Trench fever	*B. quintana*	Human body louse	Body louse infestation during outbreak
Bacteremia, endocarditis	*B. henselae*	Cat for *B. henselae*	Severely immunocompromised
	B. quintana		
	B. elizabethae		
Bacillary angiomatosis	*B. henselae*	Cat for *B. henselae*	Severely immunocompromised
	B. quintana		
Peliosis hepatis	*B. henselae*	Cat for *B. henselae*	Severely immunocompromised
	B. quintana		

vacuoles. The resultant hemolytic anemia may involve as many as 90% of the erythrocytes. Patients who survive this acute phase may or may not develop the cutaneous manifestations, which are nodular hemangiomatous lesions or verrucae ranging in size from a few millimeters to several centimeters.

Clinical Manifestations. The incubation period is 2–14 wk. Patients may be totally asymptomatic or may have nonspecific symptoms such as headache and malaise without anemia. Patients with Oroya fever are febrile, with rapid development of anemia. Clouding of the sensorium and delirium are common symptoms and may progress to overt psychosis. Physical examination demonstrates signs of severe anemia, icterus, and pallor, which may be associated with generalized lymphadenopathy.

In the pre-eruptive stage, patients may complain of arthralgias, myalgias, and paresthesias. Inflammatory reactions such as phlebitis, pleuritis, erythema nodosum, and encephalitis may develop. The appearance of verrucae is pathognomonic of the eruptive phase. They vary greatly in size and number.

Diagnosis. The diagnosis is established on clinical grounds in conjunction with a blood smear demonstrating organisms, or by blood culture. The anemia is macrocytic and hypochromic, with reticulocyte counts as high as 50%. *B. bacilliformis* may be seen on Giemsa stain as red-violet rods in the erythrocytes. In the recovery phase, these organisms change to a mere coccoid form and disappear from the blood. In the absence of anemia, the diagnosis depends on blood cultures. In the eruptive phase, the typical verruca confirms the diagnosis. Antibody testing has been used to document infection.

Treatment. *B. bacilliformis* is sensitive to many antibiotics, including rifampin, tetracycline, and chloramphenicol. Treatment is very effective in rapidly diminishing fever and eradicating the organism from the blood. Chloramphenicol (50–75 mg/kg/24 hr) is considered the drug of choice, because it also is useful in the treatment of concomitant infections such as *Salmonella*. Blood transfusions and supportive care are critical in patients with severe anemia. Treatment for verruca peruana is not necessary unless large lesions are disfiguring or interfere with function; then, surgical excision may be needed. Oral tetracycline, rifampin, or quinolones may aid in healing of lesions.

Prevention. Prevention depends on avoidance of the vector, particularly at night, by the use of protective clothing and insect repellents (Chapter 285).

192.2 Cat-Scratch Disease (*Bartonella henselae*)

The most common presentation of *Bartonella* infection is CSD, a subacute, regional lymphadenitis caused by *B. henselae*. It is the most common cause of chronic lymphadenitis that persists for >3 wk.

Etiology. In 1983, small pleomorphic gram-negative bacilli were first visualized by Warthin-Starry stain in affected lymph nodes from patients with CSD. A putative causative organism, *Afipia felis*, was cultured and initially presumed to be the agent of CSD, but most patients with CSD did not develop an immune response to this organism. *A. felis* has not been cultured from lymph node tissue of a patient with CSD. In 1992, *B. henselae* was cultured from the blood of a healthy cat and was used in serologic studies that indicated *B. henselae* as the cause of CSD. Development of serologic tests that showed prevalence of antibodies in 84–100% of cases of CSD, culturing of *B. henselae* from CSD nodes, and detection of *B. henselae* by polymerase chain reaction in the majority of lymph node samples and pus from patients with CSD confirmed the organism as the cause of CSD. Occasional cases of CSD may be caused by other organisms; one report described a veterinarian with CSD caused by *B. clarridgeiae*.

Epidemiology. CSD is common, with more than 24,000 estimated cases per year in the United States. It is transmitted by cutaneous inoculation. Most (87–99%) patients have had contact with cats, many of which are kittens younger than 6 mo. More than 50% have a definite history of a cat scratch or bite. Cats have a high-level *Bartonella* bacteremia for months without any clinical symptoms; kittens are more frequently bacteremic than adult cats. The precise mechanism of cat-to-human transmission remains unclear. Transmission between cats is arthropod-borne by the cat flea, *Ctenocephalides felis*. In temperate zones, the majority of cases occur between September and March. This may be related to the seasonal breeding of domestic cats or to close proximity to family pets in the fall and winter. In tropical zones, there is no seasonal prevalence. Distribution is worldwide and infection occurs in all races.

Cat scratches appear to be more common among children, and boys are affected more often than girls. CSD is a sporadic illness; only one family member usually is affected, even though many siblings play with the same kitten. However, clusters do occur with family cases within weeks of one another. Anecdotal reports have implicated other sources such as dog scratches, wood splinters, fishhooks, cactus spines, and porcupine quills.

Pathogenesis. The pathologic findings in the primary inoculation papule and affected lymph nodes are similar. Both show a central avascular necrotic area with surrounding lymphocytes, giant cells, and histiocytes. Three stages of involvement occur in affected nodes, although they may coexist in the same node. First is generalized enlargement with thickening of the cortex and germinal center hypertrophy. Lymphocytes predominate. Epithelioid granulomas with Langhans' giant cells are scattered throughout the node. In the middle stage, granulomas become denser, fuse, and become infiltrated with polymorphonuclear leukocytes. Central necrosis of these granulomas begins in this stage, progressing to the last stage with formation of large pus-filled sinuses. This purulent material may rupture into surrounding tissue. Similar granulomas have been found in the liver and osteolytic lesions of bone when those organs are involved.

Clinical Manifestations. After an incubation period of 7–12 days (range 3–30 days), one or more 3–5 mm red papules develop at the site of cutaneous inoculation, often reflecting a linear cat scratch. Because of their small size, these lesions are often overlooked but with careful search are found in at least two thirds of patients. Lymphadenopathy generally is evident within a period of 1–4 wk. Chronic regional lymphadenitis is the hallmark, affecting the first or second set of nodes draining the entry site. Affected lymph nodes in order of frequency include the axillary, cervical, submandibular, preauricular, epitrochlear, femoral, and inguinal nodes. Involvement of more than one group occurs in 10–20% of patients, although at a given site, half the cases involve several nodes.

Nodes involved are usually tender and have overlying erythema but without cellulitis. They usually range between 1–5 cm in size, although they can become much larger. Between 10–40% eventually suppurate. The duration of enlargement is usually 1–2 mo, with persistence up to 1 yr in rare cases. Fever, usually a temperature of 38–39°C, occurs in about 30% of patients. Other nonspecific symptoms including malaise, anorexia, fatigue, and headache affect less than one third of patients. Transient rashes may occur in about 5% of patients. These consist mainly of truncal maculopapular rashes; erythema nodosum, erythema multiforme and erythema annulare are also reported.

The most common atypical presentation, noted in 2–17% of patients, is **Parinaud occuloglandular syndrome**, which is unilateral conjunctivitis followed by preauricular lymphadenopathy. Direct eye inoculation as a result of rubbing with the hands after cat contact is the presumed mode of spread. A conjunctival granuloma may be found at the inoculation site. The involved eye is usually not painful and has little or no discharge, but it may be quite red and swollen. Submandibular or cervical lymphadenopathy may also occur. CSD is usually a self-limited infection with spontaneous resolution within a few weeks to months.

More severe, disseminated illness occurs in a small percentage of patients. These patients present with high fever often persisting for several weeks. Although systemic symptoms are usually more pronounced than with isolated lymphadenitis, they often seem mild relative to fever, the exception being abdominal pain and weight loss, both of which can be dramatic. Hepatosplenomegaly may occur, although hepatic dysfunction is rare. Granulomatous changes may be seen in the liver and spleen. Another common site of dissemination is bone, with the development of granulomatous osteolytic lesions. These are usually associated with localized pain, without erythema, tenderness, or swelling.

Diagnosis. In most cases, the diagnosis can be strongly suspected on clinical grounds with the history of exposure to a cat. Several serologic assays have been developed. The Centers for Disease Control and Prevention has developed an indirect immunofluorescent assay (IFA) that has shown good correlation with disease. Other IFA and enzyme-linked immunoassay tests are commercially available, although little comparative data are available. Most patients have elevated antibody titers at presentation; however, the timing of IgG and IgM response to *B. henselae* can be quite variable. There is cross reactivity among *Bartonella* species, particularly *B. henselae* and *B. quintana*.

If tissue specimens are obtained, bacilli may be visualized with Warthin-Starry and Brown-Hopp tissue Gram stains. *Bartonella* DNA can be identified by polymerase chain reaction, but this test is not available in most hospitals. Culturing of the organism is not practical for clinical diagnosis.

Use of a skin test antigen prepared by heat-treating purulent aspirate from a CSD node is strongly discouraged because of lack of standardization and potential transmission of infectious agents.

DIFFERENTIAL DIAGNOSIS. The differential diagnosis of CSD includes virtually all causes of lymphadenopathy (Chapter 482). The more common entities include pyogenic lymphadenitis primarily from staphylococcal or streptococcal infections, atypical mycobacterial infections, and malignancy. Less common entities include tularemia, brucellosis, or sporotrichosis. Epstein-Barr virus, cytomegalovirus, or *Toxoplasma gondii* infections usually cause more generalized lymphadenopathy.

Laboratory Findings. Routine laboratory tests are not helpful. The erythrocyte sedimentation rate is often elevated. The white blood cell count may be normal or mildly elevated. Hepatic transaminases may be elevated in systemic disease. Ultrasonography or CT may reveal many granulomatous nodules in the liver and spleen, appearing as hypodense round irregular lesions.

Treatment. Antibiotic treatment of CSD is not clearly beneficial. For most patients, treatment consists of conservative symptomatic care and observation. Studies show a significant discordance between in vitro activity of antibiotics and clinical effectiveness. For many patients, diagnosis is considered in the context of failure to respond to β-lactam antibiotic treatment of presumed staphylococcal lymphadenitis. Azithromycin, clarithromycin, trimethoprim-sulfamethoxazole, rifampin, ciprofloxacin, and gentamicin appear to be the best agents if treatment is considered. A small prospective study of oral azithromycin (500 mg on day 1, then 250 mg on days 2–5; for smaller children, 10 mg/kg/24 hr on day 1 and 5 mg/kg/24 hr day 2–5) showed a decrease in initial lymph node volume in 50% of patients during the first 30 days, but after 30 days there was no difference in lymph node volume. No other clinical benefit was found. It is clear that for the majority of patients, the disease is self-limited, with resolution occurring over weeks to months, and that treatment affords minimal, if any, clinical benefit.

Suppurative lymph nodes that become tense and extremely painful should be drained by needle aspiration, which may need to be repeated. Incision and drainage of nonsuppurative nodes should be avoided because chronic draining sinuses may result. Surgical excision of the node rarely is necessary.

Complications. Encephalopathy can occur in as many as 5% of patients, typically occurring 1–3 wk after the onset of lymphadenitis with the sudden onset of neurologic symptoms, which often include seizures, combative or bizarre behavior, and altered level of consciousness. Imaging studies are generally normal. The cerebrospinal fluid is normal or shows minimal pleocytosis and protein elevation. Recovery occurs without sequelae in nearly all patients but takes place slowly over many months.

Other neurologic manifestations include peripheral facial nerve paralysis, myelitis, radiculitis, compression neuropathy, and cerebellar ataxia. One patient with encephalopathy with persistent cognitive impairment and memory loss has been reported.

Stellate macular retinopathy has been associated with several infections, including CSD. Children and young adults present with unilateral or rarely bilateral loss of vision with central scotoma, optic disc swelling, and macular star formation from exudates radiating out from the macula. The findings resolve completely, with recovery of vision, usually within 2–3 mo.

Hematologic manifestations include hemolytic anemia, thrombocytopenic purpura, nonthrombocytopenic purpura, and eosinophilia. Leukocytoclastic vasculitis similar to Henoch-Schönlein purpura has been reported in association with CSD in one child. A systemic presentation of CSD with pleurisy, arthralgia or arthritis, mediastinal masses, enlarged nodes at the head of the pancreas, and atypical pneumonia has also been reported.

Prognosis. The prognosis for CSD in a normal host is generally excellent, with resolution of clinical findings over several months. Recovery occasionally is slower and may take as long as a year.

Prevention. Person-to-person spread of *Bartonella* infections is not known. Isolation is not necessary. Prevention would require elimination of cats from households, which is not practical or necessarily desirable. Awareness of the risk of cat (and particularly kitten) scratches should be emphasized to parents.

192.3 Trench Fever (*Bartonella quintana*)

Etiology. The causative agent of trench fever was first designated as *Rickettsia quintana*, then assigned to the genus *Rochalimaea*, which has been reassigned as *B. quintana*.

Epidemiology. Trench fever was first recognized as a distinct clinical entity during World War I, when more than a million troops in the trenches were infected. The disease became quiescent until World War II, when it again was epidemic. It is extremely rare in the United States.

Humans are the only known reservoir. No other animal is naturally infected, nor are the usual laboratory animals susceptible. The human body louse, *Pediculus humanus* var. *corporis*, is the vector, capable of transmission to a new host 5–6 days after feeding on an infected person. Lice excrete the organism for life; transovarian passage does not occur. Humans may have prolonged asymptomatic bacteremia for years.

Clinical Manifestations. The incubation period averages about 22 days (range, 4–35 days). The clinical presentation is highly variable. Symptoms can be very mild and brief. About half of infected persons have a single febrile illness with abrupt onset lasting 3–6 days. In others, prolonged, sustained fever may occur. More commonly, patients have periodic febrile illness with three to eight episodes lasting 4–5 days each, sometimes occurring over a period of a year or more. This form is reminiscent of malaria or relapsing fever (*Borrelia recurrentis*). Afebrile bacteremia can occur.

Clinical findings usually include fever (usually temperature of 38.5–40°C), malaise, chills, sweats, anorexia, and severe headache. Common findings include marked conjunctival injection, tachycardia, myalgias, arthralgias, and severe pain in the neck, back, and legs. Crops of erythematous macules or papules may occur or the trunk in as many as 80% of patients. Splenomegaly and mild liver enlargement may be noted.

Diagnosis. In nonepidemic situations, it is impossible to establish a diagnosis of trench fever on clinical grounds because the findings are not distinctive. A history of body louse infection or having been in an area of epidemic disease should heighten suspicions. *B. quintana* can be cultured from the blood with modification to include culture on epithelial cells. Serologic tests for *B. quintana* are available, but there is cross reaction with *B. henselae*.

Treatment. There are no controlled trials of treatment; however, patients with trench fever have responded dramatically to tetracycline and chloramphenicol with rapid defervescence.

192.4 Bacillary Angiomatosis and Bacillary Peliosis Hepatis (*Bartonella henselae* and *Bartonella quintana*)

Both *B. henselae* and *B. quintana* cause two vascular proliferative diseases, bacillary angiomatosis and bacillary peliosis, in severely immunocompromised persons, primarily adult patients with AIDS or cancer and organ transplant recipients. Subcutaneous and lytic bone lesions are strongly associated with *B. quintana*, whereas peliosis hepatis is associated exclusively with *B. henselae*.

Bacillary Angiomatosis. Lesions of cutaneous bacillary angiomatosis (BA), also known as epithelioid angiomatosis, are the most easily identified and recognized form of *Bartonella* infection in immunocompromised hosts. They are found primarily in patients with AIDS with very low CD4 counts. The clinical appearance can be quite diverse. The vasoproliferative lesions of BA may be cutaneous or subcutaneous and resemble the vascular lesions (verruca peruana) of *B. bacilliformis* in immunocompetent persons. They are erythematous papules on an erythematous base with a collarette of scale. They may enlarge to form large pedunculated lesions. Ulceration may occur, as can profuse bleeding after trauma.

BA may be clinically indistinguishable from Kaposi sarcoma. Other considerations in the differential diagnosis are pyogenic granuloma and verruca peruana (*B. bacilliformis*). Deep soft tissue masses caused by BA may mimic a malignancy.

Osseous BA lesions commonly involve the long bones. These lytic lesions are very painful and highly vascular. Occasionally found is an erythematous plaque over the lesion. The high degree of vascularity, which produces a very positive result on a technetium-99m methylene diphosphonate bone scan, resembles a malignant lesion.

Lesions can be found in virtually any organ, producing similar vascular proliferative lesions. They may appear raised, nodular, or ulcerative when seen on endoscopy or bronchoscopy. They may be associated with enlarged lymph nodes with or without an obvious local cutaneous lesion. Lesions in one brain parenchyma have been described.

Bacillary Peliosis. Bacillary peliosis affects the reticuloendothelial system, primarily the liver (**peliosis hepatis**) and less frequently the spleen and lymph nodes. It is a vasoproliferative disorder characterized by random proliferation of venous lakes surrounded by fibromyxoid stroma harboring numerous bacillary organisms. Clinical findings include fever and abdominal pain in association with abnormal results of liver function tests, particularly a markedly increased alkaline phosphatase level. Cutaneous BA or splenomegaly may be associated, with or without thrombocytopenia or pancytopenia. The vascular proliferative lesions in the liver and spleen appear on CT scan as hypodense lesions scattered throughout the parenchyma. The differential diagnosis includes hepatic Kaposi sarcoma, lymphoma, and disseminated infection with *Pneumocystis carinii* or *Mycobacterium avium* complex.

Bacteremia and Endocarditis. *B. henselae*, *B. quintana*, and *B. elizabethae* all have been reported to cause bacteremia or endocarditis. They are associated with symptoms of prolonged fevers, night sweats, and profound weight loss. A cluster of cases in Seattle in 1993 occurred in a homeless population with chronic alcoholism. These patients with high fever or hypothermia were thought to represent "urban trench fever," but no body louse infestation was associated. Some cases of culture-negative endocarditis may represent *Bartonella* endocarditis. One report described central nervous system involvement with *B. quintana* in two children.

Diagnosis. Diagnosis of BA is made initially by biopsy. The characteristic small vessel proliferation with mixed inflammatory response and the staining of bacilli by Warthin-Starry silver staining distinguish it from Kaposi sarcoma or pyogenic granuloma. Travel history can usually preclude verruca peruana.

Culture is impractical for CSD but is the diagnostic procedure for suspected bacteremia or endocarditis. The use of lysis-centrifugation technique or fresh chocolate or heart infusion agar with 5% rabbit blood with prolonged incubation may increase the yield of culture.

Treatment. *Bartonella* infections in immunocompromised hosts caused by both *B. henselae* and *B. quintana* have been treated successfully with antimicrobial agents. Rigorous studies have not been published; thus, therapy is guided by clinical experience. BA responds rapidly to erythromycin, azithromycin or clarithromycin, which are the drugs of choice. An alternative choice is doxycycline or tetracycline. Severely ill patients with peliosis hepatis, endocarditis, or osteomyelitis may be treated initially with intravenous erythromycin or doxycycline with the addition of rifampin or gentamicin. A Jarisch-Herxheimer reaction may occur. Relapses may follow; prolonged treatment for several months may be necessary.

Prevention. Immunocompromised persons should consider the potential risks of cat ownership because of the risks of *Bartonella* infections, as well as toxoplasmosis and enteric infections. Those who elect to obtain a cat should adopt or purchase a cat >1 yr of age and in good health.

Anderson BE, Newman NA: *Bartonella* spp. as emerging human pathogens. *Clin Microbiol Rev* 1997;10:203–19.

Baorto E, Payne M, Slater LN, et al: Culture-negative endocarditis caused by *Bartonella henselae. J Pediatr* 1998;132:1051–4.

Bass JW, Freitas BC, Freitas AD, et al: Prospective randomized double blind placebo-controlled evaluation of azithromycin for treatment of cat-scratch disease. *Pediatr Infect Dis J* 1998;17:447–52.

Bass JW, Vincent JM, Person DA: The expanding spectrum of *Bartonella* infections: I. Bartonellosis and trench fever. *Pediatr Infect Dis J* 1997;16:2–10.

Bass JW, Vincent JM, Person DA: The expanding spectrum of *Bartonella* infections: II. Cat scratch disease. *Pediatr Infect Dis J* 1997;16:163–79.

Carithers HA: Cat scratch disease: an overview based on a study of 1,200 patients. *Am J Dis Child* 1985;139:1124–33.

Carithers HA, Margileth AM: Cat scratch disease: Acute encephalopathy and other neurologic manifestations. *Am J Dis Child* 1991;145:98–101.

Dunn MW, Berkowitz FE, Miller JJ, et al: Hepatosplenic cat-scratch disease and abdominal pain. *Pediatr Infect Dis J* 1997;16:269–72.

Jacobs R, Schutze G: *Bartonella henselae* as a cause of prolonged fever and fever of unknown origin in children. *Clin Infect Dis* 1998;26:80–4.

Koehler JE, Sanchez MA, Garrido CS, et al: Molecular epidemiology of *Bartonella* infections in patients with bacillary angiomatosis-peliosis. *N Engl J Med* 1997;337:1876–86.

Maguiña C, Gotuzzo E: Bartonellosis: New and old. *Infect Dis Clin North Am* 2000;14:1–22.

Ricketts WE: Clinical manifestations of Carrión's disease. *Arch Intern Med* 1949;84:751–81.

SECTION 4 *Anaerobic Bacterial Infections*

Chapter 193
Botulism
(*Clostridium botulinum*)*

Robert Schechter and Stephen S. Arnon

Three naturally occurring forms of human botulism are known: infant botulism (the most common in the United States), foodborne (classic) botulism, and wound botulism. A fourth, manmade form, inhalational botulism, is one possible outcome of a bioterrorist attack.

Etiology. Botulism is the acute, flaccid paralysis caused by the neurotoxin produced by *Clostridium botulinum* or, rarely, an equivalent neurotoxin produced by atypical strains of *C. butyricum* and *C. baratii. C. botulinum* is a gram-positive, sporeforming obligate anaerobe whose natural habitat worldwide is soil, dust, and marine sediments. It is found in a wide variety of fresh and cooked agricultural products. Spores of some *C. botulinum* strains endure boiling for several hours, which enables the organism to survive efforts at food preservation. In contrast, botulinum toxin is heat labile and easily destroyed by heating at ≥85°C for 5 min. Neurotoxigenic *C. butyricum* has been isolated from a soybean food and from soils near Lake Weishan in China, the site of foodborne botulism outbreaks associated with this organism. Little is known about the ecology of neurotoxigenic *C. baratii.*

Botulinum toxin is the most poisonous substance known, the parenteral human lethal dose being estimated at 10^{-6} mg/kg.

The toxin blocks neuromuscular transmission and causes death through airway and respiratory muscle paralysis. Seven antigenic toxin types, assigned the letters A–G, are distinguished by the inability of neutralizing antibody against one toxin type to protect against a different toxin type. The seven toxin types serve as convenient clinical and epidemiologic markers. Toxin types A, B, E, and F are well-established causes of human botulism, whereas types C and D cause illness in other animals. Neurotoxigenic *C. butyricum* strains produce a type E toxin, whereas neurotoxigenic *C. baratii* strains produce a type F toxin. Type G has not been established as a cause of either human or animal disease.

Botulinum toxin is a simple di-chain protein consisting of a 100-kd "heavy" chain that contains the neuronal attachment sites and a 50-kd "light" chain that is taken into the cell after binding. The phenomenal potency of botulinum toxin is explained by the fact that its seven light chains are zinc-endopeptidases, whose substrates are one or two of three proteins of the docking complex by which synaptic vesicles fuse with the terminal cell membrane and release acetylcholine into the synaptic cleft.

Epidemiology. Infant botulism has been reported from all inhabited continents except Africa. Notably, the infant is the only family member who is ill. The most striking epidemiologic feature of infant botulism is its age distribution, in which in 95% of cases, the infants are between 3 wk and 6 mo of age, with a broad peak at 2–4 mo of age. This pattern is matched only by one other condition, the sudden infant death syndrome. However, cases in infants as young as 3 days or as old as 382 days at onset have been recognized. The male:female ratio of cases is essentially 1:1, and cases have occurred in most racial and ethnic groups.

Infant botulism is an uncommon and often unrecognized illness. In the United States, about 100 cases are diagnosed annually; more than 1,800 cases were reported from 1976 to 2000. Approximately 40% of U.S. cases were reported from California.

---

*All material in this chapter is in the public domain, with the exception of any borrowed figures or tables.

Consistent with the known asymmetric soil distribution of *C. botulinum* toxin types, most cases west of the Mississippi River have been caused by type A strains, and most cases east of the Mississippi River have been caused by type B strains. One case each in the states of New Mexico, Washington, and Ohio resulted from *C. baratii* and type F toxin, whereas cases in Italy resulted from *C. butyricum* and type E toxin. Identified risk factors for the illness include the ingestion of honey and a slow intestinal transit time (<1 stool/day). Breast-feeding appears to provide protection against fulminant, sudden death from infant botulism. Under rare circumstances of altered intestinal anatomy, physiology, and microflora, older children and adults may contract infant-type botulism.

Foodborne botulism results from the ingestion of a food in which *C. botulinum* has multiplied and produced its toxin. Recent outbreaks in North America associated with baked potatoes, sautéed onions, and chopped garlic served in restaurants have revised the traditional view of foodborne botulism as resulting mainly from home-canned foods. Other outbreaks in the United States have occurred from commercial foods sealed in plastic pouches that relied solely on refrigeration to prevent outgrowth of *C. botulinum* spores. Noncanned foods responsible for recent foodborne botulism episodes include peyote tea, the hazelnut flavoring added to yogurt, sweet cream cheese, sautéed onions in "patty melt" sandwiches, potato salad, and fresh and dried fish. A recent trend toward a single case per outbreak or of cases presenting separately in different cities or hospitals has meant that the physician cannot rely on the temporal and geographic clustering of illness to suggest the diagnosis.

Most preserved foods have been implicated in foodborne botulism, but the usual offenders in the United States are the "low-acid" (pH ≥ 6.0) home-canned foods such as jalapeño peppers, asparagus, olives, and beans. The potential for foodborne botulism exists throughout the world, but outbreaks occur most commonly in the temperate zones rather than the tropics, where preservation of fruits, vegetables, and other foods is less common.

In the past 10 yr, approximately nine outbreaks and 24 cases of foodborne botulism have occurred annually in the United States. Most of the continental U.S. outbreaks resulted from proteolytic type A or type B strains, which produce a strongly putrefactive odor in the food that some people find necessary to verify by tasting. In contrast, in Alaska and Canada, most foodborne outbreaks have resulted from nonproteolytic type E strains in Native American foods, such as fermented salmon eggs and seal flippers, which do not exhibit signs of spoilage. A further hazard of type E strains is their ability to grow at the temperatures (5°C) maintained by household refrigerators.

Wound botulism is an exceptionally rare disease, with less than 300 cases reported worldwide, but it is important to pediatrics because adolescents and children are disproportionately affected. Although many cases have occurred in young, physically active males at greatest risk of traumatic injury, wound botulism also occurs with crush injuries in which no break in the skin is evident. In the past 10 yr, wound botulism from injection has become increasingly common in adult heroin abusers in the western United States, not always with evident abscess formation or cellulitis.

A single outbreak of inhalational botulism was reported in 1962 in which three laboratory workers in Germany were exposed unintentionally to aerosolized botulinum toxin.

Pathogenesis. All forms of botulism produce disease through a final common pathway. Botulinum toxin is carried by the bloodstream to peripheral cholinergic synapses, where it binds irreversibly, blocking acetylcholine release and causing impaired neuromuscular and autonomic transmission. Infant botulism is an infectious disease that results from ingesting the spores of any of the three botulinum toxin-producing clostridial strains,

with subsequent spore germination, multiplication, and production of botulinum toxin in the large intestine. Foodborne botulism is an intoxication that results when preformed botulinum toxin contained in an improperly preserved or inadequately cooked food is swallowed. Wound botulism results from spore germination and colonization of traumatized tissue by *C. botulinum*; it is the analog of tetanus. Inhalational botulism occurs when aerosolized botulinum toxin is inhaled. A bioterrorist attack could result in large or small outbreaks of inhalational or foodborne botulism (Chapter 706).

Because botulinum toxin is not a cytotoxin, it causes no overt macroscopic or microscopic pathology. However, secondary pathologic changes (e.g., pneumonia, petechiae on intrathoracic organs) may be found at autopsy. No diagnostic technique is available to identify botulinum toxin bound at the neuromuscular junction. The healing process in botulism consists of sprouting of new terminal unmyelinated motor neurons. Movement resumes when these new twigs locate noncontracting muscle fibers and reinnervate them by inducing formation of a new motor end plate. In experimental animals, this process takes about 4 wk.

Clinical Manifestations. Botulinum toxin is distributed hematogenously. Because relative blood flow and density of innervation are greatest in the bulbar musculature, all forms of botulism manifest neurologically as a symmetric, descending, flaccid paralysis beginning with the cranial nerve musculature. It is not possible to have botulism without having multiple bulbar palsies, yet in infants such symptoms as poor feeding, weak suck, feeble cry, drooling, and even obstructive apnea are often not recognized as bulbar in origin. Patients with evolving illness may already have generalized weakness and hypotonia in addition to bulbar palsies when first examined. In contrast to botulism caused by *C. botulinum*, a majority of the rare cases caused by intestinal colonization with *C. butyricum* have had a Meckel diverticulum along with abdominal distention, often leading to misdiagnosis as an acute abdomen.

In older children with foodborne or wound botulism, the onset of neurologic symptoms follows a characteristic pattern of diplopia, blurred vision, ptosis, dry mouth, dysphagia, dysphonia, and dysarthria, with deceased gag and corneal reflexes. Importantly, because the toxin acts only on motor nerves, paresthesias are not seen in botulism, except when a patient hyperventilates from anxiety. The sensorium remains clear, but this may be difficult to ascertain because of the slurred speech.

Foodborne botulism begins with gastrointestinal symptoms of nausea, vomiting, or diarrhea in about one third of cases. These symptoms are thought to result from metabolic by-products of growth of *C. botulinum* or from the presence of other toxic contaminants in the food, because gastrointestinal distress is rarely observed in wound botulism. Constipation may occur in foodborne botulism once flaccid paralysis becomes evident. Illness usually begins 12–36 hr after ingestion of the contaminated food but can range from as little as 2 hr to as long as 8 days. The incubation period in wound botulism is 4–14 days. Fever may be present in wound botulism but is absent in foodborne botulism unless a secondary infection (e.g., pneumonia) is present. All forms of botulism display a wide spectrum in their clinical severity, from the very mild with minimal ptosis, flattened facial expression, minor dysphagia, and dysphonia to the fulminant, with rapid onset of extensive paralysis, frank apnea, and fixed, dilated pupils. Fatigability with repetitive muscle activity is the clinical hallmark of botulism.

Infant botulism differs in apparent initial symptoms of illness only because the infant cannot verbalize them. Usually, the first indication of illness is a decreased frequency or even absence of defecation, although this sign is frequently overlooked. Parents typically notice inability to feed, lethargy, listlessness, weak cry, and diminished spontaneous movement. Dysphagia may be evident as secretions drooling from the mouth. Gag, suck, and corneal reflexes diminish as the paralysis advances. Oculomotor palsies may be evident only with sustained observation. Paradoxically, the pupillary light reflex may be unaffected until the child is severely paralyzed, or it may be initially sluggish. Loss of head control is typically a prominent sign. Respiratory arrest may occur suddenly from airway occlusion by unswallowed secretions or from obstructive flaccid pharyngeal musculature. Occasionally, the diagnosis of infant botulism is suggested by a respiratory arrest that occurs after the infant is curled into position for lumbar puncture.

In mild cases or in the early stages of illness, the physical signs of infant botulism may be subtle and easily missed. Eliciting cranial nerve palsies and fatigability of muscular function requires careful examination. Ptosis may not be seen unless the head of the child is kept erect.

Diagnosis. Clinical diagnosis of botulism is confirmed by specialized laboratory testing that often requires days to complete. Therefore, clinical diagnosis is the foundation for early recognition of and response to all forms of botulism. Routine laboratory studies, including those of the cerebrospinal fluid (CSF), are normal in botulism unless dehydration, starvation (metabolic acidosis and ketosis), or secondary infection is present.

The classic picture of botulism is the acute onset of a symmetric flaccid descending paralysis with clear sensorium, no fever, and no paresthesias. *Suspected botulism represents a medical and public health emergency that is immediately reportable by telephone in most U.S. health jurisdictions.* State health departments (first call) and the Centers for Disease Control and Prevention (second call; 404-639-2206 workdays; 404-639-2888 at other times) can arrange for diagnostic testing, epidemiologic investigation, and provision of equine antitoxin.

The diagnosis of botulism is unequivocally established by demonstrating the presence of botulinum toxin in serum or of *C. botulinum* toxin or organisms in wound material or feces. *C. botulinum* is not part of the normal resident intestinal flora of humans, and its presence in the setting of acute flaccid paralysis is diagnostic. An epidemiologic diagnosis of foodborne botulism can be established when *C. botulinum* organisms and toxin are found in food eaten by patients.

Electromyography (EMG) can sometimes distinguish between causes of acute flaccid paralysis, although results may be variable, including normal, in patients with botulism. The distinctive EMG finding in botulism is facilitation (potentiation) of the evoked muscle action potential at high-frequency (50 Hz) stimulation. In infant botulism, a characteristic pattern, known by the acronym BSAP (brief, small, abundant motor-unit action potentials), is present only in clinically weak muscles. Nerve conduction velocity and sensory nerve function are normal in botulism.

Infant botulism requires a high index of suspicion for early diagnosis (Box 193–1). Even today, more than 25 yr after its recognition, "rule-out sepsis" is the most common admission diagnosis. If a previously healthy infant, usually 2–4 mo of age, develops weakness with difficulty in sucking, swallowing, crying, or breathing, infant botulism should be considered a likely diagnosis. A careful cranial nerve examination is then helpful.

DIFFERENTIAL DIAGNOSIS. Botulism is frequently misdiagnosed, most often as a polyradiculoneuropathy (Guillain-Barré or Miller Fisher syndrome), myasthenia gravis, or a disease of the central nervous system (Box 193–2). In the United States, botulism is more likely than Guillain-Barré syndrome, intoxication, or poliomyelitis to cause a cluster of cases of acute flaccid paralysis. Botulism differs from other flaccid paralyses in its prominent cranial nerve palsies disproportionate to milder weakness and hypotonia below the neck, in its symmetry, and in its absence of sensory nerve damage.

Additional diagnostic procedures may be useful in rapidly excluding botulism as the cause of paralysis. Cerebrospinal fluid

BOX 193–1. Differential Diagnosis of Infant Botulism

ADMISSION DIAGNOSIS	COMMON SUBSEQUENT DIAGNOSES
Suspected sepsis	Guillain-Barré syndrome
Pneumonia	Myasthenia gravis
Dehydration	Disorders of amino acid metabolism
Viral syndrome	Hypothyroidism
Hypotonia of unknown etiology	Drug ingestion
	Brainstem encephalitis
Constipation	Heavy metal poisoning (Pb, Mg, As)
Failure to thrive	Poliomyelitis
Werdnig-Hoffmann disease	Viral polyneuritis
	Hirschsprung disease
	Metabolic encephalopathy
	Medium chain acetyl-CoA dehydrogenase (MCAD) deficiency

BOX 193–2. Differential Diagnoses of Foodborne and Wound Botulism

Acute gastroenteritis	Aminoglycoside-associated paralysis
Myasthenia gravis	Tick paralysis
Guillain-Barré syndrome	Hypocalcemia
Organophosphate poisoning	Hypermagnesemia
Meningitis	Carbon monoxide poisoning
Encephalitis	Hyperemesis gravidarum
Psychiatric illness	Laryngeal trauma
Cerebrovascular accident	Diabetic complications
Poliomyelitis	Inflammatory myopathy
Hypothyroidism	Overexertion

(CSF) is unchanged in botulism but is abnormal in many central nervous system diseases. Although the CSF protein level eventually is elevated in Guillain-Barré syndrome, it may be normal early in illness. Imaging of the brain, spine, and chest may reveal hemorrhage, inflammation, or neoplasm. A test dose of edrophonium chloride briefly reverses paralytic symptoms in many patients with myasthenia gravis and, reportedly, in some with botulism. A close inspection of the skin, especially the scalp, may reveal an attached tick that is causing paralysis. Possible organophosphate intoxication should be pursued aggressively because specific antidotes (oximes) are available and because the patient may be part of a commonly exposed group, some of whom have yet to develop illness. Other tests that require days for results include stool culture for *Campylobacter jejuni* as a precipitant of Guillain-Barré syndrome and assays for the autoantibodies that cause myasthenia gravis, Lambert-Eaton syndrome, and Guillain-Barré syndrome.

Treatment. Management of botulism rests on three principles: (1) fatigability with repetitive muscle activity is the clinical hallmark of the disease; (2) complications are best avoided by anticipating them; and (3) meticulous supportive care is a necessity. The first principle applies mainly to feeding and breathing. Correct positioning is imperative to protect the airway and improve respiratory mechanics. The patient is placed face up on a rigid-bottomed crib (or bed), the head of which is tilted at 30 degrees. A small cloth roll is placed under the cervical vertebrae to tilt the head back so that secretions drain to the posterior pharynx and away from the airway. In this tilted position the abdominal viscera pull the diaphragm down, thereby improving respiratory mechanics. The patient's head and torso should not be elevated by bending the middle of the bed; if this is done, the hypotonic thorax will slump into the abdomen and breathing will be compromised.

About one half of patients require endotracheal intubation, which is best done prophylactically. The indications include diminished gag and cough reflexes and progressive airway obstruction by secretions. With meticulous management technique (especially proper tube diameter), monitoring, and positioning, patients have tolerated months of intubation without subglottic stenosis or need for tracheostomy.

Feeding should be done by a nasogastric or nasojejunal tube until sufficient oropharyngeal strength and coordination enables feeding by breast or bottle. Expressed breast milk is the most desirable food for infants, in part because of its immunologic components (e.g., sIgA, lactoferrin, leukocytes). Tube feeding also assists in the restoration of peristalsis, a nonspecific but probably essential part of eliminating *C. botulinum* from the intestinal flora. Intravenous feeding (hyperalimentation) is discouraged because of the potential for infection and the advantages to tube feeding.

Antibiotic therapy is not part of the treatment of uncomplicated infant or foodborne botulism because the toxin is primarily an intracellular molecule that is released into the intestinal lumen with vegetative bacterial cell death and lysis. Antibiotics are reserved for the treatment of secondary infections, and in the absence of antibody therapy a nonclostridiocidal antibiotic such as trimethoprim-sulfamethoxazole is preferred. Aminoglycoside antibiotics should be avoided because they may potentiate the blocking action of botulinum toxin at the neuromuscular junction. However, wound botulism requires aggressive treatment with antibiotics and antitoxin in a manner analogous to tetanus (Chapter 194). The currently licensed botulinum antitoxin used in foodborne and wound botulism is a horse serum–derived product that has side effects of serum sickness, anaphylaxis, and potential lifelong sensitization to equine proteins; its use in children requires careful consideration.

Specific treatment for infant botulism is now available. In California a 5-year, randomized, double-blind, placebo-controlled treatment trial demonstrated the apparent safety and efficacy of **human-derived botulinum antitoxin** (BIG-IV), formally known as botulism immunoglobulin intravenous (human). Use of BIG-IV reduced mean hospital stay from approximately 5.5 wk to approximately 2.5 wk and reduced mean hospitalization cost by approximately $70,000 per case. Treatment with BIG-IV should be started as early in the illness as possible. In the United States, BIG-IV may be obtained from the California Department of Health Services (24-hour telephone: 510-540-2646; http://www.infantbot.org). Older patients with suspected food, wound, or inhalational botulism may be treated with equine botulinum antitoxin, available in the United States through the Centers for Disease Control and Prevention by way of state and local health departments.

Because sensation remains intact, providing auditory, tactile, and visual stimuli is beneficial. Maintaining strong central respiratory drive is essential, so sedatives or central nervous system depressants (e.g., metoclopramide) are discouraged. Full hydration and stool softeners such as lactulose may mitigate the protracted constipation. Cathartics are not recommended. Patients with foodborne and infant botulism excrete *C. botulinum* toxin and organisms in their feces, often for weeks, and care should be taken in handling their excreta. When bladder palsy occurs in severe cases, gentle suprapubic pressure with the patient in the sitting position with the head supported may help attain complete voiding and reduce the risk of urinary tract infection. Families may require emotional and financial support, especially when the paralysis of botulism is prolonged.

Complications. Avoidance of complications is best accomplished by noting past experience (Box 193–3); all of these complications are nosocomial, and some are iatrogenic. Even so, some critically ill, paralyzed patients who must spend weeks or months on ventilators in intensive care units will inevitably develop complications. Suspected "relapses" in infant botulism usually reflect premature hospital discharge, an undiscovered underlying complication, such as pneumonia, or perhaps additional toxemia.

BOX 193–3. Complications of Infant Botulism

Adult respiratory distress syndrome	Recurrent atelectasis
Aspiration	Seizures secondary to hyponatremia
Clostridium difficile enterocolitis	Sepsis
	Subglottic stenosis
Fracture of the femur	Tension pneumothorax
Inappropriate antidiuretic hormone secretion	Transfusion reaction
	Tracheal granuloma
Misplaced or plugged endotracheal tube	Tracheitis
	Urinary tract infection
Otitis media	
Pneumonia	

Prognosis. When the regenerating nerve endings have induced formation of a new motor end plate, neuromuscular transmission is restored. In the absence of complications, particularly those related to hypoxia, the prognosis in infant botulism is for full and complete recovery. Hospital stay in untreated infant botulism averages approximately 1 mo but differs significantly by toxin type, with untreated type B patients being hospitalized a mean of 3.7 wk and untreated type A patients 5.6 wk. In the United States, the case-fatality ratio for hospitalized infant botulism is <1%. The case-fatality ratio in foodborne and wound botulism varies by age, with younger patients having the best prognosis. Some adults with botulism have reported chronic weakness and fatigue as sequelae. After recovery, untreated infant botulism patients appear to have an increased incidence of strabismus that requires timely screening and treatment.

Prevention. Foodborne botulism is best prevented by adhering to safe methods of home canning (pressure cooker and acidification), by avoiding suspicious foods, and by heating all home canned foods to 85°C for ≥5 min. Wound botulism is best prevented by not using illicit drugs and by treatment of contaminated wounds with thorough cleansing, surgical debridement, and provision of appropriate antibiotics.

Most infant botulism patients probably inhale and then swallow airborne clostridial spores; these cases cannot be prevented. The one identified, avoidable source of botulinum spores for infants is honey. Honey is an unsafe food for any child younger than 1 yr of age. Corn syrups were once thought to be a possible source of botulinum spores, but recent evidence indicates otherwise. Breast-feeding appears to slow the onset of infant botulism and to diminish the risk of sudden death in infants in whom the disease develops.

Arnon SS, Schechter R, Inglesby TV, et al: Botulinum toxin as a biological weapon: Medical and public health management. *JAMA* 2001;285:1059–70.

Arnon SS, Damus K, Thompson B, et al: Protective role of human milk against sudden death from infant botulism. *J Pediatr* 1982;100:568–73.

Arnon SS, Werner SB, Faber HK, et al: Infant botulism in 1931. Discovery of a misclassified case. *Am J Dis Child* 1979;133:580–2.

Fenicia L, Franciosa G, Pourshaban M, et al: Intestinal toxemia botulism in two young people, caused by *Clostridium butyricum* type E. *Clin Infect Dis* 1999;29:1381–7.

Hatheway CL, McCroskey LM: Examination of feces and serum for diagnosis of infant botulism in 336 patients. *J Clin Microbiol* 1987;25:2334–8.

Long SS, Gajeweski JL, Brown LW, et al: Clinical, laboratory, and environmental features of infant botulism in southeastern Pennsylvania. *Pediatrics* 1985;75:935–41.

Puig de Centorbi O, Centorbi HJ, Demo N, et al: Infant botulism during a one year period in San Luis, Argentina. *Zentralbl Bakteriol* 1998;287:61–6.

Schreiner MS, Field E, Ruddy R: Infant botulism. A review of 12 years' experience at the Children's Hospital of Philadelphia. *Pediatrics* 1991;87:159–65.

Shapiro RL, Hatheway C, Swerdlow DL: Botulism in the United States: A clinical and epidemiological review. *Ann Intern Med* 1998;129:221–8.

Werner SB, Passaro D, McGee J, et al: Wound botulism in California, 1951–1998: Recent epidemic in heroin injectors. *Clin Infect Dis* 2000;31:1018–24.

Tetanus (*Clostridium tetani*)* Stephen S. Arnon

Etiology. Tetanus, historically called **lockjaw**, is an acute, spastic paralytic illness caused by tetanus toxin, the neurotoxin produced by *Clostridium tetani*, a motile, gram-positive, spore-forming obligate anaerobe whose natural habitat worldwide is soil, dust, and the alimentary tracts of various animals. It forms spores terminally, thus producing a drumstick or tennis racket appearance microscopically. Tetanus spores can survive boiling but not autoclaving, whereas the vegetative cells are killed by antibiotics, heat, and standard disinfectants. Unlike many clostridia, *C. tetani* is not a tissue-invasive organism; instead it causes illness through the effects of a single toxin, **tetanospasmin**, more commonly referred to as tetanus toxin. Tetanus toxin (tetanospasmin) is the second most poisonous substance known, being surpassed in potency only by botulinum toxin; the human lethal dose of tetanus toxin is estimated to be 10^{-6} mg/kg.

Epidemiology. Tetanus occurs worldwide and is endemic in 90 developing countries, but its incidence varies considerably. The most common form, neonatal (umbilical) tetanus, kills approximately 500,000 infants each year because the mother was not immunized; about 80% of these deaths occur in just 12 tropical Asian and African countries. In addition, an estimated 15,000–30,000 unimmunized women worldwide die each year of maternal tetanus that results from postpartum, postabortal, or postsurgical wound infection with *C. tetani*. Approximately 50 cases of tetanus are reported each year in the United States, mostly in persons older than 60 yr of age, but toddler-aged and neonatal cases also occur. One fifth of children in the United States 10–16 yr of age lack a protective antibody level. The majority of childhood cases of tetanus in the United States during the past decade have occurred in unimmunized children whose parents objected to vaccination.

Most non-neonatal cases of tetanus are associated with a traumatic injury, often a penetrating wound inflicted by a dirty object, such as a nail, splinter, fragment of glass, or unsterile injection, but a rare case may have no history of trauma. Tetanus occurring after illicit drug injection is becoming more common, whereas uncommon settings include animal bites, abscesses (including dental abscesses), ear and other body piercing, chronic skin ulceration, burns, compound fractures, frostbite, gangrene, intestinal surgery, ritual scarification, infected insect bites, and female circumcision. The disease also occurs after the use of contaminated suture material or after intramuscular injection of medicines, most notably quinine for chloroquine-resistant falciparum malaria.

Pathogenesis. Tetanus occurs after introduced spores germinate, multiply, and produce tetanus toxin in the low oxidation-reduction potential (E_h) of an infected injury site. A plasmid carries the toxin gene; the toxin is released with vegetative bacterial cell death and subsequent lysis. Tetanus toxin (and the botulinum toxins) are 150-kd simple proteins consisting of a heavy (100 kd) and a light (50 kd) chain joined by a single disulfide bond. Tetanus toxin binds at the neuromuscular junction and enters the motor nerve by endocytosis, after which it undergoes retrograde axonal transport to the cytoplasm of the alpha-motoneuron. In the sciatic nerve, the transport rate was found to be 3.4 mm/hr. The toxin exits the motoneuron in the spinal cord and next enters adjacent spinal inhibitory interneurons, where it prevents release of the neurotransmitter α-aminobutyric acid (GABA). Tetanus toxin thus blocks the normal inhibition of antagonistic muscles, which is the basis of voluntary coordinated movement; in consequence, affected muscles sustain maximal contraction. The autonomic nervous system is also rendered unstable in tetanus.

The phenomenal potency of tetanus toxin is enzymatic in nature. The light chain of tetanus toxin (and of several of the botulinum toxins) is a zinc-containing endoprotease whose substrate is **synaptobrevin**, a constituent protein of the docking complex that enables the synaptic vesicle to fuse with the terminal cell membrane. The heavy chain of the toxin contains its binding and internalization domains.

C. tetani is not an invasive organism and its toxin-producing vegetative cells remain where introduced into the wound, which may or may not display local inflammatory changes and a mixed infectious flora.

Clinical Manifestations. Tetanus may be either generalized, which is more common, or localized. The incubation period typically is 2–14 days, but it may be as long as months after the injury. In **generalized tetanus, trismus** (masseter muscle spasm, or **lockjaw**) is the presenting symptom in about half of cases. Headache, restlessness, and irritability are early symptoms, often followed by stiffness, difficulty chewing, dysphagia, and neck muscle spasm. The so-called **sardonic smile of tetanus (risus sardonicus)** results from intractable spasm of facial and buccal muscles. When the paralysis extends to abdominal, lumbar, hip, and thigh muscles, the patient may assume an arched posture of extreme hyperextension of the body, **opisthotonos,** with the head and the heels bent backward and the body bowed forward with only the back of the head and the heels touching the supporting surface. Opisthotonos is an equilibrium position that results from unrelenting total contraction of opposing muscles, all of which display the typical **boardlike rigidity** of tetanus. Laryngeal and respiratory muscle spasm can lead to airway obstruction and asphyxiation. Because tetanus toxin does not affect sensory nerves or cortical function, the patient unfortunately remains conscious, in extreme pain, and in fearful anticipation of the next tetanic seizure. These seizures are characterized by sudden, severe tonic contractions of the muscles, with fist clenching, flexion, and adduction of the arms and hyperextension of the legs. Without treatment, the seizures range from a few seconds to a few minutes in length with intervening respite periods, but as the illness progresses, the spasms become sustained and exhausting. The smallest disturbance by sight, sound, or touch may trigger a tetanic spasm. Dysuria and urinary retention result from bladder sphincter spasm; forced defecation may occur. Fever, occasionally with a temperature as high as 40°C, is common because of the substantial metabolic energy consumed by spastic muscles. Notable autonomic effects include tachycardia, arrhythmias, labile hypertension, diaphoresis, and cutaneous vasoconstriction. The tetanic paralysis usually becomes more severe in the 1st wk after onset, stabilizes in the 2nd wk, and ameliorates gradually over the ensuing 1–4 wk.

Neonatal tetanus (tetanus neonatorum), the infantile form of generalized tetanus, typically manifests within 3–12 days of birth as progressive difficulty in feeding (i.e., sucking and swallowing), with associated hunger and crying. Paralysis or diminished movement, stiffness to the touch, and spasms, with or without opisthotonos, characterize the disease. The umbilical stump may hold remnants of dirt, dung, clotted blood, or serum, or it may appear relatively benign.

Localized tetanus results in painful spasms of the muscles adjacent to the wound site and may precede generalized tetanus. **Cephalic tetanus** is a rare form of localized tetanus involving the bulbar musculature that occurs with wounds or foreign bodies in the head, nostrils, or face. It also occurs in

---

*All material in this chapter is in the public domain, with the exception of any borrowed figures or tables.

association with chronic otitis media. Cephalic tetanus is characterized by retracted eyelids, deviated gaze, trismus, risus sardonicus, and spastic paralysis of tongue and pharyngeal musculature.

Diagnosis. The picture of tetanus is one of the most dramatic in medicine, and the diagnosis may be established clinically. The typical setting is an unimmunized patient (and/or mother) who was injured or born within the preceding 2 wk and who presents with trismus, other rigid muscles, and a clear sensorium.

Routine laboratory studies are usually normal. A peripheral leukocytosis may result from a secondary bacterial infection of the wound or may be stress induced from the sustained tetanic spasms. The cerebrospinal fluid (CSF) is normal, although the intense muscle contractions may raise intracranial pressure. Neither the electroencephalogram nor the electromyogram shows a characteristic pattern. *C. tetani* is not always visible on Gram stain of wound material, and it is isolated in only about one third of cases.

DIFFERENTIAL DIAGNOSIS. Fully developed, generalized tetanus cannot be mistaken for any other disease. However, trismus may result from parapharyngeal, retropharyngeal, or dental abscesses, or rarely, from acute encephalitis involving the brainstem. Either rabies or tetanus may follow an animal bite, and rabies may present as trismus with seizures. However, rabies may be distinguished from tetanus by its hydrophobia, marked dysphagia, predominantly clonic seizures, and CSF pleocytosis. Although strychnine poisoning may result in tonic muscle spasms and generalized seizure activity, it seldom produces trismus, and unlike tetanus, general relaxation usually occurs between spasms. Hypocalcemia may produce tetany, characterized by laryngeal and carpopedal spasms, but trismus is absent. Occasionally, epileptic seizures, narcotic withdrawal, or other drug reactions may suggest tetanus.

Treatment. Management of tetanus requires eradication of *C. tetani* and the wound environment conducive to its anaerobic multiplication, neutralization of all accessible tetanus toxin, control of seizures and respiration, palliation and provision of meticulous supportive care, and, finally, prevention of recurrences.

Surgical wound excision and debridement is often needed to remove the foreign body or devitalized tissue that created anaerobic growth conditions. Surgery should be done promptly, after the administration of human tetanus immunoglobulin (TIG) and antibiotics. Excision of the umbilical stump in neonatal tetanus is no longer recommended.

Once tetanus toxin has begun its axonal ascent to the spinal cord, it cannot be neutralized by TIG. Accordingly, TIG is given as soon as possible to neutralize toxin that diffuses from the wound into the circulation before the toxin can bind at distant muscle groups. An optimal dose of TIG has not been determined. A single intramuscular injection of 500 U of TIG is sufficient to neutralize systemic tetanus toxin, but total doses as high as 3,000–6,000 U are also recommended. Infiltration of TIG into the wound is now considered unnecessary. If TIG is unavailable, use of human intravenous immunoglobulin (IVIG), which contains 4–90 U/mL of TIG, or of equine- or bovine-derived tetanus antitoxin (TAT), may be necessary. However, the optimal dosage of IVIG is not known, and it is not approved for this indication. The usual dose of TAT is 50,000–100,000 U, with half given intramuscularly and half intravenously, but as little as 10,000 U may be sufficient. TAT is not available in the United States. Approximately 15% of patients given the usual dose of TAT experience serum sickness. When using TAT, it is essential to check for possible sensitivity to horse serum and desensitization may be needed. The human-derived immunoglobulins are much preferred because of their longer half-life (30 days) and the virtual absence of allergic and serum sickness adverse effects. Intrathecal TIG, given to neutralize tetanus toxin in the spinal cord, is not effective.

Penicillin G (100,000 U/kg/24 hr divided q 4–6 hr IV for 10–14 days) remains the antibiotic of choice because of its effective clostridiocidal action and its diffusibility, an important consideration because blood flow to injured tissue may be compromised. Metronidazole (500 mg q 8 hr IV for adults) appears to be equally effective. Erythromycin and tetracycline (for patients 8 yr old or older) are alternatives for penicillin-allergic patients.

All patients with generalized tetanus need muscle relaxants. Diazepam provides both relaxation and seizure control; the initial dose of 0.1–0.2/kg q 3–6 hr given intravenously is then titrated to control the tetanic spasms, after which it is sustained for 2–6 wk before its tapered withdrawal. Magnesium sulfate, other benzodiazepines (e.g., midazolam), chlorpromazine, dantrolene, and baclofen are also used. Intrathecal baclofen produces such complete muscle relaxation that apnea often ensues; like most other agents listed, baclofen should be used only in an intensive care unit setting. The best survival rates in generalized tetanus are achieved with neuromuscular blocking agents such as vecuronium and pancuronium, which produce a general flaccid paralysis that is then managed by mechanical ventilation. Autonomic instability is regulated with standard α- and β- (or both) blocking agents; morphine has also proved useful.

Meticulous supportive care in a quiet, dark, secluded setting is most desirable. Because tetanic spasms may be triggered by minor stimuli, the patient should be sedated and protected from all unnecessary sounds, sights, and touch; and all therapeutic and other manipulations must be carefully scheduled and coordinated. Endotracheal intubation may not be required, but it should be done to prevent aspiration of secretions before laryngospasm develops. A tracheotomy kit should be immediately at hand for unintubated patients. However, endotracheal intubation and suctioning easily provoke reflex tetanic seizures and spasms, and early tracheostomy deserves consideration in severe cases not managed by pharmacologically induced flaccid paralysis. Cardiorespiratory monitoring, frequent suctioning, and maintenance of the substantial fluid, electrolyte, and caloric needs are fundamental. Careful nursing attention to mouth, skin, bladder, and bowel function is needed to avoid ulceration, infection, and obstipation. Prophylactic subcutaneous heparin use is sensible.

Complications. The seizures and the severe, sustained rigid paralysis of tetanus predispose the patient to many complications. Aspiration of secretions and pneumonia may have begun before the first medical attention was received. Maintaining airway patency often mandates endotracheal intubation and mechanical ventilation with their attendant hazards, including pneumothorax and mediastinal emphysema. The seizures may result in lacerations of the mouth or tongue, in intramuscular hematomas or rhabdomyolysis with myoglobinuria and renal failure, or in long bone or spinal fractures. Venous thrombosis, pulmonary embolism, gastric ulceration with or without hemorrhage, paralytic ileus, and decubitus ulceration are constant hazards. Excessive use of muscle relaxants, an integral part of care, may produce iatrogenic apnea. Cardiac arrhythmias, including asystole, unstable blood pressure, and labile temperature regulation reflect disordered autonomic nervous system control that may be aggravated by inattention to maintenance of intravascular volume needs.

Prognosis. Recovery in tetanus occurs through regeneration of synapses within the spinal cord and thereby the restoration of muscle relaxation. However, because an episode of tetanus does not result in the production of toxin-neutralizing antibodies, active immunization with tetanus toxoid at discharge with provision for completion of the primary series is mandatory.

The most important factor influencing outcome is the quality of supportive care. Mortality is highest in the very young and the very old. A favorable prognosis is associated with a long incubation period, with the absence of fever, and with localized disease. An unfavorable prognosis is associated with a week or less between the injury and the onset of trismus and with 3 days or less between trismus and the onset of generalized tetanic spasms. Sequelae of hypoxic brain injury, especially in infants, include cerebral palsy, diminished mental abilities, and behavioral difficulties. Most fatalities occur within the 1st wk of illness. Reported case fatality rates for generalized tetanus range between 5% and 35% and for neonatal tetanus extend from <10% with intensive care treatment to >75% without it. Cephalic tetanus has an especially poor prognosis because of breathing and feeding difficulties.

Prevention. Tetanus is an entirely preventable disease; a serum antibody titer of ≥0.01 U/mL is considered protective. Active immunization should begin in early infancy with combined diphtheria toxoid-tetanus toxoid-pertussis vaccine at 2, 4, and 6 mo of age, with a booster at 4–6 yr of age and at 10-yr intervals thereafter throughout adult life with tetanus-diphtheria (Td) toxoids. Immunization of women with tetanus toxoid prevents neonatal tetanus, and the World Health Organization is currently engaged in a global elimination of neonatal tetanus campaign through maternal immunization with at least two doses of tetanus toxoid. For unimmunized persons 7 yr of age or older, the primary immunization series consists of three doses of Td toxoid given intramuscularly, with the second given 4–6 wk after the first and the third given 6–12 mo after the second. However, unanticipated mass immunization campaigns in developing countries may rarely provoke a widespread hysterical reaction.

WOUND MANAGEMENT. Tetanus prevention measures after trauma consist of inducing active immunity to tetanus toxin and of passively providing antitoxic antibody (Table 194–1). Tetanus prophylaxis is an essential part of all wound management, but specific measures depend on the nature of the injury and the immunization status of the patient. Tetanus toxoid should always be given after a dog or other animal bite, even though *C. tetani* is infrequently found in canine mouth flora. All nonminor wounds require human TIG except those in a fully immunized patient. In any other circumstances (e.g., patients with an unknown or incomplete immunization history; crush, puncture, or projectile wounds; wounds contaminated with saliva, soil, or feces; avulsion injuries; compound fractures; or frostbite), 250 U of TIG should be given intramuscularly, and 500 U should be given for highly tetanus-prone wounds (i.e., unable to be debrided, with substantial bacterial contamination,

or >24 hr old). If TIG is unavailable, then use of human IGIV may be considered. If neither of these products is available, then 3,000–5,000 U of equine- or bovine-derived TAT may be given intramuscularly after testing for hypersensitivity; even at this dose, serum sickness may occur.

The wound should have immediate, thorough surgical cleansing and debridement to remove foreign bodies and any necrotic tissue in which anaerobic conditions might develop. Tetanus toxoid should be given to stimulate active immunity and may be administered concurrently with TIG (or TAT) if given in separate syringes at widely separated sites. A tetanus toxoid booster (preferably Td) is given to all persons with *any* wound if their tetanus immunization status is unknown or incomplete. A booster is given to injured persons who have completed their primary immunization series if (1) the wound is clean and minor but ≥10 yr have passed since the last booster or (2) the wound is more serious and ≥5 yr have passed since the last booster. With delayed wound care, active immunization should be started at once. Although fluid tetanus toxoid produces a more rapid immune response than the adsorbed or precipitated toxoids, the adsorbed toxoid results in a more durable titer.

Bennett J, Ma C, Traverso H, et al: Neonatal tetanus associated with topical umbilical ghee: Covert role of cow dung. *Int J Epidemiol* 1999;28:1172–5.

Cook TM, Protheroe RT, Handel JM: Tetanus: A review of the literature. *Br J Anaesth* 2001;87:477–87.

Dyce O, Bruno JR, Hong D, et al: Tongue piercing: The new "rusty nail?" *Head Neck* 2000;22:728–32.

Fair E, Murphy TV, Golaz A, et al: Philosophic objection to vaccination as a risk for tetanus among children younger than 15 years. *Pediatrics* 2002;109:E2.

Farrar JJ, Yen LM, Cook T, et al: Tetanus. *J Neurol Neurosurg Psychiatry* 2000;69:292–301.

Gupta R, Vohra AK, Madaa V, et al: Mass hysteria among high school girls following tetanus toxoid immunization. *Ir J Psychol Med* 2001;18:90.

Johkura K, Kuroiwa Y, Hara M: Tetanus originating from a benign scalp tumor. *J Neurol Neurosurg Psychiatry* 1999;67:120–3.

Kara CO, Cetin CB, Yalcin N: Cephalic tetanus as a result of rooster pecking: An unusual case. *Scand J Infect Dis* 2002;34:64–6.

Kharabsheh S, Al-Otoum H, Clements J, et al: Mass psychogenic illness following tetanus-diphtheria toxoid vaccination in Jordan. *Bull WHO* 2001;79:764–70.

Lee DC, Lederman HM: Anti-tetanus antibodies in intravenous gamma globulin: An alternative to tetanus immune globulin. *J Infect Dis* 1992;166:642–5.

McQuillan G, Kruszon-Moran D, Deforrest A, et al: Serologic immunity to diphtheria and tetanus in the United States. *Ann Intern Med* 2002;136:660–6.

Miranda-Filho DB, Ximenes RA, Bernardino SN, et al: Identification of risk factors for death from tetanus in Pernambuco, Brazil: A case-control study. *Rev Inst Med Trop Sao Paulo* 2000;42:333–9.

Patel JC, Mehta BC: Tetanus: Study of 8697 cases. *Indian J Med Sci* 1999;53:393–401.

Schiavo G, Matteoli M, Montecucco C: Neurotoxins affecting exocytosis. *Physiol Rev* 2000;80:717–66.

TABLE 194–1. Tetanus Prophylaxis in Wound Management

	Clean, Minor Wounds		Other Wounds*	
Prior Tetanus Doses	Td†	TIG‡	Td†	TIG‡
Uncertain, or <3	Yes	No	Yes	Yes
Three or more	No§	No	No‖	No

*Such as, but not limited to wounds contaminated with dirt, feces, and saliva; puncture wounds; avulsions; wounds resulting from missiles, crushing, burns, and frostbite; and wounds extending into muscle.

†For children <7 yr, DTaP or DTP is preferred to tetanus toxoid alone if < 3 doses of DTaP/DTP have been previously given; if pertussis vaccine is contraindicated, DT is given. For persons ≥ 7 yr, Td is preferred to tetanus toxoid alone.

‡TIG = tetanus immune globulin. TIG should be administered for tetanus-prone wounds in HIV-1–infected patients regardless of the history of tetanus immunizations.

§Yes, if ≥ 10 yr since the last dose.

‖Yes, if ≥ 5 yr since the last dose. (More frequent boosters are not needed and can accentuate adverse events.)

Adapted from Centers for Disease Control. Diphtheria, tetanus, and pertussis: Recommendations for vaccine use and other preventive measures. Recommendations of the Immunization Practices Advisory Committee (ACIP). MMWR 1991;40(RR-10):1–28.

Chapter 195

Clostridium difficile–Associated Diarrhea

Margaret C. Fisher

Clostridium difficile–associated diarrhea, also known as **pseudomembranous colitis** or **antibiotic-associated diarrhea**, is a major cause of nosocomial diarrhea. Uncommon causes of antibiotic-associated diarrhea include the enterotoxins of *Staphylococcus aureus* and *Clostridium perfringens*.

Etiology. *C. difficile* is a ubiquitous spore-forming gram-positive anaerobic bacillus. The organism produces two toxins: **toxin A (enterotoxin)** acts on the intestinal mucosa to produce diarrhea; **toxin B (cytotoxin)** increases vascular permeability in low doses and is lethal to experimental animals in high doses. In general, strains produce either both toxins or neither toxin.

Epidemiology. *C. difficile*-associated diarrhea usually occurs in patients receiving antimicrobial therapy. In children, some cases occur without prior antibiotics in the setting of altered bowel flora. Virtually all known antibiotics have been implicated; penicillins, broad-spectrum cephalosporins, and clindamycin are the most frequent offenders.

Newborns are often colonized with *C. difficile* during the first weeks of life, and colonization has been identified in approximately half of healthy infants during the first year of life. Many of these strains produce toxin. Carriage decreases to the adult rate of 1–3% by 2 yr of age. Illness is unusual in neonates and infants; the basis for this remains unknown. The incidence of toxin-mediated diarrhea peaks in children between the ages of 6 mo and 2 yr. *C. difficile*–associated diarrhea has been reported in children of all ages. Asymptomatic carriers are not at increased risk for disease unless given antibiotics.

Pathogenesis. Normal gut flora appears to be protective. The administration of antibiotics that impair growth of normal flora but not *C. difficile* is the most common risk factor, but any process that disrupts the normal bowel flora (e.g., weaning, chemotherapy) or bowel motility (e.g., bowel stasis, bowel surgery) predisposes to *C. difficile*–associated diarrhea.

Toxin A binds to a specific receptor on the intestinal brush border; the binding site for toxin B is still undefined. Both toxins are internalized and act within cells to modify proteins, resulting in cell death. Inflammatory response contributes to the diarrhea and formation of **pseudomembranes**. Antibody to the toxins appears to prevent binding and modify or abort clinical disease.

Clinical Manifestations. Clinical symptoms vary widely. Asymptomatic colonization is common in infants and young children. Illness is commonly a mild self-limited diarrhea without pseudomembranes, or it is explosive watery diarrhea with occult blood. The classic picture of pseudomembranous colitis is diarrhea with blood and mucus accompanied by fever, cramps, abdominal pain, nausea, and vomiting. Disease occurs during and as long as weeks after antibiotic therapy. Severe and extensive colitis occurs in children undergoing chemotherapy and has been reported in a few children with cystic fibrosis. *C. difficile* disease occasionally involves the small gut; in some hosts, bacteremia and abscess formation have been reported.

Diagnosis. The diagnosis is confirmed by detecting *C. difficile* or its toxin in the stool of a patient with significant diarrhea or colitis in the setting of prior or current antimicrobial use.

It has been recommended in adult patients that the diagnosis of *C. difficile*–associated diarrhea be considered in any patient with diarrhea (≥3 watery or unformed stools in 24 hr) or abdominal pain who has received antibiotics within 2 mo or whose diarrhea began >3 days after hospitalization.

Identification of toxin in a single stool specimen is the laboratory test usually used for diagnosis. Inoculation of stool filtrates into cell culture to detect cytotoxicity is considered the reference method; however, this is a labor-intensive method that requires 24–48 hr for results. Many clinical laboratories use enzyme immunoassay tests that detect toxin A only, or toxin A plus B. Testing for both toxins increases the yield of positive studies. Culture of the stool for *C. difficile* is time consuming and does not differentiate toxin-producing from non–toxin-producing strains. The interpretation of positive *C. difficile* culture or toxin in stool from children younger than 1 yr of age requires clinical correlation.

Findings at sigmoidoscopy or colonoscopy include pseudomembranous nodules and plaques characteristic of toxin-related colitis. Fecal leukocytes are present in approximately one half of cases; occult or frank blood is common.

Treatment. The first and essential step in treatment is the discontinuation of the current antibiotics, if possible. In most instances, this course combined with appropriate fluid and electrolyte replacement is sufficient. If symptoms persist, antibiotics cannot be discontinued, or the illness is severe, then oral metronidazole (20–40 mg/kg/24 hr divided q 6–8 hr PO) or vancomycin (25–40 mg/kg/24 hr divided q 6 hr PO) should be given for a 7–10 day course. Oral metronidazole is the preferred therapy for most children; it is less expensive, has an excellent response rate, and minimizes the emergence of vancomycin-resistant *Enterococcus*, which is especially important in hospitalized or institutionalized patients (Chapter 171).

Prognosis. The initial response rate is >95%, but 5–30% of patients have clinical relapse, usually within 1–2 wk of treatment. These patients should be re-evaluated and treated again; most will respond to a second course of the original treatment. A few patients develop multiple recurrences, with short-lived responses to repeated treatment. Treatment strategies for these patients include oral cholestyramine, oral bacitracin, oral immunoglobulin, reconstitution of bowel flora with oral lactobacilli or baker's yeast, or instillation of fecal flora by tube feeding or enemas. None of these methods is effective for all cases.

Prevention. *C. difficile* is often acquired nosocomially or in child-care settings. The spores of the organism are resistant to drying and to some disinfectants and frequently contaminate bathrooms and diaper changing areas of hospital rooms or child-care areas. Electronic thermometers are easily contaminated and have been implicated in several hospital outbreaks. Prevention of *C. difficile*–associated diarrhea requires meticulous hand hygiene, use of contact isolation, appropriate environmental cleaning, and appropriate use of antimicrobial agents.

Jacobs A, Barnard K, Fishel R, et al: Extracolonic manifestations of *Clostridium difficile* infections. Presentation of 2 cases and review of the literature. *Medicine* 2001;80:88–101.

Jernigan JA, Siegman-Igra Y, Guerrant RC, et al: A randomized crossover study of disposable thermometers for prevention of *Clostridium difficile* and other nosocomial infections. *Infect Control Hosp Epidemiol* 1998;19:494–9.

Johnson S, Gerding DN: *Clostridium difficile*-associated diarrhea. *Clin Infect Dis* 1998;26:1027–36.

Kyne L, Farrell RJ, Kelly CP: *Clostridium difficile*. *Gastroenterol Clin North Am* 2001; 30:753–77.

Markowitz JE, Brown KA, Mamula P, et al: Failure of single-toxin assays to detect *Clostridium difficile* infection in pediatric inflammatory bowel disease. *Am J Gastroenterol* 2001;96:2688–90.

Mylonakis E, Ryan ET, Calderwood SB: *Clostridium difficile*-associated diarrhea. A review. *Arch Intern Med* 2001;161:525–33.

Rivlin J, Lerner A, Augarten A, et al: Severe *Clostridium difficile*-associated colitis in young patients with cystic fibrosis. *J Pediatr* 1998;132:177–9.

Chapter 196

Other Anaerobic Infections

Margaret C. Fisher

Anaerobic bacteria are the most numerous organisms colonizing humans. Anaerobes are present in soil and are normal inhabitants of all living animals, but infections caused by anaerobes are relatively uncommon. Anaerobes are relatively or entirely intolerant of exposure to oxygen. The ability to survive in the presence of oxygen varies greatly, with the majority of organisms being **facultative anaerobes**, that is, able to survive in the presence of oxygen but growing better when oxygen tension is reduced. Some anaerobes are **obligate anaerobes** and will not survive any exposure to oxygen.

Infections with anaerobes occur most commonly adjacent to mucosal surfaces and as mixed infections with aerobes. Optimal conditions for proliferation of anaerobes are circumstances with reduced oxygen tension. Traumatized areas, devascularized areas, and areas of crush injury are all ideal sites for anaerobic infections. Often both aerobic and anaerobic flora are inoculated but local extension and bacteremia are most often due to the more virulent aerobes. Abscess formation evolves over days to weeks and generally involves a mixture of aerobes and anaerobes. Examples of such infections include appendicitis and abscesses: appendiceal, perirectal, peritonsillar, retropharyngeal, parapharyngeal, lung, and dental. Septic thrombophlebitis, a consequence of appendicitis, chronic sinusitis, pharyngitis, and otitis media, provides a route for spread of the infection to vital organs such as the liver, brain, or lungs.

Anaerobic infection is due to endogenous flora. Combinations of impaired physical barriers to infection, compromised tissue viability, alterations in endogenous flora, defects in host immunity, and anaerobic bacterial virulence factors contribute to infection with these normal inhabitants of mucous membranes.

Virulence factors include capsules, toxins, enzymes, and fatty acids.

Clinical Manifestations. Anaerobic infections occur in a variety of sites throughout the body (Table 196–1). Anaerobes exist synergistically with aerobes; infections with anaerobes are almost always polymicrobial and include aerobes.

CENTRAL NERVOUS SYSTEM. Meningitis is rare, but it has occurred in neonates and as a complication of *Fusobacterium* infections of the ear and neck (Lemierre syndrome). Brain abscess and subdural empyema are usually polymicrobial, with anaerobes being commonly involved. Brain abscess occurs most commonly after spread of infection from sinuses, middle ear, or lung.

TABLE 196–1. Infections Associated with Anaerobic Bacteria

Site and Infection	Major Risk Factors	Anaerobic Bacteria*
Central Nervous System		
Cerebral abscess	Direct extension from contiguous sinusitis, otitis media, mastoiditis	(Polymicrobial)
Subdural empyema		*B. fragilis*†
Epidural abscess		*Fusobacterium*
		Peptostreptococcus
		Veillonella
Upper Respiratory Tract		
Dental abscess	Poor periodontal hygiene	*Peptostreptococcus*
Ludwig angina (cellulitis of sublingual-submandibular space)	Drugs that cause gum hypertrophy	*Fusobacterium*
Necrotizing gingivitis (Vincent stomatitis)		*P. melaninogenica*
Chronic otitis-mastoiditis-sinusitis		
Peritonsillar abscess		
Retropharyngeal abscess		
Lower Respiratory Tract		
Aspiration pneumonia	Periodontal disease	(Polymicrobial)
Necrotizing pneumonitis	Bronchial obstruction	*P. melaninogenica*
Lung abscess	Altered gag or consciousness	*B. intermedius*
Pulmonary empyema		*Fusobacterium*
		Peptostreptococcus, Eubacterium
		B. fragilis, Veillonella
Intra-abdominal		
Abscess	Appendicitis	(Polymicrobial)
Secondary peritonitis	Penetrating trauma (especially of the colon)	*B. fragilis*
		Other *Bacteroides*
		Clostridium
		Peptostreptococcus
		Eubacterium
		Fusobacterium
Female Genital Tract		
Bartholin abscess	Vaginosis	*B. fragilis*
Tubo-ovarian abscess	Intrauterine device	*B. bivius*
Endometritis		*Peptostreptococcus*
Pelvic cellulitis or thrombophlebitis		*Clostridium*
Salpingitis		*Mobiluncus*
Chorioamnionitis		Actinomycosis
Septic abortion		
Skin and Soft Tissue		
Cellulitis	Decubitus ulcers	(Varies with site and contamination with mouth or enteric flora)
Perirectal cellulitis	Abdominal wounds	
Myonecrosis (gas gangrene)	Pilonidal sinus	*Clostridium perfringens* (myonecrosis)
Necrotizing fasciitis	Trauma	*Bacteroides*
Synergistic gangrene	Human and animal bites	*Fusobacterium*
	Immunosuppressed or neutropenic patients	*Clostridium tertium*
		C. septicum
		Anaerobic streptococci
Bacteremia		
	Secondary to intra-abdominal infection, abscess, myonecrosis, or necrotizing fasciitis	*B. fragilis*
		Clostridium
		Anaerobic streptococci

*Infections may also be due to or involve aerobic bacteria as the sole or part of a mixed infection: brain abscess may contain microaerophilic streptococci; intra-abdominal infections may contain gram-negative enteric organisms and enterococci; and salpingitis may contain Neisseria gonorrhoeae, and Chlamydia trachomatis.

†Bacteroides fragilis is usually isolated from infections below the diaphragm except for brain abscesses.

UPPER RESPIRATORY TRACT. The respiratory tract is colonized by both aerobes and anaerobes. Anaerobic bacteria are involved in chronic sinusitis, chronic otitis media, peritonsillar infections, parapharyngeal and retropharyngeal abscesses, and periodontal infections. Anaerobic periodontal disease is most common in patients with poor dental hygiene and in those who are receiving drugs that result in hypertrophy of the gums. **Vincent angina,** or **trench mouth,** is an acute, fulminating, necrotizing infection of the gums and floor of the mouth. The disease is characterized by pain, foul breath, and pseudomembrane formation. Ludwig angina is a life-threatening cellulitis of the sublingual and submandibular spaces; disease spreads rapidly in the neck, and airway obstruction can occur.

Lemierre syndrome, or **postanginal sepsis**, is a suppurative infection of the lateral pharyngeal space with septic thrombophlebitis of the jugular vein leading to septic embolization to the lungs and/or central nervous system. Clinical signs include neck swelling and pain, trismus, dysphagia, and severe toxicity. *Fusobacterium necrophorum* is the most commonly involved organism; polymicrobial infection is frequent.

LOWER RESPIRATORY TRACT. Anaerobic lung abscess, empyema, and anaerobic pneumonia are most common in children with swallowing dysfunction, in those with an increased incidence of aspiration, or an increased volume of aspiration and in the presence of a foreign body occluding the airway. All children and adults aspirate during sleep or during periods of unconsciousness. In most cases, the lung cilia and phagocytes clear particulate matter and microbes. If the aspiration is of high volume or high frequency or a foreign body blocks drainage, the ability of lung clearance mechanisms is overcome and infection ensues.

INTRA-ABDOMINAL INFECTION. The digestive tract is colonized throughout by anaerobes. The density of organisms is highest in the colon, where anaerobes outnumber aerobes 1,000:1. Rupture of the gut leads to spillage of gut flora into the peritoneum, resulting in peritonitis that involves both aerobes and anaerobes. Bacteremia due to aerobes occurs early. As the infection is walled off in the peritoneum, an abscess composed of both aerobes and anaerobes is formed. Liver abscesses are rare in children; predisposing illnesses are appendicitis, inflammatory bowel disease, and biliary tract disease. In children with malignancies who are receiving chemotherapy, the gut mucosa is often damaged, leading to translocation of bacteria and focal invasion of bowel flora. Typhlitis, or necrotizing colitis, is a mixed infection of the gut wall usually beginning in the colon; abdominal pain, diarrhea, fever, and abdominal distention are common features. Empirical therapy of fever and neutropenia may not be optimal against the anaerobes involved in typhlitis.

GENITAL TRACT. Genital tract infections in women often involve anaerobes. Pelvic inflammatory disease and tubo-ovarian abscesses are frequently due to mixed aerobes and anaerobes. Vaginitis can be caused by overgrowth of anaerobic flora. Anaerobes frequently contribute to chorioamnionitis and premature labor and may result in anaerobic bacteremia in the neonate. Although most of these bacteremias are transient, anaerobes occasionally cause invasive disease in the newborn.

SKIN AND SOFT TISSUE. Anaerobic skin infections occur in the setting of bites, foreign bodies, and skin and tissue ulceration due to pressure necrosis or lack of adequate blood supply. Animal bites and human bites inoculate oral and skin flora into the subcutaneous tissues. Oral flora includes anaerobes, but the more virulent aerobic infections are responsible for most clinical infections (Chapter 707). The extent of the infection depends on the depth of the bite and the associated crush injury to the tissues. **Clostridial myonecrosis**, or **gas gangrene**, is a rapidly progressive infection associated with *Clostridium perfringens.* **Necrotizing fasciitis** is a polymicrobial infection with acute onset and rapid progression, with significant morbidity and mortality. Group A streptococcus and *Staphylococcus aureus* occa-

sionally are the sole pathogens. **Synergistic gangrene** is caused by synergistic infection between *S. aureus* or gram-negative bacilli and anaerobic streptococci. All of these are uncommon infections in healthy children. Early recognition with aggressive surgical debridement and antimicrobial therapy is necessary to limit morbidity and mortality.

OTHER SITES. Occasionally the bone adjacent to anaerobic infection becomes infected by direct extension from contiguous infections or by direct inoculation associated with trauma. Anaerobic infections of the kidneys (renal and perirenal abscesses) and heart (pericarditis) are rare. **Enteritis necroticans (pigbel)** is a rare but often fatal gastrointestinal infection, which most commonly follows ingestion of a large meal in a previously starved child or adult. Recently hemorrhagic necrosis of the jejunum due to *C. perfringens* was reported in an American child with poorly controlled diabetes following ingestion of chitterlings (pork intestines).

Diagnosis. The diagnosis of anaerobic infection requires a high index of suspicion and the collection of appropriate and adequate specimens for culture (Box 196–1). Cultures should be obtained in a manner that protects the specimen from contamination with mucosal bacteria and from exposure to ambient oxygen. Swab cultures of mucosal surfaces or of nasal secretions, respiratory specimens, and stool should not be sent for anaerobic culture because these sites normally harbor anaerobes. Aspirates of infected sites, abscess material, and biopsy specimens are ideal. The specimen should be protected from oxygen and transported to the laboratory immediately. A transport medium is used to increase the recovery of obligate anaerobes. Gram stains are useful; anaerobic infections are usually polymicrobial. Susceptibility testing of anaerobes is not always performed because it is labor intensive and time consuming. Several laboratory methods for susceptibility testing are available; a rapid and easy screening test is used to detect β-lactamase production.

BOX 196–1. Clues to Presumptive Diagnosis of Anaerobic Infections*

Infection that is contiguous to or in proximity with a mucosal surface colonized with anaerobic bacteria (oropharynx, intestinal-genitourinary tract)
Foul-smelling, putrid odor (present in 50% of anaerobic infections)
Severe tissue necrosis, abscesses, gangrene, or fasciitis
Gas formation in tissues (crepitus or on radiograph)
Failure to recover organisms using conventional aerobic microbiologic methods
Failure of organisms to grow after pretreatment with antibiotics effective against anaerobics
Failure of organisms to respond to antibiotics with poor efficacy against anaerobic bacteria (e.g., aminoglycosides)
Toxin-mediated syndromes (botulism, tetanus, gas gangrene, *Clostridium perfringens* food poisoning, *C. difficile* pseudomembranous colitis)
Typical infections associated with anaerobic bacteria (see Table 196–1)
Sterile pus
Septic thrombophlebitis
Septicemic syndrome with jaundice or intravascular hemolysis
Mixed polymorphic organisms on Gram stain
Typical Gram stain appearance:
　Bacteroides species—small, delicate, pleomorphic, pale, gram-negative bacilli
　Fusobacterium nucleatum—thin gram-negative bacilli with fusiform shape, pointed ends
　F. necrophorum—pleomorphism gram-negative bacilli with rounded ends
　Peptostreptococcus—gram-positive cocci similar to aerobic cocci
　C. perfringens—large, short, fat (boxcar-shaped) gram-positive bacilli

---

*Suspicion of anaerobic infection is critical before specimens are cultured to ensure optimal microbiologic techniques and prompt, appropriate therapy.

Treatment. Treatment of anaerobic infections requires adequate drainage and appropriate antimicrobial therapy. Antibiotic therapy varies depending on the suspected or proven anaerobe involved. Some oral anaerobic flora are susceptible to penicillins, whereas many produce β-lactamase. The drugs that are active against these organisms include metronidazole, penicillins combined with β-lactamase inhibitors (ampicillin-sulbactam, ticarcillin-clavulanate, and piperacillin-tazobactam), carbapenems (imipenem and meropenem), clindamycin, cefoxitin, and chloramphenicol. Penicillin and vancomycin are active against the gram-positive anaerobes.

Aerobes are usually present with the anaerobes, necessitating broad-spectrum antibiotic combinations for empirical therapy. Specific therapy is based on culture results and clinical course.

For soft tissue infections, providing perfusion to the area is key to success; at times, a muscle flap or skin flap procedure is needed to ensure that nutrients and antimicrobial agents are brought to the affected area. Drainage of infected areas is often necessary for cure. Bacteria may survive in abscesses due to high bacterial inoculum, lack of bactericidal activity, and local conditions that facilitate bacterial proliferation. Aspiration is sometimes effective for small collections whereas incision and drainage may be required for larger abscesses. Extensive debridement and resection of all devitalized tissue is needed to control fasciitis and myonecrosis.

COMMON ANAEROBIC PATHOGENS

Clostridium. Strains of *Clostridium* cause disease by infection, production of toxins, or both. More than 60 species have been identified, but only a few cause diseases in humans. The most commonly recovered organisms are *Clostridium difficile* (Chapter 195) and *C. perfringens*; other species encountered in human disease include *C. botulinum* (Chapter 193), *C. tetani* (Chapter 194), *C. butyricum*, *C. septicum*, *C. sordellii*, *C. tertium*, and *C. histolyticus*.

C. perfringens produces a variety of toxins and virulence factors. Strains of *C. perfringens* are designated A through E. **Alpha toxin** is a phospholipase that hydrolyzes sphingomyelin and lecithin and is produced by all strains. This toxin causes hemolysis, platelet lysis, increased capillary permeability, and hepatotoxicity. **Beta toxin**, produced by strains B and C, causes hemorrhagic necrosis of the small bowel. **Epsilon toxin**, produced by B and D strains, injures vascular endothelial cells leading to increased vascular permeability, edema, and organ dysfunction. **Iota toxin**, produced by E strains, causes dermal edema. An enterotoxin is produced by type A and some type C and D strains. Hemolysins and a variety of enzymes are produced by many *C. perfringens* strains.

MYONECROSIS. *C. perfringens* is the major cause of myonecrosis, or gas gangrene, a rapidly progressive infection of soft tissue. In compromised hosts, especially patients receiving cancer chemotherapy, *C. septicum* is a cause of rapidly fatal gas gangrene. A clue to the diagnosis is pain out of proportion to the clinical appearance of the wound. Infection progresses rapidly with edema, swelling, myonecrosis, and sometimes crepitation of the soft tissue. Hypotension, mental confusion, shock, and renal failure are common. A characteristic sweet odor is present in the serosanguineous discharge. Gram stain of the exudate reveals gram-positive rods and a few leukocytes. Early and complete debridement with excision of necrotic tissue is key to controlling the infection. High-dose penicillin (250,000 U/kg/24 hr divided q 4–6 hr IV) or clindamycin (25–40 mg/kg/24 hr divided q 6–8 hr IV) should be started immediately. The role of hyperbaric oxygen remains unclear but has been beneficial in several studies. The prognosis is poor even with early, aggressive therapy.

FOOD POISONING. *C. perfringens* type A produces an enterotoxin that causes food poisoning (Chapter 705). The intoxication results in the acute onset of watery diarrhea and crampy abdominal pain. The usual foods containing toxin are improperly prepared meats and gravies. A specific diagnosis is rarely made in children with food poisoning. Therapy consists of rehydration and electrolyte replacement if necessary. The illness resolves spontaneously within 24 hr of onset. Prevention requires the maintenance of hot food at a temperature of ≥74°C.

GASTROENTERITIS. A severe gastroenteritis, termed **enteritis necroticans** or **pigbel**, is caused by type C strains of *C. perfringens* that produce beta toxin. The disease occurs most commonly in Papua New Guinea, and is related to particular dietary habits and malnutrition. Recently, enteritis necroticans was recognized in the United States in a 12-yr-old boy with poorly controlled diabetes mellitus; the source of the infection was undercooked pork chitterlings.

Bacteroides and Prevotella. *Bacteroides fragilis* is one of the more virulent of the anaerobes. It is the anaerobic pathogen that is most frequently recovered from blood cultures and cultures of tissue or pus. The most common infection in children is infection associated with appendicitis. The organism is part of normal colonic flora but is not common in the mouth or respiratory tract. *B. fragilis* is usually found as part of a polymicrobial appendiceal and other intra-abdominal abscesses and is involved in genital tract infections such as pelvic inflammatory disease and tubo-ovarian abscess. *Prevotella* are normal oral flora; infection involves gums, teeth, tonsils, and parapharyngeal spaces. Both organisms are sometimes involved in anaerobic pneumonia and lung abscess.

Strains of *B. fragilis* and *P. melaninogenica* produce β-lactamase and thus are resistant to penicillins. Antibiotics of choice include ticarcillin-clavulanate, piperacillin/tazobactam, cefoxitin, metronidazole, clindamycin, imipenem, meropenem, and chloramphenicol. Chloramphenicol is rarely used because of toxicity and failure of therapy for intra-abdominal infection. Because infections involving these organisms are polymicrobial, therapy should include antimicrobial agents active against the probable aerobic pathogens. Drainage of abscesses and debridement of necrotic tissue are often required for control of these infections.

Fusobacterium. *Fusobacterium* inhabit the intestine, respiratory, and female genital tracts. These organisms are more virulent than most of the normal anaerobic flora and have been reported to cause bacteremia and a variety of rapidly progressive infections. Lemierre syndrome, bone and joint infection, and abdominal and genital tract infections are most common. Some strains produce β-lactamase and are thus resistant to penicillins.

Veillonella. *Veillonella* are normal flora of the mouth, upper respiratory tract, intestine, and vagina. These anaerobes rarely cause infection; strains are recovered as part of the polymicrobial flora causing abscess, chronic sinusitis, empyema, peritonitis, and wound infection. *Veillonella* are susceptible to penicillins, cephalosporins, clindamycin, metronidazole, and carbapenems.

Anaerobic Cocci. *Peptostreptococcus* are normal flora of the skin, respiratory tract, and gut. These organisms are often present in brain abscesses, chronic sinusitis, chronic otitis, and lung abscesses. Such infections are often polymicrobial, and therapy is aimed at the accompanying aerobes as well as the anaerobes. Most of the gram-positive cocci are susceptible to penicillin, cephalosporins, carbapenems, and vancomycin.

Brook I: Anaerobic infections in children. *Adv Pediatr* 2000;47:395–437.

Citron DM, Goldstein EJC, Kenner MA, et al: Activity of ampicillin/sulbactam, ticarcillin/clavulanate, clarithromycin, and eleven other antimicrobial agents against anaerobic bacteria isolated from infections in children. *Clin Infect Dis* 1995;20:S356–60.

Hecht DW: Evolution of anaerobe susceptibility testing in the United States. *Clin Infect Dis* 2002;35:S28–35.

Kristensen LH, Prag J: Human necrobacillosis, with emphasis on Lemierre's syndrome. *Clin Infect Dis* 2000;31:524–32.

Lee SS, Schwartz RH, Bahadori RS: Retropharyngeal abscess: Epiglottitis of the new millennium. *J Pediatr* 2001;138:435–7.

Petrillo TM, Beck-Sague CM, Songer JG, et al: Enteritis necroticans (pigbel) in a diabetic child. *N Engl J Med* 2000;342:1250–3.

Nichols RL, Florman S: Clinical presentations of soft-tissue infections and surgical site infections. *Clin Infect Dis* 2001;33:S84–93.

Rautio M, Saxén H, Siitonen A, et al: Bacteriology of histopathologically defined appendicitis in children. *Pediatr Infect Dis J* 2000;19:1078–83.

Sloas MM, Flynn PM, Kaste SC, et al: Typhlitis in children with cancer: A 30-year experience. *Clin Infect Dis* 1993;17:484–90.

Snydman DR, Jacobus NV, McDermott LA, et al: National survey on the susceptibility of *Bacteroides fragilis* group: Report and analysis of trends for 1997–2000. *Clin Infect Dis* 2002;35:S126–34.

Tibbles PM, Edelsberg JS: Hyperbaric-oxygen therapy. *N Engl J Med* 1996;334:1642–8.

SECTION 5 *Mycobacterial Infections*

Chapter 197

Tuberculosis (*Mycobacterium tuberculosis*) *Flor M. Munoz and*

Jeffrey R. Starke

During the last decade of the 20th century the number of new cases of tuberculosis increased worldwide. Currently, 95% of tuberculosis cases occur in developing countries, where HIV/AIDS epidemics have had the greatest impact, and where resources are often unavailable for proper identification and treatment of these diseases. In many industrialized countries, most cases of tuberculosis occur in foreign-born populations. The World Health Organization (WHO) estimates that more than 8 million new cases of tuberculosis occur and approximately 3 million people die of the disease worldwide each year. Almost 1.3 million cases and 450,000 deaths occur in children each year. More than one third of the world's population is infected with *Mycobacterium tuberculosis*. If present trends continue, 10.5 million new cases are expected to occur annually by 2005, with Africa having more cases than any other region of the world. In the United States, after a resurgence in the late 1980s, the total number of cases of tuberculosis began to decrease in 1992, but tuberculosis continues to be a public health concern.

Etiology. There are five closely related mycobacteria in the *Mycobacterium tuberculosis* complex: *M. tuberculosis*, *M. bovis*, *M. africanum*, *M. microti*, and *M. canetti*. All belong to the order Actinomycetales and the family Mycobacteriaceae. *M. tuberculosis* is the most important cause of tuberculosis disease in humans. The tubercle bacilli are non–spore-forming, non-motile, pleomorphic, weakly Gram-positive curved rods 2–4 μm long. They may appear beaded or clumped in stained clinical specimens or culture media. They are obligate aerobes that grow in synthetic media containing glycerol as the carbon source and ammonium salts as the nitrogen source (e.g., Loewenstein Jensen culture media). These mycobacteria grow best at 37–41°C, produce niacin, and lack pigmentation. A lipid-rich cell wall accounts for resistance to the bactericidal actions of antibody and complement. A hallmark of all mycobacteria is acid-fastness—the capacity to form stable mycolate complexes with arylmethane dyes such as crystal violet, carbolfuchsin, auramine, and rhodamine. Once stained, they resist decoloration with ethanol and hydrochloric or other acids.

Mycobacteria grow slowly, their generation time being 12–24 hr. Isolation from clinical specimens on solid synthetic media usu-ally takes 3–6 wk, and drug-susceptibility testing requires an additional 4 wk. However, growth can be detected in 1–3 wk in selective liquid medium using radiolabeled nutrients (the BACTEC radiometric system), and drug susceptibilities can be determined in an additional 3–5 days. The presence of *M. tuberculosis* in clinical specimens can be detected within hours using nucleic acid amplification (NAA) tests, including polymerase chain reaction, that employ a DNA probe complementary to mycobacterial DNA or RNA. Data from children are limited, but the sensitivity of some NAA techniques is similar to that for culture for pulmonary tuberculosis and is generally better than culture for extrapulmonary disease. Restriction fragment length polymorphism (RFLP) profiling of mycobacteria has become a helpful tool to study the epidemiology of tuberculosis.

Epidemiology. Latent tuberculosis infection (LTBI) occurs after the inhalation of infective droplet nuclei containing *M. tuberculosis*. A reactive tuberculin skin test and the absence of clinical and radiographic manifestations are the hallmark of this stage. Tuberculosis disease occurs when signs and symptoms or radiographic changes become apparent. The word *tuberculosis* refers to disease. Untreated infants with LTBI have up to a 40% likelihood of developing tuberculosis, with the risk of progression decreasing gradually through childhood to adult lifetime rates of 5–10%. The greatest risk for progression occurs in the first 2 yr after infection.

The WHO estimates that one third of the world's population—2 billion people—are infected with *M. tuberculosis*. Infection rates are highest in Africa, Asia, and Latin America (Fig. 197–1). The global burden of tuberculosis continues to grow due to several factors, which include the impact of HIV epidemics, population migration patterns, increasing poverty, social upheaval and crowded living conditions in developing countries and in inner city populations in developed countries, inadequate health coverage and poor access to health services, and inefficient tuberculosis control programs.

Tuberculosis case rates decreased steadily in the United States during the first half of the 20th century, long before the advent of antituberculosis drugs, as a result of improved living conditions. A resurgence of tuberculosis in the late 1980s was associated primarily with the HIV epidemic and multidrug resistance adding to increased immigration and poor tuberculosis control (Fig. 197–2). Since 1992, the number of reported cases of tuberculosis has decreased each year, reaching a record low of 15,989 cases (rate of 5.6/100,000 population) in the year 2001. Of these, only 931 (6%) cases occurred in children <15 yr of age (rate 1.5/100,000 population). The decline in overall incidence was mostly due to a substantial decrease in cases in individuals born in the United States. Forty-nine percent of all cases were among foreign-born persons, a rate of 26.6/100,000 population. The total number of cases among foreign-born individuals increased

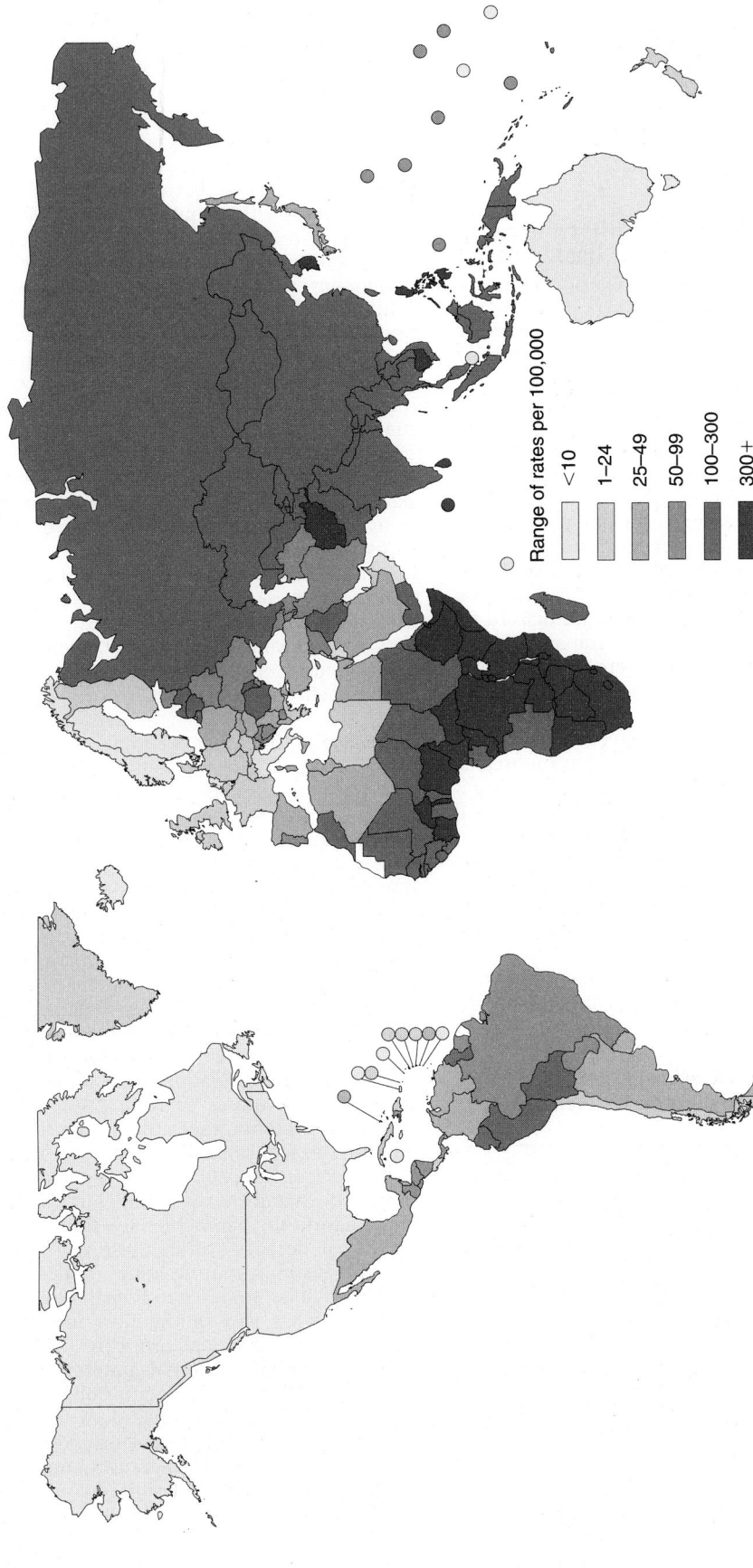

FIGURE 197–1. Estimated incidence of tuberculosis in the world, 2001. (Redrawn from World Health Organization Global Report on Tuberculosis, 2002. The designations employed and the presentation of material on this map do not imply any opinion on the part of the World Health Organization concerning the legal status of any country, city, or area or of its authorities, or concerning the delineation of its frontiers or boundaries.)

Range of rates per 100,000

<10
1–24
25–49
50–99
100–300
300+

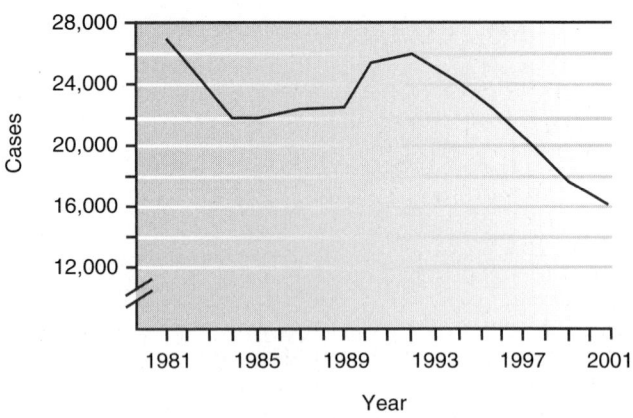

FIGURE 197–2. Observed rates of childhood tuberculosis in the United States, 1981–2001. The total number of tuberculosis cases peaked in 1992, decreasing by 5%–7% annually since. (From Centers for Disease Control and Prevention, 2002.)

4% between 1992 and 2000. In all age groups, the proportion of reported cases was strikingly higher in foreign-born and non-white individuals, even though the number of cases among foreign-born children <15 yr has declined. In white populations in the United States, tuberculosis rates are highest among the elderly who acquired the infection decades ago. In contrast, among nonwhite populations, tuberculosis is most common in young adults and children <5 yr of age. The age range of 5–14 yr is often called the "favored age" because in all human populations this group has the lowest rate of tuberculosis disease. Among adults, two thirds of cases occur in males, but there is no significant difference in gender distribution in childhood.

In the United States, most children are infected with *M. tuberculosis* in their home by someone close to them but outbreaks of childhood tuberculosis also occur in elementary and high schools, nursery schools, daycare centers, homes, churches, school buses, and sports teams. HIV-infected adults with tuberculosis can transmit *M. tuberculosis* to children, and children with HIV infection are at increased risk of developing tuberculosis after infection. Population groups at high risk for acquiring tuberculosis infection and factors that increase the risk to progress from LTBI to tuberculosis are described in Box 197–1.

The incidence of drug-resistant tuberculosis has increased dramatically throughout the world. In the United States, about

---

BOX 197–1. Groups at High Risk for Acquiring Tuberculosis Infection and Developing Disease in Developed Countries

RISK FOR TUBERCULOSIS INFECTION

Children exposed to high-risk adults
Foreign-born persons from high-prevalence countries
Poor and indigent persons, especially in large cities
Homeless persons
Persons who inject drugs
Present and former residents or employees of correctional institutions, homeless shelters, and nursing homes
Health care workers caring for high-risk patients

RISK FOR PROGRESSION TO TUBERCULOSIS DISEASE ONCE INFECTED

Infants and children ≤4 yr of age, especially those <2 yr of age
Adolescents and young adults
Persons co-infected with HIV
Persons with skin test conversion in the past 1–2 yr
Persons who are immunocompromised, especially in cases of malignancy and solid organ transplantation, immunosuppressive medical treatments, diabetes mellitus, chronic renal failure, silicosis, and malnutrition

---

8% of *M. tuberculosis* isolates are resistant to at least isoniazid, whereas 1% are resistant to both isoniazid and rifampin. Resistance to isoniazid remained relatively stable between 1992 and 2000, but the proportion of cases that were multidrug resistant decreased from 1.7% to 1%. In some countries drug resistance rates range from 20–50%. The major reasons for the development of drug resistance are poor patient adherence to treatment and provision of inadequate drug regimens by the physician or national tuberculosis program

TRANSMISSION. Transmission of *M. tuberculosis* is person to person, usually by airborne mucus droplet nuclei, particles 1–5 μm in diameter that contain *M. tuberculosis*. Transmission rarely occurs by direct contact with an infected discharge or a contaminated fomite. The chance of transmission increases when the patient has an acid-fast smear of sputum, an extensive upper lobe infiltrate or cavity, copious production of thin sputum, and severe and forceful cough. Environmental factors, especially poor air circulation, enhance transmission. Most adults no longer transmit the organism within several days to 2 wk after beginning adequate chemotherapy, but some patients remain infectious for many weeks. Young children with tuberculosis rarely infect other children or adults. Tubercle bacilli are sparse in the endobronchial secretions of children with pulmonary tuberculosis, and cough is often absent or lacks the tussive force required to suspend infectious particles of the correct size. However, children and adolescents with adult-type pulmonary tuberculosis can transmit the organism. Airborne transmission of *M. bovis* and *M. africanum* can also occur. *M. bovis* may penetrate the gastrointestinal mucosa or invade the lymphatic tissue of the oropharynx when large numbers of the organism are ingested. Human infection with *M. bovis* is rare in developed countries as a result of the pasteurization of milk and effective tuberculosis control programs for cattle.

Pathogenesis. The primary complex of tuberculosis includes local infection at the portal of entry and the regional lymph nodes that drain the area. The lung is the portal of entry in over 98% of cases. The tubercle bacilli multiply initially within alveoli and alveolar ducts. Most of the bacilli are killed, but some survive within nonactivated macrophages, which carry them through lymphatic vessels to the regional lymph nodes. When the primary infection is in the lung, the hilar lymph nodes usually are involved, although an upper lobe focus may drain into paratracheal nodes. The tissue reaction in the lung parenchyma and lymph nodes intensifies over the next 2–12 wk as the organisms grow in number and tissue hypersensitivity develops. The parenchymal portion of the primary complex often heals completely by fibrosis or calcification after undergoing caseous necrosis and encapsulation. Occasionally, this portion continues to enlarge, resulting in focal pneumonitis and pleuritis. If caseation is intense, the center of the lesion liquefies and empties into the associated bronchus, leaving a residual cavity.

The foci of infection in the regional lymph nodes develop some fibrosis and encapsulation, but healing is usually less complete than in the parenchymal lesion. Viable *M. tuberculosis* can persist for decades within these foci. In most cases of initial tuberculosis infection the lymph nodes remain normal in size. However, hilar and paratracheal lymph nodes that enlarge significantly as part of the host inflammatory reaction may encroach on a regional bronchus. Partial obstruction of the bronchus caused by external compression may cause hyperinflation in the distal lung segment. Complete obstruction results in atelectasis. Inflamed caseous nodes can attach to the bronchial wall and erode through it, causing endobronchial tuberculosis or a fistula tract. The caseum causes complete obstruction of the bronchus. The resulting lesion, a combination of pneumonitis and atelectasis, has been called a collapse-consolidation or segmental lesion (Fig. 197–3).

During the development of the primary complex, tubercle bacilli are carried to most tissues of the body through the blood

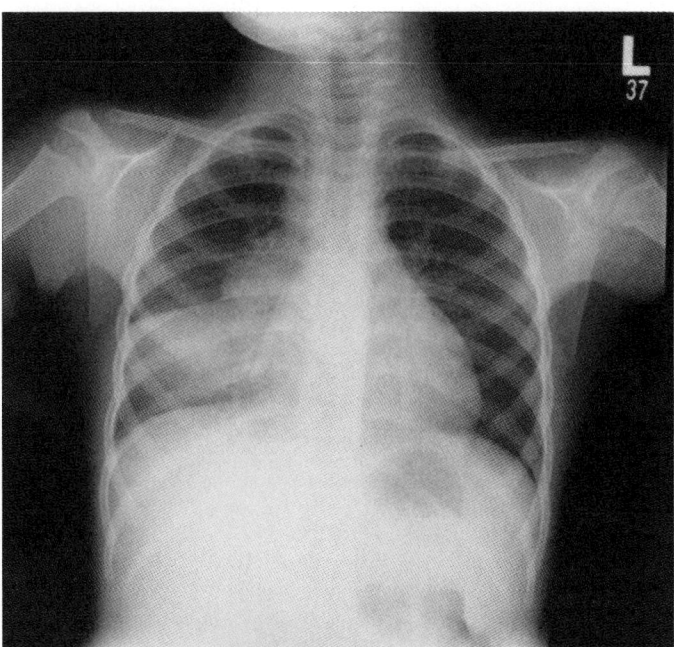

FIGURE 197–3. Right-sided hilar lymphadenopathy and collapse-consolidation lesions of primary tuberculosis in a 4-yr-old child.

and lymphatic vessels. Although seeding of the organs of the reticuloendothelial system is common, bacterial replication is more likely to occur in organs with conditions that favor their growth, such as the lung apices, brain, kidneys, and bones. Disseminated tuberculosis occurs if the number of circulating bacilli is large and the host cellular immune response is inadequate. More often the number of bacilli is small, leading to clinically inapparent metastatic foci in many organs. These remote foci usually become encapsulated, but they may be the origin of both extrapulmonary tuberculosis and reactivation tuberculosis in some individuals.

The time between initial infection and clinically apparent disease is variable. Disseminated and meningeal tuberculosis are early manifestations, often occurring within 2–6 mo of the infection. Clinically significant lymph node or endobronchial tuberculosis usually appears within 3–9 mo. Lesions of the bones and joints take several years to develop, whereas renal lesions may become evident decades after infection. From 25–35% of children with tuberculosis develop extrapulmonary manifestations compared with about 10% of immunocompetent adults.

Pulmonary tuberculosis that occurs more than a year after the primary infection is usually caused by endogenous regrowth of bacilli persisting in partially encapsulated lesions. This reactivation tuberculosis is rare in children but is common among adolescents and young adults. The most common form is an infiltrate or cavity in the apex of the upper lobes, where oxygen tension and blood flow are great.

The risk of dissemination of *M. tuberculosis* is very high in HIV-infected persons. Reinfection also can occur in persons with advanced HIV or AIDS. In immunocompetent individuals the response to the initial infection with *M. tuberculosis* usually provides protection against reinfection when a new exposure occurs. However exogenous reinfection has been reported to occur in adults without immune compromise in highly endemic areas.

PREGNANCY AND THE NEWBORN. Pulmonary and particularly extrapulmonary tuberculosis other than lymphadenitis in a pregnant woman is associated with increased risk for pre-

maturity, fetal growth retardation, low birthweight and perinatal mortality. Congenital tuberculosis is rare because the most common result of female genital tract tuberculosis is infertility. Congenital transmission usually occurs from a lesion in the placenta through the umbilical vein. Primary infection in the mother just before or during pregnancy is more likely to cause congenital infection than is reactivation of a previous infection. The tubercle bacilli first reach the fetal liver, where a primary focus with periportal lymph node involvement may occur. Organisms pass through the liver into the main fetal circulation and infect many organs. The bacilli in the lung usually remain dormant until after birth, when oxygenation and pulmonary circulation increase significantly. Congenital tuberculosis may also be caused by aspiration or ingestion of infected amniotic fluid. However, the most common route of infection for the neonate is postnatal airborne transmission from an adult with infectious pulmonary tuberculosis.

IMMUNITY. Conditions that adversely affect cell-mediated immunity predispose to progression from tuberculosis infection to disease. Rare specific genetic defects associated with deficient cell mediated immunity in response to mycobacteria include interleukin-12 receptor B1 (IL-12B1) deficiency and complete and partial interferon-γ receptor 1 chain deficiencies. Tuberculosis infection is associated with a humoral antibody response, which appears to play little role in host defense. Shortly after infection, tubercle bacilli replicate in both free alveolar spaces and within inactivated alveolar macrophages. Sulfatides in the mycobacterial cell wall inhibit fusion of the macrophage phagosome and lysosomes, allowing the organisms to escape destruction by intracellular enzymes. Cell-mediated immunity develops 2–12 wk after infection, along with tissue hypersensitivity. After bacilli enter macrophages, lymphocytes that recognize mycobacterial antigens proliferate and secrete lymphokines and other mediators that attract other lymphocytes and macrophages to the area. Certain lymphokines activate macrophages, causing them to develop high concentrations of lytic enzymes that enhance their mycobactericidal capacity. A discrete subset of regulator helper and suppressor lymphocytes modulates the immune response. Development of specific cellular immunity prevents progression of the initial infection in most individuals.

The pathologic events in the initial tuberculosis infection seem to depend on the balance among the mycobacterial antigen load; cell-mediated immunity, which enhances intracellular killing; and tissue hypersensitivity, which promotes extracellular killing. When the antigen load is small and the degree of tissue sensitivity is high, granuloma formation results from the organization of lymphocytes, macrophages, and fibroblasts. When both antigen load and the degree of sensitivity are high, granuloma formation is less organized. Tissue necrosis is incomplete, resulting in formation of caseous material.. When the degree of tissue sensitivity is low, as is often the case in infants or immunocompromised individuals, the reaction is diffuse and the infection is not well contained, leading to dissemination and local tissue destruction. Tissue necrosis factor and other cytokines released by specific lymphocytes promote cellular destruction and tissue damage in susceptible individuals.

TUBERCULIN SKIN TESTING. The development of delayed-type hypersensitivity (DTH) in most individuals infected with the tubercle bacillus makes the tuberculin skin test a useful diagnostic tool. Multipuncture tests (MPTs) are not as accurate as the Mantoux test because the exact dose of tuberculin antigen introduced into the skin cannot be controlled. The MPTs should no longer be used in pediatric practice.

The **Mantoux tuberculin skin test** is the intradermal injection of 0.1 mL containing 5 tuberculin units (TU) of purified protein derivative (PPD) stabilized with Tween 80. T cells sensitized by prior infection are recruited to the skin where they release lymphokines that induce induration through local vasodilatation, edema, fibrin deposition, and recruitment of other inflammatory cells to the area. The amount of induration in response to the test should be measured by a trained person 48–72 hr after administration. Occasional patients will have the onset of induration >72 hr after placement; this is a positive result. Immediate hypersensitivity reactions to tuberculin or other constituents of the preparation are short lived (<24 hr) and not considered a positive result. Tuberculin sensitivity develops 3 wk to 3 mo—most often in 4–8 wk—after inhalation of organisms. Host-related factors, including very young age, malnutrition, immunosuppression by disease or drugs, viral infections (e.g., measles, mumps, varicella, influenza), vaccination with live-virus vaccines, and overwhelming tuberculosis can depress the skin test reaction in a child infected with *M. tuberculosis*. Corticosteroid therapy may decrease the reaction to tuberculin, but the effect is variable. Tuberculin skin testing done at the time of initiating corticosteroid therapy is usually reliable. Approximately 10% of immunocompetent children with tuberculosis disease—up to 50% of those with meningitis or disseminated disease—do not react initially to PPD; most become reactive after several months of antituberculosis therapy. Nonreactivity may be specific to tuberculin or more global to a variety of antigens, so positive "control" skin tests with a negative tuberculin test never rule out tuberculosis. The most common reasons for a false-negative skin test are poor technique or misreading of the results.

False-positive reactions to tuberculin can be caused by cross sensitization to antigens of nontuberculous mycobacteria (NTM), which generally are more prevalent in the environment as one approaches the equator. These cross reactions are usually transient over months to years and produce less than 10–12 mm of induration. Previous vaccination with bacille Calmette-Guérin (BCG) also can cause a reaction to a tuberculin skin test. Approximately one half of infants who receive a BCG vaccine never develop a reactive tuberculin skin test, and the reactivity usually wanes in 2–3 yr in those with initially positive skin tests. Older children and adults who receive a BCG vaccine are more likely to develop tuberculin reactivity, but most lose the reactivity by 5–10 yr after vaccination. When skin test reactivity is present, it usually causes <10 mm of induration, although larger reactions occur in some individuals. In general, a tuberculin skin reaction ≥10 mm in a BCG-vaccinated child or adult indicates infection with *M. tuberculosis*, which necessitates further diagnostic evaluation and treatment. Prior vaccination with BCG is never a contraindication to tuberculin testing.

The appropriate size of induration indicating a positive Mantoux tuberculin skin test varies with related epidemiologic and risk factors. In children with no risk factors for tuberculosis skin test reactions are usually false-positive results. For this reason, the American Academy of Pediatrics (AAP) and Centers for Disease Control and Prevention (CDC) discourage routine testing of children, and recommend targeted tuberculin testing of children at risk identified through periodic screening surveys conducted by the primary care provider. Possible exposure to an adult with or at high risk for infectious pulmonary tuberculosis is the most crucial risk factor for children. Reaction size limits for determining a positive tuberculin test result vary with the individual's risk of infection (Box 197–2). For adults and children at the highest risk of having infection progress to disease—those with recent contact with infectious persons, clinical illnesses consistent with tuberculosis, or HIV infection or other immunosuppression—a reactive area ≥5 mm is classified as a positive result, indicating infection with *M. tuberculosis*. For other high-risk groups, a reactive area ≥10 mm is considered positive. For low-risk persons, especially those residing in communities where the prevalence of tuberculosis is low, the cutoff point for a positive reaction is ≥15 mm. An increase of induration of ≥10 mm within a 2-yr period is considered a tuberculin skin test conversion at any age. Classifying children with this scheme depends on the willingness and ability of the clinician and family to develop

a thorough exposure history for the child and the adults who care for the child. To interpret the tuberculin skin test correctly, the clinician must clearly understand the epidemiology of tuberculosis in the community and the correct indication for tuberculin testing of the individual.

Clinical Manifestations and Diagnosis. The majority of children with tuberculosis infection develop no signs or symptoms at any time. Occasionally, infection is marked by low-grade fever and mild cough, and rarely by high fever, cough, malaise, and flu-like symptoms that resolve within a week. The proportion of extrapulmonary tuberculosis cases has increased over the past 2 decades in the United States. About 15% of adult tuberculosis cases are extrapulmonary, and 25–30% of children with tuberculosis have an extrapulmonary presentation.

PRIMARY PULMONARY DISEASE. The primary pulmonary complex includes the parenchymal focus and the regional lymph nodes. About 70% of lung foci are subpleural, and localized pleurisy is common. The initial parenchymal inflammation usually is not visible on chest radiograph, but a localized, nonspecific infiltrate may be seen before the development of tissue hypersensitivity. All lobar segments of the lung are at equal risk of initial infection. Two or more primary foci are present in 25% of cases. The hallmark of primary tuberculosis in the lung is the relatively large size of the regional lymphadenitis compared with the relatively small size of the initial lung focus. As DTH develops, the hilar lymph nodes continue to enlarge in some children, especially infants, compressing the regional bronchus and causing obstruction. The usual sequence is hilar lymphadenopathy, focal hyperinflation, and then atelectasis. The resulting radiographic shadows have been called collapse-consolidation or segmental tuberculosis (see Fig. 197–3). Rarely, inflamed caseous nodes attach to the endobronchial wall and erode through it, causing endobronchial tuberculosis or a fistula tract. The caseum causes complete obstruction of the bronchus, resulting in extensive infiltrate and collapse. Enlargement of the subcarinal lymph nodes can cause compression of the esophagus and, rarely, a bronchoesophageal fistula.

Most cases of tuberculous bronchial obstruction in children resolve fully with appropriate treatment. Occasionally, there is residual calcification of the primary focus or regional lymph nodes. The appearance of calcification implies that the lesion has been present for at least 6–12 mo. Healing of the segment can be complicated by scarring or contraction associated with cylindrical bronchiectasis, but this is rare.

Children may have lobar pneumonia without impressive hilar lymphadenopathy. If the primary infection is progressively destructive, liquefaction of the lung parenchyma can lead to formation of a thin-walled primary tuberculosis cavity. Rarely, bullous tuberculous lesions can occur in the lungs and lead to pneumothorax if they rupture. Erosion of a parenchymal focus of tuberculosis into a blood or lymphatic vessel may result in dissemination of the bacilli and a **miliary pattern**, with small nodules evenly distributed on the chest radiograph.

The symptoms and physical signs of primary pulmonary tuberculosis in children are surprisingly meager considering the degree of radiographic changes often seen. More than 50% of infants and children with radiographically moderate to severe pulmonary tuberculosis have no physical findings and are discovered only by contact tracing. Infants are more likely to experience signs and symptoms. Nonproductive cough and mild dyspnea are the most common symptoms. Systemic complaints such as fever, night sweats, anorexia, and decreased activity occur less often. Some infants have difficulty gaining weight or develop a true failure-to-thrive syndrome that often does not improve significantly until several months of effective treatment have been taken. Pulmonary signs are even less common. Some infants and young children with bronchial obstruction have localized wheezing or decreased breath sounds that may be accompanied by tachypnea or, rarely, respiratory distress. These pulmonary symptoms and signs are occasionally alleviated by antibiotics, suggesting bacterial superinfection.

The most specific confirmation of pulmonary tuberculosis is isolation of *M. tuberculosis.* Sputum specimens for culture should be collected from adolescents and older children who are capable to expectorate. The best culture specimen in young children is the early morning gastric acid obtained before the child has arisen and peristalsis has emptied the stomach of the pooled secretions that have been swallowed overnight. Even under optimal conditions, though, three consecutive morning gastric aspirates yield the organisms in <50% of cases. The culture yield from bronchoscopy is even lower, but this procedure may demonstrate the presence of endobronchial disease or a fistula. Negative cultures never exclude the diagnosis of tuberculosis in a child. For most children, the presence of a positive tuberculin skin test, an abnormal chest radiograph consistent with tuberculosis, and history of exposure to an adult with infectious tuberculosis is adequate proof that the disease is present. The drug susceptibility test results from the adult source case's isolate can be used to determine the best therapeutic regimen for the child. Cultures should be obtained from the child whenever the source case is unknown or the source case has possible drug-resistant tuberculosis.

PROGRESSIVE PRIMARY PULMONARY DISEASE. A rare but serious complication of tuberculosis in a child occurs when the primary focus enlarges steadily and develops a large caseous center. Liquefaction may cause formation of a primary cavity associated with large numbers of tubercle bacilli. The enlarging focus may slough necrotic debris into the adjacent bronchus, leading to further intrapulmonary dissemination. Significant signs or symptoms are frequent in locally progressive disease in children. High fever, severe cough with sputum production, weight loss, and night sweats are common. Physical signs include diminished breath sounds, rales, and dullness or egophony over the cavity. The prognosis for full but usually slow recovery is excellent with appropriate therapy.

REACTIVATION TUBERCULOSIS. Pulmonary tuberculosis in adults usually represents endogenous reactivation of a site of tuberculosis infection established previously in the body. This form of tuberculosis is rare in childhood but may occur in adolescence. Children with a healed tuberculosis infection acquired before 2 yr of age rarely develop chronic reactivation pulmonary disease, which is more common in those who acquire the initial infection after 7 yr of age. The most frequent pulmonary sites

are the original parenchymal focus, lymph nodes, or the apical seedings (Simon foci) established during the hematogenous phase of the early infection. This form of disease usually remains localized to the lungs because the established immune response prevents further extrapulmonary spread. The most common radiographic presentations of this type of tuberculosis are extensive infiltrates or thick-walled cavities in the upper lobes.

Older children and adolescents with reactivation tuberculosis are more likely to experience fever, anorexia, malaise, weight loss, night sweats, productive cough, hemoptysis, and chest pain than children with primary pulmonary tuberculosis. However, physical examination findings usually are minor or absent, even when cavities or large infiltrates are present. Most signs and symptoms improve within several weeks of starting effective treatment, although the cough may last for several months. This form of tuberculosis may be highly contagious if there is significant sputum production and cough. The prognosis for full recovery is excellent when patients are given appropriate therapy.

PLEURAL EFFUSION. Tuberculous pleural effusions, which can be local or general, originate in the discharge of bacilli into the pleural space from a subpleural pulmonary focus or caseated lymph node. Asymptomatic local pleural effusion is so frequent in primary tuberculosis that it is basically a component of the primary complex. Larger and clinically significant effusions occur months to years after the primary infection. Tuberculous pleural effusion is infrequent in children <6 yr of age and rare in children <2 yr of age. Effusions are usually unilateral but can be bilateral. They are virtually never associated with a segmental pulmonary lesion and are rare in disseminated tuberculosis. Often the radiographic abnormality is more extensive than would be suggested by physical findings or symptoms (Fig. 197–4).

Clinical onset of tuberculous pleurisy is often sudden, characterized by low to high fever, shortness of breath, chest pain on deep inspiration, and diminished breath sounds. The fever and other symptoms may last for several weeks after the start of antituberculosis chemotherapy. The tuberculin skin test is positive in only 70–80% of cases. The prognosis is excellent, but radiographic resolution often takes months. Scoliosis is a rare complication from a long-standing effusion.

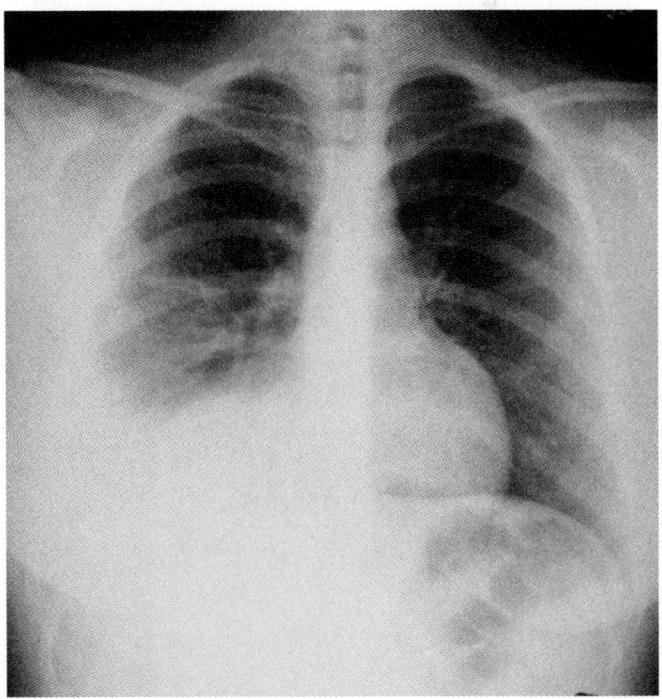

FIGURE 197–4. Pleural tuberculosis in a 16-yr-old girl.

Examination of pleural fluid and the pleural membrane is important to establish the diagnosis of tuberculous pleurisy. The pleural fluid is usually yellow and only occasionally tinged with blood. The specific gravity is usually 1.012–1.025, the protein level is usually 2–4 g/dL, and the glucose concentration may be low, although it is usually in the low-normal range (20–40 mg/dL). Typically there are several hundred to several thousand white blood cells per cubic millimeter with an early predominance of polymorphonuclear cells followed by a high percentage of lymphocytes. Acid-fast smears of the pleural fluid are rarely positive. Cultures of the fluid are positive in only <30% of cases. Biopsy of the pleural membrane is more likely to yield a positive acid-fast stain or culture, and granuloma formation usually can be demonstrated.

PERICARDIAL DISEASE. The most common form of cardiac tuberculosis is pericarditis. It is rare, occurring in 0.5–4% of tuberculosis cases in children. Pericarditis usually arises from direct invasion or lymphatic drainage from subcarinal lymph nodes. The presenting symptoms are nonspecific, including low-grade fever, malaise, and weight loss. Chest pain is unusual in children. A pericardial friction rub or distant heart sounds with pulsus paradoxus may be present. The pericardial fluid is typically serofibrinous or hemorrhagic. Acid-fast smear of the fluid rarely reveals the organism, but cultures are positive in 30–70% of cases. The culture yield from pericardial biopsy may be higher, and the presence of granulomas often suggests the diagnosis. Partial or complete pericardiectomy may be required when constrictive pericarditis develops.

LYMPHOHEMATOGENOUS (DISSEMINATED) DISEASE. Tubercle bacilli are disseminated to distant sites, including liver, spleen, skin, and lung apices, in all cases of tuberculosis infection. The clinical picture produced by lymphohematogenous dissemination depends on the quantity of organisms released from the primary focus and the adequacy of the host immune response. Lymphohematogenous spread is usually asymptomatic. Rare patients experience protracted hematogenous tuberculosis caused by the intermittent release of tubercle bacilli as a caseous focus erodes through the wall of a blood vessel in the lung. Although the clinical picture may be acute, more often it is indolent and prolonged, with spiking fever accompanying the release of organisms into the bloodstream. Multiple organ involvement is common, leading to hepatomegaly, splenomegaly, lymphadenitis in superficial or deep nodes, and papulonecrotic tuberculids appearing on the skin. Bones and joints or kidneys also may become involved. Meningitis occurs only late in the course of the disease. Early pulmonary involvement is surprisingly mild, but diffuse involvement becomes apparent with prolonged infection.

The most clinically significant form of disseminated tuberculosis is miliary disease, which occurs when massive numbers of tubercle bacilli are released into the bloodstream, causing disease in two or more organs. Miliary tuberculosis usually complicates the primary infection, occurring within 2–6 mo of the initial infection. Although this form of disease is most common in infants and young children, it is also found in adolescents and older adults, resulting from the breakdown of a previously healed primary pulmonary lesion. The clinical manifestations of miliary tuberculosis are protean, depending on the load of organisms that disseminate and where they lodge. Lesions are often larger and more numerous in the lungs, spleen, liver, and bone marrow than other tissues. Because this form of tuberculosis is most common in infants and malnourished or immunosuppressed patients, the host's immune incompetency probably also plays a role in pathogenesis.

The onset of miliary tuberculosis is sometimes explosive, and the patient may become gravely ill in several days. More often, the onset is insidious with early systemic signs, including anorexia, weight loss, and low-grade fever. At this time abnormal physical signs are usually absent. Generalized lymphadenopathy and hepatosplenomegaly develop within several weeks in about 50% of cases. The fever may then become higher and more sustained, although the chest radiograph usually is normal and respiratory symptoms are minor or absent. Within several more weeks, the lungs may become filled with tubercles, and dyspnea, cough, rales, or wheezing occurs. The lesions of miliary tuberculosis are usually smaller than 2–3 mm in diameter when first visible on chest radiograph (Fig. 197–5). The smaller lesions coalesce to form larger lesions and sometimes extensive infiltrates. As the pulmonary disease progresses, an alveolar–air block syndrome may result in frank respiratory distress, hypoxia, and pneumothorax, or pneumomediastinum. Signs or symptoms of meningitis or peritonitis are found in 20–40% of patients with advanced disease. Chronic or recurrent headache in a patient with miliary tuberculosis usually indicates the presence of meningitis, whereas the onset of abdominal pain or tenderness is a sign of tuberculous peritonitis. Cutaneous lesions include papulonecrotic tuberculids, nodules, or purpura. Choroid tubercles occur in 13–87% of patients and are highly specific for the diagnosis of miliary tuberculosis. Unfortunately, the tuberculin skin test is nonreactive in up to 40% of patients with disseminated tuberculosis.

Diagnosis of disseminated tuberculosis can be difficult, and a high index of suspicion by the clinician is required. Often the patient presents with fever of unknown origin. Early sputum or gastric aspirate cultures have a low sensitivity. Biopsy of the liver or bone marrow with appropriate bacteriologic and histologic

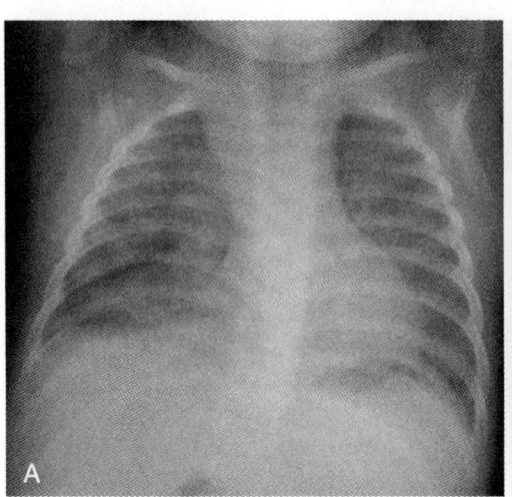
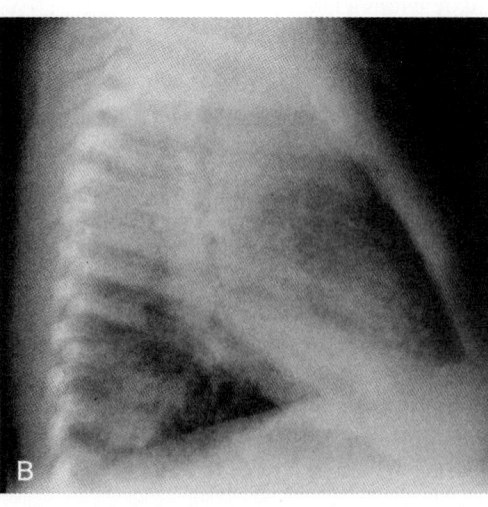

FIGURE 197–5. Posteroanterior (A) and lateral (B) chest radiographs of an infant with miliary tuberculosis. The child's mother had failed to complete treatment for pulmonary tuberculosis twice within 3 yr of this child's birth.

examinations more often yields an early diagnosis. The most important clue is usually history of recent exposure to an adult with infectious tuberculosis.

The resolution of miliary tuberculosis is slow, even with proper therapy. Fever usually declines within 2–3 wk of starting chemotherapy, but the chest radiographic abnormalities may not resolve for many months. Occasionally, corticosteroids hasten symptomatic relief, especially when air block, peritonitis, or meningitis is present. The prognosis is excellent if the diagnosis is made early and adequate chemotherapy is given.

UPPER RESPIRATORY TRACT DISEASE. Tuberculosis of the upper respiratory tract is rare in developed countries but is still observed in developing countries. Children with laryngeal tuberculosis have a croupy cough, sore throat, hoarseness, and dysphagia. Most children with laryngeal tuberculosis have extensive upper lobe pulmonary disease, but occasional patients have primary laryngeal disease with a normal chest radiograph. Tuberculosis of the middle ear results from aspiration of infected pulmonary secretions into the middle ear or from hematogenous dissemination in older children. The most common signs and symptoms are painless unilateral otorrhea, tinnitus, decreased hearing, facial paralysis, and a perforated tympanic membrane. Enlargement of lymph nodes in the preauricular or anterior cervical chains may accompany this infection. Diagnosis is difficult because stains and cultures of ear fluid are frequently negative and histology of the affected tissue often shows a nonspecific acute and chronic inflammation without granuloma formation.

LYMPH NODE DISEASE. Tuberculosis of the superficial lymph nodes, often referred to as scrofula, is the most common form of extrapulmonary tuberculosis in children. Historically, scrofula was usually caused by drinking unpasteurized cow's milk laden with *M. bovis*. Most current cases occur within 6–9 mo of initial infection by *M. tuberculosis*, although some cases appear years later. The tonsillar, anterior cervical, submandibular, and supraclavicular nodes become involved secondary to extension of a primary lesion of the upper lung fields or abdomen. Infected nodes in the inguinal, epitrochlear, or axillary regions result from regional lymphadenitis associated with tuberculosis of the skin or skeletal system. The nodes usually enlarge gradually in the early stages of lymph node disease. They are firm but not hard, discrete, and nontender. The nodes often feel fixed to underlying or overlying tissue. Disease is most often unilateral, but bilateral involvement may occur because of the crossover drainage patterns of lymphatic vessels in the chest and lower neck. As infection progresses, multiple nodes are infected, resulting in a mass of matted nodes. Systemic signs and symptoms other than a low-grade fever are usually absent. The tuberculin skin test is usually reactive. The chest radiograph is normal in 70% of cases. The onset of illness is occasionally more acute, with rapid enlargement of lymph nodes, high fever, tenderness, and fluctuance. The initial presentation is rarely a fluctuant mass with overlying cellulitis or skin discoloration.

Lymph node tuberculosis may resolve if left untreated but more often progresses to caseation and necrosis. The capsule of the node breaks down, resulting in the spread of infection to adjacent nodes. Rupture of the node usually results in a draining sinus tract that may require surgical removal. Tuberculous lymphadenitis usually responds well to antituberculosis therapy, although the lymph nodes do not return to normal size for months or even years. Surgical removal alone is not adequate therapy because the lymph node disease is but one part of a systemic infection.

A definitive diagnosis of tuberculous adenitis usually requires histologic or bacteriologic confirmation, which is best accomplished by excisional biopsy of the involved node. Culture of lymph node tissue yields the organism in only about 50% of cases. Many other conditions can be confused with tuberculous adenitis, including infection due to NTM, cat-scratch disease (*Bartonella henselae*), tularemia, brucellosis, toxoplasmosis,

tumor, branchial cleft cyst, cystic hygroma, and pyogenic infection. The most frequent problem is distinguishing infection due to *M. tuberculosis* from lymphadenitis due to NTM in geographic areas where NTM are common. Both conditions are usually associated with a normal chest radiograph and a reactive tuberculin skin test. An important clue to the diagnosis of tuberculous adenitis is an epidemiologic link to an adult with infectious tuberculosis. In areas where both diseases are common, the only way to distinguish them may be culture of the involved tissue.

CENTRAL NERVOUS SYSTEM DISEASE. Tuberculosis of the central nervous system is the most serious complication in children and is fatal without effective treatment. Tuberculous meningitis usually arises from the formation of a metastatic caseous lesion in the cerebral cortex or meninges that develops during the lymphohematogenous dissemination of the primary infection. This initial lesion increases in size and discharges small numbers of tubercle bacilli into the subarachnoid space. The resulting gelatinous exudate infiltrates the corticomeningeal blood vessels, producing inflammation, obstruction, and subsequent infarction of cerebral cortex. The brainstem is often the site of greatest involvement, which accounts for the frequently associated dysfunction of cranial nerves III, VI, and VII. The exudate also interferes with the normal flow of cerebrospinal fluid (CSF) in and out of the ventricular system at the level of the basilar cisterns, leading to a communicating hydrocephalus. The combination of vasculitis, infarction, cerebral edema, and hydrocephalus results in the severe damage that can occur gradually or rapidly. Profound abnormalities in electrolyte metabolism, due to salt wasting or the syndrome of inappropriate antidiuretic hormone secretion, also contribute to the pathophysiology of tuberculous meningitis.

Tuberculous meningitis complicates about 0.3% of untreated tuberculosis infections in children. It is most common in children between 6 mo and 4 yr of age. Occasionally, tuberculous meningitis occurs many years after the infection, when rupture of one or more of the subependymal tubercles discharges tubercle bacilli into the subarachnoid space. The clinical progression of tuberculous meningitis may be rapid or gradual. Rapid progression tends to occur more often in infants and young children, who may experience symptoms for only several days before the onset of acute hydrocephalus, seizures, and cerebral edema. More commonly, the signs and symptoms progress slowly over several weeks and can be divided into three stages. The first stage, which typically lasts 1–2 wk, is characterized by nonspecific symptoms, such as fever, headache, irritability, drowsiness, and malaise. Focal neurologic signs are absent, but infants may experience a stagnation or loss of developmental milestones. The second stage usually begins more abruptly. The most common features are lethargy, nuchal rigidity, seizures, positive Kernig or Brudzinski signs, hypertonia, vomiting, cranial nerve palsies, and other focal neurologic signs. The accelerating clinical illness usually correlates with the development of hydrocephalus, increased intracranial pressure, and vasculitis. Some children have no evidence of meningeal irritation but may have signs of encephalitis, such as disorientation, movement disorders, or speech impairment. The third stage is marked by coma, hemiplegia or paraplegia, hypertension, decerebrate posturing, deterioration of vital signs, and, eventually, death. The prognosis of tuberculous meningitis correlates most closely with the clinical stage of illness at the time treatment is initiated. The majority of patients in the first stage have an excellent outcome, whereas most patients in the third stage who survive have permanent disabilities, including blindness, deafness, paraplegia, diabetes insipidus, or mental retardation. The prognosis for young infants is generally worse than for older children. It is imperative that antituberculosis treatment be considered for any child who develops basilar meningitis and hydrocephalus, cranial nerve palsy, or stroke with no other apparent etiology. Often the key to the correct diagnosis is identifying an adult in contact with the child who has infectious tuberculosis. Because of the short incubation period of tuberculous meningitis, the ill adult has not yet been diagnosed in many cases.

The diagnosis of tuberculous meningitis can be difficult early in its course, requiring a high degree of suspicion on the part of the clinician. The tuberculin skin test is nonreactive in up to 50% of cases and 20–50% of children have a normal chest radiograph. The most important laboratory test for the diagnosis of tuberculous meningitis is examination and culture of the lumbar CSF. The CSF leukocyte count usually ranges from 10–500 cells/mm^3. Polymorphonuclear leukocytes may be present initially, but lymphocytes predominate in the majority of cases. The CSF glucose is typically <40 mg/dL but rarely <20 mg/dL. The protein level is elevated and may be markedly high (400–5,000 mg/dL) secondary to hydrocephalus and spinal block. Although the lumbar CSF is grossly abnormal, ventricular CSF may have normal chemistries and cell counts because this fluid is obtained from a site proximal to the inflammation and obstruction. The success of the microscopic examination of acid-fast stained CSF and mycobacterial culture is related directly to the volume of the CSF sample. Examinations or culture of small amounts of CSF are unlikely to demonstrate *M. tuberculosis*. When 5–10 mL of lumbar CSF can be obtained, the acid-fast stain of the CSF sediment is positive in up to 30% of cases and the culture is positive in 50–70% of cases. Cultures of other fluids, such as gastric aspirates or urine, may help confirm the diagnosis. Radiographic studies may aid in the diagnosis of tuberculous meningitis. CT or MRI of the brain of patients with tuberculous meningitis may be normal during early stages of the disease. As disease progresses, basilar enhancement and communicating hydrocephalus with signs of cerebral edema or early focal ischemia are the most common findings. Some small children with tuberculous meningitis may have one or several clinically silent tuberculomas, occurring most often in the cerebral cortex or thalamic regions.

Another manifestation of central nervous system tuberculosis is the **tuberculoma**, which usually presents clinically as a brain tumor. Tuberculomas account for up to 40% of brain tumors in some areas of the world, but they are rare in North America. In adults tuberculomas are most often supratentorial, but in children they are often infratentorial, located at the base of the brain near the cerebellum. Lesions are most often singular but may be multiple. The most common symptoms are headache, fever, and convulsions. The tuberculin skin test is usually reactive, but the chest radiograph is usually normal. Surgical excision is often necessary to distinguish tuberculoma from other causes of brain tumor. However, surgical removal is not necessary because most tuberculomas resolve with medical management. Corticosteroids are usually administered during the first few weeks of treatment or in the immediate postoperative period to decrease cerebral edema. On CT or MRI of the brain, tuberculomas usually appear as discrete lesions with a significant amount of surrounding edema. Contrast medium enhancement is often impressive and may result in a ringlike lesion. Since the advent of CT, the paradoxical development of tuberculomas in patients with tuberculous meningitis who are receiving ultimately effective chemotherapy has been recognized. The cause and nature of these tuberculomas are poorly understood, but they do not represent failure of drug treatment. This phenomenon should be considered whenever a child with tuberculous meningitis deteriorates or develops focal neurologic findings while on treatment. Corticosteroids may help alleviate the occasionally severe clinical signs and symptoms that occur. These lesions may persist for months or even years.

CUTANEOUS DISEASE. Cutaneous tuberculosis is rare in the United States but occurs worldwide and accounts for 1–2% of tuberculosis (Chapter 655).

BONE AND JOINT DISEASE. Bone and joint infection complicating tuberculosis is most likely to involve the vertebrae. The classic manifestation of tuberculous spondylitis is progression to Pott disease, in which destruction of the vertebral bodies leads to gibbus deformity and kyphosis (Chapter 669.4). Skeletal tuberculosis is a late complication of tuberculosis and although it has become a rare entity since antituberculosis therapy became available, it is more likely to occur in children than in adults. Tuberculous bone lesions may resemble pyogenic and fungal infections, or bone tumors. Multifocal bone involvement can occur. A bone biopsy is essential to confirm the diagnosis.

ABDOMINAL AND GASTROINTESTINAL DISEASE. Tuberculosis of the oral cavity or pharynx is quite unusual. The most common lesion is a painless ulcer on the mucosa, palate, or tonsil with enlargement of the regional lymph nodes. Tuberculosis of the parotid gland has been reported rarely in endemic countries. Tuberculosis of the esophagus is rare in children but may be associated with a tracheoesophageal fistula in infants. These forms of tuberculosis are usually associated with extensive pulmonary disease and swallowing of infectious respiratory secretions. However, they can occur in the absence of pulmonary disease, presumably by spread from mediastinal or peritoneal lymph nodes.

Tuberculous peritonitis, which occurs most often in young men, is uncommon in adolescents and rare in children. Generalized peritonitis may arise from subclinical or miliary hematogenous dissemination. Localized peritonitis is caused by direct extension from an abdominal lymph node, intestinal focus, or genitourinary tuberculosis. Rarely, the lymph nodes, omentum, and peritoneum become matted and can be palpated as a "doughy" irregular nontender mass. Abdominal pain or tenderness, ascites, anorexia and low-grade fever are typical manifestations. The tuberculin skin test is usually reactive. The diagnosis can be confirmed by paracentesis with appropriate stains and cultures, but this procedure must be performed carefully to avoid entering a bowel that is intertwined with the matted omentum.

Tuberculous enteritis is caused by hematogenous dissemination or by swallowing tubercle bacilli discharged from the patient's own lungs. The jejunum and ileum near Peyer patches and the appendix are the most common sites of involvement. The typical findings are shallow ulcers that cause pain, diarrhea or constipation, and weight loss with low-grade fever. Mesenteric adenitis usually complicates the infection. The enlarged nodes may cause intestinal obstruction or erode through the omentum to cause generalized peritonitis. The clinical presentation of tuberculous enteritis is nonspecific, mimicking other infections and conditions that cause diarrhea. The disease should be suspected in any child with chronic gastrointestinal complaints and a reactive tuberculin skin test. Biopsy, acid-fast stain, and culture of the lesions are usually necessary to confirm the diagnosis.

GENITOURINARY DISEASE. Renal tuberculosis is rare in children because the incubation period is several years or longer. Tubercle bacilli usually reach the kidney during lympho-hematogenous dissemination. The organisms often can be recovered from the urine in cases of miliary tuberculosis and in some patients with pulmonary tuberculosis in the absence of renal parenchymal disease. In true renal tuberculosis, small caseous foci develop in the renal parenchyma and release *M. tuberculosis* into the tubules. A large mass develops near the renal cortex that discharges bacteria through a fistula into the renal pelvis. Infection then spreads locally to the ureters, prostate, or epididymis. Renal tuberculosis is often clinically silent in its early stages, marked only by sterile pyuria and microscopic hematuria. Dysuria, flank or abdominal pain, and gross hematuria develop as the disease progresses. Superinfection by other bacteria, which often causes more acute symptoms, occurs frequently but may also delay recognition of the underlying tuberculosis. Hydronephrosis or ureteral strictures may complicate the disease. Urine cultures for *M. tuberculosis* are positive in 80–90% of cases, and acid-fast stains of large volumes of urine sediment are positive in 50–70% of cases. The tuberculin skin test is nonreactive in up to 20% of patients. An intravenous pyelogram often reveals mass lesions, dilatation of the proximal ureters, multiple small filling defects, and hydronephrosis if ureteral stricture is present. Disease is most often unilateral.

Tuberculosis of the genital tract is uncommon in both males and females before puberty. This condition usually originates from lymphohematogenous spread, although it can be caused by direct spread from the intestinal tract or bone. Adolescent girls may develop genital tract tuberculosis during the primary infection. The fallopian tubes are most often involved (90–100% of cases) followed by the endometrium (50%), ovaries (25%), and cervix (5%). The most common symptoms are lower abdominal pain and dysmenorrhea or amenorrhea. Systemic manifestations are usually absent and the chest radiograph is normal in the majority of cases. The tuberculin skin test is usually reactive. Genital tuberculosis in adolescent males causes epididymitis or orchitis. The condition usually manifests as a unilateral nodular painless swelling of the scrotum. Involvement of the glans penis is extremely rare. Genital abnormalities and a positive tuberculin skin test in an adolescent male or female should suggest the diagnosis of genital tract tuberculosis.

DISEASE IN HIV-INFECTED CHILDREN. Most cases of tuberculosis in HIV-infected children have been described in developing countries. The rate of tuberculosis disease in HIV-infected children is 30 times higher than in non–HIV-infected children in the United States. Establishing the diagnosis of tuberculosis in an HIV-infected child may be difficult because skin test reactivity can be absent, culture confirmation is difficult, and the clinical features of tuberculosis are similar to many other HIV-related infections and conditions. Tuberculosis in HIV-infected children is often more severe, progressive, and likely to occur in extrapulmonary sites. Radiographic findings are similar to those in children with normal immune systems, but lobar disease and lung cavitation are more common. Nonspecific respiratory symptoms, fever, and weight loss are the most common complaints. Rates of drug-resistant tuberculosis are higher in HIV-infected adults and, probably, are also higher in HIV-infected children. The mortality rate of HIV-infected children with tuberculosis is high, especially as the CD4 lymphocyte numbers decrease. In adults, the host immune response to tuberculosis infection appears to enhance HIV replication and accelerate the immune suppression caused by HIV. Increased mortality rates are attributed to progressive HIV infection rather than tuberculosis. Therefore, HIV-infected children with potential exposures and/or recent infection should be promptly evaluated and treated for tuberculosis. Conversely, all children with tuberculosis disease should be tested for HIV co-infection, because of the potential benefits of early diagnosis and treatment of HIV infection, and because the presence of HIV may necessitate a longer duration of treatment.

PERINATAL DISEASE. Symptoms of congenital tuberculosis may be present at birth but more commonly begin by the 2nd or 3rd wk of life. The most common signs and symptoms are respiratory distress, fever, hepatic or splenic enlargement, poor feeding, lethargy or irritability, lymphadenopathy, abdominal distention, failure to thrive, ear drainage, and skin lesions. The clinical manifestations vary in relation to the site and size of the caseous lesions. Many infants have an abnormal chest radiograph, most often a miliary pattern. Some infants with no pulmonary findings early in the course of the disease later develop profound radiographic and clinical abnormalities. Hilar and mediastinal lymphadenopathy and lung infiltrates are common. Generalized lymphadenopathy and meningitis occur in 30–50% of patients.

The clinical presentation of tuberculosis in newborns is similar to that caused by bacterial sepsis and other congenital infections, such as syphilis, toxoplasmosis, and cytomegalovirus. The diagnosis should be suspected in an infant with signs and symp-toms of bacterial or congenital infection whose response to antibiotic and supportive therapy is poor and evaluation for other infections is unrevealing. The most important clue for rapid diagnosis of congenital tuberculosis is a maternal or family history of tuberculosis. Frequently, the mother's disease is discovered only after the neonate's diagnosis is suspected. The infant's tuberculin skin test is negative initially but may become positive in 1–3 mo. A positive acid-fast stain of an early morning gastric aspirate from a newborn usually indicates tuberculosis. Direct acid-fast stains on middle-ear discharge, bone marrow, tracheal aspirate, or biopsy tissue (especially liver) can be useful. The CSF should be examined and cultured, although the yield for isolating *M. tuberculosis* is low. The mortality rate of congenital tuberculosis remains very high because of delayed diagnosis; many children will have a complete recovery if the diagnosis is made promptly and adequate chemotherapy is started.

Treatment. Tubercle bacilli can be killed only during replication. Individual organisms that are naturally resistant to each antimycobacterial drug are present within large populations of *M. tuberculosis*. All known genes that encode for drug resistance within *M. tuberculosis* are located on a chromosome; transfer between organisms does not occur. The estimated frequency of these naturally drug-resistant organisms is about 10^{-6} but varies among drugs: with streptomycin (STM) it is 10^{-5}; with isoniazid (INH), 10^{-6}; with rifampin (RIF), 10^{-8}. A cavity containing 10^9 tubercle bacilli has thousands of drug-resistant organisms, whereas a closed caseous lesion with its much smaller population contains few, if any, naturally resistant organisms. Fortunately, the natural occurrence of resistance to one drug is independent of resistance to any other drug. The chance that an organism is naturally resistant to both INH and RIF is on the order of 10^{-14}. Because populations of this size do not occur in patients, organisms naturally resistant to two drugs are essentially nonexistent.

The major biologic determinant of the success of antituberculosis chemotherapy is the size of the bacillary population within the host. For patients with large bacterial populations, such as adults with cavities or extensive infiltrates, many naturally drug-resistant organisms are present and at least two antituberculosis drugs must be used to achieve cure. Conversely, for patients with infection (reactive skin test) but no disease, the bacterial population is small, drug-resistant organisms are rare or nonexistent, and a single drug can be used. Children with pulmonary tuberculosis and most patients with extrapulmonary tuberculosis have medium-sized populations in which significant numbers of naturally drug-resistant organisms may or may not be present. In general, these patients are treated with at least two drugs. The phenomena of drug resistance mutation and microbial population size explain why poor patient adherence to treatment or an inadequate treatment regimen can lead to the development of drug-resistant tuberculosis. If a patient with extensive pulmonary tuberculosis is given a single medication, the subpopulation of bacilli susceptible to that drug will be eliminated but the subpopulation of bacilli resistant to the drug have the opportunity to multiply and become the predominant strain. The patient will temporarily improve but will suffer a relapse from tuberculosis completely resistant to that drug. With treatment using two drugs to which the *M. tuberculosis* isolate is susceptible, drug X eliminates the subpopulation of bacilli resistant to drug Y, and drug Y eliminates the subpopulation of bacilli resistant to drug X. If all the organisms have initial resistance to a certain medication (called primary resistance) and the patient is treated with that plus one other medication, only one effective medication is being used and the patient will eventually relapse with tuberculosis that is resistant to both drugs.

The various antituberculosis drugs (Table 197–1) differ in their primary site of activity and their actions. INH and RIF are highly bactericidal for *M. tuberculosis*. STM and several other aminoglycoside antibiotics are also bactericidal for extracellular

TABLE 197–1. **Most Commonly Used Antituberculosis Drugs**

Drug	Daily Dose (mg/kg/24 hr)	Twice-Weekly Dose (mg/kg/dose)	Maximum Dose
Isoniazid*	10–15	20–30	Daily: 300 mg; twice weekly: 900 mg
Rifampin*	10–20	10–20	600 mg
Pyrazinamide*	20–40	40–60	2 g
Streptomycin (IM)	20–40	20–40	1 g
Ethambutol	15–25	25–50	2.5 g
Ethionamide	15–20 (1–3 divided doses)	—	1 g
Cycloserine	10–20 (1–2 divided doses)	—	1 g
Kanamycin or capreomycin (IM)	15–30	15–30	1 g
Amikacin (IV)	15–30	15–30	1 g

IM = intramuscular; IV = intravenous.
*Isoniazid (150 mg) and rifampin (300 mg) are combined in one preparation called Rifamate. Isoniazid (50 mg), rifampin (120 mg), and pyrazinamide (300 mg) are combined in one preparation called Rifater.

tubercle bacilli, but their penetration into macrophages is poor. Pyrazinamide (PZA) cannot be shown to be bactericidal in the laboratory but clearly contributes to the killing of *M. tuberculosis* within the patient. Other antituberculosis drugs, such as ethambutol (EMB) at low doses (15 mg/kg/24 hr), ethionamide (ETH), and cycloserine, are bacteriostatic for *M. tuberculosis* and their primary purpose in the therapeutic regimen is to prevent emergence of resistance to other drugs. EMB at 25 mg/kg/24 hr has some bactericidal activity, which may be important in treating cases of drug-resistant tuberculosis. INH, RIF, and EMB are also effective in preventing emergence of resistance to other drugs, but pyrazinamide has almost no similar activity.

ISONIAZID. INH is inexpensive, diffuses into all tissues and body fluids, and has a very low rate of adverse reactions in children. It can be administered either orally or intramuscularly. At the usual daily dose of 10 mg/kg, serum concentrations greatly exceed the minimum inhibitory concentration for *M. tuberculosis*. Peak concentrations in blood, sputum, and CSF are reached within a few hours and persist for at least 6–8 hr. INH is metabolized by acetylation in the liver. Rapid acetylation is more frequent among African-Americans and Asians than among whites. There is no correlation between acetylation rate and either efficacy or adverse reactions in children.

INH has two principal toxic effects, both of which are rare in children. Peripheral neuritis results from competitive inhibition of pyridoxine utilization. Pyridoxine levels are decreased in children taking INH, but clinical manifestations are rare and pyridoxine administration is not generally recommended. However, teenagers with inadequate diets, children from groups with low levels of milk and meat intake, symptomatic HIV-infected children, and breast-feeding infants require supplemental pyridoxine. The most common physical manifestation of peripheral neuritis is numbness and tingling in the hands or feet. CNS toxicity from INH is rare, occurring usually when there is a significant overdose. The major toxic effect of INH is hepatotoxicity. As many as 3–10% of children taking INH experience transient elevated serum transaminase levels. Clinically significant hepatotoxicity is rare, being more likely to occur in adolescents or in children with severe forms of tuberculosis or underlying liver disease. For most children, routine biochemical monitoring is not necessary, and toxicity can be monitored using clinical signs and symptoms. Early manifestations include nausea, vomiting, abdominal pain, and jaundice. Serum transaminase levels usually normalize with discontinuation of INH. Allergic or hypersensitivity reactions caused by INH are rare. INH can increase phenytoin levels and lead to toxicity by blocking its metabolism. Occasionally, INH interacts with theophylline, requiring modification of the dosage. Rare side effects of INH include pellagra, hemolytic anemia in patients with glucose-6-phosphate dehy-

drogenase deficiency, and a lupus-like reaction with rash and arthritis.

RIFAMPIN. RIF is well absorbed from the gastrointestinal tract during fasting, with peak serum levels achieved within 2 hr. Oral and intravenous forms of RIF are available. Like INH, rifampin is distributed widely in tissues and body fluids, including the CSF, and it is metabolized by the liver. Whereas excretion is mainly through the biliary tract, effective levels are reached in the kidneys and urine. Side effects are more common than with INH and include orange discoloration of urine and tears (with permanent staining of contact lenses), gastrointestinal disturbances, and hepatotoxicity, usually manifested as asymptomatic elevations in serum transaminase levels. When RIF is administered with INH, there is an increased risk of hepatotoxicity, which can be minimized by lowering the daily dose of INH to 10 mg/kg/24 hr. Severe hepatotoxicity has been reported in adults treated with combination of RIF and PZA, but not in children. RIF has been associated with thrombocytopenia and influenza-like syndrome. It can render oral contraceptives ineffective and interacts with several drugs, including quinidine, cyclosporine, sodium warfarin, protease inhibitors, non-nucleoside reverse-transcriptase inhibitors, and corticosteroids. RIF is generally available in 150 mg and 300 mg capsules that, unfortunately, are inconvenient for many weight ranges of children. A suspension can be made using a variety of carriers but should not be taken with food because of malabsorption. A fixed combination preparation, Rifamate, contains both INH (150 mg) and RIF (300 mg); this preparation helps to ensure that the patient receives both INH and RIF so that selective drug resistance is not created.

PYRAZINAMIDE. In adults, a once-daily dose of PZA, 30 mg/kg/24 hr, produces serum levels of 20 μg/mL and little liver toxicity. The optimal dose in children is unknown, but this same dose causes high CSF levels, is well tolerated by children, and correlates with clinical success in treatment trials of tuberculosis in children. Extensive experience with PZA in children has verified its safety. Approximately 10% of adults treated with PZA develop arthralgias, arthritis, or gout due to hyperuricemia. Although uric acid levels are slightly elevated in children taking PZA, clinical manifestations of the hyperuricemia are extremely rare. Hypersensitivity reactions are rare in children. The only dosage form of PZA is a rather large 500-mg tablet, which produces some dosing problems for children, especially infants. These pills can be crushed and given with food in the same manner as INH, but formal pharmacokinetic studies using this method have not been reported. A fixed combination preparation, Rifater, contains INH (50 mg), RIF (120 mg), and PZA (300 mg).

STREPTOMYCIN. STM is used less frequently than in the past for the treatment of childhood tuberculosis but is important for the treatment of drug-resistant disease. It may be given intramuscularly or intravenously. Pain and induration at the injection site are common after intramuscular administration. STM penetrates inflamed meninges fairly well but does not cross uninflamed meninges. Its major current use is when initial INH resistance is suspected or when the child has a life-threatening form of tuberculosis. The major toxicity of STM is dose-related damage to the vestibular and auditory portions of the 8th cranial nerve. Renal toxicity is much less frequent. STM is contraindicated in pregnant women because up to 30% of their infants will suffer severe hearing loss.

ETHAMBUTOL. EMB has received little attention in children because of its potential toxicity to the eye. At a dose of 15 mg/kg/24 hr it is primarily bacteriostatic, and its historic purpose has been to prevent emergence of resistance to other drugs. However, at 25 mg/kg/24 hr, EMB has some bactericidal activity, which may be important in the treatment of drug-resistant disease. It is well tolerated by both adults and children when given orally as a once- or twice-a-day dose. The major potential toxicity is optic neuritis and red-green color blindness. There have been no reports of optic toxicity in children, but the drug has not been widely used because of the inability to routinely test visual fields and acuity in young children. EMB is not recommended for general use in young children for whom vision cannot be adequately examined but should be considered for children with suspected drug-resistant tuberculosis when other agents are not available or cannot be used.

ETHIONAMIDE. ETH is a bacteriostatic drug whose major purpose is treatment of drug-resistant tuberculosis. ETH penetrates into CSF very well and may be particularly useful in cases of tuberculous meningitis. It is generally well tolerated by children but often must be given in two or three divided daily doses because of gastrointestinal disturbance. ETH is chemically similar to INH and can cause significant hepatitis.

OTHER DRUGS. These drugs are used less commonly for tuberculosis because they are significantly less effective or more toxic. Several aminoglycosides, especially kanamycin and amikacin, have significant antituberculosis activity and are used in cases of streptomycin-resistant tuberculosis. A closely related drug, capreomycin, is used more commonly in adults. These drugs can be given either intramuscularly or intravenously, are bactericidal, and usually do not demonstrate cross resistance with STM. Cycloserine is an effective antituberculosis drug in adults but has been used infrequently in children because of its major side effects of impairment with thought processes and tendency to cause depression and other psychiatric abnormalities. The drug is usually given in one or two divided doses, and most experts recommend monitoring serum levels during administration. Pyridoxine supplementation should be given when cycloserine is used. Ciprofloxacin and ofloxacin are quinolones with significant antituberculosis activity that are used commonly for drug-resistant tuberculosis in adults. These drugs are generally contraindicated in children because they cause destruction of growing cartilage in some animal models. However, they have been used effectively in some cases of multidrug-resistant tuberculosis in children when few other effective agents were available.

TREATMENT REGIMENS FOR DISEASE. The basic principles of management of tuberculosis disease in children and adolescents are the same as those in adults. Several drugs are used to effect a relatively rapid cure and prevent the emergence of secondary drug resistance during therapy. The choice of regimen depends on the extent of tuberculosis disease, the host, and the likelihood of drug resistance. The standard therapy of intrathoracic tuberculosis (pulmonary disease and/or hilar lymphadenopathy) in children, recommended by the CDC and AAP, is a 6 mo regimen of INH and RIF supplemented in the first 2 mo of treatment by PZA. Several clinical trials have shown that this regimen yields a success rate approaching 100% with an inci-

dence of clinically significant adverse reactions of <2%. A regimen of INH and RIF for 9 mo is also highly effective for drug-susceptible tuberculosis, but the necessary length of treatment, the need for good adherence by the patient, and the relative lack of protection against possible initial drug resistance have led to the use of shorter regimens. Most experts recommend that all drug administration be directly observed, meaning that a health care worker is physically present when the medications are administered to the patients. When directly observed therapy is used, intermittent (twice-weekly) administration of drugs after an initial period as short as 2 wk of daily therapy is as effective in children as daily therapy for the entire course. In locales where the community rate of INH resistance is greater than 5–10%, or when the adult source case is at increased risk for drug-resistant tuberculosis, most experts recommend adding a fourth drug—usually STM, EMB, or ETH—to the initial regimen. The reason to add the fourth drug is that PZA is not effective in preventing the emergence of RIF resistance during therapy when INH resistance already exists.

Controlled clinical trials for treating various forms of extrapulmonary tuberculosis are virtually nonexistent. Extrapulmonary tuberculosis is usually caused by small numbers of mycobacteria. In general, the treatment for most forms of extrapulmonary tuberculosis in children, including cervical lymphadenopathy, is the same as for pulmonary tuberculosis. Exceptions are bone and joint, disseminated, and CNS tuberculosis for which there are inadequate data to recommend 6-mo therapy. These cases usually are treated for 9–12 mo. Surgical debridement in bone and joint disease and ventriculoperitoneal shunting in CNS disease are frequently necessary.

The optimal treatment of tuberculosis in HIV-infected children has not been established. HIV seropositive adults with tuberculosis can be treated successfully with standard regimens that include INH, RIF, and PZA. The total duration of therapy should be 6–9 mo, or 6 mo after culture of sputum becomes sterile, whichever is longer. Data for children are limited to isolated case reports and small series. Most experts believe that HIV-seropositive children with drug-susceptible tuberculosis should receive at least three drugs such as INH, RIF, and PZA for the first 2 mo followed by INH and RIF for a total duration of at least 9 mo. A fourth drug such as ETM or STM should be added for disseminated disease and when drug-resistance is suspected. Rifampin resistant tuberculosis is more common in HIV-infected patients. Children with HIV infection appear to have more frequent adverse reactions to antituberculosis drugs and must be monitored closely during therapy. Coadministration of rifampin and some antiretroviral agents results in subtherapeutic blood levels of protease inhibitors and non-nucleoside reverse transcriptase inhibitors, and toxic levels of rifampin. Concomitant administration of these drugs is not recommended. Treatment of HIV infected children is often empirical based on epidemiologic and radiographic information, because the radiographic appearance of other pulmonary complications of HIV in children, such as lymphoid interstitial pneumonitis and bacterial pneumonia, may be similar to that of tuberculosis. Therapy should be considered when tuberculosis cannot be excluded.

DRUG-RESISTANT TUBERCULOSIS. The incidence of drug-resistant tuberculosis is increasing in many areas of the world, including North America. There are two major types of drug resistance. Primary resistance occurs when an individual is infected with *M. tuberculosis* that is already resistant to a particular drug. Secondary resistance occurs when drug-resistant organisms emerge as the dominant population during treatment. The major causes of secondary drug resistance are poor adherence with the medication by the patient or inadequate treatment regimens prescribed by the physician. Nonadherence with one drug is more likely to lead to secondary resistance than failure to take all drugs. Secondary resistance is rare in children because of the small size of their mycobacterial population. Therefore, most drug resistance in children is primary, and patterns of drug resistance among children tend to mirror those found among adults in the same population. The main predictors of drug-resistant tuberculosis among adults are history of previous antituberculosis treatment, co-infection with HIV, and exposure to another adult with infectious drug-resistant tuberculosis.

Treatment of drug-resistant tuberculosis is successful only when at least two bactericidal drugs are given to which the infecting strain of *M. tuberculosis* is susceptible. When a child has possible drug-resistant tuberculosis, at least three and usually four or five drugs should be administered initially until the susceptibility pattern is determined and a more specific regimen can be designed. The specific treatment plan must be individualized for each patient according to the results of susceptibility testing on the isolates from the child or the adult source case. Treatment duration of 9 mo with RIF, PZA, and EMB is usually adequate for INH-resistant tuberculosis in children. When resistance to INH and RIF is present, the total duration of therapy often must be extended to 12–18 mo, and twice-a-week regimens should not be used. The prognosis of single- or multidrug-resistant tuberculosis in children is usually good if the drug resistance is identified early in the treatment, appropriate drugs are administered under directly observed therapy, adverse reactions from the drugs do not occur, and the child and family are in a supportive environment. The treatment of drug-resistant tuberculosis in children always should be undertaken by a clinician with specific expertise in the treatment of tuberculosis.

CORTICOSTEROIDS. These are useful in the treatment of some children with tuberculosis disease. They are most beneficial when the host inflammatory reaction contributes significantly to tissue damage or impairment of organ function. There is convincing evidence that corticosteroids decrease mortality rates and long-term neurologic sequelae in some patients with tuberculous meningitis by reducing vasculitis, inflammation, and ultimately, intracranial pressure. Lowering the intracranial pressure limits tissue damage and favors circulation of antituberculosis drugs through the brain and meninges. Short courses of corticosteroids also may be effective for children with endobronchial tuberculosis that causes respiratory distress, localized emphysema, or segmental pulmonary lesions. Several randomized clinical trials have shown that corticosteroids can help relieve symptoms and constriction associated with acute tuberculous pericardial effusion. Corticosteroids may cause dramatic improvement in symptoms in some patients with tuberculous pleural effusion and shift of the mediastinum. However, the long-term course of disease is probably unaffected. Some children with severe miliary tuberculosis have dramatic improvement with corticosteroid therapy if the inflammatory reaction is so severe that alveolocapillary block is present. There is no convincing evidence that one corticosteroid preparation is better than another. The most commonly prescribed regimen is prednisone, 1–2 mg/kg/24 hr in one to two divided doses orally for 4–6 wk, followed by gradual tapering.

SUPPORTIVE CARE. Children receiving treatment should be followed carefully to promote adherence with therapy, to monitor for toxic reactions to medications, and to ensure that the tuberculosis is being adequately treated. Adequate nutrition is important. Patients should be seen at monthly intervals and should be given just enough medication to last until the next visit. Anticipatory guidance with regard to the administration of medications to children is crucial. The physician should foresee difficulties that the family might have in introducing several new medications in inconvenient dosage forms to a young child. The clinician must report all cases of suspected tuberculosis in a child to the local health department to be sure that the child and family receive appropriate care and evaluation.

Nonadherence to treatment is the major problem in tuberculosis therapy. The patient and family must know what is expected of them through verbal and written instructions in their primary language. From 30–50% of patients taking long-term treatment are significantly nonadherent with self-administered medications, and clinicians are usually not able to determine in advance which patients will be nonadherent. Preferably, directly observed therapy should be instituted with the help of the local health department.

TREATMENT OF LATENT TUBERCULOSIS INFECTION. The treatment of children with asymptomatic tuberculosis infection (reactive tuberculin skin test, normal chest radiograph, normal physical examination) to avoid the development of tuberculosis disease is an established practice. The effectiveness of INH therapy in children has approached 100% and has lasted for at least 30 yr. INH therapy should be given to any child with a positive tuberculin skin test but no clinical or radiographic evidence of disease. The currently recommended regimen is 9 mo of daily INH therapy. INH can be given twice weekly under direct observation if adherence with daily treatment is likely to be poor. INH therapy also should be started for children <6 yr of age with a negative tuberculin skin test who have had recent exposure to an adult with infectious tuberculosis, including infants born to mothers who have tuberculosis. These children may already be infected with *M. tuberculosis* but have not yet developed delayed hypersensitivity. Significant tuberculosis disease may develop simultaneously with skin test reactivity in small children and infants, and the illness may develop before the positive skin test is recognized. In exposed children, tuberculin skin testing is repeated 3 mo after contact with the adult source case has been interrupted. If the repeat tuberculin skin test is negative, INH can be discontinued; if the second skin test is reactive (≥5 mm), the child has tuberculosis infection and a full course of INH therapy can be administered. Children with HIV infection or other causes of immune suppression should receive 12 mo of treatment.

The optimal treatment for LTBI caused by drug-resistant strains of *M. tuberculosis* has not been established. For infections with strains that are INH resistant only, most experts recommend a 6–9 mo course of RIF. No data from controlled clinical trials support this practice, however. Similarly, no data are available concerning treatment of tuberculosis infection caused by organisms that are resistant to both INH and RIF. Some experts have recommended a combination of a quinolone and PZA for 6–9 mo. An alternative regimen is high-dose EMB and PZA for a similar period of time. For infection with isolates that are resistant to many drugs, the clinician usually administers two drugs to which the organism is susceptible. The efficacy and safety of these regimens in children are not established, and an expert in pediatric tuberculosis should be consulted for treatment of multidrug-resistant tuberculosis infection in children.

Prevention. The highest priority of any tuberculosis control program should be case finding and treatment, which interrupts transmission of infection between close contacts. All children and adults with symptoms suggestive of tuberculosis disease and those in close contact with an adult suspected of having infectious pulmonary tuberculosis should be tuberculin skin tested and examined as soon as possible. On average, 30–50% of household contacts to infectious cases will be tuberculin skin test positive, and 1% of contacts already have overt disease. This scheme relies on effective and adequate public health response and resources. Children, particularly young infants, should receive high priority during contact investigations because their risk of infection is high and they are more likely to rapidly develop severe forms of tuberculosis.

Mass testing of large groups of children for tuberculosis infection is an inefficient process. When large groups of children at low risk for tuberculosis are tested, the vast majority of skin test reactions are actually false-positive reactions due to biologic variability or cross sensitization with NTM. However, testing of high-risk groups of adults or children should be encouraged because most of these individuals with positive tuberculin skin tests have tuberculosis infection. Testing should take place only if effective mechanisms are in place to ensure adequate evaluation and treatment of the individuals who test positive.

BACILLE CALMETTE-GUÉRIN VACCINATION. The only available vaccine against tuberculosis is the BCG, named for the two French investigators responsible for its development. The original vaccine organism was a strain of *M. bovis* attenuated by subculture every 3 wk for 13 yr. This strain was distributed to dozens of laboratories that continued to subculture the organism on different media under various conditions. The result has been production of many BCG vaccines that differ widely in morphology, growth characteristics, sensitizing potency, and animal virulence. The route of administration and dosing schedule for the BCG vaccines are important variables for efficacy. The preferred route of administration is intradermal injection with a syringe and needle because it is the only method that permits accurate measurement of an individual dose. The BCG vaccines are extremely safe in immunocompetent hosts. Local ulceration and regional suppurative adenitis occur in 0.1–1% of vaccine recipients. Local lesions do not suggest underlying host immune defects and do not affect the level of protection afforded by the vaccine. Most reactions are mild and they usually resolve spontaneously, but chemotherapy is needed occasionally. Surgical excision of a suppurative draining node is rarely necessary and should be avoided if possible. Osteitis is a rare complication of BCG vaccination that appears to be related to certain strains of the vaccine that are no longer in wide use. Systemic complaints such as fever, convulsions, loss of appetite, and irritability are extraordinarily rare after BCG vaccination. Profoundly immunocompromised patients may develop disseminated BCG infection after vaccination. Children with HIV infection appear to have rates of local adverse reactions to BCG vaccines that are comparable to rates in immunocompetent children. However, the incidence in these children of disseminated infection months to years after vaccination is currently unknown.

Recommended vaccine schedules vary widely among countries. The official recommendation of the WHO is a single dose administered during infancy, including in asymptomatic HIV-infected children in populations where the risk of tuberculosis is high. In some countries repeat vaccination is universal. In others it is based on either tuberculin skin testing or the absence of a typical scar. The optimal age for administration and dosing schedule are unknown because adequate comparative trials have not been performed.

Although dozens of BCG trials have been reported in various human populations, the most useful data have come from several controlled trials. The results of these studies have been disparate. Some demonstrated a great deal of protection from BCG vaccines, but others showed no efficacy at all. A recent meta-analysis of published BCG vaccination trials suggested that BCG is 50% effective in preventing pulmonary tuberculosis in adults and children. The protective effect for disseminated and meningeal tuberculosis appears to be slightly higher, with BCG preventing 50–80% of cases. A variety of explanations for the varied responses to BCG vaccines have been proposed, including methodologic and statistical variations within the trials, interaction with NTM that either enhances or decreases the protection afforded by BCG, different potencies among the various BCG vaccines, and genetic factors for BCG response within the study populations. BCG vaccination administered during infancy has little effect on the ultimate incidence of tuberculosis in adults, suggesting that the effect of the vaccine is time limited.

In summary, BCG vaccination has worked well in some situations but poorly in others. Clearly, BCG vaccination has had little effect on the ultimate control of tuberculosis throughout the world because more than 5 billion doses have been administered but tuberculosis remains epidemic in most regions. BCG

vaccination does not substantially influence the chain of transmission because those cases of contagious pulmonary tuberculosis in adults that can be prevented by BCG vaccination constitute a small fraction of the sources of infection in a population. The best use of BCG vaccination appears to be prevention of life-threatening forms of tuberculosis in infants and young children.

BCG vaccination has never been adopted as part of the strategy for the control of tuberculosis in the United States. Widespread use of the vaccine would render subsequent tuberculin skin testing less useful. However, BCG vaccination may contribute to tuberculosis control in selected population groups. BCG is recommended for tuberculin skin test-negative infants and children who (1) are at high risk of intimate and prolonged exposure to persistently untreated or ineffectively treated adults with infectious pulmonary tuberculosis and cannot be removed from the source of infection or placed on long-term preventive therapy or (2) are continuously exposed to persons with tuberculosis who have bacilli that are resistant to INH and RIF. Any child receiving BCG vaccination should have a documented negative tuberculin skin test before receiving the vaccine. After receiving the vaccine, the child should be separated from the possible sources of infection until it can be demonstrated that the child has had a vaccine response, demonstrated by tuberculin reactivity, which usually develops within 1–3 mo. Occasionally, a second BCG vaccination must be given to children who fail to develop skin test reactivity after the first dose. In the United States, BCG is contraindicated in children with primary or secondary immunodeficiencies.

Active research to develop new tuberculosis vaccines has led to the creation and preliminary testing of several vaccine candidates based on attenuated strains of mycobacteria, subunit proteins, or DNA. The genome of *M. tuberculosis* has been sequenced, allowing researchers to further study and better understand the pathogenesis and host immune responses to tuberculosis.

PERINATAL TUBERCULOSIS. The most effective way of preventing tuberculosis infection and disease in the neonate or young infant is through appropriate testing and treatment of the mother and other family members. High-risk pregnant women should be tested with a tuberculin skin test, and those with a positive test should receive a chest radiograph with appropriate abdominal shielding. If the mother has a negative chest radiograph and is clinically well, no separation of the infant and mother is needed after delivery. The child needs no special evaluation or treatment if he or she remains asymptomatic. Other household members should receive tuberculin skin testing and further evaluation as indicated.

If the mother has suspected tuberculosis at the time of delivery, the newborn should be separated from the mother until the chest radiograph is obtained. If the mother's chest radiograph is abnormal, separation should be maintained until the mother has been evaluated thoroughly, including examination of the sputum. If the mother's chest radiograph is abnormal but the history, physical examination, sputum examination, and evaluation of the radiograph show no evidence of current active tuberculosis, it is reasonable to assume that the infant is at low risk for infection. The mother should receive appropriate treatment, and she and her infant should receive careful follow-up care. In addition, all household members should be evaluated for tuberculosis.

If the mother's chest radiograph or acid-fast sputum smear shows evidence of current tuberculosis disease, additional steps are necessary to protect the infant. INH therapy for newborns has been so effective that separation of the mother and infant is no longer considered mandatory. Separation should occur only if the mother is ill enough to require hospitalization, she has been or is expected to become nonadherent with her treatment, or there is strong suspicion that she has drug-resistant tuberculosis. INH treatment for the infant should be continued until the mother has been shown to be sputum culture negative for at least 3 mo. At that time, a Mantoux tuberculin skin test should be placed on the child. If positive, INH is continued for a total duration of 9–12 mo; if negative, INH can be discontinued. Because INH resistance is increasing in the United States, it is not always clear that INH therapy will be effective for the neonate. If INH resistance is suspected or the mother's adherence to medication is in question, separation of the infant from the mother should be considered. The duration of separation must be at least as long as is necessary to render the mother noninfectious. An expert in tuberculosis should be consulted if the young infant has potential exposure to the mother or another adult with tuberculosis disease caused by an INH-resistant strain of *M. tuberculosis.*

Although INH is not thought to be teratogenic, the treatment of pregnant women with asymptomatic tuberculosis infection is often deferred until after delivery. However, symptomatic pregnant women or those with radiographic evidence of tuberculosis disease should be appropriately evaluated. Because pulmonary tuberculosis is harmful to both the mother and the fetus, and it represents a great danger to the infant after delivery, tuberculosis in pregnant women always should be treated. The most common regimen for drug-susceptible tuberculosis is INH, RIF, and EMB. The aminoglycosides and ETH should be avoided because of their teratogenic effect. The safety of PZA in pregnancy has not been established.

Al-Dossary FS, Ong LT, Correa AG, et al: Treatment of childhood tuberculosis with a six month directly observed regimen of only two weeks of daily therapy. *Pediatr Infect Dis J* 2002;21:91–7.

American Thoracic Society: Diagnostic standards and classification of tuberculosis in adults and children. *Am J Respir Crit Care Med* 2000;161:1376–95.

American Thoracic Society: Treatment of tuberculosis and tuberculosis infection in adults and children. *Am J Respir Crit Care Med* 1994;149:1359–74.

Centers for Disease Control and Prevention: Reported Tuberculosis in the United States, 2001. Division of Tuberculosis Elimination, National Center for HIV, STD and TB Prevention. See *http://www.cdc.gov/nchstp/tb/surv/surv.htm.*

Centers for Disease Control and Prevention: Initial therapy for tuberculosis in the era of multidrug resistance: Recommendations of the Advisory Council for the Elimination of Tuberculosis. *JAMA* 1993;270:694–8.

Centers for Disease Control and Prevention: Screening for tuberculosis and tuberculosis infection in high-risk populations: Recommendations of the Advisory Committee for the Elimination of Tuberculosis. *MMWR Morb Mortal Wkly Rep* 1995;44(RR-11):19–34.

Centers for Disease Control and Prevention: Prevention and treatment of tuberculosis among patients infected with human immunodeficiency virus: Principles of therapy and revised recommendations. *MMWR Morb Mortal Wkly Rep* 1998; 47(RR-20):1–58.

Centers for Disease Control and Prevention. Targeted tuberculin testing and treatment of latent tuberculosis infection. *MMWR Morb Mortal Wkly Rep* 2000;49(RR-6):1–51.

Colditz GA, Brewer TF, Berkey CS, et al: Efficacy of BCG vaccine in the prevention of tuberculosis: Meta-analysis of the published literature. *JAMA* 1994;271:698–702.

Espinal MA, Laszlo A, Simonsen L, et al: Global trends in resistance to antituberculosis drugs. *N Engl J Med* 2001;344:1294–303.

Hsu KH: Thirty years after isoniazid: Its impact on tuberculosis in children and adolescents. *JAMA* 1984;251:1283–5.

Hussey G, Chisholm T, Kibel M: Miliary tuberculosis in children: A review of 94 cases. *Pediatr Infect Dis J* 1991;10:832–6.

Lee E, Holzman RS: Evolution and current use of the tuberculin skin test. *J Clin Infect Dis* 2002;34:365–70.

Lobato MN, Mohle-Boetani JC, Royce SE: Missed opportunities for preventing tuberculosis among children younger than five years of age. *Pediatrics* 2000;106: E75.

McMaster P, Isaacs D: Critical review of evidence for short course therapy for tuberculous adenitis in children. *Pediatr Infect Dis J* 2000;19:401–4.

Mukadi Yu, Wiktor SZ, Coulibaly IM, et al: Impact of HIV infection on the development, clinical presentation and outcome of tuberculosis among children in Abidjan, Cote d'Ivoire. *AIDS* 1997;11:1151–8.

O'Brien R, Long M, Cross F, et al: Hepatotoxicity from isoniazid and rifampin among children treated for tuberculosis. *Pediatrics* 1983;72:491–9.

Salazar GE, Schmitz TL, Cama R, et al: Pulmonary tuberculosis in children in a developing country. *Pediatrics* 2001;108:448–53.

Starke JR, Correa AG: Management of mycobacterial infection and disease in children. *Pediatr Infect Dis J* 1995;14:455–69.

Starke JR: Transmission of *Mycobacterium tuberculosis* to and from children and adolescents. *Semin Pediatr Infect Dis* 2001;12:115–23.

Te Water Naude JM, Donald PR, Hussey GD, et al: Twice weekly vs. daily chemotherapy for childhood tuberculosis. *Pediatr Infect Dis J* 2000;19:405–10.

Ussery XT, Valway SE, McKenna M, et al: Epidemiology of tuberculosis among children in the United States, 1985 to 1994. *Pediatr Infect Dis J* 1996;15:697–704.

World Health Organization: Global tuberculosis control. WHO Report 2002, Geneva, Switzerland, WHO/CDS/TB/2001.287. See *http://www.who. int/gtb/publications/globrep02/index.html.*

Yaramis A, Gurkan F, Elevli M, et al: Central nervous system tuberculosis in children: A review of 214 cases. *Pediatrics* 1998;102:E49.

Chapter 198

Hansen Disease (*Mycobacterium leprae*)

Dwight A. Powell

Hansen disease (leprosy) is a chronic disease resulting from infection with *Mycobacterium leprae* and the ensuing host response. The organs most prominently affected are the respiratory mucosa, skin, and the peripheral nervous system, but testicular and ocular involvement are described. Humans were long believed to be the sole host of *M. leprae*, but naturally acquired infection has been documented in armadillos in the southeastern United States, and experimental infection has been established in primates, nude mice, and armadillos.

Chronic skin lesions, madarosis, sensory neuropathy resulting in the loss of digits or limbs, and paresis secondary to motor nerve dysfunction are among the sequelae of leprosy. The highly visible nature of these debilities led to the historical stigmatization of the "leper." The psychologic and sociologic sequelae of this stigma can be as debilitating as the disease itself and may result in delays in seeking medical attention. To combat this prejudice, the term **leprosy patient** has replaced the word leper, and **Hansen disease**, after Armauer Hansen who identified *M. leprae* as the cause of leprosy in 1873, has become an accepted designation.

Etiology. *M. leprae*, an obligate intracellular pathogen with a generation time of 14 days, is an acid-fast bacillus of the family Mycobacteriaceae. *M. leprae* grows optimally at 27–30°C and cannot be cultured in vitro. The incubation period of leprosy in humans ranges from 3 mo–20 yr (average 3–5 yr). The rare occurrence of leprosy in infants as young as 3 mo of age suggests that in utero transmission may occur or that very short incubation periods may be possible in certain situations.

Epidemiology. After the introduction of multidrug therapy (MDT) by the World Health Organization (WHO) in 1982, there has been a steady decline in the prevalence of leprosy. On a global scale, the estimated prevalence rate has been reduced 85% from >20 cases/10,000 persons in 1985 to 1.25 cases/10,000 persons in 2000. Approximately 11 million leprosy patients have been cured over the past 15 yr. However, the new case detection rate has remained nearly steady since 1985 with 750,000 new cases detected and registered for treatment in 2000. The World Health Organization estimates that an additional 2.5 million cases will be detected between the years 2000–2005. The goal by 2005 is to decrease the global prevalence rate to ≤1 case/10,000 persons. Currently, >90% of the world's leprosy patients reside in 10 major endemic countries in Africa, Southeast Asia, and Central and South America, with 70% residing in India. Approximately 100 cases are reported annually in the United States, of which 85% are immigrants. Small numbers of endemic cases are reported from Texas, Hawaii, and Louisiana.

Human-to-human transmission accounts for an overwhelming majority of cases; a high percentage of them occur in family members or in close contacts of known patients. Leprosy occurs at all ages, but infections in infants are extremely rare; incidence rates peak during childhood and early adulthood in endemic areas. HIV infection has not been documented to alter the risk of leprosy in areas of high prevalence for both pathogens.

Pathogenesis. The entry of *M. leprae* into the human host is poorly understood. Possible modes of transmission include contact with desquamated infected epidermis, ingestion of infected breast milk, and bites of mosquitos or other vectors. At present, however, the basis for most infections appears to be transmission from untreated lepromatous patients by means of prolonged contact with infected nasal secretions containing a high bacterial load. Little is known of the host immune responses in the initial period after infection, but skin testing and serologic studies suggest that up to 80–90% of those infected develop immunity without ever manifesting clinical disease. Studies in endemic areas using polymerase chain reaction (PCR) show widespread presence of the organism in nasal secretions from asymptomatic individuals.

From the nasal mucosa, *M. leprae* appears to be transported hematogenously to skin and peripheral nerves. Using the armadillo model of neuritis, *M. leprae* has been shown to colonize the perineural space and gain access to the interstitium of the endoneural space. Once there, it is available for phagocytosis by Schwann cells surrounding peripheral nerve axons and interstitial macrophages. Intracellular replication of *M. leprae* follows with varying degrees depending on the host cellular immune response. *M. leprae* attachment to and ingestion by Schwann cells has been shown to depend on receptors on the lamin-2 glycoprotein in the basal lamina and the α-dystroglycan complex in the Schwann cell basement membrane. *M. leprae* specific phenolic glycolipid-1 appears to be the ligand mediating this binding. With the recent mapping of the genome of *M. leprae*, more details of this important binding will become available.

Once *M. leprae* has colonized the surface of nerves and has infected endoneural macrophages and Schwann cells, several mechanisms of skin and nerve injury occur depending on the host immune response. One end of the spectrum is **tuberculoid leprosy**, in which there is a vigorous and specific cell-mediated immune response to *M. leprae* antigens. In tissue biopsies there are tightly organized granulomas composed of epithelioid cells and lymphocytes but bacilli are scant or absent. Macrophages, when present, do not contain intracellular organisms. Caseation is rare. Heavy cellular infiltration is found in the dermis with destruction of cutaneous nerve fibers.

At the other end of the spectrum is **lepromatous leprosy**, in which there is total and specific anergy to *M. leprae* both by skin testing and by in vitro assays of cell-mediated immunity. Large amounts of circulating and tissue-based antibody to mycobacterial antigens are present, but they afford no protective immunity. Bacilli are found in enormous numbers in the skin, nasal mucosa, and peripheral nerves. There is continual bacillemia as well as bacillary invasion of all major organs except the central nervous system. Tissue granulomas are poorly formed and are composed chiefly of loose aggregates of foamy histiocytes. Macrophages teeming with undigested bacilli are common. There is extensive, symmetric involvement of peripheral nerves, although the cutaneous nerve endings are usually spared.

An *M. leprae*–specific suppressor T-cell population is found in the circulation of patients with lepromatous leprosy, and increased numbers of suppressor T cells are found in their skin granulomas. T cells from lepromatous patients also produce less interleukin 2 and less interferon-γ after stimulation with *M. leprae* antigens than do T cells from tuberculoid patients or normal controls.

Borderline or dimorphous leprosy is subdivided into three subclasses that lie between the tuberculoid and lepromatous poles.

Clinical Manifestations

INDETERMINATE LEPROSY (IL). Indeterminate leprosy is the earliest clinically detectable form of leprosy. Although it is observed in only 10–20% of infected individuals, it is a stage through which most patients with advanced leprosy have passed. Usually there is a single hypopigmented macule, 2–4 cm in diameter, with a poorly defined border but having no erythema or induration. Anesthesia is minimal or absent, particularly if the lesion is on the face. Tissue samples may contain granulomas, but bacilli are rarely demonstrable. The histopathology is not distinctive; the diagnosis is usually made by exclusion of other skin disorders in contacts (especially children) of leprosy patients. In 50–75% of patients with indeterminate leprosy, the lesions heal spontaneously; in the remainder, they progress to one of the classic forms.

TUBERCULOID LEPROSY (TL). There is usually a single, large (often >10 cm in diameter) lesion with a well-demarcated, elevated erythematous rim. The interior of the lesion is flat, atrophic, hypopigmented, occasionally scaly, and anesthetic. Rarely, there may be as many as four lesions. The closest superficial nerve is often impressively thickened. The ulnar, posterior tibial, and great auricular nerves are most commonly affected. Periodic examination of all leprosy patients and their contacts should include palpation of these nerves. Without therapy, the skin lesion tends to enlarge slowly, but documented instances of spontaneous resolution exist. The coloration of the rim slowly fades with therapy and the induration resolves, resulting in a flat lesion with central hypopigmentation and a ring of postinflammatory hyperpigmentation. Loss of hair follicles, sweat glands, cutaneous nerve receptors, and sensation in the central portion of the lesion is irreversible. Marked improvement should be apparent within 1–2 mo after initiating therapy, but complete resolution may take up to 8–12 mo. There is an entity of "pure neural" tuberculoid leprosy, which presents as either pure sensory or combined sensory and motor nerve dysfunction with prominent nerve thickening but no cutaneous lesions. Histopathology is mandatory to establish this diagnosis. Nerve trunk size varies widely, and over diagnosis of "enlarged" nerves is common among inexperienced observers. Nodular or fusiform nerve thickening has greater diagnostic value than a palpable nerve that is smooth and symmetric.

BORDERLINE LEPROSY. The clinical and histologic criteria for the three subdivisions of borderline leprosy are less well defined than are those of the two polar categories. In contrast to the tuberculoid and lepromatous patterns, those in the borderline divisions are unstable. For example, host or bacterial factors can result in immunologic downgrading of the clinical condition toward the lepromatous pattern or upgrading it toward the tuberculoid pattern. Therapy is the most common cause of upgrading reactions; downgrading can be seen in conditions that compromise host immunity, for example, pregnancy. Clinical characteristics of the three generally accepted borderline subclasses are as follows.

In the **borderline tuberculoid (BT)** pattern, the lesions are greater in number but smaller in size than in tuberculoid leprosy. There may be small satellite lesions around older lesions, and the margins of the borderline tuberculoid lesions are less distinct. There is usually thickening of two or more superficial nerves.

In the **borderline (BB)** pattern, the lesions are more numerous and more heterogeneous in appearance. They may become confluent, and plaques may be present. The borders are poorly defined, and the erythematous rim fades into the surrounding skin. There may be anesthesia, but hypesthesia is more common. Mild to moderate nerve thickening is common, but severe muscle wasting and neuropathy are unusual.

In the **borderline lepromatous (BL)** pattern, a large number of asymmetrically distributed lesions are heterogeneous in appearance. Macules, papules, plaques, and nodules may all coexist. Individual lesions are small unless confluent. Anesthesia is mild and superficial nerve trunks are spared. The initial response to therapy is often dramatic; nodules and plaques flatten within 2–3 mo. With continued therapy, the lesions become macular and almost invisible.

LEPROMATOUS LEPROSY (LL). The lesions are innumerable, often confluent, and symmetric. Initially there may be only vague macules or even uniform, diffuse skin infiltrations without discernible lesions. As the disease progresses, the lesions become increasingly papular and nodular, so that with the diffuse thickening and infiltration of the skin, the characteristic leonine facies accompanied by loss of the eyebrows and distortion of the earlobes becomes apparent. Anesthesia of the lesions is less severe than in tuberculoid leprosy, but a symmetric peripheral sensory neuropathy usually develops late in the course of the disease. Testicular infiltration leading to azoospermia, infertility, and gynecomastia is common in adults but not in children. Bacilli are demonstrable in most internal organs other than the central nervous system, but tissue damage or interference with function is infrequent. Glomerulonephritis, when it occurs, is believed to be secondary to immune complex deposition rather than to infection per se. The initial response to therapy may be encouraging but is often followed by a long (2–5 yr) period of very slow improvement. In true lepromatous leprosy, the specific anergy to the leprosy bacillus persists despite therapy, thus making the patient theoretically susceptible to relapse if even a single viable bacillus remains at the end of therapy.

REACTIONAL STATES. Acute clinical exacerbations are common in leprosy and are believed to reflect abrupt changes in the host-parasite immunologic balance. Although these reactional states do occur in the absence of therapy, they are especially common during the initial years of treatment. Approximately 30% of patients receiving effective chemotherapy can develop reactions, and, unless adequately treated, they will result in crippling deformities. Two major variants are recognized.

Type 1 (reversal) reactions are observed predominantly in borderline leprosy and result from a sudden increase in effective cell-mediated immunity in response to *M. leprae* antigens in dermis and Schwann cells. Acute tenderness and swelling at the site of existing cutaneous and neural lesions and the development of new lesions are the major manifestations. Existing or new skin lesions often ulcerate to leave hideous scars. Fever and systemic toxicity are uncommon, but the acute neuritis that can present either as a severe painful episode or be insidious and painless can lead to irreversible nerve injury (anesthesia, facial paralysis, claw hand, footdrop) if not treated immediately. Reversal reactions constitute perhaps the only medical emergency related to leprosy per se. Patients should be instructed to contact their physicians immediately if signs of a reaction appear.

Type 2 (erythema nodosum leprosum) reactions (ENL) occur in lepromatous and borderline lepromatous cases as a systemic inflammatory response to deposition of extravascular immune complexes of antibody and *M. leprae* antigen. Tender red dermal papules or nodules, clinically resembling erythema nodosum, are the hallmarks of this syndrome. They develop in a few hours and last only a few days. High fever, migrating polyarthralgia, painful swelling of lymph nodes or spleen, orchitis, iridocyclitis, and, rarely, nephritis may occur. Leukocytosis and albuminuria may be present. Circulating and tissue-based immune complexes are frequently present and may explain the resemblance to other immune complex disorders, but the underlying mechanism appears to involve the activation of a helper T-cell subset. There is a strong tendency to recurrence (45% of patients), and there is a risk of amyloidosis and renal failure if treatment is inadequate.

Diagnosis. The critical factor in the diagnosis of leprosy is its inclusion in the differential diagnosis of a skin disorder in anyone who has resided in an endemic leprosy region. Anesthetic skin lesions with or without thickened peripheral nerves are virtually pathognomonic of leprosy. A full-thickness skin biopsy from an active lesion (stained with both a standard histologic stain and an acid-fast stain such as Fite-Faraco) is the optimal procedure for confirmation of the diagnosis and accurate disease classification. Acid-fast bacilli are rarely found in patients with indeterminate or tuberculoid disease, but the presence of granulomas and lymphocytic infiltration of nerves in anesthetic skin lesions essentially confirms the diagnosis. For purposes of assigning patients to the appropriate WHO MDT regimen, slit skin smears are assessed to determine whether patients have paucibacillary infection (≤5 skin lesions and no bacilli on skin smears) or multibacillary infection (≥6 skin lesions and bacilli on skin smears). The bacterial index can range from zero (no bacilli in 100 oil-immersion fields) to 6+ (>1,000 bacilli per field). Other routine clinical, microbiologic, and radiologic tests have little or no role in the diagnosis of leprosy, although they may be useful in the exclusion of other diagnoses. Various assays for serum antibodies directed against unique antigens of *M. leprae* have been developed, but current tests lack sufficient sensitivity and specificity for active disease to be useful for clinical diagnostic purposes. PCR analysis has been found to detect *M. leprae* only when biopsy specimens are positive for acid-fast bacilli.

DIFFERENTIAL DIAGNOSIS. Many diseases endemic in developing countries can mimic the appearance of leprosy; these include secondary syphilis, cutaneous leishmaniasis, yaws, and cutaneous fungal infections. None of these entities involve paresthesia/anesthesia localized to the skin lesions or cause thickening of peripheral nerves. The presence of nerve thickening with skin lesions also differentiates leprosy from primary neurologic disease. Indeterminate leprosy may present as minimal anesthesia, no nerve thickening, and equivocal histopathology, suggesting a superficial fungal infection, particularly tinea versicolor. The diagnosis of indeterminate leprosy should be considered one of exclusion and will rarely be established in anyone other than a close contact of a known lepromatous patient.

Treatment. Physicians in the United States considering the diagnosis or treatment of leprosy are strongly encouraged to obtain consultation and assistance in patient management from the National Hansen Disease Programs (800-642-2477; *http://bphc. hrsa.gov/nhdp/default.htm*).

Only three antimycobacterial agents have proven to be consistently effective in the treatment of leprosy. Since the early 1940s, dapsone has remained the cornerstone of therapy because of its low cost, minimal toxicity, and wide availability. However, secondary resistance develops when it is used as the sole agent. Dermatitis, hepatitis, and methemoglobinemia are the most common side effects; granulocytopenia is rare but potentially fatal. Dose-related hemolytic anemia, which can be severe, is seen in patients with glucose-6-phosphate dehydrogenase deficiency, methemoglobin reductase deficiency, or hemoglobin M. Pregnancy studies have not shown an increased risk of fetal abnormalities.

Rifampin is the most rapidly mycobactericidal drug for *M. leprae*, achieving excellent levels inside cells, where most leprosy bacilli reside. Resistance develops when Rifampin is used as the sole agent. The widespread use of rifampin has been limited by cost more than by toxicity. Hepatitis is the most common side effect that necessitates discontinuance.

Clofazimine, a phenazine dye with both antimycobacterial and anti-inflammatory activity, has been particularly useful in decreasing the incidence of reactional states. The pharmacokinetics are poorly understood, but the half-life is several days. The drug is avidly taken up by epithelial cells, a feature that may be important for its activity but also results in cutaneous hyperpigmentation, ichthyosis, xerosis, and enteritis. The intense reddish-brown discoloration of the skin is cosmetically a deterrent to use and often results in discontinuation or poor compliance.

Minocycline, certain second-generation quinolones, and some new macrolide derivatives such as clarithromycin have shown promise in experimental models but limited human treatment data exist.

Introduced by the WHO in 1982, multidrug therapy has been very successful with a high cure rate and a relapse rate of 1%/yr following a full course of therapy. For adults with multibacillary leprosy (all BL and lepromatous patients), therapy is recommended for 12–24 mo to include rifampin (600 mg once monthly PO, directly observed), dapsone (100 mg once daily PO, self-administered), and clofazimine (300 mg once monthly, directly observed, and 50 mg once daily PO, self-administered). For adults with paucibacillary leprosy (all indeterminate, TT, and most BT patients), therapy is recommended for 6 mo with rifampin (600 mg once monthly PO, directly observed) and dapsone (100 mg once daily PO, self-administered). Patients who experience relapse are re-treated with the same regimens. To date there have been no patients treated with WHO recommended MDT who have experienced secondary Rifampin resistance in contrast to those treated with Rifampin monotherapy or multidrug therapy not recommended by WHO. Resistance is difficult to determine at present, requiring an in vivo mouse footpad test of 12 mo duration. Newer genetic testing models evaluating for resistance-associated mutations in the *rpoB* gene of *M. leprae* are much faster and appear very accurate.

Patients treated in the United States may be advised to receive regimens that vary from WHO recommendations. Adults with paucibacillary disease receive dapsone (100 mg once daily PO) and rifampin (600 mg once daily PO) for 12 mo; those with multibacillary disease receive dapsone (100 mg once daily PO), rifampin (600 mg once daily PO), and clofazimine (50 mg once daily PO) for 24 mo. Daily pediatric doses are dapsone 1 mg/kg, rifampin 10 mg/kg, and clofazimine 1 mg/kg, not to exceed the recommended adult doses.

Therapy for reactional states can be complicated and generally requires expert consultation. Management depends on maintenance of antimycobacterial drugs, effective and prolonged anti-inflammatory therapy, and adequate analgesia and physical support during the phase of active neuritis. Mild ENL may respond to nonsteroidal anti-inflammatory agents. More severe ENL usually requires corticosteroid therapy (prednisolone 1 mg/kg/24 hr) but often relapses when the drug is discontinued. Clinical remission of acute or suppression of chronic ENL can be achieved with thalidomide. A dose of 100 mg qid will usually control the reaction within 48 hrs. The dose is then tapered to a maintenance level of around 100 mg/24 hr, and every few months an attempt should be made to wean patients off the drug altogether. *Thalidomide is absolutely contraindicated in women of child-bearing age;* otherwise it is much safer than corticosteroids for chronic use. The major side effect is fatigue. Pediatric dosages have not been established. Clofazimine 300 mg/24 hr tapering to 100 mg/24 hr or less for 12 mo is also useful in managing chronic ENL. Type 1 reversal reactions are optimally treated with high-dose corticosteroids (prednisolone 20–40 mg/24 hr PO in adults, and 1 mg/kg/24 hr PO in children) tapered over several months. Alternate-day regimens may be effective in patients with frequent relapses requiring prolonged treatment.

Prognosis. The prognosis for arresting progression of tissue and nerve damage is good, but recovery of lost sensory and motor function is variable and generally incomplete; hyperpigmentation, hypopigmentation, and loss of hair follicles or sweat glands persist. Intercurrent reactional states, poor compliance, and emergence of drug resistance can all lead to clinical exacerbations or relapses necessitating close follow-up of patients. Much of the chronic debility results from repeated trauma to anesthetic digits and limbs. Careful counseling of patients and consultation with physical and occupational therapy services is essential for an optimal outcome.

Prevention. Two approaches are advocated for interrupting leprosy transmission in endemic areas. The first is directed at the risk of infection among household contacts of leprosy patients, especially those with multibacillary disease. It is based on regular periodic examination of contacts and early treatment at the first evidence of leprosy. The second is the use of bacille Calmette-Guerin (BCG) vaccination. One dose of BCG appears to be 50% protective against leprosy; a second dose increases the protective benefit.

One historical practice that has fortunately been abandoned is the forcing of leprosy patients into a leprosarium. Mouse footpad inoculation studies have demonstrated that viability of *M. leprae* in skin biopsies decreases sharply within 3 wk of initiating therapy with dapsone and rifampin. This rapid decrease in infectivity combined with the high probability that family members have already had prolonged exposure to the patient before the diagnosis makes physical isolation of leprosy patients unnecessary.

Cambau E, Bonnafous P, Perani E, et al: Molecular detection of rifampin and ofloxacin resistance for patients who experience relapse of multibacillary leprosy. *Clin Infect Dis* 2002;34:39–45.

Cole ST, Eiglmeier K, Parkhill J, et al: Massive gene decay in the leprosy bacillus. *Nature* 2001;409:1007–11.

Haimanot RT, Melaku Z: Leprosy. *Curr Opin Neurol* 2000;13:317–22.

Jacobson RR, Krahenbuhl JL: Leprosy. *Lancet* 1999;353:655–60.

Marlowe SN, Lockwood DN: Update on leprosy. *Hosp Med* 2001;62:471–6.

Naafs B: Current views on reactions in leprosy. *Indian J Leprosy* 2000;72:97–122.

Ooi WW, Moschella SL: Update on leprosy in immigrants in the United States: Status in the year 2000. *Clin Infect Dis* 2001;32:930–7.

Rambukkana A: Molecular basis for the peripheral nerve predilection of *Mycobacterium leprae*. *Curr Opin Microbiol* 2001;4:21–7.

Scollard DM: Endothelial cells and the pathogenesis of lepromatous neuritis: Insights from the armadillo model. *Microbes Infect* 2000;2:1835–43.

World Health Organization, Leprosy Elimination Project: Remaining challenges toward the elimination of leprosy. *Indian J Lepr* 2000;72:33–45.

Chapter 199

Nontuberculous Mycobacteria *Dwight A. Powell*

Nonleprous, nontuberculous *Mycobacterium* (NTM), which are also referred to as **atypical mycobacteria, mycobacteria other than tuberculosis (MOTT)**, or potentially pathogenic environmental mycobacteria, are members of the family of Mycobacteriaceae. They differ from *M. tuberculosis* in their nutritional requirements, ability to produce pigments, enzymatic activity, and susceptibility patterns to antituberculous drugs. In contrast to *M. tuberculosis*, NTM are generally acquired from contact with the environment rather than by person-to-person spread.

Etiology. Fourteen strains of NTM are associated with human infections. Phenotypically, they are divided into four groups described by Runyon in 1959 (Table 199–1) based on their colony growth and morphology on solid media. Groups I, II, and III are slow growing (>7 days to detect growth); group IV is rapid growing (<7 days to detect growth). Photochromogens form pigment after exposure to light, scotochromogens form pigment in the dark, and nonchromogens fail to produce pigment. Species and serovars of NTM are now defined by biochemical reactions, antibody specificity, radiolabeled DNA probes, DNA restriction fragment length polymorphism, or ribosomal-RNA sequencing. Biochemically and immunologically related species

TABLE 199–1. Classification of Nontuberculous Mycobacteria Associated with Human Disease

Runyon Group	Mycobacteria
I. Photochromogens	*M. kansasii*
	M. marinum
	M. simiae
II. Scotochromogens	*M. scrofulaceum*
	M. xenopi
	M. szulgai
III. Nonchromogens	*M. avium*
	M. intracellulare
	M. malmoense
	M. haemophilum
	M. ulcerans
IV. Rapid growers	*M. chelonae*
	M. fortuitum
	M. abscessus

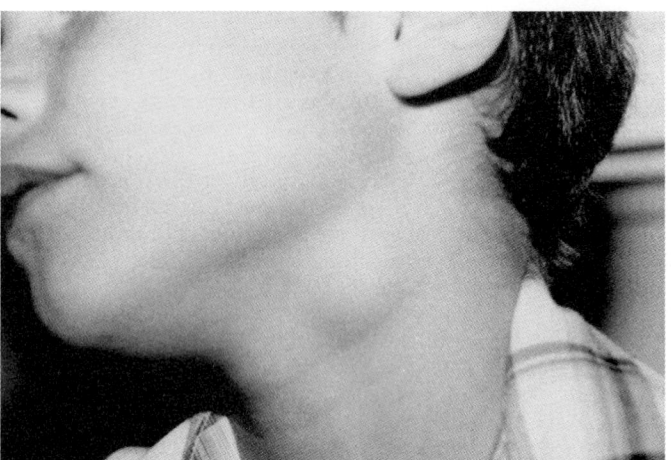

FIGURE 199–1. An enlarging cervical lymph node with nontuberculous mycobacterial infection, which is firm, painless, freely movable, and not erythematous.

that are difficult for clinical laboratories to differentiate are often referred to as "complexes," such as the **M. fortuitum complex** (*M. fortuitum* and *M. chelonae*) and the **M. avium complex** (*M. avium* and *M. intracellulare*).

Epidemiology. NTM are distributed worldwide and are ubiquitous in the environment, existing as saprophytes in soil and water; as pathogens in swine, birds, and cattle; and as part of the normal human pharyngeal flora. Some NTM have well-defined ecologic niches that help explain transmission patterns. The natural reservoir for *M. marinum* is fish and other cold-blooded animals, so infections follow injury in an aquatic environment. *M. fortuitum* and *M. chelonae* are ubiquitous in the hospital environment and have caused clusters of nosocomial surgical wound and venous catheter-related infections. *M. ulcerans* is recovered only from soils and waters of rain forests and is associated with chronic skin infections in the tropics. *M. avium* complex is found in abundance in the waters, soils, and aerosols of the acid, brown-water swamps of the southeastern United States. In rural counties in this region, asymptomatic infections with *M. avium* complex approach 70% by adulthood.

With the exception of cervical lymphadenitis, illness related to NTM infections is relatively uncommon in children. Infection with NTM, particularly *M. avium* complex, is one of the most common terminal infections in patients with AIDS.

Pathogenesis. The histologic appearances of lesions produced by *M. tuberculosis* and NTM are often indistinguishable. The classic pathologic lesion consists of caseating granulomas. However, compared with *M. tuberculosis*, NTM infections are more likely to result in granulomas that are noncaseating, ill-defined (nonpalisading), and irregular or serpiginous. Granulomas may be absent, with only chronic inflammatory changes observed. In patients with AIDS and disseminated NTM infection, the inflammatory reaction is usually scant and tissues are filled with large numbers of histiocytes packed with acid-fast bacilli.

Clinical Manifestations. Lymphadenitis of the superior anterior cervical or submandibular nodes is the most frequent manifestation of NTM infection in children. Preauricular, posterior cervical, axillary, and inguinal nodes are involved occasionally. Lymphadenitis is most common in children 1–5 yr of age because of their tendency to put objects contaminated with soil, dust, or standing water into their mouths. Affected children usually lack constitutional symptoms and present with a unilateral subacute and slowly enlarging lymph node or group of closely approximated nodes >1.5 cm that are firm, painless, freely movable, and not erythematous (Fig. 199–1). The involved nodes occasionally resolve without treatment, but most undergo rapid suppuration after several weeks. The center of the node becomes fluctuant, and the overlying skin becomes erythematous and thin. Eventually, the

nodes rupture and form cutaneous sinus tracts that drain for months or years, resembling the classic scrofula of tuberculosis (Fig. 199–2). In the United States, *M. avium* complex accounts for approximately 80% of NTM lymphadenitis in children. *M. scrofulaceum* and *M. kansasii* account for most other cases, particularly in the southwestern United States. Rarely, *M. xenopi*, *M. malmoense*, *M. haemophilum*, and *M. szulgai* are described.

Cutaneous disease due to NTM is rare in children. Infection usually follows percutaneous inoculation with fresh or salt water contaminated by *M. marinum*. Within several weeks of exposure, a solitary nodule develops at the site of minor abrasions on the elbows, knees, or feet (**swimming pool granuloma**) and on the hands and fingers of fish fanciers (**fish tank granuloma**). The lesions are usually nontender and enlarge over 3–5 wk to ulcerated granulomas or warty lesions, as seen in cutaneous tuberculosis. The lesions sometimes resemble sporotrichosis; satellite lesions near the site of entry extend along the skin following the superficial lymphatics. Lymphadenopathy is usually absent. Although most infections remain localized to skin, penetrating *M. marinum* infections may result in tenosynovitis, bursitis, osteomyelitis, or arthritis.

M. ulcerans also causes cutaneous infection in children living in tropical countries (Africa, Australia, Asia, and South America). Infection follows percutaneous inoculation and presents as a painless erythematous nodule, most frequently on a leg, which

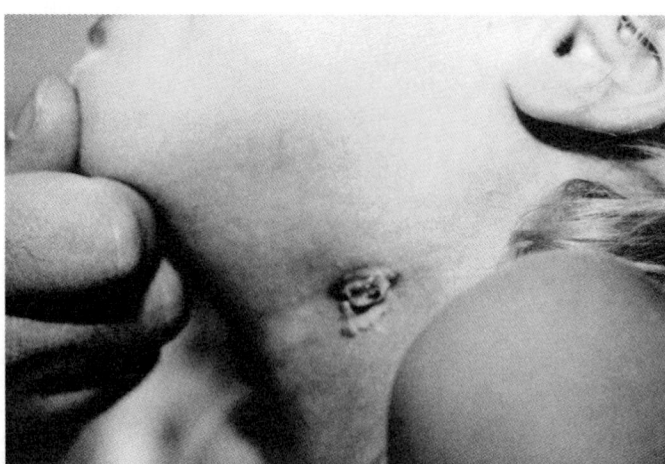

FIGURE 199–2. A ruptured cervical lymph node with nontuberculous mycobacterial infection, which resembles the classic scrofula of tuberculosis.

undergoes central necrosis and ulceration. The lesion, often called a **Buruli ulcer** after the region in Uganda where most cases are reported, has a characteristic undermined edge, gradually expands, and may result in extensive soft tissue destruction with secondary bacterial infection. The lesion may heal slowly over 6–9 mo or may continue to spread, leading to deformities and contractures.

Skin and soft tissue infections due to *M. fortuitum, M. chelonae,* or *M. abscessus* are rare in children and usually follow percutaneous inoculation due to puncture wounds and minor abrasions. Clinical disease usually arises after a 4–6 wk incubation period and presents as a localized cellulitis, painful nodules, or a draining abscess. A unique case has been described of mastitis due to *M. abscessus* following insertion of a nipple ring. *M. haemophilum* may cause painful subcutaneous nodules, which often ulcerate and suppurate in immunocompromised patients, particularly after renal transplant.

Nontuberculous mycobacteria are uncommon sources of catheter-associated infections, but are becoming increasingly recognized. These are most commonly caused by *M. fortuitum, M. chelonae,* or *M. abscessus* and may present as bacteremia or localized catheter tunnel infections.

Pulmonary infections, although the most common cause of NTM illness in adults, are uncommon in children. *M. avium* complex has been described as a cause of acute pneumonitis, chronic cough, or wheezing associated with paratracheal or peribronchial lymphadenitis and airway compression in normal children. Rare cases of progression to endobronchial granulation tissue have been reported. Chronic infections in older cystic fibrosis patients have been caused by *M. avium* complex and *M. fortuitum* complex. *M. kansasii, M. xenopi,* and *M. szulgai* are uncommon in children and usually occur in adults with underlying chronic lung disease. The onset is insidious and consists of low-grade fever, cough, night sweats, and generalized malaise. Thin-walled cavities with minimal surrounding parenchymal infiltrates are characteristic, but radiographic findings may resemble those of tuberculosis.

In unusual circumstances, NTM cause bone and joint infections that are indistinguishable from those produced by *M. tuberculosis* or bacterial agents. Such infections usually result from operative incision or accidental puncture wounds. *M. fortuitum* infections from puncture wounds of the foot resemble infections caused by *Pseudomonas aeruginosa* and *Staphylococcus aureus.*

Disseminated disease, usually associated with *M. avium* complex infections, occurs occasionally in children without any apparent immunodeficiency. Most of these patients have mutations in genes coding for the interferon-γ receptor (IFNGR) or the interleukin-12 (IL-12) receptor, or for IL-12 production. Those patients with complete IFNGR deficiency have severe disease that is difficult to treat. Those with partial IFNGR deficiency or IL-12 pathway mutations have milder disease that may respond to interferon and antimycobacterial therapy. Multifocal osteomyelitis is particularly prevalent in individuals with the IFNGR1 818del4 mutation. Recurrence, years after a course of treatment, has been well documented.

Disseminated disease due to *M. avium* complex infections is among the most common opportunistic infections in patients with AIDS, usually late in the illness when CD4 cell counts are <100 cells/mm³. Colonization of the respiratory or gastrointestinal tract probably precedes disseminated *M. avium* complex infections, but screening studies of respiratory secretions or stool samples are not useful to predict dissemination. Continuous high-grade bacteremia is usual, and multiple organs are infected, including most commonly lymph nodes, liver, spleen, bone marrow, and gastrointestinal tract. Thyroid, pancreas, adrenal gland, kidney, muscle, and brain may be involved. The most common signs and symptoms of disseminated *M. avium* complex infections in AIDS patients are fever, night sweats, chills, anorexia, marked weight loss, wasting, weakness, generalized lymphadenopathy,

and hepatosplenomegaly. Jaundice, elevated alkaline phosphatase level, anemia, and neutropenia may occur. Imaging studies usually demonstrate massive lymphadenopathy of hilar, mediastinal, mesenteric, or retroperitoneal nodes. In children with AIDS, the mean survival time after isolation of *M. avium* complex from a body source is 5–9 mo.

Diagnosis. The differential diagnosis of NTM lymphadenitis includes acute bacterial lymphadenitis, tuberculosis, cat-scratch disease (*Bartonella henselae*), mononucleosis, toxoplasmosis, brucellosis, tularemia, and malignancies, especially lymphomas. An intermediate strength tuberculin skin test (5 tuberculin units) is usually weakly positive with 5–15 mm induration. Although the Centers for Disease Control and Prevention have produced skin tests representing the different Runyon groups of NTM, these antigens are no longer available. Differentiation between NTM and *M. tuberculosis* may be difficult, but children with NTM lymphadenitis usually have a Mantoux tuberculin skin test reaction <15 mm in duration, unilateral anterior cervical node involvement, a normal lung roentgenogram, and no exposure to adult tuberculosis; children with tuberculous lymphadenitis more often have bilateral posterior cervical node involvement, a Mantoux tuberculin skin test reaction ≥15 mm in duration, an abnormal lung roentgenogram, or exposure to adult tuberculosis. Definitive diagnosis requires excision of involved nodes and recovery of the responsible pathogen.

Diagnosis of cutaneous infections depends on isolating the responsible microorganisms from an excised lesion. The diagnosis of pulmonary NTM infection in children is difficult because many species of NTM, including *M. avium* complex, can be isolated from oral and gastric secretions of healthy children. Definitive diagnosis requires invasive procedures such as bronchoscopy and pulmonary or endobronchial biopsy. Mycolic acids and other lipids in the cell wall of mycobacteria give them their hallmark trait of acid-fastness with the Ziehl-Neelsen or Kinyoun stains. They may also be identified with the fluorochrome stain auramine-rhodamine. The sensitivity of these stains for detecting NTM in tissue samples is less than with *M. tuberculosis.*

Blood cultures are 90–95% sensitive in AIDS patients with disseminated infection. *M. avium* complex may be detected within 7 days of inoculation in nearly all patients with the BACTEC radiometric blood culture system. Commercially available DNA probes differentiate NTM from *M. tuberculosis.* Identification of histiocytes containing numerous acid-fast bacilli from bone marrow and other biopsy tissues provides a rapid presumptive diagnosis of disseminated mycobacterial infection.

Treatment. Therapy for NTM infections involves medical, surgical, or combined treatment. Isolation of the infecting strain followed by susceptibility testing is ideal because susceptibility patterns vary. *M. kansasii, M. marinum, M. xenopi, M. ulcerans,* and *M. malmoense* are usually susceptible to some standard antituberculous drugs. *M. fortuitum, M. chelonae, M. scrofulaceum,* and *M. avium* complex are often resistant to standard antituberculous drugs but have variable susceptibility to newer antibiotics such as quinolones and macrolides. Multiple drug therapy is essential to avoid development of resistance.

The preferred treatment of NTM lymphadenitis is complete surgical excision. Nodes should be removed while still firm and encapsulated. Excision is more difficult if extensive caseation with extension to surrounding tissue has occurred, and complications of facial nerve damage or recurrent infection are more likely. Incomplete surgical excision is not advised because chronic drainage may develop. Standard antituberculous medications have little effect on NTM lymphadenitis and are not necessary with complete excision. If there is concern for *M. tuberculosis* infection, therapy with isoniazid, rifampin, and pyrazinamide should be given until cultures confirm the cause. If for some reason surgery of NTM lymphadenitis cannot be performed, removal of infected tissue is incomplete, or recurrence or chronic drainage develops, a 4–6 mo trial of chemotherapy is warranted. Although there are no published controlled trials, several case reports and small series have reported successful treatment with chemotherapy alone or combined with surgical excision. Clarithromycin or azithromycin combined with rifabutin or ethambutol are the most commonly reported therapy regimens.

Cutaneous NTM lesions usually heal spontaneously after incision and drainage without other therapy. *M. marinum* is susceptible to rifampin, amikacin, ethambutol, sulfonamides, trimethoprim-sulfamethoxazole, and tetracycline. Therapy with a combination of these drugs may be given for 3–4 mo. Corticosteroid injections should not be used. Superficial infections with *M. fortuitum* or *M. chelonae* usually resolve after surgical incision and open drainage, but deep-seated or catheter-related infections require removal of infected central lines and therapy with parenteral amikacin plus cefoxitin or clarithromycin. Pulmonary infections should be treated initially with isoniazid, rifampin, and pyrazinamide pending culture identification and susceptibility testing.

Patients with disseminated *M. avium* complex and IL-12 pathway defects or deficiency of IFNGR should be treated for at least 12 months with clarithromycin or azithromycin combined with one or more second-line drugs (rifabutin, clofazimine, ethambutol, or a quinolone). In vitro susceptibility testing is important. Once the clinical illness has resolved, lifelong daily prophylaxis with clarithromycin is advisable to prevent recurrent disease. The use of interferon adjunctive therapy is determined by the specific genetic defect.

In adults with AIDS, daily prophylaxis with azithromycin with or without rifabutin reduces infection with *M. avium* complex by >50%. Although pediatric studies are lacking, the U.S. Public Health Service recommends either azithromycin (20 mg/kg once weekly PO; maximum: 1200 mg/dose) or clarithromycin (7.5 mg/kg/dose bid PO; maximum: 500 mg/dose) for HIV-infected children with the following indications: for children ≥6 yr, CD4 count <50/μL; 2–6 yr, CD4 count <75/μL; 1–2 yr, CD4 count <500/μL; <1 yr, CD4 count <750 μL.

Abrams EJ: Opportunistic infections and other clinical manifestations of HIV diseases in children. *Pediatr Clin North Am* 2000;47:79–108.

Centers for Disease Control and Prevention: 2002 USPHSHS/IDSA guidelines for the prevention of opportunistic infections in persons infected with human immunodeficiency virus. *MMWR* 2002;51(RR-8):1–60.

Hazra R, Robson CD, Perez-Atayde AR, et al: Lymphadenitis due to nontuberculous mycobacteria in children: Presentation and response to therapy. *Clin Infect Dis* 1999;28:123–9.

Holland SM: Immunotherapy of mycobacterial infections. *Semin Respir Infect* 2001; 16:47–59.

Holland SM: Nontuberculous mycobacteria. *Am J Med Sci* 2001;321:49–55.

Litman DA, Shah UK, Pawel BR: Isolated endobronchial atypical mycobacterium in a child: A case report and review of the literature. *Int J Pediatr Otorhinolaryngol* 2000;55:65–8.

Palenque E: Skin disease and nontuberculous atypical mycobacteria. *Int J Dermatol* 2000;39:659–66.

Pursner M, Haller JO, Berdon WE: Imaging features of *Mycobacterium avium-intracellulare* complex (MAC) in children. *Pediatr Radiol* 2000;30:426–9.

Starke JR: Management of nontuberculous mycobacterial cervical adenitis. *Pediatr Infect Dis J* 2000;19:674–5.

Swanson DS: Central venous catheter-related infections due to nontuberculous *Mycobacterium* species. *Pediatr Infect Dis J* 1998;17:1163–4.

SECTION 6 *Spirochetal Infections*

Chapter 200

Syphilis (*Treponema pallidum*) Parvin Azimi

Etiology. Syphilis is a systemic communicable infection caused by *Treponema pallidum*, a long, slender, tightly coiled, motile spirochete with finely tapered ends belonging to the family Spirochaetaceae. The pathogenic members of this genus include *T. pallidum* (venereal syphilis), *T. pertenue* (yaws), *T. pallidum* subsp. *endemicum* (endemic syphilis), and *T. carateum* (pinta). Because these microorganisms stain poorly, detection in clinical specimens requires dark-field microscopy or direct immunofluorescent staining techniques. *T. pallidum* cannot be cultured in vitro but has been propagated by intratesticular inoculation in rabbits.

Epidemiology. Two forms of syphilis are encountered in children. Acquired syphilis is transmitted almost exclusively by sexual contact. Less frequent modes of transmission include transfusion of contaminated blood or direct contact with infected tissues. After an epidemic resurgence of primary and secondary syphilis in the 1980s in the United States that peaked in 1989, the annual rate has declined and in 1997 was the lowest since reporting for syphilis began in 1941. Rates further declined in 2000 due to targeted United States public health efforts in the racial/ethnic minority population at risk. Despite these declines, syphilis remains endemic in parts of the south, where it is more common (3.8 per 100,000 population) than in the midwest (2.0), northeast (0.7), and west (1.0). The rates for primary and secondary syphilis remain substantially higher for blacks (12.8 per 100,000 population) than for nonwhite Hispanics (1.8) and for non-Hispanic whites (0.6).

Congenital syphilis results from transplacental transmission of spirochetes. Pregnant women with primary and secondary syphilis and spirochetemia are more likely to transmit infection to the fetus than are women with latent infection. Transmission can occur at any stage of pregnancy. The incidence of congenital infection in the offspring of untreated infected women remains highest during the first 4 yr after acquisition of primary infection, secondary, and early latent disease. The risk factors most commonly associated with congenital syphilis are lack of prenatal care and cocaine drug abuse, which is associated with prostitution, unprotected sexual contact, and trading of sex for drugs, in addition to inadequate prenatal care of pregnant addicts.

Clinical Manifestations. Primary syphilis is characterized by syphilitic chancre and regional lymphadenitis. A painless papule appears at the site of inoculation 2–6 wk after *T. pallidum* has been introduced. The papule soon develops into a clean, painless ulcer with raised borders called a chancre. The chancre, usually on the genitals, contains viable *T. pallidum* and is highly contagious. Extragenital chancres can also be seen, depending on the site of primary inoculation. Adjacent lymph nodes are generally enlarged. The chancre heals spontaneously within 4–6 wk, leaving a thin scar.

Untreated patients develop manifestations of **secondary syphilis** 2–10 wk after the chancre heals. Manifestations of secondary syphilis are related to spirochetemia and include a nonpruritic maculopapular rash, which can cover the entire body, involving palms and soles; pustular lesions may also develop. **Condylomata lata** (gray-white to erythematous wartlike plaques) can occur in moist areas around the anus and vagina, and white plaques called mucous patches may be found in mucous membranes. A flulike illness with low-grade fever, headache, malaise, anorexia, weight loss, sore throat, myalgias, and arthralgias, and generalized lymphadenopathy is often present. Renal, hepatic, and ophthalmologic manifestations may be present, as may be meningitis, which occurs in 30% of patients with secondary syphilis, manifested by cerebrospinal fluid (CSF) pleocytosis and elevated protein level, although the patient may not show neurologic symptoms. Secondary infection becomes **latent** within 1–2 mo after the onset of the rash. Relapses with secondary manifestations can be seen during the 1st year of latency. This period is referred to as the **early latent period**. No relapses occur after the 1st year; what follows is late syphilis, which may be either asymptomatic (**late latent**) or symptomatic (**tertiary**). At this stage, patients may begin showing the manifestations of tertiary disease, which include neurologic, cardiovascular, and gummatous lesions. The latter are granulomas of the skin and musculoskeletal system resulting from the host's delayed hypersensitivity reaction.

CONGENITAL INFECTION. Syphilis during pregnancy has a transmission rate approaching 100%. Fetal or perinatal death occurs in 40% of affected infants. Among survivors, manifestations have traditionally been divided into early and late stages. **Early signs** appear during the first 2 yr of life, whereas **late signs** appear gradually during the first 2 decades. Early manifestations result from transplacental spirochetemia and are analogous to the secondary stage of acquired syphilis. Approximately two thirds of infected infants are asymptomatic at the time of birth and are identified only by routine prenatal screening; if they are untreated, symptoms develop within weeks or months.

The early manifestations of congenital infection are varied and involve multiple organ systems. Hepatosplenomegaly, jaundice, and elevated liver enzymes are common. Histologically, liver involvement includes bile stasis, fibrosis, and extramedullary hematopoiesis. Lymphadenopathy tends to be diffuse and resolve spontaneously; shotty nodes may persist. Coombs negative hemolytic anemia is characteristic. Thrombocytopenia is often associated with platelet trapping in an enlarged spleen. Characteristic osteochondritis and periostitis (Fig. 200–1) and mucocutaneous rash (Fig. 200–2), presenting with erythematous maculopapular or bullous lesions, followed by desquamation involving hands and feet, are common. Mucous patches, rhinitis (**snuffles**), and condylomatous lesions are highly characteristic features of mucous membrane involvement in congenital syphilis. Bone involvement occurs frequently. Roentgenographic abnormalities include multiple sites of osteochondritis at the wrists, elbows, ankles, and knees; and periostitis of the long bones, and rarely the skull. The osteochondritis is painful and often results in irritability and refusal to move the involved extremity (**pseudoparalysis of Parrot**). Central nervous system (CNS) abnormalities, failure to thrive, chorioretinitis, nephritis, and nephrotic syndrome may also be seen. Clinical manifestations of renal involvement include hypertension, hematuria, proteinuria, hypoproteinemia, hypercholesterolemia, and hypocomplementemia. They appear to be related to glomerular deposition of circulating immune complexes. Less common clinical manifestations of early congenital syphilis include gastroenteritis, peri-

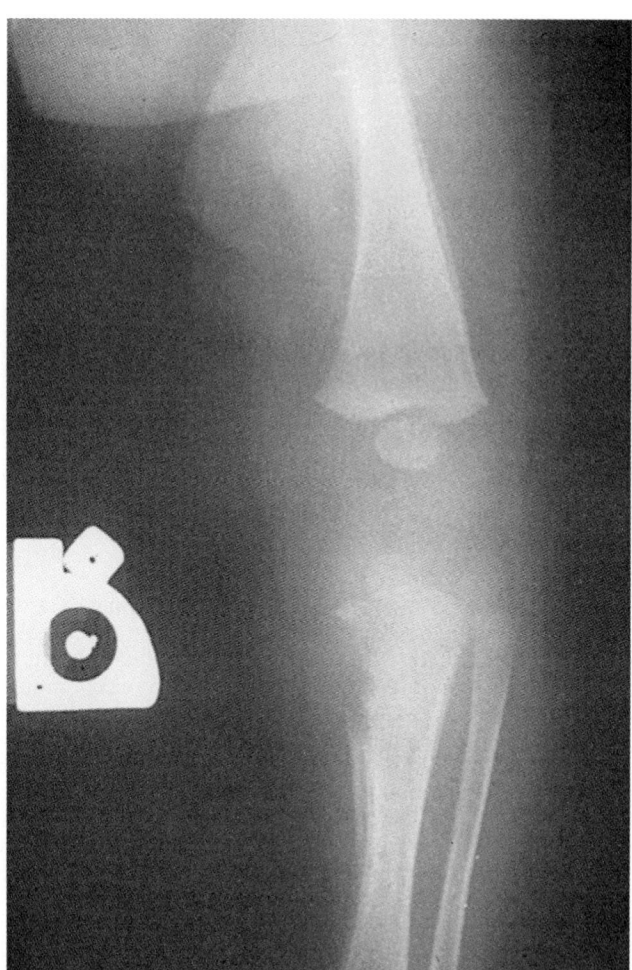

FIGURE 200–1. Osteochondritis and periostitis in a newborn with congenital syphilis.

tonitis, pancreatitis, pneumonia, eye involvement (glaucoma and chorioretinitis), nonimmune hydrops, and testicular masses.

The late manifestations result primarily from chronic inflammation of bone, teeth, and the CNS. Skeletal changes due to persistent or recurrent periostitis and associated thickening of bone include frontal bossing, a bony prominence of the forehead (**"olympian brow"**); unilateral or bilateral thickening of the sternoclavicular portion of the clavicle (**Higouménakis sign**); an anterior bowing of the midportion of the tibia (**saber shins**); and scaphoid scapula, a convexity along its medial border. Dental abnormalities are common and include (1) **Hutchinson teeth** (Fig. 200–3), which are the peg or barrel-shaped upper central incisors that erupt during the 6th yr of life; (2) abnormal enamel, which results in a notch along the biting surface; and (3) **mulberry molars**, abnormal 1st lower (6 yr) molars, characterized by a small biting surface and an excessive number of cusps. Defects in enamel formation lead to repeated caries and eventual tooth destruction.

A **saddle nose** (Fig. 200–4), a depression of the nasal root, is a result of syphilitic rhinitis that destroys the adjacent bone and cartilage. A perforated nasal septum is an associated abnormality. **Rhagades** are linear scars that extend in a spokelike pattern from previous mucocutaneous fissures of the mouth, anus, and genitalia. **Juvenile paresis**, an uncommon latent meningovascular infection, typically presents during adolescence with behavioral changes, focal seizures, or loss of intellectual function. **Juvenile tabes** with spinal cord involvement and cardiovascular involvement with aortitis are extremely rare.

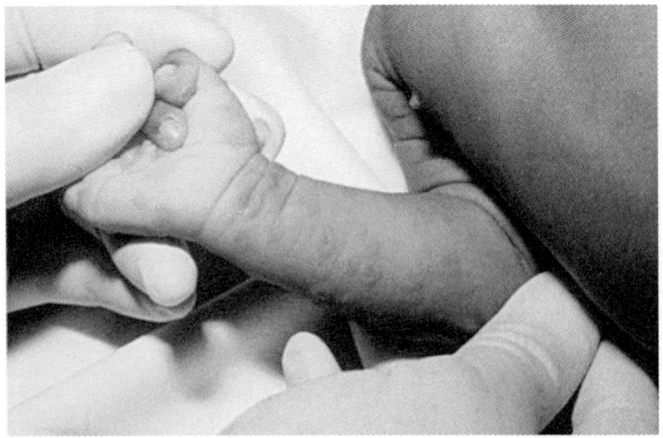

FIGURE 200–2. The mucocutaneous rash of congenital syphilis. See also color plates.

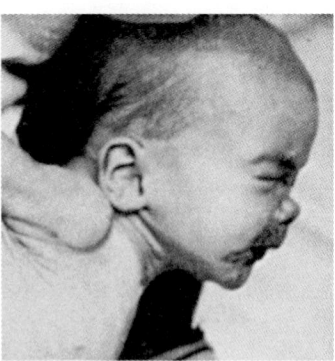

FIGURE 200–4. Saddle nose in a newborn with congenital syphilis.

Other late manifestations of congenital syphilis may represent a hypersensitivity phenomenon. These include unilateral or bilateral interstitial keratitis with symptoms such as intense photophobia and lacrimation, followed within weeks or months by corneal opacification and complete blindness. Less common ocular manifestations include choroiditis, retinitis, vascular occlusion, and optic atrophy. Eighth nerve deafness may be unilateral or bilateral, appears at any age, presents initially as vertigo and high-tone hearing loss, and progresses to permanent deafness. The **Clutton joint** represents a unilateral or bilateral synovitis involving the lower extremities (usually the knee), which presents as painless joint swelling with sterile synovial fluid; spontaneous remission usually occurs after a period of several weeks. Soft tissue gummas (identical to those of acquired disease) and paroxysmal cold hemoglobinuria are rare hypersensitivity phenomena.

Diagnosis. Diagnosis of primary syphilis is made with certainty when *T. pallidum* is demonstrated by dark-field microscopy or direct immunofluorescence on specimens from skin lesions, placenta, or umbilicus. However, serologic tests for syphilis are the principal means for diagnosis.

Nontreponemal tests, such as the **Venereal Disease Research Laboratory (VDRL)** and **rapid plasma reagin (RPR)** tests, detect antibodies against a cardiolipin-cholesterol-lecithin complex, not specific for syphilis. The quantitative results of these nontreponemal tests tend to correlate with disease activity and therefore are helpful in screening. Titers elevate when disease is active (including treatment failure or reinfection) and decline when treatment is adequate. Serum usually becomes nonreactive in the nontreponemal tests within 1 yr of adequate therapy for primary syphilis and within 2 yr of treatment for secondary disease. In congenital infection, these tests become nonreactive within a few months after adequate treatment. Certain conditions such as autoimmune diseases may give false-positive VDRL results in the serum (but not in the CSF), although false-positive results are less common because of the introduction of purified cardiolipin-lecithin-cholesterol antigen. Pregnancy itself does not give a false-positive VDRL result; all positive maternal serologic tests for syphilis, regardless of the titer, necessitate thorough investigation.

Treponemal tests, which measure antibody specific for *T. pallidum*, include the *T. pallidum* immobilization test (TPI), the fluorescent treponemal antibody absorption test (FTA-ABS), and the microhemagglutination assay for antibodies to *T. pallidum* (MHA-TP). Treponemal tests are used as confirmatory testing of positive results from the nontreponemal antibody tests. The MHA-TP has few false-positive test results (<1% of healthy persons) and is the treponemal test used by most clinical laboratories. Treponemal antibody titers become positive soon after initial infection and usually remain positive for life, even with adequate therapy. These antibody titers do not correlate with disease activity and are not quantified. They are useful for diagnosis of a first episode of syphilis and for distinguishing false-positive results of nontreponemal antibody tests but are of limited usefulness in the evaluation of response to therapy and possible reinfections.

There is limited cross-reactivity of treponemal antibody tests with the causative organisms of Lyme disease (*Borrelia burgdorferi*), yaws (*T. pallidum* subsp. *pertenue*), endemic syphilis (*T. pallidum* subsp. *endemicum*), and pinta (*T. carateum*). Only venereal syphilis (*T. pallidum*) and Lyme disease are found in the United States. The nontreponemal tests (VDRL, RPR) are uniformly nonreactive in Lyme disease.

Tests for IgM antibodies have been developed, including FTA-ABS 19S-IgM, IgM capture enzyme-linked immunosorbent assay, and Western immunoblotting assays, but these have been relatively insensitive and are not generally available. Tests for *T. pallidum* using polymerase chain reaction (PCR) amplification are also being developed.

The interpretation of nontreponemal and treponemal serologic tests in the newborn may be confounded by maternal IgG antibodies that are transferred to the fetus. Passively acquired antibody is suggested by neonatal titer at least fourfold (i.e., a two-tube dilution) less than the maternal titer. This can be verified by gradual decline in antibody in the infant, usually becoming undetectable by 3–6 mo of age.

The diagnosis of neurosyphilis in acquired disease is made by demonstrating pleocytosis and increased protein in the CSF, and

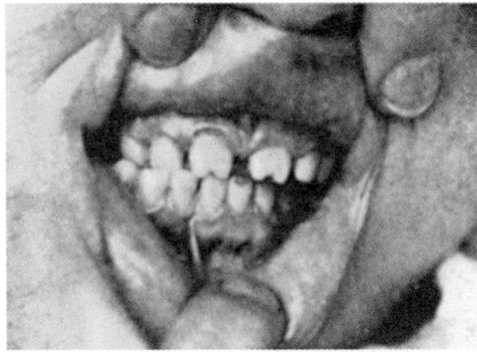

FIGURE 200–3. Hutchinson teeth as a late manifestation of congenital syphilis.

a positive CSF VDRL along with neurologic symptoms. The CSF VDRL is very specific but relatively insensitive (22–69%) for neurosyphilis.

Dark-field microscopy of scrapings from primary lesions or congenital or secondary lesions can reveal *T. pallidum*, often before serology becomes positive, but this technique is usually not available in clinical practice. Similarly, rabbit infectivity testing, used for measuring the sensitivity of investigational tests such as PCR and Western immunoblotting, is not widely available. Placental examination by gross and microscopic techniques can be useful in the diagnosis of congenital syphilis. The disproportionately large placentas are characterized histologically by focal proliferative villitis, endovascular and perivascular arteritis, and focal or diffuse immaturity of placental villi.

CONGENITAL SYPHILIS. Symptomatic infants should be thoroughly evaluated and treated. Asymptomatic infants considered at risk for congenital syphilis because the maternal non-treponemal and treponemal serology is positive should be evaluated if (1) maternal treatment was inadequate, unknown, or undocumented; (2) maternal treatment was ≤30 days before delivery; (3) the mother was treated with erythromycin or other nonpenicillin regimen; or (4) the maternal nontreponemal titers did not decrease sufficiently to demonstrate a cure (four-fold or greater). If the maternal treatment was adequate and ≥1 mo before delivery, the infant's positive nontreponemal test represents passively acquired antibody and the infant does not need treatment at delivery, but follow-up serology should be obtained. If the maternal evaluation is unable to be completed, these infants must be assumed to be infected and treated.

The diagnosis of neurosyphilis in the newborn with syphilitic infection is difficult owing to the poor sensitivity of the CSF VDRL in this age group and the lack of CSF abnormalities. In general, a positive CSF VDRL in a newborn warrants treatment for neurosyphilis, even though it might reflect passive transfer of antibodies from serum to CSF. More importantly, it is now accepted that all infants with a presumptive diagnosis of congenital syphilis should be treated with regimens effective for neurosyphilis because this cannot be reliably excluded.

The Centers for Disease Control and Prevention (CDC) recommends that infants be treated if (1) they were born to mothers who had untreated syphilis at delivery; (2) there is evidence of maternal relapse or reinfection; (3) there is physical evidence of active disease; (4) there is radiologic evidence of syphilis; (5) there is a reactive CSF VDRL or, for infants born to seropositive mothers, an abnormal CSF white blood cell count or protein, regardless of CSF serology; or (6) a serum quantitative nontreponemal serologic titer in the infant is at least fourfold greater than the mother's titer.

Treatment. *T. pallidum* is extremely sensitive to penicillin, and there is no evidence of emerging penicillin resistance. Penicillin remains the drug of choice for treatment of syphilis (Table 200–1). A concentration 0.018 μg/mL (0.03 U/mL) of penicillin is needed to ensure killing of spirochetes in serum and CSF. Although nonpenicillin regimens are available to the penicillin-allergic patient, desensitization followed by standard penicillin therapy is the most reliable strategy. An acute systemic febrile reaction, the Jarisch-Herxheimer reaction, with exacerbation of lesions, occurs in 15–20% of all patients with acquired or congenital syphilis who are treated with penicillin. It is not an indication for discontinuation of penicillin therapy.

ACQUIRED SYPHILIS. Primary, secondary, and early latent disease are treated with a single dose of benzathine penicillin G (50,000 units/kg IM; maximum: 2.4 million units). Nonpregnant penicillin-allergic patients without neurosyphilis may be treated with either doxycycline (100 mg PO bid for 2 wk) or tetracycline (500 mg PO qid for 2 wk).

Patients who are also infected with HIV are at increased risk for neurologic complications and have higher rates of treatment failures. The CDC guidelines recommend the same treatment of primary and secondary syphilis as for non–HIV-infected persons, but some experts recommend three weekly doses of benzathine penicillin G. HIV-infected patients with late latent syphilis or latent syphilis of unknown duration should have a CSF evaluation for neurosyphilis before treatment.

Incubating syphilis may be effectively treated with the currently recommended penicillin regimens for gonorrhea, and all patients treated for gonorrhea should have serologic testing for syphilis at the time of treatment and at follow-up 6–8 weeks later. Therapy with ampicillin, amoxicillin, or ceftriaxone is probably also effective. Spectinomycin therapy will not cure incubating syphilis. Because of the high risk of acquiring infection, "prophylactic treatment" should be given to sexual contacts of persons with infectious syphilis within the preceding 3 mo, regardless of serology. Three additional elements of syphilis therapy are obligatory: (1) Follow-up serology should be performed on treated individuals to establish adequacy of therapy; (2) sexual contacts should be identified and treated; and (3) testing for other sexually transmitted diseases, including HIV, should be performed on all patients.

SYPHILIS IN PREGNANCY. When clinical or serologic findings suggest active infection or when the diagnosis of active syphilis cannot be excluded with certainty, treatment is indicated. Patients should be treated with the penicillin regimen appropriate for the woman's stage of syphilis. Women who have been adequately treated in the past do not require additional therapy unless quantitative serology suggests evidence of reinfection

TABLE 200–1. Treatment of Syphilis

Stage	Treatment and Dosage	Alternatives
Primary, secondary, or early latent (<1 yr)	Penicillin G benzathine (2.4 million U IM, in one dose) For children: Penicillin G benzathine (50,000 U/kg IM, up to the adult dose in a single dose)	Tetracycline (500 mg PO qid for 2 wk) or doxycycline (100 mg PO bid for 2 wk) or erythromycin (500 mg PO qid for 2 wk)
Late latent (>1 yr), latent of unknown duration, or tertiary (gumma or cardiovascular syphilis)	Penicillin G benzathine (2.4 million U IM) weekly for 3 doses	Tetracycline (500 mg PO qid for 4 wk) or doxycycline (100 mg PO bid for 4 wk)
Neurosyphilis	Aqueous crystalline penicillin G (12–24 million U/24 hr IV given as 2.4 million U every 4 hr) for 10–14 days For children: Aqueous crystalline penicillin G (200,000–300,000 U/kg every day IV, given every 4-6 hr) for 10-14 days	Penicillin G procaine (2.4 million U/day IM) *plus* probenicid (500 mg PO qid). Both for 10–14 days
Congenital syphilis	Aqueous crystalline penicillin G (100,000–150,000 U/kg/24 hr, given as 50,000 U/kg IV every 12 hr for the first 7 days and every 8 hr thereafter) for 10–14 days or Procaine penicillin G (50,000 U/kg IM daily in a single dose) for 10–14 days	

(fourfold elevation in titer). Doxycycline and tetracycline should not be administered during pregnancy, and erythromycin does not effectively treat fetal infection.

CONGENITAL SYPHILIS. Adequate maternal therapy should eliminate the risk of congenital syphilis. All infants born to mothers with syphilis should be followed up until nontreponemal serology is negative. The infant should be treated if there is an uncertainty about the adequacy of the mother's treatment.

Current recommendations for treatment of congenital syphilis include regimens of aqueous penicillin G (100,000–150,000 U/kg/24 hr divided q 12 hr IV for the first wk of life, and q 8 hr thereafter) or procaine penicillin G (50,000 U/kg IM once daily) given for 10 days. Higher concentrations of penicillin are achieved in the CSF of infants treated with intravenous aqueous penicillin G than in those treated with intramuscular procaine penicillin. Both penicillin regimens are still recognized as adequate therapy for congenital syphilis. Treated infants should be followed up serologically to confirm decreasing nontreponemal antibody titers.

Prevention. Testing is indicated at any time for persons with suspicious lesions, a history of recent sexual exposure to a person with syphilis, or diagnosis of another sexually transmitted infection, including HIV infection.

CONGENITAL SYPHILIS. Routine prenatal screening for syphilis remains the most important factor in the identification of infants at risk for development of congenital syphilis and is legally required at the beginning of prenatal care in all states. In pregnant women without optimal prenatal care, serologic screening for syphilis should be performed at the time pregnancy is diagnosed. Any woman who is delivered of a stillbirth infant ≥20 wk of gestation should be tested for syphilis. In communities and populations with a high prevalence of syphilis, or for patients at high risk, testing should be performed at least two additional times, at the beginning of the third trimester (28 wk) and at delivery. Some states mandate repeat testing at delivery for all women. Women at high risk for syphilis should possibly be screened more frequently, either monthly or pragmatically because of inconsistent prenatal care, at every medical encounter because they may have repeat infections during pregnancy or reinfection late in pregnancy.

No newborn should leave the hospital without the maternal serologic status having been determined at least once during pregnancy. In states conducting newborn screening for syphilis, both the mother's and infant's serologic results should be known before discharge. Testing of the mother's serum is preferred to testing cord blood or the infant's serum because the titers are frequently lower in the infant and may be nonreactive if the mother was infected late in pregnancy.

Augenbraun M: The diagnosis and management of syphilis in the HIV-infected patient. *Curr Infect Dis Rep* 2000;2:10–13.

Azimi PH, Janner D, Berne P, et al: Concentrations of procaine and aqueous penicillin in the cerebrospinal fluid of infants treated for congenital syphilis. *J Pediatr* 1994;124:649–53.

Beck-Sague C, Alexander ER: Failure of benzathine penicillin G treatment in early congenital syphilis. *Pediatr Infect Dis J* 1987;6:1061–4.

Centers for Disease Control and Prevention: Sexually transmitted diseases treatment guidelines 2002. *MMWR Morb Mortal Wkly Rep* 2002;51(RR-6):1–80.

Centers for Disease Control: Congenital Syphilis—United States, 2000. *MMWR Morb Mortal Wkly Rep* 2001;50:573–7.

Centers for Disease Control and Prevention: *Sexually Transmitted Disease Surveillance, 2000.* Atlanta, GA: U.S. Department of Health and Human Services, Centers for Disease Control and Prevention, September 2001.

Moyer VA, Schneider V, Yetman R, et al: Contribution of long-bone radiographs to the management of congenital syphilis in the newborn infant. *Arch Pediatr Adolesc Med* 1998;152:353–7.

Musher DM: Syphilis, neurosyphilis, penicillin, and AIDS. *J Infect Dis* 1991;163: 1201–6.

Sison CG, Ostrea Jr EM, Reyes MP, et al: The resurgence of congenital syphilis. A cocaine-related problem. *J Pediatr* 1997;130:289–92.

Wicher K, Horowitz HW, Wicher V: Laboratory methods of diagnosis of syphilis for the beginning of the third millennium. *Microbes Infect* 1999;1:1035–49.

Zenker PN, Berman SM: Congenital syphilis. Trends and recommendations for evaluation and management. *Pediatr Infect Dis J* 1991;10:516–22.

Chapter 201
Nonvenereal Treponemal Infections *Parvin Azimi*

Several variants of nonvenereal or endemic treponematoses are recognized by their geographic distribution. These diseases, which include yaws, bejel (or endemic syphilis), and pinta, are caused by spirochetes belonging to the genus *Treponema* that are morphologically and immunologically identical to *T. pallidum* and extremely sensitive to penicillin. They cause diseases that are differentiated primarily on the basis of clinical findings. Yaws is the most common of the nonvenereal spirochetal diseases.

201.1 Yaws (*Treponema pertenue*)

Yaws is a chronic relapsing infection involving the skin and bony structures caused by the spirochete *T. pertenue*, which cannot be differentiated microscopically or serologically from *T. pallidum*. It is found in the warm, humid tropical regions of Africa, Asia, South America, and Oceania. Almost all cases occur in children. A high percentage of the population is infected in endemic areas.

T. pertenue cannot penetrate intact skin and is transmitted by direct contact from an infected lesion through a skin abrasion or laceration. Transmission is facilitated by overcrowding and poor personal hygiene. The initial papular lesion, the "mother yaw," occurs 2–8 wk after inoculation. The papule develops into a raised raspberry-like papilloma, which is often associated with regional lymphadenopathy. Secondary lesions erupt before or after the ulceration and healing of the mother yaw. With the healing of the mother yaw, there is hypopigmented scar formation. Secondary papillomas may appear anywhere and can be associated with lymphadenopathy, anorexia, and malaise. Ulcerated lesions are covered by exudates containing treponemes. Secondary lesions heal without scarring, but relapses are common within 5 yr after the primary lesion.

The lesions and exacerbations are often associated with bone pain and underlying periostitis or osteomyelitis, especially in the fingers, nose, and tibia. After the initial period of clinical activity, the patient enters a 5–10 yr period of latency. This is followed by the appearance of tertiary lesions at puberty, which are often solitary and destructive. These present as painful papillomas on the hands and feet, gummatous skin ulcerations, or osteitis. Bony destruction and deformity are common, as are juxta-articular nodules, depigmentation, and painful hyperkeratosis ("dry crab yaws") of the palms and soles.

Diagnosis depends on the clinical manifestations of the disease in an endemic area. Dark-field examination of cutaneous lesions and serologic tests for syphilis, both treponemal and nontreponemal, are confirmatory.

Treatment of patients and all contacts consists of a single dose of benzathine penicillin G (1.2 million U IM), which cures the lesions of active yaws, renders them noninfectious, and prevents relapse. Eradication of yaws from endemic foci may be accomplished by treating the entire population with penicillin. Patients allergic to penicillin may be treated with erythromycin or tetracycline.

201.2 Bejel (Endemic Syphilis) (*Treponema pallidum* subsp. *endemicum*)

Bejel, or endemic syphilis, affects children living in the Saharan regions of Africa and the Middle East. Infection with *T. pallidum* subsp. *endemicum* follows penetration of the spirochete through traumatized skin or mucous membranes. In experimental infections, a primary papule forms at the inoculation site after an incubation period of 3 wk; in human infections a primary lesion is almost never visualized.

The *clinical manifestations* of the secondary stage are confined to the skin and mucous membranes and consist of highly infectious mucous patches on the oral mucosa and condyloma-like lesions on the moist areas of the body, especially the axilla and anus. These mucocutaneous lesions resolve spontaneously over a period of several months, but recurrences are common. The secondary stage is followed by a variable latency period before the onset of late or tertiary bejel. The late complications, identical to those of yaws, include gumma formation in skin, subcutaneous tissue, and bone, resulting in painful destructive ulcerations, swelling, and deformity.

Diagnosis is suspected on epidemiologic and clinical grounds and is confirmed either by dark-field examination of cutaneous lesions or by serologic tests for syphilis, both treponemal and nontreponemal (Chapter 200).

Differentiation from venereal syphilis is extremely difficult in an endemic area. Bejel can be suspected by the absence of a primary chancre and lack of involvement of the central nervous system and cardiovascular system during the late stage.

Treatment of early injection consists of a single dose of benzathine penicillin G (1.2 million U IM); late infection is treated with 3 injections of the same dose at intervals of 7 days. Patients allergic to penicillin may be treated with erythromycin or tetracycline.

201.3 Pinta (*Treponema carateum*)

Pinta is a chronic, nonvenereally transmitted infection caused by *Treponema carateum*, a spirochete morphologically and serologically indistinguishable from other human treponemes. The disease is endemic in Mexico, Central America, South America, and parts of the West Indies. Infection follows direct inoculation of the treponeme through abraded skin. After a variable incubation period of days, a primary lesion appears at the inoculation site as a small asymptomatic erythematous papule resembling localized psoriasis or eczema. The regional lymph nodes are often enlarged, and spirochetes can be visualized on dark-field examination of skin scrapings or of the involved lymph nodes. After a period of enlargement, the primary lesion disappears. Secondary lesions follow within 6–8 mo and consist of small macules and papules on the face, scalp, and other exposed portions of the body. These pigmented lesions are scaly and nonpruritic and may coalesce to form large plaquelike elevations resembling psoriasis. In the late stage, atrophic and depigmented lesions develop on the hands, wrists, ankles, feet, face, and scalp. Hyperkeratosis of palms and soles is uncommon. *Diagnosis* is confirmed by dark-field examination of early lesions and a positive serologic test for syphilis. *Treatment* consists of a single dose of benzathine penicillin G (1.2 million U IM). Tetracycline and erythromycin are alternatives for patients allergic to penicillin.

Antal GM, Lukehart SA, Meheus AZ: The endemic treponematoses. *Microbes Infect* 2002;4:83–94.

Koff AB, Rosen T: Nonvenereal treponematoses: Yaws, endemic syphilis, and pinta. *J Am Acad Dermatol* 1993;29:519–35.

Chapter 202
Leptospira *Parvin Azimi*

Etiology. Leptospirosis is caused by spirochetes of the genus *Leptospira* and is the most widespread zoonosis in the world. The organisms are aerobic bacteria, 6–20 μm long and 0.1 μm wide with a terminal hook at one or both ends. They can be visualized by dark-field examination and by silver staining. Leptospires are cultured in liquid media; growth is slow on primary isolation and may require up to 13 weeks. Pathogenic leptospires have historically been classified as a single species, *Leptospira interrogans*, which includes more than 200 distinct serovars that have been useful for characterizing the epidemiology. Nonpathogenic leptospires were classified as *L. biflexa*, which has more than 60 serovars. More than 200 pathogenic serovars are recognized, making up the 23 serogroups. A single serovar may produce a variety of distinct syndromes, and a single clinical manifestation may be caused by multiple serotypes

Epidemiology. Leptospirosis is a zoonosis of worldwide distribution with most human cases in tropical and subtropical developing countries. Leptospires infect many species of domestic and feral animals, including pets and livestock, and have been isolated also from birds, fish, and reptiles. The rat is the principal source of human infection. Other important animal reservoirs include dogs, cats, livestock, and wild animals. Animal infection varies from inapparent to fatal. Once infected, animals excrete spirochetes in urine for an extended period of time. Leptospire survival outside the animal host is dependent on the moisture content, temperature, and pH of the soil or water into which they are shed. The majority of human cases worldwide result from occupational exposure to water or soil contaminated with rat urine. Occupational groups with a high incidence of leptospirosis include agricultural workers, veterinarians, abattoir workers, meat inspectors, rodent control workers, laboratory workers, and workers in other occupations that require contact with animals. In the United States, the major animal reservoir is the dog, and contact with spirochetes is often associated with recreational activities that result in contact with contaminated soil or water during the summer months. Transmission via contaminated water, animal bites, and directly from person-to-person, which is rare, has been reported.

Pathogenesis. Leptospires enter humans through abrasions and cuts in the skin or through mucous membranes. After penetration, leptospires circulate in the bloodstream and spread to all organs of the body. The primary lesion caused by leptospires is damage to the endothelial lining of small blood vessels with resultant ischemic damage to the liver, kidneys, meninges, and muscles.

Clinical Manifestations. The spectrum of human leptospirosis ranges from asymptomatic infection to a severe syndrome of multiorgan dysfunction with high mortality. The clinical presentation is biphasic. After an incubation period of 7–12 days, the initial or **septicemic phase** begins in which leptospires can be isolated from the blood, cerebrospinal fluid (CSF), and other tissues. Initial symptoms, which last 2–7 days, may be followed by a brief period of well-being and the second symptomatic or **immune phase**. The immune phase is associated with the appearance of circulating antibody, the disappearance of organisms from the blood and CSF, and the appearance of additional signs and symptoms associated with localization of leptospires in the tissues. Despite the presence of circulating antibody, leptospires may persist in the kidney, urine, and aqueous humor. The immune or leptospiruric phase may last for several weeks.

Most cases of human leptospirosis are subclinical or very mild, with inapparent infection particularly common in high-risk occupational groups such as farmers and their families. Symptomatic infection may present as an acute febrile illness with nonspecific signs and symptoms (70%), as aseptic meningitis (20%), or as hepatorenal dysfunction (10%). The onset is typically sudden, and the illness tends to follow a biphasic course (Fig. 202–1).

ANICTERIC LEPTOSPIROSIS. The onset of the septicemic phase is abrupt, with fever, shaking chills, lethargy, severe headache, malaise, nausea, vomiting, and severe, often debilitating myalgia. Some patients have bradycardia and hypotension but circulatory collapse is uncommon. Additional physical findings include extreme muscle tenderness, which is most prominent in the lower extremities, the lumbosacral spine, and the abdomen. Conjunctival suffusion with photophobia and orbital pain (in the absence of chemosis and purulent exudate), generalized lymphadenopathy, and hepatosplenomegaly may also be present. A transient rash, lasting <24 hr, may occur in 10% of cases, and usually consists of a truncal erythematous maculopapular rash but may be urticarial, petechial, purpuric, or desquamating. Less common manifestations include pharyngitis, pneumonitis, arthritis, carditis, cholecystitis, and orchitis. The second or immune phase may follow a brief asymptomatic interlude and is characterized by recurrence of fever and aseptic meningitis. Despite abnormal CSF profiles in 80% of infected children, only 50% have meningeal manifestations. CSF abnormalities include a modest elevation in pressure, a pleocytosis with polymorphonuclear leukocytes initially followed by mononuclear predominance and rarely exceeding 500 cells/mm³, normal or slightly elevated protein levels, and normal glucose values. Encephalitis, cranial and peripheral neuropathies, papilledema, and paralysis are uncommon. Uveitis may occur during this phase; it can be unilateral or bilateral and is usually self-limited, rarely resulting in permanent visual impairment. Symptoms referable to the central nervous system resolve spontaneously within about 1 wk, with almost no mortality.

ICTERIC LEPTOSPIROSIS (WEIL SYNDROME). This severe form of leptospirosis occurs in <10% of cases and is less common in children and more common in persons older than 30 yr of age. The initial manifestations are similar to those described for anicteric leptospirosis. The immune phase, however, is distinctive, being characterized by clinical and laboratory evidence of hepatic and renal dysfunction. In fulminating cases, hemorrhagic phenomena and cardiovascular collapse also occur. Hepatic abnor-malities include right upper quadrant pain, hepatomegaly, direct and indirect hyperbilirubinemia, and modestly elevated serum levels of hepatic enzymes. The jaundice is not the result of hepatocellular necrosis, and liver function usually returns to normal after recovery. Renal manifestations are common; all patients have abnormal findings on urinalysis (hematuria, proteinuria, and casts), and azotemia is common, often associated with oliguria or anuria. Acute renal failure occurs in 16–40% of cases and is the principal cause of death. Abnormal electrocardiograms are present in 90% of cases, but congestive heart failure is uncommon. Hemorrhagic manifestations are rare but when present may include epistaxis, hemoptysis, and gastrointestinal and adrenal hemorrhage. Thrombocytopenia occurs in >50% of cases, but is transient and does not result from disseminated intravascular coagulation. Mortality is 5–15%.

Diagnosis. Leptospirosis should be considered in the differential diagnosis of any acute febrile illness when there is a history of direct contact with animals or with soil or water contaminated with animal urine, and especially when the onset is abrupt with chills, fever, severe myalgias, conjunctival suffusion, headache, nausea, and vomiting.

The diagnosis is established most often by serologic testing, and less frequently by isolation of the infecting organism from clinical specimens. Serologic tests for *Leptospira* include genus-specific and serogroup-specific tests. The reference method is the **microscopic agglutination test**, which is a serogroup-specific assay using live antigen suspensions of leptospiral serovars. The test is read by dark-field microscopy for agglutination, and titers are determined. This test requires live cultures of all serovars for use as antigens. A fourfold or greater increase in titer in paired sera confirms the diagnosis. Agglutinins usually appear by the 12th day of illness and reach a maximum titer by the 3rd wk. Low titers may persist for years. Approximately 10% of infected persons do not have detectable agglutinins, presumably because available antisera do not identify all *Leptospira* serotypes. An adaptation of the agglutination test is the use of antigens from killed or formalinized organisms; titer results are slightly lower and more cross-reactions occur. Enzyme-linked immunosorbent assay (ELISA) methods, including an IgM-specific dot-ELISA test, have also been developed.

Warthin-Starry silver staining and immunofluorescent and immunohistochemical methods permit identification of leptospires in infected tissue or body fluids. Spirochetes may also be demonstrated by phase-contrast or dark-field microscopy, but these are insensitive.

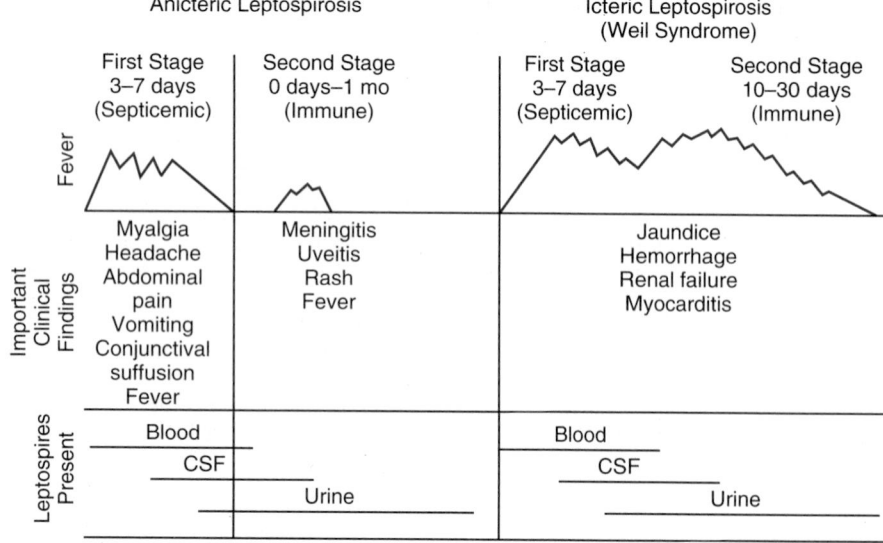

FIGURE 202–1. Stages of anicteric and icteric leptospirosis. Correlation between clinical findings and presence of leptospires in body fluids. (Reprinted with permission from Feigin RD, Anderson DC: Human leptospirosis. *CRC Crit Rev Clin Lab Sci* 1975;5: 413–67. Copyright CRC Press, Inc., Boca Raton, FL.)

Unlike other pathogenic spirochetes, leptospires are easily cultured on commercially available media containing rabbit serum or bovine serum albumin and long-chain fatty acids. Repeated blood cultures in the 1st wk of infection with very small inocula of blood are recommended. A small inoculum (i.e., one drop of blood in 5 mL of medium) is used to minimize growth inhibitory factors. Leptospires can be recovered from the blood or CSF during the first 10 days of illness and from urine after the 2nd wk. The number of leptospires in clinical specimens is small and their growth rate is slow; leptospires may be seen in several days, although cultures may not become positive for 2–4 mo. Prolonged incubation is required.

Treatment. Despite the in vitro sensitivity of *Leptospira* to penicillin and tetracycline and the efficacy of these agents in treating experimental infection, their effectiveness in human leptospirosis remains controversial. It appears that initiation of treatment before the 7th day will probably shorten the clinical course and decrease the severity of the infection, and therefore treatment with penicillin or tetracycline (in children 9 yr of age or older) should be instituted as soon as the diagnosis is suspected. Parenteral penicillin G (6–8 million $U/m^2/24$ hr divided q 4 hr IV for 7 days) is recommended, with tetracycline (10–20 mg/kg/24 hr divided q 6 hr PO or IV for 7 days) as an alternative for patients allergic to penicillin.

Prevention. Prevention of human leptospirosis is facilitated by instituting rodent control measures and avoiding contaminated water and soil. Immunization of livestock and family pets has been recommended as a means of eliminating animal reservoirs, but these programs have met with limited success. A formalin-killed polyvalent human vaccine has been used in "at risk" occupation groups in Europe and Asia; however, there have been no clinical trials to determine its efficacy. Leptospirosis has been prevented in American servicemen stationed in the tropics by administering doxycycline (200 mg PO once a week) as prophylaxis. This schedule may be similarly effective for the traveler entering a highly endemic area for a limited period of time.

Farr RW: Leptospirosis. *Clin Infect Dis* 1995;21:1–8.

Heath CW Jr, Alexander AD, Galton MM: Leptospirosis in the United States. Analysis of 483 cases in man, 1949–1961. *N Engl J Med* 1965;273:857–64.

Jackson LA, Kaufmann AF, Adams WG, et al: Outbreak of leptospirosis associated with swimming. *Pediatr Infect Dis J* 1993;12:48–54.

Levett PN: Leptospirosis. *Clin Microbiol Rev* 2001;14:296–326.

Takafnji ET, Kirkpatrick JW, Miller RN, et al: An efficacy trial of doxycycline chemoprophylaxis against leptospirosis. *N Engl J Med* 1984;310:497–500.

Vinetz JM, Glass GE, Flexner CE, et al: Sporadic urban leptospirosis. *Ann Intern Med* 1996;125:794–8.

Watt G, Alquiza LM, Padre LP, et al: The rapid diagnosis of leptospirosis. A prospective comparison of the dot enzyme-linked immunosorbent assay and the genus-specific microscopic agglutination test at different stages of illness. *J Infect Dis* 1988;157:840–2.

Wong ML, Kaplan S, Dunkle LM, et al: Leptospirosis: A childhood disease. *J Pediatr* 1977;90:532–7.

Chapter 203
Relapsing Fever (*Borrelia*)

Parvin Azimi

Etiology. Relapsing fever is an uncommon arthropod-borne infection characterized by recurrent episodes of fever. It is caused by spirochetes of the genus *Borrelia*, a fastidious microorganism with worldwide distribution that is transmitted to humans by lice or ticks.

Epidemic relapsing fever, or **louse-borne fever**, is caused by *B. recurrentis* and is transmitted from person to person by *Pediculus humanus*, the human body louse. After ingestion of an infective blood meal by the louse, the spirochetes penetrate its midgut, migrate to and multiply within the hemolymph, and remain viable throughout its lifespan (several weeks). Human infection occurs as a result of crushing lice during scratching, allowing infected hemolymph to enter through the abraded skin.

Endemic relapsing fever, or **tick-borne fever**, is caused by several species of *Borrelia* and is transmitted to humans by *Ornithodoros* ticks. *B. hermsii* is the common species in the western United States, and *B. dugesi* is the major cause of disease in Mexico and Central America. After ingestion of an infective blood meal, spirochetes invade all tissues of their arthropod hosts, including the salivary glands and reproductive tract. The latter permits transovarian passage of infected spirochetes, perpetuating arthropod infection in successive generations. Human infection occurs when saliva, coxal fluid, or excrement is released by the tick during feeding, thereby permitting spirochetes to penetrate the skin and mucous membranes.

Epidemiology. Louse-borne epidemic relapsing fever tends to occur in epidemics, often in association with typhus. Epidemics are associated with war, poverty, famine, and poor personal hygiene. This form of relapsing fever occurs more commonly during the winter. The major endemic focus of the disease is the highlands of Ethiopia.

Ornithodoros ticks, which transmit endemic relapsing fever, are distributed worldwide, including the western United States, prefer warm, humid environments and high altitudes, and are found in rodent burrows, caves, and other nesting sites. Rodents are the principal reservoirs. Infected ticks gain access to human dwellings on the rodent host. Human contact is often unnoticed because these soft ticks, unlike the hard ticks, which attach and feed over a period of days, are nocturnal feeders, have a painless bite, and detach immediately after a short blood meal.

Pathogenesis. The cyclic nature of relapsing fever is explained by the ability of *Borrelia* organisms to continually undergo antigenic (phase) variation. Multiple variants evolve simultaneously during the first relapse, with one type becoming predominant. Spirochetes isolated during the primary febrile episode differ antigenically from those recovered during a subsequent relapse. During febrile episodes, spirochetes enter the bloodstream, induce the development of specific IgM and IgG antibody, and undergo agglutination, immobilization, lysis, and phagocytosis. During remission, *Borrelia* spirochetes may remain in the bloodstream, but spirochetemia is insufficient to produce symptoms. The number of relapses in untreated patients depends on the number of antigenic variants of the infecting strain.

Clinical Manifestations. Relapsing fever is characterized by periods of fever lasting 2–9 days, separated by afebrile periods of 2–7 days. Louse-borne disease has a longer incubation period, longer periods of pyrexia, fewer relapses, and longer remission periods than tick-borne disease. The incubation period of tick-borne disease is usually 8 days, with a range of 5–15 days. Each form of relapsing fever is associated with sudden onset of high fever, lethargy, headache, photophobia, nausea, vomiting, myalgia, and arthralgia. Additional symptoms may appear later and include abdominal pain, a productive cough, and mild respiratory distress. Bleeding manifestations are common and include epistaxis, hemoptysis, hematuria, and hematemesis. A diffuse, erythematous, macular, or petechial rash may develop over the trunk and shoulders. This rash is more common in louse-borne fever (25%), is of 1–2 days' duration, and occurs almost exclusively during the end of the primary febrile episode. There may also be lymphadenopathy, pneumonia, and splenomegaly. Hepatic tenderness associated with hepatomegaly is a common sign, with jaundice in half of affected children. Central nervous system manifestations may be the principal feature of late relapses in tick-borne disease; they include lethargy, stupor, meningismus, convulsions, peripheral neuritis, focal neurologic deficits, and cranial nerve paralysis. Severe manifestations include myocarditis, hepatic failure, and disseminated intravascular coagulopathy.

The initial symptomatic period characteristically ends with a crisis in 2–9 days, marked by abrupt diaphoresis, hypothermia, hypotension, bradycardia, profound muscle weakness, and prostration. In untreated patients, the first relapse occurs within 1 wk, followed by usually 3 but up to 10 relapses with symptoms during each relapse becoming milder and shorter as the afebrile remission period lengthens.

Diagnosis. Diagnosis depends on demonstration of spirochetes in thin or thick blood smears stained with Giemsa or Wright's stain. During afebrile remissions, spirochetes are not found in the blood. Serologic tests, such as enzyme immunoassay and Western blotting, are not standardized and generally not available. Tick-borne disease produces a serologic cross reaction with other spirochetes, including *Borrelia burgdorferi*, the agent of Lyme disease.

Treatment. Oral or parenteral tetracycline is the drug of choice for louse-borne and tick-borne relapsing fever. For older children and young adults, tetracycline (500 mg PO q 6 hr) for 10 days has been effective. Single-dose treatment with tetracycline (500 mg PO) or erythromycin is efficacious in adults, but experience in children is limited. In children younger than 12 yr of age, erythromycin (50 mg/kg/24 hr divided q 6 hr PO) for a total of 10 days is recommended. Penicillin and chloramphenicol are also effective.

Resolution of each febrile episode either by natural crisis or as a result of antimicrobial treatment is usually accompanied within 2 hr by the Jarisch-Herxheimer reaction, which is associated with clearing of the spirochetemia. Attempts to control this reaction by prior treatment with corticosteroids or antipyretics have met with limited success.

Prognosis. With adequate therapy, the mortality rate for relapsing fever is <5%. A majority of patients recover from their illness with or without treatment after the appearance of anti-*Borrelia* antibodies, which agglutinate, kill, or opsonize the spirochete.

Prevention. No vaccine is available. Disease control requires avoidance or elimination of the arthropod vectors. In epidemics of louse-borne disease, dissemination can be prevented by good personal hygiene and delousing of persons, dwellings, and clothing with commercially available insecticides. The risk of tick-borne disease can be minimized in endemic areas by maintaining rodent-free dwellings.

Butler TC: Relapsing fever: New lessons about antibiotic action. *Ann Intern Med* 1985;102:397–9.

Butler TC, Jones PK, Wallace CK: *Borrelia recurrentis* infection. Single dose antibiotic regimens and management of Jarisch-Herxheimer reaction. *J Infect Dis* 1978;137:573–7.

Perine PL, Teklu B: Antibiotic treatment of louse-borne relapsing fever in Ethiopia: A report of 377 cases. *Am J Trop Med Hyg* 1983;32:1096–100.

Stoennerita DT, Dodd T, Larcen C: Antigenic variation in *Borrelia hermsii. J Exp Med* 1982;156:1297–311.

Chapter 204
Lyme Disease (*Borrelia burgdorferi*) *Eugene D. Shapiro*

Lyme disease is the most common vector-borne disease in the United States. Although Lyme disease is a public health concern, extensive publicity as well as a very high frequency of misdiagnoses have resulted in a degree of anxiety about Lyme disease that is out of proportion to the actual morbidity that it causes.

Etiology. Lyme disease is caused by the spirochete *Borrelia burgdorferi*, a fastidious, microaerophilic bacterium that replicates very slowly and requires special media for in vitro growth. *B. burgdorferi* is cylindrically shaped with a cell membrane that is covered by flagella and a loosely associated outer membrane. The three major outer-surface proteins—OspA, OspB, and OspC (which are highly charged basic proteins of molecular weights of about 31, 34, and 23 kd, respectively)—as well as the 41 kd flagellar protein, are important targets for the immune response. Differences in the molecular structure of *B. burgdorferi* strains, especially between isolates from Europe and the United States, are well documented. Clinical manifestations of Lyme borreliosis in Europe and in the United States, such as the greater frequency of radiculoneuritis in Europe, may be attributable to these differences.

Epidemiology. Lyme disease has been reported from more than 50 countries. In 2000, there were 17,730 cases reported in the United States, with most cases in southern New England, the eastern parts of the Middle Atlantic states, and the upper Midwest, with a smaller endemic focus of Lyme disease along the Pacific coast (Fig. 204–1). In Europe, most cases occur in the

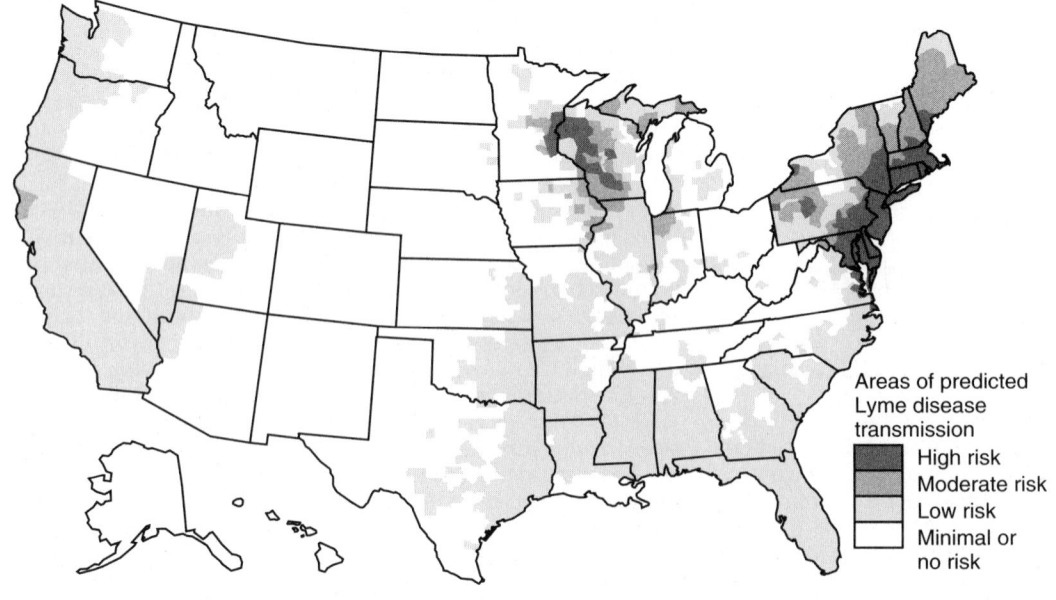

Areas of predicted
Lyme disease
transmission

■ High risk
■ Moderate risk
□ Low risk
□ Minimal or
no risk

FIGURE 204–1. The approximate distribution of predicted risk for Lyme disease in the United States. The risk varies by the distribution of *Ixodes scapularis* and *I. pacificus*, the proportion of infected ticks for each species at each stage of the tick's life cycle, and the presence of grassy or wooded locations favored by white-tailed deer. (Figure from the Centers for Disease Control and Prevention.)

Scandinavian countries and in central Europe, especially Germany, Austria, and Switzerland. Estimates of the incidence of Lyme disease are complicated by passive systems for reporting of Lyme disease and the high frequency of misdiagnosis of this illness. In endemic areas, the reported annual incidence ranges from 20–100 cases/100,000 population, although this figure may be as high as 1,000 cases/100,000 population in hyperendemic areas such as Lyme, Connecticut. The reported incidence is highest among children 5–10 yr of age, which is almost twice as high as the incidence among older children and adults.

TRANSMISSION. Lyme disease is a zoonosis caused by the transmission of *B. burgdorferi* to humans through the bite of an infected tick of the *Ixodes* species. In the eastern and midwestern United States, the vector is *Ixodes scapularis* (formerly known as *Ixodes dammini*), the black-legged tick that is commonly known as the deer tick, which is responsible for most cases of Lyme disease in the United States. The vector on the Pacific Coast is *Ixodes pacificus*, the western black-legged tick. *Ixodes* ticks have a 2-yr, three-stage life cycle. The larvae hatch in the early summer and are usually uninfected with *B. burgdorferi*. The tick may become infected at any stage of its life cycle by feeding on a host, usually a small mammal such as the white-footed mouse (*Peromyscus leucopus*), which is a natural reservoir for *B. burgdorferi*. The larvae overwinter and emerge the following spring in the nymphal stage, which is the stage of the tick that is most likely to transmit the infection. The nymphs molt to adults in the fall. The females lay their eggs the following spring before they die, and the 2-yr life cycle begins again.

Several factors are associated with increased risk of transmission of *B. burgdorferi* from ticks to humans. The proportion of infected ticks varies by geographic area and for each stage of the tick's life cycle. In endemic areas in the northeastern and midwestern United States, 15–20% of nymphal ticks and 35–40% of the adult ticks are infected with *B. burgdorferi*. There are small foci in which the rate of infection of adult deer ticks is 60–80% or even higher. By contrast, *Ixodes pacificus* often feeds on lizards, which are not a competent reservoir for *B. burgdorferi*. Only 1–3% of these ticks, even in the nymphal and adult stages, are infected with *B. burgdorferi*. The risk of transmission of *B. burgdorferi* from infected *Ixodes* ticks is related to the duration of feeding. It takes hours for the mouthparts of ticks to implant fully in the host and much longer (days) for the tick to become fully engorged. Experiments in animals have shown that infected nymphal ticks must feed for ≥36–48 hr, and infected adults must feed for ≥48–72 hr, before the risk of transmission of *B. burgdorferi* becomes substantial. Most individuals who are bitten by a tick will recognize and remove the tick before the transmission of *B. burgdorferi* can occur. Persons with increased occupational, recreational, or residential exposure to tick-infested woods or fields (the preferred habitat of ticks) in endemic areas are at increased risk of developing Lyme disease.

Pathogenesis. The skin is the initial target of infection by *B. burgdorferi*. Inflammation induced by *B. burgdorferi* leads to the development of the characteristic rash, erythema migrans. Early disseminated Lyme disease is caused by the spread of spirochetes, through the bloodstream, to tissues throughout the body. The spirochete adheres to the surfaces of a wide variety of different types of cells, which may be responsible for the involvement of many organs. Because the organism may persist in tissues for prolonged periods of time, symptoms may appear very late after initial infection.

The symptoms of early disseminated as well as of late Lyme disease are due to inflammation mediated by interleukin-1 and other lymphokines in response to the presence of the organism. It is likely that relatively few organisms actually invade the host, but cytokines serve to amplify the inflammatory response and lead to much of the tissue damage. The refractory symptoms of late Lyme disease may have an immunogenetic basis. Patients with the HLA-DR2, DR3, and DR4 allotypes may be genetically predisposed to develop chronic recurrent Lyme arthritis. These class II histocompatibility molecules located on macrophages and B cells are involved in the presentation of antigens to T-helper cells that initiate the immune response. Although rare (especially in children), in genetically susceptible individuals, *B. burgdorferi* may initiate an autoimmune response that causes persistent inflammation of the synovium and clinical symptoms long after the bacteria have been killed.

Histologically, Lyme disease is characterized by inflammatory lesions that contain both T and B lymphocytes, macrophages, plasma cells, and some mast cells. The erythema migrans rash consists of a moderately dense infiltrate of lymphocytes, plasma cells, and occasional macrophages, located around the small blood vessels of the upper dermis. Lyme myocarditis is a transmural myocarditis with widespread interstitial lymphocytic and plasma cell infiltrate. Similar infiltrates have been seen in the meninges and cerebral cortex. There are few reports of the histology of synovial tissue during the acute stages of Lyme arthritis. At this stage of the illness, the synovial fluid often has a marked predominance of polymorphonuclear cells, suggesting that the synovial tissue also will have a polymorphonuclear inflammatory infiltrate. By contrast, chronic, recurrent arthritis is characterized by a chronic hypertrophic synovitis. This nonspecific abnormality, also found in other disorders such as rheumatoid arthritis, is marked by hyperplasia of the synovial cells with varying degrees of lymphocytic infiltrates that sometimes form abortive germinal centers and follicles. Plasma cells are present at the periphery of the lymphoid aggregates. In advanced disease, neovascularization (a nonspecific response to chronic inflammation) may occur.

Clinical Manifestations. The clinical manifestations of Lyme disease are divided into early and late stages. Early Lyme disease is further classified as early localized or early disseminated disease. Untreated patients may progressively develop clinical symptoms of each stage of the disease, or they may present with early disseminated or with late disease without apparently having had any symptoms of the earlier stages of Lyme disease.

EARLY LOCALIZED DISEASE. The first clinical manifestation of Lyme disease is the typical annular rash, named **erythema migrans**. Although it usually occurs 7–14 days after the bite, the onset of the rash has been reported from 3–32 days later. The initial lesion occurs at the site of the bite. The rash may be uniformly erythematous, or it may appear as a target lesion with central clearing; rarely, there may be central vesicular or necrotic areas. Occasionally the rash may be itchy or painful. The lesion can occur anywhere on the body, although the most common locations are the axilla, the periumbilical area, the thigh, and the groin. Erythema migrans may be associated with systemic features including fever, myalgia, headache, or malaise. Without treatment, the rash gradually expands (hence the name *migrans*) to an average diameter of 15 cm and remains present for at least 1–2 wk.

EARLY DISSEMINATED DISEASE. In the United States, a substantial proportion (about 20%) of patients with acute *B. burgdorferi* infection develop secondary erythema migrans lesions, a common manifestation of early disseminated Lyme disease caused by hematogenous spread of the organisms to multiple skin sites. The secondary lesions, which may develop several days or even weeks after the first lesion, usually are smaller than the primary lesion and are often accompanied by fever, myalgia, headache, and malaise; conjunctivitis and lymphadenopathy also may develop. Occasionally, when the erythema migrans rash resolves, new evanescent lesions, which usually are small (1–3 cm), erythematous annular lesions that do not expand, continue to appear for several weeks. Other manifestations may include aseptic meningitis, with signs of meningeal irritation such as nuchal rigidity (and associated with papilledema in about 25–35% of cases); uveitis; focal neurologic findings, especially cranioneuropathies; and, rarely, carditis, with varying degrees of heart block. Paralysis of the facial (7th) cranial nerve is relatively common in children and may be the initial or the only manifestation of Lyme disease. The paralysis usually lasts 2–8 wk and resolves completely in most cases. There is no evidence that the clinical course of the facial palsy is affected by antimicrobial treatment.

LATE DISEASE. Arthritis, beginning weeks to months after the initial infection, is the usual manifestation of late Lyme disease. Arthritis typically involves the large joints, especially the knee, which is affected in >90% of cases, but any joint may be affected. The joint is swollen and tender but patients usually do not experience the exquisite pain that is typical of bacterial arthritis. Although it may last for several weeks, the joint swelling usually resolves within 1–2 wk before recurring, often in other joints. If the disease is not treated, the episodes of arthritis may increase in duration, sometimes lasting for months; but in most cases the disease eventually resolves, even in patients who are untreated and who have had many recurrences of arthritis.

Late manifestations of Lyme disease involving the central nervous system, sometimes termed **tertiary neuroborreliosis**, are rarely reported in children. In adults, chronic demyelinating encephalitis, polyneuritis, and impairment of memory have been attributed to Lyme disease.

CONGENITAL LYME DISEASE. Although *B. burgdorferi* has been identified from several abortuses and from a few liveborn children with congenital anomalies, the placentas and the abortuses in which the spirochete was identified usually did not show histologic evidence of inflammation. No consistent pattern of fetal damage has been identified to suggest a clinical syndrome of congenital infection. Furthermore, studies conducted in endemic areas have indicated that there is no difference in the prevalence of congenital malformations among the offspring of women with serum antibodies against *B. burgdorferi* and the offspring of those without such antibodies. A survey of child neurologists in endemic areas found that none had seen a credible case of a child with congenital Lyme disease. If congenital Lyme disease does exist, it must be extremely rare.

Diagnosis. The clinical manifestations of Lyme disease, other than erythema migrans, are not specific. The monoarticular or pauciarticular arthritis may mimic either an acute septic joint or other causes of arthritis in children, such as juvenile rheumatoid arthritis or rheumatic fever. Clinically, 7th nerve palsy due to Lyme disease is indistinguishable from idiopathic Bell palsy, and Lyme meningitis may mimic enteroviral meningitis. The diagnosis of erythema migrans may be difficult because the rash initially may be confused with nummular eczema, tinea, granuloma annulare, an insect bite, or cellulitis. However, the relatively rapid expansion of erythema migrans helps distinguish it from these other conditions.

Although attempts have been made to develop antigen-based diagnostic tests, including the polymerase chain reaction, all of these tests are experimental. None of the tests for *B. burgdorferi* antigens that have been adequately evaluated are sufficiently sensitive and specific to be clinically useful. Consequently, the confirmation of Lyme disease usually is based on the demonstration of antibodies to *B. burgdorferi* in the patient's serum.

SEROLOGY. Specific IgM antibodies appear first, usually at 3–4 wk, peak at 6–8 wk, and subsequently decline, although a prolonged elevation of IgM antibodies sometimes occurs despite effective antimicrobial treatment. Consequently, the results of tests for specific IgM antibodies should not be used as an indicator of either active or recent infection. Specific IgG antibodies usually appear at 6–8 wk, peak after 4–6 mo, and may remain elevated indefinitely. The antibody response to *B. burgdorferi* may be abrogated in patients with early Lyme disease who are treated promptly with an effective antimicrobial agent, but in most patients IgG antibodies remain detectable for many years after treatment and clinical resolution of the illness.

Because the immunofluorescent antibody test requires subjective interpretation and is time consuming to perform, it has been replaced by enzyme-linked immunosorbent assays (ELISA) for the detection of antibodies against *B. burgdorferi*. The ELISA method sometimes produces false-positive results because of cross-reactive antibodies to other spirochetal infections (e.g., syphilis, leptospirosis, or relapsing fever), to certain viral infections (e.g., varicella), against spirochetes that comprise part of the normal oral flora, and with certain autoimmune diseases (e.g., systemic lupus erythematosus).

Western blotting (i.e., immunoblotting) is also used as a diagnostic test for Lyme disease, although there is still some debate about its interpretation. For example, many people who do not have Lyme disease have antibodies against the 41-kd protein (the flagellar protein) of *B. burgdorferi*. Official recommendations for serologic tests for Lyme disease are to perform a quantitative test (such as ELISA) and a confirmatory Western immunoblot test if the ELISA result is either positive or equivocal.

The currently available serologic tests, especially widely used commercial kits, generally have only fair specificity. Use of these commercial diagnostic serologic tests will result in a high rate of misdiagnosis. In contrast, the serologic tests for Lyme disease performed by reference laboratories are relatively accurate. However, even with these tests, the predictive value of the result still depends primarily on the probability that the patient has Lyme disease based on the clinical and epidemiologic history and the physical examination (the "pretest probability"). With few exceptions, the pretest probability that a patient has Lyme disease will be very low in areas in which Lyme disease is rare. Even in areas with a high prevalence of Lyme disease, patients with *only* nonspecific signs and symptoms, such as fatigue, headache, or arthralgia, are not likely to have Lyme disease; virtually all positive serologic test results in such patients are false-positive results. Consequently, serologic tests for Lyme disease should not be ordered in such patients. Serologic tests for Lyme disease should only be obtained for patients with a relatively high (≥20%) probability of having Lyme disease—that is, only in patients who have objective physical signs that are suggestive of Lyme disease, in whom the predictive value of a positive test result is high.

Even though a symptomatic patient has antibodies to *B. burgdorferi*, Lyme disease may not be the cause of the patient's symptoms. The test result may be falsely positive, or the patient may have been infected previously. Once serum antibodies to *B. burgdorferi* develop, they may persist for many years despite adequate treatment and clinical cure of the disease. Because some people who become infected with *B. burgdorferi* are asymptomatic, the background rate of seropositivity among patients who have never had clinically apparent Lyme disease may be substantial in endemic areas.

CULTURE. The isolation of *B. burgdorferi* from a symptomatic patient is considered diagnostic of Lyme disease. Although *B. burgdorferi* has been isolated from blood, skin, cerebrospinal fluid (CSF), myocardium, and the synovium of patients with Lyme disease, the medium in which *B. burgdorferi* is cultured is expensive, it can take as long as 4 wk for the bacteria to grow in culture, and the frequency of isolation of *B. burgdorferi* from patients with active Lyme disease is low. It usually is necessary for patients to undergo an invasive procedure, such as a skin biopsy or a lumbar puncture, to obtain appropriate tissue or fluid for culture. *B. burgdorferi* has been identified with silver stains (Warthin-Starry or modified Dieterle) and with immunohistochemical stains (using monoclonal or polyclonal antibodies) in skin, synovial, and myocardial biopsy specimens. However, *B. burgdorferi* can be confused with normal tissue structures or it can be missed because it usually is present in low concentrations.

LABORATORY FINDINGS. Routine laboratory tests rarely are helpful in diagnosing Lyme disease because the associated laboratory abnormalities usually are nonspecific. The peripheral white blood cell count may be either normal or elevated. The erythrocyte sedimentation rate usually is elevated. The white blood cell concentration in joint fluid may range from 25,000–125,000/mL, often with a preponderance of polymorphonuclear cells. When the central nervous system is involved, there usually is a mild pleocytosis with a lymphocytic predominance. The CSF protein level may be elevated, but the glucose concentration usually is normal.

Treatment. No clinical trials of treatment for Lyme disease have been conducted in children. Recommendations for the treatment of children (Box 204–1) are extrapolated from studies of adults. Children younger than 8 yr of age should not be treated with doxycycline because it may cause permanent discoloration of their teeth. Patients who are treated with doxycycline should be alerted to the risk of developing dermatitis in sun-exposed areas while taking the medication. Cefuroxime is also licensed for the treatment of Lyme disease and is an alternative for persons who cannot take doxycycline and who are allergic to penicillin. Preliminary results with azithromycin have been disappointing. There is little need to use newer agents because the results of treatment with either amoxicillin or doxycycline have been good.

Some patients may develop a Jarisch-Herxheimer reaction soon after treatment is initiated. The manifestations of this reaction are increased temperature, sweats, and myalgia. These symptoms resolve spontaneously within 24–48 hr, although administration of nonsteroidal anti-inflammatory drugs often is beneficial. Nonsteroidal anti-inflammatory agents also may be useful in treating symptoms of early Lyme disease and of Lyme arthritis.

Fatigue, arthralgia, and myalgia, which may accompany or follow more specific symptoms and signs of Lyme disease but almost never are the sole presenting manifestations of Lyme disease, sometimes persist after treatment but generally resolve over a period of weeks to months. There is little evidence that these symptoms are related to persistence of the organism. Because antibodies against *B. burgdorferi* persist after successful treatment, there is no reason to obtain follow-up serologic tests. There is also no evidence that either repeated or prolonged courses of antimicrobial agents hasten the resolution of such symptoms. Indeed, a National Institutes of Health–sponsored double-blind, randomized, placebo-controlled clinical trial of long-term antibiotic treatment (1 mo of ceftriaxone followed by 2 mo of doxycycline) of patients with "chronic" Lyme disease was discontinued before full enrollment was reached, concluding that long-term treatment with antibiotics was no more effective than placebo. After reviewing the preliminary data, the data monitoring board concluded that the chance of finding a statistically significant difference in the outcomes of patients in the treatment group vs. the placebo group was virtually nil, even if full enrollment was reached.

Prognosis. There is a widespread misconception that Lyme disease is difficult to treat successfully and that chronic symptoms and clinical recurrences are common. In fact, the most common reason for apparent treatment failure is misdiagnosis in patients who do not have Lyme disease. The impression that Lyme disease requires prolonged treatment, including intravenous antimicrobial therapy, and that treatment is often unsuccessful can be attributed to the treatment of patients whose symptoms were not due to Lyme disease.

The prognosis for children treated for Lyme disease is excellent. Cases in children treated for erythema migrans rarely progress to late Lyme disease. The long-term prognosis for patients who are treated beginning in the late phase of Lyme disease also is excellent. Although recurrences of arthritis do occur rarely, especially among patients with the DR2, DR3, or DR4 HLA allotypes (an autoimmune process), most children who are treated for Lyme arthritis are permanently cured. Although there are rare reports of adults who have developed late neuroborreliosis after being treated for Lyme disease, no similar cases have been documented in children.

Prevention. Children in endemic areas are often bitten by deer ticks, but the overall risk of acquiring Lyme disease is low (1–3%), even in these areas. Even if the patient is bitten by a nymphal stage deer tick infected with *B. burgdorferi*, the risk of acquiring Lyme disease is only 8–10%. If infection develops, treatment of the infection is highly effective. A recent study of prophylaxis among persons 12 yr of age and older found that a single dose of doxycycline (200 mg PO) was 87% effective in preventing Lyme disease (although the lower bound of the 95% confidence interval for this estimate was only 25%). Because most people who recognize a deer tick bite remove the tick within 48 hours (before the tick can transmit Lyme disease), the overall risk of Lyme disease after a recognized bite is low and administration of antimicrobial prophylaxis is not recommended routinely. The routine testing of ticks that have been removed from humans for infection with *B. burgdorferi* also is not recommended because the predictive value of a positive test result (in the tick) for infection in the human host is unknown.

The most reasonable approach to preventing Lyme disease is to wear appropriate protective clothing when entering tick-infested areas and to check for and remove ticks after spending time in such areas. Insect repellents may provide temporary protection, but they may be absorbed from the skin and, if used frequently or in large doses, they may produce significant toxicity, especially in children.

VACCINE. A Lyme vaccine composed of recombinant OspA protein was shown to be effective and safe, and was licensed in 1998 for persons 15–70 yr of age. Local adverse effects such as pain and swelling at the site of the injection were common. Many experts had reservations about the advisability of routine use of a vaccine for a disease that is relatively rare and that is usually easily treated. These reservations, coupled with the

---

| **BOX 204–1. Antimicrobial Treatment of Lyme Disease (*Lyme borreliosis*)** |

EARLY DISEASE

Erythema migrans and disseminated early disease without focal findings
Doxycycline, 100 mg twice daily for 14–21 days (do not use in children <8 yr)
or
Amoxicillin, 50 mg/kg/24 hr divided tid (maximum: 500 mg/dose) PO for 14–21 days
Preferred alternative agent for those who cannot take either amoxicillin or doxycycline is cefuroxime, 30 mg/kg/24 hr divided bid (maximum: 500 mg/dose) PO for 14–21 days. Another alternative is erythromycin, 30–50 mg/kg/24 hr divided qid (maximum: 250 mg/dose) PO for 14–21 days.
Carditis
For mild-moderate disease, treat as for erythema migrans for 21 days. For severe disease (e.g., third degree block), treat as for meningitis.
Palsy of the cranial nerves (including 7th nerve palsy)
If no clinical evidence of meningitis, treat as for erythema migrans for 21 days. Do not use corticosteroids.
Meningitis
Ceftriaxone, 50–80 mg/kg/24 hr in a single dose (maximum: 2 g) IV or IM for 14–28 days, or penicillin G, 200,000–400,000 U/kg/24 hr (maximum: 20 million units/24 hr) divided q 4 hr IV for 14–28 days

LATE DISEASE

Arthritis
Initial treatment is the same as for erythema migrans except treatment is continued for 28 days. If symptoms fail to resolve after 2 mo or there is a recurrence, then give either a second course of an orally administered antimicrobial agent for 28 days or treat as for meningitis.

theoretical concern for potentiation of symptoms of arthritis or Lyme disease in vaccinees, resulted in low demand that led the manufacturer to withdraw the vaccine from the market in early 2002.

Gerber MA, Shapiro ED, Burke GS, et al: Lyme disease in children in Southeastern Connecticut. *N Engl J Med* 1996;335:1270–4.

Klempner MS, Hu LT, Evans J, et al: Two controlled trials of antibiotic treatment in patients with persistent symptoms and a history of Lyme disease. *N Engl J Med* 2001;345:85–92.

Nadelman RB, Nowakowski J, Fish D, et al: Prophylaxis with single-dose doxycycline for the prevention of Lyme disease after an *Ixodes scapularis* tick bite. *N Engl J Med* 2001;345:79–84.

Reid MC, Schoen RT, Evans J, et al: The consequences of overdiagnosis and overtreatment of Lyme disease. An observational study. *Ann Intern Med* 1998: 128:354–62.

Seltzer EG, Shapiro ED: Misdiagnosis of Lyme disease: When not to order serologic tests. *Pediatr Infect Dis J* 1996;15:762–3.

Seltzer EG, Gerber MA, Cartter ML, et al: Long-term outcomes of persons with Lyme disease. *JAMA* 2000;283:609–16.

Shadick NA, Liang MH, Phillips CB, et al: The cost-effectiveness of vaccination against Lyme disease. *Arch Intern Med* 2001;161:554–61.

Shapiro ED, Gerber MA: Lyme disease. *Clin Infect Dis* 2000;31:533–42.

Shapiro ED: Doxycycline for tick bites—Not for everyone. *N Engl J Med* 2001;345: 133–4.

Wormser GP, Nadelman RB, Dattwyler RJ, et al: Practice guidelines for the treatment of Lyme disease. *Clin Infect Dis* 2000;31:S1–14.

SECTION 7 *Mycoplasmal Infections*
Dwight A. Powell

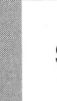

Chapter 205
Mycoplasma pneumoniae

Among the five *Mycoplasma* species isolated from the human respiratory tract, *Mycoplasma pneumoniae* is the only recognized human pathogen. It is a major cause of respiratory infections in school-aged children and young adults.

Etiology. *M. pneumoniae*, originally thought to be a virus and called the Eaton agent, was found to be a *Mycoplasma* in the early 1960s. Mycoplasmas are the smallest self-replicating biologic system and are dependent on attachment to host cells for obtaining essential precursors such as nucleotides, fatty acids, sterols, and amino acids. They contain double-stranded DNA with genomes ranging from 577–1380 Kb. *M. pneumoniae* is fastidious, and growth in commercially available culture systems is generally too slow to be of practical clinical use.

Epidemiology. *M. pneumoniae* infections occur worldwide and throughout the year. In contrast to the acute, short-lived epidemics of some respiratory agents, *M. pneumoniae* infection is endemic in larger communities, with epidemic outbreaks occurring every 4–7 yr. In smaller communities, infections are sporadic with long-lasting and smoldering outbreaks occurring at irregular intervals.

The occurrence of mycoplasmal illness is related, in part, to age and pre-exposure immunity. Overt illness is unusual before 3 yr of age; younger children appear to have frequent mild or subclinical infections, and reinfections appear to be common. The peak incidence of illness occurs in school-aged children; *M. pneumoniae* accounts for 7–30% of all community acquired pneumonias in children 3–15 yr of age. Recurrent infections occur infrequently but are well documented to occur in adults at intervals of 4–7 yr.

High rates of transmission have been documented within families, with a high proportion of secondary cases involving lower respiratory tract infections. Infection occurs through the respiratory route by large droplet spread. The incubation period is thought to be 1–3 wk. Outbreaks can occur in closed settings (e.g., military recruits, institutions, and summer camps for children) or can occur as community epidemics.

Pathogenesis. Cells of the ciliated respiratory epithelium are the target cells of *M. pneumoniae* infection. The organism is an elon-

gated snakelike structure with an attachment tip characterized by an electron-dense core and a trilaminar outer membrane. Attachment to the ciliary membrane is mediated by a complex network of interactive adhesion and adherence-accessory proteins localized to this specialized attachment tip. These proteins cooperate structurally and functionally to mobilize and concentrate adhesion proteins at the tip and permit mycoplasmal colonization of mucous membranes. Avirulent phenotypes that arise through spontaneous mutations at high frequency cannot synthesize specific cytoadherence-related proteins or are unable to stabilize them at the tip organelle.

Virulent organisms attach to ciliated respiratory epithelial cell surfaces through sialated glycoprotein receptors and burrow down between cells, resulting in ciliastasis and eventual sloughing of the cells. Although the mechanisms of cytopathology have not been determined, intracellular organisms have not been found, and *M. pneumoniae* rarely invades beyond the basement membrane.

Although the presence of circulating antibodies in humans correlates with protection against *M. pneumoniae* infections, studies in the hamster model have shown that circulating antibody alone, in the absence of other forms of immunity, provides incomplete protection. In hamsters, most of the peribronchial mononuclear cells are laden with antibody. However, ablation of the T-cell system with antithymocyte serum completely prevents the development of pneumonia. Thus, the disease produced by *M. pneumoniae* is very complex; the immunologic response of the host may be responsible for the manifestations of disease itself as well as for protection against infection, depending on the qualitative and quantitative balance of humoral and cellular immunity. Patients with immunodeficiency such as hypogammaglobulinemia and sickle cell disease may have more severe mycoplasmal pneumonia than do immunocompetent hosts. *M. pneumoniae* may persist for years in the respiratory tract of patients with hypogammaglobulinemia despite multiple courses of antibiotics. *M. pneumoniae* is one of the most common infectious causes of acute chest syndrome in sickle cell disease, but is not prevalent in patients with AIDS.

Clinical Manifestations. Bronchopneumonia is the most commonly recognized clinical syndrome associated with *M. pneumoniae* infection. Although the onset of illness may be abrupt, it is usually characterized by gradual onset of headache, malaise, fever, and sore throat, followed by progression of lower respiratory symptoms including hoarseness and cough. Coryza is unusual with *M. pneumoniae* pneumonia and usually suggests a viral etiology. Although the clinical course in untreated individuals is variable, coughing usually worsens during the first 2 wk of illness, then all symptoms gradually resolve within 3–4 wk. The cough is initially nonproductive, but older children and adolescents may produce a frothy, white sputum. The severity of symptoms is usually greater than that suggested by the physical signs, which appear later in the disease. Crackles or rales, which are fine and resemble those heard in asthma and bronchiolitis, are the most prominent sign. With progression of the disease, the fever intensifies, the cough becomes more troublesome, and the patient may become dyspneic.

Radiographic findings are not specific. Pneumonia is usually described as interstitial or bronchopneumonic; involvement is most common in the lower lobes, with unilateral, centrally dense infiltrates described in 75% of cases. Lobar pneumonia is seen infrequently. Hilar lymphadenopathy may occur in up to 33% of patients. Significant amounts of pleural fluid are unusual, but patients with large effusions due to *M. pneumoniae* have been described as having more severe and prolonged illness compared with those without pleural involvement. The white blood cell and differential counts are usually normal, whereas the erythrocyte sedimentation rate is usually elevated.

Additional respiratory illnesses caused infrequently by *M. pneumoniae* include undifferentiated upper respiratory tract infections, pharyngitis, sinusitis, croup, and bronchiolitis. *M. pneumoniae* is a common trigger of wheezing in asthmatic children. Otitis media and bullous myringitis have been described but are rarely seen without associated lower respiratory tract infection.

Diagnosis. No specific clinical, epidemiologic, or laboratory observations permit a definite diagnosis of mycoplasmal infection early in the clinical course. Certain observations, however, are suggestive and can be helpful. Pneumonia in school-aged children and young adults, especially if cough is a prominent finding, is always suggestive of *M. pneumoniae* disease. Cultures on special media of the throat or sputum may demonstrate *M. pneumoniae*, but growth is rarely detected earlier than 1 wk, and few commercial laboratories maintain the capability of culturing *M. pneumoniae*. Cold agglutinins are the result of an IgM autoantibody to the I component of the red blood cell surface membrane induced by *M. pneumoniae*. In the presence of cold agglutinins, erythrocytes agglutinate at 4°C (39.2°F) but not at room temperature. A high titer of cold agglutinins is probably responsible for the hemolytic anemia that sometimes accompanies *M. pneumoniae* infection. A cold agglutinin titer 1:32 or greater suggests *M. pneumoniae* infection. Positive IgM *M. pneumoniae* antibody identified by indirect fluorescence or enzyme-linked immune assay (EIA) more specifically supports the diagnosis. A fourfold increase in IgG *M. pneumoniae* antibody titer, by complement fixation or EIA, between acute and convalescent sera obtained 10 days to 3 wk after the onset of illness is diagnostic. Polymerase chain reaction (PCR) of a nasopharyngeal or throat swab for *M. pneumoniae* DNA has been shown to be rapid, sensitive, and specific in many studies. When *M. pneumoniae* is confirmed in the community in a few patients, the probability of the existence of other mycoplasmal illnesses is greatly increased.

Treatment. In general, *M. pneumoniae* illness is mild, and hospitalization is infrequently required. Because of the absence of a cell wall, the organism is resistant to the penicillins and cephalosporins. *M. pneumoniae* is exceptionally sensitive to erythromycin, clarithromycin, azithromycin, and the tetracyclines in vitro, which are effective in shortening the course of mycoplasmal illnesses, although they are not mycoplasmacidal. Hence, there may be delay in eradicating the organism from the respiratory tract. Two multicenter studies of pediatric community–acquired pneumonia demonstrated equal efficacy between erythromycin and clarithromycin or azithromycin. These newer macrolides were better tolerated and more effective at eradication of *M. pneumoniae* from the respiratory tract. Clarithromycin (15 mg/kg/24 hr divided bid PO for 10 days) or azithromycin (10 mg/kg PO on day 1 and 5 mg/kg/24 hr PO on days 2–5) eradicated *M. pneumoniae* in 100% of patients studied. Prophylaxis with azithromycin has been shown to substantially reduce the secondary attack rate in institutional outbreaks.

Complications. Complications, including bacterial superinfection, are unusual. Despite the reportedly rare isolation of *M. pneumoniae* from nonrespiratory sites such as joints, pleural fluid, and cerebrospinal fluid (CSF), the availability of PCR to detect specific segments of *M. pneumoniae* DNA has led to increasing identification of *M. pneumoniae* in nonrespiratory sites, particularly the central nervous system (CNS). Extra-respiratory illness may therefore involve direct invasion with *M. pneumoniae* or may involve autoimmune mechanisms, which is reflected by the frequency with which human antigens cross react with *M. pneumoniae*. Patients with or without respiratory symptoms may manifest illness involving the skin, CNS, blood, heart, gastrointestinal tract, and joints. Skin lesions include a variety of exanthems, most notably maculopapular rashes, erythema multiforme, and the Stevens-Johnson syndrome. Stevens-Johnson syndrome associated with *M. pneumoniae* usually develops 3–21 days after initial respiratory symptoms, lasts less than 14 days, and is rarely associated with severe complications (Figs. 205–1 and 205–2).

Neurologic complications include meningoencephalitis, transverse myelitis, aseptic meningitis, cerebellar ataxia, Bell palsy, deafness, brainstem syndrome, acute demyelinating encephalitis, and Guillain-Barré syndrome. Neurologic complications occur 3–28 days (mean 10 days) after respiratory illness but may not be preceded by respiratory illness in 20% of cases. Encephalitis occurring within 5 days of the onset of prodromal symptoms may be caused by direct *M. pneumoniae* infection of the CNS; encephalitis occurring >7 days after onset of prodromal symptoms is more likely to be auto-immune. *M. pneumoniae* accounts for 1–15% of all forms of childhood encephalitis and most commonly manifests as seizures, impaired consciousness, facial motor deficit, ataxia, or meningeal signs. Concomitant infection with viral agents such as HSV, HHV6, enteroviruses or respiratory viruses may be common. Involvement of the brain stem may result in severe dystonia and movement disorders. The CSF may be normal or have mild mononuclear pleocytosis. Diagnosis is confirmed with positive CSF PCR, positive PCR from a throat swab, or the presence of definitive serum antibody titers. Findings on MRI include focal ischemic changes, ventriculomegaly, diffuse edema, or multifocal white matter inflammatory lesions consistent with postinfectious demyelinating encephalomyelitis. Neurologic sequelae occur in 20–30% of patients.

Common hematologic complications include mild degrees of hemolysis with positive Coombs test and minor reticulocytosis 2–3 wk after the onset of illness. Severe hemolysis, which is associated with high titers of cold hemagglutinins (≥1:512), is rare, as are thrombocytopenia and coagulation defects. Mild hepatitis, pancreatitis, and protein-losing hypertrophic gastropathy are rarely reported gastrointestinal complications. Myocarditis, pericarditis, and a rheumatic fever-like syndrome are uncommon manifestations, but arrhythmias, ST- and T-wave changes, and cardiac dilation with heart failure may accompany *M. pneumoniae* infection in adults more commonly than children. Transient monoarticular arthritis was described in 1% of patients in one large series.

It is unclear from existing literature whether antibiotic treatment of *M. pneumoniae* infection decreases the risk of complications. There is also no specific established therapy for most of the complications. Corticosteroids have been the most frequently used agents in the management of severe *M. pneumoniae* complications, particularly neurologic complications.

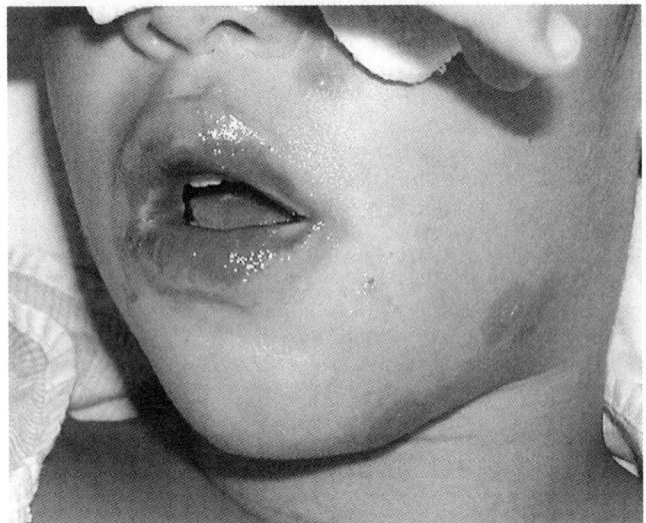

FIGURE 205–1. Lip changes found in Stevens-Johnson syndrome associated with *Mycoplasma pneumoniae* infection. See also color plates.

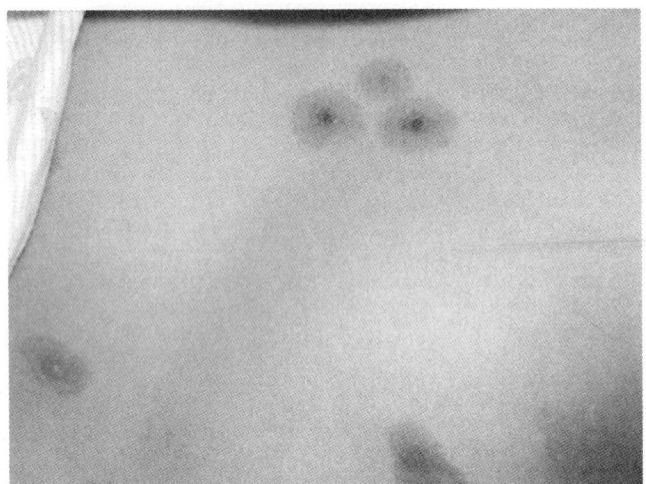

FIGURE 205–2. Classic erythema multiforme skin lesions found in Stevens-Johnson syndrome associated with *Mycoplasma pneumoniae* infection. See also color plates.

Prognosis. Fatal *M. pneumoniae* infections are very rare. Anatomic abnormalities such as altered lung perfusion, mild bronchiectasis, and bronchial wall thickening were detected by high-resolution CT in 37% of children 1–2 yr following *M. pneumoniae* pneumonia. Abnormalities in pulmonary gas diffusion have been reported in nearly half of children 6 mo after recovery from *M. pneumoniae*. Patients generally recover without complications, although sequelae of encephalitis may be severe and permanent.

Bitnun A, Ford-Jones EL, Petric M, et al: Acute childhood encephalitis and *Mycoplasma pneumoniae*. *Clin Infect Dis* 2001;32:1674–84.

Dorigo-Zetsma JW, Zaat SA, Wertheim-van Dillen PME, et al: Comparison of PCR, culture, and serological tests for diagnosis of *Mycoplasma pneumoniae* respiratory tract infection in children. *J Clin Microbiol* 1999;37:14.

Harris JA, Kolokathis A, Campbell M, et al: Safety and efficacy of azithromycin in the treatment of community-acquired pneumonia in children. *Pediatr Infect Dis J* 1998;17:865–71.

Marc E, Chaussain M, Moulin F, et al: Reduced lung diffusion capacity after *Mycoplasma pneumoniae* pneumonia. *Pediatr Infect Dis J* 2000;19:706–10.

Mezarina KB, Huffmire A, Downing J, et al: Outbreak of community-acquired pneumonia caused by *Mycoplasma pneumoniae*—Colorado, 2000. *MMWR Morb Mortal Wkly Rep* 2001;50:227–30.

Radisic M, Torn A, Gutierrez P, et al: Severe acute lung injury caused by *Mycoplasma pneumoniae*: Potential role for steroid pulses in treatment. *Clin Infect Dis* 2000;31: 1507–11.

Smith R, Eviatar L: Neurologic manifestations of *Mycoplasma pneumoniae* infections: Diverse spectrum of diseases. *Clin Pediatr* 2000;39:195–201.

Tay YK, Huff JC, Weston WL: *Mycoplasma pneumoniae* infection is associated with Stevens-Johnson syndrome, not erythema multiforme (von Hebra). *J Am Acad Dermatol* 1996;35:757–60.

Wubbel L, Muniz L, Ahmed A, et al: Etiology and treatment of community-acquired pneumonia in ambulatory children. *Pediatr Infect Dis J* 1999;18:98–104.

Chapter 206
Genital Mycoplasmas (*Mycoplasma hominis* and *Ureaplasma urealyticum*)

Two *Mycoplasma* species, *Mycoplasma hominis* and *Ureaplasma urealyticum*, are human urogenital pathogens. They are often associated with sexually transmitted diseases such as nongonococcal urethritis (NGU) or puerperal infections such as endometritis. Both organisms commonly colonize the female genital tract and are capable of causing chorioamnionitis, colonization of neonates, and perinatal infections. *M. genitalium* has been implicated as a possible cause of NGU. Two other genital *Mycoplasma* species, *M. fermentans* and *M. penetrans*, have been identified in respiratory or genitourinary secretions with greater frequency in patients infected with HIV than in those without HIV. This has led to speculation, as yet unproven, that these mycoplasmas may play a role as cofactors in progression of HIV infection.

Etiology. *M. hominis* and *U. urealyticum* require sterols for growth and can grow in cell-free media. They produce characteristic colonies on agar (*M. hominis*: 200–300 μm, with a "fried-egg" appearance; *U. urealyticum*: 16–60 μm). They are resistant to β-lactams because they lack a cell wall, and resistant to sulfonamides and trimethoprim because they do not produce folic acid. All seven serovars of *M. hominis* are susceptible to clindamycin, moderately susceptible to chloramphenicol, and resistant to erythromycin and rifampin. Aminoglycosides have limited activity, and increasing numbers of tetracycline-resistant strains are being reported. There are 14 serovars of *U. urealyticum*, and most are susceptible to erythromycin, clarithromycin, and the newer quinolones but resistant to clindamycin. Susceptibility to aminoglycosides and tetracyclines is variable.

Epidemiology. *M. hominis* and *U. urealyticum* colonize the genital and urinary tracts of postpubertal females and males. Female colonization is maximal in the vagina and less in the endocervix, urethra, or endometrium. Male colonization occurs primarily in the urethra. Colonization rates are directly related to sexual activity, with colonization occurring in <10% of prepubertal children and sexually inactive adults. Rates are highest in those with multiple sexual partners. Colonization of pregnant females varies from 40–90%, and vertical transmission rates of 25–60% are observed among neonates born to colonized women. Contamination from colonized amniotic fluid or during vaginal delivery is the usual route of neonatal acquisition. However, neonatal colonization can occur in the presence of intact amniotic fluid membranes and with delivery by cesarean section. Colonization rates are highest in infants weighing <1,500 g, in the presence of clinical chorioamnionitis, and among newborns to mothers of lower socioeconomic status. Organisms are recovered from the newborn's throat, vagina, rectum, and, occasionally, eyes for as long as 3 mo after birth.

Pathogenesis. Genital mycoplasmas can produce chronic inflammation of the genitourinary tract and amniotic fluid membranes. *U. urealyticum* may infect the amniotic sac early in gestation without rupturing the fetal membranes, resulting in a clinically silent, chronic chorioamnionitis characterized by an intense inflammatory response. Attachment to fetal human tracheal epithelium has been shown to cause ciliary disarray, clumping, and loss of epithelial cells. *U. urealyticum* induces macrophages in vitro to increase production of interleukin-6 (IL-6) and tumor necrosis factor 2. Very low birthweight infants colonized with *U. urealyticum* have been shown to have increased levels of monocyte chemoattractant protein and IL-8, which are proinflammatory agents possibly associated with development of bronchopulmonary dysplasia. Immunity appears to require serotype-specific antibody. Thus, a lack of maternal antibody may account for a higher risk of disease in premature newborns.

Clinical Manifestations. In adults and sexually active adolescents, genital mycoplasmas are associated with sexually transmitted diseases and uncommonly associated with focal infections outside the genital tract. *M. hominis* has been described causing septicemia, wound infection, osteomyelitis, lymphadenitis, meningitis, brain abscess, and arthritis. Life-threatening mediastinitis, sternal wound infections, pleuritis, and pericarditis have been reported with high mortality rates in patients following organ transplant. Extragenital *U. urealyticum* infections are rarely described but include osteomyelitis, arthritis, meningitis, mediastinitis, infection of aortic grafts, and postcesarean wound infections. Patients with hypogammaglobulinemia appear to be at high risk for chronic arthritis caused by various *Mycoplasma*.

U. urealyticum and *M. genitalium* are confirmed pathogens of NGU; approximately 30% of cases in males may be caused by these organisms either alone or together with *Chlamydia trachomatis* (see Chapter 208). Disease is most common in young adults but is also prevalent in sexually active adolescents. The average incubation period is 2–3 wk, with symptoms typically consisting of scanty, mucoid-white urethral discharge, dysuria, and penile discomfort. The discharge is often evident only in the morning or after the urethra is stripped. Rare complications of nongonococcal urethritis are epididymitis and proctitis. Approximately 20–60% of patients with acute NGU will develop recurrent or chronic urethritis despite 1–2 wk of treatment. *U. urealyticum* and *M. genitalium* appear to be the most likely agents of chronic symptomatic urethritis. Females rarely have urethritis and despite high vaginal colonization rates, vaginitis or cervicitis is uncommon. *M. hominis* is an occasional contributing cause of pelvic inflammatory disease, and both genital mycoplasmas are rarely associated with endometritis and postpartum sepsis.

NEONATES. Genital mycoplasmas are associated with a variety of fetal and neonatal infections. *U. urealyticum* may cause clinically inapparent chorioamnionitis resulting in an eightfold increase in fetal death or premature delivery. Up to 50% of infants <34 wk of gestational age may have *U. urealyticum* recovered from tracheal, blood, cerebrospinal fluid (CSF), or lung biopsy specimens. The role of these organisms causing severe respiratory insufficiency, the need for assisted ventilation, the development of bronchopulmonary dysplasia, or death remains controversial. A large number of controlled studies have investigated this question. Early studies demonstrated that infants weighing <1,000 g who had *U. urealyticum* isolated from tracheal aspirates within the first 24 hr of life were twice as likely to die or develop chronic lung disease compared with uninfected infants of similar birthweight or those weighing >1,000 g. More recent studies, controlling for gestational age and other factors, have shown no correlation between the respiratory isolation of *U. urealyticum* and development of bronchopulmonary dysplasia, duration of ventilatory support, oxygen dependency, or length of hospitalization. Furthermore, a small study of intravenous erythromycin for 1 wk after birth in infants with tra-

cheobronchial colonization of *U. urealyticum* failed to show any difference in treated versus nontreated infants in the development of chronic lung disease. Thus, although it is clear that a high percentage of premature infants are colonized with *U. urealyticum*, the pathogenicity in premature infants awaits further study.

M. hominis and *U. urealyticum* have been isolated from the CSF of premature and, in a few cases, full-term infants. Simultaneous isolation of other pathogens is unusual, and most infants have no overt signs of central nervous system infection. CSF pleocytosis is not a consistent observation, and spontaneous clearance of mycoplasmas has been documented without specific therapy. *U. urealyticum* meningitis has been associated with intraventricular hemorrhage and hydrocephalus; meningitis due to *M. hominis* may be benign. The onset of meningitis varies from 1–196 days of life; organisms may persist in the CSF without therapy for days to weeks. *M. hominis* and *U. urealyticum* have been described to cause neonatal conjunctivitis, lymphadenitis, pharyngitis, pneumonitis, osteomyelitis, and scalp abscess.

Diagnosis. Diagnosis of a genital tract infection may be difficult because of high colonization rates in the vagina and urethra. Nongonococcal urethritis is confirmed by Gram stain of urethral discharge showing at least three polymorphonuclear leukocytes/oil-immersion field and the absence of gram-negative diplococci. A urethral swab or exudate should be cultured for *C. trachomatis* and *U. urealyticum*.

NEONATES. *U. urealyticum* and *M. hominis* have been isolated from urine, blood, CSF, tracheal aspirates, pleural fluid, abscess, and lung tissue. Premature neonates who are clinically ill with pneumonitis, focal abscesses, or central nervous system disease (particularly progressive hydrocephalus with or without pleocytosis) for whom bacterial cultures are negative or in whom there is no improvement with standard antibiotic therapy warrant cultures for genital mycoplasmas. Isolation requires special media, and clinical specimens must be cultured immediately or be frozen at −80°C to avoid loss of organisms. When inoculated into broth containing arginine (*M. hominis*) or urea (*U. urealyticum*), growth is indicated by an alkaline pH. Identification of *U. urealyticum* on agar requires 1–2 days of growth and visualization with the dissecting microscope, whereas *M. hominis* is apparent to the eye but may require 1 wk to grow. Cultures from the upper respiratory tract are probably meaningless owing to high colonization rates. Cultures of the lower respiratory tract through endotracheal aspirate or biopsy are essential.

Treatment. Nongonococcal urethritis in adolescents and adults is treated with azithromycin (1 g PO as a single dose) or doxycycline (100 mg bid PO for 7 days). Sexual partners should also be treated to avoid recurrent disease. Nongenital mycoplasmal infections may require surgical drainage and prolonged antibiotic therapy. *M. hominis* is resistant to erythromycin and newer macrolide antibiotics but usually susceptible to clindamycin and variably susceptible to quinolones and tetracycline. *U. urealyticum* are susceptible to tetracycline, aminoglycosides, and quinolones.

NEONATES. Therapy for neonatal genital mycoplasma infections is indicated in infections associated with a pure growth of the organism and evidence that the disease manifestations are compatible with an infectious process rather than merely colonization. The role of therapy in preventing chronic lung disease in very low birthweight infants awaits results of further studies. Treatment is based on predictable antimicrobial sensitivities because susceptibility testing is not readily available. For symptomatic central nervous system infections, doxycycline is recommended. The long-term consequences of asymptomatic central nervous system infection with genital mycoplasmas, especially in the absence of pleocytosis, are unknown. Because mycoplasmas may spontaneously be cleared from the CSF, therapy should involve minimal risks.

Asmar BI, Andresen J, Brown WJ: Ureaplasma urealyticum arthritis and bacteremia in agammaglobulinemia. *Pediatr Infect Dis J* 1998;17:73–6.

Baier RJ, Loggins J, Kruger TE: Monocyte chemoattractant protein-1 and interleukin-8 are increased in bronchopulmonary dysplasia: Relation to isolation of *Ureaplasma urealyticum. J Invest Med* 2001;49:362–9.

Cassel GH, Waites KB, Watson HL, et al: *Ureaplasma urealyticum* intrauterine infection: Role in prematurity and disease in newborns. *Clin Microbiol Rev* 1993;6:69–87.

DaSilva O, Gregson D, Hammerberg O: Role of *Ureaplasma urealyticum* and *Chlamydia trachomatis* in development of bronchopulmonary dysplasia in very low birth weight infants. *Pediatr Infect Dis J* 1997;16:364–9.

Horner P, Thomas B, Gilroy CB, et al: Role of *Mycoplasma genitalium* and *Ureaplasma urealyticum* in acute and chronic nongonococcal urethritis. *Clin Infect Dis* 2001; 32:995–1003.

Li Y, Brauner A, Jonsson B, et al: *Ureaplasma urealyticum*-induced production of pro-inflammatory cytokines by macrophages. *Pediatr Res* 2000;48: 114–9.

Lyon AJ, McColm J, Middlemist L, et al: Randomized trial of erythromycin on the development of chronic lung disease in preterm infants. *Arch Dis Child Fetal Neonatal Ed* 1998;78:F10–4.

Mattila PS, Carlson P, Sivonen A, et al: Life-threatening *Mycoplasma hominis* mediastinitis. *Clin Infect Dis* 1999;29:1529–37.

Ollikainen J, Korppi M, Heiskanen-Kosma T, et al: Chronic lung disease of the newborn is not associated with *Ureaplasma urealyticum. Pediatr Pulmonol* 2001;32:303–7.

Taylor-Robinson D: Infections due to species of *Mycoplasma* and *Ureaplasma*: An update. *Clin Infect Dis* 1996;23:671–82.

SECTION 8 *Chlamydial Infections*

Margaret R. Hammerschlag

Chapter 207
Chlamydia pneumoniae

Chlamydia pneumoniae is increasingly recognized as a common cause of lower respiratory tract diseases, including pneumonia in children and bronchitis and pneumonia in adults. The first isolates of *C. pneumoniae* were obtained during studies of trachoma in the 1960s. Subsequent serologic studies demonstrated that the organism caused an outbreak of mild pneumonia among school children in Finland in 1978. In 1986, the organism was isolated from the respiratory tract of college students with acute respiratory disease.

Etiology. Chlamydiae are obligate intracellular pathogens that have established a unique niche within the host cell. Chlamydiae cause a variety of diseases in animal species at virtually all phylogenic levels. The order contains one genus, *Chlamydia*, with four recognized species: *C. pneumoniae, C. trachomatis, C. psittaci,* and *C. pecorum. C. pneumoniae* and *C. trachomatis* are the most significant human pathogens. *C. psittaci* is an important zoonosis. DNA hybridization studies show <5% relatedness between *C. pneumoniae, C. trachomatis,* and *C. psittaci.* Recent taxonomic analysis using the 16S and 23S rRNA genes has supported splitting the genus *Chlamydia* into two genera, *Chlamydia* and *Chlamydophila. Chlamydia* would contain *C. trachomatis* and two new species, *Chlamydia muridarum* (formerly the agent of mouse pneumonitis, MoPn) and *C. suis. Chlamydophila* would contain *C. pecorum, C. pneumoniae, C. psittaci,* and three new species split out from *C. psittaci: C. abortus, C. caviae* (formerly *C. psittaci* guinea pig conjunctivitis strain), and *C. felis.* There is continuing controversy regarding this reclassification.

Chlamydiae are characterized by a unique developmental cycle with morphologically distinct infectious and reproductive forms: **elementary body** (EB) and **reticulate body** (RB). Chlamydiae have a gram-negative envelope without detectable peptidoglycan, although recent genomic analysis has revealed that both *C. pneumonia* and *C. trachomatis* encode proteins forming a nearly complete pathway for synthesis of peptidoglycan, including penicillin-binding proteins. Chlamydiae also share a group-specific lipopolysaccharide antigen and use host adenosine triphosphate for the synthesis of chlamydial proteins. Although chlamydiae are auxotrophic for 3 of 4 nucleoside triphosphates, they do encode functional glucose-catabolizing enzymes that can be used for generation of ATP. As with peptidoglycan synthesis, for some reason these genes are turned off. All Chlamydiae also encode an abundant protein called the **major outer membrane protein** (MOMP, or OmpA) that is surface exposed in *C. trachomatis* and *C. psittaci,* but apparently not in *C. pneumoniae.* The MOMP is the major determinant of the serologic classification of *C. trachomatis* and *C. psittaci* isolates.

Epidemiology. *C. pneumoniae* appears to be a primary human respiratory pathogen. The organism has also been isolated from nonhuman species, including horse, koalas, reptiles, and amphibians, although the role these infections may play in transmission to humans is unknown. *C. pneumoniae* appears to affect individuals of all ages. The proportion of community-acquired pneumonias associated with *C. pneumoniae* infection has ranged from 2–19%, varying with geographic location, the age group examined, and the diagnostic methods used. Several studies of the role of *C. pneumoniae* in lower respiratory tract infection in pediatric populations have found evidence of infection from none to more than 18%. Most of these studies have relied entirely on serology for diagnosis. Results of a large U.S. multicenter study of community-acquired pneumonia in children 3–12 yr of age found evidence of *C. pneumoniae* infection, based on culture, in 14% and of *Mycoplasma pneumoniae* in 22%. The prevalence of *C. pneumoniae* infection in children 6 yr of age or younger was 15%; in those older than 6 yr of age it was 18%. Almost 20% of the children with *C. pneumoniae* infection were co-infected with *M. pneumoniae. C. pneumoniae* may also be responsible for 10–20% of episodes of acute chest syndrome in children with sickle cell disease, 10% of episodes of bronchitis, and 5–10% episodes of pharyngitis in children. Transmission probably occurs from person to person through respiratory droplets. Spread of the infection can occur among members in the same household.

Pathogenesis. Following infection, the infectious EBs, which are 200–400 µm in diameter, attach to the host cell by a process of electrostatic binding and are taken into the cell by endocytosis that does not depend on the microtubule system. Within the host cell, the EB remains within a membrane-lined phagosome. The phagosome does not fuse with the host cell lysosome. The inclusion membrane is devoid of host cell markers, but lipid markers traffic to the inclusion, which suggests a functional interaction with the Golgi apparatus. The EBs then differentiate into RBs that undergo binary fission. After approximately 36 hr, the RBs differentiate into EBs. At about 48 hr, release may occur by cytolysis or by a process of exocytosis or extrusion of the whole inclusion, leaving the host cell intact. Chlamydiae may also enter a persistent state after treatment with certain cytokines such as interferon-γ, treatment with antibiotics, or restriction of certain nutrients. While Chlamydiae are in the persistent state, metabolic activity is reduced. The ability to cause prolonged, often subclinical, infection is one of the major characteristics of Chlamydiae.

Clinical Manifestations. Infections caused by *C. pneumoniae* cannot be readily differentiated from those caused by other respiratory pathogens, especially *M. pneumoniae*. The pneumonia usually presents as a classic atypical (or nonbacterial) pneumonia characterized by mild to moderate constitutional symptoms including fever, malaise, headache, cough, and frequently pharyngitis. However, severe pneumonia with empyema has been described.

C. pneumoniae may serve as an infectious trigger for asthma and can cause pulmonary exacerbations in patients with cystic fibrosis. *C. pneumoniae* has been isolated from middle ear aspirates of children with acute otitis media, but is usually associated with bacterial otitis media. Asymptomatic respiratory infection has been documented in 2–5% of adults and children and may persist for a year or more.

Diagnosis. It is not possible to differentiate *C. pneumoniae* from other causes of atypical pneumonia on the basis of clinical findings. Auscultation reveals the presence of rales and often wheezing. The chest radiograph often appears worse than the patient's clinical status would indicate and may show mild, diffuse involvement or lobar infiltrates with small pleural effusions. The complete blood count may be elevated with a left shift but is usually unremarkable.

Specific diagnosis of *C. pneumoniae* infection is based on isolation of the organism in tissue culture. *C. pneumoniae* grows best in cycloheximide-treated HEp-2 and HL cells. The optimum site for culture is the posterior nasopharynx; the specimen is collected with wire-shafted swabs in the same manner as that used for *C. trachomatis*. The organism can be isolated from sputum, throat cultures, bronchoalveolar lavage fluid, and pleural fluid, but few laboratories perform such cultures because of technical difficulties.

Polymerase chain reaction (PCR) testing appears to be the most promising technology in the development of a rapid, non-culture method for detection of *C. pneumoniae*. Numerous PCR assays for detection of *C. pneumoniae* in clinical specimens have been reported but none of these assays are standardized or have been extensively validated compared with culture for detection of *C. pneumoniae* in respiratory specimens. None are commercially available or have Food and Drug Administration approval.

Serologic diagnosis can be accomplished using the microimmunofluorescence (MIF) or the complement fixation (CF) tests. The CF test is genus specific and is also used for diagnosis of lymphogranuloma venereum (Chapter 208.4) and psittacosis (Chapter 209). Its sensitivity in hospitalized patients with *C. pneumoniae* infection and children is variable. The Centers for Disease Control and Prevention (CDC) recently proposed modifications in the serologic criteria for diagnosis. Although the MIF test was considered to be the only currently acceptable serologic test, the criteria were made significantly more stringent. Acute infection, using the MIF test, was defined by a fourfold increase in IgG titer or an IgM titer of 16 or greater; use of a single elevated IgG titer was discouraged. An IgG titer of 16 or greater was thought to indicate past exposure, but neither elevated IgA titers nor any other serologic marker was thought to be a valid indicator of persistent or chronic infection. The CDC did not recommend the use of any enzyme-linked immune assay (EIA) test for detection of antibody to *C. pneumoniae* because there is concern about the inconsistent correlation of these results with culture results. Studies of *C. pneumoniae* infection in children with pneumonia and asthma show that more than 50% of children with culture-documented infection have no detectable MIF antibody.

Treatment. The optimum dose and duration of antimicrobial therapy for *C. pneumoniae* infections remain uncertain. Most treatment studies have used serology only for diagnosis, thus the microbiologic efficacy cannot be assessed. Prolonged therapy (≥2 wk) may be desirable because recrudescent symptoms and persistent positive cultures have been described following 2 wk of erythromycin and 30 days of tetracycline or doxycycline.

Tetracyclines, erythromycin, the newer macrolides (azithromycin and clarithromycin), and quinolones show in vitro activity. Like *C. psittaci*, *C. pneumoniae* is resistant to sulfonamides. The results of recent treatment studies have shown that erythromycin (40 mg/kg/24 hr divided bid PO for 10 days), clarithromycin (15 mg/kg/24 hr divided bid PO for 10 days), and azithromycin (10 mg/kg/24 PO on day 1, 5 mg/kg/24 hr PO on days 2–5) are effective for eradication of *C. pneumoniae* from the nasopharynx of children with pneumonia in approximately 80% of cases.

Prognosis. Clinical response to antibiotic therapy varies. Coughing often persists for several weeks even after therapy.

Block S, Hedrick J, Hammerschlag MR, et al: *Mycoplasma pneumoniae* and *Chlamydia pneumoniae* in pediatric community-acquired pneumonia. Comparative efficacy and safety of clarithromycin vs. erythromycin ethylsuccinate. *Pediatr Infect Dis J* 1995;14:471–7.
Boman J, Gaydos CA, Quinn TC: Molecular diagnosis of *Chlamydia pneumoniae* infection. *J Clin Microbiol* 1999;37:3791–9.
Dowell SF, Peeling RW, Boman J, et al: Standardizing *Chlamydia pneumoniae* assays: Recommendations from the Centers for Disease Control and Prevention (USA) and the Laboratory Centre for Disease Control (Canada). *Clin Infect Dis* 2001;33:492–503.
Grayston JT, Campbell LA, Kuo CC, et al: A new respiratory pathogen: *Chlamydia pneumoniae* strain TWAR. *J Infect Dis* 1990;161:618–25.
Hammerschlag MR, Roblin PM, Bébéar CM: Activity of telithromycin, a new ketolide antimicrobial, against atypical and intracellular respiratory tract pathogens. *J Antimicrob Chemother* 2001;48:25–31.
Harris J-A, Kolokathis A, Campbell M, et al: Safety and efficacy of azithromycin in the treatment of community acquired pneumonia in children. *Pediatr Infect Dis J* 1998;17:865–71.
Kutlin A, Roblin PM, Hammerschlag MR: Antibody response to *Chlamydia pneumoniae* infection in children with respiratory illness. *J Infect Dis* 1998;177:720–24.
Rockey DD, Lenart J, Stephens RS: Genome sequencing and our understanding of Chlamydiae. *Infect Immunol* 2000;68:5473–9.

Chapter 208
Chlamydia trachomatis

The organism *Chlamydia trachomatis* is subdivided into two biovars: lymphogranuloma venereum (LGV) and trachoma (the agent of human oculogenital diseases other than LGV). Although the strains of both biovars have almost complete DNA homology, they differ in growth characteristics and virulence in tissue culture and animals. In developed countries, *C. trachomatis* is the most prevalent sexually transmitted disease, causing urethritis in men, cervicitis and salpingitis in women, and conjunctivitis and pneumonia in infants.

208.1 Trachoma

Trachoma is the most important preventable cause of blindness in the world. It is caused primarily by the A, B, Ba, and C serotypes of *C. trachomatis*. It is endemic in the Middle East and Southeast Asia and among Navajo Indians in the southwestern United States. In areas that are endemic for trachoma, such as Egypt, genital chlamydial infection is caused by the serotypes responsible for oculogenital disease: D, E, F, G, H, I, J, and K. The disease is spread from eye to eye. Flies are a frequent vector.

Trachoma begins as a follicular conjunctivitis, usually in early childhood. The follicles heal, leading to conjunctival scarring that may result in an entropion, with the eyelid turning inward so that the lashes abrade the cornea. It is the corneal ulceration secondary to the constant trauma that leads to scarring and blindness. Bacterial superinfection may also contribute to scarring. Blindness occurs years after the active disease.

Trachoma can be diagnosed clinically. The World Health Organization suggests that at least two of four criteria must be present for a diagnosis of trachoma: (1) lymphoid follicles on the upper tarsal conjunctivae, (2) typical conjunctival scarring, (3) vascular pannus, and (4) limbal follicles. The diagnosis is confirmed by culture or staining tests for *C. trachomatis* performed during the active stage of disease. Serologic tests are not helpful clinically because of the long duration of the disease and the high seroprevalence in endemic populations.

Poverty and lack of sanitation are important factors in the spread of trachoma. As socioeconomic conditions improve, the incidence of the disease decreases substantially. Endemic trachoma has been controlled in most instances by administering topical tetracyclines (or, rarely, erythromycin ointment) daily for periods of 6–10 wk or intermittently over a 6-mo period. Oral doxycycline is effective but is contraindicated in children younger than 9 yr of age. Oral erythromycin requires frequent dosing, which is impractical in the control of endemic trachoma. A recent study reported that 1–6 doses of oral azithromycin was equivalent to 30 days of treatment with topical oxytetracycline/polymyxin ointment. Currently the WHO recommends single-dose azithromycin (20 mg/kg; maximum: 1 g) for the treatment of trachoma in children.

208.2 Genital Tract Infections

Epidemiology. There are an estimated 3 million new cases of chlamydial sexually transmitted infections each year in the United States. *C. trachomatis* is a major cause of epididymitis and is the cause of 23–55% of all cases of nongonococcal urethritis, although the proportion of chlamydial nongonococcal urethritis has been gradually declining. As many as 50% of men with gonorrhea may be co-infected with *C. trachomatis*. The prevalence of chlamydial cervicitis among sexually active women is 2–35%. Rates of infection among adolescent girls exceed 20% in many urban populations but can be as high as 15% in suburban populations as well (Chapter 110).

Children who have been sexually abused may acquire anogenital *C. trachomatis* infection, which is usually asymptomatic. Culture is the only method that should be used for diagnosis of *C. trachomatis* from these sites when a prepubertal child is being tested for suspected sexual abuse. However, because perinatally acquired rectal and vaginal *C. trachomatis* infections may persist for ≥3 yr, the detection of *C. trachomatis* in the vagina or rectum of a young child is not absolute evidence of sexual abuse.

Clinical Manifestations. The trachoma biovar of *C. trachomatis* causes a spectrum of disease in sexually active adolescents and adults. Up to 75% of women with *C. trachomatis* have no symptoms of infection. *C. trachomatis* can cause urethritis (acute urethral syndrome), epididymitis, cervicitis, salpingitis, proctitis, and pelvic inflammatory disease. The symptoms of chlamydial genital tract infections are less acute than those of gonorrhea, consisting of a discharge that is usually mucoid rather than purulent. Asymptomatic urethral infection is frequent in sexually active men. Autoinoculation from the genital tract to the eyes can lead to concomitant inclusion conjunctivitis.

Diagnosis. Definitive diagnosis of genital chlamydial infection is accomplished by isolation of the organism in tissue culture and confirmed by microscopic identification of the characteristic

inclusions using fluorescent antibody staining in culture specimens obtained from the urethra in men and the endocervix in women. Care should be taken to obtain epithelial cells, not only discharge. *C. trachomatis* can be cultured in cycloheximide-treated HeLa, McCoy, and HEp-2 cells. *Chlamydia* culture has been further defined by the CDC as isolation of the organism in tissue culture and as confirmation of the characteristic intracytoplasmic inclusions by fluorescent antibody staining.

Alternatively, a nonculture method, specifically a nucleic acid amplification test (NAAT) can be used. These tests have high sensitivity, perhaps even detecting 10–20% greater than culture, while retaining high specificity. There are currently four Food and Drug Administration (FDA)-approved, commercially available NAATs for *Chlamydia* using different methods: polymerase chain reaction (PCR) (Amplicor *Chlamydia* test, Roche Molecular Diagnostics, Nutley, NJ); ligase chain reaction (LCR) (LCx *Chlamydia trachomatis* assay, Abbott Diagnostics, Abbott Park, IL); strand displacement amplification (SDA) (BeAware GC/CT, BD Diagnostic Systems, Sparks, MD); and transcription mediated amplification (TMA) (Amp CT, Gen-Probe, San Diego, CA). PCR, LCR, and SDA are all DNA amplification tests that use primers that target gene sequences on the cryptogenic *C. trachomatis* plasmid, which is present at approximately 10 copies/cell. TMA is an rRNA amplification assay. The SDA test and a version of the TMA test (PACE, Gen-Probe) are a dual assay for simultaneously detecting *C. trachomatis* and *Neisseria gonorrhoeae*. Currently available commercial NAATs have FDA approval for cervical swabs from women, urethral swabs from men, and urine from men and women. The use of urine avoids the necessity for a clinical pelvic examination and may greatly facilitate screening in certain populations, especially adolescents. Data on use of NAATs for vaginal specimens or urine from children are very limited and insufficient to allow making a recommendation for their use. The CDC recommends that NAATs may be used as an alternative to culture *only* if confirmation is available. Confirmation tests should consist of a second FDA-approved NAAT that targets a different gene sequence from the initial test.

The etiology of most cases of nonchlamydial nongonococcal urethritis is unknown; *Ureaplasma urealyticum* and possibly *Mycoplasma genitalium* are implicated in up to one third of cases (see Chapter 206). Proctocolitis may develop in individuals who have a rectal infection with an LGV strain (see Subchapter 208.4).

Treatment. Recommended treatment regimens for uncomplicated *C. trachomatis* genital infection in men and nonpregnant women are azithromycin (1 g orally PO as a single dose) or doxycycline (100 mg PO bid for 7 days). Neither of these regimens can be used in pregnant women. Alternative regimens are erythromycin base (500 mg PO qid for 7 days), erythromycin ethylsuccinate (800 mg PO qid for 7 days), ofloxacin (300 mg PO bid for 7 days), and levofloxacin (500 mg PO once daily for 7 days). The high erythromycin dosages may not be well tolerated. Doxycycline and ofloxacin are contraindicated in pregnant women; quinolones are contraindicated in persons younger than 18 yr of age. For pregnant women, the recommended treatment regimen is erythromycin base (500 mg PO bid for 7 days) or amoxicillin (500 mg PO tid for 7 days). Alternative regimens are erythromycin base (250 mg PO qid for 14 days), erythromycin ethylsuccinate (800 mg PO qid for 7 days or 400 mg PO qid for 14 days), and azithromycin (1 g orally in a single dose). Amoxicillin at this dosage is as effective as any of the erythromycin regimens and is much better tolerated. However, experience with all these regimens is still limited.

Empirical treatment without microbiologic diagnosis is recommended only for patients at high risk for infection who are unlikely to return for follow-up evaluation, which includes adolescents with multiple sexual partners. These patients should be treated empirically for both *C. trachomatis* and gonorrhea (Chapter 177).

Sex partners of patients with nongonococcal urethritis should be treated if they have had sexual contact with the patient during the 60 days preceding the onset of symptoms. The most recent sexual partner should be treated even if the last sexual contact was more than 60 days from onset of symptoms.

Complications. Complications of genital chlamydial infections in women include perihepatitis (Fitz-Hugh-Curtis syndrome) and salpingitis. Of women with untreated chlamydial infection who develop pelvic inflammatory disease, up to 40% will have significant sequelae; approximately 17% will suffer from chronic pelvic pain, approximately 17% will become infertile, and approximately 9% will have an ectopic (tubal) pregnancy. Adolescent girls may be at higher risk for developing complications, especially salpingitis, than older women. Salpingitis in adolescent girls is also more likely to lead to tubal scarring, subsequent obstruction with secondary infertility, and increased risk of ectopic pregnancy. Approximately 50% of neonates born to pregnant women with chlamydial infection will acquire *C. trachomatis* infection (Chapter 208.3). Women with *C. trachomatis* infection have a threefold to fivefold increased risk of acquiring HIV infection.

Prevention. Timely treatment of sex partners is essential for decreasing risk of re-infection. Sex partners should be evaluated and treated if they had sexual contact during the 60 days preceding onset of symptoms in the patient. The most recent sex partner should be treated even if the last sexual contact was >60 days. Patients and their sex partners should abstain from sexual intercourse until 7 days after a single-dose regimen or after completion of a 7-day regimen.

Annual routine screening for *C. trachomatis* is recommended for all sexually active adolescents and females 20–25 yr of age, and older women with risk factors such as new or multiple partners or inconsistent use of barrier contraceptives. Sexual risk assessment may indicate more frequent screening of some women.

208.3 Conjunctivitis and Pneumonia in Newborns

Epidemiology. Chlamydial genital infection is reported in 5–30% of pregnant women with a risk of vertical transmission at parturition to newborn infants of about 50%. The infant may become infected at one or more sites including the conjunctivae, nasopharynx, rectum, and vagina. Transmission is rare following cesarean section with intact membranes.

Clinical Manifestations. Approximately 70% of infected infants are infected in the nasopharynx. Clinically, the infant may develop conjunctivitis or pneumonia.

INCLUSION CONJUNCTIVITIS. *C. trachomatis* is the most frequent identifiable infectious cause of neonatal conjunctivitis, the primary clinical manifestation of neonatal chlamydial infection. Approximately 30–50% of infants born to mothers with active chlamydial infection develop clinical conjunctivitis. Symptoms usually develop 5–14 days after delivery, or earlier with prolonged rupture of membranes. The presentation is extremely variable and ranges from mild conjunctival injection with scant mucoid discharge to severe conjunctivitis with copious purulent discharge, chemosis, and pseudomembrane formation. The conjunctiva may be very friable and may bleed when stroked with a swab. Chlamydial conjunctivitis must be differentiated from gonococcal ophthalmia, which is sight-threatening. At least 50% of infants with chlamydial conjunctivitis also have nasopharyngeal infection.

PNEUMONIA. Pneumonia due to *C. trachomatis* develops in 10–20% of infants born to women with chlamydial infection. Only about 25% of infants with nasopharyngeal chlamydial infection develop pneumonia. *C. trachomatis* pneumonia of infancy has a very characteristic presentation. Onset is usually between 1 and 3 mo of age and is often insidious with persistent cough, tachypnea, and absence of fever. Auscultation reveals rales; wheezing is uncommon. The absence of fever and wheezing helps to distinguish *C. trachomatis* pneumonia from respiratory syncytial virus (RSV) pneumonia. A distinctive laboratory finding is the presence of peripheral eosinophilia (>400 cells/mm^3). The most consistent finding on chest radiograph is hyperinflation accompanied by minimal interstitial or alveolar infiltrates.

INFECTIONS AT OTHER SITES. Infants born to mothers with *C. trachomatis* may develop an infection in the rectum or vagina. Although infection in these sites appears to be totally asymptomatic, it may cause confusion if it is identified at a later date. Perinatally acquired rectal, vaginal, and nasopharyngeal infections may persist for ≥3 yr. *C. pneumoniae* can also be confused with *C. trachomatis* infection in nasopharyngeal cultures if a genus-specific monoclonal antibody is used to confirm the culture.

DIAGNOSIS. Definitive diagnosis is achieved by isolation of *C. trachomatis* in cultures of specimens obtained from the conjunctiva or nasopharynx. Several nonculture methods, using DFA and EIA, are approved for diagnosis of chlamydial conjunctivitis. These tests have sensitivities of ≥90% and specificities of ≥95% for conjunctival specimens compared with culture. Their accuracy for nasopharyngeal specimens is not as good. Data on use of NAATs in children are limited. Preliminary data suggest that PCR is equivalent to culture for detection of *C. trachomatis* in the conjunctiva and nasopharynx of infants with conjunctivitis.

Nonculture methods should never be used to test rectal or vaginal specimens obtained from children. Because all available EIA tests use genus-specific antibodies, these tests also detect *C. pneumoniae* if used for tests of respiratory specimens.

Treatment. The recommended treatment regimen for *C. trachomatis* conjunctivitis or pneumonia in infants is erythromycin (base or ethylsuccinate, 50 mg/kg/24 hr divided qid PO for 14 days). The rationale for using oral therapy for conjunctivitis is that 50% or more of these infants have concomitant nasopharyngeal infection or disease at other sites, and studies have demonstrated that topical therapy with sulfonamide drops and erythromycin ointment is not effective. The failure rate with oral erythromycin remains 10–20%, and some infants require a second course of treatment. The results of one small study suggest that a short course of azithromycin (20 mg/kg/24 hr once daily PO for 3 days) was as effective as 14 days of erythromycin. Mothers (and their sexual contacts) of infants with *C. trachomatis* infections should be empirically treated for genital infection. An association between treatment with oral erythromycin and infantile hypertrophic pyloric stenosis has been reported in infants younger than 6 wk of age who were given the drug for prophylaxis after nursery exposure to pertussis. Data on use of other macrolides (azithromycin or clarithromycin) for the treatment of neonatal chlamydia infection are limited.

Prevention. Neonatal gonococcal prophylaxis with topical erythromycin or tetracycline ointment, unlike silver nitrate, does not appear to prevent chlamydial ophthalmia. Neither agent prevents nasopharyngeal colonization with *C. trachomatis* or chlamydial pneumonia. The most effective method of controlling perinatal chlamydial infection appears to be screening and treatment of pregnant women. For treatment of *C. trachomatis* infection in pregnant women, the CDC currently recommends either erythromycin base (500 mg PO qid for 7 days) or amoxicillin (500 mg PO tid for 7 days) as first line regimens. Erythromycin base (250 mg PO qid for 14 days), erythromycin ethylsuccinate (800 mg qid for 7 days, or 400 mg PO qid for 14 days), and azithromycin (1 g PO as a single dose) are listed as alternative regimens. Reasons for failure of maternal treatment to prevent infantile chlamydial infection include poor compliance and reinfection from an untreated sexual partner.

208.4 Lymphogranuloma Venereum (LGV)

LGV is a systemic sexually transmitted disease caused by the L_1, L_2, and L_3 serotypes of the LGV biovar of *C. trachomatis*. Unlike strains of the trachoma biovar, LGV strains have a predilection for lymphoid tissue. About 20 cases of LGV have been reported in children, and fewer than 1,000 cases are reported in adults in the United States each year.

Clinical Manifestations. The first stage of LGV is characterized by the appearance of the primary lesion, a painless, usually transient papule on the genitals. The second stage is characterized by usually unilaterally femoral or inguinal lymphadenitis with enlarging, painful buboes. The nodes may break down and drain, especially in males. In females, the vulvar lymph drains to the retroperitoneal nodes. Fever, myalgia, and headache are common. In the tertiary stage, a genitoanorectal syndrome occurs, with rectovaginal fistulas, rectal strictures, and urethral destruction.

Diagnosis. LGV is diagnosed by culture of *C. trachomatis* from a specimen aspirated from a bubo or by serologic testing. Most patients with LGV have complement-fixing antibody titers of >1:16. Chancroid and herpes simplex virus can be distinguished clinically from LGV by the concurrent presence of painful genital ulcers. Syphilis can be differentiated by serologic tests. However, co-infections can occur.

Treatment. Doxycycline (100 mg PO bid for 21 days) is the recommended treatment. The alternative regimen is erythromycin base (500 mg PO qid for 21 days). Azithromycin (1 g PO once weekly for 3 weeks) may also be effective but clinical data are lacking. Sex partners of patients with LGV should be treated if they have had sexual contact with the patient during the 30 days preceding the onset of symptoms.

Bell TA, Stamm WE, Wang SP, et al: Chronic *Chlamydia trachomatis* infections in infants. *JAMA* 1992;267:400–2.

Black CM, Morse SA: The use of molecular techniques for the diagnosis and epidemiologic study of sexually transmitted infections. *Curr Infect Dis Rep* 2000;2:31–43.

Centers for Disease Control and Prevention: Sexually transmitted diseases treatment guidelines 2002. *MMWR* 2002;51(RR-6):1–80.

Centers for Disease Control and Prevention: Screening tests to detect *Chlamydia trachomatis* and *Neisseria gonorrhoeae* infections—2002. *MMWR* 2002;51(RR-15):1–37.

Cohen DA, Nsuami M, Martin DH, Farley TA: Repeated school-based screening for sexually transmitted diseases: a feasible strategy for reaching adolescents. *Pediatrics* 1999;104:1281–5.

Fraser-Hurt N, Bailey RL, Cousens S, et al: Efficacy of oral azithromycin versus topical tetracycline in mass treatment of endemic trachoma. *Bull World Health Organ* 2001;79:632–40.

Hammerschlag MR, Roblin PM, Gelling M, et al: Use of polymerase chain reaction for the detection of *Chlamydia trachomatis* in ocular and nasopharyngeal specimens from infants with conjunctivitis. *Pediatr Infect Dis J* 1997;16:293–7.

Hammerschlag MR, Gelling M, Roblin PM, et al: Treatment of neonatal chlamydial conjunctivitis with azithromycin. *Pediatr Infect Dis J* 1998;17:1049–50.

Tabbara KF: Trachoma: A review. *J Chemother* 2001;13(Suppl 1):18–22.

Van der Pol B, Ferrero DV, Buck-Barrington L, et al: Multicenter evaluation of the BD ProbeTec ET System for detection of *Chlamydia trachomatis* and *Neisseria gonorrhoeae* in urine specimens, female endocervical swabs and male urethral swabs. *J Clin Microbiol* 2001;39:1008–16.

Chapter 209
Psittacosis (*Chlamydia psittaci*)

Chlamydia psittaci, the cause of psittacosis (also known as **parrot fever** and **ornithosis**), is primarily an animal pathogen and causes human disease infrequently. In birds, *C. psittaci* infection is known as **avian chlamydiosis**.

Etiology. *C. psittaci* is a diverse species that affects nonpsittacine birds and many mammalian species as well. The known host range includes 15 mammalian species and 130 avian species representing 10 orders. The life cycle of *C. psittaci* is the same as that for *C. pneumoniae* (Chapter 207). The diversity of *C. psittaci* probably is a reflection of its wide host range; recent genomic analysis has suggested reorganizing the organism into four separate species in a new genus, *Chlamydophila*. Strains of *C. psittaci* have been analyzed by patterns of pathogenicity, inclusion morphology in tissue culture, DNA restriction endonuclease analysis, and monoclonal antibodies, which indicate that there are nine mammalian serovars, seven avian serovars, and two koala biovars. The mammalian strains differ greatly from avian strains in their antigenic characteristics. Two of the avian serovars, psittacine and turkey, are of major importance in the avian population of the United States. Each is associated with important host preferences and disease characteristics.

Epidemiology. From 1988 to 1998 there were 813 cases of psittacosis reported in the United States, and 85% of cases were associated with exposure to birds; 70% of these reported cases were the result of exposure to caged pet birds, which were usually psittacine birds including cockatiels, parakeets, parrots, and macaws. Among caged nonpsittacine birds, chlamydiosis occurs most frequently in pigeons, doves, and mynah birds. Persons at highest risk of acquiring psittacosis include bird fanciers and owners of pet birds (43% of cases) and pet shop employees (10% of cases).

Inhalation of aerosols from feces, fecal dust, and secretions of animals infected with *C. psittaci* is the primary route of infection. Source birds are either asymptomatic or have anorexia, ruffled feathers, lethargy, and watery green droppings. Psittacosis is uncommon in children, in part because children may be less likely to have close contact with infected birds. Several major outbreaks of psittacosis have occurred in turkey processing plants; workers exposed to turkey viscera are at the highest risk of infection.

Clinical Manifestations. Infection with *C. psittaci* in humans ranges from clinically inapparent to severe infection involving multiple organ systems as well as pneumonia. The mean incubation period is 15 days after exposure, with a range of 5–21 days. Onset of disease is usually abrupt with fever, cough, headache, and malaise. The fever is high and often is associated with rigors and sweats. The headache can be so severe that meningitis is considered. The cough is usually nonproductive. Crackles may be heard on auscultation. Chest radiographs are usually abnormal with variable infiltrates, and pleural effusions may be present. The white blood cell count is usually not elevated, but a mild leukocytosis may be present. Elevated levels of aspartate aminotransferase, alkaline phosphatase, and bilirubin are common.

Diagnosis. The diagnosis of psittacosis can be difficult because of the varying clinical presentations. A history of exposure to birds or association with an active case are important clues, but as many as 20% of patients with psittacosis have no known contact. Person-to-person spread has been suggested but not proved. Other infections that cause pneumonia with high fever, unusually severe headache, and myalgia include *Coxiella burnetii* (Q fever), *Mycoplasma pneumoniae*, *Chlamydia pneumoniae*, tularemia, tuberculosis, fungal infections, legionnaires' disease, and, most commonly, bacterial and viral respiratory infections.

The mainstay of diagnosis remains serology using the complement-fixation (CF) test, which is genus-specific. According to the 2000 recommendations from the Centers for Disease Control and Prevention, a confirmed case of psittacosis requires a compatible clinical illness, usually with a reliable history of avian exposure. Laboratory confirmation may be by one of the three following methods: (1) culture of *C. psittaci* from respiratory secretions; (2) a fourfold or greater increase in CF or microimmunofluorescence (MIF) titer in sera collected at least 2 wk apart; or (3) a single MIF IgM titer greater than or equal to 1:16. A probable case should be epidemiologically linked to a confirmed case or have a single CF or MIF antibody titer of 1:32 or more in at least one serum sample obtained after onset of symptoms. As with use of the MIF for diagnosis of *C. pneumoniae* infections, cross reactions with other *Chlamydia* species and bacteria can occur. Early treatment of psittacosis with tetracycline may abrogate the antibody response.

The organism can be also isolated by culture from sputum or pleural fluid. Although *C. psittaci* will grow in the same culture systems used for isolation of *C. trachomatis* and *C. pneumoniae*, very few laboratories culture for *C. psittaci*, mainly because of the potential biohazard.

Treatment. Recommended treatment regimens for psittacosis are doxycycline (100 mg PO bid) or tetracycline (500 mg PO qid) for at least 10–14 days after the fever abates. The initial treatment of severely ill patients is doxycycline hyclate (4.4 mg/kg/24 hr divided q 12 hr IV; maximum: 100 mg/dose). Erythromycin (500 mg qid PO) is an alternative drug if tetracyclines are contraindicated (e.g., children younger than 9 yr of age and pregnant women), but may be less effective. Remission is usually evident within 48–72 hours. Initial infection does not appear to be followed by long-term immunity. Reinfection and clinical disease can develop within 2 mo of treatment; there are two well-documented cases of reinfection reported.

Prognosis. The mortality of untreated psittacosis is 15–20%, but is <1% with appropriate treatment. Severe illness leading to respiratory failure and fetal death has been reported among pregnant women.

Prevention. Several control measures are recommended to prevent transmission of *C. psittaci* from birds. Bird handlers and avatars should be cognizant of the potential risk. *C. psittaci* is susceptible to most disinfectants and detergents as well as heat, but is resistant to acid and alkali. Accurate records of all bird-related transactions aid in identifying sources of infected birds and potentially exposed persons. Newly acquired birds, including birds that have been to shows, exhibitions, fairs, or other events, should be isolated for 30–45 days, or tested or treated prophylactically before adding them to a group of birds. Care should be taken to prevent transfer of fecal material, feathers, food, or other materials between birdcages. Birds with signs of avian chlamydiosis (e.g., ocular or nasal discharge, watery green droppings, or low body weight) should be isolated and should neither be sold nor purchased. Their handlers should wear protective clothing and a disposable surgical cap and use a respirator with an N95 or higher-efficiency rating (not a surgical mask) when handling them or cleaning their cages. Infected birds should be isolated until fully treated, which is generally 45 days.

Centers for Disease Control and Prevention: Compendium of measures to control *Chlamydia psittaci* infection among humans (psittacosis) and pet birds (avian chlamydiosis), 2000. *MMWR* 2000; 49(RR-8):1–17.

Moroney JF, Guevara R, Iverson C, et al: Detection of chlamydiosis in a shipment of pet birds, leading to recognition of an outbreak of clinically mild psittacosis in humans. *Clin Infect Dis* 1998;26:1425–9.

Wong KH, Skelton SK, Daugharty H: Utility of complement fixation and microimmunofluorescence assays for detecting serologic responses in patients with clinically diagnosed psittacosis. *J Clin Microbiol* 1994;32: 2417–21.

Yung AP, Grayson ML: Psittacosis: A review of 135 cases. *Med J Austr* 1988;148: 228–33.

SECTION 9 *Rickettsial Infections*

J. Stephen Dumler

Chapter 210

Spotted Fever Group Rickettsioses

Many members of the spotted fever group of rickettsiae are pathogenic for humans (Table 210–1). These include the tick-borne agents *Rickettsia rickettsii* (Rocky Mountain spotted fever [RMSF]), *R. conorii* (Mediterranean spotted fever [MSF] or boutonneuse fever), *R. sibirica* (North Asian tick typhus), *R. japonica* (Oriental spotted fever), *R. australis* (Queensland tick typhus), *R. honei* (Flinders Island spotted fever), *R. africae* (African tick bite fever), the unnamed Israeli spotted fever rickettsia, and possibly others. *R. akari* (rickettsialpox) is transmitted by the bite of a mite. Infections with the uncommon members of the spotted fever group rickettsiae present with signs similar to MSF (fever, maculopapular rash, and eschar at the initial site of tick attachment). Israeli spotted fever is generally associated with a more severe course, including fatalities in children. African tick typhus (*R. africae*) is relatively mild, often lacks disseminated rash, and usually presents with multiple eschars. In recent years, new rickettsial agents have been identified as potentially important pathogenic species, including *R. slovaca*, the cause of TIBOLA (tick-borne lymphadenopathy), and *R. felis*, a flea-transmitted murine typhus-like illness.

210.1 Rocky Mountain Spotted Fever (*Rickettsia rickettsii*)

RMSF is the most frequently identified rickettsial disease and the second most common vector-borne disease in the United States. RMSF is considered uncommon, but it is probably significantly underdiagnosed. Because it is a potentially rapidly fatal infection, RMSF should be considered in the differential diagnosis of fever, headache, and rash in the summer months, especially after tick exposure.

Etiology. RMSF is caused by systemic endothelial cell infection by the obligate intracellular bacterium *R. rickettsii*.

Epidemiology. The term *Rocky Mountain* spotted fever is a misnomer because only a small percentage of all documented cases are currently reported from the Rocky Mountain region. The disease occurs in almost every state of the continental United States, southwestern Canada, Mexico, Central America, and

TABLE 210–1. Rickettsial Diseases of Humans: Selected Agents and Summary of Pertinent Features

Group Disease	Causative Agent	Arthropod Vector-Transmission	Hosts	Confirmatory Tests	Geographic Distribution
Spotted Fever					
Rocky Mountain spotted fever	*Rickettsia rickettsii*	Tick bite	Dogs, rodents	IFA, DFA, IH	Western hemisphere
Mediterranean spotted fever (Boutonneuse fever)	*Rickettsia conorii*	Tick bite	Dogs, rodents	IFA, DFA, IH	Africa, Mediterranean region, India, Middle East
African tick-bite fever	*Rickettsia africae*	Tick bite	Cattle, goats?	IFA, DFA, IH	Sub-Saharan Africa, Caribbean
Rickettsialpox	*Rickettsia akari*	Mite bite	Mice	IFA, DFA, IH	North America, Russia, Ukraine, Adriatic region, Korea, South Africa
Murine typhus-like illness	*Rickettsia felis*	Flea bite	Opossums, cats, dogs	IFA, PCR	Western Hemisphere, Europe
Typhus					
Murine typhus	*Rickettsia typhi*	Rat flea or cat flea feces	Rats	IFA, DFA	Worldwide
Epidemic typhus	*Rickettsia prowazekii*	Louse feces	Humans	IFA	Africa, South America, Central America, Mexico, Asia
Brill-Zinsser disease (recrudescent typhus)	*Rickettsia prowazekii*	Reactivation of latent infection	Humans	IFA	Potentially worldwide; United States, Canada, Eastern Europe
Flying squirrel (sylvatic) typhus	*Rickettsia prowazekii*	Louse or flea of flying squirrel	Flying squirrels	IFA	United States
Scrub Typhus					
Scrub typhus	*Orientia tsutsugamushi*	Chigger bite	Rodents?	IFA	Southern Asia, Japan, Indonesia, Australia, Korea, Asiatic Russia, India, China
Ehrlichioses and Anaplasmosis					
Human monocytic ehrlichiosis	*Ehrlichia chaffeensis*	Tick bite	Deer, dogs	IFA, PCR	United States, Europe, Africa
Anaplasmosis (human granulocytic ehrlichiosis)	*Anaplasma phagocytophilum*	Tick bite	Rodents, deer, ruminants	IFA, PCR	United States, Europe
Ehrlichiosis "ewingii"	*Ehrlichia ewingii*	Tick bite	Dogs	IFA, PCR	United States
Sennetsu ehrlichiosis	*Neorickettsia sennetsu*	Ingestion of helminth-contaminated fish?	Unknown	IFA	Japan, Malaysia
Q fever					
Q fever	*Coxiella burnetii*	Inhalation of infected aerosols, ingestion of contaminated dairy products, ticks?	Cattle, sheep, goats, cats, rabbits	IFA	Worldwide

South America. In 1999, most cases were reported from North Carolina, Tennessee, South Carolina, Georgia, Maryland, Oklahoma, Arkansas, and Virginia; however, the changing ecology of tick vectors influences the geographic prevalence over time. The incidence of RMSF varies in a cyclical pattern over decades, the last peak occurring approximately in 1981; since 1996, the average annual number of cases reported to the Centers for Disease Control and Prevention (CDC) has fluctuated around 500 cases/yr. Habitat associations with disease are predicted by those favored by tick vectors including wooded areas or coastal grassland and salt marshes. Foci of intense infection have also been well documented in rural and some urban settings such as the South Bronx, and local abundance of infected ticks may predispose to clusters of cases even in single families. In the United States, 90% of cases occur during seasons of peak tick activity and potential human exposure, between April and September. The highest age-specific incidence of RMSF is among children <10 yr of age.

TRANSMISSION. Ticks are the natural hosts, reservoirs, and vectors of *R. rickettsii*. Ticks maintain the infection naturally by **transovarial transmission** (passage of the organism from infected ticks to their progeny) with a high rate of fecundity; thus, horizontal transmission by acquisition of rickettsiae when a blood meal is taken from transiently rickettsemic animal hosts such as small mammals or dogs is a significant mechanism for enzootic maintenance of infection. Many species of ticks are capable of sustaining and transmitting the infectious agent to mammalian hosts by regurgitation of infected saliva during feeding. The principal tick hosts of *R. rickettsii* are *Dermacentor variabilis*

(the American dog tick) in the eastern United States and Canada, *D. andersoni* (the wood tick) in the western United States and Canada, *Rhipicephalus sanguineus* (the brown dog tick) in Mexico, and *Amblyomma cajennense* in Central and South America.

Dogs may also serve as reservoir hosts for *R. rickettsii* and are important vehicles for bringing potentially infected ticks into the environment shared by humans. Serologic studies of patients with RMSF indicate that a high percentage may have contracted the illness from ticks carried by the family dog. Infection is largely transmitted by way of the bite of an infected tick; however, transmission can occur by inoculation of tick fluids or feces into open wounds or conjunctivae from the fingers and hands. Fatalities have occurred in laboratory workers exposed to infectious aerosols.

Pathogenesis. Lesions are most obvious on the skin, but are systemically distributed, affecting nearly all organs and tissues. Following inoculation into the dermis, the rickettsiae attach to the vascular endothelium via protein ligands and initiate host cell membrane injury due to rickettsial phospholipase activity. The membrane damage induces phagocytosis and the internalized rickettsia then gains access to the cytosol by continued vacuolar membrane lysis. Members of the spotted fever serologic group actively initiate intracellular actin polymerization to achieve directional movement, and rickettsiae can thus easily invade neighboring cells while inducing minimal initial host cell damage. The rickettsiae proliferate and damage the host cell by peroxidative membrane alterations, protease activation, or continued phospholipase activity.

Initially, a perivascular infiltrate of lymphoid and histiocytic cells and edema without significant endothelial damage is present, coinciding with the development of macules and maculopapules. Proliferation of rickettsiae within endothelial cell cytoplasm leads to lymphohistiocytic or leukocytoclastic vasculitis of small venules and capillaries that results in the formation of petechial skin lesions and microvascular leakage, tissue hypoperfusion, and end-organ ischemic injury. Rickettsiae are localized within endothelial cells of inflamed vessels that may be eccentrically involved, including infrequent nonocclusive thrombi; small and large vessels rarely become completely obliterated by thrombosis, leading to tissue infarction or hemorrhagic necrosis. Sequelae result from interstitial pneumonitis and vascular leakage in the lungs, leading to noncardiogenic pulmonary edema, or from meningoencephalitis, leading to cerebral edema.

The presence of the infectious agent initiates the inflammatory cascade including release of cytokines such as tumor necrosis factor-α (TNFα), interleukin-1β, and interferon gamma (IFN-γ). Infection of endothelial cells by *R. rickettsii* induces surface E-selectin expression and procoagulant activity. Cytokine release and vascular selectin expression result in infiltration of the damaged endothelial cells by lymphocytes, macrophages, and occasionally neutrophils. Local inflammatory and immune responses have been suspected as contributors to vascular injury in the rickettsioses; however, the benefits of effective inflammation and immunity outweigh any potential damage mediated by host responses directed toward elimination of local infection. Blockade of TNFα and IFN-γ action in animal models diminishes survival and increases the morbidity of spotted fever group infections, probably by abrogating upregulation of nitric oxide synthase and arginine-dependent intracellular killing events. Important mediators for control of infection include direct contact of infected endothelial cells with CD8 T lymphocytes that produce perforin and NK cells that produce IFN-γ. *Rickettsia* infection leads to upregulated expression of procoagulant molecules on the surfaces of infected endothelial cells. This is associated with induction of tissue plasminogen activator inhibitor and reduction in plasminogen activator levels that promote coagulation factor consumption, platelet adhesion, and leukocyte emigration and may result in a clinical syndrome similar to disseminated intravascular coagulation.

Clinical Manifestations. The incubation period in children varies from 2–14 days, with a median of 7 days. The illness is initially nonspecific with headache, fever, anorexia, myalgias, and restlessness. Gastrointestinal symptoms including nausea, vomiting, diarrhea, and abdominal pain occur frequently (39–63%)

early in the disease. Often considered the hallmark of rickettsial infection, skin rash is detected usually after the 3rd day of illness, and the typical clinical triad of headache, fever, and rash that is observed in 44% of patients overall is documented in only 3% of all patients at presentation. Approximately 10–15% of patients never develop rash or have atypical cutaneous manifestations. The site of the tick bite is usually inapparent. Discrete, pale, rose-red blanching macules or maculopapules appear initially, characteristically on the extremities, including the ankles, wrists, or lower legs (Fig. 210–1A). The rash then spreads rapidly to involve the entire body, including the soles and palms. After several days, the rash becomes more petechial or hemorrhagic, sometimes with palpable purpura (see Fig. 210–1B). Fever and headache persist and are accompanied by severe myalgia and malaise. Splenomegaly and hepatomegaly are present in approximately 33% of patients. In severe disease, the petechiae may enlarge into ecchymoses, which may become necrotic. Severe vascular obstruction secondary to the rickettsial vasculitis and thrombosis is infrequent but may result in gangrene of the digits, earlobes, scrotum, nose, or an entire limb. Central nervous system infection often produces changes in the sensorium, and delirium or coma may supervene. In addition, patients may manifest ataxia, meningismus, or auditory deficits. Other severe manifestations include facial edema, myocarditis, acute renal failure, vascular collapse, and pneumonitis with noncardiogenic pulmonary edema.

Fulminant RMSF, defined as *R. rickettsii* infection leading to death in <5 days, may occur, especially among persons with glucose-6-phosphate dehydrogenase (G6PD) deficiency. The clinical course of fulminant RMSF is characterized by profound coagulopathy and extensive visceral thrombosis with kidney, liver, or respiratory failure. Clinical features associated with a fatal outcome include hepatomegaly, jaundice, stupor, acute renal failure, respiratory distress, and a disseminated intravascular coagulation–like syndrome in the absence of host inflammatory response.

Diagnosis. Severe or fatal rickettsial infections are associated with delays in diagnosis and treatment. The diagnosis of RMSF should be considered in patients presenting during the spring through fall with an acute febrile illness accompanied by headache and myalgia, particularly if they were exposed to ticks in known endemic regions, were in forested or tick-infested rural areas, or had contact with a dog. A history of tick exposure and the appearance of a rash, especially on the palms or soles, together with laboratory findings of normal or low leukocyte count with a marked left shift, a relatively low or decreasing

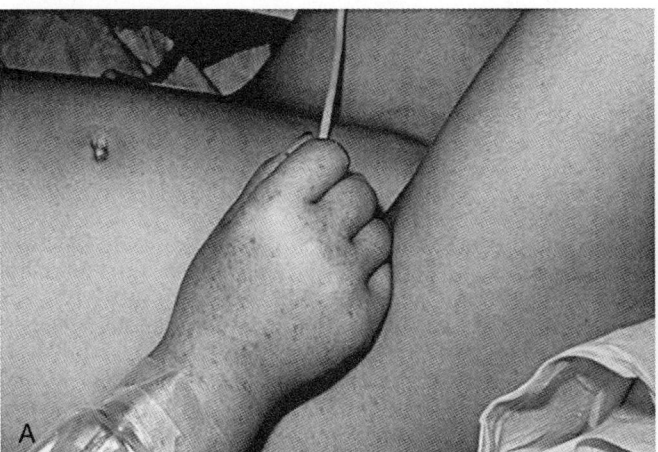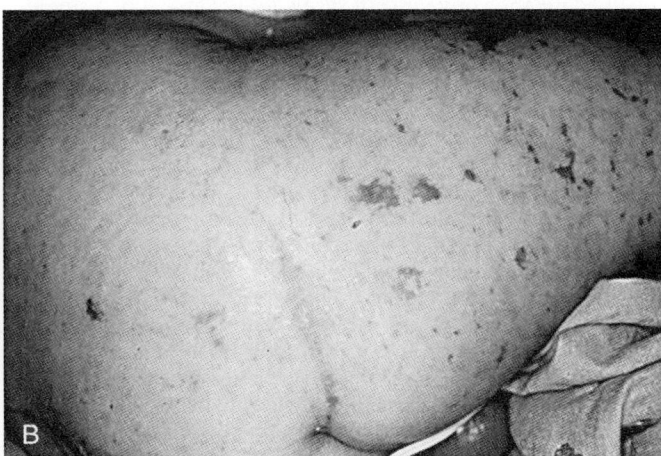

FIGURE 210–1. Patient with Rocky Mountain spotted fever. *A*, Rash early in the illness that is prominent on the extremities. *B*, Later in the course of Rocky Mountain spotted fever, the rash may become hemorrhagic or purpuric. (Courtesy of Debra Karp Skopicki, MD.) See also color plates.

platelet count, and a low serum sodium concentration, are clues that are sometimes helpful in distinguishing RMSF from some other acute infections. In patients with no rash or in dark-skinned individuals in whom a rash may be difficult to appreciate, the diagnosis may be exceptionally elusive and delayed. One half of pediatric fatalities occur within 9 days of onset of symptoms. On occasion, rickettsial vascular infection predominates in a single organ or system, erroneously suggesting a localized process such as appendicitis or cholecystitis. A thorough evaluation usually reveals evidence of a systemic process and can avoid unnecessary surgical intervention.

An abnormally low platelet count, normal to slightly low leukocyte count, and low serum sodium concentration are present in about half of patients and may be early clues to the diagnosis. Most other clinical laboratory findings are nonspecific and vary depending on the degree of specific organ involvement. RMSF may cause meningoencephalitis that presents with a cerebrospinal fluid pleocytosis with a predominance of mononuclear cells. However, no single laboratory test completely establishes an early diagnosis. Thus, treatment should not be withheld pending laboratory results for a patient with clinically suspected illness.

If a rash is present, a vasculotropic rickettsial infection can be diagnosed as early as day 3 of illness by immunohistologic demonstration of specific rickettsial antigen in the endothelium in skin biopsies of petechial lesions. The procedure may be performed by immunofluorescence or immunoperoxidase and is very specific. However, the sensitivity of this method is probably not greater than 70%, and it can be adversely influenced by prior antimicrobial therapy, suboptimal biopsy of skin lesions, and examination of insufficient tissue because the infection may be very focal. Moreover, selection of an appropriate biopsy site may be difficult because approximately 10–15% of patients with RMSF either do not have a rash or have an atypical rash. Evaluation of blood for *R. rickettsii* nucleic acids by polymerase chain reaction demonstrates little sensitivity beyond that of immunohistology, probably because the level of rickettsemia is generally very low (<6 rickettsia/mL).

Radiologic evaluations often reveal no significant abnormalities, and when present on CT or MR neuroimaging studies, the findings are generally subtle and do not alter treatment. However, in one series, 17% of patients with radiologic abnormalities (e.g., cerebral edema, meningeal enhancement, and prominent perivascular spaces) died of RMSF.

Because treatment must be initiated on the clinical diagnosis alone, confirmation is most often accomplished by serologic tests. Diagnostic serologic criteria include a fourfold increase in antibody titer, usually by indirect fluorescent antibody (IFA) assay, in acute and convalescent sera (2–4 wk apart) or a single elevated IFA titer of ≥1:64 in convalescent serum. A case is considered probable if a single titer of ≥1:128 is found. Weil-Felix antibody testing should not be performed because it lacks both sensitivity and specificity.

DIFFERENTIAL DIAGNOSIS. Other rickettsial infections are easily confused with RMSF, especially all forms of human ehrlichiosis and murine typhus. RMSF can mimic many diseases; among the most important of these are meningococcemia, measles, and enteroviral exanthemas. Negative blood cultures may aid in reaching a correct diagnosis. However, *R. rickettsii* may cause aseptic meningitis and elicit lymphocytic pleocytosis, suggesting a viral etiology and further confounding the diagnosis. Other diseases sometimes included in the differential diagnosis are typhoid fever, secondary syphilis, Lyme disease, leptospirosis, scarlet fever, toxic shock syndrome, rheumatic fever, rubella, Kawasaki disease, idiopathic thrombocytopenic purpura, thrombotic thrombocytopenic purpura, Henoch-Schönlein purpura, hemolytic uremic syndrome, aseptic meningitis, acute gastrointestinal illness, acute abdomen, hepatitis, infectious mononucleosis, dengue fever, and drug reactions.

Treatment. The time-proven effective therapies for RMSF are tetracycline and chloramphenicol. Both agents have drawbacks for pediatric therapy in that tetracycline and doxycycline may be associated with tooth discoloration, whereas chloramphenicol is associated rarely with aplastic anemia. Recent controversial evaluations reveal that mortality is significantly increased when chloramphenicol alone is used compared with tetracycline alone, even when other factors such as severity are considered. Moreover, chloramphenicol is no longer available as an oral preparation in the United States. Doxycycline can be used for RMSF safely in children younger than 9 yr of age, because tooth discoloration is dose-dependent, and it is unlikely that children younger than 9 yr of age will require multiple courses.

Greater morbidity and excess mortality are associated with sulfonamide therapy, which is discouraged. Other antibiotics including penicillins, cephalosporins, and aminoglycosides are not effective. The use of alternative antimicrobial agents such as quinolones and the new macrolides (azithromycin and clarithromycin) for RMSF has not been evaluated.

Recommended treatment regimens for RMSF are doxycycline orally or intravenously (two loading doses of 2.2 mg/kg/dose at 12-hr intervals followed by 2.2 mg/kg/24 hr divided q 12 hr PO or IV; maximum: 300 mg/dose); tetracycline orally (25–50 mg/kg/24 hr divided q 6 hr PO; maximum: 2 g/24 hr); or chloramphenicol intravenously (50–100 mg/kg/24 hr divided q 6 hr IV; maximum: 3 g/24 hr), which must be monitored to maintain serum concentrations between 10 and 30 μg/mL. Therapy should be continued for a minimum of 5 days and until the patient has been afebrile for at least 2–4 days to avoid relapse, especially in patients who were treated early. Patients treated with one of these regimens usually become afebrile within 48 hr, and thus the entire period of therapy usually lasts <10 days.

SUPPORTIVE CARE. Most infections resolve rapidly with appropriate antimicrobial therapy and do not require hospitalization or other supportive care. On occasion, severe infections require intensive care. Particular attention to hemodynamic status is required in severely ill children because iatrogenic pulmonary or cerebral edema is easy to precipitate given pre-existing diffuse microvascular lung and meningovascular and cerebrovascular injury. Judicious use of corticosteroids for meningoencephalitis has been advocated by some, although no controlled trials have been conducted.

Complications. Complications of RMSF include noncardiogenic pulmonary edema from pulmonary microvascular leakage, cerebral edema from meningoencephalitis, and multiorgan damage (hepatitis, pancreatitis, cholecystitis, epidermal necrosis, and gangrene) partly mediated by rickettsial vasculitis or the accumulated effects of hypoperfusion and ischemia (acute renal failure). Long-term neurologic sequelae are more likely to occur in patients who have been hospitalized for ≥2 weeks and include paraparesis, hearing loss, peripheral neuropathy, bladder and bowel incontinence, cerebellar, vestibular, and motor dysfunction, and language disorders.

Prognosis. Delays in diagnosis and therapy are significant factors associated with death or severe illness. Before the advent of effective antimicrobial therapy for RMSF, the case fatality rate was 10–40%. CDC statistics suggest stabilization of this rate between 2% and 7%; however, a case fatality rate of 8.5% was documented in Texas from 1986 through 1996. Evidence exists that diagnosis based upon serology alone underestimates the true mortality of RMSF. Fatalities occur despite the availability of effective therapeutic agents, indicating the need for vigilant clinical suspicion and a low threshold for early and aggressive therapy in clinically suspected cases. Even with administration of appropriate antimicrobials, delayed therapy may allow irreversible vascular or end-organ damage and long-term sequelae or death. Early therapy in uncomplicated cases ordinarily leads to rapid defervescence within 1–3 days and recovery within 7–10 days.

Prevention. No vaccines are available. Prevention of RMSF is best accomplished by eliminating tick infestations of dogs, avoiding wooded or grassy areas where ticks reside, using insect repellents containing DEET, wearing protective clothing, and carefully inspecting children who have been playing in the woods or fields.

Prompt and complete removal of attached ticks helps reduce the risk of transmission because reactivation to virulence of rickettsiae in the tick requires at least several hours to days of exposure to body heat or blood. Contrary to popular belief, the application of petroleum jelly, 70% isopropyl alcohol, fingernail polish, or a hot match are not effective in removing ticks from persons or animals. A tick can be safely removed by grasping the mouthparts with a pair of forceps at the site of cutaneous contact and applying gentle and steady retraction to remove the entire tick and mouth parts. The site of attachment should then be disinfected. Ticks should not be squeezed or crushed because their fluids may be infectious. Tick disposal should be accomplished by soaking the tick in alcohol or flushing it down the toilet, followed by good hand washing. Prophylactic antimicrobial therapy should not be administered because tetracyclines and chloramphenicol are only rickettsiostatic; such therapy simply delays the onset of illness and confuses the clinical picture by prolonging the incubation period.

210.2 Mediterranean Spotted Fever or Boutonneuse Fever (*Rickettsia conorii*)

The disease caused by *R. conorii* is known by various geographically recognized names, including Mediterranean spotted fever, or MSF, boutonneuse fever, Kenya tick typhus, and Indian tick typhus. It is a moderately severe vasculotropic rickettsiosis that is often initially associated with an eschar at the site of the tick bite

Etiology. MSF is caused by systemic endothelial cell infection by the obligate intracellular bacterium *R. conorii*. Similar illnesses are distributed globally but are caused by distinct yet related species including *R. sibirica* in Russia, China, Mongolia, and Pakistan, *R. australis* or *R. honei* in Australia, *R. japonica* in Japan, and *R. africae* in South Africa (see Table 210–1). These species are closely related to *R. rickettsii* by analysis of antigens and DNA sequences.

Epidemiology. *R. conorii* is distributed over a large geographic region including India, Pakistan, Russia, Ukraine, Georgia, Israel, Ethiopia, Kenya, South Africa, Morocco, and southern Europe.

MSF has demonstrated a steadily increasing incidence since 1980 in southern Europe and has reached seroprevalence rates of 11–26% in some areas. The peak incidence is seen during July and August in the Mediterranean basin, but in other regions it occurs during warm seasons when ticks are active. Many cases of imported infection have been documented in travelers to endemic regions, especially those who go on safari in regions with high grass and bush land.

TRANSMISSION. Transmission occurs after the bite of the brown dog tick, *R. sanguineus*, or other tick species including *Dermacentor, Haemaphysalis, Amblyomma, Hyalomma,* and *Ixodes.* A strong correlation exists among the incidence of boutonneuse fever, infected ticks, and evidence of infection in both dogs and humans, implicating the household dog as a potential vehicle for transmission.

Pathogenesis. The underlying pathology for MSF is nearly identical to that of RMSF, except that eschars are often identified at the primary site of tick bite and inoculation of the rickettsiae.

The histopathology of the tick bite lesion includes necrosis of dermal and epidermal tissues with a superficial crust, and dermal structures are densely infiltrated by lymphocytes, histiocytes, and scattered neutrophils, among damaged capillaries and venules. Immunohistochemical stains confirm that the lesions contain rickettsia-infected endothelial cells, although the remnant structure of the vasculature may not be apparent owing to the extensive inflammation and necrosis. The necrosis results from both direct rickettsia-mediated vasculitis and extensive local inflammation. Rickettsiae released at this site have ready access to lymphatics or venous blood and disseminate to cause a systemic infection.

Clinical Manifestations. Patients with MSF typically experience fever, headache, myalgias, and a maculopapular rash, which appears 3–5 days after onset of symptoms. In about 70% of patients, an eschar, the tache noire, at the initial site of tick attachment and regional lymphadenopathy are present. Although it was previously considered benign and self-limited, this infection may cause severe disease in up to 6% of infected individuals. It is characterized by findings similar to RMSF, including purpuric skin lesions, neurologic signs, respiratory distress, acute renal failure, severe thrombocytopenia, and death in 1.4–5.6% of cases. As with RMSF, a particularly malignant form occurs in patients with G6PD deficiency and in individuals with other underlying conditions such as alcoholic liver disease or diabetes mellitus.

Diagnosis. Laboratory diagnosis of MSF and the other spotted fever group rickettsioses is the same as that for Rocky Mountain spotted fever and may be accomplished by immunohistologic demonstration of rickettsiae on skin biopsy, immunocytologic demonstration of *R. conorii* (and potentially other spotted fever group rickettsiae) in circulating endothelial cells, in vitro cultivation by means of centrifugation-assisted shell vial tissue culture, or the demonstration of serum antibodies to spotted fever group rickettsiae in convalescent patients. Reagents useful for the diagnosis of RMSF in the United States or MSF in Europe, Africa, and Asia can be used effectively for the diagnosis of infections by most members of the spotted fever group of rickettsiae.

DIFFERENTIAL DIAGNOSIS. The differential diagnosis is similar to that of RMSF with the inclusion of conditions associated with single eschars that may be seen also with other rickettsioses such as rickettsialpox, African tick-bite fever, or scrub typhus. The recently described spotted fever rickettsia, *R. africae*, causes a milder illness and is often associated with multiple eschars; it may be observed in African locations where MSF also occurs.

Treatment. MSF is effectively treated with tetracycline, doxycycline, chloramphenicol, ciprofloxacin, ofloxacin, pefloxacin, levofloxacin, azithromycin, or clarithromycin. Regimens for doxycycline, tetracycline, and chloramphenicol are as described for RMSF. Azithromycin (10 mg/kg/24 hr once daily PO) and clarithromycin (15 mg/kg/24 hr divided bid PO) are alternatives. Specific quinolone regimens effective for children have not been established. Intensive care may be required for hemodynamic management of severely affected individuals.

Complications. The complications of MSF are similar to those of RMSF. The case fatality rate is approximately 2%. Particularly severe infections have been noted in patients with underlying medical conditions including G6PD deficiency and diabetes mellitus.

Prevention. MSF is transmitted by tick bites, and prevention is the same as recommended for RMSF. No vaccine is currently available.

210.3 Rickettsialpox (*Rickettsia akari*)

Rickettsialpox is caused by *R. akari*, which is transmitted by the mouse mite, *Allodermanyssus sanguineus*. The mouse host for this mite is widely distributed in cities in the United States, Europe, and Asia. Seroepidemiologic studies suggest a high prevalence for this infection in urban settings; however, the disease is usually mild and is infrequently diagnosed. Unlike most forms of spotted fever rickettsiosis, an important target cell for infection is the macrophage.

Rickettsialpox is best known because of its association with a varicelliform rash. In fact, this rash is a modified form of an antecedent typical macular or maculopapular rash like those seen in other vasculotropic rickettsioses. At presentation, most patients have fever, headache, and chills. There may be a papular or ulcerative lesion at the initial site of inoculation in up to 90% of cases, which may be associated with regional lymphadenopathy. In some patients, the maculopapular rash, which is distributed over the trunk, head, and extremities, may become vesicular. The infection resolves spontaneously even without therapy. Complications and fatalities are rare.

Abramson JS, Givner LB: Rocky Mountain spotted fever. *Pediatr Infect Dis J* 1999; 18:539–40.

Billings AN, Rawlings JA, Walker DH: Tick-borne disease in Texas: A 10-year retrospective examination of cases. *Tex Med* 1998;94:66–76.

Centers for Disease Control and Prevention: Consequences of delayed diagnosis of Rocky Mountain spotted fever in children—West Virginia, Michigan, Tennessee, and Oklahoma, May–July 2000. *MMWR Morb Mortal Wkly Rep* 2000;49:885–8.

Comer JA, Tzianabos T, Flynn C, et al: Serologic evidence of rickettsialpox (*Rickettsia akari*) infection among intravenous drug users in inner-city Baltimore, Maryland. *Am J Trop Med Hyg* 1999;60:894–8.

Holman RC, Paddock CD, Curns AT, et al: Analysis of risk factors for fatal Rocky Mountain spotted fever: Evidence for superiority of tetracyclines for therapy. *J Infect Dis* 2001;184:1437–44.

Kass EM, Szaniawski WK, Levy H, et al: Rickettsialpox in a New York City Hospital, 1980 to 1989. *N Engl J Med* 1994;331:1612–7.

Thorner AR, Walker DH, Petri WA: Rocky Mountain spotted fever. *Clin Infect Dis* 1998;27:1353–9.

Treadwell TA, Holman RC, Clarke MJ, et al: Rocky Mountain spotted fever in the United States, 1993–1996. *Am J Trop Med Hyg* 2000;63:21–6.

Walker DH: Tick-transmitted infectious diseases in the United States. *Annu Rev Public Health* 1998;19:237–69.

Chapter 211

Scrub Typhus (*Orientia tsutsugamushi*)

Scrub typhus is a common and important febrile infectious disease in many parts of the eastern hemisphere. Recent reports suggest that natural resistance to doxycycline and other antibiotics make selection of appropriate antimicrobial therapy difficult. Some evidence suggests that concurrent scrub typhus may inhibit the replication of HIV.

Etiology. The causative agent of scrub typhus, or Tsutsugamushi fever, is *Orientia tsutsugamushi*, which is distinct from other spotted fever and typhus group rickettsiae. *O. tsutsugamushi* lacks both lipopolysaccharide and peptidoglycan in its cell wall. Like other vasculotropic *Rickettsia*, *O. tsutsugamushi* infects endothelium and elicits vasculitis, the predominant clinicopathologic feature of the disease. However, the organism also infects cardiac myocytes and macrophages, raising questions about how these findings may explain the clinical manifestations.

Epidemiology. Approximately 1 million infections occur each year, and it is estimated that more than 1 billion people are at risk. Scrub typhus occurs mostly in the Far East, including areas delimited by a triangle connecting Korea, Pakistan, and northern Australia. Aside from infections in these tropical and subtropical regions, the disease occurs in Japan, the Primorye of far eastern Russia, Tajikistan, Nepal, and nontropical China includ-

ing Tibet. Cases imported to the United States and other parts of the world are reported.

TRANSMISSION. *O. tsutsugamushi* is transmitted via the bite of the larval stage (chigger) of a trombiculid mite (*Leptotrombidium*), which serves as both vector and reservoir. Transovarial transmission (passage of the organism from infected ticks to their progeny) occurs efficiently, and transmission of the organism to mites from infected animals is poor; however, a role for horizontal transmission from infected rodent hosts to uninfected mites has not been disproved. Multiple serotypes are recognized, and some share antigenic cross reactivity.

Pathogenesis. The pathogenesis of scrub typhus is uncertain. Recent studies inidicate that the process is stimulated by a disseminated rickettsial infection of vascular endothelial cells that corresponds to the distribution of disseminated vasculitic and perivascular inflammatory lesions observed in histopathologic examinations. The major result of the vascular injury appears in autopsy series to be hemorrhage. However, it is very likely that the vascular injury initiated by the rickettsial infection results in significant vascular leakage and compromise and is further confounded by the waxing immune and inflammatory reactions. The net result is significant vascular compromise and ensuing end-organ injury, most often manifest in the brain and lungs, as with other vasculotropic rickettsioses.

Clinical Manifestations. Scrub typhus may be mild or severe. After an incubation period of 6–21 days, the rickettsiae proliferate at the site of the chigger bite to form in <50% of cases a necrotic eschar with an erythematous rim. The onset of illness usually becomes manifest by fever, headache, and sometimes myalgia, cough, and gastrointestinal symptoms. Regional or generalized lymphadenopathy is common. A maculopapular rash is present in <50% of patients and involves the trunk and extremities and infrequently the hands or face. Complications include severe meningoencephalitis, myocarditis, and interstitial pneumonitis. The case fatality rate in untreated patients may be as high as 30%.

Diagnosis. The diagnosis is usually confirmed by indirect fluorescent antibody assay or immunoperoxidase serologic tests using various serotypes of *O. tsutsugamushi* as antigen. The differential diagnosis includes other rickettsioses, tularemia, anthrax, dengue, leptospirosis, typhoid fever, malaria, and infectious mononucleosis.

Treatment. Recommended treatment regimens for scrub typhus are doxycycline orally or intravenously (two loading doses of 2.2 mg/kg/dose at 12-hr intervals followed by 2.2 mg/kg/24 hr divided q 12 hr PO or IV; maximum: 300 mg/dose); tetracycline orally (25–50 mg/kg/24 hr divided q 6 hr PO; maximum: 2 g/24 hr); or chloramphenicol intravenously (50–100 mg/kg/24 hr divided q 6 hr IV; maximum: 3 g/24 hr), which must be monitored to maintain serum concentrations between 10 and 30 µg/mL. Therapy should be continued for a minimum of 5 days and until the patient has been afebrile for at least 2–4 days to avoid relapse, especially in patients who were treated early. Patients treated with one of these regimens usually become afebrile within 48 hr, and thus the entire period of therapy usually lasts <10 days.

Some reports suggest that more virulent or potentially doxycycline-resistant strains may have emerged. Recent clinical trials have shown, in regions where doxycycline resistance is frequent, that azithromycin may be as effective, and that rifampicin is superior to doxycycline. Intensive care may be required for hemodynamic management of severely affected individuals.

Complications. Serious complications of scrub typhus include pneumonitis, acute respiratory distress syndrome, acute renal failure, myocarditis, a septic shock-like syndrome, encephalomyelitis, and death.

Prevention. Prevention is based on avoidance of the chiggers that transmit *O. tsutsugamushi*. Protective clothing is the next most useful mode of prevention. No vaccine is currently available.

Pai H, Sohn S, Seong Y, et al: Central nervous system involvement in patients with scrub typhus. *Clin Infect Dis* 1997;24:436–40.

Silpapojakul K, Chupuppakam S, Yuthasompob S, et al: Scrub and murine typhus in children with obscure fever in the tropics. *Pediatr Infect Dis J* 1991;10:200–3.

Tsay RW, Chang FY: Serious complications in scrub typhus. *J Microbiol Immunol Infect* 1998;31:240–4.

Wang CL, Yang KD, Cheng SN, et al: Neonatal scrub typhus: A case report. *Pediatrics* 1992;89:965–8.

Watt G, Kantipong P, de Souza M, et al: HIV-1 suppression during acute scrub-typhus infection. *Lancet* 2000;356:475–9.

Watt G, Kantipong P, Jongsakul K, et al: Doxycycline and rifampicin for mild scrub-typhus infections in northern Thailand: A randomised trial. *Lancet* 2000; 356:1057–61.

Chapter 212
Typhus Group Rickettsioses

Members of the typhus group of rickettsiae pathogenic for humans (see Table 210–1) include *Rickettsia typhi* (murine typhus) and *R. prowazekii* (epidemic typhus). *R. typhi* is flea-transmitted, whereas *R. prowazekii* is transmitted to humans in the feces of body lice. Epidemic typhus (*R. prowazekii*) is widely considered to be the most virulent of all *Rickettsia*, with a high mortality rate even with treatment. Murine typhus is moderately severe and perhaps one of the most under-recognized infections in the world. The entire genome of *R. prowazekii* has been sequenced, allowing a number of novel observations regarding genes required for obligate intracellular bacterial life.

212.1 Murine Typhus (*Rickettsia typhi*)

Etiology. Murine typhus is caused by *Rickettsia typhi*, a rickettsia that is transmitted from infected fleas to rats or opossums and back to fleas. Transovarial transmission (passage of the organism from infected ticks to their progeny) in fleas is inefficient, and thus, transmission depends on distribution by the flea to uninfected mammals, which become transiently rickettsemic and, in turn, transmit the organism to uninfected fleas.

A novel agent within the genus *Rickettsia* has been identified as a cause of a murine typhus–like illness in south Texas and is recognized increasingly worldwide. This new rickettsia, *R. felis*, is genetically a spotted fever group rickettsia and is capable of highly efficient transovarial transmission in cat fleas. This organism is found in cat fleas obtained from areas endemic for murine typhus in the United States.

Epidemiology. Murine typhus has a worldwide distribution and occurs especially in warm coastal ports where it is maintained in a cycle involving rat fleas (*Xenopsylla cheopis*) and rats (*Rattus* species). Peak incidence occurs when rat populations are highest during spring, summer, and fall. In the United States, the disease is most prevalent in south Texas and southern California, although sporadic cases have been reported in most other states as well. In the coastal areas of south Texas, the disease is seen predominantly from March through June and is associated with opossums, cats, and cat fleas (*Ctenocephalides felis*). Seroepidemiologic testing has shown a high prevalence in southeastern U.S. urban settings, expanding the endemic areas in which pediatricians must be alert for this infection.

TRANSMISSION. Human acquisition of murine typhus occurs when rickettsiae-infected flea feces contaminate flea bite wounds.

Pathogenesis. *R. typhi* is a vasculotropic rickettsial species that causes disease in much the same way as does *R. rickettsii* (Chapter 225.1). *R. typhi* organisms in flea feces deposited on the skin as part of the flea feeding reflex are inoculated into the pruritic flea bite wound. After an interval during which local proliferation occurs, the rickettsiae spread systemically to infect the endothelium in many tissues. As with spotted fever group rickettsiae, typhus group rickettsiae infect endothelial cells but polymerize actin poorly for intracellular mobility and probably cause cellular injury by mechanical lysis owing to the accumulation of large numbers of rickettsiae within the endothelial cell cytoplasm. Intracellular infection leads to endothelial cell damage and recruitment of inflammatory cells and vasculitis. The inflammatory cell infiltrates bring in a number of effector cells, including macrophages that produce proinflammatory cytokines, and CD4, CD8, and NK lymphocytes, which may produce immune cytokines such as interferon-γ or participate in cell-mediated cytotoxic responses. Intracellular rickettsial proliferation of typhus group rickettsiae is inhibited by cytokine-mediated, nitric oxide–dependent and –independent mechanisms.

Pathologic findings include the presence of systemic vasculitis in response to the presence of rickettsiae within endothelial cells. This is manifest as interstitial pneumonitis, interstitial nephritis, myocarditis, meningitis, and mild hepatitis with periportal lymphohistiocytic infiltrates. As vasculitis and inflammatory damage accumulate, multiorgan damage may ensue.

Clinical Manifestations. Murine typhus is a moderately severe infection that is similar to other vasculotropic rickettsioses. The infection in children generally appears to be mild. The incubation period may vary from 1–2 wk. The initial presentation is often nonspecific, with fever of undetermined origin the most frequent presentation. Pediatric patients exhibit the typically important clues for murine typhus somewhat less frequently than for the other vasculotropic rickettsioses, including rash (48–80%), myalgias (29–57%), vomiting (29–45%), cough (15–40%), headache (19–77%), and diarrhea or abdominal pain (10–40%). Although neurologic involvement may be a frequent finding in adults with murine typhus, photophobia, confusion, stupor, coma, seizures, meningismus, and ataxia are seen in <17% of hospitalized and <6% of infected children treated as outpatients. A petechial rash is observed in only up to 13% of children, and the usual appearance is that of macules or maculopapules distributed on the trunk and extremities. The rash may involve both the soles and palms on rare occasions.

Diagnosis. As for other vasculotropic rickettsioses, delays in diagnosis and therapy are associated with increased morbidity and mortality; thus, diagnosis must be based on clinical suspicion. Occasionally, patients present with findings suggestive of pharyngitis, bronchitis, hepatitis, gastroenteritis, or sepsis; thus, the differential diagnosis may be extensive.

Although they are nonspecific, laboratory findings that may be helpful include mild leukopenia (36–40%) with a moderate left shift, mild to marked thrombocytopenia (43–60%), hyponatremia (20–66%), hypoalbuminemia (46–87%), and elevated aspartate aminotransferase (82%) and alanine aminotransferase (38%). Elevations in serum urea nitrogen are usually due to prerenal mechanisms.

Confirmation of the diagnosis is usually accomplished in convalescence by indirect fluorescent antibody assay serology. Research tools now being evaluated include polymerase chain reaction amplification of rickettsial nucleic acids in acute phase blood, rickettsial culture by the centrifugation-assisted shell vial assay, and immunohistology on skin biopsy.

Treatment. Therapy for murine typhus includes the use of tetracyclines or chloramphenicol and is similar to that recommended for Rocky Mountain spotted fever. No controlled trials of other antimicrobial agents have been performed; however, ciprofloxacin has been used effectively to treat murine typhus, and in vitro experiments suggest that minimal inhibitory concentrations of azithromycin and clarithromycin for *R. typhi* should be easily achieved.

Recommended treatment regimens for murine typhus include doxycycline orally or intravenously (2.2 mg/kg/24 hr divided bid PO or IV; maximum: 300 mg/dose), tetracycline orally (25–50 mg/kg/24 hr divided q 6 hr PO; maximum: 2 g/24 hr), and chloramphenicol intravenously (50–100 mg/kg/24 hr divided q 6 hr IV; maximum: 3 g/24 hr). Therapy should be continued for a minimum of 5 days or until the patient has been afebrile for at least 2–4 days to avoid relapse, especially in patients treated early.

SUPPORTIVE CARE. Although usually mild, 7% of children with murine typhus may require intensive care to manage complications such as meningoencephalitis or a disseminated intravascular coagulation–like condition. As for other rickettsial infections with significant systemic vascular injury, careful hemodynamic management is mandatory to avoid pulmonary or cerebral edema.

Complications. Complications of murine typhus in pediatric patients are infrequent; however, relapse, stupor, facial edema, dehydration, and meningoencephalitis have been reported.

Prevention. Control of murine typhus has been dependent on elimination of the rat and rat flea reservoir, and this remains an important component of control. However, with the recognition of cat fleas as potentially significant reservoirs and vectors, the presence of these flea vectors and their mammalian hosts in suburban and urban areas where close human exposures occur will probably pose increasingly important control problems.

212.2 Epidemic Typhus (*Rickettsia prowazekii*)

Etiology. Humans have long been considered the principal or only reservoir of *R. prowazekii*, the causative agent of epidemic or louse-borne typhus, and its recrudescent form, Brill-Zinsser disease, also known as Brill disease. Another reservoir has recently been identified in flying squirrels, implying that a sylvatic cycle with small rodents and their ectoparasites also exists. The rickettsia is the most pathogenic of the genus, and multiplies to very high quantities through the mechanical rupture of infected endothelial cells. The genome of *R. prowazekii* is thought to be losing functional genes as it has adapted to its unique intracellular niche. *R. prowazekii* is now clearly recognized as a genetic relative of the eukaryotic mitochondrion.

Epidemiology. The infection is characteristically seen in winter or spring or during times of poor hygienic practices associated with crowding, war, famine, extreme poverty, and civil strife. A cause of some sporadic cases of a mild, typhus-like illness has been confirmed as *R. prowazekii*; such cases are associated with exposure to flying squirrels harboring infected lice or fleas. The *R. prowazekii* organisms isolated from these squirrels appear to be genetically different from isolates obtained during typical outbreaks.

Most cases of epidemic typhus from 1981–1997 have been sporadic, but outbreaks have been identified in Africa (Ethiopia, Nigeria, Burundi), Mexico, Central America, South America, eastern Europe, Afghanistan, Russia, northern India, and China. Following the Burundi civil war in 1993, there were approximately 35,000 cases of epidemic typhus diagnosed among 764,334 displaced refugees.

TRANSMISSION. Human body lice (*Pediculus humanus* subsp. *corporis*) become infected by feeding on rickettsemic persons. The ingested rickettsiae infect the midgut epithelial cells of the lice and are passed into the feces, which are introduced in turn into a susceptible human host through abrasions or perforations in the skin, through the conjunctivae, or rarely through inhalation of dried infected louse excreta present in clothing, bedding, or furniture.

Clinical Manifestations. Epidemic typhus fever may be a mild or severe disease in children. The incubation period is usually <14 days. The typical clinical manifestations include fever, severe headache, abdominal tenderness, and rash in most patients, as well as chills (82%), myalgias (70%), arthralgias (70%), anorexia (48%), nonproductive cough (38%), dizziness (35%), photophobia (33%), nausea (32%), abdominal pain (30%), tinnitus (23%), constipation (23%) meningismus (17%), visual disturbances (15%), vomiting (10%), and diarrhea (7%). However, investigation of recent African outbreaks has shown a lower frequency of rash (25%) and a high frequency of delirium (81%) and cough associated with pneumonitis (70%). The rash is initially pink or erythematous and blanches. In one third of patients, red, nonblanching macules and petechiae appear predominantly on the trunk. Infections identified during the preantibiotic era typically produced a variety of central nervous system findings including delirium (48%), coma (6%), and seizures (1%). Estimates of case fatality rates range between 3.8% and 20% in outbreaks.

Brill-Zinsser disease is an unusual form of typhus that becomes recrudescent months to years after the primary infection. When rickettsemic, these infected individuals may transmit the agent to lice.

Treatment. Recommended treatment regimens for epidemic or sylvatic typhus are identical to those used for murine typhus: doxycycline orally or intravenously (2.2 mg/kg/24 hr divided q 12 hr PO or IV; maximum: 300 mg/dose), tetracycline orally (25–50 mg/kg/24 hr divided q 6 hr PO; maximum: 2 g/24 hr), or chloramphenicol intravenously (50–100 mg/kg/24 hr divided q 6 hr IV; maximum: 3 g/24 hr). Therapy should be continued for a minimum of 5 days and until the patient has been afebrile for at least 2–4 days to avoid relapse, especially in patients treated early. Good evidence exists that doxycycline as a single 200-mg oral dose is also efficacious.

Prevention. Immediate destruction of vectors with an insecticide is important in the control of an epidemic. For epidemic typhus, antibiotic therapy and delousing measures will interrupt transmission, reduce the prevalence of infection in the human reservoir, and diminish the impact of an outbreak. Dust containing excreta from infected lice is capable of transmitting typhus, and care must be taken to prevent its inhalation.

Bernabeu-Wittel M, Pachon J, Alarcon A, et al: Murine typhus as a common cause of fever of intermediate duration: A 17-year study in the south of Spain. *Arch Intern Med* 199l;159:872–6.

Dumler JS: Murine typhus. *Semin Pediatr Infect Dis* 1994;5:137.

Fergie JE, Purcell K, Wanat D: Murine typhus in South Texas children. *Pediatr Infect Dis J* 2000;19:535–8.

Marshall GS, Tick-Borne Infections in Children Study (TICS) Group: *Rickettsia typhi* seroprevalence among children in the Southeast United States. *Pediatr Infect Dis J* 2000;9:1103–4.

Massung RF, Davis LE, Slater K, et al: Epidemic typhus meningitis in the southwestern United States. *Clin Infect Dis* 2001;32:979–82.

Raoult D, Ndihokubwayo JB, Tissot-Dupont H, et al: Outbreak of epidemic typhus associated with trench fever in Burundi. *Lancet* 1998;352:353–8.

Silpapojakul K, Chupuppakam S, Yuthasompob S, et al: Scrub and murine typhus in children with obscure fever in the tropics. *Pediatr Infect Dis J* 1991;10:2000–3.

Tarasevich I, Rydkina E, Raoult D: Outbreak of epidemic typhus in Russia. *Lancet* 1998;352:1151.

Whiteford SF, Taylor JP, Dumler JS: Clinical, laboratory, and epidemiologic features of murine typhus in 97 Texas children. *Arch Pediatr Adolesc Med* 2001;155:396–400.

Chapter 213
Ehrlichiosis and Anaplasmosis

Etiology. In 1987, clusters of bacteria confined within cytoplasmic vacuoles of circulating leukocytes (morulae), particularly mononuclear leukocytes, were detected in the peripheral blood of a severely ill patient with suspected Rocky Mountain spotted fever (RMSF). The etiologic agent of the infection and of other cases in which serologic tests could not prove RMSF was found to be similar to a canine pathogen in the genus *Ehrlichia*. In 1990, a new species, *Ehrlichia chaffeensis*, was cultivated and identified as the predominant agent of human ehrlichiosis. Seroepidemiologic investigation has shown that in some geographic areas *E. chaffeensis* infections occur more frequently than RMSF, and the infection is strongly associated with tick bites.

In 1994, another similar species was recognized in human blood with the observation of morulae only in circulating neutrophils. Serologic investigation in these cases revealed the absence of *E. chaffeensis* antibodies, and most had serologic reactions to *E. phagocytophila* and *E. equi*, previously known only as pathogens of ruminant and horse granulocytes, respectively. DNA of these bacteria was also found in the blood of many infected persons. In 1996, the agent was cultivated in vitro, and based upon genetic studies in 2001, the human agent and the two veterinary pathogens were unified into a single species and placed into the genus *Anaplasma* under the name *Anaplasma phagocytophilum*.

In 1996, a veterinary pathogen of canine neutrophils, *Ehrlichia ewingii*, was identified as the causative agent of some human infections initially thought to be due to *E. chaffeensis*. The agent is occasionally identified in peripheral blood neutrophils and the infection is generally milder and involves children or adults with pre-existing immunosuppression, including organ transplant recipients or persons with HIV infection. Although not yet cultivated in vitro, it is serologically cross reactive with *E. chaffeensis*.

Although bacteria assigned to various genera cause these infections, the name **ehrlichiosis** is applied to all. To differentiate among these infections, disease caused by *E. chaffeensis*, which infects predominantly monocytic cells, is called **human monocytic ehrlichiosis (HME)**, disease caused by *Anaplasma phagocytophilum* is called **human anaplasmosis**, formerly **granulocytic ehrlichiosis (HGE)**, and disease caused by *E. ewingii* has received various names, including **ehrlichiosis ewingii**.

All of these bacteria are now classified in the Anaplasmataceae family, and share many characteristics including transmission by tick bite. In addition, *Neorickettsia* (formerly *Ehrlichia*) *sennetsu* is another related bacterium in this family that is a rare cause of human disease, but is not tick-transmitted. In general, these are small, pleomorphic, obligate intracellular bacteria that possess gram-negative–type cell walls. *E. chaffeensis* induces the endosome to enter a receptor recycling pathway that avoids phagosome-lysosome fusion and allows the growth of a cytoplasmic aggregate of bacteria called a morula. Little is known about the vacuoles in which *A. phagocytophila* and *E. ewingii* grow. These bacteria are pathogens of hematopoietic cells in mammals, and characteristically each species has a specific host cell affinity: *E. chaffeensis* and *N. sennetsu* infect mononuclear phagocytes, and *A. phagocytophila* and *E. ewingii* infect neutrophils. Infection leads to modifications in function of the host cell, and insufficient levels of infection are usually obtained to account directly for the severity and pathology observed. Thus, an increasing body of data suggests that host immune and inflammatory reactions may in part account for many of the clinical manifestations in all forms of ehrlichiosis.

Epidemiology. Infections with *E. chaffeensis* occur in broad areas across the southeastern, south central, and mid-Atlantic states, in a distribution that parallels that of RMSF. Although suspected cases with appropriate serologic findings have been reported in Europe, Africa, and the Far East, no other data supports the existence of this human disease outside of North America. Anaplasmosis is the most frequently recognized of all forms of ehrlichiosis and is found mostly in the northeast and upper midwestern United States, but infections have now been identified in northern California, the mid-Atlantic, and broadly across Europe, confirming that the agent is widely distributed. Human infections with *E. ewingii* have only been identified in areas where *E. chaffeensis* also exist, perhaps owing to a shared tick vector.

Although the median age of patients with ehrlichiosis and anaplasmosis is generally older (>42 yr), many infected children have been identified. Little is known about the epidemiologic aspects of *E. ewingii* infection. As expected, all infections are highly associated with tick exposure and tick bites, and are identified predominantly during May through September; a second peak of anaplasmosis occurs in late October through December because of activity of the adult stage of *Ixodes scapularis* ticks during this time.

TRANSMISSION. The predominant tick species that harbors *E. chaffeensis* and *E. ewingii* is *Amblyomma americanum*, the Lone Star tick. Additional vectors such as *Dermacentor variabilis*, the American dog tick, have not been proved but may explain the presence of HME outside the known range of *A. americanum*. The tick vectors of *A. phagocytophilum* are *Ixodes*, including *I. scapularis* (black-legged or deer tick) in the eastern United States, *I. pacificus* (western black-legged tick) in the western United States, *I. ricinus* (sheep tick) in Europe, and potentially *I. persulcatus* in Eurasia.

Ehrlichia and *Anaplasma* species are maintained in nature predominantly by horizontal transmission (tick to mammal to tick) because the organisms are not transmitted to the progeny of infected adult female ticks. The major reservoir host for *E. chaffeensis* is the white-tailed deer (*Odocoileus virginianus*), which is found abundantly in many parts of the United States. A reservoir for the *A. phagocytophilum* in the eastern United States appears to be the white-footed mouse, *Peromyscus leucopus*, but increasing evidence also implicates deer or domestic ruminants. This suggests that efficient transmission requires persistent infection of mammals, long recognized in dogs with *E. canis*, ruminants with *A. phagocytophilum*, and other hosts of various ehrlichial species. However, while *E. chaffeensis* and *A. phagocytophilum* may cause persistent infections in animals, persistence is rarely proved in humans.

Pathogenesis. Although patients with human monocytic ehrlichiosis and anaplasmosis often present with an illness that appears similar to RMSF or typhus, vasculitis is rare. Pathologic findings include diffuse but mild perivascular lymphohistiocytic infiltrates, infrequent hepatocyte apoptoses, Kupffer cell hyperplasia, mild lobular hepatitis, increases in mononuclear phagocyte infiltrates in the spleen, lymph nodes, and bone marrow in which occasional erythrophagocytic cells are present, granulomas of the liver and bone marrow in patients with *E. chaffeensis* infections, and hyperplasia of one or more bone marrow hematopoietic lineages.

The exact pathogenetic mechanisms are poorly understood, but histopathologic examinations suggest diffuse mononuclear phagocyte activation and overinduction of host immune and inflammatory reactions. This activation results in moderate to profound leukopenia and thrombocytopenia in the presence of a hypercellular bone marrow, and fatalities are often associated with severe hemorrhage or secondary opportunistic infections. Hepatic or other organ-specific injury occurs by an unknown mechanism that is apparently unrelated to direct infection. An unexplained observation in severe disease is the occurrence of diffuse alveolar damage that results in the clinical picture of adult respiratory distress syndrome (ARDS), which also appears to be unrelated to direct ehrlichial tissue damage. Meningoencephalitis with a mononuclear cell cerebrospinal fluid pleocytosis may be present in HME but is rare with anaplasmosis.

Clinical Manifestations. HME, anaplasmosis, and ehrlichiosis ewingii are distinct clinical entities caused by infection with different species that result in similar illnesses. Many well-defined cases of pediatric infection of variable severity have been reported, including one fatality from HME and anaplasmosis each. Insufficient numbers of children infected with *E. ewingii* have been identified to allow a thorough characterization. The incubation period after the last preceding tick bite or tick exposure ranges from 2 days to 3 wk. No tick bite is documented in nearly one fourth of all patients. The diseases usually present with nonspecific findings including fever and headache. A majority of patients also describe myalgias, anorexia, and nausea or vomiting. Unlike adult patients, nearly two thirds of children with HME present with a rash. The rash is usually described as macular or maculopapular, although petechial lesions may occur. Photophobia and conjunctivitis also may occur, and pharyngitis and lymphadenopathy are seen in a minority of patients.

Hepatomegaly and splenomegaly are frequent physical findings, and a systolic ejection murmur is often identified. Meningoencephalitis with a mononuclear cell-predominant cerebrospinal fluid pleocytosis is infrequently encountered but can be a severe complication in HME, but appears to be rare with anaplasmosis. The presence of arthritis or arthralgias may suggest Lyme borreliosis or meningococcemia, but this presentation appears to be infrequent. Edema of the face, hands, and feet may contribute to diagnostic uncertainty.

The illness ordinarily lasts 4–12 days, and in most published cases hospitalization was required. Well-documented cases of seroconversion in the absence of overt clinical manifestations strongly suggest the occurrence of mild or subclinical infections. Clinically evident infections of children with ehrlichiosis ewingii are infrequent; however, the clinical presentation of this illness in adults is very similar to that of adult E. chaffeensis infection.

Diagnosis. As with RMSF, a delay in diagnosis or treatment may contribute to increased morbidity or mortality; thus, an early clinical diagnosis is important. Because both HME and anaplasmosis have been associated with a fatal outcome, therapy should not be withheld while awaiting confirmatory laboratory test results.

Characteristically, most children with monocytic ehrlichiosis present with leukopenia (58–72%), lymphopenia (75–78%), or thrombocytopenia (80–92%). Leukocytosis may also occur. Despite the presence of pancytopenia, examination usually reveals a cellular or reactive bone marrow in adults. Interestingly, granulomas and granulomatous inflammation are identified in nearly 75% of bone marrow specimens examined from patients with proven cases of E. chaffeensis infection, but this finding is not present in patients with anaplasmosis. Mild to severe hepatic injury is

documented by the frequent (83–91%) finding of elevated transaminase levels. Hyponatremia is present in a minority of cases. Severely affected children may experience varying degrees of renal failure accompanied by elevated concentrations of serum creatinine and urea nitrogen. A clinical picture similar to that of disseminated intravascular coagulopathy with prolonged activated partial thromboplastin time and prothrombin time and hypofibrinogenemia has occurred in several patients.

The first patient and several subsequent pediatric patients with E. chaffeensis infection were identified presumptively on the basis of typical Ehrlichia morulae in peripheral blood leukocytes (Fig. 213–1A). This finding has been too infrequent to be considered a useful diagnostic tool. In contrast, anaplasmosis presents with a small but significant percentage (1–40%) of circulating neutrophils (see Fig. 213–1B) containing typical morulae in 20–60% of patients. The distinction between the two infections relies on polymerase chain reaction (PCR) amplification of species-specific DNA sequences or on the demonstration of specific antibodies to E. chaffeensis or A. phagocytophilum antigen.

The current diagnostic criteria for E. chaffeensis infection include a seroconversion with a titer of ≥1:64, or a single serum titer (usually convalescent serum) of ≥1:128, in the context of a clinically compatible illness. Similarly, anaplasmosis may be confirmed by a seroconversion or single high titer of A. phagocytophilum antibodies; some laboratories refer to the causative agent as the HGE agent or E. equi. E. ewingii infection induces antibodies that cross react with E. chaffeensis in routine serologic tests and can only be differentiated by identification of specific nucleic acids or by the demonstration of morulae in neutrophils where the E. chaffeensis titer is at least fourfold higher than the A. phagocytophilum titer. Patients with anaplasmosis experience serologic reactions to E. chaffeensis in up to 15% of cases, and thus serodiagnosis depends on testing with both E. chaffeensis and A. phagocytophilum antigens. During the acute phase of illness when antibodies may not be detected, PCR amplification of specific E. chaffeensis or A. phagocytophilum DNA sequences is sensitive in 50–86% of cases. E. chaffeensis and A. phagocytophilum have both been cultivated in tissue culture, but neither method provides a timely result.

DIFFERENTIAL DIAGNOSIS. Because of the nonspecific presentation, ehrlichiosis may be mimicked by other arthropod-

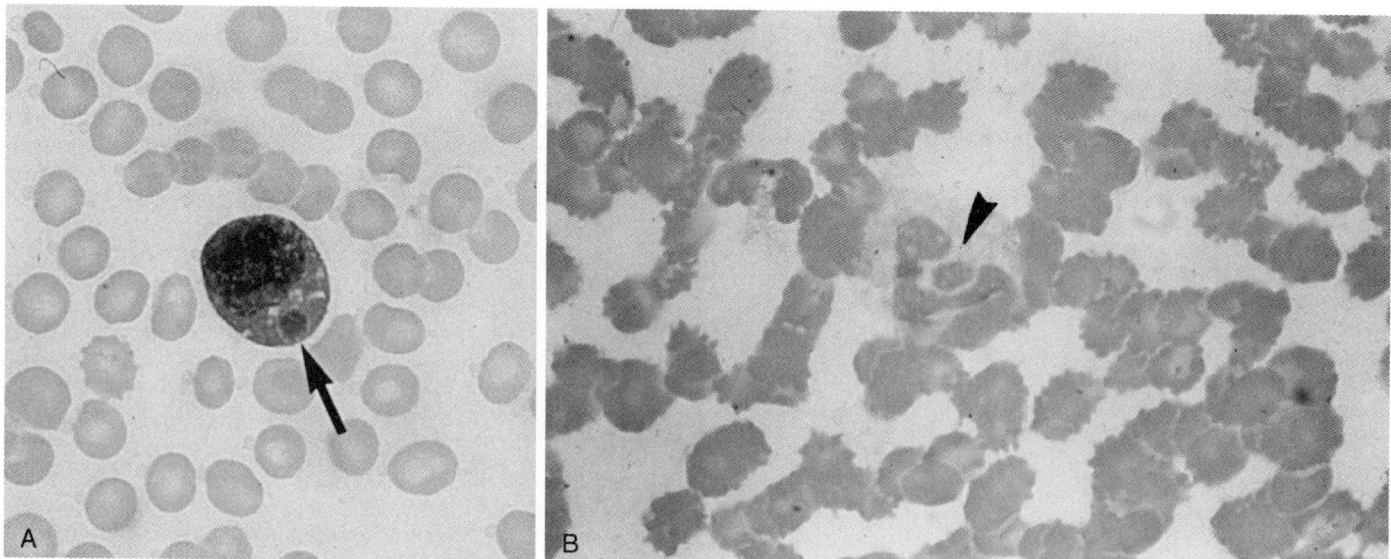

FIGURE 213–1. Morulae in peripheral blood leukocytes in patients with HME and anaplasmosis. *A,* A morula *(arrow)* containing *Ehrlichia chaffeensis* in a monocyte. *B,* A morula *(arrowhead)* containing *Anaplasma phagocytophilum* in a neutrophil. Wright stains, original magnifications ×1,200. *Ehrlichia chaffeensis* and *A. phagocytophilum* have similar morphologies but are serologically and genetically distinct. See also color plates.

borne infections such as RMSF, tularemia, babesiosis, Lyme disease, murine typhus, relapsing fever, and Colorado tick fever. Other potential diagnoses considered include otitis media, streptococcal pharyngitis, infectious mononucleosis, Kawasaki disease, endocarditis, viral syndromes, hepatitis, leptospirosis, Q fever, collagen-vascular diseases, and leukemia. When rash and disseminated intravascular coagulopathy predominate, meningococcemia, bacterial sepsis, and toxic shock syndrome should be suspected. Meningoencephalitis may suggest enterovirus or herpes simplex virus infections, bacterial meningitis, or RMSF, whereas severe respiratory disease may be confused with bacterial, viral, or fungal pneumonitis.

Treatment. Both ehrlichiosis and anaplasmosis are effectively treated with tetracyclines, especially doxycycline, and the majority of patients usually improve within 48 hr. In vitro tests document that both *E. chaffeensis* and *A. phagocytophilum* have chloramphenicol minimal inhibitory concentrations above safely achieved blood levels. Because of these findings, a short course of doxycycline is the recommended regimen. Doxycycline can be used safely in children <9 yr of age because tooth discoloration is dose dependent, and the need for multiple courses is unlikely. Little information exists to recommend alternative therapies; both *E. chaffeensis* and *A. phagocytophilum* are susceptible to rifampin in vitro, and it has been successfully used to treat anaplasmosis in pregnant women.

The recommended treatment regimen for patients with severe or complicated HME and anaplasmosis is doxycycline orally or intravenously (two loading doses of 2.2 mg/kg/dose q 12 hr followed by 2.2 mg/kg/24 hr divided q 12 hr PO or IV; maximum dose: 300 mg). The loading doses may be omitted in patients with less severe disease. An alternative regimen is tetracycline orally (25–50 mg/kg/24 hr divided q 6 hr PO; maximum: 2 g/24 hr). Therapy should be continued for a minimum of 5 days and until the patient has been afebrile for at least 2–4 days.

Other broad-spectrum antibiotics including penicillins, cephalosporins, aminoglycosides, and macrolides are not effective. *Anaplasma phagocytophilum* is not susceptible to azithromycin, but in vitro studies suggest a potential role for rifamycin in HME and anaplasmosis. In vitro studies show promising activity for quinolones against *A. phagocytophilum*; *E. chaffeensis* is naturally resistant. Increasing evidence suggests that the antecedent treatment with sulfamethoxazole-trimethoprim may result in more severe disease.

Complications. Fatal monocytic ehrlichiosis has been reported in one pediatric patient where the findings were initially dominated by pulmonary involvement with respiratory failure complicated by nosocomial bacterial pneumonia. The pattern of severe pulmonary involvement culminating in diffuse alveolar damage and ARDS and secondary nosocomial or opportunistic infections is now well documented with HME and anaplasmosis in adults. One child with anaplasmosis died after a 3-wk interval of fever, thrombocytopenia, and lymphadenopathy suspected to be a hematologic malignancy. Other severe complications include a toxic shock–like illness, meningoencephalitis with long-term neurologic sequelae, brachial plexopathy, myocarditis, rhabdomyolysis, and renal failure. Patients with underlying immune compromise (e.g., HIV infection, high-dose corticosteroid therapy, cancer chemotherapy, organ transplantation) are at high risk for fulminant infection.

Prevention. HME, anaplasmosis, and ehrlichiosis ewingii are tick-borne diseases, and any activity that allows exposure to the tick vectors increases risk. Avoidance of tick-infested areas, the wearing of appropriate light-colored clothing, tick repellents sprayed on clothing, careful inspection for ticks after exposure, and prompt removal of any attached ticks diminish the risk of acquisition of HME and anaplasmosis. The interval after tick attachment and before transmission of the infectious agents may be as short as 4 hr; thus, any attached tick should be promptly removed. The role of prophylactic therapy for ehrlichiosis and anaplasmosis after tick bites has not been investigated.

Arav-Boger R, Knepp JH, Walls JJ, et al: Human monocytic ehrlichiosis in a child with leukemia. *Pediatr Infect Dis J* 2000;19:173–5.
Berry DS, Miller RS, Hooke JA, et al: Ehrlichial meningitis with cerebrospinal fluid morulae. *Pediatr Infect Dis J* 1999;18:552–5.
Buller RS, Arens M, Hmiel SP, et al: *Ehrlichia ewingii*, a newly recognized agent of human ehrlichiosis. *N Engl J Med* 1999;341:148–55.
Dumler JS, Dey C, Meier F, et al: Human monocytic ehrlichiosis: A potentially severe disease in children. *Arch Pediatr Adolesc Med* 2000;154:847–9.
Horowitz HW, Kilchevsky E, Haber S, et al: Perinatal transmission of the agent of human granulocytic ehrlichiosis. *N Engl J Med* 1998;339:375–8.
IJdo JW, Meek JI, Cartter ML, et al: The emergence of another tick-borne infection in the 12-town area around Lyme, Connecticut: Human granulocytic ehrlichiosis. *J Infect Dis* 2000;181:1388–93.
Jacobs RF, Schutze GE: Ehrlichiosis in children. *J Pediatr* 1997;131:184–92.
Peters TR, Edwards KM, Standaert SM: Severe ehrlichiosis in an adolescent taking trimethoprim-sulfamethoxazole. *Pediatr Infect Dis J* 2000;19:170–2.
Schutze GE, Jacobs RF: Human monocytic ehrlichiosis in children. *Pediatrics* 1997;100:E10.

Chapter 214
Q Fever (*Coxiella burnetii*)

Q fever (for query fever) is a febrile disease, often with no rash, that presents in acute and chronic forms.

Etiology. The causative organism of Q fever, *Coxiella burnetii*, is genetically distinct from members of the genera *Rickettsia* and *Ehrlichia* and it is no longer classified within the order Rickettsiales, and has been assigned to the order Legionellales, family Coxiellaceae. *C. burnetii* is highly infectious for humans and animals; even a single organism can cause infection. The organism may enter a sporogenic differentiation cycle, unlike *Rickettsia*, which renders it highly resistant to chemical and physical treatments.

C. burnetii resides intracellularly within phagolysosomes. Unlike *Ehrlichia*, *Anaplasma*, and *Chlamydia*, *C. burnetii* tolerates and actively proliferates within the acidified phagolysosome to form aggregates that often contain >100 bacteria. *C. burnetii* organisms undergo a lipopolysaccharide "phase variation" similar to that described for smooth and rough strains of Enterobacteriaceae.

Epidemiology. The disease is reported worldwide. Children younger than 19 yr and adults older than 80 yr are infrequently infected, most likely reflecting infrequent exposure. Serologic surveys in the United States and elsewhere indicate that many more cases of Q fever occur each year than are recognized, which is not surprising because acute Q fever is a nonspecific illness, specialized laboratory diagnostic tests are required, and it is not currently a notifiable disease in many states. *C. burnetii* may be the cause of 0.5–3% of serologically investigated acute respiratory illnesses or suspected viral hepatitis in some areas of the United States. In Japan and parts of Europe, *C. burnetii* is implicated as a cause of atypical pneumonia in up to 40% of pediatric patients. Immune compromise secondary to cancer therapies, AIDS, organ transplantation, hemodialysis, alcoholic liver disease, chronic granulomatous disease, or underlying cardiac valve or vascular damage or prostheses is identified as an underlying factor in >20% of patients with acute or chronic Q fever.

TRANSMISSION. In contrast to other rickettsial infections, humans acquire *C. burnetii* predominantly after inhalation of infectious aerosols or by ingestion of contaminated foods; arthropod vectors are rarely implicated in human transmission. Domestic livestock (e.g., cattle, sheep, and goats), parturient cats, wild animals such as rabbits, and ticks serve as reservoirs. Frequent modes of transmission include aerosols from dust, straw, cloth contaminated with organisms from birth tissues, or processing of animal products (in abattoirs, hides, wool), or by ingestion of contaminated raw dairy products (fresh cheese or unpasteurized milk). In Nova Scotia and Maine, exposure to newborn animals, chiefly kittens, has been associated with small outbreaks of Q fever in family settings. In Europe and Australia, exposure to domestic ruminants is the major risk; however, many urban dwellers in France, who presumably lack significant exposure to farm animals, acquire Q fever. Human placental infection is sometimes associated with intrauterine growth retardation or death and may result from primary or reactivation of maternal infection. Obstetric health care workers are at risk for acquiring infection because of the quantity of *C. burnetii* released from infected products of conception.

Pathogenesis. The pathology of Q fever depends on the mode of transmission, the route of dissemination, and the specific tissues involved. After inhalation of infectious aerosols, pulmonary infection elicits a mild interstitial lymphocytic pneumonitis with a dense macrophage-rich intra-alveolar exudate that is heavily infected with *C. burnetii*. Single lesions may develop in the pulmonary parenchyma that histologically are inflammatory pseudotumors. Occasionally the characteristic fibrin-ring granulomas may be identified in liver, bone marrow, meninges, and other organs, and this finding is generally a sign of an acute, self-limited infection; with hepatic involvement, there is mild to moderate lymphocytic lobular hepatitis. Typically, infected tissues are moderately to densely infiltrated by lymphoid and histiocytic cells. Chronic Q fever endocarditis and prosthetic valve endocarditis is characterized by macrophage and lymphocyte-rich infiltrates in necrotic fibrinous valvular vegetations and by the absence of granulomas.

As with many other obligate intracellular pathogens, recovery from acute infection may result in nonsterile immunity and persistent subclinical infection. It is now recognized that development of chronic Q fever results after recovery from a mild or inapparent episode of acute Q fever, during which the agent is not cleared. The persistence of *C. burnetii* in tissue macrophages at sites of pre-existing tissue damage causes a low-grade smoldering inflammation, which eventually leads to irreversible cardiac valve damage or persistent vascular injury.

Clinical Manifestations. Two forms of Q fever occur. The most frequent is acute Q fever, a self-limited form that is usually associated with an influenza-like illness and interstitial pneumonitis, granulomatous hepatitis, or both. Chronic Q fever usually implies involvement of the heart valves and often occurs in prosthetic valves or other endovascular prostheses; it is diagnosed clinically as culture-negative endocarditis and often results in death.

ACUTE Q FEVER. Acute Q fever develops about 3 wk (range, 14–39 days) after exposure to the causative agent. The severity of illness in children ranges from subclinical infection to a systemic febrile illness characterized by severe frontal headache, arthralgia, and myalgia, often accompanied by respiratory symptoms. Fewer than half of patients have cough or pneumonia. Most pediatric patients present with fever of unknown origin. In adults, the pneumonia usually resembles primary atypical or viral pneumonitis or legionnaires' disease with a nonproductive cough. Other prominent clinical findings that may lead to diagnostic confusion include fatigue, vomiting, abdominal pain, and meningismus. Hepatomegaly and splenomegaly may be detected in some patients.

In a review of 428 French patients with acute Q fever, 40% presented with hepatitis, 20% with hepatitis and pneumonia, 17% with pneumonia only, and 14% with isolated fever; other presentations included meningitis and meningoencephalitis, pericarditis, and myocarditis. Of those with either acute or chronic Q fever, 91% had fever, 34% had respiratory involvement, 11% had rash, and 4% had neurologic findings that

required lumbar puncture for evaluation. Nearly 20% of patients with pneumonia alone were afebrile and such patients often present with one or more hepatic, pulmonic, cutaneous, or neurologic findings.

Laboratory investigations in acute Q fever are usually normal but may reveal leukopenia with a left shift (>5%) in 50% of patients and thrombocytopenia in 9–48%. Most children (62%) have elevated serum transaminase levels, which spontaneously return to normal after 20–30 days. The erythrocyte sedimentation rate is elevated in half of all Q fever cases. Chest X-ray films are abnormal in 27%, and pulmonary consolidations on radiographs become round and resolve slowly.

Acute Q fever in children is usually a self-limited illness that lasts 2–3 wk. However, severe infections including acute encephalopathy with impaired consciousness and an abnormal pattern on electroencephalogram and CT scans of the brain have been reported.

CHRONIC Q FEVER. The risk of development of chronic Q fever is strongly correlated with advancing age and underlying conditions such as cardiac valve damage or immunosuppression. Thus, children are rarely diagnosed with chronic Q fever, including endocarditis. Chronic Q fever tends to be resistant to therapy and often results in death (23–65% of cases). Endocarditis, which almost invariably develops on damaged or prosthetic valves, may occur months to years after acute Q fever, or even in the absence of any history of acute Q fever. Less frequently, chronic Q fever may present as an infection of vascular prostheses and aneurysms, osteomyelitis, myocarditis, undifferentiated fever, pneumonia, and hepatitis, placental infection, or an isolated purpuric rash. The clinical presentation in children is similar to that in adults. In Q fever endocarditis, fever may be absent in up to 15% of cases, and more than 75% of all identified patients have congestive heart failure. Other frequently observed features include marked clubbing of the fingers, hepatomegaly, and splenomegaly.

Frequent laboratory abnormalities in patients with chronic Q fever include erythrocyte sedimentation rate >20 mm/hr (80% of cases), hypergammaglobulinemia (54%), and hyperfibrinogenemia (67%). The presence of rheumatoid factor in >50% of cases and circulating immune complexes in nearly 90%, plus the frequent findings of antiplatelet antibodies, anti–smooth muscle antibodies, antimitochondrial antibodies, circulating anticoagulants, and positive direct Coombs test results suggests an autoimmune process.

Diagnosis. Although it is infrequently diagnosed, Q fever should be considered in children with fever of unknown origin, atypical pneumonia, or culture-negative endocarditis and who live in rural areas or who are in close contact with domestic livestock, cats, or animal products.

The diagnosis of Q fever is most easily confirmed serologically by testing acute and convalescent sera (2–4 wk apart), which show a fourfold increase in indirect fluorescent antibody titers to phase I and phase II antigens. Predominant, elevated, or increasing titers of phase II antibody are characteristic of acute Q fever, and the appearance and persistence of elevated titers of phase I and phase II antibody are indicative of chronic Q fever. Elevated titers of phase I immunoglobulin (Ig) A antibody are reported to be diagnostic for Q fever endocarditis; however, one evaluation showed that a phase II IgG titer of ≥1:200 is indicative of *C. burnetii* infection and that a phase I IgG titer of <1:800 is inconsistent with chronic Q fever.

C. burnetii has been cultivated in tissue culture cells, which may become positive within 48 hr, but isolation and antimicrobial susceptibility testing of *C. burnetii* should be attempted only in specialized biohazard facilities.

DIFFERENTIAL DIAGNOSIS. The differential diagnosis depends on the clinical presentation. For respiratory disease, *Mycoplasma* pneumonia, legionellosis, psittacosis, and Epstein-Barr virus infection should be considered. For granulomatous hepatitis, mycobacterial infections, salmonellosis, visceral leishmaniasis, toxoplasmosis, Hodgkin disease, ehrlichiosis, brucellosis, or autoimmune disorders including sarcoidosis should be considered. Culture-negative endocarditis also suggests infection with *Brucella* or *Bartonella*, or nonbacterial endocarditis.

Treatment. Selection of an appropriate antimicrobial regimen for children is difficult owing to the lack of thorough studies, the limited therapeutic window for drugs that are known to be efficacious, and the potential length of therapy required to preclude relapse. Most pediatric patients with Q fever experience a self-limited illness that is identified only on retrospective serologic evaluation. However, to prevent potential complications, patients with acute Q fever should be treated within 3 days of onset of symptoms with tetracycline (25–50 mg/kg/24 hr divided qid PO) or doxycycline (2.2 mg/kg/24 hr divided bid PO). Chloramphenicol is effective, but is unavailable as an oral preparation in the United States. Therapy started after 3 days of onset has little effect on the course of the acute infection. Because early laboratory confirmation is not currently available, empirical therapy is warranted in clinically suspected cases. The quinolones ofloxacin and pefloxacin have proved effective, and success with a combination of pefloxacin and rifampin has also been achieved with prolonged therapy (16–21 days). Macrolides, including erythromycin, clarithromycin, and roxithromycin, are less effective than doxycycline, but more effective than β-lactams, which are ineffective. However, the efficacy of macrolides in children has not been well studied. Individual reports document success with a wide variety of agents including chloramphenicol, trimethoprim-sulfamethoxazole, and ceftriaxone. In anecdotal cases of hepatitis associated with "autoimmune" laboratory findings, prednisone was reported to provide additional clinical benefit.

For chronic Q fever, especially endocarditis, prolonged therapy is mandatory with the bacteriostatic drugs tetracycline or doxycycline in combination with bactericidal drugs such as rifampin, ofloxacin, or pefloxacin. The use of lysosomotropic alkalinizing agents such as chloroquine aids in maintaining the activity of pH-sensitive antimicrobial agents in the phagolysosomal environment of *C. burnetii*. The addition of hydroxychloroquine allowed a significant shortening of the interval for required therapy in a recent clinical study, and no patient treated for 18 mo with a combination of doxycycline and hydroxychloroquine developed relapse. For patients with heart failure, valve replacement may be warranted and should be accompanied by an effective antibiotic regimen to avoid reinfection of the prosthetic valves. Therapy should be monitored by periodic serologic evaluation; phase I titers of <1:200 for IgG and a negative IgA titer indicate cure. Even with such evaluation, cure of chronic Q fever in less than 2 yr is unlikely; thus, therapy should be continued for at least 18 mo. Interferon-γ therapy has been used to control intractable Q fever endocarditis.

Prevention. Recognition of the disease in livestock or other domestic animals should alert communities to the risk of human infection. Milk from infected herds must be pasteurized at temperatures sufficient to destroy *C. burnetii*. *C. burnetii* is resistant to significant environmental conditions but may be inactivated with a solution of 1% Lysol, 1% formaldehyde, or 5% hydrogen peroxide. Special isolation measures are not required because person-to-person transmission is rare, except during exposure to infected products of conception. A vaccine preparation is available and provides protection against Q fever for at least 5 yr in abattoir workers. Because the vaccine is strongly reactogenic and no trials in children have been conducted, it should only be used where extreme risk is judged to exist.

Al-Hajjar S, Hussain Qadri SM, al-Sabban E, et al: *Coxiella burnetii* endocarditis in a child. *Pediatr Infect Dis J* 1997;16:911–3.

Fenollar F, Fournier PE, Carrieri MP, et al: Risk factors and prevention of Q fever endocarditis. *Clin Infect Dis* 2001;33:312–6.

Fournier PE, Etienne J, Harle JR, et al: Myocarditis, a rare but severe manifestation of Q fever: Report of 8 cases and review of the literature. *Clin Infect Dis* 2001;32:1440–7.

Gikas A, Kofteridis DP, Manios A, et al: Newer macrolides as empiric treatment for acute Q fever infection. *Antimicrob Agents Chemother* 2001;45:3644–6.

Maurin M, Raoult D: Q fever. *Clin Microbiol Rev* 1999;12:518–53.

Raoult D, Tissot-Dupont H, Foucault C, et al: Q fever 1985–1998. Clinical and epidemiologic features of 1,383 infections. *Medicine (Baltimore)* 2000;79:109–23.

Raoult D, Houpikian P, Tissot-Dupont H, et al: Treatment of Q fever endocarditis: comparison of 2 regimens containing doxycycline and ofloxacin or hydroxychloroquine. *Arch Intern Med* 1999;159:167–73.

Richardus JH, Dumas AM, Huisman J, et al: Q fever in infancy: A review of 18 cases. *Pediatr Infect Dis* 1985;4:369–73.

Ruiz-Contreras J, Montero RG, Amador JT, et al: Q fever in children. *Am J Dis Child* 1993;146:300–2.

Tissot-DuPont H, Raoult D, Brouqui P, et al: Epidemiologic features and clinical presentation of acute Q fever in hospitalized patients: 323 French cases. *Am J Med* 1992;93:427–34.

SECTION 10 *Mycotic Infections*

Chapter 215

Candida Martin E. Weisse and

Stephen C. Aronoff

Candidiasis is caused by several species of the genus *Candida*. The former genus name was *Monilia*, and the term **moniliasis** is still used occasionally to describe skin or mucous membrane infection. *Candida* exists in three morphologic forms: oval to round blastospores or yeast cells (3–6 mm in diameter); double-walled chlamydospores (7–17 mm in diameter), which are usually at the terminal end of a pseudohypha; and pseudomycelium, which is a mass of pseudohyphae and represents the tissue phase of *Candida*. Pseudohyphae are filamentous processes that elongate from the yeast cell without the cytoplasmic connection of a true hypha. *Candida* grows aerobically on routine laboratory media but may require several days for incubation.

C. albicans accounts for most human infections, but *C. parapsilosis*, *C. tropicalis*, *C. krusei*, *C. lusitaniae*, *C. glabrata* (formerly *Torulopsis glabrata*), and several other species have been reported as pathogens with increasing frequency. Because *C. albicans* is the most frequently isolated pathogen, a rapid **germ tube test** should be performed before further identification tests are ordered. *C. albicans* is the only species that forms a germ tube when suspended in rabbit or human serum and incubated for

1–2 hr. The other clinically important species can be identified within 48 hr on the basis of biochemical test results.

Treatment of invasive *Candida* infections has become complicated with the emergence of these non-*albicans* strains. Amphotericin is inactive against approximately 20% of strains of *C. lusitaniae*. Fluconazole is useful for many *Candida* infections but is inactive against all strains of *C. krusei* and approximately 20% of strains of *C. glabrata*. These species are usually susceptible to ketoconazole and itraconazole, but cross resistance to other azoles does occur. Susceptibility testing of these clinical isolates is recommended.

215.1 Neonatal Infections

Candida is a common cause of oral mucous membrane infections (thrush) and perineal skin infections (diaper dermatitis) in newborn infants. With the improved survival of very low-birthweight infants, disseminated *Candida* infections have become more frequent in special care nurseries; the incidence can be as high as 5% in very low-birthweight infants.

Epidemiology. *C. albicans* is commonly part of the gastrointestinal and vaginal flora of adults. Pregnancy increases the rate of vaginal colonization from <20% to >30%. In approximately 10% of term infants, the gastrointestinal and respiratory tracts are colonized in the first 5 days of life; the colonization rate in infants weighing <1,500 g approaches 30%. Skin colonization is common after 2 wk of age. Neonatal risk factors for invasive candidiasis include prematurity, abdominal surgery, prolonged ventilatory support, prolonged intravenous catheterization, parenteral alimentation, and especially broad-spectrum antibiotic administration.

Pathogenesis. The inability of the newborn infant to localize, control, and eradicate *Candida* infections appears to be related to the relative impairment of specific and nonspecific host defense mechanisms. Overgrowth of *Candida* on mucocutaneous surfaces and colonization of intravenous catheters favor entry and penetration; clinical infection is related to inoculum size. Hematogenous spread leads to vasculitis and miliary nodules in many organs. The liver, spleen, lungs, kidneys, gastrointestinal tract, heart, eyes, and meninges are commonly involved.

Clinical Manifestations. The manifestations of systemic neonatal candidiasis vary in acuteness and severity, from thrush and candidal diaper dermatitis (see Section 215.2) to fungemia that may be asymptomatic or may be associated with sepsis and shock indistinguishable from bacterial sepsis. *Candida* causes significant disease in 2–5% of premature infants weighing <1,500 g. Cutaneous evidence of *Candida* infection is present in as many as half of these patients and manifests as a diffuse erythroderma or vesiculopustules from which the organism can be cultured. Renal involvement is found in >50% of patients and may be subclinical with persistent candiduria or may become manifest with a flank mass, hypertension, renal failure, renal abscesses, papillary necrosis, or fungal balls in the collecting system, resulting in obstruction and hydronephrosis.

Central nervous system involvement occurs in as many as one third of cases and may involve the meninges, ventricles, or cerebral cortex with abscess formation. Clinical manifestations of central nervous system disease may be inapparent, which mandates evaluation of the cerebrospinal fluid in all neonates with disseminated candidiasis regardless of central nervous system signs or symptoms. Because endophthalmitis is seen in as many as 45% of cases, retinal examinations should be performed in neonates with systemic candidiasis; repeat examinations are necessary to monitor resolution of the retinal lesions. Endophthalmitis begins as chorioretinitis and may extend to the vitreous. Cotton ball exudates are typical of candidal retinal pathologic conditions. Osteoarthritis is a complication in 20% of cases.

Vascular disease ranges from vasculitis of the aorta or vena cava to endocarditis. Infected thrombi in vessels and the right atrium are not uncommon. Candidal endocarditis is an infrequent complication but should be considered in patients with central venous catheters that extend into the atrium as well as in those with persistent candidemia. Pneumonia occurs in as many as 70% of patients with disseminated candidemia on the basis of autopsy studies, although some patients do not have radiographic evidence of pneumonia on initial evaluation. Cultures from the endotracheal tube are not predictive of pulmonary involvement.

CONGENITAL CANDIDIASIS. Congenital candidiasis, which is rare, occurs in otherwise normal neonates and presents at birth as widespread skin involvement, especially in the intertriginous areas. The pathogenesis of congenital candidiasis is ascending infection from a mother with heavy colonization or vulvar infection with *Candida*. The newborn rash is maculopapular; *Candida* may be recovered from some vesicles and pustules. There is usually little or no mucous membrane involvement. Topical antifungal therapy is usually all that is necessary unless the neonate shows evidence of systemic infection. Congenital candidiasis in preterm infants may progress to systemic disease.

Diagnosis. Definitive diagnosis requires identification of the fungus histologically in tissue specimens or recovery of the fungus by culture of normally sterile body fluids. Buffy coat smears of blood may show yeast, allowing a preliminary diagnosis. Skin scrapings of generalized rashes in very low-birthweight infants with suspected systemic candidiasis should be examined microscopically for yeast. Because cultures of blood and cerebrospinal fluid are often intermittently positive, multiple samples should be obtained. Cerebrospinal fluid cultures are positive in one third of infants with disseminated infection. Cultures should be obtained from peripheral veins as well as catheters to differentiate systemic infection from contaminated catheters. *Candida* antigen detection from blood samples may increase detection of candidemia. Urine specimens for culture must also be obtained by catheterization or suprapubic tap to differentiate infection perineal colonization.

Radiographs of the chest may reveal pneumonia. Ultrasonography is useful for localizing *Candida* infection in the urinary tract, central nervous system, and cardiovascular system. Ultrasonography, CT, and MRI may also be helpful in identifying foci in the liver and spleen.

Treatment. Transient candidemia and disseminated candidiasis may be associated with a contaminated intravascular catheter, which must be removed. Amphotericin B (0.5–1.0 mg/kg/24 hr IV) is the drug of choice for systemic candidiasis and is active against both yeast and mycelial forms. The duration of therapy varies widely according to the extent of infection, clinical response, and drug toxicity. The total recommended dose is 20–30 mg/kg. Nephrotoxicity is common in the newborn infant and generally presents with oliguria, azotemia, and hyperkalemia. Lipid-complex formulations of amphotericin B (5 mg/kg/24 hr) are recommended for neonates with compromised renal function (including doubling of the serum creatinine with amphotericin B desoxycholate therapy), those who are receiving other nephrotoxic therapy, or those who are otherwise intolerant of amphotericin B desoxycholate. The addition of flucytosine (100–150 mg/kg/24 hr divided every 6 hr PO) is recommended for the treatment of central nervous system and parenchymal kidney infections. Patients must be observed for bone marrow, gastrointestinal, and hepatic toxicities.

Fluconazole has also been found to be useful for invasive neonatal *Candida* infections. It is inactive against all strains of *C. krusei* and approximately 20% of strains of *C. glabrata*. These are usually susceptible to ketoconazole and itraconazole, but cross resistance to other azoles does occur. The susceptibility of these clinical isolates should be tested if treatment with azoles is contemplated.

Vascular catheters associated with transient fungemia or disseminated infection should be removed, followed by treatment with amphotericin B for 2–3 wk. Infected intracardiac and intravascular thrombi usually must be resected, but resolution without surgery has been described.

215.2 Infections in Immunocompetent Children and Adolescents

Oral Candidiasis. Oral thrush, or oral pseudomembranous candidiasis, is a superficial mucous membrane infection that affects approximately 2–5% of normal newborns. Infants acquire *Candida* from their mothers at delivery and remain colonized. Thrush may develop as early as 7–10 days of age. The use of antibiotics, especially in the 1st year of life, may lead to recurrent or persistent thrush. The plaques of thrush invade the mucosa superficially and may be found on the lips, buccal mucosa, tongue, and palate. Removal of plaques from these surfaces may cause mild punctate areas of bleeding, which helps to confirm the diagnosis. Thrush may be asymptomatic or may cause pain, fussiness, and decreased feeding. It is uncommon after 12 mo of age but may occur in older children treated with antibiotics. Persistent or recurrent thrush with no obvious predisposing reason, such as recent antibiotic treatment, warrants investigation of an underlying condition such as diabetes mellitus or immunodeficiency, especially vertically transmitted HIV infection.

Treatment of mild cases may not be necessary. When treatment is warranted, the most commonly prescribed antifungal agent is nystatin. Therapeutic agents found to be effective include (in decreasing order of efficacy) miconazole gel, amphotericin B suspension, gentian violet, and nystatin suspension. Clotrimazole troches may also be effective, although clinical studies are lacking. Miconazole gel is currently unavailable in the United States. For recalcitrant or recurrent infections, a single dose of fluconazole may be useful. Fluconazole has been shown to be safe in premature infants, and effective in a single dose in HIV-infected children with oral candidiasis. In breast-fed infants, a single dose of fluconazole suspension by the mother may be adequate to treat both her and her infant.

Diaper Dermatitis. Diaper dermatitis is the most common infection caused by *Candida*. Primary infection generally occurs in the intertriginous areas of the perineum and presents as a confluent papular erythema with erythematous satellite papules. *Candida* diaper dermatitis often complicates other noninfectious diaper dermatitides and occurs as an adverse effect of oral antibiotic treatment. Many physicians presumptively treat any diaper rash that has been present for >3 days for *Candida*.

Treatment is usually with nystatin cream, powder, or ointment; clotrimazole 1% cream; miconazole 2% ointment; or amphotericin cream or ointment. If significant inflammation is present, the addition of hydrocortisone 1% may be useful for the 1st day or two. Combination drugs with topical corticosteroids, such as clotrimazole/triamcinolone, should be used cautiously or not at all in infants because the relatively potent topical corticosteroid may lead to unwanted local adverse effects. Frequent diaper changes and short periods without diapers are important adjunctive treatments.

Periungual Infections. Paronychia and onychomycosis may be due to *Candida*, although this agent is much less common than *Trichophyton* or *Epidermophyton* as a cause of periungual infection. Candidal onychomycosis differs from tinea infections by its propensity to involve the fingernails and not the toenails, and by the associated paronychia. Candidal infections often respond to treatment that consists of keeping the hands dry and using a topical antifungal agent. A short course of systemic therapy with an oral azole antifungal drug may be necessary.

Vulvovaginitis. Vulvovaginitis is a common candidal infection of pubertal and postpubertal female patients that affects as many as 75% of female patients at one time or another (see Chapter 541). Predisposing factors include pregnancy, oral contraceptive use, poor hygiene, and use of oral antibiotics. Prepubertal girls with candidal vulvovaginitis usually have a predisposing factor such as diabetes mellitus or prolonged antibiotic treatment. Clinical manifestations may include pain or itching, dysuria, vulvar or vaginal erythema, an opaque white or cheesy exudate, and thrushlike mucosal plaques.

Candidal vulvovaginitis can be effectively treated with either vaginal creams or troches of nystatin, clotrimazole, or miconazole. Oral therapy with a single dose of fluconazole has been found to be as effective as topical clotrimazole in women. Persistent vulvovaginal candidiasis can be safely and effectively treated with fluconazole.

215.3 Infections in Immunocompromised Children and Adolescents

Etiology. Most cases of candidemia in immunocompromised patients are due to *C. albicans* (70–90%). Other species commonly involved include *C. tropicalis* (5–15%), *C. parapsilosis* (3–13%), *C. glabrata* (0–4%), *C. lusitaniae*, *C. krusei*, and *C. guilliermondii* (all <2%).

Clinical Manifestations. *Candida* infections in immunocompromised patients vary from superficial mucocutaneous infections to life-threatening sepsis and shock. Evidence of *Candida* of one organ system usually belies systemic infection and multiorgan involvement.

HIV-INFECTED CHILDREN. Oral thrush and diaper dermatitis are the most common candidal infections in HIV-infected children, occurring in 50–85% of patients. Infants with symptomatic HIV infection are more than twice as likely to have thrush, which is often much more extensive in these infants than in healthy children. Besides oral candidiasis, three other clinical variants of candidal infection may be observed in HIV-infected children: **atrophic candidiasis,** which presents as a fiery erythema of the mucosa or loss of papilla of the tongue; **chronic hyperplastic candidiasis,** which presents with oral symmetric white plaques that cannot be rubbed away; and **angular cheilitis,** in which there is erythema and fissuring of the angles of the mouth. Topical therapy may be effective, but systemic treatment with fluconazole or itraconazole is usually necessary. Symptoms of dysphagia or poor oral intake may indicate that the infection has progressed to candidal esophagitis, necessitating systemic therapy with either itraconazole or fluconazole.

Candidal dermatitis and onychomycosis are also more common in HIV-infected children. These infections are generally more severe than they are in immunocompetent children and may require oral therapy or more aggressive and prolonged topical therapy.

CANCER AND TRANSPLANT PATIENTS. Fungal infections, especially *Candida* and *Aspergillus* infections, are a significant problem in oncology patients with chemotherapy-associated neutropenia (see Chapter 164). Although the greatest risk for these patients is from bacterial pathogens, the risk of candidemia increases dramatically after 5–7 days of neutropenia and fever. Accordingly, if fever and neutropenia persist for ≥5–7 days, amphotericin B is usually indicated because of the risk of systemic fungal infection. Fluconazole may be an acceptable alternative to amphotericin B for some patients in hospitals where drug-resistant *Candida* and *Aspergillus* species are uncommon.

Bone marrow transplant recipients have a much higher risk of fungal infection because of the dramatically increased duration of neutropenia. Prophylactic use of fluconazole has been shown to decrease the incidence of candidemia in bone marrow transplant recipients but not in leukemia patients undergoing chemotherapy. An increased incidence of infection with *C. krusei*, which is resistant to fluconazole, has been noted. The use of myelopoietic colony-stimulating factor affects the duration of neutropenia after chemotherapy and is associated with decreased risk for candidemia. When *Candida* infection occurs, the lung, spleen, kidney, and liver are involved in >50% of cases.

Solid organ transplant recipients are also at increased risk for superficial and invasive candidal infections. Studies in liver transplant recipients demonstrate the utility of antifungal prophylaxis with either amphotericin B or fluconazole.

CATHETER-ASSOCIATED INFECTIONS. Central venous catheter infections occur most often in oncology patients but may affect any patient with a central catheter (see Chapter 165). Neutropenia, use of broad-spectrum antibiotics, and parenteral alimentation are associated with increased risk of candidal central catheter infection. Recovery of *Candida* from the central catheter alone poses the same risk of disseminated infection as culture of the organism from both the central catheter and peripheral blood. Treatment requires removal of the catheter as well as a 2–3 wk course of amphotericin B (1 mg/kg/24 hr, total dose of 20 mg/kg).

Diagnosis. Diagnosis may be presumptive in neutropenic patients with prolonged fever because positive blood fungal cultures occur only in a minority of patients who are later found to have disseminated infection. *Candida* grows readily on routine blood culture media; 90% or more of positive cultures are identified in 72 hr or less, and 97% or more are identified in 7 days or less. *Candida* recovered from urine or tracheal secretions may represent colonization or infection.

Treatment. Amphotericin B remains the treatment of choice for systemic candidal infections, alone or with the addition of flucytosine or fluconazole, which is especially useful for central nervous system infections and parenchymal kidney infections. In one study in adults, fluconazole was as effective as amphotericin B for disseminated candidal infections and had fewer adverse effects. Fluconazole may be useful for selected candidal infections but is not effective against *C. krusei* and many strains of *C. glabrata*. Amphotericin is inactive against approximately 20% of strains of *C. lusitaniae*; susceptibility testing should be performed for all strains. Lipid-complex formulations of amphotericin B (5 mg/kg/24 hr) are recommended for persons with compromised renal function (including doubling of the serum creatinine with amphotericin B desoxycholate therapy), for those who are receiving other nephrotoxic therapy, or for those who are otherwise intolerant of amphotericin B desoxycholate.

215.4 Chronic Mucocutaneous Candidiasis

Chronic mucocutaneous candidiasis is a heterogeneous group of immune disorders, all of which involve a primary defect of T-lymphocyte responsiveness to *Candida*. Endocrinopathies (e.g., hypoparathyroidism, Addison disease) and autoimmune disorders are often associated with this disorder. Symptoms may begin in the first few months of life or as late as the 2nd decade of life. The disorder is characterized by chronic and severe skin and mucous membrane infections with *Candida* and occasionally other dermatophytes. Systemic candidiasis rarely occurs. Topical antifungal therapy may provide limited improvement early in the course of the disease, but repeated courses of ketoconazole or fluconazole, and occasionally amphotericin B, are usually necessary. The infection usually responds temporarily to treatment but is not eradicated and recurs.

Eppes SC, Troutman JL, Gutman LT: Outcome of treatment of candidemia in children whose central catheters were removed or retained. *Pediatr Infect Dis J* 1989; 8:99–104.

Hoppe JE: Treatment of oropharyngeal candidiasis and candidal diaper dermatitis in neonates and infants. Review and reappraisal. *Pediatr Infect Dis J* 1997;16: 885–96.

Makhoul IR, Kassis I, Smolkin T: Review of 49 neonates with acquired fungal sepsis: Further characterization. *Pediatrics* 2001;107:61–6.

Noyola DE, Fernandez M, Moylett EH: Ophthalmologic, visceral and cardiac involvement in neonates with candidemia. *Clin Infect Dis* 2001;32:1018–23.

Palma-Carlos AG, Palma-Carlos ML: Chronic mucocutaneous candidiasis revisited. *Allerg Immunol* 2001;33:229–32.

Rowen JL, Tate JM: Management of neonatal candidiasis. Neonatal Candidiasis Study Group. *Pediatr Infect Dis J* 1998;17:1007–11.

Saiman L, Ludington E, Pfaller M, et al: Risk factors for candidemia in neonatal intensive care unit patients. The National Epidemiology of Mycosis Survey study group. *Pediatr Infect Dis J* 2000;19:319–24.

Schwarze R, Penk A, Pittrow L: Treatment of candidal infections with fluconazole in neonates and infants. *Eur J Med Res* 2000;5:203–8.

Chapter 216
Cryptococcus neoformans
Stephen C. Aronoff

Etiology. Cryptococcosis is an invasive fungal disease caused by the monomorphic, encapsulated yeast *Cryptococcus neoformans*. *C. neoformans* var. *neoformans* predominates in temperate climates and is found in soil contaminated with avian droppings, on fruits and vegetables, and may be carried by cockroaches. It is the predominant pathogenic fungal infection among individuals infected with HIV. *C. neoformans* var. *gatti* is found mostly in the tropics under flowering river red gum trees (*Eucalyptus camaldulensis*) and causes endemic disease in the tropics in non–HIV-infected individuals. *C. albidus* and *C. laurentii* are rare human pathogens.

Epidemiology. Cryptococcosis is an unusual disease in immunocompetent persons and is rare in children. Pigeon breeders and laboratory personnel who work with *Cryptococcus* are at greatest risk. Studies of cryptococcal seroprevalence show no evidence of exposure in young infants, <5% in children older than 5 yr of age, and 60% in adults. Cryptococcosis is also rare (<1%) among HIV-infected children but occurs in 5–10% of HIV-infected adults; higher rates of infection have been reported from developing countries. Pediatric cases of cryptococcosis are evenly divided among immunocompetent and immunocompromised individuals.

Pathogenesis. In most cases *C. neoformans* is acquired by inhalation of fungal spores. Local inoculation rarely manifests into cutaneous or ophthalmic infection. Infection in immunocompetent persons is limited to the lung. When the immune system fails to contain the infection, dissemination follows with potential involvement of the brain, meninges, skin, eyes, and skeletal system.

Pulmonary cryptococcosis produces granulomas that are often subpleural in location and contain yeast forms. Cystic cryptococcomas occur in the central nervous system (CNS) in 20% of non–HIV-infected patients with disseminated disease and may be found in the absence of overt meningitis. Granulomas and microabscesses containing yeast occur in patients with cutaneous and bony infection.

Clinical Manifestations. Pneumonia is the most common form of cryptococcosis. Other manifestations include disseminated disease that may be associated with a sepsis syndrome, or focal symptoms such as meningitis, cutaneous infection, osteoarticular infection, or ocular infection that result from dissemination.

PNEUMONIA. Asymptomatic pulmonary infections occur frequently, especially among pigeon breeders, bird fanciers, and microbiology laboratory workers. Asymptomatic carriage may occur in patients with underlying chronic lung disease. Progressive pulmonary disease is symptomatic and often precedes disseminated infection in the immunocompromised host. Fever, cough, pleuritic chest pain, and constitutional symptoms occur. Chest radiographs may demonstrate a poorly localized bronchopneumonia, nodular changes, or lobar consolidations; cavities and pleural effusions are rare.

DISSEMINATED INFECTION. Disseminated infection follows primary pulmonary disease and occurs most often in immunocompromised individuals. HIV infection is the most common predisposing factor for disseminated cryptococcosis; other major predisposing conditions include hematologic malignancies, bone marrow transplantation, primary immunodeficiencies affecting both T- and B-cell lines, immunosuppression for rheumatic diseases, and celiac disease. A sepsis syndrome is a rare but often fatal manifestation of cryptococcosis that occurs almost exclusively in HIV-infected patients. Fever is followed by respiratory distress and multiorgan system disease.

MENINGITIS. Subacute or chronic meningitis is the most common clinical manifestation of disseminated cryptococcal infection. The clinical presentation is variable and prognostic. Good outcomes are associated with headache as the initial symptom, normal mental status, absence of a predisposing condition, normal cerebrospinal fluid (CSF) opening pressure, normal CSF glucose, CSF leukocyte count of <20 cells/μL, negative CSF India ink stain, absence of extraneural infection by culture, and cryptococcal antigen titers in CSF and serum of <1:32. Overt symptoms of meningitis and HIV infection are predictors of a poor outcome. HIV-infected patients typically present with unexplained fevers, headache, and malaise with cryptococcal antigen titers >1:1,024. CT of the brain identifies cryptococcomas in as many as 30% of patients with disseminated infection and no clinical signs of CNS involvement. The mortality rate for cryptococcal meningitis is 15–30%, with most deaths occurring within several weeks of diagnosis. The fatality rates are higher in HIV-infected individuals, who have relapse rates of >50%. Relapse is unusual in adequately treated, non–HIV-infected patients. Postinfectious sequelae are common and include hydrocephalus, changes in visual acuity, deafness, cranial nerve palsies, seizures, and ataxia.

CUTANEOUS INFECTION. Cutaneous disease may accompany disseminated cryptococcosis or local infection. Early lesions are erythematous, may be single or multiple, and are variably indurated and tender. Lesions often become ulcerated with central necrosis and raised borders. Cutaneous cryptococcosis in HIV-infected patients may resemble molluscum contagiosum.

OSTEOARTICULAR INFECTION. Osteoarticular infection occurs in approximately 5% of individuals with disseminated infection but rarely in HIV-infected patients. The onset of symptoms is insidious and chronic. Bony involvement is typified by soft tissue swelling and tenderness, and arthritis is characterized by effusion, erythema, and pain on motion. Skeletal disease is unifocal in approximately 75% of cases. The vertebrae are the most common sites of infection followed by the tibia, ileum, rib, femur, and humerus. Concomitant bone and joint disease results from contiguous spread.

OCULAR INFECTION. Chorioretinitis is rare, occurs primarily in adults, and is usually a manifestation of disseminated disease, although direct inoculation of the eye has been described. Eye infection is characterized by the acute loss of visual acuity, eye pain, visual floaters, and photophobia. On examination, choroiditis with or without retinitis is usually noted. Retinal and vitreal masses and anterior uveitis are seen less commonly. Because eye disease is often a manifestation of disseminated infection, the mortality rate with associated ocular infection is >20%. Only 15% of survivors recover full vision.

LYMPH NODES. Lymphonodular disease has been reported in two children, one of whom had an underlying immunodeficiency. Lymphonodular cryptococcosis is characterized by disseminated lymphadenopathy including thoracic and abdominal nodes, subcutaneous lesions, liver granulomas, and concomitant pulmonary disease.

Diagnosis. Definitive diagnosis requires identification of the fungus histologically in tissue specimens or recovery of the fungus from the site of infection by culture. A latex agglutination test, which detects cryptococcal antigen in serum and CSF, is the most useful diagnostic test. India ink preparations of CSF are useful prognostically but are less sensitive than culture and antigen detection. Skin test antigens are poorly characterized, and the sensitivity and specificity are unknown.

Treatment. Immunocompetent persons with asymptomatic or mild disease limited to the lungs may be closely observed without therapy or, alternatively, treated with oral fluconazole (200–400 mg/24 hr) for 3–6 mo. All patients with cryptococcal antigen titers >1:8 should be treated. Immunocompetent hosts with progressive pulmonary disease or immunocompromised patients, other than HIV-infected persons, with disease limited to the lungs can be treated with amphotericin B (0.7–1 mg/kg/24 hr) alone or in combination with flucytosine. Lipid-complex formulations of amphotericin B (5 mg/kg/24 hr) are recommended for persons with compromised renal function (including doubling of the serum creatinine with amphotericin B desoxycholate therapy), for those who are receiving other nephrotoxic therapy, or for those who are otherwise intolerant of amphotericin B desoxycholate.

For the treatment of CNS and other manifestations of disseminated infection in non–HIV-infected individuals, staged therapy is often used. Initial treatment consists of amphotericin B (0.7–1 mg/kg/24 hr), or lipid-complex formulations of amphotericin B (5 mg/kg/24 hr), plus flucytosine (50–150 mg/kg/24 hr) for 2 wk; the dosage of flucytosine should be adjusted to maintain serum concentrations of 50–150 μg/mL. This regimen may be continued for a total of 6–10 wk, or fluconazole alone may be given orally for an additional 10 wk. Effectiveness of therapy is monitored by serial cryptococcal antigen testing; serum or CSF values of ≥1:8 are predictive of relapse. Ventriculoperitoneal shunts may be required for patients with hydrocephalus, and aggressive medical management of increased intracranial pressure may also be required.

Cryptococcosis in HIV-infected patients is prone to relapse upon termination of treatment. HIV-infected patients with isolated pulmonary disease require lifelong therapy with fluconazole. HIV-infected patients with CNS or disseminated cryptococcal infection require induction and maintenance therapy. Induction therapy consists of amphotericin B and flucytosine for at least 2 wk; amphotericin B may given alone if flucytosine is not tolerated. Amphotericin B and flucytosine may be continued for 6–10 wk as consolidation therapy, or fluconazole may be given alone for 10 wk. After completion of consolidation therapy, fluconazole is continued for life. Cessation of maintenance therapy for individuals whose HIV infection is well controlled on antiretroviral therapy has not been studied.

Cutaneous infections are usually treated medically, although surgical biopsy may be required for diagnosis. Skeletal infections generally require surgical debridement in addition to systemic antifungal therapy. Chorioretinitis also requires systemic antifungal therapy with amphotericin B and either fluconazole or flucytosine, both of which achieve high drug concentrations in the vitreous.

Dismukes WE: Management of cryptococcosis. *Clin Infect Dis* 1993;17:507–12.
Dromer F, Mathoulin S, Dupont B, et al: Epidemiology of cryptococcosis in France: A 9-year survey (1985–1993). *Clin Infect Dis* 1996;23:82–90.

Gumbo T, Kadzirange G, Mielke J, et al: *Cryptococcus neoformans* meningoencephalitis in African children with AIDS. *Pediatr Infect Dis J* 2002;21:54–6.

Gonzalez CE, Shetty D, Lewis LL, et al: *Cryptococcus* in human immunodeficiency virus-infected children. *Pediatr Infect Dis J* 1996;15:796–800.

Leggiadro RJ, Barrett FF, Hughes WT: Extrapulmonary cryptococcosis in immunocompromised infants and children. *Pediatr Infect Dis J* 1992;11:43–7.

Leggiadro RJ, Kline MW, Hughes WT: Extrapulmonary cryptococcosis in children with acquired immunodeficiency syndrome. *Pediatr Infect Dis J* 1991;10:658–62.

Moncino MD, Gutman LT: Severe systemic cryptococcal disease in a child. Review of prognostic indicators predicting treatment failure and an approach to maintenance therapy with oral fluconazole. *Pediatr Infect Dis J* 1990;9:363–5.

Saag MS, Graybill RJ, Larsen RA, et al: Practice guidelines for the management of cryptococcal disease. *Clin Infect Dis* 2000;30:710–8.

Speed BR, Kaldor J: Rarity of cryptococcal infection in children. *Pediatr Infect Dis J* 1997;16:536.

Chapter 217

Malassezia Martin E. Weisse

Members of the genus *Malassezia* include the causative agent of the fungal dermatosis tinea versicolor and have emerged as infrequent causes of fungemia in patients with indwelling catheters. *Malassezia* is a commensal lipophilic yeast with a predilection for the sebum-rich areas of skin. Because the yeast forms may be either oval or round, they were earlier designated *Pityrosporum ovale* and *P. orbiculare*. Transformation of the yeast to hyphal forms facilitates invasive disease. The clusters of thick-walled blastospores together with the hyphae produce the characteristic "spaghetti and meatballs" appearance. *M. furfur* is the most common clinical isolate of the seven species; however, *M. pachydermatis* has been implicated in several outbreaks in neonatal intensive care units.

M. globosa is a major cause of tinea versicolor (see Chapter 656). *Malassezia* has been implicated in neonatal acne and seborrheic dermatitis. *Malassezia* may be isolated from sebum-rich skin of asymptomatic persons, emphasizing that demonstration of the fungus does not equate with infection.

Catheter-related *Malassezia* fungemia occurs almost exclusively in patients receiving intravenous lipids. The use of lipid emulsions containing medium-chain triglycerides inhibits the growth of *Malassezia*, which may prevent infection with *Malassezia*. Infection is most common in premature infants, although immunocompromised patients, especially those with malignancies, may also be infected. Symptoms of catheter-associated fungemia are indistinguishable from other causes of catheter-associated infections (see Chapter 165) but should be suspected in patients, especially neonates, receiving intravenous lipid infusions. Compared with other causes of fungal sepsis, it is unusual for catheter-related *Malassezia* fungemia to be associated with secondary focal infection.

Malassezia does not grow readily on standard fungal media, and successful culture requires overlaying the agar with olive oil. Recovery of *Malassezia* from blood culture is optimized by supplementing the media with olive oil or palmitic acid.

Fungemia due to *M. furfur* or other species can be successfully treated in most cases by immediately discontinuing the lipid infusion and removing the infected catheter. For persistent or invasive infections, amphotericin B (desoxycholate or lipid-complex formulations), fluconazole, and itraconazole are effective. Flucytosine has no activity.

Chryssanthou E, Broberger U, Petrini B: *Malassezia pachydermatis* fungaemia in a neonatal intensive care unit. *Acta Paediatr* 2001;90 323–7.

Midgley G: The lipophilic yeasts: State of the art and prospects. *Med Mycol* 2000; 38:9–16.

Nakabayashi A, Sei Y, Guillot J: Identification of *Malassezia* species isolated from patients with seborrheic dermatitis, atopic dermatitis, pityriasis versicolor and normal subjects. *Med Mycol* 2000;38:337–41.

Papavassilis C, Mach KK, Mayser PA: Medium-chain triglycerides inhibit growth of *Malassezia*: Implications for prevention of systemic infection. *Crit Care Med* 1999; 27:1781–6.

Chapter 218

Aspergillus Stephen C. Aronoff

Aspergillosis refers to a group of diseases caused by monomorphic, mycelial fungi of the genus *Aspergillus*. Most diseases in children are caused by *A. fumigatus* and less frequently by *A. flavus* and *A. niger*. Other species, including *A. nidulans* and *A. terreus*, have also been reported in pediatric infections. Aspergilli are distributed worldwide, and spores (conidia) are readily isolated from soil and decaying plants. Outbreaks of invasive disease among immunocompromised children may occur after they have been exposed to aerosolized conidia at construction sites within or near hospitals and clinics. Infection is usually acquired from inhalation of airborne spores, which colonize the upper and lower respiratory tracts. Immunocompromised persons are at risk for hematogenous dissemination. Cutaneous infection is also common and may follow wound contamination, intradermal inoculation, or hematogenous dissemination. Ingestion and aspiration may also produce disease. *Aspergillus*-associated diseases may be immunoglobulin (Ig) E mediated (hypersensitivity syndromes), saprophytic (noninvasive) syndromes, and invasive syndromes.

218.1 Hypersensitivity Syndromes

Asthma. Atopic asthma (see Chapter 134) may be precipitated by inhalation of *Aspergillus* spores, which triggers an IgE-mediated response and bronchospasm. The clinical symptoms are nonspecific and include the acute onset of wheezing in the absence of pulmonary infiltrates or fever.

Extrinsic Alveolar Alveolitis. Extrinsic alveolar alveolitis is a hypersensitivity pneumonitis that occurs in nonatopic individuals after repeated exposures to organic dust and usually with occupational exposure (malt worker's lung or farmer's lung). *Aspergillus* is one of many organic substances that produce this syndrome. The pathogenesis is unknown but is similar to the alveolitis caused by other immunogens and may represent an immune complex disease. The clinical manifestations typically follow exposure by 4–6 hr and include fever, cough, and dyspnea. Physical examination often reveals rhonchi without wheezes. Eosinophilia is absent from blood and sputum, and chest radiograph often shows diffuse interstitial infiltrates. Chronic exposure gradually leads to irreversible pulmonary fibrosis.

Allergic Bronchopulmonary Aspergillosis. Allergic bronchopulmonary aspergillosis complicates chronic pulmonary disease in approximately 10% of children with asthma or cystic fibrosis. Chronic mucosal colonization with *A. fumigatus* produces an exaggerated IgG and IgE response, which results in recurrent bronchospasm and proximal cylindrical bronchiectasis. This should be considered in patients with asthma or cystic fibrosis who have recurrent bronchospasm and transient pulmonary infiltrates. Expectoration of mucous spirals containing mycelia is a hallmark of this illness; peripheral eosinophilia is common. Diagnostic criteria for allergic bronchopulmonary aspergillosis include (1) reversible paroxysmal bronchiolar obstruction (asthma); (2) immediate cutaneous reactivity to *A. fumigatus* antigens or specific serum IgE to *A. fumigatus*, by the radioallergosorbent test; (3) elevated total serum IgE; (4) peripheral blood eosinophilia; (5) precipitating serum antibodies against *A. fumigatus*; (6) history of previous pulmonary infiltrates; and (7) proximal bronchiectasis. The disease may progress through three stages: steroid responsive, steroid dependence, and end-stage pulmonary fibrosis.

Treatment. Treatment of the hypersensitivity pulmonary syndromes focuses on anti-inflammatory agents, notably corticosteroids, and bronchodilator therapy. Acute exacerbations of disease are characterized by increased episodes of wheezing, diminished pulmonary function, and increased serum IgE concentrations. These episodes can be treated initially with prednisone 0.5 mg/kg/24 hr for 1 wk followed by 0.5 mg/kg every other day until symptoms abate and serum IgE returns to pre-illness levels. Although not studied in children, adults with allergic bronchopulmonary aspergillosis randomized to oral itraconazole for 16 wk experienced fewer symptoms, had reduced serum IgE concentrations, and required less prednisone than placebo recipients.

218.2 Saprophytic (Noninvasive) Syndromes

Otomycosis. Otomycosis is a chronic condition that is found predominantly in tropical and subtropical regions and is rare in infants and children. Most infections are due to *A. niger* or, less commonly, *A. fumigatus*; co-infection with *Staphylococcus aureus* or *Pseudomonas* occurs in one third of cases. Most cases are unilateral, with presenting symptoms of ear pain, itching of the auditory canal, and a sense of fullness. Otorrhea, decreased hearing, and tinnitus are less common. Examination of the auditory canal typically shows conidial "forests" or mycelial mats. Topical antifungal agents such as nystatin, tolnaftate, dilute acetic acid, and corticosteroids are therapeutic. Oral itraconazole has also been effective; however, experience is limited.

Sinus Disease. *Aspergillus* noninvasive sinonasal disease may present in three forms. Chronic or indolent sinusitis is confined to one sinus and presents as a chronic sinus infection that is unresponsive to antibacterial therapy. Sinus radiographs are nonspecific, showing mucosal thickening without bony changes. Endoscopic surgery is curative in most cases. Sinus aspergilloma, which is rare in children, presents with long-standing nasal symptoms. Sinus radiographs demonstrate a solitary mass in the ethmoid or maxillary sinus. Bony destruction is variable. Surgical removal of the mass, which can often be performed endoscopically, is the treatment of choice. Allergic fungal sinusitis involves multiple sinuses and occurs in immunocompetent persons who usually have a history of multiple preceding sinus surgeries and nasal polyposis. *Aspergillus* and, less often, *Curvularia lunata* are the usual etiologic agents. Histology of nasal secretions in these patients reveals thick mucin, eosinophils, and few fungal hyphae. Sinus imaging typically shows involvement of multiple sinuses with hypodense areas and occasionally calcifications and bony erosions. Criteria for the diagnosis of allergic fungal sinusitis are immunologic and are identical to those listed for allergic bronchopulmonary aspergillosis, which may complicate allergic fungal sinusitis. Treatment includes surgical drainage and debridement as well as corticosteroid therapy. Antibiotics may be required for secondary bacterial infections.

Pulmonary Aspergilloma. Pulmonary aspergillomas develop in poorly drained bronchi or pre-existing pulmonary cavities and may complicate pulmonary tuberculosis, histoplasmosis, blastomycosis, or sarcoidosis; rarely, aspergillomas complicate invasive *Aspergillus* pulmonary disease. Colonization and fungal proliferation occur in the cavity, but no vascular invasion occurs; an amorphous mycelial mass (mycetoma or fungus ball) results. Affected children are often asymptomatic or have cough and hemoptysis. Chest radiographs characteristically demonstrate the air shadow of a pulmonary cavity outlining a rounded mass; these findings may be confirmed by CT of the chest. Management is controversial and may range from watchful waiting for asymptomatic and otherwise healthy children to surgical resection for those patients with symptoms.

218.3 Invasive Disease

Pneumonia and Disseminated Infection. Invasive pulmonary aspergillosis is the most common form of *Aspergillus* infection and usually occurs in immunocompromised patients. The onset is often insidious. In both immunocompetent and immunocompromised patients, symptomatic infection presents acutely with fever, cough, dyspnea, and abnormal chest findings; pleuritic chest pain is an infrequent complaint. Chest radiographs often show nodular infiltrates. Coexisting sinusitis is a common finding in neutropenic children. In children with chronic granulomatous disease, direct extension from the lungs to the chest wall has been reported.

The diagnosis is confirmed by histologic demonstration of hyphal invasion of blood vessels and recovery of the fungus by culture of the biopsy specimen. Recovery by culture or *Aspergillus* antigen detection in bronchoalveolar lavage fluid is also diagnostic in immunosuppressed patients with new pulmonary findings. Recovery of a pure culture of a single *Aspergillus* species in two sputum samples from immunocompromised patients with nodular, cavitary, or wedge-shaped lesions seen on chest radiographs is highly suggestive of invasive disease.

Treatment with high-dose amphotericin B (1 mg/kg/24 hr) for 4–6 wk, or until the neutropenia resolves or the underlying disease goes into remission, is recommended. Lipid-complex formulations of amphotericin B (5 mg/kg/24 hr) are recommended for persons with compromised renal function (including doubling of the serum creatinine with amphotericin B desoxycholate therapy), those who are receiving other nephrotoxic therapy, or those who are otherwise intolerant of amphotericin B desoxycholate. Completion of therapy with oral itraconazole has also been suggested but definitive trials are lacking.

Invasive *Aspergillus* infection is characterized by hyphal infiltration of vascular structures, thrombosis, and focal necrosis. Invasive disease occurs most commonly in immunocompromised patients, especially among patients with cancer who are receiving chemotherapy, HIV-infected persons, bone marrow transplant recipients, and, less commonly, solid organ recipients. Primary invasive disease may occur at any site in which airborne conidia may colonize and germinate, such as the respiratory tract or skin. In the severely neutropenic child, dissemination results from direct extension from the primary site and hematogenous seeding of distant sites. Sinonasal disease, pulmonary disease, and cutaneous disease are the most common primary infections in children. Otitis media is rare. Although systemic amphotericin B (either desoxycholate or lipid-complex formulations) remains the recommended treatment for most established *Aspergillus* infections, the outcome appears to hinge on resolution of the underlying immunocompromised state. Itraconazole, a triazole antifungal agent, has appreciable in vitro activity against *Aspergillus* but experience with this agent for the treatment of aspergillosis in children is limited. Aerosolized amphotericin B is currently under investigation for prophylaxis in cancer patients during periods of profound neutropenia.

Otitis Externa. Otitis externa associated with *Aspergillus* infection is rare, occurs in immunosuppressed individuals, and is associated with hearing loss and direct extension to the petrous portion of the temporal bone and the pinna. Therapy includes surgical debridement and amphotericin B; experience with itraconazole is limited. Less invasive disease may be controlled with topical antifungal therapy, lavage, and cerumen removal.

Sinus Disease. Acute, invasive sinusitis is rare in children and occurs almost exclusively in patients with profound neutropenia associated with chemotherapy for cancer. Fever, cough, epistaxis, headache, and sinus pain are the most common clinical signs. Examination typically shows nasal crusting with rhinorrhea, sinus tenderness, nasal or oral ulceration, and duskiness or necrosis of the nasal septum or inferior turbinates. Multiple sinus involvement with opacification or air-fluid levels can be demonstrated radiographically or by CT. Endoscopic examination demonstrates mucosal necrosis. Biopsy and culture of the nasal or sinus mucosa demonstrate large numbers of hyphae, and fungal cultures typically yield *A. fumigatus, A. flavus,* or, less often, *Rhizopus* or *Candida.* The disease is characterized by rapid spread to adjacent tissues and a high mortality rate. Treatment is not standardized but often includes surgical drainage, intravenous and intranasal amphotericin B, and removal of avascular necrotic tissue. Extensive surgical procedures are often hampered by underlying thrombocytopenia with extensive and at times life-threatening hemorrhage. Sporadic treatment successes and failures have been reported with itraconazole; however, comparative data with amphotericin B are not available. Invasive sinusitis has a poor prognosis for children with leukemia in relapse; better outcomes result from resolution of the granulocytopenia or remission of the underlying disease.

Chronic invasive sinus disease occurs in immunocompetent individuals who live in arid regions where endemic mold counts are high such as the Middle East and Africa. *A. flavus* is the most common pathogen. Infected patients have a progressive course spanning months to years, with extension of the infection to the surrounding sinuses, orbits, and cranial vaults. Treatment encompasses surgical debridement and drainage. Antifungal therapy is occasionally used.

Skin. Cutaneous aspergillosis is a common manifestation of invasive aspergillosis in immunocompromised children. Cutaneous disease may result either from direct inoculation of the skin, typically at sites of local trauma such as intravenous catheter sites or complicating burn wounds or diaper dermatitis, or, more frequently, from hematogenous dissemination. The skin lesions appear initially as tender erythematous plaques that progress to hemorrhagic bullae and necrotic ulcers and eschars, termed ecthyma gangrenosum. Cutaneous aspergillosis in most children with profound neutropenia is a sentinel marker of disseminated *Aspergillus* disease and portends a poor outcome. Treatment with high-dose amphotericin B (1 mg/kg/24 hr) is recommended for 4–6 wk, or until the neutropenia resolves or the underlying disease is in remission. Lipid-complex formulations of amphotericin B (5 mg/kg/24 hr) are recommended for persons with compromised renal function (including doubling of the serum creatinine with amphotericin B desoxycholate therapy), for those who are receiving other nephrotoxic therapy, or for those who are otherwise intolerant of amphotericin B desoxycholate. Local debridement and topical amphotericin B have also been used. Experience with itraconazole is limited.

Onychomycosis due to *Aspergillus* may be treated successfully with oral itraconazole alone or combined with topical therapy.

Eye. Fungal endophthalmitis is an important diagnostic finding in immunosuppressed children with disseminated *Aspergillus* infection. Although most patients have no ocular symptoms, pain, photophobia, and diminished visual acuity may occur. Examination of the retina shows focal retinitis, an overlying vitreitis, and retinal hemorrhage. Treatment of the underlying immunosuppressive illness, systemic antifungal therapy, vitrectomy, and intraocular amphotericin B are recommended. Amphotericin B and itraconazole achieve poor intraocular concentrations.

Orbital cellulitis rarely complicates invasive sinusitis and follows destruction of the orbital walls and fungal extension into the retro-orbital space. Diplopia, periorbital edema, proptosis, and pain on lateral gaze may occur. Treatment requires a combination of surgical debridement, systemic antifungal therapy, and resolution of the underlying immunocompromised state.

Fungal keratitis and episcleritis are rare and follow direct inoculation of spores into the eye. In the absence of disseminated disease, topical and intrascleral amphotericin B therapy is recommended.

Central Nervous System. Cerebral aspergillosis is a rare and almost uniformly fatal complication of disseminated disease. In most cases, infection involves single or multiple foci within the cerebral hemispheres or cerebellum. Focal neurologic deficits begin acutely, most often hemiparesis, anterior cranial nerve palsies, or seizures; progression to herniation is rapid. Meningeal signs are rare. At autopsy arachnoiditis is limited to the area adjacent to the cerebral focus. Cerebrospinal fluid shows a mild mononuclear pleocytosis, elevated CSF protein, and variable degrees of hypoglycorrhachia. Imaging studies demonstrate focal central nervous system lesions with edema and variable enhancement. The diagnosis can be established by the acute appearance of neurologic symptoms in a patient with proven or suspected invasive aspergillosis or occasionally by cerebrospinal fluid or brain biopsy culture. High-dose amphotericin B combined with flucytosine has been effective in a paucity of cases. In recalcitrant cases, intraventricular therapy may also be required.

Epidural abscess is a rare complication of vertebral osteomyelitis caused by *Aspergillus* species. In two children with epidural abscess, vertebral osteomyelitis, and cord compression, surgical decompression and high-dose amphotericin B were curative.

Bone. Aspergillosis of the bone is an extremely rare disease and follows direct extension of infection from a surgical or traumatic wound, or hematogenous seeding. Involvement of the vertebrae is most common. Osteomyelitis of the rib is rare but occurs in children with chronic granulomatous disease and often represents extension from a pulmonary focus. Surgical drainage is often required. Although definitive studies are not available, therapy with amphotericin B plus flucytosine has been used successfully despite the poor bone penetration of amphotericin B. Itraconazole achieves good bone concentrations and has been used successfully.

Heart. Endocarditis is a rare form of aspergillosis and can follow contamination at the time of surgery or implantation of a contaminated graft, or, uncommonly, it may be a manifestation of disseminated aspergillosis. High-dose amphotericin B therapy coupled with surgical removal of infected grafts or prostheses is recommended.

Denning DW, Stevens DA: Antifungal and surgical treatment of invasive aspergillosis. Review of 2,121 published cases. *Rev Infect Dis* 1990;12:1147–201.
Horvath JA, Dummer S: The use of respiratory tract cultures in the diagnosis of invasive pulmonary aspergillosis. *Am J Med* 1996;100:171–8.
Neijens HJ, Frenkel J, de Muinck Keizer-Schrama SM, et al: Invasive *Aspergillus* infection in chronic granulomatous disease. Treatment with itraconazole. *J Pediatr* 1989;115:1016–9.
Stevens DA, Schwartz HJ, Lee JY, et al: A randomized trial of itraconazole in allergic bronchopulmonary aspergillosis. *N Engl J Med* 2000;342:756–62.
Stevens DA, Kan VL, Judson MA, et al: Practice guidelines for diseases caused by *Aspergillus. Clin Infect Dis* 2000;30:696–709.
Walmsley S, Devi S, King S, et al: Invasive *Aspergillus* infections in a pediatric hospital. A ten-year review. *Pediatr Infect Dis J* 1993;12:673–82.
Wong-Beringer A, Jacobs RA, Guglielmo BJ: Lipid formulations of amphotericin B. Clinical efficacy and toxicities. *Clin Infect Dis* 1998;27:603–18.

Chapter 219
Histoplasmosis (*Histoplasma capsulatum*)

Stephen C. Aronoff

Etiology. The etiologic agent of histoplasmosis, *Histoplasma capsulatum*, exhibits temperature dimorphism, existing as a mycelial form (mold) in nature at ambient temperatures (25°C–30°C) and as a yeast in human tissues (37°C).

Epidemiology. The saprophytic form is found in soil throughout the midwestern United States, primarily along the Ohio and Mississippi rivers; sporadic cases of human and animal histoplasmosis have been reported from 31 of the 48 contiguous states. In parts of Kentucky and Tennessee, almost 90% of the population older than 20 yr of age have positive skin tests to histoplasmin.

H. capsulatum thrives in soil rich in nitrates such as areas that are heavily contaminated with bird droppings or decayed wood. Fungal spores are often carried on the wings of birds. Focal outbreaks of histoplasmosis have been reported after aerosolization of microconidia resulting from construction in areas previously occupied by starling roosts or chicken coops or by chopping decayed wood. Unlike birds, bats are actively infected with *Histoplasma*. Outbreaks of histoplasmosis have also been reported after intense exposure to bat guano in caves and along bridges frequented by bats.

Pathogenesis. Human infection begins with inhalation of microconidia that reach the alveoli, germinate, and proliferate as yeast. The initial infection is a bronchopneumonia. As the initial pulmonary lesion matures, giant cells form, which are followed by formation of granuloma and central necrosis. At the time of spore germination, yeast cells gain access to the reticuloendothelial system by way of the pulmonary lymphatic system and hilar lymph nodes. Dissemination with splenic involvement typically follows the primary pulmonary infection. The immune response follows in approximately 2 wk. The initial pulmonary lesion resolves within 2–4 mo but may undergo calcification resembling the Ghon complex of tuberculosis; alternatively, "buckshot" calcifications involving the lung and spleen may be seen. Unlike tuberculosis, reinfection with *H. capsulatum* occurs and may lead to exaggerated host immune responses in some cases.

Clinical Manifestations. There are three forms of human histoplasmosis: acute pulmonary infection, chronic pulmonary histoplasmosis, and progressive disseminated histoplasmosis. **Acute pulmonary histoplasmosis** follows initial or recurrent respiratory exposure to microconidia. Most patients are asymptomatic. Symptomatic disease occurs more often in young children; in older individuals, symptoms follow exposure to large inocula in closed spaces (e.g., chicken coops, caves) or prolonged exposure (e.g., camping on contaminated soil, chopping decayed wood). The prodrome is nonspecific and usually consists of flulike symptoms: headache, fever, chest pain, and cough. Hepatosplenomegaly occurs more often in infants and young children. Symptomatic infections may be associated with significant respiratory distress and hypoxia and may require intubation, ventilation, and corticosteroid therapy. Acute pulmonary disease may also present with a prolonged illness (10 days to 3 wk) consisting of weight loss, dyspnea, high fever, asthenia, and fatigue. Approximately 10% of patients with acute pulmonary infection present with a sarcoid-like disease that includes arthritis or arthralgia, erythema nodosum, keratoconjunctivitis, iridocyclitis, and pericarditis. Most children with acute pulmonary disease have normal chest radiography findings. Individuals with symptomatic disease typically have a patchy bronchopneumonia; hilar lymphadenopathy is variably present. In young children, the pneumonia may coalesce. Focal or buckshot calcifications are convalescent findings in patients with acute pulmonary infection.

Exaggerated immune responses to fungal antigens within the lung parenchyma or hilar lymph nodes produce thoracic complications of acute pulmonary histoplasmosis. **Histoplasmomas** are fibroma-like lesions of parenchymal origin that are usually solitary, asymptomatic, and often concentrically calcified. Rarely, these lesions produce broncholithiasis associated with "stone spitting," wheezing, and hemoptysis. In endemic regions, these lesions may mimic parenchymal tumors and are occasionally diagnosed at lung biopsy. **Mediastinal granulomas** form when reactive hilar lymph nodes coalesce and mat together. Although these lesions are usually asymptomatic, huge granulomas may compress the mediastinal structures, producing symptoms of esophageal, bronchial, or vena caval obstruction. Local extension and necrosis may produce pericarditis or pleural effusions. **Mediastinal fibrosis** is a rare complication of mediastinal granulomas and represents an uncontrolled fibrotic reaction arising from the hilar lymph nodes. Structures within the mediastinum become encased within a fibrotic mass, producing obstructive symptoms including superior vena cava syndrome, pulmonary venous obstruction with a mitral stenosis-like syndrome, and pulmonary artery obstruction with congestive heart failure. Dysphagia accompanies esophageal entrapment, and a syndrome of cough, wheeze, hemoptysis, and dyspnea accompanies bronchial obstruction.

Chronic pulmonary histoplasmosis is an opportunistic infection in adult patients with centrilobular emphysema. This entity is rare in children.

Progressive disseminated histoplasmosis is a disease that affects infants and immunocompromised individuals. Disseminated disease of infancy occurs almost exclusively in children younger than 2 yr of age and follows primary pulmonary infection. Fever is the most common finding and may last for weeks to months before the condition is diagnosed. The majority of patients have hepatosplenomegaly, anemia, and thrombocytopenia. Pneumonia and pancytopenia are variably present. In one series, half of the infected infants had transient T-cell deficiencies and many experienced a transient hyperglobulinemia. Although chest radiographs are normal in more than half of these children, the yeast can frequently be identified on bone marrow examination.

Children who are immunocompromised from cancer and chemotherapy, organ transplant, or HIV infection are at increased risk for disseminated histoplasmosis. In non–HIV-infected persons, disseminated disease presents with unexplained fevers, weight loss, lymphadenopathy, and interstitial pulmonary disease. Extrapulmonary infection is a characteristic of disseminated disease and may include destructive bony lesions, oropharyngeal ulcers, Addison's disease, meningitis, cutaneous infection, and endocarditis. Elevated liver function test results and high serum concentrations of angiotensin-converting enzyme may be observed.

Disseminated histoplasmosis with HIV infection is an AIDS-defining disease. Disseminated disease is often preceded or followed by another opportunistic infection in this patient population. HIV-infected individuals at greatest risk for acquiring disseminated histoplasmosis are those with a history of exposure to avian excreta or bat guano, no history of antiretroviral therapy, or no history of previous antifungal prophylaxis. Fever and weight loss occur in most individuals, with pulmonary disease occurring in most patients. Hepatosplenomegaly, lymphadenopathy, skin rashes, and meningoencephalitis are variably present. A sepsis-like syndrome has been identified in HIV-infected patients with disseminated histoplasmosis, which is characterized by the rapid onset of shock, multiorgan failure, and coagulopathy.

Diagnosis. Recovery of *H. capsulatum* by culture differs with the form of infection. In immunocompetent hosts with symptomatic or asymptomatic acute pulmonary histoplasmosis, sputum cultures are variably positive; cultures of bronchoalveolar lavage fluid appear to have a slightly higher yield than sputa. Blood cultures are sterile in patients with acute pulmonary histoplasmosis. Cultures from any source are typically sterile in individuals with the sarcoid form of the disease. Yeast forms may be demonstrated histologically in tissues from patients with complicated forms of acute pulmonary disease (histoplasmoma, mediastinal granuloma, and mediastinal fibrosis). Sputum cultures are positive in 60% of adults with chronic pulmonary histoplasmosis. The yeast can be recovered from blood or bone marrow in >90% of patients with progressive disseminated histoplasmosis.

Radioimmunoassay is the most widely available diagnostic study for detection of fungal antigen in patients with suspected progressive disseminated histoplasmosis. In HIV-infected patients as well as others at risk for disseminated disease, *Histoplasma*-associated antigen can be demonstrated in the serum or urine in >90% of cases. False-positive results may occur in individuals with blastomycosis, coccidioidomycosis, and paracoccidioidomycosis. Antigen detection by enzyme immunoassay has comparable sensitivity and improved specificity but limited availability. Sequential measurement of antigen in patients with disseminated disease is useful for monitoring response to therapy. Serum and urine from individuals with acute or chronic pulmonary infections are variably antigen positive.

Seroconversion continues to be useful for the diagnosis of acute pulmonary histoplasmosis, its complications, and chronic pulmonary disease. Serum antibody to yeast and mycelium-associated antigens is classically measured by complement fixation. Titers >1:8 are found in >80% of patients with histoplasmosis, and titers of ≥1:32 are considered significant for the diagnosis of recent infection. Complement fixation antibody titers are often not significant early in the infection and do not become positive until 4–6 wk after exposure. Complement fixation titers may be falsely positive in patients with other systemic mycoses and may be falsely negative in immunocompromised patients. Antibody detection by immunodiffusion is less sensitive than complement fixation and is used to confirm questionably positive complement fixation titers. Skin testing is useful only for epidemiologic studies because cutaneous reactivity is lifelong, and intradermal injection may elicit an immune response in otherwise seronegative individuals.

Treatment. Antifungal therapy is not warranted for immunocompetent persons with asymptomatic or mildly symptomatic acute pulmonary histoplasmosis. Oral itraconazole should be considered in patients with acute pulmonary infections who fail to improve clinically over a 1-mo period. Individuals with primary or re-exposure to pulmonary histoplasmosis who become hypoxemic or require ventilatory support should receive amphotericin B desoxycholate (0.7 mg/kg/24 hr IV) or a lipid-complex amphotericin B (3–5 mg/ kg/24 hr IV), until improved; continued therapy with oral itraconazole for a minimum of 12 wk is recommended. Lipid-complex formulations of amphotericin B are recommended for persons with compromised renal function (including doubling of the serum creatinine with amphotericin B desoxycholate therapy), those who are receiving other nephrotoxic therapy, or those who are otherwise intolerant of amphotericin B desoxycholate. Patients with severe obstructive symptoms caused by granulomatous mediastinal disease can be treated initially with amphotericin B and then switched to itraconazole, which is given for 6–12 mo. Milder mediastinal disease can be treated with oral itraconazole alone. Some experts recommend that surgery be reserved for those patients who fail to improve after 1 mo of intensive amphotericin B therapy. Sarcoid-like disease with or without pericarditis may be treated with nonsteroidal anti-inflammatory agents.

Amphotericin B continues to be the cornerstone of therapy for infants with progressive disseminated histoplasmosis. In one study, sequential therapy with amphotericin B and oral ketoconazole for 3 mo was curative in 88% of patients. Alternatively, amphotericin B may be given initially followed by oral itraconazole as maintenance therapy for 6–18 mo, with the duration based on serial *Histoplasma* antigen testing.

Relapses in HIV-infected individuals with progressive disseminated histoplasmosis are common. Currently, induction therapy with amphotericin B (total dose 10–15 mg/kg in children; >500 mg in adults) or lipid-complex formulations is recommended. Lifelong suppressive therapy with daily itraconazole (200 mg/

24 hr in adults) is also required. For severely immunocompromised, HIV-infected children living in endemic regions, itraconazole (2–5 mg/kg every 12–24 hr) may be used for prophylaxis. Care must be taken to avoid interactions between antifungal azoles and protease inhibitors.

Goodwin RA, Loyd JE, Des Prez RM: Histoplasmosis in normal hosts. *Medicine* 1981;60:231–66.

Hajjeh RA, Pappas PG, Henderson H, et al: Multicenter case-control study of risk factors for histoplasmosis in HIV infected persons. *Clin Infect Dis* 2001;32:1215–20.

Leggiadro RJ, Barrett FF, Hughes WT: Disseminated histoplasmosis of infancy. *Pediatr Infect Dis J* 1988;7:799–805.

Mocherla S, Wheat LJ: Treatment of histoplasmosis. *Semin Respir Infect* 2001;16:141–8.

Odio CM, Navarrete M, Carillo JM, et al: Disseminated histoplasmosis in infants. *Pediatr Infect Dis J* 1999;18:1065–8.

Tobon AM, Franco L, Espinal D, et al: Disseminated histoplasmosis in children. The role of itraconazole therapy. *Pediatr Infect Dis J* 1996;15:1002–8.

USPHS/IDSA Working Group: 1997 USPHS/IDSA guidelines for the prevention of opportunistic infections in persons infected with HIV: Disease-specific recommendations. *Clin Infect Dis* 1997;25:313–35.

Walsh TJ, Seibel NL, Arndt L, et al: Amphotericin B lipid complex in pediatric patients with invasive fungal infection. *Pediatr Infect Dis J* 1999;18:702–8.

Wheat J, Hafner R, Wulfsohn M, et al: Prevention of relapse of histoplasmosis with itraconazole in patients with the acquired immunodeficiency syndrome. The National Institute of Allergy and Infectious Diseases Clinical Trials and Mycoses Study Group Collaborators. *Ann Intern Med* 1993;118:610–6.

Wheat LJ: Histoplasmosis in Indianapolis. *Clin Infect Dis* 1992;14:91–9.

Chapter 220
Blastomycosis (*Blastomyces dermatitidis*)
Robin B. Churchill and Stephen C. Aronoff

Etiology. The etiologic agent of blastomycosis, *Blastomyces dermatitidis*, exhibits temperature dimorphism, existing as a mycelial form (mold) in nature at ambient temperatures (25°C–30°C) and as a thick-walled yeast in human tissues (37°C).

Epidemiology. Blastomycosis is an uncommon fungal infection and among children is rare; children <15 yr of age constitute only 2–10% of reported cases. Sporadic infection in endemic regions accounts for the majority of cases. Blastomycosis occurs primarily in North America but has been encountered in Africa, India, the Middle East, Central America, and South America. The organism is found throughout the midwestern, south-central, and southeastern United States, especially along the Ohio and Mississippi River valleys and in the Great Lakes region. Although difficult to isolate from soil, *B. dermatitidis* has been recovered from earth enriched with organic material, particularly near waterways in endemic areas. Epidemics are unusual but have been described after excavation of contaminated soil in endemic regions. Individuals who spend large amounts of time in wooded areas within endemic regions, such as hunters or forestry workers, are at highest risk for infection.

Pathogenesis. The pathogenesis of blastomycosis is similar to that of histoplasmosis. The primary site of infection is the lungs. Inhalation of spores results in alveolar inoculation and germination to yeast forms. Although pulmonary macrophages eliminate the majority of spores before infection occurs, those that survive produce pneumonitis and may disseminate hematogenously. The immune response to infection consists of neutrophil and macrophage migration into infected tissues. The resulting "pyogranulomatous" response with associated necrosis and subsequent fibrosis is characteristic of the disease.

Clinical Manifestations. The clinical spectrum of disease in human blastomycosis is diverse and ranges from asymptomatic infection to disseminated disease. Lack of an inexpensive, reliable screening test prevents identification of infection in most asymptomatic individuals. Nonspecific symptoms such as weight loss, unexplained fever, night sweats, and malaise may be the initial complaints in some patients. Acute pneumonia is the most common form of blastomycosis in both adults and children. Patients usually present with the acute onset of fever, chills, and productive cough, at times with hemoptysis. The most common radiographic findings of acute pulmonary blastomycosis are nonspecific lobar and segmental consolidation. Diffuse pulmonary disease associated with adult respiratory distress syndrome has been described in immunocompetent adults with acute pneumonia. Chronic pneumonia is characterized by several months of weight loss, cough, night sweats, and chest pain. Fever is typically low grade, and hemoptysis can occur. Patients with chronic pneumonia are more likely to have masslike lesions shown on chest radiograph, but diffuse miliary patterns may be present. Cavitary disease is an uncommon complication of this form of infection.

Extrapulmonary or disseminated disease occurs in immunocompromised persons and is usually preceded by pulmonary symptoms. Dissemination to almost any organ can occur but the most common sites are skin, bone, central nervous system (CNS), and genitourinary system. Cutaneous disease follows hematogenous or direct inoculation of the subcutaneous tissue and appears as either verrucous or ulcerative lesions. Osteomyelitis occurs in 25–50% of patients with extrapulmonary infections. The long bones, skull, vertebrae, and ribs are most commonly involved, but almost any bone can be affected. Involvement of the CNS occurs in 10% of patients with extrapulmonary infections and is typified by intracranial abscesses or, rarely, meningitis. Prostatitis and orchitis can occur in male patients but is unusual. Endometrial disease in female patients is sexually transmitted. Laryngeal blastomycosis generally follows primary infection of the upper airway and presents as a laryngeal mass. Fungal abscesses may form anywhere, including the heart and its surrounding structures, the orbit, and the sinuses.

Diagnosis. Definitive diagnosis requires identification of the fungus histologically in tissue specimens or recovery of the fungus by culture. Serologic diagnosis using complement fixation or immunodiffusion is insensitive and is complicated by the high rate of cross reactivity with anti-*Histoplasma* antibody. Enzyme-linked immunosorbent assay is the most specific serologic test and has shown sensitivities of 80–88% and specificities of 98–100% in some studies. Although serologic tests can be used adjunctively to support clinical and other laboratory data, they should not be used to exclude infection or as a basis for the initiation of therapy. Skin testing is unreliable because reactivity wanes over time at an unpredictable rate.

Treatment. Because uncomplicated pneumonia may resolve spontaneously, some patients can be carefully monitored without therapy. Patients should be thoroughly evaluated for extrapulmonary disease before deciding to withhold therapy.

Treatment is required for patients who are immunocompromised or have progressive pulmonary disease, CNS disease, or disseminated disease. Specific treatment regimens are based on the location, severity, and immune status of the patient. Itraconazole (200–400 mg/24 hr) or fluconazole (400–800 mg/24 hr) for ≥6 mo is recommended for adults with mild to moderate pulmonary disease without CNS involvement. Itraconazole (5–7 mg/kg/24 hr) has been used successfully to treat a small number of children with non–life-threatening infections. Amphotericin B (total dose: ≥30 mg/kg in children; 1.5–2.5 g in adults) remains the drug of choice for life-threatening and CNS infections for adults and children, as well as blastomycosis in pregnant women and immunocompromised persons. Lipid-complex formulations

of amphotericin B (5 mg/kg/24 hr) are recommended for persons with compromised renal function (including doubling of the serum creatinine with amphotericin B desoxycholate therapy), those who are receiving other nephrotoxic therapy, or those who are otherwise intolerant of amphotericin B desoxycholate. Immunocompromised persons, especially patients with AIDS, may require chronic suppressive therapy after completion of a course of amphotericin B. In selected cases of pulmonary or extrapulmonary disease, initial therapy with amphotericin B can be switched to itraconazole or fluconazole after the patient's condition has stabilized. The role of surgery in the treatment of blastomycosis is limited.

Areno JP 4th, Campbell GD, George RB Jr: Diagnosis of blastomycosis. *Semin Respir Infect* 1997;12:252–62.
Chapman SW, Bradsher RW Jr, Campbell GD Jr, et al: Practice guidelines for the management of patients with blastomycosis. *Clin Infect Dis* 2000;30:679–83.
Lemos LL, Guo M, Baliga M: Blastomycosis: Organ involvement and etiologic diagnosis. A review of 123 patients from Mississippi. *Ann Diagn Pathol* 2000;4:391–406.
Schutze GE, Hickerson SL, Fortin EM, et al: Blastomycosis in children. *Clin Infect Dis* 1996;22:496–502.

Chapter 221
Coccidioidomycosis (*Coccidioides immitis*)

Demosthenes Pappagianis

Etiology. Coccidioidomycosis (San Joaquin fever, Valley fever, desert rheumatism, coccidioidal granuloma) is an infection caused by the fungus *Coccidioides immitis*, which is found in the soil. *C. immitis* exhibits dimorphism, existing as a filamentous mycelial form (mold) in nature and usual laboratory cultures; and, influenced by body temperature, leukocytes, increased CO_2, and surface active substances, as an endosporulating spherule in human tissues.

Epidemiology. *C. immitis* is concentrated in generally arid areas of the Western hemisphere, including California, Arizona, Texas, parts of Nevada, and Utah (including Dinosaur National Monument), Mexico, Central America, and South America (including Brazil). Longtime residents—humans, cattle, sheep, dogs, wild rodents, and other animals—have been infected; however, even transient visitors can develop the disease, which may not be considered in the differential diagnosis when they return to nonendemic areas. Many environmental influences affect the incidence of the disease. Recovery from infection generally confers permanent immunity.

Pathogenesis. The minute arthroconidia of the *C. immitis* mycelial saprophytic phase that are airborne in dust are inhaled or, rarely, enter the host through injured skin. In the infected host they round up into spherules, which develop endospores. Liberation of the endospores leads to formation of new spherules and endospores, which spread within a host but not to a new host. Viable *C. immitis* occurs in pulmonary cavities, often in the mycelial as well as spherule form. However, person-to-person transmission of infection has been documented only through organ transplantation from an infected individual. The arthroconidia that occur in nature and on the surface of cultures are highly infectious. Although isolation of the patient is unnecessary, precautions should be taken with dressings and casts over open lesions to preclude the development of infective arthroconidia, which occurs in 4–5 days on surface cultures.

Clinical Manifestations. Human infection takes three forms (Fig. 221–1): (1) a benign, self-limited, primary infection (60% of infected persons show no clinical manifestations); (2) residual pulmonary lesions; and (3) a rare, disseminating, sometimes fatal disease. The disease tends to be milder in children; however, in children requiring medical attention, dissemination to the bones and meninges is fairly common and approaches the incidence of these complications in adults. Laryngeal coccidioidomycosis, although not frequent, has been detected at a proportionately higher rate in children. Maternal-fetal and maternal-neonatal infections have been reported.

PRIMARY COCCIDIOIDOMYCOSIS. The incubation period varies from 1–4 wk, with an average of 10–16 days. Symptoms are flulike; the onset may be insidious or abrupt with malaise, chills, and fever. Chest pain is frequent and may vary from a mere sense of constriction to excruciating pain. Night sweats and anorexia are common. On occasion, there is a persistent dry cough, and the throat may be painful. There also may be headache or backache.

An evanescent generalized, fine, macular erythema or urticarial eruption may appear within the 1st day or so and may be present only in the groin. Rarely, a varicella-like rash has been noted. Most frequently, tibial erythema nodosum occurs, with or without erythema multiforme, usually when sensitivity to coccidioidin is maximal from 3–21 days after onset of symptoms. These early rashes do not contain the organism and may result from hypersensitivity to coccidioidal antigen. Skin lesions may occur, however, in persons who are otherwise asymptomatic. Arthritis and phlyctenular conjunctivitis may occur concomitantly.

Auscultation of the lungs may be unrevealing, even though radiography reveals extensive consolidation. Dullness, a friction rub, or fine crackles may be detected. Pleural effusions occasionally occur, even without preceding respiratory symptoms, and may be sufficient to compromise respiratory status. Occasionally, acute respiratory insufficiency may occur.

RESIDUAL PULMONARY COCCIDIOIDOMYCOSIS. A transient cavity may develop in an area of pulmonary consolidation during the primary infection. More often, however, after a variably prolonged period a persistent cavity may form, more often in patients with diabetes mellitus. There are often no symptoms, and the diagnosis is made radiographically. Occasionally, there is mild to moderate hemoptysis, which may recur and be alarming. Rarely, fatal hemorrhage occurs. Dissemination of the fungus from cavities to other areas is rare. Pulmonary residual "granulomas" sometimes persist. They are not harmful but are difficult to differentiate from tuberculosis or neoplasms. Infrequently, a chronic progressive fibrocavitary pulmonary disease occurs.

DISSEMINATED OR PROGRESSIVE COCCIDIOIDOMYCOSIS (COCCIDIOIDAL GRANULOMA). In certain persons, coccidioidal infection does not localize. Dissemination, which is rare and occurs mainly in male patients, especially Filipinos, other Asians, and blacks, usually follows the initial illness within 6 mo, often without any interlude. This is analogous to the course of progressive primary tuberculosis. Persons with blood group B and a certain class II human leukocyte antigen locus may

be particularly disposed to dissemination. Certain immunosuppressed states enhance dissemination or bring about relapse of apparently arrested coccidioidomycosis. Dissemination is likely if infection is acquired during pregnancy. Skin lesions and subcutaneous or osseous cold abscesses occur. Meningitis is the most serious of the disseminated lesions and is clinically similar to tuberculous meningitis. In whites, it is not unusual for meningitis to be the only extrapulmonary lesion. Miliary dissemination and peritonitis may be distinguishable from tuberculosis only by demonstration of the causative agent, although coccidioidal peritonitis may present as a very mild disease. The mortality rate of untreated meningitis is practically 100% but varies with other forms of disseminated coccidioidomycosis.

Diagnosis. Disseminated infection may be established by biopsy or at autopsy. Sputum is often scanty with the primary infection; bronchoalveolar lavage or gastric aspirates, especially in children, may be advisable. The diagnosis is confirmed by detection of the characteristic double-contoured spherules with endospores, such as in an excised pulmonary nodule. Demonstration of the fungus by culture and confirmation by DNA probe, exoantigen test, or animal inoculation is also diagnostic. *Cultures are especially hazardous* and require special precautions.

The erythrocyte sedimentation rate is elevated in patients with primary or disseminated infection and is helpful in evaluating clinical status. Eosinophilia is common and is proportionately higher in patients with more severe infections. Serum alkaline phosphatase may be elevated in acute coccidioidomycosis even in the absence of obvious systemic dissemination.

The cerebrospinal fluid (CSF) findings in coccidioidal meningitis are similar to those of tuberculous meningitis (see Chapter 197). Eosinophilic pleocytosis may occur, and in rare instances CSF leukocytes have been reported as "malignant" cells. Lumbar puncture for CSF analysis should be performed in patients with disseminated or progressive coccidioidomycosis. Concomitant coccidioidomycosis and tuberculosis can be confounding.

SKIN TEST. Intradermal tests with coccidioidin or spherulin are specific except for occasional cross-reactions in patients with histoplasmosis and blastomycosis. A positive reaction does not distinguish between a recent and an old infection unless it has been preceded within a reasonably short time by a negative test result. However, *a negative skin test does not exclude coccidioidal infection*. The reaction generally reaches its peak at 36 hr and should be read at 24 and 48 hr. An area of induration >5 mm in diameter is positive. Patients with suspected coccidioidal erythema nodosum are likely to be hypersensitive and should receive the 1:1,000 dilution. Some patients with disseminated infections are anergic; even a 1:10 dilution of antigen may not elicit a reaction. There is no danger of disseminating or activating a coccidioidal infection by producing a strong coccidioidin reaction, although there may be a local or systemic reaction. Coccidioidin does not evoke antibodies in the human; therefore, the skin test may precede serologic tests. A negative skin test should not preclude serologic tests. A positive skin test in a healthy individual indicates resistance to reinfection with *C. immitis*.

SEROLOGY. Antibodies to *C. immitis* are generally not demonstrable in persons with asymptomatic acute infections. Serum precipitins, which are immunoglobulin (Ig) M antibodies, and complement fixation (CF) antibodies, which are IgG antibodies, are detectable in early coccidioidomycosis and may persist in those with disseminated coccidioidomycosis. Higher CF antibody titers are generally associated with more severe infections. Rarely, serologic tests may be negative in patients with active coccidioidomycosis, especially if they are immunocompromised.

Antibodies detectable by CF do not pass the blood-brain barrier, although immunodiffusion and enzyme immunoassay may reveal presence of the IgG in CSF that is concentrated, and are found in cord blood at the same titer as in the mother's blood. Passively transferred antibody disappears from the infant within

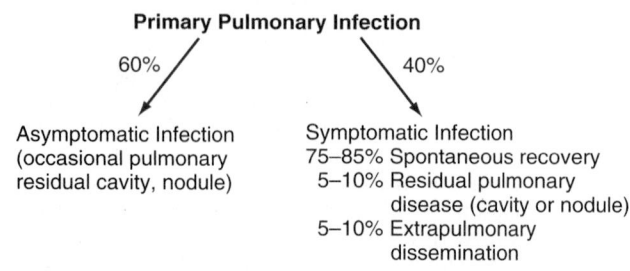

FIGURE 221–1. Natural history of coccidioidomycosis.

6 mo. Coccidioidal serum precipitins (IgM) has been detected in some neonates of mothers with coccidioidomycosis when there has been no manifestation of disease in the infants.

C. immitis antibodies in CSF, which are detectable in 95% of patients with meningitis, are usually diagnostic, although they occasionally are present in patients with epidural coccidioidal lesions. CF antibody can be detected in cisternal and lumbar CSF but may be deceptively absent from the ventricular CSF.

RADIOGRAPHY. During the primary infection, chest radiography may not reveal pulmonary changes. There may be single or multiple, sharply circumscribed or soft, feathery, small pulmonary densities or larger consolidated areas. Hilar lymphadenopathy is frequent. Miliary or reticulonodular lesions are prognostically unfavorable. Pulmonary cavities, which occur less frequently in children than in adults, tend to be thin-walled. Pleural effusions vary in extent. Osseous lesions are usually lytic and have a predilection for cancellous bone and can be single or multiple.

Treatment. Because most primary coccidioidal infections resolve spontaneously over a variable time period, they have historically been treated conservatively. The patient's activity and symptomatic measures are restricted until the erythrocyte sedimentation rate returns to normal, clinical and radiographic improvements are noted, and the serum CF (IgG) antibody titer decreases. With the advent of the relatively benign oral azoles, physicians have often initiated therapy as soon as coccidioidomycosis is suspected or confirmed. There is limited evidence that such treatment for primary coccidioidomycosis hastens recovery or decreases the risk of extrapulmonary dissemination or development of pulmonary residua (e.g., cavity or solitary nodule).

Antifungal chemotherapy is indicated for those at high risk of severe coccidioidomycosis and those who have recognized metapulmonary dissemination. Currently available chemotherapeutic agents include oral fluconazole, oral or intravenous itraconazole, and oral ketoconazole, as well as amphotericin B, both desoxycholate and lipid-complex formulations. Indications for the choice of medication are not clearly defined. Amphotericin B (up to 1 mg/kg/24 hr) should be administered for rapidly progressing coccidioidomycosis. Lipid-complex formulations of amphotericin B (5 mg/kg/24 hr) are recommended for persons with compromised renal function (including doubling of the serum creatinine resulting from amphotericin B desoxycholate therapy), those who are receiving other nephrotoxic therapy, or those who are otherwise intolerant of amphotericin B desoxycholate. Once the full dose has been achieved, it can be given every other day or 2–3 times a week to minimize renal toxicity.

Systemic amphotericin B desoxycholate does not cross the blood-brain barrier in therapeutic amounts for *C. immitis*, but it may mask the presence of meningitis. Intrathecal (cisternal or lumbar) or intraventricular administration of amphotericin B had been the mainstay of treatment of coccidioidal meningitis. However, both fluconazole and itraconazole have proved useful in the treatment of coccidioidal meningitis, although lifetime treatment may be required.

Ketoconazole (3–10 mg/kg/24 hr), fluconazole (3–12 mg/kg/24 hr), or itraconazole (3–6 mg/kg/24 hr) administered orally have been useful in treating disseminated coccidioidomycosis outside the central nervous system that is neither extensive nor progressing rapidly. The higher doses may be required for the treatment of meningitis. The azoles have increasingly been used to treat children as well as adults with coccidioidomycosis, but there is limited information about their long-term adverse effects in younger patients. While ketoconazole can cause hepatic dysfunction and inhibit testosterone synthesis in adults, these effects have not been adequately evaluated in children. Fluconazole is primarily excreted by the kidneys, and itraconazole is metabolized in the liver; these drugs do not significantly affect testosterone or adrenocorticoid synthesis. On the basis of

limited experience, coccidioidomycosis in pregnant women should be treated with amphotericin B, which has no apparent adverse effect on the fetus. Until more data are available, azoles should not be given to pregnant patients. The duration of therapy required with the azoles has not been clearly defined and must be determined individually. Relapses have occurred in some patients after favorable clinical responses have been seen following therapy for longer than 1 yr.

SURGERY. Chronic pulmonary coccidioidal disease, cavitary or fibrocavitary, has not been consistently improved by the azoles or by amphotericin B. Pulmonary cavities may close spontaneously and are often best left alone, but when a cavity persists or is located peripherally, or when there is recurrent bleeding or rupture of the cavity through the pleura, excision should be considered. Coccidioidal cavities that have a fluid level or that are accompanied by fever or hemoptysis should initially be treated with antibacterial antibiotics. Infrequently, bronchopleural fistulas or recurrent cavitation occurs as a surgical complication; rarely, dissemination may result. When thoracic surgery is required, perioperative intravenous therapy with amphotericin B may be desirable.

Surgical drainage of cold abscesses, removal of infected synovial membranes, and curettage or excision of osseous lesions is recommended for localized extrapulmonary coccidioidomycosis. Local as well as systemic administration of amphotericin B can be used to treat coccidioidal articular disease. Limited experience indicates that artificial joints may be used to replace infected joints as long as antifungal (triazole) chemotherapy continues.

Prevention. Avoidance of exposure to the arthroconidia is the only means of preventing infection. Whole killed cell vaccine did not prevent coccidioidomycosis in humans.

Bickel KD, Press BH, Hovey LM: Successful treatment of coccidioidomycosis osteomyelitis in an infant. *Ann Plast Surg* 1993;30:462–5.

Boyle JO, Coulthard SW, Mandel RM: Laryngeal involvement in disseminated coccidioidomycosis. *Arch Otolaryngol Head Neck Surg* 1991;117:433–8.

Dewsnup DH, Galgiani JN, Graybill JR, et al: Is it ever safe to stop azole therapy for *Coccidioides immitis* meningitis? *Ann Intern Med* 1996;124:305–10.

Galgiani JN, Ampel NM, Catanzaro A, et al: Practice guidelines for the treatment of coccidioidomycosis. *Clin Infect Dis* 2000;30:658–61.

Herron LD, Kissel P, Smilovitz D: Treatment of coccidioidal spinal infection: Experience in 16 cases. *J Spinal Disord* 1997;10:215–22.

Kafka JA, Catanzaro A: Disseminated coccidioidomycosis in children. *J Pediatr* 1981;98:355–61.

Linsangan LC, Ross LA: *Coccidioides immitis* infection of the neonate: Two routes of infection. *Pediatr Infect Dis J* 1999;18:171–3.

Pappagianis D: Serologic studies in coccidioidomycosis. *Seminars Resp Infect* 2001;16:242–50.

Pappagianis D: Marked increase in cases of coccidioidomycosis in California: 1991, 1992, and 1993. *Clin Infect Dis* 1994;19:S14–8.

Peterson CM, Schuppert K, Kelly PC, et al: Coccidioidomycosis and pregnancy. *Obstet Gynecol Surg* 1993;48:149–52.

Polesky A, Kirsch CM, Snyder LS: Airway coccidioidomycosis-reported cases and review. *Clin Infect Dis* 1999;28:1273–80.

Richardson V, Valenciano-Vega JI, Valenzuela-Espinoza A: Bronchoesophageal fistulas secondary to coccidioidomycosis. *Pediatr Infect Dis J* 1994;13:159–61.

Chapter 222
Paracoccidioides brasiliensis Robin B. Churchill and

Stephen C. Aronoff

Etiology. Paracoccidioidomycosis (South American blastomycosis, Brazilian blastomycosis, Lutz-Splendore-Almeida blastomycosis) is an uncommon fungal infection of Central and South America. The etiologic agent, *Paracoccidioides brasiliensis*, exhibits temperature dimorphism, existing as a mycelial form (mold) in nature at ambient temperatures (25°C–30°C) and as a yeast in human tissues (37°C).

Epidemiology. *P. brasiliensis* is ecologically unique to Central and South America. Endemic outbreaks occur mainly in the tropical rainforests of Brazil with scattered cases in Argentina, Colombia, and Venezuela. A recent epidemiologic study showed increased incidence in areas with moderately high altitude, high humidity, and high rainfall and where coffee and tobacco are grown. The most common route of infection is by inhalation of conidia. The disease is not usually thought to be contagious and person-to-person transmission has not been confirmed. No animal vectors have been described.

Clinical Manifestations. There are two clinical forms of disease. The acute form is rare, occurs almost exclusively in children and persons with impaired host defense, and targets the reticuloendothelial system. Pulmonary symptoms may be absent, although chest radiographs often show patchy, confluent, or nodular densities. Patients typically present acutely with fever, malaise, wasting, lymphadenopathy, and abdominal enlargement from intra-abdominal lymphadenopathy and hepatomegaly or splenomegaly, which are nearly constant features. Multiple areas of osteomyelitis, arthritis, and pericardial effusions can also occur. This form of the disease has a 25% mortality rate.

Adults with extensive exposure to soil, such as farmers, are most likely to develop the chronic form that presents initially with flulike symptoms, fever, and weight loss. Pulmonary infection with progressive dyspnea, cough, chest pain, and hemoptysis is most common. Findings on physical examination are scant, although chest radiographs may show infiltrates that are disproportionately greater than the clinical findings. Mucositis involving the mouth and its structures as well as the nose may become manifest with localized pain, change in voice, or dysphagia. Lesions may extend beyond the oral cavity onto the skin. Generalized lymphadenopathy, hepatosplenomegaly, and adrenal involvement leading to Addison's disease may also occur.

Diagnosis. Definitive diagnosis requires identification of the fungus histologically in tissue specimens or recovery of the fungus by culture. Demonstration of the fungus by direct (potassium hydroxide) wet mount preparation of sputum, exudate, or pus can establish the diagnosis in a high percentage of cases. Histopathologic examination of biopsy materials using special fungal stains is another effective method of diagnosis. The fungus can be recovered by culture on Sabouraud-dextrose or yeast extract agar. Antibodies to *P. brasiliensis* can be demonstrated in the sera of most patients. Serial antibody titers and lymphocyte proliferative responses to fungal antigens are useful in monitoring the response to therapy. Skin testing with paracoccidioidin is not reliable, in that one third of patients with active disease have test results that are nonreactive. Newer diagnostic methods that may prove to be very useful include polymerase chain reaction detection techniques to detect the organism in tissues and capture enzyme-linked immunosorbent assay to detect organism-specific immunoglobulin E in serum.

Treatment. Recent studies suggest that itraconazole (50–400 mg/24 hr) for a mean duration of 6 mo is the treatment of choice for paracoccidioidomycosis. Fluconazole has also been used but higher doses (600 mg/24 hr, or greater) and longer treatment periods are required. Amphotericin B (total dose 3–6 g for adults) is recommended in cases of disseminated disease and failure of other therapies. Lipid-complex formulations of amphotericin B (5 mg/kg/24 hr) are recommended for persons with compromised renal function (including doubling of the serum creatinine with amphotericin B desoxycholate therapy), for those who are receiving other nephrotoxic therapy, or for those who are otherwise intolerant of amphotericin B desoxycholate. In the past, therapy with sulfonamide compounds, including sulfadiazine, trimethoprim-sulfamethoxazole (TMP-SMZ), and dapsone, have been used. Sulfonamide therapy is inexpensive but the treatment course is prolonged, lasting months to years depending on the agent selected. Terbinafine, a broad-spectrum antifungal allylamine that has been used to treat a variety of fungal infections in patients of all ages, has also recently been reported as successful treatment for a case of paracoccidioidomycosis unresponsive to treatment with TMP-SMZ in an adult.

Benard G, Orii NM, Marques HHS, et al: Severe acute paracoccidioidomycosis in children. *Pediatr Infect Dis J* 1994;13:510–5.

Borgia G, Reynaud L, Cerini R, et al: A case of paracoccidioidomycosis: Experience with long-term therapy. *Infection* 2000;28:11920.

Diaz M, Negroni R, Montero-Gei F, et al: A Pan-American 5 - year study of fluconazole therapy for deep mycoses in immunocompetent host. Pan-American Study Group. *Clin Infect Dis* 1992;14:68–76.

Gomes GM, Cisalpino PS, Taborda CP, et al: PCR for diagnosis of paracoccidioidomycosis. *J Clin Microbiol* 2000;38:3478–80.

Lortholary O, Denning DW, Dupont B: Endemic mycoses: A treatment update. *J Antimicrob Chemother* 1999;43:321–31.

Mamoni RL, Rossi CL, Camargo ZP, et al: Capture enzyme-linked immunosorbent assay to detect specific immunoglobulin E in sera of patients with paracoccidioidomycosis. *Am J Trop Med Hyg* 2001;65:237–41.

Motoyama AB, Venancio EJ, Brandao GO, et al: Molecular identification of *Paracoccidioides brasiliensis* by PCR amplification of ribosomal DNA. *J Clin Microbiol* 2000;38:3106–9.

Ollague JM, de Zurita AM, Calero G: Paracoccidioidomycosis (South American blastomycosis) successfully treated with terbinafine: First case report. *Br J Dermatol* 2000;143:188–91.

Chapter 223

Sporotrichosis (*Sporothrix schenckii*)

Robin B. Churchill and Stephen C. Aronoff

Etiology. The etiologic agent of sporotrichosis *Sporothrix schenckii* exhibits temperature dimorphism, existing as a mycelial form (mold) in nature at ambient temperatures (25°C–30°C) and as a yeast in human tissues (37°C).

Epidemiology. Sporotrichosis is a rare fungal infection that occurs worldwide both sporadically and in outbreaks. *S. schenckii* is distributed worldwide, but most cases of sporotrichosis are reported from North and South America and Japan. Most cases in the United States occur in the Midwest, particularly in areas along the Mississippi and Missouri Rivers. The fungus occurs in decaying vegetation and has been isolated most commonly from sphagnum moss, rosebushes, barberry, straw, and some types of hay. Disease in humans usually follows cutaneous inoculation of the fungus into a minor wound. Transmission from bites and scratches of animals, most frequently cats and armadillos, has occurred. Sporotrichosis is an occupational disease among farmers, gardeners, veterinarians, and laboratory workers. Reports of human-to-human transmission are rare. Pulmonary infection may result from the inhalation of large numbers of spores. Disseminated infection is unusual but can occur in immunocompromised patients following ingestion or inhalation of spores.

Pathogenesis. The cellular immune response to *S. schenckii* infection is both neutrophilic and monocytic. T-cell–mediated immunity appears to be important in limiting infection; antibody does not protect against infection. Histologically, noncaseating granulomas and microabscess formation are characteristic. Due to the paucity of organisms, it is usually difficult to demonstrate the fungi in biopsy specimens.

Clinical Manifestations. Cutaneous sporotrichosis is the most common form of disease in all age groups. Cutaneous disease may either be **lymphocutaneous** or **fixed cutaneous**. Lymphocutaneous sporotrichosis accounts for >75% of reported cases in children and follows traumatic subcutaneous inoculation. After a variable and often prolonged incubation period (1–12 wk), an isolated, painless erythematous papule develops at the inoculation site, which is usually on an extremity but may be on the face in children. The original papule enlarges and ulcerates. Although the infection may remain limited to the inoculation site (fixed cutaneous form), satellite lesions follow lymphangitic spread and cause **nodular angiitis** with multiple tender subcutaneous nodules tracking the lymphatic channels that drain the lesion. These secondary nodules are subcutaneous granulomas that adhere to the overlying skin and subsequently ulcerate. Sporotrichosis does not heal spontaneously, and these ulcerative lesions may persist for years if they are untreated. Systemic signs and symptoms are uncommon.

Extracutaneous sporotrichosis is rare in children; most cases are reported in adults with underlying medical conditions. The most common form of extracutaneous sporotrichosis involves infection of the bones and joints. Pulmonary sporotrichosis usually presents as a chronic pneumonitis that is similar to the presentation of pulmonary tuberculosis.

Diagnosis. Definitive diagnosis requires identification of the fungus histologically in tissue specimens or recovery of the fungus from the site of infection by culture. Special histologic staining, such as periodic acid–Schiff and methenamine silver, is required to identify yeast forms in tissues. Despite special staining techniques, diagnostic yield from biopsy specimens is low due to the small number of organisms present in the tissues. In cases of disseminated disease, demonstration of serum antibody against *S. schenckii*–related antigens can be diagnostically useful. New techniques for rapid identification of dimorphic fungal pathogens using specific DNA probes have recently been introduced and may be useful in the future.

DIFFERENTIAL DIAGNOSIS. Lymphocutaneous and cutaneous sporotrichosis must be differentiated from other causes of nodular lymphangitis including atypical mycobacterial infection, nocardiosis, leishmaniasis, tularemia, melioidosis, cutaneous anthrax, and other systemic mycoses including coccidioidomycosis.

Treatment. Although comparative trials and extensive experience in children are not available, itraconazole is the recommended treatment of choice for infections outside the central nervous system. The usual dosage for children is 5 mg/kg/24 hr up to 100 mg/24 hr; the adult dosage is 100–200 mg daily. Alternatively, younger children with only cutaneous disease may be treated with a saturated solution (1 g/mL) of potassium iodide (SSKI) given orally. The dose is started at 5–10 drops three times per day and gradually advanced to 25–40 drops three times per day for children or 40–50 drops three times per day for adolescents and adults. Associated adverse effects of anorexia, nausea, a metallic taste, and rash contribute to poor patient compliance and should be managed by temporary cessation of therapy and reinstitution at a lower dosage. Therapy is continued until the cutaneous lesions have resolved, which usually takes 6–12 wk. SSKI is not effective for other forms of sporotrichosis. Terbinafine, an allylamine, also has been used successfully to treat cutaneous sporotrichosis but further data are needed before it can be recommended. Amphotericin B is the treatment of choice for pulmonary infections, disseminated infections, and infections in immunocompromised persons. Central nervous system infections should be treated with amphotericin B in combination with flucytosine. Lipid-complex formulations of amphotericin B are recommended for persons with compromised renal function (including doubling of the serum creatinine with amphotericin B desoxycholate therapy), for those who are receiving other nephrotoxic therapy, or for those who are otherwise intolerant of amphotericin B desoxycholate. Surgical debridement has a role in the treatment of some cases of sporotrichosis, particularly in osteoarticular disease. Therapy with azoles or SSKI should not be used in pregnancy. Pregnant women with pulmonary or disseminated disease should be treated with amphotericin B; pregnant women with cutaneous disease can be treated with **hyperthermic treatment** in the form of hot compresses or a hand-held heating device applied 40–60 min/24 hr, or therapy can be delayed until after delivery. Dissemination to the fetus does not occur, nor is the disease worsened by pregnancy.

Burch JM, Morelli JG, Weston WL: Unsuspected sporotrichosis in childhood. *Pediatr Infect Dis J* 2001;20:442–5.
Kauffman CA, Hajjeh R, Chapman SW, et al: Practice guidelines for the management of patients with sporotrichosis. *Clin Infect Dis* 2000;30:684–7.
Kauffman CA: Sporotrichosis. *Clin Infect Dis* 1999;29:231–6.
Lindsley MD, Hurst SF, Iqbal NJ, et al: Rapid identification of dimorphic and yeast-like fungal pathogens using specific DNA probes. *J Clin Microbiol* 2001;39:3505–11.
Pappas PG, Tellez I, Deep AE, et al: Sporotrichosis in Peru: Description of an area of hyperendemicity. *Clin Infect Dis* 2000;30:65–70.
Perez A: Terbinafine: Broad new spectrum of indications in several subcutaneous and systemic and parasitic diseases. *Mycoses* 1999;42:111–4.

Chapter 224

Zygomycosis *Robin B. Churchill and Stephen C. Aronoff*

Etiology. Zygomycosis (mucormycosis or phycomycosis) refers to a group of opportunistic fungal infections characterized by vascular invasion, thrombosis, and necrosis caused by dimorphic fungi of the order Mucorales, which is in the class Zygomycetes. Members of the genera *Absidia, Mucor, Rhizopus,* and *Rhizomucor* are the most common causative organisms; *Cunninghamella* and *Apophysomyces* are seen less frequently. These are saprobic and parasitic fungi that are ubiquitous in soil, decayed plant or animal matter, and may be found on moldy cheese, fruit, and bread.

Epidemiology. Zygomycosis is primarily a disease of persons with altered host defenses associated with underlying conditions such as diabetes mellitus, hematologic malignancies, persistent acidosis, iron overload, corticosteroid therapy, organ transplantation, and, less frequently, AIDS. Cases occur predominately in developed countries, likely related to the concentration of severely immunocompromised patients. Infections in healthy children are extremely rare but have been reported after insect bites or penetrating injuries. Person-to-person spread does not occur.

Pathogenesis. The primary mechanism of acquisition of Zygomycetes is inhalation of the spores from the environment. Percutaneous inoculation can lead to cutaneous and subcutaneous zygomycosis, and ingestion of contaminated food or drinks has been linked to gastrointestinal disease. Neutrophils appear to be the most important component of the immune response against these organisms, which may explain the predilection zygomycoses among patients with conditions associated with neutropenia or neutrophil dysfunction.

Clinical Manifestations. Zygomycosis can occur as any of several clinical syndromes including sinusitis/rhinocerebral, pulmonary, gastrointestinal, cutaneous, and disseminated disease. Rhinocerebral and pulmonary disease are most common.

Rhinocerebral zygomycosis occurs primarily in individuals with diabetes mellitus and hematologic malignancies. Initial symptoms consistent with sinusitis such as headache, retro-orbital pain, fever, and nasal discharge are followed by signs of orbital involvement including periorbital edema, proptosis, ptosis, and ophthalmoplegia. The nasal discharge is often dark and bloody; examination of the nasal mucosa reveals black, necrotic areas. Extension beyond the nasal cavity is common. Involved tissues become red, then violaceous, and finally black as vessel thrombosis and tissue necrosis occur. Destructive paranasal sinusitis with intracranial extension can be demonstrated by CT or MRI scanning. Brain abscesses can result from direct extension of rhinocerebral infection from the nasal cavity and sinuses, usually to the frontal or frontotemporal lobes, or from disseminated disease, which may involve the occipital lobe or brainstem.

Pulmonary zygomycosis usually occurs in severely immunocompromised patients and is characterized by fever, tachypnea, and productive cough with pleuritic chest pain and hemoptysis. Signs of consolidation are found on physical examination. Chest radiograph findings are nonspecific and may show parenchymal infiltrate, lobar consolidation, or a nodular mass.

Gastrointestinal zygomycosis may occur as a complication of disseminated disease or as an isolated intestinal infection associated with diabetic mellitus, immunosuppression, malnutrition, or prematurity. Abdominal pain and distention with hematemesis, hematochezia, or melena may be seen. Stomach or bowel wall perforation is not uncommon.

Cutaneous zygomycosis can complicate burns or surgical wounds. An outbreak among preterm infants followed the use of contaminated wooden tongue depressors to immobilize the extremities. Outbreaks have also been associated with contaminated elastic bandages. Infection presents as an erythematous papule that ulcerates, leaving a black necrotic center. The skin lesions are painful and usually associated with fever.

Disseminated disease manifests as involvement of two or more organs; pulmonary involvement is usually present, but any organ can be involved. This form of disease occurs in the most severely immunocompromised patients. Signs and symptoms may be nonspecific, and prognosis is generally poor.

Diagnosis. Definitive diagnosis requires identification of the fungus histologically in tissue specimens or recovery of the fungus by culture. Demonstration of fungal elements with fungal specific stains such as calcofluor white or Gomori methenamine silver is recommended. In lung biopsy specimens and other tissue samples stained with silver, Mucorales appear as thick-walled, aseptate, right angle–branched hyphae. By gastrointestinal endoscopy, the lesions appear as black ulcers with deep erythematous margins. Vascular invasion is a hallmark of the disease. These fungi may also be identified in secretions by suspending the clinical material in a solution of 20% potassium hydrochloride before microscopic examination is performed. The fungi may be grown on standard laboratory media from sputum, bronchoalveolar lavage fluid, skin lesions, or biopsy material. Serologic tests for detecting zygomycosis are not clinically useful. Diagnosis of disseminated zygomycosis using a polymerase chain reaction assay has been recently reported and may prove to be a useful adjunct to standard diagnostic techniques in the future.

Treatment. The optimal therapy for zygomycosis in children has not been established. All forms of the disease can be aggressive and difficult to treat, with high fatality rates. Correction of the underlying disease, if possible, is an essential component of management. Successful outcomes have been reported with extensive surgical debridement and high-dose amphotericin B therapy (1–1.5 mg/kg/24 hr to a total dose of 70 mg/kg, or 3–4 g in adults). Isolated pulmonary and cutaneous disease has been successfully treated with lower dosages of amphotericin B (30 mg/kg total dose). Lipid-complex formulations of amphotericin B (5 mg/kg/24 hr) are recommended for persons with compromised renal function (including doubling of the serum creatinine with amphotericin B desoxycholate therapy), those who are receiving other nephrotoxic therapy, or those who are otherwise intolerant of amphotericin B desoxycholate. Additional therapies have included rifampin and flucytosine in combination with amphotericin B, and hyperbaric oxygen and granulocyte-macrophage colony-stimulating factor as adjunctive therapies.

Garcia-Diaz JB, Palau L, Pankey GA: Resolution of rhinocerebral zygomycosis associated with adjuvant administration of granulocyte-macrophage colony-stimulating factor. *Clin Infect Dis* 2001,32:145–50.

Kontoyiannis DP, Wessel VC, Bodey GP, et al: Zygomycosis in the 1990s in a tertiary-care cancer center. *Clin Infect Dis* 2000;30:851–6.

Rickerts V, Loeffler RV, Bohme A, et al: Diagnosis of disseminated zygomycosis using a polymerase chain reaction assay. *Eur J Clin Microbiol Infect Dis* 2001;20:744–5.

Ribes JA, Vanover-Sams CL, Baker DJ: Zygomycetes in human disease. *Clin Microbiol Rev* 2000;13:236–301.

Shah PD, Peters KR, Reuman PD: Recovery from rhinocerebral mucormycosis with carotid artery occlusion. A pediatric case and review of the literature. *Pediatr Infect Dis* 1997;16:68–71.

Walsh TJ, Seibel NL, Arndt C, et al: Amphotericin B lipid complex in pediatric patients with invasive fungal infections. *Pediatr Infect Dis J* 1999;18:702–8.

SECTION 11 *Viral Infections*

Chapter 225
Measles *Yvonne Maldonado*

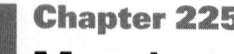

Measles (**rubeola**) is an important childhood disease that was widespread in the United States but is now very infrequent. However, in developing countries, measles is still an important cause of childhood morbidity and mortality. It is an acute viral infection characterized by a final stage with a maculopapular rash erupting successively over the neck and face, trunk, arms, and legs, and accompanied by a high fever.

Etiology. Measles virus, the cause of measles, is an RNA virus of the genus *Morbillivirus* in the family Paramyxoviridae. Only one serotype is known. During the prodromal period and for a short time after the rash appears, virus is shed in nasopharyngeal secretions, blood, and urine. Virus can remain viable for at least 34 hr at room temperature.

Epidemiology. Measles is endemic throughout the world. In the past, epidemics tended to occur irregularly, appearing in the spring in large cities at 2–4-yr intervals as new groups of susceptible children were exposed. It is rarely subclinical. Prior to the use of measles vaccine, the peak incidence was among children 5–10 yr of age. Individuals born before 1957 are considered to have had natural infection and to be immune.

During the 1980s the incidence of measles in the United States rose, probably due to inadequate vaccination as well as vaccine failure. The reported numbers of measles cases dropped from 894,134 cases in 1941 by more than 99.7% to an all-time low of 80 cases in 2000, probably as a result of intensified efforts to ensure appropriate vaccination. Measles now occurs most often among unimmunized preschool-aged children, as occasional epidemics in high schools and colleges, and as imported cases. Because measles is still a common disease in many countries, infective persons entering this country may infect United States residents, and Americans traveling abroad risk exposure there. More than half of the 108 cases reported in 2001 in the United States were imported or due to exposure to imported cases.

The Pan American Health Organization had established the goal of eliminating measles from the Western hemisphere by the year 2000. Although that goal has not been met, efforts have achieved interruption of indigenous measles transmission. During 1990–2000, measles cases in the Western Hemisphere declined 99.3%, from approximately 250,000 to 1,754 cases annually (Fig. 225-1). The many similarities among the biologic features of measles and smallpox suggest the possibility that measles might be eradicated. These features are (1) a distinctive rash as a sentinel marker; (2) no animal reservoir; (3) no vector; (4) seasonal occurrence with disease-free periods; (5) no transmissible latent virus; (6) one serotype; and (7) an effective vaccine. A prevalence of greater than 90% immunization of infants has been shown to produce disease-free zones.

TRANSMISSION. Measles is highly contagious; approximately 90% of susceptible household contacts acquire the disease. Maximal dissemination of virus occurs by droplet spray during the prodromal period (catarrhal stage). Transmission to susceptible contacts often occurs prior to diagnosis of the index case.

Infants acquire immunity transplacentally from mothers who have had measles or measles immunization. This immunity is usually complete for the first 4–6 mo of life and wanes at a variable rate. Although maternal antibody levels are generally undetectable in infants after 9 mo of age by the usual antibody tests performed, some protection persists that may interfere with immunization administered before 12 mo of age. Most women of childbearing age in the United States now have measles immunity by means of immunization rather than disease, and studies suggest that infants of mothers with measles vaccine–induced immunity lose passive antibody at a younger age than infants of mothers who had measles infection. Infants of mothers who are susceptible to measles have no measles immunity and may contract the disease simultaneously with the mother before or after delivery.

Pathogenesis. The essential lesion of measles is found in the skin, conjunctivae, and the mucous membranes of the nasopharynx, bronchi, and intestinal tract. Serous exudate and proliferation of mononuclear cells and a few polymorphonuclear cells occur around the capillaries. Hyperplasia of lymphoid tissue usually occurs, particularly in the appendix, where multinucleated giant cells of up to 100 μm in diameter (**Warthin-Finkeldey reticuloendothelial giant cells**) may be found. In the skin, the reaction is particularly notable about the sebaceous glands and hair follicles. **Koplik spots** consist of serous exudate and proliferation of endothelial cells similar to those in the skin lesions. A general inflammatory reaction of the buccal and pharyngeal mucosa extends into the lymphoid tissue and the tracheobronchial mucous membrane. Interstitial pneumonitis resulting from measles virus takes the form of **Hecht giant cell pneumonia**. Bronchopneumonia may occur from secondary bacterial infection. In fatal cases of encephalomyelitis, perivascular demyelinization occurs in areas of the brain and spinal cord. In subacute sclerosing panencephalitis (SSPE), there may be degeneration of the cortex and white matter with intranuclear and intracytoplasmic inclusion bodies (see Chapter 225.1).

Clinical Manifestations. Measles has three clinical stages: an incubation stage, a prodromal stage with an enanthem (Koplik spots) and mild symptoms, and a final stage with a maculopapular rash accompanied by high fever. The incubation period lasts approximately 10–12 days to the first prodromal symptoms and another 2–4 days to the appearance of the rash; rarely, it may be as short as 6–10 days. Body temperature may increase slightly 9–10 days from the date of infection and then subside for 24 hr or so. The patient may transmit the virus by the 9th–10th day after exposure and occasionally as early as the 7th day, before the illness can be diagnosed.

The prodromal phase usually lasts 3–5 days and is characterized by a low-grade to moderate fever, a dry cough, coryza, and conjunctivitis. These symptoms nearly always precede the appearance of Koplik spots, the pathognomonic sign of measles, by 2–3 days. An enanthem or red mottling is usually present on the hard and soft palates. **Koplik spots** are grayish white dots, usually as small as grains of sand, that have slight, reddish areolae; occasionally they are hemorrhagic. They tend to occur opposite the lower molars but may spread irregularly over the rest of the buccal mucosa. Rarely they are found within the midportion of the lower lip, on the palate, and on the lacrimal caruncle. They appear and disappear rapidly, usually within

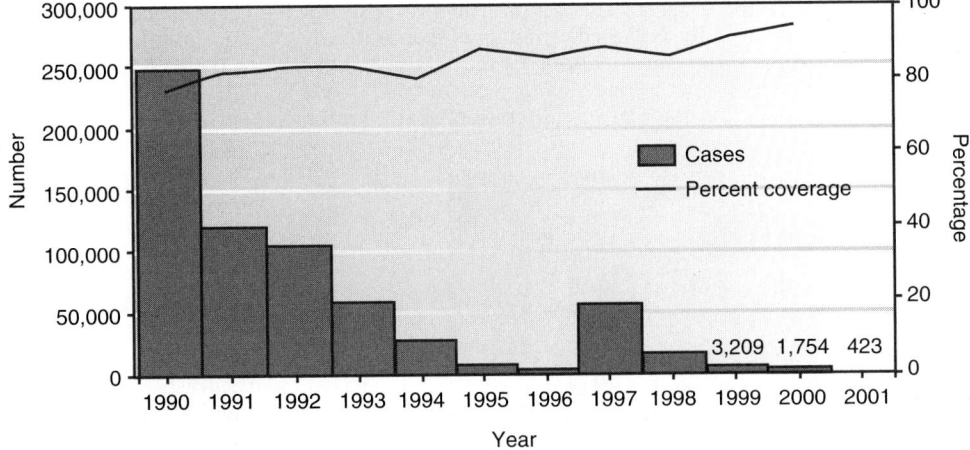

FIGURE 225–1. Reported cases of measles and percentage of routine measles vaccination coverage among infants in North, Central, and South America (combined) from 1990 to 2001. (From Centers for Disease Control and Prevention: Progress toward interrupting indigenous measles transmission—Region of the Americas, January–November 2001. *MMWR* 2001; 50:1133–7.)

1990–1994 = total number of reported cases; 1995–2001= total number of confirmed cases. As of November 26, 2001 (423 confirmed cases from nine countries).

12–18 hr. As they fade, a red, spotty discoloration of the mucosa may remain. The conjunctival inflammation and photophobia may suggest measles before Koplik spots appear. In particular, a transverse line of conjunctival inflammation, sharply demarcated along the eyelid margin, may be of diagnostic assistance in the prodromal stage. As the entire conjunctiva becomes involved, the line disappears.

Occasionally, the prodromal phase may be severe, being ushered in by a sudden high fever, sometimes with convulsions and even pneumonia. Usually the coryza, fever, and cough are increasingly severe up to the time the rash has covered the body.

The temperature rises abruptly as the rash appears and often reaches 40°C (104°F) or higher. In uncomplicated cases, as the rash appears on the legs and feet, the symptoms subside rapidly within about 2 days, usually with an abrupt drop in temperature to normal. Patients up to this point may appear desperately ill, but within 24 hr after the temperature drops, they appear well.

The rash usually starts as faint macules on the upper lateral parts of the neck, behind the ears, along the hairline, and on the posterior parts of the cheek. The individual lesions become increasingly maculopapular as the rash spreads rapidly over the entire face, neck, upper arms, and upper part of the chest within approximately the first 24 hr (Fig. 225–2). During the succeeding 24 hr the rash spreads over the back, abdomen, entire arm, and thighs. As it finally reaches the feet on the 2nd–3rd day, it begins to fade on the face. The rash fades downward in the same sequence in which it appeared. The severity of the disease is directly related to the extent and confluence of the rash. In mild measles the rash tends not to be confluent, and in very mild cases there are few, if any, lesions on the legs. In severe cases the rash is confluent, the skin is completely covered, including the palms and soles, and the face is swollen and disfigured.

The rash is often slightly hemorrhagic; in severe cases with a confluent rash, petechiae may be present in large numbers, and there may be extensive ecchymoses. Itching is generally slight. As the rash fades, branny desquamation and brownish discoloration occur and then disappear within 7–10 days.

The appearance of the rash may vary markedly. Infrequently a slight urticarial, faint macular, or scarlatiniform rash may appear during the early prodromal stage, disappearing in advance of the typical rash. Complete absence of rash is rare except in patients who have received immunoglobulin (Ig) during the incubation period, in some patients with HIV infection, and occasionally in infants younger than 9 mo of age who have appreciable levels of maternal antibody. In the hemorrhagic type of measles (**black measles**), bleeding may occur from the mouth, nose, or bowel. In mild cases the rash may be less macular and more nearly pinpoint, somewhat resembling that of scarlet fever or rubella.

Lymph nodes at the angle of the jaw and in the posterior cervical region are usually enlarged, and slight splenomegaly may be noted. Mesenteric lymphadenopathy may cause abdominal pain. Characteristic pathologic changes of measles in the mucosa of the appendix may cause obliteration of the lumen

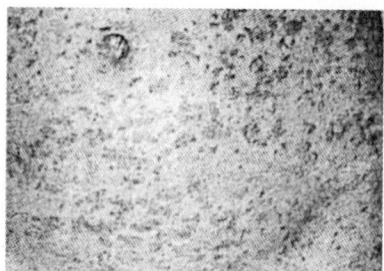

FIGURE 225–2. Maculopapular rash of measles. (From Korting GW: *Hautkrankheiten bei Kindern und Jugendlichen*, 3rd ed. Stuttgart, FK Schattauer Verlag, 1982.) See also color plates.

and symptoms of appendicitis. Changes of this type tend to subside as the Koplik spots disappear. Otitis media, bronchopneumonia, and gastrointestinal symptoms such as diarrhea and vomiting are more common in infants and small children (especially if they are malnourished) than in older children.

ATYPICAL MEASLES. Atypical measles occurs in recipients of killed measles virus vaccine, which was used from 1963 to 1967, who later come in contact with wild-type measles virus. Typical measles prodromal symptoms, except for fever, occur infrequently. Atypical measles is characterized by severe headache, severe abdominal pain, often with vomiting, myalgias, respiratory symptoms, pneumonia with pleural effusion, and an exanthem that is very different from the typical measles rash. The atypical measles rash first appears on the palms, wrists, soles, and ankles, and progresses in a centripetal direction. The lesions are initially maculopapular but become vesicular and later may become purpuric or hemorrhagic. Koplik spots rarely appear in patients with atypical measles.

Diagnosis. The diagnosis is usually apparent from the characteristic clinical picture; laboratory confirmation is rarely needed. However, because indigenous measles rarely occurs in the United States, it is important to confirm suspected infection serologically. Testing for measles IgM antibodies is recommended, which is provided free of charge by the Centers for Disease Control and Prevention or by the state health department. Measles IgM is detectable for 1 mo after illness, but sensitivity of IgM assays may be limited in the first 72 hr of the rash illness. Isolation of measles virus from clinical samples is also useful in identifying the genotype of the strain to track transmission patterns. All suspected measles cases should be reported immediately to local or state health departments. During the prodromal stage multinucleated giant cells can be demonstrated in smears of the nasal mucosa. Antibodies become detectable when the rash appears; testing of acute and convalescent sera demonstrates the diagnostic seroconversion or fourfold increase in titer. Measles virus can be isolated by tissue culture in human embryonic or rhesus monkey kidney cells. Cytopathic changes, visible in 5–10 days, consist of multinucleated giant cells with intranuclear inclusions.

The white blood cell count tends to be low with a relative lymphocytosis. Cerebrospinal fluid in patients with measles encephalitis usually shows an increase in protein and a small increase in lymphocytes. The glucose level is normal.

The diagnosis of measles is frequently delayed in adults because practitioners providing health care for adults are not used to encountering the disease and rarely include it in the differential diagnosis. The clinical picture is similar to that seen in children. Liver involvement, with abdominal pain, mild to moderate elevation of aspartate aminotransferase (AST) levels, and occasionally jaundice, is common in adults.

DIFFERENTIAL DIAGNOSIS. The rash of rubeola must be differentiated from that of rubella; roseola infantum (human herpesvirus 6); infections resulting from echovirus, coxsackievirus, and adenovirus; infectious mononucleosis; toxoplasmosis; meningococcemia; scarlet fever; rickettsial diseases; Kawasaki disease; serum sickness; and drug rashes.

Koplik spots are pathognomonic for measles. The rashes of rubella and of enteroviral and adenoviral infections tend to be less striking than that of measles, as do the degree of fever and severity of illness. The rash of roseola infantum appears as the fever disappears, whereas in measles it appears concomitantly. Although cough is present in many rickettsial infections, the rash usually spares the face, which is characteristically involved in measles. The absence of administration of a drug in the history usually serves to exclude serum sickness or drug rashes. Meningococcemia may be accompanied by a rash that is somewhat similar to that of measles, but cough and conjunctivitis are usually absent. In acute meningococcemia the rash is characteristically petechial and purpuric. The diffuse, finely papular rash of scarlet fever has a "goose flesh" texture on an erythematous base and is relatively easy to differentiate from the maculopapular rash of measles.

Treatment. There is no specific antiviral therapy; treatment is entirely supportive. Antipyretics (acetaminophen or ibuprofen) for fever, bed rest, and maintenance of an adequate fluid intake are indicated. Humidification may alleviate symptoms of laryngitis or an excessively irritating cough; it is best to keep the room comfortably warm rather than cool. Patients with photophobia should be protected from exposure to strong light. Bacterial complications of otitis media and bronchopneumonia require appropriate antimicrobial therapy.

Complications such as encephalitis, subacute sclerosing panencephalitis, giant cell pneumonia, and disseminated intravascular coagulation must be assessed individually. Good supportive care is essential. Immunoglobulin and corticosteroids are of limited value. Currently available antiviral compounds are not effective.

VITAMIN A. Hyporetinemia is present in more than 90% of cases of measles in Africa and in approximately 22–72% of children with measles in the United States; there is an apparent inverse correlation between retinol concentration and measles severity. Treatment with oral vitamin A reduces morbidity and mortality in children with severe measles in the developing world. Although data to determine the need for vitamin A supplementation for children with measles in the United States are incomplete, the American Academy of Pediatrics recommends consideration of vitamin A supplementation for children 6 mo to 2 yr of age who are hospitalized for measles and its complications and for children older than 6 mo of age with measles and immunodeficiency; ophthalmologic evidence of vitamin A deficiency (e.g., night blindness, Bitot spots, or evidence of xerophthalmia); impaired intestinal absorption (e.g., biliary obstruction, short-bowel syndrome, cystic fibrosis); moderate to severe malnutrition; or recent immigration from areas where high mortality rates from measles have been observed. The recommended regimen is a single dose of 100,000 IU orally for children 6 mo to 1 yr, and 200,000 IU for children 1 yr of age or older. Children with ophthalmologic evidence of vitamin A deficiency should be given additional doses the next day and 4 wk later.

Complications. The chief complications of measles are otitis media, pneumonia, and encephalitis. Noma of the cheeks may occur in rare instances. Gangrene elsewhere appears to be secondary to purpura fulminans or disseminated intravascular coagulation following measles. Interstitial pneumonia may be caused by the measles virus (giant cell pneumonia). Measles pneumonia in HIV-infected patients is often fatal and is not always accompanied by rash. Bacterial superinfection and bronchopneumonia are more frequent, however, usually with pneumococcus, group A *Streptococcus, Staphylococcus aureus,* and *Haemophilus influenzae* type b. Laryngitis, tracheitis, and bronchitis are common and may be due to the virus alone. Measles may exacerbate underlying *Mycobacterium tuberculosis* infection. There may also be a temporary loss of hypersensitivity reaction to tuberculin skin testing. Myocarditis is an infrequent serious complication, although transient electrocardiographic changes may be relatively common.

Neurologic complications are more common in measles than in any of the other exanthematous diseases. The incidence of encephalomyelitis is estimated to be 1–2/1,000 cases of measles. There is no correlation between the severity of the rash illness and that of the neurologic involvement, or between the severity of the initial encephalitic process and the prognosis. Infrequently, encephalitic involvement is manifest in the pre-eruptive period, but more often its onset occurs 2–5 days after the appearance of the rash. The cause of measles encephalitis remains controversial. It has been suggested that direct viral invasion may be operative for encephalitis early in the course of the disease, although

measles virus has rarely been isolated from brain tissue. Encephalitis that occurs later is predominantly demyelinating and may reflect an immunologic reaction. In this demyelinating type the symptoms and course do not differ from those of other parainfectious encephalitides. Fatal encephalitis has occurred in children receiving immunosuppressive treatment. Other central nervous system complications, including Guillain-Barré syndrome, hemiplegia, cerebral thrombophlebitis, and retrobulbar neuritis, occur rarely.

Prognosis. Case fatality rates in the United States have decreased in recent years to low levels for all age groups, largely because of improved socioeconomic conditions but also because of effective antibacterial therapy for the treatment of secondary bacterial infections. Despite the decline in measles cases and fatalities in the United States, the case fatality rate is still 1–3/1,000 cases. Deaths are primarily due to pneumonia or secondary bacterial infections. In developing countries measles frequently occurs in infants; possibly because of concomitant malnutrition, the disease is very severe in these locations and has a high mortality.

When measles is introduced into a highly susceptible population, the results may be disastrous. Such an occurrence in the Faroe Islands in 1846 resulted in the deaths of about one fourth, nearly 2,000, of the total population. At Ungava Bay, Canada, where 99% of 900 persons contracted measles, the mortality rate was 7%.

Prevention. Isolation precautions, especially in hospitals and other institutions, should be maintained from the 7th day after exposure until 5 days after the rash has appeared.

VACCINE. The initial measles immunization, usually as measles-mumps-rubella (MMR) vaccine, is recommended at 12–15 mo of age but may be given for measles postexposure and outbreak prophylaxis as early as 6 mo of age. A second immunization, also as MMR, is recommended routinely at 4–6 yr of age but may be administered at any time during childhood provided at least 4 wk have elapsed since the first dose. Children who have not previously received the second dose should be immunized by 11–12 yr of age. Adolescents entering college or the workforce should have received a second measles immunization.

The response to live measles vaccine may be abrogated if immunoglobulin has been recently administered (see Chapter 282). Anergy to tuberculin skin testing may develop and can persist for longer than 1 mo after measles vaccination. Children with active tuberculous infection should be receiving antituberculosis treatment when measles vaccine is administered. A tuberculin test prior to or concurrent with active immunization against measles is desirable if tuberculosis is under consideration.

Measles vaccine is not recommended for pregnant women, children with primary immunodeficiency, untreated tuberculosis, cancer, or organ transplantation, those receiving long-term immunosuppressive therapy, or severely immunocompromised HIV-infected children. HIV-infected children without severe immunosuppression and without evidence of measles immunity may receive measles vaccine.

POSTEXPOSURE PROPHYLAXIS. Passive immunization with immune globulin is effective for prevention and attenuation of measles within 6 days of exposure. Susceptible household and hospital contacts who are younger than 12 mo of age or who are pregnant should receive immune globulin (0.25 mL/kg; maximum: 15 mL) intramuscularly as soon as possible after exposure, but within 5 days. Immunocompromised persons should receive immune globulin (0.5 mL/kg; maximum: 15 mL) intramuscularly regardless of immunization status. Infants 6 mo of age or younger born to nonimmune mothers should receive immune globulin; infants 6 mo of age or younger born to immune mothers are considered protected by maternal antibody. Susceptible children 6–12 mo of age should also be vaccinated; this vaccination does not count as one of the two required measles vaccinations. Susceptible children 12 mo of age or older should receive vaccine alone within 72 hr. Pregnant women and immunocompromised persons should receive immune globulin but not vaccine.

225.1 Subacute Sclerosing Panencephalitis

Etiology. Subacute sclerosing panencephalitis (Dawson encephalitis) is a chronic encephalitis caused by persistent measles virus infection of the central nervous system. Dawson was the first to describe it clearly and to postulate a viral cause. Subsequently, measles virus was isolated from the brains of patients with subacute sclerosing panencephalitis (SSPE).

Epidemiology. SSPE is a rare disease that occurs worldwide. The disease has been diagnosed in patients 6 mo to older than 30 yr of age, but it affects primarily children and young adolescents. In more than 85% of cases, onset occurs from 5 to 15 yr of age. Infection with measles at younger than 18 mo of age seems to increase the risk of SSPE substantially. The risk among boys is more than twice that among girls, and it is higher among rural children than city children, children with more than two siblings, and children of lower socioeconomic status. SSPE was once especially common in the southeastern United States, the Ohio River valley, and some New England states. Recently, cases have been more common in the western United States and in New York City, especially among Hispanic immigrant children. Exposure to birds and other animals has been reported with abnormal frequency in the histories of patients with SSPE; the reason is not clear.

The annual incidence of SSPE in the United States fell markedly from 0.61 cases per 1 million persons younger than 20 yr of age in 1960 to 0.06 cases per 1 million in 1980. Since 1982, fewer than five new cases in the entire country have been registered with the U.S. National SSPE Registry each year. The decrease roughly parallels the progressive decline in the annual number of measles cases diagnosed since the introduction of live attenuated measles vaccine in the United States in 1963. The risk of SSPE has been estimated at 8.5 SSPE cases per 1 million cases of measles for a 6-yr period, during which the estimated risk after measles vaccination was only 0.7 cases per 1 million doses of vaccine. The overwhelming advantage of measles vaccination in preventing SSPE is clear.

In a recent case control study, the lack of vaccination was a highly significant risk factor for SSPE, and in a survey in England and Wales the relative risk of SSPE after measles infection was 29 times that of the risk of SSPE after measles vaccination. In cases occurring in vaccinated children, it has not been determined whether SSPE resulted from persistent infection with the attenuated measles virus of the vaccine, from undiagnosed wild-type measles infection preceding vaccination, or from vaccine failure and subsequent undiagnosed measles. SSPE continues to occur in areas of the world where measles remains unchecked and may be anticipated to increase wherever compliance with vaccination protocols diminishes.

Children with SSPE generally have a history of typical measles, which may have been either mild or severe, with full recovery several years before the onset of neurologic disease. Some patients with SSPE have had measles pneumonia, but none have had a history of typical measles encephalitis. The mean interval between measles and onset of SSPE was formerly about 7 yr, but recently it has increased to 12 yr. In vaccinated patients without a history of measles, the mean interval between vaccination and onset of SSPE was 5 yr before 1980 and 7.7 yr between 1980 and 1986.

Pathogenesis. The histopathology of SSPE consists of inflammation, necrosis, and repair. Brain biopsy performed in the early stages of SSPE shows mild inflammation of the meninges and a

panencephalitis involving cortical and subcortical gray matter as well as white matter, with cuffs of plasma cells and lymphocytes around blood vessels (Fig. 225–3) and increased numbers of glia throughout. Neuronal loss may not be marked until later in the course of the illness, when loss of myelin secondary to neuronal degeneration may be apparent. Intranuclear inclusion bodies surrounded by clear halos (**Cowdry type A**) may be seen within the nuclei of neurons, astrocytes, and oligodendrocytes. On electron microscopy, the inclusions are seen to contain tubular structures typical of the nucleocapsids of paramyxoviruses. Measles viral antigens can be demonstrated by labeled antibody techniques within the inclusions as well as in cells without inclusions. Lesions may be unevenly distributed throughout the brain, and biopsy is not always diagnostic.

The same findings of inclusion-body panencephalitis are generally present at autopsy; however, late in the disease it may be difficult to find typical areas of inflammation, and the main histopathologic changes are necrosis and gliosis. The disease is believed to begin in the cortical gray matter, progressing then to the subcortical white and gray matter (myoclonus probably results from extrapyramidal involvement) and finally to the lower structures. Although persistent infection of lymphoid tissues with measles virus has been reported, these show no pathologic changes.

It has been proposed that viral mutation may render the measles virus more likely to establish persistent central nervous system (CNS) infection, and multiple mutations have been found in isolates from patients with SSPE. However, no consistent genomic abnormalities have been identified in those isolates, and clusters of SSPE cases suggestive of strains of special virulence have been described only rarely. It has also been theorized that patients with SSPE have subtle predisposing immune deficiency; the markedly increased risk of SSPE after measles in infancy suggests that either immunologic immaturity or persistence of maternal antibodies to measles virus is involved in the later occurrence of the disease.

Complete measles virus particles are not found in the brains of patients with SSPE, and the matrix (M) protein required for the final assembly and budding of virus from the host cells is missing not only from the brain tissue of patients but also from cells cultured from their brains; however, the full complement of genetic material needed to code for all proteins, including the M protein, is present and functional. Several studies have suggested that M proteins are encoded but that because of a variety of mutations they cannot bind to nucleocapsid, resulting in

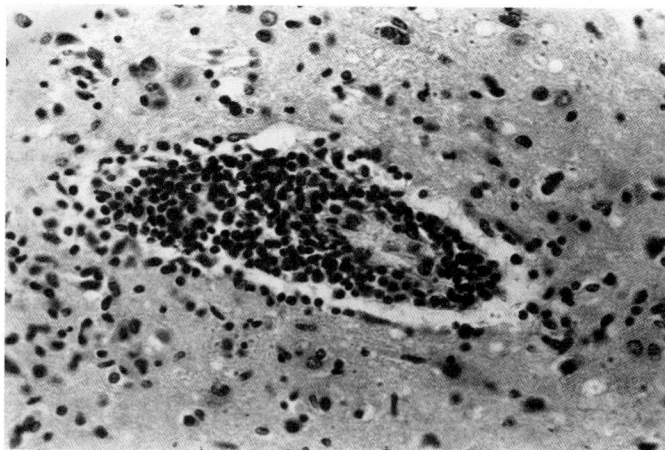

FIGURE 225–3. A cuff of inflammatory cells surrounds a blood vessel in the cerebral cortex of a child with subacute sclerosing panencephalitis. (Courtesy of Janice Stevens, MD, National Institute of Mental Health, and Peggy Swoveland, MD, University of Maryland School of Medicine.)

accumulation of incomplete measles virus that cannot be cleared either by antibodies or by cell-mediated immunity.

Clinical Manifestations. The clinical picture of SSPE tends to be quite stereotypical; almost 70% of cases have an acute, subacute, or chronic progressive course; fewer than 10% have remissions. The onset is usually insidious and is marked by subtle changes in behavior and deterioration of schoolwork; this is followed by more overtly bizarre behavior and finally by frank dementia.

There is no fever, photophobia, or other findings of acute encephalitis except for occasional complaints of headache. Diffuse neurologic disease becomes progressively more severe. The appearance of massive, repetitive myoclonic jerks, generally symmetric, involving especially the axial musculature and occurring at 5–10-sec intervals, marks the onset of the second clinical stage of SSPE. The myoclonic jerks appear to be abnormal movements rather than epileptic seizures, but true convulsions can also occur at any stage of the illness. In addition to myoclonic jerks, which tend to disappear as the disease progresses, a variety of other abnormal movements and dystonias have been observed. Cerebellar ataxia may occur. Retinopathy and optic atrophy may appear, sometimes even before the behavioral changes. Dementia progresses to stupor and coma, sometimes with autonomic insufficiency. Patients may be rigid or spastic with decorticate postures, or they may be flaccid.

The speed of progression is highly variable, but in at least 60% of patients the course is inexorable and relatively rapid. The total duration of illness may be as short as a few months, but most patients survive for 1–3 yr after diagnosis, with a mean of about 18 mo. Occasional patients show some spontaneous improvement and live for more than 10 yr. In recent years, the few patients diagnosed with SSPE in the United States have tended to have a relatively long survival, perhaps because of improvements in chronic care.

Diagnosis. Blood tests are normal except for elevated titers of antibodies to measles virus; IgG and IgM antibodies are directed against all the component proteins of measles virus except the M protein. Cell content of the cerebrospinal fluid (CSF) is generally normal, although stained sediments may show plasma cells. Total protein content of the CSF is normal or only slightly elevated; however, the gamma globulin fraction is greatly elevated (usually comprising at least 20% of total protein), resulting in a paretic type of colloidal gold curve. When the CSF is examined by electrophoresis or isoelectric focusing, oligoclonal bands of Ig are often observed. IgG and IgM antibodies to measles virus, not normally found in unconcentrated CSF, make up most of the Ig, and these can often be detected in dilutions of 1:8 or more. The complement fixation test has been especially useful for demonstrating antibodies in CSF, but hemagglutination inhibition, immunofluorescence, and other serologic tests, including enzyme-labeled immunosorbent assays (ELISA), are also satisfactory. The usual ratio of antibody in serum to CSF is reduced (<1:200) for measles antibodies, whereas the serum-to-CSF ratio is normal for other viral antibodies and for albumin, indicating that the increased amounts of measles antibodies in the CSF of patients with SSPE result from synthesis within the nervous system and that the blood-brain barrier is normal.

Early in the course of disease, the electroencephalogram (EEG) may be normal or show only moderate nonspecific slowing. In the myoclonic stage, most patients with SSPE have "suppression-burst episodes" in which high-amplitude slow and sharp waves recur at intervals of 3–5 sec on a slow background; however, this pattern is not unique to SSPE. Later in the illness, the EEG becomes increasingly disorganized and shows high-amplitude, random dysrhythmic slowing; in terminal disease, the amplitude may fall.

CT or MRI scans of patients with SSPE may show variable cortical atrophy and ventricular enlargement, and there may be focal or multifocal low-density lesions in the white matter. However, these studies may be normal, especially early in the disease.

Brain biopsy is no longer needed to diagnose SSPE. When performed, it often shows the typical histopathologic findings described earlier. Examination of frozen sections by immunofluorescence techniques may demonstrate the presence of measles viral antigens. Persistence of measles virus infection in cultures may be demonstrated by labeled antibody techniques before the complete virus appears. Many specimens fail to yield complete virus. Modifications of the polymerase chain reaction can detect various regions of the measles virus RNA in frozen and even paraffin-embedded brain tissue specimens of patients with SSPE. Nucleic acid hybridization techniques have also been used to demonstrate the measles viral genome.

DIFFERENTIAL DIAGNOSIS. It is most important to rule out potentially treatable illnesses such as bacterial infections and tumors. The diverse cerebral storage diseases and nonstorage poliodystrophies, leukodystrophies, and demyelinating diseases of childhood can also produce progressive dementia with seizures and paralysis resembling SSPE. Early in the course of illness, SSPE must be distinguished from atypical acute viral encephalitides. Other slow viral infections, such as Creutzfeldt-Jakob disease (CJD) and progressive rubella panencephalitis, must be considered in appropriate age groups. The presence of a typical EEG pattern suggests SSPE, as do unusually high levels of measles antibodies in serum. The diagnosis is practically confirmed if measles antibodies are detected in CSF.

The persistent measles infection seen in SSPE does not result in complete virus particles. Patients with SSPE, therefore, pose no hazard of infection to others, and no special precautions need ordinarily be taken. Blood precautions might be justified under special circumstances.

Treatment. Administration of inosiplex (100 mg/kg/24 hr) may prolong survival and may produce some clinical improvement in the degree of disability. Other treatments have been ineffective. The use of anticonvulsants, maintenance of nutritional status, prompt treatment of secondary bacterial infections, physical therapy, and other supportive care may also prolong survival and improve the quality of life for the patient and family. Information on current therapeutic trials can be obtained from the U.S. National SSPE Registry (Dr. Paul R. Dyken, Institute for Research in Childhood Neurodegenerative Diseases, Mobile, Alabama; Telephone 334-478-6424).

Complications. Patients with SSPE have the usual secondary complications associated with incapacitating neurologic diseases, such as recurrent pneumonias and decubitus ulcers.

Prognosis. Few patients live for longer than 3 yr after the diagnosis of SSPE, and those who do survive longer are usually disabled.

Prevention. Measles vaccination is the most important measure to prevent SSPE.

American Academy of Pediatrics, Committee on Infectious Diseases: Age of routine administration of the second dose of measles-mumps-rubella vaccine. *Pediatrics* 1998;101:129–33.

American Academy of Pediatrics, Committee on Infectious Diseases: Vitamin A treatment of measles. *Pediatrics* 1993;91:1014–5.

Alcardi J, Goutieres F, Arsenio-Nunes ML, et al: Acute measles encephalitis in children with immunosuppression. *Pediatrics* 1977;59:232–9.

Brem J: Koplik spots for the record: An illustrated historical note. *Clin Pediatr* 1972;11:161–3.

Centers for Disease Control and Prevention: Progress toward interrupting indigenous measles transmission—Region of the Americas, January–November 2001. *MMWR Morb Mortal Wkly Rep* 2001;50:1133–7.

Centers for Disease Control and Prevention: Advances in global measles control and elimination. Summary of the 1997 international meeting. *MMWR Morb Mortal Wkly Rep* 1998;47(RR-11):1–23.

Gustafson TL, Brunell PA, Lievens AW, et al: Measles outbreak in a "fully immunized" secondary school population. *N Engl J Med* 1987;316:771–4.

Hussey G, Klein N: A randomized trial of vitamin A in children with severe measles. *N Engl J Med* 1990;323:160–4.

Jabbour JT, Duenas DA, Sever JL, et al: Epidemiology of subacute sclerosing panencephalitis (SSPE). A report of the SSPE registry. *JAMA* 1972;220:959–62.

Markowitz LE, Preblud SR, Orenstein WA, et al: Patterns of transmission in measles outbreaks in the United States, 1985–1986. *N Engl J Med* 320:75–81.

Mathias RG, Meeklson WC, Arcand TA, et al: The role of secondary vaccine failures in measles outbreaks. *Am J Public Health* 1989;79:475–8.

McLaughlin M, Thomas P, Onorato I, et al: Live virus vaccines in human immunodeficiency virus-infected children. A retrospective study. *Pediatrics* 1988;82:229–33.

Modlin JF: Epidemiologic studies of measles, measles vaccine, SSPE. *Pediatrics* 1977;59:505–12.

Payne FE, Baublis JV, Itabashi HH: Isolation of measles virus from cell cultures of brain from a patient with subacute sclerosing panencephalitis. *N Engl J Med* 1969;281:585–9.

Quiambao BP, Gatchalian SR, Halonen P, et al: Coinfection is common in measles-associated pneumonia. *Pediatr Infect Dis J* 1998;17:89–93.

Vitek CR, Redd SC, Redd SB, et al: Trends in importation of measles to the United States, 1986–1994. *JAMA* 1997;277:1952–6.

Chapter 226

Rubella *Yvonne Maldonado*

Rubella (**German** or **three-day measles**) is an important childhood disease that was historically widespread but is now very infrequent. It is an acute viral infection ordinarily characterized by mild constitutional symptoms, a rash similar to that of mild rubeola or scarlet fever, and enlargement and tenderness of the postoccipital, retroauricular, and posterior cervical lymph nodes. Rubella in early pregnancy may cause the congenital rubella syndrome, a serious multisystem disease with a wide spectrum of clinical expression and sequelae.

Etiology. Rubella virus, the cause of rubella, is an RNA virus of the genus *Rubivirus* in the family Togaviridae.

Epidemiology. Humans are the only natural host of rubella virus, which is spread either by oral droplet or transplacentally to the fetus, causing congenital infection. It is distributed worldwide and affects both sexes equally. Before introduction of the rubella vaccine in 1969, pandemics of rubella occurred every 6–9 yr, with most cases occurring in the spring. In 1964–1965, an epidemic in the United States caused more than 12 million cases of rubella and an additional 20,000 infants with congenital rubella syndrome. The peak incidence of rubella was among children 5–14 yr of age but most cases now occur among susceptible teenagers and young adults. Outbreaks have been reported among college students and in unvaccinated populations, such as Amish communities, and among unvaccinated foreign-born adults. In closed populations, such as institutions and military barracks, almost 100% of susceptible individuals may become infected. In family settings, 50–60% of susceptible family members acquire the disease.

Indigenous rubella and congenital rubella syndrome were targeted for elimination in the United States by the year 2000. From a peak of 57,686 cases in 1969 through 1989, the numbers of annual reported cases have decreased, with a slight resurgence during 1990–1991, by 99.7% to 128–192 cases of rubella and 4–11 cases of congenital rubella syndrome annually from 1992 to 1997. In 2001, only 20 cases of rubella were reported in the United States. Despite these advances, outbreaks of rubella and congenital rubella still occur, primarily among unvaccinated foreign-born adults.

During clinical illness the virus is shed in nasopharyngeal secretions, blood, feces, and urine. Virus has been recovered from the nasopharynx 7 days before exanthem and 7–8 days after its disappearance. Patients with subclinical disease are also infectious.

Pathogenesis. The pathogenesis of rubella is not well understood. Virus can be found from both infected and uninfected areas of skin, suggesting that immune processes may be important.

The risk for congenital defects and disease is greatest with primary maternal infection during the first trimester. Congenital defects occur in about 90% of infants whose mothers acquire maternal infection before the 11th week of pregnancy, diminishing to about 10–20% by the end of the first trimester, with an overall risk for the trimester being about 70%. Maternal infection after the 16th week of pregnancy poses a low risk for congenital defects, although infection of the fetus may occur.

Clinical Manifestations. The incubation period is 14–21 days. The prodromal phase of mild catarrhal symptoms is shorter than that of measles and may be so mild that it goes unnoticed. Approximately two thirds of infections are subclinical.

The most characteristic sign is retroauricular, posterior cervical, and postoccipital lymphadenopathy. No other disease causes the tender enlargement of these nodes to the extent that rubella does. An enanthem appears in 20% of patients just before the onset of the skin rash. It consists of discrete rose-colored spots on the soft palate (**Forchheimer spots**) that may coalesce into a red blush and extend over the fauces.

Lymphadenopathy is evident at least 24 hr before the rash appears and may remain for 1 wk or more. The exanthem is more variable than that of rubeola. It begins on the face (Fig. 226–1) and spreads quickly. Its evolution is so rapid that the rash may be fading on the face by the time it appears on the trunk. Discrete maculopapules are present in large numbers; there are also large areas of flushing that spread rapidly over the entire body, usually within 24 hr. The rash may be confluent, particularly on the face. During the second day the rash may assume a pinpoint appearance, especially over the trunk, resembling that of scarlet fever. Mild itching may occur. The eruption usually clears by the third day. Desquamation is minimal. Rubella without a rash has been described.

The pharyngeal mucosa and the conjunctivae are slightly inflamed. In contrast to rubeola, there is no photophobia. Fever is low grade or absent during the rash and persists for 1, 2, or occasionally 3 days. Anorexia, headache, and malaise are not common.

Especially in older girls and women, polyarthritis may occur with arthralgia, swelling, tenderness, and effusion but usually

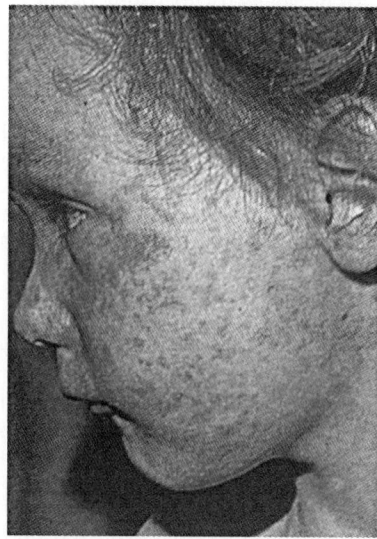

FIGURE 226–1. Rash of rubella (German measles). (From Korting GW: *Hautkrankheiten bei Kindern und Jugendlichen*, 3rd ed. Stuttgart, Germany, FK Schattauer Verlag, 1982.) See also color plates.

without any residuum. Any joint may be involved, but the small joints of the hands are affected most frequently. The duration is usually several days to 2 wk; rarely it persists for months. Paresthesia also has been reported.

CONGENITAL RUBELLA SYNDROME. See Complications.

Diagnosis. The diagnosis of rubella may be apparent from the clinical symptoms and physical examination, but it is usually confirmed by serology or virus culture. The spleen is often slightly enlarged. The white blood cell count is normal or slightly reduced; thrombocytopenia is rare, with or without purpura. Hemagglutination-inhibition (HI) antibody has been the reference method of determining immunity to rubella, but newer methods that are easier to perform are now used more commonly. Latex agglutination, enzyme immunoassay, passive hemagglutination, and fluorescent immunoassay appear to be equal or superior to the HI test in sensitivity. Immunoglobulin (Ig) M antibodies are detectable in the first few days of illness and are considered diagnostic. Detection of IgM antibodies, which do not cross the placenta, in the newborn is especially useful for the diagnosis of congenital rubella syndrome. Seroconversion, or a fourfold increase in IgG titer, is diagnostic.

Rubella virus can be cultured from the nasopharynx and blood. It is detected by the ability of rubella-infected African green monkey kidney (AGMK) cells to resist challenge with enterovirus.

DIFFERENTIAL DIAGNOSIS. Because similar symptoms and rashes can occur with many other viral infections, rubella is a difficult disease to diagnose clinically except when the patient is seen during an epidemic. A history of having had rubella or rubella vaccine is unreliable; immunity should be determined by antibody testing. Particularly in its more severe forms, rubella may be confused with the mild types of scarlet fever and rubeola. Roseola infantum (exanthem subitum) is distinguished by a higher fever and the appearance of the rash at the end of the febrile episode rather than at the height of the signs and symptoms. Infectious mononucleosis may have a rash but is associated with generalized lymphadenopathy and characteristic atypical lymphocytosis. Enteroviral infections accompanied by a rash can be differentiated in some instances by accompanying respiratory or gastrointestinal manifestations and the absence of retroauricular lymphadenopathy. Drug rashes may be extremely difficult to differentiate from the rash of rubella, but the characteristic enlargement of the lymph nodes strongly supports a diagnosis of rubella.

Treatment. There is no specific antiviral therapy; treatment is entirely supportive. Antipyretics (acetaminophen or ibuprofen) are indicated for fever.

Complications. Complications are relatively uncommon in childhood. Encephalitis similar to that seen with measles occurs in about 1 in 6,000 cases. The severity is highly variable, and there is an overall mortality rate of 20%. Symptoms in survivors usually resolve within 1–3 wk without neurologic sequelae. Thrombocytopenic purpura occurs at an overall rate of 1 in 3,000 cases.

The most important consequence of rubella in a pregnant woman is congenital rubella syndrome. Progressive rubella panencephalitis is a persistent, slowly progressive rubella infection of the central nervous system (see Chapter 226.1).

CONGENITAL RUBELLA SYNDROME. Congenital rubella affects virtually all organ systems. The most common manifestation is intrauterine growth retardation. Other common findings include cataracts, bilateral or unilateral, which are frequently associated with microphthalmia; myocarditis and structural cardiac defects (e.g., patent ductus arteriosus or pulmonary artery stenosis); "blueberry muffin" skin lesions, similar to those seen in congenital cytomegalovirus infection; hearing loss from sensorineural deafness; and meningoencephalitis. Persistent

infection leads to pneumonia, hepatitis, bone lucencies, thrombocytopenic purpura, and anemia. Later sequelae include motor and mental retardation.

The diagnosis is confirmed by finding rubella-specific IgM antibody in the neonatal serum, or by culturing rubella virus from the infant (nasopharynx, urine, or tissues). Virus can be shed in the urine for 1 yr or longer. Prenatal diagnosis of fetal rubella infection can be made either by isolating the virus from amniotic fluid or by identification of rubella-specific IgM in cord blood.

Infants with the complete spectrum of the congenital rubella syndrome have a grim prognosis, especially when the neurologic symptoms continue to progress throughout infancy. The prognosis is better for infants with fewer stigmata of the syndrome, presumably those who were initially infected later in gestation. Only about 30% of infants with encephalitis appear to escape residual neuromotor deficits, including an autistic syndrome.

Prognosis. The prognosis of rubella in childhood is excellent. Infection usually confers permanent immunity, although reinfection may occur.

REINFECTION. The incidence of reinfection on exposure to wild virus is 3–10% among those with a history of previous rubella and 14–18% among those immunized with the RA 27/3 vaccine. Reinfection may lead only to an IgG booster response, to both an IgM and IgG response, or to clinical rubella. Maternal reinfection during pregnancy has resulted in congenital rubella syndrome. The significance of rubella reinfection is controversial.

Prevention. Rubella vaccine is derived from the RA 27/3 strain of rubella virus, which is attenuated by serial passage tissue culture in WI-38 and MRC-5 human diploid cells. The vaccine induces antibody in more than 99% of seronegative recipients and has protective efficacy in more than 90%. Vaccine virus may be shed from the nasopharynx in low titers for as long as 18–25 days after vaccination, although there is no evidence of communicability.

The initial rubella immunization, usually as measles-mumps-rubella (MMR), is recommended at 12–15 mo of age. A second immunization, also as MMR, is recommended routinely at 4–6 yr of age but may be administered at any time during childhood provided at least 4 wk have elapsed since the first dose. Children who have not previously received the second dose should be immunized by 11–12 yr of age. It is especially important for girls to have immunity to rubella before they reach childbearing age.

Pregnant women should not be given live rubella virus vaccine and should avoid becoming pregnant for 3 mo after they have been vaccinated. Routine serologic testing of postpubertal women before rubella immunization is not necessary. Inadvertent immunization is not ordinarily a reason to interrupt the pregnancy. No cases of congenital rubella syndrome have been reported in more than 200 women immunized during pregnancy with RA 27/qa3 vaccine who have been studied. Other contraindications include allergy to a vaccine component (anaphylaxis to neomycin), moderate or severe acute illness with or without fever, immunodeficiency (primary immunodeficiency, cancer and cancer therapy, long-term high-dose corticosteroids, severely immunocompromised, including those with HIV infection), and recent immunoglobulin administration (see Chapter 282).

Symptoms that may follow rubella immunization include fever (5–15%), rash (5%), lymphadenopathy, and arthralgias and arthritis. Joint involvement, usually seen in the small peripheral joints 10–21 days after vaccination, is uncommon in children but occurs frequently in postpubertal females with both arthralgias (25%) and transient arthritis (10%) being reported. It may last for weeks. Transient peripheral paresthesia and pain in the arms and legs are reported rarely.

All health care workers should be immune to rubella as well as to measles and varicella. Persons born before 1957 can be considered immune to rubella, except women of childbearing age who could become pregnant. Adolescent girls and premenopausal women should either be vaccinated or have documented laboratory evidence of immunity. Maternal antibody is protective for the infant for the first 6 mo of life.

POSTEXPOSURE PROPHYLAXIS. Nonpregnant susceptible contacts of persons with rubella should be vaccinated. This does not prevent infection but ensures protection for future rubella exposures.

All pregnant women, regardless of immunization history, should make every effort to avoid exposure to rubella. If a pregnant woman whose immune status is unknown is exposed to rubella, an antibody test should be performed immediately. Immune women should be reassured. Susceptible pregnant women exposed to rubella should not receive vaccine because of the potential risk of transmission of vaccine virus to the fetus. Susceptible women should undergo repeat serologic testing 3–4 wk after exposure, and, if they are still seronegative, again 6 wk after exposure. Seroconversion on either specimen indicates infection, and the mother should be counseled about the risk of transmission to the fetus and the resulting anomalies. Routine immune globulin administration for postexposure prophylaxis in pregnancy is not recommended but should be considered if termination of the pregnancy is not an option. For the susceptible pregnant woman exposed to measles for whom termination of pregnancy is a viable option and for whom timing permits documentation of seroconversion within the period of time when abortion is possible, immune globulin is not recommended because it may provide an unjustified sense of security and precludes a positive serologic diagnosis as the basis for termination of pregnancy. However, for the susceptible pregnant woman exposed to rubella for whom abortion is not an option, immunoglobulin should be administered in a dose of 0.55 mL/kg, which reduces the attack rate but does not eliminate the risk of fetal infection. Fetal infection may occur even in the absence of clinical signs in the mother. The use of intravenous immunoglobulin (IVIG) may be an alternative but has not been studied.

226.1 Progressive Rubella Panencephalitis

Epidemiology. Progressive rubella panencephalitis is an exceedingly rare form of chronic encephalitis associated with persistent rubella virus infection of the brain. Since the disease was first recognized in 1974, 20 cases have been reported, all involving males 8–21 yr of age at onset. Most had typical stigmata of the congenital rubella syndrome including cataracts, deafness, and mental retardation, but two had apparently had childhood rubella from which they made a full recovery. No new cases have been described in the United States in recent years, presumably because of effective childhood rubella immunization programs.

Pathogenesis. Rubella virus has been isolated from brain cell cultures and from blood lymphocytes. The histopathologic changes seen in the brain are similar to those seen in SSPE, with cuffs of lymphocytes and plasma cells around blood vessels, glial nodules in the cortex, some loss of neurons, an increase in astrocytes throughout the gray matter, and an even greater increase in the white matter. However, in progressive rubella panencephalitis, there are no inclusion bodies, and deposits of material that stains with the periodic acid-Schiff reaction are found around vessels in subcortical white matter.

Clinical Manifestations. At onset, progressive rubella panencephalitis resembles subacute sclerosing panencephalitis (SSPE; see Chapter 225.1), with insidious changes in behavior and deteriorating school performance. Subsequently, frank dementia and other signs of multifocal brain disease occur, including seizures, cerebellar ataxia, and spastic weakness. Myoclonus and other abnormal movements may occur but are not as common as those seen in SSPE. Retinopathy and optic atrophy may occur.

Diagnosis. Early in the course of illness, progressive rubella panencephalitis must be distinguished from atypical acute viral encephalitides. Other slow viral infections, such as Creutzfeldt-Jakob disease (CJD) and SSPE, must be considered in appropriate age groups. Stigmata of congenital rubella syndrome or rubella infection suggest the diagnosis of progressive rubella panencephalitis.

Remarkable laboratory abnormalities include elevated antibody titers to rubella virus, a normal or slightly elevated CSF cell count, and a slightly elevated CSF protein concentration with a marked increase in globulin, which may constitute more than 50% of the total protein. Oligoclonal electrophoretic bands of globulin consist of antibodies to rubella virus antigens. Antibodies to rubella virus are readily detectable in CSF, often at dilutions of 1:8 or higher. The hemagglutination-inhibition, complement fixation, and enzyme immunoassay techniques should be satisfactory for testing the cerebrospinal fluid. Most of the rubella antibodies in the CSF are IgG, although some IgM antibodies have also been detected early in the course of progressive rubella panencephalitis. There is a high CSF:serum ratio of rubella antibody titers compared with ratio of titers to measles and other viruses. Isolation of rubella virus from blood lymphocytes may be attempted, but brain biopsy should not be needed to establish the diagnosis.

The EEG shows a generalized slowing with occasional high-voltage activity, but the suppression-burst pattern of SSPE has not been seen in progressive rubella panencephalitis. Encephalograms (computed tomography was not available when published cases were studied) show enlargement of all ventricles, especially the fourth, with prominent atrophy of the cerebellum.

Prognosis. The course of progressive rubella panencephalitis is similar to that seen in SSPE, progressing to coma, spasticity, brainstem involvement, and death in 2–5 yr.

Patients with progressive rubella panencephalitis pose no substantial risk of infection to others. Rubella viruria has not been detected.

Prevention. Rubella vaccination is the most important measure to prevent rubella panencephalitis.

Centers for Disease Control and Prevention: Measles, mumps, and rubella—vaccine use and strategies for elimination of measles, rubella, and congenital rubella syndrome and control of mumps. Recommendations of the Advisory Committee on Immunization Practices (ACIP). *MMWR* 1998;47(RR-8):1–57.

Chang TW: Editorial: Rubella reinfection and intrauterine involvement. *J Pediatr* 1974;84:617–8.

Dudgeon JA: Congenital rubella. *J Pediatr* 1975;87:1078–86.

Howson CP, Katz M, Johnston RB, et al: Chronic arthritis after rubella vaccination. *Clin Infect Dis* 1992;15:307–12.

Lee SH, Ewert DP, Frederick PD, et al: Resurgence of congenital rubella syndrome in the 1990s. Report on missed opportunities and failed prevention policies among women of childbearing age. *JAMA* 1992;267:2616–20.

Miller E, Cradock-Watson JE, Pollock TM: Consequences of confirmed maternal rubella at successive stages of pregnancy. *Lancet* 1982;2:781–4.

Rawls WE, Desmyter J, Melnick JL: Serologic diagnosis and fetal involvement in maternal rubella. Criteria for abortion. *JAMA* 1968;203:627–31.

Rawls WE, Phillips CA, Melnick JL, et al: Persistent virus infection in congenital rubella. *Arch Ophthalmol* 1967;77:430–3.

Reef SE, Frey TK, Theall K, et al: The changing epidemiology of rubella in the 1990s: On the verge of elimination and new challenges for control and prevention. *JAMA* 2002;287:464–72.

Tardieu M, Grospierre B, Durandy A, et al: Circulating immune complexes containing rubella antigens in late-onset rubella syndrome. *J Pediatr* 1980;97:370–3.

Townsend JJ: Progressive rubella panencephalitis. Late onset after congenital rubella. *N Engl J Med* 1975;292:990–3.

Weibel RE, Benor DE: Chronic arthropathy and musculoskeletal symptoms associated with rubella vaccines. A review of 124 claims submitted to the National Vaccine Injury Program. *Arthritis Rheum* 1996;39:1529–34.

Chapter 227

Mumps *Yvonne Maldonado*

Mumps is an important childhood disease that was historically widespread but now occurs very infrequently. It is an acute viral infection characterized by painful enlargement of the salivary glands, chiefly the parotids, as the usual presenting sign.

Etiology. Mumps virus, the cause of mumps, is an RNA virus of the genus *Paramyxovirus* in the family Paramyxoviridae, which also includes the parainfluenza viruses. Only one serotype is known.

Epidemiology. Mumps is endemic in most unvaccinated populations; the virus is spread from human reservoir by direct contact, airborne droplets, fomites contaminated by saliva, and possibly by urine. It is distributed worldwide and affects both sexes equally. Before introduction of the vaccine in 1967, the peak incidence of the disease occurred in children 5–9 yr of age; 85% of infections occurred in children younger than 15 yr of age. Now most cases occur in young adults, producing outbreaks in colleges or in the workplace. Outbreaks appear to be primarily related to a lack of immunization, especially in an underimmunized cohort of children born from 1967–1977, rather than to waning to immunity. Epidemics occur at all seasons but are slightly more frequent in late winter and spring.

There has been a dramatic decrease in the incidence of mumps since the introduction of the mumps vaccine in 1968. Except for a small increase in 1987, the incidence of mumps has steadily decreased in the United States. In 2001 there were 226 reported cases of mumps, a greater than 99% reduction from the 152,209 cases reported in 1968.

Virus has been isolated from saliva as long as 6 days before and up to 9 days after appearance of salivary gland swelling. Transmission does not seem to occur more than 24 hr before the appearance of the swelling or later than 3 days after it has subsided. Virus has been isolated from urine from the 1st–14th day after the onset of salivary gland swelling.

Pathogenesis. After entry into the last and initial multiplication in the cells of the respiratory tract, the virus is bloodborne to many tissues, among which the salivary and other glands are the most susceptible.

Clinical Manifestations. The incubation period ranges from 14–24 days, with a peak at 17–18 days. Approximately 30–40% of infections are subclinical. In children, prodromal manifestations are rare but may be manifest by fever, muscular pain (especially in the neck), headache, and malaise.

SALIVARY GLANDS. The onset is usually characterized by pain and swelling in one or both parotid glands. The parotid swells characteristically; it first fills the space between the posterior border of the mandible and the mastoid and then extends in a series of crescents downward and forward, being limited above by the zygoma. Edema of the skin and soft tissues usually extends further and obscures the limit of the glandular swelling, so that the swelling is more readily appreciated by sight than by palpation. Swelling may proceed extremely rapidly, reaching a maximum within a few hours, although it usually peaks in 1–3 days. The swollen tissues push the earlobe upward and outward, and the angle of the mandible is no longer visible. Swelling slowly subsides within 3–7 days but occasionally lasts longer. One parotid gland usually swells a day or two before the other, but in approximately one quarter of cases the disease remains unilateral. The swollen area is tender and painful, pain being elicited especially by tasting sour liquids such as lemon juice or vinegar. Redness and swelling about the opening of the Stensen duct are common. Edema of the homolateral pharynx and soft palate accompanies the parotid swelling and displaces the tonsil medially; acute edema of the larynx has also been described. Edema over the manubrium and upper chest wall may occur, probably because of lymphatic obstruction. The parotid swelling is usually accompanied by low-grade fever, but this may be absent.

Although the parotid glands alone are affected in the majority of patients, swelling of the submandibular glands occurs frequently and usually accompanies or closely follows that of the parotid glands. In 10–15% of patients only the submandibular gland(s) may be swollen. Little pain is associated with the submandibular infection, but the swelling subsides more slowly than that of the parotids. Redness and swelling at the orifice of the Wharton duct frequently accompany swelling of the gland. Least commonly, the sublingual glands are infected, usually bilaterally; the swelling is evident in the submental region and in the floor of the mouth.

Diagnosis. The diagnosis of mumps parotitis is usually apparent from the clinical symptoms and physical examination. When the clinical manifestations are limited to less common lesions, the diagnosis is less clear but may be suspected during an outbreak.

Routine laboratory tests are nonspecific; usually leukopenia is present with relative lymphocytosis. An elevation in serum amylase levels is common; the rise tends to parallel the parotid swelling and then to return to normal within 2 wk.

The microbiologic diagnosis is by serology or virus culture. Enzyme immunoassay for mumps immunoglobulin (Ig) G and IgM antibodies are most commonly used for diagnosis. IgM antibodies are detectable in the first few days of illness and are considered diagnostic. They may remain elevated for weeks to months. IgG antibodies are directed primarily against the fusion (F) protein; cross reactions with parainfluenza viruses may occur. Seroconversion, or a fourfold increase in IgG titer, is diagnostic.

Mumps virus can be cultured from the saliva, cerebrospinal fluid, blood, urine, brain, and other infected tissues. Primary cultures of human or monkey kidney cells are used for viral isolation. Cytopathic effect is occasionally observed, but hemadsorption is the most sensitive indicator of infection.

The mumps skin test is unreliable for diagnosis of mumps and for determination of susceptibility to infection.

DIFFERENTIAL DIAGNOSIS. Other viral causes of parotitis include HIV infection, influenza, parainfluenza viruses 1 and 3, cytomegalovirus, and coxsackieviruses. Acute suppurative parotitis is a bacterial infection usually caused by *Staphylococcus aureus* in which pus can often be expressed from the duct. A salivary calculus obstructing either a parotid or, more commonly, a submandibular duct causes intermittent swelling. Preauricular or anterior cervical lymphadenitis can be differentiated by the well-defined borders of the lymph node and a location that is completely posterior to the angle of the mandible. Orchitis may also be caused by coxsackieviruses.

Treatment. There is no specific antiviral therapy; treatment is entirely supportive. Antipyretics (acetaminophen or ibuprofen) are indicated for fever. Bed rest should be guided by the patient's needs, but no evidence indicates that it prevents complications. The diet should be adjusted to the patient's ability to chew. Orchitis should be treated with local support and bed rest. Mumps arthritis may respond to a 2-wk course of a nonsteroidal anti-inflammatory agent or corticosteroids. Salicylates do not appear to be effective.

Complications. Viremia early in the infection probably accounts for the widespread complications. There is no firm evidence that maternal infection is damaging to the fetus; a possible relationship to endocardial fibroelastosis has not been firmly established. Mumps in early pregnancy does increase the chance of abortion.

MENINGOENCEPHALOMYELITIS. This is the most frequent complication in childhood. Its true incidence is hard to estimate because subclinical infection of the central nervous system, as evidenced by cerebrospinal fluid pleocytosis, has been reported in more than 65% of patients with mumps parotitis. Clinical manifestations occur in more than 10% of patients. The incidence of mumps meningoencephalitis is approximately 250/100,000 cases; 10% of these cases occurred in patients older than 20 yr of age. The mortality rate is about 2%. Males are affected three to five times as frequently as females.

The pathogenesis of mumps meningoencephalitis may be either a primary infection of neurons or a postinfectious encephalitis with demyelination. In the first type, parotitis frequently appears at the same time or following the onset of encephalitis. In the latter type, encephalitis follows parotitis by an average of 10 days. Parotitis may in some cases be absent. Aqueductal stenosis and hydrocephalus have been associated with mumps infection. Injecting mumps virus into suckling hamsters has produced similar lesions.

Mumps meningoencephalitis is clinically indistinguishable from meningoencephalitis of other origins (see Chapter 174.2). Moderate stiffness of the neck is seen, but the remaining findings on neurologic examination are usually normal. The cerebrospinal fluid may show a lymphocytic pleocytosis of less than 500 cells/ mm^3, although occasionally the count may exceed 2,000 cells/mm^3.

ORCHITIS AND EPIDIDYMITIS. These complications rarely occur in prepubescent boys but are common (14–35%) in adolescents and adults. The testis is most often infected with or without epididymitis; epididymitis may also occur alone. Bilateral orchitis occurs in approximately 30% of patients. Rarely, there is a hydrocele. The orchitis usually follows parotitis within 8 days. Orchitis may also occur without evidence of salivary gland infection. The onset is usually abrupt, with a rise in temperature, chills, headache, nausea, and lower abdominal pain; when the right testis is implicated, appendicitis may be suggested as a diagnostic possibility. The affected testis becomes tender and swollen, and the adjacent skin is edematous and red. The average duration of illness is 4 days. Approximately 30–40% of affected testes atrophy, leaving a cosmetic imbalance. Infertility is rare even with bilateral orchitis.

OOPHORITIS. Pelvic pain and tenderness are noted in about 7% of postpubertal female patients. There is no evidence of impairment of fertility.

PANCREATITIS. Mild or subclinical pancreatic involvement is common, but severe pancreatitis is rare. It may be unassociated with salivary gland manifestations and may be misdiagnosed as gastroenteritis. Epigastric pain and tenderness, which are suggestive, may be accompanied by fever, chills, vomiting, and prostration. An elevated serum amylase value is characteristically present in patients with mumps, with or without clinical manifestations of pancreatitis.

MYOCARDITIS. Serious cardiac manifestations are extremely rare, but mild infection of the myocardium may be more common than is recognized. Electrocardiographic tracings revealed changes, mostly depression of the ST segment, in 13% of adults in one series. Such involvement may explain the precordial pain, bradycardia, and fatigue sometimes noted among adolescents and adults with mumps.

ARTHRITIS. Migratory polyarthralgia and even arthritis are occasionally seen in adults with mumps but are rare in children. The knees, ankles, shoulders, and wrists are most commonly affected. The symptoms last from a few days to 3 mo, with a median duration of 2 wk.

THYROIDITIS. Although it is uncommon in children, a diffuse, tender swelling of the thyroid may occur about 1 wk after the onset of parotitis; antithyroid antibodies subsequently develop.

DEAFNESS. Unilateral, rarely bilateral, nerve deafness may occur; although the incidence is low (1/15,000 cases), mumps was historically a leading cause of unilateral nerve deafness. The hearing loss may be transient or permanent.

OCULAR COMPLICATIONS. Dacryoadenitis may occur with painful swelling, usually bilateral, of the lacrimal glands. Optic neuritis (papillitis) may occur; symptoms vary from loss of vision to mild blurring, with recovery in 10–20 days.

Prognosis. The prognosis of rubella in childhood is excellent. Infection usually confers permanent immunity, although reinfections have been documented.

Prevention. Mumps vaccine is derived from the **Jeryl Lynn strain** of mumps virus, which is attenuated by serial passage in embryonated hens' eggs and chick embryo cell culture. The vaccine induces antibody in 96% of seronegative recipients and has 97% protective efficacy.

The initial mumps immunization, usually as measles-mumps-rubella (MMR) vaccine, is recommended at 12–15 mo of age. A second immunization, also as MMR, is recommended routinely at 4–6 yr of age but may be administered at any time during childhood provided at least 4 wk have elapsed since the first dose. Children who have not previously received the second dose should be immunized by 11–12 yr of age. Women should avoid becoming pregnant for 30 days after monovalent mumps vaccination (3 mo if vaccination was performed with rubella vaccine). Other contraindications to vaccination include allergy to a vaccine component (anaphylaxis to neomycin), moderate or severe acute illnesses with or without fever, immunodeficiency (primary immunodeficiencies, cancer and cancer therapy, long-term high-dose corticosteroid therapy, severely immunocompromised, including those with HIV infection), and recent immune globulin administration (see Chapter 282). Rarely, parotitis and low-grade fever can develop 10–14 days after vaccination. Vaccinees do not shed virus.

Persons born before 1957 can be considered immune to mumps. Maternal antibody is protective in the infant in the first 6 mo of life.

Bistrian B, Phillips CA, Kaye IS: Fatal mumps meningoencephalitis: Isolation of virus premortem and postmortem. *JAMA* 1972;222:478–9.

Centers for Disease Control and Prevention: Measles, mumps, and rubella: Vaccine use and strategies for elimination of measles, rubella, and congenital rubella syndrome and control of mumps. Recommendations of the Advisory Committee on Immunization Practices (ACIP). *MMWR* 1998;47(RR-8):1–57.

Centers for Disease Control and Prevention. Mumps surveillance—United States, 1988–1993. *MMWR* 1995;44(SS-3):1–14.

Cochi SI, Preblud SR, Orenstein WA: Perspectives in the relative resurgence of mumps in the United States. *Am J Dis Child* 1988;142:499–507.

Gordon SC, Lauter CB: Mumps arthritis. A review of the literature. *Rev Infect Dis* 1984;6:338.

Ni J, Bowles NE, Kim YH, et al: Viral infection of the myocardium in endocardial fibroelastosis. Molecular evidence for the role of mumps virus as an etiologic agent. *Circulation* 1997;95:133–9.

Quast U, Hennessen W, Widmark RM: Vaccine-induced mumps-like disease. *Dev Biol Stan* 1979;43:269–72.

Chapter 228

Polioviruses *Eric A. F. Simoes*

Etiology. The polioviruses are non-enveloped, positive-stranded RNA viruses belonging to the Picornaviridae family, in the genus *Enterovirus*, and include three antigenically distinct serotypes (types 1, 2, and 3). Polioviruses spread from the intestinal tract to the central nervous system (CNS), where they cause aseptic meningitis and poliomyelitis, or **polio**. The polioviruses are extremely hardy and can retain activity for several days at room temperature, and can be stored indefinitely frozen at −20°C. They are rapidly inactivated by heat (>56°C), formaldehyde, chlorination, and ultraviolet light. Polioviruses grow well in many cell cultures and rapidly cause cytopathic effects.

Epidemiology. In 1952 there were 57,879 reported cases of polio in the United States, including 21,269 cases of paralytic polio that resulted in more than 3,000 deaths, with similar epidemics being reported in Europe. These epidemics appeared to affect mostly adolescents and young adults and were growing at a steady pace, which spurred development of the Salk inactivated poliovirus vaccine, and Sabin, Cox, and Koprowski live attenuated vaccines. The universal use of the Salk and Sabin vaccines has resulted in the almost complete global eradication of polio.

The most devastating result of poliovirus infection is paralysis, but more than 90% of infections are asymptomatic or inapparent but do induce protective immunity. Clinically apparent but nonparalytic illness occurs in about 5% of all infections, with paralytic polio occurring in about 1 out of 1,000 infections among infants to about 1 out of 100 infections among adolescents. Prior to the introduction of vaccines in the United States and Europe, improvements in sanitation had limited the fecal-oral spread of polioviruses, resulting in epidemics of infection occurring later in life, when 1 in every 100 infections resulted in paralysis. Thus, in developed countries prior to universal vaccination, epidemics of paralytic poliomyelitis were observed among adolescents. Conversely, in developing countries where sanitation was and continues to be poor, infection early in life results in infantile paralysis. Undoubtedly, good sanitation explains the virtual eradication of polio as a disease from the United States in the early 1960s, when only about two thirds of the population was immunized with the Salk vaccine, and the subsequent absence of circulating wild-type poliovirus in the United States and Europe. In contrast, poor sanitation and crowding have permitted the continued transmission of poliovirus in certain poor countries in Africa and Asia, despite massive global efforts to eradicate polio, in some areas with an average of 12–13 doses of polio vaccine administered to children younger than 5 yr of age.

TRANSMISSION. Humans are the only known reservoir for the polioviruses. Poliovirus has been isolated from feces more than 2 wk before paralysis to several weeks after the onset of symptoms.

Pathogenesis. Polioviruses infect cells by adsorbing to specific genetically determined receptors, including poliovirus receptor (PVR). The virus penetrates the cell and is then uncoated and releases RNA. The RNA is translated to produce proteins responsible for replication of the RNA, shut-off of host-cell protein synthesis, and synthesis of structural elements that compose the capsid. Mature virus particles are produced in 6–8 hr and are released into the environment by disruption of the cell.

In the contact host, polioviruses gain entry through the gastrointestinal tract. The pathology of vaccine-associated poliomyelitis (VAPP) mimics natural disease. The primary site of replication may be in M cells lining the mucosa of the small intestine. Regional lymph nodes are infected, and primary viremia occurs after 2–3 days. The virus seeds multiple sites, including the reticuloendothelial system, the brown fat deposits, and skeletal muscle. Poliovirus probably accesses the CNS along peripheral nerves. Because poliovirus replicates in endothelial cells, the theory of viremic spread to the CNS was favored; however, poliovirus has almost never been cultured from the cerebrospinal fluid (CSF) of patients with paralytic disease, and patients with aseptic meningitis caused by poliovirus never have paralytic disease. With the first appearance of non-CNS symptoms, a secondary viremia probably occurs as a result of enormous viral replication in the reticuloendothelial system.

The exact mechanism of entry into the CNS is not known. Once entry is gained, however, the virus may traverse neural pathways, and multiple sites within the CNS are often affected. The effect on motor and vegetative neurons is most striking and correlates with the clinical manifestations. Perineuronal inflammation, a mixed inflammatory reaction with both polymorphonuclear leukocytes and lymphocytes, is associated with extensive neuronal destruction. Petechial hemorrhages and considerable inflammatory edema also occurs in areas of poliovirus infection. The poliovirus primarily infects motor neuron cells in the spinal cord (the anterior horn cells) and the medulla oblongata (the cranial nerve nuclei). Because of the overlap in muscle innervation by adjacent 2–3 segments of the spinal cord, clinical signs of weakness in the limbs develop when more than 50% of motor neurons are destroyed. In the medulla, less extensive lesions cause paralysis and involvement of the reticular formation that contains the vital centers controlling respiration and circulation, which may have a catastrophic outcome. Involvement of the intermediate and dorsal horn and dorsal root ganglia in the spinal cord cause the typical hyperesthesia and myalgias that are seen in acute poliomyelitis. Other neurons affected are the nuclei in the roof and vermis of the cerebellum, the substantia nigra, and occasionally the red nucleus in the pons; there may be variable involvement of thalamic, hypothalamic, and pallidal nuclei and the motor cortex.

Apart from the histopathology of the CNS, inflammatory changes occur generally in the reticuloendothelial system. Inflammatory edema and sparse lymphocytic infiltration are prominently associated with hyperplastic lymphocytic follicles.

Infants acquire immunity transplacentally from their mothers; the immunity disappears at a variable rate during the first 4–6 mo of life. Active immunity after natural infection is probably lifelong but protects against the infecting serotype only; infections with other serotypes are possible. Poliovirus neutralizing antibodies develop within several days after exposure as a result of replication of the virus in the M cells in the intestinal tract and deep lymphatic tissues. This early production of circulating immunoglobulin (Ig) G antibodies protects against CNS invasion. Local (mucosal) immunity, conferred mainly by secretory IgA, is an important defense against subsequent re-infection of the gastrointestinal tract.

Clinical Manifestations. The incubation period of poliovirus from contact to initial clinical symptoms is usually considered to be 8–12 days, with a range of 5–35 days. Poliovirus infections may follow one of several courses: inapparent infection, which occurs in 90–95% of cases and causes no disease and no sequelae; abortive poliomyelitis; nonparalytic poliomyelitis; or paralytic poliomyelitis. Paralysis, if it occurs, appears 3–8 days after the initial symptoms.

ABORTIVE POLIOMYELITIS. In about 5% of patients, a nonspecific influenza-like syndrome occurs 1–2 wk after infection; this is termed abortive poliomyelitis. Fever, malaise, anorexia, and headache are prominent features, and there may be sore throat and abdominal or muscular pain. Vomiting occurs irregularly. The illness is short-lived (up to 2–3 days). The physical examination may be normal or may reveal nonspecific pharyngitis, abdominal or muscular tenderness, and weakness. Recovery is complete, and no neurologic signs or sequelae develop.

NONPARALYTIC POLIOMYELITIS. In about 1% of all infected patients, the signs of abortive poliomyelitis are present but headache, nausea, and vomiting are more intense, and there is soreness and stiffness of the posterior muscles of the neck, trunk, and limbs. Fleeting paralysis of the bladder and constipation are frequent. Approximately two thirds of these children have a short symptom-free interlude between the first phase (**minor illness**) and the second phase (CNS disease or **major illness**). This two-phase course is less common in adults, in whom the evolution of symptoms is more insidious. Nuchal and spinal rigidity are the basis for the diagnosis of nonparalytic poliomyelitis during the second phase.

Physical examination reveals nuchal-spinal signs and changes in superficial and deep reflexes. In cooperative patients the nuchal-spinal signs are first sought by active tests. The patient is asked to sit up unassisted. If this causes undue effort and if the knees flex upward and the patient writhes a bit from side to side in sitting up and uses the hands on the bed to assume the tripod supporting position, spinal rigidity is unmistakable. While sitting, the patient is asked to flex the chin to the chest and is observed for nuchal rigidity. Alternatively, in the supine position, with the knees held down gently, the patient is asked to sit up and kiss his or her knees. If the knees draw up sharply or if the maneuver cannot be adequately completed, there is stiffness of the spine, which is a result of muscle spasm. If the diagnosis is still uncertain or in infants, attempts should be made to elicit the Kernig and Brudzinski signs. Gentle forward flexion of the occiput and neck will elicit nuchal rigidity. Head drop is demonstrated by placing the hands under the patient's shoulders and raising the trunk. Although normally the head follows the plane of the trunk, in poliomyelitis it often falls backward limply but is not due to true paresis of the neck flexors. In struggling infants it may be difficult to distinguish voluntary resistance from clinically important true nuchal rigidity. One may place the infant's shoulders flush with the edge of the table, support the weight of the occiput in the hand, and then flex the head anteriorly. True nuchal rigidity will persist during this maneuver. When open, the anterior fontanel may be tense or bulging.

In the early stages the reflexes are normally active and remain so unless paralysis supervenes. Changes in reflexes, either increased or decreased, may precede weakness by 12–24 hr; hence, it is important to test reflexes, especially in nonparalytic patients managed at home. The superficial reflexes, the cremasteric and abdominal reflexes, and the reflexes of the spinal and gluteal muscles are usually the first to diminish. The spinal and gluteal reflexes may disappear before the abdominal and cremasteric reflexes. Changes in the deep tendon reflexes generally occur 8–24 hr after the superficial reflexes are depressed and indicate impending paresis of the extremities. Tendon reflexes are absent with paralysis. Sensory defects do not occur in poliomyelitis.

PARALYTIC POLIOMYELITIS. Paralytic poliomyelitis develops in about 0.1% of persons infected with poliovirus, causing three clinically recognizable syndromes that represent a continuum of infection differentiated only by the portions of the CNS most severely affected. These are (1) spinal paralytic poliomyelitis, (2) bulbar poliomyelitis, and (3) polioencephalitis.

Spinal Paralytic Poliomyelitis. Spinal paralytic poliomyelitis may occur as the second phase of a biphasic illness, the first phase of which corresponds to abortive poliomyelitis. The patient then appears to recover and feels better for 2–5 days, after which severe headache and fever occur with exacerbation of the previous systemic symptoms. Severe muscle pain is present and sensory and motor phenomena (e.g., paresthesia, hyperesthesia, fasciculations, and spasms) may develop. On physical examination the distribution of paralysis is characteristically spotty. Single muscles, multiple muscles, or groups of muscles may be involved in any pattern. Within 1–2 days, asymmetric flaccid paralysis or paresis occurs. Involvement of one leg is most common, followed by involvement of one arm. The proximal areas of the extremities tend to be involved to a greater extent than the distal areas. To detect mild muscular weakness, it is often necessary to apply gentle resistance in opposition to the muscle group being tested. Examination at this point may reveal nuchal stiffness or rigidity, muscle tenderness, initially hyperactive deep tendon reflexes (for a short period) followed by absent or diminished reflexes, and paresis or flaccid paralysis. In the spinal form there is weakness of some of the muscles of the neck, abdomen, trunk, diaphragm, thorax, or extremities. Sensation is intact; sensory disturbances, if present, suggest a disease other than poliomyelitis.

The paralytic phase of poliomyelitis is extremely variable; some patients progress during observation from paresis to paralysis, whereas others recover, which may be slow or rapid. The extent of paresis or paralysis is directly related to the extent of neuronal involvement; paralysis occurs if more than 50% of the neurons supplying the muscles are destroyed. The extent of involvement is usually obvious within 2–3 days; only rarely does progression occur beyond this interval. Paralysis of the lower limbs is often accompanied by bowel and bladder dysfunction ranging from transient incontinence to paralysis with constipation and urinary retention.

The onset and course of paralysis are variable and age-related. Infants and young children most frequently manifest the biphasic course, with prominent prodromal symptoms. Older persons may have a single phase in which prodromal symptoms and paralysis occur in a continuous fashion. In developing countries, where a history of intramuscular injections precedes paralytic poliomyelitis in about 50–60% of patients, patients may present initially with fever and paralysis without the characteristic biphasic course (**provocation paralysis**). The degree and duration of muscle pain are also variable; some patients have none, and others complain for days or weeks. Spasm and increased muscle tone with a transient increase in deep tendon reflexes occur in some patients, whereas in others flaccid paralysis may occur abruptly. Once the temperature returns to normal, no further paralytic manifestations are noted in most patients. Little recovery from paralysis is noted in the first days or weeks but, if it is to occur, is usually evident within 6 mo. The return of strength and reflexes is slow and may continue to improve as long as 18 mo after the acute disease. Lack of improvement from paralysis within the first several weeks or months after onset is usually evidence of permanent paralysis. Atrophy of the limb, failure of growth, and deformity is common and is especially evident in the growing child.

Bulbar Poliomyelitis. Bulbar poliomyelitis may occur as a clinical entity without apparent involvement of the spinal cord. Yet the infection is a continuum, and designation of the disease as bulbar implies only dominance of the clinical manifestations by dysfunctions of the cranial nerves and medullary centers. The clinical findings seen with bulbar poliomyelitis with respiratory difficulty (other than paralysis of extraocular, facial, and masticatory muscles) include (1) nasal twang to the voice or cry caused by palatal and pharyngeal weakness (hard-consonant words such as "cookie" or "candy" bring this out best); (2) inability to swallow smoothly, resulting in accumulation of saliva in the pharynx, indicates partial immobility (holding the larynx lightly and asking the patient to swallow will confirm such immobility); (3) accumulated pharyngeal secretions, which may cause irregular respirations because each inspiration must be "planned" to avoid aspirating; the respirations may thus appear interrupted and abnormal even to the point of falsely simulating intercostal or diaphragmatic weakness; (4) absence of effective coughing, shown by constant fatiguing efforts to clear the throat; (5) nasal regurgitation of saliva and fluids as a result of palatal paralysis, with inability to separate the oropharynx from the nasopharynx during swallowing; (6) deviation of the palate, uvula, or tongue; (7) involvement of vital centers in the medulla, which are manifested by irregularities in rate, depth, and rhythm of respiration; by cardiovascular alterations including blood pressure changes (especially increased blood pressure), alternate flushing and mottling of the skin, and cardiac arrhythmias; and by rapid changes in body temperature; (8) paralysis of one or both vocal cords, causing hoarseness, aphonia, and ultimately asphyxia unless this is recognized by laryngoscopy and managed by immediate tracheostomy; and (9) **the rope sign,** an acute angulation between the chin and larynx caused by weakness of the hyoid muscles (the hyoid bone is pulled posteriorly, narrowing the hypopharyngeal inlet).

Uncommonly, bulbar disease may culminate in an ascending paralysis (Landry type), in which there is progression cephalad from initial involvement of the lower extremities. Hypertension and other autonomic disturbances are common in bulbar involvement and may persist for a week or more or may be transient.

Occasionally, hypertension is followed by hypotension and shock and is associated with irregular or failed respiratory effort, delirium, or coma. This kind of bulbar disease may be rapidly fatal.

The course of bulbar disease is variable; some patients die as a result of extensive, severe involvement of the various centers in the medulla; others recover partially but require ongoing respiratory support, and others recover completely. Cranial nerve involvement is seldom permanent. Atrophy of muscles may be evident, patients immobilized for long periods may develop pneumonia, and renal stones may form as a result of hypercalcemia and hypercalciuria secondary to bone resorption.

Polioencephalitis. Polioencephalitis is a rare form of the disease in which higher centers of the brain are severely involved. Seizures, coma, and spastic paralysis with increased reflexes may be observed. Irritability, disorientation, drowsiness, and coarse tremors not explained by inadequate ventilation are noted; peripheral or cranial nerve paralysis coexists or ensues. Hypoxia and hypercapnia caused by inadequate ventilation due to respiratory insufficiency may produce disorientation without true encephalitis. The manifestations are common to encephalitis of any cause and can only be attributed to polioviruses by specific viral diagnosis or if accompanied by flaccid paralysis.

Paralytic Poliomyelitis with Ventilatory Insufficiency. A number of components acting together may produce ventilatory insufficiency resulting in hypoxia and hypercapnia, which may produce profound effects on many other systems. Because respiratory insufficiency may develop rapidly, close continued clinical evaluation is essential. Despite weakness of the respiratory muscles, the patient may respond with so much respiratory effort (associated with anxiety and fear) that overventilation may occur at the outset, resulting in respiratory alkalosis. Such effort is fatiguing and contributes to respiratory failure.

There are certain characteristic patterns of disease. Pure spinal poliomyelitis with respiratory insufficiency involves tightness, weakness, or paralysis of the respiratory muscles (chiefly the diaphragm and intercostals) without discernible clinical involvement of the cranial nerves or vital centers that control respiration, circulation, and body temperature. The cervical and thoracic spinal cord segments are chiefly affected. Pure bulbar poliomyelitis involves paralysis of the motor cranial nerve nuclei with or without involvement of the vital centers. Involvement of the 9th, 10th, and 12th cranial nerves results in paralysis of the pharynx, tongue, and larynx with consequent airway obstruction. Bulbospinal poliomyelitis with respiratory insufficiency affects the respiratory muscles and results in coexisting bulbar paralysis.

The clinical findings associated with involvement of the respiratory muscles include (1) anxious expression; (2) inability to speak without frequent pauses, resulting in short, jerky, "breathless" sentences; (3) increased respiratory rate; (4) movement of the ala nasi and of the accessory muscles of respiration; (5) inability to cough or sniff with full depth; (6) paradoxical abdominal movements caused by diaphragmatic immobility due to spasm or weakness of one or both leaves; and (7) relative immobility of the intercostal spaces, which may be segmental, unilateral, or bilateral. When the arms are weak, and especially when deltoid paralysis occurs, there may be impending respiratory paralysis because the phrenic nerve nuclei are in adjacent areas of the spinal cord. Observation of the patient's capacity for thoracic breathing while the abdominal muscles are splinted manually indicates minor degrees of paresis. Light manual splinting of the thoracic cage will help to assess the effectiveness of diaphragmatic movement.

Diagnosis. Poliomyelitis should be considered in any unimmunized or incompletely immunized child with nonspecific febrile illness, aseptic meningitis, or paralytic disease. VAPP should be considered in any child with paralytic disease occurring 7–14 days after receiving oral poliovirus vaccine. VAPP can occur at later times after administration, and should be considered in any child with paralytic disease in countries or regions where wild type poliovirus has been eradicated and OPV has been administered to the child or a contact. The combination of fever, headache, neck and back pain, asymmetric flaccid paralysis without sensory loss, and pleocytosis does not regularly occur in any other illness.

The World Health Organization (WHO) currently recommends that the laboratory diagnosis of poliomyelitis be confirmed by isolation and identification of poliovirus in the stool, with specific identification of wild-type and vaccine type strains. In suspected cases of acute flaccid paralysis, 2 stool specimens should be collected 24–48 hr apart, as soon as possible after the diagnosis of poliomyelitis is suspected. Poliovirus concentrations are high in the stool in the first week after the onset of paralysis, which is the optimal time for collection of stool specimens. Polioviruses may be isolated from 80 to 90% of acutely ill patients, whereas less than 20% may yield virus within 3–4 wk after onset of paralysis. Because most children with spinal or bulbospinal poliomyelitis have constipation, rectal straws may be used to obtain specimens; ideally a minimum of 8–10 grams should be collected. In laboratories that can isolate poliovirus, isolates should be sent to either the Centers for Disease Control and Prevention or to one of the WHO-certified poliomyelitis laboratories where DNA sequence analysis can be performed to distinguish between wild poliovirus and neurovirulent, revertant oral poliovirus vaccine strains. With the current WHO global plan for eradication of poliomyelitis worldwide, most regions of the world (the Americas, Europe, and Australia) have been certified wild-poliovirus free; in these areas, poliomyelitis is most often caused by vaccine strains. Hence it is critical to differentiate between wild type and revertant vaccine type strains.

The CSF, while often normal during the minor illness, demonstrates a pleocytosis between 20 and 300 cells/mm^3 with CNS involvement; the cells in the CSF may be polymorphonuclear early in the disease but shift to mononuclear cells soon afterward. By the second week of the major illness, the CSF cell count falls to near-normal values. In contrast, the CSF protein is normal or only slightly elevated at the outset of CNS disease but usually rises to between 50–100 mg/dL by the second week of illness. In polioencephalitis the CSF may remain normal or show minor changes. Serologic testing demonstrates seroconversion or a fourfold or greater increase in antibody titers, when measured during the acute phase of illness and 3–6 wk later.

DIFFERENTIAL DIAGNOSIS. Poliomyelitis should be considered in the differential diagnosis of any case of paralysis, and is only one of many causes of acute flaccid paralysis in children and adults. The possibility of polio should be considered in any case of acute flaccid paralysis even in countries where polio has been eradicated. The diagnoses most often confused with polio are the Guillain-Barré syndrome, transverse myelitis, and traumatic paralysis due to sciatic nerve injury. In Guillain-Barré syndrome, which is the most difficult to distinguish from poliomyelitis, the paralysis is characteristically symmetric and sensory changes and pyramidal tract signs are common; these are absent in poliomyelitis. Fever, headache, and meningeal signs are less notable, and there are few cells but an elevated protein level in the CSF. Transverse myelitis progresses rapidly over hours to days, causing an acute symmetric paralysis of the lower limbs with concomitant anesthesia and diminished sensory perception. Autonomic signs of hypothermia in the affected limbs are common, and there is bladder dysfunction. The CSF is usually normal. Traumatic neuritis occurs from a few hours to a few days after the traumatic event, is asymmetric, acute, and affects only one limb. There is reduced or absent muscle tone and deep tendon reflects in the affected limb with pain in the gluteus. The CSF is normal.

There are numerous other causes of acute flaccid paralysis (Table 228–1). In most conditions, the clinical features are sufficient to differentiate between these various causes, but in

TABLE 228–1. Differential Diagnosis of Acute Flaccid Paralysis

Site, Condition, Factor, or Agent	Clinical Findings	Onset of Paralysis	Progression of Paralysis	Sensory Signs and Symptoms	Reduced or Absent Deep Tendon Reflexes	Residual Paralysis	Pleocytosis
Anterior Horn Cells of Spinal Cord							
Poliomyelitis (Wild and VAPP)	Paralysis	Incubation period 7–14 days (4–35 days)	24–48 hr to onset of full paralysis; proximal > distal, asymmetric	No	Yes	Yes	Aseptic meningitis (moderate polymorphonuclear leukocytes at 2–3 days)
Nonpolio enterovirus	Hand-foot-and-mouth disease, aseptic meningitis, AHC	As in poliomyelitis	As in poliomyelitis	No	Yes	Yes	As in poliomyelitis
Other Neurotropic Viruses							
Rabies virus		Months to years	Acute, symmetric, ascending	Yes	Yes	No	+/–
Varicella-zoster virus	Exanthematous vesicular eruptions	Incubation period 10–21 days	Acute, symmetric, ascending	Yes	+/–	+/–	Yes
Japanese encephalitis virus		Incubation period 5–15 days	Acute, proximal, asymmetric	+/–	+/–	+/–	Yes
Guillain-Barré Syndrome							
Acute inflammatory polyradiculoneuropathy	Preceding infection, bilateral facial weakness	Hours to 10 days	Acute, symmetric, ascending (days to 4 wk)	Yes	Yes	+/–	No
Acute motor axonal neuropathy	Fulminant, widespread paralysis, bilateral facial weakness, tongue involvement	Hours to 10 days	1–6 days	No	Yes	+/–	No
Acute Traumatic Sciatic Neuritis							
Intramuscular gluteal injection	Acute, asymmetrical	Hours to 4 days	Complete, affected limb	Yes	Yes	+/–	No
Acute transverse myelitis	Preceding *Mycoplasma pneumoniae*, *Schistosoma*, other parasitic or viral infection	Acute, symmetric hypotonia of lower limbs	Hours to days	Yes	Yes, early	Yes	Yes
Epidural abscess	Headache, back pain, local spinal tenderness, meningismus	Complete		Yes	Yes	+/–	Yes
Spinal cord compression; trauma		Complete	Hours to days	Yes	Yes	+/–	+/–
Neuropathies							
Exotoxin of *Corynebacterium diphtheriae*	In severe cases, palatal paralysis, blurred vision	Incubation period 1–8 wk (paralysis 8–12 wk after onset of illness)		Yes	Yes		+/–
Toxin of *Clostridium botulinum*	Abdominal pain, diplopia, loss of accommodation, mydriasis	Incubation period 18–36 hr	Rapid, descending, symmetric	+/–	No		No
Tick bite paralysis	Ocular symptoms	Latency period 5–10 days	Acute, symmetric, ascending	No	Yes		No
Diseases of the Neuromuscular Junction							
Myasthenia gravis	Weakness, fatigability, diplopia, ptosis, dysarthria		Multifocal	No	No	No	No
Disorders of Muscle							
Polymyositis	Neoplasm, autoimmune disease	Subacute, proximal > distal	Weeks to months	No	Yes		No
Viral myositis		Pseudoparalysis	Hours to days	No	No		No
Metabolic Disorders							
Hypokalemic periodic paralysis		Proximal limb, respiratory muscles	Sudden postprandial	No	Yes	+/–	No
ICU Weakness							
Critical illness polyneuropathy	Flaccid limbs and respiratory weakness	Acute, following SIRS/sepsis	Hours to days	+/–	Yes	+/–	No

AHC = acute hemorrhagic conjunctivitis; ICU = intensive care unit; SIRS = systemic inflammatory response syndrome.
Modified from Marx A, Glass JD, Sutter RW: Differential diagnosis of acute flaccid paralysis and its role in poliomyelitis surveillance. Epidemiol Rev 2000;22:298–316.

some cases nerve conduction studies and electromyograms in addition to muscle biopsies may be required.

Conditions causing pseudoparalysis do not present with nuchal-spinal rigidity or pleocytosis. These causes include unrecognized trauma, transient (toxic) synovitis, acute osteomyelitis, acute rheumatic fever, scurvy, and congenital syphilis (pseudoparalysis of Parrot).

Treatment. Inasmuch as there are no specific antiviral agents for treating poliomyelitis, the management is supportive and aimed at limiting progression of disease, prevention of ensuing skeletal deformities, and preparation of the child and family for prolonged treatment required and for permanent disability if this seems likely. Patients with the nonparalytic and mildly paralytic forms of poliomyelitis may be treated at home. All intramuscular injections and surgical procedures are contraindicated during the acute phase of the illness, especially in the first week of illness, because these may result in progression of disease.

ABORTIVE POLIOMYELITIS. Supportive treatment with analgesics, sedatives, an attractive diet, and bed rest until the child's temperature is normal for several days is usually sufficient. Avoidance of exertion for the ensuing 2 wk is desirable, and there should be careful neurologic and musculoskeletal examinations 2 mo later to detect any minor involvement.

NONPARALYTIC POLIOMYELITIS. Treatment for the nonparalytic form is similar to that for the abortive form; in particular, relief is indicated for the discomfort of muscle tightness and spasm of the neck, trunk, and extremities. Analgesics are more effective when they are combined with the application of hot packs for 15–30 min every 2–4 hr. Hot tub baths are sometimes useful. A firm bed is desirable and can be improvised at home by placing table leaves or a sheet of plywood beneath the mattress. A footboard or splint should be used to keep the feet at a right angle to the legs. Because muscular discomfort and spasm may continue for some weeks, even in the nonparalytic form, hot packs and gentle physical therapy may be necessary. Such patients should also be carefully examined 2 mo after apparent recovery to detect minor residual effects that might cause postural problems in later years.

PARALYTIC POLIOMYELITIS. Most patients with the paralytic form require hospitalization, and complete physical rest in a calm atmosphere is desirable for the first 2–3 weeks. Suitable body alignment is necessary for comfort and to avoid excessive skeletal deformity. A neutral position with the feet at a right angle to the legs, knees slightly flexed, and hips and spine straight is achieved by use of boards, sandbags, and, occasionally, light splint shells. The position should be changed every 3–6 hr. Active and passive motions are indicated as soon as the pain has disappeared. Moist hot packs may relieve muscle pain and spasm. Opiates and sedatives are permissible only if no impairment of ventilation is present or impending. Constipation is common, and fecal impaction should be prevented. When bladder paralysis occurs, a parasympathetic stimulant such as bethanechol may induce voiding in 15–30 min; some patients do not respond, and others respond with nausea, vomiting, and palpitations. Bladder paresis rarely lasts more than a few days. If bethanechol fails, manual compression of the bladder and the psychologic effect of running water should be tried. If catheterization must be performed, care must be taken to prevent urinary tract infections. An appealing diet and a relatively high fluid intake should be started at once unless the patient is vomiting. Additional salt should be provided if the environmental temperature is high or if the application of hot packs induces sweating. Anorexia is common initially. Adequate dietary and fluid intake can be maintained by placement of a central venous catheter. An orthopedist and a physiatrist should see these patients as early in the course of the illness as possible and should assume responsibility for their care before fixed deformities develop.

The management of pure bulbar poliomyelitis consists of maintaining the airway and avoiding all risk of inhalation of saliva, food, or vomitus. Gravity drainage of accumulated secretions is favored by using the head-low (foot of bed elevated 20–25 degrees) prone position with the face to one side. Patients with weakness of the muscles of respiration or swallowing should be nursed in a lateral or semi-prone position. Aspirators with rigid or semirigid tips are preferred for direct oral and pharyngeal aspiration, and soft, flexible catheters may be used for nasopharyngeal aspiration. Fluid and electrolyte equilibrium is best maintained by intravenous infusion because tube or oral feeding in the first few days may incite vomiting. In addition to close observation for respiratory insufficiency, the blood pressure should be taken at least twice daily because hypertension is not uncommon and occasionally leads to hypertensive encephalopathy. Patients with pure bulbar poliomyelitis may require tracheostomy because of vocal cord paralysis or constriction of the hypopharynx; most patients who recover have little residual impairment, although some exhibit mild dysphagia and occasional vocal fatigue with slurring of speech.

Impaired ventilation must be recognized early; mounting anxiety, restlessness, and fatigue are early indications for preemptive intervention. Tracheostomy is indicated for some patients with pure bulbar poliomyelitis, spinal respiratory muscle paralysis, and bulbospinal paralysis because these patients are generally unable to cough, sometimes for many months. Mechanical respirators are often needed.

Complications. Paralytic poliomyelitis may be associated with numerous complications. Melena severe enough to require transfusion may result from single or multiple superficial intestinal erosions; perforation is rare. Acute gastric dilatation may occur abruptly during the acute or convalescent stage, causing further respiratory embarrassment; immediate gastric aspiration and external application of ice bags are indicated. Mild hypertension of a few days' or weeks' duration is common in the acute stage, probably related to lesions of the vasoregulatory centers in the medulla and especially to underventilation. In the later stages, because of immobilization, hypertension may occur along with hypercalcemia, nephrocalcinosis, and vascular lesions. Dimness of vision, headache, and a lightheaded feeling associated with hypertension should be regarded as premonitory of a frank convulsion. Cardiac irregularities are uncommon, but electrocardiographic abnormalities suggesting myocarditis are not rare. Acute pulmonary edema occurs occasionally, particularly in patients with arterial hypertension. Pulmonary embolism is uncommon despite the immobilization. Hypercalcemia occurs due to skeletal decalcification that begins soon after immobilization and results in hypercalciuria, which in turn predisposes the patient to urinary calculi, especially when urinary stasis and infection are present. A high fluid intake is the only effective prophylactic measure.

Prognosis. The outcome of inapparent, abortive poliomyelitis and aseptic meningitis syndromes is uniformly good, with death being exceedingly rare and with no long-term sequelae. The outcome of paralytic disease is determined primarily by degree and severity of CNS involvement. In severe bulbar poliomyelitis, the mortality may be as high as 60%, whereas in less severe bulbar involvement and/or spinal poliomyelitis, mortality varies from 5 to 10%, generally from causes other than the poliovirus infection.

Maximum paralysis usually occurs 2–3 days after the onset of the paralytic phase of the illness, with stabilization followed by gradual return of muscle function. The recovery phase lasts usually about 6 mo, beyond which persisting paralysis is permanent. Male children but female adults, generally, are more likely to develop paralysis. Mortality and the degree of disability are greater after the age of puberty. Pregnancy is associated with an increased risk of paralytic disease. Tonsillectomy and intramuscular injections may enhance the risk of acquisition of bulbar or localized disease, respectively. Increased physical activity, exercise, and fatigue during the early phase of illness have been cited as factors leading to an increased risk of paralytic disease. Finally it has been clearly demonstrated that type 1 poliovirus has the greatest propensity for natural poliomyelitis and type 3 for VAPP.

Postpolio Syndrome. After an interval of 30–40 years, as many as 30–40% of persons who survived paralytic poliomyelitis in childhood may experience muscle pain and exacerbation of existing weakness, or they may develop new weakness or paralysis. This entity, which is referred to as postpolio syndrome, has been reported only in persons who were infected in the era of wild poliovirus circulation. Risk factors for postpolio syndrome include increasing length of time since acute poliovirus infection, presence of permanent residual impairment after recovery from acute illness, and female sex.

Prevention. Vaccination is the only effective method of preventing poliomyelitis. Hygienic measures help limit the spread of the infection among young children, but immunization is necessary to control transmission among all age groups. Both the inactivated polio vaccine (IPV), which is currently produced using improved methods compared with the original vaccine and is sometimes referred to as enhanced IPV, and the live, attenuated, orally administered polio vaccine (OPV) have established efficacy in preventing poliovirus infection and paralytic poliomyelitis. Both vaccines induce production of antibodies against the three strains of poliovirus. IPV elicits higher serum IgG antibody titers, but OPV also induces significantly greater mucosal IgA immunity in the oropharynx and gastrointestinal tract that limits replication of the wild poliovirus at these sites. Transmission of wild poliovirus by fecal spread is limited in OPV recipients. The immunogenicity of IPV is not affected by the presence of maternal antibodies and IPV has no adverse effects. Live vaccine may undergo reversion to neurovirulence as it multiplies in the human intestinal tract and may cause VAPP in vaccinees or in their contacts. The overall risk for recipients is 1 case/6.2 million doses. As of January 2000, the IPV-only schedule is recommended for routine polio vaccination in the United States. All children should receive four doses of IPV at 2 mo, 4 mo, 6–18 mo, and 4–6 yr of age.

In 1988, the World Health Assembly resolved to eradicate poliomyelitis globally by 2000, and remarkable progress has been made toward reaching this target. To achieve this, the WHO used four basic strategies: routine immunization, National Immunization Days (NIDs), Acute Flaccid Paralysis surveillance, and mopping up immunization. The oral polio vaccine is the only vaccine recommended by WHO for eradication. By the end of 1999, at least one set of NIDs had been conducted in every polio endemic country in the world. This strategy has resulted in a greater than 99% decline in poliomyelitis cases; as of February 2002, there are only 10 countries in the world endemic for poliomyelitis. Globally there were 542 cases of polio, of which 478 were confirmed as wild virus. Given this rapid progress, planning has begun for the "end game" for the global polio eradication initiative. The main concerns are the containment of laboratory stocks of poliovirus (since the risk of inadvertent transmission of poliovirus from a laboratory to the community is possible) and the circulation of vaccine-derived polioviruses (VDPVs). As long as OPV is being used, there is the potential that circulating VDPVs will acquire the neurovirulent and transmission characteristics of the wild type polioviruses; indeed, this occurred in Egypt in 1993, Hispaniola during 2000 to 2001, and in the Philippines in 2001. Poor vaccination coverage appeared to be the major risk factor for circulating VDPVs. There is also concern that immune-deficient persons can act as long-term poliovirus carriers and pose a threat of reseeding the population. There are no long-term carriers identified yet in developing countries, and overall 12 have been identified worldwide who have excreted poliovirus for more than 6 mo, only 4 of whom are currently excreting virus. HIV has not been found to be a cause for long-term excretion of virus.

Currently there are 10 countries that are global priorities because they face challenges in eradication. The Indian subcontinent, Nigeria, Ethiopia, and the Democratic Republic of Congo are considered poliovirus reservoirs where transmission is particularly intense due to dense populations, low immunization coverage, and poor sanitation. The second major category is those afflicted by conflict where implementation of vaccination and surveillance activities is challenging (e.g., Afghanistan, Angola, Somalia, and Sudan). All these countries require multilevel eradication activities, but they pose a problem to surrounding countries because wild type poliovirus can be imported from these countries to countries where immunization rates have dropped (but have been declared poliomyelitis free) such as China and Bulgaria. Hence to achieve global eradication, intensified activities are being conducted in all the remaining identified countries. Once eradication has been achieved, which is conceivable in the near future, there are 3 possible strategies: (1) coordinated discontinuation of OPV use worldwide; (2) replacement of OPV with IPV; and (3) development of new live vaccines that would not cause VAPP and that are not transmittable. Obviously the first strategy would be the most desirable but the debate continues and the main concerns are that a VDPV circulation may continue, especially if other enteroviruses recombine with OPV. Because the whole genetic structure of poliovirus is known, it would be easy to genetically reconstruct poliovirus for use in bioterrorism. Until such time as this decision is reached, in countries where the risk for VAPP is higher than the risk of transmission of poliomyelitis, the injectable poliovirus vaccines continue to confer immunity and are being used routinely, and in other countries that either cannot afford IPV or where transmission is endemic, the OPV will continue to be used both in routine immunization as well as in the NIDs strategy.

American Academy of Pediatrics Committee on Infectious Diseases: Prevention of poliomyelitis: Recommendations for use of only inactivated poliovirus vaccine for routine immunization. *Pediatrics* 1999;104:1404–6.

Dalakas MC, Elder G, Hallett M, et al: A long-term follow-up study of patients with post-poliomyelitis neuromuscular symptom. *N Engl J Med* 1986;314:959–63.

Hull HF, Aylward RB: Progress towards global polio eradication. *Vaccine* 2001; 19:4378–84.

Marx A, Glass JD, Sutter RW: Differential diagnosis of acute flaccid paralysis and its role in poliomyelitis surveillance. *Epidemiol Rev* 2000;22:298–316.

Nomoto A, Arita I: Eradication of poliomyelitis. *Nature Immunol* 2002;3:205–8.

Sutter RW, Suleiman AJM, Malankar P, et al: Trial of a supplemental dose of four poliovirus vaccines. *N Engl J Med* 2000;343:767–73.

Technical Consultative Group to the World Health Organization on the Global Eradication of Poliomyelitis: "Endgame" Issues for the Global Polio Eradication Initiative. *Clin Infect Dis* 2002;34:72–7.

Wattigney WA, Mootrey GT, Braun MM, et al: Surveillance for poliovirus vaccine adverse events, 1991 to 1998: Impact of a sequential vaccination schedule of inactivated poliovirus vaccine followed by oral poliovirus vaccine. *Pediatrics* 2001;107:1–7.

World Health Organization: *Global Polio Eradication Initiative Strategic Plan 2001–2005.* World Health Organization, 2000.

Chapter 229
Nonpolio Enteroviruses*

Mark J. Abzug

The genus *Enterovirus* contains a large number of viral agents that produce a broad range of clinically important illnesses. The genus name reflects the importance of the gastrointestinal tract as the primary source for transmission and primary site of viral invasion and replication. However, viremic spread to distant sites accounts for the majority of clinical manifestations associated with the enteroviruses.

---

*Includes text from the Enteroviruses chapter written by Abraham Morag and Pearay L. Ogra from the 16th edition.

Etiology. Enteroviruses are non-enveloped, single-stranded, positive-sense viruses in the Picornaviridae family, so-named because they are small RNA-containing viruses. Other members of this family include the genus *Rhinovirus*, the genus *Hepatovirus* (hepatitis A virus), and genera containing related animal viruses. The original enterovirus subgroups—polioviruses (Chapter 228), coxsackieviruses, and echoviruses—were differentiated by their replication patterns in tissue culture and animals (Box 229–1). Coxsackieviruses derive their name from Coxsackie, New York, where they were discovered; echoviruses reflect an acronym applied to a group of viruses originally without disease associations (*e*—enteric, *c*—cytopathic, *h*—human, *o*—orphan *viruses*). Newer enteroviruses are classified by numbering. Serotypes (species) are distinguished by antigenic differences. Although more than 60 different serotypes have been identified, 11 account for the majority of disease. No enterovirus disease is uniquely associated with any specific serotype; however, certain manifestations are preferentially associated with specific serotypes.

Epidemiology. Enterovirus infections are very common and have a worldwide distribution. In temperate climates, they have a distinct seasonality, with an annual epidemic peak in summer and fall. Some transmission does occur year-round, however. Enteroviruses have been found to be responsible for 33–65% of acute febrile illnesses and 55–65% of hospitalizations for suspected sepsis in infants during the summer and fall in the United States, and 25% year-round. In tropical and semitropical areas, enteroviruses frequently circulate all year-round. In general, only a few serotypes circulate simultaneously. Infections by different serotypes in the same child can occur within the same season. Factors associated with increased incidence and/or severity of enterovirus infection include young age, male sex, poor hygiene, overcrowding, and low socioeconomic status; more than 25% of symptomatic enterovirus infections occur in children younger than 1 yr of age. Breast-feeding reduces the risk of infection in infants.

Humans are the only known reservoir for the human enteroviruses. Virus is spread person-to-person by the fecal-oral and respiratory routes and vertically, from mother to neonate, either prenatally or in the peripartum period. Enteroviruses can survive on environmental surfaces, permitting transmission via fomites. Enteroviruses also can frequently be isolated from sewage and can survive for months in wet soil, but person-to-person spread is the primary mode of transmission. Environmental contamination is likely the result of, rather than the cause for, human infection. Transmission occurs within families with young children (>50% spread to susceptible household contacts), daycare centers, playgrounds, summer camps, orphanages, and hospital nurseries; severe secondary infections may occur in nursery outbreaks. Diaper changing is a risk factor for spread, whereas handwashing decreases transmission.

Large outbreaks of enterovirus infections can occur. Outbreaks of hand-foot-and-mouth disease associated with severe central nervous system (CNS) and/or cardiopulmonary disease due to enterovirus 71 have occurred in recent years in Malaysia, Japan, Taiwan, and Australia; outbreaks of acute hemorrhagic conjunctivitis due to enterovirus 70 and coxsackievirus A24 have occurred in India and tropical regions; and community outbreaks of enterovirus meningitis have been reported. Modern molecular tools such as reverse transcription polymerase chain reaction (RT-PCR), restriction fragment length polymorphism (RFLP) analysis, single-strand conformation polymorphism (SSCP) analysis, and genomic sequencing have been used to rapidly identify outbreaks, demonstrate commonality of outbreak strains, and detect differences between epidemic strains and older prototype strains. Such analyses have demonstrated that enteroviruses undergo genetic drift that can lead to changes in antigenicity.

The incubation period of enterovirus infections is typically 3–6 days, except for acute hemorrhagic conjunctivitis, which has a shorter incubation period of 1–3 days. Infected children, both symptomatic and asymptomatic, frequently shed enteroviruses from the respiratory tract for less than 1–3 wk, whereas fecal shedding continues from several weeks up to 8 wk postinfection.

Pathogenesis. Following acquisition of virus by the oral or respiratory route, initial viral replication occurs in the pharynx and intestine, possibly within mucosal M cells. The absence of an envelope favors survival of enteroviruses in the harsh conditions of the gastrointestinal tract. Cell surface macromolecules, including poliovirus receptor (PVR), integrin VLA-2, decay accelerating factor complement regulatory protein (DAF/CD55), intercellular adhesion molecule-1 (ICAM-1), and coxsackievirus-adenovirus receptor, serve as receptors in the gastrointestinal tract for enteroviruses. Two or more enteroviruses may invade and replicate in the gastrointestinal tract at the same time, but replication of one type often interferes with growth of the heterologous type (interference).

After an enterovirus attaches to its cell surface receptor, a conformational change in surface capsid proteins facilitates penetration into the cell and release of viral RNA in the cytoplasm (uncoating). Translation of the positive-sense RNA ensues, resulting in synthesis of a polyprotein that undergoes sequential cleavage by proteinases encoded in the polyprotein. Several proteins produced then guide synthesis of negative-sense RNA that serves as a template for replication of new positive-sense RNA. The genome is approximately 7500 nucleotides long and includes a highly conserved 5′ non-coding region important for replication efficiency and a 3′ polyA region, also highly conserved, that flank a continuous region that encodes viral proteins. The 5′ end is covalently linked to a small viral protein (VPg) necessary for initiation of RNA synthesis. There is significant variation in the genomic regions encoding the structural proteins (with corresponding variability in antigenicity). Replication is followed by further cleavage of proteins and assembly of the genome and the viral capsid into 30-nm icosahedral virions. Of the 4 structural proteins in the viral capsid, VP1-VP4 (additional regulatory proteins such as an RNA-dependent RNA polymerase and proteases are also present in the virion), VP1 is the most important determinant of serotype specificity. Approximately 10^4–10^5 virions are released from an infected cell by lysis within 5–10 hr of infection.

The presumed pathogenesis of enterovirus infections beyond the gastrointestinal tract is largely based on studies of animal models. Initial replication in the pharynx and intestine is followed within days by multiplication in lymphoid tissue such as tonsils, Peyer patches, and regional lymph nodes. A primary, transient viremia (**minor viremia**) results in spread to more distant parts of the reticuloendothelial system including the liver, spleen, bone marrow, and distant lymph nodes. Host immune responses may limit replication and progression beyond the

---

BOX 229–1. Classification of Human Enteroviruses

Family: Picornaviridae
Genus: Enterovirus
Subgroups: Poliovirus serotypes 1–3
         Coxsackie A virus serotypes A1–A22, A24 (A23 reclassified as echovirus 9)
         Coxsackie B virus serotypes B1–B6
         Echovirus serotypes 1–9, 11–27, 29–33 (echoviruses 10 and 28 reclassified as non-enteroviruses; echovirus 34 reclassified as coxsackievirus A24; echoviruses 22 and 23 may be reclassified to a separate genus designated parenteroviruses)
         Numbered enterovirus serotypes 68–71 (enterovirus 72 reclassified as hepatitis A virus; a new serotype, enterovirus 73, has recently been proposed)

reticuloendothelial system, resulting in subclinical infection. Clinical infection occurs if replication proceeds in the reticuloendothelial system and virus spreads via a secondary, sustained viremia (**major viremia**) to target organs such as the CNS, heart, and skin. Tropism to target organs is determined in part by the infecting serotype.

Enteroviruses can damage a wide variety of organs and systems, including the CNS, heart, liver, lungs, pancreas, kidneys, muscle, and skin. Damage is mediated both by local necrosis and the host inflammatory response. Central nervous system infections are often associated with mononuclear pleocytosis of the cerebrospinal fluid (macrophages and activated T lymphocytes) and a mixed meningeal inflammatory response. Parenchymal involvement may occur at multiple sites, including cerebral white and gray matter, cerebellum, basal ganglia, brainstem, and spinal cord; perivascular and parenchymal mixed or lymphocytic inflammation, perivascular lymphocytic cuffing, gliosis, cellular degeneration, and neuronophagocytosis may be present. Encephalitis during recent outbreaks of enterovirus 71 has been characterized by severe brainstem and spinal cord involvement. Myocarditis is characterized by perivascular and interstitial mixed inflammatory infiltrates and myocyte damage. Chronic inflammation may persist after virus has been cleared.

Severe neonatal infections can manifest hepatic necrosis with variable inflammation; myocardial mixed inflammatory infiltrates, edema, and necrosis; meningeal and brain inflammation, hemorrhage, gliosis, and necrosis; pulmonary inflammation, hemorrhage, and thrombosis; pancreatic inflammation and necrosis; adrenal inflammation, hemorrhage, infarct, and necrosis; and disseminated intravascular coagulation.

Possible persistent infection by enteroviruses, especially coxsackie B viruses, has been implicated in dilated cardiomyopathy. Enteroviral RNA sequences and/or antigens have been demonstrated in a significant percentage of cardiac tissues in some series. Other studies, however, have failed to confirm a significant association. Persistent enterovirus infection has also been implicated in other conditions such as chronic fatigue syndrome and amyotrophic lateral sclerosis. An etiologic role in these syndromes awaits definitive proof.

Infection by coxsackie B viruses, coxsackie A viruses, and echoviruses has also been implicated in the pathogenesis of type I (insulin-dependent) diabetes mellitus. These viruses can induce β cell damage in mice, and reports of human infection in utero or in early childhood in temporal relation to development of clinical diabetes or laboratory evidence of a prediabetic state suggest a possible link. Other evidence includes detection of enteroviral RNA in diabetic or prediabetic children and demonstration of altered immune responses to enteroviruses in patients with diabetes. Finally, in rare cases, enteroviruses have been recovered from affected pancreases. Enteroviruses have also been suggested as contributors to other autoimmune diseases such as Graves disease.

Development of circulating type-specific neutralizing antibodies appears to be the most important aspect of the immune response mediating prevention against and recovery from enterovirus infections. IgM antibodies, followed by long-lasting IgA and IgG antibodies, are produced. Mucosal immunity, conferred mainly by secretory IgA, is also an important defense, conferring protection against intestinal re-infection. Although local re-infection of the gastrointestinal tract can occur, replication is usually limited and not associated with disease. Evidence also suggests that cellular defenses (especially macrophage function) play an important role in recovery from infection. Altered T-lymphocyte responses to enterovirus 71 were associated with severe meningoencephalitis during recent epidemics.

Antibody deficiency states, including hypogammaglobulinemia and agammaglobulinemia, predispose to severe, often chronic enterovirus infections. Similarly, perinatally infected neonates who lack maternal type-specific antibody to the infecting virus

are at risk for severe clinical disease. Other risk factors for significant enterovirus illness include young age, immune suppression (e.g., post-transplantation), and, according to animal model studies and/or epidemiologic observations, exercise, cold exposure, malnutrition, and pregnancy.

Clinical Manifestations. The clinical manifestations of enterovirus infections are protean, ranging from asymptomatic infection or undifferentiated febrile or respiratory illnesses in the majority, to, less frequently, severe diseases such as meningoencephalitis, myocarditis, and neonatal sepsis. Symptomatic disease is generally more frequent in young children.

ASYMPTOMATIC INFECTION. A large percentage of enterovirus infections are asymptomatic. A majority of individuals shedding virus are asymptomatic or had very mild illness, yet may serve as a significant source for spread of infection.

NONSPECIFIC FEBRILE ILLNESS. Nonspecific febrile illnesses are the most common symptomatic manifestations of enterovirus infections, and are especially frequent in infants and young children. In addition to being problematic for the symptoms they cause, they are difficult to clinically differentiate from serious infections such as bacteremia and bacterial meningitis and therefore prompt diagnostic testing, presumptive therapy, and hospitalizations for suspected bacterial infection in young infants.

Illness usually begins with abrupt onset of fever, usually 38.5–40°C (101–104°F), with accompanying malaise and irritability. Other symptoms may include lethargy, anorexia, diarrhea, nausea and vomiting, abdominal discomfort, rash, sore throat, and respiratory symptoms. In older children, headache and myalgia frequently also occur. Findings on examination are generally nonspecific and may include mild conjunctivitis, mild injection of the pharynx, and cervical lymphadenopathy. Meningitis may be present but, in infants, specific clinical features distinguishing those with and without meningitis are often lacking. Fever lasts a mean of 3 days. Occasionally fever is biphasic; it is present for 1 day, absent for 2–3 days, then recurs for an additional 2–4 days. Duration of illness is usually 4–7 days but can range from 1 day to longer than 1 wk. White blood cell count and other routine laboratory tests are generally normal. Concomitant enterovirus and bacterial infection has been observed in a small number of infants.

Enterovirus illnesses may be associated with a wide variety of skin manifestations. In general, the frequency is inversely related to age. Some serotypes commonly associated with rashes are echoviruses 9, 11, 16, and 25; coxsackie A viruses 2, 4, 9, and 16; and coxsackie B viruses 3–5. Rashes vary widely in their characteristics and include macular, maculopapular, urticarial, vesicular, and petechial eruptions. Virus can occasionally be recovered from vesicular skin lesions. Fever and rash illnesses caused by enteroviruses may mimic other infections such as meningococcemia, measles, and rubella.

HAND-FOOT-AND-MOUTH DISEASE. Hand-foot-and-mouth disease is one of the more distinctive rash syndromes caused by enteroviruses. It is most frequently caused by coxsackievirus A16, but can also be caused by enterovirus 71; coxsackie A viruses 5, 7, 9, and 10; and coxsackie B viruses 2 and 5. It is usually a mild illness, with or without low-grade fever. The oropharynx is inflamed and contains scattered vesicles on the tongue, buccal mucosa, posterior pharynx, palate, gingiva, and/or lips. These may ulcerate, leaving 4–8 mm shallow lesions with surrounding erythema. Maculopapular, vesicular, and/or pustular lesions may also occur on the hands and fingers, feet, and buttocks and groin; hands are more commonly involved than the feet. Lesions on the hands and feet are usually tender and vesicular and vary in size from 3–7 mm; they are generally more common on the dorsal surfaces but frequently occur on the palms and soles as well. Vesicles resolve in about 1 wk. Buttock lesions do not usually progress to vesiculation. Disseminated vesicular rashes may complicate preexisting eczema.

Hand-foot-and-mouth disease caused by enterovirus 71 is frequently more severe than that due to coxsackievirus A16, with high rates of associated neurologic disease including aseptic meningitis, encephalitis, and paralysis. Recent outbreaks in Malaysia, Japan, and Taiwan have been notable for brainstem encephalomyelitis, neurogenic pulmonary edema, pulmonary hemorrhage, shock, and rapid death, especially in young children.

HERPANGINA. Herpangina is characterized by a sudden onset of fever, sore throat, dysphagia, and characteristic lesions in the posterior pharynx. Initial temperatures can range from normal to 41°C (106°F); fever tends to be greater in younger patients. Headache and backache may occur in older children, and vomiting and abdominal pain occur in 25%. Oropharyngeal lesions may be present on the anterior tonsillar pillars, soft palate, uvula, tonsils, posterior pharyngeal wall, and, occasionally, the posterior buccal surfaces. Characteristic lesions are discrete 1–2 mm vesicles and ulcers that enlarge over 2–3 days to 3–4 mm and are surrounded by erythematous rings that vary in size up to 10 mm. An average of 5 lesions is usually present (range, 1 to >15). The remainder of the pharynx appears normal or minimally erythematous. Most cases of herpangina are mild and have no complications; however, some are associated with aseptic meningitis or other more severe illness. Fever generally lasts 1–4 days and resolution of symptoms occurs in 3–7 days. A variety of enteroviruses can cause herpangina, although coxsackie A viruses are implicated most often. Some cases of herpangina have been noted during recent outbreaks of enterovirus 71 disease.

RESPIRATORY MANIFESTATIONS. Respiratory symptoms such as sore throat and coryza frequently accompany enterovirus illnesses. In some cases, respiratory manifestations dominate the clinical presentation. Findings may include upper respiratory symptoms, wheezing, apnea, respiratory distress, pneumonia, otitis media, bronchiolitis, croup, parotitis, and pharyngotonsillitis. In the latter, pharyngeal erythema, occasionally with exudate, may be evident.

Pleurodynia (**Bornholm disease**) is an illness characterized by paroxysmal thoracic pain, due to myositis involving chest and abdominal wall muscles. Etiologic agents are most frequently coxsackieviruses B3 and B5, as well as coxsackieviruses B1 and B2 and echoviruses 1 and 6. Disease may be epidemic or sporadic. In epidemics, children and adults are affected, but most cases occur in persons younger than 30 yr of age. Prodromal symptoms such as malaise, myalgias, and headache are followed by sudden onset of fever and pain. Pain, typically located in the chest or upper abdomen, is spasmodic and can be excruciatingly severe. It is pleuritic and aggravated by coughing, sneezing, deep breathing, or other movement. Spasms last from a few minutes to several hours. During spasms, respirations are usually rapid, shallow, and grunting, suggesting pneumonia or pleural inflammation. A pleural friction rub may be noted during pain episodes, though chest radiographs are most often normal. Pain localized to the abdomen is frequently crampy, suggesting colic in the younger child. A pale, sweaty, shock-like appearance may suggest intestinal obstruction; tenderness and guarding may also suggest appendicitis and peritonitis. Illness usually lasts 3–6 days, but can last up to a couple of weeks. The illness is frequently biphasic. Rarely, patients have several recurrent episodes over a period of a few weeks, with less prominent fever during recurrences. Pleurodynia may occasionally be associated with meningitis, orchitis, myocarditis, or pericarditis.

ACUTE HEMORRHAGIC CONJUNCTIVITIS. Enterovirus 70 and coxsackievirus A24 are the primary causes of epidemics of acute hemorrhagic conjunctivitis that have occurred in both tropical regions and temperate climates, including the United States. Epidemics are explosive, spread mainly via eye-hand-fomite-eye transmission. Teenagers and adults 20–50 yr of age have the highest attack rates, with young children less often affected. Illness is characterized by sudden onset of severe eye pain associated with photophobia, blurred vision, lacrimation, conjunctival erythema and congestion, and lid edema. Subconjunctival hemorrhages of varying size occur in a fraction of patients, and superficial punctate keratitis is frequently present. Eye discharge is initially serous but becomes mucopurulent with secondary bacterial infection. Preauricular lymphadenopathy may be found. Systemic symptoms including fever are rare, although a picture suggestive of pharyngoconjunctival fever occasionally occurs. Recovery is usually complete within 1–2 weeks. A small number of patients have polyradiculoneuropathy or paralytic disease following enterovirus 70 acute hemorrhagic conjunctivitis.

MYOCARDITIS AND PERICARDITIS. Enteroviruses are among the most frequent pathogens implicated in myocarditis and pericarditis, accounting for approximately 25–35% of cases with proven cause. Coxsackie B viruses are the most common etiologic types; coxsackie A viruses and echoviruses also may be causative. Myocarditis has been observed in enterovirus 71 outbreaks associated with hand-foot-and-mouth disease and neurologic manifestations. Adolescents and young adults, especially males, are disproportionately affected by enterovirus myocarditis. Myopericarditis may be the dominant feature of illness or it may be part of more disseminated disease, as seen in neonates. Disease ranges from relatively mild to severe and fatal. Upper respiratory symptoms frequently precede cardiac manifestations such as fatigue, dyspnea, chest pain, congestive heart failure, and dysrhythmias. Presentations may mimic myocardial infarction; in other cases, patients present with sudden death. A pericardial friction rub indicates pericardial involvement. Chest radiograph often demonstrates cardiac enlargement. Electrocardiogram frequently reveals ST segment, T wave, and/or rhythm abnormalities, and echocardiogram may confirm cardiac dilatation, reduced contractility, and/or pericardial effusion. Myocardial enzymes may be elevated. The acute mortality of enterovirus myocarditis is 0–4%. Recovery is complete without residual disability in the majority of survivors. Occasionally, however, chronic cardiomyopathy or constrictive pericarditis may result. The role of possible persistent enterovirus infection in chronic dilated cardiomyopathy is controversial.

GASTROINTESTINAL MANIFESTATIONS. Gastrointestinal symptoms are frequent with enterovirus infections but are generally not dominant features. Symptoms may include emesis (especially with meningitis), diarrhea that is rarely severe, and abdominal pain. Diarrhea, hematochezia, pneumatosis intestinalis, and necrotizing enterocolitis have been observed in premature infants infected during nursery outbreaks. Enterovirus infection has been implicated as a cause of chronic intestinal inflammation in hypogammaglobulinemic patients.

NEUROLOGIC MANIFESTATIONS. Enteroviruses are the most common cause of viral meningitis in mumps-immunized populations; they account for over 90% of cases in which a causative agent is identified. Meningitis is particularly common in infants, especially among infants younger than 3 mo of age, and disease frequently occurs as part of community epidemics. Frequently implicated serotypes include coxsackieviruses B2–B5; echoviruses 4, 6, 7, 9, 11, 16, and 30; and enteroviruses 70 and 71. Most cases in infants and young children are mild and lack specific signs and symptoms. Fever is present in 75–100%; other findings may include irritability, malaise, headache, photophobia, nausea, emesis, anorexia, lethargy, rash, cough, rhinorrhea, pharyngitis, diarrhea, and myalgia. Nuchal rigidity is apparent in more than half of children older than 1–2 yr. Some cases are biphasic, with fever and nonspecific symptoms for a few days, followed by absence of symptoms for several days, then return of fever with meningeal signs. Fever usually resolves in 3–5 days, and other symptoms in infants and young children usually resolve within 1 wk. Symptoms tend to be more severe and longer lasting in adults. Cerebrospinal fluid findings include pleocytosis that generally is less than

500 WBC/mm^3 (occasionally as high as 1000–8000 WBC/mm^3) and often consists predominantly of polymorphonuclear cells in the first 48 hr before becoming mostly mononuclear; normal or slightly low glucose, with 10% below 40 mg/dL; and normal or mildly increased protein (generally <100 mg/dL). Cerebrospinal fluid occasionally has normal parameters despite positive viral culture or polymerase chain reaction. Complications of enterovirus meningitis occur in approximately 10% of young children; these include simple and complex seizures, obtundation, increased intracranial pressure, syndrome of inappropriate antidiuretic hormone secretion, and coma. The prognosis for most children with enterovirus meningitis is good. Although earlier studies suggested developmental, language, and cognitive sequelae in young infants, recent larger, prospective, comparative studies have generally not demonstrated long-term adverse outcomes.

Enteroviruses are also responsible for 10–20% of encephalitis with identified cause. Frequently implicated serotypes include echoviruses 3, 4, 6, 9, and 11; coxsackieviruses B2, B4, and B5; coxsackievirus A9, and enterovirus 71. After initial nonspecific symptoms, encephalitis becomes apparent by progression to marked confusion, weakness, lethargy, and/or irritability. Depression is usually generalized, although focal findings such as focal motor seizures, hemichorea, acute cerebellar ataxia, focal neurologic deficits, and/or focal imaging abnormalities may occasionally occur. Encephalitis includes a spectrum of disease from altered mental status to coma to decerebrate status; long-term neurologic sequelae may follow more severe disease.

Neurologic disorders have been prominent in recent epidemics of enterovirus 71 disease. The majority of affected children had hand-foot-and-mouth disease, some had herpangina, and others had no mucocutaneous manifestations. Neurologic syndromes observed included meningitis, meningoencephalomyelitis, poliomyelitis-like paralytic disease, Guillain-Barré syndrome, transverse myelitis, cerebellar ataxia, opsoclonus-myoclonus syndrome, benign intracranial hypertension, and brainstem encephalitis (rhombencephalitis involving the midbrain, pons, and medulla). The latter is characterized by myoclonus, vomiting, ataxia, nystagmus, tremor, and cranial nerve abnormalities. Although findings were mild and reversible in some, in others rapid progression to neurogenic pulmonary edema and hemorrhage, shock, and coma developed. High mortality rates have been reported, especially in children younger than 5 yr of age. Neurologic deficits have been observed among surviving children.

Patients with antibody deficiencies are at risk for chronic meningoencephalitis characterized by persistent cerebrospinal fluid (CSF) abnormalities, viral detection by culture or polymerase chain reaction for years, and recurrent encephalitis and/or progressive neurologic deterioration. Clinical findings include altered mental status, seizures, motor weakness, and increased intracranial pressure. Although the disease may wax and wane, deficits generally become progressive, and ultimately may be fatal. A dermatomyositis-like syndrome and hepatitis may supervene in advanced stages. Fortunately, chronic enterovirus meningoencephalitis has become less common in hypogammaglobulinemic patients receiving routine antibody replacement with intravenous immunoglobulin.

Nonpolio enteroviruses, especially enteroviruses 70 and 71, coxsackievirus A7, and coxsackie B viruses, can cause poliomyelitis-like paralytic disease with acute motor weakness due to anterior horn cell involvement. Disease tends to be milder than that caused by poliovirus, with less bulbar involvement and less persistent weakness.

Other neurologic syndromes observed with enterovirus infections include cerebellar ataxia, transverse myelitis, Guillain-Barré syndrome, and peripheral neuritis.

MYOSITIS AND ARTHRITIS. Although myalgia is a common complaint accompanying enterovirus illness, direct evidence of muscle involvement has only occasionally been reported.

Several enterovirus types have been associated with focal myositis and polymyositis. A dermatomyositis-like syndrome can be seen in enterovirus-infected hypogammaglobulinemic patients. Enteroviruses have rarely been demonstrated to cause arthritis.

PANCREATITIS AND ORCHITIS. A variety of coxsackie B virus and echovirus serotypes have been reported to cause pancreatitis. Coxsackie B viruses are second only to mumps as causative agents of orchitis. The illness is frequently biphasic; fever and pleurodynia or meningitis are followed by apparent recovery and then, in about 2 weeks, by orchitis, often with epididymitis.

NEONATAL INFECTIONS. Enterovirus infections in neonates are relatively common, with an incidence of clinical disease comparable to or greater than that of symptomatic neonatal infections due to herpes simplex virus, cytomegalovirus, and group B *Streptococcus*. Infection frequently is with coxsackieviruses B2–B5 and echoviruses 6, 9, 11, and 19, although many enterovirus serotypes have been implicated. Enteroviruses may be acquired vertically before, during, or after delivery; they also may be acquired horizontally from other infected family members or by transmission in hospital nurseries (sporadic or epidemic). Infection in utero may be associated with placentitis, fetal demise, neonatal illness, and, possibly, congenital anomalies. Neonatal infection is associated with a range of clinical manifestations, from asymptomatic (the majority) to benign febrile illness to severe multisystem disease. Most affected newborns are full-term and previously well; maternal history often reveals a recent viral illness, including fever and, frequently, abdominal pain. Symptoms in the neonate may occur throughout the newborn period, with some beginning as early as day 1 of life; severe disease generally has an onset within the first 2 wk of life. Frequent findings include fever or hypothermia, irritability, lethargy, anorexia, rash (usually maculopapular, occasionally petechial or papulovesicular), jaundice, respiratory symptoms, apnea, hepatomegaly, abdominal distention, emesis, diarrhea, and decreased perfusion. Most symptomatic neonates have benign courses, with resolution of fever in an average of 3 days and of other symptoms in about 1 wk. Occasionally, a biphasic course may occur. A minority has severe disease that may be dominated by any combination of sepsis, meningoencephalitis, myocarditis, hepatitis, coagulopathy, and pneumonitis. Meningoencephalitis may be indicated by focal or complex seizures, bulging fontanelle, nuchal rigidity, or reduced level of consciousness. Myocarditis, most often associated with coxsackie B virus infection, may be suggested by tachycardia, dyspnea, cyanosis, and cardiomegaly. Hepatitis is more associated with echovirus infection, although it may occur with coxsackie B viruses; pneumonitis is also more frequently seen with echovirus infection. Laboratory evaluation may reveal leukocytosis, thrombocytopenia, pleocytosis, elevated transaminases and bilirubin, coagulopathy, pulmonary infiltrates, and electrocardiographic changes. Complications include CNS necrosis and generalized or focal neurologic compromise; arrhythmias, congestive heart failure, myocardial infarction, and pericarditis; hepatic necrosis and failure; intracranial or other bleeding; adrenal necrosis and hemorrhage; and rapidly progressive pneumonitis. Myositis, necrotizing enterocolitis, inappropriate antidiuretic hormone secretion, hemophagocytic syndrome, and sudden death are rare events. Mortality in those with severe disease is significant and is most often associated with hepatitis and associated bleeding complications, myocarditis, or pneumonitis. The majority of surviving infants have gradual resolution of hepatic and cardiac dysfunction, although chronic calcific myocarditis can occur. CNS infection, especially if clinical signs of encephalitis are present, may be associated with morbidity such as speech and language impairment; cognitive deficits; spasticity, hypotonicity, or weakness; seizure disorders; microcephaly or hydrocephaly; and ocular abnormalities. However, most survivors appear not to have long-term sequelae. Risk factors for severe disease include illness onset in the first few days of life, maternal illness just prior to or at delivery, prematurity, male sex, infection by echovirus 11 or a coxsackie B virus, positive serum viral culture, absence of neutralizing antibody to the infecting virus, and evidence of severe hepatitis and/or multisystem disease.

BONE MARROW TRANSPLANT RECIPIENTS. In recent years, a variety of severe and/or prolonged enterovirus infections have been reported in bone marrow and stem cell transplant recipients. Cases include progressive pneumonia, severe diarrhea, pericarditis and heart failure, and disseminated disease. High fatality rates have been reported.

Diagnosis. Enterovirus infection can often be suspected on clinical grounds, especially when relatively specific clinical findings such as hand-foot-and-mouth disease or herpangina lesions are present. Additional clues include consistent seasonality, known community outbreak, and exposure to enterovirus-compatible disease. In the neonate, history of maternal fever, malaise, and/or abdominal pain near delivery during enterovirus season is suggestive.

Viral culture using a combination of cell lines that support the growth of enteroviruses is the gold standard method for confirmation of infection. Sensitivity of culture is in the range of 50–75%. Sensitivity is increased by culturing multiple sites. For example, in children with meningitis, culture yield is enhanced by culturing CSF plus additional sites such as throat and rectum. In neonates, significant yields (30–70%) have been observed when blood, urine, and CSF are cultured in addition to mucosal swabs. A major limitation of culture is the inability of most coxsackie A viruses to grow in culture. Coxsackie A viruses are more readily identified by their pathologic effects in suckling mice, a technique generally available only in research laboratories. Culture yield may also be limited by the presence of neutralizing antibody in patient specimens, improper specimen handling, or insensitivity of the cell lines used. Additionally, culture is relatively slow, with 3–8 days usually required to detect growth. Antigen detection has been coupled with culture to shorten the time required for viral detection, but sensitivity has been a limiting factor. In general, cultivation of an enterovirus from any site can be considered evidence of recent infection; however, isolation from the rectum or stool can also reflect shedding from a more remote infection. Similarly, recovery from a mucosal site may suggest an association with an illness, whereas recovery from a normally sterile site such as CSF, blood, or tissue is more conclusive evidence of causation. Serotype identification can be performed in reference laboratories by testing with neutralizing antisera. This is generally only required for investigation of an outbreak or an unusual disease manifestation or to distinguish nonpolio enteroviruses from polioviruses (vaccine type or wild type).

Direct testing of patient specimens for enterovirus antigen or nucleic acid has been pursued to overcome the limitations of culture, that is, imperfect sensitivity and delayed results. Antigen detection, such as by enzyme-linked immunosorbent assay, has had some success, but sensitivity is limited by the lack of surface antigens shared by the majority of enteroviruses. Greater success has been achieved by applying reverse transcription polymerase chain reaction (PCR) to detection of highly conserved areas of the 5′ non-coding region of the enterovirus genome. This approach, which detects the majority of enteroviruses (but frequently not echoviruses 22 and 23), has been applied to a variety of specimens, including CSF, serum, urine, and conjunctival, nasopharyngeal, throat, and rectal specimens. Sensitivity and specificity are high, and testing can be accomplished in periods as short as five hours. PCR testing of CSF from children with acute aseptic meningitis and from hypogammaglobulinemic patients with chronic enterovirus meningoencephalitis are frequently positive despite negative cultures. In ill neonates, PCR testing of serum and urine specimens is associated with higher yields than culture of these fluids. Routine application of PCR to testing of CSF from infants and young children with meningitis has been demonstrated to decrease diagnostic testing, duration of hospital stay, antibiotic use, and overall costs.

Enterovirus infections can be detected serologically, either by demonstration of a rise in neutralizing, complement fixation, or other type-specific antibody or by detection of serotype-specific IgM antibody. However, serologic testing requires presumptive knowledge of the infecting serotype, either by isolation of a virus from the patient or a contact or by association with a community epidemic of a known serotype. Sensitivity may also be limited. In general, except for epidemiologic studies, serology is less useful than is viral culture or nucleic acid detection.

Enterovirus infection may be diagnosed by detection of virus in tissue specimens, such as biopsies of myocardium, liver, or brain. Detection methods include culture, nucleic acid detection by PCR or in situ hybridization, and antigen detection by immunofluorescence.

Differential Diagnosis. The differential diagnosis of enterovirus infections varies with the clinical presentation (Table 229–1).

Treatment. Newborns, infants, and children presenting with nonspecific febrile illnesses or meningitis due to enterovirus infections frequently require diagnostic evaluations for bacterial and herpes simplex virus infection. Hospitalization is often indicated for presumptive treatment of these causes until tests rule out these diagnoses. Neonates with severe disease, infants, and children with myocarditis and patients with concerning neurologic diseases may require intensive supportive care, including cardio-respiratory support and blood product administration.

Immune globulin has been used as a potential therapy for enterovirus infections for several reasons. The humoral immune response to enteroviruses is a key defense against infection, and

TABLE 229–1. Differential Diagnosis of Enterovirus Infections

Clinical Manifestation	Bacterial Pathogens	Viral Pathogens
Nonspecific febrile illness	*Streptococcus pneumoniae, Haemophilus influenzae* type b, *Neisseria meningitidis*	Influenza viruses, human herpesviruses 6 and 7
Exanthems/enanthems	Group A streptococcus, *Staphylococcus aureus, Neisseria meningitidis*	Herpes simplex virus, adenoviruses, varicella-zoster virus, Epstein-Barr virus, measles virus, rubella virus, human herpesviruses 6 and 7
Respiratory illness/conjunctivitis	*Streptococcus pneumoniae, Haemophilus influenzae* type b, *Neisseria meningitidis, Mycoplasma pneumoniae, Chlamydia pneumoniae*	Adenoviruses, influenza viruses, respiratory syncytial virus, parainfluenza viruses, rhinovirus
Myocarditis/pericarditis	*Staphylococcus aureus, Haemophilus influenzae* type b, *Mycoplasma pneumoniae*	Adenoviruses, influenza virus, other viruses
Meningitis/encephalitis	*Streptococcus pneumoniae, Haemophilus influenzae* type b, *Neisseria meningitidis, Mycobacterium tuberculosis, Borrelia burgdorferi, Mycoplasma pneumoniae, Bartonella henselae, Listeria monocytogenes*	Herpes simplex virus, influenza viruses, adenovirus, Epstein-Barr virus, mumps virus, lymphocytic choriomeningitis virus, arboviruses
Neonatal infections	Group B streptococcus, gram-negative enteric bacilli, *Listeria monocytogenes, Enterococcus*	Herpes simplex virus, adenoviruses, cytomegalovirus, rubella virus

lack of neutralizing antibody is a risk factor for symptomatic infection. Immune globulin products contain neutralizing antibodies to many of the commonly circulating serotypes, although titers vary with serotype and among products. Routine use of maintenance intravenous immune globulin for hypogammaglobulinemic patients has been associated with a decrease in chronic enterovirus disease. Therefore, anecdotal, uncontrolled use of intravenous immune globulin to treat newborns with severe disease has been reported. The one reported randomized, controlled trial was too small to demonstrate significant clinical benefits, although neonates who received immune globulin containing a high neutralizing titer to their own isolates had shorter periods of viremia and viruria. Infusion of maternal convalescent plasma has also been anecdotally reported. Intravenous and intraventricular immune globulin have been used to treat hypogammaglobulinemic patients with chronic enterovirus meningoencephalitis, with variable success. A retrospective study suggested treatment of myocarditis with immune globulin was associated with improved outcome; virologic diagnoses were not made in this study. Evaluation of corticosteroids and other immunosuppressive therapy for myocarditis has been inconclusive.

Specific antiviral therapy for enterovirus infections is being developed. Agents that act at several key steps in the enterovirus life cycle, including attachment, uncoating, protease activity, and replication, are being evaluated. The investigational agent that has advanced furthest, pleconaril, fits within a pocket beneath the floor of a canyon at the junctions of VP1 and VP3 on the viral capsid and inhibits viral attachment and uncoating. Its use was associated with modest acceleration of symptom resolution in some clinical trials involving children and adults with enterovirus meningitis and slightly faster clinical resolution of upper respiratory tract infections caused by picornaviruses (enteroviruses or rhinoviruses). Other conditions in which this generally well tolerated, oral medication is being evaluated include severe neonatal enterovirus infection, myocarditis, encephalitis, paralytic disease, and infections in immunodeficient patients. Uncontrolled experience suggests possible treatment benefits in these high-risk conditions.

Complications. Complications of enterovirus infections are primarily those associated with the clinical manifestations of myocarditis and encephalitis, and also severe neonatal infections following peripartum transmission.

Prognosis. The prognosis in the vast majority of enterovirus infections is excellent. Morbidity and mortality are primarily related to myocarditis, neurologic syndromes, severe neonatal disease, and infections in immune compromised hosts. Specific comments are included with the descriptions of these clinical manifestations.

Prevention. Vaccines for enteroviruses (other than polioviruses) are not available. The first line of defense against transmission of enteroviruses is basic hygiene such as handwashing to prevent fecal-oral and respiratory spread within families, preschools, and schools. Infection control techniques such as cohorting have proven effective in limiting nursery outbreaks. Prophylactic administration of intramuscular or intravenous immunoglobulin or convalescent plasma has been used in some nursery epidemics to prevent infection or ameliorate symptomatic disease. Simultaneous infection control interventions make it difficult to determine the efficacy of these approaches.

Pregnant women near term should avoid contact with individuals ill with probable enterovirus infections. If a pregnant woman develops an illness considered likely to be caused by an enterovirus, it is advisable not to proceed with emergent delivery unless there is concern for fetal compromise or that obstetric emergencies cannot be excluded. Rather, it may be advantageous to extend pregnancy, allowing the fetus time to passively

acquire protective antibodies. A strategy of prophylactically administering immune globulin to neonates born to mothers with enterovirus infections near delivery is untested.

Maintenance antibody replacement with intravenous immune globulin for patients with hypogammaglobulinemia has reduced the incidence of chronic enterovirus meningoencephalitis among these patients.

Abzug MJ: Prognosis for neonates with enterovirus hepatitis and coagulopathy. *Pediatr Infect Dis J* 2001;20:758–763.
Abzug MJ, Rotbart HA: Enterovirus infections of neonates and infants. *Semin Pediatr Infect Dis* 1999;10:169–176.
Byington CL, Taggart EW, Carroll KC, Hillyard DR: A polymerase chain reaction-based epidemiologic investigation of the incidence of nonpolio enteroviral infections in febrile and afebrile infants 90 days and younger. *Pediatrics* 1999;103:e27.
Ho M, Chen E, Hsu K, et al: An epidemic of enterovirus 71 infection in Taiwan. *N Engl J Med* 1999;341:929–935.
Huang C, Liu C, Chang Y, et al: Neurologic complications in children with enterovirus 71 infection. *N Engl J Med* 1999;341:936–942.
Ramers C, Billman G, Hartin M, et al: Impact of a diagnostic cerebrospinal fluid enterovirus polymerase chain reaction test on patient management. *JAMA* 2000;283:2680–2685.
Rotbart HA: Antiviral therapy for enteroviral infections. *Pediatr Infect Dis J* 1999;18:632–633.
Rotbart HA, McCracken GH Jr, Whitley J, et al: Clinical significance of enteroviruses in serious summer febrile illnesses of children. *Pediatr Infect Dis J* 1999;18:869–874.
Rotbart HA, Webster AD: Treatment of potentially life-threatening enterovirus infections with pleconaril. *Clin Infect Dis* 2001;32:228–235.
Sawyer MH: Enterovirus infections: Diagnosis and treatment. *Pediatr Infect Dis J* 1999;18:1033–1040.

Chapter 230
Parvovirus B19 *William C. Koch*

The frequency of B19 infection in the general pediatric population was not fully appreciated until 1983, when Anderson and colleagues identified B19 as the cause of **erythema infectiosum** or **fifth disease**, which is a classic, well-recognized childhood exanthem.

Etiology. Parvovirus B19 (B19) is a member of the genus *Erythrovirus* in the family Parvoviridae. Parvoviruses are small DNA viruses that infect a variety of animal species. As a group, the parvoviruses include a number of important animal pathogens including canine parvovirus and feline panleukopenia virus. Discovered in 1975, B19 is the only parvovirus that is pathogenic in humans. It does not infect other animals, and animal parvoviruses do not infect humans.

B19 is composed of an icosahedral protein capsid without an envelope that contains single-stranded DNA approximately 5.5 kb in length. It is relatively heat- and solvent-resistant. It is antigenically distinct from other mammalian parvoviruses, and there is only one known serotype. Parvoviruses replicate in mitotically-active cells. Because of their limited genome, they require host cell factors present in late S phase to replicate. B19 can be propagated only in erythropoietin-stimulated erythropoietic cells derived from human bone marrow, umbilical cord blood, or primary fetal liver culture.

Epidemiology. Infections with parvovirus B19 are common and worldwide. Clinically apparent infections, such as rash illness and transient aplastic crisis, are most prevalent in school-aged children, with 70% of cases occurring between 5 and 15 yr of age. Seasonal peaks occur in the late winter and spring; sporadic infections occur throughout the year. Seroprevalence increases with age; 40–60% of adults have evidence of prior infection.

Transmission of B19 is by the respiratory route, presumably via large droplet spread from nasopharyngeal viral shedding. The transmission rate in households ranges from 15 to 30% in susceptible contacts; mothers are more commonly infected than fathers. In outbreaks of erythema infectiosum in elementary schools, the secondary attack rates range from 10–60%. Nosocomial outbreaks are described, with secondary attack rates of 30% in susceptible health care workers.

Although respiratory spread is the primary mode of transmission, B19 is transmissible in blood and blood products, which has been documented among children with hemophilia receiving pooled donor clotting factor. Given the resistance of the virus to solvents, fomite transmission could be important in childcare and other group settings, but this mode of transmission has not been documented.

Pathogenesis. The primary target of B19 infection is the erythroid cell line, specifically erythroid precursors near the pronormoblast stage. Viral infection produces lysis of these cells, leading to a progressive depletion and a transient arrest of erythropoiesis. The virus has no apparent effect on the myeloid cell line. The tropism for erythroid cells is related to the erythrocyte P blood group antigen, which serves as a cellular receptor for the virus. Endothelial cells, placenta, and fetal myocardial cells also possess this antigen. Thrombocytopenia and neutropenia are often observed clinically, but their pathogenesis is unexplained.

Experimental infection of normal volunteers revealed a biphasic illness. From 7 to 11 days after inoculation, the subjects had viremia and nasopharyngeal viral shedding and experienced fever, malaise, and rhinorrhea. Their reticulocyte counts dropped to undetectable levels but resulted only in a mild, clinically insignificant fall in serum hemoglobin. Symptoms resolved and hemoglobin returned to normal with the appearance of specific antibodies. Several subjects experienced a rash associated with arthralgia 17–18 days after inoculation. Some manifestations of B19 infection, such as transient aplastic crisis, appear to be a direct result of viral infection, whereas others, including the exanthem and arthritis, appear to be postinfectious phenomena related to the immune response. Skin biopsy results from patients with erythema infectiosum are compatible with an immune process, showing edema in the epidermis and a perivascular mononuclear infiltrate.

Individuals with chronic hemolytic anemia and increased red cell turnover are very susceptible to perturbations in erythropoiesis. Infection with B19 leads to a transient arrest in red cell production and a precipitous fall in serum hemoglobin, often requiring transfusion. The reticulocyte count falls to near zero, reflecting the lysis of infected erythroid precursors. Humoral immunity is crucial in controlling infection. Specific immunoglobulin M (IgM) appears within 1–2 days followed by anti-B19 IgG, leading to control of the infection, restoration of reticulocytosis, and a rise in serum hemoglobin.

Individuals with impaired humoral immunity are at increased risk for more serious or persistent infection with B19, which usually manifests as chronic red cell aplasia, but neutropenia, thrombocytopenia, and marrow failure are also described. Children on chemotherapy for leukemia, those with congenital immunodeficiency states, transplant patients, and those with AIDS are at risk for chronic B19 infections.

Infections in the fetus and neonate are somewhat analogous to infections in the immunocompromised host. B19 is associated with nonimmune fetal hydrops and stillbirth in women experiencing a primary infection but does not appear to be teratogenic. Like most mammalian parvoviruses, B19 can cross the placenta and cause fetal infection during primary maternal infection. Parvovirus cytopathic effects are seen primarily in erythroblasts of the bone marrow and sites of extramedullary hematopoiesis in the liver and spleen. Fetal infection can presumably occur as early as 6 wk of gestation, when erythroblasts are first found in the fetal liver; after the 4th gestational month hematopoiesis switches to the bone marrow. In some cases, fetal infection leads to a profound fetal anemia and subsequent high-output cardiac

failure (Chapter 92). Fetal hydrops ensues, often associated with fetal mortality. There may also be a direct effect of the virus on myocardial tissue that contributes to the cardiac failure. However, most infections during pregnancy result in normal deliveries at term. Some of these asymptomatic infants have been reported to have chronic postnatal infection with B19 that is of unknown significance.

Clinical Manifestations. Many infections are clinically inapparent. Children characteristically develop erythema infectiosum. Adults, especially women, frequently develop acute arthropathy with or without the rash of erythema infectiosum.

ERYTHEMA INFECTIOSUM (FIFTH DISEASE). The most common manifestation of parvovirus B19 is erythema infectiosum, also known as fifth disease, which is a benign, self-limited exanthematous illness of childhood. It was the fifth in a classification scheme of childhood exanthems. The preceding four exanthems were measles, scarlet fever, rubella and Filatov-Dukes disease (an atypical scarlet fever), with roseola infantum as the "sixth disease."

The incubation period for erythema infectiosum ranges from 4 to 28 days (average, 16–17 days). The prodromal phase is mild and consists of low-grade fever, headache, and symptoms of mild upper respiratory tract infection. The hallmark of erythema infectiosum is the characteristic rash, which occurs in three stages that are not always distinguishable. The initial stage is an erythematous facial flushing, often described as a "slapped-cheek" appearance. The rash spreads rapidly or concurrently to the trunk and proximal extremities as a diffuse macular erythema in the second stage. Central clearing of macular lesions occurs promptly, giving the rash a lacy, reticulated appearance. Palms and soles are spared, and the rash tends to be more prominent on extensor surfaces. Affected children are afebrile and not ill-appearing. Older children and adults often complain of mild pruritus. The rash resolves spontaneously without desquamation but tends to wax and wane over 1–3 wk. It can recur with exposure to sunlight, heat, exercise, and stress. Lymphadenopathy and atypical papular, purpuric, vesicular rashes are also described.

ARTHROPATHY. Arthritis and arthralgia occur as a complication of fifth disease or as the only clinical manifestation of B19 infection. Joint symptoms are much more common in adults and older adolescents. Females are affected more frequently than males. In one outbreak of fifth disease, 60% of adults and 80% of adult women reported joint symptoms. Joint symptoms range from diffuse arthralgias with morning stiffness to frank arthritis. The joints most often affected are the hands, wrists, knees, and ankles, but practically all have been reported. The joint symptoms are self-limited and, in the majority of patients, resolve within 2–4 wk. Some patients may have a prolonged course of many months, suggesting rheumatoid arthritis. Transient rheumatoid factor positivity is reported in some of these patients but with no joint destruction.

TRANSIENT APLASTIC CRISIS. The incubation period for transient aplastic crisis is shorter than for erythema infectiosum because it occurs coincident with the viremia. The transient arrest of erythropoiesis and absolute reticulocytopenia induced by B19 infection leads to a sudden fall in serum hemoglobin in individuals with chronic hemolytic conditions. B19-induced aplastic crises occur in patients with all types of chronic hemolysis, including sickle cell disease, thalassemia, hereditary spherocytosis, and pyruvate kinase deficiency. In contrast to children with erythema infectiosum, these patients are ill with fever, malaise, and lethargy and have signs and symptoms of profound anemia, such as pallor, tachycardia, and tachypnea. Rash is rarely present. Children with sickle cell hemoglobinopathies may also have a concurrent vaso-occlusive pain crisis.

IMMUNOCOMPROMISED PERSONS. Patients with impaired humoral immunity are at risk for chronic infections with parvovirus B19. Chronic anemia is the most common manifestation, sometimes accompanied by neutropenia, thrombocytopenia, or complete marrow suppression. Chronic infections are seen in children with cancer receiving cytotoxic chemotherapy, children with congenital immunodeficiencies, patients on immunosuppressive therapy for transplants, children (and adults) with AIDS, and patients with functional defects in IgG production who are unable to generate neutralizing antibodies.

FETAL INFECTION. Primary maternal infection is associated with nonimmune fetal hydrops and intrauterine fetal demise; the risk of fetal loss after infection is estimated at <5%. The mechanism of fetal disease appears to be a viral-induced red cell aplasia at a time when the fetal erythroid fraction is rapidly expanding. This can lead to profound anemia, high-output cardiac failure, and hydrops. Viral DNA has been detected in infected abortuses. The second trimester seems to be the most sensitive period, but fetal losses are reported at every stage of gestation. Most infants infected in utero are born normally at term, even some with ultrasonographic evidence of hydrops. Some of these infants may acquire a chronic or persistent postnatal infection with B19, but its significance is unknown. Congenital anemia associated with intrauterine B19 infection has been reported in a few cases, sometimes following intrauterine hydrops. This process may mimic other forms of congenital hypoplastic anemia (i.e., Diamond-Blackfan syndrome). Fetal infection with B19 has not been associated with other birth defects. B19 is only one of many causes of hydrops fetalis (Chapter 92).

MYOCARDITIS. B19 infection has been associated with cases of myocarditis in fetuses, infants, children and a few adults. Diagnosis has often been based on serology suggestive of a concurrent B19 infection but in many cases B19 DNA has been demonstrated in cardiac tissue. This is plausible because fetal myocardial cells are known to express the receptor for the virus (P antigen). In the few cases where histology is reported, a predominantly lymphocytic infiltrate is described. Outcomes have varied from complete recovery to chronic cardiomyopathy to fatal cardiac arrest. Although B19-associated myocarditis appears to be a rare occurrence, there appears to be enough evidence to consider B19 as a potential cause of lymphocytic myocarditis, especially in infants.

OTHER CUTANEOUS MANIFESTATIONS. A variety of atypical skin eruptions have been reported in association with B19 infection. Most of these are petechial or purpuric in nature, often with evidence of vasculitis on those on which biopsies have been performed. Among these, the **papular-purpuric "gloves and socks" syndrome (PPGSS)** appears well established in the dermatologic literature as distinctly associated with B19 infection. PPGSS is characterized by fever, pruritus, and painful edema and erythema localized to the distal extremities in a distinct glove and sock distribution, followed by acral petechiae and oral lesions. The syndrome is self-limited and resolves within a few weeks. Initially described in young adults, a number of reports in children have since been published. In those linked to B19 infection, the eruption is accompanied by serologic evidence of acute infection.

Diagnosis. The diagnosis of erythema infectiosum is usually based on clinical presentation of the typical rash. Similarly, the diagnosis of a typical transient aplastic crisis in a child with sickle cell disease rarely requires virologic confirmation.

Serologic tests for the diagnosis of B19 infection are available. B19-specific IgM develops rapidly after infection and persists for 6–8 wk. Anti-B19 IgG serves as a marker of past infection or immunity. Determination of anti-B19 IgM is the best marker of recent/acute infection on a single serum sample; seroconversion of anti-B19 IgG antibodies in paired sera can also be used to confirm recent infection. Serologic diagnosis is unreliable in immunocompromised patients; diagnosis in these patients requires methods to detect viral DNA.

The virus cannot be isolated by culture. Methods to detect viral particles or viral DNA such as polymerase chain reaction (PCR) or nucleic acid hybridization are necessary to establish the diagnosis. Prenatal diagnosis of B19-induced fetal hydrops can be accomplished by detection of viral DNA in fetal blood by these methods or visualization of viral particles by immune electron microscopy.

DIFFERENTIAL DIAGNOSIS. The rash of erythema infectiosum must be differentiated from that of rubella, measles, enteroviral infections, and drug reactions. Rash and arthritis in older children should prompt consideration of juvenile rheumatoid arthritis, systemic lupus erythematosus, and other connective tissue disorders.

Treatment. There is no specific antiviral therapy. Commercial lots of intravenous immunoglobulin (IVIG) have been used with some success to treat B19-related episodes of anemia and bone marrow failure in immunocompromised children. Specific antibody may facilitate clearance of the virus; it is not always necessary, however, because cessation of cytotoxic chemotherapy will often suffice. In patients whose immune status is not likely to improve, such as patients with AIDS, administration of IVIG may give only a temporary remission, and periodic re-infusions may be required.

B19-infected fetuses with anemia and hydrops have been managed successfully with intrauterine transfusions, but this has significant attendant risks. Once fetal hydrops is diagnosed, regardless of the suspected cause, the mother should be referred to a fetal therapy center for further evaluation because of the high risk for serious complications (Chapter 92).

Complications. Erythema infectiosum is often accompanied by arthralgias or arthritis in adolescents and adults, which may persist after resolution of the rash. B19 may cause thrombocytopenic purpura and, rarely, aseptic meningitis in normal individuals after erythema infectiosum. B19 is also a cause of virus-associated hemophagocytic syndrome, usually in immunocompromised patients.

Prevention. Children with erythema infectiosum are not likely to be infectious at presentation because the rash and arthropathy represent immune-mediated, postinfectious phenomena. Isolation and exclusion from school or childcare are unnecessary and ineffective after diagnosis.

Children with B19-induced red cell aplasia (transient aplastic crisis) are infectious when they present and demonstrate a more intense viremia. Most of these children require transfusions and supportive care until their hematologic status stabilizes. They should be isolated in the hospital to prevent spread to susceptible patients and staff. Isolation should continue for at least 1 wk and until after resolution of fever. Pregnant caregivers should not be assigned to these patients. Exclusion of pregnant women from workplaces where children with erythema infectiosum may be present (e.g., schools) is not recommended as a general policy because it is unlikely to reduce their risk. There are no data to support the use of IVIG for postexposure prophylaxis in pregnant caregivers or immunocompromised children. No vaccine is available.

Anand A, Gray ES, Brown T, et al: Human parvovirus infection in pregnancy and hydrops fetalis. *N Engl J Med* 1987;316:183–6.

Anderson MJ, Jones SE, Fisher-Hoch SP, et al: Human parvovirus, the cause of erythema infectiosum (fifth disease)? Lancet 1983;1:1378.

Cherry JD: Parvovirus infections in children and adults. *Adv Pediatr* 1999;46:245–69.

Gratacos E, Torres PJ, Vidal J, et al: The incidence of human parvovirus B19 infection during pregnancy and its impact on perinatal outcome. *J Infect Dis* 1995;171:1360–3.

Koch WC, Harger JH, Barnstein B, et al: Serologic and virologic evidence for frequent intrauterine transmission of human parvovirus B19 with a primary maternal infection during pregnancy. *Pediatr Infect Dis J* 1998;17:489–94.

Koch WC, Massey G, Russell CE, et al: Manifestations and treatment of human parvovirus B19 infection in immunocompromised patients. *J Pediatr* 1990;116:355–9.

Nigro G, Bastianon V, Colloridi V, et al: Human parvovirus B19 infection in infancy associated with acute and chronic lymphocytic myocarditis and high cytokine levels: Report of 3 cases and review. *Clin Infect Dis* 2000;31:65–9.

Smith PT, Landry ML, Carey H, et al: Papular-purpuric gloves and socks syndrome associated with acute parvovirus B19 infection: Case report and review. *Clin Infect Dis* 1998;27:164–8.

Török TJ: Unusual clinical manifestations reported in patients with parvovirus B19 infection. In Anderson LJ and Young NS (editors): *Human Parvovirus B19,* Monographs in Virology, vol 20. Basel, Karger, 1997, pp 61–92.

Chapter 231
Herpes Simplex Virus *Steve Kohl*

Herpes simplex virus (HSV) infection is common among humans and has a variety of clinical manifestations involving the skin, mucous membranes, eye, central nervous system (CNS), and genital tract. It also causes generalized systemic disease. Disease manifestations are in large part determined by the immune competence of the host. Two strains of the virus are identified: HSV-1 commonly infects skin and mucous membranes above the waist, and HSV-2 commonly infects the genitals and the neonate.

Three types of infection are recognized: primary infection; first infection, nonprimary; and recurrent. **Primary infection** represents infection in HSV-seronegative persons, and is the susceptible host's first experience with the virus, which in most instances is subclinical infection or limited to local superficial lesions accompanied by varying degrees of systemic reaction. In newborns, immunocompromised persons, and severely malnourished infants, a serious systemic infection, often without superficial lesions, may occur. Circulating antibodies and a cell-mediated response develop following infection.

First infection, nonprimary, is infection in a person with immunity to one type of HSV (e.g., type 1) but infection by a second type (e.g., type 2). These infections are usually less severe than primary infection. In pregnant women near delivery, first infection nonprimary disease can lead to severe infection in the newborn owing to the absence of type-specific antibody.

Recurrent infection represents reactivation of a latent infection in an immune host with circulating antibodies. Reactivation follows such nonspecific stimuli as changes in the external milieu (e.g., cold, ultraviolet light) or in the internal milieu (e.g., menstruation, fever, or emotional stress). The lesions tend to be localized and, generally, are not associated with systemic reactions. In immunocompromised persons, especially with T- or natural killer lymphocyte defects, lesions may be progressive if untreated. Viral reactivation may take place in the absence of clinical recurrence, leading to asymptomatic viral shedding.

Etiology. HSV is a double-stranded DNA-containing enveloped virus. The icosahedral protein core is surrounded by a lipid envelope in which are embedded a number of viral glycoproteins (e.g., glycoproteins B, C, D, E, G, I, J, K, L) responsible for viral–target cell interaction and infection. These glycoproteins are also key targets for the host humoral and cellular immune response. HSV grows rapidly in human and nonhuman cell lines and produces characteristic cytopathic changes. HSV-1 and HSV-2 are about 50% homologous by nucleic acid analysis and share immunologic cross reactivity but may be differentiated by DNA analysis (endonuclease restriction analysis) and commercially by reactivity with type-specific monoclonal antibodies in a variety of fluorescent and enzyme-linked immunosorbent assays (ELISA). Several enzymes important for viral DNA synthesis, such as thymidine kinase and DNA polymerase, are targets for antiviral agents.

Epidemiology. The virus develops an extremely compatible relationship with its host. In about 85% of instances the infection is subclinical. Even when clinical manifestations are present, the host is only rarely seriously disabled. Occasionally, the primary or recurrent infection may lead to institutional or family outbreaks of stomatitis, which has been reported in orphanages and daycare center settings. HSV may also be transmitted by infection of digits (**herpetic whitlow**), during contact sports such as rugby or wrestling (**herpes gladiatorum**), and rarely in the hospital setting. The incubation period is 2–12 days (average, 6 days). The spread of infection appears to be determined by two factors: close body contact and trauma such as teething or a break in the skin.

The higher incidence of HSV antibodies in lower socioeconomic groups correlates with crowded living conditions. The epidemiology differs for the two types of HSV. In low-income socioeconomic groups, most infants have transplacental antibody for about the first 6 mo of life. There is a sharp rise in seroprevalence from 1 to 4 yr of age corresponding to antibodies to HSV-1, a much slower rate of acquisition to 14 yr of age, and then a second sharp rise in antibodies, principally to HSV-2. HSV-1 antibodies are found in 30% of university students. Recent serologic studies have indicated a rise in the prevalence of HSV-2 antibody in the United States to 21.7%. Among adults, HSV-2 antibodies are present in up to 60% of adults in lower socioeconomic groups, 10–30% of adults in higher socioeconomic groups, and 3% in nuns. Approximately 10% of HSV-2 seronegative persons with HSV-2-seropositive sexual partners will become infected each year. Approximately 2% of pregnant women in the United States acquire a new HSV infection during the 9 months of pregnancy.

Once infected, the majority of individuals continue to carry the virus in a latent state in neuronal ganglia and maintain an almost constant level of circulating antibodies. The initial level of antibodies reached after a primary infection may fall and several subclinical recurrences may occur before a stable antibody level is established. Carriers may distribute the virus without having any manifest lesion. HSV can be isolated from the oropharynx of 1–2% of asymptomatic adults.

Pathogenesis. The pathologic changes vary with the tissue infected. In general, a specific lesion is characterized by the presence of intranuclear inclusion bodies, which are homogeneous masses lying in the middle of a severely disorganized nucleus in which the basic chromatin has marginated to the nuclear membrane. Around the specific lesion there is always evidence of an acute inflammatory reaction. In the skin and mucous membranes the typical lesion is a unilocular vesicle. In the skin, the vesicle is tense. Ballooned epithelial cells containing intranuclear inclusions can best be seen at the margins of the vesicle. The vesicular fluid contains infected epithelial cells, including multinucleated giant cells and leukocytes. In the corium there is no necrosis, but capillaries are dilated and there is infiltration with mononuclear and polymorphonuclear cells. In the mucous membrane, because of maceration, there is early leakage of the vesicular fluid, resulting in a collapsed vesicle, mainly filled with fibrin. The edematous roof cells form a gray membrane over the ulcerated lesion.

In otherwise healthy persons, the lesions are confined to the skin and mucous membranes; viremia has rarely been described. Bloodstream spread of the virus with resultant widely disseminated disease occurs mainly in the newborn, in severely malnourished children, in persons with skin diseases such as eczema, and in those with defects in cell-mediated immunity. In these patients the virus spreads hematogenously from the portal of entry to susceptible organs. Virus increases within these organs, and secondary viremia occurs with evidence of extensive cell destruction. It is probable, however, that most cases of HSV-1 encephalitis other than in the newborn are caused by neurogenic transmission of the virus to the brain. Healing begins with clearing of the viremia and a decrease in the production of virus within the cells. This is accomplished by the coordinated effect of antibody and cell-mediated immunity including T and natural killer cells, as well as a variety of cytokines and complement.

Clinical Manifestations. HSV characteristically produces vesicular skin lesions. Only rarely is there a viremic distribution that results in widespread systemic disease or neurogenic transmission that leads to meningoencephalitis. Although the occurrence of primary and recurrent lesions is an accepted characteristic of herpetic infection, their distinction clinically is often not possible without knowledge of the presence or absence of homologous type-specific serum antibodies in the patient.

SKIN AND MUCOUS MEMBRANES. Skin lesions consist of aggregates of thin-walled vesicles on an erythematous base. These rupture, scab, and heal within 7–10 days without leaving a scar except after repeated attacks or secondary bacterial infections; temporary depigmentation may occur in darkly pigmented individuals. The lesions may be preceded by mild irritation or burning at the local site or by severe neuralgic pain in the region. The vesicles may become secondarily infected, introducing impetigo into the differential diagnosis. The lesions tend to recur at the same site, particularly at mucocutaneous junctions, but may occur anywhere.

Primary infection, especially in immunocompromised persons, may, uncommonly, result in a generalized vesicular eruption in which the lesions are small and may continue to appear over a period of 2–3 wk. If the systemic manifestations are mild, the infection must be differentiated from varicella.

Traumatic lesions of the skin or burns can be infected by HSV. Primary lesions can also occur on apparently unbroken skin, as, for example, on the chin of a drooling infant with herpetic stomatitis, in whom scattered isolated vesicles appear, in contrast to the grouped vesicles of recurrent attacks. When the skin of a limb is infected, vesicles appear in 2–3 days at the site of trauma. There is often centripetal spread along lymph channels, causing enlargement of regional lymph nodes and scattered vesicles on the intervening undamaged skin. This clinical picture may be mistaken for that of herpes zoster, especially if accompanied by neuralgic pain, unless the lesions are recognized as not being confined to a dermatome. The lesions heal slowly, often taking 3 wk. Recurrences at the site of local trauma are common and may assume a bullous pattern. Wrestlers, and also medical personnel, are prone to herpetic infections of superficial abrasions, which is known as **herpes gladiatorum**. HSV infection of minor trauma about the nails that leads to extremely painful, deep-seated spreading lesions with vesicles is known as **herpetic whitlow**. These lesions resolve spontaneously in 2–3 wk. Similar lesions occur on the fingers of thumb suckers who are suffering from herpetic gingivostomatitis. The lesions must be differentiated from bacterial infection. They should not be incised because incision may facilitate systemic spread of HSV.

ACUTE HERPETIC GINGIVOSTOMATITIS. Oral HSV primary infection, probably the most common cause of stomatitis in children 1–3 yr of age, can also occur in older children and adults. The symptoms may appear abruptly, with pain in the mouth, salivation, fetor oris, refusal to eat, and fever, often as high as 40–40.6°C (104–105°F). Fever and irritability may precede the oral lesions by 1–2 days. The initial lesion is a vesicle (Fig. 231–1), which is seldom seen because of its early rupture. The residual lesion is 2–10 mm in diameter and is covered with a yellow-gray membrane (Fig. 231–2). When this membrane sloughs, a true ulcer remains. Although the tongue and cheeks are most commonly involved, no part of the oral lining is exempt. Except in edentulous infants, acute gingivitis is characteristic of the disease and may precede the appearance of mucosal vesicles. Submaxillary lymphadenitis is common. The

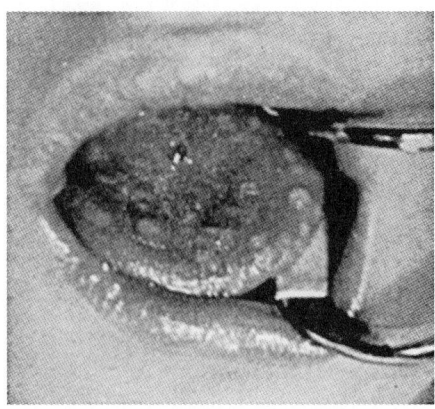

FIGURE 231–1. Vesicular lesions of herpetic stomatitis on the tongue.

acute phase lasts 4–9 days and is self-limited. Pain tends to disappear 2–4 days before healing of the ulcers is complete. In some instances the tonsillar regions are involved early and appear exudative, and acute tonsillitis of bacterial origin or enterovirus-induced herpangina may be suspected. Negative cultures for group A streptococcus and other bacterial pathogens and failure of the lesion to respond to antibiotic therapy differentiate a bacterial infection. The spread of the vesiculation to the buccal mucosa and anterior portion of the mouth is atypical for herpangina. A rare but serious complication of HSV gingivostomatitis is bacteremia with oral flora such as group A streptococcus and *Kingella*.

RECURRENT STOMATITIS AND HERPES LABIALIS. The typical oral recurrence of HSV is one or a few vesicles grouped at the mucocutaneous junction. Lesions are usually accompanied by local pain, tingling, or itching and last 3–7 days. Systemic symptoms are unusual. Less commonly, localized lesions may occur on the palate in association with a febrile illness or on the mucosa adjacent to a lesion on the lip. Recurrent aphthous ulcers, however, are not caused by HSV. In some persons a generalized stomatitis recurs consistently 7–10 days after a recurrent herpetic lesion of the lip or elsewhere and is often accompanied by skin lesions of erythema multiforme. Indeed, recurrent HSV infection is one of the most common causes of recurrent erythema multiforme.

ECZEMA HERPETICUM (KAPOSI VARICELLIFORM ERUPTION). This, the most serious manifestation of "traumatic herpes," results from a widespread infection of the eczematous skin with HSV. The severity of this complication varies; the lesion

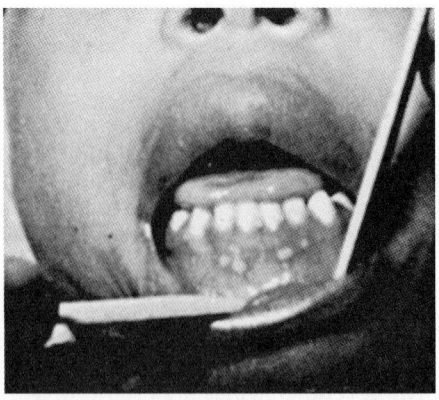

FIGURE 231–2. Herpetic stomatitis with vesicular-pustular lesions on the gingival mucosa.

may be so mild as to be overlooked, or it may be fatal. In a typical severe primary attack, vesicles develop abruptly in large numbers over the area of eczematous skin. They continue to appear in crops for as long as 7–9 days. Isolated at first, they later become grouped and may occur on adjoining areas of normal skin (Fig. 231–3). Wide denudation of the epidermis may occur. Scabs eventually form, and epithelialization occurs. The systemic reaction varies, but temperatures of 39.4–40.6°C (103–105°F) for 7–10 days are not uncommon. Recurrent attacks develop on chronic atopic skin lesions. Death may result from profound physiologic disturbances from loss of fluid, electrolytes, and protein through the skin; from dissemination of the virus to the brain and other organs; or from secondary bacterial invasion usually with *Staphylococcus* or group A streptococcus. Differentiation from eczema vaccinatum can usually be established by determining that the child has not been exposed to vaccinia and by the occurrence of crops of vesicles in herpes. The diagnosis can be confirmed by examination and culture of vesicular fluid.

OCULAR INFECTIONS. Conjunctivitis and keratoconjunctivitis may occur as manifestations of either a primary or a recurrent infection. The conjunctiva appears congested and swollen, but there is little, if any, purulent discharge. In primary infection the preauricular node is usually enlarged and tender. Cataracts, uveitis, and chorioretinitis have been described in newborns and in the immunocompromised.

Corneal lesions may be superficial, in the form of a dendritic ulcer, or deep, as a disciform keratitis. Dendritic keratitis is unique to HSV eye involvement. The diagnosis is suggested by the presence of herpetic vesicles on the lids; it is established by the isolation of the virus. Topical corticosteroid use will worsen HSV ocular disease. The highly contagious **epidemic keratoconjunctivitis** (shipyard conjunctivitis) caused by any of several serotypes of adenovirus- or enterovirus-induced conjunctivitis must be considered in the differential diagnosis. Recurrent herpetic corneal infection may result in scarring of the cornea and vision impairment.

GENITAL HERPES. Genital infections with herpesvirus occur most commonly in adolescents and young adults, are usually due to HSV-2, and are usually spread by sexual activity.

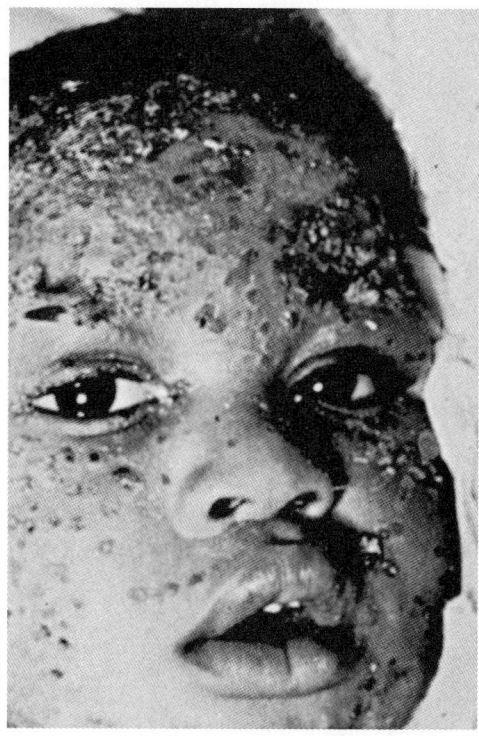

FIGURE 231–3. Eczema herpeticum (Kaposi varicelliform eruption).

Although hand-to-genital transmission and autoinoculation are possible, genital or rectal herpes in a young child warrants a sensitive and careful appraisal of the possibility of child abuse. From 10 to 25% of primary genital herpes is caused by HSV-1. Most cases of recurrent genital herpes are due to HSV-2. In primary genital infection, when the patient has no antibody to either type of herpes, systemic symptoms such as fever, regional lymphadenopathy, and dysuria are more likely to occur. In adult women, the vulva and vagina may be involved with vesicles and ulcers, but the cervix is the primary site of infection. Recurrence is common. Both primary and recurrent disease are frequently subclinical, but virus shed during this time may infect a sex partner or an infant during passage through the birth canal. In males, herpetic vesicles or ulcers are usually seen on the glans penis, prepuce, or shaft of the penis. The scrotum is less frequently involved. Genital HSV is a risk factor for HIV infection.

CENTRAL NERVOUS SYSTEM INFECTIONS. HSV has a predilection to infect the nervous system. Both types 1 and 2 may cause a meningoencephalitis as part of neonatal HSV. In patients with primary genital herpes, usually resulting from HSV-2, an aseptic meningitis syndrome may complicate the course. The cerebrospinal fluid (CSF) reveals a lymphocytic pleocytosis, and the virus may be cultured from it in patients with this self-limited syndrome. HSV-1 is an unusual cause of the aseptic meningitis syndrome, but it is the most common cause of fatal sporadic encephalitis. It has a striking predilection to involve the frontal and parietal areas. Typical signs and symptoms include fever, altered consciousness, headache, personality changes, seizures, dysphasia, and focal neurologic signs. If untreated, the mortality rate is 75%, with severe sequelae in survivors. HSV is the cause of most cases of recurrent aseptic meningitis (Mollaret meningitis), based on demonstration of HSV DNA in the CSF by polymerase chain reaction (PCR).

IMMUNOCOMPROMISED PERSONS. Unusually severe HSV infection may occur in a variety of persons, including the newborn; the severely malnourished; and children with malignancies or other conditions necessitating immunosuppressive therapy, with AIDS, with burns, or with primary immunodeficiency diseases that particularly impair cell-mediated immunity. In children receiving therapy for cancer or organ transplantation, the risk of severe HSV infection coincides with the time of maximum immunosuppression. The most common syndrome is local and chronic oral or genital mucocutaneous disease. The lesions may resemble typical vesicles and ulcers or progress to large necrotic painful erosions or atypical exophytic, wartlike lesions. Mucositis, esophagitis, proctitis, and pneumonitis are less common. The most severe manifestation, usually a result of primary infection in the immunocompromised child, is widespread disseminated disease involving the liver, lungs, adrenal gland, and CNS. These patients have a sepsis-like syndrome with leukopenia, hepatitis, disseminated intravascular coagulopathy, fever, or hypothermia and progression to death. Skin lesions may be localized to mucous membranes, widely disseminated, resembling varicella infection, or absent. This form of HSV infection has a high mortality rate even with therapy.

PERINATAL INFECTIONS. Most cases of neonatal herpes occur due to maternal infection during delivery, and approximately 75% are HSV type 2. At delivery, 0.2–0.4% of women shed HSV in their genital tract, which increases to 1–2% if there is a history of maternal genital herpes. The classification of maternal genital disease predicts the attack rate in newborns. Maternal primary or first episode genital herpes (no antibody present against the type of virus shed) has an infant attack rate of 33–50%. Recurrent maternal disease has an infant attack rate of only 1–3%. Only 15–20% of women with infants with neonatal herpes have a history of HSV infection, and only approximately 25% have some relevant symptoms at delivery. Intrapartum monitoring may be a risk factor; 40% of neonates with HSV infection had fetal scalp electrodes placed during delivery.

Rarely, in about 5% of cases, true intrauterine infection occurs. About 10% of infants acquire their infection postpartum, not necessarily from the mother, but also from another close family member shedding HSV (often type 1), from fever blisters, finger infections, or lesions at other sites.

Perinatal infection manifests in the first month of life, with 9% on the first day, and in 40% by the first week. There are 3 major categories: (1) localized skin, eye, and mouth infection; (2) CNS infection; and (3) disseminated infection. Localized skin, eye, and mouth infection and also disseminated infection occur at a mean of 5–6 days postpartum, whereas localized CNS infection occurs later at a mean of 8–12 days postpartum. The hallmark of neonatal HSV infection—the vesicular, ulcerative skin lesions (Fig. 231–4)—is present in only 30–43% of children at presentation; one third will never manifest skin lesions. Symptoms of CNS involvement are found in 48–79% and include lethargy, poor feeding, irritability, poor tone, and seizures. Fever (7–14%) and respiratory distress (5–19%) may also be present.

Particular attention should be directed to sites of fetal monitoring for the signs of pustular-vesicular infection, especially if unresponsive to antibiotics, and to the eyes for signs of herpetic keratoconjunctivitis. Approximately 70% of neonates with localized infection that is not treated will progress to CNS or disseminated disease. The typical 5–7-day delay in diagnosis of neonatal HSV must be shortened if outcome is to improve.

Neonatal HSV infection should be considered in any neonate with suggestive signs born to a parent (mother or father) with a history of genital herpes; sepsis unresponsive to antibiotics especially with thrombocytopenia, elevated liver function tests, disseminated intravascular coagulopathy, or early pneumonitis; unexplained neonatal lymphocytic meningitis; unexplained hepatitis; or unexplained vesicular-ulcerative cutaneous eruption. These neonates must be treated for HSV pending diagnostic evaluation.

The infant born with a congenital infection syndrome, especially with skin vesicles or scars, chorioretinitis, microphthalmia, and microcephaly, should be evaluated for both congenital HSV and varicella, as well as other causes of congenital infection.

The risk of mortality due to treated HSV increases with CNS (6%) or disseminated (31%) disease. It is also increased in infants with coma, disseminated intravascular coagulopathy, prematurity, and pneumonitis. Morbidity among survivors increases with CNS or disseminated diseases, seizures, infection with type 2 virus, and frequent cutaneous recurrences.

The differential diagnosis of a vesicular-ulcerative eruption in the neonate is extensive (Table 231–1). Often an experienced

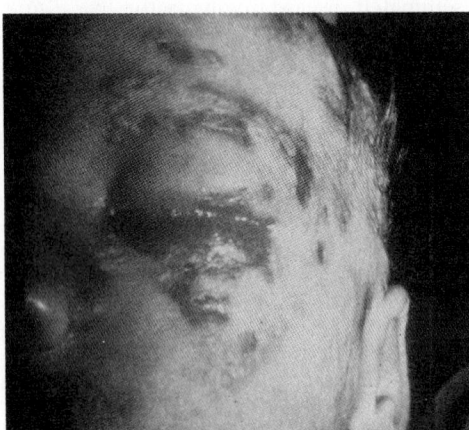

FIGURE 231–4. Vesicular-pustular lesions on the face of a neonate with herpes simplex virus infection. (From Kohl S: Neonatal herpes simplex virus infection. *Clin Perinatol* 1997;24:129–50.) See also color plates.

TABLE 231–1. Differential Diagnosis of Vesicular Eruptions in the Neonate

Infectious Etiologies

Herpes simplex virus	Aspergillus
Staphylococcus aureus	Varicella-zoster virus
Pseudomonas	Cytomegalovirus
Haemophilus influenzae type b	Listeria monocytogenes
Treponema pallidum	Group B streptococcus
Candida	

Noninfectious Conditions

Erythema toxicum	Herpes gestationis
Pustular melanosis	Incontinentia pigmenti
Miliaria	Neonatal lupus
Letterer-Siwe disease	Epidermolysis bullosa
Urticaria pigmentosa	Epidermolytic hyperkeratosis
Bullous mastocytosis	Acropustulosis
Dermatitis herpetiformis	Neonatal bullous dermatitis
Pemphigus vulgaris	Langerhans cell histiocytosis

Data from Case records of the Massachusetts General Hospital. Weekly clinicopathological exercises. N Engl J Med *1989;320:1399–410; 1996;334:1591–7.*
From Kohl S: Neonatal herpes simplex virus infection. Clin Perinatol *1997;24:129–50.*

pediatric dermatologist is invaluable help for diagnosis of some of the more arcane syndromes listed.

Diagnosis. The diagnosis is based on any two of the following: (1) a compatible clinical pattern; (2) isolation of the virus; (3) development of specific antibodies; and (4) demonstration of characteristic cells, histologic changes, viral antigen, or HSV DNA in scrapings, CSF, or biopsy material. A rise in CSF HSV antibody occurs in HSV encephalitis, but it is late in the illness and is useful only for retrospective diagnosis. HSV serologic changes (fourfold rise or seroconversion from negative to positive) usually occur after the critical period for diagnosis and therapy. Illnesses resulting from HSV recurrence may not demonstrate a diagnostic serologic rise, and neonates or severely immunocompromised individuals may fail to produce antibody during primary infection. Reliable antibody tests to differentiate serologic response to HSV-1 from HSV-2 are now commercially available. HSV-1 and HSV-2 viral isolates may be typed by a variety of readily available antigen (ELISA, fluorescent antibody) and molecular techniques. HSV isolates that are unrelated epidemiologically are all slightly different at the nucleic acid level, as discerned by DNA endonuclease restriction analysis. Using this technique, available in research laboratories only, it is possible to confirm infection of one individual by another and to demonstrate that apparent nosocomial outbreaks or viral transmission may instead represent a chance collection of unrelated cases, which could be extremely important for counseling and medicolegal reasons.

The use of PCR analysis of CSF and perhaps blood is critical to diagnose neonatal HSV infection, especially in the absence of skin lesions. The sensitivity of CSF PCR in neonatal CNS infection is 75%. Serology is not a useful tool for rapid diagnosis of HSV infection in the neonate, as in the older child, because of transplacental maternal antibodies; MRI of the brain is often abnormal in neonates with CNS involvement and suggestive of HSV infection. CSF PCR is the only practical test, short of brain biopsy, to diagnose HSV encephalitis beyond the neonatal period, with a sensitivity and specificity of over 95%.

LABORATORY FINDINGS. Microscopic examination of scrapings from lesions (Tzanck stain) reveals multinuclear giant cells and intranuclear inclusions approximately 50% of the time. Specific antigen detection methods such as ELISA and immunofluorescent techniques applied to these specimens can be useful in rapidly diagnosing herpes infection and in differentiating the two types of herpes. Virus can be readily isolated from vesicles and from conjunctival swabs in 1–4 days. The CSF is positive for virus in about one third of infected neonates but is rarely positive in older children with encephalitis. PCR permits detection of viral DNA in CSF and, if positive, will make brain biopsy unnecessary. Brain biopsy may be necessary if PCR is negative for definitive diagnosis and exclusion of other treatable entities. At this time, PCR for HSV is available through specialized laboratories only.

Moderate polymorphonuclear leukocytosis occurs in acute herpetic gingivostomatitis, eczema herpeticum, and meningoencephalitis. In meningoencephalitis there are frequently red cells in the CSF and an increase in lymphocytes, usually below $100/mm^3$ but occasionally up to $1,000/mm^3$; the protein level is elevated, and the glucose is usually within the normal range but may be reduced. Electroencephalography (EEG) and MRI may demonstrate a temporal lobe lesion in early encephalitis. CT may be normal in early encephalitis but becomes abnormal as the disease progresses. Thrombocytopenia and elevated levels of liver function tests often occur with systemic infection.

Treatment. Acyclovir (9-[2-hydroxyethoxymethyl] guanine, a purine nucleoside analog) is the mainstay of therapy for HSV. Viral thymidine kinase phosphorylates acyclovir, which is then triphosphorylated by cellular enzymes to act as an HSV DNA polymerase inhibitor and DNA chain terminator. Thymidine kinase-negative HSV isolates are resistant to acyclovir.

Two more recently licensed oral anti-herpes drugs simplify the therapy for genital herpes. Valacyclovir, a prodrug of acyclovir, and famciclovir, a prodrug of penciclovir, have excellent oral bioavailability (55–80%) and are converted in vivo to acyclovir and penciclovir, respectively. As with acyclovir, penciclovir is phosphorylated by HSV thymidine kinase and then cellular enzymes to the triphosphate active agents. Due to excellent oral adsorption these drugs may be used less frequently than acyclovir. The ease of use is offset by the increased cost compared with generic acyclovir. Ongoing studies using famciclovir in immunocompromised persons show that larger oral doses reach serum levels obtained with intravenous acyclovir, and have facilitated oral therapy and prophylaxis of more severe forms of HSV infection.

Acyclovir-resistant HSV is rare in the normal host but occurs in the immunocompromised host treated with long-term or multiple, intermittent courses of acyclovir. When immunocompromised patients have unresponsive or worsening HSV infection despite acyclovir therapy, the virus should be forwarded to reference laboratories for drug susceptibility testing. Pending laboratory results (resistance to acyclovir is associated with inhibitory levels >2 μg/mL), the drug of choice for acyclovir-resistant HSV is intravenous foscarnet (phosphonoformic acid; 40 mg/kg/dose q 8 hr IV). This drug has serious adverse effects including azotemia, electrolyte disturbance, anemia, and granulocytopenia. Cidofovir has been successfully used in a small number of cases of acyclovir- and foscarnet-resistant virus. Acyclovir and foscarnet dosages must be modified in patients with renal impairment.

Topical acyclovir therapy for oral or genital herpes may decrease the period of viral shedding but has little effect on symptoms and is not recommended. Topical penciclovir, another nucleoside analog, reduces symptoms of oral recurrent herpes only modestly.

Topical trifluorothymidine, vidarabine, and idoxuridine are all usually effective in treating herpetic keratitis but do not reduce the recurrence rate. Topical corticosteroids may increase ocular involvement, if used alone, and should only be used with antiviral therapy.

The child or adolescent with recurrent oral or genital herpes may experience psychologic problems and may benefit from anticipatory guidance or formal counseling. Genital disease should be destigmatized, and safer sex practices emphasized. Parents of children with most types of HSV infection, such as gingivostomatitis or skin infection, should be reassured that common childhood HSV infections are not related to sexual activity or abuse.

SKIN AND MUCOUS MEMBRANES. Oral acyclovir (15 mg/kg/dose five times a day with a maximum dose of 1 g/24 hr for 7 days) started within 72 hr of onset of lesions has significant benefits in children with primary herpetic gingivostomatitis by decreasing drooling, gum swelling, pain, eating and drinking difficulties, and duration of lesions. Therapy for recurrent oral herpes with oral acyclovir has limited effect.

Symptomatic and supportive therapy is of great importance. Oral lavage should be used for mouth care; Ceepryn 1:4,000 or Zephiran 1:1,000 may be useful. Local analgesics, such as viscous lidocaine or benzocaine lozenges, are not advocated because they may cause the child to damage friable and anesthetized parts of the mouth. Food and fluid intake will be facilitated by acquiescing to the child's whims. Ice-cold fluids, ice slush, or semisolids are often accepted when other food is refused. In infants especially, eczema herpeticum and stomatitis may lead to severe dehydration, shock, and hypoproteinemia, requiring intravenous replacement of fluids, electrolytes, and proteins.

Acyclovir has no effect on HSV-associated erythema multiforme. Suppression of the HSV infection by prophylactic therapy as for genital disease prevents the erythema multiforme recurrences.

Oral acyclovir is beneficial for treating primary and recurrent herpes whitlow and rectal herpes.

GENITAL HERPES. Patients with primary genital infection who are treated with oral acyclovir have significantly less pain, itching, and time to crusting; a shorter duration of viral shedding; and fewer new lesions compared with control patients. Those with recurrent genital infections who are treated similarly with oral acyclovir have a shorter duration of viral shedding and heal faster. Therapy for primary attacks does not prevent recurrences. However, daily prophylactic administration of oral acyclovir can diminish the number of recurrences and may be prescribed if recurrences are frequent or severe.

The recommended treatment regimen for initial genital herpes in older adolescents and adults is valacyclovir (1,000 mg/dose bid PO for 7–10 days) or famciclovir (250 mg/dose tid PO for 7–10 days); these are equivalent to acyclovir (200 mg/dose 5 times a day PO). For HSV genital recurrence, valacyclovir (500 mg/dose bid PO for 5 days) and famciclovir (125 mg/dose bid PO for 5 days) are equivalent to acyclovir (400 mg/dose tid or 200 mg/dose 5 times a day PO). Daily suppressive therapy reduces the frequency of genital herpes recurrences by 75% or more among persons with 6 or more recurrences per year. Recommended regimens for daily suppressive therapy in older adolescents and adults are famciclovir (125 mg/dose or 250 mg/dose bid PO), valacyclovir (500 mg/dose or 1000 mg/dose PO once daily), or acyclovir (400 mg/dose bid or tid PO). The child dose of acyclovir for primary genital HSV is 10–20 mg/kg/dose qid PO, not to exceed adult dosage. There are no pediatric dosage regimens of valacyclovir or famciclovir.

Genital lesions may be made less painful by using sitz baths. Local drying agents prolong healing and may increase secondary infection. Analgesics should be used systemically as required. Antibiotics are useful only in treating secondary bacterial infections.

CENTRAL NERVOUS SYSTEM AND SYSTEMIC INFECTIONS. Intravenously administered acyclovir (10 mg/kg/dose given over 1 hr q 8 hr IV for 14–21 days) is the treatment of choice for herpes encephalitis. The drug is well tolerated. The best results are obtained when treatment is started early. Patients younger than 30 yr of age and those who are only lethargic compared with those who have progressed to coma have a better prognosis. Supportive care to minimize increased intracranial pressure, seizure activity, and respiratory compromise requires an intensive care setting and a team of experts.

Intravenous acyclovir (5–10 mg/kg/dose given over 1 hr q 8 hr, with the duration depending on clinical response) is recommended for treatment of HSV infections in the immunocompromised host. The larger doses are used for severe and systemic infections. The lower dose may be used for localized mucocutaneous disease. As the patient responds, therapy may be switched to the oral route. Oral acyclovir, as used in genital disease, may be used to suppress HSV recurrences in seropositive patients during periods of maximum immunosuppression after organ or marrow transplantation or during induction therapy for leukemia, lymphoma, or solid tumors. Immunosuppressed patients with frequently recurring HSV infection, such as those with AIDS or primary immunodeficiencies, benefit from chronic suppressive oral therapy. Valacyclovir should not be used in immunocompromised children due to unusual adverse effects.

PERINATAL INFECTIONS. As in other serious forms of HSV infection, intravenous acyclovir (20 mg/kg/dose q 8 hr for 14–21 days) is the drug of choice for neonatal HSV infection. This high dose of acyclovir may be associated with neutropenia. For the neonate with HSV infection, intensive care is necessary initially to observe for signs of disseminated or CNS disease necessitating ventilatory control, seizure management, and intensive supportive care. There is preliminary evidence to suggest extending therapy of HSV neonatal encephalitis for longer than 21 days until the HSV CSF PCR becomes negative. Preliminary data suggest that the use of daily oral acyclovir (300 mg/m^2 tid PO) for 6 mo can suppress the common cutaneous recurrences associated with poor outcome, but the effects on central nervous system infection and long-term prognosis are unproved. Recurrence of cutaneous infection soon after cessation of suppressive therapy is frequent. Prolonged treatment has been associated with neutropenia and the rare emergence of acyclovir-resistant virus.

Prognosis. Primary localized infections with HSV in the normal host are self-limited, usually lasting 1–2 wk. Mortality rates are high in newborns who also have systemic infection and in older infants who are severely immunocompromised or malnourished. In patients with meningoencephalitis the prognosis for survival or for recovery without serious permanent residua is guarded. Outcome is improved with early diagnosis and therapy.

Attacks may frequently recur, but they seldom cause more than temporary inconvenience except in the eye, where they may eventually cause scarring of the cornea and blindness. Recurrent herpes lesions can be a significant problem in immunocompromised patients. Recurrent genital disease may be associated with significant discomfort and psychologic morbidity. The major complication of any form of genital HSV infection in a woman is infection of her newborn.

Prevention. Acyclovir administered during periods of high risk in immunocompromised hosts and administered chronically in individuals with frequently recurrent genital or oral disease markedly decreases the rate of recurrence. Acyclovir administered before a known trigger factor, such as intense sunlight, usually prevents recurrences.

HSV spread can be limited by standard methods of infection control. Open lesions on skin, hands, and mucous membranes should be well covered. Wrestlers with possible HSV cutaneous lesions should be excluded from practice and competition until they are healed. Wrestling mats should be cleansed with a bleach solution at least daily. Children with immunodeficiencies or chronic skin diseases that predispose to severe HSV infection should not be cared for by persons with herpetic whitlow or active uncovered fever blisters. Active herpes lesions that can be covered are not a reason to exclude children from daycare or school activities.

There is active research to develop a vaccine to prevent HSV infection. HSV may be prevented in some animal models by live, attenuated, naked DNA, or subunit viral particle vaccines.

Several purified HSV glycoprotein vaccines are antigenic in humans, but to date these vaccines have lacked consistent efficacy in clinical trials.

OBSTETRIC MANAGEMENT OF THE WOMAN WITH GENITAL HSV INFECTION. The major aims of obstetric care of the woman with genital HSV infection are to ameliorate the symptoms of infection in the mother and to lessen the risk of neonatal HSV infection in the neonate. A reliable history of genital HSV infections must be determined for all women presenting for prenatal care.

Acyclovir is a pregnancy category C medication (should not be used during pregnancy unless the potential benefit justifies the potential risk to the fetus). In a registry of more than 600 women exposed to acyclovir during pregnancy, no increased rate of fetal malformations or unusual pattern of malformations has been noted, although this number is too low to detect a low-level or rare teratogenic effect. It is clear that primary HSV infection in the pregnant woman carries an increased risk of life-threatening dissemination, and intravenous acyclovir should be administered if there are any signs of disseminated HSV disease.

Recommendations of both the American Academy of Pediatrics and the American College of Obstetrics and Gynecology are for a cesarean section if primary, first-episode, or recurrent HSV lesions are present at the onset of labor (Box 231–1). This recommendation for recurrent infection is controversial: Given the low attack rate of HSV to the neonate in the case of maternal recurrent disease, nearly 1,600 excess cesarean deliveries will be performed for every prevention of poor neonatal outcome, at a cost of $2.5 million per case of neonatal herpes prevented and a possible excess of maternal deaths outnumbering prevented deaths in neonates.

If no lesions can be demonstrated at delivery, the child may be delivered via the vaginal route. For women with a history of recurrent genital herpes who have no obvious lesions at the time of delivery, it is not universally agreed that routine HSV cultures taken at delivery of mother or newborn are useful, although some experts advocate routine cultures. If cultures at delivery are positive for HSV, most experts recommend obtaining cultures from the neonate at 24–48 hr of life (eyes, mouth, urine, stool) and treating with acyclovir if any cultures are positive or if the neonate has any signs of HSV infection in the ensuing 4 wk.

BOX 231–1. Management of the Child Born to a Woman with Active Genital HSV Infection

MATERNAL PRIMARY OR FIRST-EPISODE INFECTION
Cesarean section within 24 hr (preferably 4 hr) of ruptured membranes
  Culture eyes, nose, mouth, urine, and stool at 48 hr
  Treat with acyclovir if any culture is positive or there are signs of neonatal HSV*
Unavoidable vaginal delivery
  Culture eyes, nose, mouth, urine, stool, and cerebrospinal fluid
  Treat with acyclovir

RECURRENT INFECTION, ACTIVE AT DELIVERY
Cesarean section within 24 (preferably 4) hours of ruptured membranes
  Culture eyes, nose, mouth, urine, and stool at 48 hr
  Treat with acyclovir if any culture is positive or there are signs of HSV infection*
Unavoidable vaginal delivery
  Culture eyes, nose, mouth, urine, and stool at 48 hr
  Treat with acyclovir if any culture is positive or there are signs of HSV infection*

---

*If the infant is to be treated with acyclovir, cerebrospinal fluid analysis, culture, and polymerase chain reaction test for HSV DNA are indicated.
From Kohl S: Neonatal herpes simplex virus infection. *Clin Perinatol* 1997;24:129–50.

For pregnant women with a history of genital herpes, there are preliminary data to demonstrate that suppressive acyclovir therapy administered near delivery reduces viral shedding and the need for cesarean section. This strategy of prophylactic maternal acyclovir needs further confirmation before it can be universally recommended.

Primary and first-episode genital infections are probably associated with some increased risk of spontaneous abortion, and with increased risk of premature delivery of 30–50%. Intrauterine infection is a rare consequence of genital infection.

In the neonate inadvertently born vaginally to a woman with active primary or first-episode HSV infection, positive cultures at 24–48 hr of life (eyes, mouth, urine, stool, and CSF), abnormal CSF findings, or any signs of HSV in the first 4 wk of life mandate acyclovir therapy (see Box 231–1). Many experts recommend anticipatory use of acyclovir therapy after delivery in this setting because of the high attack rate, although there are no data that demonstrate reduction of neonatal infection, and several case reports had demonstrated failure of early neonatal therapy.

Cesarean section is not completely protective, because 20–30% of infants with neonatal HSV infection are born by abdominal delivery. Thus, all newborns of women with primary or first-episode genital HSV infection also should have cultures taken at 48 hr of life and be followed for signs of infection regardless of the route of delivery.

Most women who are delivered of a neonate with HSV infection are not aware of their own HSV infection and usually have no symptoms at delivery. It also may be difficult to determine clinically if a genital infection at delivery represents a recurrence or a more severe primary or first-episode infection. Determination of serologic status of these women and their partners with type-specific antibody, and a rapid antigen or PCR strategy for genital viral detection, may be useful in the future.

Chen Y, Scieux C, Garrait V, et al: Resistant herpes simplex virus type 1 infection: An emerging concern after allogeneic stem cell transplantation. *Clin Infect Dis* 2000;31:927–35.

Corey L, Langenberg A, Ashley R, et al: Recombinant glycoprotein vaccine for the prevention of genital HSV-2 infection. Two randomized controlled trials. *JAMA* 1999;282:331–40.

Kimberlin DW, Lin C-Y, Jacobs RF, et al: Safety and efficacy of high-dose intravenous acyclovir in the management of neonatal herpes simplex virus infections. *Pediatrics* 2001;108:230–8.

Kimberlin DW, Lin C-Y, Jacobs RF, et al: Natural history of neonatal herpes simplex virus infections in the acyclovir era. *Pediatrics* 2001;108:223–9.

Kohl S: Herpes simplex infections in newborn infants. *Semin Pediatr Infect Dis* 1999;10:154–60.

Wald A, Zeh J, Selke S, et al: Reactivation of genital herpes simplex virus type 2 infection in asymptomatic seropositive persons. *N Engl J Med* 2000;342:844–50.

Chapter 232
Varicella-Zoster Virus

Martin G. Myers, Lawrence R. Stanberry, and Jane F. Seward

Varicella-zoster virus (VZV) causes primary, latent, and recurrent infections. The primary infection is manifested as varicella (chickenpox) and results in establishment of a lifelong latent infection of sensory ganglion neurons. Reactivation of the latent infection causes herpes zoster (shingles). Although often a mild illness of childhood, chickenpox can cause substantial morbidity and mortality in otherwise healthy children; it causes increased morbidity and mortality in adolescents, adults and immunocompromised persons and predisposes to severe group A streptococcus and *Staphylococcus aureus* infections. Chickenpox and zoster can be treated with antiviral drugs. Infection can be prevented by immunization with live-attenuated VZV vaccine. Gestational chickenpox can be severe in the mother and can cause a rare but distinct intrauterine syndrome. Chickenpox in the newborn can be severe and life threatening.

Etiology. VZV is a neurotropic human herpesvirus with similarities to herpes simplex virus, which is also an α-herpesvirus. These viruses are enveloped with double-stranded DNA genomes that encode more than 70 proteins, including proteins that are targets of cellular and humoral immunity.

Epidemiology. Prior to the introduction of vaccine in 1995, varicella was an almost universal communicable infection of childhood in the United States. Most children were infected by 15 yr of age, with fewer than 5% of adults remaining susceptible. Annual varicella epidemics occurred in winter and spring, accounting for about 4 million cases, 11,000 hospitalizations, and 100 deaths every year. Varicella is a more serious disease with higher rates of complications and deaths among infants, adults, and immunocompromised persons. Within households, transmission of VZV to susceptible individuals occurs at a rate of 65–86%; more casual contact, such as occurs in a school classroom, is associated with lower attack rates among susceptible children. Patients with varicella are contagious from 24–48 hr before the rash appears and until vesicles are crusted, usually 3–7 days after onset of rash. Susceptible children may also acquire varicella after close, direct contact with adults or children who have herpes zoster. Varicella has declined substantially in areas with moderate to high levels of vaccine coverage; varicella that occurs among immunized children (so-called **breakthrough varicella**) is usually very mild.

Herpes zoster, because it is due to the reactivation of latent VZV, is uncommon in childhood and shows no seasonal variation in incidence. The lifetime risk for herpes zoster for individuals with a history of varicella is 10–15%, with 75% of cases occurring after 45 yr of age. Herpes zoster is very rare in healthy children younger than 10 years of age except for those infected in utero or in the first year of life; herpes zoster in children tends to be milder than disease in adults and is less frequently associated with postherpetic neuralgia. However, herpes zoster occurs more frequently, occasionally multiple times, and may be severe in children receiving immunosuppressive therapy for malignancy or other diseases and in those who have HIV infection.

Pathogenesis. VZV is transmitted in respiratory secretions and in the fluid of skin lesions either by airborne spread or through direct contact. Primary infection (varicella) results from the respiratory inoculation of virus. During the early part of the 10–21-day incubation period, virus replicates in the respiratory tract followed by a brief subclinical viremia. Widespread cutaneous lesions occur during a second viremic phase. Peripheral blood mononuclear cells carry infectious virus, generating new crops of vesicles for 3–7 days. VZV is also transported back to respiratory mucosal sites during the late incubation period, permitting spread to susceptible contacts before the appearance of rash. Host immune responses limit viral replication and facilitate recovery from infection. In the immunocompromised child, the failure of immune responses, especially cell-mediated immune responses, results in continued viral replication with resultant injury to lungs, liver, brain, and other organs.

VZV establishes latent infection in sensory ganglia cells in all individuals who experience primary infection. Subsequent reactivation of latent virus causes herpes zoster, a vesicular rash that usually is dermatomal in distribution. During herpes zoster, necrotic changes may be produced in the associated ganglia. The skin lesions of varicella and herpes zoster have identical histopathology, and infectious VZV is present in both. Varicella elicits humoral and cell-mediated immunity that is highly protective against symptomatic re-infection. Suppression of cell-mediated immunity to VZV correlates with an increased risk of VZV reactivation as herpes zoster.

Clinical Manifestations. Varicella is an acute febrile rash illness, common in children who have not been immunized. It has variable severity but is usually self-limited. It may be associated with severe complications, including bacterial super-infection, pneumonia, encephalitis, bleeding disorders, congenital infection, and life-threatening perinatal infection. Herpes zoster, uncommon in children, causes localized cutaneous symptoms, but may disseminate in immunocompromised patients.

VARICELLA. The illness usually begins 14–16 days after exposure, although the incubation period can range from 10–21 days. Subclinical varicella is rare; almost all exposed, susceptible children experience a rash, but illness may be limited to only a few lesions. Prodromal symptoms may be present, particularly in older children. Fever, malaise, anorexia, headache, and occasionally mild abdominal pain may occur 24–48 hr before the rash appears. Temperature elevation is usually moderate, usually from 100–102°F but may be as high as 106°F; fever and other systemic symptoms persist during the first 2–4 days after the onset of the rash.

Varicella lesions often appear first on the scalp, face, or trunk. The initial exanthem consists of intensely pruritic erythematous macules that evolve through the papular stage to form clear, fluid-filled vesicles. Clouding and umbilication of the lesions begin in 24–48 hr. While the initial lesions are crusting, new crops form on the trunk and then the extremities; the simultaneous presence of lesions in various stages of evolution is characteristic of varicella (Fig. 232–1). The distribution of the rash is predominantly central or centripetal in contrast to smallpox, where the rash is more prominent on the face and distal extremities. Ulcerative lesions involving the oropharynx and vagina are also common; many children have vesicular lesions on the eyelids and conjunctivae, but corneal involvement and serious ocular disease is rare. The average number of varicella lesions is about 300, but healthy children may have fewer than 10 to more than 1,500 lesions. In cases resulting from secondary household spread and in older children, more lesions usually occur, and new crops of lesions may continue to develop for a longer period of time. The exanthem may be much more extensive in children with skin disorders, such as eczema or recent sunburn. Hypopigmentation or hyperpigmentation of lesion sites persists for days to weeks in some children, but severe scarring is unusual unless the lesions were secondarily infected.

The differential diagnosis of varicella includes vesicular rashes caused by other infectious agents, such as herpes simplex virus, enterovirus, or *Staphylococcus aureus*; drug reactions; contact dermatitis; and insect bites. Severe varicella was the most common illness confused with smallpox before the eradication of this disease.

BREAKTHROUGH VARICELLA. Vaccine is more than 95% effective in preventing typical varicella and is 70–90% effective at preventing all disease. Asymptomatic infection with wild-type virus may occur frequently in the previously immunized child. Breakthrough disease is varicella in a child vaccinated more than 42 days before rash onset and is due to wild-type VZV. Rash occurring within the first 2 weeks of vaccination is most commonly wild-type VZV, rash occurring 2–6 weeks after vaccination could be due to either the wild or vaccine strains. The rash in breakthrough disease is frequently atypical, predominantly maculopapular, vesicles are uncommon, being seen in only about 6% of cases, and the illness is most commonly mild with fewer than 50 lesions and little or no fever. Children with breakthrough disease should be considered potentially infectious and excluded from school until lesions have crusted or, if there are no vesicles present, until no new lesions are occurring. Transmission has been documented to occur from breakthrough cases in household, childcare, and school settings.

PROGRESSIVE VARICELLA. Progressive varicella, with visceral organ involvement, coagulopathy, severe hemorrhage, and continued lesion development is a dreaded complication of primary VZV infection. Severe abdominal pain and the appearance of hemorrhagic vesicles in otherwise healthy adolescents and adults, immunocompromised children, pregnant women, and newborns may herald this. The risk of progressive varicella is highest in children with congenital cellular immune deficiency disorders and those with malignancy, particularly if chemotherapy was given during the incubation period and the absolute lymphocyte count is <500 cells/mm^3. In one large series, the mortality rate for children who acquired varicella while undergoing treatment for malignancy and who were not treated with antiviral therapy was 7%. In this series all varicella-related deaths occurred within 3 days after the diagnosis of varicella pneumonia. Children who acquire varicella after organ transplantation are also at risk for progressive VZV infection. Children on long-term, low-dose systemic corticosteroid therapy are not considered to be at higher risk of severe varicella, but progressive varicella does occur in patients receiving high-dose corticosteroids and has been reported in patients receiving inhaled corticosteroids. Unusual clinical findings of varicella, including lesions that develop a unique hyperkeratotic appearance and the continued new lesion formation for weeks or months, have been described in children with HIV infection.

NEONATAL CHICKENPOX. Newborns have particularly high mortality in the circumstances of a susceptible mother contracting varicella around the time of delivery. Birth within 1 wk before or after the onset of maternal varicella frequently results in the newborn developing varicella, which may be severe. The initial infection is intrauterine, although the newborn often develops clinical chickenpox postpartum. The risk to the newborn is dependent on the amount of maternal anti-VZV antibody that the fetus acquired transplacentally before birth. If there was 1 wk or greater interval between maternal chickenpox and parturition, it is likely that the newborn received sufficient transplacental antibody to VZV to ameliorate neonatal infection. Alternatively, if the interval was less than 1 wk, the newborn will be unlikely to have protective VZV antibody and neonatal chickenpox may be exceptionally severe.

The recommendations for varicella-zoster immune globulin (VZIG) reflect the differing risks to the exposed infant. Newborns whose mothers develop varicella 5 days before to 2 days after delivery should receive one vial. Although neonatal varicella may occur in about half of these infants despite administration of VZIG, it is usually mild. Every premature infant born to a mother with active chickenpox at delivery (even if present > 1 wk) should receive VZIG. Because perinatally acquired varicella may be life threatening, it should be treated with acyclovir (10 mg/kg q 8 hr IV). Neonatal chickenpox can also follow a postpartum exposure of an infant delivered to a mother who was susceptible to VZV, although the frequency of complications declines rapidly in the weeks after birth. Infants with commu-

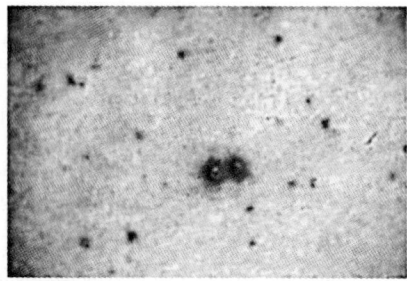

FIGURE 232–1. Skin lesions of chickenpox. Note the varying stages of development (macules, papules, and vesicles) present at the same time. See also color plates. (Courtesy of PF Lucchesi.)

nity-acquired chickenpox who develop severe varicella, especially those who develop a complication such as pneumonia, hepatitis, or encephalitis, should also receive treatment with intravenous acyclovir (10 mg/kg q 8 hr IV).

CONGENITAL VARICELLA SYNDROME. When pregnant women contract chickenpox, about 25% of the fetuses may become infected although not every infected fetus is clinically affected. However, up to 2% of fetuses whose mothers had varicella in the first 20 weeks of pregnancy may demonstrate VZV embryopathy. The period of greatest risk to the fetus correlates with the gestational period when there is major development and innervation of the limb buds and maturation of the eyes. Fetuses infected at 6–12 wk of gestation appear to have maximal interruption with limb development; fetuses infected at 16–20 wk may have eye and brain involvement. In addition, viral damage to the sympathetic fibers in the cervical and lumbosacral cord may lead to divergent effects such as Horner syndrome and dysfunction of the urethral or anal sphincters. Most of the stigmata can be attributed to virus-induced injury to the nervous system, although there is no obvious explanation why certain regions of the body are preferentially infected during fetal VZV infection. The stigmata involve mainly the skin, extremities, eyes, and brain (Box 232–1). The characteristic cutaneous lesion has been called a cicatrix, a zigzag scarring, often in a dermatomal distribution. The characteristic cicatricial scarring may represent the cutaneous residua of VZV infection of the sensory nerves, analogous to herpes zoster. The virus may select tissues that are in a rapid developmental stage, such as the limb buds. This may result in one or more shortened and malformed extremities (Fig. 232–2). Frequently, the atrophic extremity is covered with a cicatrix. The remainder of the torso may be entirely normal in appearance. Alternatively, there may be neither skin nor limb abnormalities but the infant may show cataracts or even extensive aplasia of the entire brain. Occasionally, calcifications are evident within a microcephalic head (Fig. 232–3). Histologic examination of the brain demonstrates necrotizing cerebral lesions involving the leptomeninges, the cortex, and the adjacent white matter.

Many infants with severe manifestations of congenital varicella syndrome have significant neurologic deficiencies, whereas those with only isolated stigmata, amenable to treatment, develop normally throughout childhood. Infants with neonatal chickenpox who receive prompt antiviral therapy have an excellent prognosis.

The diagnosis of VZV fetopathy is based mainly on the history of gestational chickenpox combined with the stigmata seen in the fetus. Virus cannot be cultured from the affected newborn, but viral DNA can be detected in tissue samples by PCR. Some

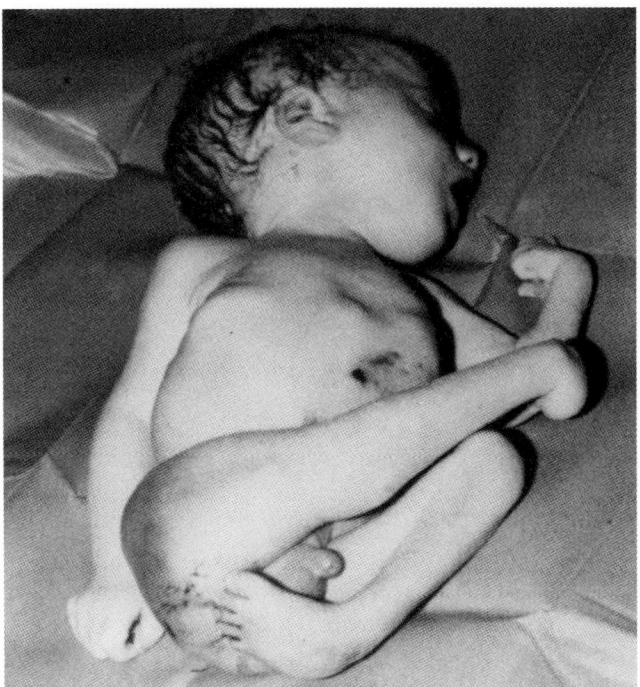

FIGURE 232–2. Newborn with congenital varicella syndrome. The infant had severe malformations of both lower extremities and cicatricial scarring over his left abdomen.

infants have VZV-specific IgM antibody detectable in the cord blood sample, although the IgM titer drops quickly postpartum. Chorionic villus sampling and fetal blood collection for the detection of viral DNA, virus, or antibody have been used in an attempt to diagnose fetal infection and embryopathy. The usefulness of these tests for patient management and counseling has not been defined. Because these tests may not distinguish between infection and disease, their utility may primarily be that of reassurance when the test is negative.

Although VZIG is often administered to the susceptible mother exposed to chickenpox, it is uncertain as to whether this modifies infection in the fetus. Similarly, acyclovir treatment may be given to the mother with severe varicella; however, neither its safety nor its efficacy for the fetus is known. The damage caused by fetal VZV infection does not progress postpartum, an indication that there is no persistent viral replication. Thus, antiviral treatment of infants with congenital VZV syndrome is not indicated.

HERPES ZOSTER. Herpes zoster is manifested as vesicular lesions clustered within one or less commonly two adjacent dermatomes (Fig. 232–4). Unlike zoster in adults, zoster in children is infrequently associated with localized pain, hyperesthesias, pruritus, and low-grade fever. In children, the rash is mild, with new lesions appearing for a few days; symptoms of acute neuritis are minimal; and complete resolution usually occurs within 1–2 wk. In contrast to adults, postherpetic neuralgia is very unusual in children. Approximately 4% of patients suffer a second episode of herpes zoster; 3 or more episodes are rare. Transverse myelitis with transient paralysis is a rare complication of herpes zoster. An increased risk of herpes zoster early in childhood has been described in children who acquire varicella in the first year of life as well as in those whose mothers have a varicella infection in the third trimester of pregnancy.

Immunocompromised children may have more severe herpes zoster, which is similar to that in adults, including postherpetic neuralgia. Immunocompromised patients may also experience disseminated cutaneous disease that mimics varicella, as well as

---

BOX 232–1. Stigmata of Varicella-Zoster Virus Fetopathy

Damage to Sensory Nerves
  Cicatricial skin lesions
  Hypopigmentation
Damage to Optic Stalk and Lens Vesicle
  Microphthalmia
  Cataracts
  Chorioretinitis
  Optic atrophy
Damage to Brain/Encephalitis
  Microcephaly
  Hydrocephaly
  Calcifications
  Aplasia of brain
Damage to Cervical or Lumbosacral Cord
  Hypoplasia of an extremity
  Motor and sensory deficits
  Absent deep tendon reflexes
  Anisocoria
  Horner syndrome
  Anal/urinary sphincter dysfunction

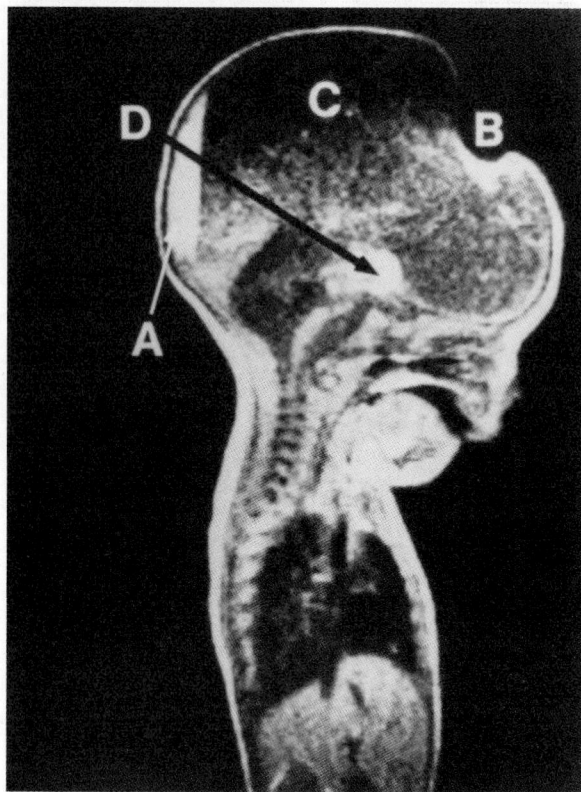

FIGURE 232–3. Magnetic resonance image of newborn with encephalitis secondary to congenital varicella syndrome. The intrauterine infection occurred about 3 mo antepartum, at which time there was extensive necrosis of the cerebral hemispheres. The image of the newborn head was taken with the patient supine; therefore, there is a fluid/fluid interface in the dependent occiput (A). The hydrocephalus (C) and calcifications in the basal ganglia (D) are visible; a cranial artifact (B) is seen secondary to a scalp vein needle.

visceral dissemination with pneumonia, hepatitis, encephalitis, and disseminated intravascular coagulopathy. Severely immunocompromised children, particularly those with HIV infection, may have unusual, chronic, or relapsing cutaneous disease, retinitis, or central nervous system disease without rash. A lower risk of herpes zoster in vaccinated children with leukemia compared with those who have had varicella disease suggests that varicella vaccine virus reactivates less commonly than wild-type VZV.

Diagnosis. Laboratory evaluation has not been considered necessary for the diagnosis or management of healthy children with

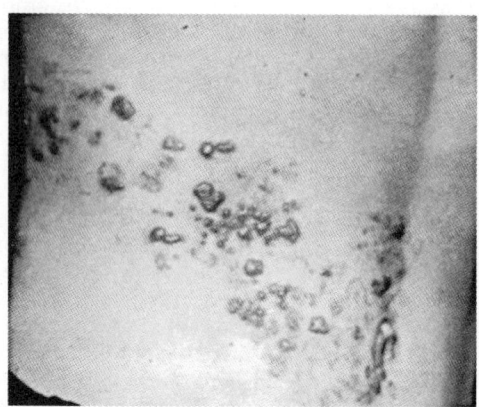

FIGURE 232–4. Herpes zoster.

varicella or herpes zoster. However, as disease declines to low levels, laboratory confirmation of all varicella cases will become necessary. Leukopenia is typical during the first 72 hours; it is followed by a relative and absolute lymphocytosis. Results of liver function tests are also usually (75%) mildly elevated. Patients with neurologic complications of varicella or uncomplicated herpes zoster have a mild lymphocytic pleocytosis and a slight to moderate increase in protein in the cerebrospinal fluid; the glucose concentration is usually normal.

Unusual or very severe varicella in otherwise immunocompetent individuals must be distinguished from smallpox, which may occur following deliberate release of smallpox virus (Chapter 706). A suspected case of smallpox should be reported immediately to the local and state health departments. A protocol for evaluating patients with acute vesicular-pustular rash illness for the possibility of smallpox is available on the CDC website at www.cdc.gov/nip/.

Rapid laboratory diagnosis of VZV is often important in high-risk patients and is sometimes important for infection control. Confirmation of varicella (or herpes simplex virus) can be accomplished by most referral hospital laboratories. VZV can be identified quickly by direct fluorescence assay (DFA) of cells from cutaneous lesions, which is widely available, and by polymerase chain reaction (PCR) amplification testing. Although multinucleated giant cells can be detected with nonspecific stains (**Tzanck smear**), they have poor sensitivity and do not differentiate VZV and herpes simplex virus infections. Infectious virus may be recovered using tissue culture methods; newer methods have decreased time needed for culture from 7–10 days to 3–4 days. VZV immunoglobulin G (IgG) antibodies can be detected by several methods and a 4-fold rise in IgG antibodies is also confirmatory of acute infection. VZV IgG antibody tests can also be valuable to determine the immune status of individuals whose clinical history of varicella is unknown or equivocal. Testing for VZV IgM antibodies is not useful for clinical diagnosis because commercially available methods are unreliable. A capture IgM assay is available at the national VZV laboratory at CDC

Treatment. Antiviral treatment modifies the course of both varicella and herpes zoster. Antiviral drug resistance is rare but has occurred in children with HIV infection who have been treated. Foscarnet is the only drug now available for the treatment of acyclovir-resistant VZV infections.

VARICELLA. The only antiviral drug available in liquid formulation and that is licensed for pediatric use is acyclovir. Given the safety profile of acyclovir and its demonstrated efficacy in the treatment of varicella, treatment of all children, adolescents, and adults with varicella is acceptable. However, acyclovir therapy is not recommended routinely by the American Academy of Pediatrics for treatment of uncomplicated varicella in the otherwise healthy child because of the marginal benefit, the cost of the drug, and the low risk of complications. Oral therapy with acyclovir (20 mg/kg/dose; maximum: 800 mg/dose) given as 4 doses per day for 5 days should be used to treat uncomplicated varicella in nonpregnant individuals 13 yr of age or older and children 12 mo of age or older with chronic cutaneous or pulmonary disorders; receiving short-term, intermittent, or aerosolized corticosteroids; receiving long-term salicylate therapy; and possibly second cases in household contacts. To be most effective, treatment should be initiated as early as possible, preferably within 24 hr of the onset of the exanthem. There is dubious clinical benefit if initiation of treatment is delayed more than 72 hr after onset of the exanthem. Acyclovir therapy does not interfere with the induction of VZV immunity. Intravenous therapy is indicated for severe disease and for varicella in immunocompromised patients. Acyclovir has been used to treat varicella in pregnant women; however, its safety for the fetus has not been established. Any patient who has signs of disseminated VZV including pneumonia, severe hepatitis, thrombocytopenia, or encephalitis should receive immediate treatment. Intravenous acyclovir (500 mg/m^2 q 8 hr IV) therapy initiated within 72 hr of development of initial symptoms decreases the likelihood of progressive varicella and visceral dissemination in high-risk patients. Treatment is continued for 7 days or until no new lesions have appeared for 48 hr. Delaying antiviral treatment until prolonged new lesion formation is evident is not advisable because visceral dissemination occurs during the same time period.

HERPES ZOSTER. Antiviral drugs are effective for treatment of herpes zoster. In healthy adults, acyclovir (800 mg 5 times a day PO for 5 days), famciclovir (500 mg tid PO for 7 days), and valacyclovir (1,000 mg tid PO for 7 days) reduce the duration of the illness and the risk of developing postherpetic neuralgia; concomitant corticosteroid usage improves the quality of life in the elderly. In otherwise healthy children, however, herpes zoster is a less severe disease, and postherpetic neuralgia is rare. Therefore, treatment of uncomplicated herpes zoster in the child with an antiviral agent may not always be necessary, although some experts would treat with oral acyclovir (20 mg/kg/dose; maximum 800 mg/dose) to shorten the duration of the illness. Use of corticosteroids for herpes zoster in otherwise healthy children is not recommended.

In contrast, herpes zoster in immunocompromised children can be severe and disseminated disease may be life threatening. Patients at high risk for disseminated disease should receive acyclovir (500 mg/m^2 or 10 mg/kg q 8 hr IV). Oral acyclovir is an option for immunocompromised patients with uncomplicated herpes zoster and who are considered at low risk for visceral dissemination.

Complications. The complications of VZV infection occur with varicella, or with reactivation of infection, more commonly in immunocompromised patients. In the otherwise healthy child, mild varicella hepatitis is relatively common but rarely clinically symptomatic. Mild thrombocytopenia occurs in 1–2% of children with varicella and may be associated with transient petechiae. Purpura, hemorrhagic vesicles, hematuria, and gastrointestinal bleeding are rare complications that may have serious consequences. Cerebellar ataxia occurs in 1 in every 4000 cases. Other complications, some of them rare, of varicella include encephalitis, pneumonia, nephritis, nephrotic syndrome, hemolytic-uremic syndrome, arthritis, myocarditis, pericarditis, pancreatitis, and orchitis.

BACTERIAL INFECTIONS. Secondary bacterial infections of the skin, usually caused by *Streptococcus* and *Staphylococcus*, may occur in up to 5% of children with varicella. These range from superficial impetigo to cellulitis, lymphadenitis, and subcutaneous abscesses. An early manifestation of secondary bacterial infection is erythema of the base of a new vesicle. Recrudescence of fever 3–4 days after the initial exanthem may also herald a secondary bacterial infection. Varicella is a well-described risk factor for serious infections caused by group A streptococcus. The more invasive infections, such as varicella gangrenosa, bacterial sepsis, pneumonia, arthritis, osteomyelitis, and necrotizing fasciitis, account for much of the morbidity and mortality of varicella in otherwise healthy children. Bacterial toxin–mediated diseases (e.g., toxic shock syndrome) also may complicate varicella.

ENCEPHALITIS AND CEREBELLAR ATAXIA. Encephalitis and acute cerebellar ataxia are well-described neurologic complications of varicella; morbidity from central nervous system complications is highest among patients younger than 5 yr or older than 20 yr of age. Nuchal rigidity, altered consciousness, and seizures characterize meningoencephalitis. Patients with cerebellar ataxia have a gradual onset of gait disturbance, nystagmus, and slurred speech. Neurologic symptoms usually begin 2–6 days after the onset of the rash but may occur during the

incubation period or after resolution of the rash. Clinical recovery is typically rapid, occurring within 24–72 hr, and is usually complete. Although severe hemorrhagic encephalitis, analogous to that caused by herpes simplex virus, is very rare in children with varicella, the consequences are similar to herpes encephalitis. Reye syndrome of encephalopathy and hepatic dysfunction associated with varicella has become rare since salicylates are no longer routinely used as antipyretics (Chapter 342).

PNEUMONIA. Varicella pneumonia is a severe complication that accounts for most of the increased morbidity and mortality in adults and other high-risk populations, but pneumonia may also complicate varicella in young children. Respiratory symptoms, which may include cough, dyspnea, cyanosis, pleuritic chest pain, and hemoptysis, usually begin within 1–6 days after the onset of the rash. Smoking has been described as a risk factor for severe pneumonia complicating varicella. The frequency of varicella pneumonia may be greater in the parturient and may lead to premature termination of pregnancy.

Prognosis. Primary varicella has a mortality rate of 2–3 per 100,000 cases with the lowest case fatality rates among children 1–4 years and 5–9 years (approximately 1 death per 100,000 cases). Compared with these age groups, infants have a 4 times greater risk of dying and adults have a 25 times greater high risk of dying. Approximately 100 deaths occurred in the United States annually before the introduction of the VZV vaccine; the most common complications among people who died from varicella were pneumonia, CNS complications, secondary infections, and hemorrhagic conditions. The mortality rate of untreated primary infection in immunocompromised children is 7–14% and may approach 50% in adults. Varicella morbidity has declined in recent years as vaccine coverage has improved. It is expected that when data are available, a decline in mortality will also be apparent.

Neuritis with herpes zoster should be managed with appropriate analgesics. Postherpetic neuralgia can be a severe problem in adults and may persist for months, requiring care by a specialist in pain management.

Prevention. VZV transmission is difficult to prevent because the infection is contagious for 24–48 hr before the rash appears. Infection control practices, including caring for infected patients in isolation rooms with filtered air systems, are essential. All health care workers should have documented VZV immunization or immunity. Susceptible health care workers who have had a close exposure to VZV should not care for high-risk patients during the incubation period.

VACCINE. Varicella is a vaccine-preventable disease. Live virus vaccine is recommended for routine administration in children at 12–18 mo of age. Older children, adolescents and adults without a history of VZV infection should also be immunized. Children 12 mo to 12 yr receive a single vaccine dose; adolescents and adults require 2 vaccine doses, a minimum of 4 wk apart. Live virus vaccine is contraindicated in children with cell-mediated immune deficiencies, although the vaccine may be administered to children with acute lymphoblastic leukemia who are in remission and who meet enrollment criteria under a research protocol, and the vaccine may also be considered for HIV-infected children with CD4% greater than 25%. Both these groups receive 2 doses of vaccine, 3 months apart. Administration of varicella vaccine within 4 wk of MMR vaccine has been associated with a higher risk of breakthrough disease; therefore, it is recommended that the vaccines either be administered simultaneously at different sites or be given at least 4 weeks apart. Vaccine virus establishes latent infection; however, the risk of developing subsequent herpes zoster is lower after vaccine than after natural VZV infection among immunocompromised children. Post-licensure data also suggest the same trend in healthy vaccinees. Post-licensure effectiveness studies and ongoing studies of the persistence of immunity after vaccination, however, may ultimately demonstrate a need for children to receive a booster dose of vaccine.

POSTEXPOSURE PROPHYLAXIS. Varicella-zoster immune globulin (VZIG) postexposure prophylaxis is recommended for immunocompromised children, pregnant women, and newborns exposed to maternal varicella. VZIG is distributed by FFF Enterprises, California. The dosage is 1 vial (125 units) for each 10 kg increment (maximum: 625 units) given intramuscularly as soon as possible but within 96 hr after exposure.

Newborns whose mothers develop varicella 5 days before to 2 days after delivery should receive one vial of VZIG. Adults should be tested for VZV IgG antibodies before VZIG administration because many adults with no clinical history of varicella are immune. VZIG prophylaxis may ameliorate disease but does not eliminate the possibility of progressive disease; patients should be monitored and treated with acyclovir if necessary. Immunocompromised patients who have received high-dose intravenous immune globulin (100–400 mg/kg) for other indications within 2–3 wk before the exposure can be expected to have serum antibodies to VZV.

Close contact between a susceptible high-risk patient and a patient with herpes zoster is also an indication for VZIG prophylaxis. Passive antibody administration or treatment does not reduce the risk of herpes zoster or alter the clinical course of varicella or herpes zoster when given after the onset of symptoms.

Vaccine given to normal children within 3–5 days exposure is effective in preventing or modifying varicella, especially in a household setting where exposure is very likely to result in infection. Varicella vaccine is now recommended for postexposure use, for outbreak control. Oral acyclovir administered late in the incubation period may modify subsequent varicella in the normal child. However, its use in this manner is not recommended until it can be further evaluated.

Arvin AM: Varicella-zoster virus. *Clin Microbiol Rev* 1996;9:361–8.

Brunell PA: Varicella in pregnancy, the fetus and the newborn. Problems in management. *J Infect Dis* 1992;(Suppl 1):S42–7.

Centers for Disease Control and Prevention: Prevention of varicella. Recommendations of the Advisory Committee on Immunization Practices (ACIP). *MMWR* 1996;45:1–36.

Centers for Disease Control and Prevention: Varicella-related deaths among adults—United States, 1997. *MMWR* 1997;46:409–12.

Choo PW, Donahue JG, Manson JE, et al: The epidemiology of varicella and its complications. *J Infect Dis* 1995;172:706–12.

Connelly BL, Stanberry LR, Bernstein DI: Detection of varicella-zoster virus DNA in nasopharyngeal secretions of immune household contacts of varicella. *J Infect Dis* 1993;168:1253–5.

Dunkle LM, Arvin AM, Whitley RJ, et al: A controlled trial of acyclovir for chickenpox in normal children. *N Engl J Med* 1991;325:1539–44.

Enders G, Miller E. Cradock-Watson J, et al: Consequences of varicella and herpes zoster in pregnancy. Prospective study of 1739 cases. *Lancet* 1994;343:1548–51.

Gershon AA, LaRussa P: Varicella vaccine. *Pediatr Infect Dis J* 1998;17:248–9.

Gershon AA, Mervish N, LaRussa P, et al: Varicella-zoster virus infection in children with underlying human immunodeficiency virus infection. *J Infect Dis* 1997;176:1496–500.

Grose C: Congenital infections caused by varicella zoster virus and herpes simplex virus. *Semin Pediatr Neurol* 1994;1:43–9.

Guess HA, Broughton DD, Melton LJ II, et al: Population-based studies of varicella complications. *Pediatrics* 1986;78:723–7.

Kustermann A, Zoppini C, Tassis B, et al: Prenatal diagnosis of congenital varicella infection. *Prenat Diagn* 1996;16:71–4.

Meyer PA, Seward JF, Jumaan AO, et al: Varicella mortality: Trends before vaccine licensure in the United States 1970–1994. *J Infect Dis* 2000;182:383–90.

Nader S, Bergen R, Sharp M, et al: Age-related differences in cell-mediated immunity to varicella zoster virus among children and adults immunized with live attenuated varicella vaccine. *J Infect Dis* 1995;171:13–7.

Pastuszak AL, Levy M, Schick B, et al: Outcome after maternal varicella infection in the first 20 weeks of pregnancy. *N Engl J Med* 1994;330:901–5.

Peterson CL, Mascola L, Chao SM, et al: Children hospitalized for varicella. A pre vaccine review. *J Pediatr* 1996;129:529–36.

Petursson G, Helgason S, Gudmundsson S, et al: Herpes zoster in children and adolescents. *Pediatr Infect Dis J* 1998;17:905–8.

Seward JF, Watson BM, Peterson CL, et al: Varicella disease after the introduction of varicella vaccine in the United States, 1995–2000. *JAMA* 2002;287:606–11.

Watson BM, Piercy SA, Plotkin SA, et al: Modified chickenpox in children immunized with the Oka/Merck varicella vaccine. *Pediatrics* 1993;91:17–22.

Wood MJ, Johnson RW, McKendrick MW, et al. A randomized trial of acyclovir for 7 days or 21 days with and without prednisolone for treatment of acute herpes zoster. *N Engl J Med* 1994;330:896–900.

Zerboni L, Nader S, Aoki K, et al: Analysis of the persistence of humoral and cellular immunity in children and adults immunized with varicella vaccine. *J Infect Dis* 1998;177:1701–4.

Chapter 233
Epstein-Barr Virus *Hal B. Jenson*

Infectious mononucleosis is the best-known clinical syndrome caused by Epstein-Barr virus (EBV). It is characterized by systemic somatic complaints consisting primarily of fatigue, malaise, fever, sore throat, and generalized lymphadenopathy. Originally described as **glandular fever**, it derives its name from the mononuclear lymphocytosis with atypical-appearing lymphocytes that accompany the illness. Other infections may cause infectious mononucleosis-like illnesses.

Etiology. EBV, a member of the γ-herpesviruses, causes more than 90% of infectious mononucleosis cases. As many as 5–10% of infectious mononucleosis-like illnesses are caused by primary infection with cytomegalovirus, *Toxoplasma gondii*, adenovirus, viral hepatitis, HIV, and possibly rubella virus. In the majority of EBV-negative infectious mononucleosis-like illnesses, the exact cause remains unknown.

Epidemiology. The epidemiology of infectious mononucleosis is related to the epidemiology and age of acquisition of EBV infection. EBV infects >95% of the world's population. It is transmitted in oral secretions by close contact such as kissing or exchange of saliva from child to child, such as occurs between children in out-of-home child care. Nonintimate contact, environmental sources, or fomites do not contribute to spread of EBV.

EBV is shed in oral secretions for >6 mo after acute infection and then intermittently for life. As many as 20–30% of healthy EBV-infected persons excrete virus at any particular time. Immunosuppression permits reactivation of latent EBV; 60–90% of EBV-infected immunosuppressed patients shed the virus. EBV is also found in the genital tract of women and may be spread by sexual contact.

Infection with EBV in developing countries and among socioeconomically disadvantaged populations of developed countries usually occurs during infancy and early childhood. In central Africa, almost all children are infected by 3 yr of age. Primary infection with EBV during childhood is usually inapparent or indistinguishable from other childhood infections; the clinical syndrome of infectious mononucleosis is practically unknown in undeveloped regions of the world. Among more affluent populations in industrialized countries, infection during childhood is still most common, but approximately one third of cases occur during adolescence and young adulthood. Primary EBV infection in adolescents and adults is manifest in >50% of cases by the classic triad of fatigue, pharyngitis, and generalized lymphadenopathy, which constitute the major clinical manifestations of infectious mononucleosis. This syndrome may be seen at all ages but is rarely apparent in children <4 yr of age, when most EBV infections are asymptomatic, or in adults >40 yr of age, when most individuals have already been infected by EBV. The true incidence of the syndrome of infectious mononucleosis is unknown but is estimated to occur in 20–70/100,000 persons/yr; in young adults, the incidence increases to about 1/1,000 persons/yr. The prevalence of serologic evidence of past EBV infection increases with age; almost all adults in the United States are seropositive.

Pathogenesis. After acquisition in the oral cavity, EBV initially infects oral epithelial cells; this may contribute to the symptoms of pharyngitis. After intracellular viral replication and cell lysis with release of new virions, virus spreads to contiguous structures such as the salivary glands, with eventual viremia and infection of B lymphocytes in the peripheral blood and the entire lymphoreticular system, including the liver and spleen. The atypical lymphocytes that are characteristic of infectious mononucleosis are CD8+ T lymphocytes, which exhibit both suppressor and cytotoxic functions that develop in response to the infected B lymphocytes. This relative as well as absolute increase in CD8+ lymphocytes results in a transient reversal of the normal 2rc1 CD4+/CD8+ (helper-suppressor) T-lymphocyte ratio. Many of the clinical manifestations of infectious mononucleosis may result, at least in part, from the host immune response, which is effective in reducing the number of EBV-infected B lymphocytes to less than 1 per 10^6 of circulating B lymphocytes.

Epithelial cells of the uterine cervix may become infected by sexual transmission of the virus, although neither local symptoms nor infectious mononucleosis have been described after sexual transmission.

EBV, like the other herpesviruses, establishes lifelong latent infection after the primary illness. The latent virus is carried in oropharyngeal epithelial cells and systemic B lymphocytes as multiple episomes in the nucleus. The viral episomes replicate with cell division and are distributed to both daughter cells. Viral integration into the cell genome is not typical. Only a few viral proteins, including the EBV-determined antigens (EBNA), are produced during latency. These proteins are important in maintaining the viral episome during the latent state. Progression to viral replication begins with production of EBV early antigens (EA), proceeds to viral DNA replication, is followed by production of viral capsid antigen (VCA), and culminates in cell death and release of mature virions. Reactivation with viral replication occurs at a low rate in populations of latently infected cells and is responsible for intermittent viral shedding in oropharyngeal secretions of infected individuals. Reactivation is apparently asymptomatic and not recognized to be accompanied by distinctive clinical symptoms.

ONCOGENESIS. EBV was the first human virus to be associated with malignancy and, therefore, was the first virus to be identified as a human tumor virus. EBV infection may result in a spectrum of proliferative disorders ranging from self-limited, usually benign disease such as infectious mononucleosis to aggressive, nonmalignant proliferations such as the virus-associated hemophagocytic syndrome to lymphoid and epithelial cell malignancies. Benign EBV-associated proliferations include oral hairy leukoplakia, primarily in adults with AIDS, and lymphoid interstitial pneumonitis, primarily in children with AIDS. Malignant EBV-associated proliferations include nasopharyngeal carcinoma, Burkitt lymphoma, Hodgkin disease, lymphoproliferative disorders, and leiomyosarcoma in immunodeficient states, including AIDS.

Nasopharyngeal carcinoma occurs worldwide but is 10 times more common in persons in southern China, where it is the most common malignant tumor among adult men. It is also common among whites in North Africa and Inuits in North America. Patients usually present with cervical lymphadenopathy and eustachian tube blockage and nasal obstruction with epistaxis. All malignant cells of undifferentiated nasopharyngeal carcinoma contain a high copy number of EBV episomes. Persons with undifferentiated and partially differentiated, nonkeratinizing nasopharyngeal carcinomas have elevated EBV antibody titers that are both diagnostic and prognostic. High levels of immunoglobulin (Ig) A antibody to EA and VCA may be detected in asymptomatic individuals and can be used to follow response to tumor therapy (Table 233–1). Cells of well-differentiated, keratinizing nasopharyngeal carcinoma contain a low or zero copy number of EBV genomes; these persons have EBV serologic patterns similar to those of the general population.

CT and MRI images are helpful in both identifying and defining masses in the head and neck. The diagnosis is established by biopsy of the mass or of a suspicious cervical lymph node. Surgery is important for staging and diagnosis. Radiation therapy is effective for control of the primary tumor and regional nodal metastases. Chemotherapy with 5-fluorouracil, cisplatin, and methotrexate is effective but not always curative. The prognosis is good if the tumor is localized.

Endemic (African) Burkitt lymphoma, often found in the jaw, is the most common childhood cancer in equatorial East Africa and New Guinea (Chapter 488.2). The median age at onset is 5 yr. These regions are holoendemic for *Plasmodium falciparum* malaria and have a high rate of EBV infection early in life.

TABLE 233–1. Correlation of Clinical Status and Serologic Responses to EBV Infection

Clinical Status	Heterophile Antibodies (Qualitative Test)	Serologic Response				
		EBV-Specific Antibody				
		IgM-VCA	IgG-VCA	EA-D	EA-R	EBNA
Negative reaction	−	<1:8*	<1:10*	<1:10*	<1:10*	<1:2.5*
Susceptible	−	−	−	−	−†	−
Acute primary infection: infectious mononucleosis	+	1:32 to 1:256	1:160 to 1:640	1:40 to 1:160	−†	− to 1:2.5
Recent primary infection: infectious mononucleosis	+/−	− to 1:32	1:320 to 1:1,280	1:40 to 1:160	−†	1:5 to 1:10
Remote infection	−	−	1:40 to 1:160	−‡	− to 1:40	1:10 to 1:40
Reactivation: immunosuppressed or immunocompromised	−	−	1:320 to 1:1,280	−‡	1:80 to 1:320	− to 1:160
Burkitt lymphoma	−	−	1:320 to 1:1,280	−‡	1:80 to 1:320	1:10 to 1:80
Nasopharyngeal carcinoma	−	−	1:320 to 1:1,280	1:40 to 1:160	−§	1:20 to 1:160

The data were obtained from numerous studies. Individual responses outside the characteristic range may occur.
*Or the lowest test dilution.
†In young children and adults with asymptomatic seroconversion, the anti–early antigen response may be mainly to the EA-R component.
‡A minority of individuals will have the anti–early antigen response mainly to the EA-D component.
§A minority of individuals will have the anti–early antigen response mainly to the EA-R component.
EBV = Epstein-Barr virus; − = negative; + = positive; IgM = immunoglobulin M; IgG = immunoglobulin G; VCA = viral capsid antigen; EA-D = diffuse staining component of EA; EA-R = cytoplasmic restricted component of early antigen; EBNA = EBV-determined nuclear antigens.
Reprinted with permission from Jenson HB, Ench Y: Epstein-Barr virus. In Rose NR, Hamilton RB, Detrick B (editors): Manual of Clinical Laboratory Immunology, 6th ed. Washington, DC, American Society for Microbiology, 2002.

The constant malarial exposure acts as a B-lymphocyte mitogen that contributes to the polyclonal B-lymphocyte proliferation with EBV infection. It also impairs the T-lymphocyte control of EBV-infected B lymphocytes. Approximately 98% of cases of endemic Burkitt lymphoma contain the EBV genome compared with only 20% of nonendemic (sporadic or American) Burkitt lymphoma cases. Individuals with Burkitt lymphoma have unusually and characteristically high levels of antibody to VCA and EA that correlate with the risk of developing tumor (see Table 233–1).

All cases of Burkitt lymphoma, including those that are EBV negative, are monoclonal and demonstrate chromosomal translocation of the c-*myc* proto-oncogene to the constant region of the immunoglobulin heavy-chain locus, t(8;14), to the kappa constant light-chain locus, t(2;8), or to the lambda constant light-chain locus, t(8;22). This results in the deregulation and constitutive transcription of the c-*myc* gene with overproduction of a normal c-*myc* product that autosuppresses c-*myc* production on the untranslocated chromosome.

The incidence of **Hodgkin disease** peaks in childhood in developing countries and in young adulthood in developed countries. Levels of EBV antibodies are consistently elevated preceding development of Hodgkin disease; only a small minority of patients are seronegative for EBV. Infection with EBV appears to increase the risk of Hodgkin disease by a factor of 2 to 4. EBV is associated with more than one half of cases of mixed cellularity Hodgkin disease and approximately one fourth of cases of the nodular sclerosing subtype and is rarely associated with lymphocyte-predominant Hodgkin disease. Immunohistochemical studies have localized EBV to the Reed-Sternberg cells and their variants, the pathognomonic malignant cells of Hodgkin disease.

Failure to control EBV infection may result from host immunologic deficits. The prototype is the **X-linked lymphoproliferative syndrome (Duncan syndrome)**, an X chromosome–linked recessive disorder of the immune system associated with severe, persistent, and sometimes fatal EBV infection (Chapter 114.7). Approximately two thirds of these male patients die of disseminated and fulminating lymphoproliferation involving multiple organs at the time of primary EBV infection. Surviving patients acquire hypogammaglobulinemia, B-cell lymphoma, or both. Most patients die within 10 yr.

A number of other congenital and acquired immunodeficiency syndromes are associated with an increased incidence of EBV-associated B-lymphocyte lymphoma, particularly central nervous system lymphoma and leiomyosarcoma. The incidence of lymphoproliferative syndromes parallels the degree of immunosuppression. A decline in T-cell function evidently permits EBV to escape from immune surveillance. Congenital immunodeficiencies predisposing to EBV-associated lymphoproliferations include the X-linked lymphoproliferative syndrome, common-variable immunodeficiency, ataxia-telangiectasia, Wiskott-Aldrich syndrome, and Chediak-Higashi syndrome. Individuals with acquired immunodeficiencies resulting from anticancer chemotherapy, immunosuppression after solid organ or bone marrow transplantation, or HIV infection have a significantly increased risk of EBV-associated lymphoproliferations. The lymphomas may be focal or diffuse, and they are usually histologically polyclonal but may become monoclonal. Their growth is not reversed on cessation of immunosuppression.

EBV has been credibly linked to leiomyosarcomas in HIV-infected patients and transplant patients, primary central nervous system lymphoma, and carcinoma of the salivary glands. Other tumors putatively associated with EBV include some T-lymphocyte lymphomas (including lethal midline), angioimmunoblastic lymphadenopathy-like lymphoma, thymomas and thymic carcinomas derived from thymic epithelial cells, supraglottic laryngeal carcinomas, lymphoepithelial tumors of the respiratory tract and gastrointestinal tract, and gastric adenocarcinoma. The precise contribution of EBV to these various malignancies is not well defined.

Clinical Manifestations. The incubation period of infectious mononucleosis in adolescents is 30–50 days. In children, it may be shorter. The majority of cases of primary EBV infection in infants and young children are clinically silent. In older patients, the onset of illness is usually insidious and vague. Patients may complain of malaise, fatigue, fever, headache, sore throat, nausea, abdominal pain, and myalgia. This prodromal period may last 1–2 wk. The complaints of sore throat and fever gradually increase until patients seek medical care. Splenic enlargement may be rapid enough to cause left upper quadrant abdominal discomfort and tenderness, which may be the presenting complaint.

The physical examination is characterized by generalized lymphadenopathy (90% of cases), splenomegaly (50% of cases), and hepatomegaly (10% of cases). Lymphadenopathy occurs most commonly in the anterior and posterior cervical nodes and the submandibular lymph nodes and less commonly in the axillary and inguinal lymph nodes. Epitrochlear lymphadenopathy is particularly suggestive of infectious mononucleosis. Symptomatic hepatitis or jaundice is uncommon. Splenomegaly to 2–3 cm below the costal margin is typical; massive enlargement is uncommon.

The sore throat is often accompanied by moderate to severe pharyngitis with marked tonsillar enlargement, occasionally with exudates (Fig. 233–1). Petechiae at the junction of the hard and soft palate are frequently seen. The pharyngitis resembles that caused by streptococcal infection. Other clinical findings may include rashes and edema of the eyelids. Rashes are usually maculopapular and have been reported in 3–15% of patients. Up to 80% of patients with infectious mononucleosis experience **"ampicillin rash"** if treated with ampicillin or amoxicillin. This vasculitic rash is probably immune-mediated and resolves without specific treatment.

Diagnosis. The diagnosis of infectious mononucleosis implies primary EBV infection. A presumptive diagnosis may be made by the presence of typical clinical symptoms with atypical lymphocytosis in the peripheral blood. The diagnosis is confirmed by serologic testing.

DIFFERENTIAL DIAGNOSIS. Infectious mononucleosis-like illnesses may be caused by primary infection with cytomegalovirus, *T. gondii*, adenovirus, viral hepatitis, HIV, or possibly rubella virus. Cytomegalovirus infection is a particularly common cause in adults. Streptococcal pharyngitis may cause sore throat and cervical lymphadenopathy indistinguishable from that of infectious mononucleosis but is not associated with hepatosplenomegaly. Approximately 5% of cases of EBV-associated infectious mononucleosis have positive throat cultures for group A β-hemolytic streptococci; this represents pharyngeal streptococcal carriage. Failure of a patient with streptococcal pharyngitis to improve within 48–72 hr should evoke suspicion of infectious mononucleosis. The most serious problem in the diagnosis of acute illness arises in the occasional patient with extremely high or low white blood cell counts, moderate thrombocytopenia, and even hemolytic anemia. In these patients, bone marrow examination

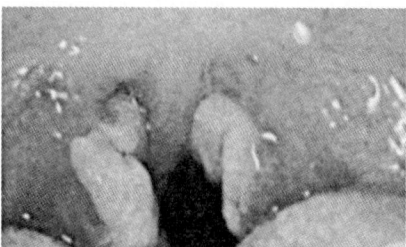

FIGURE 233–1. Tonsillitis with membrane formation in infectious mononucleosis. See also color plates. (Courtesy of Alex J. Steigman, MD)

and hematologic consultation are warranted to exclude the possibility of leukemia.

ROUTINE LABORATORY TESTS. In >90% of cases there is leukocytosis of 10,000–20,000 cells/mm³, of which at least two thirds are lymphocytes; atypical lymphocytes usually account for 20–40% of the total number. The atypical cells are mature T lymphocytes that have been antigenically activated. Compared with regular lymphocytes microscopically, atypical lymphocytes are larger overall, with larger, eccentrically placed indented and folded nuclei with a lower nuclear-to-cytoplasm ratio. Although atypical lymphocytosis may be seen with many of the infections usually causing lymphocytosis, the highest degree of atypical lymphocytes is classically seen with EBV infection. Other syndromes associated with atypical lymphocytosis include acquired cytomegalovirus infection (in contrast to congenital cytomegalovirus infection), toxoplasmosis, viral hepatitis, rubella, roseola, mumps, tuberculosis, typhoid, *Mycoplasma* infection, and malaria, as well as some drug reactions. Mild thrombocytopenia to 50,000–200,000 platelets/mm³ occurs in >50% of patients, but only rarely are values low enough to cause purpura. Mild elevation of hepatic transaminases occurs in approximately 50% of uncomplicated cases but is usually asymptomatic without jaundice.

HETEROPHILE ANTIBODY TEST. Heterophile antibodies agglutinate cells from species different from those in the source serum. The transient heterophile antibodies seen in infectious mononucleosis, also known as Paul-Bunnell antibodies, are IgM antibodies detected by the Paul-Bunnell-Davidsohn test for sheep red cell agglutination. The heterophile antibodies of infectious mononucleosis agglutinate sheep or, for greater sensitivity, horse red cells but not guinea pig kidney cells. This adsorption property differentiates this response from the heterophile response found in patients with serum sickness, rheumatic diseases, and some normal individuals. Titers greater than 1:28 or 1:40 (depending on the dilution system used) after absorption with guinea pig cells are considered positive.

The sheep red cell agglutination test is likely to be positive for several months after infectious mononucleosis; the horse red cell agglutination test may be positive for as long as 2 yr. The most widely used method is the qualitative rapid slide test using horse erythrocytes. It detects heterophile antibody in 90% of cases of EBV-associated infectious mononucleosis in older children and adults but in only up to 50% of cases in children <4 yr of age because they typically develop a lower titer. From 5–10% of cases of infectious mononucleosis are not caused by EBV and are not uniformly associated with a heterophile antibody response.

The false-positive rate is <10%, usually resulting from erroneous interpretation. If the heterophile test is negative and an EBV infection is suspected, EBV-specific antibody testing is indicated.

SPECIFIC EBV ANTIBODIES. EBV-specific antibody testing is useful to confirm acute EBV infection, especially in heterophile-negative cases, or to confirm past infection and determine susceptibility to future infection. Several distinct EBV antigen systems have been characterized for diagnostic purposes (Fig. 233–2 and see Table 233–1). The EBNA, EA, and VCA antigen systems are most useful for diagnostic purposes. The acute phase of infectious mononucleosis is characterized by rapid IgM and IgG antibody responses to VCA in all cases and an IgG response to EA in most cases. The IgM response to VCA is transient but can be detected for at least 4 wk and occasionally up to 3 mo. The laboratory must take steps to remove rheumatoid factor, which may cause a false-positive IgM VCA result. The IgG response to VCA usually peaks late in the acute phase, declines slightly over the next several weeks to months, and then persists at a relatively stable level for life.

Anti-EA antibodies are usually detectable for several months but may persist or be detected intermittently at low levels for many years. Antibodies to the diffuse-staining component of EA, EA-D, are found transiently in 80% of patients during the acute phase of infectious mononucleosis and reach high titers in patients with nasopharyngeal carcinoma. Antibodies to the cytoplasmic-restricted component of EA, EA-R, emerge transiently in the convalescence from infectious mononucleosis and often attain high titers in patients with EBV-associated Burkitt lymphoma, which in the terminal stage of the disease may be exceeded by antibodies to EA-D. High levels of antibodies to EA-D or EA-R may be found also in immunocompromised patients with persistent EBV infections and active EBV replication. Anti-EBNA antibodies are the last to develop in infectious mononucleosis and gradually appear 3–4 mo after the onset of illness and remain at low levels for life. Absence of anti-EBNA when other antibodies are present implies recent infection, whereas the presence of anti-EBNA implies infection occurring more than 3–4 mo previously. The wide range of individual antibody responses and the various laboratory methods used can occasionally make interpretation of an antibody profile difficult. The detection of IgM antibody to VCA is the most valuable and specific serologic test for the diagnosis of acute EBV infection and is generally sufficient to confirm the diagnosis.

Treatment. There is no specific treatment for infectious mononucleosis. Therapy with high doses of acyclovir, with or without

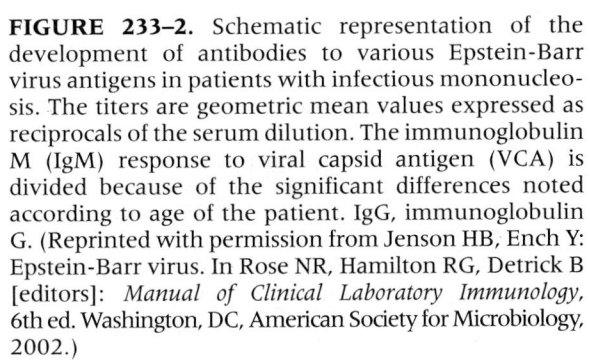

FIGURE 233–2. Schematic representation of the development of antibodies to various Epstein-Barr virus antigens in patients with infectious mononucleosis. The titers are geometric mean values expressed as reciprocals of the serum dilution. The immunoglobulin M (IgM) response to viral capsid antigen (VCA) is divided because of the significant differences noted according to age of the patient. IgG, immunoglobulin G. (Reprinted with permission from Jenson HB, Ench Y: Epstein-Barr virus. In Rose NR, Hamilton RG, Detrick B [editors]: *Manual of Clinical Laboratory Immunology*, 6th ed. Washington, DC, American Society for Microbiology, 2002.)

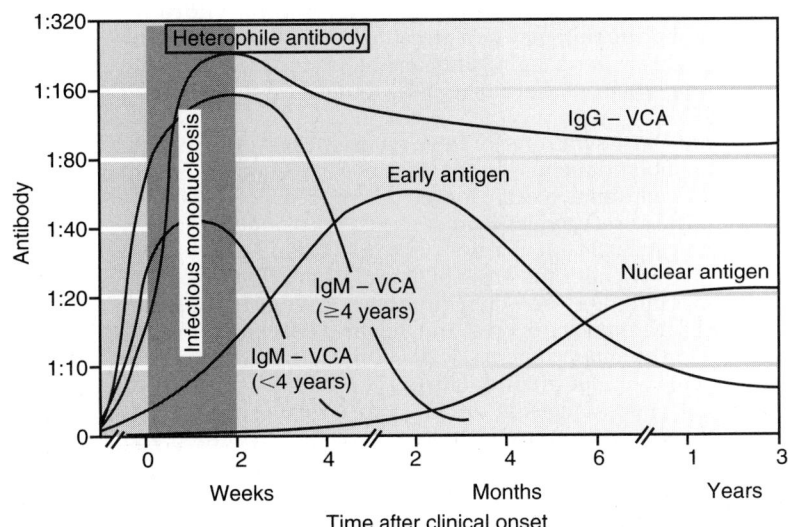

corticosteroids, decreases viral replication and oropharyngeal shedding during the period of administration but does not reduce the severity or duration of symptoms or alter the eventual outcome. Rest and symptomatic therapy are the mainstays of management. Bed rest is necessary only when the patient has debilitating fatigue. As soon as there is definite symptomatic improvement, the patient should be allowed to begin resuming normal activities. Because blunt abdominal trauma may predispose patients to splenic rupture, it is customary and prudent to advise against participation in contact sports and strenuous athletic activities during the first 2–3 wk of illness or while splenomegaly is present.

Short courses of corticosteroids (less than 2 wk) may be helpful for complications of infectious mononucleosis, but this use has not been evaluated critically. Some appropriate indications include incipient airway obstruction, thrombocytopenia with hemorrhaging, autoimmune hemolytic anemia, and seizures and meningitis. A recommended dosage is prednisone, 1 mg/kg/24 hr (maximum: 60 mg/24 hr) or equivalent, for 7 days and tapered over another 7 days. There are no controlled data to show efficacy of corticosteroids in any of these conditions. In view of the potential and unknown hazards of immunosuppression for a virus infection with oncogenic complications, corticosteroids should not be used in uncomplicated cases of infectious mononucleosis.

Complications. Very few patients with infectious mononucleosis experience complications. The most feared complication is subcapsular splenic hemorrhage or splenic rupture, which occurs most frequently during the 2nd week of the disease at a rate of <0.5% of cases in adults; the rate in children is unknown but is probably much lower. Rupture is commonly related to trauma, which often may be mild, and is rarely fatal. Swelling of the tonsils and oropharyngeal lymphoid tissue may be substantial and cause airway obstruction that is manifest by stridor and interference with breathing. Airway impairment with progressive symptoms occurs in <5% of cases and is one of the most common indications for hospitalization with infectious mononucleosis. It may be treated by administration of head-of-bed elevation, intravenous hydration, humidified air, and systemic corticosteroids. Respiratory distress with incipient or actual airway occlusion should be managed by tonsilloadenoidectomy followed by endotracheal intubation for 12–24 hr in an intensive care setting.

Many uncommon and unusual neurologic conditions have been reported to be associated with EBV infectious mononucleosis. Headache is present in about half of cases, with severe neurologic manifestations, such as seizures and ataxia, in 1–5% of cases. Perceptual distortions of sizes, shapes, and spatial relationships, known as the **Alice in Wonderland syndrome (metamorphopsia)**, may be a presenting symptom. There may be meningitis with nuchal rigidity and mononuclear cells in the cerebrospinal fluid, facial nerve palsy, transverse myelitis, and encephalitis.

Guillain-Barré syndrome or Reye syndrome may follow acute illness. Hemolytic anemia, often with a positive Coombs test and with cold agglutinins specific for red cell antigen i, occurs in 3% of cases. The onset is typically in the first 2 wk of illness and lasts for <1 mo. Aplastic anemia is a rare complication that usually presents 3–4 wk after the onset of illness, usually with recovery in 4–8 days but some cases do require bone marrow transplantation. Mild thrombocytopenia and neutropenia are common, but severe thrombocytopenia (<20,000 platelets/μL) or severe neutropenia (<1,000 neutrophils/μL) are rare. Myocarditis or interstitial pneumonia may occur, both resolving in 3–4 wk. Other rare complications include pancreatitis, parotitis, and orchitis.

Prognosis. The prognosis for complete recovery is excellent if no complications ensue during the acute illness. The major symp-

toms typically last 2–4 wk, followed by gradual recovery. Second attacks of infectious mononucleosis caused by EBV have not been documented. Fatigue, malaise, and some disability that may wax and wane for several weeks to a few months are common complaints even in otherwise unremarkable cases. Occasional persistence of fatigue for a few years after infectious mononucleosis is well recognized. At present, there is no convincing evidence linking EBV infection or EBV reactivation to chronic fatigue syndrome (Chapter 111).

Alpert G, Fleisher GR: Complications of infection with Epstein-Barr virus during childhood. A study of children admitted to the hospital. *Pediatr Infect Dis* 1984;3:304–7.

Horwitz CA, Henle W, Henle G, et al: Clinical and laboratory evaluation of cytomegalovirus-induced mononucleosis in previously healthy individuals. Report of 82 cases. *Medicine* 1986;65:124–34.

Jenson H: Acute complications of Epstein-Barr virus infectious mononucleosis. *Curr Opin Pediatr* 2000;12:263–8.

Jenson H, McIntosh K, Pitt J, et al: Natural history of primary Epstein-Barr virus infection in children of mothers infected with human immunodeficiency virus type 1. *J Infect Dis* 1999;179:1395–404.

Seemayer TA, Gross TG, Egeler RM, et al: X-linked lymphoproliferative disease. Twenty-five years after the discovery. *Pediatr Res* 1995;38:471–8.

Straus SE, Tosato G, Armstrong G, et al: Persisting illness and fatigue in adults with evidence of Epstein-Barr virus infection. *Ann Intern Med* 1985;102:7–16.

Sumaya CV, Ench Y: Epstein-Barr virus infectious mononucleosis in children I. Clinical and general laboratory findings. *Pediatrics* 1985;75:1003–10.

Sumaya CV, Ench Y: Epstein-Barr virus infectious mononucleosis in children II. Heterophil antibody and viral-specific responses. *Pediatrics* 1985;75:1011–9.

Tynell E, Aurelius E, Brandell A, et al: Acyclovir and prednisolone treatment of acute infectious mononucleosis. A multicenter, double-blind, placebo-controlled study. *J Infect Dis* 1996;174:324–31.

Chapter 234
Cytomegalovirus *Sergio Stagno*

Human cytomegalovirus (CMV) is a member of the Herpesviridae family and is widely distributed. Most CMV infections are inapparent, but the virus can cause a variety of clinical illnesses that range in severity from mild to fatal. CMV is the most common cause of congenital infection, which occasionally causes the syndrome of **cytomegalic inclusion disease** (hepatosplenomegaly, jaundice, petechia, purpura, and microcephaly). In immunocompetent adults, the infection is occasionally characterized by a mononucleosis-like syndrome. In immunosuppressed individuals, including transplant recipients and patients with AIDS, CMV pneumonitis, retinitis, and gastrointestinal disease are common and can be fatal.

Primary infection occurs in a seronegative, susceptible host. Recurrent infection represents reactivation of latent infection or reinfection of a seropositive immune host. Disease may result from primary or recurrent CMV infection, but the former is a more common cause of severe disease.

Etiology. CMV is the largest of the herpesviruses, and has a diameter of 200 nm with a double-stranded DNA viral genome of 240 kb in a 64-nm core enclosed by an icosahedral capsid composed of 162 capsomers. The core is assembled in the nucleus of the host cells. The capsid is surrounded by a poorly defined amorphous tegument, which is itself surrounded by a loosely applied, lipid-containing envelope. The envelope is acquired during the budding process through the nuclear membrane into a cytoplasmic vacuole, which contains the protein components of the envelope. Mature viruses exit the cells by reverse pinocytosis. Routine serologic tests do not define specific serotypes. In contrast, restriction endonuclease analysis of CMV DNA shows that, although all known human strains are genetically homologous, none are identical unless obtained from epidemiologically related cases.

Epidemiology. Seroepidemiologic surveys demonstrate CMV infection in every population examined worldwide. The prevalence of infection, which increases with age, is higher in developing countries and among lower socioeconomic strata of the more developed nations.

Transmission sources of CMV include saliva, breast milk, cervical and vaginal secretions, urine, semen, stools, blood, and tissue or organ transplants. The spread of CMV requires very close or intimate contact because it is very labile. Transmission occurs by direct person-to-person contact, but indirect transmission is possible via contaminated fomites.

The incidence of congenital CMV infection ranges from 0.2 to 2.4% of all live births, with the higher rates among populations with a lower economic standard of living. The risk for fetal infection is greatest with maternal primary CMV infection (30%) and much less likely with recurrent infection (<1%). In the United States, from 1 to 4% of pregnant women acquire primary CMV infection, with as many as 8,000 newborns with neurodevelopmental sequelae associated with congenital CMV infection.

Perinatal transmission is common, accounting for an incidence of 10–60% through the first 6 mo of life. The most important perinatal sources of virus are genital tract secretions at delivery and breast milk. Among CMV-seropositive mothers, virus is detectable in breast milk in 96%, with postnatal transmission occurring in approximately 38% of infants, resulting in symptomatic infection in nearly one half of preterm infants. Infected infants excrete virus for years in saliva and urine.

After the first year of life, the prevalence of infection is dependent on group activities, with childcare centers contributing to rapid spread of CMV among children. Infection rates of 50–80% during childhood are common. For children who are not exposed to other toddlers, the rate of infection increases very slowly throughout the first decade of life. A second peak occurs in adolescence as a result of sexual transmission. Seronegative childcare workers and parents of young children shedding CMV have a 10–20% annual risk of acquiring CMV, which contrasts with 1–3% per year for the general population.

CMV infection may be transmitted in transplanted organs (e.g., kidney, heart, and bone marrow). Following transplantation, many patients excrete CMV as a result of infection acquired from the donor organ or from reactivation of latent infection caused by immunosuppression. Seronegative transplant recipients of organs from seropositive donors are at greatest risk for severe disease.

Health care providers are not at increased risk for acquiring CMV infection from patients. Nosocomial infection is a hazard of transfusion of blood and blood products. In a population with a 50% prevalence of CMV infection, the risk has been estimated at 2.7% per unit of whole blood. Leukocyte transfusions pose a much greater risk. Infection is usually asymptomatic, but even in well children and adults there is a risk of disease if the recipient is seronegative and receives multiple units. Immunocompromised patients and seronegative premature infants have a much higher (10–30%) risk of disease.

Pathogenesis. Cytomegalic cells contain large intranuclear inclusions and smaller intracytoplasmic inclusions, and are pathognomonic for CMV infection. The virus induces focal mononuclear cell infiltrates, which may be present with or without cytomegalic cells. The virus may induce focal necrosis in the brain and liver, which may be extensive and accompanied by granulomatous change with calcifications. The lung, liver, kidney, gastrointestinal tract, and salivary and other exocrine glands are the most commonly affected organs, although the virus has been found in most cell types. The extent of abnormal organ function and the quantity of virus that can be recovered from infected organs are not related to the number of cytomegalic inclusion–bearing cells, which may be few or absent in each organ section examined.

Clinical Manifestations. The signs and symptoms of CMV infection vary with age, route of transmission, and immunocompetence of the patient. The infection is subclinical in most patients. In infants and young children, primary CMV infection occasionally causes pneumonitis, hepatomegaly, hepatitis, and petechial rashes. In older children, adolescents, and adults, CMV may cause mononucleosis-like syndrome characterized by fatigue, malaise, myalgia, headache, fever, hepatosplenomegaly, elevated liver enzymes, and atypical lymphocytosis. The course of CMV mononucleosis is generally mild, lasting 2–3 wk. Occasionally clinical presentations may include persistent fever, overt hepatitis, or a morbilliform rash. Recurrent infections are asymptomatic in the immunocompetent host.

IMMUNOCOMPROMISED PERSONS. The risk of CMV disease is increased in immunocompromised persons, with both primary and recurrent infections (Chapter 164). Illness with a primary infection includes pneumonitis (most common), hepatitis, chorioretinitis, gastrointestinal disease, or fever with leukopenia as isolated entities or as manifestations of generalized disease, which may be fatal. The risk is greatest in bone marrow transplant recipients and in patients with AIDS. Pneumonia, retinitis, and involvement of the central nervous system and gastrointestinal tract are usually severe and progressive. Submucosal ulcerations can occur anywhere in the gastrointestinal tract and may lead to hemorrhage and perforation. Pancreatitis and cholecystitis may also occur.

CONGENITAL INFECTION. Symptomatic congenital CMV infection was originally termed cytomegalic inclusion disease. Only 5% of all congenitally infected infants have severe cytomegalic inclusion disease, another 5% have mild involvement, and 90% are born with subclinical, but still chronic, CMV infection. The characteristic signs and symptoms include intrauterine growth retardation, prematurity, hepatosplenomegaly and jaundice, thrombocytopenia and purpura, and microcephaly and intracranial calcifications. Other neurologic problems include chorioretinitis, sensorineural hearing loss, and mild increases in cerebrospinal fluid protein. Symptomatic newborns are usually easy to identify. Most symptomatic congenital infections and those resulting in sequelae are caused by primary rather than reactivated infections in pregnant women. Re-infection with a different strain of CMV can lead to symptomatic congenital infection. Asymptomatic congenital CMV infection is likely a leading cause of sensorineural hearing loss, which occurs in approximately 7% of infected infants.

PERINATAL INFECTION. Infections resulting from exposure to CMV in the maternal genital tract at delivery or in breast milk occur despite the presence of maternally derived, passively acquired antibody. Approximately 6–12% of seropositive mothers transmit CMV to their infants by contaminated cervical-vaginal secretions and 50% by breast milk. The majority of infants remain asymptomatic and do not exhibit sequelae. Occasionally, perinatally acquired CMV infection is associated with pneumonitis and sepsis-like syndrome. Premature and ill full-term infants may have neurologic sequelae and psychomotor retardation. However, the risk of hearing loss, chorioretinitis, and microcephaly does not appear to be increased. Premature infants with transfusion-acquired CMV infection have a much greater risk of morbidity.

Diagnosis. Active CMV infection is best confirmed by virus isolation from urine, saliva, bronchoalveolar washings, breast milk, cervical secretions, buffy coat, and tissues obtained by biopsy. Rapid (24 hr) identification is now routine with the centrifugation-enhanced rapid culture system based on the detection of CMV early antigens using monoclonal antibodies. Several methods are used for rapid quantitative detection of CMV antigens, and quantitative polymerase chain reaction (PCR) assays are also available. The presence of viral shedding and active infection does not distinguish between primary and recurrent infections. A primary infection is confirmed by seroconversion or the simultaneous detection of immunoglobulin (Ig) M and IgG antibodies with low functional avidity. A simple increase in antibody titers in initially seropositive patients must be interpreted with caution because this is occasionally observed years after primary infection. IgG antibodies persist for life. For the first weeks after primary infection, the functional avidity of IgG class antibodies is very low and rises to a peak in 4–5 mo. IgM antibodies can be demonstrated transiently (4–16 wk) during the acute phase of symptomatic as well as asymptomatic primary infection in adults. IgM antibodies are occasionally found with these assays (0.2–1%) in patients with recurrent infection.

Recurrent infection is defined by the reappearance of viral excretion in a patient known to have been seropositive in the past. The distinction between reactivation of endogenous virus and re-infection with a different strain of CMV requires restriction enzyme analysis of viral DNA or the measurement of antibodies against strain-specific epitopes of CMV, such as glycoprotein H epitopes.

In immunocompromised persons, excretion of CMV, increases in IgG titers, and even the presence of IgM antibodies are common, making the distinction between primary and recurrent infections more difficult. Demonstrating viremia by buffy coat culture or detection of CMV DNA implies active disease and worse prognosis regardless of whether the type of infection is primary, recurrent, or uncertain.

CONGENITAL INFECTION. The definitive method for diagnosis of congenital CMV infection is virus isolation or PCR, which should be performed at or shortly after birth. Urine and saliva are the best specimens for culture. Infants with congenital CMV infection may excrete CMV in the urine for several years. An IgG antibody test is of little diagnostic value because a positive result also reflects maternal antibodies, although a negative result excludes the diagnosis of congenital CMV infection. Demonstration of stable or rising titers in serial specimens during the first year of life does not help because acquired infection in the first few months of life is common. In general, IgM tests lack sensitivity and specificity and are unreliable for diagnosis of congenital CMV infection. Congenital toxoplasmosis and syphilis must also be considered.

IgM antibody tests and the measurement of CMV-IgG avidity can identify women at high risk of transmitting CMV in utero. Fetal infection can be confirmed by viral isolation from amniotic fluid. The sensitivity of this method is excellent after the 22nd wk of gestation. The detection of viral genome by PCR in amniotic fluid is equally sensitive and specific; quantitative PCR demonstrating 10^5 genome equivalents per mL of amniotic fluid is a predictor of symptomatic congenital infection.

Treatment. There are limited options for treatment of CMV infection. Treatment is not indicated for immunocompetent persons, but is recommended for immunocompromised persons, and remains controversial for infants with symptomatic congenital infection.

IMMUNOCOMPROMISED PERSONS. Ganciclovir combined with immune globulin, either standard intravenous immunoglobulin (IVIG) or hyperimmune CMV IVIG, has been used to treat life-threatening CMV infections in immunocompromised hosts (e.g., bone marrow, heart, and kidney transplant recipients and patients with AIDS). Two published regimens are: ganciclovir (7.5 mg/kg/24 hr divided q 8 hr IV for 14 days) with CMV IVIG (400 mg/kg on days 1, 2, and 7, and 200 mg/kg on day 14); and ganciclovir (7.5 mg/kg/24 hr divided q 8 hr IV for 20 days with IVIG 500 mg/kg every other day for 10 doses).

CMV retinitis and gastrointestinal disease appear to be clinically responsive to therapy but, like viral excretion, often recur on cessation. Toxicity with ganciclovir is frequent and often severe and includes neutropenia, thrombocytopenia, liver dysfunction, reduction in spermatogenesis, and gastrointestinal

and renal abnormalities. Foscarnet is an alternative antiviral agent, although there is limited information on its use in children. CMV prophylaxis with ganciclovir or acyclovir reduces the risk of morbidity in solid organ transplantation. Prophylactic treatment with valacyclovir in adults (2 g q 6 hr PO for 90 days) is a safe and effective regimen to prevent CMV disease after renal transplantation.

CONGENITAL INFECTION. A randomized controlled Phase III study with ganciclovir (6 mg/kg/dose q 12 hr IV for the first 6 wk of life) concluded that treatment both prevents hearing deterioration and improves or maintains normal hearing function at 6 mo of age, and may prevent hearing deterioration at 1 yr of age or older. Drug-related toxicity was common with 63% of ganciclovir-treated patients developing significant neutropenia, compared with 21% in the untreated group. The logistic obstacles of intravenous therapy for the first 6 wk of life, limited benefit, and adverse effects have limited enthusiasm for this regimen.

Prognosis. Patients with CMV mononucleosis usually recover fully, although some have a protracted symptoms. Most immunocompromised patients also recover uneventfully, but many experience severe pneumonitis, with a high fatality rate if hypoxemia develops. CMV infection and disease may be fatal in individuals with increased susceptibility to infections such as patients with AIDS.

CONGENITAL DISEASE. Nearly 90% of children with symptomatic congenital infection demonstrate central nervous system and hearing defects in later years. Infants with subclinical infection have a much more favorable outlook. Principal concerns are the subsequent development of sensorineural hearing loss (5–10%), chorioretinitis (3–5%), and other less frequent manifestations such as developmental abnormalities, microcephaly, and neurologic deficits.

Prevention. The use of CMV-free blood products, especially for premature newborns, and, whenever possible, the use of organs from CMV-free donors for transplantation, represent important measures to prevent CMV infection and disease in patients at high risk.

Pregnant women who are CMV seropositive are at low risk of delivering a symptomatic newborn. If possible, pregnant women should have a CMV serologic test, especially if they provide care for young children who are potential CMV excreters. Pregnant women who are CMV seronegative should be counseled regarding good handwashing and other hygienic measures and avoidance of contact with oral secretions of others. Those with suspected recent CMV infection may undergo additional diagnostic evaluations to ascertain in utero transmission and fetal disease.

PASSIVE IMMUNOPROPHYLAXIS. The use of IVIG or CMV IVIG for prophylaxis of infection in solid organ and bone marrow transplant recipients reduces the risk of symptomatic disease but does not prevent infection. The efficacy of prophylaxis is more striking when the hazard of primary CMV infection is greatest, such as in bone marrow transplantation. There is no consensus for a uniform prophylaxis regimen for CMV infection. Recommended regimens include either IVIG (1,000 mg/kg) or CMV IVIG (500 mg/kg) given as a single intravenous dose beginning within 72 hr of transplantation and once weekly thereafter until 90–120 days after transplantation.

ACTIVE IMMUNIZATION. The beneficial role of immunity is substantial, as illustrated by the fact that most severe disease follows primary infection, especially with congenital infection, transfusion-acquired infection, and infection in transplant recipients. Candidates for a CMV vaccine include seronegative women of childbearing age and seronegative transplant recipients. Live, attenuated vaccines based on the Towne strain prototype are immunogenic, but immunity wanes quickly. Vaccine virus does not seem to be transmissible. The vaccine does not protect renal transplant recipients from CMV infection, but appears to reduce the virulence of primary infection. In a study of vaccine efficacy in normal adult women, the Towne strain vaccine did not provide protection against naturally acquired infection. Other types of vaccines, such as subunit and recombinant vaccines, are being evaluated in early clinical trials.

Bodeus M, Beulne D, Goubau P: Ability of three IgG-avidity assays to exclude recent cytomegalovirus infection. *Eur J Clin Microbiol Infect Dis* 2001;20:248–52.

Boppana SB, Rivera LB, Fowler KB, et al: Intrauterine transmission of cytomegalovirus to infants of women with preconceptional immunity. *N Engl J Med* 2001;344:1366–71.

Couchoud C: Cytomegalovirus prophylaxis with antiviral agents for solid organ transplantation. *Cochrane Database Syst Rev* 2000;(2):CD001320

Dumont LJ, Luka J, VandenBroeke T, et al: The effect of leukocyte-reduction method on the amount of human cytomegalovirus in blood products: A comparison of apheresis and filtration methods. *Blood* 2001;97:3640–7.

Hamprecht K, Maschmann J, Vochem M, et al: Epidemiology of transmission of cytomegalovirus from mother to preterm infant by breastfeeding. *Lancet* 2001;357:513–8.

Kimberlin DW, Lin CY, Sanchez P, et al: NIAID Collaborative Antiviral Study Group (CASG): Ganciclovir (GCV) treatment of symptomatic congenital cytomegalovirus (CMV) infections: Results of a phase III randomized trial. 40th Interscience Conference on Antimicrobial Agents and Chemotherapy (ICAAC), Toronto, Ontario, Canada, 2000; Abstract 1942.

Lazzarotto T, Varani S, Guerra B, et al: Prenatal indicators of congenital cytomegalovirus infection. *J Pediatr* 2000;137:90–5.

Lowance D, Neumayer HH, Legendre CM, et al: Valacyclovir for the prevention of cytomegalovirus disease after renal transplantation. International valacyclovir cytomegalovirus prophylaxis study group. *N Engl J Med* 1999;340:1462–70.

Noyola DE, Demmler GJ, Nelson CT, et al: Early predictors of neurodevelopmental outcome in symptomatic congenital cytomegalovirus infection. *J Pediatr* 2001;138:325–31.

Rubin RH, Kemmerly SA, Conti D, et al: Prevention of primary cytomegalovirus disease in organ transplant recipients with oral ganciclovir or oral acyclovir prophylaxis. *Transpl Infect Dis* 2000;2:112–7.

Chapter 235

Roseola (Human Herpesviruses 6 and 7)

Charles T. Leach

Human herpesvirus 6 (HHV-6) was discovered in 1986, 22 yr after the discovery of the 5th human herpesvirus (Epstein-Barr virus). Six isolates of a new virus were identified in the peripheral blood mononuclear cells (PBMCs) of adult patients with AIDS or lymphoproliferative diseases. In 1990, human herpesvirus 7 (HHV-7) was identified in the peripheral blood mononuclear cells of an HIV-uninfected adult. HHV-6 is the etiologic agent for most cases of roseola infantum (**exanthem subitum**, or **sixth disease**), and also is associated with other diseases in normal and immunocompromised patients. Disease associations for HHV-7 are fewer; only its role in some cases of roseola is well established.

Etiology. Roseola was first established as a distinct illness at the turn of the 20th century. Until recently, no pathogen could be consistently identified as the agent responsible for roseola. However, it is now clear that primary infection with HHV-6, and less frequently HHV-7, causes the majority of cases of roseola. In studies of children with roseola from Europe and Asia, HHV-6 was responsible for approximately two thirds of cases and HHV-7 caused one fourth of cases. Other viruses (e.g., echovirus 16) probably account for the remainder.

HHV-6 and HHV-7 belong to the β-herpesvirus subfamily of herpesviruses, which includes human cytomegalovirus (CMV). HHV-6 and HHV-7 share physical and biologic characteristics with other herpesviruses, including a large double-stranded DNA genome, the presence of a nucleocapsid, and the establishment of latency after primary infection. HHV-6 is essentially colinear with HHV-7, and both viruses share much homology with CMV. The principal target cells for HHV-6 and HHV-7 infection in vivo are CD4 T cells; HHV-6 can also infect other cells, including CD8 (suppressor) T cells, natural killer T cells, δγ T cells, glial cells, epithelial cells, monocytes, megakaryocytes, and endothelial cells. HHV-6 and HHV-7 are typically cultivated in vitro in mitogen-stimulated human mononuclear cells (isolated from cord blood or peripheral blood) and can be identified by the development of large balloon-like cells accompanied by cell lysis. Two distinct types of HHV-6 (types A and B) exist. Type B causes more than 99% of HHV-6–associated roseola cases. Latent type A virus can be found in immunodeficient as well as healthy patients and may reactivate in severely ill adult patients. However, it has not been consistently linked with any disease.

Epidemiology. Primary HHV-6 infection occurs early in life. More than 90% of newborn infants are HHV-6 seropositive, reflecting transplacental transfer of maternal antibodies. By 4–6 mo of age, the prevalence drops significantly (0–60%). By 12 mo of age, 60–90% of children possess antibodies to HHV-6, and by 3–5 yr, 80–100% of children are seropositive. Peak acquisition of primary HHV-6 infection, from 6–15 mo of age, corresponds with peak acquisition of roseola. Less than half of HHV-6 infections in U.S. infants are clinically recognizable as roseola, whereas 80% of Japanese infants with primary HHV-6 infection develop roseola. Primary infection with HHV-7 occurs slightly later than HHV-6 infection, with 45–75% of children infected by 2 yr of age and 90% by 7–10 yr of age.

Roseola can develop in children year-round; some series indicate a higher incidence during spring and fall months. Unlike some of the other childhood exanthems, children with roseola rarely report contact with other affected children, and outbreaks are uncommon. Sex, race, and geography do not play an important role in acquisition of roseola. The incubation period averages 10 days (range of 5–15 days).

Most adults excrete HHV-6 and HHV-7 in saliva and may serve as primary sources for virus transmission to children. Women excrete HHV-6 and HHV-7 in the genital tract at low rates, but sexual transmissibility has not been demonstrated. There is evidence that HHV-6 can be transmitted in utero, although this is a rare occurrence and no malformations have been noted. No congenital HHV-7 infections have been described. HHV-6 has been transmitted to susceptible infant transplant recipients via infected donor bone marrow or solid organ. There is no evidence that infection is spread by breast milk or blood transfusion.

Pathogenesis. Little is known regarding the pathogenesis of infections associated with HHV-6 and HHV-7, including roseola. Virus is probably acquired from the saliva of healthy persons and enters the host through the oral, nasal, or conjunctival mucosa. Cellular receptors for both viruses have been identified: HHV-6 uses the CD46 receptor (also used by measles virus), and HHV-7 uses the CD4 receptor (also used by HIV-1). Following viral replication at an unknown site, a high level of viremia develops in PBMCs. After acute infection, HHV-6 and HHV-7 establish latency in blood mononuclear cells and possibly in the salivary glands, kidneys, lungs, and central nervous system. Both viruses may evade the immune system through downregulation of the major histocompatibility complex (MHC) type I response. The basis for the unique pattern of rash after resolution of fever in children with roseola has not been established.

HHV-6 can suppress all cellular lineages within the bone marrow, and active HHV-6 infection is associated with bone marrow suppression in bone marrow transplant patients. HHV-6 infection also has significant effects on the immune system, including enhancement of natural killer (NK) T-cell activity, suppression of PBMC proliferation, and induction of a proinflammatory cytokine response.

Clinical Manifestations. Roseola is the prototypical HHV-6 and HHV-7 infection, although nonspecific infections are common.

ROSEOLA INFANTUM (EXANTHEM SUBITUM). Roseola is a mild febrile, exanthematous illness occurring almost exclusively during infancy. More than 95% of roseola cases occur in children younger than 3 yr, with a peak at 6–15 mo of age. Transplacental antibodies likely protect most infants until 6 mo of age.

Infants with classic roseola exhibit a unique constellation of findings displayed over a short period of time. Consequently, classic roseola is infrequently confused with other childhood exanthems.

The prodromal period of roseola is usually asymptomatic but may include mild upper respiratory tract signs, among them minimal rhinorrhea, slight pharyngeal inflammation, and mild conjunctival redness. Mild cervical or, less frequently, occipital lymphadenopathy may be noted. Some children may have mild palpebral edema. Physical findings during the prodromal stage have no clear relationship to roseola, and may simply reflect an accompanying respiratory viral infection.

Clinical illness is generally heralded by high temperature, usually ranging from 37.9 to 40°C (101–106°F), with an average of 39°C (103°F). Some children may become irritable and anorexic during the febrile stage, but most behave normally despite high temperatures. Seizures may occur in 5–10% of children with roseola during this febrile period. Infrequent complaints include rhinorrhea, sore throat, abdominal pain, vomiting, and diarrhea. In Asian countries, ulcers at the uvulopalatoglossal junction (**Nagayama spots**) are common in infants with roseola.

Fever persists for 3–5 days, and then typically resolves rather abruptly ("crisis"). Occasionally, the fever may gradually diminish over 24–36 hours ("lysis"). A rash appears within 12–24 hr of fever resolution. In many cases, the rash develops during defervescence or within a few hours of fever resolution. The rash of roseola is rose colored, as the name implies, and is fairly distinctive. However, it may be confused with exanthems resulting from rubella, measles, or erythema infectiosum. The roseola rash begins as discrete, small (2–5 mm), slightly raised pink lesions on the trunk and usually spreads to the neck, face, and proximal extremities. The rash is not usually pruritic, and no vesicles or pustules develop. Lesions typically remain discrete but occasionally may become almost confluent. After 1–3 days, the rash fades. Some children experience evanescent rashes that resolve within a few hours.

Subtle differences in clinical presentation have been noted between roseola associated with HHV-7 compared with HHV-6. These include a slightly older age, lower mean temperature, and shorter duration of fever in HHV-7-associated cases. However, these differences are insufficient to clinically distinguish HHV-6– from HHV-7–associated roseola. There are reports of children experiencing HHV-6–associated roseola followed later by HHV-7–associated roseola.

FEVER IN INFANTS WITHOUT CLASSIC ROSEOLA. HHV-6 and HHV-7 account for a significant proportion of nonspecific febrile illnesses in infants. Studies among infants presenting to a hospital emergency room indicate that approximately 15% had primary HHV-6 or HHV-7 infection.

CENTRAL NERVOUS SYSTEM INFECTIONS. Both HHV-6 and HHV-7 are neurotropic and can invade the CNS. Primary HHV-6 infection is responsible for one third of febrile seizures in infants. Most of these children (70–80%) do not subsequently experience a rash. Smaller studies suggest that HHV-7 also is associated with some febrile seizures. HHV-6 and HHV-7 are also associated with rare cases of encephalitis and meningoencephalitis. One large study noted HHV-6 DNA in cerebrospinal fluid from 6% of children and adults with focal encephalitis of unknown cause.

MONONUCLEOSIS-LIKE ILLNESS AND HEPATITIS. Several heterophile-negative mononucleosis-like infections associated with HHV-6 have been reported in adults. HHV-6 and HHV-7 may rarely cause clinical symptoms of hepatitis. Some infants have developed HHV-6-associated liver failure, and one fatal case of hepatitis was reported in a neonate after maternal transmission of HHV-6.

INFECTIONS IN IMMUNOCOMPROMISED PATIENTS. Numerous severe and occasionally fatal HHV-6–associated infections (encephalitis and pneumonitis) have occurred in immunocompromised patients, including patients with AIDS or organ transplants. These have occurred predominantly in stem cell transplant recipients and usually reflect reactivated HHV-6 infection. Recent studies suggest that concomitant HHV-6 and HHV-7 infections may augment CMV-associated disease following organ transplantation.

Because HHV-6 shares CD4 cell tropism with HIV, upregulates HIV, and stimulates in vitro replication of HIV, there has been considerable interest in the role of HHV-6 as a cofactor for clinical progression of AIDS. Epidemiologic studies in adults do not support a significant role for HHV-6 as a cofactor, but one small pediatric study does suggest more rapid progression of immune deficiency in HIV/HHV-6 coinfected patients. Further prospective studies are necessary to assess the impact of HHV-6 on HIV-infected children.

OTHER DISEASES POSSIBLY ASSOCIATED WITH HHV-6 OR HHV-7. Rash illness without fever has been described in a small number of infants with primary HHV-6 infection. Other small studies or case reports have suggested that HHV-6 may be associated with some cases of hemophagocytic syndrome, intussusception, idiopathic thrombocytopenic purpura, recurrent aphthous stomatitis, myocarditis, and disseminated disease. There are conflicting data linking HHV-7 and pityriasis rosea, a benign exanthematous illness. HHV-6, like several other infectious agents, has been linked to multiple sclerosis by some, but not all, investigators.

HHV-6 DNA has been detected in various malignancies, including non-Hodgkin lymphoma, Hodgkin disease, cervical and oral carcinoma, and leukemia. However, no consistent etiologic relationship has been established with any of these cancers.

Diagnosis. The most important reason for establishing the diagnosis of roseola is to differentiate this generally mild illness from other potentially more serious childhood rash illnesses such as measles. It is also important to identify other, more serious illnesses caused by HHV-6, such as encephalitis and pneumonitis, especially in immunocompromised patients, for timely consideration of antiviral therapy.

The diagnosis of roseola can be established primarily on the basis of age, history, and clinical findings. HHV-6- and HHV-7-associated roseola cases cannot be distinguished solely on clinical grounds. Specific testing for HHV-6 or HHV-7 infection may be performed using laboratory methods, including serology, virus culture, antigen detection, and polymerase chain reaction (PCR).

HHV-6 serologic testing is available from many commercial laboratories; few offer HHV-7 serology. An HHV-6 immunoglobulin (Ig) M response typically develops by the 5th–7th day of illness, peaks at 2–3 wk, and resolves within 2 mo. Unfortunately, the accuracy of currently available IgM tests varies widely, and none have been sufficiently evaluated to provide unequivocal evidence of acute HHV-6 infection. Seroconversion of HHV-6 or -7 IgG antibodies in serum samples collected 2–3 wk apart is a more reliable means of establishing primary infection, but is not timely. Fourfold increases or decreases in HHV-6 or -7 IgG antibodies also suggest active infection (primary or reactivated). Because of the high seroprevalence of HHV-6 in the general population, a single positive HHV-6 or -7 IgG test is of no diagnostic significance for diagnosis of acute infection. CMV antibodies can cross react with HHV-6 and HHV-7; therefore, diagnosis of HHV-6 and HHV-7 infections by serologic means requires exclusion of CMV infection.

Identification of HHV-6 or HHV-7 in PBMCs by virus culture firmly establishes the presence of active infection in immunocompetent hosts; association with specific disease is more problematic in immunocompromised patients as a result of a low background rate of viremia. Identification of HHV-6 and HHV-7 by culture requires incubation of PBMCs (with or without cocultivation with exogenous PBMCs) for days to several weeks, and is presently available only in research laboratories. A commercial HHV-6 rapid (shell-vial) culture is available; it appears comparable to standard virus culture for detection of active HHV-6 infection.

PCR amplification tests for HHV-6 are becoming available and may provide more timely information for diagnosis. Active, replicating infection is indicated if HHV-6 DNA is detected in acellular specimens such as serum or cerebrospinal fluid. However, detection at other sites (e.g., PBMCs, saliva, and tissues) does not necessarily indicate active infection, because HHV-6 exists in latent form in many tissues after primary infection.

Other diagnostic tests for consideration in selected circumstances include in situ hybridization and immunohistochemistry.

LABORATORY FINDINGS. White blood cell (WBC) counts of 8,000–9,000 WBCs/μL may be found during the first few days of fever in children with roseola, but by the time the exanthem appears, the WBC count falls to 4,000–6,000 WBCs/μL with a relative lymphocytosis (70–90%). The cerebrospinal fluid in children with HHV-6–associated febrile seizures typically is normal. The cerebrospinal fluid from rare cases of HHV-6–associated meningoencephalitis and encephalitis is characterized by a mild pleocytosis with predominance of mononuclear cells, normal glucose, and normal to slightly elevated protein.

DIFFERENTIAL DIAGNOSIS. Children with roseola typically present at two different stages of the illness: at the time of fever before the rash (pre-eruptive) and after the rash has appeared. During the pre-eruptive stage, many conditions may be confused with roseola. However, the pattern of fever in a generally well child without significant physical findings, rather precipitous defervescence, and a subsequent rash is unique for roseola. Nonetheless, some patients may not display all these characteristics and conditions may mimic other illnesses.

Roseola is probably most commonly confused with rubella. In contrast to the absence of a distinct prodrome in children with roseola, children with rubella invariably have a mildly symptomatic prodromal period, including prominent occipital and postauricular lymphadenopathy. Lymphadenopathy is an inconsistent finding in roseola; when lymphadenopathy does occur, occipital lymph nodes are more frequently affected than those in the postauricular region. Rubella usually causes only low-grade fever, which is coincident with the exanthem. The rubella rash is typically more extensive than that seen with roseola, and coalescence is more common. A history of exposure is frequently elicited from those in whom rubella develops. Most important, vaccinated persons rarely acquire rubella.

Roseola may be confused with measles. However, the development of an exanthem at the height of the fever, as well as the presence of cough, coryza, conjunctivitis, and Koplik spots on the buccal mucosa in the early stages of measles, differentiates these two illnesses.

Outbreaks of roseola-like illnesses have been associated with many different viruses, most commonly enteroviruses. In summer and fall months, some cases of roseola-like illnesses may be attributable to enteroviruses.

Scarlet fever may also resemble roseola. Important features of scarlet fever are its rarity in infancy, the simultaneous presence of fever and rash, and the discrete, small, sandpaper-like rash lesions.

Drug hypersensitivity is a common condition resembling roseola. Antibiotics are frequently prescribed to children with roseola during the febrile phase before onset of the rash. A child who acquires a drug rash may do so soon after resolution of the fever, which is the characteristic pattern for children with roseola. However, the usually morbilliform nature, pruritus, and resolution after discontinuation of the implicated drug should distinguish a drug rash.

It may be difficult to distinguish central nervous system disease caused by HHV-6 from other causes. Development of a roseola-like illness in association with febrile seizures, meningoencephalitis, or encephalitis makes HHV-6 infection more likely; however, this occurs infrequently.

Hepatitis and heterophile-negative mononucleosis are rarely associated with HHV-6, and other causes for these infections should first be sought.

Treatment. HHV-6 is inhibited by ganciclovir, cidofovir, and foscarnet (but not acyclovir) at levels that are achievable in serum; HHV-7 is inhibited by cidofovir and foscarnet. Case reports have indicated successes and failures with these drugs; however, prospective trials evaluating the clinical efficacy of antiviral agents for HHV-6 or HHV-7 infections have not been performed.

The generally benign nature of roseola precludes consideration of antiviral therapy. However, future studies may address the need for specific antiviral therapy in those unusual cases of roseola or other forms of HHV-6 infection in which significant morbidity exists, such as children with neurologic complications of roseola or immunocompromised children with severe HHV-6 or HHV-7 infection.

Children in the febrile, pre-eruptive phase of roseola usually are quite comfortable and require little supportive therapy. Those children who are uncomfortable and irritable, or in whom histories of febrile convulsions exists, may benefit from treatment with acetaminophen or ibuprofen. Adequate fluid balance should be maintained in all affected children. Referral should be considered in those unusual circumstances in which serious disease develops, such as encephalitis, hepatitis, or pneumonitis.

Prognosis. The prognosis for the great majority of children with roseola is excellent, with no obvious sequelae. Before the discoveries of HHV-6 and HHV-7, rare complications of roseola (hemiparesis, mental retardation) were attributable to brain anoxia during prolonged febrile seizures. However, damage resulting from direct viral invasion of the brain, liver, and other organs has been demonstrated for HHV-6. Deaths directly attributable to HHV-6 have been reported in normal as well as immunocompromised patients in whom encephalitis, hepatitis, pneumonitis, disseminated disease, or hemophagocytosis syndrome developed.

Prevention. Very little information is available on which to base guidelines for prevention of HHV-6 or HHV-7 infection. Experimental evidence suggests that roseola may be transmitted via blood or saliva, and both HHV-6 and HHV-7 are shed in the saliva. It is likely that healthy immune carriers with latent viral infections transmit infection to susceptible infants and children. No specific recommendations for prevention can be made until proper studies have been conducted. No vaccine has been developed.

Black JB, Pellett PE: Human herpesvirus 7. *Rev Med Virol* 1999;9:245–62.

Caserta MT, Hall CB, Schnabel K, et al: Primary human herpesvirus 7 infection: A comparison of human herpesvirus 7 and human herpesvirus 6 infections in children. *J Pediatr* 1998;133:386–9.

Caserta MT, Mock DJ, Dewhurst S: Human herpesvirus 6. *Clin Infect Dis* 2001;33: 829–33.

Chua KB, Lam SK, AbuBakar S, et al: The predictive value of uvulo-palatoglossal junctional ulcers as an early clinical sign of exanthem subitum due to human herpesvirus 6. *J Clin Virol* 2000;17:83–90.

Desachy A, Ranger-Rogez S, Francois B, et al: Reactivation of human herpesvirus type 6 in multiple organ failure syndrome. *Clin Infect Dis* 2001;32:197–203.

Hall CB, Long CE, Schnabel KC, et al: Human herpesvirus-6 infection in children: A prospective study of complications and reactivation. *N Engl J Med* 1994;331: 432–8.

Kositanont U, Wasi C, Wanprapar N, et al.: Primary infection of human herpesvirus 6 in children with vertical infection of human immunodeficiency virus type 1. *J Infect Dis* 1999;180:50–5.

Lanphear BP, Hall CB, Black J, Auinger P: Risk factors for the early acquisition of human herpesvirus 6 and human herpesvirus 7 infections in children. *Pediatr Infect Dis J* 1998;17:792–5.

Leach CT: Human herpesvirus-6 and -7 infections in children: Agents of roseola and other syndromes. *Curr Opin Pediatr* 2000;12:269–74.

Leach CT, Pollock BH, McClain KL, et al: Human herpesvirus 6 (HHV-6) and cytomegalovirus (CMV) infections in children with acquired immunodeficiency syndrome (AIDS) and cancer. *Pediatr Infect Dis J* 2002;21:125–32.

Mendez JC, Dockrell DH, Espy MJ, et al: Human ß-herpesvirus interactions in solid organ transplant recipients. *J Infect Dis* 2001;183:179–84.

Yamanishi K, Okuno T, Shiraki K, et al: Identification of human herpesvirus-6 as a causal agent for exanthem subitum. *Lancet* 1988;1:1065–7.

Chapter 236

Human Herpesvirus 8

Charles T. Leach

The identification of the newest human herpesvirus, human herpesvirus 8 (HHV-8; also known as **Kaposi sarcoma (KS)– associated herpesvirus**), in 1994 resulted from a search for an infectious agent responsible for KS in patients with AIDS. Further studies have revealed its strong association with KS as well as other rarer malignancies.

Etiology. HHV-8 is a member of the γ-herpesviruses, which includes Epstein-Barr virus. HHV-8 is an enveloped DNA virus of approximately 165,000 base pairs, and has an overall genomic structure typical for other human herpesviruses. However, unlike most other viruses, the HHV-8 genome contains viral homologues of several human proteins important in regulation of cellular proliferation. It is postulated that these viral proteins contribute to the pathogenesis of HHV-8–associated malignancies.

Epidemiology. HHV-8 infection is uncommon in healthy children and adults in most developed countries. Rates of HHV-8 infection in HIV-uninfected persons and blood donors in the United States are generally less than 10%, but may be higher in specific areas. HHV-8 infection is more common (15–20%) in certain areas of Greece and Italy. HHV-8 seroprevalence rates are much higher in Brazil, Egypt, and Central Africa, where 40–60% of children are infected.

Approximately one third of HIV-infected homosexual males and more than 80% of HIV-infected homosexual males who acquire KS are infected with the virus. Patients with HIV infection acquired in another manner (e.g., vertically from an HIV-positive mother or through transfusion of blood or blood products) have low rates (0–5%) of HHV-8 infection that are similar to those observed in HIV-uninfected persons and blood donors.

HHV-8 is shed in the saliva of most HHV-8–infected persons, and probably serves as a major source for intrafamilial transmission. Sexual transmission also is important, especially among homosexual males. Rarely, HHV-8 has been transmitted vertically and via blood transfusion. Most HHV-8–associated disease in transplant recipients is caused by reactivated virus, although some infections have been transmitted via the donor organ.

Clinical Manifestations. Rare reports describe immunocompromised adults with symptoms developing in conjunction with primary HHV-8 infections. In children, one report describes fever and rash in immunocompetent Egyptian infants 1–4 yr of age undergoing primary HHV-8 infection.

Three malignancies occurring primarily in adults with AIDS are strongly associated with HHV-8: KS, multicentric Castleman disease, and primary effusion lymphoma. KS is the most common neoplasm associated with AIDS but also occurs in HIV-uninfected persons living in the Mediterranean region (**classic KS**), in equatorial Africa (**endemic KS**), and in organ trans-

plant recipients (post-transplant KS). Multicentric Castleman disease and primary effusion lymphoma are much rarer lymphoproliferative diseases. Although HHV-8 can be identified in malignant tissue from most patients with these disorders, a clear etiologic link has not yet been firmly established. It has been suggested that HHV-8 may play an indirect role in these malignancies by providing viral analogs of cellular growth factors. There is controversy regarding the role of HHV-8 in development of multiple myeloma in elderly adults.

Diagnosis. HHV-8 infection can be demonstrated by serologic testing (enzyme immunoassay, immunofluorescence, and Western immunoblotting) or detection of HHV-8 DNA sequences by polymerase chain reaction amplification. Combinations of tests are often used, to maximize accuracy. However, tests are available from only a limited number of commercial laboratories. The virus is not easily cultivated.

Treatment. Several antiviral compounds inhibit HHV-8 in vitro, including ganciclovir, foscarnet, and cidofovir. However, the benefit of specific antiviral therapy for HHV-8–associated disease has not yet been established. Introduction of highly active antiretroviral therapy has dramatically improved survival for AIDS patients with KS. Other treatment options for KS include cryotherapy, phototherapy, topical retinoic acid, chemotherapy, radiation therapy, and surgery.

Andreoni M, Sarmati L, Nicastri E, et al: Primary human herpesvirus 8 infection in immunocompetent children. *JAMA* 2002;287:1295–300.

Baillargeon J, Deng JH, Hettler E, et al: Seroprevalence of Kaposi's sarcoma-associated herpesvirus infection among blood donors from Texas. *Ann Epidemiol* 2002;11:512–8.

Baillargeon J, Leach CT, Deng JH, et al: High prevalence of human herpesvirus 8 (HHV-8) infection in South Texas children. *J Med Virol* 2002;67:542–8.

Boshoff C, Chang Y: Kaposi's sarcoma-associated herpesvirus: A new DNA tumor virus. *Annu Rev Med* 2001;52:453–70.

Mantina H, Kankasa C, Klaskala W, et al: Vertical transmission of Kaposi's sarcoma-associated herpesvirus. *Int J Cancer* 2001;94:749–52.

Plancoulaine S, Abel L, van Beveren M, et al: Human herpesvirus 8 transmission from mother to child and between siblings in an endemic population. *Lancet* 2000;356:1062–5.

Singh N: Human herpesviruses-6,-7 and -8 in organ transplant recipients. *Clin Microbiol Infect* 2000;6:453–9.

Spira TJ, Lam L, Dollard SC, et al: Comparison of serologic assays and PCR for diagnosis of human herpesvirus 8 infection. *J Clin Microbiol* 2000;38:2174–80.

Chapter 237

Influenza Viruses *Peter Wright*

Influenza viral infections cause a broad array of respiratory illnesses that are responsible for significant morbidity and mortality in children.

Etiology. Influenza viruses are members of the family Orthomyxoviridae. They are large, single-stranded RNA viruses with a segmented genome encased in a lipid-containing envelope. The two major surface proteins that determine the serotype of influenza, hemagglutinin and neuraminidase, project as spikes through the envelope. Influenza viruses are divided into three types: A, B, and C. Influenza types A and B are the primary influenzal pathogens and causes of epidemic disease. Influenza type C is a sporadic cause of predominantly upper respiratory tract disease. Influenza types A and B are further divided into serotypically distinct strains that circulate on a yearly basis through the population.

Epidemiology. Influenza A viruses have a complex epidemiology involving animal hosts that serve as a reservoir for diverse strains with potential for infecting the human population. The segmented nature of the influenza genome allows reassortment to occur between an animal and human virus when co-infection occurs. Thus, potentially any of 15 hemagglutinins (H) and 9 neuraminidases (N) residing in animal reservoirs may be introduced into humans; influenza A viruses behave epidemiologically as though there were many serotypes. Minor changes within a serotype are termed antigenic drift; major changes in serotype are termed antigenic shift. In addition, migratory avian hosts may be responsible for spread of disease. Recent examples have occurred in Hong Kong with H5N1 and H9N2 viruses. For example, in the winter of 1997, a small outbreak of a virulent avian H5N1 influenza in humans was associated with a high mortality; 6 of 18 patients died. Influenza B has much less capacity for major antigenic change and no identified animal reservoir.

The worldwide epidemiology of influenza viruses demonstrates annual spread between the Northern and Southern hemispheres with the origins of new strains often traced to Asia. When a virus identified by a novel and serologically distinct hemagglutinin or neuraminidase enters the population, there is potential for a pandemic of influenza with excess morbidity and mortality on a global scale in a largely nonimmune population. The most dramatic pandemic in recent history occurred in 1918, when influenza was estimated to have killed more than 20 million people. More common is the almost yearly variation in the antigenic composition of the surface proteins, which confers a selective advantage to a new strain and results in localized epidemics of disease with mortality largely confined to the elderly and to those with underlying cardiopulmonary disease. Each year's strain is novel for infants because they have no pre-existing antibody except for maternally transferred antibody in the very young.

The attack rate and frequency of isolation of influenza is highest in young children. As many as 30–50% of children have serologic evidence of infection in a typical year. Children undergoing primary exposure to an influenza strain have higher levels and more prolonged shedding of the virus than adults, making them extremely effective transmitters of infection. Influenza is a disease of the colder months of the year in temperate climates; spread appears to occur by small-particle aerosol. Transmission through a community is rapid; the highest incidence of illness occurs within 2–3 wk of introduction. Influenza is marked by increased school absenteeism and a yearly peak in sick visits to the pediatrician. Influenza has been implicated in hospital spread of infection and may complicate the original illness that required hospitalization.

On a country or global basis, one or two predominant strains spread to create the annual epidemic. At present, influenza type A strains with the H1N1 and H3N2 serotypes and type B strains are co-circulating, and either type may be predominant in any one year, making predictions about the serotype and severity of the upcoming influenza season difficult. Strain variants are identified by their hemagglutinin and neuraminidase serotypes, by the geographic area from which they were originally isolated, by their isolate number, and by year of isolation. Thus, the influenza vaccine for 2002–2003 was trivalent, having strains identified as A/New Caledonia/20/99 (H1N1), A/Moscow/10/99 (H3N2), and B/Hong Kong/330/01.

Pathogenesis. The virus attaches to sialic acid residues on cells via the hemagglutinin and, via endocytosis, makes its way into vacuoles, where, with progressive acidification, there is fusion to the endosomal membrane and release of the viral RNA into the cytoplasm. The RNA is transported to the nucleus and transcribed. Newly synthesized RNA is returned to the cytoplasm and translated into proteins, which are transported to the cell membrane. This is followed by budding of virus through the cell membrane. The packaging mechanisms for the segmented genome are not well understood. A proteolytic cleavage of the hemagglutinin occurs at some point in the assembly and release

of the virus, which is essential for successful reinfection and amplification of virus titer. In humans, this replicative cycle is confined to the respiratory epithelium. With primary infection, virus replication continues for 10–14 days. Implicit in successful replication in the respiratory tract is the assumption that key proteolytic enzymes exist at this site. The effective cleavage of hemagglutinin has been demonstrated by respiratory secretions, but the cellular origin of the enzyme remains undefined.

Influenza causes a lytic infection of the respiratory epithelium with loss of ciliary function, decreased mucus production, and desquamation of the epithelial layer. These changes permit secondary bacterial invasion either directly through the epithelium or, in the case of the middle ear space, through obstruction of the normal drainage through the eustachian tube. Influenza types A and B have been reported to cause myocarditis, and influenza type B can cause myositis. Reye syndrome can result with the use of salicylates for influenza type B infection (Chapter 342).

The exact immune mechanisms involved in termination of primary infection and protection against reinfection are not well understood but may correspond to the induction of cytokines which inhibit viral replication such as interferon and tumor necrosis factor-α. The incubation period of influenza can be as short as 48–72 hr. The extremely short incubation period of influenza and its growth on the mucosal surface pose particular problems for invoking a protective immune response. Antigen presentation must be primarily at mucosal sites acting through the bronchial associated lymphoid tract. The major humoral response is directed against the hemagglutinin. High serum antibody levels generated by inactivated vaccine correlate with protection. Mucosally produced immunoglobulin (IgA) antibodies are presumably directed at the same antigenic sites and are thought to be the most effective and immediate response that can be generated to protect against influenza. Unfortunately, measurable IgA antibodies against influenza persist for a relatively short period, and symptomatic reinfection with influenza can be seen at intervals of 3–4 yr. Although heterotypic immunity can be demonstrated in the mouse through cell-mediated immune mechanisms directed toward common internal proteins, heterotypic immunity has not been shown in humans.

Clinical Manifestations. Influenza types A and B cause predominantly a respiratory illness. The onset of illness is abrupt and is marked by coryza, conjunctivitis, pharyngitis, and dry cough (Table 237–1). The predominant symptoms may localize anywhere in the respiratory tract, producing an isolated upper respiratory tract illness, croup, bronchiolitis, or pneumonia. More so than any of the other respiratory viruses, influenza is accompanied by systemic signs of high temperature, myalgia, malaise, and headache. Many of these symptoms may be mediated through cytokine production by the respiratory tract epithelium instead of reflecting systemic spread of the virus. The typical duration of the febrile illness is 2–4 days. Cough may persist for longer periods of time, and evidence of small airway dysfunction is often found weeks later. Other family members or close contacts often have a similar illness. Influenza is a less distinct illness in younger children and infants; manifestations may be localized to any region of the respiratory tract. The children may be highly febrile and toxic in appearance, prompting a full diagnostic work-up. Despite the distinctive features of influenza, the illness is often indistinguishable from that caused by other respiratory viruses such as respiratory syncytial virus, parainfluenza viruses, and adenoviruses.

Diagnosis. The diagnosis of influenza depends on epidemiologic and clinical considerations. In the context of an epidemic, the clinical diagnosis of influenza in a young child with fever, malaise, and respiratory symptoms can be made with some certainty. The laboratory confirmation of influenza can be made in three ways. If seen early in the illness, virus can be isolated from

TABLE 237–1. Relative Frequency of Symptoms and Signs During Classic Influenza in Older Children and Adolescents

Variable	Occurrence
Symptoms	
Chilly sensation	++++
Cough	+++
Headache	+++
Sore throat	+++
Prostration	++
Nasal stuffiness	++
Diarrhea	++
Dizziness	+
Eye irritation or pain	+
Vomiting	+
Myalgia	+
Signs	
Fever	++++
Pharyngitis	+++
Conjunctivitis (mild)	++
Rhinitis	++
Cervical lymphadenopathy	+
Pulmonary rales, wheezes, or rhonchi	+

++++ = 76–100%; +++ = 51–75%; ++ = 26–50%; + = 1–25%.

the nasopharynx by inoculation of the specimen into embryonated eggs or a limited number of cell lines that support the growth of influenza. The presence of influenza in the culture is confirmed by hemadsorption, which depends on the capacity of the hemagglutinin to bind red cells. Rapid diagnostic tests for influenza A are available that use variations on antigen capture such as an enzyme-linked immunosorbent assay. The diagnosis can be confirmed serologically with acute and convalescent sera drawn around the time of the illness and tested by hemagglutination inhibition.

LABORATORY FINDINGS. The clinical laboratory abnormalities associated with influenza are nonspecific. A relative leukopenia is frequently seen. Chest radiographs show evidence of atelectasis or infiltrate in about 10% of children.

Treatment. Two classes of antiviral drugs are effective in the treatment of influenza (Table 237–2). Guidelines for the use of the neuraminidase inhibitors, zanamivir and oseltamivir, are now available for children down to the ages of 7 years and 1 year, respectively. These drugs, given either as an inhalation in the case of zanamivir or orally in the case of oseltamivir, are effective against both influenza A and B strains. The second class of drugs, amantadine and rimantadine, can be used in influenza type A outbreaks. These two antivirals are not effective against influenza B and are not approved for use in children <1 yr of age. Each class of drug must be given within the first 48 hr of symptoms to decrease the severity and duration of influenza. Confusion and inability to concentrate or sleep are seen in some patients given amantadine. Drug resistance develops fairly

quickly during a course of amantadine or rimantadine therapy, but it is not widespread among circulating viruses. Partial resistance to the neuraminidase inhibitors may occur but is less common. All of these drugs are an adjunct to a strong vaccination program. A family home or schoolroom may be appropriate places to try to prevent secondary illness, particularly where individuals have underlying conditions that predispose them to severe or complicated influenza infection.

Adequate fluid intake and rest are important components in the management of influenza. Acetaminophen or ibuprofen, but not salicylates because of the risk of Reye syndrome (Chapter 342), should be used as antipyretics to control fever. The most difficult question for parents is the appropriate timing of consultation with a health care provider. Bacterial superinfections are relatively common, and in that case antibiotic therapy should be administered. Bacterial superinfections should be suspected with recrudescence of fever, prolonged fever, or deterioration in clinical status. With uncomplicated influenza, children should feel better after the first 48–72 hr.

Complications. Otitis media and pneumonia are common complications of influenza in young children. Acute otitis media may be seen in up to 25% of cases of culture-documented influenza. Pneumonia accompanying influenza may be a primary viral process. An acute hemorrhagic pneumonia may be seen in the most severe cases, as may have been frequent with the highly virulent strain seen in 1918. The more common cause of pneumonia is probably secondary bacterial infection through the damaged epithelial layer. Unusual clinical manifestations of influenza include acute myositis seen with influenza type B, which follows the acute respiratory illness by 5–7 days and is marked by muscle weakness and pain, particularly in the thigh muscles, and myoglobinuria. Myocarditis also follows influenza, and toxic shock syndrome is associated with influenza type B and staphylococcal colonization. Influenza is particularly severe in children with underlying cardiopulmonary disease, including congenital and acquired valvular disease, cardiomyopathy, bronchopulmonary dysplasia, asthma, cystic fibrosis, and neuromuscular diseases affecting the accessory muscles of breathing. Virus is shed for longer periods of time in children receiving cancer chemotherapy and children with immunodeficiency.

Prognosis. The prognosis for recovery is excellent, although full return to normal levels of activity and freedom from cough usually requires weeks rather than days.

Prevention. Influenza vaccine of targeted populations is the best means of prevention of severe disease from influenza. Recommendations for use of influenza vaccine have become progressively broader as the impact of influenza is appreciated in such groups as pregnant mothers and young children. Chemoprophylaxis with the drugs discussed under treatment is a secondary means of prevention.

VACCINE. An inactivated influenza vaccine becomes available each summer, incorporating changes in formulation that

TABLE 237–2. Recommended Daily Dosage of Influenza Antiviral Medications for Treatment and Prophylaxis*

Antiviral Agent	Route	Treatment	Prophylaxis	Age Group (yr)		
				1–6	7–9	>10
Zanamivir[†]	Inhaled	Yes	Not indicated	Not indicated	10 mg bid	10 mg bid
Oseltamivir[†]	Oral	Yes	Yes[§]	Dose varies from 30–75 mg bid by child's weight		
Amantadine[‡]	Oral	Yes	Yes	5 mg/kg/24 hr (maximum dose, 150 mg)		100 mg bid
Rimantadine[‡]	Oral	Yes	No	5 mg/kg/24 hr (maximum dose, 150 mg)		100 mg bid

*For details, consult annually updated recommendations from the Advisory Committee on Immunization Practices of the Centers for Disease Control and Prevention.
[†]Effective against both influenza A and B strains.
[‡]Effective only against influenza A strains.
[§]Over 12 yr of age with a single daily dose of 75 mg.

reflect the strains anticipated to circulate in the coming winter. The American Committee on Immunization Practices publishes guidelines for their use each year when the vaccines are formulated and released. Current guidelines include the administration of vaccine intramuscularly to children ≥6 mo of age as well as adults in groups at high risk for complications of influenza, including residents of long-term care facilities; patients with chronic disorders of the pulmonary or cardiovascular system, including asthma; patients with chronic metabolic diseases (including diabetes mellitus), renal dysfunction, hemoglobinopathies, or immunosuppression (including immunosuppression caused by medications and HIV); and patients receiving long-term aspirin therapy who may be at risk for Reye syndrome after influenza. Vaccination is also recommended for women who will be in the second or third trimester (≥14 wk gestation) of pregnancy during the influenza season (October–March). In addition, vaccine is recommended for individuals who may transmit influenza to persons at high risk, including all health care workers and household members of persons in groups at high risk. More recently the recommendations have been extended to encourage vaccination "to the extent logistically and economically feasible" of all healthy children who will be 6–23 months of age during influenza season (October–March) because their risk of hospitalization is similar to the elderly. Annual influenza vaccine is also recommended for all adults over 50 years of age, and all members of households, including children, with persons in groups at high risk.

Because of the decreased potential for causing febrile reactions, only the split-virus vaccine is recommended for children <12 yr of age. Two doses of vaccine (0.25 mL for 6–36 mo of age; 0.5 mL for 3–8 yr of age) at least 1 mo apart are recommended for primary immunization of children <9 yr of age. Live attenuated vaccines that are administered intranasally are in clinical trials and have been demonstrated to have an efficacy comparable to that of inactivated vaccine in adults. Trials in children have shown efficacy of 90%. These vaccines are likely to be licensed soon. Their ease of administration could serve to increase influenza vaccination among children.

CHEMOPROPHYLAXIS. Amantadine and zanamivir are licensed for prophylaxis of influenza A infections (see Table 237–2). They are recommended for prophylaxis for vaccinated and unvaccinated high-risk patients and their unvaccinated health care providers during influenza A outbreaks in closed settings, for unvaccinated persons and health care providers during community influenza A outbreaks and during the period of peak influenza A activity, for immunodeficient persons, and for those for whom the influenza vaccine is contraindicated.

Belshe RB, Mendelman PM, Treanor J, et al: The efficacy of live attenuated, cold-adapted, trivalent, intranasal influenza virus vaccine in children. *N Engl J Med* 1998;338:1405–12.

Centers for Disease Control and Prevention: Prevention and control of influenza: Recommendations of the Advisory Committee on Immunization Practices (ACIP). *MMWR Morb Mortal Wkly Rep* 2002;51(RR-3):1–31.

Couch RB: Prevention and treatment of influenza. *N Engl J Med* 2000;343:1778–87.

Glezen PW, Couch RB: Interpandemic influenza in the Houston area (1974–76). *N Engl J Med* 1978;298:587–92.

Neuzil KM, Mellen BG, Wright PF, et al: The effect of influenza on hospitalizations, outpatient visits, and courses of antibiotics in children. *N Engl J Med* 2001;343:225–31.

Subbarao K, Klimov A, Katz J, et al: Characterization of an avian influenza A (H5N1) virus isolated from a child with a fatal respiratory illness. *Science* 1998;279:393–6.

Reichert TA, Sugaya N, Fedson DS, et al: The Japanese experience with vaccinating schoolchildren against influenza. *N Engl J Med* 2002;344:889–96.

Wright PF, Bryant JD, Karzon DT: Comparison of influenza B/Hong Kong virus infections among infants, children, and young adults. *J Infect Dis* 1980;141:430–5.

Wright PF, Ross KB, Thompson J, et al: Influenza A infections in young children. *N Engl J Med* 1977;296:829–34.

Chapter 238
Parainfluenza Viruses
Peter Wright

Viruses in the parainfluenza family are common causes of respiratory illness in infants and young children. They cause a spectrum of upper and lower respiratory tract illnesses, but are particularly associated with laryngotracheitis, bronchitis, and croup.

Etiology. The parainfluenza viruses are members of the Paramyxoviridae family. There are four viruses in the parainfluenza group that cause illness in humans; they are designated types 1–4. The viruses have a nonsegmented, single-stranded RNA genome with a lipid-containing envelope derived from budding through the cell membrane. The major antigenic moieties are envelope spike proteins that exhibit hemagglutinating (HN protein) and cell fusion (F protein) properties.

Epidemiology. Parainfluenza viruses are spread from the respiratory tract by aerosolized secretions or direct hand contact with secretions. By 3 yr of age, most children have experienced infection with types 1, 2, and 3. Type 3 is endemic and can cause disease in the infant younger than 6 mo. Serious illness is seen with parainfluenza type 3 in immunocompromised patients. Types 1 and 2 occur in a seasonal pattern in the summer and fall and alternate years in which their serotype is most prevalent. Parainfluenza type 4 is more difficult to grow in tissue culture; thus, its epidemiology is less well defined. However, it does not appear to be a major cause of illness.

Pathogenesis. Parainfluenza viruses replicate in the respiratory epithelium without evidence of systemic spread. The propensity to cause illness in the upper large airways is presumably related to enhanced replication in the larynx, trachea, and bronchi compared with other viruses. The destruction of cells in the upper airways can lead to secondary bacterial invasion and resultant bacterial tracheitis. Eustachian tube obstruction can lead to secondary bacterial invasion of the middle-ear space and acute otitis media.

Illness caused by parainfluenza occurs shortly after inoculation with the virus. The mechanisms by which viral injury occurs are not known. Some parainfluenza viruses induce cell-to-cell fusion. During the budding process, cell membrane integrity is lost, and viruses can induce cell death through the process of apoptosis. The severity of illness correlates with the amount of viral shedding. Immune destruction of virally infected cells may also occur, but appears to be less important with mucosal than systemic infection. The level of immunoglobulin A antibody is the best predictor of susceptibility to infection. Reinfection is seen particularly with parainfluenza type 3 as mucosal immunity wanes. The inability of children with serious T-cell defects to clear parainfluenza type 3 suggests a cell-mediated component of immunity.

Clinical Manifestations. Most parainfluenza virus infections are confined to the upper respiratory tract (Table 238–1). This relatively mild-appearing illness is belied by a spectrum of rarer but more serious illnesses that result in hospitalization. The parainfluenza viruses account for 50% of hospitalizations for croup and 15% of cases of bronchiolitis and pneumonia. Parainfluenza type 1 causes more cases of croup, whereas parainfluenza type 3 causes a broad spectrum of lower respiratory tract diseases.

Parainfluenza virus infections are not associated with fever. Aside from low-grade fever, systemic complaints are rare. The illness usually lasts 4–5 days; however, virus may be recovered in low titers for 2–3 wk. Rarely, parainfluenza viruses have been implicated in parotitis.

TABLE 238–1. Diagnoses and Signs and Symptoms of Children Younger than 5 Yr of Age with Parainfluenza Infections

Diagnoses	Type 1 (n = 77)	Type 2 (n = 33)	Type 3 (n = 157)	Other (n = 19)
Upper Respiratory	90%	94%	89%	84%
Common cold	31%	42%	32%	42%
Pharyngitis	21%	18%	10%	11%*
Acute otitis media	38%	30%	52%	32%†
Lower Respiratory	17%	15%	15%	21%
Croup (laryngotracheobronchitis)	16%	6%	5%	21%‡
Bronchiolitis	1%	9%	6%	0%
Signs and Symptoms				
Coryza	74%	75%	83%	83%
Conjunctivitis	36%	36%	36%	44%
Cough	73%	67%	81%	77%
Hoarseness	28%	18%	11%	39%§
Rales or rhonchi	6%	15%	15%	11%
Wheezing	9%	12%	4%	5%
Temperature > 38°C	33%	16%	38%	6%‖
Temperature > 39°C	8%	6%	10%	0%
Irritability	47%	30%	54%	72%¶
Anorexia	36%	36%	36%	44%
Vomiting	15%	15%	24%	22%
Diarrhea	21%	15%	14%	22%

Note that p values are for Fisher's exact test for the null hypothesis that all types are alike.

*p = .09
†p = .03
‡p = .01
§p = .001
‖p = .004
¶p = .02

From Reed G, Jewett PH, Thompson J, et al: Epidemiology and clinical impact of parainfluenza virus infections in otherwise healthy infants and young children < 5 years old. J Infect Dis 1997; 175:808. Used with permission.

Diagnosis. The diagnosis of parainfluenza virus infection in children is usually based only on clinical and epidemiologic criteria. The virus should be specifically sought in persistent pneumonias in immunosuppressed children. The radiographic "steeple sign" of progressive narrowing of the subglottic region is characteristic of parainfluenza virus respiratory tract infections.

LABORATORY FINDINGS. There are no distinctive laboratory findings. The laboratory diagnosis of parainfluenza virus infection can be accomplished by inoculation of nasal secretions into tissue culture, with presumptive diagnosis based on finding a hemadsorbent agent and final serologic diagnosis based on hemadsorption inhibition. Direct immunofluorescent staining is available in some centers for rapid identification of virus antigen in oropharyngeal sections.

Treatment. The possibility of rapid respiratory compromise during severe croup should influence the level of care given (Chapter 371). Careful attention to symptomatic care is important. Parents should be provided a description of the signs of increasing respiratory distress that should lead to reassessment by a health care provider. Humidification and exposure to cold air are both classically associated with a decrease in mucosal edema and liquefaction of secretions that may help to relieve obstruction; however, their value has not been shown in controlled trials. Aerosolized racemic epinephrine may temporarily improve aeration, but has the possibility of rebound. Aerosolized or systemic corticosteroids should be part of the management of croup in the emergency room setting and after hospitalization. The indications for antibiotics are limited to well-documented secondary bacterial infections of the middle ears or lower respiratory tract.

Ribavirin has some antiviral activity against parainfluenza virus, and should be considered in the immunocompromised child with persistent parainfluenza viral pneumonia.

Complications. In children with fever or more severe respiratory compromise, the possibility of a bacterial tracheitis with purulent infection below the epiglottis and vocal cords should be considered. The high frequency of otitis media complicating parainfluenza virus indicates that careful pneumatic otoscopy should be performed in all children with suspected parainfluenza virus infection.

Prognosis. The prognosis for full recovery is excellent in the normal child. No long-term pulmonary residua of parainfluenza virus infection have been described.

Prevention. Work is progressing with both live and subunit parainfluenza type 3 vaccines. The live vaccine candidates include a cold-adapted virus of human origin and a bovine parainfluenza virus, which is attenuated because of host range adaptation. The measure of protection afforded by vaccines will be difficult to assess because symptomatic reinfection is seen and the frequency of serious infection in the general population is low. Nonetheless, it is clear that prevention of acute respiratory illness that results from parainfluenza virus is a worthwhile goal.

Denny FW, Murphy TF, Clyde WA Jr, et al: An 11-year study in a pediatric practice. *Pediatrics* 1983;71:871–6.

Hall CB, Geiman JM, Breese BB, et al: Parainfluenza infections in children: Correlation of shedding with clinical manifestations. *J Pediatr* 1977;91:194–8.

Hall CB: Respiratory syncytial virus and parainfluenza virus. *N Engl J Med* 2001;344:1917–28.

Henrickson KJ, Kuhn SM, Savatski LL: Epidemiology and cost of infection with human parainfluenza virus types 1 and 2 in young children. *Clin Infect Dis* 1994; 18:770–9.

Knott AM, Long CE, Hall CB: Parainfluenza viral infections in pediatric outpatients: Seasonal patterns and clinical characteristics. *Pediatr Infect Dis J* 1994;13: 269–73.

Landau LI, Geelhoed GC: Aerosolized steroids for croup. *N Engl J Med* 1994;331: 322–3.

Orelicek SL: Management of acute laryngotracheobronchitis. *Pediatr Infect Dis J* 1998;17:1164–65.

Reed G, Jewett PH, Thompson J, et al: Epidemiology and clinical impact of parainfluenza virus infections in otherwise healthy infants and young children <5 years old. *J Infect Dis* 1997;175:807–13.

Chapter 239
Respiratory Syncytial Virus

Kenneth McIntosh

Respiratory syncytial virus (RSV) is the major cause of bronchiolitis (Chapter 371) and pneumonia in children younger than 1 yr of age (Chapter 389). It is the most important respiratory tract pathogen of early childhood.

Etiology. RSV is a medium-sized, membrane-bound RNA virus that develops in the cytoplasm of infected cells and matures by budding from the plasma membrane. It belongs to the family Paramyxoviridae, along with parainfluenza, mumps, and measles viruses, but is the sole member of the genus *Pneumovirus* that infects human beings. Although different strains of RSV show some antigenic heterogeneity, this variation is primarily in one of the two surface glycoproteins (G protein), and it is not clear that this degree of difference is clinically or epidemiologically significant. RSV grows in a number of types of tissue culture, in which it produces characteristic syncytial cytopathology.

Epidemiology. The occurrence of annual outbreaks and the high incidence of infection during the first months of life are unique among human viruses. RSV is distributed worldwide and appears in yearly epidemics. In temperate climates, these epidemics occur each winter and last 4–5 mo. During the remainder of the year, infections are sporadic and uncommon. In the Northern Hemisphere, epidemics usually peak in January, February, or March, but peaks have been recognized as early as December and as late as June. At these times, hospital admissions for bronchiolitis and pneumonia of children younger than 1 yr increase and decrease in proportion to the number of RSV infections in the community. In the tropics, the epidemic pattern is less clear.

Transplacentally transmitted anti-RSV antibody, when present in high concentration, has some protective effect. This probably accounts for the low frequency of severe infections in the first 4–6 wk of life, except in infants born prematurely who receive less than a full complement of maternal immunoglobulin (Ig) G. Nevertheless, serum antibody is not fully protective, and the age at which an infant undergoes first infection depends also on the opportunities for exposure. It is estimated that in an urban setting about half of the susceptible infants undergo primary infection in each epidemic. Thus, infection is almost universal by the 2nd birthday. Reinfection occurs at a rate of 10–20% per epidemic throughout childhood; the frequency is lower in adults. In situations of high exposure such as daycare centers, attack rates are higher: nearly 100% for first infections and 60–80% for second and subsequent infections.

Estimates of the severity of primary infections have emerged from studies of outbreaks in nurseries and institutions. Under these circumstances, asymptomatic infection is rare. Most infants experience coryza and pharyngitis, usually with fever and occasionally with otitis media. In 10–40% of patients, the lower respiratory tract is involved to a varying degree. Bronchitis, bronchopneumonia, and bronchiolitis all occur. Calculations based on hospital admissions in the United States and Britain yield a ratio of 1–3 infants hospitalized with bronchiolitis or pneumonia for every 100 primary infections with the virus.

Reinfection may occur as early as a few weeks after recovery, but usually takes place during subsequent annual outbreaks. The severity of illness during reinfection is usually lower, and appears to be a function of both partial immunity and increased age. Nevertheless, instances of severe RSV bronchiolitis occurring twice in succession have been documented.

Bronchiolitis is the most common clinical diagnosis in infants hospitalized with RSV infections, although the syndrome is often indistinguishable from RSV pneumonia in infants, and, indeed, the two frequently coexist. All RSV diseases of the lower respiratory tract (excluding croup) have their highest incidence from 2–7 mo of age and decrease in frequency thereafter. The syndrome of bronchiolitis becomes uncommon after the 1st birthday; acute infective wheezing attacks after that age are often termed "wheezy bronchitis," "asthmatoid bronchitis," or simply asthma attacks. Viral pneumonia is a persistent problem throughout childhood, although RSV becomes less prominent as the etiologic agent after the 1st year. RSV is responsible for 45–75% of cases of bronchiolitis, 15–25% of childhood pneumonias, and 6–8% of cases of croup.

Bronchiolitis and pneumonia resulting from RSV are more common in boys than in girls by a ratio of about 1.5:1. Racial factors make little difference. Lower respiratory tract involvement occurs more often and earlier in life in lower socioeconomic groups and in crowded living conditions.

The incubation period from exposure to first symptoms is about 4 days. The virus is excreted for variable periods, probably depending on severity of illness and immunologic status. Most infants with lower respiratory tract illness shed virus for 5–12 days after hospital admission. Excretion for 3 wk and longer has been documented. Spread of infection occurs when large, infected droplets, either airborne or conveyed on hands, are inoculated in the nose or conjunctiva of a susceptible subject. RSV is probably introduced into most families by schoolchildren undergoing reinfection. Typically, in the space of a few days, older siblings and one or both parents acquire colds, but the infant becomes more severely ill with fever, otitis media, or lower respiratory tract disease.

Nosocomial infection during RSV epidemics is an important concern. Virus is usually spread from child to child on the hands of caregivers. Adults undergoing reinfection have also been implicated in spread of the virus.

Pathogenesis. Bronchiolitis is characterized by virus-induced necrosis of the bronchiolar epithelium, hypersecretion of mucus, and round cell infiltration and edema of the surrounding submucosa. These changes result in formation of mucous plugs obstructing bronchioles with consequent hyperinflation or collapse of the distal lung tissue. In interstitial pneumonia, infiltration is more generalized, and epithelial necrosis may extend to both the bronchi and the alveoli. Infants are particularly apt to experience small airway obstruction because of the small size of the normal bronchioles.

Immunologic injury is likely a factor in the pathogenesis of bronchiolitis caused by RSV. A large number of soluble factors (interleukins, leukotrienes, and chemokines) with the potential to stimulate inflammation and tissue damage are liberated during RSV infection. In animal models, reactive T cells are involved both in the pathogenesis of lung damage and in recovery from infection. In many children, RSV bronchiolitis is followed by recurrent wheezing episodes, and certain markers found during the acute episode, particularly the presence of eosinophils and eosinophilic cationic protein in blood, appear to be associated with such recurrences.

It is not clear how often superimposed bacterial infection plays a pathogenic role in RSV lower respiratory tract disease. The present view is that RSV-induced bronchiolitis in infants is an exclusively viral disease and that bacteria are of little importance even when the disease is accompanied by atelectasis or interstitial pneumonia.

Clinical Manifestations. The first signs of infection of the infant with RSV are rhinorrhea and pharyngitis. Cough may appear simultaneously but more often after an interval of 1–3 days, at which time there may also be sneezing and a low-grade fever. Soon after the cough develops, the child begins to wheeze audibly. If the disease is mild, the symptoms may not progress beyond this stage. Auscultation often reveals diffuse rhonchi, fine rales or crackles, and wheezes. Abundant, clear rhinorrhea usually persists throughout the illness, with intermittent fever. Roentgenograms of the chest at this stage are frequently normal.

If the illness progresses, cough and wheezing increase and air hunger ensues with increased respiratory rate, intercostal and subcostal retractions, hyperexpansion of the chest, restlessness, and peripheral cyanosis. Signs of severe, life-threatening illness are central cyanosis, tachypnea of more than 70 breaths/min, listlessness, and apneic spells. At this stage, the chest may be greatly hyperexpanded and almost silent to auscultation because of poor air exchange.

Chest radiographs of infants hospitalized with RSV bronchiolitis are normal in about 10% of cases; air trapping or hyperexpansion of the chest is evident in about 50%. Peribronchial thickening or interstitial pneumonia is seen in 50–80%. Segmental consolidation occurs in 10–25%. Pleural effusion is rarely, if ever, seen.

In some infants, the course of the illness may be more like that of pneumonia with the prodromal rhinorrhea and cough followed by dyspnea, poor feeding, and listlessness, with a minimum of wheezing and hyperexpansion. Although the clinical diagnosis is pneumonia, wheezing is often present intermittently and the chest roentgenogram may show air trapping.

Fever is an inconstant sign in RSV infection. Otitis media, with viral nucleic acid detectable in middle ear fluids, is common. Rash and conjunctivitis each occur in a few cases. In young infants, particularly those who were born prematurely, periodic breathing and apneic spells have been distressingly frequent signs, even with relatively mild bronchiolitis. It is likely that a small portion of deaths included in the category of sudden infant death syndrome are due to RSV infection.

RSV infections in profoundly immunocompromised hosts may be severe at any age. The mortality associated with RSV pneumonia after bone marrow or solid organ transplantation is 50% or higher. RSV infection does not seem to be severe in HIV-infected patients.

Diagnosis. Bronchiolitis is a clinical diagnosis. Causation by RSV can be suspected with varying degrees of certainty from the clinical picture, the season of the year, and the presence of a typical outbreak at the time. Another helpful epidemiologic feature is the presence of colds in older household contacts, because RSV frequently reinfects and produces symptoms in older children and adults.

Routine laboratory tests offer little helpful information in most cases of bronchiolitis or pneumonia caused by RSV. The white cell count is normal or elevated, and the differential count may be normal with either a neutrophilic or mononuclear predominance. Bacterial cultures of the throat grow normal flora. Hypoxemia is frequent and tends to be more marked than anticipated on the basis of the clinical findings. When it is severe, it may be accompanied by hypercapnia and acidosis.

The diagnostic dilemma of greatest import is the question of possible bacterial or chlamydial involvement, because such presence dictates the possible use of antimicrobials. When bronchiolitis is clinically mild or when infiltrates are absent by roentgenogram, there is little likelihood of a bacterial component. In infants 1–4 mo of age, interstitial pneumonitis may be caused by *Chlamydia trachomatis* (Chapter 208.3). In *C. trachomatis* pneumonia, there may be a history of conjunctivitis, and the illness tends to be of subacute onset. Coughing and rales are prominent; wheezing is not. There may also be eosinophilia. Fever and rhinorrhea are usually absent.

Consolidation without other signs or with pleural effusion is considered of bacterial origin until proved otherwise. Other signs suggesting bacterial pneumonia are elevation of the neutrophil count, depression of the white cell count in the presence of severe disease, ileus or other abdominal signs, pleuritic pain, high temperature, and circulatory collapse. In such instances, there is rarely any doubt about the need for antibiotics.

Definitive diagnosis of RSV infection is based on the detection of virus or viral components in respiratory secretions. An aspirate of mucus or a nasopharyngeal wash from the child's posterior nasal cavity is the optimal specimen. A nasopharyngeal swab is also acceptable. A tracheal aspirate is unnecessary. The specimen should be placed on ice, taken directly to the laboratory, and processed for antigen detection or inoculated onto susceptible cell monolayers.

Treatment. In uncomplicated cases of bronchiolitis, treatment is symptomatic. Humidified oxygen is usually indicated for hospitalized infants because most are hypoxic. Many infants are slightly to moderately dehydrated; therefore, fluids should be carefully administered in amounts somewhat greater than maintenance. Often intravenous or tube feeding is helpful when sucking is difficult due to tachypnea. Infants may breathe more easily when propped up at an angle of 10–30 degrees.

A trial of epinephrine administered either parenterally or by aerosol may relieve wheezing and improve clinical status, and should be repeated if initial benefit is shown. Corticosteroids are not indicated except in older children with an established diagnosis of asthma.

In most instances antibiotics are not useful, and their indiscriminate use in presumed viral bronchiolitis and pneumonia should be discouraged. Interstitial pneumonia in infants 1–4 mo old may be chlamydial; therefore, erythromycin (40 mg/kg/24 hr) or azithromycin (10mg/kg on day 1, 5 mg/kg on days 2–5) may be beneficial. Parenteral antibiotics are indicated for older infants with interstitial pneumonia, when consolidation is found, and for critically ill children.

The antiviral drug ribavirin, delivered by **small-particle aerosol** for 3–5 days, probably has a modest beneficial effect on the course of RSV pneumonia. Shortened hospital stay and reduced mortality have not been demonstrated, however, and trials in intubated infants have not shown efficacy. Its use is, therefore, rarely indicated except for selected cases of severe immunodeficiency, in which unrestricted viral replication is clearly important in the pathogenesis of severe disease.

Intravenous immunoglobulin prepared from plasma with high neutralization antibody titers (RSV-IGIV), as well as humanized monoclonal antibody, palivizumab, have been used to treat severely immunodeficient patients with pneumonia and RSV infection. Although there is no clear evidence of efficacy, such treatment does reduce the titer of virus in the respiratory tract and may offer a rational therapeutic approach in situations in which the prognosis is otherwise poor.

Prognosis. The mortality of hospitalized infants with RSV infection of the lower respiratory tract is about 2%. Almost all deaths occur in young, premature infants or those with underlying disease of the neuromuscular, pulmonary, cardiovascular, or immunologic system.

Many children with asthma have a history of bronchiolitis in infancy. There is recurrent wheezing in 33–50% of children with typical RSV bronchiolitis in infancy. In patients older than 1 yr with bronchiolitis, there is an increasing probability that, although the episode may be virus induced, this is the first of multiple wheezing attacks that will later be called asthma.

As mentioned, RSV infection in profoundly immunodeficient or immunosuppressed individuals of any age may, if clinical pneumonia occurs, carry a mortality rate as high as 50%.

Prevention. Within the hospital, the most important preventive measures are aimed at blocking nosocomial spread. During RSV season, high-risk infants should be separated from infants with respiratory symptoms. Separate gowns and gloves and careful handwashing should be used for the care of all infants with suspected or established RSV infection.

PASSIVE IMMUNOPROPHYLAXIS. Administration of either palivizumab (15 mg/kg intramuscularly), a monoclonal antibody against RSV, or high-titered RSV intravenous immunoglobulin (RSV-IVIG; 750 mg/kg) is recommended for protecting high-risk children against serious complications from RSV disease. Immunoprophylaxis reduces the frequency and total days of hospitalization for RSV infections in high-risk infants. These agents are administered monthly from the beginning (October–December) to the end (March–May) of the RSV season. Palivizumab is preferred for most children because of ease of intramuscular administration and lack of interference with live virus vaccinations (measles-mumps-rubella and varicella). RSV-IVIG provides some protection against other respiratory pathogens and may be substituted for IVIG during the RSV season for children with immunodeficiency receiving monthly IVIG.

The cost-effectiveness of prophylaxis depends on the health care setting and the risk of the individual child. In the United States, candidates for immunoprophylaxis include infants with lung disease and infants who were born very prematurely. Children younger than 2 yr with bronchopulmonary dysplasia requiring supplemental oxygen therapy currently or within the 6 mo before the RSV season should receive prophylaxis for the first two RSV seasons if they have severe lung disease and only the first RSV season for less severe lung disease. Infants without bronchopulmonary dysplasia should receive prophylaxis up to 12 mo of age if they were born at 28 wk of gestation or earlier and up to 6 mo of age if they were born at 29–32 wk of gestation. One dose of immunoprophylaxis may be considered for premature infants to be discharged from the hospital during the RSV season. RSV-IVIG is contraindicated and palivizumab is not recommended for children with cyanotic congenital heart disease. Adverse events with palivizumab are uncommon.

VACCINE. There is not currently a vaccine against RSV. Vaccine development for RSV has proceeded cautiously since the experience in the 1960s with an alum-precipitated formalin-inactivated vaccine. This vaccine was excellent for inducing serum antibodies, but vaccinees had augmented disease after natural infection. Live, attenuated vaccines have produced unacceptable symptoms or reverted to wild-type virus. Current candidate vaccines are either purified subunit vaccines against one of the surface proteins or attenuated, cold-adapted live vaccines.

American Academy of Pediatrics, Committee on Infectious Diseases and Committee on Fetus and Newborn: Prevention of respiratory syncytial virus infections: Indications for the use of palivizumab and update on the use of RSV-IGIV. *Pediatrics* 1998;102:1211–6.

Glezen WP, Paredes A, Allison JE, et al: Risk of respiratory syncytial virus infection for infants from low-income families in relationship to age, sex, ethnic group and maternal antibody level. *J Pediatr* 1981;98:708–15.

Guerguerian AM, Gauthier M, Lebel MH, et al: Ribavirin in ventilated respiratory syncytial virus bronchiolitis. A randomized, placebo-controlled trial. *Am J Respir Crit Care Med* 1999;160:829–34.

Hall CB, Douglas RG Jr, Geiman JM, et al: Nosocomial respiratory syncytial virus infections. *N Engl J Med* 1975;293:1343–6.

Henderson FW, Collier AM, Clyde WA Jr, et al: Respiratory-syncytial-virus infections, reinfections and immunity: A prospective, longitudinal study in young children. *N Engl J Med* 1979;300:530–4.

Hertz MI, Englund JA, Snover D, et al: Respiratory syncytial virus-induced acute lung injury in adult patients with bone marrow transplants. A clinical approach and review of the literature. *Medicine* 1989;68:269–81.

Holberg CJ, Wright AL, Martinez FD, et al: Risk factors for respiratory syncytial virus-associated lower respiratory illnesses in the first year of life. *Am J Epidemiol* 1991;133:1135–51.

Impact-RSV Study Group: Palivizumab, a humanized respiratory syncytial virus monoclonal antibody, reduces hospitalization from respiratory syncytial virus infection in high-risk infants. The Impact-RSV Study Group. *Pediatrics* 1998;102:531–7.

Simpson W, Hacking PM, Court SDM, et al: Radiological findings in respiratory syncytial virus infection in children: II. The correlation of radiological categories with clinical and virological findings. *Pediatr Radiol* 1974;2:155–60.

Welliver RC: Immunology of respiratory syncytial virus infection: Eosinophils, cytokines, chemokines and asthma. *Pediatr Infect Dis J* 2000;19:780–3.

Chapter 240
Adenoviruses *Kenneth McIntosh*

Adenoviruses cause 5–8% of acute respiratory disease in infants, plus a wide array of other syndromes, including pharyngoconjunctival fever, follicular conjunctivitis, epidemic keratoconjunctivitis, myocarditis, hemorrhagic cystitis, acute diarrhea, intussusception, and encephalomyelitis. Adenoviral pneumonia may have serious long-term sequelae, including bronchiolitis obliterans. Only one third of the 49 serotypes have been associated with disease.

Etiology. The Adenoviridae are DNA viruses of intermediate size, which are classified into subgenera A to F. The virion has an icosahedral coat (capsid) made up of 252 subunits (capsomers) of which 240 are "hexons" and 12 are "pentons." The hexons have a cross reacting antigen common to all mammalian adenoviruses. The penton confers type specificity, and antibody to it is protective. Adenoviruses can also be classified by their characteristic DNA "fingerprints" on gels after being digested with restriction endonucleases, and this classification generally conforms to their antigenic types.

All adenovirus types, except types 40 and 41, grow in primary human embryonic kidney cells, and most grow in HEp-2 or HeLa cells, producing a typical destructive cytopathic effect. Types 40 and 41 (and other serotypes as well) grow in 293 cells, a line of human embryonic kidney cells into which certain "early" adenovirus genes have been introduced.

Many adenovirus types, but particularly the common childhood types (1, 2, and 5), are shed for prolonged periods from both the respiratory and gastrointestinal tracts. These types also establish low-level and chronic infection of the tonsils and adenoids.

Epidemiology. Adenoviral infections are distributed worldwide. They occur year-round but are most prevalent in spring or early summer and again in midwinter in temperate climates. Certain types tend to occur in epidemics, notably types 4 and 7 in outbreaks of febrile respiratory disease, types 3, 7, and 21 in severe pneumonia; type 3 in pharyngoconjunctival fever; type 11 in hemorrhagic cystitis; and types 8, 19, and 37 in epidemic keratoconjunctivitis. For unexplained reasons, adenovirus types 3 and 7 cause severe epidemics of pneumonia in the children of northern China and Korea, with mortality rates in hospitalized cases of 5–15%.

More than 60% of school-aged children have antibodies to the common respiratory types. Almost all adults have serum antibody to types 1–7. Spread occurs by the respiratory and fecal-oral routes, although it is not clear whether spread is by large- or small-particle aerosol. Hospital outbreaks of respiratory disease and keratoconjunctivitis have been described.

Pathogenesis. Adenoviruses are among the few "respiratory" viruses that grow well in the epithelium of the small intestine. Although mucosal surfaces are the primary target early in infection and typically the site of the most common pathology, viremia probably occurs frequently, with accompanying fever.

Adenoviral pneumonia produces characteristic microscopic changes, with dense lymphocytic infiltrates, destruction of the bronchial and bronchiolar epithelium, focal necrosis of mucous glands, hyaline membrane formation, and several types of nuclear inclusion bodies.

Clinical Manifestations. Adenoviruses cause a wide array of clinical syndromes.

ACUTE RESPIRATORY DISEASE. This is the most common manifestation of adenovirus infection in children and adults. Acute adenovirus respiratory tract infections in infants and children are not clinically distinctive and are usually caused by types 1, 2, 3, 5, or 6. Primary infections in infants are frequently associated with fever and respiratory symptoms and are complicated by otitis media in more than half of the patients. Adenovirus respiratory infections are associated with a significant incidence of diarrhea.

Pharyngitis due to adenovirus typically has symptoms of coryza, sore throat, and fever. Adenoviruses can be identified in 15–20% of children with isolated pharyngitis, mostly in preschoolers and infants.

Pneumonia is uncommon, but 7–9% of hospitalized children with acute pneumonia have adenovirus infection. Any of the "respiratory" types can cause pneumonia, but severe infections are most likely due to type 3, 7, or 21. Such infections have a mortality as high as 10%, and survivors may have residual airway damage, manifested by bronchiectasis, bronchiolitis obliterans, or, rarely, pulmonary fibrosis. Neonatal adenovirus pneumonia occurs rarely, but may be severe or fatal.

A *pertussis-like syndrome* has been described in association with adenovirus infections. In these cases, adenoviruses frequently accompany *Bordetella pertussis* as co-infecting agents, but occasionally they may be causative on their own.

Pharyngoconjunctival fever is a clinically distinct syndrome that occurs particularly in association with type 3 adenovirus. Features include a high temperature that lasts 4–5 days, pharyngitis, conjunctivitis, preauricular and cervical lymphadenopathy, and rhinitis. Nonpurulent conjunctivitis occurs in 75% of patients and is manifested by inflammation of both the bulbar and palpebral conjunctivae of one or both eyes; it often persists after the fever and other symptoms have resolved. Headache, malaise, and weakness are common, and there is considerable lethargy after the acute stage.

CONJUNCTIVITIS AND KERATOCONJUNCTIVITIS. Adenovirus is one of the most common causes of follicular conjunctivitis, which is a relatively mild illness, and keratoconjunctivitis, which may occur in epidemics and is associated with infection by adenovirus types 8, 19, and 37. Keratitis begins as the conjunctivitis wanes, and may cause corneal opacities that last several years.

MYOCARDITIS. In several series of acute myocarditis or idiopathic cardiomyopathy, investigated by the application of polymerase chain reaction (PCR) in the search for microbial agents, adenovirus has been found as commonly as, or more commonly than, nonpolio enteroviruses. It is widely assumed that adenovirus has an important etiologic role in this disease. It has also been associated with heart transplant rejection and with some cases of endocardial fibroelastosis.

GASTROINTESTINAL INFECTIONS. Adenoviruses can be found in the stools of 5–9% of children with acute diarrhea. About one half of these are the "enteric" types, 40 or 41. It is also clear that enteric infection with any adenovirus serotype is often asymptomatic, so the causative role in these episodes is frequently uncertain.

The pathogenesis of intussusception is thought by many to include enlarged lymph nodes as an initiating factor. Adenoviruses have been recovered from mesenteric lymph nodes or appendices at surgery and also from surface cultures in a higher percentage of children with intussusception than of controls. Adenoviruses have also been found in the appendices of children with appendicitis.

HEMORRHAGIC CYSTITIS. This syndrome has a sudden onset of bacteriologically sterile hematuria, dysuria, frequency, and urgency lasting 1–2 wk. Infection with adenovirus types 11 and 21 has been found in some affected children and young adults.

REYE SYNDROME AND REYE-LIKE SYNDROMES. Typical Reye syndrome has followed confirmed adenovirus infection of several serotypes, particularly in very young children. In addition, several cases of a Reye-like syndrome have been reported, all of which are caused by infection with adenovirus type 7. The latter disease, which is frequently fatal, is characterized by severe bronchopneumonia, hepatitis, seizures, and disseminated intravascular coagulation. Circulating adenovirus penton antigen has been found in several patients and has been implicated in the pathogenesis.

INFECTIONS IN IMMUNOCOMPROMISED HOSTS. Adenoviruses are important pathogens in immunocompromised hosts with either B- or T-cell deficiencies. In B-cell–deficient (hypogammaglobulinemic) patients, a chronic meningoencephalitis similar to that caused by enteroviruses has been described. In T-cell–deficient patients, regardless of whether this deficiency is congenital, acquired, or iatrogenic, prolonged diarrhea is common, and fulminant hepatitis and pneumonia, frequently with a fatal outcome, have been described. There is also a close association between adenovirus infection and both hemorrhagic cystitis and tubulointerstitial nephritis in immunocompromised children, particularly following bone marrow transplantation.

Diagnosis. The laboratory diagnosis of adenovirus infection in children may be made by immunohistology or suggestive pathologic changes in biopsy material, detection of virus by culture or PCR, demonstration of an increase in antibody titers, or a combination of virus detection and serologic testing. PCR is a very useful method in the detection of adenovirus in biopsy tissues. If virus is found in a "privileged" site, such as blood, urine, or cerebrospinal fluid, or in a biopsy of the lung or liver, the implication of infection with disease and organ damage is strong. Likewise,

detection of certain adenovirus types in respiratory secretions (type 7 or 21) probably indicates their etiologic involvement. The presence of untyped virus or the common childhood types (1, 2, and 5) in respiratory secretions or stool does not, however, indicate clinical adenovirus infection because these viruses may be excreted chronically and asymptomatically. In these instances, discovery of a coincident increase in antibody is helpful in assigning a specific adenovirus type to disease. Adenovirus infection may also be considered etiologic if an increase in antibody is found between sera drawn in the acute stage and in convalescence from a patient with an appropriate illness. Adenovirus infection often results in a high erythrocyte sedimentation rate and white blood cell count.

Treatment. There is interest in the possible role of cidofovir, a renal-toxic antiviral drug that requires intravenous administration, in treatment of severe adenovirus infections. Ribavirin can inhibit viral growth of some strains in vitro, but evidence of its clinical efficacy is lacking.

Prevention. Vaccines that contain either killed or live virus have been developed to prevent type 4 and 7 infections in military recruits. These vaccines have not, however, been used in children.

Brandt CD, Kim HW, Jeffries BC, et al: Infections in 18,000 infants and children in a controlled study of respiratory tract disease: II. Adenovirus pathogenicity in relation to serologic type and illness syndrome. *Am J Epidemiol* 1969;90: 484–500.

Hale GA, Heslop HE, Krance RA, et al: Adenovirus infection after pediatric bone marrow transplantation. *Bone Marrow Transplant* 1999;23:277–82.

Hong JY, Lee HJ, Piedra PA, et al. Lower respiratory tract infections due to adenovirus in hospitalized Korean children: Epidemiology, clinical features, and prognosis. *Clin Infect Dis* 2001;32:1423–9.

Ladisch S, Lovejoy FH, Hierholzer JC, et al: Extrapulmonary manifestations of adenovirus type 7 pneumonia simulating Reye syndrome and the possible role of an adenovirus toxin. *Pediatrics* 1979;95:348–55.

Martin AB, Webber S, Fricker FJ, et al: Acute myocarditis: Rapid diagnosis by PCR in children. *Circulation* 1994;90:330–9.

Michaels MG, Green M, Wald ER, et al: Adenovirus infection in pediatric liver transplant recipients. *J Infect Dis* 1992;165:170–4.

Nelson KE, Gavitt F, Batt MD, et al: The role of adenoviruses in the pertussis syndrome. *J Pediatr* 1975;86:335–41.

Numazaki Y, Kumasaka T, Yano N, et al: Further study on acute hemorrhagic cystitis due to adenovirus type 11. *N Engl J Med* 1973;289:344–7.

Ruuskanen O, Meurman O, Sarkkinen H: Adenoviral diseases in children: A study of 105 hospital cases. *Pediatrics* 1985;76:79–83.

Similau S, Ylikorkala O, Wasz-Hockert O: Type 7 adenovirus pneumonia. *J Pediatr* 79:605–11.

Van R, Wun CC, O'Ryan ML, et al: Outbreaks of human enteric adenovirus types 40 and 41 in Houston day care centers. *J Pediatr* 1992;120:516–21.

Chapter 241

Rhinoviruses *Kenneth McIntosh*

Rhinoviruses are collectively the most common cause of the "common cold" in adults. They are also very common in young children, but because of the frequency of other viral respiratory tract infections in this age group, their relative importance is somewhat less than in adults. They are difficult to grow in tissue culture, however, and studies using polymerase chain reaction (PCR) indicate that their frequency and importance in respiratory illnesses are considerably greater than was thought.

Etiology. There are 101 serologically distinct rhinoviruses (numbered 1–100, and subtype 1A), members of the Picornaviridae family of small RNA viruses. They are best identified in clinical samples by PCR performed on nasal secretions from infected individuals. Tissue culture is approximately one third as sensitive as PCR. Routine serologic testing for development of antibody is not practical because of the multiplicity of serotypes.

Not all rhinovirus infections are associated with symptoms, even in infants and children. In longitudinal studies, 75% of pediatric rhinovirus infection (detected by culture) is associated with illness, usually rhinitis or pharyngitis. Rhinoviruses have been found in middle ear fluids during acute otitis media, and they can also be associated with serious lower respiratory tract disease, particularly in very young infants and those with underlying illnesses. They are frequent precipitators of asthmatic attacks.

Epidemiology. Rhinoviruses are distributed worldwide with no predictable pattern of infection by serotype. Multiple types may be present in a community at one time.

In temperate climates, the incidence of rhinovirus infection peaks in September and again in April or May, but infections occur year-round. The peak incidence in the tropics occurs during the rainy season.

Rhinoviruses are recovered in highest concentration in nasal secretions, and experimental infection is most easily accomplished by nasal or conjunctival instillation. Virus persists for several hours in secretions on hands or other surfaces. Transmission occurs when infected secretions carried on contaminated fingers are rubbed into the nasal or conjunctival mucosa. Evidence also implicates spread through prolonged contact with aerosols produced by talking, coughing, or sneezing.

Pathogenesis. Rhinoviruses, like other picornaviruses, infect cells only after interaction with specific cell receptors. For most rhinovirus types, this is ICAM-1, an intercellular adhesion molecule present on the epithelium covering the adenoids (lymphoepithelium) and on other epithelial cells of the nose after stimulation by various interleukins (interferon-α, tumor necrosis factor, interleukin 1). Thus, for these types, infection probably begins in the nasopharynx and then, as interleukins are produced, spreads forward to the nasal mucosa. The peak nasal inflammatory response occurs when virus growth is at its greatest, 2–4 days after experimental infection, and is accompanied by the production of multiple proinflammatory mediators. Immune responses include specific nasal immunoglobulin (Ig) A and serum IgG antibody, which may contribute to modifying the illness and limiting viral shedding.

Clinical Manifestations. The primary clinical response to rhinovirus infection is the common cold (see Chapter 364). There is an incubation period of 2–4 days; then sneezing, nasal obstruction and discharge, and sore throat ensue. Cough and hoarseness occur in 30–40% of cases. Fever is neither as frequent nor as high as in primary infections with respiratory syncytial virus, parainfluenza virus, influenza virus, or adenovirus. Symptoms are worse in the first 2–3 days of illness and last for 1 wk in a majority of patients; they persist for more than 14 days in 35% of young children.

Rhinovirus RNA has been found in the middle-ear fluid of 24% of children with acute otitis media, often in conjunction with bacteria.

Diagnosis. Because other viral agents can produce the same manifestations, a clinical diagnosis is only presumptive but is usually adequate. Bacterial antigen testing or cultures should be performed to exclude streptococcal nasopharyngitis if this is suspected (see Chapter 366). PCR is the most sensitive method for identifying rhinoviruses in respiratory samples, but laboratory diagnosis is not practical under ordinary circumstances.

Treatment. Relief of acute symptoms may be provided by acetaminophen or ibuprofen for antipyresis and mild analgesia and by saline or decongestant (for children >6 mo of age) nose drops used for a short time for nasal discharge and obstruction.

Several antiviral drugs have been developed with potent activity against rhinoviruses, such as pleconaril. Although these drugs reduce the titer of virus in the nose, they do not lessen symptoms or decrease the duration of illness. It seems likely that successful treatment will have to target the host response as well as the virus.

Complications. Otitis media and sinusitis are common complications. In one study, rhinoviruses were the most common virus recovered from the middle-ear fluids of infants and children with otitis media. In very young infants, bronchiolitis may occur. Rhinoviruses are the most common cause of acute exacerbations of asthma in school-aged children.

Prevention. The best approach to reducing spread includes careful handwashing and avoidance of manual nose and eye manipulation.

Dick EC, Jennings LC, Mink KA, et al: Aerosol transmission of rhinovirus colds. *J Infect Dis* 1987;156:442–8.

Hendley JO, Wenzel RP, Gwaltney JM Jr: Transmission of rhinovirus colds by self-inoculation. *N Engl J Med* 1973;288:1361–4.

Johnston SL, Pattemore PK, Sanderson G, et al: Community study of role of viral infections in exacerbations of asthma in 9–11 year old children. *Br Med J* 1995;310:1225–9.

Juven T, Mertsola J, Waris M, et al. Etiology of community-acquired pneumonia in 254 hospitalized children. *Pediatr Infect Dis J* 2000;19:293–8.

Ketler A, Hall CE, Fox JP, et al: The Virus Watch Program: A continuing surveillance of viral infections in metropolitan New York families: VIII. Rhinovirus infections: Observations of virus excretion, intrafamilial spread and clinical response. *Am J Epidemiol* 1969;90:244–54.

Pitkaranta A, Virolainen A, Jero J, et al. Detection of rhinovirus, respiratory syncytial virus, and coronavirus infections in acute otitis media by reverse transcriptase polymerase chain reaction. *Pediatrics* 1998;102:291–5.

Chapter 242

Rotavirus and Other Agents of Viral Gastroenteritis

Dorsey M. Bass

Diarrhea is probably the leading cause of childhood mortality in the world, accounting for 5–10 million deaths per year. In early childhood, the single most important cause of severe dehydrating diarrhea is rotavirus infection. Rotavirus and other gastroenteritis viruses not only are major causes of pediatric mortality but also lead to significant morbidity as a result of malnutrition.

Etiology. Rotavirus, astrovirus, adenovirus, and caliciviruses, such as the Norwalk agent, are the medically important pathogens of human viral gastroenteritis.

Rotaviruses cause disease in virtually all mammals and birds. The virus is a wheel-like, double-shelled icosahedron containing 11 segments of double-stranded RNA. The diameter of the particles by electron microscopy is approximately 80 nm. Rotaviruses are classified by group (A, B, C, D, E), subgroup (I or II), and serotype. Group A, which has no antigenic relationship to the other groups, includes the common human pathogens as well as a variety of animal viruses. Group B rotavirus is reported as a cause of severe disease in infants and adults in China but not elsewhere. Occasional human outbreaks of group C rotavirus are reported. The other groups are limited to animal strains. Rotavirus strains are species-specific and do not cause disease in heterologous hosts. Subgrouping of rotaviruses is determined by the antigenic structure of the inner capsid protein, VP6. Serotyping of rotaviruses, as determined by classic cross-neutralization serology, depends on the outer capsid glycoproteins, VP7 and VP4. The VP7 serotype is referred to as the G type (for glycoprotein). The VP4 serotype is referred to as the P type. Although both VP4 and VP7 can elicit neutralizing immunoglobulin (Ig) G antibodies, the relative role of these systemic antibodies compared with mucosal IgA antibodies and cellular responses in protective immunity remains unclear.

Astroviruses are the second most important agent of viral gastroenteritis in young children, with a high incidence in both the developing and the developed worlds. Astroviruses are positive-sense, single-stranded RNA viruses. They are small, approximately 30-nm diameter particles with a characteristic central five- or six-pointed star when viewed by electron microscopy. The capsid consists of three structural proteins. There are eight known human serotypes.

Enteric adenoviruses are another common cause of viral gastroenteritis in infants and children. Although many adenovirus serotypes exist and are found in stool, especially during and after typical upper respiratory tract infections (Chapter 240), only serotypes 40 and 41 cause gastroenteritis. These strains do not cause respiratory symptoms and are very difficult to grow in tissue culture. They are 80-nm diameter icosahedral viruses with a relatively complex single-stranded DNA genome.

Caliciviruses are small 27- to 35-nm viruses that are the most common cause of gastroenteritis outbreaks in older children and adults. They are positive-sense, single-stranded RNA viruses with a single structural protein. Variant but closely related caliciviruses have been named for locations of initial outbreaks: **Norwalk**, Snow Mountain, Montgomery County, Sapporo, and others. Caliciviruses also cause a rotavirus-like illness in young infants. Caliciviruses and astroviruses are sometimes referred to as small, round viruses on the basis of appearance on electron microscopy.

Several other viruses that may cause diarrheal disease in animals have been postulated but not well established as human gastroenteritis viruses. These include coronaviruses, toroviruses, and pestiviruses. Picobirnaviruses, another group of small 30-nm, double-stranded RNA viruses, have been reported to be found in 10% of patients with HIV-associated diarrhea.

Epidemiology. Worldwide, rotavirus is estimated to cause more than 125 million cases of diarrhea annually in children younger than 5 yr of age. Of these, 18 million cases are considered at least moderately severe, with approximately 600,000 deaths per year. Rotavirus causes 3 million cases of diarrhea, 50,000 hospitalizations, and 20–40 deaths annually in the United States.

Rotavirus infection is most common in winter months in temperate climates. In the United States, the annual winter peak spreads from west to east (Fig. 242–1). Unlike other winter viruses such as influenza, this wave of increased incidence is not due to a single prevalent strain or serotype. Typically, several serotypes predominate in a given community for one or two seasons while nearby locations may harbor unrelated strains. Disease tends to be most severe in patients 3–24 mo of age, although 25% of the cases of severe disease occur after 2 yr of age, with serologic evidence of infection developing in virtually all children by 4–5 yr of age. Infants younger than 3 mo of age are relatively protected by transplacental antibody and possibly breast-feeding. Infections in neonates and in adults in close contact with infected children are generally asymptomatic. Some rotavirus strains have stably colonized newborn nurseries for years, infecting virtually all newborns without any overt illness.

Rotavirus and the other gastroenteritis viruses spread efficiently via a fecal-oral route, and outbreaks are common in children's hospitals and child-care centers. The virus is shed in stool at very high concentration before and for days after the clinical illness. Very few infectious virions are needed to cause disease in a susceptible host.

The epidemiology of astroviruses is not as thoroughly studied as rotavirus, but it is a common cause of mild to moderate watery winter diarrhea in children and infants and an uncommon pathogen in adults. Hospital outbreaks are common. Enteric adenovirus gastroenteritis occurs year-round, mostly in

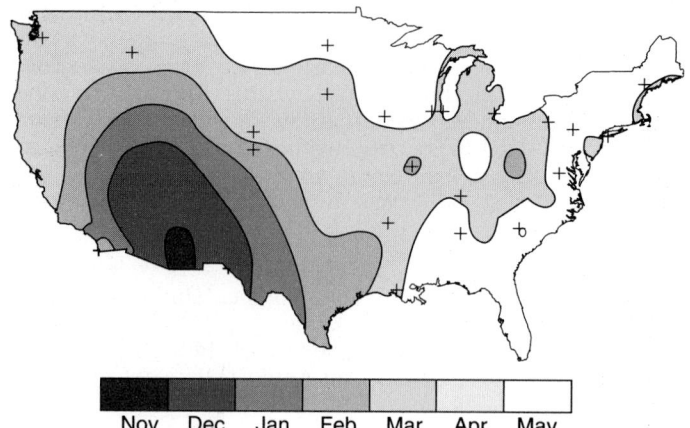

Nov Dec Jan Feb Mar Apr May

FIGURE 242–1. Peak rotavirus activity by month in the United States for July 1996 to June 1997. This pattern is typical of the annual rotavirus activity each year. (From Centers for Disease Control and Prevention: Laboratory-based surveillance for rotavirus—United States, July 1996–June 1997. *MMWR* 1997; 46:1092–4. A short animation showing rotavirus activity by week from July 1996–1997 is available online (ftp://ftp.cdc.gov/pub/publications/mmwr/wk/rota9697.gif).

children younger than 2 yr. Nosocomial outbreaks occur but are less common than with rotavirus and astrovirus. Calicivirus is best known for causing large, explosive outbreaks among older children and adults, particularly in settings such as schools, cruise ships, and hospitals. Often a single food, such as shellfish or water used in food preparation, is identified as a source.

Pathogenesis. Viruses that cause human diarrhea selectively infect and destroy villus tip cells in the small intestine. Biopsies of the small intestines show variable degrees of villus blunting and round cell infiltrate in the lamina propria. Pathologic changes may not correlate with the severity of clinical symptoms and usually resolve before the clinical resolution of diarrhea. The gastric mucosa is not affected despite the commonly used term "gastroenteritis," although delayed gastric emptying has been documented during Norwalk virus infection.

In the small intestine, the upper villus enterocytes are differentiated cells, which have both digestive functions, such as hydrolysis of disaccharides, and absorptive functions, such as the transport of water and electrolytes via glucose and amino acid co-transporters. The crypt enterocytes are undifferentiated cells, which lack the brush border hydrolytic enzymes and are net secretors of water and electrolytes. Selective viral infection of intestinal villus tip cells thus leads to (1) an imbalance in the ratio of intestinal fluid absorption to secretion and (2) malabsorption of complex carbohydrates, particularly lactose. Most evidence supports the first mechanism as the more important factor in the genesis of viral diarrhea. It has been proposed that a rotavirus nonstructural protein may function as an enterotoxin.

In the normal host, extraintestinal infection is rare, although immunocompromised patients may experience hepatic and renal involvement. The increased vulnerability of infants (compared with older children and adults) to severe morbidity and mortality from gastroenteritis viruses may relate to a number of factors, including decreased intestinal reserve function, lack of specific immunity, and decreased nonspecific host defense mechanisms such as gastric acid and mucus. Viral enteritis greatly enhances intestinal permeability to luminal macromolecules and has been postulated to increase the risk of food allergies.

Clinical Manifestations. Rotavirus infection typically begins after an incubation period of less than 48 hr, with mild to moderate fever and vomiting followed by the onset of frequent, watery stools. Vomiting and fever typically abate during the second day of illness, but diarrhea often continues for 5–7 days. The stool is without gross blood or white cells. Dehydration may develop and progress rapidly, particularly in infants. Malnourished children and children with underlying intestinal disease such as short-bowel syndrome are particularly likely to acquire severe rotavirus diarrhea. Rarely, immunodeficient children experience severe and prolonged illness. Although most newborns infected with rotavirus are asymptomatic, some outbreaks of necrotizing enterocolitis have been associated with the appearance of a new rotavirus strain in the affected nurseries.

The clinical course of astrovirus appears to be similar to that of rotavirus, with the notable exception that the disease tends to be milder, with less significant dehydration. Adenovirus enteritis tends to cause diarrhea of longer duration, often 10–14 days. The Norwalk virus has a short (12 hr) incubation period. Vomiting and nausea tend to predominate in illness associated with the Norwalk virus, and the duration is brief, usually 1–3 days of symptoms. The clinical and epidemiologic picture of Norwalk virus often closely resembles so-called food poisoning from preformed toxins such as *Staphylococcus aureus* and *Bacillus cereus*.

Diagnosis. In most cases, a satisfactory diagnosis can be made on the basis of the clinical and epidemiologic features. Enzyme immunoassays, which offer approximately 90% specificity and sensitivity, are available for detection of group A rotavirus and enteric adenovirus in stool samples. More obscure cases can be studied by electron microscopy of stools, RNA electrophoresis, nucleic acid hybridization, and polymerase chain reaction assays. The diagnosis of viral gastroenteritis should always be questioned in patients with persistent high temperature, blood or white cells in the stool, or persistent severe or bilious vomiting (especially in the absence of diarrhea).

LABORATORY FINDINGS. Isotonic dehydration with acidosis is the most common finding in children with severe viral enteritis. The stools are free of blood and leukocytes. Although the white blood cell count may be moderately elevated secondary to stress, the marked left shift seen with invasive bacterial enteritis is absent.

DIFFERENTIAL DIAGNOSIS. The differential diagnosis includes other infectious causes of enteritis such as bacteria and protozoa. Occasionally, surgical conditions such as appendicitis, bowel obstruction, and intussusception may initially mimic viral gastroenteritis.

Treatment. Avoiding and treating dehydration are the main goals in treatment of viral enteritis. A secondary goal is maintenance of the nutritional status of the patient.

There is no role for antiviral drug treatment of viral gastroenteritis. Controlled studies have shown no benefit from antiemetics or antidiarrheal drugs, and there is a significant risk of serious side effects. Antibiotics are similarly of no benefit. Immunoglobulins have been administered orally to both normal and immunodeficient patients with severe rotavirus gastroenteritis, but this treatment is currently considered experimental. Therapy with probiotic organisms such as *Lactobacillus* species has been shown to reduce somewhat the intensity and duration of illness.

SUPPORTIVE TREATMENT. Rehydration can be accomplished in most patients via the oral route. Modern rehydration solutions containing appropriate quantities of sodium and glucose promote optimum absorption of fluid from the intestine (see Table 47.1). There is no evidence that a particular carbohydrate source (e.g., rice) or addition of amino acids improves the efficacy of these solutions for children with viral enteritis. Other clear liquids such as flat soda, fruit juice, and sports drinks are inappropriate for rehydration of young children with significant stool loss. Rehydration via the oral (or nasogastric) route should

be done over 6–8 hr and feedings begun immediately thereafter. Providing the rehydration fluid at a slow, steady rate, typically 5 mL/min, reduces vomiting and improves the success of oral therapy. Rehydration solution should be continued as a supplement to make up for ongoing excessive stool losses. Initial intravenous fluids are required for the infant in shock or the occasional child with intractable vomiting.

After rehydration has been achieved, resumption of a normal diet for age has been shown to result in a more rapid recovery from viral gastroenteritis. Prolonged (>12 hr) administration of exclusive clear liquids or dilute formula is without clinical benefit and actually prolongs the duration of diarrhea. Breast-feeding should be continued even during rehydration. Selected infants may benefit from lactose-free feedings (such as soy formula or lactose-free cow's milk) for several days, although this is not necessary for most children. Hypocaloric diets low in protein and fat such as BRAT (**b**ananas, **r**ice, cereal, **a**pplesauce, and **t**oast) have not been shown to be superior to a regular diet.

Prognosis. Most fatalities occur in infants with poor access to medical care and are attributed to dehydration. Children may be infected with rotavirus several times during their lives but with decreasing severity of subsequent infections. After the initial natural infection, children have limited protection against any subsequent infection (38%) and diarrhea (77%) but have protection against severe diarrhea (87%).

Prevention. Good hygiene reduces the transmission of viral gastroenteritis, but even in the most hygienic societies virtually all children become infected as a result of the efficiency of infection of the gastroenteritis viruses. Good handwashing and isolation procedures can help control nosocomial outbreaks. The role of breast-feeding in prevention or amelioration of rotavirus infection may be small given the variable protection observed in a number of studies.

VACCINE. A rotavirus vaccine was licensed in 1998 for oral administration to infants at 2, 4, and 6 mo of age. The vaccine offered >80% protection against severe disease. In 1999, preliminary analysis of ongoing post-licensure surveillance of adverse events identified several cases of intussusception among recipients of rotavirus vaccine, usually occurring during the 1st wk after immunization and usually after the first dose. Use of the vaccine was suspended in July 1999 and the manufacturer has removed it from the market. Subsequent analysis has suggested that infants receiving the vaccine had an approximate 1 in 10,000 risk of developing intussusception. Several new rotavirus vaccine candidates are under development.

Ball JM, Tian P, Zeng CQ, et al: Age-dependent diarrhea induced by a rotaviral nonstructural glycoprotein. *Science* 1996;272:101–4.

Blacklow NR, Greenberg HB: Viral gastroenteritis. *N Engl J Med* 1991;325:252–64.

Gore SM, Fontaine O, Pierce NF: Impact of rice based oral rehydration solution on stool output and duration of diarrhea. Meta-analysis of 13 clinical trials. *Br Med J* 1992;304:287–91.

Guandalini S, Pensabene L, Zikri MA, et al: Lactobacillus GG administered in oral rehydration solution to children with acute diarrhea: A multicenter European trial. *J Pediatr Gastroenterol Nutr* 2000;30:54–60.

Guerrero ML, Noel JS, Mitchell DK, et al: A prospective study of astrovirus diarrhea of infancy in Mexico City. *Pediatr Infect Dis J* 1998;17:723–7.

Murphy TV, Gargiullo PM, Massoudi MS, et al: Intussusception among infants given an oral rotavirus vaccine. *N Engl J Med* 2001;344:564–72.

Parashar UD, Holman RC, Clarke MJ, et al: Hospitalizations associated with rotavirus diarrhea in the United States, 1993 through 1995. Surveillance based on the new ICD-9-CM rotavirus-specific diagnostic code. *J Infect Dis* 1998;77:13–7.

Shastri S, Doane AM, Gonzales J, et al: Prevalence of astroviruses in a children's hospital. *J Clin Microbiol* 1998;36:2571–4.

Simonsen L, Morens D, Elixhauser A, et al: Effect of rotavirus vaccination programme on trends in admission of infants to hospital for intussusception. *Lancet* 2001;358:1224–9.

Tucker AW, Haddix AC, Bresee JS, et al: Cost-effectiveness analysis of a rotavirus immunization program for the United States. *JAMA* 1998;279:1371–6.

Chapter 243

Human Papillomaviruses

Anna-Barbara Moscicki

Human papillomaviruses (HPVs) cause a variety of proliferative cutaneous and mucosal lesions, including common skin warts, benign and malignant ano-genital tract lesions, and life-threatening respiratory papillomas. Most HPV-related infections in children and adolescents who come to medical attention are benign.

Etiology. The papillomaviruses are small (55 nm), DNA-containing viruses that are ubiquitous in nature, infecting most mammalian and many nonmammalian animal species. Strains are almost always species-specific. More than 100 different types of HPVs have been identified by sequence homology. The different HPV types typically cause disease in specific anatomic sites; about 30 of the HPV types have been identified from genital tract specimens.

The difficulty to propagate these pathogens in tissue culture has prevented the application of traditional virologic culture methods to their study and slowed progress in the field, but newer molecular techniques have spawned a dramatic increase in current understanding.

Epidemiology. HPV infections of the skin are common, and most individuals are probably infected with one or more HPV types at some time. There are no animal reservoirs for HPV, and all transmission is presumably person-to-person. There is little evidence to suggest that HPV is transmitted by fomites. Common warts including palmar and plantar warts are frequently seen in children and adolescents, where they infect the hands and feet, common areas of frequent minor trauma.

Human papillomavirus is the most prevalent viral sexually transmitted infection in the United States. Although up to 70% of sexually active women eventually acquire HPV through sexual transmission, the infection is rare among preadolescent children. The greatest risk for HPV in sexually active adolescents is exposure to new sexual partners, underscoring the ease of transmission of this virus through sexual contact. As with many other genital pathogens, perinatal transmission to newborns also occurs but the transmission of genital types appears to be relatively inefficient.

The most common manifestation of HPV is latent infection defined by the detection of HPV DNA in the absence of any detectable HPV-associated lesion. Approximately 20% of sexually active adolescents have detectable HPV at any one point in time without detectable lesions. In contrast, external genital warts are much less common, occurring in <1% of adolescents.

The most common clinically detected lesion in adolescent women is the cervical lesion termed **low-grade squamous intraepithelial lesion (LSIL)** (Table 243–1). This appears to occur in 25–50% of adolescents infected with HPV. LSILs are considered benign cellular changes associated with HPV infection. As with HPV DNA detection, most LSILs regress spontaneously and do not require any intervention or therapy. Less common, HPV can induce more severe cellular changes termed **high-grade squamous intraepithelial lesions (HSIL)**. Although HSILs are considered true precancerous lesions, these lesions rarely progress to invasive cancer. HSIL occurs in approximately 0.4–3% of sexually active women, whereas invasive cervical cancer occurs in less than 14 cases per 100,000 adult women. In true virginal populations, including children who are not sexually abused, rates of both clinical disease and HPV detection are very low to zero.

Some infants may acquire papillomaviruses during passage through an infected birth canal, leading to recurrent respiratory papillomatosis. Cases have been reported after cesarean section. The maximum incubation period for emergence of clinically apparent lesions (genital warts or laryngeal papillomas) after perinatally acquired infection is unknown, but appears to be around 6 mo of age. Genital warts appearing in later childhood often result from sexual abuse, with papillomavirus transmission during the abusive contact. Genital warts may represent a sexually transmitted disease even in some very young children. Their presence is cause to suspect that possibility. A child with genital warts should, therefore, be provided with a complete evaluation for possible abuse (Chapter 35.1), including the presence of other sexually transmitted diseases (Chapter 110).

Pathogenesis. Initial infection of the cervix with HPV is thought to begin by viral invasion of the basal cells of the epithelium, which is enhanced by disruption of the epithelium caused by trauma or inflammation. It is thought that, at first, the virus remains relatively dormant, because the virus is present without any evidence of clinical disease. The life cycle of HPV is dependent on the differentiation program of keratinocytes. The pattern of HPV transcription varies throughout the epithelial layer as well as through different stages of disease (i.e., LSIL, HSIL, invasive cancer). Understanding of HPV transcription enhances understanding of its ability to behave as an oncovirus. Much of the research has focused on the early region proteins, E6 and E7. These proteins function as trans-activating factors that regulate cellular transformation. Complex interactions between E6 and E7 transcribed proteins and host proteins result in the perturbation of normal processes that regulate cellular DNA synthesis. The perturbations caused by E6 and E7 are primarily through disruption of the anti-oncoproteins, p53 and retinoblastoma protein (Rb), respectively, contributing to the development of anogenital cancers.

TABLE 243–1. Bethesda System for Reporting Cervical/Vaginal Cytology

Descriptive Diagnosis of Epithelial Cell Abnormalities	Equivalent Terminology
Squamous Cell	
Atypical squamous cells of undetermined significance (ASC-US)	Squamous atypia
Atypical squamous cells, cannot exclude HSIL (ASC-H)	
Low-grade squamous intraepithelial lesion (LSIL)	Mild dysplasia, condylomatous atypia, HPV-related changes, koilocytic atypia, cervical epithelial neoplasia (CIN) 1
High-grade squamous intraepithelial lesion (HSIL)	Moderate dysplasia, CIN 2, severe dysplasia, CIN 3, carcinoma in situ
Glandular Cell	
Endometrial cells, cytologically benign, in a postmenopausal woman	
Atypical glandular cells of undetermined significance	
Endocervical adenocarcinoma	
Endometrial adenocarcinoma	
Extrauterine adenocarcinoma	
Adenocarcinoma, not otherwise specified	

Evidence of productive viral infection occurs in benign lesions such as external genital warts and LSIL with the abundant expression of viral capsid proteins in the superficial keratinocytes. The appearance of the HPV-associated koilocyte is due to the expression of E4, a structural protein that causes collapse of the cytoskeleton. Although not as abundant, mild expression of E6 and E7 proteins results in cell proliferation seen in the basal cell layer of LSIL. Most researchers conclude that LSIL is a manifestation of active viral replication and protein expression. However, as the lesions advance in grade, expression of those products important in the process of cell transformation, such as E6 and E7, now predominate, rather than structural proteins, resulting in the chromosomal abnormalities and aneuploidy characteristic of the higher grade lesions.

Cutaneous lesions (e.g., common warts) are not associated with malignant HPV types nor do they have any malignant potential except in the rare skin disorder epidermodysplasia verruciformis. Genital lesions caused by HPV may be broadly grouped into those with little to no malignant potential (i.e., low risk) and those with greater malignant potential (i.e., high risk). Low-risk HPV types 6 and 11 are most commonly found in genital warts and are rarely to never found isolated in malignant lesions. Whereas high-risk types, including types 16 and 18 but also 31, 33, 35, 45, and 56, are commonly found in SIL and invasive anogenital cancers. These types are also most commonly found in women without lesions as well. Lesions may also be infected simultaneously with multiple HPV types. Almost all latent infections with low-risk types spontaneously resolve over time. Genital and common warts in general resolve without therapy but may take years. Although most latent high-risk type infections resolve as well, they are more likely than low-risk types to persist. Persistent high risk type infections are associated with increased risk of developing HSIL and invasive cancer.

Most infants with recognized genital warts are infected with the low-risk types. In contrast, children with a history of sexual abuse have a picture more like adult genital warts with mixed low- and high-risk types. There have been only rare reports of HPV-associated genital malignancies occurring in preadolescent children and adolescents. On the other hand, HSIL does occur in sexually active adolescents. There is also a concern that younger age of sexual debut has contributed to the increase of invasive cervical cancer seen in women <50 yr in the United States. Prevention of adolescent sexually transmitted diseases, including HPV infections, is a major goal of current public health initiatives.

Clinical Manifestations. The clinical findings depend on the site of epithelial infection.

SKIN LESIONS. The typical HPV-induced lesions of the skin are proliferative, papular, and hyperkeratotic. Common warts are raised circinate lesions with a keratinized surface. Plantar and palmar warts are the results of pressure and are therefore practically flat. Multiple warts are common and may create a mosaic pattern. Flat warts appear as small, 1–5 mm flat flesh-colored papules.

GENITAL WARTS. Genital warts may be found throughout the perineum around the anus, vagina, and urethra, as well as the cervical, intravaginal, and intra-anal areas. Intra-anal warts occur predominantly in patients who have had receptive anal intercourse, as contrasted with perianal warts that may occur in men and women without a history of anal sex. Although rare, lesions caused by genital genotypes can also be found on other mucosal surfaces such as conjunctivae, gingiva, and nasal mucosa. They may be single or multiple lesions and are frequently found in multiple anatomic sites. External genital warts can be flat, dome-shaped, keratotic, pedunculated, and cauliflower-shaped; they may occur singly, in clusters, or as plaques. On mucosal epithelium, the lesions are softer. Depending on the size and anatomic location, lesions may be pruritic and painful, cause burning with urination, be friable and bleed, or become superinfected. Children may be very disturbed by the development of genital lesions. Other rarer lesions caused by HPV of the external genital area include Bowen disease, Bowenoid papulosis, squamous cell carcinomas, Buschke-Löwenstein tumors, and vulvar intraepithelial neoplasias (VIN).

Squamous intraepithelial lesions detected by cytology are usually invisible to the naked eye and require the aid of colposcopic magnification and acetic acid. With aid, the lesions appear white and show evidence of neovascularity. SIL can occur on the cervix, vagina, vulva, and intra-anus. Invasive cancers tend to be more exophytic with aberrant appearing vasculature. These lesions are rarely found in non-sexually active individuals.

LARYNGEAL PAPILLOMATOSIS. The median age of onset of recurrent laryngeal papillomatosis is 3 yr of age. Children present with hoarseness or, in infants, an altered cry and sometimes stridor. Rapid growth of respiratory papillomas can occlude the upper airway, causing respiratory compromise. These lesions may recur within weeks of removal, requiring frequent surgery. The lesions do not become malignant.

Diagnosis. The diagnosis of external genital warts and common warts may be reliably determined by visual inspection of a lesion by an experienced observer and does not require additional tests for confirmation. A biopsy should be considered if the diagnosis is uncertain, the lesions do not respond to therapy, or the lesions worsen during therapy.

The diagnosis for cervical SIL or cancer is initiated by screening with cytology. The most recent recommended terminology for cytologic evaluation is listed in Table 243–1. Although the purpose of screening is to identify the significant precancer HSIL, the majority of confirmed HSIL is found in women who were referred for ASC-US or LSIL. Therefore, cytologic evaluation of cervical cells is a screening test and not confirmatory. Current recommendations for triage to colposcopy and biopsy for women with ASC-US is to repeat a Papanicolaou smear in 4–6 mo and refer only those women with persistent abnormal cytology. Because of the high rate of LSIL regression in adolescents and young women, clinicians may also choose to repeat cytologic study with LSIL within 6–12 mo for young women diagnosed with LSIL. For persistent LSIL, referral to colposcopy can be deferred up to 24 months. However, close follow-up of these women is critical because 17% of young women with LSIL have HSIL confirmed on histology. All women with cytologically identified HSIL should be referred for colposcopy and biopsy.

The majority of recommendations agree that cytologic screening should be initiated after the onset of sexual activity. Although the recommended interval between first sexual intercourse and first annual Papanicolaou smear is debatable, evidence suggests that screening may begin within the first 3 yr after intercourse. Screening earlier than 3 yr is more likely to result in overreferrals for colposcopy because most lesions in this group are likely to be LSIL. Upper age limit for screening is 18–21 yr in order to capture those women who have not revealed their sexual activity.

There are no commercially available serologic tests to assist in the diagnosis of HPV infection. During the past decade, very sensitive tests for the presence of HPV DNA, RNA, and proteins have been developed. These tests are becoming generally available, although they are not required for the diagnosis of external genital warts or related conditions. Recent application of HPV DNA testing assists in the triage of atypical cells of undetermined significance. Because half of patients with ASC-US do not require any further evaluation, HPV testing can assist in triage. Women with ASC-US and a positive HPV test for high-risk types are more likely to have significant underlying disease (i.e., HSIL) than women with a negative HPV test, and they may benefit from referral for colposcopy rather than waiting another 6 mo for repeat cytology. Another indication for HPV testing is follow-up of LSIL. At 12 mo follow-up of LSIL, a positive test for high-risk HPV types indicates referral for colposcopy.

DIFFERENTIAL DIAGNOSIS. A number of other conditions should be considered including condyloma latum, seborrheic keratoses, dysplastic and benign nevi, molluscum contagiosum, pearly penile papules, and neoplasms. Condyloma latum is due to secondary syphilis and can be diagnosed using dark-field microscopy and standard serologic tests for syphilis. Seborrheic keratoses are common, localized hyperpigmented lesions that are rarely associated with malignancy. Molluscum contagiosum is caused by a poxvirus, is highly infectious, and is often umbilicated. Pearly penile papules occur at the penile corona and are normal variants that require no treatment.

Treatment. Most common warts eventually resolve spontaneously. Symptomatic lesions should be removed. Removal includes a variety of self-applied therapies including salicylic acid preparations and provider-applied therapies (e.g., cryotherapy, laser therapy, and electrosurgery). Genital warts of children and adolescents are benign and usually remit, but only over an extended period of time. It is recommended that genital lesions be treated if the patient or the parent requests therapy. Similar to common warts, treatment is categorized into self-applied and provider applied. No one therapy has been shown to be more efficacious than any other. Provider-applied therapies include surgical treatments (e.g., electrosurgery, surgical excision, and laser surgery) and office-based treatment (e.g., cryotherapy with liquid nitrogen or a cryoprobe, podophyllin resin 10–25%, and bi- and tri-chloroacetic acid). Podophyllin resins have lost favor to other methods because of the variability in preparations. Intralesional, but not systemic, interferon is no more effective than other therapies and is associated with significant adverse effects. This therapy is reserved for treatment of recalcitrant cases.

Many therapies are painful, and children should not undergo painful genital treatments unless adequate pain control is provided. Parents and patients should not be expected to apply painful therapies themselves. In adolescents and adults, recommended patient-applied treatment regimens for external genital warts include topical podofilox and imiquimod. Podofilox 0.5% solution (using a cotton swab) or gel (using a finger) is applied to visible warts in a cycle of applications twice a day for 3 days followed by 4 days of no therapy, repeated for up to a total of four cycles. Imiquimod 5% cream is applied at bedtime, three times a week, every other day, for up to 16 wk; the treated area should be washed with mild soap and water 6–10 hr after treatment. Neither podofilox nor imiquimod is recommended during pregnancy. For any of the nonsurgical treatments, prescription is contraindicated when there is any history of hypersensitivity to any product constituents.

If exposure as a result of sexual abuse is suspected or known, the clinician should ensure that the child's safety has been achieved and is maintained.

Ablative treatment including cryotherapy, loop electrosurgical excisional procedure, and laser therapy for HSIL is universally recommended. LSIL can be observed for up to 24 mo before treatment is offered.

Complications. The presence of these lesions in the genital area may be a cause of profound embarrassment to a child or parent. Complications of therapy are uncommon; chronic pain (vulvodynia) or hypoesthesia may occur at the treatment site. Lesions may heal with hypopigmentation or hyperpigmentation and less commonly with depressed or hypertrophic scars. Surgical therapies can lead to infection and scarring. Repeated procedures of the cervix may lead to problems with infertility.

Numerous epidemiologic studies of adults, but not children, have demonstrated that papillomavirus infection, especially with types 16 and 18, is a strong risk factor for precancerous lesions and cancer. Respiratory papillomas also may become malignant, especially if they have been treated with radiation.

Prognosis. With all forms of therapy, lesions very commonly recur, and approximately one half of children require a second or third treatment. This appears to be especially true for respiratory papillomatosis. Patients and parents should be warned of this likelihood. Combination therapy does not improve response but may increase complications. Prognosis of cervical disease is better, with 85–90% cure rates after a single treatment. Recalcitrant disease should prompt an evaluation and is common in immunocompromised individuals, specifically men and women infected with HIV.

Prevention. The only means to prevent infection is to avoid direct contact with lesions. Condoms have not been shown universally to prevent HPV transmission, although condoms prevent other sexually transmitted infections, which are risk factors associated with SIL development. In addition, avoiding smoking cigarettes is important in preventing cervical cancer.

American Academy of Pediatrics, Committee on Child Abuse and Neglect: Guidelines for the evaluation of sexual abuse of children. *Pediatrics* 1991;87: 254–60.

Beutner KR, Reitano MV, Richwald GA, et al: External genital warts: Report of the American Medical Association Consensus Conference. AMA Expert Panel on External Genital Warts. *Clin Infect Dis* 1998;27:796–806.

Centers for Disease Control and Prevention: Sexually transmitted diseases treatment guidelines 2002. *MMWR* 2002;51(RR-6):1–78.

Gutman LT, St. Claire KK, Herman-Giddens ME, et al: Evaluation of intravaginal specimens from sexually abused and unabused girls for human papillomavirus infection. *Am J Dis Child* 1992;146:694–9.

Ho GYF, Birman R, Beardsley L, et al. Natural history of cervicovaginal papillomavirus infection in young women. *N Engl J Med* 1998;338:423–8.

Moscicki AB, Shiboski S, Broering J, et al: The natural history of human papillomavirus infection as measured by repeated DNA testing in adolescent and young women. *J Pediatr* 1998;132:277–84.

Moscicki AB, Hills N, Shiboski S, et al: Risks for incident human papillomavirus infection and low-grade squamous intraepithelial lesion development in young females. *JAMA* 2001;285:2995–3002.

Siegfried E, Rasnick-Conley J, Cook S, et al: Human papillomavirus screening in pediatric victims of sexual abuse. *Pediatrics* 1998;101:43–7.

Wright TC Jr, Cox JT, Massad LS, et al: 2001 consensus guidelines for the management of women with cervical cytological abnormalities. *JAMA* 2002;287:2120–9.

Chapter 244
Arboviral Encephalitis in North America *Scott B. Halstead*

The *arthropod-borne* (*arbo*virus) viral encephalitides are a group of clinically similar severe neurologic infections caused by several different viruses. They are transmitted by mosquitoes during warm weather and are incurred by outdoor exposure in overlapping regions across most of the United States and much of southern Canada.

Etiology. The principal causes of the arthropod-borne encephalitides of North America include the newly introduced West Nile encephalitis (WNE), St. Louis encephalitides (SLE), the complex of viruses included in the California (CE) encephalitis group of viruses, and, less frequently, western equine encephalitis (WEE), eastern equine encephalitis (EEE), and Colorado tick fever. The etiologic agents belong to different viral taxa: alphaviruses of the family Togaviridae (EEE and WEE), Flaviviridae (WNE, SLE), the California complex of the Bunyaviridae (CE), and Reoviridae (Colorado tick fever virus). Alphaviruses are 69-nm enveloped positive-strand RNA viruses that evolved from a common Venezuelan equine encephalitis-like viral ancestor in the Western Hemisphere. Flaviviruses are 40- to 50-nm enveloped positive-strand RNA viruses evolved from a common ancestor, globally distributed, and responsible for many important human viral diseases. The California serogroup, one of 16 Bunyavirus groups, are 75- to 115-nm enveloped viruses possessing a three-segment negative-strand RNA genome. Reoviruses are 60- to 80-nm double-stranded RNA viruses.

Epidemiology. Viral encephalitis cases and outbreaks were only recognized during the 20th century, when human population densities across the United States became relatively high, public health disease reporting systems were maturing, and laboratories were able to discriminate viral from bacterial infections. From the mid-19th century, epizootics of equine encephalitis were observed in the United States. In 1931, WEE was isolated from horse cases in the Central Valley of California. In 1938, the same virus was recovered from the central nervous system from fatal human cases. In the summer of 1932, an epidemic of human encephalitis, first regarded as Von Economo's disease, was recognized in Paris, IL. The next year, more than 1,000 cases

were reported from St. Louis County, and several SLE viruses were isolated. In 1933, EEE virus was isolated from a horse epizootic, which occurred in Virginia, Maryland, Delaware, and New Jersey. The same virus was isolated from human cases in 1938. The first CE virus, now called La Crosse virus, was isolated in 1960 from a fatal case of encephalitis in a 4-yr-old girl in rural Wisconsin. Colorado tick fever was first described as a nosologic entity in 1930.

EASTERN EQUINE ENCEPHALITIS. In the United States, EEE is a very low incidence disease, with a median of three cases occurring annually in the Atlantic and Gulf states (Fig. 244–1). Transmission occurs often in focal endemic areas of the coast of Massachusetts, the six southern counties of New Jersey, and northeastern Florida. In North America, the virus is maintained in freshwater swamps in a zoonotic cycle involving *Culiseta melanura* and birds. Various other mosquito species obtain viremic

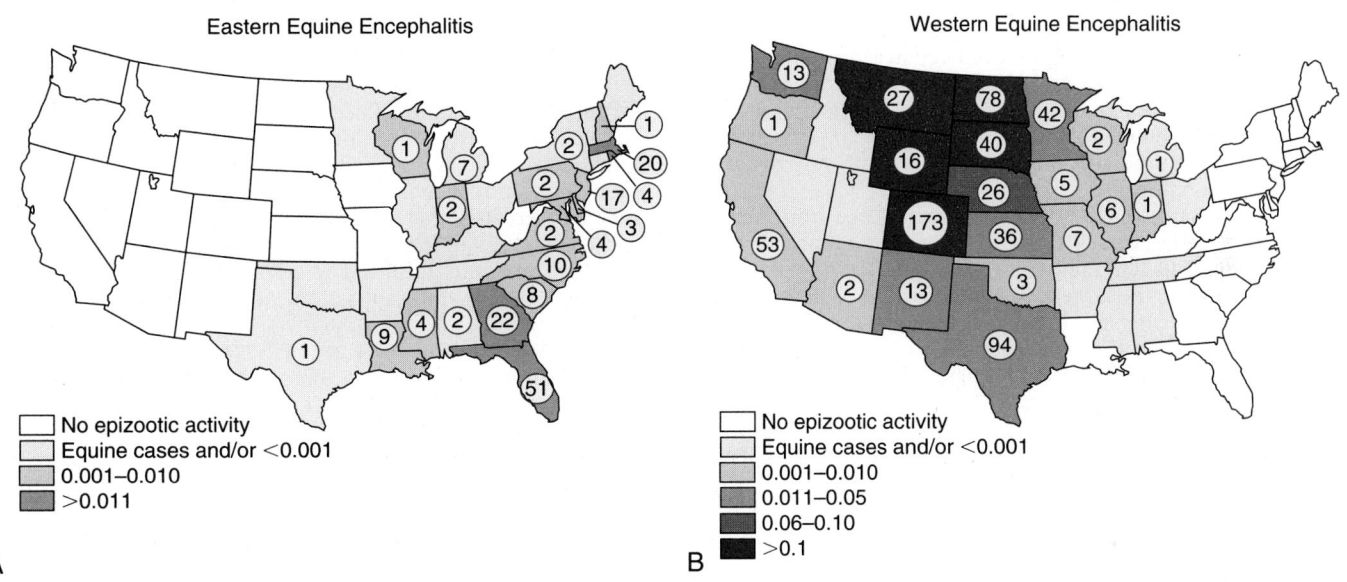

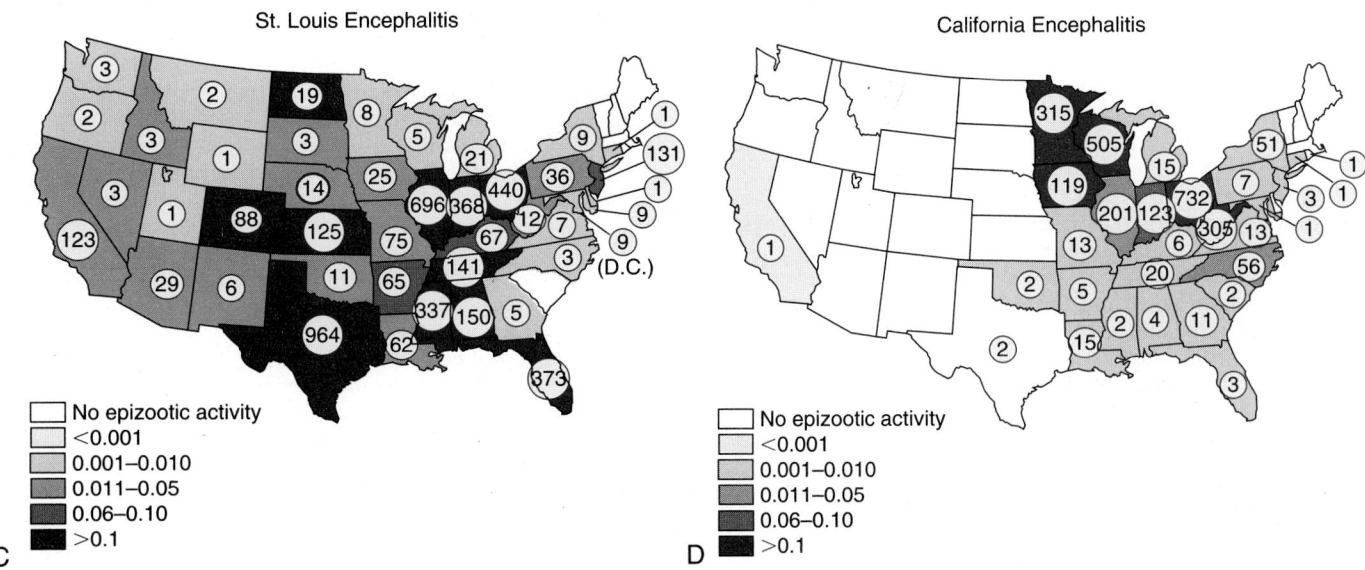

FIGURE 244–1. The incidence of reported cases of Eastern equine encephalitis (*A*), Western equine encephalitis (*B*), St. Louis encephalitis (*C*), and California encephalitis (*D*) reported to the Centers for Disease Control and Prevention in 1997.

meals from birds and transmit the virus to horses and humans. Virus activity varies markedly from year to year in response to still unknown ecologic factors. Most infections in birds are silent, but infections in pheasants are often fatal, and epizootics in these species are used as sentinels for periods of increased viral activity. Cases have been recognized on Caribbean islands. The case to infection ratio is lowest in children (1:8) and somewhat higher in adults (1:29).

WESTERN EQUINE ENCEPHALITIS. Infections occur principally in the United States and Canada west of the Mississippi River (see Fig. 244–1) mainly in rural areas where water impoundments, irrigated farmland, and naturally flooded land provide breeding sites for *Culex tarsalis*. The virus is transmitted in a cycle involving mosquitoes, birds, and other vertebrate hosts. Humans and horses are susceptible to encephalitis. The case to infection ratio varies by age, having been estimated at 1:58 in children younger than 4 yr and 1:1,150 in adults. Infections are most severe at the extremes of life; one third of cases occur in children younger than 1 yr. Recurrent human epidemics have been reported from the Yakima Valley in Washington State and the Central Valley of California; the largest outbreak on record—3,400 cases—occurred in Minnesota, North and South Dakota, Nebraska, and Montana and Alberta, Manitoba, and Saskatchewan, Canada. Epizootics in horses precede human epidemics by several weeks. For the past 20 years, possibly as a result of successful mosquito abatement, few cases of WEE have been reported.

ST. LOUIS ENCEPHALITIS. Cases are reported from nearly all states; the highest attack rates occur in the Gulf and central states (see Fig. 244–1). Epidemics frequently occur in urban and suburban areas; the largest, in 1975, involved 1,800 persons living in Houston, Chicago, Memphis, and Denver. Cases often cluster in areas where there is ground water or septic systems, which support mosquito breeding. The principal vectors are *Culex pipiens* and *C. quinquefasciatus* in the central Gulf states, *C. nigripalpus* in Florida, and *C. tarsalis* in California. SLE virus is maintained in nature in a bird-mosquito cycle. Viral amplification occurs in bird species abundant in residential areas (e.g., sparrows, blue jays, and doves). Virus is transmitted in the late summer and early fall. The case to infection ratio may be as high as 1:300. Age-specific attack rates are lowest in children and highest in individuals older than 60 yr.

WEST NILE ENCEPHALITIS. During the past decade, WNE virus has been implicated as the cause of sporadic summer time human cases of encephalitis and meningitis in Israel, India, Pakistan, Romania, and Russia. West Nile virus belonging to lineage I was introduced into the United States in 1999. It was initially isolated from a cluster of patients in Queens, NY, in September 1999 following an earlier die-off of crows and exotic birds at the Bronx Zoo. All American WNE viruses are genetically similar and are related to a virus recovered from a goose in Israel in 1998. WNE virus survives in a broad enzootic cycle in the United States and within 4 yr has spread to most states east of the Rocky Mountains plus California. A nationwide epidemic, particularly in the central states, occurred in 2002. Throughout its range, the virus is maintained in nature by transmission between mosquitoes of the *Culex* genus and various species of birds. In the United States, human infections are largely acquired from *Culex pipiens*. Horses are the nonavian vertebrates most likely to exhibit disease with WNE infection. In New York in 1999, 25 equine cases were observed.

Disease occurs predominantly in individuals over the age of 50 yr.

LA CROSSE/CALIFORNIA ENCEPHALITIS. La Crosse viral infections are endemic in the United States, occurring annually from July to September, principally in the north central and central states (see Fig. 244–1). Infections occur in peridomestic environments as the result of bites from *Aedes triseriatus* mosquitoes, which often breed in tree holes. The virus is maintained vertically in nature by transovarial transmission and can be spread between mosquitoes by copulation and amplified in mosquito populations by viremic infections in various vertebrate hosts. Amplifying hosts include chipmunks, squirrels, foxes, and woodchucks. A case:infection ratio of 1:22–300 has been surmised. La Crosse encephalitis is principally a disease of children, who may constitute up to 75% of cases.

COLORADO TICK FEVER. Colorado tick fever virus is transmitted by the wood tick *Dermacentor andersoni*, which inhabits high-elevation areas of states extending from the central plains to the Pacific coast. The tick is infected with the virus at the larval stage and remains infected for life. Squirrels and chipmunks serve as primary reservoirs. Human infections typically occur in hikers and campers in indigenous areas during the spring and early summer.

Clinical Manifestations. With the exception of EEE, these arboviruses produce similar symptoms of encephalitis.

EASTERN EQUINE ENCEPHALITIS. Infections result in a fulminant encephalitis with a rapid progression to coma and death in one third of cases. In infants and children, abrupt onset of fever, irritability, and headache are followed by lethargy, confusion, seizures, and coma. High temperature, bulging fontanel, stiff neck, and generalized flaccid or spastic paralysis are observed. There may be a brief prodrome of fever, headache, and dizziness. Unlike most other viral encephalitides, the peripheral white blood cell count usually demonstrates a marked leukocytosis, and the cerebrospinal fluid may show marked pleocytosis. Pathologic changes are found in the cortical and gray matter, with viral antigens localized to neurons. There is necrosis of neurons, neutrophilic infiltration, and perivascular cuffing by lymphocytes.

WESTERN EQUINE ENCEPHALITIS. There may be a prodrome with symptoms of an upper respiratory tract infection. The onset is usually sudden with chills, fever, dizziness, drowsiness, increasing headache, malaise, nausea and vomiting, stiff neck, and disorientation. Infants typically present with the sudden cessation of feeding, fussiness, fever, and protracted vomiting. Convulsions and lethargy develop rapidly. On physical examination, patients are somnolent, exhibit meningeal signs, and have generalized motor weakness and reduced deep tendon reflexes. In infants, a bulging fontanel, spastic paralysis, and generalized convulsions may be observed. On pathologic examination, disseminated small focal abscesses, small focal hemorrhages, and patchy areas of demyelination are distinctive.

ST. LOUIS ENCEPHALITIS. Clinical manifestations vary from a mild flulike illness to fatal encephalitis. There may be a prodrome of nonspecific symptoms with subtle changes in coordination or mentation of several days to 1 wk in duration. Early signs and symptoms include fever, photophobia, headache, malaise, nausea, vomiting, and neck stiffness. About one half of patients exhibit abrupt onset of weakness, incoordination, disturbed sensorium, restlessness, confusion, lethargy, and delirium or coma. The peripheral white blood cell count is modestly elevated, with 100–200 cells/mm^3 found in the cerebrospinal fluid. On autopsy, the brain shows scattered foci of neuronal damage and perivascular inflammation.

WEST NILE ENCEPHALITIS. In the early literature, WNE in adults was described as a dengue-like syndrome. Disease in the United States has been accompanied by prolonged lymphopenia and the syndromes of encephalitis or meningitis.

CALIFORNIA ENCEPHALITIS. The clinical spectrum includes a mild febrile illness, aseptic meningitis, and fatal encephalitis. Children typically present with a prodrome of 2–3 days with fever, headache, malaise, and vomiting. The disease evolves with clouding of the sensorium, lethargy, and, in severe cases, focal or generalized seizures. On physical examination, children are lethargic but not disoriented. Focal neurologic signs, including weakness, aphasia, and focal or generalized seizures, have been reported in 16–25% of cases. Cerebrospinal fluid shows low to moderate leukocyte counts. On autopsy, the brain shows focal areas of neuronal degeneration, inflammation, and perivascular cuffing.

COLORADO TICK FEVER. The illness begins with the abrupt onset of a flulike illness, including high temperature, malaise, arthralgias and myalgia, vomiting, headache, and decreased sensorium. Rash is uncommon. The symptoms rapidly disappear after 3 days of illness. However, in approximately one half of patients, a second, identical episode recurs 24–72 hr after the first, producing the typical "saddle-back" temperature curve of Colorado tick fever. Complications, including encephalitis or meningoencephalitis or a bleeding diathesis, develop in 3–7% of infected persons and may be more common in children younger than 12 yr.

Diagnosis. The etiologic diagnosis of a specific arboviral infection is established by testing an acute-phase serum ≥5 days after onset of illness for the presence of virus-specific immunoglobulin (Ig) M antibodies using an indirect immunofluorescence test or an enzyme-linked immunosorbent assay (ELISA) IgM-capture test. Alternatively, acute and convalescent sera can be tested for a fourfold or greater increase in ELISA, hemagglutination inhibition, or neutralizing IgG antibody titers. The diagnosis may also be established by isolation in cell cultures of virus in brain tissue, obtained by brain biopsy or at autopsy, or by identification of viral RNA reverse transcriptase/polymerase chain reactions.

The diagnosis of encephalitis may be aided by CT or MRI and by electroencephalography. Focal seizures or focal findings on CT or MRI or electroencephalogram should suggest the possibility of herpes simplex encephalitis, which should be treated with acyclovir (Chapter 231).

Treatment. There is no specific treatment for arboviral encephalitides. The treatment of acute arboviral encephalitis is intensive supportive care (Chapter 57), including control of seizures (Chapter 586).

Prognosis. With the exception of EEE, the arboviral encephalitides are self-limited and resolve without residua in most, but not all, patients.

EASTERN EQUINE ENCEPHALITIS. The prognosis is better for patients with a prolonged prodrome; the occurrence of convulsions conveys a poor prognosis. Patient fatality rates are 33–75% and are highest in the elderly. Residual neurologic defects are common, especially in children.

WESTERN EQUINE ENCEPHALITIS. Patient fatality rates are 3–9%, and are highest in the elderly. Major neurologic sequelae have been reported in up to 13% of cases and may be as high as 30% in infants. Parkinsonian syndrome has been reported as a residual in adult survivors.

ST. LOUIS ENCEPHALITIS. The principal risk factor for fatal outcome is advanced age, with patient fatality rates being as high as 80% in early outbreaks. In children, mortality rates are 2–5%. In adults, underlying hypertensive cardiovascular disease has been a risk factor for fatal outcome. Recovery from SLE is usually complete, but serious neurologic sequelae have been reported to be as high as 10% in children.

WEST NILE ENCEPHALITIS. Cases and deaths occurred mainly in the elderly, although serologic surveys in 1999 and 2000 showed evidence that 2.6% and 1% of the population in focal areas of New York City were infected, respectively. The mortality rate was approximately 10%; in 1999, there were 7 fatalities among 62 cases; in 2002, 263 deaths among 4,007 cases.

CALIFORNIA ENCEPHALITIS. Recovery from CE is usually complete. The case fatality rate is about 1%.

COLORADO TICK FEVER. Recovery from Colorado tick fever is usually complete. Three deaths have been reported, all in persons with hemorrhagic signs.

Prevention. A killed EEE vaccine is available for horses, and an experimental killed vaccine is administered to human laboratory workers who handle EEE virus. Flocks of sentinel chickens or pheasants have been stationed at various locations along the Atlantic coast during the late summer or early fall to obtain early warning of increased transmission of EEE virus.

No human vaccine is available for the other arboviral encephalitides, although WNE vaccines are being developed. Extensive water management and mosquito abatement programs in California have reduced transmission of WEE and the incidence of human infections. Urban WNE and SLE outbreaks in the Eastern United States, Texas, and the Midwest have been controlled by the application of ultra low-volume adulticide chemicals applied from trucks or low-flying aircraft.

Because infections in children may occur as the result of summer daytime mosquito biting in residential areas, sealing mosquito breeding sites, using insect repellents, and instructing children to play in open, sunny areas away from forest fringe may help prevent disease.

Balfour HH Jr, Siem RA, Bauer H, et al: California arbovirus (La Crosse) infections. I. Clinical and laboratory findings in 66 children with meningoencephalitis. *Pediatrics* 1973;52:680–91.

Cunha BA, Minnaganti V, Johnson DH, et al: Profound and prolonged lymphocytopenia with West Nile encephalitis. *Clin Infect Dis* 2000;31:1116–7.

Earnest MP, Goolishian HA, Calverley JR, et al: Neurologic, intellectual, and psychologic sequelae following western encephalitis: A follow-up study of 35 cases. *Neurology* 1971;21:969–74.

Griffen DE, Levine B, Ubol S, et al: The effects of alphavirus infection on neurons. *Ann Neurol* 1994;35:S23–7.

Komar N, Spielman A: Emergence of eastern encephalitis in Massachusetts. *Ann N Y Acad Sci* 1995;740:157–68.

Kulasekera V, Kramer LD, Nasci RS et al: West Nile virus infection in mosquitoes, birds, horses and humans, Staten Island, New York, 2000. *Emerg Infect Dis* 2001; 7:722–5.

Marfin AA, Bleed DM, Lofgren JP, et al: Epidemiological aspects of a St. Louis encephalitis epidemic in Jefferson County, Arkansas. *Am J Trop Med Hyg* 1993; 49:30–7.

Monath TP, Tsai TF: St. Louis encephalitis: Lessons from the last decade. *Am J Trop Med Hyg* 1987;37:40S–59S.

Przelomski MM, O'Rourke E, Grady GE, et al: Eastern equine encephalitis in Massachusetts: A report of 16 cases, 1970–1984. *Neurology* 1988;38:736–9.

Spruance SL, Bailey A: Colorado tick fever: A review of 115 laboratory confirmed cases. *Arch Intern Med* 1973;131:288–93.

Tsai TF: Arboviral infections in the United States. *Infect Dis Clin North Am* 1991; 5:73–102.

Chapter 245
Arboviral Encephalitis Outside North America

Scott B. Halstead

The principal causes of arboviral encephalitides outside North America are Venezuelan equine encephalitis (VEE) virus, Japanese encephalitis (JE) virus, tick-borne encephalitis (TBE), and West Nile (WN) virus (see Chapter 244) (Table 245–1).

245.1 Venezuelan Equine Encephalitis

The VEE virus was isolated from an epizootic in Venezuelan horses in 1938. Human cases were first identified in 1943. Hundreds of thousands of equine and human cases have occurred over the past 70 yr. During 1971, epizootics moved through Central America and Mexico to southern Texas. After 2 decades of quiescence, epizootic disease emerged again in Venezuela and Colombia in 1995.

TABLE 245–1. Vectors and Geographic Distribution of Arboviral Encephalitis Outside North America

Genus	Virus and Disease	Vector	Geographic Distribution
Flavivirus	Japanese encephalitis	Culex tritaeniorhynchus	Asia/Japan to Sri Lanka
Flavivirus	Murray Valley encephalitis	Culex annulirostris	Eastern Australia
Flavivirus	Rocio	Psorophora or Aedes	Sao Paulo, Brazil
Flavivirus	West Nile	Culex and others	Europe to Australia
Flavivirus	Tick-borne encephalitis	Ixodes ricinus I. persulcatus	Europe Russia
Togavirus	Venezuelan equine encephalitis	Culex and others	Northern South America

Etiology. VEE is an alphavirus of the genus Togaviridae. VEE circulates in nature in six subtypes. Types I and III viruses have multiple antigenic variants. Types IAB and IC have caused epizootics and human epidemics.

Epidemiology. The majority of epizootics resulting from types IAB and IC have occurred in Venezuela and Colombia. The virus resides in ill-defined sylvatic reservoirs in the South American rain forests. Known hosts include rodents and aquatic birds with transmission by *Culex melaconion* species. Vectors for horse-to-horse and horse-to-human transmission include *Aedes taeniorhynchus* and *Psorophora confinnis*. Epizootics move rapidly, up to several miles per day. Human cases are proportional to and follow epizootic occurrences. Viremia levels in human blood are high enough to infect mosquitoes. Because virus can be recovered from human pharyngeal swabs, and household attack rates are often as high as 50%, it is widely believed that person-to-person transmission occurs, although direct evidence is lacking. Types II–VI viruses are restricted to relatively small foci; each has a unique vector-host relationship and rarely results in human infections.

Clinical Manifestations. The incubation period is 2–5 days followed by the abrupt onset of fever, chills, headache, sore throat, myalgia, malaise, prostration, photophobia, nausea, vomiting, and diarrhea. In 5–10% of cases, there is a biphasic illness; the second phase is heralded by seizures, projectile vomiting, ataxia, confusion, agitation, and mild disturbances in consciousness. On physical examination, there is cervical lymphadenopathy and conjunctival suffusion. Cases of meningoencephalitis may demonstrate cranial nerve palsy, motor weakness, paralysis, seizures, and coma. Microscopic examination of tissues reveals inflammatory infiltrates in lymph nodes, spleen, lung, liver, and brain. Lymph nodes show cellular depletion, necrosis of germinal centers, and lymphophagocytosis. The liver shows patchy hepatocellular degeneration, the lungs demonstrate a diffuse interstitial pneumonia with intra-alveolar hemorrhages, and the brain shows patchy cellular infiltrates.

Diagnosis. The etiologic diagnosis of VEE is established by testing an acute-phase serum collected early in the illness for the presence of virus-specific immunoglobulin (Ig) M antibodies or, alternatively, demonstrating a fourfold or greater increase in IgG antibody titers by testing paired acute and convalescent sera. The virus can also be identified by polymerase chain reaction (PCR).

Treatment. There is no specific treatment for VEE. The treatment is intensive supportive care (Chapter 57), including control of seizures (Chapter 586).

Prognosis. In patients with meningoencephalitis, the fatality rate ranges from 10–25%. Sequelae include nervousness, forgetfulness, recurrent headache, and easy fatigability.

Prevention. Several veterinary vaccines are available to protect equines. VEE virus is highly infectious in laboratory settings, and BL-3 containment should be used. An experimental vaccine is available for use in laboratory workers.

245.2 Japanese Encephalitis

Epidemics of encephalitis were reported in Japan from the late 1800s. The JE virus was first isolated by Japanese workers by intracerebral inoculation of monkeys in 1934 and subsequently in mice in 1936. The virus was initially called Japanese B encephalitis to distinguish it from an unusual epidemic of von Economo (type A) encephalitis that occurred in Japan in the 1920s.

Etiology. JE virus is a positive-sense single-stranded RNA virus and a member of the family Flaviviridae.

Epidemiology. JE is a mosquito-borne viral disease of humans as well as horses, swine, and other domestic animals that causes human infections and acute disease in a vast area of Asia, northern Japan, Korea, China, Taiwan, Philippines, and the Indonesian archipelago and from Indochina through the Indian subcontinent. *Culex tritaeniorhynchus summarosus*, a nighttime-biting mosquito that feeds preferentially on large domestic animals and birds but only infrequently on humans, is the principal vector of zoonotic and human JE in northern Asia. A more complex ecology prevails in southern Asia. From Taiwan to India, *C. tritaeniorhynchus* and members of the closely related *Culex vishnui* group are vectors. Before the introduction of JE vaccine, summer outbreaks of JE occurred regularly in Japan, Korea, China, Okinawa, and Taiwan. Over the past decade, there has been a pattern of steadily enlarging recurrent seasonal outbreaks in Vietnam, Thailand, Nepal, and India, with small outbreaks in the Philippines, Indonesia, and the northern tip of Queensland, Australia. Seasonal rains are accompanied by increases in mosquito populations and increased transmission. Pigs serve as amplifying host.

The annual incidence in endemic areas ranges from 1–10/10,000 population. Children younger than 15 yr are principally affected, with nearly universal exposure by adulthood. The case to infection ratio for JE virus has been variously estimated at 1:25–1:1,000. Higher ratios have been estimated for populations indigenous to enzootic areas. JE occurs in travelers visiting Asia; therefore, a travel history in the diagnosis of encephalitis is critical.

Clinical Manifestations. After a 4–14 day incubation period, cases typically progress through four stages: prodromal illness (2–3 days), acute stage (3–4 days), subacute stage (7–10 days), and convalescence (4–7 wk). Onset may be characterized by abrupt onset of fever, headache, respiratory symptoms, anorexia, nausea, abdominal pain, vomiting, and sensory changes, including psychotic episodes. Grand mal seizures are seen in 10–24% of children; parkinsonian-like nonintention tremor and cogwheel rigidity are seen less frequently. Particularly characteristic are rapidly changing central nervous system signs (e.g., hyperreflexia followed by hyporeflexia or plantar responses that change). The sensory status of the patient may vary from confusion, disorientation, delirium, or somnolence, progressing to coma. There is usually a mild pleocytosis (100–1,000 leukocytes/mm^3) in the cerebrospinal fluid, initially polymorphonuclear but in a few days predominantly lymphocytic. Albuminuria is common. Fatal cases usually progress rapidly to coma, and the patient dies within 10 days.

Diagnosis. JE should be suspected in patients reporting exposure to night-biting mosquitoes in endemic areas during the transmission season. The etiologic diagnosis of JE is established by testing an acute-phase serum collected early in the illness for the presence of virus-specific IgM antibodies or, alternatively, demonstrating a four-fold or greater increase in IgG antibody titers by testing paired acute and convalescent sera. The virus can also be identified by PCR.

Treatment. There is no specific treatment for JE. The treatment is intensive supportive care (Chapter 57), including control of seizures (Chapter 586).

Prognosis. Patient fatality rates are 24–42% and are highest in children aged 5–9 yr and in persons older than 65 yr. The frequency of sequelae is 5–70% and is directly related to age of the patient and to the severity of disease. Sequelae are most common in patients younger than 10 yr at the onset of disease. The more common sequelae are mental deterioration, severe emotional instability, personality changes, motor abnormalities, and speech disturbances.

Prevention. Travelers to endemic countries staying ≥1 mo in rural areas of the endemic region during the expected period of seasonal transmission, or those traveling in areas experiencing endemic transmission, should receive JE vaccine. The JE vaccine is given in a 3-dose series (0.5 mL for 1–3 yr of age; 1 mL for >3 yr of age) subcutaneously; the first two doses are given 1 wk apart and the third dose 30 days later. Booster doses are given every 2 yr while risk of exposure continues. Reactions to vaccination, including headache, malaise, myalgia, tenderness, redness, and swelling, occur in about 20% of vaccines. Serious generalized urticaria, facial angioedema, and respiratory distress have been observed in adults. Because vaccine is prepared in mouse brain, surveillance should be maintained for central nervous system disease after JE vaccination. In humans, prior dengue virus infection provides partial protection from clinical JE.

Personal measures should be taken to reduce exposure to mosquito bites, especially for short-term residents in endemic areas. This consists of avoiding evening outdoor exposure, using insect repellents, covering the body with clothing, and using bed nets or house screening.

Commercial pesticides, widely used by rice farmers in Asia, are effective in reducing populations of *C. tritaeniorhynchus*. Fenthion, fenitrothion, and phenthoate are effectively adulticidal and larvicidal. Insecticides may be applied from portable sprayers or from helicopters or light aircraft.

245.3 Tick-Borne Encephalitis

TBE was identified by Russian scientists in 1937 and was subsequently shown to be widespread in Europe, where it was identified as the cause of milk-borne encephalitis.

Etiology. TBE virus is a positive-sense, single-stranded RNA virus and a member of the family Flaviviridae.

Epidemiology. Tick-borne encephalitis refers to neurotropic tick-transmitted flaviviral infections occurring across the Eurasian land mass. In the Far East, the disease is called Russian spring-summer encephalitis; the milder, often biphasic form in Europe is simply called tick-borne encephalitis. TBE is found in all countries of Europe except Portugal and the Benelux countries. The incidence is particularly high in Austria, Poland, Hungary, Czech Republic, Slovakia, former Yugoslavia, and Russia. The incidence tends to be very focal. Seroprevalence is as high as 50% in farm and forestry workers. The majority of cases occur in adults, but even young children may be infected while playing in the woods

or on picnics or camping trips. The seasonal distribution of cases is midsummer in southern Europe, with a longer season in Scandinavia and the Russian Far East. TBE can be excreted from the milk of goats, sheep, or cows. Before World War II, when milk was consumed unpasteurized, milk-borne cases were common.

Viruses are transmitted principally by hard ticks of *Ixodes ricinus* in Europe and *Ixodes persulcatus* in the Far East. Viral circulation is maintained by a combination of transmission from ticks to birds, rodents, and larger mammals and transtadial transmission from larval to nymphal and adult stages. In some parts of Europe and Russia, ticks feed actively during the spring and early fall, giving rise to the name spring-summer encephalitis.

Clinical Manifestations. After an incubation period of 7–14 days, the European form begins as an acute nonspecific febrile illness followed in 5–30% of cases by meningoencephalitis. The Far Eastern variety more often results in encephalitis with higher case fatality and sequelae rates. The first phase of illness is characterized by fever, headache, myalgia, malaise, nausea, and vomiting for 2–7 days. Fever disappears and after 2–8 days may return accompanied by vomiting, photophobia, and signs of meningeal irritation in children and more severe encephalitic signs in adults. This phase rarely lasts more than 1 wk.

Diagnosis. The diagnosis of TBE should be suspected in patients reporting a tick bite in endemic areas during the transmission season. The etiologic diagnosis of TBE is established by testing an acute-phase serum collected early in the illness for the presence of virus-specific IgM antibodies or, alternatively, demonstrating a fourfold or greater increase in IgG antibody titers by testing paired acute and convalescent sera. The virus can also be identified by PCR.

Treatment. There is no specific treatment for TBE. The treatment is intensive supportive care (Chapter 57), including control of seizures (Chapter 586).

Prognosis. The main risk for fatal outcome is advanced age; the fatality rate in adults is about 1%, but sequelae in children are rare. Transient unilateral paralysis of an upper extremity is a common finding in adults. Common sequelae include chronic fatigue, headache, sleep disorders, and emotional disturbances.

Prevention. Specific Ig has been given to persons with seasonal tick bite exposure, although efficacy of this preventive therapy is not well studied. Effective inactivated vaccines for human use, made from virus grown in tissue culture, are licensed in Russia and Europe. They are administered in a three-dose series, as described for JE vaccine.

Centers for Disease Control: Inactivated Japanese encephalitis virus vaccine. Recommendations of the Advisory Committee on Immunization Practices (ACIP). *MMWR Morb Mortal Wkly Rep* 1993;42(RR-1):1–15.

Innis BL, Nisalak A, Nimmannitya S, et al: An enzyme-linked immunosorbent assay to characterize dengue infections where dengue and Japanese encephalitis co-circulate. *Am J Trop Med Hyg* 1989;40:418–27.

Kluger G, Schottler A, Waldvogel K, et al: Tickborne encephalitis despite specific immunoglobulin prophylaxis. *Lancet* 1995;346:1502.

McNeil JG, Lednar WM, Stansfield SK, et al: Central European tick-borne encephalitis: Assessment of risk for persons in the Armed Forces and vacationers. *J Infect Dis* 1985;152:650–1.

Paul WS, Moore PS, Karabatsos N, et al: Outbreak of Japanese encephalitis on the island of Saipan, 1990. *J Infect Dis* 1993;167:1053–8.

Poland JD, Cropp CB, Craven RB, et al: Evaluation of the potency and safety of inactivated Japanese encephalitis vaccine in U.S. inhabitants. *J Infect Dis* 1990;161:878–82.

Rico-Hesse R, Weaver SC, de Siger J, et al: Emergence of a new epidemic/epizootic of Venezuelan equine encephalitis virus in South America. *Proc Natl Acad Sci U S A* 1995;92:5278–81.

Siegel-Itzkovich J: Twelve die of West Nile virus in Israel. *Br Med J* 2000;321:724.

Tsai TF: Arboviral infections: General considerations for prevention, diagnosis and treatment in travelers. *Semin Pediatr Infect Dis* 1992;3:62–9.

Tsai TF, Popovici F, Cerescu C, et al: West Nile encephalitis epidemic in southeastern Romania. *Lancet* 1998;352:767–71.

Chapter 246
Dengue Fever and Dengue Hemorrhagic Fever

Scott B. Halstead

Dengue fever, a benign syndrome caused by several arthropod-borne viruses, is characterized by biphasic fever, myalgia or arthralgia, rash, leukopenia, and lymphadenopathy. **Dengue hemorrhagic fever** (Philippine, Thai, or Singapore hemorrhagic fever; hemorrhagic dengue; acute infectious thrombocytopenic purpura) is a severe, often fatal, febrile disease caused by dengue viruses. It is characterized by capillary permeability, abnormalities of hemostasis, and, in severe cases, a protein-losing shock syndrome (**dengue shock syndrome**). It is currently thought to have an immunopathologic basis.

Etiology. There are at least four distinct antigenic types of dengue virus, members of the family Flaviviridae. In addition, three other *arthropod-borne* (*arbo*viruses) cause similar or identical febrile diseases with rash (Table 246–1).

Epidemiology. Dengue viruses are transmitted by mosquitoes of the *Stegomyia* family. *Aedes aegypti*, a daytime biting mosquito, is the principal vector, and all four virus types have been recovered from it. In most tropical areas, *A. aegypti* is highly urbanized, breeding in water stored for drinking or bathing and in rainwater collected in any container. Dengue viruses have also been recovered from *Aedes albopictus*, as in the 2001 Hawaiian epidemic, while outbreaks in the Pacific area have been attributed to several other *Aedes* species. These species breed in water trapped in vegetation. In Southeast Asia and West Africa, dengue may be maintained in a cycle involving canopy-feeding jungle monkeys and *Aedes* species, which feed on monkeys.

Epidemics were common in temperate areas of the Americas, Europe, Australia, and Asia until early in the 20th century. Dengue fever and dengue-like disease are now endemic in tropical Asia, the South Pacific Islands, northern Australia, tropical Africa, the Caribbean, and Central and South America. Dengue fever occurs frequently among travelers to these areas.

Dengue outbreaks in urban areas infested with *A. aegypti* may be explosive; up to 70–80% of the population may be involved. Most disease occurs in older children and adults. Because *A. aegypti* has a limited range, spread of an epidemic occurs mainly through viremic human beings and follows the main lines of transportation. Sentinel cases may infect household mosquitoes; a large number of nearly simultaneous secondary infections give the appearance of a contagious disease. Where dengue is endemic, children and susceptible foreigners may be the only persons to acquire overt disease, adults having become immune.

DENGUE-LIKE DISEASES. Dengue-like diseases may also occur in epidemics. Epidemiologic features depend on the vectors and their geographic distribution (see Table 246–1). Chikungunya virus is widespread in the most populous areas of the world. In Asia, *A. aegypti* is the principal vector; in Africa, other *Stegomyia* may be important vectors. In Southeast Asia, dengue and chikungunya outbreaks occur concurrently. Outbreaks of o'nyong-nyong and West Nile fever usually involve villages or small towns, in contrast to the urban outbreaks of dengue and chikungunya.

DENGUE HEMORRHAGIC FEVER. Dengue hemorrhagic fever occurs where multiple types of dengue virus are simultaneously or sequentially transmitted. Currently, it is endemic in all of tropical America and Asia, where warm temperatures and the practices of water storage in homes plus outdoor breeding sites result in large, permanent populations of *A. aegypti*. Under these conditions, infections with dengue viruses of all types are common, and second infections with heterologous types are frequent.

Second dengue infections are relatively mild in the majority of instances, ranging from an inapparent infection through an undifferentiated upper respiratory tract or dengue-like disease, but may also progress to dengue hemorrhagic fever. Nonimmune foreigners, adults and children, exposed to dengue virus during outbreaks of hemorrhagic fever have classic dengue fever or even milder disease. The differences in clinical manifestations of dengue infections between natives and foreigners in Southeast Asia are related more to immunologic status than to racial susceptibility. Dengue hemorrhagic fever can occur during primary dengue infections, most frequently in infants whose mothers are immune to dengue.

Dengue 3 virus strains circulating in mainland Southeast Asia since 1983 are associated with a particularly severe clinical syndrome, characterized by encephalopathy, hypoglycemia, markedly elevated liver enzymes, and, occasionally, jaundice.

Pathogenesis. The pathogenesis of dengue fever is not clear. Fatalities with chikungunya and West Nile fever infections have been ascribed to viral encephalitis or hemorrhage.

The pathogenesis is incompletely understood, but epidemiologic studies suggest that it is usually associated with second infections with dengue types 1–4. In the Americas, dengue hemorrhagic fever and dengue shock syndrome have been associated only with dengue 2 strains of recent Southeast Asian origin. Recent occurrences of sizable dengue hemorrhagic fever outbreaks in India, Pakistan, and Bangladesh also appear to be related to imported dengue strains. Dengue viruses demonstrate enhanced growth in cultures of human mononuclear phagocytes prepared from dengue-immune donors or in cultures supplemented with non-neutralizing dengue antibodies. Retrospective studies of sera from human mothers whose infants acquired dengue hemorrhagic fever or prospective studies in children acquiring sequential dengue infections have shown that the circulation of infection-enhancing antibodies at the time of infection is the strongest risk factor for development of severe disease. Monkeys infected sequentially or receiving small quantities of enhancing antibodies have enhanced viremias. In humans studied early during the course of secondary dengue infections, viremia levels directly predicted disease severity. Early in the acute stage of secondary dengue infections, there is rapid activation of the complement system. Shortly before or during shock, blood levels of soluble tumor necrosis factor receptor, interferon-γ, and interleukin 2 are elevated. C1q, C3, C4, C5–C8, and C3 proactivators are depressed, and C3 catabolic rates are elevated. These factors may interact at the endothelial cell to produce increased vascular permeability through the nitric oxide final pathway. The blood clotting and fibrinolytic systems are activated, and levels of factor XII (Hageman factor) are depressed. The mechanism of bleeding in dengue hemorrhagic fever is not known, but a mild degree of disseminated intravascular coagulation, liver damage, and thrombocytopenia

TABLE 246–1. Vectors and Geographic Distribution of Dengue-Like Diseases

Genus	Virus and Disease	Vector	Geographic Distribution
Togavirus	Chikungunya	*Aedes aegypti* *Aedes africanus*	Africa, India, Southeast Asia
Togavirus	O'nyong-nyong	*Anopheles funestus*	East Africa
Flavivirus	West Nile fever	*Culex molestus* *Culex univittatus*	Europe, Africa, Middle East, India

may operate synergistically. Capillary damage allows fluid, electrolytes, small proteins, and, in some instances, red cells to leak into extravascular spaces. This internal redistribution of fluid, together with deficits caused by fasting, thirsting, and vomiting, results in hemoconcentration, hypovolemia, increased cardiac work, tissue hypoxia, metabolic acidosis, and hyponatremia.

Usually no pathologic lesions are found to account for death. In rare instances, death may be due to gastrointestinal or intracranial hemorrhages. Minimal to moderate hemorrhages are seen in the upper gastrointestinal tract, and petechial hemorrhages are common in the interventricular septum of the heart, on the pericardium, and on the subserosal surfaces of major viscera. Focal hemorrhages are occasionally seen in the lungs, liver, adrenals, and subarachnoid space. The liver is usually enlarged, often with fatty changes. Yellow, watery, and at times blood-tinged effusions are present in serous cavities in about three fourths of patients.

Microscopically, there is perivascular edema in the soft tissues and widespread diapedesis of red cells. There may be maturational arrest of megakaryocytes in bone marrow, and increased numbers of them are seen in capillaries of the lungs, in renal glomeruli, and in sinusoids of the liver and spleen.

Dengue virus is usually absent in tissues at the time of death; rare isolations have been reported from liver and lymphatic tissues, most often in children <1 yr of age with primary infection.

Clinical Manifestations. The incubation period is 1–7 days. The clinical manifestations are variable and are influenced by the age of the patient. In infants and young children, the disease may be undifferentiated or characterized by fever for 1–5 days, pharyngeal inflammation, rhinitis, and mild cough. A majority of infected older children and adults experience sudden onset of fever, with temperature rapidly increasing to 39.4–41.1°C (103–106°F), usually accompanied by frontal or retro-orbital pain, particularly when pressure is applied to the eyes. Occasionally, severe back pain precedes the fever (back-break fever). A *transient*, macular, generalized rash that blanches under pressure may be seen during the first 24–48 hr of fever. The pulse rate may be slow relative to the degree of fever. Myalgia and arthralgia occur soon after the onset and increase in severity. Joint symptoms may be particularly severe in patients with chikungunya or o'nyong-nyong infection. From the 2nd–6th days of fever, nausea and vomiting are apt to occur, and generalized lymphadenopathy, cutaneous hyperesthesia or hyperalgesia, taste aberrations, and pronounced anorexia may develop.

About 1–2 days after defervescence, a generalized, morbilliform, maculopapular rash appears that spares the palms and soles. It disappears in 1–5 days; desquamation may occur. Rarely there is edema of the palms and soles. About the time this second rash appears, the body temperature, which has previously decreased to normal, may become slightly elevated and demonstrate the characteristic biphasic temperature pattern.

DENGUE HEMORRHAGIC FEVER. Differentiation between dengue fever and dengue hemorrhagic fever is difficult early in the course of illness. A relatively mild first phase with abrupt onset of fever, malaise, vomiting, headache, anorexia, and cough is followed after 2–5 days by rapid clinical deterioration and collapse. In this second phase, the patient usually has cold, clammy extremities, a warm trunk, flushed face, diaphoresis, restlessness, irritability, and midepigastric pain. Frequently, there are scattered petechiae on the forehead and extremities; spontaneous ecchymoses may appear, and easy bruising and bleeding at sites of venipuncture are common. A macular or maculopapular rash may appear, and there may be circumoral and peripheral cyanosis. Respirations are rapid and often labored. The pulse is weak, rapid, and thready and the heart sounds faint. The liver may enlarge to 4–6 cm below the costal margin and is usually firm and somewhat tender. Approximately 20–30% of cases of

dengue hemorrhagic fever are complicated by shock (dengue shock syndrome). Fewer than 10% of patients have gross ecchymosis or gastrointestinal bleeding, usually after a period of uncorrected shock. After a 24–36 hr period of crisis, convalescence is fairly rapid in the children who recover. The temperature may return to normal before or during the stage of shock. Bradycardia and ventricular extrasystoles are common during convalescence.

Diagnosis. A clinical diagnosis of dengue fever derives from a high index of suspicion and a knowledge of the geographic distribution and environmental cycles of causal viruses. Because clinical findings vary and there are many possible causative agents, the term "dengue-like disease" should be used until a specific diagnosis is established.

The World Health Organization criteria for **dengue hemorrhagic fever** are fever, minor or major hemorrhagic manifestations, thrombocytopenia ($\leq$100,000/mm^3), and objective evidence of increased capillary permeability (hematocrit increased $\geq$20%), pleural effusion (by chest radiograph), or hypoalbuminemia. **Dengue shock syndrome** criteria include those for dengue hemorrhagic fever as well as hypotension or narrow pulse pressure ($\leq$20 mm Hg).

Virologic diagnosis can be established by serologic tests or by isolation of the virus from blood leukocytes or serum. In both primary and secondary dengue infections, there is a relatively transient appearance of antidengue immunoglobulin (Ig) M antibodies. These disappear after 6–12 wk, which can be used to time a dengue infection. In second primary dengue infections, most antibody is of the IgG class. Serologic diagnosis depends on a fourfold or greater increase in IgG antibody titer in paired sera by hemagglutination inhibition, complement fixation, enzyme immunoassay, or neutralization test. Carefully standardized immunoglobulin IgM- and IgG-capture enzyme immunoassays are now widely used to identify acute-phase antibodies from patients with primary or secondary dengue infections in single-serum samples. Usually such samples should be collected not earlier than 5 days nor later than 6 wk after onset. It may not be possible to distinguish the infecting virus by serologic methods alone, particularly when there has been prior infection with another member of the same arbovirus group. Virus can be recovered from acute-phase serum after inoculating tissue culture or living mosquitoes. Viral RNA can be detected in blood or tissues by specific complementary DNA probes or amplified first by the polymerase chain reaction.

DIFFERENTIAL DIAGNOSIS. The differential diagnosis of dengue fever includes viral respiratory and influenza-like diseases, the early stages of malaria, mild yellow fever, scrub typhus, viral hepatitis, and leptospirosis.

Four arboviral diseases have dengue-like courses but without rash: Colorado tick fever, sandfly fever, Rift Valley fever, and Ross River fever. Colorado tick fever occurs sporadically among campers and hunters in the western United States; sandfly fever in the Mediterranean region, the Middle East, southern Russia, and parts of the Indian subcontinent; and Rift Valley fever in North, East, Central, and South Africa. Ross River fever is endemic in much of eastern Australia with epidemic extension to Fiji. In adults, Ross River fever often produces protracted and crippling arthralgia involving weight-bearing joints.

Because meningococcemia, yellow fever (Chapter 247), other viral hemorrhagic fevers (Chapter 248), many rickettsial diseases, and other severe illnesses caused by a variety of agents may produce a clinical picture similar to dengue hemorrhagic fever, the etiologic diagnosis should be made only when epidemiologic or serologic evidence suggests the possibility of a dengue infection.

LABORATORY FINDINGS. In dengue fever, pancytopenia may occur after the 3–4 days of illness. Neutropenia may persist or reappear during the latter stage of the disease and may continue into convalescence with white blood cell counts as low as 2,000/mm³. Platelets rarely fall below 100,000/mm³. Venous clotting, bleeding and prothrombin times, and plasma fibrinogen values are within normal ranges. The tourniquet test infrequently is positive. Mild acidosis, hemoconcentration, increased transaminase values, and hypoproteinemia may occur during some primary dengue virus infections. The electrocardiogram may show sinus bradycardia, ectopic ventricular foci, flattened T waves, and prolongation of the P-R interval.

The most common hematologic abnormalities during dengue hemorrhagic fever and dengue shock syndrome are hemoconcentration with an increase of >20% in hematocrit, thrombocytopenia, prolonged bleeding time, and moderately decreased prothrombin level that is seldom <40% of control. Fibrinogen levels may be subnormal and fibrin split products elevated. Other abnormalities include moderate elevations of the serum transaminase levels, consumption of complement, mild metabolic acidosis with hyponatremia, and occasionally hypochloremia, slight elevation of serum urea nitrogen, and hypoalbuminemia. Roentgenograms of the chest reveal pleural effusions (left > right) in nearly all patients.

Treatment. Treatment of uncomplicated dengue fever is supportive. Bed rest is advised during the febrile period. Antipyretics should be used to keep body temperature less than 40°C (104°F). Analgesics or mild sedation may be required to control pain. Aspirin is contraindicated and should not be used because of its effects on hemostasis. Fluid and electrolyte replacement is required for deficits caused by sweating, fasting, thirsting, vomiting, and diarrhea.

DENGUE HEMORRHAGIC FEVER. Management of dengue hemorrhagic fever and dengue shock syndrome includes immediate evaluation of vital signs and degrees of hemoconcentration, dehydration, and electrolyte imbalance. Close monitoring is essential for at least 48 hr because shock may occur or recur precipitously early in the disease. Patients who are cyanotic or have labored breathing should be given oxygen. Rapid intravenous replacement of fluids and electrolytes can frequently sustain patients until spontaneous recovery occurs. Normal saline is more effective in treating shock than the more expensive Ringer lactated saline. When pulse pressure is ≤10 mmHg, or when elevation of the hematocrit persists after replacement of fluids, plasma or colloid preparations are indicated.

Care must be taken to avoid overhydration, which may contribute to cardiac failure. Transfusions of fresh blood or platelets suspended in plasma may be required to control bleeding; they should not be given during hemoconcentration but only after evaluation of hemoglobin or hematocrit values. Salicylates are contraindicated because of their effect on blood clotting.

Paraldehyde or chloral hydrate may be required for children who are markedly agitated. Use of vasopressors has not resulted in a significant reduction of mortality compared with that observed with simple supportive therapy. Disseminated intravascular coagulation may require treatment (Chapter 475). Corticosteroids do not shorten the duration of disease or improve prognosis in children receiving careful supportive therapy.

Hypervolemia during the fluid reabsorptive phase may be life-threatening and is heralded by a decrease in hematocrit with wide pulse pressure. Diuretics and digitalization may be necessary.

Complications. Primary infections with dengue fever and dengue-like diseases are usually self-limited and benign. Fluid and electrolyte losses, hyperpyrexia, and febrile convulsions are the most frequent complications in infants and young children. Epistaxis, petechiae, and purpuric lesions are uncommon but may occur at any stage. Swallowed blood from epistaxis, vomited or passed by rectum, may be erroneously interpreted as gastrointestinal bleeding. In adults and possibly in children, underlying conditions may lead to clinically significant bleeding.

Convulsions may occur during high temperature especially with chikungunya fever. Infrequently, after the febrile stage, prolonged asthenia, mental depression, bradycardia, and ventricular extrasystoles may occur in children.

In endemic areas, dengue hemorrhagic fever should be suspected in children with a febrile illness suggestive of dengue fever who experience hemoconcentration and thrombocytopenia.

Prognosis. The prognosis of dengue fever may be adversely affected by passively acquired antibody or by prior infection with a closely related virus that predisposes to development of dengue hemorrhagic fever.

DENGUE HEMORRHAGIC FEVER. Death has occurred in 40–50% of patients with shock, but with adequate intensive care deaths should occur in less than 1% of cases. Survival is directly related to early and intense supportive treatment. Infrequently, there is residual brain damage caused by prolonged shock or occasionally by intracranial hemorrhage.

Prevention. Several types of dengue types 1, 2, 3, and 4 vaccines are under development, and a killed vaccine for chikungunya is efficacious but not generally available. Prophylaxis consists of avoiding mosquito bites by use of insecticides, repellents, body covering with clothing, screening of houses, and destruction of *A. aegypti* breeding sites (Chapter 285). If water storage is mandatory, a tight-fitting lid or a thin layer of oil may prevent egg laying or hatching. A larvicide, such as Abate [O,O′-(thiodi-*p*-phenylene) O,O,O,O′-tetramethyl phosphorothioate], available as a 1% sand-granule formation and effective at a concentration of 1 ppm, may be added safely to drinking water. Ultra-low-volume spray equipment effectively dispenses the adulticide malathion from truck or airplane for rapid intervention during an epidemic. Only personal antimosquito measures are effective against mosquitoes in the field, forest, or jungle.

The possibility exists that dengue vaccination may sensitize a recipient so that ensuing dengue infection could result in hemorrhagic fever. Vaccination with yellow fever 17D strain has no effect on the severity of dengue illness, although seroconversion rates to a dengue 2 vaccine were enhanced in persons immune to yellow fever.

Bethell DB, Gamble J, Pham PL, et al: Noninvasive measurement of microvascular leakage in patients with dengue hemorrhagic fever. *Clin Infect Dis* 2001;32: 243–53.

Bhamarapravati N, Yoksan S, Chayaniyayothin T, et al: Immunization with a live attenuated dengue-2 virus candidate vaccine (16681-PDK 53): Clinical, immunological and biological responses in adult volunteers. *Bull World Health Organ* 1987;65:189–95.

Burke DS, Nisalak A, Johnson DE, et al: A prospective study of dengue infections in Bangkok. *Am J Trop Med Hyg* 1988;38:172–80.

Cohen SN, Halstead SB: Shock associated with dengue infection. I. The clinical and physiologic manifestations of dengue hemorrhagic fever in Thailand, 1964. *J Pediatr* 1966;68:448–56.

Dung NM, Day NP, Tam DT, et al: Fluid replacement in dengue shock syndrome: A randomized, double-blind comparison of four intravenous-fluid regimens. *Clin Inf Dis* 1999;29:787–94.

Guirakhoo F, Weltzin R, Chambers TJ, et al: Recombinant chimeric yellow fever-dengue type 2 virus is immunogenic and protective in nonhuman primates. *J Virol* 2000;74:5477–85.

Guzman Mg, Kouri G, Valdes L, et al: Epidemiological studies on dengue in Santiago de Cuba, 1997. *Am J Epidemiol* 2000;152: 793–9.

Halstead SB: Pathogenesis of dengue: Challenges to molecular biology. *Science* 1988;239:476–81.

Kliks SC, Nisalak A, Brandt WE, et al: Evidence that maternal dengue antibodies are important in the development of dengue hemorrhagic fever in infants. *Am J Trop Med Hyg* 1988;38:411–9.

Sangkawibha N, Rojanasuphot S, Ahandrik S, et al: Risk factors in dengue shock syndrome: A prospective epidemiological study in Rayong, Thailand. *Am J Epidemiol* 1984;120:653–69.

Vaughn DW, Green S, Kalayanarooj S, et al: Dengue viremia titer, antibody response pattern and virus serotype correlate with disease severity. *J Infect Dis* 2000;181:2–9.

Watts D, Porter K, Putvatana R, et al: Failure of secondary infections with American genotype dengue 2 viruses to cause dengue haemorrhagic fever. *Lancet* 1999; 354:1431–4.

Chapter 247
Yellow Fever *Scott B. Halstead*

Yellow fever is an acute infection characterized in its most severe form by fever, jaundice, proteinuria, and hemorrhage. The virus is mosquito-borne and occurs in epidemic or endemic form in South America and Africa. Seasonal epidemics occurred in cities located in temperate areas of Europe and the Americas until 1900; epidemics continue to occur in West, Central, and East Africa.

Etiology. Yellow fever is the prototype of the *Flavivirus* genus of the family Flaviviridae, which are enveloped single-stranded RNA viruses 35–50 nm in diameter.

Yellow fever circulates zoonotically as three genotypes: type I and IIA in Central and West Africa, respectively, and type IIB in South America. The type IIA virus is capable of urban transmission between human beings by *Aedes aegypti*. Sometime in the 1600s, this virus was brought to the American tropics through the African slave trade. Subsequently, yellow fever caused enormous coastal and riverine epidemics until the 20th century, when the virus and its urban and sylvan mosquito cycles were identified and a vaccine and mosquito control developed.

Epidemiology. Human and nonhuman primate hosts acquire the infection by the bite of infected mosquitoes. After an incubation period of 3–6 days, virus appears in the blood and may serve as a source of infection for other mosquitoes. The virus must replicate in the gut of the mosquito and pass to the salivary gland before the mosquito can transmit the virus. Yellow fever virus is transmitted in an urban cycle—human to *A. aegypti* to human—and a jungle cycle—monkey to jungle mosquitoes to monkey. Classic yellow fever epidemics in the United States, South America, the Caribbean, and parts of Europe were of the urban variety. Present-day African epidemics are primarily urban. Most of the approximately 200 cases reported each year in South America are jungle yellow fever. In colonial times, attack rates in white adults were very high, suggesting that subclinical infections are uncommon in this age group. Yellow fever may be less severe in children, with subclinical infections to clinical case ratios of ≥2:1. In areas where outbreaks of urban yellow fever are common, most cases involve children because many adults are immune. Transmission in West Africa is highest during the rainy season, from July to November. The migration of nonimmune laborers into endemic regions is a significant factor in some outbreaks.

In tropical forests, yellow fever virus is maintained in a transmission cycle involving monkeys and tree hole–breeding mosquitoes (*Haemagogus* in Central and South America, *Aedes africanus* in Africa). In the Americas, most cases involve men who work in forested areas and are exposed to infected mosquitoes. In Africa, the virus is prevalent in moist savanna and savanna transition areas where other tree hole–breeding *Aedes* vectors transmit the virus between monkeys and humans and between humans.

Pathogenesis. Pathologic changes seen in the liver include (1) coagulative necrosis of hepatocytes in the midzone of the liver lobule, with sparing of cells around the portal areas and central veins; (2) eosinophilic degeneration of hepatocytes (**Councilman bodies**); (3) microvacuolar fatty change; and (4) minimal inflammation. The kidneys show acute tubular necrosis. In the heart, myocardial fiber degeneration and fatty infiltration are seen. The brain may show edema and petechial hemorrhages. Direct viral injury to the liver results in impaired ability to perform functions of biosynthesis and detoxication; this is the central pathogenic event of yellow fever. Hemorrhage is thought to result from decreased synthesis of vitamin K–dependent clotting factors and, in some cases, disseminated intravascular clotting. Renal dysfunction has been attributed to hemodynamic factors (prerenal failure progressing to acute tubular necrosis). The pathogenesis of shock in patients with yellow fever appears to be similar to that described in dengue shock syndrome and the other viral hemorrhagic fevers.

Clinical Manifestations. In Africa, inapparent, abortive, or clinically mild infections are frequent; some studies suggest that children experience a milder disease than adults do. Abortive infections, characterized by fever and headache, may be unrecognized except during epidemics.

In its classic form, yellow fever begins with sudden onset of fever, headache, myalgia, lumbosacral pain, anorexia, nausea, and vomiting. Physical findings during the early phase of illness, when virus is present in the blood, include prostration, conjunctival injection, flushing of face and neck, reddening of the tongue at the tip and edges, and relative bradycardia. After 2–3 days, there may be a brief period of remission, followed in 6–24 hr by reappearance of fever with vomiting, epigastric pain, jaundice, dehydration, gastrointestinal and other hemorrhages, albuminuria, hypotension, signs of renal failure, delirium, convulsions, and coma. Death may occur between the 7th and 10th days. The fatality rate in severe cases approaches 50%. Some patients who survive the acute phase of illness later succumb to renal failure or myocardial damage. Laboratory abnormalities include leukopenia; prolonged clotting, prothrombin, and partial thromboplastin times; thrombocytopenia; hyperbilirubinemia; elevated serum transaminases; albuminuria; and azotemia. Hypoglycemia may be present in severe cases. Electrocardiogram abnormalities characterized by bradycardia and ST-T changes are described.

Diagnosis. Yellow fever should be suspected when fever, headache, vomiting, myalgia, and jaundice appear in residents of endemic areas or in unimmunized visitors who have recently traveled (within 2 wk before onset of symptoms) to endemic areas. Clinically, yellow fever is quite similar to dengue hemorrhagic fever. In contrast to the gradual onset of acute viral hepatitis resulting from types hepatitis A, B, C, D, or E viruses, jaundice in yellow fever appears after 3–5 days of high temperature and is often accompanied by severe prostration. Mild yellow fever is dengue-like and cannot be distinguished from a wide variety of other infections. Jaundice and fever may occur in any of several other tropical diseases, including malaria, viral hepatitis, louse-borne relapsing fever, leptospirosis, typhoid fever, rickettsial infections, certain systemic bacterial infections, sickle cell crisis, Rift Valley fever, Crimean-Congo hemorrhagic fever, and other viral hemorrhagic fevers. Outbreaks of yellow fever always include cases with severe gastrointestinal hemorrhage.

Specific diagnosis depends on detection of virus or viral antigen in acute-phase blood samples or antibody assays. The immunoglobulin M enzyme immunoassay is particularly useful. Sera obtained during the first 10 days after onset of symptoms should be kept in an ultra-low-temperature freezer (–70°C) and shipped on dry ice for virus testing. Convalescent-phase samples for antibody tests are managed by conventional means. In handling acute-phase blood specimens, medical personnel must take care to avoid contaminating themselves or others on the evacuation trail (laboratory personnel and others). Postmortem diagnosis is based on virus isolation from liver or blood, identification of Councilman bodies in liver tissue, or detection of antigen or viral genome in liver tissue.

Treatment. It is customary to keep yellow fever patients in a mosquito-free area, using mosquito nets if necessary. Patients are viremic during the febrile phase of the illness. Although there is no specific treatment for yellow fever, medical care is directed at maintaining physiologic status: (1) sponging and acetaminophen to reduce high temperature, (2) vigorous fluid replacement of losses resulting from fasting, thirsting, vomiting, or plasma leakage, (3) correcting acid-base imbalance, (4) maintaining nutritional intake to lessen the severity of hypoglycemia, and (5) avoiding drugs that are either metabolized by the liver or toxic to the liver, kidney, or central nervous system.

Complications. Complications of acute yellow fever include severe hemorrhage, liver failure, and acute renal failure. Bleeding should be managed by transfusion of fresh whole blood or fresh plasma with platelet concentrates if necessary. Renal failure may require peritoneal dialysis or hemodialysis.

Prevention. Yellow fever 17D is a live, attenuated vaccine with a long record of safety and efficacy. It is administered as a single 0.5-mL subcutaneous injection at least 10 days before arrival in a yellow fever endemic area. All persons traveling to endemic areas in South America and Africa should be considered for vaccination, but length of stay, exact locations to be visited, and environmental or occupational exposure may determine the specific risk and individual need for vaccination. Persons traveling from yellow fever–endemic to yellow fever–receptive countries may be required to obtain a yellow fever vaccine (e.g., from South America or Africa to India). Usually countries that require travelers to obtain a yellow fever immunization do not issue a visa without a valid immunization certificate. Vaccination is valid for 10 yr for international travel certification, although immunity lasts at least 40 yr and probably for life.

Yellow fever vaccine should not be administered to persons with symptomatic immunodeficiency diseases and those taking immunosuppressant drugs. Although the vaccine is not known to harm fetuses, its administration during pregnancy is not advised. In very young children, there is a small risk of encephalitis and death after yellow fever 17D vaccination. The 17D vaccine should not be administered to infants younger than 4 mo because nearly all neurologic complications occur in this age group. Questions have been raised about the safety of 17D vaccine in older individuals. Several cases of fatal yellow fever–like disease have been reported in elderly recipients of 17D vaccine. Residence or travel to areas of known or anticipated yellow fever activity (e.g., forested areas in the Amazon basin), which places an individual at high risk, warrants immunization of infants 4–9 mo of age. Immunization of children ≥9 mo of age is routinely recommended before entry into endemic areas. Vaccination should be avoided for persons with a history of egg allergy. Alternatively, a skin test can be performed to determine whether a serious allergy exists that would preclude vaccination.

Centers for Disease Control: Yellow fever vaccine. Recommendations of the Advisory Committee on Immunization Practices (ACIP). *MMWR Morb Mortal Wkly Rep* 1990;39(RR-6):1–6.

Chang GJ, Cropp BC, Kinney RM, et al: Nucleotide sequence variation of the envelope protein gene identifies two distinct genotypes of yellow fever virus. *J Virol* 1995;69:5773–80.

Martin M, Weld LH, Tsai TF et al: Advanced age as a risk factor for illness temporally associated with yellow fever vaccination. *Emerg Infect Dis* 2001;7:945–51.

Monath TP: Yellow fever: A medically neglected disease. Report on a seminar. *Rev Infect Dis* 1987;9:165–75.

Monath TP: Yellow fever and dengue: The interactions of virus, vector and host in the re-emergence of epidemic disease. *Semin Virol* 1994;5:133.

Monath TP, Nasidi A: Should yellow fever vaccine be included in the expanded program of immunization in Africa? A cost-effectiveness analysis for Nigeria. *Am J Trop Med Hyg* 1993;48:274–99.

Yellow fever: The global situation. *Bull WHO* 1992;70:667.

Chapter 248
Other Viral Hemorrhagic Fevers *Scott B. Halstead*

Viral hemorrhagic fevers are a loosely defined group of clinical syndromes in which hemorrhagic manifestations are either common or especially notable in severe illness. Both the etiologic agents and clinical features of the syndromes differ, but disseminated intravascular coagulopathy may be a common pathogenetic feature.

Etiology. Six of the viral hemorrhagic fevers are caused by *ar*thropod-*bo*rne (arboviruses) viruses (Table 248–1). Four are togaviruses of the family Flaviviridae, including Kyasanur Forest disease, Omsk, dengue (Chapter 246), and yellow fever (Chapter 247) viruses. Three are of the family Bunyaviridae, including Congo, Hantaan, and Rift Valley fever viruses. Four are of the family Arenaviridae, including Junin, Machupo, Guanarito, and Lassa viruses. Two are of the family Filoviridae, including Ebola and Marburg viruses. The Filoviridae are enveloped, filamentous RNA viruses, which are sometimes branched, unlike any other known virus.

Epidemiology and Clinical Manifestations. With some exceptions, the viruses causing viral hemorrhagic fevers are transmitted to humans via a nonhuman entity. The specific ecosystem required for viral survival determines the geographic distribution of disease. Although it is commonly thought that all viral hemorrhagic fevers are arthropod-borne, seven may be contracted from environmental contamination caused by animals or animal cells or from infected humans (see Table 248–1). Laboratory and hospital infections have occurred with many of these agents. Lassa fever and Argentine and Bolivian hemorrhagic fevers are reportedly milder in children than in adults.

CRIMEAN-CONGO HEMORRHAGIC FEVER. Sporadic human infection in Africa provided the original virus isolation. Natural foci are recognized in Bulgaria, western Crimea, and the Rostov-on-Don and Astrakhan regions; a somewhat similar disease occurs in Kazakhstan and Uzbekistan. Index cases were followed by nosocomial transmission in Pakistan and Afghanistan

TABLE 248–1. Viral Hemorrhage Fevers

Mode of Transmission	Disease	Virus
Tick borne	Crimean-Congo HF*	Congo
	Kyasanur Forest disease	Kyasanur Forest disease
	Omsk HF	Omsk
Mosquito borne†	Dengue HF	Dengue (four types)
	Rift Valley fever	Rift Valley fever
	Yellow fever	Yellow fever
Infected animals or materials to humans	Argentine HF	Junin
	Bolivian HF	Machupo
	Lassa fever*	Lassa
	Marburg disease*	Marburg
	Ebola HF*	Ebola
	Hemorrhagic fever with renal syndrome	Hantaan

*Patients may be contagious; nosocomial infections are common.
†Chikungunya virus is associated at low frequency with petechiae, petechial hemorrhages, and epistaxis. More severe hemorrhagic manifestations have been reported in some studies.
HF = hemorrhagic fever.

in 1976, in the Arabian Peninsula in 1983, and in South Africa in 1984. Recent outbreaks have been reported from Pakistan, Oman, and southern Russia. In the Russian Federation, the vectors are *Hyalomma marginatum* and *Hyalomma anatolicum*, which, along with hares and birds, may serve as viral reservoirs. Disease occurs from June to September, largely among farmers and dairy workers.

KYASANUR FOREST DISEASE. Human cases occur chiefly in adults in an area of Mysore State, India. The main vectors are two *Ixodidae* ticks, *Haemaphysalis turturis* and *Haemaphysalis spinigera*. Monkeys and forest rodents may be amplifying hosts. Laboratory infections are common.

OMSK HEMORRHAGIC FEVER. The disease occurs throughout south central Russia and northern Romania. Vectors may include *Dermacentor pictus* and *Dermacentor marginatus*, but direct transmission from moles and muskrats to humans seems well established. Human disease occurs in a spring-summer-autumn pattern, paralleling the activity of vectors. This infection occurs most frequently in persons with outdoor occupational exposure. Laboratory infections are common.

RIFT VALLEY FEVER. The virus causing Rift Valley fever is responsible for epizootics involving sheep, cattle, buffalo, certain antelopes, and rodents in North, Central, East, and South Africa. The virus is transmitted to domestic animals by *Culex theileri* and several *Aedes* species. Mosquitoes may serve as reservoirs by transovarial transmission. An epizootic in Egypt in 1977–78 was accompanied by thousands of human infections, principally among veterinarians, farmers, and farm laborers. Smaller outbreaks occurred in Senegal in 1987, Madagascar in 1990, and Saudi Arabia and Yemen in 2000–2001. Humans are most often infected during the slaughter or skinning of sick or dead animals. Laboratory infection is common.

ARGENTINE HEMORRHAGIC FEVER. Before introduction of vaccine, hundreds to thousands of cases occurred annually from April through July in the maize-producing area northwest of Buenos Aires that reaches to the eastern margin of the Province of Cordoba. Junin virus has been isolated from the rodents *Mus musculus*, *Akodon arenicola*, and *Calomys laucha laucha*. It infects migrant laborers who harvest the maize and who inhabit rodent-contaminated shelters.

BOLIVIAN HEMORRHAGIC FEVER. The recognized endemic area consists of the sparsely populated province of Beni in Amazonian Bolivia. Sporadic cases occur in farm families who raise maize, rice, yucca, and beans. In the town of San Joaquin, a disturbance in the domestic rodent ecosystem may have led to an outbreak of household infection caused by *Calomys callosus*, ordinarily a field rodent. Mortality rates are high in young children.

VENEZUELAN HEMORRHAGIC FEVER. In 1989, an outbreak of hemorrhagic illness occurred in the farming community of Guanarito, Venezuela, 200 miles south of Caracas. Subsequently, in 1990–1991, there were 104 cases reported with 26 deaths. Cotton rats (*Sigmodon alstoni*) and cane rats (*Zygodontomys brevicauda*) have been implicated as likely reservoirs.

LASSA FEVER. Lassa virus has an unusual potential for human-to-human spread and has resulted in many small epidemics in Nigeria, Sierra Leone, and Liberia. Medical workers in Africa and the United States have also contracted the disease. Patients with acute Lassa fever have been transported by international aircraft, necessitating extensive surveillance among passengers and crews. The virus is probably maintained in nature in a species of African peridomestic rodent, *Mastomys natalensis*. Rodent-to-rodent transmission and infection of humans probably operate via mechanisms established for other arenaviruses.

MARBURG DISEASE. Until recently, the world experience has been limited to 26 primary and five secondary cases in Germany and Yugoslavia in 1967, to small outbreaks in Zimbabwe in 1975, Kenya in 1980 and 1988, South Africa in 1983, and a large outbreak in Congo Republic in 1999. Transmission occurs by direct contact with tissues of the African green monkey, with infected blood, or with human semen. The reservoir and mode of transmission of the virus in nature are unknown.

EBOLA HEMORRHAGIC FEVER. Ebola virus was isolated in 1976 from a devastating epidemic involving small villages in northern Zaire and southern Sudan; smaller outbreaks have occurred subsequently. Outbreaks initially have been nosocomial. Attack rates have been highest in the birth–1 yr and 15–50 yr old age groups. The virus resembles Marburg virus. Ebola virus has been particularly active recently, with a well-known outbreak in Kikwit, Zaire, in 1995, followed recently by scattered outbreaks in Uganda and Central and West Africa. The virus has been recovered from chimpanzees, but the vertebrate reservoir and mode of transmission to humans are unknown. Reston virus, related to Ebola, has been recovered from Philippine monkeys and has caused subclinical infections in workers in monkey colonies in the United States.

HEMORRHAGIC FEVER WITH RENAL SYNDROME (HFRS). The endemic area of HFRS, also known as **epidemic hemorrhagic fever** and **Korean hemorrhagic fever**, includes Japan, Korea, Far Eastern Siberia, north and central China, European and Asian Russia, Scandinavia, Czechoslovakia, Romania, Bulgaria, Yugoslavia, and Greece. Although the incidence and severity of hemorrhagic manifestations and the mortality are lower in Europe than in northeastern Asia, the renal lesion is the same. Disease in Scandinavia, **nephropathia epidemica,** is caused by a different although antigenically related virus, Puumala virus, associated with the bank vole, *Clethrionomys glareolus*. Cases occur predominantly in the spring and summer. There appears to be no age factor in susceptibility, but because of occupational hazards, young adult men are most frequently attacked. Rodent plagues and evidence of rodent infestation have accompanied endemic and epidemic occurrences. Hantaan virus has been detected in lung tissue and excreta of *Apodemus agrarius coreae*. Antigenically related agents have been detected in laboratory rats and in urban rat populations around the world, including Prospect Hill virus in the wild rodent *Microtus pennsylvanicus* in North America and Sin Nombre virus in the deer mouse in southern and southwestern United States; these viruses are causes of hantavirus pulmonary syndrome (Chapter 250). Rodent-to-rodent and rodent-to-human transmission presumably occurs via the respiratory route.

Clinical Manifestations. Dengue hemorrhagic fever (Chapter 246) and yellow fever (Chapter 247) are more frequent causes of similar diseases in children in endemic areas.

CRIMEAN-CONGO HEMORRHAGIC FEVER. The incubation period of 3–12 days is followed by a febrile period of 5–12 days and a prolonged convalescence. Illness begins suddenly with fever, severe headache, myalgia, abdominal pain, anorexia, nausea, and vomiting. After 1–2 days, fever may subside until the patient experiences an erythematous facial or truncal flush and injected conjunctivae. A second febrile period of 2–6 days then develops, with a hemorrhagic enanthem on the soft palate and a fine petechial rash on the chest and abdomen. Less frequently, there are large areas of purpura and bleeding from gums, nose, intestine, lungs, or uterus. Hematuria and proteinuria are relatively rare. During the hemorrhagic stage, there is usually tachycardia with diminished heart sounds and occasionally hypotension. The liver is usually enlarged, but there is no icterus. In protracted cases, central nervous system signs may include delirium, somnolence, and progressive clouding of consciousness. Early in the disease, leukopenia with relative lymphocytosis, progressively worsening thrombocytopenia, and gradually increasing anemia occur. In convalescence there may be hearing and memory loss. The mortality rate is 2–50%.

KYASANUR FOREST DISEASE AND OMSK HEMORRHAGIC FEVER. After an incubation period of 3–8 days, both diseases begin with sudden onset of fever and headache. Kyasanur Forest disease is characterized by severe myalgia, prostration, and bronchiolar involvement; it often presents without hemorrhage but occasionally with severe gastrointestinal bleeding. In Omsk hemorrhagic fever, there is moderate epistaxis, hematemesis, and a hemorrhagic enanthem but no profuse hemorrhage; bronchopneumonia is common. In both diseases, severe leukopenia and thrombocytopenia, vascular dilatation, increased vascular permeability, gastrointestinal hemorrhages, and subserosal and interstitial petechial hemorrhages occur. Kyasanur Forest disease may be complicated by acute degeneration of renal tubules and focal liver damage. In many patients, recurrent febrile illness may follow an afebrile period of 7–15 days. This second phase takes the form of a meningoencephalitis.

RIFT VALLEY FEVER. Most infections have occurred in adults with disease similar to dengue fever (Chapter 246). Onset is acute, with fever, headache, prostration, myalgia, anorexia, nausea, vomiting, conjunctivitis, and lymphadenopathy. The fever lasts 3–6 days and is often biphasic. Convalescence is often prolonged. In the 1977–1978 outbreak, many patients died after showing signs that included purpura, epistaxis, hematemesis, and melena. At autopsy, there was extensive eosinophilic degeneration of the parenchymal cells of the liver.

ARGENTINE, VENEZUELAN, AND BOLIVIAN HEMORRHAGIC FEVER AND LASSA FEVER. The incubation period is commonly 7–14 days; the acute illness lasts for 2–4 wk. Clinical illnesses range from undifferentiated fever to the characteristic severe illness. Lassa fever is most often clinically severe in whites. Onset is usually gradual, with increasing fever, headache, diffuse myalgia, and anorexia. During the 1st wk, signs frequently include a sore throat, dysphagia, cough, oropharyngeal ulcers, nausea, vomiting, diarrhea, and pains in chest and abdomen. Pleuritic chest pain may persist for 2–3 wk. In Argentine and Bolivian hemorrhagic fevers, and less frequently in Lassa fever, a petechial enanthem appears on the soft palate 3–5 days after onset and at about the same time on the trunk. The tourniquet test may be positive. The clinical course of Venezuelan hemorrhagic fever has not been well described.

In 35–50% of all patients, these diseases may become severe, with persistent high temperature, increasing toxicity, swelling of face or neck, microscopic hematuria, and frank hemorrhages from the stomach, intestines, nose, gums, and uterus. A syndrome of hypovolemic shock is accompanied by pleural effusion and renal failure. Respiratory distress resulting from airway obstruction, pleural effusion, or congestive heart failure may occur. A total of 10–20% of patients experience late neurologic involvement characterized by intention tremor of the tongue and associated speech abnormalities. In severe cases, there may be intention tremors of the extremities, seizures, and delirium. The cerebrospinal fluid is normal. In Lassa fever, nerve deafness occurs in early convalescence in 25% of cases. Prolonged convalescence is accompanied by alopecia, and in Argentine and Bolivian hemorrhagic fevers by signs of autonomic nervous system lability, such as postural hypotension, spontaneous flushing or blanching of the skin, and intermittent diaphoresis.

Laboratory studies reveal marked leukopenia, mild to moderate thrombocytopenia, proteinuria, and, in Argentine hemorrhagic fever, moderate abnormalities in blood clotting, decreased fibrinogen, increased fibrinogen split products, and elevated serum transaminases. Pathologically, there is focal, often extensive eosinophilic necrosis of liver parenchyma, focal interstitial pneumonitis, focal necrosis of the distal and collecting tubules, and partial replacement of splenic follicles by amorphous eosinophilic material. Usually bleeding occurs by diapedesis with little inflammatory reaction. The mortality rate is 10–40%.

MARBURG DISEASE AND EBOLA HEMORRHAGIC FEVER. After an incubation period of 4–7 days, illness begins abruptly with severe frontal headache, malaise, drowsiness, lumbar myalgia, vomiting, nausea, and diarrhea. A maculopapular eruption begins 5–7 days later on the trunk and upper arms. It becomes generalized, often hemorrhagic, and exfoliates during convalescence. The exanthem is accompanied by a dark red enanthem on the hard palate, conjunctivitis, and scrotal or labial edema. Gastrointestinal hemorrhage occurs as the severity of illness increases. Late in the illness, the patient may become tearfully depressed with marked hyperalgesia to tactile stimuli. In fatal cases, patients become hypotensive, restless, and confused and lapse into coma. Convalescent patients may experience alopecia and have paresthesias of the back and trunk. There is a marked leukopenia with necrosis of granulocytes. Disseminated intravascular coagulation and thrombocytopenia are universal and correlate with severity of disease; there are moderate abnormalities in clotting proteins and elevated serum transaminases and amylase. The mortality rate of Marburg disease is 25% and of Ebola hemorrhagic fever, 50–90%.

HEMORRHAGIC FEVER WITH RENAL SYNDROME. In most cases, HFRS is characterized by fever, petechiae, mild hemorrhagic phenomena, and mild proteinuria, followed by relatively uneventful recovery. In 20% of recognized cases, the disease may progress through four rather distinct phases. The *febrile phase* is ushered in with fever, malaise, and facial and truncal flushing. It lasts 3–8 days and ends with thrombocytopenia, petechiae, and proteinuria. The *hypotensive phase* of 1–3 days follows defervescence. Loss of fluid from the intravascular compartment may result in marked hemoconcentration. Proteinuria and ecchymoses increase. The *oliguric phase*, usually 3–5 days in duration, is characterized by a low output of protein-rich urine, increasing nitrogen retention, nausea, vomiting, and dehydration. Confusion, extreme restlessness, and hypertension are common. The *diuretic phase*, which may last for days or weeks, usually initiates clinical improvement. The kidneys show little concentrating ability, and rapid loss of fluid may result in severe dehydration and shock. Potassium and sodium depletion may be severe. Fatal cases manifest abundant protein-rich retroperitoneal edema and marked hemorrhagic necrosis of the renal medulla. The mortality rate is 5–10%.

Diagnosis. Diagnosis depends on a high index of suspicion in endemic areas. In nonendemic areas, histories of recent travel, recent laboratory exposure, or exposure to an earlier case should evoke suspicion of a viral hemorrhagic fever.

In all viral hemorrhagic fevers, the viral agent circulates in the blood at least transiently during the early febrile stage. Togaviruses and bunyaviruses can be recovered from acute-phase serum by inoculation into tissue culture or living mosquitoes. Argentine, Bolivian, and Venezuelan hemorrhagic fever viruses can be isolated from acute-phase blood or throat washings by inoculation intracerebrally into guinea pigs, infant hamsters, or infant mice. Lassa virus may be isolated from acute-phase blood or throat washings by inoculation into tissue cultures. For Marburg disease and Ebola hemorrhagic fever, acute-phase throat washings, blood, and urine may be inoculated into tissue culture, guinea pigs, or monkeys. The viruses are readily identified by electron microscopy, with a filamentous structure differentiating them from all other known agents. Specific complement-fixing and immunofluorescent antibodies appear during convalescence. The virus of HFRS is recovered from acute-phase serum or urine by inoculation into tissue culture. A variety of antibody tests using viral subunits are becoming available. Serologic diagnosis depends on demonstrating seroconversion, or a fourfold or greater increase in immunoglobulin G antibody titer in acute and convalescent sera taken 3–4 wk apart. Viral RNA may also be detected in blood or tissues using reverse-transcriptase polymerase chain reactions.

Handling blood and other biologic specimens is hazardous and must be performed by specially trained personnel. Blood and autopsy specimens should be placed in tightly sealed metal containers, wrapped in absorbent material inside a sealed plastic bag, and shipped on dry ice to laboratories with biocontainment safety level 4 facilities. Even routine hematologic and biochemical tests should be done with extreme caution.

DIFFERENTIAL DIAGNOSIS. Mild cases of hemorrhagic fever may be confused with almost any self-limited systemic bacterial or viral infection. More severe cases may suggest typhoid fever; epidemic, murine, or scrub typhus; leptospirosis; or a rickettsial spotted fever, for which effective chemotherapeutic agents are available. Many of these may be acquired in geographic or ecologic locations endemic for a viral hemorrhagic fever.

Treatment. Ribavirin administered intravenously is effective in reducing mortality in Lassa fever and HFRS. Further information and advice about management, control measures, diagnosis, and collection of biohazardous specimens can be obtained from Centers for Disease Control and Prevention, National Center for Infectious Diseases, Special Pathogens Branch, Atlanta, Georgia 30333 (404-639-1115).

The principle involved in all these diseases, especially HFRS, is the reversal of dehydration, hemoconcentration, renal failure, and protein, electrolyte, or blood losses. The contribution of disseminated intravascular coagulopathy to the hemorrhagic manifestations is unknown, and the management of hemorrhage should be individualized. Transfusions of fresh blood and platelets are frequently given. Good results have been reported in a few patients after the administration of clotting factor concentrates. The efficacy of corticosteroids, ε-aminocaproic acid, pressor amines, or α-adrenergic blocking agents has not been established. Sedatives should be selected with regard to the possibility of kidney or liver damage. The successful management of HFRS may require renal dialysis.

Prevention. A live, attenuated vaccine (Candid-I) for Argentine hemorrhagic fever is highly efficacious. A form of inactivated mouse brain vaccine is reported to be effective in preventing Omsk hemorrhagic fever. Inactivated Rift Valley fever vaccines are widely used to protect domestic animals and laboratory workers. HFRS inactivated vaccine is licensed in Korea, and killed and live, attenuated vaccines are widely used in China. A vaccinia-vector glycoprotein vaccine provides protection against Lassa fever in monkeys. VEE replicon Ebola envelope glycoprotein and DNA-adenovirus Ebola glycoprotein vaccines have provided protection in experimental animals.

Prevention of mosquito-borne and tick-borne infections includes use of repellents, tight-fitting clothing that fully covers the extremities, careful examination of the skin after exposure with removal of any vectors found. Diseases transmitted from a rodent-infected environment can be prevented through methods of rodent control; elimination of refuse and breeding sites is particularly successful in urban and suburban areas.

Crimean-Congo hemorrhagic fever, Lassa fever, Marburg disease, and Ebola hemorrhagic fever may be transmitted in hospital settings. Patients should be isolated until they are virus-free or for 3 wk after illness. Patients' urine, sputum, blood, clothing, and bedding should be disinfected. Disposable syringes and needles should be used. Prompt and strict enforcement of barrier nursing may be lifesaving. The mortality rate among medical workers contracting these diseases is 50%. Recent studies show that a few entirely asymptomatic Ebola infections result in strong antibody production.

Centers for Disease Control and Prevention: Update: Management of patients with suspected viral hemorrhagic fever. *MMWR Morb Mortal Wkly Rep* 1995;44:475–79.
Centers for Disease Control and Prevention: Update: outbreak of Rift Valley fever—Saudi Arabia, August–November 2000. *MMWR Morb Mortal Wkly Rep* 2000;49:982–5.
Fisher-Hoch SP, Platt GS, Neild GH, et al: Pathophysiology of shock and hemorrhage in a fulminating viral infection (Ebola). *J Infect Dis* 1985;152:887–94.
Huggins JW, Hsiang CM, Cosgriff TM, et al: Prospective, double-blind, concurrent, placebo-controlled trial of intravenous ribavirin therapy of hemorrhagic fever with renal syndrome. *J Infect Dis* 1991;164:1119–27.
Isaacson M: Viral hemorrhagic fever hazards for travelers in Africa. *Clin Infect Dis* 2001;33:1707–12.
Leroy EM, Baize S, Volchkov VE, et al: Human asymptomatic Ebola infection and strong inflammatory response. *Lancet* 2000;355:2210–5.
McCormick JB, King IJ, Webb PA, et al: A case-control study of the clinical diagnosis and course of Lassa fever. *J Infect Dis* 1987;155:445–55.
McCormick JB, King IJ, Webb PA, et al: Lassa fever: Effective therapy with ribavirin. *N Engl J Med* 1986;314:20–6.
Pushko P, Bray M, Ludwig GV et al: Recombinant RNA replicons derived from attenuated Venezuelan equine encephalitis virus protect guinea pigs and mice from Ebola hemorrhagic fever virus. *Vaccine* 2000;19:142–53.
Sullivan NJ, Sanchez A, Rollin PE, et al: Development of a preventive vaccine for Ebola virus infection in primates. *Nature* 2000;408:605–9.

Chapter 249
Lymphocytic Choriomeningitis Virus
Hal B. Jenson

Etiology. Lymphocytic choriomeningitis virus was discovered in 1933 but not classified until the late 1960s as a member of the family Arenaviridae, which are negative-sense single-stranded RNA viruses. These enveloped viruses are round, oval, or pleomorphic, averaging 110–130 nm in diameter, with a range of 50–300 nm.

Rodents are the primary reservoir. A study in Baltimore found 9% prevalence among house mice. The virus establishes persistent infection in utero from maternal viremia that occurs in chronically infected rodents, including the common house mouse, *Mus musculus*, and pet hamsters. Their infected offspring do not develop an effective immune response and excrete virus continuously throughout life in saliva, nasal secretions, semen, milk, urine, and feces.

Epidemiology. The virus has been found in temperate regions of Europe and the Americas. The epidemiology of rodent infection is highly focal. Human cases are sporadic and are least common during the summer. Outbreaks have been reported after exposure to infected pet hamsters. A serologic survey of adults attending a sexually transmitted disease clinic in Baltimore found that 4.7% of adults had evidence of past infection.

Transmission from rodents to humans is by aerosol, by direct contact with rodents or contaminated food and fluids, and infrequently by rodent bites. There is no evidence of chronic infection in humans or of person-to-person transmission.

Pathogenesis. Viral infection of rodents is chronic and appears to lead to chronic glomerulonephritis. After inhalation of virus by humans, there is pulmonary and hilar lymph node viral replication with viremia within 48 hr. The liver, spleen, and lymph nodes are most affected and show lymphoid hyperplasia. The kidneys, heart, skeletal muscle, epididymis, and other organs may show mononuclear infiltration.

Clinical Manifestations. Infection in humans is inapparent in approximately one third of cases. Symptomatic cases may include a nonspecific flulike illness that is unrecognized as lymphocytic choriomeningitis virus infection, or may be characterized by lymphocytic meningitis or meningoencephalitis of varying severity. The classic course is a biphasic illness with usually 3–5 days of nonspecific illness with fever, malaise, myalgias, nausea and vomiting, sore throat and cough, lymphadenopathy, and occasionally a maculopapular rash. There is defervescence for 2–4 days followed by recurrence of fever and headache. In a small proportion of patients, signs of meningoencephalitis develop, sometimes without the prodromal symptoms. The cerebrospinal fluid pressure is elevated, and shows elevated protein (50–300 mg/dL) with several hundred lymphocytes per microliter. There may be papilledema. Transverse myelitis has also been reported. Extraneural manifestations include arthritis, parotitis, orchitis, rash, and myocarditis.

Leukopenia and thrombocytopenia are typical. There are no associated bleeding diatheses, as occur with other arenaviruses (Junin, Machupo, Guanarito, and Lassa) that are associated with viral hemorrhagic fevers (Chapter 248).

CONGENITAL INFECTION. Approximately 32 cases of congenital lymphocytic choriomeningitis virus infection have been reported. Only one half of mothers relate illnesses compatible with lymphocytic choriomeningitis virus during pregnancy, usually with only flulike symptoms but occasionally compatible with aseptic meningitis. Only one fourth of mothers have known exposure to rodents.

The affected offspring typically have chorioretinitis, encephalomalacia, microcephaly, hydrocephalus, punctate intracranial calcifications, and developmental delay. The neonatal presentation is similar to congenital cytomegalovirus and toxoplasmosis, but typically without hepatosplenomegaly, and should be considered if there is a history of maternal rodent exposure. Other ophthalmologic manifestations may include optic atrophy, microphthalmia, vitreitis, leukokoria, and cataracts. Unlike congenital cytomegalovirus infection, hearing loss has not been reported.

The cerebrospinal fluid shows a mild pleocytosis (<70 white blood cells/μL) and mildly elevated protein (average of 67 mg/dL; range of 9–477 mg/dL). CT and MRI reveal encephalomalacia, ventricular enlargement, and calcifications (by CT) adjacent to the lateral ventricles or in the periventricular white matter.

Diagnosis. The diagnosis is usually suspected by the clinical manifestations after exposure to rodents. Serologic tests using immunofluorescent antibody and enzyme-linked immunosorbent assay methods can confirm the clinical diagnosis. The virus can also be isolated from the blood and cerebrospinal fluid during the first week of illness.

Treatment. There is no specific treatment for lymphocytic choriomeningitis virus. Ribavirin is active against lymphocytic choriomeningitis virus and other arenaviruses in vitro. Supportive care includes headache control and intravenous hydration, if necessary.

Prognosis. The illness is usually self-limited without sequelae. Hydrocephalus, probably resulting from arachnoidal and ependymal inflammation, is a characteristic complication of congenital infection and has been reported rarely after lymphocytic choriomeningitis virus infection in older children and adults.

Prevention. Minimizing direct contact with the rodent hosts, especially excreta, is the best means of prevention. This precaution is especially important for pregnant women and should be emphasized. The prevalence of lymphocytic choriomeningitis virus in laboratory animals and household pets, primarily hamsters, is variable and depends on the breeding and handling conditions. Routine monitoring of rodents for infection is not uniformly practiced or mandated.

Biggar RJ, Woodall JP, Walter PD, et al: Lymphocytic choriomeningitis outbreak associated with pet hamsters. Fifty-seven cases from New York State. *JAMA* 1975;232:494–500.

Childs J, Glass G, Korch G, et al: Lymphocytic choriomeningitis virus infection and house mouse (*Mus musculus*) distribution in urban Baltimore. *Am J Trop Med* 1992;47:27–34.

Childs JE, Glass GE, Ksiazek TG, et al: Human-rodent contact and infection with lymphocytic choriomeningitis and Seoul viruses in an inner-city population. *Am J Trop Med Hyg* 1991;44:117–21.

Enders G, Barho-Gobel M, Lohler J, et al: Congenital lymphocytic choriomeningitis virus infection: An underdiagnosed disease. *Pediatr Infect Dis J* 1999;18:652–5.

Farmer TW, Janeway CA: Infection with the virus of lymphocytic choriomeningitis. *Medicine (Baltimore)* 1942;21:1–63.

Larsen PD, Chartrand SA, Tomashek KM, et al: Hydrocephalus complicating lymphocytic choriomeningitis virus infection. *Pediatr Infect Dis J* 1993;12:528–31.

Mets MB, Barton LL, Khan AS, et al: Lymphocytic choriomeningitis virus: An underdiagnosed cause of congenital chorioretinitis. *Am J Ophthalmol* 2000;130: 209–15.

Wright R, Johnson D, Neumann M, et al: Congenital lymphocytic choriomeningitis virus syndrome. A disease that mimics congenital toxoplasmosis or cytomegalovirus infection. *Pediatrics* 1997;100:E9.

Chapter 250

Hantaviruses *Scott B. Halstead*

In June 1993, a newly recognized hantavirus was identified as the etiologic agent of an outbreak of severe respiratory illness in the southwestern United States. Now called the **hantavirus pulmonary syndrome (HPS)**, hundreds of cases caused by multiple closely related hantaviruses have been identified from the Western United States, with sporadic cases reported from Eastern United States, Canada, and several countries in South America. HPS is characterized by a febrile prodrome followed by the rapid onset of noncardiogenic pulmonary edema and hypotension or shock. More than half of patients diagnosed with HPS have died.

Etiology. Hantaviruses are a genus in the family Bunyaviridae, which are lipid-enveloped viruses with a negative-stranded RNA genome composed of three unique segments. Several pathogenic viruses that have been recognized within the genus include **Hantaan virus,** which causes the most severe form of hemorrhagic fever with renal syndrome (HFRS) seen primarily in mainland Asia; **Dobrava virus,** which causes the most severe form of HFRS seen primarily in the Balkans; **Puumala virus,** which causes a milder form of HFRS with a high proportion of subclinical infections and is prevalent in northern Europe; and **Seoul virus,** which results in moderate HFRS and is transmitted predominantly in Asia by urban rats or worldwide by laboratory rats. **Prospect Hill virus,** a Hantavirus that is widely disseminated in U.S. meadow voles, is not known to cause human disease.

Cases of HPS identified in 1993 were associated with **Sin Nombre virus,** isolated from deer mice, *Peromyscus maniculatus,* in New Mexico. Multiple HPS agents isolated to date belong to a single genetic group of hantaviruses and are associated with rodents of the family *Muridae,* subfamily *Sigmodontinae.* These rodent species are restricted to the Americas, suggesting that HPS may be a Western Hemisphere disease.

Epidemiology. Persons acquiring HPS generally have a history of recent outdoor exposure or live in an area with large populations of deer mice. Clusters of cases have occurred among individuals who have cleaned houses that were rodent infested. *P. maniculatus* is one of the most common North American mammals and, where found, is frequently the dominant member of the rodent community. About half of cases occur between the months of May and July. Patients are almost exclusively from 12–70 yr of age; 60% of patients are 20–39 yr of age. Rare cases are reported in children <12 yr of age. Two thirds of patients are male, probably reflecting greater outdoor activities. It is not known whether almost complete absence of disease in young children is a reflection of innate resistance or simply lack of exposure. Evidence of human transmission has been obtained in Argentine outbreaks.

Hantaviruses do not cause apparent illness in their reservoir hosts, which remain asymptomatically infected for life. Infected rodents shed virus in saliva, urine, and feces for many weeks, but the duration of shedding and the period of maximum infectivity are unknown. The presence of infectious virus in saliva, the sensitivity of these animals to parenteral inoculation with hantaviruses, and field observations of infected rodents indicate that biting is important for rodent-to-rodent transmission. Aerosols from infective saliva or excreta of rodents are implicated in the transmission of hantaviruses to humans. Persons visiting animal care areas housing infected rodents have been infected after exposure for as little as 5 min. It is possible that hantaviruses are spread through contaminated food and breaks in skin or mucous membranes; transmission to humans has occurred by rodent bites. Person-to-person transmission is distinctly uncommon but has been documented in Argentina.

Pathogenesis. HPS is characterized by sudden and catastrophic pulmonary edema, resulting in anoxia and acute heart failure. The virus is detected in pulmonary capillaries, suggesting that pulmonary edema is the direct consequence of virus-induced capillary damage. Disease severity is predicted by level of acute phase viremia titer.

Clinical Manifestations. HPS is characterized by a prodrome and a cardiopulmonary phase. The mean duration after the onset of prodromal symptoms to hospitalization is 5.4 days. The mean duration of symptoms to death is 8 days (median of 7 days; range of 2–16 days). The most common prodromal symptoms are fever and myalgia (100%); cough or dyspnea (76%); gastrointestinal symptoms, including vomiting, diarrhea, and midabdominal pain (76%); and headache (71%). The cardiopulmonary phase is heralded by progressive cough and shortness of breath. The most common initial physical findings are tachypnea (100%), tachycardia (94%), and hypotension (50%). Rapidly progressive acute pulmonary edema, anoxemia, and shock develop in most severely ill patients. The clinical course of the illness in patients who die is characterized by pulmonary edema accompanied by severe hypotension, frequently terminating in sinus bradycardia, electromechanical dissociation, ventricular tachycardia, or fibrillation. Hypotension may be progressive even with adequate oxygenation.

Diagnosis. The diagnosis of HPS should be considered in a previously healthy patient presenting with a febrile prodrome and acute respiratory distress. Occurrence of thrombocytopenia with the febrile prodrome and outdoor exposure in the spring and summer months are strongly suggestive of HPS. Specific diagnosis of HPS is made by serologic tests that detect hantavirus immunoglobulin M antibodies. Hantavirus antigen can be detected in tissue by immunohistochemistry and amplification of hantavirus nucleotide sequences detected by reverse transcriptase polymerase chain reaction. The state health department or the Centers for Disease Control and Prevention should be consulted to assist in diagnosis, epidemiologic investigations, and outbreak control.

LABORATORY FINDINGS. Laboratory findings include leukocytosis (median of 26,000 cells/μL), an increased hematocrit (resulting from hemoconcentration), thrombocytopenia (median of 64,000/μL), prolonged prothrombin and partial thromboplastin times, elevated serum lactate dehydrogenase concentration, decreased serum protein concentrations, and proteinuria.

DIFFERENTIAL DIAGNOSIS. The differential diagnosis includes adult respiratory distress syndrome, pneumonic plague, psittacosis, severe mycoplasmal pneumonia, influenza, leptospirosis, inhalation anthrax, rickettsial infections, pulmonary tularemia, atypical bacterial and viral pneumoniae, legionellosis, meningococcemia, and other sepsis syndromes.

Treatment. Management of patients with hantavirus infection requires maintenance of adequate oxygenation and careful monitoring and support of cardiovascular function. The pathophysiology of HPS resembles that of dengue shock syndrome (Chapter 246). Pressor or inotropic agents should be administered in combination with judicious volume replacement to treat symptomatic hypotension or shock while avoiding exacerbating the pulmonary edema. Intravenous ribavirin, which is lifesaving if given early in the course of HFRS, has been shown to be of no value in HPS.

Further information and advice about management, control measures, diagnosis, and collection of biohazardous specimens can be obtained from Centers for Disease Control and Prevention, National Center for Infectious Diseases, Special Pathogens Branch, Atlanta, Georgia 30333 (404-639-1115).

Prognosis. Patient fatality rates are about 50%. Severe abnormalities in hematocrit, white blood cell count, lactate dehydrogenase, and partial thromboplastin time predict mortality with high specificity and sensitivity.

Prevention. Avoiding contact with rodents is the only preventive strategy. Rodent control in and around the home is important. Biosafety level 2 facilities and practices are recommended for laboratory handling of blood, body fluids, and tissues from suspect patients or rodents because the virus may be aerosolized. Barrier nursing is advised.

Armstrong LR, Bryan RT, Sarisky J, et al: Mild hantaviral disease caused by Sin Nombre virus in a four-year-old-child. *Pediatr Infect Dis J* 1995;12:1108–10.

Bryan RT, Doyle TJ, Moolenaar RL, et al: Hantavirus pulmonary syndrome in children. *Semin Pediatr Infect Dis* 1997;8:44–9.

Centers for Disease Control and Prevention: Hantavirus pulmonary syndrome: United States, 1995 and 1996. *MMWR Morb Mortal Wkly Rep* 1996;45:291–5.

Centers for Disease Control and Prevention: Laboratory management of agents associated with hantavirus pulmonary syndrome: Interim biosafety guidelines. *MMWR Morb Mortal Wkly Rep* 1994;43(RR-7):1–7.

Childs JE, Ksiazek TG, Spiropoulou CF, et al: Serologic and genetic identification of Peromyscus maniculatus as the primary rodent reservoir for a new hantavirus in the southwestern United States. *J Infect Dis* 1994;169:1271–80.

Hughes JM, Peters CJ, Cohen ML, et al: Hantavirus pulmonary syndrome. An emerging infectious disease. *Science* 1993;262:850–1.

Khan AS, Khabbaz RF, Armstrong LR, et al: Hantavirus pulmonary syndrome: The first 100 U.S. cases. *J Infect Dis* 1996;173:1297–303.

Peters CJ, Simpson GL, Levy H: Spectrum of hantavirus infection: Hemorrhagic fever with renal syndrome and hantavirus pulmonary syndrome. *Annu Rev Med* 1999;50:531–45.

Terajima M, Hendershot JD 3rd, Kariwa H, et al: High levels of viremia in patients with the Hantavirus pulmonary syndrome. *J Infect Dis* 1999;180:2030–4.

Chapter 251
Rabies *William G. Adams*

Human rabies is a viral infection of the central nervous system usually transmitted by contamination of a wound with saliva from a rabid animal. Rabies transmission can be prevented with postexposure prophylaxis; however, the disease is virtually 100% fatal once symptoms develop.

Etiology. Rabies virus is a member of the family Rhabdoviridae. Rabies and several closely related rabies-like viruses are classified in the genus *Lyssavirus*. Rabies-related viruses are found in Europe and Africa and are relatively rare. The viral particles resemble striated bullets, 70–85 nm in diameter and 130–380 nm in length. They have a lipid-containing envelope with a helical nucleocapsid containing one molecule of the negative-sense single-stranded RNA genome. The envelope contains a glycoprotein that elicits neutralizing antibodies and acts as a protective antigen in animal experiments.

Epidemiology. Rabies infection occurs in warm-blooded animals throughout the world. In the United States, rabies occurs principally in skunks, raccoons, foxes, and bats. Skunks are the principal vectors in the Midwest, Southwest, and California, with distinct northern and southern virus strains. Raccoon rabies is found throughout the eastern United States. Fox rabies is found in Alaska and the northeastern United States, with a separate strain in the Southwest. Bat rabies is found in practically every state. In Central and South America, dogs are the usual source of exposure. Vampire bats, which bite cattle, are an important part of the cycle of rabies in Latin America. Europe has had an epizootic of fox rabies. In Asia and Africa, the principal problem is the rabid dog.

Monoclonal antibody analysis and reverse transcriptase(RT) followed by polymerase chain reaction (PCR) of rabies virus strains has revealed considerable antigenic variation of the virus. The result has been the identification of variant strains, called **rabies-related viruses**, and antigenic differences among true rabies viruses that correlate with host species or geographic location. Strains isolated from cattle rabies in South America resemble bat strains, confirming the transmission of virus from the vampire bat to the cow.

The existence of rabies-free land areas permits health authorities in certain locations to omit postexposure prophylaxis of humans after most dog bites on the grounds that terrestrial rabies has been unknown there for years. The continent of Australia and many islands, including those of the United Kingdom and Hawaii, are free of rabies.

Human rabies is a rare disease in the United States and western Europe, where domestic animals are routinely vaccinated and animal control efforts have been successful. Most human cases in these areas are imported from other countries or follow bat exposure. Rabies continues to be a major public health problem in areas where dogs are not controlled. Human rabies occurs routinely in India, Southeast Asia, and Africa. The annual global incidence of human rabies is unknown, but is likely between 40,000–100,000 cases. Children are at particularly high risk for rabies exposure and infection because of their shorter stature, fearlessness of animals, and inability to protect themselves.

TRANSMISSION. In animals, as in humans, rabies produces encephalitis as the principal symptom followed by spread of virus down nerves away from the brain. It multiplies in many organs, but those most important to transmission are the salivary glands. However, not all rabid animals have virus in the saliva, and even when it is present, the quantity is variable. The incubation period for rabies in infected dogs is variable, from 14–180 days. However, viral shedding in saliva of dogs occurs for only 3–6 days before visible symptoms begin. Rabies transmission to humans from dogs that appeared normal for ≥10 days after a biting incident has not been reported. The variability of virus in saliva explains the low transmissibility; less than half of untreated bites by proven rabid animals result in rabies.

Transmission of rabies can also occur from nonbite exposures. Scratches by the claws of rabid animals are dangerous because animals lick their claws. Saliva applied to a mucosal surface such as the conjunctiva may be infectious. Furthermore, several cases of human rabies in the United States appear to have been caused by bats without any visible sign of direct contact. Bat excreta contain enough rabies virus to pose a danger of rabies to those who enter infested caves and inhale aerosols created by bats or with insignificant physical contact. Aerosols of rabies virus inadvertently produced in laboratories are dangerous to laboratory workers. Transmission of rabies by corneal transplant from patients with undiagnosed rabies encephalitis to healthy recipients has been recorded with sufficient frequency to warrant exclusion of donors dead from unexplained neurologic disease. Human-to-human transmission is theoretically possible but is poorly documented and occurs rarely, if at all.

Pathogenesis. The means by which rabies virus travels from the wound to the brain are only partially understood. Because the virus attaches to and penetrates cells rapidly in vitro, it is unlikely that it remains dormant in the wound for long periods of time.

Although the virus ascends along axons from the distal extremities to the spinal cord, the speed of spread (3 mm/hr) is far too rapid to account for the long incubation period of the disease.

After inoculation with contaminated saliva from a bite or scratch, the virus infects and multiplies in striated muscle cells, to which it attaches via several receptors, probably including the nicotinic acetylcholine receptor. It is hypothesized that antibody, interferon, and other host factors act on the virus as it leaves striated muscle; if these factors are insufficiently protective, virus eventually attaches to the nerve. At this stage, the development of rabies may be inevitable. The possibility that the virus must overcome another barrier in passing from the first infected neuron to other neurons is indicated by electron microscopic studies of the brain, which demonstrate contiguous viral passage from cell to cell.

Rabies virus causes neuronal destruction in the brainstem and medulla. The cerebral cortex is usually normal in the absence of prolonged anoxia before death. The hippocampus, thalamus, and basal ganglia often show neuronal destruction and glial infiltrates. The most severe disease is evident in the pons and the floor of the fourth ventricle. The inspiratory muscle spasms that result in the striking symptom of hydrophobia may be due to destruction of brainstem neurons inhibitory to the neurons of the nucleus ambiguus, which control inspiration. Hydrophobia does not occur in other diseases because only rabies combines brainstem encephalitis with an intact cortex and maintenance of consciousness.

The **Negri body**, long the pathologic hallmark of rabies, is a cytoplasmic inclusion found in neurons; it consists of clumped viral nucleocapsid. The absence of Negri bodies does not exclude rabies; fluorescent antibody stains of brain sections or smears may be positive in their absence.

Clinical Manifestations. The incubation period of rabies in humans is extremely variable. Exceptionally long incubation periods have been described, including a 7-yr incubation period that was confirmed by strain identification. Conversely, an incubation period of as little as 9 days has followed severe exposure. Usually, the incubation period is 20–180 days, with the peak at 30–60 days. The incubation period tends to be shorter in children.

There is usually a prodromal phase of rabies lasting 2–10 days. Pain, pruritus, or paresthesia at the site of the wound is common. Nonspecific symptoms such as fever, malaise, headache, anorexia, and vomiting are often seen. The patient may also have apprehension, anxiety, agitation, or depression.

The illness then enters an acute neurologic phase, of either the **furious variety** or **paralytic variety**, which lasts 2–21 days. In the former, **hydrophobia** is a pathognomonic sign. Attempts to swallow liquids, including saliva, result in aspiration into the trachea. Hydrophobia appears to be an exaggerated respiratory tract protective reflex, perhaps mediated by neuronal dysfunction in the brainstem. Eventually, a psychological component exacerbates the spasms, and even the sight of water evokes terror. **Aerophobia** may be present and is considered by some also to be pathognomonic of rabies. Aerophobia is elicited by fanning a current of air across the face, which causes violent spasms of the pharyngeal and neck muscles.

The neurologic picture in the typical case may consist of bursts of hyperactivity, disorientation, and bizarre combative behavior, alternating with periods of lucidity. During the lucid periods, the patient may be aware of what is happening and may be able to articulate his or her fears. The facial expression is one of grim hopelessness. Patients may also complain of pharyngeal pain, difficulty in swallowing, and hoarseness. Seizures are common, perhaps on the basis of hypoxia compounded by hyperventilation.

In about 20% of patients, an ascending symmetric paralysis with flaccidity and decreased tendon reflexes dominates the entire acute phase. This course is particularly common after bat bites. In the remainder of patients, paralysis develops toward the end of the acute neurologic phase.

Some rabid patients experience meningism or even opisthotonos. The cerebrospinal fluid may be normal or may reflect meningeal irritation, with varying elevations of cells (predominantly lymphocytes) and protein. The peripheral white blood cell count often shows a polymorphonuclear leukocytosis.

If the patient does not die of cardiorespiratory arrest during the acute stage, coma ensues. With modern intensive care, life may be prolonged, but numerous complications occur during this stage. Most significant is myocarditis, manifested by hypotension and arrhythmias. Rabies virus has been recovered from the heart, which shows inflammation at autopsy. Also prominent is pituitary dysfunction expressed clinically as either diabetes insipidus or inappropriate secretion of antidiuretic hormone.

Humans infected with rabies are infectious for about 1 wk before onset of symptoms and can continue to be infectious for up to 5 wk afterward.

Diagnosis. Rabies should be suspected in patients with a history of an animal bite or proximity to bats, especially involving wounds complicated by paresthesia or dysesthesia surrounding the wound site, central nervous system changes, hydrophobia, or aerophobia.

Laboratory diagnosis is possible before death. The virus may be demonstrated by fluorescent antibody stain or reverse-transcriptase polymerase chain reaction (RT-PCR) of smears of corneal epithelial cells or sections of skin from the neck at the hairline. These are sensitive tests because virus migrates down the nerves from the brain, and both the cornea and hair follicles are richly innervated. Virus can also be isolated or identified in saliva. Autopsy examination of the brains of patients with fatal encephalitis should include fluorescent antibody test or RT-PCR for rabies.

Serologic diagnosis is also possible if the patient survives beyond the acute period. Neutralizing antibodies develop eventually in both serum and cerebrospinal fluid and rapidly increase to extremely high levels, usually more than 100 IU/mL. Vaccination, even with potent vaccine, is unlikely to raise titers above 20 IU/mL.

DIFFERENTIAL DIAGNOSIS. Any disease in which there is encephalitis may occasionally cause mental status changes and confusion, such as the encephalitides caused by arboviruses, enteroviruses, and herpes simplex. Other diagnoses can usually be set aside with signs of brainstem involvement in a patient whose sensorium is basically clear and who has no signs of a space-occupying lesion. Paralytic rabies may be misdiagnosed as Guillain-Barré syndrome, poliomyelitis, or postrabies vaccine encephalomyelitis. Careful neurologic examination and analysis of the cerebrospinal fluid distinguish these diagnoses. The

spasms of tetanus may represent a diagnostic dilemma, but trismus is not seen in rabies, and hydrophobia is not seen in tetanus. Botulism (wound or ingestion) causes paralysis, but the absence of sensorineural changes excludes rabies. Perhaps the most confusing differential problem is hysteria in an individual who thinks that he or she has rabies. Normal blood gases and the absence of variation in bizarre behavior suggest pseudorabies.

Treatment. There is no specific treatment available. Intensive supportive care is often required but is insufficient for recovery. Therapies with antiviral agents, interferon, and high-dose rabies immunoglobulin have only prolonged the clinical course. It is doubtful that any treatment can affect mortality once the virus has already spread to the brain.

Prognosis. Recovery from symptomatic rabies in humans is extremely rare. Several persons in the United States have survived rabies infection, but all appear to have been partially immunized before exposure.

Prevention. Primary prevention of rabies infection includes avoiding contact with potentially rabid animals and vaccination of all domestic animals. Special efforts should be made to teach children to avoid wild animals, stray animals, and animals with unusual behavior.

LOCAL WOUND CARE. Regardless of the decision whether to provide immunoprophylaxis, local wound management after exposure to a potentially rabid animal is important. All postexposure treatment begins with immediate thorough cleansing of all wounds with soap and water. Vigorous cleansing has been shown to effectively prevent infection in countries with endemic rabies. Wounds should be irrigated for at least 10 min, preferably with a virucidal agent such as povidone-iodine. Catheters should be used for irrigation of puncture wounds. If the mechanical trauma of the local treatment is painful, local anesthetics (e.g., lidocaine) may be used to infiltrate the area without adding risk.

EVALUATION OF EXPOSURES. Human exposure to a potentially rabid animal is considered to be present if the person (1) is bitten or scratched (with penetration of skin) by a potentially rabid animal or (2) has contamination of a scratch, abrasion, mucous membranes, or open wound with potentially infectious material such as saliva or central nervous system tissue from a potentially rabid animal. The evaluation of human exposures to potentially rabid animals can be complex and is often compounded by a high degree of anxiety. The decision to give postexposure rabies prophylaxis should be based on several factors (Table 251–1). The local epidemiology of rabies should be considered. The type of animal is important because some animals such as raccoons, skunks, bats, woodchucks, and unvaccinated domestic animals are more likely to be infected with

TABLE 251–1. **Rabies Postexposure Prophylaxis Guide for the United States**

Animal	Evaluation and Disposition of Animal	Postexposure Prophylaxis Recommendations
Dogs, cats, ferrets	Healthy and available for 10-day observation	Should not begin prophylaxis unless signs of rabies develop in animal*
	Rabid or suspected rabid	Immediately vaccinate
	Unknown (e.g., escaped)	Consult public health officials
Skunks, racoons, foxes, most other carnivores; bats	Regarded as rabid unless animal proven negative by laboratory tests†	Consider immediate vaccination
Livestock, small rodents, lagomorphs (rabbits and hares), large rodents (woodchucks and beavers), other mammals	Consider individually	Consult public health officials; bites of squirrels, hamsters, guinea pigs, gerbils, chipmunks, rats, mice, other small rodents, rabbits, and hares almost never require antirabies prophylaxis

Modified from Centers for Disease Control: Human rabies prevention—United States, 1999. Recommendations of the Advisory Committee on Immunization Practices (ACIP). MMWR 1999;48(RR-1):1–21.
During the 10-day holding period, begin postexposure prophylaxis with human rabies immune globulin (HRIG) and rabies vaccine (HDCV, PCEC, or RVA) at first sign of rabies in a dog or cat that has bitten someone. If the animal exhibits clinical signs of rabies, it should be euthanized immediately and tested.
†The animal should be euthanized and tested as soon as possible. Holding for observation is not recommended. Discontinue vaccine if immunofluorescence test results of the animal are negative.

rabies virus in certain areas than other animals, such as vaccinated dogs and cats or small wild animals such as squirrels or rodents. The availability of the responsible animal for testing or quarantine is an important consideration and can determine whether or not postexposure prophylaxis is necessary. The circumstances around the exposure, namely whether the attack was provoked or unprovoked, can be considered, especially in situations involving animals rarely infected with rabies virus such as squirrels or mice.

Postexposure rabies prophylaxis is indicated for all persons with a history of a bat bite, scratch, or mucous membrane exposure unless the bat is available for testing or is negative for evidence of rabies. Postexposure prophylaxis is appropriate after bat exposure even in the absence of known direct contact, when there is a reasonable probability that such contact occurred, such as when a sleeping person awakes to find a bat in the room or when an adult witnesses a bat in the room with a previously unattended child, mentally disabled person, or intoxicated person.

Evaluation of secondary or indirect exposure can be more difficult than the evaluation of the direct exposures outlined previously. Secondary contact is typically considered to occur when a domestic animal has had direct contact with a potentially rabid animal and a human then handles or is licked by the domestic animal. The factors that should be considered include the interval since the pet's exposure, the ambient temperature, and whether the domestic animal's contact with the human involved an open wound or mucous membranes.

POSTEXPOSURE PROPHYLAXIS. If rabies prophylaxis is to be given after exposure, prevention depends on three complementary means of reducing the risk. Local wound care is designed to remove or kill the virus by mechanical and virucidal action. Passive immunization with human rabies immunoglobulin (HRIG) then provides immediate blockage of attachment of virus to the nerve endings. However, passive antibody ultimately disappears and must be replaced by the active immune response induced by vaccine. The vaccine must not only produce a primary antibody response but also overcome the depressive effect of passive antibody on the immune response. When given according to currently recommended protocols, no failure of combined HRIG and approved rabies vaccine has been reported in the United States.

Passive Immunization. Passive antibody is available as HRIG; the two available formulations are considered equivalent. The dose for HRIG is 20 IU/kg with as much as possible of the full dose of HRIG thoroughly infiltrated into and around the wounds. Any remaining volume should be administered intramuscularly at a site distant from vaccine inoculation. In some countries, rabies antibody is in the form of purified equine immunoglobulin, which is associated with serum sickness reactions in about 1% of recipients. Anaphylaxis is a rare possibility with the equine product, but tests for hypersensitivity should be carried out in the usual manner (consult package insert). The dose for equine immunoglobulin is 40 IU/kg delivered in the same manner as for HRIG.

HRIG is effective if given within 7 days of the bite and ideally should be given with rabies vaccine on the day of the exposure. If vaccine was started previously, passive immunization should not be given after 7 days have elapsed. Corticosteroids should be avoided if possible in the treatment of reactions because they cause activation of rabies virus in experimental animals.

Active Immunization. Early rabies vaccines were prepared in the central nervous systems of animals. Their antigenicity was poor, and multiple injections were required. As a result, postvaccination encephalitis was a frequent problem. Animal nerve tissue vaccines are still in use in many places in the world, in particular, suckling mouse brain vaccine, which gives fewer neurologic reactions than sheep brain vaccines because it contains less myelin.

The major advance in rabies vaccine was the development of cell culture technology, which permitted the production of concentrated vaccines with high antigenic potency and low contamination with cellular proteins. Thus, immunogenicity was improved, allowing reduced numbers of doses and adverse reactions. Two cell culture rabies vaccines are available in the United States: **human diploid cell vaccine (HDCV)** and **purified chick embryo cell culture vaccine (PCECV)**. Outside the United States, vaccines produced in monkey kidney, chick embryo, duck embryo, and other cultured cells are also available.

For previously unvaccinated persons, the schedule for postexposure vaccination is five doses given intramuscularly in the deltoid on days 0, 3, 7, 14, and 28. The dose is not reduced for children, although the anterolateral thigh can be used instead of the deltoid if necessary. Administration of rabies vaccine in the gluteus muscle has been associated with vaccine failure and is to be avoided. Immune responses to the postexposure schedule are regularly seen by the 14th day. However, for effective postexposure prophylaxis to rabies, it is mandatory to provide passive as well as active immunization.

For previously fully vaccinated persons after rabies exposure, two vaccine doses are given at an interval of 3 days. HRIG is not given.

Determination of postvaccination antibody titers is not needed unless the patient is immunosuppressed or is receiving antimalarial therapy, which may suppress the response.

Adverse reaction rates to cell culture vaccines have been low, and neurologic reactions have been rare because no nerve tissue is present in the cell cultures used to grow the virus. Allergic reactions occur in less than 0.1% of cases after primary vaccination with HDCV, and systemic symptoms such as malaise and fever occur in only 5–15%. Administration of boosters is associated with an allergic reaction rate of up to 6%. Individuals at continued risk of rabies exposure should have antibody titers determined every 2 yr, and if inadequate, should be given a booster dose. PCECV may be useful in those who have reactions to HDCV. Although no controlled study has been done, the efficacy of rabies vaccination is evidently high, judging from the known incidence of disease after untreated bites by infected animals (approximately 15%) and the paucity of vaccine failures. When seen, vaccine failure has usually followed incomplete immunizations schedules or incorrect use of HRIG.

PREEXPOSURE PROPHYLAXIS. Persons at risk for rabies, such as veterinarians, laboratory workers, spelunkers, and travelers to rabies-enzootic areas, should be immunized before exposure. For preexposure immunization, a three-dose vaccination schedule is followed, consisting of intramuscular doses (1.0 mL) given on days 0, 7, and 21 or 28.

Baer GM (editor): *The Natural History of Rabies,* 2nd ed. Boca Raton, FL, CRC Press, 1991.

Centers for Disease Control and Prevention: Compendium of animal rabies prevention and control, 2001. National Association of State Public Health Veterinarians, Inc. *MMWR* 2001;50(RR-8):1–9.

Centers for Disease Control and Prevention: Human rabies prevention-United States, 1999. Recommendations of the Advisory Committee on Immunization Practices (ACIP). *MMWR* 1999;48(RR-1):1–21.

Centers for Disease Control and Prevention rabies website: *http://www.cdc.gov/nci-dod/dvrd/rabies/.*

Fishbein DB, Robinson LE: Rabies. *N Engl J Med* 1993;329:1632–8.

Houff SA, Burton RC, Wilson RW, et al: Human-to-human transmission of rabies virus by corneal transplant. *N Engl J Med* 1979;300:603–4.

Krebs JW, Rupprecht CE, Childs JE: Rabies surveillance in the United States during 1999. *J Am Vet Med Assoc* 2000;217:1799–811.

Lontai I: The current state of rabies prevention in Europe. *Vaccine* 1997;15: S16–9.

Sureau P, Rollin P, Wiktor TJ: Epidemiologic analysis of antigenic variations of street rabies virus: Detection by monoclonal antibodies. *Am J Epidemiol* 1983; 117:605–9.

Tsiang H: Pathophysiology of rabies virus infection of the nervous system. *Adv Virus Res* 1993;42:375–412.

Chapter 252
Polyomaviruses *Hal B. Jenson*

The polyomaviruses, which with the papillomaviruses constitute the Papovaviridae family, are small, nonenveloped, double-stranded circular DNA viruses. The two polyomaviruses that infect humans, JC virus and BK virus, share 75% genome homology but are antigenically distinct. Both viruses are tropic for renal epithelium; JC virus also infects brain oligodendrocytes and is the etiologic agent of **progressive multifocal leukoencephalopathy (PML)**, a fatal demyelinating disease. Several million persons in the United States were exposed to simian virus 40, an oncogenic polyomavirus of Asian macaques, from contaminated inactivated poliovirus vaccines administered between 1955 and 1963, without recognized sequelae and with no demonstrable increased risk of cancer.

Approximately one half of children in the United States are infected with BK virus by 3–4 yr of age and with JC virus by 10–14 yr of age, and approximately 60–80% of adults are seropositive for one or both viruses. Infection persists throughout life, with the viruses remaining latent in renal epithelium, oligodendrocytes, and peripheral blood lymphocytes. Reactivation and viruria occur with increased frequency with advancing age and are more common in immunocompromised persons. BK and JC viruria, as detected by polymerase chain reaction (PCR), occurs in 2.6% and 13.2%, respectively, of persons <30 yr of age and in approximately 9% and 50%, respectively, of persons >60 yr of age.

Reactivation of BK virus and JC virus with asymptomatic viruria occurs in 10–50% of bone marrow transplant patients and in 20% of renal transplant patients. The direct cytopathic effect of reactivated BK virus on donor ureter has caused localized ureteral ulceration and ureteral stenosis in a few renal transplant patients. BK virus has also been associated with prolonged hemorrhagic cystitis in bone marrow transplant recipients.

PML is a rare central nervous system demyelinating disease resulting from viral lytic infection of myelin-producing oligodendrocytes and an abortive infection of astrocytes. It occurs almost exclusively in immunocompromised persons. More than one half of cases occur in HIV-infected persons, and PML is found in approximately 5% of autopsied AIDS patients. PML characteristically presents with motor weakness, visual field deficits (typically a homonymous hemianopsia), and speech and cognitive impairment (dementia, confusion, personality change). Less frequent symptoms include ataxia, cranial nerve deficits, and extrapyramidal symptoms. The brain shows multifocal, asymmetric, coalescing focal demyelination of white matter with a characteristic cytologic appearance of hyperchromatic enlarged oligodendroglial nuclei and bizarre astrocytes with enlarged multilobulated nuclei. The lesions on CT scan appear as hypodense, nonenhancing focal lesions without surrounding edema or inflammation. On MRI the lesions are hyperintense on T2 weighted images. The cerebrospinal fluid (CSF) is typically normal, but may show mild elevation of protein and less frequently a mononuclear pleocytosis, usually less than 25 cells/μL. JC virus DNA may be detected by PCR in the CSF. Confirmation of the diagnosis requires brain biopsy for histopathologic examination. Patients rapidly experience severe neurologic deficits, including cortical blindness and quadriparesis, with death ensuing usually within 6 months of initial presentation. There is no specific treatment.

Polyomavirus sequences have been identified in human tumors, including osteosarcomas, mesotheliomas, and brain tumors (ependymomas, glioblastomas, oligodendrogliomas, and others). The etiologic role of these viruses in human oncogenesis remains uncertain.

Bergsagel DJ, Finegold MJ, Butel JS, et al: DNA sequences similar to those of simian virus 40 in ependymomas and choroid plexus tumors of childhood. *N Engl J Med* 1992;326:988–93.

Elsner C, Dörries K: Evidence of human polyomavirus BK and JC infection in normal brain tissue. *Virology* 1992;191;72–80.

Hirsch HH, Knowles W, Dickenmann M, et al: Prospective study of polyomavirus type BK replication and nephropathy in renal-transplant patients. *N Engl J Med* 2002;347:488–96.

Strickler HD, Rosenberg PS, Devesa SS, et al: Contamination of poliovirus vaccines with simian virus 40 (1955–1963) and subsequent cancer rates. *JAMA* 1998; 279:292–5.

Sundsfjord A, Flaegstad T, Flø R, et al: BK and JC viruses in human immunodeficiency virus type 1-infected persons: Prevalence, excretion, viremia, and viral regulatory regions. *J Infect Dis* 1994;169:485–90.

Chapter 253
Transmissible Spongiform Encephalopathies*
David M. Asher

The transmissible spongiform encephalopathies (TSEs) are slow infections of the human nervous system, consisting of at least four diseases of humans (Table 253–1): kuru; Creutzfeldt-Jakob disease (CJD) with its variants—**sporadic CJD (sCJD), familial CJD (fCJD), iatrogenic CJD (iCJD),** and **new-variant or variant CJD (vCJD); Gerstmann—Sträussler-Scheinker syndrome (GSS);** and **fatal familial insomnia (FFI),** or the even more rare **sporadic fatal insomnia syndrome**. TSEs also affect animals; the most common and best-known TSEs of animals are **scrapie** in sheep, **bovine spongiform encephalopathy (BSE or "mad cow disease")** in cattle, and a **chronic wasting disease (CWD)** of deer and elk found in parts of the United States and Canada. All TSEs have similar clinical manifestations and histopathology, and all are "slow" infections with very long asymptomatic incubation periods of at least a year, durations of several months or more, and overt disease (although not infection) restricted to the nervous system. The most striking neuropathologic change that occurs in each TSE, to a greater or lesser extent, is spongy degeneration of the cerebral cortical gray matter.

Etiology. The TSEs are all transmissible to susceptible animals by inoculation of tissues from affected subjects. Although the infectious agents replicate in some cell cultures, they do not achieve the high titers of infectivity found in brain tissues or cause recognizable cytopathic effects in cultures. Most studies of TSE agents have used in vivo assays, using the appearance of typical neurologic disease in animals as evidence that the agent was present and intact. Inoculation of susceptible recipient animals with small amounts of infectious TSE agent results, months later, in the accumulation in tissues of large amounts of agent with the same physical and biologic properties as the original agent. The TSE agents display a spectrum of extreme resistance to inactivation by a variety of chemical and physical treatments that is unknown among conventional pathogens. This characteristic, as well as their partial sensitivity to protein-disrupting treatments and their consistent association with an abnormal amyloid protein stimulated the hypothesis that the TSE agents are probably subviral in size, composed of protein, and devoid of nucleic acid.

In 1982, S. B. Prusiner suggested the term **prion** (for proteinaceous infectious agent) as an appropriate name for such

---

*All material in this chapter is in the public domain, with the exception of any borrowed figures or tables.

TABLE 253–1. Transmissible Spongiform Encephalopathies (TSEs; Prion Diseases) of Humans and Animals

Disease	Naturally Infected Hosts
Creutzfeldt-Jakob disease (CJD)	Humans
Sporadic CJD	
Iatrogenic CJD	
(New) Variant CJD (vCJD)	
Fatal insomnia syndromes	Humans
Fatal familial insomnia	
Sporadic fatal insomnia	
Gerstmann-Sträussler-Scheinker syndrome	Humans
Kuru	Humans
Bovine spongiform encephalopathy ("mad cow" disease)	Cattle, zoo ungulates; zoo felines and domestic cats as feline spongiform encephalopathy; humans as vCJD
Chronic wasting disease	American, Canadian deer, elk
Scrapie	Sheep, goats
Transmissible mink encephalopathy	Mink

agents. The prion hypothesis, in its most recent form, proposes that the molecular mechanism by which the pathogen-specific information of TSE agents is propagated involves a self-replicating change in the folding of a host-encoded protein associated with a transition from an α-helix–rich structure in the native protease-sensitive conformation to a β-sheet–rich structure in the protease-resistant conformation associated with infectivity. The existence of a second host-encoded protein—termed "protein X"—that participates in the transformation was also postulated to explain certain otherwise puzzling findings.

The prion hypothesis has been widely accepted and was recognized by the awarding of the Nobel Prize in physiology and medicine to Prusiner in 1997. However, the prion hypothesis has not been universally accepted; it relies on the postulated existence of a genome-like coding mechanism based on differences in protein folding that have not been satisfactorily explained at a molecular level. In addition, it has yet to account for the many biologic strains of TSE agent that have been observed, although strain-specific differences in the abnormal forms of the prion protein (PrP) have been found and proposed as providing a molecular basis for the coding. It fails to explain why pure PrP uncontaminated with nucleic acid from an uninfected host has not transmitted a typical spongiform encephalopathy associated with a serially self-propagating agent. If the TSE agents ultimately prove to consist of protein and only protein, without any nucleic acid component, then the term prion will indeed be appropriate. If the agents are ultimately found to contain small nucleic acid genomes, then they might better be considered atypical viruses for which the term **virino** has been suggested. Until the actual molecular structure of the infectious TSE pathogens and the presence or absence of a nucleic acid genome are rigorously established, it seems less contentious to continue calling them TSE agents.

The first evidence that abnormal proteins are associated with the TSE was morphologic: **Scrapie-associated fibrils (SAFs)** were found in extracts of tissues from a variety of patients and animals with spongiform encephalopathies but not in normal tissues. SAFs resemble but are distinguishable from the amyloid fibrils that accumulate in the brains of patients with Alzheimer disease. A group of antigenically related, protease-resistant proteins, now designated **PrP^Sc (scrapie-type prion protein) or PrP-res (protease-resistant prion protein)**, proved to be components of SAF and to be present in the amyloid plaques found in the brains of patients and animals with TSE.

It is not yet clear whether abnormal PrP constitutes the complete infectious particle of spongiform encephalopathies or a component of those particles, or is simply a pathologic host protein not usually separated from the actual infectious entity by currently used techniques. The demonstration that PrP is encoded by a normal host gene seemed to favor the last possibility. However, several studies have suggested that agent-specific pathogenic information can be transmitted and replicated by different conformations of a protein with the same primary amino acid sequence in the absence of agent-specific nucleic acids. (Properties of two fungal proteins were found to be heritable without encoding in nucleic acid, although those properties have not been transmitted to recipient fungi as infectious elements.) Whatever its relationship to the actual infectious TSE particles, PrP clearly plays a central role in infection, because the normal prion protein must be expressed in mice if they are to acquire a TSE or to sustain replication of the infectious agents.

PrPs are glycoproteins; protease-resistant PrPs have the physical properties of amyloid proteins. The PrPs of several species of animals are very similar in their amino acid sequences and antigenicity, but are not identical in structure. The primary structure of PrP is encoded by the host and is not altered by the source of the infectious agent provoking its formation. The function of the ubiquitous protease-sensitive **PrP precursor (designated PrP^C for "cellular" PrP or PrP-sen for protease-sensitive PrP)** in normal cells is unknown; it binds copper and may play some role in normal synaptic transmission, but it is not required for life or for relatively normal cerebral function. As noted, expression of PrP is clearly required both for development of scrapie disease and for replication of the transmissible agent in mice. The degree of homology between amino acid sequences of PrPs in different animal species may correlate with the "species barrier" that affects susceptibility of animals of one species to infection with a TSE agent adapted to grow in another species.

Attempts to find particles resembling those of viruses or virus-like agents in brain tissues of humans or animals with spongiform encephalopathies have generally been unsuccessful. Peculiar tubulovesicles have been seen in thin sections of infected brain tissue. However, it has never been established that those structures are associated with infectivity.

It has been claimed that two other human diseases—*familial Alzheimer disease* of adults and *Alpers disease* of young children—may be caused by infections with agents similar to those causing the spongiform encephalopathies. The latter is a convulsive disorder associated with hemiatrophy and status spongiosus of the cerebral gray matter. Attempts to confirm these claims have failed.

Epidemiology. Kuru once affected many children ≥4 yr of age, adolescents, and young adults—mainly women—living in one area of Papua New Guinea. Transmission of the infection was interrupted more than 40 years ago, and kuru is now extremely rare and recognized only in older adults born before 1958. The complete disappearance of kuru among young people suggests that the practice of ritual cannibalism was the most important mechanism—probably the only mechanism—by which the infection spread in Papua New Guinea.

CJD, the most common human spongiform encephalopathy, was formerly thought to occur only in older adults; however, iCJD and, much more rarely, sCJD have affected adolescents and young adults. GSS and the insomnia syndromes have not been diagnosed in children or adolescents. Variant CJD has a peculiar predilection for younger people; only one patient with vCJD has been older than 55 years. CJD has been recognized worldwide, at yearly rates of 0.25–2 cases/million population (not age adjusted), with foci of considerably higher incidence among Libyan Jews in Israel, in isolated villages of Slovakia, and in other limited areas. Epidemiologic surveys have investigated several hypothetical mechanisms of spread of CJD. Person-to-person spread has been confirmed only for iatrogenic cases. The striking resemblance of CJD to scrapie prompted the suggestion that infected sheep tissues might be a source of spongiform encephalopathy in humans. However, no reliable epidemiologic evidence suggests that exposure to potentially scrapie-contaminated animals, meat, meat products, or experimental preparations of the scrapie agent have transmitted a TSE to humans.

The same can no longer be said about BSE. The outbreak of BSE among cattle (probably infected by eating scrapie agent–contaminated meat and bone meal) was first recognized in the United Kingdom in 1986 and from there spread to native cattle in at least 21 other countries (not the United States). The finding of a new TSE in ungulate and feline animals in British zoos and then in domestic cats there raised a fear that some strain of the scrapie agent, having crossed the species barrier from sheep to cattle, had acquired a broadened range of susceptible hosts, posing a potential danger for humans. That seems to be the most plausible explanation for the occurrence of vCJD, first recognized in adolescents in 1995 and now affecting more than 130 people in the United Kingdom, six in France, and one in Italy as well as a small number of former UK residents living in Canada, Hong Kong, Ireland, and the United States. The potential of the CWD agent, now known to have infected wild deer as well as farmed deer and elk in at least five states and in Canada, to infect human beings is unknown but is currently under investigation. Preliminary epidemiologic studies have not suggested that a history of eating either venison in general or venison from animals in areas where CWD occurs is a risk factor for the later development of CJD. However, it has long seemed prudent to avoid exposing children to meat or other products likely to be contaminated with any TSE agent, including the agents of scrapie and CWD; the BSE agent clearly poses a special danger.

Iatrogenic transmission of CJD has been recognized for >25 yr (Table 253–2). Accidental transmissions of CJD have occurred by means of contaminated neurosurgical instruments or operating facilities, cortical electrodes contaminated during epilepsy surgery, injections of human cadaveric pituitary growth hormone and gonadotropin, and transplantation of contaminated corneas and allografts of human dura mater. Pharmaceuticals and tissue grafts derived from or contaminated with human neural tissues, particularly when obtained from unselected donors and large pools of donors, pose special risks. Studies of animals experimentally infected with TSE agents suggest that blood and blood components from humans in whom CJD later develops may pose a theoretical risk of transmitting disease to recipients (and such blood components are withdrawn as a precaution), but no epidemiologic study has identified any subject exposed to such products who was later diagnosed with a TSE.

Spouses and household contacts of patients are at very low risk of acquiring CJD, although two instances of conjugal CJD have been reported. However, medical personnel exposed to brains of patients with CJD may be at increased risk; at least 20 health care workers have been recognized with the disease.

Pathogenesis. The probable portal of entry for the kuru agent has been thought to be either through the gastrointestinal tract or

TABLE 253–2. Iatrogenic Transmission of Creutzfeldt-Jakob Disease by Products of Human Origin

Product	No. of patients	Incubation time	
		Mean	*Range*
Cornea	3	17 mo	16–18 mo
Dura mater allograft	>100	7.4 yr	1.3–16 yr
Pituitary extract			
Growth hormone	>100*	12 yr	5–38.5 yr
Gonadotropin	4	13 yr	12–16 yr

Twenty-nine cases /≈8,000 estimated recipients in the United States (the rest in other countries).

lesions in the mouth or integument incidentally exposed to the agent during cannibalism. Subjects with vCJD (and animals with BSE and related infections) are thought to have been similarly infected with the BSE agent through exposure to some contaminated beef product, possibly through the intestinal tract. The first site of replication of the TSE agents appears to be in tissues of the reticuloendothelial system.

The TSE agents have been detected in low titers in blood of experimentally infected animals (mice, monkeys, hamsters, and sheep), mainly, though not exclusively, associated with nucleated cells. Circulating lymphoid cells seem to be required to infect mice by peripheral routes. Limited evidence suggests that the scrapie agent also spreads to the central nervous system of mice by ascending peripheral nerves. Several researchers claim to have detected the CJD agent in human blood, although most attempts have failed.

In human kuru, it seems probable that the only portal of exit of the agent from the body, at least in quantities sufficient to infect others, was through infected tissues exposed during cannibalism. In iatrogenically transmitted CJD, the brain and eyes of patients with CJD have been the probable sources of contamination. Kidney, liver, lung, lymph node, spleen, and cerebrospinal fluid (CSF) may also contain the CJD agent. At no time during the course of any TSE have antibodies or cell-mediated immunity to the infectious agents been convincingly demonstrated in either patients or animals. However, mice must be immunologically competent to be infected with the scrapie agent by peripheral routes of inoculation.

Typical changes in TSE include vacuolation and loss of neurons with hypertrophy and proliferation of glial cells, most pronounced in the cerebral cortex in patients with CJD and in the cerebellum in those with kuru. The CNS lesions are usually most severe in or even confined to gray matter, at least early in the disease. Loss of myelin appears to be secondary to degeneration of neurons. There generally is no inflammation, but usually a marked increase in the number and size of astrocytes is noted. Status spongiosus is not a striking autopsy finding in patients with FFI, and neuronal degeneration is largely restricted to thalamic nuclei.

"Amyloid" plaques are found in the brains of all patients with GSS and in at least 70% of those with kuru; they are less common in those with CJD. Amyloid plaques are most commonly found in the cerebellum but occur elsewhere in the brain as well. In brains of patients with vCJD, plaques surrounded by halos of vacuoles (described as flower-like or "florid" plaques) have been a consistent finding. TSE plaques react with antiserum prepared against PrP, and, even in the absence of plaques, extracellular PrP can be detected in the brain parenchyma by immunostaining.

Clinical Manifestations. Kuru is a progressive degenerative disease of the cerebellum and brainstem with less obvious involvement of the cerebral cortex. The first sign of kuru is usually cerebellar ataxia followed by progressive incoordination. Coarse, shivering tremors are characteristic. Variable abnormalities in cranial nerve function appear, frequently with impairment in conjugate gaze and swallowing. Patients die of inanition and pneumonia or of burns from cooking fires, usually 1 yr after onset. Although changes in mentation are common, there is no frank dementia or progression to coma, as in CJD. There are no signs of acute encephalitis such as fever, headaches, and convulsions.

CJD occurs throughout the world. Patients initially have either sensory disturbances (most often visual) or confusion and inappropriate behavior, with progression over weeks or months to frank dementia and ultimately coma. Some patients have cerebellar ataxia early in disease, and most experience myoclonic jerking movements. Mean survival of patients with sCJD has been <1 yr from the earliest signs of illness, although about 10% live for 2 yr. Variant CJD (Table 253–3) differs from

TABLE 253–3. Clinical and Histopathologic Features of Patients with Variant and Typical Sporadic Creutzfeldt-Jakob Disease

Feature	Variant CJD (>10 patients)	Sporadic CJD (185 patients)
Age at death (yr)*, (range)*	29 (19–74)	65
Duration of illness (mo)*, (range)*	12 (8–23)	4
Presenting signs	Abnormal behavior, dysesthesia	Dementia
Later signs	Dementia, ataxia, myoclonus	Ataxia, myoclonus
Periodic complexes on EEG	None	Most
PRNP 129 Met/Met	100%	83%
Histopathologic changes	Vacuolation, neuronal loss, astrocytosis, plaques (100%)	Vacuolation, neuronal loss, astrocytosis, plaques (≈15%)
Florid PrP plaques[†]	100%	0
PrP glycosylation	BSE-like[‡]	Not BSE-like

Modified from Will RG, Ironside JW, Zeidler M, et al: A new variant of Creutzfeldt-Jakob disease in the UK. Lancet 1996;347:921–5.
*Median age and duration for vCJD; averages for typical sporadic CJD.
[†]Dense plaques, pale periphery, surrounded by vacuolated cells.
[‡]Characterized by an excess of high-molecular-mass band and 19-kilodalton non-glycosylated band ("type 4") glycoform of PrP-res (Collinge et al., 1996).
BSE = bovine spongiform encephalopathy; EEG = electroencephalogram; PRNP = prion-protein-encoding gene; Met = codon 129 of one PRNP gene encoding for methionine.

the more common sCJD: Patients with vCJD are much younger at onset, and they more often present with complaints of dysesthesia and more subtle behavioral changes, often mistaken for psychiatric illness, than those seen in sCJD. Severe mental deterioration occurs later in the course of vCJD. Patients with vCJD have survived substantially longer than those with sCJD.

GSS is a familial disease resembling CJD but with more prominent cerebellar ataxia and amyloid plaques; dementia may appear only late in the course, and the average duration of illness is longer than that in typical sCJD. FFI and sporadic fatal insomnia are characterized by progressively severe insomnia and dysautonomia as well as ataxia, myoclonus, and other signs resembling those of CJD and GSS. Neither GSS nor an insomnia syndrome has been diagnosed in children or adolescents.

Diagnosis. Diagnosis of spongiform encephalopathies is most often determined on clinical grounds after excluding other diseases. The presence of 14-3-3 protein in CSF may aid in distinguishing between CJD and Alzheimer disease, although this is not a consideration in children. Brain biopsy may be diagnostic of CJD, but it can be recommended only if a potentially treatable disease remains to be excluded or if there is some other compelling reason to make an antemortem diagnosis. Definitive diagnosis requires microscopic examination of brain tissue obtained at autopsy. The demonstration of protease-resistant PrP proteins in brain extracts has been useful to confirm histopathologic diagnosis. Accumulation of the abnormal PrP in lymphoid tissues, even before the onset of neurologic signs, is typical of vCJD; tonsil biopsy may replace the need for brain biopsy when antemortem diagnosis of vCJD is indicated. Transmission of disease to susceptible animals by inoculation of brain suspension must be reserved for cases of special research interest.

LABORATORY FINDINGS. Virtually all patients with typical sporadic, iatrogenic, and familial forms of CJD have abnormal electroencephalograms (EEGs) as the disease progresses; the background becomes slow and irregular with diminished amplitude. A variety of paroxysmal discharges may also appear—slow waves, sharp waves, spike and wave complexes—and these may sometimes be unilateral or focal as well as bilaterally synchronous. Paroxysmal discharges may be precipitated by loud noise. Many patients have typical periodic suppression-burst complexes of high-voltage slow activity on EEG at some time during the illness. Patients with the vCJD had only generalized slowing, without periodic bursts of high-voltage discharges on EEG. CT or MRI may show cortical atrophy and large ventricles late in the course of CJD; many patients with vCJD have an increase in density of the pulvinar on MRI, something not typical of sCJD.

There may be modest elevation of CSF protein content in patients with TSE. Unusual protein spots were observed in CSF specimens after two-dimensional separation in gels and silver staining; the spots were identified as 14-3-3 proteins, normal proteins abundant in neurons but not ordinarily detected in CSF. (The 14-3-3 protein is not related to PrP.) However, the finding of 14-3-3 protein in CSF is not specific to CJD; it has also been detected in CSF specimens from some patients with acute viral encephalitides and recent cerebral infarctions. In clinical practice, the usual diagnostic problem is to differentiate between CJD and Alzheimer disease, and the presence of 14-3-3 proteins in CSF, while neither sensitive nor specific, militates against the latter. Finding the 14-3-3 protein in CSF has also been of some help in confirming the diagnosis of vCJD.

Treatment. No treatment has proven to be effective. Recent studies of cell cultures and rodents experimentally infected with TSE agents suggested that treatment with chlorpromazine, quinacrine, and tetracyclines might be of benefit, especially during the incubation periods of TSEs; early reports of clinical trials based on those studies have not been encouraging, and it seems unlikely that the severe brain damage found in late disease can be reversed by such treatment. Appropriate supportive care should be provided as for other progressive fatal neurologic diseases. On the basis of experimental studies in animals, several prophylactic postexposure treatment regimens have been suggested, but none has been widely accepted.

GENETIC COUNSELING. TSE sometimes occurs in families with a pattern of occurrence consistent with an autosomal dominant mode of inheritance. In patients with a family history of CJD, the clinical and histopathologic findings are similar to those seen in sporadic cases. In the United States, only about 10% of cases of CJD are familial. GSS and FFI are always familial. In some affected families, about 50% of siblings and children of a patient with a familial TSE eventually acquire the disease; in other families, the "penetrance" of illness may be less.

The gene coding for PrP is closely linked if not identical to that controlling the incubation periods of scrapie in sheep and both scrapie and CJD in mice. The gene encoding the PrP in humans, currently designated the *PRNP* gene, is located on the short arm of chromosome 20. It has an open reading frame of 759 nucleotides (253 codons), in which 12 different point mutations, as well as a variety of inserted sequences encoding extra tandem-repeated octapeptides, have been linked to the occurrence of spongiform encephalopathy in families.

Although the interpretation of these findings in regard to the prion hypothesis is in dispute, in affected families with an autosomal dominant pattern of CJD or GSS, individuals who are heterozygous for linked mutations in the *PRNP* gene clearly have a high probability of acquiring spongiform encephalopathy. The significance of mutations in the *PRNP* genes of individuals from families with no history of spongiform encephalopathy is not known. It seems wise to avoid alarming those who have miscellaneous mutations—several of which appear to represent normal polymorphisms—in the *PRNP* gene and their families because the implications are not yet clear.

The same nucleotide substitution at codon 178 of the *PRNP* gene associated with CJD in some families has been found in all patients with FFI; however, it is linked to a different amino acid–encoding sequence at codon 129, a site that is polymorphic in normal individuals. Homozygosity for methionine or for valine at codon 129, especially for methionine, seems to increase susceptibility to iCJD and sCJD, although methionine-valine heterozygotes are also susceptible to both diseases. So far, all patients with vCJD to be genotyped have been homozygous for methionine at codon 129 of the PRNP gene.

Prognosis. The prognosis of spongiform encephalopathies is uniformly poor. About 10% of patients may survive for ≥1 yr, but the quality of life is poor.

Prevention. Standard precautions should be used for handling all human tissues, blood, and body fluids. Materials and surfaces known to be contaminated with tissues or fluids from patients suspected of having CJD must be treated with great care. Whenever possible, contaminated instruments should be discarded by careful packaging and incineration. Contaminated tissues and biologic products probably cannot be completely freed of infectivity without destroying their structural integrity and biologic activity; therefore, the medical and family histories of individual tissue donors should be carefully reviewed to exclude a diagnosis of TSE. Histopathologic examination of brain tissues of donors and testing for abnormal PrP should be performed where feasible. Although no method of sterilization can be relied on to remove all infectivity from contaminated surfaces, exposure to moist heat, sodium hydroxide, chlorine bleach, concentrated formic acid, and guanidine salts markedly reduces infectivity.

Asher DM: Transmissible spongiform encephalopathies. In Yolken R (editor). *Manual of Clinical Microbiology,* 8th ed. Washington, DC: American Society for Microbiology, 2003.

Brown P: Transfusion medicine and spongiform encephalopathy. *Transfusion* 2001; 41:433–6.

Brown P, Gibbs CJ Jr, Rodgers-Johnson P, et al: Human spongiform encephalopathy: The NIH series of 300 cases of experimentally transmitted disease. *Ann Neurol* 1994;35:513–29.

Brown P, Will RG, Bradley R, et al. Bovine spongiform encephalopathy and variant Creutzfeldt-Jakob disease: Background, evolution, and current concerns. *Emerg Infect Dis* 20017:6–16.

Bruce ME, Will RG, Ironside JW, et al: Transmissions to mice indicate that 'new variant' CJD is caused by the BSE agent. *Nature* 1997;389:498–501.

Chesebro B. Prion protein and the transmissible spongiform encephalopathy diseases. *Neuron* 1999;24:503–6.

Collinge J, Sidle KC, Meads J, et al: Molecular analysis of prion strain variation and the aetiology of 'new variant' CJD. *Nature* 1996;383:685–90.

Hsich G, Kenney K, Gibbs CJ Jr, et al: The 14-3-3 brain protein in cerebrospinal fluid as a marker for transmissible spongiform encephalopathies. *N Engl J Med* 1996;335:924–30.

Oldstone MB, Race R, Thomas D, et al. Lymphotoxin-alpha- and lymphotoxin-beta–deficient mice differ in susceptibility to scrapie: Evidence against dendritic cell involvement in neuroinvasion. *J Virol* 2002;76:4357–63.

Occupational Safety and Health Administration, U.S. Department of Labor: Occupational Exposure to Bloodborne Pathogens; Final Rule (29 CFR Part 1910.1030). *Fed Reg U S A* 1991;56:64175.

Otto M, Wiltfang J, Cepek L, et al. Tau protein and 14-3-3 protein in the differential diagnosis of Creutzfeldt-Jakob disease. *Neurology* 2002;58:192–7.

Prusiner SB. Shattuck lecture-neurodegenerative diseases and prions. *N Engl J Med* 2001;344:1516–26.

Schonberger LB: New variant Creutzfeldt-Jakob disease and bovine spongiform encephalopathy. *Infect Dis Clin North Am* 1998;12:111–21.

Spencer MD, Knight RS, Will RG. First hundred cases of variant Creutzfeldt-Jakob disease: Retrospective case note review of early psychiatric and neurological features. *Br Med J* 2002;324:1479–82.

Taylor DM. Inactivation of transmissible degenerative encephalopathy agents: A review. *Vet J* 2000;159:10–7.

van Duijn CM, Delasnerie-Lauprêtre N, Masullo C, et al: Case-control study of risk factors of Creutzfeldt-Jakob disease in Europe during 1993–95. European Union (EU) Collaborative Study Group of Creutzfeldt-Jakob disease. *Lancet* 1998; 351:1081–5.

Will RG, Ironside JW, Zeidler M, et al: A new variant of Creutzfeldt-Jakob disease in the UK. *Lancet* 1996;347:921–5.

Will RG. Variant Creutzfeldt-Jakob disease. *J Neurol Neurosurg Psychiatry* 2002; 72:285–6.

Williams ES, Miller MW. Chronic wasting disease in deer and elk in North America. *Rev Sci Tech* 2002;21:305–16.

World Health Organization. Infection Control Guidelines for Transmissible Spongiform Encephalopathies. Report of a WHO Consultation, Geneva, Switzerland, 23–26 March 1999, WHO Communicable Disease Surveillance and Control. (Available at *http://www.who.int/emc-documents/tse/docs/whocdscsraph 20003.pdf*)

Chapter 254

Acquired Immunodeficiency Syndrome (Human Immunodeficiency Virus)

Ram Yogev and Ellen Gould Chadwick

Recent advances in research and major improvements in the treatment and management of HIV infection have brought about a substantial decrease in the incidence of new infections and AIDS in children born in the United States and Western Europe. However, most HIV-infected children are born in developing countries. It is estimated that in 2001, 800,000 children <15 yr of age were newly infected with HIV and that 2.7 million children were living with HIV or AIDS. In addition, because HIV-infected mothers are likely to die of AIDS, 10 million children have been orphaned thus far and an estimated 20 million will be orphaned by 2010. HIV infection in children progresses more rapidly than in adults, and some untreated children die within the first 2 yr of life. In general, this rapid progression is correlated with higher viral burden and faster depletion of infected CD4 lymphocytes in infants and children than in adults. Newer diagnostic tests and the availability of potent drugs to inhibit HIV replication have dramatically increased our ability to prevent and control this devastating disease.

Etiology. HIV-1 and HIV-2 are members of the Retroviridae family and belong to the *Lentivirus* genus, which includes cytopathic viruses causing diverse diseases in several animal species. Each virus particle contains two copies of the genome. The HIV-1 genome is single-stranded RNA that is 9.2 kb in size. At both ends of the genome there are identical regions, called **long terminal repeats,** which contain the regulation and expression genes of HIV. The remainder of the genome includes three major sections: the **GAG** region, which encodes the viral core proteins (e.g., p24, p17, p9, p6, which are derived from the precursor p55), the **POL** region, which encodes the viral enzymes (i.e., reverse transcriptase [p51], protease [pl0], and integrase [p32]); and the **ENV** region, which encodes the viral envelope proteins (i.e., gp120 and gp41, which are derived from the precursor gp160). Other regulatory proteins such as tat (pl4), rev (p19), nef (p27), vpr (pl5), and vif (p23) are involved in transactivation, viral mRNA expression, viral replication, induction of cell-cycle arrest, promotion of nuclear import of viral reverse transcription complexes, downregulation of cell surface receptors CD4 and class I major histocompatibility complex, proviral DNA synthesis, and virus release (Fig. 254–1).

The major external viral protein of HIV-1 is a heavily glycosylated gp120 protein that is associated with the transmembrane glycoprotein gp41; gp41 is very immunogenic and is used to detect HIV-1 antibodies in diagnostic assays; gp120 is a complex

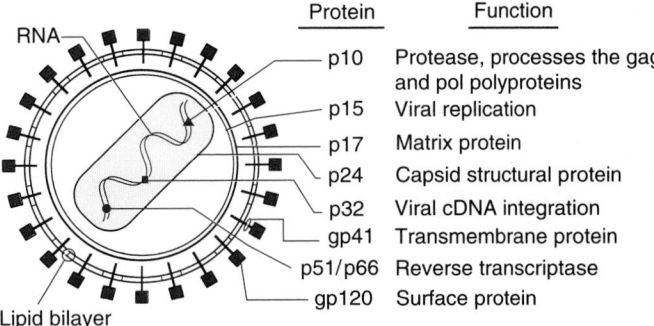

Protein	Function
p10	Protease, processes the gag and pol polyproteins
p15	Viral replication
p17	Matrix protein
p24	Capsid structural protein
p32	Viral cDNA integration
gp41	Transmembrane protein
p51/p66	Reverse transcriptase
gp120	Surface protein

FIGURE 254–1. The HIV virus and associated proteins and their functions.

molecule that includes the highly variable **V3 loop**. This region is immunodominant for neutralizing antibodies. The heterogeneity of gp120 presents major obstacles in establishing an effective HIV vaccine. The gp120 also carries the binding site for the CD4 molecule, the most common host cell surface receptor of T lymphocytes. Several chemokines serve as co-receptors for the envelop glycoproteins permitting membrane fusion and entry into the cell. Most HIV strains have a specific tropism for one of the chemokines: the fusion-inducing molecule, CXCR-4, which has been shown to act as a co-receptor for HIV attachment to lymphocytes, and CCR-5, a β chemokine receptor that facilitates HIV entry into macrophages. Several other chemokine receptors (e.g., CCR-3) have been shown in vitro to also serve as co-receptors.

Other mechanisms of attachment of HIV to cells use nonneutralizing antiviral antibodies and complement receptors. The Fab portion of these antibodies attaches to the virus surface, and the Fc portion binds to cells that express Fc receptors (i.e., macrophages, fibroblasts), thus facilitating virus transfer into the cell. Other cell surface receptors such as mannose-binding protein on macrophages and DC-specific C-type lectin (DC-SIGN) on dendritic cells also bind to the HIV-1 envelope glycoprotein and increase the efficiency of the virus infectivity. Following viral attachment, gp120 and the CD4 molecule undergo conformational changes, and gp41 interacts with the fusion receptor on the cell surface. Viral fusion with the cell membrane allows entry of viral RNA into the cell cytoplasm. Viral DNA copies are then transcribed from the virion RNA through viral reverse transcriptase enzyme activity, and duplication of the DNA copies produces double-stranded circular DNA. The HIV-1 reverse transcriptase is error-prone and lacks error-correcting mechanisms. Thus, many mutations arise, creating wide genetic variation in HIV-1 isolates even within an individual patient. The circular DNA is transported into the cell nucleus where it is integrated into chromosomal DNA and referred to as the provirus. The provirus can remain dormant for extended periods. Depending on the relative expression of the viral regulatory genes (e.g., tat, rev, nef), the proviral DNA may encode production of the viral RNA genome, which in turn leads to production of viral proteins necessary for viral assembly.

HIV-1 transcription is followed by translation. A capsid polyprotein is cleaved to produce, among others, the virus-specific protease (p10). This enzyme is critical for HIV-1 assembly. Several HIV-1 antiprotease drugs have been developed, targeting the increased sensitivity of the viral protease, which differs from the cellular proteases. The RNA genome is then incorporated into the newly formed viral capsid. As the new virus is formed, it buds through the cell membrane and is released.

The HIV diversity (e.g., groups M [main], O [outlier], N [non M, non O]) probably occurred from multiple zoonotic infections from primates in different geographic regions. Group M diversi-

fied to several subtypes (or clades A to H). In each region of the world certain clades predominate. For example, clade B is found in South America, clade E in Thailand, and clade C in South Africa. Clades are mixed in some patients due to HIV recombination, and some crossing between groups (i.e., M and O) has been reported.

HIV-2 is a rare cause of infection in children. It is most prevalent in Western and Southern Africa. The diagnosis of HIV-2 infection is more difficult because the standard antibody assays are HIV-1–specific and may give indeterminate results in those with HIV-2 infection. If HIV-2 is suspected, a specific test that detects antibody to HIV-2 peptides should be used.

Epidemiology. The World Health Organization (WHO) estimated that more than 40 million persons worldwide were living with HIV infection at the end of 2001; 2.7 million of these were children <15 yr of age. In 2001 alone, 5 million people acquired HIV and 3 million died, including 580,000 children. More than 90% of HIV-infected individuals live in developing nations where an estimated 720,000 infants were infected through perinatal transmission in 2001. Sub-Saharan Africa accounts for the fastest growing epidemic, with almost 90% of the world's total population of HIV-infected children. India and Thailand dominate the epidemic in Southeast Asia, with more recent expansion into Vietnam, China, and Cambodia.

Worldwide, 60% of HIV-infected individuals are women, and heterosexual transmission accounts for most HIV spread. In the United States, women account for 26% of AIDS cases reported to the CDC in 2000. In 2000, the percentage of American women whose exposure category was heterosexual contact (38%) surpassed that of injecting drug use (IDU) (25%). However, heterosexual transmission is probably even more common because further investigation of the category "risk not reported or identified" (36%) often leads to reclassification as heterosexual transmission. These are women who have been infected heterosexually by men unrecognized to be infected or to be in a high-risk group. Among mothers giving birth to children with AIDS, heterosexually acquired infection and "risk not reported" are the most common exposure categories, accounting for approximately 80% of the total. The estimated number of U.S. children with AIDS diagnosed each year increased from 1984 to 1992, then declined by 75% by 2000. This decline most likely reflects the effectiveness of zidovudine (ZDV) and other antiretroviral drugs in reducing perinatal HIV transmission. However, while the number of HIV-infected infants is decreasing in industrialized nations, the worldwide number of HIV-infected children is increasing dramatically because of lack of funds to provide medications to prevent perinatal transmissions.

In the United States, virtually all HIV infections in children <13 yr of age are the result of vertical transmission from an HIV-infected mother. A vanishing minority of children were infected through receipt of contaminated blood products and/or clotting factors (2%), primarily before 1985 when screening of the blood supply was instituted. Children of racial and ethnic minority groups are disproportionally over-represented, in particular non-Hispanic African-Americans and Hispanics. Race/ethnicity is not a risk factor for HIV infection per se but more likely reflects other factors that may be predictive of increased risk for HIV infection, such as lack of educational and economic opportunities and higher rates of IDU. The Northeast (44%) and the South (36%) account for most U.S. pediatric cases; 85% were diagnosed in metropolitan areas with populations >500,000 persons and 9% in metropolitan areas with populations of 50,000–500,000 persons.

Although adolescents (13–19 yr of age) with AIDS represent only 0.5% of U.S. cases, they constitute one of the fastest growing groups of newly infected persons in the country. Considering the long latency period between the time of infection and the development of clinical symptoms, reliance on AIDS case definition surveillance data severely under-represents the impact of the disease in adolescents. Based on a median incubation period of 8–12 yr, it has been estimated that 15–20% of all AIDS cases were acquired between 13–19 yr of age. Risk factors for HIV infection vary by gender in adolescents. Whereas 36% of the cumulative number of teenaged males with AIDS were infected by contaminated blood or blood products (primarily patients with hemophilia), only 7% of females were infected via this route. As in the adult population, the majority of teenaged males with AIDS who acquired HIV through sexual contact had male-to-male transmission. In contrast, more than half of adolescent females with AIDS were infected through heterosexual contact and one-sixth through IVDU, compared with 5% and 6%, respectively, in teenaged males.

As in the pediatric population, adolescent racial and ethnic minority populations are over-represented, especially among females. In addition, a greater proportion of female adolescents have AIDS (male:female ratio 1.2:1) than do female adults >25 yr of age (male:female ratio 4.5:1).

TRANSMISSION. Transmission of HIV-1 occurs via sexual contact, parenteral exposure to blood, or vertical transmission from mother to child. The primary route of infection in the pediatric population is vertical transmission, accounting for virtually all new cases. Rates of transmission of HIV from mother to child have varied in different parts of the United States and among countries. Most large studies in the United States and Europe have documented transmission rates in untreated women between 12–30%. In contrast, transmission rates in Africa and Haiti are higher (25–52%). Perinatal treatment of HIV-infected mothers with antiretroviral drugs has dramatically decreased these rates.

Vertical transmission of HIV can occur before (intrauterine), during (intrapartum), or after (through breast-feeding) delivery. Intrauterine transmission has been suggested by identification of HIV by culture or polymerase chain reaction (PCR) in fetal tissue as early as 10 weeks' gestation. In addition, first-trimester placental tissue from HIV-infected women has been demonstrated to contain HIV by in situ hybridization and immunocytochemistry. It is generally accepted that 30% to 40% of infected newborns are infected in utero, because this percentage of infants has laboratory evidence of infection (positive viral culture or PCR) within the 1st wk of life. Some studies have found that viral detection soon after birth also correlates with early onset of symptoms and rapid progression to AIDS, consistent with more long-standing infection during gestation.

The highest percentage of HIV-infected children acquire the virus intrapartum, evidenced by the fact that 60–70% of infected infants do not demonstrate detectable virus before 1 wk of age. The mechanism of transmission appears to be exposure to infected blood and cervicovaginal secretions in the birth canal, where HIV is found in high titers during late gestation and delivery. Furthermore, the international registry of HIV-exposed twins found that first-born twins were three times more likely to be infected, reflecting the longer time that twin A is exposed to the birth canal.

The least common route of vertical transmission in industrialized nations is breast-feeding; however, this is an important transmission route in developing countries. Both free and cell-associated virus have been detected in breast milk from HIV-infected mothers. A meta-analysis of prospective studies found that the additional risk of transmission through breast-feeding in women with HIV infection before pregnancy was 14% compared with a 29% increase in breast-feeding women who acquired HIV postnatally. This suggests that the viremia experienced by the mother during primary infection doubles the risk of transmission. It therefore seems reasonable for women to substitute infant formula for breast milk if they are known to be HIV-infected or are at risk for ongoing sexual or parenteral exposure to HIV. However, the WHO recommends that in devel-

oping countries where other diseases (e.g., diarrhea, pneumonia, and malnutrition) substantially contribute to a high infant mortality rate, the benefit of breast-feeding outweighs the risk of HIV transmission, and HIV-infected women should breast-feed their infants.

Several risk factors influence the rate of vertical transmission: preterm delivery (<34 wk gestation), a low maternal antenatal CD4 count, and use of illicit drugs during pregnancy. The most important variables appear to be >4 hr duration of ruptured membranes and birthweight <2500 g, each of which doubles the transmission rate. A meta-analysis of more than 1,000 pregnancies demonstrated that elective cesarean delivery decreased transmission by 87% if used in conjunction with zidovudine therapy in the mother and infant. However, because these data predated the advent of **highly active antiretroviral therapy (HAART)**, the additional benefit of cesarean section is probably negligible if the mother's viral load is <500 copies/mL. Although several studies have shown an increased rate of transmission in women with advanced disease (i.e., AIDS) or high viral load (>50,000 copies/mL), some transmitting mothers in each group were asymptomatic or had a low, but detectable, viral load.

Transfusions of infected blood or blood products have accounted for 3–6% of all pediatric AIDS cases. The period of highest risk was between 1978 and 1985, before the availability of HIV antibody–screened blood products. Whereas the prevalence of HIV infection in individuals with hemophilia treated before 1985 was as high as 70%, heat treatment of factor VIII concentrate and HIV antibody screening of donors has virtually eliminated HIV transmission in this population. Blood donor screening has dramatically reduced, but not eliminated, the risk of transfusion-associated HIV infection. The rate of HIV transmission through antibody-screened blood in the United States is estimated to be approximately 1/60,000 transfused units. In many developing countries, screening of blood donors is not uniform, and the risk of transmitting HIV infection via transfusion is still substantial.

Although HIV can be isolated rarely from saliva, it is in very low titers (<1 infectious particle/mL) and has not been implicated as a transmission vehicle. Studies of hundreds of household contacts of HIV-infected individuals have found that the risk of HIV transmission is practically nonexistent. Only a few cases have been reported in which urine or feces (possibly devoid of visible blood) have been proposed as a possible vehicle of HIV transmission.

In the pediatric population, sexual transmission is infrequent, but a small number of cases resulting from sexual abuse have been reported. In contrast, sexual contact is a major route of transmission in the adolescent population, accounting for most of the cases.

Pathogenesis. When the mucosa serves as the portal of entry for the HIV, the first cells to be infected are the dendritic cells. These cells are in charge of collecting and processing antigens introduced from the periphery and transporting them to the lymphoid tissue. The HIV does not infect the dendritic cell but it binds to its DC-SIGN surface molecule, which allows the virus to survive until it reaches the lymphatic tissue. In the lymph node, the HIV selectively binds to cells expressing CD4 molecules on their surface, primarily helper T lymphocytes (CD4 cells) and cells of the monocyte-macrophage lineage. Other cells bearing CD4, such as microglia, astrocytes, oligodendroglia, and placental tissue containing villous Hofbauer cells, may also be infected by HIV. Usually, CD4 lymphocytes, recruited to respond to viral antigen, migrate to the lymph nodes where they become activated and proliferate, making them highly susceptible to HIV infection. This antigen-driven migration and accumulation of CD4 cells within the lymphoid tissue may contribute to the generalized lymphadenopathy characteristic of the acute retroviral syndrome in adults and adolescents. Recently it was shown that the HIV preferentially infects the very cells that respond to it (i.e., HIV-specific memory CD4 cells), which accounts for the progressive loss of these cells' response and the subsequent loss of control of HIV replication. When the HIV replication reaches a threshold (usually within 3–6 wk from the time of infection), a burst of plasma viremia occurs. This intense viremia cause flu-like symptoms (i.e., fever, rash, lymphadenopathy, and arthralgia) in 50–70% of infected adults. With establishment of a cellular and humoral immune response within 2–4 mo, the viral load in the blood declines substantially, and patients enter a phase characterized by a lack of symptoms and a return of CD4 cells to only moderately decreased levels.

Early HIV-1 replication in children has no apparent clinical manifestations. Whether tested by virus isolation or by PCR for viral nucleic acid sequences, fewer than 50% of HIV-1–infected infants demonstrate evidence of the virus at birth. The virus load increases by 1–4 mo, and almost all HIV-infected infants have detectable HIV-1 in peripheral blood by 4 mo of age.

In adults, the long period of clinical latency (up to 8–12 yr) is not indicative of viral latency. In fact, there is a very high turnover of virus and CD4 lymphocytes (more than a billion cells per day), which gradually causes deterioration of the immune system, evidenced particularly by depletion of CD4 cells. These cells may be destroyed by multiple mechanisms: HIV-mediated single cell killing, formation of multinucleated giant cells of infected and uninfected CD4 cells (**syncytia formation**), virus-specific immune responses, superantigen-mediated activation of T cells (rendering them more susceptible to infection with HIV), and programmed cell death (apoptosis). The viral burden in the lymphoid organs is greater than that in the peripheral blood during the asymptomatic period. As HIV virions and their immune complexes migrate through the lymph nodes, they are trapped in the network of dendritic follicular cells. Because the ability of HIV to replicate in T cells depends on the state of activation of the cells, the immune activation that takes place within the microenvironment of the nodes in HIV disease serves to promote infection of new CD4 cells as well as subsequent viral replication within the cells. Viral replication in monocytes, which can be infected productively yet resist killing, explains their role as reservoirs of HIV and as effectors of tissue damage in organs such as the brain.

Cell-mediated and humoral responses occur early in the infection. The CD8 T cells play an important role in containing the infection. HIV-specific cytotoxic T lymphocytes (CTLs) develop against both the structural (i.e., ENV, POL, GAG) and regulatory (e.g., tat) viral proteins. The CTL cells appear at the end of the acute retroviral infection as the viral replication is controlled. The CTL cells control the infection by killing HIV-infected cells before new viruses are produced and by secreting potent antiviral factors that compete with the virus for its receptors (e.g., CCR5). Neutralizing antibodies appear later during the infection and seem to help in the continued suppression of viral replication during clinical latency. There are at least two possible mechanisms that control the steady-state viral load level during the chronic clinical latency. One mechanism may be the limited availability of activated CD4 cells which prevent further increase in viral load due to a set point (i.e., controlled) replication. The other mechanism, the immune-control, suggests that the development of active immune response (whose magnitude is controlled by the amount of the viral antigen) limits the viral replication at a steady state. There is no general consensus about which of these two mechanisms is more important. The CD4–cell limitation mechanism accounts for the effect of antiretroviral therapy, whereas the immune-control mechanism emphasizes the importance of immune-modulation treatment (e.g., cytokines, vaccines) to increase the efficiency of the immune response, which, in turn, slows the disease progression.

A group of cytokines, such as tumor necrosis factor α (TNFα), TNFβ, interleukin 1 (IL-1), IL-3, IL-6, interferon-γ, granulocyte-macrophage colony-stimulating factor (GM-CSF), and macrophage colony-stimulating factor, play an integral role in upregulating HIV expression from a state of quiescent infection to active viral replication. Other cytokines such as interferon γ (INFγ), INF-β, and transforming growth factor D exert a suppressive effect on HIV replication. The interactions among these cytokines influence the concentration of viral particles in the tissues. Plasma concentrations of cytokines need not be elevated for them to exert their effect, because they are produced and act locally in the tissues. Thus, even during states of apparent immunologic quiescence, the complex interaction of cytokines sustains a constant level of viral expression, particularly in the lymph nodes.

Commonly the phenotypic HIV isolated during the clinical latency period grows slowly in culture and produces low titers of reverse transcriptase. These isolates are called **non–syncytium-inducing (NSI) viruses**, which use CCR5 as their co-receptor. By the late stages of the clinical latency, the isolated virus is phenotypically different. It grows rapidly and to high titers in culture and it uses CXCR4 as its co-receptor. These isolates are called **syncytium-inducing (SI) viruses**. The switch from NSI to SI increases the capacity of the virus to replicate, to infect a broader range of target cells (CXCR4 is more widely expressed on resting and activated immune cells), and to kill T cells more rapidly and efficiently. As a result, the clinical latency phase is over and progression toward AIDS is noted. The progression of disease is related temporally to the gradual disruption of lymph node architecture and degeneration of the follicular dendritic cell network with loss of its ability to trap HIV particles. This frees the virus to recirculate, producing high levels of viremia and an increased disappearance of CD4 T cells during the later stages of disease.

Before HAART was available, three distinct patterns of disease were described in children. Approximately 15–25% of HIV-infected newborns in developed countries present with a rapid disease course, with onset of AIDS and symptoms during the first few months of life and, if untreated, a median survival time of 6–9 mo. In resource-poor countries, >85% of the HIV-infected newborns will have such rapidly progressing disease. It has been suggested that if intrauterine infection coincides with the period of rapid expansion of CD4 cells in the fetus, it could effectively infect the majority of the body's immunocompetent cells. The normal migration of these cells to the marrow, spleen, and thymus would result in efficient systemic delivery of HIV, unchecked by the immature immune system of the fetus. Thus infection would be established before the normal ontogenic development of the immune system, causing more severe impairment of immunity. Most children in this group have a positive HIV-1 culture and/or detectable virus in the plasma (median level 11,000 copies/mL) in the first 48 hr of life. This early evidence of viral presence suggests that the newborn was infected in utero. The viral load rapidly increases and peaks by 2–3 mo of age (median 750,000 copies/mL) and subsequently declines slowly. In contrast to the viral load in adults, the viral load in infants stays high for at least the first 2 yr of life.

The majority of perinatally infected newborns (60–80%) present with a second pattern, that of a much slower progression of disease with a median survival time of 6 yr. Many patients in this group have a negative viral culture or PCR in the 1st wk of life and are therefore considered to be infected intrapartum. In a typical patient, the viral load rapidly increases by 2–3 mo of age (median 100,000 copies/mL) and slowly declines over a period of 24 mo. The slow decline in viral load is in sharp contrast to the rapid decline after primary infection seen in adults. This observation can be explained only partially by the immaturity of the immune system in newborns and infants.

The third pattern of disease (i.e., long-term survivors) occurs in a small percentage (<5%) of perinatally infected children who have minimal or no progression of disease with relatively normal CD4 counts and very low viral loads for longer than 8 yr.

HIV-infected children have changes in the immune system that are similar to those in HIV-infected adults. CD4 cell depletion may be less dramatic because infants normally have a relative lymphocytosis. Therefore, for example, a value of 1,500 CD4 cells/mm^3 in children <1 yr of age is indicative of severe CD4 depletion and is comparable to <200 CD4 cells/mm^3 in adults. Lymphopenia is relatively rare in perinatally infected children and is usually only seen in older children or those with end-stage disease. Although cutaneous anergy is common during HIV infection, it is also frequent in healthy children <1 yr of age and thus its interpretation is difficult in infected infants.

B-cell activation occurs in most children early in the infection as evidenced by hypergammaglobulinemia (>1.750 g/L) with high levels of anti–HIV-1 antibody. This response may reflect both dysregulation of T-cell suppression of B-cell antibody synthesis and active CD4 enhancement of B-lymphocyte humoral response. In some children, evidence of specific antibody production does not occur and in others adequate antibody levels do not confer protection. Because hypergammaglobulinemia is so common in HIV-infected children, it may serve as a surrogate marker of HIV infection in symptomatic children in whom specific diagnostic tests (e.g., PCR, culture) are not available or are too expensive. Hypogammaglobulinemia is very rare (<1%). Central nervous system (CNS) involvement is more common in pediatric patients than in adults. Macrophages and microglia play an important role in HIV neuropathogenesis, and data suggest that astrocytes may also be involved. Although the specific mechanisms for encephalopathy in children are not yet clear, the developing brain in young infants, with its delayed myelinization, is more vulnerable to invasion by HIV.

Understanding the complex relationship between the virus-specific immune responses and the mechanisms used by the virus to survive are crucial for therapeutic strategies. Even though viral replication currently can be suppressed by antiretroviral drugs, it is important to develop strategies to modulate the immune response.

Clinical Manifestations. The clinical manifestations of HIV infection vary widely among infants, children, and adolescents. In most infants, physical examination at birth is normal. Initial symptoms may be subtle, such as lymphadenopathy and hepatosplenomegaly, or nonspecific, such as failure to thrive, chronic or recurrent diarrhea, interstitial pneumonia, or oral thrush, and may be distinguishable only by their persistence. Whereas systemic and pulmonary findings are common in the United States and Europe, chronic diarrhea, wasting, and severe malnutrition predominate in Africa. Symptoms found more commonly in children than adults with HIV infection include recurrent bacterial infections, chronic parotid swelling, lymphocytic interstitial pneumonitis (LIP), and early onset of progressive neurologic deterioration.

The HIV classification system is used to categorize the stage of pediatric disease by using two parameters: clinical status, and degree of immunologic impairment (Table 254–1). Among the clinical categories, category A (mild symptoms) includes children with at least two mild symptoms such as lymphadenopathy, parotitis, hepatomegaly, splenomegaly, dermatitis, and recurrent or persistent sinusitis or otitis media. Category B (moderate symptoms) includes, for example, children with LIP, oropharyngeal thrush persisting for >2 mo, recurrent or chronic diarrhea, persistent fever >1 mo, hepatitis, recurrent herpes simplex stomatitis or HSV esophagitis or pneumonitis, disseminated varicella (i.e., with visceral involvement), cardiomegaly, or nephropathy. Category C (severe symptoms) includes, for example, children with two serious bacterial infections (e.g., sepsis, meningitis, pneumonia) in a 2-yr period, esophageal or lower respiratory tract candidiasis, cryptococcosis, cryptosporidiosis (>1 mo), encephalopathy, malignancies, disseminated mycobacterial infection, *Pneumocystis carinii* pneumonia (PCP), cerebral toxoplasmosis (onset after 1 mo of age) and severe weight loss.

The immune classification is based on the absolute CD4 lymphocyte count or the percentage of CD4 cells (CD4%) (Table 254–2). Age adjustment of the absolute CD4 count is necessary because counts that are relatively high in normal infants decline steadily until 6 yr of age, when they reach adult norms. If there is a discrepancy between the CD4 count and percentage, the disease is classified into the more severe category.

INFECTIONS. Approximately 20% of AIDS-defining illnesses in children are recurrent bacterial infections caused primarily by encapsulated organisms such as *Streptococcus pneumoniae* and *Salmonella*. Other pathogens including *Staphylococcus, Enterococcus, Pseudomonas aeruginosa, Haemophilus influenzae*, and other gram-positive and gram-negative organisms may also be seen. Most of these infections are the result of HIV-related disturbances in humoral immunity. The most common serious infections are bacteremia, sepsis, and pneumonia, accounting for more than 50% of infections in HIV-infected children. Meningitis, urinary tract infections, deep-seated abscesses, and bone/joint infection occur less frequently. Milder recurrent infections, such as otitis media, sinusitis, and skin and soft tissue infections are very common and may be chronic with atypical presentations.

Opportunistic infections are generally seen in children with severe depression of the CD4 count. In adults, these infections usually represent reactivation of a latent infection acquired early in life. In contrast, young children generally have primary infection and, lacking prior immunity, often have a more fulminant course of disease. This principle is best illustrated by PCP, the most common opportunistic infection in the pediatric population. The peak incidence of PCP occurs at age 3–6 mo with the highest mortality rate in children <1 yr of age. However, newer, more aggressive approaches to treatment have improved the outcome substantially.

The classic clinical presentation of PCP includes acute onset of fever, tachypnea, dyspnea, and marked hypoxemia; however, in some children more indolent development of hypoxemia may precede other clinical or roentgenographic manifestations. Chest radiography findings most commonly consist of interstitial infiltrates or diffuse alveolar disease, which rapidly progresses. Nodular lesions, streaky or lobar infiltrates, or pleural effusions

TABLE 254–1. CDC Pediatric HIV Classification*

	Clinical Categories			
Immune Categories	N—No Signs/Symptoms	A—Mild Signs/Symptoms	B—Moderate Signs/Symptoms†	C—Severe Signs/Symptoms†
1. No evidence of suppression	N1	A1	B1	C1
2. Evidence of moderate suppression	N2	A2	B2	C2
3. Severe suppression	N3	A3	B3	C3

*Children whose HIV infection status is not confirmed are classified by using the above grid with a letter E (for perinatally exposed) placed before the appropriate classification code (e.g., EN2).
†Category C and lymphoid interstitial pneumonitis (LIP) in category B are reportable to state and local health departments as AIDS.
From Centers for Disease Control and Prevention: 1994 revised classification system for human immunodeficiency virus infection in children less than 13 years of age. MMWR 1994;43 (RR-12):1–10.

TABLE 254–2. CDC Revised Pediatric HIV Classification: Immune Categories Based on CD4 Count or CD4 Percentage

Immune Categories	<12 Months		1–5 Years		≥6 Years	
	Cells/μL	%	Cells/μL	%	Cells/μL	%
1. No evidence of suppression	≥1500	≥25	≥1000	≥25	≥500	≥25
2. Evidence of moderate suppression	750–1499	15–24	500–999	15–24	200–499	15–24
3. Severe suppression	<750	<15	<500	<15	<200	<15

may occasionally be seen. Diagnosis is established by demonstration of *P. carinii* with appropriate staining of bronchoalveolar fluid lavage; rarely, an open lung biopsy is necessary.

The first-line therapy for PCP is intravenous trimethoprim (TMP)-sulfamethoxazole (SMZ) (15–20 mg/kg/24 hr of TMP and 75–100 mg/kg/24 hr of SMZ q 6 hr IV) with adjunctive corticosteroids. When the patient has improved, therapy with oral TMP-SMZ should be continued for a total of 21 days. Historically, up to one third of HIV-infected children have had allergic reactions to TMP-SMZ that have required desensitization. However, because of the use of adjunctive corticosteroid therapy, this is considerably less frequent. Alternative therapy for PCP includes intravenous administration of pentamidine (4 mg/kg/24 hr). Other regimens such as TMP plus dapsone, clindamycin plus primaquine, or atovaquone are used as alternatives in adults but have not been widely used in children to date.

Atypical mycobacterial infection, particularly with *Mycobacterium avium-intracellulare* complex (MAC), may cause disseminated disease in HIV-infected children who are severely immunosuppressed. The incidence of MAC infection in children with <100 CD4 cells/mm^3 who were not treated with antiretroviral drugs was estimated to be 10%. Effective antiretroviral combination therapies that result in viral suppression have made MAC infections rare. Disseminated MAC infection is characterized by fever, malaise, weight loss and night sweats; diarrhea, abdominal pain, and rarely intestinal perforation or jaundice (due to biliary tract obstruction by lymphadenopathy) may also be present. Diagnosis is made by isolation of MAC from blood, bone marrow, or tissue; the isolated presence of MAC in the stool does not confirm a diagnosis of disseminated MAC. Treatment can reduce symptoms and prolong life but is only capable of suppressing the infection as long as severe CD4 depletion persists. Therapy should include at least two drugs: clarithromycin (or azithromycin) and ethambutol. A third drug (e.g., rifabutin, rifampin, ciprofloxacin, or amikacin) is generally added to decrease the emergence of drug-resistant isolates. Careful consideration of possible drug-drug interactions with antiretroviral agents is necessary before initiation of disseminated MAC therapy. Drug susceptibilities should be ascertained and the treatment regimen adjusted accordingly in the event of inadequate clinical response to therapy. Because of the great potential for toxicity with most of these medications, surveillance for side effects should be ongoing.

Oral candidiasis is the most common fungal infection seen in HIV-infected children. Oral nystatin suspension (2–5 mL qid) is often effective. Clotrimazole troches are an effective alternative. In refractory cases, oral amphotericin suspension should be considered. Oral thrush progresses to involve the esophagus in as many as 20% of children, presenting with symptoms such as anorexia, dysphagia, vomiting, and fever. Treatment with oral fluconazole (4–6 mg/kg/24 hr) for 14 days generally results in rapid improvement in symptoms. Disseminated histoplasmosis and coccidiomycosis or cryptococcosis are rare in pediatric patients but may occur in endemic areas. Parasitic infections such as intestinal cryptosporidiosis and microsporidiosis and rarely isosporiasis or giardiasis are other opportunistic infections that cause significant morbidity. Although usually self-limiting diseases in healthy hosts, they cause severe chronic diarrhea

often leading to malnutrition in HIV-infected children with low CD4 counts. Until recently, there was no effective therapy for cryptosporidiosis, which generally resulted in lifelong infection. However, preliminary data on an investigational agent, nitazoxanide, has been promising, with clearance of the infection in some patients. Albendazole was reported to be effective in a few cases of chronic microsporidiosis, and TMP-SMZ seems to be effective for isosporiasis.

Viral infections, especially with the herpesvirus group, pose significant problems for HIV-infected children. Herpes simplex virus causes recurrent gingivostomatitis, which may be complicated by local and distant cutaneous dissemination. Primary varicella-zoster virus (VZV) infection (chickenpox) may be prolonged and complicated by bacterial infections or visceral dissemination, including pneumonitis. Recurrent, atypical, or chronic episodes of herpes zoster are often debilitating and require prolonged therapy with acyclovir; in rare instances, VZV has developed resistance to acyclovir, requiring the use of foscarnet. Disseminated cytomegalovirus (CMV) infection can occur with severe CD4 depletion (<50 CD4 cells/mm^3) and may involve single or multiple organs. Retinitis, pneumonitis, esophagitis, gastritis with pyloric obstruction, hepatitis, colitis, and encephalitis have been reported, but these complications are rarely seen if HAART is given. Ganciclovir (5 mg/kg bid IV) or foscarnet (60 mg/kg tid IV) are the drugs of choice. Measles may occur despite immunization and may present without the typical rash. It often disseminates to the lung or brain with a high mortality rate. Respiratory viruses such as respiratory syncytial virus (RSV) and adenovirus may present with prolonged symptoms and persistent viral shedding.

CENTRAL NERVOUS SYSTEM. The incidence of central nervous system (CNS) involvement in perinatally infected children is 50–90% in developing countries but lower in developed countries, with a median onset at 19 mo of age. The most common presentation is progressive encephalopathy with loss or plateau of developmental milestones, cognitive deterioration, impaired brain growth resulting in acquired microcephaly, and symmetric motor dysfunction. Encephalopathy may be the initial manifestation of the disease or may present much later when severe immune suppression occurs. With progression, marked apathy, spasticity, hyperreflexia, and gait disturbance may occur, as well as loss of language, oral, fine, and/or gross motor skills. The encephalopathy may progress intermittently, with periods of deterioration followed by transiently stable plateaus. Older children may exhibit behavioral problems and learning disabilities. Associated abnormalities identified by neuroimaging techniques include cerebral atrophy in up to 85% of children with neurologic symptoms, increased ventricular size, basal ganglia calcifications, and, less frequently, leukomalacia.

Focal neurologic signs and seizures are unusual and may imply a comorbid pathologic process such as a CNS tumor, opportunistic infection, or stroke. CNS lymphoma may present with a new onset of focal neurologic findings, headache, seizures, and mental status changes. Characteristic findings on neuroimaging studies include a hyperdense or isodense mass with variable contrast enhancement or a diffusely infiltrating contrast-enhancing mass. CNS toxoplasmosis is exceedingly rare in young infants, but may occur in HIV-infected adolescents; the overwhelming majority of these cases have presence of serum IgG antitoxoplasma as a marker of infection. Other opportunistic infections of the CNS are rare and include CMV, JC virus (causing progressive multifocal leukoencephalopathy), herpes simplex virus, and cryptococcal or coccidioides meningitis. Although the true incidence of cerebrovascular disorders (both hemorrhagic and nonhemorrhagic strokes) is unclear, 6–10% of children from large clinical series have been affected.

RESPIRATORY TRACT. Recurrent upper respiratory tract infections such as otitis media and sinusitis are very common. Although the typical pathogens (e.g., *S. pneumoniae, H. influenzae, Moraxella catarrhalis*) are most common, unusual pathogens, such as *P. aeruginosa,* yeast and anaerobes, may be present in chronic infections and result in complications such as invasive sinusitis and mastoiditis.

LIP is the most common chronic lower respiratory tract abnormality, occurring in approximately 25% of HIV-infected children. LIP is a chronic process with nodular lymphoid hyperplasia in the bronchial and bronchiolar epithelium, often leading to progressive alveolar capillary block over months to years. It has a characteristic chronic diffuse reticulonodular pattern on chest radiograph (rarely with hilar lymphadenopathy), which allows a presumptive diagnosis to be made radiographically before the onset of symptoms. Clinically, there is an insidious onset of tachypnea, cough, and mild to moderate hypoxemia with normal auscultatory findings or minimal rales. Progressive disease may be accompanied by digital clubbing and symptomatic hypoxemia, which usually resolves with oral corticosteroid therapy. The etiology of LIP has not been proven, although several studies suggest LIP is associated with a primary Epstein-Barr virus infection in the setting of HIV infection.

Most symptomatic HIV-infected children experience at least one episode of pneumonia during the course of their disease. *S. pneumoniae* is the most common bacterial pathogen, but gram-negative bacteria may also be problematic; *P. aeruginosa* pneumonia occurs most commonly in severely symptomatic children (CDC C3 category) and is often associated with acute respiratory failure and death. Rarely, bronchiectasis can develop and cause recurrent secondary infections. PCP is the most common opportunistic infection, but other pathogens, including CMV, *Aspergillus, Histoplasma,* and *Cryptococcus,* can cause pulmonary disease. Infection with common respiratory viruses, including respiratory syncytial virus, parainfluenza, influenza, and adenovirus, may occur simultaneously and have a protracted course and period of viral shedding from the respiratory tract. Pulmonary and extrapulmonary tuberculosis has been reported with increasing frequency in HIV-infected children, although it is considerably more common in HIV-infected adults.

CARDIOVASCULAR SYSTEM. Subclinical cardiac abnormalities in HIV-infected children are common, persistent, and often progressive. A prospective study of young children with symptomatic HIV infection revealed that dilated cardiomyopathy and left ventricular hypertrophy were common; the 2-yr cumulative incidence of congestive heart failure was almost 5%. Children with encephalopathy or other AIDS-defining conditions have the highest rate of adverse cardiac outcomes. Resting sinus tachycardia has been reported in up to 64% and marked sinus arrhythmia in 17% of HIV-infected children. Hemodynamic instability occurs more frequently with advanced HIV disease and relates to the high frequency of severe autonomic neuropathy in patients with AIDS (up to 88%). Gallop rhythm with tachypnea and hepatosplenomegaly appear to be the best clinical indicators of CHF in HIV-infected children; anticongestive therapy is generally very effective, especially when initiated early. Electrocardiography and echocardiography are helpful in assessing cardiac function before the onset of clinical symptoms.

GASTROINTESTINAL AND HEPATOBILIARY TRACT. Oral manifestations of HIV disease include erythematous or pseudomembranous candidiasis, periodontal disease (e.g., ulcera-

tive gingivitis or periodontitis), salivary gland disease (i.e., swelling, xerostomia), and rarely ulcerations or oral hairy leukoplakia and ulcerations. Gastrointestinal tract involvement is common in HIV-infected children. A variety of pathogens can cause gastrointestinal disease, including bacteria (*Salmonella, Campylobacter,* MAC), protozoa (*Giardia, Cryptosporidium, Isospora,* microsporidia), viruses (CMV, HSV, rotavirus), and fungi (*Candida*). MAC and the protozoal infections are most severe and protracted in patients with severe CD4 cell depletion. Infections may be localized or disseminated and affect any part of the gastrointestinal tract from the oropharynx to the rectum. Oral or esophageal ulcerations, either viral in origin or idiopathic, are painful and often interfere with eating. Lesions that have negative viral cultures may respond to thalidomide, which is currently investigational, or to short courses of prednisone. **AIDS enteropathy,** a syndrome of malabsorption with partial villous atrophy not associated with a specific pathogen, has been postulated to be a result of direct HIV infection of the gut. Disaccharide intolerance is common in HIV-infected children with chronic diarrhea.

The most common symptoms of gastrointestinal disease are chronic or recurrent diarrhea with malabsorption, abdominal pain, dysphagia, and failure to thrive (FTT). Prompt recognition of weight loss or poor growth velocity in the absence of diarrhea is critical. Linear growth impairment is often correlated with the level of HIV viremia. Supplemental enteral feedings should be instituted, either by mouth or with nighttime nasogastric tube feedings in cases associated with more chronic growth problems; placement of a gastrostomy tube for nutritional supplementation may be necessary. The **wasting syndrome**, defined as a loss of >10% of body weight, is not as common as FTT in pediatric patients. However, the resulting malnutrition is associated with a grave prognosis and generally requires parenteral hyperalimentation.

Chronic liver inflammation evidenced by fluctuating serum levels of transaminases with or without cholestasis is relatively common, often without identification of an etiologic agent. Cryptosporidial cholecystitis is associated with abdominal pain, jaundice, and elevated gamma GT. In some patients, chronic hepatitis caused by CMV, hepatitis B or C, or MAC may lead to portal hypertension and liver failure. Several of the antiretroviral drugs or other drugs such as didanosine, protease inhibitors, and dapsone may also cause reversible elevation of transaminases.

Pancreatitis with increased pancreatic enzymes with or without abdominal pain, vomiting, and fever may be the result of drug therapy, e.g., pentamidine, didanosine, and lamivudine, or, rarely, opportunistic infections such as MAC or CMV.

RENAL DISEASE. Nephropathy is an unusual presenting symptom of HIV infection, more commonly occurring in older symptomatic children. A direct effect of HIV on renal epithelial cells has been suggested as the cause, but immune complexes, hyperviscosity of the blood (secondary to hyperglobulinemia), and nephrotoxic drugs are other possible factors. A wide range of histologic abnormalities has been reported, including focal glomerulosclerosis, mesangial hyperplasia, segmental necrotizing glomerulonephritis, and minimal change disease. Focal glomerulosclerosis generally progresses to renal failure within 6–12 mo, but other histologic abnormalities in children may remain stable without significant renal insufficiency for prolonged periods. Nephrotic syndrome is the most common manifestation of pediatric renal disease, with edema, hypoalbuminemia, proteinuria, and azotemia with normal blood pressure. Cases resistant to steroid therapy may benefit from cyclosporin therapy. Polyuria, oliguria, and hematuria have also been observed in some patients.

SKIN MANIFESTATIONS. Many cutaneous manifestations seen in HIV-infected children are inflammatory or infectious disorders that are not unique to HIV infection. These disorders tend to be more disseminated and respond less consistently to conventional therapy than in the uninfected child. Seborrheic dermatitis or eczema that is severe and unresponsive to treatment may be an early nonspecific sign of HIV infection. Recurrent or chronic episodes of herpes simplex virus, herpes zoster, molluscum contagiosum, flat warts, anogenital warts, and candidal infections are common and may be difficult to control.

Allergic drug eruptions are also common, in particular related to sulfonamides, and generally respond to withdrawal of the drug or to desensitization. Epidermal hyperkeratosis with dry, scaling skin is frequently observed, and sparse hair or hair loss may be seen in the later stages of the disease.

HEMATOLOGIC AND MALIGNANT DISEASES. Anemia occurs in 20–70% of HIV-infected children, more commonly in children with AIDS. The anemia may be due to chronic infection, poor nutrition, autoimmune factors, virus-associated conditions (e.g., hemophagocytic syndrome, parvovirus B19 red cell aplasia), or adverse effect of drugs (e.g., zidovudine). In children with low erythropoietin levels, subcutaneous recombinant erythropoietin may be successful in treating the anemia.

Leukopenia occurs in almost one third of untreated HIV-infected children, and neutropenia often occurs. In some cases, antineutrophil antibodies are the cause, and treatment with intravenous immunoglobulin (IVIG) has been successful. Multiple drugs used for treatment or prophylaxis for opportunistic infections such as PCP, MAC, and CMV or antiretroviral drugs (e.g., zidovudine) may also cause leukopenia and/or neutropenia. In many cases, treatment with subcutaneous granulocyte colony-stimulating factor (GCSF) is successful.

Thrombocytopenia has been reported in 10–20% of patients. The etiology may be immunologic (i.e., circulating immune complexes or antiplatelet antibodies) or due to drug toxicity, or the cause may be unknown. Treatment with IVIG or anti-D offers temporary improvement in most cases. If ineffective, a 2–3 day course of high dose steroids (30 mg/kg/24 hr) may be an alternative. Antiretroviral therapy may also reverse thrombocytopenia. Deficiency of clotting factors (e.g., factors II, VII, IX) is not rare in children with advanced HIV disease and is often easy to correct (i.e., vitamin K). A novel disease of the thymus has been observed in a few HIV-infected children. These patients were found to have characteristic anterior mediastinal multilocular thymic cysts without clinical symptoms. Histologic examination shows focal cystic changes, follicular hyperplasia, and diffuse plasmocytosis and multinucleated giant cells. Spontaneous involution occurred in some cases.

In contrast to the more frequent occurrence in adults, malignant diseases have been reported infrequently in HIV-infected children, representing only 2% of AIDS-defining illnesses. Non-Hodgkins lymphoma, primary central nervous system lymphoma, and leiomyosarcoma are the most commonly reported neoplasms among HIV-infected children. Epstein-Barr virus is associated with most lymphomas and with all leiomyosarcomas. Kaposi sarcoma, which is caused by human herpesvirus 8 (Chapter 236), occurs frequently among HIV-infected adults but is exceedingly uncommon among HIV-infected children.

Diagnosis. All infants born to HIV-infected mothers test antibody-positive at birth because of passive transfer of maternal HIV antibody across the placenta during gestation. Most uninfected infants (seroreverters) lose maternal antibody between 6–12 mo of age. Because a small proportion of uninfected infants continues to test HIV antibody–positive for up to 18 mo of age, positive IgG antibody tests cannot be used to make a definitive diagnosis of HIV infection in infants younger than this age. The presence of IgA or IgM anti-HIV in the infant's circulation can indicate HIV infection, because these immunoglobulin classes do not cross the placenta; however, detectable quantities of IgA anti-HIV are not generally produced until 3–6 mo of age, limiting its utility in young infants (sensitivity is 50–60% at 3 mo of age and 60–100% at 6 mo of age). IgM anti-HIV assays have been both insensitive and nonspecific and therefore are not valuable for clinical use. In any child >18 mo of age, demonstration of IgG antibody to HIV by a repeatedly reactive enzyme immunoassay (EIA) and confirmatory test (e.g., Western blot or immunofluorescence assay) establishes the diagnosis of HIV infection.

Several new rapid HIV tests are currently available with sensitivity and specificity similar to those of the standard EIA. Many of these new tests require only a single step that allows test results to be reported within 1–2 hr. Because the false-positive result of each test alone is high, the World Health Organization has recommended specific combinations of different rapid tests to confirm reactive HIV test results. Incorporating rapid HIV testing during delivery or immediately after birth allows HIV prevention counseling to those whose HIV status is unknown during pregnancy. Viral diagnostic assays, such as HIV DNA or RNA PCR, HIV culture, or HIV p24 antigen immune dissociated p24 (ICD-p24), are considerably more useful in young infants, allowing a definitive diagnosis in most infected infants by 1–6 mo of age. By 6 mo of age, the HIV culture and/or PCR identifies all infected infants. HIV DNA PCR is the preferred virologic assay in developed countries. Almost 40% of infected newborns have positive tests in the first 2 days of life, with >90% testing positive by 2 wk of age. Plasma HIV RNA assays, which detect viral replication, may be more sensitive than DNA PCR for early diagnosis, but data are limited. HIV culture has similar sensitivity to HIV DNA PCR; however, it is more technically complex and expensive, and results are often not available for 2–4 wk compared to 2–3 days with PCR. The p24 antigen assay is cheaper, highly specific, and easy to perform, but it is less sensitive than the other virologic tests. It is not recommended for diagnosis of infection in infants <1 mo of age because of the high rate of false-positive results. In developing countries, the ICD-p24 test may be considered for older infants; however, if results are negative, it does not rule out infection.

Viral diagnostic testing should be performed within the first 2 days of life, at 1–2 mo of age, and at 4–6 mo of age; some also favor testing at age 14 days to maximize early detection of infected infants, if initiation of antiretroviral therapy is desired. A positive virologic assay (i.e., detection of HIV by PCR, culture, or p24 antigen) suggests HIV infection and should be confirmed by a repeat test on a second specimen as soon as possible. A diagnosis of HIV infection can be made with two positive virologic tests obtained from different blood samples.

Infants who have negative virologic assays initially should be retested at the intervals outlined above. Although the perinatal use of prophylactic zidovudine to prevent vertical transmission has not affected the predictive value of viral diagnostic testing, the effect of more intensive antiviral combinations (e.g., protease inhibitors) in pregnant women on the accuracy of the infant's viral tests is unknown. HIV infection can be reasonably excluded if an infant has had at least two negative virologic tests at age ≥1 mo of age with at least one test performed at ≥4 mo of age. In older infants and children, two or more negative HIV antibody tests performed at least 1 mo apart past 6 mo of age in the absence of hypogammaglobulinemia or clinical evidence of HIV disease can reasonably exclude HIV infection. The infection can be excluded definitively if the same parameters are met when the infant is at least 18 mo of age.

For infants born to HIV-infected mothers, who should be prescribed zidovudine perinatal prophylaxis, a complete blood count, differential leukocyte count, and platelet count should be performed at 4 wk of age. If the child is found to be HIV-infected or if the HIV status is not clear, these tests should be continued every 1–3 mo to assess the hematologic effect of the disease and its treatment (e.g., prophylactic TMP-SMZ and antiretroviral therapy). CD4 and CD8 lymphocyte counts should be performed at 1 and 3 mo of age. If the child is HIV-infected or the HIV status is not clear, the test should be repeated every 3 mo starting at 6 mo of age. The frequency of the test should be increased (i.e., every 4–6 wk) if the CD4 lymphocyte count or percentage declines rapidly.

Treatment. The currently available therapy does not eradicate the virus and cure the patient; it only suppresses the virus for extended periods of time and changes the course of the disease to a chronic process. Decisions about antiretroviral therapy for pediatric HIV-infected patients are based on the magnitude of viral replication (i.e., viral load), CD4 lymphocyte count or percentage, and clinical condition. Because antiretroviral therapy changes as new drugs become available, decisions regarding therapy should be made in consultation with an expert in pediatric HIV infection. Although early treatment trials consisted of single or dual drug therapy, more recent trials have uniformly confirmed the superiority of three or more drug combination therapy using virologic, immunologic, and clinical end-points. Plasma viral load monitoring and measurement of CD4 values have made it possible to implement rational treatment strategies for viral suppression as well as to assess the efficacy of a particular drug combination. The following principles form the basis for antiretroviral treatment: (1) uninterrupted HIV replication causes destruction of the immune system and progression to AIDS; (2) the magnitude of the viral load predicts the rate of disease progression, and the CD4 cell count reflects the risk of opportunistic infections and HIV infection complications; (3) potent combination therapy that suppresses HIV replication to an undetectable level restricts the selection of antiretroviral-resistant mutants; drug-resistant strains are the major factor limiting successful viral suppression and delay of disease progression; (4) the goal of sustainable suppression of HIV replication is best achieved by the simultaneous initiation of combinations of antiretroviral agents to which the patient has not been exposed previously and which are not cross-resistant to drugs with which the patient has been treated previously; (5) adherence to the complex drug regimens is crucial for a successful outcome.

COMBINATION THERAPY. Antiretroviral drugs licensed as of 2002 (Table 254–3) are categorized based on their ability to inhibit the HIV reverse transcriptase or protease enzymes. Within the reverse transcriptase inhibitors, a further subdivision can be made: nucleoside (or nucleotide) reverse transcriptase inhibitors (NRTIs) and non-nucleoside reverse transcriptase inhibitors (NNRTIs). The NRTIs have a similar structure to the building blocks of the DNA (e.g., thymidine, cytosine). By incorporating themselves into the DNA, they act like a chain terminator and block further incorporation of nucleosides, which prevent viral DNA synthesis. Among the NRTIs, thymidine analogs (stavudine [d4T] and zidovudine [ZDV]) are found in higher concentrations in activated or dividing cells, and nonthymidine analogs (didanosine [ddI], lamivudine [3TC], and dideoxycytidine [ddC]) have more activity in resting cells. Activated cells are thought to produce >99% of the population of HIV virons. In contrast, resting cells account for <1% of the population, but may serve as a reservoir of HIV. Suppression of replication in both populations is thought to be an important component of long-term viral control. NNRTIs (e.g., nevirapine and efaverenz) act differently than the NRTIs. They attach to the reverse transcriptase and restrict its motility, which reduces the activity of the enzyme. Protease inhibitors (e.g., ritonavir, nelfinavir, saquinavir) are potent agents that are active farther along in the viral life cycle. They bind to the site where the viral long polypeptides are cut to individual, mature, and functional core proteins, which produces the infectious virons before they leave the cell.

While the principal site of viral replication is lymphoid tissue, sanctuary sites such as the CNS may harbor residual virons with the potential of being a source of local or persistent disease. Impaired penetration of drugs to these compartments could result in development of resistance. Although data on CNS penetration of antiviral agents are presently limited, ZDV, d4T, and 3TC appear to achieve inhibitory concentrations in the CNS. Indinavir and nevirapine also penetrate the CSF, but other protease inhibitors are actively transported out of the CNS, thereby limiting their potential efficacy.

By targeting different points in the viral life cycle and stages of cell activation, and delivering drug to all tissue sites, maximal viral suppression may be feasible. Combinations of three drugs, such as a thymidine analog NRTI, a nonthymidine analog NRTI (to suppress replication in both active and resting cells), and a protease inhibitor or an NNRTI have been shown in adults and in children to produce prolonged viral suppression. Additional regimens such as triple NRTIs (i.e., abacavir, zidovudine, and

TABLE 254–3. Antiretroviral Drugs Available in 2003 and Some of Their Toxicities*

	Drug Toxicity	
	Most frequent	*Unusual*
Reverse Transcriptase Inhibitors (NRTI)†		
Abacavir (ABC)	Gastrointestinal intolerance, headache, rash	Hypersensitivity, pancreatitis
Didanosine (ddI)	Gastrointestinal intolerance, abdominal pain	peripheral neuropathy, pancreatitis, lactic acidosis
Lamivudine (3TC)	Headache, fatigue, gastrointestinal intolerance, rash	Pancreatitis, peripheral neuropathy, neutropenia, lactic acidosis
Stavudine (d4T)	Headache, gastrointestinal intolerance	Rash, peripheral neuropathy, pancreatitis, lactic acidosis
Tenofavir (TNF)	Gastrointestinal complaints, asthenia, headache	Hepatomegaly, lactic acidosis, bone abnormalities
Zalcitabine (ddC)	Gastrointestinal intolerance, headache, malaise	Pancreatitis, oral/esophageal ulcers, peripheral neuropathy, lactic acidosis
Zidovudine (ZDV)	Anemia, granulocytopenia, headache	Hepatotoxicity, myopathy, lactic acidosis
Non-nucleoside Reverse Transcriptase Inhibitors (NNRTI)		
Delavirdine§ (DLV)	Rash, gastrointestinal complaints, headache, fatigue	Abdominal pain, headache, fatigue
Efavirenz (EFV)	Rash, CNS symptoms	Hepatotoxicity, pancreatitis
Nevirapine§ (NVP)	Rash, gastrointestinal complaints, headache, fatigue	Hepatotoxicity, hypersensitivity
Protease Inhibitors (PI)‡		
Amprenavir (APV)	Gastrointestinal intolerance, rash	Perioral paresthesia, headache
Indinavir§ (IDV)	Gastrointestinal intolerance, hyperbilirubinemia	Nephrolithiasis, dizziness
Lopinavir¶ (LPV)	Gastrointestinal intolerance, headache, asthenia	Rash, hepatotoxicity
Nelfinavir§ (NFV)	Diarrhea, abdominal pain	Asthenia, rash, exacerbation of chronic liver disease
Ritonavir§ (RTV)	Gastrointestinal intolerance, abdominal pain, anorexia, headache	Elevated transaminases, perioral paresthesias, hepatotoxicity
Saquinavir§ (SQV)	Diarrhea, abdominal pain, headache, nausea	Exacerbation of chronic liver disease, perioral paresthesia, rash

*Not all adverse effects are listed. See prescribing information in package inserts.
†Combinations of ZDV and 3TC (Combivir) and ZDV, 3TC, and ABC (Trizivir) are available for adolescents and adults.
‡All the protease inhibitors can cause hyperglycemia, diabetes, lipodystrophy, hemolytic anemia, and spontaneous bleeding episodes in hemophiliacs.
§Significant drug-drug interactions; some may be life-threatening.
¶Always in combination with a low-dose ritonavir.

lamivudine) or lopinavir/ritonavir in combination with two NRTIs or one NRTI and an NNRTI are also recommended as alternatives. Although not ideal, less potent combinations (e.g., dual NRTIs, ritonavir with stavudine, amprenavir with abacavir) may be considered in special situations when there are concerns about adherence to a complex drug regimen or when the patient and/or family prefer an alternative regimen. Combination treatment increases the rate of toxicities (see Table 254–3), and complex drug-drug interactions exist among many of the antiretroviral drugs. Most NNRTI and protease inhibitor drugs are inducers or inhibitors of the cytochrome P450 system. The protease inhibitors are particularly likely to have serious interactions with multiple drug classes, including nonsedating antihistamines, psychotropic, vasoconstrictor, antimycobacterial, cardiovascular, analgesic, and gastrointestinal drugs (e.g., cisapride). Whenever new medications are added to an antiretroviral treatment, especially a protease inhibitor-containing regimen, a pharmacist and/or HIV specialist should be consulted to address possible drug interactions. Recently the inhibitory effect of ritonavir (a protease inhibitor) on the cytochrome P450 system was exploited, and small doses of the drug are added to several other protease inhibitors (e.g., lopinavir, indinavir, saquinavir) to slow their metabolism by the P450 system and to improve their pharmacokinetic profile. This provides more effective drug levels with less toxicity and less frequent dosing.

ADHERENCE. Assessment of the likelihood of adherence to treatment is an important factor in deciding whether and when to initiate therapy. Numerous studies have shown that compliance of <80–90% results in less successful suppression of the viral load. In addition, poor adherence to prescribed medication regimens results in subtherapeutic drug concentrations and enhances development of resistance, particularly with protease inhibitors and NNRTI drugs. Combination antiretroviral regimens require multiple daily doses and are often unpalatable, requiring extreme dedication on the part of the care provider and child; this makes participation of the family in the decision to initiate therapy essential. Intensive education on the relationship of drug adherence to viral suppression, training on drug administration, frequent follow-up visits, and commitment of the caregiver and the patient (despite the inconvenience of side effects, dosing schedule, and so on) are critical for successful antiviral treatment.

INITIATION OF THERAPY. HIV-infected children with symptoms (clinical category A, B, or C) or with evidence of immune dysfunction (immune category 2 or 3) should be treated with antiretroviral therapy, regardless of age or viral load. Children <1 yr of age are at high risk for disease progression, and immunologic and virologic tests to identify those likely to develop rapidly progressive disease are less predictive than in older children. Therefore, such infants should be treated with antiretroviral agents as soon as the diagnosis of HIV infection has been confirmed, regardless of clinical or immunologic status, or viral load. Data suggest that HIV-infected infants who are treated before the age of 3 mo of age control their HIV infection better than infants whose antiretroviral therapy started later than 3 mo of age.

Many clinicians advocate treating asymptomatic children ≥1 yr of age to prevent immunologic deterioration. However, when there are concerns regarding drug adherence, safety, and durability of antiretroviral response, some providers elect to delay treatment in the immunologically normal child >1 yr with a low viral load (<50,000 copies/mm^3) for whom the risk for clinical progression is low. Such children should be monitored regularly for evidence of virologic, immunologic, or clinical progression, at which point therapy should be initiated.

DOSING. Data on antiretroviral drug dosages for neonates are often limited. Because of the immaturity of the neonatal liver, premature infants and newborns often require an increase in the dosing interval of drugs primarily cleared through hepatic metabolism (glucuronidation).

Adolescents should have antiretroviral dosages prescribed on the basis of Tanner staging of puberty rather than on the basis of age. During early puberty (Tanner stage I, II, and III), pediatric dosing ranges should be used, whereas adolescents in late puberty (Tanner stage IV and V) should follow adult dosing schedules.

CHANGING ANTIRETROVIRAL THERAPY. Therapy should be changed when the current regimen is judged ineffective as evidenced by increase in viral load, deterioration of the CD4 cell count, or clinical progression. Development of toxicity or intolerance to drugs is another reason to consider a change in therapy. When a change is considered, the patient and family should be reassessed for adherence problems. While considering possible new drug choices, potential cross-resistance should be addressed. In addition, few patients who have virologic failure may still demonstrate elevated CD4 cell counts (**discordant response**). Impaired replication ability of the resistant virus and autoimmunization with enhanced cytotoxic T lymphocyte (CTL) effect are some of the reasons for this discordant response. Ideally, all drugs should be changed. However, in many situations (e.g., previous antiretroviral experience, intolerance, toxicity) this is not possible, and, therefore, at least two drugs should be changed. If an alternative regimen that is likely to suppress the viral load is not available in patients with discordant response, the same regimen should be continued to maximize the clinical and immunologic benefits.

MONITORING ANTIRETROVIRAL THERAPY. Virologic and immunologic surveillance (using HIV RNA copy number and CD4 lymphocyte count or percentage) as well as clinical assessment should be performed regularly in children taking antiretroviral therapy. Initial virologic response (i.e., at least five fold [0.7 log$_{10}$] reduction in viral load) should be achieved within 4 wk of initiating antiretroviral therapy. The maximum response to therapy usually occurs within 12–16 wk. Thus, HIV RNA levels should be measured at 4 wk and 3–4 mo after therapy initiation. Once an optimal response has occurred, viral load should then be measured at least every 3–6 mo. If the response is unsatisfactory, another viral load should be performed as soon as possible to verify the results before a change in therapy is considered. The CD4 cells respond more slowly to successful treatment and, therefore, can be monitored less frequently (i.e., every 3–4 mo). Potential toxicity should be monitored closely for the first 8–12 wk, and if no clinical or laboratory toxicity is documented, a follow-up every 2–3 mo is adequate. Several toxicities have been causing increasing concern regarding antiretroviral use (especially protease inhibitors). These toxicities include lipodystrophy (e.g., redistribution of body fat and elevation of cholesterol and triglyceride concentrations), insulin intolerance, lactic acidosis, and severe hepatomegaly with steatosis.

RESISTANCE TO ANTIRETROVIRAL THERAPY. The high mutation rate of HIV (mainly due to the absence of error-correcting mechanisms) severely impairs the success of antiretroviral therapy. Failure to reduce the viral load to less than 50 copies/mL increases the risk of developing resistance. Recent data suggest that even effectively treated patients are not completely suppressing viral replication and that persistence of HIV transcription and evolution of envelope sequences continue in the latent cellular reservoirs. The accumulation of resistance mutation progressively diminishes the potency of the antiretroviral therapy and challenges the physician to find new regimens. Testing for drug resistance when devising a new regimen is rapidly becoming the standard of care. Two types of tests are available. The **phenotypic assay** that measures the virus susceptibility in various concentrations of the drug and the **genotypic assay** that predicts the virus susceptibility from mutations identified on the HIV genome isolated from the patient. Several studies have shown that the treatment success was higher in patients whose antiretroviral therapy was guided by genotype or phenotype testing.

SUPPORTIVE CARE. Even before the new antiretroviral drugs were available, a significant impact on the quality of life and survival of HIV-infected children was achieved when supportive care was given. A multidisciplinary team approach is desirable for successful management. Close attention should be paid to nutrition status, which is often delicately balanced and may require aggressive preemptive intervention (e.g., nasogastric or gastric feedings or parenteral nutrition) to achieve adequate caloric and protein intake. Painful oropharyngeal lesions and dental caries are frequent and may interfere with eating; routine dental evaluations and careful attention to oral hygiene should be encouraged. Development should be evaluated regularly with provision of necessary physical, occupational, and/or speech therapy. Recognition of pain in the young child may be difficult, and effective pharmacologic and nonpharmacologic protocols for pain management should be instituted, especially during the terminal phase of the disease.

All HIV-exposed and infected children should receive standard pediatric immunizations. In general, live oral polio vaccine and live bacterial vaccines (e.g., BCG) should not be given (Fig. 254–2). Varicella and MMR vaccines are recommended for children in immune categories 1 and 2, but neither varicella nor MMR should be given to severely immunocompromised children (immune category 3). Of note, prior immunizations do not always provide protection, as evidenced by outbreaks of measles and pertussis in immunized HIV-infected children.

Prophylactic regimens are integral for the care of HIV-infected children. All infants between 6 wk–1 yr of age either (1) born to HIV-infected mothers or (2) proved to be HIV-infected should receive prophylaxis regardless of the CD4 count or percentage (see Table 254–3). When the child is >1 yr of age, prophylaxis should be given according to the CD4 lymphocyte count (Table 254–4). The best prophylactic regimen is $150/750$ mg/m^2/24 hr of TMP-SMZ given as one or two daily doses 3 days per week. If the patient experiences a mild allergic reaction (e.g., rash), desensitization is usually successful to allow daily TMP-SMZ prophylaxis. For severe adverse reactions to TMP-SMZ, alternative therapies include dapsone, atovaquone, or aerosolized or intravenous pentamidine.

Prophylaxis against MAC should be offered to HIV-infected children with advanced immunosuppression (i.e., CD4 lymphocyte count <500 cells/mm^3 in children <1 yr of age, <75 cells/ mm^3 in children 1–6 yr of age, and <50 cells/mm^3 in children >6 yr of age). The drugs of choice are clarithromycin (7.5 mg/kg bid PO) or azithromycin (20 mg/kg once a week PO or 5 mg/kg once daily PO).

Primary prophylaxis against opportunistic infections may be discontinued if patients have experienced sustained (>6 mo duration) immune reconstitution with HAART. Even if patients have had opportunistic infections such as PCP or DMAC, it may also be possible to discontinue secondary prophylaxis if immune reconstitution has been sustained.

Some experts recommend IVIG to prevent recurrent serious bacterial infections for HIV-infected children who (1) have suffered from at least two documented serious bacterial infections within 1 yr, (2) have laboratory-documented inability to make antigen-specific antibodies, or (3) are hypogammaglobulinemic. The dose is 400 mg/kg every 4 wk.

All HIV-exposed children should have skin testing (i.e., 5TU PPD) for tuberculosis at 1 yr of age and be retested every 2 yr. If the child is living in close contact with a person with tuberculosis, he or she should be tested annually. To reduce the incidence of other potential infections, parents should be counseled about (1) the importance of good hand washing, (2) avoiding raw or undercooked food (salmonella), (3) avoiding drinking or swimming in lake or river water or being in contact with young farm animals (*Cryptosporidium*), and (4) the risk of playing with pets (e.g., *Toxoplasma* and *Bartonella* from cats, *Salmonella* from reptiles).

Because of the frequent changes in these guidelines, physicians providing care to few HIV-exposed or infected children should periodically consult physicians with expertise in pediatric HIV infection.

Prognosis. The improved understanding of the pathogenesis of HIV infection in children and the availability of more effective antiretroviral drugs have changed the prognosis considerably. In developed countries where early diagnosis leads to prompt antiretroviral therapy, progression of the disease and mortality rate have diminished. HIV-infected children live longer with improved quality of life. In general, the best single prognostic indicator is the plasma viral load. Although there is no threshold above which rapid progression can be predicted, it is unusual to see rapid progression in an infant with a viral load <100,000 copies/mL. In addition, a high viral load (>100,000 copies/mL)

Vaccine	Birth	1 mo	2 mo	4 mo	6 mo	12 mo	15 mo	18 mo	24 mo	4–6 yr	11–12 yr	14–16 yr
Measles, Mumps Rubella*						MMR§				MMR§		
Influenza					Influenza†							
Pneumococcal Conjugate			PCV	PCV	PCV	PCV					Pneumococcal‡	
Varicella						Varicella§						
Hepatitis A								Hepatitis A‖				

FIGURE 254–2. Differences in immunization schedule for HIV-infected children from the routine childhood immunization schedule.

* See text.
† Revaccination is recommended every year.
‡ Revaccination with pneumococcal polysaccharide vaccine (PPV) every 5 yr.
§ Contraindicated in children with AIDS or immune category 3 (see Table 254–1).
‖ Recommended routinely for all HIV-infected children.

TABLE 254–4. Recommendations for PCP Prophylaxis and CD4 Monitoring for Human Immunodeficiency Virus (HIV)-Exposed Infants and HIV-Infected Children, By Age and HIV-Infection Status

Age/HIV-infection Status	PCP Prophylaxis	CD4 Monitoring
Birth to 4–6 wk, HIV exposed	No prophylaxis	1 mo
4–6 wk to 4 mo or HIV exposed 4–12 mo	Prophylaxis	3 mo
HIV-infected or indeterminate	Prophylaxis	6, 9, and 12 mo
HIV infection reasonably excluded*	No prophylaxis	None
1–5 yr, HIV infected	Prophylaxis if: CD4 count is <500 cells/μL or CD4 percentage is <15%[‡§]	Every 3–4 mo[†]
6–12 yr, HIV infected	Prophylaxis if: CD4 count is <200 cells/μL or CD4 percentage is <15%[§]	Every 3–4 mo[†]

*HIV infection can be reasonably excluded among children who have had 2 or more negative HIV diagnostic tests (i.e., HIV culture or PCR), both of which are performed at ≥ 1 mo of age and one of which is performed at ≥ 4 mo of age, or 2 or more negative HIV IgG antibody tests performed at > 6 mo of age among children who have no clinical evidence of HIV disease.

[†]More frequent monitoring (e.g., monthly) is recommended for children whose CD counts or percentages are approaching the threshold at which prophylaxis is recommended.

[‡]Children 1–2 yr of age who were receiving PCP prophylaxis and had a CD4 count of <750 cells/μL or percentage of <15% at <12 mo of age should continue prophylaxis.

[§]Prophylaxis should be considered on a case-by-case basis for children who might otherwise be at risk for PCP, such as children with rapidly declining CD4 counts or percentages or children with Category C conditions. Children who have had PCP should receive lifelong PCP prophylaxis.

From Centers for Disease Control and Prevention: 1995 revised guidelines for prophylaxis against Pneumocystis carinii pneumonia for children infected with or perinatally exposed to human immunodeficiency virus. MMWR 1995; 44(RR-4):1–18.

over time is associated with greater risk for disease progression and death. CD4 lymphocyte percentage is another prognostic indicator and the mortality rate is higher in patients with CD4 lymphocyte percentage <15%. To define prognosis more accurately, the use of changes in both markers (i.e., CD4 lymphocyte percentage and plasma viral load) is recommended.

In developing countries where antiretroviral therapy and sophisticated diagnostic tests are scarce, a clinical staging system can be used to predict progression of disease. The suggested clinical staging is quite similar to the classification recommended in the 1994 revised CDC classification. Children with opportunistic infections (e.g., PCP, MAC), encephalopathy, or wasting syndrome have the worst prognosis, with 75% dying before 3 yr of age. Persistent fever and/or oral thrush, serious bacterial infections (e.g., meningitis, pneumonia, sepsis), hepatitis, persistent anemia (<8.0 g/dL), and/or thrombocytopenia (<100,000/mm^3) also suggest a poor outcome, with >30% of such children dying before age 3 yr of age. In contrast, lymphadenopathy, splenomegaly, hepatomegaly, lymphoid interstitial pneumonitis, and parotitis are indicators of a better prognosis.

Prevention. Interruption of perinatal transmission from mother-to-child has been achieved by administering ZDV chemoprophylaxis to the pregnant woman (100 mg five times/24 hr PO, started as early as 4 wk of gestation) and continued during delivery (2 mg/kg loading dose IV followed by 1 mg/kg/hr IV) and in the newborn for the first 6 wk of life (2 mg/kg q 6 hr PO). In the developed world, such therapy has been documented to decrease the rate of perinatal HIV-1 transmission to <8%. Toxicity from ZDV therapy in both mothers and infants is minimal. Although this treatment was first given to untreated, asymptomatic, and immunologically intact women, epidemiologic data have confirmed the efficacy of ZDV chemoprophylaxis for reduction of perinatal transmission to offspring of women with advanced disease, low CD4 counts, and prior ZDV therapy. Rates of perinatal transmission have been as low as 2% among women who received HAART and all three components of the ZDV regimen, even in women with advanced HIV-1 disease. Even though this regimen is effective, it is logistically complex and expensive. A short-term regimen (300 mg twice daily from

36 wk gestation and 300 mg every 3 hr during delivery) offers a simpler, effective (almost 50% reduction in transmission), and less expensive regimen that can be used in areas where the long-term regimen is difficult to implement. Retrospective data suggest that even if a mother has received no antiretroviral therapy during gestation or delivery, the 6-wk component of the ZDV prophylactic regimen instituted for the newborn as soon as possible after delivery and preferably within 12–24 hr of birth results in a meaningful reduction of transmission rate. Full-term infants should be given ZDV at a dose of 2 mg/kg q 6 hr for 6 wk. For preterm infants, the dose should be 1.5 mg/kg orally or intravenously q 12 hr for the first 2 wk of life and then increased to 2 mg/kg q 8 hr.

A study evaluating the efficacy of oral nevirapine, a non-nucleoside reverse transcriptase inhibitor, given once to women in labor and once to the infant during the first 48–72 hr of life, capitalizes on the prolonged half-life of this drug. It has been shown to reduce perinatal transmission by 50% in Africa, providing a simple and highly cost-effective regimen for developing countries. Combinations of drugs more potent than ZDV are being used for treatment of HIV-1 infection in non-pregnant women; the role of these agents in prevention of perinatal transmission is under investigation. Decisions regarding use and choice of antiretroviral drugs during pregnancy are complex and require coordination between the HIV-specialist and the obstetrician. However, ZDV should be included as a component of all perinatal regimens, because ZDV is the only drug that has been demonstrated to prevent perinatal transmission.

Now that it is clear that perinatal transmission can be reduced dramatically by treating pregnant mothers, a compelling argument can be made for prenatal identification of HIV-1 infection in the mother. The benefit of therapy, both for the mother's health and to prevent transmission to the infant, cannot be overemphasized. The recommended universal prenatal HIV-1 counseling and HIV-1 testing with consent for all pregnant women has reduced the number of new infections dramatically in many areas of the United States. When risk assessment alone is used to decide which women warrant perinatal counseling and testing, a substantial number of women do not receive these services. For women not tested during pregnancy, the use of rapid HIV antibody testing during labor, or in the first day of life for the infant is a way to provide perinatal prophylaxis to an additional group of at-risk infants.

Prevention of sexual transmission involves avoiding the exchange of bodily fluids. In sexually active adolescents, condoms should be an integral part of programs to reduce sexually transmitted diseases. Unprotected sex with older partners or with multiple partners and use of illicit drugs is common among HIV-1–infected adolescents, which increases their risk. Educational efforts about avoidance of risk factors are essential for older school-aged children and adolescents and should begin before the onset of sexual activity.

American Academy of Pediatrics, Committee on Pediatric AIDS: Evaluation and medical treatment of the HIV-exposed infant. *Pediatrics* 1997;99:909–17.

Centers for Disease Control and Prevention: 1994 Revised classification system for human immunodeficiency virus infection in children less than 13 years of age. *MMWR* 1994;43:1–10.

Centers for Disease Control and Prevention: 1995 Revised guidelines for prophylaxis against *Pneumocystis carinii* pneumonia for children infected with or perinatally exposed to human immunodeficiency virus. *MMWR* 1995;44(RR-4):1–18.

Centers for Disease Control and Prevention: Revised guidelines for HIV counseling, testing, and referral. *MMWR* 2001;50:1–110.

Centers for Disease Control and Prevention: Revised recommendations for HIV screening of pregnant women. *MMWR* 2001;50:1–20.

Clapham PR, McKnight A: HIV-1 receptors and cell tropism. *Br Med Bull* 2001; 58:43–59.

Department of Health and Human Services (DHHS): Guidelines for the use of antiretroviral agents in HIV-infected adults and adolescents, 2000. HIV/AIDS Treatment Information Service (ATIS) website at *www.aidsinfo.nih.gov*

Emini EA (editor): The Human Immunodeficiency Virus: Biology, Immunology, and Therapy. Princeton, NJ, Princeton University Press, 2002.

Foster G, Williamson J: A review of current literature on the impact of HIV/AIDS on children in sub-Saharan Africa. *AIDS* 2000;14:275–84.

Goulder PJR, Jeena P, Tudor-Williams G: Paediatric HIV infection: Correlates of protective immunity and global perspectives in prevention and management. *Br Med Bull* 2001;58:89–108.

National Pediatric and Family HIV Resource Center (NPHRC) and Health Resources and Services Administration (HRSA): Guidelines for the use of antiretroviral agents in pediatric HIV infection, 2001. (Available at www.aidsinfo.nih.gov)

U.S. Public Health Service Task Force recommendations for use of antiretroviral drugs in pregnant HIV-1 infected women for maternal health and interventions to reduce perinatal HIV-1 transmission in the United States, 2002. *MMWR* 2002;51 (RR-18):1–38.

U.S. Public Health Service (USPHS) and Infectious Diseases Society of America (IDSA): 1999 USPCH/IDSA guidelines for the prevention of opportunistic infections in persons infected with human immunodeficiency virus. *MMWR Morb Mortal Wkly Rep* 1999;48(RR-10):1–59. (Available at *www.aidsinfo.nih.gov*)

Chapter 255
Human T-Cell Lymphotropic Viruses Types I and II

Hal B. Jenson

Human T-cell lymphotropic viruses type I (HTLV-I) and type II (HTLV-II), members of the *Oncovirinae* subfamily of the Retroviridae family, are single-stranded RNA viruses that encode reverse-transcriptase, an RNA-dependent DNA polymerase that transcribes the single-stranded viral RNA into a double-stranded DNA copy. The circular DNA is transported into the nucleus, where it is integrated into chromosomal DNA (provirus), evading the usual mechanisms of immune surveillance and resulting in lifelong infection. HTLV-I and HTVL-II both transform lymphocytes in vitro and share approximately 65% genome homology. Serologic assays used in early epidemiologic studies were unable to differentiate between the two viruses, but more recent Western immunoblot assays as well as polymerase chain reaction may be used to discriminate infection with these two viruses.

Epidemiology and Clinical Manifestations. HTLV-I was the first human retrovirus to be associated with cancer, as the cause of adult T-cell leukemia/lymphoma (ATL). HTLV-I is also associated with several nonmalignant conditions including the neurodegenerative disorder **HTLV-I-associated myelopathy (HAM),** also known as **tropical spastic paraparesis (TSP)** and currently termed HAM/TSP. The geographic epidemiology of ATL and HAM/TSP are similar. HTLV-I is endemic in southern Japan (where more than 25% of adults are seropositive), Asia, areas of the Caribbean, and in parts of sub-Saharan Africa and Central and South America. There is microclustering with marked variability within small geographic regions. The seroprevalence of HTLV-I and HTLV-II in the United States in the general population is 0.01% for each virus, with higher rates with increasing age. HTLV-I infection correlates greatest with birth from or sexual contact with persons from endemic areas of Japan or the Caribbean, with overall higher prevalence in females and African-American and Hispanic persons. HTLV-II infection correlates with intravenous illicit drug use, with an overall prevalence of approximately 18% in one study of drug users in the United States, often with concomitant HTLV-I or HIV infection.

HTLV-I and II are transmitted as cell-associated viruses through sexual contact, contaminated blood products, intravenous illicit drug use, and perinatally, usually via breast milk. Studies in Japan have shown that approximately 25% of children born to infected mothers become infected; more than 90% of HTLV-I–infected children have HTLV-I–infected mothers. Perinatal HTLV-I transmission occurs primarily via breast-feeding from infected mothers, with a threefold increased risk of transmission with breast-feeding for more than 6 mo. Intrauterine and intrapartum transmission probably account for less than 5% of vertical transmission. HTLV-II, like HTLV-I, may also be transmitted via breast-feeding but has a lower breast milk transmission rate of approximately 14%.

T-CELL LEUKEMIA/LYMPHOMA. The age distribution of ATL peaks at approximately 50 yr, underscoring the long latent period of HTLV-I infection. HTLV-I–infected persons remain at risk for ATL even if they move to an area of low HTLV-I prevalence, with a lifetime risk of ATL of 2–4%. HTLV-I infects CD4$^+$ lymphocytes with a spectrum of disease from subclinical lymphoproliferation that may spontaneously resolve in approximately half of cases, or progress to chronic leukemia, lymphoma, and culminate in acute ATL. Chronic, low-grade, HTLV-I–associated lymphoproliferation (pre-ATL) may persist for years with abnormal lymphocytes with or without peripheral lymphadenopathy before progressing to the acute form. Most cases of ATL are associated with monoclonal integration of HTLV-I provirus into the cellular genome. ATL is characterized by hypercalcemia, lytic bone lesions, lymphadenopathy that spares the mediastinum, hepatomegaly, splenomegaly, cutaneous lymphomas, and opportunistic infections. Leukemia may occur with circulating polylobulated malignant lymphocytes possessing mature T-cell markers, called flower cells. Conventional chemotherapy is not curative, and relapses are common, with median survival of 11 mo from diagnosis.

Sequences of the HTLV-I tax gene have been found in lesions of mycosis fungoides, a T-cell lymphoma characterized by proliferation of atypical lymphocytes preferentially in the skin. Patients are usually middle-aged and present with diffuse hypopigmented plaques and patches. Mycosis fungoides may be caused by HTLV-I or a closely related virus.

MYELOPATHY. HAM/TSP occurs in <1% of persons with HTLV-I infection, usually developing during middle age. It is characterized by gradual onset and slowly progressive neurologic degeneration of the corticospinal tracts and, to a lesser extent, the sensory system. Approximately 50% of patients with HAM/TSP have HTLV-I infection; other postulated causes include chronic intoxication of cyanogenic glycosides from the consumption of cassava or from amino acid dietary deficiencies.

HAM/TSP is more common in women than in men, and has a relatively short incubation period after HTLV-1 infection: 1–4 yr compared with 40–60 yr for ATL. Clinical manifestations include permanent evolution of lower extremity spasticity or weakness, lower back pain, and hyperreflexia of the lower extremities with an extensor plantar response. The bladder and intestines may become dysfunctional, and men may become impotent. Some patients may have dysesthesias of the lower extremities with diminished sensation to vibration and pain. Upper extremity function and sensation, cranial nerves, and cognitive function are usually preserved. The cerebrospinal fluid may have a mildly elevated protein and a mild monocytic pleocytosis. Neuroimaging studies are normal or show periventricular lesions in the white matter. Treatment with corticosteroids or danazol, a synthetic androgen, has been reported to benefit some patients.

HTLV-II. HTLV-II was originally identified in patients with hairy cell leukemia, although most patients with hairy cell leukemia are seronegative for HTLV-II infection. HTLV-II has been rarely isolated from patients with leukemias or with myelopathies resembling HAM/TSP, but there is limited evidence of disease specifically associated with HTLV-II infection.

Prevention. Routine antibody testing of all blood products using HTLV-I viral lysate began in the United States in 1988, which missed 30–58% of HTLV-II infections, but combination HTLV-I/II antibody testing was implemented in 1997. Formula feeding of infants of HTLV-I–infected mothers is an effective means to control endemic HTLV-I transmission in developed countries. No vaccine is available.

Bucher B, Poupard JA, Vernant JC, et al: Tropical neuromyelopathies and retroviruses: A review. *Rev Infect Dis* 1990;12:890–9.

Centers for Disease Control and Prevention: Recommendations for counseling persons infected with human T-lymphotropic virus, types I and II. *MMWR* 1993;42 (RR-):1–28.

Hollsberg P, Hafler DA: Pathogenesis of diseases induced by human lymphotropic virus type I infection. *N Engl J Med* 1993;328:1173–82.

Kaplan JE, Abrams E, Schaffer N, et al: Low risk of mother-to-child transmission of human lymphotropic virus type II in non-breast-fed infants. *J Infect Dis* 1992;166:892–5.

Manns A, Hisada M, La Grenade L: Human T-lymphotrophic virus type I infection. *Lancet* 1999;353:1951–8.

Manns A, Miley WJ, Wilks RJ, et al: Quantitative proviral DNA and antibody levels in the natural history of HTLV-I infection. *J Infect Dis* 1999;180:1487–93.

Van Dyke RB, Heneine W, Perrin ME, et al: Mother-to-child transmission of human T-lymphotropic virus type II. *J Pediatr* 1995;127:924–8.

Zucker-Franklin D, Kosann MK, Pancake BA, et al: Hypopigmented mycosis fungoides associated with human T cell lymphotropic virus type I tax in a pediatric patient. *Pediatrics* 1999;103:1039–45.

SECTION 12 *Protozoan Diseases*

Chapter 256
Primary Amebic Meningoencephalitis

Martin E. Weisse and Stephen C. Aronoff

Naegleria, Acanthamoeba, and *Balamuthia* are small free-living amebas that cause human amebic meningoencephalitis. Amebic meningoencephalitis has two distinct clinical presentations. The more common is an acute, usually fatal **amebic meningitis** that is caused by *Naegleria* and that occurs in previously healthy children and young adults. The second form, **granulomatous amebic meningoencephalitis**, is caused by *Acanthamoeba* and *Balamuthia* and is a more indolent infection that is more likely to occur in immunocompromised individuals.

Etiology. *Naegleria* is an ameboflagellate that can exist as cysts, trophozoites, and transient flagellate forms. Temperature and environmental nutrient and ion concentrations are the major factors determining which stage of the ameba is found in the environment. Trophozoites are the only stages that are invasive, although cysts are potentially infective because they can convert to the vegetative form very quickly under the proper environmental stimuli. There are several species of *Naegleria*, of which only *N. fowleri* has been shown to be pathogenic for humans.

In contrast to *Naegleria* organisms, *Acanthamoeba* has only a cyst and trophozoite form, of which only the trophozoite form is invasive. Of the 13 species of *Acanthamoeba*, 7 are human pathogens. *A. castellani, A. culbertsoni, A. polyphaga,* and *A. rhysodes* have all been recovered from human infections of both the eye and the central nervous system (CNS). *A. astronyxis* and *A. palestinensis* have only been implicated in CNS infections. *A. hatchetti* has only been isolated from the eye. Granulomatous amebic encephalitis from *Acanthamoeba* has been reported worldwide. Most of the cases reported have been associated with immunomodulating conditions such as HIV infection, diabetes mellitus, alcoholism, or radiation therapy. Cases of *Acanthamoeba* keratitis have usually followed incidents of corneal trauma involving flushing with contaminated water or have occurred in contact lens wearers whose lenses have been contaminated with *Acanthamoeba*.

In 1990 the ameba *Balamuthia mandrillaris* was isolated from the brain of a mandrill baboon that died of meningoencephalitis. On the basis of immunofluorescent staining results, this same organism has been implicated in 35 cases of granulomatous amebic encephalitis that had formerly been without definitive diagnosis but were attributed to *Acanthamoeba*. Although the clinical presentation is similar to infection with *Acanthamoeba*, most patients have no known immunocompromising condition.

Epidemiology. The free-living amebas have a worldwide distribution. *Naegleria* has been isolated from a variety of freshwater sources, including ponds and lakes, domestic water supplies, hot springs and spas, thermal discharge of power plants, and groundwater and occasionally from the nasal passages of healthy children. *Acanthamoeba* has been isolated from soil, mushrooms and vegetables, brackish water, and seawater, as well as most of the freshwater sources for *Naegleria*.

Naegleria meningoencephalitis was first reported in the United States in 1966, and since that time infection has been reported from every continent. Most of the cases have been contracted during the summer months by previously healthy individuals with a history of swimming in or contact with fresh water before their illness. Usually only 1–2 cases are reported per year in the United States, with a peak of 8 cases reported in 1980. Most of the reports have come from the southern and southwestern states, with occasional infections occurring in the Midwest and East.

Pathogenesis. The free-living amebas enter the nasal cavity by inhalation or aspiration of dust or water contaminated with trophozoites or cysts. *Naegleria* gains access to the CNS through the olfactory epithelium and migration via the olfactory nerve to the olfactory bulbs, which are located in the subarachnoid space bathed by the cerebrospinal fluid (CSF). This space is richly vascularized and is the route of spread to other areas of the CNS. In addition to evidence of widespread cerebral edema and hyperemia of the meninges, the olfactory bulbs are necrotic, hemorrhagic, and surrounded by a purulent exudate. Microscopically, the gray matter is the most severely affected, with severe involvement in all cases. Fibrinopurulent exudate may be found throughout the cerebral hemispheres, brain stem, cerebellum, and upper portions of the spinal cord. Pockets of trophozoites may be seen in necrotic neural tissue, usually in the perivascular spaces of arteries and arterioles. No cysts are present in the CNS.

The route of invasion and penetration in cases of granulomatous amebic meningoencephalitis, caused by *Acanthamoeba* and *Balamuthia*, is hematogenous, probably originating from a primary focus in the skin or lungs. Pathologic examination reveals granulomatous encephalitis, with multinucleated giant cells mainly in the posterior fossa structures, basal ganglia, bases of the cerebral hemispheres, and cerebellum. Both trophozoites and cysts may be found in the CNS lesions, primarily located in the perivascular spaces and invading blood vessel walls. The olfactory bulbs and spinal cord are usually spared.

Clinical Manifestations. The incubation of *Naegleria* infection may be as short as 2 days or as long as 15 days. Symptoms have an acute onset and are rapidly progressive. There is a sudden onset of severe headache, fever, nausea, and vomiting; signs of meningitis; and then encephalitis. Most cases end in death within 1 wk of onset of symptoms.

Granulomatous amebic meningoencephalitis may occur weeks to months after acquiring the organism. The presenting signs and symptoms are often those of single or multiple CNS space-occupying lesions; they include hemiparesis, personality changes, seizures, and drowsiness. Altered mental status is often a prominent symptom. Headache and fever occur only sporadically, but stiff neck is seen in a majority of cases. Palsies of the cranial nerves may be present. There is also one report of acute hydrocephalus and fever with *Balamuthia*. Results of neuroimaging studies of the brain usually demonstrate multiple low-density lesions resembling infarcts.

Diagnosis. The CSF in *Naegleria* infection may mimic that of herpes simplex encephalitis early in the disease and, later, of acute bacterial meningitis, with a neutrophilic pleocytosis, elevated protein level, and low glucose level. The amebas, which may be motile, may be seen on a wet mount of the CSF but are often mistaken for lymphocytes. A hanging drop examination of CSF and a strong clinical suspicion early in the course of disease affords the best chance for early treatment and cure. *Naegleria* can be grown on agar enriched with gram-negative bacteria, on which they feed.

In granulomatous meningoencephalitis, findings of examination of the CSF resemble those of aseptic meningitis. The isolation and identification of *Acanthamoeba* from the CNS are the best methods of diagnosis. Brain tissue and CSF may be cultured for *Acanthamoeba* using the same agar used for growing *Naegleria*, but *Balamuthia* must be grown on mammalian cell cultures. Pediatric cases of *Balamuthia* meningoencephalitis

have been diagnosed post mortem or by brain biopsy ante mortem. Immunofluorescence staining of brain tissue can differentiate between *Acanthamoeba* and *Balamuthia*.

Treatment. *Naegleria* infection is nearly always fatal, and early recognition and early treatment are crucial to successful therapy. There have only been six treatment survivors, five of whom apparently recovered fully. *Naegleria* infections have been successfully treated with regimens of amphotericin B, rifampin, and chloramphenicol; amphotericin B, oral rifampin, and oral ketoconazole; and amphotericin alone. The duration of treatment is uncertain.

Trophozoites and cysts from *Acanthamoeba* keratitis are usually susceptible in vitro to chlorhexidine, polyhexamethyl biguanide (PHMB), propamidine, pentamidine, diminazene, and neomycin, and especially to combinations of these drugs.

There is no satisfactory treatment for granulomatous amebic meningoencephalitis. Strains of *Acanthamoeba* isolated from fatal cases are usually susceptible in vitro to pentamidine, ketoconazole, flucytosine, and less so to amphotericin B. One patient has been successfully treated with sulfadiazine and fluconazole and another with intravenous pentamidine, topical chlorhexidine, and 2% ketoconazole cream, followed by oral itraconazole. Limited success has been demonstrated in *Balamuthia* infection with systemic azole therapy combined with flucytosine. Corticosteroids appear to have a detrimental effect, with rapid progression of disease, and should be avoided.

Denney CF, Iragui VJ, Uber-Zak LD, et al: Amebic encephalitis caused by *Balamuthia mandrillaris*: Case report and review. *Clin Infect Dis* 1997;25:1354–8.
Kidney DD, Kim SH: CNS infections with free-living amebas: Neuroimaging findings. *AJR Am J Roentgenol* 1998;171:809–12.
Seijo Martinez M, Gonzalez-Medeiro G, Santiago P, et al: Granulomatous amebic encephalitis in a patient with AIDS: Isolation of *Acanthamoeba* sp. Group II from brain tissue and successful treatment with sulfadiazine and fluconazole. *J Clin Microbiol* 2000;38:3892–5.

Chapter 257
Amebiasis
Chandy C. John and Robert A. Salata

Human infection with *Entamoeba* is prevalent worldwide; endemic foci are particularly common in the tropics, especially in areas with low socioeconomic and sanitary standards. *Entamoeba* parasitizes the lumen of the gastrointestinal tract and causes few or no symptoms or sequelae in most infected subjects. In a small proportion of individuals the organisms invade the intestinal mucosa or may disseminate to other organs, especially the liver.

Etiology. There are two morphologically identical but genetically distinct species of *Entamoeba* that commonly infect humans. *Entamoeba dispar*, the more prevalent species, is associated only with an asymptomatic carrier state. *Entamoeba histolytica*, the pathogenic species, can become invasive, causing symptomatic disease. Five other species of nonpathogenic *Entamoeba* infrequently colonize the human gastrointestinal tract: *E. coli*, *E. hartmanni*, *E. gingivalis*, *E. moshkovskii*, and *E. polecki*.

Infection is established by ingestion of parasite cysts, measuring 10–18 μm, that contain four nuclei. Cysts are resistant to environmental conditions such as low temperature and the concentrations of chlorine commonly used in water purification; the parasite can be killed by heating to 55°C. On ingestion, the cyst, which is resistant to gastric acidity and digestive enzymes, excysts in the small intestine to form eight trophozoites. These are large, actively motile organisms that colonize the lumen of the large intestine and may invade its mucosal lining under conditions that are currently unknown. Infection is not transmitted by trophozoites because of their rapid degeneration outside the body or in the low pH environment of normal gastric contents. Trophozoites have an average diameter of 25 μm, with a single spherical nucleus containing fine peripheral chromatin and a central nucleolus. The endoplasm also contains vacuoles, where, in cases of invasive amebiasis, erythrocytes may be seen.

Epidemiology. The regional prevalence of amebic infections worldwide varies from 5–81%, with the highest frequency in the tropics. Humans are the major reservoir. It is estimated that 10%, approximately 480 million people, of the population worldwide is infected with *E. dispar* or *E. histolytica*. This infection is associated with 50 million cases of symptomatic disease and an annual mortality of 40,000–110,000 deaths; amebiasis is the third leading parasitic cause of death worldwide. *E. dispar* is 10-fold more common than is *E. histolytica*. Symptomatic disease occurs in about 10% of individuals with *E. histolytica* infection. Therefore, invasive disease occurs in approximately 1% of persons determined to be infected with *Entamoeba* by light microscopy. Dissemination of the parasites to internal organs such as the liver occurs in an even smaller fraction of infected individuals and is less common in children than in adults.

Although highly endemic in Africa, Latin America, India, and Southeast Asia, amebiasis is not exclusively limited to the tropics. In the United States, amebiasis has been estimated to occur with a prevalence of 1–4% in certain high-risk groups, including chronically institutionalized persons, mentally retarded children, promiscuous homosexual males, emigrants from and travelers to endemic areas, migrant workers, and individuals in lower socioeconomic groups. Most children infected with *Entamoeba* fall into these risk groups.

Food or drink contaminated with *Entamoeba* cysts and direct fecal-oral contact are the most common means of infection. Untreated water and human feces used as fertilizer are important sources of infection. Food handlers carrying amebic cysts may, therefore, play a role in spreading the infection. Direct contact with infected feces also may be responsible for person-to-person transmission.

Pathogenesis. Trophozoites, which are responsible for tissue invasion and destruction, attach to the colonic mucosa by a galactose-specific lectin receptor. This receptor is also thought to be responsible for resistance to complement-mediated lysis. Once attached to the colonic mucosa, amebas release a cysteine-rich proteinase that allows for penetration through the epithelial layer. *E. histolytica* trophozoites require direct contact with target cells to cause cell death. Host cells are destroyed by trophozoite release of spore-forming peptides, phospholipases, and hemolysins. Once *E. histolytica* trophozoites invade the intestinal mucosa, they produce tissue destruction (ulcers) with little local inflammatory response because of the cytolytic capacity of the organism. The organisms multiply and spread laterally underneath the intestinal epithelium to produce characteristic flask-shaped ulcers. These lesions are commonly seen in the cecum, transverse colon, and sigmoid colon. Amebae may produce similar lytic lesions if they reach the liver; these lesions are commonly called abscesses, although they contain no granulocytes. The disparity between the extent of tissue destruction by amebae and the absence of a local host inflammatory response in the presence of systemic humoral (antibody) and cell-mediated responses remains a major scientific puzzle.

Clinical Manifestations. Clinical presentations range from asymptomatic cyst passage to amebic colitis, amebic dysentery, ameboma, and extraintestinal disease. To date, *E. dispar* has not been associated with symptomatic disease. *E. histolytica* infection is asymptomatic in 90% of persons, but it has the potential to become invasive and thus should be treated. Severe disease is more common in young children, pregnant women, malnourished individuals, and person using corticosteroids.

Extraintestinal disease usually involves only the liver, but rare extraintestinal manifestations include amebic brain abscess, pleuropulmonary disease, and ulcerative skin and genitourinary lesions.

INTESTINAL AMEBIASIS. Intestinal amebiasis may occur within 2 wk of infection or be delayed for months. The onset is usually gradual with colicky abdominal pains and frequent bowel movements (6–8/day). Diarrhea is frequently associated with tenesmus. Stools are blood stained and contain a fair amount of mucus with few leukocytes. Generalized constitutional symptoms and signs are characteristically absent, with fever documented in only one third of patients. Amebic colitis affects all age groups, but its incidence is strikingly high in children 1–5 yr of age. Severe amebic colitis in infants and young children tends to be rapidly progressive with frequent extraintestinal involvement and high mortality rates, particularly in tropical countries. Occasionally, amebic dysentery is associated with sudden onset of fever, chills, and severe diarrhea, which may result in dehydration and electrolyte disturbances. In a few patients complications such as ameboma, toxic megacolon, extraintestinal extension, or local perforation and peritonitis may occur.

Uncommonly, a chronic form of amebic colitis develops, which can mimic inflammatory bowel disease with bouts of abdominal pain and bloody diarrhea, often recurring over several years. An **ameboma** is a nodular focus of proliferative inflammation sometimes developing in chronic amebiasis, usually in the wall of the colon. Chronic amebiasis should be excluded before initiating corticosteroid treatment for inflammatory bowel disease.

HEPATIC AMEBIASIS. Hepatic amebiasis is a very serious manifestation of disseminated infection. Although diffuse liver enlargement has been associated with intestinal amebiasis, liver abscess occurs in less than 1% of infected individuals and may appear in patients with no clear history of intestinal disease. In children, fever is the hallmark of amebic liver abscess and is frequently associated with abdominal pain, distention, and enlargement and tenderness of the liver. Changes at the base of the right lung, such as elevation of the diaphragm and atelectasis or effusion, may also occur. Laboratory examination findings are a slight leukocytosis, moderate anemia, high erythrocyte sedimentation rate, and nonspecific elevations of hepatic enzyme (particularly alkaline phosphatase) level. Stool examination for amebae yields negative results in more than 50% of patients with documented amebic liver abscess. In most cases, CT, MRI, or isotope scans can localize and delineate the size of the abscess cavity. Most patients have a single cavity in the right hepatic lobe, although results of recent studies employing CT have shown an increased rate of multiple abscesses and left lobe involvement. Amebic liver abscess may be associated with rupture into the peritoneum or thorax or through the skin when diagnosis and therapy are delayed.

Diagnosis. Diagnosis is based on detecting the organisms in stool samples, sigmoidoscopically obtained smears, tissue biopsy samples, or, rarely, aspirates of a liver abscess. Examination of three fresh stool samples by experienced laboratory personnel has a sensitivity of 90% for detecting *Entamoeba*. Fresh stool samples should be examined within 30 min of passage and screened for motile trophozoites containing erythrocytes. Whenever amebiasis is suspected, an additional stool sample should be preserved in polyvinyl alcohol for further examination. Endoscopy and biopsies of suspicious areas should be performed when stool sample results are negative and the index of suspicion for amebiasis remains high. Unfortunately, unless phagocytized erythrocytes are seen, microscopy findings do not distinguish between *E. histolytica* and *E. dispar*. Patients with invasive amebic colitis have positive test results for fecal occult blood.

Various serum antiamebic antibody tests are available. Serologic results are positive in 95% of patients with symptomatic disease of more than 7 days and in most asymptomatic carriers of pathogenic strains of *Entamoeba. E. dispar* does not elicit a humoral response. The most sensitive serologic test, indirect hemagglutination, yields a positive result years after invasive infection. Antigen detection in stool or serum can establish a diagnosis while also distinguishing *E. dispar* from *E. histolytica*. Antigen detection tests are not yet routinely available.

Treatment. Two types of drugs are used to treat infection with *E. histolytica*. The luminal amebicides, such as iodoquinol, paromomycin, and diloxanide furoate, are primarily effective in the gut lumen. Metronidazole or other nitroimidazoles, chloroquine, and dehydroemetine are effective in the treatment of invasive amebiasis. All individuals with *E. histolytica* trophozoites or cysts in their stools, whether symptomatic or not, should be treated. The recommended regimen for treating asymptomatic cyst carriers is iodoquinol (30–40 mg/kg/24 hr divided tid PO for 20 days; maximum: 650 mg/dose). Paromomycin (25–35 mg/kg/24 hr divided tid PO for 7 days), a nonabsorbable aminoglycoside, is an alternative. Diloxanide furoate is only available through the Centers for Disease Control and Prevention (CDC). Toxicity is rare, but the drug should not be used in children younger than 2 yr of age.

Invasive amebiasis of the intestine, liver, or other organs requires the use of metronidazole (30–50 mg/kg/24 hr divided tid PO for 10 days; maximum: 500–750 mg/dose), a tissue amebicidal drug. Two related nitroimidazoles, tinidazole and ornidazole, are available and have been used outside the United States. Adverse effects of metronidazole include nausea, abdominal discomfort, and metallic taste; these are uncommon and disappear after completion of therapy. Metronidazole is also a luminal amebicide but is less effective for this purpose and should be followed by a luminal agent. Metronidazole-resistant *E. histolytica* has not been reported. Nevertheless, for fulminant cases, some experts suggest adding dehydroemetine (1 mg/kg/24 hr subcutaneously or IM, never IV), which is available only through the CDC. Patients should be hospitalized when dehydroemetine is given, and the drug should be discontinued if tachycardia, T-wave depression, arrhythmias, or proteinuria develops. Chloroquine, which concentrates in the liver, may be useful in the treatment of amebic hepatic abscess. Aspiration of large lesions or left lobe abscesses may be necessary if rupture is imminent or if the patient shows a poor clinical response 4–6 days after administration of amebicidal drugs.

Stool examination should be repeated every 2 wk until the result is negative after completion of antiamebic therapy to confirm cure.

Prognosis. Most infections evolve to either an asymptomatic carrier state or eradication. Death occurs in about 5% of persons having extraintestinal infection.

Prevention. Control of amebiasis can be achieved by exercising proper sanitary measures and avoiding fecal-oral contact. Regular examination of food handlers and thorough investigation of diarrheal episodes may identify the source of infection in some communities. No prophylactic drug or vaccine is available for amebiasis.

Adams EB, MacLeod IN: Invasive amebiasis: I. Amebic dysentery and its complications. *Medicine* 1997;56:315–23.
Haque R, Neville LM, Hahn O, et al: Rapid diagnosis of *Entamoeba* infection using *Entamoeba* and *Entamoeba histolytica* stool antigen detection kits. *J Clin Microbiol* 1995;33:2558–61.
Li E, Stanley SL: Protozoa, amebiasis. *Gastroenterol Clin North Am* 1996;25:471–92.
Merritt RJ, Coughlin E, Thomas DW, et al: Spectrum of amebiasis in children. *Am J Dis Child* 1982;136:785–9.
Nazir Z, Moazam F: Amebic liver abscess in children. *Pediatr Infect Dis J* 1993; 12:929–32.
Ravdin JI: Amebiasis. *Clin Infect Dis* 1995;20:1453–64.
Reed SL: New concepts regarding the pathogenesis of amebiasis. *Clin Infect Dis* 1995;21:S182–5.

Chapter 258
Giardiasis and Balantidiasis
Larry K. Pickering

258.1 *Giardia lamblia*

Giardia lamblia (also referred to as *G. intestinalis* and *G. duodenalis*) is a flagellated protozoan that infects the duodenum and small intestine. Infection results in a wide variety of clinical manifestations, ranging from asymptomatic colonization to acute or chronic diarrhea and malabsorption. Infection is more prevalent in children than in adults. *Giardia* organisms are endemic in areas of the world with poor levels of sanitation and also are an important cause of morbidity in developed countries, where they are associated with urban child-care centers, residential institutions for the mentally delayed, and waterborne and foodborne outbreaks. *Giardia* is a particularly significant pathogen in people with malnutrition, certain immunodeficiencies, and cystic fibrosis.

Etiology. The life cycle of *Giardia* is composed of two stages: trophozoites and cysts. *Giardia* infects humans after ingestion of as few as 10–100 cysts. Ingested cysts, which measure 8–10 μm, each produce two trophozoites in the duodenum. After excystation, trophozoites colonize the lumen of the duodenum and proximal jejunum, where they attach to the brush border of the intestinal epithelial cells and multiply by binary fission. The body of the trophozoite is teardrop shaped, measuring 10–20 μm in length and 5–15 μm in width. *Giardia* trophozoites contain two oval nuclei anteriorly, a large ventral disk, a curved median body posteriorly, and four pair of flagella. As detached trophozoites pass down the intestinal tract, they encyst to form oval cysts that contain four nuclei. Cysts are passed in stools of infected individuals and may remain viable in water for as long as 2 mo. Their viability often is not affected by the usual concentrations of chlorine used to purify water for drinking.

Giardia strains that infect humans are diverse biologically, as shown by differences in antigens, restriction endonuclease patterns, DNA fingerprinting, isoenzyme patterns, and pulsed-field gel electrophoresis. Differences in clinical manifestations and antimicrobial susceptibility patterns of various strains remain unknown.

Epidemiology. *Giardia* occurs worldwide and is the most common intestinal parasite identified in public health laboratories in the United States. *Giardia* infection usually occurs sporadically but is a frequently identified etiologic agent of outbreaks associated with drinking water. The age-specific prevalence of giardiasis is high during childhood and begins to decline after adolescence. The asymptomatic carrier rate of *G. lamblia* in the United States is estimated to be 3–7%, and as high as 20% in southern regions and in children younger than 36 mo of age attending child-care centers. Asymptomatic carriage may persist for several months.

Transmission of *Giardia* is common in certain high-risk groups, including children and employees in child-care centers, consumers of contaminated water, travelers to certain areas of the world, male homosexuals, and persons exposed to certain animals. The major reservoir and vehicle for spread of *Giardia* appears to be water contaminated with *Giardia* cysts, but foodborne transmission occurs. The seasonal peak in age-specific case reports coincides with the summer recreational water season and might be a result of the extensive use of communal swimming venues by young children, the low infectious dose, and the extended periods of cyst shedding that can occur. In addition, *Giardia* cysts are relatively resistant to chlorination and to ultraviolet light irradiation. Boiling is effective for inactivating cysts.

Person-to-person spread also occurs, particularly in areas of low hygiene standards, frequent fecal-oral contact, and crowding. Individual susceptibility, lack of toilet training, crowding, and fecal contamination of the environment all predispose to transmission of enteropathogens, including *Giardia*, in child-care centers. Child-care centers play an important role in transmission of urban giardiasis, with secondary attack rates in families as high as 17–30%. Children in child-care centers may pass cysts for several months.

Humoral immunodeficiencies including common variable hypogammaglobulinemia and X-linked agammaglobulinemia predispose humans to chronic symptomatic *Giardia* infection, suggesting the importance of humoral immunity in controlling giardiasis. There is no convincing evidence that patients with acquired immunodeficiency syndrome (AIDS) or selective immunoglobulin A (IgA) deficiency have more severe or prolonged disease. There is a higher incidence of *Giardia* infection in patients with cystic fibrosis, probably owing to local factors such as the increased amount of mucus, which may protect the organism against host factors in the duodenum. Human milk contains glycoconjugates and secretory IgA antibodies that may provide protection to nursing infants.

Clinical Manifestations. The incubation period of *Giardia* infection usually is 1–2 wk but may be longer. A broad spectrum of clinical manifestations occurs, depending on the interaction between *G. lamblia* and the host. Children who are exposed to *G. lamblia* may experience asymptomatic excretion of the organism, acute infectious diarrhea, or chronic diarrhea with persistent gastrointestinal tract signs and symptoms, including failure to thrive. Most infections in both children and adults are asymptomatic. There usually is no extraintestinal spread, but occasionally trophozoites may migrate into bile or pancreatic ducts.

Symptomatic infections occur more frequently in children than in adults. Most symptomatic patients usually have a limited period of acute diarrheal disease with or without low-grade fever, nausea, and anorexia; in a small proportion an intermittent or more protracted course characterized by diarrhea, abdominal distention and cramps, bloating, malaise, flatulence, nausea, anorexia, and weight loss develops (Table 258–1). Initially, stools may be profuse and watery and later become greasy and foul smelling and may float. Stools do not contain blood, mucus, or fecal leukocytes. Varying degrees of malabsorption may occur. Abnormal stool patterns may alternate with periods of constipation and normal bowel movements. Malabsorption of sugars, fats, and fat-soluble vitamins has been well documented and may be responsible for substantial weight loss.

Diagnosis. Giardiasis should be considered in young children in child care or in any person who has had contact with an index case or a history of recent travel to an endemic area who has persistent diarrhea, intermittent diarrhea and constipation,

malabsorption, crampy abdominal pain and bloating, or failure to thrive or weight loss.

A definitive diagnosis of giardiasis is established by documentation of trophozoites, cysts, or *Giardia* antigens in stool specimens or duodenal fluid. Several types of specimens from the gastrointestinal tract can be used to diagnose *Giardia* infection. For both trophozoites and cysts of *Giardia* organisms, identification can be made on direct smears of stool or after concentration of stool specimens. Stool specimens should be examined within 1 hr of passage or should be preserved in vials containing polyvinyl alcohol (PVA) or 10% formalin, both of which preserve parasite morphologic characteristics. Trophozoites may be present in unformed stools as a result of rapid bowel transit; they are not stable outside the gastrointestinal tract. Cysts are stable outside the gastrointestinal tract and are the infectious form.

In patients in whom the diagnosis is suspected but in whom examination of stool specimens for *Giardia* yields a negative result, aspiration or biopsy of the duodenum or upper jejunum should be performed. In a fresh specimen, trophozoites usually can be visualized by direct wet mount. An alternate method of directly obtaining duodenal fluid is the commercially available Entero-Test (Hedeco Corp, Mountain View, CA). The biopsy can be used to make touch preparations and tissue sections for identification of *Giardia* and other enteric pathogens, as well as to visualize changes in histologic features. Biopsy of the small intestine should be considered in patients with characteristic clinical symptoms, negative stool and duodenal fluid specimen findings, and one of the following: abnormal radiographic findings, such as edema and segmentation in the small intestine; abnormal lactose tolerance test result; absent secretory IgA level; hypogammaglobulinemia; or achlorhydria.

Medications, including antimicrobial agents, antacids, antidiarrheals, and enema and laxative preparations, can interfere with identification of the organism by altering their morphologic characteristics or by causing a temporary disappearance of parasites from stool specimens. Patients should not take these compounds for 48–72 hr before collection of stool for identification of *Giardia*. Contrast material such as barium also will mask the presence of parasites.

Appropriately conducted direct examination of stool will establish the diagnosis in up to 70% of patients by a single examination, 85% by examination of a second stool specimen, and more than 90% by examination of three specimens. Comparison of stool examination results with small bowel aspiration results in patients with diarrhea revealed that parasites were detected in 50% of stools of patients in whom a small bowel focus of infection was documented by aspiration. Laboratories can reduce reagent and personnel costs by pooling specimens submitted for detection of *Giardia* before evaluation by either microscopy or by enzyme immunoassay (EIA).

Efforts to improve diagnostic testing include the use of polyclonal antisera or monoclonal antibodies against *Giardia* organism–specific antigens in EIA or immunofluorescent assays. Polymerase chain reaction and gene probe–based detection systems specific for *Giardia* have been used in environmental monitoring.

Radiographic contrast studies of the small intestine may show nonspecific findings such as irregular thickening of the mucosal folds. Blood cell counts usually are normal. Giardiasis is not associated with eosinophilia.

Treatment. Children with acute diarrhea in whom *Giardia* organisms are identified should receive therapy. In addition, children who manifest failure to thrive or exhibit malabsorption or gastrointestinal tract symptoms such as chronic diarrhea should be treated.

Asymptomatic excreters generally are not treated except in specific instances such as in outbreak control, for prevention

TABLE 258–1.	Clinical Signs and Symptoms of Giardiasis
Symptom	**Frequency (%)**
Diarrhea	64–100
Malaise, weakness	72–97
Abdominal distention	42–97
Flatulence	35–97
Abdominal cramps	44–81
Nausea	14–79
Foul-smelling, greasy stools	15–79
Anorexia	41–73
Weight loss	53–73
Vomiting	14–35
Fever	0–28
Constipation	0–27

TABLE 258–2. Oral Antimicrobial Therapy for Giardiasis

Antiprotozoal Agent	Pediatric Dose	Adult Dose
Albendazole (Albenza)	400 mg once a day for 5 days PO	400 mg once a day PO for 5 days
Furazolidone (Furoxone)	6 mg/kg/24 hr divided qid PO for 10 days (maximum: 400 mg/24 hr)	100 mg qid PO for 10 days
Metronidazole (Flagyl)	15 mg/kg/24 hr divided tid PO for 5 days (maximum: 750 mg/24 hr)	250 mg tid PO for 5 days
Paromomycin	Not recommended	30 mg/kg/24 hr tid PO for 7 days (maximum: 1500 mg/24 hr)
Quinacrine* (Atabrine)	6 mg/kg/24 hr divided tid PO for 5 days (maximum: 300 mg/24 hr)	100 mg tid PO for 7 days
Tinidazole	50 mg/kg once (maximum: 2 g). Not available in the United States	2 gm PO once. Not available in the United States

Can be compounded by Medical Center Pharmacy in New Haven, CT (203-785-6818) or Panorama Compounding Pharmacy in Van Nuys, CA (800-247-9767).

of household transmission by toddlers to pregnant women and patients with hypogammaglobulinemia or cystic fibrosis, and in situations requiring oral antibiotic treatment where *Giardia* may have produced malabsorption of the antibiotic.

There are several drugs available in the United States that are effective in the treatment of patients with giardiasis, including albendazole, furazolidone, metronidazole, paromomycin, and quinacrine (Table 258–2). Tinidazole is used in other countries as single-dose therapy but is not available in the United States. Metronidazole is the treatment most often prescribed in the United States for adults. Furazolidone is less effective than metronidazole but is often prescribed in children because it is available in liquid form. Furazolidone is the only drug approved by the U.S. Food and Drug Administration for treatment of giardiasis. Quinacrine is effective and inexpensive but is not available from any U.S. manufacturer. Albendazole appears to be as effective as metronidazole with fewer adverse effects among children 2–12 yr of age and is effective against many helminths, making it useful for treatment when multiple intestinal parasites are identified or suspected. Paromomycin, a nonabsorbable aminoglycoside, is less effective than other agents but is recommended for treatment of pregnant women with giardiasis because of potential teratogenic effects of other agents. A combination of metronidazole and quinacrine has been used to treat refractory cases.

Prognosis. Symptoms recur in some patients, in whom reinfection cannot be documented and in whom an immune deficiency such as an immunoglobulin abnormality is not present, despite use of appropriate therapy. Several studies have demonstrated that variability in antimicrobial susceptibility exists among strains of *Giardia,* and in some instances resistant strains have been demonstrated. Combined therapy may benefit patients in whom infection persists after single-drug therapy, assuming reinfection has not occurred and the medication was taken as prescribed.

Prevention. Infected persons and persons at risk should practice strict handwashing after any contact with feces. This is especially important for caregivers of diapered infants in child-care centers, where diarrhea is common and *Giardia* organism carriage rates are high.

Methods to purify public water supplies adequately include chlorination, sedimentation, and filtration. Inactivation of *Giardia* cysts by chlorine requires the coordination of multiple variables such as chlorine concentration, water pH, turbidity, temperature, and contact time. These variables cannot be appropriately controlled in all municipalities and are difficult to control in swimming pools. People, especially children in diapers, should avoid swimming if they have diarrhea. People should avoid swallowing recreational water and drinking untreated water from shallow wells, lakes, springs, ponds, streams and rivers.

Travelers to endemic areas are advised to avoid uncooked foods that might have been grown, washed, or prepared with water that was potentially contaminated. Purification of drink-ing water can be achieved by a filter with a pore size of 1 μm or less or one that has been National Sanitation Foundation-rated for cyst removal, or by brisk boiling of water for at least 1 min. Treatment of water with chlorine or iodine is somewhat less effective but may be used as an alternate method when boiling or filtration is not possible.

258.2 Balantidiasis

Balantidium coli is a ciliated protozoan and is the largest protozoan that parasitizes humans. Both trophozoites and cysts may be identified in feces. Disease caused by this organism is uncommon in the United States and generally is reported where there is a close association of humans with pigs, which are the natural hosts of the organism. Because the organism infects the large intestine, symptoms are consistent with large bowel disease, similar to those associated with amebiasis and trichuriasis, and include nausea, vomiting, lower abdominal pain, tenesmus, and bloody diarrhea. Symptoms associated with chronic infection include abdominal cramps, watery diarrhea with mucus, occasionally bloody diarrhea, and colonic ulcers similar to those associated with *Entamoeba histolytica.* Extraintestinal spread of *B. coli* does not occur, and most infections are asymptomatic.

Diagnosis using direct saline mounts is established by identification of trophozoites (50–100 μm long) or spherical or oval cysts (50–70 μm in diameter) in stool specimens. Trophozoites usually are more numerous than cysts. The recommended treatment regimen is metronidazole (45 mg/kg/24 hr divided tid PO; maximum: 750 mg/dose) for 5 days, or tetracycline (40 mg/kg/24 hr divided qid PO; maximum: 500 mg/dose) for 10 days for persons 8 yr of age or older; an alternative is iodoquinol (40 mg/kg/24 hr divided tid PO; maximum: 650 mg/dose) for 20 days. Prevention of contamination of the environment by pig feces is the important means for control.

Adam RD: The biology of *Giardia* spp. *Microbiol Rev* 1991;55:706–32.

Brodsky RE, Spencer HC Jr, Schultz MG: Giardiasis in American travelers to the Soviet Union. *J Infect Dis* 1974;130:319–23.

Burke JA: Giardiasis in childhood. *Am J Dis Child* 1975;129:1304–10.

Centers for Disease Control and Prevention: Giardiasis surveillance. United States, 1992–1997. *MMWR Morbid Mortal Wkly Rep* 2000;49:1–24.

Craft JC, Holt EA, Tan SH: Malabsorption of oral antibiotics in humans and rats with giardiasis. *Pediatr Infect Dis J* 1987;6:832–6.

Davidson RA: Issues in clinical parasitology: The treatment of giardiasis. *Am J Gastroenterol* 1984;79:256–61.

Garcia LS, Shimizu RY: Evaluation of nine immunoassay kits (enzyme immunoassay and direct fluorescence) for detection of *Giardia lamblia* and *Cryptosporidium parvum* in human fecal specimens. *J Clin Microbiol* 1997;35:1526–9.

Gardner TB, Hill DR: Treatment of giardiasis. *Clin Microbiol Rev* 2001;14:114–28.

Morrow AL, Reves RR, West MS, et al: Protection against infection with *Giardia lamblia* by breastfeeding in a cohort of Mexican infants. *J Pediatr* 1992;121:363–70.

Ortega YR, Adam RD: *Giardia:* Overview and update. *Clin Infect Dis* 1997;25:545–9.

Pickering LK, Woodward WE, DuPont HL, et al: Occurrence of *Giardia lamblia* in children in day care centers. *J Pediatr* 1984;104:522–6.

Rauch AM, Van R, Bartlett AV, et al: Longitudinal study of *Giardia lamblia* infection in a day care center population. *Pediatr Infect Dis J* 1990;9:186–9.

Chapter 259
Spore-Forming Intestinal Protozoa *Patricia M. Flynn*

The spore-forming intestinal protozoa—*Cryptosporidium, Isospora, Cyclospora,* and microsporidia—have become increasingly important intestinal pathogens in both immunocompetent and immunocompromised hosts during the past decade. The severity of illness in HIV-infected patients and those with AIDS and improved diagnostic capabilities have helped elucidate the epidemiologic characteristics and clinical manifestations of these organisms. *Cryptosporidium, Isospora,* and *Cyclospora* are coccidian parasites that predominantly infect the epithelial cells lining the digestive tract. Microsporidia are ubiquitous, obligate intracellular protozoa that infect many other organ systems in addition to the gastrointestinal tract and cause a broader spectrum of disease.

CRYPTOSPORIDIUM

Initially, *Cryptosporidium* was thought to be pathogenic almost exclusively in immunocompromised persons. It is now recognized to be a leading protozoal cause of diarrhea in children worldwide and is a common cause of outbreaks in child-care centers.

Etiology. Infection with *Cryptosporidium parvum,* the cause of cryptosporidiosis in humans, is initiated by ingestion of infectious oocysts. The oocyst releases four sporozoites that invade enterocytes, primarily in the small intestine. The infection progresses through two stages: the asexual, which allows autoinfection at the luminal surface of the epithelium, and the sexual, which results in production of oocysts that are shed in the stools. The cysts are immediately infectious to other hosts or can reinfect the same host. Ingestion of very few cysts is required to produce infection, even in immunocompetent hosts.

Epidemiology. Cryptosporidiosis is associated with diarrheal illness worldwide and is more prevalent in developing countries and in children younger than 2 yr of age. It has been implicated as an etiologic agent of persistent diarrhea in the developing world and as a cause of significant morbidity and mortality from malnutrition, including permanent effects on growth.

Transmission of *Cryptosporidium* to humans can occur by close association with infected animals, via person-to-person transmission, or from environmentally contaminated water. Although zoonotic transmission, especially from cows, occurs in persons in close association with animals, person-to-person transmission is probably responsible for cryptosporidiosis outbreaks within hospitals and child-care centers, where rates as high as 67% have been reported. Recommendations to prevent outbreaks in child-care centers include strict handwashing, use of protective clothes or diapers capable of retaining liquid diarrhea, and separation of diapering and food handling areas and responsibilities.

Outbreaks of cryptosporidial infection have been associated with contaminated community water supplies and recreational waters in several states in the United States and in Great Britain. Wastewater, in the form of raw sewage, and runoff from dairies and grazing lands can contaminate both drinking and recreational water sources. It is estimated that *Cryptosporidium* oocysts are present in 65–97% of the surface water in the United States. The organism's small size (4–6 μm in diameter), resistance to chlorination, and ability to survive for long periods outside a host create problems in public water supplies. A waterborne outbreak in 1993 in Milwaukee, Wisconsin, caused more than 400,000 cases of diarrhea.

Clinical Manifestations. The incubation period is 2–14 days. Infection with *Cryptosporidium* is associated with profuse, watery, nonbloody diarrhea that can be accompanied by diffuse crampy abdominal pain, nausea, vomiting, and anorexia. Although less common in adults, vomiting occurs in more than 80% of children with cryptosporidiosis. Nonspecific symptoms such as myalgia, weakness, and headache also may occur. Fever occurs in 30–50% of cases. Malabsorption, lactose intolerance, dehydration, weight loss, and malnutrition often occur in severe cases.

In immunocompetent hosts, the disease is usually self-limiting, although diarrhea may persist for several weeks and oocyst shedding may persist many weeks after symptoms resolve. Chronic diarrhea is common in individuals with immunodeficiency, such as congenital hypogammaglobulinemia or HIV infection. Symptoms and oocyst shedding can continue indefinitely and may lead to severe malnutrition, wasting, anorexia, and even death.

Cryptosporidiosis in immunocompromised hosts is often associated with biliary tract disease, characterized by fever, right upper quadrant pain, nausea, vomiting, and diarrhea. It also has been associated with pancreatitis. Respiratory tract disease, with symptoms of cough, shortness of breath, wheezing, croup, and hoarseness, is very rare.

Diagnosis. Infection is best diagnosed by identifying oocysts in feces or other body fluids or tissues. In stool, they appear as small, spherical bodies (2–6 μm) and stain red when using modified acid-fast staining. Staining for *Cryptosporidium* should be specifically requested so that appropriate concentration and staining techniques can be employed. Because *Cryptosporidium* does not invade below the epithelial layer of the mucosa, fecal leukocytes are not found in stool specimens.

Because oocyst shedding in feces can be intermittent, several fecal specimens (at least three for an immunocompetent host) should be collected for microscopic examination. In addition to the modified acid-fast staining procedure, enzyme immunoassay, indirect immunofluorescence, and polymerase chain reaction testing are available. Serologic diagnosis is not helpful in acute cryptosporidiosis.

In tissue sections, *Cryptosporidium* organisms can be found along the microvillus region of the epithelia that line the gastrointestinal tract. The highest concentration usually is detected in the jejunum. Histologic section results reveal villus atrophy and blunting, epithelial flattening, and inflammation of the lamina propria.

Treatment. Because the diarrheal illness due to cryptosporidiosis is self-limited in immunocompetent patients, no specific antimicrobial therapy is required. Treatment should focus on supportive care, consisting of rehydration orally, or, if fluid losses are severe, intravenously.

Immunocompromised patients with severe cryptosporidial enteritis have been treated with a variety of antibiotics, none of which has been consistently effective. Nitazoxanide (100 mg bid PO for 3 days) was effective in children in Egypt; it is only available on an investigative basis in the United States. Combination therapy with paromomycin (1 g bid PO) and azithromycin (600 mg/day PO) for 4 wk followed by paromomycin monotherapy for 8 wk has also been used in adult patients with AIDS. Treatment with orally administered human serum immunoglobulin or bovine colostrum has been successful in several anecdotal reports.

ISOSPORA

Like *Cryptosporidium, Isospora belli* has been implicated as a cause of diarrhea in institutional outbreaks and in travelers and has also been linked with contaminated water and food. *Isospora* appears to be more common in tropical and subtropical climates and in developing areas, including South America, Africa, and Southeast Asia. *Isospora* has not been associated with animal contact. It is also an infrequent cause of diarrhea in patients with AIDS in the United States but may infect up to 15% of AIDS patients in Haiti.

The life cycle and pathogenesis of infection with *Isospora* species are similar to those of *Cryptosporidium* organisms except that oocysts excreted in the stool are not immediately infectious and must undergo further maturation below 37°C. Histologic appearance of gastrointestinal epithelium reveals blunting and atrophy of the villi, acute and chronic inflammation, and crypt hyperplasia.

The clinical manifestations are indistinguishable from those of cryptosporidiosis, although fever may be a more common finding. Eosinophilia, not found with other enteric protozoan infections, may be present. The diagnosis is established by detecting the oval, 22–33 μm long by 10–19 μm wide, oocysts by using modified acid-fast staining of the stool. Each oocyst contains two sporocysts with four sporozoites in each. Fecal leukocytes are not detected.

Unlike cryptosporidiosis, isosporiasis responds promptly to treatment with oral trimethoprim-sulfamethoxazole (TMP-SMZ) (5 mg TMP, 25 mg SMZ/kg/dose; maximum: 160 mg TMP, 800 mg SMZ/dose qid for 10 days, then bid for 3 wk). In patients with AIDS, relapses are common and often necessitate maintenance therapy. Ciprofloxacin, or a regimen of pyrimethamine alone or with folinic acid, is effective in patients intolerant of sulfonamide drugs.

CYCLOSPORA

Cyclospora cayetanensis is a coccidian parasite similar to but larger than *Cryptosporidium parvum*. Cyclosporiasis is endemic in Nepal, Peru, and Haiti but may be found throughout the world. The organism infects both immunocompromised and immunocompetent individuals and is more common in children younger than 18 mo of age. The pathogenesis and pathologic findings of cyclosporiasis are similar to those of isosporiasis. Asymptomatic carriage of the organism has been found, but travelers who harbor the organism almost always have diarrhea. Outbreaks of cyclosporiasis have been linked with contaminated food and water. After fecal excretion, the oocysts must sporulate to become infectious. This finding explains the lack of person-to-person transmission.

The clinical manifestations of cyclosporiasis are similar to those of cryptosporidiosis and isosporiasis and follow an incubation period of approximately 7 days. Moderate *Cyclospora* illness is characterized by a median of 6 stools/day with a median duration of 10 days (range, 3–25 days). The duration of diarrhea in immunocompetent persons is characteristically longer in cyclosporiasis than in the other intestinal protozoan illnesses. Associated symptoms frequently include fatigue; abdominal bloating or gas; abdominal cramps or pain; nausea; muscle, joint, or body aches; fever; chills; headache; and weight loss. Vomiting may occur. Bloody stools are uncommon. Biliary disease has been reported.

The diagnosis is established by identification of oocysts in the stool. Oocysts are wrinkled spheres, measure 8–10 μm in diameter, and resemble large *Cryptosporidium* organisms. Each oocyst contains two sporocysts, each with two sporozoites. The organisms can be seen by using modified acid-fast staining but stain less consistently than *Cryptosporidium*. They can also be detected with phenosafranin stain and by autofluorescence using strong green or intense blue under ultraviolet (UV) epifluorescence. Fecal leukocytes are not present.

The treatment of choice for cyclosporiasis, as for isosporiasis, is trimethoprim-sulfamethoxazole (5 mg TMP, 25 mg SMZ/kg/dose bid PO for 7 days; maximum: 160 mg TMP, 800 mg SMZ/dose). Ciprofloxacin is effective in patients intolerant of sulfonamide drugs.

MICROSPORIDIA

Microsporidia are ubiquitous and infect most animal groups, including humans. At least seven genera and unclassified organisms of the order Microsporidia have been linked with human disease in both immunocompetent and immunocompromised hosts. The microsporidian organisms best associated with gastrointestinal disease are *Enterocytozoon bieneusi* and *Encephalitozoon intestinalis*.

Little is known about the epidemiologic characteristics of these organisms, but they are likely similar to that of the other spore-forming intestinal protozoa. There have been recent reports of waterborne outbreaks. Unlike *Cryptosporidium* and the other protozoa, spores of microsporidia inject their contents into the host cell to establish infection. Intracellular division produces new spores that can spread to nearby cells, disseminate to other host tissues, or be passed into the environment via feces. Spores also have been detected in urine and respiratory epithelium, suggesting that some body fluids may also be infectious. Once in the environment, microsporidial spores remain infectious for up to 4 mo.

Microsporidial intestinal infection has been almost exclusively reported in patients with AIDS, but this finding may be due to the difficulty in diagnosing the infection. Microsporidia-associated diarrhea is intermittent, copious, watery, and non-bloody. Abdominal cramping and weight loss may be present; fever is unusual. Disseminated disease, involving liver, kidney, bladder, biliary tract, lung, bone, and sinuses, has been reported.

Microsporidia stain with hematoxylin-eosin, Giemsa, Gram, periodic acid–Schiff, and acid-fast stains but are often overlooked because of their small size (1–2 μm) and the absence of associated inflammation in surrounding tissues. Electron microscopy remains the reference method of detection, but success with modified trichrome stains and polymerase chain reaction is encouraging.

There is no proven therapy for microsporidial intestinal infections. *E. intestinalis* infection usually responds to albendazole (adult dose: 400 mg bid PO for 3 wk). Fumagillin (adult dose: 20 mg tid PO for 2 wk) was effective in a small controlled study. Atovaquone and nitazoxanide have also been reported to decrease symptoms, but controlled clinical trials have not been performed. Improvement in underlying HIV infection with aggressive antiviral therapy also improves microsporidiosis symptoms.

Chen X-M, Keithly JS, Paya CV, et al: Cryptosporidiosis. *N Engl J Med* 2002; 346: 1723–31.
Conteas CN, Berlin OG, Ash LR, Pruthi JS: Therapy for human gastrointestinal microsporidiosis. *Am J Trop Med Hyg* 2000;63:121–7.
Didier ES: Microsporidiosis. *Clin Infect Dis* 1998;27:1–7.
Franzen C, Muller A: Cryptosporidia and microsporidia—waterborne diseases in the immunocompromised host. *Diagn Microbiol Infect Dis* 1999;34:245–62.
Herwaldt BL: *Cyclospora cayetanensis*: A review, focusing on the outbreaks of cyclosporiasis in the 1990s. *Clin Infect Dis* 2000;31:1040–57.
Mota P, Rauch CA, Edberg SC: *Microsporidia* and *Cyclospora*: Epidemiology and assessment of risk from the environment. *Crit Rev Microbiol* 2000;26:69–90.
Okhuysen PC: Traveler's diarrhea due to intestinal protozoa. *Clin Infect Dis* 2001; 33:110–4.

Chapter 260

Trichomoniasis (*Trichomonas vaginalis*)

Chandy C. John and Robert A. Salata

Trichomonas vaginalis is a sexually transmitted protozoan parasite that primarily causes symptomatic vaginitis in women.

Epidemiology. An estimated 3 million American women have trichomoniasis each year; the occurrence in males is unknown. The incidence of trichomoniasis is highest among females with multiple sexual partners and in groups with the highest rates of other sexually transmitted infections. Thus, patients found to harbor *T. vaginalis* should be screened for other sexually transmitted infections. *T. vaginalis* is recovered from more than 60% of female partners of infected men and 30–80% of male sexual partners of infected women. Trichomonads can survive for several hours in moist environments, but no case of transmission by indirect exposure has been documented. Vaginal trichomoniasis is rare until menarche; diagnosis in a younger child should raise the possibility of sexual abuse.

Trichomoniasis may be transmitted to neonates during passage through an infected birth canal. Neonatal infection is usually self-limited, but rare cases of neonatal vaginitis and respiratory infection have been reported.

Pathogenesis. Infected vaginal secretions contain 10^1–10^5 or more protozoa/mL. In fresh preparations, *T. vaginalis* are highly motile and pear shaped and are most easily recognized by their characteristic twitching motility. The organisms reproduce by binary fission and exist only as vegetative cells; cyst forms have not been described. *T. vaginalis* activates the alternative pathway of complement, attracting polymorphonuclear neutrophils, which in turn can kill the protozoon. Monocytes and macrophages have been shown to kill trichomonads in vitro, but their role in natural infection is uncertain. Durable protective immunity does not occur.

Clinical Manifestations. The incubation period in females is 5–28 days. Symptoms may begin or exacerbate during menses. About 10–50% of women asymptomatically harbor the organism. Signs and symptoms most commonly associated with trichomoniasis include copious malodorous yellow vaginal discharge, vulvovaginal irritation, dysuria, and dyspareunia. On physical examination, a frothy discharge with vaginal erythema and cervical hemorrhages (**"strawberry cervix"**) may be seen. The vaginal discharge has a pH greater than 4.5. Unfortunately, none of these signs and symptoms alone or in combination is sensitive or specific enough to confidently establish a diagnosis of trichomoniasis. Abdominal discomfort is unusual and should prompt evaluation for pelvic inflammatory disease.

Most males carrying *T. vaginalis* are asymptomatic. The organism can be isolated in 5–15% of men with nongonococcal urethritis; these patients have symptoms that are indistinguishable from those of nongonococcal urethritis of other causes. Symptomatic males usually have dysuria and scant urethral discharge. Trichomonads occasionally cause epididymitis, prostatic involvement, and superficial penile ulceration. Infection in men is often self-limited, spontaneously resolving in 36% of men.

There is growing evidence that trichomoniasis is associated with poor pregnancy outcomes and gynecologic complications. In various studies, trichomoniasis has been shown to be associated with premature rupture of membranes, preterm labor, low birthweight, tubal infertility, and vaginal cuff cellulitis after hysterectomy. There is some evidence to suggest trichomoniasis increases the risk of HIV transmission.

Diagnosis. The accurate diagnosis of trichomoniasis in both sexes is dependent on the demonstration of the protozoan in genital secretions. Trichomonads may be recognized in vaginal secretions by using the wet mount technique, which will identify 60–70% of infected females. Endocervical specimens are unreliable for diagnosis. Wet mount examination of material obtained by platinum loop from the anterior urethra will reveal the organism in 50–90% of infected men. Microscopic examination of urine sediment after prostatic massage is also of high yield in infected men. A negative wet mount finding does not exclude the diagnosis of trichomoniasis. Culture of the organism is the most sensitive (>95%) method of detection, especially for asymptomatic carriers, but is not routinely available. Enzyme-linked immunosorbent assay and direct fluorescence antigen testing of vaginal secretions are more sensitive than wet mount

testing but less sensitive than culture for detection of *T. vaginalis* infection. DNA immunoblot and polymerase chain reaction testing of vaginal secretions appear to be highly sensitive and specific for detection of *T. vaginalis* infection but are not yet widely available.

Treatment. Trichomoniasis is treated with a nitroimidazole. In the United States, metronidazole is used; in other countries tinidazole or ornidazole has been used with similar efficacy. Numerous studies have substantiated the efficacy of metronidazole as a single large dose (2 g PO) in adolescent females; an alternative regimen is metronidazole, 250 mg tid PO, or 375 mg bid PO, for 7 days. All regimens are equally efficacious, eradicating more than 90% of *T. vaginalis* infections. The single-dose regimen is associated with more frequent gastrointestinal side effects, but it ensures compliance. The recommended regimen for infected children is metronidazole, 15 mg/kg/24 hr (maximum 1 g) divided tid PO, for 7 days. Topical metronidazole gel is not efficacious when used as the sole therapy for *T. vaginalis* infection, but it may decrease symptoms in individuals with severe infection when used in conjunction with oral metronidazole. All sexual partners should be treated simultaneously to prevent reinfection.

Meta-analyses suggest that metronidazole therapy is safe in the first trimester of pregnancy, and several studies have reported the safety of this drug in the last two trimesters. *T. vaginalis* infection in any trimester of pregnancy should be treated with the 2-g oral single-dose regimen for metronidazole.

The number of putative metronidazole failures appears to be increasing. In some cases, metronidazole-resistant *T. vaginalis* has been documented. In most cases, failure is a consequence of reinfection from an untreated sexual partner or of noncompliance with multidose therapy. Options for cases of truly metronidazole-resistant *T. vaginalis* infection include higher-dose metronidazole, tinidazole, and topical paromomycin. Tinidazole appears to be the most effective treatment for resistant infection, but it is not available in the United States; topical paromomycin is less effective and has been associated with severe local side effects.

Cotch MF, Pastorek JG, Nugent RP, et al: *Trichomonas vaginalis* associated with low birth weight and preterm delivery. *Sex Transm Dis* 1997;24:353–60.
Forna F, Gulmezoglu AM: Interventions for treating trichomoniasis in women. *Cochrane Database Syst Rev* 2000;CD000218.
Patel SR, Wiese W, Patel SC, et al: Systematic review of diagnostic tests for vaginal trichomoniasis. *Infect Dis Obstet Gynecol* 2000;8:248–57.
Petrin D, Delgaty K, Bhatt R, et al: Clinical and microbiological aspects of *Trichomonas vaginalis*. *Clin Microbiol Rev* 1998;11:300–17.

Chapter 261

Leishmaniasis (*Leishmania*)

Peter C. Melby

The leishmaniases are a diverse group of diseases caused by intracellular protozoan parasites of the genus *Leishmania*, which are transmitted by phlebotomine sandflies. Multiple species of *Leishmania* organisms are known to cause human disease involving the skin and mucosal surfaces and the visceral reticuloendothelial organs. Cutaneous disease is generally mild but may cause cosmetic disfigurement. Mucosal and visceral leishmaniasis is associated with significant morbidity and mortality rates.

Etiology. *Leishmania* are members of the Trypanosomatidae family and include two subgenera, *L. (Leishmania)* spp. and *L. (Viannia)* spp. The parasite is dimorphic, existing as a flagellate promastigote in the insect vector and as an aflagellate amastigote that resides and replicates only within mononuclear phagocytes of the vertebrate host. Within the sandfly vector the promastigote changes from a noninfective procyclic form to an infective metacyclic stage. Fundamental to this transition are changes that take place in the terminal polysaccharides of the surface lipophosphoglycan (LPG), which allow forward migration of the infective parasites from the sandfly midgut to the mouth parts, from which they are inoculated into the host during a blood meal. The metacyclic LPG also plays an important role in the entry and survival of *Leishmania* in the mammalian host by conferring complement resistance and by facilitating entry into the macrophage by way of complement receptor 1. Once within the macrophage the promastigote transforms to an amastigote and resides and replicates within a phagolysosome. The parasite is resistant to the acidic, hostile environment of the macrophage and eventually ruptures the cell and goes on to infect other macrophages. Infected macrophages have a diminished capacity to initiate and respond to an inflammatory response, thus providing a safe haven for the intracellular parasite.

Epidemiology. The leishmaniases are estimated to affect 10–50 million people in endemic tropical and subtropical regions on all continents except Australia and Antarctica. The different forms of the disease are distinct in their causes, epidemiologic characteristics, transmission, and geographic distribution. Localized cutaneous leishmaniasis (LCL) is caused by *L. (Leishmania) major* and *L. (L.) tropica* in North Africa, the Middle East, central Asia, and the Indian subcontinent. *L. (L.) aethiopica* is a cause of LCL and diffuse cutaneous leishmaniasis (DCL) in Kenya and Ethiopia. Visceral leishmaniasis (VL) in the Old World is caused by *L. (L.) donovani* in Kenya, Sudan, India, Pakistan, and China and by *L. (L.) infantum* in the Mediterranean basin, Middle East, and central Asia. *L. infantum* is also a cause of LCL (without visceral disease) in this same geographic distribution. *L. tropica* also has been recognized as an uncommon cause of visceral disease in the Middle East and India. In the New World, *L. (L.) mexicana* causes LCL in a region stretching from southern Texas through Central America. *L. (L.) amazonensis, L. (L.) pifanoi, L. (L.) garnhami,* and *L. (L.) venezuelensis* are causes of LCL in South America, in the Amazon basin, and northward. Members of the *Viannia* subgenus (*L. [V.] braziliensis, L. [V.] panamensis, L. [V.] guyanensis,* and *L. [V.] peruviana*) are causes of LCL from the northern highlands of Argentina northward to Central America. Members of the *Viannia* subgenus also cause mucosal leishmaniasis (ML) in a similar geographic distribution. VL in the New World is caused by *L. (L.) chagasi* (now considered by most taxonomists to be the same organism as *L. infantum),* which is distributed from Mexico (rare) through Central and South America. Like *L. infantum, L. chagasi* can also cause LCL in the absence of visceral disease. The leishmaniases may occur sporadically throughout an endemic region or may occur in epidemic focuses. With only rare exceptions, the *Leishmania* that primarily cause cutaneous disease do not cause visceral disease.

The maintenance of *Leishmania* in most endemic areas is through a zoonotic cycle in which humans are only incidentally infected. In general, the dermotropic strains in both the Old and New Worlds are maintained in rodent reservoirs, and the domestic dog is the usual reservoir for members of the *L. donovani* complex. The transmission between reservoir and sandfly is highly adapted to the specific ecologic characteristics of the endemic region. Human infections occur when human activities bring them in contact with the zoonotic cycle. Anthroponotic transmission, in which humans are the presumed reservoir, occurs with *L. tropica* in some urban areas of the Middle East and with *L. donovani* in India.

Over the past decade an increased number of cases have been reported from a number of long-standing endemic focuses, and large numbers of cases have been recognized in some new focuses. Severe epidemics with more than 100,000 deaths from VL have occurred in India and Sudan. The emergence of the leishmaniases in new focuses is the result of (1) movement of a susceptible population into existing endemic areas, usually because of agricultural or industrial development or timber harvesting; (2) increase in vector and/or reservoir populations as a result of agriculture development projects; (3) increase in anthroponotic transmission owing to rapid urbanization in some focuses; and (4) increase in sandfly density resulting from a reduction in malaria vector control programs.

Pathogenesis. Cellular immune mechanisms determine resistance or susceptibility to infection with *Leishmania*. Resistance is mediated by expansion of the T helper 1 (Th1) cell population, with interferon-γ production resulting in macrophage activation and parasite killing. Interleukin 12 (IL-12) plays a central role in the development of the protective Th1 response. Susceptibility is associated with expansion of IL-4–producing Th2 cells and/or the production of IL-10 and transforming growth factor-β, which are potent inhibitors of macrophage activation. Patients with ML exhibit a hyperresponsive cellular immune reaction that may contribute to the prominent tissue destruction seen in this form of the disease. Patients with DCL or active VL demonstrate minimal or absent *Leishmania*-specific cellular immune responses, but these responses resume after successful therapy.

Within endemic areas people who have had a subclinical infection can be identified by a positive delayed-type hypersensitivity response to leishmanial antigens (**Montenegro skin test**). Subclinical infection occurs considerably more frequently than does active cutaneous or visceral disease. Host factors (genetic background, concomitant disease, nutritional status), parasite factors (virulence, size of the inoculum), and possibly vector-specific factors (vector genotype, immunomodulatory salivary constituents) influence the expression as either subclinical infection or active disease. Within endemic areas the prevalence of skin test result positivity increases with age and the incidence of clinical disease decreases with age, indicating that immunity is acquired in the population over time. Individuals with prior active disease or subclinical infection are usually immune to a subsequent clinical infection.

Clinical Manifestations. The different forms of the disease are distinct in their causes, epidemiologic features, transmission, and geographic distribution.

LOCALIZED CUTANEOUS LEISHMANIASIS. LCL (**Oriental sore**) can affect individuals of any age, but children are the primary victims in many endemic regions. It typically presents as one or a few papular, nodular, plaquelike, or ulcerative lesions that are usually located on exposed skin, such as the face and extremities. Rarely, more than 100 lesions have been recorded. The lesions typically begin as a small papule at the site of the sandfly bite, which enlarges to 1–3 cm in diameter and may ulcerate over the course of several weeks to months. The shallow ulcer is usually nontender and surrounded by a sharp, indurated, erythematous margin. There is no drainage unless a bacterial superinfection develops. Lesions caused by *L. major* and *L. mexicana* usually heal spontaneously after 3–6 mo, leaving a depressed scar. Lesions on the ear pinna caused by *L. mexicana,* called **chiclero ulcer** because they were common in chicle harvesters in Mexico and Central America, often follow a chronic, destructive course. In general, lesions caused by *L. (Viannia)* spp. tend to be larger and more chronic. Regional lymphadenopathy and palpable subcutaneous nodules or lymphatic cords, the so-called **sporotrichoid** appearance, are also more common when the patient is infected with organisms of the *Viannia* subgenus. If lesions do not become secondarily infected, there are usually no complications aside from the residual cutaneous scar.

DIFFUSE CUTANEOUS LEISHMANIASIS. DCL is a rare form of leishmaniasis caused by organisms of the *L. mexicana* complex in the New World, and *L. aethiopica* in the Old World. DCL manifests as large nonulcerating macules, papules, nodules, or plaques that often involve large areas of skin and may resemble lepromatous leprosy. The face and extremities are most commonly involved. Dissemination from the initial lesion usually takes place over several years. It is thought that an immunologic defect underlies this severe form of cutaneous leishmaniasis.

MUCOSAL LEISHMANIASIS. ML (espundia) is an uncommon but serious manifestation of leishmanial infection resulting from hematogenous metastases to the nasal or oropharyngeal mucosa from a cutaneous infection. It is usually caused by parasites in the *L. (Viannia)* complex. Approximately half of the patients with mucosal lesions will have had active cutaneous lesions within the preceding 2 yr, but ML may not develop until years after resolution of the primary lesion. ML occurs in less than 5% of individuals who have, or have had, LCL caused by *L. (V.) braziliensis*. Patients with ML most commonly have nasal mucosal involvement and present with nasal congestion, discharge, and recurrent epistaxis. Oropharyngeal and laryngeal involvement is less common but associated with severe morbidity. Marked soft tissue, cartilage, and even bone destruction occurs late in the course of disease and may lead to visible deformity of the nose or mouth, nasal septal perforation, and tracheal narrowing with airway obstruction.

VISCERAL LEISHMANIASIS. VL (kala-azar) typically affects children younger than 5 yr of age in the New World (*L. chagasi*) and Mediterranean region (*L. infantum*) and older children and young adults in Africa and Asia (*L. donovani*). Elegant epidemiologic studies performed in Brazil have defined the clinical evolution of this disease. After inoculation of the organism into the skin by the sandfly, the child may have a completely asymptomatic infection or an oligosymptomatic illness that either resolves spontaneously or evolves into active kala-azar. Children with asymptomatic infection are transiently seropositive but show no clinical evidence of disease. Children who are oligosymptomatic have mild constitutional symptoms (malaise, intermittent diarrhea, poor activity tolerance) and intermittent fever; most will have a mildly enlarged liver. In most of these children illness will resolve without therapy, but in approximately one fourth it will evolve to active kala-azar within 2–8 mo. Extreme incubation periods of several years have rarely been described. During the first few weeks to months of disease evolution the fever is intermittent, there is weakness and a loss of energy, and the spleen begins to enlarge. The classic clinical features of high fever, marked splenomegaly, hepatomegaly, and severe cachexia typically develop approximately 6 mo after the onset of the illness, but a rapid clinical course over 1 mo has been noted in up to 20% of patients in some series. At the terminal stages of kala-azar the hepatosplenomegaly is massive, there is gross wasting, the pancytopenia is profound, and jaundice, edema, and ascites may be present. Anemia may be severe enough to precipitate heart failure. Bleeding episodes, especially epistaxis, are frequent. The late stage of the illness is often complicated by secondary bacterial infections, which frequently are a cause of death. A younger age at the time of infection and underlying malnutrition may be risk factors for the development and more rapid evolution of active VL. Death occurs in more than 90% of patients without specific antileishmanial treatment.

VL has been increasingly recognized as an opportunistic infection associated with HIV infection. Most cases have occurred in southern Europe and Brazil, but there is potential for many more cases as the endemic regions for HIV and VL converge. Leishmaniasis may also result from reactivation of a long-standing subclinical infection. Frequently there is an atypical clinical presentation of VL in HIV-infected individuals with prominent involvement of the gastrointestinal tract and absence of the typical hepatosplenomegaly.

A small percentage of patients who have previously been treated for VL will have diffuse skin lesions, a condition called **post–kala-azar dermal leishmaniasis (PKDL)**. These lesions may appear during or shortly after therapy (Africa) or up to several years later (India). The lesions of PKDL are hypopigmented, erythematous, or nodular and commonly involve the face and torso. They may persist for several months or for many years.

Diagnosis. The development of one or several slowly progressive, nontender, nodular, or ulcerative lesions in a patient who had potential exposure in an endemic area should raise suspicion of LCL. Other diseases that should be considered include sporotrichosis, blastomycosis, chromomycosis, lobomycosis, cutaneous tuberculosis, atypical mycobacterial infection, leprosy, ecthyma, syphilis, yaws, and neoplasms. Histopathologic analysis of the LCL lesion shows intense chronic granulomatous inflammation involving the epidermis and dermis. Occasionally, neutrophils and even microabscesses can be seen. The lesions of DCL are characterized by dense infiltration with vacuolated macrophages containing abundant amastigotes.

ML is characterized by an intense granulomatous reaction with prominent tissue necrosis, which may include adjacent cartilage or bone. Other infections such as syphilis, tertiary yaws, histoplasmosis, paracoccidioidomycosis, as well as sarcoidosis, Wegener granulomatosis, midline granuloma, and carcinoma may have clinical features similar to those of ML.

A definitive diagnosis of leishmaniasis is established by the demonstration of amastigotes in tissue specimens or isolation of the organism by culture. Amastigotes can be identified in Giemsa-stained tissue sections, aspirates, or impression smears in about half of the cases of LCL but only rarely in the lesions of ML. Serologic tests for diagnosis of ML or LCL generally have a low sensitivity and specificity and offer little for diagnosis. Culture of a tissue biopsy or aspirate, best performed by using Novy-McNeal-Nicolle (NNN) biphasic blood agar medium, yields a positive finding in only about 65% of cases. A positive culture result allows speciation of the parasite (usually by isoenzyme analysis by a reference laboratory), which may have therapeutic and prognostic significance. Identification of parasites in impression smears, histopathologic sections, or culture medium is more readily accomplished in DCL than in LCL.

VL should be strongly suspected in the patient with prolonged fever, weakness, cachexia, marked splenomegaly, hepatomegaly, cytopenias, and hypergammaglobulinemia who has had potential exposure in an endemic area. The clinical picture may also be consistent with that of malaria, typhoid fever, miliary tuberculosis, schistosomiasis, brucellosis, amebic liver abscess, infectious mononucleosis, lymphoma, and leukemia. In VL there is prominent reticuloendothelial cell hyperplasia in the liver, spleen, bone marrow, and lymph nodes. Amastigotes are abundant in the histiocytes and Kupffer cells. Late in the course of disease, splenic infarcts are common, centrilobular necrosis and fatty infiltration of the liver occur, the normal marrow elements are replaced by parasitized histiocytes, and erythrophagocytosis is present. Results of smears or cultures of material from splenic, bone marrow, or lymph node aspirations are usually diagnostic. In experienced hands, splenic aspiration has a higher diagnostic sensitivity, but it is rarely performed in the United States because of the risk of bleeding complications. Serologic testing by enzyme immunoassay, indirect fluorescence assay, or direct agglutination is very useful in VL because of the very high level of antileishmanial antibodies. An enzyme-linked immunosorbent assay (ELISA) using a recombinant (K39) antigen has a sensitivity and specificity close to 100%. A negative serologic test result in an immunocompetent individual is strong evidence against a diagnosis of VL. Serodiagnostic tests have positive findings in only about half of the patients who are co-infected with HIV.

Laboratory Findings. Patients with cutaneous or mucosal leishmaniasis generally do not have abnormal laboratory results unless the lesions are secondarily infected with bacteria. Laboratory findings associated with classic kala-azar include anemia (hemoglobin 5–8 mg/dL), thrombocytopenia, leukopenia (2,000–3,000 cells/μL), elevated hepatic transaminase levels, and hyperglobulinemia (>5 g/dL) that is mostly immunoglobulin G (IgG).

Treatment. Specific antileishmanial therapy is not routinely indicated for uncomplicated LCL caused by strains that have a high rate of spontaneous resolution and self-healing (*L. major, L. mexicana*). Lesions that are extensive, severely inflamed, or located where a scar would result in disability (near a joint) or cosmetic disfigurement (face or ear); that involve the lymphatics; or that do not begin healing within 3–4 mo should be treated. Cutaneous lesions suspected or known to be caused by members of the *Viannia* subgenus (New World) should be treated because of the low rate of spontaneous healing and the potential risk of development of mucosal disease. Similarly, patients with lesions caused by *L. tropica* (Old World), which are typically chronic and nonhealing, should be treated. All patients with VL or ML should receive therapy.

The pentavalent antimony compounds (sodium stibogluconate [Pentostam, Wellcome Foundation, United Kingdom] and meglumine antimoniate [Glucantime, Rhafone-Poulenc, France]) have been the mainstay of antileishmanial chemotherapy for more than 40 yr. These drugs have similar efficacies, toxicities, and treatment regimens. Currently, for sodium stibogluconate (available in the United States from the Centers for Disease Control and Prevention, Atlanta, GA) the recommended regimen is 20 mg/kg/24 hr intravenously or intramuscularly for 20 days (for LCL and DCL) or 28 days (for ML and VL). Repeated courses of therapy may be necessary in patients with severe cutaneous lesions, ML, or VL. An initial clinical response to therapy usually occurs in the 1st week of therapy, but complete clinical healing (re-epithelialization and scarring for LCL and ML and regression of splenomegaly and normalization of cytopenias for VL) is usually not evident for weeks to a few months after completion of therapy. Cure rates with this regimen of 90–100% (LCL), 50–70% (ML), and 80–100% (VL) can be expected. Lower initial cure rates have been noted in patients from regions where clinical resistance to antimony therapy is common, such as India, East Africa, or some parts of Latin America. Relapses are common in patients who do not have an effective antileishmanial cellular immune response, such as those who have DCL or are co-infected with HIV. These patients often require multiple courses of therapy or a chronic suppressive regimen. When clinical relapses occur, they are usually evident within 2 mo after completion of therapy. Adverse effects of antimony therapy are dose and duration dependent and commonly include fatigue, arthralgias and myalgias (50%), abdominal discomfort (30%), elevated hepatic transaminase level (30–80%), elevated amylase and lipase levels (almost 100%), mild hematologic changes (slightly decreased leukocyte count, hemoglobin level, and platelet count) (10–30%), and nonspecific T-wave changes on electrocardiography (30%). Sudden death due to cardiac toxicity is extremely rare and usually associated with use of very high doses of pentavalent antimony.

Several other therapies have been used increasingly in the treatment of the leishmaniases. Amphotericin B desoxycholate and the newer lipid formulations are very useful in the treatment of antimony-unresponsive VL or ML. Amphotericin B desoxycholate at doses of 0.5–1.0 mg/kg each day or every other day for 14–20 doses achieved a cure rate for VL of close to 100%,

but the renal toxicity commonly associated with amphotericin B was evident. The lipid formulations of amphotericin B are especially attractive for treatment of leishmaniasis because the drugs are concentrated in the reticuloendothelial system and are less nephrotoxic. Liposomal amphotericin B (3 mg/kg on days 1–5, and again on day 10) has been shown to be highly effective (90–100% cure rate) for treatment of VL in immunocompetent children, some of whom were refractory to antimony therapy. Treatment of VL with parenteral paromomycin has also shown some success, although it does not appear to be superior to either antimony or amphotericin B. Recombinant human interferon-γ has been successfully used as an adjunct to antimony therapy in treatment of refractory cases of ML and VL. It is not effective alone and has the frequent side effects of fever and flu-like symptoms. A phase II trial of miltefosine given orally at 50–150 mg/day for 4–6 weeks demonstrated a cure rate of more than 90%. Gastrointestinal side effects were frequent but did not require discontinuation of the drug. This may become the first oral drug that is effective in the treatment of VL. Pentamidine is an effective alternative treatment for LCL (especially in cases unresponsive to antimony) when given at 2–3 mg/kg every other day for four to seven doses. Treatment of ML and VL with pentamidine requires high doses and a long duration of therapy, making this drug less attractive than amphotericin B desoxycholate and the lipid formulations. Treatment of LCL with oral drugs has had only modest success. Ketoconazole has been effective in treating adults with LCL caused by *L. major, L. mexicana,* and *L. panamensis* but not *L. tropica* or *L. braziliensis.* Allopurinol has been used for many years in the treatment of CL, but recent controlled trials indicate that it is probably not effective as monotherapy. It may have a role as adjunct therapy with standard treatment regimens.

Prevention. Personal protective measures should include avoidance of exposure to the nocturnal sandflies and, when necessary, the use of insect repellent and permethrin-impregnated mosquito netting. Where peridomiciliary transmission is present, community-based residual insecticide spraying has had some success in reducing the prevalence of leishmaniasis, but long-term effects are difficult to maintain. Control or elimination of infected reservoir hosts (e.g., seropositive domestic dogs) has had limited success. Where anthroponotic transmission is thought to occur, early recognition and treatment of cases are essential. A number of vaccines have been demonstrated to have efficacy in experimental models; vaccination of humans or domestic dogs may have a role in the control of the leishmaniases in the future.

Alvar J, Canavate C, Gutierrez-Solar B, et al: *Leishmania* and human immunodeficiency virus coinfection: The first 10 years. *Clin Microbiol Rev* 1997;10:298–319.

Badaro R, Jones TC, Carvalho EM, et al: New perspectives on a subclinical form of visceral leishmaniasis. *J Infect Dis* 1986;154:1003–11.

Badaro R, Falcoff E, Badaro F, et al: Treatment of visceral leishmaniasis with pentavalent antimony and interferon gamma. *N Engl J Med* 1990;322:16–21.

Berman JD: Human leishmaniasis: Clinical, diagnostic, and chemotherapeutic developments in the last 10 years. *Clin Infect Dis* 1997;24:684–703.

di Martino L, Davidson RN, Giacchino R, et al: Treatment of visceral leishmaniasis in children with liposomal amphotericin B. *J Pediatr* 1997;131:271–7.

Dye C, Williams BG: Malnutrition, age, and the risk of parasitic disease: Visceral leishmaniasis revisited. *Proc R Soc Lond* 1993-254:33–39.

Jha TK, Sundar S, Thakur CP, et al: Miltefosine, an oral agent, for the treatment of Indian visceral leishmaniasis. *N Engl J Med* 1999;341:1795–1800.

Magill AJ, Grogl M, Gasser RA, et al: Visceral infection caused by *Leishmania tropica* in veterans of Operation Desert Storm. *N Engl J Med* 1993;328:1383–7.

Melby PC: Vaccination against cutaneous leishmaniasis: Current status. *Am J Clin Dermatol* 2002;3:557–70.

Sundar S, Murray HW: Cure of antimony-unresponsive Indian visceral leishmaniasis with amphotericin B lipid complex. *J Infect Dis* 1996;173:762–5.

Sundar S, Jha TK, Thakur CP, et al: Oral miltefosine for Indian visceral leishmaniasis. *N Engl J Med* 2002;347:1736–46.

Chapter 262

African Trypanosomiasis (Sleeping Sickness; *Trypanosoma brucei* complex) *Robert A. Bonomo and Robert A. Salata*

There are more than 66 million men, women, and children in close to 40 countries throughout sub-Saharan Africa who suffer from African trypanosomiasis, or sleeping sickness. The two forms of African trypanosomiasis are each caused by a protozoan parasite that causes a specific illness. One form, *Trypanosoma brucei gambiense*, causes a chronic infection lasting years and mostly affecting people who live in western and central Africa (**West African sleeping sickness**). A second form, *Trypanosoma brucei rhodesiense*, is an acute illness lasting several weeks and usually occurring in residents of eastern and southern Africa (**East African sleeping sickness**). Each year nearly 20,000–25,000 people are newly infected and 50,000 deaths from sleeping sickness occur. The greatest risk of contracting disease occurs in Uganda, Kenya, Tanzania, Malawi, Ethiopia, Zaire, and Botswana. It is at epidemic levels in Angola, the Democratic Republic of the Congo, Sudan, Cameroon, Ivory Coast, Tanzania, and Chad. In the Democratic Republic of the Congo, where 70% of the cases occur, the prevalence of African sleeping sickness has nearly reached that of AIDS. The length of time the insect vector is able to transmit disease is up to 6 mo, which is unappreciated. So far, 21 cases of East African sleeping sickness have been diagnosed in the United States since 1967.

Etiology. Human trypanosomiasis, or African sleeping sickness, is a vector-borne disease caused by a parasitic trypanosome that is transmitted to humans through the bite of a tsetse fly of the genus *Glossina*, which is found only in Africa. The range of the tsetse fly includes watercourses, lakes, forests, and the savanna.

The tsetse fly feeds on the blood of humans and wild game animals and penetrates intact mucous membranes or skin. Humans usually contract the East African form of disease *(Trypanosoma brucei rhodesiense)* when they venture from towns to rural areas to visit woodlands or livestock. Once inoculated in the skin, the trypanosomes proliferate and gradually invade all organs.

The West African form *(Trypanosoma brucei gambiense)* is usually contracted close to settlements. This latter form only requires a small vector population and thus will be particularly difficult to eradicate. The infective metacyclic forms of the trypanosomes possess no free flagella. After a period of local multiplication in the skin for 1–3 wk, long and slender forms can be seen in the peripheral blood; intermediate and stumpy forms also occur. These are flagellated forms with a well-developed undulating membrane. In the early stages of human infection, the organisms multiply rapidly in the blood and lymph nodes. They appear in waves in the peripheral blood, with each wave followed by a febrile crisis. The reappearance of another population of organisms in the blood heralds the formation of a new antigenic variant. Invasion of the central nervous system (CNS) occurs early in *T. brucei rhodesiense* infection but late in the Gambian form.

The insect intermediate vectors are species of the tsetse flies of the genus *Glossina*. Inside the flies, the organisms localize in the posterior part of the midgut, where they multiply for about 10 days and then gradually migrate anteriorly, where they attach to the walls of the salivary ducts and complete the final stages of development into the infective metacyclic forms. The life cycle within the tsetse fly takes 15–35 days.

Direct transmission to humans has also been reported, which occurs either mechanically through contact with the contaminated mouth parts of tsetse flies during feeding or congenitally to infants by way of the placenta of infected mothers.

Epidemiology. Trypanosomiasis is one of the major public health problems in Africa. Unfortunately, data regarding the true incidence of the infection are unreliable. Political unrest and social change create favorable conditions for the emergence and resurgence of trypanosomiasis. Epidemics in rural areas pose a serious handicap to developing communities. Human trypanosomiasis in Africa occurs primarily in the region between latitudes 15 degrees north and 15 degrees south, which corresponds roughly to the area where the annual rainfall creates optimal climatic conditions for *Glossina* flies.

T. brucei rhodesiense infection is restricted to the eastern third of the endemic area in tropical Africa, stretching from Ethiopia to the northern boundaries of South Africa; *T. brucei gambiense* occurs mainly in the western half of the continent's endemic region. African trypanosomiasis affects more than 1 million people.

The insect intermediate vector plays a major role in determining the epidemiologic pattern of trypanosomiasis. Several *Glossina* species transmit the infection in different parts of tropical Africa. *Glossina* captured in endemic foci show a low rate of infection, usually less than 5%. In the Rhodesian form, which usually has an acute and often fatal course, chances of transmission to tsetse flies are greatly reduced. However, the ability of *T. brucei rhodesiense* to multiply enormously in the bloodstream of humans and to infect other species of mammals helps to maintain its life cycle.

T. brucei gambiense infection usually has a chronic protracted course with very low levels of parasitemia. Because of low rates of infection in tsetse flies, the life cycle of the Gambian form necessitates close and repeated contact between humans and insects to permit frequent biting. *T. brucei gambiense* is found in a variety of animal reservoirs that may play an important role in the endemic nature of the Gambian form of infection.

Pathogenesis. The initial entry site of the organisms soon develops into a hard, painful, red nodule known as a **trypanosomal chancre**. Histologically, it contains long, thin trypanosomes multiplying beneath the dermis and is surrounded by a lymphocytic cellular infiltrate. Dissemination into the blood and lymphatic systems follows, with subsequent localization in the CNS. The histopathologic findings in the brain are those of meningoencephalitis, with increased cellularity of the pia-arachnoid owing to lymphocyte infiltration and perivascular cuffing. In chronic cases the appearance of **morular cells** (large, strawberry-like cells, supposedly derived from plasma cells) is the most characteristic finding.

A key feature of trypanosomiasis is the ability of the parasite to evade the immune system by antigenic variation. *T. brucei gambiense* regulates internal genetic switches to avoid immunologic attack by the host.

Clinical Manifestations. The clinical presentations vary not only because of the two subspecies of organisms but also because of differences in host response in the indigenous population of endemic areas and in newcomers or visitors. Visitors usually suffer more from the acute symptoms, but in untreated cases death is inevitable for natives and visitors alike. Symptoms usually occur within 1–4 wk of infection. Initially, these are nonspecific and include personality changes, weight loss, ataxia, fatigue during the day, and insomnia at night. The clinical syndromes of African trypanosomiasis are best described as the trypanosomal chancre, hemolymphatic stage, and meningoencephalitic stage.

TRYPANOSOMAL CHANCRE. The site of the tsetse fly bite may be the first presenting feature. A nodule or chancre develops in 2–3 days and within 1 wk becomes a painful, hard, red nodule surrounded by an area of erythema and swelling. Nodules are commonly seen on the lower limbs but sometimes also on the head. They subside spontaneously in about 2 wk, leaving no permanent scar.

HEMOLYMPHATIC STAGE. The most common presenting features of acute African trypanosomiasis occur at the time of invasion of the bloodstream by the parasites, 2–3 wk after infection. Irregular episodes of fever, each lasting 1–7 days, are the usual early feature, frequently accompanied by headache, sweating, and generalized lymphadenopathy. Attacks may be separated by symptom-free intervals of days or even weeks. Painless, nonmatted lymphadenopathy, most commonly of the posterior cervical and supraclavicular nodes, is one of the most constant signs, particularly in the Gambian form. A common feature of trypanosomiasis in whites is the presence of blotchy, irregular, nonpruritic, erythematous macules, which may appear any time after the first febrile episode, usually within 6–8 wk. The majority of macules have a normal central area, giving the rash a circinate outline. This rash is seen mainly on the trunk and is evanescent, fading in one place only to appear at another site. Examination of the blood during this stage may show anemia, leukopenia with relative monocytosis, and elevated levels of immunoglobulin M (IgM).

MENINGOENCEPHALITIC STAGE. Neurologic symptoms and signs are generally nonspecific, including irritability, insomnia, and irrational and inexplicable anxieties with frequent changes in mood and personality. Neurologic symptoms may precede invasion of the CNS by the organisms. In untreated *T. brucei rhodesiense* infections, CNS invasion occurs within 3–6 wk and is associated with recurrent bouts of headache, fever, weakness, and signs of acute toxemia. Tachycardia may be evidence of myocarditis. Death occurs in 6–9 mo as a result of secondary infection or cardiac failure.

In the Gambian form, cerebral symptoms can be expected to appear within 2 yr after the onset of acute symptoms. A general increase in drowsiness during the day and insomnia at night reflect the continuous progression of infection, which may be further evidenced by increasing anemia, leukopenia, and wasting of body musculature. Patients with chronic Gambian trypanosomiasis have an increased susceptibility to secondary infections.

The chronic, diffuse meningoencephalitis without localizing symptoms is the form commonly known as **sleeping sickness.** Drowsiness and an uncontrollable urge to sleep are the major features of this stage of the disease and may become almost continuous in the terminal stages. Associated signs and symptoms, including tremor or rigidity with stiff and ataxic gait, suggest involvement of the basal ganglia. Psychotic changes occur in almost one third of untreated patients.

Diagnosis. Definitive diagnosis can be established during the early stages by examination of a fresh, thick blood smear, which permits visualization of the motile active forms. In the bloodstream, the parasite can be detected using a variety of sensitive techniques: quantitative buffy coat smears and mini anion exchange resins are common examples. The **Card Agglutination Trypanosomiasis Test (CATT)** is of value for epidemiologic purposes and to screen for *T. brucei gambiense*. Dried, Giemsa-stained smears should be examined for the detailed morphologic features of the organisms. If a thick blood or buffy-coat smear yields a negative finding, a simple concentration method may help; 10 mL of heparinized blood is added to 30 mL of 0.87% ammonium chloride, the mixture is centrifuged at 1,000 g for 15 min, and the sediment is examined fresh or by staining dried smears. Aspiration of an enlarged lymph node can also be used to obtain material for parasitologic examination. For every positive result a sample of cerebrospinal fluid should also be examined for the organisms.

Treatment. The choice of chemotherapeutic agents for treatment depends on the stage of the infection and the causative organ-

isms. The hematogenous forms of both Rhodesian and Gambian trypanosomiasis are susceptible to the action of suramin, which is available as a 10% solution for intravenous administration. A test dose (10 mg for children; 100–200 mg for adults) should first be administered intravenously to detect the rare idiosyncratic reactions of shock and collapse. The dose for subsequent IV injections is 20 mg/kg (maximum: 1 g) administered on days 1, 3, 7, 14, and 21. Suramin is nephrotoxic; therefore, urine should be examined before each administration. The presence of marked proteinuria, blood, or casts is a contraindication to continuation of therapy with suramin. Pentamidine isethionate (4 mg/kg/24 hr IM for 10 days) is better tolerated than suramin.

If CNS invasion is present, melarsoprol should be used. Melarsoprol is an investigational arsenical compound with trypanosomicidal effects. It has been used outside the United States for the treatment of late hemolymphatic and CNS African trypanosomiasis. Treatment of children is initiated with melarsoprol 0.36 mg/kg/24 hr IV, with the dose gradually increased every 1–5 days to 3.6 mg/kg IV; treatment usually necessitates 10 doses (18–25 mg/kg total dose). Treatment of adults is by melarsoprol, 2–3.6 mg/kg IV for 3 days, and, after 1 wk, 3.6 mg/kg IV for 3 days, which is repeated after 10–21 days. Recommended guidelines suggest 18–25 mg/kg total over 1 month. Mild reactions such as fever and pains in the chest or abdomen may rarely occur immediately or very soon after administration. The most important and serious toxic effects are encephalopathy and, less commonly, exfoliative dermatitis.

Eflornithine has been reported to be effective in late-stage West African sleeping sickness or in instances where CNS involvement is suspected or present. It is more effective against *T. brucei gambiense* and variably effective against *T. brucei rhodesiense*. It is in short supply and is given as 400 mg/kg/24 hr divided q6h IV. The World Health Organization has contacted with a number of pharmaceutical corporations to produce and donate large quantities of eflornithine. Pentamidine has been used successfully as a prophylactic drug. A single injection of pentamidine (3–4 mg/kg IM) will provide protection against Gambian trypanosomiasis for at least 6 mo, although the effect against the Rhodesian form is uncertain.

Prevention. Currently, an effective vaccine or prophylactic therapy is not available. The control of trypanosomiasis in endemic areas of Africa depends on recognition, effective therapy of human infections, and control of the vector. This is complicated by the logistics of applying the available preventive measures in areas of political conflicts and massive population movements.

The World Health Organization and the Centers for Disease Control and Prevention have recommended several measures. Vector control programs to control *Glossina* is critical. The use of screens, traps, and sanitary measures is fundamental. Encouraging neutral colored clothing that is not attractive to the tsetse fly may reduce bites. Using serology and parasitologic methods, mobile medical surveillance of the population at risk by specialized staff is critical. The creation of referral centers for evaluation and treatment is needed. Ground spraying of insecticides, aerial spraying, and the use of cloth and live animal baits are successful. Transgenic techniques to restrict the ability of the tsetse fly to survive and transmit pathogens are also being developed.

Difficulties to be anticipated in the treatment of sleeping sickness are drug resistance and continued change in range of antigenic expression. Vector control strategies are potentially the most promising but most difficult to implement.

Allsop R: Options for vector control against trypanosomiasis in Africa. *Trends Parasitol* 2001;17:15–19.

Askoy S, Maudlin I, Dale C, et al: Prospects for control of African trypanosomiasis by tsetse vector manipulation. *Trends Parasitol* 2001;17:29–34.

Chapter 263

American Trypanosomiasis (Chagas Disease; *Trypanosoma cruzi*)

Robert A. Bonomo and Robert A. Salata

Chagas disease (American trypanosomiasis) is a zoonotic illness caused by the blood-sucking triatomine insects, or **kissing bugs,** that transmit the parasitic, hemoflagellate protozoan *Trypanosoma cruzi*. This illness is found only in the Western hemisphere. Chagas first described this illness in 1911 in a Brazilian child who had fever, anemia, and lymphadenopathy.

Etiology. There are nearly 20 species of *Trypanosoma*. Only 4 species infect humans: *Trypanosoma brucei rhodesiense* and *Trypanosoma brucei gambiense* (the agents of African sleeping sickness), *Trypanosoma cruzi* (the agent of Chagas disease), and *Trypanosoma rangeli*. *T. cruzi* has three recognizable morphogenetic phases: amastigotes, trypomastigotes, and epimastigotes. **Amastigotes** are the intracellular forms found in mammalian tissues and are spherical and have a short flagellum but form clusters of oval shapes **(pseudocysts)** within infected tissues. **Trypomastigotes** are the extracellular nondividing forms and are spindle shaped, are 20 μm long, and possess a large **kinetoplast,** which is a large complex mitochondrion containing DNA that stains darkly on routine smears. A flagellum arises from the blepharoplast and extends along the outer edge of the undulating membrane until it reaches the anterior end of the body. Trypomastigotes are found in blood and are responsible for transmission of infection to the insect vector and for cell-to-cell spread of infection. **Epimastigotes** are found in the midgut of the blood-sucking insects *Triatoma infestans, Rhodnius prolixus,* and *Panstrongylus megistus*. Epimastigotes multiply in the midgut and rectum of arthropods and differentiate into metacyclic trypomastigotes. Metacyclic trypomastigotes, the infectious form for humans, are released onto the skin of a human when the insect defecates close to the site of a bite. Hence, this is an infection caused by contamination, not inoculation. The trypomastigotes enter the skin or damaged mucous membranes and either enter host cells or are phagocytized by macrophages. Once in the host, they multiply intracellularly as amastigotes and are released into the host's circulation when the cell dies. The bloodborne trypomastigotes circulate until they enter another host cell or are taken up by the bite of another insect, completing the life cycle.

Epidemiology. Chagas disease is endemic in Mexico and South America, particularly Brazil, Argentina, Uruguay, Chile, and Venezuela. The World Health Organization estimates that Chagas disease affects close to 20 million people, primarily children and young adults. This insect-transmitted illness frequently is asymptomatic and is essentially untreatable, with infection persisting for life. Because of its prevalence, infection by *T. cruzi* is regarded as the most important endemic disease in South America. From 45,000–70,000 individuals die annually as a result of this infection. Up to 30% of persons with chronic *T. cruzi* infection will acquire symptomatic disease. It is still unclear how this parasitic protozoan escapes the immune system because antigenic variation is not reported.

Although reduviid insects can be found in warmer regions of the United States as far north as Maryland, cases of Chagas disease are extremely rare, owing to the higher standard of domestic housing. Most U.S. cases are associated with laboratory accidents. Approximately 100,000 immigrants living in the United States from endemic countries may be infected with *T. cruzi*, and several cases in immigrants have been reported in American cities.

T. cruzi infection is primarily a zoonosis. Humans are not absolutely required to maintain the parasite in nature. *T. cruzi* has been isolated from numerous species of animals (large sylvan reservoir). The vectors transmitting this disease are found in rural, wooded areas and become infected by ingesting blood from humans or animals that possess circulating trypomastigotes. Humans become infected when land in enzootic areas is opened up for agricultural or commercial purposes. As the natural reservoir is disrupted, vectors take up residence in domestic areas and establish a cycle of transmission to animals and humans.

The presence of reservoirs and vectors of *T. cruzi* and the socioeconomic and educational levels of the population are the most important risk factors in disease transmission to humans, which occurs by means of insect vectors. The arthropod vectors for *T. cruzi* are the reduviid insects, variably known as wild bedbugs, assassin bugs, or kissing bugs. Housing conditions are very important in the transmission chain; the incidence and prevalence of infection depend on the adaptation of the triatomids to human dwellings as well as the vector capacity of the species. The animal reservoirs of reduviid bugs are dogs, cats, rats, opossum, guinea pigs, monkeys, bats, and raccoons. In South America, uncontrolled deforestation, increased migration of infected humans from endemic to nonendemic areas, and the presence of domestic reservoir hosts facilitate spread.

Humans can be infected transplacentally, as occurs in 10.5% of infected mothers, causing congenital Chagas disease that is associated with premature birth, fetal wastage, and placentitis. Disease transmission may also occur through blood transfusions in endemic areas from asymptomatic blood donors. Seropositivity rates in blood donors from endemic areas are more than 20%. The risk of transmission through a single blood transfusion from a chagasic donor is 13–23%. Currently, blood in the southern United States is not screened for *T. cruzi*. Percutaneous injection as a result of laboratory accidents is also a documented mode of transmission. Oral transmission through contaminated food has been reported. Although breast-feeding is a very uncommon mode of transmission, women with acute infections should not nurse until they have been treated.

Pathogenesis. Although the pathogenesis of chronic Chagas disease is unknown, two main mechanisms have been proposed: (1) direct tissue destruction by the parasite and (2) development of an inflammatory reaction resulting from an allergic response to parasitic antigens absorbed by host cells or an autoimmune reaction resulting from shared antigens between host and parasite.

At the site of entry (puncture site), polymorphonuclear neutrophils, lymphocytes, macrophages, and monocytes infiltrate. *T. cruzi* are engulfed by macrophages and are sequestered in membrane-bound vacuoles. Parasite attachment and phagocytosis by macrophages are mediated by protease-sensitive receptors on the surface of the macrophage. Trypanosomes lyse the phagosome membrane, escape into the cytoplasm, and replicate. A local tissue reaction develops (the **chagoma**), and the process extends to a local lymph node. Blood forms appear next, and the process disseminates.

T. cruzi strains demonstrate selective parasitism for certain tissues. Most strains are myotropic, invading smooth, skeletal, and heart muscle cells. Attachment is mediated by specific receptors on the trypomastigotes that attach to complementary glycoconjugates on the host cell surface. Attachment to cardiac muscle results in inflammation of the endocardium and myocardium, edema, focal necrosis in the contractile and conducting systems, periganglionitis, and lymphocytic inflammation. The heart becomes enlarged, and endocardial thrombosis or aneurysm may result. Right bundle branch block is also common. Trypanosome parasites also attach to neural cells and reticuloendothelial cells. In patients with gastrointestinal tract involvement, myenteric plexus destruction leads to organ dilatation (megaesophagus and megacolon).

Immunologic mechanisms for control of parasitism and resistance are not completely understood. Despite strong acquired immunity, there is no parasitologic cure. Antigenic variation that is typical of African trypanosomiasis is not seen with American trypanosomiasis. Antibodies involved with resistance to *T. cruzi* are related to the phase of infection. Immunoglobulin G (IgG) antibodies, probably to several major surface antigens, mediate immunophagocytosis of the parasite by macrophages. Conditions associated with depression of cell-mediated immunity increase the severity of infection with *T. cruzi*. Macrophages probably play a major role in protection against *T. cruzi* infection, especially in the acute phase. Interferon-γ stimulates macrophage killing of amastigotes through oxidative mechanisms.

Clinical Manifestations. Chagas disease occurs in acute and chronic forms. **Acute Chagas disease** in children is usually asymptomatic or is associated with a mild febrile illness characterized by malaise, facial edema, and lymphadenopathy. Infants often demonstrate local signs of inflammation at the site of parasite entry (chagomas). Approximately 50% of children come to medical attention with Romaña sign (unilateral, painless eye swelling), conjunctivitis, and preauricular lymphadenitis. Patients complain of fatigue and headache. Fever can persist for 4–5 wk. More severe systemic presentations can occur in children younger than 2 yr of age and include lymphadenopathy, hepatosplenomegaly, and meningoencephalitis. A cutaneous morbilliform eruption can accompany the acute syndrome. Anemia, lymphocytosis, hepatitis, and thrombocytopenia have been described.

The heart, central nervous system, peripheral nerve ganglia, and reticuloendothelial system are often heavily parasitized. The heart is the primary target organ. The intense parasitism can result in acute inflammation and in four-chamber cardiac dilatation. Diffuse myocarditis and inflammation of the conduction system lead to the development of fibrosis. Histologic examination reveals the characteristic pseudocysts, which are the intracellular aggregates of amastigotes.

Intrauterine infection in pregnant women can cause spontaneous abortion or premature birth. In children with congenital infection, severe anemia, hepatosplenomegaly, jaundice, and convulsions can mimic congenital cytomegalovirus infection, toxoplasmosis, and erythroblastosis fetalis. *T. cruzi* can be visualized in the cerebrospinal fluid in meningoencephalitis. Children usually undergo spontaneous remission in 8–12 wk and enter an indeterminate phase with lifelong low-grade parasitemia and development of antibodies to many *T. cruzi* cell surface antigens. Mortality rate is 5–10%; deaths are caused by acute myocarditis with resultant heart failure, or meningoencephalitis. Acute Chagas disease must be differentiated from malaria, schistosomiasis, visceral leishmaniasis, brucellosis, typhoid fever, and infectious mononucleosis.

Chronic Chagas disease may be asymptomatic or symptomatic. The most common presentation of chronic *T. cruzi* infection is cardiomyopathy, manifested by congestive heart failure, arrhythmia, and thromboembolic events. Abnormalities detected electrocardiographically include partial or complete atrioventricular block and right bundle branch block. Left bundle branch block is unusual. Pathologic examination of infected heart muscle reveals muscle atrophy, myonecrosis, myocytolysis, fibrosis, and lymphocytic infiltration. Myocardial infarction has been reported and may be secondary to left apical aneurysm embolization or necrotizing arteriolitis of the microvasculature. Left ventricular apical aneurysms are pathognomonic of chronic chagasic cardiomyopathy.

Autonomic nervous system abnormalities have also been implicated in Chagas cardiomyopathy. The reduction in acetylcholine and choline acetyltransferase levels in experimental *T. cruzi* infection lends support to this notion.

Autoimmune abnormalities have been reported in Chagas cardiomyopathy. Depletion of CD8 cells accelerates infection. *T. cruzi*–infected human peripheral blood mononuclear and endothelial cells synthesize increased levels of interleukin 1β (IL-1β), IL-6, and tumor necrosis factor (TNF). These cytokines result in increasing leukocyte recruitment and smooth muscle cell proliferation, which may be responsible for some of the manifestations of the disease. Viral myocarditis, rheumatic heart disease, and endomyocardial fibrosis can mimic chronic chagasic cardiomyopathy.

The gastrointestinal manifestations of chronic Chagas disease occur in 8–10% of patients and involve a diminution in Auerbach plexus and Meissner plexus. There are also preganglionic lesions and a reduction in the number of dorsal motor nuclear cells of the vagus nerve. Characteristically, this involvement presents clinically as megaesophagus and megacolon. Sigmoid dilatation, volvulus, and fecalomas are often found in megacolon. Loss of ganglia in the esophagus results in abnormal dilatation (megaesophagus); the esophagus can reach up to 26 times its normal weight and hold up to 2 L of excess fluid. Megaesophagus presents as dysphagia, odynophagia, and cough. Esophageal body abnormalities occur independently of lower esophageal dysfunction. Megaesophagus can lead to esophagitis and cancer of the esophagus. Aspiration pneumonia and pulmonary tuberculosis are more common in patients with megaesophagus.

Autonomic dysfunction and peripheral neuropathy can occur. Central nervous system involvement in Chagas disease is uncommon. If granulomatous encephalitis occurs in the acute infection it is usually fatal.

IMMUNOCOMPROMISED PERSONS. *T. cruzi* infections in immunocompromised persons are caused by transmission from an asymptomatic donor of blood products or activation of prior infection by immunosuppression. Organ donation to allograft recipients can result in a devastating form of the illness. Cardiac transplantation for Chagas cardiomyopathy has resulted in reactivation, despite prophylaxis and postoperative treatment with benznidazole. HIV infection also leads to reactivation; cerebral lesions are more common in these patients and can mimic those of toxoplasmic encephalitis. In immunocompromised patients at risk for reactivation, serologic testing and close monitoring are necessary.

Diagnosis. A careful history with attention to geographic origin and travel is important. Microscopic examination of a fresh preparation of a peripheral blood smear or a Giemsa-stained smear during the acute phase of illness will demonstrate motile trypanosomes, which is diagnostic for Chagas disease. These are only seen in the peripheral blood in the first 6–12 wk of the illness. Buffy coat smears may improve yield.

Most persons seek medical attention during the chronic phase of the disease, when parasites are not found in the bloodstream and clinical symptoms are not diagnostic. Serologic testing is also a good means of diagnosis. Complement fixation is considered the most reliable immunodiagnostic method for establishing the diagnosis. Specific IgM antibodies can be detected using an enzyme-linked immunosorbent assay (ELISA) and indirect fluorescent antibody test. Indirect fluorescent antibody testing is also very accurate and can be used to distinguish acute chagasic infection, with IgM antibodies, from chronic infection, with only IgG antibodies. These tests are available from the Centers for Disease Control and Prevention (CDC). Because false-positive reactions can result from other infections (e.g., malaria, syphilis, and leishmaniasis), it is recommended that a minimum of two independent serologic tests be performed.

Nonimmunologic methods of diagnosis are also available. Mouse inoculation has been used when repeated peripheral smear results are negative. Xenodiagnosis, allowing uninfected reduviid bugs to feed on a patient's blood and examining the intestinal contents of those bugs 30 days after the meal, detects 100% of cases. Detection assays using polymerase chain reaction (PCR) amplification of nuclear and kinetoplast DNA (kDNA) sequences are in development. Parasites may be cultivated in Nicole-Novy-MacNeal (NNN) media. PCR has a sensitivity of 96–100% and is able to detect a single parasite in 20 mL of blood. Chemiluminescent ELISAs are being developed and are also reported to be highly sensitive and specific.

Treatment. Drug treatment for *T. cruzi* infection is generally limited to two drugs: nifurtimox and benznidazole. Both are effective against trypomastigotes and amastigotes and have been used to eradicate parasites in the acute stages of infection. The results vary according to the phase of Chagas disease, the period of treatment, the dose, the age of the patient, and the geographic origin of the patient. Neither drug is safe in pregnancy.

Nifurtimox has been used most extensively, but whether it is effective in the chronic phase of the illness is uncertain. The treatment regimen for children 1–10 yr of age is 15–20 mg/kg/24 hr divided qid PO for 90 days; for children, 11–16 yr of age, 12.5–15 mg/kg/24 hr divided qid PO for 90 days; and for children older than 16 yr of age, 8–10 mg/kg/24 hr divided tid–qid PO for 90–120 days. Nifurtimox interferes with the carbohydrate metabolism of the parasite by disrupting pyruvic acid synthesis. Because *T. cruzi* is partially deficient in free radical detoxification mechanisms it is susceptible to such intermediates. Nifurtimox has been associated with weakness, anorexia, gastrointestinal disturbances, toxic hepatitis, tremors, seizures, and hemolysis in patients with glucose-6-phosphate dehydrogenase (G6PD) deficiency. The mode of action of nifurtimox involves generation of nitro-anion radicals by nitroreductases that lead to reactive intermediates. Nifurtimox is available from the CDC.

Benznidazole is a nitroimidazole derivative that is also used and may be more effective than nifurtimox. The mode of action of benznidazole is more complex than that of nifurtimox. The recommended treatment regimen for children younger than 12 yr of age is 10 mg/kg/24 hr divided bid PO for 60 days, and for those 12 yr of age or older, 5–7 mg/kg/24 hr PO for 60 days. In one randomized, double-blind, placebo-controlled trial in a rural area of Brazil, a 60-day course of benznidazole was studied in the treatment of early chronic phase *T. cruzi* infection in schoolchildren 7–12 yr of age. The efficacy of benznidazole was 55.8% in producing negative seroconversion. This drug is also associated with significant toxicities, including rash, photosensitivity, peripheral neuritis, and granulocytopenia and thrombocytopenia. Of some concern are the reports that detail the development of lymphomas in laboratory animals treated with benznidazole. This finding has not been reported in humans.

Regardless of the clinical status or the time elapsed since infection, patients with chronic asymptomatic Chagas disease should be treated with nifurtimox or benznidazole. Nitroimidazolic derivatives substantially reduced and significantly modified parasite related outcomes compared with placebo. Benznidazole has the greatest effect. It is yet unclear if recombinant interferon-γ should be used in immunocompromised patients.

A number of other agents have also been tried. Allopurinol, a drug that inhibits hypoxanthine oxidase, has also been used and has been shown to reduce parasitemia. It is ineffective in the acute phase. Many other drugs that are directed against novel targets are in experimental trials.

Biochemical differences between the metabolism of American trypanosomes and that of mammalian hosts may be exploited for chemotherapy. These trypanosomes are very sensitive to oxidative radicals, and they do not possess catalase or glutathione reductase/glutathione peroxidase, which are key enzymes in scavenging free radicals. All trypanosomes also have an unusual reduced nicotinamide-adenine dinucleotide phosphate (NADPH)–dependent disulfide reductase. For this reason, drugs that stimulate H_2O_2 generation or prevent its utilization are potential trypanocidal agents.

Treatment of heart failure and arrhythmia, as well as prevention of thromboembolism, requires the use of diuretics, antiarrhythmics, and anticoagulants. Digitalis toxicity occurs frequently in patients with Chagas cardiomyopathy. Pacemakers may be necessary in cases of severe heart block. A light, balanced diet is recommended for megaesophagus. Surgery or dilation of the lower esophageal sphincter treats megaesophagus; pneumatic dilation is the superior mode of therapy. Nitrates and nifedipine have been used to reduce lower esophageal sphincter pressure in patients with megaesophagus. Treatment of megacolon is surgical and symptomatic. Treatment of meningoencephalitis is also supportive.

In accidental infection when parasitic penetration is certain, treatment should be immediately initiated and continued for 10–15 days. Blood is usually collected and serologic samples tested for seroconversion at 15, 30, and 60 days.

Prevention. No vaccine or prophylactic therapy is available. Education of residents in endemic areas, use of bed nets, use of insecticides such as dieldrin or lindane, and destruction of adobe houses that harbor reduviid bugs are effective methods to control the bug population. Synthetic pyrethroid insecticides help keep houses free of vectors for 2 yr and have low toxicity for humans. Paints incorporating insecticides have also been used. Vaccine development has been fruitless. Prophylactic therapy with nifurtimox or benznidazole should be considered only for laboratory accidents. Because immigrants can carry this disease to nonendemic areas, serologic testing should be performed in blood donors from high-risk populations. Potential seropositive donors can be identified by determining whether they have been or have spent extensive time in an endemic area. Questionnaire-based screening of potentially infected blood donors from areas endemic for infection can reduce the risk of transmission.

Blood transfusions in endemic areas are a significant risk. Gentian violet, an amphophilic cationic agent that acts photodynamically, has been used to kill the parasite in blood. Photoirradiation of blood containing gentian violet and ascorbate generates free radicals and superoxide anions that are trypanocidal. Mepacrine and maprotiline have also been used to eradicate the parasite in blood transfusions. Potential organ donors from endemic areas should also be screened; seropositivity should be considered a contraindication to organ donation. Although cardiac transplantation has been successful in chagasic patients, further study is needed. An international program has been established in endemic areas (Argentina, Bolivia, Brazil, Uruguay, Paraguay, and Chile) to help eliminate transmission. Screening of emigrants from endemic areas may significantly reduce transmission.

Almeida IC, Covas DT, Soussumi LM, et al: A highly sensitive and specific chemiluminescent enzyme linked immunoabsorbent assay for the diagnosis of acute *Trypanosoma cruzi* infection. *Transfusion* 1997;37:850–57.

de Andrade AL, Zicker F, de Oliveira RM, et al: Randomized trial of the efficacy of benznidazole in the treatment of early *Trypanosoma cruzi* infection. *Lancet* 1996; 348:1407–13.

Docampo R, Moreno SN, Cruz FS: Enhancement of the cytotoxicity of crystal violet against *Trypanosoma cruzi* in blood by ascorbate. *Mol Biochem Parasitol* 1988; 27:241–47.

Prata A: Clinical and epidemiological aspects of Chagas' disease. *Lancet Infect Dis* 2001;l:92–100.

Rodrigues Coura JR, de Castro SL: A critical review on Chagas disease chemotherapy. *Mem Inst Oswaldo Cruz* 2002;97:3–24.

Villar JC, Marin-Neto JA, Ebrahim S, et al: Trypanocidal drugs for chronic asymptomatic *Trypanosoma cruzi* infection (Cochrane Review). *Cochrane Database Syst Rev* 2002:CD003463.

Chapter 264
Malaria (*Plasmodium*)

Peter J. Krause

Malaria is an acute and chronic illness characterized by paroxysms of fever, chills, sweats, fatigue, anemia, and splenomegaly. It has played a major role in human history, having arguably caused more harm to more people than any other infectious disease. Malaria is of overwhelming importance in the developing world today, with an estimated 300 million cases and more than 1 million deaths each year. Most malarial deaths occur in infants and young children. Although there is no endemic malaria in the United States, approximately 1,000 imported cases are recognized each year. Physicians practicing in nonendemic areas should consider the diagnosis of malaria in any febrile child who has returned from a malaria-endemic area within the previous year because delay in diagnosis and treatment can result in severe illness or death.

Etiology. Malaria is caused by intracellular *Plasmodium* protozoa transmitted to humans by female *Anopheles* mosquitoes. Four species of *Plasmodium* cause malaria in humans: *P. falciparum, P. malariae, P. ovale,* and *P. vivax.* Malaria also can be transmitted through blood transfusion, by use of contaminated needles, and from a pregnant woman to her fetus. The risk of blood transmission is small and decreasing in the United States but may occur by way of whole blood, packed red blood cells, platelets, leukocytes, and organ transplantation.

Epidemiology. Malaria is a worldwide problem with transmission occurring in over 100 countries with a combined population of over 1.6 billion people. The principal areas of transmission are Africa, Asia, and South America. *P. falciparum* and *P. malariae* are found in most malarious areas. *P. falciparum* is the predominant species in Africa, Haiti, and New Guinea. *P. vivax* predominates in Bangladesh, Central America, India, Pakistan, and Sri Lanka. *P. vivax* and *P. falciparum* predominate in Southeast Asia, South America, and Oceania. *P. ovale,* the rarest species, is transmitted primarily in Africa. Transmission of malaria has been eliminated in most of North America (including the United States), Europe, and the Caribbean, as well as Australia, Chile, Israel, Japan, Korea, Lebanon, and Taiwan.

Most cases of malaria in the United States or Europe consist of previously infected visitors from endemic areas, citizens who travel to endemic areas without taking appropriate chemoprophylactic drugs, and a small number of transfusion-associated and congenital cases. Since 1986, 11 indigenous cases have been documented in the United States. It is likely that untreated patients with malaria acquired in an endemic country traveled to the United States and infected local mosquitoes that subsequently transmitted the disease to others.

Pathogenesis. *Plasmodium* species exist in a variety of forms and have a complex life cycle that enables them to survive in different cellular environments in the human host (asexual phase) and the mosquito vector (sexual phase). A marked amplification of *Plasmodium* organisms from approximately 10^2 to as many as 10^{14} occurs during a two-step process in humans. The first occurs in the cells of the liver **(exoerythrocytic phase)** and the second in the red cells **(erythrocytic phase)**. The exoerythrocytic phase begins with inoculation of sporozoites into the bloodstream by a female *Anopheles* mosquito. Within minutes, the sporozoites enter the hepatocytes of the liver, where they develop and multiply asexually. The parasite is referred to as a **schizont** at this stage. After 1–2 wk, the hepatocytes rupture and release thousands of merozoites into the circulation. The tissue schizonts of *P. falciparum* and *P. malaria* rupture once, and

none persists in the liver. There are two types of tissue schizonts for *P. ovale* and *P. vivax.* The primary type ruptures in 6–9 days while a secondary type remains dormant in the liver cell for weeks, months, or as long as 5 yr before releasing merozoites, and thereby causing *relapses* of infection. The erythrocytic phase of *Plasmodium* asexual development begins when the merozoites from the liver penetrate erythrocytes. Once inside the erythrocyte, the parasite transforms into the **ring form,** which then enlarges to become a trophozoite. These latter two forms can be identified with Giemsa stain on blood smear, the primary means of confirming the diagnosis of malaria (Fig. 264–1). The trophozoite multiplies asexually to produce a number of small erythrocytic merozoites. Merozoites are released into the bloodstream when the erythrocyte membrane ruptures, a process associated with the production of fever. Over time, some of the merozoites develop into male and female gametocytes. It is the gametocytes that complete the *Plasmodium* life cycle when they are ingested during a blood meal by the female *Anopheline* mosquito. The male and female gametocytes fuse to form a zygote in the stomach cavity of the mosquito. After a series of further transformations, sporozoites enter the salivary gland of the mosquito and are inoculated into a new host with the next blood meal.

Four important pathologic processes have been identified in patients with malaria: (1) fever, (2) anemia, (3) immunopathologic events, and (4) tissue anoxia resulting from cytoadherence of infected erythrocytes. Fever occurs when erythrocytes rupture and release merozoites into the circulation. Anemia is caused by hemolysis, sequestration of erythrocytes in the spleen and other organs, and bone marrow depression. Immunopathologic events that have been documented in patients with malaria include polyclonal activation resulting in both hypergammaglobulinemia and the formation of immune complexes, immunodepression, and release of cytokines such as tumor necrosis factor that may be responsible for much of the pathology of the disease. Cytoadherence of infected erythrocytes to vascular endothelium occurs in *P. falciparum* malaria. It may lead to obstruction of blood flow and capillary damage with resultant vascular leakage of protein and fluid, edema, and tissue anoxia in the brain, heart, lung, intestine, and kidney.

Immunity after *Plasmodium* species infection is incomplete so that severe disease is averted but complete eradication or prevention of future infection is not achieved. In some cases parasites circulate in small numbers for a long time but are prevented from rapidly multiplying and causing severe illness. Repeated episodes of infection occur because the parasite has developed a number of immune evasive strategies, such as intracellular replication, rapid antigenic variation, and alteration of the host immune system that includes partial immune

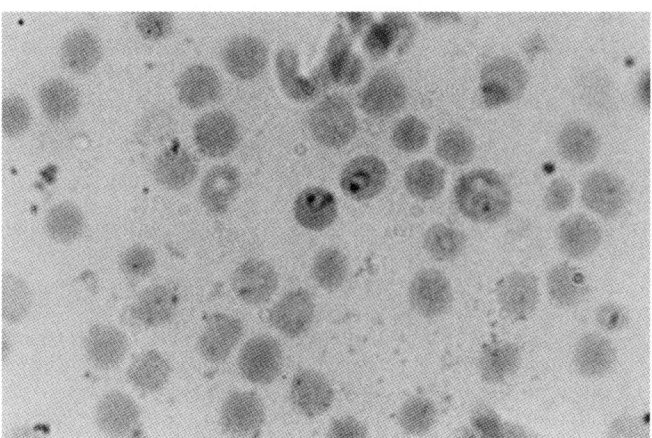

FIGURE 264–1. Ring forms of *Plasmodium falciparum* within two erythrocytes *(center).*

suppression. The human host response to *Plasmodium* species infection includes natural immune mechanisms that prevent infection by other *Plasmodium* species, such as those of birds or rodents, as well as several alterations in erythrocyte physiology that prevent or modify malarial infection. Erythrocytes containing hemoglobin S (sickle erythrocytes) resist malaria parasite growth, erythrocytes lacking Duffy blood group antigen are resistant to *P. vivax*, and erythrocytes containing hemoglobin F (fetal hemoglobin) and ovalocytes are resistant to *P. falciparum*. In hyperendemic areas, newborns rarely become ill with malaria, in part owing to passive maternal antibody and high levels of fetal hemoglobin. Children 3 mo to 2–5 yr of age have little specific immunity to malaria species and therefore suffer yearly attacks of debilitating and potentially fatal disease. Immunity is subsequently acquired, and severe cases of malaria become less common. Severe disease may occur during pregnancy or after extended residence outside the endemic region. In general, extracellular *Plasmodium* organisms are targeted by antibody, whereas intracellular organisms are targeted by cellular defenses such as T lymphocytes, macrophages, polymorphonuclear leukocytes, and the spleen.

Clinical Manifestations. Children and adults are asymptomatic during the initial phase, the **incubation period** of malaria infection. The usual incubation periods follow: *P. falciparum*, 9–14 days; *P. vivax*, 12–17 days; *P. ovale*, 16–18 days, and *P. malariae*, 18–40 days. The incubation period can be prolonged for any *Plasmodium* species in patients with partial immunity or incomplete chemoprophylaxis and as long as 6–12 mo for *P. vivax*. A prodrome lasting 2–3 days is noted in some patients before parasites are detected in the blood. Prodromal symptoms include headache, fatigue, anorexia, myalgia, slight fever, and pain in the chest, abdomen, or joints.

The classic presentation of malaria, seldom noted with other infectious diseases, consists of **paroxysms** of fever alternating with periods of fatigue but otherwise relative wellness. Symptoms associated with febrile paroxysms include high fever, rigors, sweats, and headache, as well as myalgia, back pain, abdominal pain, nausea, vomiting, diarrhea, pallor, and jaundice. Paroxysms coincide with the rupture of schizonts that occurs every 48 hr with *P. vivax* and *P. ovale* and results in daily fever spikes and every 72 hr with *P. malariae* resulting in every other or every third day fever spikes. Periodicity is less apparent with *P. falciparum* and mixed infections. Patients with primary infection, such as travelers from nonendemic regions, also may have irregular symptomatic episodes for 2–3 days before regular paroxysms begin. Children with malaria often have special clinical features that differ from those of adults. In children older than 2 mo of age who are nonimmune, symptoms of malaria vary widely from low-grade fever and headache to a temperature greater than 104°F with headache, drowsiness, anorexia, nausea, vomiting, diarrhea, pallor, cyanosis, splenomegaly, hepatomegaly, anemia, thrombocytopenia, a normal or low leukocyte count, or any combination of these manifestations.

Recrudescence after a primary attack may occur from the survival of erythrocyte forms in the bloodstream. Long-term relapse is caused by release of merozoites from an exoerythrocytic source in the liver (*P. vivax* and *P. ovale*) or persistence within the erythrocyte (*P. malariae*). A history of typical symptoms in a person more than a few weeks after return from an endemic area therefore indicates *P. vivax*, *P. ovale*, or *P. malariae* infection.

P. falciparum is the most severe form of malaria and is associated with more intense parasitemia. Fatality rates of up to 25% in nonimmune adults and 30% in nonimmune infants may occur if appropriate therapy is not instituted promptly. For this reason, *the diagnosis of P. falciparum malaria constitutes a medical emergency.* Malaria caused by *P. ovale*, *P. vivax*, and *P. malariae* usually result in parasitemias of less than 2%. Malaria caused by

P. falciparum, however, can reach 60% or more because *P. ovale* and *P. vivax* primarily infect immature erythrocytes, *P. malariae* infects only mature erythrocytes, while *P. falciparum* infects immature and mature erythrocytes. *P. falciparum* is most commonly associated with serious complications, although milder or asymptomatic infections occur in those who are partially immune.

P. vivax malaria generally is less severe than *P. falciparum* malaria but may cause death from ruptured spleen or in association with reticulocytosis after anemia. Relapse of *P. vivax* malaria may occur if antihepatic malaria treatment is not given and is common within 6 mo after an acute attack but may occur as long as 5 yr after initial infection.

P. malariae is the mildest and most chronic of all malaria infections. Recrudescence has been observed 30–50 yr after an acute attack. Although parasitemia is often low, untreated *P. malariae* can cause chronic ill health in addition to acute febrile illness.

P. ovale malaria is the least common type of malaria. It is similar to *P. vivax* malaria and commonly is found in conjunction with *P. falciparum* malaria.

Congenital malaria (malaria acquired from the mother prenatally or perinatally) is a serious problem in tropical areas but is rarely reported in the United States. In endemic areas, congenital malaria is an important cause of abortions, miscarriages, stillbirths, premature births, intrauterine growth retardation, and neonatal deaths. Congenital malaria usually occurs in a nonimmune mother with *P. vivax* or *P. malariae*, although it can be observed with any of the human malaria species. The first sign or symptom most commonly occurs between 10–30 days of age (range, 14 hr to several months of age). Signs and symptoms include fever, restlessness, drowsiness, pallor, jaundice, poor feeding, vomiting, diarrhea, cyanosis, and hepatosplenomegaly. Malaria is often severe during pregnancy and may have an adverse effect on the fetus or neonate owing to maternal illness or placental infection even in the absence of transmission from mother to child.

Diagnosis. Any child who presents with fever or unexplained systemic illness and has traveled or had residence in a malaria-endemic area within the previous year should be assumed to have life-threatening malaria until proven otherwise. Malaria illness should be considered regardless of the use of chemoprophylaxis. Important criteria that suggest *P. falciparum* malaria include symptoms occurring less than 1 mo after return from an endemic area, intense parasitemia (>2%), ring forms with double chromatin dots, and erythrocytes infected with more than one parasite.

The diagnosis of malaria is established by identification of organisms on Giemsa-stained smears of peripheral blood. Giemsa stain is superior to Wright stain or Leishman stain. Both thick and thin blood smears should be examined. The concentration of erythrocytes on a thick smear is 20–40 times that on a thin smear and is used to quickly scan large numbers of erythrocytes. The thin smear allows for positive identification of the malaria species and determination of the percentage of infected erythrocytes. The latter is useful in following the response to therapy. Identification of the species is best made by an experienced microscopist and checked against color plates of the various *Plasmodium* species. Although *P. falciparum* is most likely to be identified from blood just after a febrile paroxysm, the timing of the smears is less important than their being obtained several times a day over a period of 3 successive days. A single negative blood smear does not exclude malaria; it may be necessary to repeat the smears as often as every 4–6 hr a day to make a diagnosis. Most symptomatic patients with malaria will have detectable parasites on thick blood smears within a 48-hr period. It is important to realize that in nonimmune persons symptoms typically occur 1–2 days before parasites are detectable on blood smear. A new monoclonal antibody test that is incorporated in a test strip for fingerprick blood samples is as sensitive as a thick smear for detection of *P. falciparum*. Polymerase chain reaction is even more sensitive but technically more complex.

DIFFERENTIAL DIAGNOSIS. The differential diagnosis of malaria is broad and includes viral infections such as influenza and hepatitis, sepsis, pneumonia, meningitis, encephalitis, endocarditis, gastroenteritis, pyelonephritis, babesiosis, brucellosis, leptospirosis, tuberculosis, relapsing fever, typhoid fever, yellow fever, amebic liver abscess, Hodgkin disease, and collagen vascular disease.

Treatment. Physicians caring for patients with malaria or traveling to endemic areas need to be aware of current information regarding malaria because the problem of resistance to antimalarial drugs is ongoing and has greatly complicated therapy and prophylaxis. The best source for such information is the CDC Malaria Hotline, which is available to physicians 24 hr a day (770-488-7788 from 8:00 AM to 4:30 PM EST and 404-639-2888 from 4:30 PM to 8:00 AM EST weekends and holidays). Fever without an obvious cause in any patient who has left a *P. falciparum*– endemic area within the incubation period of 9–14 days and is nonimmune should be considered a medical emergency. Thick and thin blood smears should immediately be obtained and, if positive, the patient should be hospitalized and begun on therapy. If blood films are negative, they should be repeated every few hours; but if the patient is severely ill, antimalarial therapy should be initiated immediately.

P. FALCIPARUM **MALARIA.** Malaria acquired in *P. falciparum* areas with known chloroquine resistance or where there is any doubt about chloroquine sensitivity after checking the CDC Malaria Hotline should generally be treated with drugs other than chloroquine (Table 264–1). Intravenous quinidine or quinine* should be administered for patients who cannot retain oral fluids and medication because of vomiting; have neurologic dysfunction, pulmonary edema, or renal failure; have a peripheral asexual parasitemia more than 5%; or have a peripheral asexual parasitemia of 1–4% with a severe attack. Such patients should be admitted to the intensive care unit for electrocardiographic monitoring to detect arrhythmias, widening QRS complex, or prolonged QT interval. Patients also should be monitored for hypotension and other complications and for plasma quinidine levels. Parenteral therapy should be continued until the parasitemia is less than 1%, which usually occurs within 48 hr, and/or until oral medication can be tolerated. Quinine sulfate (30 mg/kg/24 hr PO in 3 doses) is then given for a total of 3 days of combined quinidine/quinine therapy, with completion of therapy by either tetracycline 6.25 mg/kg PO qid for 7 days or Fansidar (25 mg pyrimethamine and 500 mg sulfadoxine per tablet) in one oral dose (1/4–3 tablets according to age) on the last day of therapy. Use of Fansidar is contraindicated in patients with a history of sulfonamide or pyrimethamine intolerance, in infants younger than 2 mo of age, and in pregnant women at term.

Patients with mild to moderate infection, parasitemia less than 5%, and any doubt about chloroquine sensitivity should be given oral quinine sulfate (30 mg/kg/24 hr in 3 doses) for 3–7 days with an additional antimalarial drug consisting of any one of the following: a single treatment dose of Fansidar on the last day of quinine; doxycycline or tetracycline qid for 7 days; or clindamycin for 5 days. Alternatives to these regimens include mefloquine given in two doses 12 hr apart, atovaquone and proguanil (Malarone) for 3 days, or atovaquone and doxycycline for 3 days (see Table 264–1). Exceptions to the just mentioned regimens include quinine treatment for 7 consecutive days for patients who acquire *P. falciparum* in Thailand and the avoidance of Fansidar for patients who acquire *P. falciparum*

infections in Thailand, Burma, Cambodia, or the Amazon basin. Mefloquine is contraindicated for use in patients with a known hypersensitivity to mefloquine or with a history of epilepsy or severe psychiatric disorders. Mefloquine may be administered to persons concurrently receiving β–blockers if they have no underlying arrhythmia; however, mefloquine is not recommended for persons with cardiac conduction abnormalities. Quinidine or quinine may exacerbate the known side effects of mefloquine; patients not responding to mefloquine therapy or failing mefloquine prophylaxis should be monitored closely if they are treated with quinidine or quinine.

Patients with uncomplicated *P. falciparum* malaria acquired in areas without chloroquine resistance should be treated with oral chloroquine; however, if the parasite count does not drop rapidly (within 24–48 hr) and become negative after 4 days, chloroquine resistance should be assumed and the patient begun on a different antimalarial drug. Supportive therapy is very important and includes red blood cell transfusion(s) to maintain the hematocrit more than 20%, exchange transfusion in life-threatening *P. falciparum* malaria with parasitemia more than 5%, supplemental oxygen and ventilatory support for pulmonary edema or cerebral malaria, careful intravenous rehydration for severe malaria, intravenous glucose for hypoglycemia, anticonvulsants for cerebral malaria with seizures, and dialysis for renal failure. Corticosteroids are no longer recommended for cerebral malaria.

P. VIVAX, P. OVALE, OR *P. MALARIAE* **MALARIA.** If malaria was acquired in areas where *P. falciparum* is not endemic, the treatment is with chloroquine even though a few rare cases of chloroquine-resistant *P. vivax* malaria have been described from Indonesia and New Guinea. Clinical and blood smear response to therapy should be monitored. If vomiting precludes oral administration, chloroquine can be given by nasogastric tube, or, in rare cases and with great care, by intramuscular administration. Sudden death has been attributed to parenteral administration of chloroquine to children. Intravenous quinidine or quinine is given in severe cases. Patients with *P. vivax* or *P. ovale* malaria should be given primaquine once daily for 14 days to prevent relapse. Some strains may require two courses of primaquine. Patients given primaquine must be checked for glucose-6-phosphate dehydrogenase deficiency before initiation of the drug because it can cause hemolytic anemia in such patients. Patients with malaria of any type need to be monitored for possible recrudescence with repeat blood smears at the end of therapy because recrudescence may occur 90 or more days after therapy with low-grade resistant organisms. For children living in endemic areas, mothers should be encouraged to treat fever with an antimalarial drug. If such children are severely ill, they should be given the same therapy as nonimmune children.

Complications. Cerebral malaria is a serious complication of *P. falciparum* infection that is especially common in children and nonimmune adults. Cerebral malaria is associated with a fatality rate of 20–40% but rarely causes long-term sequelae if it is treated appropriately. It usually develops after the patient has been ill for several days but may develop precipitously. As with other complications, cerebral malaria is more likely in patients with parasitemia greater than 5%. The symptoms always include decreased level of consciousness and range in severity from drowsiness and severe headache to confusion, delirium, hallucinations, or deep coma. Physical findings may be normal or may include fever to 106–108°F, seizures, muscular twitching, rhythmic movement of the head or extremities, contracted or unequal pupils, retinal hemorrhages, hemiplegia, absent or exaggerated deep tendon reflexes, and a positive Babinski sign. Lumbar puncture reveals increased pressure and cerebrospinal fluid protein with minimal or no pleocytosis and a normal glucose concentration. There are no specific electroencephalographic findings with cerebral malaria.

---

*Quinine is not available in the United States.

TABLE 264–1. Treatment of Malaria in Children

Drug*	Dosage
All Plasmodium Species Except Chloroquine-Resistant Plasmodium falciparum	
Oral Drug of Choice	
Chloroquine phosphate	10 mg base/kg (maximum: 600 mg base) then 5 mg base/kg (maximum: 300 mg base), 6 hr later, and 5 mg base/kg/24 hr (maximum: 300 mg base) at 24 and 48 hr
Parenteral Drug of Choice	
Quinidine gluconate	10 mg/kg loading dose (maximum: 600 mg) over 1–2 hr, then 0.02 mg/kg/min continuous infusion until oral therapy can be started
or	
Quinine dihydrochloride (not available in the USA)	20 mg/kg loading dose over 4 hr, then 10 mg/kg over 2–4 hr q8h (maximum: 1,800 mg/24 hr) until oral therapy can be started
P. falciparum *Acquired in Areas of Known Chloroquine Resistance*	
Oral Regimen of Choice	
Quinine sulfate†	30 mg/kg/24 hr divided in three doses for 3–7 days (maximum: 650 mg/dose)
plus	
Tetracycline‡	20 mg/kg/24 hr divided in four doses for 7 days (maximum: 250 mg/dose)
or plus	
Pyrimethamine-sulfadoxine (Fansidar)§	<1 yr, single dose of 1/4 tablet 1–3 yr, single dose of 1/2 tablet 4–8 yr, single dose of 1 tablet 9–14 yr, single dose of 2 tablets >14 yr, single dose of 3 tablets
or	
Mefloquine hydrochloride‖	15 mg PO followed by 10 mg/kg PO 8–12 hours later (maximum: 1,250 mg) for 1 day
Parenteral	
Quinidine gluconate	Same as for chloroquine-sensitive *P. falciparum*
or	
Quinine dihydrochloride	Same as for chloroquine-sensitive *P. falciparum*
Prevention of Relapses: **Plasmodium vivax** *and* **Plasmodium ovale** *Only*	
Primaquine phosphate¶	0.3 mg base/kg/24 hr for 14 days (maximum: 15 mg base [26.3 mg salt])

*Review contraindications and adverse effects before use (see text).

†For treatment of P. falciparum infections acquired in Southeast Asia, and possibly in other areas including South America, quinine sulfate should be continued for 7 days.

‡Physicians must weigh the benefits of tetracycline therapy against the possibility of dental staining in children younger than 8 yr of age.

§Fansidar (25 mg pyrimethamine and 500 mg sulfadoxine per tablet) should not be used for treatment of malaria acquired in Southeast Asia and the Amazon basin because of possible resistance. Carry a single dose for treatment of febrile illness when medical care is not immediately available.

‖Mefloquine is not licensed by the U.S. Food and Drug Administration (FDA) for children who weigh less than 15 kg, but recent Centers for Disease Control and Prevention (CDC) recommendations allow use of the drug to be considered in children without weight restrictions when travel to chloroquine-resistant P. falciparum areas cannot be avoided. For most patients, 15 mg/kg (maximum: 750 mg) in a single dose is effective therapy, except for those who acquired infection in the areas of the Amazon basin, or the Thailand-Cambodia and Thailand-Myanmar borders. If the 25 mg/kg/24 hr dose is used, 15 mg/kg (maximum: 750 mg) is given followed 8–12 hr later by 10 mg/kg (maximum: 500 mg).

¶Primaquine phosphate can cause hemolytic anemia in patients with glucose-6-phosphate dehydrogenase (G6PD) deficiency. A G6PD screening test should be performed before intiating treatment. Pregnant women should not be administered primaquine.

Renal failure is a common complication of severe *P. falciparum* malaria. It results from deposition of hemoglobin in renal tubules, decreased renal blood flow, and acute tubular necrosis. **Blackwater fever** is a clinical syndrome that consists of severe hemolysis, hemoglobinuria, and renal failure. It is a rare complication that occurs when the combination of antibody directed against parasite-laden erythrocytes and complement result in severe hemolytic anemia, hemoglobinuria, oliguria, and jaundice. Renal failure usually requires peritoneal dialysis or hemodialysis.

Pulmonary edema may occur several days after therapy has begun and is commonly associated with excessive intravenous therapy. It can develop rapidly and may be fatal. Thus, great care should be taken not to overhydrate patients with *P. falciparum* malaria.

Hypoglycemia is a complication of malaria that is more common in children, pregnant women, and patients receiving quinine therapy. Patients may have a decreased level of consciousness that can be confused with cerebral malaria. Hypoglycemia is associated with increased mortality and neurologic sequelae.

Thrombocytopenia is a common complication of *P. falciparum* and *P. vivax* malaria. Although significant bleeding is uncommon without DIC, platelet counts can decrease to 10,000–20,000/mm³.

Splenic rupture is a rare complication that may occur with acute infection owing to any malaria species. Splenic rupture can occur spontaneously but is usually the result of trauma that includes overly vigorous palpation on physical examination. It causes severe internal hemorrhage and may result in death if removal of the spleen and blood transfusion are not performed in a timely manner.

Algid malaria is a rare form of *P. falciparum* malaria that occurs with overwhelming infection, hypotension, hypothermia, rapid weak pulse, shallow breathing, pallor, and vascular collapse. Death may occur within a few hours.

Prevention. Malaria prevention consists of reducing exposure to infected mosquitoes and chemoprophylaxis. The most accurate and current information on areas in the world where malaria risk and drug resistance exist can be obtained by contacting local and state health departments or the Centers for Disease Control and Prevention or consulting the United States Public Health Service's annual publication *Health Information for International Travel.*

Travelers to endemic areas should remain in well-screened areas from dusk to dawn when the risk of transmission is highest. They should sleep under permethrin-treated mosquito netting and spray insecticides indoors at sundown. During the day the travelers should wear clothing that covers the arms and legs with trousers tucked into shoes or boots. Mosquito repellent should be applied to thin clothing and exposed areas of the skin with repeated applications every 1–2 hr. A child should not be taken outside from dusk to dawn but, if absolutely necessary, diethyltoluamide (DEET) in a 10–15% solution should be applied to exposed areas except for the eyes, mouth, or hands (hands are often placed in the mouth). The DEET should then be washed off as soon as the child comes back inside. Adverse reactions to DEET include rashes, toxic encephalopathy, and seizures. Even with these precautions, a child should be taken to a physician immediately if the child develops illness when traveling to a malarious area.

Chemoprophylaxis is necessary for all visitors to and residents of the tropics who have not lived there since infancy (see Table 285–2). Children of nonimmune women should have chemoprophylaxis from birth. Chemoprophylaxis should be started 1–2 wk before entering the endemic area (except for doxycycline administration, which can begin 1–2 days before departure) and continue for at least 4 wk after leaving. Chloroquine is given in the few remaining areas of the world free of chloroquine-resistant malaria strains (as of January 1992, Hispaniola, Central America north of Panama, and the Middle East). In areas where chloroquine-resistant *P. falciparum* exists, chemoprophylaxis is complicated. Children who travel to areas where chloroquine-resistant strains are transmitted should be given mefloquine. An alternative regimen should be given to children if they have a known hypersensitivity to mefloquine, are receiving cardiotropic drugs, especially β-blockers, or have a history of convulsive or certain psychiatric disorders. Such children should be given chloroquine. In addition, if they weigh more than 30 pounds, they should bring Fansidar tablets to be taken if fever develops and medical care is not available within 24 hr. An alternative combination that could be considered for sulfa-sensitive individuals older than 8 yr of age is chloroquine and, in place of Fansidar, doxycycline. Doxycycline is equivalent to mefloquine for short-term prophylaxis, but for long-term prophylaxis doxycycline is not as good because of side effects associated with its long-term use. There have been several reports of both mefloquine and Fansidar resistance. The combination of atovaquone and proguanil (Malarone) has been approved for prophylaxis of malaria in areas where chloroquine resistance exists, although dosing is uncertain in children who weigh less than 30 pounds. Finally, extensive efforts have been made to develop a malaria vaccine but results to date have been disappointing.

Centers for Disease Control and Prevention: *Health Information for International Travel, 2001–2002.* Atlanta, US Department of Health and Human Services, Public Health Service, 2001. (Available at http://www.cdc.gov/travel/yb/index.htm)

Centers for Disease Control and Prevention: Malaria surveillance—United States, 1998. *MMWR Morb Mortal Wkly Rep* 2001;50:1–20.

Taylor TE, Strickland GT: Malaria. In Strickland GT (editor): *Hunter's Tropical Medicine,* 8th ed. Philadelphia, WB Saunders, 2000.

Viani RM, Bromberg K: Pediatric imported malaria in New York: Delayed diagnosis. *Clin Pediatr* 1999;38:333–37.

Zucker JR, Campbell CC: Malaria: Principles of prevention and treatment. *Infect Dis Clin North Am* 1993;7:547–67.

Chapter 265
Babesiosis (*Babesia*)

Peter J. Krause

Babesiosis is an emerging malaria-like disease caused by an intraerythrocytic protozoan that is transmitted by ticks. The clinical manifestations of babesiosis range from subclinical illness to fulminant disease resulting in death.

Etiology. The causative protozoan was first described in cattle in 1891 by the Hungarian microbiologist Babes. Since then, more than 90 species of *Babesia* have been described that infect a wide variety of wild and domestic animals throughout the world.

The primary reservoir for *Babesia microti* is the white-footed mouse *(Peromyscus leucopus),* and the primary vector is the deer tick *(I. dammini,* also known as *I. scapularis).* Deer ticks also transmit the etiologic agents of Lyme disease and human granulocytic ehrlichiosis and may simultaneously transmit both microorganisms. Deer *(Odocoileus virginianus)* serve as the host on which adult ticks most abundantly feed but are incompetent reservoirs.

Epidemiology. Since the first documented case of human babesial infection was reported in 1957, infection by *B. divergens* has been demonstrated in Europe and infection by *B. microti* has become endemic in the northeastern and upper midwestern United States. A parasite very closely related to *B. gibsoni* (WA-1) appears to infect humans along the Pacific coast, whereas another that is closely related to *B. divergens* (MO-1) has been reported in Missouri. Human babesiosis cases also have been documented in Asia and Africa.

Rarely, babesiosis is acquired through blood transfusions or by transplacental transmission.

Pathogenesis. Erythrocyte lysis is responsible for many of the clinical manifestations and complications of the disease, including fever, hemolytic anemia, jaundice, hemoglobinemia, hemoglobinuria, and renal insufficiency. Obstruction of blood vessels by parasitized erythrocytes causes ischemia and necrosis that may result in splenomegaly, hepatomegaly and hepatic dysfunction, and cerebral abnormalities. The spleen has an important role in clearing parasitemia along with antibody, T and B cells, complement, cytokines, macrophages, and polymorphonuclear leukocytes. Immunity is sometimes incomplete because low-level parasitemia may exist for as long as 26 mo after symptoms have resolved and recrudescence may occur.

Clinical Manifestations. The clinical severity of babesiosis ranges from subclinical infection to fulminating disease resulting in death. Although infection is common in endemic areas, many are mild or asymptomatic. In some highly endemic areas, moderate to severe disease is frequently observed. Nantucket Island reported 21 cases in 1994, which translates to 280 cases/100,000 population, placing the community burden of disease in a category with gonorrhea as "moderately common." The case fatality rate was estimated at 5% in a retrospective study of 136 New York cases. Thus, in certain sites, in certain years of high transmission, babesiosis may constitute a significant public health burden.

There is often no recollection of a tick bite because the unengorged *I. dammini* nymph is only about 2 mm long. In clinically apparent cases, symptoms of babesiosis begin after an incubation period of 1–9 wk from the beginning of tick feeding or 6–9 wk after transfusion. Typical symptoms in moderate to severe infection include intermittent temperature to as high as 40°C (104°F) and one or more of the following: chills, sweats, myalgia, arthralgia, nausea, and vomiting. Less commonly noted are emotional lability, hyperesthesia, headache, sore throat, abdominal pain, conjunctival injection, photophobia, weight loss, and nonproductive cough. The findings on physical examination generally are minimal, often consisting only of fever. Mild splenomegaly, hepatomegaly, or both are noted occasionally but rash seldom is reported. Abnormal laboratory findings include moderately severe hemolytic anemia, an elevated reticulocyte count, thrombocytopenia, proteinuria, and elevated blood urea nitrogen and creatinine levels. The leukocyte count is normal to slightly decreased, with a "left shift." Babesiosis usually lasts for a few weeks to several months, with prolonged recovery of up to 18 mo in severe cases.

Patients at increased risk for severe disease include those who lack a spleen, are on immunosuppressive drugs, are infected with *B. divergens*, are older than age 40 yr, or with concomitant HIV infection or Lyme disease. Concurrent babesiosis and Lyme disease infection occurs in approximately 15% of patients experiencing Lyme disease in parts of southern New England and results in more severe illness than with either disease alone. Moderate to severe babesiosis may occur in children, but infection generally is less severe than in adults. Several cases of neonatal babesiosis have been described. Neonates usually are infected from blood transfusion and may develop severe illness.

Diagnosis. Diagnosis of *B. microti* infection in human hosts is made by microscopic demonstration of the organism using Giemsa-stained thin blood films. Parasitemias may be exceedingly sparse, especially early in the course of illness. Thick blood smears may be used, but the organisms appear as simple chromatin dots that might be mistaken for stain precipitate or iron inclusion bodies. Subinoculation of a sample of patient's blood into hamsters or gerbils or in vitro cultivation are too specialized for all but the most experienced laboratories. The polymerase chain reaction (PCR) is a sensitive and specific test for detection of *Babesia* DNA that should supplant the hamster inoculation test. Serologic testing is useful, particularly in diagnosing *B. microti* infection. The indirect immunofluorescence serologic assay (for both IgG and IgM antibodies) is sensitive and specific and may quickly confirm a diagnosis of babesiosis when parasites are scarce or not detectable.

Treatment. The combination of clindamycin (20–40 mg/kg/day divided tid PO) and quinine (25 mg/kg/day divided tid PO) for 7 to 10 days is the therapy of choice for babesiosis in children. Adverse reactions are common, however, especially tinnitus and abdominal distress. In addition, treatment failures have been reported, particularly in patients with HIV infection. The combination of atovaquone (40 mg/kg/day divided bid PO) and azithromycin (12 mg/kg/day as a single dose PO) is an alternative antibabesial combination that has been shown in adults to be as effective as clindamycin and quinine but with fewer adverse effects. Exchange blood transfusion can decrease parasitemia rapidly and remove toxic by-products of babesial infection but should be reserved for patients with severe infections.

Prevention. Prevention of babesiosis can be accomplished by avoiding areas where ticks, deer, and mice are known to thrive. Use of clothing that covers the lower part of the body and that is sprayed or impregnated with diethyltoluamide (DEET), dimethyl phthalate, or permethrin (Permanone) is recommended for those who travel in the foliage of endemic areas. A search for ticks on people and pets should be carried out and the ticks removed using tweezers to grasp the mouth parts without squeezing the body of the tick.

Prospective blood donors with a history of babesiosis are excluded from giving blood to prevent transfusion-related cases.

Herwaldt BL: Babesiosis. In Strickland GT (editors): *Hunter's Tropical Medicine*, 8th ed. Philadelphia, WB Saunders, 2000.

Krause PJ, Lepore T, Sikand VK, et al: Atovaquone and azithromycin for the treatment of babesiosis. *N Engl J Med* 2000;343:1454–58.

Krause PJ, Telford SR III, Pollack RJ, et al: Babesiosis: An underdiagnosed disease of children. *Pediatrics* 1992;89:1045–48.

Krause PJ, Telford SR III, Spielman A, et al: Concurrent Lyme disease and babesiosis: Evidence for increased severity and duration of illness. *JAMA* 1996;275:1657–60.

Chapter 266

Toxoplasmosis (*Toxoplasma gondii*) *Rima McLeod and Jack S. Remington*

Toxoplasma gondii, an obligate intracellular protozoan, is acquired perorally, transplacentally, or, rarely, parenterally in laboratory accidents; by transfusion; or from a transplanted organ. In immunologically normal children, acute acquired infection may be asymptomatic, cause lymphadenopathy, or damage almost any organ. Once acquired, latent encysted organisms persist for the lifetime of the host. In immunocompromised infants or children, either initial acquisition or recrudescence of latent organisms often causes signs or symptoms related to the central nervous system (CNS). Infection acquired congenitally, if untreated, almost always causes signs or symptoms in the perinatal period or later in life. The most frequent of these signs are due to chorioretinitis and CNS lesions. However, other manifestations, such as intrauterine growth retardation, fever, lymphadenopathy, rash, hearing loss, pneumonitis, hepatitis, and thrombocytopenia, also occur. Congenital toxoplasmosis in infants with HIV infection may be fulminant.

Etiology. *T. gondii* is a coccidian protozoan that multiplies only in living cells. The tachyzoites are oval or crescent-like, measuring $2–4 \times 4–7$ μm. Tissue cysts, which are 10–100 μm in diameter, may contain thousands of parasites and remain in tissues, especially the CNS and skeletal and heart muscle, for the life of the host. *Toxoplasma* can multiply in all tissues of mammals and birds.

Newly infected cats and other Felidae excrete infectious *Toxoplasma* oocysts in their feces. *Toxoplasma* are acquired by susceptible cats by ingestion of infected meat containing encysted bradyzoites or by ingestion of oocysts excreted by other recently infected cats. The parasites then multiply through schizogonic and gametogonic cycles in the distal ileal epithelium of the cat intestine. Oocysts containing two sporocysts are excreted, and, under proper conditions of temperature and moisture, each sporocyst matures into four sporozoites. For about 2 wk the cat excretes $10^5–10^7$ oocysts/day, which, in a suitable environment, may retain their viability for more than 1 yr. Oocysts sporulate 1–5 days after excretion and are then infectious. Oocysts are killed by drying, boiling, and exposure to some strong chemicals, but not to bleach. Oocysts have been isolated from soil and sand frequented by cats, and outbreaks associated with contaminated water have been reported. Oocysts and tissue cysts are sources of animal and human infections (Fig. 266–1). There are three clonal types of *T. gondii* that have different virulence for mice (and perhaps for humans) and different capacity to form large numbers of cysts.

Epidemiology. *Toxoplasma* infection is ubiquitous in animals and is one of the most common latent infections of humans throughout the world. Incidence varies considerably among people and animals in different geographic areas. In many areas of the world, approximately 5.35% of pork, 9–60% of lamb, and 0–9% of beef contain *T. gondii* organisms. Significant antibody titers have been detected in 50–80% of residents of some localities and in less than 5% in others. A higher prevalence of infection usually occurs in warmer, more humid climates.

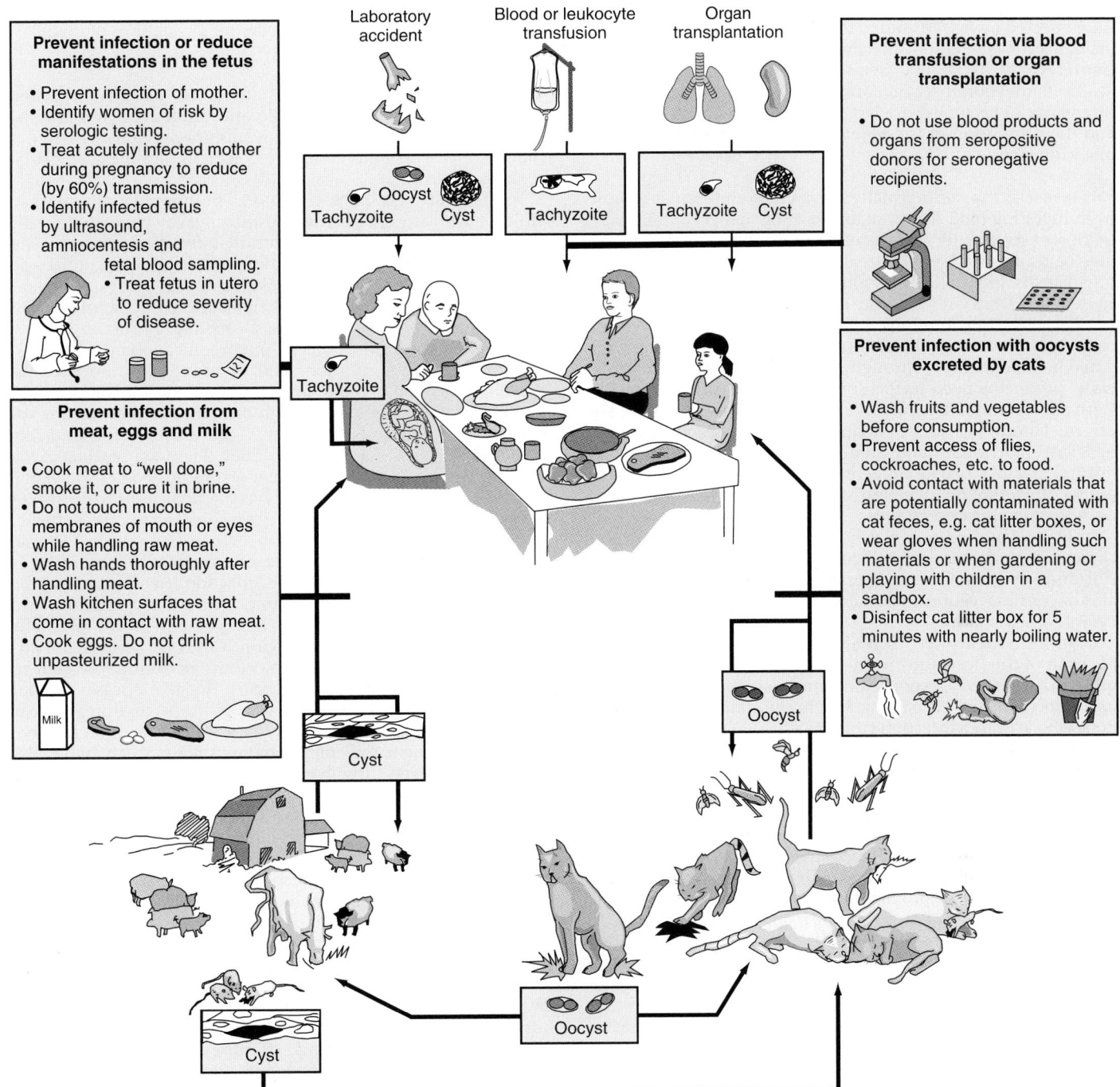

Prevent infection or reduce manifestations in the fetus

- Prevent infection of mother.
- Identify women of risk by serologic testing.
- Treat acutely infected mother during pregnancy to reduce (by 60%) transmission.
- Identify infected fetus by ultrasound, amniocentesis and fetal blood sampling.
  - Treat fetus in utero to reduce severity of disease.

Prevent infection from meat, eggs and milk

- Cook meat to "well done," smoke it, or cure it in brine.
- Do not touch mucous membranes of mouth or eyes while handling raw meat.
- Wash hands thoroughly after handling meat.
- Wash kitchen surfaces that come in contact with raw meat.
- Cook eggs. Do not drink unpasteurized milk.

Prevent infection via blood transfusion or organ transplantation

- Do not use blood products and organs from seropositive donors for seronegative recipients.

Prevent infection with oocysts excreted by cats

- Wash fruits and vegetables before consumption.
- Prevent access of flies, cockroaches, etc. to food.
- Avoid contact with materials that are potentially contaminated with cat feces, e.g. cat litter boxes, or wear gloves when handling such materials or when gardening or playing with children in a sandbox.
- Disinfect cat litter box for 5 minutes with nearly boiling water.

FIGURE 266–1. Life cycle of *Toxoplasma gondii* and prevention of toxoplasmosis by interruption of transmission to humans.

Human infection is usually acquired by the oral route by eating undercooked or raw meat that contains cysts or by ingestion of oocysts. Freezing meat to −20°C or heating it to 66°C renders the cysts noninfectious. Outbreaks of acute acquired infection have occurred in families who have consumed the same infected food. Except for transplacental infection from mother to fetus and, rarely, by organ transplantation or transfusion, *Toxoplasma* organisms are not transmitted from person to person.

Seronegative transplant recipients who receive an organ (e.g., heart or kidney) from seropositive donors have experienced life-threatening illness requiring therapy. Seropositive recipients may have increased serologic titers without associated disease.

CONGENITAL TOXOPLASMOSIS. Transmission to the fetus usually occurs when infection is acquired by an immunologically normal mother during gestation. Congenital transmission from immunologically normal women infected before pregnancy is extremely rare. Immunocompromised women who are chronically infected have transmitted the infection to their fetuses. The incidence of congenital infection in the United States ranges from 1/1,000 to 1/8,000 live births. The incidence of newly acquired infection in a population of pregnant women depends on the risk of becoming infected in that specific geographic area and the proportion of the population that has not been previously infected.

Pathogenesis. *T. gondii* is usually acquired by children and adults from ingesting food that contains cysts or that is contaminated with oocysts usually from acutely infected cats. Oocysts also may be transported to food by flies and cockroaches. When the organism is ingested, bradyzoites are released from cysts or sporozoites from oocysts, and organisms then enter gastrointestinal cells. They multiply, rupture cells, and infect contiguous cells. They are transported through lymphatics and disseminated hematogenously throughout the body. Tachyzoites proliferate, producing necrotic foci surrounded by a cellular reaction. With development of a normal immune response (humoral and cell-mediated), tachyzoites disappear from tissues. In immunodeficient individuals and some apparently immunologically normal patients, acute infection progresses and may cause potentially lethal involvement such as pneumonitis, myocarditis, or necrotizing encephalitis.

In acute acquired toxoplasmosis, characteristic lymph node changes include reactive follicular hyperplasia with irregular clusters of epithelioid histiocytes that encroach on and blur margins of germinal centers. Focal distention of sinuses with monocytoid cells also occurs.

Cysts form as early as 7 days after infection and remain for the life span of the host. During latent infection they produce little or no inflammatory response but cause recrudescent disease in immunocompromised patients or chorioretinitis in older children who acquired infection congenitally.

CONGENITAL TOXOPLASMOSIS. When a mother acquires infection during gestation, organisms may disseminate hematogenously to the placenta. When this occurs, infection may be transmitted to the fetus transplacentally or during vaginal delivery. Of untreated maternal infections acquired in the first trimester, approximately 17% of fetuses are infected, usually with severe disease. Of untreated maternal infection acquired in the third trimester, approximately 65% of fetuses are infected, usually with disease that is mild or inapparent at birth. These different rates of transmission and outcomes are most likely related to placental blood flow, virulence and amount of *T. gondii* acquired, and immunologic capacity of the mother to limit parasitemia.

Examination of the placenta of infected newborns may reveal chronic inflammation and cysts. Tachyzoites can be seen with Wright or Giemsa stains but are best demonstrated with immunoperoxidase technique. Tissue cysts stain well with periodic acid–Schiff (PAS) and silver stains as well as with immunoperoxidase technique. Gross or microscopic areas of necrosis may be present in many tissues, especially CNS, choroid and retina, heart, lungs, skeletal muscle, liver, and spleen. Areas of calcification occur in brain.

Almost all congenitally infected individuals manifest signs or symptoms of infection, such as chorioretinitis, by adolescence if they are not treated in the newborn period. Some severely involved infants with congenital infection appear to have *Toxoplasma* antigen–specific anergy of their lymphocytes, which may be important in pathogenesis of their disease. Predilection to predominant involvement of the CNS and eye in congenital infection has not been fully explained.

IMMUNITY. There are profound and prolonged alterations of T-lymphocyte populations during acute acquired *T. gondii* infections, but they have not correlated with outcome. Lymphocytosis, increased CD8 count, and decreased CD4:CD8 ratio are commonly present. Depletion of CD4 cells in patients with AIDS may contribute to severe manifestations of toxoplasmosis seen in these patients.

Clinical Manifestations. Manifestations of primary infection with *T. gondii* are highly variable and influenced primarily by host immunocompetence. Reactivation of previously asymptomatic congenital toxoplasmosis is usually manifest as ocular toxoplasmosis.

ACQUIRED TOXOPLASMOSIS. Immunologically normal children who acquire infection postnatally may have no clinically recognizable disease. When clinical manifestations are apparent, they may include almost any combination of fever, stiff neck, myalgia, arthralgia, maculopapular rash that spares the palms and soles, localized or generalized lymphadenopathy, hepatomegaly, hepatitis, reactive lymphocytosis, meningitis, brain abscess, encephalitis, confusion, malaise, pneumonia, polymyositis, pericarditis, pericardial effusion, and myocarditis. Chorioretinitis, usually unilateral, occurs in approximately 1% of cases. In Erecim, Brazil, an unusually high incidence of presumed toxoplasmic chorioretinitis, believed to be associated with acute acquired infection, has been described. Eighteen percent of the 80% of the population who have serum antibodies indicating they are infected with *T. gondii* have retinal lesions consistent with *T. gondii* chorioretinitis or scars. Two additional series of cases have been reported, one in France and one in Victoria, British Columbia, clearly documenting toxoplasmic chorioretinitis as part of the acute acquired infection. Symptoms may be present for a few days only or may persist many months. The most common manifestation is enlargement of one or a few lymph nodes in the cervical region. Cases of *Toxoplasma* lymphadenopathy rarely resemble infectious mononucleosis (due to Epstein-Barr virus or cytomegalovirus), Hodgkin disease, or other lymphadenopathies (see Chapter 482). In the pectoral area in older girls and women, the nodes may be confused with breast neoplasms. Mediastinal, mesenteric, and retroperitoneal lymph nodes may be involved. Involvement of intra-abdominal lymph nodes may be associated with fever and mimic appendicitis. Nodes may be tender but do not suppurate. Lymphadenopathy may appear and disappear for as long as 1–2 yr.

Most patients with malaise and lymphadenopathy recover spontaneously without antimicrobial therapy. Significant organ involvement in immunologically normal individuals is uncommon; however, some individuals have suffered significant morbidity (e.g., with rare instances of encephalitis, brain abscesses, hepatitis, myocarditis, pericarditis, or polymyositis).

OCULAR TOXOPLASMOSIS. In the United States and Western Europe, *T. gondii* has been estimated to cause 35% of cases of chorioretinitis (Fig. 266–2). In Brazil, retinal lesions with the appearance of toxoplasmic chorioretinitis have occurred in multiple members of the same family. Retinal lesions are present in 18% of those who are seropositive for *T. gondii* infection in Erecim, Brazil. Manifestations include blurred vision, photophobia, epiphora, and, with macular involvement, loss of central vision. Findings due to congenital ocular toxoplasmosis also include strabismus, microphthalmia, microcornea, cataract, anisometropia, and nystagmus. Episodic recurrences are common, but precipitating factors have not been defined.

IMMUNOCOMPROMISED PERSONS. Congenital *T. gondii* infection in infants with AIDS is usually a fulminant, rapidly fatal disorder, involving brain and other organs such as the lung and heart. Disseminated *T. gondii* infections also occur in older children who are immunocompromised by AIDS, by malignancies and cytotoxic therapy or corticosteroids, or by immunosuppressive drugs given for organ transplantation. Immunocompromised individuals experience the clinical forms of *Toxoplasma* infection that occur in immunologically normal individuals. Signs and symptoms that are referable to the CNS are the most frequent manifestations of severe disease (occurring in 50% of patients),

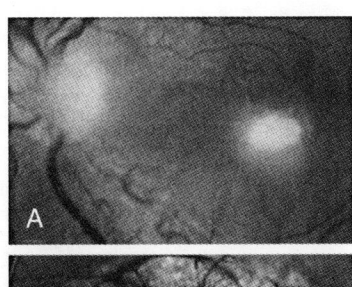

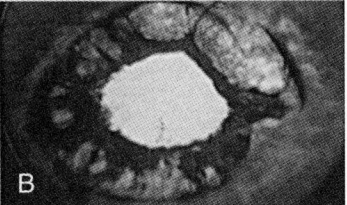

FIGURE 266–2. Toxoplasmic chorioretinitis. *A,* Active acute lesion by indirect ophthalmoscopy. *B,* The healed foci of toxoplasmic chorioretinitis may resemble a colobomatous defect (macular pseudocoloboma). (*B,* adapted from Desmonts G, Remington J: Congenital toxoplasmosis. In Remington JS, Klein JO [editors]: *Infectious Diseases of the Fetus and Newborn Infant,* 5th ed. Philadelphia, WB Saunders, 2001.) See also color plates.

although other organs also may be involved, including the heart, gastrointestinal tract, and testes.

Bone marrow transplant recipients present a special problem because active infection in these patients is difficult to diagnose. After transplantation, specific antibody level may remain the same, increase, or decrease and can become negative. Active infection often is fulminant and rapidly fatal.

Individuals who have antibodies to *T. gondii* and HIV infection are at significant risk of development of toxoplasmic encephalitis, which may be the presenting manifestation of AIDS. Although HAART and trimethoprim-sulfamethoxazole prophylaxis have diminished the incidence of toxoplasmosis in patients with HIV infection, toxoplasmic encephalitis remains the presenting manifestation in 20% of patients with AIDS. In patients with AIDS, toxoplasmic encephalitis is fatal if not treated. Typical findings of CNS toxoplasmosis in patients with AIDS include fever, headache, altered mental status, psychosis, cognitive impairment, seizures and focal neurologic defects, including hemiparesis, aphasia, ataxia, visual field loss, cranial nerve palsies, and dysmetria or movement disorders. Uncommon findings of CNS involvement include meningismus, panhypopituitarism, and the syndrome of inappropriate secretion of antidiuretic hormone. In adult patients with AIDS, toxoplasmic retinal lesions are often large with diffuse necrosis and contain many organisms but little inflammatory cellular infiltrate.

Toxoplasmic encephalitis and congenital toxoplasmosis are a particular problem in immunocompromised individuals from areas where the incidence of latent infection is high. From 25–50% of patients with AIDS and *Toxoplasma* antibodies ultimately experience toxoplasmic encephalitis in the absence of prophylaxis with trimethoprim-sulfamethoxazole and treatment of HIV infection with protease inhibitors. The reason why only a subpopulation of latently infected individuals experiences toxoplasmic encephalitis is unknown. A diagnosis of presumptive toxoplasmic encephalitis in patients with AIDS should prompt a therapeutic trial of medications effective against *T. gondii*. Clear clinical improvement within 7–14 days and improvement in findings of neuroradiologic studies within 3 wk after therapy is initiated make the presumptive diagnosis almost certain.

CONGENITAL TOXOPLASMOSIS. The signs and symptoms associated with acute acquired *T. gondii* infection in the pregnant woman are the same as those seen in the immunologically nor-

mal child, most commonly lymphadenopathy. Most often, the acute acquired infection occurs without recognized symptoms or signs. Congenital infection also may be transmitted by an asymptomatic immunocompromised woman (e.g., those treated with corticosteroids and those with HIV infection).

Genetics. In monozygotic twins the clinical pattern of involvement is most often similar, whereas in dizygotic twins manifestations often differ. In dizygotic twins severe manifestations in one twin have led to a diagnosis of subclinical disease in the other twin. Also, congenital infection has occurred in only one twin of a pair of dizygotic twins. The major histocompatibility complex (MHC) class II gene DQ3 appears to be more frequent in patients seropositive for *T. gondii* infection with AIDS and toxoplasmic encephalitis than in patients seropositive for *T. gondii* infection with AIDS who do not have toxoplasmic encephalitis, and in children with congenital toxoplasmosis and hydrocephalus as compared with those without hydrocephalus. There were no children who were homozygous for the HLA-DQ3 allele with hydrocephalous, in contrast to the expected prevalence of homozygosity for this allele. This finding suggests that presence of HLA-DQ3 might be particularly detrimental to the fetus when toxoplasmosis is transmitted early in gestation.

Spectrum and Frequency of Signs and Symptoms. Congenital infection may present as a mild or severe neonatal disease, with onset during the 1st mo of life, or with sequelae or relapse of a previously undiagnosed infection at any time during infancy or later in life. A wide variety of manifestations of congenital infection occur in the perinatal period. These range from relatively mild signs, such as small size for gestational age, prematurity, peripheral retinal scars, persistent jaundice, mild thrombocytopenia, and cerebrospinal fluid pleocytosis, to the classic triad of signs consisting of chorioretinitis, hydrocephalus, and cerebral calcifications. Infection may result in erythroblastosis, hydrops fetalis, and perinatal death. More than half of congenitally infected infants are considered normal in the perinatal period, but almost all such children will have ocular involvement later in life. Neurologic signs in neonates, which include convulsions, setting-sun sign, and an increase in head circumference due to hydrocephalus, may be associated with substantial cerebral damage. However, such signs also may occur in association with encephalitis without extensive destruction or with relatively mild inflammation adjacent to and obstructing the aqueduct of Sylvius. If such infants are treated promptly, signs and symptoms may resolve, and they may develop normally.

The spectrum and frequency of manifestations that develop in the perinatal period in infants with congenital *Toxoplasma* infection are presented in Table 266–1. Infection in most of these 210 infants was initially suspected because their mothers were identified by a serologic screening program that detected pregnant women with acute acquired *T. gondii* infection. Twenty-one infants (10%) had severe congenital toxoplasmosis with CNS involvement, eye lesions, and general systemic manifestations. Seventy-one (34%) had mild involvement with normal clinical examination results other than retinal scars or isolated intracranial calcifications. In 116 (55%) there were no detectable manifestations; this may reflect the difficulties associated with funduscopic examination of the peripheral retina in infants and young children. These numbers represent an underestimation of the relative frequency of severe congenital infection for several reasons: the most severe cases, including most of those individuals who died, were not referred; therapeutic abortion was often performed when acute acquired infection of the mother was diagnosed early during pregnancy; in utero spiramycin therapy may have diminished the severity of infection; and only 13 infants had CT brain scans and 23% did not have a cerebrospinal fluid examination. Routine newborn examinations often yield normal findings for congenitally infected infants, but more careful evaluations may reveal significant abnormalities: specifically, of

TABLE 266–1. Signs and Symptoms in 210 Infants with Proved Congenital Toxoplasma Infection*

Finding	No. Examined	No. Positive (%)
Prematurity	210	
Birthweight <2,500 g		8 (3.8)
Birthweight 2,500–3,000 g		5 (7.1)
Intrauterine growth retardation		13 (6.2)
Icterus	201	20 (10)
Hepatosplenomegaly	210	9 (4.2)
Thrombocytopenic purpura	210	3 (1.4)
Abnormal blood count (anemia, eosinophilia)	102	9 (4.4)
Microcephaly	210	11 (5.2)
Hydrocephaly	210	8 (3.8)
Hypotonia	210	12 (5.7)
Convulsions	210	8 (3.8)
Psychomotor retardation	210	11 (5.2)
Intracranial calcification x-ray	210	24 (11.4)
Ultrasound	49	5 (10)
Computed tomography	13	11 (84)
Abnormal electroencephalogram	191	16 (8.3)
Abnormal cerebrospinal fluid	163	56 (34.2)
Microphthalmia	210	6 (2.8)
Strabismus	210	111 (5.2)
Chorioretinitis	210	
Unilateral		34 (16.1)
Bilateral		12 (5.7)

*Infants were identified by prospective study of infants born to women who acquired Toxoplasma gondii infection during pregnancy.

Data adapted from Couvreur J, Desmonts G, Tournier G, et al: A homogeneous series of 210 cases of congenital toxoplasmosis in 0–11 mo old infants detected prospectively. Ann Pediatr (Paris) 1984;31:815–9.

TABLE 266–2. Signs and Symptoms Occurring Before Diagnosis or During the Course of Untreated Acute Congenital Toxoplasmosis in 152 Infants (A) and in 101 of These Same Children After They Had Been Followed 4 yr or More (B)

Signs and Symptoms	Frequency of Occurrence in Patients with	
	"Neurologic" Disease*	"Generalized" Disease†
A. Infants	**108 Patients (%)**	**44 Patients (%)**
Chorioretinitis	102 (94)	29 (66)
Abnormal cerebrospinal fluid	59 (55)	37 (84)
Anemia	55 (51)	34 (77)
Convulsions	54 (50)	8 (18)
Intracranial calcification	54 (50)	2 (4)
Jaundice	31 (29)	35 (80)
Hydrocephalus	30 (28)	0 (0)
Fever	27 (25)	34 (77)
Splenomegaly	23 (21)	40 (90)
Lymphadenopathy	18 (17)	30 (68)
Hepatomegaly	18 (17)	34 (77)
Vomiting	17 (16)	21 (48)
Microcephalus	14 (13)	0 (0)
Diarrhea	7 (6)	11 (25)
Cataracts	5 (5)	0 (0)
Eosinophilia	6 (4)	8 (18)
Abnormal bleeding	3 (3)	8 (18)
Hypothermia	2 (2)	9 (20)
Glaucoma	2 (2)	0 (0)
Optic atrophy	2 (2)	0 (0)
Microphthalmia	2 (2)	0 (0)
Rash	1 (1)	11 (25)
Pneumonitis	0 (0)	18 (41)
B. Children ≥4 yr of age	**70 Patients (%)**	**31 Patients (%)**
Mental retardation	62 (89)	25 (81)
Convulsions	58 (83)	24 (77)
Spasticity and palsies	53 (76)	18 (58)
Severely impaired vision	48 (69)	13 (42)
Hydrocephalus or microcephalus	31 (44)	2 (6)
Deafness	12 (17)	3 (10)
Normal	6 (9)	5 (16)

*Patients with otherwise undiagnosed central nervous system disease in the 1st yr of life.

†Patients with otherwise undiagnosed non-neurologic diseases during the first 2 mo of life.

Adapted from Eichenwald H: A study of congenital toxoplasmosis. In Siim JC (editor): Human Toxoplasmosis. Copenhagen, Munksgaard, 1960, pp 41–49. Study performed in 1947. The most severely involved institutionalized patients were not included in the later study of 101 children.

28 infants who were detected by a universal state mandated serologic screening program for *T. gondii*–specific immunoglobulin M (IgM), 26 had normal findings on routine newborn examinations and 14 had significant abnormalities detected with more careful evaluation. These abnormalities included retinal scars (7 infants), active chorioretinitis (3 infants), and CNS abnormalities (8 infants).

There is a wide clinical spectrum of untreated congenital toxoplasmosis that is clinically apparent in the first year of life (Table 266–2). More than 80% of these children had an IQ of less than 70, and many had convulsions and severely impaired vision.

Skin. Cutaneous manifestations in infants with congenital toxoplasmosis include rashes, petechiae, ecchymoses, or large hemorrhages secondary to thrombocytopenia. Rashes may be fine punctate, diffuse maculopapular, lenticular, deep blue-red, sharply defined macular, and diffuse blue and papular. Macular rashes involving the entire body, including the palms and soles; exfoliative dermatitis; and cutaneous calcifications have been described. Jaundice due to hepatic involvement with *T. gondii* and/or hemolysis, cyanosis due to interstitial pneumonitis from congenital infection, and edema secondary to myocarditis or nephrotic syndrome may be present. Jaundice and conjugated hyperbilirubinemia may persist for months.

Systemic Signs. From 25% to more than 50% of infants with clinically apparent disease at birth are born prematurely. Low Apgar scores also are common. Intrauterine growth retardation and instability of temperature regulation may occur. Other systemic manifestations include lymphadenopathy, hepatosplenomegaly, myocarditis, pneumonitis, nephrotic syndrome, vomiting, diarrhea, and feeding problems. Bands of metaphyseal lucency and irregularity of the line of provisional calcification at the epiphyseal plate may occur without periosteal reaction in the ribs, femurs, and vertebrae. Congenital toxoplasmosis may be confused with isosensitization causing erythroblastosis fetalis; the Coombs test result is usually negative with congenital *T. gondii* infection.

Endocrine Abnormalities. Endocrine abnormalities may occur secondary to hypothalamic or pituitary involvement or end-organ involvement. Reported endocrinopathies include myxedema, persistent hypernatremia with vasopressin-sensitive diabetes insipidus without polyuria or polydipsia, sexual precocity, and partial anterior hypopituitarism.

Central Nervous System. Neurologic manifestations of congenital toxoplasmosis vary from massive acute encephalopathy to subtle neurologic syndromes. Toxoplasmosis should be considered as a cause of any undiagnosed neurologic disease in children younger than 1 yr of age, especially if retinal lesions are present.

Hydrocephalus may be the sole clinical neurologic manifestation of congenital toxoplasmosis and may either be compensated or require shunt placement. Hydrocephalus may present in the perinatal period, progress after the perinatal period, or, less commonly, present later in life. Patterns of seizures are protean and have included focal motor seizures, petit and grand mal seizures, muscular twitching, opisthotonus, and hypsarrhythmia (which may resolve with corticotropin [ACTH] therapy). Spinal or bulbar involvement may be manifested by paralysis of the extremities, difficulty in swallowing, and respiratory distress. Microcephaly usually reflects severe brain damage, but some children with microcephaly caused by congenital toxoplasmosis who have been treated appear to function normally in the early years of life. Untreated congenital toxoplasmosis that is symptomatic in the 1st yr of life can cause substantial diminution in cognitive function and developmental delays. Intellectual impairment also occurs in some children with subclinical infection despite treatment with pyrimethamine and sulfonamides. Seizures and focal motor defects may become apparent after the newborn period, even when infection is subclinical at birth.

Cerebrospinal fluid (CSF) abnormalities occur in at least one third of infants with congenital toxoplasmosis. Local production of *T. gondii*–specific antibodies may be demonstrated in CSF of congenitally infected individuals. CT of the brain with con-

trast medium enhancement is useful to detect calcifications, determine ventricular size, image active inflammatory lesions, and demonstrate porencephalic cystic structures (Fig. 266–3). Calcifications occur throughout the brain, but there appears to be a special propensity for development of such lesions in the caudate nucleus (i.e., especially basal ganglia area), choroid plexus, and subependyma. Ultrasonography may be useful for following ventricular size in congenitally infected infants. MRI, enhanced CT, and radionuclide brain scans may be useful for detecting active inflammatory lesions.

Eyes. Almost all untreated congenitally infected individuals will develop chorioretinal lesions by adulthood, and about 50% will have severe visual impairment. *T. gondii* causes a focal necrotizing retinitis in congenitally infected individuals (see Fig. 266–2). Retinal detachment may occur. Any part of the retina

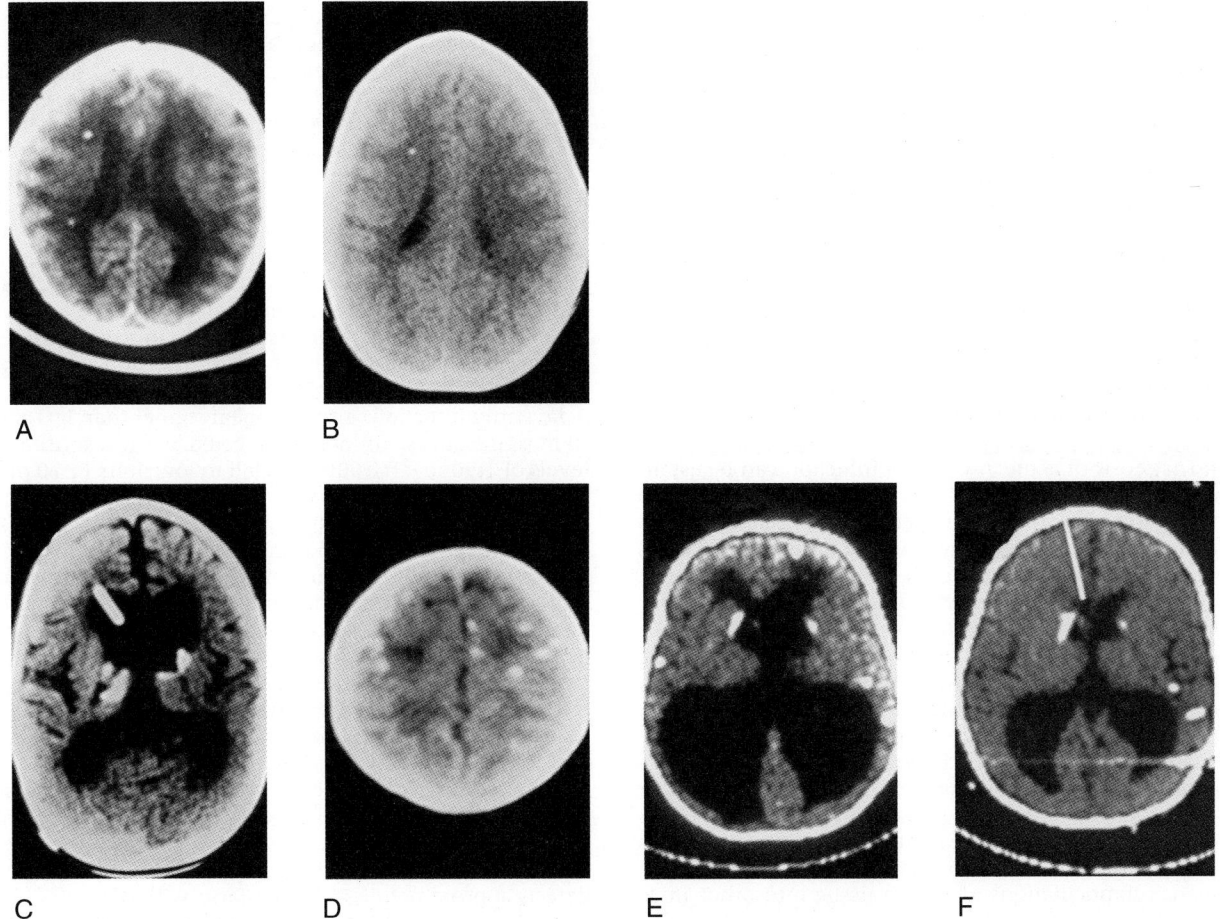

FIGURE 266–3. Head CT scans of infants with congenital toxoplasmosis. *A,* CT scan at birth that has areas of hypolucency, mildly dilated ventricles, and small calcifications. *B,* CT scan of the same child at 1 yr of age (after antimicrobial therapy for 1 yr). This scan is normal with the exception of two small calcifications. This child's Mental Development Index (MDI) at 1 yr of age was 140 by the Bayley Scale of Infant Development. *C,* CT scan from a 1-yr-old infant who was normal at birth. His meningoencephalitis became symptomatic in the 1st weeks of life but was not diagnosed correctly and remained untreated during his 1st 3 mo of life. At 3 mo of age, development of hydrocephalus and bilateral macular chorioretinitis led to the diagnosis of congenital toxoplasmosis, and antimicrobial therapy was initiated. This scan shows significant residual atrophy and calcifications. This child has substantial motor dysfunction, development delays, and visual impairment. *D,* CT scan obtained during the 1st mo of life of a microcephalic child. Note the numerous calcifications. This child's IQs (i.e., using the Stanford-Binet Intelligence Scale for children when she was 3 yr old and the Wechsler Preschool and Primary Scale Intelligence when she was 5 yr old) were 100 and 102, respectively. She received antimicrobial therapy during her 1st yr of life. *E,* CT scan with hydrocephalus owing to aqueductal stenosis (before shunt). *F,* Scan from the same patient as the scan in *E,* after shunt. This child's IQ (i.e., using the Stanford-Binet Intelligence Scale for children) was approximately 100 when she was 3 and 6 yr old. (Adapted from McAuley J, Boyer K, Patel D, et al: Early and longitudinal evaluations of treated infants and children and untreated historical patients with congenital toxoplasmosis: The Chicago Collaborative Treatment Trial. *Clin Infect Dis* 1994;18:38–72.)

may be involved, either unilaterally or bilaterally, including the maculae. The optic nerve may be involved, and toxoplasmic lesions that involve projections of the visual pathways in the brain or the visual cortex also may lead to visual impairment. In association with retinal lesions and vitritis, the anterior uvea may be intensely inflamed, leading to erythema of the external eye. Other ocular findings include cells and protein in the anterior chamber, large keratic precipitates, posterior synechiae, nodules on the iris, and neovascular formation on the surface of the iris, sometimes with an associated increase in intraocular pressure and development of glaucoma. The extraocular musculature may also be involved directly. Other manifestations include strabismus, nystagmus, visual impairment, and microphthalmia. The differential diagnosis of lesions resembling those of ocular toxoplasmosis includes congenital colobomatous defect and other inflammatory lesions due to cytomegalovirus, *Treponema pallidum, Mycobacterium tuberculosis,* or vasculitis. Ocular toxoplasmosis is a recurrent and progressive disease that requires multiple courses of therapy. There are limited data that suggest that occurrence of lesions in the early years of life may be prevented by instituting antimicrobial treatment (with pyrimethamine and sulfonamides in alternate months with spiramycin) during the 1st yr of life and that treatment of the infected fetus in utero followed by treatment in the 1st yr of life with pyrimethamine, sulfadiazine, and leukovorin reduces the incidence and the severity of the retinal disease.

Ears. Sensorineural hearing loss, both mild and severe, may occur. It is not known whether this is a static or progressive disorder. Treatment in the 1st yr of life is associated with diminished occurrence of this sequela.

Concomitant Infections. Congenital toxoplasmosis in infants with HIV infection usually presents as a severe and fulminant illness with substantial CNS involvement but also may be more indolent in its presentation with focal neurologic deficits or systemic manifestations such as pneumonitis.

Diagnosis. Diagnosis of acute *Toxoplasma* infection can be established by isolation of *T. gondii* from blood or body fluids and also by demonstration of tachyzoites in sections or preparations of tissues and body fluids, cysts in the placenta or tissues of a fetus or newborn, and characteristic lymph node histologic features. Serologic tests also are very useful for diagnosis.

CULTURE. Organisms are isolated by inoculation of body fluids, leukocytes, or tissue specimens into mice or tissue cultures. Body fluids should be processed and inoculated immediately, but *T. gondii* has been isolated from tissues and blood that have been stored at 4°C overnight. Freezing or treatment of specimens with formalin kills *T. gondii.* From 6–10 days after inoculation into mice, or earlier if mice die, peritoneal fluids should be examined for tachyzoites. If they survive for 6 wk and there is antibody in sera of the inoculated mouse, definitive diagnosis is made by visualization of *Toxoplasma* cysts in mouse brain. If cysts are not seen, subinoculations of mouse tissue into other mice are performed.

Microscopic examination of tissue culture inoculated with *T. gondii* shows necrotic, heavily infected cells with numerous extracellular tachyzoites. Isolation of *T. gondii* from blood or body fluids reflects acute infection. Except in the fetus or neonate it is usually not possible to distinguish acute from past infection by isolation of *T. gondii* from tissues such as skeletal muscle, lung, brain, or eye obtained by biopsy or at autopsy.

Diagnosis of acute infection can be established by demonstration of tachyzoites in biopsy tissue sections, bone marrow aspirate, or body fluids such as CSF or amniotic fluid. Immunofluorescent antibody and immunoperoxidase staining techniques may be necessary because it is often difficult to see the tachyzoite with ordinary stains. Tissue cysts are diagnostic of infection but do not differentiate between acute and chronic infection; the presence of many cysts suggests recent acute infection. Cysts

in the placenta or tissues of the newborn infant establish the diagnosis of congenital infection. Characteristic histologic features strongly suggest the diagnosis of toxoplasmic lymphadenitis.

SEROLOGIC TESTING. Multiple serologic tests may be necessary to confirm the diagnosis of congenital or acutely acquired *Toxoplasma* infection. Each laboratory that reports serologic test results must have established values for their tests that diagnose infection in specific clinical settings, provide interpretation of their results, and ensure appropriate quality control before therapy is based on serologic test results. Serologic test results used as the basis for therapy should be confirmed in a reference laboratory.

The **Sabin-Feldman dye test** is sensitive and specific. It measures primarily IgG antibodies. Results should be expressed in international units (IU/mL), based on international standard reference sera available from the World Health Organization.

The **IgG indirect fluorescent-antibody (IgG-IFA) test** measures the same antibodies as the dye test, and the titers tend to be parallel. These antibodies usually appear 1–2 wk after infection, reach high titers (≥1:1,000) after 6–8 wk, and then decline over months to years. Low titers (1:4–1:64) usually persist for life. Antibody titer does not correlate with severity of illness. Approximately half of the commercially available IFA kits for *T. gondii* have been found to be improperly standardized and may yield significant numbers of false-positive and false-negative results.

An **agglutination test** (Bio-Mérieux, Lyon, France) that is available commercially in Europe uses formalin-preserved whole parasites to detect IgM antibodies. This test is accurate, simple to perform, and inexpensive.

The **IgM indirect fluorescent antibody (IgM-IFA) test** is useful for the diagnosis of acute infection with *T. gondii* in the older child because IgM antibodies appear earlier (often by 5 days after infection) and disappear sooner than IgG antibodies. In most instances, antibodies detected by the test rise rapidly (to levels of 1:50 to <1:1,000) and fall to low titers (1:10 or 1:20) or disappear after weeks or months. However, some patients continue to have positive results at low titers for as long as several years. The IgM-IFA test detects *Toxoplasma*-specific IgM in only approximately 25% of congenitally infected infants at birth. IgM antibodies also are often not present in sera of immunodeficient patients with acute toxoplasmosis or in most patients with active toxoplasmosis present only in the eye. The IgM-IFA test may yield false-positive results as a result of rheumatoid factor.

The **double-sandwich enzyme-linked immunosorbent assay (ELISA)** is more sensitive and specific than the IgM-IFA test for detection of *Toxoplasma* IgM antibodies. In the older child, a level of IgM antibodies against *Toxoplasma* in serum of 2.0 or greater (value of one reference laboratory; each laboratory must establish its own values) indicates that *Toxoplasma* infection has most likely been acquired recently. The IgM-ELISA detects approximately 75% of infants with congenital infection. IgM-ELISA avoids both the false-positive results from rheumatoid factor and false-negative results from high levels of passively transferred maternal IgG antibody in fetal serum, as occurs in the IgM-IFA test. Results obtained with commercial kits must be interpreted with caution because false-positive reactions are not infrequent. Care must also be taken to determine whether kits have been standardized for diagnosis of infection in specific clinical settings (e.g., in the newborn infant). The **IgA-ELISA** is a more sensitive test than the IgM ELISA for detection of congenital infection in the fetus and newborn as well as for detection of acute infection in some pregnant women.

The **immunosorbent agglutination assay (ISAGA)** combines trapping of a patient's IgM to a solid surface and use of formalin-fixed organisms or antigen-coated latex particles. It is read as an agglutination test. There are no false-positive results from rheumatoid factor or antinuclear antibodies. IgM antibodies to *Toxoplasma* are detected by the IgM-IFA test for a shorter time than they are by the IgM-ELISA. The IgM-ISAGA is more sensitive than the IgM-ELISA and may detect specific IgM antibodies before and for longer periods than the IgM-ELISA. At present, IgM-ISAGA is the best test for diagnosis of congenital infection in the newborn. The IgE-ELISA and IgE-ISAGA are also useful in establishing the diagnosis of congenital toxoplasmosis or acute acquired *T. gondii* infection.

The **differential agglutination test (HS/SC)** compares antibody titers obtained with formalin-fixed tachyzoites (**HS antigen**) with titers obtained using acetone- or methanol-fixed tachyzoites (**AC antigen**) to differentiate recent and remote infections in adults and older children. This method may be particularly useful in differentiating remote infection in pregnant women, because levels of IgM and IgA antibodies detectable by ELISA or ISAGA may remain elevated for prolonged periods (e.g., months to years in adults and older children).

The **avidity test** can be used to determine whether acute infection began more than 12–16 wk earlier (high avidity test result).

The **indirect hemagglutination (IHA) test** measures different *T. gondii* antibodies from those measured in IFA and dye tests. They may persist for years. However, the IHA test should not be used in infants with suspected congenital infection or in screening for infection acquired during pregnancy because it may be negative for too long a period early during infection.

A relatively higher level of *Toxoplasma* antibody in the aqueous humor or in cerebrospinal fluid demonstrates local production of antibody during active ocular or CNS toxoplasmosis. This comparison is calculated as follows:

$$C = \frac{\text{Antibody titer in body fluid}}{\text{Antibody titer in serum}} \times \frac{\text{Concentration of IgG in serum}}{\text{Concentration of IgG in body fluid}}$$

Significant correlation coefficients [C] are more than or equal to 8 for ocular infection, more than or equal to 4 for CNS for congenital infection, and more than 1 for CNS infection in patients with AIDS. If the serum dye test titer is more than or equal to 300 IU/mL, most often it is not possible to demonstrate significant local antibody production using this formula with either the dye test or the IgM-IFA test titer. IgM antibody may be present in CSF.

Toxoplasma antigen has been detected during acute *Toxoplasma* infection but not in sera of uninfected or chronically infected individuals. Antigen was present in the serum, amniotic fluid, and CSF in the few infants tested with congenital infections.

Comparative **Western immunoblot** tests of sera from a mother and infant may detect congenital infection. Infection is suspected when the mother's serum and her infant's serum contain antibodies that react with different *Toxoplasma* antigens.

Enzyme-linked immunofiltration assay (ELIFA), using micropore membranes, permits simultaneous study of antibody specificity by immunoprecipitation and characterization of antibody isotypes by immunofiltration with enzyme-labeled antibodies. This method may be capable of detecting 85% of cases of congenital infection in the first few days of life. It is still being evaluated.

Polymerase chain reaction (PCR) is used to amplify the DNA of *T. gondii,* which then can be detected by using a DNA probe. Detection of a repetitive *T. gondii* gene, the *B1* gene, in amniotic fluid is the procedure of choice for establishing the diagnosis of congenital *Toxoplasma* infection in the fetus. Sensitivity and specificity of this test using amniotic fluid obtained at 18 wk of gestation or later are approximately 95%. Before and after that time, PCR is less sensitive for detection of congenital infec-

tion. PCR of vitreous fluid has been used to diagnose ocular toxoplasmosis. PCR of peripheral white blood cells, CSF, and urine has detected congenital infection.

Lymphocyte blastogenesis to *Toxoplasma* antigens has been used to diagnose congenital toxoplasmosis if a question persists concerning the diagnosis and other test results are negative. However, a negative result does not exclude the diagnosis, because many infected infants do not respond to *T. gondii* antigens in the newborn period.

ACQUIRED TOXOPLASMOSIS. Recent infection is diagnosed by seroconversion from a negative to a positive IgG antibody titer (in the absence of transfer of antibody by transfusion); a serial two-tube rise in *Toxoplasma*-specific IgG titer when sera are obtained 3 wk apart and tested in parallel; or the presence of *Toxoplasma*-specific IgM antibody.

OCULAR TOXOPLASMOSIS. IgG antibody titers of 1:4 to 1:64 are usual in older children with active toxoplasmic chorioretinitis. When the retinal lesions are characteristic and serologic tests findings are positive, the diagnosis is likely. PCR of vitreous fluid has been used to diagnose ocular toxoplasmosis but is infrequently performed because of risks associated with obtaining vitreous fluid.

IMMUNOCOMPROMISED PERSONS. IgG antibody titers may be low, and *Toxoplasma*-specific IgM is often absent in immunocompromised patients with toxoplasmosis. Demonstration of *Toxoplasma* antigens or DNA in serum, blood, and CSF may identify disseminated *Toxoplasma* infection in immunocompromised persons.

Resolution of CNS lesions during a therapeutic trial of pyrimethamine and sulfadiazine has been useful in patients with AIDS. Brain biopsy has been used to establish the diagnosis of toxoplasmic encephalitis when there is no response to this therapeutic trial or to exclude other likely diagnoses.

CONGENITAL TOXOPLASMOSIS. Fetal ultrasound examination, performed every 2 wk during gestation, and PCR analysis of amniotic fluid are used for prenatal diagnosis. *T. gondii* may also be isolated from the placenta.

Serologic tests are the most useful in establishing a diagnosis of congenital toxoplasmosis. Either persistent or rising titers in the dye or IFA test or a positive IgM ELISA or ISAGA result is diagnostic of congenital toxoplasmosis. The half-life of IgM is 3–5 days, so if there is a placental leak, the level of IgM antibodies in the infant's serum decreases significantly within 1–2 wk. Passively transferred maternal IgG antibodies may require many months to a year to disappear from the infant's serum, depending on the magnitude of the original titer. Synthesis of *Toxoplasma* antibody is usually demonstrable by the 3rd mo of life if the infant is untreated. If the infant is treated, synthesis may be delayed until the 9th mo of life, and, infrequently, it may not occur at all. When an infant begins to synthesize antibody, infection may be documented serologically even without demonstration of IgM antibodies by an increase in the ratio of specific serum antibody titer to the total IgG, whereas the ratio will decrease if the specific antibody has been passively transferred from the mother.

At birth, when a diagnosis of congenital toxoplasmosis is suspected, the following diagnostic studies should be performed: general, ophthalmologic, and neurologic examinations; head CT scan; attempt to isolate *T. gondii* from placenta and infant's leukocytes from umbilical cord blood and buffy coat; measurement of serum *Toxoplasma*-specific IgG, IgM, IgA, and IgE antibodies and the total amount of IgM and IgG in serum; lumbar puncture including analysis of CSF for cells, glucose, protein, *Toxoplasma*-specific IgG and IgM antibodies, and total amount of IgG; and evaluations of CSF for *T. gondii* by PCR and inoculation into mice. Presence of *Toxoplasma*-specific IgM in CSF that is not contaminated with blood or local antibody production of Toxoplasma-specific IgG antibody demonstrated in CSF establishes the diagnosis of congenital *Toxoplasma* infection.

Many manifestations similar to those of congenital toxoplasmosis occur in other perinatal diseases, especially disease caused by cytomegalovirus. Neither cerebral calcification nor chorioretinitis is pathognomonic. Fewer than 50% of children younger than 5 yr of age with chorioretinitis satisfy the serologic criteria for congenital toxoplasmosis; the causes of most of the other cases are unknown. The clinical picture in the newborn infant may also be compatible with sepsis, aseptic meningitis, syphilis, or hemolytic disease.

Treatment. Pyrimethamine plus sulfadiazine or trisulfapyrimidines act synergistically against *Toxoplasma*. Combined therapy is indicated to treat many of the forms of toxoplasmosis. However, use of pyrimethamine is contraindicated during the 1st trimester of pregnancy. Spiramycin should be used to prevent transmission of infection to the fetus of acutely infected pregnant women and to treat congenital toxoplasmosis. Pyrimethamine inhibits the enzyme dihydrofolate reductase (DHFR), and thus the synthesis of folic acid, and therefore produces a dose-related, reversible, and usually gradual depression of the bone marrow, resulting in thrombocytopenia, leukopenia, and anemia. Neutropenia is the most common side effect in treated infants. All patients treated with pyrimethamine should have platelet and leukocyte counts twice weekly. Seizures may occur with overdosage of pyrimethamine. Folinic acid (calcium leukovorin) should always be administered concomitantly with pyrimethamine to prevent suppression of the bone marrow. Potential toxic effects of sulfonamides (e.g., crystalluria, hematuria, and rash) should be monitored. Hypersensitivity reactions occur, especially in patients with AIDS.

ACQUIRED TOXOPLASMOSIS. Patients with lymphadenopathy do not need specific treatment unless they have severe and persistent symptoms or evidence of damage to vital organs. If such signs and symptoms occur, treatment with pyrimethamine, sulfadiazine, and leukovorin should be initiated. Patients who appear to be immunologically normal but have severe and persistent symptoms or damage to vital organs (e.g., chorioretinitis, myocarditis) need specific therapy until these specific symptoms resolve, followed by therapy for an additional 2 wk. This therapy usually lasts for at least 4–6 wk; the optimal duration of therapy is unknown. A loading dose of pyrimethamine for older children is 2 mg/kg/24 hr (maximum: 50 mg/24 hr), given for the first 2 days of treatment. The maintenance dose is 1 mg/kg/24 hr (maximum: 50 mg/24 hr). Folinic acid is administered orally at a dosage of 5–20 mg three times a week (or even daily depending on the leukocyte count). Sulfadiazine or trisulfapyrimidine is administered to children older than 1 yr of age at a dosage of 100 mg/kg/24 hr (maximum: 4 g/24 hr).

OCULAR TOXOPLASMOSIS. Patients with ocular toxoplasmosis are usually treated with pyrimethamine, sulfadiazine, and leukovorin for approximately 1 wk after the lesion develops a quiescent appearance (i.e., sharp borders and associated inflammatory cells in the vitreous resolve), which usually occurs in 2–4 wk. Within 7–10 days the borders of the retinal lesions sharpen, and visual acuity usually returns to that noted before development of the acute lesion. Systemic corticosteroids have been administered concomitantly with antimicrobial treatment when lesions involve the macula, optic nerve head, or papillomacular bundle. Most new lesions appear contiguous to old ones). Occasionally, vitrectomy and removal of the lens are needed to restore visual acuity.

IMMUNOCOMPROMISED PERSONS. Serologic evidence of acute infection in an immunocompromised patient, regardless of whether signs and symptoms of infection are present or tachyzoites are present in tissue, are indications for therapy similar to that described for immunocompetent children with symptoms of organ injury. It is important to establish the diagnosis as rapidly as possible and institute treatment early. In immunocompromised patients other than those with AIDS, therapy should be continued for at least 4–6 wk beyond complete resolution of all signs and symptoms of active disease.

Careful follow-up observation of these patients is imperative because relapse may occur, requiring prompt reinstitution of therapy. Relapse is frequent in patients with AIDS, and suppressive therapy with pyrimethamine and sulfonamides traditionally has been continued for life. One study suggests that it may be possible to discontinue maintenance therapy when the CD4 count has remained at more than 200 cells/μL for 4–6 mo and all lesions have resolved. Therapy usually induces a beneficial response clinically, but it does not eradicate cysts. Treatment of patients with AIDS and *T. gondii* seropositively should be continued as long as CD4 counts remain at less than 200 cells/μL. Prophylactic treatment with trimethoprim-sulfamethoxazole for *Pneumocystis carinii* pneumonia appears to reduce the incidence of toxoplasmosis in patients with AIDS.

CONGENITAL TOXOPLASMOSIS. All infected newborns should be treated, whether or not they have clinical manifestations of the infection. In infants with congenital infection, treatment may be effective in interrupting acute disease that damages vital organs. Infants should be treated for 1 yr with oral pyrimethamine (2 mg/kg/24 hr for 2 days, then 1 mg/kg/24 hr for 2 or 6 mo, then 1 mg/kg/ given on Monday, Wednesday, and Friday), sulfadiazine or triple sulfonamides (100 mg/kg/24 hr divided bid), and calcium leukovorin (5–10 mg/kg/24 hr given on Monday, Wednesday, and Friday). In the U.S. National Collaborative Study, the relative efficacy in reducing sequelae of infection and the safety of treatment with 2 versus 6 mo of the higher dosage of pyrimethamine are being compared.* Pyrimethamine and sulfadiazine are available only in tablet form and can be prepared as suspensions. Prednisone (1 mg/kg/24 hr divided bid PO) has been utilized in addition when active chorioretinitis involves the macula or otherwise threatens vision or the CSF protein is 1,000 mg/dL or more at birth, but its efficacy also is not established.

PREGNANT WOMEN WITH *T. GONDII* INFECTION. The immunologically normal pregnant woman who acquired *T. gondii* before conception does not need treatment to prevent congenital infection of her fetus. Although data are not available to allow for a definitive time interval, if infection occurs during the 6 mo prior to conception, it is reasonable to evaluate the fetus and treat to prevent congenital infection in the fetus in the same manner as described for the acutely infected pregnant patient.

Treatment of a pregnant woman who acquires infection at any time during pregnancy reduces the chance of congenital infection in her infant. The medications used are spiramycin† for prevention and pyrimethamine in combination with sulfadiazine when the fetus is found or it is highly likely to be infected. Because pyrimethamine is potentially teratogenic, spiramycin is administered in the 1st trimester. The dose of spiramycin is 1 g every 8 hr given without food; lower doses are less effective. Toxicity is infrequent. Adverse reactions include paresthesias, rash, nausea, vomiting, and diarrhea. Fetal infection is treated with pyrimethamine (50 mg once daily PO) and sulfadiazine (2 g bid PO). Leukovorin (10 mg once daily PO) is administered with pyrimethamine. Treatment of the mother of an infected fetus with pyrimethamine and sulfadiazine reduces infection in the placenta and the severity of disease in the newborn. Delay in maternal treatment during gestation results in more brain and eye disease in the infant. Diagnostic amniocentesis should not be limited to 17–18 wk gestation pregnancies when there is high suspicion that the fetus may be infected. Overall sensitivity of PCR with amniotic fluid is at 85%: sensitivity of PCR using amniotic fluid is less in early and late gestation than in mid gestation.

---

*Information concerning the U.S. National Collaborative Study evaluating these regimens can be obtained by calling 773-834-4152.

†Spiramycin is available in the United States through the FDA (telephone: 302-443-7580) when diagnosis of acute infection is confirmed in a reference laboratory (telephone: 650-326-8120).

The approach in France to congenital toxoplasmosis includes systematic serologic screening of all women of childbearing age and again intrapartum. Mothers with acute infection are treated with spiramycin, which decreases the transmission from 60% to 23%. Ultrasonography and amniocentesis for PCR at approximately 18 wk gestation are used for fetal diagnosis; they have 97% sensitivity and 100% specificity. Fetal infection is treated with pyrimethamine and sulfadiazine, or by termination of pregnancy. This strategy has an excellent outcome with normal development of children. Only 19% have subtle findings of congenital infection, including intracranial calcifications (13%) and chorioretinal scars (6%), although 39% have chorioretinal scars detected at follow-up observation during later childhood.

Chronically infected pregnant women who have been immunocompromised by cytotoxic drugs or corticosteroid therapy have transmitted *T. gondii* to their fetuses. Such women should be treated with spiramycin throughout gestation. The best approach to prevention of congenital toxoplasmosis in the fetus of a pregnant woman with HIV infection and inactive *T. gondii* infection is unknown. If the pregnancy is not terminated, the mother should be treated with spiramycin during the first 17 wk of gestation and then with pyrimethamine and sulfadiazine until term. In a study of adult patients with AIDS, pyrimethamine (75 mg/24 hr Po) combined with high dosages of intravenously administered clindamycin (1,200 mg every 6 hr IV) appeared equal in efficacy to sulfadiazine and pyrimethamine. Other currently experimental agents include the macrolides roxithromycin and azithromycin.

Prognosis. Early institution of specific treatment for congenitally infected infants usually cures the manifestations of toxoplasmosis, including active chorioretinitis, meningitis, encephalitis, hepatitis, splenomegaly, and thrombocytopenia. Hydrocephalus due to aqueductal obstruction may develop or become worse during therapy. Such treatment also may reduce the incidence of some sequelae, such as diminished cognitive or abnormal motor function. Without therapy, chorioretinitis often recurs. Children with extensive involvement at birth may function normally later in life or have mild to severe impairment of vision, hearing, cognitive function, and other neurologic functions. Delays in diagnosis and therapy, perinatal hypoglycemia, hypoxia, hypotension, repeated shunt infections, and severe visual impairment are associated with a poorer prognosis. The prognosis is guarded but is not necessarily poor for infected babies. Treatment with pyrimethamine and sulfadiazine does not eradicate the encysted parasite. No protective vaccine is available.

Prevention. Counseling pregnant women about the methods of preventing transmission of *T. gondii* (see Fig. 266–1) during pregnancy can substantially reduce acquisition of infection during gestation. Women who do not have specific antibody to *T. gondii* before pregnancy should only eat well-cooked meat during pregnancy and avoid contact with oocysts excreted by cats. Cats that are kept indoors, maintained on prepared food, and not fed fresh, uncooked meat should not contact encysted *T. gondii* or shed oocysts. Serologic screening, ultrasound monitoring, and treatment of pregnant women during gestation can also reduce the incidence and manifestations of congenital toxoplasmosis.

Bretagne S, Costa JM, Vidaud M, et al: Detection of *Toxoplasma gondii* by competitive DNA amplification of bronchoalveolar lavage samples. *J Infect Dis* 1993;168:1585–8.

Brooks RG, McCabe RE, Remington JS: Role of serology in the diagnosis of toxoplasmic lymphadenopathy. *Rev Infect Dis* 1987;9:1055–62.

Couvreur J, Desmonts G, Tournier G, et al: A homogeneous series of 210 cases of congenital toxoplasmosis in 0 to 11-month-old infants detected prospectively. *Ann Pediatr (Paris)* 1984;31:815–9.

Daffos F, Forestier F, Capella-Pavlovsky M, et al: Prenatal management of 746 pregnancies at risk for congenital toxoplasmosis. *N Engl J Med* 1988;318:271–5.

Dannemann BR, Vaughan WC, Thulliez P, et al: The differential agglutination test for diagnosis of recently acquired infection with *Toxoplasma gondii*. *J Clin Microbiol* 1990;28:1928–33.

Derouin F, Devergie A, Auber P, et al: Toxoplasmosis in bone marrow transplant recipients: Report of seven cases and review. *Clin Infect Dis* 1992;15:267–70.

Desmonts G, Couvreur J: Natural history of congenital toxoplasmosis. *Ann Pediatr* 1984;31:799–802.

Desmonts G, Daffos F, Forestier F, et al: Prenatal diagnosis of congenital toxoplasmosis. *Lancet* 1985;1:500–4.

Foulon W, Villena E, Stray-Pedersen B, et al: Treatment of toxoplasmosis during pregnancy: A multicenter study of impact on fetal transmission and children's sequelae at age 1 year. *Am J Obstet Gynec* 180;410–15.

Foulon W, Naessens A, Ho-Yen D: Prevention of congenital toxoplasmosis. *J Perinat Med* 2000;28:337–45.

Grover CM, Thulliez P, Remington JS, et al: Rapid prenatal diagnosis of congenital *Toxoplasma* infection by using polymerase chain reaction and amniotic fluid. *J Clin Microbiol* 1990;28:2297–301.

Guerrina NG, Hsu HW, Meissner HC, et al: Neonatal serologic screening and early treatment for congenital *Toxoplasma gondii* infection. *N Engl J Med* 1994;330:1858–63.

Haentjens M, Sacre L, Demeuter F: Congenital toxoplasmosis after maternal infection before or slightly after conception. *Acta Paediatr Scand* 1986;75:343–5.

Hohlfeld P, Daffos F, Thulliez P, et al: Fetal toxoplasmosis: Outcome of pregnancy and infant follow-up after in utero treatment. *J Pediatr* 1989;115:765–69.

Ives NJ, Gazzard BG, Easterbrook PJ: The changing pattern of AIDS-defining illnesses with the introduction of highly active anti-retroviral therapy (HAART) in a London clinic. *J Infect* 2001;42:134–9.

Jenum PA, Stray-Pedersen B, Gundersen AG: Improved diagnosis of primary *Toxoplasma gondii* infection in early pregnancy by determination of anti-*Toxoplasma* immunoglobulin G avidity. *J Clin Microbiol* 1997;35:1972–9.

Koppe JG, Loewer-Sieger DH, de Roever-Bonnet H: Results of 20-year follow-up of congenital toxoplasmosis. *Lancet* 1986;1:254–6.

Luft BJ, Remington JS: Toxoplasmic encephalitis in AIDS. *Clin Infect Dis* 1992;15:211–22.

McAuley J, Boyer K, Patel D, et al: Early and longitudinal evaluations of treated infants and children and untreated historical patients with congenital toxoplasmosis. The Chicago Collaborative Treatment Trial. *Clin Infect Dis* 1994;18:38–72.

McCabe RE, Brooks RG, Dorfman RF, et al: Clinical spectrum in 107 cases of toxoplasmic lymphadenopathy. *Rev Infect Dis* 1987;9:754–74.

McCabe RE, Remington JS: Toxoplasmosis: The time has come. *N Engl J Med* 1988;318:313–5.

McGee T, Wolters C, Stein L, et al: Absence of sensorineural hearing loss in treated infants and children with congenital toxoplasmosis. *Otolaryngol Head Neck Surg* 1992;106:75–80.

McLeod R, Boyer K, Roizen N, et al: The child with congenital toxoplasmosis. *Curr Clin Top Infect Dis* 2000;20:189–208.

Mets MB, Holfels E, Boyer KM, et al: Eye manifestations of congenital toxoplasmosis. *Am J Ophthalmol* 1997;123:1–16.

Mitchell CD, Erlich SS, Mastrucci MT, et al: Congenital toxoplasmosis occurring in infants perinatally infected with human immunodeficiency virus. *J Pediatr Infect Dis* 1990;9:512–6.

Mitchell W: Neurological and developmental effects of HIV and AIDS in children and adolescents. *Ment Retard Dev Disabil Res Rev* 2001;7:211–6.

Minkoff H, Remington JS, Holman S, et al: Vertical transmission of *Toxoplasma* by human immunodeficiency virus–infected women. *Am J Obstet Gynecol* 1997;176:555–9.

Montoya JG, Jordan R, Lingamneni S, et al: Toxoplasmic myocarditis and polymyositis in patients with acute acquired toxoplasmosis diagnosed during life. *Clin Infect Dis* 1997;24:676–83.

Montoya JG, Remington JS: Studies on the serodiagnosis of toxoplasmic lymphadenitis. *Clin Infect Dis* 1995;20:781–9.

Montoya JG: Laboratory diagnosis of *Toxoplasma gondii* infection and toxoplasmosis. *J Infect Dis* 2002;1855:S73–82.

Montoya JG, Remington JS: Toxoplasmic chorioretinitis in the setting of acute acquired toxoplasmosis. *Clin Infect Dis* 1996;23:277–82.

Patel DV, Holfels EM, Vogel NP, et al: Resolution of intracerebral calcifications in infants with treated congenital toxoplasmosis. *Radiology* 1996;199:433–40.

Remington JS, McLeod R, Thulliez P, et al: Toxoplasmosis. In Remington J, Klein J (editors): *Infectious Diseases of the Fetus and Newborn Infant*, 5th ed. Philadelphia, WB Saunders, 2001.

Roberts F, McLeod R: Pathogenesis of toxoplasmosis retinochoroiditis. *Parasitol Today* 1999;15:51–7.

Roberts F, Mets MB, Ferguson DJP, et al: Histopathological feature of ocular toxoplasmosis in the fetus and infant. *Arch Ophthalmol* 2001;119:1–58.

Roizen N, Swisher C, Boyer K, et al: Developmental and neurologic outcome in congenital toxoplasmosis. *Pediatrics* 1995;95:11–20.

Romand S, Wallon J, Franck J, et al: Prenatal diagnosis using polymerase chain reaction on amniotic fluid for congenital toxoplasmosis. *Obstet Gynecol* 2001;97:296–300.

Saxon SA, Knight W, Reynolds DW, et al: Intellectual deficits in children born with subclinical congenital toxoplasmosis: A preliminary report. *J Pediatr* 1973;82:792–7.

Silveira C, Belfort R Jr, Burnier M Jr, et al: Acquired toxoplasmic infection as the cause of toxoplasmic retinochoroiditis in families. *Am J Ophthalmol* 1988;106:362–4.

Vogel N, Kirisits J, Michael E, et al: Congenital toxoplasmosis transmitted from an immunologically competent mother infected before conception. *Clin Infect Dis* 1996;23:1055–60.

Wilson CB, Remington JS, Stagno S, et al: Development of adverse sequelae in children born with subclinical congenital *Toxoplasma* infection. *Pediatrics* 1980; 66:767–74.

Chapter 267
Pneumocystis carinii
Walter T. Hughes

Pneumocystis carinii pneumonia (interstitial plasma cell pneumonitis) in an immunocompromised host is a life-threatening infection. It is believed to result in part from activation of latent organisms acquired in early childhood, de novo infection acquired later in life, or both. Even in the most severe cases, with rare exceptions, the organisms and the disease remain localized to the lungs.

Etiology. *P. carinii* is a common extracellular parasite found in the lungs of mammals worldwide. The taxonomic placement of this organism has not been established, but it has attributes of fungi and protozoa. Although *P. carinii* DNA has genomic homology closer to those of fungi, its morphologic features and susceptibility to drugs are similar to those of protozoa.

Epidemiology. Serologic surveys show most humans become infected with *P. carinii* before 4 yr of age. In the healthy host, these infections are usually asymptomatic. *P. carinii* DNA can often be detected in nasopharyngeal aspirates of normal infants. Pneumonia caused by *P. carinii* occurs almost exclusively in severely immunocompromised hosts, including those with congenital or acquired immunodeficiency disorders or malignancies, and in organ transplant recipients.

Without prophylaxis, approximately 40% of infants and children and 70% of adults with AIDS, 12% of children with leukemia, and 10% of patients with organ transplants experience *P. carinii* pneumonia. Epidemics that occurred among debilitated infants in Europe during and after World War II have been attributed to malnutrition.

The natural habitat and mode of transmission to humans are unknown. Experiments in rats have demonstrated animal-to-animal transmission by the airborne route, but animal-to-human transmission is unlikely because of the host-specific nature of *P. carinii*. Person-to-person transmission has been suggested from a few studies but has not been conclusively demonstrated.

Pathogenesis. Two forms of *P. carinii* are found in the alveolar spaces: cysts that are 5–8 μm in diameter and may contain up to eight pleomorphic intracystic sporozoites, and the extracystic trophozoites, which are 2–5 μm delicate cells derived from excysted sporozoites. *P. carinii* attaches to type I alveolar epithelial cells by adhesive proteins such as fibronectin and mannose-dependent ligand. Alveolar macrophages phagocytize and kill opsonized *P. carinii* organisms, releasing tumor necrosis factor. The inflammatory process is associated with disruption of surfactant function and respiratory impairment. The histopathologic features of *P. carinii* pneumonia are of two types. The first type is infantile interstitial plasma cell pneumonitis, which is seen in epidemic outbreaks in debilitated infants at 3–6 mo of age. Extensive infiltration with thickening of the alveolar septum occurs, and plasma cells are prominent. The second type is a diffuse desquamative alveolar disease found in immunocompromised children and adults. The alveoli contain large numbers of *P. carinii* in a foamy exudate with alveolar macrophages active in the phagocytosis of organisms. The alveolar septum is not infiltrated to the extent it is in the infantile type, and plasma cells are usually absent.

Cell-mediated immunity has the major role in defense against *P. carinii* pneumonia. This is evidenced by the high frequency of *P. carinii* pneumonia in severe combined immunodeficiency disorder, with attack rates greater than 40%, and the infrequency of its occurrence in X-linked agammaglobulinemia. Studies in patients with AIDS show an increase in the occurrence of *P. carinii* pneumonia in the presence of markedly decreased CD4 T-lymphocyte counts. The CD4 cell count provides a useful indicator in both older children and adults of the necessity of prophylaxis for *P. carinii* pneumonia.

Clinical Manifestations. The epidemic infantile form of *P. carinii* interstitial plasma cell pneumonitis is seen predominantly in infants 3–6 mo of age. The onset of hypoxia and symptoms is subtle with tachypnea but without fever, progressing to intercostal, suprasternal, and infrasternal retractions, nasal flaring, and cyanosis. In the sporadic form of *P. carinii* pneumonia occurring in children and adults with underlying immunodeficiency, the onset of hypoxia and symptoms is usually abrupt with fever, tachypnea, dyspnea, and cough, progressing to nasal flaring and cyanosis. This latter type accounts for the majority of cases, although the severity of clinical expression may vary. Rales are usually not detected on physical examination.

The chest radiograph reveals bilateral diffuse alveolar disease with a granular pattern. The earliest densities are perihilar, and progression proceeds peripherally, sparing the apical areas until last.

Diagnosis. A definitive diagnosis requires the demonstration of *P. carinii* in the lung in the presence of clinical signs and symptoms of the infection. Methods for obtaining appropriate specimens for detecting organisms include bronchoalveolar lavage, tracheal aspirate, transbronchial lung biopsy, bronchial brushings, percutaneous transthoracic needle aspiration, and open lung biopsy. Induced sputum samples are helpful if *P. carinii* is found, but the absence of the organisms in induced sputum does not exclude the infection. The open lung biopsy is the most reliable method, although bronchoalveolar lavage is more practical in most cases. Four stains are in general use: Grocott-Gomori stain and toluidine blue stain for the cyst form, polychrome stains such as Giemsa stain for the trophozoites and sporozoites, and the fluorescein-labeled monoclonal antibody stains for both trophozoites and cysts. Polymerase chain reaction analysis of respiratory specimens offers promise as a rapid diagnostic method, but a standardized system for clinical use has not been established.

Treatment. The recommended therapy is trimethoprim-sulfamethoxazole (TMP-SMZ) (15–20 mg TMP, 75–100 mg SMZ/kg/24 hr divided qid) administered intravenously, or orally if there is mild disease and no malabsorption or diarrhea. The duration of treatment is about 3 wk for patients with AIDS and 2 wk for other patients. Unfortunately, adverse reactions frequently occur with trimethoprim-sulfamethoxazole, including rash and neutropenia in patients with AIDS but are less common in non–AIDS patients. For patients who cannot tolerate or fail to respond to trimethoprim-sulfamethoxazole after 5–7 days, pentamidine isethionate (4 mg/kg/24 hr as a single dose IV) may be used. Adverse reactions are frequent and include renal and hepatic dysfunction, hyperglycemia or hypoglycemia, rash, and thrombocytopenia. Atovaquone and trimetrexate glucuronate are alternative treatments that have been used primarily in adults with mild to moderate disease. Pharmacokinetic studies of atovaquone show that a dose of 30 mg/kg/24 hr divided bid PO for children 2 yr of age or older is adequate and safe; a dose of 45 mg/kg/24 hr divided bid PO is needed for children younger than 2 yr of age. Other effective therapies include combinations of trimethoprim plus dapsone and of clindamycin plus primaquine.

Some studies in adults suggest that administration of corticosteroids in addition to anti–*P. carinii* drugs increases the chances for survival in moderate and severe cases of *P. carinii* pneumonia. The recommended regimen of corticosteroids for adolescents older than 13 yr of age and for adults is oral prednisone, 80 mg/24 hr divided bid PO on days 1–5, 40 mg/24 hr once daily PO on days 6–10, and 20 mg/24 hr once daily PO on days 11–21. A regimen for children is oral prednisone, 2 mg/kg/24 hr for the first 7–10 days, followed by a tapering regimen for the next 10–14 days.

Complications. Most complications occur as adverse events associated with the drugs used for treatment. Rarely, *P. carinii* infection affects extrapulmonary sites (e.g., retina, spleen, and bone marrow), but such infections are usually not symptomatic and also respond to treatment.

Prognosis. Without treatment, *P. carinii* pneumonitis is fatal in almost all immunocompromised hosts within 3–4 wk of onset. The mortality rate is 10–30% if treatment is initiated early in the course of the pneumonia. Patients remain at risk for *P. carinii* pneumonia as long as they are immunocompromised. Continuous prophylaxis should be initiated or reinstituted at the end of therapy for patients with AIDS.

Prevention. Patients at high risk for *P. carinii* pneumonia should be placed on chemoprophylaxis. Prophylaxis of infants born to HIV-infected mothers, and for HIV-infected infants and children, are based on age and CD4 cell counts (see Table 254–4). Patients with severe combined immunodeficiency syndrome, those with organ transplants, and those receiving intensive immunosuppressive therapy for cancer or other diseases are also candidates for prophylaxis. Trimethoprim-sulfamethoxazole (5 mg TMP, 25 mg SMZ/kg/24 hr once daily PO) is the drug of choice and may be given for 3 consecutive days each week, or, alternatively, each day. Alternatives for prophylaxis include dapsone (2 mg/kg/24 hr once daily PO; maximum: 100 mg/dose; or 4 mg/kg once weekly PO; maximum: 200 mg), atovaquone (30 mg/kg/24 hr once daily PO for 1–3 mo and infants older than 24 mo of age; 45 mg/kg/24 hr for infants 4–23 mo of age), and aerosolized pentamidine (300 mg monthly by Respirgard II nebulizer). The prophylaxis must be continued as long as the patient remains immunocompromised. Some AIDS patients who reconstitute adequate immune response during highly active antiretroviral therapy (HAART) may have prophylaxis withdrawn.

Centers for Disease Control and Prevention: Guidelines for preventing opportunistic infections among HIV-infected persons-2002: Recommendations of the U.S. Public Health Service and the Infectious Diseases Society of America. *MMWR* 2002;51(RR-8):1–46.

Hughes WT: *Pneumocystis carinii* pneumonia. *Semin Pediatr Infect Dis* 2001;12: 309–14.

Hughes WT, Leoung G, Kramer F, et al: Comparison of atovaquone (566C80) with trimethoprim-sulfamethoxazole to treat *Pneumocystis carinii* pneumonia in patients with AIDS. *N Engl J Med* 1993;328:1521–7.

Ledergerber B, Mocroft A, Reiss P, et al: Discontinuation of secondary prophylaxis against *Pneumocystis carinii* pneumonia in patients with HIV infection who have a response to antiretroviral therapy. Eight European Study Groups. *N Engl J Med* 2001;344:168–74.

McIntosh K, Cooper E, Xu J, et al: Toxicity and efficacy of daily vs. weekly dapsone for prevention of *Pneumocystis carinii* pneumonia in children infected with human immunodeficiency virus. *Pediatr Infect Dis J* 1999;18:432–39.

Poulsen A, Demeny AK, Bang Plum C, et al: *Pneumocystis carinii* pneumonia during maintenance treatment of childhood acute lymphocytic leukemia. *Med Pediatr Oncol* 2001;37:20–3.

Torres J, Goldman M, Wheat LJ, et al: Diagnosis of *Pneumocystis carinii* pneumonia in human immunodeficiency virus-infected patients with polymerase chain reaction: A blinded comparison to standard methods. *Clin Infect Dis* 2000;30: 141–5.

Vargas SL, Hughes WT, Santolaya ME, et al: Search for primary infection by *Pneumocystis carinii* in a cohort of normal, healthy infants. *Clin Infect Dis* 2001;32: 855–61.

Wright TW, Notter RH, Wang Z, et al: Pulmonary inflammation disrupts surfactant function during *Pneumocystis carinii* pneumonia. *Infect Immun* 2001;69:758–64.

SECTION 13 *Helminthic Diseases*

Chapter 268

Ascariasis (*Ascaris lumbricoides*)

Sheral S. Patel and James W. Kazura

Etiology. Ascariasis is caused by the nematode, or roundworm, *Ascaris lumbricoides*. Adult worms of *A. lumbricoides* inhabit the lumen of the small intestine and have a lifespan of 10–24 mo. The reproductive potential of *Ascaris* is prodigious in that a gravid female worms produces 200,000 eggs/24 hr. The fertile ova are oval in shape with a thick mammillated covering measuring 45–70 μm in length and 35–50 μm in breadth (Fig. 268–1). After passage in the feces, the eggs embryonate and become infective in 5–10 days under favorable environmental conditions.

Epidemiology. Ascariasis occurs globally and is the most prevalent human helminthiasis in the world. It is most common in tropical areas of the world where environmental conditions are optimal for maturation of ova in the soil. Approximately 1 billion persons are estimated to be infected, with 4 million cases in the United States. Key factors linked with a higher prevalence of infection include poor socioeconomic conditions, use of human feces as fertilizer, and geophagia. Even though infection can occur at any age, the highest rate is in children of preschool or early school age. Transmission is primarily hand-to-mouth but may also involve ingestion of contaminated raw fruits and vegetables. Transmission is enhanced by the high output of eggs by fecund female worms and resistance of ova to the outside environment. *Ascaris* eggs can remain viable at 5–10°C for as long as 2 yr.

Pathogenesis. *Ascaris* ova hatch in the small intestine after ingestion by the human host. Larvae are released, penetrate the intestinal wall, and migrate to the lungs by way of the venous circulation. The parasites then cause **pulmonary ascariasis** as they enter into the alveoli and migrate through the bronchi and trachea. They are subsequently swallowed and return to the intestines, where they mature into adult worms. Female *Ascaris* begin depositing eggs in 8–10 wk.

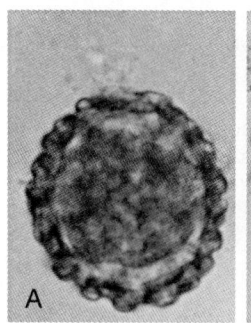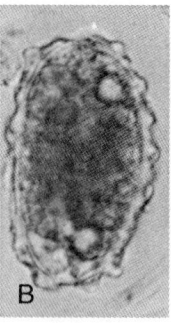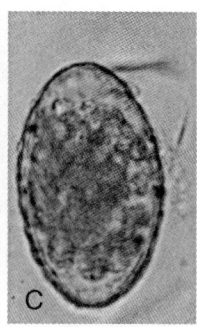

FIGURE 268–1. Fertilized (*A*) and unfertilized (*B, C*) eggs of *Ascaris lumbricoides* (×400). The egg illustrated in *C* may be mistaken for that of a different nematode or of a trematode.

Clinical Manifestations. The clinical presentation depends on the intensity of infection and the organs involved. Most individuals have low to moderate worm burdens and have no symptoms or signs. The most common clinical problems are due to pulmonary disease and obstruction of the intestinal or biliary tract. Larvae migrating through these tissues may cause allergic symptoms, fever, urticaria, and granulomatous disease. The pulmonary manifestations resemble Löffler syndrome and include transient respiratory symptoms such as cough and dyspnea, pulmonary infiltrates, and blood eosinophilia. Larvae may be observed in the sputum. Vague abdominal complaints have been attributed to the presence of adult worms in the small intestine, although the precise contribution of the parasite to these symptoms is difficult to ascertain. A more serious complication occurs when a large mass of worms leads to acute bowel obstruction. Children with heavy infections may present with vomiting, abdominal distention, and cramps. In some cases, worms may be passed in the vomitus or stools. *Ascaris* worms occasionally migrate into the biliary and pancreatic ducts, where they cause cholecystitis or pancreatitis. Dead worms can serve as a nidus for stone formation. It is unclear whether infection with *A. lumbricoides* affects growth and nutrition. Some studies suggest that worm burden and poor growth status are independent, whereas others conclude that children with recurrent heavy infection are at risk of protein-energy malnutrition.

Diagnosis. Microscopic examination of fecal smears can be used for diagnosis because of the high number of eggs excreted by adult female worms (see Fig. 268–1). A high index of suspicion in the appropriate clinical context is needed to diagnose pulmonary ascariasis or obstruction of the gastrointestinal tract.

Treatment. Although several chemotherapeutic agents are effective against ascariasis, none have documented utility during the pulmonary phase of infection. Treatment options for gastrointestinal ascariasis include albendazole (400 mg PO once, for all ages), mebendazole (100 mg bid PO for 3 days or 500 mg PO once for all ages), or pyrantel pamoate (11 mg/kg PO once; maximum: 1 g). Piperazine citrate (150 mg/kg PO initially, followed by six doses of 65 mg/kg at 12-hr intervals PO), which causes neuromuscular paralysis of the parasite and rapid expulsion of the worms, is the treatment of choice for intestinal or biliary obstruction and is administered as a syrup through a nasogastric tube. Surgery may be required for cases with severe obstruction.

Prevention. Although ascariasis is the most prevalent worm infection in the world, little attention has been given to its control because of controversy surrounding its public health significance and the likelihood of recurrent infections in epidemiologic settings where transmission rates are high. Short-term preventive measures include chemotherapy. Anthelmintic chemotherapy programs can be implemented in one of three ways: (1) offering universal treatment to all individuals in an area of high endemicity; (2) offering treatment targeted to groups with high frequency of infection, such as children attending primary school; (3) offering individual treatment based on intensity of current or past infection. Improving sanitary conditions and sewage facilities, discontinuing the practice of using human feces as fertilizer, and education are the most effective long-term preventive measures.

Crompton DW: *Ascaris* and ascariasis. *Adv Parasitol* 2001;48:285–375.

Hall A, Holland C: Geographical variation in *Ascaris lumbricoides* fecundity and its implications for helminth control. *Parasitol Today* 2000;16:540–4.

O'Lorcain P, Holland CV: The public health importance of *Ascaris lumbricoides*. *Parasitology* 2000;121:S51–71.

Chapter 269
Hookworms (*Ancylostoma* and *Necator americanus*)
Peter J. Hotez

Etiology. Two major genera of hookworms, which are nematodes or roundworms, infect humans. Hookworms of the genus *Ancylostoma* include the major anthropophilic hookworm *Ancylostoma duodenale*, which causes classic hookworm infection, and the less common zoonotic species *A. ceylanicum*, *A. caninum*, and *A. braziliense*. Human zoonotic infection with the dog hookworm, *A. caninum*, has been linked to an eosinophilic enteritis syndrome. The larval stage of *A. braziliense*, whose definitive hosts include dogs and cats, is the principal cause of cutaneous larva migrans. *Necator americanus*, the only representative of its genus, is also a major anthropophilic hookworm and causes classic hookworm infection.

The infective larval stages of the anthropophilic hookworms live in a developmentally arrested state in warm, moist soil. The larvae infect humans either by penetrating through the skin (*N. americanus* and *A. duodenale*) or when they are ingested (*A. duodenale*). Larvae entering the human host by skin penetration undergo **extraintestinal migration** through the venous circulation and lungs before they are swallowed, whereas orally ingested larvae may either undergo extraintestinal migration or remain in the gastrointestinal tract. Larvae returning to the small intestine undergo two molts to become adult sexually mature male and female worms ranging in length from 5–13 mm. The buccal capsule of the adult hookworm is armed with teeth (*A. duodenale*) or cutting plates (*N. americanus*) to facilitate attachment to the mucosa and submucosa of the small intestine. Hookworms can remain in the intestine for 1–5 yr, where they mate and produce eggs. Although approximately 2 mo is required for the larval stages of hookworms to undergo extraintestinal migration and develop into mature adults, *A. duodenale* larvae may remain developmentally arrested for many months before resuming development in the intestine. Mature *A. duodenale* female worms produce about 30,000 eggs/24 hr; daily egg production by *N. americanus* is less than 10,000/24 hr. The eggs are thin-shelled and ovoid, measuring approximately 40×60 µ. Eggs that are deposited on soil with adequate moisture and shade develop into first-stage larvae and hatch. Over the ensuing several days, under appropriate conditions, the larvae molt twice to the infective stage. Infective larvae are developmentally arrested and nonfeeding. They migrate vertically in the soil until they either infect a new host or exhaust their lipid metabolic reserves and die.

Epidemiology. Hookworm infection is one of the most prevalent infectious diseases of humans, affecting an estimated 1 billion individuals worldwide. Because of the requirement for adequate soil moisture, shade, and warmth, hookworm infection is usually confined to rural areas, especially where human feces are used for fertilizer or where sanitation is inadequate. For that reason, hookworm is an infection associated with economic underdevelopment and poverty throughout the tropics and subtropics. High rates of infection are often associated with cultivation of certain agricultural products such as tea in India; sweet potato, corn, cotton, and mulberry trees in China; coffee in Central and South America; and rubber in Africa. China and India have the highest prevalence of hookworm infection. Wherever hookworm occurs, it is not uncommon to find patients with mixed *N. americanus* and *A. duodenale* infections. *N. americanus* predominates in Central and South America, as well as in South China and southeast Asia, whereas *A. duodenale* predominates in North Africa, in northern India, in China north of the Yangtze River, and among aboriginal people in western Australia. The ability of *A. duodenale* to withstand somewhat harsher environmental and climactic conditions may reflect its ability to undergo arrested development in human tissues. *A. ceylanicum* infection occurs in India and Southeast Asia.

Eosinophilic enteritis caused by *A. caninum* was first described in Queensland, Australia, with two reported cases in the United States. Because of its global distribution in dogs, it is anticipated that human *A. caninum* infections will be identified in many locales.

Pathogenesis. The major morbidity of human hookworm infection is a direct result of intestinal blood loss. Adult hookworms adhere tenaciously to the mucosa and submucosa of the proximal small intestine by using their teeth (or cutting plates) and a muscular esophagus that creates negative pressure in their buccal capsules. At the attachment site, hookworms downregulate host inflammation by releasing anti-inflammatory polypeptides. Rupture of capillaries in the lamina propria is followed by blood extravasation; some of the blood is directly ingested by the hookworms, which anticoagulate blood through the release of peptides that block factor Xa and VIIa/tissue factor. Each adult *A. duodenale* hookworm causes loss of an estimated 0.2 mL of blood/24 hr; blood loss is less for *N. americanus*. Individuals with light infections suffer from very little blood loss and, consequently, may have *hookworm infection* but not *hookworm disease.* Hookworm disease results only when individuals with moderate and heavy infections experience sufficient blood loss to develop iron deficiency and anemia. Hypoalbuminemia and consequent edema and anasarca from the loss of intravascular oncotic pressure can also occur. These features depend heavily on the dietary reserves of the host.

Clinical Manifestations. Heavily infected children suffer from intestinal blood loss resulting in iron deficiency, which can lead to anemia as well as protein malnutrition. Prolonged iron deficiency associated with hookworms in childhood can lead to physical growth retardation and cognitive and intellectual deficits.

Anthropophilic hookworm larvae elicit dermatitis sometimes referred to as **ground itch** when they penetrate human skin. The vesiculation and edema of ground itch are exacerbated by repeated infection. Infection with a zoonotic hookworm, especially *A. braziliense,* can result in lateral migration of the larvae to cause the characteristic cutaneous tracts of cutaneous larva migrans (see later text). Cough subsequently occurs in *A. duodenale* and *N. americanus* hookworm infection when larvae migrate through the lungs to cause laryngotracheobronchitis, usually about 1 wk after exposure. Pharyngitis also can occur.

Intestinal hookworm infection may occur without specific gastrointestinal complaints, although pain, anorexia, and diarrhea have been attributed to the presence of hookworms.

Eosinophilia is often first noticed in the context of asymptomatic infection. The major clinical manifestations are related to intestinal blood loss. Heavily infected children exhibit all of the signs and symptoms of iron deficiency anemia and protein malnutrition. In some cases, children with chronic hookworm disease acquire a yellow-green pallor known as **chlorosis**.

An infantile form of ancylostomiasis resulting from heavy *A. duodenale* infection has been described. Affected infants experience diarrhea, melena, failure to thrive, and profound anemia. Infantile ancylostomiasis has significant mortality.

Eosinophilic enteritis caused by *A. caninum* is associated with colicky abdominal pain, usually exacerbated by food, which begins in the epigastrium and radiates outward. Extreme cases may mimic acute appendicitis.

Diagnosis. Children with hookworm release eggs that can be detected by direct fecal examination (Fig. 269–1). Quantitative methods are available to determine whether a child has a heavy worm burden that can cause hookworm disease. The eggs of *A. duodenale* and *N. americanus* are morphologically indistinguishable. Species identification typically requires egg hatching and differentiation of third-stage infective larvae; newer methods using polymerase chain reaction methods are under development.

In contrast, eggs are generally not present in the feces of patients with eosinophilic enteritis caused by *A. caninum.* Eosinophilic enteritis is often diagnosed by demonstrating ileal and colonic ulcerations by colonoscopy in the presence of significant blood eosinophilia. An adult canine hookworm may occasionally be recovered during colonoscopic biopsy. Patients with this syndrome develop IgG and IgE serologic responses.

Treatment. The goals of therapy are removal of the adult hookworms with an anthelmintic drug in addition to nutritional support for children with hookworm-associated iron deficiency and protein malnutrition. The benzimidazole anthelmintics, mebendazole and albendazole, are highly effective at eliminating hookworms from the intestine. Albendazole (400 mg PO once for all ages) achieves cure rates of up to 95%, although *N. americanus* adult hookworms are sometimes more refractory and require additional doses. Mebendazole (100 mg bid PO for 3 days or 500 mg PO once for all ages) is equally effective. Mebendazole is recommended for *A. caninum*-associated eosinophilic enteritis, although recurrences are common. Because the benzimidazoles have been reported to be embryotoxic and teratogenic in laboratory animals, their safety in young children is a potential concern. However, benzimidazole treatment of thousands of children in developing countries indicates that these agents are safe. Pyrantel pamoate (11 mg/kg PO once daily for 3 days; maximum dose: 1 g) is available in liquid form and is an effective alternative to the benzimidazoles. Replacement therapy with an iron salt preparation is often required to correct hookworm-associated iron deficiency.

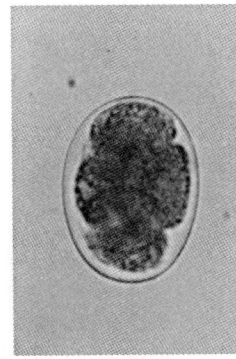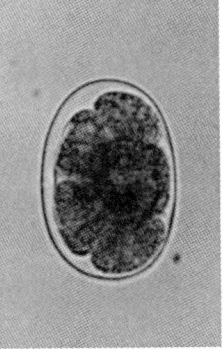

FIGURE 269–1. Eggs of hookworm *Necator americanus* in early cleavage, as seen in freshly passed feces (×400).

Prevention. Although anthelmintic drugs are effective at eliminating hookworms from the intestine, the high rates of reinfection among children suggest that drug chemotherapy alone is not effective for controlling hookworm in highly endemic areas. Improved sanitation, health education, avoidance of human feces as fertilizer, and economic development are still critical for reducing endemicity. Work is in progress to genetically engineer hookworm antigens to use as vaccines in humans.

269.1 Cutaneous Larva Migrans

Etiology. Cutaneous larva migrans (creeping eruption) is caused by the larvae of several nematodes, primarily hookworms, which are not usually parasitic for humans. *A. braziliense,* a hookworm of dogs and cats, is the most common cause, but other animal hookworms (*A. caninum, Uncinaria stenocephala,* and *Bunostomum phlebotomum*) and human parasites (*N. americanus, A. duodenale,* and *Strongyloides stercoralis*) may also produce the disease.

Epidemiology. Cutaneous larva migrans, which is usually caused by *A. braziliense,* is endemic to the southeastern United States and Puerto Rico.

Clinical Manifestations. After penetrating the skin, larvae localize at the epidermal-dermal junction and migrate in this plane, moving at a rate of 1–2 cm/24 hr. The response to the parasite is characterized by raised, erythematous, serpiginous tracks, which occasionally form bullae (Fig. 269–2). These lesions may be single or numerous and are usually localized to an extremity, although any area of the body may be affected. As the organism migrates, new areas of involvement may appear every few days. Intense localized pruritus, without any systemic symptoms, may be associated with the lesions.

Diagnosis. Cutaneous larva migrans is diagnosed by clinical examination of the skin. Patients are often able to recall the exact time and location of exposure because the larvae produce intense itching at the site of penetration. Eosinophilia may occur but is uncommon.

Treatment. If left untreated, the larvae die, and the syndrome resolves within a few weeks to several months. Topical application of thiabendazole (10% of the oral suspension applied topically qid) or oral treatment with ivermectin (200 µg/kg daily PO for 1–2 days), or albendazole (400 mg daily PO for 3 days, for all

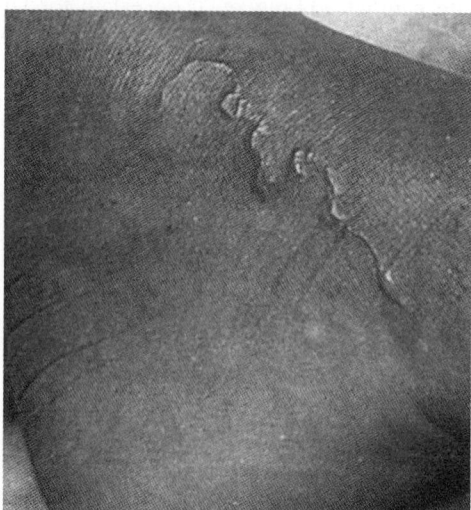

FIGURE 269–2. Creeping eruption of cutaneous larva migrans. (From Korting GW: *Hautkrankheiten bei Kindern und Jugendlichen.* Stuttgart, FK Schattauer Verlag, 1969.) See also color plates.

ages), hastens resolution and may be used if symptoms warrant treatment. Nausea and vomiting frequently preclude repeated administration of oral thiabendazole.

Cowden J, Hotez PJ: Mebendazole and albendazole treatment of geohelminth infections in children and pregnant women. *Pediatr Infect Dis J* 2000;19:659–60.
Davies HD, Sakuls S, Keystone JS: Creeping eruption. A review of clinical presentation and management of 60 cases presenting to a tropical disease unit. *Arch Dermatol* 1993;129:588–91.
Hotez PJ, Ghosh K, Hawdon JM, et al: Experimental approaches to the development of a recombinant hookworm vaccine. *Immunol Rev* 1999;171:163–71.
Jelinek T, Maiwald H, Nothdurft HD, et al: Cutaneous larva migrans in travelers: Synopsis of histories, symptoms, and treatment of 98 patients. *Clin Infect Dis* 1994;19:1062–6.

Chapter 270
Trichuriasis (*Trichuris trichiura*)

Sheral S. Patel and James W. Kazura

Etiology. Trichuriasis is caused by the **whipworm**, *Trichuris trichiura*, a nematode, or roundworm, that inhabits the cecum and ascending colon of humans. The principal hosts of *T. trichiura* are humans who acquire infection by ingesting embryonated, barrel-shaped eggs (Fig. 270–1). The larvae escape from the shell in the upper small intestine and penetrate the intestinal villi. The worms slowly move toward the cecum where the anterior three-fourths whiplike portion remains within the superficial mucosa and the short posterior end is free in the lumen. In 1–3 mo, egg deposition by the adult female worm begins producing 5,000–20,000 eggs/24 hr. After excretion in the feces, embryonic development occurs in 2–4 wk with optimal temperature and soil conditions.

Epidemiology. Trichuriasis occurs throughout the world and is especially common in poor rural communities with inadequate sanitary facilities and soil contaminated with human or animal feces. Trichuriasis is one of the most prevalent human helminthiases, with an estimated one billion infected individuals worldwide. In many parts of the world where protein-energy malnutrition and anemia are common, the prevalence of *T. trichiura* infection can be as high as 95%. It is estimated that 2.2 million people are infected in the rural southeastern United States. The highest rate of infection occurs among children 5–15 yr of age. Infection develops after ingesting embryonated ova by direct contamination of hands, food (raw fruits and vegetables fertilized with human feces), or drink. Transmission can also occur indirectly through flies or other insects.

Clinical Manifestations. Most persons harbor low worm burdens and do not have symptoms. Some individuals may have a history of right lower quadrant or vague periumbilical pain. Adult *Trichuris* suck approximately 0.005 mL of blood/worm/24 hr. Children, who are most likely to be heavily infected, frequently suffer from disease. Clinical manifestations include chronic dysentery, rectal prolapse, anemia, poor growth, as well as developmental and cognitive deficits. There is no significant eosinophilia even though a portion of the worms is embedded in the mucosa of the large bowel.

Diagnosis. Because egg output is so high, fecal smears frequently reveal the characteristic barrel-shaped ova of *T. trichiura.*

Treatment. Mebendazole (100 mg bid PO for 3 days or 500 mg PO once for all ages) is a safe and effective drug, in part because it is poorly absorbed from the gastrointestinal tract. It reduces egg

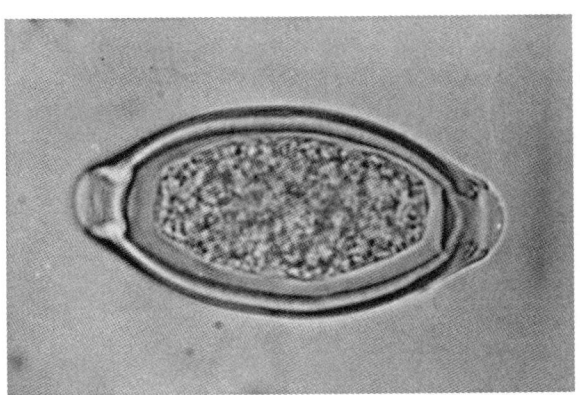

FIGURE 270–1. Egg of *Trichuris trichiura*, as seen in freshly passed feces (× 1,000).

output by 90–99% and has cure rates of 70–90%. Albendazole (400 mg PO once for all ages) is an alternative but with heavy infections the daily dose of albendazole may have to be administered for 3 days.

Prevention. Disease can be prevented by personal hygiene, improved sanitary conditions, and eliminating the use of human feces as fertilizer.

Bundy DA, Cooper ES, Thompson DE, et al: Effect of age and initial infection intensity on the rate of reinfection with *Trichuris trichiura* after treatment. *Parasitology* 1988;97:469–76.
Bundy DA, Cooper ES: *Trichuris* and trichuriasis in humans. *Adv Parasitol* 1989; 28:107–73.
Stephenson LS, Holland CV, Cooper ES: The public health significance of *Trichuris trichiura*. *Parasitology* 2000;121:S73–95.

Chapter 271
Enterobiasis (*Enterobius vermicularis*)

Sheral S. Patel and James W. Kazura

Etiology. The cause of enterobiasis, or **pinworm** infection, is *Enterobius vermicularis*, which is a small (1 cm in length), white, threadlike nematode, or roundworm, that typically inhabits the cecum, appendix, and adjacent areas of the ileum and ascending colon. Gravid females migrate at night to the perianal and perineal regions where they deposit eggs. Ova are convex on one side and flattened on the other and have diameters of ~30 × 60 μm. Eggs embryonate within 6 hr and remain viable for 20 days. Human infection occurs by ingestion of embryonated eggs that are carried on fingernails, clothing, bedding, or house dust. After ingestion, the larvae mature to form adult worms in 36–53 days.

Epidemiology. Enterobiasis infection occurs in individuals of all ages and socioeconomic levels. It is prevalent in regions with temperate climates and is the most common helminth infection in the United States. Infection occurs primarily in institutional or family settings that include children. The prevalence of pinworm infection is highest in children from 5–14 yr of age. It is common in areas where children live, play, and sleep close together, thus facilitating egg transmission. Because the life span of the adult worm is short, chronic parasitism is likely due to

repeated cycles of reinfection. Autoinoculation can occur in individuals who habitually put their fingers in their mouth.

Pathogenesis. *Enterobius* infection may cause symptoms by mechanical stimulation and irritation, allergic reactions, and migration of the worms to anatomic sites where they become pathogenic.

Clinical Manifestations. Pinworm infection is innocuous and rarely causes serious medical problems. The most common complaints include itching and restless sleep secondary to nocturnal perianal or perineal pruritus. The precise cause and incidence of pruritus are unknown. They may be related to the intensity of infection, psychological profile of the infected individual and his or her family, or allergic reactions to the parasite. Eosinophilia is not observed in most cases because tissue invasion does not occur. Perianal granulomas containing live or dead worms or eggs develop rarely but may require surgical excision. Aberrant migration to ectopic sites occasionally may lead to appendicitis, chronic salpingitis, peritonitis, hepatitis, and ulcerative lesions in the large or small bowel.

Diagnosis. A history of nocturnal perianal pruritus in children strongly suggests enterobiasis. Definitive diagnosis is established by identification of parasite eggs or worms. Microscopic examination of adhesive cellophane tape pressed against the perianal region early in the morning frequently demonstrates eggs (Fig. 271–1). Repeated examinations increase the chance of detecting ova; a single examination detects 50% of infections, three examinations 90%, and five examinations 99%. Worms seen in the perianal region should be removed and preserved in 75% ethyl alcohol until microscopic examination can be performed. Digital rectal examination may also be used to obtain samples for a wet mount. Routine stool samples rarely demonstrate *Enterobius* ova.

Treatment. Anthelmintic drugs should be administered to infected individuals and their family members. A single oral dose of mebendazole (100 mg PO for all ages) repeated in 2 wk results in cure rates of 90–100%. Alternative regimens include a single oral dose of albendazole (400 mg PO for all ages) repeated in 2 wk or a single dose of pyrantel pamoate (11 mg/kg PO, maximum: 1 g).

Prevention. Repeated treatments every 3–4 mo may be required in circumstances with repeated exposure, such as with institutionalized children. Although personal cleanliness is a useful general principle, there is no evidence that it has a role in the control or prevention of enterobiasis.

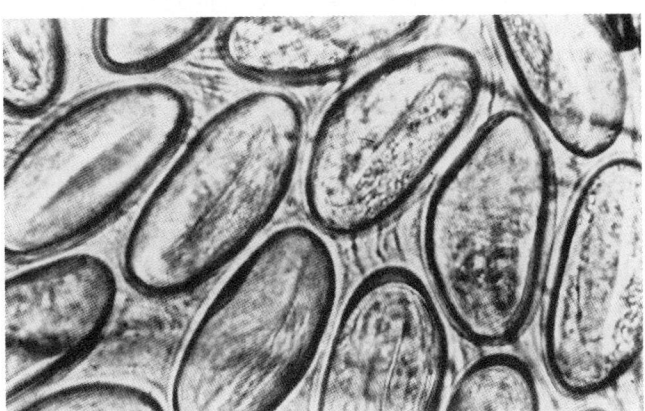

FIGURE 271–1. Eggs of *Enterobius vermicularis* adherent to cellulose acetate tape. (From Guerrant et al: *Tropical Infectious Diseases.* Churchill Livingstone, 1999, p. 949.)

Avolio L, Avoltini V, Ceffa F, et al: Perianal granuloma caused by *Enterobius vermicularis*: Report of a new observation and review of the literature. *J Pediatr* 1998; 132:1055–6.

Jones JE: Pinworms. *Am Fam Physician* 1988;38:159–64.

Tandan T, Pollard AJ, Money DM, et al: Pelvic inflammatory disease associated with *Enterobius vermicularis*. *Arch Dis Child* 2002;86:439–40.

Tanowitz HB, Weiss LM, Wittner M: Diagnosis and treatment of common intestinal helminths II: Common intestinal nematodes. *Gastroenterologist* 1994;2:39–49.

Weller TH, Sorensen CW: Enterobiasis: Its incidence and symptomatology in a group of 505 children. *N Engl J Med* 1941;224:143–6.

Chapter 272

Strongyloidiasis (*Strongyloides stercoralis*)

Sheral S. Patel and James W. Kazura

Etiology. Strongyloidiasis is caused by the nematode, or roundworm, *Strongyloides stercoralis*. Only adult female worms inhabit the small intestine. The nematode reproduces in the human host by parthenogenesis and releases eggs containing mature larvae into the intestinal lumen. Rhabditiform larvae immediately emerge from the ova and are passed in feces, where they can be visualized by stool examination. Rhabditiform larvae either differentiate into free-living adult male and female worms or metamorphose into the infectious filariform larvae. Humans are usually infected through skin contact with soil contaminated with infectious larvae. Larvae penetrate the skin, enter the venous circulation and then pass to the lungs, break into alveolar spaces, and migrate up the bronchial tree. They are then swallowed and pass through the stomach, and adult female worms develop in the small intestine. Egg deposition begins about 28 days after initial infection.

The **hyperinfection syndrome** occurs when large numbers of larvae transform into infective organisms during their passage in feces and then reinfect (i.e., autoinfect) the host by way of the lower gastrointestinal tract or perianal region. This cycle may be accelerated in immunocompromised persons, particularly those with depressed T-cell function.

Epidemiology. *S. stercoralis* infection is prevalent in tropical and subtropical regions of the world and endemic in several areas of Europe, the southeastern United States, and Puerto Rico. Transmission requires appropriate environmental conditions, particularly warm, moist soil. Poor sanitation and crowded living conditions are conducive to high levels of transmission. The highest prevalence of infection in the United States (4% of the general population) is in impoverished rural areas of Kentucky and Tennessee. Infection may be especially common among residents of mental institutions, veterans who were prisoners of war in areas of high endemicity, and refugees and immigrants. Individuals with hematologic malignancies, autoimmune diseases, malnutrition, and drug-induced immunosuppression are at high risk of the hyperinfection syndrome. Patients with AIDS may experience a rapid course of disseminated strongyloidiasis with a fatal outcome.

Pathogenesis. The initial host immune response to infection is production of IgE and eosinophilia in blood and tissues, which presumably prevents dissemination and hyperinfection in the immunocompetent host. Adult female worms in otherwise healthy and asymptomatic individuals may persist in the gastrointestinal tract for years. If infected persons become immunocompromised, the reduction in cellular and humoral immunity may lead to an abrupt and dramatic increase in parasite load with systemic dissemination.

Clinical Manifestations. Approximately one third of infected individuals are asymptomatic. The remaining two thirds have symptoms that correlate with the three stages of infection: invasion of the skin, migration of larvae through the lungs, and parasitism of the small intestine by adult worms. **Larva currens** is the manifestation of an allergic reaction to filariform larvae that migrate through the skin, where they leave pruritic, tortuous, urticarial tracks. The lesions may recur and are typically found over the lower abdominal wall, buttocks, or thighs. Pulmonary disease secondary to larval migration through the lung rarely occurs and may resemble Löffler's syndrome (cough, wheezing, shortness of breath, and transient pulmonary infiltrates accompanied by eosinophilia). Gastrointestinal strongyloidiasis is characterized by indigestion, crampy abdominal pain, vomiting, diarrhea, steatorrhea, protein-losing enteropathy, and weight loss. Edema of the duodenum with irregular mucosal folds, ulcerations, and strictures can be seen radiographically.

Strongyloidiasis is potentially lethal because of the ability of the parasite to cause overwhelming hyperinfection in immunocompromised persons. The **hyperinfection syndrome** is characterized by an exaggeration of the clinical features that develop in symptomatic immunocompetent individuals. The onset is usually sudden with generalized abdominal pain, distention, and fever. Multiple organs can be affected as massive numbers of larvae disseminate throughout the body and introduce bowel flora. The latter may result in bacteremia and septicemia. Cutaneous manifestations may include petechiae and purpura. Cough, wheezing, and hemoptysis are indicative of pulmonary involvement. Whereas eosinophilia is a prominent feature of strongyloidiasis in immunocompetent persons, this sign may be absent in immunocompromised persons.

Diagnosis. Intestinal strongyloidiasis is diagnosed by examining feces or duodenal fluid for the characteristic larvae (Fig. 272–1). Several stool samples should be examined either by direct smear or a concentration method such as formaldehyde-ether or the Baermann test. Alternatively, duodenal fluid can be sampled by the **enteric string test** (Entero-Test) or aspiration. In children with the hyperinfection syndrome, larvae may be found in sputum, gastric aspirates, and rarely in small intestinal biopsy specimens. An enzyme-linked immunosorbent assay for IgE antibody to *Strongyloides* may be more sensitive than parasitologic methods for diagnosing intestinal infection in the immunocompetent host. The utility of the assay in diagnosing infection in immunocompromised subjects with the hyperinfection syndrome has not been determined.

Treatment. Treatment is directed at eradication of infection. A recent study showed that ivermectin (200 μg/kg/24 hr once daily PO for 1–2 days), which is the drug of choice for uncomplicated strongyloidiasis, is equally effective and associated with fewer adverse effects than thiabendazole (50 mg/kg bid PO for 2 days; maximum: 3 g/24 hr), which is the traditional treatment. Patients with the hyperinfection syndrome should be treated with ivermectin for 7–10 days and may require repeated courses. Reducing the dose of immunosuppressive therapy and treatment of concomitant bacterial infections are essential in the management of the hyperinfection syndrome. Close follow-up with repeated stool examination is necessary to ensure complete elimination of the parasite.

Prevention. Sanitary practices designed to prevent soil and person-to-person transmission are the most effective control measures. Wearing shoes is a main preventive strategy. Reduction in transmission in institutional settings can be achieved by decreasing fecal contamination of the environment such as by the use of clean bedding. Because infection is uncommon in most settings, case detection and treatment are advisable. Individuals who will be given immunosuppressive drugs before organ transplantation or cancer chemotherapy should have a

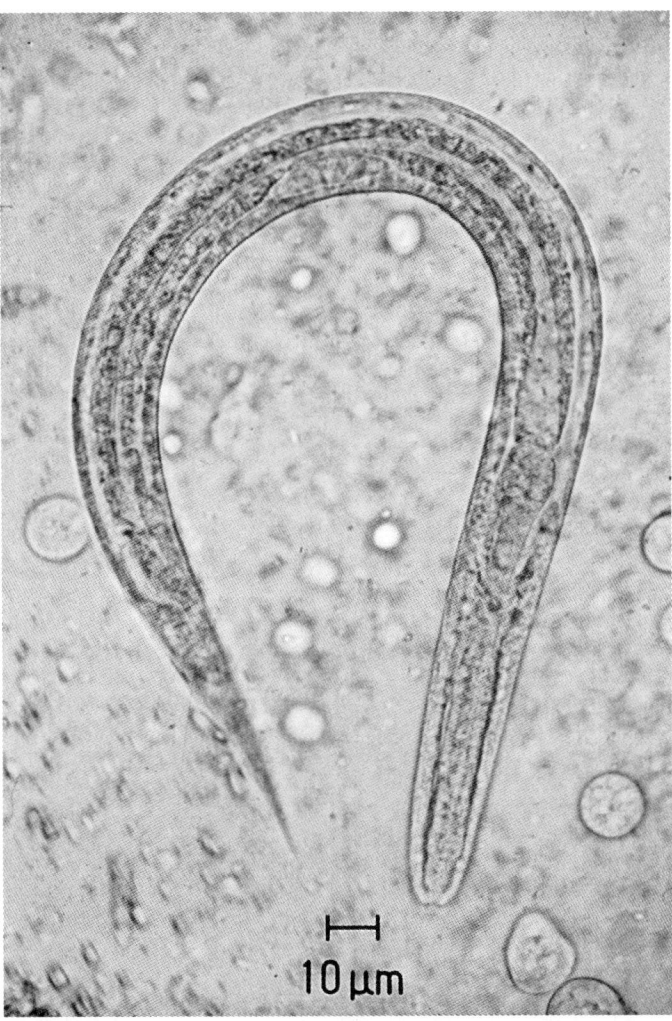

FIGURE 272–1. Larvae of intestinal strongyloidiasis. See also color plates.

screening examination for *S. stercoralis*. If infected, they should be treated before immunosuppression is induced.

Burke JA: Strongyloidiasis in childhood. *Am J Dis Child* 1978;132:1130–8.
Mahmoud AA: Strongyloidiasis. *Clin Infect Dis* 1996;23:949–53.
Sarangarajan R, Ranganathan A, Belmonte AH, et al: *Strongyloides stercoralis* infection in AIDS. *AIDS Patient Care STDs* 1997;11:407–14.
Zaha O, Hirata T, Kinjo F: Strongyloidiasis—Progress in diagnosis and treatment. *Intern Med* 2000;39:695–700.

Chapter 273

Lymphatic Filariasis (*Brugia malayi, Brugia timori, Wuchereria bancrofti*)

Sheral S. Patel and James W. Kazura

Etiology. The filarial worms *Brugia malayi* (**Malayan filariasis**), *Brugia timori*, and *Wuchereria bancrofti* (**bancroftian filariasis**) are threadlike nematodes that cause similar infections. Infective larvae are introduced into humans during blood feeding by the mosquito vector. Over a period of 4–6 mo, the larval forms develop into adult worms that reside in the afferent lymphatic vessels. Sexually mature adult female worms release large numbers of microfilariae that circulate in the bloodstream. The life cycle of the parasite is completed when mosquitoes ingest microfilariae in a blood meal and molt to form infective larvae over a period of 10–14 days.

Epidemiology. More than 120 million people living in tropical Africa, Asia, and Latin America are infected; approximately 10–20% of these individuals have clinically significant morbidity attributable to filariasis. *W. bancrofti* is transmitted in Africa, Asia, and Latin America. *B. malayi* is restricted to the South Pacific and Southeast Asia, and *B. timori* is restricted to several islands of Indonesia. Travelers from nonendemic areas of the world who spend brief periods of time in endemic areas are rarely infected.

Clinical Manifestations. The clinical manifestations of *B. malayi*, *B. timori*, and *W. bancrofti* infection are similar; manifestations of acute infection include transient, recurrent lymphadenitis and lymphangitis, whereas chronic filariasis is characterized by lymphatic obstruction with hydrocele and elephantiasis. The early signs and symptoms include episodic fever, lymphangitis of an extremity, lymphadenitis (especially the inguinal and axillary areas), headaches, and myalgia that last a few days to several weeks. The syndrome is most frequently observed in young persons 10–20 yr of age. Manifestations of chronic lymphatic filariasis, such as hydrocele and elephantiasis, occur mostly in adults 30 yr of age or older and result from anatomic and functional obstruction to lymph flow. Elephantiasis may involve one or more limbs, the scrotum, the breasts, or the vulva. It is uncommon for children to have overt signs of chronic filariasis.

TROPICAL PULMONARY EOSINOPHILIA. The presence of microfilariae in the body has no apparent pathologic consequences except in persons with tropical pulmonary eosinophilia, a syndrome of filarial etiology in which microfilariae are found in the lungs and lymph nodes but not bloodstream. It occurs only in individuals who have lived for years in endemic areas. Men 20–30 yr of age are most likely to be affected, although the syndrome occasionally occurs in children. The presentation includes paroxysmal nocturnal cough with dyspnea, fever, weight loss, and fatigue. Rales and rhonchi are found on auscultation of the chest. The roentgenographic findings may occasionally be normal but increased bronchovascular markings, discrete opacities in the middle and basal regions of the lung, or diffuse miliary lesions are usually present. Recurrent episodes may result in interstitial fibrosis and chronic respiratory insufficiency in untreated individuals. Hepatosplenomegaly and generalized lymphadenopathy are often seen in children. The diagnosis is suggested by residence in a filarial endemic area, eosinophilia (>2,000/μL), compatible clinical symptoms, increased serum IgE (>1,000 IU/mL), and high titers of antimicrofilarial antibodies in the absence of microfilaremia. Although microfilariae may be found in sections of lung or lymph node, biopsy of these tissues is unwarranted in most situations. The clinical response to diethylcarbamazine (5 mg/kg/24 hr PO for 10 days) is the final criterion for diagnosis; the majority of patients improve with this therapy. If symptoms recur, a second course of the anthelmintic should be administered. Patients with chronic symptoms are less likely to show improvement than those who have been ill for a short time.

Diagnosis. Demonstration of microfilariae in the blood is the primary means for confirming the diagnosis of lymphatic filariasis. Because microfilaremia is nocturnal in most cases, blood samples should be obtained between 10 o'clock at night and 2 o'clock in the morning. Anticoagulated blood is passed through a Nuclepore filter that is stained and examined microscopically for microfilariae. Infection with *W. bancrofti* in the absence of blood-borne microfilariae may be diagnosed by detection of parasite antigen in the serum.

Treatment. The use of antifilarial drugs in the management of acute lymphadenitis and lymphangitis is controversial. No controlled studies demonstrate that administration of drugs such as diethylcarbamazine modifies the course of acute lymphangitis. Diethylcarbamazine may be given to asymptomatic microfilaremic persons to lower the intensity of parasitemia. The drug also kills a proportion of the adult worms. Because treatment-associated complications such as pruritus, fever, generalized body pain, hypertension, and even death may occur, especially with high microfilarial levels, the dose of diethylcarbamazine should be increased gradually (children: 1 mg/kg PO as a single dose on day 1; 1 mg/kg tid PO on day 2; 1–2 mg/kg tid PO on day 3; and 6 mg/kg/24 hr divided tid PO on days 4–14; adults: 50 mg PO on day 1; 50 mg tid PO on day 2; 100 mg tid PO on day 3; and 6 mg/kg/24 hr divided tid PO on days 4–14). For patients with no microfilaria in the blood, the full dose (6 mg/kg/24 hr divided tid PO) can be given beginning on day 1. Repeat doses may be necessary to reduce further the microfilaremia and kill lymph-dwelling adult parasites. *W. bancrofti* is more sensitive than *B. malayi* to diethylcarbamazine.

Addiss DG, Beach MJ, Streit TG, et al: Randomised placebo-controlled comparison of ivermectin and albendazole alone and in combination for *Wuchereria bancrofti* microfilaraemia in Haitian children. *Lancet* 1997;350:480–4.

Bockarie MH, Alexander ND, Hyun P, et al: Randomised community-based trial of annual single-dose diethylcarbamazine with or without ivermectin against *Wuchereria bancrofti* infection in human beings and mosquitoes. *Lancet* 1998; 351:162–8.

Brown KR, Ricci FM, Ottesen EA: Ivermectin: Effectiveness in lymphatic filariasis. *Parasitology* 2000;121:S133–46.

Dreyer G, Norões J, Figueredo-Silva J: New insights into the natural history and pathology of bancroftian filariasis: Implications for clinical management and filariasis control programmes. *Trans R Soc Trop Med Hyg* 2000;94:594–6.

Horton J, Witt C, Ottesen EA, et al: An analysis of the safety of the single dose, two drug regimens used in programmes to eliminate lymphatic filariasis. *Parasitology* 2000;121:S147–S160.

Molyneux DH, Neira M, Liese B: Lymphatic filariasis: Setting the scene for elimination. *Trans R Soc Trop Med Hyg* 2000;94:589–91.

Ottesen EA: Filarial infections. *Infect Dis Clin North Am* 1993;7:619–33.

Chapter 274
Other Tissue Nematodes

Sheral S. Patel and James W. Kazura

ONCHOCERCIASIS (*ONCHOCERCA VOLVULUS*)

Infection with *Onchocerca volvulus* leads to onchocerciasis or river blindness. Onchocerciasis occurs primarily in West Africa but also Central and East Africa. There are scattered foci in Central and South America. *O. volvulus* larvae are transmitted to humans by way of the bite of *Simulium* blackflies that breed in fast-flowing streams. The larvae penetrate the skin and migrate through the connective tissue and eventually develop into adult worms that can be found tangled in fibrous tissue. Female worms produce large numbers of microfilariae that migrate through the skin and connective tissue. Most infected individuals are asymptomatic. In heavily infected subjects, clinical manifestations are due to localized host inflammatory reactions to dead or dying microfilariae. These reactions produce pruritic dermatitis, punctate keratitis, corneal pannus formation, and chorioretinitis. Adult worms in subcutaneous nodules are not painful and tend to occur over bony prominences of the hip. The diagnosis can be established by obtaining snips of skin covering the scapulae, iliac crests, buttocks, or calves. The snips are immersed in saline for several hours and examined microscopically for microfilariae that have emerged into the fluid. The diagnosis can also be established by demonstrating microfilariae in the cornea or anterior chamber on slit-lamp examination or finding adult worms on a nodule biopsy specimen. Ophthalmology consultation should be obtained before treatment of eye lesions. A single dose of ivermectin (150 µg/kg PO) is the drug of choice and clears microfilariae from the skin for several months, but it has no effect on the adult worm. Treatment with ivermectin should be repeated at 3–6 mo intervals if there are continuing symptoms or evidence of eye infection. Adverse effects of ivermectin therapy include fever, urticaria, and pruritus and are more frequent in individuals not born in endemic areas who acquired the infection following periods of intense exposure, such as Peace Corps volunteers. Patients with concurrent loiasis may develop encephalopathy with ivermectin therapy. Personal protection includes avoiding areas where biting flies are numerous, wearing protective clothing, and using insect repellant. Vector control and mass ivermectin distribution programs have been implemented in Africa in an effort to eradicate onchocerciasis.

LOIASIS (*LOA LOA*)

Loiasis is caused by infection with the tissue nematode *Loa loa*. The parasite is transmitted to humans via diurnally biting flies (*Chrysops*) that live in the rain forests of West and Central Africa. Migration of adult worms through skin, subcutaneous tissue, and subconjunctivae can lead to transient episodes of pruritus, erythema, localized edema known as **Calabar swellings**, which are nonerythematous areas of subcutaneous edema 10–20 cm in diameter that are typically found around joints such as the wrist or the knee (Fig. 274–1), or eye pain. They resolve over several days to weeks and may recur at the same or different sites. Although lifelong residents of endemic regions may have microfilaremia and eosinophilia, these individuals are often asymptomatic. In contrast, travelers to endemic regions may have a hyperreactive response to *L. loa* infection characterized by frequent recurrences of swelling, high level eosinophilia, debilitation, and serious complications such as glomerulonephritis and encephalitis. Diagnosis is usually established on clinical grounds. Microfilariae may be detected in blood smears collected between 10 o'clock in the morning and 2 o'clock in the afternoon. Adult worms should be surgically excised when possible. Diethylcarbamazine is the agent of choice for eradication of microfilaremia but the drug does not kill adult worms. Because treatment-associated complications such as pruritus, fever, generalized body pain, hypertension,

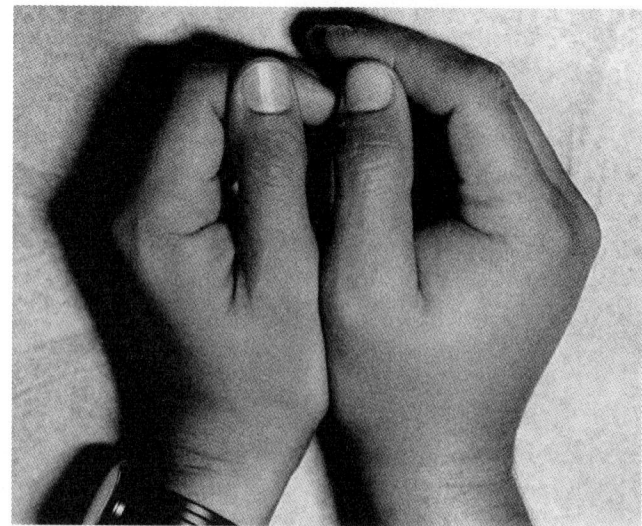

FIGURE 274–1. Calabar swelling of the right hand. (From Guerrant et al: *Tropical Infectious Diseases.* Churchill Livingstone, 1999, p. 863.)

and even death may occur, especially with high microfilarial levels, the dose of diethylcarbamazine should be increased gradually (children: 1 mg/kg PO on day 1; 1 mg/kg tid PO on day 2; 1–2 mg/kg tid PO on day 3; 9 mg/kg/24 hr divided tid PO on days 4–21; adults: 50 mg PO on day 1; 50 mg PO on day 2; 100 mg tid PO on day 3; 9 mg/kg/24 hr divided tid PO on days 4–21). Full doses can be instituted on day 1 in persons without microfilaremia. Individuals concurrently infected with *O. volvulus* are at increased risk of developing encephalopathy with ivermectin treatment. A single dose of ivermectin (200 μg/kg) decreases microfilarial densities in the blood in persons with high-density microfilaremia. A 3-wk course of albendazole can also be used to slowly reduce microfilarial levels as a result of embryotoxic effects on the adult worms. Antihistamines or corticosteroids may be used to limit allergic reactions secondary to killing of microfilariae. Personal protective measures include avoiding areas where biting flies are present, wearing protective clothing, and using insect repellants. Diethylcarbamazine (300 mg PO once weekly) prevents infection in travelers who spend prolonged periods of time in endemic areas.

INFECTION WITH ANIMAL FILARIAE

The most commonly recognized zoonotic filarial infections are caused by members of the genus *Dirofilaria*. The worms are introduced into humans by the bites of mosquitoes containing third-stage larvae. The most common filarial zoonosis in the Unites States is *Dirofilaria tenuis*, a parasite of raccoons. In Europe, Africa, and Southeast Asia, infections are most commonly caused by the dog parasite *Dirofilaria repens*. The **dog heartworm**, *Dirofilaria immitis*, is the second most commonly encountered filarial zoonosis worldwide. Other genera including *Dipetalonema*-like worms, *Onchocerca*, and *Brugia* are rare causes of zoonotic filarial infections.

Animal filariae do not undergo normal development in the human host. The clinical manifestations and pathologic findings correspond to the anatomic site of infection and can be categorized into four major groups: subcutaneous, lung, eye, and lymphatic. Pathologic examination of affected tissue reveals a localized foreign body reaction around a dead or dying parasite. The lesion consists of granulomas with eosinophils, neutrophils, and tissue necrosis. *D. tenuis* does not leave the subcutaneous tissues, whereas *B. beaveri* eventually localizes to superficial lymph nodes. Infections may be present for up to several months. *D. immitis* larvae migrate for several months in subcutaneous tissues and most frequently result in a well-circumscribed coinlike lesion in a single lobe of the lung. The chest radiograph typically reveals a solitary pulmonary nodule 1–3 cm in diameter. Definitive diagnosis and cure depend on surgical excision and identification of the nematode within the surrounding granulomatous response. *D. tenuis* and *B. beaveri* infections present as painful 1–5 cm rubbery nodules in the skin of the trunk, extremities, and around the orbit. Patients often report having been engaged in activities predisposing to exposure to infected mosquitoes, such as working or hunting in swampy areas. Diagnosis and management is by surgical excision.

ANGIOSTRONGYLUS CANTONENSIS

Angiostrongylus cantonensis, the **rat lungworm**, is the most common cause of eosinophilic meningitis worldwide. Rats are the definitive host. Human infection follows ingestion of third-stage larvae in raw or undercooked intermediate hosts such as snails and slugs, or transport hosts such as freshwater prawns, frogs, and fish. Most cases are sporadic but clusters have been reported, including consumption of lettuce contaminated with intermediate or transport hosts. Even though most infections have been described in Southeast Asia, the South Pacific, and Taiwan, shipboard travel of infected rats has spread the parasite

to Madagascar, Africa, Caribbean, and, most recently, Australia and North America. Larvae penetrate the vasculature of the intestinal tract and migrate to the meninges, where they usually die but induce eosinophilic aseptic meningitis. Patients present 2–35 days after ingestion of larvae with severe headache, neck pain or nuchal rigidity, hyperesthesias and paresthesias, fatigue, fever, rash, pruritus, nausea, and vomiting. Neurologic involvement varies from asymptomatic to paresthesias, severe pain, weakness, and focal neurologic findings such as cranial nerve palsies. Coma and death due to hydrocephalus occur rarely in heavy infections. Peripheral blood eosinophilia is not always present on initial examination, but peaks about 5 wk after exposure, often when symptoms are improving. Cerebrospinal (CSF) fluid analysis reveals pleocytosis with >10% eosinophils in more than half of patients, with mildly elevated protein and normal glucose levels. The diagnosis is established clinically with supporting travel and diet history. A sensitive and specific enzyme-linked immunosorbent assay (ELISA) is available on a limited basis from the Centers for Disease Control and Prevention for testing either CSF or serum. Treatment is primarily supportive because the majority of infections are mild and most patients recover within 2 mo without neurologic residua. Analgesics should be given for headache. Careful, repeated lumbar punctures should be performed to relieve hydrocephalus. Anthelmintic drugs have not been shown to influence the outcome and may exacerbate neurologic symptoms. The use of corticosteroids may shorten the duration of symptoms for persistent and severe headaches. There is a higher incidence of permanent neurologic sequelae and mortality among children than among adults. Infection can be avoided by not eating raw or undercooked crabs, prawns, or snails.

ANGIOSTRONGYLUS COSTARICENSIS

Angiostrongylus costaricensis is a nematode that infects several species of rodents and causes abdominal angiostrongyliasis, which has been described predominantly in Latin America and the Caribbean. The mode of transmission to humans, who are accidental hosts, is unknown. It is speculated that infectious larvae from a molluscan intermediate host, such as the slug *Vaginulus plebeius*, contaminate water or vegetation that are inadvertently consumed (e.g., chopped up in salads or on vegetation contaminated with their mucus secretions). Although this slug is not indigenous to the continental United States, it has been found on imported flowers and produce. A study of 116 Costa Rican children with clinical abdominal angiostrongyliasis reported that the disease was twice as frequent in males as females and occurred predominantly during the rainy season in children 6–13 yr of age and of relatively high socioeconomic status. The incubation period for abdominal angiostrongyliasis is unknown but limited data suggest it ranges from 2 wk to several months after ingestion of larvae. Third-stage larvae migrate from the gastrointestinal tract to the mesenteric arteries where they mature into adults. These eggs degenerate and elicit an eosinophilic granulomatous reaction. The clinical findings of abdominal angiostrongyliasis mimic appendicitis although the former are typically more indolent. Children can have fever, right lower quadrant pain, a tumor-like mass, abdominal rigidity, and painful rectal examination. Most patients have leukocytosis with eosinophilia. Radiologic examination may show bowel wall edema, spasticity, or filling defects in the ileocecal region and the ascending colon. Examination of stool for ova and parasites is not useful for *A. costaricensis* but is useful for evaluating the presence of other intestinal parasites. An ELISA is available for diagnosis on a limited basis from the Centers for Disease Control and Prevention but the specificity of the test is low and it is known to cross-react with *Toxocara, Strongyloides,* and *Paragonimus.* Many patients undergo laparotomy for suspected appendicitis and are found to have a mass in the terminal ileum to the ascending colon. No specific treatment is known for abdominal angiostrongyliasis. Even though the use of anthelmintic therapy has not been studied systematically, thiabendazole or diethylcarbamazine has been suggested. The prognosis is generally good. Most cases are self-limited, although surgery may be required in some patients. Cornerstones of prevention include avoidance of slugs and not ingesting raw food and water that may be contaminated with imperceptible slugs or slime from slugs. Rat control is also important in preventing the spread of infection.

DRACUNCULIASIS (*DRACUNCULUS MEDINENSIS*)

Dracunculiasis is caused by the guinea worm, *Dracunculus medinensis*. The infection is confined to 13 countries in Africa with approximately 61% of the 79,000 annual reported cases occurring in Sudan. Humans become infected by drinking contaminated stagnant water containing immature forms of the parasite in the gut of tiny crustaceans (copepods). Larvae are released in the stomach, penetrate the mucosa, mature, and mate. About 1 yr later, the adult female worm (1–2 mm in diameter and up to 1 m long) migrates and partially emerges through the skin, usually of the legs. Thousands of immature larvae are released when the affected body part is immersed in the water. The cycle is completed when larval forms are ingested by the crustaceans. Infected humans have no symptoms until the worm reaches the subcutaneous tissue, causing a stinging papule that may be accompanied by urticaria, nausea, vomiting, diarrhea, and dyspnea. The lesion vesiculates, ruptures, and forms a painful ulcer in which a portion of the worm is visible. Diagnosis is established clinically. Larvae can be identified by microscopic examination of the discharge fluid. Metronidazole (25 mg/kg tid PO for 10 days: maximum dose: 750 mg) decreases local inflammation. Although the drug does not kill the worm, it facilitates its removal by a process rolling the emerging 1-m long parasite onto a thin stick over a week. Topical corticosteroids shorten the time to complete healing while topical antibiotics decrease the risk of secondary bacterial infection. Dracunculiasis can be prevented by boiling or chlorinating drinking water or passing the water through a cloth sieve before consumption.

GNATHOSTOMA SPINIGERUM

Gnathostoma spinigerum is a dog and cat nematode endemic to Southeast Asia, Japan, China, Bangladesh, and India. Infection is acquired by ingesting intermediate hosts containing larvae of the parasite such as raw or undercooked freshwater fish, chickens, pigs, snails, or frogs. Penetration of the skin by larval forms and prenatal transmission has also been described. Nonspecific signs and symptoms such as generalized malaise, fever, urticaria, anorexia, nausea, vomiting, diarrhea, and epigastric pain develop 24–48 hr after ingestion of *G. spinigerum*. Moderate to severe eosinophilia develops as larvae penetrate the gastric or intestinal wall and migrate through various tissues. Cutaneous gnathostomiasis is manifest as intermittent episodes of localized, migratory nonpitting edema associated with pain, pruritus, or erythema. Central nervous system involvement in gnathostomiasis is suggested by focal neurologic findings, initially neuralgia followed within a few days by paralysis or changes in mental status. Multiple cranial nerves may be involved, and the cerebrospinal fluid typically shows an eosinophilic pleocytosis. Diagnosis of gnathostomiasis is based on clinical presentation and epidemiologic background. Serologic testing varies in sensitivity and specificity and is not widely available. There is no well-documented effective chemotherapy, although albendazole (400 mg PO bid for 21 days) has been suggested to be useful. Surgical resection of the *Gnathostoma* is the major mode of therapy and the treatment of choice. Blind surgical resection of subcutaneous areas of diffuse swelling is not recommended because the worm can rarely be located. Prevention through the avoidance of ingestion of poorly cooked or raw fish, poultry, or pork should be emphasized for individuals living in or visiting endemic areas.

Onchocerciasis (*Onchocerca volvulus*)
Burnham G: Onchocerciasis. *Lancet* 1998;351:1341–6.
Van Laethem Y, Lopes C: Treatment of onchocerciasis. *Drugs* 1996;52:861–9.

Loiasis (*Loa loa*)
Hayden MK, Trenholme GM: Photo quiz. Loiasis. *Clin Infect Dis* 1998;27:429, 634–5.
Boussinesq M, Gardon, J: Prevalence of *Loa loa* microfilaremia throughout the area endemic for the infection. *Ann Trop Med Parasitol* 1997;91:573–89.

Infection with Animal Filariae
Baird JK, Alpert LI, Friedman R, et al: North American brugian filariasis: Report of nine infections of humans. *Am J Trop Med Hyg* 1986;35:1205–9.
Orihel TC, Eberhard ML. Zoonotic filariasis. *Clin Microbiol Rev* 1998;11:366–77.
Pampiglione S, Rivasi F, Angeli G, et al: Dirofilariasis due to *Dirofilaria repens* in Italy, an emergent zoonosis: Report of 60 new cases. *Histopathology* 2001;38:344–54.
Vakalis NC, Himonas CA: Human and canine dirofilariasis in Greece. *Parasitology* 1997;39:389–91.

Angiostrongylus cantonensis
Chotmongkol V, Sawanyawisuth K, Thavornpitak Y: Corticosteroid treatment of eosinophilic meningitis. *Int J Parasitol* 2000;30:1295–303.
Pien FD, Pien BC: Angiostrongylus cantonensis eosinophilic meningitis. *Int J Infect Dis* 1999;3:161–3.
Slom TJ, Crotese MM, Gerber SI, et al: An outbreak of eosinophilic meningitis caused by *Angiostrongylus cantonensis* in travelers returning from the Caribbean. *N Engl J Med* 2002;346:668–75.
Tsai HC, Liu YC, Kunin CM, et al: Eosinophilic meningitis caused by *Angiostrongylus cantonensis*: Report of 17 cases. *Am J Med* 2001;111:109–14.

Angiostrongylus costaricensis
Hulbert TV, Larsen RA, Chandrasoma PT: Abdominal angiostrongyliasis mimicking acute appendicitis and Meckel's diverticulum: Report of a case in the United States and review. *Clin Infect Dis* 1992;14:836–40.
Kramer MH, Greer GJ, Quinonez JF, et al: First reported outbreak of abdominal angiostrongyliasis. *Clin Infect Dis* 1998;26:365–72.
Loria-Cortes R, Lobo-Sanahuja JF: Clinical abdominal angiostrongyliasis. A study of 116 children with intestinal granulomas caused by *Angiostrongylus costaricensis*. *Am J Trop Med Hyg* 1980;29:538–44.

Dracunculiasis (*Dracunculus medinensis*)
Hopkins DR, Ruiz-Tiben E, Ruebush TK, et al: Dracunculiasis eradication: Delayed, not denied. *Am J Trop Med Hyg* 2000;62:163–8.
Sing A, Wienert P, Sabisch P, et al: Photo quiz. Infection due to *Dracunculus medinensis*. *Clin Infect Dis* 1998;27:1361,1508–9.

Gnathostoma spinigerum
Rusnak JM, Lucey DR: Clinical gnathostomiasis: Case report and review of the English-language literature. *Clin Infect Dis* 1993;16:33–50.

Chapter 275

Toxocariasis (Visceral and Ocular Larva Migrans)

Sheral S. Patel and James W. Kazura

Etiology. Most cases of human toxocariasis are caused by the **dog roundworm**, *Toxocara canis*. Adult female *T. canis* worms live in the intestinal tracts of young puppies and their lactating mothers. Large numbers of eggs are passed in the feces of dogs and embryonate under optimal soil conditions. *Toxocara* eggs can survive relatively harsh environmental conditions and are resistant to freezing and extremes of moisture and pH. Humans ingest embryonated eggs contaminating soil, hands, or fomites. The larvae hatch and penetrate the intestinal wall and travel by way of the circulation to the liver, lung, and other tissues. Humans do not excrete *T. canis* eggs because the larvae are unable to complete their maturation to adult worms in the intestine. The **cat roundworm**, *T. cati*, is responsible for far fewer cases of visceral larva migrans than *T. canis*. Ingestion of infective larvae of the raccoon and opossum ascarids *Baylisascaris procyonis* and *Lagochilascaris minor* can rarely lead to visceral larva migrans.

Epidemiology. Human *T. canis* infections have been reported in nearly all parts of the world, primarily in temperate and tropical areas where dogs are popular household pets. Young children are at highest risk because of their unsanitary play habits and tendency to place fingers in the mouth. Other behavioral risk factors include pica, contact with puppy litters, and institutionalization. In North America, the highest prevalences of infection are in the southeastern United States and Puerto Rico, particularly among socially disadvantaged African-American and Hispanic children. The highest reported frequency of infection in the world is in a village in Saint Lucia where 86% of children between the ages 6 mo and 6 yr were found to be seropositive. The high rate of infection in this community was attributed to a high prevalence of canine toxocariasis, widespread contamination of peridomestic areas with infective eggs, and pica. Assuming an unrestrained and untreated dog population, toxocariasis is prevalent in settings where other geohelminth infections such as ascariasis, trichuriasis, and hookworm infections are common.

Pathogenesis. *T. canis* larvae secrete large amounts of immunogenic glycosylated proteins. These antigens induce immune responses that lead to eosinophilia and polyclonal and antigen-specific IgE production. The characteristic histopathologic lesions are granulomas containing eosinophils, multinucleated giant cells (histiocytes), and collagen. Granulomas are typically found in the liver but may also occur in the lungs, central nervous system, and ocular tissues. Clinical manifestations reflect the intensity and chronicity of infection, anatomic localization of larvae, and host granulomatous responses.

Clinical Manifestations. There are three major clinical syndromes associated with human toxocariasis: visceral larva migrans (VLM), ocular larva migrans (OLM), and covert toxocariasis (Table 275–1). The classic presentation of VLM includes eosinophilia, fever, and hepatomegaly, and occurs most commonly in toddlers with a history of pica and exposure to puppies. The findings include fever, cough, wheezing, bronchopneumonia, anemia, hepatomegaly, leukocytosis, eosinophilia, and positive *Toxocara* serology. OLM tends to occur in older children without signs or symptoms of VLM. Presenting symptoms include unilateral visual loss, eye pain, white pupil, or strabismus that develops over a period of weeks. Granulomas occur on the posterior pole of the retina and may be mistaken for retinoblastoma. Serologic testing for *Toxocara* has allowed the identification of individuals with less obvious or covert symptoms of infection. These children may have nonspecific complaints that do not constitute a recognizable syndrome. Common findings include hepatomegaly, abdominal pain, cough, sleep disturbance, failure to thrive, and

headache with elevated *Toxocara* antibody titers. Eosinophilia may be present in only 50–75% of cases. The prevalence of positive *Toxocara* serology in the general population supports the notion that most children with *T. canis* infection are asymptomatic and will not develop overt clinical sequelae over time. A correlation between positive *Toxocara* serology and allergic asthma has also been described.

Diagnosis. A presumptive diagnosis can be established in a young child with eosinophilia, leukocytosis, hepatomegaly, fevers, wheezing, and a history of geophagia and exposure to puppies or unrestrained dogs. Supportive laboratory findings include hypergammaglobulinemia and elevated isohemagglutinin titers to A and B blood group antigens. Most patients with VLM have an absolute eosinophil count of 500/μL or greater. Eosinophilia is less common in subjects with OLM. An enzyme-linked immunosorbent assay using excretory-secretory proteins harvested from *T. canis* larvae maintained in vitro is the standard serologic test used to confirm toxocariasis. The sensitivity is >75% and specificity >90% using a cutoff dilution of 1:32. The diagnosis of OLM can be established in patients with typical clinical findings of a retinal or peripheral pole granuloma or endophthalmitis with elevated antibody titers. Vitreous and aqueous humor fluid anti-*Toxocara* titers are usually greater than serum titers. The diagnosis of covert toxocariasis should be considered in individuals with chronic weakness, abdominal pain, or allergic signs with eosinophilia and increased IgE. In temperate regions of the world, nonparasitic causes of eosinophilia that should be considered in the differential diagnosis include allergies, drug hypersensitivity, lymphoma, vasculitis, and the idiopathic hypereosinophilic syndrome (see Chapter 119).

Treatment. Most cases do not require treatment because signs and symptoms are mild and subside over a period of weeks to months. Several anthelmintic drugs have been used for symptomatic cases, often with adjunctive corticosteroids to limit inflammatory responses that presumably result from release of *Toxocara* antigens by dying parasites. Albendazole (400 mg once daily PO for 5 days for all ages) has demonstrated efficacy in both children and adults. Mebendazole (100–200 mg bid PO for 5 days for all ages) is also useful. Even though there are no clinical trials regarding therapy of OLM, a course of oral corticosteroids such as prednisone (1 mg/kg/24 hr PO for 2–4 wk) has been recommended to suppress local inflammation while treatment with anthelmintic agents is initiated.

Prevention. Transmission can be minimized by public health measures that prevent dog feces from contaminating the environment. These include keeping dogs on leashes and excluding pets from playgrounds and sandboxes that toddlers use. Children should be discouraged from putting dirty fingers in their mouth and eating dirt. Vinyl covering of sandboxes reduces the viability

TABLE 275–1. Clinical Syndromes of Human Toxocariasis

Syndrome	Clinical Findings	Average Age	Infectious Dose	Incubation Period	Laboratory Findings	ELISA
Visceral larva migrans	Fevers, hepatomegaly, asthma	5 yr	Moderate to high	Weeks to months	Eosinophilia, leukocytosis, elevated IgE	High (≥1:16)
Ocular larva migrans	Visual disturbances, retinal granulomas, endophthalmitis, peripheral granulomas	12 yr	Low	Months to years	Usually none	Low (<1:512)
Covert toxocariasis	Abdominal pain, gastrointestinal symptoms, weakness, hepatomegaly, pruritus, rash	School age to adult	Low to moderate	Weeks to years	± Eosinophilia, ± elevated IgE	Low to moderate

ELISA, enzyme-linked immunosorbent assay; ±, with or without.
Adapted from Liu LX: Toxocariasis and larva migrans syndrome. In Guerrant RL, Walker DH, Weller PF (editors): Tropical Infectious Diseases: Principles, Pathogens & Practice. Philadelphia, Churchill-Livingstone, 1999, p. 908.

of *T. canis* eggs. Widespread veterinary use of broad-spectrum anthelmintics effective against *Toxocara* may lead to a decline in parasite transmission to humans.

Gillespie SH: Human toxocariasis. *Communicable Disease Report CDR Rev* 1993;3: R140–3.

Glickman LT, Magnaval JF: Zoonotic roundworm infections. *Infect Dis Clin North Am* 1993;7:717–32.

Mok CH: Visceral larva migrans: A discussion based on review of the literature. *Clin Pediatr* 1968;7:565–73.

Molk R: Ocular toxocariasis: A review of the literature. *Ann Ophthalmol* 1983; 15:216–31.

Schantz PM, Glickman LT: Toxocaral visceral larva migrans. *N Engl J Med* 1978; 298:436–9.

Chapter 276
Trichinosis (*Trichinella spiralis*) *Sheral S. Patel and James W. Kazura*

Etiology. Human trichinosis is caused by consumption of meat containing encysted larvae of *Trichinella spiralis*, a tissue-dwelling nematode with a worldwide distribution. After ingestion of raw or inadequately cooked meat containing viable *Trichinella* larvae, the organisms are released from the cyst by acid-pepsin digestion of the cyst walls in the stomach and then pass into the small intestine. The larvae invade the small intestine columnar epithelium at the villi base and develop into adult worms. The adult female produces about 500 larvae over 2 wk and is then expelled in the feces. The larvae seed striated muscle via the bloodstream and burrow into individual muscle fibers. Over a period of 3 wk, they coil as they increase about 10 times in length and become capable of infecting a new host if ingested. The larvae eventually become encysted and can remain viable for years.

Epidemiology. Despite veterinary public health efforts to control and eradicate the parasite, reemergence of the disease has been observed in many areas of the world in the past 10–20 yr. Trichinosis is most common in Asia, Latin America, and Central Europe. Swine fed with garbage may become infected when given uncooked trichinous scraps, usually pig meat, or when the carcasses of infected wild animals such as rats are eaten. Prevalence rates of *T. spiralis* in domestic swine range from 0.001% in the United States to 25% or greater in China. The recent resurgence of this disease can be attributed to translocations of animal populations, human travel, and export of food as well as ingestion of sylvatic *Trichinella* through game meat. Most outbreaks occur from the consumption of *T. spiralis*–infected pork (or horse meat in areas of the world where horse is eaten) obtained from a single-source.

Pathogenesis. During the first 2–3 wk after infection, pathologic reactions to infection are limited to the gastrointestinal tract and include a mild, partial villous atrophy with an inflammatory infiltrate of neutrophils, eosinophils, lymphocytes, and macrophages in the mucosa and submucosa. Larvae are released by female worms and disseminate over the next several weeks. Skeletal muscle fibers show the most striking changes with edema and basophilic degeneration. The muscle fiber may contain the typical coiled worm, the cyst wall derived from the host cell, and the surrounding lymphocytic and eosinophilic infiltrate.

Clinical Manifestations. The development of symptoms depends on the number of viable larvae ingested. Most infections are asymptomatic or mild. Diarrhea is the most common symptom corresponding to maturation of the adult worms in the gastrointestinal tract, which occurs during the first 1–2 wk after inges-

tion. Patients may also complain of abdominal discomfort and vomiting. Fulminant enteritis may develop in individuals with extremely high worm burdens. The classic symptoms of periorbital edema, fever, and myalgia peak about 2–3 wk after the infected meat is ingested as the larvae encyst in the muscle. Headache, cough, dyspnea, dysphagia, subconjunctival and splinter hemorrhages, and a macular or petechial rash may occur. Patients with high intensities of infection may die from myocarditis, encephalitis, or pneumonia.

Diagnosis. The Centers for Disease Control and Prevention diagnostic criteria for trichinosis requires positive serology or muscle biopsy for *Trichinella* with one or more compatible clinical symptoms such as eosinophilia, fever, myalgia, and periorbital edema. In a discrete outbreak, at least one person must have positive serology or muscle biopsy. Antibodies to *Trichinella* are detectable about 3 wk after infection. Severe muscle involvement can result in elevated serum creatine phosphokinase and lactic dehydrogenase levels. Muscle biopsy is not usually necessary, but if needed, a sample should be obtained from a tender swollen muscle. A history of eating undercooked meat supports the diagnosis.

Treatment. Mebendazole (200–400 mg tid PO for 3 days then 400–500 mg tid PO for 10 days for all ages) should be administered to eradicate the adult worms if a patient has ingested contaminated meat within the previous week. An alternative regimen is albendazole (400 mg bid PO for 8–14 days for all ages). There is no consensus for treatment of muscle-stage trichinosis. Systemic corticosteroids with mebendazole may be used, although evidence for their efficacy is anecdotal. A recent study demonstrated that both thiabendazole (25 mg/kg bid PO for 10 days) and mebendazole (200 mg bid PO for 10 days) are effective against muscle larvae although mebendazole may have been less active but thiabendazole was poorly tolerated.

Prevention. *Trichinella* larvae can be killed by cooking meat (55°C or more) until there is no trace of pink fluid or flesh, or storage in a freezer (-15°C) for 3 weeks or longer. Smoking, salting, and drying meat are unreliable methods of killing *Trichinella*. Strict adherence to pubic health measures can reduce infection with *Trichinella*. These measures include following garbage feeding regulations, stringent rodent control, prevention of exposure of pigs and other livestock to animal carcasses, constructing barriers between livestock, wild animals, and domestic pets, and proper handling of wild animal carcasses by hunters.

Ko RC: A brief update on the diagnosis of trichinellosis. *Southeast Asian J Trop Med Public Health* 1997;28:91–8.

Moorhead A, Grunenwald PE, Dietz VJ, et al: Trichinellosis in the United States, 1991–1996: Declining but not gone. *Am J Trop Med Hyg* 1999;60:66–9.

Murrell KD, Pozio E: Trichinellosis: The zoonosis that won't go quietly. *Int J Parasitol* 2000;30:1339–49.

Watt G, Saisorn S, Jongsakul K, et al: Blinded, placebo-controlled trial of anti-parasitic drugs for trichinosis myositis. *J Infect Dis* 2000;182:371–4.

Chapter 277
Schistosomiasis (*Schistosoma*) *Charles H. King*

Etiology. *Schistosoma* organisms are the flukes, or trematodes, that parasitize the bloodstream. Five schistosome species infect humans: *Schistosoma haematobium*, *S. mansoni*, *S. japonicum*, *S. intercalatum*, and *S. mekongi*. Humans are infected through contact with water contaminated with **cercariae**, the free-living infective stage of the parasite. These motile, forked-tail organisms emerge from infected snails and are capable of penetrating intact human skin. In the subcutaneous tissues, cercariae change into the next developmental stage, the **schistosomula**, and migrate to the lungs and finally the liver. As they reach sexual maturity, adult worms migrate to specific anatomic sites characteristic of each schistosome species: *S. haematobium* adults are found in the perivesical and periureteral venous plexus, *S. mansoni* in the inferior mesenteric, and *S. japonicum* in the superior mesenteric veins. *S. intercalatum* and *S. mekongi* are found in the mesenteric vessels. Adult schistosome worms (1–2 cm long) are clearly adapted for an intravascular existence. Unlike the other flukes, *Schistosoma* organisms are diecious, and the two sexes are dissimilar in appearance. The female accompanies the male in a groove formed by the lateral edges of its body. On fertilization, female worms begin oviposition in the small venous tributaries. The eggs of the three main schistosome species have characteristic morphologic features: *S. haematobium* has a terminal spine, *S. mansoni* has a lateral spine, and *S. japonicum* has a smaller size with a short, curved spine (Fig. 277–1). Eggs reach the lumen of the urinary tract or intestines and are carried to the outside environment, where they hatch if deposited in fresh water. Motile **miracidia** emerge; they infect specific freshwater snail intermediate hosts and divide asexually. In 4–6 wk, the infective cercariae are released in the water.

Epidemiology. Schistosomiasis infects >200 million people worldwide, primarily children and young adults. Prevalence is increasing in many areas as population density increases and new irrigation projects provide broader habitats for vector snails. Humans are the definitive host for the five clinically important species of schistosomes, although *S. japonicum* may infect some animals such as dogs and cattle. *S. haematobium* is prevalent in Africa and the Middle East; *S. mansoni* in Africa, the Middle East, the Caribbean, and South America; and *S. japonicum* in China, the Philippines, and Indonesia, with some sporadic foci in parts of Southeast Asia. The other two species are less prevalent. *S. intercalatum* is found in West and Central Africa, and *S. mekongi* is found in the Far East.

Transmission depends on disposal of excreta, the presence of specific intermediate snail hosts, and the patterns of water contact and social habits of the population. The distribution of infection in endemic areas shows that prevalence increases with age to a peak at 10–20 yr of age. Measuring intensity of infection (by quantitative egg count in urine or feces) demonstrates that the heaviest worm loads are found in the younger age groups. Schistosomiasis, therefore, is most prevalent and most severe in children and young adults, who are at maximal risk of suffering from its acute and chronic sequelae.

Pathogenesis. The early manifestations of schistosomiasis are immunologically mediated. Acute schistosomiasis, Katayama fever, is a febrile illness that represents an immune complex disease associated with early infection and oviposition. The major pathology of infection is with chronic schistosomiasis, in which retention of eggs in the host tissues is associated with chronic granulomatous injury. Eggs may be trapped at sites of deposition (urinary bladder, ureters, intestine) or be carried by the bloodstream to other organs, most commonly the liver and less often the lungs and central nervous system. The host response to these eggs involves local as well as systemic manifestations. The cell-mediated immune response leads to granulomas composed of lymphocytes, macrophages, and eosinophils that surround the trapped eggs and add significantly to the degree of tissue destruction. Granuloma formation in the bladder wall and at the ureterovesical junction results in the major disease manifestations of schistosomiasis haematobia: hematuria, dysuria, and obstructive uropathy. Intestinal as well as hepatic granulomas underlie the pathologic sequelae of the other schistosome infections: ulcerations and fibrosis of intestinal wall, hepatosplenomegaly, and portal hypertension due to presinusoidal obstruction of blood flow. Protective immunity against schistosomiasis has been demonstrated in some animal species and may occur in humans.

Clinical Manifestations. Most infected individuals suffer no apparent ill health; symptoms occur mainly in those who are heavily infected. Cercarial penetration of human skin may result in a papular pruritic rash known as **schistosomal dermatitis** or **swimmer's itch**. It is more pronounced in previously exposed individuals and is characterized by edema and massive cellular infiltrates in the dermis and epidermis. Acute schistosomiasis, **Katayama fever**, may occur, particularly in heavily infected individuals 4–8 wk after exposure; this is a serum sickness–like syndrome manifested by the acute onset of fever, chills, sweating, lymphadenopathy, hepatosplenomegaly, and eosinophilia. Acute schistosomiasis most commonly presents in first-time visitors to endemic areas who experience primary infection at an older age.

Symptomatic children with chronic schistosomiasis haematobia usually complain of frequency, dysuria, and hematuria. Urine examination shows erythrocytes, parasite eggs, and occasional leukocytes. In endemic areas, moderate to severe pathologic lesions have been demonstrated in the urinary tract of >50% of infected children. The extent of disease correlates with the intensity of infection, but significant morbidity can occur even in lightly infected children. The terminal stages of schistosomiasis haematobia are associated with chronic renal failure, secondary infections, and cancer of the bladder.

Children with chronic schistosomiasis mansoni, japonica, intercalatum, or mekongi may have intestinal symptoms; colicky abdominal pain and bloody diarrhea are the most common. The intestinal phase may, however, pass unnoticed, and the syndrome of hepatosplenomegaly, portal hypertension, ascites, and hematemesis may be the initial presentation. Liver disease is due to granuloma formation and subsequent fibrosis; no appreciable liver cell injury occurs, and hepatic function may be preserved for a long time. Schistosome eggs may escape into the lungs, causing pulmonary hypertension and cor pulmonale. *S. japonicum* worms may migrate to the brain vasculature and produce localized lesions that cause seizures. Transverse myelitis rarely has been reported in children or young adults with chronic *S. haematobium* or *S. mansoni* infection.

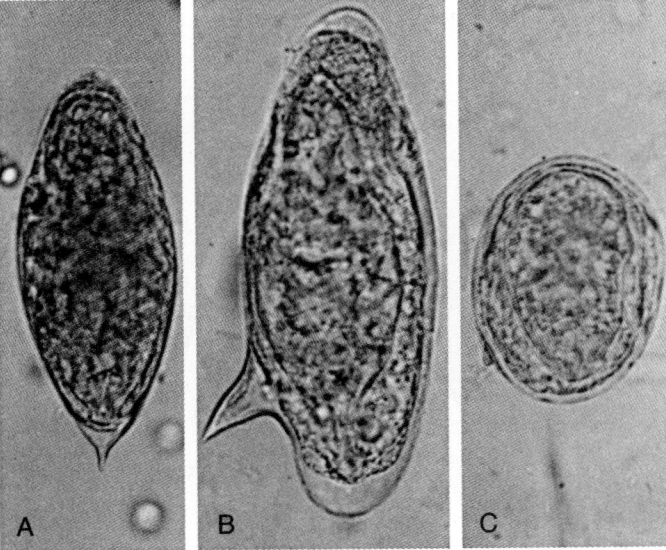

FIGURE 277–1. Eggs of *Schistosoma haematobium* (A), *Schistosoma mansoni* (B), and *Schistosoma japonicum* (C) (×320).

Diagnosis. Schistosome eggs are found in the excreta of infected individuals; quantitative methods should be used to provide an indication of the intensity of infection. For diagnosis of schistosomiasis haematobia, a volume of 10 mL of urine should be collected around midday, which is the time of maximal egg excretion, and filtered for microbiological examination. Stool examination by the Kato thick smear procedure is the method of choice for diagnosis and quantification of other schistosome infections.

Treatment. Treatment of children with schistosomiasis should be based on an appreciation of the intensity of infection and the extent of disease. The recommended treatment for schistosomiasis is praziquantel (40 mg/kg/24 hr divided bid for 1 day for schistosomiasis haematobia, mansoni, and intercalatum; 60 mg/kg/24 hr divided tid for 1 day for schistosomiasis japonica and mekongi).

Prevention. Transmission in endemic areas may be decreased by reducing the parasite load in the population. The availability of oral, single-dose, effective chemotherapeutic agents may help achieve this goal. Other measures, particularly improved sanitation and focal application of molluscicides, may be useful. Control of schistosomiasis is closely linked to economic and social development.

Case records of the Massachusetts General Hospital: Weekly clinicopathological exercises. Case 31-2000. A 32-year-old man with a lesion of the urinary bladder. *N Engl J Med* 2000;343:1105–11.

Centers for Disease Control and Prevention: Schistosomiasis. Health Topics A to Z (available at *http://www.cdc.gov/ncidod/dpd/parasites/schistosomiasis/default.htm*).

Hatz CF: The use of ultrasound in schistosomiasis. Adv Parasitol 2001;48:225–84.

King CH, Mahmoud AA: Schistosomiasis. In Guerrant RL, Walker DH, Weller PF (editors): *Tropical Infectious Diseases, Principles, Pathogens and Practice.* New York, Churchill Livingstone, 1999, pp. 1031–8.

Mahmoud AA (editor): *Schistosomiasis.* London, Imperial College Press, 2001.

Medical Letter on Drugs and Therapeutics: Drugs for parasitic infections. Med Lett Drugs Therapeut April 2000 (available at *http://www.medletter.com/freedocs/parasitic.pdf*).

Saconato H, Atallah A: Interventions for treating schistosomiasis mansoni. *Cochrane Database Syst Rev* 2000:CD000528.

Squires N: Interventions for treating schistosomiasis haematobium. *Cochrane Database Syst Rev* 2000:CD000053.

Chapter 278
Flukes (Liver, Lung, and Intestinal) *Charles H. King*

Several different **trematodes**, or **flukes**, can parasitize humans and cause disease. Flukes are endemic worldwide but are more prevalent in the less developed parts of the world. They include *Schistosoma*, the blood flukes (Chapter 277), as well as fluke species that cause infection in the human biliary tree, lung tissue, and intestinal tract. These latter trematodes are characterized by their complex life cycles. Sexual reproduction of adult worms in the definitive host produces eggs that are passed in the stool. Larvae, called **miracidia**, develop in fresh water. These, in turn, infect certain species of molluscs (snails or clams), in which asexual multiplication by parasite larvae produces **cercariae**. Cercariae then seek a second intermediate host such as an insect, crustacean, or fish or attach to vegetation to produce infectious **metacercariae**. Humans acquire liver, lung, and intestinal fluke infections by eating uncooked, lightly cooked, pickled, or smoked foods containing these infectious parasite cysts. The "alternation of generations" requires that flukes parasitize more than one host (often three) to complete their life cycle. Because parasitic flukes are dependent on these nonhuman species for transmission, the distribution of human fluke infection closely matches their ecologic range.

LIVER FLUKES

Fascioliasis (*Fasciola hepatica*). *Fasciola hepatica,* the **sheep liver** fluke, infects cattle, other ungulates, and occasionally humans. Infection has been reported in many different parts of the world, particularly South America, Europe, Africa, China, Australia, and Cuba. Although *F. hepatica* is enzootic in North America, reported cases are extremely rare. Humans are infected by ingestion of metacercariae attached to vegetation, especially wild watercress. In the duodenum, the parasites excyst and penetrate the intestinal wall, liver capsule, and parenchyma. They wander for a few weeks before entering the bile ducts, where they mature. Adult *F. hepatica* (1 × 2.5 cm) commence oviposition approximately 12 wk after infection; the eggs are large (75 × 140 μm) and operculated. They pass to the intestines with bile and exit the body in the feces (Fig. 278–1). On reaching fresh water, the eggs mature and hatch into miracidia, which infect specific snail intermediate hosts to multiply into many cercariae. These then emerge from infected snails and encyst on aquatic grasses and plants.

Clinical manifestations usually occur either during the liver migratory phase of the parasites or after their arrival at their final habitat in bile canaliculi. Fever, right upper quadrant pain, and hepatosplenomegaly characterize the first phase of illness. Peripheral blood eosinophilia is usually marked. As the worms enter bile ducts, most of the acute symptoms subside. On rare occasions, patients may suffer from obstructive jaundice or biliary cirrhosis. *F. hepatica* infection is diagnosed by identifying the characteristic eggs in fecal smears or duodenal aspirates.

Bithionol (30–50 mg/kg once daily PO on alternate days for a total of 10–15 doses) is the recommended treatment. In the United States, bithionol is available from the Centers for Disease Control and Prevention (telephone: 404-639-3670). The investigational drug triclabendazole (Ciba-Geigy) may also be used to treat fascioliasis.

Clonorchiasis (*Clonorchis sinensis*). Infection of bile passages with *Clonorchis sinensis,* the **Chinese or oriental liver fluke,** is endemic in China, other parts of East Asia, and Japan. Humans acquire infection by ingestion of raw or inadequately cooked freshwater fish carrying the encysted metacercariae of the parasite under their scales or skin. Metacercariae excyst in the duodenum and pass through the ampulla of Vater to the common bile duct and bile capillaries, where they mature into hermaphroditic adult worms (3 × 15 mm). *C. sinensis* worms deposit small operculated eggs (14 × 30 μm), which are discharged by way of the bile duct to the intestine and feces (see Fig. 278–1). The eggs mature and hatch outside the body, releasing motile miracidia into local

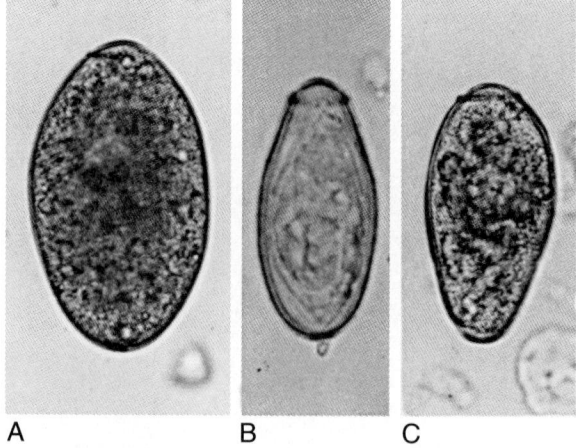

FIGURE 278–1. Eggs of liver flukes. *A, Fasciola hepatica* (× 400). *B, Clonorchis sinensis* (×1,000). *C,* A lung fluke, *Paragonimus westermani* (×400).

freshwater streams, rivers, or ponds. If these are ingested by the appropriate snails, they develop into cercariae, which are in turn released from the snail to encyst under the skin or scales of freshwater fish.

Most individuals with *C. sinensis* infection, particularly those with few organisms, are asymptomatic. In heavily infected individuals, who tend to be older (>30 yr of age), localized obstruction of a bile duct results from repeated local trauma and inflammation. In these cases, cholangitis and cholangiohepatitis may lead to liver enlargement and jaundice. In Hong Kong, Korea, and other parts of Asia, cholangiocarcinoma is associated with chronic *C. sinensis* infection.

Clonorchiasis is diagnosed by examination of feces or duodenal aspirates for the parasite eggs. The recommended treatment of clonorchiasis is praziquantel (75 mg/kg/24 hr divided tid PO for 1 day). An alternative, used in adults, is albendazole (10 mg/kg once daily PO for 7 days).

Opisthorchiasis (*Opisthorchis*). Infections with species of *Opisthorchis* are clinically similar to those by *C. sinensis*. *O. felineus* and *O. viverrini* are liver flukes of cats and dogs that infect humans through ingestion of metacercariae in freshwater fish. Infection with *O. felineus* is endemic in Eastern Europe and Southeast Asia, and *O. viverrini* is found mainly in Thailand. Most individuals are asymptomatic; liver enlargement, relapsing cholangitis, and jaundice may occur in heavily infected individuals. Diagnosis is based on recovering eggs from stools or duodenal aspirates. The recommended treatment of opisthorchiasis is praziquantel (75 mg/kg/24 hr divided tid PO for 1 day).

LUNG FLUKES

Paragonimiasis (*Paragonimus*). Human infection by the **lung fluke** *Paragonimus westermani,* and less frequently other species of *Paragonimus,* occurs throughout the Far East, in localized areas of West Africa, and in several parts of Central and South America. The highest incidence of paragonimiasis occurs in older children and adolescents 11–15 yr of age. Although *P. westermani* is found in many carnivores, human cases are relatively rare and seem to be associated with specific dietary habits, such as eating raw freshwater crayfish or crabs. These crustaceans contain the infective metacercariae in their tissues. After ingestion, the metacercariae excyst in the duodenum, penetrate the intestinal wall, and migrate to their final habitat in the lungs. Adult worms (5 × 10 mm) encapsulate within the lung parenchyma and deposit brown operculated eggs (60 × 100 μm), which pass into the bronchioles and are expectorated by coughing (see Fig. 278–1). Ova can be detected in the sputum of infected individuals or in their feces. If eggs reach fresh water, they hatch and undergo asexual multiplication in specific snails. The cercariae encyst in the muscles and viscera of crayfish and freshwater crabs.

Most individuals infected with *P. westermani* harbor low or moderate worm loads and are asymptomatic. The *clinical manifestations* include hemoptysis, which is the principal manifestation and occurs in 98% of symptomatic children, cough, and production of rust-colored sputum. There are no characteristic physical findings, but laboratory examination usually demonstrates marked eosinophilia. Chest radiography often reveals small patchy infiltrates or radiolucencies in the middle lung fields; however, the radiograph may appear normal in one fifth of infected individuals. In rare circumstances, lung abscess, pleural effusion, or bronchiectasis may develop. Extrapulmonary localization of *P. westermani* in the brain, peritoneum, intestines, or pleura may rarely occur. Cerebral paragonimiasis is encountered primarily in heavily infected individuals living in highly endemic areas of the Far East; the clinical presentation resembles jacksonian epilepsy or cerebral tumors.

Definitive diagnosis of paragonimiasis is established by identification of eggs in fecal or sputum smears. The recommended treatment of paragonimiasis is praziquantel (75 mg/kg/24 hr divided tid PO for 2 days).

INTESTINAL FLUKES

Several wild and domestic animal intestinal flukes, such as *Fasciolopsis buski, Nanophyetus salmincola,* and *Heterophyes heterophyes,* may accidentally infect humans. *F. buski* is endemic in the Far East. Humans who ingest metacercariae encysted on aquatic plants become infected. These develop into large flukes (1 × 5 cm) that inhabit the duodenum and jejunum. Mature worms produce operculated eggs that pass with feces; the organism completes its life cycle through specific snail intermediate hosts. Individuals with *F. buski* infection are usually asymptomatic; heavily infected subjects complain of abdominal pain and diarrhea and show signs of malabsorption. Diagnosis of fasciolopsiasis and other intestinal fluke infections is established by fecal examination and identification of the eggs. As for other fluke infections, praziquantel (75 mg/kg/24 hr divided tid PO for 1 day) is the drug of choice.

King CH: Pulmonary flukes. In Mahmoud AA (editor): *Parasitic Lung Diseases.* New York, Marcel Dekker, 1997.

Liu LX, Harinasuta KT: Liver and intestinal flukes. *Gastroenterol Clin North Am* 1996;25:627–36.

MacLean JD, Cross J, Mahanty S: Liver, lung and intestinal fluke infections. In Guerrant RL, Walker DH, Weller PF (editors): *Tropical Infectious Diseases, Principles, Pathogens and Practice.* New York, Churchill Livingstone, 1999.

Medical Letter on Drugs and Therapeutics: Drugs for parasitic infections. *Med Lett Drugs Ther,* April 2000. (Available at *http://www.medletter.com/freedocs/parasitic.pdf*)

Millan JC, Mull R, Freise S, et al: The efficacy and tolerability of triclabendazole in Cuban patients with latent and chronic *Fasciola hepatica* infection. *Am J Trop Med Hyg* 2000;63:264–9.

Price TA, Tuazon CU, Simon GL: Fascioliasis: Case reports and review. *Clin Infect Dis* 1993;17:426–30.

World Health Organization: Triclabendazole and fascioliasis—A new drug to combat an age-old disease. WHO Fact Sheet No. 191, April 1998. (Available at *http://www.who.int/inf-fs/en/fact191.html*)

Chapter 279
Adult Tapeworm Infections
Ronald Blanton

Infections with **cestodes**, or **tapeworms**, are prevalent on every continent except Antarctica. Unlike many parasites that strictly segregate their developmental stages in different host species, some tapeworms can infect humans with the adult worm stage, the invasive intermediate stage, or both. The intermediate stages of some tapeworms, such as with cysticercosis (Chapter 280) and echinococcosis (Chapter 281), are invasive and form cystic structures that produce tissue damage from mass effect or inflammatory reactions. No signs or symptoms can clearly be attributed to infection with any adult tapeworm except for *Diphyllobothrium latum.* Infection with the adult worm can be easily diagnosed by finding eggs or segments of adult worms in the stool, whereas the invasive stage of the parasite cannot be observed in any easily sampled fluid. Infection with an intermediate stage, therefore, must be diagnosed by serologic tests, imaging, or invasive procedures.

TAENIASIS (*TAENIA SAGINATA* AND *TAENIA SOLIUM*)

Etiology. The **beef tapeworm**, *T. saginata,* and the **pork tapeworm**, *T. solium,* are large parasites (4–10 m) named for their intermediate hosts. The adult stages are only found in the human intestine. The body of the adult stage is a connected series of hundreds or thousands of flattened segments, called **proglot-**

tids, whose most anterior segment, the **scolex**, anchors the parasite to the bowel wall. New segments arise at the caudal end of the scolex followed by progressively more mature ones. The gravid terminal segments are each packed with 50,000–100,000 eggs, and the eggs or these intact proglottids pass in the stool. These two tapeworms differ most significantly in that the intermediate stage of the pork tapeworm (cysticercus) can also infect humans and cause significant morbidity (Chapter 280).

Epidemiology. Both *Taenia* species are distributed worldwide, with the highest risk of infection in Central America, Africa, India, Southeast Asia, and China. The prevalence in adults may not reflect the prevalence in young children, because cultural practices may dictate how well meat is cooked and how much is served to children.

Pathogenesis. Uncomplicated infection with the adult beef or pork tapeworm by itself is an infrequent source of symptoms. When children ingest raw or undercooked infected meat, gastric acid and bile facilitate release of the immature scolex that attaches to the lumen of the small intestine. The parasite adds new segments, and after 2–3 mo the terminal segments mature and become gravid.

Clinical Manifestations. Adult beef and pork tapeworms cause very little overt morbidity apart from nonspecific abdominal symptoms. The proglottids of these tapeworms are visually striking. They are also motile and sometimes produce anal pruritus. They can often be felt as they pass and are thus likely to be noticed and cause a strong emotional reaction in older children and parents when discovered. The adult beef and pork tapeworms are rare causes of intestinal obstruction, cholangitis, and appendicitis.

Diagnosis. It is important to identify the infecting species of tapeworm. Carriers of adult pork tapeworms are at increased risk of transmitting eggs with the pathogenic intermediate stage (cysticercus) to themselves or others, whereas children infected with the beef tapeworm are a risk only to livestock. Because proglottids are generally passed intact, visual examination for gravid proglottids in the stool is a sensitive test; these segments may be used to identify species. Eggs, by contrast, are often absent from stool and cannot reliably distinguish between *T. saginata* and *T. solium* (Fig. 279–1). If the parasite is completely expelled, the scolex of each species is diagnostic. The scolex of *T. saginata* has only a set of four anteriorly oriented suckers, whereas *T. solium* is armed with a double row of hooks in addition to suckers. The proglottids of *T. saginata* have more than 20 uterine branches from a central uterine structure, and those of *T. solium* have 10 or fewer. When in doubt, more proglottids should be obtained or the sample should be referred to a laboratory with parasitologic expertise.

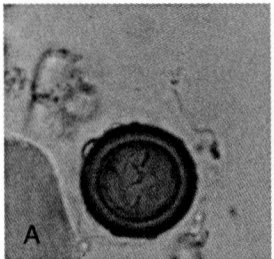 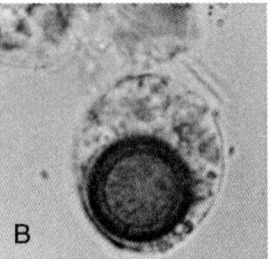

FIGURE 279–1. Eggs of *Taenia saginata* recovered from feces (×400). The eggs are generally bile-stained, dark, and prismatic. There is occasionally some surrounding cellular material from the proglottid in which the egg develops, which is more evident in *B* than in *A*. The larva within the egg show three pairs of hooklets *(A)*, which may occasionally be seen in motion.

DIFFERENTIAL DIAGNOSIS. Anal pruritus may mimic symptoms of pinworm (*Enterobius vermicularis*) infection. *D. latum* or even *Ascaris lumbricoides* might be mistaken for *T. saginata* or *T. solium* in stools.

Treatment. Infections with all adult tapeworms respond to praziquantel (5–10 mg/kg PO once), which is the recommended treatment for taeniasis. Praziquantel tends to cause parasite death and subsequent resorption unless purged. An alternative treatment is niclosamide (50 mg/kg PO once for children, 2g PO once for adults). The parasite is usually expelled on the day of administration.

Prevention. Prolonged freezing or thorough cooking of beef and pork kills the parasite. Appropriate human sanitation can interrupt transmission by preventing infection in livestock.

DIPHYLLOBOTHRIASIS (*DIPHYLLOBOTHRIUM LATUM*)

Etiology. The **fish tapeworm**, *D. latum*, is the longest human tapeworm (10–20 m) and has an organization similar to that of other adult cestodes. An elongated scolex equipped with slits, called **bothria**, along each side, but no suckers or hooks, is followed by thousands of segments looped in the small bowel. The terminal gravid proglottid detaches periodically but tends to disintegrate before expulsion, thus releasing its eggs into the feces. In contrast to taeniids, the life cycle of *D. latum* requires two intermediate hosts. Eggs hatch in fresh water and release embryos that are swallowed by small crustaceans (copepods). The parasite passes up the food chain as small fish eat the copepods and are in turn eaten by larger fish. In this way, the juvenile parasite becomes concentrated in pike, walleye, perch, salmon, and similar fish. Consumption of raw or undercooked fish leads to human infection with adult fish tapeworms.

Epidemiology. The fish tapeworm is most prevalent in the temperate climates of Europe, North America, and Asia but may be found in cold lakes at high altitudes in South America and Africa. In North America, the prevalence is highest in Alaska, Canada, and the northern United States, and the tapeworm is found in fish from those areas brought to market in the continental United States. Persons who prepare raw fish for home or commercial use or who sample fish before cooking are particularly at risk for infection.

Pathogenesis. The adult worm efficiently scavenges vitamin B_{12} for its own use in the constant production of large numbers of segments and as many as 1 million eggs per day. The parasite also inhibits vitamin B_{12} uptake by uncoupling the B_{12}-intrinsic factor complex. As a result, diphyllobothriasis causes megaloblastic anemia in 2–9% of infections. Children with other causes of vitamin B_{12} or folate deficiency such as chronic infectious diarrhea, celiac disease, or congenital malabsorption are more likely to develop symptomatic infection.

Clinical Manifestations. Infection is largely asymptomatic except in those who develop B_{12} or folate deficiency. Megaloblastic anemia with leukopenia, thrombocytopenia, glossitis, and signs of spinal cord posterior column degeneration (loss of vibratory sense, proprioception, and coordination) can be evidence of advanced nutritional deficiency due to diphyllobothriasis. The hematologic and neurologic signs may present independently or as a cluster.

Diagnosis. Parasitologic examination of the stool is useful because eggs are abundant in the feces and have a morphology distinct from that of all other tapeworms. The eggs are ovoid and have an operculum, which is a cap structure at one end that opens to release the embryo (Fig. 279–2). The worm itself has a distinct scolex and proglottid morphology; however, these are not likely to be passed spontaneously.

DIFFERENTIAL DIAGNOSIS. A segment or a whole section of the worm might be confused with *Taenia* or *Ascaris* after it is

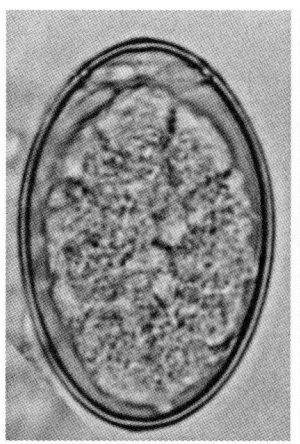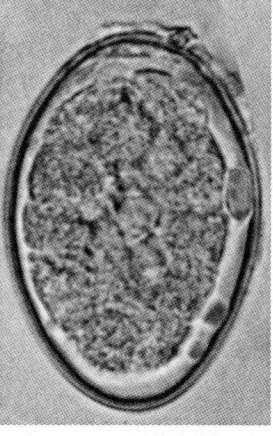

FIGURE 279–2. Eggs of *Diphyllobothrium latum* as seen in feces (×400). The caplike operculum is at the upper end of the egg here.

passed. Pernicious anemia, bone marrow toxins, and dietary restrictions may contribute to or mimic diphyllobothriasis.

Treatment. Infections with all adult tapeworms respond to praziquantel (5–10 mg/kg PO once), which is the recommended treatment for diphyllobothriasis.

Prevention. The intermediate stage is easily eliminated by brief cooking or prolonged freezing. Because humans are the major reservoir for adult worms, health education is one of the most important tools for preventing transmission, together with improved human sanitation.

HYMENOLEPIASIS (*HYMENOLEPIS*)

Infection with *Hymenolepis nana*, the dwarf tapeworm, is very common in developing countries. It is a major cause of eosinophilia, and although it rarely causes overt disease, the presence of *H. nana* eggs in stool may serve as a marker for exposure to poor hygienic conditions. Although the intermediate stage develops in various hosts (rodents, ticks, and fleas), the entire life cycle can be completed in humans. Hyperinfection with thousands of small adult worms in a single child is thus a potential. Less commonly, a similar infection may occur with the species *H. diminuta*. Eggs but not segments may be found in the stool. *H. nana* infection responds to praziquantel (25 mg/kg PO once) or niclosamide (1 g PO for children 11–34 lb, 1.5 g PO for ≥35 lb for 6 days).

DIPYLIDIASIS (*DIPYLIDIUM CANINUM*)

Dipylidium caninum is a common tapeworm of domestic dogs and cats, yet human infection is relatively rare. Direct transmission between pets and humans does not occur; human infection requires ingestion of the parasite's intermediate host, the dog or cat flea. Infants and small children are particularly susceptible because of their level of hygiene, generally more intimate contact with pets, and activities in areas where fleas can be encountered. Eosinophilia may occur, but no symptoms clearly result from infection. Anal pruritus, vague abdominal pain, and diarrhea have at times been associated with dipylidiasis. Dipylidiasis may be confused with pinworm (*E. vermicularis*). Dipylidiasis is effectively treated with praziquantel (5–10 mg/kg PO once) or niclosamide (1 g for 11–34 lb, 1.5 g for ≥35 lb PO once). Deworming pets and flea control are the best preventive measures.

Schantz PM: Tapeworms (cestodiasis). *Gastroenterol Clin North Am* 1996;25:637–53.
Weisse ME; Raszka WV Jr: Cestode infection in children. *Adv Pediatr Infect Dis* 1996;12:109–53.

Chapter 280
Cysticercosis *Ronald Blanton*

Etiology. Cysticercosis is caused by infection with the intermediate stage of *Taenia solium*, the **pork tapeworm**, and is the most common and serious parasitic infection of the central nervous system (CNS). Unlike the beef tapeworm (see Chapter 279), the intermediate stage of *Taenia solium* is infectious for humans and preferentially invades the CNS, causing **neurocysticercosis**. Whereas consumption of infected undercooked pork produces intestinal infection with the adult worm, humans acquire the intermediate form by ingestion of food or water contaminated with the eggs of *T. solium*. Cysticercosis may, therefore, develop even in individuals who do not eat pork. Individuals infected with an adult *T. solium* may infect themselves with the eggs by the fecal-oral route. Reverse peristalsis in the small intestine has also been implicated as a means of autoinfection.

In the small intestine, the egg releases an **oncosphere** that crosses the gut wall and spreads hematogenously to many tissues, primarily brain and muscle. Wherever the eggs lodge, they produce small (0.2–0.5 cm) fluid-filled bladders containing a single **protoscolex**, the juvenile-stage parasite.

Epidemiology. The pork tapeworm is distributed worldwide wherever pigs are raised. Intense transmission occurs in Central and South America, India, Indonesia, Korea, and China as well as some areas of Africa. In these areas, 20–50% of cases of epilepsy may be due to cysticercosis. Most cases of cysticercosis in the United States are imported; transmission is uncommon but occurs on occasion.

Pathogenesis. The cystic stages of most tapeworms do not provoke a strong immunologic response while they remain alive and intact. Intact viable cysts can be associated with disease when the initial parasite invasion of the brain is massive or when they obstruct the flow of cerebrospinal fluid (CSF). Most cysts remain viable for 5–10 yr and then begin to degenerate, followed by a vigorous host response. The natural history of cysts is to resolve by complete resorption or calcification.

Clinical Manifestations. Seizures are the presenting finding in >70% of cases, although any cognitive or neurologic abnormality from psychosis to stroke may be a manifestation of cysticercosis. Neurocysticercosis can be classified as parenchymal, intraventricular, meningeal, spinal, or ocular on the basis of anatomic location, clinical presentation, and radiologic appearance.

Parenchymal neurocysticercosis produces seizures as well as focal neurologic deficits. The seizures are generalized in 80% of cases but frequently begin as simple or complex partial seizures. Rarely, cerebral infarction can result from obstruction of small terminal arteries or vasculitis. With extensive frontal lobe disease, symptoms of intellectual deterioration with dementia or Parkinsonism may obfuscate diagnosis until focal signs appear. A fulminant encephalitis-like presentation also occurs, most frequently in children who have had a massive initial infection. **Intraventricular neurocysticercosis** (5–10% of all cases) is associated with hydrocephalus and acute, subacute, or intermittent signs of increased intracranial pressure without localizing signs. The fourth ventricle is the most common site for obstruction and symptoms; cysts in the lateral ventricles are less likely to cause obstruction. **Meningeal neurocysticercosis** is associated with signs of meningeal irritation and also increased intracranial pressure that results from edema, inflammation, or the presence of a cyst obstructing flow of CSF. Chronic basilar meningitis is associated with many forms of neurocysticercosis, but predominantly meningeal presentations. **Racemose**

neurocysticercosis is a meningeal form of disease in which large, lobulated cysts appear in the basal cisterns. **Spinal neurocysticercosis** presents with evidence of spinal cord compression, nerve root pain, transverse myelitis, or meningitis. **Ocular neurocysticercosis** causes decreased visual acuity due to cysticerci floating in the vitreous, retinal detachment, or iridocyclitis. Outside of the CNS, cysts can sometimes be palpated under the skin, and very heavy infections in skeletal or heart muscle can result in myositis or carditis.

Diagnosis. Neurocysticercosis should be suspected in any child with any onset of a neurologic, cognitive, or personality disorder and also a history of residence in an endemic area or a care provider from an endemic area. Seizures, hydrocephalus, unilateral visual impairment, or symptoms of encephalitis are particularly suspicious. Proglottids (segments) or eggs are observed in feces from only 25% of cases of neurocysticercosis; therefore, imaging studies and serologic tests are necessary to confirm a clinical suspicion.

The most useful diagnostic study for parenchymal disease is CT. A solitary parenchymal cyst, with or without contrast enhancement, and numerous calcifications are the most common findings in children (Fig. 280–1). Intraventricular cysts are found in 11–17% of cases of neurocysticercosis. MRI better detects intraventricular cysts as well as those in the spinal cord by delineating parasite membranes and differences in signal intensity between the fluids and tissues of the cysticercus. The protoscolex may even be visible within the cyst by MRI, which provides a pathognomonic sign of cysticercosis. MRI is also more sensitive for detecting evidence of inflammation surrounding a cyst. Plain films may reveal calcifications in muscle or brain consistent with cysticercosis, but these are often nondiagnostic in children.

Serologic diagnosis using the enzyme-linked immunotransfer blot (EITB) is available commercially in the United States and through the Centers for Disease Control and Prevention. Serum antibody testing has >90% sensitivity and specificity; testing of CSF is not required. Persons with many parenchymal cysts almost always have a positive serum EITB test result. Cases with solitary lesions or old calcified disease may not have detectable antibodies. Neurocysticercosis is the most important and most frequent cause of eosinophilia in CSF, but this is not a reliable finding and if absent does not preclude the diagnosis.

DIFFERENTIAL DIAGNOSIS. Neurocysticercosis can be confused clinically with encephalitis, stroke, meningitis, and many other conditions. Clinical suspicion is based on travel history or a history of contact with an individual who might carry an adult tapeworm. On imaging studies, cysticerci can be difficult to distinguish from tuberculomas, histoplasmosis, blastomycosis, toxoplasmosis, sarcoidosis, vasculitis, and tumor.

Treatment. The specific treatment of neurocysticercosis depends on disease presentation. Many issues concerning whether, when, and how to treat are still not resolved. Observation, symptomatic treatment, antiparasitic drugs, and surgery all may have a role. Children with seizures, no hydrocephalus, and only calcified, inactive lesions on CT do not require therapy other than anticonvulsant medications. If no anticysticercal drugs are administered, however, it is also necessary to determine whether these patients carry adult worms, which poses a public health risk. Niclosamide used in the treatment of adult worms is not absorbed and does not provoke an inflammatory response to cysticerci. Most seizures that are associated with inflammation, as demonstrated by CT or MRI, can be controlled using standard anticonvulsants. If seizures are recurrent or associated with inactive lesions, treatment should be continued for 2–3 yr before attempting weaning from anticonvulsants.

Active parenchymal lesions usually resolve spontaneously, and some experts do not treat with anticysticercal drugs. Some studies indicate, however, that anticysticercal chemotherapy is associated with fewer residual seizures on long-term follow-up. Two effective drugs are available: albendazole (15 mg/kg/24 hr divided bid PO for 28 days; maximum: 800 mg/24 hr) taken with a fatty meal to improve absorption and praziquantel (50–100 mg/kg/24 hr divided tid PO for 30 days). Several studies indicate that albendazole produces a somewhat better outcome than praziquantel. A worsening of symptoms can follow the use of either drug as the host responds to the dying parasite with increased inflammation. Corticosteroids for 2–3 days before and during drug therapy can ameliorate these effects but may decrease praziquantel levels by as much as 50%. An increase of praziquantel (to 100 mg/kg/24 hr divided tid PO) or administration of cimetidine, an inhibitor of the cytochrome P450 system, has been advocated when both praziquantel and corticosteroids are used. Albendazole levels, in contrast, increase in the presence of corticosteroids.

Antiparasitic therapy may convert quiescent parenchymal lesions to active lesions or may worsen ventricular, spinal, or ocular disease. A ventricular shunt must be placed before medical therapy whenever there is evidence of hydrocephalus or ventricular or spinal disease. Surgery should be limited to placement of shunts, removal of large solitary cysts for decompression, removal of mobile cysts causing ventricular obstruction, and some cases that fail to respond to medical therapy. Neuroendoscopy may be used to remove some ventricular cysts. Spillage of cyst contents during surgery is not associated with dissemination of the parasite, in contrast with echinococcosis. Ocular cysticercosis is essentially a surgical disease, although there are reports of cure using medical therapy alone. The outcome is not good in most cases, and enucleation is frequently required. Most treatment options remain controversial and expert consultation is recommended.

Prevention. All family members of index cases of cysticercosis, as well as persons handling their food, should be examined for signs of disease or evidence of adult worms. Attention to personal hygiene, proper handwashing by food handlers, and avoidance of fresh fruits and vegetables in areas endemic for *T. solium* help prevent ingestion of eggs. All pork should be cooked thoroughly.

Carpio A, Escobar A, Hauser WA: Cysticercosis and epilepsy: A critical review. *Epilepsia* 1998;39:1025–40.

Garcia HH, Del Brutto OH: *Taenia solium* cysticercosis. *Infect Dis Clin North Am* 2000; 14:97–119.

Monteiro L, Nunes B, Mendonca D, et al: Spectrum of epilepsy in neurocysticercosis: A long-term follow-up of 143 patients. *Acta Neurol Scand* 1995;92: 33–40.

Singhi P, Ray M, Singhi S, et al: Clinical spectrum of 500 children with neurocysticercosis and response to albendazole therapy. *J Child Neurol* 2000;15: 207–13.

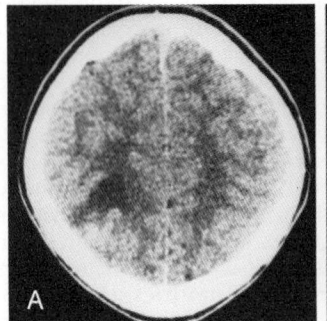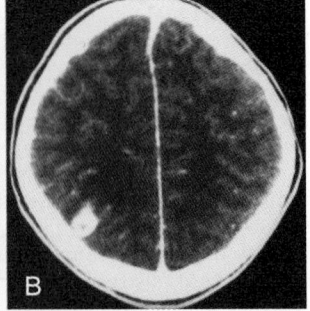

FIGURE 280–1. CT image of a solitary lesion of neurocysticercosis with *(A)* and without *(B)* contrast, showing contrast enhancement. (Courtesy of Dr. Wendy G. Mitchell and Dr. Marvin D. Nelson, Children's Hospital, Los Angeles.)

Echinococcosis (*Echinococcus granulosus* and *E. multilocularis*)

Ronald Blanton

Etiology. Echinococcosis (**hydatid disease** or **hydatidosis**) is the most widespread, serious human cestode infection in the world. It is a zoonosis that is transmitted from domestic and wild members of the canine family. Two major *Echinococcus* species are responsible for distinct clinical presentations, *E. granulosus* (**unilocular** or **cystic hydatid disease**) and the more malignant *E. multilocularis* (**alveolar hydatid disease**). Dogs, wolves, dingoes, jackals, coyotes, and foxes become infected after eating infected viscera and are the hosts of the small adult worms (2–7 mm). The adult worms are composed of 2–6 proglottids and have a life span of about 5 mo. Eggs from adult worms are passed in stool and contaminate the soil and water, as well as the coats of dogs themselves.

Domestic animals such as sheep, goats, cattle, and camels ingest *E. granulosus* eggs while grazing. Humans are infected with the intermediate stage of the parasite by ingesting food or water contaminated with eggs or by direct contact with infected dogs. The intermediate forms penetrate the gut and are carried by the vascular or lymphatic systems to the liver, lungs, and less commonly to other tissues. A sylvatic cycle also exists for *E. granulosus* in a wolf/moose cycle in North America, but it is of less importance for transmission to humans. The transmission cycle of *E. multilocularis* is similar to that of *E. granulosus*, except that this species is mainly sylvatic and uses small rodents as its natural intermediate host. The rodents are consumed by foxes, their natural predators, and sometimes by dogs and cats.

Epidemiology. *E. granulosus* thrives in environments as diverse as arctic tundra and the deserts of North Africa. There is potential for transmission of this parasite to humans wherever animals are herded by humans with the help of dogs. In urban areas, dogs may be infected by eating entrails after home slaughter of domestic animals. Cysts have been detected in up to 10% of the human population in northern Kenya and Western China. In South America, the disease is prevalent in sheep-herding areas of the Andes, the beef-herding areas of the Brazilian/Argentine Pampas, and Uruguay. Among developed countries, the disease is recognized in Italy, Greece, Portugal, Spain, and Australia. In North America, transmission occurs by way of the sylvatic cycle in Alaska, Canada, and Isle Royale on Lake Superior, as well as in foci of the domestic cycle in sheep-raising areas of the western United States.

Transmission of *E. multilocularis* occurs primarily in temperate climates of Northern Europe, Siberia, Turkey, and China. There is also an extensive area of transmission in Alaska, Canada, and the central United States as far south as Nebraska. Alveolar echinococcosis is, fortunately, uncommon. A separate species, *E. vogeli*, causes polycystic disease similar to alveolar hydatidosis in South America.

Pathogenesis. In areas endemic for *E. granulosus*, the parasite is often acquired in childhood, but liver cysts require many years to become large enough to detect or cause symptoms. In children, the lungs appear to be the most common site, whereas 70% of adults have disease in the right lobe of the liver. Cysts can also develop in bone, the genitourinary system, bowels, subcutaneous tissues, and brain. The host surrounds the primary cyst with a tough, fibrous capsule. Inside this capsule, the

parasite produces a thick lamellar layer that supports a thin germinal layer of cells responsible for production of thousands of juvenile-stage parasites (protoscolices) that remain attached to the wall or float free in the cyst fluid. With cystic hydatidosis from *E. granulosus* infection, the established cyst may also produce smaller daughter cysts that remain contained within the primary cysts. The fluid in a healthy cyst is clear and watery. After medical treatment, it may become thick and bile stained.

Active infection with *E. multilocularis* resembles a malignancy. The secondary reproductive units bud externally and are not confined within a single well-defined structure. Furthermore, the cyst tissues are poorly demarcated from those of the host, which makes these cysts unsuitable for surgical removal. The secondary cysts are also capable of distant metastatic spread of the parasite. The growing cyst mass eventually replaces a significant portion of the liver and compromises adjacent tissues and structures.

Clinical Manifestations. The majority of cysts occur in the liver. Many cysts never become symptomatic and regress spontaneously. Those that become symptomatic initially have relatively nonspecific symptoms. Later, increased abdominal girth, hepatomegaly, a palpable mass, vomiting, or abdominal pain ensues. The more serious complications, however, result from compression of adjacent structures, spillage of cyst contents, and location of cysts in sensitive areas such as the reproductive tract, brain, and bone. Anaphylaxis can occur with cyst rupture or spillage of cyst fluid intraoperatively. Spillage can be catastrophic, in that each protoscolex can form a new cyst. Jaundice due to cystic hydatid disease is rare. The second most common site is the lung, where cysts produce chest pain, coughing, or hemoptysis. Bone cysts may cause pathologic fractures, and in the genitourinary system they can produce hematuria or infertility.

In alveolar hydatid disease, cyst tissue continues to proliferate and may separate and metastasize distantly. The proliferating mass compromises hepatic tissue or the biliary system and causes progressive obstructive jaundice and hepatic failure. Symptoms also occur from expansion of extrahepatic foci.

Diagnosis. On physical examination, subcutaneous nodules, hepatomegaly, or a palpable abdominal mass may be found. The parasite cannot be recovered from any easily accessible body fluid unless a lung cyst ruptures, after which protoscolices may briefly be seen in sputum. Ultrasonography has proved a very valuable tool in the diagnosis of hydatid disease. Portable machines and generators have made office diagnosis or survey of even isolated populations possible. Benign, simple cysts of the liver are relatively common, but the presence of internal membranes and floating echogenic cyst material (hydatid sand) strongly suggests hydatid disease. Alveolar disease is less cystic in appearance and resembles a diffuse solid tumor. CT findings (Fig. 281–1) are similar to those of ultrasonography and can at times be useful in distinguishing alveolar from cystic hydatid disease in geographic regions where both occur.

Serologic studies can be useful in confirming a diagnosis of echinococcosis, but the false-negative rate may be as high as 50% in cystic hydatid disease of the lungs or when only young, intact liver cysts are present. Most patients with alveolar hydatidosis, however, develop detectable antibody responses. Current tests use crude or partially purified antigens that can cross react in individuals infected with other parasites, such as in cysticercosis or schistosomiasis.

DIFFERENTIAL DIAGNOSIS. Cystic hydatid disease can usually be distinguished from benign hepatic cysts on ultrasonography by the presence of either internal structures or hydatid sand. The density of bacterial hepatic abscesses is distinct from the watery cystic fluid characteristic of *E. granulosus* infection, but hydatid cysts may be complicated by secondary bacterial infection. Alveolar echinococcosis is often confused

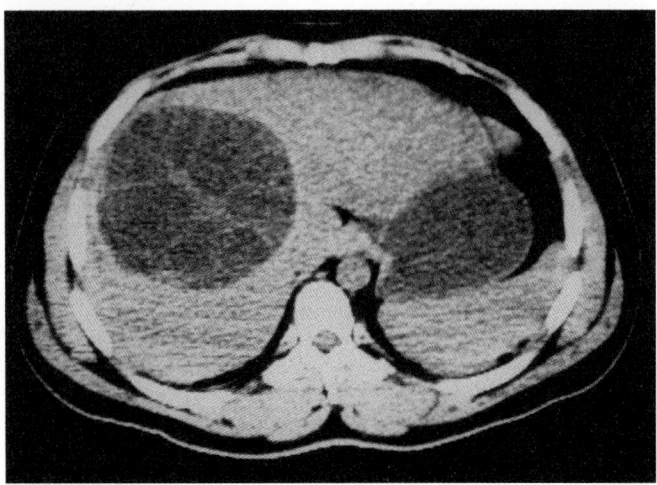

FIGURE 281–1. CT image of a hepatic *Echinococcus granulosus* hydatid cyst. The membranes of multiple internal daughter cysts are visible within the primary cyst structure. (Courtesy of Dr. John R. Haaga, University Hospitals, Cleveland, Ohio.)

with hepatoma and cirrhosis and presents features suggestive of pancreatic carcinoma, metastatic liver disease, and cholangitis.

Treatment. Hydatidosis is still primarily a surgical disease. For *E. granulosus* disease, open surgical procedures are rapidly being replaced by ultrasound- or CT-guided *p*ercutaneous *a*spiration, *i*nstillation of hypertonic saline or another scolicidal agent, and *r*easpiration (PAIR) after 15 min. Spillage with PAIR is surprisingly uncommon, but prophylactic albendazole therapy is recommended. At present, PAIR is appropriate for small simple cysts of the liver, but larger more complicated cysts, lung cysts, and renal cysts have been successfully treated. Cysts found to have bile-stained fluid should not be injected with a scolicidal agent because toxicity is increased.

For conventional surgery, the inner cyst wall (laminate and germinal layers) can be easily peeled from the fibrous layer, and only these inner layers need be removed. The cavity is then topically sterilized and either closed or filled with omentum. Considerable care must be taken to avoid spillage of cyst contents, because cyst fluid contains viable protoscolices, each capable of producing secondary cysts wherever it lodges. An additional risk

is development of anaphylaxis to spilled cyst fluid as a result of surgery, spontaneous rupture, or trauma.

For *E. granulosus* cysts not amenable to PAIR or surgery, albendazole (15 mg/kg/24 hr divided bid PO for 1–6 mo; maximum: 800 mg/24 hr) is the preferred drug for treatment. A positive response occurs in 40–60% of patients. There are few adverse effects except for occasional mild gastrointestinal disturbance and elevated transaminases on prolonged use. Morbid inflammatory response to chemotherapy is not common, as it is in cysticercosis, and corticosteroids thus are not indicated unless patients have anaphylaxis or another allergic response. Ultrasonographic indications of successful therapy are a change in shape from spherical to elliptic or flat, progressive increase in echogenicity, and detachment of membranes from the capsule (water lily sign). Additional CT criteria are reduction in diameter and augmented density of cyst fluid up to that of other tissues.

Alveolar hydatidosis is frequently incurable by any modality, but radical surgery such as partial hepatectomy or lobectomy may cure early limited disease. Medical therapy with albendazole may slow the progression of alveolar hydatidosis, but if at all feasible, removal of the infected tissue is indicated.

Prognosis. Factors predictive of success with chemotherapy are age of the cyst (<2 yr), low internal complexity of the cyst, and small size. The site of the cyst is not important, although cysts in bone respond poorly. For alveolar hydatidosis, if surgical removal is successful, the average mortality is 92% by 10 yr after diagnosis.

Prevention. Important measures to interrupt transmission include, above all, thorough handwashing, avoiding contact with dogs in endemic areas, boiling or filtering water when camping, proper disposal of animal carcasses, and proper meat inspection. Strict procedures for proper disposal of refuse from slaughterhouses must be instituted and followed so that dogs or wild carnivores do not have access to entrails. Other useful measures are control or treatment of the feral dog population and regular praziquantel treatment of pets and working dogs in endemic areas.

Akhan O, Ozmen MN: Percutaneous treatment of liver hydatid cysts. *Eur J Radiol* 1999;32:76–85.
Kammerer WS, Schantz PM: Echinococcal disease. *Infect Dis Clin North Am* 1993;7: 605–18.
Khuroo MS, Wani NA, Javid G, et al: Percutaneous drainage compared with surgery for hepatic hydatid cysts. *N Engl J Med* 1997;337:881–7.
Venkatesan P: Albendazole. *J Antimicrob Chemother* 1998;41:145–7.
WHO Working Group on Echinococcosis: Guidelines for treatment of cystic and alveolar echinococcosis in humans. *Bull World Health Org* 1996;74: 231–42.

SECTION 14 *Preventive Measures*

Chapter 282
Immunization Practices

Georges Peter

Immunization is a remarkably successful and very cost-effective means of preventing infectious diseases and is one of the leading achievements of public health and pediatrics. As a result of routine childhood immunizations, the occurrence of once common contagious diseases declined markedly in the United States and

other countries in the second half of the 20th century. Public health programs based on vaccination have led to global eradication of smallpox, elimination of wild-type polioviruses from the Americas and likely from the world in the near future, and more than 95% reduction in the United States of invasive *Haemophilus influenzae* type b (Hib) disease. In addition, congenital rubella syndrome, tetanus, and diphtheria have been nearly eliminated and the incidence of rubella and measles has been reduced to record low rates in the United States.

Infants and children in the United States routinely receive vaccines against 11 diseases: diphtheria, tetanus, pertussis, poliomyelitis, measles, mumps, rubella, Hib infection, pneumococcal infection, hepatitis B, and varicella. Hepatitis A and influenza vaccines are recommended for some groups of children.

DEFINITIONS AND GENERAL CONCEPTS

Vaccination is administration of any vaccine or **toxoid** (inactivated toxin) for prevention of disease. **Immunization** is the process of inducing immunity artificially by either vaccination **(active immunization)** or administration of antibody **(passive immunization)**. Active immunization involves stimulating the immune system to produce antibodies and cellular immune responses that protect against the infectious agent. Passive immunization provides temporary protection through administration of exogenously produced antibody, such as immune globulin. Passive immunization also occurs naturally through transplacental transmission of antibodies to a fetus, which provides protection against many infectious diseases for the first several months of the infant's life.

Immunizing agents include vaccines, toxoids, antitoxins, and immune globulins derived from human or animal donors (Table 282–1); more than 50 immunobiologic products are licensed in the United States. Immune globulins for passive immunization now can be prepared from monoclonally produced antibody. Most immunizing agents contain preservatives, stabilizers, antibiotics, adjuvants, and a suspending fluid (Table 282–2).

The current approaches to active immunization are the use of (1) live-attenuated infectious agents and (2) inactivated or detoxified agents, their extracts, or specific recombinant products (e.g., hepatitis B vaccine). For many diseases, such as poliomyelitis and typhoid fever, both approaches have been used. Live-attenuated vaccines are more likely than killed vaccines to induce an immunologic response simulating the response to natural infection. Inactivated or killed vaccines include inactivated whole organisms (e.g., whole-cell pertussis and hepatitis A vaccines), detoxified exotoxins (e.g., tetanus and diphtheria toxoids), purified protein antigens (e.g., acellular pertussis and hepatitis B vaccines), polysaccharides (e.g., capsular meningococcal vaccine), capsular polysaccharides conjugated to carrier proteins (e.g., Hib and pneumococcal conjugate vaccines), and components of the organism (e.g., subunit influenza vaccine).

Organisms in live vaccines multiply in the recipient until the desired immune response occurs, similar to that which occurs in natural infection. Thus, live-attenuated viral vaccines (e.g., measles, rubella, and mumps) are likely to confer lifelong protection with a single immunizing dose. In contrast, many inactivated or killed vaccines, which have a lesser antigenic mass, require booster vaccinations to provide protection.

Determinants of the Immune Response. Responses of individuals to the same vaccine vary because the immune response to specific

TABLE 282–1. Immunizing Agents

Agent	Definition
Vaccine	A preparation of proteins, polysaccharides, or nucleic acids of pathogens that are delivered to the immune system as single entities, as part of complex particles, or by live-attenuated agents or vectors, to induce specific responses that inactivate, destroy, or suppress the pathogen
Toxoid	A modified bacterial toxin that has been made nontoxic but retains the capacity to stimulate the formation of antitoxin
Immune globulin	An antibody-containing solution derived from human blood obtained by cold ethanol fractionation of large pools of plasma and used primarily for the maintenance of immunity of immunodeficient persons or for passive immunization; available in intramuscular and intravenous preparations
Antitoxin	An antibody derived from the serum of humans or animals after stimulation with specific antigens; used to provide passive immunity

TABLE 282–2. Constituents of Vaccines

Component	Use and Examples
Preservatives, stabilizers, antibiotics	Constituents can inhibit or prevent bacterial growth or stabilize the antigen. Materials such as mercurials or antibiotics are used. Allergic reactions to any of the additives may occur.
Adjuvants	An aluminum salt is used in some vaccines to enhance the immune response (e.g., toxoids, hepatitis B).
Suspending fluid	Sterile water, saline, or more complex fluids derived from the growing media or biologic system in which the agent is produced (e.g., egg antigens, cell culture ingredients, serum proteins).

antigens is genetically determined. The extensive polymorphism of the major histocompatibility complex (MHC) in humans results in recognition by different individuals of different epitopes within a complex protein antigen. To vaccinate a population effectively, a vaccine must contain epitopes that are processed and bound to the product of at least one MHC allele in most individuals.

The nature and magnitude of the response to vaccines or toxoids are determined by many factors, including the chemical and physical state of the antigen, the mode of administration, the catabolic rate of the antigen, host factors (e.g., age, nutrition, gender, and pre-existing antibody), and antigen processing as well as the genetic determinants of the host. The age-dependent differences in immune responses are a critically important consideration in the routine immunization schedule of infants and young children. The presence of high concentrations of maternal antibody in the first few months of life and the relative immaturity of the immune response impair the initial immune response to some vaccines.

The route of administration is another important factor in the immune response. Parenterally administered vaccines may not induce mucosal secretory IgA, whereas vaccines given orally are likely to do so. The immunogenicity of some vaccines is reduced when not given by the proper route. For example, subcutaneous administration of hepatitis B vaccine into the fatty tissue of the buttock of adults rather than intramuscularly in the deltoid results in substantially lower seroconversion rates.

Immune Response to Vaccine Antigens. Antibodies produced in response to vaccine constituents may be of any immunoglobulin class. Important protective antibodies include those that inactivate soluble toxic protein products of bacteria (i.e., antitoxins), facilitate phagocytosis and intracellular digestion of bacteria (i.e., opsonins), interact with components of serum complement to damage the bacterial membrane with resultant bacteriolysis (i.e., lysins), prevent proliferation of infectious virus (i.e., neutralizing antibodies), and interact with components of the bacterial surface to prevent adhesion to mucosal surfaces (i.e., antiadhesins). Antibodies function alone or in conjunction with other components of the immune system by participating directly in the neutralization of a toxin (e.g., diphtheria); opsonization of virus (e.g., poliovirus); initiating or combining with complement and promoting phagocytosis (e.g., pneumococcus); reacting with nonsensitized lymphocytes to stimulate phagocytosis; or sensitizing macrophages to stimulate phagocytosis.

Many of the structural constituents of microorganisms and exotoxins are antigenic. Most antigens require the interaction of B lymphocytes and T lymphocytes to generate an immune response and, thus, are termed T (thymus)-dependent antigens. However, some antigens initiate B-cell proliferation and antibody production without the help of T cells and, thus, are T-independent antigens. In contrast to T-dependent antigens, most T-independent antigens are poor immunogens in children younger than 2 yr of age. Because many purified polysaccharides are T-independent antigens, vaccines composed of these antigens are often ineffective in infants and young children. Examples include the first generation of Hib and pneumococcal vaccines. By conjugation to a protein carrier, however, a polysaccharide can acquire the antigenic properties of the protein and resulting characteristics of a T-dependent antigen, including immunogenicity in infants. This phenomenon is the basis of the development of Hib and pneumococcal conjugate vaccines. Meningococcal conjugate vaccines also have been developed and are now available in several countries, including Great Britain and Canada.

Induction of a T-dependent antibody response initially requires activation of T-helper (CD4) lymphocytes by presentation of an antigen to mononuclear phagocytes or dendritic cells, a process that may be facilitated by an adjuvant. Antigen presentation triggers the secretion of a cascade of mediators, called cytokines, which stimulate the maturation of naive T-helper cells and communication between leukocytes, using interleukins to regulate the immune response.

In the primary response to a vaccine antigen, a latent period of several days elapses before humoral and cell-mediated immunity can be detected. Serum antibodies initially are detected usually 7–10 days or more after vaccination. The immunoglobulin class of the response evolves and varies with the type of antigen. The initial antibodies are usually IgM; subsequent antibodies are usually IgG. The early IgM and IgG antibodies are secreted by B lymphocytes in response to T-dependent antigens. IgM antibodies are detectable first and fix complement, which facilitates lysis and phagocytosis of microorganisms. The IgM titer diminishes and the IgG titer rises during the 2nd wk or later. IgG responses peak within 2–6 wk. The change from IgM synthesis to predominately IgG synthesis in B lymphocytes requires T-lymphocyte cooperation. IgG antibodies are produced in high concentrations and are critical to resistance to infections. Their functions include affinity to microorganisms, viral neutralization, precipitation of antigens, and fixation of complement.

Live-virus vaccines given orally (e.g., oral poliovirus and investigational influenza) replicate at mucosal surfaces before host invasion and induce secretory IgA at respiratory, gastrointestinal, and other local sites. IgA antibodies neutralize viruses efficiently, fix complement through the alternative pathway, prevent absorption of organisms to the intestinal wall, and lyse gram-negative bacteria with complement and lysozyme. Most other types of vaccines do not effectively induce secretory IgA antibodies.

Heightened humoral or cell-mediated responses are elicited by a second exposure to the same T-dependent antigen. Secondary responses occur rapidly and usually within 4–5 days, result from immunologic memory mediated by T and B lymphocytes, and are characterized by a marked proliferation of antibody-producing B lymphocytes or effector T lymphocytes. However, T-independent antigens such as purified polysaccharide vaccines do not evoke these heightened secondary immune responses.

The response to vaccines in clinical practice is assessed by the serum concentration of specific antibody. The presence of circulating antibodies usually correlates with protection, and for some vaccines (e.g., tetanus, diphtheria, and Hib) the specific antibody titers that correlate with protection have been established. However, antibody seroconversion and concentrations are only one parameter of the host response. Cellular immunity also is important but is much more difficult to measure and to correlate with protection. Amnestic responses on revaccination, which indicate immunologic memory, suggest that immunity may be persistent. Accordingly, the lack of detectable serum antibody may not mean that the individual is unprotected, particularly with infections that have a long incubation period, such as hepatitis B.

Stimulation of the immune system by vaccination, independent of antibody production, may elicit unanticipated responses, especially hypersensitivity reactions. For example, killed measles vaccine induced incomplete humoral immunity and cell-mediated hypersensitivity, resulting in the development of a syndrome of atypical measles (see Chapter 225) in some children after subsequent infection by wild-type virus.

VACCINE RECOMMENDATIONS

Many factors are considered in the development of recommendations and schedules for vaccine administrations, including the epidemiology of the disease, age-specific morbidity and mortality, vaccine immunogenicity, risks of vaccine-related adverse reactions, cost effectiveness, and the ages of recommended routine health care visits. In general, vaccines for universal administration to children are recommended at the youngest age at which significant risk of disease and its complications exist and at which a protective immunologic response can be expected. Other vaccines are recommended only in special circumstances, such as for children at increased risk for infection during foreign travel (e.g., typhoid vaccine), those at increased risk of severe infections (e.g., pneumococcal polysaccharide vaccine for children with sickle cell disease), and those after exposure (e.g., rabies vaccine in children bitten by a potentially rabid animal).

In the United States, recommendations for childhood immunization are formulated by two committees, the Advisory Committee on Immunization Practices (ACIP) of the Centers for Disease Control and Prevention (CDC) and the American Academy of Pediatrics (AAP) Committee on Infectious Diseases. These two committees and the American Academy of Family Physicians (AAFP) issue an annual national schedule for routinely recommended childhood vaccinations.

Vaccines for Routine Use in Children and Adolescents. All children should be vaccinated against diphtheria, tetanus, pertussis, poliomyelitis, measles, mumps, rubella, Hib, *Streptococcus pneumoniae*, hepatitis B, and varicella unless contraindicated (Fig. 282–1). As of 2002, completion of this schedule by 18 mo of age necessitates 16–20 injections in four to five visits. However, introduction of new combination vaccine is anticipated in the near future and will reduce the number of injections for routine vaccine administration.

The first dose of hepatitis must be given at birth to infants of hepatitis B surface antigen (HBsAg)-positive mothers for optimal prevention of maternal-fetal viral transmission (see Chapter 339). All infants should receive the first dose soon after birth and before hospital discharge, but it also may be given in the first 2 mo of life if the mother is HBsAg negative.

For poliomyelitis immunization in the United States, inactivated poliovirus vaccine (IPV) now is recommended to eliminate the risk of vaccine-associated paralytic poliomyelitis associated with oral poliovirus vaccine (OPV). The recommended regimen for IPV, which is the same as that for OPV, is 2, 4, and 6–18 mo and 4–6 yr of age. OPV, if available, is indicated for unvaccinated children who will be traveling within 4 wk to areas where polio is endemic. OPV remains the vaccine of choice for global eradication of poliomyelitis and is recommended for areas with continued or recent circulation of wild-type poliovirus, most developing countries because of its lower cost than IPV, and areas with inadequate sanitation that necessitate an optimal mucosal barrier to wild-type virus circulation.

Acellular pertussis vaccine, combined with diphtheria and tetanus toxoids (DTaP), is now the recommended vaccine for pertussis immunization in the United States and many countries in Europe. Whole-cell pertussis vaccine, although no longer available in the United States, is still routinely given in many areas, including the United Kingdom and developing countries. After the 7th birthday, combined tetanus and diphtheria toxoids in the adult formulation (Td), which contains a lesser amount of diphtheria toxoid, are recommended for both primary and booster

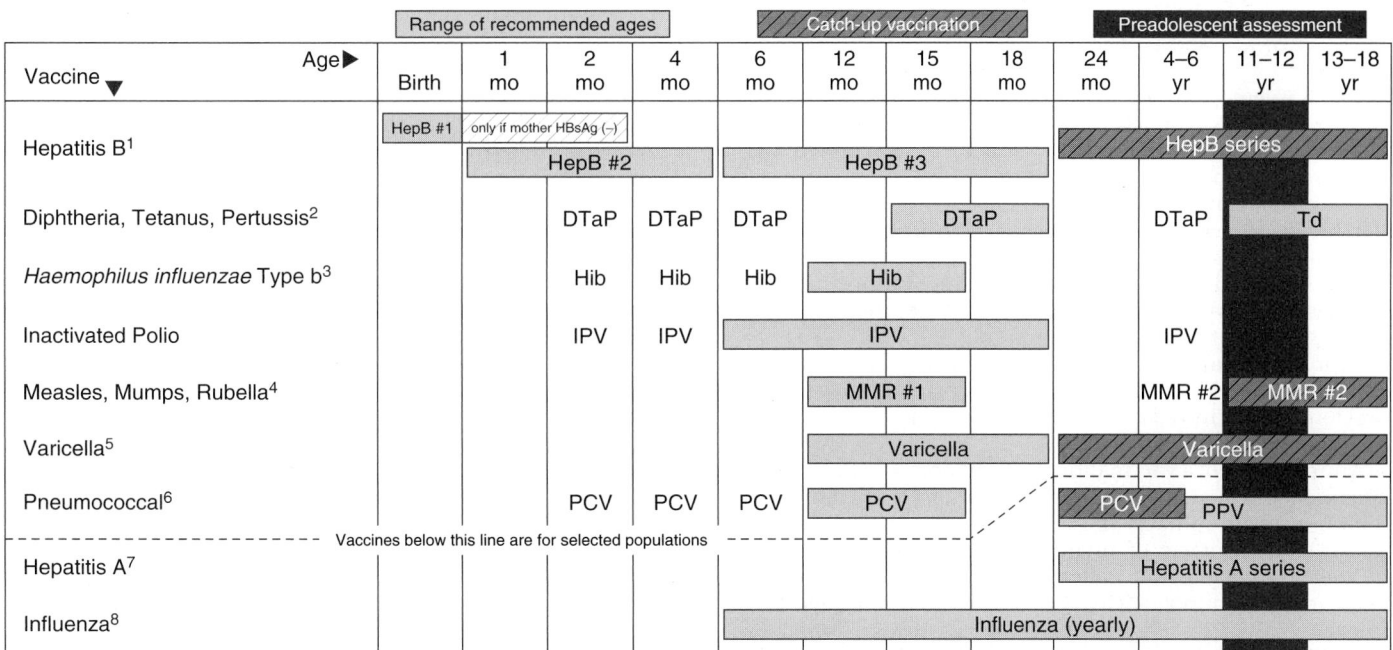

FIGURE 282–1. Recommended childhood and adolescent immunization schedule, United States, 2003.

---

[1]**Hepatitis B vaccine (HepB).** All infants should receive the first dose of hepatitis B vaccine soon after birth and before hospital discharge; the first dose may also be given by age 2 mo if the infant's mother is HBsAg-negative. Only monovalent HepB can be used for the birth dose. Monovalent or combination vaccine containing HepB may be used to complete the series. Four doses of vaccine may be administered when a birth dose is given. The second dose should be given at least 4 wk after the first dose, except for combination vaccines which cannot be administered before age 6 wk. The third dose should be given at least 16 wk after the first dose and at least 8 wk after the second dose. The last dose in the vaccination series (third or fourth dose) should not be administered before age 6 mo.

Infants born to HBsAg-positive mothers should receive HepB and 0.5 mL Hepatitis B Immune Globulin (HBIG) within 12 hr of birth at separate sites. The second dose is recommended at age 1–2 mo. The last dose in the vaccination series should not be administered before age 6 mo. These infants should be tested for HBsAg and anti-HBs at 9–15 mo of age.

Infants born to mothers whose HBsAg status is unknown should receive the first dose of the HepB series within 12 hr of birth. Maternal blood should be drawn as soon as possible to determine the mother's HBsAg status; if the HBsAg test is positive, the infant should receive HBIG as soon as possible (no later than age 1 wk). The second dose is recommended at age 1–2 mo. The last dose in the vaccination series should not be administered before age 6 mo.

[2]**Diphtheria and tetanus toxoids and acellular pertussis vaccine (DTaP).** The fourth dose of DTaP may be administered as early as age 12 mo, provided 6 mo have elapsed since the third dose and the child is unlikely to return at age 15–18 mo. **Tetanus and diphtheria toxoids (Td)** is recommended at age 11–12 yr if at least 5 yr have elapsed since the last dose of tetanus and diphtheria toxoid-containing vaccine. Subsequent routine Td boosters are recommended every 10 yr.

[3]*Haemophilus influenzae* **type b (Hib) conjugate vaccine.** Three Hib conjugate vaccines are licensed for infant use. If PRP-OMP (PedvaxHIB® or ComVax® [Merck]) is administered at ages 2 and 4 mo, a dose at age 6 mo is not required. DTaP/Hib combination products should not be used for primary immunization in infants at ages 2, 4 or 6 mo, but can be used as boosters following any Hib vaccine.

[4]**Measles, mumps, and rubella vaccine (MMR).** The second dose of MMR is recommended routinely at age 4–6 yr but may be administered during any visit, provided at least 4 wk have elapsed since the first dose and that both doses are administered beginning at or after age 12 mo. Those who have not previously received the second dose should complete the schedule by the 11–12 year old visit.

[5]**Varicella vaccine.** Varicella vaccine is recommended at any visit at or after age 12 mo for susceptible children, i.e., those who lack a reliable history of chickenpox. Susceptible persons aged ≥13 yr should receive two doses, given at least 4 wk apart.

[6]**Pneumococcal vaccine.** The heptavalent **pneumococcal conjugate vaccine (PCV)** is recommended for all children age 2–23 mo. It is also recommended for certain children age 24–59 mo. **Pneumococcal polysaccharide vaccine (PPV)** is recommended in addition to PCV for certain high-risk groups. See *MMWR* 2000;49(RR-9);1–38.

[7]**Hepatitis A vaccine.** Hepatitis A vaccine is recommended for children and adolescents in selected states and regions, and for certain high-risk groups; consult your local public health authority. Children and adolescents in these states, regions, and high-risk groups who have not been immunized against hepatitis A can begin the hepatitis A vaccination series during any visit. The two doses in the series should be administered at least 6 months apart. See *MMWR* 1999;48(RR-12);1–37.

[8]**Influenza vaccine.** Influenza vaccine is recommended annually for children age ≥6 mo with certain risk factors (including but not limited to asthma, cardiac disease, sickle cell disease, HIV, diabetes, and household members of persons in groups at high risk; see *MMWR* 2002;51(RR-3);1–31), and can be administered to all others wishing to obtain immunity. In addition, healthy children age 6–23 mo are encouraged to receive influenza vaccine if feasible because children in this age group are at substantially increased risk for influenza-related hospitalizations. Children aged ≤12 yr should receive vaccine in a dosage appropriate for their age (0.25 mL if age 6–35 mo or 0.5 mL if aged ≥3 yr). Children aged ≤8 yr who are receiving influenza vaccine for the first time should receive two doses separated by at least 4 wk.

This immunization schedule is updated annually. The current recommended schedule is available at www.nelsonpediatrics.com. For additional information about vaccines, including precautions and contraindications for immunization and vaccine shortages, please visit the National Immunization Program Website at *www.cdc.gov/nip* or call the National Immunization Information Hotline at 800-232-2522 (English) or 800-232-0233 (Spanish).

vaccination. The first booster dose of Td is recommended at 11–12 yr of age and is followed by boosters at 10-yr intervals thereafter.

The 7-valent pneumococcal polysaccharide-protein conjugate vaccine (PCV-7) is routinely recommended for all children 2–23 mo of age in a four-dose schedule at 2, 4, 6, and 12–15 months of age. It also is recommended for older children, 24–59 mo of age, at high risk of invasive pneumococcal infection, such as those with sickle cell disease, asplenia, or HIV infection who have not previously been immunized.

The second dose of measles-containing vaccine (given as measles-mumps-rubella [MMR]) should be routinely given before school entry at 4–6 yr of age.

Varicella vaccine is recommended beginning at 12 mo of age and for older children through 12 yr of age if they have not been previously immunized or if they lack a reliable history of chickenpox.

Annual influenza vaccination of all children 6–23 mo of age is encouraged, when feasible. Vaccination also is encouraged for their household contacts and out-of-home caretakers, and particularly for contacts of infants younger than 6 mo of age. Influenza vaccine is not indicated for these infants because of inadequate immunogenicity. Children 0–23 mo of age are at substantially increased risk for influenza-related hospitalizations. Routine influenza immunization of all young children may be recommended in the near future.

Hepatitis A vaccine is recommended at 24 mo of age in states and regions with an increased incidence of disease. A second dose is administered 6–12 mo later to complete the series.

To enhance the delivery of vaccines to adolescents, a routine visit at 11–12 yr of age has been established for administration of the first Td booster and, if not already immunized, for hepatitis B and varicella vaccination and the second dose of MMR if not previously administered.

Simultaneous Administration of Multiple Vaccines. Most vaccines can be given simultaneously without impairment of effectiveness or safety. Simultaneous administration of vaccines is particularly important for inadequately immunized children to ensure timely completion of the recommended schedule. New combination products facilitate administration of multiple vaccines by reducing the number of necessary injections.

Interchangeability of Vaccine Products. Vaccines made by different manufacturers but directed against the same infections are generally considered interchangeable for the primary series and recommended booster doses. Because data are limited on the safety, immunogenicity, and efficacy of different DTaP vaccines, the same product should be used, whenever feasible, in the pertussis vaccination schedule. However, in circumstances in which the specific DTaP product received previously is not known or the previously administered product is not readily available, any licensed product may be used. Vaccination should not be deferred in these situations.

Lapsed Immunizations. In general, intervals between vaccine doses that exceed those that are recommended do not adversely affect the immunologic response, provided the immunization series is completed. Hence, restarting the immunization series or giving additional doses is not indicated under these circumstances.

Vaccines with Selective Indications. Vaccines with selected indications for children include influenza, pneumococcal polysaccharide, hepatitis A, meningococcal polysaccharide, rabies, and those given primarily for international travel.

Influenza vaccine should be given annually in the fall to those children 6 mo of age or older who are at increased risk for severe influenza disease or its complications. Major risk factors are asthma and other chronic pulmonary diseases (e.g., cystic fibrosis), congenital heart disease, HIV infection, other immunosuppressive disorders and therapy, sickle cell disease, and aspirin

therapy. Vaccination also should be considered for children with diabetes mellitus, other chronic metabolic disorders, and chronic renal disease and for those traveling to foreign countries where influenza may be occurring.

Pneumococcal polysaccharide vaccine is a 23-valent formulation with limited but important indications for children with sickle cell disease, functional or anatomic asplenia, nephrotic syndrome, renal failure, HIV infection, or organ transplants. It is given in addition to routine PCV-7 immunization. Because the polysaccharide vaccine is composed of T-independent antigens, it is not given until 2 yr of age. A single revaccination is recommended 3–5 yr later if the child remains at increased risk of severe or frequent infections. For older children who were initially immunized 5 yr or more before, revaccination also is indicated.

Meningococcal polysaccharide quadrivalent vaccine is recommended for children 2 yr of age or older who are at increased risk of infection. Indications include functional or anatomic asplenia, terminal complement component or properdin deficiency, travel to geographic areas where disease is hyperendemic or epidemic, and for control of outbreaks as determined by public health officials. Vaccination also should be considered for students entering college, especially those students who will be living in dormitories. These students and their parents should be informed about the increased risk of meningococcal disease in college freshman living in dormitories and the potential benefits of immunization. Vaccine should be made available both by their physician and by college and university health services and may be required by some states. Other college students, although not at increased risk, also may be immunized if they desire.

International travel is a common indication for many vaccines that are not otherwise routinely given to children, because of increased risk of exposure to the diseases. For children living in North America, vaccines for travel may include hepatitis A, typhoid fever, meningococcal disease, yellow fever, and Japanese encephalitis, depending on the location and circumstances of the travel (see Chapter 285). In addition, children and adolescents before departure should have received all routinely recommended vaccines for their age. The risk of exposure to cases of measles may be substantial in some countries. Hence, the second dose of measles vaccine, given as MMR, should be given to children and adolescents who have received only one dose irrespective of age, provided an interval of 4 wk or more has elapsed since the first dose. Influenza vaccine should be considered for children traveling to areas where influenza outbreaks are occurring. Some countries may require yellow fever vaccination for entry.

ADVERSE EVENTS AFTER VACCINATION

Modern vaccines, although safe and effective, can be associated with adverse events ranging in severity from mild to life threatening. In addition, because no vaccine can be expected to be completely effective, some persons may develop disease after exposure despite vaccination.

Vaccine components can cause allergic reactions in some recipients. These components include the protective antigens, other components of the microorganisms, animal proteins introduced during vaccine production, antibiotics and other preservatives, or stabilizers such as gelatin. Reactions may be local or systemic, including anaphylaxis and urticaria. Local or systemic reactions result from too frequent administration of some vaccines, such as tetanus toxoids or rabies, and are probably caused by antigen-antibody complexes.

Some adverse events, however, occur coincidentally in temporal association with vaccination and are not caused by the vaccine. Determination of causality of an adverse event in a single child may be difficult. Epidemiologic and related studies are necessary to ascertain the incidence and nature of adverse reactions to vaccines and are important in ensuring a scientific rationale for vaccine recommendations. The decision to use a vaccine involves assessment of the risk of disease, the benefit of vaccination, and the risk associated with vaccination. Continued reassessment of vaccine indications and safety is necessary. Precautions and contraindications are based on these factors, which may be modified with new information. Physicians delivering vaccines should be knowledgeable about indications, vaccine risks, and parental and public misconceptions about alleged vaccine-related adverse events.

PRECAUTIONS AND CONTRAINDICATIONS

Knowledge of vaccine contraindications and precautions is an important aspect of immunization practice (Table 282–3). A pre-

caution specifies a circumstance in which a vaccine may be indicated if the benefit to an individual is judged to outweigh the risk and consequences of an adverse event. In contrast, a contraindication indicates that the vaccine should not be administered. Applying valid contraindications and precautions helps to minimize the occurrence of adverse reactions and maintain the health of children. Deciding not to vaccinate a child because of an inappropriate contraindication or precaution denies the child the benefit of immunization and is a missed opportunity for vaccination.

Generic contraindications to vaccination are an anaphylactic reaction to a previous dose of the same vaccine and an anaphylactic reaction to a vaccine constituent, such as egg proteins, gelatin, or an antibiotic. Viral vaccines that contain egg proteins, associated with vaccine production using embryonated chicken

TABLE 282–3. Guide to contraindications and precautions* to commonly used vaccines

Vaccine	True Contraindications and Precautions*	Untrue (Vaccines Can Be Administered)
General for all vaccines, including diphtheria and tetanus toxoids and acellular pertussis vaccine (DTaP); pediatric diphtheria-tetanus toxoid (DT); adult tetanus-diphtheria toxoid (Td); inactivated poliovirus vaccine (IPV); measles-mumps-rubella vaccine (MMR); *Haemophilus influenzae* type b vaccine (Hib); hepatitis A vaccine; hepatitis B vaccine; varicella vaccine; pneumococcal conjugate vaccine (PCV); influenza vaccine; and pneumococcal polysaccharide vaccine (PPV)	**Contraindications** Serious allergic reaction (e.g., anaphylaxis) after a previous vaccine dose Serious allergic reaction (e.g., anaphylaxis) to a vaccine component **Precautions** Moderate or severe acute illness with or without fever	Mild acute illness with or without fever Mild to moderate local reaction (i.e., swelling, redness, soreness); low-grade or moderate fever after previous dose Lack of previous physical examination in well-appearing person Current antimicrobial therapy Convalescent phase of illness Premature birth (hepatitis B vaccine is an exception in certain circumstances)[†] Recent exposure to an infections disease History of penicillin allergy, other nonvaccine allergies, relatives with allergies, receiving allergen extract immunotherapy
DTaP	**Contraindications** Severe allergic reaction after a previous dose or to a vaccine component Encephalopathy (e.g., coma, decreased level of consciousness; prolonged seizures) within 7 days of administration of previous dose of DTP or DTaP Progressive neurologic disorder, including infantile spasms, uncontrolled epilepsy, progressive encephalopathy: defer DTaP until neurologic status clarified and stabilized. **Precautions** Fever of >40.5˚C ≤48 hours after vaccination with a previous dose of DTP or DTaP Collapse or shock-like state (i.e., hypotonic hyporesponsive episode) ≤48 hours after receiving a previous dose of DTP/DTaP Seizure ≤3 days of receiving a previous dose of DTP/DTaP[§] Persistent, inconsolable crying lasting ≥3 and hours and ≤48 hours after receiving a previous dose of DTP/DTaP Moderate or severe acute illness with or without fever	Temperature of <40.5˚C, fussiness or mild drowsiness after a previous dose of diphtheria toxoid-tetanus toxoid-perfussis vaccine (DTP)/DTaP Family history of seizures[§] Family history of sudden infant death syndrome Family history of an adverse event after DTP or DTaP administration Stable neurologic conditions (e.g., cerebral palsy, well-controlled convulsions, developmental delay)
DT, Td	**Contraindications** Severe allergic reaction after a previous dose or to a vaccine component **Precautions** Guillain-Barré syndrome ≤6 weeks after previous dose of tetanus toxoid-containing vaccine Moderate or severe acute illness with or without fever	
IPV	**Contraindications** Severe allergic reaction to previous dose or vaccine component **Precautions** Pregnancy Moderate or severe acute illness with or without fever	—
MMR[¶]	**Contraindications** Severe allergic reaction after a previous dose or to a vaccine component Pregnancy Known severe immunodeficiency (e.g., hematologic and solid tumors; congenital immunodeficiency; long-term immunosuppressive therapy,** or severely symptomatic human immunodeficiency virus [HIV] infection) **Precautions** Recent (≤11 months) receipt of antibody-containing blood product (specific interval depends on product)[§§] History of thrombocytopenia or thrombocytopenic purpura Moderate or severe acute illness with or without fever	Positive tuberculin skin test Simultaneous TB skin testing[††] Breast-feeding Pregnancy of recipient's mother or other close or household contact Recipient is child-bearing–age female Immunodeficient family member or household contact Asymptomatic or mildly symptomatic HIV infection Allergy to eggs

Table continued on following page

TABLE 282–3. Guide to contraindications and precautions* to commonly used vaccines *Continued*

Vaccine	True Contraindications and Precautions*	Untrue (Vaccines Can Be Administered)
Hib	**Contraindications** Severe allergic reaction after a previous dose or to a vaccine component Age <6 weeks **Precaution** Moderate or severe acute illness with or without fever	—
Hepatitis B	**Contraindication** Severe allergic reaction after a previous dose or to a vaccine component **Precautions** Infant weighing <2,000 grams† Moderate or severe acute illness with or without fever	Pregnancy Autoimmune disease (e.g., systemic lupus erythematosis or rheumatoid arthritis)
Hepatitis A	**Contraindications** Severe allergic reaction after a previous dose or to a vaccine component **Precautions** Pregnancy Moderate or severe acute illness with or without fever	—
Varicella¶	**Contraindications** Severe allergic reaction after a previous dose or to a vaccine component Substantial supression of cellular immunity Pregnancy **Precautions** Recent (≤11 months) receipt of antibody-containing blood product (specific interval depends on product)§§ Moderate or severe acute illness with or without fever	Pregnancy of recipient's mother or other close or household contact Immunodeficient family member or household contact Asymptomatic or mildly symptomatic HIV infection Humoral immunodeficiency (e.g., agammaglobulinemia)
PCV	**Contraindication** Severe allergic reaction after a previous dose or to a vaccine component **Precaution** Moderate or severe acute illness with or without fever	—
Influenza	**Contraindication** Severe allergic reaction to previous dose or vaccine component, including egg protein **Precautions** Moderate or severe acute illness with or without fever	Nonsevere (e.g., contact) allergy to latex or thimeros Concurrent administration of coumadin or aminophyl line
PPV	**Contraindication** Severe allergic reaction after a previous dose or to a vaccine component **Precaution** Moderate or severe acute illness with or without fever	—

*Events or conditions listed as precautions should be reviewed carefully. Benefits and risks of administering a specific vaccine to a person under these circumstances should be considered. If the risk from the vaccine is believed to outweight the benefit, the vaccine should not be administered. If the benefit of vaccination is believed to outweigh the risk, the vaccine should be administered. Whether and when to administer DTaP to children with proven or suspected underlying neurologic disorders should be decided on a case-by-case basis.

†Hepatitis B vaccination should be deferred for infants weighing <2,000 grams if the mother is documented to be hepatitis B surface antigen (HBsAg)-negative at the time of the infant's birth. Vaccination can commence at chronological age 1 month. For infants born to HBsAg-positive women, hepatitis B immunoglobulin and hepatitis B vaccine should be administered at or soon after birth regardless of weight. See text for details.

§Acetaminophen or other appropriate antipyretic can be administered to children with a personal or family history of seizures at the time of DTaP vaccination and every 4–6 hours for 24 hours thereafter to reduce the possibility of postvaccination fever (Source: American Academy of Pediatrics. Active immunization. In: Pickering LK, ed. 2000 red book: report of the Committee on Infectious Diseases. 25th ed. Elk Grove Village, IL: American Academy of Pediatrics, 2000).

¶MMR and varicella vaccines can be administered on the same day. If not administered on the same day, these vaccines should be separated by ≥28 days.

**Substantially immunosuppressive steroid dose is considered to be ≥2 wk of daily receipt of 20 mg or 2 mg/kg body weight of prednisone or equivalent.

††Measles vaccination can suppress tuberculin reactivity temporarily. Measles-containing vaccine can be administered on the same day as tuberculin skin testing. If testing cannot be performed until after the day of MMR vaccination, the test should be postponed for ≥4 wk after the vaccination. If an urgent need exists to perform skin test, do so with the understanding that reactivity might be reduced by the vaccine.

§§See text for details.

¶¶If a vaccinee experiences a presumed vaccine-related rash 7–25 days after vaccination, avoid direct contact with immunocompromised persons for the duration of the rash.

From Centers for Disease Control and Prevention: General recommendations on immunization: Recommendations of the Advisory Committee on Immunization Practices (ACIP) and the American Academy of Family Physicians (AAFP). MMWR 2002; 51 (RR-2):1–35.

eggs or chicken embryo fibroblast tissue culture, include those for measles, mumps, influenza, and yellow fever. Measles and mumps vaccines, however, contain insignificant amounts of egg proteins, and persons with hypersensitivity to eggs are at negligible risk of anaphylactic reactions from these vaccines. As a result, skin testing with measles vaccine is not predictive of a subsequent allergic reaction to vaccination. Hypersensitivity reactions to MMR that were previously attributed to egg protein may have been caused by allergic reactions to the gelatin stabilizer in the vaccine.

A generic precaution is moderate or severe acute illness, regardless of the presence or absence of fever. A mild illness does

not impair the immunogenicity and safety of vaccines. Failure to vaccinate children with minor, acute illness is a missed opportunity and can seriously impede immunization delivery.

Administration of live-virus vaccines (e.g., MMR, OPV, and varicella) generally is contraindicated in immunocompromised persons, including recipients of high-dose corticosteroids. The exception is measles vaccine, which is recommended for HIV-infected persons who are not severely immunosuppressed (see Chapter 254).

Because of the theoretical risk to a developing fetus, live-virus vaccines in most cases are not recommended during pregnancy. However, inadvertent vaccination is not necessarily a reason for termination of pregnancy and some live-virus vaccines (e.g., OPV, influenza, and yellow fever) can be given to pregnant women. Influenza vaccine is specifically recommended for all pregnant women who will be in the 2nd or 3rd trimester (≥14 wk gestation) during the influenza season (late November through March) because of the increased morbidity of influenza in pregnant women.

In some recipients, vaccines can cause severe reactions that may constitute contraindications or precautions to subsequent administration of the specific vaccine. An example is the contraindication to further doses of DTP or DTaP if encephalopathy occurs within 7 days of administration of a previous dose of either DTP or DTaP. In contrast, a history of a temperature of 40.5°C or greater (≥105°F) within 48 hr of a prior dose is a precaution. In most cases in this circumstance, further doses of DTaP or DTP would not be given. However, if an epidemic of pertussis were occurring in the community, the potential benefit to the child of completing the immunization series may be greater than the risk of recurrence of a severe febrile reaction attributed to pertussis vaccine, the consequences of which are unknown.

VACCINES IN SPECIAL CIRCUMSTANCES

Indications for vaccination also involve considerations of the immunologic status of a child and exposure to infection. As a result, in special circumstances, immunization recommendations may be different from those for most other children.

Immunodeficiency. Recommendations for vaccination of immunocompromised persons vary according to the degree and cause of the immunodeficiency, risk of exposure to the disease, and the type of vaccine (Table 282–4). Specific recommendations for HIV-infected children are given in Figure 254–2. Live-bacteria (e.g., oral typhoid) and live-virus vaccines (e.g., MMR, varicella, and rotavirus) are contraindicated in most circumstances involving clinically significant immunosuppression. An exception is

TABLE 282–4. Recommendations for Immunization of Immunocompromised Infants and Children

Vaccine	Routine (not Immunocompromised)	HIV Infection/ AIDS	Severely Immunocompromised (Non–HIV Related)*†	Asplenia	Renal Failure	Diabetes
Routine Infant Immunizations						
DTaP (DT/T/Td)	Recommended	Recommended	Recommended	Recommended	Recommended	Recommended
Hepatitis B	Recommended	Recommended	Recommended	Recommended	Recommended	Recommended
Hib	Recommended	Recommended	Recommended	Recommended	Recommended	Recommended
IPV	Recommended	Recommended	Recommended	Recommended	Recommended	Recommended
MMR (MR/M/R)	Recommended	Recommended/Consider‡	**Contraindicated**	Recommended	Recommended	Recommended
Pneumococcal (PCV7)	Recommended	Recommended	Recommended	Recommended	Recommended	Recommended
Varicella	Recommended	Consider§	**See Note‖**	Recommended	Recommended	Recommended
Other Childhood Immunizations						
Hepatitis A	Use if indicated	Use if indicated	Use if indicated	Use if indicated	Use if indicated	Use if indicated
Influenza	Use if indicated	Recommended	Recommended	Recommended	Recommended	Recommended
Pneumococcal (PPV23)¶	Use if indicated	Recommended	Recommended	Recommended	Recommended	Recommended
Nonroutine Live Vaccines†						
BCG	Use if indicated	**Contraindicated**	**Contraindicated**	**Contraindicated**	**Contraindicated**	Use if indicated
Typhoid, Ty21a	Use if indicated	**Contraindicated**	**Contraindicated**	**Contraindicated**	**Contraindicated**	Use if indicated
Vaccinia	Use if indicated	**Contraindicated**	**Contraindicated**	**Contraindicated**	**Contraindicated**	Use if indicated
Yellow Fever**	Use if indicated	**Contraindicated**	**Contraindicated**	**Contraindicated**	**Contraindicated**	Use if indicated
Nonroutine Killed (Inactivated) Vaccines						
Anthrax	Use if indicated	Use if indicated	Use if indicated	Use if indicated	Use if indicated	Use if indicated
Plague	Use if indicated	Use if indicated	Use if indicated	Use if indicated	Use if indicated	Use if indicated
Rabies	Use if indicated	Use if indicated	Use if indicated	Use if indicated	Use if indicated	Use if indicated
Typhoid, inactivated	Use if indicated	Use if indicated	Use if indicated	Use if indicated	Use if indicated	Use if indicated

*Severe immunosuppression can be the result of congenital immunodeficiency, HIV infection, leukemia, lymphoma, aplastic anemia, generalized malignancy or therapy with alkylating agents, antimetabolites, radiation, or large amounts of corticosteroids.

†Live vaccines are contraindicated in solid organ transplant recipients and with chronic immunosuppressive therapy.

‡MMR vaccination is recommended for all **asymptomatic** HIV-infected persons who do not have evidence of severe immunosuppression for whom measles vaccination would otherwise be indicated. MMR vaccination should be considered for all **symptomatic** HIV-infected persons who do not have evidence of severe immunosuppression or of measles immunity (see Chapter 254).

§Two doses of varicella vaccine, administered 3 mo apart, should be considered for asymptomatic or mildly symptomatic HIV-infected children in CDC class N1 or A1 with age-specific T-cell percentages of ≥25%.

‖Varicella vaccine is not licensed for use in persons who have any malignant condition, including blood dyscrasias, leukemia, lymphomas of any type, or other malignant neoplasms affecting the bone marrow or lymphatic systems. Varicella vaccine should not be administered to persons who have cellular immunodeficiencies, but persons with impaired humoral immunity may be vaccinated. An investigational protocol exists for use of varicella vaccine in patients with acute lymphoblastic leukemia. Varicella vaccine should not be administered to persons who have a family history of congenital or hereditary immunodeficiency in first-degree relatives unless the immune competence of the potential vaccine recipient has been clinically substantiated or verified by a laboratory. Varicella vaccine should not be administered to persons receiving immunosuppressive therapy (except children who have ALL in remission, as noted above), including systemic corticosteroids, ≥2 mg/kg or 20 mg/day of prednisone or its equivalent.

¶Children who have completed the PCV7 vaccination series before age 2 yr and who are among risk groups for which PPV23 is already recommended should receive one dose of PPV23 at age 2 yr (≥2 mo after the last dose of PCV7). These groups at high risk include children with sickle cell disease, functional or anatomic asplenia, HIV infection, and immunocompromising or chronic diseases.

**Yellow fever vaccine should be considered for patients when exposure to yellow fever cannot be avoided.

Adapted from Centers for Disease Control and Prevention: Recommendations of the Advisory Committee on Immunization Practices (ACIP): Use of vaccines and immune globulino in persons with altered immunocompetence. MMWR Morbid Mortal Wkly Rop 1993;42(RR-4):1–18.

MMR and varicella vaccination of HIV-infected children who are not severely immunosuppressed (see Chapter 254). Children and adolescents with acute lymphocytic leukemia in remission can receive varicella vaccine under an investigational protocol provided appropriate institutional review board approval and informed consent have been obtained. The vaccine in this circumstance is available without cost from the manufacturer. OPV is contraindicated in households with immunocompromised persons because of a risk of vaccine-associated paralytic poliomyelitis.

Influenza and pneumococcal vaccines are indicated at the appropriate ages for household contacts of immunocompromised persons to help prevent spread of infection among these high-risk patients. Although bacillus of Calmette-Guérin vaccine (BCG) is contraindicated in HIV-infected children in the United States, the World Health Organization (WHO) recommends giving BCG to asymptomatic HIV-infected children in areas with a high incidence of tuberculosis.

Live-virus vaccines should be administered with caution to children receiving corticosteroids. Children receiving physiologic or low doses of corticosteroids, defined as less than 2 mg/kg/24 hr of prednisone or its equivalent, or less than 20 mg/24 hr if they weigh more than 10 kg, can be immunized while on treatment. Children receiving 2 mg/kg/24 hr or more of daily, alternate-day prednisone or its equivalent, or 20 mg or more daily if they weigh more than 10 kg, for fewer than 14 days should have live-virus immunizations deferred until at least discontinuation of corticosteroids. If the duration is 14 days or more, immunization should be deferred for at least 1 month.

PRETERM INFANTS. The immune response to vaccination is a function of postnatal rather than gestational age. Prematurity does not increase the incidence of vaccine-related adverse events. Hence, preterm infants, including those of very low birthweight, should be vaccinated at the same chronologic age as full-term infants and according to the routine childhood immunization schedule (see Fig. 282–1). One exception to this recommendation is hepatitis B vaccination of those born of HBsAg-negative mothers with low birthweights (i.e., <2 kg). Initiation of vaccination in this case should be delayed until the infant is 1 mo of age. Vaccine in conjunction with hepatitis B immunoglobulin (HBIG) should be given to low birthweight infants born of HBs-positive mothers at birth but the vaccine dose is not counted in the completion of a three-dose primary hepatitis B vaccine schedule. The dose for preterm infants should not be reduced for any vaccine.

Breast-Feeding. Human milk does not adversely affect the immune response of infants and breast-feeding is not a contraindication to any vaccine, including OPV. Most live-virus vaccines, although they replicate in the mother, are not excreted in human milk. Breast-feeding women also may safely receive vaccines without interrupting breast-feeding, and their infants should be vaccinated according to routinely recommended vaccines.

Internationally Adopted Children. Determination of whether a child has been adequately vaccinated on the basis of their country of origin and records alone is limited. Adopted children should receive vaccines according to the recommended schedules for children in the United States. Only written documentation should be accepted as evidence of prior vaccination. These records are more likely to predict protection if the vaccines, dates of administration, intervals between doses, and the child's age at the time of administrations are comparable to current recommendations in the United States. The majority of vaccines used worldwide are produced with adequate quality controls and standards and are potent.

Given the limitations in determining whether a child's prior vaccination history is reliable, one of several approaches can be followed. An acceptable one is repeating the vaccinations. Doing so is usually safe and avoids the need to obtain and interpret serologic antibody tests. If avoiding unnecessary injections is desired, judicious use of serologic testing may be helpful in determining which immunizations are needed.

POSTEXPOSURE IMMUNOPROPHYLAXIS

For certain infections, active or passive immunization shortly after exposure can prevent or ameliorate disease. For example, postexposure active immunization with rabies vaccine combined with passive immunization with rabies immune globulin (RIG) is highly effective in preventing rabies (see Chapter 251). Varicella-zoster immune globulin (VZIG) is indicated after susceptible persons who are immunocompromised are exposed to varicella (see Chapter 232). VZIG also is recommended for a newborn infant whose mother had onset of chickenpox within 5 days before to 2 days after delivery (see Chapter 232). For otherwise healthy, susceptible children exposed to varicella, administration of varicella vaccine within 72 hr of exposure is recommended to prevent or significantly modify disease (see Chapter 232). After a susceptible person is exposed to measles, either measles vaccine given within 72 hr or immune globulin given within 6 days can prevent or modify disease (see Chapter 225). Other infections for which passive immunization of a susceptible person is indicated after exposure are tetanus in wound management (see Chapter 194) and hepatitis A and hepatitis B (see Chapter 339).

PASSIVE IMMUNIZATION

Administration of an immune globulin is indicated in some circumstances for preventing specific infections. The different preparations include intramuscular immune globulin (IG), intravenous immune globulin (IVIG), and immune globulin preparations (termed *hyperimmune globulin*) that have high concentrations of specific antibody against a particular pathogen. These products, which historically were prepared from animal sera but today are derived from human sera, include VZIG, RIG, hepatitis B immune globulin (HBIG), cytomegalovirus immune globulin, and respiratory syncytial virus (RSV) immune globulin for intravenous administration (RSV-IGIV).

A monoclonal antibody against RSV, palivizumab, administered intramuscularly at monthly intervals during the RSV season, also is available. Either palivizumab or RSV-IGIV is recommended for protecting high-risk children against serious complications of RSV disease (see Chapter 239). Other monoclonal antibody products may supplant hyperimmune globulins in the future.

Prevention of hepatitis A during foreign travel is another indication for passive immunization with IG. For children age 2 yr of age and older, however, active immunization with hepatitis A vaccine is preferred because the protection is prolonged, if not lifelong, in contrast to the temporary protection afforded by passive immunoprophylaxis.

ADVERSE EVENTS

Record Keeping and Reporting. Accurate record keeping by physicians is required. Parents also should keep up- to-date immunization records for their children. In the United States, the **National Childhood Vaccine Injury Act** requires for childhood-mandated vaccines (i.e., those routinely recommended for all children) that health care providers record in a child's medical record the date of administration of the vaccine, manufacturer, lot number, and the name of the health care provider administering the vaccines.

All children and their parents or guardians should be informed about the benefits and risks of vaccines to be administered and the provisions of the National Vaccine Injury Compensation Program. The discussion should be in language understood by the recipient or parent or guardian, and ample opportunity for questions and discussion should be provided. A **Vaccine Information Statement** for each vaccine has been prepared for this purpose by the Department of Health and Human Services; its use is required before each dose of vaccine.

Under the National Childhood Vaccine Injury Act, all temporally associated events severe enough for a patient to seek medical attention should be reported to the **Vaccine Adverse Events Reporting System (VAERS)**. In addition, specific adverse events occurring in recipients of childhood-mandated vaccines are required to be reported. Forms, instructions on reporting, and additional information can be obtained from the **National Vaccine Injury Compensation Program** (800-338-2382 and http://www.vaers.org/).

Compensation for Vaccine Injuries. The Vaccine Injury Compensation Program (VICP) is a no-fault federal program that ensures fairness to persons who have suffered certain vaccine-related injuries and protects federal, state, and local immunization programs, private immunization providers, and vaccine manufacturers. The program is designed to provide prompt and fair compensation to the families of children who have died or have been injured as a result of routinely required immunization and to reduce the adverse impact of the tort judicial system on vaccine supply, cost, innovation, and development. This program provides no-fault compensation for specific adverse events associated with vaccines. These events can be accessed at the VICP Internet site (http://www.vaers.org).

DELIVERY OF VACCINES

Success of vaccination in preventing childhood infectious diseases necessitates effective means of vaccine delivery so that children receive recommended immunizations on schedule. In the United States, high rates of immunization in school-aged children have been achieved for the past 2 decades, in part because of state laws requiring immunization for school entry. In contrast to current rates of approximately 95% or higher in school-aged children, immunization rates in infants and young children in the 1980s were significantly lower; rates ranged from 18–79% for completed vaccinations by the 2nd birthday. This failure to immunize young children was a major factor in the 1989–1991 measles outbreaks in urban areas. Major barriers to successful infant and childhood immunization that were identified in these outbreaks include the following: inadequate access to immunization services, missed opportunities to administer vaccines, inadequate resources for public health and preventive programs, and low public awareness and resulting lack of public demand for immunization.

This recognition of low immunization rates prompted a national campaign to achieve the goal of 90% vaccine coverage of children by 2 yr of age. Initiatives included improved access to vaccines, education of health care providers, and the development of standards for pediatric immunization practices. These standards serve as guidelines for improving the delivery of vaccines and have recently been updated by the National Vaccine Advisory Committee of the Department of Health and Human Services (Box 282–1). They include readily available vaccination services, evaluation of immunization status of patients at all medical visits, effective communication with vaccine recipients about vaccine benefits and risks, use of valid contraindications, simultaneous administration of all indicated vaccines, and routine patient record reviews and assessments by providers of the immunization status of their patients. An important principle in these standards is the need to eliminate missed opportunities to vaccinate infants and children.

These and other initiatives have resulted in increasing immunization rates of young children in recent years. Since 1995, composite vaccination coverage rates for preschool-aged children have been approximately 75% or greater. According to the National Immunization Survey, coverage rates among children 19–35 mo of age in 2001 were 73.7% for completion of the schedule of four doses of DTaP/DTP/DT, three doses of poliovirus vaccines, three doses of Hib vaccine, three doses of hepatitis B vaccine, and one dose of measles-containing vaccine. All of the national coverage goals for specific vaccines established in the Childhood Immunization Initiative have been met, and vaccination rates are the highest ever recorded in the United States for preschool children. The rate for varicella vaccination rose from 67% in 2000 to 76% in 2001. This success reflects the collaborative efforts of the public and private sectors in public health.

INTERNATIONAL CONSIDERATIONS

Since the establishment of the Expanded Programme on Immunization (EPI) of the WHO, immunization rates for the basic children's vaccines increased from 5% to as high as approximately 80% worldwide. At least 2.7 million deaths due to measles, neonatal tetanus, and pertussis and 200,000 cases of paralysis due to poliomyelitis are prevented each year. Despite the successes of the EPI, which include elimination of poliomyelitis from the Americas, some vaccine-preventable diseases such as measles, pertussis, and neonatal tetanus remain prevalent in the developing world.

Vaccines against seven diseases are currently recommended by the EPI for routine use in the developing world and are BCG, DTP, OPV, measles, and hepatitis B vaccines for children and tetanus toxoid for pregnant women. Hib, Yellow fever, Japanese encephalitis, group A meningococcus, mumps, and rubella vaccines are used regionally, depending on the disease epidemiology and resources. Poliomyelitis has been targeted for global eradication by 2003.

Because infectious diseases know no geographic or political boundaries, uncontrolled disease anywhere in the world poses

---

BOX 282–1. Standards for Child and Adolescent Immunization Practices

1. Vaccination services are readily available.
2. Vaccinations are coordinated with other health care services and provided in a medical home when possible.
3. Barriers to vaccination are identified and minimized.
4. Patient costs are minimized.
5. Health care professionals review the vaccination and health status of patients at every encounter to determine which vaccines are indicated.
6. Health care professionals assess for and follow only medically accepted contraindications.
7. Parents/guardians and patients are educated about the risks and benefits of vaccination in a culturally appropriate manner and in easy-to-understand language.
8. Health care professionals follow appropriate procedures for vaccine storage and handling.
9. Up-to-date, written vaccination protocols are accessible at all locations where vaccines are administered.
10. Persons who administer vaccines and staff who manage or support vaccine administration are knowledgeable and receive on-going education.
11. Health care professionals simultaneously administer as many indicated doses as possible.
12. Vaccination records for patients are accurate, complete, and easily accessible.
13. Health care professionals report adverse events following vaccination promptly and accurately to the Vaccine Adverse Event Reporting System (VAERS) and are aware of a separate program, the National Vaccine Injury Compensation Program (VICP).
14. All personnel who have contact with patients are appropriately vaccinated.
15. Systems are used to remind parents/guardians, patients, and health care professionals when vaccines are due and to recall those who are overdue.
16. Office-or clinic-based patient record reviews and vaccination coverage assessments are performed annually.
17. Health care professionals practice community-based approaches.

a threat to the United States. Vaccines offer the opportunity to control and even eradicate some diseases. Successful eradication means that vaccines are no longer needed. The experience with smallpox demonstrates that the eradication of disease is a remarkably sound economic investment. The total sum spent by the United States for the global smallpox eradication campaign has been recouped in 1968 dollars every 2.5 months since 1971. A similar achievement with poliomyelitis would save the United States more than $300 million each year in vaccine and associated delivery costs.

Abramsom JS, Pickering LK: US Immunization Policy. *JAMA* 2002:287;505–9.
Ada G: Vaccines and vaccination. *N Engl J Med* 2001;345:1042–53.
Atkinson WL, Pickering LK, Watson JC, et al: General immunization practices. In Plotkin SA, Orenstein WA (editors): *Vaccines*, 4th ed. Philadelphia, WB Saunders, in press.
Centers for Disease Control and Prevention: General recommendations on immunizations: Recommendations of the Advisory Committee on Immunization Practices and the American Academy of Family Physicians. *MMWR* 2002:51(RR-2):1–35.
Centers for Disease Control and Prevention: *Health Information for International Travel 2001–2002*. Atlanta; US Department of Health and Human Services, Public Health Service, 2001.
Peter G: Childhood immunizations. *N Engl J Med* 1992;327:1794–1800.
Pickering L (editor): *2003 Red Book: Report of the Committee on Infectious Diseases*, 26th ed. Grove Village, IL, American Academy of Pediatrics (in press).
Plotkin SA, Orenstein WA (editors): *Vaccines*, 4th ed. Philadelphia, WB Saunders, in press.

Chapter 283

Infection Control and Prophylaxis *Margaret C. Fisher*

Infection control is a vital part of pediatric medicine. Controlling infections requires an intact and active public health system, universal immunizations, optimal nutrition, and use of specific methods to prevent transmission of infection from child to child, child to adult, and adult to child. Infection control is the responsibility of every health care provider.

Nosocomial infections are those acquired during hospitalization. An estimated 3–5% of children admitted to hospitals acquire a nosocomial infection; rates are much higher in intensive care units. Infections are also acquired in emergency departments, physicians' offices, and long-term care settings. Medical devices are increasingly used in the home, and they also require appropriate infection control techniques. Education of home health care providers as well as of families is essential.

Determinants of infection include host factors, prior invasive procedures, use of catheters, use of antibiotics, and exposure to other patients, visitors, or health care providers with contagious diseases. Host factors that increase the risk for infection include anatomic abnormalities (e.g., dermoid sinuses, cleft palate, obstructive uropathy), damage to skin, organ dysfunction, malnutrition, and underlying diseases or co-morbidities. Diseases and therapies that alter immunity are most likely to predispose to infection. Prior procedures may introduce pathogens and damage anatomic host defenses. Intravenous and other catheters bypass host defenses, provide direct access to sterile sites, provide adherence sites for microbes, and may occlude normal ostia such as the eustachian tubes. Antibiotics often alter normal bowel flora and encourage colonization by resistant flora, and they may suppress hematopoiesis. Exposure to adults or children with contagious diseases is a clear risk for nosocomial transmission of disease.

Transmission of infectious agents occurs by various routes, but by far the most common and important route is via the hands. Children are constantly placing their own hands in their noses, eyes, and mouths; thus, child-to-child exchange of secretions is common whenever children are together. Bacteria, fungi, viruses, and parasites often travel on hands from one person to another. Medical equipment, toys, and hospital and office furnishings can be contaminated and thus have a role as fomites for transmission of potential pathogens. Thermometers and other equipment that come into contact with mucous membranes are special risks. Some agents are disseminated by airborne transmission, such as varicella virus, measles virus, and *Mycobacterium tuberculosis*. Food and water can be contaminated and have been involved in hospital outbreaks.

Common causes of nosocomial infections in children are seasonal viruses, staphylococci, and gram-negative bacilli. Fungi and resistant bacteria are frequent causes of infection in immunocompromised children and in those who require intensive care and prolonged hospitalization. Common sites of infection are the respiratory tract, gastrointestinal tract, bloodstream, skin, and urinary tract.

Nosocomial infections cause considerable morbidity and occasional mortality; infections prolong hospital stays and increase health care costs. Surveillance for infection is the first step in identifying nosocomial infections and suggesting methods for prevention. Within hospitals, surveillance is the responsibility of the Infection Control Committee, a multidisciplinary group that collects and reviews surveillance data, establishes policy, and investigates outbreaks. Surveillance within outpatient settings and during home care is often less well established but no less important. Local, state, and federal health departments play important roles in identifying and controlling outbreaks and in establishing public health policy.

Prevention. Prevention of infection is the goal.

HAND HYGIENE. The most important measure in any infection control program is hand hygiene. Although much attention is directed at the types of soap used, the important component of handwashing is placement of the hands under water and use of friction with or without soap. Studies show that a 15-sec scrub removes the majority of transient flora but does not alter the permanent flora. A variety of hand gels and rubs can be used in place of handwashing. Waterless hand hygiene products have been shown to increase compliance and save time; these agents are now the preferred agents for routine hand hygiene. These products are effective in killing microbes; however, they will not remove dirt or debris. Hands should be cleaned before and after every patient encounter. Studies in child-care settings and schools have determined that handwashing can be taught to children and that the rates of infection are decreased when children as well as caregivers regularly clean their hands.

STANDARD PRECAUTIONS. Standard precautions, formerly known as universal precautions, are intended to protect health care workers from blood and body fluids and should be used whenever providing care. Infected individuals are often contagious before symptoms of disease develop, and asymptomatic carriers are capable of transmitting the agent. Standard precautions involve the use of barriers—gloves, gowns, masks, goggles, and face shields—as needed to prevent transmission of microbes associated with contact with blood or body fluids.

ISOLATION. Isolation of patients infected with certain pathogens decreases the risk of nosocomial transmission. The type of isolation depends on the infecting agent and the route of transmission. Contact transmission is the most frequent mode and involves direct contact or contact with a contaminated intermediate object. Droplet transmission is by droplets propelled a short distance through the air and deposited on mucous membranes. Airborne transmission occurs by dissemination of droplet nuclei (≤5 μm) of evaporated droplets or dust particles carrying the infectious agent.

Standard precautions are indicated for all patients and are appropriate in the office as well as the hospital. In addition, for hospitalized patients, transmission-based precautions are indicated for certain diseases (Table 283–1). Contact precautions include gowns and gloves and single room isolation. Droplet precautions include masks for close contact (<3 ft) and single room isolation. For both contact and droplet precautions, a single room is preferred but is not required. Cohorting of children infected with the same pathogen is acceptable. Airborne precautions include masks and single room isolation with negative-pressure ventilation. Transmission-based precautions are continued for as long as a patient is considered to be contagious.

The use of isolation techniques in an outpatient setting has not been studied. Each office must establish policies to ensure that the proper cleaning, disinfection, and sterilization methods are used. Many practices and clinics provide separate waiting areas for sick and well children. Triage of patients is essential to ensure that contagious children or adults are not present in waiting areas.

Outbreaks of measles in patients within the waiting area have been reported where airflow allowed the exhaust from the examination room to enter the waiting area. Cleaning the environment is important. Toys and items that are shared between patients should be cleaned between uses; soap and water are sufficient for these items. More complete disinfection or sterilization is required for items that encounter mucous membranes and for all reusable items used for body fluid sampling.

ADDITIONAL MEASURES. Other preventive measures include aseptic technique, catheter care, prudent use of antibiotics, isolation of contagious patients, cleaning of the environment, disinfection and sterilization of medical equipment, reporting of infections, safe handling of needles and other sharp instruments, and establishment of employee health services. Aseptic technique must be used for all invasive procedures; this is especially important during catheter placement and manipulation. Catheter care also includes limiting the duration and number of catheters as much as possible and removing catheters as soon as they become unnecessary. Prudent use of antibiotics is important.

TABLE 283–1. Selected Diseases and Indications for Transmission-Based Isolation in Addition to Standard Precautions

Clinical Syndrome or Condition	Potential Pathogens	Empirical Precautions
Diarrhea		
Acute diarrhea with a likely infectious cause in an incontinent or diapered patient	*Salmonella, Shigella, Escherichia coli* O157:H7, rotavirus, hepatitis A	Contact
Diarrhea in any patient, especially an adult, with a history of recent antibiotic use	*Clostridum difficile*	Contact
Meningitis		
	Neisseria meningitidis, Haemophilus influenzae type b	Droplet
	Streptococcus pneumoniae	Standard
Rash or Exanthems		
Petechial/ecchymotic with fever	*N. meningitidis*	Droplet
Vesicular		
Chickenpox	Varicella-zoster virus	Airborne and contact
Zoster (localized in an immunocompetent patient)	Varicella-zoster virus	Standard
Zoster (disseminated or in an immunocompromised patient)	Varicella-zoster virus	Airborne and contact
Maculopapular with coryza and fever	Measles virus	Airborne
Erythema infectiosum	Parvovirus B19	Standard
Parvovirus B19 in an immunocompromised patient	Parvovirus B19	Droplet
Roseola	Human herpesvirus 6	Standard
Rubella	Rubella virus	Droplet
Respiratory Tract Infections		
Paroxysmal or severe persistent cough during periods of pertussis activity	*Bordetella pertussis*	Droplet
Bronchiolitis and croup, other lower respiratory tract infections in infants and young children	Respiratory syncytial or parainfluenza virus	Contact
Influenza	Influenza virus	Droplet
Atypical pneumonia	*Mycoplasma pneumoniae*	Droplet
Afebrile pneumonia in young infants	*Chlamydia trachomatis*	Standard
Diphtheria (pharyngeal)	*Corynebacterium diphtheriae*	Droplet
Pneumonic plague	*Yersinia pestis*	Droplet
Pneumococcal pneumonia	*Streptococcus pneumoniae*	Standard
Group A streptococcal pharyngitis, pneumonia, or scarlet fever in infants and young children	Group A streptococcus	Droplet
Skin Diseases		
Skin infections that are highly contagious or that may occur on dry skin (cutaneous diphtheria; herpes simplex virus, neonatal or mucocutaneous; impetigo; major or draining abscesses; cellulitis; decubiti; staphylococcal furunculosis; zoster disseminated or in an immunocompromised host)		Contact
Urinary Tract Infections		Standard
Other Infections		
Infection or colonization with multidrug-resistant organisms	Resistant bacteria	Contact
Invasive *Neisseria meningitidis* disease (meningitis, pneumonia, and sepsis)	*N. meningitidis*	Droplet
Invasive *Haemophilus influenzae* type b disease (meningitis, pneumonia, epiglottitis, and sepsis)	*H. influenzae* type b	Droplet
Viral infections spread by droplet transmission (adenovirus, influenza, mumps, parvovirus B19 in an immunocompromised patient, rubella)		Droplet

Adapted from Garner JS: The Hospital Infection Control Practices Advisory Committee: Guidelines for isolation precautions in hospitals. Infect Control Hosp Epidemiol *1996;17:53–80.*

Surgical Prophylaxis. Surgical prophylaxis is appropriate when there is a high risk of postoperative infection or when the consequences of infection are catastrophic. The choice of antibiotic depends on the site and type of surgery (Table 283–2). A useful classification of surgical procedures based on this risk recognizes four categories: clean wounds, clean contaminated wounds, contaminated wounds, and dirty and infected wounds. Clinical recommendations are standards of the American College of Surgeons, the Surgical Infection Society, and the American Academy of Pediatrics.

Clean wounds are uninfected operative wounds in which no inflammation is noted and the respiratory, alimentary, and genitourinary tracts and the oropharynx are not entered. In addition, the procedure is elective and is performed as primarily closed or drained with closed drainage. Operative incisional wounds after nonpenetrating trauma are included in this category. For clean wounds, prophylactic antimicrobial therapy is not recommended, except in patients at high risk for infection and in circumstances in which the consequences of infection are potentially life threatening (e.g., implantation of a prosthetic foreign body such as a prosthetic heart valve; open heart surgery for repair of structural defects; surgery in patients who are immunocompromised as a result of an inherited disease or are receiving corticosteroids or chemotherapy for malignancy; and newborn infants). Systemic antimicrobial agents have been recommended empirically for a clean procedure in patients with infection at another site.

Clean contaminated wounds are operative wounds in which the respiratory, alimentary, or genitourinary tract is entered under controlled conditions and does not have unusual contamination preoperatively. These wounds occur in operations that involve the biliary tract, appendix, vagina, and oropharynx and in which no evidence of infection or major break in technique is encountered, as well as in urgent or emergency surgery in an otherwise clean procedure. In clean but potentially contaminated procedures, the risk of contamination is variable. Recommendations for pediatric patients derived from data on adults suggest that prophylaxis be provided for procedures in patients with obstructive jaundice, certain alimentary tract procedures, and urinary tract surgery or instrumentation in the presence of bacteriuria or obstructive uropathy.

Contaminated wounds include open, fresh, and accidental wounds; major breaks in otherwise sterile operative technique; gross spillage from the gastrointestinal tract; penetrating trauma occurring less than 4 hr earlier; and incisions in which acute nonpurulent inflammation is encountered.

Dirty and infected wounds include penetrating traumatic wounds longer than 4 hr earlier, those with retained devitalized tissue, and those in which clinical infection is apparent or in which the viscera have been perforated. In contaminated and dirty or infected wound procedures, antimicrobial therapy is indicated and may need to be continued for 5–10 days.

In the truest sense, antimicrobial prophylaxis refers to the use of antibiotics before attachment of contaminating bacteria to the host tissues, as in the clean and potentially contaminated categories. Antibiotics given after the microbial attachment constitute therapy, as in the case of contaminated and dirty wounds.

When used, prophylactic antibiotics should be administered, preferably intravenously, approximately 30 min before the skin incision is made, with the intent of having peak concentrations of the drug at this time. Adequate plasma and tissue concentration of the drugs should be maintained until the incision is closed. Repeat doses are necessary only if the surgery lasts longer than 6 hr. Postoperative therapy is usually not necessary; in cases of contaminated surgery, antibiotics are continued as therapy for infection at the site. Drugs administered postoperatively for prophylaxis do not reduce the infection rate. For patients undergoing colonic procedures, additional oral antibiotics may be used and should also be given on the day before surgery.

The selection of antibiotic regimen for prophylaxis is based on the procedure, the expected contaminating organisms, and safety of the drugs. Because of the vast array of antibiotics available now, more than one regimen may be acceptable (see Table 283–2). Knowledge of the susceptibilities of the prevalent bacterial causes of nosocomial infections in each hospital is especially important in choosing drugs.

Employee Health. Employee health is important because employees are at risk for acquiring infection from patients. This risk is minimized by use of standard precautions and hand hygiene before and after all patient contacts. Infected employees also pose a risk to patients. Within hospitals, personnel health services or departments of occupational safety and health manage employee health issues. New employees should be screened for the presence of infectious diseases. Their immunization history should be noted and necessary immunizations offered.

All health care workers (medical or nonmedical, paid or volunteer, full time or part time, student or nonstudent, with or without patient care responsibilities) who work in facilities that provide health care to patients (inpatient or outpatient, public or private) should be immune to measles, rubella, and varicella.

TABLE 283–2. **Common Surgical Procedures for Which Perioperative Prophylactic Antibiotics Are Recommended**

Surgical Procedure	Likely Pathogens	Suggested Drug
Clean Wounds		
Cardiac surgery (e.g., open heart surgery) Vascular surgery Neurosurgery Orthopedic surgery (e.g., joint replacement)	Skin flora, enteric gram-negative bacilli	Cefazolin or vancomycin
Clean Contaminated Wounds		
Head and neck surgery entering the oral cavity or pharynx	Skin flora, oral anaerobes, oral streptococci	Cefazolin or clindamycin
Gastrointestinal and genitourinary surgery	Enteric gram-negative bacilli, anaerobes, gram-positive cocci	Cefazolin; if colon involved, consider oral decontamination with neomycin and erythromycin
Contaminated Wounds		
Traumatic wounds (e.g., compound fracture)	Skin flora	Cefazolin
Dirty Wounds		
Appendectomy Colorectal surgery	Enteric gram-negative bacilli, anaerobes, gram-positive cocci	Cefoxitin, or clindamycin plus gentamicin

All employees who might be exposed to blood or body fluids should be immunized against hepatitis B. Annual influenza immunizations are recommended for all health care workers who have contact with patients at risk for influenza or its complications. This program lessens staff illness and absenteeism during the influenza season and reduces nosocomial infections. Immunizations should be encouraged and whenever possible should be provided free of charge. Each office and hospital must comply with the rules developed by the Occupational Safety and Health Administration. Furthermore, each office and hospital should have written policies about exclusion of infected staff. Regular educational sessions should be performed to ensure that the staff is aware of infection control methods and that they adhere to infection control policies.

Abrutyn E, Goldman DA, Scheckler WE (editors): Saunders Infection Control Reference Service: *The Experts' Guide to the Guidelines*, 2nd ed. Philadelphia, WB Saunders, 2001.

American Academy of Pediatrics, Committee on Infectious Diseases and Committee on Hospital Care: The revised CDC guidelines for isolation precautions in hospitals: Implications for pediatrics. *Pediatrics* 1998;101:E3.

Bennett JV, Brachman PS (editors): *Hospital Infections*, 3rd ed. Boston, Little, Brown, 1992.

Centers for Disease Control and Prevention: Recommendations of the Advisory Committee on Immunization Practices (ACIP) and the Hospital Infection Control Practices Advisory Committee (HICPAC): Immunization of health-care workers. *MMWR* 1997;46(RR-18):1–42.

Centers for Disease Control and Prevention: Guideline for hand hygiene in health-care settings: Recommendations of the Healthcare Infection Control Practices Advisory Committee and the HICPAC/SHEA/APIC/ISDA Hand Hygiene Task Force. *MMWR* 2002;51(RR-16):1–56.

Herwaldt LA, Decker MD (editors): The Society for Healthcare Epidemiology of America: *A Practical Handbook for Hospital Epidemiologists*. Thorofare, NJ, Slack, 1998.

Lohr JA, Ingram DL, Dudley SM, et al: Hand washing in pediatric ambulatory settings: An inconsistent practice. *Am J Dis Child* 1991;145:1198–9.

Chapter 284

Child Care and Communicable Diseases

Larry K. Pickering

An estimated 13 million children age 5 yr and younger and 60% of school-aged children younger than age 13 yr attend some form of child-care facility on a regular basis (see Chapter 32). Child-care facilities can be classified on the basis of size of enrollment, ages of attendees, health status of the children enrolled, and type of setting. As defined in the United States, child-care facilities consist of child-care centers, small and large family child-care homes, and facilities for ill children or children with special needs. Child-care centers are facilities where care and education are provided to any number of children in a nonresidential setting and the facility is open on a regular basis (i.e., not a drop-in facility). Centers are licensed and regulated by state governments and care for a larger number of children than are cared for in family homes. In contrast, family child-care homes are designated as small (1–6 children) or large (7–12 children), may be full day or part day, may expect regular daily attendance, or may be designed for sporadic use. Family homes generally are not licensed or registered, depending on state requirements.

Most studies of infectious diseases have been conducted in child-care centers among infant (birth–12 mo of age) and toddler (13–36 mo of age) groups. Almost any organism has the potential to be spread and cause disease in a child-care setting. Epidemiologic studies have established that children in child-care facilities are 2–18 times more likely to acquire certain infectious diseases than children not enrolled in child-care (Table 284–1). In addition, children in child-care facilities are at risk of receiving more courses of antimicrobial agents for longer periods and of acquiring antibiotic-resistant organisms. Transmission of organisms and illness in group care depends on the age and immune status of children involved, the season, hygiene practices, crowding, environmental characteristics of the facilities, and characteristics of particular organisms, including infectivity, survivability in the environment, and virulence. Rates of infection, duration of illness, and risk of hospitalization tend to decrease among children in child-care facilities after the first 6 mo of attendance and decline to levels observed among homebound children after 3 yr of age.

Epidemiology. There are several different patterns of occurrence of infectious diseases among children in child care and their contacts. Respiratory tract infections and diarrhea are the most common diseases associated with child care. These infections occur in children, child-care staff, and household contacts and may spread into the community. Organisms such as enteric pathogens (see Chapter 321), which are transmitted by the fecal-oral route, and respiratory tract pathogens can infect both children and adults. Infections caused by hepatitis A virus may

TABLE 284–1. Infectious Diseases in the Child-Care Setting

Disease	Increased Incidence with Child Care
Respiratory Tract Infections	
Otitis media	Yes
Sinusitis	Probably
Pharyngitis	Probably
Pneumonia	Yes
Gastrointestinal Tract Infections	
Diarrhea (rotavirus, calicivirus, astrovirus, enteric adenovirus, *Giardia lamblia*, *Cryptosporidium*, *Shigella*, *Escherichia coli* O157:H7, and *Clostridium difficile*)	Yes
Hepatitis A	Yes
Skin Diseases	
Impetigo	Probably
Scabies	Probably
Pediculosis	Probably
Tinea (ringworm)	Probably
Invasive Bacteria Infections	
Haemophilus influenzae type b	No*
Neisseria meningitidis	Probably
Streptococcus pneumoniae	Yes
Aseptic Meningitis	
Enteroviruses	Probably
Herpesvirus Infections	
Cytomegalovirus	Yes
Varicella-zoster virus	Yes
Herpes simplex virus	Probably
Bloodborne Infections	
Hepatitis B	Few case reports
HIV	No cases reported
Hepatitis C	No cases reported
Vaccine-Preventable Diseases	
Measles, mumps, rubella, diphtheria, pertussis, tetanus	Not established
Polio	No
H. influenzae type b	No*
Varicella	Yes

Not in the postvaccine era; yes in the prevaccine era.

not be apparent in young children attending child care but may have a major clinical impact on older children and adult contacts, including child-care staff and household contacts. Other diseases, such as otitis media, varicella, and invasive *Haemophilus influenzae* type b disease, usually affect children rather than adults. Some infections, such as cytomegalovirus (CMV) and parvovirus B19, may have serious consequences for the fetuses of pregnant women or for certain immunosuppressed hosts. Bloodborne pathogens such as hepatitis B virus and HIV (see Chapter 254) can infect all ages but have rarely (hepatitis B) or never (HIV) been reported to be transmitted in a child-care setting. Skin infections and infestations are acquired through close personal contact and contaminated linens or clothing and more often affect children older than 2 yr of age.

RESPIRATORY TRACT INFECTIONS. Respiratory tract infections account for the majority of child care–related illness. Children younger than 2 yr of age and who attend child-care centers have more upper and lower respiratory tract infections than age-matched children not in child care. The organisms responsible for illness are similar to those that circulate in the community and include respiratory syncytial virus, parainfluenza viruses, adenoviruses, rhinoviruses, coronaviruses, influenza viruses, parvovirus B19, *Streptococcus pneumoniae*, and, infrequently, *Bordetella pertussis* and *Mycobacterium tuberculosis*. The risk of developing otitis media is two to three times greater in children attending child-care centers than in children receiving home-based care. Otitis media is responsible for most of the antibiotic use in children younger than 3 yr of age in child care. These children also are at increased risk for recurrent otitis media, further increasing use of antimicrobial agents in this population. Although children in child care show earlier acquisition of pharyngeal carriage of group A *Streptococcus*, outbreaks of this organism are uncommon.

GASTROINTESTINAL TRACT INFECTIONS. Acute infectious diarrhea is two to three times more common in children in child care than in children cared for in their homes. Outbreaks of diarrhea occur frequently in child-care centers and generally are caused by enteric viruses such as rotaviruses, enteric adenoviruses, astroviruses, and caliciviruses or by enteric parasites such as *Giardia lamblia* or *Cryptosporidium*. Low infective doses and high asymptomatic excretion rates characterize the more common enteropathogens, such as rotavirus and *G. lamblia*. Bacterial enteropathogens, such as *Shigella* and *Escherichia coli* O157:H7, and, less commonly, *Campylobacter, Clostridium difficile*, and *Bacillus cereus* (from contaminated fried rice) also have caused outbreaks of diarrhea in child-care settings. *Salmonella* rarely is associated with outbreaks of diarrhea in child-care settings. Hepatitis A in children enrolled in child-care facilities has resulted in community-wide outbreaks. Hepatitis A usually is mild or asymptomatic in young children and is identified when illness becomes manifested in older children or adults. Enteropathogens and hepatitis A virus are transmitted in child-care facilities by the fecal-oral route and rarely by contaminated food or water. Enteric illness and hepatitis A are more common in centers that care for children who are not toilet trained and where proper hygienic practices are lacking.

SKIN DISEASES. The most commonly recognized skin infections or infestations in children in child care are impetigo caused by staphylococcus *aureus* or group A streptococcus, pediculosis, scabies, tinea capitis, and tinea corporis (ringworm). The magnitude of these infections and infestations in children in child care is not known. Parvovirus B19, which causes erythema infectiosum (fifth disease), is spread through the respiratory route, and outbreaks have occurred in child-care centers. As with CMV, the greatest health hazard is for pregnant women and immunocompromised hosts owing to their respective risks of fetal loss and aplastic crisis.

INVASIVE ORGANISMS. Primary invasive disease caused by *H. influenzae* type b has been shown to be more common in children in child care; evidence for increased risk of subsequent or secondary disease from *H. influenzae* type b in a child-care setting is less convincing. Routine immunization against *H. influenzae* type b has reduced greatly the risk of primary invasive infection. There is an indication that the risk of primary disease caused by *Neisseria meningitidis* is higher among children in child care than among children cared for at home. Child-care attendance is associated with nasopharyngeal carriage of penicillin-resistant *Streptococcus pneumoniae* and invasive pneumococcal disease, especially among children with a history of recurrent otitis media and antibiotic use. Secondary spread of *S. pneumoniae* and *N. meningitidis* has been reported, indicating the potential for outbreaks to occur in this setting. Use of *S. pneumoniae* conjugate vaccine will reduce the incidence of invasive disease and reduce carriage of serotypes of *S. pneumoniae* contained in the vaccine.

Outbreaks of aseptic meningitis from echovirus 30 have been reported among children in child-care centers, their parents, and their teachers.

HERPESVIRUSES. Studies of CMV infection in child-care centers have shown that as many as 70% of diapered children continuously shed CMV in urine and saliva after acquisition. CMV-infected children often transmit the virus to other children with whom they have contact, as well as to 8–20% of their care providers and mothers per year. Transmission occurs as a result of contact with infected saliva or urine. Varicella frequently has been transmitted in child-care centers, but routine varicella immunization should reduce this risk. The role of child-care facilities in the spread of herpes simplex virus, especially during episodes of gingivostomatitis, requires further clarification.

BLOODBORNE ORGANISMS. Hepatitis B virus (HBV), HIV, and hepatitis C virus (HCV) are bloodborne pathogens. Hepatitis B transmission among children in child care has been documented in a few instances, but the potential for transmission of this infection has declined with implementation of universal immunization of infants with HBV vaccine. Issues about HIV in child care include the potential risk of HIV transmission within the child-care setting and risks to HIV-infected children associated with acquisition of infectious agents. No cases of HIV transmission in out-of-home child care have been reported. Children with HIV infection enrolled in child-care facilities should be monitored for exposure to infectious diseases, and their health and immune status should be evaluated frequently. Transmission risks of HCV infection in child-care settings have not been reported.

ANTIBIOTIC USE AND BACTERIAL RESISTANCE. Antibiotic resistance has become an alarming problem in child-care facilities because the frequency of infection by organisms resistant to frequently used antimicrobial agents has increased dramatically. The estimated annual rate of antibiotic use in children in child care is from two to four times higher than in age-matched children cared for at home. In addition, the mean duration of antibiotic treatment is four times longer in children in child care. This frequency of antibiotic use combined with the propensity for person-to-person transmission of pathogens in a crowded environment has resulted in an increased prevalence of antibiotic-resistant bacteria in the respiratory and intestinal tracts, including *S. pneumoniae, H. influenzae, Moraxella catarrhalis, E. coli* O157:H7, and *Shigella* species.

Prevention. Written child-care center policies designed to prevent or control the spread of infectious agents should be available and reviewed regularly. Standards for environmental and personal hygiene should include maintenance of current immunization records for children and staff, appropriate exclusion policies, targeting frequently contaminated areas for environmental cleaning, adherence to appropriate diaper changing procedures, appropriate handling of food, management of pets, and communicable disease surveillance and reporting. Educational strategies for improving adherence to these standards should be implemented. Appropriate and thorough hand hygiene is the most important factor for reducing infectious diseases in the child-care setting.

In the United States, there are 11 diseases and organisms for which all children should be immunized unless there are contraindications: diphtheria, pertussis, tetanus, measles, mumps, rubella, polio, hepatitis B, varicella, *H. influenzae* type b, and *S. pneumoniae*. Immunization against hepatitis A is routinely recommended for children 2 yr of age and older in high-risk groups and in certain geographic areas, including 11 western states. Immunization against influenza of children 6–23 mo of age is recommended, when feasible. High levels of immunization exist among children in licensed child-care facilities, in part because of laws in almost all states requiring age-appropriate immunizations of children attending licensed child-care programs and in part because of the increased rates of immunization of all children in the United States. The use of vaccines has had a significant beneficial effect on the health of children in child-care settings. Use of *H. influenzae* type b conjugate vaccines has practically eliminated disease associated with invasive *H. influenzae* type b organisms. HBV, varicella, conjugate pneumococcal vaccines, and hepatitis A vaccine in certain geographic locations should also benefit children in child-care centers. The role of influenza vaccine among children and adults in child-care settings requires further evaluation.

Child-care providers should receive all immunizations that are recommended routinely for adults. Local public health authorities should be notified about cases of communicable disease involving children or providers in child-care settings.

Standards. Every state has specific standards for licensing and reviewing child-care centers and family child-care homes. The American Academy of Pediatrics and the American Public Health Association jointly publish comprehensive health and safety performance standards that can be used by pediatricians and other health care professionals to guide decisions about infectious diseases and other health care related matters in child-care facilities (available in print form and at http://nrc.uchsc.edu/).

Alho O-P, Laara E, Oja H: Public health impact of various risk factors for acute otitis media in Northern Finland. *Am J Epidemiol* 1996;143:1149–56.

American Academy of Pediatrics and the American Public Health Association: *Caring for Our Children: National Health and Safety Performance Standards: Guidelines for Out-of-Home Childcare Programs,* 2nd ed. Elk Grove, IL, American Academy of Pediatrics, 2002.

Carabin H, Gyorkos TW, Soto JC, et al: Estimation of direct and indirect costs because of common infections in toddlers attending day care centers. *Pediatrics* 1999;103:556–64.

Churchill RB, Pickering LK: Infection control challenges in childcare centers. *Infect Dis Clin North Am* 1997;11:347–65.

Dagan, R, Sikuler-Cohen M, Zamir O, et al: Effect of a conjugate pneumococcal vaccine on the occurrence of respiratory infections and antibiotic use in day-care center attendees. *Pediatr Infect Dis J* 2001;20:951–58.

Helfand RF, Khan AS, Pallansch MA, et al: Echovirus 30 infection and aseptic meningitis in parents of children attending a childcare center. *J Infect Dis* 1994; 169:1133–37.

Holmes SJ, Morrow AL, Pickering LK: Childcare practices: Effects of social changes on epidemiology of infectious diseases and antibiotic resistance. *Epidemiol Rev* 1996;18:10–28.

Hurwitz ES, Haber M, Chang A, et al: Effectiveness of influenza vaccination of day care children in reducing influenza-related morbidity among household contacts. *JAMA* 284:1677–82.

Louhiala PJ, Jaakkola N, Ruotsalainen R, et al: Day-care centers and diarrhea: A public health perspective. *J Pediatr* 1997;131:476–79.

MacDonald JK, Boase J, Stewart LK, et al: Active and passive surveillance for communicable diseases in childcare facilities, Seattle-King County, Washington. *Am J Public Health* 1997;87:1951–55.

Nafstad P, Hagen JA, Øie L, et al: Day care centers and respiratory health. *Pediatrics* 1999;103:753–58.

National Institute of Child Health and Human Development Early Childcare Research Network: Childcare and common communicable illnesses. Results from the National Institute of Child Health and Human Development Study of Early Child Care. *Arch Pediatr Adolesc Med* 2001;155:481–88.

Pass RF: Day care centers and the spread of cytomegalovirus and parvovirus B19. *Pediatr Ann* 1991;20:419–26.

Reves RR, Pickering LK: Impact of child day care on infectious diseases in adults. *Infect Dis Clin North Am* 1992;6:239–50.

Roberts L, Smith W, Jorm L, et al: Effect of infection control measures on the frequency of upper respiratory infection in childcare: A randomized, controlled trial. *Pediatrics* 105:738–42.

Shah S, Hoffman R, Shillam P, et al: Prolonged fecal shedding of *Escherichia coli* O157:H7 during an outbreak at a day care center. *Clin Infect Dis* 1996;23: 835–36.

Thrane N, Olesen C, Mortensen JT, et al: Influence of day care attendance on the use of systemic antibiotics in 0- to 2-year-old children. *Pediatrics* 2001;107: E76.

Chapter 285

Health Advice for Children Traveling Internationally

Chandy C. John and Robert A. Salata

The health risks and pre-travel requirements of children traveling internationally, particularly those who are younger than 2 years of age, differ from those of adults. Many physicians trained in developed countries are unfamiliar with the health hazards of international travel and with the frequently changing recommendations of measures to prevent illness during international travel. In the United States, recommendations and vaccine requirements for travel to different countries are provided in publications by the Centers for Disease Control and Prevention (CDC), including *Health Information for International Travel* (available from the Superintendent of Documents, U.S. Government Printing Office, Washington, DC 20402-9235, and also at www.cdc.gov/travel/yb/index.htm).

General Travel Preparation. Parents of traveling children should seek medical consultation at least 4–6 wk before departure to obtain a realistic assessment of health risks, a schedule of vaccinations and list of medications, and instructions on dealing with disease during travel.

HEALTH INSURANCE. Parents should be encouraged to ask their insurers whether their health care plan covers health care internationally. If it does, parents should ask about the need for preauthorization for medical treatment, the level of co-payment required, and whether emergency medical evacuation is covered. Additional travel insurance that covers emergency medical evacuation and the costs of local care is available at reasonable rates through various providers, and parents should be made aware of this option.

UNDERLYING MEDICAL ILLNESS. Parents of traveling children should be asked whether the child has any current health problems or has had any problems in the past that have required medical evaluation or medication. Children with medical conditions should take with them a brief medical summary. Parents should be counseled to take a sufficient supply of prescription medications for their children and to ensure that the bottles are clearly identified. For children requiring care by specialists, an international directory for that specialty can be consulted. A directory of physicians worldwide who speak English and who have met certain qualifications is available from the

International Association for Medical Assistance to Travelers (736 Center Street, Lewiston, NY 14092; telephone: 716-754-4883). If medical care is needed urgently when abroad, sources of information include the American embassy or consulate, hotel managers, travel agents catering to foreign tourists, and missionary hospitals. Children with chronic cardiopulmonary disease, diabetes, allergies, and gastrointestinal problems, especially diarrhea associated with malabsorption or inflammatory bowel disease, are at particular risk for health problems when traveling. Patients with insulin-dependent diabetes or hemophilia should carry an adequate supply of sterile needles, syringes, and disinfectant swabs. Special arrangements should be made for patients with bleeding disorders, those on anticoagulation therapy, and those who require hemodialysis. Biologic products such as clotting factor concentrates or immune globulin should be avoided if manufactured abroad. A travel health kit consisting of prescription medications and nonprescription items such as acetaminophen, an antihistamine, oral rehydration solution packets, antibiotic ointment, bandages, insect repellent, and sunscreen is highly recommended for all children.

SAFETY. Injuries and motor vehicle accidents are the major causes of serious disability and loss of life during travel. The use of safety belts for children, preferably sitting in the rear seat, should be emphasized. When possible, child safety-restraint seats should be taken on the trip. Travelers to remote areas should be warned about the risks of contact with stray dogs (rabies), rodents (plague), and venomous animals (snake and scorpion bites can be fatal in infants). Swimming or diving in contaminated water can result in serious injury and can increase the risk of infections, including schistosomiasis, leptospirosis, and primary amebic meningoencephalitis. Many illnesses that develop in traveling children are related to risks that can be modified with proper advice and supervision by parents.

INFECTIOUS DISEASE PRECAUTIONS. Infectious disease risks to traveling children can generally be divided into three categories: those that are foodborne, those that are transmitted by insects, and those from contact with an infected person or by needle or blood exposure.

Ingestion of contaminated food or water makes travel-associated diarrhea the most common health complaint among international travelers. Among the bacterial and protozoan infections children can acquire from contaminated water are shigellosis, salmonellosis, *Escherichia coli* infections, cholera, giardiasis, amebiasis, and cryptosporidiosis. Viral infections, particularly rotavirus infections, are also a major cause of travel-associated diarrhea in children. Boiled water, hot beverages made with boiled water, and canned or bottled carbonated beverages are generally safest. Ice should be avoided, and tap water should not be used when brushing teeth. Boiling water for at least 1 minute is the most reliable method of water disinfection. An acceptable alternative is the use of a micropore filter with an on-demand iodine release system. Unpeeled fruit, uncooked vegetables, unpasteurized milk, milk products such as cheese, and undercooked meat or fish may all be contaminated and should be avoided. Fish, especially reef fish, red snapper, and barracuda, are of particular concern because they may possess toxins. Breast-feeding should be encouraged for young children, especially infants younger than 6 mo.

Insect-borne infections for which traveling children are at risk include malaria, yellow fever, dengue, Japanese encephalitis, filariasis, trypanosomiasis, and onchocerciasis, depending on the area of travel. Malaria, yellow fever, Japanese encephalitis, and filariasis are typically caused by night-biting mosquitoes, whereas dengue is usually caused by day-biting mosquitoes. Exposure to insect bites can be avoided by restricting high-risk activities, staying indoors in a screened and protected area from dusk to dawn, wearing appropriate attire, and using insect repellents containing permethrin or N,N-diethyl-M-toluamide (DEET). Rare instances of toxic encephalopathy have been reported in young children with exposure to high concentrations of DEET, but use of repellent with no more than 30% DEET and avoidance of repeated applications minimizes the risk of this complication. Bed nets, particularly permethrin-impregnated bed nets, also decrease the risk of insect bites.

Many of the infections that may be acquired by children traveling internationally through contact with other individuals are preventable by routine childhood immunizations. Other diseases transmitted through human contact include viral respiratory and gastrointestinal infections, hepatitis, and sexually transmitted diseases, including HIV infection. Many of these diseases are more prevalent in developing countries than in the United States. Adolescent travelers should be reminded that sexual encounters and needle or blood exposure (including tattooing and body piercing) carry a significant risk of HIV and hepatitis infection. Systematic screening of blood donations for HIV and other blood-borne infections is not yet feasible in many developing countries, so the safety of transfusion services in these countries cannot be ensured. Travelers may wish to have their blood typed before departure to determine whether family members or travel companions have similar blood types and might be able to donate blood for transfusion in an emergency situation.

Immunizations. Parents should allow 4–6 wk before departure for optimal administration of vaccines to their children, because some immunizations require repeated doses for full protection and some vaccines and medications require either simultaneous or staggered dosing for optimal efficacy. The vaccines currently indicated for children traveling internationally, whether part of routine childhood immunization or travel-related, can be given concurrently with no decrease in safety or efficacy. Live-attenuated viral vaccines should be administered concurrently or at least 30 days apart to minimize interference. Intramuscular immune globulin (IG) interferes with the immune response to measles immunization and possibly to varicella immunization. If a child requires measles or varicella immunization, the vaccines should be given either 2 wk before or 3 mo after IG administration. IG does not interfere with the immune response to oral typhoid, oral poliovirus, or yellow fever vaccines.

Vaccine products produced in eggs (e.g., yellow fever, influenza) may contain an allergenic substance that causes hypersensitivity responses, including anaphylaxis in persons with known severe egg sensitivity. Screening by inquiring about adverse effects when eating eggs is a reasonable way to identify those at risk for anaphylaxis from receiving influenza or yellow fever vaccines. Although measles and mumps vaccines are produced in chick embryo cell cultures, children with egg allergy are at very low risk for anaphylaxis with these vaccines. Most hypersensitivity reactions to measles-containing vaccines have been attributed to trace amounts of gelatin or neomycin.

In general, live-virus vaccines (e.g., oral poliovirus, measles, varicella) and live bacterial vaccines (e.g., bacille Calmette-Guérin [BCG], oral typhoid) are contraindicated in immunocompromised persons (see Table 282–5). However, HIV-infected children who are not severely immunocompromised (see Chapter 254) should receive measles and varicella vaccines. Asymptomatic HIV-infected children may also be vaccinated against yellow fever if the risk is significant, but children with symptomatic HIV infection should not receive yellow fever vaccine. Inactivated vaccines and toxoids are not contraindicated in immunocompromised children but may be associated with diminished immune responses.

ROUTINE CHILDHOOD VACCINATIONS. All children who travel should be immunized according to the routine childhood immunization schedule with all vaccines appropriate for their age (see Chapter 282). The immunization schedule can be accelerated to maximize protection for traveling children, especially for unvaccinated or incompletely vaccinated children (see Table 282–1).

Diphtheria, Tetanus, and Pertussis. Diphtheria is endemic in many developing countries. After the disintegration of the Soviet Union in 1991, diphtheria re-emerged in the new independent states. The highest incidence of diphtheria has been reported from Azerbaijan, Tajikistan, and Latvia. Tetanus is a major cause of worldwide neonatal mortality and is most prevalent in tropical countries. Neonatal tetanus usually occurs in infants born to inadequately vaccinated mothers in unhygienic conditions. Pertussis is common in developing countries and in some developed nations where pertussis immunization is less widespread than in the United States because of earlier concerns about pertussis vaccine side effects.

Protection is attained with four doses of DTaP, a booster at 4–6 yr of age, and subsequent tetanus boosters (with adult-type diphtheria and tetanus toxoids [dT]) every 10 yr (see Chapter 282). The schedule can be accelerated for children traveling internationally (Table 285–1). DT should be used for children younger than 7 yr of age and who have a contraindication to pertussis vaccine. Pertussis vaccination is not recommended for persons 7 yr of age or older.

Haemophilus influenzae type b. Severe *H. influenzae* type b infection is most common in children 6 mo–1 yr of age, but one third of cases of invasive infection are found in children 18 mo of age or older. Before they travel, all unimmunized children younger than 60 mo and all children with chronic illness at risk for *H. influenzae* type b infections should be vaccinated (see Chapter 282).

Hepatitis B. Hepatitis B is highly prevalent in eastern and southeastern Asia, sub-Saharan Africa, and the Pacific basin. In certain parts of the world, 8–15% of the population may be chronically infected. Situations in which disease transmission can occur include receipt of blood transfusions not screened for hepatitis B surface antigen, exposure to unsterilized needles, close contact with local children who have open skin lesions, and sexual exposure. Exposure to hepatitis B is more likely for travelers residing for prolonged periods in endemic areas. Vaccination for hepatitis B is recommended for all children in the United States. The hepatitis B schedule can be accelerated (see Table 285–1). Partial protection may be provided by one or two doses.

Measles, Mumps, and Rubella. Measles is still endemic in many developing countries and in some industrialized nations. Measles vaccine, preferably in combination with mumps and rubella vaccines (MMR), should be given to all children at 12–15 mo of age and at 4–6 yr of age, unless there is a contraindication (see Chapter 301). In children traveling internationally, the second vaccination can be given as soon as 4 wk after the first. In the accelerated schedule the first MMR vaccination can be given to children as early as 6 mo of age, but if the vaccine is given at earlier than 12 mo of age, two additional doses should be given at least 4 wk apart after 12 mo of age (see Table 285–1). Infants younger than 6 mo of age are protected by maternal antibodies. HIV-infected children who travel abroad should be vaccinated unless severely immunocompromised (see Table 254–2), because measles in HIV-infected children can be a devastating illness.

Pneumococcus. *Streptococcus pneumoniae* is the leading cause of bacterial pneumonia and among the leading causes of bacteremia and bacterial meningitis in children in developing and industrialized nations. Immunization against *S. pneumoniae* with a protein-conjugated 7-valent pneumococcal vaccine is now part of routine childhood immunization in the United States. The four-dose schedule starts at 2 mo of age but can be accelerated for children preparing to travel (see Table 285–1). Unimmunized children older than 2 yr of age should be immunized only if they are at high risk, such as children with sickle cell disease, asplenia, HIV infection, congenital immunodeficiency, nephrotic syndrome, chronic cardiac or pulmonary disease, and those on immunosuppressive medication (see Chapter 282).

Poliomyelitis. Poliomyelitis was eradicated from the Western hemisphere in 1991, but it remains endemic in several developing countries. The poliovirus vaccination schedule in the United States is now a four-dose, all inactivated poliovirus (IPV) regimen (see Chapter 282). Immunization can be started as early as 4–6 wk of age (see Table 285–1). In the United States, oral poliovirus vaccine (OPV) is now recommended only for children who will be traveling in less than 4 wk to an area where polio is endemic or epidemic, that is, those who

TABLE 285–1. Accelerated Schedule of Routine Childhood Immunizations if Necessary for Travel

Vaccine	Routine Schedule	Accelerated Schedule
Diphtheria, tetanus, pertussis	DTaP: 2, 4, 6, and 15–18 mo of age DTaP: 4–6 yr of age (booster) dT every 10 yr	DTaP: 6, 10, and 14 wk of age; 4th dose 6 mo after 3rd dose DTaP: 4 yr of age (booster) dT every 5 yr if at high risk
Haemophilus influenzae type b	HbOC or PRP-T: 2, 4, 6, and 12–15 mo of age PRP-OMP: 2, 4, and 12 mo of age	HbOC or PRP-T: 6, 10, and 14 wk and 12 mo of age PRP-OMP: 6 and 10 wk and 12 mo of age
Hepatitis B	Birth, 1–2 mo and 6 mo of age	Birth, 1 and 2 mo of age; booster at 12 mo of age
Measles, mumps, rubella	MMR: 12–15 mo and 4–6 yr of age Not routinely recommended for children <12 mo of age	MMR: Two doses at ≥12 mo of age, ≥4 wk apart May give first measles dose as early as 6 mo of age, with additional two doses age ≥12 mo, 4 wk apart
Poliomyelitis	IPV: 2, 4, and 6 mo of age; booster at 4–6 yr of age No additional boosters unless traveling to an endemic area	IPV: 6, 10, and 14 wk of age; booster at 4–6 yr of age A single IPV lifetime booster for adolescents and adults who have completed primary immunization
Pneumococcus	Pneumococcal conjugate (PCV): 2, 4, 6, and 12–15 mo of age	PCV7: 6, 10, and 14 wk of age; 4th dose 2 mo after 3rd dose
Varicella	12–18 mo of age	12 mo (two doses 1 mo apart for persons ≥13 yr of age)

cannot receive two doses of IPV before departure. Individuals who are immunocompromised or contacts of an immunocompromised person should never receive OPV. Unvaccinated adults who are at increased risk of exposure to poliovirus and who cannot complete the recommended IPV regimen (0, 1–2, and 6–12 mo) should receive three doses of IPV given at least 4 wk apart.

Varicella. All children 12 mo of age or older who have no history of varicella vaccination or chickenpox should be vaccinated unless there is a contraindication to vaccination (see Chapter 282). Infants younger than 6 mo of age are generally protected by maternal antibodies. Children younger than 13 yr of age require only one dose; children 13 yr of age or older require two doses separated by 4–8 wk.

SPECIAL VACCINATIONS FOR TRAVEL

Cholera. Cholera is present in many developing countries, but the risk of infection among travelers to these countries is very low. The killed cholera vaccine formerly used in the United States has less than 50% efficacy and is not recommended by the CDC or the World Health Organization (WHO) for travel to or from cholera-infected areas. It is no longer generally available. No country or territory currently requires cholera vaccination, but rarely a local authority may require documentation of vaccination; in such cases, a single dose is sufficient to satisfy local requirements. If cholera vaccine is given, it should be given at least 3 wk apart from yellow fever vaccination. A new oral live cholera vaccine is available in Canada and many European countries for use in children age 2 yr and older; it is not currently available in the United States.

Hepatitis A. Hepatitis A virus is endemic in most of the world, and travelers are at risk even if their travel is restricted to the usual tourist routes. Hepatitis A infection can occur as a result of eating shellfish harvested from sewage-contaminated waters, eating unwashed vegetables or fruits, or eating food prepared by an asymptomatic carrier of hepatitis A virus. Young children infected with hepatitis A are often asymptomatic, but they may transmit infection to older children and adults, who are more likely to develop clinical hepatitis. Hepatitis A immunization or immune globulin prophylaxis is recommended for children traveling to a developing country and should probably be given to all traveling children regardless of destination, because few areas carry no risk of this infection.

The two inactivated hepatitis A vaccines currently available in the United States are approved by the Food and Drug Administration only for children 2 yr of age and older. Hepatitis A vaccine in two doses intramuscularly (0.5 mL for 2–17 yr of age; 1 mL for ≥18 yr of age), given 6–12 mo apart, is recommended for children traveling to countries with intermediate or high hepatitis A endemicity (areas other than the United States, Canada, Australia, New Zealand, Japan, Western Europe, and Scandinavia). Protective immunity develops 2–4 wk after receiving the initial vaccine dose. A combined, three-dose hepatitis A and hepatitis B vaccine is now available in the United States, but it is licensed for use only in adults older than 18 yr of age.

Children younger than 2 yr of age and children who will be traveling to an endemic area in less than 2 wk should receive intramuscular immune globulin (IG). For short-term protection (1–2 mo), 0.02 mL/kg of IG is given IM; for long-term protection (3–5 mo), 0.06 mL/kg of IG is given IM and repeated every 5 mo while exposure to hepatitis A continues. Immune globulin can be administered at the same time as the inactivated vaccine but should be given at a separate site and in a separate syringe. If a child requires MMR or varicella immunization, these live-attenuated viral vaccines should be given either 2 wk before or 3 mo after IG administration.

Influenza. The risk for exposure to influenza during international travel varies depending on the time of year, destination, and intermingling of persons from different parts of the world where influenza may be circulating. In the tropics, such as the Caribbean, influenza can occur throughout the year. In the temperate regions of the Southern Hemisphere, including Australia and South America, most activity occurs from April through September. In the Northern Hemisphere, including the United States and Canada, influenza generally occurs from November through March. Influenza vaccination is recommended for children ≥ 6 mo of age at increased risk for complications of influenza, including children of any age with chronic medical conditions such as chronic cardiac, renal or pulmonary disease, immunosuppressive conditions or therapy, HIV infection, sickle cell disease, and diabetes mellitus (see Chapter 282).

Japanese Encephalitis. Japanese encephalitis is a disease transmitted by mosquitoes in rural areas of Asia, where people are in close proximity to livestock. Asymptomatic cases outnumber symptomatic cases by at least 200 to 1, but when symptomatic the disease has a 10–70% case fatality rate. The risk in travelers is extremely low, less than 1 case/million travelers, but the risk is highest in children. The disease occurs primarily from June to September in temperate zones and throughout the entire year in tropical zones. Vaccination is recommended for travelers planning visits of greater than 1 mo to rural areas of Asia where the disease is endemic, especially areas of rice or pig farming, or shorter visits to such an area if the traveler will frequently be outdoors (e.g., camping or hiking). Risk of infection can be greatly reduced by following the standard precautions to avoid mosquito bites. Parents of very young children should be discouraged from traveling with their children to high-risk areas.

The inactivated Japanese encephalitis vaccine is licensed for children 1 yr of age and older. It is administered in three doses (0.5 mL for 1–3 yr of age; 1 mL for 3 yr of age and older) subcutaneously on days 0, 7, and 30, or on days 0, 7, and 14 in an accelerated dosing schedule. The vaccine has an efficacy of more than 95%, but hypersensitivity reactions occur in up to 0.6% of vaccine recipients; 1 in 1,000 vaccinees have urticarial reactions or facial or oropharyngeal angioedema that may occur within minutes or up to 2 wk after vaccination. The series should be completed 2 wk before travel so that any adverse reactions to the vaccine can be observed and treated.

Meningococcus. *Neisseria meningitidis* causes epidemic and endemic disease worldwide (see Chapter 176). Most cases occur in the "meningitis belt" of sub-Saharan Africa between December and June. Epidemics have also occurred in the Indian subcontinent and Saudi Arabia. Cases in American travelers are rare, and vaccination is indicated primarily in travelers to an area with an active outbreak or those who may have prolonged contact with the local population in an endemic area, especially in crowded conditions. Saudi Arabia requires all pilgrims to Mecca to have documentation of meningococcal vaccination 10 or more days but less than 3 yr before arrival. Serogroup A is the most common cause of epidemics outside the United States, but serogroup C and, rarely, serogroup B have also been associated with epidemics.

The only meningococcal vaccine currently available in the United States is the quadrivalent polysaccharide A/C/Y/W-135 vaccine. The vaccine is ineffective against serogroup A in infants younger than 3 mo of age and may be only partially effective against this serogroup in children 3–11 mo of age. Children younger than 2 yr of age are not protected against the other serogroups. The meningococcus vaccine (0.5 mL SC) is recommended for children age 2 yr and older who are at risk for meningococcal disease caused by a vaccine serogroup, as well as for children 3 mo of age and older who are at risk for serogroup A meningococcal disease. Children vaccinated before 4 yr of age should be revaccinated after 2–3 yr if they remain in an endemic area. Highly effective meningococcal conjugate vaccines against serogroups A and C are available in Europe but have not yet been licensed for use in the United States.

Rabies. The risk of rabies is currently the highest in countries where rabies in dogs is uncontrolled, including Colombia, Ecuador, El Salvador, Guatemala, India, Mexico, Nepal, Philippines, Thailand, and Vietnam. Rabies is also endemic in most other countries of Africa, Asia, and Central and South America. Children are at particular risk because facial bites are more common in children. Pre-exposure prophylaxis should be considered if a child will be in an endemic area for longer than 1 mo or will be traveling to an area where rapid, effective post-exposure prophylaxis may not be available. An animal bite in a rabies-endemic area is a medical emergency. Immediate medical care should be sought at a facility that can administer appropriate postexposure rabies prophylaxis. If possible, the animal in question should be caught and quarantined for 10 days of observation for signs of rabies. Postexposure prophylaxis is required even for individuals who received pre-exposure vaccination.

Three inactivated rabies vaccines are available in the United States for pre-exposure vaccination: the human diploid cell vaccine (HDCV), the rabies vaccine absorbed (RVA), and the purified chick embryo cell vaccine (PCEC). Pre-exposure prophylaxis is given either intramuscularly (HDCV, RVA, or PCEC) as three doses (1 mL) on days 0, 7, and 28, or intradermally (HDCV) as three doses (0.1 mL) on days 0, 7 and 28. Postexposure prophylaxis is given as five doses (1 mL) of HDCV, RVA, or PCEC vaccine intramuscularly on days 0, 3, 7, 14, and 28 if previously unvaccinated and two doses (1 mL) intramuscularly on days 0 and 3 if previously vaccinated. Previously unvaccinated individuals should receive rabies immune globulin (RIG) (20 IU/ kg, with as much of the dose as possible infiltrated around the wound site) at the time of initial postexposure prophylaxis. Previously vaccinated individuals should not receive RIG. Children receiving mefloquine or chloroquine may have limited immune reactions to intradermal rabies vaccine and should be vaccinated intramuscularly. Purified cell culture–derived vaccines are not always available abroad; travelers should be aware that rabies vaccines derived from neural tissue carry an increased risk of adverse reactions, often with neurologic sequelae. Unpurified or purified equine RIG preparations are still used in some developing countries and are also associated with a higher risk of severe reactions, including serum sickness and anaphylaxis. If rabies prophylaxis is initiated abroad, neutralizing titers should be checked on return and immunization completed with a cell culture–derived vaccine.

Tuberculosis. The risk of tuberculosis in the typical traveler is low. All children traveling for prolonged periods to high-risk areas should have tuberculin skin testing done before and after travel. Immunization with bacille Calmette-Guérin (BCG) is controversial. It is not frequently used in the United States, but some authorities believe it should be given to children, especially infants, who will reside for a long time in an area with a high prevalence of tuberculosis or with multidrug-resistant tuberculosis because it is highly protective against meningeal and miliary tuberculosis in children.

Typhoid. *Salmonella* ser. Typhi (*Salmonella typhi*) infection, or typhoid fever, is common in many developing countries in Asia, Africa, and Latin America (see Chapter 181.2). Typhoid vaccination is recommended for children traveling to the Indian subcontinent, the area of highest risk, and for individuals traveling to endemic areas who are at higher risk of infection: long-term travelers (those traveling for >4 wk), backpackers, and travelers staying with friends or relatives in developing countries. Vaccination should be strongly considered for all children traveling to endemic areas, especially if exposure to contaminated food and water is likely.

Two typhoid vaccines, the intramuscular Vi-polysaccharide vaccine and oral Ty21a strain live-attenuated vaccine, are recommended for use in children in the United States. The intramuscular Vi-polysaccharide vaccine is licensed for use in children 2 yr of age and older. It is given as a single dose (0.5 mL IM), with a booster every 2 yr. It can be given any time before departure, but it should ideally be administered 1 mo or more before travel. The oral Ty21a vaccine can only be used in children 6 yr of age and older. The oral vaccine is given in four doses over a 1-wk period: one enteric-coated capsule is swallowed whole with a cool drink, at least 1 hour before a meal, every other day until the four doses are completed. The course should be repeated as a booster every 5 yr if there is continued exposure to typhoid. Antibiotics and the antimalarial drugs mefloquine and chloroquine inhibit the immune response to the oral Ty21a vaccine. The vaccine should not be given for 24 hr after the most recent dose of antibiotic or mefloquine or chloroquine. Oral Ty21a vaccine should not be given to immunocompromised children; these children should receive the intramuscular Vi-polysaccharide vaccine. An early-generation heat-phenol–inactivated vaccine (strain Ty2) is efficacious and remains available, but use of this vaccine is no longer recommended owing to the high incidence of adverse reactions.

Yellow Fever. Yellow fever (see Chapter 247) is a mosquito-borne viral illness resembling other viral hemorrhagic fevers (see Chapter 248) but with more prominent hepatic involvement. Yellow fever is present in tropical areas of South America and Africa. In the past 15 years, Nigeria and Peru have reported the greatest number of cases.

Yellow fever vaccination is indicated in children older than 9 months traveling to an endemic area. Some countries require yellow fever vaccination by law for travelers arriving from endemic areas. Some African countries require evidence of vaccination from all entering travelers. Current recommendations can be obtained by contacting state or local health departments or the Division of Vector-Borne Infectious Diseases of the CDC (telephone: 404-332-4555; or website: www.cdc. gov). Most countries accept a medical waiver for children who are too young to be vaccinated (<4 mo of age) and for individuals with a contraindication to vaccination, such as immunodeficiency. Children with asymptomatic HIV infection may be vaccinated if exposure to yellow fever virus cannot be avoided.

Yellow fever vaccine (0.5 mL SC), a live-attenuated vaccine (17D strain) developed in chick embryos, is safe and highly effective in children older than 9 mo of age, but in young infants it is associated with an increased risk of encephalitis (0.4%) and other severe reactions. Yellow fever vaccine should never be administered to infants younger than 4 mo of age; infants 4–6 mo of age should be vaccinated only in consultation with the CDC; infants 6–9 mo of age should be vaccinated only if they cannot avoid traveling to areas with an ongoing epidemic. Children with a history of anaphylactic reactions to eggs should also not receive yellow fever vaccine. Long-lived, perhaps life-time immunity develops to this vaccine; however, international travel certificates require proof of immunization within 10 yr. Cholera vaccination is not currently recommended in the United States but if given should be given 3 wk apart from yellow fever vaccination.

Traveler's Diarrhea. Traveler's diarrhea, characterized by a twofold or greater increase in the frequency of unformed bowel movements, occurs in as many as 40% of all travelers overseas. Children, especially those younger than 3 yr of age, have a higher incidence of diarrhea, more severe symptoms, and more prolonged symptoms than adults. Traveler's diarrhea is usually acquired through ingestion of fecally contaminated food and water. Diverse infectious agents (bacteria, viruses, and parasites) have been associated with traveler's diarrhea; enterotoxigenic *E. coli* is still the most frequent cause. Other bacterial causes include *Shigella, Salmonella, Campylobacter, Vibrio cholerae, Vibrio parahaemolyticus, Aeromonas hydrophilia,* and *Plesiomonas shigelloides.* Protozoan infections such as *Entamoeba histolytica, Giardia lamblia, Cryptosporidium parvum,* and *Isospora* are more common in long-term travelers. Rotavirus has also been associated with traveler's diarrhea. The most important risk factor for traveler's diarrhea is the country of destination. High-risk areas (attack rates of 25–50%) include developing countries of Latin America, Africa, the Middle East, and Asia. Intermediate risk occurs in the Mediterranean, China, and Israel. Low-risk areas include North America, Northern Europe, Australia, and New Zealand. Immunocompromised children, including children with HIV, are at increased for complications from bacterial causes of traveler's diarrhea, particularly *Salmonella.* Careful selection and preparation of food and water can significantly reduce the risk of developing traveler's diarrhea (see "General Travel Preparation"). Chemoprophylactic agents for traveler's diarrhea are not recommended for children.

Dehydration is the greatest threat presented by a diarrheal illness in a small child. Parents should be made aware of the symptoms and signs of dehydration. Prepackaged WHO/UNICEF oral rehydration solution (ORS) packets, which are available at stores or pharmacies in almost all developing countries, should be part of a child's travel kit. ORS should be mixed as directed with bottled or boiled water and given slowly, as tolerated, to the child. Antimotility agents such as diphenoxylate (Lomotil) and loperamide (Imodium) should be avoided in young children; loperamide (2 mg tid PO) may be useful for children older than 8 yr of age if they do not have fever or bloody stools. Bismuth subsalicylate (5 mL for 3–5 yr of age; 10 mL for 6–8 yr of age; 15 mL for 9–11 yr of age; 30 mL for ≥12 yr of age) as often as every 30 min for eight doses, with no more than eight doses/24 hr, decreases the rate of stooling and shortens the duration of illness. Higher doses of bismuth subsalicylate should be avoided because of concerns of salicylate toxicity. Bismuth subsalicylate should not be used if the child may have influenza or is in an area experiencing an influenza outbreak, because there is an increased risk of Reye syndrome in children with influenza who receive salicylate therapy.

Increased antibiotic resistance among the organisms that cause traveler's diarrhea has led to new recommendations for presumptive treatment of traveler's diarrhea. Presumptive self-treatment is usually recommended for adults, and most experts agree that it should also be given to children. For adults 18 yr of age and older the recommended regimen is ciprofloxacin (500 mg), norfloxacin (400 mg), or ofloxacin (300 mg) orally twice daily for 3 days. The recommended drug for children age 2 mo or older was formerly trimethoprim-sulfamethoxazole (TMP-SMZ), but increased bacterial resistance has diminished its efficacy. Azithromycin (either 10 mg/kg/day for 3 days or 10 mg/kg/day 1, 5 mg/kg days 2–5) is not specifically approved

for the treatment of diarrhea, but it is highly effective against most pathogens that cause traveler's diarrhea and is probably the drug of choice for children with traveler's diarrhea. Antimicrobial therapy for traveler's diarrhea in infants and young children should be administered in consultation with a physician. This is particularly true if the illness is severe, persists for longer than 3 days, or is associated with bloody stools, temperature greater than 102°F, chills, vomiting, or moderate to severe dehydration.

Malaria Chemoprophylaxis. Malaria, a mosquito-borne infection, is the leading parasitic cause of death in children worldwide (see Chapter 264). Of the four *Plasmodium* species that infect humans, *P. falciparum* causes the greatest morbidity and mortality. Each year, more than 8 million U.S. citizens visit parts of the world where malaria is endemic (sub-Saharan Africa, Central and South America, India, Southeast Asia, Oceania). Given the major resurgence of malaria, physicians in developed countries are increasingly required to give advice on prevention, diagnosis, and treatment of malaria. The CDC maintains updated information at www.cdc.gov/travel/index. htm, as well as a malaria hotline for physicians (770-488-7788). It is important to check this updated information because continuing changes in the risk of developing malaria in many areas of the world, changing *Plasmodium* resistance patterns, and the availability of new antimalarial medications result in regular modifications of recommendations for prophylaxis and treatment.

Avoidance of mosquitoes and barrier protection from mosquitoes are an important part of malaria prevention for travelers to endemic areas. The *Anopheles* mosquito feeds from dusk to dawn. Travelers should remain in well-screened areas, wear clothing that covers most of the body, sleep under a bed net (ideally one impregnated with permethrin), and use insect repellents with DEET during these hours. Parents should be discouraged from taking a young child on a trip that will entail evening or night-time exposure in rural areas of countries with chloroquine- or multidrug-resistant *P. falciparum.*

Chemoprophylaxis is the cornerstone of malaria prevention for nonimmune children and adults who travel to malaria endemic areas, but it is not a replacement for other protective measures because no chemoprophylaxis regimen guarantees complete protection against malaria. Travelers often do not take malaria prophylaxis as prescribed; frequently they do not take it at all. They are more likely to use prophylactic antimalarial drugs if their physicians provide appropriate recommendations and education before departure. However, in one survey, only 14% of persons who sought medical advice obtained correct information about malaria prevention and prophylaxis.

Resistance of *P. falciparum* to the traditional chemoprophylactic agent, chloroquine, is rapidly increasing worldwide, and in most areas of the world other agents must be used (Table 285–2). Factors that must be considered in choosing appropriate chemoprophylaxis medications and dosing schedules include age of the child, travel itinerary (including whether the child will be traveling to areas of risk within a particular country and whether chloroquine-resistant *P. falciparum* is present in the country), vaccinations being given (particularly rabies and oral typhoid, see earlier), allergic or other known adverse reactions to antimalarial agents, and the availability of medical care during travel.

Weekly mefloquine is the drug of choice for malaria chemoprophylaxis in children and adults traveling to areas with chloroquine-resistant *P. falciparum.* Although mefloquine is FDA-approved only for children weighing more than 15 kg, the CDC recommends mefloquine prophylaxis for all children

TABLE 285–2. Chemoprophylaxis of Malaria in Children

Area	Drug	Dosage (Oral)
Chloroquine-resistant area	Mefloquine*	<15 kg: 4.6 mg base (5 mg salt)/kg/wk 15–19 kg: ¼ tablet/wk 20–30 kg: ½ tablet/wk 31–45 kg: ¾ tablet wk >45 kg: 1 tablet/wk (228-mg base)
	Doxycyline† Atovaquone/proguanil‡ (Malarone)	2 mg/kg/24 hr (maximum: 100 mg) Pediatric tablets: 62.5 mg atovaquone/25 mg proguanil Adult tablets: 250 mg proguanil/100 mg proguanil 11–20 kg: 1 *pediatric* tablet once daily 21–30 kg: 2 *pediatric* tablets once daily 31–40 kg: 3 *pediatric* tablets once daily >40 kg: 1 *adult* tablet once daily 5 mg base/kg/wk (maximum: 300 mg base)
Chloroquine-sensitive area	Chloroquine phosphate *plus* Pyrimethamine/sulfadoxine for presumptive treatment§	<1 yr: ¼ tablet 1–3 yr: ½ tablet 4–8 yr: 1 tablet 9–14 yr: 2 tablets >14 yr: 3 tablets

*Chloroquine and mefloquine should be started 1 wk before departure and continued 4 wk after last exposure.
†Doxycycline should be started 1 day before departure and continued for 4 wk after last exposure. Do not use in children <8 yr old or pregnant women.
‡Atovaquone/proguanil (Malarone) should be started 1 to 2 days before departure and continued for 7 days after last exposure.
§Sulfadoxine/pyrimethamine resistance is present in South America, Africa, and Asia. It can be used for presumptive treatment if medical care is not available within 24 hr, while promptly seeking medical care.

regardless of weight because the risk of acquiring severe malaria outweighs the risk of potential mefloquine toxicity. Adults have 10–25% incidence of sleep disturbance and dysphoria with mefloquine, but these side effects appear to be less common in children. Other potential side effects of mefloquine therapy include nausea and vomiting. The lack of a liquid or suspension formulation sometimes makes chloroquine and mefloquine administration difficult; they are better tolerated by children if they are "disguised" in other foods. Individuals with epilepsy or neuropsychiatric disorders should not take mefloquine. A fixed combination of atovaquone and proguanil (trade name: Malarone) was recently approved by the FDA for the prophylaxis and treatment of chloroquine-resistant *P. falciparum* malaria in adults and children. Atovaquone/proguanil is highly effective chemoprophylaxis for travelers to chloroquine-resistant malaria endemic areas. Adverse effects are infrequent, mild (abdominal pain, vomiting, and headache) and rarely result in discontinuation of the medication. Atovaquone/proguanil prophylaxis must be taken every day, so it is better suited for prophylaxis during short periods of exposure. Daily doxycycline is an alternative chemoprophylaxis regimen for chloroquine-resistant *P. falciparum* malaria that is considerably less expensive than atovaquone/proguanil. Doxycycline has been used extensively and is highly effective, but it cannot be used in children younger than 8 years old, and side effects (nausea, vomiting, photosensitivity, vaginal candidiasis) are not uncommon. Individuals given doxycycline prophylaxis should be warned to decrease exposure to direct sunlight to minimize the possibility of photosensitivity. Primaquine has also been used successfully as chemoprophylaxis, but there are limited data about its use in nonimmune children. Chloroquine, chloroquine-proguanil, and azithromycin do not provide adequate protection for children traveling to a chloroquine-resistant malaria endemic area.

Weekly chloroquine is the drug of choice for malaria chemoprophylaxis in those areas of the world where *P. falciparum* remains fully chloroquine-sensitive (Haiti, the Dominican Republic, Central America north of the Panama Canal, and some countries in the Middle East). Updated information is available at www.cdc.gov/travel.

On leaving a malaria-endemic area after a prolonged visit, travelers may require treatment with primaquine (0.3 mg/kg base or 0.5 mg/kg salt daily for 14 days) to eliminate the extraerythrocytic forms of *P. vivax* and *P. ovale* to prevent relapses. Primaquine can cause severe hemolysis in G6PD-deficient individuals. Individuals must always be screened for G6PD-deficiency before primaquine is prescribed.

Small amounts of antimalarial drugs are secreted into breast milk of lactating women. The amounts of transferred drug are not considered to be either harmful or sufficient to provide adequate prophylaxis against malaria. Prolonged infant exposure to doxycycline via breast milk is not advisable.

The Returning Traveler. Post-travel evaluations are part of travel medicine and continuing care. Children who will be traveling abroad for a prolonged period of time (>6 mo) should receive tuberculin skin testing before and after travel and should be tested for asymptomatic gastrointestinal parasitic infections on their return. Physicians unfamiliar with diseases that occur in developing countries often misdiagnose the cause of illness in a child returning from travel abroad. Fever is a particularly worrisome symptom: malaria and typhoid are the two most common causes of fever in children returning from travel to developing countries, but dozens of other illnesses acquired in these countries may cause fever. Malaria must be considered in the evaluation of any fever that develops within 1 yr, and particularly within the first 2 mo, after travel to malaria-endemic areas. Children returning from international travel who have specific signs and symptoms of illness, such as fever, rash, or chronic diarrhea, should see a pediatric travel medicine or infectious disease specialist.

Adachi JA, Ostrosky-Zeichner L, et al: Empirical antimicrobial therapy for traveler's diarrhea. *Clin Infect Dis* 2000;31:1079–83.

Centers for Disease Control and Prevention: *Health Information for International Travel 2001–2002.* Washington, DC, US Department of Health and Human Services, Public Health Services, 2001.

Fisher PR: Travel with infants and children. *Infect Dis Clin North Am* 1998;12: 355–68.

Jong EC: Travel immunizations. *Med Clin North Am* 1999;83:903–22.

Kain KC, Keystone JS: Malaria in travelers: Epidemiology, diseases, and prevention. *Infect Dis Clin North Am* 1998;12:267–84.

Kain KC, Shanks GD, Keystone JS: Malaria chemoprophylaxis in the age of drug resistance: I. Currently recommended drug regimens. *Clin Infect Dis* 2001;33: 226–34.

Ryan ET, Kain KC: Health advice and immunizations for travelers. *N Engl J Med* 2000;342:1716–25.

Schuman AJ: Preparing children and families to travel overseas. *Contemp Pediatr* 2001;18:45–59.

Sood SK: Immunization for children traveling abroad. *Pediatr Clin North Am* 2000;47:435–48.

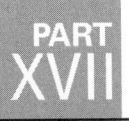
The Digestive System

SECTION 1 *Clinical Manifestations of Gastrointestinal Disease*

Robert Wyllie

Chapter 286

Normal Digestive Tract Phenomena

Gastrointestinal function varies with maturity; a symptom that might be abnormal at an older age, such as regurgitation, is normal in an infant. A fetus can swallow amniotic fluid as early as 12 wk gestation, but nutritive sucking in neonates first develops at about 34 wk gestation. The coordinated oral and pharyngeal movements necessary for swallowing solids develop within the first few months of life in term infants. Before this time, the tongue thrust is upward and outward to express milk from the nipple instead of a backward motion, which propels solids toward the esophageal inlet. By 1 mo of age, infants appear to show preferences for sweet and salty foods. Infants' interest in solids increases at about 4 mo of age. The current recommendation to begin solids at 6 mo of age is based on nutritional concepts rather than maturation of the swallowing process (see Chapter 41). Infants swallow air during feeding and must be stimulated to burp to prevent gaseous distention of the stomach.

A number of normal anatomic variations may be noted in the mouth. A short lingual frenulum ("tongue-tie") may be worrisome to parents but only rarely interferes with eating or speech, generally requiring no treatment. Surface furrowing of the tongue (i.e., a geographic or scrotal tongue) is usually a normal finding. A bifid uvula may be normal or associated with a submucous cleft of the soft palate.

Regurgitation, the result of gastroesophageal reflux, occurs commonly in the first year of life. Effortless regurgitation may dribble out of an infant's mouth but also may be forceful. In an otherwise healthy infant with regurgitation, volumes of emesis are commonly about 15–30 mL but may occasionally be larger. Most often, the infant remains happy, although possibly hungry, after an episode of regurgitation. Episodes may occur from less than one to several times per day. Regurgitation gradually resolves in 80% of infants by 6 mo of age and in 90% by 12 mo. If complications develop or regurgitation persists, gastroesophageal reflux is considered pathologic rather than merely developmental and deserves further evaluation and treatment. Complications include failure to thrive, pulmonary disease (apnea or aspiration pneumonitis), and esophagitis with its sequelae (see Chapters 304 and 305).

Infants and young children may be erratic eaters; this may be a worry to parents. A toddler may eat insatiably or refuse to consume food during a meal. There is also a tendency for toddlers and young children to eat only a limited variety of foods. Parents should be encouraged to view nutritional intake over several days and not be overly concerned about individual meals. Infancy and adolescence are periods of rapid growth; high nutrient requirements for growth may be associated with voracious appetites. The reduced appetite of toddlers and preschool children is often a worry to parents who are used to the relatively greater dietary intake during infancy. Demonstration of age-appropriate growth on a growth curve is reassuring.

The *number, color,* and *consistency of stools* may vary greatly in the same infant and between infants of similar age without apparent explanation. The earliest stools after birth consist of meconium, a dark, viscous material that is normally passed within the first 48 hr of life. With the onset of feeding, meconium is replaced by green-brown transition stools, often containing curds, and, after 4–5 days, by yellow-brown milk stools. Stool frequency is extremely variable in normal infants and may vary from none to seven per day. Breast-fed infants may have frequent small, loose stools early (transition stools) and then after 2–3 wk may have very infrequent soft stools. It is possible for a nursing infant not to pass any stool for 1–2 wk and then to have a normal soft bowel movement. The color of stool has little significance except for the presence of blood or absence of bilirubin products (white-gray rather than yellow-brown). The presence of vegetable matter, such as peas or corn, in the stool of an older infant or toddler ingesting solids is normal and suggests poor chewing and not malabsorption. A pattern of intermittent loose stools, known as "toddler's diarrhea," occurs commonly between 1 and 3 yr of age. These otherwise healthy growing children often drink excessive carbohydrate-containing beverages and eat snacks throughout the day. The stools typically occur during the day and not overnight. The volume of fluid intake is often excessive; limiting sugar-containing beverages and increasing fat in the diet often leads to resolution of the pattern of loose stools.

A *protuberant abdomen* is often noted in infants and toddlers, especially after large feedings. This may result from the combination of weak abdominal musculature, relatively large abdominal organs, and lordotic stance. In the 1st yr of life, it is common to palpate the liver 1 to 2 cm below the right costal margin. The normal liver is soft in consistency and percusses to normal size for age. A Riedel lobe is a thin projection of the right lobe of the liver that may be palpated low in the right lateral abdomen. A soft spleen tip may also be palpable as a normal finding. In thin young children, the vertebral column is easily palpable and an overlying structure may be mistaken for a mass. Commonly, pulsation of the aorta can be appreciated. Normal stool can often be palpated in the left lower quadrant in the descending or sigmoid colon.

Blood loss from the gastrointestinal tract is never normal, but swallowed blood may be misinterpreted as gastrointestinal bleeding. Maternal blood may be ingested at the time of birth or later by a nursing infant if there is bleeding near the mother's nipple. Nasal or oropharyngeal bleeding is occasionally mistaken for gastrointestinal bleeding (see Chapter 92.4). Red dyes in foods or drinks may turn the stool red but do not produce a positive test result for occult blood.

Jaundice is common in neonates, especially among premature infants, and usually results from the inability of an immature liver to conjugate bilirubin, leading to an elevated indirect component (see Chapter 91.3). Persistent elevation of indirect bilirubin levels in nursing infants may be a result of breast milk jaundice, which is usually a benign entity in full-term infants. Elevated direct bilirubin is never normal and suggests liver disease, although in infants it may be a result of extrahepatic infection (e.g., urinary tract infection). The direct bilirubin fraction should account for no more than 15% to 20% of the total bilirubin content. Indirect hyperbilirubinemia, which occurs commonly in normal newborns, tends to tint the sclerae and skin golden yellow, whereas direct hyperbilirubinemia produces a greenish yellow hue.

Chapter 287
Major Symptoms and Signs of Digestive Tract Disorders

Disorders of organs outside the gastrointestinal tract can produce symptoms and signs that mimic digestive tract disorders and should be considered in the differential diagnosis (Box 287–1). Understanding the potential pathogenesis of symptoms will allow rational diagnosis and management decisions. In children with normal growth and development, treatment may be initiated without a formal evaluation based on a presumptive diagnosis after taking a history and performing a physical examination. Poor weight gain or weight loss is often associated with a significant pathologic process and usually necessitates a more formal evaluation.

Dysphagia. Dysphagia, or difficulty swallowing, may be caused by a structural defect or motility disorder. Structural defects that cause a fixed impediment to the food bolus arise from narrowing within the esophagus, such as a stricture, web, or tumor. Extrinsic obstruction is most often caused by a vascular ring. Structural defects typically cause more problems swallowing solids than liquids. Most nonstructural causes of dysphagia are caused by motility abnormalities of the oropharynx or the esophagus. Swallowing is a complex process that starts in the mouth with mastication and lubrication of food that is formed into a bolus. The bolus is pushed to the pharynx by the tongue. The pharyngeal phase of swallowing is rapid and involves protective mechanisms to prevent food from entering the airway. The epiglottis is lowered over the larynx while the soft palate is elevated against the nasopharyngeal wall; there is a temporary arrest of respiration while the upper esophageal sphincter opens to allow the bolus to enter the esophagus. In the esophagus, peristaltic coordinated muscular contractions push the food bolus toward the stomach. The lower esophageal sphincter relaxes shortly after the upper esophageal sphincter so liquids that rapidly clear the esophagus enter the stomach without resistance.

Dysphagia during the oropharyngeal phase of swallowing is termed *transfer dysphagia* and is usually associated with neuromuscular disorders (cerebral palsy). The sensation that something is stuck in the upper esophagus is globus (formerly termed *globus hystericus*). Globus is usually associated with gastroesophageal reflux.

BOX 287–1. Some Nondigestive Tract Causes of Gastrointestinal Symptoms in Children

ANOREXIA
Systemic disease (e.g., inflammatory, neoplastic)
Cardiorespiratory compromise
Iatrogenic—drug therapy, unpalatable therapeutic diets
Depression
Anorexia nervosa

VOMITING
Inborn errors of metabolism
Medications (erythromycin, chemotherapy)
Increased intracranial pressure
Brain tumor
Infection (e.g., urinary tract)
Labyrinthitis
Adrenal insufficiency
Pregnancy
Psychogenic
Abdominal migraine
Toxins

DIARRHEA
Infection (e.g., otitis media, urinary)
Uremia
Medications (antibiotics, cisapride)
Tumors (neuroblastoma)
Pericarditis

CONSTIPATION
Hypothyroidism
Spina bifida
Psychomotor retardation
Dehydration (e.g., diabetes insipidus, renal tubular lesions)
Medications (narcotics)
Lead poisoning
Infant botulism

ABDOMINAL PAIN
Pyelonephritis, hydronephrosis, renal colic
Pneumonia
Pelvic inflammatory disease
Porphyria
Angioedema
Endocarditis
Abdominal migraine
Familial Mediterranean fever
Sexual or physical abuse
Systemic lupus erythematosus
School phobia
Sickle cell crisis
Vertebral disk inflammation
Medications (NSAIDs)
Pelvic osteomyelitis

ABDOMINAL DISTENTION OR MASS
Ascites (e.g., nephrotic syndrome, neoplasm, heart failure)
Discrete mass (e.g., Wilms' tumor, hydronephrosis, neuroblastoma, mesenteric cyst, hepatoblastoma, lymphoma)
Pregnancy

JAUNDICE
Hemolytic disease
Urinary tract infection
Sepsis
Hypothyroidism
Panhypopituitarism

When dysphagia is associated with a delay in passage through the esophagus, a child may be able to point to the level of the chest where the delay occurs; esophageal symptoms may be referred to the suprasternal notch. Therefore, when a child points to the suprasternal notch, the impaction may be found anywhere in the esophagus.

TRANSFER DYSPHAGIA. A complex sequence of neuromuscular events is involved in the transfer of foods to the upper esophagus. Suckling requires the lips to form a tight seal about the nipple while the tongue is displaced posteriorly. As the glottis closes to guard the airway, the soft palate rises to close the nasopharynx, the cricopharyngeal muscles relax, and food passes to the back of the pharynx. Solids similarly require coordinated actions; for large chunks of solid food, jaw movement and teeth become factors to consider. Salivary secretions, stimulated by the anticipation and act of ingestion, lubricate foods as they pass through the mouth. It is abnormalities of the muscles involved in the ingestion process, their innervation, strength, or coordination that usually cause transfer dysphagia in infants and children. In such cases, an oropharyngeal problem is almost always part of a more generalized neurologic or muscular problem (botulism, diphtheria, cerebral palsy). Painful oral lesions, such as acute viral stomatitis or trauma, occasionally interfere with ingestion. If the nasal air passage is seriously obstructed, the need for air causes severe distress when suckling. Although severe structural, dental, and salivary abnormalities would be expected to create difficulties, ingestion proceeds relatively well in most affected children if they are hungry.

NONTRANSFER DYSPHAGIA. Primary motility disorders causing impaired peristaltic function and dysphagia are rare in children. Motility of the distal esophagus is disordered after repair of tracheoesophageal fistula. Abnormal motility may accompany collagen vascular disorders. Achalasia rarely occurs in children. Esophageal web, tracheobronchial remnant, or vascular ring may cause dysphagia in infancy. An esophageal stricture secondary to chronic gastroesophageal reflux and esophagitis occasionally presents with dysphagia as the first manifestation. A Schatzki ring is another mechanical cause of recurrent dysphagia presenting after infancy. An esophageal foreign body or a stricture secondary to a caustic ingestion also causes dysphagia.

Regurgitation. Regurgitation is the effortless movement of stomach contents into the esophagus and mouth. It is not associated with distress, and infants with regurgitation are often hungry immediately after an episode. The lower esophageal sphincter prevents reflux of gastric contents into the esophagus (see Chapter 304). Regurgitation is a result of gastroesophageal reflux through an incompetent or, in infants, immature lower esophageal sphincter. This is often a developmental process, and regurgitation or "spitting" resolves with maturity. Regurgitation should be differentiated from vomiting, which denotes an active reflex process with a different differential diagnosis (Table 287–1).

Anorexia. Hunger and satiety centers are located in the hypothalamus; it seems likely that afferent nerves from the gastrointestinal tract to these brain centers are important determinants of the anorexia that characterizes many diseases of the stomach and intestine. Satiety is stimulated by distention of the stomach or upper small bowel, the signal being transmitted by sensory afferents, which are especially dense in the upper gut. Chemoreceptors in the intestine, influenced by the assimilation of nutrients, also affect afferent flow to the appetite centers. Impulses reach the hypothalamus from higher centers, possibly influenced by pain or the emotional disturbance of an intestinal disease. Other regulatory factors include hormones, leptin, and plasma glucose, which in turn reflect intestinal function.

Vomiting. Vomiting is a highly coordinated reflex process that may be preceded by increased salivation and begins with involuntary retching. Violent descent of the diaphragm and constriction of the abdominal muscles with relaxation of the gastric cardia actively force gastric contents back up the esophagus. This process is coordinated in the medullary vomiting center, which is influenced directly by afferent innervation and indirectly by the chemoreceptor trigger zone and higher central

TABLE 287–1. Differential Diagnosis of Emesis During Childhood

Infant	Child	Adolescent
Common		
Gastroenteritis	Gastroenteritis	Gastroenteritis
Gastroesophageal reflux	Systemic infection	GERD
Overfeeding	Gastritis	Systemic infection
Anatomic obstruction	Toxic ingestion	Toxic ingestion
Systemic infection	Pertussis syndrome	Gastritis
Pertussis syndrome	Medication	Sinusitis
Otitis media	Reflux (GERD)	Inflammatory bowel disease
	Sinusitis	Appendicitis
	Otitis media	Migraine
		Pregnancy
		Medication
		Ipecac abuse/bulimia
Rare		
Adrenogenital syndrome	Reye syndrome	Reye syndrome
Inborn error of metabolism	Hepatitis	Hepatitis
Brain tumor (increased intracranial pressure)	Peptic ulcer	Peptic ulcer
	Pancreatitis	Pancreatitis
Subdural hemorrhage	Brain tumor	Brain tumor
Food poisoning	Increased intracranial pressure	Increased intracranial pressure
Rumination	Middle ear disease	Middle ear disease
Renal tubular acidosis	Chemotherapy	Chemotherapy
	Achalasia	Cyclic vomiting (migraine)
	Cyclic vomiting (migraine)	Biliary colic
	Esophageal stricture	Renal colic
	Duodenal hematoma	
	Inborn error of metabolism	

GERD = gastroesophageal reflux disease.

nervous system (CNS) centers. Many acute or chronic processes can cause vomiting (Boxes 287–1 and 287–2).

Vomiting caused by obstruction of the gastrointestinal tract is probably mediated by intestinal visceral afferent nerves stimulating the vomiting center (see Box 287–1). If obstruction occurs below the second part of the duodenum, vomitus is usually bile stained. With repeated vomiting in the absence of obstruction, however, duodenal contents are refluxed into the stomach and the emesis may become bile stained. Nonobstructive lesions of the digestive tract can also cause vomiting; most diseases of the upper bowel, pancreas, liver, or biliary tree are capable of provoking emesis. CNS or metabolic derangements may lead to severe, persistent emesis.

Cyclic vomiting is a syndrome with numerous episodes of vomiting (about nine episodes/mo) interspersed with well intervals. The onset is usually between 3–5 yr of age; the episodes last 2–3 days, with four or more emesis episodes per hour. Patients may have a prodrome of nausea, lethargy, and headache or fever. Precipitants include stress and excitement. Idiopathic cyclic vomiting may be a migraine equivalent (abdominal migraine), or it may result from altered intestinal motility or mutations in mitochondrial DNA. The *differential diagnosis* includes gastrointestinal anomalies (malrotation, duplication cysts, choledochal cysts), CNS disorders (neoplasm, epilepsy, vestibular pathology), nephrolithiasis, cholelithiasis, hydronephrosis, metabolic-endocrine disorders (urea cycle, fatty acid metabolism, Addison disease, porphyria, hereditary angioedema, familial Mediterranean fever), chronic appendicitis, and inflammatory bowel disease. Laboratory evaluation is based on a careful history and physical examination and may include, if indicated, endoscopy, contrast gastrointestinal radiography, brain MRI, and metabolic studies (lactate, organic acids, ammonia). *Treatment* includes hydration and ondansetron. *Prevention* may be possible with the antimigraine agent amitriptyline or cyproheptadine.

BOX 287–2. Causes of Gastrointestinal Obstruction

ESOPHAGUS

Congenital

Esophageal atresia
Vascular rings
Schatzki ring
Tracheobronchial remnant

Acquired

Esophageal stricture
Foreign body
Achalasia
Chagas disease
Collagen vascular disease

STOMACH

Congenital

Antral webs
Pyloric stenosis

Acquired

Bezoars/foreign body
Pyloric stricture (ulcer)
Chronic granulomatous
    disease of childhood
Eosinophilic gastroenteritis
Crohn disease
Epidermolysis bullosa

SMALL INTESTINE

Congenital

Duodenal atresia
Annular pancreas
Malrotation/volvulus
Malrotation/Ladd bands

Ileal atresia
Meconium ileus
Meckel diverticulum with
    volvulus or intussusception
Inguinal hernia
Intestinal duplication

Acquired

Postsurgical adhesions
Crohn disease
Intussusception
Distal ileal obstruction
    syndrome (cystic fibrosis)
Duodenal hematoma
Superior mesenteric artery
    syndrome

COLON

Congenital

Meconium plug
Hirschsprung disease
Colonic atresia, stenosis
Imperforate anus
Rectal stenosis
Pseudo-obstruction
Volvulus
Colonic duplication

Acquired

Ulcerative colitis (toxic
    megacolon)
Chagas disease
Crohn disease
Fibrosing colonopathy (cystic
    fibrosis)

Diarrhea. Diarrhea is best defined as excessive loss of fluid and electrolyte in the stool. Normally, a young infant has about 5 g/kg of stool output per day; the volume increases to 200 g/24 hr in an adult. The greatest volume of intestinal water is absorbed in the small bowel; the colon concentrates intestinal contents against a high osmotic gradient. The small intestine of an adult may absorb 10–11 L/day of a combination of ingested and secreted fluid, whereas the colon absorbs about 0.5 L. Disorders that interfere with absorption in the small bowel tend to produce voluminous diarrhea, whereas disorders compromising colonic absorption produce lower volume diarrhea. Dysentery (i.e., small-volume, frequent bloody stools with mucus, tenesmus, and urgency) is the predominant symptom of colitis.

The basis for all diarrhea is disturbed intestinal solute transport; water movement across intestinal membranes is passive and is determined by both active and passive fluxes of solutes, particularly sodium, chloride, and glucose. The pathogenesis of most episodes of diarrhea can be explained by secretory, osmotic, or motility abnormalities or a combination of these (Table 287–2).

Secretory diarrhea is often caused by a secretagogue, such as cholera toxin, binding to a receptor on the surface epithelium of the bowel and thereby stimulating intracellular accumulation of cyclic adenosine monophosphate or cyclic guanosine monophosphate. Some intraluminal fatty acids and bile salts cause the colonic mucosa to secrete through this mechanism. Diarrhea not associated with an exogenous secretagogue may also have a secretory component (e.g., congenital microvillus inclusion disease). Secretory diarrhea tends to be watery and of large volume; the osmolality of the stool can be accounted for by the presence of electrolytes. Secretory diarrhea generally persists even when no feedings are given by mouth.

Osmotic diarrhea occurs after ingestion of a poorly absorbed solute. The solute may be one that is normally not well absorbed (e.g., magnesium, phosphate, lactulose, or sorbitol) or one that is not well absorbed because of a disorder of the small bowel (e.g., lactose with lactase deficiency or glucose with rotavirus diarrhea). Malabsorbed carbohydrate is fermented in the colon, and short-chain fatty acids (SCFAs) are produced. Although SCFAs can be absorbed in the colon and used as an energy source, the net effect is to increase the osmotic solute load. This form of diarrhea is usually of lesser volume than a secretory diarrhea and stops with fasting. The osmolality of the stool will not be explained by the electrolyte content, because another osmotic component is present [the difference between electrolyte content (sum of [NA$^+$], [K$^+$], and associated anions) and stool osmolality is >50 mOsm] (see Chapter 321). Motility disorders may be associated with rapid or delayed transit and generally are not associated with large volume diarrhea. Slowed motility may be associated with bacterial overgrowth as a cause of diarrhea. The differential diagnosis of common causes of acute and chronic diarrhea is noted in Table 287–3.

Constipation. Any definition of constipation is relative and depends on stool consistency, stool frequency, and difficulty in passing the stool. A normal child may have a soft stool only every 2nd or 3rd day without difficulty; this is not constipation. However, a hard stool passed with difficulty every 3rd day should be treated as constipation. Constipation may arise from defects either in filling or emptying the rectum (Box 287–3).

TABLE 287–2. Mechanisms of Diarrhea

Primary Mechanism	Defect	Stool Examination	Examples	Comment
Secretory	Decreased absorption, increased secretion: electrolyte transport	Watery, normal osmolality; osmols = 2 × (Na$^+$ + K$^+$)	Cholera, toxigenic *Escherichia coli*; carcinoid, VIP, neuroblastoma, congenital chloride diarrhea, *Clostridium difficile, cryptosporidiosis* (AIDS)	Persists during fasting; bile salt malabsorption also may increase intestinal water secretion; no stool leukocytes
Osmotic	Maldigestion, transport defects, ingestion of unabsorbable solute	Watery, acidic, + reducing substances; increased osmolality; osmosis >2 × (Na$^+$ + K$^+$)	Lactase deficiency, glucose-galactose malabsorption, lactulose, laxative abuse	Stops with fasting, increased breath hydrogen with carbohydrate malabsorption, no stool leukocytes
Motility				
Increased motility	Decreased transit time	Loose to normal-appearing stool, stimulated by gastrocolic reflex	Irritable bowel syndrome, thyrotoxicosis, postvagotomy dumping syndrome	Infection also may contribute to increased motility
Decreased motility	Defect in neuromuscular unit(s) Stasis (bacterial overgrowth)	Loose to normal-appearing stool	Pseudo-obstruction, blind loop	Possible bacterial overgrowth
Mucosal inflammation	Inflammation, decreased mucosal surface area and/or colonic reabsorption, increased motility	Blood and increased WBCs in stool	Celiac disease, *Salmonella, Shigella*, amebiasis, *Yersinia, Campylobacter*, rotavirus enteritis	Dysentery = blood, mucus, and WBCs

VIP = vasoactive intestinal peptide; WBC = white blood cell.
Adapted from Behrman RE, Kliegman RM (editors): Nelson Essentials of Pediatrics, 3rd ed. Philadelphia, WB Saunders, 1998.

TABLE 287–3. **Differential Diagnosis of Diarrhea**

	Infant	Child	Adolescent
Acute			
Common	Gastroenteritis Systemic infection Antibiotic associated	Gastroenteritis Food poisoning Systemic infection Antibiotic associated	Gastroenteritis Food poisoning Antibiotic associated
Rare	Primary disaccharidase deficiency Hirschsprung toxic colitis Adrenogenital syndrome	Toxic ingestion	Hyperthyroidism
Chronic			
Common	Postinfectious secondary lactase deficiency Cow's milk/soy protein intolerance Chronic nonspecific diarrhea of infancy Celiac disease Cystic fibrosis AIDS enteropathy	Postinfectious secondary lactase deficiency Irritable bowel syndrome Celiac disease Lactose intolerance Giardiasis Inflammatory bowel disease AIDS enteropathy	Irritable bowel syndrome Inflammatory bowel disease Lactose intolerance Giardiasis Laxative abuse (anorexia nervosa)
Rare	Primary immune defects Familial villous atrophy Secretory tumors Congenital chloridorrhea Acrodermatitis enteropathica Lymphangiectasia Abetalipoproteinemia Eosinophilic gastroenteritis Short bowel syndrome Intractable diarrhea syndrome Autoimmune enteropathy Factitious Microvillus inclusion disease	Acquired immune defects Secretory tumors Pseudo-obstruction Factitious	Secretory tumor Primary bowel tumor Gay bowel disease

From Behrman RE, Kliegman RM (editors): Nelson Essentials of Pediatrics, *3rd ed.* Philadelphia, WB Saunders, 1998.

A nursing infant may have very infrequent stools of normal consistency; this is usually a normal pattern. True constipation in the neonatal period is most likely secondary to Hirschsprung disease, intestinal pseudo-obstruction, or hypothyroidism.

Defective rectal filling occurs when colonic peristalsis is ineffective (e.g., in cases of hypothyroidism or opiate use and when bowel obstruction is caused either by a structural anomaly or by Hirschsprung disease). The resultant colonic stasis leads to excessive drying of stool and a failure to initiate reflexes from the rectum that normally trigger evacuation. Emptying the rectum by spontaneous evacuation depends on a defecation reflex initiated by pressure receptors in the rectal muscle. Stool retention, therefore, may also result from lesions involving these rectal muscles, the sacral spinal cord afferent and efferent fibers, or the muscles of the abdomen and pelvic floor. Disorders of anal sphincter relaxation may also contribute to fecal retention.

Constipation tends to be self-perpetuating, whatever its cause. Hard, large stools in the rectum become difficult and even painful to evacuate; thus, more retention occurs and a vicious circle ensues. Distention of the rectum and colon lessens the sensitivity of the defecation reflex and the effectiveness of peristalsis. Eventually, watery content from the proximal colon may percolate around hard retained stool and pass per rectum unperceived by the child. This involuntary *encopresis* may be mistaken for diarrhea. Constipation does not per se have deleterious systemic organic effects. Urinary tract stasis may accompany severe long-standing cases. Constipation may generate anxiety, having a marked emotional impact on the patient and family.

Abdominal Pain. Individual children differ greatly in their perception of and tolerance for abdominal pain. This is one reason the evaluation of chronic abdominal pain is difficult. A child with functional abdominal pain (i.e., no identifiable organic cause) may be as uncomfortable as one with an organic cause. This distinction is an extremely important part of the medical evalua-

tion, guiding how the work-up is approached and the child is treated. The more specific the pain and the more suggestive of a particular diagnosis, the more likely it will have an organic basis. Normal growth and physical examination (including a rectal examination) are reassuring in a child who is suspected of having functional pain.

A specific cause may be difficult to find, but the nature and location of a pain-provoking lesion can usually be determined from the clinical description. Two types of nerve fibers transmit painful stimuli in the abdomen. In skin and muscle, A fibers mediate sharp localized pain; and C fibers from viscera, peritoneum, and muscle transmit poorly localized, dull pain. These afferent fibers have cell bodies in the dorsal root ganglia, and some axons cross the midline and ascend to the medulla, midbrain, and thalamus. Pain is perceived in the cortex of the postcentral gyrus, which can receive impulses arising from both sides of the body.

Visceral pain tends to be experienced in the dermatome from which the affected organ receives innervation. Painful stimuli originating in the liver, pancreas, biliary tree, stomach, or upper bowel are felt in the epigastrium; pain from the distal small bowel, cecum, appendix, or proximal colon is felt at the umbilicus; and pain from the distal large bowel, urinary tract, or pelvic organs is usually suprapubic. When pain is referred to remote areas supplied by the same neurologic segment as the diseased organ, the phenomenon usually means an increased intensity of the provoking stimuli. Parietal pain impulses travel in C fibers of nerves corresponding to dermatomes T6–L1; such pain tends to be more localized and intense than visceral pain.

In the gut, the usual stimulus provoking pain is tension or stretching. Inflammatory lesions may lower the pain threshold, but the mechanisms producing pain of inflammation are not clear. Tissue metabolites released near nerve endings probably account for the pain caused by ischemia. Perception of these painful stimuli can be modulated by input from both cerebral and peripheral sources. Psychologic factors are particularly

BOX 287–3. Causes of Constipation

NONORGANIC (FUNCTIONAL)—RETENTIVE

ORGANIC

Anatomic

Anal stenosis
Imperforate anus
Anteriorly displaced anus
Intestinal stricture (post necrotizing enterocolitis)

Abnormal Musculature

Prune belly syndrome
Gastroschisis
Down syndrome

Intestinal Nerve or Muscle Abnormalities

Hirschsprung disease
Pseudo-obstruction (visceral myopathy or neuropathy)
Intestinal neuronal dysplasia

Spinal Cord Defects

Tethered cord
Spinal cord trauma
Spina bifida

Drugs

Anticholinergics
Narcotics
Antidepressants
Chemotherapeutic agents (vincristine)
Pancreatic enzymes (fibrosing colonopathy)
Lead
Vitamin D intoxication

Metabolic Disorders

Hypokalemia
Hypercalcemia
Hypothyroidism
Diabetes mellitus

Intestinal Disorders

Celiac disease
Cow's milk protein intolerance
Cystic fibrosis (meconium ileus equivalent)
Inflammatory bowel disease (stricture)
Tumor

Connective Tissue Disorders

Systemic lupus erythematosus
Scleroderma

Psychiatric Diagnosis

Anorexia nervosa

important. Features of abdominal pain are noted in Tables 287–4 and 287–5.

Gastrointestinal Hemorrhage. Bleeding may occur anywhere along the gastrointestinal tract, and identification of the site may be challenging (Table 287–6). The small intestine, which is most difficult to study, is the least likely site of bleeding. The only exception is the painless bleeding of a Meckel diverticulum, which is not difficult to identify. Erosive damage to the mucosa of the gastrointestinal tract is the most common cause of bleeding, although variceal bleeding secondary to portal hypertension occurs frequently enough to require consideration. Vascular malformations are a rare cause in children; they are difficult to identify. The swallowed capsule-size mini camera assists in identifying small vascular lesions.

When bleeding originates in the esophagus, stomach, or duodenum, it may cause *hematemesis*. When exposed to gastric or intestinal juices, blood quickly darkens to resemble coffee grounds; massive bleeding is likely to be red. Red or maroon blood in stools, *hematochezia*, signifies either a distal bleeding site or massive hemorrhage above the distal ileum. Moderate to mild bleeding from sites above the distal ileum tends to cause blackened stools of tarry consistency *(melena)*; major hemorrhages in the duodenum or above can cause melena.

Children can develop iron-deficiency anemia from chronic enteric blood loss even when occult blood is not found in stools on random testing. Gastrointestinal hemorrhage may produce hypotension and tachycardia but rarely causes gastrointestinal symptoms; brisk duodenal or gastric bleeding may lead to nausea, vomiting, or diarrhea. The breakdown products of intraluminal blood may tip patients into hepatic coma if liver function is already compromised and lead to elevation of serum bilirubin.

Abdominal Distention and Abdominal Masses. Enlargement of the abdomen can result from diminished tone of the wall musculature or from increased content: fluid, gas, or solid. Ascites, the accumulation of fluid in the peritoneal cavity, distends the abdomen both in the flanks and anteriorly when it is large in volume. This fluid shifts with movement of the patient and conducts a percussion wave.

Ascitic fluid is usually a transudate with a low-protein concentration resulting from reduced plasma colloid osmotic pressure of hypoalbuminemia, from raised portal venous pressure, or from both. In cases of portal hypertension, the fluid leak probably occurs from lymphatics on the liver surface and from

TABLE 287–4. Recurrent Abdominal Pain in Children

Disorder	Characteristics	Key Evaluations
Nonorganic		
Recurrent abdominal pain syndrome (functional abdominal pain)	Nonspecific pain, often periumbilical	Hx and PE; tests as indicated
Irritable bowel syndrome	Intermittent cramps, diarrhea, and constipation	Hx and PE
Nonulcer dyspepsia	Peptic ulcer–like symptoms without abnormalities on evaluation of the upper gastrointestinal tract	Hx; esophagogastroduodenoscopy
Gastrointestinal Tract		
Chronic constipation	Hx of stool retention, evidence of constipation on examination	Hx and PE; plain x-ray of abdomen
Lactose intolerance	Symptoms may be associated with lactose ingestion; bloating, gas, cramps, and diarrhea	Trial of lactose-free diet; lactose breath hydrogen test
Parasite infection (especially *Giardia*)	Bloating, gas, cramps, and diarrhea	Stool evaluation for O & P; specific immunoassays for *Giardia*
Excess fructose or sorbitol ingestion	Nonspecific abdominal pain, bloating, gas, and diarrhea	Large intake of apples, fruit juice, or candy/chewing gum sweetened with sorbitol
Crohn disease	See Chapter 317	
Peptic ulcer	Burning or gnawing epigastric pain; worse on awakening or before meals; relieved with antacids	Esophagogastroduodenoscopy or upper GI contrast x-rays
Esophagitis	Epigastric pain with substernal burning	Esophagogastroduodenoscopy
Meckel's diverticulum	Periumbilical or lower abdominal pain; may have blood in stool	Meckel scan or enteroclysis
Recurrent intussusception	Paroxysmal severe cramping abdominal pain; blood may be present in stool with episode	Identify intussusception during episode or lead point in intestine between episodes with contrast studies of gastrointestinal tract
Internal, inguinal, or abdominal wall hernia	Dull abdomen or abdominal wall pain	PE, CT of abdominal wall
Chronic appendicitis or appendiceal mucocele	Recurrent RLQ pain; often incorrectly diagnosed, may be rare cause of abdominal pain	Barium enema, CT

TABLE 287–4. Recurrent Abdominal Pain in Children *Continued*

Disorder	Characteristics	Key Evaluations
Gallbladder and Pancreas		
Cholelithiasis	RUQ pain, may worsen with meals	Ultrasound of gallbladder
Choledochal cyst	RUQ pain, mass ± elevated bilirubin	Ultrasound or CT of RUQ
Recurrent pancreatitis	Persistent boring pain, may radiate to back, vomiting	Serum amylase and lipase ± serum trypsinogen; ultrasound or CT of pancreas
Genitourinary Tract		
Urinary tract infection	Dull suprapubic pain, flank pain	Urinalysis and urine culture; renal scan
Hydronephrosis	Unilateral abdominal or flank pain	Ultrasound of kidneys
Urolithiasis	Progressive, severe pain: flank to inguinal region to testicle	Urinalysis, ultrasound, IVP, CT
Other genitourinary disorders	Suprapubic or lower abdominal pain; genitourinary symptoms	Ultrasound of kidneys and pelvis; gynecologic evaluation
Miscellaneous Causes		
Abdominal migraine	See text; nausea, family Hx migraine	Hx
Abdominal epilepsy	May have seizure prodrome	EEG (may require more than one study, including sleep-deprived EEG)
Gilbert syndrome	Mild abdominal pain (causal or coincidental?); slightly elevated unconjugated bilirubin	Serum bilirubin
Familial Mediterranean fever	Paroxysmal episodes of fever, severe abdominal pain, and tenderness with other evidence of polyserositis	Hx and PE during an episode, DNA diagnosis
Sickle cell crisis	Anemia	Hematologic evaluation
Lead poisoning	Vague abdominal pain ± constipation	Serum lead level
Henoch-Schönlein purpura	Recurrent, severe crampy abdominal pain, occult blood in stool, characteristic rash, arthritis	Hx, PE, urinalysis
Angioneurotic edema	Swelling of face or airway, crampy pain	Hx, PE, upper gastrointestinal contrast x-rays, serum C1 esterase inhibitor
Acute intermittent porphyria	Severe pain precipitated by drugs, fasting, or infections	Spot urine for porphyrins

O & P = ova and parasites; Hx = history; PE = physical exam; RUQ = right upper quadrant; RLQ = right lower quadrant; IVP = intravenous pyelography; EEG = electroencephalogram; abd = abdominal.

TABLE 287–5. Distinguishing Features of Acute Gastrointestinal Tract Pain in Children

Disease	Onset	Location	Referral	Quality	Comments
Pancreatitis	Acute	Epigastric, left upper quadrant	Back	Constant, sharp, boring	Nausea, emesis, tenderness
Intestinal obstruction	Acute or gradual	Periumbilical—lower abdomen	Back	Alternating cramping (colic) and painless periods	Distention, obstipation, emesis, increased bowel sounds
Appendicitis	Acute	Periumbilical, then localized to lower right quadrant; generalized with peritonitis	Back or pelvis if retrocecal	Sharp, steady	Anorexia, nausea, emesis, local tenderness, fever with peritonitis
Intussusception	Acute	Periumbilical—lower abdomen	None	Cramping, with painless periods	Hematochezia, knees in pulled-up position
Urolithiasis	Acute, sudden	Back (unilateral)	Groin	Sharp, intermittent, cramping	Hematuria
Urinary tract infection	Acute, sudden	Back	Bladder	Dull to sharp	Fever, costochondral tenderness, dysuria, urinary frequency

TABLE 287–6. Differential Diagnosis of Gastrointestinal Bleeding in Childhood

Infant	Child	Adolescent
Common		
Bacterial enteritis	Bacterial enteritis	Bacterial enteritis
Milk protein allergy	Anal fissure	Inflammatory bowel disease
Intussusception	Colonic polyps	Peptic ulcer/gastritis
Swallowed maternal blood	Intussusception	Mallory-Weiss syndrome
Anal fissure	Peptic ulcer/gastritis	Colonic polyps
Lymphonodular hyperplasia	Swallowed epistaxis	
	Mallory-Weiss syndrome	
Rare		
Volvulus	Esophageal varices	Hemorrhoids
Necrotizing enterocolitis	Esophagitis	Esophageal varices
Meckel diverticulum	Meckel diverticulum	Esophagitis
Stress ulcer, stomach	Lymphonodular hyperplasia	Telangiectasia-angiodysplasia
Coagulation disorder (hemorrhagic disease of newborn)	Henoch-Schönlein purpura	Gay bowel disease
	Foreign body	Graft versus host disease
	Hemangioma, arteriovenous malformation	
	Sexual abuse	
	Hemolytic-uremic syndrome	
	Inflammatory bowel disease	
	Coagulopathy	

visceral peritoneal capillaries, but ascites does not usually develop until the serum albumin level falls. Sodium excretion in the urine decreases greatly as the ascitic fluid accumulates, and thus additional dietary sodium goes directly to the peritoneal space, taking with it more water. When ascitic fluid contains a high protein concentration, it is usually an exudate caused by an inflammatory or neoplastic lesion.

When fluid distends the gut, either obstruction or imbalance between absorption and secretion should be suspected. The factors causing fluid accumulation in the bowel lumen frequently cause gas to accumulate, too. The result may be audible gurgling noises. The source of gas is usually swallowed air, but endogenous flora may increase considerably in malabsorptive states and produce excessive gas when substrate reaches the lower intestine. Gas in the peritoneal cavity (pneumoperitoneum), perhaps signaled by a tympanitic percussion note even over solid organs such as the liver, indicates a perforated viscus.

An abdominal organ may enlarge diffusely or be affected by a discrete mass. In the digestive tract, such discrete masses may occur in the lumen, in the wall, or in the mesentery. In a constipated child, mobile, nontender fecal masses are often found. Anomalies, cysts, or inflammatory disease can affect the wall of the gut; gut wall neoplasms are extremely rare in children. The liver may enlarge diffusely in response to many disorders. Discrete liver masses may be islands of regenerating liver tissue in a cirrhotic liver or may be inflammatory or neoplastic in origin.

Jaundice. See Chapters 91.3, 91.4, and 337.

Baker SS, Liptak GS, Colletti RB, et al: Constipation in infants and children: Evaluation and treatment: A medical position statement of the North American Society for Pediatric Gastroenterology and Nutrition. *J Pediatr Gastroenterol Nutr* 1999;29:612–26.

Castro-Rodriguez JA, Salazar-Lindo E, Leon-Barua R: Differentiation of osmotic and secretory diarrhea by stool carbohydrate and osmolar gap measurements. *Arch Dis Child* 1997;77:201–5.

Croffie JM, Fitzgerald JF, Chong SK: Recurrent abdominal pain in children—a retrospective study of outcome in a group referred to a pediatric gastroenterology practice. *Clin Pediatr* 2000;39:267–74.

Felt B, Wise CG, Olson A, et al: Guideline for the management of pediatric idiopathic constipation and soiling: Multidisciplinary team from the University of Michigan Medical Center in Ann Arbor. *Arch Pediatr Adolesc Med* 1999;153:380–85.

Hyams JS, Burke G, Davis PM, et al: Abdominal pain and irritable bowel syndrome in adolescents: A community-based study. *J Pediatr* 1996;129:220–26.

Hyams JS, Treem WR, Etienne NL, et al: Effect of infant formula on stool characteristics of young infants. *Pediatrics* 1995;95:50–4.

Li BUK, Murray RD, Heitlinger LA, et al: Heterogeneity of diagnoses presenting as cyclic vomiting: Effective prophylactic therapy for cyclic vomiting syndrome in children using amitriptyline or cyproheptadine. *Pediatrics* 1998;102:583–87.

Meropol SB, Luberti AA, De Jong AR: Yield from stool testing of pediatric inpatients. *Arch Pediatr Adolesc Med* 1997;151:142–45.

Pfau BT, Li BU, Murray RD, et al: Differentiating cyclic from chronic vomiting patterns in children: Quantitative criteria and diagnostic implications. *Pediatrics* 1996;97:364:8.

Wewer V, Strandberg C, Paerregaard A, Krasilnikoff PA: Abdominal ultrasonography in the diagnostic work-up in children with recurrent abdominal pain. *Eur J Pediatr* 1997;156:787–88.

Withers GD, Silburn SR, Forbes DA: Precipitants and aetiology of cyclic vomiting syndrome. *Acta Paediatr* 1998;87:272–77.

Youssef NN, Di Lorenzo C: Childhood constipation: Evaluation and treatment. *J Clin Gastroenterol* 2001;33:199–205.

SECTION 2 *The Oral Cavity*

Norman Tinanoff

Oral health is integral to the physical and psychologic health of children. Timely diagnosis and treatment require close cooperation between physicians and dentists. Disorders of the teeth and surrounding structures may occur in isolation or in combination with other systemic conditions. Dental caries is the most common chronic disease of childhood, and children identified at high risk for caries should be referred for dental care by 1 yr of age. Approximately 10% of children sustain significant trauma to their teeth.

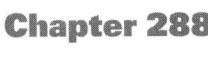

Chapter 288

Development and Developmental Anomalies of the Teeth

INITIATION

The primary teeth form in dental crypts that arise from a band of epithelial cells incorporated into each developing jaw. By the 12th wk of fetal life, each of these epithelial bands (the dental laminae) has five areas of rapid growth on each side of the maxilla and the mandible, seen as rounded, budlike enlargements. Organization of adjacent mesenchyme takes place in each area of epithelial growth, and the two elements together are the beginning of a tooth.

After the formation of these crypts for the 20 primary teeth, another generation of tooth buds forms lingually (toward the tongue), which will develop into the succeeding permanent incisors, canines, and premolars that eventually replace the primary teeth. This process takes place from about the 5th gestational month for the central incisors to about the 10th mo of age for the second premolars. The permanent first, second, and third molars, on the other hand, arise from extension of the dental laminae distal to the second primary molars. Buds for these teeth develop at approximately 4 mo of gestation, 1 yr of age, and 4 to 5 yr of age, respectively.

Histodifferentiation-Morphodifferentiation. As the epithelial bud proliferates, the deeper surface invaginates and a mass of mesenchyme becomes partially enclosed. The epithelial cells differentiate into the ameloblasts that lay down an organic matrix that forms enamel; the mesenchyme forms the dentin and dental pulp.

Calcification. After the organic matrix has been laid down, the deposition of the inorganic mineral crystals takes place from several sites of calcification that later coalesce. The characteristics of the inorganic portions of a tooth can be altered by (1) disturbances in formation of the matrix, (2) decreased availability of minerals, or (3) the incorporation of foreign materials. Such disturbances may affect the color, texture, or thickness of the tooth surface. Calcification of primary teeth begins at 3 to 4 mo in utero and concludes postnatally at approximately 12 mo with mineralization of the second primary molars (Table 288–1).

Eruption. At the time of tooth bud formation, each tooth begins a continuous movement toward the oral cavity. The times of eruption of the primary and permanent teeth are listed in Table 288–1.

ANOMALIES ASSOCIATED WITH TOOTH DEVELOPMENT

Both failures and excesses of tooth initiation are observed. *Developmentally missing teeth* may result from environmental insult, a genetic defect involving only teeth, or the manifestation of a syndrome. *Anodontia*, or absence of teeth, occurs when no tooth buds form (ectodermal dysplasia, or familial missing teeth) or when there is a disturbance of a normal site of initiation (the area of a palatal cleft). The teeth that are most commonly absent include the third molars, the maxillary lateral incisors, and the mandibular second premolars.

If the dental lamina produces more than the normal number of buds, supernumerary teeth occur, most often in the area between the maxillary central incisors. Because they

tend to disrupt the position and eruption of the adjacent normal teeth, their identification by radiographic examination is important. Supernumerary teeth also occur with cleidocranial dysplasia (see Chapter 292) and in the area of cleft palates.

Twinning, in which two teeth are joined together, is most often observed in the mandibular incisors of the primary dentition. It may result from gemination, fusion, or concrescence. Gemination is the result of the division of one tooth germ to form a bifid crown on a single root with a common pulp canal; an extra tooth appears to be present in the dental arch. Fusion is the joining of incompletely developed teeth that, owing to pressure or trauma or crowding, continue to develop as one tooth. Fused teeth are sometimes joined through their entire length; in other cases, a single wide crown is supported on two roots. Concrescence is the attachment of the roots of closely approximated adjacent teeth by an excessive deposit of cementum. This type of twinning, unlike the others, is found most often in the maxillary molar region.

Disturbances during differentiation may result in alterations in dental morphology, such as *macrodontia* (large teeth) or *microdontia* (small teeth). The maxillary lateral incisors may assume a slender, tapering shape ("peg-shaped laterals").

Amelogenesis imperfecta represents a group of hereditary conditions that manifest in enamel defects of the primary and permanent teeth without evidence of systemic disorders. The teeth are covered by only a thin layer of abnormally formed enamel through which the yellow underlying dentin is seen. The primary teeth are generally affected more than the permanent teeth. Susceptibility to caries is low, but the enamel is subject to destruction from abrasion. Complete coverage of the crown may be indicated for dentin protection, to reduce tooth sensitivity, and for improved appearance.

Dentinogenesis imperfecta, or hereditary opalescent dentin, is an analogous condition to amelogenesis imperfecta in which the odontoblasts fail to differentiate normally, resulting in poorly calcified dentin. This autosomal dominant disorder may also occur in patients with osteogenesis imperfecta. The enamel-dentin junction is altered, causing enamel to break away. The exposed dentin is then susceptible to abrasion, in some cases worn to the gingiva. The teeth are opaque and pearly, and the pulp chambers are generally obliterated by calcification. Both primary and permanent teeth are usually involved.

Localized disturbances of calcification that correlate with periods of illness, malnutrition, premature birth, or birth trauma are common. Hypocalcification appears as opaque white patches or horizontal lines on the tooth; hypoplasia is more severe and manifests as pitting or areas devoid of enamel. Systemic conditions, such as renal failure and cystic fibrosis, are associated with enamel defects. Local trauma to the primary incisors also can affect calcification of permanent incisors.

Fluorosis (mottled enamel) may result from systemic fluoride consumption above 0.05 mg/kg/day during enamel formation. This high fluoride consumption may be caused by residing in an area of high fluoride content of the drinking water (greater than 2.0 ppm), swallowing excessive fluoridated toothpaste, or inappropriate fluoride prescriptions. Excessive fluoride during enamel formation affects ameloblastic function, resulting in inconspicuous white, lacy patches on the enamel to severe, brownish discoloration and hypoplasia. The latter changes are usually seen with fluoride concentrations in the drinking water greater than 5.0 ppm.

Discolored teeth may result from incorporation of foreign substances into developing enamel. Neonatal *hyperbilirubinemia* may produce blue to black discoloration of the primary teeth. Porphyria produces a red-brown discoloration. *Tetracyclines* are extensively incorporated into bones and teeth and, if administered during the period of formation of enamel, may result

TABLE 288–1. Calcification, Crown Completion and Eruption

Tooth	First Evidence of Calcification	Crown Completed	Eruption
Primary Dentition			
Maxillary			
Central incisor	3–4 mo in utero	4 mo	7½ mo
Lateral incisor	4½ mo in utero	5 mo	8 mo
Canine	5½ mo in utero	9 mo	16–20 mo
First molar	5 mo in utero	6 mo	12–16 mo
Second molar	6 mo in utero	10–12 mo	20–30 mo
Mandibular			
Central incisor	4½ mo in utero	4 mo	6½ mo
Lateral incisor	4½ mo in utero	4¼ mo	7 mo
Canine	5 mo in utero	9 mo	16–20 mo
First molar	5 mo in utero	6 mo	12–16 mo
Second molar	6 mo in utero	10–12 mo	20–30 mo
Permanent Dentition			
Maxillary			
Central incisor	3–4 mo	4–5 yr	7–8 yr
Lateral incisor	10 mo	4–5 yr	8–9 yr
Canine	4–5 mo	6–7 yr	11–12 yr
First premolar	1½–1¾ yr	5–6 yr	10–11 yr
Second premolar	2–2¼ yr	6–7 yr	10–12 yr
First molar	At birth	2½–3 yr	6–7 yr
Second molar	2½–3 yr	7–8 yr	12–13 yr
Third molar	7–9 yr	12–16 yr	17–21 yr
Mandibular			
Central incisor	3–4 mo	4–5 yr	6–7 yr
Lateral incisor	3–4 mo	4–5 yr	7–8 yr
Canine	4–5 mo	6–7 yr	9–10 yr
First premolar	1¾–2 yr	5–6 yr	10–12 yr
Second premolar	2¼–2½ yr	6–7 yr	11–12 yr
First molar	At birth	2½–3 yr	6–7 yr
Second molar	2½–3 yr	7–8 yr	11–13 yr
Third molar	8–10 yr	12–16 yr	17–21 yr

Modified from Logan WHG, Kronfeld R: Development of the human jaws and surrounding structures from birth to age fifteen years. J Am Dent Assoc 1993;20:379.

in brown-yellow discoloration and hypoplasia of the enamel. Such teeth fluoresce under ultraviolet light. The period at risk extends from about the 4th mo of gestation to the 7th yr of life. Repeated or prolonged therapy with tetracycline carries the highest risk.

Delayed eruption of the 20 primary teeth may be familial or indicate systemic or nutritional disturbances such as hypopituitarism, hypothyroidism, cleidocranial dysplasia, trisomy 21, progeria, Albright osteodystrophy, incontinentia pigmenti, rickets, or multiple syndromes. Failure of eruption of single or small groups of teeth may arise from local causes such as malpositioned teeth, supernumerary teeth, cysts, or retained primary teeth. Premature loss of primary teeth is most commonly caused by premature eruption of the permanent teeth. If the entire dentition is advanced for age and sex, precocious puberty or hyperthyroidism should be considered.

Natal teeth are observed in approximately 1 in 2,000 newborn infants; usually there are two in the position of the mandibular central incisors. Natal teeth are present at birth, whereas neonatal teeth erupt in the 1st mo of life. Attachment of natal/neonatal teeth is generally limited to the gingival margin, with little root formation or bony support. They may be a supernumerary or a prematurely erupted primary tooth. A radiograph can easily differentiate between the two conditions. Natal teeth are associated with cleft palate, Pierre Robin syndrome, Ellis-van Creveld syndrome, Hallermann-Streiff syndrome, pachyonychia congenita, and other anomalies. A family history of natal teeth or premature eruption is present in 15–20% of affected children.

Natal/neonatal teeth may occasionally result in pain and refusal to feed and at times may produce maternal discomfort because of abrasion or biting of the nipple during nursing. There is a remote danger of detachment, with aspiration of the tooth. Because the tongue lies between the alveolar processes during birth, it may become lacerated, and occasionally the tip is amputated (Riga-Fede disease). Decisions regarding extraction of prematurely erupted primary teeth must be made on an individual basis.

Exfoliation failure occurs when a primary tooth is not shed before the eruption of its permanent successor. Most often the primary tooth will eventually exfoliate, but in some cases the primary tooth may need to be extracted. This occurs most commonly in the mandibular incisor region.

Chapter 289
Disorders of the Oral Cavity Associated with Other Conditions

Disorders of the teeth and surrounding structures may occur in isolation or in combination with other systemic conditions. Most commonly, medical conditions that occur during tooth development may affect tooth formation or appearance. Damage to teeth during their development is permanent. Some of the disorders of the oral cavity associated with medical conditions are noted in Table 289–1.

TABLE 289–1. Dental Problems Associated with Selected Medical Conditions

Medical Condition	Common Associated Dental or Oral Findings
Cleft lip and palate	Missing teeth, extra (supernumerary) teeth, shifting of arch segments, feeding difficulties, speech problems
Kidney failure	Mottled enamel (permanent teeth), facial dysmorphology
Cystic fibrosis	Stained teeth with extensive medication, mottled enamel
Immunosuppression	Oral candidiasis with potential for systemic candidiasis, cyclosporine-induced gingival hyperplasia
Low birthweight with prolonged oral intubation	Palatal groove, narrow arch
Heart defects with susceptibility for bacterial endocarditis	Bacteremia from dental procedures or trauma
Neutrophil chemotactic deficiency	Juvenile periodontitis (loss of supporting bone around teeth)
Juvenile diabetes (uncontrolled)	Juvenile periodontitis
Neuromotor dysfunction	Oral trauma from falling; malocclusion (open bite); gingivitis from lack of hygiene
Prolonged illness (generalized) during tooth formation	Enamel hypoplasia of crown portions forming during illness
Seizures	Gingival enlargement if phenytoin is used
Maternal infections	Syphilis—abnormally shaped teeth
Vitamin D–dependent rickets	Enamel hypoplasia

Chapter 290
Malocclusion

The oral cavity is essentially a masticatory instrument. The purpose of the anterior teeth is to bite off portions of large food. The posterior teeth reduce foodstuffs to a soft, moist bolus. The cheeks and tongue force the food onto the areas of tooth contact. Establishing a proper relationship between the mandibular and maxillary teeth is important for physiologic and cosmetic reasons.

Variations in Growth Patterns. Growth patterns are classified into three main types of occlusion, determined when the jaws are closed and the teeth are held together (Fig. 290–1). According to the Angle Classification of Malocclusion, in Class I (normal) the cusps of the posterior mandibular teeth interdigitate ahead of and inside the corresponding cusps of the opposing maxillary teeth. This relationship provides a normal facial profile. In Class II malocclusion, "buck teeth," the cusps of the posterior mandibular teeth are behind and inside the corresponding cusps of the maxillary teeth. This common occlusal disharmony is found in approximately 45% of the population. The facial profile may give the appearance of a "receding chin" (retrognathia) or protruding front teeth. The resultant increased space between upper and lower anterior teeth encourages finger sucking and tongue-thrust habits. Additionally, children with pronounced Class II malocclusions are at greater risk of damage to the incisors due to trauma. In Class III malocclusion, "underbite," the cusps of the posterior mandibular teeth interdigitate a tooth or more ahead of their opposing maxillary counterparts. The anterior teeth appear in "cross bite," with the mandibular incisors protruding beyond the maxillary incisors. The facial profile gives the appearance of a "protruding chin" (prognathia).

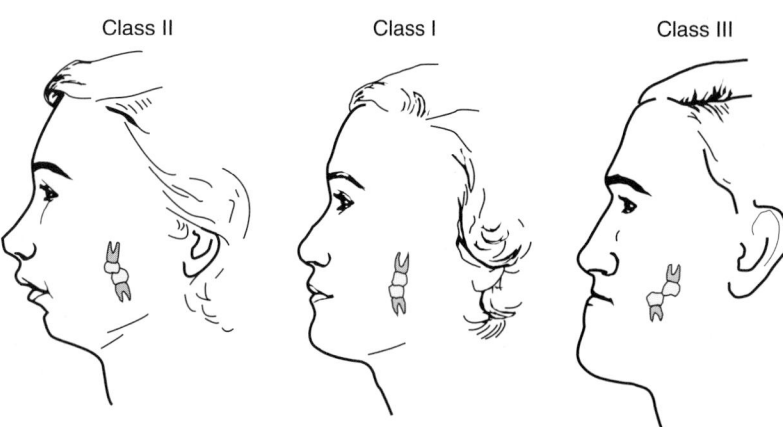

Class II   Class I   Class III

FIGURE 290–1. Angle classification of occlusion. The typical correspondence between the facial-jaw profile and molar relationship is shown.

Cross Bite. Normally, the mandibular teeth are in a position just inside the maxillary teeth, so that the outside mandibular cusps or incisal edges meet the central portion of the opposing maxillary teeth. A reversal of this relation is referred to as a *cross bite*. Cross bites may be anterior, involving the incisors; may be posterior, involving the molars; or may involve single or multiple teeth.

Open and Closed Bites. If the posterior mandibular and maxillary teeth make contact with each other but the anterior teeth are still apart, the condition is called an *open bite*. Open bites may be due to skeletal growth pattern or digit sucking. If digit sucking is terminated before skeletal and dental growth is complete, natural resolution of the open bite may occur. If mandibular anterior teeth occlude inside the maxillary anterior teeth in an overclosed position, the condition is referred to as a *closed or deep bite*. Treatment of open and closed bites consists of orthodontic correction, generally performed in the preteen or teenage years. Some cases require orthognathic surgery to optimally position the jaws in a vertical direction.

Dental Crowding. Overlap of incisors can result when the jaws are too small or the teeth are too large for adequate alignment of the teeth. Growth of the jaws is mostly in the posterior aspects of the mandible and maxilla, and therefore inadequate space for the teeth at 7 or 8 yr of age will not resolve with growth of the jaws. Spacing in the primary dentition is normal and favorable for adequate alignment of successor teeth.

Digit Sucking. Various and conflicting etiologic theories and recommendations for correction have been proposed for digit sucking in children. Prolonged digit sucking can cause flaring of the maxillary incisor teeth, an open bite, as well as a posterior cross bite. The prevalence of digit sucking decreases steadily from the age of 2 yr to approximately 10% by the age of 5. The earlier the habit is discontinued after the eruption of the permanent maxillary incisors (age 7–8 yr), the greater the likelihood that there will be lessening effects on the dentition. A variety of treatments have been suggested, from behavioral modification to insertion of an appliance with extensions that serves as a reminder when the child attempts to insert the digit. The greatest likelihood of success occurs in cases in which the child desires to stop. Stopping of the habit, however, will not rectify a malocclusion caused by a deviant growth pattern.

Cleft Lip and Palate

Clefts of the lip and palate are distinct entities closely related embryologically, functionally, and genetically. Although there are a variety of theories, it is commonly thought that cleft of the lip appears because of hypoplasia of the mesenchymal layer, resulting in a failure of the medial nasal and maxillary processes to join. Cleft of the palate appears to represent failure of the palatal shelves to approximate or fuse.

Incidence and Epidemiology. The incidence of cleft lip with or without cleft palate is about 1 in 750 white births; the incidence of cleft palate alone is about 1 in 2,500 white births. Clefts of the lip are more common in males. Possible causes include maternal drug exposure, a syndrome-malformation complex, or genetic factors. Although both may appear to occur sporadically, the presence of susceptibility genes appears important. There are families in which a cleft lip or palate, or both, is inherited in a dominant fashion (van der Woude syndrome), and careful examination of parents is important to distinguish this type from others, because the recurrence risk is 50%. Ethnic factors also affect the incidence of cleft lip and palate. Clefts are highest among Asians and lowest among blacks. The incidence of associated congenital malformations and of impairment in development is increased in children with cleft defects, especially in those with cleft palate alone. These findings are partially explained by an increased incidence of conductive hearing impairment in children with cleft palate, owing in part to repeated middle ear infections, and by the increased frequency of cleft defects among children with chromosomal abnormalities. The risks of recurrence of cleft defects within families are discussed in Chapters 69 and 72.

Clinical Manifestations. Cleft lip may vary from a small notch in the vermilion border to a complete separation extending into the floor of the nose. Clefts may be unilateral (more often on the left side) or bilateral and may involve the alveolar ridge. Deformed, supernumerary, or absent teeth are associated findings. The nasal alar cartilage clefts of the lip are frequently associated with deficiency of the columella and elongation of the vomer, producing a protrusion of the anterior aspect of the cleft premaxillary process.

Isolated cleft palate occurs in the midline and may involve only the uvula or may extend into or through the soft and hard palates to the incisive foramen. When associated with cleft lip, the defect may involve the midline of the soft palate and extend into the hard palate on one or both sides, exposing one or both of the nasal cavities as a unilateral or bilateral cleft palate.

Treatment. A complete program of habilitation for the child with a cleft lip or palate may require years of special treatment by a team consisting of a pediatrician, plastic surgeon, otolaryngologist, pediatric dentist, prosthodontist, orthodontist, speech therapist, geneticist, medical social worker, psychologist, and public health nurse. The child's physician should be responsible for seeking the coordinated use of specialists and for parental counseling and guidance.

The immediate problem in an infant born with a cleft lip or palate is feeding. Although some may advocate the construction of a plastic obturator to assist in feedings, most believe that with the use of soft artificial nipples with large openings, a squeezable bottle, and proper instruction, feeding of infants with clefts can be achieved with relative ease and effectiveness.

Surgical closure of a cleft lip is usually performed by 3 mo of age, when the infant has shown satisfactory weight gain and is free of any oral, respiratory, or systemic infection. Z-plasty is the most commonly used technique; a staggered suture line minimizes notching of the lip from retraction of scar tissue. The initial repair may be revised at 4 or 5 yr of age. Corrective surgery on the nose may be delayed until adolescence. Nasal surgery can also be performed at the time of the lip repair. Cosmetic results depend on the extent of the original deformity, healing potential of the individual, absence of infection, and the skill of the surgeon.

Because clefts of the palate vary considerably in size, shape, and degree of deformity, the timing of surgical correction should be individualized. Criteria such as width of the cleft, adequacy of the existing palatal segments, morphology of the surrounding areas (e.g., width of the oropharynx), and neuromuscular function of the soft palate and pharyngeal walls affect the decision. The goals of surgery are the union of the cleft segments, intelligible and pleasant speech, reduction of nasal regurgitation, and avoidance of injury to the growing maxilla.

In an otherwise healthy child, closure of the palate is usually done before 1 yr of age to enhance normal speech development. When surgical correction is delayed beyond the 3rd yr, a contoured speech bulb can be attached to the posterior of a maxillary denture so that contraction of the pharyngeal and velopharyngeal muscles can bring tissues into contact with the bulb to accomplish occlusion of the nasopharynx and help the child develop intelligible speech.

A cleft palate usually crosses the alveolar ridge and interferes with the formation of teeth in the maxillary anterior region. Teeth in the cleft area may be displaced, malformed, or missing. Missing teeth or teeth that are nonfunctional are replaced by prosthetic devices.

Postoperative Management. During the immediate postoperative period, special nursing care is essential. Gentle aspiration of the nasopharynx minimizes the chances of the common complications of atelectasis or pneumonia. The primary considerations in postoperative care are maintenance of a clean suture line and avoidance of tension on the sutures. For these reasons, the infant is fed with a Mead Johnson bottle and the arms are restrained with elbow cuffs. A fluid or semifluid diet is maintained for 3 wk; feeding is continued with a Mead Johnson bottle or a cup. The patient's hands, toys, and other foreign bodies must be kept away from the surgical site.

Sequelae of Cleft Lip and Palate. Recurrent otitis media and hearing loss are frequent with cleft palate. Displacement of the maxillary arches and malposition of the teeth usually require orthodontic correction.

Speech defects are often associated with cleft lip and palate and may be present or persist because of inadequate surgical closure of the palate. Such speech is characterized by the emission of air from the nose and by a hypernasal quality with certain sounds. Both before and sometimes after palatal surgery, the speech defect is caused by inadequacies in function of the palatal and pharyngeal muscles. The muscles of the soft palate and the lateral and posterior walls of the nasopharynx constitute a valve that separates the nasopharynx from the oropharynx during swallowing and in the production of certain sounds. If the valve does not function adequately, it is difficult to build up enough pressure in the mouth to make such explosive sounds as *p, b, d, t, h, y,* or the sibilants *s, sh,* and *ch,* and such words as "cats," "boats," and "sisters" are not intelligible. After operation or the insertion of a speech appliance, speech therapy is necessary.

Palatopharyngeal Incompetence. The speech disturbance characteristic of the child with a cleft palate can also be produced by other osseous or neuromuscular abnormalities where there is an inability to form an effective seal between oropharynx and nasopharynx during swallowing or phonation. The abnormality may be in the structure of the palate or pharynx or in the muscles attached to these structures. In a child who has the potential for abnormal speech, adenoidectomy may precipitate overt hypernasality. A submucous cleft palate may be the cause of this problem. In such cases, the adenoid mass may have facilitated velopharyngeal closure when the elevated soft palate contacted it. If the neuromuscular function is adequate, compensation in palatopharyngeal movement may take place and the speech defect may improve, although speech therapy is necessary. In other cases, slow involution of the adenoids may allow for gradual compensation in palatal and pharyngeal muscular function. This may explain why a speech defect does not become apparent in some children who have a submucous cleft palate or similar anomaly predisposing to palatopharyngeal incompetence. Velopharyngeal incompetency (VPI) can also occur in children with an inherent palatal abnormality (velocardiofacial syndrome). VPI should be evaluated by a craniofacial disorders team or a geneticist.

CLINICAL MANIFESTATIONS. Although clinical signs vary, the symptoms of palatopharyngeal incompetence are similar to those of a cleft palate. There may be hypernasal speech (especially noted in the articulation of pressure consonants such as *p, b, d, t, h, v, f,* and *s*); conspicuous constricting movement of the nares during speech; inability to whistle, gargle, blow out a candle, or inflate a balloon; loss of liquid through the nose when drinking with the head down; otitis media; and hearing loss. Oral inspection may reveal a cleft palate or a relatively short palate with a large oropharynx; absent, grossly asymmetric, or minimal muscular activity of the soft palate and pharynx during phonation or gagging; or a submucous cleft. The latter is suggested by a bifid uvula, by a translucent membrane in the midline of the soft palate (revealing lack of continuity of muscles), by palpable notching in the posterior border of the hard palate instead of a posterior nasal spinous process, or by forward or V-shaped displacement or grooving on the soft palate during phonation or gagging.

Palatopharyngeal incompetence may also be demonstrated radiographically. The head should be carefully positioned to obtain a true lateral view; one film is obtained with the patient at rest and another during continuous phonation of the vowel *u* as in "boom." The soft palate contacts the posterior pharyngeal wall in normal function, whereas in palatopharyngeal incompetence such contact is absent. Most accurate evaluations of VPI are accomplished by the use of nasoendoscopy.

TREATMENT. In selected cases, the palate may be repositioned or pharyngoplasty performed using a flap of tissue from the posterior pharyngeal wall. Dental speech appliances have also been used successfully. The type of surgery used is best tailored to the findings on nasoendoscopy.

Chapter 292
Syndromes with Oral Manifestations

Many syndromes have distinct or accompanying facial, oral, and dental manifestations (e.g., Apert syndrome, see Chapter 585; Crouzon disease, see Chapter 585; Down syndrome, see Chapter 70). The conditions described here are examples of some of the common occurring conditions.

Osteogenesis imperfecta often is accompanied by effects on the teeth, termed *dentinogenesis imperfecta* (see Chapter 288). Depending on the severity of presentation, treatment of the dentition varies from routine preventive and restorative monitoring to covering affected posterior teeth with stainless steel crowns, to reduce abrasion from chewing. Dentinogenesis imperfecta can also occur in isolation without the bony effects.

Another syndrome, *cleidocranial dysplasia*, has orofacial variations such as frontal bossing, mandibular prognathism, and a broad nasal base. Tooth eruption is often delayed. In addition, the primary teeth can be abnormally retained while the permanent teeth remain unerupted. Supernumerary teeth are common, especially in the premolar area. Although the erupted teeth are usually free of hypoplasia, variations in the size and shape of the teeth are common. Restoration of the erupted primary and permanent teeth should be performed when carious lesions are present. It is common to see extensive dental rehabilitation therapy in individuals with this disorder to maintain effective mastication.

Ectodermal dysplasia (see Chapter 639) is a heterogeneous group of conditions in which oral manifestations range from little or no involvement (the dentition is completely normal) to cases in which the teeth can be totally or partially absent or malformed. Because alveolar bone does not develop in the absence of teeth, the alveolar processes can be either totally or partially absent, and the resultant overclosure of the mandible causes the lips to protrude. Facial development is otherwise not disturbed. Teeth, when present, can range from normal to small and conical. If aplasia of the buccal and labial mucous glands is present, dryness and irritation of the oral mucosa can occur. People with ectodermal dysplasia may need either partial or full dentures, even at a very young age. The vertical height between the jaws is thus restored, improving the position of the lips and facial contours. Masticatory function is restored, and eating habits are therefore improved.

Pierre Robin sequence consists of micrognathia usually accompanied by a high arched or cleft palate. The tongue is usually of normal size, but the floor of the mouth is foreshortened. Obstruction of the air passages may occur, particularly on inspiration, and usually requires treatment to prevent suffocation. The infant should be maintained in a prone or partially prone position so that the tongue falls forward to relieve respiratory obstruction. Some patients may require endotracheal intubation or tracheostomy. Sufficient mandibular growth often takes place within a few months to relieve the potential airway obstruction. Often the growth of the mandible will achieve a normal profile within 4–6 yr. The feeding of infants with mandibular hypoplasia requires great care and patience but can usually be accomplished without resorting to gavage. Dental anomalies usually require individualized treatment. Thirty to 50 per cent of children with Pierre Robin syndrome have Stickler syndrome, an autosomal dominant condition that includes other findings such as early arthritis and ocular problems.

In *mandibulofacial dysostosis* (Treacher Collins syndrome or Franceschetti syndrome), the facial appearance is characterized by downward sloping palpebral fissures, colobomas of the lower eyelids, sunken cheekbones, blind fistulas opening between the angles of the mouth and the ears, deformed pinnae, atypical hair growth extending toward the cheeks, receding chin, and large mouth. Facial clefts, abnormalities of the ears, and deafness are common. The disorder is autosomal dominant, often with incomplete penetrance. The mandible is usually hypoplastic; the ramus may be deficient, and the coronoid and condylar processes are flat or even aplastic. The palatal vault may be either high or cleft. Infrequently, unilateral or bilateral macrostomia, or failure of embryonic fusion of the maxillary and mandibular processes, may occur. Dental malocclusions are frequent. The teeth may be widely separated, hypoplastic, or displaced or have an open bite. Orthodontic and routine dental treatments are indicated.

Hemifacial microsomia is usually characterized by unilateral hypoplasia of the mandible and can be associated with partial paralysis of the facial nerve, macrostomia, blind fistulas between the angles of the mouth and the ears, and deformed external ears. Severe facial asymmetry and malocclusion can develop because of the absence or hypoplasia of the mandibular condyle on the affected side. Congenital condylar deformity tends to increase with age. Early craniofacial surgery may be indicated to minimize the deformity. This disorder can be associated with ocular and vertebral anomalies (oculo-auriculo-vertebral spectrum, including Goldenhar syndrome); therefore, radiographs of the vertebrae and ribs should be considered to determine the extent of skeletal involvement.

Chapter 293
Dental Caries

Etiology. The development of dental caries depends on interrelationships between the tooth surface, dietary carbohydrates, and specific oral bacteria. Organic acids produced by bacterial fermentation of dietary carbohydrates reduce the pH of dental plaque adjacent to the tooth to a point at which demineralization occurs. The initial carious lesion appears as an opaque white spot on the enamel; and with progressive loss of tooth mineral, cavitation occurs.

A group of microorganisms, *mutans streptococci*, are associated with the development of dental caries. These bacteria have the ability to adhere to enamel, produce abundant acid, and survive at low pH. Once the enamel surface cavitates, other oral bacteria (lactobacilli) colonize the tooth, produce acid, and foster further tooth demineralization. Demineralization from bacterial acid production is determined by the frequency of carbohydrate consumption and by the type of carbohydrate. Sucrose is the most cariogenic sugar because one of its by-products during bacterial metabolism is glucan, a polymer that enables bacteria to adhere more readily to tooth structures. With regard to frequency of consumption, the cariogenic potential of a nursing bottle of a sweetened beverage that is consumed throughout the night or at nap times is much greater than that of the same volume of drink consumed at a single meal. Similarly, sticky candies retained orally for long periods (sucrose in sticky candies) is more cariogenic than the sugar in food products retained for short times.

Epidemiology. The incidence of dental caries has decreased in developed countries in the past 30 yr but still remains highly prevalent in low-income children and children from developing countries. The decrease is thought to be due to advances in prevention, particularly in the use of fluorides. Still, over half of the children in the United States have dental caries, with most of those having caries primarily in the pits and fissures of the occlusal (biting) surfaces of the molar teeth.

Clinical Manifestations. The age-related epidemiology is noted in Figure 293–1. Dental caries of the primary dentition usually begin in the pits and fissures. Small lesions may be difficult to diagnose by visual inspection, but larger lesions present as cavitations of the occlusal surface. The second most frequent sites of caries occur on approximal sites (contact surfaces between the teeth), which in many cases can only be detected by intraoral radiographs. Caries lesions of the exposed smooth (buccal and lingual) surfaces are generally found only in children with rampant caries (Fig. 293–2).

Rampant caries in infants and toddlers, referred to as early childhood caries (ECC), nursing bottle caries, or baby bottle tooth decay, was ascribed to inappropriate bottle-feeding. Although the combination of a child infected with cariogenic bacteria and the frequent ingestion of sugar, either in the bottle or in solid foods, is critical, other factors such as enamel hypoplasia of primary teeth because of nutritional deficiencies during pregnancy or because of premature birth may play a role. Reports have also associated "at will" breast-feeding in older infants with caries of the maxillary anterior teeth, but the possibility of cariogenic dietary practices other than breast-feeding, in such cases, needs further exploration.

Early childhood caries are common, with a reported prevalence of 30–50% in children from low socioeconomic backgrounds and as high as 70% in some Native American groups. It may occur as early as 12 mo of age, long before children visit a dentist. Pediatricians have the responsibility to both examine the child's teeth for caries and to refer to a dentist those children who they consider at risk for ECC. Risk factors include high-frequency sugar consumption (prolonged and frequent drinking from bottle or sippy cup, frequent eating of sugar-containing snacks); children of low socioeconomic status; immigrant children; parents or siblings with high caries rates; and evidence of defects on the teeth.

Children who develop caries at a young age are known to be at high risk for developing further caries as they get older. Therefore, the appropriate prevention of ECC can result in the elimination of major dental problems in toddlers and less decay in later childhood.

Complications. If left untreated, dental caries usually destroy most of the tooth and invade the dental pulp (Fig. 293–3), leading to an inflammation of the pulp (pulpitis) and significant pain. Pulpitis can progress to necrosis, with bacterial invasion of the alveolar bone causing a dental abscess. Infection of a primary tooth may disrupt normal development of the successor permanent tooth. In a small percentage of cases this process may lead to sepsis and facial space infection (Fig. 293–4).

Treatment. The age at which caries occurs is important in dental management. Children younger than 3 yr of age lack the developmental ability to cooperate with dental treatment and often require restraint, sedation, or general anesthesia to repair carious teeth. After age 4, children generally can cope with dental restorative care with the use of local anesthesia.

Dental treatment, using silver amalgam, plastic composite restorations, or stainless steel crowns, can restore most teeth affected with dental caries. If caries involve the dental pulp, a partial removal of the pulp (pulpotomy) or complete removal of the pulp (pulpectomy) may be required. If a tooth requires extraction, a space maintainer may be indicated to prevent migration of teeth that subsequently leads to malposition of permanent successor teeth.

Clinical management of the pain and infection associated with untreated dental caries varies with the extent of involvement and the medical status of the patient. Dental infection localized to the dentoalveolar unit can be managed by local measures (extraction, pulpectomy). Oral antibiotics are indicated for dental infections associated with cellulitis, facial swelling, or if it is difficult to anesthetize the tooth in the presence of inflammation. Penicillin is the antibiotic of choice, except in patients with a history of allergy to this agent; clindamycin and erythromycin are suitable alternatives. Oral analgesics, such as ibuprofen, are usually adequate for the pain control. If the infection involves a vital

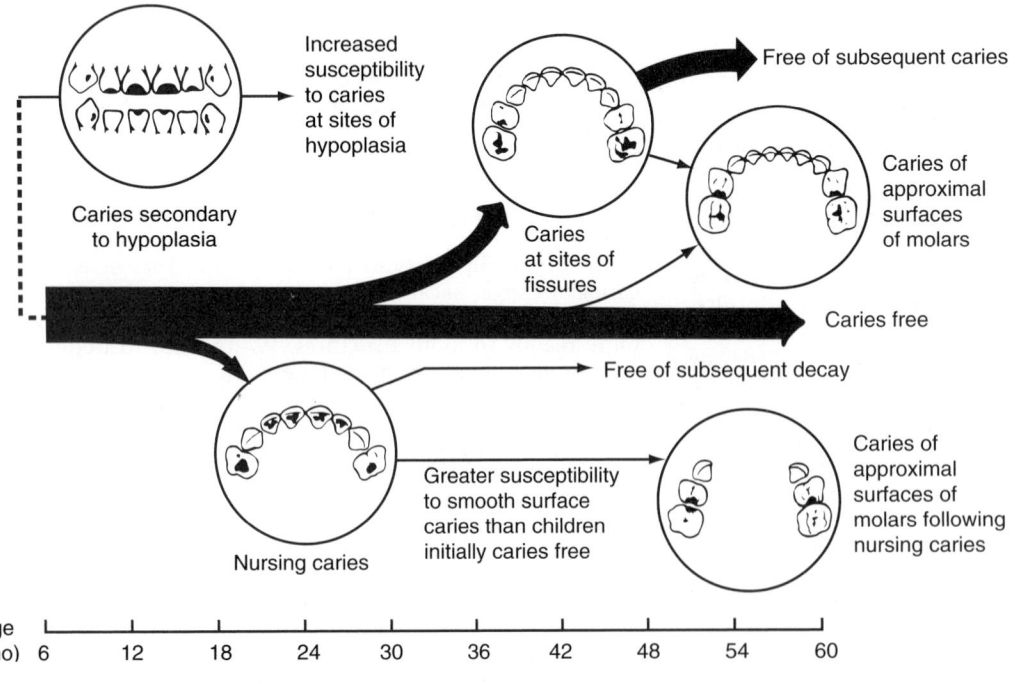

FIGURE 293–1. Schematic for different kinds of caries and ages when each can start. A significant percentage of children remain caries free. Nursing caries (early childhood caries [ECC]) begins between 1 and 2 yr of age; children with ECC are at significantly greater risk for future caries than are caries-free children. Pit and fissure caries usually begins after about age 3, with caries of approximating tooth surfaces beginning shortly after. (From Johnsen DC: The role of the pediatrician in identifying and treating dental caries. *Pediatr Clin North Am* 1991;38: 1173.)

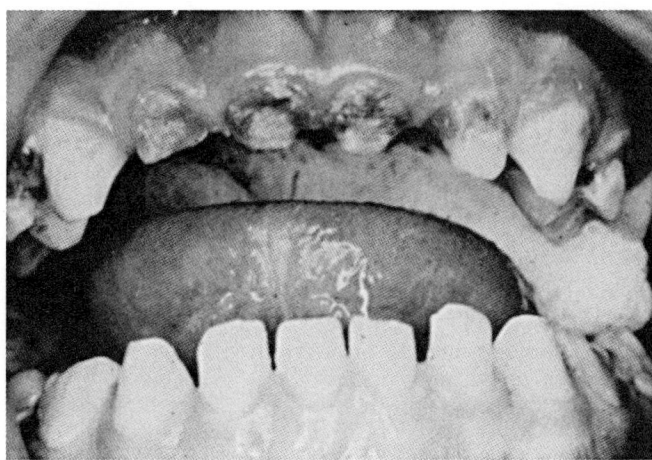

FIGURE 293–2. Early childhood caries, also called nursing bottle caries or baby bottle tooth decay.

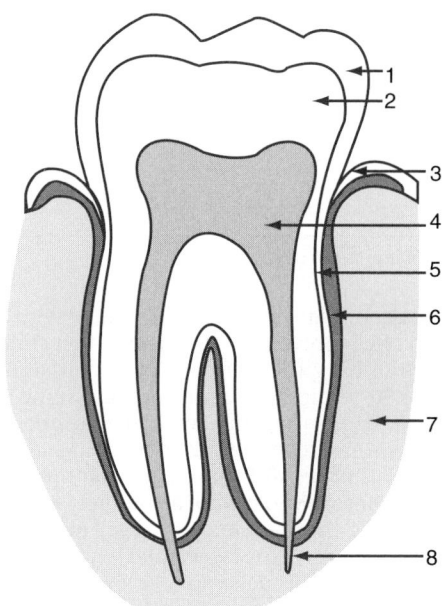

FIGURE 293–3. Basic dental anatomy: 1 = enamel; 2 = dentin; 3 = gingival margin; 4 = pulp; 5 = cementum; 6 = periodontal ligament; 7 = alveolar bone; 8 = neurovascular bundle.

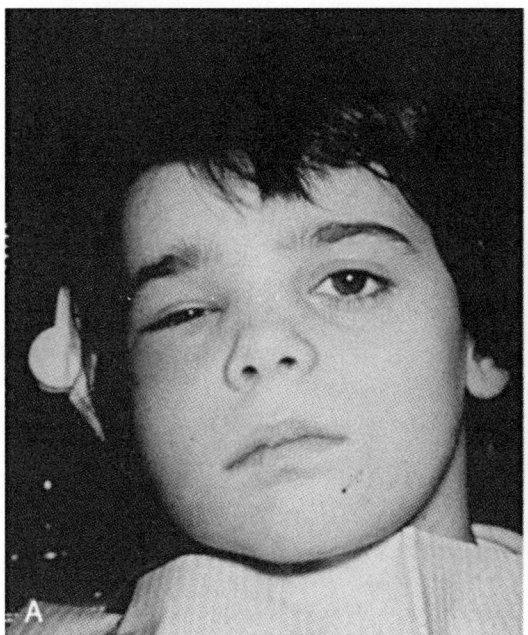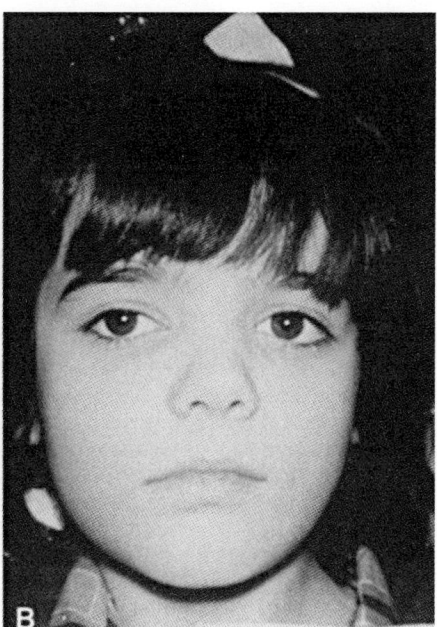

FIGURE 293–4. *A,* Facial inflammation-infection from the abscess of a maxillary primary molar. *B,* Resolution of the inflammation in 1 wk with a course of antibiotics and extraction of the tooth.

area (submandibular space, which can lead to Ludwig angina; facial triangle, which can lead to cavernous sinus thrombosis; or periorbital space, which can rarely lead to orbital involvement), parenteral antibiotics are indicated.

Prevention

FLUORIDE. The most effective preventive measure against dental caries is optimizing the fluoride content of communal water supplies to 1 ppm. Children who reside in areas with fluoride-deficient water supplies and are at caries risk will benefit from dietary fluoride supplements (Table 293–1). The fluoride level of public water supplies can usually be obtained by calling the local health department. If the patient uses a private water supply, it is necessary to get the water tested for fluoride levels before prescribing fluoride supplements. To avoid potential overdoses, no fluoride prescription should be written for more than a total of 120 mg of fluoride. Significant acute overdose of fluoride (greater than 5 mg/kg) needs immediate medical attention. The use of topical fluoride agents, applied professionally or by the patient, is beneficial to children at risk for caries.

TABLE 293–1. Supplemental Fluoride Dosage Schedule

	Fluoride in Home Water (ppm)		
Age	<0.3	0.3–0.6	>0.6
6 mo–3 yr	0.25*	0	0
3–6 yr	0.50	0.25	0
6–16 yr	1.00	0.50	0

Milligrams of fluoride per day.

ORAL HYGIENE. Daily brushing, especially with fluoridated toothpaste, will help prevent dental caries. Most children under 8 yr of age do not have the coordination required for adequate tooth brushing. Accordingly, parents should assume responsibility for the child's oral hygiene, with the degree of parental involvement appropriate to the child's changing abilities. Only a pea-sized amount, or less, of fluoridated toothpaste should be used in young children who cannot adequately expectorate.

DIET. Decreasing the frequency of sugar ingestion prevents dental caries. Therefore, using sweetened beverages in the nursing bottle and bedtime bottle should be discouraged, and children at risk for dental caries should reduce between-meal sugar-containing snacks.

DENTAL SEALANTS. Plastic dental sealants have been shown to be effective in the prevention of caries on the pit and fissure of the primary and permanent molars. Sealants are most effective when placed soon after teeth erupt (usually within 1–2 yr) and when used in children with deep grooves and fissures in the molar teeth.

Chapter 294
Periodontal Diseases

The periodontium includes the gingiva, alveolar bone, cementum, and periodontal ligament (see Fig. 293–3).

Gingivitis. Poor oral hygiene results in the accumulation of a dental plaque at the tooth-gingival interface that activates an inflammatory response, expressed as localized or generalized reddening and swelling of the gingiva. Over half of American schoolchildren experience gingivitis. In severe cases, the gingiva spontaneously bleeds and there is oral malodor. *Treatment* is with proper oral hygiene (careful tooth brushing and flossing); complete resolution can be expected. Gingivitis in healthy prepubertal children is unlikely to progress to periodontitis (inflammation of the periodontal ligament resulting in loss of alveolar bone). Inability to resolve gingivitis by oral hygiene measures necessitates considering other problems in which gingivitis may be a presenting component (leukemia, diabetes mellitus, neutropenia, thrombocytopenia, scurvy, and hormonal changes associated with puberty and pregnancy).

Prepubertal Periodontitis. Periodontitis in children before puberty, leading to premature loss of primary teeth, is often associated with systemic problems, including neutropenia, leukocyte adhesion or migration defects, hypophosphatasia, Papillon-Lefèvre syndrome, and histiocytosis X. In many cases, however, there is no apparent underlying medical problem. *Treatment* includes aggressive professional tooth cleaning, strategic extraction of affected teeth, and antibiotic therapy. Although there are few reports of long-term successful treatment to reverse bone loss surrounding primary teeth, diagnostic work-ups are necessary to rule out underlying systemic disease.

Localized Juvenile Periodontitis. Localized juvenile periodontitis is characterized by rapid alveolar bone loss, especially around the permanent incisors and first molars. It is associated with a strain of *Actinobacillus*. In addition, the neutrophils of patients with localized juvenile periodontitis may have chemotactic and phagocytic defects. If left untreated, affected teeth lose their attachment and may exfoliate. *Treatment* varies with the degree of involvement. Patients diagnosed at the onset of the disease are usually managed by local debridement, antibiotic therapy, and meticulous oral hygiene. Patients who have extensive alveolar bone loss at the time of initial diagnosis require extensive periodontal therapy that may include autologous osseous grafting. Prognosis depends on the degree of initial involvement and compliance with therapy.

Teething. Teething can lead to intermittent localized discomfort in the area of erupting primary teeth, irritability, low-grade fevers, and excessive salivation; many children have no apparent difficulties. *Symptomatic treatment* includes chewing on ice rings and oral analgesics. Similar manifestations can also arise when the first permanent molars erupt at about age 6 yr.

Cyclosporine- or Phenytoin-Induced Gingival Overgrowth. The use of cyclosporine to suppress organ rejection or phenytoin for anticonvulsant therapy, and in some cases calcium channel blockers, is associated with generalized enlargement of the gingiva. Phenytoin and its metabolites have a direct stimulatory action on gingival fibroblasts, resulting in accelerated synthesis of collagen. Clinical studies indicate that phenytoin induces less gingival hyperplasia in patients who maintain meticulous oral hygiene.

Gingival hyperplasia occurs in 10–30% of patients treated with phenytoin. Severe manifestations may include (1) gross enlargement of the gingiva, sometimes covering the teeth; (2) edema and erythema of the gingiva; (3) secondary infection, resulting in abscess formation; (4) migration of teeth; and (5) inhibition of exfoliation of primary teeth and subsequent impaction of permanent teeth. *Treatment* should be directed toward prevention and, if possible, discontinuation of cyclosporine or phenytoin. Patients undergoing long-term treatment with these drugs should receive frequent dental examinations and oral hygiene care. Severe forms of gingival overgrowth are treated by gingivectomy, but the lesion recurs if drug use is continued.

Acute Pericoronitis. Acute inflammation of the flap of gingiva that partially covers the crown of an incompletely erupted tooth is common in mandibular permanent molars. Accumulation of debris and bacteria between the gingival flap and tooth precipitates the inflammatory response. A variant of this condition is a gingival abscess due to entrapment of bacteria because of orthodontic bands or crowns. Trismus and severe pain may be associated with the inflammation. Untreated cases may result in facial space infections and facial cellulitis.

Treatment includes local debridement and irrigation, warm saline rinses, and antibiotic therapy. When the acute phase has subsided, extraction of the tooth or resection of the gingival flap prevents recurrence. Early recognition of the partial impaction of mandibular third molars and their subsequent extraction will prevent these areas from having pericoronitis.

Acute Necrotizing Ulcerative Gingivitis. Acute necrotizing ulcerative gingivitis (ANUG), also called Vincent stomatitis and trench mouth, is a distinct periodontal disease associated with oral spirochetes and fusobacteria. It is not clear, however, whether bacteria initiate the disease or are secondary. ANUG develops primarily in young adults and adolescents. It rarely develops in healthy children in developed countries. It occurs frequently among children in southern India and certain African countries where affected children usually have protein malnutrition. In such children, the lesion may extend into adjacent tissues, causing necrosis of facial structures (cancrum oris, or noma).

Clinical manifestations of ANUG include (1) necrosis and ulceration of gingiva between the teeth, (2) an adherent grayish pseudomembrane over the affected gingiva, (3) oral malodor,

(4) cervical lymphadenopathy, (5) malaise, and (6) fever. The condition may be mistaken for acute herpetic gingivostomatitis. Dark-field microscopy of debris obtained from ANUG lesions will demonstrate dense spirochete populations.

Treatment of ANUG is divided into an acute management with antibiotics (penicillin or erythromycin), local debridement, oxygenating agents (direct application of 10% carbamide peroxide in anhydrous glycerol qid), and analgesics. Dramatic resolution usually occurs within 48 hr. A second phase of treatment may be necessary if the acute phase of the disease has caused irreversible morphologic damage to the periodontium. The disease is not contagious.

Chapter 295
Dental Trauma

Traumatic oral injuries may be categorized into three groups: (1) injuries to teeth, (2) injuries to soft tissue (contusions, abrasions, lacerations, punctures, avulsions, and burns), and (3) injuries to jaw (mandibular or maxillary fractures or both).

Injuries to Teeth. Approximately 10% of children between 18 mo and 18 yr of age will sustain significant tooth trauma. There appear to be three age periods of greatest predilection: (1) toddlers (1–3 yr), usually due to falls or child abuse; (2) school-aged (7–10 yr), usually from bicycle and playground accidents; and (3) adolescents (16–18 yr), often the result of fights, athletic injuries, and automobile accidents. Injuries to teeth are more frequent among children with protruding front teeth. Children with craniofacial abnormalities or neuromuscular deficits are also at increased risk for dental injury. Injuries to teeth may involve the hard dental tissues, the dental pulp (nerve), and injuries to the periodontal structure (surrounding bone and attachment apparatus) (Fig. 295–1; Table 295–1).

Fractures of teeth may be uncomplicated (confined to the hard dental tissues) or complicated (involving the pulp). Exposure of the pulp will result in its bacterial contamination, which can lead to infection and pulp necrosis. Such pulp exposure complicates therapy and may lower the likelihood of a favorable outcome.

The teeth most often affected are the maxillary incisors. Uncomplicated crown fractures are treated by covering exposed dentin and by placing an aesthetic restoration. Complicated crown fractures usually require endodontic (root canal) therapy. Crown-root fractures and root fractures usually require extensive dental therapy. Such injuries in the primary dentition may interfere with normal development of the permanent dentition, and, therefore, significant injuries of the primary incisor teeth are usually managed by extraction.

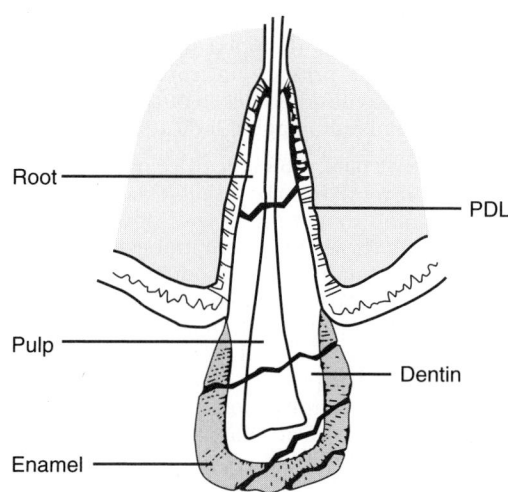

FIGURE 295–1. Tooth fractures may involve enamel, dentin, or pulp and may occur in the crown or root of a tooth. (From Pinkham JR: *Pediatric Dentistry: Infancy Through Adolescence.* Philadelphia, WB Saunders, 1988, p 172.)

Traumatic oral injuries should be referred to a dentist as soon as possible. Even when the teeth appear intact, a dentist should evaluate the patient promptly. Baseline data (radiographs, mobility patterns, responses to specific stimuli) enable the dentist to assess the likelihood of future complications.

Injuries to Periodontal Structures. Trauma to teeth with associated injury to periodontal structures that hold the teeth usually presents as mobile or displaced teeth. Such injuries are more frequent in the primary than in the permanent dentition. Categories of trauma to the periodontium include (1) concussion, (2) subluxation, (3) intrusive luxation, (4) extrusive luxation, and (5) avulsion.

CONCUSSION. Injuries that produce minor damage to the periodontal ligament are termed *concussions*. Teeth sustaining such injuries are not mobile or displaced but react markedly to percussion (gentle hitting of the tooth with an instrument). This type of injury usually requires no therapy and resolves without complication. Primary incisors that sustain concussion may change color, indicating pulpal degeneration, and should be evaluated by a dentist.

SUBLUXATION. Subluxated teeth exhibit mild to moderate horizontal mobility, vertical mobility, or both. Hemorrhage is usually evident around the neck of the tooth at the gingival margin. There is no displacement of the tooth. Many subluxated teeth need to be immobilized by splints to ensure adequate repair of the periodontal ligament. Some of these teeth will develop pulp necrosis.

TABLE 295–1. Injuries to Crowns of Teeth

Type of Trauma	Description	Treatment and Referral
Enamel infraction (crazing)	Incomplete fracture of enamel without loss of tooth structure.	Initially may not require therapy but should be assessed periodically by dentist.
Enamel fractures	Fracture of only the tooth enamel.	Tooth may be smoothed or treated to replace fragment.
Enamel and dentin fracture	Fracture of enamel and dentinal layer of the tooth. Tooth may be sensitive to cold or air. Pulp may become necrotic, leading to periapical abscess.	Refer as soon as possible. Area should be treated to preserve the integrity of the underlying pulp.
Enamel, dentin fracture involving the pulp	Bacterial contamination may lead to pulpal necrosis and periapical abscess. The tooth may have the appearance of bleeding or may display a small red spot.	Refer immediately. The dental therapy of choice depends on the extent of injury, the condition of the pulp, the development of the tooth, time elapsed from injury, and any other injuries to the supporting structures. Therapy is directed toward minimizing contamination in an effort to improve the prognosis.

From Jossell SD, Abrams RG: Managing common dental problems and emergencies. Pediatr Clin North Am 1991;38:1325.

INTRUSIVE LUXATION. Intruded teeth are pushed up into their socket, sometimes to the point where they are not clinically visible. Intruded primary incisors may give the false appearance of being avulsed (knocked out) (Fig. 295–2). To rule out avulsion, a dental radiograph is indicated (Fig. 295–3).

EXTRUSIVE LUXATION. This type of injury is characterized by displacement of the tooth from its socket. The tooth is usually displaced to the lingual (tongue) side, with fracture of the wall of the alveolar socket. These teeth need immediate treatment; the longer the delay, the more likely the tooth will be fixed in its displaced position. Therapy is directed at reduction (repositioning the tooth) and fixation (splinting). In addition, the pulp of such teeth often becomes necrotic and requires endodontic therapy. Extrusive luxation in the primary dentition is usually managed by extraction because complications of reduction and fixation may result in problems with development of permanent teeth.

AVULSION. If avulsed permanent teeth are replanted within 20 min after injury, good success may be achieved; if the delay exceeds 2 hr, however, failure (root resorption, ankylosis) is frequent. The likelihood that normal reattachment will follow replantation of the tooth is related to the viability of the periodontal ligament. Parents confronted with this emergency situation can be instructed to do the following:

1. Find the tooth.
2. Rinse the tooth. (Do not scrub the tooth. Do not touch the root. After plugging the sink drain, hold the tooth by the crown and rinse it under running tap water.)
3. Insert the tooth into the socket. (Gently place it back into its normal position. Do not be concerned if the tooth extrudes slightly. If the parent or child is too apprehensive for replanta-tion of the tooth, the tooth should be placed in cold cow's milk or other cold isotonic solutions).
4. *Go directly to the dentist.* (In transit, the child should hold the tooth in place with a finger. The parent should buckle a seatbelt around the child and drive safely.)

After the tooth is replanted, it must be immobilized to facilitate reattachment; endodontic therapy is always required. The initial signs of complications associated with replantation may appear as early as 1 wk post trauma or as late as several years later. Close dental follow-up is indicated for at least 1 yr.

PREVENTION

To minimize the likelihood of dental injuries:

1. Every child or adolescent who engages in contact sports should wear a mouth guard, which may be constructed by a dentist or purchased at any athletic goods store.
2. Helmets with face guards should be worn by children or adolescents with neuromuscular problems or seizure disorders to protect the head and face during falls.
3. Helmets should also be used during biking, roller blading, and skateboarding.
4. All children or adolescents with protruding incisors should be evaluated by a pediatric dentist or orthodontist.

Additional Considerations. Children who experience dental trauma may also have sustained head or neck trauma, and therefore neurologic assessment is warranted. Tetanus prophylaxis should be considered with any injury that disrupts the integrity of the oral tissues. The possibility of child abuse should always be considered.

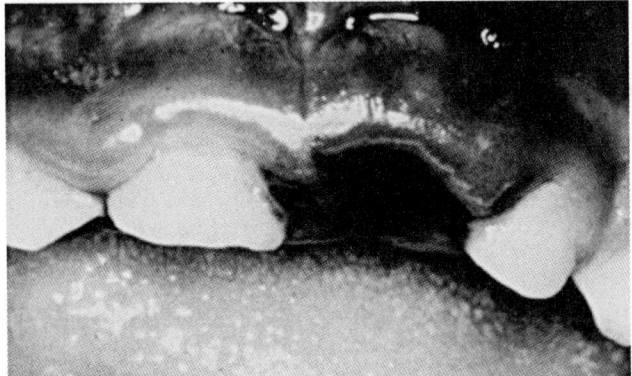

FIGURE 295–2. Intruded primary incisor that appears avulsed (knocked out).

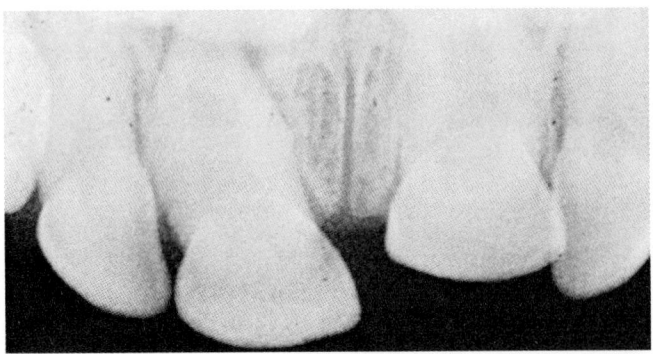

FIGURE 295–3. Occlusal radiograph documents intrusion of "missing tooth" presented in Figure 295–2.

Chapter 296

Common Lesions of the Oral Soft Tissues

Oropharyngeal Candidiasis (see Chapter 215.1). Oropharyngeal infection with *Candida albicans* (thrush, moniliasis) is common in neonates from contact with the organism in the birth canal. The lesions of oropharyngeal candidiasis (OPC) appear as white plaques covering all or part of the oropharyngeal mucosa. These plaques are removable from the underlying surface, which is characteristically inflamed with pinpoint hemorrhages. The diagnosis is confirmed by direct microscopic examination on potassium hydroxide smears and culture of scrapings from lesions. OPC is usually self-limited in the healthy newborn infant, but treatment with nystatin will hasten recovery and reduce the risk of spreading to other infants. Persistent infections should be treated with fluconazole therapy.

Oropharyngeal candidiasis is also a major problem during myelosuppressive therapy. Systemic candidiasis (SC), a major cause of morbidity and mortality during myelosuppressive therapy, develops almost exclusively in patients who have had prior oropharyngeal, esophageal, or intestinal candidiasis. This observation implies that prevention of OPC should reduce the incidence of SC. The use of a multiagent regimen, 0.2% chlorhexidine solution and fluconazole, for OPC prophylaxis in children receiving bone marrow transplants may be effective in preventing OPC, SC, or candidal esophagitis.

Aphthous Ulcers. The aphthous ulcer (canker sore) is a distinct oral lesion, prone to recurrence. The differential diagnosis is noted in Table 296–1. Aphthous ulcers are reported to develop in 20% of the population. Their etiology is unclear, but infectious causes, such as *Helicobacter pylori,* herpes simplex virus, and even measles are have been implicated. Clinically, they are characterized by well-circumscribed, ulcerative lesions with a white necrotic base surrounded by a red halo. The lesions last 10 to 14 days and heal without scarring. Expensive prescription medications appear to offer little advantage over readily available over-the-counter palliative therapies.

Herpetic Gingivostomatitis (see Chapter 231). After an initial incubation period of approximately 1 wk, the initial infection with herpes simplex virus manifests as fever and malaise. The oral cavity may show various expressions, including the gingiva becoming erythematous and clusters of small vesicles erupting throughout the mouth. The symptoms usually regress within 2 wk without scarring. Fluids should be encouraged because the child may become dehydrated. Analgesics and anesthetic rinses may make the child more comfortable. Caution should be exercised to prevent autoinoculation or transmission of infection to the eyes.

Recurrent Herpes Labialis. Approximately 90% of the population develops antibodies to herpes simplex virus. In periods of quiescence, the virus is thought to remain latent in sensory neurons. Unlike primary herpetic gingivostomatitis, which manifests as multiple painful vesicles on the lips, tongue, palate, gingiva, and mucosa, recurrent herpes is generally limited to the lips. Other than the annoyance of causing pain and an unattractive appearance, there are generally no systemic symptoms. Reactivation of the virus is thought to be the result of exposure to ultraviolet light, tissue trauma, stress, or fevers. There is little advantage of antiviral therapy over palliative therapies in an otherwise healthy patient affected by recurrent herpes.

Bohn Nodules. Bohn nodules are small developmental anomalies located along the buccal and lingual aspects of the mandibular and maxillary ridges and in the hard palate of the neonate. These lesions arise from remnants of mucous gland tissue. Treatment is not necessary, as the nodules disappear within a few weeks.

Dental Lamina Cysts. Dental lamina cysts are small cystic lesions located along the crest of the mandibular and maxillary ridges of the neonate. These lesions arise from epithelial remnants of the dental lamina. Treatment is not necessary; they will disappear within a few weeks.

TABLE 296–1. Differential Diagnosis of Oral Ulceration

Condition	Comment
Common	
Aphthous (canker sore)	Painful, circumscribed lesions
Traumatic	Accidents, chronic cheek biter or after dental local anesthesia
Hand, foot, mouth disease	Painful, lesions on tongue, anterior oral cavity, hands and feet
Herpangina	Painful, lesions confined to soft palate and oropharynx
Herpetic gingivostomatitis	Vesicles on mucocutaneous borders; painful, febrile
Recurrent herpes labialis	Vesicles on lips; painful
Chemical burns	Alkali, acid, aspirin; painful
Heat burns	Hot food, electrical
Uncommon	
Neutrophil defects	Agranulocytosis, leukemia, cyclic neutropenia; painful
Systemic lupus erythematosus	Recurrent, may be painless
Behçet's syndrome	Resembles aphthous lesions; associated with genital ulcers, uveitis, etc.
Necrotizing ulcerative gingivostomatitis	Vincent stomatitis; painful
Syphilis	Chancre or gumma; painless
Oral Crohn disease	Aphthous-like; painful
Histoplasmosis	Lingual

Fordyce Granules. Almost 80% of adults have multiple, yellow-white granules in clusters or plaquelike areas on the oral mucosa, most commonly on the buccal mucosa or lips. They are aberrant sebaceous glands. The glands are present at birth, but they may hypertrophy and first appear as discrete yellowish papules during the preadolescent period in approximately 50% of children. No treatment is necessary.

Parulis. The parulis (gum boil) is a soft, reddish papule located adjacent to the root of a chronically abscessed tooth. It occurs at the endpoint of a draining dental sinus tract. Treatment consists of diagnosing which tooth is abscessed and extracting it or root canal treatment of the offending tooth.

Cheilitis. Dryness of the lips, followed by scaling and cracking and accompanied by a characteristic burning sensation, is common in children. It is usually caused by sensitivity to contact substances (from toys and foods) plus photosensitivity to the sun's rays. It is aggravated by the alternation of wetting with the tongue and drying by the wind, especially in cold weather. Cheilitis often occurs in association with fever. Frequent application of petroleum jelly facilitates healing and is also preventative.

Ankyloglossia. Ankyloglossia or "tongue-tie" is characterized by an abnormally short lingual frenum that hinders the tongue movement. The frenum may lengthen as the child gets older. If the extent of the ankyloglossia is severe, speech may be affected and surgical correction indicated.

Geographic Tongue. Geographic tongue (migratory glossitis) is a benign and asymptomatic lesion and is characterized by one or more smooth, bright-red patches, often showing a yellow, gray, or white membranous margin on the dorsum of an otherwise normally roughened tongue. The condition has no known cause and no treatment is indicated (see Chapter 654).

Fissured Tongue. The fissured tongue (scrotal tongue) is a malformation manifested clinically by numerous small furrows or grooves on the dorsal surface (see Chapter 654). If the tongue is painful, the bacteria in the fissures can be reduced by brushing the tongue or use of water irrigation.

Chapter 297
Diseases of the Salivary Glands and Jaws

With the exception of mumps (see Chapter 227), disease of the salivary glands is rare in children. Bilateral enlargement of the submaxillary glands may occur in AIDS, cystic fibrosis, and malnutrition and, transiently, during acute asthmatic attacks. Chronic vomiting may be accompanied by enlargement of the parotid glands. Benign salivary gland hypertrophy has been associated with endocrinopathies: thyroid disease, diabetes, and disorders of the pituitary-adrenal axis.

Recurrent Parotitis. Recurrent idiopathic swelling of the parotid gland may occur in otherwise healthy children. The swelling is usually unilateral, but both glands may be involved simultaneously or alternately. There is little pain; the swelling is limited to the gland and usually lasts 2–3 wk. The incidence appears to be higher in the spring.

Suppurative Parotitis. This is usually due to *Staphylococcus aureus* and may be primary or a complication of parotitis from another cause. It is usually unilateral and may be accompanied by fever. The gland becomes swollen, tender, and painful. Suppurative parotitis responds to appropriate antibacterial therapy based on culture obtained from the Stensen duct or by surgical drainage, which is infrequently required.

Ranula. Ranula is a cyst associated with a major salivary gland in the sublingual area. A ranula is a large, soft, mucus-containing swelling in the floor of the mouth. It occurs at any age, including infancy. The cyst should be excised, and the severed duct should be exteriorized.

Mucocele. A mucocele is a salivary gland lesion caused by a blockage of a salivary gland duct. They are most common on the lower lip and have the appearance of a fluid-filled vesicle or a fluctuant nodule with the overlying mucosa normal in color. Treatment is by surgical excision with removal of the involved accessory salivary gland.

Congenital Lip Pits. Lip pits are caused by fistulous tracts that lead to imbedded mucus glands in the lower lip. They leak saliva, especially with salivary stimulation. Lip pits may be isolated anomalies, or they may be found in patients with cleft lip or palate. Treatment is by surgical excision of the glandular tissue.

Eruption Cyst. An eruption cyst is a smooth painless swelling over the erupting tooth. If bleeding occurs in the cyst space, it may appear blue or blue-black. In most cases, no treatment is indicated and the cyst will resolve with the full eruption of the tooth.

Xerostomia. Xerostomia (or dry mouth) may be associated with fever, dehydration, anticholinergic drugs, chronic graft versus host disease, Mikulicz disease (leukemia infiltrates), Sjögren syndrome, or tumoricidal doses of radiation when the salivary glands are within the field. Long-term xerostomia is a high risk factor for dental caries.

Salivary Gland Tumors. See Chapter 492.1.

Histiocytosis X (see Chapter 499). The etiology and pathogenesis of histiocytosis remains obscure. In the severe form there are oral lesions with pain, swelling, gingival necrosis, and destruction of alveolar bone resulting in premature exfoliation of teeth. Treatment will vary according to the extent of the disease, with surgical curettage or radiation therapy being used to treat the focal disease. Multiagent chemotherapy is successful in treating the disseminated disease.

Tumors of the Jaws. Ossifying fibroma is a common benign tumor of the jaw. It is often asymptomatic, being discovered on routine radiographic examinations. Treatment is by enucleation or curettage. Central giant cell granuloma is another common lesion thought to be reactive rather than neoplastic. Although usually asymptomatic, it may be expansile with or without divergence of teeth. Treatment is by complete curettage or surgical excision. Dentigerous cysts are common lesions associated with the crown of an impacted or unerupted tooth. Although usually asymptomatic they may become large and destructive. Treatment is by surgical removal.

The malignant primary tumors of the jaws in children include Burkitt lymphoma, osteogenic sarcoma, lymphosarcoma, ameloblastoma, and, more rarely, fibrosarcoma.

Chapter 298
Diagnostic Radiology in Dental Assessment

The *panoramic radiograph* provides a single tomographic image of the upper and lower jaw, including all the teeth and supporting structures. The x-ray tube rotates about the patient's head with reciprocal movement of the film or image receptor during the exposure. The panoramic image shows the mandibular bodies,

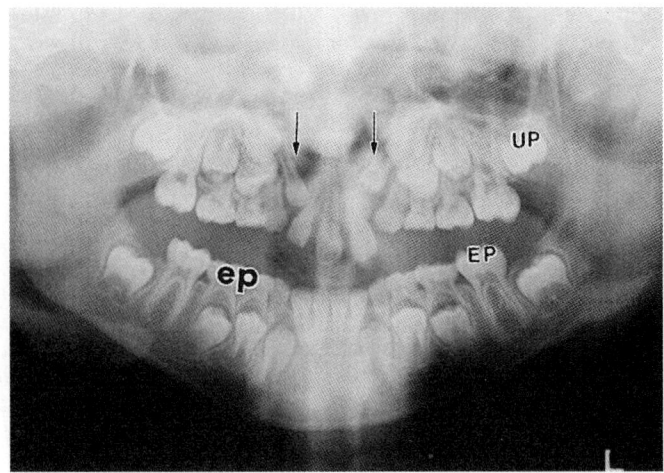

FIGURE 298–1. A panoramic radiograph of an 8-yr-old patient with a cleft palate showing abnormal numbers and position of teeth in the area of the cleft *(arrows)*. Also shown are erupted primary teeth (ep), erupted permanent teeth (EP), and unerupted permanent teeth (UP).

rami, and condyles; maxillary sinuses; and a majority of the facial buttresses. Such images are used to show abnormalities of tooth number, development and eruption pattern, cystic and neoplastic lesions, extensive bone infections, and fractures (Fig. 298–1).

Cephalometric radiographs are posteroanterior and lateral skull films that are taken using a head positioner (cephalostat) and employ techniques that clearly demonstrate the facial skeleton and soft facial tissues. Similar protocols for positioning children are used throughout the world. From these images, cranial and facial points and planes can be determined and compared with standards derived from thousands of images. A child's facial growth can be assessed serially when cephalometric radiographs are taken sequentially. Relationships among the maxilla, mandible, cranial base, and facial skeleton can be determined in a quantitative manner. Additionally, the alignment of the teeth and the relation of the teeth to the supporting bone can be serially measured.

Intraoral dental radiographs are highly detailed, direct exposure films that demonstrate sections of the child's teeth and supporting bone structures. The film or image receptor is placed lingual to the teeth, and the x-ray beam is directed through the teeth and supporting structures. The resulting images are used to detect dental caries, loss of alveolar bone (periodontal disease), abscesses at the roots of the teeth, and trauma to the teeth and alveolar bone and to demonstrate the developmental status of permanent teeth within the bone.

Andreasen JO, Andreasen FM: *Essentials of Traumatic Injuries to the Teeth.* Copenhagen, Munksgaard, 1990.

Flaitz CM: Oral pathologic conditions and soft tissue anomalies. In Pinkham JR (editor): *Pediatric Dentistry: Infancy Through Adolescence,* 3rd ed. Philadelphia, WB Saunders, 1999, p 12.

Griffen AL (editor): Pediatric oral health. *Pediatr Clin North Am* 2000;47.

Johnsen DC, Tinanoff N (editors): Dental care for the preschool child. *Dent Clin North Am* 1995.

Josell SD, Abrams RG (editors): Pediatric oral health. *Pediatr Clin North Am* 1991; 38.

Kalsbeek H, Verrips GH: Consumption of sweet snacks and caries experience of primary school children. *Caries Res* 1994;28:447.

Nakata M: Genetics in oral-facial growth and disease. *Int Dent J* 1995;45:227.

Nelson LP, Shusterman S: Emergency management of oral trauma in children. *Curr Opin Pediatr* 1997;9:242.

Sonis A, Zaragoza S: Dental health for the pediatrician. *Curr Opin Pediatr* 2001;13: 289.

Tinanoff N: Dental caries: Etiology, pathogenesis, clinical manifestations, and management. In Wei SHY (editor): *Pediatric Dentistry: Total Patient Care.* Philadelphia, Lea & Febiger, 1988, p 9.

SECTION 3 *The Esophagus*

Susan Orenstein, John Peters, Seema Khan, Nader Youssef, and Sunny Zaheed Hussain

Chapter 299

Embryology, Anatomy, and Function of the Esophagus

The esophagus is a hollow muscular tube, separated from the pharynx above and the stomach below by two tonically closed sphincters. Its primary function is to convey ingested material from the mouth to the stomach. Largely lacking digestive glands and enzymes, and exposed only briefly to nutrients, it has no active role in digestion.

Embryology. The esophagus develops from the postpharyngeal foregut and can be distinguished from the stomach in the 4-week (5-mm) embryo. At the same time, the trachea begins to bud just anterior to the developing esophagus; the resulting laryngotracheal groove extends and becomes the lung. Disturbances in this stage may result in congenital anomalies such as tracheoesophageal fistula. The length of the esophagus is 2.5 mm in a 13.5-mm embryo, is 8–10 cm at birth, and doubles during the first 2–3 yr of life, reaching approximately 25 cm in an adult. The abdominal portion of the esophagus is as large as the stomach in an 8-wk old fetus but gradually shortens to a few millimeters at birth, attaining a final length of about 3 cm by a few years of age. This intra-abdominal location of both the distal esophagus and the lower esophageal sphincter (LES) is an important antireflux mechanism, because increase in intra-abdominal pressure is also transmitted to the sphincter, augmenting its defense. Swallowing can be seen in utero as early as 16–20 wk of gestation, helping to circulate the amniotic fluid; polyhydramnios is thus a hallmark of lack of normal swallowing or of esophageal or gastrointestinal obstruction. Sucking and swallowing are not fully coordinated before 34 wk of gestation, a contributing factor for feeding difficulties in premature infants.

Anatomy. The luminal aspect of the esophagus is covered by thick, protective, nonkeratinized stratified squamous epithelium, which abruptly changes to simple columnar epithelium at the stomach's upper margin at the gastroesophageal junction (GEJ). This squamous epithelium is relatively resistant to damage by gastric secretions (in contrast to the ciliated columnar epithelium of the respiratory tract), but chronic irritation by gastric contents may result in morphometric changes (see morphometric esophagitis, later) and subsequent metaplasia of the cells lining the lower esophagus from squamous to columnar. Deeper layers of the esophageal wall are composed successively of lamina propria, muscularis mucosae, submucosa, and the two layers of muscularis propria (circular surrounded by longitudinal). The two delimiting sphincters of the esophagus, the upper esophageal sphincter (UES) at the cricopharyngeus muscle and the LES at the GEJ, narrow the caliber of the esophageal lumen at its proximal and distal boundaries. The muscularis propria of the upper third of the esophagus is predominantly striated, and that of the lower two thirds is smooth muscle. Clinical conditions involving striated muscle (cricopharyngeal dysfunction, cerebral palsy) affect the upper esophagus, whereas those involving smooth muscle (achalasia, reflux esophagitis) affect the lower esophagus. The muscular LES and the mucosal "Z-line" of the GEJ may be discrepant up to several centimeters.

Function. The esophagus can be divided into three areas: the UES, the esophageal body, and the LES. At rest, the tonic LES pressure is normally about 20 mm Hg; values below 10 mm Hg are usually considered abnormal, although it seems that competence against retrograde flow of gastric material is maintained if the LES pressure is above 5 mm Hg. The LES pressure rises during intragastric pressure amplifications, whether caused by gastric contractions, abdominal wall muscle contractions ("straining"), or external pressure applied to the abdominal wall. It also rises in response to cholinergic stimuli, gastrin, gastric alkalization, and certain drugs (bethanechol, metoclopramide, cisapride). The UES pressure is more variable and often higher than that of the LES; it decreases almost to zero during deep sleep but increases markedly during stress and straining.

Swallowing is initiated by elevation of the tongue, propelling the bolus into the pharynx. The larynx elevates and moves anteriorly, pulling open the relaxing UES, while the epiglottis drops back to cover the larynx and direct the bolus over the larynx and into the UES and the soft palate occludes the nasopharynx. The primary peristalsis thus initiated is a contraction originating in the oropharynx that clears the esophagus aborally (Fig. 299–1). The LES, tonically contracted as a barrier against gastroesophageal reflux, relaxes as swallowing is initiated, at nearly the same time as the UES relaxation. However, the LES relaxation persists considerably longer, until the peristaltic wave traverses it and closes it. The normal esophageal peristaltic speed is about 3 cm/s; the wave takes at least 4 s to traverse the 12-cm esophagus of a young infant and considerably longer in a larger child. Facial stimulation by a puff of air can induce swallowing and esophageal peristalsis in healthy young infants, a reflex termed the *Santmyer swallow.*

In addition to relaxing to move swallowed material past the GEJ into the stomach, the LES normally relaxes to vent swallowed air or to allow retrograde expulsion of material from the stomach. Perhaps as an extension of these functions, the normal LES also permits physiologic reflux episodes that are brief and occur approximately five times in the first postprandial hour but uncommonly otherwise. Transient LES relaxation, not associated with swallowing, comprises the major mechanism underlying pathologic reflux (see Fig. 299–1).

The close linkage of the anatomy of the upper digestive and respiratory tracts has mandated intricate functional protections of the respiratory tract during retrograde movement of gastric contents as well as during swallowing. The protective functions include the LES tone, the bolstering of the LES by the surrounding diaphragmatic crura, and the "backup protection" of the UES tone. In addition, secondary ("esophageal") peristalsis, akin to primary peristalsis but without an oral component, clears refluxed gastric contents from the esophagus. Another protective reflex is the "pharyngeal swallow" (initiated above the esophagus, but without lingual participation). Multiple levels of protection against aspiration include the rhythmic coordination of swallowing and breathing as well as a series of protective reflexes with esophagopharyngeal afferents and efferents that close the UES or larynx. These reflexes include the esophago-UES contractile reflex, the pharyngo-UES contractile reflex, the esophagoglottal closure reflex, and two pharyngoglottal adduction reflexes. The latter two reflexes have chemoreceptors on the laryngeal surface of the epiglottis and mechanoreceptors on the aryepiglottic folds as their sites of stimulus. It is likely that interactions between the esophagus and the respiratory tract, which cause extraesophageal manifestations of gastroesophageal reflux

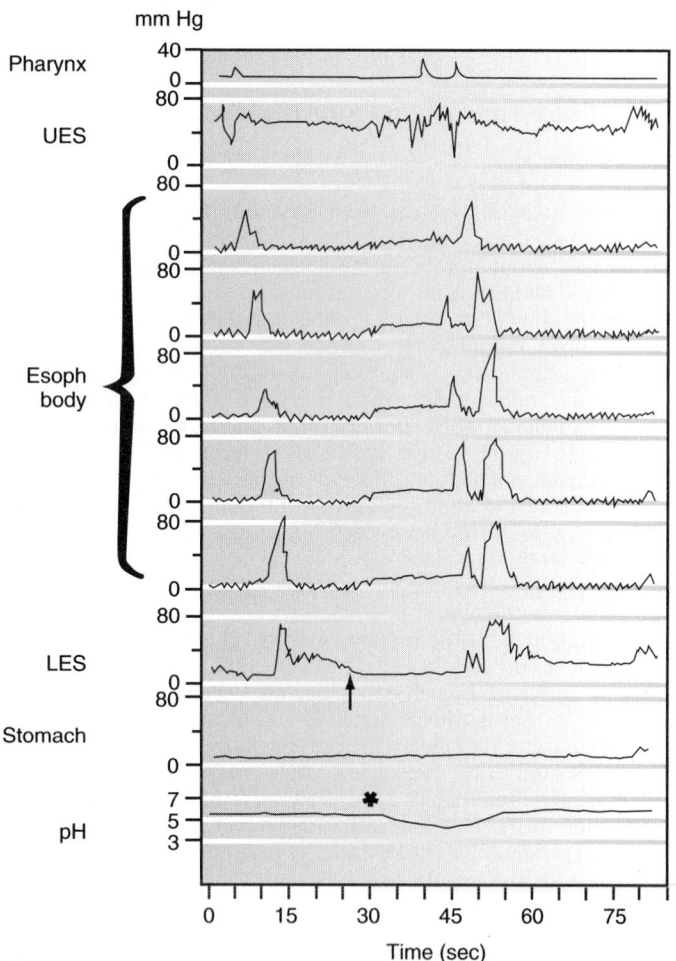

FIGURE 299–1. A continuous tracing of esophageal motility showing 2 swallows, as indicated by the pharyngeal contraction associated with relaxation of the UES and followed by peristalsis in the body of the esophagus. The LES also displays a transient relaxation *(arrow)* unassociated with a swallow. There is an episode of gastroesophageal reflux (*) recorded by a pH probe at the time of the transient LES relaxation. (Courtesy of John Dent, FRACP, PhD, and Geoffrey Davidson, MD.)

disease, will be explained by subtle abnormalities in these protective reflexes.

299.1 Common Clinical Manifestations and Diagnostic Aids

Common Clinical Manifestations. Manifestations of esophageal disease may be categorized as pain, obstruction or difficulty swallowing, abnormal retrograde movement of gastric contents (reflux, regurgitation, or vomiting), or bleeding; esophageal disease may also engender respiratory symptoms. Pain in the chest unrelated to swallowing ("heartburn") can be a sign of esophagitis, but similar pain may also represent cardiac, pulmonary, or musculoskeletal disease. Pain during swallowing (odynophagia) localizes the disease more discretely to the pharynx and esophagus and often represents inflammatory mucosal disease. Complete esophageal obstruction may be produced acutely by esophageal foreign bodies, including food impactions; may be congenital, as in esophageal atresia; or may evolve over time as a peptic stricture occludes the esophagus. Difficulty swallowing (dysphagia) may be produced by incompletely occlusive

esophageal obstruction (by extrinsic compression, intrinsic narrowing, or foreign bodies) but also may result from dysmotility of the esophagus (whether primary/idiopathic or secondary to systemic disease). Inflammatory lesions of the esophagus without obstruction or dysmotility are a third cause of dysphagia; eosinophilic esophagitis, most often afflicting older male children, is a relatively common cause. The most common esophageal disorder in children is gastroesophageal reflux disease (GERD), which is retrograde return of gastric contents. Esophagitis may be caused by GERD, by eosinophilic disease, by infection, or by caustic substances. Esophageal bleeding may result from severe esophagitis that produces erosions or ulcerations and may manifest as anemia or Hemoccult-positive stools. More acute or severe bleeding may be due to ruptured esophageal varices. The resulting hematemesis must be differentiated from more distal bleeding (gastric ulcer) and from more proximal bleeding (a nosebleed or hemoptysis). Respiratory symptoms of esophageal disease may result from luminal contents incorrectly being directed into the respiratory tract or to reflexive respiratory responses to esophageal stimuli.

Diagnostic Aids. The esophagus may be evaluated by radiography, endoscopy, histology, scintigraphy, manometry, pH-metry (linked as indicated with other polysomnography), and intraluminal impedance. Contrast (usually barium) radiographic study of the esophagus usually incorporates fluoroscopic imaging over time so that motility, as well as anatomy, can be assessed. Although most often requested to evaluate for GERD, it is neither sensitive nor specific for this purpose; however, it can detect complications of GERD (stricture or hiatal hernia) or conditions mimicking GERD (pyloric stenosis or malrotation with intermittent volvulus). Barium fluoroscopy is optimal to evaluate for structural anomalies, such as duplications, strictures, or external esophageal compression by an aberrant blood vessel, or for causes of dysmotility, such as achalasia. Modifications of the routine barium fluoroscopic study are used in special situations. When an "H-type" tracheoesophageal fistula is suspected, the test is most sensitive if the radiologist distends the esophagus with barium via a nasogastric tube with the patient prone. A "modified barium swallow" performed with varying consistencies of barium (oropharyngeal video-esophagogram or "cookie swallow") optimally evaluates children with dysphagia by demonstrating incoordination in the pharyngeal and esophageal phases of swallowing. In some centers videofluoroscopy is combined with fiberoptic (naso)pharyngeal endoscopy to provide exquisite detail when UES dysfunction is suspected. Endoscopy allows direct visualization of esophageal mucosa and helps therapeutically in the removal of foreign bodies and treatment of esophageal varices. Endoscopy also allows biopsy samples to be taken, thus improving the diagnosis of "endoscopy-negative" GERD, differentiating GERD from eosinophilic esophagitis, and identifying viral or fungal causes of esophagitis. Radionuclide scintigraphy scans are helpful in evaluating the efficiency of peristalsis and demonstrating reflux episodes. They can be specific, although not very sensitive, for aspiration and can quantify gastric emptying, thus hinting at a cause for GERD. Esophageal manometry evaluates for dysmotility from the pharynx to the stomach; by synchronized quantitative pressure measurements along the esophagus it detects dysfunctions sometimes missed radiographically. Manometry is often challenging in young infants, and sphincters are optimally evaluated with a special Dent sleeve. Extended pH monitoring of the distal esophagus is a quantitative and sensitive test for acidic GER episodes. It is linked with polysomnography (a pneumogram) when GER is suspected to cause apnea or similar symptoms. Intraluminal electric impedance is a method for pH-independent detection of bolus movements in the esophagus and can distinguish between acid and nonacid liquid and gaseous reflux.

Chapter 300

Congenital Anomalies: Esophageal Atresia and Tracheoesophageal Fistula

Esophageal atresia (EA) is the most frequent congenital anomaly of the esophagus, affecting about 1 in 4,000 neonates. Of these, more than 90% have an associated tracheoesophageal fistula (TEF). In the most common form of EA, the upper esophagus ends in a blind pouch and the TEF is connected to the distal esophagus. The types of EA and TEF and their relative frequencies are shown in Figure 300–1. This defect now has survival rates of greater than 90%, owing largely to improved neonatal intensive care, earlier recognition, and appropriate intervention. Infants weighing less than 1,500 g at birth have the highest risk for mortality. Fifty per cent of infants have associated anomalies, most often associated with the VATER/VACTERL (*V*ertebral, *A*norectal, *T*rachea, *E*sophagus, *C*ardiac, *R*enal, *R*adial, and *L*imb) syndrome.

Presentation. The neonate with EA typically has frothing and bubbling at the mouth and nose, episodes of coughing, cyanosis, and respiratory distress. Feeding exacerbates these symptoms, causes regurgitation, and may precipitate aspiration. Aspiration of gastric contents via a distal fistula causes more damaging pneumonitis than aspiration of pharyngeal secretions from the blind upper pouch. The infant with an isolated TEF in the absence of EA ("H-type" fistula) may come to medical attention later in life with chronic respiratory problems, including refractory bronchospasm and recurrent pneumonias.

Diagnosis. In the setting of early-onset respiratory distress, the inability to pass a nasogastric or orogastric tube in the newborn is suggestive of esophageal atresia. Prenatally, maternal polyhydramnios may alert the physician to EA. Plain radiography in the evaluation of respiratory distress may reveal a coiled feeding tube in the esophageal pouch and/or an air-distended stomach indicating the presence of a coexisting TEF (Fig. 300–2). Conversely, pure EA may present as an airless, scaphoid abdomen. In isolated TEF, an esophagogram with contrast medium injected under pressure may demonstrate the defect. Alternatively, the orifice may be detected at bronchoscopy or when methylene blue dye injected into the endotracheal tube during endoscopy is observed in the esophagus during forced inspiration.

Management. Initially, maintaining a patent airway and preventing aspiration of secretions is paramount. Prone positioning minimizes movement of gastric secretions into a distal fistula, and esophageal suctioning minimizes aspiration from a blind pouch. Endotracheal intubation is avoided because it may worsen distention of abdominal viscera. Surgical ligation of the TEF and primary end-to-end anastomosis of the esophagus are performed when feasible. In the premature or otherwise complicated infant, a primary closure may be delayed by temporizing with fistula ligation and gastrostomy tube placement. If the gap between the atretic ends of the esophagus is greater than 3–4 cm, primary repair cannot be done; options include using gastric, jejunal, or colonic segments interposed as a neo-esophagus. Careful search must be undertaken for the common associated cardiac and other anomalies.

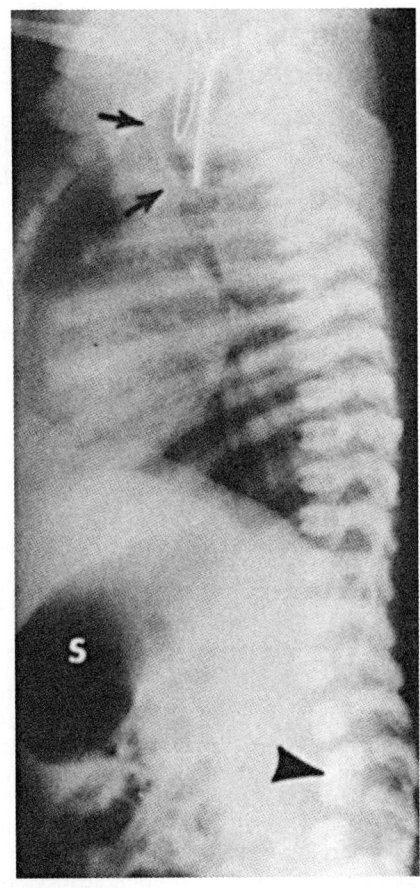

FIGURE 300–2. Tracheoesophageal fistula. Lateral radiograph demonstrating a nasogastric tube coiled *(arrows)* in the proximal segment of an atretic esophagus. The distal fistula is suggested by gaseous dilatation of the stomach (S) and small intestine. The *arrowhead* depicts vertebral fusion, whereas a heart murmur and cardiomegaly suggest the presence of a ventricular septal defect. This patient demonstrated elements of the VATER anomalad. (From Balfe D, Ling D, Siegel M: The esophagus. In Putman CE, Ravin CE [editors]: *Textbook of Diagnostic Imaging.* Philadelphia, WB Saunders, 1988.)

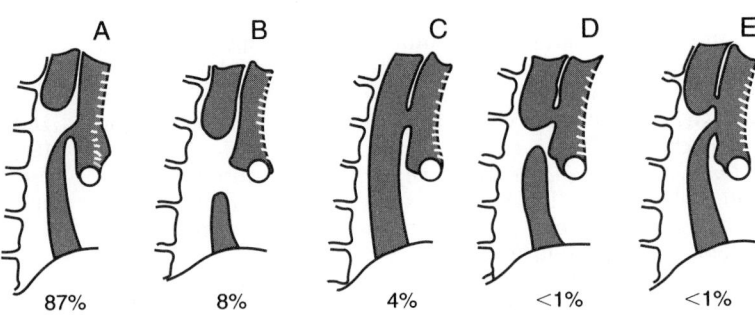

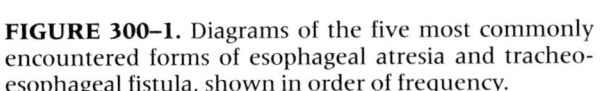

FIGURE 300–1. Diagrams of the five most commonly encountered forms of esophageal atresia and tracheoesophageal fistula, shown in order of frequency.

Outcome. The majority of infants grow up to lead normal lives, but complications are frequently challenging, particularly during infancy. Complications of surgery include anastomotic leak, re-fistulization, and anastomotic stricture. Gastroesophageal reflux disease (GERD), resulting from intrinsic abnormalities of esophageal function, often combined with delayed gastric emptying, contributes to management challenges in many cases. GERD contributes significantly to the respiratory disease (reactive airway disease) that often complicates EA and TEF and also worsens the frequent anastomotic strictures after repair of EA.

300.1 Congenital Anomalies: Laryngotracheoesophageal Clefts

These uncommon anomalies result when the septum between the esophagus and trachea fails to develop fully, leading to a common channel defect between the pharyngoesophagus and laryngotrachea, and thus making the laryngeal closure incompetent during swallowing or reflux. Early in life, the infant presents with stridor, choking, cyanosis, aspiration of feedings, and recurrent chest infections. The diagnosis is difficult and usually requires direct visualization of the larynx and esophagus endoscopically. When contrast radiography is used, material is often seen in the esophagus and trachea. Treatment is by surgical repair, which can be complex if the defects are long.

Chapter 301

Obstructing and Motility Disorders of the Esophagus

Obstructing lesions classically produce dysphagia to solids earlier and more noticeably than to liquids and may manifest when the infant liquid diet begins to incorporate solids; this is in contrast to dysphagia from dysmotility, in which swallowing of liquids is affected as early as, or earlier than, solids. In most instances of dysphagia, evaluation begins with fluoroscopy. Secondary studies are often endoscopic, if intrinsic obstruction is suspected; manometric, if dysmotility is suspected; and other imaging studies in particular cases. Congenital lesions may require surgery, whereas webs and peptic strictures may respond adequately to endoscopic (or bougie) dilation. Peptic strictures, once dilated, should prompt consideration of fundoplication for ongoing prophylaxis.

Extrinsic. *Esophageal duplication cysts* comprise the most frequently encountered foregut duplications. These cysts are lined by intestinal epithelium, have a well-developed smooth muscle wall, and are attached to the normal gastrointestinal tract. Two thirds occur on the right side of the esophagus. The most common presentation is respiratory distress caused by compression of the adjacent airways. Dysphagia is a common symptom in older children. Upper gastrointestinal bleeding may occur as a result of acid-secreting gastric mucosa in the duplication wall. Neuroenteric cysts may contain glial elements and are associated with vertebral anomalies. Diagnosis is made either on barium swallow or chest CT. Treatment is surgical; laparoscopic approach to excision is possible.

Enlarged mediastinal or subcarinal lymph nodes, caused by infection (tuberculosis, histoplasmosis) or neoplasm (lymphoma), are the most common external masses that may compress the esophagus and produce obstructive symptoms. *Vascular anomalies* may also compress the esophagus; *dysphagia lusoria* is a term denoting the dysphagia produced by a developmental anomaly,

which is often an aberrant right subclavian artery or right-sided or double aortic arch (see Chapter 425.1).

Intrinsic. Intrinsic narrowing of the esophageal lumen may be congenital or acquired. The etiology is suggested by the location, the character of the lesion, and the clinical situation. The lower esophagus is the most common location for *peptic strictures*, which are generally somewhat ragged and several centimeters long. *Thin membranous rings*, including the Schatzki ring at the squamocolumnar junction, may also occlude this area. In the mid esophagus, congenital narrowing may be associated with the esophageal atresia/tracheoesophageal fistula complex, in which some of the lesions may incorporate cartilage and be impossible to dilate safely; alternatively, reflux esophagitis may induce a ragged and extensive narrowing that is more proximal than the usual peptic stricture, sometimes in conjunction with hiatal hernia or Barrett esophagus. *Congenital webs or rings* may narrow the upper esophagus by a postinflammatory stricture resulting from caustic ingestion or epidermolysis bullosa or posteriorly by a cricopharyngeal "bar" in the upper esophagus.

Chapter 302

Dysmotility

Upper Esophageal and Upper Esophageal Sphincter (UES) Dysmotility (Striated Muscle). *Cricopharyngeal achalasia* signifies a failure of complete relaxation of the UES, whereas *cricopharyngeal incoordination* implies full relaxation of the UES but incoordination of the relaxation with the pharyngeal contraction. These entities are usually detected on videofluoroscopic evaluation of swallowing (sometimes accompanied by visible cricopharyngeal prominence, termed a *bar*), but often the most precise definition of the dysfunction is obtained with manometry. A self-limited form of cricopharyngeal incoordination occurs in infancy and remits spontaneously during the first year of life if nutrition is maintained despite the dysphagia. In older children, idiopathic cricopharyngeal spasm is usually treated by myotomy of the UES. It is important, however, to evaluate such children thoroughly, including cranial MRI to detect Arnold Chiari malformations, which may present in this way but are best treated by cranial, rather than esophageal, surgery. Cricopharyngeal spasm may be severe enough to produce posterior pharyngeal (Zenker) diverticulum above the obstructive sphincter, but this entity occurs rarely in children.

Systemic causes of swallowing dysfunction that may affect the oropharynx, UES, and upper esophagus include cerebral palsy, Arnold Chiari malformations, syringomyelia, bulbar palsy or cranial nerve defects (Möbius syndrome, transient infantile paralysis of the superior laryngeal nerve), transient pharyngeal muscle dysfunction, spinal muscular atrophy (including Werdnig-Hoffmann disease), muscular dystrophy, infections (botulism, tetanus, poliomyelitis, diphtheria), inflammatory and connective tissue diseases (dermatomyositis, myasthenia gravis, polyneuritis, scleroderma), and familial dysautonomia. All of these may produce dysphagia. Medications (nitrazepam and benzodiazepines) and tracheostomy can adversely affect the function of the UES and thereby produce dysphagia.

Lower Esophageal and Lower Esophageal Sphincter (LES) Dysfunction (Smooth Muscle). Causes of dysphagia due to more distal primary esophageal dysmotility include achalasia, diffuse esophageal spasm, nutcracker esophagus, and hypertensive LES; all but achalasia are rarely described in children.

Achalasia is a primary esophageal motor disorder of unknown etiology characterized by loss of LES relaxation and loss of esophageal peristalsis, both contributing to a functional obstruction of the distal esophagus. Degenerative, autoimmune, and infectious factors are possible causes. Pathologically, inflammation surrounds ganglion cells, which are decreased in number. There is selective loss of postganglionic inhibitory neurons that normally lead to sphincter relaxation, leaving postganglionic cholinergic neurons unopposed. This imbalance produces high basal LES pressures and insufficient LES relaxation. The loss of esophageal peristalsis may be a secondary phenomenon. Achalasia presents as dysphagia for solids and liquids and may be accompanied by undernutrition or respiratory symptoms; retained esophageal food may produce esophagitis. The mean age in children is 8.8 yr with a mean duration of symptoms before diagnosis of 23 mo; it is uncommon before school age. Chest radiograph shows an air-fluid level in a dilated esophagus. Barium fluoroscopy reveals a smooth tapering of the lower esophagus leading to the closed LES, resembling a "bird's beak" (Fig. 302–1). Loss of primary peristalsis in the distal esophagus with retained food and poor emptying are often present. Manometry confirms the diagnosis and reveals incomplete relaxation of a high-pressure LES during swallowing, often accompanied by nonpropulsive simultaneous contractions in the distal esophagus. The two most effective treatment options are pneu-

matic dilatation and surgical (Heller) myotomy. Surgeons often supplement a myotomy with an antireflux procedure to prevent the gastroesophageal reflux disease that otherwise often ensues when the sphincter is rendered less competent. Calcium channel blockers (e.g., nifedipine) and phosphodiesterase inhibitors offer temporary relief of dysphagia. Endoscopic injection of the LES with botulinum toxin counterbalances the selective loss of inhibitory neurotransmitters by inhibiting the release of acetylcholine from nerve terminals. Botulinum toxin is expensive; half the patients may require a repeat injection within 1 yr.

Diffuse esophageal spasm causes chest pain and dysphagia and affects adolescents and adults. It is diagnosed manometrically and may be treated with nitrates or calcium channel blocking agents.

Gastroesophageal reflux disease constitutes the most common cause of nonspecific abnormalities of esophageal motor function, probably through the effect of the esophageal inflammation on the musculature.

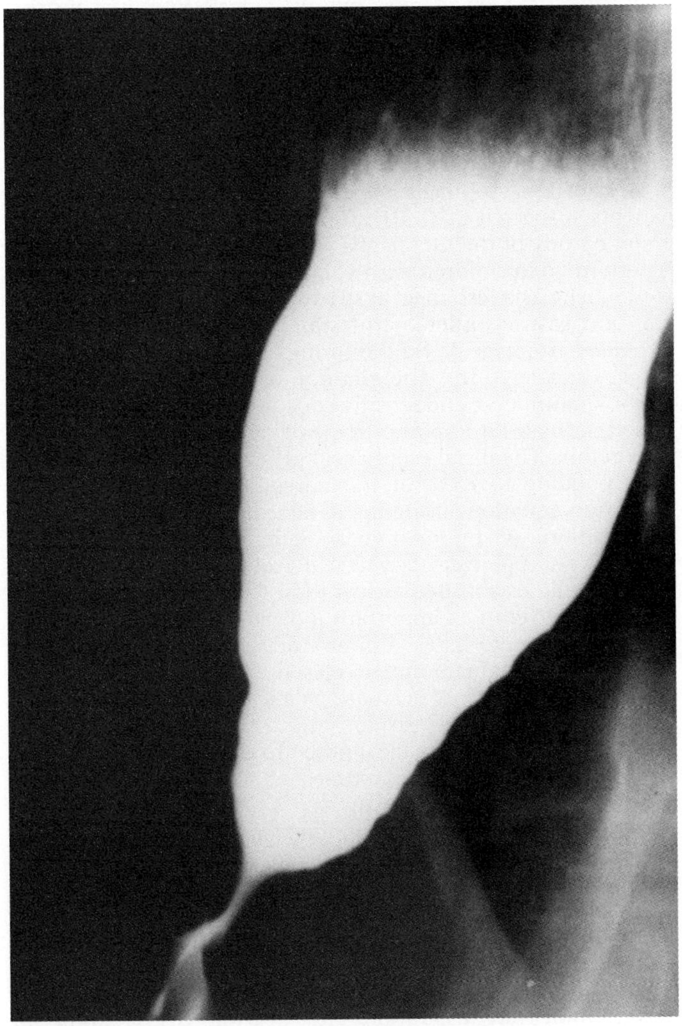

Chapter 303
Hiatal Hernia

Herniation of the stomach through the esophageal hiatus may occur as a common sliding hernia, in which the gastroesophageal junction slides into the thorax, or it may be paraesophageal, in which a portion of the stomach (usually the fundus) is insinuated inside the gastroesophageal junction in the hiatus (Fig. 303–1). Sliding hernias are frequently associated with gastroesophageal reflux, especially in retarded children. The relationship to hiatal hernias in adults is unclear. Medical treatment is not directed at the hernia but at the gastroesophageal reflux.

Paraesophageal hernias may be encountered after fundoplication for gastroesophageal reflux, especially if the edges of a dilated esophageal hiatus have not been approximated. Fullness after eating and upper abdominal pain are the usual symptoms. Infarction of the herniated stomach is rare.

FIGURE 302–1. Barium esophagogram of a patient with achalasia demonstrating dilated esophagus and narrowing at the lower esophageal sphincter. Note retained secretions layered on top of barium in the esophagus.

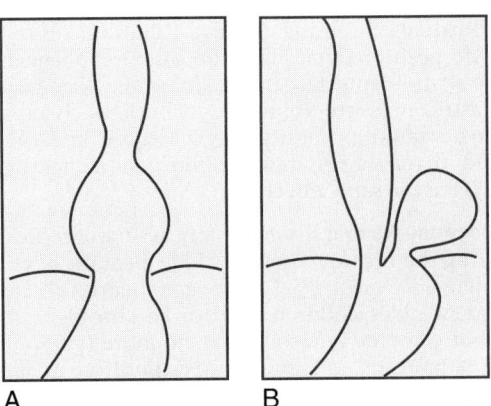

FIGURE 303–1. Types of esophageal hiatal hernia. *A,* Sliding hiatal hernia, the most common type. *B,* Paraesophageal hiatal hernia.

Chapter 304

Gastroesophageal Reflux Disease (GERD)

GERD is the most common esophageal disorder in children of all ages. Gastroesophageal reflux (GER) signifies the retrograde movement of gastric contents across the lower esophageal sphincter (LES) into the esophagus. Although occasional episodes of reflux are physiologic, exemplified by the regurgitation of normal infants, the phenomenon becomes pathologic (GERD) in children who have episodes that are more frequent or persistent, and thus produce esophagitis or esophageal symptoms, or in those who have respiratory sequelae.

Pathophysiology. Factors determining the esophageal manifestations of reflux include the duration of esophageal exposure (a product of the frequency and duration of reflux episodes), the causticity of the refluxate, and the susceptibility of the esophagus to damage. The LES, supported by the crura of the diaphragm at the gastroesophageal junction, together with valvelike functions of the esophagogastric junction anatomy, form the antireflux barrier. In the context of even the normal intra-abdominal pressure augmentations that occur during daily life, the frequency of reflux episodes is increased by insufficient LES tone, by abnormal frequency of LES relaxations (see later), and by hiatal herniation that prevents the LES pressure from being proportionately augmented during abdominal straining. Normal intra-abdominal pressure augmentations may be further exacerbated by straining or respiratory efforts. The duration of reflux episodes is increased by lack of swallowing (during sleep) and by defective esophageal peristalsis. Vicious cycles ensue because chronic esophagitis produces esophageal peristaltic dysfunction (low amplitude waves and propagation disturbances), decreased LES tone, and inflammatory esophageal shortening that induces hiatal herniation, all of them worsening reflux.

Transient LES relaxation (TLESR) is the major primary mechanism allowing reflux to occur. TLESRs occur independent of swallowing, reducing LES pressure to 0–2 mm Hg (above gastric), and last more than 10 s; they appear by the 26 wk of gestation. A vagovagal reflex, composed of afferent mechanoreceptors in the proximal stomach, a brain stem pattern generator, and efferents in the LES, regulates TLESRs. Gastric distention (postprandially, or due to abnormal gastric emptying or air swallowing) is thus the main stimulus for TLESRs. Whether GERD is caused by a higher frequency of TLESRs or by a greater incidence of reflux during TLESRs is debated; both are likely in different individuals. Straining during a TLESR makes reflux more likely, as do positions that place the gastroesophageal junction below the air-fluid interface in the stomach. Other factors influencing gastric pressure-volume dynamics, such as increased movement, straining, obesity, large volume or hyperosmolar meals, and increased respiratory effort (e.g., coughing, wheezing) may have the same effect.

Epidemiology and Natural History. Infant reflux becomes symptomatic during the first few months of life, peaking at about 4 mo and resolving in most by 12 mo and nearly all by 24 mo. Symptoms in older children tend to be chronic, waxing and waning, but completely resolving in no more than half, resembling adult patterns. A genetic predisposition as an autosomal dominant form is located on chromosome 13q14 and chromosome 9.

Clinical Manifestations. Most of the common clinical manifestations of esophageal disease can signify the presence of GERD.

Infantile reflux manifests more often with regurgitation (especially postprandially), signs of esophagitis (irritability, arching, choking, gagging, feeding aversion), and resulting failure to thrive; symptoms resolve spontaneously in the majority by 12 to 24 mo. Older children, in contrast, may have regurgitation during the preschool years; complaints of abdominal and chest pain supervene during later childhood and adolescence. Occasional children present with neck contortions designated Sandifer syndrome. The respiratory (extraesophageal) presentations are also age dependent: GERD in infants may manifest as obstructive apnea or as stridor or lower airway disease in which reflux complicates primary airway disease such as laryngomalacia or bronchopulmonary dysplasia. In contrast, airway manifestations in older children are more frequently related to asthma or to otolaryngologic disease such as laryngitis or sinusitis.

Diagnosis. For most of the typical GERD presentations, a thorough history and physical examination suffice to reach the diagnosis initially. This initial evaluation aims to identify the pertinent positives in support of GERD and its complications and the negatives that make other diagnoses unlikely. The history may be facilitated and standardized by questionnaires (the Infant Gastroesophageal Reflux Questionnaire, the I-GERQ), which also permit quantitative scores to be evaluated for their diagnostic discrimination. Important diagnoses to consider in the evaluation of an infant or a child with chronic vomiting are milk and other food allergies, pyloric stenosis, intestinal obstruction (especially malrotation with intermittent volvulus), nonesophageal inflammatory diseases, infections, inborn errors of metabolism, hydronephrosis, increased intracranial pressure, rumination, and bulimia. Focused diagnostic testing, depending on the presentation and the differential diagnosis, may then supplement the initial examination.

Most of the esophageal tests are of some use in particular patients suspected of GERD. Contrast (usually barium) radiographic study of the esophagus and upper gastrointestinal tract is performed in children with vomiting and dysphagia to evaluate for achalasia, esophageal strictures and stenosis, hiatal hernia, and gastric outlet or intestinal obstruction (Fig 304–1). Extended esophageal pH monitoring of the distal esophagus, no longer considered the sine qua non of a GERD diagnosis, provides a quantitative and sensitive documentation of acidic reflux episodes, the most important type of reflux episodes for pathologic reflux. The distal esophageal pH probe is placed at a level corresponding to 87% of the nares-LES distance, based on regression equations using the patient's height, by fluoroscopic visualization, or by manometric identification of the LES. Normal values of distal esophageal acid exposure (i.e., pH < 4) are generally established as less than 5–8% of the total monitored time. The most important indications for esophageal pH monitoring are to assess efficacy of acid suppression during treatment, to evaluate apneic episodes in conjunction with a pneumogram, and to evaluate atypical GERD presentations such as chronic cough, stridor, and asthma. Dual pH probes, adding a proximal esophageal probe to the standard distal one, are used in the diagnosis of extraesophageal GERD, identifying upper esophageal acid exposure times of about 1% of the total time to be threshold values for abnormality. Endoscopy allows diagnosis of erosive esophagitis and complications such as strictures or Barrett esophagus; esophageal biopsies may diagnose histologic reflux esophagitis in the absence of erosions while simultaneously eliminating allergic and infectious causes. Endoscopy is also used therapeutically to dilate reflux-induced strictures. Radionucleotide scintigraphy using technetium may demonstrate aspiration and delayed gastric emptying when these are suspected. The intraluminal impedance testing is a cumbersome test, infrequently used clinically, but can document nonacid reflux. Laryngotracheobronchoscopy evaluates for visible airway signs that are associated with extra-

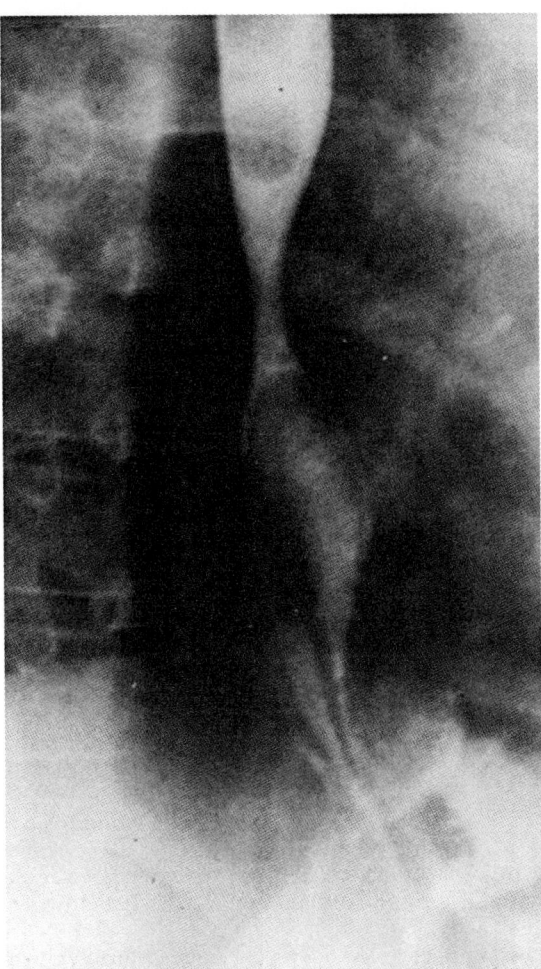

FIGURE 304–1. Barium esophagogram demonstrating free gastroesophageal reflux. Note stricture caused by peptic esophagitis. Longitudinal gastric folds above the diaphragm indicate the unusual presence of an associated hiatal hernia.

esophageal GERD, such as posterior laryngeal inflammation and vocal nodules; it may permit diagnosis of silent aspiration (during swallowing or during reflux) by bronchoalveolar lavage with subsequent quantification of lipid-laden macrophages in airway secretions. Esophageal manometry permits evaluation for dysmotility, particularly in preparation for antireflux surgery.

Empirical antireflux therapy, using a time-limited trial of high-dose proton pump inhibitor (PPI), has been demonstrated in adults to be a cost-effective strategy for diagnosis; although not formally evaluated in older children, it has also been applied to this age group. However, failure to respond to such empirical treatment, or a requirement for the treatment for prolonged periods, mandates formal diagnostic evaluation.

Management. Conservative therapy and lifestyle modification form the foundation of GERD therapy. *Dietary measures* for infants include normalization of feeding techniques, volumes, and frequency if abnormal. Thickening of formula with a tablespoon of rice cereal per ounce of formula results in fewer regurgitation episodes, greater caloric density (30 kcal/oz), and reduced crying time, although it may not modify the number of nonregurgitant reflux episodes. A short trial of a hypoallergenic diet may be used to exclude milk or soy protein allergy before pharmacotherapy. Older children and adults should be counseled to avoid acidic foods (tomatoes, chocolate, mint) and beverages (juices, carbonated and caffeinated drinks, alcohol). Weight reduction for obese patients and elimination of smoke exposure are other crucial measures at all ages.

Positioning measures are particularly important for infants, who cannot control their positions independently. Seated position worsens infant reflux and should be avoided in infants with GERD. Esophageal pH monitoring has shown significantly more reflux episodes in infants in supine and side positions compared with the prone position, but evidence supporting the supine position to reduce the risk of sudden infant death syndrome has led the American Academy of Pediatrics and the North American Society of Pediatric Gastroenterology and Nutrition to recommend nonprone positioning during sleep. During awake periods when the infant is observed, prone position and upright carried position may be used to minimize reflux. The efficacy of positioning for older children is unclear, but some evidence suggests a benefit to left side position and head elevation during sleep. Head elevation should utilize elevation of the head of the bed, rather than excess pillows, to avoid abdominal flexion and compression that might worsen reflux.

Pharmacotherapy is directed at ameliorating the acidity of the gastric contents or at promoting its aboral movement.

Antacids are the most commonly used antireflux therapy and are readily available over-the-counter. They provide rapid but transient relief of symptoms by acid neutralization. The long-term regular use of antacids cannot be recommended because of side effects of diarrhea (magnesium) and constipation (aluminum) and rare reports of more serious side effects of chronic use.

Histamine-2 receptor antagonists (H2RAs)—cimetidine, famotidine, nizatidine, and ranitidine—are widely used antisecretory agents and act by selective inhibition of histamine receptors on gastric parietal cells. There is a definite benefit of H2RAs in treatment of mild-to-moderate reflux esophagitis. H2RAs are recommended as first-line therapy because of their excellent overall safety profile.

Proton pump inhibitors (PPIs)—omeprazole, lansoprazole, pantoprazole, rabeprazole, and esomeprazole—provide the most potent antireflux effect by blocking the hydrogen-potassium ATPase channels of the final common pathway in gastric acid secretion. PPIs are superior to H2RAs in the treatment of severe and erosive esophagitis. Doses of omeprazole for children have been established (0.7–3.3 mg/kg/day), higher than those used in adults on a dose per weight basis.

Prokinetic agents available in the United States include metoclopramide (dopamine-2 and 5HT-3 antagonist), bethanechol (cholinergic agonist), and erythromycin (motilin receptor agonist). Most of these increase LES pressure; some improve gastric emptying or esophageal clearance. None affects the frequency of TLESRs. The available controlled trials have not demonstrated much efficacy for GERD.

Surgery, usually fundoplication, is effective therapy for intractable GERD in children, particularly those with refractory esophagitis or strictures and those at risk for significant morbidity from chronic pulmonary disease. It may be combined with a gastrostomy for feeding or venting. The current availability of potent acid-suppressing medication mandates more rigorous analysis of the relative risks (or costs) and benefits of this relatively irreversible therapy in comparison to long-term pharmacotherapy. Some of the risks of fundoplication include a wrap that is "too tight" (producing dysphagia or gas-bloat) or "too loose" (and thus incompetent). Surgeons may choose to perform a "tight" (360°, Nissen) or "loose" (<360°, Thal, etc.) wrap or to add a gastric drainage procedure (e.g., pyloroplasty) to improve gastric emptying, based on their experience and the patient's disease. Preoperative accuracy of diagnosis of GERD and the skill of the surgeon are two of the most important predictors of successful outcome.

304.1 Complications of GERD

Esophageal: Esophagitis and Sequelae—Stricture, Barrett Esophagus, Adenocarcinoma. Esophagitis may manifest as irritability, arching, and feeding aversion in infants; chest or epigastric pain in older children; and rarely as hematemesis, anemia, or Sandifer syndrome at any age. Prolonged and severe esophagitis leads to formation of strictures, generally located in the distal esophagus, producing dysphagia, and requiring repeated esophageal dilations and often fundoplication. Long-standing esophagitis predisposes to metaplastic transformation of the normal esophageal squamous epithelium into intestinal columnar epithelium, termed *Barrett esophagus*, a precursor of esophageal adenocarcinoma. Both Barrett esophagus and adenocarcinoma occur more in white males and in those with increased duration, frequency, and severity of reflux symptoms. This transformation thus increases with age to plateau in the 5th decade; adenocarcinoma is thus rare in childhood. Barrett esophagus warrants periodic surveillance biopsies, aggressive pharmacotherapy, and fundoplication for progressive lesions.

Nutritional. Esophagitis and regurgitation may be severe enough to induce failure to thrive because of caloric deficits. Enteral (nasogastric or nasojejunal, or percutaneous gastric or jejunal) or parenteral feedings are sometimes required to treat such deficits.

Extraesophageal: Respiratory ("Atypical") Presentations. It is important to include GERD in the differential diagnosis of children with unexplained or refractory otolaryngologic and respiratory complaints. GERD may produce respiratory symptoms by direct contact of the refluxed gastric contents with the respiratory tract (aspiration or microaspiration) or by reflexive interactions between the esophagus and respiratory tract (inducing laryngeal closure or bronchospasm). Frequently, GERD and a primary respiratory disorder interact, and a vicious cycle between them worsens both diseases. Many children with these extraesophageal presentations do not have typical GERD symptoms, making the diagnosis difficult. These atypical GERD presentations require a thoughtful approach to the differential diagnosis that considers a multitude of primary otolaryngologic (infections, environmental allergies, postnasal drip, voice overuse) and pulmonary (asthma, cystic fibrosis) disorders. Therapy for the GERD must be more intense (usually incorporating a PPI) and prolonged (usually at least 3 to 6 mo). Subspecialist assistance from the perspective of the airway disease (otolaryngology, pulmonology) and the reflux disease (gastroenterology) is often warranted and useful, both for specialized diagnostic testing and for optimizing intensive management.

APNEA AND STRIDOR. These upper airway presentations have been linked with GERD in case reports and epidemiologic studies; temporal relationships between them and reflux episodes have been demonstrated in some patients by esophageal pH probe monitoring; and a beneficial response to therapy for GERD provides further support in a number of case series. A comprehensive evaluation of 1,400 infants with apnea attributed the apnea to GERD in 50%. Apnea due to reflux is generally obstructive, owing to laryngospasm that may be conceived of as an abnormally intense protective reflex. Infants with such apnea are often provocatively positioned (supine or flexed seated), are recently fed, and show signs of obstructive apnea, with unproductive respiratory efforts. Stridor triggered by reflux generally occurs in infants anatomically predisposed toward stridor (by laryngomalacia or micrognathia). Spasmodic croup, an episodic frightening upper airway obstruction, may be an analogous condition in older children. Esophageal pH probe studies that fail to demonstrate linkage of these manifestations with reflux may not exclude reflux as a cause owing to the buffering of gastric contents by infant formula and the episodic nature of the conditions.

Reflux laryngitis and other otolaryngologic manifestations are now widely attributed to GERD. Hoarseness, voice fatigue,

throat clearing, chronic cough, pharyngitis, sinusitis, otitis media, and a sensation of globus have been cited in this context. The paucity of well-controlled evaluations of the association contributes to the skepticism with which the associations may be considered. Other risk factors irritating the upper respiratory passages may predispose some patients with GERD to present predominantly with these complaints.

Asthma may co-occur with GERD in about 50% of asthmatic children, which contrasts to the prevalence of each condition independently in about 10% of children. Asthmatics who may be particularly likely to have GERD as a provocative factor are those with symptoms of reflux disease, those with refractory or steroid-dependent asthma, and those with nocturnal worsening. Endoscopic evaluation that discloses esophageal sequelae of GERD provides an impetus to embark on the aggressive (high dose and many months duration) therapy of GERD.

Dental erosions constitute the most common oral lesion of GERD, the lesions being distinguished by their location on the lingual surface.

Chapter 305
Non–GERD Esophagitis

Eosinophilic Esophagitis. The esophageal epithelium is infiltrated by eosinophils, typically in a density exceeding 15 per high-power field. Presenting symptoms include vomiting, chest or abdominal pain, and dysphagia with occasional food impactions or strictures. Most patients are male. The mean age at diagnosis is 7 yr with the duration of symptoms of 3 yr. Patients often have atopy, associated food allergies, peripheral eosinophilia (~50% of patients), and elevated IgE levels. Endoscopically the esophagus presents a granular, furrowed, or ringed appearance; esophageal histology reveals eosinophilia. It is differentiated from GERD by its general lack of erosive esophagitis, by its greater eosinophil density, and by its refractoriness to antireflux therapies. Treatment involves elimination diets for those with proven allergies, whereas inhaled and systemic corticosteroids have been used successfully for nonresponders and for nonallergic ("primary") eosinophilic esophagitis. Little is known about its natural history, but it seems that eosinophilic esophagitis left untreated may result in stricture formation.

Infective Esophagitis. Uncommon, and most often afflicting immunocompromised children, infective esophagitis is caused by fungal agents, such as *Candida* and *Torulopsis glabrata*; viral agents, such as herpes simplex, cytomegalovirus, and varicella zoster; and bacterial infections, including diphtheria and tuberculosis. The typical presenting signs and symptoms are odynophagia, dysphagia, and retrosternal pain; there may also be fever, nausea, and vomiting. Esophageal candidiasis commonly, but not always, presents as concurrent oropharyngeal infection and may affect immunocompetent as well as immunocompromised children. Esophageal viral infections may also present in immunocompetent hosts as an acute febrile illness. Infectious esophagitis, like other forms of esophageal inflammation, may occasionally progress to esophageal stricture. Diagnosis of infectious esophagitis is made by endoscopy and histopathologic examination; adding polymerase chain reaction, tissue-viral culture, and immunocytochemistry enhances the diagnostic sensitivity. Treatment is with appropriate antimicrobial agents, analgesics, and antacids.

"Pill" Esophagitis. These acute injuries are produced by contact with a damaging agent. Medications implicated in "pill" esophagitis include tetracycline, potassium chloride, ferrous sulfate, and nonsteroidal anti-inflammatory medications, with the tablet most often ingested at bedtime with inadequate water. This practice often produces acute discomfort followed by progressive retrosternal pain, odynophagia, and dysphagia; endoscopy shows a focal lesion often localized to one of the anatomic narrowed regions of the esophagus or to an unsuspected pathologic narrowing. Treatment is supportive; lacking much evidence, antacids, topical anesthetics, and bland or liquid diets are often used.

Chapter 306
Esophageal Perforation

The majority of esophageal perforations in children either are from blunt trauma (automobile accidents, gunshot wounds, child abuse) or are iatrogenic. Cardiac massage, the Heimlich maneuver, nasogastric tube placement, traumatic laryngoscopy or endotracheal intubation, excessively vigorous postpartum suctioning of the airway during neonatal resuscitation, difficult upper endoscopy, sclerotherapy of esophageal varices, esophageal compression by a cuffed endotracheal tube, and pneumatic dilatation for therapy of achalasia have all been implicated. Esophageal rupture has also followed forceful vomiting in patients with anorexia or caustic ingestion.

Spontaneous esophageal rupture *(Boerhaave syndrome)* is less frequent and is associated with sudden increases in intra-esophageal pressure wrought by situations such as vomiting, coughing, or straining at stool. In children and adults, the tear occurs on the distal left lateral esophageal wall, because the smooth muscle layer here is weakest; in neonates *(neonatal Boerhaave syndrome)*, spontaneous rupture is on the right.

Symptoms of esophageal perforation include pain, neck tenderness, dysphagia, crepitus, fever, and tachycardia; several patients with cervical perforations have displayed cold water polydipsia in an attempt to soothe pain in the throat. Perforations in the proximal thoracic esophagus tend to create signs (pneumothorax, effusions) in the left chest, whereas the signs of distal tears are more often on the right. Cervical spine and chest radiographs are frequently diagnostic, showing mediastinal widening or paracervical free air. If normal, an esophagogram utilizing water-soluble contrast media should be performed next but may miss more than one third of cervical perforations. Therefore, a negative water-soluble contrast esophagogram should be followed by a barium study, the greater density of which may better demonstrate a small defect, though with a higher risk of inflammatory mediastinitis. Endoscopy may also be useful but carries a 30% false-negative rate. CT of the chest may assist in difficult cases.

Treatment must be individualized. Although small tears and minimal mediastinal contamination may be handled conservatively with broad-spectrum antibiotics, nothing by mouth, gastric drainage, and parenteral nutrition, the majority of pediatric esophageal perforations require surgical management.

Chapter 307
Esophageal Varices

Portal hypertension is defined as an elevation of portal venous pressure to levels 10 to 12 mm Hg higher than pressures present in the inferior vena cava (see Chapter 348). Decompression of this hypertension through portosystemic collateral circulation via the coronary vein, in conjunction with the left gastric veins, gives rise to esophageal varices. Most esophageal varices are "uphill varices"; less commonly, those that arise in the absence of portal hypertension and with superior vena cava (SVC) obstruction are termed "downhill varices." Their treatment is directed at the underlying cause of the SVC abnormality. Hemorrhage from esophageal varices is the major cause of morbidity and mortality due to portal hypertension. Presentation is with significant hematemesis and melena; whereas most patients have liver disease, some children with entities such as extrahepatic portal venous thrombosis may have been asymptomatic. Any child with hematemesis and splenomegaly should be presumed to have esophageal variceal bleeding until proven otherwise.

Varices occasionally may be seen on fluoroscopic barium contrast studies, but upper endoscopy is preferred because it provides definitive diagnosis as well as therapy for acute bleeding episodes via either sclerotherapy or band ligation.

Treating children with varices with prophylactic sclerotherapy with the goal of preventing an initial hemorrhage can decrease the incidence of esophageal bleeding. Treated patients are likely to bleed from congestive gastropathy, and no improvement in survival rate may be seen. Nonselective β-blockade, such as with propranolol, has also been used in pediatrics to achieve prevention of variceal bleeding. Endoscopic variceal ligation in adults reduces the risk of first-time variceal bleeding when compared with untreated controls as well as patients treated with β-blockade; a decrease in mortality is only noted versus the control group (see Chapter 348).

Chapter 308
Ingestions

308.1 Foreign Bodies in the Esophagus

The majority (80%) of foreign body ingestions occur in children, most of whom are between 6 mo and 3 yr of age. Youngsters with developmental delays as well as those with psychiatric disorders are at increased risk. Coins are the most commonly ingested foreign bodies. Food impactions are less common in children than in adults and usually occur in children with an underlying structural anomaly or motility disorder, such as repair of esophageal atresia or eosinophilic esophagitis. Most esophageal foreign bodies lodge at either the level of the cricopharyngeus (upper esophageal sphincter [UES]), the aortic arch, or just superior to the diaphragm at the gastroesophageal junction (lower esophageal sphincter [LES]).

At least 30% of children with esophageal foreign bodies may be totally asymptomatic, so any history of foreign body ingestion should be taken seriously and investigated. An initial bout of choking, gagging, and coughing may be followed by excessive salivation, dysphagia, food refusal, emesis, or pain in the neck, throat, or sternal notch regions. Respiratory symptoms such as stridor, wheezing, cyanosis, or dyspnea may be encountered if the foreign body impinges on the larynx or membranous posterior tracheal wall. Cervical swelling, erythema, or crepitations point to perforation of the oropharynx or proximal esophagus.

Diagnostic evaluation of the child with a history of foreign body ingestion starts with plain anteroposterior radiographs of the neck, chest, and abdomen, along with lateral views of the neck and chest. The flat surface of a coin in the esophagus is seen on the anteroposterior view and the edge on the lateral view. The reverse is true for coins lodged in the trachea; here, the edge is seen anteroposteriorly and the flat side is seen laterally (Fig. 308–1). Materials such as plastic, wood, glass, aluminum, and bones may be radiolucent; therefore, failure to visualize the object with plain films in a symptomatic patient warrants urgent endoscopy. Although barium contrast studies may be helpful in the occasional asymptomatic patient with negative plain films, their use is to be discouraged because of the potential of aspiration as well as making subsequent visualization and object removal more difficult.

Treatment of esophageal foreign bodies generally merits endoscopic visualization of the object and underlying mucosa and removal of the object; this therapeutic endoscopy is most conservatively done with an endotracheal tube protecting the airway. Sharp objects in the esophagus, disc button batteries, or foreign bodies associated with respiratory symptoms mandate urgent removal. Button batteries in particular must be expediently removed, because they may induce mucosal injury with as little as 1 hr of contact time and involve all esophageal layers within 4 hr. Asymptomatic blunt objects and coins lodged in the esophagus may be observed for up to 24 hr in anticipation of passage into the stomach. If there are no problems in handling secretions, meat impactions can be observed for up to 12 hr. In patients without prior esophageal surgeries, glucagon (0.05 mg/kg intravenously) may sometimes be useful in facilitating passage of distal esophageal food boluses by decreasing the LES pressure. The use of meat tenderizers or gas-forming agents may lead to perforation and are not recommended. An alternative technique for removing esophageal coins impacted for under 24 hr, performed most safely by experienced radiology personnel, consists of passage of a Foley catheter beyond the coin at fluoroscopy, inflating the balloon, and then pulling the catheter and coin back simultaneously with the patient in a prone oblique position.

308.2 Caustic Ingestions

Ingestion of caustic substances results in esophagitis, necrosis, perforation, and stricture formation (see Chapter 704.7). Most cases (70%) are accidental ingestions of liquid alkali substances that produce severe, deep liquefaction necrosis; drain decloggers are most common and because they are tasteless more is ingested. Acidic agents (20% of cases) are bitter, so less may be consumed; they produce coagulation necrosis and a somewhat protective thick eschar. They may produce severe gastritis, and volatile acids may result in respiratory symptoms. Caustic ingestions produce signs and symptoms such as vomiting, drooling, refusal to drink, oral burns, dysphagia, abdominal pain, and stridor. Twenty percent of patients develop esophageal strictures. Absence of oropharyngeal lesions does not exclude the possibility of significant esophagogastric injury, which may lead to perforation or stricture. The absence of symptoms is usually associated with no or minimal lesions; in contrast, hematemesis, respiratory distress, or presence of at least three symptoms predict severe lesions. An upper endoscopy is recommended as the most efficient means of rapid identification of tissue damage and must be undertaken in symptomatic children. Dilution by water or milk is recommended as acute treatment, but neutralization, induced emesis, and gastric lavage are contraindicated. Treatment depends on the severity and extent of damage. Stricture risk is increased by circumferential ulcerations, white plaques, and sloughing of the mucosa. They may require treatment with dilation, and in some severe cases surgical resection and colon or small bowel interposition are needed. Rare late cases of superimposed esophageal carcinoma are reported.

Embryology, Anatomy, and Function of the Esophagus
Shaker R, Hogan WJ: Reflex-mediated enhancement of airway protective mechanisms. *Am J Med* 2000;108:8S–14S.

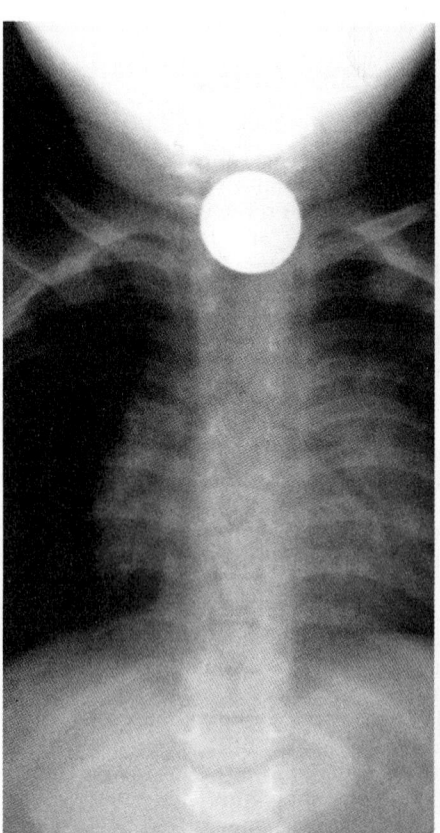
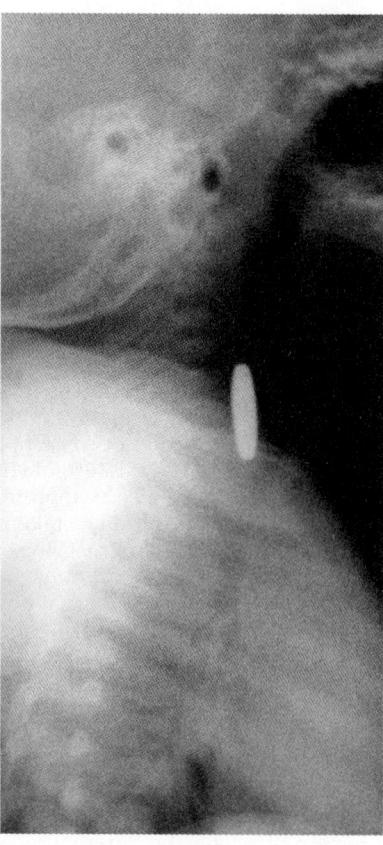

A   B

FIGURE 308–1. Radiographs of a coin in the esophagus. When foreign bodies lodge in the esophagus, the flat surface of the object is seen in the anteroposterior view *(A)* and the edge is seen in the lateral view *(B)*. The reverse is true for objects in the trachea. (Courtesy of Beverley Newman, MD.)

Congenital Anomalies: Esophageal Atresia and Tracheoesophageal Fistula

Adzick NS, Nance ML: Pediatric surgery: I. *N Engl J Med* 2000;342:1651–57.

Carr MM, Clark KD, Webber E, et al: Congenital laryngotracheoesophageal cleft. *J Otolaryngol* 1999;28:112–17.

Romeo C, Bonanno N, Baldari S, et al: Gastric motility disorders in patients operated on for esophageal atresia and tracheoesophageal fistula: Long-term evaluation. *J Pediatr Surg* 2000;35:740–44.

Sharma AK, Shekhawat NS, Agrawal LD, et al: Esophageal atresia and tracheoesophageal fistula: A review of 25 years' experience. *Pediatr Surg Int* 2000;16:478–82.

Gastroesophageal Reflux Disease

Benhamou PH, Francoual C, Glangeaud MC, et al: Risk factors for severe esophageal and gastric lesions in term neonates: A case-control study. Groupe Francophone d'Hepato-Gastroenterologie et Nutrition Pediatrique. *J Pediatr Gastroenterol Nutr* 2000;31:377–80.

Davidson G, Omari TI: Pathophysiological mechanisms of gastroesophageal reflux disease in children. *Curr Gastroenterol Rep* 2001;3:257–62.

Fonkalsrud E, Ashcraft K, Coran A, et al: Surgical treatment of gastroesophageal reflux in children: A combined hospital study of 7467 patients. *Pediatrics* 1998;101:419.

Lehman GA: Endoscopic and endoluminal techniques for the control of gastroesophageal reflux: Are they ready for widespread clinical application? *Gastrointest Endosc* 2000;52:808–11.

Lidums I, Lehmann A, Checklin H, et al: Control of transient lower esophageal sphincter relaxations and reflux by the GABA$_B$ agonist baclofen in normal subjects. *Gastroenterology* 2000;118:7–13.

Nelson SP, Chen EH, Syniar GM, et al: Prevalence of symptoms of gastroesophageal reflux during childhood: A pediatric practice–based survey. *Arch Pediatr Adolesc Med* 2000;154:150–54.

Orenstein SR, Di Lorenzo C: Postfundoplication complications in children. *Curr Treat Options Gastroenterol* 2001;4:441–49.

Orenstein SR, Peters JM: Vomiting and regurgitation. In Kleigman RM (editor): *Practical Strategies in Pediatric Diagnosis and Therapy*, 2nd ed. Philadelphia, WB Saunders, in press.

Orenstein SR, Shalaby TM, Barmada MM, et al: Genetics of gastroesophageal reflux disease: A review. *J Pediatr Gastroenterol Nutr* 2002;34:506–10.

Orenstein SR: Pediatric gastroesophageal reflux disease. In Orland RC (editor): *Gastroesophageal Reflux Disease*. New York, Marcel Dekker, 2000.

Rudolph CD, Mazur LJ, Liptak GS, et al: Pediatric gastroesophageal reflux clinical practice guidelines: Guidelines for evaluation and treatment of gastroesophageal reflux in infants and children. *J Pediatric Gastroenterol Nutr* 2001;32:S1–S31.

Salvia G, De Vizia B, Manguso F, et al: Effect of intragastric volume and osmolality on mechanisms of gastroesophageal reflux in children with gastroesophageal reflux disease. *Am J Gastroenterol* 2001;96:1725–32.

Complications of Gastroesophageal Reflux Disease

Bagucka B, Badriul H, Vandemaele K, et al: Normal ranges of continuous pH monitoring in the proximal esophagus. *J Pediatr Gastroenterol Nutr* 2000;31:244–47.

Bauman NM, Bishop WP, Sandler AD, et al: Value of pH probe testing in pediatric patients with extraesophageal manifestations of gastroesophageal reflux disease: A retrospective review. *Ann Otol Rhinol Laryngol* 2000;109:18–24.

Black DD, Haggitt RC, Orenstein SR, et al: Esophagitis in infants: Morphometric histologic diagnosis and correlation with measures of gastroesophageal reflux. *Gastroenterology* 1990;98:1408–14.

El-Serag HB, Gilger MA, Kuebeler M, et al: Extraesophageal associations of gastroesophageal reflux disease in children without neurologic defects. *Gastroenterology* 2001;121:1294–99.

Fuloria M, Hiatt D, Dillard RG, et al: Gastroesophageal reflux in very low birth weight infants: Association with chronic lung disease and outcomes through 1 year of age. *J Perinatol* 2000;4:235–39.

Goldenhersh MJ, Ament M: Asthma and gastroesophageal reflux in infants and children. *Immunol Allergy Clin North Am* 2001;21:439–48.

Harding SM, Sontag SJ: Asthma and gastroesophageal reflux. *Am J Gastroenterol* 2000;95:S23–32.

Irwin RS, Madison JM: Anatomical diagnostic protocol in evaluating chronic cough with specific reference to gastroesophageal reflux disease. *Am J Med* 2000;108:126S–130S.

Kimball AL, Carlton DP: Gastroesophageal reflux medications in the treatment of apnea in premature infants. *J Pediatr* 2001;138:355–60.

Linnett V, Seow WK: Dental erosion in children: A literature review. *Pediatr Dent* 2001;23:37–43.

Menges M, Muller M, Zietz M: Increased acid and bile reflux in Barrett's esophagus compared to reflux esophagitis and effect of proton pump inhibitor therapy. *Am J Gastroenterol* 2000;96:331–37.

Nostrant TT: Gastroesophageal reflux and laryngitis: A skeptic's view. *Am J Med* 2000;108:149S–52S.

Orenstein SR: Update on gastroesophageal reflux and respiratory disease in children: A review. *Can J Gastroenterol* 2000;14:131–35.

Orlando RC: Mechanisms of reflux-induced epithelial injuries in the esophagus. *Am J Med* 2000;108:104S–8S.

Sacco O, Fregonese B, Silvestri M, et al: Bronchoalveolar lavage and esophageal pH monitoring data in children with "difficult to treat" respiratory symptoms. *Pediatr Pulmonol* 2000;30:313–19.

Suskind DL, Zeringue GP III, Kluka EA, et al: Gastroesophageal reflux and pediatric otolaryngologic disease: The role of anti-reflux surgery. *Arch Otolaryngol Head Neck Surg* 2001;127:511–14.

Non-GERD Esophagitis

Arora AS, Murray JA: Iatrogenic esophagitis. *Curr Gastroenterol Rep* 2000;2:224–29.

Diaz M, et al: Infectious strictures requiring esophageal replacement in children. *J Pediatr Gastroenterol Nutr* 2001;32:611–13.

Hill DJ, Heine RG, Cameron DJ, et al: Role of food protein intolerance in infants with persistent distress attributed to reflux esophagitis. *J Pediatr* 2000;136:641–47.

Orenstein SR, Shalaby TM, Di Lorenzo C, et al: The spectrum of pediatric eosinophilic esophagitis beyond infancy: A clinical series of 30 children. *Am J Gastroenterol* 2000;95:1422–30.

Ramanathan J, Rammouni M, Baran J Jr, et al: Herpes simplex virus esophagitis in the immunocompetent host: An overview. *Am J Gastroenterol* 2000;95:2171–76.

Vodonik A, Cerar A: Synchronous herpes simplex virus and cytomegalovirus esophagitis. *Z Gastroenterol* 2000;38:491–94.

Dysphagia—Obstruction

Enterline H, Thompson J: *Pathology of the Esophagus*. New York, Springer-Verlag, 1984.

Janssen M, et al: Dysphagia lusoria: Clinical aspects, manometric findings, diagnosis, and therapy. *Am J Gastroenterol* 2000;95:1411–16.

Dysmotility

Cook IJ: Diagnosis and management of cricopharyngeal achalasia and other upper esophageal sphincter opening disorders. *Curr Gastroenterol Rep* 2000;2:191–95.

Hurwitz M, Bahar RJ, Ament ME, et al: Evaluation of the use of botulinum toxin in children with achalasia. *J Pediatr Gastroenterol Nutr* 2000;30:509–14.

Imperiale TF, O'Connor JB, Vaezi MF, et al: A cost-minimization analysis of alternative treatment strategies for achalasia. *Am J Gastroenterol* 2000;95:2737–45.

Massey BT: Management of idiopathic achalasia: Short-term and long-term outcomes. *Curr Gastroenterol Rep* 2000;2:196–200.

Pineiro-Carrero VM, Sullivan CA, Rogers PL: Etiology and treatment of achalasia in the pediatric age group. *Gastrointest Endosc Clin North Am* 2001;2:387–408.

Putnam PE, Orenstein SR, Pang D, et al: Cricopharyngeal dysfunction associated with Chiari malformations. *Pediatrics* 1992;89:871–76.

Scolapio JS, et al: Dysphagia without endoscopically evident disease: To dilate or not? *Am J Gastroenterol* 2001;96:327–30.

Miscellaneous Esophageal Disorders

Arana A, Hauser B, Hachimi-Idrissi S, et al: Management of ingested foreign bodies in childhood review of the literature. *Eur J Pediatr* 2001;160:468–72.

Byrne WJ: Caustic ingestion and foreign bodies. In Wyllie R, Hyams JS (editors): *Pediatric Gastrointestinal Disease: Pathophysiology, Diagnosis, Management*, 2nd ed. Philadelphia, WB Saunders, 1999.

de Jong AL, Macdonald R, Ein S, et al: Corrosive esophagitis in children: A 30-year review. *Int J Pediatr Otorhinolaryngol* 2001;57:203–11.

Goncalves MEP, Cardoso SR, Maksoud JG: Prophylactic sclerotherapy in children with esophageal varices: Long-term results of a controlled prospective randomized trial. *J Pediatr Surg* 2000;35:401–5.

Gupta SK, Croffie JM, Fitzgerald JF: Is esophagogastroduodenoscopy necessary in all caustic ingestions? *J Pediatr Gastroenterol Nutr* 2001;32:50–53.

Imperiale TF, Chalasani N: A meta-analysis of endoscopic variceal ligation for primary prophylaxis of esophageal variceal bleeding. *Hepatology* 2001;33:802–7.

Karjoo M: Caustic ingestion and foreign bodies in the gastrointestinal system. *Curr Opin Pediatr* 1998;10:516–22.

Lamireau T, Rebouissoux L, Denis D, et al: Accidental caustic ingestion in children: Is endoscopy always mandatory? *J Pediatr Gastroenterol Nutr* 2001;33:81–4.

Soprano JV, Fleisher GR, Mandl KD: The spontaneous passage of esophageal coins in children. *Arch Pediatr Adolesc Med* 1999;153:1073–76.

Chapter 309

Normal Development, Structure, and Function

Robert Wyllie

Development. The primitive gut is recognizable by the 4th wk of gestation and is composed of the foregut, midgut, and hindgut. The foregut gives rise to the upper gastrointestinal tract including the esophagus, stomach, and duodenum to the level of the insertion of the common bile duct. The midgut gives rise to the rest of the small bowel and the large bowel to the level of the mid-transverse colon. The hindgut forms the remainder of the colon and upper anal canal. The rapid growth of the midgut causes it to protrude out of the abdominal cavity through the umbilical ring during fetal development. The midgut subsequently returns to the peritoneal cavity and rotates counterclockwise until the cecum lies in the right lower quadrant. The process is normally complete by the 8th wk of gestation. The liver derives from the hepatic diverticulum that evolves into parenchymal cells, bile ducts, vascular structures, and hematopoietic and Kupffer cells. The extrahepatic bile ducts and gallbladder develop first as solid cords that canalize by the 3rd mo of gestation. The dorsal and ventral pancreatic buds grow from the foregut by the 4th wk of gestation. The two buds fuse by the 6th wk. Exocrine secretory capacity is present by the 5th mo. *Cis*-regulatory genomic sequences govern gene expression during development. Modules of *cis* sequences are linked and allow a cascade of gene regulation that controls functional development. Extrinsic factors have the capacity to influence gene expression. In the gut, several growth factors, including growth factor-β, insulin-like growth factor, and growth factors found in human colostrum (human growth factor and epidermal growth factor) influence gene expression.

Propulsion of food down the gastrointestinal tract relies on the coordinated action of muscles in the bowel wall. The contractions are regulated by the enteric nervous system under the influence of a variety of peptides and hormones. The enteric nervous system is derived from neural crest cells that migrate in a cranial to caudal fashion. Migration of the neural crest tissue is complete by the 24th wk of gestation. Interruption of the migration results in Hirschsprung disease. Bowel motor patterns in the newborn differ from adults. Normal fasting upper gastrointestinal motility is characterized by a triphasic pattern known as the migrating motor complex. Migrating motor complexes occur less often in neonates and they have more nonmigrating phasic activity. This leads to ineffective propulsion, particularly in premature infants. Motility in the fed state consists of a series of ring contractions that spread caudad over variable distances.

Digestion and Absorption. The wall of the stomach, small bowel, and colon consists of four layers: the mucosa, submucosa, muscularis, and serosa. Eighty-five percent of the gastric mucosa is lined by oxyntic glands that contain cells that secrete hydrochloric acid, pepsinogen, intrinsic factor, and mucous and endocrine cells that secrete peptides that have paracrine and endocrine effects. Pepsinogen is a precursor of the proteolytic enzyme pepsin, and

intrinsic factor is required for the absorption of vitamin B_{12}. Pyloric glands are located in the antrum and contain gastrin-secreting cells. Acid production and gastrin levels are inversely related to each other except in pathologic secretory states. Acid secretion is low at birth but increases dramatically by 24 hr. Acid and pepsin secretion peak during the first 10 days and decrease from 10–30 days after birth. Intrinsic factor secretion rises slowly during the first 2 wk of life.

The small bowel is approximately 270 cm in length at birth in a term neonate and grows to an adult length of 450 to 550 cm by 4 yr of age. The mucosa of the small intestine is composed of villi, which are finger-like projections of the mucosa into the bowel lumen that significantly expand the absorptive surface area. The mucosal surface is further expanded by a brush border containing digestive enzymes and transport mechanisms for monosaccharides, amino acids, dipeptides and tripeptides, and fats. The cells of the villi originate in adjacent crypts and become functional as they migrate from the crypt up the villus. The small bowel mucosa is completely renewed in 4–5 days, providing a mechanism for rapid repair after injury; but in young infants or malnourished children the process may be delayed. Crypt cells also secrete fluid and electrolytes. The villi are present by 8 wk gestation in the duodenum and by 11 wk in the ileum. Disaccharidase activities are measurable at 12 wk, but lactase activity does not reach maximal levels until 36 wk. Even premature infants usually tolerate lactose-containing formulas because of carbohydrate salvage by colonic bacteria. In African and Asian people lactase levels may begin to fall at 4 yr of age leading to intolerance to mammalian milk. Mechanisms to digest and absorb protein are in place by the 20th wk of gestation including pancreatic enzymes and mucosal mechanisms to transport amino acids and dipeptides and tripeptides. Carbohydrate, protein, and fat are normally absorbed by the upper half of the small intestine; the distal segments represent a vast reserve of absorptive capacity. Most of the sodium, potassium, chloride, and water are absorbed in the small bowel. Bile salts and vitamin B_{12} are selectively absorbed in the distal ileum, and iron is absorbed in the duodenum and proximal jejunum. Intraluminal digestion depends on the exocrine pancreas. Secretin and cholecystokinin stimulate synthesis and secretion of bicarbonate and digestive enzymes, which are released by the upper intestinal mucosa in response to various intraluminal stimuli, among them components of the diet.

Carbohydrate digestion is normally an efficient process that is completed in the distal duodenum. Starches are broken down to glucose and oligosaccharides and disaccharides by pancreatic amylase. Residual glucose polymers are broken down at the mucosal level by glucoamylase. Lactose is broken down at the brush border by lactase, forming glucose and galactose, while sucrose is broken down by sucrase isomaltase to fructose and glucose. Galactose and glucose are primarily transported into the cell by a sodium- and energy-dependent process, whereas fructose is transported by facilitated diffusion.

Proteins are hydrolyzed by pancreatic enzymes, including trypsin, chymotrypsin, elastase, and carboxypeptidases, into individual amino acids and oligopeptides. The pancreatic enzymes are secreted as proenzymes, which are activated by release of the mucosal enzyme enterokinase. Oligopeptides are further broken down at the brush border by peptidases into dipeptides and tripeptides and amino acids. Protein can enter the cell by separate noncompetitive carriers that can transport individual amino acids or dipeptides and tripeptides similar to those in the renal tubule. The human gut is capable of absorbing antigenic intact proteins during the first few weeks of life because of "leaky" junctions between enterocytes. Entry of potential protein antigens through the mucosal barrier may have a role in later food- and microbe-induced symptoms.

Fat absorption occurs in two phases. Dietary triglycerides are broken down into monoglycerides and free fatty acids by pancreatic lipase and colipase. The free fatty acids are subsequently emulsified by bile acids forming micelles with phospholipids and other fat-soluble substances and are transported to the cell membrane where they are absorbed. The fats are re-esterified in the enterocyte, forming chylomicrons that are transported through the intestinal lymphatics to the thoracic duct. Medium-chain fats are absorbed more efficiently and may directly enter the cell. They are subsequently transported to the liver via the portal system. Fat absorption may be affected at any stage of the digestion and absorption process. Decreased pancreatic enzymes occur in cystic fibrosis, cholestatic liver disease leads to poor bile salt production and micelle formation, celiac disease affects mucosal surface area, abnormal chylomicron formation occurs in abetalipoproteinemia, and intestinal lymphangiectasia affects transport of the chylomicrons.

Fat absorption is less efficient in the neonate compared with adults. Premature infants may lose up to 20% of their fat calories compared with 6% or less in the adult. Decreased synthesis of bile acids and pancreatic lipase and decreased efficiency of ileal absorption are contributing factors. Fat digestion in the neonate is facilitated by lingual and gastric lipases. Bile salt–stimulated lipase in human milk augments the action of pancreatic lipase. Infants with malabsorption of fat are usually placed on formulas that have a greater percentage of medium-chain triglycerides, which are absorbed independently of bile salts.

The colon is a 75–100 cm sacculated tube due to three strips of longitudinal muscle called taenia coli that traverse its length and fold the mucosa into haustra. Haustra and taenia appear by the 12th wk of gestation. The most common motor activity in the colon is nonpropulsive rhythmic segmentation that acts to mix the chyme and expose the contents to the colonic mucosa. Mass movement within the colon typically occurs after a meal. The colon extracts additional water and electrolytes from the luminal contents to render the stools partially or completely solid. The colon also acts to scavenge byproducts of bacterial degradation of carbohydrates. Stool is stored in the rectum until distention triggers a defecation reflex that, when assisted by voluntary relaxation of the external sphincter, permits evacuation.

Chapter 310
Pyloric Stenosis and Congenital Anomalies of the Stomach *Robert Wyllie*

The hallmark of gastric obstruction is nonbilious vomiting. Other symptoms include abdominal pain and nausea. Signs of gastric outlet obstruction include abdominal distention and bleeding from secondary inflammation of the gastric or esophageal mucosa.

The most common cause of nonbilious vomiting is infantile hypertrophic pyloric stenosis. Similar symptoms may be associated with various other gastric malformations, including pyloric atresia, antral webs, gastric duplications, and gastric volvulus. The differential diagnosis includes gastroesophageal reflux, peptic ulcer disease, salt-wasting adrenogenital syndrome, eosinophilic gastroenteritis, bezoars, and various other metabolic and motility abnormalities.

310.1 Hypertrophic Pyloric Stenosis

Hypertrophic pyloric stenosis occurs in approximately 3 in 1,000 infants in the United States; its frequency may be increasing. It is more common in whites of northern European ancestry, less common in blacks, and rare in Asians. Males (especially first-borns) are affected approximately four times as often as females. The offspring of a mother and to a lesser extent the father who had pyloric stenosis are at higher risk for pyloric stenosis. Pyloric stenosis develops in approximately 20% of the male and 10% of the female descendants of a mother who had pyloric stenosis. The incidence of pyloric stenosis is increased in infants with type B and O blood groups. Pyloric stenosis is associated with other congenital defects, including tracheoesophageal fistula.

Etiology. The cause of pyloric stenosis is unknown, but many factors have been implicated. Pyloric stenosis is usually not present at birth and is more concordant in monozygotic than dizygotic twins. Abnormal muscle innervation has been implicated. In addition, elevated serum levels of prostaglandins, reduced levels of pyloric nitric oxide synthase, and infant hypergastrinemia have been found. It is unusual in stillbirths and probably develops after birth. Pyloric stenosis has been associated with eosinophilic gastroenteritis, Apert syndrome, Zellweger syndrome, trisomy 18, Smith-Lemli-Opitz syndrome, and Cornelia de Lange syndrome. There is an association between the use of erythromycin in neonates, which is administered for pertussis postexposure prophylaxis and pyloric stenosis. Erythromycin is a motilin agonist and at doses used as an antibiotic can result in strong, nonpropagated contractions that may lead to hypertrophy of the pylorus. Intravenous prostaglandins may be associated with the development of pyloric obstruction.

Clinical Manifestations. Nonbilious vomiting is the initial symptom of pyloric stenosis. The vomiting may or may not be projectile initially but is usually progressive, occurring immediately after a feeding. Emesis may follow each feeding, or it may be intermittent. The vomiting usually starts after 3 wk of age, but symptoms may develop as early as the 1st wk of life and as late as the 5th mo. After vomiting, the infant is hungry and wants to feed again. As vomiting continues, a progressive loss of fluid, hydrogen ion, and chloride leads to hypochloremic metabolic alkalosis. Serum potassium levels are usually maintained, but there may be a total body potassium deficit. Greater awareness of pyloric stenosis has led to earlier identification of patients with fewer instances of chronic malnutrition and severe dehydration.

Jaundice associated with a decreased level of glucuronyl transferase is seen in approximately 5% of affected infants. The indirect hyperbilirubinemia usually resolves promptly after relief of the obstruction.

The *diagnosis* has traditionally been established by palpating the pyloric mass. The mass is firm, movable, approximately 2 cm in length, olive shaped, hard, best palpated from the left side, and located above and to the right of the umbilicus in the mid epigastrium beneath the liver edge. In healthy infants, feeding can be an aid to the diagnosis. After feeding, there may be a visible gastric peristaltic wave that progresses across the abdomen (Fig. 310–1). After the infant vomits, the abdominal musculature is more relaxed and the "olive" easier to palpate. Sedation may be used to facilitate examination but is usually unnecessary. The diagnosis can be established clinically 60–80% of the time by an experienced examiner.

Ultrasound examination confirms the diagnosis in the majority of cases, allowing an earlier diagnosis in infants with

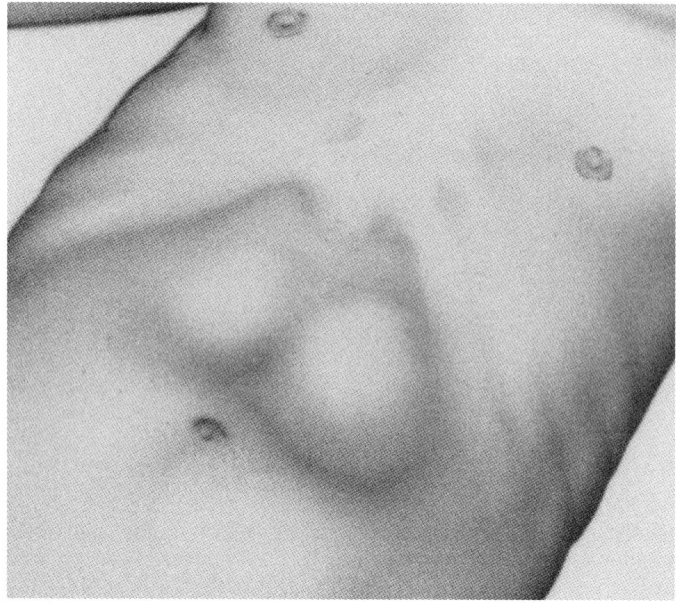

FIGURE 310–1. Gastric peristaltic wave in an infant with pyloric stenosis.

suspected disease but no pyloric mass on physical examination. Criteria for diagnosis include pyloric thickness greater than 4 mm or an overall pyloric length greater than 14 mm (Fig. 310–2). Ultrasonography has a sensitivity of approximately 95%. When barium studies are performed, they demonstrate an elongated pyloric channel, a bulge of the pyloric muscle into the antrum (shoulder sign), and parallel streaks of barium seen in the narrowed channel, producing a "double tract sign" (Fig. 310–3).

Differential Diagnosis. The usual patient can be diagnosed by the characteristic clinical pattern and the identification of a pyloric mass on physical examination or ultrasonography. Infants who are exceptionally reactive to external stimuli, those fed by inexperienced or anxious caretakers, or those for whom an adequate maternal-infant bonding relationship has not been established may vomit frequently in the early weeks of life. Such infants may come to resemble infants with pyloric stenosis; the vomiting may be persistent and even projectile. Gastric waves are occasionally visible in small, emaciated infants who do not have pyloric stenosis. Infrequently, gastroesophageal reflux, with or without a hiatal hernia, may be confused with pyloric stenosis. Gastroesophageal reflux disease can be differentiated from pyloric stenosis by radiographic studies. Adrenal insufficiency may simulate pyloric stenosis, but the absence of a metabolic acidosis and elevated serum potassium and urinary sodium concentrations of adrenal insufficiency aid in differentiation. Inborn errors of metabolism may produce recurrent emesis with alkalosis (urea cycle) or acidosis (organic acidemia) and lethargy, coma, or seizures. Vomiting with diarrhea suggests gastroenteritis, but patients with pyloric stenosis occasionally have diarrhea. Very rarely, a pyloric membrane or pyloric duplication may result in projectile vomiting, visible peristalsis, and, in the case of a duplication, a palpable mass. Duodenal stenosis proximal to the ampulla of Vater results in the clinical features of pyloric stenosis but can be differentiated by the presence of a pyloric mass on physical examination or ultrasonography.

Treatment. The preoperative treatment is directed toward correcting the fluid, acid-base, and electrolyte losses. Intravenous fluid therapy is begun with 0.45–0.9% saline, in 5–10% dextrose, with the addition of potassium chloride in concentrations of 30–50 mEq/L. Fluid therapy should be continued until the infant is rehydrated and the serum bicarbonate concentration is less than 30 mEq/dL, which implies that the alkalosis has been corrected. Correction of the alkalosis is essential to prevent postoperative apnea, which may be associated with anesthesia. Most

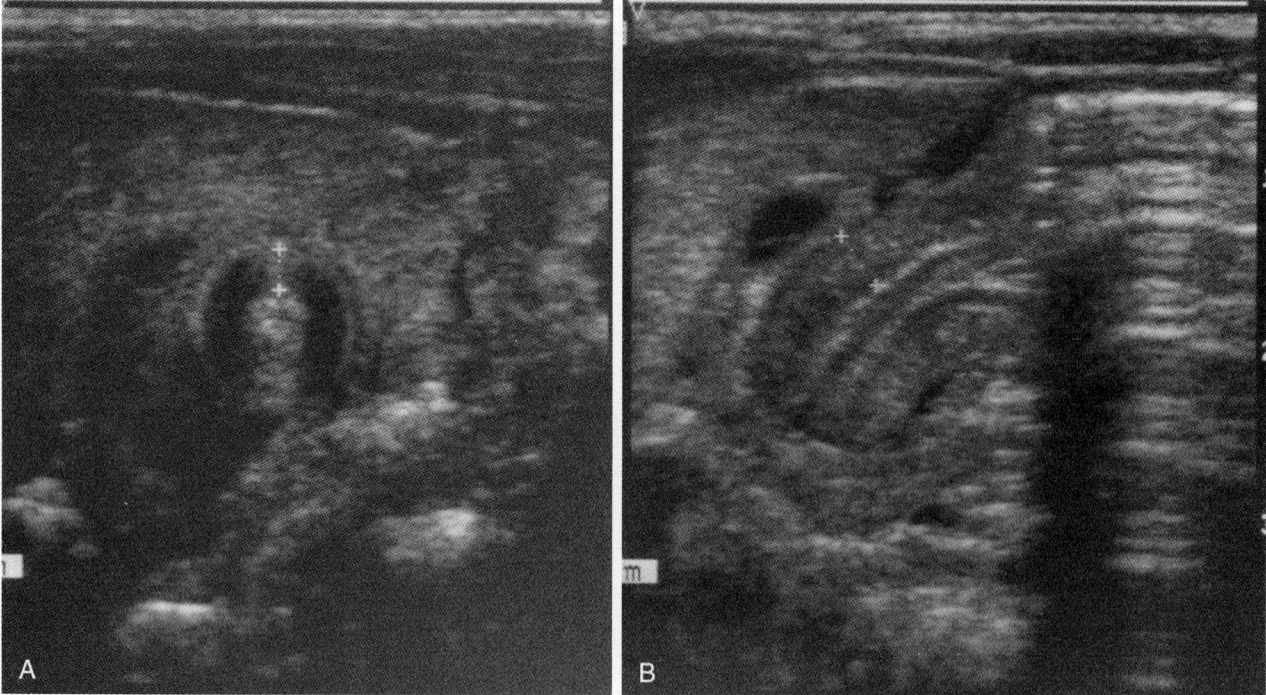

FIGURE 310–2. *A,* Transverse sonogram demonstrating a pyloric muscle wall thickness of greater than 4 mm *(distance between crosses).* *B,* Horizontal image demonstrating a pyloric channel length greater than 14 mm *(wall thickness outlined between crosses)* in an infant with pyloric stenosis.

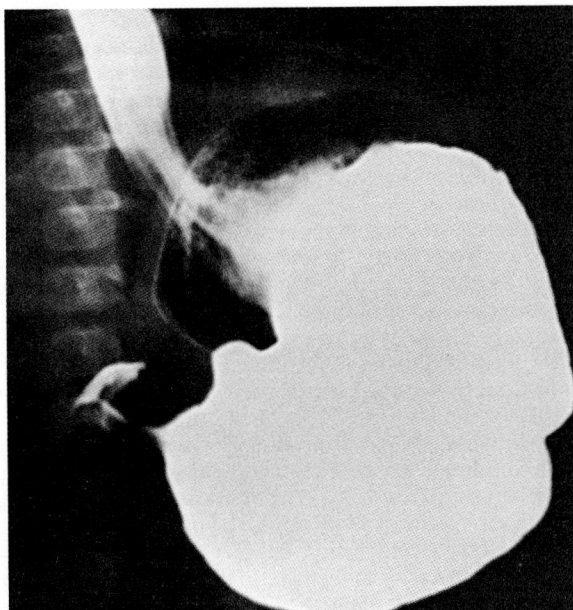

FIGURE 310–3. Barium in the stomach of an infant with projectile vomiting. The attenuated pyloric canal is typical of congenital hypertrophic pyloric stenosis.

infants can be successfully rehydrated within 24 hr. Vomiting usually stops when the stomach is empty, and only an occasional infant requires nasogastric suction.

The surgical procedure of choice is the Ramstedt pyloromyotomy. The procedure is performed through a short transverse incision or laparoscopically. The underlying pyloric mass is split without cutting the mucosa, and the incision is closed. Postoperative vomiting may occur in half the infants and is thought to be secondary to edema of the pylorus at the incision site. In most infants, however, feedings can be initiated within 12–24 hr after surgery and advanced to maintenance oral feedings within 36–48 hr of the surgery. Persistent vomiting suggests an incomplete pyloromyotomy, gastritis, gastroesophageal reflux disease, or another cause of the obstruction.

The surgical treatment of pyloric stenosis is curative, with an operative mortality of 0–0.5%. Conservative medical therapy (small frequent feedings, atropine) has been attempted in the past but is associated with slow improvement and a higher mortality. Endoscopic balloon dilation has been successful in infants with persistent vomiting secondary to incomplete pyloromyotomy.

310.2   Congenital Gastric Outlet Obstruction

Gastric outlet obstruction resulting from pyloric atresia and antral webs is uncommon and accounts for less than 1% of all the atresias and diaphragms of the alimentary tract. The cause of the defects is unknown. Pyloric atresia has been associated with epidermolysis bullosa and usually presents in early infancy. The sex distribution is equal.

Clinical Manifestations. Infants with pyloric atresia present with nonbilious vomiting, feeding difficulties, and abdominal distention during the 1st day of life. Polyhydramnios occurs in the majority of cases, and low birthweight is common. Rupture of the stomach may occur as early as the 1st 12 hr of life. Infants with antral web may present with less dramatic symptoms, depending on the degree of obstruction. Older children with antral webs present with nausea, vomiting, abdominal pain, and weight loss.

Diagnosis. The diagnosis of congenital gastric outlet obstruction is suggested by the finding of a large, dilated stomach on abdominal plain radiographs. Upper gastrointestinal contrast series is usually diagnostic and demonstrates a pyloric dimple. An antral web may appear as a thin septum near the pyloric channel. In older children, endoscopy has been helpful in identifying antral webs.

Treatment. The treatment of gastric outlet obstruction in neonates starts with the correction of dehydration and hypochloremic alkalosis. Persistent vomiting should be relieved with nasogastric decompression. Surgical or endoscopic repair should be undertaken when a patient is stable.

310.3   Gastric Duplication

Gastric duplications are uncommon cystic or tubular structures that usually occur within the wall of the stomach. Most are smaller than 12 cm in diameter and do not usually communicate with the stomach lumen. Associated anomalies occur in as many as 35% of patients. Duplications have been attributed to a failure of recanalization after the solid stage of intestinal development.

The most common *clinical manifestations* are associated with partial or complete gastric outlet obstruction. In 33% of patients, the cyst may be palpable. Communicating duplications may cause gastric ulceration and be associated with hematemesis or melena.

Gastric duplications are visualized on upper gastrointestinal series as an extrinsic defect usually located along the lesser curve of the stomach. CT or ultrasonography may be helpful in defining a cystic structure. Surgical excision is the treatment for symptomatic gastric duplications.

310.4   Gastric Volvulus

Gastric volvulus presents as a triad of a sudden onset of severe epigastric pain, intractable retching with emesis, and inability to pass a tube into the stomach. The stomach is tethered longitudinally by the gastrohepatic, gastrosplenic, and gastrocolic ligaments. In the transverse axis, it is tethered by the gastrophrenic ligament and the retroperitoneal attachment of the duodenum. A volvulus occurs when one of these attachments is absent or stretched, allowing the stomach to rotate around itself. In most children, other associated defects are present, including intestinal malrotation, diaphragmatic defects, or asplenia. Volvulus may occur along the longitudinal axis, producing organoaxial volvulus, or along the transverse axis, producing mesenteroaxial volvulus.

Clinical Manifestations. The clinical presentation of gastric volvulus is nonspecific and suggests high intestinal obstruction. Gastric volvulus in infancy is usually associated with nonbilious vomiting. Acute volvulus may advance rapidly to strangulation and perforation. Chronic gastric volvulus is more common in older children; the children present with a history of emesis, abdominal pain, and early satiety.

The *diagnosis* is suggested in plain abdominal radiographs by the presence of a dilated stomach. Erect abdominal films demonstrate a double fluid level with a characteristic "beak" near the lower esophageal junction in mesenteroaxial volvulus. In organoaxial volvulus, a single air-fluid level is seen without the characteristic beak. *Treatment* of acute gastric volvulus is emergent surgery once a patient is stabilized. In selected cases of chronic volvulus in older patients, endoscopic correction has been successful.

310.5   Hypertrophic Gastropathy

Hypertrophic gastropathy in children is uncommon and, in contrast to that in adults (Ménétrier disease), is usually a transient, benign, self-limited condition, possibly initiated by an infectious agent (cytomegalovirus, herpes simplex virus, *Giardia, Helicobacter pylori*). Clinical manifestations include vomiting, anorexia, upper abdominal pain, diarrhea, edema (hypoproteinemic protein-losing enteropathy), ascites, and, rarely, hematemesis if ulceration occurs. Endoscopy with biopsy confirms the diagnosis. The mean age at diagnosis is 5 yr (range: 2 days–17 yr); the illness usually lasts 2–4 wk, with complete resolution the rule. The differential diagnosis includes eosinophilic gastroenteritis, gastric lymphoma or carcinoma, Crohn disease, and inflammatory pseudotumor.

Chen EA, Luks FI, Gilchrist BF, et al: Pyloric stenosis in the age of ultrasonography: Fading skills, better patients? *J Pediatr Surg* 1996;31:829–30.

Honein MA, Paulozzi LJ, Himelright IM, et al: Infantile hypertrophic pyloric stenosis after pertussis prophylaxis with erythromycin: A case review and cohort study. *Lancet* 1999;354:2101–15.

Jacobe S, Lam A, Elliott E: Transient hypertrophic gastropathy. *J Pediatr Gastroenterol Nutr* 1998;26:211–15.

McLeary MS, Thomas RD, Young LW: Imaging of congenital and acquired gastric abnormalities in children. *Acad Radiol* 2000;7:117–27.

Rogers IM: The enigma of pyloric stenosis: Some thoughts on the etiology. *Acta Paediatr* 1997;86:6–9.

Chapter 311
Intestinal Atresia, Stenosis, and Malrotation *Robert Wyllie*

General Considerations. Intestinal obstruction occurs in approximately 1 in 1,500 live births. Obstruction may be partial or complete and may arise from intrinsic or extrinsic abnormalities of the gut. Obstruction can be further classified as simple or strangulating. Simple obstruction is associated with the failure of progression of aboral flow of luminal contents. Strangulating obstruction is associated with impaired blood flow to the intestine in addition to obstruction of the flow of luminal contents. If strangulating obstruction is not promptly relieved, it may lead to bowel infarction and perforation.

Obstruction is typically associated with an accumulation of ingested food, gas, and intestinal secretions proximal to the point of obstruction, leading to distention of the bowel. As the bowel dilates, intestinal absorption decreases and secretion of fluid and electrolytes increases. The shift in fluid and electrolytes results in isotonic intravascular depletion usually associated with hypokalemia. The gut proximal to the obstruction initially demonstrates an increase in contractile activity, which is followed by a marked decrease with hypoactive bowel sounds. The combination of fluid accumulation and hypomotility is associated with nausea and vomiting.

Congenital obstructive lesions of the intestines can be viewed as *intrinsic* (e.g., atresia, stenosis, meconium ileus, and aganglionic megacolon) or *extrinsic* (e.g., malrotation, constricting bands, intra-abdominal hernias, and duplications). An attempt should be made to locate the lesion preoperatively to guide the surgical approach.

When the obstruction is *complete*, there should be little difficulty in clinical recognition, but when it is *incomplete,* diagnosis may pose considerable difficulty. Polyhydramnios frequently accompanies high intestinal obstruction, as it does in esophageal atresia. When polyhydramnios has been noted, the infant's stomach should be aspirated immediately after birth. Aspiration of 15–20 mL or more of gastric fluid, especially if it is bile stained, is suggestive of a high intestinal obstruction.

Meconium stools may be passed initially if the obstruction is in the upper part of the small intestine or if the obstruction developed late in intrauterine life.

When obstruction is *incomplete* (e.g., as with intestinal stenosis, constricting bands, duplications, and incomplete volvulus), signs (vomiting, abdominal distention, obstipation) may appear shortly after birth or may be delayed an indeterminate time. They may approach in severity those of a completely obstructive lesion, or they may be sufficiently mild and infrequent as to be overlooked until either an acute episode or diagnostic studies disclose the lesion.

Atresia refers to complete obstruction of the bowel lumen, and stenosis refers to a partial block of luminal contents. Intestinal atresia is common in the duodenum, jejunum, and ileum and rare in the colon. Intestinal atresia accounts for approximately 33% of all cases of neonatal intestinal obstruction. Atresias affect males and females equally.

Blood flow to the obstructed bowel decreases as the bowel dilates. Blood flow is shifted away from the mucosa, with loss of mucosal integrity. Bacteria proliferate in the stagnant bowel, with a predominance of coliforms and anaerobes. The rapid proliferation of bacteria coupled with the loss of mucosal integrity allows bacterial translocation across the bowel wall, resulting in endotoxemia, bacteremia, and sepsis.

The *clinical presentation* of intestinal obstruction varies with the cause, level of obstruction, and time between the obstructing event and the patient's evaluation. The classic symptoms of obstruction include nausea and vomiting, abdominal distention, and obstipation. Obstruction high in the intestinal tract involving the duodenum or proximal jejunum results in large-volume, frequent, bilious emesis. Pain is intermittent and is usually relieved by vomiting. The pain is localized to the epigastrium or periumbilical area, and there is little abdominal distention. Obstruction in the distal small bowel leads to moderate or marked abdominal distention with emesis that is progressively feculent. Pain is usually diffuse over the entire abdomen.

No laboratory studies are diagnostic of obstruction or differentiate simple obstruction from obstruction associated with bowel infarction. Obstruction high in the gastrointestinal tract is often associated with hypochloremic metabolic alkalosis. Marked leukocytosis with or without thrombocytopenia, metabolic acidosis, and hematochezia suggests bowel infarction. Serum amylase and lipase determinations should be performed to rule out pancreatitis.

Bowel obstruction is usually suggested on the basis of history and physical examination. Imaging is used to confirm the diagnosis and localize the area of obstruction. Plain supine and erect or decubitus radiographs are the initial studies.

Valuable information on the location of congenital obstructive lesions in the intestine may often be obtained from flat and upright radiographs of the abdomen taken without use of contrast media. With completely obstructing lesions, distention of the bowel is noted above the obstruction and a series of fluid levels with superimposed gas in the distended loops may be observed in the upright or cross-table lateral position. Pneumoperitoneum may be seen if there is a perforation with free air in the subphrenic regions or over the liver in the left lateral decubitus position. Calcification within the peritoneal cavity usually indicates meconium peritonitis. Rarely, obstruction with intraluminal calcification may be associated with rectourinary fistula, colonic aganglionosis, or intestinal atresia. A characteristic ground-glass appearance in the right lower quadrant with trapped bubbles of air within the obstructing meconium may be seen in patients with meconium ileus. Air is usually demonstrable radiographically in the stomach of a normal infant immediately after birth; within 1 hr air may reach the proximal portion of the small intestine and segments of the colon; air may become visible in the distal parts of the colon as early as the 3rd hr or as late as 18 hr. It is difficult to accurately differentiate small from large bowel obstruction in children younger than 2 yr.

Ultrasonography is helpful in identifying pyloric stenosis, malrotation, and volvulus or intussusception and in differentiating pyloric stenosis from other causes of proximal obstruction. Contrast studies of the bowel are indicated when plain films or sonograms fail to identify the source of obstruction. Water-soluble contrast studies avoid the risk of barium contamination of the peritoneum when there is a significant chance of perforation not detected by the presence of pneumoperitoneum on plain films. Water-soluble contrast enemas are useful in diagnosing malrotation, meconium ileus, meconium plug, and intussusception. In meconium ileus, meconium plug, and intussusception the enema may be diagnostic and relieve the obstruction. Oral or nasogastric contrast medium is used to identify obstructing lesions in the proximal bowel (atresia, volvulus, malrotation). Water-soluble agents are used if perforation is suspected.

Management. Infants and children with bowel obstruction have mechanical obstruction and loss of fluid and electrolytes. Those with strangulating vascular obstruction may also develop intestinal ischemia with sepsis and shock. Initial treatment must be directed at fluid resuscitation and stabilizing the patient. Nasogastric decompression usually provides relief of pain and vomiting. After appropriate cultures, broad-spectrum antibiotics are usually started in neonates with bowel obstruction and those with suspected strangulating infarction. Patients with strangulation must have immediate surgical relief before the bowel infarcts, resulting in gangrene and intestinal perforation. Extensive intestinal necrosis results in short-gut syndrome (see Chapter 320.7). Nonoperative conservative management is usually limited to children with suspected adhesions or inflammatory strictures that may resolve with nasogastric decompression or anti-inflammatory medications. If clinical signs of improvement are not evident within 12–24 hr, then operative intervention is usually indicated.

311.1 Duodenal Obstruction

Duodenal atresia is thought to arise from failure to recanalize the lumen after the solid phase of intestinal development during the 4th and 5th wk of gestation. The incidence of duodenal atresia is 1 in 10,000 births and accounts for 25–40% of all intestinal atresias. Half the patients are born prematurely. Duodenal atresia may take several forms, including an intact membrane obstructing the lumen, a short fibrous cord connecting two blind duodenal pouches, or a gap between the nonconnecting ends of the duodenum. An unusual cause of obstruction is a "windsock" web, which is a distensible flap of tissue associated with anomalies of the biliary tract. The membranous form of atresia is most common, with obstruction occurring distal to the ampulla of Vater in the majority of patients. Duodenal obstruction may also be a result of an extrinsic compression such as an annular pancreas or from Ladd bands in patients with malrotation. Down syndrome occurs in 20–30% of patients with duodenal atresia. Other congenital anomalies that are associated with duodenal atresia include malrotation (20%), esophageal atresia (10–20%), congenital heart disease (10–15%), and anorectal and renal anomalies (5%).

Clinical Manifestations. The hallmark of duodenal obstruction is bilious vomiting without abdominal distention, which is usually noted on the 1st day of life. Peristaltic waves may be visualized early in the disease process. A history of polyhydramnios is present in half the pregnancies and is caused by a failure of absorption of amniotic fluid in the distal intestine. Jaundice is present in one third of the infants. The diagnosis is suggested by the presence of a "double-bubble sign" on plain abdominal radiographs (Fig. 311–1). The appearance is caused by a distended and gas-filled stomach and proximal duodenum. Contrast

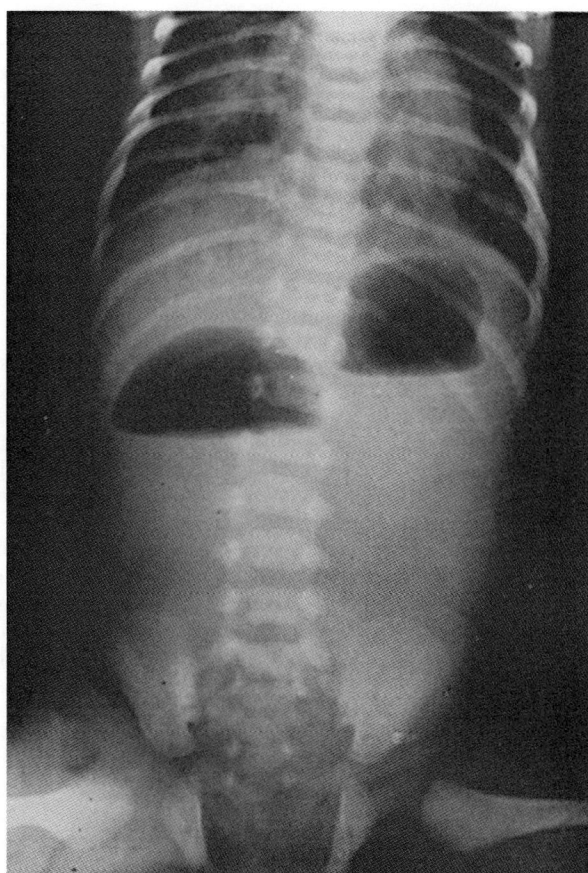

FIGURE 311–1. Abdominal radiograph of a newborn infant held upright. Note the "double bubble" gas shadow above and the absence of gas in the distal bowel in this case of congenital duodenal atresia.

studies are usually not necessary and may be associated with aspiration if attempted. Contrast studies may occasionally be needed to exclude malrotation and volvulus because intestinal infarction may occur within 6–12 hr if the volvulus is not relieved. Prenatal diagnosis of duodenal atresia is readily detected by fetal ultrasonography.

Treatment. The initial treatment of infants with duodenal atresia includes nasogastric or orogastric decompression with intravenous fluid replacement. Echocardiogram and radiology of the chest and spine should be performed to evaluate for associated anomalies. Approximately one third of infants with duodenal atresia have associated life-threatening congenital anomalies. Definitive correction of duodenal atresia is usually postponed to evaluate and treat these life-threatening anomalies.

The usual surgical repair for duodenal atresia is duodenoduodenostomy. The dilated proximal bowel may be tapered in an attempt to improve peristalsis. A gastrostomy tube may be placed to drain the stomach and protect the airway. Intravenous nutritional support or a transanastomotic jejunal tube is needed until infants start to feed orally. The prognosis is primarily dependent on the presence of associated anomalies.

If obstruction is due to Ladd bands with malrotation, an operation is necessary without delay. After division of the abnormal peritoneal folds or bands, the entire large intestine is placed within the left side of the abdomen, after first removing the appendix, with the small bowel on the right—the fetal position of nonrotation. Appendectomy is performed to avoid later misdiagnosis of appendicitis. Malrotation may also coexist with an intrinsic duodenal obstruction, such as a membrane or stenosis;

this may be identified by passing a balloon-tipped catheter into the jejunum below the site of obstruction, inflating the balloon, and slowly withdrawing the catheter. Annular pancreas is best treated by duodenoduodenostomy without dividing the pancreas, leaving as short a defunctioned loop as possible. Duodenal diaphragmatic obstruction is managed by duodenoplasty. The possibility exists that the common bile duct may open on the diaphragm itself.

311.2 Jejunal and Ileal Atresia and Obstruction

Jejunoileal atresias have been attributed to intrauterine vascular accidents leading to ischemic necrosis of the sterile bowel and resorption of the affected segments. Four different types of jejunal and ileal atresia are encountered (Fig. 311–2). Type I accounts for 20% of the atresias and is an intraluminal diaphragm that obstructs the lumen while continuity is maintained between the proximal and distal bowel. In type II, a small-diameter solid cord connects the proximal and distal bowel, accounting for about 35% of defects. Type III is divided into two subtypes. Type IIIa accounts for approximately 35% of all atresias and occurs when both ends of the bowel end in blind loops accompanied by a small mesenteric defect. Type IIIb is associated with an extensive mesenteric defect and a loss of the normal blood supply to the distal bowel. The distal ileum coils around the ileocolic artery, from which it derives its entire blood supply, producing an "apple-peel" appearance. This anomaly is associated with prematurity, an unusually short distal ileum, and significant foreshortening of the bowel. Type IV is multiple segments of bowel atresia and accounts for approximately 5% of all bowel atresias. Colon atresia has similarities to jejunoileal atresia but is much less common.

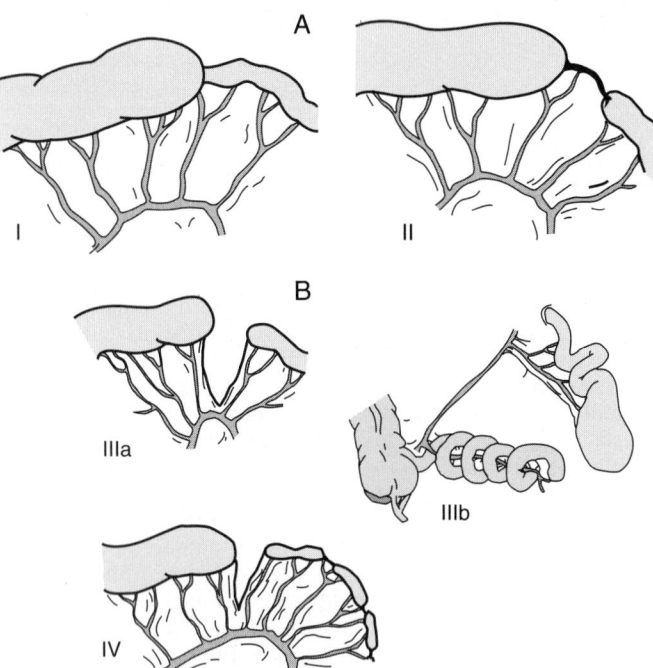

FIGURE 311–2. *A* and *B*, Classification of intestinal atresia. Type I: Mucosal obstruction caused by an intraluminal membrane with intact bowel wall and mesentery. Type II: Blind ends are separated by a fibrous cord. Type IIIa: Blind ends are separated by a V-shaped mesenteric defect. Type IIIb: "Apple peel" appearance. Type IV: Multiple atresias. (From Grosfeld J: Jejunoileal atresia and stenosis. In Welch KJ, et al [editors]: *Pediatric Surgery*, 4th ed. Chicago, Year Book Medical Publishers, 1986.)

Meconium ileus occurs primarily in newborn infants with cystic fibrosis. Approximately 10% of infants with cystic fibrosis will develop meconium ileus; 80–90% of infants presenting with meconium ileus have cystic fibrosis. *In simple meconium ileus*, the last 20–30 cm of ileum is collapsed and filled with pellets of pale-colored stool, above which a dilated loop of varying length appears obstructed by meconium with the consistency of thick syrup or glue. Peristalsis fails to propel this very viscid material forward, and it becomes impacted in the ileum. Volvulus, atresia, or perforation of the bowel accompanies *complicated* meconium ileus. Perforation in utero produces meconium peritonitis. Intraperitoneal meconium can cause dense adhesions, leading postnatally to adhesive intestinal obstruction, and may rapidly become calcified.

In 5% of patients with *Hirschsprung disease*, the aganglionic segment involves not only the entire colon but also terminal ileum. This condition causes a dilated small intestine with ganglionated but somewhat hypertrophied walls, a funnel-shaped transitional hypoganglionic zone, and a collapsed distal aganglionic bowel.

Clinical Manifestation. In contrast to duodenal atresia, extragastrointestinal anomalies are less common in atresias of the distal intestine. The diagnosis of jejunoileal atresia may be made by prenatal ultrasonograms. Polyhydramnios occurs in 25% of affected patients. Monozygotic twins are at higher risk for atresias than are dizygotic twins or singletons. Premature birth occurs in one third of infants. Most infants become symptomatic during the 1st day of life with abdominal distention and bile-stained emesis or gastric aspirate. Sixty to 75% of the infants fail to pass meconium. Jaundice has been found in 20–30% of the patients. Plain radiographs demonstrate many air-fluid levels or peritoneal calcification associated with meconium peritonitis. Contrast studies of the upper and lower bowel can delineate the level of obstruction and differentiate atresia from meconium ileus, meconium plug, and Hirschsprung disease. Abdominal ultrasound can distinguish meconium ileus from ileal atresia and identify intestinal malrotation.

In meconium ileus, plain films of the abdomen show a typical hazy or ground-glass appearance in the right lower quadrant. Small bubbles of gas trapped in meconium are dispersed within this area (see Chapter 91.1). Furthermore, owing to their viscid contents, moderately dilated loops of bowel do not have the air-fluid levels usually seen radiographically on the erect projection. If there is meconium peritonitis, patchy calcification may be noted, usually in the flanks. Pneumoperitoneum is most readily seen as free air between the liver and the diaphragm on an upright radiograph of the abdomen; if there is a large amount of free air, the entire abdomen may look like a football from distention with air; the ligamentum teres is sometimes clearly visible in the midline.

It is impossible to consistently distinguish small bowel from large bowel by studying plain radiographs of the abdomen in newborns and infants. If plain radiographs are nonspecific, a water-soluble contrast (Gastrografin, Hypaque) study of the colon may be needed to distinguish small from large intestine obstructions. A small colon, "microcolon," suggests disuse and the presence of obstruction proximal to the ileocecal valve. Water-soluble enemas should be used with caution in the diagnosis and treatment of meconium ileus because their hyperosmolality may result in dehydration; the enema pressure may result in perforation.

Treatment. Patients with small bowel obstruction should be stable and in adequate fluid and electrolyte balance before operation or radiographic attempts at disimpaction unless volvulus is suspected. Infections should be treated with appropriate antibiotics. Prophylactic antibiotics are usually given before surgery.

Ileal or jejunal atresia requires resection of the dilated proximal portion of the bowel followed by end-to-end anastomosis. If a simple mucosal diaphragm is present, jejunoplasty or ileoplasty with partial excision of the web is an acceptable alternative to resection. In uncomplicated meconium ileus Gastrografin enemas will diagnose the obstruction and wash out the inspissated material. Gastrografin is hypertonic and care must be taken to avoid dehydration, shock, and bowel perforation. The enema may have to be repeated after 8–12 hr. Resection after reduction is not needed if there have been no ischemic complications.

About 50% of patients with simple meconium ileus do not adequately respond to water-soluble enemas and need laparotomy. Operative management is indicated when the obstruction cannot be relieved by repeated attempts at nonoperative management and for infants with complicated meconium ileus. The extent of surgical intervention depends on the degree of pathology. In simple meconium ileus, the plug can be relieved by manipulation or direct enteral irrigation with *N*-acetylcysteine following an enterotomy. In complicated cases, bowel resection, peritoneal lavage, abdominal drainage, and stoma formation may be necessary. Total parenteral nutrition will be required.

311.3 Malrotation

Malrotation is incomplete rotation of the intestine during fetal development. The gut starts as a straight tube from stomach to rectum. The midbowel (distal duodenum to midtransverse colon) begins to elongate and progressively protrudes into the umbilical cord until it lies totally outside the confines of the abdominal cavity. As the developing bowel rotates in and out of the abdominal cavity, the superior mesenteric artery, which supplies blood to this section of gut, acts as an axis. The duodenum, on re-entering the abdominal cavity, moves to the region of the ligament of Treitz, and the colon that follows is directed to the left upper quadrant. The cecum subsequently rotates counterclockwise within the abdominal cavity and comes to lie in the right lower quadrant. The duodenum becomes fixed to the posterior abdominal wall before the colon is completely rotated. After rotation, the right and left colon and the mesenteric root become fixed to the posterior abdomen. These attachments provide a broad base of support to the mesentery and the superior mesenteric artery, thus preventing twisting of the mesenteric root and kinking of the vascular supply. Abdominal rotation and attachment are completed by 3 mo gestation.

Nonrotation occurs when the bowel fails to rotate after it returns to the abdominal cavity. The first and second portions of the duodenum are in their normal position, but the remainder of the duodenum, jejunum, and ileum occupy the right side of the abdomen while the colon is located on the left. Malrotation and nonrotation are associated with abdominal heterotaxia and the asplenia-polysplenia congenital heart malformation syndrome anomalad (see Chapter 424.11).

The most common type of malrotation involves failure of the cecum to move into the right lower quadrant (Fig. 311–3). The usual location of the cecum is in the subhepatic area. Failure of the cecum to rotate properly is associated with failure to form the normal broad-based adherence to the posterior abdominal wall. The mesentery including the superior mesenteric artery is tethered by a narrow stalk, which may twist around itself, producing a midgut volvulus. In addition, bands of tissue (Ladd bands) may extend from the cecum to the right upper quadrant, crossing and possibly obstructing the duodenum.

Clinical Manifestation. The majority of patients present within the 1st yr of life with symptoms of acute or chronic obstruction. Infants often present within the 1st wk of life with bilious emesis and acute bowel obstruction. Older infants present with episodes of recurrent abdominal pain that may mimic colic. Malrotation in older children may present with recurrent episodes of vomiting, abdominal pain, or both. Patients

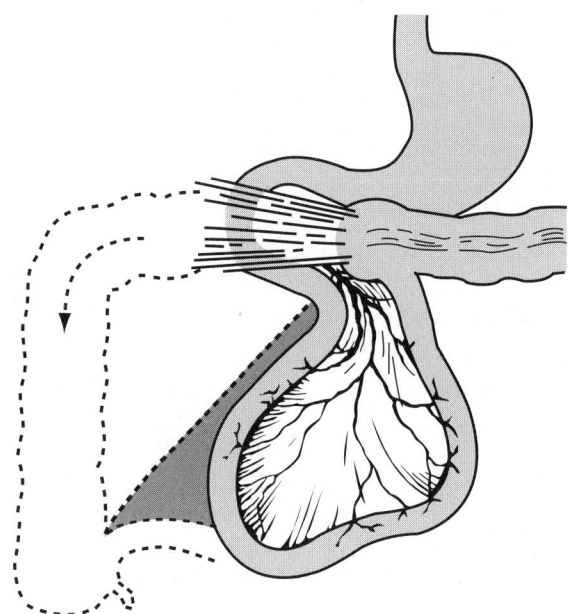

FIGURE 311–3. The mechanism of intestinal obstruction with incomplete rotation of the midgut (malrotation). The *dotted lines* show the course the cecum should have taken. Failure to rotate has left obstructing bands across the duodenum and a narrow pedicle for the midgut loop, making it susceptible to volvulus. (From Nixon HH, O'Donnell B: *The Essentials of Pediatric Surgery*. Philadelphia, JB Lippincott, 1961.)

occasionally present with malabsorption or protein-losing enteropathy associated with bacterial overgrowth. Symptoms are caused by intermittent volvulus or duodenal compression by Ladd bands or other adhesive bands affecting the small and large bowel. Twenty-five to 50% of adolescents with malrotation are asymptomatic. Adolescents who become symptomatic present with acute intestinal obstruction or history of recurrent episodes of abdominal pain with less frequent vomiting and diarrhea. Patients of any age with a rotational anomaly can develop volvulus without pre-existing symptoms.

An acute presentation of small bowel obstruction in a patient without previous bowel surgery is usually a result of volvulus associated with malrotation. This is a life-threatening complication of malrotation and the main reason that symptoms suggestive of malrotation should be investigated. The diagnosis is by ultrasound or contrast radiographic studies. The abdominal plain film is usually nonspecific but may demonstrate evidence of duodenal obstruction with a double-bubble sign. Barium enema usually demonstrates malposition of the cecum but may be normal in 10% of patients. Upper gastrointestinal series demonstrates malposition of the ligament of Treitz. Ultrasonography demonstrates inversion of the superior mesenteric artery and vein. A superior mesenteric vein located to the left of the superior mesenteric artery is suggestive of malrotation. Malrotation with volvulus is suggested by duodenal obstruction, thickened bowel loops to the right of the spine, and free peritoneal fluid.

Surgical intervention is recommended for any patient with a significant rotational abnormality, regardless of age. If a volvulus is present, it is reduced and the duodenum and upper jejunum are freed of any bands and remain in the right abdominal cavity. The colon is freed of adhesions and placed in the right abdomen with the cecum in the left lower quadrant, usually accompanied by incidental appendectomy. Extensive intestinal ischemia from volvulus produces the short-gut syndrome (see Chapter 320.7). Persistent symptoms after repair of malrotation should suggest a pseudo-obstruction–like motility disorder.

Chao HC, Kong MS, Chen JY, et al: Sonographic features related to volvulus in neonatal intestinal malrotation. *J Ultrasound Med* 2000;19:371–76.

Coutts JA, Docherty JG, Carachi R, et al: Clinical course of patients with cystic fibrosis presenting with meconium ileus. *Br J Surg* 1997;84:555.

Dalla Vecchia LK, Grosfeld JL, West KW, et al: Intestinal atresia and stenosis: A 25-year experience with 277 cases. *Arch Surg* 1998;133:490–96.

Fuchs JR, Langer JC: Long-term outcome after neonatal meconium obstruction. *Pediatrics* 1998;101:E7.

Kao SC, Franken EA, Franken EA Jr: Nonoperative treatment of simple meconium ileus: A survey of the Society for Pediatric Radiology. *Pediatr Radiol* 1995;25:97–100.

Kimble RM, Harding J, Kolbe A: Additional congenital anomalies in babies with gut atresia or stenosis: When to investigate, and which investigation. *Pediatr Surg Int* 1997;12:565–70.

Murshed R, Spitz L, Kiely E, et al: Meconium ileus: A ten-year review of thirty-six patients. *Eur J Pediatr Surg* 1997;7:275–77.

Neal MR, Seibert JJ, Vanderzalm T, et al: Neonatal ultrasonography to distinguish between meconium ileus and ileal atresia. *J Ultrasound Med* 1997;16:263–66.

Prasil P, Flageole H, Shaw KS, et al: Should malrotation in children be treated differently according to age? *J Pediatr Surg* 2000;35:756–58.

Sato S, Nishijima E, Muraji T, et al: Jejunoileal atresia: A 27-year experience. *J Pediatr Surg* 1998;33:1633–35.

Shimotake T, Go S, Tsuda T, et al: Ultrasonographic detection of intrauterine intussusception resulting in ileal atresia complicated by meconium peritonitis. *Pediatr Surg Int* 2000;16:43–44.

Velasco B, Lassaletta L, Gracia R, et al: Intestinal lengthening and growth hormone in extreme short bowel syndrome: A case report. *J Pediatr Surg* 1999;34:1423–24.

Chapter 312

Intestinal Duplications, Meckel Diverticulum, and Other Remnants of the Omphalomesenteric Duct

Robert Wyllie

312.1 Intestinal Duplication

Duplications of the intestinal tract are rare anomalies that consist of well-formed tubular or spherical structures firmly attached to the intestine with a common blood supply. The lining of the duplications resembles that of the gastrointestinal tract. Duplications are located on the mesenteric border and may communicate with the intestinal lumen. Duplications can be classified into three categories: localized duplications, duplications associated with spinal cord defects and vertebral malformations, and duplications of the colon. Occasionally (10–15%), multiple duplications are found.

Localized duplications may occur in any area of the gastrointestinal tract but are most common in the ileum and jejunum. They are usually cystic or tubular structures within the wall of the bowel. The cause is unknown, but their development has been attributed to defects in recanalization of the intestinal lumen after the solid stage of embryologic development. Duplication of the intestine occurring in association with vertebral and spinal cord anomalies (hemivertebra, anterior spina bifida, band connection between lesion and cervical or thoracic spine) is thought to arise from splitting of the notochord in the developing embryo. Duplication of the colon is usually associated with anomalies of the urinary tract and genitals. Duplication of the entire colon, rectum, anus, and terminal ileum may occur. The defects are thought to be secondary to caudal twinning, with duplication of the hindgut, genital, and lower urinary tracts.

Clinical Manifestations. Symptoms depend on the size, location, and mucosal lining. Duplications may cause bowel obstruction by compressing the adjacent intestinal lumen, or they may act as the lead point of an intussusception or a site for a volvulus. If they are lined by acid-secreting mucosa, they may cause ulceration, perforation, and hemorrhage of the adjacent bowel. Patients may present with abdominal pain, vomiting, palpable mass, or acute gastrointestinal hemorrhage. Intestinal duplications in the thorax (neuroenteric cysts) may present as respiratory distress. Duplications of the lower bowel may cause constipation or diarrhea or be associated with recurrent prolapse of the rectum.

The *diagnosis* is suspected on the basis of the history and physical examination. Radiologic studies such as barium studies, ultrasonography, CT, and MRI are helpful but usually nonspecific, demonstrating cystic structures or mass effects. Radioisotope technetium scanning may localize ectopic gastric mucosa. The *treatment* of duplications is surgical resection and management of associated defects.

312.2 Meckel Diverticulum and Other Remnants of the Omphalomesenteric Duct

A Meckel diverticulum is a remnant of the embryonic yolk sac, which may also be referred to as the omphalomesenteric duct or vitelline duct. The omphalomesenteric duct connects the yolk sac to the gut in a developing embryo and provides nutrition until the placenta is established. Between the 5th and 7th wk of gestation, the duct attenuates and separates from the intestine. Just before this involution, the epithelium of the yolk sac develops a lining similar to that of the stomach. Partial or complete failure of involution of the omphalomesenteric duct results in various residual structures. Meckel diverticulum is the most common of these structures and is the most frequent congenital gastrointestinal anomaly, occurring in 2–3% of all infants. A typical Meckel diverticulum is a 3–6 cm outpouching of the ileum along the antimesenteric border 50–75 cm from the ileocecal valve (Fig. 312–1). The distance from the ileocecal valve depends on the age of the patient. Other omphalomesenteric duct remnants occur infrequently, including a persistently patent duct, a solid cord, or a cord with a central cyst or a diverticulum associated with a persistent cord between the diverticulum and the umbilicus.

Clinical Manifestations. Symptoms of a Meckel diverticulum usually arise within the 1st 2 yr of life, but initial symptoms are common during the 1st decade. The majority of symptomatic Meckel diverticula are lined by an ectopic mucosa, including an acid-secreting mucosa that causes intermittent painless rectal bleeding by ulceration of the adjacent normal ileal mucosa. Unlike the upper duodenal mucosa, the acid is not neutralized by pancreatic bicarbonate.

The stool is typically described as brick colored or currant jelly colored. Bleeding may cause significant anemia but is usually self-limited because of contraction of the splanchnic vessels, as patients become hypovolemic. Bleeding from a Meckel diverticulum can also be less dramatic, with melanotic stools.

Less often, a Meckel diverticulum may be associated with partial or complete bowel obstruction. The most common mechanism of obstruction occurs when the diverticulum acts as the lead point of an intussusception. This presentation is more common in older male children. Other causes of obstruction may result from intraperitoneal bands connecting residual omphalomesenteric duct remnants to the ileum and umbilicus. These bands cause obstruction by internal herniation or volvulus of the small bowel around the band. A Meckel diverticulum may occasionally become inflamed (diverticulitis) and present similarly to acute appendicitis. Diverticulitis may lead to perforation and peritonitis.

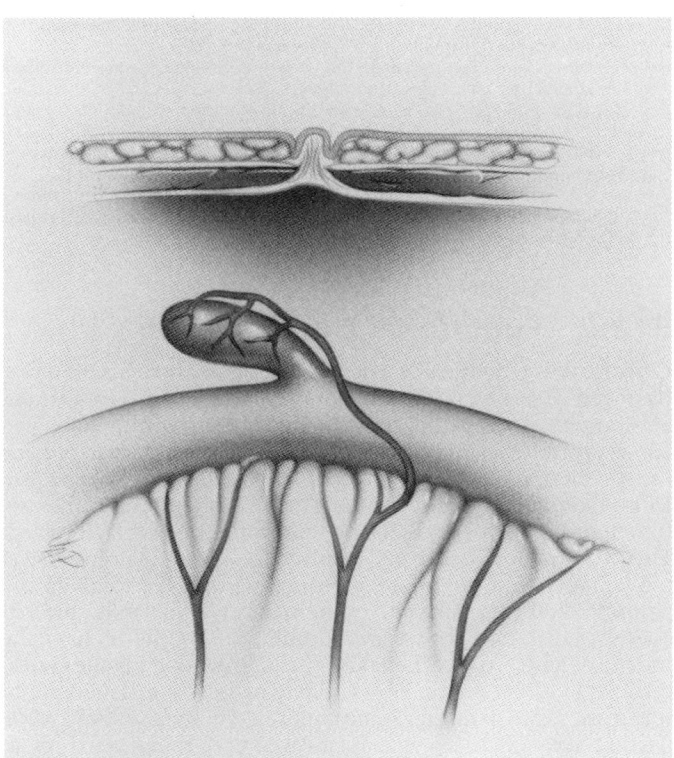

FIGURE 312–1. Typical Meckel diverticulum located on the antimesenteric border.

20 min.

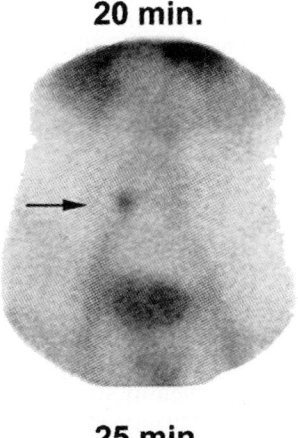

25 min.

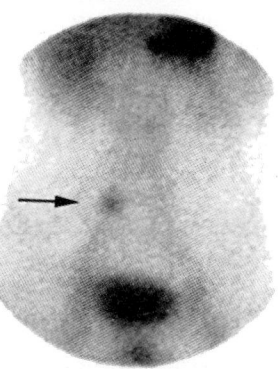

FIGURE 312–2. Meckel scan demonstrating accumulation of technetium in the stomach superior bladder (inferior) and in the acid-secreting mucosa of a Meckel diverticulum.

Diagnosis. The diagnosis of omphalomesenteric duct remnants depends on their clinical presentation. If an infant or child presents with significant painless rectal bleeding, the presence of a Meckel diverticulum should be suspected. Confirmation of a Meckel diverticulum can be difficult. Plain abdominal radiographs are of no value, and routine barium studies rarely fill the diverticulum. The most sensitive study is a Meckel radionuclide scan, which is performed after intravenous infusion of technetium-99m pertechnetate. The mucus-secreting cells of the ectopic gastric mucosa take up pertechnetate, permitting visualization of the Meckel diverticulum (Fig. 312–2). The uptake can be enhanced with various agents, including cimetidine, glucagon, and gastrin. The sensitivity of the enhanced scan is approximately 85%, with a specificity of approximately 95%. Other methods of detection include abdominal ultrasound, superior mesenteric angiography, abdominal CT scan, and exploratory laparoscopy. In patients who present with intestinal obstruction or a picture of appendicitis with omphalomesenteric duct remnants, the diagnosis is rarely made before surgery. The treatment of a symptomatic Meckel diverticulum is surgical excision.

Brown RL, Azizkhan RG: Gastrointestinal bleeding in infants and children: Meckel's diverticulum and intestinal duplication. *Semin Pediatr Surg* 1999;8:202–9.

Emamian SA, Shalaby-Rana E, Majd M: The spectrum of heterotopic gastric mucosa in children detected by Tc-99m pertechnetate scintigraphy. *Clin Nucl Med* 2001;26:529–35.

Lee KH, Yeung CK, Tam YH, et al: Laparoscopy for definitive diagnosis and treatment of gastrointestinal bleeding of obscure origin in children. *J Pediatr Surg* 2000;35:1291–93.

Mitchell AW, Spencer J, Allison DJ, et al: Meckel's diverticulum: Angiographic findings in 16 patients. *AJR Am J Roentgenol* 1998;170:1329–33.

Swaniker F, Soldes O, Hirschl RB: The utility of technetium 99m pertechnetate scintigraphy in the evaluation of patients with Meckel's diverticulum. *J Pediatr Surg* 1999;34:760–64.

Chapter 313
Motility Disorders and Hirschsprung Disease

Robert Wyllie

313.1 Chronic Intestinal Pseudo-Obstruction

Chronic intestinal pseudo-obstruction comprises a group of disorders characterized by signs and symptoms of intestinal obstruction in the absence of an anatomic lesion. Pseudo-obstruction may occur as a primary disease or may be secondary to a large number of conditions that may transiently or permanently alter bowel motility. Pseudo-obstruction represents a wide spectrum of pathologic disorders from abnormal myoelectric activity to abnormalities of the nerves (intestinal neuropathy) or musculature (intestinal myopathy) of the gut. The organs involved may include the entire gastrointestinal tract or may be limited to certain components, such as the stomach or colon. The distinctive pathologic abnormalities are considered together because of their clinical similarities.

Most congenital forms of pseudo-obstruction occur sporadically. A few clusters of autosomal dominant or recessive individuals have been reported as having cases associated with abnormal gut muscle or nerves. Patients with autosomal dominant forms of pseudo-obstruction have variable expressions of the disease. Acquired pseudo-obstruction may follow episodes of acute gastroenteritis, presumably resulting in injury to the myenteric plexus.

In congenital pseudo-obstruction, abnormalities of the muscle or nerves can be demonstrated in most cases. In muscular disease, the outer longitudinal muscle layer is replaced by fibrous material. In neuronal disease, there may be disorganized or hypoganglionosis or hyperganglionosis. Abnormalities in the interstitial cells of Cajal have been demonstrated in some children and mitochondrial defects found in others.

Clinical Manifestations. More than half the children with congenital pseudo-obstruction experience symptoms within the first few months of life. Two thirds of the infants presenting within the first few days of life are born prematurely, and about 40% have malrotation of the intestine. In 75% of these children symptoms occur during the 1st yr of life, and the remainder become symptomatic in the next several years. The most common symptoms are abdominal distention and vomiting, which are present in 75% of affected infants. Constipation, growth failure, and abdominal pain occur in approximately 60% of patients, and diarrhea occurs in 30–40%. The symptoms wax and wane in the majority of the patients; poor nutrition and intercurrent illness tend to exacerbate symptoms. Urinary tract involvement is not uncommon and may present as recurrent urinary tract infection or mimic obstructive symptoms.

The diagnosis of pseudo-obstruction is based on the presence of compatible symptoms in the absence of anatomic obstruction. Plain abdominal radiographs demonstrate air-fluid levels in the small intestine. Neonates with evidence of obstruction at birth have a microcolon. Contrast studies demonstrate slow passage of barium; consideration should be given to using water-soluble agents.

Other studies may provide information on the underlying pathophysiology. Esophageal motility is abnormal in about half the patients. Antroduodenal motility and gastric emptying studies have abnormal results if the upper gut is involved. Manometric evidence of a normal migrating motor complex should redirect the diagnostic evaluation. Anorectal motility is normal and differentiates pseudo-obstruction from Hirschsprung disease. Full-thickness intestinal biopsy may show involvement of the muscle layers or abnormalities of the intrinsic intestinal nervous system.

The *differential diagnosis* includes Hirschsprung disease, other causes of mechanical obstruction, psychogenic constipation, neurogenic bladder, and superior mesenteric artery syndrome. Secondary causes of ileus or pseudo-obstruction, such as hypothyroidism, narcotics, scleroderma, Chagas disease, hypokalemia, diabetic neuropathy, amyloidosis, porphyria, angioneurotic edema, and radiation must be excluded.

Treatment. Nutritional support is the mainstay of treatment for pseudo-obstruction. Thirty to 50% require partial or complete parenteral nutrition. Some patients can be treated with intermittent enteral supplementation, whereas others may maintain themselves on selective oral diets. Prokinetic drugs are generally not useful. Isolated gastroparesis may follow episodes of viral gastroenteritis and spontaneously resolves usually within 6–24 mo. Cisapride (a 5-hydroxytryptamine receptor antagonist) and erythromycin (a motilin receptor agonist) may enhance gastric emptying and proximal small bowel motility and may be of use in this selected group of patients.

Symptomatic small bowel bacterial overgrowth is usually treated with oral antibiotics. Bacterial overgrowth may be associated with steatorrhea and malabsorption. Antibiotics should be used judiciously, however, because they may lead to the emergence of drug-resistant bacteria. Patients with acid peptic symptoms are treated with acid suppressors (see Chapter 316). Some children benefit from decompressive ileostomies or colostomies. Colectomy with ileorectal anastomosis is beneficial if the large bowel is the primary site of the motility abnormality. Bowel transplantation may benefit selected patients.

Goulet O, Jobert-Giraud A, Michel JL, et al: Chronic intestinal pseudo-obstruction syndrome in pediatric patients. *Eur J Pediatr Surg* 1999;9:83–89.

Haftel LT, Lev D, Barash V, et al: Familial mitochondrial intestinal pseudo-obstruction and neurogenic bladder. *J Child Neurol* 2000;15:386–89.

Heneyke S, Smith VV, Spitz L, et al: Chronic intestinal pseudo-obstruction: Treatment and long-term follow-up of 44 patients. *Arch Dis Child* 1999;81:21–27.

Iyer K, Kaufman S, Sudan D, et al: Long-term results of intestinal transplantation for pseudo-obstruction in children. *J Pediatr Surg* 2001;36:174–77.

Rudolph CD, Hyman PE, Altschuler SM, et al: Diagnosis and treatment of chronic intestinal pseudo-obstruction in children: Report of consensus workshop. *J Pediatr Gastroenterol Nutr* 1997;24:102–12.

313.2 ■ Functional Constipation

Constipation is defined by a delay or difficulty in defecation that has been present for 2 wk or longer. Functional constipation, also known as idiopathic constipation or fecal withholding, can usually be differentiated from constipation secondary to organic causes on the basis of a history and physical examination. Unlike anorectal malformations and Hirschsprung disease, functional constipation typically starts after the neonatal period. The constipation is caused by the passage of painful bowel movements with voluntary withholding of feces to avoid the painful stimulus. Perianal inflammation from milk protein allergy may initiate the painful stimuli. When children have the urge to defecate, typical behaviors include contracting the gluteal muscles by stiffening the legs while lying down or holding onto furniture while standing. Some children will squat or hide while passing stool. Caregivers may misinterpret these activities as straining. Daytime encopresis is common, and some children will have a history of blood in the stool noted with the passage of a large bowel movement. Findings suggestive of underlying pathology include failure to thrive, weight loss, abdominal pain, vomiting, or persistent anal fissure or fistula.

The physical examination often demonstrates a large volume of stool palpated in the suprapubic area; rectal examination demonstrates a dilated rectal vault filled with guaiac-negative stool. The presence of a hair tuft over the spine, spinal dimple, or failure to elicit a cremasteric reflex or anal wink is suggestive of spinal pathology. A tethered cord is suggested by decreased or absent lower leg reflexes. Urinary tract symptoms include recurrent urinary tract infection; evidence of obstruction may occur in constipated children and those with spinal disorders. Children with no evidence of abnormalities on physical examination rarely require radiologic evaluation. In refractory patients, specialized testing should be considered to rule out conditions such as hypothyroidism, hypocalcemia, lead toxicity, and celiac disease. Selected children may benefit from MRI of the spine to identify an intraspinal process, motility studies to identify underlying myopathy or neuropathic bowel abnormalities, or a barium enema to identify structural abnormalities.

Therapy for functional constipation includes patient education, relief of impaction, and softening of the stool. The parents must understand that soiling associated with overflow incontinence is associated with loss of normal sensation and not a willful act. A regular bowel training program including sitting on the toilet for 5–10 min after meals and keeping track of the frequency of bowel movements is often helpful in establishing a regular bowel habit. If an impaction is present on the initial physical examination, an enema is usually required to clear the impaction while bowel softeners are started as maintenance medications. Typical regimens include the use of mineral oil, lactulose, and polyethylene glycol preparation. Prolonged use of stimulants such as senna or bisacodyl should be avoided. Children with behavioral problems that are interfering with successful treatment may benefit from a referral to a mental health care provider. Maintenance therapy is generally continued until a regular bowel pattern has been established for several months. Children with spinal problems can be successfully managed with low volumes of fluid through a cecostomy tube.

Baker SS, Liptak GS, Colletti RB, et al: Constipation in infants and children: Evaluation and treatment: A medical position statement of the North American Society for Pediatric Gastroenterology and Nutrition. *J Pediatr Gastroenterol Nutr* 1999;29:612–26.

Brooks RC, Copen RM, Cox DJ, et al: Review of the treatment literature for encopresis, functional constipation, and stool-toileting refusal. *Ann Behav Med* 2000;22:260–67.

Chait PG, Shandling B, Richards HM, et al: Fecal incontinence in children: Treatment with percutaneous cecostomy tube placement—a prospective study. *Radiology* 1997;203:621–24.

Corazziari E, Badiali D, Bazzocchi G, et al: Long-term efficacy, safety, and tolerability of low daily doses of isosmotic polyethylene glycol electrolyte balanced solution (PMF-100) in the treatment of functional chronic constipation. *Gut* 2000;46:522–26.

Emmanuel AV, Kamm MA: Response to a behavioral treatment, biofeedback, in constipated patients is associated with improved gut transit and autonomic innervation. *Gut* 2001;49:214–19.

Kim HL, Gow KW, Penner JG, et al: Presentation of low anorectal malformations beyond the neonatal period. *Pediatrics* 2000;105:E68.

Penning C, Gielkens HA, Hemelaar M, et al: Prolonged ambulatory recording of antroduodenal motility in slow-transit constipation. *Br J Surg* 2000;87:211–17.

Youssef NN, Di Lorenzo C: Childhood constipation: Evaluation and treatment. *J Clin Gastroenterol* 2001;33:199–205.

313.3 Congenital Aganglionic Megacolon (Hirschsprung Disease)

Hirschsprung disease, or congenital aganglionic megacolon, is caused by abnormal innervation of the bowel, beginning in the internal anal sphincter and extending proximally to involve a variable length of gut. Hirschsprung disease is the most common cause of lower intestinal obstruction in neonates, with an overall incidence of 1 in 5,000 live births. Males are affected more often than females (4:1); prematurity is uncommon. There is an increased familial incidence in long segment disease. Hirschsprung disease may be associated with other congenital defects, including Down, Smith-Lemli-Opitz, Waardenburg, cartilage-hair hypoplasia, and congenital hypoventilation ("Ondine curse") syndromes and urogenital or cardiovascular abnormalities.

Pathology. Hirschsprung disease is result of an absence of ganglion cells in the bowel wall, extending proximally and continuously from the anus for a variable distance. The absence of neural innervation is a consequence of an arrest of neuroblast migration from the proximal to distal bowel. Hirschsprung disease is usually sporadic; however, dominant and recessive patterns of inheritance have been demonstrated in family groups. Genetic defects have been identified most often on the *RET* gene localized on chromosome 10q11 and the *EDNRB* gene located on 13q22. Defects in *SOX10* (22q13) have been associated with Hirschsprung disease and Waardenburg syndrome. Other mutations that have been identified include gene defects in *GDNF* and *NTN*, which are involved in *RET* activation, and defects in *EDN3* and *ECE1*, which are involved in *EDNRB* initiation. The aganglionic segment is limited to the rectosigmoid in 75% of patients; in 10% the entire colon lacks ganglion cells. Total bowel aganglionosis is rare. Observed histologically is an absence of Meissner and Auerbach plexus and hypertrophied nerve bundles with high concentrations of acetylcholinesterase between the muscular layers and in the submucosa.

Clinical Manifestations. The clinical symptoms of Hirschsprung disease usually begin at birth with the delayed passage of meconium. In 99% of full-term infants, meconium is passed within 48 hr of birth. Hirschsprung disease should be suspected in any full-term infant (the disease is unusual in preterm infants) with delayed passage of stool. Some infants pass meconium normally but subsequently present with a history of chronic constipation. Failure to thrive, with hypoproteinemia from a protein-losing enteropathy, is a less common presentation now that Hirschsprung disease is usually recognized early in the course of the illness. Breast-fed infants may not suffer as severe a disease as formula-fed infants.

Failure to pass stool leads to dilatation of the proximal bowel and abdominal distention. As the bowel dilates, intraluminal pressure increases, resulting in decreased blood flow and deterioration of the mucosal barrier. Stasis allows proliferation of bacteria, which may lead to enterocolitis (*Clostridium difficile, Staphylococcus aureus*, anaerobes, coliforms) with associated sepsis and signs of bowel obstruction. Early recognition of Hirschsprung disease before the onset of enterocolitis is essential in reducing morbidity and mortality.

Hirschsprung disease in older patients must be distinguished from other causes of abdominal distention and chronic constipation (Table 313–1; Fig. 313–1). The history often reveals increasing difficulty with the passage of stools, starting in the 1st few weeks of life. A large fecal mass is palpable in the left lower abdomen, but on rectal examination the rectum is usually empty of feces. The stools, when passed, may consist of small pellets, may be ribbon-like, or may have a fluid consistency; the large stools and fecal soiling of patients with functional constipation are absent. In neonates, Hirschsprung disease must be differentiated from meconium plug syndrome, meconium ileus, and intestinal atresia. In older patients, the Currarino triad must be considered (anorectal malformations—ectopic, anus, rectal stenosis; sacral bone anomalies—hypoplasia, poor segmentation; or presacral masses—anterior meningoceles, teratoma, cysts).

Rectal examination demonstrates normal anal tone and is usually followed by an explosive discharge of foul-smelling feces and gas. Intermittent attacks of intestinal obstruction from retained feces may be associated with pain and fever.

Diagnosis. Rectal manometry and rectal suction biopsy are the easiest and most reliable indicators of Hirschsprung disease. Anorectal manometry measures the pressure of the internal anal sphincter while a balloon is distended in the rectum. In normal individuals, rectal distention initiates a reflex decline in internal sphincter pressure. In patients with Hirschsprung disease, the pressure fails to drop or there is a paradoxical rise in pressure with rectal distention. The accuracy of this diagnostic test is more than 90%, but it is technically difficult in young infants. A normal response in the course of manometric evaluation precludes a diagnosis of Hirschsprung disease; an equivocal or paradoxical response requires a rectal biopsy.

TABLE 313–1. Distinguishing Features of Hirschsprung Disease and Functional Constipation

Variable	Functional (Acquired)	Hirschsprung Disease
History		
Onset of constipation	After 2 yr of age	At birth
Encopresis	Common	Very rare
Failure to thrive	Uncommon	Possible
Enterocolitis	None	Possible
Forced bowel training	Usual	None
Examination		
Abdominal distention	Uncommon	Common
Poor weight gain	Rare	Common
Anal tone	Normal	Normal
Rectal examination	Stool in ampulla	Ampulla empty
Malnutrition	None	Possible
Laboratory		
Anorectal manometry	Distention of the rectum causes relaxation of the internal sphincter	No sphincter relaxation or paradoxical increase in pressure
Rectal biopsy	Normal	No ganglion cells Increased acetylcholinesterase staining
Barium enema	Massive amounts of stool, no transition zone	Transition zone, delayed evacuation (>24 hr)

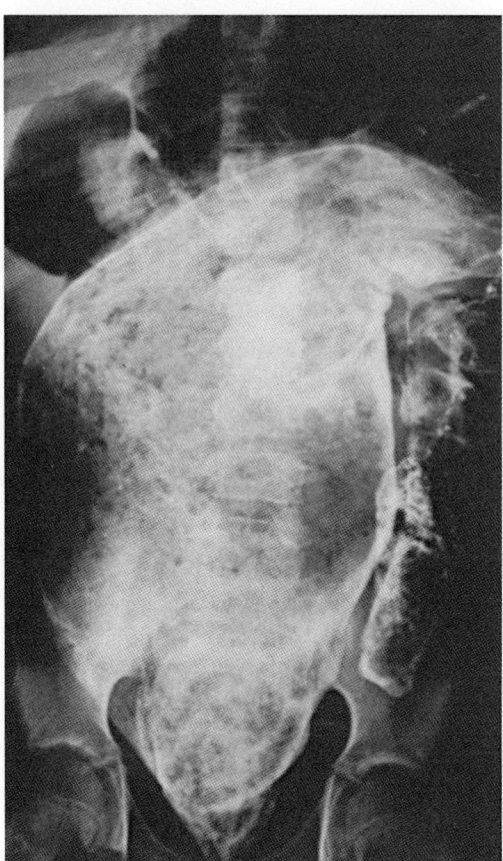

FIGURE 313–1. Barium enema in a 14-yr-old boy with severe constipation. The enormous dilatation of the rectum and distal colon is typical of acquired functional megacolon.

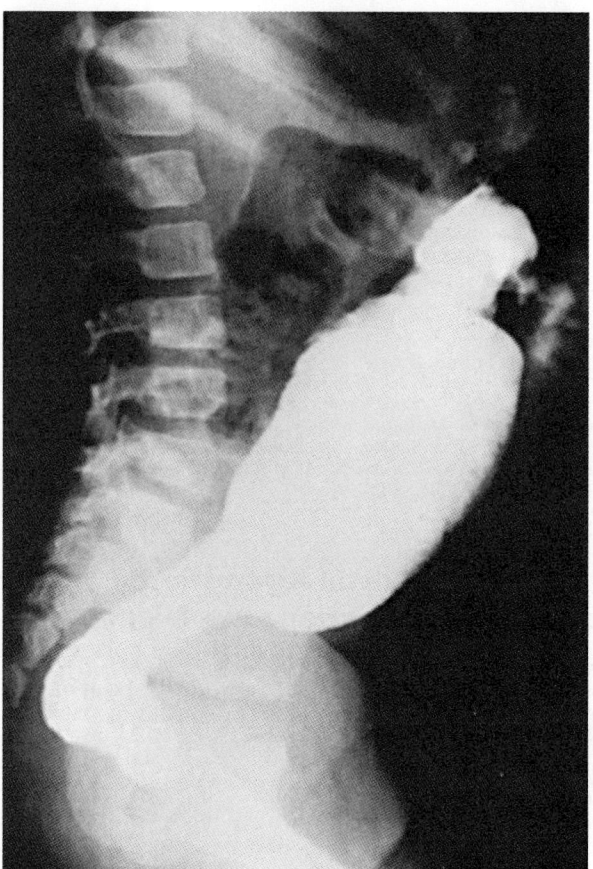

FIGURE 313–2. Lateral view of a barium enema in a 3-yr-old girl with Hirschsprung disease. The aganglionic distal segment is narrow, with distended normal ganglionic bowel above it.

Rectal suction biopsies should be performed no closer than 2 cm to the dentate line to avoid the normal area of hypoganglionosis at the anal verge. The biopsy material should contain an adequate sample of submucosa to evaluate for the presence of ganglion cells. The biopsy specimen can be stained for acetylcholinesterase, which may facilitate interpretation. Patients with aganglionosis demonstrate a large number of hypertrophied nerve bundles that stain positively for acetylcholinesterase with an absence of ganglion cells.

The radiographic diagnosis of Hirschsprung disease is based on the presence of a transition zone between normal dilated proximal colon and a smaller-caliber obstructed distal colon caused by the nonrelaxation of the aganglionic bowel. The transition zone is not usually present before 1–2 wk of age and on a radiograph is a funnel-shaped area of intestine between the proximal dilated colon and the constricted distal bowel. Radiologic evaluation should be performed without preparation to prevent transient dilatation of the aganglionic segment. Twenty-four-hour delayed films are helpful (Fig. 313–2). If significant barium is still present in the colon, it increases the suspicion of Hirschsprung disease even if a transition zone is not identified. Barium enema examination is useful in determining the extent of aganglionosis before surgery and in evaluating other diseases that present as lower bowel obstruction in a neonate. Full-thickness rectal biopsy may be performed at the time of surgery to confirm the diagnosis and level of involvement.

Treatment. Once the diagnosis is established, the definitive treatment is operative intervention. The operative options are to perform a definitive procedure as soon as the diagnosis is established or perform a temporary colostomy and wait until the infant is 6–12 mo old to perform definitive repair. There are three basic surgical options. The first successful surgical procedure, described by Swenson, was to excise the aganglionic segment and anastomose the normal proximal bowel to the rectum 1–2 cm above the dentate line. The operation is technically difficult and led to the development of two other procedures. Duhamel described a procedure to create a neorectum, bringing down normally innervated bowel behind the aganglionic rectum. The neorectum created in this procedure has an anterior aganglionic half with normal sensation and a posterior ganglionic half with normal propulsion. The endorectal pull-through procedure described by Boley involves stripping the mucosa from the aganglionic rectum and bringing normally innervated colon through the residual muscular cuff, thus bypassing the abnormal bowel from within. Advances in techniques have led to successful laparoscopic pull-through.

In ultrashort segmental Hirschsprung disease or internal sphincter achalasia, the aganglionic segment is limited to the internal sphincter. The clinical symptoms are similar to those of children with functional constipation. Ganglion cells are present on rectal suction biopsy, but the rectal motility is abnormal. Excision of a strip of rectal muscle usually leads to a more regular bowel pattern.

Long-segment Hirschsprung disease involving the entire colon and part of the small bowel represents a difficult problem. Rectal motility studies and rectal suction biopsy demonstrate findings of Hirschsprung disease, but radiologic studies are difficult to interpret because no colonic transition zone can be identified. The extent of aganglionosis can be determined accurately by biopsy at the time of laparotomy. When the entire colon is aganglionic, often together with a length of terminal ileum, ileal-anal anastomosis is the treatment of choice, preserving part of the aganglionic colon to facilitate water absorption, which helps the stools to become firm.

The prognosis of surgically treated Hirschsprung disease is generally satisfactory; the great majority of patients achieve fecal continence. Postoperative problems include recurrent enterocolitis, stricture, prolapse, perianal abscesses, and fecal soiling.

Baker SS, Liptak GS, Colletti RB, et al: Constipation in infants and children: Evaluation and treatment: A medical position statement of the North American Society for Pediatric Gastroenterology and Nutrition. *J Pediatr Gastroenterol Nutr* 1999;29:612–26.

Coran AG, Teitelbaum DH: Recent advances in the management of Hirschsprung's disease. *Am J Surg* 2000;180:382–87.

De Caluwe D, Yoneda A, Akl U, et al: Internal anal sphincter achalasia: Outcome after internal sphincter myectomy. *J Pediatr Surg* 2001;36:736–38.

Gereige RS, Frias JL: Is it more than just constipation? *Pediatrics* 2001;109:961–65.

Makitie O, Kaitila I, Rintala R: Hirschsprung disease associated with severe cartilage-hair hypoplasia. *J Pediatr* 2001;138:929–31.

McCabe ERB: Hirschsprung's disease: Dissecting complexity in a pathogenetic network. *Lancet* 2002;359:1169–70.

Parisi MA, Kapur R: Genetics of Hirschsprung disease. *Curr Opin Pediatr* 2000;12:610–17.

Teitelbaum DH, Cilley RE, Sherman NJ, et al: A decade of experience with the primary pull-through for Hirschsprung disease in the newborn period: A multicenter analysis of outcomes. *Ann Surg* 2000;232:372–80.

Van Kuyk EM, Brugman-Boezeman ATM, Wissink-Essink M, et al: Defecation problems in children with Hirschsprung's disease: A prospective controlled study of a multidisciplinary behavioural treatment. *Acta Paediatr* 2001;90:1153–59.

313.4 Superior Mesenteric Artery Syndrome (Wilkie Syndrome, Cast Syndrome, Arteriomesenteric Duodenal Compression Syndrome)

The superior mesenteric artery syndrome describes an extrinsic compression of the duodenum in children after rapid weight loss and in a supine position. The compression is thought to occur as the mesentery loses its fat and allows the superior mesenteric artery to collapse on the duodenum, compressing it between the superior mesenteric artery anteriorly and the aorta posteriorly. Alternatively, the cause may be that the loss of supporting fat in the second and third portions of the duodenum allows the duodenum to collapse against the spine.

The classic example is an adolescent who starts vomiting after application of a body cast for orthopedic surgery. Other associated factors include anorexia, prolonged bed rest, weight loss, abdominal surgery, and exaggerated lumbar lordosis. The *diagnosis* is established radiologically with the demonstration of a cutoff of the duodenum just to the right of the midline. The duodenal obstruction may be accompanied by proximal duodenal and gastric dilatation.

Treatment of the acute syndrome involves relief of the obstruction and improved nutrition to alter the anatomic relationships of the duodenum with surrounding structures. Positioning patients in a lateral or prone position shifts the duodenum away from potential obstructing structures and may allow resumption of oral intake. Prokinetic agents such as metoclopramide or cisapride may be helpful. If repositioning is unsuccessful in relieving symptoms, a nasojejunal tube may be placed past the point of obstruction and feedings begun. Some patients require total parenteral nutrition to replete lost body fat, and occasional patients may need surgical intervention.

Chapter 314
Ileus, Adhesions, Intussusception, and Closed-Loop Obstructions

Robert Wyllie

314.1 Ileus

Ileus is the failure of intestinal peristalsis without evidence of mechanical obstruction. Lack of normal gut motility interferes with aboral movement of intestinal contents and in children is most often associated with abdominal surgery or infection (pneumonia, gastroenteritis, peritonitis). Ileus also accompanies metabolic abnormalities, such as uremia, hypokalemia, or acidosis, and occurs with administration of certain drugs, such as opiates and vincristine. Ileus may also occur when antimotility drugs such as loperamide are used during episodes of gastroenteritis.

Ileus presents as increasing abdominal distention and initially minimal pain. Pain increases with increasing distention. Bowel sounds are minimal or absent, in contrast to early mechanical obstruction, when they are hyperactive. Plain abdominal radiographs demonstrate many air-fluid levels throughout the abdomen. Serial radiographs usually do not show progressive distention as they do in mechanical obstruction. Contrast radiographs, if performed, demonstrate slow movement of the barium through a patent lumen.

Treatment of ileus involves correction of the underlying abnormality. Nasogastric decompression is used if abdominal distention is associated with pain or to relieve recurrent vomiting. Ileus after abdominal surgical procedures usually results in return of normal intestinal motility within 24–72 hr. Prokinetic agents such as metoclopramide or erythromycin may stimulate the return of normal bowel motility and be of assistance to children with prolonged ileus. Oral administration of drugs that block gastrointestinal opiate receptors but do not block central nervous system opiate action may reduce the ileus in postoperative patients receiving narcotics.

314.2 Adhesions

Adhesions are fibrous bands of tissue that are a common cause of postoperative small bowel obstruction after abdominal surgery. The risk of forming an adhesion that causes obstructive symptoms in childhood has not been well studied but seems to occur in 2–3% of patients after abdominal surgery. The majority of obstructions are associated with single adhesions and can occur at any time after the 2nd postoperative week.

The *diagnosis* is suspected in patients with abdominal pain, constipation, emesis, and a history of intraperitoneal surgery. Nausea and vomiting quickly follow the development of pain. Bowel sounds initially are hyperactive, and the abdomen is flat. The bowel subsequently dilates, producing abdominal distention in most patients, and bowel sounds disappear. Fever and leukocytosis are suggestive of necrotic bowel and peritonitis. Plain radiographs demonstrate obstructive features, and contrast studies may be needed to define the cause of obstruction.

Patients with suspected obstruction should have nasogastric decompression, intravenous fluid resuscitation, and broad-spectrum antibiotics in anticipation of surgery. Nonoperative intervention is contraindicated unless a patient is stable with clear evidence of clinical improvement.

314.3 Intussusception

Intussusception occurs when a portion of the alimentary tract is telescoped into an adjacent segment. It is the most common cause of intestinal obstruction between 3 mo and 6 yr of age. Sixty per cent of patients are younger than 1 yr, and 80% of the cases occur before 24 mo; it is rare in neonates. The incidence varies from 1–4 in 1,000 live births. The male:female ratio is 4:1. A few intussusceptions reduce spontaneously, but if left untreated, most will lead to peritonitis, perforation, and death.

Etiology and Epidemiology. The cause of most intussusceptions is unknown. The seasonal incidence has peaks in spring and autumn. Correlation with adenovirus infections has been noted, and the condition may complicate otitis media, gastroenteritis, Henoch-Schönlein purpura, or upper respiratory tract infections. The risk of intussusception in infants 1 yr of age or younger after receiving the tetravalent rhesus-human reassortant rotavirus vaccine within 2 wk of immunization is substantially increased (odds ratio: 21:7). The risk is much greater after the first dose of the vaccine compared with the risk after the second dose. The Advisory Committee on Immunization Practices no longer recommends this vaccine. Although wild-type human rotavirus produces an enterotoxin, it is rarely detected in cases of spontaneous intussusception.

It is postulated that gastrointestinal infection or the introduction of new food proteins results in swollen Peyer patches in the terminal ileum. The prominent mounds of tissue lead to mucosal prolapse of the ileum into the colon, thus causing an intussusception. In 2–8% of patients, recognizable lead points for the intussusception are found, such as a Meckel diverticulum, intestinal polyp, neurofibroma, intestinal duplication, hemangioma, or malignant conditions such as lymphoma. Intussusception may complicate mucosal hemorrhage as in Henoch-Schönlein purpura or hemophilia. Cystic fibrosis is another risk factor. Postoperative intussusception is ileoileal and usually occurs within 5 days of an abdominal operation. Lead points are more common in children older than 2 yr of age. Intrauterine intussusception is associated with the development of intestinal atresia.

Pathology. Intussusceptions are most often ileocolic and ileoileocolic, less commonly cecocolic, and rarely exclusively ileal. Very rarely, the appendix forms the apex of an intussusception. The upper portion of bowel, the intussusceptum, invaginates into the lower, the intussuscipiens, dragging its mesentery along with it into the enveloping loop. Constriction of the mesentery obstructs venous return; engorgement of the intussusceptum follows, with edema, and bleeding from the mucosa leads to a bloody stool, sometimes containing mucus. The apex of the intussusception may extend into the transverse, descending, or sigmoid colon, even to and through the anus in neglected cases. This presentation must be distinguished from rectal prolapse. Most intussusceptions do not strangulate the bowel within the first 24 hr but may later eventuate in intestinal gangrene and shock.

Clinical Manifestations. In typical cases there is sudden onset, in a previously well child, of severe paroxysmal colicky pain that recurs at frequent intervals and is accompanied by straining efforts with legs and knees flexed and loud cries. The infant may initially be comfortable and play normally between the paroxysms of pain; but if the intussusception is not reduced, the infant becomes progressively weaker and lethargic. At times, the lethargy is out of proportion to the abdominal signs. Eventually a shocklike state may develop with fever. The pulse becomes weak and thready, the respirations become shallow and grunt-ing, and the pain may be manifested only by moaning sounds. Vomiting occurs in most cases and is usually more frequent early. In the later phase, the vomitus becomes bile stained. Stools of normal appearance may be evacuated during the first few hours of symptoms. After this time, fecal excretions are small or more often do not occur and little or no flatus is passed. Blood generally is passed in the first 12 hr but at times not for 1–2 days and infrequently not at all; 60% of infants pass a stool containing red blood and mucus, the *currant jelly stool.* Some patients have only irritability and alternating or progressive lethargy.

Palpation of the abdomen usually reveals a slightly tender sausage-shaped mass, sometimes ill defined, which may increase in size and firmness during a paroxysm of pain and is most often in the right upper abdomen, with its long axis cephalocaudal. If it is felt in the epigastrium, the long axis is transverse. About 30% of patients do not have a palpable mass. The presence of bloody mucus on the finger as it is withdrawn after rectal examination supports the diagnosis of intussusception. Abdominal distention and tenderness develop as intestinal obstruction becomes more acute. On rare occasions, the advancing intestine prolapses through the anus. This prolapse can be distinguished from prolapse of the rectum by the separation between the protruding intestine and the rectal wall, which does not exist in prolapse of the rectum.

Ileoileal intussusception may have a less typical clinical picture, the symptoms and signs being chiefly those of small intestinal obstruction. *Recurrent intussusception* is noted in 5–8% and is more common after hydrostatic than surgical reduction. *Chronic intussusception,* in which the symptoms exist in milder form at recurrent intervals, is more likely to occur with or after acute enteritis and may arise in older children as well as in infants.

Diagnosis. The clinical history and physical findings are usually sufficiently typical for diagnosis. Plain abdominal radiographs may show a density in the area of the intussusception. A barium enema shows a filling defect or cupping in the head of barium where its advance is obstructed by the intussusceptum (Fig. 314–1). A central linear column of barium may be visible in the compressed lumen of the intussusceptum, and a thin rim of barium may be seen trapped around the invaginating intestine in the folds of mucosa within the intussuscipiens (coiled-spring sign), especially after evacuation. Retrogression of the intussusceptum under the pressure of the enema and gaseous distention of the small intestine from obstruction are also useful radiographic signs. Ileoileal intussusception is usually not demonstrable by barium enema but is suspected because of gaseous distention of the intestine above the lesion. The use of "air" enemas in the diagnosis and treatment of intussusception has supplanted hydrostatic reduction. Reflux of air into the terminal ileum and the disappearance of the mass at the ileocecal valve document successful reduction. Air reduction is associated with fewer complications and lower radiation exposure than traditional hydrostatic techniques.

Ultrasonography is a sensitive diagnostic tool in the diagnosis of intussusception. The diagnostic findings of intussusception include a tubular mass in longitudinal views and a doughnut or target appearance in transverse images (Fig. 314–2). Ultrasonography is also useful in demonstrating reduction of the intussusception by hydrostatic or air techniques.

DIFFERENTIAL DIAGNOSIS. It may be particularly difficult to diagnose intussusception in a child who already has *gastroenteritis;* a change in the pattern of illness, in the character of pain, or in the nature of vomiting or the onset of rectal bleeding should alert the physician. The bloody stools and abdominal cramps that accompany *enterocolitis* can usually be differentiated from intussusception because the pain is less severe and less

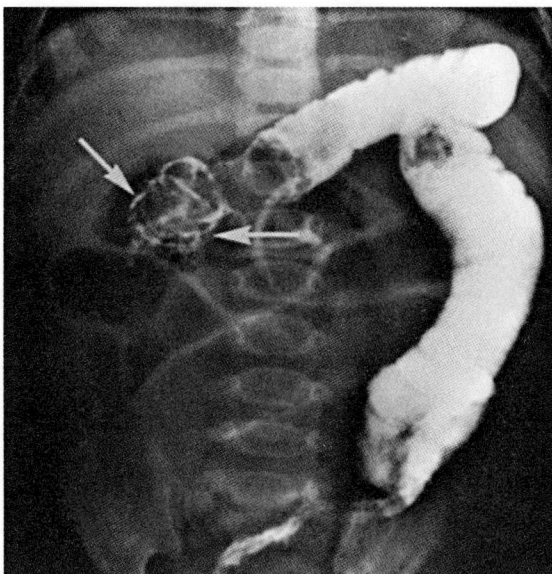

FIGURE 314–1. Intussusception in an infant. The obstruction is evident in the proximal transverse colon. Contrast material between the intussusceptum and the intussuscipiens is responsible for the coil-spring appearance.

regular, there is diarrhea, and the infant is recognizably ill between pains. Bleeding from *Meckel diverticulum* is usually painless. Joint symptoms or purpura usually but not invariably accompanies the intestinal hemorrhage of Henoch-Schönlein purpura. Because intussusception may be a complication of this disorder, ultrasonography may be needed to distinguish the conditions.

Treatment. Reduction of an acute intussusception is an emergency procedure and performed immediately after diagnosis in preparation for possible surgery. In patients with prolonged

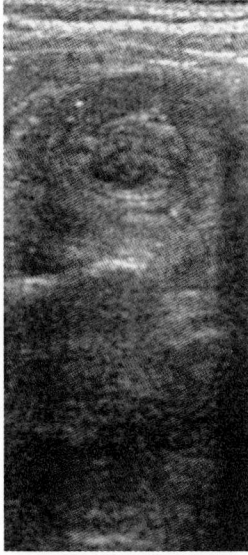

FIGURE 314–2. Transverse image of an ileocolic intussusception. Note the loops within the loops of bowel.

intussusception with signs of shock, peritoneal irritation, intestinal perforation, or pneumatosis intestinalis, reduction should not be attempted.

The success rate of radiologic reduction under fluoroscopic or ultrasonic guidance is approximately 50% if symptoms are present longer than 48 hr and 70–90% if reduction is done within the first 48 hr. Bowel perforations occur in 0.5–2.5% of attempted barium and hydrostatic (saline) reductions. The perforation rate with air reduction ranges from 0.1–0.2%.

An ileoileal intussusception is best demonstrated by abdominal ultrasonography. Reduction by instillation of barium, saline, or air may not be possible. Such intussusceptions may develop insidiously after bowel surgery and require reoperation if they do not spontaneously reduce. If manual operative reduction is impossible or the bowel is not viable, resection of the intussusception is necessary, with end-to-end anastomosis.

Prognosis. Untreated intussusception in infants is almost always fatal; the chances of recovery are directly related to the duration of intussusception before reduction. Most infants recover if the intussusception is reduced within the first 24 hr, but the mortality rate rises rapidly after this time, especially after the 2nd day. Spontaneous reduction during preparation for operation is not uncommon.

The recurrence rate after barium enema reduction of intussusceptions is about 10%, and after surgical reduction it is 2–5%; none has recurred after surgical resection. The administration of dexamethasone has been reported to reduce the frequency of recurrent intussusception. Recurrent intussusception can usually be reduced radiologically. It is unlikely that an intussusception caused by a lesion such as lymphosarcoma, polyp, or Meckel diverticulum will be successfully reduced by radiologic intervention. With adequate surgical management, operative reduction carries a very low mortality rate in early cases.

314.4 Closed-Loop Obstructions

Intestinal obstruction may be caused by defects in the mesentery ("internal hernias") through which loops of small bowel may pass and become trapped. Vascular engorgement of the trapped bowel results in intestinal ischemia and gangrene unless promptly relieved. Symptoms include bilious vomiting, abdominal distention, and abdominal pain. Peritoneal signs suggest ischemic bowel. Plain radiographs demonstrate signs of small bowel obstruction or free air if the bowel has perforated. Supportive management includes intravenous fluids, antibiotics, and nasogastric decompression. Prompt surgical relief of the obstruction is indicated if intestinal gangrene is to be prevented. Symptoms can occasionally be transient or recurrent if the herniated bowel slides out of the mesenteric defect, spontaneously relieving the obstruction.

de Vries S, Sleeboom C, Aronson DC: Postoperative intussusception in children. *Br J Surg* 1999;86:81–83.

Hadidi AT, El Shal N: Childhood intussusception: A comparative study of nonsurgical management. *J Pediatr Surg* 1999;34:304–7.

Lin SL, Kong MS, Houng DS: Decreasing early recurrence rate of acute intussusception by the use of dexamethasone. *Eur J Pediatr* 2000;159: 551–52.

Murphy TV, Gargiullo PM, Massoudi MS, et al: Intussusception among infants given an oral rotavirus vaccine. *N Engl J Med* 2001;344:564–72.

Navarro O, Dugougeat F, Kornecki A, et al: The impact of imaging in the management of intussusception owing to pathologic lead points in children: A review of 43 cases. *Pediatr Radiol* 2000;30:594–603.

Taguchi A, Sharma N, Saleem RM, et al: Selective postoperative inhibition of gastrointestinal opioid receptors. *N Engl J Med* 2001;345:935–40.

Weber P, Von Lengerke HJ, Oleszczuk-Rascke K, et al: Internal abdominal hernias in childhood. *J Pediatr Gastroenterol Nutr* 1997;25:358–62.

Yoon CH, Kim HJ, Goo HW: Intussusception in children: US-guided pneumatic reduction—initial experience. *Radiology* 2001;218:85–88.

Chapter 315
Foreign Bodies and Bezoars

Robert Wyllie

315.1   Foreign Bodies in the Stomach and Intestine

Eighty percent of all foreign body ingestions occur in children, with a peak incidence between the ages of 6 mo and 3 yr. Coins are the most common foreign body ingested by young children. In older children, teenagers, and adults, fish or chicken bones are the most common objects accidentally ingested. The risk of ingestion increases after alcohol consumption or cold liquids because of a decrease in oral sensory acuity. Repeat ingestion may occur in young children and psychiatrically impaired patients. Of the foreign bodies that come to medical attention, 80–90% pass through the gastrointestinal tract without difficulty. Ten to 20% require endoscopic removal or other conservative management, whereas 1% or less require surgical intervention. Once in the stomach, 95% of all ingested objects pass without difficulty through the remainder of the gastrointestinal tract. Perforation after ingestion of a foreign body is estimated to be less than 1% of all objects ingested. Perforation tends to occur in areas of physiologic sphincters (pylorus and ileocecal valve), acute angulation (such as the duodenal sweep), congenital gut malformations (webs, diaphragms, or diverticula), or areas of previous bowel surgery.

Patients with nonfood foreign bodies often describe a history of ingestion. Young children may have a witness to ingestion. Approximately 90% of foreign bodies are opaque. Radiologic examination is routinely performed to determine the type, number, and location of the suspected objects. Contrast radiographs may be necessary to demonstrate some objects such as plastic parts or toys.

Conservative management is indicated in most foreign bodies that have passed through the esophagus and entered the stomach. Most objects pass though the intestine in 4–6 days, although some may take as long as 3–4 wk. While waiting for the object to pass, parents are instructed to continue a regular diet and to observe the stools for the appearance of the ingested object. Cathartics should be avoided. Exceptionally long or sharp objects are usually monitored radiologically. Parents or patients should be instructed to report abdominal pain, vomiting, persistent fever, and hematemesis or melena immediately to their physician. Failure of the object to progress over a 3- to 4-wk period seldom implies an impeding perforation but may be associated with a congenital malformation or acquired bowel abnormality.

In older children and adults, oval objects greater than 5 cm in diameter or 2 cm in thickness tend to lodge in the stomach and should be endoscopically retrieved. Thin objects greater than 10 cm in length fail to negotiate the duodenal sweep and should also be removed. In infants and toddlers, objects longer than 3 cm or larger than 20 mm in diameter usually do not pass through the pylorus and should be removed. Open safety pins should also be endoscopically retrieved, but other sharp objects can be managed conservatively. Drugs (aggregated iron pills, cocaine packing) may need to be surgically removed; initial management may include oral polyethylene glycol lavage.

Children occasionally place objects in their rectum. Small, blunt objects usually pass spontaneously, but large or sharp objects usually need to be retrieved. Adequate sedation is essential to relax the anal sphincter before attempted endoscopic or speculum removal. If the object is proximal to the rectum,

observation for 12–24 hr usually allows the object to descend into the rectum.

315.2   Bezoars

A bezoar is an accumulation of exogenous matter in the stomach or intestine. Most bezoars have been found in females with underlying personality problems or in neurologically impaired individuals. Patients who have undergone abdominal surgery are at higher risk for the development of bezoars. The peak age at onset of symptoms is the second decade of life. Bezoars are classified on the basis of their composition. Trichobezoars are composed of the patient's own hair, and phytobezoars are composed of a combination of plant and animal material. Lactobezoars were previously found most often in premature infants and may be attributed to the high casein or calcium content of some premature formulas. Swallowed chewing gum may occasionally lead to a bezoar.

Trichobezoars can become large and form casts of the stomach; they may enter into the proximal duodenum. They present as symptoms of gastric outlet or partial intestinal obstruction including vomiting, anorexia, and weight loss. Patients may complain of abdominal pain, distention, and severe halitosis. Physical examination may demonstrate patchy baldness and a firm mass in the left upper quadrant. Patients may occasionally have iron-deficiency anemia, hypoproteinemia, or steatorrhea caused by an associated chronic gastritis. Phytobezoars present in a similar manner.

An abdominal plain film may suggest the presence of a bezoar, which can be confirmed on ultrasound or CT examination. Bezoars in the stomach can usually be removed endoscopically. If endoscopy is unsuccessful, surgical intervention may be needed. Lactobezoars usually resolve when feedings are withheld for 24–48 hr.

Efrati Y, Freud E, Serour F, et al: Phytobezoar-induced ileal and colonic obstruction in childhood. *J Pediatr Gastroenterol Nutr* 1997;25:214–16.

Karjoo M: Caustic ingestion and foreign bodies in the gastrointestinal system. *Curr Opin Pediatr* 1998;10:516–22.

Kim JK, Kim SS, Kim JI, et al: Management of foreign bodies in the gastrointestinal tract: An analysis of 104 cases in children. *Endoscopy* 1999;31:302–4.

Milov DE, Andres JM, Erhart NA, et al: Chewing gum bezoars of the gastrointestinal tract. *Pediatrics* 1998;102:e22.

Ripolles T, Garcia-Aguayo J, Martinez MJ, et al: Gastrointestinal bezoars: Sonographic and CT characteristics. *AJR Am J Roentgenol* 2001;177:65–69.

Stack LB, Munter DW: Foreign bodies in the gastrointestinal tract. *Emerg Med Clin North Am* 1996;14:493–521.

Chapter 316
Peptic Ulcer Disease

Francisco A. Sylvester

Ulcers are deep lesions that breech the integrity of the epithelium and penetrate through the muscularis mucosae, whereas *erosions* are superficial and stop short of the muscularis propria. Both lesions often occur in the presence of gastric inflammation or *gastritis*.

Gastric and duodenal ulcers occur infrequently in children; the precise prevalence is unknown. Gastritis and ulcers of the duodenum or stomach can be classified either as primary or secondary. This classification is arbitrary and predates the knowledge of the association between *Helicobacter pylori* infection and duodenal and gastric ulcers.

The majority of children with active gastritis and ulcers in the stomach or duodenum will have an associated systemic condition, such as overwhelming sepsis, severe head or body trauma, or burns, or be on medications such as nonsteroidal anti-inflammatory drugs. Other conditions associated with upper gastrointestinal inflammation include inflammatory bowel disease (particularly Crohn disease), eosinophilic gastroenteritis, allergic enteropathy, hypertrophic gastritis (Ménétrier disease), autoimmune gastritis, varioliform (lymphocytic) gastritis, and Zollinger-Ellison syndrome. In addition, although uncommon, secondary ulcers have been reported as sequelae to hepatic disease, cystic fibrosis, and sickle cell anemia.

Children who do not have any obvious systemic disease who present with gastritis and/or ulcers are said to have "primary" gastroduodenal inflammation. In most of these patients, the inflammation is caused by *Helicobacter pylori*. *H. pylori* is a gram-negative spiral organism with polar flagellae that lives primarily in the mucus layer covering gastric epithelial cells. A portion of the bacterial population attaches to gastric epithelial cells via specific adhesins. To survive in the harsh environment of the acidic stomach, *H. pylori* produces urease, an enzyme that catalyzes the conversion of urea in the gastric juice to ammonia and bicarbonate. These products buffer the gastric acid and create a friendly microenvironment for *H. pylori*. This property is the basis for several diagnostic tests, such as rapid urease tests and the urea breath test (see later). Humans appear to be the primary natural reservoir of *H. pylori* infection. There is no known animal or insect reservoir of *H. pylori*. *Helicobacter* species are present in many animals. Humans occasionally can become infected with *Helicobacter* species harbored in domestic animals (e.g., *H. heilmanii*).

In most individuals, *H. pylori* is acquired early in life (before 5 yr). Although the precise mechanism of transmission is not yet known, person-to-person contagion in close contacts and family members is strongly suspected. The route of transmission may involve fecal-oral, gastric-oral (in vomitus), or oral-oral routes. Crowding and poor sanitary conditions are risk factors for acquisition of *H. pylori*. *H. pylori* infection is more common in Third World countries, where over 90% of adults may be infected. In North America, it is estimated that about one third of the adult population is infected; the prevalence of infection may be decreasing.

Based on epidemiologic and animal studies, colonization with *H. pylori* may predispose to the development of gastric adenocarcinoma and mucosal associated lymphoid tissue (MALT) lymphoma, particularly when the infection is acquired early in life. It is likely that other factors (e.g., high-salt diet, diet with low consumption of fresh fruits and vegetables, and other environmental factors) need to occur concurrently for cancer to evolve. Studies showing that *H. pylori* eradication during childhood prevents subsequent development of gastric malignancies have yet to be performed.

Although colonization with *H. pylori* leads to a vigorous immune response in the stomach, once acquired the infection tends to be permanent, unless it is treated with antibiotics. In the vast majority of individuals, *H. pylori* infection is silent, even in the presence of chronic active gastritis. Serologic surveys, endoscopic evaluations, and treatment trials conducted in adults with dyspepsia (pain or discomfort in the upper abdomen) suggest that in the absence of a peptic ulcer *H. pylori* probably does not cause abdominal pain. Studies in children also have questioned the role of *H. pylori* as a cause of abdominal pain in the absence of peptic ulceration. Guidelines by the North American Society for Pediatric Gastroenterology, Hepatology, and Nutrition (NASPGHAN) suggest that the goal of diagnostic testing in children with abdominal pain should be to determine the cause of presenting symptoms rather than the presence of *H. pylori* infection.

Pathogenesis. The pathogenesis of peptic ulcer disease is incompletely understood. Ulceration occurs when aggressive factors (e.g., gastric acid, digestive enzymes, *H. pylori* bacterial products) overwhelm the natural barriers that protect the gastroduodenal lining (bicarbonate-mucus barrier, gastric epithelial cells, mucosal blood flow, prostaglandins). Patients with duodenal ulceration may have increased acid secretion, whereas patients with gastric ulcers may have reduced acid output. Drugs such as nonsteroidal anti-inflammatory agents inhibit protective prostaglandin synthesis and reduce the mucosal production of bicarbonate. *H. pylori* colonization leads to a blunted response of duodenal bicarbonate secretion in response to intraluminal acidification in adults. Also, the ability of mucins (mucus glycoprotein) to normally polymerize may be altered in patients with duodenal ulcers. Patients who develop ulcers may be genetically predisposed; increased levels of pepsinogen I are seen in children with duodenal ulcers and their parents. Peptic ulcer disease may be present in either parent of an affected child.

Clinical Manifestations. The classic symptom of peptic ulceration, epigastric pain alleviated by the ingestion of food, is present only in a minority of children. Most pediatric patients will present with poorly localized abdominal pain, which may be periumbilical. However, the vast majority of patients with periumbilical or epigastric pain or discomfort will not have a peptic ulcer but rather a functional gastrointestinal disorder, such as irritable bowel syndrome or functional dyspepsia, respectively. Patients with peptic ulceration rarely present with acute abdominal pain from perforation or symptoms and signs of pancreatitis from a penetrating ulcer. Patients can also present with gastrointestinal bleeding, with hematemesis and/or melena. Occasionally, bright red blood per rectum may be seen if the rate of bleeding is brisk and the intestinal transit time is short. Vomiting may be a sign of gastric outlet obstruction.

In the 1st mo of life, the two main manifestations are gastrointestinal hemorrhage and perforation. Between the neonatal period and 2 yr of age, recurrent vomiting, slow growth, and gastrointestinal hemorrhage are the major symptoms. In preschool-aged children, periumbilical postprandial pain is often elicited whereas vomiting and hemorrhage remain common. After 6 yr of age, the clinical features of ulcer disease are similar to those in adults and commonly include epigastric abdominal pain, acute or chronic gastrointestinal blood loss (hematemesis, hematochezia, or melena) often leading to iron-deficiency anemia, predominantly male gender, and a strong family history of ulcer disease. The pain is often described as dull or aching rather than sharp or burning, as in adults. It may last from minutes to hours, and patients have frequent exacerbations and remissions lasting from weeks to months. Nocturnal pain is common. A history of typical ulcer pain with prompt relief after taking antacids is found in fewer than 33% of patients. Rarely, in patients with acute or chronic blood loss, penetration of the ulcer into the abdominal cavity or adjacent organs produces shock, anemia, peritonitis, or pancreatitis. If inflammation and edema are extensive, acute or chronic gastric obstruction may occur.

Diagnosis. Endoscopy is the method of choice to diagnose peptic ulcer disease in children. It provides an opportunity to examine the upper gastrointestinal tract for the presence of inflammation, erosion, and ulceration and to take biopsy samples for microscopic examination and other tests. Endoscopy can also be used therapeutically. Endoscopic accessories can be used to clip, ligate, cauterize, or resect bleeding tissues. An experienced therapeutic endoscopist is required to perform these procedures. The disadvantages of endoscopy include cost and the need for sedation or anesthesia.

Contrast radiography is of limited value in the diagnosis of peptic ulcers in children, with both false-positive and false-negative findings. These studies are helpful, however, in determining the anatomy of the upper gastrointestinal tract.

There are several invasive and noninvasive tests available to detect *H. pylori* infection. Testing for *H. pylori* is recommended only when there is a documented duodenal or gastric ulcer and when there is MALT lymphoma. There are no convincing data to support routine testing of children with recurrent abdominal pain or children who are asymptomatic. The accuracy of a specific diagnostic test is greatly impacted by the prevalence of *H. pylori* in the community. In areas of low prevalence, such as North America, endoscopy is the most reliable test to establish not only the presence of infection but also its consequences in children. Endoscopy frequently shows antral micronodules that represent lymphoid follicles in *H. pylori*–infected children. To confirm the presence of infection, biopsy specimens should be obtained from the antrum, the body, and the transition zones of the stomach. This is especially important in patients who have been on antacid therapy, because *H. pylori* will migrate proximally, away from the antrum in such patients. Tissue samples can then be stained to detect *H. pylori* and to examine the severity and chronicity of the gastritis. Rapid urease tests can be performed in biopsy samples. In this test, biopsy specimens are placed in a well containing agar with a pH-sensitive dye. Presence of urease-producing organisms in the sample is signaled by a color change. Specimens can also be cultured in microaerophilic conditions to establish patterns of antibiotic sensitivity, especially in patients in whom treatment has failed to eradicate the bacteria. *H. pylori* is a fastidious organism, and cultures are best performed by a skilled microbiologist. Noninvasive tests include *H. pylori* antibody detection in serum, whole blood, urine, or saliva and antigen detection in stool. These tests have low sensitivity and specificity in low prevalence areas, especially in children. Treatment based on the results of these tests cannot be recommended. Most of these tests do not distinguish between past and present infection and therefore are not reliable to document eradication. The urea breath test (UBT) is another noninvasive method in which urea labeled with an isotope of carbon (either ^{14}C or ^{13}C) is ingested by the patient. Samples of exhaled air are then collected to detect the presence of labeled carbon dioxide released from the breakdown of urea in the stomach. The UBT is highly sensitive and specific, but the methodology has not yet been standardized for children. This test requires a cooperative child to provide adequate samples of exhaled air and thus is generally not suitable for very young patients. Concerns about exposure to radioactivity in growing individuals dictate that the test be performed with a nonradioactive isotope of carbon, such as ^{13}C. The methodology to analyze samples containing ^{13}C is not widely available, and detection can be expensive. Samples may need to be sent promptly to a reference laboratory. Prior antibiotic exposure and treatment with proton-pump inhibitors and other antacids can influence the test. A promising modality is the detection of *H. pylori* antigens in stool. This test is both sensitive and specific in children. Potential disadvantages include the need for a fresh stool specimen, reluctance of some patients to collect a stool sample, and prolonged shedding of *H. pylori* antigens for several weeks, even after successful eradication.

Treatment. Treatment should be offered to patients with *H. pylori* who have ulcers (both duodenal and gastric) and have a history of ulcers, MALT lymphoma, and atrophic gastritis with intestinal metaplasia. In the absence of compelling data, the decision to treat the patient with gastritis but without ulcer rests with the clinician and the informed patient. The potential benefits of eradication have to be weighed against the side effects of therapy, its cost, and the emergence of resistant strains. Several treatment regimens are available to treat *H. pylori* infection. They consist of at least two antibiotics and a potent antacid (Table 316–1) given for 1–2 wk and result in eradication rates of more than 80% in adults.

316.1 Secondary or Stress (Peptic) Ulcer Disease

The underlying causes of secondary peptic ulcer disease are not fully understood; multiple factors that interfere with host defense mechanisms are involved. Mucosal blood flow is thought to be important in acute stress ulcers; other factors include mucus production, prostaglandin synthesis, acid production, and cell proliferation.

Clinical Manifestations. In infants, stress ulcers are usually caused by sepsis, respiratory or cardiac insufficiency, trauma, or

TABLE 316–1. Recommended Eradication Therapies for *H. pylori* Disease in Children

Medications	Dosage
First-Line Options	
Amoxicillin	50 mg/kg/day up to 1 g bid
Clarithromycin	15 mg/kg/day up to 500 mg bid
Proton pump inhibitor: omeprazole (or comparable acid inhibitory doses of another PPI)	1 mg/kg/day up to 20 mg bid
Amoxicillin	50 mg/kg/day up to 1 g bid
Metronidazole	20 mg/kg/day up to 500 mg bid
Proton pump inhibitor: omeprazole (or comparable acid inhibitory doses of another PPI)	1 mg/kg/day up to 20 mg bid
Clarithromycin	15 mg/kg/day up to 500 mg bid
Metronidazole	20 mg/kg/day up to 500 mg bid
Proton pump inhibitor: omeprazole (or comparable acid inhibitory doses of another PPI)	1 mg/kg/day up to 20 mg bid
Second-Line Options	
Bismuth subsalicylate	1 tablet (262 mg) qid *or* 15 mL (17.6 mg/mL qid)
Metronidazole	20 mg/kg/day up to 500 mg bid
Proton pump inhibitor: omeprazole (or comparable acid inhibitory doses of another PPI) *plus* an additional antibiotic:	1 mg/kg/day up to 20 mg bid
Amoxicillin	50 mg/kg/day up to 1 g bid
or Tetracycline	50 mg/kg/day up to 1 g bid
or Clarithromycin	15 mg/kg/day up to 500 mg bid
Ranitidine bismuth-citrate	1 tablet qid
Clarithromycin	15 mg/kg/day up to 500 mg bid
Metronidazole	20 mg/kg/day up to 500 mg bid

From Gold BD, et al: Medical position statement: The North American Society for Pediatric Gastroenterology and Nutrition. Helicobacter pylori infection in children: Recommendations for diagnosis and treatment. J Pediatr Gastroenterol Nutr 2000;31:490–97.

dehydration. In older children, they are related to trauma or other life-threatening conditions. Stress ulcers and erosions associated with burns are also known as *Curling ulcers*. They are associated with normal gastric secretions and are common in patients with more than 25% body burns. *Cushing ulcers* follow head trauma or surgery and are associated with gastric hypersecretion. Most stress ulcers are asymptomatic, are often multiple, and may be terminal events. They can be associated with severe hemorrhage or perforation. Coagulopathy, hypotension, and need for mechanical respiration are important risk factors for overt clinically important gastrointestinal bleeding. Perforation and, more often, massive hemorrhage are often the initial symptoms.

Drug-Related Peptic Disease. Nonsteroidal anti-inflammatory drugs, including aspirin, are common causes of gastritis and erosions. These drugs are thought to damage the mucosa by inhibiting prostaglandin synthesis, thereby inhibiting cell proliferation as well as mucosal bicarbonate and mucus secretion. Cyclooxygenase-2–specific inhibitors have a lower incidence of gastric ulceration.

Alcohol and smoking are known to affect gastroduodenal mucosa adversely. Although results of studies are conflicting, a meta-analysis of available studies indicates a statistical association between corticosteroid use and ulcer disease in children. An inhibitory effect on local production of mucus and prostaglandin is postulated. Other agents that may rarely cause gastritis include iron, calcium salts, potassium chloride, and antibiotics, including chloramphenicol, penicillins, tetracyclines, and cephalosporins.

Treatment. Treatment of secondary ulcers is similar to that of primary ulcers. The inciting cause should be removed if possible. Bleeding and, less often, perforation are common presentations and must be addressed immediately. Maintaining gastric pH at more than 3.5 in critically ill patients helps to prevent ulcer formation. Control of gastric acidity is a cornerstone of continuing therapy and should continue for 6 wk if the patient has active disease.

Antacids have been used to neutralize acid once it is secreted. The buffering ability of antacids varies, as do recommendations for their use. The aim is to increase the pH to more than 5. The full adult dose of the concentrated liquids is 15 mL per dose. The optimal pediatric dose of antacids is controversial and varies with acid secretion and the buffering capacity of the antacid. Doses of as much as 1 mL/kg/dose have been recommended. Most antacids are mixtures of magnesium and aluminum salts. The magnesium ion causes diarrhea, whereas the aluminum salts may cause constipation. Aluminum hydroxide binds with dietary phosphates and interferes with their absorption. If large doses of aluminum hydroxide are used over a period of time, complications of phosphate depletion and aluminum toxicity including anorexia, osteomalacia, and osteoporosis may occur. Patients with renal disease are especially prone to aluminum toxicity. Calcium antacids can cause increased acid secretion after the buffering effect has stopped.

Histamine (H_2)-receptor blockers that suppress acid secretion are widely used even though they are not approved for children. Cimetidine (20–40 mg/kg/24 hr in four doses) and ranitidine (4–6 mg/kg/24 hr in two doses) are the most frequently used liquid preparations. They are rapidly absorbed and may be taken with meals. They can also be administered intravenously or added to parenteral nutrition solutions.

Hydrogen pump inhibitors (e.g., omeprazole and lansoprazole) are the most potent inhibitors of gastric acid secretion and have raised concerns about achlorhydria-related bacterial overgrowth. In adults, healing of ulcers occurs with 4 wk of therapy; hydrogen pump inhibitors are a component of several schemes to eradicate *H. pylori*.

Sucralfate forms a white pastelike substance in an acid environment that adheres to inflamed mucosa and ulcers. Experience in children is limited. The adult dose is 10 mL (1 g) of the suspension four times a day on an empty stomach.

Misoprostol, a prostaglandin analogue, has been shown in adults to be effective in preventing and treating ulcers associated with the use of nonsteroidal anti-inflammatory drugs. Its use is limited by gastrointestinal side effects (abdominal pain, diarrhea). Studies in adults indicate that omeprazole is superior in treating erosions and ulcers associated with the use of nonsteroidal anti-inflammatory drugs. Octreotide reduces splanchnic blood flow and may stop active bleeding. Endoscopy can be used therapeutically to control bleeding not responding to medical therapy.

316.2 Zollinger-Ellison Syndrome

This rare syndrome can cause multiple recurrent duodenal and jejunal ulcers and is occasionally associated with diarrhea. Gastric secretion is markedly stimulated by serum gastrin and other hormones secreted by an islet cell tumor or hypertrophy. Hypergastrinemia, albeit lower than Zollinger-Ellison syndrome, may be noted in pyloric stenosis, short bowel syndrome, hyperparathyroidism, pheochromocytoma, and multiple endocrine neoplasia. Therapy with H_2-receptor blockers or omeprazole can control gastric acid secretion and can improve symptoms when these slow-growing tumors cannot be entirely removed.

Blaser MJ: *Helicobacter pylori* and gastric diseases. *BMJ* 1998;316:1507.

Bode G, Rothenbacher D, Brenner H, et al: *Helicobacter pylori* and abdominal symptoms: A population-based study among preschool children in southern Germany. *Pediatrics* 1998;101:634.

Braden B, Posselt HG, Ahrens P, et al: New immunoassay in stool provides an accurate noninvasive diagnostic method for *Helicobacter pylori* screening in children. *Pediatrics* 200;106:115.

Brown LM: *Helicobacter pylori*: Epidemiology and routes of transmission. *Epidemiol Rev* 2000;22:283.

Cook D, Guyatt G, Marshall J, et al: A comparison of sucralfate and ranitidine for the prevention of upper gastrointestinal bleeding in patients requiring mechanical ventilation. *N Engl J Med* 1998;338:791.

Dohil R, Hassall E, Jevon G, Dimmick J: Gastritis and gastropathy of childhood. *J Pediatr Gastroenterol Nutr* 1999;29:378.

Gold BD, Colletti RB, Abbott M, et al: The North American Society for Pediatric Gastroenterology and Nutrition. *Helicobacter pylori* infection in children: Recommendations for diagnosis and treatment. *J Pediatr Gastroenterol Nutr* 2000;31:490.

Hassall E: Peptic ulcer disease and current approaches to *Helicobacter pylori*. *J Pediatr* 2001;138:462.

Hawkey CJ, Karrasch JA, Szczepanski L, et al: Omeprazole compared with misoprostol for ulcers associated with nonsteroidal anti-inflammatory drugs. *N Engl J Med* 1998;338:727.

Imrie C, Rowland M, Bourke B, Drumm B: Is *Helicobacter pylori* infection in childhood a risk factor for gastric cancer? *Pediatrics* 2001;107:373.

Moshkowitz M, Reif S, Brill S, et al: One-week triple therapy with omeprazole, clarithromycin, and nitroimidazole for *Helicobacter pylori* infection in children and adolescents. *Pediatrics* 1998;102:64. http:www.pediatrics.org/cgi/ content/ full/10211/e14.

Rauws BAJ, van der Hulst RWM: The management of *H. pylori* infection. *BMJ* 1998;316:162.

Rowland M, Lambert L, Gormally S, et al: Carbon 13–labeled urea breath test for the diagnosis of *Helicobacter pylori* infection in children. *J Pediatr* 1997;131:815.

Silverstein FE, Faich G, Goldstein JL, et al: Gastrointestinal toxicity with celecoxib vs nonsteroidal anti-inflammatory drugs for osteoarthritis and rheumatoid arthritis. *JAMA* 2000;284:1247.

Stringer, Veysi VT, Puntis JW, et al: Gastroduodenal ulcers in the *Helicobacter pylori* era. *Acta Paediatr* 2000;89:1181.

Tobin JM, Sinha B, Ramani P, et al: Upper gastrointestinal mucosal disease in pediatric Crohn disease and ulcerative colitis: A blinded, controlled study. *J Pediatr Gastroenterol Nutr* 2001;32:443.

Torres J, Perez-Perez G, Goodman KJ, et al: A comprehensive review of the natural history of *Helicobacter pylori* infection in children. *Arch Med Res* 2000;31:431.

Yanez P, la Garza AM, Perez-Perez G, et al: Comparison of invasive and noninvasive methods for the diagnosis and evaluation of eradication of *Helicobacter pylori* infection in children. *Arch Med Res* 2001;31:415.

Yeomans ND, Tulassay Z, Juhasz L, et al: A comparison of omeprazole with ranitidine for ulcers associated with nonsteroidal anti-inflammatory drugs. *N Engl J Med* 1998;338:719.

Chapter 317

Inflammatory Bowel Disease *Jeffrey Hyams*

The term *inflammatory bowel disease* (IBD) is used to represent two distinctive disorders of idiopathic chronic intestinal inflammation: Crohn disease and ulcerative colitis. Their respective etiologies are poorly understood, and both disorders are characterized by unpredictable exacerbations and remissions. The most common time of onset of IBD is during adolescence and young adulthood. A bimodal distribution has been shown with an early onset at 15–25 yr of age and a second smaller peak at 50–80 yr of age. Nonetheless, IBD may begin as early as the 1st yr of life. IBD is more common in urban areas than in rural areas. In developed countries, these disorders are the major causes of chronic intestinal inflammation in children beyond the 1st few yr of life.

Both *genetic and environmental influences* are involved in the pathogenesis of IBD. The incidence among Jews is high but varies geographically. Although incidence rates are low among blacks in Africa, in the United States they are similar to those of whites. The prevalence of Crohn disease in the United States is much lower for Hispanics and Asians than for whites and blacks. The risk of IBD in family members of an affected individual has been reported in the range of 7–22%; a child whose parents both have IBD has a greater than 35% chance of acquiring the disorder. Relatives of an individual with ulcerative colitis have a greater risk of acquiring ulcerative colitis than Crohn disease, whereas relatives of an individual with Crohn disease have a greater risk of acquiring this disorder; the two diseases may occur in the same family. The risk of occurrence of IBD among relatives of individuals with Crohn disease is somewhat greater than for individuals with ulcerative colitis. Within a family, Crohn disease may demonstrate anticipation, developing at an earlier age among the 2nd generation.

The importance of genetic factors in the development of IBD is noted by a higher chance that both twins will be affected if they are monozygotic rather than dizygotic. The concordance rate in twins is higher in Crohn disease than in ulcerative colitis. Genetic disorders that have been associated with IBD include Turner syndrome, the Hermansky-Pudlak syndrome, glycogen storage disease type Ib, and various immunodeficiency disorders. It has been suggested that the susceptibility loci for Crohn disease may exist on chromosomes 5 and 16. A possible gene on chromosome 6, *NOD2* (also called *CARD15*—capase activation and recruitment domain), is expressed in macrophages and may be involved in bacterial lipopolysaccharide–host interactions. *NOD2*-positive patients that have homozygous mutations have a 20-fold risk of Crohn disease. Only 20% of patients are homozygous for *NOD2* variants. A perinuclear antineutrophil antibody (pANCA) is found in about 70% of individuals with ulcerative colitis compared with less than 20% of those with Crohn disease and is believed to represent a marker of genetically controlled immunoregulatory disturbance.

Environmental factors are also important and presumably explain discordance among twins and changes in risk among the same race in different geographic regions; the precise factors remain unknown. Individuals migrating to developed countries often appear to acquire the higher rates of IBD associated with these regions. Cigarette smoking is a risk factor for Crohn disease but paradoxically protects against ulcerative colitis. No specific infectious agent has been reproducibly associated with IBD.

An abnormality in intestinal mucosal immunoregulation may be of primary importance in the pathogenesis of IBD. The gut is under constant immunologic stimulation from microbial agents and dietary antigens. In response, the mucosa normally displays "physiologic" inflammation. In IBD, the mechanisms that keep "physiologic" inflammation in check fail and pathologic inflammation ensues. It is not clear if this represents an abnormal response to customary enteric antigens or a normal response to an as yet unidentified microbe. Mediators of inflammation (cytokines, arachidonic acid metabolites, reactive oxygen metabolites, growth factors) are involved, leading to tissue destruction and remodeling with fibrosis. Most therapies are aimed at interfering with these mediators.

It is usually possible to distinguish between ulcerative colitis and Crohn disease by the clinical presentation and radiologic, endoscopic, and histopathologic findings (Table 317–1). It is not possible to make a definitive diagnosis in about 10% of individuals with chronic colitis; this disorder is called *indeterminate colitis*. Occasionally, a child initially believed to have ulcerative colitis on the basis of clinical findings is subsequently diagnosed with Crohn colitis. The treatments of Crohn disease and ulcerative colitis overlap.

Extraintestinal manifestations occur slightly more commonly with Crohn disease than with ulcerative colitis. Growth retardation may be seen in 15–35% of individuals with Crohn disease at diagnosis. Of the extraintestinal manifestations that occur with IBD, joint, skin, eye, mouth, and hepatobiliary involvement tend to be associated with colitis, whether ulcerative or Crohn colitis. For some manifestations, activity correlates with activity of the bowel disease, including peripheral arthritis, erythema nodosum, and anemia. Activity of pyoderma gangrenosum correlates less well with activity of the bowel disease, whereas activities of sclerosing cholangitis, ankylosing spondylitis, and sacroiliitis do not correlate with intestinal disease. Arthritis occurs in three patterns: migratory peripheral arthritis involving primarily large joints, ankylosing spondylitis, and sacroiliitis. The peripheral arthritis of IBD tends to be nondestructive. Ankylosing spondylitis begins in the 3rd decade and occurs most commonly in individuals with ulcerative colitis who have the human leukocyte antigen B27 phenotype.

TABLE 317–1. Comparison of Crohn Disease and Ulcerative Colitis

Feature	Crohn Disease	Ulcerative Colitis
Rectal bleeding	Sometimes	Common
Diarrhea	Variable	Common
Abdominal pain	Common	Variable
Abdominal mass	Common	Not present
Growth failure	Common	Variable
Perianal disease	Common	Unusual
Rectal disease	Occasional	Universal
Pyoderma gangrenosum	Rare	Present
Erythema nodosum	Common	Less common
Mouth ulceration	Common	Rare
Thrombosis	Less common	Present
Colonic disease	50–75%	100%
Ileal disease	Common	None except backwash ileitis
Stomach-esophageal disease	Uncommon	None
Strictures	Common	Unusual
Fissures	Common	None
Fistulas	Common	Unusual
Toxic megacolon	None	Present
Sclerosing cholangitis	Less common	Present
Risk for cancer	Increased	Greatly increased
Discontinuous (skip) lesions	Common	Not present
Transmural involvement	Common	Unusual
Crypt abscesses	Less common	Common
Granulomas	Common	Unusual
Linear ulcerations	Uncommon	Common
Perinuclear antineutrophil cytoplasmic antibodies (pANCA)	Uncommon	Common
Anti-*Saccharomyces cerevisiae* antibodies	Common	Uncommon

Symptoms include low back pain and morning stiffness; back, hips, shoulders, and sacroiliac joints are typically affected. Isolated sacroiliitis is usually asymptomatic but is common when a careful search is performed. Among the skin manifestations, erythema nodosum is most common. Individuals with erythema nodosum or pyoderma gangrenosum have a high likelihood of having arthritis as well. Glomerulonephritis and a hypercoagulable state are other rare manifestations that occur in childhood. Cerebral thromboembolic disease has been described in children with IBD. Uveitis occurs in about 5% of children with IBD and is usually asymptomatic and transient; its occurrence does not correlate with activity of bowel disease.

317.1 Chronic Ulcerative Colitis

Ulcerative colitis, an idiopathic chronic inflammatory disorder, is localized to the colon and spares the upper gastrointestinal tract. Disease usually begins in the rectum and extends proximally for a variable distance. When it is localized to the rectum, the disease is ulcerative proctitis, whereas disease involving the entire colon is pancolitis. The former disorder is less likely to be associated with systemic manifestations, although it may be less responsive to treatment than more diffuse disease. About 30% of children who present with ulcerative proctitis experience proximal spread of the disease. Ulcerative colitis has rarely been noted to present in infancy. Dietary protein intolerance may be easily misdiagnosed as ulcerative colitis in this age group. Dietary protein intolerance (e.g., cow's milk protein) is a transient disorder; symptoms are directly associated with the intake of the offending antigen.

The incidence of ulcerative colitis has remained constant, in contrast to an increase in Crohn disease, but varies with country of origin. Incidence rates are highest in northern European countries and the United States (15/100,000) and lowest in Japan and South Africa (1/100,000). The incidence of ulcerative colitis in Israel varies with the country of origin; those born in Asia or Africa have the lowest risk. The prevalence of ulcerative colitis in northern European countries and the United States varies from 100–200/100,000 population. Men are slightly more likely to acquire ulcerative colitis than are women; the reverse is true for Crohn disease.

Clinical Manifestations. Blood in the stool and diarrhea are the typical presentation of ulcerative colitis. Constipation may be observed in those with proctitis. Symptoms such as tenesmus, urgency, cramping abdominal pain (especially with bowel movements), and nocturnal bowel movements suggest more extensive disease. The mode of onset may range from insidious with gradual progression of symptoms to fulminant. Fever, severe anemia, hypoalbuminemia, leukocytosis, and greater than five bloody stools per day for 5 days is what defines fulminant colitis. Chronicity is an important part of the diagnosis; it is difficult to know whether one is dealing with a subacute, transient infectious colitis or ulcerative colitis when a child has had 1–2 wk of symptoms. Symptoms beyond this duration often prove to be secondary to IBD. Anorexia, weight loss, and growth failure may be present, although these complications are more typical of Crohn disease.

Extraintestinal manifestations that tend to occur more commonly with ulcerative colitis than with Crohn disease include pyoderma gangrenosum, sclerosing cholangitis, chronic active hepatitis, and ankylosing spondylitis. Any of the extraintestinal disorders described previously for IBD may occur with ulcerative colitis. Iron deficiency may result from chronic blood loss as well as decreased intake. Folate deficiency is unusual but may be accentuated in children treated with sulfasalazine, which interferes with folate absorption. Chronic inflammation and the elaboration of a variety of inflammatory cytokines may interfere with erythropoiesis and result in the anemia of chronic disease.

Secondary amenorrhea is common during periods of active disease in older girls.

The clinical course of ulcerative colitis is marked by exacerbations, often without apparent explanation. The disease may be quieted with medication, but eventually it recurs. After initial symptoms, about 5% of children with ulcerative colitis have a prolonged remission (>3 yr). About 25% of children presenting with severe ulcerative colitis will require colectomy within 5 years of diagnosis, compared with only 5% of those presenting with mild disease. It is important to consider the possibility of enteric infection with recurrent symptoms; these infections may mimic a flare-up or actually provoke a recurrence. The use of nonsteroidal anti-inflammatory drugs is considered by some to predispose to exacerbation.

It is generally believed that the risk of colon cancer begins to increase after 8–10 yr of disease and may then increase by 0.5–1% per yr. The risk is delayed by about 10 yr in individuals with colitis limited to the descending colon. Proctitis alone is associated with virtually no increase in risk over the general population. Because colon cancer is usually preceded by changes of mucosal dysplasia, it is recommended that patients who have had ulcerative colitis for more than 10 yr be screened with colonoscopy and biopsy every 1–2 yr. Although this is the current standard of practice it is not clear if morbidity and mortality are changed by this approach. Two competing concerns about this plan of management remain unresolved: (1) the original studies may have overestimated the risk of colon cancer and, therefore, the need for surveillance has been overemphasized and (2) screening for dysplasia may not be adequate for the prevention of colon cancer in ulcerative colitis if some cancers are not preceded by dysplasia.

Differential Diagnosis. The major conditions to exclude are infectious colitis, allergic colitis, and Crohn colitis. Every child with a new diagnosis of ulcerative colitis should have stool cultured for enteric pathogens, stool evaluation for ova and parasites, and perhaps serologic studies for amebae (Table 317–2). In the setting of antibiotic use, pseudomembranous colitis secondary to *Clostridium difficile* should be considered. The most difficult distinction is from Crohn disease because the colitis of Crohn disease may initially appear identical to that of ulcerative colitis. The gross appearance of the colitis or development of small bowel disease eventually leads to the correct diagnosis; this may occur years after the initial presentation.

At the onset, the colitis of hemolytic-uremic syndrome may be identical to that of early ulcerative colitis. Ultimately, signs of microangiopathic hemolysis (the presence of schistocytes on blood smear), thrombocytopenia, and subsequent renal failure should confirm the diagnosis of hemolytic-uremic syndrome. Although Henoch-Schönlein purpura may present as abdominal pain and bloody stools, it is not usually associated with colitis. Behçet syndrome can be distinguished by its typical features (see Chapters 151 and 317.3). Other considerations are radiation proctitis, viral colitis in immunocompromised individuals, and ischemic colitis. In infancy, dietary protein intolerance may be confused with ulcerative colitis, although this disorder is a transient problem that resolves on removal of the offending protein. Hirschsprung disease may produce a colitis before or within months after surgical correction; this is unlikely to be confused with ulcerative colitis.

Diagnosis. The diagnosis of ulcerative colitis or ulcerative proctitis requires a typical presentation in the absence of an identifiable specific cause (Box 317–1; also see Table 317–2) and typical endoscopic and histologic findings (see Table 317–1). One should be hesitant to make a diagnosis of ulcerative colitis in a child who has experienced symptoms for fewer than 2–3 wk until infection has been excluded. When the diagnosis is suspected in a child with subacute symptoms, the physician should make a firm diagnosis only when there is evidence of chronicity

TABLE 317–2. Infectious Agents Mimicking Inflammatory Bowel Disease

Agent	Manifestations	Diagnosis	Comments
Bacterial			
Campylobacter jejuni	Acute diarrhea, fever, fecal blood, and leukocytes	Culture	Common in adolescents, may relapse
Yersinia enterocolitica	Acute→chronic diarrhea, right lower quadrant pain, mesenteric adenitis—pseudoappendicitis, fecal blood, and leukocytes	Culture	Common in adolescents as FUO, weight loss, abdominal pain
	Extraintestinal manifestations, mimics Crohn disease		
Clostridium difficile	Postantibiotic onset, watery → bloody diarrhea, pseudomembrane on sigmoidoscopy	Cytotoxin assay	May be nosocomial Toxic megacolon possible
Escherichia coli 0157:H7	Colitis, fecal blood, abdominal pain	Culture and typing	Hemolytic-uremic syndrome
Salmonella	Watery→bloody diarrhea, food borne, fecal leukocytes, fever, pain, cramps	Culture	Usually acute
Shigella	Watery→bloody diarrhea, fecal leukocytes, fever, pain, cramps	Culture	Dysentery symptoms
Edwardsiella tarda	Bloody diarrhea, cramps	Culture	Ulceration on endoscopy
Aeromonas hydrophila	Cramps, diarrhea, fecal blood	Culture	May be chronic Contaminated drinking water
Plesiomonas	Diarrhea, cramps	Culture	Shellfish source
Tuberculosis	Rarely bovine, now Mycobacterium tuberculosis Ileocecal area, fistula formation	Culture, PPD, biopsy	May mimic Crohn disease
Parasites			
Entamoeba histolytica	Acute bloody diarrhea and liver abscess, colic	Trophozoite in stool, colonic mucosal flask ulceration, serologic tests	Travel to endemic area
Giardia lamblia	Foul-smelling, watery diarrhea, cramps, flatulence, weight loss; no colonic involvement	"Owl"-like trophozoite and cysts in stool; rarely duodenal intubation	May be chronic
AIDS-Associated Enteropathy			
Cryptosporidium	Chronic diarrhea, weight loss	Stool microscopy	Mucosal findings not like IBD
Isospora belli	As in Cryptosporidium		Tropical location
Cytomegalovirus	Colonic ulceration, pain, bloody diarrhea	Culture, biopsy	

FUO = fever of unknown origin; PPD = purified protein derivative; AIDS = acquired immunodeficiency syndrome; IBD = inflammatory bowel disease.

on colonic biopsy. Laboratory studies may demonstrate evidence of anemia (either iron deficiency or the anemia of chronic disease) or hypoalbuminemia. Although the sedimentation rate is often elevated, it may be normal even with fulminant colitis.

BOX 317–1. Chronic Inflammatory-like Intestinal Disorders

INFECTION—see Table 317–2
Bacterial
Parasite
AIDS-associated
Toxin

IMMUNE-INFLAMMATORY
Congenital immunodeficiency disorders
Acquired immunodeficiency diseases
Dietary protein enterocolitis
Behçet syndrome
Lymphoid nodular hyperplasia
Eosinophilic gastroenteritis
Graft-versus-host disease

VASCULAR-ISCHEMIC DISORDERS
Systemic vasculitis (SLE, dermatomyositis)
Henoch-Schönlein purpura
Hemolytic-uremic syndrome

OTHER
Prestenotic colitis
Diversion colitis
Radiation colitis
Neonatal necrotizing enterocolitis
Typhlitis
Hirschsprung colitis
Intestinal lymphoma
Laxative abuse

AIDS = acquired immunodeficiency syndrome; SLE = systemic lupus erythematosus.

An elevated white blood cell count is usually seen only with more severe colitis.

Findings of ulcerative colitis can be identified by endoscopic and histologic examination of the colon. Barium enema has no place in the diagnosis of this disorder. Classically, disease starts in the rectum with a gross appearance characterized by erythema, edema, loss of vascular pattern, granularity, and friability. There may be a "cut off" demarcating the margin between inflammation and normal colon, or the entire colon may be involved. There may be some variability in the intensity of inflammation even in those areas involved. One can use flexible sigmoidoscopy to confirm the diagnosis or colonoscopy to evaluate the extent of disease and to rule out evidence of Crohn colitis. A colonoscopy should *not* be performed when fulminant colitis is suspected because of the risk of provoking toxic megacolon or causing a perforation during the procedure. The degree of colitis can be evaluated by the gross appearance of the mucosa. Despite the name, one does not generally see discrete ulcers, which would be more suggestive of Crohn colitis. The endoscopic findings of ulcerative colitis result from microulcers, which give the appearance of a diffuse abnormality. With very severe chronic colitis, pseudopolyps may be seen. Biopsy of involved bowel demonstrates evidence of acute and chronic mucosal inflammation. Typical findings are cryptitis, crypt abscesses, separation of crypts by inflammatory cells, foci of acute inflammatory cells, edema, mucus depletion, and branching of crypts. The last finding is a feature not seen in infectious colitis. Granulomas, fissures, or full-thickness involvement of the bowel wall (usually on surgical rather than endoscopic biopsy) suggest Crohn disease. Rectal biopsy can also distinguish chronic IBD from acute self-limiting colitis.

Perianal disease, with the exception of mild local irritation or anal fissures associated with diarrhea, should make one think of Crohn disease. Plain radiographs of the abdomen may demonstrate loss of haustral markings in an air-filled colon or marked dilatation with toxic megacolon. With severe colitis, the colon may become dilated; a diameter of greater than 6 cm, determined radiographically, in an adult suggests toxic megacolon. If it is necessary to examine the colon radiologically in a child with severe colitis (to evaluate the extent of involvement or to try to rule out Crohn disease), it is sometimes helpful to perform an upper gastrointestinal contrast series with small bowel follow-through and then look at delayed films of the colon. A barium enema is contraindicated in the setting of a potential toxic megacolon.

Treatment. A medical cure for ulcerative colitis is not available; treatment is aimed at controlling symptoms and reducing the risk of recurrence. The intensity of treatment varies with the severity of the symptoms. Twenty to 30% of individuals with ulcerative colitis have spontaneous improvement in symptoms. The first drug class to be used with mild colitis is an aminosalicylate. Sulfasalazine is composed of a sulfur moiety linked to the active ingredient 5-aminosalicylate. This linkage prevents the premature absorption of the medication in the upper gastrointestinal tract, allowing it to reach the colon, where the two components are separated by bacterial cleavage. The dose of sulfasalazine is 50–75 mg/kg/24 hr (divided into two to four doses). Generally, the dose is not more than 2 to 3 g/24 hr. It is recommended that the dosage gradually increase to full dose over the 1st wk of treatment to avoid gastrointestinal symptoms (e.g., nausea and abdominal pain) and headache and to detect sulfa hypersensitivity. Onset of action may take several weeks. Sulfasalazine treats colitis; recurrences may be prevented with its use. It is recommended that the medication be continued even when the disorder is in remission. Hypersensitivity to the sulfa component is the major side effect of sulfasalazine and may occur in 10–20% of individuals. Other less allergenic preparations of 5-aminosalicylate (mesalamine, 40–60 mg/kg/day) have been shown to treat ulcerative colitis and prevent recurrences with efficacy equal to that of sulfasalazine.

Perhaps 10–20% of individuals who have an allergic reaction to sulfasalazine will have a similar reaction to another 5-aminosalicylate product. On rare occasions, these medications cause exacerbation of colitis. Aminosalicylate may also be given in enema form and is especially useful for proctitis. Hydrocortisone enemas (100 mg) are used to treat proctitis as well. Either form of enema may be administered to older children and is given once a day (usually bedtime) for 2–3 wk. Many children prefer oral medication to enemas.

Children with moderate to severe pancolitis or colitis that is unresponsive to 5-aminosalicylate therapy should be treated with oral corticosteroids, most commonly prednisone. The usual starting dose of prednisone is 1–2 mg/kg/24 hr (40–60 mg maximal dose). If symptoms are not severe, this medication may be given in a single morning dose to lessen adrenal suppression. With severe colitis, the dose may be divided twice daily and may be given intravenously. The goal is to taper to an alternate-day dose within 1–3 mo. Persistence of symptoms despite steroid treatment or the inability to taper the dose is an indication for the use of other medications or for surgical management. Prolonged use of daily steroids beyond this period is to be avoided because of the many side effects, including growth retardation, adrenal suppression, cataracts, osteopenia, aseptic necrosis of the head of the femur, glucose intolerance, risk of infection, and cosmetic effects. With medical management, most children are in remission within 3 mo; however, 5–10% continue to have symptoms unresponsive to treatment beyond 6 mo. Many children with disease requiring frequent corticosteroid therapy are started on immunomodulators such as azathioprine (1.5–2.5 mg/kg/day) or 6-mercaptopurine (1–1.5 mg/kg/day). Uncontrolled data suggest a corticosteroid-sparing effect in many treated individuals. Cyclosporine, which has

been shown to be associated with improvement in many children with severe symptoms, does not appear to change the natural history of the disease. Anecdotal observations suggest a potential role for infliximab, a chimeric monoclonal antibody to tumor necrosis factor-α, in fulminant colitis.

Colectomy is performed for intractable disease, complications of therapy, and fulminant disease that is unresponsive to medical management. No clear benefit of the use of total parenteral nutrition or a continuous enteral elemental diet in the treatment of severe ulcerative colitis has been noted. Nevertheless, parenteral nutrition is often used so that the patient will be nutritionally ready for surgery if medical management fails. With any medical treatment for ulcerative colitis, one should always weigh the risk of the medication or therapy against the fact that colitis may be successfully treated surgically.

Surgical treatment for intractable or fulminant colitis is total colectomy. The optimal approach is to combine colectomy with an endorectal pull-through. In this procedure, the surgeon retains a segment of distal rectum and strips the mucosa from this region. The distal ileum is pulled down and sutured at the internal anus with a J pouch created from ileum immediately above the rectal cuff. This procedure allows the child to maintain continence. Commonly, a temporary ileostomy is created to protect the delicate anastomosis between the sleeve of the pouch and the rectum. The ileostomy is usually closed within several months, restoring bowel continuity. At that time stool frequency is often increased but may be improved with loperamide. The major complication of this operation is "pouchitis," which is a chronic inflammatory reaction in the pouch, leading to bloody diarrhea, abdominal pain, and occasionally low-grade fever. The cause of this complication is unknown, although it is more frequent when the ileal pouch has been constructed for ulcerative colitis than for other indications (familial polyposis coli). Pouchitis is seen in 30–40% of patients who had ulcerative colitis. It commonly responds to treatment with oral metronidazole.

The concept that ulcerative colitis is primarily a psychogenic disorder is false. However, emotional stresses may contribute to exacerbations. Difficulty adjusting to a chronic disorder is common, and distorted body image should be considered when evaluating the psychologic profile of a child with this disorder. Psychosocial support is an important part of therapy for this disorder. This may include adequate discussion of the disease manifestations and management between patient and physician, psychologic counseling for the child when necessary, and family support from a social worker or family counselor. Patient support groups have proved helpful for some families. Children with ulcerative colitis should be encouraged to participate fully in age-appropriate activities; however, activity may need to be reduced during periods of disease exacerbation.

Prognosis. The course of ulcerative colitis is marked by remissions and exacerbations. Most children with this disorder respond initially to medical management. Many children with mild manifestations continue to respond well to medical management and may stay in remission on a prophylactic 5-aminosalicylate preparation for long periods. However, an occasional child with mild onset experiences intractable symptoms at a later time. Beyond the 1st decade of disease, the risk of development of colon cancer begins to increase rapidly. The risk of colon cancer may be diminished with surveillance colonoscopies beginning after 8–10 yr of disease. Detection of significant dysplasia on biopsy would prompt colectomy.

Bridger S, Evans N, Parker A, et al: Multiple cerebral venous thromboses in a child with inflammatory bowel disease. *J Pediatr Gastroenterol Nutr* 1997;25:533.
Dolgin SE, Shlasko E, Gorfine S, et al: Restorative proctocolectomy in children with ulcerative colitis utilizing rectal mucosectomy with or without diverting ileostomy. *J Pediatr Surg* 1999;34:837.

Dubinsky MC, Ofman JJ, Urman M, et al: Clinical utility of serodiagnostic testing in suspected pediatric inflammatory bowel disease. *Am J Gastroenterol* 2001;96:758.

Dundas SA, Dutton J, Skipworth P: Reliability of rectal biopsy in distinguishing between chronic inflammatory bowel disease and acute self-limiting colitis. *Histopathology* 1997;31:60.

Hyams J, Davis P, Lerer T, et al: Clinical outcome of ulcerative proctitis in children. *J Pediatr Gastroenterol Nutr* 1997;25:149.

Hyams JS, Davis P, Grancher K, et al: Clinical outcome of ulcerative colitis in children. *J Pediatr* 1996;129:81.

Hyams JS, Markowitz J, Treem W, et al: Characterization of hepatic abnormalities in children with inflammatory bowel disease. *Inflamm Bowel Dis* 1995;1:27.

Kader HA, Mascarenhas MR, Piccoli DA, et al: Experience with 6-mercaptopurine and azathioprine therapy in pediatric patients with severe ulcerative colitis. *J Pediatr Gastroenterol Nutr* 1999;28:54.

Keene DL, Matzinger MA, Jabob PJ, et al: Cerebral vascular events associated with ulcerative colitis in children. *Pediatr Neurol* 2001;24:238–43.

Oral balsalazide (Colazal) for ulcerative colitis. *Med Lett* 2001;43:62–63.

Podolsky DK: Inflammatory bowel disease. *N Engl J Med* 2002;347:417–29.

Sawczenko A, Sandhu BK, Logan RFA, et al: Prospective survey of childhood inflammatory bowel disease in the British Isles. *Lancet* 2001;357:1093.

Treem WR, Cohen J, Davis PM, et al: Cyclosporin for the treatment of fulminant ulcerative colitis in children: Immediate response, long-term results, and impact on surgery. *Dis Colon Rectum* 1995;38:474.

317.2 Crohn Disease (Regional Enteritis, Regional Ileitis, Granulomatous Colitis)

Crohn disease, an idiopathic, chronic inflammatory disorder of the bowel, involves any region of the alimentary tract from the mouth to the anus. Although there are many similarities between ulcerative colitis and Crohn disease, there are also major differences in the clinical course and distribution of the disease in the gastrointestinal tract (see Table 317–1). The inflammatory process tends to be eccentric and segmental, often with skip areas (normal regions of bowel between inflamed areas). Although inflammation in ulcerative colitis is limited to the mucosa (except in toxic megacolon), gastrointestinal involvement in Crohn disease is transmural. Among children with Crohn disease, the initial presentation most commonly involves ileum and colon (ileocolitis) but may involve the small bowel alone in about 30% (70% of these patients have terminal ileitis alone) or colon alone in 10%–15%. Upper gastrointestinal involvement (esophagus, stomach, duodenum) is seen in up to 30% of children. As with ulcerative colitis, Crohn disease tends to have a bimodal age distribution, with the 1st peak beginning in the late teens. Diagnosis before 20 yr of age is associated with a greater chance of small bowel disease, development of stricture, and eventual need for surgery when compared with diagnosis after 40 yr. Likelihood of Crohn disease in family members is doubled with early diagnosis.

The incidence of Crohn disease has been increasing over the past 10 yr, whereas that of ulcerative colitis has been stable. The reported incidence of Crohn disease is about 3–4/100,000, and the prevalence is 30–100/100,000. The prevalence of Crohn disease in whites and blacks appears to be 3–10 times that of Hispanics and Asians living in the United States.

Clinical Manifestations. Crohn disease presents in many forms; the manifestations tend to be dictated by the region of bowel involved, the degree of inflammation, and the presence of complications such as stricture or fistula. Children with ileocolitis typically have cramping, abdominal pain, and diarrhea, sometimes with blood. Ileitis may present as right lower quadrant abdominal pain alone. Crohn colitis may be associated with bloody diarrhea, tenesmus, and urgency. Systemic signs and symptoms are more common in Crohn disease than in ulcerative colitis. Fever, malaise, and easy fatigability are common. Growth failure with delayed bone maturation and delayed sexual development may precede other symptoms by 1 or 2 yr and are at least twice as likely to occur with Crohn as with ulcera-

tive colitis. Children may present with growth failure as the only manifestation of Crohn disease. Growth retardation is associated with a decrease in lean body mass but preservation of body fat; enteric protein loss and the rate of body protein turnover are increased. Primary or secondary amenorrhea occurs frequently. In contrast to ulcerative colitis, perianal disease is common (tags, fistula, abscess). Gastric or duodenal involvement may be associated with recurrent vomiting and epigastric pain. Partial small bowel obstruction, usually secondary to narrowing of the bowel lumen from inflammation or stricture, may cause symptoms of cramping abdominal pain (especially with meals), borborygmus, and intermittent abdominal distention. Stricture should be suspected if the child notes relief of symptoms in association with a sudden sensation of gurgling of intestinal contents through a localized region of the abdomen. Ureteral obstruction (usually right-sided) secondary to extension of the inflammatory process is a rare complication of Crohn disease.

Enteroenteric or enterocolonic fistulas (between segments of bowel) are often asymptomatic but may contribute to malabsorption if they have high output or result in bacterial overgrowth. Enterovesical fistulas (between bowel and urinary bladder) originate from ileum or sigmoid colon and present as signs of urinary infection, pneumaturia, or fecaluria. Enterovaginal fistulas originate from the rectum, cause feculent vaginal drainage, and are difficult to manage. Enterocutaneous fistulas (between bowel and abdominal skin) often are caused by prior surgical anastomoses with leakage. Intra-abdominal abscess may be associated with fever and pain but may have relatively few symptoms. Hepatic or splenic abscess may occur with or without a local fistula. Anorectal abscesses often originate immediately above the anus at the crypts of Morgagni. The patterns of perianal fistulas are complex because of the different tissue planes. Perianal abscess is usually painful, but perianal fistulas tend to produce fewer symptoms than might be anticipated. Purulent drainage is commonly associated with perianal fistulas. Psoas abscess secondary to intestinal fistula may present as hip pain, decreased hip extension (psoas sign), and fever.

Extraintestinal manifestations occur more commonly with Crohn disease than with ulcerative colitis; those that are especially associated with Crohn disease include oral aphthous ulcers, peripheral arthritis, erythema nodosum, digital clubbing, episcleritis, renal stones (uric acid, oxalate), and gallstones. Any of the extraintestinal disorders described in the section on IBD may occur with Crohn disease. The peripheral arthritis is nondeforming. In general, the occurrence of extraintestinal manifestations correlates with the presence of colitis. During periods of active disease, secondary amenorrhea is common in older girls.

Extensive involvement of small bowel, especially in association with surgical resection, may lead to short-bowel syndrome, which is rare in children. Complications of terminal ileal dysfunction or resection include bile acid malabsorption with secondary diarrhea and vitamin B_{12} malabsorption. Chronic steatorrhea may lead to oxaluria with secondary renal stones. The risk of cholelithiasis is also increased secondary to bile acid depletion.

A disorder with this diversity of manifestations can have a major impact on an affected child's lifestyle. Fortunately, the majority of children with Crohn disease are able to continue with their normal activities, having to limit activity only during periods of increased symptoms.

Differential Diagnosis. As in patients with ulcerative colitis, the most common diagnoses to be distinguished from Crohn disease are the infectious enteropathies (in the case of Crohn disease: acute terminal ileitis, infectious colitis, enteric parasites, and periappendiceal abscess) (see Table 317–2 and Box 317–1). *Yersinia* may cause many of the radiologic and endoscopic findings in the distal small bowel that are seen in Crohn disease. The symptoms of bacterial dysentery are more likely to be mistaken for ulcerative colitis than for Crohn disease. *Giardia* has been noted to produce a Crohn-like presentation including protein-losing enteropathy. Gastrointestinal tuberculosis is rare but can mimic Crohn disease. Foreign-body perforation of the bowel (toothpick) may mimic a localized region with Crohn disease. Small bowel lymphoma may mimic Crohn disease but tends to be associated with nodular filling defects of the bowel without ulceration or narrowing of the lumen. Bowel lymphoma is much less common in children than is Crohn disease. Recurrent functional abdominal pain may mimic the pain of small bowel Crohn disease. Lymphoid nodular hyperplasia of the terminal ileum (a normal finding) may be mistaken for Crohn ileitis. Right lower quadrant pain or mass with fever may be the result of periappendiceal abscess. This entity may occasionally be associated with diarrhea as well. Necrotizing jejunitis is a rare condition of transient, acute inflammation of jejunum (or less commonly ileum or colon), which may recur.

Growth failure may be the only manifestation of Crohn disease; other disorders such as growth hormone deficiency or gluten-sensitive enteropathy (celiac disease) must be considered. If arthritis precedes the bowel manifestations, an initial diagnosis of juvenile rheumatoid arthritis may be made. Refractory anemia may be the presenting feature and may be mistaken as a primary hematologic disorder. Leukemia may present with abdominal pain in association with an abnormal blood cell count and initially may be mistaken for Crohn disease. Chronic granulomatous disease of childhood may cause inflammatory changes in the bowel with granulomas seen at biopsy. Antral narrowing in this disorder may be mistaken for a stricture secondary to Crohn disease.

Diagnosis. Crohn disease may present as a variety of symptom combinations. At the onset, symptoms may be subtle (growth retardation or abdominal pain alone); this explains why the diagnosis may not be made until 1 or 2 yr after the start of symptoms. The diagnosis of Crohn disease depends on finding typical clinical features of the disorder (history, physical examination, laboratory studies, and endoscopic or radiologic findings), ruling out specific entities that mimic Crohn disease, and demonstrating chronicity. The history may include any combination of abdominal pain (especially right lower quadrant), diarrhea, vomiting, anorexia, weight loss, growth retardation, and extraintestinal manifestations.

Children with Crohn disease often appear chronically ill. They commonly have weight loss and are often malnourished. Linear growth retardation frequently precedes clinical presentation by as much as 1–2 yr; this manifestation may not have been appreciated until the diagnosis is established. Children with Crohn disease often appear pale with decreased energy level and poor appetite; the latter finding sometimes results from an association between meals and abdominal pain or diarrhea. There may be abdominal tenderness that is either diffuse or localized to the right lower quadrant. A tender mass or fullness may be palpable in the right lower quadrant. Perianal disease, when present, may be characteristic. Large anal skin tags (1–3 cm diameter) or perianal fistulas with purulent drainage are suggestive of Crohn disease. Digital clubbing, findings of arthritis, and skin manifestations may be present. A complete blood cell count commonly demonstrates an anemia, often with a component of iron deficiency. Although the sedimentation rate is often elevated, it may be normal; an elevated platelet count ($>600,000/mm^3$) is common. The white blood cell count may be normal or mildly elevated. The serum albumin level may be low, and the stool α_1-antitrypsin level may be elevated, consistent with a protein-losing enteropathy. Anti-*Saccharomyces cerevisiae* antibodies are identified in 55% of children with Crohn disease but in only 5% of children with ulcerative colitis.

The small and large bowel should be examined in the child with suspected Crohn disease. The initial choice of colonoscopy or a radiologic study partly depends on the anticipated location of disease. For small bowel involvement, an upper gastrointestinal contrast examination with small bowel follow-through would be the initial study. A variety of findings may be apparent on radiologic studies. Plain films of the abdomen may be normal or may demonstrate findings of partial small bowel obstruction or thumbprinting of the colon wall. An upper gastrointestinal contrast study with small bowel follow-through may show aphthous ulceration and thickened, nodular folds as well as narrowing of the lumen anywhere in the gastrointestinal tract. Linear ulcers may give a cobblestone appearance to the mucosal surface. Bowel loops are often separated as a result of thickening of bowel wall and mesentery. Terminal ileum is most commonly involved. Diseased regions tend to be eccentric, and normal regions may be found between diseased segments (skip areas).

Other manifestations on radiographic studies that suggest more severe Crohn disease are fistulas between bowel (enteroenteric or enterocolonic), sinus tracts, and strictures. Following the flow of barium antegrade into the colon may reveal right-sided colonic disease. Ultrasonography and contrast CT are most useful in identifying intra-abdominal abscess. Thickened bowel wall may be seen on CT. MRI can localize areas of active bowel disease, although this study is probably no better for identifying an abscess. MRI is also useful in evaluating Crohn disease during pregnancy because it does not use ionizing radiation. Radionuclide scans utilizing white blood cells tagged with indium may help locate affected areas.

Colonoscopy with biopsy can be more helpful than radiologic or radionuclide studies in evaluating colon disease and in establishing a diagnosis. It is sometimes possible to enter the terminal ileum during colonoscopy; this maneuver may be helpful in clarifying an equivocal diagnosis of ileal Crohn disease. Findings on colonoscopy may include patchy, nonspecific inflammatory changes (erythema, friability, loss of vascular pattern), aphthous ulcers, linear ulcers, nodularity, and strictures. Findings on biopsy may be only nonspecific inflammatory changes. Noncaseating granulomas, similar to those of sarcoidosis, are the most characteristic histologic findings, although often they are not present. Transmural inflammation is also characteristic but can be identified only in surgical specimens.

Treatment. Crohn disease cannot be cured by either medical or surgical therapy. The aim of treatment is to relieve symptoms and prevent complications of chronic inflammation (anemia, growth failure), prevent relapse, and, if possible, effect mucosal healing. The specific therapeutic modalities used depend on geographic localization of disease, severity of inflammation, age of the patient, and the presence of complications (abscess). For mild terminal ileal disease or mild Crohn disease of the colon, an initial trial of mesalamine (40–60 mg/kg/day, maximum 3 g) may be attempted. Specific pharmaceutical preparations have been formulated to release the active 5-ASA compound in the ileum and colon. Sulfasalazine may be effective for mild Crohn colitis but will not be helpful for small bowel disease. For more extensive or severe small bowel or colonic disease, most clinicians will initiate therapy with corticosteroids (prednisone, 1–2 mg/kg/day, maximum 40–60 mg). The goal is to taper to a single morning alternate-day dose as soon as the disease becomes quiescent. Typically, tapering can begin by 3–4 wk and continue over several months. Clinicians vary in their tapering schedules, but most will decrease the daily dose by 2.5–5 mg every 6–8 days until the daily dose is about 0.5 mg/kg, and then a similar decrease is effected on alternate days in 6–8 day cycles (e.g., 25 mg alternating with 20 mg for 8 days, followed by 25 mg alternating with 15 mg for 8 days, etc.). Eventually the prednisone is given on alternate days only and then that dose is tapered as tolerated. This approach is well tolerated, but the disease may flare during the process. Continuing daily or alternate-day prednisone as maintenance therapy to prevent relapse has not been shown to be effective.

Growth is impaired with either active disease or daily corticosteroid therapy. Growth is not impaired by alternate-day therapy. Side effects of daily steroid treatment tend to occur more rapidly and be more severe when the serum albumin level is reduced. Steroid enemas have been used for distal colon disease. Budesonide is being tried in enema and oral form because of its lower potential for systemic side effects.

Unfortunately, up to 40% of children with Crohn disease will either become refractory to corticosteroid therapy or become dependent on daily dosing and quickly experience flare of the disease when the dose is decreased. Immunomodulators such as azathioprine (1.5–2.5 mg/kg/day) or 6-mercaptopurine (1.0–1.5 mg/kg/day) may be effective in some individuals who have a poor response to prednisone or who are steroid dependent. Because a beneficial effect of these drugs may be delayed for 3–6 mo after starting therapy they are not helpful acutely. The early use of these agents may decrease cumulative prednisone dosages over the first 1–2 yr of therapy. Infliximab (5 mg/kg given intravenously), a chimeric monoclonal antibody to tumor necrosis factor-α, will be associated with marked symptom improvement in 50–70% of patients and may serve as a bridge until the immunomodulators take effect. The durability of response to infliximab is variable and may be as short as 4–8 wk, making repeated dosing necessary in some patients. Side effects include allergic reactions, increased incidence of infections (especially tuberculosis), and the development of autoantibodies. Long-term safety of this biologic therapy appears good but awaits further study. A purified protein derivative (PPD) test for tuberculosis 1 should be done before starting infliximab.

There are several therapies available to treat perirectal fistula. Metronidazole (10–20 mg/dL/day) is often effective, but long-term therapy can cause neuropathy with paresthesias requiring cessation of therapy. Azathioprine and 6-mercaptopurine have succeeded in this situation. Infliximab is also useful, although recurrence is common.

Nutritional therapy is an effective primary as well as adjunctive treatment. The enteral nutritional approach (elemental or polymeric diets) is both as rapid in onset of response and as effective as the other treatments. Others suggest prednisone is more effective for the acute control of disease. Because these diets are relatively unpalatable, they are administered via a nasogastric or gastrostomy infusion. With severe, acute disease, they may be given continuously as a 24-hr infusion; the treatment may then be cycled to overnight infusion at home. Repletion should be planned for ideal weight to allow for catch-up growth. Most children are hesitant to use nasogastric infusion, but once it is begun most find it is not difficult. The advantages are that it (1) is relatively free of side effects, (2) avoids the problems associated with corticosteroid therapy, and (3) simultaneously addresses the nutritional rehabilitation. Children may participate in normal daytime activities. A major disadvantage of this approach is similar to that of other therapies: early relapse on discontinuing treatment. In addition, perianal and colon disease does not respond well. For children with growth failure this approach may be ideal.

High-calorie oral supplements, although effective, often are not tolerated because of early satiety or exacerbation of symptoms (abdominal pain, vomiting, or diarrhea). Nonetheless, they should be offered to children whose weight gain is suboptimal. The continuous administration of nocturnal nasogastric feedings for chronic malnutrition and growth failure has been effective with a much lower risk of complications than parenteral hyperalimentation. Complex formula may be given at 500–1,000 kcal nightly; treatment with 50–80 kcal/kg/night monthly every 4 mo has been considered equally effective by some.

The initial onset or a recurrence of Crohn disease may be acute, with severe pain, anorexia, fever, abdominal tenderness, and an elevated white blood cell count. In this situation, it is difficult to rule out an infectious process involving the bowel wall (microperforation). In addition to the use of intravenous corticosteroids, broad-spectrum intravenous antibiotic coverage for bowel flora (gram-negative bacteria and anaerobes) should be started initially and discontinued only if it appears that there is not an infectious process. An ultrasonogram or contrast CT study of the abdomen is necessary to rule out an intra-abdominal abscess. The development of an enteroenteric or colonic fistula may be identified on CT, although it is best seen on a conventional small bowel contrast study.

Surgical therapy should be reserved for very specific indications. Recurrence rate after bowel resection is high (>50% by 5 yr); the risk of requiring additional surgery increases with each operation. Potential complications of surgery include development of fistula or stricture, anastomotic leak, postoperative partial small bowel obstruction secondary to adhesions, and short-bowel syndrome. Surgery is the treatment of choice with localized disease of small bowel or colon that is unresponsive to medical treatment, bowel perforation, fibrosed stricture with symptomatic partial small bowel obstruction, and intractable bleeding. Intra-abdominal or liver abscess may sometimes be successfully treated by ultrasonographic or CT-guided catheter drainage and concomitant intravenous antibiotic treatment. Open surgical drainage is necessary if this approach is not successful. Perianal abscess often requires drainage unless it drains spontaneously. In general, perianal fistulas should be managed medically. However, a severely symptomatic perianal fistula may require fistulotomy; this procedure should be considered only if the location allows the sphincter to remain undamaged. Growth retardation was once considered an indication for resection; without other indications, this approach has not been shown to be beneficial, and medical or nutritional therapy, or both, is preferred.

The surgical approach for Crohn disease is to remove as small a region of bowel as possible. There is no evidence that removing bowel up to margins that are free of histologic disease has a better outcome than removing only grossly involved areas. The latter approach reduces the risk of short-bowel syndrome. One approach to symptomatic small bowel stricture has been to perform a strictureplasty rather than resection. The surgeon makes a longitudinal incision across the stricture but then closes the incision with sutures in a transverse fashion. This is ideal for short strictures without active disease. The reoperation rate is no higher with this approach than with resection, whereas bowel length is preserved.

Severe perianal disease may be incapacitating and difficult to treat if unresponsive to medical management. Colon diversion may allow the area to be less active; but on reconnection of the colon, disease activity usually recurs. Therefore, surgical treatment of severe perianal disease may require colectomy. Procedures that create a continent ileostomy or endorectal pull-through are generally discouraged in Crohn disease because of the risk of recurrence of the disease in remaining bowel. With colectomy, a conventional ileostomy is performed.

Psychosocial issues for the child with Crohn disease include a sense of being different, concerns about body image, difficulty in not participating fully in age-appropriate activities, and family conflict brought on by the added stress of this disease. Social support is an important component of the management of Crohn disease. Parents are often interested in learning about other children with similar problems, but children may be hesitant to participate. Social support and individual psychologic counseling are important in the adjustment to a difficult problem at an age that by itself often has difficult adjustment issues. Patients who are socially "connected" fare better. Ongoing education about the disease is an important aspect of management because children generally fare better if they understand and anticipate problems. The Crohn and Colitis Foundation of America has local chapters throughout the United States.

Prognosis. Crohn disease is a chronic disorder that is associated with high morbidity but low mortality. Symptoms tend to recur despite treatment and often without apparent explanation. One exception is that symptoms of partial small obstruction may occur after a high-residue meal in the presence of a small bowel stricture. Weight loss and growth failure can usually be improved with treatment and attention to nutritional needs. Up to 15% of individuals with early growth retardation secondary to Crohn disease have a permanent decrease in linear growth. Osteopenia is particularly common in those with chronic poor nutrition and frequent exposure to high doses of corticosteroids. Some of the extraintestinal manifestations may, in themselves, be major causes of morbidity, including sclerosing cholangitis, chronic active hepatitis, pyoderma gangrenosum, and ankylosing spondylitis.

The region of bowel involved may increase with time, although rapid progression typically occurs early and subsequently is slow. Complications of the inflammatory process tend to increase with time and include bowel strictures, fistulas, perianal disease, and intra-abdominal or retroperitoneal abscess. Nearly all individuals with Crohn disease eventually require surgery for one of its many complications; the rate of reoperation is high. The time between the onset of symptoms and the need for surgery appears to be shorter in children than in adults. Surgery is unlikely to be curative and should be avoided except for the specific indications noted previously. Repeated small bowel resection, which may be unavoidable, can lead to malabsorption secondary to short-bowel syndrome (see Chapter 320.7). Resection of terminal ileum may result in bile acid malabsorption with diarrhea and vitamin B_{12} malabsorption. The risk of colon cancer in individuals with long-standing Crohn colitis may approach that associated with ulcerative colitis, and screening colonoscopy after 10 years of colonic disease is indicated.

Despite these complications, most children with Crohn disease lead active, full lives with intermittent flare-up in symptoms.

Baldassano RN, Han PD, Jeshion WC, et al: Pediatric Crohn's disease: Risk factors for postoperative recurrence. *Am J Gastroenterol* 2001;196:2169.

Cortot A, Colomberl JF, Rutgeerts P, et al: Switch from systemic steroids to budesonide in steroid dependent patients with inactive Crohn's disease. *Gut* 2001;48:186.

D'Haens G, Van Deventer S, Van Hogezand R, et al: Endoscopic and histological healing with infliximab anti-tumor necrosis factor antibodies in Crohn's disease: A European multicenter trial. *Gastroenterology* 1999;116:1029.

Dietz DW, Laureti S, Strong SA, et al: Safety and long-term efficacy of stricture plasty in 314 patients with obstructing small bowel Crohn's disease. *J Am Coll Surg* 2001;192:330.

Feagan BG, Fedorak RN, Irvine EJ, et al: A comparison of methotrexate with placebo for the maintenance of remission in Crohn's disease. *N Engl J Med* 2000;342:1627.

Friedman S, Rubin P, Bodian C, et al: Screening and surveillance colonoscopy in chronic Crohn's colitis. *Gastroenterology* 2001;120:820.

Griffiths AM, Nguyen P, Smith C, et al: Growth and clinical course of children with Crohn's disease. *Gut* 1993;34:939.

Heikenen JB, Werlin SL, Brown CW, et al: Presenting symptoms and diagnostic lag in children with inflammatory bowel disease. *Inflamm Bowel Dis* 1999;5:158.

Heuschkel RB, Menache CC, Megerian JT, et al: Enteral nutrition and corticosteroids in the treatment of acute Crohn's disease in children. *J Pediatr Gastroenterol Nutr* 2000;31:8.

Hyams JS: Extraintestinal manifestations of inflammatory bowel disease. *J Pediatr Gastroenterol Nutr* 1994;19:7.

Hyams JS, Markowitz J, Wyllie R: Use of infliximab in the treatment of Crohn's disease in children and adolescents. *J Pediatr* 2000;137:192.

Keane J, Gershon S, Wise RP, et al: Tuberculosis associated with infliximab, a tumor necrosis factor α–neutralizing agent. *N Engl J Med* 2001;345:1098–1104.

Kugathasan S: Prolonged duration of response to infliximab in early pediatric Crohn's disease. *J Pediatr Gastroenterol Nutr* 2001;33:S40–43.

Markowitz J, Grancher K, Kohn N, et al: A multicenter trial of 6-mercaptopurine and prednisone in children with newly diagnosed Crohn's disease. *Gastroenterology* 2000;119:895.

Ogura Y, Bonen DK, Inohara N, et al: A frameshift mutation in *NOD2* associated with susceptibility to Crohn's disease. *Nature* 2001;411:603.

Pittock S, Drumm B, Fleming P, et al: The oral cavity in Crohn's disease. *J Pediatr* 2001;138:767–71.

Rioux JD, Daly MJ, Silverberg MS, et al: Genetic variation in the 5q31 cytokine gene cluster confers susceptibility to Crohn disease. *Nat Genet* 2001;29:223.

Ruemmele FM, Roy CC, Levy E, Seidman EG: Nutrition as primary therapy in pediatric Crohn's disease: Fact or fantasy? *J Pediatr* 2000;136:285.

Sartor RB: New therapeutic approaches to Crohn's disease. *N Engl J Med* 2000;342:1664.

Semeao EJ, Jawad AF, Stouffer NO, et al: Risk factors for low bone mineral density in children and young adults with Crohn's disease. *J Pediatr* 1999;135:593.

Sentongo TA, Semeao EJ, Piccoli DA, et al: Growth, body composition, and nutritional status in children and adolescents with Crohn's disease. *J Pediatr Gastroenterol Nutr* 2002;31:33.

Shanahan F: Crohn disease. *Lancet* 2002;359:62–68.

Tobin JM, Sinha B, Ramiani P, et al: Upper gastrointestinal mucosal disease in pediatric Crohn disease and ulcerative colitis: A blinded, controlled study. *J Pediatr Gastroenterol Nutr* 2001;32:443.

317.3 Behçet Syndrome

Behçet syndrome is a systemic vasculitis that is rare in children (see Chapter 162). Aphthous stomatitis, erythema nodosum, and arthritis are among the most common manifestations. The ulcers are 2–10 mm in diameter and occur anywhere in the mouth or posterior pharynx; intestinal ulceration may mimic Crohn disease. The ulcers are covered by white-yellow membranes, have red borders, and are painful. Other signs are genital ulcers, central nervous system involvement, and myositis. Ocular findings (iridocyclitis) are less common in children than in adults. Immunosuppressive drugs have been used with mixed success. There appears to be significant familial aggregation.

Kone-Paut I, Geisler I, Wechsler B, et al: Familial aggregation in Behçet's disease: High frequency in siblings and parents of pediatric probands. *J Pediatr* 1999;135:89.

Kone-Paut I, Yurdakul S, Bahabri AS, et al: Clinical features of Behçet's disease in children: An international collaborative study of 86 cases. *J Pediatr* 1998;132:721.

Kontogiannis V, Powell RJ. Behçet's disease. *Postgrad Med J* 2000;76:629.

Chapter 318
Food Allergy (Food Hypersensitivity) *Jeffrey Hyams*

Food allergy is a group of disorders in which symptoms result from immunologic responses to specific food antigens. Food allergy occurs in as many as 6% of children during the first 3 yr of life, including the 2–3% of infants and toddlers with cow's milk allergy. Reactions are classified as IgE mediated and non–IgE mediated. IgE-mediated reactions are caused by inflammatory mediators released when food antigen binds to specific IgE antibody on mast cells and basophils. These reactions are associated with rapid development of symptoms. Non–IgE-mediated reactions are cell mediated and develop over hours to days. For some clinical conditions there appear to be multiple mechanisms involved.

Clinical Manifestations. Food antigen may provoke respiratory, skin, or gastrointestinal symptoms. Gastrointestinal manifestations can occur anywhere in the alimentary tract and often dominate. Behavioral manifestations have been described but are controversial.

IgE-Mediated Food Hypersensitivity
ORAL ALLERGY SYNDROME. Contact with the allergen on the oropharynx causes itching or tingling and angioedema of the lips, tongue, palate, and throat. These symptoms may precede other IgE-mediated manifestations of food allergy. Allergy

to pollen (hay fever) is also common in these patients. Facial erythema from contact with citrus and tomato products is not considered an immune response.

GASTROINTESTINAL ANAPHYLAXIS. Rapid onset of nausea, cramping abdominal pain, vomiting, or diarrhea, or a combination of these conditions occurs after ingestion of an allergen. The most common proteins implicated include milk, egg, peanut, soy, cereal, and fish.

OTHER NONGASTROINTESTINAL MANIFESTATIONS. These include cutaneous—urticaria, angioedema, and atopic dermatitis (eczema); respiratory—asthma and rhinoconjunctivitis; and systemic anaphylaxis. Life-threatening reactions typically are associated with ingestion of peanuts, nuts, fish, and shellfish. These subjects often have a concomitant history of asthma.

Mixed (IgE- and Non–IgE-Mediated) Food Hypersensitivity. These disorders are characterized by intense eosinophilic infiltration of the specific organ involved. The inflammatory infiltrate may involve the mucosa, muscularis, or serosa of the stomach or small intestine. Eosinophilic infiltration of the muscularis leads to thickening and nodularity, causing symptoms of obstruction (e.g., pain and vomiting), whereas serosal infiltration leads to eosinophilic ascites. Many patients with these disorders respond to removal of certain dietary antigens from the diet (e.g., milk), whereas others require a more drastic whole protein restriction with the concomitant use of hydrolyzed protein or amino acid–based formulas. Occasional patients also require corticosteroid therapy.

ALLERGIC EOSINOPHILIC ESOPHAGITIS. This disorder is characterized by intense eosinophilic infiltration of the esophageal mucosa. In infants and toddlers vomiting is the most common symptom, whereas in older children dysphagia and abdominal pain or heartburn are more common (see Chapter 305). Rarely esophageal strictures may be present in older children and adolescents. Clinicians mistakenly diagnose these patients with gastroesophageal reflux but they do not respond to usual therapies, and intraesophageal pH probe testing is normal. Treatment usually involves dietary modification in younger patients, with the occasional temporary need for an amino acid–based diet; older patients are usually treated with corticosteroids.

ALLERGIC EOSINOPHILIC GASTRITIS. This disorder is more common in infancy and adolescence and presents as abdominal pain, vomiting, anorexia, hematemesis, poor weight gain, and, rarely, gastric outlet obstruction. It may mimic pyloric stenosis in young infants. Atopic features, elevated serum IgE levels, and peripheral eosinophilia are seen in about 50% of patients. Gastric biopsy reveals intense eosinophilic infiltration of the mucosa and submucosa, particularly in the antrum.

ALLERGIC EOSINOPHILIC GASTROENTEROCOLITIS. These patients have similar symptoms to those described for allergic esophagitis and gastritis. Failure to thrive is common, and the majority of affected individuals have atopic symptoms. Marked protein-losing enteropathy may present as generalized edema and hypogammaglobulinemia.

Non–IgE-Mediated Disorders

ALLERGIC PROCTOCOLITIS. Infants may present between 1 day and 3 mo of age with spots or streaks of blood and mucus in stool and occasional mild diarrhea. Increased numbers of white blood cells in stool and peripheral eosinophilia may be present. Typically, a patchy, mild colitis is present; nodular lymphoid hyperplasia occurs in about 25% of cases. Most often, proctocolitis results from hypersensitivity to cow's milk; soy sensitivity is less common. This disorder also occurs in exclusively breast-fed patients and occasionally abates with maternal diet modification with elimination of milk products. Non–breast-fed infants can be treated with protein hydrolysate formulas.

FOOD-INDUCED ENTEROCOLITIS. Protracted vomiting and diarrhea begin between 1 wk and 3 mo of age. Less severe reactions can occur in older children and adults. Stools contain occult blood, neutrophils, and eosinophils. Jejunal biopsy demonstrates flattened villi, edema, and inflammatory cells. Symptoms resolve within 72 hr of removal of the offending food and recur within 1–6 hr of reintroduction. The blood neutrophil count increases by at least 3.5×10^9/L at 4–6 hr after a food challenge. Older infants may develop a poorly characterized syndrome of anemia, hypoproteinemia, and failure to thrive when weaned from nursing or formula to ordinary cow's milk. Eosinophilia is common. Casein hydrolysate or amino acid–based formulas successfully treat most patients.

FOOD-INDUCED ENTEROPATHY. Malabsorption, protracted diarrhea, vomiting, and failure to thrive caused by food hypersensitivity occur most often during the 1st mo of life. Small bowel biopsy shows patchy villus atrophy with mononuclear cell inflammatory response. Reaction to food challenge as well as resolution of symptoms on removal of the offending food may take several days to weeks.

CELIAC DISEASE (GLUTEN-SENSITIVE ENTEROPATHY) AND DERMATITIS HERPETIFORMIS. Both entities occur as an immunologic response to gluten ingestion, and the two can occur together. See Chapter 320.8.

PULMONARY HEMOSIDEROSIS (HEINER SYNDROME). A combination of pulmonary infiltrates from pulmonary hemorrhage, gastrointestinal bleeding, iron-deficiency anemia, peripheral eosinophilia, and failure to thrive secondary to food intolerance (often cow's milk protein) resolves on removal of the offending food from the diet.

Diagnosis. Food allergy is suspected when typical symptoms occur with the introduction of specific foods. Other nonallergic mechanisms of food intolerance should be ruled out (compromised digestive or absorptive processes, contamination with microbes or toxins, or pharmacologic activity of foods). Lactose intolerance should be considered when cow's milk allergy is suspected. Elimination diet and subsequent double-blind, placebo-controlled food challenge (DBPCFC) are the gold standard for diagnosis of food allergy. In DBPCFC, suspected foods are administered in capsules in progressively increasing amounts, alternating with placebo, and reactions are evaluated in a blinded fashion. Open food challenges, although commonly performed, are less reliable (except in young infants). Symptoms can be reproduced by DBPCFC in only 40% of children with suspected food allergy. When anaphylaxis has followed ingestion of a food, challenge should not be performed, and an allergist should evaluate the child.

The judicious use of a skin prick test or radioallergosorbent test (RAST) can be very useful in determining whether an IgE allergic reaction is the cause of a food allergy. Children can be tested for IgE reactions to foods at any age because IgE is made by 24 wk gestation. A negative IgE test, especially if the patient is older than 1 yr of age, is very accurate in predicting that the reaction is not IgE mediated. The significance of a positive IgE test has to be determined by the history and the age of the patient. A positive skin test is found in nearly 100% of children 3 yr of age or older who have a positive DBPCFC. Total-serum IgE is unreliable in diagnosing food allergy.

In infancy, hypersensitivity is most often associated with ingestion of cow's milk or soy protein. Although nursing may prevent the development of food allergy, manifestations of food allergy, especially proctocolitis, can occur while nursing. Cow's milk in the mother's diet is the most common identifiable cause of food-allergic reactions in nursing infants; reaction to peanut, soy, or egg in the mother's diet occurs less often.

Among infants and children with food allergy, 90% of reactions are to egg, milk, peanuts, soy, and wheat. Seventy-five per cent of children with proven food allergy react only to a single food. Children with allergic eosinophilic gastroenteritis are the exception, often reacting to multiple foods.

Treatment and Prognosis. The only therapy proved effective for food allergy is an elimination diet. Most gastrointestinal manifestations resolve within several days, although some may take weeks (food-induced enteropathy). A child at risk for a severe and life-threatening IgE-mediated reaction should have access to injectable epinephrine and an antihistamine.

At least 30% of infants with cow's milk allergy also demonstrate sensitivity to soy protein. Generally, these infants improve with protein hydrolysate formula; less than 5% have persistent symptoms and these cases resolve with the use of amino acid–based formulas. Re-lactation is an alternative when cow's milk allergy presents early. About 50% of infants who experience proctocolitis while nursing improve with removal of cow's milk from the mother's diet. In the others, one must decide whether the symptoms are severe enough (anemia and hypoproteinemia) to warrant a change in the infant's diet to a protein hydrolysate formula.

Eighty-five per cent of infants with non–IgE-mediated food hypersensitivity to milk proteins no longer have symptoms on food challenge by 3 yr of age. Resolution of symptoms from cow's milk or soy protein hypersensitivity is common by 1 yr of age. When milk is reintroduced, only a teaspoon or less should be offered at first and then increased progressively over a few days if tolerated. Even older children and adults may lose their sensitivity to an offending food when it is eliminated from the diet for 1 to 2 yr. Symptoms from IgE-mediated allergy to peanut, nuts, fish, or shellfish are the exception and do not resolve.

Kokkonem J, Haapalabit M, Laurila K, et al: Cow's milk protein-sensitive enteropathy at school age. *J Pediatr* 2001;139:797–803.
Odze RD, Wershil BK, Leichtner AM, et al: Allergic colitis in infants. *J Pediatr* 1995;126:163.
Sampson HA, Anderson JA: Summary and recommendations: Classification of gastrointestinal manifestations due to immunologic reactions to foods in infants and young children. *J Pediatr Gastroenterol Nutr* 2000;30:S87.
Sicherer SH, Noone SA, Koerner CB, et al: Hypoallergenicity and efficacy of an amino acid–based formula in children with cow's milk and multiple food hypersensitivities. *J Pediatr* 2001;138:688.
Sicherer SH: Food protein–induced enterocolitis syndrome: Clinical perspective. *J Pediatr Gastroenterol Nutr* 2000;30:S45.
Snyder JD, Rosenblum N, Wershil B, et al: Pyloric stenosis and eosinophilic gastroenteritis in infants. *J Pediatr Gastroenterol Nutr* 1987;6:543.
Walsh SV, Antonioli DA, Goldman H, et al: Allergic esophagitis in children: A clinicopathologic entity. *Am J Surg Pathol* 1999;23:390.
Williams LW, Bock SA: Skin testing and food challenges for evaluation of food allergy. *Immunol Allergy Clin North Am* 1999;19:479.

Chapter 319
Eosinophilic Gastroenteritis
Jeffrey Hyams

This entity consists of a group of rare and poorly understood disorders that have in common gastric and small intestine infiltration with eosinophils and peripheral eosinophilia. The esophagus and large intestine may also be involved. Tissue eosinophilic infiltration can be seen in mucosa, muscularis, or serosa. Mucosal involvement may produce nausea, vomiting, diarrhea, abdominal pain, gastrointestinal bleeding, protein-losing enteropathy, or malabsorption. Involvement of the muscularis may produce obstruction (especially of the pylorus), whereas serosal activity produces eosinophilic ascites.

This condition clinically overlaps the dietary protein hypersensitivity disorders of the small bowel and colon (see Chapter 318). Allergies to multiple foods are often seen, and serum IgE is commonly elevated. Peripheral eosinophilia is present in more than 50% of individuals with this disorder. The mucosal form is most frequent and is diagnosed by identifying large numbers of eosinophils in biopsy specimens of gastric antrum or small bowel.

The disease usually runs a chronic, debilitating course with sporadic severe exacerbations. Rare patients are helped by elimination diets or the use of cromolyn, but most require systemic administration of corticosteroids. Isolated eosinophilic esophagitis, unresponsive to gastroesophageal reflux therapy, may improve with an elimination diet; in the absence of stomach or small bowel involvement, this may be a separate entity.

Katz AJ, Goldman H, Grand RJ: Gastric mucosal biopsy in eosinophilic (allergic) gastroenteritis. *Gastroenterology* 1977;73:705.
Kelly KJ, Lazenby AJ, Rowe PC, et al: Eosinophilic esophagitis attributed to gastroesophageal reflux: Improvement with an amino acid-based formula. *Gastroenterology* 1995;109:1503.
Whitington PF, Whitington GL: Eosinophilic gastroenteropathy in childhood. *J Pediatr Gastroenterol Nutr* 1988;7:379.

Chapter 320
Malabsorptive Disorders*
Manuel Garcia-Careaga and John A. Kerner

Intestinal malabsorption can be part of many childhood diseases. It is a condition rather than a diagnosis. Malabsorption may present as watery diarrhea, acidic diarrhea, or steatorrhea. The absence of diarrhea and even the presence of a normal stool do not rule out a malabsorptive disorder.

Malabsorptive syndromes are conditions that cause insufficient assimilation of ingested nutrients as a result either of maldigestion or of malabsorption (Table 320–1). Children with disorders that cause generalized defects in assimilation of nutrients tend to present with similar signs and symptoms: abdominal distention; pale, foul-smelling, bulky stools; muscle wasting; poor weight gain or weight loss; and growth retardation (Fig. 320–1).

Congenital disorders affecting individual intestinal digestive enzymes or transport processes have also been identified. Some of these disorders may present as early as the 1st wk of neonatal life and can be life threatening. The clinical features of these disorders typically differ from those of the generalized malabsorption syndromes. Some present without gastrointestinal symptoms (Table 320–2). The disaccharidase deficiencies are the most common of these entities.

320.1 Evaluation of Children with Suspected Intestinal Malabsorption

Clinical Manifestations. Although many disorders of malabsorption are inherited, the child without a family history presents the greatest diagnostic challenge. Presentation of congenital disorders may include diarrhea and malabsorption from birth (congenital microvillus inclusion disease, tufting enteropathy, glucose-galactose transport defect, congenital chloride diarrhea, congenital bile acid malabsorption, congenital enterokinase deficiency). Alternatively, the symptoms may not present until the introduction of a new food (gluten in gluten-sensitive enteropathy, sucrose in congenital sucrase-isomaltase deficiency, lactose in congenital lactase deficiency). A careful history of the time of onset of symptoms and the relation to diet is helpful. Often, well-intended parents may assume that symptoms are

---

*Adapted from a chapter by M. Ulshen (16th Edition).

TABLE 320–1. Generalized Malabsorptive States in Childhood

Site	More Common	Less Common
Exocrine pancreas	Cystic fibrosis Chronic protein-calorie malnutrition	Shwachman-Diamond syndrome Chronic pancreatitis Pearson syndrome
Liver, biliary tree	Biliary atresia	Other cholestatic states (including Alagille syndrome, familial neonatal hepatitis)
Intestine		
Anatomic defects	Massive resection Stagnant loop syndrome	Congenitally short gut
Chronic infection	Giardiasis	Immune deficiency
Others	Celiac disease Dietary protein intolerance (milk, soy)	Tropical sprue Idiopathic diffuse mucosal lesions

TABLE 320–2. Specific Defects of Digestive-Absorptive Function in Children

Variable	Disease
Intestinal	
Fat	Abetalipoproteinemia
Protein	Enterokinase deficiency
	Amino acid transport defects (cystinuria, Hartnup disease, methionine malabsorption, blue diaper syndrome)
Carbohydrate	Disaccharidase deficiencies (congenital: sucrase-isomaltase, lactase; developmental: lactase, acquired)
	Glucose-galactose malabsorption (congenital, acquired)
	Glucoamylase deficiency (starch malabsorption)
Vitamin	Vitamin B_{12} malabsorption (juvenile pernicious anemia, transcobalamin II deficiency, Imerslund syndrome)
	Folic acid malabsorption
Ions, trace elements	Chloride-losing diarrhea
	Congenital sodium diarrhea
	Acrodermatitis enteropathica (zinc)
	Menkes syndrome (copper)
	Vitamin D–dependent rickets
	Primary hypomagnesemia
Drug-induced	
	Sulfasalazine (folic acid malabsorption)
	Cholestyramine (calcium, fat malabsorption)
	Phenytoin (calcium malabsorption)
Pancreatic	
	Specific enzyme deficiencies
	Lipase
	Trypsinogen

associated with events that may, in fact, be coincidental. If a dietary component is important in the cause of the malabsorption, repetition of symptoms should occur on re-introduction of the substance and improvement should be reproducibly associated with removal of the offending agent. Frequency, looseness, and quantity of stool can be helpful in formulating a differential diagnosis; however, color, other than the pale stool of fat malabsorption, typically does not provide a clue. Failure to thrive can be caused by many systemic or psychosocial disorders, and one must keep this possibility in mind before making a diagnosis of malabsorption. A common example is the child with chronic, nonspecific diarrhea (toddler's diarrhea) who may unadvisedly receive frequent periods of a clear-liquid diet and may lose weight as a result. These children can appear on examination to have a malabsorption syndrome such as gluten-sensitive

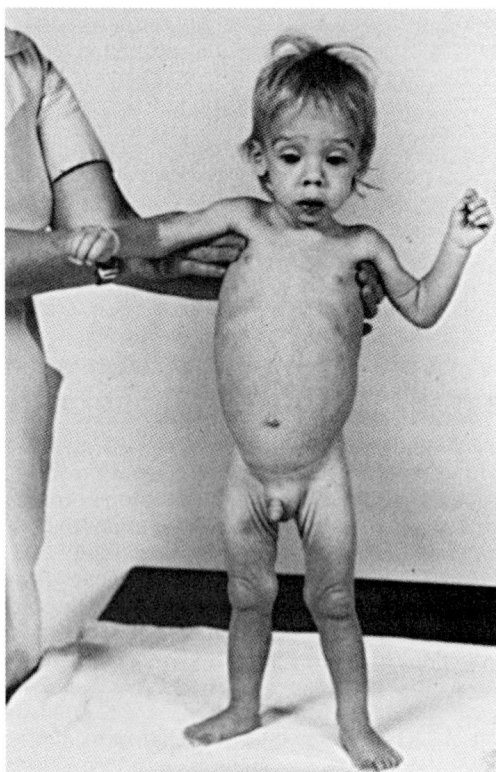

FIGURE 320–1. An 18-mo-old boy with active celiac disease. Note the loose skinfolds, marked proximal muscle wasting, and full abdomen. The child looks ill.

enteropathy. They typically respond to a return to a regular diet with improved weight gain.

The usual growth pattern associated with malabsorption and malnutrition demonstrates an initial decrease in weight followed by a deceleration in height velocity (Fig. 320–2). To make this assessment, it is essential to obtain serial weights and heights. The head circumference is usually normal, and growth of the head will be compromised when malnutrition becomes chronic. Signs of malnutrition may include lethargy, decreased subcutaneous tissue, muscle wasting, edema, clubbing, depigmentation of skin and hair, hemorrhagic diathesis, eczema, and follicular hyperkeratosis. Patients may also present with cheilosis, stomatitis, glossitis, and diffuse abdominal pain.

Initially, many infants with fat malabsorption have a voracious appetite. Other offending foods may produce avoidance behaviors if malabsorption produces gaseous distention (carbohydrates); gluten enteropathy frequently produces anorexia. The examination is typically not helpful in making a specific diagnosis, although occasionally features such as digital clubbing (cystic fibrosis, gluten-sensitive enteropathy), severe growth retardation of Shwachman syndrome, or the facial features of the Johannson-Blizzard syndrome can be helpful. A carotenemic infant or toddler is unlikely to have fat malabsorption.

Laboratory Findings. The most useful screening test for malabsorption is a microscopic examination of stool for fat. This test can be performed by mixing a small amount of stool with several drops of water or Sudan red stain. Fat droplets separate and can be easily identified, especially with a Sudan III stain. The presence of more than six to eight droplets per low-power field is abnormal. Droplets tend to accumulate at the edges of the coverslip. The addition of acetic acid is thought to protonate ionized fatty acids and to increase the number of droplets identified with Sudan stain. Castor oil, mineral oil, physiologic low levels of pancreatic enzymes in the neonate, extremely high fiber diets, and consumption of the nonabsorbable dietary additive Olestra can give a false-positive result. False-negative results may be seen with inadequate dietary fat intake. A positive test

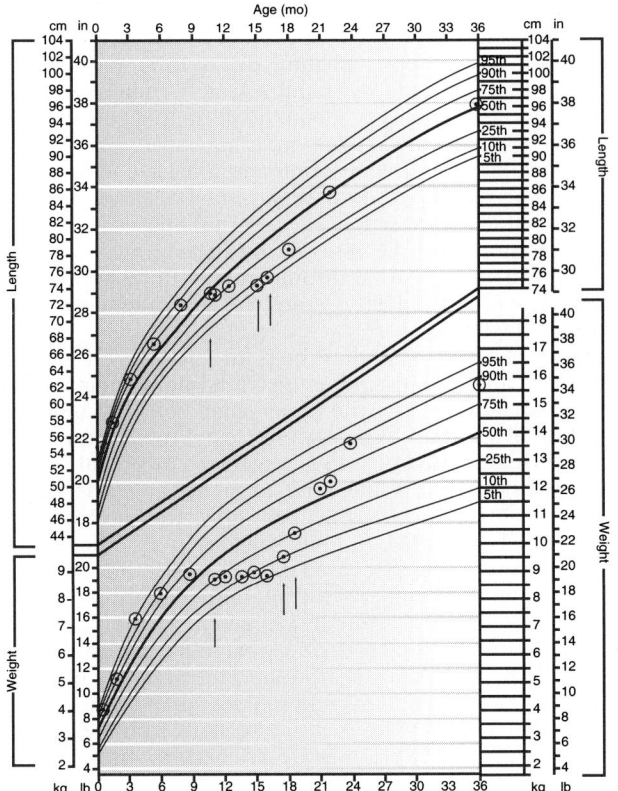

FIGURE 320–2. Gluten-sensitive enteropathy. Growth curve demonstrates initial normal growth from 0–9 mo, followed by onset of poor appetite with intermittent vomiting and diarrhea after initiation of gluten-containing diet *(single arrow)*. After biopsy-confirmed diagnosis and treatment with gluten-free diet *(double arrow)*, growth improves.

should be confirmed with a 72-hr quantitative fecal fat test, which remains the gold standard for assessing steatorrhea. Excretion of more than 7% of the total fat intake is abnormal and suggests the presence of malabsorption. Fecal fat concentration lacks the sensitivity and specificity to differentiate between the different causes of fat malabsorption. False-negative and false-positive results may occur under the same circumstances as with the use of the Sudan stain.

A dietary record during this period is used to calculate the fat intake. Many clinicians use the diet history as an average 3-day intake and collect stools from the beginning to the end of this period. Fat absorption is calculated by subtracting fat excretion from intake and dividing by fat intake; this fraction is multiplied by 100 to give the percentage of intake that is assimilated, known as the *coefficient of fat absorption.*

The ability to assimilate dietary fat varies with the maturity of the infant and the type of fat offered in the diet. A premature infant may absorb only 65–75% of dietary fat, whereas a full-term infant absorbs 90%. Therefore, the finding of fat in the stool on microscopic examination in young infants is not necessarily abnormal. Older children and adults should absorb at least 95% of the fat in a typical diet. Butterfat is absorbed less well than vegetable fat, although human milk fat is absorbed best of all. The mild decreased ability to assimilate fat by infants reflects a decrease in pancreatic enzyme secretion or a decrease in duodenal bile acid levels. In disorders with pancreatic insufficiency (cystic fibrosis or Shwachman syndrome), the fat droplets number in the hundreds to thousands. Some malabsorption syndromes, such as gluten-sensitive enteropathy, may not always be associated with fat in the stool. Serum carotene levels have

also been used as a screening test for fat malabsorption, but false-negative and false-positive results are common. The child must be receiving carotene in the diet for the test to be valid.

Steatorrhea is most prominent in disorders associated with pancreatic insufficiency; this finding warrants a sweat chloride test for cystic fibrosis as one of the initial studies. Three categories of exocrine pancreatic tests have been described: direct, indirect, and blood tests. The *direct tests* (secretin, cholecystokinin stimulation tests) assess the secretory capacity of the exocrine pancreas. The *indirect tests* detect abnormalities secondary to a loss of pancreatic function. These tests depend on the ability of the pancreatic secretagogue to break down substrate, which will provide an end product that could be recovered in the breath (carbon-13 lipids), serum and urine (bentiromide test, pancreolauryl), or stools (72-hr fecal fat, stool spot fat, trypsin chymotrypsin, elastase). The fecal elastase 1 is also useful. An enzyme-linked immunosorbent assay (ELISA) assesses elastase 1 as an indirect method of pancreatic function. Elastase 1 is an endoprotease, and it is both a human and pancreas specific protein. It is stable during conditions of abnormal intestinal transport, and it is not altered by supplementation of pancreatic enzymes. It is more sensitive than fecal chymotrypsin and will remain viable after up to 1 wk at room temperature. Its storability and the absolute specificity make this test a very attractive option to assess pancreatic function. *Blood tests* will detect pancreatic enzymes and hormones that are synthesized by the pancreas and which are normally found in the serum (trypsinogen). Measurement of serum levels of trypsinogen has proven to be a good screening test for pancreatic insufficiency in that it reflects residual exocrine pancreatic function. In cystic fibrosis with pancreatic insufficiency, the level is greatly elevated early in life but then falls, so that by 5–7 yr of age most patients have subnormal values. The levels in children with cystic fibrosis and pancreatic sufficiency are more variable but tend to be normal or elevated. In such children the trend over time is more helpful than a single value in monitoring pancreatic function. In Shwachman syndrome the serum trypsinogen level is low. The gold standard for determining pancreatic function resides in the ability to analyze duodenal contents after administration of a direct test, most commonly secretin and cholecystokinin stimulation tests. The procedure is cumbersome and involves intubation of the duodenum to aspirate its contents and avoiding direct contact with the stomach acid secretions. Few centers in the United States perform this analysis with reliable results. All the available tests to assess pancreatic function have at least one drawback.

Other initial studies should include a complete blood cell count, serum albumin determination, and measurement of serum immunoglobulin levels. Many different gastrointestinal disorders can cause hypoproteinemia as a result of decreased ability to assimilate dietary protein, inadequate protein intake, or protein-losing enteropathy (Box 320–1).

Measurement of carbohydrate in the stool using the Clinitest reagent for reducing substances is a simple screening test and can be performed at the bedside. The test is easily performed by combining 10 drops of water with 5 drops of stool and then adding a Clinitest tablet. The color change can be quantified as trace to 4+ using a color sheet provided by the manufacturer. Only 2+ or higher should raise the possibility of sugar malabsorption. Sucrose is not a reducing sugar and requires hydrolysis with hydrochloric acid before analysis.

If carbohydrates are not digested and absorbed in the small bowel, when they reach the colon they undergo degradation, where the final products are lactic acid and short-chain fatty acids such as butyrate, acetate, and propionate. There is production of methane, carbon dioxide, and hydrogen gases. Excess of carbohydrate spillage in the colon will lead to acidic stools and flatulence, which potentially could cause abdominal distention, discomfort, and a perineal chemical burn. Stool pH, obtained

---

BOX 320–1. Gastrointestinal Causes of Hypoproteinemia

Inflammatory bowel disease
Gluten-sensitive enteropathy
Cystic fibrosis
Shwachman syndrome
Disorders with secondary small-bowel mucosal damage
    (e.g., infectious disorders)
Intestinal lymphangiectasia (primary or secondary)
Hypertrophic gastropathy
Eosinophilic gastroenteropathy
Milk protein sensitivity
Trypsinogen or enterokinase deficiency

---

easily with pH paper, lower than 5.6 is also suggestive of carbohydrate malabsorption. Osmotic diarrhea may be seen with carbohydrate malabsorption. Calculation of the "stool osmotic gap": osmotic gap (mOsm/L) = 290 − 2 (Stool Na$^+$ + Stool K$^+$). A stool Na$^+$ level less than 70 mEq/L and an osmotic gap more than 100 mOsm/L suggest malabsorption from an excessive osmotic load (e.g., malabsorbed carbohydrate). The breath hydrogen test can also be used to evaluate carbohydrate malabsorption. The gas produced by bacterial degradation of carbohydrates is largely absorbed in the colon, enters the portal and systemic venous return, goes to the lung, and is then released in the breath. The child ingests a load of carbohydrate (1–2 g/kg, maximum 50 g), and the breath is collected in sealed plastic containers at timed intervals up to 2 hr after ingestion. The hydrogen content of the gas can be easily measured and is reported in parts per million (ppm). Malabsorption of any carbohydrate can be evaluated. The child should not be taking antibiotics at the time of the study because these drugs alter the colon flora and suppress hydrogen gas production. If a question exists about the ability of the colonic flora to produce hydrogen gas, the child can ingest the nonabsorbable disaccharide lactulose. A lack of hydrogen production with lactulose implies that the breath hydrogen test is not reliable in the child at that time. The major problem with the breath hydrogen study is that it is so sensitive that it identifies carbohydrate malabsorption that may not be clinically important (asymptomatic). A rise in hydrogen excretion of greater than 20 ppm from baseline is consistent with carbohydrate malabsorption.

Protein loss caused by maldigestion or malabsorption cannot be evaluated directly because bacterial protein accounts for such a large proportion of the stool nitrogen. Dietary protein is almost completely absorbed before reaching the terminal ileum. Endogenous intestinal proteins in the small bowel lumen are normally digested as well; less than 1 g of endogenous protein and products of digestion of exogenous protein pass into the colon. As a result, most of the colonic protein content is of bacterial origin.

A low serum albumin level may be the result of difficulty assimilating dietary protein, but it can also occur as a result of protein-losing enteropathy, inadequate protein intake, liver disease (reduced production), or renal disease. With protein-losing enteropathy, the peptide and amino acid products of digestion of the protein that enters the bowel lumen can be reabsorbed. Therefore, the child is not actually in negative nitrogen balance, even though levels of serum proteins including albumin and immunoglobulins are reduced.

Measurement of spot stool α_1-antitrypsin levels is helpful in establishing a diagnosis of protein-losing enteropathy. This serum protein is resistant to digestion and therefore can be measured in stool in contrast to albumin. One- or 2-day collections of stool for α_1-antitrypsin measurement or clearance studies are much more difficult to complete and do not appear to improve the test's reliability.

Nutrients that may be measured in blood include the following: iron, the level of which depends on transferrin concentra-

tion as well as on absorption; folic acid, the red cell concentration being a more accurate reflection of nutritional status than the serum concentration; calcium, zinc, and magnesium; vitamin D and its metabolites; vitamin A; and vitamin B$_{12}$. If the intake of these nutrients is adequate, decreased concentrations will suggest inadequate absorption. It may take years to deplete stores of vitamin B$_{12}$ after absorption is impaired. Vitamin E levels should be measured simultaneously with serum lipid levels and the value expressed as a ratio to lipid concentration. Vitamin K stores can be assessed by measuring prothrombin (more sensitive) and partial thromboplastin times because these times will be prolonged if the vitamin K–dependent coagulation factors are depleted.

Certain absorptive studies help to localize an intestinal lesion. Iron and D-xylose, a pentose minimally metabolized in humans, are absorbed by the upper small bowel. A blood concentration of less than 25 mg/dL of xylose 1 hr after a 14.5 g/m^2 oral dose (maximum dose: 25 g) suggests a proximal intestinal mucosal lesion, but some false-negative and false-positive results are obtained using this technique. In the distal bowel, vitamin B$_{12}$ is absorbed and bile salts are reabsorbed. *Vitamin B$_{12}$* absorption can be measured directly using the *Schilling test,* in which, after body stores of the vitamin are saturated, a tracer dose of radioactive vitamin B$_{12}$ is given by mouth, with or without intrinsic factor, and urinary excretion is measured over the next 24 hr. Defective absorption in the presence of intrinsic factor, shown by urinary excretion of less than 5% of the dose, occurs when an extensive length of distal ileum is resected or diseased or when bacterial overgrowth occurs within the bowel lumen.

Diagnosis

MICROBIOLOGIC. The only common primary infection causing chronic malabsorption is giardiasis (see Chapter 258 and Table 317–2). Techniques to fix and stain specimens have greatly improved the diagnostic value of examining stools for *Giardia* cysts. The trophozoite may be identified in fresh duodenal contents or the duodenal mucosa. Immunoassay techniques are also available to identify *Giardia* antigen in the stool and antibody in the serum. These tests appear sensitive and specific. When enteric clearing of bacteria is impaired, either from stasis of luminal contents or impaired immune function, colony counts from bacterial cultures of proximal intestinal juice may be very high.

Failure to thrive with chronic diarrhea may be the first sign of HIV infection (AIDS) (see Chapter 254) and congenital T- or B-cell defects. The cause may be primary infection or parasitic, bacterial, or viral opportunistic enteric pathogens.

SMALL BOWEL BIOPSY. Small bowel biopsy identifies diseases of the small bowel mucosa that are associated with histologic findings, including gluten-sensitive enteropathy, abetalipoproteinemia, lymphangiectasia, congenital microvillus inclusion disease, eosinophilic gastroenteritis, infectious disorders, and Whipple disease (rare in children). The biopsy can be safely performed by upper gastrointestinal endoscopy. At the time of biopsy, in addition to mucosa, it is possible to collect aspirates for examination for *Giardia* or bacterial culture. Mucosal samples can be frozen to assay for disaccharidase activities later. Depression of activities of all enzymes tested suggests a secondary deficiency associated with mucosal damage. Reduction of a specific enzyme or group of enzymes is consistent with a specific deficiency (lactase or sucrase-isomaltase deficiency).

HEMATOLOGIC. A hypochromic, microcytic blood smear indicates iron deficiency; a macrocytic smear suggests deficiency and therefore malabsorption of folic acid or vitamin B$_{12}$. Acanthocyte transformation of erythrocytes occurs in abetalipoproteinemia. A blood smear may also suggest a lymphocyte defect or neutropenia associated with Shwachman-Diamond syndrome.

IMAGING PROCEDURES. Used primarily to identify local lesions in the abdomen, these procedures have limited application to the study of children with malabsorptive disorders. *Plain radiographs* and *barium contrast studies* may suggest a site and cause of intestinal stasis. The most common anomaly causing incomplete bowel obstruction is intestinal malrotation, which can be diagnosed with barium contrast studies. Although flocculation of normal barium and dilated bowel with thickened mucosal folds have been attributed to diffuse malabsorptive lesions such as celiac disease, these abnormalities are nonspecific. The presence of multiple ulcerations in the duodenum with proximal small bowel edema suggests Zollinger-Ellison syndrome, a rare cause of malabsorption in children. *Ultrasound* can detect alterations in pancreatic mass, biliary tree abnormalities, and stones. *Retrograde studies* of the *pancreatic* and *biliary tree* using contrast medium injection by means of endoscopy are reserved for rare cases requiring careful delineation of the biliary and pancreatic ducts.

320.2   Chronic Malnutrition

Chronic protein-calorie malnutrition can lead to compromise of pancreatic and small bowel function. In developed countries, primary malnutrition is rare and chronic digestive disorders account for many cases of malnutrition in children. Environmental deprivation is also an important cause, as are feeding disorders (improper volume or dilution of formula). Protein-calorie malnutrition appears to contribute to the cycle of protracted diarrhea of infancy, perhaps through impairment of the functional capacity of the bowel, impairment of immune function, or the development of small bowel bacterial overgrowth. Worldwide, exocrine pancreatic insufficiency is most often attributable to malnutrition, not to a primary pancreatic disease.

The intestine is remarkably resistant to the effects of protein-calorie malnutrition. Patients with *kwashiorkor* may have a severely flattened small intestinal villi (see Chapter 42); these abnormalities are probably attributable to coexisting infections and infestations. In *marasmus*, villus structure is relatively well preserved, although microvillus changes and intracellular electron microscopic abnormalities are observed (see Chapter 42). Chronic malnutrition can lead to impaired immune function; bacterial overgrowth of the upper intestine is seen in malnourished subjects (see Chapter 42). When oral intake is withheld in experimental animals, intestinal mucosal mass and absorptive function diminish even if nutrient is supplied by the intravenous route. These changes can be reversed by small amounts of oral nutrient. Accordingly, a theoretical advantage exists in delivering nutrients via the gut. Recovery from injury to the gastrointestinal tract (viral gastroenteritis) may be prolonged by chronic malnutrition. Certain nutrients, such as glutamine, soluble fiber, short-chain fatty acids, and short-chain triglycerides, may promote small bowel mucosal growth.

Little is known about the *effect of specific nutritional deficiencies* on the pancreas or intestine; apart from potassium depletion causing ileus and severe dehydration causing constipation, available data suggest a relatively minor clinical effect of a wide range of specific deficiencies. Iron deficiency is associated with enhanced iron uptake at the mucosa and, in a few severe cases, occurrence of mucosal flattening. Deficiencies of vitamin B_{12} and folic acid may cause distortion of enterocyte morphology but no known serious functional abnormalities of the gut. Some hypocalcemic states may be accompanied by steatorrhea and even by ion and water secretion, but this poorly understood relationship is not constant.

Vitamin A supplementation reduces childhood mortality in developing countries. Improved survival during measles and a reduction in relative risk of contracting diarrheal and respiratory diseases have been identified. The explanation for this finding is uncertain, but children with vitamin A deficiency may have T-cell defects (including a low CD4:CD8 ratio), which can be reversed with vitamin supplementation.

320.3   Liver and Biliary Disorders

Cholestatic liver disease and biliary disorders may lead to fat malabsorption by reducing the duodenal bile acid concentration to less than the critical micellar concentration. In addition to steatorrhea, patients with these disorders have a propensity to acquire deficiencies of fat-soluble vitamins (vitamins A, D, E, and K). These deficiencies have no consistent pattern, except vitamin A is least likely to be problematic.

Vitamin E deficiency in patients with chronic cholestasis has been associated with a progressive neurologic syndrome, which includes peripheral neuropathy (presenting as loss of deep tendon reflexes and ophthalmoplegia), cerebellar ataxia, and posterior column dysfunction. Early in the course findings are partially reversible with treatment; late features may not be reversible. It can be difficult to identify vitamin E deficiency because the elevated blood lipid levels of cholestasis can falsely elevate the serum level of vitamin E. Therefore, it is important to measure the ratio of serum vitamin E to total serum lipids if one suspects this deficiency; the normal level for patients younger than 12 yr is greater than 0.6 and for patients 12 yr and older, greater than 0.8. The neurologic disease can be prevented with the use of an oral water-soluble vitamin E preparation (d-α-tocopherol polyethylene glycol-1,000 succinate [TPGS], Liqui-E) at 25–50 IU/24 hr in neonates and 1 IU/kg/24 hr in children.

Metabolic bone disease can develop secondary to vitamin D deficiency. Simultaneous administration of vitamin D with the water-soluble vitamin E preparation (TPGS) enhances absorption of vitamin D. In young infants, oral vitamin D_3 is given at 1,000 IU/kg/24 hr. After 1 mo, if the serum 25-hydroxyvitamin D level is low, the same dose of oral vitamin D is mixed with TPGS. 25-Hydroxyvitamin D is then monitored every 3 mo, with adjustment of doses as necessary.

Vitamin K deficiency can occur as a result of cholestasis and poor fat absorption. Easy bleeding may be the first sign, or a child may be identified before symptoms develop through routine screening of prothrombin (a more sensitive test) and partial thromboplastin times. It is possible for a patient taking the standard oral preparation to acquire vitamin K–deficient coagulopathy because the currently available oral preparation of vitamin K is not well absorbed.

320.4   Intestinal Infections

Malabsorption is a rare consequence of primary intestinal infection in immunocompetent children. Giardiasis is the most common infectious cause of chronic malabsorption (see Chapter 258). Factors that regulate the range of host response to *Giardia* (asymptomatic, acute, or chronic infection) remain to be explained. Symptoms may include diarrhea, vomiting, bloating, and gas. Giardiasis should be suspected if a child with persistent acquired malabsorption has family members who have had transient gastroenteritis symptoms at the onset of the child's illness. Children in daycare (especially toddlers) are at special risk for *Giardia*, although they may be asymptomatic and may pass it on to family members. Other common microorganisms that can lead to intestinal mucosal lesions and, hence, malabsorption are rotavirus, *Campylobacter, Shigella,* and *Salmonella.* Cryptosporidiosis can also occur in immunocompetent persons, as can coccidioidosis. Infectious causes of malabsorption are especially common in immunocompromised persons (see Chapters 164, 317, and 320.5).

320.5 Immunodeficiency

Gastrointestinal symptoms are a common manifestation of many immune deficiency states, including AIDS, congenital neutrophil and T- and B-cell immune deficiencies, and conditions of medical immune suppression (cancer and transplantation therapy). Most children with AIDS have diarrhea at some time. The more common congenital disorders associated with bowel disease include severe combined immunodeficiency, agammaglobulinemia, Wiskott-Aldrich syndrome, common variable immunodeficiency disease, and chronic granulomatous disease. Gastrointestinal symptoms of congenital X-linked hypogammaglobulinemia tend to be milder (chronic rotavirus or enterovirus infection or giardiasis). Malabsorption occurs in about 10% of patients with late-onset common variable hypogammaglobulinemia, a primary disorder that presents later in life. Nodular lymphoid hyperplasia may be noted on small bowel radiographs. T-cell abnormalities can also be associated with malabsorption. Selective immunoglobulin (Ig) A deficiency is common and may not always be associated with gastrointestinal symptoms, but it may be associated with an increased incidence of gluten-sensitive enteropathy, nodular lymphoid hyperplasia, inflammatory bowel disease, and giardiasis.

Chronic giardiasis and rotavirus infection have been noted to cause malabsorption in children with immune deficiencies. Small bowel bacterial overgrowth and infections with *Yersinia* and *Campylobacter* are seen in immunodeficient patients, leading to chronic diarrhea and malabsorption.

In addition, in children with AIDS, other organisms, including opportunistic infections, that can interfere with bowel function include *Cryptosporidium parvum*, cytomegalovirus, *Mycobacterium avium-intracellulare*, *Isospora belli*, *Enterocytozoon bieneusi*, *Candida albicans*, astrovirus, calicivirus, adenovirus, and the usual bacterial enteropathogens. Likelihood of infection is related to the CD4 count. *Cryptosporidium* can cause chronic secretory diarrhea and can be carried chronically in the gallbladder. HIV itself appears to be a primary bowel pathogen. Disaccharide intolerance is common in HIV-infected children but does not correlate well with enteric infection. Pancreatic insufficiency with steatorrhea and vitamin B_{12} malabsorption have been described to occur in patients with AIDS. Malnutrition and failure to thrive occur in the majority of untreated children with AIDS; diarrhea is common, although frequently pathogens are not identified. In addition to the range of infectious causes in immunosuppressed children, diarrhea can be a presentation of toxicity to the drug tacrolimus or of immunosuppression-induced lymphoproliferative disease.

Deficiency of neutrophils, congenital cyclic neutropenia, or, more commonly, the neutropenia associated with cancer chemotherapy predisposes children to neutropenic enterocolitis. The colitis can be manifested as mild bloody diarrhea, or it may present as fever, severe right lower quadrant pain, bloody stools, and diarrhea. The latter disorder, known as typhlitis, occurs most often in the lower ileum, cecum, and proximal colon, where vascular compromise, mucosal ulceration, and perforation carry a high mortality. Children with neutropenia are also at risk for fungal infections of the gastrointestinal tract including infections with *Histoplasma*, *Aspergillus*, and *Mucor*. Enterocolitis may be caused by *Clostridium difficile* in children receiving chemotherapy or long-term antibiotic therapy. In patients with chronic granulomatous disease, phagocytic function is impaired and granulomas may develop throughout the intestine, thus causing diarrhea and malabsorption and mimicking Crohn disease. Inflammation with granulomas, characterized by giant cells and lipid-containing histiocytes, may obstruct the gastric antrum. Children with chronic granulomatous disease are at risk for *Salmonella* infections as well.

320.6 Stagnant Loop Syndrome (Blind Loop Syndrome: Bacterial Overgrowth Syndrome)

These syndromes are characterized by an abnormally high bacterial population in the small bowel, exceeding 10^5 organisms/mL; they are associated with stasis of small intestinal contents, particularly in the upper regions. Incomplete bowel obstruction, either congenital (malrotation with duodenal bands, stenosis, intestinal duplications, duodenal webs, or a diverticulum) or acquired (postoperative intestinal adhesions, long-standing Crohn disease), impairs intestinal motility or causes loss of the normal intestinal mucosal barrier to microorganisms, allowing enteric bacteria to colonize the upper small bowel. Primary dysmotility disorders of the gastrointestinal tract, such as intestinal pseudo-obstruction and systemic disorders like diabetes mellitus, and scleroderma could result in bacterial overgrowth. Prematurity, immunodeficiency, and malnutrition are other factors that could lead to bacterial overpopulation of the small bowel. Bacteria deconjugate bile salts, a process that leads to inefficient intraluminal processing of dietary fat and to steatorrhea; they bind vitamin B_{12}, interfering with its absorption; and they may damage the microvillus brush border membrane, diminishing disaccharidase activities.

In addition to symptoms of chronic incomplete bowel obstruction such as distention, pain, and vomiting, the patient may have pale, foul-smelling, bulky stools typical of steatorrhea, megaloblastic anemia from vitamin B_{12} deficiency, or diarrhea from disaccharidase deficiency. Clinical manifestations often do not suggest chronic intestinal obstruction, but laboratory investigations find the aforementioned functional abnormalities as well as bacterial colonization of the upper intestine and deconjugated bile salts in the upper intestinal juice after a fatty meal. Barium contrast radiographs may reveal neither the existence nor the cause of obstruction.

Oral administration of antibiotics may be sufficient to control the problem temporarily. Metronidazole has been used for the treatment of bacterial overgrowth. An initial course of 2–4 wk may give relief for many months. If there is a relapse of symptoms, a longer treatment period (4–8 wk) is recommended. At times, cycling of antibiotics may be effective for a longer period of management. Other alternatives are oral nonabsorbable antibiotics for gram-negative bacteria (gentamicin, colistin) and trimethoprim-sulfamethoxazole. In older teenagers, tetracycline or ciprofloxacin may be used. Operative correction of a persistent partial small bowel obstruction is the ideal approach.

320.7 Short Bowel Syndrome

Short bowel syndrome produces malabsorption and malnutrition after congenital or postnatal loss of at least 50% of the small bowel, with or without loss of a portion of the large intestine. Traditional teaching is that the presence of a functioning ileocecal valve appears to have a prognostic value in short bowel syndrome. An infant with as little as 15 cm of bowel with an ileocecal valve, or 20 cm without, has the potential to survive and eventually to be weaned from total parenteral nutrition (TPN). These numbers are only applicable to the patients who had their resection as neonates. Older children can also adapt in spite of significant intestinal resection. The advances in TPN and better understanding of this condition have made predicting outcomes more difficult.

Short bowel results in inadequate absorptive surface and compromised bowel function. The condition may not be permanent because the intestine has the capacity for adaptive growth and increase in functional capacity. Adaptation is a gradual process associated with increase in villus height and small bowel surface, rather than lengthening of the bowel.

The small intestine may be congenitally short in conditions in which bowel is lost in utero (malrotation, gastroschisis, and, in some cases, atresia). Multiple atresias may be the result of anomalies in the superior mesenteric artery, and these produce an "apple peel" deformity of the small bowel. Most cases involve some surgical resection of the small intestine. Most occur in the neonatal period (necrotizing enterocolitis), although Crohn disease or trauma can account for later onset.

Clinical Manifestations. The major clinical manifestations are malabsorption and diarrhea. The ability to assimilate nutrients correlates with the length and location as well as the quality of the residual bowel. Carbohydrate malabsorption and steatorrhea are common features resulting in diarrhea and failure to thrive. Large volumes of fluid and electrolyte are normally secreted into the upper gastrointestinal tract and must be reabsorbed. The capacity to reabsorb fluid and electrolyte is usually inadequate in the short bowel syndrome and results in loss from the gastrointestinal tract with the potential for dehydration, hyponatremia, hypokalemia, and acidosis. The extent of loss is influenced by the presence or absence of the colon in continuity with the small bowel. Trace elements are also poorly absorbed and are lost in excess. D-Lactic acidosis may occur rarely as a result of fermentation of dietary carbohydrate by luminal bacteria in the small bowel caused by bacterial overgrowth. Patients with this manifestation experience confusion, hyperventilation, and acidosis with an anion gap in the absence of elevated serum lactate as measured by standard techniques, which measure L-lactate. Rapid enantiomeric differentiation of urinary metabolites can help diagnose D-lactic acidosis. Routine qualitative urinary organic acid analysis may reveal increased excretion of lactate, 3-hydroxypropionate, phenylacetate, and 4-hydroxyphenylacetate, which is a urinary pattern, found in bacterial overgrowth syndrome. Hypersecretion of acid in the stomach occurs as a result of hypergastrinemia for a transient period after small bowel resection. However, this condition does not appear to cause problems in infants and children. These patients often have associated cholestasis resulting from hyperalimentation and other factors. Cholestasis may contribute to ongoing malabsorption of fat and fat-soluble vitamins and lead to cirrhosis.

Treatment. More than 90% survive. The use of parenteral nutrition dramatically improves the outcome. These infants cannot maintain adequate nutrition by the enteral route alone and initially must have most of their nutrition given intravenously. Very small amounts of enteral nutrients are given at first as a continuous gastric infusion (1–5 mL/hr depending on the size of the infant). Usually an elemental diet is used at regular strength (20 kcal/oz). Exposure to enteral nutrients contributes to adaptive growth of the small bowel. As tolerated, the quantity can be slowly advanced, perhaps by 1–2 mL/hr/24 hr, as the amount of parenteral nutrition is simultaneously decreased. A level is reached at which diarrhea and malabsorption increase, and progression of enteral feedings must be delayed. Although the residual small bowel length remains an important predictor of duration of TPN, other factors such as the early introduction of maternal breast milk or amino acid–based formula are important in intestinal adaptation. The use of breast milk has correlated with shorter use of TPN. Breast milk contains high levels of IgA, nucleotides, and leukocytes that may enhance the protective mechanisms of the bowel. Other beneficial components of breast milk include long-chain fats, epidermal growth factor, growth hormone, glutamine, and free amino acids.

Bloody diarrhea secondary to patchy, mild colitis may develop during the progression of enteral feedings. The pathogenesis of this "feeding colitis" is unknown, but it is usually benign. It may respond to a hypoallergenic diet or to sulfasalazine. Strictures after neonatal necrotizing enterocolitis may also produce bloody stools (see Chapter 91.2).

When possible, an infant may be given a small amount of formula by mouth to maintain an interest in oral feeding and minimize or avoid the development of oral aversions. As children age beyond the 1st year, it is sometimes possible to add a small amount of solids by mouth (cereal, pureed chicken). For infants with an extremely short bowel, it may take several years or more until parenteral nutrition can be stopped.

Certain factors appear to influence the length of time until a child is independent of parenteral nutrition. Infants with less than 40 cm of small bowel take twice as long as infants with 40–80 cm of bowel (average of slightly more than 2 yr versus slightly more than 1 yr). The absence of an ileocecal valve doubles the time to complete adaptation, all other factors being equal. The length of residual ileum is inversely correlated with the time until adaptation. The presence of the ileocecal valve is not always associated with better outcome than is the absence of the valve. A better outcome is associated with breast milk, amino acid–based formula, percentage of kilocalories taken enterally by 6 wk of life, and residual small bowel length at the time of surgery. Identification of small bowel bacterial overgrowth has been associated with prolonged dependence on parenteral nutrition.

Bacterial overgrowth is common in infants with a short bowel and may delay progression of enteral feedings (see Chapter 320.6). Metronidazole is used empirically, as are nonabsorbable antibiotics that cover anaerobic and gram-negative bacteria. Occasionally, a drug that slows gastrointestinal motility, such as loperamide, can be helpful. However, these drugs often do not appear to alter the course. When the small bowel is in continuity with the colon, bile acid malabsorption can cause colonic fluid secretion. In this situation, cholestyramine, 0.25–1 g every 6–8 hr, may be helpful in reducing the watery diarrhea.

Long-Term Complications. Long-term complications include those of parenteral nutrition: central catheter infection, thrombosis, hepatotoxicity, and gallstones. For this reason, a continual effort to advance enteral feedings slowly but aggressively must be considered. Enteral nutrition, even in small amounts, is extremely important in not only promoting intestinal adaptation but also preventing or minimizing the numerous complications associated with long-term TPN. Other long-term complications of short bowel include the potential for late vitamin B_{12} deficiency. Stores of vitamin B_{12} acquired in utero are so great that deficiency may not appear until 1–2 yr of age. Therefore, it is important to periodically check vitamin B_{12} levels during and after the 1st yr of life. Gallstones are found in 60% of infants receiving chronic parenteral nutrition who had had terminal ileal resection but in none of the children with an intact ileum. Renal stones can occur as a result of hyperoxaluria secondary to steatorrhea (calcium binds to the excess fat instead of to oxalate so more oxalate is reabsorbed and excreted in urine). Venous thrombosis and vitamin deficiency have been associated with hyperhomocystinemia in short bowel syndrome.

Future Directions in Management. Certain nutrients have been considered potential stimulants of adaptive growth in experimental animals, but their role in humans remains to be determined. These include glutamine, soluble fiber, short-chain fatty acids, and short-chain triglycerides. Another area of interest is the role of peptide growth factors in promoting adaptive growth of the bowel. Bowel-lengthening surgical procedures have been performed with mixed results. A select group of children with intestinal failure, dependent on TPN, will develop life-threatening complications that would warrant intestinal transplantation. These complications are parenteral nutrition associated liver disease, recurrent events of septicemia, and loss of central vein access. Children with liver dysfunction should be considered for isolated intestinal transplant before terminal damage to the liver occurs. Combined small bowel and liver transplantation can be performed and is a particular consideration for the child with severe TPN hepatotoxicity.

320.8 Gluten-Sensitive Enteropathy (Celiac Disease, Celiac Sprue)

Celiac disease is a disorder in which the proximal small bowel mucosa is damaged as a result of dietary exposure to gluten. It mostly affects people of northern Europe and their descendants in other parts of the world. It is not exclusive in whites because it has been also documented in Hispanics, Indians, Sudanese, Chinese, Afro-Caribbean, and Middle Eastern people. The disorder does not present until gluten products have been introduced into the diet. The most common period of presentation is between 6 mo and 2 yr of age, and it is a permanent intolerance to gluten. Prevalence varies in different regions of the world. The average incidence of celiac disease in Europe is 1 case in every 1,000 live births with a range of 1:250 in Sweden to 1:4,000 in Denmark. In the United Kingdom, the use of serologic screening, followed by diagnostic confirmation with a small bowel biopsy, showed a prevalence of 1:300. In Ireland the prevalence is higher than previously recognized, 1:150. Screening of 2,000 blood donors in the United States found a prevalence of elevated antiendomysial antibodies of 1:250. In Sweden, serologic screening test of a healthy pediatric population 2.5 yr of age, living in a suburban population with high incidence of celiac disease, showed a prevalence of at least 1% and may be as high as 2% counting "silent" celiac disease. These findings suggest that celiac disease may be one of the most common chronic disorders.

Pathogenesis. The disorder develops only after long-term dietary exposure to the protein gluten, which is found in wheat, rye, and barley. The activity of gluten resides in the gliadin fraction, which contains certain repetitious amino acid sequences (motifs) that lead to sensitization of lamina propria lymphocytes. There is a genetic predisposition, as suggested by concordance in monozygotic twins approaching 100%. Two to 5% of 1st-degree relatives have symptomatic gluten-sensitive enteropathy, and as many as 10% of first-degree relatives have asymptomatic damage to small bowel mucosa consistent with this disorder. The disorder is associated with major histocompatibility complex class II alleles DQA1*0501 and DQB1*0201. This HLA-DQ2 allelic combination is found in 98% of celiac patients in Northern Europe. In Southern Europe, DQ2 is present in 92% of confirmed celiac disease patients. Celiac disease is associated with certain human leukocyte antigen (HLA) types (B8, DR7, DR3, and DQw2). Even though not all monozygotic twins have 100% concordance, those who are followed develop the disease at a later age. Other genetic influences, not linked to HLA, may be required for the development of the disease given that the rate of discordance in HLA-identical siblings is reported to be 30–50% and the risk in 1st-degree relatives is between 10–20%. It is estimated that around 25% of the normal Northern European population carries DQ2. Environmental factors may also play a role in the expression of this genetic predisposition.

The immunologic response involves the activation of a Th1/Th0 type of inflammatory response by CD4+ gluten-sensitive T cells. The inflammatory response results in villus atrophy, crypt hyperplasia, and damage to the surface epithelium in the small bowel. The injury is greatest in the proximal small bowel and extends distally for a variable distance. The latter observation is undoubtedly the explanation for the variable degree of symptoms and findings of malabsorption among persons with gluten-sensitive enteropathy. Large-scale screening studies in the adult population suggest that the diagnosed celiac population may represent a small fraction of a bigger problem,

the undiagnosed population. The "asymptomatic" form of the disease, with typical serologic markers and histologic findings, may be five to seven times more common than the symptomatic disease. Four categories have been described for the undiagnosed population: (1) *undiagnosed celiac sprue* (these patients have the classic mucosal lesions and clinical symptoms but are undiagnosed); (2) *silent celiac sprue* (small bowel biopsy have characteristic findings but there is absence of clinical symptoms); (3) *latent celiac sprue* (there is genetic susceptibility but patients do not manifest histologic or clinical signs of the disease); and (4) *true normals* (lack genetic susceptibility and show no symptoms or signs of the disease). The intestinal lesion end product results in a decrease in the absorptive and digestive capacity of the small intestinal surface area and a relative increase in immature epithelial cells. Pancreatic secretion is decreased as a result of lowered serum cholecystokinin and secretin levels.

A 33-mer peptide has been identified that may be the primary initiation of the inflammatory response in susceptible individuals. It reacts with transglutaminase and is a potent inducer of gut derived human T-cell lines. If this peptide can be detoxified, an additional therapy may be developed.

Clinical Manifestations. The mode of presentation is variable; most patients present with diarrhea (Table 320–3). Children can have failure to thrive or vomiting as the only manifestation. Perhaps as many as 10% of children referred to endocrinologists for growth retardation without an endocrine or overt gastrointestinal disorder have gluten sensitivity. Anorexia is common and may be the major cause of weight loss or lack of weight gain (see Fig. 320–2). Infants with gluten-sensitive enteropathy are often clingy, irritable, unhappy children who are difficult to comfort. In contrast to infants with cystic fibrosis, they are not interested in food, although this is not always the case. Pallor and abdominal distention are common (see Fig. 320–1). Large, bulky stools suggestive of constipation have been described in some children with this condition. Digital clubbing can occur. An increased prevalence of gluten-sensitive enteropathy has been noted in children with selective IgA deficiency, diabetes mellitus, chronic rheumatoid arthritis, thyroiditis, hypothyroidism, Addison disease, pernicious anemia, alopecia, and Down syndrome. Lymphocytic gastritis occurs in rare children with gluten-sensitive enteropathy. Pancreatic insufficiency is present in about one third of children with newly diagnosed celiac disease, usually resolving within the first months of treatment. Isolated idiopathic transaminasemia without other hepatic or enteric symptoms may be a manifestation of occult celiac disease. Macroamylasemia associated with celiac disease

TABLE 320–3. **Active Childhood Celiac Disease: 42 Cases**

	No. of Patients
Symptoms	
Failure to thrive	36
Diarrhea	30
Irritability	30
Vomiting	24
Anorexia	24
Foul stools	21
Abdominal pain	8
Excessive appetite	6
Rectal prolapse	3
Signs	
Height <25th percentile	30
Body weight <25th percentile	37
Wasted muscles	40
Abdominal distention	33
Edema	14
Finger clubbing	11

and autoimmune thyroiditis has been reported. Ataxia has been described as the most common neurologic manifestation of celiac disease. It is seen in the adult population and presents as gait and limb ataxia due to cerebellar involvement. The gastrointestinal manifestations are negligible, and these patients could fall in the category of latent celiac disease. The ataxia in these patients seems to be a clinical manifestation of an immunologic reaction, with some of these patients having resolution of symptoms after a gluten-free diet. It has been recommended that in patients who present with ataxia, the possibility of celiac disease should be considered. It has not been described in the pediatric population, but it should be considered as a possibility even in childhood. Microcephaly, developmental delay, and areflexia have been described in a 15-mo-old female with celiac disease whose symptoms resolved after a gluten-free diet. Seizures may occur as childhood partial epilepsy with occipital paroxysms. Dermatitis herpetiformis has been associated with celiac disease in that some degree of gluten-sensitive enteropathy is common to both conditions. It manifests as a maculopapular rash localized to the extremities, buttocks, face, neck, and trunk. Oral involvement has been described. It shares the constitutional and gastrointestinal symptoms found with celiac enteropathy. Almost 100% of these patients show patchy small bowel mucosal atrophy and inflammation.

Evaluation. Screening tests for malabsorption are not particularly helpful because results may be normal in a child with gluten-sensitive enteropathy. Anemia and hypoproteinemia may be present. There may be a mild dimorphic anemia; the blood smear may show target cells, Howell-Jolly bodies, Heinz bodies, siderocytes, and irregular and crenated cells with signs of hyposplenism. Splenic atrophy occurs commonly in celiac sprue in the adult. The incidence of iron deficiency with microcytic anemia is variable. Although rare, a macrocytic megaloblastic anemia can occur. Hypoprothrombinemia can occur as a result of malabsorption. Serologic markers include antibodies to gliadin, reticulin, endomysium, and tissue transglutaminase (tTG). The antigliadin antibodies are in the form of IgG and IgA. The sensitivity of IgG and IgA antigliadin antibodies is believed to be 100% and 89%, respectively, in children with celiac disease. The specificity was 95.5% for IgA and 86% for IgG antigliadin antibodies. It is estimated that 2–3% of celiac disease patients are IgA deficient. Antigliadin antibodies can also be present in other conditions such as cow's milk protein enteropathy, Crohn disease, IgA nephropathy eosinophilic enteritis, tropical sprue, and dermatitis herpetiformis. Antiendomysial antibodies (EMAs) also belong to the family of the IgA antibodies. The sensitivity is reported to be nearly 100%, and the specificity is around 98%. The use of the antigliadin antibodies and antiendomysial antibody together in screening of celiac disease patients confers positive and negative predictive values of almost 100%. The antigen for antiendomysial antibody is tissue transglutaminase. An ELISA for both IgA and IgG tTG is an attractive screening test in that it has high specificity and sensitivity equivalent to the antiendomysial test, is easier to standardize, and does not require the use of human or animal tissue. The tTG IgA assay has a specificity of 95–98% and a sensitivity of 92–94%. Patients with celiac disease who are IgA deficient are positive for the IgG tTG ELISA. Tissue transglutaminase is also valuable in screening *asymptomatic* patients who have type 1 diabetes, history of a 1st-degree relative with type 1 diabetes, and a family member with celiac disease. It has a positive predictive value between 70–83% for biopsy evidence of celiac disease. This may identify children who are at risk of developing symptomatic celiac disease and allows early intervention.

The combination of clinical symptoms and serologic markers may suggest the diagnosis of celiac disease, but histologic confirmation is mandatory, because it remains the gold standard. In 1969, the European Society of Pediatric Gastroenterology and Nutrition (ESPGAN) recommended that the diagnosis be confirmed by showing that the small bowel biopsy returned to normal within 1–2 yr after starting a gluten-free diet and then to rechallenge the patient with a gluten diet and repeat the biopsy to demonstrate the return of the intestinal lesion. ESPGAN now recommends the following: For children older than 2 yr, it is not necessary to rechallenge if the gluten-free diet has produced resolution of symptoms and normalized the specific celiac disease serologies (EMAs, Ab to tTG). For children younger than 2 yr, and when the diagnosis is in question, a rechallenge is recommended. In this age group, other conditions can lead to a flattened small bowel mucosa.

Pathology. The diffuse lesion of the upper small intestinal mucosa that characterizes celiac disease is seen on small bowel biopsy. Short, flat villi, deepened crypts, and irregular vacuolated surface epithelium with increased numbers of lymphocytes in the epithelial layer and crypt hyperplasia are seen by light microscopy. Similar abnormalities occur in other conditions, but none is likely to be confused with celiac disease. Infections such as rotavirus enteritis, *Giardia lamblia*, or tropical sprue can cause villus flattening and elongated crypts but not the marked abnormalities of enterocytes. Flat mucosa occurs in kwashiorkor but may represent a response to infestation rather than to undernutrition. Tropical sprue, a poorly understood tropical enteropathy, can cause a lesion that is indistinguishable from that of celiac disease. Some cases of cow's milk protein or soy protein intolerance are associated with lesions similar to those of celiac disease in children. In immune deficiency, eosinophilic gastroenteritis, and autoimmune enteropathy, villi can be partially shortened. Infants with familial enteropathy have short villi, but the crypt dimensions are normal.

Treatment. Treatment requires a lifelong, strict gluten-free diet. All wheat, rye, and barley products should be eliminated from the diet. Counseling from an experienced dietitian should be provided. There is disagreement about the toxicity of oats, and some physicians will allow oats in the diet of the child. A note of caution should be exercised since oats may be processed in the same mill where wheat is processed, leading to contamination. Initially, vitamin and iron supplementation is advisable. National celiac support groups provide much specific information about the gluten content of foods and medications. Processed foods must be considered carefully because they commonly contain some gluten. Gluten-free foods are commercially available. Poor weight gain in the first months after diagnosis may improve with pancreatic enzyme treatment.

Celiac disease can also present as severe diarrhea, weight loss, hypocalcemia, and hypoproteinemia, a condition known as a celiac crisis. Treatment of a celiac crisis is supportive and includes the use of corticosteroids. Osteopenia is a frequent complication of celiac disease, and it is usually reversed with a strict gluten-free diet.

Compliance with a strict gluten-free diet can be followed with the serologic markers. The antibodies will decrease to normal levels on a strict gluten-free diet. Small amounts of gluten in the diet, owing to less than optimal compliance, will result in elevation of tTG in serum.

Prognosis. The clinical response to a gluten-free diet of a child with celiac disease is gratifying. Improvement of mood and appetite is followed by lessening of diarrhea. In most cases, changes occur within 1 wk of starting therapy, but the response may occasionally be delayed. Older patients and extremely ill patients tend to respond slowly, but once in remission the celiac child should be treated as a well child. Teenagers often become noncompliant. Unfortunately, this is an age when the disorder tends to be symptomatically quiescent, and a teenager may believe that the disorder has resolved. Nevertheless, mucosal damage is present. Subtle manifestations of growth failure or delayed sexual maturation may take place when these patients ingest a gluten-containing diet. Appropriately diagnosed gluten-sensitive enteropathy is a lifelong condition requiring lifelong treatment. The development of malignancy secondary to long-standing celiac disease, especially with poor adherence to the strict gluten-free diet, is mostly a problem seen in the adult population. Malignancy affecting the esophagus, stomach, pharynx, and intestines is increased in patients with celiac disease. Intestinal lymphoma occurring in a 10-yr-old child with celiac disease has been reported. The observation that T-cell lymphoma can arise from long-standing celiac disease makes a gluten-free diet the best possible prophylaxis. Strict adherence to a gluten-free diet reduced the risk of all disease-associated cancers, including enteropathy-associated T-cell lymphoma. No complications from long-term gluten-free diet treatment are recognized.

320.9 Immunoproliferative Small Intestinal Disease

Immunoproliferative small intestinal disease (Mediterranean lymphoma) occurs most often in 10–30 yr olds in the Mediterranean basin, Mideast, Far East, and Africa. This is an IgA lymphoproliferative disorder that may progress to a B-cell lymphoma. Poverty and frequent episodes of gastroenteritis during infancy are antecedent social and medical problems. In some areas, as socioeconomic conditions have improved, the incidence of this disorder has decreased. Sporadic cases occur in Europe and North and South America, predominantly in immigrants from developing countries, although occasionally in native citizens. A similar disorder has been described in patients with AIDS.

Clinical Manifestations. Initially, patients have intermittent diarrhea and abdominal pain. Later stages demonstrate persistent chronic diarrhea, malabsorption, protein-losing enteropathy, weight loss, digital clubbing, and growth failure.

Diagnosis. Endoscopic biopsies of multiple duodenal and jejunal mucosal sites aid in the diagnosis. In addition, a serum marker (α heavy-chain paraprotein) of IgA is present in most cases. *Giardia lamblia* may also be present but is not responsible for the lymphoproliferative disorder. Immunosuppressed organ transplant recipients may develop a lymphoproliferative disorder manifesting diarrhea.

Treatment. The earliest lesions respond to prolonged (~6 mo) tetracycline or metronidazole therapy. Prelymphomatous stages and lymphomas are treated with combination chemotherapy. Lymphoproliferative disorders in immunosuppressed transplant recipients usually improve with reduction of the immunosuppressive drug dose.

Prognosis. Early therapy for antibiotic responsive lesions produces an excellent outcome. Treatment of the later lymphomatous lesions has resulted in a variable but usually poor outcome.

320.10 Other Malabsorptive Syndromes

Exocrine Pancreatic Insufficiency. Cystic fibrosis is the most common congenital disorder associated with malabsorption. The next most common cause of pancreatic insufficiency in children, although much rarer, is Shwachman syndrome (see Chapters 330 and 331). Other rare disorders causing exocrine pancreatic insufficiency are Johanson-Blizzard syndrome (severe steatorrhea, aplasia of alae nasi, deafness, hypothyroidism, scalp defects), Pearson bone marrow syndrome (sideroblastic anemia, variable degree of neutropenia, thrombocytopenia), and isolated pancreatic enzyme deficiency (lipase, colipase, trypsinogen, amylase, lipase-colipase).

Intestinal Lymphangiectasia. This group of disorders is characterized by dilatation of intestinal lymphatic vessels and leakage of lymph into the intestinal lumen and, at times, the peritoneal cavity. Because absorbed fat is normally transferred from the intestine through the lymphatic vessels, children with this disorder have steatorrhea with protein-losing enteropathy and may have lymphocyte depletion. Manifestations may include any combination of hypoalbuminemia, hypogammaglobulinemia, edema, lymphocytopenia, fat malabsorption, and chylous ascites. Intestinal lymphangiectasia can be primary or can result from abdominal or thoracic surgical damage to lymphatic vessels, chronic right-sided heart failure, constrictive pericarditis, retroperitoneal tumor, or malrotation with lymphatic obstruction. Primary intestinal lymphangiectasia is the result of a congenital abnormality of lymphatic drainage from the intestine and may be associated with abnormalities in lymphatic drainage from other regions of the body. Turner and Noonan syndromes have been associated with intestinal lymphangiectasia. Congenital intestinal lymphangiectasia in a premature infant presented as the cause of protein-losing enteropathy with hypoalbuminemia and generalized edema. It has also presented as a case of isolated fetal ascites. Intestinal lymphangiectasia should be included in the differential diagnosis when there is a history of peripheral edema and low serum albumin in a premature infant and when fetal ascites has occurred.

A few cases of intestinal B-cell lymphoma have been reported in adult patients with long-standing lymphangiectasia. The lymphoma responds well to surgery and postoperative chemotherapy.

The diagnosis is suggested by the typical findings described previously in association with an elevated fecal α_1-antitrypsin level consistent with protein-losing enteropathy. The characteristic radiologic findings of uniform, symmetric thickening of mucosal folds throughout the small intestine are usually, although not always, present on small bowel contrast radiographs. The diagnosis is confirmed by the presence of collections of abnormal dilated lacteals with distortion of villi on per oral small bowel biopsy. The disorder may be seen only in the submucosa, thus requiring surgical biopsy of the intestine. Treatment is usually dietetic, limiting the amount of long-chain fat in the diet, which is normally absorbed by means of the intestinal lymphatics. This therapy reduces the volume of intestinal lymph and decreases the pressure within the dilated lymphatics. Patients are placed on a low-fat, high-protein, medium-chain triglyceride (MCT) diet. MCTs bypass the enteric lymphatics and directly enter the portal venous system. Special MCT-containing formulas can be used during infancy. Supplementing a low-fat diet with MCT oil used in cooking can be used in older children and adolescents.

Microvillus Inclusion Disease (Congenital Microvillus Atrophy). Diarrheal diseases presenting in the neonatal period are listed in Table 320–4.

Microvillus inclusion disease is a disorder that presents at birth with intractable, secretory, watery diarrhea and severe malabsorption. It appears to be the most common cause of persistent diarrhea that begins in the neonatal period. It has presented prenatally as what appeared to be a bowel obstruction in an ultrasound, with multiple fluid-filled dilated loops of bowel and with polyhydramnios. Postnatally there was no bowel obstruction, and the diagnosis was confirmed by electron microscopy (EM) of a small bowel biopsy.

The disorder seems to be inherited in an autosomal recessive pattern. The findings on small bowel biopsy are the key to the diagnosis and include villus atrophy, crypt hypoplasia, and the specific EM findings of microvillus inclusions (involutions) and increased secretory granules in enterocytes. The EM findings can also be seen in colonocytes. The somatostatin analogue octreotide has been used as treatment and may reduce the

TABLE 320–4. **Diarrheal Diseases Presenting in the Neonatal Period**

Condition	Clinical Features
Congenital microvillus atrophy	Intractable watery diarrhea
Tufting enteropathy	Intractable watery diarrhea
Intractable diarrhea with phenotypic abnormalities	Intractable watery diarrhea Low birth weight
Congenital glucose-galactose malabsorption	Acidic diarrhea
Congenital lactase deficiency	Acidic diarrhea
Congenital chloride diarrhea	Hydramnios, intractable watery diarrhea
Congenital defective jejunal Na^+/H^+ exchange	Hydramnios, intractable watery diarrhea
Congenital bile acid malabsorption	Steatorrhea
Congenital enterokinase deficiency	Failure to thrive, edema

Adapted from Schmitz J: Maldigestion and malabsorption. In Walker WA, Durie PR, Hamilton JR, et al (editors): Pediatric Gastrointestinal Disease, 3rd ed. Hamilton, Ontario, BC Decker, 2000, p 55.

volume of stool output in some infants. Epidermal growth factor has been used with equivocal results. The disease is fatal without long-term TPN. Even so, most children die in infancy or early childhood. Intestinal transplantation has become the only definitive treatment of this rare disease. A hepatic adenoma has been reported in a 14-yr-old patient with microvillous inclusion disease on life-long TPN. The patient eventually had a right hepatic lobectomy. There was a large 5 × 6-cm adenoma and six tiny 0.4–2.0 cm adenomas. Interestingly, liver histopathology revealed no significant fibrosis and no evidence of TPN liver disease in the noninvolved liver.

Autoimmune Enteropathy. Autoimmune enteropathy is a poorly characterized syndrome of chronic diarrhea and malabsorption. If symptoms initially develop after the first 6 mo of life, the disorder is likely to be mistaken for gluten-sensitive enteropathy. Typically, the lack of response to a gluten-free diet leads to further evaluation. Histologic findings in the small bowel include partial or complete villous atrophy, crypt hyperplasia, and an increase in chronic inflammatory cells in the lamina propria. Specific serum antienterocyte antibodies may be identified in 50% or more of patients by indirect immunofluorescent staining of normal small bowel mucosa and the kidney. The colon can also be involved. Extraintestinal autoimmune disorders are usual and include arthritis, membranous glomerulonephritis, insulin-dependent diabetes, thrombocytopenia, autoimmune hepatitis, hypothyroidism, and hemolytic anemia. Treatment has included prednisone, azathioprine, cyclophosphamide (Cytoxan), cyclosporine, and tacrolimus.

Tufting Enteropathy. Tufting enteropathy (intestinal epithelial dysplasia) is a disorder that presents in the first weeks of life with persistent watery diarrhea and appears to account for a small fraction of infants with protracted diarrhea of infancy. Onset of symptoms is not immediately after birth as in microvillus inclusion disease. On small bowel biopsy, the distinctive feature is that 80–90% of the epithelial surface contains focal epithelial "tufts" (teardrop-shaped groups of closely packed enterocytes with apical rounding of the plasma membrane). In other known enteropathies, tufts are seen on 15% or less of the epithelial surface. In this disorder, colonic epithelium shows no abnormality. On electron microscopy of small bowel epithelium, the major finding is shortening of the microvilli. This does not appear to be an autoimmune enteropathy, and no known enteropathogens have been isolated. The intestinal lesion has not responded to removal of dietary antigens or use of immunosuppressive therapy. This may be a disorder of cell-cell and cell matrix interactions. This neonatal diarrhea that resists all treatments requires permanent parenteral nutrition; it is another indication for intestinal transplantation.

Endocrine Disorders. Steatorrhea may occur with a number of endocrine disorders, including adrenal insufficiency, hypoparathyroidism, and diabetes mellitus.

Tropical Sprue. This syndrome is characterized by generalized malabsorption associated with a diffuse lesion of the small intestinal mucosa that occurs only in persons who have lived in or visited certain tropical regions. The disease is rare in children. Tropical sprue is endemic in numerous locales in the tropics extending from the equator to both the north and south slightly more than 30° latitude to include the Caribbean, India, and southern Africa. The disease is particularly present in Cuba, the Dominican Republic, Haiti, and Puerto Rico, yet it has not been observed in Jamaica. It has also been well described in Colombia and Venezuela. Perhaps the most extensive documentation of tropical sprue has been that in India. Besides occurring in indigenous populations, tropical sprue is contracted by those who visit the tropics for a month or longer. Although most cases tend to arise sporadically in endemic form, a significant proportion of individuals in the tropical regions (5–10%) may contract the disease. Epidemics have been reported, particularly from India, and are said to occur as a sequela of an outbreak of acute diarrheal disease. The available evidence suggests that this disorder is an infectious disease resulting from persistent contamination of the small bowel by strains of *Klebsiella pneumoniae*, or less often by *Escherichia coli* or *Enterobacter cloacae*. Their eradication by antimicrobial therapy cures the intestinal abnormalities. Fever and malaise precede the onset of watery diarrhea. In about 1 wk, acute features subside and chronic malabsorption, intermittent diarrhea, and anorexia lead eventually to severe malnutrition. Signs of malnutrition may include night blindness, glossitis, stomatitis, cheilosis, hyperpigmentation, and edema. Muscle wasting is marked, and the abdomen is often distended. Patients have evidence of diffuse malabsorption, abnormal exocrine pancreatic function contributing to the steatorrhea, and carbohydrate intolerance. Megaloblastic anemia is the result of folate and vitamin B_{12} deficiencies. Small bowel biopsy abnormalities are more prominent in the jejunum than in the ileum early on, but subsequently the entire bowel is affected (unlike in celiac disease). Histology is similar to celiac disease, but completely flat mucosa is observed in only 10% of cases. There are reports of a thickened basement membrane and the accumulation of triglycerides subjacent to the surface epithelium. This feature is quite typical and differs from the intraenterocyte accumulation of lipid droplets observed in celiac disease and in patients with marasmus or kwashiorkor. Treatment includes folate and vitamin B_{12} therapy. To reverse all aspects of the malabsorption syndrome and prevent recurrence requires 6 months of therapy with oral folic acid (5 mg) and tetracycline or sulfonamides. Relapses, requiring additional courses of therapy, will occur in 10–20% of patients who continue to reside in an endemic tropical region.

Wolman Disease. This rare lethal lipid storage disease leads to lipid accumulation in many organs, including the small intestine. In addition to vomiting, severe diarrhea, and hepatosplenomegaly, patients may have steatorrhea as the result of lymphatic obstruction. Deficiency of lysosomal acid lipase is the cause of the disease (see Chapter 75). Successful long-term bone marrow engraftment has resulted in the normalization of peripheral leukocyte lysosomal acid lipase enzyme activity with subsequent resolution of the diarrhea and restoration of developmental milestones.

320.11 Enzyme Deficiencies

Enterokinase Deficiency. Congenital deficiency of this small intestinal enzyme has been reported in a few children. The disease results in a complete absence of pancreatic proteolytic activity because enterokinase is an essential activator of pancreatic trypsinogens. Affected patients are ill from very early life with severe diarrhea and failure to thrive. Hypoproteinemia is common and may lead to edema. In duodenal fluid, tryptic activity is missing, whereas lipase and amylase are normal; in vitro tryptic activity of the fluid can be restored by the addition of enterokinase. Malabsorption of protein is the major defect, although mild steatorrhea has been reported. Pancreatic enzyme replacements restore normal digestive function; much smaller amounts are needed compared with those required for pancreatic insufficiency.

Disaccharidase Deficiencies. The disaccharidases are located on the brush border membrane surface of the small bowel. Occasionally, congenital deficiencies occur, but abnormal disaccharidase activities in infants and young children have most often been the result of diffuse acquired lesions of the intestinal epithelium, such as those of infection or celiac disease. In older children and adults, late-onset genetic lactase deficiency is the most common condition associated with reduced disaccharidase activity.

The *clinical manifestations* of significant disaccharidase deficiency (disaccharide intolerance) are similar whatever its cause or the enzymes involved. If disaccharide hydrolysis at the brush border is incomplete, the sugar accumulates in the distal intestinal lumen, where organic acids and hydrogen gas are produced by bacteria. The excess intraluminal sugar and organic acids draw water into the lumen, leading to watery osmotic diarrhea with stools that are of low pH (pH < 5.6), contain excess sugar, and tend to excoriate the buttocks. Patients may have bloating and borborygmi, but steatorrhea is rare. In some cases, particularly those beyond infancy, gas production causing crampy abdominal pain is the dominant problem, rather than diarrhea.

If the disaccharide involved is a reducing sugar (lactose), the standard Clinitest examination will be 2+ or greater in most cases. Disaccharidase activities can be assayed in mucosal biopsy specimens. Breath hydrogen excretion after an oral sugar load is a useful noninvasive technique for detecting disaccharide intolerance (see Chapter 320.1).

Lactase Deficiency. *Congenital* absence of lactase has been reported in a few cases. The usual mechanism for primary lactose intolerance relates to the *developmental* pattern of lactase activity. Because lactase activity rises relatively late in fetal life and begins to fall after the age of 3 yr, intolerance to lactose can be anticipated in extremely premature infants and in some older children and adults. Approximately 15% of adult whites, 40% of adult Asians, and 85% of adult blacks in the United States are deficient in intestinal lactase; this is known as "adult-onset hypolactasia" and is an autosomal recessive characteristic. Because lactase activity in the mucosa is at best marginal, this enzyme is particularly likely to be depleted *secondary to diffuse mucosal diseases.*

Clinical manifestations occur in response to ingestion of lactose, the sugar in milk. Explosive watery diarrhea is associated with abdominal distention, borborygmi, flatulence, and an excoriated diaper area. A syndrome of recurrent, vague, crampy abdominal pain has also been attributed to lactose intolerance. School-aged and preschool-aged children experience episodic mid-abdominal pain. Usually, their general health is unaffected, and they may have no obvious temporal relationship of pain or diarrhea with milk ingestion.

Treatment consists of removal of milk from the diet. In most cases the elimination need not be total; stopping ingestion of milk as a beverage is important. A lactase preparation is available in prepackaged milk with 100% of the lactose predigested; it allows asymptomatic consumption of modest quantities of milk incubated with the added enzyme. A tablet with lactase activity can also be ingested with meals. Live culture yogurt con-

tains bacteria that produce lactase enzyme and is, thus, frequently tolerated by lactase-deficient individuals.

Sucrase-Isomaltase Deficiency. The only relatively common congenital deficiency of disaccharidase activities, a combined deficiency of sucrase and isomaltase, is inherited as an autosomal recessive trait and has been mapped to chromosome 3. Prevalence is the highest in the native populations of Alaska, Canada, and Greenland. It occurs in about 0.2% of North Americans. Symptoms usually begin when a sucrose or glucose polymer-containing diet is started. Patients may be intolerant to starch, but because isomaltase acts only on the branch points of the starch molecule, isomaltase deficiency itself is relatively asymptomatic. The symptoms are bloating, watery diarrhea, and failure to thrive. Recurrent abdominal pain has not been attributed to sucrose-isomaltose intolerance. Because sucrose is not a reducing sugar, its presence is not detected in the stool by Clinitest unless the specimen is first hydrolyzed with hydrochloric acid. The morphologic features of the small intestinal mucosa are normal, but enzyme assays show specific deficiencies of sucrase and isomaltase with normal levels of lactase and maltase. Breath testing usually demonstrates increased hydrogen gas after sucrose ingestion. Affected patients improve quickly after dietary sucrose is reduced to minimal amounts.

Oral replacement of genetically determined sucrase deficiency, which is part of congenital sucrase isomaltase deficiency (CSID) is available as Sucraid (sacrosidase), an oral solution, which is the only therapy approved by the U.S. Food and Drug Administration.

Sacrosidase significantly decreased breath H_2 excretion in CSID patients. Higher concentrations of sacrosidase were associated with fewer stools, fewer symptoms of gas, abdominal cramps, and bloating compared with lower concentrations and with placebo. Sacrosidase is safe and effective in preventing gastrointestinal symptoms in patients with CSID consuming a normal diet.

320.12 Defects of Absorption or Transport

Glucose-Galactose Malabsorption. More than 30 different mutations of the sodium/glucose co-transporter gene *(SGLT1)* have been identified to cause this rare autosomal recessive, congenital disorder of intestinal glucose-galactose absorption. *SGLT1* couples glucose and galactose transport to the sodium gradients across intestinal and renal brush borders. Renal tubular epithelium is affected to a lesser degree. The identification of mutations of *SGLT1* makes it possible to carry out prenatal screening in families at risk for the disease.

The selective defect in the intestinal glucose and galactose/Na$^+$ co-transport systems leads to osmotic diarrhea, which follows the ingestion of glucose, breast milk, or conventional formulas soon after birth, because most dietary sugars are polysaccharides or disaccharides with glucose or galactose moieties. The patient may be bloated; and, if diarrhea persists, dehydration and acidosis can be severe, resulting in death. The stools are acidic and contain sugar. Patients with the defect have normal absorption of fructose; their small bowel function and structure are normal in all other aspects. Intermittent or permanent glycosuria after fasting or after a glucose load is a frequent finding. Thus, the finding of positive reducing substances in watery stools and slight glycosuria despite low blood sugar levels is highly suggestive of glucose-galactose malabsorption. Malabsorption of glucose and galactose is easily identified using the breath hydrogen test. It is safe to perform the first test with a dose of 0.5 gm/kg of glucose; if necessary, a second test can be performed using 2 g/kg. Breath H_2 will rise more than 20 ppm if a patient has this defect. The diagnosis can be confirmed later by small intestinal biopsy showing (1) normal villous architecture, (2) normal disaccharidase activities, and (3) an absorptive defect confined to glucose and galactose. *Treatment* consists of rigorous restriction of glucose and galactose. Fructose, the only carbohydrate that can be given safely, should be added to a carbohydrate free formula at a concentration of 6–8%. Diarrhea immediately ceases when infants are given such a formula. Although the defect is permanent, later in life limited amounts of glucose (e.g., in starches) or sucrose may be tolerated.

Severe diffuse mucosal damage, particularly in a young infant, may also impair the glucose-galactose carrier sufficiently to cause intolerance to these sugars. Usually, if mucosal damage is severe enough to impair glucose transport, other absorptive processes are affected.

Abetalipoproteinemia (see Chapter 75.3). This rare autosomal recessive disorder of lipoprotein metabolism is associated with severe fat malabsorption from birth. Children fail to thrive during the 1st yr of life, and their stools are pale, foul smelling, and bulky. The abdomen is distended, and deep tendon reflexes are absent as a result of peripheral neuropathy.

Intellectual development tends to be slow. After 10 yr of age, intestinal symptoms are less severe, ataxia develops, and one sees a loss of position and vibration senses and the onset of intention tremors. These last symptoms reflect involvement of the posterior columns, cerebellum, and basal ganglia. In adolescence, atypical retinitis pigmentosa develops.

Diagnosis rests on finding acanthocytes in the peripheral blood and extremely low plasma levels of cholesterol (<50 mg/dL); triglycerides are very low (<20 mg/dL). Chylomicrons and very-low-density lipoproteins are not detectable, and the low-density lipoprotein (LDL) fraction is virtually absent from the circulation; marked triglyceride accumulation in villus enterocytes occurs in the fasting duodenal mucosa. Usually, steatorrhea occurs in younger patients but other processes of assimilation are intact. Rickets may be an unusual initial manifestation of abetalipoproteinemia and hypobetalipoproteinemia. Rickets is caused by steatorrhea-induced calcium losses. Patients have mutations of the microsomal triglyceride transfer protein (MTP) gene, resulting in absence of MTP function in the small bowel. This protein is required for normal assembly and secretion of very-low-density lipoproteins and chylomicrons. The neuropathy is the result of vitamin E deficiency.

Specific *treatment* is not available. Large supplements of the fat-soluble vitamins A, D, E, and K should be given. Vitamin E (100–200 mg/kg/24 hr) and vitamin A (10,000–25,000 IU/day) may arrest the neurologic and retinal degeneration. Limiting long-chain fat intake may alleviate intestinal symptoms; medium-chain triglycerides can be used to supplement the fat intake.

Homozygous Hypobetalipoproteinemia. This disorder is transmitted as an autosomal dominant trait; the homozygous form is indistinguishable from abetalipoproteinemia. However, the parents of these patients, as heterozygotes, have reduced plasma low-density lipoprotein and apoprotein-β concentrations, unlike the parents of patients with abetalipoproteinemia, who have normal levels. On EM of small bowel biopsies, the general size of the lipid vacuoles can differentiate between abetalipoproteinemia and hypobetalipoproteinemia: many small vacuoles are present in hypobetalipoproteinemia, and large vacuoles are seen in abetalipoproteinemia.

Chylomicron Retention Disease. In this rare recessive disorder, the processes leading up to the release of chylomicrons from enterocytes appear to be defective. These patients have severe intestinal symptoms with steatorrhea, chronic diarrhea, and failure to thrive. Acanthocytosis is rare, and neurologic manifestations are less severe than those observed in abetalipoproteinemia. Plasma cholesterol levels are reduced, but moderately so

(<75 mg/dL); fasting triglycerides are normal; but the fat-soluble vitamins, particularly A and E, rapidly deplete. Early aggressive therapy with fat-soluble vitamins and modification of dietary fat intake is indicated, identical to the treatment for abetalipoproteinemia.

Amino Acid Transport Defects. In several of the specific congenital disorders of amino acid transport (see Chapter 74), defective intestinal amino acid transport occurs. At least three specific small bowel carriers appear to be involved in active transport of amino acids. Amino acid uptake into the intestinal mucosa is defective in *cystinuria,* but these patients have no gastrointestinal symptoms. In *Hartnup disease,* malabsorption of neutral amino acids including tryptophan leads to ataxia, intellectual deterioration, a pellagra-like rash, and, at times, diarrhea. The clinical manifestations are due to the malabsorption of tryptophan, producing nicotinamide deficiency. Administration of nicotinamide, given orally, leads to a dramatic clinical improvement. *Methionine malabsorption* is associated with episodes of diarrhea in fair-complexioned, retarded children whose urine has a sweet odor and contains excess β-hydroxybutyric acid. In the *blue diaper syndrome,* tryptophan absorption is defective.

Vitamin B$_{12}$ Malabsorption. Causes of vitamin B$_{12}$ deficiency fall into three categories: (1) decreased intake (e.g., breast-fed babies whose mothers have undiagnosed vitamin B$_{12}$ deficiency because of strict vegetarian diets); (2) abnormal absorption (e.g., absence/dysfunction of intrinsic factor [past gastric resection, autoimmune pernicious anemia]; decreased gastric acid secretion secondary to H$_2$ receptor antagonists, proton-pump inhibitors; competition for B$_{12}$ in the intestine [bacterial overgrowth]; disruption of absorption across the ileal surface [Crohn disease, tropical sprue]); and (3) inborn errors of vitamin B$_{12}$ transport and metabolism.

Several rare congenital defects may affect assimilation of vitamin B$_{12}$. These conditions are much less common than dietary vitamin B$_{12}$ deficiency or malabsorption secondary to terminal ileal resection or dysfunction. In *juvenile pernicious anemia,* intrinsic factor production in the stomach is defective. Vitamin B$_{12}$ malabsorption results, leading to megaloblastic anemia and growth failure. Gastric structure and function are otherwise normal.

Transcobalamin II deficiency is an inherited defect of a protein necessary for intestinal transport of vitamin B$_{12}$. The result is severe megaloblastic anemia, diarrhea, and vomiting.

Imerslund syndrome occurs in patients in whom ileal absorption of vitamin B$_{12}$ is defective. Ileal structure and function are otherwise normal. Megaloblastic anemia develops toward the end of the 1st yr. Proteinuria is commonly associated.

Treatment of these disorders is to administer vitamin B$_{12}$ by injection: 1,000 μg/twice weekly for transcobalamin II deficiency and 100 μg/mo for the others. Once patients are in hematologic remission after intramuscular vitamin B$_{12}$ therapy, they can receive *intranasal* vitamin B$_{12}$, 500 μg, in once weekly metered doses.

Congenital Malabsorption of Folic Acid. Isolated congenital folate malabsorption, described in fewer than 20 patients, may be the consequence of a selective defect in intestinal and blood-brain barrier folate transport. Inheritance studies suggest an autosomal recessive disorder.

The main constant clinical feature is severe megaloblastic anemia that may begin by the age of 3 mo. Neurologic symptoms may include ataxia, convulsions, mental retardation, and intracranial calcifications. Gastrointestinal symptoms may present in the 1st week of life and include mouth ulcers, diarrhea, and failure to thrive. Diagnosis is made by lack of an increase in serum or cerebrospinal fluid (CSF) folate after a loading test with oral folic acid (5 mg). Early and aggressive use of parenteral folinic acid is the treatment of choice, and documentation of improvement of CSF folate is critical if a good outcome is possible. Subsequent treatment, aimed at maintaining levels of folate in serum, red blood cells, and CSF, is by using large (up to 100 mg/day) oral doses of folic, folinic, or methyltetrahydrofolic acid.

Chloride-Losing Diarrhea. This rare recessive inherited disorder caused by mutations in a chromosome 7 gene, first known as *DRA* (for Down Regulated in Adenoma), involves an abnormality of the chloride/bicarbonate transport mechanism in the cell surface. This congenital defect of distal ileal and colonic chloride transport is associated with maternal polyhydramnios. The dominant symptom is severe watery diarrhea beginning at birth, the result of accumulation of chloride ion in the intestinal lumen. Watery diarrhea leads to dehydration and a severe electrolyte disturbance characterized by hypokalemia, hypochloremia, and alkalosis, a most unusual pattern for a child with chronic diarrhea. Other aspects of intestinal absorption are normal. Stools contain chloride in excess of the sum of sodium and potassium (125–150 mEq/L). Treatment does not alter diarrhea but diminishes complications. All losses of electrolytes and water are replaced intravenously at first; oral solutions are usually tolerated after a month. If the diagnosis is made early in the neonatal period and adequate therapy started immediately, the affected infant will show perfect growth and development.

Congenital Sodium Diarrhea. A few patients have been described with profuse watery, secretory diarrhea from birth. There was maternal polyhydramnios and neonatal abdominal distention; however, unlike chloride diarrhea, this condition was characterized by acidosis and fecal chloride concentration less than sodium concentration (as high as 145 mEq/L). *Treatment* with oral hydration solution was effective in maintaining normal growth. The apparent basis for this rare syndrome is a defect in sodium-hydrogen exchange in the small intestine and colon.

Vitamin D–Dependent Rickets. In this autosomal recessive disorder, a specific defect in the metabolism of vitamin D causes malabsorption of calcium (see Chapter 697). Intestinal function is otherwise normal.

Primary Hypomagnesemia. This specific intestinal transport defect in magnesium transport causes severe hypomagnesemia and, secondarily, hypocalcemic tetany in infancy. Other aspects of intestinal function are normal. The findings are reversed by large supplements of magnesium, which must be continued indefinitely.

Acrodermatitis Enteropathica (see also Chapter 649). This unusual constellation of clinical findings is due to zinc deficiency secondary to zinc malabsorption. Early in life, the patient experiences rashes around mucocutaneous junctions and on the extremities; alopecia, chronic diarrhea, and sometimes steatorrhea may occur. If not treated, the patient fails to thrive. Serum zinc concentration and alkaline phosphatase activity are low. Intestinal mucosal biopsy specimens show Paneth cell inclusions that disappear after treatment. An oral supplement of zinc sulfate, 1–2 mg elemental zinc/kg/24 hr, causes rapid healing of the skin lesions and improvement of diarrhea.

Menkes (Kinky Hair) Syndrome. This rare recessively inherited disorder is characterized by growth retardation, abnormal hair, cerebellar degeneration, severe vasculopathy, fractures, and early death (see Chapter 592.5). Orally ingested copper accumulates in the intestines, and there is defective copper absorption. Its pathogenesis is unclear, but a widespread defect in cellular copper transport affects the intestine as well as other tissues. There is decrease of the cuproenzyme activities. The blood, liver, and brain are deprived of copper and, thus, are in a state of copper deficiency. Serum copper and ceruloplasmin levels are low, but cellular copper content is increased. The currently accepted treatment is the administration of parenteral copper; few patients avoid the neurologic sequelae.

Bile Acid Malabsorption. Primary bile acid malabsorption caused by mutations in the ileal sodium-dependent bile acid transporter gene results in diarrhea and steatorrhea from early infancy. These patients have reduced plasma cholesterol levels and severe growth retardation as well.

Drug-Induced Absorptive Defects. Some drugs have a diffuse impact on the small intestinal epithelium. For example, methotrexate can cause arrest of enterocyte mitoses and can result in a mucosal lesion; large doses of neomycin also affect mucosal structure. *Sulfasalazine* interferes with folic acid absorption. *Cholestyramine* binds bile salts and calcium in the intestinal lumen to cause hypocalcemia and steatorrhea. *Phenytoin* interferes with calcium absorption and can cause rickets.

Enterocyte Heparan Sulfate Deficiency and the Carbohydrate-Deficient Glycoprotein Syndrome. Congenital enterocyte heparan deficiency (CEHD) is a rare cause of intractable diarrhea with protein-losing enteropathy. Heparan sulfate is a glycosaminoglycan; such glycosaminoglycans have multiple roles within the intestine, including restriction of charged macromolecules, such as albumin, within the vascular lumen.

CEHD may be an unusual presentation of the carbohydrate deficient glycosylation syndrome (CDGS) type 1 (also known as Jaeken syndrome) (see Chapter 76.6). This latter condition in which glycan chain formation is impaired can be detected by aberrant glycosylation of serum transferrin. The disorder normally presents as mental retardation, but there is a highly variable phenotype. CDGS is usually accompanied by severe neurologic abnormalities (hypotonia, muscular weakness, developmental retardation). Blood coagulation disorders are a common feature of CDGS type 1a. One child with CDGS type 1b had no neurodevelopmental problems but rather predominantly intestinal problems (protein-losing enteropathy). She responded to oral mannose treatment, whereas other forms of CDGS have no known treatment. Any child with unexplained protein-losing enteropathy, or when there is an abnormality in another system (e.g., severe neurodevelopmental delay; altered blood clotting parameters), should have transferrin glycosylation checked.

Malabsorption Syndromes

Branski D, Lerner A, Lebenthal E: Chronic diarrhea and malabsorption. *Pediatr Clin North Am* 1996;43:307.

Hill RE, Hercz A, Corey MD, et al: Fecal clearance of alpha-1-antitrypsin: A reliable measure of protein loss in children. *J Pediatr* 1981;99:416.

Huynh H, Couper R: Pancreatic function tests. In Walker A (editor): *Pediatric Gastrointestinal Disease*, 3rd ed. Hamilton, Ontario, BC Decker, 2000, pp 1515–1528.

Jamieson D, Stringer D: Small bowel. In Stringer D, Babyn P (editors): *Pediatric Gastrointestinal Imaging and Intervention*, 2nd ed. Hamilton, Ontario, BC Decker, 2000, p 409.

Khouri M, Huang G, Shiau Y: Sudan stain of fecal fat: New insight into an old test. *Gastroenterology* 1989;96:421.

Kleinman RE, Klish W, Lebenthal E, et al: Role of juice carbohydrate malabsorption in chronic nonspecific diarrhea in children. *J Pediatr* 1992;120:825.

Murphy MS, Eastham EJ, Nelson R, et al: Non-invasive assessment of intraluminal lipolysis using a $^{13}CO_2$ breath test. *Arch Dis Child* 1990;65:574.

Riby JE, Fujisawa T, Kretchmer N: Fructose absorption. *Am J Clin Nutr* 1993;58:748S.

Riddlesberger MM: Evaluation of the gastrointestinal tract in the child: CT, MRI, and isotopic studies. *Pediatr Clin North Am* 1988;35:281.

Shams T, Ingram M: Malabsorption and malnutrition. *Prim Care Clin Office Pract* 2001;28:505–22.

Digestive Tract in Chronic Malnutrition

Durie PR, Forstner GG, Gaskin KJ, et al: Elevated serum immunoreactive pancreatic cationic trypsinogen in acute malnutrition: Evidence of pancreatic damage. *J Pediatr* 1985;106:233.

Romer H, Cerbach R, Gomez MA, et al: Moderate and severe protein-energy malnutrition in childhood: Effects on jejunal mucosal morphology and disaccharidase activities. *J Pediatr Gastroenterol Nutr* 1983;2:459.

Liver and Biliary Disorders

Argao EA, Heubi JE: Fat-soluble vitamin deficiency in infants and children. *Curr Opin Pediatr* 1993;5:562.

Hadorn B, Hess J, Troesch V, et al: Role of bile acids in the activation of trypsinogen by enterokinase: Disturbance of trypsinogen activation in patients with intrahepatic biliary atresia. *Gastroenterology* 1974;66:548.

Kooh SW, Jones G, Reilly BJ, et al: Pathogenesis of rickets in chronic hepatobiliary disease in children. *J Pediatr* 1979;94:870.

Short Bowel Syndrome

Andorsky D, Lund D, Lillehei C, et al: Nutritional and other postoperative management of neonates with short bowel syndrome correlates with outcomes. *J Pediatr* 2001;139:27–31.

Bines J, Francis D, Hill D, et al: Reducing parenteral requirement in children with short bowel syndrome: Impact of an amino acid-based complete infant formula. *J Pediatr Gastroenterol Nutr* 1998;26:123.

Caniano DA, Kanoti GA: Newborns with massive intestinal loss: Difficult choices. *N Engl J Med* 1988;318:703.

Compher C: Hyperhomocysteinemia is associated with venous thrombosis in patients with short bowel syndrome. *J Parenter Enteral Nutr* 2001;25:1–7.

Goulet O: Recent studies on small intestinal transplantation. *Curr Opin Gastroenterol* 1997;13:500.

Kauffman S: Indications for pediatric intestinal transplantation: A position paper of the American Society of Transplantation. *Pediatr Transplant* 2000;5:80–87.

Kaufman SS, Loseke CA, Lupo JV, et al: Influence of bacterial overgrowth and intestinal inflammation on duration of parenteral nutrition in children with short bowel syndrome. *J Pediatr* 1997;131:356.

Kocoshis S: Evolving concepts and improving prospects for neonates with short bowel syndrome. *J Pediatr* 2001;139:5–7.

Leonberg BL, Chuang E, Eicher P, et al: Long-term growth and development in children after home parenteral nutrition. *J Pediatr* 1998;132:461.

Taylor SF, Sondheimer JM, Sokol RJ, et al: Noninfectious colitis associated with short gut syndrome in infants. *J Pediatr* 1991;119:24.

Stagnant Loop Syndrome

Gracey M: Intestinal microflora and bacterial overgrowth in early life. *J Pediatr Gastroenterol Nutr* 1982;1:13.

Lichtman S: Bacterial overgrowth. In Walker WA, Durie PR, Hamilton JR, et al (editors): *Pediatric Gastrointestinal Disease*, 3rd ed. Hamilton, Ontario, BC Decker, 2000, pp 569–82.

Ruckebush Y: Development of digestive motor complexes during prenatal life: Mechanism and significance. *J Pediatr Gastroenterol Nutr* 1986;5:523–26.

Infections Causing Malabsorption

Farthing MJG: The molecular pathogenesis of giardiasis. *J Pediatr Gastroenterol Nutr* 1997;24:79.

Liebman WM, Thaler MM, Dehorimier A, et al: Intractable diarrhea of infancy due to intestinal coccidiosis. *Gastroenterology* 1980;78:579.

Sood M, Booth I: Is prolonged rotavirus infection a common cause of protracted diarrhoea? *Arch Dis Child* 1999;80:309.

Immunodeficiency States and the Intestine

Kotler DP, Francisco A, Clayton F, et al: Small intestinal injury and parasitic diseases in AIDS. *Ann Intern Med* 1990;113:444.

Weikel CS, Gaynes BN, Roche JK: Diarrheal disease in the immunocompromised host. In Guerrant R (editor): *Baillière's Clinical Tropical Medicine and Communicable Diseases*, vol 3. London, Baillière Tindall, 1988, p 401.

Winter H, Chang TI: Gastrointestinal and nutritional problems in children with immunodeficiency and AIDS. *Pediatr Clin North Am* 1996;43:573.

Woroniecka M, Ballow M: Primary immune deficiencies: Presentation, diagnosis and management. *Pediatr Clin North Am* 2000;47:6.

Yolken RH, Hart W, Oung I, et al: Gastrointestinal dysfunction and disaccharide intolerance in children infected with human immunodeficiency virus. *J Pediatr* 1991;118:359.

Celiac Disease

Barera G, Bazzigaluppi E, Viscaro M, et al: Macroamylasemia attributable to gluten-related amylase autoantibodies: A case report. *Pediatrics* 2001;107:1413–14.

Barera G, Bonfanti R, Viscardi M, et al: Occurrence of celiac disease after onset of type 1 diabetes: A 6-year prospective longitudinal study. *Pediatrics* 2002;109:833–38.

Bostwick H, Berezin S, Halata M, et al: Celiac disease presenting with microcephaly. *J Pediatr* 2001;138:589–92.

Bouhnik Y, Etienney I, Nemeth J, et al: Very late onset small intestinal B cell lymphoma associated with primary intestinal lymphangiectasia and diffuse cutaneous warts. *Gut* 2000;47:296–300.

Carlsson A, Axellson I, Borulf S, et al: Serological screening for celiac disease in healthy 2.5-year-old children in Sweden. *Pediatrics* 2001;107:42–45.

Carroccio A, Iacono G, Lerro P, et al: Role of pancreatic impairment in growth recovery during gluten-free diet in childhood celiac disease. *Gastroenterology* 1997;112:1839.

Catassi C, Fabiani E, Corraco G, et al: Risk of non-Hodgkin lymphoma in celiac disease. *JAMA* 2002;287:1412–18.

Ciclitira P: American Gastroenterological Association Practice Guidelines: AGA technical review on celiac sprue. *Gastroenterology* 2001;120:1526–40.

Dieterich W, Laag E, Schöpper H, et al: Autoantibodies to tissue transglutaminase as predictors of celiac disease. *Gastroenterology* 1998;115:1317.

Farrell R, Kelly C: Current concepts: Celiac sprue. *N Engl J Med* 2002;346:180–88.

Hadjivassiliou M, Grunwald R, Chattopadhyay A, et al: Clinical radiological, neurophysiological, and neuropathological characteristics of gluten ataxia. *Lancet* 1998;352:1582–85.

Hoffenberg E, Haas J, Drescher A, et al: A trial of oats in children with newly diagnosed celiac disease. *J Pediatr* 2000;137:361–66.

Hoffenberg E, Bao F, Eisenbarth G, et al: Transglutaminase antibodies in children with a genetic risk for celiac disease. *J Pediatr* 2000;137:356–60.

Janatuinen EK, Pikkarainen PH, Kemppainen TA: A comparison of diets with and without oats in adults with celiac disease. *N Engl J Med* 1995;333:1033.

Labate A, Gambardella A, Messina D, et al: Silent celiac disease in patients with childhood localization-related epilepsies. *Epilepsia* 2001;42:1153–55.

Larizza D, Calcaterra V, De Giacomo C, et al: Celiac disease in children with autoimmune thyroid disease. *J Pediatr* 2001;139:738–40.

Lepore L, Martelossi S, Pennesi M, et al: Prevalence of celiac disease in patients with juvenile chronic arthritis. *J Pediatr* 1996;129:311.

Mäki M, Collin P: Coeliac disease. *Lancet* 1997;349:1755.

Mora S, Barera G, Beccio S, et al: A prospective longitudinal study of the long-term effect of treatment on bone density in children with celiac disease. *J Pediatr* 2001;139:516–21.

Pellechia M: Idiopathic cerebellar ataxia associated with celiac disease: Lack of distinctive neurological features. *J Neurol Neurosurg Psychiatry* 1999;66:32–35.

Pueschel S, Romano C, Failla P, et al: A prevalence study of celiac disease in persons with Down's syndrome residing in the United States of America. *Acta Paediatr* 1999;88:953–56.

Report to Working Group of European Society of Paediatric Gastroenterology and Nutrition: Revised criteria for diagnosis of coeliac disease. *Arch Dis Child* 1990;65:909.

Rossi TM, Albini CH, Kumar V: Incidence of celiac disease identified by the presence of serum endomysial antibodies in children with chronic diarrhea, short stature, or insulin-dependent diabetes mellitus. *J Pediatr* 1993;123:262.

Rossi TM, Tjota A: Serologic indicators of celiac disease. *J Pediatr Gastroenterol Nutr* 1998;26:205.

Shaw L, Molberg O, Khosta C, et al: Structural basis for gluten intolerance in celiac sprue. *Science* 2002;297:2275–9.

Visakorpi J, Mäki M: Changing clinical features of coeliac disease. *Acta Paediatr Suppl* 1994;395:10.

Volta U, De Franceschi L, Lari F, et al: Coeliac disease hidden by cryptogenic hypertransaminasemia. *Lancet* 1998;352:26.

Zachor DA, Mroczek-Musulman E, Brown P: Prevalence of celiac disease in Down syndrome in the United States. *J Pediatr Gastroenterol Nutr* 2000;31:275–79.

Other Syndromes

Bell S, Kerner J, Sibley R: Microvillous inclusion disease: The importance of electron microscopy for diagnosis. *Am J Surg Path* 1991;15:1157–64.

Bousvaros A, Leichtner AM, Book L, et al: Treatment of pediatric autoimmune enteropathy with tacrolimus (FK506). *Gastroenterology* 1996;111:237.

Gray G: Tropical sprue: Chronic intestinal malabsorption in the tropics. In Blaser M, Smith P, Pavdin J, et al (editors): *Infections of the Gastrointestinal Tract*. New York, Raven Press, 1995, pp 333–341.

Kennea N, Norbury R, Anderson G, Tekay A: Congenital microvillous inclusion disease presenting as antenatal bowel obstruction. *Ultrasound Obstet Gynecol* 2001;17:172–74.

Kerner JA, Millan M, Garcia M, et al: Development of hepatic adenoma in a 14 yr old with microvillus inclusion disease (MID) on lifelong TPN. *J Pediatr Gastroenterol Nutr* 2000;31:S41.

Mack DR, Forstner GG, Wilschanski M, et al: Shwachman syndrome: Exocrine pancreatic dysfunction and variable phenotypic expression. *Gastroenterology* 1996;111:1593.

Patey N, Scoazec JY, Cuenod-Jabri B, et al: Distribution of cell adhesion molecules in infants with intestinal epithelial dysplasia (tufting enteropathy). *Gastroenterology* 1997;113:833.

Reifen RM, Cutz E, Griffiths AM, et al: Tufting enteropathy: A newly recognized clinicopathological entity associated with refractory diarrhea in infants. *J Pediatr Gastroenterol Nutr* 1994;18:379.

Salvia G, Cascioli C, Ciccimarra F, et al: A case of protein losing enteropathy caused by intestinal lymphangiectasia in a preterm infant. *Pediatrics* 2001;107:416–17.

Schmider A, Henrich W, Reles A, et al: Isolated fetal ascites caused by primary lymphangiectasia: A case report. *Am J Obstrt Gynecol* 2001;184:227–28.

Vardy PA, Lebenthal E, Shwachman H: Intestinal lymphangiectasis: A reappraisal. *Pediatrics* 1975;55:842.

Defects of Absorption or Transport

Levy E, Chouraqui JP, Ray CC: Steatorrhea and disorders of chylomicron synthesis and secretion. *Pediatr Clin North Am* 1988;35:53.

Narchi H, Amr SS, Mathew PM, El Jamil MR: Rickets as an unusual initial presentation of abetalipoproteinemia and hypobetalipoproteinemia. *J Pediatr Endocrinol Metab* 2001;14:329–33.

Rader DJ, Brewer B: Abetalipoproteinemia: New insights into lipoprotein assembly and vitamin E metabolism from a rare genetic disease. *JAMA* 1993;270:865.

Scott BB, Miller JP, Losowsky MS: Hypobetalipoproteinemia: A variant of the Bassen-Kornzweig syndrome. *Gut* 1979;20:163.

Enterokinase Deficiency

Hadorn B, Tarlow M, Lloyd JD, et al: Intestinal enterokinase deficiency. *Lancet* 1969;1:812.

Disaccharidase Deficiencies

Ament ME, Perera DR, Esther L: Sucrase-isomaltase deficiency: A frequently misdiagnosed disease. *J Pediatr* 1973;83:721.

Flats G: The genetics of lactose digestion in humans. *Adv Hum Genet* 1987;16:1.

Newton T, Murphy MS, Booth IW: Glucose polymer as a cause of protracted diarrhea in infants with unsuspected congenital sucrase-isomaltase deficiency. *J Pediatr* 1996;128:753.

Ouwendijk J, Moolenaar CE, Peters WJ, et al: Congenital sucrase-isomaltase deficiency: Identification of a glutamine to proline substitution that leads to a transport block of sucrase-isomaltase in a pre-Golgi compartment. *J Clin Invest* 1996;97:633.

Treem WR: Congenital sucrase-isomaltase deficiency. *J Pediatr Gastroenterol Nutr* 1995;21:1.

Treem WR, McAdams L, Stanford L, et al: Sacrosidase therapy for congenital sucrase-isomaltase deficiency. *J Pediatr Gastroenterol Nutr* 1999;28:137–42.

Glucose-Galactose Malabsorption

Evans L, Grasset E, Heyman M, et al: Congenital selective malabsorption of glucose and galactose. *J Pediatr Gastroenterol Nutr* 1985;4:878.

Fairclough PD, Clark ML, Dawson AM, et al: Absorption of glucose and maltose in congenital glucose-galactose malabsorption. *Pediatr Res* 1978;12:1112.

Martin MG, Turk E, Lostao MP: Defects in Na$^+$/glucose cotransporter (SGLT1) trafficking and function cause glucose-galactose malabsorption. *Nat Genet* 1996;12:216.

Vitamin B$_{12}$ Malabsorption

Hall CA: Congenital disorders of vitamin B$_{12}$ transport and their contribution to concepts. *Gastroenterology* 1973;65:684.

Hitzig WH, Dohmann V, Pluss HJ, et al: Hereditary transcobalamin II deficiency: Clinical findings in a new family. *J Pediatr* 1974;85:622.

Imerslund O: Idiopathic chronic megaloblastic anaemia in children. *Acta Paediatr Suppl* 1960;49:119.

MacKenzie IL, Donaldson RM, Trier JS, et al: Ileal mucosa in familial selective vitamin B$_{12}$ malabsorption. *N Engl J Med* 1972;286:1021.

Folate Malabsorption

Malatack J, Moran M, Moughan B: Isolated congenital malabsorption of folic acid in a male infant: Insights into treatment and mechanism of defect. *Pediatrics* 1999;104:1133–7.

Urbach J, Abrahamov A, Grossowicz N: Congenital isolated folic acid malabsorption. *Arch Dis Child* 1987;62:78.

Chloride-Losing Diarrhea

Holmberg C, Perheentupa J, Launiala K, et al: Congenital chloride diarrhea. *Arch Dis Child* 1977;52:255.

Kere J, Lohi H, Höglund P: Genetic disorders of membrane transport III. Congenital chloride diarrhea. *Am J Physiol* 1999;276:G7–G13.

Congenital Sodium Diarrhea

Booth IW, Murer H, Strange G, et al: Defective jejunal brush border Na$^+$/H$^+$ exchange: A cause of congenital secretory diarrhea. *Lancet* 1985;1:1066.

Holmberg C, Perheentupa J: Congenital Na$^+$ diarrhea: A new type of secretory diarrhea. *J Pediatr* 1985;106:56.

Primary Hypomagnesemia

Romero R, Meacham LR, Winn KT: Isolated magnesium malabsorption in a 10-year-old boy. *Am J Gastroenterol* 1996;91:611.

Stromme JH, Nesbakken R, Normann T, et al: Familial hypomagnesemia. *Acta Paediatr Scand* 1969;58:433.

Acrodermatitis Enteropathica

Bohane TD, Cutz E, Hamilton JR, et al: Acrodermatitis enteropathica, zinc and the Paneth cell. *Gastroenterology* 1977;73:587.

Moynahan EJ: Acrodermatitis enteropathica: A lethal inherited human zinc-deficiency disorder. *Lancet* 1974;2:399.

Menkes Syndrome

Danks DM: Of mice and men, metals and mutations. *J Med Genet* 1986;23:99.

Jankov RP, Boerkoel CF, Hellman J, et al: Lethal neonatal Menkes' disease with severe vasculopathy and fractures. *Acta Paediatr* 1998;87:1297–1300.

Kodama H, Murata Y, Kobayashi M: Clinical manifestation and treatment of Menkes disease and its variants. *Pediatr Int* 1999;41:423–29.

Primary Bile Acid Malabsorption

Heubi JE, Balistreri WF, Fondacaro JD, et al: Primary bile acid malabsorption: Defective in vitro ileal active bile acid transport. *Gastroenterology* 1982;83:804.

Oelkers P, Kirby LC, Heubi JE, et al: Primary bile acid malabsorption caused by mutations in the ileal sodium-dependent bile acid transporter gene (SLC10A2). *J Clin Invest* 1997;99:1880.

Drug-Induced Malabsorption

Franklin JL, Rosenberg HH: Impaired folic acid absorption in inflammatory bowel disease: Effects of salicylazosulfapyridine (Azulfidine). *Gastroenterology* 1973;64:517.

Morijiri Y, et al: Factors causing rickets in institutionalized handicapped children on anti-convulsant therapy. *Arch Dis Child* 1981;56:446.

Rogers AL, Vloedman DA, Bloom EC, et al: Neomycin-induced steatorrhea. *JAMA* 1966;197:185.

Trier JS: Morphologic alterations induced by methotrexate in the mucosa of human proximal intestine: I. Serial observations by light microscopy. *Gastroenterology* 1962;42:295.

Enterocyte Heparan Sulfate Deficiency and Carbohydrate-Deficient Glycoprotein Syndrome

Murch SH, Winyard PJ, Koletko S, et al: Congenital enterocyte heparan sulphate deficiency with massive albumin loss, secretory diarrhea, and malnutrition. *Lancet* 1996;347:1299–1301.

Walker-Smith J, Murch S: Miscellaneous disorders of the small intestine. In: *Diseases of the Small Intestine in Childhood*, 4th ed. Oxford, England, Isis Medical Media, 1999, pp 380–381.

Chapter 321

Gastroenteritis *Larry K. Pickering and John D. Snyder*

Infections of the gastrointestinal tract are caused by a wide variety of enteropathogens, including bacteria, viruses, and parasites. Clinical manifestations depend on the organism and host response to infection and include asymptomatic infection, watery diarrhea, bloody diarrhea, chronic diarrhea, and extraintestinal manifestations of infection. A presumptive etiologic diagnosis can be established from epidemiologic clues, clinical manifestations, physical examination, and knowledge of the pathophysiologic mechanisms of enteropathogens. Laboratory studies used to identify diarrheal pathogens are often not required because most episodes are self-limited. All patients with diarrhea require fluid and electrolyte therapy, a few need other nonspecific support, and some may benefit from antimicrobial therapy.

Etiology. The two basic types of acute infectious diarrhea are noninflammatory and inflammatory. Enteropathogens elicit **noninflammatory diarrhea** through enterotoxin production by some bacteria, destruction of villus (surface) cells by viruses, adherence by parasites, and adherence and/or translocation by bacteria. In contrast, **inflammatory diarrhea** usually is caused by bacteria that invade the intestine directly or produce cytotoxins. Some enteropathogens possess more than one virulence property.

Acute diarrhea or diarrhea of short duration may be associated with any of the recognized bacterial, viral, or parasitic causes of enteritis (Box 321–1). Chronic or persistent diarrhea lasting 14 days or more may be due to (1) an infectious agent such as *Giardia lamblia, Cryptosporidium parvum,* and enteroaggregative or enteropathogenic *Escherichia coli;* (2) any enteropathogen that infects an immunocompromised host; or (3) residual symptoms due to damage to the intestine by an enteropathogen after an acute infection. There also are many noninfectious causes of diarrhea in children (Box 321–2).

BACTERIAL ENTEROPATHOGENS. Bacterial enteropathogens may cause either inflammatory or noninflammatory diarrhea, and specific enteropathogens may be associated with either clinical form. Generally, inflammatory diarrhea is associated with *Aeromonas, Campylobacter jejuni, Clostridium difficile,* enteroinvasive *E. coli,* Shiga toxin–producing *E. coli* (*E. coli* O157:H7), *Plesiomonas shigelloides, Salmonella, Shigella, Vibrio parahaemolyticus,* and *Yersinia enterocolitica.* Noninflammatory diarrhea may be caused by enteropathogenic *E. coli,* enterotoxigenic *E. coli, Vibrio cholerae,* and several of the pathogens associated with inflammatory diarrhea. Antimicrobial therapy is administered to select patients with bacterial enteritis to shorten the clinical course, to

BOX 321–1. Causative Agents of Gastroenteritis

BACTERIA

Aeromonas
Bacillus cereus
Campylobacter jejuni
Clostridium perfringens
Clostridium difficile
Escherichia coli
Plesiomonas shigelloides
Salmonella
Shigella
Staphylococcus aureus
Vibrio cholerae 01 and 0139
Vibrio parahaemolyticus
Yersinia enterocolitica

VIRUSES

Astroviruses
Caliciviruses
Norovirus**
Enteric adenoviruses
Rotavirus
Cytomegalovirus*
Herpes simplex viruses*

PARASITES

Balantidium coli
Blastocystis hominis
Cryptosporidium parvum
Cyclospora cayetanensis
*Encephalitozoon intestinalis**
Entamoeba histolytica
*Enterocytozoon bieneusi**
Giardia lamblia
Isospora belli
Strongyloides stercoralis
Trichuris trichiura

*Generally associated with disease only among immunocompromised persons.
** Norwalk-like viruses

BOX 321–2. Other Causes of Diarrhea

FEEDING DIFFICULTY

ANATOMIC DEFECTS

Malrotation
Intestinal duplications
Hirschsprung disease
Fecal impaction
Short bowel syndrome
Microvillus atrophy
Strictures

MALABSORPTION

Disaccharidase deficiencies
Glucose-galactose malabsorption
Pancreatic insufficiency
  Cystic fibrosis
  Shwachman syndrome
Reduced intraluminal bile salts
  Cholestasis
Hartnup disease
Abetalipoproteinemia
Celiac disease

ENDOCRINOPATHIES

Thyrotoxicosis
Addison disease
Adrenogenital syndrome

FOOD POISONING

Heavy metals
Scombroid
Ciguatera
Mushrooms

NEOPLASMS

Neuroblastomas
Ganglioneuromas
Pheochromocytomas
Carcinoid
Zollinger-Ellison syndrome
Vasoactive intestinal peptide syndrome

MISCELLANEOUS

Nongastrointestinal infections
Milk allergy
Crohn disease (regional enteritis)
Familial dysautonomia
Immune deficiency disease
Protein-losing enteropathy
Ulcerative colitis
Acrodermatitis enteropathica
Laxative abuse
Motility disorders
Pellagra

decrease excretion of the causative organism, or to prevent complications (Table 321–1). *Helicobacter pylori* infects gastric mucosa and is associated with gastritis, peptic ulcer disease, and gastric cancer (see Chapter 316).

VIRAL ENTEROPATHOGENS. The main causes of viral gastroenteritis include rotavirus, enteric adenovirus, astrovirus, Norwalk agent–like virus, and calicivirus. Cytomegalovirus and herpes simplex virus have been associated with diarrhea and other gastrointestinal tract signs and symptoms, generally in immunocompromised hosts.

PARASITIC ENTEROPATHOGENS. *G. lamblia* is the most common parasitic cause of diarrhea in the United States; other parasitic pathogens include *Entamoeba histolytica, Strongyloides stercoralis, Balantidium coli,* and spore-forming protozoa, which include *Cryptosporidium parvum, Cyclospora cayetanensis, Isospora belli, Enterocytozoon bieneusi,* and *Encephalitozoon intestinalis.* The latter three agents have been found most often in persons with AIDS. The role of *Dientamoeba fragilis* and *Blastocystis hominis* as causes of diarrhea has not been defined fully. *Balantidium coli, Trichuris trichiura,* and *E. histolytica* can produce bloody diarrhea in humans.

Patients with diarrhea normally do not need to have their stools examined for ova and parasites unless they (1) have a history of recent travel to an endemic area, stool cultures are negative for other enteropathogens, and diarrhea persists for more than 1 wk; (2) are part of an outbreak of diarrhea; or (3) are immunocompromised. Examination of more than one

stool specimen may be necessary to establish a diagnosis. Certain medications, antidiarrheal compounds, and barium may interfere with identification of parasitic enteropathogens.

TABLE 321–1. Antimicrobial Therapy for Bacterial Enteropathogens in Children

Organism*	Antimicrobial Agent	Indication for Antimicrobial Therapy
Aeromonas	TMP/SMZ	Dysentery-like illness, prolonged diarrhea
Campylobacter	Erythromycin† or azithromycin	Early in the course of illness
Clostridium difficile	Metronidazole or vancomycin	Moderate to severe disease
Escherichia coli		
Enterotoxigenic	TMP/SMZ†	Severe or prolonged illness
Enteropathogenic	TMP/SMZ†	Nursery epidemics, life-threatening illness
Enteroinvasive	TMP/SMZ†	All cases if organism susceptible
Salmonella	Cefotaxime or ceftriaxone or ampicillin or chloramphenicol or TMP/SMZ†	Infants <3 mo patients, typhoid fever (*Salmonella typhi*), bacteremia, dissemination with localized suppuration
Shigella	Ampicillin or ciprofloxacin† or ofloxacin or ceftriaxone	All cases if organism susceptible
Vibrio cholerae	Doxycycline or tetracycline	All cases

*Susceptibility testing should be performed on all organisms
†Quinolones (ciprofloxacin or ofloxacin) may be used for persons ≥18 yr of age.
TMP/SMZ = trimethoprim and sulfamethoxazole.

Treatment of these infections depends on the clinical condition and availability of effective therapy (Table 321–2). Antimicrobial resistance is present in many parts of the world.

Epidemiology. Diarrheal diseases are one of the leading causes of morbidity and mortality in children worldwide, causing 1 billion episodes of illness and 3–5 million deaths annually. The relative importance and epidemiologic characteristics of diarrheal pathogens vary by geographic location. In the United States each year, 20–35 million episodes of diarrhea occur among the 16.5 million children younger than 5 yr of age, resulting in 2.1–3.7 million physician visits, 220,000 hospitalizations, 924,000 hospital days, and 300–400 deaths. Children in developing countries become infected with a diverse group of bacterial and parasitic pathogens, whereas all children in developed as well as developing countries acquire rotavirus and, in many cases, other viral enteropathogens, *G. lamblia*, and *C. parvum* during their first 5 yr of life.

The major mechanisms of transmission for diarrheal pathogens are person to person through the fecal-oral route or by ingestion of contaminated food or water. Enteropathogens that are infectious in a small inoculum (*Shigella, E. coli* O157:H7, enteric viruses, *G. lamblia, C. parvum*, and *E. histolytica*) may be transmitted by person-to-person contact. Factors that increase susceptibility to infection with enteropathogens include young age, immune deficiency, measles, malnutrition, travel to an endemic area, lack of breast-feeding, exposure to unsanitary conditions, ingestion of contaminated food or water, level of maternal education, and attendance at a childcare center.

General Approach to Children with Acute Diarrhea. Enteric infections cause gastrointestinal tract signs and symptoms as well as extraintestinal complications, including neurologic manifestations. Gastrointestinal tract involvement may include diarrhea, abdominal cramps, and vomiting. Systemic manifestations are varied and associated with a variety of causes. Extraintestinal infections related to bacterial enteric pathogens include vulvovaginitis, urinary tract infection, endocarditis, osteomyelitis, meningitis, pneumonia, hepatitis, peritonitis, chorioamnionitis, soft tissue infection, and septic thrombophlebitis. Neurologic manifestations of infectious enteritis include paresthesias (from ingestion of fish, shellfish, monosodium glutamate), hypotonia and descending muscle weakness *(C. botulinum)*, and a variety of other signs and symptoms (from ingestion of fish, shellfish, and mushrooms). Immune-mediated extraintestinal manifestations of enteric pathogens usually occur after diarrhea has resolved (Table 321–3). Hemolytic uremia syndrome may follow infection with *E. coli* or *Shigella* (Chapter 510).

The main objectives in the approach to a child with acute diarrhea are to (1) assess the degree of dehydration and provide fluid and electrolyte replacement, (2) prevent spread of the enteropathogen, and (3) in select episodes determine the etiologic agent and provide specific therapy if indicated. Information about oral intake, frequency and volume of stool output, general appearance and activity of the child, and

TABLE 321–3. Immune-Mediated Extraintestinal Manifestations of Enteric Pathogens

Manifestation	Related Enteric Pathogen(s)
Reactive arthritis	*Salmonella, Shigella, Yersinia, Campylobacter, Cryptosporidium, Clostridium difficile*
Guillain-Barré syndrome	*Campylobacter*
Glomerulonephritis	*Shigella, Campylobacter, Yersinia*
IgA nephropathy	*Campylobacter*
Erythema nodosum	*Yersinia, Campylobacter, Salmonella*
Hemolytic anemia	*Campylobacter, Yersinia*
HUS	*S. dysenteriae 1, E. coli*

HUS = hemolytic uremia syndrome.

frequency of urination must be obtained. Data should be obtained about childcare center attendance, recent travel to a diarrhea endemic area, use of antimicrobial agents, exposure to contacts with similar symptoms, and intake of seafood, unwashed vegetables, unpasteurized milk, contaminated water, or uncooked meats. The duration and severity of diarrhea, stool consistency, presence of mucus and blood, and other associated symptomatology, such as fever, vomiting, and seizures, should be determined. Fever is suggestive of an inflammatory process and also occurs as a result of dehydration. Nausea and emesis are nonspecific symptoms, but vomiting suggests organisms that infect the upper intestine, such as enteric viruses, enterotoxin-producing bacteria, *Giardia*, and *Cryptosporidium*. Fever is common in patients with inflammatory diarrhea, abdominal pain is more severe, and tenesmus may occur in the lower abdomen and rectum, indicating involvement of the large intestine. Emesis is common in noninflammatory diarrhea; fever usually is absent or low grade; pain is crampy, periumbilical, and not severe; and diarrhea is watery, indicating upper intestinal tract involvement. Because immunocompromised patients require special consideration, information about an underlying immunodeficiency or chronic disease is important. **Chronic diarrhea** is defined as diarrhea lasting more than 14 days.

EXAMINATION OF STOOL. Stool specimens should be examined for mucus, blood, and leukocytes, the presence of which indicates colitis. Fecal leukocytes are produced in response to bacteria that diffusely invade the colonic mucosa. A positive fecal leukocyte examination indicates the presence of an invasive or cytotoxin-producing organism such as *Shigella, Salmonella, C. jejuni*, invasive *E. coli, C. difficile, Y. enterocolitica, V. parahaemolyticus*, and possibly *Aeromonas* or *P. shigelloides*. Not all patients with colitis have positive results on fecal leukocyte examination. Patients infected with Shiga toxin–producing *E. coli* and *E. histolytica* generally have minimal fecal leukocytes.

Stool cultures should be obtained as early in the course of disease as possible from patients in whom the diagnosis of hemolytic-uremic syndrome (HUS) is suspected, in patients with bloody diarrhea, if stools contain fecal leukocytes, during outbreaks of diarrhea, and in persons who have diarrhea and are immunosuppressed. Fecal specimens that cannot immediately be plated for culture can be transported to the laboratory in a non–nutrient–holding medium such as Cary-Blair to prevent drying.

Because certain bacterial agents, including *Y. enterocolitica, V. cholerae, V. parahaemolyticus, Aeromonas, C. difficile, E. coli* O157: H7, and *Campylobacter*, require modified laboratory procedures for identification, laboratory personnel should be notified when one of these organisms is the suspected etiologic agent. Serotype and toxin assays are available for further characterization of *E. coli*. Detection of *C. difficile* toxins is valuable in the diagnosis of antimicrobial-associated colitis. Proctosigmoidoscopy may be helpful in establishing a diagnosis in patients in whom symptoms of colitis are severe or the cause of an inflammatory enteritis syndrome remains obscure after initial laboratory evaluation.

TABLE 321–2. Antimicrobial Therapy for Enteric Parasites in Children

Organism	Antimicrobial Agent
Giardia lamblia	Furazolidone or metronidazole or albendazole or quinacrine or paromomycin (pregnancy)
Entamoeba histolytica	Metronidazole followed by iodoquinol
Blastocystis hominis	Metronidazole or iodoquinol
Cryptosporidium parvum	Paromomycin or azithromycin may be indicated in immunocompromised hosts.
Cyclospora cayetanensis	Trimethoprim/sulfamethoxazole (TMP/SMZ)
Isospora belli	TMP/SMZ
Enterocytozoon bieneusi	Albendazole
Encephalitozoon intestinalis	Albendazole (minimally effective)
Strongyloides stercoralis	Ivermectin or thiabendazole

MANAGEMENT OF FLUIDS AND ELECTROLYTES AND REFEEDING (also see Chapters 47 and 48.1). Management of dehydration remains the cornerstone in the approach to patients with diarrhea. Children, especially infants, are more susceptible than adults to dehydration because of the greater basal fluid and electrolyte requirements per kilogram and because they are dependent on others to meet these demands. Patients with diarrhea and possible dehydration should be evaluated to assess the degree of dehydration as evident from clinical signs and symptoms, ongoing losses, and daily requirements.

Oral hydration usually is the treatment of choice for all but the most severely dehydrated patients whose caretakers cannot administer fluids. Rapid rehydration with replacement of ongoing losses during the first 4–6 hr should be carried out using an appropriate oral rehydration solution. Once a patient is rehydrated, an orally administered maintenance solution should be used (see Table 48–1). Home remedies including decarbonated soda beverages, fruit juices, Jell-O, Kool-Aid, and tea are not suitable for use because they have inappropriately high osmolalities owing to excessive carbohydrate concentrations, which may exacerbate diarrhea; low sodium concentrations, which may cause hyponatremia; and inappropriate carbohydrate to sodium ratios. Once rehydration is complete, food should be reintroduced while the oral electrolyte solution is continued to replace ongoing losses from stools and for maintenance. Breastfeeding of infants should be resumed as soon as possible. Older children should be re-fed as soon as they can tolerate feeding. Foods with complex carbohydrates (e.g., rice, wheat, potatoes, bread, and cereals), lean meats, yogurt, fruits, and vegetables are better tolerated. Fatty foods or foods high in simple sugars (including juices and carbonated sodas) should be avoided.

ANTIDIARRHEAL COMPOUNDS. These agents are classified by their mechanism of action, which includes alteration of intestinal motility, adsorption of fluid or toxins, alteration of intestinal microflora, and alteration of fluid and electrolyte secretion. Antidiarrheal compounds generally are not recommended for use in children with diarrhea because of their minimal benefit and potential for side effects.

Prevention. Patients who are hospitalized should be placed under contact precautions, including handwashing before and after patient contact, gowns when soiling is likely, and gloves when touching contaminated material. Patients and their families should be educated about the mode of acquisition of enteropathogens and methods to decrease transmission. Patients who attend childcare centers should be excluded from the center or cared for in a separate area until diarrhea has subsided. Cases of diarrhea caused by *C. botulinum, E. coli* O157:H7, *Salmonella, Shigella, V. cholerae, Cryptosporidium,* and *Cyclospora* are nationally notifiable diseases and should be reported to personnel at the local health department. Other enteric pathogens associated with outbreaks (e.g., in childcare centers) or food borne or water borne disease also should be reported.

Vaccines are available to prevent or modify infection by *Salmonella typhi* (see Chapter 181). A rotavirus vaccine was briefly available in the United States but has been removed from the market because of the association with intussusception. Other vaccines to prevent rotavirus infection are in clinical trials.

Acute Food Borne and Water Borne Disease. Food borne and water borne disease is a major cause of morbidity and mortality in all developed countries, including the United States. Changes in food production, flaws in inspection systems, rapid international distribution of food, alterations in dietary habits, and lack of recognition of methods of prevention magnify these problems. Food borne illness in the United States is estimated to cause millions of cases of gastroenteritis yearly, which results in thousands of deaths and is associated with billions of dollars in medical costs and lost productivity.

The diagnosis of a food borne or water borne illness should be considered when two or more persons who have ingested common food or water develop a similar acute illness that usually is characterized by nausea, emesis, diarrhea, or neurologic symptoms. Pathogenesis and severity of bacterial disease depend on whether organisms have preformed toxins (e.g., *Staphylococcus aureus, Bacillus cereus*), produce toxins, or are invasive and whether they replicate in food. The severity of disease due to viral, parasitic, and chemical causes depends on the amount inoculated into the food or water, whereas bacteria have the potential to replicate in food once introduced. The epidemiology of outbreaks often suggests specific etiologic agents. Determination of the incubation period and the specific clinical syndrome often leads to the correct diagnosis. Confirmation is established by specific laboratory testing of food, stool, or emesis. As a general rule, when outbreaks are grouped by incubation period of illness, those occurring in less than 1 hr are associated with chemical poisoning, toxins from fish or shellfish, or preformed toxins of *S. aureus* or *B. cereus.* Enterotoxin-producing bacteria, invasive bacteria, calicivirus, and some forms of mushroom poisoning have longer incubation periods.

CLINICAL SYNDROMES. Several clinical syndromes follow ingestion of contaminated food or water, including nausea and vomiting within 6 hr; paresthesia within 6 hr; neurologic and gastrointestinal tract symptoms within 2 hr; abdominal cramps and watery diarrhea within 16–48 hr; fever, abdominal cramps, and diarrhea within 8–72 hr; abdominal cramps and bloody diarrhea without fever within 72–120 hr; neurologic signs and symptoms within 6–24 hr; and nausea, vomiting, and paralysis within 18–48 hr (Table 321–4).

TABLE 321–4. Clinical Manifestations, Incubation Periods, and Major Causes of Foodborne Disease

Clinical Manifestations	Incubation Periods (hr)	Main Causative Agents
Gastrointestinal tract		
Vomiting	<1	Chemical
Vomiting and diarrhea	1–6	*Bacillus cereus* and *Staphylococcus aureus* preformed toxins
Watery diarrhea, abdominal cramps	8–72	Many organisms including *Salmonella*
Bloody diarrhea	≥15	Many organisms including *Salmonella*
Neurologic	0–6	Fish, shellfish, monosodium glutamate
	0–24	Mushrooms
	18–24	*Clostridium botulinum*
Systemic	Varied	*Listeria monocytogenes*
		Brucella
		Trichinella
		Toxoplasma gondii
		Vibrio vulnificus
		Hepatitis A

Short incubation periods with vomiting as the major sign are associated with toxins that produce direct gastric irritation, such as heavy metals, or with preformed toxins of *B. cereus* or *S. aureus*; *B. cereus* also produces an enterotoxin. Paresthesias after a brief incubation period are suggestive of scombroid (histamine) fish poisoning, paralytic or neurotoxic shellfish poisoning, Chinese restaurant syndrome (monosodium glutamate poisoning), niacin poisoning, or ciguatera fish poisoning. The early-onset syndrome associated with ingestion of toxic mushrooms ranges from gastroenteritis to neurologic symptoms that include parasympathetic hyperactivity, confusion, visual disturbances, and hallucinations to hepatic or hepatorenal failure, which occurs after a 6–24 hr incubation period.

Watery diarrhea and abdominal cramps after an 8–16 hr incubation period are associated with enterotoxin-producing *Clostridium perfringens* and *B. cereus*. Abdominal cramps and watery diarrhea after a 16–48 hr incubation period can be associated with calicivirus, several enterotoxin-producing bacteria, *Cryptosporidium*, and *Cyclospora*. Several organisms including *Salmonella, Shigella, C. jejuni, Y. enterocolitica*, enteroinvasive *E. coli*, and *V. parahaemolyticus* are associated with diarrhea that may contain fecal leukocytes, abdominal cramps, and fever, although these organisms can cause watery diarrhea without fever. Bloody diarrhea and abdominal cramps after a 72–120 hr incubation period are associated with Shiga toxin–producing *E. coli*, such as *E. coli* O157:H7. Hemolytic-uremic syndrome (see Chapter 510) is a sequela of infection with Shiga toxin–producing *E. coli*. The combination of gastrointestinal tract symptoms followed by blurred vision, dry mouth, dysarthria, diplopia, or descending paralysis suggests *Clostridium botulinum*.

Therapy for most persons with food borne disease is supportive, because the majority of these illnesses are self-limited. Exceptions are botulism, paralytic shellfish poisoning, and long-acting mushroom poisoning, all of which may be fatal in previously healthy persons. If a food borne or water borne outbreak is suspected, public health officials should be notified.

American Academy of Pediatrics, Subcommittee on Acute Gastroenteritis: Practice parameter: The management of acute gastroenteritis in young children. *Pediatrics* 1996;97:424–35.

Barwick RS, Levy DA, Craun GF, et al: Surveillance for waterborne disease outbreaks—United States, 1997–1998. *MMWR Morbid Mortal Wkly Rep* 2000;49:1–35.

Brown KH, Peerson JM, Fontaine O: Use of nonhuman milks in the dietary management of young children with acute diarrhea: A meta-analysis of clinical trials. *Pediatrics* 1994;93:17–27.

Centers for Disease Control and Prevention: Diagnosis and management of foodborne illnesses: A primer for physicians. *MMWR Morbid Mortal Wkly Rep* 2001;50:1–69.

Goodgame RW: Understanding intestinal spore-forming protozoa: Cryptosporidia, microsporidia, *Isospora*, and *Cyclospora*. *Ann Intern Med* 1996;124:429–41.

Guerrant RL, Van Gilder T, Steiner TS, et al: Practice guidelines for the management of infectious diarrhea. *Clin Infect Dis* 2001;32:331–51.

Nataro JP, Kaper JB: Diarrheogenic *Escherichia coli. Clin Microbiol Rev* 1998;11:142–201.

Olsen SJ, MacKinon LC, Goulding JS, et al: Surveillance for foodborne disease outbreaks—United States, 1993–1997. *MMWR Morbid Mortal Wkly Rep* 2000;49:1–51.

Pickering LK: Emerging antibiotic resistance in enteric bacterial pathogens. *Semin Pediatr Infect Dis* 1996;7:272–80.

Pickering LK: Food safety. In Kleinman RE (editor): *AAP Nutrition Handbook*, 5th ed (in press).

Pickering LK, Cleary TG: Therapy for diarrheal illness in children. In Blaser MJ, Smith PD, Ravdin JI, et al (editors): *Infections of the Gastrointestinal Tract*, 2nd ed. New York, Raven Press, 2002, pp 1225–40.

Sears CL, Kaper JB: Enteric bacterial toxins: Mechanisms of action and linkage to intestinal secretion. *Microbiol Rev* 1996;60:167–215.

Snyder J: The continuing evolution of oral therapy for diarrhea. *Semin Pediatr Infect Dis* 1994;5:231–35.

Chapter 322
Chronic Diarrhea *Fayez K. Ghishan*

Diarrhea in children accounts for approximately 5 million deaths per year in the developing world (see Chapter 321). In the United States, diarrhea accounts for 10% of all outpatient visits and 14 hospital admissions each year per 1,000 children younger than 1 yr of age.

Definition. Diarrhea, defined as increased total daily stool output, is usually associated with increased stool water content (see Chapters 287 and 321). For infants and children, this would result in stool output greater than 10 g/kg/24 hr or more than the adult limit of 200 g/24 hr. Diarrhea lasting longer than 2 wk is considered chronic. Diarrhea results from altered intestinal water and electrolyte transport. The gastrointestinal tract of the infant handles approximately 285 mL/kg/24 hr of fluid (intake plus intestinal secretion) with a stool output of 5–10 g/kg/24 hr. The efficient mechanisms responsible for this absorptive capacity are caused by the function of several transport proteins located at the brush border membrane of the small and large intestine. The transport of electrolytes across the gastrointestinal tract contributes to the overall absorptive process of the small and large intestine. The stool output in infants and children contains approximately, per liter, 20–25 mEq of sodium, 50–70 mEq of potassium, and 20–25 mEq of chloride. The normal cellular mechanisms responsible for the transport of nutrients and electrolytes across the gastrointestinal tract are noted in Figure 322–1.

Functional Anatomy of the Intestinal Mucosa. The villus, the functional unit of the small intestine, greatly amplifies the absorptive and digestive surface of the intestinal mucosa. The tip of the villus represents the highly differentiated absorptive cells, whereas the crypt epithelia represent undifferentiated secretory cells. The epithelial cells at the tip of the villus are continually renewed every 4–5 days from the undifferentiated crypt cells. Digestive enzymes and the transport proteins responsible for the movements of electrolytes across the intestinal mucosa are located at the brush border membrane of the villus cells. The gastrointestinal epithelia are leaky epithelia that adjust the osmotic load presented to the small intestine. Tight junctions, dynamic structures that occur between the epithelial cells, contribute to overall movement of water and electrolytes. Transport of electrolytes across the intestinal epithelia occurs through several mechanisms, including the glucose-sodium co-transporter. This transport protein requires the presence of a sodium gradient across the brush border membrane that is maintained by the sodium-potassium adenosine triphosphatase (Na^+, K^+ ATPase) pump at the basolateral membranes of the enterocyte. The defect in glucose-galactose malabsorption is a missense mutation in the sodium-glucose co-transporter gene (see Chapter 320.12).

A second mechanism of electrolyte transport across the intestinal epithelia is the electroneutral NaCl-coupled pathway that involves the double exchange mechanism by the Na^+-H^+ exchanger and the Cl^--HCO_3^- exchanger. Two Na^+-H^+ exchangers (NHE-2 and 3) located at the apical membrane appear to be involved in the transport of Na^+. Defects of the genes of Na^+-H^+ and Cl^--HCO_3^- exchangers are candidates for congenital Na^+ and Cl^- diarrhea, respectively. Na^+ is absorbed in the colon by the electroneutral NaCl-coupled pathway and by an electrogenic mechanism, which is regulated by aldosterone. Intestinal secretion occurs primarily from the crypt cells and is stimulated by an increase in the intracellular level cyclic adenosine

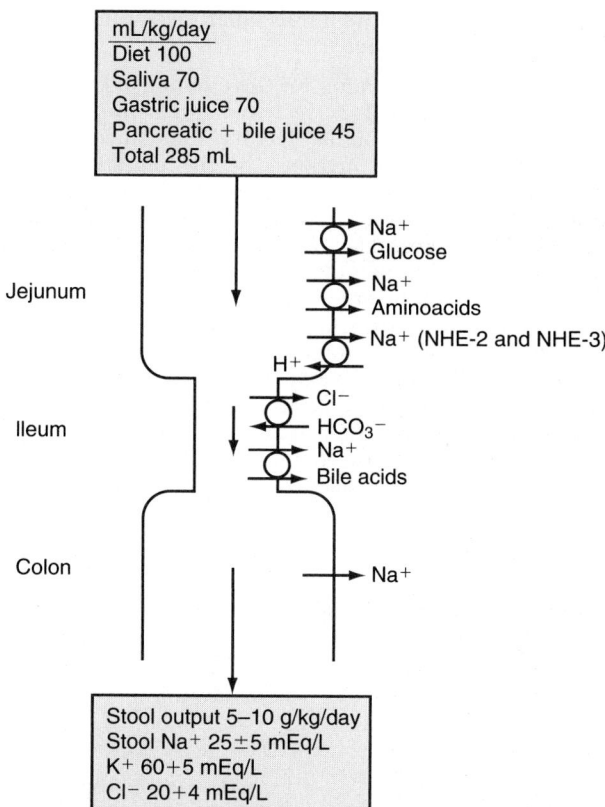

FIGURE 322–1. Normal transport of nutrients and electrolytes across the gastrointestinal (GI) tract of an infant. The GI tract of the infant handles 285 mL/kg/day of dietary and endogenous fluids. Most of the nutrients and fluids are absorbed by means of transport protein, depicted schematically. NHE-2 and NHE-3 indicate Na$^+$/H$^+$ exchanger isoforms 2 and 3. The colon absorbs mainly water and electrolytes through the electroneutral NaCl and the electrogenic Na+ process.

monophosphate (AMP), cyclic guanosine monophosphate (GMP), and Ca^{2+}. These mediators inhibit the neutral NaCl entry and permit the entry of Cl$^-$ into the cells through the basolateral membrane via the Na$^+$-K$^+$-2Cl$^-$ transporter. Cl$^-$ is then secreted through the opening of Cl$^-$ channels at the apical membrane of the crypt cells. Na$^+$ and thus water secretion will result in secretory diarrhea. The Na$^+$-glucose co-transporter is not altered by the intracellular mediators, and, thus, this concept forms the basis of oral rehydration solutions. Figure 322–2 depicts a model for intestinal secretion induced by enterotoxins.

Pathophysiology. The pathophysiologic mechanisms of diarrhea include osmotic diarrhea, secretory diarrhea, mutations in apical membrane transport proteins, a reduction in anatomic surface area, and alteration in intestinal motility (see Table 287–4).

OSMOTIC DIARRHEA. Osmotic diarrhea is caused by the presence of nonabsorbable solutes in the gastrointestinal tract (Box 322–1). The classic example of osmotic diarrhea is lactose intolerance caused by lactase enzyme deficiency in which lactose is not absorbed in the small intestine and reaches the colon intact (see Chapter 320.11). The colonic bacteria ferment the nonabsorbed lactose to short-chain organic acids, generating an osmotic load causing water to be secreted into the lumen. Other examples include ingestion of excessive amounts of sugar-containing carbonated fluids that exceed the transport capacity, especially in toddlers, and ingestion of magnesium salts and sorbitol; both are not absorbed, resulting in an osmotic load. Lactulose, a synthetic therapeutic disaccharide, is not digested in

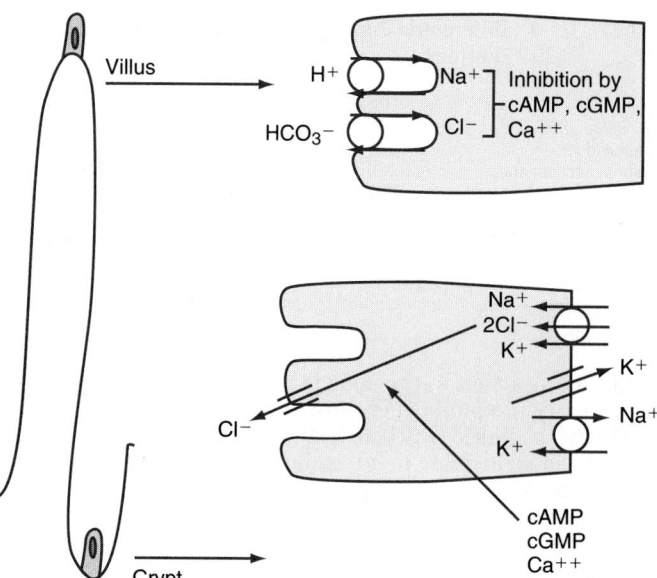

FIGURE 322–2. Model for intestinal secretion: Enterotoxins increase intracellular mediators (cAMP, cGMP, Ca2+), which open chloride channels in the crypt cells and inhibit the neutral NaCl coupled pathway at the villus cells.

the small intestine and is fermented by the colonic bacteria to form organic acids resulting in osmotic diarrhea. Osmotic diarrhea stops with fasting, has a low pH, and is positive for reducing substances. The sum of sodium plus potassium multiplied by 2 in the stools will be less than the measured stool osmolarity, a finding suggesting the presence of other osmols in the stool. The main diagnostic points that differentiate osmotic from secretory diarrhea are noted in Table 322–1.

SECRETORY DIARRHEA. The major causes of secretory diarrhea are depicted in Box 322–2. The mechanisms for secretory diarrhea include activation of the intracellular mediators such as cyclic AMP, cyclic GMP, and intracellular Ca^{2+}, which stimulate active Cl$^-$ secretion from the crypt cells and inhibit the neutral coupled sodium chloride absorption. These mediators alter the paracellular ion flux because of toxin-mediated injury to the tight junctions. The classic example of secretory diarrhea is that induced by cholera and *Escherichia coli* enterotoxins that bind to a specific enterocyte surface receptor (the monosialo-ganglioside GM$_1$); a fragment of the toxin then enters the cell, where it activates adenylate cyclase on the basolateral membrane through interaction with a stimulatory G protein. This increases intracellular cyclic AMP. The enterotoxigenic *E. coli* mediates secretory diarrhea by producing heat-labile toxin (LT) and heat-stable toxin (ST) in the small bowel. The labile toxin is

---

BOX 322–1. Causes of Osmotic Diarrhea

Malabsorption of water-soluble nutrients
    Glucose-galactose malabsorption
        Congenital
        Acquired
    Disaccharidase deficiencies (lactase and sucrase-isomaltase)
        Congenital
        Acquired
Excessive intake of carbonated fluids
Excessive intake of nonabsorbable solutes
    Sorbitol
    Lactulose
    Magnesium hydroxide

TABLE 322–1. Differential Diagnosis of Osmotic versus Secretory Diarrhea

	Osmotic Diarrhea	Secretory Diarrhea
Volume of stool	<200 mL/24 hr	>200 mL/24 hr
Response to fasting	Diarrhea stops	Diarrhea continues
Stool Na$^+$	<70 mEq/L	>70 mEq/L
Reducing substances*	Positive	Negative
Stool pH	<5	>6

*Sucrose is not a reducing agent. Add 5 drops of 0.1 N HCl to a stool sample before adding reducing agent (Clinitest tablet).

similar in its action to the cholera toxin and binds to the same GM$_1$ surface receptor. Other causes of secretory diarrhea include vasoactive peptides, which activate G protein–coupled receptors resulting in an increase in intracellular mediators causing secretory diarrhea.

Secretory diarrhea is characterized by high volume; the stools are extremely watery. Stool analysis reveals high sodium and chloride content (>70 mEq/L). Secretory diarrhea continues with fasting.

MUTATIONAL DEFECTS IN ION TRANSPORT PROTEINS. Congenital defects of Na$^+$-H$^+$ exchange, Cl$^-$-HCO$_3^-$ exchange, and Na$^+$-bile acid transport proteins result in secretory diarrhea presenting at birth (see Chapter 320.12). The defects in Cl$^-$-HCO$_3^-$ exchange and Na$^+$-bile acid transporters have gene mutations that encode their corresponding transport proteins. The defect in Na$^+$-H$^+$ exchange is believed to represent defects in the apical Na$^+$-H$^+$ exchanger (NHE-2 or NHE-3). Patients with these defects present with secretory diarrhea and failure to thrive during the neonatal period. The defect in Cl$^-$-HCO$_3^-$ exchange is well characterized and is more common compared with the defects in Na$^+$-H$^+$ exchange and Na$^+$-bile acid transporter (see Chapter 320.2). Patients with Cl$^-$ diarrhea have hypochloremic metabolic alkalosis with low serum Cl$^-$ concentration, high stool Cl$^-$ content coupled with Cl$^-$–free urine, low serum K$^+$, and high serum HCO$_3^-$. Hydramnios is present in the mothers.

REDUCTION IN ANATOMIC SURFACE AREA. Short bowel syndrome results from resection of the bowel secondary to surgical indications such as necrotizing enterocolitis, midgut volvulus, or intestinal atresia (see Chapter 320.7). Celiac disease results in flattening of the proximal intestinal surface area with marked decrease in the digestive and absorptive function of the villus epithelium (see Chapter 320.8). Diarrhea is characterized by loss of fluids, electrolytes, macronutrients, and micronutrients.

ALTERATION IN INTESTINAL MOTILITY. The causes of altered intestinal motility include malnutrition, scleroderma, intestinal pseudo-obstruction syndromes, and diabetes mellitus. Malnutrition, in general, results in hypomotility, allowing bacterial overgrowth that leads to deconjugation of bile salts and

BOX 322–2. Causes of Secretory Diarrhea

Activation of cyclic adenosine monophosphate
  Bacterial toxins: enterotoxins of cholera, *Escherichia coli* (heat-labile), *Shigella*, *Salmonella*, *Campylobacter jejuni*, *Pseudomonas aeruginosa*
  Hormones: vasoactive intestinal peptide, gastrin, secretin
  Anion surfactants: bile acids, ricinoleic acid
Activation of cyclic guanosine monophosphate
  Bacterial toxins: *E. coli* (heat-stable) enterotoxin, *Yersinia enterocolitica* toxin
Calcium-dependent
  Bacterial toxins: *Clostridium difficile* enterotoxin
  Neurotransmitters: acetylcholine, serotonin
  Paracrine agents: bradykinin

results in an increase in the intracellular mediator cyclic AMP, leading to secretory diarrhea.

Etiology. A simple classification for the etiology of chronic diarrhea is shown in Table 322–2. The two major factors resulting in diarrhea include intraluminal factors and mucosal factors. Intraluminal factors are involved in the digestion process, whereas mucosal factors are involved in the digestion and transport of nutrients across the mucosa. In many situations, both intraluminal and mucosal factors cause diarrhea. The intraluminal factors involve disorders of the pancreas, liver, and the brush border membrane of the enterocytes. In approximately 85% of patients with cystic fibrosis, pancreatic insufficiency results in malabsorption of fats and proteins. Short stature, exocrine pancreatic hypoplasia, normal sweat Cl$^-$ concentrations, and the variable features of neutropenia and skeletal changes characterize *Shwachman syndrome* (see Chapter 330). *Johannson-Blizzard syndrome* is characterized by anal imperforation, agenesis of the nasal cartilage, hair anomalies, mental retardation, deafness,

TABLE 322–2. Etiology of Chronic Diarrhea

INTRALUMINAL FACTORS	MUCOSAL FACTORS
Pancreatic Disorders	*Altered Integrity*
Cystic fibrosis	Infections: bacterial, viral, fungal
Shwachman-Diamond syndrome	Infestations: parasitic
Johannson-Blizzard syndrome	Cow's and soy protein intolerance
Isolated pancreatic enzyme deficiencies	Inflammatory bowel disease (ulcerative
Chronic pancreatitis	colitis, microscopic colitis, Crohn)
Pearson syndrome	
Bile Acid Disorders	*Altered Immune Function*
Chronic cholestasis	Autoimmune enteropathy
Terminal ileum resection	Eosinophilic gastroenteropathy
Bacterial overgrowth	AIDS
Chronic use of bile acid sequestrants	Combined immunodeficiency
Primary bile acid malabsorption	Immunoglobulin A and G deficiencies
Intestinal Disorders	*Altered Function*
Intraluminal osmolarity	Defects in Cl$^-$/HCO$_3^-$, Na$^+$/H$^+$, bile acids,
Carbohydrate malabsorption	acrodermatitis enteropathica,
Congenital and acquired sucrase, lactase	selective folate deficiency,
deficiencies	abetalipoproteinemia
Congenital and acquired monosaccharide	
malabsorption	
Excessive carbonated fluid intake	
Excessive intake of sorbitol, Mg (OH)$_2$ and	
lactulose	
	Altered Digestive Function
	Enterokinase deficiency
	Glucoamylase deficiency
	Altered Surface Area
	Celiac disease
	Postgastroenteritis syndrome
	Microvillus inclusion disease
	Short bowel syndrome
	Altered Secretory Function
	Enterotoxin-producing bacteria
	Tumors secreting vasoactive peptides
	Altered Anatomic Structures
	Hirschsprung disease
	Partial small bowel obstruction
	Malrotation

hypothyroidism, and pancreatic insufficiency (see Chapter 330). The isolated pancreatic enzyme defects are congenital and result in malabsorption of fat or proteins, depending on the defect. These defects include congenital lipase/colipase deficiency and congenital trypsinogen deficiency. Patients with chronic pancreatitis can present with pancreatic insufficiency and insulin-dependent diabetes. Familial pancreatitis, secondary to a mutation in the trypsinogen gene, can result in chronic pancreatitis and pancreatic insufficiency. *Pearson syndrome* is characterized by refractory sideroblastic anemia with vacuolization of bone marrow precursors, exocrine pancreatic insufficiency, and mitochondrial DNA deletions and duplications. Disorders of the liver, such as cholestasis, result in a decrease in bile acid pool size with malabsorption of fats. Bile acid loss with fat malabsorption can occur with terminal ileum disease such as Crohn disease or with terminal ileum resection. Primary bile acid malabsorption is a rare disorder secondary to a mutation in the ileal bile acid transporter. Patients present with fat malabsorption and diarrhea. Bacterial overgrowth in the gastrointestinal tract results in deconjugation and dehydroxylation of bile salts, resulting in diarrhea. Long-term use of bile acid sequestrants such as cholestyramine can lead to a decrease in bile acid pool size because of the continued loss of bile acids in the stools. Intraluminal osmolarity, resulting from malabsorption of carbohydrates, presents as an osmotic type of diarrhea. The causes of carbohydrate malabsorption include congenital and acquired causes of monosaccharide and disaccharidase deficiencies. Excessive sugar-containing carbonated fluid or fruit juice intake, which exceeds the transport capacity of the small intestine in younger infants, results in *nonspecific diarrhea.* Excessive intake of nonabsorbable solutes such as sorbitol, magnesium hydroxide, and lactulose results in osmotic diarrhea.

The mucosal factors that lead to chronic diarrhea could be secondary to altered mucosal integrity from infections such as bacterial, viral, parasitic, and fungal agents. Parasitic infestations such as with *Giardia* or cryptosporidia can present as chronic diarrhea. Inflammatory bowel disease such as ulcerative colitis, Crohn disease, and microscopic colitis can lead to the alteration in the mucosal integrity resulting in the decreased absorption of water electrolyte through the gastrointestinal tract. Cow's milk and soy protein intolerance can present with diarrhea secondary to partial villus atrophy or allergic colitis. Altered immune function as seen in patients with agammaglobulinemia, isolated immunoglobulin A deficiency, and combined immunodeficiency disorders can result in diarrhea. Patients with AIDS are more predisposed to bacterial, viral, and fungal infections. Similarly, autoimmune enteropathy and eosinophilic gastroenteropathy are believed to be disorders involving alteration of the mucosal immune function and can result in diarrhea. Altered mucosal transport function, as seen in congenital disorders involving Na$^+$-H$^+$ exchange, Cl$^-$HCO$_3^-$ exchange, bile acid transport, and glucose-galactose transport, results in diarrhea early in the neonatal period. Similarly, defects in the absorption of zinc, such as acrodermatitis enteropathica and folate transport, can result in diarrhea.

Abetalipoproteinemia is characterized by fat malabsorption, neurologic lesions, and ocular abnormalities such as retinitis pigmentosa (see Chapter 75.3). The diagnosis is confirmed by the typical hematologic finding of acanthocytosis and the appearance of the small bowel biopsy specimen in which the tip enterocytes are filled with lipid droplets. Altered mucosal digestive function includes congenital enterokinase deficiency that results in loss of activation of trypsinogen to trypsin with protein malabsorption (see Chapter 322.11). Glucoamylase deficiency is rare and results in loss of hydrolysis of glucose polymers.

Altered mucosal surface area is seen in celiac disease, partial villus atrophy secondary to postgastroenteritis malabsorption syndrome, tropical sprue, microvillus inclusion disease, Whipple disease, and short bowel syndrome. In these disorders, the height and structure of the villi are altered so that the absorptive capacity of the mucosal surface area is markedly decreased. Celiac disease occurs secondary to gluten sensitivity (see Chapter 320.8). Postgastroenteritis syndrome is a nutritional disorder that occurs after a prolonged episode of gastroenteritis and decreased energy intake. Microvillus inclusion disease is characterized with diarrhea, failure to thrive, and histologic picture of microvillus inclusions (see Chapter 320). The mucosal surface lacks brush border membranes or possesses irregular blunted microvilli. Whipple disease is mainly seen in adults and is secondary to an actinomycete, *Tropheryma whippelii.* Patients present with weight loss, diarrhea, and arthropathy. The diagnosis is established by a small bowel biopsy, and patients respond to prolonged administration of trimethoprim-sulfamethoxazole. Tropical sprue is commonly seen in patients living or returning from trips to developing countries (see Chapter 320.4). Patients present with diarrhea and nutritional deficiencies, especially of folate. Alteration in the anatomic structure as seen in Hirschsprung disease, malrotation, and partial small bowel obstruction can result in diarrhea secondary to bacterial overgrowth. Altered mucosal secretory function includes enterotoxin-producing bacteria and tumor-secreting vasoactive peptides. Box 322–3 summarizes the most common causes of chronic diarrhea at various ages.

Evaluation. The evaluation of patients with chronic diarrhea is depicted in Box 322–4. It is important to determine that the patient indeed has diarrhea, because patients with encopresis may be mistakenly considered to have diarrhea secondary to constant fecal soiling. In phase I, the history and physical examination, which includes a nutritional assessment, is the initial step. The clinical history should include the amount and type of fluids ingested per day. If the patient's clinical history suggests excessive carbonated drinks or fruit juices of more than 150 mL/kg/24 hr, with normal growth and height parameters, chronic nonspecific diarrhea needs to be considered. A decrease in the amount of fluid to no more than 90 mL/kg/24 hr will result in resolution of the diarrhea. If the patient is ingesting nonabsorbable nutrients in excessive amounts such as sorbitol, a dietary adjustment needs to be made before extensively investigating the patient.

The stool examination is an integral step in investigating a patient with chronic diarrhea. The most recently evacuated stool, including its liquid content, is useful for diagnostic purposes. Various collection techniques are helpful, including the placement of a urine collection bag over the anus and everting a disposable diaper to collect the stool. Once collected, the stool specimen should be stored in a refrigerator until the examination is performed. Specimens for bacterial culture should

---

BOX 322–3. Common Causes of Chronic Diarrhea

INFANCY

Postgastroenteritis malabsorption syndrome
Cow's milk/soy protein intolerance
Secondary disaccharidase deficiencies
Cystic fibrosis

CHILDHOOD

Chronic nonspecific diarrhea
Secondary disaccharidase deficiencies
Giardiasis
Postgastroenteritis malabsorption syndrome
Celiac disease
Cystic fibrosis

ADOLESCENCE

Irritable bowel syndrome
Inflammatory bowel disease
Giardiasis
Lactose intolerance

PHASE I	Clinical history including specific amounts of fluids ingested per day
	Physical examination including nutritional assessment
	Stool exam (pH, reducing substances, smear for white blood cell count, fat, ova, and parasites)
	Stool cultures
	Stool for *Clostridium difficile* toxin
	Blood studies (complete blood cell count, erythrocyte sedimentation rate, electrolytes, blood urea nitrogen, creatinine)
PHASE II	Sweat chloride
	72-Hr stool collection for fat determination
	Stool electrolytes, osmolality
	Stool for phenolphthalein, magnesium sulfate, phosphate
	Breath H_2 tests
PHASE III	Endoscopic studies
	Small bowel biopsy
	Sigmoidoscopy or colonoscopy with biopsies
	Barium studies
PHASE IV	Hormonal studies vasoactive intestinal polypeptide, gastrin, secretin, 5-hydroxyindoleacetic assays

be transported immediately to the bacteriology laboratory for inoculation into growth media. The gross examination of the stool should allow the physician to determine whether the patient has diarrhea and whether blood or mucus is present in the stool, a finding suggesting inflammation of the colon. The color of the stool is rarely helpful unless it is bloody. Occult testing for blood is useful to determine whether the patient has microscopic blood loss. Carbohydrate malabsorption is detected by analysis of the liquid fraction of a fresh specimen. A pH lower than 5 or the presence of moderate reducing substances indicates the presence of reducing carbohydrates (sucrose is not a direct reducing substance). The stools should be sent for electrolytes and osmolality testing if secretory diarrhea is considered (see Table 322–1).

Microscopic examination of the stool helps to determine the presence of white blood cells, which signifies colonic inflammation. The stools could be examined for ova and parasites such as *Giardia*, amebae, or cryptosporidia. Trichrome stain or acid-fast stain can be of value in identifying *Cryptosporidium* species. Stools should be examined for the presence of *Giardia* antigen. Sudan stain can be used either on a plain stool smear or with the addition of acetic acid and heat to determine the presence of triglycerides and split fats.

In the event that phase I investigation has failed to reveal a cause, a phase II work-up is indicated and includes a sweat chloride test to rule out cystic fibrosis. A 72-hr stool collection for fat determination is the standard to determine whether the patient does have fat malabsorption in the setting of a negative sweat chloride test. Stools could also be checked for phenolphthalein, magnesium sulfate, and phosphate to determine whether the diarrhea is secondary to the ingestion of laxatives *(factitious diarrhea)*. Breath hydrogen tests can be used to determine a specific carbohydrate malabsorption. A breath hydrogen test for glucose can be used to diagnose bacterial overgrowth.

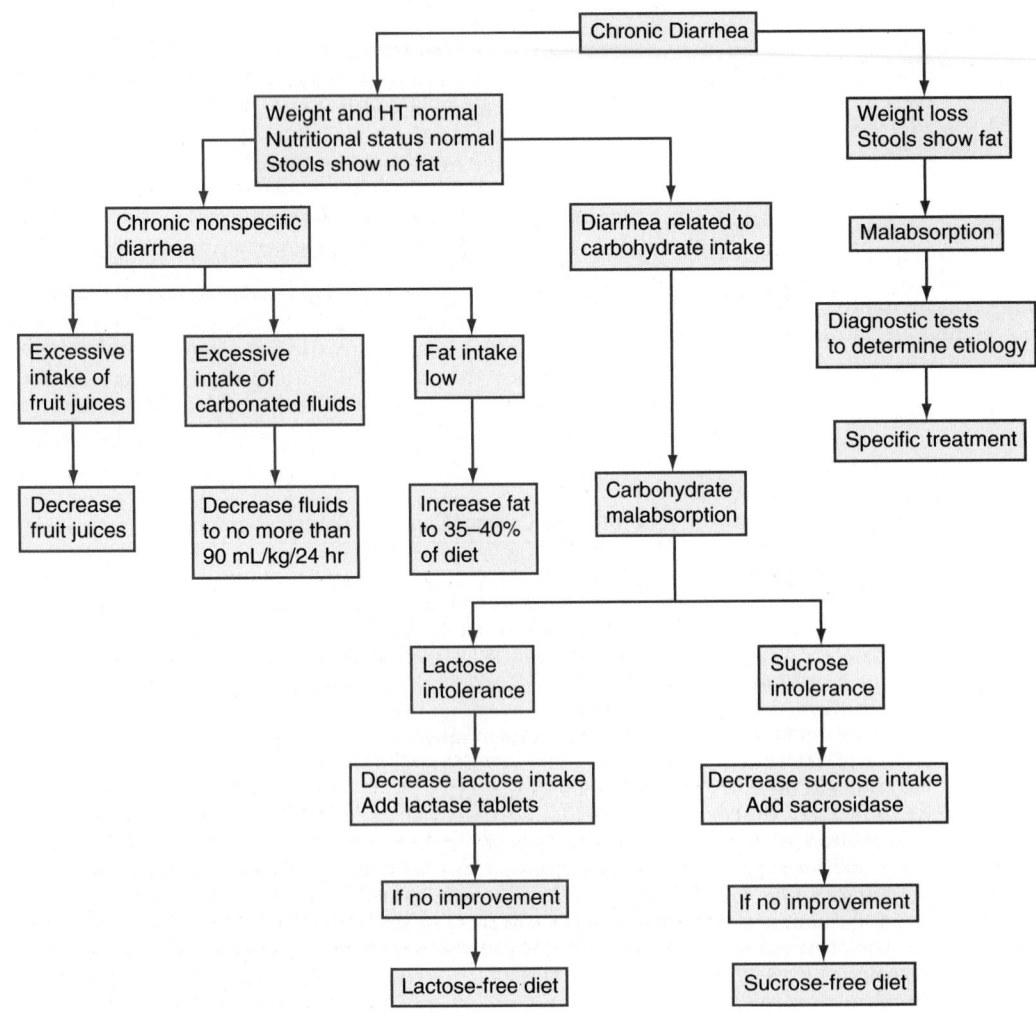

FIGURE 322–3. General therapeutic approaches to management of chronic diarrhea.

Phase III investigation includes endoscopic studies for small bowel and colonic biopsies. Barium studies, such an upper gastrointestinal series or a barium enema, can be used to rule out anatomic lesions in the gastrointestinal tract. If none of these tests is revealing, phase IV evaluation includes hormonal studies and neurohormonal and neurotransmittal studies such as vasoactive intestinal polypeptide, gastrin, secretin, and 5-hydroxyindoleacetic assays.

Treatment. Figure 322–3 depicts the general therapeutic approaches to the management of chronic diarrhea. The first principle is to maintain adequate nutritional intake to permit normal growth and development. The height, weight, and nutritional status of the patient must be documented. If nutritional parameters, including weight and height, are normal and the stool examination does not show any fat, the possibility of chronic nonspecific diarrhea needs to be considered. The pathogenesis of this condition includes excessive carbonated fluid intake, nondigestible carbohydrate malabsorption from excessive fruit juice ingestion, and low fat intake.

Chronic nonspecific diarrhea generally presents in well-appearing toddlers between 1 and 3 yr (toddler's diarrhea). The diarrhea is often brown and watery, at times containing undigested food particles. If the child's fluid intake is more than 150 mL/kg/24 hr, fluid intake should be reduced to no more than 90 mL/kg/24 hr. Parents may note that the child is irritable in the first 2 days after the fluid restriction; however, persistence in this approach for several more days results in a decrease in the stool frequency and volume. If the dietary history suggests that the child is ingesting significant amounts of fruit juices, then the offending juices should be decreased. Sorbitol, which is a nonabsorbable sugar, is found in apple, pear, and prune juices and can cause diarrhea in toddlers. Moreover, apple and pear juices contain higher amounts of fructose in excess of glucose concentration, a feature postulated to cause diarrhea in toddlers. White grape juice is the best alternative.

Levels of dietary fat intake may also play a role in chronic diarrhea. If the child's fat intake has been restricted by the parents, then fat intake can be increased to be approximately 40% of the total calories per day.

If the diarrhea is secondary to carbohydrate intolerance, then a trial period of decreased lactose or sucrose may be initiated. Lactase (LactAid) can be used to aid in the digestion of lactose. If diarrhea persists, a trial of a lactose-free or sucrose-free diet is indicated. Alternatively, breath hydrogen tests can document the presence of lactose or sucrose intolerance. A glucose breath hydrogen test can be used for the diagnosis of bacterial overgrowth.

If the patient presents with weight loss and the stool examination shows fat, the possibility of chronic diarrhea secondary to a malabsorption syndrome needs to be considered. The most common cause of chronic diarrhea associated with the malabsorption is postgastroenteritis malabsorption syndrome. These patients respond well to a predigested formula. In the event that the patient shows intolerance to oral feeding with a predigested formula, such as Pregestimil or Alimentum, nasogastric dripfeeding with an elemental formula should be considered for a period of 3–4 wk.

A patient presenting with suspected small intestinal bacterial overgrowth should undergo evaluation for surgical, medical, and nutritional support. Surgical treatment is indicated if the patient has malrotation or partial small bowel obstruction. Antibiotic therapy is usually initiated with metronidazole in combination with ampicillin or trimethoprim-sulfamethoxazole.

Patients presenting with secretory diarrhea, especially during the 1st mo of life, need to be considered for nutritional support, because the most likely cause is a congenital defect in transport proteins. In older children with secretory diarrhea, the cause needs to be identified first, and therapeutic consideration is directed toward the cause of the secretory diarrhea.

Acra S, Ghishan FK: Electrolyte fluxes in the gut and oral rehydration solutions. *Pediatr Clin North Am* 1996;43:433.

Bhutta ZA, Hendricks KM: Nutritional management of persistent diarrhea in childhood: A perspective from the developing world. *J Pediatr Gastroenterol Nutr* 1996;22:17.

Boissieu D, Chaussain M, Badoual J, et al: Small-bowel bacterial overgrowth in children with chronic diarrhea, abdominal pain, or both. *J Pediatr* 1996;128:203.

Castro-Rodriguez JA, Salazar-Lindo E, Leon-Barua R: Differentiation of osmotic and secretory diarrhea by stool carbohydrate and osmolar gap measurements. *Arch Dis Child* 1997;77:201.

Cutz E, Sherman PM, Davidson GP: Enteropathies associated with protracted diarrhea of infancy: Clinicopathological features, cellular and molecular mechanisms. *Pediatr Pathol Lab Med* 1997;17:335.

Dellert SF, Cohen MB: Diarrheal disease. *Pediatr Gastroenterol* 1994;23:637.

Donowitz M, Kokke FT, Saidi R: Evaluation of patients with chronic diarrhea. *N Engl J Med* 1995;332:725.

Duggan C, Nurko S: Feeding the gut: The scientific basis for continued enteral nutrition during acute diarrhea. *J Pediatr* 1997;131:801.

Greene HL, Ghishan FK: Excessive fluid intake as a cause of chronic diarrhea in young children. *J Pediatr* 1983;102:836.

Kneepkens CM, Hoekstra JH: Chronic nonspecific diarrhea of childhood: Pathophysiology and management. *Pediatr Clin North Am* 1996;43:375.

Chapter 323
Recurrent Abdominal Pain of Childhood *Robert Wyllie*

Chronic abdominal pain can be classified as either organic or nonorganic depending on whether a specific cause of the pain is identified. Nonorganic pain or "functional" abdominal pain refers to pain that cannot be explained on a structural or biochemical basis. Recurrent abdominal pain (RAP) in children is defined as episodes of pain occurring at least monthly for 3 consecutive months with a severity that interrupts routine functioning. RAP affects about 15% of middle and high school students. Approximately 10% of students who experience abdominal pain seek medical evaluation. The likelihood of seeking medical attention is proportional to the severity and frequency of abdominal pain and its impact on school attendance.

Early investigators found an organic cause for RAP in 5–10% of children. With advancement in medical technology, including endoscopic techniques, breath hydrogen testing, and radiographic analysis, the percentage of patients with unexplained pain is decreasing. However, for the majority of teenagers with RAP no specific cause can be found with current diagnostic techniques.

Periumbilical abdominal pain is the most common location for children with RAP. Epigastric pain is frequently associated with symptoms of early satiety, nausea, bloating, or belching and, in the presence of a negative evaluation and no response to acid-blocking medication, is referred to as nonulcer dyspepsia. Pain below the umbilicus is often accompanied by abdominal cramps, bloating, and distention with an altered bowel pattern. This complex of symptoms is consistent with irritable bowel syndrome (IBS) in the adult population. IBS-type symptoms have been documented in about one third of the children with RAP. Gastrointestinal tract symptoms are positively related to both anxiety and depression, particularly in children with IBS-type symptoms. Improvement in symptoms during weekends and school vacations suggests functional pain, but the absence of this pattern does not rule out this diagnosis.

Investigations into the etiology of RAP have focused on the autonomic nervous system and intestinal motility abnormalities. The dorsal horn of the spinal cord regulates conduction of impulses from peripheral nociceptive receptors to the spinal cord and brain, and the pain experience is further influenced by cognitive and emotional centers. Chronic peripheral pain can produce increased neural activity in higher central nervous system centers, leading to perpetuation of pain. Psychosocial stress can affect pain intensity and quality through these mechanisms. Manometric studies suggest altered motility in combination with heightened awareness in certain children may cause abdominal pain. Differences in visceral sensation may lead to differences in perception of pain.

The child's response to pain can be influenced by stress, by personality type, and by the reinforcement of illness behavior within the family. A significantly higher proportion of children with RAP have relatives with somatization disorders, alcoholism, and antisocial behavior problems. Parents and siblings are more likely to have complaints of abdominal pain, nervous breakdown, and migraine headaches. Children with functional abdominal pain are more likely to experience stressors. Sexual abuse as a child may be associated with RAP. This possibility should always be considered, especially in a girl whose abdominal symptoms begin in the pre-teenage or teenage years.

Diagnosis. A wide range of potential organic causes of RAP (see Table 287–4) must be considered before establishing a diagnosis of functional pain. Among the more common causes are chronic constipation, parasitic infection (*Giardia*), gastroesophageal reflux, and lactase deficiency. Lactose intolerance is so common that the finding may be coincidental; therefore, one must be cautious in attributing chronic abdominal pain to this condition. Pinworms are unlikely to be the cause of abdominal pain.

The characteristic presentation of children with RAP includes onset later than 6 yr of age and midline paroxysmal pain, most often periumbilical but also localized to the epigastric or suprapubic area. The pain interrupts normal activity, but there is usually no relationship with meals. Children with IBS typically have abdominal pain relieved by defecation. They may notice mucus in their stools and looser or more frequent stools at the outset of their pain. Bloating or the sense of incomplete evacuation may also be present.

Symptoms suggestive of an organic etiology include age younger than 6 yr, fever, weight loss, joint symptoms, or abnormal growth. Organic pain is usually localized away from the umbilicus and may wake the patient from sleep. Vomiting, diarrhea, and blood in the stool are more suggestive of an organic etiology. Children with RAP have a normal physical examination, whereas those with organic etiology may have fissures or evidence of occult blood in the stool. Serial growth points should be plotted if available because growth deceleration is frequently associated with organic causes of abdominal pain.

Evaluation. The laboratory, radiologic, or endoscopic evaluation of children with chronic abdominal pain should be individualized, depending on the findings suggested by a detailed history and physical examination. Laboratory studies may be unnecessary if the history and physical examination clearly lead to a diagnosis of functional abdominal pain. However, a complete blood cell count, sedimentation rate, stool test for parasites (especially *Giardia*), and urinalysis are reasonable screening studies. If inflammatory bowel disease is suspected the sedimentation rate is often elevated. The finding of an abnormal sedimentation rate would make one look further for an inflammatory, infectious, or neoplastic disorder. If indicated, an ultrasound examination of the abdomen can give information about kidneys, gallbladder, and pancreas; with lower abdominal pain, a pelvic ultrasonogram may be indicated. An upper gastrointestinal tract x-ray series is indicated if one suspects a disorder of the stomach or small intestine. *Helicobacter pylori* infection does not seem to be associated with RAP. In patients with symptoms suggestive of gastritis or ulcer an *H. pylori* test (serum or fecal) may be performed to document the infection. Esophagogastroduodenoscopy is indicated with symptoms suggestive of persistent upper gastrointestinal pathology. In the absence of this suspicion, esophagogastroduodenoscopy is unlikely to identify an abnormality and is usually not necessary.

Treatment. The family and the child with functional RAP may worry about the inability to identify an organic cause and may be resistant to a diagnosis of nonorganic disease. After a thorough history and physical examination the most important component of the treatment is reassurance of the children and family members. Specifically, they need to be reassured that no evidence of a serious underlying disorder is present. Cancer is often an unspoken concern. Anxiety about the symptom may contribute to focusing on the symptom as well as to reducing the threshold for discomfort. The parents should be instructed to avoid reinforcing the symptom with secondary gain. Furthermore, if children have missed school or have been removed from routine activities because of the pain, it is important that they return to regular activities. Medications are generally unhelpful or, at best, offer transient placebo effect. Gastric acid blockers or visceral muscle relaxants (anticholinergics) may be tried empirically, but they are most often not helpful in the absence of specific indication. Biofeedback and relaxation techniques have been useful in some children with functional pain.

If lactose intolerance is suspected, the diagnosis can be documented by breath hydrogen testing. Institution of a lactose-free diet usually results in resolution of the pain. Symptoms of gastroesophageal reflux will generally subside with the use of acid blockers. Recurrent symptoms are usually an indication for formal testing before instituting chronic therapy. Children with symptoms of irritable bowel and loose stools will often benefit from fiber supplementation. Anticholinergics or tricyclic antidepressants may be useful in some patients. If chronic constipation is identified, it should be treated in the standard fashion (see Chapters 20.4 and 313).

Successful management depends on close follow-up. The parents can try new approaches to the child's symptoms without fear that the physician is abandoning them if they know that follow-up by telephone or office visit has been arranged. Often it is during the follow-up visits that one truly comes to know the child and understand the symptoms. It is possible that an organic problem may not have been apparent on the initial visit but, with time, the symptom-complex becomes more typical. Adult patients with irritable bowel disease and constipation have been treated with tegaserod, whereas those with diarrhea have been treated with alosetron. The latter drug has serious complications; there is little experience with its use in children.

These approaches often result in reduction or elimination of the abdominal symptoms. However, children with functional abdominal pain are likely to become adults with functional disorders, although the nature of the symptoms may change.

Boey CC, Goh KL, Hassall E, et al: Endoscopy in children with recurrent abdominal pain. *Gastrointest Endosc* 2001;53:142–43.

Chong SK, Lou Q, Asnicar MA, et al: *Helicobacter pylori* infection in recurrent abdominal pain in childhood: Comparison of diagnostic tests and therapy. *Pediatrics* 1995;96:211–15.

Croffie JM, Fitzgerald JF, Chong SK: Recurrent abdominal pain in children—a retrospective study of outcome in a group referred to a pediatric gastroenterology practice. *Clin Pediatr* 2000;39:267–74.

Duarte MA, Goulart EM, Penna FJ: Pressure pain threshold in children with recurrent abdominal pain. *J Pediatr Gastroenterol Nutr* 2000;31:280–85.

Garber J, Van Slyke DA, Walker LS: Concordance between mother's and children's reports of somatic and emotional symptoms in patients with recurrent abdominal pain or emotional disorders. *J Abnorm Child Psychol* 1998;26:381–91.

Hyams JS, Hyman PE, Rasquin-Weber A: Childhood recurrent abdominal pain and subsequent adult irritable bowel syndrome. *J Dev Behav Pediatr* 1999;20:318–19.

Hyams JS, Hyman PE: Recurrent abdominal pain and the biopsychosocial model of medical practice. *J Pediatr* 1998;133:473–78.

Stordal K, Nygaard EA, Bentsen B: Organic abnormalities in recurrent abdominal pain in children. *Acta Paediatr* 2001;90:638–42.

Walker LS, Guite JW, Duke M, et al: Recurrent abdominal pain: A potential precursor of irritable bowel syndrome in adolescents and young adults. *J Pediatr* 1998;132:1010–15.

Walker LS, Garber J, Smith CA, et al: The relation of daily stressors to somatic and emotional symptoms in children with and without recurrent abdominal pain. *J Consult Clin Psychol* 2001;69:85–91.

Wewer V, Strandberg C, Paerregaard A, et al: Abdominal ultrasonography in the diagnostic work-up in children with recurrent abdominal pain. *Eur J Ped* 1997; 156:737-88.

Chapter 324

Acute Appendicitis

Gary E. Hartman

Acute appendicitis is the most common condition requiring emergency abdominal operation in childhood. Diagnosis is difficult in young children, a factor contributing to perforation rates of 30–60%. Fifty per cent of children with perforated appendicitis have been seen by a physician before the diagnosis. The risk of perforation is greatest in 1- to 4-yr-old children (70–75%) and is lowest in the adolescent age group (30–40%), which has the highest age-specific incidence of appendicitis in childhood. The difficulty in distinguishing appendicitis from other common causes of abdominal pain and the increase in morbidity and mortality accompanying perforation keep appendicitis an important concern of clinicians.

Epidemiology. Approximately 80,000 children experience appendicitis in the United States annually, a rate of 4/1,000 children younger than age 14 yr. Appendicitis is rare in developing countries, where diets are high in fiber. However, no causal relationship has been established between lack of dietary fiber and appendicitis. The incidence of appendicitis increases with age, peaking in adolescence and rarely occurring in children younger than 1 yr old. A familial predilection to appendicitis has been reported. Cases occur more often in males, clustering of cases has occurred, and cases occur more often in the autumn and spring.

Etiology. Experimentally, ligation (obstruction) of the appendix results in a marked increase of intraluminal pressure, which rapidly exceeds systolic blood pressure. Initial venous congestion progresses to thrombosis, necrosis, and perforation. Clinically, obstruction of the lumen is the prime cause of appendicitis. The obstruction is caused by inspissated fecal material (fecalith). The inspissated material may calcify, leading to a radiographically visible appendicolith (15–20%). Obstruction resulting from mucosal edema may be associated with systemic or enteric viral or bacterial *(Yersinia, Salmonella, Shigella)* infections. Abnormal mucus has been suggested as the cause of the increased incidence of appendicitis in children with cystic fibrosis. Carcinoid tumors, foreign bodies, and *Ascaris* have rarely been implicated as causes of appendicitis. Neuroproliferation of the appendix may explain some instances of right lower quadrant pain that resolves with appendectomy, although no inflammation of the appendix is identifiable grossly at operation or on routine pathologic examination.

Pathology. The pathologic changes in appendicitis progress through three predictable phases. Initially, with luminal obstruction, venous congestion progresses to mucosal ischemia, necrosis, and ulceration. Bacterial invasion with inflammatory infiltrate through all layers of the appendiceal wall characterizes the second phase. Organisms can be cultured from the serosal surface before microscopic perforation. Finally, necrosis of the wall results in perforation and contamination of the peritoneum. The perforation usually occurs at the tip of the appendix, distal to the obstructing fecalith.

Subsequent to perforation, the microbiologic fecal contamination may be confined to the pelvis or the right iliac fossa by the omentum and adjacent loops of small bowel, or it may spread throughout the peritoneal cavity. Young children have a poorly developed omentum, and local perforation is not usually confined. Bacterial invasion of the mesenteric veins may result in portal vein sepsis (pylephlebitis) and subsequent liver abscess formation. The inflammatory process associated with perforation may lead to intestinal obstruction or paralytic ileus.

Clinical Manifestations. The clinical signs and symptoms depend on the pathologic phase of appendicitis at examination. The classic triad consists of pain, nausea with vomiting, and fever. In the initial stage of appendiceal obstruction, the pain is periumbilical. Emesis usually follows the onset of pain and is infrequent. Anorexia is more common. Fever is low grade unless perforation with peritonitis has occurred. The sequence of symptoms with pain preceding emesis and fever is important in distinguishing appendicitis from infectious enteritis, which usually begins with vomiting followed by the cramping pain of hyperperistalsis. Diarrhea, if it occurs, is infrequent and consists of small, mucous stools caused by irritation of the sigmoid colon. Similarly, irritation of the bladder may produce urinary symptoms such as frequency and urgency.

As the inflammation progresses to involve the serosa and overlying peritoneum, the pain migrates to the area of peritoneal irritation, usually the right lower quadrant. If the appendix is retrocecal, the pain will be lateral or posterior and may mimic the symptoms associated with septic arthritis of the hip or psoas abscess. With perforation, the pain becomes generalized unless the contamination is well localized to produce a discrete abscess, usually of the right lower quadrant. Palpation of an abdominal or rectal mass indicates abscess formation.

The progression from onset of symptoms to perforation usually occurs over 36–48 hr. If the diagnosis is delayed beyond 36–48 hr, the perforation rate exceeds 65%.

Diagnosis

PHYSICAL EXAMINATION. History and physical examination should be directed at establishing findings consistent with appendicitis and excluding alternative diagnoses such as viral gastroenteritis, constipation, urinary tract infection, hemolytic-uremic syndrome, Henoch-Schönlein purpura, mesenteric adenitis, pelvic osteomyelitis, psoas abscess, and tubo-ovarian diseases (ectopic pregnancy, ovarian cyst, pelvic inflammatory disease, ovarian torsion).

Pertinent aspects of the history favoring a diagnosis of appendicitis include onset of pain before vomiting or diarrhea, loss of appetite, migration of pain from periumbilical to right lower quadrant, and aggravation of pain during the trip to office or hospital. In excluding alternative diagnoses, it is essential to question the history of constipation, urinary tract symptoms, cough and fever suggesting lower lobe pneumonia, profuse diarrhea, headache, myalgias or other constitutional symptoms of viral syndromes, and similar symptoms in other household members. Untreated appendicitis proceeds to perforation within 48–72 hr; therefore, duration of symptoms is important in the interpretation of physical findings and in the determination of a treatment strategy.

Physical examination should begin with inspection of the child's demeanor as well as the appearance of the abdomen. The child with appendicitis frequently moves tentatively and slowly, hunched forward, and often with a slight limp. The child may protect the right lower quadrant with a hand and may be reluctant to climb onto the examining table. Early in appendicitis, the abdomen is flat. Discoloration or bruises should suggest abdominal trauma. Abdominal distention indicates a complication such as perforation or obstruction. Auscultation may reveal normal or hyperactive bowel sounds in early appendicitis, to be replaced with hypoactive bowel sounds as it progresses to perforation. Severe gastroenteritis usually produces persistently hyperactive bowel sounds.

Palpation of the abdomen should be gentle after the establishment of rapport and is aided by distraction with conversation or the assistance of a parent. The right lower quadrant (McBurney point) should be palpated last, after the examiner has had an opportunity to judge the response to examination of quadrants that should not be painful. The McBurney point is the junction of the lateral and middle thirds of the line joining the right anterior-superior iliac spine and the umbilicus. The most important physical finding in appendicitis is persistent direct tenderness to palpation and rigidity of the overlying rectus muscle. If the child is apprehensive or agitated from prior examination, the abdominal muscles may be diffusely tense, making interpretation of this finding impossible.

Testing for rebound tenderness must be done carefully to be meaningful. Deep abdominal palpation with sudden withdrawal of the examining hand causes pain or fear in all children and is not recommended. Gentle finger percussion in all four quadrants is a better test of rebound peritoneal irritation in all age groups but particularly in the frightened child. Testing for rebound tenderness and rectal examination should be the final aspects of the abdominal examination. The value of rectal examination in the diagnosis of appendicitis has been questioned. If the history and abdominal examination are convincing for appendicitis, the rectal examination adds little information. However, if the diagnosis is in doubt, particularly in the very young (younger than 4 yr) or in the female adolescent, rectal examination often yields important information.

After the focused abdominal examination, careful examination of the other body regions, including ears, mucous membranes, lungs, and skin, for signs of other diseases should be noted. Careful attention should be made to identify shock from sepsis, dehydration, or both.

LABORATORY FINDINGS. Laboratory evaluation of children with suspected appendicitis usually consists of complete blood cell count and urinalysis. Although many children with appendicitis have leukocytosis or shift in differential, many do not. The primary role of laboratory studies is to exclude alternative diagnoses such as urinary tract infection, hemolytic-uremic syndrome, Henoch-Schönlein purpura, and so on. The proximity of the appendix to the ureter may result in inflammatory cells in the urine. Up to 30 white blood cells per high-power field and 20 red blood cells have been reported in suppurative appendicitis. The presence of bacteria or pyuria greater than 30 white blood cells per high-power field suggests true urinary tract infection. Similarly, the presence of significant proteinuria or cast formation argues against appendicitis. Review of the complete blood cell count is directed at identification of microangiopathic anemia, thrombocytosis, or thrombocytopenia, all suggesting diagnoses other than appendicitis.

IMAGING STUDIES. The imaging studies that may be helpful in evaluating children with suspected appendicitis include plain radiographs of the abdomen or chest, ultrasonography, CT, and rarely barium enema. Findings of appendicitis on abdominal films include calcified appendicolith, small bowel distention or obstruction, and soft tissue mass effect. Severe constipation or lower lobe pneumonia may establish an alternative diagnosis. Graded compression ultrasonography is a noninvasive study with false-negative and false-positive rates of 8–10% (Fig. 324–1). It is particularly helpful in adolescent girls, whose symptoms may be due to pelvic inflammatory disease, ovarian cysts, or torsion. CT of the abdomen and pelvis has been used for complicated perforation with intra-abdominal abscesses but now is the standard for early diagnostic imaging. Early CT can improve diagnostic accuracy and can reduce hospitalization in patients with a normal scan. CT is more sensitive and specific than ultrasonography and more likely to change patient management. The value of CT in the diagnosis, localization, and percutaneous drainage of abscesses occurring in the postoperative period is well established. Barium enema findings are those of

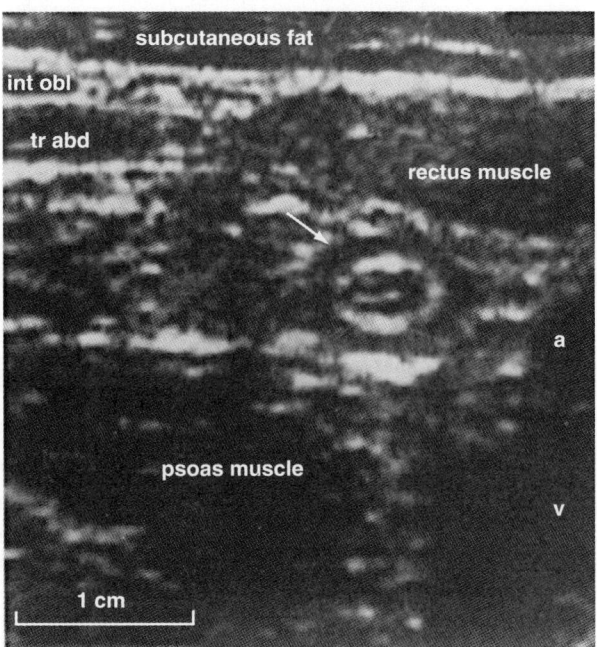

FIGURE 324–1. Graded compression ultrasonogram of acute appendicitis demonstrating edematous enlarged appendix compressed between the abdominal wall and the psoas muscle. int obl, internal oblique muscle; tr abd, transverse abdominis muscle; a, right iliac artery; v, right iliac vein. (From Puylaert JB, Rutgers PH, Laisang RI, et al: A prospective study of ultrasonography in the diagnosis of appendicitis. *N Engl J Med* 1987;317: 666.)

mass effect on the cecum from the inflammatory process and nonfilling or partial filling of the appendiceal lumen. However, many healthy children have nonfilling of the appendix, and this finding must be interpreted with caution.

DIFFERENTIAL DIAGNOSIS. Accurate diagnosis of children with abdominal pain is facilitated by a thorough and systematic approach. At the conclusion of the history, physical examination, and initial laboratory studies (complete blood cell count, urinalysis), patients fall into three groups: those with definite or highly likely appendicitis, those with a definite alternate diagnosis, and those in whom the diagnosis remains uncertain.

Vomiting preceding the pain, large-volume diarrhea, and high fever suggest gastroenteritis caused by viral or bacterial (*Yersinia*, *Campylobacter*) agents. Localized right lower quadrant pain in this setting may be mesenteric adenitis. An abnormal hemogram combined with hemorrhagic skin lesions suggests Henoch-Schönlein purpura or hemolytic-uremic syndrome if renal function and findings of urinalysis are abnormal. Weight loss and prolonged symptoms, especially in a teenager, makes inflammatory bowel disease a serious consideration. Torsion of an undescended testis is common, and particular note should be made of testicular location. Follicular cysts of the ovary occur in midcycle and may be painful as a result of rupture, rapid enlargement, or hemorrhage. In pelvic inflammatory disease, the pain is usually suprapubic, bilateral, and of longer duration.

Children with cystic fibrosis have a high incidence of appendicitis, but they also have a high incidence of intussusception, constipation, and meconium ileus equivalent. Children with malignancies may experience abdominal pain as a result of their chemotherapy, constipation, typhlitis, or appendicitis. If their malignancy is in remission, the signs and symptoms of appendicitis should be the same as those for healthy children. If the malignancy is not controlled, typhlitis is likely if the child is neutropenic. This entity results from necrotizing enterocolitis involving the terminal ileum and cecum and usually resolves with recovery of the neutrophil count and conservative management.

Those children with an uncertain diagnosis require either further diagnostic studies or observation, depending on the likelihood of appendicitis and the duration of symptoms. Observation may be done at home or in the hospital. If the diagnosis ultimately is appendicitis, the incidence of perforation is significantly higher (60% vs. 30%) if observation is carried out at home.

Once the diagnosis of appendicitis is made or highly suspect, the treatment is surgical appendectomy. Meckel diverticulitis may mimic appendicitis and is usually diagnosed at surgery (see Chapter 312.2).

Treatment. Children with nonperforated appendicitis require minimal preoperative preparation with intravenous fluids and antibiotics. Although the use of antibiotics in uncomplicated appendicitis is controversial, it has decreased the incidence of postoperative wound infections. Pain should be managed effectively with intravenous morphine even before the diagnosis is confirmed because such therapy does not adversely affect the examination or delay the diagnosis. Appendectomy should be done within a few hours of establishing the diagnosis and is usually performed through a right lower quadrant incision. Laparoscopic appendectomy has been used in children, although some studies have reported complication rates (intra-abdominal abscess formation) higher than those for open appendectomy. Further evaluation is needed before a definitive comparison of open and laparoscopic appendectomy can be made. In children with an uncertain diagnosis, particularly adolescent females, the laparoscopic approach has the advantage of allowing wider intraperitoneal exploration. Laparoscopy is associated with a shorter recovery period and a lower incidence of wound infection without a longer operative time. Appendectomy for nonperforated appendicitis is associated with a low complication rate, rapid recovery, and short (2–3 days) hospitalization.

If the appendix has perforated, especially with generalized peritonitis, significant fluid resuscitation and broad-spectrum antibiotics may be required a few hours before appendectomy. Nasogastric suction should be used if the patient has significant vomiting or abdominal distention. Antibiotics should cover the commonly encountered organisms (*Bacteroides, Escherichia coli, Klebsiella,* and *Pseudomonas* species). The commonly used intravenous regimens include ampicillin (100 mg/kg/24 hr), gentamicin (5 mg/kg/24 hr), and clindamycin (25–40 mg/kg/24 hr) or metronidazole (Flagyl) (30 mg/kg/24 hr). Appendectomy is performed with or without drainage of the peritoneal cavity, and antibiotics are continued for 7–10 days. Occasionally, a localized abscess is treated with antibiotics with or without open or percutaneous drainage with appendectomy scheduled as a second elective procedure in 4–6 wk. If antibiotics are successful, some clinicians question the need for a planned appendectomy. In perforated appendicitis, the postoperative course is characterized by continued fluid requirement, fever, intra-abdominal abscess formation, sepsis, and prolonged (4–5 days) paralytic ileus.

Complications. Complications occur in 25–30% of children with appendicitis, primarily those with perforation. The most effective method of reducing complications of appendicitis is to reduce the incidence of perforation. Mortality from appendicitis is low (0.5–1%). The complications are primarily infectious. Wound infection complicates recovery in 0–2% of children with nonperforated appendicitis and in 10–15% of those with perforated appendicitis. Treatment consists of opening the wound with healing by secondary intention. Further antibiotics are not necessary unless the patient has associated cellulitis or systemic signs of toxicity. Intra-abdominal abscess is rare in simple appendicitis but occurs in 4–6% of children with perforation.

Usually, the abscess in the right lower quadrant is solitary and, if needed, can be drained by a CT-guided or ultrasonogram-guided percutaneous approach. Multiple intra-abdominal abscesses are best treated by open laparotomy with drainage. Liver abscess from portal vein sepsis is uncommon but may require multiple drainage procedures.

Intestinal obstruction is a common complication and is usually managed with nasogastric suction if it occurs in the early postoperative period. Infertility caused by adhesions or obstruction of the distal fallopian tube is not associated with simple appendicitis but is three to four times more likely after perforation.

Applegate KE, Sivit CJ, Salvator AE, et al: Effect of cross-sectional imaging on negative appendectomy and perforation rates in children. *Radiology* 2001;220: 103–7.
Benjamin IS, Patel AG: Managing acute appendicitis. *BMJ* 2002;325:505–6.
Cobben LPJ, de Van Otterloo AM, Puylaert JB: Spontaneously resolving appendicitis: Frequency and natural history in 60 patients. *Radiology* 2000;215:349–50.
Flum DR, Morris A, Koepsell T, et al: Has misdiagnosis of appendicitis decreased over time? *JAMA* 2001;286:1748–53.
Huang MT, Wei PL, Wu CC, et al: Needlescopic, laparoscopic, and open appendectomy: A comparative study. *Surg Laparosc Endosc Percutan Tech* 2001;11:306–12.
Kim MK, Strait RT, Sato TT, et al: A randomized clinical trial of analgesia in children with acute abdominal pain. *Acad Emerg Med* 2002;9:281–87.
Murch SH: Diarrhoea, diagnostic delay, and appendicitis. *Lancet* 2000;356:787.
Sebastiano PD, Fink T, di Mola FF, et al: Neuroimmune appendicitis. *Lancet* 1999;354:461–66.
Soda K, Nemoto K, Yoshizawa S, et al: Detection of pinpoint tenderness on the appendix under ultrasonography is useful to confirm acute appendicitis. *Arch Surg* 2001;136:1136–40.

Chapter 325
Surgical Conditions of the Anus, Rectum, and Colon

Alberto Peña

In infants and children, close inspection of the anal area is as valuable as a digital rectal examination. *Fissures* can be best identified by having a parent hold the infant's hips in acute flexion so that the examiner can separate the patient's buttocks, using both thumbs, gently stretching the anus and everting the lining to expose the fissure. In all cases of constipation, especially when an obstruction is possible, a digital examination is indicated, after assessing perianal sensation. Properly done, this examination should cause little or no discomfort to the patient. A well-lubricated finger is passed over the anus a few times to accustom the patient to the unusual sensation. Then the pulp of the index or fifth finger is pressed against the anus with increasing flexion of the interphalangeal joints and the finger slips easily into the anal canal.

325.1 Anorectal Malformations

Anorectal malformations include a spectrum of defects. Some are complex, difficult to manage, and associated with important anatomic deficiencies and therefore have a poor functional prognosis. Others are minor and easily treated, having an excellent functional prognosis. The main concerns are future bowel control and urinary and sexual function. Anorectal anomalies occur in about 1/4,000 live births and manifest various grades from anal stenosis to agenesis or from rectal agenesis to atresia.

Embryology and Pathogenesis. The origin of the anus and the rectum is an embryologic structure called the cloaca. Lateral ingrowths of this structure form the urorectal septum, separating the rectum dorsally from the urinary tract ventrally. Both systems (rectum and urinary tract) become completely separated by the 7th wk of gestation. At this same time, the urogenital portion of the original cloaca already has an external opening, whereas the anal portion is closed by a membrane that opens by the 8th wk of gestation.

Abnormalities in the development of these processes at varying stages provoke a spectrum of anomalies, most of which affect the lower intestinal tract and the genitourinary structures. Persistence of communication between the genitourinary and rectal portions of the cloaca results in fistulas.

Pathology and Classification
MALE PATIENTS

Perineal Fistula. Perineal (cutaneous) fistula is the simplest defect in both sexes. Patients have a small orifice located in the perineum, anterior to the center of the external sphincter, close to the scrotum in the male or to the vulva in the female. Male patients frequently have in their perineum a "bucket handle"-type malformation or a "black ribbon"-type structure that represents a subepithelial fistula filled with meconium. These patients usually have a well-formed sacrum, a prominent midline groove, and a prominent anal dimple. The frequency of associated defects affecting other organs is less than 10%. The diagnosis is established by simple perineal inspection. Unfortunately, the diagnosis of this particular defect is frequently missed, owing to an inadequate neonatal examination. A missed or delayed diagnosis may have significant clinical implications, mainly involving exacerbation of constipation. No further investigations are required, and this defect can be repaired without a protective colostomy.

Rectourethral Fistula. In cases of rectourethral fistula, the rectum communicates with the lower part of the urethra (bulbar urethra) or the upper part of the urethra (prostatic urethra). The sphincteric mechanism usually is satisfactory; a few patients have poor perineal muscles and a flat-looking perineum. The sacrum may have different degrees of hypodevelopment, particularly in cases of rectourethral prostatic fistula. Most of these patients have a well-formed midline perineal groove and an anal dimple. Those with a rectoprostatic fistula have a poorly developed sacrum, frequently a flat perineum, a bifid scrotum, and an anal dimple located very close to the scrotum. These patients require a protective colostomy during the newborn period. The complete surgical repair is performed later in life. Rectourethral fistula represents the most frequent anorectal defect seen in male patients.

Rectovesical Fistula. In patients having rectovesical fistulas, the rectum communicates with the urinary tract at the level of the bladder neck. The rectal sphincteric mechanism is usually poorly developed. The sacrum is frequently deformed and is often absent. The perineum looks flat. This defect represents 10% of the total number of affected male patients. The prognosis for bowel function is usually poor. A colostomy is mandatory during the newborn period, followed by corrective surgical repair later in life.

Imperforate Anus Without Fistula. This defect has the same characteristics in both sexes. The rectum is completely blind and is usually found approximately 2 cm above the perineal skin. The sacrum and the sphincteric mechanism are usually well developed. The functional prognosis is usually good and is similar to that in those male patients with a rectourethral bulbar fistula. A colostomy is indicated during the newborn period. This defect is frequently associated with Down syndrome. When properly operated on, patients who have this defect and Down syndrome have the same good prognosis for bowel function as chromosomally normal children.

Rectal Atresia. Rectal atresia is a rare defect occurring in only 1% of anorectal anomalies. It has the same characteristics in both sexes. The unique feature of this defect is that affected patients have a normal anal canal and a normal anus. The defect is frequently discovered while a rectal temperature is being taken. An obstruction is present about 2 cm above the skin level. These patients need a protective colostomy. The functional prognosis is excellent because they have a normal sphincteric mechanism (and normal sensation), which resides in the anal canal.

FEMALE PATIENTS

Vestibular Fistula. Vestibular fistula is the most frequent defect seen in females. The rectum opens in the vestibule of the female genitalia immediately outside the hymen orifice. Patients are frequently mislabeled as having "rectovaginal fistula." The functional prognosis is excellent. The sacrum is usually normal, and the perineum shows a prominent midline groove and a noticeable anal dimple, all of which indicate that the sphincteric mechanism is intact. A protective colostomy is needed before the corrective surgical procedure, although this colostomy does not need to be performed on an emergency basis because the fistula is frequently competent to decompress the intestinal tract.

Persistent Cloaca. In cases of persistent cloaca, the rectum, vagina, and urinary tract meet and fuse into a single common channel. The perineum shows a single orifice located immediately behind the clitoris. The length of the common channels varies from 1–10 cm; this has important technical and prognostic implications. Patients with short common channels (<3 cm) usually have well-developed sacrums and good sphincters. A common channel longer than 3 cm usually suggests that the patient has a more complex defect and, frequently, has a poor sphincteric mechanism and a poor sacrum. Most patients with cloacas have an abnormally large vagina filled with mucous secretions (hydrocolpos). Different degrees of vaginal and uterine septation also are present. A diverting colostomy is indicated at birth; in addition, patients with a cloaca represent a urologic emergency because approximately 90% have associated urologic defects. Before the colostomy, the urologic diagnosis must be established to decompress the urinary tract, if necessary, at the same time the colostomy is created.

The term *rectovaginal fistula* is not used in this classification because true rectovaginal fistulas are extremely unusual defects.

Diagnosis and Early Management. Two important questions must be answered during the first 24 hours of life for neonates with anorectal malformations:

1. Does the neonate suffer from a serious associated defect that endangers life and requires urgent treatment?
2. Can the neonate be treated with an anoplasty or pull-through without a colostomy or is a colostomy needed?

The associated defects represent the main risk for the patient's life. The infant needs kidney, spinal, and pelvic ultrasonograms, an echocardiogram, a radiograph of the sacrum and lumbar spine, and close clinical observation for signs and symptoms of esophageal atresia and/or intestinal obstruction. The second question is answered after 24 hr because before that period imaging studies are not accurate.

MALE PATIENTS. Good clinical evaluation and a urinalysis provide sufficient information in 80–90% of patients to decide whether a colostomy is needed. If a patient has a perineal or rectourinary fistula, meconium may not be seen at the perineum or in the urine before 16–24 hr after birth. The most distal part of the bowel, in cases of perineal and rectourethral fistulas, is surrounded by voluntary sphincteric muscles; the intraluminal bowel pressure must be high enough to overcome the tone of those muscles before one can see meconium in the urine or in the perineum. At birth, the bowel is not distended; therefore, clinical and radiologic evaluations are not reliable during the first 16–24 hr of life. A piece of gauze is placed around the tip of the penis, and the nurse is instructed to check for particles of meconium filtered through this gauze. The presence of meconium in the urine and a flat bottom are considered indications to create a protective colostomy. Clinical findings consistent with the diagnosis of a perineal fistula represent an indication for an anoplasty without a protective colostomy. Sometimes none of the clinical signs already described becomes evident after 24 hr of observation; a radiologic evaluation is then indicated. A cross-table lateral film with the patient in a prone position taken after 16–24 hr of life is valuable for determining the position of the rectal pouch. When this pouch is separated from the skin by more than 1 cm, the patient needs a colostomy. During the first 24 hr of life, all these patients need renal and bladder ultrasound evaluation to identify an obstructive uropathy.

FEMALE PATIENTS. More than 90% of the time, the diagnosis can be established by a meticulous perineal inspection. These patients must be observed during the first 16–24 hr of life. The presence of a single perineal orifice is pathognomonic of a cloaca. A palpable pelvic mass (hydrocolpos) reinforces the suspicion of a cloaca. The diagnosis of a vestibular fistula can be established by careful separation of the labia to see the vestibule. The rectal orifice is located immediately behind the hymen within the female genitalia and in the vestibule. A perineal fistula is easy to diagnose. The rectal orifice is located somewhere between the female genitalia and the center of the sphincter and is surrounded by skin; the term *anterior anus*, which is sometimes used for this defect, is inadequate because these are abnormal fistula orifices not surrounded by a normal sphincteric mechanism. Fewer than 10% of these patients fail to pass meconium through the genitalia or perineum after 24 hr of observation. Those patients may require a cross-table lateral film. They also need a renal and bladder ultrasound study of the abdomen during the first 24 hr of life, because patients with persistent cloaca have the highest incidence of urologic defects.

Associated Defects. About 50% of children with anorectal anomalies have a urologic problem. The more serious and complex the anorectal defect, the more frequently it is associated with a urologic anomaly. Male patients with a rectovesical fistula and patients with a persistent cloaca have a 90% chance of having a urologic defect. On the other hand, patients with a rectoperineal fistula have less than a 10% chance. Urologic evaluation must be established before performing a colostomy. Untreated acidosis and sepsis resulting from an undetected obstructive uropathy are risks.

A good correlation exists between the degree of sacral development and the final functional prognosis. Patients with an absent sacrum have permanent fecal and urinary incontinence. Different degrees of sacral malformations are associated with important functional sequelae. Spinal abnormalities and different degrees of dysraphism are frequently associated with these defects. Tethered cord occurs in approximately 25% of patients with anorectal malformations; severe anorectal defects have a poor prognosis. It is important to establish the diagnosis to aid neurosurgical treatment. The diagnosis of spinal defects can be established during the first 3 mo of life by spinal ultrasound; in older patients, it is necessary to use magnetic resonance imaging. Other associated congenital malformations include esophageal atresia, duodenal atresia, and cardiovascular defects.

Treatment. Perineal fistulas are treated by a simple anoplasty without a protective colostomy; the operation is performed during the newborn period. The fistula orifice is moved back to the center of the external sphincter. Anal dilations are started 2 wk after the operation and are gradually increased to reach the size of a normal anus. All other defects are best managed during the newborn period with a protective colostomy. Later in life (1–12 mo), corrective surgical repair is performed. Lately, the tendency is toward the repair of most malformations during the newborn period without a protective colostomy. This approach could save these patients two operations (colostomy opening and colostomy closure). Serious complications and sequelae may occur after these operations; therefore, experienced surgeons, under controlled circumstances, should perform the neonatal approach without a colostomy. The patients must be carefully followed, and the results as well as the complications must be reported.

A posterior sagittal approach uses an electric muscle stimulator to identify the sphincteric mechanism. This approach allows a direct exposure to the internal anatomy, thus avoiding potential damage to important structures and nerves. A midline incision between both buttocks is used to split all the muscle structures in the midline. The rectum is separated from the genitourinary tract and, in cases of cloaca, the vagina and the urinary tract. The rectum is placed within the limits of the electrically determined sphincteric mechanism. The vagina and urinary tract are also reconstructed in cases of cloaca. Sometimes the rectum is too ectatic to be accommodated within the available space; therefore, the rectum has to be tailored accordingly. In male patients, the malformation can be repaired posterosagittally 90% of the time. The remaining 10% of patients have a rectovesical fistula because the rectum cannot be reached posterosagittally; a combined posterior sagittal and abdominal approach is needed. In cases of persistent cloaca, the abdomen must be opened in addition to the posterior sagittal approach, in 30–40% of patients, to mobilize a high rectum or high vagina. Laparoscopy has also been used to repair anorectal malformations. This novel form of treatment can conceivably avoid a laparotomy in those patients who would normally require such an approach. Larger series of patients and long-term follow-up of them are expected to determine the value of this therapeutic modality.

Two weeks after corrective surgery, the patients must be subjected to a protocol of anal dilations. These are done twice per day; every week a larger size dilator is passed to stretch the anus to normal size.

Prognosis. Patients of both sexes with perineal fistula and rectal atresia should have excellent functional results after the repair of their defects; they should be fully continent. Male patients with rectourethral bulbar fistula and patients of both sexes with imperforate anus without a fistula also have good prognosis. About 80% achieve bowel control between 3 and 4 yr of age. A significant number may occasionally suffer from minimal soiling.

Male patients with rectourethral prostatic fistula have about a 60% chance of having bowel control by the age of 3 yr. Male patients with rectovesical fistula have a poor functional prognosis. Only about 20% have voluntary bowel movements by the age of 3 yr.

An extremely abnormal sacrum usually means that the patient will have *fecal incontinence*. An extremely abnormal sacrum is most often associated with rectovesical fistula or rectoprostatic fistula. One rarely finds a good prognostic type of defect, such as perineal or vestibular fistula, associated with a poor sacrum. More than 90% of female patients with rectovestibular fistula have voluntary bowel movements by the age of 3 yr; few have occasional soiling.

Patients with a persistent cloaca with a common channel of less than 3 cm have about an 80% chance of having voluntary bowel movements by the age of 3 yr; most are urine continent. When the common channel is longer than 3 cm, most are fecal incontinent and require intermittent catheterization to empty their bladder. Patients with a persistent cloaca with a common channel longer than 3 cm usually have an extremely abnormal sacrum.

Approximately 25% of all patients have fecal incontinence, and about 70% of those with a cloaca with a long common channel need intermittent catheterization to empty the bladder. When these patients are old enough to be socially active, a medical program for bowel management and urinary control must be implemented. The use of enemas, suppositories, colonic irrigations, specific diets, and sometimes medications to regulate the motility of the colon will allow them to keep clean for 24 hr, thus improving their quality of life. Patients with fecal incontinence who have intractable diarrhea are usually refractory to medical management and require a permanent colostomy.

Most patients subjected to an operation to repair an imperforate anus have varying degrees of constipation. This symptom is more severe in patients with lower and simpler defects. Patients who had inadequate colostomies (loop colostomies that allow the passing of stool from the proximal into the distal limb of the bowel) may subsequently have constipation. These patients need a diet rich in fiber and, sometimes, laxatives to empty the rectum daily. Ineffective medical treatment may exacerbate the problem; the rectosigmoid colon continues to enlarge and becomes inefficient in emptying, making treatment a more difficult task.

Albanese CT, Jennings RW, Lopoo JB, et al: One-stage correction of high imperforate anus in the male neonate. *J Pediatr Surg* 1999;34:834.
Boemers TML, Beek FJA, Bax NMA: Guidelines for the urological screening and initial management of lower urinary tract dysfunction in children with anorectal malformations—the ARGUS protocol. *BJU Int* 1999;83:662.
Diseth T, Emblem R, Solbraa I, et al: A psychological follow-up of ten adolescents with low anorectal malformation. *Acta Paediatr* 1994;83:216.
Georgeson KE, Inge TH, Albanese CT: Laparoscopically assisted anorectal pull-through for high imperforate anus—A new technique. *J Pediatr Surg* 2000;35:927.
Levitt MA, Patel M, Rodriguez G, et al: The tethered spinal cord in patients with anorectal malformations. *J Pediatr Surg* 1997;32:462.
Miller OF, Kolon TF: Prenatal diagnosis of VACTERL association. *J Urol* 2001;166:2389.
Peña A, Hong AR: Advances in the management of anorectal malformations. *Am J Surg* 2000;180:370.
Peña A, Guardino K, Tovilla JM, et al: Bowel management for fecal incontinence in patients with anorectal malformations. J Pediatr Surg 1998;33:133.
Rich MA, Brock WA, Peña A: Spectrum of genitourinary malformations in patients with imperforate anus. *Pediatr Surg Int* 1988;3:110.
Torres R, Levitt MA, Tovilla JM, et al: Anorectal malformations and Down's syndrome. *J Pediatr Surg* 1998;33:194.
Tsakayannis DE, Shamberger RC: Association of imperforate anus with occult spinal dysraphism. *J Pediatr Surg* 1995;30:1010.

325.2 Anal Fissure

Anal fissure is a small laceration of the mucocutaneous junction of the anus. It is an acquired lesion secondary to the forceful passage of a hard stool, mainly seen in infancy. Fissures may be the consequence and not the cause of constipation.

Clinical Manifestations. Usually, a history of constipation is elicited. At some point, the patient had a painful bowel movement, which may correspond to the actual event of fissure formation after the passing of hard stool. Then, in addition to the primary cause of constipation, the patient retains stool voluntarily to avoid a painful bowel movement. This exacerbates the constipation, and, eventually, the passing of harder and larger stools creates a vicious cycle. Pain on defecation and bright red blood on the surface of the stool may be observed. The diagnosis is established by inspection of the anal area. For this examination, the infant's hips are held in acute flexion, the buttocks are separated to expand the folds of the perianal skin, and the fissure becomes evident as a minor laceration. Sometimes, peripheral to the laceration, the patient has a little skin appendage that actually represents epithelialized granulomatous tissue, secondary to the chronic inflammation; this is usually known as a "tag."

Treatment. The most important element in the treatment of this condition is for the parents to understand the origin of the laceration and the mechanism of the cycle of constipation. The goal of the treatment is to reverse this cycle, which can be achieved only by guaranteeing that the patient has soft stools to avoid overstretching the anus. The healing process may take several days or even several weeks. One single episode of impaction with passing of a hard piece of stool may exacerbate the problem. A stool softener is indicated, but the parents must adjust the dose to the response of the patient. The goal is to avoid both hard stools and diarrhea. Simultaneously, the primary cause of the constipation must be treated when present. No scientific basis supports other types of treatments, including stretching of the anus, "internal" anal sphincterotomy, or excision of the fissure. Chronic anal fissures in older patients have been managed with the local injection of botulinum toxin to treat the associated contraction of the sphincter. The role of this agent in young children is not defined.

325.3 Perianal Abscess and Fistula

Perianal abscess and fistula can be seen in two different groups of pediatric patients with different cause, pathogenesis, and treatment. These include (1) infants with no predisposing conditions and (2) older children with predisposing conditions. This disorder is relatively common in the first group, which includes infants, usually boys younger than 2 yr. This is usually a benign, self-limited condition; the abscess has a communication with one of the crypts of the pectinate line of the anal canal. It is believed that the crypt is the source of contamination; the exact mechanism is unknown. The abscess eventually drains through an orifice in the perianal area. After this drainage, the inflammation subsides, but a fistula remains that communicates with the affected crypt to the perianal external orifice. This condition can be demonstrated during surgical treatment. The fistula becomes chronic but usually disappears spontaneously before 2 yr of age. This fistula is located close to the lumen of the anus, a feature that makes this a very benign condition because the sphincteric mechanism is not affected.

The second group includes patients older than 2 yr with perianal or perirectal abscess and with a predisposing illness, including drug-induced or autoimmune neutropenia, leukemia, AIDS, diabetes mellitus, Crohn disease, prior rectal surgery (Hirschsprung disease, imperforate anus), or sequelae from the use of immunosuppressant drugs. This is considered a much more serious condition; the prognosis is intimately related to that of the predisposing disease. The abscess may be deep and may rapidly expand with severe toxic symptoms, particularly when the predisposing illness is associated with immunosuppression or neutropenia. Bacteriologic examination of abscess material reveals mixed aerobic (*Escherichia coli, Klebsiella pneumoniae, Staphylococcus aureus*) and anaerobic (*Bacteroides* species, *Clostridium, Veillonella*) flora. Ten to 15% yield pure growth of *E. coli, S. aureus,* or *Bacteroides fragilis.* Neutropenic patients may also have bacteremia that inconsistently has the same organism as the abscess.

Clinical Manifestations. The infants with no predisposing conditions have mild clinical manifestations, sometimes including low-grade fever, mild rectal pain, and an area of perianal cellulitis. Subsequently, a pustule is formed and the abscess drains through that orifice. This alleviates the symptoms. The inflammation disappears and the pustule heals. However, one or several weeks later, the draining of pus reappears and continues in an intermittent, chronic way. Left alone, this condition usually heals spontaneously before 2 yr of age.

Children with predisposing conditions have a much more serious clinical course. They may or may not have fever depending on their immunologic status. Cellulitis may rapidly expand with warmth, erythema, induration, tenderness, and fluctuation over the ischiorectal fossa, requiring aggressive treatment. Patients may experience severe toxicity and may become septic. In addition, they may show symptoms of the predisposing illness.

Treatment. Infants with no predisposing disease usually do not require any treatment because this condition is self-limited. No evidence indicates that antibiotics are useful in these patients. Occasionally, when the patient is extremely uncomfortable, the abscess can be drained under local anesthesia. This alleviates the symptoms of pain and fever but does not eliminate the possibility of a fistula formation. Once a chronic fistula has formed, most clinicians recommend a *fistulotomy* under general anesthesia. The anal canal and lower part of the rectum are exposed with an adequate retractor, and a lacrimal probe is passed through the external orifice of the fistula, coming out through one of the crypts. The tissue between the fistula and the lumen of the anal canal is divided with cautery. The wound is left open to granulate spontaneously. This treatment usually runs a 20% chance of recurrence. Conservative management (observation) is also accepted because in most cases the fistula disappears spontaneously before 2 yr of age.

Older children with predisposing diseases may require more aggressive treatment and treatment of the predisposing condition. Antibiotics must be administered, including a combination that covers enteric gram-negative organisms, *S. aureus,* and fecal anaerobic flora. Wide excision and drainage are mandatory in cases of sepsis and expanding cellulitis.

Fistulas in older patients are mainly associated with Crohn disease or with a history of pull-through surgery for the treatment of Hirschsprung disease. Those fistulas are difficult to treat. The treatment is the same as that of the predisposing condition.

325.4 Hemorrhoids

Hemorrhoids in children are uncommon and are usually benign. When a hemorrhoid is seen, one must suspect portal hypertension. Infants are sometimes brought for consultation after an incidental finding of a hemorrhoid. These follow a benign course. No reports of thrombosis or other complications of hemorrhoids exist in children; therefore, they should be managed conservatively. Chronic constipation, fecal impaction, or any other kind of irritating local factors must be treated to avoid exacerbation of this condition.

325.5 Rectal Prolapse

Rectal prolapse refers to the exteriorization of the rectal mucosa through the anus. When this extrusion includes all the layers of the rectal wall, it is called *procidentia.* Most cases of rectal tissue protruding through the anus are prolapse and not polyps, intussusception, or other tissue.

Most cases of prolapse are idiopathic. The onset is often between age 1 and 5 yr (mean, age 3 yr). Predisposing factors include intestinal parasites (particularly in endemic areas), malnutrition, diarrhea, ulcerative colitis, pertussis, Ehlers-Danlos syndrome, meningocele (more frequently associated with procidentia owing to the lack of perineal muscle support), cystic fibrosis, and chronic constipation. Patients treated surgically for imperforate anus may have different degrees of rectomucosal prolapse. This is particularly common in patients with poor sphincteric development.

Clinical Manifestations. Prolapse of the rectum usually occurs during defecation. Afterward, the prolapse is reduced sometimes spontaneously or manually by the patient or parent. In very severe cases, the prolapsed rectum remains chronically exteriorized, becoming congested and edematous, which makes it more difficult to reduce. Rectal prolapse is usually painless or is associated with a mild discomfort. When the rectum remains prolapsed after defecation, it may be traumatized by underwear and may produce bleeding and wetness. Eventually, the exposed rectum becomes ulcerated. The protruding mass varies from bright red to dark red; it may be as long as 10–12 cm. See Chapter 326 for a distinction from a prolapsed polyp.

Treatment. The evaluation should include all the necessary tests to rule out the already stated predisposing conditions. *Reduction of protrusion* is aided by pressure with warm compresses. An easy method of reduction is to cover the finger with a piece of toilet paper, introduce it into the lumen of the mass, and gently push it into the patient's rectum. The finger is then immediately withdrawn. The toilet paper adheres to the mucous membrane, permitting release of the finger; the paper, when softened, is later expelled.

General measures should include careful manual reduction of the prolapse after an episode of defecation, attempts to avoid excessive pushing during bowel movements (with patient's feet off the floor), use of laxatives and stool softeners in cases of constipation, avoidance of inflammatory conditions of the rectum, and treatment of intestinal parasitosis when present. If all this fails, surgical treatment may be indicated. None of the existing operations is considered ideal because each has risks and disadvantages. Therefore, medical treatment should always be tried first. Operations include the placement of a subcutaneous, ring-like band in the perianal area to decrease the diameter of the anus. Significant numbers of patients become asymptomatic with this treatment; some may experience megacolon, owing to a mechanical anal obstruction. Injection of sclerosing substances in the perirectal area has been reported but has the risk of nerve damage and infection. A posterior incision of the rectum, with anchoring of the rectum to the presacral periosteum, represents a useful alternative in severe cases. In cases of procidentia associated with myelomeningocele, patients may require laparotomy and internal fixation of the rectum to the presacral fascia.

325.6 Pilonidal Sinus and Abscess

A dimple located in the midline intergluteal cleft, at the level of the coccyx, is seen relatively frequently in normal infants. No evidence indicates that this little pilonidal sinus provokes any problems for the patient. Malignant degeneration of pilonidal sinus cyst has been reported only in patients with chronic infections and abscesses. An open dermal sinus is a benign condition and is usually asymptomatic.

Pilonidal abscesses occur in adolescent patients. Why this condition is not seen in younger patients is unknown. The abscess may require incision and drainage during the acute stage, and, subsequently, it requires en bloc resection to remove all the epithelial tract that caused the problem.

Ashcraft KW, Garred JL, Holder TM, et al: Rectal prolapse: 17 year experience with the posterior repair and suspension. *J Pediatr Surg* 1990;15:992.
Longo WE, Touloukian RJ, Seashore JN: Fistula in ano in infants and children: Implications and management. *Pediatrics* 1991;87:737.
Maria G, Cassetta E, Gui D, et al: A comparison of botulinum toxin and saline for the treatment of chronic anal fissure. *N Engl J Med* 1998;338:217.
Piazza DJ, Radhakrishnan J: Perianal abscess and fistula-in-ano in children. *Dis Colon Rectum* 1990;12:1014.
Pearl RH, Ein SH, Churchill B: Posterior sagittal anorectoplasty for pediatric recurrent rectal prolapse. *J Pediatr Surg* 1989;24:1100.
Rakhimov S: Treatment of rectal prolapse in children. *Vestn Khir* 1989;142:72.

Chapter 326
Tumors of the Digestive Tract *Joel Shilyansky*

Familial Polyposis Syndromes. The familial syndromes associated with intestinal polyps are particularly important because of the malignant potential of the lesions. Children need to be followed regularly, and a plan for appropriate intervention should be formulated in advance (Table 326–1).

TABLE 326–1. Gastrointestinal Polyps in Children

Syndrome	Gene Defect	Histology	Frequency	Gastrointestinal Cancer Risk
Common juvenile polyps	Unknown	Hamartoma	1:100 to 1:50	None*
FAP coli (including Gardner's and Turcot's variants)	APC	Adenoma	1:17,000 to 1:5,000	100%
PJS	LKB1 (STK11); ? others	Hamartoma	1:120,000	Increased
CS	PTEN; ? others	Hamartoma	Rare	Uncertain
BRRS	PTEN; ? others	Hamartoma	Rare	None
Juvenile polyposis	SMAD4; ? PTEN; ? others	Hamartoma	Rare	50%

*If solitary.

FAP = familial adematous polyposis; APC = adenomatous polyposis coli; PJS = Peutz-Jeghers syndrome; CS = Cowden syndrome; BRRS = Bannayan-Riley-Ruvalcaba syndrome; PTEN = protein tyrosine phosphatase and tensin homolog.

From Corredor J, et al: Gastrointestinal polyps in children: Advances in molecular genetics, diagnosis and management. J. Pediatr 2001;138:621–28.

Juvenile colonic polyps, also known as retention or inflammatory polyps, are the most common childhood bowel tumors, present in 1–3% of people younger than 21 yr old. Polyps rarely appear before 1 yr of age, and most present between 2–10 yr of age. Juvenile polyps are uncommon beyond age 15 yr. The polyps are evenly distributed through the colon. Solitary polyps are common; two or more may occur. Most juvenile polyps are erythematous, friable, and pedunculated and range in size from a few millimeters to 3 cm. Histologic examination demonstrates hamartomatous proliferation of mucus-filled glandular and stromal elements, marked vascularity, and infiltration with lymphocytes, eosinophils, and polymorphonuclear and plasma cells. The polyps have characteristic mucus-filled cystic glands and are covered by a fragile, single layer of epithelium. The typical juvenile polyp with no adenomatous change has no potential for malignancy. Juvenile polyps with an adenomatous component have rarely been reported (see Table 326–1).

Clinical manifestations usually include bright red, painless, rectal bleeding during or immediately after defecation. Exsanguinating hemorrhage is rare; bleeding often stops spontaneously. Iron-deficiency anemia is present in 30% of children, but it is rarely the initial chief complaint. Lower abdominal pain and cramps are uncommon and are associated with intussusception. Prolapsed polyps appear as dark, beefy red, pedunculated masses, in distinction to the lighter pink mucosal appearance of rectal prolapse. Perianal pruritus and mucous discharge are often associated with prolapse. Spontaneous polyp infarction and self-amputation are common; diarrhea and obstruction are uncommon. The differential diagnosis includes other forms of intestinal polyposis, Meckel diverticulum, anal fissure, inflammatory bowel disease, intestinal infections, Henoch-Schönlein purpura, and coagulation disorders.

The *diagnosis* is usually made by colonoscopy. Polyps appear as smooth, pedunculated lesions. Air-contrast barium enema can demonstrate polyps, but colonoscopy would still be required for treatment. *Treatment* includes the removal of the polyp at colonoscopy by snare cautery or, rarely, by transabdominal polypectomy. Retrieval of polyps for histologic confirmation of the diagnosis should always be performed. Recurrences occasionally are seen.

Multiple juvenile colonic polyps (more than three to five) occur in families as an autosomal dominant trait and are associated with congenital anomalies (20% of new cases are sporadic). In a subset of families, inactivating mutations are found in the SMAD4 and bone morphogenetic protein receptor 1A genes, resulting in interruption of intracellular signaling of the transforming growth factor-β. These polyps are identical to solitary polyps; however, afflicted individuals are at greatly increased risk for gastrointestinal cancer (~50%). Children can present with painless bleeding or, rarely, when the entire gastrointestinal tract is involved, with failure to thrive, malabsorption, anemia, hypoalbuminemia, and abdominal pain.

The risk of cancer is low in patients without a family history of cancer and two or fewer polyps, whereas patients with three or more polyps are at increased risk for malignancy. Patients with multiple juvenile polyps or a family history of juvenile polyposis should undergo colonoscopy every 3 yr. The frequency of examinations should increase in adult patients (see Table 326–1).

Cowden syndrome (CS) and **Bannayan-Riley-Ruvalcaba syndrome (BRRS)** are rare autosomal dominant syndromes associated with multiple, distinct anomalies and hamartomas in skin (99% of patients), breast, thyroid, endometrium, brain, and the gastrointestinal tract (60% of patients). Both syndromes are associated with mutations in a tumor suppressor gene termed *protein tyrosine phosphatase and tensin homologue (PTEN)*. Affected individuals are at increased risk for cancer of the thyroid and breast, whereas the risk of gastrointestinal neoplasms is uncertain (see Table 326–1).

Familial Adenomatous Polyposis Coli (FAP). Large numbers of adenomatous lesions throughout the colon characterizes these autosomal dominant, premalignant conditions. All are caused by germ line mutations in the adenomatous polyposis coli *(APC)* gene, a tumor suppressor gene localized to chromosome 5q21. *APC* gene mutations result in truncation of the cytoplasmic protein, which is responsible for binding and regulating the degradation of β-catenin. Intracellular accumulation of β-catenin may have a role in the formation of adenomas. The incidence of FAP is 1 in 5,000 to 17,000 persons, with usual onset of polyp development late in the 1st decade of life or during adolescence. By definition, more than five adenomatous polyps are present in the colon at the time of diagnosis. Usually more than 100 (often 1,000) visible adenomas are present when the patient is in the 2nd or 3rd decade. Congenital hypertrophy of retinal pigment epithelial cells is also present from birth in most patients. Variability in the clinical features, including extracolonic manifestations, depends on the location of the mutation on the *APC* gene. Thus, mutations of the *APC* gene are also responsible for **Gardner syndrome** (multiple colorectal polyps, periampullary polyps, osteomas [mandibular], lipomas, fibromas, epidermoid cysts, and desmoid tumors) and some but not all cases of **Turcot syndrome** (primary brain tumor/medulloblastoma and multiple colorectal polyposis). The soft tissue lesions (desmoid tumors) and osteomas may appear during childhood, whereas intestinal polyps may not become apparent until adolescence or early adult life. These premalignant polyps may develop anywhere along the digestive tract, but colonic and duodenal (periampullary) lesions predominate. The relative risk of hepatoblastoma, thyroid carcinoma, and cholangiocarcinoma is also increased. Some families who do not meet the criteria for familial adenomatous polyposis coli but who have a high frequency of adenomatous polyps and colonic cancer may also have a mutation of the *APC* gene (see Table 326–1).

Clinically, initially, the polyps are asymptomatic; many often remain so. When symptomatic, adenomatous polyps cause hematochezia, occasionally cramps, or, rarely, diarrhea. Malignancy arising from pre-existing adenomatous polyps has been reported in children as young as 10 yr of age, although these lesions more commonly appear in young adults. Most affected individuals will have cancer by age 40 yr.

The *diagnosis* should be suspected from the family history and confirmed by colonoscopy. The polyps are numerous; biopsies demonstrate the adenomatous nature in contrast to the inflammatory and cystic finding of juvenile polyps. *APC* gene mutations are detected in 80–90% of families with FAP, a finding allowing for presymptomatic testing in association with genetic counseling. If a mutation is identified in the index patient, affected family members can be differentiated from unaffected members by gene testing. If the index patient is among the 10–20% of individuals with this disorder in whom the mutation is not defined, genetic testing of family members may identify novel mutations in the *APC* gene. Because a negative result can be misleading, caution should be exercised in counseling families. A child with diagnosed FAP or family history of FAP and a positive gene test should be followed with colonoscopy every 6–12 mo until definitive surgical treatment is undertaken. If genetic testing is negative in a family with an identified mutation, the child is likely not to have FAP. Patients with Gardner syndrome should also undergo regular gastroduodenoscopy and removal of gastric and duodenal polyps. Premalignant lesions of the ampulla of Vater occur in adulthood and can be usually treated with local resection.

Definitive *treatment* of FAP requires prophylactic proctocolectomy to prevent cancer. Ileoanal pull-through restores bowel continuity with excellent functional results. Although controversy regarding the timing of surgery exists, the success of reconstruction has allowed earlier resection, thus averting the risk of invasive carcinoma. Nonsteroidal anti-inflammatory drugs, such as sulindac, and more selective cyclooxygenase-2 inhibitors, such as celecoxib, may slow polyp development; however, their efficacy in preventing malignant transformation is currently unknown and their use remains investigational.

Peutz-Jeghers Syndrome (PJS). This rare, autosomal dominant inherited syndrome is characterized by mucosal pigmentation of the lips and gums and hamartomas of the gastrointestinal tract. Deeply pigmented discrete freckles are seen at birth or appear during infancy on the lips and buccal mucosa and even around the mouth. Evidence of intestinal lesions may come from bleeding but more commonly may arise from crampy pain associated with obstruction due to recurrent intussusception.

Polyps in PJS are benign hamartomas characterized by a "frondlike" core of stromal tissue and smooth muscle surrounded by normal-appearing intestinal epithelium. Intestinal lesions should be excised if they are causing significant and persistent symptoms; involvement is usually too extensive to remove all the polyps.

Family studies and genetic counseling may reveal relatives with either partial or complete manifestations of the syndrome. Fifty per cent of patients, however, have no family member with the disorder, a finding suggesting a high rate of new mutations. Inactivating mutations in a gene located on chromosome 19p13.3, *LKB1* (*STK11*) encoding a serine/threonine kinase has been implicated in the pathogenesis of PJS. Cancer develops in up to 50% of people having PJS, most commonly middle-aged adults. Colorectal, breast, and gynecologic tumors are seen most frequently. Mammography, gynecologic examination, and colonoscopy starting in the late 20s or early 30s are recommended (see Table 326–1).

Hemangioma. These rare benign lesions can cause massive, even fatal, hemorrhage. The usual clinical manifestation is painless bleeding beginning in childhood. The blood loss can be subtle and chronic or sudden and massive. Usually, the patient has

no additional intestinal symptoms, but intussusception with obstructive symptoms may occur. About 50% of patients have cutaneous hemangiomas; some have a family history of similar lesions. About half of these lesions are in the colon, where they may be seen by colonoscopy. Lesions that are more difficult to locate may be seen with the capsule-size ingested camera. During a period of bleeding, selective mesenteric arteriography may be useful in locating a lesion.

Leiomyoma. This rare benign tumor occurs most commonly in the stomach, jejunum, and distal ileum. It can remain asymptomatic for long periods. Symptoms may result from intussusception, volvulus, central necrosis, and obstruction. Leiomyoma may be difficult to differentiate from leiomyosarcoma, a malignant tumor that occurs rarely in the gastrointestinal tract in children. Smooth muscle tumors occur at increased frequency in children with AIDS or immunosuppression after transplantation.

Carcinoma. Epithelial tumors of the digestive tract are rare in children. Several childhood conditions predispose to development of gastrointestinal adenocarcinoma in early adulthood, for example, FAP, hereditary nonpolyposis colon carcinoma (HNPCC), Peutz-Jeghers syndrome, juvenile polyposis coli, ulcerative colitis, and, to a lesser extent, Crohn disease and disorders associated with chromosomal fragility. The usual site is the colon, but gastric and duodenal lesions are reported. Diagnosis is made based on family history, endoscopic findings, gastrointestinal bleeding, or obstruction. Symptoms are nonspecific abdominal pain, an abdominal mass, and, less frequently, hemorrhage. The tumors are relatively undifferentiated and highly malignant. The treatment of colorectal carcinoma is primarily surgical. Prognosis is related to stage of disease. Carcinoma of the colon without any known predisposing factors is an extremely rare occurrence in children. Thus it is important to obtain a complete family history and provide effective genetic screening and counseling to cancer patients (index cases) and their families to identify family members at risk. Mutations in the *APC* gene, leading to FAP and DNA mismatch repair genes (*hMSH2, hMSH6, PMS1, PMS2 and hMLH1*), leading to HNPCC are most commonly associated with colorectal carcinoma in children and young adults. Diagnosis of HNPCC should be suspected in the presence of family history of early-onset colon carcinoma and could be confirmed by genetic analysis. While the great majority of patients with HPNCC do not develop cancers until adulthood, the author has encountered two cases of colon carcinoma in teenagers. The age to begin endoscopic surveillance remains controversial and should be tailored to the individual patient. In addition, the risk of uterine, ovarian, pancreatic, biliary, and gastric cancer is also increased. Ethical, social, and psychological impact must be considered when genetic screening is contemplated. Carcinoma of the stomach is very rare, mimics the disease in adults, and may be associated with HNPCC and hereditary diffuse gastric cancer syndrome (HDGC). HDGC, an autosomal dominant inherited disorder, is caused by inactivating germline mutations in *CDH1*, a gene encoding E-cadherin, a calcium dependent adhesion protein that regulates the localization and function of the catenins. Genetic screening for *CDH1* mutations and prophylactic gastrectomy for carriers are controversial.

Lymphoma. Lymphoma is the most common malignancy of the gastrointestinal tract in children (see Chapter 488). About 30% of children with non-Hodgkin lymphoma present with abdominal tumors. Disorders that predispose to lymphoma include AIDS, ataxia-telangiectasia, Wiskott-Aldrich syndrome, agammaglobulinemia, severe combined immunodeficiency syndrome, bone marrow or solid organ transplantation, and long-standing celiac disease. Lymphoma can arise in the stomach, distal ileum, cecum, or appendix and may present as crampy abdominal pain, vomiting,

TABLE 326-2. Diarrhea Caused by Hormone-Secreting Tumors

Name	Site	Hormone	Manifestations	Therapy
Carcinoid	Intestinal argentaffin cells Appendix, ileum, colon, jejunum, rectum Bronchial tree	Serotonin	Diarrhea, crampy abdominal pain, flushing, wheezing, cardiac valve damage	Somatostatin analogues; resection
Gastrinoma	Pancreas	Gastrin	Peptic ulcer, diarrhea	H$_2$-blocking agents; omeprazole; tumor resection; gastrectomy
Mastocytoma	Cutaneous, intestine, liver, spleen	Histamine, VIP	Pruritus, flushing, apnea, if VIP(+) diarrhea	H$_1$- and H$_2$-blocking agents, cromolyn, steroids; resection if solitary
Medullary carcinoma	Thyroid	Calcitonin, VIP, prostaglandins	Watery diarrhea	Thyroidectomy
Ganglioneuroma, ganglioneuroblastoma, neuroblastoma, pheochromocytoma	Chromaffin cells; abdominal > other sites; extra-adrenal or adrenal	Catecholamines, VIP	Hypertension, tachycardia, sweating, anxiety, watery diarrhea*	α-Adrenergic blockade for BP control; β-adrenergic blockade for tachycardia; resection
Somatostatinoma	Pancreas	Somatostatin	Massive diarrhea	Resection
VIPoma	Pancreas	VIP	Watery diarrhea, achlorhydria, hypokalemia	Somatostatin analogues; resection

*Diarrhea has been reported only in adult patients with pheochromocytoma.
VIP = vasoactive intestinal polypeptide, BP = blood pressure, H$_1$ = histamine receptor type 1, H$_2$ = histamine receptor type 2.

distention, or a palpable abdominal mass. Perforation is uncommon. Bowel lymphoma should be ruled out in children older than 3 yr of age presenting with an acute intussusception. It may be difficult to differentiate symptoms of small bowel lymphoma from Crohn disease.

Carcinoid Tumors. These tumors of the enterochromaffin cells of the intestine usually occur in the appendix in children and are very low-grade malignancies. They may be found incidentally in the appendix at appendectomy. Complete resection with clear surgical margins of a carcinoid tumor of the appendix less than 1 cm in size is usually curative. Carcinoid tumors outside the appendix (ileojejunum, colon, and rectum in order of frequency) commonly metastasize; lesions metastatic to the liver can give rise to the carcinoid syndrome, which is the result of pharmacologically active hormones produced by the tumor. These produce episodic intestinal hypermotility and diarrhea, vasomotor disturbances (flushing), bronchoconstriction (wheezing), and right-sided heart failure. The most important active agent is serotonin; and finding high urinary levels of its metabolite, 5-hydroxyindoleacetic acid (5-HIAA), usually makes the diagnosis. The functional neoplasms are rare in children. Carcinoid may also spread to the small bowel mesentery, inducing severe retroperitoneal and mesenteric fibrosis. Treatment with long-acting somatostatin analogues can provide significant palliation.

Nodular Lymphoid Hyperplasia (NLH). Lymphoid follicles in the lamina propria of the gut normally aggregate in Peyer patches, which are more prominent in the distal ileum. When hyperplastic they appear as submucosal nodules on contrast radiographs and may be mistaken for an abnormality. NLH may occur in the colon or the small bowel. Diffuse small bowel NLH may be seen in cases of immunoglobulin deficiency, with and without *Giardia lamblia* infestation. Patients may have rectal bleeding, diarrhea, and abdominal cramps, but symptoms are generally mild. In infants with dietary-protein hypersensitivity, NLH may occur in association with enterocolitis. NLH also has been noted to occur in inflammatory bowel disease and Castleman disease. The major importance of this entity is the similarity of its manifestations to more serious disorders. NLH usually resolves spontaneously and rarely requires specific treatment. Cyproheptadine or prednisone has been used for extreme bleeding or abdominal pain.

326.1 Diarrhea from Hormone-Secreting Tumors

Certain hormone-producing tumors cause a marked increase in intestinal secretion leading to severe chronic watery diarrhea (Table 326–2). The secretory diarrhea persists even if food is withheld. These tumors originate in the neural crest–derived APUD cells (*a*mine content, *p*recursor *u*ptake, amino acid *d*ecarboxylation) of the gastroenteropancreatic endocrine system and in adrenal or extra-adrenal neurogenic sites.

Diarrhea is massive and results in fluid and electrolyte imbalance and weight loss. Diagnosis is based on the presence of secretory watery diarrhea, extraintestinal manifestations, measurement of the suspected hormone or its metabolites in serum or urine, and various imaging techniques. If possible, tumor resection is the treatment of choice. Pharmacologic therapy with hormone antagonists such as long-acting synthetic somatostatin analogues may be palliative (see Table 326–2). Radioactively labeled somatostatin analogues have also been used as part of experimental treatment approaches.

Tumors of the Digestive Tract
Attard TM, Giardiello FM, Argani P, et al: Fundic gland polyposis with high-grade dysplasia in a child with attenuated familial adenomatous polyposis and familial gastric cancer. *J Pediatr Gastroenterol Nutr* 2001;32:215.
Bethel CA, Bhattacharyya N, Hutchinson C, et al: Alimentary tract malignancies in children. *Pediatr Surg* 1997;32:1004.
Bond JH: Colorectal cancer update: Prevention, screening, treatment, and surveillance for high-risk groups. *Med Clin North Am* 2000;84:1163–82.
Colon AR, DiPalma JS, Leftridge CA: Intestinal lymphonodular hyperplasia of childhood: Patterns of presentation. *J Clin Gastroenterol* 1991;13:163–66.
Corredor J, Wambach J, Barnard J: Gastrointestinal polyps in children: Advances in molecular genetics, diagnosis, and management. *J Pediatr* 2001;138:621–28.
Entius MM, Westerman AM, van Velthuysen ML, et al: Molecular and phenotypic markers of hamartomatous polyposis syndromes in the gastrointestinal tract. *Hepatogastroenterology* 1999;46:661–66.
Gupta SK, Fitzgerald JF, Croffie JM, et al: Experience with juvenile polyps in North American children: The need for pancolonoscopy. *Am J Gastroenterol* 2001;96:1695-97.
Howe JR, Bair JL, Sayed MG, et al: Germline mutations of the gene encoding bone morphogenetic protein receptor 1A in juvenile polyposis. *Nat Genet* 2001;28:184–87.
Huang SC, Lavine JE, Boland PS, et al: Germline characterization of early-aged onset of hereditary non-polyposis colorectal cancer. *J Pediatr* 2001;138:629–35.
Lipsky PE. Recommendations for the clinical use of cyclooxygenase-2-specific inhibitors. *Am J Med* 2001;110:3S–5S.
Liu H, Ruskon-Fourmestraux A, Lavergne-Slove A, et al: Resistance of t(11;18) positive gastric mucosa-associated lymphoid tissue lymphoma to *Helicobacter pylori* eradication therapy. Lancet 2001;357:39–40.

Molle ZL, Moallem H, Desai N, et al: Endoscopic features of smooth muscle tumors in children with AIDS. *Gastrointest Endosc* 2000;52:91–94.

Petersen GM. Genetic testing. *Hematol Oncol Clin North Am* 2000;14:939–52.

Reut J, Russell JC, Weiss R, et al: Adenocarcinoma of the stomach in an adolescent presenting as pneumoperitoneum. *Conn Med* 2001;65:131.

Samowitz WS, Curtin K, Lin HH, et al: The colon cancer burden of genetically defined hereditary nonpolyposis colon cancer. *Gastroenterology* 2001;121: 830–38.

Tomassetti P, Migliori M, Lalli S, et al: Epidemiology, clinical features and diagnosis of gastroenteropancreatic endocrine tumours. *Ann Oncol* 2001;12:S95–99.

Tonelli F, Valanzano R, Messerini L, et al: Long-term treatment with sulindac in familial adenomatous polyposis: Is there an actual efficacy in prevention of rectal cancer? *J Surg Oncol* 2000;74:15–20.

Tonelli F, Valanzano R, Monaci I, et al: Restorative proctocolectomy or rectum-preserving surgery in patients with familial adenomatous polyposis: Results of a prospective study. *World J Surg* 1997;21:653–58.

Vasen HFA: Clinical diagnosis and management of hereditary colorectal cancer syndromes. *J Clin Oncol* 2000;18:81s–92.

Wanner M, Celebi JT, Peacocke M: Identification of a *PTEN* mutation in a family with Cowden syndrome and Bannayan-Zonana syndrome. *J Am Acad Dermatol* 2001;44:183–87.

Diarrhea from Hormone-Secreting Tumors

Doede T, Foss HD, Waldschmidt J: Carcinoid tumors of the appendix in children—epidemiology, clinical aspects and procedure. *Eur J Pediatr Surg* 2000;10:372–77.

Oberg K: Chemotherapy and biotherapy in the treatment of neuroendocrine tumours. *Ann Oncol* 2001;12:S111–14.

Chapter 327

Inguinal Hernias *John J. Aiken*

Most inguinal hernias in infants and children are congenital indirect hernias caused by a patent processus vaginalis. Approximately 50% of inguinal hernias will present in the 1st year of life, most in the first 6 mo. Other types of inguinal hernias include direct (0.5–1%) and femoral (<0.5%). Risk factors for the development of an inguinal hernia include prematurity, developmental urogenital anomalies, conditions associated with abnormal abdominal fluid or increased intra-abdominal pressure, chronic respiratory disease, and inherited connective tissue disorders. Potential morbidity includes incarceration, strangulation, and gonadal or bowel infarction.

Embryology and Pathogenesis. Most inguinal hernias in infants and children result from a persistent patency of the processus vaginalis. Based on their location in the inguinal canal (lateral to the inferior epigastric vessels) they are *indirect* hernias but are rarely associated with a muscular weakness or defect as would be typical of an adult hernia. The pertinent embryology of the inguinal region relates to the development and descent of the intra-abdominal testes and their relation to the processus vaginalis. Differentiation into testes or ovary occurs by 7 or 8 wk gestation. The processus vaginalis is present in the fetus at 12 wk gestation as a peritoneal outpouching that extends through the internal inguinal ring. The gubernaculum forms from the caudal end of the mesonephros and is attached to the lower pole of the testes. The processus vaginalis accompanies the testis as it exits the abdomen and descends into the scrotum under direction by the gubernaculum. The cordlike structures of the gubernaculum occasionally pass to ectopic locations (perineum or femoral region), resulting in ectopic testes. The testes descend from the urogenital ridge in the retroperitoneum to the area of the internal ring by about 28 wk gestation. Both androgenic hormones and mechanical factors such as increased intra-abdominal pressure influence further descent through the inguinal canal. The testis passes through the inguinal canal in a few days but takes about 4 wk to migrate from the external ring to the scrotum. The ovaries also descend into the pelvis from the urogenital ridge, but they do not exit from the abdominal cavity. During the last few weeks' of gestation or shortly after birth, the layers of the processus vaginalis normally fuse together and obliterate the

opening from the peritoneal cavity to the inguinal canal in the area of the internal ring. The processus vaginalis also obliterates just above the testes, with the portion of the processus vaginalis that envelops the testis becoming the tunica vaginalis. In girls, the processus vaginalis obliterates earlier, at about 7 mo gestation. Failure of closure of the processus vaginalis permits fluid or abdominal viscera to escape the peritoneal cavity and accounts for a variety of inguinal-scrotal abnormalities seen in infancy and childhood (Fig. 327–1). Complete failure of obliteration of the processus predisposes to a complete inguinal hernia characterized by a protrusion of abdominal contents into the inguinal canal and possibly extending into the scrotum. Obliteration of the processus vaginalis distally (around the testis) with patency proximally results in the classic indirect inguinal hernia with the protrusion in the inguinal canal. Obliteration proximally with patency distally leads to an isolated hydrocele, also known as a scrotal hydrocele (hydrocele of the tunica vaginalis). If only fluid leaves the peritoneal cavity and enters the sac the condition is termed a *communicating* hydrocele. Obliteration of the processus vaginalis proximally and distally but patency and retained fluid in the midportion along the spermatic cord is termed a *hydrocele of the cord*. Although reasons for failure of closure of the processus vaginalis are unknown, it is more common in cases of testicular nondescent and prematurity. Persistent patency of the processus vaginalis is twice as common on the right side, presumably related to later descent of the right testis.

Pathology. Patency of the processus vaginalis after birth is a potential hernia, but not all patients with a patent processus vaginalis will develop a clinical hernia. An indirect inguinal hernia occurs when intra-abdominal contents escape the abdominal cavity and enter the inguinal region through a patent processus vaginalis. Depending on the extent of patency of the distal processus, the hernia may be confined to the inguinal region or pass down into the scrotum.

Incidence. The incidence of congenital indirect inguinal hernia in full-term newborn infants is 3.5–5.0%. The incidence in preterm infants is higher, ranging from 9.0–11.0%, and it approaches 30% in very low birthweight infants. Inguinal hernia is much more common among boys than girls (6:1). Sixty per cent of inguinal hernias occur on the right side, 30% are on the left side, and 10% are bilateral. Bilateral inguinal hernia is more common in premature infants, low birthweight infants, and females. There is an increased incidence of congenital inguinal hernias in twins and in individual families of patients with inguinal hernia. There is a history of another inguinal hernia in the family in 11.5% of patients.

Clinical Manifestations. An inguinal hernia appears as a bulge in the inguinal region that extends toward and possibly into the scrotum. The bulge is most visible at times of increased intra-abdominal pressure (crying, straining, coughing). It may be present at birth or may not appear until weeks, months, or years later. The bulge is most often first noted by the parents or on routine examination by the primary physician. The classic history from the parents is of intermittent groin, labial, or scrotal swelling that spontaneously reduces but that is gradually enlarging or is more persistent and is becoming more difficult to reduce. The hallmark signs of an inguinal hernia on physical examination are a smooth, firm mass that emerges through the external inguinal ring lateral to the pubic tubercle and enlarges with increased intra-abdominal pressure. Occasionally, an infant presents with a swelling of the scrotum without a prior bulge in the inguinal region. When the child relaxes, the hernia either reduces spontaneously or can be reduced by gentle pressure first posteriorly to free it from the external ring and then upward toward the peritoneal cavity. Methods used to demonstrate the hernia on examination vary depending on the age of the child. A quiet infant can be made to strain the abdominal

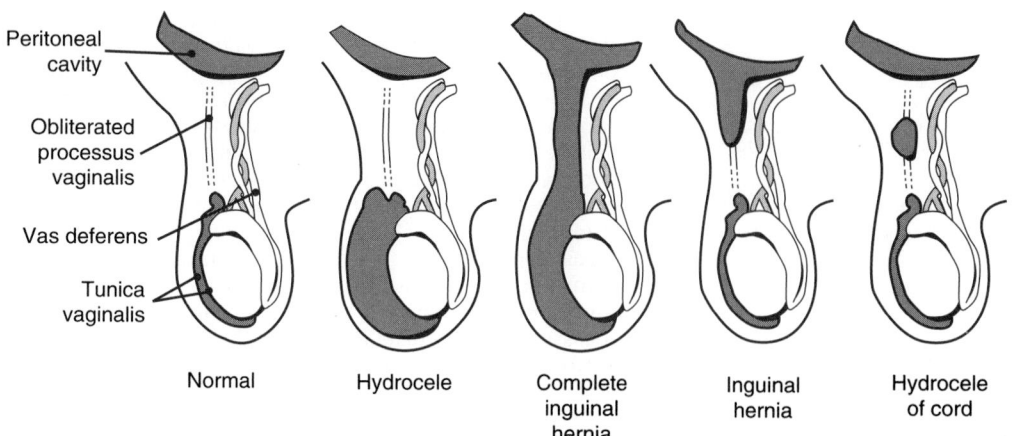

Peritoneal cavity

Obliterated processus vaginalis

Vas deferens

Tunica vaginalis

Normal   Hydrocele   Complete inguinal hernia   Inguinal hernia   Hydrocele of cord

FIGURE 327–1. Hernia and hydroceles. (Modified from Scherer LR III, Grosfeld JL: Inguinal and umbilical anomalies. *Pediatr Clin North Am* 1993;40:1122.)

muscles by stretching out supine on the bed with legs extended and arms held straight above the head. Most infants struggle to get free, thus increasing the intra-abdominal pressure and pushing out the hernia. Older patients can be asked to perform the Valsalva maneuver by blowing up a balloon or coughing. The older child should be examined while standing; examination after voiding can also be helpful. If the bulge is located below the inguinal canal on the medial aspect of the thigh, a femoral hernia should be suspected. In the absence of a bulge, the finding of increased thickness of the inguinal canal structures on palpation will suggest the diagnosis of an inguinal hernia. Another test is the "silk glove sign," which describes the feeling of the layers of the hernia sac (processus vaginalis) as they slide over the cord structures with rolling of the cord beneath the index finger at the pubic tubercle. It is important on examination to note the position of the testes because retractile testes are common in infants and young children and can mimic an inguinal hernia with a bulge in the region of the external ring. In the female patient, 20–25% of inguinal hernias are sliding hernias (the contents of the hernia sac are adherent within the sac and therefore not reducible); a fallopian tube or ovary may be palpated in the inguinal canal.

Occasionally, an inguinal mass appears suddenly in an infant or child and is associated with discomfort. The differential diagnosis includes incarcerated inguinal hernia, acute hydrocele of the cord, torsion of an undescended testis, and suppurative inguinal lymphadenitis. Differentiation between the incarcerated inguinal hernia and the acute hydrocele is probably the most difficult. The infant or child with an incarcerated inguinal hernia is likely to have associated findings suggestive of intestinal obstruction such as abdominal distention, vomiting, and multiple air-fluid levels evident on plain radiographs. On examination of the child with acute hydrocele, one may note that the mass is somewhat mobile. In addition, in the area between the suspected hydrocele mass and the internal ring, the cord structures may appear only slightly thickened. With the incarcerated hernia there is a lack of mobility of the groin mass as well as marked increased thickness extending from the mass up to and including the internal ring. An experienced clinician may use a bimanual examination to help differentiate groin abnormalities. The examiner palpates the internal ring per rectum with the other hand placing gentle pressure on the inguinal region over the internal ring. In cases of an indirect inguinal hernia, an intra-abdominal organ can be palpated extending through the internal ring. Another method is transillumination. It must be noted that transillumination may be misleading because the thin wall of the infants' intestine may approximate that of the hydrocele wall and both may transilluminate. This is also the reason why aspiration to determine the contents of a groin mass is discouraged.

The occurrence of suppurative adenopathy in the inguinal region can be confused with an incarcerated inguinal hernia. Examination of the drainage area of the regional inguinal lymph node may reveal a superficial infected or crusted lesion. In addition, the swelling associated with inguinal adenopathy is typically located more inferior and lateral than the mass of an inguinal hernia. There may be other associated nodes in the area. Torsion of an undescended testis may present as a painful erythematous mass in the groin. The absence of a gonad in the scrotum in the ipsilateral side should clinch this diagnosis.

An *incarcerated inguinal hernia* is one in which the contents of the sac cannot be reduced into the abdominal cavity. Contained structures can include small bowel, appendix, omentum, colon, or, rarely, Meckel diverticulum. In girls, the ovary, fallopian tube, or both are commonly incarcerated. A *strangulated hernia* is one that is tightly constricted in its passage through the inguinal canal and the hernia contents have become ischemic or gangrenous. Although incarceration may be tolerated in adults for years, most nonreducible inguinal hernias in children, unless treated, rapidly progress to strangulation with infarction of the hernia contents. Initially, there is pressure on the herniated viscera as they pass through the internal ring, inguinal canal, and external ring, leading to impaired lymphatic and venous drainage. This pressure leads to swelling of the herniated viscera, which further increases the compression in the inguinal canal, ultimately resulting in total occlusion of the arterial supply to the trapped viscera. Progressive ischemic changes take place, culminating in gangrene and/or perforation of the herniated viscera. The testis is also at risk of ischemia because of compression of the spermatic cord structures by the strangulated hernia. In girls, the ovary may herniate and become strangulated or undergo torsion. The incidence of incarceration of an inguinal hernia is between 12–17%. Two thirds of incarcerated hernias occur during the 1st yr of life. The greatest risk is in infancy, with reported incidences of between 25–30% for infants aged younger than 6 mo. The incidence of incarceration is slightly less in premature infants. The symptoms of an incarcerated hernia are irritability, pain in the groin and abdomen, and vomiting. A somewhat tense, nonfluctuant mass is present in the inguinal region and may extend down into the scrotum. The mass is well defined, may be tender, and does not reduce. With the onset of ischemic changes, the pain intensifies, and the vomiting becomes bilious or feculent. Blood may be noted in the stools. The mass typically is tender, and often there is edema and reddening of the overlying skin, with fever and signs of intestinal obstruction. The testes may be normal but also may be swollen and hard on the affected side because of venous congestion resulting from compression of the spermatic veins and lymphatic channels at the inguinal ring by the tightly strangulated hernia mass. Abdominal radiographs demonstrate features of partial or complete intestinal obstruction, and gas within the incarcerated bowel segments may be seen below the inguinal ligament or within the scrotum. Ultrasonography may help distinguish between a hernia and a hydrocele.

Infants with *intersex problems* frequently present with inguinal hernias, often containing a gonad and requiring special consideration. Female infants with inguinal hernias, particularly if the presentation is bilateral inguinal masses, should be suspected of having testicular feminization syndrome because more than 50% of patients with testicular feminization have an inguinal hernia. Conversely, the true incidence of testicular feminization in all female infants with inguinal hernias is difficult to determine but is approximately 1%. In phenotypic females, if the diagnosis of testicular feminization is suspected, the child should be screened with a buccal smear for Barr bodies and appropriate genetic evaluation before the hernia repair. The diagnosis of testicular feminization can also be made at the time of operation by identifying an abnormal gonad (testis) within the hernia sac, by performing rectal examination to palpate a uterus, or by pelvic ultrasonography. In the normal female infant, the uterus is easily palpated as a distinct midline structure beneath the symphysis pubis on rectal examination. Preoperative diagnosis of testicular feminization syndrome or other intersex disorders such as mixed gonadal dysgenesis and selected pseudohermaphroditism enables the family to receive counseling, and gonadectomy can be accomplished at the time of the hernia repair.

Management. The presence of an inguinal hernia in the pediatric age group constitutes the indication for operative repair. An inguinal hernia does not resolve spontaneously, and early repair eliminates the risk of incarceration and the associated potential complications, particularly in the first months of life. As many as 70% of incarcerated hernias requiring emergency operation for reduction and repair occur in the 1st yr of life. In addition, the incidence of testicular atrophy after incarceration in this setting is as high as 30%. For the routine reducible hernia, the operation should be carried out electively shortly after diagnosis. The younger the child, the more urgency with which the repair should be performed to avoid incarceration. Elective inguinal hernia repair can be safely performed in an outpatient setting with an expectation of full recovery within 48 hr. Certain conditions may dictate postponement of repair, such as marked prematurity, intercurrent pneumonia (especially respiratory syncytial virus), other infections, or severe congenital heart disease. In cases of marked prematurity, typically repair is performed before discharge home from the nursery (1800–2000 g). The operation is most often performed with the infant under general anesthesia, but it can be performed with spinal or caudal anesthesia if avoidance of intubation is preferable because of bronchopulmonary dysplasia. Preterm infants mandate special consideration because of their higher risk for apnea after general anesthesia. Preterm infants younger than 44 wk post conceptual age and full-term infants younger than 3 mo of age and with comorbid conditions are typically observed overnight with appropriate apnea and cardiorespiratory monitors.

An incarcerated, irreducible hernia without evidence of strangulation in a clinically stable patient should initially be managed nonoperatively. Reduction by gentle compression of the hernia may be attempted. The attempt should not be continued if the infant is crying and resisting the pressure on the hernia. The use of sedation or analgesia before attempting reduction may be helpful; this reduces intra-abdominal pressure and relieves the pressure on the neck of the hernia sac at the inguinal ring. Care must be taken to avoid respiratory depression, especially in the premature infant. Other techniques advocated to assist in the nonoperative reduction of an incarcerated inguinal hernia include elevation of the lower torso and legs and brief exposure to an ice pack. Many practitioners do not favor the use of an ice pack in infants because of the risk of hypothermia. Manual reduction is performed first with traction caudad and downward to free the mass from the external inguinal ring and then upward to reduce the contents back into the peritoneal cavity. If the reduction is successful, elective repair is performed 48 hr later, by which time there is less edema, handling of the sac is easier, and the risk of complications is reduced. A common presentation in female patients is the presence of an irreducible ovary in the inguinal hernia in an otherwise asymptomatic patient. The inguinal mass is soft and nontender to gentle examination, and there is no swelling or edema and thus no findings suggestive of strangulation. This represents a "sliding" hernia with the fallopian tube and ovary fused to the posterior wall of the hernia sac. Overzealous attempts to reduce the hernia are unwarranted and potentially harmful to the tube and ovary. The risk that incarceration of the ovary in this setting will lead to strangulation is not known. Most pediatric surgeons recommend elective repair of the hernia within 48–72 hr. For any patient who presents with a prolonged history, signs of peritoneal irritation, or small bowel obstruction, surgery and operative reduction of the hernia should be performed.

OPERATIVE MANAGEMENT. When the hernia cannot be reduced or is strangulated, immediate operation is indicated to prevent further damage to the contents of the hernia sac or testis. If there are signs of intestinal obstruction or strangulation, initial management includes nasogastric intubation, intravenous fluids, and broad-spectrum antibiotic therapy. When fluid and electrolyte imbalance has been corrected and the child's condition is satisfactory, exploration is undertaken. The operation consists of reduction of the contents of the hernia sac, separation of the hernia sac from the spermatic cord vessels and vas deferens in the inguinal canal, and high ligation of the hernia sac at the internal ring. Resection of nonviable structures within the hernia sac or of an infarcted testis may be indicated based on the experience and judgment of the surgeon.

CONTRALATERAL EXPLORATION. Controversy exists regarding when to proceed with contralateral groin exploration in infants and children with a unilateral indirect inguinal hernia. The incidence of a contralateral patent processus vaginalis is approximately 60% at 2 mo of age and 40% at 2 yr of age. A patent processus represents only a potential hernia, and many risk factors influence the likelihood of development of an actual inguinal hernia. The advantages of contralateral exploration include avoidance of (1) parental anxiety and possibly a second anesthesia, (2) the cost of additional surgery, and (3) the risk of contralateral incarceration. The disadvantages include (1) potential injury to the spermatic cord vessels, vas deferens, and testis, (2) increased operative time, and (3) the fact that in many infants it is an unnecessary procedure. There is a chance of developing a contralateral hernia in 10–40% in children younger than 2 yr of age. In girls, because of the higher incidence of bilateral inguinal hernias and elimination of concern for injury to the spermatic cord or testis, routine contralateral exploration has been recommended up to age 5 or 6 yr. Infants and children with risk factors for development of an inguinal hernia or with medical conditions that increase the risk of anesthesia should be approached with a low threshold for routine contralateral exploration. Laparoscopy enables the assessment of the contralateral side without the risk of injury to the spermatic cord structures or testis. This procedure can be performed through an umbilical incision or by passing a 30- or 70-degree oblique scope through the open hernia sac just before ligation of the hernia sac on the involved side. If patency of the contralateral side is demonstrated, the surgeon can proceed with bilateral hernia repair, and if the contralateral side is properly obliterated, exploration and potential complications are avoided (Figs. 327–2 and 327–3).

DIRECT INGUINAL HERNIA. Direct inguinal hernias are rare in children. Direct hernias appear as groin masses that

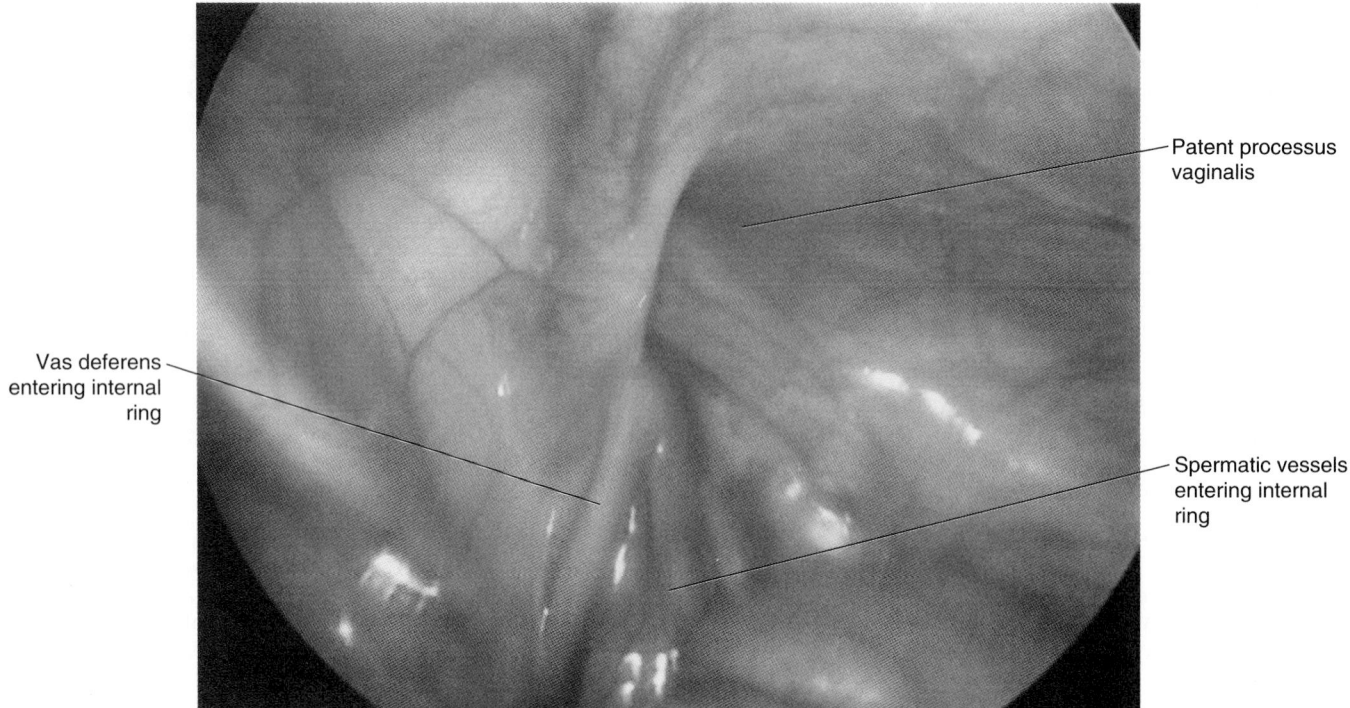

FIGURE 327–2. Image on laparoscopy of patent processus vaginalis on right side. See also color plates.

extend toward the femoral vessels with exertion or straining. The etiology is from a muscular defect or weakness in the floor of the inguinal canal medial to the epigastric vessels. Direct inguinal hernias in children are considered an *acquired* defect. In one third of cases, the patient has a history of a prior indirect hernia repair on the side of the direct hernia, which suggests a possible injury to the floor muscles of the inguinal canal at the time of the first herniorrhaphy. In addition, patients with con-

nective tissue disorders such as Ehlers-Danlos syndrome or Marfan syndrome are at increased risk for the development of direct inguinal hernias either independently or after indirect inguinal hernia repair. Operative repair of a direct inguinal hernia involves strengthening of the floor of the inguinal canal. Recurrence after repair, in contrast to that in adults, is extraordinarily rare. Prosthetic material for direct hernia repair or other approaches, such as preperitoneal repair, are rarely required in

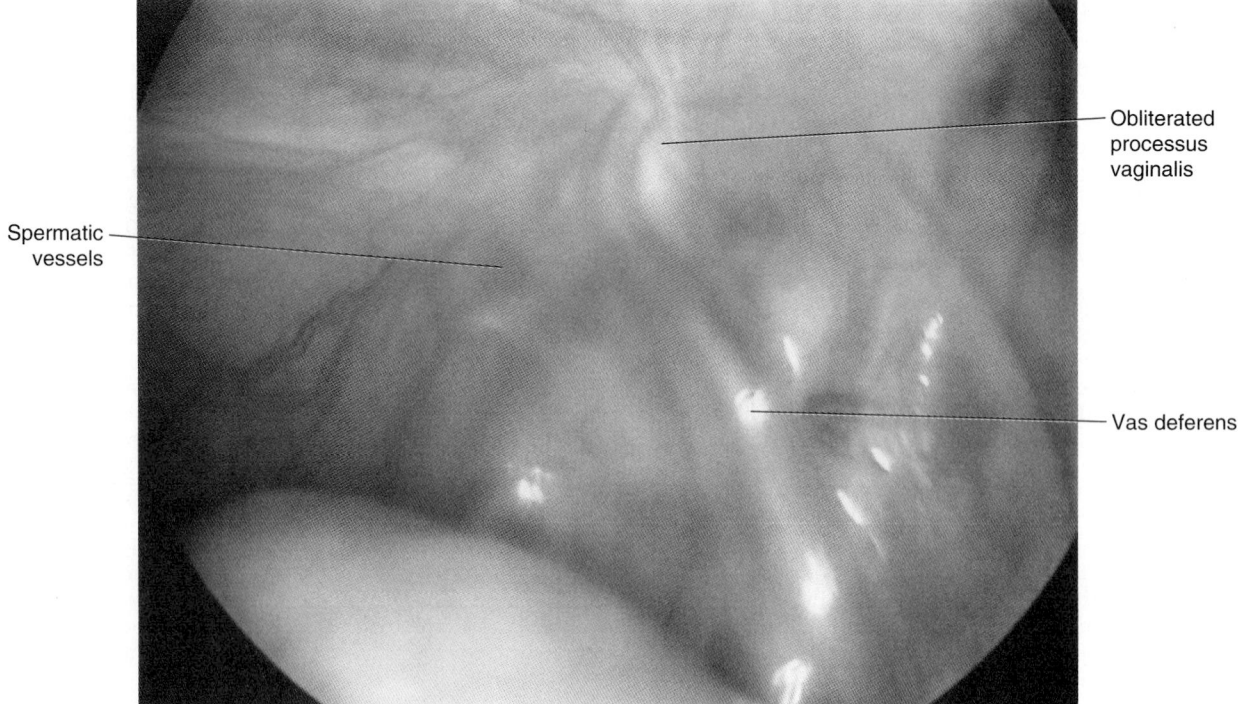

FIGURE 327–3. Image on diagnostic laparoscopy of obliterated processus vaginalis on left side. See also color plates.

the pediatric age group. The older child with a direct inguinal hernia and a connective tissue disorder may be the exception, and a prosthetic material may be useful for repair.

FEMORAL HERNIA. Femoral hernias are rare in children. They are more common in girls than boys, with a ratio of 2:1. The bulge of a femoral hernia is located below the inguinal ligament and typically projects toward the medial aspect of the thigh. Femoral hernias are more often missed than direct hernias on physical examination or at the time of indirect hernia repair. Repair of a femoral hernia involves closure of the defect at the femoral canal, generally suturing the inguinal ligament to the pectineal ligament and pectineal fascia.

Complications.

Complications after inguinal hernia repair are uncommon. Some complications are related to technical factors (recurrence, iatrogenic cryptorchidism), whereas others are related to the underlying process, such as bowel ischemia, gonadal infarction, and testicular atrophy related to an incarcerated hernia. Wound infection occurs in less than 1%. The majority of complications are related to episodes of incarceration or occur after emergency operative reduction and hernia repair.

RECURRENT HERNIA. The recurrence rate of inguinal hernias after elective inguinal hernia repairs is 0.5–1%, with rates as high as 2% for premature infants. The rate of recurrence after emergency repair of an incarcerated hernia is significantly higher, reported as 3–6%. In the group of patients who develop recurrent inguinal hernia, the recurrence occurs in 50% within 1 yr of the initial repair and in 75% by 2 yr.

Recurrence of an indirect hernia is most likely caused by a technical problem at the original procedure, such as failure to properly identify the sac, failure to perform high ligation of the sac at the level of the internal ring, or a tear in the sac that leaves a strip of peritoneum along the cord structures. Recurrence as a direct hernia can result from injury to the inguinal floor at the original procedure or failure to identify a direct hernia at the original exploration. Patients with connective tissue disorders or conditions that cause increased intra-abdominal pressure (ventriculoperitoneal shunts, ascites) are at increased risk for recurrence.

IATROGENIC CRYPTORCHIDISM. Iatrogenic cryptorchidism describes malposition of the testis after inguinal hernia repair. This complication is usually related to disruption of the testicular attachment or failure to recognize an undescended testis at the original procedure, allowing the testis to retract typically to the region of the external ring. At the completion of inguinal hernia repair, the testis should be placed in a dependent intrascrotal position. If the testis will not remain in this position, an orchiopexy should be performed at the time of the hernia repair.

INCARCERATION. Incarceration of an inguinal hernia can result in injury to the intestines, the fallopian tube and ovary, or the ipsilateral testis. Intestinal injury requiring bowel resection is uncommon, occurring in 1–2% of incarcerated hernias. In cases of incarceration in which the hernia is reduced nonoperatively, the likelihood of intestinal injury is low, but these patients should be observed closely for persistent signs and symptoms of intestinal obstruction, such as fever, vomiting, abdominal distention, or bloody stools.

The reported incidence of testicular infarction and subsequent atrophy with incarceration ranges from 4–12%, with higher rates among the irreducible cases. The testicular insult may be caused from compression of the gonadal vessels by the incarcerated hernia mass or as a result of damage incurred during repair of a difficult incarcerated hernia. Young infants are at higher risk, with testicular infarction rates reported as high as 30% in infants younger than 2–3 mo.

INJURY TO THE VAS DEFERENS AND MALE FERTILITY. Similar to the gonadal vessels, the vas deferens may be injured as a consequence of compression from an incarcerated hernia or during operative repair. This injury is almost certainly underreported because it is unlikely to be recognized until adulthood and even then possibly only if the injury is bilateral. One review reported an incidence of injury to the vas deferens of 1.6% based on pathology demonstrating segments of the vas deferens in the hernia sac specimen. The relationship between male fertility and previous inguinal hernia repair is also unknown. Male patients with infertility have an association of testicular atrophy and abnormal sperm counts with a previous hernia operation. There is an association in infertile males with spermatic autoagglutinating antibodies and previous inguinal hernia repair. Operative injury to the vas deferens during inguinal hernia repair may result in obstruction of the vas with diversion of spermatozoa to the testicular lymphatics; this breach of the blood-testis barrier may produce spermatic autoagglutinating antibodies.

Ballantyne A, Jawaheer F, Munro FD: Contralateral groin exploration is not justified in infants with a unilateral inguinal hernia. *Br J Surg* 2001;88:720–23.

Cox JA: Inguinal hernia of childhood. *Surg Clin North Am* 1985;65:1331–42.

Gallagher TM: Regional anesthesia for surgical treatment of inguinal hernia in preterm babies. *Arch Dis Childhood* 1993;69:623.

Grosfeld JL: Current concepts in inguinal hernia in infants and children. *World J Surg* 1989;13;506–15.

Holcomb GW: Laparoscopic evaluation for a contralateral inguinal hernia or a nonpalpable testis. *Pediatr Ann* 1993;22:678.

Lloyd DA, Rintala RJ: In Oneill JA Jr, Rowe MI, Grosfeld JL, et al (editors): *Pediatric Surgery*, 5th ed. St. Louis, CV Mosby, 1986, pp 1071–86.

Lobe TL, Schropp KP: Inguinal hernias in pediatrics: Initial experience with laparoscopic inguinal exploration of the asymptomatic contralateral side. *J Laparoendosc Surg* 1992;2:3:135–40.

Rescorla FJ: In Oldham KT, Colambani PM, Foglia RP (editors): *Surgery of Infants and Children: Scientific Principles and Practice*. Philadelphia, Lippincott-Raven, 1997, pp 1069–81.

Rowe MI, Clatworthy HW: Incarcerated and strangulated hernias in children. *Arch Surg* 1970;101:136.

Rowe MI, Copelson LW, Clatworthy HW: The patent processus vaginalis and the inguinal hernia. *J Pediatr Surg* 1969;4:102–7.

Weber TR, Tracy TF Jr: Groin hernias and hydroceles. In Holder TM, Ashcraft KW (editors): *Textbook of Pediatric Surgery*. Philadelphia, WB Saunders, pp 562-70.

SECTION 5 *Exocrine Pancreas*

Steven L. Werlin

Excluding cystic fibrosis, diabetes mellitus, and pancreatitis, disorders of the exocrine pancreas are uncommon in childhood. Pancreatic disease may be based on traumatic, anatomic (annular pancreas, pancreas divisum), metabolic (organic acidoses, Reye syndrome, α_1-antitrypsin deficiency), congenital (Shwachman syndrome, enzyme defects), autoimmune (diabetes mellitus), or inflammatory pathology. A comprehensive discussion of cystic fibrosis is found in Chapter 402.

Chapter 328
Embryology, Anatomy, and Physiology

The human pancreas develops from evaginations of primitive duodenum beginning at about the 5th wk of gestation. The larger dorsal anlage, which develops into the tail, body, and part of the head of the pancreas, grows directly from the duodenum. The smaller ventral anlage develops as one or two buds from the primitive liver and eventually forms the major portion of the head of the pancreas. At about the 17th wk of gestation, the dorsal and ventral anlagen fuse as the buds develop and the gut rotates. The ventral duct forms the proximal portion of the major pancreatic duct of Wirsung, which opens into the ampulla of Vater. The dorsal duct forms the distal portion of the duct of Wirsung and the accessory duct of Santorini, which may empty independently in about 15% of people. Variations in fusion account for pancreatic developmental anomalies. Pancreatic agenesis has been associated with a base pair deletion in the *ipf1* HOX gene, PDX1. Other genes involved in pancreatic organogenesis include the sonic hedgehog and TGF-1-beta genes.

The pancreas lies transversely in the upper abdomen between the duodenum and the spleen in the retroperitoneum. The head, which rests on the vena cava and renal vein, is adherent to the C-loop of the duodenum and surrounds the distal common bile duct. The tail of the pancreas reaches to the left splenic hilum and passes above the left kidney. The lesser sac separates the tail of the pancreas from the stomach.

By the 13th wk of gestation, exocrine and endocrine cells can be identified. Primitive acini containing immature zymogen granules are found by the 16th wk. Mature zymogen granules containing amylase, trypsinogen, chymotrypsinogen, and lipase are present at the 20th wk. Centroacinar and duct cells, which are responsible for water, electrolyte, and bicarbonate secretion, are also found by the 20th wk. The final three-dimensional structure of the pancreas consists of a complex series of branching ducts surrounded by grapelike clusters of epithelial cells. Cells containing glucagon are present at the 8th wk. Islets of Langerhans appear between the 12th and 16th wks.

328.1 Anatomic Abnormalities

Complete and partial *pancreatic agenesis* are rare conditions. Complete agenesis is associated with severe neonatal diabetes and usually death at an early age. Partial or dorsal pancreatic agenesis is often asymptomatic but may be associated with diabetes, congenital heart disease, polysplenia, and recurrent pancreatitis. Pancreatic agenesis is also associated with malabsorption

An *annular pancreas* results from incomplete rotation of the left (ventral) pancreatic anlage. Patients usually present in infancy with symptoms of complete or partial bowel obstruction. There is frequently a history of maternal polyhydramnios. Some children present with chronic vomiting, pancreatitis, or biliary colic. The treatment of choice is duodenojejunostomy. Division of the pancreatic ring is not attempted, because a duodenal diaphragm or duodenal stenosis frequently accompanies annular pancreas. Annular pancreas may be associated with Down syndrome, intestinal atresia, imperforate anus, pancreatitis, and malrotation.

Ectopic pancreatic rests in the stomach or small intestine occur in approximately 3% of the population. Most cases (70%) are found in the upper intestinal tract. Recognized on barium contrast studies by their typical umbilicated appearance, they are rarely of clinical importance. On endoscopy they are irregular, yellow nodules 2 to 4 mm in diameter. A pancreatic rest may occasionally be the lead point of an intussusception, produce hemorrhage, or cause bowel obstruction.

Pancreas divisum, which occurs in 5 to 15% of the population, is the most common pancreatic developmental anomaly. As the result of failure of the dorsal and ventral pancreatic anlagen to fuse, the tail, body, and part of the head of the pancreas drain through the small accessory duct of Santorini rather than the main duct of Wirsung. This anomaly may be associated with recurrent pancreatitis when there is relative obstruction of the outflow of the ventral pancreas. The treatment of choice of recurrent pancreatitis associated with pancreas divisum is endoscopic insertion of an endoprosthesis. If the episodes stop, surgical sphincterotomy is indicated.

Choledochal cysts are dilatations of the biliary tract and usually cause biliary tract symptoms, such as jaundice, pain, and fever. On occasion, the presentation may be pancreatitis. The diagnosis is usually easily made with ultrasonography, CT scanning, or biliary tract scan. Similarly, a choledochocele, an intraduodenal choledochal cyst, may present with pancreatitis. The diagnosis may be difficult and require endoscopic retrograde cholangiopancreatography (ERCP) or magnetic resonance cholangiopancreatography (MRCP).

A number of rare conditions, such as *Ivemark* and *Johanson-Blizzard syndromes*, include pancreatic dysgenesis or dysfunction among their features. Many of these syndromes include renal and hepatic dysgenesis along with the pancreatic anomalies. Absence of islet cells and agenesis of the pancreas produce permanent diabetes mellitus, which begin in the neonatal period (Chapter 583).

Hill ID, Lebenthal E: Congenital abnormalities of the exocrine pancreas. In Go ELW, et al (editors): *The Exocrine Pancreas: Biology, Pathology, and Diseases*, 2nd ed. New York, Raven Press, 1993, pp 1029–1040.
Narshney S, Johnson CD: Pancreas divisum. *Int J Pancreatol* 1999;25:135.

328.2 Physiology

The acinus is the functional unit of the exocrine pancreas. Acinar cells are arrayed in a semicircle around a lumen. Ducts that drain the acini are lined by centroacinar and ductular cells. This arrangement allows the secretions of the various cell types to mix.

The acinar cell synthesizes, stores, and secretes more than 20 enzymes. These enzymes are stored in zymogen granules, some in inactive forms. The relative concentration of the various enzymes in pancreatic juice is affected and perhaps controlled by the diet, probably by regulating the synthesis of specific messenger RNA. As a general rule, diets high in fat increase the concentration of lipase; a high-protein diet increases pancreatic content of proteases; and a high-carbohydrate diet leads to increased content of amylase in the pancreatic juice. *Amylase* splits starch into maltose, isomaltose, maltotriose, and dextrins. *Trypsin* and *chymotrypsin,* both endopeptidases, and *carboxypeptidase,* an exopeptidase, are secreted by the pancreas as the inactive proenzymes trypsinogen and chymotrypsinogen. Trypsinogen is activated in the gut lumen by *enterokinase,* a brush border enzyme. Trypsin can then activate trypsinogen, chymotrypsinogen, and procarboxypeptidase into their respective active forms. Enterokinase is thus a key enzyme for exocrine pancreatic function.

Pancreatic *lipase* requires colipase, a coenzyme also found in pancreatic fluid, for activity. Lipase liberates fatty acids from the one and three positions of triglycerides, leaving two monoglycerides. The stimuli for *exocrine pancreatic secretion* are neural and hormonal. Acetylcholine mediates the cephalic phase; cholecystokinin (CCK) mediates the intestinal phase. CCK is released from the duodenal mucosa by luminal amino acids and fatty acids. Feedback regulation of pancreatic secretion is mediated by pancreatic proteases in the duodenum. Secretion of CCK is inhibited by the digestion of a trypsin-sensitive, CCK-releasing peptide released in the lumen of the small intestine or by a monitor peptide released in pancreatic fluid.

Centroacinar and duct cells secrete water and bicarbonate. Bicarbonate secretion is under feedback control and is regulated by duodenal intraluminal pH. The stimulus for bicarbonate production is *secretin* in concert with CCK. Secretin cells are abundant in the duodenum.

Although normal pancreatic function is required for digestion, maldigestion occurs only after considerable reduction in pancreatic function; lipase and colipase secretion must be decreased by 90 to 98% before fat maldigestion occurs.

Although amylase and lipase are present in the pancreas early in gestation, secretion of both amylase and lipase is low in the infant. Adult levels of these enzymes are not reached in the duodenum until late in the 1st yr of life. Digestion of the starch found in many infant formulas depends on the low levels of salivary amylase that reach the duodenum. This explains the diarrhea that may be seen in infants who are fed formulas high in glucose polymers or starch. Neonatal secretion of trypsinogen and chymotrypsinogen is at about 70% of the level found in the 1-yr-old infant. The low levels of amylase and lipase in duodenal contents of infants may be partially compensated by salivary amylase and lingual lipase. This explains the relative starch and fat intolerance of premature infants.

Christian M, Edwards C, Weaver LT: Starch digestion in infancy. *J Pediatr Gastroenterol Nutr* 1999;29:116.
Werlin SL, Lee PC: Development of the exocrine pancreas. In Polin RA, Fox WW (editors): *Fetal and Neonatal Physiology,* 3rd ed. Philadelphia, WB Saunders, 2003 (in press).

Chapter 329
Pancreatic Function Tests

Pancreatic function can be measured by direct and indirect methods. Direct stimulation of the pancreas with a test (Lundh) meal of corn oil, skimmed milk powder, and dextrose or with secretin plus cholecystokinin can be performed. Classically a triple-lumen tube is used to isolate the pancreatic secretions in the duodenum. Measurement of bicarbonate concentration and enzyme activity (trypsin, chymotrypsin, lipase, and amylase) is performed on the aspirated secretions. The most commonly used test today is collection of pancreatic juice following stimulation with secretin and cholecystokinin at endoscopy. Pancreatic enzyme activities can be measured in stool. Stool trypsin has been the most commonly measured but is not as reliable as stool chymotrypsin. Neither test is as reliable as stool collection with fecal fat analysis.

A qualitative examination of the stool for *microscopic fat* globules is the most widely practiced screening test for malabsorption (also see Chapter 320). Analysis of random stool specimens by this method may give both false-positive and false-negative results. A 72-hr collection for *quantitative analysis of fat content* is preferable. The collection is usually performed at home, and the parent is asked to keep a careful dietary record, from which fat intake is calculated. A preweighed, sealable plastic container is used, which the parent keeps in the freezer. Freezing helps preserve the specimen and reduce the odor. Infants are dressed in disposable diapers with the plastic side facing the skin so that the complete sample can be transferred to the container. Normal fat absorption is greater than 93% of intake.

The elevated serum levels of trypsinogen found in neonates with cystic fibrosis form the basis of the newborn screening test being adapted in many states. With advancing pancreatic damage serum trypsinogen levels eventually fall below normal.

Pancreatic function can also be measured by *breath tests.* A labeled triglyceride, most commonly ^{14}C-triolein, is ingested and digested by pancreatic lipase in the duodenum, liberating $^{14}CO_2$, which is detected in the expired air. Because of the radioactivity and long half-life of ^{14}C, this test is not appropriate for use in children. Use of triolein labeled with ^{13}C, a stable, nonradioactive isotope, is safe for pediatric use. It has not gained widespread acceptance because detection of $^{13}CO_2$ requires a mass spectrophotometer that is not generally available.

Del Rosario MAF, Fitzgerald JF, Gupta SK, et al: Direct pancreatic measurement of pancreatic enzymes after stimulation with secretin vs. secretin plus cholecystokinin. *J Pediatr Gastroenterol Nutr* 2000;31:28.

Chapter 330
Disorders of the Exocrine Pancreas

Disorders Associated with Pancreatic Insufficiency. Other than cystic fibrosis, conditions that cause pancreatic insufficiency are rare in children. They include Shwachman-Diamond syndrome, isolated enzyme deficiencies, enterokinase deficiency (Chapter 320.11), chronic pancreatitis, and protein-calorie malnutrition (Chapter 320.2).

CYSTIC FIBROSIS (see Chapter 402). Cystic fibrosis is the most common lethal genetic disease and the most common cause of malabsorption among white American children. By the end of the 1st year of life, 85–90% of children with cystic fibrosis have pancreatic insufficiency, which if untreated will lead to malnutrition in many cases. Treatment of the associated pancreatic insufficiency leads to improvement in absorption, better growth, and normalized stools. Certain mutations in the cystic fibrosis gene have been associated with idiopathic chronic pancreatitis.

SHWACHMAN-DIAMOND SYNDROME (see Chapter 121.1). This is an autosomal recessive syndrome (1:20,000 births), consisting of pancreatic insufficiency; neutropenia, which may be intermittent; neutrophil chemotaxis defects; metaphyseal dysostosis; failure to thrive; and short stature. Patients present in infancy with poor growth and greasy, foul smelling stools that are characteristic of malabsorption. These children can be readily differentiated from those with cystic fibrosis by their normal sweat chloride levels, lack of the cystic fibrosis gene, characteristic metaphyseal lesions, and fatty pancreas on CT examination. Despite adequate pancreatic replacement therapy, poor growth frequently continues. Pancreatic insufficiency is often transient, and steatorrhea may spontaneously improve with age. The neutropenia may be cyclic. Recurrent pyogenic infections (otitis media, pneumonia, osteomyelitis, dermatitis, sepsis) are common and are a frequent cause of death. Thrombocytopenia is found in 70% of patients and anemia in 50%. Development of a myelodysplastic syndrome may occur and transformation to acute myeloid leukemia has been reported in up to 33% and 24% of patients respectively. Pathologically, the pancreatic acini are replaced by fat with little fibrosis. Islet cells and ducts are normal. The fatty pancreas has a characteristic hypodense appearance on computed tomographic and magnetic resonance scans. A candidate gene has been identified on chromosome 7.

PEARSON SYNDROME. This is a sporadic mitochondrial DNA mutation affecting oxidative phosphorylation that manifests in infants with severe macrocytic anemia and variable thrombocytopenia. The bone marrow demonstrates vacuoles in erythroid and myeloid precursors as well as ringed sideroblasts. In addition to severe bone marrow failure, pancreatic insufficiency will contribute to growth failure. Other mitochondrial DNA mutations are associated with the development of diabetes mellitus (Kearns-Sayre, chronic progressive external ophthalmoplegia, diabetes with deafness syndromes). Mitochondrial DNA mutations are transmitted through maternal inheritance to both sexes or are sporadic.

ISOLATED ENZYME DEFICIENCIES. Isolated deficiencies of trypsinogen, enterokinase, lipase, and colipase have been reported. Although enterokinase is a brush border enzyme, deficiency causes pancreatic insufficiency because pancreatic proteases remain inactive. Deficiencies of trypsinogen or enterokinase manifest with failure to thrive, hypoproteinemia, and edema. Isolated amylase deficiency, is typically developmental, resolving by age 2–3 ys. Amylase deficiency has not been shown to exist as a primary, permanent enzyme deficiency.

Syndromes Associated with Pancreatic Insufficiency. Pancreatic agenesis, the *Johanson-Blizzard syndrome* (pancreatic insufficiency, deafness, low birthweight, microcephaly, midline ectodermal scalp defects, psychomotor retardation, hypothyroidism, dwarfism, absent permanent teeth, and aplasia of the alae nasae), congenital pancreatic hypoplasia, and congenital rubella are rare causes of pancreatic insufficiency. Some children with both syndromic (Alagille) and nonsyndromic paucity of intrahepatic bile ducts may also have pancreatic insufficiency associated with their liver disease. Pancreatic insufficiency has also been reported in duodenal atresia and stenosis and may also be seen in the infant with familial or nonfamilial hyperinsulinemic hypoglycemia (formerly called nesidioblastosis) who requires 95–100% pancreatectomy to control hypoglycemia.

Ginzberg H, Shin J, Ellis L, et al: Shwachman syndrome: Phenotypic manifestations of sibling sets and isolated cases in a large patient cohort. *J Pediatr* 1999;135:81.

Toth T, Bokay J, Szonyi L, Detection of mtDNA deletion in Pearson syndrome by two independent PCR assays from Guthrie card. *Clin Genet* 1998;53:210.

Weizman Z: An update on diseases of the pancreas in children. *Curr Opin Pediatr* 1997;9:484.

Chapter 331
Treatment of Pancreatic Insufficiency

Treatment of exocrine pancreatic insufficiency by oral enzyme replacement appears simple. However, in practice, although creatorrhea can usually be corrected, steatorrhea is difficult to completely correct. This is due to variability of lipase activity in different commercial preparations, inadequate dosage, incorrect timing of doses, lipase inactivation by gastric acid, and the observation that chymotrypsin in the enzyme preparation digests and thus inactivates lipase. Pancrease, Creon, and Ultrase are the preparations most widely used. These products are enteric-coated preparations that resist gastric acid inactivation.

The dosage of pancreatic replacement for children depends on the amount of food eaten and is established by trial and error. Because these products contain excess protease compared with lipase, the dosage is estimated from the lipase requirement of 500–1,500 IU/kg/meal. An adequate dose is one that is followed by the return of the stools to normal fat content, size, color, and odor. Enzyme replacement should be given at the beginning of and with the meal. Tablets should be chewed; powder can be mixed with a small quantity of food. Enzyme must also be given with snacks. Increasing enzyme supplements beyond the recommended doses not only may not improve absorption but may also retard growth and cause *fibrosing colonopathy* (see following discussion).

When adequate fat absorption is not achieved, gastric acid neutralization with an H_2-receptor blocking agent or a proton pump inhibitor will prevent gastric acid enzyme inactivation and improve delivery of lipase into the intestine. The coating of enteric-coated preparations also protects lipase from acid inactivation.

Untoward effects secondary to pancreatic enzyme replacement therapy include allergic reactions, increased uric acid levels, and kidney stones. *Fibrosing colonopathy*, consisting of colonic fibrosis and strictures, occurs 7–12 mo following high-dose pancreatic supplement therapy (ranging from 6,500 to 58,000 IU lipase/kg/meal).

Anthony H, Collins SE, Davidson G, et al: Pancreatic enzyme replacement therapy in cystic fibrosis: Australian guidelines. *J Paediatr Child Health* 1999;35:125.

FitzSimmons SC, Burkhart GA, Borowitz, D et al: High-dose pancreatic-enzyme supplements and fibrosing colonopathy in children with cystic fibrosis. *N Engl J Med* 1997;336:1283.

Leus J, Van Biervliet S, Robberecht E: Detection and follow up of exocrine pancreatic insufficiency in cystic fibrosis: A review. *Eur J Pediatr* 2000;159:563.

Chapter 332
Pancreatitis

332.1 Acute Pancreatitis

Acute pancreatitis is the most common pancreatic disorder in children. Blunt abdominal injuries, mumps and other viral illnesses, multisystem disease, congenital anomalies, and biliary microlithiasis (sludging) account for most known etiologies; other causes are uncommon (Box 332–1). Many cases are of unknown etiology or are secondary to a systemic disease process. Child abuse is recognized with increased frequency as a cause of traumatic pancreatitis in young children.

DRUGS AND TOXINS

Alcohol
Acetaminophen overdose
Azathioprine
L-Asparaginase
Cimetidine
Corticosteroids
DDC
DDI
Enalapril
Erythromycin
Estrogen
Furosemide
6-Mercaptopurine
Mesalamine
Methyldopa
Pentamidine
Sulfonamides
Sulindac
Tetracycline
Thiazides
Valproic acid
Venom (spider, scorpion)
Vincristine

HEREDITARY PANCREATITIS

Hereditary pancreatitis gene
Cystic fibrosis gene
SPINK 1 gene

INFECTIOUS

Ascariasis
Coxsackie B virus
Epstein-Barr virus
Hepatitis A, B
Influenza A, B
Leptospirosis
Malaria
Measles
Mumps
Mycoplasma
Rubella
Rubeola
Reye syndrome: varicella, influenza B

OBSTRUCTIVE

Ampullary disease
Ascariasis
Biliary tract malformations
Cholelithiasis, microlithiasis and choledocholithiasis (stones or sludge)
Chlonorchis
Duplication cyst
ERCP complication
Pancreas divisum
Pancreatic ductal abnormalities
Postoperative
Sphincter of Oddi dysfunction
Tumor

SYSTEMIC DISEASE

Alpha$_1$-antitrypsin deficiency
Brain tumor
Collagen vascular diseases
Cystic fibrosis
Diabetes mellitus
Head trauma
Hemochromatosis
Hemolytic uremic syndrome
Hyperlipidemia: types I, IV, V
Hyperparathyroidism
Kawasaki disease
Malnutrition
Organic acidemia
Periarteritis nodosa
Peptic ulcer
Renal failure
Systemic lupus erythematosus
Transplantation: bone marrow, heart, liver, kidney, pancreas
Vasculitis

TRAUMATIC

Blunt injury
Burns
Child abuse
Surgical trauma
Total body cast

Clinical Manifestations. The patient with acute pancreatitis has abdominal pain, persistent vomiting, and fever. The pain is epigastric and steady, often resulting in the child's assuming an antalgic position with hips and knees flexed, sitting upright, or lying on the side. The child is very uncomfortable and irritable and appears acutely ill. The abdomen may be distended and tender. A mass may be palpable. The pain increases in intensity for 24–48 hr, during which time vomiting may increase and the patient may require hospitalization for dehydration and may need fluid and electrolyte therapy. The prognosis for the acute uncomplicated case is excellent.

Severe acute pancreatitis is rare in children. In this life-threatening condition, the patient is acutely ill with severe nausea, vomiting, and abdominal pain. Shock, high fever, jaundice, ascites, hypocalcemia, and pleural effusions may occur. A bluish discoloration may be seen around the umbilicus (Cullen sign) or in the flanks (Grey Turner sign). The pancreas is necrotic and may be transformed into an inflammatory hemorrhagic mass. The mortality rate, which is approximately 50%, is related to the *systemic inflammatory response syndrome* with multiple organ dysfunction: shock, renal failure, acute respiratory distress syndrome, disseminated intravascular coagulation, massive gastrointestinal bleeding, and systemic or intra-abdominal infection. Also see Chapter 57.2.

Diagnosis. Acute pancreatitis is usually diagnosed by measurement of serum amylase and lipase activities. The serum amylase level is typically elevated for up to 4 days. A variety of other conditions may also cause hyperamylasemia without pancreatitis (Box 332–2). Elevation of salivary amylase may mislead the clinician into making the diagnosis of pancreatitis in a child with abdominal pain, but the laboratory can separate amylase isoenzymes into pancreatic and salivary fractions. Initially, serum amylase levels are normal in 10–15% of patients. Serum lipase is more specific than amylase for acute inflammatory pancreatic disease and should be determined when pancreatitis is suspected and the amylase level is normal. The serum lipase typically remains elevated 8–14 days longer than serum amylase. Serum lipase may also be elevated in nonpancreatic diseases.

Other laboratory abnormalities that may be present in acute pancreatitis include hemoconcentration, coagulopathy, leukocytosis,

Pathogenesis. The precise sequence of events leading to pancreatitis has not been completely defined. The classic theory suggests that following an initial insult, such as ductal obstruction, lysosomal hydrolase co-localizes with pancreatic proenzymes within the acinar cell. Pancreastasis (similar in concept to cholestasis) with continued synthesis of enzymes occurs.

The pancreatic proenzymes are then activated by cathepsin leading to autodigestion, further activation and release of active proteases. Lecithin is activated by phospholipase A2 into the toxic lysolecithin. Prophospholipase is unstable and can be activated by minute quantities of trypsin. A newer theory suggests that following an insult, release of cytokines and subsequent depletion of antioxidants leads to pancreastasis and the further activation of pancreatic proenzymes. The healthy pancreas is protected by several factors: (1) the process by which pancreatic proteases are synthesized as inactive proenzymes; (2) the process by which digestive enzymes are segregated into secretory granules at pH 6.2 with low calcium concentration, which minimizes trypsin activity; (3) the presence of protease inhibitors both in the cytoplasm and zymogen granules; and (4) the process by which enzymes are secreted directly into the ducts. Histopathologically, interstitial edema appears early. Later, as the episode of pancreatitis progresses, localized and confluent necrosis, blood vessel disruption leading to hemorrhage, and an inflammatory response in the peritoneum may develop.

PANCREATIC PATHOLOGY

Acute or chronic pancreatitis
Complications of pancreatitis (pseudocyst, ascites, abscess)
Factitious pancreatitis

SALIVARY GLAND PATHOLOGY

Parotitis (mumps, *Staphylococcus aureus*, CMV, HIV, EBV)
Sialadenitis (calculus, radiation)
Eating disorders (anorexia nervosa, bulimia)

INTRA-ABDOMINAL PATHOLOGY

Biliary tract disease (cholelithiasis)
Peptic ulcer perforation
Peritonitis
Intestinal obstruction
Appendicitis

SYSTEMIC DISEASES

Metabolic acidosis (diabetes mellitus, shock)
Renal insufficiency, transplantation
Burns
Pregnancy
Drugs (morphine)
Head injury
Cardiopulmonary bypass

CMV = cytomegalovirus; HIV = human immunodeficiency virus; EBV = Epstein-Barr virus.

hyperglycemia, glucosuria, hypocalcemia, elevated gamma glutamyl transpeptidase, and hyperbilirubinemia.

Roentgenography of the chest and abdomen may demonstrate nonspecific findings. The chest roentgenogram may demonstrate platelike atelectasis, basilar infiltrates, elevation of the hemidiaphragm, left- (rarely right-) sided pleural effusions, pericardial effusion, and pulmonary edema. Abdominal roentgenograms may demonstrate a sentinel loop, dilatation of the transverse colon (cutoff sign), ileus, pancreatic calcification (if recurrent), blurring of the left psoas margin, a pseudocyst, diffuse abdominal haziness (ascites), and peripancreatic extraluminal gas bubbles.

Ultrasound and *computed tomography (CT) scanning* have major roles in the diagnosis and follow-up of children with pancreatitis. Findings may include pancreatic enlargement, a hypoechoic, sonolucent edematous pancreas, pancreatic masses, fluid collections, and abscesses (Fig. 332–1); at least 20% of children with acute pancreatitis initially have normal imaging studies. Endoscopic retrograde cholangiopancreatography (ERCP) or magnetic resonance cholangiopancreatography (MRCP) are essential in the investigation of recurrent pancreatitis, pancreas divisum, sphincter of Oddi dysfunction, and disease associated with gallbladder pathology. Endoscopic ultrasonography helps visualize the pancreaticobiliary system.

Treatment. The aims of medical management are to relieve pain and restore metabolic homeostasis. Analgesia should be given in adequate doses. Fluid, electrolyte, and mineral balance should be restored and maintained. Nasogastric suction is useful in patients who are vomiting. While vomiting, the patient should be maintained with nothing by mouth. Prophylactic antibiotics are useful in severe cases to prevent infected pancreatic necrosis. The response to treatment is usually complete over 2–5 days. Refeeding may commence when vomiting has resolved, the serum amylase is falling, and clinical symptoms are resolving.

The treatment of severe acute pancreatitis may involve enteral or total parenteral nutrition, antibiotics, gastric acid suppression and peritoneal lavage to reduce the risk of secondary infection. Endoscopic therapy may be of benefit when pancreatitis is caused by anatomic abnormalities, such as strictures or stones. Surgical therapy of acute pancreatitis is rarely required, but may include drainage of necrotic material or abscesses.

Prognosis. Children with uncomplicated acute pancreatitis do well and recover over a period of 2–5 days. When pancreatitis is associated with trauma or systemic disease, the prognosis is typically related to the associated medical conditions. Prognostic systems widely used in adults such as *Ranson's criteria* and the *APACHE score* are inappropriate for use in children. Measurement of urinary trypsin activation peptide (TAP), the amino terminus peptide split when trypsinogen is activated to trypsin, and activation peptide of carboxypeptidase B (CAPAP), which may be the most sensitive diagnostic tests for determining the severity of an episode of acute pancreatitis, are under study and have not been evaluated in children.

Baron T, Morgan D: Acute necrotizing pancreatitis. *N Engl J Med* 1999;340: 1412.
Braganza JM: Towards a novel tretment strategy for acute pancreatitis. 1. Reappraisal of the evidence for aetiogenesis. *Digestion* 2001;63:69.
Pietzak MM, Thomas DW: Pancreatitis in childhood. *Pediatr Rev* 2000;21:406.
Werlin SL: Pancreatitis. In Wyllie R, Hyams JS (editors): *Pediatric Gastrointestinal Disease*. Philadelphia, WB Saunders, 1999, pp 681–694.
Werlin SL: Acute pancreatitis in children. *Current Treatment Options in Gastroenterology* 2001;4:403–8.

332.2   Chronic Pancreatitis

Chronic, relapsing pancreatitis in children is frequently hereditary or due to congenital anomalies of the pancreatic or biliary ductal system. Hereditary pancreatitis (HP) is transmitted as an autosomal dominant trait with incomplete penetrance but variable expressivity. Symptoms frequently begin in the first decade but are usually mild at the onset. Although spontaneous recovery from each attack occurs in 4–7 days, episodes become progressively severe. HP may be clinically diagnosed by the presence of the disease in successive generations of a family. An evaluation during symptom-free intervals may be unrewarding until calcifications, pseudocysts, or pancreatic insufficiency develop. The gene for HP has been cloned and mapped to the cationic trypsinogen gene on the long arm of chromosome 7. Multiple mutations of the HP gene associated with hereditary pancreatitis have been described. The pathophysiology of HP is unclear. One theory states that cationic trypsinogen has a tendency to autoactivate but has a trypsin-sensitive cleavage site. Loss of this cleavage site in the abnormal protein permits autodigestion of the pancreas. The other theory states that mutated cationic trypsinogen autoactivates at a faster rate than normal trypsinogen. Mutations of other genes including *cystic fibrosis* gene *(CFTR,)* typically in the 5T promoter region, and the *SPINK 1 gene (pancreatic trypsin inhibitor)* have also been associated with recurrent or chronic pancreatitis.

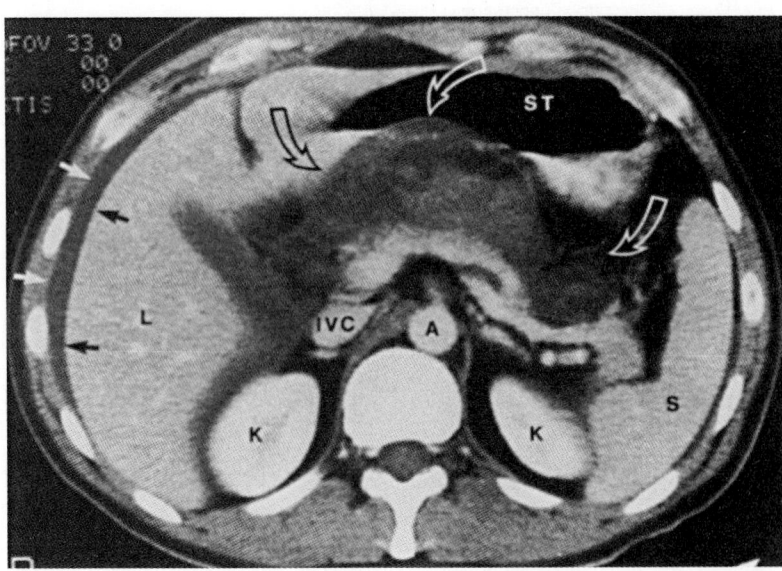

FIGURE 332–1. Acute pancreatitis. Computed tomography (CT) through the body of the pancreas demonstrates a halo of decreased attenuation around the pancreas that represents a peripancreatic zone of edema and fluid *(curved arrows)*. Note the pancreatic ascites most obvious lateral to the liver *(small arrows)*. If intravenous contrast was administered before the CT scan, the inflamed pancreas would appear more dense (whiter). (L = liver; A = aorta; K = kidney; S = spleen; IVC = inferior vena cava; ST = stomach.) (From Freeny P, Lawson T: The pancreas. In Putman CE, Ravin CE [editors]: *Textbook of Diagnostic Imaging*. Philadelphia, WB Saunders, 1988.)

Other conditions associated with chronic, relapsing pancreatitis are hyperlipidemia (types I, IV, and V), hyperparathyroidism, and ascariasis. In the past most cases of recurrent pancreatitis in childhood were considered idiopathic; however, with the discovery of at least three gene families associated with recurrent pancreatitis, this will probably change. Congenital anomalies of the ductal systems, such as pancreas divisum, are probably more common than previously recognized.

A thorough diagnostic *evaluation* of every child with more than one episode of pancreatitis is indicated. Serum lipid, calcium, and phosphorus levels are determined. Stools are evaluated for *Ascaris,* and a sweat test is performed. Evaluation of the HP, SPINK 1, and the CFTR genes is performed. Plain abdominal films are evaluated for the presence of pancreatic calcifications. Abdominal ultrasound or CT scanning is performed to detect the presence of a pseudocyst. The biliary tract is evaluated for the presence of stones.

ERCP and *MRCP* are techniques that can be used to define the anatomy of the gland and are mandatory whenever surgery is considered. One of these studies should be performed as part of the evaluation of any child with idiopathic, nonresolving, or recurrent pancreatitis and in patients with a pseudocyst before surgery. In these cases, ERCP or MRCP may detect a previously undiagnosed anatomic defect that may be amenable to endoscopic or surgical therapy. Endoscopic treatments include sphincterotomy, stone extraction, and insertion of pancreatic or biliary endoprostheses. These treatments allow for successful nonsurgical management of conditions previously requiring surgical intervention. As more experience is gained, MRCP may supplement or replace ERCP.

Mcloy R: Chronic pancreatitis at Manchester, UK. *Digestion* 1998;59:36.

Sharer N, Schwarz M, Malone G, et al: Mutations of the cystic fibrosis gene in patients with chronic pancreatitis. *N Engl J Med* 1998;339:645.

Werlin SL, Taylor A: ERCP. In Howard ER, Stringer MD, Colombani PM (editors): *Surgery of the Liver, Bile Ducts and Pancreas in Children,* 2nd ed. London, STM Publishing, 2002, pp 509–20.

Whitcomb DC: Genetic predispositions to acute and chronic pancreatitis. *Med Clin North Am* 2000;84:531.

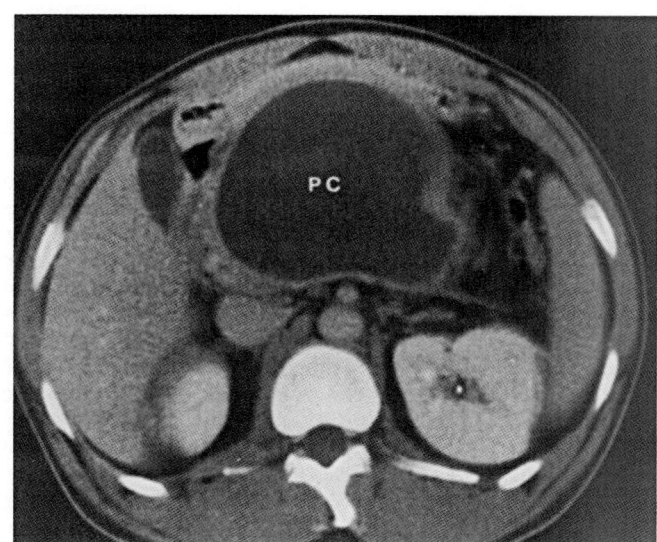

FIGURE 333–1. Pseudocyst. Follow-up computed tomographic scan 5 mo after the episode of acute pancreatitis demonstrates a large pseudocyst (PC). This large pseudocyst will probably not resolve spontaneously and may need drainage. (From Freeny P, Lawson T: The pancreas. In Putman CE, Ravin CE [editors]: *Textbook of Diagnostic Imaging.* Philadelphia, WB Saunders, 1988.)

of pseudocysts have replaced surgical drainage except for complicated or recurrent pseudocysts.. A pseudocyst must be allowed to mature for 4–6 wk before surgical drainage is attempted; percutaneous or endoscopic drainage may be attempted earlier. ERCP or MRCP should precede surgical treatment to help the surgeon plan the approach and define anatomic abnormalities.

Cooperman AM: An overview of pancreatic pseudocysts: The emperor's new clothes revisited. *Surg Clin North Am* 2001;81:391.

Chapter 333
Pseudocyst of the Pancreas

Pancreatic pseudocyst formation is an uncommon sequela to acute or chronic pancreatitis. Pseudocysts are sacs delineated by a fibrous wall in the lesser peritoneal sac. They may enlarge or extend in almost any direction, thus producing a wide variety of symptoms (Fig. 333–1).

A pancreatic pseudocyst is suggested when an episode of pancreatitis fails to resolve or when a mass develops after an episode of pancreatitis. Clinical features usually include pain, nausea, and vomiting. The most common signs are a palpable mass in 50% of patients and jaundice in 10%. Other findings include ascites and pleural effusions (usually left-sided).

The most useful diagnostic techniques are ultrasonography, computed tomography (CT) scanning, endoscopic retrograde cholangiopancreatography (ERCP) and magnetic resonance cholangiopancreatography (MRCP). Because of its ease, availability, and reliability, ultrasonography is the first choice. Sequential ultrasonography studies have demonstrated that most small pseudocysts (<6 cm) resolve spontaneously. It is recommended that the patient with acute pancreatitis undergo an ultrasonographic evaluation 2–4 wk after resolution of the acute episode for an evaluation of possible pseudocyst formation.

The treatment for nonresolving, symptomatic pseudocysts used to be surgery. Now percutaneous and endoscopic drainage

Chapter 334
Pancreatic Tumors

Neoplasia. Pancreatic tumors may be of either endocrine or nonendocrine origin. Tumors of endocrine origin include *insulinomas* and *gastrinomas*. These and other functioning tumors occur in the autosomal dominantly inherited multiple endocrine neoplasia type 1 (MEN-1). Hypoglycemia accompanied by higher than expected (for serum glucose) insulin levels or refractory gastric ulcers (Zollinger-Ellison syndrome) indicate the possibility of a pancreatic tumor (see Chapter 326). Most gastrinomas arise outside the pancreas. The treatment of choice is surgical removal. If the primary tumor cannot be found or if it has metastasized, cure may not be possible. Treatment with a proton pump inhibitor to inhibit gastric acid secretion is then indicated. Gastrectomy is no longer recommended.

The *watery diarrhea–hypokalemia–acidosis syndrome* is usually produced by the secretion of vasoactive intestinal peptide (VIP) by a non-α-cell tumor (VIPoma) (see Table 326–2). VIP levels are frequently, but not always, increased in the serum. Treatment is surgical removal of the tumor. When this is not possible, symptoms may be controlled by the use of octreotide acetate (cyclic somatostatin, Sandostatin), a synthetic analog of somatostatin. Pancreatic tumors secreting a variety of hormones, including glucagon, somatostatin, and pancreatic polypeptide, have also been described.

Pancreatoblastomas, pancreatic adenocarcinomas, cystadenomas, and rhabdomyosarcomas are rarely encountered. Peculiar to childhood are *pancreatoblastomas*, which are embryonal tumors that secrete α-fetoprotein and may contain both endocrine and exocrine elements. Their clinical behavior is malignant but not well characterized owing to their rarity. Presurgical chemotherapy should be considered for lesions not primarily resectable. Resection can be curative; adjuvant chemotherapy has been used, but its effectiveness is not established. Carcinoma of the exocrine pancreas is a major problem in adults, accounting for 2% of diagnoses and 5% of deaths due to cancer. It is very rare in childhood. No definite causes are known. Several genetic syndromes including hereditary pancreatitis and MEN-1 lead to an increased incidence of pancreatic cancer in adult life. The *Frantz tumor* is a papillary cystic tumor that is usually found in girls and young women. Presenting symptoms are usually abdominal pain, mass, or jaundice. The treatment of choice is total surgical removal.

Insulinomas and persistent hyperinsulinemic hypoglycemia of infancy (nesidioblastosis) produce symptomatic hypoglycemia. Massive subtotal or total pancreatectomy is the treatment of choice when medical treatment fails (Chapter 81). These children may then develop pancreatic insufficiency and diabetes as a complication of treatment.

Cysts of the pancreas occur in von Hippel-Lindau disease. Solid and cystic papillary tumors mimic pancreatic ontogeny. Their natural history is still being determined. Metastases have been reported, but adjuvant therapy following surgical excision cannot yet be recommended.

The diagnosis is suggested by CT scanning. Surgery is the only known effective therapy. Prognosis is good for completely resected endocrine tumors but very poor for carcinomas, even with extensive surgery. Children who survive partial or complete pancreatectomy may have decreased pancreatic exocrine and endocrine reserve.

Johnson PR, Spitz L: Cysts and tumors of the pancreas. *Semin Pediatr Surg* 2000;9:209.

Montemarano H, Lonergan GJ, Bulas DI, et al: Pancreatoblastoma: Imaging findings in 10 patients and review of the literature. *Radiology* 2000;214:476.

SECTION 6 *The Liver and Biliary System*

Chapter 335

Development and Function of the Liver and Biliary System *Michael D. Bates and*

William F. Balistreri

During the early embryonic process of gastrulation, the three embryonic germ layers (endoderm, mesoderm, and ectoderm) are formed. The liver and biliary system arise from cells of the ventral foregut endoderm; their development can be divided into three distinct processes (Fig. 335–1). First, through unknown mechanisms, ventral foregut endoderm acquires *competence* to receive signals arising from the cardiac mesoderm. These mesodermal signals, in the form of various fibroblast growth factors and bone morphogenetic proteins, result in *specification* of cells that will form the liver and activation of liver-specific genes. This specification occurs in animal models just before visible budding of the liver. These newly specified cells then migrate in a cranial ventral direction into the septum transversum in the 4th wk of gestation to initiate liver *morphogenesis*. The growth and development of the newly budded liver requires interactions with endothelial cells. Proteins that are important for mammalian liver development are listed in Table 335–1.

Within the ventral mesentery, proliferation of migrating cells form anastomosing hepatic cords, with the network of primitive liver cells, sinusoids, and septal mesenchyme establishing the basic architectural pattern of the liver lobule (Fig. 335–2). The solid *cranial* portion of the hepatic diverticulum (pars hepatis)

eventually forms the hepatic parenchyma and the intrahepatic bile ducts; the *caudal* portion (pars cystica) becomes the gallbladder, cystic duct, and common bile duct. The hepatic lobules are identifiable in the 6th gestational wk. The bile canalicular structures that include microvilli and junctional complexes are specialized loci of the liver cell membrane; these appear very early in gestation; by 6–7 wk large canaliculi bounded by several hepatocytes are seen. The intrahepatic bile ducts are derived through branching and remodeling of the hepatic duct; formation is complete by the 3rd mo. The cystic duct and the gallbladder are fully recanalized by the 7th–8th wk (see Fig. 335–2*C*).

In the hepatic excretory (biliary) system, intercellular bile canaliculi empty into the smallest bile ductules, which unite to form interlobular bile ducts that follow the terminal branches of the portal vein. At the hilum of the liver, the intrahepatic ducts leave the branches of the portal vein and merge to form the extrahepatic biliary system. The ducts of the right and left lobes form the common hepatic duct. The common bile duct is formed from the merger of the common hepatic duct and cystic duct; it extends along the right edge of the lesser omentum, terminating as the intramural papilla of Vater. Union of the biliary tract with the pancreatic ducts forms the ampulla of Vater, which, with the sphincter of Oddi, regulates the flow of bile into the intestine, prevents entry of bile into the pancreatic duct, and inhibits reflux of intestinal contents into the ducts.

Fetal hepatic blood flow is derived from the hepatic artery and from the portal and umbilical veins, which form the portal sinus. The portal venous inflow is directed mainly to the right lobe of the liver; umbilical flow is primarily to the left. The ductus venosus shunts blood from the portal and umbilical veins to the hepatic vein, bypassing the sinusoidal network. The ductus venosus becomes obliterated when oral feedings are initiated. The oxygen saturation is lower in portal than in umbilical venous blood; accordingly, the right hepatic lobe has lower

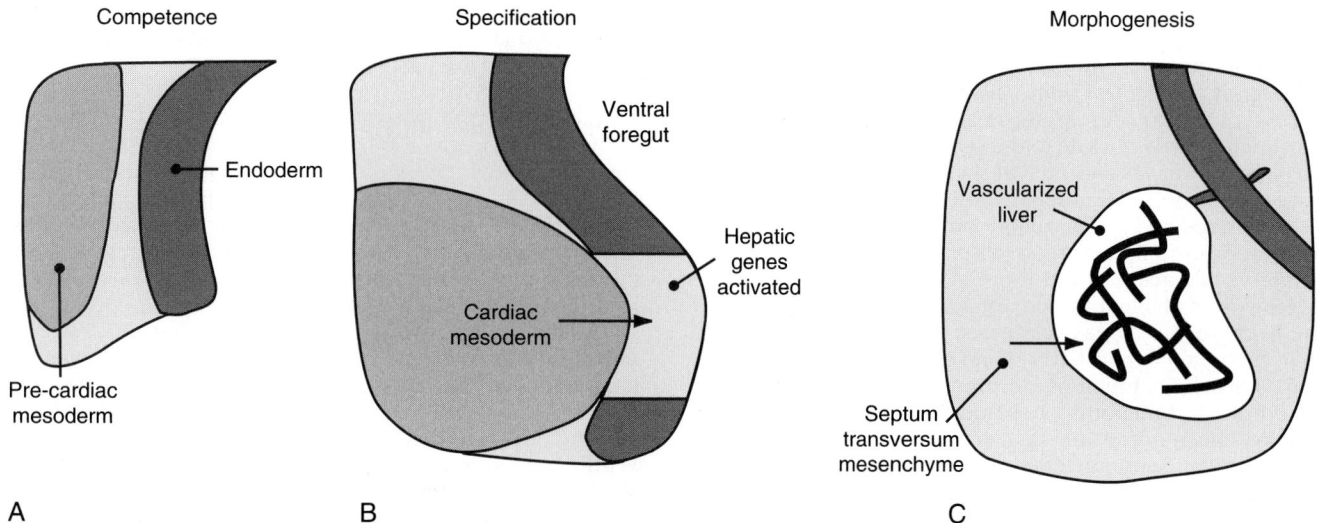

FIGURE 335–1. Processes involved in early liver development. *A,* The ventral foregut endoderm acquires *competence* to receive signals arising from the cardiac mesoderm. *B,* Specific cells of the ventral foregut endoderm undergo *specification* and activation of liver-specific genes under the influence of mesodermal signals. *C,* The newly specified cells migrate into the septum transversum to initiate liver *morphogenesis.* (Reprinted from Zaret KS: Liver specification and early morphogenesis. Mech Dev 2000;92:83–88, with permission. ©2000.)

oxygenation and greater hematopoietic activity than the left hepatic lobe. The fetal sinusoidal endothelium is the site of large macrophages, which become the Kupffer (reticuloendothelial) cell network.

The transport and metabolic activities of the liver are facilitated by the structural arrangement of liver cell cords, which are formed by rows of hepatocytes, separated by sinusoids that converge toward the tributaries of the hepatic vein (the central vein) located in the center of the lobule (see Fig. 335–2*D*). This establishes the pathways and patterns of flow for substances to and from the liver. In addition to arterial input from the systemic circulation, the liver also receives venous input from the gastrointestinal tract via the portal system. The products of the hepatobiliary system are released by two different paths: through the hepatic vein, and through the biliary system back into the intestine. Plasma proteins and other plasma compo-

TABLE 335–1. Proteins Required for Normal Liver Development in Animal Models

Function; Protein	Family/Function
Growth Factors	
Bone morphogenetic proteins 2, 4, 7	Transforming growth factor-β family
FGF-1, FGF-2, FGF-8	Fibroblast growth factor family
Hepatocyte growth factor	Kringle-containing family
Protein Kinases	
IκB kinase 2 (IKKβ)	Serine-threonine protein kinase
NF-κB essential modulator (NEMO/IKKγ)	Protein kinase modulator
Mitogen-activated kinase 4	Serine-threonine protein kinase
Receptors	
Flk-1	Vascular endothelial growth factor receptor
Met	Hepatocyte growth factor receptor
Transcription Factors	
GATA-4	Zinc finger family
Hepatocyte nuclear factor-3β	Winged helix family
Hepatocyte nuclear factor-4α	Orphan nuclear receptor
Hex	Homeobox family
Hlx	Homeobox family
Jun/AP-1	bZIP family
Metal regulatory transcription factor-1	Zinc finger family
NF-κB p65 subunit (RelA)	Transcription factor
N-myc	Basic helix-loop helix family
Prox1	Homeobox family
X-box binding protein-1	bZIP family

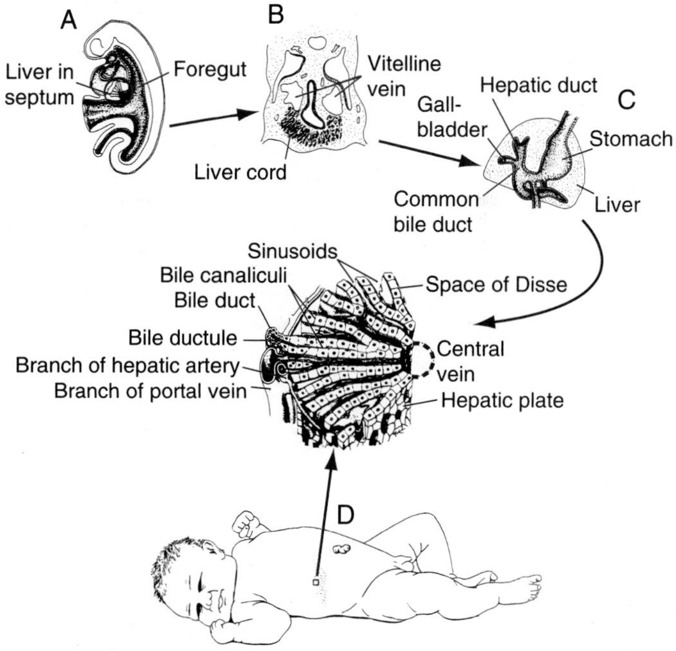

FIGURE 335–2. Hepatic morphogenesis. *A,* Ventral outgrowth of hepatic diverticulum from foregut endoderm in the 3.5-wk embryo. *B,* Between the two vitelline veins, the enlarging hepatic diverticulum buds off epithelial (liver) cords that become the liver parenchyma, around which the endothelium of capillaries (sinusoids) align (4-wk embryo). *C,* Hemisection of embryo at 7.5 wk demonstrating recanalization of the biliary tract. *D,* Three-dimensional representation of the hepatic lobule as present in the newborn. (Reprinted from Andres JM, Mathis RK, Walker WA: Liver disease in infants. Part I: Developmental hepatology and mechanisms of liver dysfunction. *J Pediatr* 1977;90:686–697.)

nents are secreted by the liver. Absorbed and circulating nutrients arrive through the portal vein or the hepatic artery and pass through the sinusoids and past the hepatocytes to the systemic circulation at the central vein. Biliary components are transported via the series of enlarging channels from the bile canaliculi through the bile ductule to the common bile duct.

Bile secretion has been noted at the 12th gestational wk. The major components of bile vary with stage of development. Near term, cholesterol and phospholipid content is relatively low; low concentrations of bile acids, the absence of bacterially derived (secondary) bile acids, and the presence of unusual bile acids reflect low rates of bile flow and immature bile acid synthesis.

The liver reaches a peak relative size at the 9th wk at about 10% of the fetal weight. Early in development, the liver is the primary site of hematopoiesis; during the 7th wk, hematopoietic cells outnumber functioning hepatocytes in the hepatic anlage. These early hepatocytes are smaller than at maturity (~20 μm vs. 30–35 μm) and contain less glycogen. Near term, the hepatocyte mass expands to dominate the organ, as cell size and glycogen content increase. Hematopoiesis is virtually absent by the 2nd postnatal month in full-term infants. As the density of hepatocytes increases with gestational age, the relative volume of the sinusoidal network decreases. The liver constitutes 5% of body weight at birth but only 2% in an adult.

Several metabolic processes are immature in a healthy newborn infant, owing in part to the fetal patterns of activity of various enzymatic processes. Many hepatic functions are carried out for a fetus by the maternal liver, which provides nutrients and serves as a route of elimination of metabolic end products and toxins. Fetal liver metabolism is devoted primarily to the production of proteins for growth requirements. Toward term, primary functions become production and storage of essential nutrients, excretion of bile, and establishment of processes of elimination. Extrauterine adaptation requires de novo enzyme synthesis. Modulation of these processes depends on substrate and hormonal input via the placenta and on dietary and hormonal input in the postnatal period.

HEPATIC ULTRASTRUCTURE

Hepatocytes exhibit various ultrastructural features that reflect their biologic functions (Fig. 335–3). First, hepatocytes, like other epithelial cells, are polarized; their structure and function are directionally oriented. One result of this polarity is that various regions of the hepatocyte plasma membrane exhibit specialized functions. Bidirectional transport can occur at the sinusoidal surface, where materials reaching the liver via the portal system enter and compounds secreted by the liver leave the hepatocyte. Canalicular membranes of adjacent hepatocytes form bile canaliculi, which are bounded by tight junctions preventing transfer of secreted compounds back into the sinusoid. Within hepatocytes, a number of different cell organelles are the sites of hepatic metabolic and synthetic activity. Abundant mitochondria are the sites of oxidation and metabolism of heterogeneous classes of substrates, of fatty acid oxidation, of key processes in gluconeogenesis, and of storage and release of energy. The endoplasmic reticulum, a continuous network of rough- and smooth-surfaced tubules and cisternae, is the site of various processes, including protein and triglyceride synthesis and drug metabolism. The endoplasmic reticulum is the major component of the microsomal fraction obtained by ultracentrifugation of liver homogenate. Low fetal activity of microsomal-bound enzymes accounts for a relative inefficiency of xenobiotic (drug) metabolism. The Golgi apparatus is active in protein packaging and possibly in bile secretion. Hepatocyte peroxisomes are single-membrane-limited cytoplasmic organelles that contain enzymes such as oxidases and catalase and those that have a role in lipid and bile acid metabolism. Lysosomes

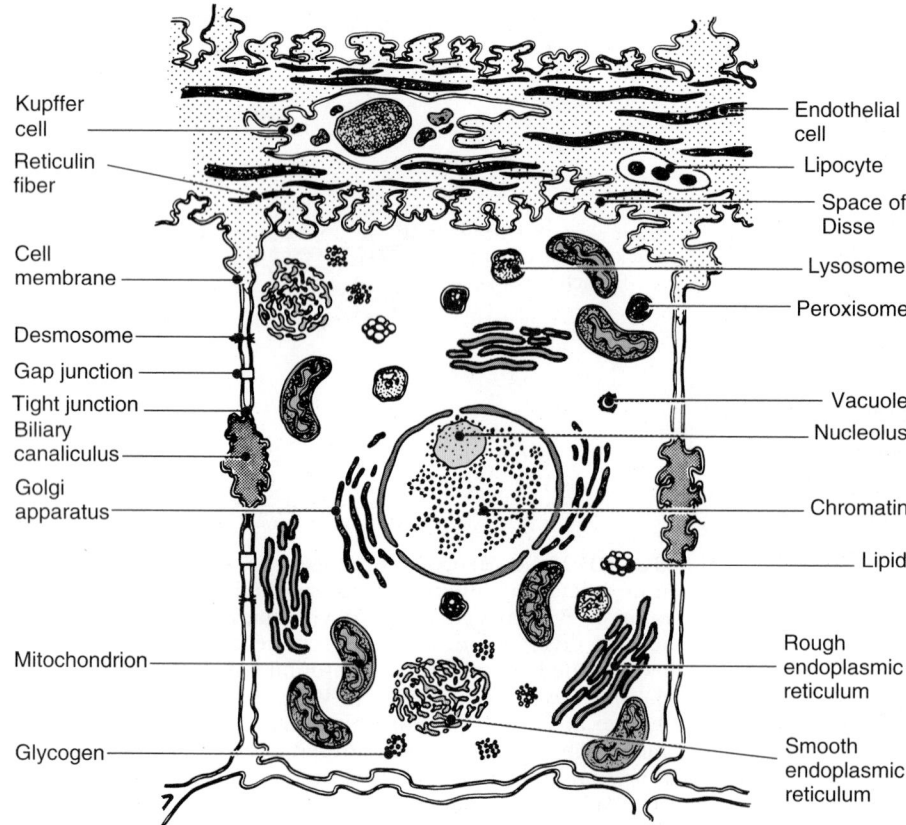

FIGURE 335–3. Schematic view of the ultrastructure and organelles of hepatocytes. (Reprinted from Sherlock S: Hepatic cell structure. In Sherlock S [editor]: *Diseases of the Liver and Biliary System*, 6th ed. Oxford, Blackwell Scientific, 1981, p 10, with permission from Blackwell Scientific.)

contain numerous hydrolases that have a role in intracellular digestion. The hepatocyte cytoskeleton, composed of actin and other filaments, is distributed throughout the cell and concentrated near the plasma membrane. Microfilaments and microtubules may have a role in receptor-mediated endocytosis, in bile secretion, and in maintaining the architecture and motility of the cell.

METABOLIC FUNCTIONS OF THE LIVER

Carbohydrate Metabolism. The liver regulates serum glucose levels closely. The liver stores excess carbohydrate as glycogen, a polymer of glucose readily hydrolyzed to glucose during fasting. To maintain serum glucose, hepatocytes produce free glucose by either gluconeogenesis or glycogenolysis. Gluconeogenic activity is present in the fetal liver but increases rapidly after birth. Immediately after birth, an infant is dependent on hepatic glycogenolysis; thereafter, an infant is capable of both glycogenolysis and gluconeogenesis. Fetal glycogen synthesis begins at about the 9th wk of gestation, with glycogen stores most rapidly accumulated near term, when the liver contains two to three times the amount of glycogen of adult liver. Most of this stored glycogen is used in the immediate postnatal period. Reaccumulation is initiated at about the 2nd wk of postnatal life, and glycogen stores reach adult levels at approximately the 3rd wk in healthy full-term infants. The fluctuations in serum glucose levels in preterm infants are due in part to the fact that efficient regulation of the synthesis, storage, and degradation of glycogen develops only near the end of full-term gestation. Dietary carbohydrates such as galactose are converted to glucose, but there is a substantial dependence on gluconeogenesis during fasting for glucose in early life, especially if glycogen stores are limited.

Protein Metabolism. During the rapid fetal growth phase, specific decarboxylases that are rate-limiting in the biosynthesis of physiologically important polyamines have higher activities than in the mature liver. The rate of synthesis of albumin and secretory proteins in the developing liver parallels the quantitative changes in endoplasmic reticulum. Synthesis of albumin appears at approximately the 7th–8th wk in a human fetus and increases in inverse proportion to that of α-fetoprotein, which is a dominant early fetal protein. By the 3rd–4th mo of gestation, the fetal liver is able to produce fibrinogen, transferrin, and low-density lipoproteins. From this period on, fetal plasma contains each of the major protein classes, at concentrations considerably below those achieved at maturity.

The *postnatal* patterns of development of various proteins are heterogeneous. Lipoproteins of each class rise abruptly in the 1st wk after birth to reach levels that vary little until puberty. Albumin concentrations are low in a neonate (~2.5 g/dL), reaching adult levels (~3.5 g/dL) after several months. Levels of ceruloplasmin and complement factors increase slowly to adult values during the first year. In contrast, transferrin levels at birth are similar to those of an adult, decline for 3–5 mo, and rise thereafter to achieve their final concentrations. Low levels of activity of specific proteins have implications for the nutrition of an infant; for example, a low level of cystathionine γ-lyase (cystathionase) activity impairs the trans-sulfuration pathway by which dietary methionine is converted to cysteine; accordingly, the latter must be supplied exogenously. Similar dietary requirements may exist for other sulfur-containing amino acids, such as taurine.

Lipid Metabolism. Fatty acid oxidation provides a major source of energy in early life, complementing glycogenolysis and gluconeogenesis. Newborn infants are relatively intolerant of prolonged fasting, owing in part to a restricted capacity for hepatic ketogenesis. Rapid maturation of the ability of the liver to oxidize fatty acid occurs during the 1st few days of life. Milk provides the major source of calories in early life; this high-fat, low-carbohydrate diet mandates active gluconeogenesis to maintain blood sugar levels. When the glucose supply is limited, ketone body production from endogenous fatty acids may provide energy for hepatic gluconeogenesis and an alternative fuel for brain metabolism. When carbohydrates are in excess, the liver produces triglycerides. Metabolic processes involving lipids and lipoprotein are predominantly hepatic; liver immaturity or disease affects lipid concentrations and lipoproteins.

Biotransformation. Newborn infants have a decreased capacity to metabolize and detoxify certain drugs, owing to underdevelopment of the hepatic microsomal component that is the site of the specific oxidative, reductive, hydrolytic, and conjugation reactions required for these biotransformations. The major components of the mono-oxygenase system, such as cytochrome P_{450}, the reduced form of nicotinamide-adenine dinucleotide phosphate, and cytochrome c reductase, are present in low concentrations in fetal microsomal preparations. In full-term infants, hepatic uridine diphosphate (UDP) glucuronosyltransferase and enzymes involved in the oxidation of polycyclic aromatic hydrocarbons have very low activities. Age-related differences in pharmacokinetics vary. For example, the half-life of acetaminophen in a newborn is similar to that of an adult, whereas theophylline has a half-life of approximately 100 hr in a premature infant, as compared to 5–6 hr in an adult. These differences in metabolism as well as factors such as binding to plasma proteins and renal clearance determine appropriate drug dosage to avoid toxicity. Dramatic examples of the susceptibility of newborn infants to drug toxicity are the responses to chloramphenicol ("gray baby" syndrome) or to benzoyl alcohol and its metabolic products, which involve ineffective glucuronide and glycine conjugation, respectively. The low concentrations of antioxidants (vitamin E, superoxide dismutase, and glutathione peroxidase) in the fetal and early newborn liver lead to increased susceptibility to deleterious effects of oxygen toxicity and oxidant injury through lipid peroxidation.

Conjugation reactions (which convert drugs or metabolites into forms that can be eliminated in bile) are also catalyzed by hepatic microsomal enzymes. Newborn infants have decreased activity of UDP glucuronosyltransferase, which converts unconjugated bilirubin to the readily excreted glucuronide conjugate and is the rate-limiting enzyme in the excretion of bilirubin. There is rapid postnatal development of transferase activity, even in prematurely born infants, irrespective of gestational age; this suggests that birth-related rather than age-related factors are of primary importance in the postnatal development of activity of this enzyme. Microsomal activity can be stimulated by administration of phenobarbital, rifampin, or other inducers of cytochrome P_{450}. Alternatively, drugs such as cimetidine may inhibit microsomal P_{450} activity.

Hepatic Excretory Function. Hepatic excretory function and bile flow are closely related to bile acid excretion and recirculation. Bile acids are the major product of degradation of cholesterol. Their incorporation into mixed micelles with cholesterol and phospholipid creates an efficient vehicle for solubilization and intestinal absorption of lipophilic compounds, such as dietary fats and fat-soluble vitamins. Secretion of bile acids is the major determinant of bile flow in the mature animal. Accordingly, maturity of bile acid metabolic processes affects overall hepatic excretory function, including biliary excretion of endogenous and exogenous compounds.

In humans, the two primary bile acids, cholic acid and chenodeoxycholic acid, are synthesized in the liver. Before excretion, they are conjugated with glycine and taurine. In response to a meal, contraction of the gallbladder delivers bile acids to the intestine to assist in fat digestion and absorption. After mediating fat digestion, the bile acids themselves are reabsorbed from the terminal ileum through specific active transport processes.

Meier PJ, Stieger B: Molecular mechanisms of bile formation. *News Physiol Sci* 2000;15:89–93.
Rudolph AM: Hepatic and ductus venosus blood flows during fetal life. *Hepatology* 1983;3:254–8.
Shneider BL: Intestinal bile acid transport: Biology, physiology, and pathophysiology. *J Pediatr Gastroenterol Nutr* 2001;32:407–417.
Zaret KS: Liver specification and early morphogenesis. *Mech Dev* 2000;92:83–88.
Zaret KS: Hepatocyte differentiation: from the endoderm and beyond. *Curr Opin Genet Dev* 2001;11:568–574.

BOX 335–1. Causes of Impaired Bile Acid Metabolism and Enterohepatic Circulation

DEFECTIVE BILE ACID SYNTHESIS/TRANSPORT

Inborn errors of bile acid synthesis: reductase deficiency, isomerase deficiency
Intrahepatic cholestasis (neonatal hepatitis)
Progressive familial intrahepatic cholestasis (PFIC)
Acquired defects in bile acid synthesis secondary to severe liver disease

ABNORMALITIES OF BILE ACID DELIVERY TO THE BOWEL

Celiac sprue (sluggish gallbladder contraction)
Extrahepatic bile duct obstruction (biliary atresia)

LOSS OF ENTEROHEPATIC CIRCULATION OF BILE ACIDS

External bile fistula
Cystic fibrosis
Contaminated small bowel syndrome (with bile acid precipitation, increased jejunal absorption, and "short circuiting")
Drug-induced entrapment of bile acids in intestinal lumen (cholestyramine)

BILE ACID MALABSORPTION

Primary bile acid malabsorption (absent or inefficient ileal active transport)
Secondary bile acid malabsorption
    Ileal disease or resection
    Cystic fibrosis

DEFECTIVE UPTAKE OR ALTERED INTRACELLULAR METABOLISM

Parenchymal disease (acute hepatitis, cirrhosis)
Regurgitation from cells
Portosystemic shunting
Cholestasis

They return to the liver via portal blood, are taken up by liver cells, and are re-excreted in bile. In an adult, this enterohepatic circulation involves 90–95% of the circulating bile acid pool. Bile acids that escape ileal reabsorption reach the colon, where the bacterial flora, through dehydroxylation and deconjugation, produces the secondary bile acids, deoxycholate and lithocholate. In an adult, the composition of bile reflects the excretion of the primary and also the secondary bile acids, which are reabsorbed from the distal intestinal tract.

Neonates have inefficient ileal bile acid reabsorption and a low rate of hepatic clearance of bile acids from portal blood. The latter results in elevated serum concentrations of bile acids in healthy newborns, often to levels that would suggest liver disease in older individuals. The size of the bile acid pool in a neonate is about half that of an adult, and the bile acid concentration in the proximal intestinal lumen is similarly decreased to levels that are frequently below the concentration required for micelle formation (2 mM); accordingly, absorption of dietary fats and fat-soluble vitamins is reduced but not sufficiently to produce malabsorption. Transient phases of "physiologic cholestasis" and "physiologic steatorrhea" have a role in the nutrition of low birthweight infants but are of minor importance to healthy full-term newborns. Beyond the neonatal period, disturbances in bile acid metabolism may be responsible for diverse effects on hepatobiliary and intestinal function (Box 335–1).

Bates MD, Balistreri WF: The gastrointestinal tract: Development of the human digestive system. In Fanaroff AA, Martin RJ (editors): *Neonatal-Perinatal Medicine: Diseases of the Fetus and Infant*, 7th ed. St. Louis, Mosby, 2002, pp 1255–1263.
Bezerra JA: Liver development: A paradigm for hepatobiliary disease in later life. *Sem Liver Dis* 1998;18:203–216.
Desmet VJ: Congenital diseases of intrahepatic bile ducts: Variations on the theme "ductal plate malformation." *Hepatology* 1992;16:1069–83.
Duncan SA: Transcriptional regulation of liver development. *Dev Dyn* 2000;219:131–142.
Karpen SJ, Suchy FJ: Structural and functional development of the liver. In Suchy FJ, et al (editors): *Liver Disease in Children*, 2nd ed. Philadelphia, Lippincott Williams & Wilkins, 2001, pp 3–21.

Chapter 336

Manifestations of Liver Disease *Vicky Lee Ng and William Balistreri*

Pathologic Manifestations. Alterations in hepatic structure and function can be *acute* or *chronic*, with varying patterns of reaction of the liver to cell injury. Hepatocyte injury may result in inflammation or cell death (necrosis), which may be followed by a healing process of scar formation (fibrosis), and potentially nodule formation (regeneration). Cirrhosis is the end result of virtually any progressive liver disease.

Inflammation or necrosis, or both, of individual hepatocytes can result from viral infection, drugs or toxins, hypoxia, immunologic disorders, or inborn errors of metabolism. The evolving process leads to repair, continuing injury with chronic changes, or in rare cases to massive hepatic damage.

Cholestasis is an alternative or concomitant response to injury caused by extrahepatic or intrahepatic obstruction to bile flow. Accumulation in serum of substances normally excreted in bile such as direct-reacting bilirubin, cholesterol, bile acids, and trace elements occurs. Bile pigment in liver parenchyma can be seen in a liver biopsy specimen. In extrahepatic obstruction, bile pigment may be visible in the intralobular bile ducts or throughout the parenchyma as bile lakes or infarcts. In intrahepatic cholestasis, an injury to hepatocytes or an alteration in hepatic physiology leads to a reduction in the rate of secretion of solute and water. Likely causes include alterations in (1) ultrastructure or cytoskeleton of the hepatocyte; (2) organelles responsible for bile secretion; (3) enzymatic or transporter activity; or (4) permeability of the bile canalicular apparatus. The end result may be clinically indistinguishable from obstructive cholestasis.

Cirrhosis, defined histologically by the presence of bands of fibrous tissue that link central and portal areas and form parenchymal nodules, is a potential end stage of any acute or chronic liver disease. Cirrhosis may be posthepatitic (after acute or chronic hepatitis) or postnecrotic (after toxic injury), or it may follow chronic biliary obstruction (biliary cirrhosis). Cirrhosis may be **macronodular,** with nodules of various sizes (up to 5 cm) separated by broad septa, or **micronodular,** with nodules of uniform size (<1 cm) separated by fine septa. Mixed forms also occur. The progressive scarring of cirrhosis results in altered hepatic blood flow, with further impairment of liver cell function. In addition, the increased intrahepatic resistance to portal blood flow leads to portal hypertension.

Primary tumors of the liver are discussed in Chapter 496. The liver may be **secondarily** involved in neoplastic (metastatic) and non-neoplastic (storage diseases and fat infiltration) processes as well as a number of systemic conditions and infectious processes. The liver may also be affected by chronic passive congestion or acute hypoxia, with hepatocellular damage.

Clinical Manifestations

HEPATOMEGALY. Enlargement of the liver can be due to several mechanisms (Box 336–1). Concepts of normal liver size have been based on age-related clinical indices, such as (1) the degree of extension of the liver edge below the costal margin;

BOX 336–1. Mechanisms of Hepatomegaly

INCREASE IN THE NUMBER OR SIZE OF THE CELLS IN THE LIVER
Storage
Fat: malnutrition, obesity, metabolic liver disease (e.g.,
   diseases of fatty acid oxidation and Reye syndrome–like
   illnesses), lipid infusion (total parenteral nutrition),
   cystic fibrosis, diabetes mellitus, medication related,
   pregnancy
Specific lipid storage diseases: Gaucher, Niemann-Pick, Wolman
   disease
Glycogen: glycogen storage diseases (multiple enzyme defects);
   total parenteral nutrition; infant of diabetic mother, Beckwith
   syndrome
Miscellaneous: α_1-antitrypsin deficiency, Wilson disease,
   hypervitaminosis A, neonatal iron storage disease

INFLAMMATION
Hepatocyte enlargement (hepatitis)
   Viral—acute and chronic
   Bacterial—sepsis, abscess, cholangitis
   Toxic—drugs
Kupffer cell enlargement
Autoimmune
   Chronic hepatitis
   Sarcoidosis
   Systemic lupus erythematosus
   Sclerosing cholangitis

INFILTRATION
Primary liver tumors
   Benign
      Hepatocellular
         Focal nodular hyperplasia
         Nodular regenerative hyperplasia
         Hepatocellular adenoma
      Mesodermal
         Infantile hemangioendothelioma
         Mesenchymal hamartoma

Cystic masses
   Choledochal cyst
   Hepatic cyst
   Hematoma
   Parasitic cyst
   Pyogenic or amebic abscess
Malignant
   Hepatocellular
      Hepatoblastoma
      Hepatocellular carcinoma
   Mesodermal
      Angiosarcoma
      Undifferentiated embryonal sarcoma
Secondary or metastatic tumors
   Lymphoma
   Leukemia
   Histiocytosis
   Neuroblastoma
   Wilms tumor

INCREASED SIZE OF VASCULAR SPACE
Intrahepatic obstruction to hepatic vein outflow
   Veno-occlusive disease
   Hepatic vein thrombosis (Budd-Chiari syndrome)
   Hepatic vein web
Suprahepatic
   Congestive heart failure
   Pericardial disease
   Tamponade
   Constrictive pericarditis
   Hematopoietic: sickle cell anemia, thalassemia

INCREASED SIZE OF BILIARY SPACE
   Congenital hepatic fibrosis
   Caroli disease
   Extrahepatic obstruction

IDIOPATHIC (? "BENIGN")

---

(2) the span of dullness to percussion; or (3) the length of the vertical axis of the liver, as estimated from imaging techniques. In children, the normal liver edge can be felt up to 2 cm below the right costal margin. In a newborn infant, extension of the liver edge more than 3.5 cm below the costal margin in the right midclavicular line suggests hepatic enlargement. Measurement of *liver span* is carried out by percussing the upper margin of dullness and by palpating the lower edge in the right midclavicular line; it may be more reliable than an extension of the liver edge alone; the two measurements may correlate poorly.

The liver span increases linearly with body weight and age in both sexes, ranging from about 4.5–5 cm at 1 wk of age to approximately 7–8 cm in boys and 6–6.5 cm in girls by 12 yr of age. The lower edge of the right lobe of the liver extends downward **(Riedel lobe)** and may be palpable as a broad mass in some normal people. An enlarged left lobe of the liver may be palpable in the epigastrium of some patients with cirrhosis. Downward displacement of the liver by the diaphragm or thoracic organs can create an erroneous impression of hepatomegaly.

Examination of the liver should note the consistency, contour, tenderness, or the presence of any masses or bruits, as well as assessment of spleen size. Documentation of the presence of ascites and any stigmata of chronic liver disease is important.

Ultrasonography is useful in assessment of **liver size and consistency**, as well as **gallbladder size**. Hyperechogenic hepatic parenchyma can be seen with metabolic disease (glycogen storage disease) or fatty liver (from obesity, malnutrition, hyperalimentation, corticosteroids). Gallbladder distention may be seen in infants with sepsis. The gallbladder is often absent in infants with biliary atresia. Gallbladder length normally varies from 1.5 to 5.5 cm (average, 3.0) in infants to 4 to 8 cm in adolescents; width ranges from 0.5 to 2.5 cm for all ages.

JAUNDICE (ICTERUS). Yellow discoloration of the sclera, skin, and mucous membranes is a sign that hyperbilirubinemia exists (Chapter 91.3). Clinically apparent jaundice in children and adults occurs when the serum concentration of bilirubin reaches 2–3 mg/dL (34–51 µmol/L); however, the neonate may not appear icteric until the bilirubin level is over 5 mg/dL (85 µmol/L). Jaundice may be the earliest and only sign of hepatic dysfunction. Liver disease must be suspected in the infant who may appear only mildly jaundiced, but has dark urine or acholic (light-colored) stools. Immediate evaluation to establish the cause is required.

Measurement of the total serum bilirubin concentration allows quantitation of jaundice. Bilirubin occurs in plasma in four forms: (1) *unconjugated bilirubin* tightly bound to albumin; (2) *free* or *unbound bilirubin* (the form responsible for kernicterus, because it can cross cell membranes); (3) *conjugated bilirubin* (the only fraction to appear in urine); and (4) *delta* (δ) *fraction* (bilirubin covalently bound to albumin), which appears in serum when hepatic excretion of conjugated ·bilirubin is impaired in patients with hepatobiliary disease. The δ fraction permits conjugated bilirubin to persist in the circulation and delays resolution of jaundice. Although the terms *direct* and *indirect* bilirubin are used equivalently with *conjugated* and *unconjugated* bilirubin, this is not quantitatively correct, because the direct fraction includes both conjugated bilirubin and δ bilirubin. An elevation of serum bile acids is frequently seen in the presence of any form of cholestasis.

Investigation of jaundice in an infant or older child must include determination of the accumulation of either unconjugated or conjugated bilirubin. An unconjugated hyperbilirubinemia may indicate increased production, hemolysis, reduced hepatic removal, or altered metabolism of bilirubin (Box 336–2). A conjugated bilirubinemia (>20% of total) reflects

BOX 336–2. Differential Diagnosis of Unconjugated Hyperbilirubinemia

INCREASED PRODUCTION OF UNCONJUGATED BILIRUBIN FROM HEME
Hemolytic disease (hereditary of acquired)
  Isoimmune hemolysis (neonatal; acute or delayed transfusion reaction; autoimmune)
    Rh incompatibility
    ABO incompatibility
    Other blood group incompatibilities
  Congenital spherocytosis
  Hereditary elliptocytosis
  Infantile pyknocytosis
  Erythrocyte enzyme defects
  Hemoglobinopathy
    Sickle cell anemia
    Thalassemia
    Others
  Sepsis
  Microangiopathy
    Hemolytic-uremic syndrome
    Hemangioma
    Mechanical trauma (heart valve)
Ineffective erythropoiesis
Drugs
Infection
Enclosed hematoma
Polycythemia
  Diabetic mother
  Fetal transfusion (recipient)
  Delayed cord clamping

DECREASED DELIVERY OF UNCONJUGATED BILIRUBIN (IN PLASMA) TO HEPATOCYTE
Right-sided congestive heart failure
Portacaval shunt

DECREASED BILIRUBIN UPTAKE ACROSS HEPATOCYTE MEMBRANE
Presumed enzyme transporter deficiency
Competitive inhibition
  Breast milk jaundice
  Lucey-Driscoll syndrome
  Drug inhibition (radiocontrast material)
Miscellaneous
  Hypothyroidism
  Hypoxia
  Acidosis

DECREASED STORAGE OF UNCONJUGATED BILIRUBIN IN CYTOSOL (DECREASED Y AND Z PROTEINS)
Competitive inhibition
Fever

DECREASED BIOTRANSFORMATION (CONJUGATION)
Neonatal jaundice (physiologic)
Inhibition (drugs)
Hereditary (Crigler-Najjar)
  Type I (complete enzyme deficiency)
  Type II (partial deficiency)
Gilbert disease
Hepatocellular dysfunction

ENTEROHEPATIC RECIRCULATION
Intestinal obstruction
  Ileal atresia
  Hirschsprung disease
  Cystic fibrosis
  Pyloric stenosis
Antibiotic administration

BREAST MILK JAUNDICE

---

decreased excretion by damaged hepatic parenchymal cells or disease of biliary tract, which may be due to sepsis, endocrine or metabolic disease, inflammation of the liver, or obstruction (Box 336–3).

PRURITUS. Intense generalized itching may occur in patients with cholestasis (conjugated hyperbilirubinemia). Pruritus is unrelated to the degree of hyperbilirubinemia; deeply jaundiced patients may be asymptomatic, and vice versa. Although retained components of bile are important, the cause is probably multifactorial as evidenced by the symptomatic relief of pruritus following administration of various therapeutic agents including bile acid–binding agents such as cholestyramine; choleretic agents such as phenobarbital or ursodeoxycholic acid; opiate antagonists; antihistamines; and antibiotics such as rifampin. Surgical diversion of bile via a procedure called partial external biliary diversion has provided relief for medically refractory pruritus.

SPIDER ANGIOMAS. Vascular spiders (telangiectasias), characterized by central pulsating arterioles from which small, wiry venules radiate, may be seen in patients with chronic liver disease, usually most prominent in the face and chest. These are presumably reflective of altered estrogen metabolism in the presence of hepatic dysfunction.

PALMAR ERYTHEMA. Blotchy erythema, most noticeable over the thenar and hypothenar eminences and on the tips of the fingers, is also noted in patients with chronic liver disease. These may be due to vasodilation and increased blood flow.

XANTHOMAS. The marked elevation of serum cholesterol (to levels > 500 mg/dL) associated with chronic cholestasis may cause the deposition of lipid in the dermis and subcutaneous tissue. Brown nodules may develop first over the extensor surfaces of the extremities; rarely, xanthelasma of the eyelids develops.

PORTAL HYPERTENSION. The portal vein drains the splanchnic area (abdominal portion of the gastrointestinal tract, pancreas, and spleen) into the hepatic sinusoids. Normal portal pressure gradient, the pressure difference between the portal vein and the systemic veins (hepatic veins or inferior vena cava), is 3–6 mm Hg, with "clinically significant portal hypertension" being a threshold above 10 mm Hg. Portal hypertension is the main complication of cirrhosis, directly responsible for two of its most common and potentially lethal complications—ascites and variceal hemorrhage.

ASCITES. Ascites may be associated with urinary tract abnormalities, metabolic diseases (such as lysosomal storage diseases), congenital or acquired heart disease, and hydrops fetalis. Factors favoring the intra-abdominal accumulation of fluid include (1) decreased plasma colloid osmotic pressure; (2) increased capillary hydrostatic pressure; (3) increased ascitic colloid osmotic fluid pressure; and (4) decreased ascitic fluid hydrostatic pressure. Abnormal renal sodium retention must be considered (Chapter 351). The onset of ascites in the child with chronic liver disease means that the two prerequisite conditions for ascites are present—portal hypertension and hepatic insufficiency.

VARICEAL HEMORRHAGE. Gastroesophageal varices are the more clinically significant portosystemic collaterals because of their propensity to rupture and cause life-threatening hemorrhage. Variceal hemorrhage results from increased pressure within the varix, which leads to changes in the diameter of the varix and increased wall tension. When the variceal wall strength is exceeded, physical rupture of the varix results, and given the high blood flow and pressure in the portosystemic collateral system coupled with the lack of a natural mechanism to tamponade variceal bleeding, the rate of hemorrhage can be striking.

ENCEPHALOPATHY. Hepatic encephalopathy can involve any neurologic function, and may be prominent, or it may present in subtle forms such as deterioration of school performance, depression, or emotional outbursts. It may be recurrent and precipitated by intercurrent illness, drugs, bleeding, or electrolyte

BOX 336–3. Differential Diagnosis of Neonatal and Infantile Cholestasis

INFECTIOUS

Generalized bacterial sepsis
Viral hepatitis
  Hepatitis A, B, C (rare)
  Cytomegalovirus
  Rubella virus
  Herpes virus HSV, HHV 6 and 7
  Varicella virus
  Coxsackievirus
  Echovirus
  Reovirus type 3
  Parvovirus B19
  HIV
Others
  Toxoplasmosis
  Syphilis
  Tuberculosis
  Listeriosis

TOXIC

Parenteral nutrition related
Sepsis (e.g., urinary tract) with endotoxemia
Drug related

METABOLIC

Disorders of amino acid metabolism
  Tyrosinemia
Disorders of lipid metabolism
  Wolman disease
  Niemann-Pick disease (type C)
  Gaucher disease
Disorders of carbohydrate metabolism
  Galactosemia
  Fructosemia
  Glycogenosis IV
Disorders of bile acid biosynthesis
Other metabolic defects
  α_1-Antitrypsin deficiency
  Cystic fibrosis
  Idiopathic hypopituitarism
  Hypothyroidism
  Zellweger (cerebrohepatorenal) syndrome

Neonatal iron storage disease
Indian childhood cirrhosis/infantile copper overload
Hemophagocytic lymphohistiocytosis (HLH)
Congenital disorders of glycosylation
Mitochrondrial hepatopathies

GENETIC/CHROMOSOMAL

Trisomy E
Down syndrome
Donahue syndrome (leprechaunism)

INTRAHEPATIC DISEASES

Intrahepatic cholestasis—persistent
  "Idiopathic" neonatal hepatitis
  Alagille syndrome (arteriohepatic dysplasia)
  Intrahepatic biliary hypoplasia or paucity of intrahepatic bile ducts
    (nonsyndromic)
  Progressive familial intrahepatic cholestasis (PFIC)
Intrahepatic cholestasis—recurrent
  Familial benign recurrent cholestasis associated with lymphedema
    (Aagenaes)
Congenital hepatic fibrosis
Caroli disease (cystic dilatation of intrahepatic ducts)

EXTRAHEPATIC DISEASES

Biliary atresia
Sclerosing cholangitis
Bile duct stenosis
Choledochal-pancreaticoductal junction anomaly
Spontaneous perforation of the bile duct
Choledochal cyst
Mass (neoplasia, stone)
Bile/mucous plug ("inspissated bile")

MISCELLANEOUS

Langerhans cell histiocytosis
Shock and hypoperfusion
Associated with enteritis
Associated with intestinal obstruction
Neonatal lupus erythematosus
Myeloproliferative disease (21-trisomy)

---

and acid-base disturbances. The appearance of hepatic encephalopathy depends on the presence of portosystemic shunting, alterations in the blood-brain barrier, and the interactions of toxic metabolites with the central nervous system. Postulated causes include altered ammonium metabolism, synergistic neurotoxins, or "false neurotransmitters" with plasma amino acid imbalance (Chapter 345).

ENDOCRINE ABNORMALITIES. Endocrine abnormalities are more common in adults with hepatic disease than in children. They reflect alterations in hepatic synthetic, storage, and metabolic functions, including those concerned with hormonal metabolism in the liver. Proteins that bind hormones in plasma are synthesized in the liver, and steroid hormones are conjugated in the liver and excreted in the urine; failure of such functions may have clinical consequences. Endocrine abnormalities may also result from malnutrition or specific deficiencies.

RENAL DYSFUNCTION. There is a close relationship between hepatic and renal dysfunction. Systemic disease or toxins may affect both organs simultaneously, or parenchymal liver disease may produce secondary impairment of renal function, and vice versa. In hepatobiliary disorders, there may be renal alterations in sodium and water economy, impaired renal concentrating ability, and alterations in potassium metabolism. Ascites in patients with cirrhosis may be related to inappropriate retention of sodium by the kidneys, with expansion of plasma volume, or to sodium retention mediated by diminished effective plasma volume. *Hepatorenal syndrome* is defined as functional renal failure in patients with end-stage liver disease. The pathophysiol-

ogy is poorly defined but the hallmark is intense renal vasoconstriction (mediated by hemodynamic, humoral, or neurogenic mechanisms) with coexistent systemic vasodilation. The diagnosis is supported by the findings of oliguria (<1 mL/kg/day); a characteristic pattern of urine electrolyte abnormalities (urine sodium of <10 mEq/L, fractional excretion of sodium of <1%, urine:plasma creatinine ratio < 10 and normal urinary sediment), absence of hypovolemia and exclusion of other kidney pathology. The best treatment is timely liver transplantation, as complete renal recovery can be expected.

PULMONARY INVOLVEMENT. *Hepatopulmonary syndrome* is characterized by the typical triad of hypoxemia, intrapulmonary vascular dilations, and liver disease. In this entity, there is intrapulmonic right-to-left shunting of blood, which results in systemic desaturation. It should be suspected and investigated in the child with chronic liver disease with history of shortness of breath or exercise intolerance and clinical examination findings of cyanosis (particularly of the lips and fingers), digital clubbing, and oxygen saturations below 96%, particularly in the upright position. Treatment is timely liver transplantation; successful pulmonary resolution follows.

RECURRENT CHOLANGITIS. Ascending infection of the biliary system is most often seen in pediatric cholestatic liver disease, due most commonly to gram-negative enteric organisms, such as *E. coli, Klebsiella, Pseudomonas,* and *Enterococcus.* Liver transplantation is the definitive effective treatment for recurrent cholangitis in the child with chronic cholestatic liver disease, especially when medical therapy is not effective.

Miscellaneous Manifestations of Liver Dysfunction. Nonspecific signs of acute and chronic liver disease include (1) *anorexia,* which often affects patients with anicteric hepatitis and with cirrhosis associated with chronic cholestasis; (2) *abdominal pain or distention* resulting from ascites, spontaneous peritonitis, or visceromegaly; (3) *malnutrition and growth failure;* and (4) *bleeding,* which may be due to altered synthesis of coagulation factors (biliary obstruction with vitamin K deficiency or excessive hepatic damage) or to portal hypertension with hypersplenism. In the presence of hypersplenism, there may be decreased synthesis of specific clotting factors, production of qualitatively abnormal proteins, or alterations in platelet number and function. Altered drug metabolism may prolong the biologic half-life of commonly administered medications.

336.1 Evaluation of Patients with Possible Liver Dysfunction

Adequate evaluation of an infant, child, or adolescent with suspected liver disease involves an appropriate and accurate history, a carefully performed physical examination, and skillful interpretation of signs and symptoms. Further evaluation is aided by judicious selection of diagnostic tests, followed by a liver biopsy or the use of imaging modalities. Most of the so-called liver function tests do not measure specific hepatic functions; a rise in serum aminotransferase (transaminase) level reflects liver cell injury; an increase in immunoglobulin level reflects an immunologic response to injury; or an elevation in serum bilirubin level may reflect any of several disturbances of bilirubin metabolism outlined in Boxes 336–2 and 336–3. Any single biochemical assay provides limited information, which must be placed in the context of the entire clinical and historic picture. The most cost-efficient approach is to become familiar with the rationale, implications, and limitations of a selected group of tests so that specific questions can be answered.

For a patient with suspected liver disease, evaluation addresses the following issues in sequence: (1) Is liver disease present? (2) If so, what is its nature? (3) What is its severity? (4) Is specific treatment available? (5) How can we monitor the response to treatment? and (6) What is the prognosis?

Biochemical Tests. Laboratory tests commonly used to screen for or to confirm a suspicion of liver disease include measurements of serum transaminase, bilirubin (total and fractionated) and alkaline phosphatase (AP) levels, as well as determinations of prothrombin time (PT) or international normalized ratio (INR) and albumin level. These tests are complementary and provide an estimation of synthetic and excretory functions and may suggest the nature of the disturbance (e.g., inflammation or cholestasis).

Acute liver cell injury (parenchymal disease) in viral hepatitis, drug- or toxin-induced liver disease, shock, hypoxemia, or metabolic disease is best reflected by marked increases in serum aminotransferase levels. Cholestasis (obstructive disease) involves regurgitation of bile components into serum; the serum levels of total and conjugated bilirubin and serum bile acids are elevated. Elevations in serum alkaline phosphatase, 5′ nucleotidase (5′ NT), and γ-glutamyl transpeptidase (GGT) levels are also sensitive indicators of obstruction or inflammation of the biliary tract.

The severity of the liver disease may be reflected in (1) *clinical signs* (occurrence of encephalopathy, variceal hemorrhage, worsening jaundice, apparent shrinkage of liver mass owing to massive necrosis, or onset of ascites) or in (2) *biochemical alterations* (hypoglycemia, hyperammonemia, electrolyte imbalance, continued hyperbilirubinemia, marked hypoalbuminemia, or prolonged PT or INR unresponsive to parenteral administration of vitamin K).

Fractionation of the total serum bilirubin level into *conjugated and unconjugated bilirubin fractions* helps to distinguish between elevations caused by hemolysis and those caused by hepatic dysfunction. A predominant elevation in the conjugated bilirubin level provides a relatively sensitive index of hepatocellular disease and hepatic excretory dysfunction, whereas elevation in transaminase levels are more highly sensitive indices of hepatocellular damage.

Alanine aminotransferase (ALT, serum glutamate pyruvate transaminase) is liver specific, whereas *aspartate aminotransferase* (AST, serum glutamic-oxaloacetic transaminase) is derived from other organs in addition to the liver. The most marked rises of both AST and ALT levels may occur with acute hepatocellular injury—a several thousand-fold elevation may result from acute viral hepatitis, toxic injury, hypoxia or hypoperfusion. After blunt abdominal trauma, parallel elevations in transaminase levels may provide an early clue to hepatic injury. A differential rise or fall in AST and ALT levels can sometimes provide useful information. In acute hepatitis, the rise in ALT may be greater than the rise in AST. In alcohol-induced liver injury, fulminant echovirus infection, and various metabolic diseases, more predominant rises in AST have been reported. In chronic liver disease or in intrahepatic and extrahepatic biliary obstruction, AST and ALT elevations may be less marked. *Nonalcoholic steatohepatitis (NASH),* also known as nonalcoholic fatty liver disease, is a chronic liver disorder that is seen in obese children presenting with elevated serum transaminase levels. Its notable characteristic is the similar histology to alcoholic-induced liver injury in the absence of alcohol abuse.

Hepatic synthetic function is reflected in *serum albumin* and *protein* levels and in the *PT* or *INR.* Examination of *serum globulin* concentration and of the relative amounts of the globulin fractions may be helpful. Gamma-globulin levels are often high, and increased titers of smooth muscle antibody as well as antinuclear antibodies, anti–liver-kidney-microsome (LKM) antibody, and antimitochondrial antibodies may be found in patients with autoimmune hepatitis. A resurgence in α-fetoprotein levels may suggest hepatoma or hereditary tyrosinemia. Hypoalbuminemia caused by depressed synthesis may complicate severe liver disease and serve as a prognostic factor. Deficiencies of *factor V* and of the *vitamin K–dependent factors (II, VII, IX, and X)* may occur in patients with severe liver disease or fulminant hepatic failure. If the PT or INR is prolonged as a result of intestinal malabsorption of vitamin K (resulting from cholestasis) or decreased nutritional intake of vitamin K, then parenteral administration of vitamin K should correct the coagulopathy, leading to normalization within 24 hr. Unresponsiveness to vitamin K would suggest hepatic disease. Persistently low levels of factor VII are evidence of a poor prognosis in fulminant liver disease.

Interpretation of results of biochemical tests of hepatic structure and function must be made in the context of age-related changes. The activity of *alkaline phosphatase (AP)* varies considerably with age. Normal growing children have significant elevations of serum AP activity originating from influx into serum of the isoenzyme that originates in bone, particularly in rapidly growing adolescents. Therefore, an isolated increase in AP does not indicate hepatic or biliary disease if other liver function test results are normal. Other enzymes such as *5′ NT and GGT* are increased in cholestatic conditions, and may be more specific for hepatobiliary disease. 5′ NT is located in both sinusoidal and canalicular membranes, and is not found in bone. GGT exhibits high enzyme activity in early life that declines rapidly with age. Cholesterol concentrations increase throughout life. *Cholesterol levels* may is markedly elevated in patients with cholestasis, whether the cause is intrahepatic or extrahepatic. On the other hand, with acute liver disease, such as hepatitis, serum cholesterol levels may be depressed.

Interpretation of *serum ammonia* values must be carried out with caution because of variability in their physiologic determinants and the inherent difficulty in laboratory measurement.

Liver Biopsy. Liver biopsy combined with clinical data can suggest a cause in most cases. Specimens of liver tissue can be used (1) to provide a precise histology diagnosis in patients with neonatal cholestasis, chronic active hepatitis, metabolic liver disease, suspected Reye syndrome, intrahepatic cholestasis (paucity of bile ducts), congenital hepatic fibrosis, or undefined portal hypertension; (2) for enzyme analysis to detect inborn errors of metabolism; and (3) for analysis of stored material such as iron, copper, or specific metabolites. Liver biopsies can monitor responses to therapy or detect complications of treatment with potentially hepatotoxic agents, including but not exclusively, aspirin, anti-infectives (erythromycin, minocycline, ketoconazole, isoniazid), antimetabolites, anti-neoplastics, or anticonvulsant agents.

In infants and children, needle biopsy of the liver is easily accomplished through the percutaneous approach. The amount of tissue obtained, even in small infants, is usually sufficient for histologic interpretation and for biochemical analyses, if the latter are deemed necessary. Percutaneous liver biopsy can be performed safely in infants as young as 1 wk. Patients usually require only sedation and *local* anesthesia. Contraindications include prolonged PT or INR; thrombocytopenia; suspicion of a vascular, cystic, or infectious lesion in the path of the needle; and severe ascites. Therefore, if administration of fresh frozen plasma or of platelet transfusions fails to correct a prolonged PT, INR, or thrombocytopenia, a tissue specimen may be obtained via alternative techniques. Considerations include either the open laparotomy (wedge) approach by a general surgeon, or the transjugular approach under ultrasound and fluoroscopic guidance by an experienced pediatric interventional radiologist in an appropriately equipped fluoroscopy suite. The risk of development of a complication such as hemorrhage, hematoma, creation of an arteriovenous fistula, pneumothorax, or bile peritonitis is very small.

Hepatic Imaging Procedures. Various techniques help define the size, shape, and architecture of the liver and the anatomy of the intrahepatic and extrahepatic biliary trees. Although imaging may not provide a precise histologic and biochemical diagnosis, specific questions can be answered, such as whether hepatomegaly is related to accumulation of fat or glycogen or is due to a tumor or cyst. These studies may direct further evaluation such as percutaneous biopsy and make possible prompt referral of patients with biliary obstruction to a surgeon. Choice of imaging procedure should be part of a carefully formulated diagnostic approach, with avoidance of redundant demonstrations by several techniques.

A *plain roentgenographic study* may suggest hepatomegaly, but a carefully performed physical examination gives a more reliable assessment of liver size. The liver may appear less dense than normal in patients with fatty infiltration or more dense with deposition of heavy metals such as iron. A hepatic or biliary tract mass may displace an air-filled loop of bowel. Calcifications may be evident in the liver (parasitic and neoplastic disease), in the vasculature (with portal vein thrombosis), or in the gallbladder or biliary tree (gallstones). Collections of gas may be seen within the liver (abscess), biliary tract, or portal circulation (necrotizing enterocolitis).

Ultrasonography (US) provides information about the size, composition, and blood flow of the liver. Increased echogenicity is observed with fatty infiltration, and mass lesions as small as 1–2 cm may be shown. US has replaced cholangiography in detecting stones in the gallbladder or biliary tree. Even in neonates, US can assess gallbladder size, detect dilatation of the biliary tract, and define a choledochal cyst. In infants with biliary atresia, US findings may include small or absent gallbladder; nonvisualization of the common duct; and presence of the "triangular cord sign," a triangular/tubular-shaped echogenic density in the bifurcation of the portal vein, representing fibrous remnants at the porta hepatis. In patients with portal hypertension, Doppler US can evaluate patency of the portal vein, demonstrate collateral circulation, and assess size of spleen and amount of ascites. Relatively small amounts of ascitic fluid can also be detected. The use of Doppler US has been helpful in determining vascular patency after orthotopic liver transplantation.

Computed tomography (CT) scanning provides information similar to that obtained by US but is less suitable for use in patients younger than 2 yr of age because of the small size of structures, the paucity of intra-abdominal fat for contrast, and the need for heavy sedation or general anesthesia. *Magnetic resonance imaging (MRI)* is a useful alternative. Magnetic resonance cholangiography can be of value in differentiating biliary tract lesions. CT scan or MRI may be more accurate than US in detecting focal lesions such as tumors, cysts, and abscesses. When enhanced by contrast medium, CT scanning may reveal a neoplastic mass density only slightly different from that of a normal liver. When a hepatic tumor is suspected, CT scanning is the best method to define anatomic extent, solid or cystic nature, and vascularity. CT scanning can also reveal subtle differences in density of liver parenchyma, the average liver attenuation coefficient being reduced with fatty infiltration. Increases in density may occur with diffuse iron deposition or with glycogen storage. In differentiating obstructive from nonobstructive cholestasis, CT scanning or MRI identifies the precise level of obstruction more frequently than US. Either CT scanning or US may be used to guide percutaneously placed fine needles for biopsies, aspiration of specific lesions, or cholangiography.

Radionuclide scanning relies on selective uptake of a radiopharmaceutical agent. Commonly used agents include (1) technetium 99m-labeled sulfur colloid, which undergoes phagocytosis by Kupffer cells; (2) ^{99m}Tc-iminodiacetic acid agents, which are taken up by hepatocytes and excreted into bile in a fashion similar to bilirubin; and (3) gallium 67, which is concentrated in inflammatory and neoplastic cells. The anatomic resolution possible with hepatic scintiscans is generally less than that obtained with CT scanning, MRI, or US.

The ^{99m}Tc-sulfur colloid scan may detect focal lesions (tumors, cysts, or abscesses) greater than 2–3 cm in diameter. This modality may help to evaluate patients with possible cirrhosis and with patchy hepatic uptake and a shift of colloid uptake from liver to bone marrow.

The ^{99m}Tc-substituted iminodiacetic acid dyes may differentiate intrahepatic cholestasis from extrahepatic obstruction in neonates. Imaging results are best when scanning is preceded by a 5–7-day period of treatment with phenobarbital to stimulate bile flow. After intravenous injection, the isotope is normally detected in the bowel within 1–2 hr. In the presence of extrahepatic obstruction, excretion of the isotope is delayed; accordingly, serial scans should be made for up to 24 hr after injection. Early in the course of biliary atresia, hepatocyte function is usually good; uptake (clearance) occurs rapidly, but excretion into the intestine is absent. In contrast, uptake is poor in parenchymal liver disease, such as neonatal hepatitis, but excretion into the bile and intestine eventually ensues.

Cholangiography, direct visualization of the intrahepatic and extrahepatic biliary tree after injection of opaque material, may be required in some patients to evaluate the cause, location, or extent of biliary obstruction. Percutaneous transhepatic cholangiography with a fine needle is the technique of choice in infants and young children. The likelihood of opacifying the biliary tract is excellent in patients in whom CT scanning, MRI, or ultrasonography has shown dilated ducts. Percutaneous transhepatic cholangiography has been used to outline the biliary ductal system.

Endoscopic retrograde cholangiopancreatography (ERCP) is an alternative method of examining the bile ducts in older children. The papilla of Vater is cannulated under direct vision through a fiberoptic endoscope, and contrast material is injected into the biliary and pancreatic ducts to outline the anatomy.

Selective angiography of the celiac, superior mesenteric, or hepatic artery may be used to visualize the hepatic or portal circulation. Both arterial and venous circulatory systems of the liver can be examined. Angiography is frequently required to define the blood supply of tumors before surgery and is useful in the study of patients with known or presumed portal hypertension. The patency of the portal system, the extent of collateral circulation, and the caliber of vessels under consideration for a shunting procedure can be evaluated. MRI can provide similar information.

Balistreri WF: Pediatric hepatology. A half-century of progress. *Clin Liver Dis* 2000;4:191–210.

Balistreri WF: Bile acid therapy in pediatric hepatobiliary disease: The role of ursodeoxycholic acid. *J Pediatr Gastroenterol Nutr* 1997;24:573–89.

Batres LA, Maller ES: Laboratory assessment of liver function and injury in children: In Suchy FS, Sokol RJ, Balistreri WF (editors): *Liver Disease in Children,* 2nd ed. Philadelphia, Lippincott, Williams & Wilkins, 2001, pp 155–170.

Bezerra JA, Balistreri WF: Cholestatic syndromes of infancy and childhood. *Semin Gastrointest Dis* 2001;12:54–65.

Feranchak AP, Ramirez RO, Sokol RJ: Medical and nutritional management of cholestasis: In Suchy FS, Sokol RJ, Balistreri WF (editors): *Liver Disease in Children,* 2nd ed. Philadelphia, Lippincott, Williams & Wilkins, 2001, pp 195–238.

Garcia-Tsao G: Current management of the complications of cirrhosis and portal hypertension: Variceal hemorrhage, ascites and spontaneous bacterial peritonitis. *Gastroenterology* 2001;120:726–48.

Ryckman FC, Alonso MH: Causes and management of portal hypertension in the pediatric population. *Clin Liver Dis* 2001;5:789–818.

Ryckman FC, Alonso MH, Bucuvalas JC, Balistreri WF: Liver transplantation in children: In Suchy FS, Sokol RJ, Balistreri WF (editors): *Liver Disease in Children,* 2nd ed. Philadelphia, Lippincott, Williams & Wilkins, 2001, pp 949–974.

Squires RH: End-stage liver disease in children. *Curr Treat Options Gastroenterol* 2001;4:409–21.

Trauner M, Meier PJ, Boyer JL: Molecular pathogenesis of cholestasis. *N Engl J Med* 1998;339:1217.

Chapter 337

Cholestasis

Hassan H. A-Kader and William F. Balistreri

337.1 Neonatal Cholestasis

Neonatal cholestasis is defined as prolonged elevation of serum levels of conjugated bilirubin beyond the first 14 days of life. Jaundice that appears after 2 wk of age, progresses after this time, or does not resolve at this time should be evaluated and a direct bilirubin level determined. Cholestasis in a newborn may be due to infectious, genetic, metabolic, or undefined abnormalities giving rise either to mechanical obstruction of bile flow or to functional impairment of hepatic excretory function and bile secretion (see Box 336–3). An example of the former is stricture or obstruction of the common bile duct; biliary atresia is the prototypic obstructive abnormality. Functional impairment of bile secretion may result from congenital defects or damage to liver cells or to the biliary secretory apparatus. Neonatal cholestasis may be divided into extrahepatic and intrahepatic disease (Fig. 337–1). The clinical features of any form of cholestasis are similar. In an affected neonate, the diagnosis of certain entities, such as galactosemia, sepsis, and hypothyroidism, is relatively simple. In most cases, however, the cause of cholestasis is more obscure. Differentiation among *biliary atresia,* idiopathic *neonatal hepatitis,* and *intrahepatic cholestasis* is particularly difficult.

MECHANISMS. The two most likely pathogenetic mechanisms are virus-induced liver injury or metabolic liver disease.

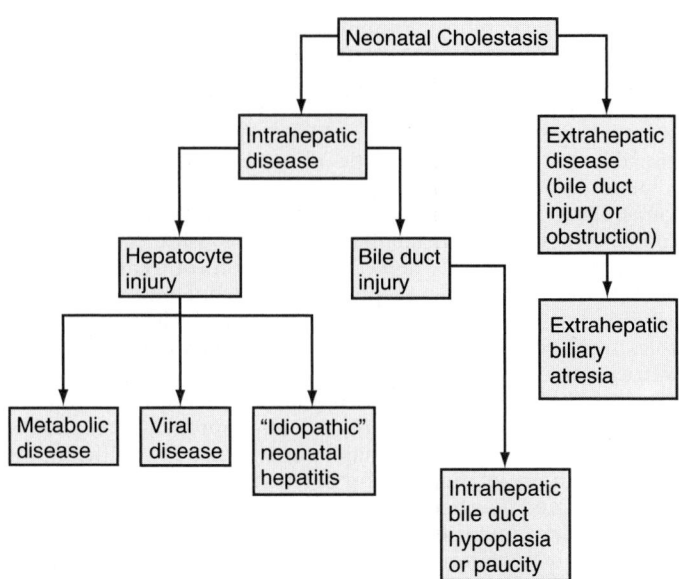

FIGURE 337–1. Neonatal cholestasis. Conceptual approach to the group of diseases presenting as cholestasis in the neonate. There are areas of overlap—patients with extrahepatic biliary atresia may have some degree of intrahepatic injury. Patients with "idiopathic" neonatal hepatitis may in the future be determined to have a primary metabolic or viral disease.

Metabolic liver disease caused by inborn errors of bile acid metabolism is associated with accumulation of toxic primitive bile acids and failure to produce normal choleretic and trophic bile acids. The clinical and histologic manifestations are nonspecific and are similar to those in other forms of neonatal hepatobiliary injury. It is also possible that autoimmune mechanisms may be responsible for some of the enigmatic forms of neonatal liver injury. Overall, the mechanisms are not well documented. Some of the histologic manifestations of hepatic injury in early life are not common in older individuals. Giant cell transformation of hepatocytes occurs frequently in infants with cholestasis and may occur in any form of neonatal liver injury. It is more frequent and more severe, however, in intrahepatic forms of cholestasis (neonatal hepatitis or intrahepatic bile duct paucity). The clinical and histologic findings thought to exist in patients with neonatal hepatitis and in those with biliary atresia have suggested that these diseases are manifestations of a single basic process, with an undefined initiating insult causing inflammation of the liver cells or of the cells within the biliary tract. If bile duct epithelium is the predominant site of disease, cholangitis may result and lead to progressive sclerosis and narrowing of the biliary tree, the ultimate state being complete obliteration *(biliary atresia).* Injury to liver cells may present the clinical and histologic picture of *neonatal hepatitis.* This concept does not account for all phenomena but offers an explanation for well-documented cases of unexpected postnatal evolution of these disease processes; infants initially regarded as having neonatal hepatitis, with a patent biliary system shown on cholangiography, have later been found to have biliary atresia.

Functional abnormalities in the generation of bile flow may also have a role in neonatal cholestasis. Bile flow is directly dependent on effective hepatic bile acid excretion. During the phase of relatively inefficient liver cell transport and metabolism of bile acids in early life, minor degrees of hepatic injury may further decrease bile flow and lead to production of abnormal toxic bile acids. Selective impairment of a single step in the series of events involved in hepatic excretion may produce the full expression of a cholestatic syndrome. A small number of cholestatic syndromes have a familial pattern. Byler disease (progressive familial intrahepatic cholestasis [PFIC]) and benign recurrent cholestasis are presumably related to impaired membrane transport of bile acids. Specific defects in bile acid synthesis have been found in infants with intrahepatic cholestasis and in infants with Zellweger syndrome. Severe forms of familial cholestasis have been associated with neonatal hemochromatosis and an aberration in the contractile proteins that compose the cytoskeleton of the hepatocyte. Sepsis is known to cause cholestasis, presumably mediated by an endotoxin produced by *Escherichia coli*.

EVALUATION. The evaluation of the infant with jaundice should follow a logical, cost-effective sequence in a multistep process (Table 337–1). Although cholestasis in the neonate may be the initial manifestation of numerous disorders, the clinical manifestations are usually similar and provide very few clues about etiology. Affected infants have icterus, dark urine, light or acholic stools, and hepatomegaly, all resulting from decreased bile flow due to either hepatocyte injury or bile duct obstruction. Hepatic synthetic dysfunction may lead to hypoprothrombinemia and a bleeding disorder. Therefore, administration of vitamin K should be the initial treatment of cholestatic infants to prevent hemorrhage.

In contrast to unconjugated hyperbilirubinemia, which may be physiologic, cholestasis in the neonate is always pathologic and prompt differentiation is imperative. The initial step in identification of cholestasis is the finding that more than 20% of the hyperbilirubinemia is conjugated bilirubin. The next step is to recognize conditions that cause cholestasis and for which specific therapy is available to prevent further damage and avoid long-term complications such as *sepsis*, an *endocrinopathy* (hypothyroidism or panhypopituitarism), *nutritional hepatotoxicity* caused by a specific metabolic illness (galactosemia), or other *metabolic diseases* (tyrosinemia).

Hepatobiliary disease may be the initial manifestation of homozygous α_1-antitrypsin deficiency or of cystic fibrosis. Neonatal liver disease may also be associated with congenital syphilis and specific viral infections notably echo virus and herpesviruses including cytomegalovirus (CMV). The hepatitis viruses (A, B, C) rarely cause neonatal cholestasis.

The final step in evaluating neonates with cholestasis is to differentiate extrahepatic biliary atresia from neonatal hepatitis.

Neonatal Hepatitis Syndrome (Intrahepatic Cholestasis). The term *neonatal hepatitis* implies intrahepatic cholestasis (see Fig. 337–1), which has various forms:

Idiopathic neonatal hepatitis, which can occur in either a sporadic or a familial form, is a disease of unknown cause. These patients presumably are afflicted with a specific yet undefined metabolic or viral disease. In the past, patients with α_1-antitrypsin deficiency were included in this category; after char-

acterization of this specific metabolic disease, it is possible to define this subgroup of patients precisely.

Infectious hepatitis in a neonate may be shown to be due to a specific virus, such as herpes simplex, enteroviruses, CMV, or, rarely, hepatitis B. This accounts for a small percentage of cases of neonatal hepatitis syndrome.

Cases of **intrahepatic cholestasis,** a heterogeneous subset of cholestatic diseases due to congenital defects in hepatic excretory function that may present as neonatal cholestasis.

Intrahepatic Bile Duct Paucity. Some syndromes characterized morphologically by intrahepatic cholestasis may be clinically manifested either as neonatal hepatitis or as cholestasis in an older child. As patients mature, clinical and histologic features may suggest a specific syndrome. Certain cases are associated with bile duct "paucity" (often erroneously called intrahepatic biliary atresia), which designates an absence or marked reduction in the number of interlobular bile ducts in the portal triads, with normal-sized branches of portal vein and hepatic arteriole. This unusual histologic feature may represent either congenital bile duct absence, partial failure of bile duct development, progressive bile duct atrophy, or disappearance of the bile ducts due to segmental destructive processes. Biopsy in early life often reveals an inflammatory process involving the bile ducts; subsequent biopsy specimens then show subsidence of the inflammation with residual reduction in the number and diameter of bile ducts, analogous to the "disappearing bile duct syndrome" noted in adults with immune-mediated disorders.

Observations suggest that it is possible to identify distinctive syndromes of isolated intrahepatic bile duct paucity and an intact extrahepatic biliary tree.

Alagille syndrome (arteriohepatic dysplasia) is the most common syndrome incorporating intrahepatic bile duct paucity. Serial assessment of hepatic histology often suggests progressive destruction of bile ducts. Clinical manifestations of Alagille syndrome are expressed in various degrees and may be nonspecific; they include unusual *facial characteristics* (broad forehead; deep-set, widely spaced eyes; long, straight nose; and an underdeveloped mandible). There may also be *ocular* abnormalities (posterior embryotoxon), *cardiovascular* abnormalities (usually peripheral pulmonic stenosis, sometimes tetralogy of Fallot), *vertebral* arch defects and failure of anterior vertebral arch fusion (butterfly vertebrae), and tubulointerstitial *nephropathy*. Other findings such as growth retardation and defective spermatogenesis may reflect nutritional deficiency. The prognosis for prolonged survival is good, but patients are likely to have pruritus, xanthomas with markedly elevated serum cholesterol levels, and neurologic complications of vitamin E deficiency if untreated. Mutations in human Jagged 1 gene *(JAG1)*, which encodes a ligand for the notch receptor, are linked to Alagille syndrome.

TABLE 337–1. Value of Specific Tests in the Evaluation of Patients with Suspected Neonatal Cholestasis

Test	Rationale
Serum bilirubin fractionation	Documents cholestasis
Assessment of stool color	Indicates bile flow into intestine
Urine/serum bile acids measurement	Confirms cholestasis; may indicate inborn error of bile acid biosynthesis
Hepatic synthetic function (albumin, coagulation profile)	Indicates severity of hepatic dysfunction
α_1-antitrypsin phenotype	Suggests (or excludes) PiZZ
Thyroxine and TSH	Suggests (or excludes) endocrinopathy
Sweat chloride/mutation analysis	Suggests (or excludes) cystic fibrosis
Urine/serum amino acids and urine reducing substances	Suggests (or excludes) metabolic liver disease
Ultrasonography	Suggests (or excludes) choledochal cyst; may detect the triangular cord (TC) sign suggesting biliary atresia
Hepatobiliary scintigraphy	Documents bile duct patency or obstruction
Liver biopsy	Distinguishes biliary atresia from neonatal hepatitis; suggests alternative diagnosis

Modified from Balistreri WF, Schubert WK: Liver disease in infancy and childhood. In Schiff L, Schiff ER (editors): Diseases of the Liver, *8th ed. Philadelphia, Lippincott, 1999.*

There are several forms of intrahepatic cholestasis due to defects in specific transport proteins involved in bile formation (Table 337–2). **Byler disease,** a severe form of *progressive intrahepatic cholestasis* (PFIC type 1), was initially described in the Amish kindred of Jacob Byler. The disease is characterized by unique structural abnormalities in the bile canicular membrane. Affected patients present with failure to thrive, steatorrhea, pruritus, rickets, and low γ-glutamyl transpeptidase levels. Cirrhosis gradually develops. The major clinical differentiation from Alagille syndrome is the absence of bile duct paucity and extrahepatic features.

PFIC type 1 (Byler disease) is mapped to chromosome 18q12. Affected patients have low serum levels of γ-glutamyltransferase, normal serum cholesterol, and high serum bile acid levels. A mutation in P-type membrane adenosine triphosphatase is the responsible mechanism in Amish families.

PFIC type 2 is similar to Byler disease but is present in non-Amish families (Middle Eastern Europeans) and has a gene locus at chromosome 2q24. Mutations of BSEP gene, which codes for a bile canicular adenosine triphosphate-dependent bile acid transporter, may be responsible.

PFIC type 3 is characterized by high serum levels of α-glutamyl-transferase and histologically by portal bile duct inflammation and proliferation. There is complete absence of the multidrug resistance 3 P glycoprotein, with deficient translocation of phosphatidylcholine across the canicular membrane. Mothers who are heterozygous for this gene are at risk for intrahepatic cholestasis of pregnancy.

Aagenaes syndrome is a form of idiopathic familial intrahepatic cholestasis associated with lymphedema of the lower extremities. The relation between the liver disease and lymphedema is not understood and may be attributable to decreased hepatic lymph flow or hepatic lymphatic hypoplasia. Affected patients usually present with episodic cholestasis with elevation of serum aminotransferases, alkaline phosphatase, and bile acids. Between the episodes the patients are usually asymptomatic and the biochemical indices improve. The locus for Aagenaes syndrome has been mapped to a 6.6-cM interval on chromosome 15q.

Zellweger (cerebrohepatorenal) syndrome is a rare autosomal recessive genetic disorder marked by progressive degeneration of the liver and kidneys (Chapter 75.2). The incidence is estimated to be 1/100,000 births; the disease is usually fatal within 6–12 mo. Affected infants have severe, generalized hypotonia and markedly impaired neurologic function with psychomotor retardation. Patients have an abnormal head shape and unusual facies, hepatomegaly, renal cortical cysts, stippled calcifications of the patellas and greater trochanter, and ocular abnormalities. Hepatic cells on ultrastructural examination show an absence of peroxisomes.

Neonatal iron storage disease (NISD) is a rapidly progressive disease characterized by increased iron deposition in the liver, heart, and endocrine organs without increased iron stores in the reticuloendothelial system. Patients have multiorgan failure and shortened survival. Familial cases have been reported and the disease is most likely transmitted in an autosomal recessive or codominant pattern. Laboratory findings include hypoglycemia, hyperbilirubinemia, hypoalbuminemia and profound hypoprothrombinemia. Serum aminotransferases may be high initially but normalize with the progression of the disease. The diagnosis is usually confirmed by buccal mucosal biopsy or magnetic resonance imaging demonstrating extrahepatic siderosis. The prognosis is poor; liver transplantation can be curative. Despite initially encouraging reports, the use of a combination of antioxidants and prostaglandin infusion with chelation may not uniformly improve outcome in the patients with NISD.

Defective bile acid biosynthesis has been postulated to be an initiating or perpetuating factor in neonatal cholestatic disorders; the hypothesis is that inborn errors in bile acid biosynthesis lead to absence of normal trophic or choleretic primary bile acids and accumulation of primitive (hepatotoxic) metabolites. **Inborn errors of bile acid biosynthesis** is a recognizable cause of acute and chronic liver disease; early recognition allows institution of targeted bile acid replacement, which reverses the hepatic injury. Several specific defects have been described:

Deficiency of Δ^4-3-oxosteroid-5β reductase, the fourth step in the pathway of cholesterol degradation to the primary bile acids is manifested as significant cholestasis and liver failure

---

TABLE 337–2. **Genetic Forms of Intrahepatic Cholestasis or Hyperbilirubinaemia**

Disease	Chromosome	Gene	Defect	Phenotype
PFIC type 1	18q21	*FIC1*, P type ATPase with homology to a putative aminophospholipid translocator	Pathogenetic mechanism unknown	First recurrent, later permanent and progressive cholestasis, no bile duct proliferation, normal gamma-GT, extrahepatic manifestations in some patients
BRIC	18q21	*FIC1*	Unknown but most likely a regulatory defect of bile salt secretion	Recurrent attacks of severe cholestasis, pruritus, jaundice, steatorrhea, and weight loss. Normal liver function in intervals between the attacks
PFIC type 2	2q24	*BSEP*, bile salt export pump	Deficient canalicular bile salt transport	Progressive cholestasis, no bile duct proliferation, giant cell transformation, lobular and portal fibrosis, normal gamma-GT
PFIC type 3	7q21	*PGY3*	Deficient canalicular phosphatidylcholine transport	Cholestasis, jaundice less prominent, extensive bile duct proliferation and periportal fibrosis, elevated gamma-GT
ICP	e.g., 7q21 heterozygosity	e.g., *PGY3*	May be associated with, e.g., PFIC type 3 but is also associated with other PFIC types	Cholestasis in third trimester of pregnancy, therapeutic effect of ursodeoxycholic acid, associated with increased fetal loss and prematurity
Bile acid synthesis defects	e.g., 8q2.3	e.g., *CYP7B1*	Bile acid synthesis enzyme defects with accumulation of toxic intermediates and deficiency of normal bile acids	Cholestasis since birth, failure to thrive, low to normal gamma-GT
Dubin-Johnson syndrome	10q24	*MRP2/cMOAT*, canalicular multispecific organic anion transporter	Deficient canalicular organic anion transport, including that of bilirubin conjugates	Conjugated hyperbilirubinaemia, increased urinary coproporphyrin isomer I, hepatic lysosomal pigment, normal life span

PFIC = progressive familial intrahepatic cholestasis; BRIC = benign recurrent intrahepatic cholestasis; ICP = intrahepatic cholestasis of pregnancy; PGY = P-glycoprotein; CYP = cytochrome P-450; gamma-GT = gamma-glutamyltransferase.
Not mentioned in the table is Aagenaes syndrome (intrahepatic cholestasis with lymphedema) because the gene defect underlying this disease is unknown.
From Jansen PLM, Muller M: The molecular genetics of familial intrahepatic cholestasis. Gut 2000; 47: 1–5.

developing shortly after birth with coagulopathy and metabolic liver injury resembling tyrosinemia. Hepatic histology is characterized by lobular disarray with giant cells, pseudoacinar transformation, and canalicular bile stasis. Mass spectrometry is required to document increased urinary bile acid excretion and the predominance of oxo-hydroxy and oxo-dihydroxy cholenoic acids. Treatment with cholic acid and ursodeoxycholic acid is associated with normalization of biochemical, histologic, and clinical features.

Deficiency of **3β-hydroxy C_{27}-steroid dehydrogenase (3-HSD) isomerase,** the second step in bile acid biosynthesis, causes **progressive familial intrahepatic cholestasis**. Affected patients usually have jaundice with increased aminotransferase levels and hepatomegaly; γ-glutamyl transpeptidase levels and serum cholylglycine levels are normal. The histology is variable, ranging from giant cell hepatitis to chronic hepatitis. The diagnosis, suggested by mass spectrometry detection of C^{24} bile acids in urine, which retain the 3β-hydroxy-Δ^5 structure, can be confirmed by determination of 3-HSD activity in cultured fibroblasts using 7α-hydroxy-Δ^5 cholesterol as a substrate. Primary bile acid therapy, administered orally to downregulate cholesterol 7α-hydroxylase activity, limit the production of 3β-hydroxy-Δ^5 bile acids, and facilitate hepatic clearance, has been effective in reversing hepatic injury.

Another metabolic defect in bile acid synthesis involves a deficiency in 7α-hydroxylation due to a mutation in the gene for the microsomal **oxysterol 7α-hydroxylase** enzyme, active in the acidic pathway for bile acid synthesis. The defect presents with severe cholestasis, cirrhosis, and liver synthetic failure. Diagnosis is established by fast atom bombardment ionization–mass spectrometry, which reveals elevated urinary excretion of sulfate and glycosulfate conjugates of unsaturated monohydroxy-cholenoic acids, and an absence of primary bile acids. The biochemical findings are consistent with a deficiency in 7α-hydroxylation, leading to the accumulation of hepatotoxic unsaturated monohydroxy bile acids.

BILIARY ATRESIA

The term *biliary atresia* is imprecise because the anatomy of abnormal bile ducts in affected patients varies markedly. A more appropriate terminology would reflect the pathophysiology—namely, *progressive obliterative cholangiopathy*. Patients may have distal segmental bile duct obliteration with patent extrahepatic ducts up to the porta hepatis. This is a surgically correctable lesion, but it is uncommon. However, the most common form of biliary atresia, accounting for approximately 85% of the cases, is obliteration of the entire extrahepatic biliary tree at or above the porta hepatis. This presents a much more difficult problem in surgical management.

Incidence. Biliary atresia has been detected in 1/10,000–15,000 live births, idiopathic neonatal hepatitis in 1/5,000–10,000. Intrahepatic bile duct paucity appears much less commonly, in about 1/50,000–75,000 live births.

Differentiation of Idiopathic Neonatal Hepatitis from Biliary Atresia. It may be difficult to clearly differentiate infants with biliary atresia, who require surgical correction, from those with intrahepatic disease (neonatal hepatitis) and patent bile ducts. No single biochemical test or imaging procedure is entirely satisfactory. Diagnostic schemas incorporate clinical, historical, biochemical, and radiologic features.

Idiopathic neonatal hepatitis has a familial incidence of approximately 20%, whereas biliary atresia is unlikely to recur within the same family. A few infants with biliary atresia have an increased incidence of other abnormalities, such as the polysplenia syndrome with abdominal heterotaxia, malrotation, levocardia, and intra-abdominal vascular anomalies. Neonatal hepatitis appears to be more common in premature or small for gestational age infants. Persistently acholic stools suggest biliary obstruction (biliary atresia), but patients with severe idiopathic neonatal hepatitis may have a transient severe impairment of bile excretion. Consistently pigmented stools rule against biliary atresia. The finding of bile-stained fluid on duodenal intubation also excludes biliary atresia. Palpation of the liver may find an abnormal size or consistency in patients with extrahepatic biliary atresia; this is less common with neonatal hepatitis.

Abdominal ultrasound is a helpful diagnostic tool in the evaluation of neonatal cholestasis because it will identify choledocholithiasis, perforation of the bile duct, or other structural abnormalities of the biliary tree such as a choledochal cyst. In patients with biliary atresia, ultrasound may detect associated anomalies such as abdominal polysplenia and vascular malformations. The gallbladder is either not visualized or a micro-gallbladder is seen in patients with biliary atresia. Children with intrahepatic cholestasis caused by idiopathic neonatal hepatitis, cystic fibrosis, or total parenteral nutrition may have similar ultrasonographic findings. Ultrasonographic *triangular cord (TC) sign*, which represents a cone-shaped fibrotic mass cranial to the bifurcation of the portal vein, may be seen in patients with biliary atresia. The echogenic density, which represents the fibrous remnants at the porta hepatis of biliary atresia cases at surgery, may be a helpful diagnostic tool in the evaluation of patients with neonatal cholestasis.

Hepatobiliary scintigraphy with technetium-labeled iminodiacetic acid derivatives is used to differentiate biliary atresia from nonobstructive causes of cholestasis. The hepatic uptake of the agent is normal in patients with biliary atresia but excretion into the intestine is absent. Although the uptake may be impaired in neonatal hepatitis, excretion into the bowel will eventually occur. Obtaining a follow-up scan after 24 hr is of value to determine the patency of the biliary tree. The administration of phenobarbital (5 mg/kg/day) for 5 days before the scan is recommended because it may enhance biliary excretion of the isotope. Hepatobiliary scintigraphy is a sensitive but not specific test for biliary atresia. It fails to identify other structural abnormalities of the biliary tree or vascular anomalies. The lack of the specificity of the test and the need to wait for 5 days makes this procedure less practical and of limited usefulness in the evaluation of children suspected to have biliary atresia.

Percutaneous liver biopsy is a valuable procedure in the evaluation of neonatal hepatobiliary diseases and provides the most reliable discriminatory evidence. Biliary atresia is characterized by bile ductular proliferation, the presence of bile plugs, and portal or perilobular edema and fibrosis, with the basic hepatic lobular architecture intact. In neonatal hepatitis, there is severe, diffuse hepatocellular disease, with distortion of lobular architecture, marked infiltration with inflammatory cells, and focal hepatocellular necrosis; the bile ductules show little alteration. Giant cell transformation is found in infants with either condition and has no diagnostic specificity.

The histologic changes seen in patients with idiopathic neonatal hepatitis may also occur in various diseases, including α_1-antitrypsin deficiency, galactosemia, and, various forms of intrahepatic cholestasis. Although paucity of intrahepatic bile ductules may be detected on liver biopsy even within the first few weeks of life, later biopsies in such patients reveal a more characteristic pattern.

Management of Patients with Suspected Biliary Atresia. All patients suspected of having biliary atresia should undergo exploratory laparotomy and direct cholangiography to determine the presence and site of obstruction. Direct drainage can be accomplished in patients with correctable lesion. When no correctable lesion is found, an examination of frozen sections obtained from the transected porta hepatis can detect the presence of biliary epithelium and determine the size and patency of the residual bile ducts. In some cases, the cholangiogram indicates that the biliary tree is patent but of diminished caliber, suggesting that the cholestasis is not due to biliary tract obliteration but to bile duct paucity or markedly diminished flow in the presence of intrahepatic disease. In these cases, transection of or further dissection into the porta hepatis should be *avoided*.

For patients in whom no correctable lesion is found, the hepatoportoenterostomy procedure of Kasai can be carried out. The rationale for this operation is that minute bile duct remnants, representing residual channels, may be present in the fibrous tissue of the porta hepatis; such channels may be in direct continuity with the intrahepatic ductule system. In such cases, transection of the porta hepatis with anastomosis of bowel mucosa to the proximal surface of the transection may allow bile drainage. If flow is not rapidly established within the first months of life, progressive obliteration and cirrhosis ensue. If microscopic channels of patency greater than 150 μm in diameter are found, postoperative establishment of bile flow is likely. The success rate for establishing good bile flow following the Kasai operation is much higher (90%) if performed before 8 wk of life. Therefore, the importance of early referral and prompt evaluation of infants with suspected biliary atresia is emphasized.

Some patients with biliary atresia, even of the "non-correctable" type, derive long-term benefits from interventions such as the Kasai procedure. In most, however, a degree of hepatic dysfunction persists. Patients with biliary atresia usually have persistent inflammation of the intrahepatic biliary tree, which suggests that biliary atresia reflects a dynamic process involving the entire hepatobiliary system. This may account for the ultimate development of complications such as portal hypertension. The short-term benefit of hepatoportoenterostomy is decompression and drainage sufficient to forestall the onset of cirrhosis and sustain growth until a successful liver transplantation can be done (Chapter 349).

MANAGEMENT OF CHRONIC CHOLESTASIS

With any form of neonatal cholestasis, whether the primary disease is idiopathic neonatal hepatitis, intrahepatic bile duct paucity, or biliary atresia, affected patients are at increased risk for chronic complications. These reflect various degrees of residual hepatic functional capacity and are due directly or indirectly to diminished bile flow:

1. Any substance normally excreted into bile is retained in the liver, with subsequent accumulation in tissue and in serum. Involved substances include bile acids, bilirubin, cholesterol, and trace elements.

2. Decreased delivery of bile acids to the proximal intestine leads to inadequate digestion and absorption of dietary long-chain triglycerides and fat-soluble vitamins.

3. Impairment of hepatic metabolic function may alter hormonal balance and utilization of nutrients.

4. Progressive liver damage may lead to biliary cirrhosis, portal hypertension, and liver failure.

Treatment of such patients (Table 337–3) is empirical, and is guided by careful monitoring. No therapy is known to be effective in halting the progression of cholestasis or in preventing further hepatocellular damage and cirrhosis.

Growth failure is a major concern and is related in part to malabsorption and malnutrition resulting from ineffective digestion and absorption of dietary fat. Use of a medium-chain triglyceride–containing formula may improve caloric balance.

With chronic cholestasis and prolonged survival, children with hepatobiliary disease may experience deficiencies of the fat-soluble vitamins (A, D, E, and K). Inadequate absorption of fat and fat-soluble vitamins may be exacerbated by administration of the bile acid binder cholestyramine. Metabolic bone disease is common.

Serum vitamin A concentration can usually be maintained at normal levels in patients who have chronic cholestasis and who received oral supplementation of vitamin A esters. It is essential to monitor the vitamin A status in such patients.

A degenerative neuromuscular syndrome is found with chronic cholestasis caused by malabsorption and vitamin E deficiency; affected children experience progressive areflexia, cerebellar ataxia, ophthalmoplegia, and decreased vibratory sensation. Specific morphologic lesions have been found in the central nervous system, peripheral nerves, and muscles. These lesions are potentially reversible in young children (<3–4 yr old). Affected children have low serum vitamin E concentrations, increased hydrogen peroxide hemolysis, and low ratios of serum vitamin E to total serum lipids (<0.6 mg/g for children younger than 12 yr and <0.8 mg/g for older patients). Vitamin E deficiency may be prevented by oral administration of large doses (up to 1,000 IU/day); patients unable to absorb sufficient quantities may require administration of D-tocopherol polyethylene glycol-1000 succinate orally. Serum levels may be monitored as a guide to efficacy.

Pruritus is a particularly troublesome complication of chronic cholestasis, often with the appearance of xanthomas. Both features seem to be related to the accumulation of cholesterol and bile acids in serum and in tissues. Elimination of these retained compounds is difficult when bile ducts are obstructed, but if there is any degree of bile duct patency, administration of ursodeoxycholic acid may increase bile flow or interrupt the enterohepatic circulation of bile acids and thus decrease the xanthomas and ameliorate the pruritus (see Table 337–3). Ursodeoxycholic acid therapy may also lower serum cholesterol levels. The recommended dose is 15 mg/kg/24 hr.

Progressive fibrosis and cirrhosis will lead to the development of portal hypertension and consequently to ascites and variceal hemorrhage. The presence of ascites is a risk factor for the development of spontaneous bacterial peritonitis (SBP). The first step in the management of patients with ascites is to rule out SBP and restrict sodium intake to 0.5 g (~1–2 mEq/kg/24 hr). There is no need for fluid restriction in patients with adequate renal output. Should this be ineffective, diuretics may be helpful. The

TABLE 337–3. Suggested Medical Management of Persistent Cholestasis

Clinical Impairment	Management
Malnutrition resulting from malabsorption of dietary long-chain triglycerides	Replace with dietary formula or supplements containing medium-chain triglycerides
Fat-soluble vitamin malabsorption:	
Vitamin A deficiency (night blindness, thick skin)	Replace with 10,000–15,000 IU/day as Aquasol A
Vitamin E deficiency (neuromuscular degeneration)	Replace with 50–400 IU/day as oral α-tocopherol or TPGS
Vitamin D deficiency (metabolic bone disease)	Replace with 5,000–8,000 IU/day of D_2 or 3–5 μg/kg/day of 25-hydroxycholecalciferol
Vitamin K deficiency (hypoprothrombinemia)	Replace with 2.5–5.0 mg every other day as water-soluble derivative of menadione
Micronutrient deficiency	Calcium, phosphate, or zinc supplementation
Deficiency of water-soluble vitamins	Supplement with twice the recommended daily allowance
Retention of biliary constituents such as cholesterol (itch or xanthomas)	Administer choleretic bile acids and ursodeoxycholic acid, 15–20 mg/kg/day
Progressive liver disease; portal hypertension (variceal bleeding, ascites, hypersplenism)	Interim management (control bleeding; salt restriction; spironolactone)
End-stage liver disease (liver failure)	Transplantation

TPGS = D-tocopherol polyethylene glycol-1000 succinate.

diuretic of choice is spironolactone (3–5 mg/kg/24 hr in four doses). If spironolactone alone does not control ascites, the addition of another diuretic such as thiazide or furosemide may be beneficial. Patients with ascites but without peripheral edema are at risk for reduced plasma volume and decreased urine output during diuretic therapy. Tense ascites alters renal blood flow and systemic hemodynamics. Paracentesis and intravenous albumin infusion may improve hemodynamics, renal perfusion, and symptoms. Follow-up includes dietary counseling and monitoring of serum and urinary electrolyte concentrations (Chapters 345 and 348).

In patients with portal hypertension, variceal hemorrhage and the development of hypersplenism are common. It is important to ascertain the cause of bleeding because episodes of gastrointestinal hemorrhage in patients who have chronic liver disease may be due to gastritis or peptic ulcer disease. Because the management of these various complications differs, differentiation perhaps via endoscopy is necessary before treatment is initiated (Chapter 348). If the patient is volume depleted, blood transfusion should be carefully administered avoiding overtransfusion, which may precipitate further bleeding. The use of balloon tamponade is not recommended in children because it may be associated with significant complications. On the other hand, sclerotherapy or endoscopic variceal ligation may be useful palliative measures in the management of bleeding varices and may be superior to surgical alternatives.

In patients with advanced liver disease, hepatic transplantation may have a success rate greater than 85% (Chapter 349). If the operation is technically feasible, it will prolong life and may correct the metabolic error in diseases such as α_1-antitrypsin deficiency, tyrosinemia, and Wilson disease. Success depends on adequate intraoperative, preoperative, and postoperative care and on cautious use of immunosuppressive agents. Scarcity of donors of small livers severely limits the application of liver transplantation for infants and children. The use of *reduced*-size transplants and living donors increases the ability to treat small children successfully.

PROGNOSIS

For patients with idiopathic neonatal hepatitis, the variable prognosis may reflect the heterogeneity of the disease. In **sporadic** cases, 60–70% recover with no evidence of hepatic structural or functional impairment. Approximately 5–10% have persistent fibrosis or inflammation, and a smaller percentage have more severe liver disease, such as cirrhosis. Death of infants usually occurs early in the course of the illness, owing to hemorrhage or sepsis. Of infants with idiopathic neonatal hepatitis of the **familial** variety, only 20–30% recover; 10–15% acquire chronic liver disease with cirrhosis. Liver transplantation may be required.

337.2 Cholestasis in the Older Child

Most cases of cholestasis with onset after the neonatal period are due to acute viral hepatitis or drug-induced. Many of the conditions causing neonatal cholestasis may also cause chronic cholestasis in older patients. Adolescents with conjugated hyperbilirubinemia should be evaluated for acute and chronic hepatitis, α_1-antitrypsin deficiency, Wilson disease, liver disease associated with inflammatory bowel disease, autoimmune hepatitis, and the syndromes of intrahepatic cholestasis (with or without bile duct paucity). Other causes include obstruction caused by cholelithiasis, abdominal tumors, enlarged lymph nodes, or hepatic inflammation resulting from drug ingestion. Management of cholestasis in the older child is similar to that proposed for neonatal cholestasis (see Table 337–3).

Aagenaes O: Hereditary recurrent cholestasis with lymphedema: Two new families. *Acta Pediatr Scand* 1974;63:465.

Alagille D, Estrada A, Hadchovel M, et al: Syndromic paucity of interlobular bile ducts (Alagille syndrome or arteriohepatic dysplasia): Review of 80 cases. *J Pediatr* 1987;110:195.

Arrese M, Ananthananarayanan M, Suchy FJ: Hepatobiliary transport: Mechanisms of development and cholestasis. *Pediatr Res* 1998;44:141.

Bull LN, van Eijk MJT, Pawlikowska L, et al: A gene encoding a P-type ATPase mutated in two forms of hereditary cholestasis. *Nat Genet* 1998;18:219.

Bull LN, Roche E, Song EJ, et al: Mapping of the locus for cholestasis-lymphedema syndrome (Aagenaes syndrome) to a 6.6-cM interval on chromosome 15q. *Am J Hum Genet* 2000;67:994–9.

Chardot C, Carton M, Spire-Bendelac N, et al: Is the Kasai operation still indicated in children older than 3 months diagnosed with biliary atresia? *J Pediatr* 2001;138:224–8.

Chen HL, Chang PS, Hsu HC, et al: Progressive familial intrahepatic cholestasis with high γ-glutamyltranspeptidase levels in Taiwanese infants: Role of MDR3 gene defect? *Pediatr Res* 2001;50:50–5.

Danks DM, Campbell PE, Smith AL, et al: Prognosis of babies with neonatal hepatitis. *Arch Dis Child* 1977;52:368.

Debray D, Pariente D, Gauthier F, et al: Cholelithiasis in infancy: A study of 40 cases. *J Pediatr* 1993;122:385.

Hoffenberg EJ, Narkewicz MR, Sondheimer JM, et al: Outcome of syndromic paucity of interlobular bile ducts (Alagille syndrome) with onset of cholestasis in infancy. *J Pediatr* 1995;127:220.

Jacquemin E, Hadchouel M: Genetic basis of progressive familial intrahepatic cholestasis. *J Hepatol* 1999;31:377–81.

Jansen PLM, Muller M: The molecular genetics of familial intrahepatic cholestasis. *Gut* 2000;47:1–5.

Kasai M, Mochizuki I, Ohkohchi N, et al: Surgical limitations for biliary atresia: Indications for liver transplantation. *J Pediatr Surg* 1989;24:851.

Kotb MA, Sheba M, El Koofy N, et al: Evaluation of the "Triangular Cord Sign" in the diagnosis of biliary atresia. *Pediatrics* 2001;108:416–20.

Miga D, Sokol RJ, MacKenzie T, et al: Survival after first esophageal variceal hemorrhage in patients with biliary atresia. *J Pediatr* 2001;139:291–6.

Milkiewicz P, Elias E: Obstetric cholestasis. *BMJ* 2002;324:123–4.

Mowat AP, Psacharopoulos HT, Williams R: Extrahepatic biliary atresia versus neonatal hepatitis: Review of 137 prospectively investigated infants. *Arch Dis Child* 1976;51:763.

Oda T, Elkahloun AG, Pike BL, et al: Mutations in the human *Jagged1* gene are responsible for Alagille syndrome. *Nat Genet* 1997;16:235.

Ryckman FC, Fisher RA, Pedersen SH, et al: Improved survival in biliary atresia patients in the present era of liver transplantation. *J Pediatr Surg* 1993;28:382.

Sokol RJ, Heubi JE, Butler-Simon N, et al: Treatment of vitamin E deficiency during chronic childhood cholestasis with oral D-tocopheryl polyethylene glycol-1000 succinate. *Gastroenterology* 1987;93:975.

Setchell KD, Schwarz M, O'Connell NC, et al: Identification of a new inborn error in bile acid synthesis: Mutation of the oxysterol 7alpha-hydroxylase gene causes severe neonatal liver disease. *J Clin Invest* 1998;102:1690–703.

Stringer MD, Dhawan A, Davenport M, et al: Choledochal cysts: Lessons from a 20 year experience. *Arch Dis Child* 1995;73:528.

Trauner M, Meier PJ, Boyer JL: Molecular pathogenesis of cholestasis. *N Engl J Med* 1998;339:1217.

Yoon PW, Bresee JS, Olney RS, et al: Epidemiology of biliary atresia: A population-based study. *Pediatrics* 1997;99:376.

Chapter 338

Metabolic Diseases of the Liver *Jeffrey A. Rudolph and*

William F. Balistreri

See also Chapters 73 and 91.3.

Because the liver has a central role in synthetic, degradative, and regulatory pathways involving carbohydrate, protein, lipid, trace element, and vitamin metabolism, many metabolic abnormalities or specific enzyme deficiencies affect the liver primarily or secondarily (Box 338–1). Liver disease may arise when absence of an enzyme produces a block in a metabolic pathway, when unmetabolized substrate accumulates proximal to a block, when deficiency of an essential substance produced distal to an aberrant chemical reaction develops, or when synthesis of an abnormal metabolite occurs. The spectrum of pathologic

BOX 338–1. Inborn Errors of Metabolism Manifested as Hepatobiliary Dysfunction

I. Disorders of Carbohydrate Metabolism
  A. Disorders of **galactose** metabolism
    1. Galactosemia *(76.2)**
  B. Disorders of **fructose** metabolism *(76.3)*
    1. Hereditary fructose intolerance (aldolase deficiency)
    2. Fructose-1,6 diphosphatase deficiency
  C. **Glycogen storage** diseases *(76.1)*
    1. Type I
      a. Von Gierke (Ia)
      b. Type Ib
    2. Type III (Cori/Forbes)
    3. Type IV (Andersen)
    4. Type VI (Hers)
  D. Disorders of carbohydrate glycosylation *(76.6)*
II. Disorders of Amino Acid and Protein Metabolism
  A. Disorders of **tyrosine** metabolism *(74.2)*
    1. Hereditary tyrosinemia (type I)
    2. Tyrosinemia, type II
  B. Inherited **urea cycle** enzyme defects *(74.11)*
    1. CPS deficiency
    2. OTC deficiency (X-linked dominant)
    3. Citrullinemia
    4. Argininosuccinic aciduria
    5. Argininemia
    6. N-AGS deficiency

III. Disorders of Lipid Metabolism *(75)*
  A. Wolman disease
  B. Cholesteryl ester storage disease
  C. Gaucher disease
  D. Niemann-Pick type C
IV. Disorders of Bile Acid Metabolism
  A. Isomerase deficiency
  B. Reductase deficiency
  C. Zellweger syndrome (cerebrohepatorenal)
V. Disorders of Metal Metabolism
  A. Wilson disease
  B. Hepatic copper overload
  C. Indian childhood cirrhosis
  D. Neonatal iron storage disease (perinatal hemochromatosis)
VI. Disorders of Bilirubin Metabolism
  A. Crigler-Najjar
    1. Type I
    2. Type II
  B. Gilbert disease
  C. Dubin-Johnson syndrome
  D. Rotor syndrome
VII. Miscellaneous
  A. α_1-Antitrypsin deficiency
  B. Cystic fibrosis
  C. Erythropoietic protoporphyria

CPS = Carbamoyl phosphate synthetase; OTC = ornithine transcarbamoylase; N-AGS = *N*-acetylglutamate synthetase.
*See chapters in parentheses.

changes includes (1) *hepatocyte injury,* with subsequent failure of other metabolic functions, often eventuating in cirrhosis, liver tumors, or both; (2) *storage* of lipid, glycogen, or other products manifested as hepatomegaly, often with complications specific to deranged metabolism (decreased blood glucose in patients with glycogen storage disease); and (3) absence of structural change despite profound metabolic effects, as with urea cycle defects. The clinical manifestations of metabolic diseases of the liver mimic infections, intoxications, and hematologic and immunologic diseases (Box 338–2). Further clues are provided by family history of a similar illness or by the observation that the onset of symptoms is closely associated with a change in dietary habits (initiation of ingestion of fructose). In most cases, clinical and laboratory evidence guide the evaluation. Liver biopsy offers morphologic study and permits enzyme assays, as well as quantitative and qualitative assays of various other constituents. Such studies require cooperation of experienced laboratories and careful attention to collection and handling of specimens.

BOX 338–2. Clinical Manifestations That Suggest the Possibility of Metabolic Disease

- Recurrent vomiting, failure to thrive, short stature, dysmorphic features
- Jaundice, hepatomegaly (± splenomegaly), fulminant hepatic failure
- Hypoglycemia, organic acidemia, lactic acidemia, hyperammonemia, bleeding (coagulopathy)
- Recurrent vomiting, failure to thrive, short stature, dysmorphic features
- Developmental delay/psychomotor retardation, hypotonia, progressive neuromuscular deterioration, seizures
- Cardiac dysfunction/failure, unusual odors, rickets, cataracts

338.1 Inherited Deficient Conjugation of Bilirubin (Familial Nonhemolytic Unconjugated Hyperbilirubinemia)

Hepatic glucuronyl transferase activity (Chapter 91.3) is deficient in two genetically and functionally distinct disorders (Crigler-Najjar syndromes, type I and II), producing congenital nonobstructive, nonhemolytic, unconjugated hyperbilirubinemia. The molecular mechanism of the various Crigler-Najjar syndromes is complex. This is partly because the activity of multiple glucuronyl transferase isoforms is deficient in various phenotypes of the Crigler-Najjar syndrome. Low enzyme levels with unconjugated hyperbilirubinemia also occur in **Gilbert syndrome,** a benign disorder, commonly caused by a polymorphism in the promoter region of the transferase gene.

Crigler-Najjar Syndrome (Type I Glucuronyl Transferase Deficiency). This form is inherited as an autosomal recessive trait and is due to mutations in the UDP(B)-GT gene. Parents of affected children have partial defects in conjugation as determined by hepatic enzyme assay or by measurement of glucuronide formation, but their serum bilirubin concentrations are normal.

CLINICAL MANIFESTATIONS. Severe unconjugated hyperbilirubinemia develops in homozygous infants during the first 3 days of life, and without treatment, serum concentrations of 25–35 mg/dL are reached during the 1st mo. Kernicterus, an almost universal complication of this disorder, is usually first noted in the early neonatal period, but some treated infants have survived childhood without clinical sequelae. Stools are pale yellow. Persistence of unconjugated hyperbilirubinema at levels above 20 mg/dL after the 1st wk of life in the absence of hemolysis should suggest the syndrome.

DIAGNOSIS. The diagnosis of Crigler-Najjar syndrome is based on the early age of onset and the extreme level of bilirubin elevation in the absence of hemolysis. In the bile, bilirubin concentration is less than 10 mg/dL compared with normal concentrations of 50–100 mg/dL, and there is no bilirubin glucuronide. Definitive diagnosis is established by measuring hepatic glucuronyl transferase activity in a liver specimen obtained by a closed biopsy; open biopsy should be avoided because surgery and anesthesia may precipitate kernicterus. DNA diagnosis is also available. Identification of the heterozygous state in the parents is also strongly suggestive of the diagnosis. Differential diagnosis is discussed in Chapter 91.3. Type II disease may be distinguished from type I by the marked decline in serum bilirubin level that occurs in type II disease after 1 wk of treatment with phenobarbital.

TREATMENT. Serum bilirubin concentration should be kept below 20 mg/dL for at least the first 2–4 wk of life; in low birth-weight infants, the levels should be kept lower. This usually requires repeated exchange transfusions and phototherapy. Phenobarbital therapy should be considered to determine responsiveness and differentiation between type I and II. Because the risk of kernicterus persists into adult life, although the serum bilirubin levels required to produce brain injury beyond the neonatal period are considerably higher (usually >35 mg/dL), phototherapy is generally continued throughout the early years of life. In older infants and children, phototherapy is used mainly during sleep in order not to interfere with normal activities. However, despite the administration of increasing intensities of light for longer periods, the serum bilirubin decrement response to phototherapy decreases with age. Adjuvant therapy using agents that bind photobilirubin products such as calcium phosphate, cholestyramine, or agar may be used to interfere with the enterohepatic recirculation of bilirubin. Prompt treatment of intercurrent infections, febrile episodes, and other types of illness may help prevent the later development of kernicterus, which may occur at bilirubin levels of 45–55 mg/dL. All patients with type I have eventually experienced severe kernicterus by young adulthood, despite vigorous continuous management that maintained neurologic normality during childhood. Orthotopic hepatic transplantation cures the disease and has been successful in a small number of patients, and isolated hepatocyte transplantation has been reported in one patient. Other therapeutic modalities have included plasmapheresis and limitation of bilirubin production. The latter option, inhibiting bilirubin generation, is possible via inhibition of heme oxygenase using metalloporphyrin therapy. Genetically engineered enzymatic replacement therapy and liver-directed gene therapy remain potential therapeutic options in the future.

Crigler-Najjar Syndrome (Type II Glucuronyl Transferase Deficiency). This autosomal dominant disease with marked variability of penetrance may present in a manner similar to type I syndrome, or it may be a less severe disorder, occasionally even without neonatal manifestations. Crigler-Najjar syndrome type II is caused by homozygous missense mutation in glucuronyl transferase isoform I resulting in only partial enzymatic activity.

CLINICAL MANIFESTATIONS. When this disorder presents in the neonatal period, unconjugated hyperbilirubinemia usually occurs during the first 3 days of life; serum bilirubin concentrations may be in a range compatible with physiologic jaundice or may be at pathologic levels. The concentrations characteristically remain elevated into and after the 3rd wk of life, persisting in a range of 1.5–22 mg/dL; concentrations in the lower part of this range may create uncertainty about whether chronic hyperbilirubinemia is present. The onset of kernicterus is unusual. Stool color is normal, and the infants are without clinical signs or symptoms of disease. There is no evidence of hemolysis.

DIAGNOSIS. Concentration of bilirubin in bile is nearly normal in type II syndrome. Jaundiced infants and young children having type II syndrome respond readily to 5 mg/kg/24 hr of oral phenobarbital with a decrease in serum bilirubin concentration to 2–3 mg/dL within 7–10 days. Those with type I syndrome do not respond.

TREATMENT. Long-term reduction in serum bilirubin levels can be achieved with continued administration of phenobarbital

at 5 mg/kg/24 hr. The cosmetic and psychosocial benefit should be weighed against the risks of an effective dose of the drug because there is a small long-term risk of kernicterus in the absence of hemolytic disease.

INHERITED CONJUGATED HYPERBILIRUBINEMIA

In inherited conjugated hyperbilirubinemias (see also Chapter 337), which are autosomal recessive disorders characterized by mild jaundice, the transfer of bilirubin and other organic anions from liver to bile is defective. Chronic mild conjugated hyperbilirubinemia is usually detected during adolescence or early adulthood but may occur as early as the 2nd year of life. The results of routine liver function tests are normal. Jaundice may be exacerbated with infection, pregnancy, oral contraceptives, alcohol consumption, or surgery. There is usually no morbidity, and life expectancy is normal; but these disorders may initially present difficult problems in the differential diagnosis of more serious diseases.

Dubin-Johnson Syndrome. Dubin-Johnson syndrome is considered to be an autosomal recessive inherited defect in hepatocyte secretion of bilirubin glucuronide. The defect in hepatic excretory function is not limited to conjugated bilirubin excretion but also involves several organic anions normally excreted from the liver cell into bile. Absent function of multiple drug-resistant protein (MRP2), an adenosine triphosphate (ATP)-dependent canalicular transporter, is the responsible defect. Bile acid excretion is normal, and serum bile acid levels are normal. Urinary coproporphyrin excretion is normal in quantity; however, due to a defect in porphyrin excretion, coproporphyrin I constitutes 80% of the total. Coproporphyrin III is normally greater than 75% of the total. Cholangiography fails to visualize the biliary tract and roentgenography of the gallbladder is also abnormal. The liver cells contain black pigment similar to melanin.

Rotor Syndrome. These patients have an additional deficiency in organic anion uptake. Total urinary coproporphyrin excretion is elevated, with a relative increase in the amount of the coproporphyrin I isomer. The gallbladder is normal by roentgenography, and liver cells contain no black pigment. Sulfobromophthalein excretion is often abnormal.

338.2 Wilson Disease

Wilson disease (hepatolenticular degeneration) is an autosomal recessive disorder characterized by degenerative changes in the brain, liver disease, and Kayser-Fleischer rings in the cornea (Chapter 592). The incidence is 1/500,000–100,000 births. It is fatal if untreated; however, specific effective treatment is available. Rapid diagnostic investigation of the possibility of Wilson disease in a patient presenting with any form of liver disease, particularly if older than 5 yr, not only facilitates early institution of management of Wilson disease and related genetic counseling but also allows appropriate treatment of non-Wilson liver disease once copper toxicosis is ruled out.

Pathogenesis. Defective mobilization of copper from lysosomes in liver cells for excretion into bile is the basis for the multiorgan damage in patients with Wilson disease. Relentless accumulation of copper in the liver reaches the point at which the retention capacity is exceeded. Copper then escapes the liver to damage other organs, particularly the brain and kidneys, and accumulates in the cornea, visible as Kayser-Fleischer rings. The underlying mechanism of liver damage in Wilson disease is presumably oxidant injury to the hepatocyte mitochondria, which is the target organelle in copper-induced toxicity. Lipid peroxidation of the mitochondria resulting from copper overload leads to functional alterations.

The abnormal gene for Wilson disease is on chromosome 13; linkage studies have assigned the Wilson disease locus to chromosome 13 at q14–q21. The gene encodes amino acid structural motifs consistent with a role in copper transport. The Wilson disease gene, like the Menkes disease gene, is predicted to encode a copper-binding, cation-transporting P-type ATPase and acts as a copper pump with ATP as an energy source. More than 100 mutations in the gene have been identified, making diagnosis by DNA mutational analysis a difficult task unless a proband mutation is known. Mutations that completely destroy gene function are associated with an onset of disease symptoms as early as 2–3 yr of age, when Wilson's disease may not typically be considered in the differential diagnosis. Milder mutations can be associated with neurologic symptoms or liver disease as late as 50 yr of age. Cloning of the gene for Wilson disease raises the prospect of precise presymptomatic detection of Wilson disease, timely initiation of therapy, and ultimately gene therapy.

Fetal and neonatal liver normally contains relatively high concentrations of sulfur-rich copper-binding protein (metallothionein) and of copper; serum ceruloplasmin and copper levels are relatively low. The mechanisms responsible for copper homeostasis in older children reach maturity by 2 yr of age. The wilsonian trait may be expressed after this time, but Wilson disease is not clinically manifested before age 5 yr.

Altered incorporation of copper into hepatic proteins such as ceruloplasmin is associated with diffuse accumulation of copper in the cytosol of hepatocytes. Later, as liver cells are overloaded, copper is distributed to other tissues, to which it is toxic, primarily as a potent inhibitor of enzymatic processes. Ionic copper inhibits pyruvate oxidase in brain and ATPase in membranes, leading to decreased ATP-phosphocreatine and potassium content of tissue. The glycolytic pathway and microsomal membrane ATPases are inhibited.

Clinical Manifestations. Copper enters the circulation in a non-ceruloplasmin-bound form and accumulates in many organs, inducing injury resulting in the various symptoms of Wilson disease. Manifestations are variable, with a tendency to familial patterns. The younger the patient, the more likely hepatic involvement will be the predominant manifestation. After 20 yr of age, neurologic symptoms predominate. Forms of hepatic disease include asymptomatic hepatomegaly (with or without splenomegaly), subacute or chronic hepatitis, and fulminant hepatic failure. Cryptogenic cirrhosis, portal hypertension, ascites, edema, variceal bleeding, or other effects of hepatic dysfunction (delayed puberty, amenorrhea, or coagulation defect) may be manifestations of Wilson disease.

Neurologic and psychiatric disorders may develop insidiously or precipitously, with intention tremor, dysarthria, dystonia, deterioration in school performance, or behavioral changes. Kayser-Fleischer rings may be absent in young patients with liver disease but are always present in patients with neurologic symptoms. Hemolysis may be an initial manifestation, possibly related to the release of large amounts of copper from damaged hepatocytes; this form of Wilson disease is usually fatal without transplantation. During hemolytic episodes, urinary copper excretion and serum copper levels (non-ceruloplasmin-bound) are markedly elevated. Manifestations of Fanconi syndrome and progressive renal failure with alterations in tubular transport of amino acids, glucose, and uric acid may be present. Unusual manifestations include arthritis and endocrinopathies, such as hypoparathyroidism.

Pathology. All grades of hepatic injury occur, with fatty change, ballooned hepatocytes, glycogen granules, minimal inflammation, and enlarged Kupffer cells. The lesion may be indistinguishable from that of chronic hepatitis. Ultrastructural changes include large, dense mitochondria with altered smooth endoplasmic reticulum.

Diagnosis. Wilson disease should be considered in children and teenagers with unexplained acute or chronic liver disease, neurologic symptoms of unknown cause, acute hemolysis, psychiatric illnesses, behavioral changes, Fanconi syndrome, or unexplained bone disease. The clinical suspicion is confirmed by study of indices of copper metabolism.

The best screening test is to measure the serum ceruloplasmin level. Most patients with Wilson disease have decreased ceruloplasmin levels. Serum copper level may be elevated in early Wilson disease, and urinary copper excretion (usually <40 μg/day) is increased to greater than 100 μg/day and often up to 1,000 μg or more per day. In equivocal cases, the response of urinary copper output to chelation may be of diagnostic help; after a 1-g oral dose of D-penicillamine, affected patients excrete 1,200–2,000 μg/24 hr.

Liver biopsy is of value for examination of the histology and for measurement of the hepatic copper content (normally <10 μg/g dry weight). In Wilson disease, hepatic copper content exceeds 250 μg/g dry weight. In healthy heterozygotes, levels may be intermediate.

Family members of patients with proven cases require screening for presymptomatic Wilson disease. Such screening should include determination of the serum ceruloplasmin level and urinary copper excretion. If these results are abnormal or equivocal, liver biopsy should be carried out to determine morphology and hepatic copper content. Genetic screening by either linkage analysis or direct DNA mutation analysis is possible, especially if the mutation for the proband case is known.

Treatment. Administration of copper-chelating agents leads to rapid excretion of excess deposited copper in patients with Wilson disease. A major attempt should be made to restrict copper intake to less than 1 mg/day. Foods such as liver, shellfish, nuts, and chocolate should be avoided. If the copper content of the water exceeds 0.1 mg/L, it may be necessary to demineralize the water. Chelation therapy is currently best managed with oral administration of penicillamine (β, β-dimethylcysteine) in a dose of 1 g/day in two doses before meals for adults and 0.5–0.75 g/day for patients younger than 10 yr. In response to D-penicillamine, urinary copper excretion markedly increases and there may be slow clinical improvement. Urinary copper levels may become normal with continued administration of D-penicillamine, with marked improvement in hepatic and neurologic function and the disappearance of Kayser-Fleischer rings. Toxic effects of penicillamine are uncommon and consist of hypersensitivity reactions (Goodpasture syndrome, systemic lupus erythematosus, polymyositis), interaction with collagen and elastin, deficiency of other elements such as zinc, as well as aplastic anemia and nephrosis. Because penicillamine is an antimetabolite of vitamin B_6, additional amounts of this vitamin are necessary. For those patients who are unable to tolerate penicillamine, triethylene tetramine dihydrochloride (Trien, TETA, trientine) at a dose of 0.5–2 g/24 hr is an acceptable alternative. Zinc has also been used as adjuvant therapy or as maintenance therapy owing to its unique ability to impair the gastrointestinal absorption of copper. Zinc acetate is given in adults at a dose of 25 to 50 mg three times a day. Pediatric dosing guidelines have not been established.

Prognosis. Untreated patients with Wilson disease die of the hepatic, neurologic, renal, or hematologic complications. The prognosis for patients receiving prompt and continuous D-penicillamine is variable and depends on the time of initiation of and the individual responsiveness to chelation. Liver transplantation should be considered for patients with fulminant liver disease, decompensated cirrhosis, or progressive neurologic disease; the latter indication remains controversial. In asymptomatic siblings of affected patients, early institution of chelation therapy can prevent expression of the disease.

338.3 Hepatic Copper Overload Syndrome

Another form of childhood cirrhosis apparently associated with a genetic disturbance in copper metabolism has been described. This syndrome differs from Wilson disease in its earlier onset. Affected children experience progressive lethargy, abdominal distention, and jaundice and die before 6 yr of age. The hepatic histopathology resembles that of Indian childhood cirrhosis. Variants of this syndrome have been named according to the population where it has been described, such as Tyrolean childhood cirrhosis and North American Indian cirrhosis.

338.4 Indian Childhood Cirrhosis

Indian childhood cirrhosis is a fatal familial disorder that occurs predominantly in rural India in middle income Hindu families. It has been reported also in the Middle East, in West Africa, and in Central America. It affects children of both sexes, with onset usually at 1–3 yr of age. Hepatomegaly is often the first sign; fever, anorexia, and jaundice occur. There is in most cases rapid evolution to cirrhosis and liver failure. Serum immunoglobulin levels and hepatic copper concentrations are markedly elevated. No effective therapy is known.

It has been suggested that excessive dietary copper may have a role in the cause, owing to the use of copper and brass in cooking and for storage of water and milk. However, there may be a predisposing inherited susceptibility. Early introduction of copper-contaminated milk into infant diets may explain the epidemiologic features.

338.5 Neonatal Iron Storage Disease (NISD)

NISD is a rare form of fulminant liver disease of unknown cause characterized by diffuse increased iron deposition in the liver, pancreas, heart, and endocrine organs without evidence of increased iron intake (ingestion or transfusion). Inheritance may be autosomal recessive in some cases. Affected infants may be born prematurely, or with intrauterine growth retardation. A large placenta is found, and a rapidly fatal progressive illness characterized by hepatomegaly, hypoglycemia, hypoprothrombinemia, hypoalbuminemia, and hyperbilirubinemia follows. Symptoms begin in utero or in the 1st wk of life. The coagulopathy is refractory to therapy with vitamin K. The diagnosis can be confirmed through documentation of extrahepatic siderosis (biopsy material of buccal mucosal glands is laden with iron) or magnetic resonance imaging determination of iron storage in organs such as the pancreas.

The hepatic pathology reveals fibrosis, regenerative nodules, giant cell formation, necrosis, and hepatocellular hemosiderin deposits not unlike those in adult-type hereditary hemochromatosis. Hyperferritinemia is present.

Treatment with chelating agents (deferoxamine) alone is ineffective. Preliminary studies suggest that aggressive antioxidant therapy, combined with iron chelation, may be effective if initiated very early. Liver transplantation should also be an early consideration.

338.6 Miscellaneous Metabolic Diseases of the Liver

α-ANTITRYPSIN DEFICIENCY

A small percentage of individuals homozygous for deficiency of the major serum protease inhibitor, α_1-antitrypsin, have neonatal cholestasis and later childhood cirrhosis (see also Chapter 393.4). α_1-Antitrypsin, a protease inhibitor synthesized by the liver, accounts for 80% of the serum α_1-globulin fraction. α_1-Antitrypsin is present in more than 20 different co-dominant alleles, only a few of which are associated with defective protease inhibitors. The most common allele of the protease inhibitor (Pi) system is M, and the normal phenotype is PiMM. The Z allele predisposes to clinical deficiency; patients with liver disease are usually PiZZ and have serum α_1-antitrypsin levels less than 2 mg/mL (approximately 10–20% of normal). The incidence of the PiZZ genotype in the white population is estimated at 1/2,000–4,000. Intermediate phenotypes PiMS, PiMZ, and PiSZ are not definitively associated with liver disease. The null genotype has no periodic acid-Schiff (PAS)-positive inclusions and is not associated with liver disease. Of all PiZZ persons, fewer than 20% develop neonatal cholestasis. These patients are indistinguishable from other infants with "idiopathic" neonatal hepatitis, of whom they constitute approximately 5–10%.

In affected patients, the course of liver disease is highly variable. Jaundice, acholic stools, and hepatomegaly are present during the 1st wk of life, but the jaundice usually clears during the 2nd–4th mo. Complete resolution, persistent liver disease, or the development of cirrhosis may follow. Older children may present with manifestations of chronic liver disease or cirrhosis, with evidence of portal hypertension.

The fact that liver disease is not universal suggests a complex pathogenesis. The liver disease may be secondary to retention of α_1-antitrypsin in the liver with failure of degradation.

The diagnosis is best made by determination of an α_1-antitrypsin (Pi) phenotype and confirmed by liver biopsy. PAS-positive disease-resistant intracytoplasmic globules are seen in periportal hepatocytes. Immunofluorescence and immunocytochemical studies have shown this material to be antigenically related to α_1-antitrypsin. It has been suggested that abnormal biosynthesis of the protein or defective glycosylation may interfere with excretion of the product from the rough endoplasmic reticulum into the extracellular space. Electron microscopy shows amorphous deposits (glycoprotein) within dilated rough endoplasmic reticulum.

The pattern of neonatal liver injury may be highly variable. Hepatocellular damage with giant cell transformation, minimal inflammation, and bile stasis may be noted. Various degrees of portal fibrosis with biliary duct proliferation occur.

Liver transplantation has been curative. There is no other effective therapy for liver disease yet, but in the future, gene therapy will be possible.

CYSTIC FIBROSIS

Cystic fibrosis (CF) (see also Chapter 402) is a multiorgan disease caused by a mutation in the cystic fibrosis transmembrane conductance regulator (CFTR) gene, a cAMP dependent chloride transporter found in epithelial cells. The cholangiocytes, which line the bile ducts of the liver, express CFTR to enable electrolyte transport necessary for the efficient flow of bile. Therefore, cystic fibrosis is a defect of the cholangiocytes. Liver disease may affect from 17 to 25% of all CF patients. The liver lesions include cholestasis, steatosis, focal biliary cirrhosis, multilobular cirrhosis, and biliary tract abnormalities such as microgallbladder and gallstones. Diagnosis of liver disease in CF is made by biochemical analysis, hepatic ultrasound, or liver biopsy in patients with a positive sweat test or known genetic mutation of CFTR. Liver biopsy is controversial in that there is no curative therapy and should be considered only to stage fibrosis or exclude other lesions. Although no therapy has proved useful to reverse liver disease, ursodeoxycholic acid, given at a dose of 10–15 mg/kg/day has been shown to improve bile flow.

NONALCOHOLIC STEATOHEPATITIS

Obesity may lead to nonalcoholic steatohepatitis (NASH; see also Chapter 43), an acquired metabolic disease of the liver characterized by steatosis, and in some cases, inflammation and fibrosis. The pathogenic mechanisms leading to NASH are not well characterized but may involve increased oxidative stress leading to adipose tissue synthesis of tumor necrosis factor and activation of hepatic stellate cells resulting in increased deposition of extracellular matrix leading to inflammation and fibrosis. NASH appears to be associated with obesity, insulin resistance, and hyperlipidemia. Patients are often asymptomatic but will have hepatomegaly. Diagnosis can be made by an elevation of aminotransaminase levels (aspartate aminotransferase > alanine aminotransferase), ultrasound changes suggestive of fat accumulation, and the exclusion of infectious, toxic, or metabolic causes. Other causes of fatty liver disease include intestinal bypass surgery for obesity, drugs (steroids, estrogens, valproic acid, zidovudine, methotrexate, tetracycline, aspirin), pregnancy, lipid metabolic disorders, hepatotoxins, human immunodeficiency virus, and inflammatory bowel disease. Liver biopsy can be considered, but is not necessary as long as other etiologies for fatty accumulation can be discarded. Treatment consists of dietary counseling; improvement has been noted in patients after weight reduction or vitamin E therapy. Attempts to manage patients with diet often fail and the symptoms persist.

Angulo P: Nonalcoholic fatty liver disease. *N Engl J Med* 2002;346:1221–31.

Arias IM: New genetics of inheritable jaundice and cholestatic liver disease. *Lancet* 1998;352:82.

Balistreri WF: Nontransplant options for the treatment of metabolic liver disease: Saving livers while saving lives. *Hepatology* 1994;19:782.

Bavdekar AR, Bhave SA, Pradhan AM, et al: Long term survival in Indian childhood cirrhosis treated with D-penicillamine. *Arch Dis Child* 1996;74:32.

Bove KE, Daugherty CC, Tyson W, et al: Bile acid synthetic defects and liver disease. *Pediatr Dev Pathol* 2000;3:1.

Bull PC, Thomas GR, Rommens JM, et al: The Wilson disease gene is a putative copper transporting P-type ATPase similar to the Menkes gene. *Nat Genet* 1993;5:327.

Brewer GJ, Dick RD, Johnson VD, et al: Treatment of Wilson's disease with zinc: XV long-term follow-up studies. *J Lab Clin Med* 1998;132:264.

Burchell B, Hume R: Molecular genetic basis of Gilbert's syndrome. *J Gastroenterol Hepatol* 1999;14:960.

Feranchak AP, Sokol RJ: Cholangiocyte biology and cystic fibrosis liver disease. *Semin Liver Dis* 2001;21:471.

Fox IJ, Chowdhury JR, Kaufman SS, et al: Treatment of the Crigler-Najjar syndrome type I with hepatocyte transplantation. *N Engl J Med* 1998;338:1422.

Grompke M: The pathophysiology and treatment of hereditary tyrosinemia type 1. *Semin Liver Dis* 2001;21:563.

Gu M, Cooper JM, Butler P, et al: Oxidative-phosphorylation defects in liver of patients with Wilson's disease. *Lancet* 2000;356:469–74.

James OF, Day CP: Non-alcoholic steatohepatitis (NASH): A disease of emerging identity and importance. *J Hepatol* 1998;29:495.

Jansen, PLM: Diagnosis and management of Crigler-Najjar syndrome. *Eur J Pediatr* 1999;158:S89.

Kelley AL, Lunt PW, Rodrigues F, et al: Classification and genetic features of neonatal haemochromatosis: A study of 27 affected pedigrees and molecular analysis of genes implicated in iron metabolism. *J Med Genet* 2001;38: 599.

Lee WS, McKiernan PJ, Beath SV, et al: Bile bilirubin pigment analysis in disorders of bilirubin metabolism in early infancy. *Arch Dis Child* 2001;85:38.

Lefkowitch JH, Honig CL, King ME, et al: Hepatic copper overload and features of Indian childhood cirrhosis in an American sibship. *N Engl J Med* 1982;307:271.

Loudinos G, Gitlin JD: Wilson's Disease. *Semin Liver Dis* 2000;20:353.

Manton ND, Lipsett J, Moore DJ, et al: Non-alcoholic steatohepatitis in children and adolescents. *Med J Aust* 2000;173:476.

Singh JH: Biochemistry of peroxisomes in health and disease. *Mol Cell Biochem* 1997;167:1.

Tanner MS: Indian childhood cirrhosis and Tyrollean childhood cirrhosis. Disorders of a copper transport gene? *Adv Exp Med Biol* 1999;448:127.

Teckman JH, Qu DF, Perlmutter DH: Molecular pathogenesis of liver disease in alpha(1)-antitrypsin deficiency. *Hepatology* 1996;24:1504.

van der Veere CN, Sinaasappel M, McDonagh AF, et al: Current therapy for Crigler-Najjar syndrome type 1: Report of a world registry. *Hepatology* 1996;24:311.

Vennarecci G, Gunson BK, Ismail T, et al: Transplantation for end stage liver disease related to alpha$_1$-antitrypsin. *Transplantation* 1996;61:1488.

Chapter 339

Viral Hepatitis *John D. Snyder and Larry K. Pickering*

Viral hepatitis is a major health problem in developing and developed countries. Hepatotropic viruses are designated hepatitis A, B, C, D, E, and G viruses (Table 339–1). Many other viruses can cause hepatitis as one component of a multi-system disease, including herpes simplex virus (HSV), cytomegalovirus (CMV), Epstein-Barr virus, varicella-zoster virus, human immunodeficiency virus (HIV), rubella, adenoviruses, enteroviruses, parvovirus B19, and arboviruses.

The six hepatotropic viruses are a heterogeneous group that cause similar acute clinical illness, except for HGV, which appears to cause no or mild disease. HBV is a DNA virus, whereas HAV, HCV, HDV, HEV, and HGV are RNA viruses representing four different families (Table 339–2). HAV and HEV are not known to cause chronic illness, whereas HBV, HCV, and HDV viruses can cause important morbidity and mortality through chronic infections. HGV can cause chronic infections but with little morbidity or mortality yet reported. In the United States, HAV appears to cause most cases of hepatitis in children. HBV probably accounts for about one third of symptomatic cases in children, whereas HCV is found in approximately 20%. HDV, which occurs only in the presence of HBV, occurs in only a small percentage of children. HEV has not been reported in children who have lived and traveled only in the United States. HGV's role is not yet completely known, but the virus appears to account for a small percentage of cases of non–HAV-HEV infections.

Differential Diagnosis. The probable causes of hepatitis vary somewhat by age. In the newborn period, infection remains an important cause of hyperbilirubinemia but metabolic and anatomic causes (e.g., biliary atresia and choledochal cysts) also must be considered. The introduction of pigmented vegetables into an infant's diet may result in carotenemia, which may be mistaken for jaundice.

In later infancy and childhood, hemolytic-uremic syndrome may be initially mistaken for hepatitis (Chapter 449). Reye and Reye-like syndromes present in a similar fashion to acute fulminating hepatitis (Chapter 342). Jaundice also may occur with malaria, leptospirosis, and brucellosis and with severe infection in older children, particularly in children with malignancy or immunodeficiency. Gallstones may obstruct biliary drainage and cause jaundice in adolescents as well as in children with chronic hemolytic processes. Hepatitis may be the initial presentation of Wilson disease, cystic fibrosis, and Jamaican vomiting sickness. The liver may also be involved in collagen diseases including systemic lupus erythematosus.

TABLE 339–1. Viral Hepatitis Nomenclature

Hepatotropic Viruses	Antigens	Identified Antibodies
Hepatitis A virus (HAV)	HAV	anti-HAV*
		IgM anti-HAV
Hepatitis B virus (HBV)	HBsAg*	anti-HBsAg*
		IgM anti-HBsAg*
	HBcAg	anti-HBcAg*
	HBeAg*	anti-HBeAg*
Hepatitis C virus (HCV)		anti-HCV*
Hepatitis D virus (HDV)	HDAg	anti-HDV*
Hepatitis E virus (HEV)		anti-HEV
		IgM anti-HEV
Hepatitis G virus (HGV)		anti-HGV

Assays are commercially available.

TABLE 339–2. Features of the Six Hepatotropic Viruses

	HAV	HBV	HCV	HDV	HEV	HGV
Nucleic acid	RNA	DNA	RNA	RNA	RNA	RNA
Incubation (mean)	30 days	100–120 days	7–9 wk	2–4 mo	40 days	Unknown
Transmission						
Percutaneous	Rare	Common	Common	Common	No	Common
Fecal-oral	Common	No	No	No	Common	No
Sexual	Rare	Common	Rare	Rare	Rare	Rare
Transplacental	No	Common	Rare	No	Probably no	Rare
Chronic infection	No	Yes	Yes	Yes	No	Yes
Fulminant disease	Rare	Yes	Rare	Yes	Rare	Probably no

Medications, including acetaminophen overdose, valproic acid, and various hepatotoxins, including long-acting mushroom toxins, can be associated with a hepatitis-like picture (Chapter 344). Drugs well tolerated in healthy children may cause problems in children with certain illnesses.

HEPATITIS A

Etiology. HAV is a 27-nm-diameter, RNA-containing virus that is a member of the Picornavirus family. Acute infection is diagnosed by detecting immunoglobulin M (IgM) antibodies (anti-HAV) by radioimmunoassay or, rarely, by identifying viral particles in stool.

Epidemiology. HAV infections occur throughout the world but are found most commonly in developing countries, where the prevalence rate approaches 100% in children by 5 yr of age. In the United States, approximately 30–40% of the adult population has evidence for previous HAV infection, with the rates of infection being similar in the first, second, and third decades of life. Hepatitis A causes only acute hepatitis and accounts for approximately 50% of clinically apparent acute viral hepatitis in the United States. Most infections in children younger than 5 yr of age are asymptomatic or have mild, nonspecific manifestations; the illness is much more likely to be symptomatic in adults than in children. Prior to 1997, approximately half of cases in the United States occurred in 11 western states (Alaska, Arizona, California, Idaho, Nevada, New Mexico, Oklahoma, Oregon, South Dakota, Utah, and Washington), which account for only 22% of the population, with prevalence rates of ≥20 cases/100,000 population. With routine hepatitis A vaccination in these and all or part of 6 other states (Arkansas, Colorado, Missouri, Montana, Texas, and Wyoming) with intermediate prevalence of 10–20 cases/100,000 population, the incidence is changing, with many eastern and southern states now showing the highest rates of HAV in the United States.

Transmission of HAV is almost always by person-to-person contact. Spread is predominantly by the fecal-oral route; percutaneous transmission occurs rarely, and maternal-neonatal transmission is not recognized. HAV infection during pregnancy or at the time of delivery does not appear to result in increased complications of pregnancy or increased clinical disease in the newborn. The infectivity of human saliva, urine, and semen is unknown. In the United States, increased risk of infection is found in contacts of infected persons, child-care centers, household contacts of children in child care, and homosexual populations and is associated with contact with contaminated food or water and travel to endemic areas. However, no known source is found in about half of the cases. Common source food-borne and water-borne outbreaks have occurred, including several due to contaminated shellfish, frozen berries, and raw produce. Fecal excretion of the virus occurs late in the incubation period, reaches its peak just before the onset of symptoms, and is minimal in the week after the onset of jaundice (Fig. 339–1). The mean incubation period for HAV is about 4 wk, with a range of 15–50 days.

Pathogenesis. The acute response of the liver to HAV is similar to that of the other hepatotropic viruses (HBV-HEV). The entire liver is involved with necrosis, most markedly in the centrilobular areas, and increased cellularity, which is predominant in the portal areas. The lobular architecture remains intact, although balloon degeneration and necrosis of single or groups of parenchymal cells occur initially. Fatty change is rare. A diffuse mononuclear cell inflammatory reaction causes expansion in the portal tracts; bile duct proliferation is common, but bile duct damage is not often found. Diffuse Kupffer cell hyperplasia is present in the sinusoids, along with infiltration of polymorphonuclear leukocytes and eosinophils. Neonates respond to hepatic injury by forming giant cells. In fulminant hepatitis, total destruction of the parenchyma occurs, leaving only connective tissue septa. By 3 mo after the onset of acute hepatitis due to HAV, the liver usually is normal morphologically.

Other organ systems can be affected during HAV infection. Regional lymph nodes and the spleen may be enlarged. The bone marrow may be moderately hypoplastic, and aplastic anemia has been reported. Small intestine tissue may show changes in villous structure, and ulceration of the gastrointestinal tract can occur, especially in fatal cases. Acute pancreatitis and myocarditis have been reported rarely, and nephritis, arthritis, vasculitis, and cryoglobulinemia may result from circulating immune complexes.

Injury in acute hepatitis caused by hepatotropic viruses is evidenced in three main ways. The first is a reflection of cytopathic injury to the hepatocytes, which release alanine aminotransferase (ALT, formerly serum glutamic-pyruvic transaminase) and aspartate aminotransferase (AST, formerly serum glutamic-oxaloacetic transaminase) into the bloodstream. ALT is more specific to the liver than AST, which also can be elevated after injury to erythrocytes, skeletal muscle, or myocardial cells. The height of elevation does not correlate with the extent of hepatocellular necrosis and has little prognostic value. In some cases, a

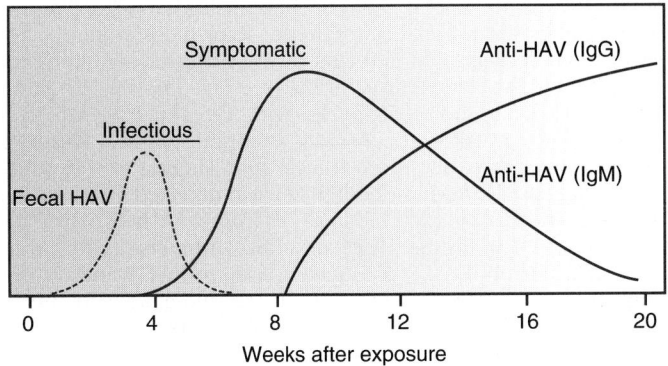

FIGURE 339–1. Pattern of response to hepatitis A virus (HAV) infection. (IgM = immunoglobulin M; IgG = immunoglobulin G.)

falling aminotransferase level may predict a poor outcome if the decline occurs in conjunction with a rising bilirubin level and prolonged prothrombin time (PT). This combination of findings indicates that massive hepatic injury has occurred, resulting in few functioning hepatocytes. Another enzyme, lactic dehydrogenase (LDH), is even less specific to liver than AST and usually is not helpful in evaluating liver injury. The second mechanism of injury in viral hepatitis results from cholestatic jaundice, in which both direct and indirect bilirubin levels are elevated. Jaundice results from obstruction of biliary flow and damage to hepatocytes. Elevations of serum alkaline phosphatase (ALP), 5'-nucleotidase, γ-glutamyl transpeptidase (GGT), and urobilinogen all can reflect injury to the biliary system. Abnormal protein synthesis is reflected by increased PT. Because of the short half-life of these proteins, the PT is a sensitive indicator of damage to the liver. Serum albumin is another liver-manufactured serum protein, but its longer half-life limits its role in monitoring acute liver injury. Cholestasis results in a decreased intestinal bile acid pool and decreased absorption of fat-soluble vitamins. The third mechanism of hepatic injury by HAV is related to changes that occur in carbohydrate, ammonia, and drug metabolism. Although circulating immune complexes commonly occur in HAV infection, no direct evidence shows that they induce hepatic necrosis or viral clearance.

Clinical Manifestations. The onset of HAV infection usually is abrupt and is accompanied by systemic complaints of fever, malaise, nausea, emesis, anorexia, and abdominal discomfort. This prodrome may be mild and often goes unnoticed in infants and preschool-aged children. Diarrhea often occurs in children, but constipation is more common in adults. Jaundice may be so subtle in young children that it can be detected only by laboratory tests. When jaundice and dark urine occur, they usually develop after the systemic symptoms. In contrast to infections in children, most HAV infections in adults are symptomatic and can be severe. Symptoms of HAV infection include right upper quadrant pain, dark-colored urine, and jaundice. The duration of symptoms usually is less than 1 mo, and appetite, exercise tolerance, and a feeling of well-being gradually return. Almost all patients with HAV infection recover completely, but a relapsing course can occur for several months. Fulminant hepatitis leading to death is uncommon in children; co-infection with HCV increases the risk for fulminant hepatitis. HAV is not associated with chronic liver disease, persistent viremia, or an intestinal carrier state.

Treatment. There is no specific treatment for hepatitis A. Most children are asymptomatic or only mildly symptomatic. Treatment is supportive and consists of intravenous hydration as needed.

Diagnosis. The diagnosis of HAV infection should be considered when a history of jaundice exists in family contacts, friends, schoolmates, or childcare playmates or personnel or if the child or family have traveled to an area endemic for HAV. The diagnosis is established by serologic criteria; liver biopsies rarely are performed. Anti-HAV is detected at the onset of symptoms of acute hepatitis A and persists for life (see Fig. 339–1). The acute infection is diagnosed by the presence of IgM anti-HAV, which is present at the onset of illness and usually disappears within 4 mo but may persist for more than 6 mo. Thereafter, IgG anti-HAV is detectable. IgM antibody is seldom detected after immunization. The virus is excreted in stools from 2 wk before to 1 wk after the onset of illness. Rises are almost universally found in ALT, AST, bilirubin, ALP, 5'-nucleotidase, and GGT and do not help to differentiate the cause. The PT should always be measured in a child with hepatitis to help assess the extent of liver injury; prolongation is a serious sign mandating hospitalization.

Complications. Children almost universally recover from HAV infections. Rarely, fulminant hepatitis (see Chapter 345) can

occur, in which a progressive rise in serum bilirubin is accompanied by an initial rise in aminotransferases followed by a fall to normal or low values despite disease progression. Hepatic synthetic function decreases, and the PT becomes prolonged and is often accompanied by bleeding. The serum albumin level falls, causing edema and ascites. The ammonia level usually rises, and the sensorium becomes altered, progressing from drowsiness to stupor and then deep coma. End-stage disease and death can occur in less than 1 wk or can develop more insidiously.

Prevention. Persons infected with HAV are contagious for about 7 days after the onset of jaundice and should be excluded from school, child care, or work during this period. Careful handwashing is necessary, particularly after changing diapers and before preparing or serving food. In hospital settings, contact as well as standard precautions, including strict handwashing, are recommended for diapered or incontinent patients for 1 wk after onset of symptoms.

VACCINE. The availability of two inactivated, highly immunogenic and safe HAV vaccines is having a major impact on the prevention of HAV infection. Both vaccines are approved for children older than 2 yr of age. They are administered intramuscularly in a two-dose schedule, with the second dose given 6–12 mo after the first dose. Seroconversion rates in children exceed 90% after an initial dose and approach 100% after the second dose. The immune response in immunocompromised persons may be suboptimal. HAV vaccine may be administered simultaneously with other vaccines at separate sites. Because the financial, social, and clinical impact of hepatitis A is so substantial in the United States, with indirect costs estimated to be in the hundreds of millions of dollars annually, more widespread vaccination is being recommended. A major obstacle to universal immunization is the lack of a vaccine licensed for children younger than 2 yr of age. Recommended use of HAV vaccine in the United States has been primarily for susceptible persons traveling to or working in countries where HAV is endemic. For persons older than 2 yr of age, vaccine is preferable to immunoglobulin (IG) for pre-exposure prophylaxis (Table 339–3). However, greater consideration is being given to other at-risk groups including (1) children older than 2 yr of age in defined and circumscribed communities with endemic rates or periodic outbreaks of HAV infection (e.g., Native Americans or Alaskan Natives); (2) patients with chronic liver disease; (3) men who have sex with men; (4) users of injection and illicit drugs; (5) individuals at occupational risk of exposure; and (6) persons with clotting factor disorders.

TABLE 339–3. **Hepatitis A Virus Prophylaxis**

Age	Exposure	Dose
Pre-Exposure Prophylaxis (Travelers to Endemic Regions)		
<2 yr	Expected <3 mo	IG 0.02 mL/kg
	Expected 3–5 mo	IG 0.06 mL/kg
	Expected long term	IG 0.06 mL/kg at departure and every 5 mo thereafter
≥2 yr	Expected <3 mo	HAV vaccine* or IG 0.02 mL/kg
	Expected 3–5 mo	HAV vaccine* or IG 0.06 mL/kg
	Expected long term	HAV vaccine*
Postexposure Prophylaxis		
	Future exposure likely	
≥2 yr	≤2 wk since exposure	IG 0.02 mL/kg and HAV vaccine
	>2 wk since exposure	HAV vaccine*
	Future exposure unlikely	
All ages	≤2 wk since exposure	IG 0.02 mL/kg and HAV vaccine should be considered (if ≥2 years)
	>2 wk since exposure	No prophylaxis

*Two inactivated vaccines are approved for use in persons ≥2 yr of age.
IG = immunoglobulin.

IMMUNOGLOBULIN. Indications for intramuscular administration of IG include pre-exposure and postexposure prophylaxis (see Table 339–3). Intravenous IG (IVIG) is likely to be effective against HAV infection, but appropriate dose, efficacy, and duration of protection have not been defined. IG is recommended for pre-exposure prophylaxis for all susceptible travelers to countries where HAV is endemic. For children older than 2 yr of age, HAV immunization is preferred if the interval before departure is more than 1 mo after dose one. IG as prophylaxis in postexposure situations is used in (1) household and sexual contacts of HAV cases; (2) newborn infants of HAV-infected mothers; (3) child-care center staff, employees, children and their household contacts during an outbreak; and (4) outbreaks in institutions and hospitals. The use of IG more than 2 wk after exposure is not indicated.

IG is not recommended routinely for sporadic nonhousehold exposure (e.g., protection of hospital personnel or school-mates). Mass immunization of school children has been used when epidemics have been school centered. Available data are not sufficient to recommend HAV vaccine alone for postexposure prophylaxis.

HEPATITIS B

Etiology. HBV is a 42-nm-diameter member of the Hepadnaviridae family, a noncytopathogenic, hepatotropic group of DNA viruses. HBV has a circular, partially double-stranded DNA genome composed of approximately 3,200 nucleotides. Four genes have been identified, the S (surface), C (core), X, and P (polymer) genes. The surface of the virus includes two particles designated **hepatitis B surface antigen (HBsAg)**: a 22-nm-diameter spherical particle and a 22-nm-wide tubular particle with a variable length of up to 200 nm. The inner portion of the virion contains **hepatitis B core antigen (HBcAg)**, the nucleocapsid that encodes the viral DNA, and a nonstructural antigen called **hepatitis B e antigen (HBeAg)**, a nonparticulate soluble antigen derived from HBcAg by proteolytic self-cleavage. HBeAg serves as a marker of active viral replication. Replication of HBV occurs predominantly in the liver but also occurs in the lymphocytes, spleen, kidney, and pancreas.

Epidemiology. Worldwide, the areas of highest prevalence of HBV infection are sub-Saharan Africa, China, parts of the Middle East, the Amazon basin, and the Pacific Islands. In the United States, the Eskimo population in Alaska has the highest prevalence rate. An estimated 6 million persons in the United States are infected, with approximately 300,000 new cases of HBV occurring each year with the highest incidence among adults ages 20–39 yr. The number of new cases in children reported each year is thought to be low but is difficult to estimate because the majority of infections in children are asymptomatic. The risk of chronic infection is related inversely to age; although less than 10% of infections occur in children, these infections account for 20–30% of all chronic cases.

The most important risk factor for acquisition of HBV in children is perinatal exposure to an HBsAg-positive mother. The risk of transmission is greatest if the mother also is HBeAg positive; 70–90% of their infants become chronically infected if untreated. During the neonatal period, hepatitis B antigen is present in blood of 2.5% of infants born to affected mothers, indicating that intrauterine infection occurred. In most cases, antigenemia appears later, suggesting that transmission occurred at the time of delivery; virus contained in amniotic fluid or in maternal feces or blood may be the source. Although most infants born to infected mothers become antigenemic by 2–5 mo of age, some infants of HBsAg-positive mothers are not affected until later ages. Of the 22,000 infants born each year to HBsAg-positive mothers in the United States, more than 98% receive immunoprophylaxis and are protected from infection.

HBsAg has been demonstrated inconsistently in human milk of infected mothers. Breast-feeding of unimmunized infants by infected mothers does not appear to confer a greater risk of hepatitis on offspring than does formula feeding, despite the possibility that cracked nipples may result in ingestion of contaminated maternal blood by a nursing infant. Routine immunoprophylaxis of infants born to HBsAg-positive mothers with HB vaccine and HBIG may eliminate theoretical risks.

Other important risk factors for HBV infection in children and adolescents include intravenous acquisition by drugs or blood products, sexual contact, institutional care, and contact with carriers. No risk factors are identified in about 40% of cases.

The risk of developing chronic HBV infection, defined as being positive for HBsAg for more than 6 mo or being negative for IgM anti-HBc and positive for HBsAg, is related inversely to age; the older the age of acquisition, the lower the risk of chronic disease. Chronic infection is associated with chronic liver disease and primary hepatocellular carcinoma, which is the most important cause of cancer-related death in Asia.

HBV is present in high concentrations in blood, serum, and serous exudates and in moderate concentrations in saliva, vaginal fluid, and semen. For these reasons, efficient transmission occurs through blood exposure and sexual contact. The incubation period ranges from 45 to 160 days, with a mean of about 120 days.

Pathogenesis. The acute response of the liver to HBV is the same as for all hepatotropic viruses. Persistence of histologic changes in patients with hepatitis B, C, or D indicates development of chronic liver disease (Chapter 343).

HBV, unlike the other hepatotropic viruses, is a noncytopathogenic virus that causes injury by immune-mediated processes. The severity of hepatocyte injury reflects the degree of the immune response, with the most complete immune response being associated with the greatest likelihood of viral clearance and the most severe injury to hepatocytes. The first step in the process of acute hepatitis is infection of hepatocytes by HBV, resulting in viral antigens on the cell surface. The most important of these viral antigens may be the nucleocapsid antigens, HBcAg and HBeAg. These antigens, in combination with class I major histocompatibility (MHC) proteins, make the cell a target for cytotoxic T-cell lysis.

The mechanism for development of chronic hepatitis is less well understood. To permit hepatocytes to continue to be infected, the core protein or MHC class I protein may not be recognized, the cytotoxic lymphocytes may not be activated, or some other yet unknown mechanism may interfere with destruction of hepatocytes. For cell-to-cell infection to continue, some virus-containing hepatocytes must remain alive.

Immune-mediated mechanisms also are involved in the extrahepatic conditions that can be associated with HBV infections. Circulating immune complexes containing HBsAg can occur in patients who develop associated polyarteritis nodosa, membranous or membranoproliferative glomerulonephritis, polymyalgia rheumatica, leukocytoclastic vasculitis, and Guillain-Barré syndrome.

Mutations of HBV are more common than for the usual DNA viruses, and a series of mutant strains has been recognized. The most important mutation, which does not affect replication, is one that results in failure to express HBeAg and has been associated with development of severe hepatitis and perhaps more severe exacerbations of chronic HBV infection. Other core-related mutations yielding similar results have been noted.

Clinical Manifestations. Many cases of HBV infection are asymptomatic, as evidenced by the high carriage rate of serum markers in persons who have no history of acute hepatitis. The usual acute symptomatic episode is similar to that of HAV and HCV infections but may be more severe and is more likely to include involvement of skin and joints. The first clinical evidence of HBV infection is elevation of ALT levels, which begin to rise just before development of lethargy, anorexia, and malaise, which occurs about 6–7 wk after exposure. The illness may be preceded in a few children by a serum sickness–like prodrome marked by arthralgia or skin lesions, including urticarial, purpuric, macular, or maculopapular rashes. Papular acrodermatitis, the Gianotti-Crosti syndrome, also may occur. Other extrahepatic conditions associated with HBV infections in children can include polyarteritis, glomerulonephritis, and aplastic anemia. Jaundice, which may be present in about 25% of infected individuals, usually begins about 8 wk after exposure and lasts for about 4 wk. In the usual course of resolving HBV infection, symptoms are present for 6–8 wk. The percentage of children in whom clinical evidence of hepatitis develops is higher for HBV than for HAV, and the rate of fulminant hepatitis also is greater. Chronic hepatitis also occurs, and the chronic active form can result in cirrhosis and hepatocellular carcinoma, which occurs almost exclusively in patients with cirrhosis, typically 25–30 yr after HBV infection.

On physical examination, symptomatic infection results in skin and mucous membranes that are icteric, especially the sclera and the mucosa under the tongue. The liver usually is enlarged and tender to palpation. When the liver is not palpable below the costal margin, tenderness can be demonstrated by gently striking the rib cage over the liver with a closed fist. Splenomegaly and lymphadenopathy are common.

Diagnosis. The serologic pattern for HBV is more complex than for HAV and differs depending on whether the disease is acute, subclinical, or chronic (Fig. 339–2). Several antigens and antibodies are used to confirm the diagnosis of acute HBV infection (see Table 339–1). Routine screening for HBV infection requires assay of at least two serologic markers. HBsAg is the first serologic marker of infection to appear and is found in almost all infected persons; its rise closely coincides with the onset of symptoms. HBeAg is often present during the acute phase and indicates a highly infectious state. Because HBsAg levels fall before the end of symptoms, IgM antibody to HBcAg (IgM anti-HBcAg) also is required because it rises early after infection and persists for many months before being replaced by IgG anti-HBcAg, which persists for years. IgM anti-HBcAg usually is not present in perinatal HBV infections. Anti-HBcAg is the most valuable single serologic marker of acute HBV infection because it is present almost as early as HBsAg and continues to be present later in the course of the disease when HBsAg has disappeared. Only anti-HBsAg is present in persons immunized with hepatitis B vaccine, whereas anti-HBsAg and anti-HBcAg are detected in persons with resolved infection.

Treatment. No available medical therapy is successful in the majority of persons infected with HBV. Interferon-α-2b (IFN-α2b) and lamivudine are the current therapies for treatment of chronic hepatitis B in adults older than 18 yr of age with compensated liver disease and HBV replication. IFN-α2b also has been used in children, with long-term eradication rates similar to the 25% rate reported in adults. Recombinant interferons have immunomodulatory and antiviral effects whereas lamivudine, a nucleoside analog, inhibits the viral enzyme reverse transcriptase. Persons most likely to respond have low serum HBV DNA titers, HBeAg, active inflammation, and recently acquired disease. Sustained response to treatment is not attained in most patients receiving these drugs alone or in combination. Research efforts are being focused on developing methods to stimulate a successful immune response that could result in long-term viral clearance and avoid the need for maintenance therapy. Liver transplantation also has been used to treat patients with end-stage HBV infection.

Complications. Acute fulminant hepatitis with coagulopathy, encephalopathy, and cerebral edema occurs more frequently with HBV than with the other hepatotropic viruses, and the risk of fulminant hepatitis is further increased when there is co-infection or superinfection with HDV. Mortality due to fulminant hepatitis is more than 30%. Liver transplantation is the only effective intervention; supportive care aimed at sustaining patients while providing the time needed for regeneration of hepatic cells is the only other option.

HBV infections also can result in chronic hepatitis, which can lead to cirrhosis and primary hepatocellular carcinoma (Chapter 496). Membranous glomerulonephritis with deposition of complement and HBeAg in glomerular capillaries is a rare complication of HBV infection. Immunization to decrease the carrier rate in the population has resulted in a marked decline in the incidence of hepatocellular carcinoma in children in Taiwan.

Prevention. Hepatitis B vaccine and hepatitis B immunoglobulin (HBIG) are available for prevention of HBV infection. Two recombinant DNA vaccines are available in the United States, and both are highly immunogenic in children. Universal immunization of all infants with hepatitis B vaccine is recommended in both pre-exposure and postexposure situations and provides long-term protection. In addition, all children who have not previously received the vaccine should be immunized by 11–12 yr of age, and catch-up programs should be implemented for unimmunized adolescents and high-risk adults. To help increase coverage, many states have made immunization a requirement for entry into junior high school. HBIG is indicated only for specific postexposure circumstances and provides only temporary protection.

Infants born to HBsAg-positive women should receive vaccine at birth, 1–2 mo, and 6 mo of age (see Table 282–4). The first dose should be accompanied by administration of 0.5 mL of HBIG as soon after delivery as possible, because the effectiveness decreases rapidly with increased time after birth. Postvaccination testing for HBsAg and anti-HBs should be at 9–15 mo. If the result is positive for anti-HBs, the child is immune to HBV. If the result is positive for HBsAg only, the parent should be counseled and the child evaluated by a pediatric hepatologist. If the result is negative for both HBsAg and anti-HBs, a second complete hepatitis B vaccine series should be administered, followed by testing for anti-HBs to determine if subsequent doses are needed.

Infants born to HBsAg-negative women should receive the vaccine at 0–2 mo, 1–4 mo, and at 6–18 mo of age. Routine postvaccination testing of immunized infants born to HBsAg-negative women or with anti-HBs is not recommended. The

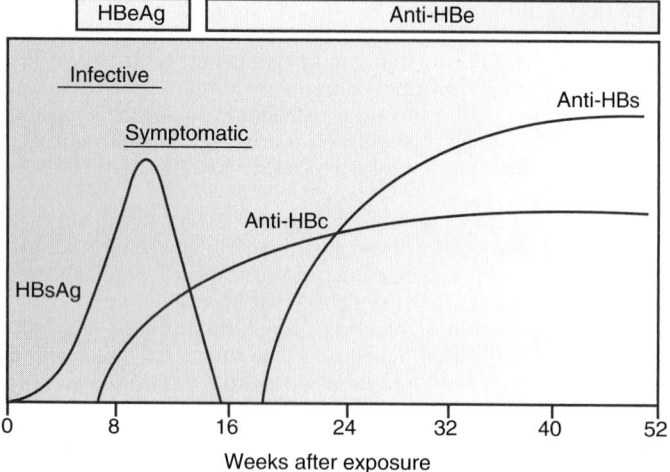

FIGURE 339–2. Pattern of response to hepatitis B virus infection. (HBeAg = hepatitis B e antigen; HBsAg = hepatitis B surface antigen; HBc = hepatitis B core antigen.)

three-dose series can be completed even if the interval between doses is longer than recommended.

Recommendations for postexposure prophylaxis for prevention of hepatitis B infection depend on the conditions under which the person is exposed to HBV (Table 339–4).

HEPATITIS C

Etiology. HCV is recognized as the cause of almost all parenterally acquired cases of what was previously known as non-A, non-B hepatitis. The virus has not been isolated but was cloned in 1988 using recombinant DNA technology. HCV is a single-stranded RNA virus, classified as a separate genus within the Flaviviridae family, with marked genetic heterogeneity. It has six major genotypes and numerous subtypes and quasi-species, which may permit it to escape host immune surveillance. Genetic variation may partially explain the differences in clinical course.

Epidemiology. HCV infection is the most common cause of chronic liver disease in the United States and causes 8,000–10,000 deaths per year. About 4 million people in the United States are estimated to be infected with HCV. Approximately 85% of infected individuals remain persistently infected, even in the absence of biochemical evidence of liver disease. Risk factors for HCV transmission in the United States have changed dramatically over the past two decades. Previously, blood transfusion was the most common route of infection but with the current screening practices, the risk of HCV is now about 0.001% per unit transfused. Illegal drug use with exposure to blood or blood products from HCV-infected persons now accounts for more than half of the cases in the United States. Sexual transmission, especially through multiple sexual partners, is the second most common cause of infection but the rate of transmission between long-term steady partners is very low. Other risk factors include imprisonment, and occupational exposure. Approximately 10% of new infections are unexplained. Perinatal transmission has been described but is uncommon except when the mother is HIV infected or has a high titer of HCV RNA. Genotypes may also be risk factors for outcome because patients with genotype 2 or 3 respond better to ribavirin or interferon therapy than those with genotype 1. Type 1b is the most common genotype in the United States. The incubation period is 7–9 wk (range of 2–24 wk).

Pathogenesis. The pattern of acute hepatic injury is similar to that of the other hepatotropic viruses. In chronic cases, lymphoid aggregates or follicles in portal tracts are found, either alone or as part of a general inflammatory infiltration of the tracts. HCV appears to cause injury primarily by cytopathic mechanisms, but immune-mediated injury also may occur. The cytopathic component appears to be mild, because the acute illness is typically the least severe of all hepatotropic virus infections except HGV.

Clinical Manifestations. The clinical pattern of the acute infection is similar to that of the other hepatitis viruses. Acute disease tends to be mild and insidious in onset in adults and children. Fulminant liver failure rarely occurs. HCV is the most likely hepatotropic virus to cause chronic infection; about 85% of cases become chronic, with a fluctuating pattern of elevated hepatic transaminases. After approximately 20–30 yr, about 25% ultimately progress to cirrhosis, liver failure, and occasionally primary hepatocellular carcinoma. The clinical disease in children appears to be milder with a slower progression to cirrhosis than in adults. However, cirrhosis for HCV has been reported in children. Hepatocellular carcinoma associated with HCV, which is less effective than HBV in causing primary hepatocellular carcinoma, almost always occurs in the presence of cirrhosis and probably results from chronic inflammation and necrosis rather than an oncogenic effect of the virus.

Chronic HCV infection may be associated with small vessel vasculitis and is a common cause of essential mixed cryoglobulinemia. Other extrahepatic manifestations include cutaneous vasculitis, peripheral neuropathy, cerebritis, membranoproliferative glomerulonephritis, and nephrotic syndrome. The complications of chronic HCV infection have become one of the most common causes of liver transplantation in adults.

Diagnosis. The clinically available assays for detection of HCV infection are based on detection of antibodies to HCV antigens or testing directly for viral RNA or DNA. These are diagnostic tests and neither the serologic nor the virologic tests can predict the severity of liver disease. The most widely used tests are the three generations of enzyme immunoassays (EIAs) that have increasing sensitivity. The predictive value of these assays is greatest in high-risk populations but the false-positive rate can be as high as 50–60% in low-risk populations. False-negative results also occur because antibodies remain negative for as long as 1–3 mo after clinical onset of illness. Anti-HCV antibody is not a protective antibody, does not confer immunity, and is usually present simultaneously with the virus. The other serologic test is the high sensitivity recombinant immunoblot assay (RIBA) which is used primarily to confirm a positive EIA result in a low-risk patient.

TABLE 339–4. Indications and Dosing Schedule for Hepatitis B Vaccine and Hepatitis B Immune Globulin

	Vaccine			HBIG	
Groups	Recombivax HB (μg)	Engerix-B (μg)	Schedule	Dose (μL)	Schedule
Neonates					
Infants of HBsAg-positive women	5	10	Birth, 1, 6 mo	0.5	Within 12 hr of birth
Infants of HBsAg-negative women	5	10	Birth, 1–2, 6–18 mo	None	
Children and adolescents (11–19 yr)	5	10	0, 1, and 6 mo	None	
Contact with acute HBV					
Intimate					
0–19 yr old	5	10	Exposure, 1 and 6 mo	0.06/kg	At exposure
>19 yr old	10	20	Exposure, 1 and 6 mo	0.06/kg	At exposure
Household	None	None	None	None	
Casual	None	None	None	None	
Contact with chronic HBV					
Intimate and household					
0–19 yr old	5	10	Exposure, 1 and 6 mo	None	
>19 yr old	10	20	Exposure, 1 and 6 mo	None	
Casual	None	None		None	
Immunosuppressed or hemodialysis patients	40	40	Exposure, 1 and 6 mo	None	

The virologic assays for HCV are the polymerase chain reaction (PCR) and the branched-chain DNA (bDNA test), which permit detection of small amounts of HCV RNA in serum and tissue samples within days of infection. The qualitative PCR detection is especially useful in patients with recent or perinatal infection, hypogammaglobulinemia, or immunosuppression and is very sensitive. The quantitative PCR and bDNA tests measure the viral load and are currently considered research tools but may aid in monitoring therapy in the future. Methods for determining HCV genotype are available, and can be helpful in assessing the response to therapy. The presence of HCV-associated liver disease is indicated by an elevated serum ALT level and confirmed by histologic examination of liver biopsy. Chronic HCV infection in patients with anti-HCV is defined by persistently elevated levels of ALT in the presence of hepatic fibrosis and by the presence of HCV RNA in blood. Currently there is no means to identify patients who will have progressive disease; a liver biopsy is the only means to assess the presence and extent of hepatic fibrosis. Most patients with chronic HCV hepatitis have 10^{5-7} genome copies/mL of HCV RNA in their serum.

Individuals with HCV risk factors should be screened, including persons who have used any illegal drugs (even if only once); recipients of clotting factors made before 1987 (when inactivation procedures were introduced); patients undergoing hemodialysis; persons with persistently abnormal (even slightly) ALT levels; persons who have been notified that they received blood from an HCV-positive donor; and recipients of any blood transfusion, blood component, or organ transplant before 1992. Persons with clinical hepatitis not due to hepatitis A or hepatitis B should be tested for anti-HCV. Routine screening of all pregnant women is not recommended. Children born to HCV-infected women should be tested for anti-HCV after 12 mo of age by EIA but qualitative PCR can be done in infancy. Neither national nor international adoptees are at increased risk, although adoptees should be tested if the mother was known to be at high risk.

Treatment. Effective therapy to prevent the progression of HCV infection to cirrhosis, liver failure, or hepatocellular cancer is not yet available for the majority of patients. The Food and Drug Administration–approved monotherapy with IFN-α2b has resulted in sustained response in 10–15% of patients, defined as having normal ALT levels and negative PCR results 6 mo after completion of therapy. Combination therapy with interferon and ribavirin has yielded sustained response in about one third of patients and is now considered first-line therapy. Factors associated with improved response include mild liver histopathologic abnormalities, low serum HCV RNA levels, and infection with a genotype other than genotype 1, which is the predominant type in the United States. Preliminary experience with the use of pegylated interferon has demonstrated some improvement over IFN-α2b, but rates of sustained response are still low. Most treatment studies have been done in adults but the limited data in children have shown similar rates of success. Future treatment strategies are likely to include development of more effective protease and helicase inhibitors and drugs that can disrupt the HCV RNA genome.

Complications. The risk of fulminant hepatitis is low with HCV, but the risk of chronic hepatitis is the highest of the hepatotropic viruses. Risk factors for progression to hepatic fibrosis include older age, male sex, and even moderate alcohol ingestion (two 1-oz drinks per day). Infected adults should refrain from using alcohol to prevent additional hepatic injury. Persons infected with HCV should be immunized with hepatitis A and hepatitis B vaccines to minimize further hepatic injury and to reduce the chance for fulminant hepatitis. The usual chronic course is a mild one even when cirrhosis develops; long-term follow-up indicates that the overall mortality of persons with transfusion-acquired HCV is no different from that of noninfected controls.

Prevention. No vaccine is available to prevent HCV. Immunoglobulin has not proved to be of benefit. Immunoglobulin produced in the United States does not contain antibodies to HCV because blood and plasma donors are screened for anti-HCV and excluded from the donor pool.

To minimize transmission, persons with HCV should use condoms, not share toothbrushes or razors, and not donate blood or organs.

HEPATITIS D

Etiology. HDV, the smallest known animal virus, is considered defective because it cannot produce infection without a concurrent HBV infection. The 36-nm-diameter virus is incapable of making its own coat protein; its outer coat is composed of excess HBsAg from HBV. The inner core of the virus is single-stranded circular RNA that expresses the HDV antigen.

Epidemiology. HDV cannot produce infection without HBV as a helper virus. HDV can cause an infection at the same time as the initial HBV infection (co-infection), or HDV can infect a person who is already infected with HBV (superinfection). Transmission usually occurs by intrafamilial or intimate contact in areas of high prevalence, which are primarily developing countries. In areas of low prevalence, such as the United States, the percutaneous route is far more common. HDV infections are uncommon in children in the United States but must be considered when fulminant hepatitis occurs. In the United States, HDV infection is found most frequently in parenteral drug abusers, the developmentally disabled, patients with hemophilia, and persons emigrating from areas that include southern Italy, parts of eastern Europe, South America, Africa, and the Middle East. HDV is uncommon in the Far East, where HBV infection is common. The incubation period for HDV superinfection is about 2–8 wk; with co-infection, the incubation period is similar to that of HBV infection.

Pathogenesis. Liver pathology in HDV hepatitis has no distinguishing features except that damage is usually more severe. In contrast to HBV, HDV causes injury directly by cytopathic mechanisms. Many of the most severe cases of HBV infection appear to be a result of co-infection of HBV and HDV. HDV superinfection of a person who has chronic HBV infection is more common in developed countries.

Clinical Manifestations. The symptoms of hepatitis D infection are similar to but usually more severe than those of the other hepatotropic viruses. The clinical outcome for HDV infection depends on the mechanism of infection. In co-infection, acute hepatitis, which is much more severe than for HBV alone, is common but the risk of developing chronic hepatitis is low. In superinfection, acute illness is rare and chronic hepatitis is common. However, the risk of fulminant hepatitis is highest in superinfection. Hepatitis D should be considered in any child who experiences acute hepatic failure.

Diagnosis. HDV has not been isolated, and no circulating antigen has been identified. The diagnosis is made by detecting IgM antibody to HDV; the antibodies to HDV develop about 2–4 wk after co-infection and about 10 wk after a superinfection. A test for anti-HDV antibody is commercially available. PCR assays for viral RNA are available only as a research tool.

Complications. HDV must be considered in all cases of fulminant hepatitis.

Prevention. There is no vaccine for hepatitis D. However, because HDV replication cannot occur without hepatitis B co-infection, immunization against HBV also prevents HDV infection.

Hepatitis B vaccines and HBIG are used for the same indications as for hepatitis B alone.

HEPATITIS E

Etiology. HEV has not been isolated but has been cloned using molecular techniques. This RNA virus has a nonenveloped sphere shape with spikes and is similar in structure to the caliciviruses.

Epidemiology. Hepatitis E is the epidemic form of what was formally called non-A, non-B hepatitis. Transmission is associated with shedding of 27–34-nm particles in the stool. The highest prevalence of HEV infection has been reported in the Indian subcontinent, the Middle East, Southeast Asia, and Mexico, especially in areas with poor sanitation. In the United States, the only reported cases have been in persons who have visited or emigrated from endemic areas. The mean incubation period is about 40 days (range of 15–60 days).

Pathogenesis. HEV appears to act as a cytopathic virus. The pathologic findings are similar to those of the other hepatitis viruses.

Clinical Manifestations. The clinical illness associated with HEV infection is similar to HAV, the other enterically transmitted virus, but is often more severe. Both viruses produce only acute disease; chronic illness does not occur. In addition to often causing a more severe episode than HAV, HEV affects older patients with a peak age between 15 and 34 yr. Another important clinical difference is that HEV has a high case fatality rate in pregnant women.

Diagnosis. Recombinant DNA technology has resulted in development of antibodies to HEV particles, and IgM and IgG assays are available to distinguish between acute and resolved infections. IgM antibody to viral antigen becomes positive after about 1 wk of illness. Viral RNA can be detected in stool and serum by PCR.

Complications. HEV is associated with a high prevalence of death in pregnant women.

Prevention. No vaccines are available, and no evidence shows that immunoglobulin is effective in preventing HEV infections. However, immunoglobulin pooled from patients in endemic areas may prove to be effective.

HEPATITIS F

In 1994, French researchers reported the isolation of an enteric agent responsible for sporadic cases of non-A-E hepatitis and named the virus hepatitis F (HFV), for hepatitis French virus. However, their findings have not been confirmed by others and the term HFV is currently unclaimed.

HEPATITIS G

Etiology. Hepatitis G virus (HGV), which includes HGV and GBV-C virus, was identified by PCR of the plasma of a patient with chronic hepatitis. HGV is a single-stranded RNA virus that is included in the Flaviviridae family and shares a 27% homology with HCV. The virus has not yet been isolated, but PCR testing indicates that it has a worldwide distribution and can cause chronic infection and viremia.

Epidemiology. HGV has been reported in adults and children from all population groups, and GBV-C RNA is found in about 1.5% of blood donors and 15–20% of injection drug users in the United States. Even higher rates are found when serologic testing is used. Infection is found in many patients with HIV and has been reported in 10–20% of adults with chronic hepatitis B and hepatitis C, indicating that co-infection is a common occurrence. The primary route of spread is thought to be through transfusions, but HGV also can be transmitted by organ transplantation. Other important risk factors for infection include injection drug use, hemodialysis, and homosexual and bisexual relationships, indicating that sexual transmission also occurs. Vertical transmission also may occur.

Pathogenesis. Most infected persons have evidence of persistent viremia, but histologic evidence of HGV infection is rare and ALT values usually are normal. To date, little evidence shows that infections with HGV cause symptomatic disease. The detection of HGV in lymphocytes suggests that the virus may behave biologically like Epstein-Barr virus or CMV. No cases of chronic hepatitis have developed in patients infected with HGV alone.

Clinical Manifestations. HGV accounts for only a small proportion of cases of non-A-E hepatitis. Most HGV infections are not associated with hepatic inflammation, and co-infection does not seem to worsen the course of concurrent HBV or HCV infection. Because the virus is distributed so widely and is associated with only mild or no disease, it is not yet clear whether HGV is a pathogen.

Diagnosis. The only diagnostic tests for HGV infection are PCR assays used to detect HGV RNA. Development of serologic tests will greatly improve our understanding of this virus.

Complications. No conclusive evidence shows that HGV causes fulminant or chronic disease. Recent data indicate that patients infected with both HIV and GBV-C have a more favorable prognosis and delayed development of AIDS.

Prevention. There is currently no method to prevent infection with HGV.

339.1 Hepatitis in Neonates

Various infectious agents have been implicated in hepatic inflammation in neonates, including bacterial and viral pathogens. Hepatitis in neonates due to specific causes usually is distinguished from the term *neonatal hepatitis*, which has been used to designate hepatic inflammation of unknown cause.

Etiology. The six hepatotropic viruses that cause hepatitis as their primary disease manifestation rarely cause clinical hepatitis in neonates. Transplacental and perinatal transmission of HAV, HDV, and HEV is rare. The greatest risk of perinatal transmission of any hepatotropic virus occurs with HBV, but almost all neonates infected with HBV are asymptomatic. Perinatal transmission rarely is associated with HCV, but the risk is increased in neonates of HIV-infected mothers or mothers with high titers of HCV; symptomatic infection is rare. HGV infection has been reported in neonates, but clinical illness has not been associated with infection.

Most cases of neonatal hepatitis are a result of systemic disease. Sepsis caused by systemic and extrahepatic bacterial and viral infections must always be considered when hepatitis is present in a newborn infant. Gram-negative bacterial infections are especially important causes of sepsis in newborn infants and require immediate, appropriate therapy. The pathogenesis of hepatic involvement is not understood completely, but the cholestatic effects of bacterial endotoxins appear to have an important role. Sepsis caused by gram-positive organisms and viruses can also be associated with hepatitis. In most infants, bilirubin elevation, predominantly conjugated, is of much greater magnitude than that of the aminotransferases. Syphilis also causes neonatal hepatitis.

Many other viruses, including enteroviruses, CMV, HSV, and HIV, must be considered in the etiology of neonatal hepatitis. Hepatitis associated with these viruses occurs as part of a systemic illness. Nonviral infectious causes of hepatitis in neonates include congenital syphilis and congenital toxoplasmosis.

Clinical Manifestations. Hepatitis in neonates may be characterized by jaundice, vomiting, poor feeding, and elevated hepatic enzyme levels. When infection is caused by an organism other than one of the six hepatotropic viruses, evidence of diffuse illness usually is present and may involve the skin, central nervous, cardiorespiratory, and musculoskeletal systems. A spectrum of illness, ranging from mild to fulminant disease, can occur with any of the infecting agents listed. Fulminant hepatitis is characterized by rapid progression to very high hepatic enzyme levels, decreased production of coagulation proteins, elevated serum ammonia level, shock, coma, or death. The levels of the serum bilirubin and aminotransferase levels are poor predictors of outcome. Because of the short half-life of the coagulation proteins, the PT is the best prognostic indicator.

HBV, the most common hepatotropic virus that infects neonates, usually results in an asymptomatic infection. The most common sequence of events is for an infant to have no clinical evidence of disease and to become chronically infected and positive for HBsAg. These children often have normal or only mildly abnormal hepatic enzyme values. Liver biopsy findings may be normal initially, but chronic infection can lead to cirrhosis usually in the 3rd to 4th decades of life, greatly increasing the risk of developing primary hepatocellular carcinoma.

The differential diagnosis of hepatitis in neonates must include infectious causes, many of which are treatable, and non-infectious causes including anatomic (e.g., intrahepatic and extrahepatic biliary atresia and choledochal cyst), metabolic (e.g., cystic fibrosis, disorders of bile acid metabolism, galactosemia, tyrosinosis, and α_1-antitrypsin deficiency), and toxic (e.g., drugs, hyperalimentation) disorders.

Treatment. In addition to effective antimicrobial therapy for bacteria-associated hepatitis, acyclovir is effective against HSV and varicella virus, and ganciclovir and foscarnet can be used to treat CMV infections. Pleconaril is effective against enteroviruses.

Prevention. Women should be tested for HBsAg during routine prenatal care, and infants born to women who are HBsAg positive should receive hepatitis B vaccine and HBIG (see Table 339–4) within 12 hr of birth. Additional doses of vaccine are administered 1–2 mo and 6 mo of age. Hepatitis B vaccine should be administered to all other infants, beginning in the first 2 mo of life. After administration of the first dose to infants born to HBsAg-negative mothers, the second dose should be administered at least 1 mo after the first dose, and the third dose at least 4 months after the first dose and at least 2 months after the second dose and not before 6 months of age. Routine postvaccination testing of infants to determine the presence of anti-HBs is not recommended. However, testing is advised 1–2 mo after the third vaccine dose for infants born to HBsAg-positive mothers.

Aach RD, Yomatovian RA, Hack M: Neonatal and pediatric posttransfusion hepatitis C: A look back and a look forward. *Pediatrics* 2000;105:836–42.

Abiad H, Ramani R, Currie JB, et al: The natural history of hepatitis D virus infection in Illinois state facilities for the developmentally disabled. *Am J Gastroenterol* 2001;96:534–40.

Alter MJ, Gallagher M, Morris TT, et al: Acute non-A-E hepatitis in the United States and the role of hepatitis G virus infection. Sentinel counties viral hepatitis study team. *N Engl J Med* 1997;336:741–6.

Alter MJ, Kruszon-Moran D, Nainan OV, et al: The prevalence of hepatitis C virus infection in the United States, 1988 through 1994. *N Engl J Med* 1999;341:556–62.

Alter MJ, Mast EE: The epidemiology of viral hepatitis in the United States. *Gastroenterol Clin North Am* 1994;23:437–55.

American Academy of Pediatrics Committee on Infectious Diseases: Prevention of hepatitis A infections: Guidelines for use of hepatitis A vaccine and immune globulin. *Pediatrics* 1996;98:1207–15.

American Academy of Pediatrics Committee on Infectious Diseases: Hepatitis C virus infection. *Pediatrics* 1998;101:481–5.

Armstrong G, Alter MJ, McQuillan GM, et al: The past incidence of hepatitis C virus infection: Implications for the future burden of chronic liver disease in the United States. *Hepatology* 2000;31:777–82.

Centers for Disease Control and Prevention: Recommendations for prevention and control of hepatitis C virus (HCV) infection and HCV-related chronic disease. *MMWR Morb Mortal Wkly Rep* 1998;47:1–39.

Fishman LN, Jonas MM, Lavine JE: Update on viral hepatitis in children. *Pediatr Clin North Am* 1996;43:57–74.

Francavilla R, Mieli-Vergani G: Treatment of hepatitis C virus infection in children. *Can J Gastroenterol* 2000;14:41B–4B.

Hochman JA, Balistreri WF: Viral hepatitis: Expanding the alphabet. *Adv Pediatr* 1999;46:207–43.

Hoofnagle JH, di Bisceglie AM: The treatment of chronic viral hepatitis. *N Engl J Med* 1997;336:347–56.

Hutin YJ, Pool V, Cramer EH, et al: A multistate, foodborne outbreak of hepatitis A. National Hepatitis A Investigation Team. *N Engl J Med* 1999;340:595–602.

Jacobs RJ, Margolis HS, Coleman PJ: The cost-effectiveness of adolescent hepatitis A vaccination in states with the highest disease rates. *Arch Pediatr Adolesc Med* 2000;154:763–70.

Lee WM: Hepatitis B virus infection. *N Engl J Med* 1997;337:1733–45.

McHutchison JG, Gordon SC, Schiff ER, et al: Interferon alfa-2b alone or in combination with ribavirin as initial treatment for chronic hepatitis C. Hepatitis Interventional Therapy Group. *N Engl J Med* 1998;339:1485–92.

Ohto H, Terazawa S, Sasaki N, et al: Transmission of hepatitis C virus from mothers to infants. *N Engl J Med* 1994;330:744–50.

Pianko S, McHutchison J: Chronic hepatitis B: New therapies on the horizon? *Lancet* 1999;354:1662–3.

Polish LB, Gallagher M, Fields HA, et al: Delta hepatitis: Molecular biology and clinical and epidemiological features. *Clin Microbiol Rev* 1993;6:211–29.

Rizetto M, Durazzo M: Hepatitis delta virus (HDV) infections: Epidemiological and clinical heterogeneity. *J Hepatol* 1991;13:S116–8.

Rosenberg, PM. Hepatitis C: Hepatologist's approach to an infectious disease. *Clin Infect Dis* 2001;33:1728–32.

Shamoun DK, Anania FA: Which patients with hepatitis C virus should be treated? *Semin Gastrointest Dis* 2000;11:84–95.

Sjogren MH: Serologic diagnosis of viral hepatitis. *Med Clin North Am* 1996;80:929–56.

Thomas DL, Astemborski J, Rai RM, et al: The natural history of hepatitis C virus infection: Host, viral, and environmental factors. *JAMA* 2000;284:450–6.

Tung J, Hadzic N, Layton M, et al: Bone marrow failure in children with acute liver failure. *J Pediatr Gastroenterol Nutr* 2000;31:557–61.

Wilson ME: Travel-related vaccines. *Infect Dis Clin North Am* 2001;15:231–51.

Zwiener RJ, Fielman BA, Cochran C, et al: Interferon-α-2b treatment of chronic hepatitis C in children with hemophilia. *Pediatr Infect Dis J* 1996;15:906–8.

Chapter 340
Liver Abscess
Jeffrey Schwimmer and William F. Balistreri

Hepatic abscesses occur in infants in association with sepsis, umbilical vein infection, or vessel cannulation. Beyond infancy, hepatic abscesses occur most commonly in immunosuppressed patients. Of a large series of hepatic abscesses, 40% were found in patients with chronic granulomatous disease, and 20% in otherwise immunosuppressed patients (e.g., leukemia). Pyogenic hepatic abscesses may arise from the portal circulation in patients with pylephlebitis or intra-abdominal sepsis (appendicitis, inflammatory bowel disease) or generalized sepsis; cholangitis associated with biliary tract obstruction, such as by gallstones, in inflammatory bowel disease, after a Kasai procedure, and with choledochal cysts; systemic spread from an intra-abdominal infection or contiguous spread, which usually produces large abscesses; and cryptogenic biliary tract infections. Small abscesses (microabscesses) are most commonly secondary to bacteremia, candidemia, or cat-scratch disease. Implicated organisms include predominantly *Staphylococcus aureus*, *Escherichia coli*, *Salmonella*, and anaerobic organisms. Symptoms are nonspecific and may suggest systemic infection. Patients may have fever and pain in the right upper quadrant, and the liver is enlarged and may be tender to percussion. Jaundice is uncommon; serum aminotransferase and alkaline phosphatase levels may be mildly elevated. The erythrocyte sedimentation rate is high, and leukocytosis is noted. The results of blood cultures are not always positive. Roentgenographic study of the chest may show elevation of the right hemidiaphragm with decreased mobility. Ultrasound or nuclear scans or both may indicate the site of the abscess. In most cases, treatment requires percutaneous ultrasonogram- or CT-guided needle aspiration or surgical drainage. Antibiotic therapy is based on the culture results and Gram stain of the abscess fluid. *Entamoeba histolytica* may also cause hepatic abscesses in symptomatic or asymptomatic patients with amebic infection of the gastrointestinal tract. Multiple infectious hepatic (and/or splenic) granulomas may be seen with cat scratch disease or fungi.

Chambon M, Delage C, Bailly JL, et al: Fatal hepatic necrosis in a neonate with echovirus 20 infection: Use of the polymerase chain reaction to detect enterovirus in liver tissue. *Clin Infect Dis* 1997;24:523.
Pineiro-Carrero VM, Andres JM: Morbidity and mortality in children with pyogenic liver abscess. *Am J Dis Child* 1989;143:1424.

Chapter 341
Liver Disease Associated with Systemic Disorders

Jeffrey Schwimmer and William F. Balistreri

Inflammatory Bowel Disease (IBD). Hepatobiliary disease may complicate ulcerative colitis and Crohn disease (see Chapter 317). Both the manifestations and the severity vary. Fatty liver, cholangitis, drug-induced injury, chronic hepatitis, portal fibrosis, cirrhosis, hepatic abscesses, infarction, portal vein thrombosis, sclerosing cholangitis, carcinoma of the biliary tract, and cholelithiasis all have been associated with IBD. These complications are more likely to occur in patients with other extraintestinal complications, but there is no correlation with the severity of the IBD. The cause of abnormalities in liver function in patients with ulcerative colitis or Crohn disease is unknown. Total colectomy has not been beneficial in preventing or managing hepatobiliary complications in patients with ulcerative colitis.

Extensive fatty change in the liver has been found, especially in malnourished or chronically incapacitated patients with IBD. Most patients have no symptoms; hepatomegaly is the only sign. The chemical abnormalities are mild. The fatty infiltration usually subsides with therapy.

Sclerosing cholangitis may be difficult to distinguish from chronic hepatitis in patients with inflammatory bowel disease. Patients may be asymptomatic or may have jaundice, pruritus, or abdominal pain. Elevation of alkaline serum phosphatase (ALP), 5′-nucleotidase, or γ-glutamyltransferase activities is almost universal. This complication can occur any time in the course of IBD. Sclerosing cholangitis (fibrosing inflammation of various segments of the bile ducts) may lead to obliteration of the duct lumen. The clinical and biochemical picture is that of cholestasis, often with intermittent attacks of acute cholangitis (fever, jaundice, right upper quadrant pain, anorexia, weight loss, and pruritus), followed by portal hypertension. This complication occurs in 1–3% of patients with ulcerative colitis and Crohn disease.

Primary sclerosing cholangitis (not associated with inflammatory bowel disease) is uncommon in children. Cholangiography reveals beading and irregularity of the intrahepatic and extrahepatic bile ducts. Treatment is aimed at improving biliary drainage and attempting to halt progression of the obliterative process. Symptomatic treatment is required for such complications as pruritus, malnutrition, and infection. There is no definitive treatment. Ursodeoxycholic acid, in a dose of 15 mg/kg/ 24 hr, may lead to amelioration of pruritus and a decrease in abnormal biochemical values. Oral vancomycin may also improve serum ALT and GGT. The course is usually slowly progressive to a fatal outcome if liver transplantation is not carried out.

Bacterial Sepsis. (See Chapters 98 and 163.) Sepsis may be complicated by liver disease. The most frequently associated organisms are *Escherichia coli*, *Klebsiella pneumoniae*, and *Pseudomonas aeruginosa*. It is postulated that bacterial endotoxin directly inhibits bile formation by altering the structure or function of bile canalicular membrane. Clinical manifestations may be subtle and difficult to differentiate from other causes of cholestasis. The serum bilirubin level is elevated, usually predominantly in the conjugated fraction. Serum ALP and aminotransferase activities may be elevated. Liver biopsy shows intrahepatic cholestasis with little or no hepatocyte necrosis. Kupffer cell hyperplasia and an increase in inflammatory cells are also common. Similar findings may occur with urosepsis.

Cardiac Disease. Hepatic congestion and injury may occur as a complication of severe *chronic* or *acute congestive heart failure* (Chapter 434) or *cyanotic heart disease* (Chapters 422–424). Hepatic dysfunction derives from hypoxemia, systemic venous congestion, and low cardiac output. Hepatic manifestations of left-and right-sided heart failure are similar. With decreased cardiac output, there is decreased hepatic blood flow and centrizonal hypoxia. Hepatic necrosis leads to lactic acidosis, elevated aminotransferase activities, jaundice, prolonged partial thromboplastin time, and possibly hypoglycemia. With right-sided heart failure, increases in right atrial and hepatic venous pressures lead to centrizonal sinusoidal distention that presents a barrier to oxygen diffusion. Hemorrhage, pressure atrophy, and necrosis follow. Jaundice and tender hepatomegaly occur. Ascites may also occur with chronic right-sided congestive heart failure. In patients with shock liver, elevated aminotransferase activities may return rapidly to normal when perfusion and cardiac function improve. A syndrome of acute liver failure may occur, particularly in patients with aortic coarctation. Hepatic necrosis may be found in patients with hypoplastic left-sided heart syndrome.

Hemoglobinopathies. Patients with *sickle cell anemia* (Chapter 454.1) or *sickle cell thalassemia* (Chapter 454.1) may have hepatic dysfunction owing to acute or chronic virus-associated hepatitis, iron overload, hepatic crises related to severe intrahepatic cholestasis, sequestration, and ischemic necrosis. In addition, cholelithiasis and a benign form of extreme hyperbilirubinemia have been noted. Hepatic sickle cell crisis or "sickle hepatopathy" may produce intense right upper quadrant pain, fever, leukocytosis, right upper quadrant tenderness, and jaundice. Bilirubin levels may be markedly elevated; serum ALP levels may be only moderately elevated.

On occasion, children with sickle cell disease experience bilirubin levels exceeding 20 mg/dL; these levels are unaccompanied by severe pain or fever. There is no change in hematocrit or reticulocyte count nor any association with a hemolytic crisis. The clinical course is benign.

Cholestasis Associated with Total Parenteral Nutrition. The most common metabolic complication of *total parenteral nutrition* (TPN) in premature infants is the development of various degrees of liver dysfunction. Cholestasis is the most severe form and is potentially fatal. It is the major factor limiting effective long-term use of TPN (Chapter 91.3).

In *low birthweight infants*, the incidence of TPN-associated cholestasis is inversely correlated with birthweight. It develops with TPN in almost half of infants with birthweights less than 1,000 g, in 20% of those 1,000–1,500 g, and in 5–10% of those 1,500–2,000 g. The incidence of cholestasis also correlates with the duration of TPN, with onset usually after 2 wk. Respiratory distress, acidosis, hypoxia, necrotizing enterocolitis, short-bowel syndrome, and sepsis enhance the likelihood and severity of cholestasis. Associated illness, the exclusion of enteral intake, and the nature of the underlying disorder that necessitates TPN may also affect the incidence.

The onset is usually insidious, with progressive jaundice and hepatic enlargement or splenomegaly. In low birthweight infants, the onset of jaundice may overlap the phase of physiologic unconjugated hyperbilirubinemia. Any icteric infant who has received TPN for more than 1 wk should have all bilirubin determinations fractionated. Cholestasis is frequently first detected through routine monitoring of infants receiving TPN. A slow progression of abnormalities is found in biochemical measurements of hepatic function. Serum bile acid concentrations may increase. Rises in serum aminotransferase activities may be a late finding. An elevation in serum ALP activity may be due to rickets, a common complication of TPN in low birthweight infants.

In addition to cholestasis, biliary complications of intravenous nutrition include cholelithiasis and the development of biliary sludge, associated with thick, inspissated gallbladder contents. These may be asymptomatic.

An effort must be made to differentiate TPN-associated hepatic dysfunction from benign causes of hepatomegaly, such as the deposition of glycogen or fat, which is common with TPN. Serum bilirubin and bile acid levels remain within the normal range in the latter situation. Consideration of other causes of cholestasis is also appropriate. The group in which TPN-associated cholestasis most frequently occurs (i.e., infants in a neonatal intensive care unit) often receives blood products or drugs. Therefore, hepatic disease related to drug-induced liver disease is a consideration.

The most striking histologic finding in TPN-associated liver disease is canalicular cholestasis, which may begin after less than 2 wk of TPN. Bile duct proliferation may resemble that seen in patients with biliary atresia. Portal fibrosis is a late finding. Progression of injury to cirrhosis is possible. Milder changes may be reversible with discontinuation of TPN and initiation of oral feedings.

The pathogenesis of TPN-associated cholestasis is most likely multifactorial. Affected infants are of low birthweight, are receiving nothing by mouth, may have significant gastrointestinal disease, and often have other systemic complications. The administered nutrient solution has potential toxicity and may induce specific deficiencies. The omission of oral feedings and the absence of intraluminal nutrients blunt the output of the gastrointestinal hormones, which are normal stimulants to bile flow and to development of the hepatobiliary system. Potential hepatotoxins include bacterial endotoxins, specific amino acids or metabolic or degradation products, aluminum, copper, or manganese; the last two are particularly hepatotoxic.

The goal in treatment of infants with TPN-associated cholestasis is to avoid progressive liver injury. The administration of oral feedings will produce gradual resolution of the liver disease. Initiation of oral feedings of small volume or infusion of nutrients by continuous nasogastric drip may enhance biliary flow and intestinal motility while reducing bacterial translocation. This effect may occur even when the enteral intake does not provide the total caloric needs. Improved solutions that meet the specific needs of neonates may prevent deficiencies and avoid toxicities. In the decision to continue TPN, one must weigh the risk of further hepatic injury against the risk of malnutrition.

In *older children,* TPN-associated cholestasis is less common and less severe than in infants. Hepatic steatosis without cholestasis is often the only abnormality. However, biochemical abnormalities are not uncommon in older patients who are maintained on TPN for prolonged periods, either at home or in the hospital. Patients with chronic intestinal disease, which may be complicated by infection or bacterial overgrowth, are particularly susceptible to hepatic dysfunction. In most such patients, partial enteral alimentation reverses the abnormalities. It may be necessary at any age, when serum ALP or aminotransferase levels are elevated, to evaluate the underlying liver disease by liver biopsy.

Bone Marrow Transplantation. Hepatic dysfunction is common in patients who have undergone *bone marrow transplantation.* The genesis is multifactorial and may be related to: (1) infections (viral, bacterial, or fungal), drugs, parenteral nutrition, chemotherapy, or radiation; (2) veno-occlusive disease (VOD); or (3) graft versus host disease (GVHD); or any combination of these. Candidates for bone marrow transplantation have often had pre-existing liver disease, such as viral hepatitis, drug-related injury, or malignant infiltration. Percutaneous liver biopsy in such patients may show extensive bile duct injury in GVHD, viral inclusions in cytomegalovirus disease, or the characteristic endothelial lesion in VOD; the histologic distinction is often unclear. This presents a dilemma because treatment of one suspected complication (e.g., initiation of immunosuppressive therapy for GVHD) may have a deleterious effect if the symptoms are due to another (e.g., fungal or viral infection).

VOD of the liver usually has its onset 1–3 wk after bone marrow transplantation but may appear up to 6 wk afterward. The most characteristic presentation is onset of rapid weight gain, with ascites, hepatomegaly, right upper quadrant pain, jaundice, and oliguria. Hepatic encephalopathy and fulminant hepatic failure may follow. Less severe forms may be characterized by jaundice and ascites with a slow resolution; a mild form of VOD has histologic changes as the sole manifestation. The diagnosis rests on the exclusion of other diseases, such as congestive cardiomyopathy, constrictive pericarditis, and venous thrombosis (Budd-Chiari syndrome).

Pathologic changes in patients with VOD are best demonstrated using special (trichrome) stains to highlight the central veins. An early lesion is concentric narrowing of the lumina of small central veins, owing to edema in the subendothelial zone. There is a dense, wavy continuous band of collagen in the central veins and centrilobular hemorrhagic necrosis. The lesions may be patchy. The venular changes may progress to complete obliteration. The cause of VOD following bone marrow transplantation is not clear; it may be related to radiation, antineoplastic drugs, or both. Risk factors for VOD include high-dose conditioning regimens, leukemia, advanced age, and pre-existing liver disease.

Budd-Chiari syndrome involves occlusion of the inferior vena cava or hepatic veins and tributaries; it may be caused by obstruction resulting from a web, mass, or thrombus. The disease has rarely been noted in children. Risk factors include trauma, coagulopathies, sickle cell anemia, leukemia, polycythemia vera, hepatic abscesses, irradiation, and GVHD. The syndrome is to be regarded as distinct from VOD, which affects the centrilobular and sublobular hepatic veins, sparing the larger veins; it is not associated with thrombosis.

GVHD of the liver may be acute or chronic and is generally concomitant with GVHD in other target organs (Chapter 127). Cholestasis and hepatic injury of various degrees occur; there may be hepatic tenderness, dark urine, acholic stools, itching, and anorexia. There are parallel rises in the serum bilirubin level and the ALP activity; aspartate aminotransaminase elevation is less striking. GVHD is characterized histologically by degeneration and loss of small bile ducts and sparse inflammation, along with cholestasis.

Collagen Vascular Disease. Hepatic involvement in patients with *collagen vascular disease* is uncommon. It has been noted especially in patients with systemic lupus erythematosus. Reactive hepatitis, chronic hepatitis, steatosis, and hepatic infarction have also been described. The association of hepatic injury with drug therapy, such as salicylate use, must be differentiated.

Obesity. Nonalcoholic steatohepatitis (NASH) is a chronic condition of the liver, seen in obese patients, characterized by fatty infiltration, inflammation and fibrosis in an individual with little or no exposure to ethanol. See Chapter 338.

Balistreri WF: The liver—the next frontier in the treatment of patients with cystic fibrosis. In Reyes HB, Leuschner U, Arias I (editors): *Pregnancy, Sex Hormones, and the Liver. Proceedings of the 89th Falk Symposium.* Lancaster, UK, Kluwer Academic Publishers, 1996, pp 114–135.

Buchanan GR, Glader BE: Benign course of extreme hyperbilirubinemia in sickle cell anemia: Analysis of six cases. *J Pediatr* 1977;91:21.

Cohen JA, Kaplan MM: Left sided heart failure presenting as hepatitis. *Gastroenterology* 1978;74:583.

Colombo C, Battezzati PM, Podda M, et al: Ursodeoxycholic acid for liver disease associated with cystic fibrosis: A double-blind multicenter trial. *Hepatology* 1996;23:1484.

Duthie A, Doherty DG, Donaldson PT, et al: The major histocompatibility complex influences the development of chronic liver disease in male children and young adults with cystic fibrosis. *J Hepatol* 1995;23:532.

El-Shabrawi M, Wilkinson ML, Portmann B, et al: Primary sclerosing cholangitis in childhood. *Gastroenterology* 1987;92:1226.

Gentile-Kocher S, Bernard O, Brunnelle F, et al: Budd Chiari syndrome in children: Report of 22 cases. *J Pediatr* 1988;113:30.

Hofmann AF: Defective biliary secretion during total parenteral nutrition: Probable mechanisms and possible solutions. *J Pediatr Gastroenterol Nutr* 1995;20:376.

Kawasaki T, Hashimoto N, Kikuchi T, et al: The relationship between fatty liver and hyperinsulinemia in obese Japanese children. *J Pediatr Gastroenterol Nutr* 1997;24:317.

Lavine JE: Vitamin E treatment of nonalcoholic steatohepatitis in children: A pilot study. *J Pediatr* 2000;136:734–8.

McDonald GB, Sharma P, Matthews DE, et al: Veno-occlusive disease of the liver after bone marrow transplantation: Diagnosis, incidence, and predisposing factors. *Hepatology* 1984;4:116.

Moseley RH: Sepsis-associated cholestasis. *Gastroenterology* 1997;112:302.

Mullick FG, Moran CA, Ishak KG: Total parenteral nutrition: A histopathologic analysis of the liver changes in 20 children. *Mod Pathol* 1994;7:190.

Narkewicz MR, Sokol RJ, Beckwith B, et al: Liver involvement in Alpers disease. *J Pediatr* 1991;119:260.

Nemeth A, Ejderhamm J, Glaumann H, et al: Liver damage in juvenile inflammatory bowel disease. *Liver* 1990;10:239.

Sale GE, Shulman HM: Liver disease after marrow transplantation. In Sale GE, Shulman HM (editors): *The Pathology of Bone Marrow Transplantation.* Chicago, Year Book Medical Publishers, 1984.

Sisto A, Feldman P, Garel L, et al: Primary sclerosing cholangitis in children: Study of five cases and review of the literature. *Pediatrics* 1987;80:818.

Snover DC, Weisdorf SA, Ramsay NK, et al: Hepatic graft-versus-host disease: A study of the predictive value of the liver biopsy in diagnosis. *Hepatology* 1984;4:123.

Strauss RS, Barlow SE, Dietz WH: Prevalence of abnormal serum aminotransferase values in overweight and obese adolescents. *J Pediatr* 2000;136:727.

Chapter 342

Reye Syndrome and the Mitochondrial Hepatopathies

Jeffrey A. Rudolph and William F. Balistreri

Reye syndrome is characterized by acute encephalopathy and fatty degeneration of the liver. Investigation of this syndrome has uncovered a wide variety of previously undefined metabolic diseases whose clinical picture is similar and need to be considered in the differential diagnosis (Box 342–1). The pathophysiology involves generalized loss of mitochondrial function, leading to disturbances in fatty acid and carnitine metabolism. There is an entire class of mitochondrial hepatopathies—inherited disorders that are characterized by defects in fatty acid oxidation, oxidative phosphorylation, and general mitochondrial dysfunction.

BOX 342–1. Diseases That Present a Clinical/Pathologic Picture Resembling Reye Syndrome

Metabolic disease

- Organic acidurias
- Disorders of oxidative phosphorylation
- Urea cycle defects (carbamoyl phosphate synthetase, ornithine transcarbamylase)
- Defects in fatty acid oxidation metabolism
- Acyl-CoA dehydrogenase deficiencies
- Systemic carnitine deficiency
- Hepatic carnitine palmitoyltransferase deficiency
- 3-OH, 3-methylglutaryl-CoA lyase deficiency
- Fructosemia

Central nervous system infections or intoxications (meningitis, encephalitis, toxic encephalopathy)
Hemorrhagic shock with encephalopathy
Drug or toxin ingestion (salicylate, valproate)

CoA = coenzyme A.

"CLASSIC" REYE SYNDROME

Epidemiology. Case reports of Reye syndrome were sporadic until 1974, when almost 400 cases were reported in the United States, with a mortality rate of more than 40%. The incidence was increased in direct temporal and geographic relationship to viral epidemics, especially those caused by influenza B and varicella. By 1988, the incidence had declined dramatically; only 20 cases were reported; today this disorder is rare.

Reye syndrome presented most commonly at approximately 6 yr of age, with most cases in the 4–12-yr age range. There was no gender difference in incidence, but rural and suburban populations appeared to be more frequently affected than urban populations. It is very likely that mild cases were missed and that patients recovered without event. In the late 1970s, Reye syndrome was the most common potentially lethal virus-associated encephalopathy in the United States.

Clinical Manifestations. Classic Reye syndrome exhibits a stereotypic, biphasic course. It usually occurs in a previously healthy child. A prodromal febrile illness, an upper respiratory tract infection (in 90% of the cases), or chickenpox (in 5–7%) is followed by an interval in which the child has seemingly recovered. The abrupt onset of protracted vomiting then occurs, usually within 5–7 days after the onset of the viral illness. Delirium, combative behavior, and stupor may occur simultaneously or within a few hours after the onset of vomiting. Neurologic symptoms may rapidly progress to seizures, coma, and death; focal neurologic signs are absent. The clinical features are best reflected in the system of clinical staging that has been proposed (Box 342–2); grades I through III represent mild to moderate illness and grades IV and V represent severe illness. The majority of affected children have mild illness without

---

BOX 342–2. Clinical Staging of Reye Syndrome

SYMPTOMS AT TIME OF ADMISSION

I. Usually quiet, **lethargic** and sleepy, vomiting, laboratory evidence of liver dysfunction

II. Deep lethargy, **confusion,** delirium, combative, hyperventilation, hyper-reflexic

III. Obtunded, **light coma** ± seizures, decorticate rigidity, intact pupillary light reaction

IV. Seizures, deepening coma, **decerebrate rigidity,** loss of oculocephalic reflexes, fixed pupils

V. Coma, loss of deep tendon reflexes, respiratory arrest, fixed dilated pupils, **flaccidity/decerebrate** (intermittent); isoelectric electroencephalogram

progression. There is a slight to moderate liver enlargement with abnormalities of hepatic function; patients remain anicteric. Cerebrospinal fluid (CSF) is normal except for elevated pressure.

Diagnosis. There is explosive release from liver and muscle of such enzymes as aminotransferases, creatine kinase, and lactic dehydrogenase. The activity of the mitochondrial enzyme serum glutamate dehydrogenase is greatly increased. Patients who are not in coma but who have a threefold or higher elevation in serum ammonia level are more likely to progress to coma, as are patients who have hypoprothrombinemia unresponsive to vitamin K. Younger patients may have hypoglycemia; however, these patients should be carefully screened for the presence of metabolic disease (see Box 342–1).

Pathology. The striking and characteristic gross pathologic feature of Reye syndrome is a yellow to white liver, reflective of a high content of triglyceride. Light microscopy shows a uniform foaminess of liver cell cytoplasm with microvesicular fatty accumulation, which may be concealed in routine preparations. Electron microscopic changes include a unique alteration of mitochondrial morphology. At present, biopsy should be carried out to rule out metabolic or toxic liver disease, especially in patients younger than 1–2 yr. Histologic examination of brain tissue reveals a similar pattern of injury; grossly, marked edema is noted.

Pathogenesis. The major site of injury is the mitochondria. The activities of hepatic intramitochondrial enzymes, including ornithine transcarbamylase (OTC), carbamoylphosphate synthetase (CPS), and pyruvate dehydrogenase, are reduced, often to less than half of their normal values. Hyperammonemia may result from acquired decreases in the activities of OTC and CPS.

The reasons for mitochondrial dysfunction are unknown. No toxic factor has yet been conclusively identified, but studies have suggested an etiologic link among Reye syndrome; the use of aspirin and/or anti-emetics, and viral infections. **It is prudent to avoid the use of aspirin as an antipyretic in pediatric patients with influenza or varicella.**

Treatment. Successful management of Reye syndrome requires precise diagnostic evaluation to preclude disorders resembling Reye syndrome; those disorders, which are more likely to be encountered, include defects in fatty acid oxidation, oxidative phosphorylation, and other metabolic injuries presenting as acute liver failure (see Box 342–1). Control of increased intracranial pressure (ICP) secondary to cerebral edema is also imperative since this is the major lethal factor.

Early diagnosis may be aided by a high level of clinical suspicion and by assessment of hepatic function in suspected cases. Marked elevation of serum aminotransferase levels, prolongation of prothrombin time, and elevation of the serum ammonia level suggest the diagnosis. It is imperative that cerebral edema is identified and counteracted and that aerobic metabolism is maintained.

Management varies with the severity of the illness. Whereas observation alone may suffice in patients with grade I severity, more aggressive therapy is needed in patients with more severe neurologic deterioration. All patients should initially receive glucose (10–15%) intravenously, because glycogen depletion is common. In patients with cerebral edema, the amount of fluid administered should be restricted to approximately 1500 mL/m^2 day. Hyperthermia should be avoided. Coagulopathy is managed with vitamin K, fresh frozen plasma, and platelet transfusions.

In more severely ill, comatose patients, endotracheal intubation permits adequate oxygenation; hyperventilation induces hypocarbia, which decreases cerebral blood flow by cerebral vasoconstriction. Close monitoring of ICP assists in decisions about management. Stimulation of patients should be minimized because procedures such as suctioning may generate increases in ICP.

An indwelling arterial catheter permits continuous assessment of cerebral perfusion pressure. The ICP should be held to less than 20 mm Hg and the cerebral perfusion pressure to greater than 50 mm Hg. Pressure (CSF) monitoring provides an effective guide to therapy. Pentobarbital (2.5 mg/kg) to maintain a serum barbiturate level of 20–30 μg/mL may have a protective effect on the central nervous system by decreasing cerebral metabolic demands, decreasing cerebral blood flow, and causing cerebral vasoconstriction. Excessive pentobarbital may reduce cardiac function, lowering blood pressure and, therefore, cerebral perfusion pressure. Orthotopic liver transplantation is not indicated due to the reversible nature of the liver pathology.

Prognosis. The duration of disordered cerebral function during the acute stage of illness is the best predictor of eventual outcome. In patients with grade I disease, recovery is rapid and complete. In patients with more severe disease there may be subsequent subtle neuropsychologic defects noted (in intelligence, school achievement, visuomotor integration, and concept formation).

THE MITOCHONDRIAL HEPATOPATHIES

With the advances in the identification and diagnosis of specific enzyme defects in complex metabolic disease, there has been increasing recognition that functional alterations in the mitochondria, organelles responsible for the production of cellular energy, can lead to disease. The hepatocytes, rich in mitochondria due to the energy required for the process of metabolism, are a target organ for this type of disease. The mitochondrial hepatopathies can be roughly divided into three categories: disorders of fatty acid oxidation (see Chapter 75), disorders of oxidative phosphorylation, and the mitochondrial depletion syndromes.

Disorders of Oxidative Phosphorylation

Oxidative phosphorylation (OXPHOS) includes the oxidation of fuel molecules by oxygen and the concomitant energy transduction into adenosine triphosphate. During the oxidation process, reducing equivalents are transferred from respiratory substrates to oxygen with the resultant production of ATP via five multienzyme complexes: reduced nicotinamide-adenine dinucleotide (NAD) coenzyme Q reductase (*complex I*), coenzyme Q succinate dehydrogenase (*complex II*), coenzyme Q H$_2$-cytochrome c reductase (*complex III*), cytochrome c oxidase (*complex IV*), and ATP synthetase (*complex V*). Genetic defects of the OXPHOS pathway have been described in isolation or combination with complexes I, III, IV, and V. For example, Pearson's marrow-pancreas syndrome, a disease characterized by a variable pancytopenia, pancreatic fibrosis, and hepatic steatosis and cirrhosis, has been ascribed to large deletions in complex I. Because mitochondria are maternally inherited and affected mitochondria co-segregate with normal mitochondria asymmetrically (heteroplasmy), presentation of an OXPHOS defect can occur in a single organ such as the liver or in combination with other organs. In addition, the disorders can present at any age. Most often, they are a cause of rapidly fatal hepatic failure in neonates. Children affected later in life usually present with hepatomegaly and jaundice, and often with neurologic involvement. While mitochondrial DNA defects have been the most common mutations described in OXPHOS disease, nuclear DNA mutations have also been implicated as the OXPHOS complexes are derived from both nuclear and mitochondrial gene products. A complex III deficiency is secondary to a defect in the nuclear DNA gene BCS1L and presents as a tubulopathy, encephalopathy, and liver failure. Diagnosis of OXPHOS mutation relies on enzymatic analysis or tests of mitochondrial respiration performed on fresh or fresh frozen liver samples, available at a very

only 10–20% of patients with liver failure caused by non-A, non-B, non-C hepatitis or an acute onset of Wilson's disease. In patients who progress to stage IV coma (see Table 345–1), the prognosis is extremely poor. Major complications such as sepsis, severe hemorrhage, or renal failure increase the mortality. The prognosis is particularly poor in patients with liver necrosis and multiorgan failure. Studies indicate that jaundice for more than 7 days before the onset of encephalopathy, a prothrombin time more than 50 sec, and a serum bilirubin level more than 17.5 mg/dL (300 μmol/L) indicate a poor prognosis irrespective of the initial stage of hepatic coma. Survival of 50–75% is being achieved in patients with the poorest prognosis after orthotopic liver transplantation. Patients who recover from fulminant hepatic failure with only supportive care do not usually experience cirrhosis or chronic liver disease. Aplastic anemia is a common and usually fatal complication of fulminant hepatic failure secondary to sporadic non-A, non-B, non-C hepatitis.

Anand AC, Nightengale P, Neuberger JM: Early indicators of prognosis in fulminant hepatic failure: An assessment of the King's criteria. *J Hepatol* 1997; 26:62.

Dubern B, Broue P, Dubuisson C, et al: Orthotopic liver transplantation for mitochondrial respiratory chain disorders: A study of 5 children. *Transplantation* 2001;71:633–7.

Emre S, Schwartz ME, Shneider B, et al: Living related liver transplantation for acute liver failure in children. *Liver Transpl Surg* 1999;5:161–5.

Lee WM: Management of acute liver failure. *Semin Liver Dis* 1996;16:369.

Nora DB, Amaral OB, Busnello JV, et al: Usefulness of plasma exchange plus continuous hemodiafiltration to reduce adverse effects associated with plasma exchange in patients with acute liver failure. *Crit Care Med* 2001;29: 1386–92.

Rivera-Penera T, Moreno J, Skaff C, et al: Delayed encephalopathy in fulminant hepatic failure in the pediatric population and the role of liver transplantation. *J Pediatr Gastroenterol Nutr* 1997;24:128.

Schiodt FV, Atillasoy E, Shakil AO, et al: Etiology and outcome for 295 patients with acute liver failure in the United States. *Liver Transpl Surg* 1999;5: 29–34.

Singer AL, Olthoff KM, Kim H, et al: Role of plasmapheresis in the management of acute hepatic failure in children. *Ann Surg* 2001;234:418–24.

Teo EK, Ostapowicz G, Hussain M, et al: Hepatitis B infection in patients with acute liver failure in the United States. *Hepatology* 2001;33:972–6.

Ting PP, Demetriou AA: Clinical experience with artificial liver support systems. *Can J Gastroenterol* 2000;14:79D–84D.

Chapter 346
Cystic Diseases of the Biliary Tract and Liver

Frederick J. Suchy

Cystic lesions of liver parenchyma or of the biliary system may be recognized initially during infancy and childhood. Their classification is not yet satisfactory. Pathologic features may be found in common among several of these disorders, but different patterns of inheritance indicate that their etiology is heterogeneous.

Choledochal Cysts. These are congenital dilatations of the common bile duct that may cause progressive biliary obstruction and biliary cirrhosis. Cylindrical and spherical cysts of the extrahepatic ducts are the most common types. Segmental or diffuse dilatation can be observed. A diverticulum of the common bile duct or dilatation of the intraduodenal portion of the common duct (choledochocele) is a variant. Cystic dilatation of the intrahepatic bile ducts may be associated with a choledochal cyst.

The pathogenesis of choledochal cysts remains uncertain. Some reports have suggested that junction of the common bile duct and the pancreatic duct before their entry into the sphincter of Oddi may allow reflux of pancreatic enzymes into the common bile duct, causing inflammation, localized weakness, and dilatation of the duct. Other possibilities are that choledochal cysts represent malformations of the common duct or that they occur as part of the spectrum of an infectious disease that includes neonatal hepatitis and biliary atresia. Consistent with this theory, reovirus RNA has been detected in liver and biliary tissues of some infants with choledochal cysts.

Approximately 75% of cases appear during childhood. The infant typically presents with cholestatic jaundice; severe liver dysfunction including ascites and coagulopathy can rapidly evolve if biliary obstruction is not relieved. An abdominal mass is rarely palpable. In an older child, the classic triad of abdominal pain, jaundice, and mass occurs in fewer than 33% of patients. Features of acute cholangitis (fever, right upper quadrant tenderness, jaundice, leukocytosis) may be present. The diagnosis is made by ultrasonography; choledochal cysts have been identified prenatally using this technique. Magnetic resonance cholangiography is useful in the preoperative assessment of choledochal cyst anatomy.

The treatment of choice is primary excision of the cyst and a Roux-en-Y choledochojejunostomy. Simple drainage into the small bowel is less satisfactory owing to a risk for development of carcinoma in the residual cystic tissue. The postoperative course may be complicated by recurrent cholangitis or stricture at the anastomotic site.

Cystic Dilatation of the Intrahepatic Bile Ducts (Caroli Disease). Congenital, saccular dilatation may affect several segments of the intrahepatic bile ducts; the dilated ducts are lined by cuboidal epithelium and are in continuity with the main duct system, which is usually normal. Caroli actually described two variants: *Caroli disease*, characterized by ectasias of the intrahepatic bile ducts without other abnormalities, and *Caroli syndrome*, in which congenital ductal dilatation is associated with features of congenital hepatic fibrosis and the renal lesion of autosomal recessive polycystic renal disease. Caroli syndrome is more common, but both varieties may occur in the same family and are inherited in an autosomal recessive fashion. Choledochal cysts have also been associated with Caroli disease. There is a marked predisposition to ascending cholangitis and calculus formation within the abnormal bile ducts.

Affected patients usually experience symptoms of acute cholangitis as children or young adults. Fever, abdominal pain, mild jaundice, and pruritus occur; and a slightly enlarged, tender liver is palpable. Elevated alkaline phosphatase (ALP) activity, direct-reacting bilirubin levels, and leukocytosis may be observed during episodes of acute infection. In patients with Caroli syndrome, clinical features may be due to a combination of recurring bouts of cholangitis reflecting the intrahepatic ductal abnormalities and portal hypertensive bleeding resulting from hepatic fibrosis. Ultrasonography shows the dilated intrahepatic ducts, but definitive diagnosis and extent of disease must be determined by percutaneous transhepatic, endoscopic, or magnetic resonance cholangiography.

Cholangitis and sepsis are treated with appropriate antibiotics. Calculi may require surgery. Partial hepatectomy may be curative in rare cases when disease is confined to a single lobe. The prognosis is otherwise guarded, largely owing to difficulties in controlling cholangitis and biliary lithiasis and to a significant risk for developing cholangiocarcinoma. Liver transplantation may be required.

Congenital Hepatic Fibrosis. This is an autosomal recessive disorder characterized pathologically by diffuse periportal and perilobular fibrosis in broad bands that contain distorted bile ductlike structures and that often compress or incorporate central or sublobular veins. The ductlike structures may become dilated to the point of microcyst formation but do not communicate with the biliary tract. Irregularly shaped islands of liver parenchyma contain normal-appearing hepatocytes. Caroli disease and choledochal cysts have been associated (see earlier discussion). About 75% of patients have renal disease, such as renal tubular ectasia, nephronophthisis, or autosomal recessive polycystic renal disease. Congenital hepatic fibrosis also occurs as part of the COACH syndrome (*C*erebellar vermis hypoplasia, *O*ligophrenia, congenital *A*taxia, *C*oloboma, and *H*epatic fibrosis). Congenital hepatic fibrosis has been described in children with a congenital disorder of glycosylation caused by mutations in the gene encoding phosphomannose isomerase (Chapter 76.6).

The disorder usually has its clinical onset in childhood, with hepatosplenomegaly or with bleeding secondary to portal hypertension. Cholangitis may occur in patients who have associated abnormalities of bile ducts.

Hepatocellular function is well preserved. Serum aminotransferase activities and bilirubin levels are usually normal; serum ALP activity may be slightly elevated. The serum albumin level and prothrombin time are normal. Liver biopsy is usually required for diagnosis.

Treatment of this disorder should focus on control of bleeding from esophageal varices. Infrequent mild bleeding episodes may be managed by endoscopic sclerotherapy or band ligation of the varices. After more severe hemorrhage, portacaval anastomosis may bring relief of portal hypertension. The prognosis may be greatly improved by a shunting procedure, but survival in some patients may be limited by renal failure.

A **solitary liver cyst** (nonparasitic) rarely occurs in childhood. Abdominal distention and pain may be present, and a poorly defined right upper quadrant mass may be palpable. These benign lesions are best left undisturbed unless they compress adjacent structures or a complication occurs, such as hemorrhage into the cyst.

Autosomal Dominant Polycystic Kidney Disease (ADPKD) (Chapter 513.2). ADPKD, a common inherited disease, affects 1/1,000 live births. It is characterized by progressive renal cyst development and enlargement and an array of extrarenal manifestations. There is a high degree of intrafamilial and interfamilial variability in the clinical expression of the disease.

At least three genetic loci are seen in ADPKD. The PKD 1 gene (accounting for 85% of cases) is on chromosome 16p13.3 and encodes for a novel protein called *polycystin*, which may have a potential role in cell-cell and cell-matrix interactions. The PKD 2 gene (~15% of cases) is on chromosome 4q13–23 and encodes for a protein thought to interact in some fashion with polycystin. A third locus for autosomal dominant polycystic liver disease not associated with kidney cysts has been found on chromosome 19p13.2–13.1.

Multiple hepatic lesions have been associated with ADPKD and include the ductal plate malformation with cystic communicating duct elements, dilated and apparently noncommunicating cysts, and biliary microhamartomas (the so-called von Meyenburg complexes). Segmental dilatation of the intrahepatic ducts (Caroli disease) and congenital hepatic fibrosis have been reported. Approximately 50% of patients with renal failure have demonstrable hepatic cysts that are not in continuity with the biliary tract. The hepatic cysts increase with age but are extremely uncommon before the age of 16 yr. Hepatic cystogenesis appears to be influenced by estrogens. Although the frequency of cysts is similar in males and females, the development of large hepatic cysts is largely a complication in females. Hepatic cysts are often asymptomatic but may cause pain and are occasionally complicated by hemorrhage, infection, jaundice from bile duct compression, portal hypertension with variceal bleeding, or hepatic venous outflow obstruction from mechanical compression of hepatic veins, resulting in tender hepatomegaly and exudative ascites. Cholangiocarcinoma may occur. Selected patients with severe symptomatic polycystic liver disease and favorable anatomy benefit from liver resection or fenestration.

Subarachnoid hemorrhage may result from the associated cerebral arterial aneurysms.

Autosomal Recessive Polycystic Kidney Disease (ARPKD) (Chapter 513.1). ARPKD presents predominantly in childhood. Bilateral enlargement of the kidneys is caused by a generalized dilatation of the collecting tubules. The disorder is invariably associated with congenital hepatic fibrosis and various degrees of biliary ductal ectasia. The gene responsible for ARPKD has been localized to chromosome 6p21, with no evidence for genetic heterogeneity among the different clinical phenotypes.

ARPKD normally presents in early life, often shortly after birth, and is generally more severe than ADPKD. Patients with ARPKD may die in the perinatal period owing to renal failure or lung dysgenesis. The kidneys in these patients are usually markedly enlarged and dysfunctional. Respiratory failure may result from compression of the chest by grossly enlarged kidneys, from fluid retention, or from concomitant pulmonary hypoplasia. The clinical pathologic findings within a family tend to breed true, although there has been some variability in the severity of the disease and the time for presentation within the same family.

The liver in patients with ARPKD demonstrates various degrees of periportal fibrosis, bile ductular hyperplasia, and biliary dysgenesis. Liver disease and complications from hepatic fibrosis are most likely to be clinically significant in patients whose kidney disease allows prolonged survival. The most prominent clinical problem in older patients with ARPKD and congenital hepatic fibrosis is portal hypertension. Although portal hypertensive bleeding may occur during the first year of life, it more commonly presents in older children with hematemesis or melena. Firm or hard hepatomegaly is usually present. Splenomegaly is a frequent finding accompanied by hypersplenism. Owing to dilatation of the intrahepatic bile ducts, these patients are at increased risk of bacterial cholangitis. Caroli disease or a congenital, segmental, saccular dilatation of the intrahepatic bile ducts may coexist with congenital hepatic fibrosis and ARPKD.

Hemorrhage from esophageal varices may be initially managed by using endoscopic sclerotherapy or banding. Some patients with well-preserved hepatic function may benefit from a selective portacaval shunt. Biliary sepsis should be aggressively treated. Recurrent bouts of bacterial cholangitis can lead to progressive loss of hepatic function. Rare patients may have unilateral involvement that can be treated by hepatic resection. Hepatic transplantation may be required for patients with hepatic failure.

Variable abnormalities of bile ducts (irregular dilatation, proliferation, cysts) and portal fibrosis may be associated with Meckel's syndrome, 17–18 trisomy, tuberous sclerosis, and asphyxiating thoracic dystrophy.

Choledochal Cysts
Miyano T, Yamataka, A: Choledochal cysts. *Curr Opin Pediatr* 1997;9:283.
Stringer MD, Dhawan A, Davenport M, et al: Choledochal cysts: Lessons from a 20 year experience. *Arch Dis Child* 1995;73:528.

Caroli Disease

Asselah T, Ernst O, Sergent G, et al: Caroli's disease: A magnetic resonance cholangiopancreatography diagnosis. *Am J Gastroenterol* 1998;93;109.

Desmet VJ: Ludwig symposium on biliary disorders—part I. Pathogenesis of ductal plate abnormalities. *Mayo Clin Proc* 1998;73:80.

Keane F, Hadzic N, Wilkinson ML, et al: Neonatal presentation of Caroli's disease. *Arch Dis Child Fetal Neonatal Ed* 1997;77:F145.

Congenital Hepatic Fibrosis

Desmet VJ: What is congenital hepatic fibrosis? *Histopathology* 1992;20:465–77.

Perisic VN: Long-term studies on congenital hepatic fibrosis in children. *Acta Paediatr* 1995;84:695.

Polycystic Diseases of the Liver and Kidney

Calvet JP, Grantham JJ: The genetics and physiology of polycystic kidney disease. *Semin Nephrol* 2001;21:107–23.

Chauveau D, Fakhouri F, Grunfeld JP: Liver involvement in autosomal-dominant polycystic kidney disease: Therapeutic dilemma. *J Am Soc Nephrol* 2000;11:1767–75.

Griffin MD, Torres VE, Kumar R: Cystic kidney diseases. *Curr Opin Nephrol Hypertens* 1997;6:276.

Zerres K, Rudnik-Schoneborn S, Deget F, et al: Autosomal recessive polycystic kidney disease in 115 children: Clinical presentation, course and influence of gender. Arbeitsgemeinschaft fur Pädiatrische, Nephrologie. *Acta Paediatr* 1996; 85: 437.

Chapter 347
Diseases of the Gallbladder

Frederick J. Suchy

Anomalies. The gallbladder is congenitally absent in about 0.1% of the population. Hypoplasia or absence of the gallbladder may be associated with extrahepatic biliary atresia or cystic fibrosis. Duplication of the gallbladder occurs rarely.

Acute Hydrops (Box 347–1). Acute noncalculous, noninflammatory distention of the gallbladder may occur in infants and children. It is defined by the absence of calculi, bacterial infection, or congenital anomalies of the biliary system. The disorder may complicate acute infections, but the cause is often not identified. Hydrops of the gallbladder may also develop in patients receiving long-term parenteral nutrition, presumably as a result of gallbladder stasis during the period of enteral fasting. Hydrops is distinguished from acalculous cholecystitis by the absence of a significant inflammatory process and a generally benign prognosis.

Affected patients usually have right upper quadrant pain with a palpable mass. Fever, vomiting, and jaundice may be present and are usually associated with a systemic illness such as streptococcal infection. Ultrasonography shows a markedly distended, echo-free gallbladder, without dilatation of the biliary tree. Acute hydrops is usually treated conservatively and rarely needs cholecystostomy and drainage. At laparotomy, a large, edematous gallbladder is found to contain white, yellow, or green bile.

Obstruction of the cystic duct by mesenteric adenopathy is occasionally observed. Cholecystectomy is required if the gallbladder is gangrenous. Pathologic examination of the gallbladder wall shows edema and mild inflammation. Cultures of bile are usually sterile. Treatment of gallbladder hydrops is usually nonsurgical, with a focus on supportive care and managing the intercurrent illness. Spontaneous resolution and return of normal gallbladder function usually occur over a period of several weeks.

Cholecystitis and Cholelithiasis. *Acute acalculous cholecystitis* is uncommon in children and is usually caused by infection. Pathogens include streptococci (groups A and B), gram-negative organisms, particularly *Salmonella*, and *Leptospira interrogans*. Parasitic infestation with ascaris or *Giardia lamblia* may be found. Acalculous cholecystitis may rarely follow abdominal trauma or burn injury or may be associated with a systemic vasculitis, such as periarteritis nodosa.

Clinical features include right upper quadrant or epigastric pain, nausea, vomiting, fever, and jaundice. Right upper quadrant guarding and tenderness are present. Ultrasonography discloses an enlarged, thick-walled gallbladder, without calculi. Serum alkaline phosphatase activity and direct-reacting bilirubin levels are elevated. Leukocytosis is usual.

The diagnosis is confirmed at laparotomy. Cholecystectomy and treatment of the systemic infection are required.

Cholelithiasis is relatively rare in otherwise healthy children, occurring more commonly in patients with various predisposing disorders (Box 347–2). Gallstones, composed of a mixture of cholesterol, bile pigment, calcium, and inorganic matrix, are common. In children, more than 70% of gallstones are the pigment type, 15–20% are cholesterol stones, and the remainder is of unknown composition. Stones of pure cholesterol or bile pigment may also occur. Biliary dyskinesia, a disorder of impaired gallbladder contractility, is an abnormality predisposing to gallstones in late childhood and teenage years.

Acute or chronic cholecystitis is often associated with gallstones. The acute form may be precipitated by impaction of a stone in the cystic duct. Proliferation of bacteria within the obstructed gallbladder lumen can contribute to the process and lead to biliary sepsis. Chronic calculous cholecystitis is more common. It may develop insidiously or follow several attacks of acute cholecystitis. The gallbladder epithelium commonly becomes ulcerated and scarred.

The most important clinical feature of cholelithiasis is recurrent abdominal pain, which is often colicky and localized to the right upper quadrant. An older child may have intolerance for fatty foods. Acute cholecystitis may be the first manifestation, with fever, pain in the right upper quadrant, and often a palpable mass. Pain may radiate to an area just below the right scapula. A plain roentgenogram of the abdomen may reveal opaque calculi, but radiolucent (cholesterol) stones are not visualized. Accordingly, ultrasonography is the method of choice for gallstone detection. Hepatobiliary scintography is a valuable

---

BOX 347–1. Conditions Associated with Hydrops of the Gallbladder

Kawasaki disease	Thalassemia
Streptococcal pharyngitis	Total parenteral nutrition
Staphylococcal infection	Prolonged fasting
Leptospirosis	Viral hepatitis
Ascariasis	Sepsis
Threadworm	Henoch-Schönlein purpura
Sickle cell crisis	Mesenteric adenitis
Typhoid fever	Necrotizing enterocolitis

BOX 347–2. Conditions Associated with Cholelithiasis

Chronic hemolytic disease (sickle cell anemia, spherocytosis)
Obesity
Ileal resection or disease
Cystic fibrosis
Chronic liver disease
Crohn disease
Prolonged parenteral nutrition
Prematurity with complicated medical or surgical course
Prolonged fasting or rapid weight reduction
Treatment of childhood cancer
Abdominal surgery
Pregnancy

adjunct in that failure to visualize the gallbladder provides evidence of cholecystitis.

Cholecystectomy is usually curative; operative cholangiography should be done at the time of surgery to preclude common duct calculi. Dissolution of cholesterol gallstones with oral ursodeoxycholic acid is ineffective in the treatment of gallstones in children, except in terms of relieving symptoms while on treatment.

Laparoscopic cholecystectomy is commonly performed in symptomatic infants and children with cholelithiasis. Common bile duct stones are unusual in children, occurring in 2–6% of cases with cholelithiasis, often in association with obstructive jaundice and pancreatitis. Endoscopic retrograde cholangiography with stone extraction performed before or after laparoscopic cholecystectomy is the procedure of choice in this setting.

Patients with hemolytic disease (including sickle cell anemia, the thalassemias, and red blood cell enzymopathies) and Wilson disease are at increased risk for black pigment cholelithiasis. In sickle cell disease, pigment gallstones may develop before age 4 yr and have been reported in 17% to 33% of patients aged 2 to 18 yr.

Cirrhosis and chronic cholestasis also increase the risk for pigment gallstones. Increasing numbers of sick premature infants are being found to have gallstones; their treatment is often complicated by such factors as bowel resection, necrotizing enterocolitis, prolonged parenteral nutrition without enteral feeding, cholestasis, frequent blood transfusions, and use of diuretics. Cholelithiasis in premature infants is often asymptomatic and may resolve spontaneously. Brown pigment stones have been found in patients with obstructive jaundice and infected intra- and extrahepatic bile ducts. These stones are usually radiolucent, owing to a lower content of calcium phosphate and carbonate and a higher amount of cholesterol than in black pigment stones.

Cholesterol cholelithiasis in children most frequently affects obese adolescent girls. Cholesterol gallstones are found also in children with disturbances of the enterohepatic circulation of bile acids, including patients with ileal disease and bile acid malabsorption, such as those with ileal resection, ileal Crohn disease, and cystic fibrosis. Pigment stones may also occur in these patients.

Cholesterol gallstone formation seems to result from an excess of cholesterol in relation to the cholesterol-carrying capacity of micelles in bile. Supersaturation of bile with cholesterol leading to crystal and stone formation could result from decreased bile acid or from an increased cholesterol concentration in bile. Other initiating factors that may be important in stone formation include gallbladder stasis or the presence in bile of abnormal mucoproteins or bile pigments that may serve as a nidus for cholesterol crystallization.

Barton LL, Luisiri A, Dawson JE: Hydrops of the gallbladder in childhood infections. *Pediatr Infect Dis J* 1995;14:163.

Lobe TE: Cholelithiasis and cholecystitis in children. *Semin Pediatr Surg* 2000;9:170–6.

McEvoy CF, Suchy FJ: Biliary tract disease in children. *Pediatr Clin North Am* 1996;43:75.

Rescorla FJ: Cholelithiasis, cholecystitis, and common bile duct stones. *Curr Opin Pediatr* 1997;9:276.

Suchy FJ: Anatomy, anomalies and pediatric disorders of the biliary tract. In Feldman M, Scharschmidt BF, Sleisenger MH (editors): *Gastrointestinal and Liver Disorders*, 6th ed. Philadelphia, WB Saunders, 1998, pp 905–928.

Walker TM, Hambleton IR, Serjeant GR: Gallstones in sickle cell disease: Observations from the Jamaican Cohort study. *J Pediatr* 2000;136:80–5.

Chapter 348
Portal Hypertension and Varices *Frederick J. Suchy*

Portal hypertension—defined as an elevation of portal pressure above 10–12 mm Hg—is a major cause of morbidity and mortality in children with liver disease. The normal portal venous pressure is approximately 7 mm Hg. The clinical features of the various forms of portal hypertension may be similar, but the associated complications, management, and prognosis can vary significantly and depend on whether the process is complicated by hepatic insufficiency.

Etiology. Numerous causes of portal hypertension result from obstruction to portal blood flow anywhere along the course of the portal venous system. The various disorders associated with portal hypertension are outlined in Box 348–1. Portal hypertension may occur as a result of prehepatic, intrahepatic, or posthepatic obstruction to the flow of portal blood.

Extrahepatic portal vein obstruction is an important cause of portal hypertension in childhood. The obstruction may occur at any level of the portal vein. Umbilical infection with or without a history of catheterization of the umbilical vein may be causal in neonates. The infection can spread potentially from the umbilical vein to the left branch of the portal vein and eventually to the main portal venous channel. Intra-abdominal infec-

---

BOX 348–1. Causes of Portal Hypertension

EXTRAHEPATIC PORTAL HYPERTENSION

Portal Vein Obstruction

Portal vein thrombosis or cavernous transformation
Splenic vein thrombosis

Increased Portal Flow

Arteriovenous fistula

INTRAHEPATIC PORTAL HYPERTENSION

Hepatocellular Disease

Acute and chronic viral hepatitis
Cirrhosis
Congenital hepatic fibrosis
Wilson disease
α_1-Antitrypsin deficiency
Glycogen storage disease type IV
Hepatotoxicity
    Methotrexate
    Parenteral nutrition

Biliary Tract Disease

Extrahepatic biliary atresia
Cystic fibrosis
Choledochal cyst
Sclerosing cholangitis
Intrahepatic bile duct paucity

Idiopathic Portal Hypertension

Postsinusoidal Obstruction

Budd-Chiari syndrome
Veno-occlusive disease

tions including acute appendicitis and primary peritonitis can be causal in older children. Portal vein thrombosis has also been associated with neonatal dehydration and systemic infection. In older children, inflammatory bowel disease can be associated with a hypercoagulable state and portal venous obstruction. Thrombosis of the portal vein has also occurred in association with biliary tract infections and primary sclerosing cholangitis. Portal vein thrombosis has also been associated with hypercoagulable states such as factor V Leiden deficiency or protein C and protein S deficiencies. The portal vein can be replaced by a fibrous remnant or contain an organized thrombus. Obstruction by a web or diaphragm can also occur. At least half of reported cases have no defined cause.

Uncommonly, presinusoidal hypertension can be caused by increased flow through the portal system as a result of a congenital or acquired arteriovenous fistula.

The intrahepatic causes of portal hypertension are numerous. Obstruction to flow can occur on the basis of a presinusoidal process including acute and chronic hepatitis, congenital hepatic fibrosis, or schistosomiasis. Portal infiltration with malignant cells or granulomas can also contribute. An idiopathic form of portal hypertension characterized by splenomegaly, hypersplenism, and portal hypertension without occlusion of portal or splenic veins and with no obvious disease in the liver has been described. In some patients, noncirrhotic portal fibrosis has been observed.

Cirrhosis is the predominant cause of portal hypertension and is related to obstruction of blood through the portal vein. The numerous causes of cirrhosis include recognized disorders such as extrahepatic biliary atresia, metabolic liver disease such as α_1-antitrypsin deficiency, Wilson's disease, glycogen storage disease type IV, hereditary fructose intolerance, and cystic fibrosis.

Postsinusoidal causes of portal hypertension are also observed during childhood. The Budd-Chiari syndrome occurs with obstruction to hepatic veins anywhere between the efferent hepatic veins and the entry of the inferior vena cava into the right atrium. In most cases, no specific cause can be found, but the thrombosis can complicate neoplasms, collagen vascular disease, infection, and trauma. Veno-occlusive disease is the most frequent cause of hepatic vein obstruction in children. In this disorder, occlusion of the centrilobular venules or sublobular hepatic veins occurs. The disorder occurs after total body irradiation with or without cytotoxic drug therapy that is commonly used before bone marrow transplantation. The disease has also occurred after ingestion of herbal remedies containing the pyrrolizidine alkaloids, which are sometimes taken as medicinal teas.

Pathophysiology. The primary hemodynamic abnormality in portal hypertension is increased resistance to portal blood flow. This is the case whether the resistance to portal flow has an intrahepatic cause such as cirrhosis or is due to portal vein obstruction. Portosystemic shunting should decompress the portal system and thus significantly lower portal pressures. However, despite the development of significant collaterals deviating portal blood into systemic veins, portal hypertension is maintained by an overall increase in portal venous flow and thus maintenance of portal hypertension. A hyperdynamic circulation is achieved by tachycardia, an increase in cardiac output, and decreased systemic vascular resistance. Splanchnic dilatation also occurs. Overall, the increase in portal flow likely contributes to an increase in variceal transmural pressure. The increase in portal blood flow is related to the contribution of hepatic and collateral flow; the actual portal blood flow reaching the liver is reduced. It is also likely that hepatocellular dysfunction and portosystemic shunting lead to the generation of various humoral factors that cause vasodilatation and an increase in plasma volume.

Many of the portal hypertension complications can be accounted for by the development of a remarkable collateral circulation. Collateral vessels may form prominently in areas in which absorptive epithelium joins stratified epithelium, particularly in the esophagus or anorectal region. The superficial submucosal collaterals, especially those in the esophagus and stomach and to a lesser extent those in the duodenum, colon, or rectum, are prone to rupture and bleeding under increased pressure. In portal hypertension, the vascularity of the stomach is also abnormal and demonstrates prominent submucosal arteriovenous communications between the muscularis mucosa and dilated precapillaries and veins. The resulting lesion—a vascular ectasia—has been called *congestive gastropathy* and contributes to a significant risk of bleeding from the stomach.

Clinical Manifestations. Bleeding from esophageal varices is the most common presentation. In patients with underlying hepatic disease, physical examination may show jaundice and stigmata of cirrhosis such as palmar erythema and vascular telangiectasias. Ascites may be present in patients with intrahepatic causes of portal hypertension but is uncommon with portal vein obstruction. Dilated cutaneous collateral vessels carrying blood from the portal to systemic circulation may be apparent in the periumbilical region. In the absence of clinical or biochemical features of liver disease and a liver of normal size, portal vein obstruction is most likely. However, well-compensated cirrhosis cannot be completely ruled out under these conditions. An enlarged, hard liver with minimal disturbance of hepatic function suggests the possibility of congenital hepatic fibrosis. Hemorrhage, particularly in children with portal vein obstruction, may be precipitated by minor febrile, intercurrent illness. The mechanism is often unclear; aspirin or other nonsteroidal anti-inflammatory drugs may be a contributing factor by damaging the integrity of a congested gastric mucosa or interfering with platelet function. Coughing during a respiratory illness can also increase intravariceal pressure. The bleeding may become apparent with hematemesis or with melena. Gastrointestinal hemorrhage can also originate from portal hypertensive gastropathy or from gastric, duodenal, peristomal, or rectal varices. Splenomegaly, sometimes with hypersplenism, is the next most common presenting feature in portal vein obstruction and may be discovered first on routine physical examination. Because more than half of patients in many series with portal vein obstruction do not experience bleeding until after age 6 yr, the diagnosis should be suggested in a child without hepatocellular disease who had a complicated neonatal course and in whom asymptomatic splenomegaly later developed.

Children with portal hypertension, regardless of the underlying cause, may have recurrent bouts of life-threatening hemorrhage. In patients with portal vein obstruction and normal hepatic function, the bleeding usually stops spontaneously. In patients with intrahepatic disease, the combination of portal hypertension and poor liver synthetic ability (coagulopathy) can make bleeding much more difficult to control. Moreover, esophageal hemorrhage and cirrhosis may have injurious effects on the liver, further impairing hepatic function and sometimes precipitating jaundice, ascites, and encephalopathy.

Diagnosis. In patients with established chronic liver disease or in those in whom portal vein obstruction is suspected, an experienced ultrasonographer should be able to demonstrate the patency of the portal vein. In addition, the use of Doppler flow ultrasonography may demonstrate the direction of flow within the portal system. The pattern of flow correlates with the severity of cirrhosis and encephalopathy. Hepatopetal flow is more likely to be associated with variceal bleeding. Ultrasonography is also effective in detecting the presence of esophageal varices. Another important feature of extrahepatic portal vein obstruction is so-called cavernous transformation of the portal vein in which an extensive complex of small collateral vessels has formed to bypass the obstruction. Various other imaging techniques also contribute to further definition of the portal vein anatomy but are required less often; computed tomography and magnetic resonance imaging provide similar information to ultrasonography. Selective arteriography of the celiac axis, superior mesenteric artery, and splenic vein may be useful in precise mapping of the extrahepatic vascular anatomy. This is not required to establish a diagnosis but may prove valuable in planning surgical decompression of portal hypertension.

Endoscopy is the most reliable method for detecting esophageal varices and for identifying the source of gastrointestinal bleeding. Although bleeding from esophageal or gastric varices is most common in children with portal hypertension, up to one third of patients, particularly those with cirrhosis, may have bleeding from some other source such as portal hypertensive gastropathy or gastric or duodenal ulcerations. There is a strong correlation between variceal size as assessed endoscopically and the probability of hemorrhage. Red spots apparent over varices at the time of endoscopy are a strong predictor of imminent hemorrhage.

Treatment. The therapy of portal hypertension can be divided into emergency treatment of potentially life-threatening hemorrhage and prophylaxis directed at prevention of initial or subsequent bleeding. It must be emphasized that many trials of therapy are based on experience with adults with portal hypertension.

Treatment of patients with variceal hemorrhage must focus on fluid resuscitation initially in the form of crystalloid infusion followed by the replacement of red blood cells. Correction of coagulopathy by administration of vitamin K or the infusion of platelets or fresh frozen plasma, or both therapies, may be required. A nasogastric tube should be placed to document the presence of blood within the stomach and to monitor for ongoing bleeding. An H_2 receptor blocker such as ranitidine should be given intravenously to reduce the risk of bleeding from gastric erosions. In most patients, particularly those with extrahepatic portal hypertension and with normal hepatic synthetic function, bleeding usually stops spontaneously. Care should be taken in fluid resuscitation of children after bleeding to avoid producing an excessively high venous pressure and an increased risk for further bleeding.

Pharmacologic therapy to decrease portal pressure may be considered in patients with continued bleeding. Vasopressin or one of its analogs has been commonly used and is thought to act by increasing splanchnic vascular tone and thus decreasing portal blood flow. Vasopressin is administered initially with a bolus of 0.33 U/kg over 20 min followed by a continued infusion of the same dose on an hourly basis or a continuous infusion of 0.2 U/1.73 m^2/min. The drug has a half-life of approximately 30 min. Its use may be limited by the side effects of vasoconstriction, which can impair cardiac function and perfusion to the heart, bowel, and kidneys and may also, as a result, exacerbate fluid retention. Nitroglycerin, usually given as a portion of a skin patch, has also been used to decrease portal pressure and, when

used in conjunction with vasopressin, may ameliorate some of its untoward effects. The somatostatin analog octreotide decreases splanchnic blood flow with fewer side effects. Although studies in adults are promising, its use and efficacy in children have not been well evaluated.

After an episode of variceal hemorrhage or in patients in whom bleeding cannot be controlled, endoscopic sclerosis of esophageal varices is an important option. In this technique, sclerosants are injected either intravariceally or paravariceally until bleeding has stopped. Although bleeding may be controlled acutely in most cases, further sessions of sclerotherapy are required to achieve temporary obliteration of the varices. Treatments may be associated with further bleeding, bacteremia, esophageal ulceration, and stricture formation. Most centers do not perform endoscopic sclerotherapy of varices prophylactically but use the procedure as a bridge to the time of liver transplantation or until collateral circulation develops in extrahepatic portal vein obstruction. Endoscopic elastic band ligation of varices has been introduced as a safer and potentially as effective therapy for obliteration of varices.

In patients who continue to bleed despite pharmacologic and endoscopic methods to control hemorrhage, a Sengstaken-Blakemore tube may be placed to stop hemorrhage by mechanically compressing esophageal and gastric varices. The device may be the only option to control life-threatening hemorrhage but carries a significant rate of complications and a high rate of bleeding when the device is removed. It poses a particularly high risk for pulmonary aspiration, and the tube is not well tolerated in children without significant sedation.

Various surgical procedures have been devised to divert portal blood flow and to decrease portal pressure. A portacaval shunt diverts nearly all of the portal blood flow into the subhepatic inferior right vena cava. Although portal pressure is significantly reduced, because of the significant diversion of blood from the liver, patients with parenchymal liver disease have a marked risk for hepatic encephalopathy. More selective shunting procedures, such as mesocaval or distal splenorenal shunt, may effectively decompress the portal system while allowing a greater amount of portal blood flow to the liver. The small size of the vessels makes these operations technically challenging in infants and small children, and there is a significant risk of failure as a result of shunt thrombosis. Therefore, orthotopic liver transplantation represents a much better therapy for portal hypertension resulting from intrahepatic disease. A prior portosystemic shunting operation does not preclude a successful liver transplantation but makes the operation technically more difficult. Portosystemic shunting may remain an option in children with extrahepatic portal hypertension, particularly in those patients who are suffering from potentially life-threatening hemorrhage not effectively controlled by other measures and who reside a great distance from emergency medical care. A transjugular intrahepatic portosystemic shunt (TIPS), in which a stent is placed by an interventional radiologist between the right hepatic vein and the right or left branch of the portal vein, can aid in the management of portal hypertension in children, especially in those needing temporary relief before liver transplantation. However, the TIPS procedure may precipitate hepatic encephalopathy and is prone to thrombosis.

Long-term treatment with nonspecific β-blockers such as propanolol has been used extensively in adults with portal hypertension. These agents may act by lowering cardiac output and portal perfusion. Evidence in adult patients shows that β-blockers may reduce the incidence of variceal hemorrhage and improve long-term survival. A therapeutic effect is thought to result when the pulse rate is reduced by at least 25%. There is limited published experience with the use of this therapy in children.

Prognosis. Portal hypertension secondary to intrahepatic disease has a poor prognosis. Portal hypertension is usually progressive in these patients and is often associated with deteriorating liver function. Efforts should be directed toward prompt treatment of acute bleeding and prevention of recurrent hemorrhage with available methods. Patients with progressive liver disease and significant esophageal varices ultimately require orthotopic liver transplantation. Liver transplantation might also be considered for patients with portal hypertension secondary to hepatic vein obstruction or resulting from severe veno-occlusive disease.

In patients with portal vein obstruction, episodes of bleeding may become less frequent and severe with age as a collateral circulation develops. Most patients can be treated conservatively with endoscopic sclerotherapy when necessary. However, children may continue to experience significant bleeding during adolescence and may eventually require a portosystemic shunting procedure.

Alvarez F, Bernard O, Brunelle F, et al: Portal obstruction in children: I. Clinical investigation and hemorrhage risk. *J Pediatr* 1983;103:696.

Alvarez F, Bernard O, Brunelle F, et al: Portal obstruction in children: II. Results of surgical portosystemic shunts. *J Pediatr* 1983;103:703.

Gentil-Kocher S, Bernard O, Brunelle F, et al: Budd-Chiari syndrome in children: Report of 22 cases. *J Pediatr* 1988;113:30.

Heyman MB, LaBerge JM, Somberg KA, et al: Transjugular intrahepatic portosystemic shunts (TIPS) in children. *J Pediatr* 1997;131:914.

Lykavieris P, Gauthier F, Hadchouel P, et al: Risk of gastrointestinal bleeding during adolescence and early adulthood in children with portal vein obstruction. *J Pediatr* 2000;136:805–8.

Miga D, Sokol RJ, Mackenzie T, et al: Survival after first esophageal variceal hemorrhage in patients with biliary atresia. *J Pediatr* 2001;139:291–6.

Ryckman FC, Alonso MH: Causes and management of portal hypertension in the pediatric population. *Clin Liver Dis* 2001;5:789–818.

Shashidhar H, Langhans N, Grand RJ: Propranolol in prevention of portal hypertensive hemorrhage in children: A pilot study. *J Pediatr Gastroenterol Nutr* 1999;29:12–7.

Stringer MD, McClean P: Treatment of esophageal varices. *Arch Dis Child* 1997;77:476.

Chapter 349
Liver Transplantation

Kenneth L. Cox

Liver transplantation is standard therapy for children with end-stage liver disease, life-threatening hepatic metabolic disorders, and cancers of the liver. With current immunosuppression and surgical techniques, 1- and 5-yr survival rates for children after liver transplantation are 84% and 79%, respectively. One half of pediatric liver transplant recipients are younger than 2 yr of age at the time of transplant and have a significantly poorer 1-yr survival rate (81%) as compared with older children (87%). Approximately, 500 children in the United States undergo liver transplantation each year with 10% having more than one organ transplanted simultaneously, which usually includes either a kidney or small intestine. The most frequent indication is extrahepatic biliary atresia after a failed portoenterostomy (Kasai) procedure. Metabolic liver disease and acute hepatic necrosis are next in frequency (Table 349–1). The decision to transplant in patients with metabolic liver disease includes the following considerations: Is it hepatic in origin, can it be successfully treated medically, and are the extrahepatic manifestations reversible?

Early referral to a transplant center is important so that patients and their families may be evaluated and treated in a timely fashion. Medical and psychological issues are assessed to determine the appropriateness of transplant, optimal manage-

TABLE 349–1. Indications for Pediatric Liver Transplantation

Indications	Cases
Biliary atresia	43
Metabolic liver disease	13
α_1-Antitrypsin deficiency	6
Tyrosinemia	2
Wilson's disease	1
Other	4
Acute hepatic necrosis (idiopathic)	11
Idiopathic cirrhosis	6
Biliary hypoplasia (Alagille)	5
Neonatal hepatitis	3
Hyperalimentation	3
Autoimmune hepatitis	2
Tumors (hepatoblastoma)	2
Cystic fibrosis	2
Primary sclerosing cholangitis	1
Congenital hepatic fibrosis	1
Familial cholestasis	1
Miscellaneous	7

Data are from the United Network for Organ Sharing Data Base for 3,595 pediatric liver transplants performed on children who were 0–17 yrs of age.

ment, and urgency. Age (<1 yr), growth failure (defined as height or weight 2 standard deviations below normal), hyperbilirubinemia, hypoalbuminemia, and coagulopathy as indicated by prolonged international normalized ratio (INR) have been predictive of increased morbidity and mortality from liver disease and are used to determine the urgency for liver transplantation. Other variables that also indicate the need for liver transplantation are ascites, encephalopathy, variceal bleeding, and renal failure. Prompt referral of patients with fulminant hepatic failure is critical because a majority quickly die without liver transplantation. Counseling families about the special needs of children with chronic illness improves the psychosocial outcome. Early evaluation allows sufficient time to find a donor and for families to learn about liver transplantation.

Pretransplantation management is critical to the success of the procedure and to limiting morbidity from the liver disease. Portoenterostomies (the Kasai operation) should be performed in children with biliary atresia because it often delays and occasionally obviates the need for liver transplantation. Even children with biliary atresia who are over 3 mo of age may benefit from this procedure. Areas of major importance are nutrition and immunizations. Patients with liver disease have malabsorption as well as anorexia, which lead to growth retardation. Growth retardation is inversely correlated with age and is reversible in a majority of children after liver transplantation. Formula containing medium-chain triglycerides is helpful because bile salts are not necessary for their absorption. Caloric requirements may be as high as 150 kcal/kg/24 hr. Nocturnal nasogastric tube feedings and intravenous nutrition, especially lipids, may be required because of the anorexia and malabsorption. Fat-soluble vitamin deficiencies must be prevented by providing vitamin supplements. Vitamin E deficiency (ataxia, peripheral neuropathy, gross motor delay) is best avoided by using a well-absorbed preparation containing D-α-tocopherol polyethylene glycol succinate. Vitamin D deficiency–associated bone disease is prevented with oral preparations of 25-hydroxyvitamin D_3. Early changes of vitamin A deficiency appear in the conjunctiva and cornea; they are prevented by using an oral, water-soluble preparation of vitamin A. Vitamin K deficiency is commonly encountered as a prolonged prothrombin time, which may respond to oral supplementation, but often requires parenteral vitamin K. Vitamin and fat absorption may be enhanced with oral ursodeoxycholic acid as a choleretic (increases bile flow into the intestine) and an intraluminal bile acid. Prothrombin time and serum levels of vitamins E, D, and A should be monitored. Iron deficiency due to occult blood loss and zinc deficiency associated with chronic diarrhea may occur. Immunizations should be given for hepatitis A and B to avoid additional hepatic injury caused by these infections, and those containing live viruses (measles-mumps-rubella, varicella) should be given on schedule because immunosuppression after transplantation may prevent administration.

Medical management should also be directed toward control of variceal bleeding, ascites, encephalopathy, coagulopathy, and sepsis. While waiting for transplantation, morbidity and mortality from liver failure can be reduced by prompt diagnosis and aggressive treatment of these complications.

The success of *transplantation* has been enhanced by better preservation of the organ (up to 18 hr ex vivo with <2% primary non-function), refinement of surgical techniques, and advances in immunosuppressive therapy. In pediatrics, the donor pool size has been expanded by using a lobe or segment of the liver from a cadaver or living donor and by using ABO blood type mismatch. Living related donation using the right lobe of the liver has recently been successful in adolescent and adult recipients. Most frequently, the biliary tract in young children is connected to a Roux-en-Y loop of jejunum and direct vascular connections are made. Donor venous grafts are occasionally used if pretransplant portal vein thrombosis is present. Steroids and either cyclosporine (Sandimmune or Neoral) or tacrolimus (Prograf, FK506) are standard therapies to prevent rejection. Many children are weaned off steroids within 1 yr of the transplant. Compared with cyclosporine (Sandimmune), tacrolimus has been associated with lower rates of acute and chronic rejection. The water-soluble microemulsion of cyclosporine (Neoral) has been better absorbed than the bile salt-dependent, fat soluble form (Sandimmune) and may be more comparable to tacrolimus in the prevention of rejection. Hirsutism and gingival hyperplasia are specific side effects of cyclosporine. Post-transplant lymphoproliferative disease (PTLD) occurs in 4–11% of children, is associated with high doses of immunosuppression and Epstein-Barr virus (EBV) infection, and has resulted a 10–20% mortality rate. The morbidity and mortality from PTLD has been reduced by early diagnoses with frequent monitoring of EBV serology and blood EBV PCR and by lowering immunosuppression as soon as infection is detected. Blood pressure and creatinine clearance should be monitored because hypertension and renal failure are common long-term complications, especially in children on high doses of cyclosporine or tacrolimus. When rejection has required high doses of cyclosporine or tacrolimus and/or continued use of steroids, azathioprine (Imuran), sirolimus (Rapamune), or mycophenolate mofetil (Cellcept) may control rejection and allow reduction of the doses of these more toxic drugs. Mouse anti-T cell monoclonal antibodies (OKT3) have been used to treat severe, steroid-resistant rejection. Less toxic, genetically engineered monoclonal anti-interleukin-2 (IL-2)-receptor antibodies can be used instead of OKT3.

Early *complications* include fluid shifts, electrolyte imbalance, renal dysfunction, and hypertension. Primary nonfunction of the graft or vascular complications, such as thrombosis of graft vessels, are ominous early problems that often result in death unless the graft is replaced within 48 hr. After this early phase, infection and organ rejection are the most frequent problems. Bacterial infections are most common, followed by viral (especially cytomegalovirus and adenovirus), fungal, and rarely parasitic (*Pneumocystis carinii*) infections. Hospital stays are usually 2–3 wk but may be several months. Late complications may arise (rejection, cyclosporine- or tacrolimus-induced renal dysfunction, EBV-associated PTLD). The latter may progress to lymphoma. Rejection in older children is often due to poor compliance in taking medications.

The *prognosis* for survivals is very encouraging. Most children have improvement in growth and development and the stigmata of chronic liver disease resolve. Children and their families resume more normal lives. Close follow-up of medical and psychosocial issues is necessary. Though some children may become tolerant of their graft and not need immunosuppression, many will reject up to 4 yr after immunosuppression has been discontinued. As a result, children are left on immunosuppression indefinitely until methods are developed that will identify those who are tolerant.

Bartosh, S, Thomas SE, Sutton MM, et al: Linear growth after pediatric liver transplantation. *J Pediatr* 1999;135:624.

Cacciarelli TV, Reyes J, Jaffe R, et al: Primary tacrolimus (FK506) therapy and the long-term risk of post-transplant lymphoproliferative disease in pediatric liver transplant recipients. *Pediatr Transplantation* 2001;5:359.

Chardot C, Carton M, Spire-Bendelac N, et al: Is the Kasai operation still indicated in children older than 3 months diagnosed with biliary atresia? *J Pediatr* 2001;138:224.

Cherqui D, Soubrane O, Husson E, et al: Laparoscopic living donor hepatectomy for liver transplantation in children. *Lancet* 2002;359:392–6.

Cox KL, Rodriguez-Baez N, Nasr A, et al: Mortality rate correlated with the number of pediatric liver transplants performed at a center. *Transplant Proceedings* 2001;33:1512.

Marariegos GV, Reyes J, Marino IR, et al: Weaning of immunosuppression in liver recipients. *Transplantation* 1997;63:243.

McDiarmid SV: Liver transplantation: The pediatric challenge in Clinics in Liver Disease 2000;4:1–46.

Split Research Group: Studies of pediatric liver transplantation (SPLIT): Year 2000 outcomes. *Transplantation* 2001;72:463–76.

United Network for Organ Sharing (UNOS) Scientific Registry data as of June 17, 2000.

Van Mourik IDM, Beath SV, Brook GA, et al: Long-term nutritional and neurodevelopmental outcomes of liver transplantation in infants aged less than 12 month. *J Pediatr Gastroenterol Nutr* 2000;30:269–75.

Wayman KI, Cox KL, Esquivel CO: Neurodevelopmental outcome of young children with extrahepatic biliary atresia 1 year after liver transplantation. *J Pediatr* 1997;131:894.

SECTION 7 *Peritoneum*

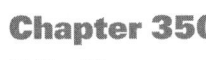

Chapter 350

Malformations *Jeffrey S. Hyams*

Congenital peritoneal bands may be responsible for intestinal obstruction; numerous other anomalies may occur in the course of the development of the peritoneum but are rarely of clinical importance. Intra-abdominal herniations infrequently occur through ring-like formations produced by anomalous peritoneal bands. Absence of the omentum or its duplication occurs rarely. Omental cysts arise in obstructed lymphatic channels within the omentum. They may be congenital or may result from trauma and are usually asymptomatic. Abdominal pain or partial small bowel obstruction may result from compression or torsion of the small bowel from traction on the omentum.

Chapter 351

Ascites *Jeffrey S. Hyams*

Ascites is an accumulation of serous fluid within the peritoneal cavity. Multiple causes of ascites have been described (Box 351–1). In children, hepatic, renal, and cardiac disease are the most common causes.

The clinical hallmark of ascites is abdominal distention, but this may also be caused by other conditions, including gaseous distention, fecal retention, tumor masses, peritoneal hemorrhage, extreme bladder distention, pregnancy, and obesity. Considerable intraperitoneal fluid may accumulate before ascites is detectable by the five classic physical signs: bulging flanks, flank dullness, shifting dullness, fluid wave, and the "puddle sign" (decreased auscultation of high-frequency vibrations in central abdomen when flicking side of abdomen with patient on hands and knees). Umbilical herniation may be associated with tense ascites. Ultrasound examination can detect small amounts of ascites.

The course, prognosis, and treatment of ascites depend entirely on the cause. Patients with any type of ascites are at increased risk for spontaneous bacterial peritonitis.

351.1 Chylous Ascites

Chylous ascites can result from an anomaly, injury, or obstruction of the intra-abdominal portion of the thoracic duct. Although uncommon, it can occur at any age. Causes include congenital malformations, peritoneal bands, generalized lymphangiomatosis, chronic inflammatory processes of the bowel, tumors, enlarged lymph nodes, previous abdominal surgery, and trauma.

In neonates, rapidly progressing abdominal distention is noted along with poor weight gain and loose stools. Peripheral edema is common. Massive chylous ascites may result in scrotal edema, inguinal and umbilical herniation, and respiratory embarrassment.

Diagnosis of chylous ascites depends on the demonstration of milky ascitic fluid obtained via paracentesis after a fat-containing feeding. Fluid analysis will reveal a high protein content, elevated triglycerides, and lymphocytosis. If the patient has had nothing by mouth, the fluid will appear serous. Hypoalbuminemia, hypogammaglobulinemia, and lymphopenia are common.

Treatment includes the provision of a high-protein, low-fat diet supplemented with medium-chain triglycerides that are absorbed directly into the portal circulation. Parenteral alimentation may be necessary if nutrition remains impaired on oral feedings and also in order to decrease lymph flow to facilitate sealing at the point of lymph leakage. Paracentesis should be repeated only if abdominal distention causes respiratory distress. Laparotomy may be indicated to search for the site of the leak if a trial of dietary management has been unsuccessful.

Browse NL, Wilson NM, Russo F, et al: Aetiology and treatment of chylous ascites. *Br J Surg* 1992;79:1145.
Griscom NT, Colodny AH, Rosenberg HK, et al: Diagnostic aspects of neonatal ascites: Report of 27 cases. *AJR Am J Roentgenol* 1977;128:961.
Unger SW, Chandler JG: Chylous ascites in infants and children. *Surgery* 1983;93:455.

Chapter 352

Peritonitis *Jeffrey S. Hyams*

Inflammation of the peritoneal lining of the abdominal cavity may result from infectious, autoimmune, and chemical processes. Infectious peritonitis is usually defined as primary (spontaneous) or secondary. In primary peritonitis, the source of infection originates outside the abdomen and seeds the

---

BOX 351–1. Causes of Ascites

HEPATIC
Cirrhosis
Congenital hepatic fibrosis
Portal vein obstruction
Fulminant hepatic failure
Budd-Chiari syndrome
Lysosomal storage disease

RENAL
Nephrotic syndrome
Obstructive uropathy
Perforation of urinary tract
Peritoneal dialysis

CARDIAC
Heart failure
Constrictive pericarditis
Inferior vena cava web

INFECTIOUS
Abscess
Tuberculosis
Chlamydia
Schistosomiasis

GASTROINTESTINAL
Infarcted bowel
Perforation

NEOPLASTIC
Lymphoma
Neuroblastoma

GYNECOLOGIC
Ovarian tumors
Ovarian torsion, rupture

PANCREATIC
Pancreatitis
Ruptured pancreatic duct

MISCELLANEOUS
Systemic lupus erythematosus
Ventriculoperitoneal shunt
Eosinophilic ascites
Chylous ascites
Hypothyroidism

peritoneal cavity via hematogenous or lymphatic spread. Secondary peritonitis arises from the abdominal cavity itself through either extension from or rupture of an intra-abdominal viscus or an abscess within an organ.

Peritonitis in the neonatal period may arise from a transplacental in utero infection; more frequently, it is the result of infection acquired during or shortly after birth. It may be a manifestation of septicemia, a direct extension from an umbilical infection or from perforation of the intestine, necrotizing enterocolitis, or, rarely, the sequela of a ruptured appendix or Meckel diverticulum. Meconium peritonitis is described in Chapters 91.1 and 311.2.

352.1 Acute Primary Peritonitis

Etiology and Epidemiology. Primary peritonitis usually refers to bacterial infection of the peritoneal cavity without a demonstrable intra-abdominal source. Most cases occur in children with ascites resulting from nephrotic syndrome or cirrhosis. Rarely, it may occur in previously healthy children. Most frequently, isolated bacteria include pneumococci, group A streptococci, enterococci, staphylococci, and gram-negative enteric bacteria, especially *Escherichia coli* and *Klebsiella pneumoniae*. The genders are affected equally; most cases occur before 6 yr of age. *Mycobacterium tuberculosis* and *M. bovis* are rare causes of peritonitis.

Clinical Manifestations. Onset may be insidious or rapid and is characterized by fever, abdominal pain, vomiting, diarrhea, and a "toxic appearance." Hypotension and tachycardia are common along with shallow, rapid respirations because of discomfort associated with breathing. Abdominal palpation may demonstrate rebound tenderness and rigidity. Bowel sounds are hypoactive or absent. The prior use of corticosteroids may diminish the clinical expression of peritonitis and delay diagnosis.

Diagnosis and Treatment. Leukocytosis (on complete blood count) with a marked predominance of polymorphonuclear cells is common, although the level of the white cell count may be affected by pre-existing hypersplenism in patients with cirrhosis. Proteinuria is present in subjects with nephrotic syndrome. Roentgenographic examination of the abdomen reveals dilatation of the large and small intestines, with increased separation of loops secondary to bowel wall thickening. Distinguishing primary peritonitis from appendicitis may be impossible in patients without a history of nephrotic syndrome or cirrhosis; accordingly, the diagnosis of primary peritonitis is made only at laparotomy. In a child with known renal or hepatic disease and ascites, the presence of peritoneal signs should prompt a diagnostic paracentesis. Infected fluid usually reveals a white cell count of 250 cells/mm^3 or greater, with more than 50% polymorphonuclear cells.

Other peritoneal fluid findings suggestive of primary peritonitis include a pH less than 7.35, arterial-ascitic fluid pH gradient greater than 0.1, and elevated lactate. Gram stain of the ascitic fluid characteristically reveals a single species of gram-positive or, less often, gram-negative bacteria. The presence of mixed bacterial flora on ascitic fluid examination or free air on abdominal roentgenogram in children with presumed primary peritonitis mandates laparotomy to localize a perforation as a likely intra-abdominal source of the infection. Inoculation of ascitic fluid obtained at paracentesis directly into blood culture bottles will increase the yield of positive cultures. Parenteral antibiotic therapy with cefotaxime and an aminoglycoside should be started promptly, with subsequent changes dependent on sensitivity testing (vancomycin for resistant pneumococci). Therapy should be continued for 10–14 days.

Culture-negative neutrocytic ascites is a variant of primary peritonitis with a cell count of 500 cells/mm^3, a negative culture, no intra-abdominal source of infection, and no prior treatment with antibiotic. It should be treated in a similar manner as primary peritonitis.

Bhuva M, Ganger D, Jensen D: Spontaneous bacterial peritonitis: An update on evaluation, management and prevention. *Am J Med* 1994;97:169.
Gorensek MJ, Lebel MH, Nelson JD: Peritonitis in children with nephrotic syndrome. *Pediatrics* 1988;81:849.
Nohr CW, Marshall BG: Primary peritonitis in children. *Can J Surg* 1984;27:179.

352.2 Acute Secondary Peritonitis

This is most often due to the entry of enteric bacteria into the peritoneal cavity through a necrotic defect in the wall of the intestines or other viscus as a result of obstruction or infarction or after rupture of an intra-abdominal visceral abscess. It commonly follows perforation of the appendix. Other gastrointestinal causes include incarcerated hernias, rupture of a Meckel diverticulum, midgut volvulus, intussusception, hemolytic uremic syndrome, peptic ulceration, inflammatory bowel disease, necrotizing cholecystitis, necrotizing enterocolitis, typhlitis, and traumatic perforation. Peritonitis in the neonatal period most often occurs as a complication of necrotizing enterocolitis but may be associated with meconium ileus or spontaneous (or indomethacin-induced) rupture of the stomach or intestines. In postpubertal females, bacteria from the genital tract *(Neisseria gonorrhoeae, Chlamydia trachomatis)* may gain access to the peritoneal cavity via the fallopian tubes, causing secondary peritonitis. The presence of a foreign body, such as a ventriculoperitoneal catheter or peritoneal dialysis catheter, can predispose to peritonitis, with skin microorganisms, such as *Staphylococcus epidermidis, S. aureus,* and *Candida albicans,* contaminating the shunt.

Clinical Manifestations. Similar to primary peritonitis, characteristic symptoms include fever (39.5°C or more), diffuse abdominal pain, nausea, and vomiting. Physical findings of peritoneal inflammation include rebound tenderness, abdominal wall rigidity, a paucity of body motion (lying still), and decreased or absent bowel sounds from a paralytic ileus. Massive exudation of fluid into the peritoneal cavity, along with the systemic release of vasodilatory substances, can lead to the rapid development of shock. A "toxic appearance," irritability, and restlessness are common. Basilar atelectasis as well as intrapulmonary shunting may develop with progression to acute respiratory distress syndrome.

Laboratory studies reveal a peripheral white cell count greater than 12,000 cells/mm^3 with a marked predominance of polymorphonuclear forms. Roentgenograms of the abdomen may reveal free air in the peritoneal cavity, evidence of ileus or obstruction, peritoneal fluid, and obliteration of the psoas shadow.

Treatment. Aggressive fluid resuscitation and support of cardiovascular function should begin immediately. Stabilization of the patient before surgical intervention is mandatory. Antibiotic therapy must provide coverage for those organisms that predominate at the site of presumed origin of the infection. For perforation of the lower gastrointestinal tract, a regimen of ampicillin, gentamicin, and clindamycin will adequately address infection by *E. coli, Klebsiella,* and *Bacteroides* species, and enterococci. Alternative therapy could include ticarcillin-clavulanic acid and an aminoglycoside. Surgery to repair a perforated viscus should proceed after the patient is stabilized and antibiotic therapy initiated. Intraoperative peritoneal fluid cultures will indicate whether a change in the antibiotic regimen is warranted.

Furth SL, Donaldson LA, Sullivan EK, et al: Peritoneal dialysis catheter infections and peritonitis in children: A report of the North American Pediatric Renal Transplant Cooperative Study. *Pediatr Nephrol* 2000;15:179.

Haecker FM, Berger D, Schumacher U, et al: Peritonitis in childhood: Aspects of pathogenesis and therapy. *Pediatr Surg Int* 2000;16:182.

352.3 Acute Secondary Localized Peritonitis (Peritoneal Abscess)

Etiology. Intra-abdominal abscesses may develop within visceral intra-abdominal organs (hepatic, splenic, renal, pancreatic, tubo-ovarian abscesses) or in the interintestinal, periappendiceal, subdiaphragmatic, subhepatic, pelvic, and retroperitoneal spaces. Most commonly, periappendiceal and pelvic abscesses arise from a perforation of the appendix. Transmural inflammation with fistula formation may result in intra-abdominal abscess formation in children with Crohn disease.

Clinical Manifestations. Prolonged fever, anorexia, vomiting, and lassitude are suggestive of the development of an intra-abdominal abscess. The peripheral white cell count is elevated, as is the erythrocyte sedimentation rate. With an appendiceal abscess, there is localized tenderness and a palpable mass in the right lower quadrant.

A pelvic abscess is suggested by abdominal distention, rectal tenesmus with or without the passage of small-volume mucous stools, and bladder irritability. Rectal examination may reveal a tender mass anteriorly. Subphrenic gas collection, basal atelectasis, elevated hemidiaphragm, and pleural effusion may be present with a subdiaphragmatic abscess. Psoas abscess can develop from extension of infection from a retroperitoneal appendicitis, Crohn disease, or a perirenal or intrarenal abscess. Abdominal findings may be minimal, and presentation may include a limp, hip pain, and fever. Both ultrasound examination and computed tomography (CT) scanning can be used to localize intra-abdominal abscesses. Gallium scanning is usually not needed.

Treatment. An abscess should be drained and appropriate antibiotic therapy provided. Drainage may be performed under radiologic control (ultrasonogram or CT guidance) and an indwelling drainage catheter left in place. Initial broad-spectrum antibiotic coverage with ampicillin, gentamicin, and clindamycin should be started and can be modified depending on the results of sensitivity testing. The treatment of appendiceal rupture complicated by abscess formation may be problematic because intestinal phlegmon formation can make surgical resection more difficult. Intensive antibiotic therapy for 4–6 wk followed by an interval appendectomy is often the treatment course followed.

Schwartz MZ, Tapper D, Solenberger RI: Management of perforated appendicitis in children: The controversy continues. *Ann Surg* 1983;197:407.
Wilson-Storey D, Scobie WG: Appendix masses—A 15 year review. *Pediatr Surg Int* 1989;4:165.

Chapter 353

Diaphragmatic Hernia

Gary E. Hartman

Herniation of abdominal contents into the thoracic cavity may occur as a result of a congenital or traumatic defect in the diaphragm. Symptomatology and prognosis depend on the location of the defect and associated anomalies. The defect may be at the esophageal hiatus (hiatal), adjacent to the hiatus (paraesophageal), retrosternal (Morgagni), or posterolateral (Bochdalek). Although all these defects are congenital, the term *congenital diaphragmatic hernia* (CDH) has become synonymous with herniation through the posterolateral foramen of Bochdalek. These lesions usually present with profound respiratory distress in the neonatal period, may be associated with anomalies of other organ systems, and have a significant (40–50%) mortality.

Epidemiology. Reports of the incidence of CDH vary from 1 in 5,000 live births to 1 in 2,000 if stillbirths are included. Defects are more common on the left (70–85%) and are occasionally (5%) bilateral. Malrotation of the intestine and some degree of pulmonary hypoplasia occur in virtually all cases and are considered components of the lesion and not associated anomalies. True associated anomalies have been recognized in 20–30% and include central nervous system lesions, esophageal atresia, omphalocele, cardiovascular lesions, and recognized syndromes. In addition to trisomy 21, the lethal syndromes of trisomy 13, trisomy 18, Fryn, Brachmann–de Lange, and Pallister-Killian have been described. Tetrasomy 12p mosaicism (Pallister-Killian syndrome) may have a normal peripheral blood karyotype as a result of infrequent involvement of lymphocytes. This lethal syndrome can be diagnosed by karyotype from amniocentesis or neonatal bone marrow or fibroblasts. Reports of occurrence of CDH in twins, siblings, and offspring are sporadic. An autosomal recessive inheritance mode has been suggested in families with complete agenesis of the diaphragm.

Etiology. Separation of the developing thoracic and abdominal cavities is accomplished by closure of the posterolateral pleuroperitoneal canals during the 8th wk of gestation. Failure of this canal to close has been the postulated mechanism for the development of congenital posterolateral diaphragmatic hernia. This may be the mechanism in patients with a small diaphragmatic defect. Production of unilateral or bilateral diaphragmatic defects in experimental animals by in utero drug exposure suggests an additional mechanism that may explain larger defects. Portions of the diaphragm and the pulmonary parenchyma arise from the developing thoracic mesenchyme, which, if disrupted, may explain the absence of the major portion of a hemidiaphragm and the severe pulmonary hypoplasia that usually accompanies such a large defect.

Pathology. The pathologic changes in infants with congenital diaphragmatic hernia are not limited to the diaphragm. The diaphragmatic defect may be small and slitlike or include the entire hemidiaphragm. Both lungs are small compared with those of age- and weight-matched controls, with the lung on the side of the defect more severely affected. There is a decrease in the number of alveoli and bronchial generations. The pulmonary vasculature is abnormal, with a decrease in volume and marked increase in muscular mass in the arterioles. Although there is some evidence that the pulmonary abnormalities are due to compression by the intrathoracic abdominal viscera, it is not accepted that physical compression is the sole or primary cause.

Clinical Manifestations. Although many cases are identified by prenatal ultrasonography, the majority of infants with CDH experience severe respiratory distress within the first hours of life. A small group will present beyond the neonatal period. Patients with a delayed presentation may experience vomiting as a result of intestinal obstruction or mild respiratory symptoms. Delayed presentation of right diaphragmatic hernia after a documented episode of group B streptococcal sepsis is well described. Occasionally, incarceration of the intestine will proceed to ischemia with sepsis and cardiorespiratory collapse. Unrecognized diaphragmatic hernia is a rare cause of sudden death in infants and toddlers.

Diagnosis. Prenatal diagnosis by ultrasonography is common. Careful evaluation for other anomalies should include echocardiography and amniocentesis. Occasionally, a fetus with ultrasonographic diagnosis in utero will have no abnormality on postnatal x-ray film. Parents with the ultrasonographic diagnosis of diaphragmatic hernia must be counseled carefully by a multidisciplinary group with significant experience with this condition if unnecessary terminations and unrealistic expectations are to be avoided.

After birth most infants with diaphragmatic hernia will experience severe respiratory collapse within the first 24 hr. The absence of breath sounds and shift of heart sounds common to CDH and pneumothorax will be accompanied by a scaphoid abdomen in infants with CDH. Thoracentesis or tube thoracostomy should be withheld if CDH is considered a possibility. Chest roentgenogram is usually diagnostic (Fig. 353–1). The lateral view frequently demonstrates the intestine passing through the posterior portion of the diaphragm. Occasionally, congenital cystic lesions of the lung may produce a similar radiographic appearance. Differentiation from diaphragmatic hernia may be accomplished by postnatal ultrasonography or injection of contrast into the stomach or umbilical artery catheter to identify intestine above the diaphragm. In older children with atypical symptoms, contrast studies of the gastrointestinal tract are usually required. Ultrasonography and fluoroscopy are helpful in distinguishing eventration from true hernia, and computed tomography may be necessary to exclude pneumatoceles or complicated effusions.

Treatment. The availability of extracorporeal membrane oxygenation (ECMO) and the utility of preoperative stabilization have been the major stimuli to aggressive therapy (Chapter 90.7). Diaphragmatic hernia was once considered a surgical emergency. Recognition of the role of pulmonary hypertension in addition to pulmonary hypoplasia and the adverse effects of operative repair on pulmonary function has caused a policy of delayed repair. The postnatal mass effect of the herniated viscera is a minor factor in the cardiorespiratory compromise compared with the pulmonary hypertension and hypoplasia.

Initial resuscitation has traditionally consisted of attempted stabilization with sedation and paralysis and modest hyperventilation (partial pressure of carbon dioxide of 25–30 mm Hg). Permissive hypercapnia with gentle ventilation has been proposed by a number of centers with reports of equal or improved survival and decreased incidence of need for ECMO. Volume resuscitation, dopamine, and bicarbonate (to maintain pH > 7.50) may also be helpful. If the infant stabilizes and demonstrates stable pulmonary vascular resistance without significant right-to-left shunting, repair of the diaphragm is performed at 24–72 hr of age. If stabilization is not possible or significant shunting persists, most infants will require ECMO support. Vasoactive drugs (dopamine) and inhaled nitric oxide may provide some improvement but have been disappointing as definitive therapy for the pulmonary hypertension associated with diaphragmatic hernia. Dipyridamole has been reported to facilitate weaning from inhaled nitric oxide in refractory pulmonary hypertension. Surfactant administration has also been shown to produce a transient improvement in oxygenation in some infants with CDH.

ECMO with paralysis and nasogastric suction may produce a dramatic reduction of the volume of herniated viscera. The duration of ECMO for neonates with diaphragmatic hernia is significantly longer (7–14 days) than for those with persistent fetal circulation or meconium aspiration and may last up to 2–4 wk. Timing of repair of the diaphragm on ECMO is controversial; some centers prefer early repair to allow a greater duration of postrepair ECMO, whereas many centers defer repair until the infant has demonstrated the ability to tolerate weaning from ECMO. In either case, recurrence of pulmonary hypertension carries a high mortality, and weaning from ECMO support should be cautious. If the patient cannot be weaned from ECMO after repair, options include discontinuing support or therapies such as nitric oxide or lung transplantation. High-frequency jet ventilation and oscillatory ventilation have had limited success in newborns with CDH.

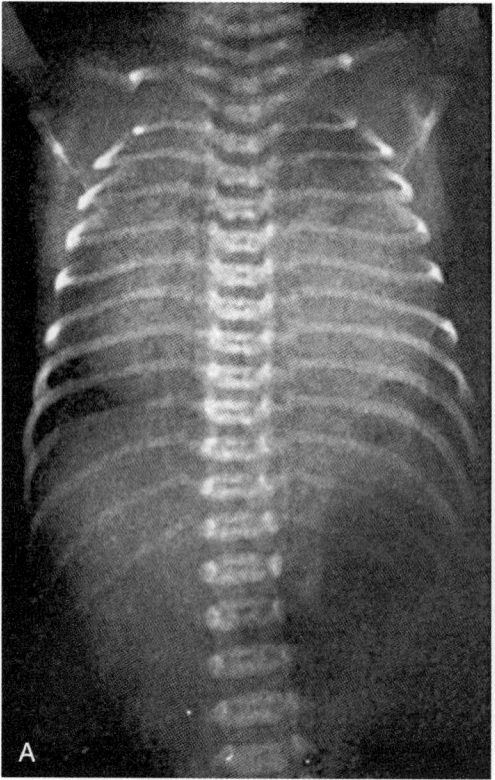
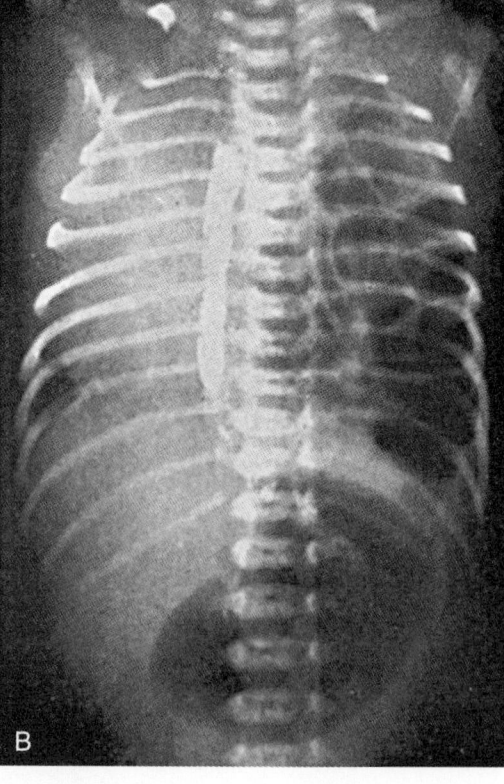

FIGURE 353–1. Congenital diaphragmatic hernia. *A,* Film exposed shortly after birth: Distortion of shadow of the left leaf of the diaphragm with huge, masslike density in left hemithorax displacing the heart to the right. *B,* Film exposed about 20 min after *A.* As the result of swallowed air, coils of air-filled small bowel are now demonstrated in the left hemithorax. The esophagus is outlined by swallowed contrast material. Operative correction was attempted because of extreme dyspnea. Infant died 5.5 hr after birth.

The abdominal surgical approach is favored because the accompanying malrotation may be addressed if necessary, and the abdominal wall may be left open with skin only closed or a Silastic pouch applied if abdominal pressure is considered excessive. Synthetic patch (polytetrafluoroethylene) is now preferred over autologous muscle transfer or tight primary closure for large defects.

The appreciation of the compressive effects of the herniated viscera and the availability of prenatal diagnosis suggested the utility of in utero measures directed at potentially reversing the pulmonary hypoplasia and, it is hoped, the pulmonary vascular changes. Prenatal treatment with glucocorticoids has stimulated pulmonary maturity in experimental animals with diaphragmatic hernia. In utero reduction of the herniated viscera also has been successsfully performed. In experimental animals, occluding the trachea in utero enhances lung growth by preventing lung fluid egress. Randomized trials comparing in utero repair or tracheal occlusion with standard postnatal therapy has been discontinued because there was no difference in mortality or morbidity between treatment groups.

Prognosis. Studies of infants with CDH identified in utero report lower survival (27–55%) than noted in reports limited to live births (42–75%). It appears that many fetuses with the diagnosis of CDH who do not survive pregnancy die as a result of elective termination. The incidence of spontaneous fetal demise among fetuses diagnosed as having CDH appears to be 7–10%. Of those surviving to delivery, survival appears to range from 42–75% despite current modalities including ECMO. Factors associated with a poor prognosis include associated major anomaly, symptoms before 24 hr of age, severe pulmonary hypoplasia and herniation to the contralateral lung, distress severe enough to require ECMO, and delivery in a nontertiary center. Initial attempts at intrauterine repair were associated with a low survival (29%), although current results are more encouraging.

A significant number of survivors are being identified with serious sequelae, primarily pulmonary, neurologic, and growth retardation. These long-term sequelae are probably the result of survival of infants with severe pulmonary compromise. Ten to 20% of CDH survivors require oxygen therapy at discharge.

Studies have documented abnormalities of pulmonary function in the perioperative period and years after repair. Survivors of CDH repair studied at 6–11 yr of age demonstrate significant decreases in forced expiratory flow at 50% of vital capacity and peak expiratory flow. The lung on the affected side is larger than predicted, suggesting hyperinflation, and has reduced perfusion. These patients had undergone repair before the availability of ECMO. In studies of neonatal pulmonary function, neonates with CDH requiring ECMO demonstrate significantly decreased compliance, dynamic compliance, and tidal volume when compared with those not requiring ECMO. After repair, infants with CDH also have evidence of reactive airway disease. Survivors of CDH have evidence of restrictive lung disease and airway reactivity, which are related to the severity of their initial respiratory failure.

Neurologic abnormalities have been identified in survivors of CDH. The incidence of neurologic abnormalities is higher in those infants requiring ECMO (67% vs 24%). The abnormalities are similar to those seen in neonates treated with ECMO for other diagnoses and include transient and permanent developmental delay, abnormal hearing or vision, seizures, and abnormal CT. The majority of neurologic abnormalities are classified as mild or moderate.

Growth and nutrition are compromised in CDH survivors who require ECMO. Forty to 50% are at less than the 5th percentile for weight at 2 yr of age. Weight-to-length ratio is less than the 5th percentile in 40% of survivors at 1 yr and at the 21st percentile at 2 yr. Nearly all ECMO survivors demonstrate clinical evidence of gastroesophageal reflux, and 20% or more

have required fundoplication. Dilation of the esophagus with altered motility that resolves during the 1 yr of life has been correlated with a prenatal history of polyhydramnios.

Other long-term problems occurring in this population include pectus excavatum, scoliosis, fixed pulmonary hypertension, and recurrent herniation. Recurrent hernia formation is common in newborns with large defects requiring synthetic patch repair. Reherniation, which occurs within the 1st yr, has been reported in 20–40% of those requiring patch repair.

Survivors of CDH repair, particularly those requiring ECMO support, have a variety of long-term abnormalities that appear to improve with time but require close monitoring and multidisciplinary support.

353.1 Foramen of Morgagni Hernia

The anteromedial diaphragmatic defect through the foramen of Morgagni accounts for 2% or less of diaphragmatic hernias. The transverse colon or small intestine is usually contained in the hernia sac. Symptoms are gastrointestinal and typically occur beyond the neonatal period. Repair is recommended for all patients and can be accomplished by laparotomy.

353.2 Paraesophageal Hernia

Paraesophageal hernia is differentiated from hiatal hernia in that the gastroesophageal junction is in the normal location. The herniation of the stomach alongside or adjacent to the gastroesophageal junction is prone to incarceration with strangulation and perforation. This unusual diaphragmatic hernia should be repaired promptly after identification.

353.3 Eventration

Eventration of the diaphragm consists of a thinned diaphragmatic muscle producing elevation of the entire hemidiaphragm or, more commonly, the anterior aspect of the hemidiaphragm. Most eventrations are asymptomatic and do not require repair. Large or symptomatic eventrations may be repaired by plication through an abdominal or a thoracic approach.

Muratore CS, Utter S, Jaksic T, et al: Nutritional morbidity in survivors of congenital diaphragmatic hernia. *J Pediatr Surg* 2001;36:1171–6.

Rasheed A, Tindall S, Cueny DL, et al: Neurodevelopmental outcome after congenital diaphragmatic hernia: Extracorporeal membrane oxygenation before and after surgery. *J Pediatr Surg* 2001;36:539–44.

Sbragia L, Paek BW, Filly RA, et al: Congenital diaphragmatic hernia without herniation of the liver: Does lung to head ratio predict survival? *J Ultrasound Med* 2000;19(12):845–8.

Thibeault DW, Haney B: Lung volume, pulmonary vasculature, and factors affecting survival in congenital diaphragmatic hernia. *Pediatrics* 1998;101:289.

Van Meurs KP, Robbins ST, Reed VL, et al: Congenital diaphragmatic hernia: Long-term outcome in neonates treated with extracorporeal membrane oxygenation. J Pediatr 1993;122:893.

Chapter 354
Epigastric Hernia *Gary E. Hartman*

Epigastric hernias are defects in the linea alba between the xyphoid and the umbilicus. They are uncommon in childhood, constituting less than 1% of hernias requiring operation. Similar defects below the umbilicus are even more uncommon. These hernias usually contain preperitoneal fat and rarely cause symptoms. They may appear as an intermittent bulge or a midline mass if the fat is incarcerated. Herniation of intestine or other viscera is extremely rare. Repair is indicated for symptomatic hernias or for diagnosis in the case of a mass. Treatment of asymptomatic hernias of the linea alba is less clear. Some believe that many will resolve spontaneously and discourage elective repair. Others believe that they never resolve and will eventually require repair. Abdominal symptoms other than local pain and tenderness should prompt further diagnostic study rather than repair of the epigastric hernia.

354.1 ■ Incisional Hernia

Hernia formation at the site of a previous laparotomy is uncommon in childhood. Factors associated with an increased risk of incisional hernia include increased intra-abdominal pressure, wound infection, and midline incision. Transverse abdominal incisions are favored because of their increased strength and blood supply, which reduce the likelihood of wound infection and incisional hernia. Although most incisional hernias will require repair, operation should be deferred until the child is in optimal medical condition. Some incisional hernias will resolve, especially those occurring in infants. Some recommend elastic bandaging to discourage enlargement of the hernia and to promote spontaneous healing. Newborns with abdominal wall defects represent the largest group of children with incisional hernias. Initial management should be conservative, with repair deferred until about 1 yr of age. Incarceration is very uncommon but is an indication for prompt repair.

Coats RD, Helikson MA, Burd RS: Presentation and management of epigastric hernias in children. *J Pediatr Surg* 2000;35:1754–6.
Neblett KW, Holcomb TM: Umbilical and other abdominal wall hernias. In Ashcraft KW, Holder TM (editors): *Pediatric Surgery.* Philadelphia, WB Saunders, 1993, pp 557–561.

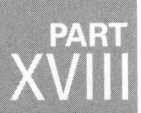
The Respiratory System

SECTION 1 *Development and Function*

Chapter 355

Development of the Respiratory System

Gabriel G. Haddad and J. Julio Pérez Fontán

The development of the respiratory system encompasses three distinct processes: morphogenesis or formation of all the necessary structures, adaptation to postnatal atmospheric breathing, and dimensional growth. The first two processes take place primarily before or shortly after birth of an infant. Growth, in contrast, continues after birth at a pace that is generally dictated by the functional needs of the other growing organs and metabolic activity of the child. The effects of an injury to the respiratory system depend, therefore, not only on the severity and chronicity of the injury but also on the timing of the injury in relation to the developmental timetable of the lungs. Insults occurring during morphogenesis, for instance, tend to produce severe and irreversible disruptions of respiratory structure and function, often incompatible with survival. In contrast, injuries that take place during later stages of lung growth are frequently reversible and, if not, can be compensated for by the growth process itself.

Prenatal Development: Morphogenesis. In humans and other mammals, the morphogenesis of the respiratory system is divided into five periods (Fig. 355–1). The first, or *embryonic period*, begins at approximately 4 wk of gestation, when the primitive airways appear as a ventral outpouching on the endodermal epithelium of the foregut. This outpouching divides almost immediately into two main stem bronchial buds, which burrow rapidly into the mesenchyme separating the foregut from the coelomic cavity. The bronchial buds start to branch, first by monopodal outgrowth (secondary branches grow out of a main branch) and then by asymmetric dichotomy (two secondary branches originate from one main branch).

The peribronchial mesenchyme or *splanchnopleura* plays an essential role in shaping the lungs during the embryonic period. Close contact between this mesenchyme and the epithelium of the bronchial buds is essential for the continued branching of the airways. Although the factors that promote bronchial division are not fully identified, steroid-induced secretion of growth factors by the mesenchymal fibroblasts, specific interactions with acellular components of the mesenchyme, and even direct molecular communications between fibroblasts and endodermal cells across gaps in the basal membrane may be signaling mechanisms. The interactions between mesenchyme and the bronchial bud endoderm are organ specific.

The pulmonary vasculature is a mesenchymal derivative. Soon after their appearance, the bronchial buds are surrounded by a vascular plexus, which originates from the aorta and drains into the major somatic veins. This vascular plexus connects with the pulmonary artery and veins to complete the pulmonary circulation at the 7th wk of gestation but retains some aortic connections that form the bronchial arteries. All the supporting structures of the lungs, including the pleura, the septal network of the lungs, and the smooth muscle, cartilage, and connective covers of the airways, originate from the mesenchyme.

Toward the 6th wk of gestation, at the beginning of the second or *pseudoglandular period*, the lungs resemble an exocrine gland with a thick stroma crossed by narrow ducts lined by an epithelium of tall cells that almost fill the lumen. The major airways are already present and are in close association with pulmonary arteries and veins. The trachea and the foregut are now separated after the progressive fusion of epithelial ridges growing from the primitive airway. The incomplete fusion of these ridges results in a **tracheoesophageal fistula,** a common congenital malformation. During the pseudoglandular period, the airways continue to branch until the entire conducting airway system is formed, including the primitive bronchioles that eventually give rise to the air-exchanging portions of the lungs. Simultaneously, the pluripotential cells that line the airways differentiate, starting from the trachea and main bronchi. They soon form a thinner, pseudostratified epithelium containing ciliated, secretory (Clara), globular, and neuroendocrine (Kulchitsky) cells of neuroectodermal origin. Mucus glands, cartilage, and smooth muscle can be easily distinguished by the 16th wk of gestation.

The diaphragm is formed during this period. Its central tendon originates from the transverse septum, a plate of mesodermal tissue located between the pericardium and the stalk of the yolk sac. Its lateral portions are formed by the pleuroperitoneal folds, which grow from the body wall until they fuse with the esophageal mesentery and the transverse septum. The fusion eliminates the communication between thorax and abdomen and establishes a barrier to the caudal growth of the lungs. Its failure, usually on the left side, causes the **congenital diaphragmatic hernia of Bochdalek** (see Chapter 353). This defect allows the abdominal organs to enter the primitive pleural cavity and interferes with airway and pulmonary vascular branching. The result is severe hypoplasia of the lung, particularly on the side of the hernia.

During the third or *canalicular period*, between the 16th and 26–28th wk of gestation, epithelial growth predominates over mesenchymal growth. As a result, the bronchial tree develops a more tubular appearance, whereas its distal regions subdivide further to lay the structural foundations of the pulmonary acinus. The epithelial cells in these regions become more cuboidal and start to express some of the antigen markers that characterize cells as type II pneumocytes. Some cells become flatter and can be identified as potential type I pneumocytes by the presence of a sparse endoplasmic reticulum and abundant cytoplasmic glycogen. The capillaries contained in the distal bronchial mesenchyme form a denser network and grow closer to the

1357

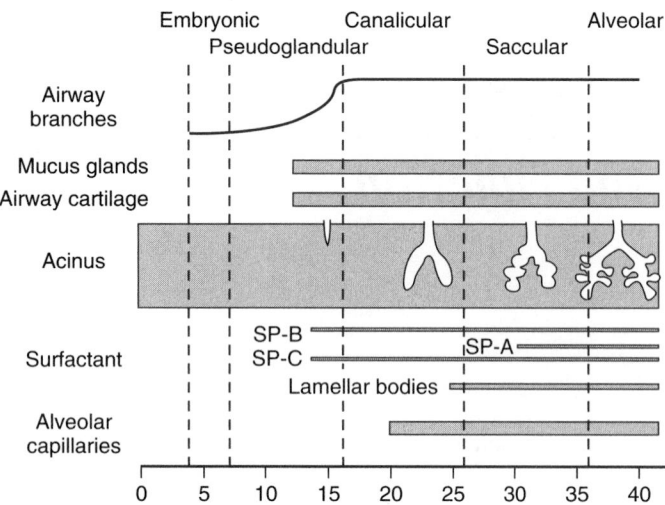

FIGURE 355–1. Development of various pulmonary structures during the five stages of prenatal lung development (see text).

potential air spaces, making limited gas exchange possible by 22 wk of gestation.

Between the 26–28th wk of gestation, lung morphogenesis enters its *saccular period*, during which the terminal airways continue to widen and form cylindrical structures known as saccules. Initially smooth, the internal surface of the saccules soon develops ridges or secondary crests, which originate as folds of the epithelium and peribronchial mesenchyme and contain a double capillary layer. The distance between the capillaries and the potential air spaces narrows further until eventually only a thin basal membrane separates them.

Exactly when the saccular period ends and the *alveolar period* begins depends on the definition of what constitutes an alveolus. Formation of alveoli before birth is not a requisite for survival. In the human fetus, the saccular septation initiated with the appearance of the secondary crests continues at a rapid rate so that multifaceted structures analogous to the alveoli of the mature lung can be seen at 32 wk of gestation. There is substantial evidence that the timing and progression of alveolar septation is under endocrine regulation. Thyroid hormones stimulate septation, whereas glucocorticoids impair it in a fashion that, at least in the rat, can be irrevocable (even though they accelerate the thinning of the alveolar capillary membranes). Alveolarization is also influenced by physical stimuli. Both the stretch by the liquid contained in the fetal lung and the periodic distention provided by the action of the respiratory muscles during fetal breathing, for instance, appear to be necessary for the development of the acini. Their absence when the lungs or chest are compressed (as in the case of a diaphragmatic hernia or oligohydramnios) or when fetal breathing is abolished (e.g., by spinal cord lesions) results in **pulmonary hypoplasia** with reduced numbers of alveoli.

A number of gene families have been identified as being essential for development. The homeodomain or homeobox (hox) gene family is critical in mammalian organ development, including that of the respiratory system. Hoxa-1,2,3,5, and Hoxb-3,4,6,7,8 mRNA transcripts have been identified using molecular biologic techniques in branching regions of the developing mouse lung. These *Hox* genes were differentially expressed in time and space in early lung development, indicating that they play a role in the differentiation, maturation, and proliferation of various lung cells throughout the various phases of lung development. Hoxa-2 seems to be tied to a proximal role in branching and differentiation, whereas Hoxb-6 is involved in distal airway branching. Also of importance is the fact that the expression of some of these genes is controlled by retinoic acid.

This may be related to a possible therapeutic role of retinoic acid at later stages of lung development or in injured lungs.

Adaptation to Air Breathing. The transition from placental dependence to autonomous gas exchange requires adaptive changes in the lungs. These changes include the production of surfactant in the alveoli, the transformation of the lung from a secretory to a gas-exchanging organ, and the establishment of parallel pulmonary and systemic circulations.

As soon as the newborn infant takes the first breath of air, an air-liquid interface becomes established inside the lungs. Unless the surface tension generated at this interface is reduced, the walls of the air spaces would tend to stick together and collapse, threatening the geometric stability of the lungs. The pulmonary surfactant makes such a reduction possible by forming a hydrophobic lipid monolayer at the very surface of the liquid film that lines the air spaces (see Chapters 90.3 and 397). Pulmonary surfactant is a heterogeneous mixture of phospholipids and proteins secreted into the saccular or alveolar subphase by the type II pneumocytes. Its presence is first recognized in characteristic secretory organelles known as lamellar bodies as early as the 24th wk of gestation. However, surfactant lipids, of which the most abundant is phosphatidylcholine, are not detectable in the amniotic fluid until the 30th wk of gestation, suggesting that there is a chronologic gap between surfactant synthesis and secretion. Labor probably shortens this gap because phospholipids are consistently found in the air spaces of infants born before the 30th wk of gestation. Three apoproteins (SP-A, SP-B, SP-C) identified in pulmonary surfactant (a fourth lectin-like glycoprotein, SP-D, has been isolated, but its function and regulation are still poorly understood) promote the spreading of the surfactant layer and are therefore essential for the effective reduction of surface tension. Apoproteins also appear to be important for the reuptake and recycling of surfactant products and for the formation of tubular myelin (the structures in which surfactant is stored in the liquid subphase).

Surfactant apoproteins and phospholipids share some, but not all, of their regulatory influences. Glucocorticoids, for instance, increase the synthesis of both apoproteins and lipids; accordingly, their prenatal administration has been used to prevent the respiratory distress syndrome associated with prematurity. Because many actions of the steroids involve direct stimulation of response elements in apoprotein and phospholipid enzyme genes and therefore require messenger RNA production, sufficient time must elapse between steroid administration and birth. Thyroid hormones also enhance the synthesis of phospholipids by a receptor-mediated mechanism, but, unlike the glucocorticoids, have little or no effect on surfactant apoprotein synthesis. Conversely, β-adrenergic agonists and other agents that raise cellular cyclic adenosine monophosphate content increase apoprotein synthesis and phosphatidylcholine secretion into the air spaces but have no effect on phospholipid synthesis. Insulin, hyperglycemia, ketosis, and androgens may have negative effects on the production of surfactant proteins and phospholipids, thus explaining the high incidence of respiratory distress syndrome in infants of diabetic mothers and the slight maturational delay of the lungs of male fetuses compared with female fetuses.

Surfactant proteins and lipids also may play an important role in lung immunity, although the molecular details are not known. Surfactant proteins A and D are lectins (bind to carbohydrates) and belong to the collectins family of genes. These proteins, present in the serum and lungs, stimulate phagocytosis and chemotaxis, produce reactive oxygen species, and regulate the production and release of cytokines by immune cells. Alternatively, surfactant lipids can suppress immunity. It is possible that the ratio between surfactant lipids and proteins is important in regulating the immune status of the lungs. This may be critical in premature infants and in newborns who lack surfactant proteins; knockout mice with SP-A deficiency have a major problem with infections.

The fetal lung is a secretory organ. Throughout gestation, a Cl^-, K^+-, and H^+-enriched fluid is produced in its peripheral air spaces with the help of a Cl^- pump. The presence of this fluid appears to be important for the development of the acinus because chronic drainage of the trachea in experimental animals results in lung hypoplasia. Fluid secretion, however, is incompatible with air breathing. Accordingly, and in preparation for birth, lung fluid production decreases slowly at the end of gestation. This decrease, which is accelerated by the beginning of labor, denotes a transformation in the ion transfer activities of the pulmonary epithelium from Cl^- (and water) secretion to Na^+ (and water) absorption. In experimental animals, such a transformation can be precipitated by the administration of β-adrenergic agonists at doses that result in serum levels comparable to those found during labor. Stimulation of β-adrenergic receptors is not the only labor-related signal because fluid clearance in the fetal lung is delayed by the Na^+ channel blocker amiloride but not by β-blockers. After birth, the still substantial amount of fluid left in the lungs is absorbed over several hours into the circulation either directly through pulmonary vessels or indirectly through an already very effective lymphatic system. The cellular elements responsible for fluid secretion and absorption in the lungs are not fully identified. It is obvious that a mature alveolar epithelium is not essential for fluid secretion, which is already taking place before alveoli or even saccules exist. Alveolar cells, in contrast, probably play a protagonistic role in fluid absorption. Type II pneumocytes may be involved because they cover a larger portion of the air space surface in the newborn than in the adult and their metabolic machinery appears to be particularly well adapted to active ion transport.

A number of transporters and channels that are important to water and solute transport in early life have been cloned and identified in the past decade. Most prominent has been the epithelial sodium channel (ENaC). It is the amiloride-sensitive and apical channel that is responsible for sodium and water absorption in the luminal surface of the airways and renal tubular cells. This channel seems to be critical in early life.

At birth, the pulmonary circulation changes from a high-resistance to a low-resistance system and, as a consequence, pulmonary blood flow becomes capable of accommodating systemic venous return. The change in resistance is brought about by the combined effects of the mechanical forces applied on the pulmonary vascular walls by the expanding lung tissue and the relaxation of the pulmonary arterial smooth muscle caused by the increased alveolar concentrations of oxygen and probably by endogenous release of vasodilators. The subsequent closure of the foramen ovale and the ductus arteriosus completely separates the pulmonary from the systemic circulation. Arterial oxygen tension then rises sharply and becomes homogeneous throughout the body. Pulmonary vascular resistance continues to decrease gradually during the first few weeks after birth through a process of structural remodeling of the pulmonary vessel musculature.

Postnatal Development. The postnatal development of the lungs can be divided into two phases depending on the relative rates of development of the various components of the lungs. During the first phase, which extends to the first 18 mo after birth, there is a disproportionate increase in the surface and volume of the compartments involved in gas exchange. Capillary volume increases more rapidly than air space volume, which, in turn, increases more rapidly than solid tissue volume. These changes are accomplished primarily through a process of alveolar septation. This process is particularly active during early infancy and may reach completion within the first 2 yr of life. The configuration of the air spaces becomes progressively more complex, not only because of the development of new septa but

also because of the lengthening and folding of the existing alveolar structures. Soon after birth, the double capillary system contained in the alveolar septa of the fetus fuses into one single, denser system. At the same time, new arterial and venous branches develop within the circulatory system of the acinus and muscle starts to appear in the medial layer of the intra-acinar arteries.

During the second phase, all compartments grow more proportionately to each other. Although new alveoli may still be formed, the majority of the growth occurs through an increase in the volume of existing alveoli. Alveolar and capillary surfaces expand in parallel with somatic growth. As a result, taller individuals tend to have larger lungs. However, the final size of the lungs and, ultimately, the dimensions of the individual constituents of the acinus are also influenced by factors such as the subject's level of activity and prevailing state of oxygenation (altitude), which allow for a better adaptation of lung structure and function. The same factors are probably operative in the compensatory responses to pulmonary disease and injury.

Bucher U, Reid L: Development of the intrasegmental bronchial tree: The pattern of branching and development of cartilage at various stages of intrauterine life. *Thorax* 1961;16:207.
Gross I: Regulation of fetal lung maturation. *Am J Physiol* 1990;259:L337.
Langston C, Kida K, Reed M, et al: Human lung growth in late gestation and in the neonate. *Am Rev Respir Dis* 1984;129:607.
O'Brodovich H: Epithelial ion transport in the fetal and perinatal lung. *Am J Physiol* 1991; 261:C555.
Tchepichev S, Ueda J, Canessa C, et al: Lung epithelial Na channel subunits are differentially regulated during development and by steroids. *Am J Physiol* 1995; 269:C805.

Chapter 356
Regulation of Respiration
Gabriel G. Haddad

Pediatricians need to be familiar with the general principles of the regulation of respiration because (1) clinical situations involving one or more elements of the respiratory control system are prevalent, especially in critically ill patients (e.g., apnea, upper airway obstruction, severe asthma, hypoventilation, and heart failure, or hypoxemia from various causes); (2) transition from fetal to neonatal life is an extremely complex process during which there are major changes in almost every aspect of respiratory control; and (3) understanding of the neural control of respiration is likely to increase significantly from advances in understanding brain function in general.

The Respiratory Control System is a Negative Feedback System with a Central Controller. The overall aim of the respiratory feedback system is to keep blood gas homeostasis in a normal range in the most economical way, from an energy consumption and mechanical standpoint. The term *negative* in this concept refers to the fact that the controller attempts to rectify the deviation from normality. If CO_2 increases, for example as a result of airway obstruction, the output of the controller is increased in an attempt to increase alveolar ventilation and decrease CO_2. To accomplish this, the feedback system makes use of both an afferent limb and an efferent limb. The afferent limb is made up of tissues (e.g., the airways) that have receptor endings and can send information to the central controller about certain functional parameters, such as the magnitude of stretch of the airways. The carotid bodies that inform the central controller of the status of O_2 and pH represent another important part of the afferent system. Both airway and carotid body sensors have a way to compare signals, the inherent set point signal and the real actual one, note differences, and translate these differences into information (e.g., a decrease or increase in action potential volleys) to the central nervous system (CNS). The efferent loop is the part of the feedback system that is responsible for the execution of the decision made centrally to increase or decrease central respiratory output (i.e., increase or decrease respiratory muscle output). There are many muscles of respiration, the intercostal muscles and the diaphragm being only two of them. Activity and timing of the airway muscles, as is seen later, are crucial in determining airway resistance and, therefore, the magnitude of ventilation.

The Central Controller Integrates Incoming Afferent Information and Generates and Maintains Respiration. It is not known in precise mechanistic and cellular terms how and where integration and generation of breathing take place. Two groups of medullary neurons have been considered as potential sites for the initiation of respiration, namely, the nucleus tractus solitarius and the nucleus ambiguus (and retroambiguus). Another area in the medulla (pre-Botzinger complex) has been implicated as a major site for the generation of respiration. This region is essential for the respiratory rhythm generation and could constitute the "sinus node" of respiration. There are neurons in this complex that have pacemaker-like membrane properties. However, the nature of the central respiratory rhythm generator is not yet fully clear. The respiratory controller may be a group of neurons that either form an emergent network or are endogenous or conditional bursters. In the first case, respiratory neurons would not have special properties (e.g., bursting properties) that would make their membrane potential oscillate. This type of a respiratory rhythm generator would *not* be like the sinus node cells of the heart. Rather, the output of the network that they form would oscillate because of the special interconnections and synaptic interactions among these respiratory neurons. In the second case, in a manner similar to that of the heart, the respiratory neurons would have special properties that make individual neurons "burst" or oscillate (pacemaker), even if they are disconnected from any other neurons (endogenous burster). A conditional burster neuron is a neuron that oscillates only when exposed to certain chemicals (e.g., neurotransmitters). It is likely that, independent of the location of the central pattern generator, a respiratory oscillatory output takes place by virtue of the synaptic and cellular-molecular properties of the neurons in all of these locations. This oscillatory output from the brainstem then drives the phrenic motor neurons in the spinal cord that, in turn, stimulate the diaphragm and other respiratory muscles to contract and move air in the lungs. One issue regarding the activation (or inactivation) of various respiratory muscles is how the central output gets "distributed" on muscles to ensure patency of airways and contraction of the appropriate muscles in order to optimize the work of breathing and lessen the energy needed to move a certain volume of air and ensure alveolar ventilation. This issue is important in some pathologic states during which airway muscle activation may not be well coordinated with chest wall muscle activation, leading to lack of airway patency and inefficient gas exchange.

Afferent Information is Not Necessary for Initiating Respiration but Plays an Important Role in Modulating Breathing. A multitude of afferent messages converge on the brainstem at any one time. Chemoreceptors and mechanoreceptors in the larynx and upper airways sense stretch, air temperature, and chemical changes over the mucosa and relay this information to the brainstem. Afferent impulses from these areas travel through the superior laryngeal nerve and the 10th cranial (vagus) nerve. The superior laryngeal nerve joins and becomes part of the vagal trunk at the nodose ganglion. Changes in O_2 or CO_2 tensions are sensed at the carotid and aortic bodies, and afferent impulses travel

through the carotid and aortic sinus nerves. Thermal or metabolic changes are sensed by skin or mucosal receptors or by hypothalamic neurons and are carried through spinal or central tracts to the brainstem for integrative purposes. Furthermore, afferent information to the brainstem need not be only formulated and sensed by the peripheral nervous system. For example, (1) sensors of CO_2 lie on the ventral surface of the medulla oblongata and therefore feedback about CO_2 levels comes from the brainstem itself and (2) emotions and changes in mood that result from CNS processing in the limbic system influence respiration through pathways connecting higher brain centers to the brainstem.

Afferent information from the peripheral or central nervous system is not a prerequisite for generating and maintaining respiration. When the brainstem and spinal cord are removed from the body and maintained in vitro, rhythmic phrenic activity can be detected and measured for hours. Other experiments in vivo in which several sensory systems are blocked simultaneously indicate that afferent information is not necessary to initiate an inherent respiratory rhythm in brainstem respiratory networks. However, both in vitro and in vivo studies demonstrate that in the absence or elimination of afferent information regarding CO_2 levels, O_2 levels, a wakeful stimulus, and so on, the inherent rhythm of the central generator (respiratory frequency) is slow. Hence, chemoreceptors, temperature receptors, mechanoreceptors, and laryngeal receptors and their afferents play an important part in *modulating* respiration and rhythmic behavior.

The neonate is more exquisitely sensitive to afferent input than is the adult. Laryngeal reflexes are extremely potent in inhibiting respiration in the newborn. Aspiration and stimulation of laryngeal chemoreceptors in premature infants (who lack the ability of a strong cough), especially when these infants are anemic or hypoglycemic or even during normal sleep, can cause life-threatening respiratory events.

Central Integration and Processing in the Brainstem is Hierarchical. Respiratory muscles can be recruited to perform different tasks at different times. For example, the diaphragm and some abdominal muscles are activated not only during tidal breathing but also during expulsive maneuvers such as coughing and straining. In other conditions, respiratory muscles can be totally inhibited. For example, when delivering a speech, CO_2 responsiveness is decreased substantially because speech muscles are recruited mostly at the expense of other respiratory muscles. Bottle- or breast-feeding in the young is often associated with a reduction in ventilation and a drop in Pao_2 because of partial inhibition of respiratory muscles and breathing efforts. Presented with a number of neurophysiologic signals (representing options about various needs), the central controller responds differently to various stimuli and can enhance or reduce the effect of certain stimuli. Therefore, there is a hierarchy that is used by brainstem networks for determining the response of the respiratory system at any one time.

Changes in the state of consciousness modulate the ability of the brainstem to respond to afferent stimuli. For example, trigeminal afferent impulses are less inhibited by cortical influences during quiet sleep than during rapid eye movement (REM) sleep or wakefulness. Thus, the effect of trigeminal stimulation on respiration is more pronounced in quiet sleep. Similarly, age is important. The response of the brainstem to stimuli varies with maturation and thus with cortical input to brainstem structures.

The idea of hierarchical responses is important also because some of the afferent inputs to the CNS have a major impact on the respiratory output whereas others do not. For example, many experiments have shown that the laryngeal afferent input into the brainstem is an extraordinarily potent inhibitory reflex to breathing and its effect on the CNS integrator/pattern generator is instantaneous, taking place in a few milliseconds! This reflex is also very powerful during anesthesia when cortical input to the brainstem is attenuated. This becomes especially important in infants who show frequent apnea and whose apnea gets exaggerated when they are sedated or anesthetized.

Respiratory Muscles and Chest Wall Properties Undergo Postnatal Maturation and Can Fatigue. Effective ventilation requires *coordinated interaction* between the respiratory muscles of the chest wall (including the diaphragm and intercostals) and those of the upper airway (including the pharynx and the larynx) under various conditions of altered respiratory drive. In infants, a specific sequential pattern of nerve and muscle activation occurs so that some upper airway muscles contract before and during the early part of inspiratory flow: the genioglossus muscle contracts, moving the tongue forward, which prevents pharyngeal obstruction, and the vocal cords abduct, reducing inspiratory laryngeal resistance. Laryngeal muscles also modulate expiratory flow and thus may influence lung volume. Imbalance of pharyngeal and diaphragmatic activities or their responses to chemoreceptor or mechanoreceptor stimulation may contribute to obstructive apnea in infants and children.

Because the *respiratory muscles* are responsible for executing central neural responses and because muscle and chest wall properties change with age in early life, it is likely that neural responses can be influenced by pump properties. Thus, it is important to consider the maturational changes of respiratory muscles and the chest wall. For example, one of the important maturational aspects of respiratory muscles (e.g., in skeletal muscles) is their pattern of innervation. In the adult, one muscle fiber is innervated by one motor neuron. Therefore, if a motor neuron innervates certain muscle fibers (e.g., about 200 muscle fibers in the case of the diaphragm), these fibers do not receive innervation from any other motor neuron. In the newborn, however, each fiber is innervated by two or more motor neurons, and the axons of different motor neurons can synapse on the same muscle fiber, hence the term *polyneuronal innervation*. Synapse elimination takes place postnatally and, in the case of the diaphragm, the adult type of innervation is reached by several weeks of age depending on the animal species. The time course of polyneuronal innervation of the diaphragm in the human newborn is not known.

The neuromuscular junctional folds, postsynaptic membranes, and acetylcholine receptors and metabolism undergo major postnatal maturational changes. The acetylcholine quantal content per end plate potential is lower in the newborn than in the adult rat diaphragm. The newborn diaphragm is also more susceptible to neuromuscular transmission failure than is that of the adult, especially at higher frequencies of stimulation. Whether this is the result of differences in acetylcholine metabolism between the newborn and the adult or is related to the neuromuscular junction itself is not known.

In addition to an increase in cross-sectional area and muscle mass, *muscle fiber types* in the diaphragm change as a function of gestational and postnatal age. It is not known whether human newborn muscles are more oxidative or fatigue resistant than those of the adult. The sarcoplasmic reticulum of the premature diaphragm is, however, underdeveloped compared with that of the adult. This is one major reason for the delay in the release and uptake of calcium, which may have functional significance. The poorly developed sarcoplasmic reticulum in the newborn causes increased contraction and relaxation time in neonatal muscle fibers. This increased relaxation time may be an important factor in impeding blood flow and limiting oxidative metabolism when the muscle is under a load.

The *chest wall* in newborn infants is highly compliant. Because of this and because young infants spend a large proportion of time in REM sleep, during which the intercostal muscles are inhibited, there is little splinting of the chest wall for diaphragmatic action. Therefore, with every breath in supine infants

(especially in REM sleep), the chest wall is sucked in paradoxically at a time when the abdomen expands. This creates an additional load on the respiratory system and results in a higher work of breathing per minute ventilation in the infant than in the adult. This may be an important reason for the newborn's susceptibility to muscle fatigue and respiratory failure.

The Newborn Infant and Young Child Respond Differently to Stimuli Compared with the Mature Individual. The young child and neonate respond to various stimuli in a different way than does the adult. In response to low O_2, the newborn infant does not sustain an increase in ventilation, and often ventilation decreases to below baseline levels. CO_2 levels do not increase at a time when ventilation is decreasing, suggesting that ventilation is matching metabolic needs. This neonatal response to low O_2 can be considered an intermediate response between those of the fetus and the adult; the fetus shuts off all respiratory efforts in response to O_2 deprivation, and the adult hyperventilates as long as the stimulus is present. The mechanism or mechanisms for the lack of sustained increase in ventilation during hypoxia in the newborn are not well understood. In addition to differences in metabolic rate during hypoxemia among neonates and adults, changes in the mechanical properties of the lung and airways, maturation of carotid chemoreceptors, and alterations in the cellular and membrane properties of central neurons have all been proposed as potential individual or combined mechanisms. It is clinically important that neonatal tissues (especially heart, brain, and kidneys) resist O_2 deprivation and do not injure as easily as those of the adult. These differences between newborn and adult sensitivity to anoxic injury are not well understood but possibly relate to the ability of the newborn cell to metabolize lactate and ketone, to downregulate metabolism during severe O_2 deprivation, and to regulate certain protein synthesis (e.g., heat-shock proteins) differently from the adult.

CO_2 response is also reduced in the young. Whether this is a reflection of an inherent difference in sensitivity or the result of differences in mechanical function is not known and, presumably, is related to both mechanical and central differences.

Although alterations in responsiveness can be secondary to a number of differences between the young and the mature organism, the central neuronal changes with maturation seem especially important. For example, the soma of lumbar and phrenic motor neurons increases with age, and their input resistance (or inverse of membrane conductance) decreases with age. The decrease in input resistance results in major part from the increase in soma size, but other mechanisms, such as a change in the geometry of the dendrites and their outgrowth, a change in the number of ion channels per surface area, and an increase in the number of synapses onto motor neurons, cannot be ruled out. Axonal velocity also increases with age, and action potentials of phrenic and hypoglossal motoneurons decrease in duration. There are also major maturational changes in active cellular properties in some motor neurons or premotor neurons. For example, with increasing postnatal age, neurons in the area of the nucleus tractus solitarius develop cellular properties important for repetitive firing. Changes in neuronal properties could play an important role in the integrative abilities of neuronal cells and, therefore, in their response to stimulation.

Clinical Implications

APNEA (see Chapter 90.2). Apnea can be defined statistically as the respiratory pause that exceeds 3 SD of the mean breath time for an infant or a child at any particular age. This definition requires data from a population of infants at a particular age, lacks physiologic value, and does not differentiate between relatively shorter or longer respiratory pauses. Alternatively, the definition of apnea may be based on the fact that respiratory pauses are associated with cardiovascular or neurophysiologic changes. Such definition relies on the functional assessment of pauses and is therefore more relevant clinically. Because infants have higher O_2 consumption (per unit weight) than the adult and relatively smaller lung volume and O_2 stores, it is possible that short (e.g., seconds) respiratory pauses that may not be clinically important in the adult may present serious consequences in the very young or premature infant. Independent of age group, respiratory pauses are more prevalent during sleep than during the waking state. The frequency and duration of respiratory pauses depend on the sleep state in human infants. Respiratory pauses are more frequent and shorter in REM than in quiet sleep and are more frequent in younger than in older infants.

Although there is controversy regarding the pathogenesis of respiratory pauses, there is a consensus about certain observations. Normal full-term infants, children, and adult humans exhibit respiratory pauses during sleep. Paradoxically, some believe that the presence of respiratory pauses and breathing irregularity is a "healthy" sign and that the complete absence of such pauses may be indicative of abnormalities. However, prolonged apnea can be life threatening. The pathogenesis of these apneas may relate to the clinical condition of the patient at the time of the apnea, associated cardiovascular (systemic or pulmonary) changes, the chronicity of the clinical condition, the perinatal history, and whether the cause is central or peripheral. Prolonged apneic spells require therapy and, optimally, treatment should be targeted to the underlying pathophysiology.

UPPER AIRWAY OBSTRUCTION (see Chapters 20.5 and 369). Upper airway obstruction (UAO) during sleep is recognized with increasing frequency in children. Many of these children have anatomic abnormalities. A common cause of UAO in children is tonsillar and adenoidal hypertrophy caused by repeated upper respiratory tract infections. Other associated abnormalities include craniofacial malformations, micrognathia, and muscular hypotonia. The usual site of obstruction in UAO in both infants and adults is the oropharynx, between the posterior pharyngeal wall, the soft palate, and the genioglossus. During sleep (especially REM sleep), upper airway muscles, including those of the oropharynx, lose tone and trigger an episode of UAO. The treatment should be targeted primarily at the underlying cause of obstruction.

Haddad GG: Cellular and membrane properties of brainstem neurons in early life. In Haddad GG, Farber J (editors): *Lung Biology in Health and Disease*, Vol 53, *Developmental Neurobiology of Breathing*. New York, Marcel Dekker, 1991, pp 591–614.

Haddad GG, Donnelly DF, Bazzy AR: Developmental control of respiration: Neurobiologic basis. In Dempsey JA, Pack AI (editors): *Lung Biology in Health and Disease*, Vol 79, *Regulation of Breathing*. New York, Marcel Dekker, 1994, pp 743–85.

Smith JC, Ellenberger HH, Ballanyi K, et al: Pre-Botzinger complex: A brainstem region that may generate respiratory rhythm in mammals. *Science* 1991;254: 726–29.

Chapter 357

Respiratory Pathophysiology

J. Julio Pérez Fontán and Gabriel G. Haddad

In humans, the respiratory system consists of a pumping mechanism (the respiratory muscles, the chest wall, and the conducting airways), a membrane gas exchanger (the interface between the air spaces and the pulmonary circulation), and a central neural control connected to a network of chemical and mechanical sensors distributed throughout the circulation and the components of the respiratory system itself. Basic to this arrangement is the close integration of respiratory and circulatory functions, which ensures not only the efficiency of gas exchange but also the ability to adapt oxygen uptake and carbon dioxide elimination to the variable demands of life. Alterations in the components of the respiratory system or its interaction with the circulatory system give rise to a variety of clinical manifestations. The most severe of these manifestations is the development of abnormal partial pressures of carbon dioxide (Pco_2) and oxygen (Po_2) in the arterial blood, a situation known as respiratory failure.

Respiratory Distress and Respiratory Failure. The function of the respiratory pump is regulated by a highly responsive neuronal network that integrates chemical signals from chemoreceptors located in the ventral reticular nuclei of the medulla (central chemoreceptors sensitive to pH and Pco_2) and carotid bodies (peripheral chemoreceptors, sensitive to Po_2) and from mechanoreceptors located in the lungs to influence the neural output to the respiratory muscles. Increases in arterial Pco_2 (hypercapnia) and decreases in arterial Po_2 (hypoxemia) trigger an immediate increase in this output, which is distributed primarily to various spinal nuclei innervating either the diaphragm or muscles such as the scalenes and abdominal muscles, the latter being muscles that do not participate in normal breathing at rest (accessory muscles). The result is an increase in minute ventilation (the product of tidal volume and breathing frequency), which may return, under some circumstances, the Pco_2 and Po_2 to the physiologic range. Consequently, even before respiratory failure occurs, respiratory disease is usually detected either as an apparent or a subjective increase in the effort that the individual makes during breathing or as a limitation in the respiratory system's ability to accommodate increased demands for gas exchange, such as those created by exercise or fever. The development of arterial hypoxemia and especially hypercapnia without increase in the respiratory effort should always raise strong suspicion of an anomaly in the neural control of breathing, which can be the result of a central nervous system (CNS) injury (e.g., trauma, intracranial hemorrhage), drug-induced inhibition of the inspiratory neuronal network (e.g., opioid intoxication), or dysfunction/injury of the spinal motor neurons or nerve fibers that innervate the respiratory muscles (e.g., polyneuritis).

The timing and force of the respiratory effort elicited by a chemoreceptor stimulus and the specific muscles that participate in this effort are influenced by sensory inputs from mechanoreceptors distributed throughout the conducting airways, lung parenchyma, and chest wall. These inputs act through a system of neuronal relays to modulate the activity of inspiratory and expiratory premotor neurons in the medulla, modifying the duration of inspiration and expiration (and thus the breathing frequency), the tidal volume, and the specific sequence in which the respiratory muscles become recruited. This results in the adoption of a breathing pattern that is best suited for the specific mechanical conditions of the respiratory system. By observing the characteristics of this pattern, the experienced clinician can often infer a substantial amount of information about the nature of a respiratory impairment.

Work and Energy Cost of Breathing. Most forms of respiratory disease involve anomalies in the mechanical function of the lungs or chest wall. From a physiologic point of view, the effect of these anomalies is an increase in the work that the respiratory muscles must do to keep up with the body's demands for gas exchange. The increased work is frequently accommodated through an increase in the neural drive to the respiratory muscles, which may be perceived by the patient as shortness of breath *(dyspnea)* or by an observer as *respiratory distress*. On occasion, however, the workload demands cannot be met by the contractile machinery of the respiratory muscles and *respiratory failure* ensues (see Chapter 357.1).

In the case of breathing movements, work is defined as the product of lung volume change by the pressure that the respiratory muscles must generate to produce that volume change. This product is graphically represented by the area enclosed between the volume-pressure relationships of the lungs and chest wall and the volume axis (Fig. 357–1). Volume-pressure relationships are determined by properties that define the ease with which the lung tissue is stretched or the amount of resistance that the airways oppose to the passage of air. Thus, the work of breathing describes in one single value the overall mechanical behavior of the respiratory system, providing in the process a valuable account of the energy cost of the breathing activity.

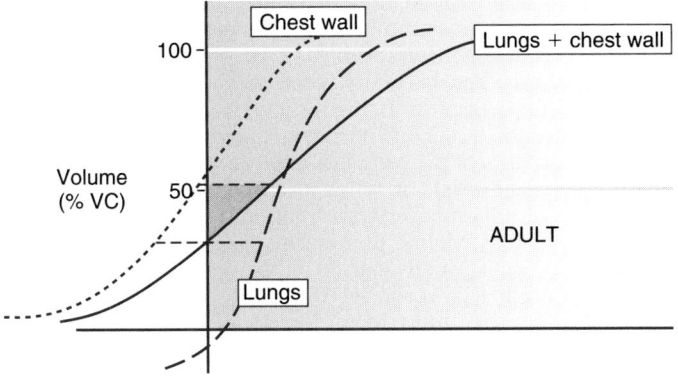

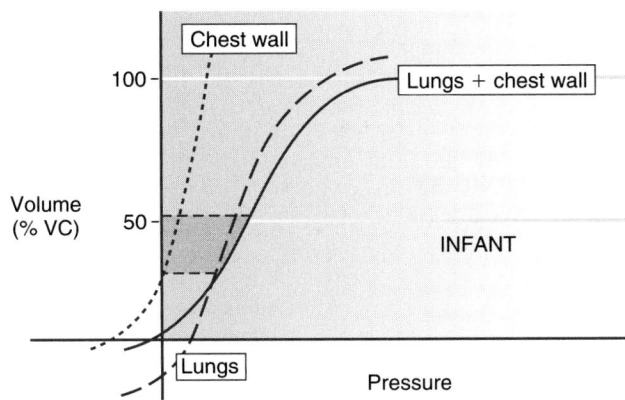

FIGURE 357–1. Idealized elastic volume-pressure relationships of the lungs, chest wall, and respiratory system in the adult and the infant. Volume is expressed as a proportion of vital capacity (VC). At any volume, the pressure that the respiratory muscles generate to oppose the elastic recoil of the respiratory system is equivalent to the sum of the recoil pressures of lungs and chest wall. The intersection of each relationship with the volume axis corresponds to the relaxation volume of each component (the volume at which the elastic recoil is zero). The volume-elastic pressure relationships of the lungs are similar in the adult and infant. The volume-elastic pressure relationship of the chest wall is steeper in the infant, causing the relaxation volume of the respiratory system to be lower than in the adult. The *shaded area* represents the elastic work done by the respiratory muscles for a characteristic tidal volume. Note that this work is greater in the infant because the recoil of the chest wall does not contribute to inflate the lungs as it does in the adult. (From Pérez Fontán JJ: Mechanics of breathing. In Gluckman PD, Heymann MA [editors]: *Perinatal and Pediatric Pathophysiology: A Clinical Perspective*. London, Edward Arnold, 1993.)

Restrictive and Obstructive Respiratory Dysfunction. The respiratory muscles extract energy from the metabolic substrates that are brought to them by the blood. Energy is then transformed into physical work or is otherwise dissipated as heat. Depending on how energy is handled after its transformation into work, it is possible to divide the work of breathing into two components.

First, an important portion of the work of breathing produces reversible rearrangements of the alveolar gas-liquid interface and tissue molecular structures as the lungs and chest wall are stretched during inflation. As a result of their reversible nature, the energy stored in such rearrangements remains available to be used during deflation. These types of processes are responsible for the *elastic* properties of lung tissue. They are exemplified by the behavior of a rubber band, which stores energy when stretched and returns it when allowed to recover its original shape.

Another large portion of the work of breathing produces nonreversible molecular rearrangements or interactions. The energy so spent is permanently lost, usually by being converted into heat, which is then dissipated into the atmosphere or carried away by the circulating blood. All the mechanical processes that result in energy dissipation take place only in the presence of movement. As a result, the magnitude of the work done in connection with these processes bears a relationship to the rate at which gas flows in and out of the lungs. The decrease in alveolar pressure produced by the action of the inspiratory muscles is the reason why gas flows into the lungs during inspiration. The rate of flow is directly proportional to the pressure gradient and inversely proportional to the resistance of the conducting airways.

Establishing a diagnosis and formulating a therapy for children with respiratory disease is greatly aided by the clinician distinguishing between conditions that alter primarily the *elastic (restrictive respiratory disease)* and *resistive (obstructive respiratory disease)* properties of the respiratory system. This distinction is facilitated by an understanding of how these properties influence the physiologic behaviors of the lungs and chest wall.

Elastic Properties of the Respiratory System: Restrictive Respiratory Disease. There are two primary structural reasons why the lungs and chest wall exhibit elastic behavior. First, the surface tension generated by the liquid film that lines the alveoli opposes lung inflation, particularly at low lung volumes when the air spaces are smaller and, in fulfillment of Laplace's law, the same surface tension causes the inward-acting pressure to increase. By coating the surface of the alveolar film with a monolayer of hydrophobic molecules, alveolar surfactant diminishes this pressure. Surfactant is less spread out when the surface area of the alveolar film contracts, and therefore it is more effective in reducing surface tension at low than at high lung volumes. Even in the presence of normal amounts of surfactant in the air spaces, surface tension is responsible for approximately 65% of the elastic recoil of the lungs. When surfactant is absent or dysfunctional *(respiratory distress syndrome of the newborn)* (see Chapter 90.3), elastic recoil becomes markedly increased and alveolar collapse ensues.

The fibrous scaffolding of the lungs and chest wall also imparts substantial elasticity to each of these components of the respiratory system. Particularly in the lungs, collagen and elastin fibers form a supportive web embedded in the alveolar walls and lung septa. This web is organized in a fashion that confers the tissues with a much greater ability to stretch and recoil than would be expected from the behavior of isolated fibers. In addition to allowing these tissues to expand and retract during breathing without generating undue tension, both the alveolar surfactant and the fibrous scaffolding play a critical role in preserving alveolar and airway stability. By reducing surface tension homogeneously throughout the lung, alveolar surfactant prevents small alveoli from emptying into larger ones, as it happens with soap bubbles over time. By anchoring different intrapulmonary structures to each other, septal fibers ensure that the recoil forces generated within the lungs by the action of the respiratory muscles are evenly transmitted to alveolar walls, airways, and vessels. The ensuing *mechanical interdependence* between alveoli, airways, and pulmonary vessels keeps lung inflation homogeneous within the constraints imposed by the shape of the chest wall.

Both surface tension and elastic forces generated by lung fibers depend on the dimensions of the air spaces. Thus, it is not surprising that the overall elastic recoil of the lungs is highly dependent on lung volume just like, in the example of the rubber band, tension depends on the extent to which the rubber band is stretched. The relationship between volume and elastic pressure can be obtained easily for the lungs and the chest wall together or independently by measuring the corresponding pressure changes while the lungs are passively inflated and deflated in a stepwise manner (see Fig. 357–1). All three relationships are sigmoid. Volume therefore increases much less for a given pressure change at low and high volumes than at the intermediate volumes at which normal breathing takes place. In this range, the relationship is steeper and relatively linear and can therefore be described accurately by a fixed ratio of volume to pressure changes, which defines the concept of *compliance*.

Two premises define these interactions. First, at any volume the elastic recoil of the respiratory system is equal to the sums of the individual elastic recoils of the lungs and chest wall. Second, the volume changes experienced by the lungs, the chest wall, and the respiratory system are identical. Thus, pleural pressure (which, when the respiratory muscles are relaxed, represents the elastic recoil of the chest wall) may be high in a patient with asthma who has no intrinsic chest wall anomalies but whose lung volume is markedly increased by gas trapping. Because the heart and vessels inside the thorax are exposed to pleural pressure, cardiac output and arterial blood pressure often undergo an exaggerated decrease during inspiration as lung volume increases even further *(pulsus paradoxus)*.

A similar analysis also demonstrates some other principles that regulate lung volume. Each relationship crosses the volume axis at a different point, regardless of age (see Fig. 357–1). This point defines the *relaxation volume*, which is the volume at which no elastic recoil is generated. Under normal conditions, the relaxation volume of the lungs is considerably smaller than that of the chest wall, a discrepancy that has several important consequences. First, it forces the respiratory system as a whole to adopt a relaxation volume intermediate between that of the lungs and that of the chest wall. After the newborn period, this volume coincides with the *functional residual capacity*, the gas volume of the lungs at the end of a tidal expiration (Fig. 357–2). In addition, the opposing recoils of the lungs and the chest wall at the relaxation volume of the respiratory system create a negative pleural pressure; this pressure promotes the return of venous blood into the heart and keeps the lung and chest wall attached to each other. If the pleural space were open to the atmosphere and the lungs and the chest wall were allowed to change volume freely, the lungs would collapse and the chest wall would expand. This is precisely what happens when a *pneumothorax* develops (see Chapter 403). Finally, for at least a portion of the volume range, the outward-acting recoil of the chest wall helps the expansion of the lungs, thereby reducing energy expenditure during inspiration.

Restrictive lung disease occurs when surface tension is abnormally high (e.g., respiratory distress syndrome of the newborn) (see Chapter 90.3), when the geometry or composition of the solid constituents of the lung is altered (e.g., interstitial edema, pneumonitis, fibrosis), or when the alveolar spaces are filled with liquid or inflammatory cells that limit their ability to admit gas (e.g., alveolar edema, pneumonia). *Restrictive chest wall disease*, in contrast, is usually caused by structural anomalies of the chest wall itself (e.g., scoliosis, rib cage dystrophy), neuromuscular disease, or, most commonly, abdominal distention. Whether originating in the lungs or the chest wall, restrictive respiratory disease has some unique clinical characteristics (Table 357–1). First, only the work performed during inspiration increases, and thus the extra load is carried almost exclusively by the inspiratory muscles, the diaphragm in particular. Second, the patient typically tries to minimize energy demands by adopting a pattern of rapid and shallow breathing, which, when present, almost always indicates a restrictive derangement. Last, the increased elastic recoil of the lungs or the chest wall lowers the relaxation volume of the respiratory system as a whole. Consequently, the functional residual capacity and, to a more variable extent, the forced vital capacity are reduced in all forms of restrictive disease (see Fig. 357–2). Because the recoil forces

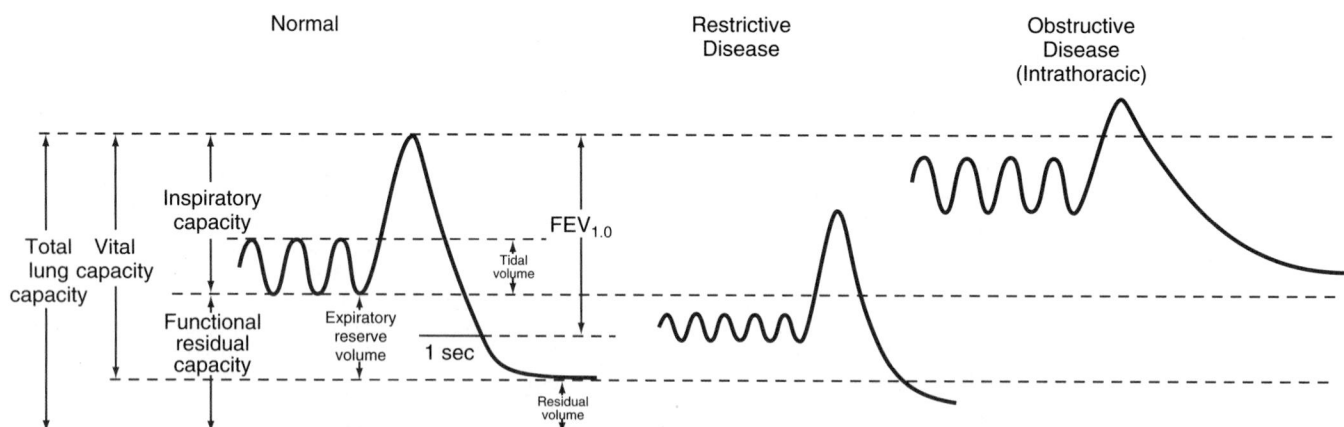

FIGURE 357–2. Effects of restrictive and intrathoracic obstruction on the divisions of total lung capacity. Functional division of total lung capacity. Restrictive disease is usually characterized by a pattern of shallow, rapid breaths. All lung capacities (total lung capacity, functional residual capacity, and vital capacity) are reduced owing either to the increased recoil of the lungs or to the presence of a space-occupying lesion that limits lung inflation. Residual volume is often decreased (as shown in the illustration) but may also be increased if an abnormal configuration of the chest prevents the lungs from deflating completely. Intrathoracic obstruction impairs the ability of the lungs to deflate and thus causes gas trapping, increasing functional residual capacity and residual volume at the expense of vital capacity. The volume exhaled in the first second of a forced expiration ($FEV_{1.0}$) is reduced in both restrictive and obstructive disease. The ratio of $FEV_{1.0}$ to vital capacity, however, is maintained in the former and decreased in the latter.

TABLE 357-1. Characteristic Clinical Findings of Restrictive and Obstructive Lung Disease in Infants and Children

Finding	Restrictive Disease	Obstructive Disease Extrathoracic	Obstructive Disease Intrathoracic
Breathing rate	Increased	Decreased	Normal or increased
Duration of inspiration	Reduced	Prolonged	Unchanged
Duration of expiration	Reduced	Unchanged	Prolonged
Accessory respiratory muscles	Inspiratory	Inspiratory	Inspiratory and expiratory (abdominal)
Rib cage distortion (retractions)	Present	Present	Often present
Amplitude of breathing movements	Shallow	Normal or reduced	Normal or reduced
Auscultatory findings	Crackles, grunting	Inspiratory stridor	Expiratory wheezing
Radiographic appearance of lungs	Decreased lung volume, alveolar densities	Normal	Increased lung volume

transmitted through the fibrous network of the lungs are minimal at low lung volumes, alveoli become unstable and alveolar collapse tends to complicate the situation by further decreasing ventilation-perfusion ratios and causing hypoxemia.

Resistive Properties of the Respiratory System: Obstructive Respiratory Disease. The resistive behavior of the respiratory system results from molecular rearrangements and interactions initiated by motion. The most important of these interactions results from the collision of air molecules against the airway walls, a phenomenon that gives rise to friction. When friction is the only factor, Poiseuille's law predicts that the pressure losses are directly proportional to the viscosity of the gas, the length of the pipe, and the rate of airflow, and inversely proportional to the fourth power of the airway's radius. Thus, it is easy to understand how airway diseases such as *croup* or *viral bronchiolitis* increase the work of breathing more in newborns and small infants, who have smaller radius airways, than in older children. However, friction is not the only source of resistive work. Molecular interactions and velocity changes within the breathing gas itself, particularly when the flow becomes turbulent in pathologically narrow portions of the airways, can result in considerable energy dissipation. Unlike wall friction, the pressure needed to overcome turbulence depends on the density and not on the viscosity of the gas. This is the reason why children with *croup* have less respiratory difficulty and stridor when the air they breathe is replaced with a mixture of oxygen and helium, which has a lower density than air or oxygen (even if its viscosity is slightly higher). Finally, nonreversible molecular rearrangements within the tissue or the gas-liquid interface play an important role in the resistive properties of the lungs and the respiratory system as a whole.

The resistive behavior of the respiratory system can also be analyzed graphically (Fig. 357-3). The volume-pressure relationships of the lungs, chest wall, and respiratory system as a whole form characteristic loops; they show *hysteresis*, which means that the relationships have different courses during inspiration and expiration. The presence of hysteresis always denotes that there is an energy loss from the system. Moreover, the greater the hysteresis, the larger is this energy loss. Accordingly, the width of the loop formed by the pressure-volume relationships of the respiratory system or its components (which has the units of pressure) can be used as a quantitative estimate of resistive behavior. When divided by the rate of gas flow, it yields the *resistance* of each component, a measurement that summarizes various properties that cause resistive energy dissipation. The graphic analysis of the volume-pressure relationships of the respiratory system also reveals that, even though resistive work is done during inspiration and expiration, usually the inspiratory portion of the work is the only one that represents an energy burden. Under normal circumstances, expiration does not require the contraction of any muscles and all expiratory resistive work is performed by the elastic recoil accumulated during inspiration in the lungs and chest wall. However, when expira-

tory resistance is elevated by disease (e.g., asthma, bronchiolitis) or when the individual needs to accelerate the emptying of the lungs to increase ventilation (e.g., during exercise or when the intrathoracic airways are obstructed), abdominal and other accessory muscles of expiration become engaged. This engagement in a resting child is usually a good indication of the presence of obstructive respiratory disease.

Proper diagnosis and evaluation of airway obstruction require additional understanding of the relationships between airway caliber and lung volume. Airway caliber is determined by the coupling of airway wall elasticity and airway transmural pressure. The former depends on the state of health and maturity of the airway tissue (immature airways tend to collapse more easily) and is influenced by the tone of the muscles contained in the airway wall. This tone is, in turn, regulated by neural efferents, which are activated by the CNS to stiffen the airway walls, particularly under conditions in which breathing activity must increase (during exercise, hypoxia, or hypercarbia).

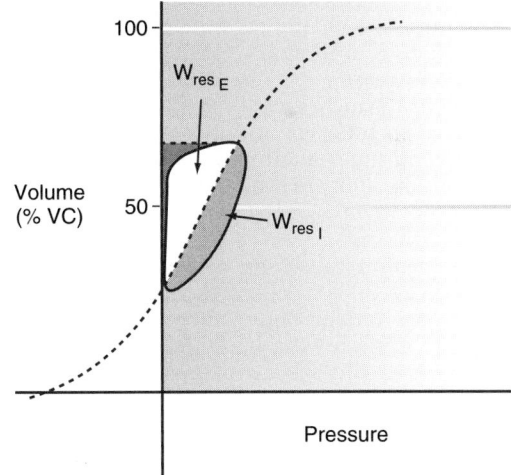

FIGURE 357-3. Graphic analysis of the resistive behavior of the respiratory system during a tidal breath. In the presence of airway flow, energy dissipation causes the relationship between lung volume (expressed as a proportion of vital capacity) and the pressure that the respiratory muscles must generate to form a loop (hysteresis). The area enclosed by this loop represents the work done to overcome resistive pressures such as those caused by the friction of the air against the airway walls. Only the inspiratory portion of this work (W_{resI}), however, is performed by the respiratory muscles. The expiratory portion (W_{resE}) is done by the energy accumulated in elastic elements of the respiratory system during inspiration. (From Pérez Fontán JJ: Mechanics of breathing. In Gluckman PD, Heymann MA [editors]: *Perinatal and Pediatric Pathophysiology: A Clinical Perspective*. London, Edward Arnold, 1993.)

Airway transmural pressure is the difference between the pressures acting on the inside and outside surfaces of the airway wall. It varies during the respiratory cycle in a fashion that depends on whether the airways are intrathoracic or extrathoracic. Extrathoracic airways (nose, pharynx, larynx, the extrathoracic portion of the trachea) are exposed to atmospheric pressure on the outside. Because the pressure acting on the inside surface is subatmospheric during inspiration and supra-atmospheric during expiration, the transmural pressure in this portion of the airway is always negative (narrowing or even collapsing the airway) during inspiration and always positive (dilating the airway) during expiration. The outside surface of the intrathoracic airways is exposed either to pleural pressure (trachea and main bronchi) or to the stresses generated by lung inflation within the lung tissue (intrapulmonary bronchi, bronchioles, and alveolar ducts). These stresses are transmitted to the airway walls by their tissue attachments to the alveolar septa and, when averaged, they add up to a value close to the pleural pressure. During inspiration, the pressure inside the airways is greater than the pressure inside the alveoli. Alveolar pressure, in turn, is always greater than pleural pressure (otherwise, the lungs would have a negative elastic recoil). Consequently, the transmural pressure of the intrathoracic airways always becomes more positive (dilating the airways) as the lungs inflate. During expiration, in contrast, the pressure at all points inside the airways must be lower than alveolar pressure. Whether the pressure inside a certain point in the airways is higher or lower than pleural pressure, however, depends on how much pressure has been lost upstream from the point in question. If the loss is large, the pressure inside the intrathoracic airways can become lower than pleural pressure. The transmural pressure then becomes negative and the airway tends to collapse, a problem that is compounded further if the airway wall is abnormally soft (in the premature infant or in children who suffer from *tracheobronchomalacia*). The more the subject tries to overcome the resultant increase in expiratory resistance by making use of the expiratory muscles, the more the pleural pressure increases and the more the airway collapses, leading to a situation in which outward airflow cannot increase any more regardless of the effort. The expiratory flow at which such *flow limitation* occurs is reproducible for a given lung volume. Determinations of maximal expiratory flow during respiratory function testing take advantage of this reproducibility to evaluate and follow the function of the intrathoracic airways over time or in response to specific therapies.

Airway obstruction causes an exaggeration of the normal changes in airway caliber. When the extrathoracic airway is obstructed (croup, foreign body), the pressure inside the airways distal to the narrowing becomes more negative during inspiration through the actions of the diaphragm and other inspiratory muscles to overcome the increased resistance at the point of obstruction. Therefore, the extrathoracic airway collapses downstream from the level of the obstruction, usually causing an audible vibration or inspiratory *stridor* as the gas rushes through the obstruction. When the intrathoracic airway is obstructed (asthma, foreign body), the pleural pressure must become more positive during expiration. Because the inside pressure beyond the obstruction decreases, the intrathoracic airways downstream from the obstruction tend to collapse, producing an exacerbation of the obstruction, audible expiratory *wheezes*, and flow limitation at low expiratory flows.

Distinction between Restrictive and Obstructive Respiratory Dysfunction: Pulmonary Function Testing.
A careful physical examination frequently yields sufficient information to establish whether an infant or child is suffering from a predominantly restrictive or obstructive ailment (see Table 357–1). However, complicated diagnostic problems and the follow-up of those patients for whom a diagnosis has already been made are aided greatly by the performance of pulmonary function tests. These tests combine gas flow and lung volume measurements to characterize in detail each patient's physiologic derangement. Gas flows rates are most informative if measured during a forced expiratory maneuver generated either voluntarily, if the patient is old enough to cooperate, or by wrapping the chest in an inflatable jacket, when the patient is too young or uncooperative. In addition to being relatively simple to determine, gas flow rates obtained under conditions of flow limitation in the airways are highly reproducible and thus can be compared over time.

Expiratory flow measurements are easier to interpret if flow is plotted against lung volume, forming characteristic flow-volume loops (Fig. 357–4). As a basic principle in the interpretation of these loops, restrictive disease causes proportional decreases in flow rate and lung volume; obstructive disease decreases flow rate but not lung volume.

Lung volume measurements can be obtained either with a body plethysmograph or by combining spirometry and gas dilution or washout techniques (see Fig. 357–2). Typically, both intrathoracic airway obstruction and restrictive respiratory disease reduce vital capacity, but as indicated in Figure 357–2, testing usually distinguishes the two disease categories.

Combinations of restrictive and obstructive disease are not uncommon and, when present, are difficult to diagnose by pulmonary function testing alone. The presence of restrictive disease should be suspected whenever gas flow rates are decreased out of proportion with the FEV_1/vital capacity ratio or when the total lung capacity is reduced.

Response to Respiratory Disease: Efficiency of the Developing Respiratory System.
When the respiratory workload increases in the course of an illness, the respiratory system initiates two responses. The most immediate is to increase the output of the respiratory muscles at the cost of increased energy expenditure. This response is limited not only by substrate availability but also by the ability of the muscles to generate a maximal contraction force. The second response is usually an attempt to improve the efficiency of respiration by changing the respiratory pattern.

The respiratory system is inherently inefficient with values as low as 8% (indicating that only 8% of the energy consumed by the muscles is transformed into actual volume-pressure work) reported in resting adults. Even lower values have been suggested in term newborn and premature infants. Because the baseline values are so low, disease-induced changes in efficiency usually have a large effect on the energy required for breathing. Factors that determine respiratory system efficiency include the breathing pattern; the configuration, length, and functional state of the diaphragm; and the degree of chest wall distortion that occurs with each breath.

Each *breathing pattern* is a unique combination of breathing frequency and tidal volume. Different breathing patterns can yield the same minute ventilation, but there is only one specific respiratory pattern that results in minimal energy expenditure at any time. This optimal pattern varies predictably depending on the mechanical characteristics of the respiratory system. Breathing frequency, for instance, increases when elastic recoil becomes greater in the course of a restrictive derangement. In contrast, the frequency decreases when the resistive properties of the respiratory system become exaggerated by airway obstruction. It is therefore possible to categorize respiratory disease as primarily restrictive or obstructive, depending on whether the patient breathes rapidly and shallowly or slowly and more deeply. It is important to remember, however, that breathing pattern is regulated by influences other than energetic considerations. It is common for children with respiratory disease to breathe transiently at frequencies that depart substantially from optimum. Crying and agitation can in this manner reduce the efficiency of the respiratory system and, in extreme circumstances, precipitate respiratory failure.

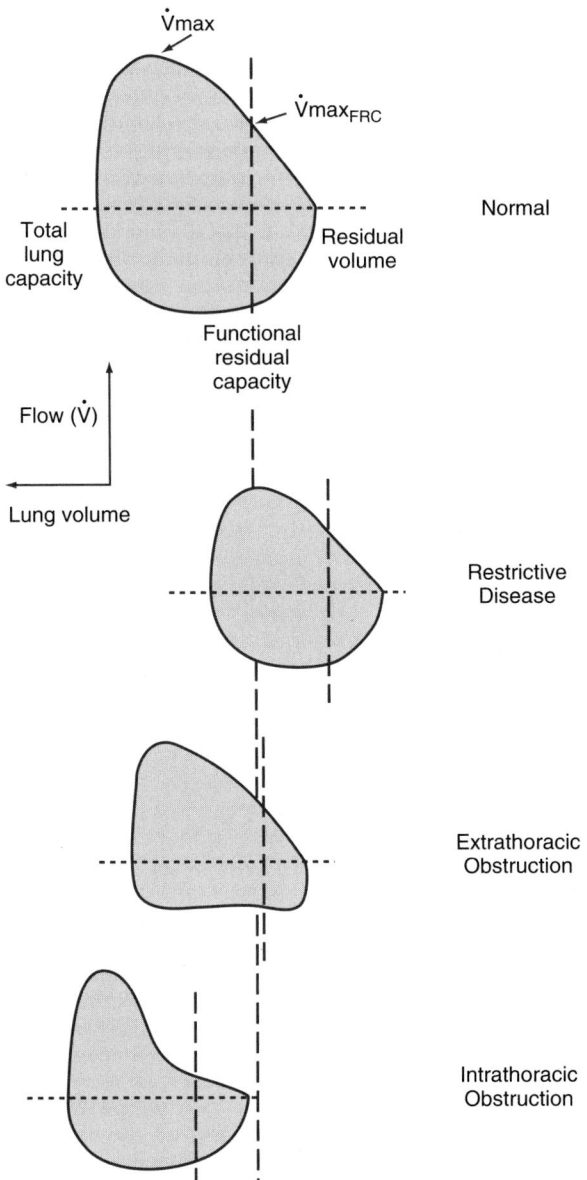

FIGURE 357–4. Flow volume loops obtained by plotting the gas flow generated during a forced vital capacity maneuver in which, after a forced exhalation, the subject inhales to vital capacity and exhales to residual volume. The direction of the loops is clockwise. Inspiration is downward; expiration is upward. $\dot{V}_{max}$ represents peak expiratory flow. $\dot{V}_{maxFRC}$ is the maximal flow recorded at functional residual capacity. Restrictive disease reduces lung volumes and both inspiratory and expiratory flow rates without changing the shape of the loop. Extrathoracic obstruction is exacerbated during inspiration and thus flattens the inspiratory limb of the loop without altering the expiratory limb. Intrathoracic obstruction increases functional residual capacity and reduces all expiratory flows. The flow reduction becomes more severe as lung volume decreases, creating a characteristic concavity or "scoop" in the expiratory limb of the loop.

Like other skeletal muscles, the *diaphragm* can develop its maximal force only if it starts its contraction from an optimal length. This length is attained when the lungs approximate their functional residual capacity (see Fig. 357–2). At this volume, the diaphragm adopts the shape of a dome-capped cylinder. In addition to increasing the volume displaced for a given fiber shortening, this shape allows for a certain area of the diaphragm's thoracic surface to be in direct apposition to the rib cage. This allows the abdominal contents to push the lower ribs forward and laterally during inspiration, increasing the volume of the lungs. The less steep dome shape of the diaphragm in the infant, particularly in the newborn, may not take advantage of these features. The lower portion of the rib cage has large anteroposterior and lateral diameters. As a result, the diaphragmatic insertions are spread out, limiting the range of lengths of the diaphragmatic fibers.

Chest wall distortion can occur at all ages and results primarily from the fact that the chest wall does not have a homogeneous structure or expand uniformly during lung inflation. Areas with no bony support, like the intercostal spaces, tend to move inward under the effects of negative pleural pressure during inspiration. This movement is exaggerated whenever the pleural pressure becomes more negative than normal in the presence of lung disease, creating visible *retractions*. The limited ossification of the ribs and sternum makes the chest walls of newborns and infants very compliant (see Fig. 357–1), a feature that facilitates the birth process but also creates some mechanical liabilities. First, it decreases the relaxation volume of the respiratory system, forcing the newborn to acquire strategies to maintain the functional residual capacity within acceptable limits. These strategies, which are generally based on delaying expiration, are easily overwhelmed when lung compliance is reduced by disease, when neurologic control is impaired by CNS injury or sedation, or when the tone of the chest wall muscles is decreased during rapid eye movement sleep. Because the functional residual capacity represents the largest oxygen store in the body, its reduction in infants can easily lead to hypoxemia because of the high oxygen consumption rates characteristic at an early age. In addition, a high chest wall compliance promotes increased regional distortion of the rib cage. The clinician must be aware that rib cage retractions are not only a sign of disease but also represent a form of work and may have a substantial energy cost. This is particularly true in premature infants, whose diaphragms may do more work to distort the rib cage than to inflate the lungs, even in the absence of lung disease.

The Lung as a Gas Exchanger

SPECIAL CHARACTERISTICS OF THE PULMONARY CIRCULATION. Gas exchange in the lungs takes place in millions of small units, each consisting of a pulmonary capillary and the neighboring portion of the air space. Before arriving there, the venous blood returning to the heart is propelled by the right ventricle into a branching network of pulmonary vessels.

After the adaptations that take place during the newborn period (see Chapter 90.1), the pulmonary circulation offers a much lower resistance to the passage of blood than does the systemic circulation. As a result, the pulmonary blood flow can be accommodated with relatively low blood pressures in the pulmonary artery, allowing the right ventricle to lose part of its muscle mass to become a chamber more adapted to handle volume than pressure loads. Reversal of this situation occurs in a variety of clinical situations, which, as a common denominator, cause *pulmonary arterial hypertension* (defined as an abnormal increase in pulmonary arterial pressure). Physiologic stimuli such as chronic hypoxemia and increased shear stress or tension in the vascular walls can produce smooth muscle hypertrophy and deposition of elastin and type I collagen, leading eventually to the obliteration of pulmonary vessels in experimental animals. Similar stimuli and possibly a failure to curtail the cell and fibroproliferative response that they induce in the vascular wall are the origin of many cases of pulmonary hypertension complicating parenchymal lung disease, left ventricular inflow or outflow obstructions, or left-to-right shunts in childhood.

Pulmonary arterioles (the resistance vessels in the pulmonary circulation) are considerably more reactive to changes in Po_2 and Pco_2 in their environment than are systemic arterioles. Even small fluctuations in these partial pressures can cause marked changes in pulmonary vascular tone. Alveolar hypoxemia is a particularly powerful vasoconstrictive stimulus, which provides the lungs with a local regulatory system to minimize arterial hypoxemia by directing nonoxygenated blood away from areas where ventilation-perfusion ratios are low. Hypercarbia produces pulmonary vasoconstriction; hypocarbia causes pulmonary vasodilation. The effects of oxygen and carbon dioxide on the pulmonary circulation are opposite to those on the cerebral circulation.

Pulmonary capillaries also have a distinctive structural characteristics that reflect their gas exchanging function. Their wall is formed by extraordinarily thin projections from endothelial cells. Because the alveolar epithelium is also very thin, blood and alveolar gas are only separated by less than 1 μm, a feature that explains the ease with which oxygen and carbon dioxide diffuse from one space to the other. In addition, rather than displaying the treelike distribution found in the vascular beds of other organs, pulmonary capillaries form a dense lattice of intercommunicating short segments. Blood circulates through these circuitous pathways, forming a continuous sheet interrupted only by small islands of connective intercapillary tissue. This arrangement enhances the contact surface between the blood and the alveolar gas, minimizes vascular obstruction when the alveoli become distended, and can accommodate easily the increased blood flow needed during exercise or disease. Alveolar capillary growth lags behind alveolar development, and newborn animals have a limited ability to expand their pulmonary capillary bed much beyond the resting state. This may promote pulmonary hypertension when pulmonary blood flow is increased (e.g., left-to-right shunts) or when disease or developmental abnormalities reduce the cross section of the capillary bed (e.g., unilateral lung hypoplasia or after lobectomy or pneumonectomy).

Extra-alveolar vessels (arteries and veins) are for the most part intrapulmonary structures (arteries follow the airways into the acinus whereas veins are interacinary) and, as such, are subjected to the forces generated inside the lungs during breathing. These forces are transmitted to the vessel wall by the vessel's attachments to the fibrous scaffolding of the lung. Alveolar vessels, in contrast, are contained entirely in the alveolar walls and therefore become compressed as the lungs inflate and the alveolar pressure rises relative to pleural pressure (which is the pressure to which the heart and major vessels are exposed). Because the effect of inflation over the extra-alveolar vessels predominates at low lung volumes and the effect over the alveolar vessels predominates at high lung volumes, the total resistance of the pulmonary circulation follows a biphasic U-shaped relationship with respect to lung volume, decreasing at low lung volumes and increasing at higher lung volumes. The inflection point of the relationship, where resistance is minimal, coincides with the functional residual capacity, which therefore represents the point at which pulmonary blood flow is maximal for any given pulmonary arterial pressure. Decreases in lung volume (e.g., alveolar collapse) and lung overinflation (e.g., asthma or excessive distention during mechanical ventilation) increase pulmonary vascular resistance and the afterload to the right ventricle.

Finally, the pulmonary circulation is the site of an active exchange of water and solutes between the vascular space and the interstitium of the lung (the continuous space that exists between alveolar epithelium and endothelium and around airways and pulmonary vessels). The exchange occurs across the endothelial cells or the interendothelial cell junctions and is regulated by a balance of hydrostatic and protein osmotic (oncotic) forces. Increases in fluid filtration, leading to pulmonary edema, occur either when the microvascular pressures increase relative to the protein osmotic pressures (e.g., left ventricular failure, pul-

monary venous obstruction) or when the water and solute permeability of the endothelium is increased (in virtually any form of lung injury). Confined initially to the pulmonary interstitium, fluid is removed by an effective system of lymphatic vessels. When the capacity of these vessels is exceeded, however, fluid can penetrate the alveolar spaces, interfering even further with both the mechanical function of the lungs and gas exchange.

FACTORS DETERMINING THE EFFICIENCY OF GAS EXCHANGE IN THE LUNGS. The arterial blood is a weighted mixture of the blood that passes through all the alveolar-capillary units of the lungs. Even under normal circumstances, there are substantial differences in the composition of the capillary blood emerging from different units. These differences are greatly exaggerated by disease, which, no matter how diffuse and apparently homogeneous, tends to affect the microscopic elementary units of the lung in an uneven manner. Thus, it is not surprising that ventilation-perfusion inequalities are the main mechanism of hypoxemia in most children with lung disease. To understand in more detail how this happens, however, it is important to know the individual processes involved in the transfer of oxygen and carbon dioxide from the atmosphere to the blood.

Ventilation is the process by which the alveolar gas is renewed during breathing. It involves a reciprocating movement of fresh or inspired gas (typically air) into the distal portions of the lung and expired gas into the atmosphere. Only a portion of the gas that enters or leaves the lungs in a unit of time (minute ventilation), however, participates in gas exchange. This portion, known as the alveolar ventilation, is defined as a function of the ratio of carbon dioxide production (or elimination) and alveolar Pco_2 (e.g., alveolar Pco_2 or, by extension, arterial Pco_2 is proportional to carbon dioxide production and inversely proportional to minute alveolar ventilation). The difference between minute ventilation and minute alveolar ventilation is known as the *dead space ventilation* and represents the part of the minute ventilation that does not take part in gas exchange. It includes both gas that remains in the conducting airways (anatomic dead space) and gas that reaches alveolar spaces but does not equilibrate its composition with capillary blood (alveolar dead space). Dead space ventilation is usually increased by respiratory disease because of the presence of a large number of gas exchange units with high ventilation-perfusion ratios.

Oxygen and carbon dioxide enter the pulmonary capillary blood by a process of diffusion driven by the partial pressures of these gases in the capillary blood and the alveolar gas. The blood that enters the pulmonary capillaries is venous blood and has a relatively fixed composition, dictated primarily by the transformations that have occurred in the once arterial blood as a result of tissue respiration. The composition of the alveolar gas, on the other hand, is dictated by the efficiency with which alveolar gas is renewed by ventilation and the efficiency with which oxygen and carbon dioxide are transported in and out of the alveoli by the blood. With other factors being constant, increases in gas flow (ventilation) with respect to blood flow (perfusion) augment alveolar and pulmonary capillary Po_2 and decrease alveolar and pulmonary capillary Pco_2. Conversely, a reduction in the ventilation-perfusion ratio decreases alveolar and pulmonary capillary Po_2. Alveolar Po_2 and Pco_2 (and arterial Po_2 and Pco_2) are bound, both at the level of each alveolus and for the lung as a whole, by a mathematical relationship (the alveolar gas equation) that takes into account the composition of the inspired gas and the relative flows of carbon dioxide and oxygen across the alveolar-capillary membrane (the quotient known as the *respiratory exchange ratio*, R):

$$Pao_2 = Pio_2 - Paco_2/R + Fio_2 Paco_2 (1 - R)/R$$

where Pao_2 represents the alveolar Po_2, Pio_2 the partial pressure of inspired oxygen (calculated by multiplying the inspired oxygen concentration, Fio_2, by the difference between the atmospheric pressure and the water vapor pressure at body temperature), and P_{ACO_2} is the alveolar P_{CO_2} (replaced in practice with the arterial P_{CO_2}). The last term of this equation is small when the subject is breathing room air; under those circumstances:

$$P_{AO_2} \cong P_{IO_2} - P_{ACO_2}/R$$

Global decreases in ventilation or *hypoventilation* are relatively rare in a pure form and are usually caused by CNS dysfunction, impaired nerve conduction, or muscle weakness or fatigue. These conditions reduce the rate at which the alveolar gas is renewed, and therefore they increase alveolar P_{CO_2} and decrease alveolar P_{O_2}, each by a magnitude predicted by the alveolar gas equation. Because hypoventilation interferes only with the composition of the alveolar gas, there is very little difference between the alveolar and the end-capillary P_{O_2}. Thus, the difference between the alveolar P_{O_2} (estimated by the alveolar gas equation) and the arterial P_{O_2} remains small, a characteristic that is unique to the hypoxemia caused by hypoventilation. Administration of supplemental oxygen increases the inspired P_{O_2} and corrects the hypoxemia readily.

From the alveoli, oxygen and carbon dioxide diffuse into the alveolar capillaries along their respective partial pressure gradients. In this process, an oxygen molecule crosses a portion of the alveolar space, the cytoplasms and basal membranes of the alveolar epithelium and endothelium, a certain distance within the plasma, and the membrane and cytoplasm of the erythrocyte, where it enters a chemical reaction with a hemoglobin molecule. This complex diffusion process occurs rapidly enough for all hemoglobin molecules to be saturated with oxygen by the time the erythrocyte has traveled one third of its trajectory within the alveolar wall. Because of the high diffusivity of both oxygen and carbon dioxide, diffusion defects are a very rare cause of hypoxemia and never a cause of hypercapnia in children at rest, even when there is substantial infiltration of the alveolar interstitium by fluid, inflammatory cells, or connective tissue. Occasionally, diffusion abnormalities become manifest as an increased alveolar-arterial P_{O_2} gradient under conditions that raise pulmonary blood flow (exercise, fever), leaving less time for equilibration of alveolar and capillary P_{O_2}.

Ventilation and diffusion define the potential for oxygen uptake and carbon dioxide elimination by individual alveolar-capillary units. Whether this potential can be reached is determined by blood flow. The terms *venous admixture* and *shunt* are used, often interchangeably, to describe a situation in which a portion of the blood that reaches the systemic circulation does not equilibrate its P_{O_2} with the alveolar gas. In a strict sense, these terms define an index calculated as the volume of venous blood that would have to be added to ideal capillary blood to reproduce the P_{O_2} of the arterial blood. Venous admixture can be caused by diffusion defects, ventilation-perfusion inequality, or true shunting of venous blood either through pulmonary blood vessels that supply nonventilated areas or through pathways that bypass the alveolar spaces altogether. The hypoxemia caused by diffusion defects and ventilation-perfusion inequality is responsive to oxygen supplementation. The hypoxemia produced by true shunts, in contrast, cannot be corrected by oxygen administration because the increase in oxygen content of the blood that is exposed to the alveoli is usually insufficient to compensate for the shunt. A small amount of venous admixture is found in all normal individuals. It accounts for a small alveolar-arterial P_{O_2} difference, which varies with age and is usually less than 5–6 mm Hg in room air for the adolescent and is slightly larger for the infant. This difference is caused by normal shunt pathways between the pulmonary and systemic circulations and small inequalities in ventilation-perfusion matching. In the term newborn, and particularly in the premature infant, the alveolar-arterial P_{O_2} difference is even greater. Possible explanations are the larger diffusion distance between the immature

saccules and saccular capillaries, heterogeneity of ventilation-perfusion ratios, and airway closure in the supine position.

Ventilation-perfusion inequality or *mismatch* has long been recognized as the main mechanism of the hypoxemia and hypercapnia in patients with lung disease. Two concepts are basic to the understanding of this mechanism. First, the oxygen and carbon dioxide contents of the blood that exits each individual alveolar-capillary unit depend on the relationship between the unit's ventilation and perfusion. In addition, the oxygen and carbon dioxide contents of the arterial blood are equivalent to the sum of the products of the oxygen and carbon dioxide contents by the blood flow through all the units that form the lungs. Areas with a low ventilation-perfusion ratio cause more of a decrease in arterial oxygenation than areas with a high ventilation-perfusion ratio increase it (Fig. 357–5). The reason is that in areas with a low ventilation-perfusion ratio, the hemoglobin-oxygen dissociation curve favors large decreases in the oxygen saturation and content of the capillary blood with small decrements in P_{O_2}. Conversely, in areas with a high ventilation-perfusion ratio, the oxygen saturation and content in the capillaries changes little, even with large increases in P_{O_2}. As a result, when the oxygen-desaturated blood from areas with a low ventilation-perfusion ratio mixes with oxygenated blood from other areas in the pulmonary veins, the overall oxygen saturation and P_{O_2} are lower than normal.

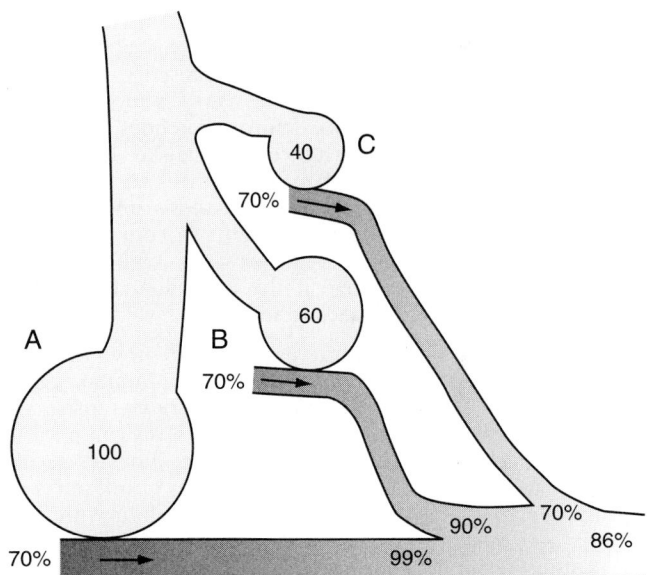

FIGURE 357–5. Diagram demonstrating the effects of decreased ventilation-perfusion ratios on arterial oxygenation in the lungs. Three alveolar-capillary units are illustrated. Unit A has normal ventilation and an alveolar P_{O_2} of 100 mm Hg (shown by the number in the middle of the air space). The blood that circulates through this unit raises its oxygen saturation from 70% (the saturation of mixed venous blood) to 99%. Unit B has a lower ventilation-perfusion ratio and a lower alveolar P_{O_2} of 60 mm Hg. The blood that circulates through this unit reaches a saturation of only 90%. Finally, unit C is not ventilated at all. Its alveolar P_{O_2} is equivalent to that of the venous blood, which travels through the unit unaltered. The oxygen saturation of the arterial blood reflects the weighted contributions of these three units. If it is assumed that each unit has the same blood flow, the arterial blood would have a saturation of only 86%. Ventilation-perfusion mismatch is the most common mechanism of arterial hypoxemia in lung disease. Supplemental oxygen increases the arteriol P_{O_2} by raising the alveolar P_{O_2} in lung units that, like B, have a ventilation-perfusion ratio greater than zero.

Bryan AC, Wohl MEB: Respiratory mechanics in children. In Macklem PT, Mead J (editors): *The Respiratory System: Mechanics of Breathing*. Bethesda, MD, American Physiological Society, 1986, p 179.

Fineman JR, Soifer SJ, Heymann MA: Regulation of pulmonary vascular tone in the perinatal period. *Annu Rev Physiol* 1995;57:115.

Joint Committee of the American Thoracic Society Assembly on Pediatrics and the European Respiratory Society Pediatrics Assembly: Respiratory mechanics in infants: Physiologic evaluation in health and disease. *Am Rev Respir Dis* 1993;147:474.

Pérez Fontán JJ: Pulmonary gas exchange. In Haddad GG, Abman SH, Chernick V (editors): *Chernick-Mellins Basic Mechanisms of Pediatric Respiratory Disease*. Philadelphia, BC Decker, 2002.

Rysconi F, Castagneto M, Gagliardi L, et al: Reference values for respiratory rate in the first 3 years of life. *Pediatrics* 1994;94:350.

West JB: *Ventilation/Blood Flow and Gas Exchange*. Oxford, Blackwell Scientific, 1990.

357.1 Respiratory Failure

J. Julio Pérez Fontán and Gabriel G. Haddad

Respiratory failure is defined in general terms as the situation in which the respiratory system cannot fulfill the gas exchange needs of the patient. Specifically, respiratory failure is defined by the presence of abnormalities in the arterial Po_2 and Pco_2 (also see Chapter 57). Po_2 and Pco_2 are tightly regulated by the central nervous system (CNS), and any alterations in their values can be taken as an indication that either the regulatory system (the breathing control) or its effector organs (the respiratory muscles and the lungs) have become impaired or overwhelmed. However, blood gas analysis requires time and should never delay the institution of lifesaving measures when the physical examination suggests that blood gas abnormalities are present or imminent. Moreover, the presence of an alteration in either the arterial Po_2 or Pco_2 is not sufficient for the diagnosis of respiratory failure, nor does its absence exclude this diagnosis. For instance, Po_2 can be decreased in patients with intracardiac right-to-left shunts and Pco_2 can be increased in patients with metabolic alkalosis, in both cases without intrinsic respiratory impairment. In contrast, arterial Po_2 may be normal even in the presence of a substantial derangement in gas exchange if the individual is breathing increased inspired oxygen concentrations.

Etiology. Acute respiratory failure may occur de novo as a complication of diseases as varied as pneumonia, pulmonary edema caused by congestive heart failure, or airway obstruction (epiglottitis, asthma). It also frequently occurs as a complication of a chronic respiratory disease. Intercurrent illnesses such as those caused by the respiratory syncytial virus or influenza frequently overcome the ability of an infant or child with bronchopulmonary dysplasia or cystic fibrosis to compensate for a pre-existing respiratory dysfunction. In some patients with compensated respiratory disease, even the relatively small increase in ventilatory demands created by an increase in temperature may be sufficient to precipitate worsening hypoxemia and hypercarbia.

Diagnosis. Although the diagnosis of respiratory failure must ultimately rely on the demonstration of gas exchange abnormalities, these are rarely the first manifestations of respiratory impairment. In most instances, the infant or child is brought to medical attention because of other symptoms or physical signs, which sometimes are unrelated to the respiratory system. In evaluating these symptoms and signs, the clinician should always start by considering whether they correspond to one of three distinctive possible clinical profiles (Fig. 357–6). A rapid assignment to one of these profiles facilitates the identification of the cause of the respiratory failure and a more rational approach for the initial treatment.

The most common profile results from alterations in the mechanical function of the conducting airways, the lung parenchyma, or the chest wall. Airway dysfunction is usually manifested as obstructive disease, whereas lung parenchymal and chest wall dysfunctions are predominantly restrictive (see Chapter 357). Mechanical alterations do not impair the ability of the breathing control to increase neural output to the respiratory muscles in response to chemical or mechanical stimuli. Consequently, they are accompanied both by the patient's subjective perception of "air hunger" (dyspnea) and by an increase in respiratory muscle effort. The latter is responsible for the constellation of signs that define respiratory distress: tachypnea, intercostal and subcostal retractions caused by decreased pleural pressure during inspiration; recruitment of muscles that do not participate in normal breathing at rest (accessory muscles); and activation of the dilator muscles of the upper airway (most visible as nasal flaring). Depending on the specific mechanical alteration and the age of the patient, additional signs such as grunting (usually present when lung volume is rendered unstable by restrictive disease), stridor (indicative of extrathoracic airway obstruction), and expiratory prolongation and wheezing (indicative of intrathoracic airway obstruction) may be prominent.

The second profile results from alterations of the respiratory muscles (myopathy involving the respiratory muscles) or their innervation (polyneuropathy or phrenic nerve injuries). These are also associated with an increased neural output, but this cannot be conducted to the muscles or translated into effective respiratory contractions. Tachypnea with shallow respiratory efforts and profound dyspnea are characteristic, but intercostal or subcostal retractions may be absent.

The third profile results from alterations in the control of breathing itself (see Chapter 357.2), usually as a consequence of developmental anomalies (e.g., Ondine's course, apnea of prematurity), CNS injury (trauma, meningoencephalitis, or brainstem compression), or the effects of inhibitory drugs (opioids). These alterations are associated with decreased neural output to the respiratory muscles and therefore produce few or no signs of respiratory distress, even in the presence of considerable derangement in gas exchange.

MECHANICAL DYSFUNCTION AND COMPENSATION ABNORMALITIES. Both restrictive and obstructive disease increase the work of breathing and therefore raise the energy demands of the respiratory muscles. If these demands are met, the mechanical abnormality remains compensated. If the demands exceed the capabilities of the respiratory muscles, respiratory failure develops. Under normal circumstances, energy availability greatly exceeds energy demands, and even substantial increases in the breathing workload can be compensated. However, when efficiency is reduced by rib cage distortion, abdominal distention, overinflation of the lungs, respiratory muscle fatigue, or malnutrition, insufficient energy is transformed into work and respiratory failure may result.

Recognizing the mechanisms that compensate for the increases in the work of breathing is just as important as blood gas analysis for the diagnosis and management of respiratory failure. These mechanisms involve an increased effort on the part of the respiratory muscles, which, similar to other skeletal muscles, can become fatigued when subjected to excessive demands over time. Respiratory muscle fatigue reduces the force generated by each contraction and impairs the ability of the respiratory system to sustain the compensatory response. Newborn infants have an increased propensity for respiratory muscle fatigue. This probably relates to decreased breathing efficiency (see Chapter 357) caused by mechanical factors such as the high compliance of the chest wall and the small surface of apposition of the diaphragm to the rib cage, rather than to maturational changes in the intrinsic properties of the respiratory muscles themselves. Other conditions frequently found in association with respiratory disease such as malnutrition, decreased perfusion, electrolyte disorders, and hypophosphatemia increase the vulnerability of the respiratory muscles to fatigue

Mechanical Dysfunction   Muscle Dysfunction   Control Dysfunction

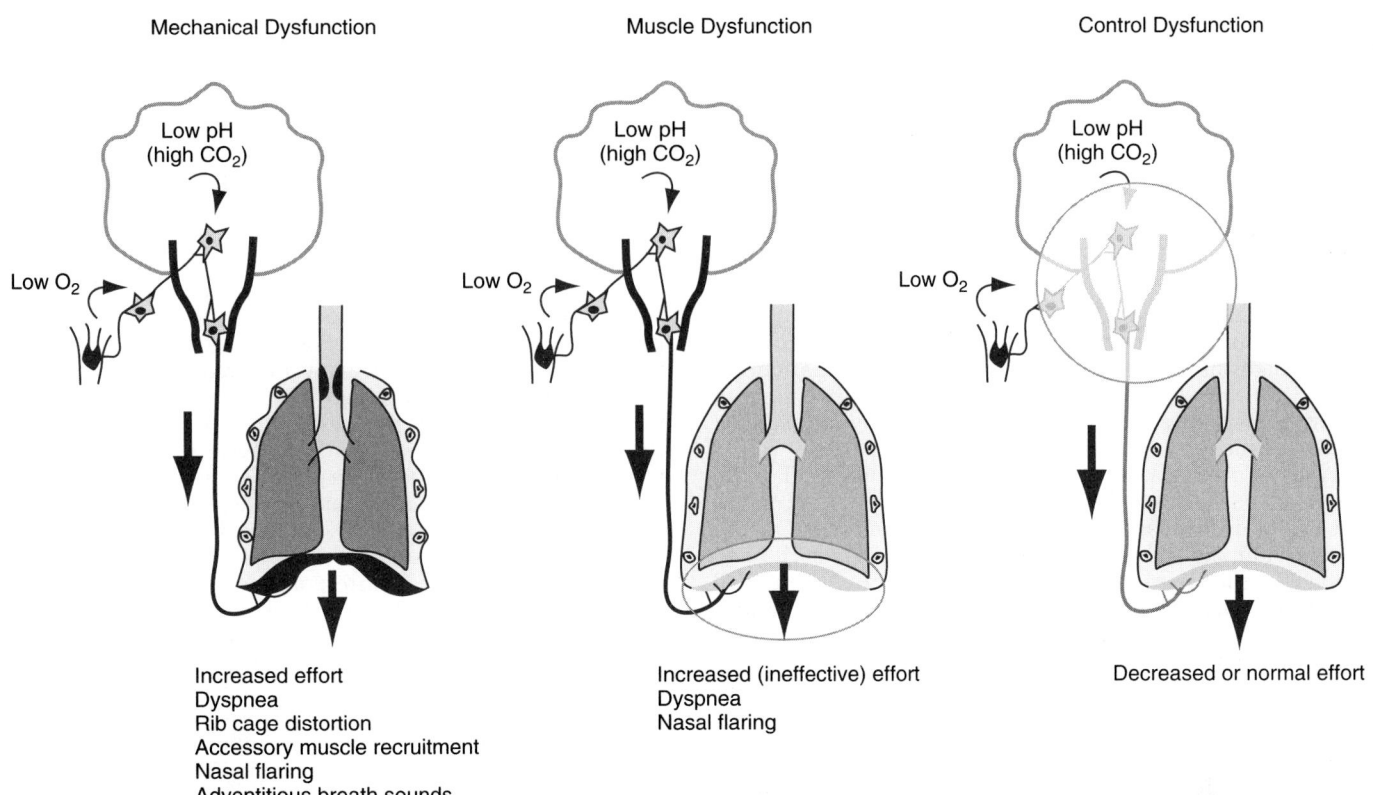

Increased effort
Dyspnea
Rib cage distortion
Accessory muscle recruitment
Nasal flaring
Adventitious breath sounds

Increased (ineffective) effort
Dyspnea
Nasal flaring

Decreased or normal effort

FIGURE 357–6. Presentation profiles of respiratory failure in childhood. When a mechanical dysfunction is present (by far, the most common circumstance), arterial hypoxemia and hypercapnia (and hence pH) are sensed by peripheral (carotid bodies) and central (medullary) chemoreceptors. After being integrated with other sensory information from the lungs and chest wall, chemoreceptor activation triggers an increase in the neural output to the respiratory muscles *(vertical arrows)*, which results in the physical signs that characterize respiratory distress. When the problem resides with the respiratory muscles (or their innervation), the same increase in neural output occurs *(arrow)*, but the respiratory muscles cannot increase their effort as demanded; therefore, the physical signs of distress are more subtle. Finally, when the control of breathing is itself affected by disease, the neural response to hypoxemia and hypercapnia is absent or blunted and the gas exchange abnormalities are not accompanied by respiratory distress.

and failure. Reversing malnutrition, improving blood flow and substrate delivery, and correcting electrolyte abnormalities are therefore important steps to maintain the force-generating ability of the respiratory muscles and to delay respiratory failure. Such considerations are critical in chronic diseases, such as asthma, cystic fibrosis, and bronchopulmonary dysplasia, and in patients being weaned from prolonged ventilatory support.

CHRONIC RESPIRATORY FAILURE. Independent of its etiology, the abnormalities in the arterial Po_2 and Pco_2 initiate a repertoire of physiologic responses directed at making the gas exchange derangement more tolerable for the patient. Most of these responses require days to weeks and, therefore, their detection in the physical or laboratory examinations indicates the chronic course of the failure. Arterial hypoxemia, for instance, induces a number of genes. The best characterized is the hypoxia-inducible factor-1 (HIF-1), a transcription factor implicated in the induction of a variety of other hypoxia-regulated genes. Among these is the erythropoietic factor, responsible for the development of polycythemia in patients with chronic arterial hypoxemia (although this may not be found in an infant or in a nutritionally impaired child). Other HIF-1–regulated genes include those encoding glycolytic enzymes, whose induction optimizes energy metabolism in the presence of reduced oxygen supply and angiogenesis (VEGF) and vasodilator factors (I-NOS), which activate biologic programs directed at raising the ability of tissues to extract oxygen from the blood.

Arterial hypercapnia stimulates H^+ secretion by the renal tubules, resulting in the addition of HCO_3^- ions to the extracellular fluid (approximately 3.5 mEq/L for every 10 mm Hg increment in the Pco_2). The increase in the serum HCO_3^- levels returns the arterial pH toward normality (without ever normalizing it), lessens the decrease in arterial pH produced by a further rise in arterial Pco_2, and reduces the stimulus for increased ventilation and the dyspnea associated with it. Infants and children with chronic respiratory failure may therefore depend on the stimulation of peripheral chemoreceptors by arterial hypoxemia to drive their breathing more than normal individuals, a feature that needs to be taken into account (but that does not contraindicate) in the administration of supplemental oxygen to these patients.

Clinical Manifestations. The limited ability of the developing respiratory system to compensate for disease-induced mechanical abnormalities makes the early recognition of respiratory failure critical. Respiratory failure should be anticipated rather than recognized so that alterations in gas exchange can be prevented (see Chapter 57.3).

During physical examination, the clinician should avoid interfering with the patient's own mechanisms of compensation. An awake child with upper airway obstruction caused by croup or epiglottitis, for instance, may be more stable in a mother's arms because the increased gas flows and the increased forces generated during crying worsen the obstruction and can precipitate failure. Similarly, most patients with severe restrictive and obstructive disease tolerate the supine position poorly because it promotes gravity-dependent perfusion of poorly ventilated areas and the weight of the abdominal organs imposes an additional burden on the diaphragm.

In a child suspected of respiratory failure, this evaluation should always start with a rapid assessment of the adequacy of ventilation, including the presence and vigor of the respiratory movements, breathing rate, the presence of cyanosis, and the presence of signs of upper airway obstruction (see Chapter 57.3). A child with grossly inadequate respiratory efforts or complete airway obstruction will die unless ventilation of the lungs is restored immediately. Special attention must be paid to the patient's state of consciousness. Hypoxemia and hypercarbia frequently cause lethargy and confusion, sometimes alternating with agitation. Whether resulting from these or other concurrent mechanisms, CNS depression requires immediate attention because it further limits the ability of the respiratory system to deal with mechanical loads and leaves the airway unprotected against obstruction and aspiration of foreign materials.

Acute hypoxemia and hypercapnia result in dilatation of the cerebral blood vessels and increased blood flow, often accompanied by severe headache. The sudden increased work of the accessory muscles of breathing may result in lower back pain. Although moderate to severe hypercapnia can cause peripheral vasodilation, mild to moderate hypoxemia can cause peripheral vasoconstriction, and the patient may have cold extremities, a finding that may divert attention toward a circulatory dysfunction when the main problem is respiratory. Other symptoms of hypoxia include restlessness, dizziness, and impaired thought.

Treatment. The goal of treatment is the restoration of adequate gas exchange with a minimum of complications. This is achieved by eliminating the initiating factors as quickly as possible. Thus, respiratory failure caused by cardiogenic pulmonary edema is treated with inotropic medications and diuretics. The child with asthma should be managed with bronchodilators and anti-inflammatory medications. Unfortunately, even in acute illnesses such as these, the response to treatment is not immediate, and frequently the entire function of the respiratory system must be artificially supported (see also Chapter 57.4).

Hypoxemia is more dangerous than hypercarbia and may be easier to correct. Administration of supplemental oxygen is a safe and wise precaution in all patients at risk for respiratory failure, even if there is no initial evidence of hypoxemia. Oxygen can be administered with face masks, nasal cannulae, hoods, or tents. Face masks are usually not well tolerated by frightened infants and children. Hoods provide more consistent inspired oxygen concentrations than any other device, but they are bulky and limit access to the patient. For this reason, they have limited applicability in the initial treatment in the emergency department.

The indication for ventilatory support in a child with respiratory failure is usually based on the persistence or worsening of gas exchange (see Chapters 57.3 and 57.4). Mechanical ventilation is necessary in a child with pneumonia in whom severe hypoxemia and hypercarbia develops because even the most effective antibiotic therapy requires time. On occasion, ventilatory support must be instituted in the absence of alterations in the arterial Pco_2 when the dysfunction of other systems places gas exchange at jeopardy by limiting the compensatory ability of the respiratory system; cardiovascular shock is a typical example. In this latter condition, decreased blood flow and substrate delivery to the respiratory muscles may reduce the force that these muscles can develop and can precipitate respiratory failure, even in the absence of substantial mechanical abnormalities of the respiratory system.

Ventilatory support often requires intubation of the trachea with an endotracheal tube or, less often, a tracheostomy cannula (see Chapters 57.3 and 57.4). Regardless of the type of ventilator, the objective of mechanical ventilation is not to normalize arterial blood gas tensions but rather to provide "ade-quate" gas exchange. The definition of what is "adequate" has changed substantially; some degree of hypercarbia and hypoxemia is acceptable to minimize oxygen- and stretch-induced lung injury of the lungs. Moderate hypercarbia (arterial Pco_2 of 60–80 mm Hg) has no detectable negative consequences over short periods, especially if the rise in Pco_2 is not very acute, in part because its effects on the arterial pH are eventually minimized through renal retention of bicarbonate. Moderate hypoxemia (oxygen saturation 85–90%) is similarly well tolerated in otherwise stable patients, particularly if the hemoglobin concentration and the cardiac output are maintained at physiologic values and conditions such as fever and agitation, which increase tissue oxygen demands, are avoided. Artificial-mechanical ventilation is usually initiated with conventional volume-driven ventilators; high-frequency jet or oscillator ventilators are often used as rescue therapy if conventional ventilators fail to improve oxygenation, but their efficacy is not proven in many circumstances (see Chapters 57.3 and 57.4).

Extracorporeal membrane oxygenation (ECMO) or carbon dioxide removal, or both, are employed in the treatment of newborns and small infants with life-threatening, refractory respiratory failure that is unresponsive to mechanical ventilation and is expected to resolve in a short time (see Chapter 90.7). Because of its risks (from vascular cannulation and anticoagulation) and the fact that its benefits over conventional management in non-neonatal patients have not been unequivocally demonstrated, indications for ECMO require considerable experience, caution, and judgment. Inhaled nitric oxide may acutely improve oxygenation by reducing increased pulmonary vascular resistance and has replaced the use of ECMO in many intensive care situations.

DeBruin W, Notterman DA, Magid M, et al: Acute hypoxemic respiratory failure in infants and children: Clinical and pathologic characteristics. *Crit Care Med* 1992;20:1223.

Guillemin K, Krasnow MA: The hypoxic response: Huffing and HIFing. *Cell* 1997;89:9.

Third European Consensus Conference in Intensive Care Medicine: Tissue hypoxia: How to detect, how to correct, how to prevent. *Am J Respir Crit Care Med* 1996;154:1573.

357.2 Congenital Central Hypoventilation Syndrome (Ondine Curse)

Gabriel G. Haddad

In children having congenital central hypoventilation syndrome (CCHS), there are usually no detectable *gross* anatomic abnormalities, although brainstem tumors and arteriovenous malformations have been described and other neurologic diseases must be considered. The primary defect is in the central nervous system (CNS), but there may also be abnormalities in other elements of the respiratory feedback loop (e.g., carotid bodies, peripheral chemosensitivity).

Pathogenesis and Pathophysiology. The cause and pathogenesis of CCHS are unknown. Although there are reports of familial cases, the specific mode of inheritance is unknown. A rare association of Hirschprung disease was first described with Ondine curse in 1978 (Haddad syndrome). In one such case, a missense mutation in exon 12 of the *RET* proto-oncogene has been reported. Evaluation of the brain-derived neurotrophic factor (BDNF) genomic DNA sequence variation revealed that 1 in 19 children with CCHS screened for mutations in that gene showed a discrete mutation in BDNF; the unaffected father of the child showing the mutation also exhibited that mutation. Case control family studies have also shown that CCHS patients, their parents, and relatives were more likely to be affected than controls and their parents and relatives in terms of an imbalance in the autonomic nervous system (ANS). The best-fitting genetic model of CCHS is that of a mendelian inheritance of a major gene disturbing the ANS.

Patients with CCHS or CCHS with Hirschsprung disease have no carbon dioxide sensitivity and no ventilatory response to carbon dioxide during sleep. During wakefulness, the carbon dioxide set point is much lower, and they respond to it, unless the condition is severe enough for hypoventilation to occur even in the awake state. These children also have been shown to have no sensitivity to hypoxia. This lack of sensitivity to carbon dioxide and the respiratory failure do not improve with time, and the oldest patients with CCHS still show the same failures. Older children with CCHS show an increase in ventilation when they are exercised at various work rates, and the increase in ventilation they exhibit may not be related to anaerobic stimuli (lactate or pH) but rather to neural reflexes (e.g., limb movements) or hormonal cues.

In CCHS, the condition expresses itself best during sleep, at which time sensory feedback plays a relatively minor role. The defect may be in the automatic control system, which resides mostly in the brainstem. Although physiologic evidence indicates that the respiratory failure in these children is mostly based on defects in central mechanisms, rather than on peripheral (carotid) mechanisms, the interactions between peripheral and central mechanisms also may be important. It is also important that premotor neurons, which communicate with phrenic or intercostal motor neurons, can be excited enough to drive the respiratory musculature in certain instances (e.g., wakefulness).

On postmortem examination of some CCHS patients, absence of the arcuate nucleus has been seen, but the relation of this anomaly to the disease is not clear. Gliosis in brainstem structures has also been noted, but this could be part of a more generalized response of the CNS to hypoxia and ischemia resulting from long-term and intermittent respiratory failure.

Clinical Manifestations. Patients with CCHS usually present early in life, often in the first few hours after delivery. Most children are the products of uneventful pregnancies and are term infants with appropriate weight for gestational age; Apgar scores have been variable. Symptoms of respiratory failure, with slow and irregular respiratory efforts, long respiratory pauses (lasting up to 40 sec), and cyanosis, appear in the first day of life. Cardiac, respiratory, infectious, and metabolic diseases, including intrauterine drug exposure, should be ruled out. One hallmark of this condition is that patients *fail* to respire adequately during sleep, not during wakefulness, although children with the most severe respiratory failure may hypoventilate in the waking state as well. In most neonates with CCHS, the $Paco_2$ accumulates to very high levels, sometimes up to 80–90 mm Hg, during sleep and drops to normal levels soon after the infants awaken. Infants in the first few weeks of life have been shown to have long respiratory pauses, a relatively normal tidal volume, and a very low respiratory rate (dropping to as low a level as 8–10 breaths/min during sleep) with interspersed respiratory pauses. Respiratory rates are generally normal during wakefulness, and the lowest respiratory rates have been found in non–rapid eye movement or quiet sleep.

Because respiratory failure in these infants has a central cause, the hypoxemia that ensues is commensurate with hypoventilation with little or no abnormality in the arterial-alveolar (A-a) gradient. However, in some children, the hypoventilation may be severe enough to produce airway closure, microatelectasis, and an increase in the A-a gradient.

In a sizable subset of these infants, abdominal distention, constipation, or complete failure to pass meconium occurs. Rarely, a child with CCHS also has diagnosed Hirschsprung disease with variable aganglionosis of the colon and small intestine. Whether all patients with congenital CCHS have some degree of aganglionosis of the large bowel is unknown.

Patients with CCHS also have a faster heart rate than normal for their age and low heart rate variability, an almost fixed heart rate with little sinus arrhythmia. Other anomalies found on autopsy suggesting abnormalities in the autonomic regulation of vital functions include multiple ganglioneuroblastomas of the sympathetic chain and the adrenal medulla.

Differential Diagnosis. Other neurologic diseases or conditions have to be excluded before this diagnosis is made. Brainstem infarction, tumors, arteriovenous malformations, syringomyelia, Leigh necrotizing encephalomyelopathy, olivopontocerebellar degeneration, and Möbius syndrome should be considered.

Treatment. Management should include general and nutritional care, ventilatory support, and prevention of acidosis, cerebral hypoxia, and ischemia. Some of these infants can grow and gain developmental and neurologic milestones that are close to normal for age, although hypoventilation abnormalities persist. These abnormalities may be a result of episodes of hypoxia or part of the spectrum of CCHS. Attempts at pharmacologic respiratory stimulation have been unsuccessful.

Phrenic nerve pacing has been used in patients after the age of 2 yr. Although there are complications related to pacing, including phrenic nerve fibrosis, infections, and multiple surgeries, a number of these patients have eventually become independent of mechanical ventilators.

Bolk S, Angrist M, Schwartz S, et al: Congenital central hypoventilation syndrome mutation analysis of the receptor tyrosine kinase RET. *Am J Med Genet* 1996;63:603.

Croaker GD, Shi E, Simpson E, et al: Congenital central hypoventilation syndrome and Hirschsprung's disease. *Arch Dis Child* 1998;78:316–22.

Haddad GG, Mazza NM, Defendini R, et al: Congenital failure of automatic control of ventilation, gastrointestinal motility and heart rate. *Medicine* 1978;57:517.

Marazita ML, Maher BS, Cooper ME, et al: Genetic segregation analysis of autonomic nervous system dysfunction in families of probands with idiopathic congenital central hypoventilation syndrome. *Am J Med Genet* 2001;100:229–36.

Mellins RB, Balfour HH, Turino GM, et al: Failure of automatic control of ventilation (Ondine's curse). *Medicine* 1990;49:487.

Sakai T, Wakizakas A, Matsuda H, et al: Point mutation in exon 12 of the receptor tyrosine kinase proto-oncogene RET in Ondine-Hirschsprung syndrome. *Pediatrics* 1998;101:924.

Weese-Mayer DE, Bolk S, Silvestri JM, et al: Idiopathic congenital central hypoventilation syndrome: Evaluation of brain-derived neurotrophic factor genomic DNA sequence variation. *Am J Med Genet* 2002;107:306–10.

Weese-Mayer DE, Silvestri JM, Huffman AD, et al: Case/control family study of autonomic nervous system dysfunction in idiopathic congenital central hypoventilation syndrome. *Am J Med Genet* 2001;100:237–45.

Chapter 358

Defense Mechanisms and Metabolic Functions of the Lung *Gabriel G. Haddad and J. Julio Pérez Fontán*

358.1 Defense Mechanisms

Overview. Effective and multiple defense mechanisms in the lungs are especially important because the respiratory system is constantly exposed to a changing and often "polluted" environment containing irritants, pathogens, and allergens. The defense system is composed of three limbs: (1) the cough reflex, which relies on the integrity of the airways, (2) the respiratory muscles, and (3) the central nervous system control centers. The cilia and mucociliary apparatus rely on the morphologic and functional integrity of the cilia and the respiratory epithelium (see Chapter 394). The mechanical defenses of the respiratory system that protect the lung include the filtering of particles, the warming and humidification of inspired air, and the absorption of noxious fumes and gases by the vascular upper airway. The temporary cessation of breathing, reflexly shallow breathing, laryngospasm, or even bronchospasm limits the depth and amount of penetration of foreign matter. Spasm or decreased breathing can provide only brief protection. Cough also is an important mechanism. Aspiration of food, secretions, and foreign bodies is prevented by swallowing and closure of the epiglottis. The respiratory tract distal to the larynx is normally sterile. The immune system is important in determining the propensity of individuals to lung infections.

The *upper airway* includes the nose, paranasal sinuses, and pharynx; the *lower airway* consists of the remainder of the system from the larynx peripherally. The nose has a relatively large surface area lined with a richly vascular, ciliated epithelium; and by the time the air column reaches the bifurcation of the trachea, up to 75% of the warming and humidification of the inspired air has occurred. During exhalation, heat and moisture are removed from the air stream. Gross filtering of particles larger than 10–15 mm is achieved by the coarse hairs at the nasal orifices, and most inhaled particles larger than 5 mm are impacted on the nasal surface (see Section 2).

Because the larynx is relatively narrow and ringed with cartilage, it is relatively susceptible to obstruction in young children, particularly by inflammation, because the resultant swelling of tissues rapidly encroaches on the lumen and produces inspiratory stridor.

The trachea and bronchi are lined with pseudostratified, ciliated, columnar epithelium and occasional goblet cells. Mucous glands occupy approximately one third of the thickness of the airway wall and for the most part lie between the epithelial surface and the cartilage. The trachea is supported by incomplete rings of cartilage with a muscular membrane posteriorly. Irregular plates of cartilage support the bronchi, especially at bifurcations. These diminish and finally disappear in the smallest bronchi. The goblet cells and principally the submucosal glands secrete the mucous layer, which is 2–5 mm in depth and rests on the tips of the cilia. Each ciliated cell has about 275 cilia; movement results from action by microtubules within each cilium. The cilia beat within a periciliary fluid layer at about 1,000 beats/min, moving the mucous blanket toward the pharynx at a rate of approximately 10 mm/min in the trachea. In the respiratory portion of the lung, the surface cells gradually become cuboidal and then flat; ciliated cells and goblet cells are usually absent.

The final 25% of the warming and humidifying of the inspired air stream occurs in the trachea and large bronchi. Failure of humidification permits dry air to reach more distal airways. Particles 1–5 mm in size precipitate out on the tracheobronchial mucous blanket so that only particles of 1 mm or less reach the respiratory bronchioles and air spaces, where some may deposit and many will be exhaled.

Respiratory tract secretions are derived primarily from mucous (glycoproteins) and serous cells of the submucosal glands that empty onto the surface epithelium; from goblet cells and Clara cells, the special secreting cells in the surface epithelium of bronchi and bronchioles, respectively; from transudation from the vascular space; and from alveolar fluid, which contributes most of the phospholipid found in tracheobronchial mucus. This mucus is about 95% water.

Beyond infancy, collateral alveolar ventilation can occur increasingly with development of the *pores of Kohn* between alveoli, which provide a means for gas to pass from one lobule to another, perhaps even between segments of lung. Bronchiolar-alveolar communications, known as the *canals of Lambert*, are also found. These anatomic connections may be helpful in preventing or delaying atelectasis.

Clearance of Particles. Particles deposited in conducting airways are cleared within hours by the mucociliary mechanism, whereas clearance of those reaching the alveoli may take several days to months. The latter may be phagocytized by alveolar macrophages and removed from lungs by the mucociliary system or carried into the interstitium for clearance by the lymphocytes into regional nodes or the blood. Some particles penetrate into the interstitium without phagocytosis. Mucociliary clearance may be aided by cough, which propels excess mucus up the airways at high pressures and flows.

Cough is characterized by four specific phases: (1) a very deep and rapid inspiratory effort, having the effect of achieving a high and optimal thoracic volume for the subsequent phases of the cough; (2) compression, which is characterized by closure of the glottis, activation of the diaphragm and chest wall muscles and, consequently, compression and building of pleural, alveolar, and abdominal pressures; (3) expression of the cough marked by a sudden opening of the glottis, high expiratory airflow, and an explosive sound; and (4) relaxation of the musculature and reversal of pressures. Although such events occur in the characteristic cough, they may not occur in every cough.

The effect of cough on mucus clearance depends on a number of factors. These are the gas-fluid interactions, the rheology of mucus, the respiratory pattern, and the cough pump structure. With very "slow" airflows, air is so sluggish that it moves through mucus without affecting its transport. This occurs during obstructive disease and when the nature of the mucus is affected by inflammation, debris, cellular material, and increased amount of secretion. Higher airflows can, on the other hand, be very effective. The rheology of mucus is important; consider for instance the severe viscous and highly elastic nature of the secretions in cystic fibrosis. The breathing pattern is also critical because the higher the volume inspired and the shorter the expiratory time, the higher the airflow and the higher the probability for the cough to clear secretions. Moreover, because the strength of cough depends on the structure of the airways and their integrity, airway pathology will affect the strength of the cough. For example, any exaggerated collapse of the airways during expiration severely limits the forcefulness of the cough, as occurs with tracheomalacia in the premature, tracheal stenosis, and extrinsic compression of the airways. Cough can also be jeopardized when respiratory muscles do not generate the necessary pressures (i.e., weak, paralyzed, fatigued) and when the airways cannot be well splinted.

Defense Against Microbial Agents. Phagocytosis and mucociliary clearance may not be sufficient protection from living agents, such as bacteria and viruses. Additional factors include cellular killing of organisms and immune responses to assist in the phagocytosis-killing process. Alveolar and interstitial macrophages, derived from monocytes, are an essential component of the defense system of the lung. The engulfment and killing of living particles by these macrophages may be enhanced by opsonins or by small lymphocytes. The principal antibody in respiratory secretions is secretory IgA, which is produced by plasma cells in the submucosa of the airways (see Chapter 114.3) and is highly resistant to digestion by proteolytic enzymes released after lysis of bacteria and dead cells. IgA can neutralize certain viruses and toxins and helps in the lysis of bacteria. IgA may also prevent antigenic substances from penetrating the epithelial surfaces. Pulmonary secretory IgA reaches adult levels in the first month of life. IgG and IgM are also found in the secretions when lung inflammation occurs.

Lysozyme, lactoferrin, and interferon may also play a defensive role in respiratory secretions. In addition, a small fraction of the antibodies of the respiratory surface is made up of IgE, which plays an important role in allergic reactions (see Chapter 130).

The phagocytic ability of alveolar macrophages and, in most cases, the mucociliary mechanism can be impaired by ethanol ingestion, cigarette smoke, hypoxemia, starvation, chilling, corticosteroids, nitrogen dioxide, ozone, increased oxygen concentration, narcotics, and some anesthetic gases. The antibacterial killing capacity of the macrophages can be decreased by acidosis, azotemia, and recent acute viral infections, especially rubeola and influenza. Beryllium and asbestos, organic dust from cotton and sugar cane, and gases such as sulfur, nitrogen dioxide, ozone, chlorine, ammonia, and cigarette smoke are toxic to epithelial cells.

Mucociliary clearance can be reduced by hypothermia, hyperthermia, morphine, codeine, and hypothyroidism. Inhalation of dry gas by mouth breathing during periods of nasal obstruction, after performance of a tracheostomy, or during use of poorly humidified oxygen results in drying of the mucous membranes and slowing of the ciliary beat. Cold air may irritate the tracheobronchial tree.

Damage to the respiratory epithelium may be reversible with rhinitis, sinusitis, bronchitis, bronchiolitis, acute respiratory infections associated with high levels of air pollution, and the epithelial shedding that can occur in asthma, or with some irritants, bronchospasm, edema, congestion, and perhaps mild surface ulceration. However, severe ulceration, bronchiectasis, bronchiolectasis, squamous cell metaplasia, and fibrosis may cause serious injury and permanent impairment of the normal clearance mechanism. Other events that can adversely affect the lung include hyperventilation, alveolar hypoxia, pulmonary thromboembolism, pulmonary edema, hypersensitivity reactions, and certain drugs, such as salicylates.

Newhouse MT, Bienenstock J: Respiratory tract defense mechanisms. In Baum GL, Wolinsky E (editors): *Textbook of Pulmonary Diseases*. Boston, Little, Brown, 1989, pp 21–47.

Wilmott RW, Fiedler MA, Stark JM: Host defense mechanisms. In Chernick V, Boat T (editors): *Kendig's Textbook on Disorders of the Respiratory Tract in Children*, 6th ed. Philadelphia, WB Saunders, 1998, pp 238–64.

358.2 Metabolic Functions

The lung contains more than 40 separate cell types; the type I and II pneumocytes, alveolar macrophages, and Clara cells are unique to the lung. The lung can synthesize lipids and proteins, including glycoproteins, secretory antibodies, interferon, proteolytic and fibrinolytic enzymes and activators, collagen, and elastin. Tissue factors such as thromboplastin are found in higher concentration in the lung than in any other organ. Megakaryocytes are concentrated in the lung.

The large alveolar type II pneumocyte synthesizes and releases lung surfactant. Injury to this cell or deficiency in this surfactant pathway results in neonatal respiratory distress syndrome and other disorders (see Chapters 90.3, 396, and 397). A major function of surfactant is to stabilize alveolar air spaces by attenuating surface forces and decreasing their unevenness. Another cell type, the neuroepithelial cell, is present at the airway bifurcation and is found in larger proportion in early life. These cells are serotonin-rich and have transmitter vesicles that are depleted when exposed to low inhaled oxygen concentration. These cells sense oxygen in the airways through plasma membrane K^+ channels and can send afferent information to the central nervous system via the vagus nerve.

Because the lung has the only capillary bed through which the entire blood flow must pass in the normal state, the pulmonary capillary circulation is ideally positioned to control circulating vasoactive hormones. Angiotensin II, up to 50 times more active than its precursor, is converted from angiotensin I during one passage through the pulmonary circulation. Some vasoactive materials, including serotonin, bradykinin, adeno-

sine triphosphate, and prostaglandins E_1, E_2, and F_2, are almost completely removed or inactivated by one passage through the pulmonary circulation, whereas others, such as epinephrine, prostaglandins A_1 and A_2, angiotensin II, and vasopressin, may be minimally affected. Norepinephrine and histamine are taken up to a moderate degree. Failure of inactivation or periodic release of substances such as serotonin, bradykinin, histamine, slow-reacting substance of anaphylaxis (SRS-A), eosinophil chemotactic factor, platelet aggregation factor, endocrine substances, and so forth, may be important in the pathogenesis of some pulmonary diseases or as mediators of secondary effects. These chemicals can contribute to systemic and pulmonary hypertension, systemic hypotension, and pulmonary edema.

The lung epithelium is also endowed with a variety of receptors and membrane proteins that are important for processes such as lung fluid absorption in early life and after lung injury or infections. The epithelium indeed has many channel species: the cystic fibrosis transmembrane conductance regulator, Na^+ and K^+ channels, exchangers (e.g., Na^+-K^+ ATPase, Na^+/K^+/2Cl$^-$, Na^+/H^+), and other membrane proteins such as aquaporins. Dopamine agonists, working through dopamine D_1 receptors, seem also to be involved in enhancing the expression of the Na^+-K^+ ATPase on the plasma membrane and hence increasing the ability of the alveolar epithelial cells to absorb fluids. High-altitude edema may also involve Na^+-dependent proteins because the expression of these is generally decreased in cells exposed to low O_2 conditions.

Barnard ML, Ridge KM, et al: Stimulation of the dopamine 1 receptor increases lung edema clearance. *Am J Respir Crit Care Med* 1999;160:982–86.

Said S: Metabolic and endocrine functions of the lung. In Chernick V, Boat T (editors): *Kendig's Textbook on Disorders of the Respiratory Tract in Children*, 6th ed. Philadelphia, WB Saunders, 1998, pp 74–85.

Towne JE, Harrod KS, Krane CM, et al: Decreased expression of aquaporin (AQP)1 and AQP5 in mouse lung after acute viral infection. *Am J Respir Cell Mol Biol* 2000;22:34–44.

Chapter 359

Diagnostic Approach to Respiratory Disease

Gabriel G. Haddad and Regina M. Palazzo

The history and physical examination are the most important first steps in diagnosing respiratory disease. The observed signs and symptoms significantly influence the direction of the subsequent investigations.

History. Family and personal histories are essential for interpreting physical findings and diagnosing respiratory system disease. The history should include questions about respiratory symptoms, their chronicity, their timing during day or night, and whether they are associated with any activity such as exercise or food intake. In addition, the respiratory system interacts with a number of other systems, and questions related to cardiac, gastrointestinal, central nervous system, hematologic, and immune systems may be relevant. For example, questions related to gastrointestinal reflux or immune status may be important in a patient with repeated pneumonias.

Physical Examination. Respiratory dysfunction usually produces detectable alterations in the pattern of breathing. Values for normal respiratory rates are presented in Table 57–1 and depend on many factors, including age. It is important at the bedside not to be satisfied with one respiratory rate measurement because respiratory rates, especially in the young, are exquisitely sensitive to extraneous stimuli. These rates vary among infants but average 40–50 breaths/min in the first weeks of life and usually less than 60 breaths/min in the first few days of life. Respiratory control abnormalities may cause the child to breathe at a low rate or periodically. Mechanical abnormalities produce compensatory changes that are generally directed at maintaining or increasing ventilation. These changes include variable increases in the breathing rate, chest wall retractions, and nasal flaring. Children with restrictive disease breathe at faster rates, and their respiratory excursions are shallow. An expiratory grunt is common as the child attempts to raise the functional residual capacity (FRC) by closing the glottis at the end of expiration. Children with obstructive disease take slower, deeper breaths. When the obstruction is extrathoracic (from the nose to the midtrachea), inspiration is more prolonged than is expiration, and an inspiratory stridor can usually be heard. When the obstruction is intrathoracic, expiration is more prolonged than is inspiration, and the patient often has to make use of accessory expiratory muscles. Lung percussion is usually dull in restrictive lung disease and tympanitic in obstructive disease but has limited value in small infants because it cannot discriminate between noises originating from tissues that are close to each other. Auscultation confirms the presence of inspiratory or expiratory prolongation and provides information about the symmetry and quality of air movement. In addition, it often detects abnormal or adventitious sounds such as *stridor* (a predominant inspiratory monophonic noise), *rales* or *crackles* (high pitch, interrupted sounds found during inspiration and more rarely during early expiration, which denote opening of previously closed air spaces), or *wheezes* (musical, continuous sounds usually caused by the development of turbulent flow in narrow airways).

Blood Gas Analysis. An arterial blood gas analysis is probably the single most useful test of pulmonary function. Because cyanosis is influenced by skin perfusion and blood hemoglobin concentration, it is an unreliable sign of hypoxemia. Arterial hypertension, tachycardia, and diaphoresis are late, and by no means exclusive, signs of hypoventilation. Blood gas exchange is evaluated most accurately by the *direct* measurement of arterial P_{O_2}, P_{CO_2}, and pH (see Chapters 55 and 90.3). The blood specimen is best collected *anaerobically* in a heparinized syringe containing only enough heparin solution to displace the air from the syringe. The syringe should be sealed, placed in ice, and carried to the laboratory for immediate analysis. Although these measurements have no substitute in many conditions, they require arterial puncture and have been replaced to a great extent by noninvasive monitoring.

The age and clinical condition of the patient need to be taken into account when interpreting blood gas tensions. With the exception of neonates, values of arterial P_{O_2} lower than 85 mm Hg are usually abnormal for a child breathing room air at sea level. Calculation of the alveolar-arterial oxygen gradient is useful in the analysis of arterial oxygenation, particularly when the patient is not breathing room air or in the presence of hypercarbia. Values of arterial P_{CO_2} exceeding 45 mm Hg usually indicate hypoventilation or a severe ventilation-perfusion mismatch, unless they reflect respiratory compensation for metabolic alkalosis (see Chapter 45).

Transillumination of the Chest. In infants up to at least 6 mo of age, a pneumothorax may often be diagnosed by transillumination of the chest wall using a fiberoptic light probe. Free air in the pleural space often results in an unusually large halo of light in the skin surrounding the probe. This test is unreliable in older patients or in those with subcutaneous emphysema or atelectasis.

RADIOGRAPHIC TECHNIQUES

Chest Roentgenograms. Whenever possible, a posteroanterior and a lateral view (upright and in full inspiration) should be obtained. Portable films, although useful, may give a somewhat distorted image. Expiratory films may easily be misinterpreted, although a comparison of expiratory and inspiratory films may be useful in the evaluation of a child with suspected foreign body (localized failure of the lung to empty reflects bronchial obstruction). If pleural fluid is suspected, decubitus films are indicated. Films taken in a recumbent position are difficult to interpret if there is fluid within the pleural space or a cavity.

Upper Airway Films. A lateral view of the neck can yield invaluable information about upper airway obstruction and particularly about the condition of the retropharyngeal, supraglottic, and subglottic spaces (which should also be viewed in an anteroposterior projection). Knowing the phase of respiration during which the film was taken is often essential for accurate interpretation. Magnified airway films are often helpful in delineating the upper airways. Patients with suggested obstruction should not be sent unattended to the radiology department.

Sinus and Nasal Films. Roentgenographic examination of the sinuses is indicated when sinus disease is suspected. A coronal CT scan gives the most information. Because of the small size and slow development of the frontal and maxillary sinus cavities in children, transillumination is not as successful in documenting sinus disease as are roentgenograms. Sinus roentgenograms are particularly useful in patients with suspected continuous sinus infection. The need for examining the nasal passages in children is unusual and occurs most often when the neonate presents with obstruction or when a tumor or occult foreign body is suggested.

CT and MRI. CT delineates the internal structure of the thorax in much greater detail than is possible with plain roentgenograms. Technical advances have greatly enhanced the utility of this diagnostic modality (three-dimensional reconstruction is often feasible), whereas scan times and radiation exposure have been markedly reduced. CT scans are of particular importance in the evaluation of mediastinal and pleural lesions, solid or cystic parenchymal lesions, and suggested bronchiectasis. Intravenous contrast material can be infused during the scan to enhance vascular structures.

MRI may be useful for the same disease entities as CT. MRI is an excellent procedure to delineate hilar and vascular anatomy associated with vascular rings or slings.

Fluoroscopy. Fluoroscopy is especially useful for evaluating stridor and abnormal movement of the diaphragm or mediastinum. Many procedures, such as needle aspiration or biopsy of a peripheral lesion, are also best accomplished with the aid of fluoroscopy. Videotape recording, which does not increase radiation exposure, may allow detailed study through "replay" capability during a brief exposure to fluoroscopy.

Contrast Studies

BARIUM SWALLOW. This study, performed with fluoroscopy and spot films, is indicated in the evaluation of patients with recurrent pneumonia, persistent cough of undetermined cause, stridor, or persistent wheezing. The technique may be modified by using barium of different textures and thicknesses, ranging from thin liquid to solids, to evaluate swallowing mechanics, the presence of vascular rings, and tracheoesophageal fistulas, especially when aspiration is suspected. A contrast esophagram has been used in the evaluation of newborns with suggested esophageal atresia, but this procedure entails a high risk of pulmonary aspiration and is not usually recommended. Barium swallows are useful in the evaluation of suggested gastroesophageal reflux, but the interpretation may not be straightforward.

BRONCHOGRAMS. The details of smaller bronchi that cannot be easily evaluated by plain films or even bronchoscopy may be delineated by instilling contrast material directly into the airway. This is indicated in patients with suspected bronchiectasis or airway anomalies who may need surgery, although CT and MRI have largely supplanted bronchography, which requires sedation and topical anesthesia, or even general anesthesia.

PULMONARY ARTERIOGRAMS. These studies allow detailed evaluation of the pulmonary vasculature and are helpful in assessing pulmonary blood flow and in diagnosing congenital anomalies, such as lobar agenesis, unilateral hyperlucent lung, vascular rings, and arteriovenous malformations and are sometimes useful in evaluating solid or cystic lesions. Real-time and Doppler echocardiography are noninvasive methods that often reveal similar information and should be performed before arteriography.

AORTOGRAMS. Thoracic aortograms demonstrate the aortic arch and its major vessels and the systemic (bronchial) pulmonary circulation. They are useful in evaluating vascular rings and suspected pulmonary sequestration. Although most hemoptysis is from the bronchial arteries, bronchial arteriography is seldom helpful in diagnosing or treating intrapulmonary bleeding in children. Echocardiography with or without CT or MRI is helpful in delineating some of these lesions and should be performed before aortography.

PNEUMOPERITONEUM AND PNEUMOTHORAX. In selected situations, such as in the evaluation of diaphragmatic eventration, it may be advantageous to inject a small amount of air into the pleural or peritoneal cavity, outlining the limits of the diaphragm or pleural surfaces by air contrast. Rapidly absorbed, the air causes no functional impairment.

RADIONUCLIDE LUNG SCANS. The usual scan uses intravenous injection of material (macroaggregated human serum albumin labeled with ^{99m}Tc) that will be trapped in the pulmonary capillary bed. The distribution of radioactivity, proportional to pulmonary capillary blood flow, is useful in evaluating pulmonary embolism and congenital cardiovascular and pulmonary defects. Acute changes in the distribution of pulmonary perfusion may reflect alterations of pulmonary ventilation.

The distribution of pulmonary ventilation also may be determined by scanning after the inhalation of a radioactive gas such as xenon-133. After the intravenous injection of xenon-133 dissolved in saline, both pulmonary perfusion and ventilation can be evaluated by continuous recording of the rate of appearance and disappearance of the xenon over the lung. Appearance of xenon early after injection is a measure of perfusion, whereas the rate of washout during breathing is a measure of ventilation in the pediatric population. The most important indication for this test is to demonstrate defects in the pulmonary arterial distribution that may occur with congenital malformations or pulmonary embolism. Spiral reconstruction CT with contrast medium enhancement is being increasingly used in the evaluation of pulmonary thrombi and emboli. Abnormalities in regional ventilation are also easily demonstrable in congenital lobar emphysema, cystic fibrosis, and asthma.

PULMONARY FUNCTION TESTING

Overview. The measurement of respiratory function in infants and young children may be difficult because of the lack of cooperation. Attempts have been made to overcome this limitation by creating standard tests that do not require the patient's active participation. Respiratory function tests still provide only a partial insight into the mechanisms of respiratory disease at early ages.

Whether restrictive or obstructive, most forms of respiratory disease cause alterations in lung volume and its subdivision (see Fig. 357–2). Restrictive diseases typically decrease total lung capacity (TLC). TLC includes residual volume, which is not accessible to direct determinations. It must therefore be measured indirectly by gas dilution methods or, preferably, by

plethysmography. Restrictive disease also decreases vital capacity (VC). VC can be measured by spirometry and is commonly used at the bedside to assess the progression of neuromuscular disorders. Obstructive diseases produce gas trapping and thus increase residual volume and FRC, particularly when these measurements are considered with respect to TLC.

Airway obstruction is most frequently evaluated from determinations of gas flow in the course of a forced expiratory maneuver. The peak expiratory flow is reduced in advanced obstructive disease. The wide availability of simple devices that perform this measurement at the bedside makes it useful for assessing children with airway obstruction. Evaluation of peak flows requires a voluntary effort, and peak flows may not be altered when the obstruction is moderate or mild. Other gas flow measurements require that the child inhale to TLC and then exhale as far and as fast as possible for several seconds. Cooperation and good muscle strength are therefore necessary for the measurements to be reproducible. The forced expiratory volume in 1 sec (FEV$_1$) correlates well with the severity of obstructive diseases. The maximal midexpiratory flow rate, the average flow greater than the middle 50% of the forced vital capacity, is a more reliable indicator of mild airway obstruction. Its sensitivity to changes in residual volume and vital capacity, however, limits its use in children with more severe disease. The construction of flow-volume relationships during the forced vital capacity maneuvers overcomes some of these limitations by expressing the expiratory flows as a function of lung volume (see Chapter 357).

Practical Issues. A *spirometer* is used to measure VC and its subdivisions and expiratory (or inspiratory) flow rates (see Fig. 357–2). A simple *manometer* can measure the maximal inspiratory and expiratory force a subject generates, normally at least 30 cm H$_2$O, which is useful in evaluating the neuromuscular component of ventilation. Expected normal values for VC, FRC, TLC, and residual volume are obtained from prediction equations based on body height.

Flow rates measured by spirometry usually include the FEV$_1$ and the maximal midexpiratory flow rate. More information results from a maximal expiratory flow-volume curve, in which expiratory flow rate is plotted against expired lung volume (expressed in terms of either VC or TLC). Flow rates at lung volumes less than about 75% VC are relatively independent of effort. Expiratory flow rates at low lung volumes (less than 50% VC) are influenced much more by small airways than are flow rates at high lung volumes (FEV$_1$). The flow rate at 25% VC (V$_{25}$) is a useful index of small airway function. Low flow rates at high lung volumes associated with normal flow at low lung volumes suggest upper airway obstruction (see Chapters 356 and 357).

Airway resistance (R$_{AW}$) is measured in a plethysmograph and is expressed as centimeters of water/liter/second. Alternatively, the reciprocal of R$_{AW}$, *airway conductance* (G$_{AW}$), may be used. Because airway resistance measurements vary with the lung volume at which they are taken, it is convenient to use specific airway resistance, SR$_{AW}$ (SR$_{AW}$ = R$_{AW}$/lung volume), which is nearly constant in subjects older than 6 yr (normally less than 7 sec/cm H$_2$O).

The *diffusing capacity for carbon monoxide* is related to oxygen diffusion and is measured by rebreathing from a container having a known initial concentration of carbon monoxide or by using a single breath technique. Decreases in diffusing capacity for carbon monoxide reflect decreases in effective alveolar capillary surface area or decreases in diffusibility of the gas across the alveolar-capillary membrane. Primary diffusion abnormalities are unusual in children; therefore, this test is most frequently employed in children exposed to toxic drugs to the lungs (e.g., oncology patients) or chest wall radiation. *Regional gas exchange* may be conveniently estimated with the perfusion-ventilation xenon scan. Determining *arterial blood gas* levels also disclose the effectiveness of alveolar gas exchange (see earlier).

Clinical Uses. Pulmonary function testing, although rarely resulting in a diagnosis, is helpful in *defining the type of process* (e.g., obstruction, restriction) and the *degree of functional impairment,* in *following the course and treatment of disease,* and in *estimating the prognosis.* It is also useful in *preoperative evaluation* and in confirmation of functional impairment in patients having subjective complaints but a normal physical examination. In most patients with obstructive disease, a repeat test after administering a bronchodilator is warranted.

Most tests require some cooperation and understanding by the patient, and interpretation is greatly facilitated if the test conditions and the patient's behavior during the test are known. Accurate testing of children aged 3–6 yr requires great patience by the physician and training of the patient, whereas most children aged 6 yr or older can be tested reliably without excessive difficulty. Infants and young children who cannot or will not cooperate with test procedures can be studied in a limited number of ways, which often require sedation. Flow rates and pressures during tidal breathing, with or without transient interruption of the flow, may be useful to assess some aspects of airway resistance or obstruction and to measure compliance of the lungs and thorax. Expiratory flow rates may be studied in sedated infants with passive compression of the chest and abdomen with a rapidly inflatable jacket. Gas dilution or plethysmographic methods may also be used in sedated infants to measure FRC and R_{AW}.

MICROBIOLOGY: EXAMINATION OF SECRETIONS

The specific diagnosis of infection in the lower respiratory tract depends on the proper handling of an adequate specimen obtained in an appropriate fashion. Nasopharyngeal or throat cultures are often used but may not correlate with cultures obtained by more direct techniques from the lower airways. Sputum specimens are preferred and are often obtained from patients who do not expectorate by deep throat swab immediately after coughing. Specimens may also be obtained directly from the tracheobronchial tree by nasotracheal aspiration (usually heavily contaminated), by transtracheal aspiration through the cricothyroid membrane (useful in adults and adolescents but hazardous in children), and in infants and children by a sterile catheter inserted into the trachea either during direct laryngoscopy or through an endotracheal tube. A specimen also may be obtained at bronchoscopy. A percutaneous lung tap or an open biopsy is the only way to obtain a specimen that may be absolutely free of oral flora.

A specimen obtained by direct expectoration is usually assumed to be of tracheobronchial origin, but often, especially in children, it is not from this source. The presence of alveolar macrophages—large, mononuclear cells—is the hallmark of tracheobronchial secretions. Both nasopharyngeal and tracheobronchial secretions may contain ciliated epithelial cells, which are more commonly found in sputum. Nasopharyngeal and oral secretions often contain large numbers of squamous epithelial cells. Sputum may contain both ciliated and squamous epithelial cells.

During sleep, mucociliary transport continually brings tracheobronchial secretions to the pharynx, where they are swallowed. An early morning fasting gastric aspirate often contains material from the tracheobronchial tract that is suitable for culture for acid-fast bacilli.

The absence of polymorphonuclear leukocytes in a Wright-stained smear of sputum or bronchoalveolar lavage (BAL) fluid containing adequate numbers of macrophages may be significant evidence against a bacterial infectious process in the lower respiratory tract, assuming that the patient has normal neutrophil counts and function. Eosinophils suggest allergic

disease. Iron stains may reveal hemosiderin granules within macrophages, suggesting pulmonary hemosiderosis. Specimens should also be examined by Gram stain. Bacteria within or near macrophages and neutrophils can be significant. Viral pneumonia may be accompanied by intranuclear or cytoplasmic inclusion bodies visible on Wright-stained smears, and fungal forms may be identifiable on Gram or silver stains.

EXERCISE TESTING

Exercise testing (also see Chapter 416.5) is a more direct approach for detecting diffusion impairment as well as other forms of respiratory disease. Measurements of heart and respiratory rate, minute ventilation, oxygen consumption, carbon dioxide production, and arterial blood gases during incremental exercise loads often provide invaluable information about the functional nature of the disease. Often a simple assessment of the patient's exercise tolerance in conjunction with other more static forms of respiratory function testing may allow a distinction between respiratory and nonrespiratory disease in children.

SLEEP STUDIES

The sleep state has an important influence on respiratory function, particularly in the newborn and young infant. Polysomnographic studies are often helpful when abnormalities of central respiratory control, muscular disorders, or respiratory complications from gastroesophageal reflux are suspected. For the latter condition, pH probe studies are indicated in which a pH probe is placed in the esophagus and prolonged (usually over several hours) monitoring is undertaken (see Chapter 304). These studies, which usually include the simultaneous assessment of ventilatory effort, airway gas flow, gas exchange, and sleep state, are also useful in the diagnosis and management of nocturnal hypoxemia and hypercarbia in children with chronic respiratory disease (see Chapter 357.2).

LUNG VISUALIZATION AND LUNG SPECIMEN–BASED DIAGNOSTIC TESTS

Endoscopy

LARYNGOSCOPY. The evaluation of stridor, problems with vocalization, and other upper airway abnormalities usually require direct inspection. Although indirect (mirror) laryngoscopy may be reasonable in older children and adults, it is rarely feasible in infants and small children. Direct laryngoscopy may be performed with either a rigid or a flexible instrument. The safe use of the rigid scope for examination of the upper airway requires topical anesthesia and either sedation or general anesthesia, whereas the flexible laryngoscope can often be used in the office setting with or without sedation. Further advantages to the flexible scope include the ability to assess the airway without the distortion that may be introduced by the use of the rigid scope and the ability to assess airway dynamics more accurately. Because there is a relatively high incidence of concomitant lesions in the upper and lower airways, it is often prudent to examine the airways above and below the glottis, even when the primary indication is in the upper airway (stridor).

BRONCHOSCOPY AND BRONCHOALVEOLAR LAVAGE (BAL). Bronchoscopy is the inspection of the airways. BAL is a method used to obtain a representative specimen of fluid and secretions from the lower respiratory tract, which is useful for the cytologic and microbiologic diagnosis of lung diseases, especially in those who are unable to expectorate sputum. Commonly, BAL is performed after the general inspection of the airways and before tissue sampling with a brush or biopsy forceps. BAL is accomplished by gently wedging the scope into a lobar, segmental, or subsegmental bronchus and sequentially instilling and withdrawing sterile nonbacteriostatic saline in a volume sufficient to ensure that some of the aspirated fluid contains material that originated from the alveolar space. Nonbronchoscopic BAL can be performed in intubated patients by instilling and withdrawing saline through a catheter passed though the artificial airway and blindly wedged into a distal airway. In either case, the presence of alveolar macrophages documents that an alveolar sample has been obtained. Because the methods used to perform BAL involve passage of the equipment through the upper airway, there is a risk of contamination of the specimen by upper airway secretions. Careful cytologic examination and quantitative microbiologic cultures are important for correct interpretation of the data. BAL can often obviate the need for more invasive procedures such as open lung biopsy, especially in immunocompromised individuals.

Indications for diagnostic bronchoscopy and BAL include recurrent or persistent pneumonia or atelectasis, unexplained or localized and persistent wheeze, the suspected presence of a foreign body, hemoptysis, suspected congenital anomalies, mass lesions, interstitial disease, and pneumonia in the immunocompromised host. Indications for therapeutic bronchoscopy and BAL include bronchial obstruction by mass lesions, foreign bodies or mucus plugs, and general bronchial toilet and bronchopulmonary lavage. The individual undergoing bronchoscopy ventilates around the flexible scope, whereas with the rigid scope ventilation is accomplished through the scope. Rigid bronchoscopy is preferentially indicated for the extraction of foreign bodies and the removal of tissue masses and in patients with massive hemoptysis. In other cases, the flexible scope offers the advantages that it can be passed through endotracheal or tracheostomy tubes, can be introduced into bronchi that come off the airway at acute angles, and can be safely and effectively inserted with topical anesthesia and conscious sedation.

Regardless of the instrument used, the procedure performed, or its indications, the most common *complications* are related to sedation. The relatively more common complications include transient hypoxemia, laryngospasm, bronchospasm, and cardiac arrhythmias. Iatrogenic infection, bleeding, pneumothorax, and pneumomediastinum are rare but reported complications of bronchoscopy or BAL. Subglottic edema is a more common complication of rigid bronchoscopy than of flexible procedures, in which the scopes are smaller and less likely to traumatize the mucosa. Postbronchoscopy croup is treated with oxygen, mist, vasoconstrictor aerosols, and corticosteroids as necessary.

THORACOSCOPY. The pleural cavity may be examined through a thoracoscope, which is similar to a rigid bronchoscope. The thoracoscope is inserted through an intercostal space and the lung is partially deflated, thus allowing the operator to view the surface of the lung, the pleural surface of the mediastinum and diaphragm, and the parietal pleura. Multiple thoracoscopic instruments can be inserted, allowing endoscopic lung or pleural biopsy, bleb resection, pleural abrasion, and ligation of vascular rings.

Purcutaneous Taps

THORACENTESIS. For diagnostic or therapeutic purposes, fluid may be removed from the pleural space by needle. Generally, as much fluid as possible should be withdrawn, and an *upright* chest roentgenogram should be obtained after the procedure. Complications of thoracentesis include infection, pneumothorax, and bleeding. Thoracentesis on the right may be complicated by puncture or laceration of the capsule of the liver and, on the left, by puncture or laceration of the capsule of the spleen. Specimens obtained should always be cultured, examined microscopically for evidence of bacterial infection, and evaluated for total protein and total differential cell counts. Lactic acid dehydrogenase, glucose, cholesterol, triglyceride (chylous), and amylase determinations may also be useful. If malignancy is suspected, cytologic examination is imperative.

Transudates result from mechanical factors influencing the rate of formation or reabsorption of pleural fluid and generally require no further diagnostic evaluation. *Exudates* result from inflammation or other disease of the pleural surface and underlying lung and require a more complete diagnostic evaluation. In general, transudates have a total protein of less than 3 g/dL or a ratio of pleural protein to serum protein less than 0.5, a total leukocyte count of fewer than 2,000/mm^3 with a predominance of mononuclear cells, and low lactate dehydrogenase levels. Exudates have high protein levels and a predominance of polymorphonuclear cells (although malignant or tuberculous effusions may have a higher percentage of mononuclear cells). Complicated exudates often require continuous chest tube drainage and have a pH less than 7.20. Tuberculous effusions may have low glucose and high cholesterol content.

LUNG TAP. Using a technique similar to that used for thoracentesis, a percutaneous lung tap is the most direct method of obtaining bacteriologic specimens from the pulmonary parenchyma and is the only technique other than open lung biopsy not associated with at least some risk of contamination by oral flora. After local anesthesia, a needle attached to a syringe containing nonbacteriostatic sterile saline is inserted using aseptic technique through the inferior aspect of an intercostal space in the area of interest. The needle is rapidly advanced into the lung; the saline is injected and reaspirated, and the needle is withdrawn. These actions are performed as quickly as possible. This procedure usually yields a few drops of fluid from the lung, which should be cultured and examined microscopically.

Major indications for a lung tap are roentgenographic infiltrates of undetermined cause, especially those unresponsive to therapy in immunosuppressed patients who are susceptible to unusual organisms. Complications are the same as for thoracentesis, but the incidence of pneumothorax is higher and somewhat dependent on the nature of the underlying disease process. In patients with poor pulmonary compliance, such as children with *Pneumocystis* pneumonia, the rate may approach 30%, with 5% requiring chest tubes. Bronchopulmonary lavage has replaced lung taps for most purposes.

Lung Biopsy. Lung biopsy may be the only way to establish a diagnosis, especially in protracted, noninfectious disease. In infants and small children, thoracoscopic or open surgical biopsies are the procedures of choice, and in expert hands there is low morbidity. Biopsy through the 3.5-mm diameter pediatric bronchoscopes limits the sample size and diagnostic abilities. As well as ensuring that an adequate specimen is obtained, the surgeon can inspect the lung surface and choose the site of biopsy. In older children, transbronchial biopsies can be performed using flexible forceps through a bronchoscope, an endotracheal tube, a rigid bronchoscope, or an endotracheal tube, usually with fluoroscopic guidance. This technique is most appropriately used when the disease is diffuse, such as *Pneumocystis* pneumonia, or after rejection of a transplanted lung. The diagnostic limitations related to the small size of the biopsy specimens can be mitigated by the ability to obtain several samples. The risk of pneumothorax related to bronchoscopy is increased when transbronchial biopsies are part of the procedure; however, the ability to obtain biopsy specimens in a procedure performed with topical anesthesia and conscious sedation offers advantages to the select population for whom this procedure offers a reasonable diagnostic yield.

Sweat Testing. See Chapter 393.

Baughman RP (editor): *Bronchoalveolar Lavage.* St. Louis, Mosby–Year Book, 1992.
Margolis P, Ferkol T, Marsocci S, et al: Accuracy of the clinical examination in detecting hypoxemia in infants with respiratory illness. *J Pediatr* 1994;124:552.
Saccomanno G: *Diagnostic Pulmonary Cytology.* Chicago, American Society of Clinical Pathologists Press, 1986.

Chapter 360

Sudden Infant Death Syndrome *Carl E. Hunt and Fern R. Hauck*

Sudden infant death syndrome (SIDS) is defined as the sudden death of an infant that is unexpected by history and unexplained by a thorough postmortem examination, which includes a complete autopsy, investigation of the scene of death, and review of the medical history. An autopsy is essential to identify natural causes of death such as congenital anomalies or infection and to diagnosis traumatic child abuse (Table 360–1). The autopsy cannot distinguish between SIDS and intentional suffocation, but the scene investigation and medical history may be of some help if inconsistencies are evident.

Epidemiology. SIDS is the third leading cause of infant mortality in the United States and the most common cause of postneonatal infant mortality (1 mo–1 yr of age). The annual rate of SIDS in the United States was stable at 1.3–1.4/1,000 live births (about 7,000 infants/yr) before 1992, the year in which the American Academy of Pediatrics first recommended that infants sleep nonprone as a way to reduce the risk of SIDS. Since then, particularly after initiation of the national Back to Sleep campaign in 1994, the rate of SIDS progressively declined to 0.70/1,000 in 1999 (2,648 infants). The decline in the number of SIDS deaths in the United States and other countries around the world has been attributed to the decreasing use of the prone position for sleep. Several other countries have decreased prone sleeping prevalence to 2% or less, but in the United States 12–35% of infants (depending on other characteristics) are still being placed prone for sleeping.

Pathology. There is no autopsy finding pathognomonic of SIDS and no finding required for the diagnosis. There are, however, some common observations. Petechial hemorrhages are found in more than 90% of cases and may be more extensive than in other causes of infant mortality. Pulmonary edema is often present and may be substantial.

There are tissue markers indicative of pre-existing, chronic low-grade asphyxia in nearly two thirds of SIDS subjects, including persistence of adrenal brown fat, hepatic erythropoiesis, brainstem gliosis, and other structural abnormalities. In addition to astrogliosis, the brainstem abnormalities include hypomyelination and persistent dendritic spines, especially in the magnocellular nucleus of the reticular formation and dorsal

and solitary nuclei of the vagal nerve. Significant increases in the number of reactive astrocytes in the medulla have also been observed; these increases are not confined to areas related to respiratory neuroregulation. Substance P, a neuropeptide transmitter found in selected sensory neurons of the central nervous system, is present in increased amounts in the pons of SIDS victims. Quantitative three-dimensional anatomic studies indicate that a small subset of SIDS victims have hypoplasia of the arcuate nucleus; this region is a site of cardiorespiratory control in the ventral medulla and is integrated with other regions that regulate arousal, autonomic, and chemosensory function. Neurotransmitter studies have also identified receptor abnormalities in the arcuate nucleus in some SIDS victims, including significant decreases in binding to kainate receptors, muscarinic cholinergic receptors, and serotonergic receptors. There is a positive correlation between decreased density of muscarinic cholinergic and kainate receptors. The neurotransmitter deficits in the arcuate nucleus thus involve more than one receptor type relevant to autonomic control overall and especially to cardiorespiratory control, including arousal responsiveness. Finally, tyrosine hydroxylase immunoreactivity in two brainstem areas, vagal nuclei and reticularis superficialis ventrolateralis, suggests that epinephrine and norepinephrine neurons are altered in SIDS victims.

Postmortem observations are also consistent with pre-existing, low-grade, chronic asphyxia. SIDS infants as a group have both prenatal and postnatal growth retardation and elevated blood cortisol levels. Elevated levels of hypoxanthine in vitreous humor have been reported, suggesting a relatively long period of tissue hypoxia preceding the death. Because adenosine, a precursor of hypoxanthine, is a respiratory inhibitor, these observations suggest a potentially important interaction between asphyxia and hypoventilation; in response to asphyxia from any cause, the secondary acceleration of adenosine monophosphate catabolism and adenosine accumulation will create a vicious cycle, leading to progressive hypoventilation.

Polymorphisms in the serotonin transporter gene have been studied in genomic DNA from Japanese SIDS victims. The L and XL alleles were found more frequently in SIDS than in healthy control infants. These findings suggest higher reuptake activity in SIDS victims than in controls and hence lower serotonin concentrations in the extracellular space. Because serotonin exerts potent excitatory effects on respiratory control in the brain, these findings are consistent with impaired cardiorespiratory control in affected infants.

Postmortem molecular analyses in SIDS cases have identified mutations on the cardiac sodium-channel gene *(SCN5A)*; some SIDS cases, therefore, might be related to a lethal arrhythmia

TABLE 360–1. Differential Diagnosis of Sudden Unexpected Death in Infancy

Cause of Death	Primary Diagnostic Criteria	Confounding Factor(s)	Frequency Distribution
Explained at Autopsy			
Natural			18–20%*
Infections	History, autopsy, and cultures	If minimal findings: SIDS	35–46%†
Congenital anomaly	History and autopsy	If minimal findings: SIDS or intentional suffocation	14–24%†
Unintentional injury	History, scene investigation, autopsy	Traumatic child abuse	15%*
Traumatic child abuse	Autopsy and scene investigation	Unintentional injury	13–24%*
Other natural causes	History and autopsy	If minimal findings: SIDS or intentional suffocation	12–17%*
Unexplained at Autopsy			
Sudden infant death syndrome (SIDS)	History, scene investigation, absence of explainable cause at autopsy	Intentional suffocation	80–82%
Intentional suffocation (filicide)	Perpetrator confession, absence of explainable cause at autopsy	SIDS	Unknown

*As a percentage of all sudden, unexpected infant deaths explained at autopsy.
†As a percentage of all natural causes of sudden, unexpected infant deaths explained at autopsy.
Adapted from Hunt CE: Sudden infant death syndrome and other causes of infant mortality: Diagnosis, mechanisms and risk for recurrence in siblings. Am J Respir Crit Care Med *2001;164:346–57.*

associated with prolonged QT interval caused by an identifiable sodium channel genetic abnormality. Clinical studies have also implicated prolongation of the QT interval as a cause of SIDS (Box 360–1). The prevalence of prolonged QT interval (>440 msec) among all SIDS deaths has not been determined, but a prolonged QT interval during the first week of life increases the risk of SIDS.

Environmental Risk Factors. Declines of 50% or more in rates of SIDS around the world after national education campaigns directed at the risk factors associated with SIDS have occurred during the past decade. These declines in SIDS rates can be attributed largely to reductions in placing infants prone for sleep and increases in placing them supine. A number of other risk factors also have significant associations with SIDS (Box 360–2).

NONMODIFIABLE RISK FACTORS. Although SIDS affects infants from all social strata, lower socioeconomic status has been consistently associated with higher risk. In the United States, African-American and Native American infants are two to three times more likely than white infants to die of SIDS, whereas Asian, Pacific Islander, and Hispanic infants have the lowest incidence of SIDS. Some of this disparity may be related to the higher concentration of poverty and other adverse environmental factors found within African-American and Native American communities.

Infants are at highest risk of SIDS at 2–4 mo of age, with most deaths having occurred by 6 mo. However, this characteristic age has decreased in some countries as SIDS incidence has declined, with deaths occurring at earlier ages and a flattening of the peak incidence. Similarly, the commonly found winter seasonal predominance of SIDS has declined or disappeared in some countries as prone prevalence has decreased, supporting prior findings of an interaction between sleep position and factors more common in colder months (e.g., overheating and infection). Male infants have been found to be 30–50% more likely to be affected than females.

MODIFIABLE RISK FACTORS

Pregnancy-Related Factors. An increased SIDS risk is associated with numerous obstetric factors, suggesting that the in utero environment of future SIDS victims is suboptimal. SIDS infants are more commonly of higher birth order, independent of maternal age, and of gestations following shorter interpregnancy intervals. Mothers of SIDS infants generally receive less prenatal care and initiate care later in pregnancy. Additionally, low birth weight, preterm birth, and slower intrauterine and postnatal growth rates are risk factors.

Maternal smoking during pregnancy significantly increases the risk for SIDS. The incidence of SIDS was about three times greater among infants of smokers in studies conducted before SIDS risk reduction campaigns and five times higher after implementation of campaigns, implying that smoking has become an

---

BOX 360–1. Genetic or Biologic Risk Factors That Have Been Associated with SIDS

Deficient regulation of brainstem autonomic control:
  Arousal/gasping
  Ventilatory responsiveness
  Respiratory pattern
  Heart rate
  Temperature
  Vagal tone
  Blood pressure
  Sleep/circadian rhythm
Family history of SIDS in a sibling
Idiopathic apparent life-threatening event
Prematurity
Metabolic (e.g., fatty acid defects)
Abnormal inflammatory/immune response to infection
Prolonged QT syndrome

BOX 360–2. Environmental Factors Associated with Increased Risk for SIDS

MATERNAL AND ANTENATAL RISK FACTORS

Smoking
Drug exposure (e.g., cocaine, heroin)
Nutritional deficiency
Inadequate prenatal care
Low socioeconomic status
Decreased age, education
Single marital status
Increased parity
Shorter interpregnancy interval
Intrauterine hypoxia
Fetal growth retardation

INFANT RISK FACTORS:

Age (peak 2–4 mo, but may be decreasing)
Male gender
Race/ethnicity (e.g., African-American and Native American)
Growth failure
No pacifier (dummy)
Prematurity
Prone (and side) sleep position
Recent (febrile) illness
Smoking exposure (prenatal and postnatal)
Soft sleeping surface, soft bedding
Thermal stress/overheating
Colder season, no central heating

---

increasingly important risk factor as prone prevalence rates have declined. Most studies have shown that the risk of death is progressively greater as daily cigarette use increases, but the accuracy of self-reported cigarette use data is uncertain. The effects of smoking by the father and other household members are more difficult to interpret because they are highly correlated with maternal smoking. There appears to be a small independent effect of paternal smoking, but data on other household members have been inconsistent.

The evidence linking prenatal illegal drug use and SIDS is conflicting. Overall, the studies do link maternal prenatal drug use with an increased risk of SIDS. The majority of published studies have not found an association between maternal alcohol use prenatally or postnatally and SIDS. In one study of Northern Plains Indians, however, drinking and, particularly, binge drinking were more common among mothers of SIDS infants.

Infant Sleep Environment. Sleeping prone has consistently been shown to increase the risk of SIDS. As rates of prone positioning have decreased in the general population, the odds ratios for SIDS in infants still sleeping prone have increased. The highest risk of SIDS may occur in infants who are usually placed nonprone but were placed prone for last sleep ("unaccustomed prone") or were found prone ("secondary prone"). The "unaccustomed prone" position is more likely to occur in daycare or other settings outside the home and highlights the need for all persons caring for infants to be educated about appropriate sleep positioning.

The initial SIDS risk reduction campaign recommendations considered side sleeping to be nearly equivalent to the supine position in reducing the risk of SIDS. Subsequent studies, however, have indicated that, although much safer than the prone position, side-sleeping infants are twice as likely to die of SIDS compared with infants sleeping supine. This increased risk may relate to the relative instability of the position, with some infants placed in the side rolling to the prone position. Thus, the current recommendations call for supine position for sleeping for all infants except the few infants with a specific medical contraindication such as micrognathia, macroglossia, or perhaps severe gastroesophageal reflux.

Many parents and health care providers were initially concerned that supine sleeping would be associated with an increase in adverse consequences, such as trouble sleeping, vomiting, or aspiration, even though some evidence suggests that the risk of regurgitation and choking are highest for prone-sleeping infants. Infants sleeping on their backs do not have more episodes of cyanosis or apnea, and reports of apparent life-threatening events decreased in Scandinavia after increased use of the supine position. Among infants in the United States who maintained the same sleep position at 1, 3, and 6 months of age, no clinical symptoms or reasons for outpatient visits (including fever, cough, wheezing, trouble breathing or sleeping, vomiting, diarrhea, or respiratory illness) were significantly more common in infants sleeping on their side or supine compared with infants sleeping prone. Three symptoms were actually less common in infants sleeping supine or on their side: fever at 1 mo, stuffy nose at 6 mo, and trouble sleeping at 6 mo. Outpatient visits for ear infection were less common at 3 and 6 mo for infants sleeping supine and less common at 3 mo for infants sleeping on their side. These results provide reassurance for parents and practitioners and will hopefully lead to progressively greater acceptance of supine as the safest and most appropriate sleep position for infants.

Soft sleep surfaces or bedding, such as comforters, pillows, sheepskins, polystyrene bean pillows, and older or softer mattresses are associated with increased risk of SIDS. Head and face covering by loose bedding, particularly heavy comforters, is also associated with increased risk. Overheating has been associated with increased risk for SIDS based on indicators such as higher room temperature, high body temperature, sweating, and excessive clothing or bedding. Some studies have identified an interaction between overheating and prone sleeping, with overheating increasing the risk of SIDS only when infants were sleeping prone.

A few studies have implicated bed sharing as a risk factor for SIDS. In seven early case-controlled studies, five showed an increased risk of SIDS, one showed a trend toward increased risk, and one small study showed a trend toward lower risk. Case-controlled studies in England and New Zealand found increased risk associated with bed sharing only among smoking mothers. Bed sharing has been found to be particularly hazardous when other children are in the same bed, when parents are co-sleeping on a couch or other soft or confining sleeping surface, and for infants younger than 4 mo of age. Some authors have hypothesized potentially protective effects among infants who are bed sharing and breast-feeding based on observational sleep laboratory studies, including improved maternal inspections, more infant arousals, and less deep sleep. However, no epidemiologic studies have reported a protective effect from bed sharing, and bed sharing hence should not be encouraged as a method to reduce the incidence of SIDS.

Infant Feeding Care Practices and Exposures. The association between breast-feeding and SIDS is inconclusive. A number of studies have demonstrated a protective effect of breast-feeding that was not present after adjusting for potentially confounding factors. This suggests that it is a marker for lifestyle or socioeconomic status rather than having an independent effect. Although the benefits of breast-feeding are many, data are inadequate to recommend it as a strategy to reduce SIDS.

Pacifier (dummy) use has been found to significantly lower the risk of SIDS in every reported study, both when used routinely and for last/reference sleep. It is not known if this is a direct effect of the pacifier itself or from associated infant or parental behaviors. Concerns have been expressed about recommending pacifiers as a means of reducing the risk of SIDS for fear of creating adverse consequences, particularly interference with breast-feeding. However, no association between pacifiers and breast-feeding duration has been found. An increased incidence of otitis media and of respiratory and gastrointestinal illness has been reported for pacifier users compared with nonusers. The Netherlands (for bottle-fed babies) and Germany have recommended pacifier use as a way to potentially reduce the risk of SIDS.

Upper respiratory tract infections have not been found to be an independent risk factor. These and other minor infections, however, may play a role in the pathogenesis of SIDS. Risk for SIDS, for example, was found to be increased after illness only among prone sleepers or among those who were heavily wrapped.

No association between immunizations and SIDS has been found. However, SIDS infants are less likely to be immunized than control infants and no temporal relationship between vaccine administration and death has been identified. Parents should be reassured that immunizations do not present a risk for SIDS.

There is a major association between intrauterine exposure to cigarette smoking and risk for SIDS. It is very difficult to assess the independent effect of infant exposure to environmental tobacco smoke (ETS) because parental smoking behaviors during and after pregnancy are highly correlated. Only one study examined the effect of maternal smoking after the birth of the infant in the absence of maternal smoking during pregnancy; an increased risk of SIDS was found for infants exposed to maternal ETS. In one U.S. study, an independent effect of postnatal ETS was found by controlling for maternal prenatal smoking; additionally, a dose response was found for the number of household smokers, number of people smoking in the same room as the infant, and the number of cigarettes smoked, although confidence intervals were large in some categories owing to small sample size. A British study also found a dose response of ETS to the number of household smokers, cigarettes smoked, and hours the infant was exposed. The data suggest that keeping the infant free of ETS may potentially further reduce an infant's risk of SIDS.

Parental smoking is the most important risk factor for SIDS on a population basis. The population attributable risk (i.e., proportion of cases that would not have occurred had the risk factor been eliminated in the population) is 48% assuming a 25% prevalence of maternal smoking. Motivating families to quit smoking (particularly during pregnancy) is much more difficult than asking them to change behaviors related to infant sleeping position or other factors associated with a safe sleep environment, however, making this endeavor a major challenge for the professional health community.

Disparities in SIDS rates among some ethnic-racial groups have increased in recent years. This may be due to group differences in adopting nonprone sleeping or other risk reduction behaviors. For example, 32% of African-American infants but only 17% of white infants were usually placed prone for sleep as reported by parents responding to a 1998 national survey of infant care practices. Greater efforts are needed to address this growing disparity and to ensure that SIDS risk reduction education reaches all parents. Further, the messages must reach all care providers, including grandparents, other relatives, and personnel at daycare centers.

Genetic Risk Factors. Data are accumulating that link specific genotypes to impaired brainstem regulation of breathing or other autonomic control as a risk factor for SIDS (see Box 360–1 and Table 360–2). Neural control of breathing and sleep are closely integrated, and abnormalities in regulation of sleep and circadian rhythmicity can hence impair cardiorespiratory integration and arousal responsiveness from sleep. Homologous counterparts of essential circadian clock genes isolated in Drosophilae have been identified in mammals. Because the sleep-wake cycle is under control of the circadian clock, these circadian master genes, as well other sleep-related genes, likely influence sleep regulation.

Furthermore, targeted gene inactivation studies in animals have identified several genes involved with prenatal brainstem

TABLE 360–2. Summary of Data Providing Direct or Indirect Evidence for Genetic Susceptibility to SIDS

Category of Data	Primary Limitations(s)
Infant Mortality Studies	
Increased risk for recurrent SIDS in siblings	Unknown number of intentional suffocations
	May include some explained causes
	Scant data about environmental risk factors
Increased risk for recurrent non-SIDS causes of infant mortality in siblings	Unable to quantify contributions from common environmental risk factors
Neuropathology Studies in SIDS Victims and Animals	Causal relationship of these abnormalities to pathophysiology of SIDS not established
Physiologic Studies	
Subsequent siblings of SIDS	Unknown role of intentional suffocation in index cases and in surviving siblings
	Causal relationship of these abnormalities to pathophysiology of SIDS not established
Parents of SIDS	Small studies with variable results
	Causal relationship of these abnormalities to pathophysiology of SIDS not established
Genetic Studies of Sleep Regulation	Unknown if SIDS is exclusively a sleep-related disorder
	Causal importance to SIDS of sleep state and arousability from sleep not fully established
Family Studies	
Obstructive sleep apnea syndrome (OSAS) or sleep-disordered breathing (SDB)	Unclear relationship of apparent life-threatening event to SIDS
	Genetic risk factors for OSAS (SDB) not fully delineated
	Limited information about the SIDS cases in these kindreds

development of respiratory control, including arousal responsiveness. During embryogenesis, for example, the survival of specific cellular populations composing the respiratory neuronal network is regulated by neurotrophins, a multigene family of growth factors and receptors. Brain-derived neurotrophic factor is required for development of normal breathing behavior in mice, and newborn mice lacking functional brain-derived neurotrophic factor exhibit ventilatory depression associated with apparent loss of peripheral chemoafferent input. Ventilation is depressed, and hypoxic ventilatory drive is deficient or absent. *Krox-20*, a homeobox gene important for hindbrain morphogenesis, also appears to be required for normal development of the respiratory central pattern generator. *Krox-20* null mutants exhibit an abnormally slow respiratory rhythm and increased incidence of respiratory pauses, and this respiratory depression can be further modulated by endogenous enkephalins. Inactivation of *Krox-20* may result in absence of a rhythm-promoting reticular neuron group localized in the caudal pons and could thus be a cause of life-threatening apnea.

Brainstem muscarinic cholinergic pathways are important in ventilatory responsiveness to CO_2. The muscarinic system develops from the neural crest, and the *ret* proto-oncogene is important for this development. *Ret* knockout mice have a depressed ventilatory response to hypercarbia, implicating absence of the *ret* gene as a cause of impaired hypercarbic responsiveness. Diminished ventilatory responsiveness to hypercarbia has also been demonstrated in male newborn mice heterozygous for *Mash-1*. There is a molecular link between *ret* and *Mash-1*, and the latter is expressed in embryonic neurons before the former is expressed in vagal neural crest derivatives and in brainstem locus coeruleus neurons, an area involved with arousal responsiveness. *Mash-1* thus appears to be involved in respiratory control development through mechanisms linked to the X chromosome. Abnormality of this gene identifies one possible genetic basis for the increased frequency of SIDS in males and for the impaired arousal responsiveness thought to be critically important in the pathophysiology of SIDS.

Gene-Environment Interaction. Based on the abundant evidence for environmental risk factors for SIDS (see Box 360–2) and the emerging evidence for genetic risk factors, the mechanism for SIDS in individual infants may best be understood as a consequence of one or more environmental risk factors interacting with one or more genetic risk factors. There appears to be an interaction between prone/side sleep position and impaired car-

diorespiratory control, for example, especially impaired ventilatory and arousal responsiveness. Face-down or nearly face-down sleeping does occasionally occur in healthy prone-sleeping infants and can result in episodes of airway obstruction and asphyxia in healthy full-term infants, especially if they are sleeping on a very soft surface. Although healthy infants will arouse before the face-down or face-nearly-down position becomes life threatening, infants with insufficient arousal responsiveness to asphyxia would be at risk for fatal asphyxia. In addition, prone sleeping may cause a clinically significant degree of thermal stress, which could further compromise infants with deficient cardiorespiratory control. There thus may be links between modifiable risk factors such as soft bedding, prone sleep position, and thermal stress and links between genetic risk factors such as cardiorespiratory control deficits (ventilatory and arousal abnormalities) and temperature/metabolic regulation deficits.

The increased risk for SIDS associated with fetal and postnatal exposure to cigarette smoke also appears at least in part to depend on genetic factors affecting brainstem autonomic control. Animal studies demonstrate impaired ventilatory and arousal responsiveness to hypoxia associated with fetal exposure and impaired autoresuscitation after apnea in association with postnatal nicotine exposure. In addition, fetal rat exposure to maternal smoking reduces protein kinase C within the dorsocaudal brainstem, which would impair ventilatory and arousal responsiveness to hypoxia.

INFANT GROUPS AT INCREASED RISK FOR SIDS

Unexplained Apparent Life-Threatening Events. Infants with an unexplained apparent life-threatening event (ALTE) are at increased risk for SIDS. A history of an unexplained ALTE has been reported in about 5% of SIDS victims, and the risk of SIDS may be higher with two or more unexplained ALTEs. Compared with healthy control infants, the risk for SIDS after an ALTE may be as much as three to five times greater.

Subsequent Siblings of a SIDS Victim. The extent to which risk for SIDS may be increased in subsequent siblings is controversial, owing in part to uncertainty about the frequency with which intentional suffocation is misclassified as SIDS. Clarification of the role of intentional suffocation has been impaired by the lack of objective criteria for diagnosis. Based on a few families with multiple sudden, unexpected infant/child fatalities and later parental confession or conviction, however, some health professionals have stated that only homicide runs in families and all second cases of SIDS in a family should be investigated for possible homicide. However, there are also substantial data in support of genetic as well as environmental factors leading to increased risk of death from natural causes in siblings in some families. The next-born siblings of first-born infants dying of any noninfectious cause are at significantly increased risk for infant death from the same cause, including SIDS (see Table 360–2). The relative risk for recurrence of each cause of infant death is similar for SIDS and for each of the explainable natural causes. Compared with first-born infants in families, subsequent siblings of a previous SIDS victim appear to be approximately five times more likely to die of SIDS. Although many of the studies have limitations (see Table 360–2), when considered in the aggregate, the evidence is strong that recurrent infant mortality in families can be due to a combination of genetic and environment risk factors, in addition to intentional suffocation.

Prematurity. Many studies have identified an inverse relationship between risk for SIDS and birthweight/gestational age. The environmental risk factors associated with SIDS in preterm infants are not substantially different than those observed in full-term infants, including prone and side sleeping. However, the postnatal age of preterm infants dying of SIDS is 5–7 wk older than full-term infants, and the postconceptional age is 4–6 wk younger than full-term infants. Compared with infants with birth weight greater than 2500 g, infants with birth weights of 1000–1499 g and 1500–2499 g are approximately four and three times more likely to die of SIDS, respectively.

Physiologic Studies. Physiologic studies have been performed in infants at increased risk for SIDS, a few of whom later died of SIDS. These studies are most consistent with a brainstem abnormality related to neuroregulation of cardiorespiratory control or other brainstem autonomic functions (see Box 360–1).

RESPIRATORY PATTERN AND CHEMORECEPTOR SENSITIVITY. The respiratory pattern abnormalities have included prolonged apnea, excess brief apneas, periodic breathing, and decreased breath-to-breath respiratory rate variability at slow respiratory rates. Some infants at increased risk for SIDS have diminished ventilatory responsiveness to hypercarbia and/or to hypoxia, but there is a high degree of individual overlap between normal and at-risk infants.

AROUSAL RESPONSES. Absent arousal responsiveness renders infants incapable of responding effectively to sleep-related asphyxia from any cause. Infants at increased risk for SIDS who have diminished ventilatory responsiveness to hypercarbia and/or hypoxia generally have a concomitant abnormality in hypercarbic and/or hypoxic arousal responsiveness. A deficit in arousal responsiveness may be a necessary prerequisite for SIDS to occur but may be insufficient to cause SIDS in the absence of other genetic or environmental risk factors. Victims of SIDS may also have deficient autoresuscitation (gasping) as a component of the asphyxic arousal response deficit; this would be the final and most devastating physiologic failure

In full-term infants with ALTE, the occurrence and severity of recurrent symptoms correlate with arousal responsiveness. Most full-term infants younger than 9 wk of age arouse in response to mild hypoxia, but only 10–15% of normal infants greater than 9 wk of age arouse. This suggests that as full-term infants mature, their ability to arouse to mild-moderate hypoxic stimuli diminishes as they reach the age range of greatest risk for SIDS. However, there is significant overlap in individual values between healthy term controls and infants in groups at increased risk for SIDS.

TEMPERATURE REGULATION. Sweating during sleep has been observed in some infants who have had an idiopathic ALTE or have died of SIDS. Although overheating may be the cause of this sweating, it may also be caused by alveolar hypoventilation and secondary asphyxia or by autonomic dysfunction as part of a more generalized deficiency in brainstem function.

CARDIAC CONTROL. The ability to shorten QT interval as heart rate increases is impaired in some SIDS infants, and some have prolongation of the QT interval (>440 msec), suggesting that such infants may be predisposed to ventricular arrhythmia. The prevalence of prolonged QT interval among all SIDS deaths has not been determined, but a prolonged QT interval during the first week of life does increase the risk of SIDS. Infants later dying of SIDS compared with normal infants also have higher heart rates in all sleep-waking states, diminished heart rate variability during wakefulness, and lower heart rate variation at a given respiratory frequency across all sleep-waking cycles. Thus, future SIDS victims differ from normal in the extent to which cardiac and respiratory activities are coupled.

Part of the decreased heart rate variability and increased heart rate observed in infants who later die of SIDS may be related to decreased vagal tone. This could be caused by vagal neuropathy, brainstem damage in areas responsible for parasympathetic cardiac control, or other factors. Furthermore, because the greatest reduction in all types of heart rate variability occurs while awake, these reductions may be related to the reduced motility retrospectively reported in SIDS victims and also observed in some infants at increased risk for SIDS. Comparing heart rate power spectra before and after obstructive apneas in infants, future SIDS victims did not have the decreases in low-frequency to high-frequency power ratios observed in control infants. Some future SIDS victims thus have different autonomic responsiveness to obstructive apneas, perhaps indicating a dysautonomia that could be associated with higher vulnerability to external or endogenous stress factors and result in reduced electrical stability of the heart and hence ventricular fibrillation.

TERMINAL RECORDINGS IN SIDS VICTIMS. Home cardiorespiratory monitors with memory capability have recorded some terminal events in SIDS victims. All of these terminal recordings utilized transthoracic impedance for breath detection, which cannot detect obstructed breaths, and most did not include pulse oximetry recordings of O_2 saturation. Therefore, one cannot reach any conclusions from these recordings as to whether the terminal event was initiated by apnea, bradycardia, desaturation, or a combination of these findings. In most instances, there has been sudden and rapid progression of severe bradycardia either preceding or at the onset of central apnea and hence too soon to be explained by the prolonged central apnea. These recordings are consistent with an abnormality in autonomic control of heart rate variability or with hypoxemia (not recorded) secondary to obstructive apnea (not recorded) as the precipitating mechanism for the severe bradycardia and fatal outcome.

CLINICAL STRATEGIES

Monitoring. SIDS cannot be prevented in individual infants because it is not possible currently to prospectively identify future SIDS victims or effectively intervene. Studies of respiratory pattern and/or cardiac abnormalities do not have sufficient sensitivity and specificity to be clinically useful as a screening test. Home electronic surveillance does not reduce the risk of SIDS. It might have a preventive role in the future, however, if obstructed breaths, central apnea, bradycardia, or oxygen desaturation occurring as part of the terminal event could be reliably detected sufficiently early so as to be amenable to intervention. Although prolonged QT interval in an infant may be treated if diagnosed, neither the role of routine postnatal electrocardiographic (ECG) screening nor the safety of treatment has been established. Parental ECG screening is not likely to be helpful because spontaneous mutations are common.

Reducing the Risk of SIDS. This goal is achievable, as evidenced by the dramatic decreases in SIDS rates in association with reduction in nonsupine sleeping. The American Academy of Pediatrics guidelines to reduce the risk of SIDS in individual infants are appropriate for most infants, but physicians and other health care providers may on occasion need to consider alternative approaches. The major components are as follows:

1. Full-term and premature infants should be placed for sleep in the supine position. There are no adverse health outcomes from supine sleeping. Side sleeping is not recommended.

2. A crib meeting federal safety standards is a desirable sleeping environment for infants. Safety standards have not been established for bassinets and cradles. Sleep surfaces designed for adults may pose hazards to infants, such as entrapment.

3. Infants should not be put to sleep on waterbeds, sofas, soft mattresses, or other soft surfaces.

4. Soft materials in the infant's sleep environment should be avoided, either over, under, or near the infant. These include pillows, comforters, quilts, sheepskins, and stuffed toys. Because loose bedding may be hazardous, blankets, if used, should be tucked in around the crib mattress. Sleeping clothing (such as a sleep sack) may be used in place of blankets.

5. Bed sharing or co-sleeping may be hazardous under some conditions. Adults (other than parents) and children or other siblings should not share a bed with an infant. The parents should not share a bed with their infant if they smoke or use substances such as drugs or alcohol that impair parental arousal. The other risk reduction recommendations should be followed, such as placing the infant supine and avoiding soft bedding. As an alternative to bed sharing, parents may wish to place the crib near their bed.

6. Avoid overheating and overbundling. The infant should be lightly clothed for sleep and the thermostat set at a comfortable temperature.

7. Infants should have some time in the prone position while awake and observed. Alternating the placement of the infant's head as well as his or her orientation in the crib can also minimize the risk of head flattening from supine sleeping.

8. Devices advertised to maintain sleep position or reduce the risk of rebreathing are not recommended.

9. Home respiratory, cardiac, and O_2 saturation monitoring may be of value for selected infants who have extreme instability, but there is no evidence that its use decreases the incidence of SIDS and it is, therefore, not recommended for this purpose.

10. The national Back to Sleep campaign should continue and be expanded to emphasize the multiple characteristics of a safe sleeping environment and to focus on the groups who continue to have higher prevalence rates for placing infants prone for sleeping. Educational strategies must be tailored to different racial-ethnic groups to ensure acceptance within diverse cultural contexts. Other risk reduction messages also should be included.

General

American Academy of Pediatrics Task Force on Infant Sleep Position and Sudden Infant Death Syndrome: Changing concepts of sudden infant death syndrome: Implications for infant sleeping environment and sleep position. *Pediatrics* 2000;105:650–6.

Byard RW, Krous HF (editors): *Sudden Infant Death Syndrome. Problems, Progress & Possibilities.* London, Arnold, 2001.

Hauck FR, Hunt CE: Sudden infant death syndrome in 2000. *Curr Probl Pediatr* 2000;30:241–61.

Ramanathan R, Corwin MJ, Hunt CE, et al and the CHIME Study Group: Cardiorespiratory events recorded on home monitors: Comparison of healthy infants with those at increased risk for SIDS. *JAMA* 2001;285:2199–2207.

Environmental Risk Factors

Arnestad M, Andersen M, Vege A, et al: Changes in the epidemiological pattern of sudden infant death syndrome in southeast Norway, 1984–1998: Implications for future prevention and research. *Arch Dis Child* 2001;85:108–115.

Corwin MJ, Lesko SM, Heeren T, et al: Secular changes in sleep position during infancy. *Pediatrics*, in press.

Gessner BD, Ives GC, Perham-Hester KA: Association between SIDS and prone sleep position, bed sharing, and sleeping outside an infant crib in Alaska. *Pediatrics* 2001;108:923–27.

Hoyert DL, Freedman MA, Strobino DM, et al: Annual summary of vital statistics. *Pediatrics* 2001;108:1241–55.

Hunt CE, Lesko SM, Vezina RM, et al: Effects of infant sleep position on health outcomes. *Arch Pediatr Adolesc Med*, in press.

Lesko SM, Corwin MJ, Vezina RM, et al: Changes in sleep position during infancy: A prospective longitudinal assessment. *JAMA* 1998;280:336–40.

MacDorman MF, Cnattingius S, Hoffman HJ, et al: Sudden infant death syndrome and smoking in the United States and Sweden. *Am J Epidemiol* 1997;146:249–57.

Malloy MH, Freeman DH: Birth weight- and gestational age-specific sudden infant death syndrome mortality: United States, 1991 versus 1995. *Pediatrics* 2000;105:1227–31.

McCoy RC, Hunt CE, Lesko SM, et al: Population-based study of bed sharing and breastfeeding. *Pediatr Res* 2000;47:154A.

Moon RY, Patel KM, Shaefer SJM: Sudden infant death syndrome in child care settings. *Pediatrics* 2000;106:295–300.

Oyen N, Markestad T, Skjaerven R, et al: Combined effects of sleeping position and prenatal risk factors in sudden infant death syndrome: The Nordic epidemiological SIDS study. *Pediatrics* 1997;100:613–21.

Willinger M, Ko C-W, Hoffman HJ, et al: Factors associated with caregivers' choice of infant sleep position, 1994–1998. The National Infant Sleep Position Study. *JAMA* 2000;283:2135–42.

Genetic Risk Factors

Ackerman MJ, Siu BL, Sturner WQ, et al: Postmortem molecular analysis of SCN5A defects in SIDS. *JAMA* 2001;286:2264–9.

Hunt CE: Sudden infant death syndrome and other causes of infant mortality: Diagnosis, mechanisms and risk for recurrence in siblings. *Am J Resp Crit Care Med* 2001;164:346–57.

Narita N, Narita M, Takashima S, et al: Serotonin transporter gene variation is a risk factor for SIDS in the Japanese population. *Pediatrics* 2001;107:690–702.

Children and adults preferentially breathe through their nose unless nasal obstruction interferes. However, most newborn infants are obligate nasal breathers, and significant nasal obstruction presenting at birth, such as choanal atresia, may be a life-threatening situation for the infant unless an alternative to the nasal airway is established.

Physiology. In addition to olfaction, the nose provides initial warming and humidification of inspired air. In the anterior nasal cavity, turbulent airflow and coarse hairs enhance the deposition of large particulate matter; the remaining nasal airways filter out particles as small as 6 μm in diameter. In the turbinate region, the airflow becomes laminar and the air stream is narrowed and directed superiorly, enhancing particle deposition, warming, and humidification. Nasal passages contribute as much as 50% of the total resistance of normal breathing. *Nasal flaring*, a sign of respiratory distress, reduces the resistance to inspiratory airflow through the nose and may improve ventilation.

The nasal mucosa is more vascular, especially in the turbinate region, than in the lower airways; however, the surface epithelium is similar, with ciliated cells, goblet cells, submucosal glands, and a covering blanket of mucus. In addition to mucous glycoproteins, which provide viscoelastic properties, the nasal secretions contain lysozyme and secretory IgA, both of which have antimicrobial activity, and IgG, IgE, albumin, histamine, bacteria, lactoferrin, and cellular debris. Aided by the ciliated cells, mucus flows toward the nasopharynx, where the air stream widens, the epithelium becomes squamous, and secretions are wiped away by swallowing; replacement of the mucous layers occurs about every 10–20 min. Estimates of daily mucus production vary from 0.1–0.3 mg/kg/24 hr, with most of the mucus being produced by the submucosal glands.

Anatomy. The *paranasal sinuses* develop in the facial bones as air cells lined with ciliated, mucus-secreting epithelium. The frontal, maxillary, and anterior ethmoid sinuses drain into the middle meatus, whereas the posterior ethmoid cells and sphenoidal sinus drain into the superior meatus of the nose. Development of the sinuses begins at 3–5 mo of gestation but occurs mostly after birth, with the maxillary and ethmoidal sinuses being the earliest to form (see Chapter 365). Growth of the sinuses continues through adolescence, with the frontal and sphenoidal sinuses often being somewhat asymmetric; up to 5% of the population has no significant frontal sinus development. Hypoplasia of the maxillary sinuses, or the presence of septa within the maxillary sinuses, is seen occasionally.

The adenoids on the posterior nasopharyngeal wall and the tonsils at the base of the tongue are directly in line with the mucociliary flow and the air stream, enhancing the protective function of this lymphoid tissue. The eustachian tubes, also lined with mucus-secreting, ciliated epithelium, enter the lateral walls of the nasopharynx and connect the nasopharynx to the middle ear.

Acquired anatomic abnormalities suggestive of sinusitis seen on plain sinus radiographs include mucosal thickening greater than 4 mm, air-fluid levels, or opacification; plain sinus radiographs in children younger than 7 yr of age may be difficult to interpret. High-resolution CT of the paranasal sinuses, the current gold standard for evaluation of disease of the paranasal sinuses, often reveals abnormalities, either congenital or acquired, that are not seen on plain films.

Chapter 361

Congenital Disorders of the Nose *Joseph Haddad Jr.*

Congenital *structural nasal malformations* are uncommon compared with acquired abnormalities. The nasal bones may be congenitally absent so that the bridge of the nose fails to develop, resulting in nasal hypoplasia. Congenital absence of the nose (arhinia), complete or partial duplication, or a single centrally placed nostril may occur in isolation but are usually a part of malformation syndromes. Rarely, supernumerary teeth may be found in the nose, or teeth may grow into it from the maxilla.

On occasion, nasal bones are sufficiently malformed to produce severe narrowing of the nasal passages. Often such narrowing is associated with a high and narrow hard palate. Children with these defects may have significant obstruction to airflow during infections of the upper airways and are more susceptible to the development of chronic or recurrent hypoventilation (see Chapter 369). Rarely, the alae nasi may be sufficiently thin and poorly supported to result in inspiratory obstruction, or there may be congenital nasolacrimal duct obstruction with cystic extension into the nasopharynx causing respiratory distress.

Nasal congestion with obstruction is common during the first year of life and may affect the quality of breathing during sleep; it may be associated with a narrow nasal airway, viral or bacterial infection with congestion, enlarged adenoids, or maternal estrogenic stimuli similar to rhinitis of pregnancy. The internal nasal airway doubles in size during the first 6 mo of life, leading to resolution of symptoms in many infants. Supportive care with a bulb syringe and saline nose drops, topical nasal decongestants, and antibiotics, when indicated, will improve symptoms in affected infants.

A wide variety of nasal and midface abnormalities exist that may be part of more extensive craniofacial anomalies. These children are best treated by a team consisting of experienced pediatric, surgical, dental, and rehabilitation specialists.

Choanal Atresia. This is the most common congenital anomaly of the nose and has a frequency of approximately 1/7,000 live births. It consists of a unilateral or bilateral bony (90%) or membranous (10%) septum between the nose and the pharynx; most cases are a combination of bony and membranous atresia. Nearly 50% of affected infants have other congenital anomalies, with the anomalies occurring more frequently in bilateral cases. The CHARGE syndrome—*C*oloboma; *H*eart disease; *A*tresia choanae; *R*etarded growth and development or CNS anomalies, or both; *G*enital anomalies or hypogonadism, or both; and *E*ar anomalies or deafness, or both—is one of the more common anomalies associated with choanal atresia.

CLINICAL MANIFESTATIONS. Newborn infants have a variable ability to breathe through their mouths, so nasal obstruction does not produce the same symptoms in every infant. When unilateral, the infant may be asymptomatic for a prolonged period, often until the first respiratory infection, when the diagnosis may be suggested by nasal discharge or persistent nasal obstruction. Infants with bilateral choanal atresia who have difficulty with mouth breathing make vigorous attempts to inspire, often suck in their lips, and develop cyanosis. Distressed children then cry (which relieves the cyanosis) and become more calm with normal skin color, only to repeat the cycle after closing their mouths. Those who are able to breathe through their mouths at once experience difficulty when sucking and swallowing, becoming cyanotic when they attempt to feed.

DIAGNOSIS. This is established by the inability to pass a firm catheter through each nostril 3–4 cm into the nasopharynx. The atretic plate may be seen directly with fiberoptic rhinoscopy. The anatomy is best evaluated by using high-resolution CT.

TREATMENT. Initially, this consists of prompt placement of an oral airway, maintaining the mouth in an open position, or intubation. A standard oral airway may be used (such as that used in anesthesia), or a feeding nipple may be fashioned with large holes at the tip to facilitate air passage. Once an oral airway is established, the infant can be fed by gavage until breathing and eating without the assisted airway is possible. In bilateral cases, intubation or tracheotomy may be indicated. If the child is free of other serious medical problems, operative intervention is considered in the neonate; transnasal repair is now more common with the introduction of small magnifying endoscopes and smaller surgical instruments and drills. Stents are usually left in place for weeks after the repair to prevent closure or stenosis. Tracheotomy should be considered in cases of bilateral atresia in which the child has other potentially life-threatening problems and in whom early surgical repair of the choanal atresia may not be appropriate or feasible. Operative correction of unilateral obstruction may be deferred for several years. In both unilateral and bilateral cases, re-stenosis necessitating dilation or reoperation, or both, is common. Mitomycin-C has been used to help prevent the development of granulation tissue and stenosis.

Congenital defects of the nasal septum, such as *perforation* or *deviation*, are rare. Perforation can be developmental (very rare) but, more commonly, is acquired after birth secondary to infection, such as syphilis, tuberculosis, or trauma. Continuous positive airway pressure cannulas are a cause of iatrogenic perforation. Trauma from delivery is the most common cause of septal deviation noted at birth. When recognized early, it may be corrected with immediate realignment using blunt probes, cotton applicators, and topical anesthesia. Formal surgical correction, when required, is usually postponed to avoid disturbance of midface growth. Mild septal deviations are common and usually asymptomatic; abnormal formation of the septum is infrequent unless other malformations are present, such as cleft lip or palate.

Pyriform aperture stenosis is a bony abnormality of the anterior nasal aperture. These infants present with severe nasal obstruction at birth or shortly thereafter. Diagnosis is made by CT of the nose; surgical repair by means of an anterior, sublabial approach may be needed if the child cannot feed or breathe without difficulty.

Congenital midline nasal masses include *dermoids, gliomas,* and *encephaloceles* (in descending order of frequency). They present intranasally or extranasally and may have intracranial connections. Nasal dermoids often have a dimple or pit on the nasal dorsum, sometimes with hair being present, and may predispose to intracranial infections if an intracranial connection is present. Recurrent infection of the dermoid itself is common. Gliomas or heterotopic brain tissue are firm, whereas encephaloceles are soft and enlarge with crying or the Valsalva maneuver. Diagnosis is based on physical examination findings and results from imaging studies. CT provides the best bony detail, but MRI allows sagittal views, which may be needed to further define intracranial extension. Surgical excision of these masses is generally required, with the extent and surgical approach based on the type and size of the mass.

Other nasal masses include hemangiomas, congenital nasolacrimal duct obstruction (which may present as an intranasal mass), nasal polyps, and tumors such as rhabdomyosarcoma. Nasal polyps are rarely present at birth, but the others often present at birth or in early infancy (see Chapter 363).

Poor development of the paranasal sinuses and a narrow nasal airway are associated with recurrent or chronic upper airway infection in Down syndrome.

Brown OE, Myer CM, Manning SC: Congenital nasal pyriform aperture stenosis. *Laryngoscope* 1989;99:86.

Hughes GB, Sharpino G, Hunt W, et al: Management of the midline nasal mass: A review. *Head Neck Surg* 1980;2:222.

Maniglia AJ, Goodwin WJ, Arnold JE, et al: Intracranial abscesses secondary to nasal sinus and orbital infections in adults and children. *Arch Otolaryngol Head Neck Surg* 1989;115:1424.

Richardson M, Osguthorpe JD: Surgical management of choanal atresia. *Laryngoscope* 1988;98:915.

Schwartz DA, Lieberman SA, Viles PH, et al: An unusual cause of respiratory distress in a neonate. *Pediatrics* 1988;101:479.

Stankiewicz JA: The endoscopic repair of choanal atresia. *Otolaryngol Head Neck Surg* 1990;103:931.

Chapter 362
Acquired Disorders of the Nose *Joseph Haddad Jr.*

362.1 Foreign Body

Food, crayons, small toys, erasers, paper wads, beads, beans, stones, pieces of sponge, and other foreign bodies are frequently introduced into the nose by children. Initial symptoms are local obstruction, sneezing, relatively mild discomfort, and, rarely, pain. Irritation results in mucosal swelling; and, because some foreign bodies are hygroscopic and increase in size as water is absorbed, signs of local obstruction and discomfort may increase with time. Infection usually follows and gives rise to a purulent, malodorous, or bloody discharge. The patient may also present with a generalized body odor known as bromhidrosis. **Disk batteries** are dangerous when placed in the nose; they leach base, which causes pain and local tissue destruction within a matter of hours.

Diagnosis. Unilateral nasal discharge and obstruction should suggest the presence of a foreign body, which can often be seen on examination with a nasal speculum or otoscope placed in the nose. Purulent secretions must often be removed so that the foreign object can actually be seen; often a headlight, suction, and topical decongestants may be needed. The object is usually situated anteriorly at first, but through unskilled attempts at removal it may be forced deeper into the nose. When of long standing, a foreign body may become embedded in granulation tissue or mucosa and appear as a nasal mass. A lateral skull radiograph assists in diagnosis if the foreign body is metallic or radiopaque.

Treatment. Removal should be carried out promptly to minimize the danger of aspiration and prevent local tissue necrosis. This can usually be performed with topical anesthesia, using either forceps or nasal suction. If there is marked swelling, bleeding, or tissue overgrowth, general anesthesia may be needed to remove the object. Infection usually clears promptly after the removal of the object, and generally no further therapy is necessary.

Complications. Tetanus is a rare complication of long-standing nasal foreign bodies in nonimmunized children. Toxic shock syndrome is also rare and most commonly occurs from nasal surgical packing (see Chapter 166.2).

Haddad J, Jr: Foreign bodies of the ear, nose and pharynx. In Burg FD, Gershon A, Indelfinger JR, Polin RA (editors): *Current Pediatric Therapy 17.* Philadelphia, WB Saunders, 2002, p 23.

362.2 Epistaxis

Nosebleeds are rare in infancy and common in childhood; their incidence decreases after puberty. Diagnosis and treatment depend on the location and cause of the bleeding.

Anatomy. The most common site of bleeding is the Kiesselbach plexus, an area in the anterior septum where vessels from both the internal carotid (anterior and posterior ethmoid arteries) and external carotid (sphenopalatine and terminal branches of the internal maxillary arteries) converge. The thin mucosa in this area, as well as the anterior location, make it prone to exposure to dry air and trauma.

Etiology. Common causes of nosebleeds from the anterior septum include digital trauma, foreign bodies, dry air, and inflammation, including upper respiratory tract infections, sinusitis, and allergic rhinitis. Nasal steroid sprays are commonly used in children, and their chronic use may be associated with bleeding. Young infants with significant gastroesophageal reflux into the nose may occasionally present with epistaxis secondary to mucosal inflammation. In many children, there is frequently a family history of childhood epistaxis. Susceptibility is increased during respiratory infections and in the winter when dry air irritates the nasal mucosa, resulting in formation of fissures and crusting. Severe bleeding may be encountered with congenital vascular abnormalities, such as hereditary hemorrhagic telangiectasia, varicosities, hemangiomas, and, in children with thrombocytopenia, deficiency of clotting factors, hypertension, renal failure, or venous congestion. Nasal polyps or other intranasal growths may be associated with epistaxis. Recurrent, and frequently severe, nosebleeds may be the initial presenting symptom in juvenile nasal angiofibromas, which occur in adolescent males. The incidence of Kiesselbach plexus bleeding seems to decrease during adolescence.

Clinical Manifestations. Epistaxis usually occurs without warning, with blood flowing slowly but freely from one nostril or occasionally from both. In children with nasal lesions, bleeding may follow physical exercise. When bleeding occurs at night, the blood may be swallowed and may become apparent only when the child vomits or passes blood in the stools. Posterior epistaxis may manifest as anterior nasal bleeding or, if copious, the patient may vomit blood as the initial symptom.

Treatment. Most nosebleeds stop spontaneously in a few minutes. The nares should be compressed and the child kept as quiet as possible, in an upright position with the head tilted forward to avoid blood trickling back into the throat. Cold compresses applied to the nose may also help. If these measures do not stop the bleeding, local application of a solution of oxymetazoline (Afrin) or Neo-Synephrine (0.25–1%) may be useful. If bleeding persists, an anterior nasal pack may need to be inserted; if bleeding originates in the posterior nasal cavity, combined anterior and posterior packing is necessary. After bleeding has been controlled, and if a bleeding site is identified, its obliteration by cautery with silver nitrate may prevent further difficulties. Because the septal cartilage derives its nutrition from the overlying mucoperichondrium, only one side of the septum should be cauterized at a time to reduce the chance of a septal perforation. During the winter, or in a dry environment, a room humidifier, saline drops, and petrolatum (Vaseline) applied to the septum may help to prevent epistaxis.

In patients with severe or repeated epistaxis, blood transfusions may be necessary. Otolaryngologic evaluation is indicated for these children and for those with bilateral bleeding or with hemorrhage that does not arise from the Kiesselbach plexus. Hematologic evaluation (for coagulopathy and anemia), along with nasal endoscopy and diagnostic imaging, may be needed to make a definitive diagnosis in cases of severe recurrent epistaxis. Replacement of deficient clotting factors may be required for patients who have an underlying hematologic disorder (see Chapter 468). Profuse epistaxis associated with a nasal mass in a boy near puberty may signal a **juvenile nasopharyngeal angiofibroma.** This unusual tumor has been reported in a 2 yr old and in 30 to 40 yr olds, but the incidence peaks in adolescent and preadolescent boys. CT with contrast medium enhancement and MRI are part of the initial evaluation; arteriography, embolization, and extensive surgery may be needed.

Surgical intervention may also be needed for bleeding from the internal maxillary artery or other vessels that may cause bleeding in the posterior nasal cavity.

Other Acquired Abnormalities of the Nose. Many acquired abnormalities of the nose and paranasal sinuses, such as tumors and septal perforations, present as epistaxis; midface trauma with a nasal or facial fracture may be accompanied by epistaxis. Trauma to the nose can cause a septal hematoma to form; if treatment is delayed, this may lead to death of nasal septal cartilage and a resultant saddle-nose deformity. Other abnormalities that may cause a change in the shape of the nose and paranasal bones, with obstruction but few other symptoms, include fibro-osseous lesions (ossifying fibroma, fibrous dysplasia, and cementifying fibroma) and mucoceles of the paranasal sinuses. These conditions may be suspected on physical examination and confirmed by CT scan and biopsy. Although these are considered benign lesions, they may all greatly change the anatomy of surrounding bony structures and often require surgical intervention for management.

Wurman LH: Epistaxis. In Gates GA (editor): *Current Therapy in Otolaryngology Head and Neck Surgery,* 5th ed. St Louis, CV Mosby, 1994, p 354.

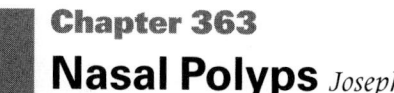

Chapter 363
Nasal Polyps *Joseph Haddad Jr.*

Etiology. Nasal polyps are benign pedunculated tumors formed from edematous, usually chronically inflamed nasal mucosa. They usually originate from the ethmoidal sinus and present in the middle meatus. Occasionally, they appear within the maxillary antrum and can extend to the nasopharynx (antrochoanal polyp). Large or multiple polyps may completely obstruct the nasal passage. The polyps originating from the ethmoidal sinus are usually smaller and multiple, as compared with the large and usually single antral choanal polyp.

Cystic fibrosis is the most common childhood cause of nasal polyposis and should be suspected in any child younger than age 12 yr with nasal polyps, even in the absence of typical respiratory and digestive symptoms; as many as 30% of children with cystic fibrosis acquire nasal polyps. Nasal polyposis is also associated with chronic sinusitis and allergic rhinitis. In the uncommon *Samter triad,* nasal polyps are associated with aspirin sensitivity and asthma.

Clinical Manifestations. Obstruction of nasal passages is prominent, with associated hyponasal speech and mouth breathing. Profuse mucoid or mucopurulent rhinorrhea may also be present. An examination of the nasal passages shows glistening, gray, grapelike masses squeezed between the nasal turbinates and the septum. Ethmoidal polyps can be readily distinguished from the well-vascularized turbinate tissue, which is pink or red; antrochoanal polyps may have a more fleshy appearance. Prolonged presence of ethmoidal polyps in a child may widen the bridge of the nose and erode adjacent osseous structures.

Treatment. Local or systemic decongestants are not usually effective in shrinking the polyps, although they may provide symptomatic relief from the associated mucosal edema. Intranasal steroid sprays, and sometimes systemic steroids, may provide some shrinkage of nasal polyps with symptomatic relief and have proved useful in children with cystic fibrosis. Polyps should be removed surgically if complete obstruction, uncontrolled rhinorrhea, or deformity of the nose appears. If the underlying pathogenic mechanism cannot be eliminated (e.g., cystic fibrosis), the polyps may soon return. Functional endoscopic sinus surgery may provide more complete polyp removal and treatment of other associated nasal disease; in some cases this has reduced the need for frequent surgeries. Nasal steroid sprays should also be started preventively, once postsurgical healing occurs.

Antral choanal polyps do not respond to medical measures and must be surgically removed. Because these types of polyps are not generally associated with any other underlying disease process, the recurrence rate is much less than for other types of polyps.

Magit AE: Tumors of the nose, paranasal sinuses, and nasopharynx. In Bluestone CD, Stool SE, Kenna MA (editors): *Pediatric Otolaryngology*, 3rd ed. Philadelphia, WB Saunders, 1996, pp 893–904.

Chapter 364
The Common Cold
Ronald B. Turner and Gregory F. Hayden

The common cold is a viral illness in which the symptoms of rhinorrhea and nasal obstruction are prominent and systemic symptoms and signs such as myalgia and fever are absent or mild. It is often termed *rhinitis* but includes self-limited involvement of the sinus mucosa and is more correctly termed *rhinosinusitis*.

Etiology. The most common pathogens associated with the common cold are the rhinoviruses (see Chapter 241), but the syndrome may be caused by many different viruses (Table 364–1).

Epidemiology. Colds occur year round, but the incidence is greatest from the early fall until the late spring, reflecting the seasonal prevalence of the viral pathogens associated with cold symptoms. The highest incidence of rhinovirus infection occurs in the early fall (August–October) and in the late spring (April–May). The seasonal incidence for parainfluenza viruses usually peaks in the late fall, and for respiratory syncytial virus (RSV) and influenza viruses it is highest between December and April.

Young children have an average of six to seven colds per year but 10–15% of children have at least 12 infections per year. The incidence of illness decreases with age, with two to three illnesses per year by adulthood. Children in out-of-home daycare centers during the first year of life have 50% more colds than children cared for only at home. The difference in the incidence of illness between these groups of children decreases as the length of time spent in daycare increases, although the incidence of illness remains higher in the daycare group through at least the first 3 yr of life.

Pathogenesis. Viruses causing the common cold are spread by small-particle aerosols, large-particle aerosols, and direct contact. Although the different common cold pathogens may presumably be spread by any of these mechanisms, some routes of transmission appear be more efficient than others for particular viruses. Studies of rhinoviruses and RSV suggest that direct contact is an efficient mechanism of transmission of these viruses, although transmission by large particle aerosols may also occur. In contrast to rhinoviruses and RSV, influenza viruses appear to be most efficiently spread by small particle aerosols.

TABLE 364–1. Pathogens Associated with the Common Cold

Association	Pathogens	Relative Frequency of Colds Caused
Agents primarily associated with colds	Rhinoviruses	Frequent
	Coronaviruses	Occasional
Agents primarily associated with other clinical syndromes that also cause common cold symptoms	Respiratory syncytial virus	Occasional
	Influenza viruses	Uncommon
	Parainfluenza viruses	Uncommon
	Adenoviruses	Uncommon
	Enteroviruses	Uncommon

The respiratory viruses have evolved different mechanisms to avoid host defenses. Infections with rhinoviruses and adenoviruses result in the development of serotype-specific protective immunity. Repeated infections with these pathogens occur because there are a large number of distinct serotypes of each virus. Similarly, influenza viruses have the ability to change the antigens presented on the surface of the virus and thus behave as though there were multiple virus serotypes. The interaction of coronaviruses with host immunity is not well defined, but it appears that there are multiple distinct strains of coronavirus that are capable of inducing at least short-term protective immunity. In contrast, the parainfluenza viruses and RSV each have a small number of distinct serotypes. Re-infection with these viruses occurs because protective immunity to these pathogens does not develop after an infection. Although re-infection is not prevented by the adaptive host response to these viruses, the severity of subsequent illness is moderated by pre-existing immunity.

Viral infection of the nasal epithelium may be associated with destruction of the epithelial lining, as with influenza viruses and adenoviruses, or there may be no apparent histologic damage, as with rhinoviruses, RSV, and coronavirus 229E. Regardless of the histopathologic findings, infection of the nasal epithelium is associated with an acute inflammatory response characterized by release of a variety of inflammatory cytokines and infiltration of the mucosa by inflammatory cells. This acute inflammatory response appears to be responsible at least in part for many of the symptoms associated with the common cold.

Clinical Manifestations. The onset of common cold symptoms typically occurs 1–3 days after viral infection. The first symptom noted is frequently sore or "scratchy" throat, followed closely by nasal obstruction and rhinorrhea. The sore throat usually resolves quickly, and by the second and third day of illness nasal symptoms predominate. Cough is associated with approximately 30% of colds and usually begins after the onset of nasal symptoms. Influenza viruses, RSV, and adenoviruses are more likely than are rhinoviruses or coronaviruses to be associated with fever and other constitutional symptoms. The usual cold persists about 1 wk, although 10% last 2 wk.

The physical findings of the common cold are limited to the upper respiratory tract. Increased nasal secretion is frequently obvious to the examiner. A change in the color or consistency of the secretions is common during the course of the illness and is not indicative of sinusitis or bacterial superinfection. Examination of the nasal cavity may reveal swollen, erythematous nasal turbinates, although this finding is nonspecific and of limited diagnostic usefulness.

Diagnosis. The most important task of the physician caring for a patient with a cold is to exclude other conditions that are potentially more serious or treatable. The differential diagnosis of the common cold includes noninfectious disorders as well as other upper respiratory tract infections (Table 364–2).

Laboratory Findings. Routine laboratory studies are not helpful for the diagnosis and management of the common cold. A nasal smear for eosinophils may be useful if allergic rhinitis is

TABLE 364–2. Conditions That May Mimic the Common Cold

Condition	Differentiating Features
Allergic rhinitis	Prominent itching and sneezing
	Nasal eosinophilia
Foreign body	Unilateral, foul-smelling discharge
	Bloody nasal secretions
Sinusitis	Headache, facial pain, or periorbital edema
	Persistence of rhinorrhea or cough for longer than 10–14 days
Streptococcal nasopharyngitis	Nasal discharge that excoriates the nares
Pertussis	Onset of persistent or paroxysmal cough
Congenital syphilis	Persistent rhinorrhea (snuffles) with onset in the first 3 mo of life

suspected. A predominance of polymorphonuclear leukocytes in the nasal secretions is characteristic of uncomplicated colds and does not indicate bacterial superinfection.

The viral pathogens associated with the common cold may be detected by culture, antigen detection, or serologic methods. These studies are generally not indicated in patients with colds because a specific etiologic diagnosis is useful only when treatment with an antiviral agent is contemplated. Bacterial cultures or antigen detection are useful only when group A *Streptococcus*, *Bordetella pertussis*, or nasal diphtheria is suspected. The isolation of other bacterial pathogens is not an indication of bacterial nasal infection and is not a specific predictor of the etiologic agent in sinusitis.

Treatment. The management of the common cold consists primarily of symptomatic treatment.

ANTIVIRAL TREATMENT. Specific antiviral therapy is not currently available for rhinovirus infections. Ribavirin, which is approved for treatment of RSV infections, has no role in the treatment of the common cold. The neuraminidase inhibitors oseltamivir and zanamivir have a modest effect on the duration of symptoms associated with influenza virus infections in children. Oseltamivir has also been shown to reduce the frequency of influenza-associated otitis media. The difficulty of distinguishing influenza from other common cold pathogens and the necessity that therapy be started early in the illness (within 48 hr of onset of symptoms) to be beneficial are practical limitations to the use of these agents for mild upper respiratory tract infections. Newer antiviral agents such as pleconaril for treatment of rhinovirus infections are being developed, although the role, if any, of these agents in routine treatment of the common cold remains to be determined. Antibacterial therapy is of no benefit in the treatment of the common cold.

SYMPTOMATIC TREATMENT. The use of symptomatic therapies in children has been the subject of some controversy because, although some of these medications have been found to be effective in adults, no studies have demonstrated a significant effect in children. The studies in children are limited because assessment of common cold therapies generally relies on subjective and objective measurements that require the cooperation of the research subject. Young children cannot assist in these measurements so studies of these treatments in children have generally been based on observations by parents or other observers. Until more definitive results are available, the use of symptomatic therapies in children can only be based on an assumption that the effects of symptomatic treatments may be similar in adults and children. A decision to use these medications in children must be balanced against the potential adverse effects of each drug. The prominent or most bothersome symptoms of colds vary during the course of the illness and, therefore, if symptomatic treatments are used, it is reasonable to target therapy to specific bothersome symptoms. If symptomatic treatments are recommended, care should be taken to assure that caregivers understand the intended effect and can determine the proper dosage of the medications.

Fever. Fever is infrequently associated with an uncomplicated common cold and antipyretic treatment is generally not indicated.

Nasal Obstruction. Either topical or oral adrenergic agents may be used as nasal decongestants. Effective topical adrenergic agents such as xylometazoline, oxymetazoline, or phenylephrine are available as either intranasal drops or nasal sprays. Reduced-strength formulations of these medications are available for use in younger children, although they are not approved for use in children younger than 2 yr old. Systemic absorption of the imidazolines (e.g., oxymetazoline and xylometazoline) has very rarely been associated with bradycardia, hypotension, and coma. Prolonged use of the topical adrenergic agents should be avoided to prevent the development of **rhinitis medicamentosa,** an apparent rebound effect that causes the sensation of nasal obstruction when the drug is discontinued. The oral adrenergic agents are less effective than the topical preparations and are associated with systemic effects such as central nervous system stimulation, hypertension, and palpitations.

Rhinorrhea. The first-generation antihistamines reduce rhinorrhea by 25–30%. The effect of the antihistamines on rhinorrhea appears to be related to the anticholinergic rather than the antihistaminic properties of these drugs and therefore the second-generation or "nonsedating" antihistamines have no effect on common cold symptoms. The major adverse effect associated with the use of the antihistamines is sedation, although there is some evidence that this adverse effect is less bothersome in children than in adults. Rhinorrhea may also be treated with ipratropium bromide, a topical anticholinergic agent. This drug produces an effect comparable to the antihistamines but is not associated with sedation. The most common side effects of ipratropium are nasal irritation and bleeding.

Sore Throat. The sore throat associated with colds is generally not severe, but treatment with mild analgesics is occasionally indicated, particularly if there is associated myalgia or headache. The use of acetaminophen during rhinovirus infection has been associated with suppression of neutralizing antibody responses, but this observation has no apparent clinical significance. Aspirin should not be given to children with respiratory infections because of the risk of Reye syndrome in children with influenza.

Cough. Cough suppression is generally not necessary in patients with colds. Cough in some patients appears to be due to upper respiratory tract irritation associated with postnasal drip. Cough in these patients is most prominent during the time of greatest nasal symptoms, and treatment with a first-generation antihistamine may be helpful. In other patients, cough may be a result of virus-induced reactive airway disease. These patients may have cough that persists for days to weeks after the acute illness and may benefit from bronchodilator therapy. Studies of codeine or dextromethorphan hydrobromide have failed to show an effect of these agents on cough in colds. Expectorants such as guaifenesin are not effective antitussive agents.

INEFFECTIVE TREATMENTS. Many common cold remedies popularized in both the lay and the medical press have no significant effect on cold symptoms in carefully controlled studies. *Vitamin C, guaifenesin,* and *inhalation of warm, humidified air* have all been found to be no more effective than placebo for the symptomatic treatment of colds.

Zinc, given as oral lozenges, has been evaluated in several studies as a treatment for common cold symptoms. The function of the rhinovirus 3C protease, an essential enzyme for rhinovirus replication, is inhibited by zinc, but there has been no evidence of an antiviral effect of zinc in vivo. The effect of zinc on symptoms has been inconsistent, with some studies reporting dramatic treatment effects whereas other studies find no beneficial effect. A synthesis of these disparate results is difficult, but it appears unlikely that zinc has a clinically significant impact on common cold symptoms.

Echinacea is a popular herbal treatment for the common cold. Although echinacea extracts have been shown to have biologic effects, the effectiveness of echinacea as a common cold treatment has not been adequately studied. The lack of standardization of commercial products containing echinacea presents a formidable obstacle to the rational evaluation or use of this therapy. Until these problems are resolved there is insufficient evidence to support a recommendation of echinacea as a common cold treatment.

Complications. The most common complication of a cold is *otitis media*, which is reported in 5–30% of children who have a cold, with the higher incidence occurring in children cared for in a group daycare setting. Symptomatic treatment has no effect on the development of acute otitis media, but treatment with oseltamivir reduced the incidence of otitis media from 19% to 9% in patients with influenza.

Sinusitis also appears to be a relatively frequent complication of the common cold (see Chapter 365). Self-limited sinus involvement is a part of the pathophysiology of the common cold, but 0.5–2% of viral upper respiratory tract infections in adults, and 5–13% in children, are complicated by acute bacterial sinusitis. The differentiation of common cold symptoms from bacterial sinusitis may be difficult. The diagnosis of bacterial sinusitis should be considered if rhinorrhea or daytime cough persists without improvement for at least 10–14 days or if signs develop of more severe sinus involvement such as fever, facial pain, or facial swelling. There is no evidence that symptomatic treatment of the common cold alters the frequency of development of bacterial sinusitis.

Exacerbation of *asthma* is a relatively uncommon but potentially serious complication of colds. The majority of asthma exacerbations in children are associated with the common cold. There is no evidence that treatment of common cold symptoms prevents this complication.

Although not a complication, another important consequence of the common cold is the inappropriate use of antibiotics for these illnesses and the associated contribution to the problem of increasing antibiotic resistance of pathogenic respiratory bacteria. In the United States in 1998 there were an estimated 25 million primary care office visits for the common cold, with 30% of these visits resulting in a prescription for antibiotics.

Prevention. Chemoprophylaxis or immunoprophylaxis is generally not available for the common cold. Immunization or chemoprophylaxis against influenza may be useful for prevention of colds caused by this pathogen; however, influenza is responsible for only a small proportion of all colds. Both vitamin C and echinacea have been reported to prevent the common cold but no significant effect has been detected in carefully controlled studies.

Colds can be prevented by interrupting the chain involved in the spread of virus by direct contact. In the hospital setting, prevention of transmission of respiratory viruses has been achieved by personnel wearing protective face shields to prevent hand-to-eye or hand-to-nose contact. Prevention of the spread of viruses by direct contact can be most readily accomplished by good handwashing by the infected individual and/or the susceptible contact.

Barrett B, Vohmann M, Calabrese C: Echinacea for upper respiratory infection. *J Fam Pract* 1999;48:628–35.

Gonzales R, Malone DC, Maselli JH, et al: Excessive antibiotic use for acute respiratory infections in the United States. *Clin Infect Dis* 2001;33:757–62.

Gwaltney JM Jr, Druce HM: Efficacy of brompheniramine maleate for the treatment of rhinovirus colds. *Clin Infect Dis* 1997;25:1188–94.

Gwaltney JM Jr, Phillips CD, Miller DR, et al: Computed tomographic study of the common cold. *N Engl J Med* 1994;33:25–30.

Hedrick JA, Barzilai A, Behre U, et al: Zanamivir for treatment of symptomatic influenza A and B infection in children five to twelve years of age: A randomized controlled trial. *Pediatr Infect Dis J* 2000;19:410–17.

Jackson JL, Peterson C, Lesho E: A meta-analysis of zinc salts lozenges and the common cold. *Arch Intern Med* 1997;157:2373–76.

Simon HK, Weinkle DA: Over-the-counter medications. Do parents give what they intend to give? *Arch Pediatr Adolesc Med* 1997;151:654–56.

Taverner D, Danz C, Economos D: The effects of oral pseudoephedrine on nasal patency in the common cold: A double-blind single-dose placebo-controlled trial. *Clin Otolaryngol* 1999;24:47–51.

Turner RB: The treatment of rhinovirus infections: Progress and potential. *Antiviral Res* 2001;49:1–14.

Turner RB, Sperber SJ, Sorrentino JV, et al: Effectiveness of clemastine fumarate for treatment of rhinorrhea and sneezing associated with the common cold. *Clin Infect Dis* 1997;25:824–30.

Chapter 365
Sinusitis *Diane E. Pappas and J. Owen Hendley*

Sinusitis is a common illness of childhood and adolescence with significant morbidity and the potential for serious complications. There are two types of acute sinusitis: viral and bacterial. The common cold produces a viral, self-limited rhinosinusitis (see Chapter 364). One-half to 2% of viral upper respiratory tract infections in children and adolescents are complicated by acute bacterial sinusitis. Some children with underlying predisposing conditions may have chronic sinus disease that does not appear to be infectious. The means for appropriate diagnosis and optimal treatment of sinusitis remain controversial.

Both the ethmoidal and maxillary sinuses are present at birth, but only the ethmoidal sinuses are pneumatized. The maxillary sinuses are not pneumatized until 4 yr of age. The sphenoidal sinuses are present by 5 yr of age, whereas the frontal sinuses begin development at age 7–8 yr and are not completely developed until adolescence. The ostia draining the sinuses are narrow (1–3 mm) and drain into the **ostiomeatal complex** in the middle meatus. The paranasal sinuses are normally sterile, maintained by the mucociliary clearance system.

Etiology. The bacterial pathogens causing acute bacterial sinusitis in children and adolescents include *Streptococcus pneumoniae* (about 30%), nontypable *Haemophilus influenzae* (about 20%), and *Moraxella catarrhalis* (about 20%). At present, approximately 50% of *H. influenzae* and 100% of *M. catarrhalis* are β-lactamase positive. About 25% of *S. pneumoniae* may be penicillin resistant. *Staphylococcus aureus*, other streptococci, and anaerobes are uncommon causes of acute bacterial sinusitis in children. *H. influenzae*, α-hemolytic streptococci, *M. catarrhalis*, *S. pneumoniae*, and coagulase-negative staphylococci are commonly recovered from children with chronic sinus disease.

Epidemiology. Acute bacterial sinusitis may occur at any age. Predisposing conditions include viral upper respiratory tract infections (which in turn are associated with out-of-home daycare or a school-aged sibling), allergic rhinitis, and cigarette smoke exposure. Children with immune deficiencies, cystic fibrosis, ciliary dysfunction, abnormalities of phagocyte function, gastroesophageal reflux, anatomic defects (e.g., cleft palate), nasal polyps, and nasal foreign bodies (including nasogastric tubes) may develop chronic sinus disease.

Pathogenesis. Acute bacterial sinusitis typically follows a viral upper respiratory tract infection. Initially, the viral infection produces a viral rhinosinusitis; CT scans have demonstrated fluid in the sinuses during the normal course of the common cold in healthy young adults. Nose blowing has been demonstrated to generate sufficient force to propel nasal secretions into the sinus cavities. Bacteria from the nasopharynx that enter the sinuses are normally cleared readily, but during viral rhinosinusitis the inflammation and edema may block sinus drainage and impair mucociliary clearance of bacteria. The growth conditions are favorable, and high titers of bacteria are produced.

Clinical Manifestations. Children and adolescents with sinusitis may present with nonspecific complaints, including nasal congestion, nasal discharge (unilateral or bilateral), fever, and cough. Less common symptoms include bad breath (halitosis), a decreased sense of smell, and periorbital edema. Complaints of headache and facial pain are rare in children. Physical examination may reveal mild erythema and swelling of the nasal mucosa with nasal discharge. Sinus tenderness may be detectable in adolescents and adults.

Diagnosis. The clinical diagnosis of acute bacterial sinusitis is based solely on history. Persistent symptoms of upper respiratory tract infection, including nasal discharge and cough, for longer than 10–14 days without improvement, or severe respiratory symptoms, including temperature of at least 102°F (39°C) and purulent nasal discharge for 3–4 consecutive days, are suggestive of a complicating acute bacterial sinusitis. Bacteria were recovered from maxillary sinus aspirates in 70% of children with such persistent or severe symptoms studied. Children with **chronic sinusitis** have a history of persistent respiratory symptoms, including cough, nasal discharge, or nasal congestion, lasting more than 90 days.

Sinus aspirate culture is the only accurate method of diagnosis but is not practical for routine use. **Transillumination** of the sinus cavities may demonstrate the presence of fluid but cannot reveal whether it is viral or bacterial in origin. In children, transillumination is difficult to perform and has been shown to be unreliable. Findings on radiographic studies (e.g., sinus plain films and CT scans) including **opacification, mucosal thickening,** or presence of an **air-fluid level** are not diagnostic. Such findings can confirm the presence of sinus inflammation but cannot be used to differentiate between viral, bacterial, or allergic causes of inflammation.

Given the nonspecific clinical picture, differential diagnostic considerations include viral upper respiratory tract infection, allergic rhinitis, nonallergic rhinitis, and nasal foreign body. Viral upper respiratory tract infections are characterized by nasal discharge, cough, and initial fever; symptoms do not usually persist beyond 10–14 days. Allergic rhinitis may be seasonal; evaluation of nasal secretions should reveal significant eosinophilia.

Treatment. It is unclear whether antimicrobial treatment of clinically diagnosed acute bacterial sinusitis offers any substantial benefit. A recent randomized, placebo-controlled trial comparing 14-day treatment of children with clinically diagnosed sinusitis with amoxicillin, amoxicillin-clavulanate, or placebo found that antimicrobial therapy did not affect symptom resolution, duration of symptoms, or days missed from school. However, the current guidelines from the American Academy of Pediatrics recommend antimicrobial treatment for acute bacterial sinusitis to promote resolution of symptoms and prevent suppurative complications, although 50–60% of children with acute bacterial sinusitis will recover without antimicrobial therapy. Initial therapy with amoxicillin (45 mg/kg/day) is adequate for the majority of children with uncomplicated acute bacterial sinusitis. Alternative treatments for the penicillin-allergic patient include cefuroxime axetil, cefpodoxime, clarithromycin, or azithromycin. For children with risk factors (i.e., antibiotic treatment in the preceding 1–3 mo, daycare attendance, or age younger than 2 yr) for the presence of resistant bacterial species, and for children who fail to respond to initial therapy with

amoxicillin within 72 hr, treatment with "high dose" amoxicillin-clavulanate (80–90 mg/kg/day of amoxicillin and 6.4 mg/kg/day of clavulanate) should be initiated. Failure to respond to this regimen necessitates referral to an otolaryngologist for further evaluation because maxillary sinus aspiration for culture and susceptibility testing may be necessary. The appropriate duration of therapy for sinusitis has yet to be determined; individualization of therapy is a reasonable approach, with treatment recommended for 7 days after resolution of symptoms.

Frontal sinusitis can rapidly progress to serious intracranial complications and necessitates initiation of parenteral ceftriaxone until substantial clinical improvement is achieved. Treatment is then completed with oral antibiotic therapy.

The use of decongestants, antihistamines, mucolytics, and intranasal corticosteroids has not been adequately studied in children and is not recommended for the treatment of acute bacterial sinusitis. Likewise, saline nasal washes or nasal sprays may help to liquefy secretions and act as a mild vasoconstrictor, but the effects have also not been systematically evaluated in children.

Complications. Because of the close proximity of the paranasal sinuses to the brain and eyes, serious orbital and/or intracranial complications may result from acute bacterial sinusitis and progress rapidly. Orbital complications, including periorbital cellulitis and orbital cellulitis, are most often secondary to acute bacterial ethmoiditis. Infection may spread directly through the lamina papyracea, the thin bone that forms the lateral wall of the ethmoidal sinus. **Periorbital cellulitis** produces erythema and swelling of the tissues surrounding the globe, whereas **orbital cellulitis** involves the intraorbital structures and produces proptosis, chemosis, decreased visual acuity, double vision and impaired extraocular movements, and eye pain. Evaluation should include CT scan of the orbits and sinuses with ophthalmology and otolaryngology consultations. Treatment with intravenous antibiotics should be initiated. Orbital cellulitis may require surgical drainage of the ethmoidal sinuses.

Intracranial complications may include meningitis, cavernous sinus thrombosis, subdural empyema, epidural abscess, and brain abscess. Children with altered mental status, nuchal rigidity, or signs of increased intracranial pressure (headache and vomiting) require immediate CT scan of the brain, orbits, and sinuses to evaluate for the presence of intracranial complications of acute bacterial sinusitis. Treatment with broad-spectrum intravenous antibiotics (usually cefotaxime or ceftriaxone combined with vancomycin) should be initiated immediately pending culture and susceptibility results. Abscesses may require surgical drainage. Other complications include osteomyelitis of the frontal bone **(Pott puffy tumor),** which is characterized by edema and swelling of the forehead, and **mucoceles,** which are chronic inflammatory lesions commonly located in the frontal sinuses that can expand, causing displacement of the eye with resultant diplopia. Surgical drainage is usually required.

Prevention. Prevention is best accomplished by frequent hand-washing and avoiding persons with colds. Because acute bacterial sinusitis may complicate influenza infection, prevention of influenza infection by yearly influenza vaccine will prevent some cases of complicating sinusitis. Immunization or chemoprophylaxis against influenza with oseltamivir or zanamivir may be useful for prevention of colds caused by this pathogen and the associated complications; however, influenza is responsible for only a small proportion of all colds.

American Academy of Pediatrics, Subcommittee on Management of Sinusitis and Committee on Quality Improvement: Clinical practice guideline: Management of sinusitis. *Pediatrics* 2001;108:798–808.

Brook I, Gooch WM III, Jenkins SG, et al: Medical management of acute bacterial sinusitis: Recommendations of a clinical advisory committee on pediatric and adult sinusitis. *Ann Otol Rhinol Laryngol* 2000;109(Suppl 1):1–20.

Don DM, Yellon RF, Casselbrant ML, et al: Efficacy of a stepwise protocol that includes intravenous antibiotic therapy for the management of chronic sinusitis in children and adolescents. *Arch Otolaryngol Head Neck Surg* 2001;127:1093–98.

Garbutt JM, Goldstein M, Gellman, E, et al: A randomized, placebo-controlled trial of antimicrobial treatment for children with clinically diagnosed acute sinusitis. *Pediatrics* 2001;107:619–24.

Gwaltney JM Jr, Phillips CD, Miller DR, et al: Computed tomographic study of the common cold. *N Engl J Med* 1994;33:25–30.

Gwaltney JM Jr, Hendley JO, Phillips CD, et al: Nose-blowing propels nasal fluid into the paranasal sinuses. *Clin Infect Dis* 2000;30:387–91.

Kaiser L, Keene ON, Hammond JM, et al: Impact of zanamivir on antibiotic use for respiratory events following acute influenza in adolescents and adults. *Arch Intern Med* 2000;160:3234–40.

Kakish KS, Mahafza T, Batieha A, et al: Clinical sinusitis in children attending primary care centers. *Pediatr Infect Dis J* 2000;19:1071–74.

Phipps CD, Wood WE, Gibson WS, et al: Gastroesophageal reflux contributing to chronic sinus disease in children: A prospective analysis. *Arch Otolaryngol Head Neck Surg* 2000;126:831–36.

Sinus and Allergy Health Partnership: Antimicrobial treatment guidelines for acute bacterial rhinosinusitis. *Otolaryngol Head Neck Surg* 2000;123:S4–S32.

Wald ER: Sinusitis in children. *N Engl J Med* 1992;326:319–23.

Chapter 366
Acute Pharyngitis

Gregory F. Hayden and Ronald B. Turner

Upper respiratory tract infections account for a substantial proportion of visits to pediatricians. Approximately one third of such illnesses feature sore throat as the primary symptom.

Etiology. The most important agents causing pharyngitis are viruses and group A β-hemolytic *Streptococcus* (GABHS). Other organisms sometimes associated with pharyngitis include group C *Streptococcus*, *Arcanobacterium haemolyticum*, *Francisella tularensis*, *Mycoplasma pneumoniae*, *Neisseria gonorrhoeae*, and *Corynebacterium diphtheriae*. Other bacteria, such as *Haemophilus influenzae* and *Streptococcus pneumoniae*, may be cultured from the throats of children with pharyngitis, but their role in causing pharyngitis has not been established.

Epidemiology. Viral upper respiratory tract infections occur most commonly in winter and spring and are spread by close contact. Streptococcal pharyngitis is uncommon before 2–3 yr of age. The incidence increases among children and then declines in late adolescence and adulthood. It occurs throughout the year but is reported most often during winter and spring. Illness often spreads among siblings and classmates. Pharyngitis from group C *Streptococcus* and *A. haemolyticum* occurs most frequently among adolescents and adults.

Pathogenesis. Colonization of the pharynx by GABHS may result in either asymptomatic carriage or acute infection. The **M protein** is the major virulence factor of GABHS and facilitates resistance to phagocytosis by polymorphonuclear neutrophils. Type-specific immunity develops during infection and provides protective immunity to subsequent infection with that particular M serotype.

Scarlet fever is caused by GABHS that produces one of three **streptococcal pyrogenic exotoxins** (SPEs)—A, B, and C—that can induce a fine papular rash. SPE-A appears to be most strongly associated with scarlet fever. Exposure to each SPE confers specific immunity only to that toxin, and therefore scarlet fever can occur up to three times.

Clinical Manifestations. The onset of streptococcal pharyngitis is often rapid with prominent sore throat and fever. Headache and gastrointestinal symptoms are frequent. The pharynx is red, and the tonsils are enlarged and classically covered with a yellow, blood-tinged exudate. There may be petechiae or "doughnut" lesions on the soft palate and posterior pharynx, and the uvula may be red, stippled, and swollen. The anterior cervical lymph nodes are enlarged and tender. Some patients demonstrate the additional stigmata of scarlet fever: circumoral pallor, strawberry tongue, and a red, finely papular rash that feels like sandpaper and resembles sunburn with goose pimples.

The onset of viral pharyngitis may be more gradual, and symptoms more often include rhinorrhea, cough, and diarrhea. Adenovirus pharyngitis may feature concurrent conjunctivitis and fever **(pharyngoconjunctival fever).** Coxsackievirus pharyngitis may produce small (1–2 mm), grayish vesicles and punched-out ulcers in the posterior pharynx **(herpangina),** or small (3–6 mm), yellowish white nodules in the posterior pharynx **(acute lymphonodular pharyngitis).** In Epstein-Barr virus (EBV) pharyngitis, there may be prominent tonsillar enlargement with exudate, cervical lymphadenitis, hepatosplenomegaly, rash, and generalized fatigue as part of the infectious mononucleosis syndrome. Primary herpes simplex virus infections in young children often present as high fever and gingivostomatitis.

The illnesses attributed to group C *Streptococcus* and *A. haemolyticum* are generally similar to those caused by GABHS. Infections with *A. haemolyticum* are sometimes accompanied by a blanching, erythematous, maculopapular rash. Gonococcal pharyngeal infections are usually asymptomatic but can cause acute pharyngitis with fever and cervical lymphadenitis.

Diagnosis. The goal of specific diagnosis is to identify GABHS infection. The clinical presentations of streptococcal and viral pharyngitis show considerable overlap. Physicians using clinical judgment often overestimate the likelihood of a streptococcal etiology, so laboratory testing is useful to identify children who are most likely to benefit from antibiotic therapy. Throat culture remains an imperfect gold standard for diagnosing streptococcal pharyngitis. False-positive cultures can occur if other organisms are misidentified as GABHS, and children who are streptococcal carriers may also have positive cultures. False-negative cultures are attributed to a variety of causes, including an inadequate throat swab specimen and patients' surreptitious use of antibiotic. The specificity of rapid tests to detect group A streptococcal antigen is high, so if a rapid test is positive, throat culture is unnecessary and appropriate treatment is indicated. Rapid tests are generally less sensitive than culture, however, so that confirming a negative rapid test with a throat culture is recommended, especially if the clinical suspicion of GABHS is high. Special culture media and a prolonged incubation are required to detect *A. haemolyticum*. Viral cultures are often unavailable and are generally too expensive and slow to be clinically useful. A complete blood cell count (CBC) showing many atypical lymphocytes and a positive slide agglutination (or "spot") test can help to confirm a clinical diagnosis of EBV infectious mononucleosis.

Treatment. Most untreated episodes of streptococcal pharyngitis resolve uneventfully in a few days, but early antibiotic therapy hastens clinical recovery by 12–24 hr. The primary benefit of treatment is the prevention of acute rheumatic fever, which is almost completely successful if antibiotic treatment is instituted within 9 days of illness. Antibiotic therapy should be started immediately without culture for children with symptomatic pharyngitis and a positive rapid streptococcal antigen test; clinical diagnosis of scarlet fever; a household contact with documented streptococcal pharyngitis; a past history of acute rheumatic fever; or a recent history of acute rheumatic fever in a family member.

A variety of antimicrobial agents are effective. GABHS remains universally susceptible to penicillin, which has a narrow spectrum and few adverse effects. Penicillin V is inexpensive and is given bid or tid for 10 days: 250 mg/dose for children and 250–500 mg/dose for adolescents and adults. Oral amoxicillin is often preferred for children because of taste and availability as chewable tablets. Studies suggest that a once-daily 750 mg dose of amoxicillin given orally for 10 days is as effective as 250 mg of penicillin given tid for 10 days. Another study suggests that a shorter, 6 day course of oral amoxicillin (50 mg/kg/day divided bid) is as effective as a 10 day course of penicillin V given tid. If confirmed, these advantages will make amoxicillin an even more popular option. A single intramuscular dose of benzathine penicillin (600,000 U for children < 27 kg [60 lb]; 1.2 million U for larger children and adults), or a benzathine-procaine penicillin G combination, is painful but assures compliance and provides adequate blood levels for more than 10 days. Erythromycin (erythromycin ethyl succinate 40 mg/kg/day divided tid or qid orally for 10 days; or erythromycin estolate 20–40 mg/kg/day divided bid, tid, or qid orally for 10 days) is recommended for patients allergic to β-lactam antibiotics. Reports that a high proportion of patients treated with oral or intramuscular penicillin remain culture positive after treatment deserve further evaluation. Based on the proportion of cultures that remain positive for GABHS after therapy, some drugs (e.g., first-generation cephalosporins) appear to be as good as, or better than, penicillin, perhaps because these drugs are more effective in eradicating streptococcal carriage. Some newer drugs such as azithromycin offer the convenience of once-daily administration or shorter length of therapy, which may improve compliance, but these drugs are generally more expensive than penicillin and have more frequent adverse effects. Evidence is not sufficient to recommend shorter courses of cephalosporins for routine therapy at this time.

Follow-up cultures are unnecessary unless symptoms recur. Some treated patients continue to harbor GABHS in their pharynx and become streptococcal carriers. Carriage generally poses little risk to patients and their contacts, but it may confound the test results used to determine the etiology of subsequent episodes of sore throat. The treatment regimen most effective for eradicating streptococcal carriage is clindamycin, 20 mg/kg/day divided in three doses (adult dose: 150–300 mg tid) orally for 10 days

Specific therapy is unavailable for most viral pharyngitis. On the basis of in vitro susceptibility data, oral penicillin is often suggested for patients with group C streptococcal isolates and oral erythromycin is recommended for patients with *A. haemolyticum*, but the clinical benefit of such treatment is uncertain.

Nonspecific, symptomatic therapy can be an important part of the overall treatment plan. An oral antipyretic/analgesic agent (e.g., acetaminophen or ibuprofen) may relieve fever and sore throat pain. Gargling with warm salt water is often comforting, and anesthetic sprays and lozenges (often containing benzocaine, phenol, or menthol) may provide local relief.

RECURRENT PHARYNGITIS. Recurrent streptococcal pharyngitis may represent relapse with an identical strain. If antibiotic compliance has been poor, intramuscular benzathine penicillin is suggested. The possibility of resistance should be considered if a nonpenicillin treatment such as erythromycin was given. Recurrences may also be caused by a different strain resulting from new exposures or may represent pharyngitis of another cause accompanied by streptococcal carriage. This last possibility is likely if the illnesses are mild and otherwise atypical for streptococcal pharyngitis. If GABHS is detected by repeat culture a few days after completing treatment, therapy to eliminate carriage is recommended.

Tonsillectomy lowers the incidence of pharyngitis for 1–2 yr among children with recurrent, culture-positive, GABHS pharyngitis that has been severe and frequent (more than seven episodes in the previous year, or more than five in each of the preceding 2 yr). Most children spontaneously have fewer episodes over time, however, so the anticipated clinical benefit must be balanced against the risks of anesthesia and surgery. Undocumented histories of recurrent pharyngitis are an inadequate basis for recommending tonsillectomy.

Complications and Prognosis. Viral respiratory tract infections may predispose to bacterial middle ear infections. The complications of streptococcal pharyngitis include local suppurative complications, such as parapharyngeal abscess, and later non-suppurative illnesses, such as acute rheumatic fever and acute postinfectious glomerulonephritis (see Chapter 168.1).

Prevention. Multivalent streptococcal vaccines based on M protein peptides are under development. Antimicrobial prophylaxis with daily oral penicillin prevents recurrent GABHS infections but is recommended only to prevent recurrences of acute rheumatic fever (see Chapter 168.1).

Bisno AL: Acute pharyngitis. *N Engl J Med* 2001;344:205–11.

Bisno AL, Gerber MA, Gwaltney JM Jr, et al: Practice guidelines for the diagnosis and management of group A streptococcal pharyngitis. *Clin Infect Dis* 2002;35:113–25.

Feder HM Jr, Gerber MA, Randolph MF, et al: Once-daily therapy for streptococcal pharyngitis with amoxicillin. *Pediatrics* 1999;103:47–51.

Gerber MA, Tanz RR: New approaches to the treatment of group A streptococcal pharyngitis. *Curr Opin Pediatr* 2001;13:51–5.

Gerber MA, Tanz RR, Kabat W, et al: Potential mechanisms for failure to eradicate group A streptococci from the pharynx. *Pediatrics* 1999;104:911–17.

Pichichero ME, Green JL, Francis AB, et al: Recurrent group A streptococcal tonsillopharyngitis. *Pediatr Infect Dis J* 1998;17:809–15.

Pichichero ME, Casey JR, Mayes T, et al: Penicillin failure in streptococcal tonsillopharyngitis: Causes and remedies. *Pediatr Infect Dis J* 2000;19:917–23.

Chapter 367

Retropharyngeal Abscess, Lateral Pharyngeal (Parapharyngeal) Abscess, and Peritonsillar Cellulitis/Abscess

Diane E. Pappas and J. Owen Hendley

The neck contains deeply located lymph nodes including retropharyngeal nodes and lateral pharyngeal nodes that drain the mucosal surfaces of the upper airway and digestive tracts. These nodes lie within the retropharyngeal space (located between the pharynx and the cervical vertebrae and extending down into the superior mediastinum) and the lateral pharyngeal space (bounded by the pharynx medially, the carotid sheath posteriorly, and the muscles of the styloid process laterally), which are interconnected. The lymph nodes in these deep neck spaces communicate with each other, allowing bacteria from either cellulitis or node abscess to spread to other nodes. Infection of the nodes usually occurs as a result of extension from a localized infection of the oropharynx. Retropharyngeal abscess may result from penetrating trauma to the oropharynx, dental infection, and vertebral osteomyelitis. Once infected, the nodes may progress through three stages: cellulitis, phlegmon, and abscess. Infection in the retropharyngeal and lateral pharyngeal spaces may result in airway compromise or posterior mediastinitis, making timely diagnosis important.

Retropharyngeal and Lateral Pharyngeal Abscess. Retropharyngeal abscess occurs most commonly in children younger than 3–4 yr of age, with boys affected more often than girls. The retropharyngeal nodes involute after 5 yr of age, and therefore infection in older children and adults is much less common.

Clinical manifestations of retropharyngeal abscess are nonspecific and include fever, irritability, decreased oral intake, and drooling. Neck stiffness, torticollis, and refusal to move the neck may also be present. The verbal child may complain of sore throat and neck pain. Other signs may include muffled voice, stridor, and respiratory distress. Physical examination may reveal bulging of the posterior pharyngeal wall, although this is present in less than 50% of infants with retropharyngeal abscess. Cervical lymphadenopathy may also be present. Lateral pharyngeal abscess commonly presents as fever, dysphagia, and a prominent bulge of the lateral pharyngeal wall, sometimes with medial displacement of the tonsil.

The *differential diagnosis* includes acute epiglottitis and foreign body aspiration. In the young child with limited neck mobility, meningitis must also be considered. Other possibilities include lymphoma, hematoma, and vertebral osteomyelitis.

Incision for drainage and culture of an abscessed node provides the definitive diagnosis, but CT can be useful to identify the presence of a retropharyngeal or lateral pharyngeal abscess (Fig. 367–1). Soft tissue neck films taken during inspiration with the neck extended may show increased width or an air-fluid level in the retropharyngeal space. CT with contrast medium enhancement may reveal central lucency, ring enhancement, or scalloping of the walls of a lymph node.

Retropharyngeal and lateral pharyngeal infections are most often polymicrobial; the usual pathogens include group A *Streptococcus*, oropharyngeal anaerobic bacteria, and *Staphylococcus aureus*. Studies have documented an increased incidence of group A *Streptococcus* recovered from such abscesses. Other pathogens may include *Haemophilus influenzae*, *Klebsiella*, and *Mycobacterium avium-intracellulare*.

Treatment options include intravenous antibiotics with or without surgical drainage. A third-generation cephalosporin combined with ampicillin-sulbactam or clindamycin to provide anaerobic coverage is effective. Studies have shown that more than 50% of children with retropharyngeal or lateral pharyngeal abscess as identified by CT can be successfully treated without surgical drainage. Drainage is necessary, however, in the patient with respiratory distress or failure to improve with intravenous antibiotic treatment. The optimal duration of treatment is unknown, but therapy for several days with intravenous antibiotics until the patient has begun to improve followed by a course of oral antibiotic is typically utilized.

Complications of retropharyngeal or lateral pharyngeal abscess include significant upper airway obstruction, rupture leading to aspiration pneumonia, and extension to the mediastinum. Thrombophlebitis of the internal jugular vein and erosion of the carotid artery sheath may also occur.

An uncommon but characteristic infection of the parapharyngeal space is **Lemierre disease,** in which infection from the oropharynx extends to cause septic thrombophlebitis of the internal jugular vein and metastatic abscesses in the lungs. The causative pathogen is *Fusobacterium necrophorum*, an anaerobic bacterial constituent of the oropharyngeal flora. The typical presentation is that of a previously healthy adolescent or young adult with a history of recent pharyngotonsillar disease who becomes acutely ill with fever and pulmonary symptoms. Chest radiography demonstrates multiple cavitary nodules, often bilateral, and often accompanied by pleural effusion. Blood culture may be positive. Treatment involves prolonged intravenous antibiotic therapy with penicillin or cefoxitin; surgical drainage of extrapulmonary metastatic abscesses may be necessary.

Peritonsillar Cellulitis/Abscess. Peritonsillar cellulitis/abscess, which is relatively common compared with the deep neck infections, is caused by bacterial invasion through the capsule of the tonsil, leading to cellulitis and/or abscess formation in the surrounding tissues. The typical patient with a peritonsillar abscess is an adolescent with a recent history of acute pharyngotonsillitis. *Clinical manifestations* include sore throat, fever, trismus, and dysphagia. Physical examination reveals an asymmetric tonsillar bulge with displacement of the uvula. An asymmetric tonsillar bulge is diagnostic, but it may be poorly visualized because of trismus. CT is helpful to reveal the abscess. Group A *Streptococcus* and mixed oropharyngeal anaerobes are the most common pathogens, with more than four bacterial isolates per abscess typically recovered by needle aspiration.

Treatment includes surgical drainage and antibiotic therapy effective against group A *Streptococcus* and anaerobes. Surgical drainage may be accomplished through needle aspiration, incision and drainage, or tonsillectomy. Needle aspiration may involve aspiration of the superior, middle, and inferior aspects of the tonsil to locate the abscess. General anesthesia may be required for the uncooperative patient. Approximately 95% of peritonsillar abscesses resolve after needle aspiration and antibiotic therapy. A small percentage of these patients require a repeat needle aspiration. The 5% who fail to resolve after needle aspiration require incision and drainage. Tonsillectomy should be considered if there is failure to improve within 24 hours of antibiotic therapy and needle aspiration, history of recurrent peritonsillar abscess or recurrent tonsillitis, or complications from peritonsillar abscess. The feared, albeit rare, complication is rupture of the abscess with resultant aspiration pneumonitis. There is a 10% recurrence risk for peritonsillar abscess.

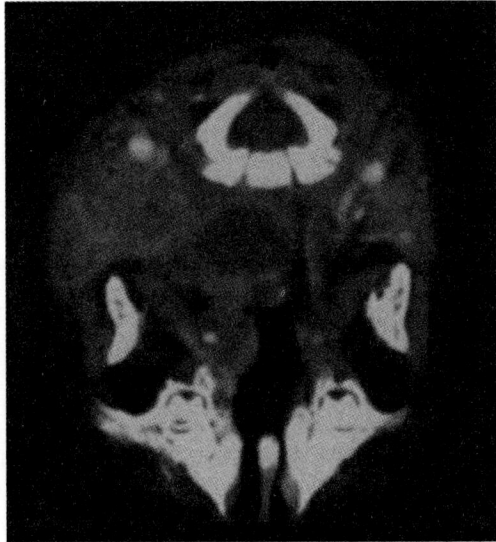

FIGURE 367–1. Retropharyngeal abscess in a 7-mo-old boy, with associated cellulitis and another involved node in the right lateral neck. The abscess was successfully treated with surgical drainage and antibiotics.

Azimi PH, Grossman M: Irritability and neck stiffness in a five-month-old infant. *Pediatr Infect Dis J* 2001;20:724, 728–29.

Blotter JW, Yin L, Glyn M, et al: Otolaryngology consultation for peritonsillar abscess in the pediatric population. *Laryngoscope* 2000;110:1698–1701.

Choi SS, Vezina LG, Grundfast KM: Relative incidence and alternative approaches for surgical drainage of different types of deep neck abscesses in children. *Arch Otolaryngol Head Neck Surg* 1997;123:1271–75.

Conway JH, Nyquist AC, Goldson E: Posterior mediastinal abscess caused by invasive group A *Streptococcus* infection. *Pediatr Infect Dis J* 1996;15:547–49.

Friedman NR, Mitchell RB, Pereira KD, et al: Peritonsillar abscess in early childhood: Presentation and management. *Arch Otolaryngol Head Neck Surg* 1997;123:630–32.

Herzon FS: Peritonsillar abscess: Incidence, current management practices, and a proposal for treatment guidelines. *Laryngoscope* 1995;105:1–17.

Jousimies-Somer H, Savolainen S, Mäkitie A, et al: Bacteriologic findings in peritonsillar abscesses in young adults. *Clin Infect Dis* 1993;16:S292–98.

Kirse DJ, Roberson DW: Surgical management of retropharyngeal space infections in children. *Laryngoscope* 2001;111:1413–22.

Lee SS, Schwartz RH, Bahadori RS: Retropharyngeal abscess: Epiglottitis of the new millennium. *J Pediatr* 2001;138:435–37.

Moreno S, Garcia Altozano J, Pinilla JC, et al: Lemierre's disease: Postanginal bacteremia and pulmonary involvement caused by *Fusobacterium necrophorum*. *Rev Infect Dis* 1989;11:319–24.

Weinberg E, Brodsky L, Stanievich J, et al: Needle aspiration of peritonsillar abscess in children. *Arch Otolaryngol Head Neck Surg* 1993;119:169–72.

Chapter 368

Tonsils and Adenoids

Ralph F. Wetmore

Because of the large number of upper respiratory infections that afflict children, especially young children, infectious and inflammatory processes of the pharynx play a significant role in their health. In this chapter the focus is on diseases of the tonsils and adenoids in children, specifically infection, airway obstruction, and, rarely, neoplastic disease.

Definitions. *Waldeyer ring* consists of lymphoid tissue that surrounds the opening of the oral and nasal cavities into the pharynx and includes the palatine tonsils, the pharyngeal tonsil or adenoid, lymphoid tissue surrounding the eustachian tube orifice in the lateral walls of the nasopharynx, the lingual tonsil at the base of the tongue, and scattered lymphoid tissue throughout the remainder of the pharynx but especially behind the posterior pharyngeal pillars and along the posterior pharyngeal wall.

Lymphoid tissue located between the palatoglossal fold (anterior tonsillar pillar) and the palatopharyngeal fold (posterior tonsillar pillar) forms the *palatine tonsil*. This lymphoid tissue is separated from the surrounding pharyngeal musculature by a thick fibrous capsule. The *adenoid* is a single aggregation of lymphoid tissue that occupies the space between the nasal septum and the posterior pharyngeal wall. A thin fibrous capsule separates it from the underlying structures; the adenoid does not contain the complex crypts that are found in the palatine tonsils but rather more simple crypts. Lymphoid tissue at the base of the tongue forms the *lingual tonsil* that also contains simple tonsillar crypts.

Normal Function. Approximately two thirds of the lymphocytes that make up the lymphoid tissue of Waldeyer ring are B lymphocytes, the remainder being either T lymphocytes or plasma cells (see Chapter 113). The immunologic role of the tonsils and adenoid is to induce secretory immunity and to regulate the production of the secretory immunoglobulins. Situated at the opening of the pharynx to the external environment, the tonsils and adenoid are in a position to provide primary defense against foreign matter. Deep crevices within tonsillar tissue form tonsillar crypts that are lined with squamous epithelium but that have a concentration of lymphocytes at the base of the crypt. Lymphoid tissue of Waldeyer ring is most immunologically active between 4–10 yr of age with a decrease after puberty. No major immunologic deficiency has been demonstrated after removal of either or both of the tonsils and adenoid.

Pathology

ACUTE INFECTION. Most episodes of acute pharyngotonsillitis are viral (see Chapter 366). Group A β-hemolytic *Streptococcus* (GABHS) is the most common cause of bacterial infection in the pharynx (see Chapter 168). Additional bacterial organisms may include other β-hemolytic streptococcal species (i.e., group C), *Staphylococcus aureus*, gram-negative organisms, *Mycoplasma pneumoniae*, and, rarely, *Neisseria gonorrhoeae* and *Corynebacterium diphtheriae*. Oral candidiasis may occur in immunocompromised patients or children who have been treated chronically with antibiotics.

CHRONIC INFECTION. The tonsils and adenoid may be infected chronically in a polymicrobial manner that may include a high incidence of β-lactamase–producing organisms. Both aerobic species, such as streptococci and *Haemophilus influenzae*, and anaerobic species, such as *Peptostreptococcus, Prevotella, and Fusobacterium,* predominate. The tonsillar crypts may accumulate desquamated epithelial cells, lymphocytes, bacteria, and other debris, causing cryptic tonsillitis. With time, these cryptic plugs may calcify into tonsillar concretions or tonsillolith.

AIRWAY OBSTRUCTION. Both the tonsils and adenoid are a major cause of upper airway obstruction in children. Airway obstruction in children is typically manifested in sleep-disordered breathing, including obstructive sleep apnea, obstructive sleep hypopnea, and upper airway resistance syndrome (see Chapter 369).

TONSILLAR NEOPLASM. Rapid enlargement of one tonsil is highly suggestive of a tonsillar malignancy, typically lymphoma in children.

Clinical Manifestations

ACUTE INFECTION. Symptoms of GABHS infection include dry throat, malaise, fever and chills, odynophagia, dysphagia, referred otalgia, headache, muscular aches, and enlarged cervical nodes. Signs include dry tongue, erythematous enlarged tonsils, tonsillar or pharyngeal exudate, and enlargement and tenderness of the jugulodigastric lymph nodes. See Chapters 168 and 366.

CHRONIC INFECTION. Children with chronic or cryptic tonsillitis frequently present with halitosis, chronic sore throats, foreign body sensation, or a history of expelling foul-tasting and smelling cheesy lumps. Examination may reveal tonsils of almost any size and frequently they contain copious debris within the crypts. Because the offending organism is not usually GABHS, streptococcal culture is usually negative.

AIRWAY OBSTRUCTION. In many children the diagnosis of airway obstruction (see Chapters 357 and 369) may be made by history and physical examination. Daytime symptoms of airway obstruction, secondary to adenotonsillar hypertrophy, include chronic mouth breathing, nasal obstruction, hyponasal speech, hyposmia, decreased appetite, poor school performance, and, rarely, symptoms of right-sided heart failure. Nighttime symptoms consist of loud snoring, choking, gasping, frank apneas, restless sleep, abnormal sleep positions, somnambulism, night terrors, diaphoresis, enuresis, and sleep talking. Large tonsils are typically seen on examination, although the absolute size may not be indicative of the degree of obstruction. The size of the adenoid tissue may be demonstrated on a lateral neck radiograph or with flexible endoscopy. Other signs that may contribute to airway obstruction include the presence of a craniofacial syndrome or hypotonia.

TONSILLAR NEOPLASM. The rapid unilateral enlargement of a tonsil, especially if accompanied by systemic signs of fever, weight loss, and lymphadenopathy, is highly suggestive of a tonsillar malignancy. The diagnosis of a tonsillar malignancy should also be entertained if the tonsil appears grossly abnormal.

Treatment

MEDICAL MANAGEMENT. The treatment of acute pharyngotonsillitis is discussed in Chapter 366. For antibiotic treatment of GABHS see Chapter 168. Because co-pathogens such as staphylococci or anaerobes may produce β-lactamase that may inactivate penicillin, the use of cephalosporins or clindamycin may be more efficacious in the treatment of chronic throat infections. Children with cryptic tonsillitis may be able to manually express tonsillolith or debris with either a cotton-tipped applicator or a water jet. Chronically infected tonsillar crypts may be cauterized using silver nitrate.

TONSILLECTOMY. Tonsillectomy alone is usually performed for recurrent or chronic pharyngotonsillitis. Although there are no strict criteria for number of infections, many experts support the criteria developed for the Children's Hospital of Pittsburgh study: seven or more throat infections treated with antibiotics in the preceding year, five or more throat infections treated in each of the preceding 2 yr, or three or more throat infections treated with antibiotics in each of the preceding 3 yr. Clinical indicators developed by the American Academy of Otolaryngology and Head and Neck Surgery suggest the occurrence of three or more treated infections per year as sufficient to warrant surgical intervention. Tonsillectomy has been shown to be effective in reducing the number of infections and the symptoms of chronic tonsillitis such as halitosis, persistent or recurrent sore throats, and recurrent cervical adenitis. In resistant cases of cryptic tonsillitis, tonsillectomy may be curative. Rarely in children, tonsillectomy may be indicated for biopsy of a unilaterally enlarged tonsil to exclude a neoplasm or to treat recurrent hemorrhage from superficial tonsillar blood vessels.

ADENOIDECTOMY. Adenoidectomy alone may be indicated for the treatment of chronic nasal infection (chronic adenoiditis), chronic sinus infections that have failed medical management, and recurrent bouts of acute otitis media, including those in children with tympanostomy tubes who suffer from recurrent otorrhea. In addition, adenoidectomy may be helpful in children with chronic or recurrent otitis media with effusion. Adenoidectomy alone may be curative in the management of patients with nasal obstruction, chronic mouth breathing, and loud snoring suggestive of sleep-disordered breathing. Adenoidectomy may also be indicated in those children in whom upper airway obstruction is suspected of causing craniofacial or occlusive developmental abnormalities.

TONSILLECTOMY AND ADENOIDECTOMY. The criteria for both tonsillectomy and adenoidectomy for recurrent infection are the same as those for tonsillectomy alone. The other major indication for performing both procedures together is upper airway obstruction secondary to adenotonsillar hypertrophy that results in sleep-disordered breathing, failure to thrive, craniofacial or occlusive developmental abnormalities, speech abnormalities, or, rarely, cor pulmonale.

Complications

ACUTE PHARYNGOTONSILLITIS. The two major complications of untreated GABHS infection are post-streptococcal glomerulonephritis and acute rheumatic fever (see Chapters 503 and 168, respectively).

PERITONSILLAR INFECTION. Peritonsillar infection may occur as either cellulitis or a frank abscess in the region superior and lateral to the tonsillar capsule (see Chapter 367). These infections usually occur in children with a history of recurrent tonsillar infection and are polymicrobial, including both aerobes and anaerobes. Unilateral throat pain, referred otalgia, drooling, and trismus are presenting symptoms. On examination, the affected tonsil is displaced down and medial by swelling of the anterior tonsillar pillar and palate. The diagnosis of an abscess may be confirmed by CT or by needle aspiration, the contents of which should be sent for culture. See Chapter 367 for treatment.

RETROPHARYNGEAL SPACE INFECTION. Infections in the retropharyngeal space develop in the lymph nodes that drain the oropharynx, nose, and nasopharynx (see Chapter 367).

PARAPHARYNGEAL SPACE INFECTION. Tonsillar infection may extend into the parapharyngeal space causing symptoms of fever, neck pain, and neck stiffness and signs of swelling of the lateral pharyngeal wall and neck on the affected side. The diagnosis is confirmed by contrast medium–enhanced CT, and treatment includes intravenous antibiotics and external incision and drainage if an abscess is demonstrated on CT. See Chapter 367.

CHRONIC PHARYNGOTONSILLITIS. Because GABHS can be found incidentally in many children, controversy exists over whether to treat those children who have been shown to be carriers. Medical management of streptococcal carriage includes (1) clindamycin (20 mg/kg/day in four divided doses), (2) amoxicillin with clavulanate (40–45 mg/kg/day in two or three divided doses), or (3) penicillin V (250 mg tid for 10 days) plus rifampin (20 mg/kg/day during the last 4 days of treatment). Tonsillectomy is usually also curative.

CHRONIC AIRWAY OBSTRUCTION (also see Chapter 369). Although rare, children with chronic airway obstruction from enlarged tonsils and adenoids may present with cor pulmonale.

The effects of chronic airway obstruction and mouth breathing on facial growth remain controversial. Studies of chronic mouth breathing, both in humans and animals, have shown changes in facial development, including prolongation of the total anterior facial height and a tendency toward a retrognathic mandible, the so-called adenoid facies. Adenotonsillectomy may reverse some of these abnormalities. Other studies have disputed these findings.

TONSILLECTOMY AND ADENOIDECTOMY. Bleeding may occur in the immediate postoperative period or may be delayed after separation of the eschar. Swelling of the tongue and soft palate may lead to acute airway obstruction in the first few hours after surgery. Children with underlying hypotonia or craniofacial anomalies are at greater risk to suffer this complication. Dehydration from odynophagia is not uncommon during the first postoperative week. Rare complications include velopharyngeal insufficiency, nasopharyngeal or oropharyngeal stenosis, and psychological problems.

Brook I, Shah K: Bacteriology of adenoids and tonsils in children with recurrent adenotonsillitis. *Ann Otol Rhinol Laryngol* 2001;110:844–48.

Gates GA, Avery CA, Prihoda TJ, et al: Effectiveness of adenoidectomy and tympanostomy tubes in the treatment of chronic otitis media with effusion. *N Engl J Med* 1987;317:1444–51.

Gozal D: Sleep-disordered breathing and school performance in children. *Pediatrics* 1998;102:616–20.

Herzon FS: Peritonsillar abscess: Incidence, current management practices, and a proposal for treatment guidelines. *Laryngoscope* 1995;105:1–17.

Paradise JL, Bluestone CD, Bachman RZ, et al: Efficacy of tonsillectomy for recurrent throat infection in severely affected children: Results of parallel randomized and nonrandomized clinical trials. *N Engl J Med* 1984;310:674–83.

Paradise JL, Bluestone CD, Rogers KD, et al: Efficacy of adenoidectomy for recurrent otitis media in children previously treated with tympanostomy tube placement. Results of parallel randomized and nonrandomized trials. *JAMA* 1990;263:2066–73.

Sie KC, Perkins JA, Clarke WR: Acute right heart failure due to adenotonsillar hypertrophy. *Int J Pediatr Otorhinolaryngol* 1997;41:53–58.

Chapter 369

Obstructive Sleep Apnea and Hypoventilation

Carol L. Rosen, Lewis J. Kass, and Gabriel G. Haddad

Obstructive sleep apnea and hypoventilation (OSA/H) (see also Chapters 57.3 and 368) is a common medical problem in adults that is increasingly recognized in children. It is a disorder of breathing during sleep characterized by prolonged partial upper airway obstruction and/or intermittent complete obstruction (obstructive apnea) that disrupts normal ventilation during sleep and normal sleep patterns (see Chapter 20.5). If unrecognized and untreated, it can lead to impaired daytime functioning as well as more serious complications, such as heart failure, developmental delay, poor growth, and death.

Etiology. Anatomic factors that increase resistance to airflow predispose to upper airway collapse and OSA/H. The most common anatomic predisposing condition in children is adenotonsillar hypertrophy. Many other predisposing nasal, pharyngeal, and craniofacial abnormalities occur less frequently (Box 369–1). Functional abnormalities also contribute to OSA/H in children. Even when the structure of the upper airway is normal, if coordinated activation of inspiratory and oropharyngeal dilator muscles do not occur, then OSA/H will develop. The most common functional process contributing to OSA/H is rapid eye movement (REM) sleep, present during one fourth of a typical night's sleep. Apnea frequency, apnea duration, and levels of hypoxemia are almost always more severe during REM sleep in both children and adults with OSA/H. Other functional abnormalities contributing to OSA/H include abnormalities of neural respiratory control and drugs that depress the central nervous system (Box 369–2). Childhood conditions associated with either anatomic and/or functional causes of OSA/H include craniofacial abnormalities (e.g., Pierre Robin sequence and Crouzon and Apert syndromes), genetic syndromes (e.g., trisomy 21), skeletal disorders (e.g., achondroplasia), storage diseases (e.g., Hunter syndrome), children with morbid obesity or Prader-Willi syndrome, and other neurologic disorders (e.g., cerebral palsy). Children with these types of problems should be periodically assessed for the development of signs and symptoms of OSA/H.

Epidemiology. OSA/H occurs in children of all ages, from newborns to young adults, with estimates of prevalence rates ranging from 0.7–3%. The peak incidence is in the preschool age group (2–5 yr), a period when adenotonsillar tissue is greatest in relationship to airway size. The incidence in males and females is similar in prepubertal children, which is in contrast to OSA/H in adults, where the disorder is more common in males. Among otherwise healthy children, obesity, upper and lower respiratory problems (e.g., chronic rhinitis and asthma), and African-American race are independent risk factors for OSA/H. For obese children in general, the severity of OSA/H correlates with the severity of obesity. Positive family history of OSA/H in another family member(s) also is a risk factor for OSA/H in childhood.

Pathogenesis. OSA/H occurs when there is failure to maintain upper airway patency, usually during sleep, which in turn affects blood gas homeostasis and sleep continuity. Two

---

BOX 369 –1. Anatomic Factors That Predispose to Obstructive Sleep Apnea and Hypoventilation in Children

NOSE
Anterior nasal stenosis
Choanal stenosis/atresia
Deviated nasal septum
Seasonal or perennial rhinitis
Nasal polyps, foreign body, hematoma, mass lesion

NASOPHARYNGEAL AND OROPHARYNGEAL
Adenotonsillar hypertrophy
Macroglossia
   Cystic hygroma
   Velopharyngeal flap repair
   Cleft palate repair
   Pharyngeal mass lesion

CRANIOFACIAL
Micrognathia/retrognathia
Midface hypoplasia (trisomy 21, Crouzon, Apert syndrome, etc.)
Mandibular hypoplasia (Pierre Robin sequence, Treacher Collins, Cornelia de Lange)
Craniofacial trauma
Skeletal and storage diseases
Achondroplasia
Glycogen storage disease (Hunter, Hurler syndrome, etc.)

BOX 369–2. Functional Factors That Predispose to Obstructive Sleep Apnea and Hypoventilation in Children

Rapid eye movement sleep–related pharyngeal hypotonia
Abnormal neural control
  Generalized hypotonia (e.g., trisomy 21)
  Global CNS injury (e.g., birth asphyxia, cerebral palsy)
  Brainstem dysfunction
    Chiari malformation (II or I)
    Foramen magnum stenosis (e.g., achondroplasia)
    Injury (e.g., anoxia, tumor, infection)
Drugs
  Sedative: chloral hydrate, benzodiazepines, phenothiazines
  Anesthetics
  Narcotics
Other
  Autonomic dysfunction
  Dysphagia
  Excess oral secretions
  Obesity
  Prematurity

---

hypotheses suggest an explanation for the pathogenesis of OSA/H in children and adults. *The Starling resistor principle* has been proposed to explain the frequent occurrence of partial upper airway obstruction associated with flow limitation. During inspiratory flow limitation, airflow is determined by pressure-generating changes in resistance upstream (e.g., at the adenoid-palate level) from the collapsible segment (pharynx). Airflow is not augmented by increased negative pressure downstream (esophageal pressure), even when inspiratory pressure-generating muscles contract more forcefully. During inspiration, a negative pressure is generated within the pharynx owing to activation of the diaphragm and intercostal muscles and mucosal adhesion forces. Collapse of the upper airway from the force of this negative pressure is prevented by simultaneous activations of the oropharyngeal dilator muscles such as the genioglossus muscle that protrudes the tongue. According to the *balance of forces hypothesis*, OSA/H occurs when an imbalance in these forces favors negative oropharyngeal pressures during inspiration. Upper airway muscle tone (oropharyngeal muscle) decreases during sleep, then to a greater degree during rapid-eye-movement (REM) sleep, thus explaining the increased vulnerability of the upper airway to collapse during this sleep state.

It is the combination of neuromuscular inactivation (or lack of full activation) superimposed on structural narrowing that contributes to the development of OSA/H. For example, the presence of adenotonsillar hypertrophy does not ordinarily cause airflow obstruction during wakefulness. Decreased airway tone that occurs when a child goes to sleep, superimposed on adenotonsillar hypertrophy, can lead to significant airway obstruction. Conditions that decrease caliber, increase collapsibility, or alter neural control of the upper airway or central ventilatory drive contribute to the development of obstruction, which, in turn, affects blood gas homeostasis and sleep quality. In normal children, arterial oxygen decreases and carbon dioxide increases only slightly during sleep. Episodes of partial or complete airway obstruction result in impaired gas exchange with hypoxemia and hypercapnia. The impaired gas exchange in conjunction with decreased airflow is potent stimuli for increased ventilatory effort and upper airway muscle activity. Arousal from sleep is associated with increased respiratory effort and airway muscle tone, which leads to resumption of airway patency. Arousals may appear in the form of movement, increased muscle tone, or changes in the electroencephalogram (EEG). Following the arousal, airflow is restored, blood gases are normalized, and sleep resumes, but the cycle of airway collapse starts again. Compared with adults with OSA/H, fewer cyclic arousals are seen in children in spite of continued hypoventilation and blood gas disturbances throughout the night. This may, in part, explain the relatively low incidence of daytime sleepiness in young children with OSA/H.

Although there is no direct correlation between tonsil size and severity of OSA/H, enlarged tonsils and adenoids are still the most common risk factors for OSA/H. Other anatomic factors such as micrognathia, retrognathia, or macroglossia may force the tongue into the oropharyngeal portion of the airway and cause airway occlusion. Fat deposition from morbid obesity or a congenitally small midface or nasopharynx also narrows the airway. Increased resistance from swollen nasal turbinates or choanal stenosis places a greater negative collapsing pressure on the pharyngeal airway and may lead to worsening obstruction. Diminished arousal responses can impair the ability to restore upper airway patency. Children with central nervous system abnormalities associated with impaired ventilatory or arousal responses to hypoxemia, hypercapnia, and/or airflow obstruction (e.g., Chiari II malformations) have increased vulnerability to severe OSA/H and cardiorespiratory failure. Finally, sedative medication or general anesthesia can further compromise neural control of the upper airway.

The development of OSA/H can have serious cardiorespiratory and neurobehavioral consequences. Chronic hypoxemia can lead to polycythemia, growth failure, increased pulmonary artery pressure and pulmonary hypertension, right-sided heart failure, arrhythmias, or even death. Recurrent arousals can lead to sleep fragmentation, loss of normal sleep patterns, and excessive daytime sleepiness. OSA/H has been associated with other daytime sequelae, including inattentiveness and hyperactivity, behavioral problems, impaired school performance, and accidents. Finally, sleep fragmentation itself can suppress arousal responses and further impair the ability to re-establish upper airway patency and restore gas exchange.

Clinical Manifestations. Common clinical manifestations of OSA/H include chronic mouth breathing, snoring, and restlessness during sleep with or without frequent awakenings. Children may sleep in unusual positions to help maintain a patent upper airway, for example, with the neck hyperextended or prone with the bottom up in the air. Typically, loud snoring is the symptom that most disturbs, and therefore alerts, the parents. Most children with OSA/H breathe normally while awake.

Habitual snoring, the most common symptom of OSA/H, ranges from 3–12% in children. However, not all habitually snoring children have or are at risk for the development of OSA/H. The spectrum of severity (ranging from snoring to congestive heart failure) is related to the degree of upper airway narrowing and resistance, duration of the disease, the presence or absence of hypoxemia episodes, and other sequelae. Primary snoring, upper airway resistance syndrome, obstructive hypoventilation, and OSA represent a spectrum of clinical manifestations associated with increasing severity of upper airway obstruction. However, the majority of children with OSA/H do not present with dramatic, repetitive obstructive apneas terminated by arousals. Instead, OSA/H presents as partial continuous obstructive hypoventilation with fewer discrete obstructive apneas, fewer arousals, and less disturbance of sleep architecture. For this reason, daytime hypersomnolence is much less frequent in children than adults. Because of this more subtle presentation, children often have an unexpected degree of airway obstruction, impairment of gas exchange, and sleep disturbance that is difficult to predict from the clinical history and physical examination alone.

Children with the more severe presentation also have noisy, mildly labored awake breathing that clearly worsens with sleep. Parents describe that cyclically the snoring becomes very loud, followed by silence, a snort, an arousal, and resumption of snoring. When snoring is associated with nocturnal breathing difficulties and witnessed respiratory pauses, this triad of symptoms is highly suggestive of OSA/H in children. However, some children with serious OSA/H have minimal noisy breathing, and diagnosis depends on the physician's high index of suspicion.

Less common symptoms include daytime hypersomnolence resulting from sleep fragmentation that occurs when OSA is repeatedly terminated by arousals. However, it is difficult to recognize excessive sleepiness in young children, who normally have daytime naps and early bedtimes. Poor school performance is increasingly recognized as being associated with OSA/H. Lower academic performance has been described in young children as well as in adolescents who suffer from OSA/H or from primary snoring. There is debate as to whether these neurocognitive deficits are the result of a poor night's sleep secondary to frequent arousal and hence inability to concentrate in school or the result of spending every night in relative hypoxemia that could be predisposing the child to cerebral ischemia. Additionally, the possible association of inattentiveness, hyperactivity, and behavioral problems with OSA/H highlights the importance of investigating whether unrecognized OSA/H may be playing a role in children diagnosed with attention deficit disorder with hyperactivity (ADHD).

Although obesity is a risk factor for OSA/H in children, most children with OSA/H are not obese. In fact, some children, especially children younger than 3 yr of age, are underweight or present with failure to thrive. Several factors might contribute to this growth retardation: dysphagia from large tonsils, nasal obstruction from enlarged adenoids that interferes with breathing during eating, chronic hypoxemia, higher metabolic expenditure from increased work of breathing, and insufficient growth hormone release in the absence of deep REM sleep. Children may also present with unexplained right-sided heart failure, but other cardiovascular complications, such as systemic hypertension or life-threatening cardiac arrhythmias, are rarely seen, except in the most long-standing and neglected cases. In the more severe cases, a relatively minor respiratory illness or infection can trigger an acute episode of respiratory failure. Finally, secondary enuresis that disappears after surgical relief of the upper airway obstruction is occasionally seen, but the mechanisms are poorly understood.

Clinical examination features associated with OSA/H include dysmorphic facies, mouth breathing, hyponasal speech, macroglossia, cleft palate, or enlarged tonsils. Specific craniofacial anomalies may be apparent. A pectus excavatum deformity can develop in long-standing upper airway obstruction. Morbid obesity mechanically loads the chest wall and narrows the upper airway, but OSA/H is not a consistent feature of obesity. The presence of excessive somnolence during the examination requires urgent evaluation. The presence of stridor or hoarse voice can indicate cranial nerve dysfunction and should prompt a meticulous neurologic examination.

Laboratory Findings. Polycythemia and respiratory acidosis with a metabolic alkalosis support the diagnosis of OSA/H when present but are absent in the majority of pediatric patients. Right ventricular hypertrophy on electrocardiography and dysfunction on echocardiography are seen only in severe OSA/H. A lateral soft tissue radiograph of the neck can identify adenoidal tissue. When procedures require sedation or anesthesia, extreme caution is required if OSA/H is suspected. Such medications have profound effects on upper airway muscle tone, and sudden respiratory decompensation can occur in these children.

Diagnosis. The diagnosis is often delayed, despite years of symptoms, for several reasons: (1) there may be absence of awake symptoms; (2) a sleep history was not obtained; (3) symptoms of snoring or restless sleep are considered inconsequential; (4) parents may be unaware of the problem because the child's most severe symptoms appear during REM sleep in the last third of the night when parents are asleep; and (5) young children may not generate the loud, disruptive snoring noises of an adult. The diagnosis should be suggested by the clinical presentation.

Parental reports of habitual snoring should be investigated. A sleep and breathing history is mandatory for any child with a medical condition that is at risk for OSA/H, especially trisomy 21, craniofacial anomalies, achondroplasia, or other neuromuscular disorders.

However, OSA/H cannot be diagnosed from clinical history alone. Snoring, reports of difficulty breathing, and enlarged tonsils can be unreliable predictors of the presence or severity of OSA/H in children. The physical examination performed during wakefulness may be entirely normal and cannot be used to exclude OSA/H when the clinical history suggests otherwise. Pulse oximetry is insensitive. Other diagnostic methods, including audio/videotaping and nap or home polysomnography (PSG), remain investigational techniques. An overnight recording of multiple physiologic sensors during sleep is considered the gold standard for the diagnosis of OSA/H (see Chapter 359). It provides a powerful, quantitative, noninvasive assessment of frequency and severity of sleep-disordered breathing and sleep disruption. PSG is especially useful in confirming the diagnosis, in determining the severity of OSA/H, and in documenting the efficacy of treatment. PSG in children, especially very young or special needs children, requires skilled, well-trained, child-friendly sleep technicians in family-centered environments. However, PSG may not be required for diagnostic purposes in all patients. For example, PSG may not be necessary when a child has noisy, awake mouth breathing and tonsils that occlude most of the pharyngeal space; is excessively sleepy; and is observed by skilled personnel to have signs of airway obstruction and hypoxemia.

PSG can confirm the presence and severity of airflow obstruction. Because patients with severe OSA/H are at increased risk for perioperative and postoperative complications from adenotonsillectomy, prior knowledge of severity can help determine the appropriateness of same-day outpatient surgery vs. overnight in-hospital observation and monitoring. PSG is required to determine the optimal level of continuous positive airway pressure (CPAP) needed to manage OSA/H when adenotonsillectomy is not a therapeutic option. Other children considered "high risk" are those younger than 3 yr of age and children with morbid obesity, craniofacial anomalies, genetic disorders, or other complex medical conditions.

Several other disorders should be considered in the *differential diagnosis* of OSA/H or may coexist with this problem. Occasionally, breathing difficulty associated with nocturnal asthma or upper airway obstruction from gastroesophageal reflux may be confused with OSA/H. New-onset dysphagia and swallowing difficulties associated with an esophageal foreign body that compresses the airway can masquerade as OSA/H. Stridor caused by anatomic airway problems, such as laryngomalacia, vascular ring, intraluminal masses, and vocal cord dysfunction, should be considered. Parasomnia events, such as night terrors or even nocturnal seizures, may be mistaken for arousals associated with OSA/H. Narcolepsy and periodic limb movement disorder should be considered when PSG fails to document OSA/H in a child with daytime hypersomnolence.

Complications. Early reports of untreated OSA/H highlighted the most severe cases with sequelae that included failure to thrive, pulmonary hypertension, and/or cor pulmonale. Such severe complications are now rare owing to increased awareness of OSA/H among primary care providers, recognition of high-risk subgroups such as trisomy 21 or craniofacial disorders, and earlier diagnosis and treatment. Many of the children who come to medical attention and consideration of surgical intervention today have much less severe OSA/H and symptoms of shorter duration.

Failure to diagnose and treat OSA/H can result in serious but generally reversible consequences for the child. Whereas the sequelae of cor pulmonale and growth and developmental

impairment are well documented, the potential negative impact of OSA/H on neurocognitive and behavioral dysfunction has not been well characterized but may include attentional capacity, memory, and cognitive function and increased behavior problems.

Prevention. Because obesity is a risk factor for the increased severity of OSA/H, the persistence of OSA/H after adenotonsillectomy, and the development of OSA/H in adulthood, weight management should be a long-term goal in a child at risk or diagnosed with OSA/H.

Treatment. Adenotonsillectomy is the most common therapy for OSA/H in children with adenotonsillar hypertrophy. However, the treatment for a particular child depends on the underlying abnormalities, the site of obstruction, and the presence or absence of contributing neurologic or functional abnormalities. Box 369–3 lists possible treatments. When adenotonsillar hypertrophy is present, the majority of otherwise healthy children without major risk factors experience resolution or significant improvement after adenotonsillectomy. Children with severe OSA/H who benefit from surgery often demonstrate "catch-up" growth. However, children with underlying problems, such as trisomy 21, craniofacial disorders, extreme obesity, or neuromuscular disorders such as cerebral palsy or Chiari malformation, or who present before 2 yr of age are at risk for incomplete resolution of OSA/H after adenotonsillectomy. Even without these risk factors, the parents and physicians of children who have had adenotonsillectomy should be aware that either persistent or recurring symptoms of OSA/H need re-evaluation, including reassessment for adenoidal regrowth and possible need for repeat adenoidectomy or other treatments.

Medical management with nasal CPAP is an option in children in whom adenotonsillectomy fails, thus avoiding the need for a tracheostomy. CPAP is safe and well tolerated but requires a motivated family for compliance. PSG is required to select the appropriate pressure level to relieve obstruction. Follow-up PSG should be performed at regular intervals because the long-term stability of CPAP requirements in the growing child is not known. CPAP should not be first-line treatment when adenotonsillar hypertrophy is present and there are no absolute contraindications to surgery. CPAP can be useful in the obese child in whom weight loss is desirable but difficult to achieve. Supplemental oxygen may relieve the hypoxemia associated with OSA/H but is clearly insufficient to address the underlying obstruction and hypoventilation. A nasopharyngeal tube may be a short- or long-term adjunct to care in selected patients.

BOX 369–3. Treatment of Obstructive Sleep Apnea and Hypoventilation in Childhood

Adenotonsillectomy
Medical therapies
   Nasopharyngeal airway
   Continuous positive airway pressure via nasal mask
   Supplemental oxygen to minimize hypoxemia
   Pharmacologic
      Topical nasal steroids
      Antibiotics
      Nasal decongestants (short-term only)
Weight loss
Other surgical therapies
   Craniofacial surgical procedures
      Mandibular distraction osteogenesis
      Mandibular/maxillary plastic surgical procedures
      Stenting procedures for nasal stenosis/atresia
      Cleft palate revision procedures
   Uvulopalatopharyngoplasty
   Correction of deviated septum, nasal polypectomy
   Tracheostomy

Pharmacologic management has only a limited role in pediatric OSA/H patients. Treatment of nasal obstruction with topical nasal steroids can reduce snoring and OSA/H severity in some children. However, significant residual obstruction from unrelieved adenotonsillar hypertrophy requires adenotonsillectomy for definitive management. Steroids and antibiotics may be a useful adjunct in the acute management of infected pharyngeal tissues that have compromised upper airway patency, but adenotonsillectomy is the definitive management once the acute processes have resolved sufficiently to allow safe surgical management. Medroxyprogesterone acetate augments ventilatory drive and has been used in the management of the daytime hypoventilation associated with the obesity-hypoventilation syndrome. However, this drug fails to improve nocturnal obstructive symptoms and has adverse effects on growth and pubertal development. Protriptyline is a nonsedating antidepressant with REM suppressant activity that has been tried in adult OSA/H patients but is not recommended for children.

If severe upper airway obstruction is present in both wakefulness and sleep, then tracheostomy is the treatment of choice, particularly when vocal cord dysfunction, impaired swallowing, or absent laryngeal protective reflexes exist. Tracheostomy may be necessary for severe OSA/H complicated by cor pulmonale when CPAP is unsuccessful or not tolerated.

There is increasing pediatric experience with treatment by mandibular distraction osteogenesis as an alternative to long-term tracheostomy. Definitive maxillomandibular reconstructive surgery for children with craniofacial disorders is another therapeutic option but is usually postponed until facial growth is complete. Uvulopalatopharyngoplasty, the resection of redundant pharyngeal tissue, has been used to eliminate snoring in adults, but the failure rate is high. Pediatric experience with this surgery has been limited to children with muscular hypotonia and oropharyngeal tissue redundancy, but no controlled studies using objective measures of efficacy have been performed.

Prognosis. Failure to diagnose and treat OSA/H can result in serious, but generally reversible, consequences for the child, including impaired growth and cardiorespiratory failure. However, the impact of OSA/H and its treatment on neurocognitive and behavioral dysfunction is unknown.

American Academy of Pediatrics Guideline: Diagnosis and management of childhood obstructive sleep apnea. *Pediatrics* 2002;109:704–12.
Cardiorespiratory sleep studies in children: Establishment of normative data and polysomnographic predictors of morbidity. American Thoracic Society. *Am J Respir Crit Care Med* 1999;160:1381–87.
Arens R, McDonough JM, Costarino AT, et al: Magnetic resonance imaging of the upper airway structure of children with obstructive sleep apnea syndrome. *Am J Respir Crit Care Med* 2001;164:698–703.
Brouillette RT, Manoukian JJ, Ducharme FM, et al: Efficacy of fluticasone nasal spray for pediatric obstructive sleep apnea. *J Pediatr* 2001;138:838–44.
Chervin RD, Archbold KH: Hyperactivity and polysomnographic findings in children evaluated for sleep-disordered breathing. *Sleep* 2001;24:313–20.
Goh DY, Galster P, Marcus CL: Sleep architecture and respiratory disturbances in children with obstructive sleep apnea. *Am J Respir Crit Care Med* 2000;162:682–86.
Gozal D, Wang M, Pope DW Jr: Objective sleepiness measures in pediatric obstructive sleep apnea. *Pediatrics* 2001;108:693–97.
Gozal D, Pope DW Jr: Snoring during early childhood and academic performance at ages thirteen to fourteen years. *Pediatrics* 2001;107:1394–99.
Marcus CL: Sleep-disordered breathing in children. *Am J Respir Crit Care Med* 2001;164:16–30.
Redline S, Tishler PV, Schluchter M, et al: Risk factors for sleep-disordered breathing in children: Associations with obesity, race, and respiratory problems. *Am J Respir Crit Care Med* 1999;159:1527–32.
Scholle S, Zwacka G: Arousals and obstructive sleep apnea syndrome in children. *Clin Neurophysiol* 2001;112:984–91.

SECTION 3 *Disorders of the Lungs and Lower Airways*

Thomas P. Green and Susanna A. McColley

Virtually every child experiences lower respiratory tract disease; for most, the disorder is mild and self-limited as often occurs with viral bronchitis. For a small but growing minority of children, recurrent respiratory disease, such as asthma, produces periods of significant respiratory dysfunction interspersed with times of relatively normal lung function. In a few children, chronic respiratory disease, as seen in cystic fibrosis or primary ciliary dyskinesia, requires constant medical supervision and may dramatically affect the quality and duration of life.

The chapters in this section deal with disorders of the lungs and the large airways below the larynx. Chapters in other sections of this book deal with important topics in lower respiratory tract disease, and this material is not duplicated here. These include acute respiratory distress and respiratory failure (see Chapters 57.3, 58, and 357.1), drowning and near-drowning (see Chapter 61), neonatal respiratory tract disorders (see Chapter 90), asthma (see Chapter 134), and sarcoidosis (see Chapter 155). Diseases of other organ systems also may result in pulmonary dysfunction. These issues are considered in this section (see Chapter 411).

Chapter 370

Chronic or Recurrent Respiratory Symptoms

Thomas F. Boat

Respiratory tract symptoms such as cough, wheeze, and stridor may occur frequently or persist for long periods in a substantial number of children; others may have persistent or recurring lung infiltrates with or without symptoms. Determining the cause of these chronic findings can be difficult because symptoms may be caused by a rapid succession of unrelated acute respiratory tract infections or by a single pathophysiologic process, and there is a paucity of easily performed, specific diagnostic tests for many acute and chronic respiratory conditions. Pressure from the affected child's family for a quick remedy because of concern over symptoms related to breathing may complicate diagnostic and therapeutic efforts.

A systematic approach to the diagnosis and treatment of these children consists of assessing whether the symptoms are the manifestation of a minor problem or a life-threatening process; determining the most likely underlying pathogenic mechanism; selecting the simplest effective therapy for the underlying process, which may often be only symptomatic therapy; and carefully evaluating the effect of therapy. Failure of this approach to identify the process responsible or to effect improvement signals the need for more extensive and perhaps invasive diagnostic efforts, including bronchoscopy.

Judging the Seriousness of Chronic Respiratory Complaints. Clinical manifestations suggesting that a respiratory tract illness may be life threatening or associated with the potential for chronic disability are listed in Box 370–1. If none of these findings is detected, the chronic respiratory process is usually benign. For example, active, well-nourished, and appropriately growing infants who present with intermittent noisy breathing but no other physical or laboratory abnormalities require only symptomatic treatment and parental reassurance. However, benign-appearing but persistent symptoms occasionally may be the harbinger of a serious lower respiratory tract problem and, conversely, a few children (e.g., those with infection-related asthma) may have recurrent life-threatening episodes but few or no symptoms in the intervals. Repeated examinations over an extended period, both when the child appears healthy and when the child is symptomatic, are often helpful in sorting out the severity and chronicity of lung disease.

Recurrent or Persistent Cough. Cough is a reflex response of the lower respiratory tract to stimulation of irritant or cough receptors in the airways' mucosa. The most common cause in children is reactive airways (asthma). Because cough receptors also reside in the pharynx, paranasal sinuses, stomach, and external auditory canal, the source of a persistent cough may need to be sought beyond the lungs. Specific lower respiratory stimuli include excessive secretions, aspirated foreign material, inhaled dust particles or noxious gases, and an inflammatory response to infectious agents or allergic processes. Some of the conditions responsible for chronic cough are listed in Box 370–2.

Characteristics of cough that may aid in distinguishing its origin are presented in Table 370–1. Additional useful information may include a history of atopic conditions (e.g., asthma, eczema, urticaria, allergic rhinitis), a seasonal or environmental variation in frequency or intensity of cough, and a strong family history of atopic conditions, all suggesting an allergic cause; symptoms of malabsorption or family history indicative of cystic fibrosis; symptoms related to feeding, suggesting aspiration; a choking episode, suggesting foreign body aspiration; headache or facial edema associated with sinusitis; and a smoking history in older children and adolescents or the presence of a smoker in the house.

Considerable information pertaining to the cause of chronic cough can be obtained during the *physical examination*. Posterior pharyngeal drainage combined with a nighttime cough suggests chronic upper airway disease such as sinusitis. An overinflated chest suggests chronic airway obstruction, as in asthma or cystic fibrosis. An expiratory wheeze, with or without diminished intensity of breath sounds, strongly suggests asthma or asthmatic bronchitis but may also be consistent with a diagnosis of cystic fibrosis, vascular ring, aspiration of foreign material, or pulmonary hemosiderosis. Careful auscultation during forced expiration may reveal expiratory wheezes that are otherwise undetectable and that are the only indication of underlying

reactive airways. Coarse crackles suggest bronchiectasis, including cystic fibrosis, but may also occur with an acute or subacute exacerbation of asthma. Clubbing of the digits is seen in most patients with bronchiectasis but in only a few other respiratory conditions with chronic cough. Tracheal deviation suggests foreign body aspiration or a mediastinal mass.

It is essential to allow sufficient examination time to detect a spontaneous cough. If not spontaneous, most children by 4–5 yr of age can cough on request. Asking the child to take a maximal breath and forcefully exhale repeatedly usually induces a cough reflex. Children who cough as often as several times a minute with regularity are likely to have a habit (tic) cough. If the cough is loose, every effort should be made to obtain sputum; most older children can comply. It is sometimes possible to pick up small bits of sputum with a throat swab quickly inserted into the lower pharynx while the child coughs with the tongue protruding. Clear mucoid sputum is most often associated with an allergic reaction or asthmatic bronchitis. Cloudy (purulent) sputum

---

BOX 370–2. Differential Diagnosis of Recurrent and Persistent Cough in Children

RECURRENT COUGH

Bronchial reactivity, including allergic asthma
Drainage from upper airways
Aspiration syndromes
Frequently recurring respiratory tract infections
Idiopathic pulmonary hemosiderosis

PERSISTENT COUGH

Hypersensitivity of cough receptors following infection
Reactive airways disease (asthma)
Chronic sinusitis
Bronchitis, tracheitis owing to chronic infection, smoking (in older children)
Bronchiectasis, including cystic fibrosis, primary ciliary dyskinesia, immunodeficiency
Foreign body aspiration
Recurrent aspiration owing to pharyngeal incompetence, tracheolaryngoesophageal cleft, tracheoesophageal fistula
Gastroesophageal reflux, with or without aspiration
Pertussis syndrome
Extrinsic compression of the tracheobronchial tract (vascular ring, neoplasm, lymph node, lung cyst)
Tracheomalacia, bronchomalacia
Endobronchial or endotracheal tumors
Endobronchial tuberculosis
Habit cough
Hypersensitivity pneumonitis
Fungal infections
Inhaled irritants, including tobacco smoke
Irritation of external auditory canal

BOX 370–1. Indicators of Serious Chronic Lower Respiratory Tract Disease in Children

Persistent fever
Ongoing limitation of activity
Failure to grow
Failure to gain weight appropriately
Clubbing of the digits
Persistent tachypnea and labored ventilation
Chronic purulent sputum
Persistent hyperinflation
Substantial and sustained hypoxemia
Refractory roentgenographic infiltrates
Persistent pulmonary function abnormalities
Family history of heritable lung disease
Cyanosis and hypercarbia

TABLE 370–1. Characteristics of a Chronic Cough and Their Etiologic Significance

Type of Cough	Likely Responsible Condition
Loose (discontinuous), productive	Bronchitis, asthmatic bronchitis, cystic fibrosis, bronchiectasis
Brassy	Tracheitis, habit cough
With stridor	Laryngeal obstruction, pertussis
Paroxysmal (with or without gagging and vomiting)	Cystic fibrosis, pertussis syndrome, foreign body
Staccato	Chlamydial pneumonitis
Nocturnal	Upper or lower respiratory tract allergic reaction, or both, sinusitis
Most severe on awakening in morning	Cystic fibrosis, bronchiectasis, chronic bronchitis
With vigorous exercise	Exercise-induced asthma, cystic fibrosis, bronchiectasis
Disappears with sleep	Habit cough, mild hypersecretory states such as in cystic fibrosis and asthma
Tight (wheezy)	Reactive airways

suggests a respiratory tract infection but may also reflect increased cellularity (eosinophilia) due to an asthmatic process. Very purulent sputum is characteristic of bronchiectasis. Malodorous expectorations suggest anaerobic infection of the lungs. In cystic fibrosis, the sputum, even when purulent, is rarely foul smelling.

Laboratory tests may help in the evaluation of a chronic cough. Only sputum specimens containing alveolar macrophages should be used for studying lower respiratory tract processes. Sputum eosinophilia suggests asthma, asthmatic bronchitis, or hypersensitivity reactions of the lung, but a polymorphonuclear cell response suggests infection; if sputum is unavailable, the presence of eosinophilia in nasal secretions also suggests atopic disease. If most of the cells in sputum are macrophages, postinfectious hypersensitivity of cough receptors should be suspected. Sputum macrophages can be stained for hemosiderin content, which is diagnostic of pulmonary hemosiderosis, or for lipid content, which in large amounts suggests, but is not specific for, repeated aspiration. Children whose coughs persist longer than 6 wk should be tested for cystic fibrosis. Sputum culture is helpful for diagnosis of cystic fibrosis but less so for other conditions because throat flora may contaminate the sample.

Hematologic assessment may reveal anemia that is the result of pulmonary hemosiderosis or eosinophilia that accompanies asthma and other hypersensitivity reactions of the lung. Infiltrates on the chest radiograph suggest cystic fibrosis, bronchiectasis, foreign body, hypersensitivity pneumonitis, or tuberculosis. When asthma-equivalent cough is suggested, a trial of bronchodilator therapy may be diagnostic. After the initial evaluation, especially if the cough does not respond to initial therapeutic efforts, more specific diagnostic procedures may be indicated, including an immunologic or allergic evaluation, chest and paranasal sinus imaging, esophagograms, tests for gastroesophageal reflux, special microbiologic studies including rapid viral testing, evaluation of ciliary morphologic features, and bronchoscopy.

Habit cough ("psychogenic cough tic") must be considered in any child with a cough that has lasted for weeks or months, that has been refractory to treatment, that disappears with sleep, and that typically has a harsh, "barking" quality. This cough may be absent if the physician listens outside the examination room but will reliably appear immediately on direct attention to the child and the symptom. It typically begins with an upper respiratory infection but then lingers. The child misses many days of school because the cough disrupts the classroom. This disorder accounts for many unnecessary medical procedures and courses of medication. It is treatable with assurance that a lung pathologic condition is absent and that the child should resume full activity, including school. This assurance, together with speech therapy techniques that allow the child to reduce musculoskeletal tension in the neck and chest and that increase the child's awareness of the initial sensations that trigger cough, has been very successful. This approach does not depend on deception, unlike a reportedly successful technique that involves wrapping the child's chest with a bedsheet to "strengthen weakened muscles" until the coughing stops. The designation "habit cough" is preferable to "psychogenic cough" because it carries no stigma and because most of these children do not have significant emotional problems. When the cough disappears, it does not re-emerge as another symptom.

Recurrent or Persistent Wheeze. Wheezing is a relatively frequent and particularly troublesome manifestation of obstructive lower respiratory tract disease in children. The site of obstruction may be anywhere from the intrathoracic trachea to the small bronchi or large bronchioles, but the sound is generated by turbulence in larger airways that collapse with forced expiration. Children younger than 2–3 yr of age are especially prone to wheezing, because bronchospasm, mucosal edema, and accumulation of excessive secretions have a relatively greater obstructive effect on their smaller airways. In addition, the compliant airways in young children collapse more readily with active expiration. Isolated episodes of acute wheezing, such as may occur with bronchiolitis, are not uncommon, but wheezing that recurs or persists for longer than 4 wk suggests other diagnoses (see Table 379–2). Most recurrent or persistent wheezing in children is the result of reactive airways disease. Nonspecific environmental factors such as cigarette smoke may be important contributors.

Frequently recurring or persistent wheezing starting at or soon after birth suggests a variety of other diagnoses, including congenital structural abnormalities involving the lower respiratory tract or tracheobronchomalacia. Wheezing that attends cystic fibrosis is most common in the first year of life. Sudden onset of severe wheezing in a previously healthy child should suggest foreign body aspiration.

Repeated examination may be required to verify a history of wheezing in a child with episodic symptoms and should be directed toward assessing air movement, ventilatory adequacy, and evidence of chronic lung disease, such as fixed overinflation of the chest, growth failure, and digital clubbing. Clubbing suggests chronic lung infection and is rarely prominent in uncomplicated asthma. Tracheal deviation from foreign body aspiration should be sought. It is essential to rule out wheezing secondary to congestive heart failure. Allergic rhinitis, urticaria, eczema, or evidence of ichthyosis vulgaris suggests asthma or asthmatic bronchitis. The nose should be examined for polyps, which may exist with allergic conditions or cystic fibrosis.

Sputum eosinophilia and elevated serum IgE levels suggest allergic reactions. An FEV_1 increase of 15% in response to bronchodilators is confirmatory of reactive airways. Specific microbiologic studies, special imaging studies of the airways and cardiovascular structures, diagnostic studies for cystic fibrosis, and bronchoscopy should be considered if the response is unsatisfactory.

Frequently Recurring or Persistent Stridor. Stridor, a harsh, medium-pitched, inspiratory sound associated with obstruction of the laryngeal area or the extrathoracic trachea, is often accompanied by a croupy cough and hoarse voice. Stridor is most commonly observed in children with croup; foreign bodies and trauma may also cause acute stridor. However, a small number of children acquire recurrent stridor or have persistent stridor from the first days or weeks of life (Box 370–3). Most congenital anomalies of large airways that produce stridor become symptomatic soon after birth. Increase of stridor when a child is supine suggests laryngomalacia or tracheomalacia. An accompanying history of hoarseness or aphonia suggests involvement of the vocal cords.

Physical examination for recurrent or persistent stridor is usually unrewarding, although changes in its severity and intensity due to changes of body position should be assessed. Anteroposterior and lateral roentgenograms, contrast esophagography, fluoroscopy, CT, and MRI are potentially useful diagnostic tools. In most cases, direct observation is necessary for diagnosis. Undistorted views of the larynx are best obtained with fiberoptic laryngoscopy.

Recurrent and Persistent Lung Infiltrates. Radiographic lung infiltrates resulting from acute pneumonia usually resolve within 1–3 wk, but a substantial number of children, particularly infants, fail to completely clear infiltrates within a 4-wk period. They may be febrile or afebrile and may display a wide range of respiratory symptoms and signs. Persistent or recurring infiltrates present a diagnostic challenge (Box 370–4).

Symptoms associated with chronic lung infiltrates during the first several weeks of life (but not related to neonatal respiratory distress syndrome) suggest infection acquired in utero or during descent through the birth canal. Early appearance of chronic infiltrates may also be associated with cystic fibrosis or congenital

BOX 370–3. Causes of Recurrent or Persistent Stridor in Children

RECURRENT

Allergic (spasmodic) croup
Respiratory infections in a child with otherwise asymptomatic
anatomic narrowing of the large airways
Laryngomalacia

PERSISTENT

Laryngeal obstruction
Laryngomalacia
Papillomas, other tumors
Cysts and laryngoceles
Laryngeal webs
Bilateral abductor paralysis of the cords
Foreign body
Tracheobronchial disease
Tracheomalacia
Subglottic tracheal webs
Endotracheal, endobronchial tumors
Subglottic tracheal stenosis
Congenital
Acquired
Extrinsic masses
Mediastinal masses
Vascular ring
Lobar emphysema
Bronchogenic cysts
Thyroid enlargement
Esophageal foreign body
Tracheoesophageal fistulas

OTHER

Gastroesophageal reflux
Macroglossia, Pierre Robin syndrome
Cri-du-chat syndrome
Hysterical stridor
Hypocalcemia

BOX 370–4. Diseases Associated with Recurrent, Persistent or Migrating Lung Infiltrates beyond the Neonatal Period

Asthma*
Repeated aspiration*
Hypersensitivity pneumonitis
Pulmonary hemosiderosis*
Foreign body
Sickle cell disease
Cystic fibrosis*
Congenital infection*
Cytomegalovirus
Rubella
Syphilis
Acquired infection
Cytomegalovirus*
Tuberculosis*
HIV
Other viruses*
Chlamydia*
Mycoplasma, Ureaplasma*
Pertussis*
Fungal organisms
Pneumocystis carinii*
Inadequately treated bacterial infection
Congenital anomalies
Lung cysts*
Pulmonary sequestration
Bronchial stenosis
Vascular ring
Congenital heart disease with large left-to-right shunt
Aspiration
Pharyngeal incompetence (e.g., cleft palate)*
Laryngotracheoesophageal cleft*
Tracheoesophageal fistula*
Gastroesophageal reflux*
Foreign body
Lipid aspiration
Immunodeficiency, phagocytic deficiency*
Humoral, cellular, combined immunodeficiency states*
Chronic granulomatous disease and related phagocytic defects*
Complement deficiency states*
Allergy-hypersensitivity
Pulmonary hemosiderosis (cow's milk–related, other*)
Asthma
Hypersensitivity pneumonitis (allergic alveolitis)
Cystic fibrosis*
Primary ciliary dyskinesia (Kartagener syndrome)
Other bronchiectases
Sarcoidosis
Neoplasms (primary, metastatic)
Interstitial pneumonitis and fibrosis*
Usual (Hamman-Rich syndrome)
Desquamative
Lymphoid (AIDS)
Alveolar proteinosis
Pulmonary lymphangiectasia*
α_1-Antitrypsin deficiency
Drug-induced, radiation-induced inflammation and fibrosis
Collagen-vascular diseases
Eosinophilic pneumonias
Visceral larva migrans
Histiocytosis
Leukemia

---

*Conditions likely to cause chronic lung infiltrates in infants.

---

anomalies, which result in aspiration or airway obstruction. A history of recurrent infiltrates, wheezing, and cough may reflect asthma, even in the first year of life.

One uncommon but characteristic syndrome appearing in the first year of life with recurrent lung infiltrates is pulmonary hemosiderosis related to cow's milk hypersensitivity. Children with a history of bronchopulmonary dysplasia frequently have episodes of respiratory distress attended by wheezing and new lung infiltrates. Recurrent pneumonia in a child with frequent otitis media, nasopharyngitis, adenitis, or dermatologic manifestations suggests an immunodeficiency state, complement deficiency, or phagocytic defect. Particular attention must be directed to the possibility that the infiltrates represent lymphocytic interstitial pneumonitis or opportunistic infection associated with human immunodeficiency virus infection. A history of paroxysmal coughing in an infant suggests pertussis syndrome or cystic fibrosis. Persistent infiltrates, especially with loss of volume, in a toddler should suggest foreign body aspiration.

Overinflation and infiltrates suggest cystic fibrosis or chronic asthma. A "silent chest" with infiltrates should arouse suspicion of alveolar proteinosis, *Pneumocystis carinii* infection, desquamative interstitial pneumonitis, or tumors. Growth should be carefully assessed to determine whether the lung process has had systemic effects, indicating substantial severity and chronicity as in cystic fibrosis or alveolar proteinosis. Cataracts, retinopathy, or microcephaly suggest in utero infection. Chronic rhinorrhea may be associated with atopic disease, cow's milk intolerance, cystic fibrosis, or congenital syphilis. The absence of tonsils and cervical lymph nodes suggests an immunodeficiency state.

Diagnostic studies should be performed selectively, based on information obtained from history and physical examination and on a thorough understanding of the conditions listed in Box 370–4. Cytologic evaluation of sputum, if available, may be helpful. Chest CT often provides more precise anatomic detail concerning the infiltrate. Bronchoscopy is indicated for detect-ing foreign bodies, congenital or acquired anomalies of the tracheobronchial tract, and obstruction by endobronchial or extrinsic masses. Bronchoscopy provides access to secretions that can be studied cytologically and microbiologically. Alveolar lavage fluid is diagnostic for alveolar proteinosis and persistent pulmonary hemosiderosis and may suggest aspiration syndromes. If all appropriate studies have been completed and the condition remains undiagnosed, lung biopsy may yield a definitive diagnosis.

Optimal medical or surgical treatment of chronic lung infiltrates frequently depends on a specific diagnosis, but chronic conditions may be self-limiting (e.g., severe and prolonged viral infections in infants); in these cases, symptomatic therapy may maintain adequate lung function until spontaneous improvement occurs. Helpful measures include inhalation and physical therapy for excessive secretions, antibiotics for bacterial infections, supplementary oxygen for hypoxemia, and maintenance of adequate nutrition. Because the lung of a young child has remarkable recuperative potential, normal lung function may ultimately be achieved with treatment despite the severity of pulmonary insult occurring during infancy or early childhood.

Anderson VM, Haesoon L: Lymphocytic interstitial pneumonitis in pediatric AIDS. *Pediatr Pathol* 1988;8:417.

Blager F, Gay M, Wood R: Voice therapy techniques adapted to treatment of habit cough: A pilot study. *J Commun Disord* 1988;21:393.

Holberg CJ, Wright AL, Martinez FD, et al: Child day care, smoking by caregivers, and lower respiratory tract illness in the first 3 years of life. *Pediatrics* 1993;91:885.

Irwin RS, Madison JM: The diagnosis and treatment of cough. *N Engl J Med* 2000;343:1715.

Lokshin B, Lindgren S, Weinberger M, et al: Outcome of habit cough in children treated with a brief session of suggestion therapy. *Ann Allergy* 1991;67:579.

Mamlock R: A cost-effective approach to the diagnosis and treatment of the wheezing infant. *Allergy Asthma Proc* 1997;18:149.

Mancuso RF: Stridor in neonates. *Pediatr Clin North Am* 1996;43:1339.

Martinez FD, Wright AL, Taussig LM, et al: Asthma and wheezing in the first six years of life. *N Engl J Med* 1995;332:133.

Morgan WJ, Taussig LM: The child with persistent cough. *Pediatr Rev* 1987;8:249.

Orenstein SR, Orenstein DM: Gastroesophageal reflux and respiratory disease in children. *J Pediatr* 1988;112:847.

Schellhase DE, Fawcett DD, Schutze GE, et al: Clinical utility of flexible bronchoscopy and broncho-alveolar lavage in young children with recurrent wheezing. *J Pediatr* 1988;132:312.

Stagno S, Brasfield DM, Brown MB, et al: Infant pneumonitis associated with cytomegalovirus, *Chlamydia*, pneumocystis, and *Ureaplasma*: A prospective study. *Pediatrics* 1981;68:322.

Chapter 371
Acute Inflammatory Upper Airway Obstruction

Genie E. Roosevelt

General Considerations. Acute inflammation of the upper airway is of great importance in infants and small children. Airway resistance is inversely proportional to the fourth power of the radius; therefore, minor reductions in cross-sectional area due to mucosal edema or other inflammatory processes cause an exponential increase in airway resistance and a significant increase in the work of breathing. The larynx is composed of four major cartilages (epiglottic, arytenoid, thyroid, and cricoid cartilages, from superior to inferior, respectively) and the soft tissues that surround them. The cricoid cartilage encircles the airway just below the vocal cords and defines the narrowest portion of the upper airway in children younger than 10 yr of age.

Inflammation involving the vocal cords and structures inferior to the cords is called laryngitis, laryngotracheitis, or laryngotracheobronchitis, and inflammation of the structures superior to the cords (i.e., arytenoids, aryepiglottic folds ["false cords"], epiglottis) is called supraglottitis. The term *croup* refers to a heterogeneous group of mainly acute and infectious processes that are characterized by a barklike or brassy cough and may be associated with hoarseness, inspiratory stridor, and respiratory distress. Stridor is a harsh, high-pitched respiratory sound, usually inspiratory but may be biphasic, produced by turbulent airflow; it is not a diagnosis but a sign of upper airway obstruction (also see Chapter 370). Croup usually affects to some degree the larynx, trachea, and bronchi. When the involvement of the larynx is sufficient to produce symptoms,

they dominate the clinical picture over the tracheal and bronchial signs. Traditionally, a distinction has been made between spasmodic or recurrent croup and laryngotracheobronchitis. Some clinicians believe that spasmodic croup may have an allergic component and improves rapidly without treatment whereas laryngotracheobronchitis is always associated with a viral infection of the respiratory tract. Others believe that the signs and symptoms are similar enough to consider them within the spectrum of a single disease.

371.1 Infectious Upper Airway Obstruction

Etiology and Epidemiology. Viral agents account for most acute infectious upper airway obstructions. The exceptions are diphtheria, bacterial tracheitis, and epiglottitis. The parainfluenza viruses (types 1, 2, and 3) account for approximately 75% of cases; other viruses associated with this disease include influenza A and B, adenovirus, respiratory syncytial virus (RSV), and measles. Influenza A has been associated with severe laryngotracheobronchitis. *Mycoplasma pneumoniae* rarely has been isolated from children with croup and causes mild disease. Most patients with croup are between the ages of 3 mo and 5 yr, with the peak in the second year of life. The incidence of croup is higher in males, and it occurs most commonly during the winter but may occur throughout the year. Recurrences are frequent from 3–6 yr of age and decrease with growth of the airway. Approximately 15% of patients have a strong family history of croup.

In the past, *Haemophilus influenzae* type b was the most commonly identified etiology of acute epiglottitis. Since the widespread use of the HiB vaccine in the United States, invasive disease due to *H. influenzae* type b in pediatric patients has been reduced by 80–90%. Therefore, other agents, such as *Streptococcus pyogenes*, *S. pneumoniae*, and *Staphylococcus aureus*, now represent a larger proportion of pediatric cases of epiglottitis. In the pre-vaccine era, the typical patient was 2–4 yr of age, although cases were seen in the first year of life and in patients as old as 7 yr of age. Currently, the typical patient with epiglottitis is an adult with a sore throat, although cases still do occur in underimmunized children.

Clinical Manifestations

CROUP (LARYNGOTRACHEOBRONCHITIS). Primarily, viruses cause croup, the most common form of acute upper respiratory obstruction. The term *laryngotracheobronchitis* refers to this viral infection of the glottic and subglottic regions. However, some clinicians use the term *laryngotracheitis* for the most common and most typical form of croup and reserve the term laryngotracheobronchitis for the more severe form that is considered an extension of laryngotracheitis associated with bacterial superinfection that occurs 5 to 7 days into the clinical course.

Most patients have an upper respiratory tract infection with some combination of rhinorrhea, pharyngitis, mild cough, and low-grade fever for 1 to 3 days before the signs and symptoms of upper airway obstruction become apparent. The child then develops the characteristic "barking" cough, hoarseness, and inspiratory stridor. The low-grade fever may persist, although temperatures may reach 39–40°C (102.2–104°F); some children are afebrile. Symptoms are characteristically worse at night and often recur with decreasing intensity for several days and resolve completely within a week. Agitation and crying greatly aggravate the symptoms and signs. The child may prefer to sit up in bed or be held upright. Older children usually are not seriously ill. Other family members may have mild respiratory illnesses. Most patients with croup progress only as far as stridor and slight dyspnea before they start to recover.

Physical examination may reveal a hoarse voice, coryza, normal to moderately inflamed pharynx, and a slightly increased respiratory rate. Patients may vary substantially in their degree of respiratory distress. Rarely, the upper airway obstruction progresses and is accompanied by an increasing respiratory rate; nasal flaring; suprasternal, infrasternal, and intercostal retractions; and continuous stridor. Croup is a disease of the upper airway, and alveolar gas exchange is usually normal. Hypoxia and low oxygen saturation are seen only when complete airway obstruction is imminent. The child who is hypoxic, cyanotic, pale, or obtunded needs immediate airway management. Occasionally, the pattern of severe laryngotracheobronchitis may be difficult to differentiate from epiglottitis despite the usually more acute onset and rapid course of the latter.

Croup is a clinical diagnosis and does not require a radiograph of the neck. Radiographs of the neck may show the typical subglottic narrowing or "steeple sign" of croup on the posteroanterior view (Fig. 371–1). However, the "steeple sign" may be absent in patients with croup, may be present in patients without croup as a normal variant, and may be present in patients with epiglottitis. In addition, the radiographs do not correlate well with disease severity. Radiographs should be considered only after airway stabilization in children who have an atypical presentation or clinical course. Radiographs may be helpful in distinguishing between severe laryngotracheobronchitis and epiglottitis, but airway management should always take priority.

ACUTE EPIGLOTTITIS (SUPRAGLOTTITIS). This dramatic, potentially lethal condition is characterized by an acute fulminating course of high fever, sore throat, dyspnea, and rapidly progressing respiratory obstruction. The degree of respiratory distress at presentation is variable. The initial lack of respiratory distress may deceive the unwary clinician, although respiratory distress may be the first manifestation. Often the otherwise healthy child suddenly develops a sore throat and fever. Within a matter of hours, the patient appears toxic, swallowing is difficult, and breathing is labored. Drooling is usually present and the neck is hyperextended in an attempt to maintain the airway. The child may assume the tripod position sitting upright and leaning forward with the chin up and mouth open while bracing on the arms. A brief period of air hunger with restlessness may be followed by rapidly increasing

cyanosis and coma. Stridor is a late finding and suggests near-complete airway obstruction. Complete obstruction of the airway and death may ensue unless adequate treatment is provided. The barking cough typical of croup is rare. Usually no other family members are ill with acute respiratory symptoms.

The *diagnosis* requires visualization of a large, "cherry-red" swollen epiglottis by laryngoscopy. Occasionally, the other supraglottic structures, especially the aryepiglottic folds, may be more involved than the epiglottis itself. In a patient in whom the diagnosis is certain or probable based on clinical grounds, laryngoscopy should be performed expeditiously in a controlled environment such as an operating room or intensive care unit depending on the institution. Anxiety provoking interventions such as phlebotomy, intravenous line placement, placing the child supine, or direct inspection of the oral cavity should be avoided until the airway is secure. If epiglottitis is thought to be possible, although not probable, in a patient with acute upper airway obstruction, the patient may undergo lateral radiographs of the upper airway first. Classic radiographs of a child who has epiglottitis show the "thumb sign" (Fig. 371–2). If the concern for epiglottitis still exists after the radiographs, visualization should be performed as described previously. Regardless, a physician skilled in airway management and use of intubation equipment should accompany patients with suspected epiglottitis at all times. Occasionally, an older cooperative child may voluntarily open the mouth wide enough for a direct view of the inflamed epiglottis.

Establishing an airway by nasotracheal intubation or, less often, by tracheostomy is indicated in patients with epiglottitis, regardless of the degree of apparent respiratory distress, because as many as 6% of children with epiglottitis without an artificial airway die, compared with less than 1% of those with an artificial airway. No clinical features have been recognized that predict mortality. Pulmonary edema may be associated with acute airway obstruction. The duration of intubation depends on the clinical course of the patient and the duration of epiglottic swelling, as determined by frequent examination using direct laryngoscopy or flexible fiberoptic laryngoscopy. In general, children with acute epiglottitis are intubated for 2–3 days, because the response to antibiotics is usually rapid (see later). Most patients have concomitant bacteremia; occasionally, other infections may be present, such as pneumonia, cervical adenopathy, or otitis media. Meningitis, arthritis, and other invasive infections with *H. influenzae* type b are rarely found in conjunction with epiglottitis.

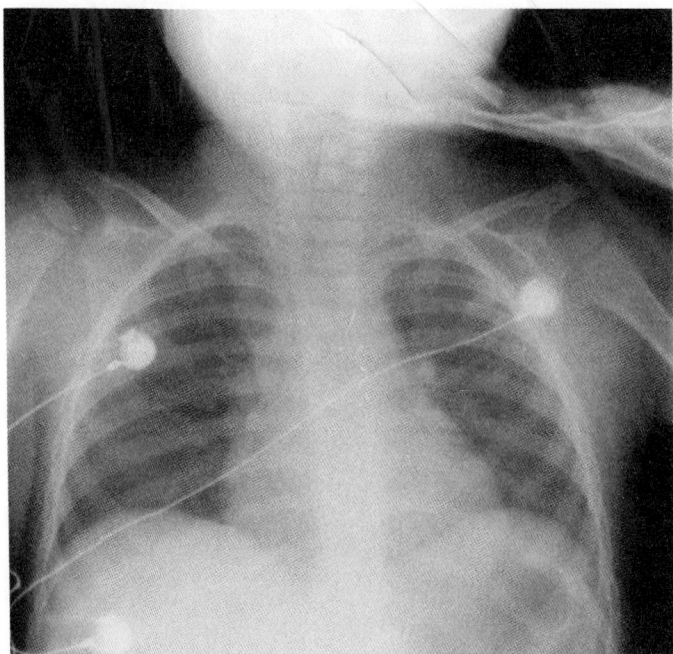

FIGURE 371–1. Radiograph of an airway of a patient with croup, showing typical subglottic narrowing ("steeple sign").

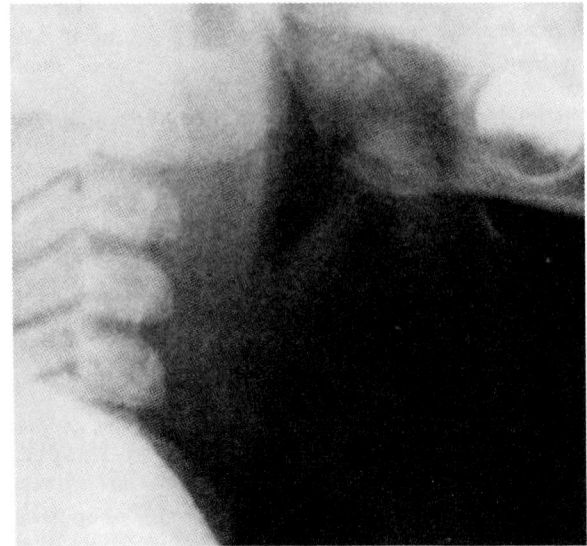

FIGURE 371–2. Epiglottitis. Lateral roentgenogram of the upper airway reveals the swollen epiglottis ("thumb sign").

ACUTE INFECTIOUS LARYNGITIS. Laryngitis is a common illness; viruses cause most cases; diphtheria is an exception but is extremely rare in developed countries. The onset is usually characterized by an upper respiratory tract infection during which sore throat, cough, and hoarseness appear. The illness is generally mild; respiratory distress is unusual except in the young infant. Hoarseness and loss of voice may be out of proportion to systemic signs and symptoms. The physical examination is usually not remarkable except for evidence of pharyngeal inflammation. Inflammatory edema of the vocal cords and subglottic tissue may be demonstrated laryngoscopically. The principal site of obstruction is usually the subglottic area.

SPASMODIC CROUP. Spasmodic croup occurs most often in children 1–3 yr of age and is clinically similar to acute laryngotracheobronchitis, except that the history of a viral prodrome and fever in the patient and family are frequently absent. The cause is viral in some cases, but allergic and psychological factors may be important in others. Laryngoscopy reveals pale, watery edema with preservation of the epithelium (unlike the erythematous edema and destruction of the epithelium of acute infectious laryngotracheobronchitis).

Occurring most frequently in the evening or nighttime, spasmodic croup begins with a sudden onset that may be preceded by mild to moderate coryza and hoarseness. The child awakens with a characteristic barking, metallic cough, noisy inspiration, and respiratory distress and appears anxious and frightened. The patient is usually afebrile. Usually, the severity of the symptoms diminishes within several hours and, the following day, the patient often appears well except for slight hoarseness and cough. Similar, but usually less severe, attacks without extreme respiratory distress may occur for another night or two. Such episodes often recur several times. Spasmodic croup may represent more of an allergic reaction to viral antigens than direct infection, although the pathogenesis is unknown.

Differential Diagnosis. These four syndromes must be differentiated from one another and from a variety of other entities that may present as upper airway obstruction. *Bacterial tracheitis* is the most important differential diagnostic consideration. **Diphtheritic croup** is extremely rare in North America, although a major epidemic of diphtheria occurred in countries of the former Soviet Union beginning in 1990 from the lack of routine immunization of adults (see Chapter 172). Early symptoms include malaise, sore throat, anorexia, and low-grade fever. Within 2–3 days, pharyngeal examination reveals the typical gray-white membrane, which may vary in size from covering a small patch on the tonsils to covering most of the soft palate. The membrane is adherent to the tissue, and forcible attempts to remove it cause bleeding. The course is usually insidious, but respiratory obstruction may occur suddenly. *Measles croup* almost always coincides with the full manifestations of systemic disease and the course may be fulminant (see Chapter 225).

Sudden onset of respiratory obstruction may be caused by *aspiration of a foreign body* (see Chapter 373). The child is usually 6 mo to 2 yr of age. Choking and coughing occur suddenly, usually without prodromal signs of infection, although children with a viral infection can also aspirate a foreign body. A *retropharyngeal or peritonsillar abscess* may mimic respiratory obstruction (see Chapter 367). Radiographs of the upper airway and chest are essential in evaluating these possibilities. Other possible causes of upper airway obstruction include *extrinsic compression* of the airway (e.g., laryngeal web, vascular ring) and *intraluminal obstruction* from masses (e.g., laryngeal papilloma, subglottic hemangioma).

Upper airway obstruction is occasionally associated with angioedema of the subglottic areas as part of anaphylaxis and generalized allergic reactions, edema after endotracheal intubation for general anesthesia or respiratory failure, *hypocalcemic tetany, infectious mononucleosis*, trauma, and tumors or malforma-

tions of the larynx. A croupy cough may be an early sign of asthma. Vocal cord dysfunction can also occur. Epiglottitis, with the characteristic manifestations of drooling or dysphagia and stridor, can also result from the accidental ingestion of very hot liquid.

Complications. Complications occur in approximately 15% of patients with viral croup. The most common is extension of the infectious process to involve other regions of the respiratory tract, such as the middle ear, the terminal bronchioles, or the pulmonary parenchyma. Bacterial tracheitis may be a complication of viral croup rather than a distinct disease. Pneumonia, cervical lymphadenitis, otitis media, or, rarely, meningitis or septic arthritis may occur during the course of epiglottitis. Mediastinal emphysema and pneumothorax are the most common complications of tracheotomy.

Treatment. The mainstay of treatment for children with **croup** is airway management. Treatment of the respiratory distress should take priority over any testing. However, most children with either acute spasmodic croup or infectious croup can be managed at home safely. Mist was first used in the 19th century when physicians anecdotally witnessed an improvement in the symptoms of croup with the steam from teapots and hot tubs. Given the risk of burns and the observation that cold night air is also beneficial led to the use of *cool mist*. The proposed mechanisms to explain the beneficial effect of cool mist are that it (1) moistens airway secretions to facilitate clearance, (2) soothes inflamed mucosa, and (3) provides comfort and reassurance to the child, lessening any anxiety. Two studies tested the efficacy of moist air in patients with croup. Neither study showed a beneficial effect, although the sample sizes were small. In a study comparing nebulized saline placebo to racemic epinephrine, croup scores significantly improved after the administration of the placebo, although there was no control group. Improvement may be explained by spontaneous recovery with time. Current recommendations are to provide cool mist through a tube held in front of the patient by the parent. Children with both wheezing and croup concomitantly may experience worsening of their bronchospasm with cool mist.

The marked decrease in the need for tracheotomies in **croup** has been attributed to the use of *nebulized epinephrine*. Although initially used with intermittent positive pressure ventilation, subsequent studies showed effectiveness with simple nebulization. The mechanism of action is believed to be constriction of the precapillary arterioles through the α-adrenergic receptors causing fluid resorption from the interstitial space and a decrease in the laryngeal mucosal edema. Traditionally, racemic epinephrine, a 1:1 mixture of the *d*- and *l*-isomers of epinephrine, has been administered. A dose of 0.25 to 0.75 mL of 2.25% racemic epinephrine in 3 mL of normal saline can be used as often as every 20 min. Racemic epinephrine was initially chosen over the more active and more readily available *l*-epinephrine to minimize anticipated cardiovascular side effects such as tachycardia and hypertension. However, there is evidence that *l*-epinephrine (5 mL of 1:1,000 solution) is equally effective as racemic epinephrine and does not carry the risk of additional adverse effects. This information is both practical and important, because racemic epinephrine is not available outside the United States.

The indications for the administration of nebulized epinephrine include moderate to severe stridor at rest, the need for intubation, respiratory distress, hypoxia, and when stridor does not respond to cool mist. The duration of activity of racemic epinephrine is less than 2 hr. The symptoms of croup may reappear, but racemic epinephrine does not cause rebound worsening of the obstruction. Therefore, observation is mandated. Patients may be safely discharged home after a 2–3 hr period of observation provided they have no stridor at rest, normal air entry, normal color, and normal level of consciousness and have received steroids (see later). Nebulized epinephrine should still be used cautiously in patients with tachycardia, heart conditions such as tetralogy of Fallot, or ventricular outlet obstruction because of possible side effects.

After several decades of debate about the effectiveness of corticosteroids in viral croup, there is now clear evidence of their benefit. *Corticosteroids* decrease the edema in the laryngeal mucosa through their anti-inflammatory action. Studies have demonstrated that steroids are beneficial, as measured by reduced hospitalization, shorter duration of hospitalization, and reduced need for subsequent interventions such as epinephrine administration. Most studies that demonstrated the efficacy of dexamethasone used a single dose of 0.6 mg/kg; however, there is some evidence that a dose as low as 0.15 mg/kg may be just as effective. Intramuscular dexamethasone and nebulized budesonide have an equivalent clinical effect, and oral dosing of dexamethasone is as effective as intramuscular administration. The only adverse effect described in the treatment of croup with corticosteroids was the development of *Candida albicans* laryngotracheitis in a patient who received dexamethasone, 1 mg/kg/24 hr, for 8 days. Corticosteroids should not be administered to children with varicella or tuberculosis (unless the patient is receiving appropriate anti-tuberculosis therapy) because they worsen the clinical course.

Antibiotics are not indicated in croup. Preliminary studies with a helium-oxygen mixture (Heliox) have shown similar clinical improvements in children with croup when compared with responses in children given racemic epinephrine.

Children with croup should be *hospitalized* for any of the following: progressive stridor, severe stridor at rest, respiratory distress, hypoxia, cyanosis, depressed mental status, or the need for reliable observation.

Epiglottitis is a medical emergency and warrants immediate treatment with an *artificial airway* placed under controlled conditions, either in an operating room or intensive care unit. All patients should receive *oxygen* en route unless the mask causes excessive agitation. Racemic epinephrine and corticosteroids are ineffective. Cultures of blood, epiglottic surface, and, in selected cases, cerebrospinal fluid, should be collected at the time of airway stabilization. *Ceftriaxone, cefotaxime,* or a combination of ampicillin and sulbactam should be given parenterally pending culture and susceptibility reports because from 10–40% of *H. influenzae* type b cases are resistant to ampicillin. After insertion of the artificial airway, the patient should improve immediately, and respiratory distress and cyanosis should disappear. Epiglottitis resolves after a few days of antibiotics, and the patient may be extubated; antibiotics should be continued for 7–10 days. Chemoprophylaxis is not recommended for household contacts of patients with invasive *H. influenzae* type b infections unless there is a child younger than 48 mo in the home who has not completed the HiB immunization series. Rifampin prophylaxis (20 mg/kg orally once a day for 4 days; maximum dose, 600 mg) should be given to all household members if there is one contact younger than 48 mo of age who is incompletely immunized or if there is an immunocompromised child in the household.

Acute laryngeal swelling on an *allergic basis* responds to epinephrine (1:1,000 dilution in dosage of 0.01 mL/kg to a maximum of 0.5 mL/dose) administered subcutaneously or racemic epinephrine (dose of 0.25–0.75 mL of 2.25% racemic epinephrine in 3 mL of normal saline). Corticosteroids are frequently required (2–4 mg/kg/24 hr of prednisone). After recovery, the patient and parents should be discharged with a preloaded syringe of epinephrine to be used in emergencies. Reactive mucosal swelling, severe stridor, and respiratory distress unresponsive to mist therapy may follow *endotracheal intubation* for general anesthesia in children. Racemic epinephrine and corticosteroids are helpful.

TRACHEOTOMY AND ENDOTRACHEAL INTUBATION (see Chapter 57.1). With the introduction of routine nasotracheal intubation or tracheotomy for epiglottitis, the mortality rate has dropped to almost zero. Both procedures should always be performed in an operating room or intensive care unit if time permits; prior intubation and general anesthesia greatly facilitate performing a tracheotomy without complications. The use of a nasotracheal tube that is 0.5–1.0 mm smaller than estimated by age is recommended to facilitate intubation and reduce long-term sequelae. The choice of procedure should be based on the local expertise and experience with the procedure and the postoperative care involved with each.

Endotracheal intubation or tracheotomy is required for all patients with epiglottitis, but for patients with laryngotracheobronchitis, spasmodic croup, or laryngitis, it is rarely required. Severe forms of laryngotracheobronchitis that require tracheotomy in a high proportion of patients have been reported during severe measles and influenza A virus epidemics. Assessing the need for these procedures requires experience and judgment because they should not be delayed until cyanosis and extreme restlessness have developed (see Chapters 55, 57.3, and 58).

The endotracheal tube or tracheostomy must remain in place until edema and spasm have subsided and the patient is able to handle secretions satisfactorily. It should be removed as soon as possible, usually within a few days. Adequate resolution of epiglottic inflammation that has been accurately confirmed by fiberoptic laryngoscopy, permitting much more rapid extubation, often occurs within 24 hr. Racemic epinephrine and dexamethasone (0.5 mg/kg/dose every 6 hr as needed) may be useful in the treatment of croup associated with extubation.

Prognosis. In general, the length of hospitalization and the mortality rate for cases of acute infectious upper airway obstruction increase as the infection extends to involve a greater portion of the respiratory tract, except in epiglottitis, in which the localized infection itself may prove to be fatal. Most deaths from croup are caused by a laryngeal obstruction or by the complications of tracheotomy. Untreated epiglottitis has a mortality rate of 6% in some series, but if the diagnosis is made and appropriate treatment is initiated before the patient is moribund, the prognosis is excellent. The outcome of acute laryngotracheobronchitis, laryngitis, and spasmodic croup is also excellent. As a group, children who need to be hospitalized for croup have somewhat increased bronchial reactivity compared with normal children when tested several years later but the significance is uncertain.

Laryngotracheobronchitis

Fogel JM, Berg IJ, Gerber MA, et al: Racemic epinephrine in the treatment of croup: Nebulization alone versus nebulization with intermittent positive pressure breathing. *J Pediatr* 1982;101:1028–31.

Geelhoed GC, Turner J, MacDonald WB: Efficacy of a small single dose of oral dexamethasone for outpatient croup: A double blind placebo controlled trial. *BMJ* 1996;313:140–42.

Johnson DW, Jacobson S, Edney PC, et al: A comparison of nebulized budesonide, intramuscular dexamethasone, and placebo for moderately severe croup. *N Engl J Med* 1998;339:498–503.

Klassen TP, Craig WR, Moher D, et al: Nebulized budesonide and oral dexamethasone for treatment of croup: A randomized controlled trial. *JAMA* 1998;279:1629–32.

Kristjansson S, Berg-Kelly K, Winso E: Inhalation of racemic adrenaline in the treatment of mild and moderately severe croup: Clinical symptom score and oxygen saturation measurements for evaluation of treatment effects. *Acta Pediatr* 1994;83:1156–60.

Ledwith CA, Shea LM, Mauro RD: Safety and efficacy of nebulized racemic epinephrine in conjunction with oral dexamethasone and mist in the outpatient treatment of croup. *Ann Emerg Med* 1995;25:331–337.

Luria JW, Gonzalez-del-Rey JA, DiBiulio GA, et al: Effectiveness of oral or nebulized dexamethasone for children with mild croup. *Pediatr Adolesc Med* 2001;155:1340–45.

Rittichier KK, Ledwith CA: Outpatient treatment of moderate croup with dexamethasone: Intramuscular versus oral dosing. *Pediatrics* 2000;106:1344–48.

Waisman Y, Klein BL, Boenning DA, et al: Prospective randomized double-blind study comparing L-epinephrine and racemic epinephrine aerosols in the treatment of laryngotracheitis. *Pediatrics* 1992;89:302–6.

Walner DL, Ouanounou S, Donnelly LF, et al: Utility of radiographs in the evaluation of pediatric upper airway obstruction. *Ann Otol Rhinol Laryngol* 1999;108:378–83.

Weber JE, Chudnofsky CR, Younger JG, et al: A randomized comparison of helium-oxygen mixture (Heliox) and racemic epinephrine for the treatment of moderate to severe croup. *Pediatrics* 2001;107:E96.

Epiglottitis

Adams WG, Deaver KA, Cochi SL, et al: Decline in childhood *Haemophilus influenzae* type b (HiB) in the HiB vaccine era. *JAMA* 1993;269:221–26.

Frantz TD, Rasgon BM: Acute epiglottitis: Changing epidemiologic patterns. *Otolaryngol Head Neck Surg* 1993;109:457–60.

Gorelick MH, Baker MD: Epiglottitis in children, 1979 through 1992: Effects of *Haemophilus influenzae* type b immunization. *Arch Pediatr Adolesc Med* 1994;148:47–50.

Hickerson SL, Kirby RS, Wheeler JG, et al: Epiglottitis: A 9-year case review. *South Med J* 1996;89:487–90.

Kulick RM, Selbst SM, Baker MD, et al: Thermal epiglottitis after swallowing hot beverages. *Pediatrics* 1988;81:441–44.

Murrage KJ, Janzen VD, Ruby RR: Epiglottitis: Adult and pediatric comparisons. *J Otolaryngol* 1988;17:194–98.

Schuller DE, Birck HG: The safety of intubation in croup and epiglottitis: An eight-year follow-up. *Laryngoscope* 1975;85:33–46.

Senior BA, Radkowski D, MacArthur C, et al: Changing patterns in pediatric epiglottis: A multi-institutional review, 1980 to 1992. *Laryngoscope* 1994;104:1314–22.

371.2 Bacterial Tracheitis

Bacterial tracheitis, an acute bacterial infection of the upper airway, does not involve the epiglottitis but, like epiglottitis and croup, is capable of causing life-threatening airway obstruction. *Staphylococcus aureus* is the most commonly isolated pathogen. *Moraxella catarrhalis*, nontypable *H. influenzae*, and anaerobic organisms have also been implicated. Most patients are younger than 3 yr of age, although older children may be affected. There are no clear sex differences in incidence or severity. Bacterial tracheitis often follows a viral respiratory infection (especially laryngotracheitis) so it may be considered a bacterial complication of a viral disease, rather than a primary bacterial illness. This life-threatening entity is now more common than epiglottitis.

Clinical Manifestations. Typically, the child has a brassy cough, apparently as part of a viral laryngotracheobronchitis. High fever and "toxicity" with respiratory distress may occur immediately or after a few days of apparent improvement. The patient with bacterial tracheitis can lie flat, does not drool, and does not have the dysphagia associated with epiglottitis. The usual treatment for croup (e.g., mist, racemic epinephrine) is ineffective. Intubation or tracheostomy may be necessary. The major pathologic feature appears to be mucosal swelling at the level of the cricoid cartilage, complicated by copious thick, purulent secretions, sometimes causing pseudomembranes. Suctioning these secretions, although occasionally affording temporary relief, usually does not sufficiently obviate the need for an artificial airway.

Diagnosis. The diagnosis is based on evidence of bacterial upper airway disease, which includes high fever, purulent airway secretions, and an absence of the classic findings of epiglottitis.

Treatment. Appropriate antimicrobial therapy, which usually includes antistaphylococcal agents, should be instituted in any patient whose course suggests bacterial tracheitis. When bacterial tracheitis is diagnosed by direct laryngoscopy or is strongly suspected on clinical grounds, an artificial airway is indicated. Supplemental oxygen may be necessary.

Complications. Chest radiographs often show patchy infiltrates and may show focal densities. Subglottic narrowing and a rough and ragged tracheal air column can often be demonstrated radiographically. If airway management is not optimal, cardiorespiratory arrest can occur. Toxic shock syndrome has been associated with tracheitis (see Chapter 166.2).

Prognosis. The prognosis for most patients is excellent. Patients usually become afebrile within 2–3 days of the institution of

appropriate antimicrobial therapy, but prolonged hospitalization may be necessary. With a decrease in mucosal edema and purulent secretions, extubation can be accomplished safely, and the patient should be observed carefully while antibiotics and oxygen therapy are continued.

Berstein T, Brilli R, Jacobs B: Is bacterial tracheitis changing? A 14-month experience in a pediatric intensive care unit. *Clin Infect Dis* 1998;27:458–62.

Brook I: Aerobic and anerobic microbiology of bacterial tracheitis in children. *Pediatr Emerg Care* 1997;13:16–18.

Eckel HE, Wideman B, Damm M, et al: Airway endoscopy in the diagnosis and treatment of bacterial tracheitis in children. *Int J Pediatr Otorhinolaryngol* 1993;27:147–57.

Chapter 372

Congenital Anomalies of the Larynx *Lauren D. Holinger*

Because the larynx functions as a breathing passage, a valve to protect the lungs, and the primary organ of communication, symptoms of laryngeal anomalies are those of airway obstruction, difficulty feeding, and abnormalities of phonation.

With airway obstruction, the severity of the obstructing lesion determines the necessity for diagnostic procedures and surgical intervention. Obstructive symptoms vary from mild stridor to severe obstruction, with episodes of apnea, cyanosis, suprasternal (tracheal tugging) and subcostal retractions, dyspnea, and tachypnea. Chronic obstruction may cause failure to thrive.

372.1 Laryngomalacia

Laryngomalacia is the most common congenital laryngeal anomaly and the most frequent cause of stridor in infants and children. Of congenital laryngeal anomalies in children with stridor, 60% are caused by laryngomalacia. Typically, stridor is inspiratory, low pitched, and exacerbated by any exertion (i.e., crying, agitation, feeding). Stridor results from the collapse of supraglottic structures inward during inspiration. Symptoms usually appear within the first 2 wk of life and increase in severity for up to 6 mo, although gradual improvement may begin at any time. Laryngopharyngeal reflux is commonly associated with laryngomalacia.

The diagnosis is confirmed by flexible laryngoscopy in the office. When the work of breathing is moderate to severe, airway films and chest radiographs are indicated. With associated dysphagia, a contrast swallow study and esophagogram may be indicated. Because 15–60% of infants with laryngomalacia have synchronous airway anomalies, complete bronchoscopy is undertaken for patients with moderate to severe obstruction.

Expectant observation is suitable for most infants because most symptoms resolve spontaneously. Laryngopharyngeal reflux is managed aggressively. For those few patients who have such severe obstruction that surgical intervention is unavoidable—patients with apparent life-threatening events, cor pulmonale, cyanosis, failure to thrive—endoscopic supraglottoplasty can be used to avoid tracheotomy.

372.2 Congenital Subglottic Stenosis

Congenital subglottic stenosis is the second most common cause of stridor. Stridor is biphasic or primarily inspiratory. Recurrent or persistent croup is typical. First symptoms often occur with a respiratory tract infection as edema and thickened secretions of a common cold narrow an already compromised airway.

The diagnosis made by airway radiographs is confirmed by direct laryngoscopy. As with all cases of upper airway obstruction, tracheostomy is avoided when possible. Dilation and endoscopic laser surgery are rarely effective because most congenital stenoses are cartilaginous. Anterior laryngotracheal decompression (cricoid split) or laryngotracheal reconstruction with cartilage grafting is usually effective in avoiding tracheostomy (also see Chapter 374).

372.3 Vocal Cord Paralysis

Vocal cord paralysis is the third most common congenital laryngeal anomaly producing stridor in infants and children. Congenital central lesions such as myelomeningocele, Arnold-Chiari malformation, and hydrocephalus are often associated. Paralysis may occur as a result of surgical correction of congenital cardiac anomalies or tracheoesophageal fistula.

Bilateral vocal cord paralysis typically produces airway obstruction manifested by high-pitched inspiratory stridor: a phonatory sound or inspiratory cry. Unilateral paralysis causes aspiration, coughing, and choking. The cry is weak and breathy, but stridor and other symptoms of airway obstruction are less common.

The diagnosis of vocal cord paralysis is made by awake flexible laryngoscopy. A thorough investigation for the underlying cause is indicated. Because of the association with other congenital lesions, evaluation includes neurology and cardiology consultations as well as diagnostic endoscopy of the larynx, trachea, and bronchi.

Vocal cord paralysis in infants usually resolves spontaneously within 6–12 mo. Bilateral paralysis may require temporary tracheotomy. For unilateral vocal cord paralysis with aspiration, the paralyzed vocal cord is injected laterally so that it touches the now paralyzed cord medially, reducing aspiration and related complications.

372.4 Congenital Laryngeal Webs and Atresia

Most congenital laryngeal webs are glottic with subglottic extension and associated subglottic stenosis. The cry may be high pitched. Airway obstruction is not always present and may be related to the subglottic stenosis. Thick webs may be suspected in lateral radiographs of the airway. Diagnosis is made by direct laryngoscopy. Treatment may require only incision or dilation. Webs with associated subglottic stenosis are likely to require cartilage augmentation of the cricoid (laryngotracheal reconstruction).

Laryngeal atresia occurs as a complete glottic web and commonly is associated with tracheal agenesis and tracheoesophageal fistula. It is not compatible with long-term survival.

372.5 Congenital Subglottic Hemangioma

See Chapter 377.3.

372.6 Laryngoceles and Saccular Cysts

A laryngocele is an abnormal air-filled dilation of the laryngeal saccule. It communicates with the laryngeal lumen and, when intermittently filled with air, causes hoarseness and dyspnea. A saccular cyst (congenital cyst of the larynx) is distinguished from the laryngocele in that its lumen is isolated from the interior of the larynx and it contains mucus, not air. A saccular cyst may be visible on radiography, but the diagnosis is made by laryngoscopy. Needle aspiration of the cyst confirms the diagnosis but rarely provides a cure. Endoscopic CO_2 laser excision may suffice, but external excision is often necessary.

372.7 Posterior Laryngeal Cleft and Laryngotracheoesophageal Cleft

The rare posterior laryngeal cleft (PLC) is characterized by deficiency in the midline of the posterior larynx. In severe cases the cleft extends inferiorly into the cervical or thoracic trachea so there is no separation between the trachea and esophagus—laryngotracheoesophageal cleft (LTEC). Laryngeal clefts may occur in families and are likely to be associated with tracheal agenesis, tracheoesophageal fistula, and multiple congenital anomalies, as with G syndrome, Opitz-Frias syndrome, and Pallister-Hall syndrome.

Initial symptoms are those of aspiration and respiratory difficulties. The cry may be weak or absent. An esophagogram is done with extreme caution. Confirmation of the diagnosis is made by direct laryngoscopy and bronchoscopy. Stabilization of the airway is the first priority. Gastroesophageal reflux must be controlled, and a careful assessment for other congenital anomalies should be undertaken.

Belmont JR, Grundfast K: Congenital laryngeal stridor (laryngomalacia): Etiologic factors, associated disorders. *Ann Otol Rhinol Laryngol* 1984;93:430.

Civantos FJ, Holinger LD: Laryngoceles and saccular cysts in infants and children. *Arch Otolaryngol Head Neck Surg* 1992;118:296.

Gonzalez C, Riley JS, Bluestone CD: Synchronous airway lesions in infancy. *Ann Otol Rhinol Laryngol* 1987;96:77.

Holinger LD: Etiology of stridor in the neonate, infant, and child. *Ann Otol Rhinol Laryngol* 1980;89:397–400.

Holinger LD: Histopathology of congenital subglottic stenosis. *Ann Otol Rhinol Laryngol* 1999;108:101–11.

Holinger LD, Konior RJ: Surgical management of severe laryngomalacia. *Laryngoscope* 1989;99:136.

Hughes CA, Rezaee A, Ludemann JP, et al: Management of congenital subglottic hemangioma. *J Otolaryngol* 1999;28:223–28.

Manroudis C, Holinger LD: Laryngotracheoesophageal clefts. *Ann Otol Rhinol Laryngol* 1997;106:1002–11.

Myers CM III, O'Connor DM, Cotton RT: Proposed grading system for subglottic stenosis based on endotracheal tube size. *Ann Otol Rhinol Laryngol* 1994;108:319.

Chapter 373

Foreign Bodies of the Airway *Lauren D. Holinger*

Epidemiology and Etiology. Although there has been a decrease in childhood deaths from asphyxiation by ingested objects, the incidence of foreign body aspiration has not changed significantly and is unlikely to do so as long as children continue to use their mouths to explore their surroundings. Most victims of foreign body aspiration are older infants and toddlers. Children younger than 3 yr of age account for 73% of cases. One third of aspirated objects are nuts, particularly peanuts. Fragments of raw carrot, apple, dried beans, popcorn, and sunflower or watermelon seeds are also common.

Clinical Manifestations. A positive history must never be ignored. A negative history may be misleading. Choking or coughing episodes accompanied by wheezing are highly suggestive of an airway foreign body. Because nuts are the most common bronchial foreign body, the physician specifically questions the toddler's parents about nuts. If there is any history of eating nuts, bronchoscopy is carried out promptly.

The most serious complication of foreign body aspiration is complete obstruction of the airway. Globular food objects such as hot dogs, grapes, nuts, and candies are the most frequent offenders. Hot dogs are rarely seen as airway foreign bodies because toddlers who choke on hot dogs asphyxiate on the spot unless treated immediately. Complete airway obstruction is recognized in the conscious child as sudden respiratory distress followed by inability to speak or cough.

Three stages of symptoms result from aspiration of an object into the airway:

1. Initial Event: Violent paroxysms of coughing, choking, gagging, and possibly airway obstruction occur immediately when the foreign body is aspirated.

2. Asymptomatic Interval: The foreign body becomes lodged, reflexes fatigue, and the immediate irritating symptoms subside. This stage is most treacherous and accounts for a large percentage of delayed diagnoses and overlooked foreign bodies. It is during this second stage that the physician may minimize the possibility of a foreign body accident, being reassured by the absence of symptoms that no foreign body is present.

3. Complications: In this third stage, obstruction, erosion, or infection develops to again direct attention to the presence of a foreign body. Complications include fever, cough, hemoptysis, pneumonia, and atelectasis.

Treatment. The treatment of choice for airway foreign bodies is prompt endoscopic removal with rigid instruments. Bronchoscopy is deferred only until preoperative studies have been obtained and the patient has been prepared by adequate hydration and emptying of the stomach. Airway foreign bodies are usually removed the same day the diagnosis is first considered (also see Chapter 57.1).

373.1 Laryngeal Foreign Bodies

Complete obstruction asphyxiates the child unless promptly relieved with the Heimlich maneuver (see Chapter 57.1).

Objects that are partially obstructive are usually flat and thin. They lodge between the vocal cords in the saggital plane, causing symptoms of croup, hoarseness, cough, stridor, and dyspnea.

373.2 Tracheal Foreign Bodies

Choking and aspiration occurs in 90% of patients with tracheal foreign bodies, stridor in 60%, and wheezing in 50%. Posteroanterior and lateral soft tissue neck radiographs (airway films) are abnormal in 92% of children, whereas chest radiographs are abnormal in only 58%.

373.3 Bronchial Foreign Bodies

Posteroanterior and lateral chest radiographs are indicated for the assessment of infants and children suspected of having aspirated a foreign object. The abdomen should be included in the field. During expiration the bronchial foreign body obstructs the exit of air from the obstructed lung, producing obstructive emphysema (air trapping) with persistent inflation of the obstructed lung and shift of the mediastinum toward the opposite side (Fig. 373–1). Air trapping is an immediate complication, in contrast to atelectasis, which is a late finding. Lateral decubitus chest films or fluoroscopy may provide the same information but are unnecessary. History and physical examination determine the indication for bronchoscopy.

Esclamato RN, Richardson MA: Laryngotracheal foreign bodies in children. *Am J Dis Child* 1987;41:259.

Holinger LD: Foreign bodies of the airway and esophagus. In Holinger LD, Lusk RP, Green CG (editors): *Pediatric Laryngology and Bronchoesophagology.* Philadelphia, Lippincott–Raven, 1997, pp 233–251.

Nova A, Muntz H, Clary R: Utility of conventional radiography in pediatric airway foreign bodies. *Ann Otol Rhinol Laryngol* 1998;107:834–38.

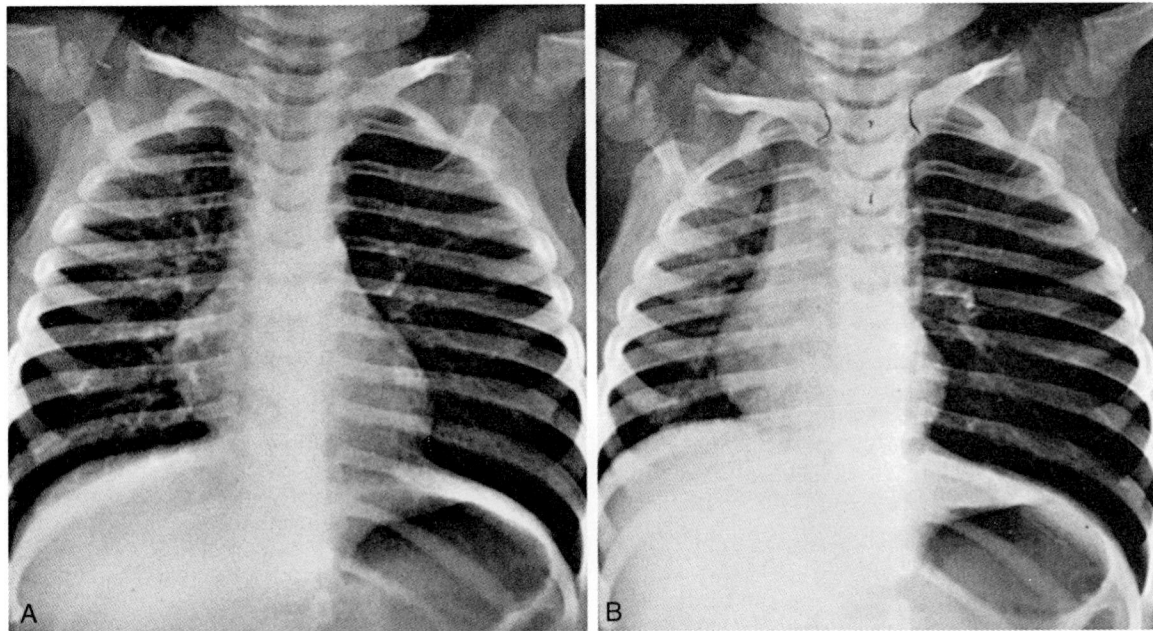

FIGURE 373–1. *A,* Normal inspiratory chest radiograph in a toddler with a peanut fragment in the left main bronchus. *B,* Expiratory radiograph of the same child showing the classic obstructive emphysema (air trapping) on the involved (left) side. Air leaves the normal right side, allowing the lung to deflate. The medium shifts toward the unobstructed side.

Chapter 374

Laryngotracheal Stenosis, Subglottic Stenosis

Lauren D. Holinger

Laryngotracheal stenosis is the most frequent cause of airway obstruction requiring tracheostomy in infants. The glottis (vocal cords) and the upper trachea are also compromised in most laryngeal stenoses, particularly those resulting from endotracheal intubation. Subglottic stenosis is considered to be congenital when there is no other apparent cause, such as a history of laryngeal trauma.

374.1 Congenital Subglottic Stenosis

See Chapter 372.2.

374.2 Acquired Laryngotracheal Stenosis

Ninety per cent of acquired stenoses are related to endotracheal intubation. When the pressure of the endotracheal tube against the mucosa is greater than the capillary pressure, ischemia occurs, followed by necrosis and ulceration. Secondary infection and perichondritis develop with exposure of cartilage. Granulation tissue forms around the ulcerations. These changes and edema throughout the larynx usually resolve spontaneously after extubation. Fortunately, chronic edema and fibrous stenosis develop in only a small percentage.

Factors that predispose to the development of laryngeal stenosis include the following:

1. Laryngopharyngeal reflux of acid and pepsin from the stomach exacerbates endotracheal tube trauma. More damage is caused in areas left unprotected, owing to loss of mucosa.

2. Congenital subglottic stenosis narrows the larynx and is more likely to be traumatized by an endotracheal tube of age-appropriate size.

3. Other patient factors include sepsis and infection, dehydration, malnutrition, chronic inflammatory disorders, and immunosuppression.

4. An oversized endotracheal tube is the most common cause of laryngeal injury. A tube that allows a small air leak at the end of the inspiratory cycle minimizes potential trauma.

5. Other extrinsic factors include traumatic intubation, multiple reintubations, movement of the endotracheal tube, and duration of intubation.

The *clinical manifestations* of acquired and congenital stenosis (see Chapter 372.2) are similar. Spasmodic croup, the sudden onset of severe croup in the early morning hours, may occur owing to an episode of laryngopharyngeal reflux with transient laryngospasm and subsequent laryngeal edema. These frightening episodes resolve rapidly, often before the family and child reach the emergency department.

The *diagnosis* is confirmed by bronchoscopy.

Treatment is based on the severity, location, and type (cartilaginous or soft tissue) of the stenosis. Mild cases can be managed without operative intervention because the airway will improve as the child grows. Moderate soft tissue stenosis is treated by endoscopy using gentle dilations or CO_2 laser. Severe laryngotracheal stenosis is likely to require laryngotracheal expansion

surgery or resection of the narrowed portion of the laryngeal and tracheal airway (cricotracheal resection). Every effort should be made to avoid tracheotomy using endoscopic techniques or open surgical procedures such as the anterior laryngotracheal decompression (cricoid split).

Benjamin B: Prolonged intubation. Injuries of the larynx: Endoscopic diagnosis, classification, and treatment. *Ann Otol Rhinol Laryngol* 1993;160(Suppl):1.

Cotton RT, Gray SD, Miller RP, et al: Update of the Cincinnati experience in pediatric laryngotracheal reconstruction. *Laryngoscope* 1989;99:1111.

Gerber M, Stern Y, Walner D, et al: Role of laryngoscopy, dual pH probe monitoring, and laryngeal mucosa biopsy in the diagnosis of pharyngoesophageal reflux. *Ann Otol Rhinol Laryngol* 2001;110:299–304.

Holinger LD, Stankiewicz JA, Livingston GL: Anterior cricoid split: The Chicago experience with an alternative to tracheotomy. *Laryngoscope* 1987;97:19.

Liu H, Chen J, Holinger L, et al: Histopathologic fundamentals of acquired laryngeal stenosis. *Pediatr Pathol Lab Med* 1995;15:55.

Chapter 375

Congenital Anomalies of the Trachea and Bronchi

Lauren D. Holinger

Congenital anomalies of the trachea, bronchi, and lungs can create serious respiratory difficulties from the first minutes of life. These intrathoracic lesions typically cause obstructive emphysema, atelectasis, or expiratory wheezing, frequently masquerading as asthma. The expiratory wheezing contrasts to the inspiratory stridor caused by extrathoracic lesions such as congenital anomalies of the larynx. See Chapter 376 for discussion of bronchomalacia and tracheomalacia.

375.1 Vascular and Cardiac Anomalies

The *aberrant innominate artery* is the most common cause of secondary tracheomalacia. Expiratory wheezing and cough occur and, rarely, reflex apnea or "dying spells." Surgical intervention is rarely necessary. Infants are treated expectantly because the problem is self-limited.

The term *vascular ring* is used to describe vascular anomalies that result from abnormal development of the aortic arch complex (see Chapter 425).

Congenital cardiac defects may compress the left main bronchus or lower trachea. Any condition that produces significant pulmonary hypertension increases the size of the pulmonary arteries, which in turn cause compression of the left main bronchus. Correction of the underlying pathology relieves the airway compression.

375.2 Tracheal Stenoses, Webs, and Atresia

Congenital soft tissue stenoses and thin webs are rare. Dilation may be all that is required. Long-segment congenital tracheal stenosis with complete tracheal rings typically presents within the first year of life, usually after a crisis has been precipitated by an acute respiratory illness. The diagnosis may be suggested by plain radiographs. CT with contrast medium enhancement delineates associated intrathoracic anomalies such as the pulmonary artery sling, which occurs in one third of patients; one fourth have associated cardiac anomalies. Bronchoscopy is the best method to define the extent of the stenosis. With an adequate airway, surgical intervention is not necessary. When the severity of obstruction dictates surgical intervention, resection of the narrowed segment and re-anastomosis will suffice for short segments. For long-segment congenital tracheal stenosis with complete tracheal rings, tracheoplasty or free tracheal autograft is undertaken with cardiopulmonary bypass.

Tracheal agenesis and atresia are rare anomalies that are incompatible with life. They are often associated with other congenital anomalies, particularly laryngeal conditions and tracheoesophageal fistula. The diagnosis is made by bronchoscopy in the newborn with severe respiratory distress.

375.3 Foregut Cysts

The bronchogenic cyst, intramural esophageal cyst (esophageal duplication), and enteric cyst may all produce symptoms of respiratory obstruction and dysphagia. The diagnosis is suspected when chest radiographs or CT scan delineate the mass and, in the case of enteric cyst, the associated vertebral anomaly. The treatment of all foregut cysts is surgical excision.

Backer CM, Mavroudis, C, Dunham ME, et al: Free tracheal autograft for long segment congenital tracheal stenosis. *J Pediatr Surg* 2000;35:813–19.
Cacciari A, Ceccarelli PL, Pilug L, et al: A series of 17 cases of congenital cystic adenoid malformation of the lung. *Eur J Pediatr Surg* 1997;7:84.
Holinger LD: Etiology of stridor in the neonate infant and child. *Ann Otol Rhinol Laryngol* 1980;89:397.
Mavroudis C, Backer CL: Vascular rings and pulmonary artery sling. In Mavroudis C, Backer CL (editors): *Pediatric Cardiac Surgery*, Chicago, Mosby, 1994 p 147.

Chapter 376
Bronchomalacia and Tracheomalacia *Jonathan D. Finder*

Chondromalacia of the trachea or of a main bronchus, in which there is insufficient cartilage to maintain the airway patency, is a common cause of persistent wheezing in infancy. Primary tracheomalacia and bronchomalacia is more common than secondary tracheomalacia and bronchomalacia, in which the chondromalacia is secondary to compression by adjacent structure (e.g., vascular ring) or to tracheoesophageal fistula. Laryngomalacia may accompany primary bronchomalacia or tracheomalacia (see also Chapter 372.1). Involvement of the entire central airway (laryngotracheobronchomalacia) is also seen.

Clinical Manifestations. Primary tracheomalacia and bronchomalacia is principally a disease of infants. The dominant finding, low-pitched wheezing, is most prominent over the central airways. When the lesion involves only one main bronchus (commonly the left), the wheezing is louder on that side, and delayed air entry can be detected with a double-headed stethoscope. In cases of tracheomalacia, the wheeze is loudest over the trachea. Hyperinflation and/or subcostal retraction do not occur unless the patient also has asthma or another cause of small airways obstruction. Thus, most patients do not improve with use of bronchodilators. It is common for β-adrenergic agents to cause worsening. Acquired tracheomalacia and bronchomalacia is seen in association with vascular rings, following repair of tracheoesophageal fistula, cardiomegaly, and after lung transplantation.

Diagnosis. Pulmonary function testing may show flattening of the flow-volume loop, but this is not a constant feature. The lesion is difficult to detect on plain radiographs, but fluoroscopy may demonstrate dynamic collapse and can avoid the need for invasive diagnostic techniques. Definitive diagnosis is by flexible bronchoscopy. Other important diagnostic modalities include MRI and CT scanning. MRI is especially useful when there is a possibility of vascular ring and should be performed when a right aortic arch is seen on plain film radiography.

Treatment. Postural drainage may help with clearance of secretions. β-adrenergic agents should be avoided, but nebulized ipratropium bromide may be useful. Endobronchial stents have been used in severely affected patients but have a high incidence of complications, ranging from airway obstruction from granulation tissue to erosion into adjacent vascular structures. Constant positive airway pressure (CPAP) or mechanical ventilation via tracheostomy may be indicated for severe cases.

Prognosis. Primary bronchomalacia and tracheomalacia has a good prognosis, because airflow improves as the airways grow. Wheezing at rest is usually gone by age 5 yr. Patients with concurrent asthma need considerable supportive treatment.

Finder JD: Primary bronchomalacia in infants and children. *J Pediatr* 1997;130:59.
Panitch HB, Keklikian EN, Motley RA, et al: Effect of altering smooth muscle tone on maximal expiratory flows in patients with tracheomalacia. *Pediatr Pulmonol* 1990;9:170.

Chapter 377
Neoplasms of the Larynx, Trachea, and Bronchi
Lauren D. Holinger

377.1 Vocal Nodules

Although vocal nodules are not true neoplasms, they are mentioned here because they are the most common cause of chronic hoarseness in children. Chronic vocal abuse or misuse produces nodules at the junction of the anterior and middle thirds of the phonating edge of the vocal cords. These symmetric, bilateral swellings interfere with voice production and cause children to strain the voice. Vocal nodules can occur in infants and are exacerbated by laryngopharyngeal reflux.

Voice therapy may be effective in the cooperative child, but for most toddlers and older children behavioral therapy is necessary. Nodules usually resolve by early teenage years as the child matures and vocal abuse is moderated. Surgical excision is rarely indicated but may be necessary if the child is unable to communicate adequately or becomes aphonic or if tension and straining is necessary to make any utterances.

Laryngopharyngeal reflux commonly exacerbates vocal abuse, adding to swelling of the vocal cords. When vocal abuse is the main factor, the voice is worse in the evenings; with laryngopharyngeal reflux, hoarseness is worse in the morning. An antireflux regimen is indicated.

377.2 Recurrent Respiratory Papillomatosis (RRP)

Epidemiology and Etiology. Papillomas are the most common respiratory tract neoplasms in children, occurring in 4.3 per 100,000. They are simply warts—benign tumors—caused by the human papillomavirus (HPV); the same pathology is found in condylomata acuminata (vaginal warts). HPV types 6 and 11 are most commonly associated with laryngeal disease. Fifty per cent occur in children younger than 5 yr, but the diagnosis may be made at any age. Of children with RRP, 67% are born to mothers who had condylomata during pregnancy or parturition. The risk for transmission is about 1 in 500 vaginal births in mothers with active condylomata. Neonates have been reported to have RRP, which suggests intrauterine transmission of HPV.

Clinical Manifestations. These benign squamous lesions can produce chronic hoarseness in the infant. Most occur in the larynx, specifically on the vocal cords, but in 31% these lesions occur in other areas of the respiratory tract: nose, pharynx (especially the uvula and posterior soft palate), trachea, bronchi, and lungs. As growth on the vocal cords progresses, hoarseness increases and communication becomes difficult. Respiratory distress develops. Symptoms often occur first during sleep with symptoms typical of obstructive sleep apnea. Progressive respiratory distress with sleep, exertion, daily activities, and finally at rest indicates the need for surgical intervention.

Treatment. The treatment of RRP is endoscopic surgical removal. Most surgeons in North America prefer excision with the CO_2 laser. Surgical excision is a quality of life issue warranting removal to improve the voice. Intervention becomes a medical necessity when airway obstruction progresses. Laryngopharyngeal reflux may require treatment when reflux laryngitis is a factor. Other types of medical management including injection of cidofovir may have some benefit.

377.3 Congenital Subglottic Hemangioma

Typically, hemangiomas are symptomatic within the first 2 mo of life, with almost all presenting before 6 mo of age. Stridor is biphasic but usually more prominent during inspiration. The infant may be hoarse, have a barking cough, and present with croup. Of congenital subglottic hemangiomas, 50% are associated with cutaneous lesions. Radiographs classically delineate an asymmetric subglottic narrowing. The diagnosis is made by direct laryngoscopy.

Medical management includes systemic steroids. Prednisone, 2–4 mg/kg/24 hr, is given orally for 4–6 wk, less if the lesions stabilize sooner. The dosage is then tapered. If there is no response, the drug is discontinued. Interferon alfa-2a has also been recommended for the treatment of life-threatening corticosteroid-resistant hemangiomas that involve the airway and endanger vital structures.

Although tracheostomy establishes a safe airway, every effort should be made to find an alternative. Corticosteroids can be injected directly into the lesion. Endoscopic excision with the CO_2 laser is effective. Combining several modalities increases the possibility of avoiding tracheotomy. External surgical excision is suitable for some lesions.

377.4 Vascular Anomalies

Vascular malformations are not true neoplastic lesions. They have a normal rate of endothelial turnover and various channel abnormalities. They are categorized by their predominant type (capillary, venous, arterial, lymphatic, or a combination). Slow-flow malformations have capillary, lymphatic, or venous components. These were incorrectly called capillary hemangiomas, cystic hygromas or lymphangiomas, and cavernous hemangiomas, respectively.

Lymphatic malformations (cystic hygromas) rarely occur in the larynx. When they do, they are invariably an extension of disease from the head and neck. Airway obstruction may necessitate tracheostomy. The lesion can be debulked with the CO_2 laser.

377.5 Other Laryngeal Neoplasms

Neurofibromatosis rarely involves the larynx. When children are affected, limited local resection is undertaken to maintain an airway and optimize the voice. Complete surgical extirpation is virtually impossible without debilitating resection of vital laryngeal structures. Most surgeons select the option of less aggressive symptomatic surgery because of the poorly circumscribed and infiltrative nature of these fibromas. Rhabdomyosarcoma and other malignant tumors of the larynx are rare. Symptoms of hoarseness and progressive airway obstruction prompt initial evaluation by flexible laryngoscopy in the office.

377.6 Tracheal Neoplasms

The majority of tracheal tumors are benign; the two most common are inflammatory pseudotumor and hamartoma. The inflammatory pseudotumor is probably a reaction to a previous bronchial infection or traumatic insult. Growth is slow, and the tumor may be locally invasive. Hamartomas are tumors of primary tissue elements that are abnormal in proportion and arrangement.

Tracheal neoplasms present with stridor, wheezing, cough, or pneumonia and are rarely diagnosed until 75% of the lumen has been obstructed. Symptoms mimic asthma and are frequently misdiagnosed as such. Chest radiographs or airway films may identify the obstruction. Pulmonary function studies demonstrate an abnormal flow-volume loop. A mild response to bronchodilator therapy may be misleading.

377.7 Bronchial Tumors

Bronchial tumors are rare; two thirds are malignant. Bronchial "adenomas" are the most common, representing 30% of all lung tumors. Bronchogenic carcinoma is the second most common and occurs in approximately 20% of cases. The diagnosis is confirmed at bronchoscopy and biopsy; treatment depends on the histopathology.

Derkay CS: Task force on recurrent respiratory papillomatosis. *Arch Otol Laryngol Head Neck Surg* 1995;121:1386–91.

Desai DP, Maddalozzo J, Holinger LD: Granular cell tumor of the trachea. *Otolaryngol Head Neck Surg* 1999;120:595–98.

Desai DP, Mahoney EM, Miller RP, et al: Case report: Mucoepidermoid carcinoma of the trachea in a child. *Int J Pediatr Otorhinolaryngol* 1998;45:259–63.

Hartman GE, Shochat SJ: Primary pulmonary neoplasms of childhood: A review. *Ann Thorac Surg* 1982;36:108.

Hughes CA, Rezaee A, Ludemann JP, et al: Management of congenital subglottic hemangioma. *J Otolaryngol* 1999;28:223–28.

Kashima H, Mounts P, Leventhal B, et al: Sites of predilection in recurrent respiratory papillomatosis. *Ann Otol Rhinol Laryngol* 1993;102:580–83.

Chapter 378

Inflammatory Disorders of the Small Airways *Denise Goodman*

378.1 Bronchitis

Bronchitis refers to nonspecific bronchial inflammation and is associated with a number of childhood conditions. *Acute bronchitis* is a syndrome, usually viral in origin, with cough as a prominent feature.

Acute tracheobronchitis is a term used when the trachea is prominently involved. Nasopharyngitis may also be present, and a variety of viral and bacterial agents, such as those causing influenza, pertussis, and diphtheria, may be responsible. Isolation of common bacteria such as pneumococcus, *Staphylococcus,* and *Streptococcus* from the sputum may not imply a bacterial cause requiring antibiotic therapy.

Asthmatic bronchitis is an obsolete term; wheezing and bronchial inflammation are integral findings of asthma, and asthma exacerbations are commonly triggered by upper respiratory tract infections. Thus, use of the term *asthmatic bronchitis* may obscure the understanding on the part of patient and family that this is asthma.

ACUTE BRONCHITIS

Clinical Manifestations. Acute bronchitis is commonly preceded by a viral upper respiratory tract infection. Thus, it is more common in the winter when respiratory viral syndromes predominate. The tracheobronchial epithelium is invaded by the infectious agent, leading to activation of inflammatory cells and release of cytokines. Constitutional symptoms, such as fever and malaise, follow. The tracheobronchial epithelium may become significantly damaged or hypersensitized, leading to a protracted cough lasting 1–3 wk.

Commonly, the child first presents with nonspecific upper respiratory infectious symptoms, such as rhinitis. Three to 4 days later, a frequent, dry, hacking cough develops, which may or may not be productive. After several days, the sputum may become purulent, but purulent sputum indicates leukocyte migration and does not necessarily imply bacterial infection. Many children swallow their sputum, and this may produce emesis. Chest pain may be a prominent complaint in older children, exacerbated by coughing. The mucus gradually thins, usually within 5–10 days, and then the cough gradually abates. The entire episode usually lasts about 2 wk and seldom longer than 3 wk.

Findings on physical examination vary with age of the patient and stage of the disease. Early findings are absent or low-grade fever and upper respiratory signs such as nasopharyngitis, conjunctivitis, and rhinitis. Auscultation of the chest may be unremarkable at this early phase. As the syndrome progresses and cough worsens, breath sounds become coarse, with coarse and fine crackles and scattered high-pitched wheezing. Chest radiographs are normal or may have increased bronchial markings.

The principal objective of the clinician is to exclude pneumonia, which is more likely caused by bacterial agents requiring antibiotic therapy. In at least one study of adults, absence of abnormality of vital signs (tachycardia, tachypnea, fever) and chest examination reduced the likelihood of pneumonia.

Differential Diagnosis. Persistent or recurrent symptoms should lead the clinician to consider entities other than acute bronchitis. Many entities may manifest with cough as a prominent symptom. See also Chapter 370 and Box 370–2.

Treatment. There is no specific therapy for acute bronchitis. The disease is self-limited, and antibiotics, although frequently prescribed, do not hasten improvement in uncomplicated acute bronchitis. Frequent shifts in position may facilitate pulmonary drainage in infants. Older children are sometimes more comfortable with humidity, but this does not shorten the disease course. Cough suppressants may produce symptomatic relief but may also increase the risk of suppuration and inspissated secretions and therefore should be used judiciously. Antihistamines dry secretions and are not helpful, and expectorants are likewise not indicated.

CHRONIC BRONCHITIS

Chronic bronchitis is well recognized in adults, formally defined as 3 mo or more of productive cough each year for 2 yr or more. The disease may develop insidiously, with episodes of acute obstruction alternating with quiescent periods. A number of predisposing conditions may lead to progression of airflow obstruction or chronic obstructive pulmonary disease (COPD), with smoking as the major factor (up to 80% of patients have a smoking history). Other conditions include air pollution, occupational exposures, and repeated infections.

The applicability of this definition to children is unclear. The existence of chronic bronchitis as a distinct entity in children is controversial. However, like adults, children with chronic inflammatory diseases or those with toxic exposures may develop damaged pulmonary epithelium. Thus, chronic or recurring cough in children should guide the clinician to search for underlying pulmonary or systemic disorders such as those summarized earlier in Box 370–2.

CIGARETTE SMOKING AND AIR POLLUTION

Exposure to environmental irritants, such as tobacco smoke and air pollution, can incite or aggravate cough. There is a well-established association between tobacco exposure and pulmonary disease, including bronchitis and wheezing. This may occur either through cigarette smoking or by exposure to passive smoke. Marijuana smoke is another irritant sometimes overlooked when eliciting a history.

A number of pollutants are also likely candidates as precipitants of lung disease, including particulate matter, ozone, and nitrogen dioxide. Because these substances coexist in the atmosphere, the relative contribution of any one to pulmonary symptoms is difficult to discern.

Arroll B, Kenealy T: Antibiotics for acute bronchitis. *BMJ* 2001;322:939–40.

Gergen PJ, Fowler JA, Maurer KR, et al: The burden of environmental tobacco smoke exposure on the respiratory health of children 2 months through 5 years of age in the United States: Third national health and nutrition examination survey, 1988 to 1994. *Pediatrics* 1998;101:e8.

Gold DR, Wang X, Wypij D, et al: Effect of cigarette smoking on lung function in adolescent boys and girls. *N Engl J Med* 1996;335:931–37.

Gonzales R, Sande MA: Uncomplicated acute bronchitis. *Ann Intern Med* 2000;133:981–91.

Heinrich J, Hoelscher B, Wichmann HE: Decline of ambient air pollution and respiratory symptoms in children. *Am J Respir Crit Care Med* 2000;161:1930–36.

Irwin RS, Madison JM: The diagnosis and treatment of cough. *N Engl J Med* 2000;343:1715–21.

Nyquist A-C, Gonzales R, Steiner JF, et al: Antibiotic prescribing for children with colds, upper respiratory tract infections, and bronchitis. *JAMA* 1998;279:875–77.

Pershagen G: Accumulating evidence on health hazards of passive smoking. *Acta Paediatr* 1999;88:490–92.

Peters JM, Avol E, Gauderman WJ, et al: A study of twelve Southern California communities with differing levels and types of air pollution: II. Effects on pulmonary function. *Am J Respir Crit Care Med* 1999;159:768–75.

Peters JM, Avol E, Navidi W, et al: A study of twelve Southern California communities with differing levels and types of air pollution: I. Prevalence of respiratory morbidity. *Am J Respir Crit Care Med* 1999;159:760–67.

Sethi S: Infectious exacerbations of chronic bronchitis: Diagnosis and management. *J Antimicrob Chemother* 1999;43(Suppl A):97–105.

Snow V, Mottur-Pilson C, Gonzales R for the American College of Physicians–American Society of Internal Medicine: Principles of appropriate antibiotic use for treatment of acute bronchitis in adults. *Ann Intern Med* 2001;134:518–20.

Yaari E, Yafe-Zimerman Y, Schwartz SB, et al: Clinical manifestations of *Bordetella pertussis* infection in immunized children and young adults. *Chest* 1999;115:1254–58.

378.2 Bronchiolitis

Acute bronchiolitis is a common disease of the lower respiratory tract in infants, resulting from inflammatory obstruction of the small airways. By age 2 yr nearly all children have been infected, with severe disease more common among infants aged 1–3 mo. Bronchiolitis is seasonal, with peak activity during winter and early spring.

Etiology and Epidemiology. Acute bronchiolitis is predominantly a viral disease. Respiratory syncytial virus (RSV) is responsible for more than 50% of cases. Other agents include parainfluenza, adenovirus, *Mycoplasma,* and occasionally other viruses. There is no evidence of a bacterial cause for bronchiolitis, although bacterial pneumonia is sometimes confused clinically with bronchiolitis and bronchiolitis may be followed by bacterial superinfection.

Estimates suggest that 50,000–80,000 of hospitalizations annually among children younger than 1 yr are attributable to RSV infection, representing an increase over the past decade. This increase may reflect increased attendance of infants in day-care centers, changes in criteria for hospital admission, and/or improved survival of premature infants and others at risk for severe RSV-associated disease.

Bronchiolitis is more common in males, in those who have not been breast-fed, and in those who live in crowded conditions. Older family members are a common source of infection but may experience only minor respiratory symptoms. The clinical manifestations of lower respiratory tract illness (LRTI) seen in young infants may be minimal in older patients, in whom bronchiolar edema is better tolerated.

Pathophysiology. Not all infected infants develop LRTI. Host anatomic and immunologic factors seem to play a significant role in the severity of the clinical syndrome. Infants with pre-existent smaller airways and diminished lung function have a more severe course. In addition, RSV infection incites a complex immune response. Eosinophils degranulate and release eosinophil cationic protein, which is cytotoxic to airway epithelium. IgE antibody release may be related to wheezing. Other mediators invoked in the pathogenesis of airway inflammation include chemokines such as interleukin-8 (IL-8), macrophage-inflammatory protein (MIP) 1α, and RANTES (Regulated on Activation, Normal T-cell Expressed and Secreted). RSV-infected infants who wheeze express higher levels of interferon-γ in the airway as well as leukotrienes. Additionally, altered regulation of surfactant proteins A and B may exacerbate the abnormal lung function of infants with bronchiolitis. These findings suggest a complex cellular dysregulation producing the clinical syndrome.

Acute bronchiolitis is characterized by bronchiolar obstruction with edema, mucus, and cellular debris. Even minor bronchiolar wall thickening significantly affects airflow because resistance is inversely proportional to the fourth power of the radius of the bronchiolar passage. Resistance in the small air passages is increased during both inspiration and exhalation, but because the radius of an airway is smaller during expiration, the resultant ball valve respiratory obstruction leads to early air trapping and overinflation. If obstruction is complete with resorption of trapped air, the child will develop atelectasis.

These cellular and pathologic processes impair normal pulmonary gas exchange. Hypoxemia is a consequence of ventilation-perfusion mismatch early in the course. With severe disease, hypercapnia develops.

Clinical Manifestations. The illness is usually preceded by exposure to an older contact with a minor respiratory syndrome within the previous week. The infant first develops a mild upper respiratory tract infection with sneezing and clear rhinorrhea. This may be accompanied by diminished appetite and fever of 38.5–39°C (101–102°F), although the temperature may range from subnormal to markedly elevated. Gradually, respiratory distress ensues, with paroxysmal wheezy cough, dyspnea, and irritability. The infant is often tachypneic, which interferes with feeding. The child does not usually have other systemic complaints, such as diarrhea or vomiting. Apnea may be more prominent than wheezing early in the course of the disease, particularly with very young infants.

The physical examination is characterized most prominently by wheezing. The degree of tachypnea does not always correlate with the degree of hypoxemia or hypercarbia, so the use of pulse oximetry and noninvasive carbon dioxide determination is essential. Work of breathing may be markedly increased, with nasal flaring and retractions. Auscultation may reveal fine crackles or overt wheezes, with prolongation of the expiratory phase of breathing. Barely audible breath sounds suggest very severe disease with nearly complete bronchiolar obstruction. Hyperinflation of the lungs may permit palpation of the liver and spleen.

Chest radiography reveals hyperinflated lungs with patchy atelectasis. This may be difficult to distinguish from early bacterial pneumonia.

The white blood cell and differential counts are usually normal, without the lymphopenia seen with other viral illnesses. The utility of viral testing (usually rapid immunofluorescence, polymerase chain reaction, or viral culture) is debatable. The diagnosis is clinical, particularly in a previously healthy infant presenting with a first-time wheezing episode during a community outbreak. However, because concurrent bacterial infection is highly unlikely, confirmation of viral bronchiolitis may obviate the need for a sepsis evaluation in a febrile infant.

Differential Diagnosis. The condition most commonly confused with acute bronchiolitis is asthma. The two conditions may not be distinguishable during the first episode, but repeated episodes of wheezing, absence of a viral prodrome, and presence of a family history of atopy or asthma supports a diagnosis of asthma. Other entities that may be confused with bronchiolitis in young infants include foreign body in the trachea, tracheo- or bronchomalacia, vascular rings, congestive heart failure, cystic fibrosis, or pertussis.

Course and Prognosis. During the first 48–72 hr after onset of cough and dyspnea the infant is at highest risk for further respiratory compromise; he or she may be desperately ill with air hunger, apnea, and respiratory acidosis. The case fatality rate is less than 1%, with death attributable to apnea, uncompensated respiratory acidosis, or severe dehydration. After this critical period, symptoms may persist. In one study of ambulatory children in South Africa, the median duration of symptoms was 12 days. Infants with conditions such as congenital heart disease, bronchopulmonary dysplasia, and immunodeficiency often have more severe disease, with higher morbidity and mortality.

Recurrent Wheezing after Bronchiolitis. Epidemiologic studies with several year follow-up of index and control children show a higher incidence of wheezing and asthma in children with a history of bronchiolitis, unexplained by family history or other atopic syndromes. It is unclear whether bronchiolitis incites an immune response that manifests as asthma later or whether those infants have an inherent predilection for asthma that is merely unmasked by their episode of RSV.

Treatment. Infants with respiratory distress should be *hospitalized*; the mainstay of treatment is supportive. If hypoxemic, the child should receive *cool humidified oxygen.* Sedatives are to be avoided because they may depress respiratory drive. The infant is sometimes more comfortable if *sitting with head and chest elevated at a 30-degree angle with neck extended.* The risk of aspiration of oral feedings may be high in infants with bronchiolitis owing to tachypnea and the increased work of breathing. The infant may be fed through a nasogastric tube. However, if there is any risk for further respiratory decompensation potentially necessitating tracheal intubation, the infant should be kept *NPO and maintained with parenteral fluids.*

A number of agents have been proposed as adjunctive therapies for bronchiolitis. *Bronchodilators* produce modest short-term improvement in clinical features, but the statistical improvement in clinical scoring systems seen with them is not always clinically significant. Several studies have included both infants with first-time and recurrent wheezing, complicating interpretation of the data. Nebulized epinephrine may be more effective than β-agonists. A trial dose of inhaled bronchodilator may be reasonable, with further therapy predicated on response in the individual patient.

Corticosteroids, whether parenteral, oral, or inhaled, are widely used despite conflicting studies. Differences of diagnostic criteria, measures of effect, timing and route of administration, and severity of illness complicate these studies. In a meta-analysis of steroid use, pooling of all studies and length-of-stay (LOS) plus duration-of-symptoms as outcomes yielded mean reduction in LOS of less than 1 day per patient. This effect disappeared if studies were used measuring LOS only or clearly excluding patients with previous episodes of wheezing. Thus, the theoretical benefits of corticosteroids do not outweigh their risks, side effects, and expense, and they are not indicated for previously healthy infants with RSV.

Ribavirin, an antiviral agent administered by aerosol, has been used for infants with congenital heart disease or chronic lung disease. There is no convincing evidence of a positive impact on clinically important outcomes such as mortality and duration of hospitalization. *Antibiotics* have no value unless there is secondary bacterial pneumonia. Likewise, there is no support for *RSV immune globulin* administration during acute episodes of RSV bronchiolitis.

Prevention. Pooled hyperimmune RSV intravenous immunoglobulin (RSV-IVIG, RespiGam) and palivizumab, (Synagis) an intramuscular monoclonal antibody to the RSV F protein are effective in preventing severe RSV disease in high-risk infants when given before and during RSV season. Palivizumab is recommended for infants younger than age 2 yr with chronic lung disease (bronchopulmonary dysplasia) or prematurity. Because of increased mortality after RespiGam administration to infants with symptomatic cyanotic congenital heart disease, the best approach to this population is still under investigation. Meticulous handwashing is the best measure to prevent nosocomial transmission.

Bertrand P, Aranibar H, Castro E, Sanchez I: Efficacy of nebulized epinephrine versus salbutamol in hospitalized infants with bronchiolitis. *Pediatr Pulmonol* 2001;31:284–88.

Bulow SM, Nir M, Levin E, et al: Prednisolone treatment of respiratory syncytial virus infection: A randomized controlled trial of 147 infants. *Pediatrics* 1999;104:e77.

Denny FW, Collier AM, Henderson FW, et al: The epidemiology of bronchiolitis. *Pediatr Res* 1977;11:234–36.

Garrison MM, Christakis DA, Harvey E, et al: Systemic corticosteroids in infant bronchiolitis: A meta-analysis. *Pediatrics* 2000;105:e44.

Hall CB: Respiratory syncytial virus and parainfluenza virus. *N Engl J Med* 2001;344:1917–28.

The Impact-RSV Study Group: Palivizumab, a humanized respiratory syncytial virus monoclonal antibody, reduces hospitalization from respiratory syncytial virus infection in high-risk infants. *Pediatrics* 1998;102:531–37.

Kellner JD, Ohlsson A, Gadomski AM, et al: Efficacy of bronchodilator therapy in bronchiolitis: A meta-analysis. *Arch Pediatr Adolesc Med* 1996; 150:1166–72.

Law BJ, Wang EEL, MacDonald N, et al: Does ribavirin impact on the hospital course of children with respiratory syncytial virus (RSV) infection? An analysis using the pediatric investigators collaborative network on infections in Canada (PICNIC) RSV database. *Pediatrics* 1997;99:e7.

Panitch HB: Bronchiolitis in infants. *Curr Opin Pediatr* 2001;13:256–60.

Perlstein PH, Kotagal UR, Bolling C, et al: Evaluation of an evidence-based guideline for bronchiolitis. *Pediatrics* 1999;104:1334–41.

Pickering LK (editor): *Respiratory Syncytial Virus in 2000 Red Book: Report of the Committee on Infectious Diseases,* 25th ed. Elk Grove Village, IL, American Academy of Pediatrics, 2000, pp 483–487.

Rodriguez WJ, Gruber WC, Groothuis JR, et al: Respiratory syncytial virus immune globulin treatment of RSV lower respiratory tract infection in previously healthy children. *Pediatrics* 1997;100:937–42.

Shay DK, Holman RC, Roosevelt GE, et al: Bronchiolitis-associated mortality and estimates of respiratory syncytial virus-associated deaths among US children, 1979–1997. *J Infect Dis* 2001;183:16–22.

Sigurs N: Epidemiologic and clinical evidence of a respiratory syncytial virus–reactive airway disease link. *Am J Respir Crit Care Med* 2001:163:s2–s6.

Swingler GH, Hussey GD, Zwarenstein M: Duration of illness in ambulatory children diagnosed with bronchiolitis. *Arch Pediatr Adolesc Med* 2000;154:997–1000.

Welliver RC: Immunology of respiratory syncytial virus infection: Eosinophils, cytokines, chemokines and asthma. *Pediatr Infect Dis J* 2000;19:780–83.

Chapter 379
Wheezing in Infants

Marzena Krawiec and Robert F. Lemanske, Jr.

In infants and young children, wheezing is common owing to unique age-specific anatomic and physiologic properties and gender-specific intrinsic lung characteristics (Table 379–1). The etiology of wheezing involves any pathophysiologic process resulting in impaired airflow mediated by a reduction in airway diameter. This pathophysiologic end-point encompasses a variety of causes and therefore poses diagnostic difficulties in the evaluation of the young wheezing child younger than age 5 yr (Table 379–2). Nonetheless, the most common causes of infantile wheezing are viral respiratory infections and asthma (for a fuller discussion of asthma, see Chapter 134).

Factors contributing to the development of asthma in early wheezing children are poorly understood. Based both on the onset and the pattern of wheezing, young children have been grouped into three wheezing phenotypes (see Table 379–2). The most important distinction among these groups is lower morbidity in the transient wheezing phenotype compared with the child with persistent wheezing. Children in this latter group have significantly higher morbidity, including irreversible loss of lung function by age 6 yr. In addition, significant airway inflammation can be found in the airways of recurrent wheezing infants, suggesting that pathophysiologic features associated with adult asthma may be starting at a very young age. However, although 20% of all children will have had at least one wheezing illness by 1 yr of age, almost 33% by 3 yr of age, and nearly 50% by 6 yr, less than 15% of children are subsequently diagnosed with asthma based on symptoms of recurrent wheezing, airway obstruction, and hyperresponsiveness. Nevertheless, asthma is the most common disease of childhood and confers a significant degree of morbidity, thereby demanding early evaluation and management in the predisposed persistently wheezing infant.

Pathophysiology. Both virus-specific and host-specific factors are likely to contribute to the clinical expression of the different wheezing phenotypes during early childhood. Virus-specific factors include the ability to preferentially affect the lower airway, to generate virus-specific IgE antibody (e.g., respiratory syncytial virus [RSV]), and to induce specific cytokine responses to various viruses and viral proteins. Host-specific factors vary based on the wheezing phenotype. Specifically, lung size is the primary factor associated with the transient wheezing phenotype, whereas parental history of asthma, elevated serum IgE levels, and the presence of atopic dermatitis are associated with the persistent wheezing phenotype. Exposure to passive smoke is a significant risk factor for both phenotypes.

The presence of atopy in the host and the development of lower respiratory tract infections are the two most important independent risk factors for the development of persistent wheezing and asthma. In addition, the atopic state can influence lower airway response to viral infections, whereas viral infections may influence the development of allergy, and interactions can occur based on simultaneous exposure to both allergens and viruses. Infection with RSV is the cause of the majority of lower respiratory tract illnesses with wheezing during the first 3 yr of life and may increase the risk of allergic sensitization later in childhood. Furthermore, diminished levels of lung function have been found years later after only a single episode of lower respiratory tract infection during infancy. The variability in clinical outcomes concerning the inception of allergic respiratory diseases may be related to the severity, viral pathogen, and/or

TABLE 379–1. Pathophysiologic Properties Predisposing Infants and Young Children to Wheeze

	Effect
Physiologic Properties in Infants Relative to Older Children/Adults	
↓Bronchial smooth muscle content	↓Structural support
	↑Risk of atelectasis
Hyperplasia of bronchial mucus glands	↑Mucus production
	↑Risk of obstruction
↓Radius of conducting airways resulting in overall ↓ turbulent flow*	↓Conductance
	↓Filtration of particles
	↑Risk of obstruction
	↑Risk of atelectasis
↑Resistance in peripheral airways due to decreased airway size†	↑Risk of obstruction
	↑Work of breathing
↑Chest wall compliance	↑Work of breathing
Diaphragm	
Horizontal insertion of the diaphragm to the rib cage	
↓ Number of fatigue-resistant skeletal muscle fibers	↑Risk of atelectasis
Deficient collateral ventilation	distal to obstruction
Gender-Based Properties Related to Infantile Wheeze	
Females	↓Lung size
Males	↓Airway conductance
	($↓V_{max}$ FRC)

*Airflow occurs in three forms: laminar, turbulent, and transitional based on the size of the airway. Laminar flow occurs primarily in the small airways, whereas turbulent flow occurs in the central airways. Turbulent flow facilitates the filtration of inhaled particles in conjunction with mucociliary clearance mechanisms. Because of the marked decrease in radial size of the proximal airways in infants compared with adults, there is less turbulent flow in infants, predisposing them to less effective filtration and clearance of particles, resulting in airflow obstruction.

†Poiseuille's equation states that resistance to airflow through a tube is inversely related to the radius to the fourth power. Therefore, any disease that decreases the diameter of the small airways can lead to increased obstruction owing to heightened airflow resistance.

timing of the initial infection and its relationship to concurrent or subsequent allergen exposures.

Clinical Manifestations. A careful history and physical examination are critical in the approach to the child with recurrent wheezing in infancy. In terms of a potential predisposition to clinical asthma, findings on history include the number and frequency of wheezing episodes, the relationship of the episode to viral infection and/or aeroallergen exposures, the presence of allergic diseases such as conjunctivitis, rhinitis, and/or eczema, and parental history of asthma. On physical examination, the following points deserve emphasis: (1) the overall appearance of the child based on an assessment of respiratory distress and the work of breathing; (2) whether there is wheezing, transmitted upper airway nasal congestion, stridor and wheezing (suggestive of both an upper and lower airway process such as croup, tracheomalacia, or bronchomalacia), or wheezing and crackles (suggestive of an interstitial lung component including infection, bronchopulmonary dysplasia [BPD], or pulmonary edema with congestive heart disease [CHD]); and (3) the location of wheezing (unilateral, suggestive of a foreign body or bronchomalacia, or bilateral, suggestive of a more generalized process).

Any young child with increased work of breathing manifested by an increased respiratory rate and/or intercostal/subcostal retractions should raise concern. More commonly in infants, respiratory distress may manifest as "abdominal or belly breathing" along with chest wall retractions. In general, children who will ultimately fall in the transient wheezing category will not have wheezing episodes associated with significant respiratory distress and/or hypoxia. Additional findings on physical examination that may provide insight into the etiology of infantile wheeze include (1) the child's growth curve (evidence of poor weight gain suggests other causes of wheezing such as cystic fibrosis, immunodeficiency, and/or gastroesophageal reflux disease [GERD]), (2) clinical features such as rhinitis and/or conjunctivitis and the presence of eczema (findings suggestive of

atopy, a risk factor for the development of persistent wheezing), and (3) the presence of a central or midline structural or cutaneous lesion such as a hemangioma (associated with an increased risk of an intrathoracic lesion).

Laboratory Findings. Radiologic assessment should vary based on the initial presentation of the child. Most infants with a single episode of wheezing will not require a chest radiograph, other than to confirm positive additional findings and/or to alleviate parental anxieties. In contrast, any child with recurrent episodes of wheezing or congenital anomalies should have anteroposterior and lateral radiographic views taken to ascertain the presence of hyperinflation and/or structural abnormalities, respectively. Furthermore, suspicion of structural abnormalities may warrant additional imaging studies such as a CT or MRI and/or direct visualization using laryngobronchoscopy. Additional laboratory considerations in the patient with an atopic family history and/or physical findings include immediate hypersensitivity skin and/or radioimmune allergosorbent (RAST) tests. Finally, infant pulmonary function testing may be utilized to assess decreased lung function. However, the degree of air flow limitation in the first 3 mo of life is not an informative predictor of children at risk for the subsequent development of asthma. Additional evaluations establishing the presence of airway hyperresponsiveness during this time period may be associated with an increased risk of asthma by 6 yr of age.

Treatment. The treatment of infantile wheeze should be based on the underlying etiology. For viral-induced wheezing (e.g., with infection with RSV or parainfluenza virus), management involves the use of supplemental oxygen to treat hypoxemia and a trial of bronchodilators including acute support with racemic epinephrine. Systemic corticosteroids are not indicated for the treatment of acute viral bronchiolitis, and the role of inhaled corticosteroids used acutely remains controversial. Because many infants experience airway hyperresponsiveness for months to years after RSV infection, treatment with bronchodilators (in the clinically responsive child) and possibly a

TABLE 379–2. Differential Diagnosis of Wheezing in Infancy

Infection
Viral
   Respiratory syncytial virus (RSV)
   Parainfluenza
   Adenovirus
   Influenza
   Rhinovirus
Other
   Chlamydia trachomatis
   Tuberculosis
   Histoplasmosis

Asthma: Three Phenotypes in Children ≤5 yr
Transient wheezer (onset ≤ 3 yr of age, then resolving)
   Initial risk factor is primarily diminished lung size
   Normal lung function by 6 yr of age
   Not associated with increased risk of developing clinical asthma
Persistent wheezers (onset ≤ 3 yr of age and then persisting)
   Initial risk factors include passive smoke exposure, maternal asthma history, and
     an elevated IgE level in the first year of life
   Irreversible reduction in lung function at 6 yr of age
   At increased risk of developing clinical asthma
Late-onset wheezer (onset of wheeze between 3 and 6 yr of age)

Anatomic Abnormalities
Central airway abnormalities
   Malacia of the larynx, trachea, and/or bronchi
   Tracheoesophageal fistula (specifically H-type fistula)
   Laryngeal cleft (resulting in aspiration)
Extrinsic airway anomalies resulting in airway compression
   Vascular ring or sling
   Mediastinal lymphadenopathy from infection or tumor
   Mediastinal mass/tumor
Intrinsic airway anomalies
   Airway hemangioma
   Cystic adenomatoid malformation
   Bronchial/lung cyst
   Congenital lobar emphysema
   Aberrant tracheal bronchus
   Sequestration
   Congenital heart disease with left-to-right shunt (increased pulmonary edema)

Inherited
Cystic fibrosis
Immunodeficiency states
   IgA deficiency
   B-cell deficiencies
   Primary ciliary dyskinesia
   Neonatal AIDS
   Bronchiectasis

Bronchopulmonary Dysplasia

Aspiration Syndromes
Gastroesophageal reflux disease
Pharyngeal/swallow dysfunction

Interstitial Lung Disease, Including Bronchiolitis Obliterans
Foreign Body

long-term medication such as an inhaled corticosteroid (nebulized or using a metered-dose inhaler with face mask) or a leukotriene-modifying agent may be considered.

Prognosis. Although the majority (~60%) of children with early-onset wheezing will stop wheezing, a minority (~14%) are at significant risk for persistent asthma. Based on the Tucson Children's Respiratory Study's asthma predictive index (API), young children with frequent wheezing episodes may be identified who are potentially at increased risk for the development of persistent asthma. During the first 3 yr of life, children with a positive API, defined as frequent episodes of wheezing and one major criterion (parent with asthma or eczema) or two minor criteria (serum eosinophilia [≥ 4%], wheezing not associated with an upper respiratory infection, and/or physician diagnosed allergic rhinitis), have been shown to have 48% and 67% positive predictive values for asthma and persistent wheezing, respectively, at age 6 yr. Conversely, a negative API inferred

92% and 77% negative predictive values for asthma and persistent wheezing, respectively. This index may be helpful (1) to facilitate early intervention (see Chapter 134) for the wheezing infant at heightened risk for the development of chronic asthma and (2) to provide reassurance in the management of the child with a negative API. Whether early identification leading to early intervention can modify asthma expression and/or progression is unclear.

Alwan WH, Kozlowska WJ, Openshaw PJ: Distinct types of lung disease caused by functional subsets of antiviral T cells. *J Exp Med* 1994;179:81.

Castro-Rodriguez JA, Holberg CJ, Wright AL, et al: A clinical index to define risk of asthma in young children with recurrent wheezing. *Am J Respir Crit Care Med* 2000;162:1403.

Frick OL: Effect of respiratory and other virus infections on IgE immunoregulation. *J Allergy Clin Immunol* 1986;78:1013.

Hesselmar B, Adolfsson S: Inhalation of corticosteroids after hospital care for respiratory syncytial virus infection diminishes development of asthma in infants. *Acta Pediatr* 2001;90:260.

Kajosaari M, Syvanen P, Forars M, et al: Inhaled corticosteroids during and after respiratory syncytial virus-bronchiolitis may decrease subsequent asthma. *Pediatr Allergy Immunol* 2000;11:198.

Kraweic ME, Westcott JY, Chu HW, et al: Persistent wheezing in very young children is associated with lower respiratory inflammation. *Am J Respir Crit Care Med* 2001;163:1338.

Martinez FD, Morgan WJ, Wright AL, et al: Diminished lung function as a predisposing factor for wheezing respiratory illness in infants. *N Engl J Med* 1988;319:1112.

Martinez FD, Wright AL, Taussig LM, et al: Asthma and wheezing in the first six years of life. *N Engl J Med* 1995;332:133.

Sheikh S, Goldsmith LJ, Howell L, et al: Lung function in infants with wheezing and gastroesophageal reflux. *Pediatr Pulmonol* 1999;27:236.

Stein RT, Sherrill D, Morgan WJ, et al: Respiratory syncytial virus in early life and risk of wheeze and allergy by age 13 years. *Lancet* 1999;354:54.

Taussig LM, Wright AL, Morgan WJ, et al: The Tucson Children's Respiratory Study: I. Design and implementation of a prospective study of acute and chronic respiratory illness in children. *Am J Epidemiol* 1989;129:1219.

van Schaik SM, Tristam DA, Nagpal IS, et al: Increased production of IFN-gamma and cysteinyl leukotrienes in virus-induced wheezing. *J Allergy Clin Immunol* 1999;103:630.

Wright AL, Taussig LM, Ray CG, et al: The Tucson Children's Respiratory Study: II. Lower respiratory tract illness in the first year of life. *Am J Epidemiol* 1989;129:1232.

Chapter 380
Emphysema and Overinflation

Steven Boas and Glenna B. Winnie

Pulmonary emphysema is distention of air spaces with irreversible disruption of the alveolar septa. It may be generalized or localized, involving part or all of a lung. Overinflation is distention with or without alveolar rupture and is often reversible.

Compensatory overinflation may be acute or chronic and occurs in normally functioning pulmonary tissue when, for any reason, a sizable portion of the lung is removed or becomes partially or completely airless, which may occur with pneumonia, atelectasis, empyema, and pneumothorax.

Obstructive overinflation results from partial obstruction of a bronchus or bronchiole, when it becomes more difficult for air to leave the alveoli than to enter; there is a gradual accumulation of air distal to the obstruction, the so-called bypass, ball valve, or check valve type of obstruction (see Chapter 373).

LOCALIZED OBSTRUCTIVE OVERINFLATION

When a ball-valve type of obstruction partially occludes the mainstem bronchus, the entire lung becomes overinflated; individual lobes are affected when the obstruction is in lobar bronchi. Segments or subsegments are affected when their individual bronchi are blocked. Localized obstructions that may be responsible for overinflation include foreign bodies and the inflammatory reaction to them, abnormally thick mucus (e.g., asthma, cystic fibrosis), endobronchial tuberculosis or tuberculosis of the tracheobronchial lymph nodes, and endobronchial or mediastinal tumors. When most or all of a lobe is involved, the percussion note is hyperresonant over the area, and the breath sounds are decreased in intensity. The distended lung may extend across the mediastinum into the opposite hemithorax. Under fluoroscopic scrutiny during exhalation, the overinflated area does not decrease in size, and the heart and the mediastinum shift to the opposite side because the unobstructed lung empties normally.

Unilateral hyperlucent lung may be associated with a variety of cardiac and pulmonary diseases of children, but in some patients, it occurs without easily demonstrable underlying active disease. More than half the cases follow one or more episodes of pneumonia; a rising titer to adenovirus has been documented in several children. This condition may follow bronchiolitis obliterans and may include obliterative vasculitis as well, accounting for the greatly diminished perfusion and vascular marking on the affected side.

Patients may present with *clinical manifestations* of pneumonia, but some are discovered only when a chest radiograph is obtained for an unrelated reason. A few patients have hemoptysis. Physical findings may include hyperresonance and a small lung with the mediastinum shifted toward the more abnormal lung. This condition has been labeled **Swyer-James** or **Macleod syndrome**. Some patients show a mediastinal shift away from the lesion with exhalation. CT scanning or bronchography may demonstrate bronchiectasis. In some patients, previous chest radiographs have been normal or have shown only an acute pneumonia, suggesting that a hyperlucent lung is an acquired lesion. No specific *treatment* is known; it may become less symptomatic with time.

Congenital lobar emphysema (CLE) may result in severe respiratory distress in early infancy and may be caused by localized obstruction. Familial occurrence has been reported. In 50% of cases, a cause of CLE can be identified. Congenital deficiency of the bronchial cartilage, external compression by aberrant vessels, bronchial stenosis, redundant bronchial mucosal flaps, and kinking of the bronchus caused by herniation into the mediastinum have been described as leading to bronchial obstruction and subsequent CLE.

Clinical manifestations usually become apparent in the neonatal period but may be delayed for as long as 5–6 mo in 5% of patients. Some patients remain undiagnosed until school age or beyond. Signs range from mild tachypnea and wheeze to severe dyspnea with cyanosis. CLE affects the upper and middle lobes, with the left upper lobe the most common site. The affected lobe is essentially nonfunctional because of the overdistention, and atelectasis of the ipsilateral normal lung may ensue. With further distention, the mediastinum is shifted to the contralateral side with impaired function seen as well (Fig. 380–1). A radiolucent lobe and a mediastinal shift are often revealed by radiographic examination.

Treatment by immediate surgery and excision of the lobe may be lifesaving when cyanosis and severe respiratory distress are present, but some patients respond to medical treatment. Some children with apparent congenital lobar emphysema have reversible overinflation, without the classic alveolar septal rupture implied in the term *emphysema*.

Overinflation of all three lobes of the right lung has been produced by anomalous location of the left pulmonary artery, which impinges on the right main stem bronchus. Hyperinflation also occurs in patients with the absent pulmonary valve type of tetralogy of Fallot and secondary aneurysmal dilatation of the pulmonary artery, which partially compresses the main stem bronchi. A number of neonates have

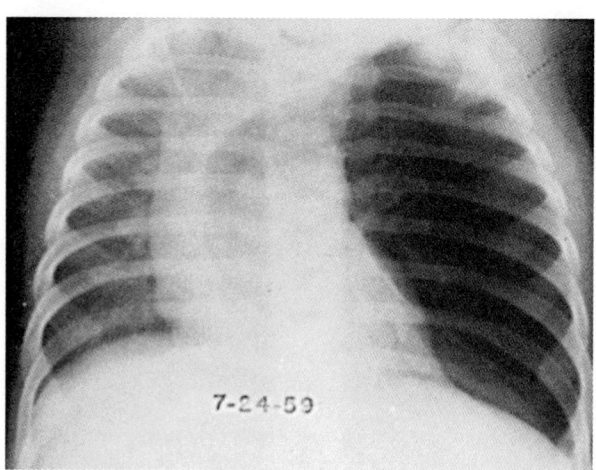

FIGURE 380–1. Congenital left upper lobe emphysema. Note the extension of the emphysematous lobe into the left lower lobe and its displacement of the mediastinum toward the right.

lobar overinflation while being treated for hyaline membrane disease with assisted ventilation, suggesting an acquired cause. Medical management with selective intubation of the unaffected bronchus or high-frequency ventilation has occasionally been successful and lobectomy avoided.

GENERALIZED OBSTRUCTIVE OVERINFLATION

Acute generalized overinflation of the lung results from widespread involvement of the bronchioles and is usually reversible. It occurs more commonly in infants than in children and may be secondary to a number of clinical conditions, including asthma, cystic fibrosis, acute bronchiolitis, interstitial pneumonitis, atypical forms of acute laryngotracheobronchitis, aspiration of zinc stearate powder, chronic passive congestion secondary to a congenital cardiac lesion, and miliary tuberculosis.

Pathology. In chronic overinflation, many of the alveoli are ruptured and communicate with one another, producing distended saccules. Air may also enter the interstitial tissue (i.e., interstitial emphysema), resulting in pneumomediastinum and pneumothorax (see Chapters 403 and 404).

Clinical Manifestations. Generalized obstructive overinflation is characterized by dyspnea, with difficulty in exhaling. The lungs become increasingly overdistended, and the chest remains expanded during exhalation. An increased respiratory rate and decreased respiratory excursion result from the overdistention of the alveoli and their inability to be emptied normally through the narrowed bronchioles. Air hunger is responsible for forced respiratory movements. Overaction of the accessory muscles of respiration results in retractions at the suprasternal notch, the supraclavicular spaces, the lower margin of the thorax, and the intercostal spaces. Unlike the flattened chest during inspiration and exhalation in cases of laryngeal obstruction, minimal reduction in the size of the overdistended chest during exhalation is observed. The percussion note is hyperresonant. On auscultation, the inspiratory phase is usually less prominent than the expiratory phase, which is prolonged and roughened. Fine or medium crackles may be heard. Cyanosis is more common in the severe cases.

Diagnosis. Radiographic and fluoroscopic examinations of the chest assist in establishing the diagnosis. Both leaves of the diaphragm are low and flattened, the ribs are farther apart than usual, and the lung fields are less dense. The movement of the diaphragm during exhalation is decreased, and the excursion of the low, flattened diaphragm in severe cases is barely discernible. The anteroposterior diameter of the chest is increased, and the sternum may be bowed outward.

BULLOUS EMPHYSEMA. Bullous emphysematous blebs or cysts (pneumatoceles) result from overdistention and rupture of alveoli during birth or shortly thereafter, or they may be sequelae of pneumonia and other infections. They have been observed in tuberculosis lesions during specific antibacterial therapy. These emphysematous areas presumable result from rupture of distended alveoli, forming a single or multiloculated cavity. The cysts may become large and may contain some fluid; an air fluid level may be demonstrated on the radiograph. The cysts should be differentiated from pulmonary abscesses. In most cases, the cysts disappear spontaneously within a few months, although they may persist for a year or more. Aspiration or surgery is not indicated except in cases of severe respiratory and cardiac compromise.

SUBCUTANEOUS EMPHYSEMA. Subcutaneous emphysema results from any process that allows free air to enter into the subcutaneous tissue. The most common causes include pneumomediastinum or pneumothorax. Additionally, it may be a complication of fracture of the orbit, permitting free air to escape from the nasal sinuses. In the neck and thorax, subcutaneous emphysema may follow tracheotomy, deep ulceration in the pharyngeal region, esophageal wounds, or any perforating lesion of the larynx or trachea. It is occasionally a complication of thoracentesis, asthma, or abdominal surgery. Air rarely may be formed in the subcutaneous tissues by gas-producing bacteria.

Tenderness over the site of emphysema and "crepitant" quality on palpation of the skin are classic manifestations. Subcutaneous emphysema is usually a self-limited process and requires no specific treatment. Minimization of activities that may increase airway pressure (i.e., cough, performance of high-pressure pulmonary function testing maneuvers) is recommended. Resolution occurs by resorption of subcutaneous air after elimination of its source. Rarely, dangerous compression of the trachea by air in the surrounding soft tissue requires surgical intervention.

Cumming GR, Macpherson RI, Chernick V: Unilateral hyperlucent lung syndrome in children. *J Pediatr* 1971;78:250.

McKenzie SA, Allison DJ, Singh MP, et al: Unilateral hyperlucent lung: The case for investigation. *Thorax* 1980;35:745.

Nuchtern JG, Harberg FJ. Congenital lung cysts. *Semin Pediatr Surg* 1994;3:233–43.

Shannon DC, Todres ID, Moylan FMB: Infantile lobar hyperinflation: Expectant treatment. *Pediatrics* 1977;39(Suppl):1012–18.

Chapter 381
α₁-Antitrypsin Deficiency and Emphysema

Glenna B. Winnie and Steven Boas

Homozygous deficiency of α₁-antitrypsin (α-AT) is an important cause of the early onset of severe panacinar emphysema in adults in the third and fourth decades of life and an important cause of liver disease in children, but it rarely causes pulmonary diseases in children (see Chapter 338.6). α₁-Antitrypsin and other serum antiproteases are important in the inactivation of proteolytic enzymes released from dead bacteria or leukocytes in the lung. Deficiency of these antiproteases leads to an accumulation of proteolytic enzymes in the lung, resulting in destruction of pulmonary tissue with subsequent development of emphysema. The concentration of proteases (e.g., elastase) in the patients' leukocytes may also be an important factor in determining the severity of clinical pulmonary disease with a given level of α₁-antitrypsin.

Clinical Manifestations. The type and concentration of α₁-antitrypsin are inherited as a series of codominant alleles on chromosomal segment 14q32.1. See Chapter 338.6 for discussion of genotypes and liver disease. Early adult-onset emphysema associated with α₁-antitrypsin deficiency occurs most frequently with PiZZ, although Pi(null) (null) and, to a lesser extent, other mutant Pi types such as SZ have been associated with emphysema. Most patients who have the PiZZ defect have little or no detectable pulmonary disease during childhood. A few have very early onset of chronic pulmonary symptoms, including dyspnea, wheezing, and cough, and panacinar emphysema has been documented by lung biopsy results. Smoking greatly increases the risk of emphysema developing in mutant Pi types. Newborn screening to identify children with PiZZ phenotype does not affect parental smoking habits but does decrease smoking rates for affected adolescents.

Physical examination may reveal growth failure, an increased anteroposterior diameter of the chest with a hyperresonant percussion note, crackles if there is active infection, and clubbing. Severe emphysema may depress the diaphragm, making the liver and spleen more easily palpable. Chest radiograph reveals overinflation with depressed diaphragms; chest CT may show more hyperexpansion in the lower lung zones and, occasionally, bronchiectasis. Serum immunoassay measures the low level of α₁-antitrypsin, and electrophoresis reveals the phenotype. Genotype can be determined by polymerase chain reaction.

Treatment. Therapy for α₁-antitrypsin deficiency is replacement with enzyme derived from pooled human plasma. Normal serum levels are 180–280 mg/dL, but a level of 80 mg/dL is protective for emphysema, and this target level for augmentation therapy results in the appearance of the transfused antiprotease in pulmonary lavage fluid. This treatment is safe, because α₁-antitrypsin is relatively heat-resistant and inactivation of hepatitis and other viruses is easily accomplished; severe toxicity has not been reported. The Food and Drug Administration has approved the use of purified blood-derived human enzyme for ZZ and null/null patients. However, the benefit of this therapy has not yet been clearly established, owing to lack of placebo-controlled trials demonstrating efficacy. Replacement therapy appears most beneficial for those with moderately severe obstructive lung disease (FEV₁ 30–65% of predicted) or those with mild lung disease experiencing a rapid decline in lung function. Treatment has been hampered by limited supply of the enzyme, although α₁-antitrypsin produced by recombinant DNA technology is also available and could alleviate the shortage. Direct delivery to the lung by aerosol appears to be effective and might decrease the total dose required, but controversy continues over its clinical use. Gene therapy offers promise, although the vectors tested either result in levels too low to be of clinical benefit or in only transient correction.

Nonspecific therapy includes aggressive treatment of pulmonary infection, routine use of pneumococcal and influenza vaccines, bronchodilators, and advice about the risks of smoking. Such treatment is also indicated for other members of the family found to have PiZZ phenotypes or null/null, even if they are asymptomatic. Persons with the MZ Pi type do not have an increased risk for the development of pulmonary disease. The clinical significance of the SZ Pi type is unknown, but nonspecific treatment seems reasonable. All persons with low levels of serum antiprotease should be warned that the eventual development of emphysema is partially related to environmental factors, including exposure to industrial fumes, respiratory tract infections, and particularly cigarette smoking. Although identification of affected individuals could help prevent development of obstructive lung disease, screening programs are suspended, owing to concerns about employment and health care insurance discrimination.

Abboud RT, Ford GT, Chapman KR: Standards Committee of the Canadian Thoracic Society. Alpha₁-antitrypsin deficiency: A position statement of the Canadian Thoracic Society. *Can Respir J* 2001;8:81–8.

Burrows JA, Willis LK, Perlmutter DH: Chemical chaperones mediate increased secretion of mutant alpha 1-antitrypsin (alpha 1-AT) Z: A potential pharmacological strategy for prevention of liver injury and emphysema in alpha 1-AT deficiency. *Proc Natl Acad Sci USA* 2000;97:1796–801.

Cox DW, Levison H: Emphysema of early onset associated with a complete deficiency of alpha-1-antitrypsin (null homozygotes). *Am Rev Respir Dis* 1988;137:371–75.

Hubbard RC, Crystal RG: Strategies for aerosol therapy of alpha 1-antitrypsin deficiency by the aerosol route. *Lung* 1990;168(Suppl):565–78.

Schievink WI, Puumala MR, Meyer FB, et al: Giant intracranial aneurysm and fibromuscular dysplasia in an adolescent with alpha 1-antitrypsin deficiency. *J Neurosurg* 1996;85:503–6.

Thelin T, Sveger T, McNeil TF: Primary prevention in a high-risk group: Smoking habits in adolescents with homozygous alpha-1-antitrypsin deficiency (ATD). *Acta Paediatr* 1996;85:1207–12.

Wiebicke W, Niggemann B, Fischer A: Pulmonary function in children with homozygous alpha1-protease inhibitor deficiency. *Eur J Pediatr* 1996;155:603–7.

Chapter 382

Other Distal Airway Diseases *Steven Boas*

382.1 Bronchiolitis Obliterans

Bronchiolitis obliterans (BO) is a rare, chronic lung disease of the bronchioles and smaller airways. BO most commonly occurs in the pediatric population after respiratory infections (i.e., adenovirus, *Mycoplasma*, measles, influenza, pertussis). Other causes include connective tissue disease (i.e., juvenile rheumatoid arthritis, systemic lupus erythematosus, scleroderma), toxin fume inhalation, as well as a manifestation after lung and bone marrow transplantation. BO occurs in all age groups, and the prevalence in one pediatric autopsy series was 2 in 1,000.

Pathogenesis. After the initial insult, inflammation affecting terminal bronchioles, respiratory bronchioles, and alveolar ducts may result in the obliteration of the airway lumen. Epithelial damage resulting in abnormal repair is characteristic of BO. Complete or partial obstruction of the airway lumen may result in air trapping or atelectasis. Bronchiolitis obliterans organizing pneumonia (BOOP) is a fibrosing lung disease that includes the histologic features of BO with extension of the inflammatory process from distal alveolar ducts into alveoli with proliferation of fibroblasts. Bronchiolitis obliterans syndrome (BOS) is a clinical entity that relates to graft deterioration after transplantation due to progressive airway disease that appears histologically similar to BO. However, the etiology of BOS is unclear and may be unrelated to the mechanisms responsible for BO in nontransplant patients.

Clinical Manifestations/Diagnosis. Cough, fever, cyanosis, and respiratory distress followed by initial improvement may be the initial signs of BO. In this phase, BO is easily confused with pneumonia, bronchitis, or bronchiolitis. Progression of the disease may ensue with increasing dyspnea, cough, sputum production, and wheezing. Chest radiographs may be relatively normal compared with the extent of physical findings but may demonstrate hyperlucency and patchy infiltrates. Occasionally, a Swyer-James syndrome (unilateral hyperlucent lung) has developed. Pulmonary function tests demonstrate variable findings but typically show signs of airway obstruction. Ventilation-perfusion scans reveal a typical motheaten appearance of multiple matched defects in ventilation and perfusion. Chest CT often demonstrates patchy areas of hyperlucency and bronchiectasis. Open lung biopsy or transbronchial biopsy

remain the best means of establishing the diagnosis of BO or BOOP.

Treatment. No definitive therapy exists for BO. Administration of corticosteroids may be beneficial. Immunomodulatory agents such as tacrolimus and antithymocyte globulin have been utilized in post–lung transplant recipients with BO with variable success. For BOOP, use of oral corticosteroids for up to 1 yr has been advocated as first-line therapy for symptomatic and progressive disease. Patients with asymptomatic or nonprogressive BOOP can be observed.

Prognosis. Some patients with BO experience rapid deterioration in their condition and die within weeks of the initial symptoms, but most nontransplant patients survive with chronic disability. Unlike in BO, total recovery is seen in 60–80% of patients with BOOP, although this depends on the underlying systemic disease. Relapse of BOOP can occur, especially if treatment is less than 1 yr and is amenable to repeat courses of oral corticosteroids. Unlike the more common idiopathic BOOP, progressive BOOP characterized by acute respiratory distress syndrome (ARDS) is rare but is aggressive in its clinical course leading to death.

Epler GR: Bronchiolitis obliterans organizing pneumonia. *Arch Intern Med* 2001;161;158–64.

Epler GR, Colby TV, McLoud TC, et al: Bronchiolitis obliterans organizing pneumonia. *N Engl J Med* 1985;312:152–58.

Hardy KA, Schidlow DV, Zaeri N: Obliterative bronchiolitis in children. *Chest* 1988;93:460–66.

Zhang L, Irion K, Kozakewich H, et al: Clinical course of postinfectious bronchiolitis obliterans. *Pediatr Pulmonol* 2000;29:341–50.

382.2 Follicular Bronchitis

Follicular bronchitis (FB) is a lymphoproliferative lung disorder characterized by the presence of lymphoid follicles coursing alongside the airways (bronchi or bronchioles). FB is rare in children. Although the cause is unknown, an infectious etiology (viral) has been proposed. Onset of symptoms generally occurs by 6 wk of age and peaks between 6 and 18 mo. Cough, moderate respiratory distress, fever, and fine crackles are common clinical findings. Fine crackles generally persist over time, and recurrence of symptoms is common. Chest radiographs may be relatively benign initially (air trapping, peribronchial thickening) but evolve into the typical interstitial pattern. Chest CT may show a fine reticular pattern. Definitive diagnosis is made by open lung biopsy. Some individuals with FB may respond to therapy with corticosteroids. Prognosis is variable, with some individuals having significant progression of pulmonary disease and others developing only mild obstructive airway disease.

Bramson RT, Cleveland R, Blickman JG, et al: Radiographic assessment of follicular bronchitis in children. *AJR Am J Roentgenol* 1996;166:1447–50.

Kinane BT, Mansell AL, Zwerdling RG, et al: Follicular bronchitis in the pediatric population. *Chest* 1993;104:1183–86.

Yousem SA, Colby TV, Carrington CB: Follicular bronchitis/bronchiolitis. *Hum Pathol* 1985;16:700–6.

382.3 Pulmonary Alveolar Microlithiasis

Approximately 400 cases of this unusual disorder have been reported. Although the underlying cause of pulmonary alveolar microlithiasis (PAM) is unknown, the disease is characterized by the formation of lamellar concretions of calcium phosphate or "microliths" within the alveoli, creating a classic pattern on the radiograph (Fig. 382–1).

Epidemiology and Etiology. Although the mean age at time of diagnosis is in the mid 30s, the onset of the disease can occur during childhood. A strong familial association is seen in half of the

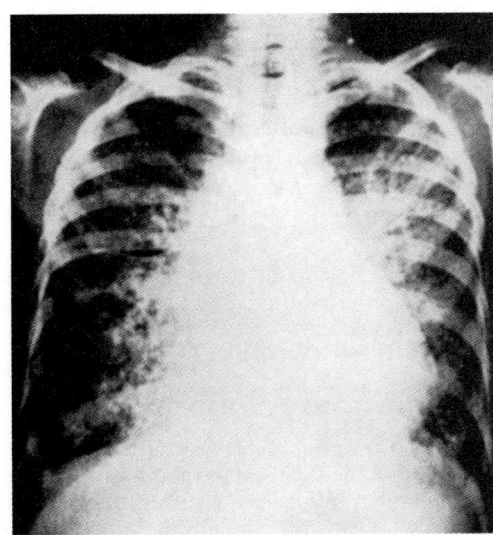

FIGURE 382–1. Radiograph of the chest of a 7-yr-old boy with pulmonary alveolar microlithiasis. (From Clark RB III, Johnson FC: Idiopathic pulmonary alveolar microlithiasis: A case report and brief review of the literature. *Pediatrics* 1961;28:650.)

reported cases, with a probable autosomal recessive pattern of inheritance. In some families a rapid progression of disease occurs. Environmental factors (i.e., sand) may play a role as well. An equal male and female frequency is noted. A relatively large proportion of patients with PAM have Turkish ancestry.

Clinical Manifestations. When symptomatic, individuals with PAM usually complain of dyspnea on exertion and nonproductive cough. Physical examination of the lungs may reveal fine inspiratory crackles and diminished breath sounds. Clubbing occurs, although this is usually a more advanced sign. Discordance between the clinical and radiographic manifestations is common. Children are often asymptomatic on initial presentation. Complications of pneumothorax, pleural adhesions and calcifications, pleural fibrosis, apical bulla, and extrapulmonary sites of microliths have been reported (i.e., kidneys, prostate, sympathetic chain, and testes).

Diagnosis. Chest radiography typically reveals bilateral infiltrates with a fine sandlike micronodular appearance or "sandstorm" appearance with greater density in the lower and middle lung fields (see Fig. 382–1). CT of the chest shows diffuse micronodular calcified densities with thickening of the microliths along the septa and around distal bronchioles, especially in the inferior and posterior regions. Diffuse uptake of technetium Tc 99m diphosphonate by nuclear scan has been reported. Open lung and transbronchial lung biopsy reveal 0.1–0.3 mm laminated calcific concretions within the alveoli. Although the alveoli are often normal initially, progression to pulmonary fibrosis with advancing disease usually ensues. Sputum expectoration may reveal small microliths, although this finding is not diagnostic for PAM and is not typically seen in children. Pulmonary function testing reveals restrictive lung disease with impaired diffusing capacity as the disease progresses, whereas exercise testing demonstrates arterial oxygen desaturation. The differential diagnosis includes sarcoidosis, miliary tuberculosis, hemosiderosis, healed disseminated histoplasmosis, pulmonary calcinosis, and metastatic pulmonary calcifications.

Treatment. No specific treatment is effective, although some have used glucocorticosteroids, etidronate disodium, and bronchopulmonary lavage with limited success. Lung transplantation has been performed for this condition, although it is unknown whether the disease recurs after transplantation.

Prognosis. Progressive cardiopulmonary disease may ensue leading to cor pulmonale, superimposed infections, and subsequent death in mid adulthood. Because of the familial nature of this disease, counseling and chest radiographs of family members are indicated.

Edelman, JD, Bavaria J, Kaiser LR, et al: Bilateral sequential lung transplantation for pulmonary alveolar microlithiasis. *Chest* 1997;112:1140–44.

Erelel M, Kiyan E, Cuhadaroglu C, et al: Pulmonary alveolar lithiasis in two siblings. *Respiration* 2001;68:327–30.

Helbich TH, Wojnarovsky C, Wunderbaldinger P, et al: *AJR Am J Roentgenol* 1997;168:635.

Schmidt H, Lorcher U, Kitz R, et al: Pulmonary alveolar microlithiasis in children. *Pediatr Radiol* 1996;26:33–36.

Volle E, Kaufmann HJ: Pulmonary alveolar microlithiasis in pediatric patients—review of the world literature and two new observations. *Pediatr Radiol* 1987;17:439–42.

Wallis C, Whitehead B, Malone M, et al: Pulmonary alveolar microlithiasis in childhood: Diagnosis by transbronchial biopsy. *Pediatr Pulmonol* 1996;21:62–64.

Chapter 383
Congenital Disorders of the Lung *Thomas P. Green and Jonathan D. Finder*

383.1 Pulmonary Agenesis and Aplasia

Pulmonary agenesis differs from hypoplasia by the complete absence of a lung, whereas it differs from aplasia by the absence of a bronchial stump or carina with agenesis. Bilateral pulmonary agenesis is incompatible with life, presenting as severe respiratory distress and failure. Pulmonary agenesis is thought to be an autosomal recessive trait based on reports of patients with parental consanguinity. Unilateral agenesis or hypoplasia may have few symptoms and nonspecific findings, resulting in only one third of the cases being diagnosed during life. Symptoms tend to be related to central airway complications of stenosis and/or tracheobronchomalacia. In patients in whom the right lung is absent, the aorta can compress the trachea and lead to symptoms of central airway compression. For this reason, right lung agenesis has a higher morbidity and mortality than left lung agenesis. Pulmonary agenesis is often seen in association with other congenital anomalies, such as the VACTERL sequence, ipsilateral facial and skeletal malformations, and central nervous system and cardiac malformations. Compensatory growth of the remaining lung allows for improved gas exchange, but the mediastinal shift can lead to scoliosis and airway compression.

383.2 Pulmonary Hypoplasia

Pulmonary hypoplasia almost always occurs secondary to other intrauterine disorders that produce an impairment of normal lung development. Conditions such as deformities of the thoracic spine and rib cage (thoracic dystrophy), pleural effusions with fetal hydrops, cystic adenomatoid malformation, and congenital diaphragmatic hernia physically constrain the developing lung. Any condition that produces oligohydramnios (e.g., fetal renal insufficiency or prolonged premature rupture of membranes) may also lead to diminished lung growth. In these conditions, airway and arterial branching are inhibited, thereby limiting the capacity for capillary and gas exchange surface area. Pulmonary hypoplasia involves a decrease in both the number of alveoli (up to 67%) and the number of airway generations (up to 50%). In some conditions, the hypoplasia is bilateral because of the presence of bilateral lung constraint, as occurs in oligohydramnios or thoracic dystrophy. However, large, unilateral lesions, such as congenital diaphragmatic hernia and cystic adenomatoid malformation, may displace the mediastinum and thereby produce a contralateral hypoplasia, although usually not as severe as that seen on the ipsilateral side.

Pulmonary hypoplasia is recognized in the newborn period either because the degree of hypoplasia is quite severe or because of the presentation of persistent pulmonary hypertension. In either case, mechanical ventilation and oxygen may be required to support gas exchange because of respiratory distress and hypoxia. Specific therapy to control the pulmonary hypertension, such as inhaled nitric oxide, may be useful. However, in cases of severe hypoplasia the limited capacity of the pulmonary circulation may be inadequate to sustain life. Occasionally, in circumstances that are not amenable to less invasive treatment and support, extracorporeal membrane oxygenation may provide gas exchange for a critical period of time and permit survival.

383.3 Cystic Adenomatoid Malformation

Cystic adenomatoid malformation is one of the most common pulmonary congenital anomalies. This disorder consists of hamartomatous or dysplastic lung tissue mixed with more normal lung and is usually confined to one lobe.

Pathology. Three histologic patterns have been described, although the relationship between the histologic appearance and outcome is controversial. Type 1 is macrocystic and consists of a single or several large (greater than 2 cm in diameter) cysts lined with ciliated pseudostratified epithelium. The wall of the cyst contains smooth muscle cells and elastic tissue. One third of cases have mucus-secreting cells. Cartilage is rarely seen in the wall of the cyst. This type has a good prognosis for survival. Type 2 is microcystic and consists of multiple small cysts with similar histology to that of the type 1 lesion. Type 2 is associated with other congenital anomalies and carries a poor prognosis. In type 3, the lesion is solid with bronchiole-like structures lined with cuboidal ciliated epithelium and separated by areas of nonciliated cuboidal epithelium. This lesion carries the worst prognosis and may be incompatible with life.

The lesion probably results from an embryologic insult, before the 35th day of gestation, with maldevelopment of terminal bronchiolar structures. Histologic examination reveals little normal lung and many glandular elements. Cysts are very common; cartilage is rare. The presence of cartilage may indicate a somewhat later embryologic insult, perhaps extending into the 10th–24th wk.

Diagnosis. The size and progression of this lesion during fetal life and early postnatal life are more important than the histologic picture. Cystic adenomatoid malformations can be diagnosed in utero by ultrasonography. In one series of 16 such cases, the diagnosis was almost always made at 21–23 wk of gestation (range, 18–36 wk). Polyhydramnios was common (25%). Lesions that cause progressive mediastinal shift and fetal hydrops are almost always fatal. Large lesions, by compressing adjacent lung, may produce pulmonary hypoplasia in nonaffected lobes (see Chapter 383.2). However, even lesions that appear large in early gestation may regress considerably or decrease in relative size and be associated with good pulmonary function in childhood.

Clinical Manifestations. Patients who present in the newborn period or early infancy have respiratory distress, recurrent respiratory infection, and pneumothorax. The lesion may be confused with diaphragmatic hernia. Patients with smaller lesions are asymptomatic until mid childhood, when brief episodes of recurrent or persistent pulmonary infection or relatively acute chest pain occur. Breath sounds may be diminished with mediastinal shift away from the lesion on physical examination. Chest radiographs reveal a cystic mass, sometimes with mediastinal shift. Occasionally, an air-fluid level suggests a lung abscess.

Treatment. Surgical excision of the affected lobe is indicated, because there is a reported increased incidence of primary pulmonary neoplasms in long-term survivors.

383.4 Pulmonary Sequestration

A pulmonary sequestration is a congenital anomaly of lung development and is defined as intrapulmonary or extrapulmonary, depending on location within the visceral pleura or without. These terms are preferred, rather than "intralobar" and "extralobar." The majority of sequestrations are intrapulmonary.

Pathophysiology. The lung tissue in a sequestration receives its arterial supply from the systemic arteries (commonly off the aorta) and returns its venous blood to the right side of the heart, usually through the inferior vena cava. As a result, the sequestration functions as a space-occupying lesion within the chest that does not function in gas exchange and does not contribute to left-to-right shunt. Most sequestrations do not have a communication with the airway, and thus do not contribute to dead space. Communication with the airway may occur as the result of rupture of infected material into an adjacent airway. In addition, collateral ventilation within intrapulmonary lesions via pores of Kohn may occur. Intralobar and extralobar sequestrations may arise through the same pathoembryologic mechanism as a remnant of a diverticular outgrowth of the esophagus. However, some propose that intralobar sequestration is an acquired lesion primarily caused by infection and inflammation, which leads to cystic changes and hypertrophy of a feeding systemic artery. This is consistent with the rarity of this lesion in autopsy series of newborns. Gastric or pancreatic tissue may be found within the sequestration. Cysts may also be present. Other congenital anomalies, including diaphragmatic hernia and esophageal cysts, are not uncommon. Some believe that intralobar sequestration is often a manifestation of cystic adenomatoid malformation and have questioned the existence of intralobar sequestration as a separate entity.

Clinical Manifestations and Treatment. *Intrapulmonary sequestration* is generally found in a lower lobe and does not have its own pleura. Patients usually present with infection. In older patients, hemoptysis is fairly common. A chest radiograph during a period when there is no active infection reveals a mass lesion; an air-fluid level may be present. During infection, the margins of the lesion may be blurred. There is no difference in the incidence of this lesion in each lung. Treatment is surgical removal of the lesion, a procedure that usually requires excision of the entire involved lobe. Segmental resection occasionally suffices.

Extrapulmonary sequestration is much more common in males and almost always involves the left lung. This lesion is enveloped by a pleural covering and is associated strongly with diaphragmatic hernia. Patients may also have other associated abnormalities, such as colonic duplication, vertebral abnormalities, and pulmonary hypoplasia. Many of these patients are asymptomatic when the mass is discovered by routine chest radiography performed for another reason. Other patients present with respiratory symptoms or heart failure. Surgical resection of the involved area is recommended. Subdiaphragmatic extrapulmonary sequestration may present as an abdominal mass on prenatal ultrasonography. In addition, with the advent of prenatal ultrasonography, fetal pulmonary sequestrations have been shown to spontaneously regress.

Physical findings in patients with sequestration include an area of dullness to percussion and decreased breath sounds over the lesion. During infection, crackles may also be present. A continuous or purely systolic murmur may be heard over the back. If findings on routine chest radiographs are consistent with the diagnosis, other procedures are indicated before surgical intervention. Bronchography reveals a mass of intrathoracic tissue without connection to the airways. Ultrasonography can help rule out a diaphragmatic hernia. Surgical removal is recommended. Preoperative aortography can be done to confirm the diagnosis and to delineate the blood supply of the lesion. However, some now believe that Doppler ultrasonography and MRI are sufficient in most cases. Identifying the blood supply before surgery avoids inadvertently severing this systemic artery, an event that has accounted for much of the intraoperative mortality in the past.

383.5 Bronchogenic Cysts

Bronchogenic cysts arise from abnormal budding of the tracheal diverticulum of the foregut before the 16th wk of gestation and are originally lined with ciliated epithelium. They are most commonly found on the right and near a midline structure (e.g., trachea, esophagus, carina), but peripheral lower lobe and perihilar intrapulmonary cysts are not infrequent. Diagnosis may be precipitated by enlargement of the cyst, which causes symptoms by pressure on an adjacent airway. When the diagnosis is delayed until infection occurs, the ciliated epithelium may be lost, and accurate pathologic diagnosis is then impossible. Cysts are rarely demonstrable at birth. Later, some cysts become symptomatic by becoming infected or by enlarging in size and compromising the function of an adjacent airway. Fever, chest pain, and productive cough are the most common presenting symptoms. A chest radiograph reveals the cyst, which may contain an air-fluid level. Additional information can be obtained by CT scan or barium esophagography. Treatment of symptomatic cysts is surgical excision after appropriate antibiotic management. Even asymptomatic cysts discovered incidentally by chest roentgenogram taken for another reason should probably be treated by surgical excision, in view of the 75–90% rate of infection.

383.6 Congenital Pulmonary Lymphangiectasia

This disease, characterized by greatly dilated lymphatic ducts throughout the lung, can occur in several pathologic circumstances. Pulmonary venous obstruction produces an elevated transvascular pressure and engorges the pulmonary lymphatics. Generalized lymphangiectasis is a generalized disease of several organ systems, predominantly the intestines, and may affect the lungs, as well. Finally, lymphangiectasis may occur only in the lung.

Children with pulmonary venous obstruction or severe pulmonary lymphangiectasis present with dyspnea and cyanosis in the newborn period. Chest radiographs reveal diffuse, dense, reticular densities. If the lung is not completely involved, the spared areas appear hyperlucent. Respiration is compromised because of the space-occupying nature of the lesion and possibly because pulmonary compliance is reduced, increasing the work of breathing. The diagnosis can be made from right-sided heart catheterization, CT scans, and open lung biopsy. Treatment is only supportive and includes administration of oxygen, mechanical ventilation, and careful fluid management with

diuretics. Primary pulmonary lymphangiectasia and pulmonary venous obstruction produce severe pulmonary dysfunction and are usually fatal in infancy. Occasionally, the pulmonary venous obstruction is secondary to left-sided cardiac lesions, and relief of the latter can produce improvement in pulmonary dysfunction. Generalized lymphangiectasis generally produces milder pulmonary dysfunction, and survival to mid childhood and beyond is not unusual.

383.7 Lung Hernia

A lung hernia is a protrusion of the lung beyond its normal thoracic boundaries. About 20% of instances of this disorder are congenital; the balance of cases are noted after chest trauma or thoracic surgery or in patients with pulmonary diseases such as cystic fibrosis and asthma, which cause frequent cough and generate high intrathoracic pressure. A congenital weakness of the suprapleural membranes or musculature of the neck may play a role in the appearance of a lung hernia. More than half of congenital lung hernias and almost all acquired hernias are cervical. Congenital cervical hernias usually occur anteriorly through a gap between the scalenus anterior and sternocleidomastoid muscles. Elsewhere, cervical herniation is prevented by the trapezius muscle (posteriorly, at the thoracic inlet) and the three scalene muscles (laterally).

The presenting sign of a cervical hernia is usually a neck mass noticed while straining or coughing. Some lesions are asymptomatic and detected only when a chest film is taken for another reason. Findings on physical examination are normal except during Valsalva maneuver, when a soft bulge may be noticed in the neck. In most cases, no treatment is necessary. However, these hernias may cause problems during attempts to place a central venous catheter through the jugular or subclavian veins. Spontaneous resolution can occur.

Paravertebral or parasternal hernias are usually associated with rib anomalies. Intercostal hernias usually occur parasternally, where the external intercostal muscle is absent. Posteriorly, despite the seemingly inadequate internal intercostal muscle, the paraspinal muscles usually prevent herniation. Straining, coughing, or playing a musical instrument may have a role in causing intercostal hernias, but in most cases, there is probably a pre-existing defect in the thoracic wall.

Surgical treatment for lung hernia is occasionally justified for cosmetic reasons. In patients with severe chronic pulmonary disease and chronic cough and for whom cough suppression is contraindicated, permanent correction may not be achieved.

383.8 Other Congenital Malformations of the Lung

Congenital Lobar Emphysema and Pulmonary Cysts. See Chapter 380.

Pulmonary Arteriovenous Malformation. See Chapters 425 and 436.

Bronchobiliary Fistula. This rare anomaly usually presents life-threatening problems during early infancy, but diagnosis occasionally has been delayed until adulthood. Females are more commonly affected. The bronchobiliary fistula consists of a fistulous connection between the right middle lobe bronchus and the left hepatic ductal system. All patients have recurrent severe bronchopulmonary infection starting in early infancy. Definitive diagnosis requires endoscopy and bronchography or exploratory surgery. Treatment includes surgical excision of the entire intrathoracic portion of the fistula. If the hepatic portion of the fistula does not communicate with the biliary system or duodenum, the involved segment may also have to be resected. Bronchobiliary communications also occur as acquired lesions resulting from hepatic disease complicated by infection.

Bagolan P, Nahom A, Giorlandino C, et al: Cystic adenomatoid malformation of the lung: Clinical evolution and management. *Eur J Pediatr* 1999;158:879–82.

Bhalla M, Leitman BS, Forcade C, et al: Lung hernia: Radiographic features. *AJR Am J Roentgenol* 1990;154:51.

Carpentieri DF, Guttenberg M, Quinn TM, Adzick NS: Subdiaphragmatic pulmonary sequestration: A case report with review of the literature. *J Perinatol* 2000;20:60.

Case Records of the Massachusetts General Hospital: Case 20-1996. *N Engl J Med* 1996;334:1726.

Case Records of the Massachusetts General Hospital: Case 14-1991. *N Engl J Med* 1991;324:980.

Case Records of the Massachusetts General Hospital: Case 31-1989. *N Engl J Med* 1989;321:309.

Fokstuen S, Schinzel A: Unilateral lobar pulmonary agenesis in sibs. *J Med Genet* 2000;37:557.

Garcia-Pena P, Lucaya J, Hendry GM, et al: Spontaneous involution of pulmonary sequestration in children: A report of two cases and review of the literature. *Pediatr Radiol* 1998;28:266–70.

Gauderer MWL, Oiticica C, Bishop HC: Congenital bronchobiliary fistula: Management of the involved hepatic segment. *J Pediatr Surg* 1993;28:452.

Glenn C, Bonekat W, Cua A, et al: Lung hernia. *Am J Emerg Med* 1997;15:260.

Hernanz-Schulman M: Cysts and cystlike lesions of the lung. *Radiol Clin North Am* 1993;31:631.

Huber A, Schranz D, Blaha I, et al: Congenital pulmonary lymphangiectasia. *Pediatr Pulmonol* 1991;10:310.

Husain AN, Hessel RG: Neonatal pulmonary hypoplasia: An autopsy study of 25 cases. *Pediatr Pathol* 1993;13:475.

Mardini MK, Nyhan WL: Agenesis of the lung: Report of four patients with unusual anomalies. *Chest* 1985;87:522.

Nicolette LA, Kosloske AM, Bartow SA, et al: Intralobar pulmonary sequestration: A clinical and pathological spectrum. *J Pediatr Surg* 1993;28:802.

Rubin EM, Garcia H, Horowitz MD, et al: Fatal massive hemoptysis secondary to intralobar sequestration. *Chest* 1994;106:954.

Schwartz D, Reyes-Mugica M, Keller M: Imaging of surgical diseases of the newborn chest. *Radiol Clin North Am* 1999;37:1067–78.

Verlaat CWM, Peters HM, Semmekrot BA, et al: Congenital pulmonary lymphangiectasis presenting as a unilateral hyperlucent lung. *Eur J Pediatr* 1994;153:202.

Zach MS: Adult outcome of congenital lower respiratory tract malformations. *Thorax* 2001;56:65–72.

Chapter 384
Pulmonary Edema

Robert Mazor and Thomas P. Green

Pulmonary edema is an excessive accumulation of fluid in the cells, interstitium, and air spaces of the lung. It is a common problem in the acutely ill child as a sequela of several different pathologic processes.

Pathophysiology. The pressure and osmolarity on either side of a pulmonary capillary, as well as the capillary permeability, are the physical factors that determine fluid movement through the capillary wall. Baseline conditions lead to a net filtration of fluid from the intravascular space into the interstitium. This "extra" interstitial fluid is rapidly reabsorbed by pulmonary lymphatics. Conditions that lead to altered capillary permeability, increased pulmonary capillary pressure, or decreased intravascular oncotic pressure will increase the flow out of the capillary (Box 384–1) and thereby lead to water accumulation in the lung

To understand the sequence of lung water accumulation, it is helpful to consider its distribution among four distinct compartments.

1. *The vascular compartment:* This compartment consists of all blood vessels that participate in fluid exchange with the interstitium. The vascular compartment is separated from the interstitium by capillary endothelial cells. Several endogenous inflammatory mediators, as well as exogenous toxins, are implicated in the pathogenesis of pulmonary capillary endothelial damage, leading to the "leakiness" seen in several systemic processes.

BOX 384–1. Etiology of Pulmonary Edema

INCREASED PULMONARY CAPILLARY PRESSURE
Cardiogenic, such as left ventricular failure
Noncardiogenic, as in pulmonary veno-occlusive disease, pulmonary venous fibrosis, mediastinal tumors

INCREASED CAPILLARY PERMEABILITY
Bacterial and viral pneumonia
Acute respiratory distress syndrome (ARDS)
Inhaled toxic agents
Circulating toxins
Vasoactive substances such as histamine, leukotrienes, thromboxanes
Diffuse capillary leak syndrome, as in sepsis
Immunologic reactions, such as transfusion reactions
Smoke inhalation
Aspiration pneumonia/pneumonitis
Drowning and near-drowning
Radiation pneumonia
Uremia

LYMPHATIC INSUFFICIENCY
Congenital and acquired

DECREASED ONCOTIC PRESSURE
Hypoalbuminemia, as in renal and hepatic diseases, protein-losing states, and malnutrition

INCREASED NEGATIVE INTERSTITIAL PRESSURE
Upper airway obstructive lesions, such as croup and epiglottitis
Re-expansion pulmonary edema

MIXED OR UNKNOWN CAUSES
Neurogenic pulmonary edema
High-altitude pulmonary edema
Eclampsia
Pancreatitis
Pulmonary embolism
Heroin (narcotic) pulmonary edema

Modified from Robin E, Carroll C, Zelis R: Pulmonary edema. *N Engl J Med* 1973; 288:239, 292 (2 parts) and Desphande J, Wetzel R, Rogers M: In Rogers M (editor): *Textbook of Pediatric Intensive Care*, 3rd ed. Baltimore, Williams & Wilkins, 1996, pp 432–42.

---

2. *The interstitial compartment:* The importance of this space lies in its interposition between the alveolar and vascular compartments. As fluid leaves the vascular compartment it collects in the interstitium before overflowing into the air spaces of the alveolar compartment.

3. *The alveolar compartment:* This compartment is lined with type 1 and type 2 epithelial cells. A growing body of evidence exists outlining the role of these epithelial cells in active fluid transport from the alveolar space.

4. *The pulmonary lymphatic compartment:* There is an extensive network of pulmonary lymphatics. Excess fluid present within the alveolar and interstitial compartments is drained via the lymphatic system. When the capacity for drainage of the lymphatics is surpassed, fluid accumulation occurs.

Etiology. Box 384–1 lists the etiology of pulmonary edema. The specific clinical findings vary according to the underlying mechanism.

Increases in pulmonary vascular pressure *(capillary hydrostatic pressure)* lead to increased flow from the vessel. Cardiac processes that lead to failure of left-sided forward flow (e.g., myocarditis) or increased left-sided back flow (e.g., valvular regurgitation) increase pulmonary capillary pressure. In addition, there are noncardiac causes involving abnormalities of the pulmonary veins that obstruct venous drainage, leading to an increase in capillary pressure.

Increased capillary permeability is usually secondary to damage to the endothelium. Because of the large amount of pulmonary blood flow, the lung is especially susceptible to circulating toxins. Endogenous substances such as inflammatory mediators (e.g., tumor necrosis factor-α, leukotrienes, thromboxanes) and vasoactive agents (e.g., nitric oxide, histamine) formed during pulmonary and systemic processes play a role in the endothelial damage, and, therefore, the altered capillary permeability that occurs with many disease processes.

Fluid homeostasis in the lung is dependent largely on drainage via the lymphatics. Experimentally, pulmonary edema occurs with obstruction of the lymphatic system. Increased lymph flow and dilation of lymphatic vessels occur in chronic edematous states.

By decreasing the forces promoting fluid re-entry into the vascular space, decreases in intravascular oncotic pressure lead to pulmonary edema. This occurs in dilutional disorders such as fluid overload with hypotonic solutions and in protein-losing states such as nephrotic syndrome and malnutrition.

Increased negative interstitial pressure is invoked in disorders in which upper airway obstruction exists, such as croup. Other mechanisms may also be involved. Theories implicate an increase in CO_2 tension, decreased O_2 tension, and extreme increases in cardiac afterload, leading to transient cardiac insufficiency.

The mechanism causing neurogenic pulmonary edema is not clear. A massive sympathetic discharge secondary to a cerebral insult may produce increased pulmonary and systemic vasoconstriction, resulting in a shift of blood to the pulmonary vasculature, an increase in capillary pressure, and edema formation. The mechanism causing high-altitude pulmonary edema is unclear, but it may also be related to sympathetic outflow, increased pulmonary vascular pressures, and hypoxia-induced increases in capillary permeability.

Clinical Manifestations. The clinical features that arise depend on the mechanism of edema formation. In general, the interstitial and alveolar edema prevent the inflation of alveoli, leading to atelectasis and decreased surfactant production, resulting in decreased pulmonary compliance and decreased tidal volumes. In an effort to maintain adequate minute ventilation, the patient must increase respiratory effort to preserve tidal volume and/or increase respiratory rate. With the accumulation of fluid in the alveolar space, auscultation reveals fine crackles and wheezing, especially in dependent lung fields.

Chest radiographs can provide useful ancillary data. Early radiographic signs include peribronchial and perivascular cuffing representing accumulation of interstitial edema. Diffuse streakiness reflects interlobular edema and distended pulmonary lymphatics. Diffuse, patchy densities secondary to alveolar filling are a late sign. Cardiomegaly and increased pulmonary vascular markings are seen with causes involving left ventricular dysfunction. Chest tomography demonstrates that edema accumulates in the dependent areas of the lung. Therefore, changing the patient position can alter regional differences in lung compliance and alveolar ventilation.

Treatment. The treatment of a patient with pulmonary edema should be directed toward the underlying cause. Patients should receive supplemental oxygen in an effort to increase alveolar oxygen tension and decrease pulmonary vasoconstriction. Patients with cardiogenic causes should be managed with inotropes, afterload-reducing agents, and diuretic agents. Several groups have questioned the universal use of diuretics in adults with pulmonary edema stating that the pulmonary edema is not, in general, associated with fluid retention but, rather, is associated with fluid redistribution. However, diuretics are valuable in the treatment of pulmonary edema associated with total-body fluid overload (e.g., sepsis, renal insufficiency). Morphine is often helpful as a vasodilator and a mild sedative.

Several studies have demonstrated the effectiveness of positive airway pressure such as positive end-expiratory pressure (PEEP) and continuous positive airway pressure (CPAP). The mechanism by which positive airway pressure improves pulmonary edema is not entirely clear but does not seem to be associated with decreasing lung water. Rather, CPAP prevents closure of alveoli and may reopen collapsed alveolar units. This leads to increased functional residual capacity (FRC). Increased FRC leads to improved pulmonary compliance, improved surfactant function, and decreased pulmonary vascular resistance. The net effect is to decrease the work of breathing, improve oxygenation, and decrease cardiac afterload.

Cotter G, Kaluski E, Moshkoviz Y, et al: Pulmonary edema: New insight on pathogenesis and treatment. *Curr Opin Cardiol* 2001;16:159–63.

Crandall E, Matthay M: Alveolar epithelial transport: Basic science to clinical medicine. *Am J Respir Crit Care Med* 2001; 162:1021–29.

Deshpande J, Wetzel R, Rogers M: Unusual causes of myocardial ischemia, pulmonary edema, and cyanosis. In Rogers M (editor): *Textbook of Pediatric Intensive Care*, 3rd ed. Baltimore, Williams & Wilkins, 1996, pp 432–42.

Gattinoni L, Pesenti A, Bombino M, et al: Relationships between lung computed tomographic density, gas exchange, and PEEP in acute respiratory failure. *Anesthesiology* 1988;69:824–32.

Robin E, Carroll C, Zelis R: Pulmonary edema. *N Engl J Med* 1973; 288:239, 292 (2 parts).

Tilden S, Logan J: Lung parenchyma. In Holbrook (editor): *Textbook of Pediatric Critical Care*. Philadelphia, WB Saunders, 1993, pp 526–29.

Chapter 385
Aspiration Syndromes
John L. Colombo

A child with aspiration of foreign materials into the lungs may present with obvious acute lung injury from massive or highly toxic substance aspiration, mechanical obstruction of large or intermediate-sized airways, infectious complications of aspiration, or recurrent microaspiration, such as may occur with gastroesophageal reflux or mild dysphagia. The first presentation listed is the focus of this chapter.

Occult aspiration of nasal pharyngeal secretions into the lower respiratory tract has been shown to be a normal event in healthy people, usually without apparent clinical significance. The spectrum of aspiration extends from this asymptomatic group to acute life-threatening events, such as with massive aspiration of gastric contents or hydrocarbon products. Most patients suffering with a syndrome of aspiration have disorders that lie between the ends of this spectrum and present a tremendous challenge in both diagnosis and treatment.

LARGE VOLUME OR TOXIC ASPIRATIONS

Gastric Contents. Aspiration of large volumes most commonly occurs with aspiration after vomiting. The pathologic and physiologic consequences can vary depending on the pH and volume of the aspirate and the amount of particulate material. Increased clinical severity should be expected with volumes greater than approximately 0.8 mL/kg and/or pH less than 2.5. Hypoxemia, hemorrhagic pneumonitis, atelectasis, intravascular fluid shifts, and pulmonary edema all occur rapidly with massive aspiration. These will occur earlier, become more severe, and last longer with acid aspiration. Most clinical changes are present within minutes to 1–2 hr after aspiration. Over the next 24–48 hr there is a marked increase in lung parenchymal neutrophil infiltration, mucosal sloughing, and alveolar consolidation that often correlates with increasing infiltrates on chest radiographs. These changes tend to occur significantly later and are more prolonged after aspiration of small particles. Infection usually does not play a role in initial lung injury after aspiration of gastric contents. However, such aspiration may impair pulmonary defenses, predisposing to later secondary bacterial pneumonia.

Hydrocarbon Aspiration. The most dangerous consequence of acute hydrocarbon ingestion is usually aspiration and resulting pneumonitis. Fortunately, significant pneumonitis is a relatively infrequent event, occurring in less than 2% of all hydrocarbon ingestions. However, the outcome can be severe. There are an estimated 20 deaths annually from hydrocarbon aspiration in both children and adults. Of these, several represent successful suicide attempts. Hydrocarbons with lower surface tensions (gasoline, turpentine, naphthalene) have more potential for aspiration toxicity than heavier mineral or fuel oils. Ingestion of more than 30 mL (approximate volume of an adult swallow) of hydrocarbon is associated with an increased risk of severe pneumonitis. Patients presenting with shortness of breath or hypoxemia are at high risk for severe pneumonitis. Other organ systems also may suffer serious injury, especially the liver, central nervous system, and heart. Cardiac dysrhythmias may occur and be exacerbated by hypoxia and acid-base or electrolyte disturbances.

Certain hydrocarbons have more inherent system toxicity. These are referred to collectively by the mnemonic CHAMP: *c*amphor, *h*alogenated hydrocarbons, *a*romatic hydrocarbons, and those associated with *m*etals and *p*esticides. Patients who ingestion these compounds in volumes greater than 30 mL, such as may occur especially with intentional overdose, may benefit from gastric emptying. However, as a general rule, gastric emptying is contraindicated because of further risk of aspiration. If gastric emptying is utilized, it must be done cautiously to avoid aspiration. If a cuffed endotracheal tube can be placed without inducing vomiting, this should be considered, especially in the presence of altered mental status. Treatment of each case should be considered individually with guidance from a poison control center.

Other substances that are particularly toxic and occasionally aspirated, causing significant lung injury, include baby powder, chlorine, shellac, beryllium, and mercury vapors. Repeated exposures to lower concentrations of these agents may lead to chronic lung disease, such as interstitial pneumonitis and granuloma formation. Corticosteroids may help reduce fibrosis development.

Treatment. If the patient has an artificial airway it is important to perform immediate suctioning of the airway. However, bronchoscopy is usually of limited therapeutic value unless it can be performed very soon after massive aspiration, or significant particle aspiration is suspected. If bronchoscopy is performed, findings of localized carinal erythema and microscopic or macroscopic food particles may be helpful if the diagnosis is in doubt. Attempts at acid neutralization are not warranted because acid is neutralized by the respiratory epithelium very rapidly. Patients with potential massive aspiration or hydrocarbon aspiration should be observed, have oxygenation measured (by oximetry or blood gas analysis), and have a chest radiograph taken, even if asymptomatic. If the chest radiograph and oxygen saturation are normal, and the patient remains asymptomatic, the patient may usually be observed at home after an observation period in the hospital or office. No therapy at that time would be indicated, but the parents should be instructed to bring their child for medical attention if respiratory symptoms or fever develops.

For those patients with abnormal findings, oxygen therapy is necessary to correct hypoxemia. Endotracheal intubation and mechanical ventilation are often necessary for more severe cases. Bronchodilators may be given, although they are usually of limited benefit. Treatment with corticosteroids does not appear to have any benefit unless they can be given nearly simultaneously with the time of aspiration (based primarily on animal studies), and their use may increase the risk of secondary

infection. As a general rule, prophylactic antibiotics are not indicated. However, risk-benefit must be assessed and, in the patient with very limited reserve, antibiotic coverage, especially for mixed anaerobes, may be appropriate. If the aspiration occurs in a hospitalized or chronically ill patient, coverage for *Pseudomonas* and enteric gram-negative organisms should also be considered. With massive aspiration, mortality rates as high as 40–80% have been reported. More recent reports indicate a mortality rate of 5%, and even lower if three or fewer lobes are involved. Unless complications develop, such as infection, most patients will recover in 2–3 wk, but prolonged lung damage may persist with scarring and bronchiolitis obliterans.

Feeding with enteral tubes passed beyond the pylorus and elevating the head of the bed of mechanically ventilated patients have been shown to reduce the incidence of aspiration complications.

Bynum L, Pierce A: Pulmonary aspiration of gastric contents. *Am Rev Respir Dis* 1976;114:1129–36.

Campinos L, Duval G, Couturier M, et al: The value of early fiberoptic bronchoscopy after aspiration of gastric contents. *Br J Anaesth* 1983;55:1103–5.

Gleeson K, Eggli D, Maxwell S: Quantitative aspiration during sleep in normal subjects. *Chest* 1997;111:1266–72.

Hickling KG, Howard R: A retrospective survey of treatment and mortality in aspiration pneumonia. *Intensive Care Med* 1988;14:617–22.

Mickiewicz M, Gomez HF: Hydrocarbon toxicity: General review and management guidelines. *Air Med J* 2001;20:8–11.

Radio DM, Rocke DA, Brock-Utne JG, et al: Critical volume for pulmonary acid aspiration: Reappraisal in a primate model. *Br J Anaesth* 1990;65:248–50.

Chapter 386
Chronic Recurrent Aspiration *John L. Colombo*

The recurrent aspiration of gastric, nasal, or oral contents can lead to several clinical presentations, including recurrent bronchitis or bronchiolitis, recurrent pneumonia, atelectasis, wheezing, cough, apnea, or laryngospasm. Pathologic outcomes include granulomatous inflammation, interstitial inflammation, fibrosis, lipoid pneumonia, and bronchiolitis obliterans. Underlying disorders that are frequently associated with recurrent aspiration are listed in Box 386-1.

In a series of 238 children hospitalized with recurrent pneumonia, the most common underlying problem was oropharyngeal incoordination present in 48% of these patients. Gastroesophageal reflux (GER) is also a common underlying problem that may predispose to recurrent respiratory disease but is less commonly associated with recurrent pneumonia. GER is discussed in Chapter 387 (see also Chapter 304).

Clinical Manifestations and Diagnosis. Underlying predisposing factors, such as those mentioned in Box 386-1, although frequently obvious, sometimes may require further evaluation. Initial assessment begins with a detailed history and physical examination. The caregivers should be asked about the timing of symptoms in relation to feedings, positional changes, spitting, vomiting, arching, or epigastric discomfort in an older child and nocturnal symptoms with coughing or wheezing. Coughing or gagging may be minimal or absent in a child with a depressed cough or gag reflex. Observation of a feeding is essential when considering a diagnosis of recurrent aspiration. Particular attention should be given to nasopharyngeal reflux, difficulty with sucking or swallowing, and associated coughing and choking. Oral cavities should be inspected for gross abnormalities and

BOX 386–1. Conditions Predisposing Children to Aspiration Lung Injury

ANATOMICAL AND MECHANICAL

Tracheoesophageal fistula
Laryngeal cleft
Vascular ring
Cleft palate
Micrognathia
Macroglossia
Achalasia
Esophageal foreign body
Tracheostomy
Endotracheal tube
Nasoenteric tube
Collagen vascular disease (scleroderma, dermatomyositis)
Gastroesophageal reflux disease
Obesity

NEUROMUSCULAR

Altered consciousness
Immaturity of swallowing
Dysautonomia
Increased intracranial pressure
Hydrocephalus
Vocal cord paralysis
Cerebral palsy
Muscular dystrophy
Myasthenia gravis
Guillain-Barré syndrome
Werdnig-Hoffmann disease
Ataxia-telangiectasia
Cerebrovascular accident

MISCELLANEOUS

Poor oral hygiene
Gingivitis
Prolonged hospitalization
Gastric outlet or intestinal obstruction
Poor feeding techniques (bottle propping, overfeeding, inappropriate foods for toddlers)

stimulated to assess the gag reflex. Drooling or excessive accumulation of secretions in the mouth suggest dysphagia. Lung auscultation may reveal transient wheezes or crackles after feeding, particularly in the dependent lung segments.

Laboratory Findings. A plain chest radiograph is the usual initial study for a child suspected of having recurrent aspiration. The classic findings of segmental or lobar infiltrates localized in dependent areas may be found, but there are a wide variety of radiographic findings. These findings include diffuse infiltrates, lobar infiltrates, bronchial wall thickening, hyperinflation, and normal findings. CT scans may show infiltrates with decreased attenuation suggestive of lipoid pneumonia. CT scans are not commonly indicated to establish a diagnosis of aspiration, but the diagnosis may be an incidental finding when such imaging is done for other reasons.

Numerous other tests are available for detecting aspiration or GER. A carefully performed barium esophagram is very useful in looking for anatomic abnormalities such as vascular ring, stricture, hiatal hernia, or tracheoesophageal fistula. It also yields qualitative information about esophageal motility and, when extended, of gastric emptying. However, the esophagogram is quite insensitive and nonspecific for aspiration or GER. A modified barium swallow with videofluoroscopy is generally considered the gold standard for evaluating the swallowing mechanism. The study is preferably done with assistance of a pediatric feeding specialist and a parent. The child should be seated in a normal eating position, and various consistencies of barium or barium-impregnated foods are offered. This is significantly more sensitive for demonstrating aspiration than

bedside assessment or traditional barium swallow. The sensitivity of this modified barium swallow is such that it occasionally detects aspiration in patients without abnormal respiratory findings.

A gastroesophageal ("milk") scintiscan offers theoretical advantages of being more physiologic and giving a longer window of viewing than the barium esophagram for detecting GER and aspiration. However, in most studies this has been relatively insensitive for detection of aspiration. Another radionuclide scan termed the *salivagram* is also useful to assess aspiration of oropharyngeal contents. The fiberoptic endoscopic evaluation of swallowing has been used primarily in adult patients but may have some utility in pediatric patients, especially when combined with laryngopharyngeal sensory testing.

Tracheobronchial aspirates also can be examined for numerous entities to evaluate for aspiration. For patients with artificial airways, the use of an oral dye and visual examination of tracheal secretions is commonly used. This test should not be done on a chronic basis owing to possible dye toxicity. In using this test acutely, it is important to administer an adequate volume of dye, but even this may be relatively insensitive compared with measuring lactose or glucose in appropriately fed patients. Quantitation of lipid-laden alveolar macrophages from bronchial aspirates is a sensitive and relatively specific test for lipid aspiration, but false-positive tests undoubtedly occur, especially with endobronchial obstruction and use of intravenous lipids. Bronchial washings may also be examined for various food substances, including lactose, glucose, food fibers, and milk antigens. Specificity and sensitivity of these tests have not been well delineated.

Treatment. If chronic aspiration is associated with another underlying medical condition, treatment should be directed toward that problem. The frequency and severity of respiratory problems will determine the level of intervention. Often mild dysphagia can be treated with alteration of feeding position or giving thickened foods. Nasogastric tube feedings can be utilized temporarily during periods of transient vocal cord dysfunction or other dysphagia. Postpyloric feedings may also be helpful, especially when GER is a concern.

Several surgical procedures may be considered. Tracheostomy, although sometimes actually predisposing to aspiration, may provide overall benefit from improved bronchial hygiene. Fundoplication with a gastrostomy or jejunostomy feeding tube will reduce the probability of GER-induced disease, but recurrent pneumonias often persist because of dysphagia and presumed aspiration of upper airway secretions. Medical treatment with anticholinergics, such as glycopyrrolate, may significantly reduce salivation and morbidity from salivary aspiration but often has side effects. Aggressive surgical intervention with salivary gland excision, ductal ligation, or laryngotracheal separation may be considered in severe, unresponsive cases. Surgical therapy usually is reserved for the most severe cases but may be associated with significant improvement of quality of life.

Blitzer A, Krespi YP, Oppenheimer RW, et al: Surgical management of aspiration. *Otolaryngol Clin North Am* 1988;21:743–50.

Colombo J, Hallberg T: Recurrent aspiration in children: Lipid-laden alveolar macrophage quantitation. *Pediatr Pulmonol* 1987;3:86–9.

Colombo JL, Sammut PH: Aspiration syndromes. In Taussig LM, Landau LI (editors): *Pediatric Respiratory Medicine*. St. Louis, CV Mosby, 1999, pp 439–41.

Cook SP, Lawless S, Mandell GA, et al: The use of the salivagram in the evaluation of severe and chronic aspiration. *Int J Pediatr Otorhinolaryngol* 1997;41:353–61.

Gerber ME, Gaugler MD, Myer CM, et al: Chronic aspiration in children: When are bilateral submandibular gland excision and parotid duct ligation indicated? *Arch Otolaryngol Head Neck Surg* 1996;122:1368–71.

Link DT, Willging JP, Miller CK, et al: Pediatric laryngopharyngeal sensory testing during flexible endoscopic evaluation of swallowing: Feasible and correlative. *Ann Otol Rhinol Laryngol* 2000;109:899–905.

Owayaed AF, Campbell DM, Wang EE: Underlying causes of recurrent pneumonia in children. *Arch Pediatr Adolesc Med* 2000;154:190–4.

Chapter 387

Gastroesophageal Reflux and Respiratory Disorders

John L. Colombo

Over 50% of children with chronic asthma and/or recurrent pneumonia also have excessive gastroesophageal reflux (GER). In addition to these disorders, GER has been associated with apnea (both central and obstructive), stridor, and recurrent cough. It also is found to an excess degree in bronchopulmonary dysplasia and cystic fibrosis. Although respiratory disease can induce GER by increasing abdominothoracic pressure gradients, there is substantial evidence suggesting that the more common pathway is that for GER to trigger respiratory symptoms, particularly of asthma. This may occur from microaspiration with resultant direct inflammation and bronchoconstriction, from vagally mediated effects from stimulation of upper airway receptors, or from esophageal afferent irritation causing a neurogenic reflex.

Clinical Manifestations and Diagnosis. The initial diagnostic approach follows that outlined in Chapter 386 for chronic, recurrent aspiration. It is not always possible to ascertain whether a patient is having microaspiration with GER, and it is often easier to demonstrate GER than aspiration. Barium esophagogram may be warranted with the same caveats noted in Chapter 386. Esophageal pH monitoring is widely considered the gold standard for detecting GER. This test is discussed in Chapter 304, but it should be mentioned here that the definition of pathologic GER used by gastroenterologists may be very different than that which is necessary to provoke respiratory disease. In susceptible individuals, even a normal degree of acid GER may cause respiratory illness, although esophagitis would not be expected. Post-prandial, non-acid GER also will not be detected. Because of this, as well as lack of strong criteria for determining which children with respiratory disease should be evaluated for GER, and given cost-efficacy considerations, an empirical diagnostic/therapeutic trial of anti-GER therapy is often warranted.

Treatment. See Chapter 304. However, control of GER does not necessarily alleviate respiratory symptoms, especially in children with neurologic impairment. This likely relates to the additional problems of these children who have poor airway protection, dysphagia, and aspirate oral contents.

Balson BM, Kravitz EK, McGeady SJ: Diagnosis and treatment of gastroesophageal reflux in children and adolescents with severe asthma. *Ann Allergy Asthma Immunol* 1998;81:159–64.

O'Connor JF, Singer ME, Richter JE: The cost-effectiveness of strategies to assess gastroesophageal reflux as an exacerbating factor in asthma. *Am J Gastroenterol* 1999;94:1472–80.

Smith CD, Othersen HB, Gogan NJ, Walker JD: Nissen fundoplication in children with profound neurologic disability: High risks and unmet goals. *Ann Surg* 1992;215:654–58.

Chapter 388

Parenchymal Disease with Prominent Hypersensitivity, Eosinophilic Infiltration, or Toxin-Mediated Injury

Oren Lakser

388.1 Hypersensitivity to Inhaled Materials

Hypersensitivity pneumonitis (HP) or extrinsic allergic alveolitis is an immunologically mediated diffuse inflammatory disease of the pulmonary interstitium caused by inhalation of a variety of organic antigens. Usually these antigens are of animal or vegetable origin and are typically between 1–5 μm and therefore deposit in the alveoli. Reactive antigens, such as a variety of drugs, can occasionally cause HP.

Etiology. Although typically an adult disease, HP has been reported in children and even infants. There are many types of HP related to the offending antigen. The most common forms in the United States include *farmer's lung* (from moldy hay; antigen is thermophilic actinomycetes), *bird fancier's* or *breeder's lung* (from feces or urine of a wide variety of species), and *ventilation* or *humidifier HP* (from contaminated humidifiers or air conditioners; also caused by thermophilic actinomycetes). Most case reports of HP in children have been the result of antigens inhaled during avian exposure or exposure to molds. There has been one report of HP after exposure to cat hair antigen.

Pathology and Pathogenesis. HP can present as an acute, subacute, or chronic illness. These forms can be distinguished based on the morphologic features of the pulmonary involvement. In the *acute* stage, alveolar walls are infiltrated with neutrophils, lymphocytes, plasma cells, and macrophages. The alveolar lumen may contain a proteinaceous exudate mixed with inflammatory cells. Repeated or continuous exposure may result in a *subacute* presentation. This stage is characterized by the classic non-caseating granuloma associated with HP. Often, there is an associated terminal and respiratory bronchiolitis and alveoli may have pale foamy macrophages. The *chronic* form demonstrates further progression of the granulomatous alveolitis resulting in interstitial fibrosis and honeycombing, primarily affecting the upper lobes.

The immune mechanisms involved with inducing these morphologic changes may include immune complex (type III) hypersensitivity (particularly in the acute presentation), delayed cellular (type IV) hypersensitivity, and the alternate complement pathway.

Clinical Manifestations. *Acute* attacks generally occur 4–8 hr after an exposure. Typical symptoms include fever, chills, cough, dyspnea, myalgia, and malaise that can persist for up to 48 hr. Physical examination usually reveals an ill-appearing, dyspneic child with bibasilar crackles or normal lung examination. Chest radiographs may also be normal or may demonstrate bilateral ground-glass haziness, often sparing the lung apices and bases. These patients may progress to the *subacute* presentation if exposure continues or recurs. The cough worsens, dyspnea becomes more prominent, and anorexia and weight loss may occur. The chest radiograph at this stage takes on a more reticulonodular appearance. Long-term exposure can lead to the *chronic* presentation. Dyspnea and cough are severe, with weight loss, weakness, and hypoxemia. These patients eventually develop chronic alveolitis and fibrosis that can lead to cor pulmonale. Chest radiographs show coarse reticulonodular infiltrates and bronchiectasis primarily in the upper and mid-lung zones.

Diagnosis. The diagnosis of HP is based primarily on the clinical presentation in association with a suspicious exposure. Because the clinical presentation is nonspecific, a high index of suspicion is crucial. A number of laboratory tests may be helpful in confirming a clinical suspicion. HP patients often demonstrate a modest leukocytosis with neutrophilia and a left shift and modest elevation of the erythrocyte sedimentation rate. Serum levels of immunoglobulins (IgG, IgM, and IgA) are often elevated. Skin testing to particular antigens lacks sensitivity and specificity, as do serum precipitins to specific antigens. Both these tests may indicate exposure, but without disease. Bronchoalveolar lavage (BAL) fluid typically demonstrates a marked lymphocytosis (often up to 70%) particularly of the CD8$^+$ suppressor T-cells. BAL fluid may also contain higher levels of immunoglobulins. Pulmonary function tests classically demonstrate a restrictive pattern with impaired gas exchange (diffusion capacity). The presence of a mild obstructive pattern during the acute stage is a poor prognostic indicator. Lastly, some have advocated an inhalational challenge either in the laboratory or by re-exposure to the environment. Challenge testing can be dangerous and therefore should be undertaken only in appropriately equipped diagnostic centers.

Treatment. The single most effective therapeutic approach is complete avoidance of the suspected antigen. Corticosteroids (1–2 mg/kg/24 hr) are of some benefit, but an extended course, perhaps up to 6 mo, is required. In general, prognosis is quite good, but if exposure persists, pulmonary fibrosis may occur and patients may not completely recover their baseline lung function.

Craig TJ, Richardson HB: Update on hypersensitivity pneumonitis. *Compr Ther* 1996;22:559–64.
Daroowalla F, Raghu G: Hypersensitivity pneumonitis. *Compr Ther* 1999;23:244–48.
Fink JW: Hypersensitivity pneumonitis. *Clin Chest Med* 1992;13:303–9.
Grech U, Vella C, Lenicker H: Pigeon breeder's lung in childhood: Varied clinical picture at presentation. *Pediatr Pulmonol* 2000;30:145–8.
Hogan MB, Patterson R, Pore RS, et al: Basement shower hypersensitivity pneumonitis secondary to *Epicoccum nigrum*. *Chest* 1996;110:855–56.
Krasnick J, Patterson R, Stillwell PC, et al: Potentially fatal hypersensitivity pneumonitis in a child. *Clin Pediatr* 1995; 34:388–91.
Olesen HU, Thelle T, Møller JCF: Childhood hypersensitivity pneumonitis probably caused by cat hair. *Acta Pediatr* 1998;87:811–13.
Pitcher WD: Southwest internal medicine conference: Hypersensitivity pneumonitis. *Am J Med Sci* 1990;300:251–66.
Sharma OP: Hypersensitivity pneumonitis. *Dis Mon* 1991;37:409–71.

388.2 Silo Filler Disease

Silo filler disease is also known as silage gas poisoning, or silo filler pneumoconiosis, and is typically caused by nitrogen dioxide toxicity. Nitrogen dioxide is produced in silos (particularly corn silos) within a few hours of filling and reaches a maximum concentration within about 2 days. Dangerous concentrations of gas can remain in a closed silo for as long as 2 wk.

Clinical Manifestations and Diagnosis. Cough and dyspnea typically occur immediately on entering the silo and are often associated with wheezing, nausea, a choking sensation, and fatigue. Rarely, symptoms may be delayed days or even weeks after exposure. Radiologic manifestations include pulmonary edema in the perihilar areas and bases. Some patients may recover and the pulmonary edema clears rapidly. However, often this initial phase is followed by a period of remission for 2–3 wk. This quiescent period gives way to a second phase characterized by fever, progressive dyspnea, cyanosis, and cough associated with

widespread, scattered miliary opacities that could become confluent and take on a more patchy and nodular appearance. These patients may suffer from methemoglobinemia.

Biopsy or autopsy findings include diffuse pulmonary edema, hyperplastic airway epithelium, widened intralobular septa, and bronchiolitis obliterans.

Treatment. Although no controlled trial has been conducted, high-dose corticosteroids have been reported to be of some benefit in reducing the severity and duration of the symptoms. Bronchodilators may also be of some limited benefit. Methemoglobinemia is treated with methylene blue in severe cases. Silo filler disease may be fatal, result in complete recovery, or leave patients with chronic lung disease associated with fibrosis and emphysema.

Dambro MR: Silo filler disease. In Griffith JA: *5 Minute Clinical Consult*. Philadelphia, Lippincott Williams & Wilkins, 2001.
Harrison RJ: Occupational and environmental medicine: Chemicals and gases. *Prim Care* 2000;27:917–82.
Juhl JH, Kuhlman JE: Diseases of occupational, chemical, and physical origin. In Juhl JH, Crummy AB, Kuhlman JE (editors): *Juhl, Paul, and Juhl: Essentials of Radiographic Imaging*, 7th ed. Philadelphia, Lippincott Williams & Wilkins, 1998.

388.3 Paraquat Lung

Paraquat is the most toxic dipyridilium herbicide. Concentrated solutions (12–20%) tend to be more dangerous than dilute solutions. Its toxic effects result from the production of superoxides and other highly reactive free radicals that cause the peroxidation of cell membranes and selective mitochondrial damage, resulting in cell death. Paraquat selectively concentrates in the lungs because of an amine uptake process that exists in alveolar epithelial cells. Additionally, paraquat-induced injury is significantly increased in the presence of high concentrations of oxygen.

Pathophysiologically, there is direct injury to the alveolar-capillary membrane and surfactant loss, adult respiratory distress syndrome, progressive intra-alveolar pulmonary fibrosis, and respiratory failure.

Clinical Manifestations. There are three degrees of paraquat intoxication that appear to be dose related. Patients with mild poisoning after ingestion of less than 20 mg of paraquat ion/kg body weight are usually asymptomatic or may develop vomiting, diarrhea, and mild impairment of gas exchange. Moderate to severe poisoning follows ingestion of 20–40 mg of paraquat ion/kg. These patients typically suffer from vomiting, diarrhea, and caustic injury to the oral or esophageal mucosa and may develop renal failure, hepatic dysfunction, and progressive pulmonary fibrosis, resulting in respiratory failure and death. Acute fulminant poisoning follows ingestion of more than 40 mg of paraquat ion/kg. Marked ulceration of the oropharynx and esophagus occurs, with multiorgan failure and 100% mortality within hours of ingestion.

Treatment. Treatment is generally supportive because no antidote exists. Gastric lavage, activated charcoal, hemoperfusion, and hemodialysis are of limited value in significant poisoning. There have been rare individual case reports of successful treatment of paraquat poisoning with antioxidant therapy consisting of deferoxamine infusion and acetylcysteine. In general, results from lung transplantation are dismal, likely related to long-term storage of paraquat in muscle and eventual reaccumulation in the transplanted lungs. One patient survived transplant when the transplant was delayed more than 40 days after the ingestion.

Overall prognosis is poor. Survivors generally suffer from a persistent restrictive defect with impaired diffusion capacity on tests of pulmonary function.

Ellenhorn MJ, Schonwald S, Ordog J, et al: Pesticides. In Ellenhorn MJ (editor): *Medical Toxicology: Diagnosis and Treatment of Human Poisoning*, 2nd ed. Baltimore, Williams & Wilkins, 1997.

Lheureux P, Leduc D, Vanbust R, et al: Survival in a case of massive paraquat ingestion. *Chest* 1995;107:285–89.

Vance MV: Pesticides. In Rosen P (editor): *Emergency Medicine Concepts and Clinical Practice*, 4th ed. St. Louis, Mosby–Year Book, 1998.

Walder B, Bründler MA, Spilopoulos A, et al: Successful single-lung transplant after paraquat intoxication. *Transplantation* 1997;64:789–91.

Yamada I Snito T, Harunari N, et al: Correlating the severity of paraquat poisoning with special hemodynamic and oxygen metabolic variables. *Crit Care Med* 2000;28:1877–83.

388.4 Eosinophilic Lung Disease (Formerly Löffler Syndrome)

Eosinophilic lung diseases are a heterogeneous group of disorders linked by the common findings of pulmonary infiltrates and circulating or tissue eosinophilia. Recently, many have adopted the term *pulmonary infiltrates with eosinophilia* (PIE) as better terminology for these disorders. There are numerous classification schemes for these types of lung disease. In general, PIE syndromes can be divided into simple pulmonary eosinophilia (Löffler syndrome), prolonged pulmonary eosinophilia, tropical pulmonary eosinophilia, pulmonary eosinophilia with asthma, polyarteritis nodosa, chronic eosinophilic pneumonia, and acute eosinophilic pneumonia. Others have included **Churg-Strauss syndrome**, allergic bronchopulmonary aspergillosis (ABPA), and idiopathic hypereosinophilia syndrome. Other lung diseases such as idiopathic pulmonary fibrosis, Langerhan cell granuloma, and other interstitial lung diseases may have associated eosinophilia but are better classified elsewhere.

Löffler syndrome, the most common PIE syndrome reported in children, is characterized by migrating pulmonary infiltrates accompanied by peripheral blood eosinophilia but minimal respiratory symptoms. This term is rarely used today, and it is likely that most patients with this diagnosis have allergic bronchopulmonary helminthiasis (parasites), medication reactions, or ABPA.

Epidemiology. PIE syndromes appear to be much less common in the pediatric population than in adults. There have been scattered case reports of acute eosinophilic pneumonia and chronic eosinophilic pneumonia in children. However, children previously classified as having Löffler syndrome make up the majority of pediatric cases. Most pediatric case reports suggest an equal number of males and females being affected; however, there may be geographic differences because one group reports a female preponderance in children, similar to adult patients with PIE syndromes. Age at presentation ranges from infancy to adolescence.

Pathology and Pathogenesis. In the pediatric population the most common etiology of PIE syndromes includes parasite infections and drug reactions. The prevalence of individual parasite infections varies geographically. The most common parasite causing PIE syndromes in the United States is *Ascaris lumbricoides*. The eggs are ingested. After the larva hatch, they pass through the intestinal wall and migrate to the lungs, causing an intense inflammatory reaction. Alveolar macrophages, lymphocytes, neutrophils, and eosinophils are the most striking inflammatory cells. Other common parasites include *Strongyloides* species, *Toxocara canis* (dog roundworm, visceral larva migrans), and *Ancylostoma braziliense* ("creeping eruption"). In Africa, South America, and Southeast Asia the filarial worms *Wuchereria bancrofti* and *Brugia malayi* cause tropical pulmonary eosinophilia.

Several drugs have also been reported to cause PIE syndromes. Sulfasalazine, penicillin, ampicillin, ibuprofen, and cromolyn are a few of these drugs that are of common use in pediatric patients. Immunologic mechanisms may be the means by which these drugs result in an intense pulmonary inflammatory reaction.

Clinical Manifestations. In general, patients with PIE syndromes caused by *parasites* or *drugs* present with chronic cough, intermittent fevers, dyspnea, wheezing, and occasionally abdominal pain and weight loss. Symptom duration varies. In *acute eosinophilic pneumonia*, symptoms are usually present for less than a month. In *chronic eosinophilic pneumonia*, symptoms are present for more than 6 mo. Results of physical examination vary but often show tachypnea, crackles, and wheezing.

Diagnosis. The diagnosis of a PIE syndrome is made by clinical manifestations with associated blood eosinophilia and chest radiographic findings. Radiologically, these patients present with nonspecific interstitial, alveolar, or mixed infiltrates. The infiltrates tend to be bilateral and diffuse. Patients with chronic eosinophilic pneumonia demonstrate peripheral infiltrates with central sparing ("photographic negative of pulmonary edema"). In addition, eosinophilic lung diseases can be diagnosed by the presence of pulmonary infiltrates and eosinophilia on bronchoalveolar lavage. Lastly, lung biopsy can be used to make the diagnosis.

Treatment. Therapy varies with the type of PIE syndrome. In general, parasite and drug-induced PIE syndromes carry a good prognosis and resolve spontaneously with supportive care and removal of exposure. Rarely, medications to eradicate the parasites may be warranted. Patients with other forms of eosinophilic lung diseases including acute eosinophilic pneumonia and chronic eosinophilic pneumonia may require a course of corticosteroids. Prognosis for patients with most forms of eosinophilic lung disease is good. Acute eosinophilic pneumonia, however, may be life threatening.

Allen JN, Davis WB: Eosinophilic lung diseases. *Am J Respir Crit Care Med* 1994;150:1423–38.

Fujimura J: A neonate with Löffler syndrome. *J Perinatol* 2001; 21:207–8.

Oermann CM, Panesar KS, Langston C, et al: Pulmonary infiltrates with eosinophilia syndromes in children. *J Pediatr* 2000;136:351–58.

Ong RKC, Doyle RL: Tropical pulmonary eosinophilia. *Chest* 1998;113:1673–79.

Sarniak AP, Heidemann SM: Acute eosinophilic pneumonia: A treatable cause of severe acute respiratory failure. *Crit Care Med* 1999;27:2069–71.

Chapter 389

Pneumonia *Theodore C. Sectish and Charles G. Prober*

Pneumonia is an inflammation of the parenchyma of the lungs. Most cases of pneumonia are caused by microorganisms, but there are several noninfectious causes, which include but are not limited to aspiration of food or gastric acid, foreign bodies, hydrocarbons, and lipoid substances; hypersensitivity reactions; and drug- or radiation-induced pneumonitis. Infections in neonates (see Chapter 98) and other immunocompromised hosts (see Chapter 164) are distinct from infections occurring in otherwise normal infants and children.

Pneumonia is a significant cause of mortality in childhood throughout the world, particularly in developing countries. It causes approximately 4 million deaths among children worldwide. In the United States from 1939 to 1996, mortality caused by pneumonia in children declined by 97%. It is hypothesized that this decline is attributable to the introduction of antibiotics and the expansion of medical insurance coverage for children

Etiology. The cause of pneumonia in an individual patient is often difficult to determine because direct culture is invasive and usually not indicated. Bacterial and viral causes are found in 44–85% of children with community-acquired pneumonia, with more than one pathogen in 25–40%. The most common combination of pathogens is *Streptococcus pneumoniae* (pneumococcus) with either respiratory syncytial virus (RSV) or *Mycoplasma pneumoniae.*

Specific risk factors for the development of pneumonia include (1) lung disease, such as asthma or cystic fibrosis; (2) anatomic problems, such as tracheoesophageal fistula; (3) gastroesophageal reflux disease with aspiration; (4) neurologic disorders that interfere with protection of the airway or compromise clearing of the airway; and (5) diseases that alter the immune system, such as immunodeficiency diseases or hemoglobinopathies.

Epidemiology. Epidemiologic factors are useful in determining the etiology of pneumonia. Age, season of the year, immunization status, and health status of the child are helpful in narrowing the list of possible causes. Viral pathogens are the predominant cause of lower respiratory tract infections in infants and children younger than 5 yr of age. Unlike bronchiolitis, for which the peak attack rate is within the 1st yr of life, the peak attack rate for viral pneumonia is between the ages of 2 and 3 yr and decreases slowly thereafter.

Of the respiratory viruses, RSV is the major pathogen, especially in children younger than 3 yr of age. Other common viruses causing pneumonia include parainfluenza viruses, influenza viruses, and adenoviruses. Nonviral pathogens including *S. pneumoniae, M. pneumoniae,* and *Chlamydia pneumoniae* are more common in children older than 5 yr of age. Other bacterial causes of pneumonia in normal children are group A *Streptococcus* (*Streptococcus pyogenes*) and *Staphylococcus aureus. Haemophilus influenzae* type b was an important cause of bacterial pneumonia in young children in the past but has become uncommon with the routine use of effective vaccines. Similarly, the overall incidence of disease caused by *S. pneumoniae* should decline with the introduction of the heptavalent conjugated pneumococcal vaccine. For example, in one study conducted in a daycare center in Israel, there was a 16% reduction in the incidence of lower respiratory tract infections in vaccine recipients.

Lower respiratory tract viral infections in the United States are much more common in the fall and winter, related to the seasonal epidemics of respiratory viral infection that occur each year. The typical pattern of these epidemics usually begins in the fall when parainfluenza infections appear and are most often manifest as croup. Later in winter, RSV and influenza virus cause widespread infection, including upper respiratory tract infections, bronchiolitis, and pneumonia. RSV attacks infants and young children, whereas influenza virus causes disease and excess hospitalization for acute respiratory illness in all age groups. The knowledge of the prevailing viral epidemic may lead to a presumptive initial diagnosis.

Immunization status is relevant because children fully immunized against *H. influenzae* type b and *S. pneumoniae* are less likely to be infected with these pathogens. Children who are immunosuppressed or who have an underlying illness are at risk for specific pathogens, such as *Pseudomonas* in patients with cystic fibrosis.

Pathogenesis. The lower respiratory tract is normally kept sterile by physiologic defense mechanisms, including the mucociliary escalator, the properties of normal secretions such as secretory IgA, and clearing of the airway by coughing. Immunologic defense mechanisms of the lung that limit invasion by pathogenic organisms include macrophages that are present in alveoli and bronchioles, secretory IgA, and other immunoglobulins.

Viral pneumonia usually results from spread of infection along the airways, accompanied by direct injury of the respiratory epithelium resulting in airway obstruction from swelling, abnormal secretions, and cellular debris. The small caliber of airways in young infants makes them particularly susceptible to severe infection. Atelectasis, interstitial edema, and ventilation-perfusion mismatch causing significant hypoxemia often accompany airway obstruction. Viral infection of the respiratory tract also can predispose to secondary bacterial infection by disturbing normal host defense mechanisms, altering secretions, and modifying the bacterial flora.

When bacterial infection is established in the lung parenchyma, the pathologic process varies according to the invading organism. *M. pneumoniae* attaches to the respiratory epithelium, inhibits ciliary action, and leads to cellular destruction and an inflammatory response in the submucosa. As the infection progresses, sloughed cellular debris, inflammatory cells, and mucus cause airway obstruction, with spread of infection occurring along the bronchial tree similar to that of viral pneumonia.

S. pneumoniae produces local edema that aids in the proliferation of organisms and spread into adjacent portions of lung, often resulting in the characteristic focal lobar involvement.

Group A *Streptococcus* infection of the lower respiratory tract results in more diffuse infection with interstitial pneumonia. The pathology includes necrosis of tracheobronchial mucosa; formation of large amounts of exudate, edema, and local hemorrhage with extension into the interalveolar septa; and involvement of lymphatic vessels and the increased likelihood of pleural involvement.

S. aureus pneumonia is manifest by confluent bronchopneumonia, which is often unilateral and characterized by the presence of extensive areas of hemorrhagic necrosis and irregular areas of cavitation of the lung parenchyma, resulting in pneumatoceles, empyema, or, at times, bronchopulmonary fistulas.

An underlying disorder should be considered if a child experiences recurrent bacterial pneumonia. Defects to consider include abnormalities of antibody production (e.g., agammaglobulinemia, hypogammaglobulinemia, or IgG subclass deficiencies), granulocyte defects (e.g., chronic granulomatous disease), cystic fibrosis, ciliary dyskinesia, congenital bronchiectasis, tracheoesophageal fistula, increased pulmonary blood flow, or a deficient gag reflex. Additional factors that promote pulmonary infection include trauma, anesthesia, and aspiration.

Clinical Manifestations. Viral and bacterial pneumonias are most often preceded by several days of symptoms of an upper respiratory tract infection, typically rhinitis and cough. In viral pneumonia, fever usually is present; however, temperatures are generally lower than in bacterial pneumonia. Tachypnea is the most consistent clinical manifestation of pneumonia. Increased work of breathing accompanied by intercostal, subcostal, and suprasternal retractions, nasal flaring, and use of accessory muscles is common. Severe infection may be accompanied by cyanosis and respiratory fatigue, especially in infants. Auscultation of the chest may reveal crackles and wheezing, but it often is difficult to localize the source of these adventitious sounds in very young children with hyperresonant chests. It is difficult to clinically distinguish viral pneumonia from disease caused by *Mycoplasma* and other bacterial pathogens.

Bacterial pneumonia in adults and older children typically begins suddenly with a shaking chill followed by a high fever, cough, and chest pain. In older children and adolescents, a brief upper respiratory tract illness is followed by the abrupt onset of shaking chills and high fever accompanied by drowsiness with intermittent periods of restlessness; rapid respirations; a dry, hacking, unproductive cough; anxiety; and occasionally delirium. Circumoral cyanosis may be observed. Many children are noted to be splinting on the affected side to minimize pleuritic pain and improve ventilation; they may lie on their side with their knees drawn up to their chest.

Physical findings depend on the stage of pneumonia. Early in the course of illness, diminished breath sounds, scattered crackles, and rhonchi are commonly heard over the affected lung field. With the development of increasing consolidation or complications of pneumonia such as effusion, empyema, or pyopneumothorax, dullness on percussion is noted and breath sounds are markedly diminished. A lag in respiratory excursion often occurs on the affected side. Abdominal distention may be prominent because of gastric dilation from swallowed air or ileus. The liver may seem enlarged because of downward displacement of the diaphragm secondary to hyperinflation of the lungs or superimposed congestive heart failure. Nuchal rigidity, in the absence of meningitis, may also be prominent, especially with involvement of the right upper lobe.

Symptoms described in adults with pneumococcal pneumonia may be noted in older children but are rarely observed in infants and young children, in whom the clinical pattern is considerably more variable. In infants, there may be a prodrome of upper respiratory tract infection and diminished appetite leading to the abrupt onset of fever, restlessness, apprehension, and respiratory distress. These infants appear ill with respiratory distress manifest by grunting; nasal flaring; retractions of the supraclavicular, intercostal, and subcostal areas; tachypnea; tachycardia; air hunger; and often cyanosis. Results of physical examination may, however, be misleading, particularly in young infants, with meager findings disproportionate to the degree of tachypnea. Some infants with bacterial pneumonia may have associated gastrointestinal disturbances characterized by vomiting, anorexia, diarrhea, and abdominal distention secondary to a paralytic ileus. Rapid progression of symptoms is characteristic in the most severe cases of bacterial pneumonia.

Diagnosis. The chest radiograph confirms the diagnosis of pneumonia and may indicate a complication such as a pleural effusion or empyema. In general, viral pneumonia is characterized by hyperinflation with bilateral interstitial infiltrates and peribronchial cuffing (Fig. 389–1). Confluent lobar consolidation is typically seen with pneumococcal pneumonia (Fig. 389–2). However, the radiographic appearance alone is not diagnostic and other clinical features must be considered.

The peripheral white blood cell (WBC) count may be useful in differentiating viral from bacterial pneumonia. In viral pneumonia, the WBC count may be normal or elevated but usually not higher than 20,000/mm³ with a lymphocyte predominance. Bacterial pneumonia is often associated with an elevated WBC count in the range of 15,000–40,000/mm³ and a predominance of granulocytes.

The definitive diagnosis of a viral infection rests on the isolation of a virus or detection of viral antigens in respiratory tract secretions. Growth of respiratory viruses in tissue culture usually requires 5–10 days. Reliable reagents for the rapid detection of RSV, parainfluenza, influenza, and adenoviruses are available. Serologic techniques also can be used to diagnose a recent respiratory viral infection but generally require testing of acute and convalescent serum samples for a rise in antibodies to a specific viral agent. This diagnostic technique is laborious, slow, and not gener-

ally clinically useful because the infection usually resolves by the time it is confirmed serologically. Nevertheless, serologic testing may be valuable as an epidemiologic tool to define the incidence and prevalence of the various respiratory viral pathogens.

The definitive diagnosis of a bacterial infection requires isolation of an organism from the blood, pleural fluid, or lung. Culture of sputum is of no value in the diagnosis of pneumonia in children. Blood cultures are positive in only 10–30% of children with pneumococcal pneumonia. In *M. pneumoniae* infections, cold agglutinins at titers greater than 1:64 are found in the blood in about 50% of patients. However, cold agglutinins are nonspecific because other infections such as influenza may also cause increases. Serologic evidence such as the anti–streptolysin O (ASO) titer is useful in the diagnosis of group A streptococcal pneumonia.

Treatment. Treatment of suspected bacterial pneumonia is based on the presumptive cause and the clinical appearance of the child. For mildly ill children who do not require hospitalization, amoxicillin is recommended. In communities with a high percentage of penicillin-resistant pneumococci, high doses of amoxicillin (80–90 mg/kg/24 hr) should be prescribed. Therapeutic alternatives include cefuroxime axetil or amoxicillin/clavulanate. For school-aged children and in those in whom infection with *M. pneumoniae* is suggested, a macrolide antibiotic such as azithromycin is an appropriate therapeutic choice.

The empirical treatment of suspected bacterial pneumonia in a hospitalized child requires an approach based on the clinical manifestations at the time of presentation. Parenteral cefuroxime (75–150 mg/kg/24 hr) is the mainstay of therapy when bacterial pneumonia is suggested. If features suggest staphylococcal pneumonia (e.g., pneumatoceles, empyema), initial therapy should also include vancomycin or clindamycin.

If viral pneumonia is suggested, it is reasonable to withhold antibiotic therapy. However, this option should be reserved for those patients who are mildly ill, have clinical evidence suggesting viral infection, and are in no respiratory distress. Up to 30% of patients with known viral infection may have co-existing bacterial pathogens; therefore, if the decision is made to withhold antibiotic therapy based on presumptive diagnosis of a viral infection, deterioration in clinical status should signal the possibility of superimposed bacterial infection and antibiotic therapy should be initiated.

Complications. Complications of pneumonia are usually the result of direct spread of bacterial infection within the thoracic cavity (e.g., pleural effusion, empyema, and pericarditis) or bacteremia and hematologic spread. Meningitis, suppurative arthritis, and osteomyelitis are rare complications of hematologic spread of infection.

S. aureus and *S. pneumoniae* are the most common causes of empyema. The treatment of empyema is based on the stage (e.g., exudative, fibrinopurulent, or organizing). Imaging studies including ultrasonography and CT are helpful in deter-

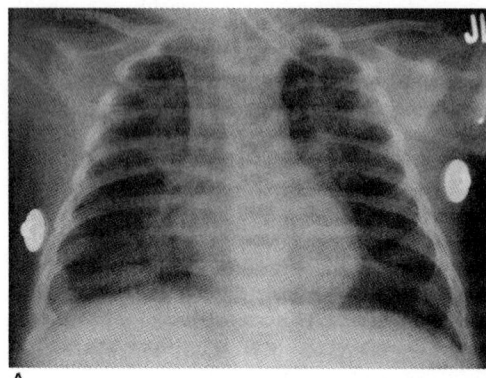
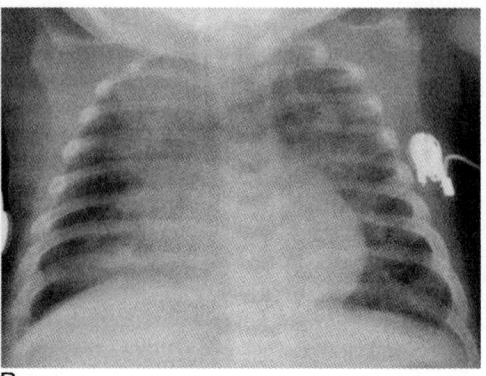

A B

FIGURE 389–1. *A,* Radiographic findings characteristic of RSV pneumonia in a 6-mo-old infant with rapid respirations and fever. Anteroposterior (AP) radiograph of the chest shows hyperexpansion of the lungs with bilateral fine air space disease and streaks of density, indicating the presence of both pneumonia and atelectasis. An endotracheal tube is in place. *B,* One day later the AP radiograph of the chest shows increased bilateral pneumonia.

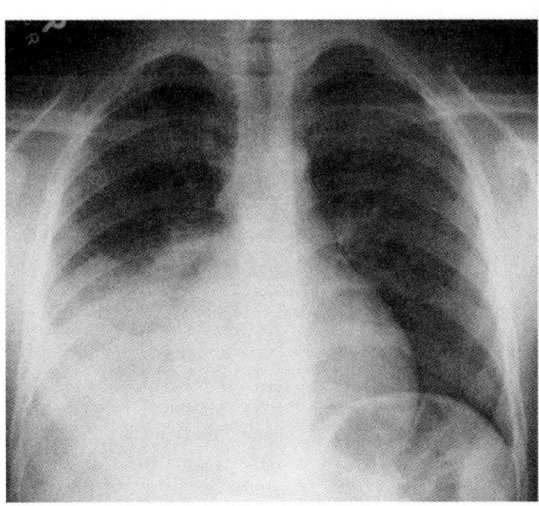
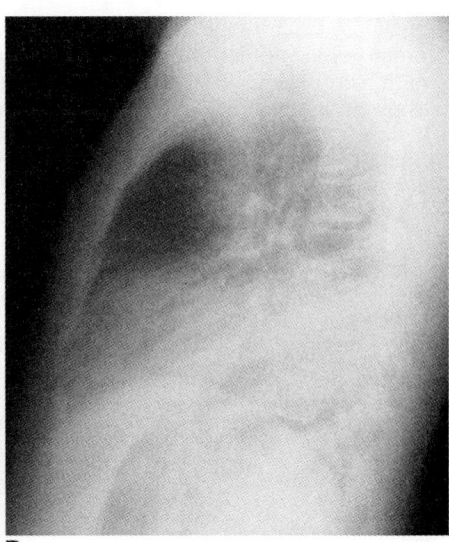

FIGURE 389–2. Radiographic findings characteristic of pneumococcal pneumonia in a 14-yr-old boy with cough and fever. Posteroanterior *(A)* and lateral *(B)* chest radiographs reveal consolidation in the right lower lobe, strongly suggesting bacterial pneumonia.

A   B

mining the stage of empyema. The mainstays of therapy include antibiotic therapy and drainage with tube thoracostomy. Newer approaches also include the use of fibrinolytic therapy and selected thoracoscopy to debride, lyse adhesions, and drain loculated areas of pus. Early diagnosis and intervention may obviate the need for thoracotomy and open debridement.

Campbell JD, Nataro JP: Pleural empyema. *Pediatr Infect Dis J* 1999;18:725–26.

Dagan R, Sikuler-Cohen M, Zamir O, et al: Effect of conjugate pneumococcal vaccine on the occurrence of respiratory infections and antibiotic use in day-care center attendees. *Pediatr Infect Dis J* 2001;20:951–58.

Davies HD, Wang EEL, Manson D, et al: Reliability of the chest radiograph in the diagnosis of lower respiratory infections in young children. *Pediatr Infect Dis J* 1996;15:600–4.

Dowell SF, Kupronis BA, Zell ER, et al: Mortality from pneumonia in children in the United States, 1939 through 1996. *N Engl J Med* 2000;342:1399–407.

Glezen WP, Loda FA, Clyde WA, et al: Epidemiologic patterns of acute lower respiratory disease of children in a pediatric group practice. *J Pediatr* 1971;78:397–406.

Heiskanen-Kosma T, Korppi M, Jokinen C, et al: Etiology of childhood pneumonia: Serological results of a prospective, population-based study. *Pediatr Infect Dis J* 1998;17:986–91.

Izurieta HS, Thompson WW, Kramarz P, et al: Influenza and the rates of hospitalization for respiratory disease among infants and young children. *N Engl J Med* 2000;342:232–39.

McCracken GH Jr: Diagnosis and management of pneumonia. *Pediatr Infect Dis J* 2000;19:924–28.

Mimica I, Donoso E, Howard JE, et al: Lung puncture in the etiologic diagnosis of pneumonia: A study of 543 infants and children. *Am J Dis Child* 1971;122:278–82.

Nelson JD: Community-acquired pneumonia in children: Guidelines for treatment. *Pediatr Infect Dis J* 2000;19:251–53.

Nohynek H, Valkeila E, Leinonen M, et al: Erythrocyte sedimentation rate, white blood cell count and serum C-reactive protein in assessing etiologic diagnosis of acute lower respiratory infections in children. *Pediatr Infect Dis J* 1995;14:484–90.

Wubbell L, Muniz L, Ahmed A, et al: Etiology and treatment of community-acquired pneumonia in ambulatory children. *Pediatr Infect Dis J* 1999;18:98–104.

Chapter 390
Slowly Resolving
Pneumonia *Oren Lakser*

Slowly resolving pneumonia refers to persistence of symptoms or radiographic abnormalities beyond the expected time course. The time course, however, will vary, depending on the organism involved, the extent of disease, and the presence of associated complicating conditions, such as pleural effusion, empyema, or lung abscess. In this chapter the focus is on the approach to the patient with delayed resolution of pneumonia; pneumonia is covered in Chapter 389.

Typically, patients with uncomplicated community acquired bacterial pneumonia respond to therapy with improvement in clinical symptoms (e.g., fever, cough, dyspnea, chest pain) within 48–96 hr of initiation of antibiotics. Changes in empirical antibiotic therapy should be delayed for 2–4 days, unless the patient's condition worsens. In general, there should be radiographic evidence of improvement within 4–6 wk, but time to complete resolution varies depending on the etiologic organism. *Pneumococcal* pneumonias often require 1–3 mo for complete radiographic clearing. Similarly, chlamydial pneumonia can require 1–3 mo for complete resolution radiographically. *Mycoplasma pneumoniae* tends to clear more rapidly, with radiographic improvement occurring within 2 wk to 2 mo. Conversely, staphylococcal, *Legionella*, and enteric gram-negative pneumonias can take as long as 3–6 mo to resolve radiographically. Children with *viral* pneumonia may have positive radiographic findings for many months.

A number of factors must be considered when confronted with a patient with slowly resolving pneumonia. *Inadequate therapy* due to inappropriate antibiotic choice, inappropriate dose, or poor compliance is a common cause for slow or lack of improvement. In addition, the development of *resistant* organisms or *impaired host defenses* (immunodeficiencies, ciliary dyskinesia, or other co-existing illnesses) often results in a slower than expected time course for resolution. The possibility of a *nonbacterial* cause for the pneumonia should also be considered in patients who fail to demonstrate appropriate improvement. Viruses, fungi, parasites, and *Mycobacteria* all have longer time courses for improvement than expected for uncomplicated community acquired bacterial pneumonia. *Obstructing endobronchial lesions* (congenital and acquired) must also be considered. Foreign bodies, pulmonary sequestration, cystic adenomatoid malformations, and postinfectious bronchiectasis are a few conditions that can result in impaired clearance of a pulmonary infiltrate. Finally, a number of *noninfectious causes* can mimic community-acquired pneumonia, both symptomatically and radiographically, but resolve slowly. These include such entities as bronchiolitis obliterans, hypersensitivity pneumonitis, eosinophilic pneumonia, aspiration, and Wegener granulomatosis. Sarcoidosis and pulmonary alveolar proteinosis may also produce a similar picture but are rare in children.

Initially, evaluation of a patient with slowly resolving pneumonia should include an attempt to identify the offending organism. Blood, sputum, pleural, bronchoalveolar lavage, or lung biopsy can provide tissue for Gram stain and/or culture and thereby guide antibiotic choice. If these do not provide an explanation, serologic testing may be helpful (anti-neutrophil cytoplasmic antibodies [ANCA] for Wegener granulomatosis). Chest CT scans (thin-cut and/or high-resolution), flexible fiberoptic bronchoscopy, and lung biopsy (transbronchial, percutaneous, video-assisted thorascopic, or open) may also be helpful.

Cassiere H, Rodrigues JC, Fen AM: Delayed resolution of pneumonia: When is slow resolving too slow? *Postgrad Med* 1996;99:151–58.

Johnson JL: Slowly resolving and nonresolving pneumonia: Questions to ask when response is delayed. *Postgrad Med* 2000; 108:115–22.

Kuru T, Lynch JP: Nonresolving or slowly resolving pneumonia. *Clin Chest Med* 1999;20:623–51.

Orens JB, Sitrin RG, Lynch JP: The approach to nonresolving pneumonia. *Med Clin North Am* 1994;78:1143–72.

Schidlow DV, Callahan CW: Pneumonia. *Pediatr Rev* 1996;17:300–10.

Chapter 391
Bronchiectasis *Oren Lakser*

Bronchiectasis is a disease characterized by irreversible abnormal dilatation of the bronchial tree and likely represents a common end stage of a number of nonspecific and unrelated antecedent events. Its incidence has been decreasing, especially in developed countries.

Pathophysiology and Pathogenesis. In the developed world, cystic fibrosis is the most common cause of clinically significant bronchiectasis. Other conditions associated with bronchiectasis include ciliary dyskinesia, immune deficiency syndromes, and infection, especially pertussis, measles, and tuberculosis. Bronchiectasis can also be congenital. *Williams-Campbell syndrome,* in which there is an absence of annular bronchial cartilage, and *Marnier-Kuhn syndrome* (congenital tracheobronchomegaly), in which there is a connective tissue disorder, are two such examples. Other disease entities associated with bronchiectasis include *right middle lobe syndrome* (chronic extrinsic compression of right middle lobe bronchus by hilar lymph nodes) and *yellow nail syndrome* (pleural effusion, lymphedema, discolored nails).

In general, three basic mechanisms are involved in the pathogenesis of bronchiectasis. Obstruction can occur because of tumor, foreign body, impacted mucus caused by poor mucociliary clearance, external compression, bronchial webs, and atresia. Infections due to *Bordetella pertussis,* measles, rubella, togavirus, respiratory syncytial virus, and *Mycobacterium tuberculosis* induce chronic inflammation, progressive bronchial wall damage, and dilatation. Chronic inflammation, similarly, contributes to the mechanism by which obstruction leads to bronchiectasis. The mechanism by which bronchiectasis occurs in congenital forms is likely related to abnormal cartilage formation, as described earlier. The common thread in the pathogenesis of bronchiectasis is difficulty clearing secretions and recurrent infections.

Bronchiectasis can present in any combination of three pathologic forms. In *cylindrical* bronchiectasis the bronchial outlines are regular but there is diffuse dilatation of the bronchial unit. The bronchial lumen ends abruptly because of mucus plugging. In *varicose* bronchiectasis the degree of dilatation is greater and local constrictions cause an irregularity of outline resembling varicose veins. There may also be small sacculations. In *saccular* (cystic) bronchiectasis, bronchial dilatation progresses and results in ballooning of bronchi that end in fluid- or mucus-filled sacs. This is the most severe form of bronchiectasis.

Clinical Manifestations. The most common complaints in patients with bronchiectasis are cough and copious purulent sputum production. Younger children may swallow the sputum. Hemoptysis is seen with some frequency. Fever can occur with infectious exacerbations. Anorexia and poor weight gain may occur as time passes. Physical examination typically reveals crackles localized to the affected area, but wheezing may also occur. In severe cases, dyspnea and hypoxemia may occur. Pulmonary function studies may demonstrate an obstructive, restrictive, or mixed pattern. Typically impaired diffusion capacity is a late finding.

Diagnosis. Chest radiographs of patients with bronchiectasis tend to be nonspecific. Typical findings may include increase in size and loss of definition of bronchovascular markings, crowding of bronchi, and loss of lung volume. In more severe forms, cystic spaces, occasionally with air-fluid levels and honeycombing, may occur. Compensatory overinflation of unaffected lung may be seen.

Bronchography was formerly the best technique to demonstrate bronchiectasis. This technique requires sedation and airway administration of a radiographic contrast agent. Today, bronchography may still be used before surgery for lung biopsy or resection to provide better localization.

Thin-section high-resolution CT scanning has replaced bronchography as the gold standard, because it has equal or better sensitivity and specificity and is less invasive. CT provides further information on disease location, presence of mediastinal lesions, and the extent of segmental involvement. The addition of radiolabeled aerosol inhalation to CT scanning can provide further information. The CT findings in patients with bronchiectasis typically include cylindrical ("tram lines," "signet ring appearance"), varicose (bronchi with "beaded contour"), cystic (cysts in "strings and clusters"), or mixed forms.

Treatment. The initial therapy for patients with bronchiectasis is medical and aims at decreasing airway obstruction and controlling infection. Chest physiotherapy (postural drainage), antibiotics, and bronchodilators are essential. It is not unusual that 2–4 wk of parenteral antibiotics are necessary to adequately manage acute exacerbations. Antibiotic choice is dictated by the identification and sensitivity of organisms found on deep throat, sputum, or bronchoalveolar fluid cultures. Chronic prophylactic oral antibiotics may be beneficial. Any underlying disorder (e.g., immunodeficiency, aspiration) that may be contributing must also be addressed. When localized bronchiectasis becomes more severe or resistant to medical management, segmental or lobar resection may be warranted. Lung transplantation has also been performed in patients with bronchiectasis.

Prognosis. Overall, the prognosis for patients with bronchiectasis has improved considerably over the past few decades. Earlier recognition or prevention of predisposing conditions, more powerful and wide-spectrum antibiotics, and improved surgical outcomes are likely reasons.

Barker AF: Bronchiectasis. *N Engl J Med* 2002;346:1383–93.

Galvin JR, D'Alessandro MP: Electric diffuse lung: The diagnosis of diffuse lung disease, bronchiectasis. University of Iowa Virtual Hospital web site. (www.vh.org/)

Herman M, Michálková K, Kopriva F: High-resolution CT in the assessment of bronchiectasis in children. *Pediatr Radiol* 1993;23:376–79.

Karakoc GB, Yilmaz M, Altintas DU, et al: Bronchiectasis: Still a problem. *Pediatr Pulmonol* 2001;32:175–78.

Kornreich L, Horev G, Ziv N, et al: Bronchiectasis in children: Assessment by CT. *Pediatr Radiol* 1993;23:120–23.

Pifferi m, Caramella D, Bartolozzi C, et al: CT-guided radiolabelled aerosol studies for assessing pulmonary impairment in children with bronchiectasis. *Pediatr Radiol* 2000;30:632–37.

Sethi GR, Batra V: Bronchiectasis: Causes and management. *Indian J Pediatr* 2000;67:133–39.

Singleton R, Morris A, Redding G, et al: Bronchiectasis in Alaska native children: Causes and clinical courses. *Pediatr Pulmonol* 2000;29:182–87.

Chapter 392
Pulmonary Abscess *Oren Lakser*

Pulmonary abscesses are composed of thick-walled purulent material formed as a result of lung infection and lead to destruction of lung parenchyma, cavitation, and central necrosis. Lung abscesses are much less common in children than in adults. A *primary* lung abscess occurs in a previously healthy patient with no underlying medical disorders. A *secondary* lung abscess occurs in a patient with underlying or predisposing conditions.

Pathology and Pathogenesis. A number of conditions predispose children to the development of pulmonary abscesses, including pneumonia, cystic fibrosis, gastroesophageal reflux, tracheoesophageal fistula, immunodeficiencies, postoperative complications of tonsillectomy and adenoidectomy, seizures, and a variety of neurologic diseases. In children, aspiration of infected materials is the predominant source of the organisms causing abscesses. Initially, a pneumonitis impairs drainage of fluid or the aspirated material. Inflammatory vascular obstruction occurs, leading to tissue necrosis, liquefaction, and abscess formation. Abscess can also occur as a result of pneumonia and hematogenous seeding from another site.

If the aspiration event occurred in the recumbent position, the right and left upper lobes and apical segment of the right lower lobes are the dependent areas most likely to be affected. If the child was upright, the posterior segments of the upper lobes are dependent and therefore most likely to be affected. Primary abscesses are found most often on the right side, whereas secondary lung abscesses, particularly in immunocompromised patients, have a predilection for the left side.

Both anaerobic and aerobic organisms can cause lung abscesses. Common anaerobic bacteria that can cause a pulmonary abscess include *Bacteroides* species, *Fusobacterium* species, and *Peptostreptococcus* species. Abscesses may be caused by aerobic organisms such as *Streptococcus* species, *Staphylococcus aureus*, *Escherichia coli*, *Klebsiella pneumoniae*, and *Pseudomonas aeruginosa*. All patients with a lung abscess should have aerobic and anaerobic cultures as part of their work-up.

Clinical Manifestations. The most common symptoms of pulmonary abscess in the pediatric population include cough, fever, tachypnea, dyspnea, chest pain, vomiting, sputum production, weight loss, and hemoptysis. Physical examination typically reveals tachypnea, dyspnea, retractions with accessory muscle use, decreased breath sounds, and dullness to percussion in the affected area. Crackles and occasionally a prolonged expiratory phase may be heard on lung examination.

Diagnosis. Diagnosis is most commonly made on chest radiography. Classically, the chest radiograph shows a parenchymal inflammation with a cavity containing an air-fluid level. A chest CT scan can provide better anatomic definition, including location and size. The determination of the etiologic bacteria can be very helpful in guiding antibiotic choice. Gram stain of sputum may provide an early clue as to the class of bacteria involved. However, sputum cultures typically yield mixed bacteria and therefore are not always reliable. Attempts to avoid contamination from oral flora include direct lung puncture and percutaneous (aided by CT guidance), bronchoscopic, and transtracheal aspiration, now the primary diagnostic procedure. Bronchoscopic aspiration may be complicated by massive intrabronchial aspiration, and therefore great care should be taken during the procedure.

Treatment. Conservative management is recommended. Most experts advocate a 2–3 wk course of parenteral antibiotics for uncomplicated cases, followed by a course of oral antibiotics to complete a total of 4–6 wk. Antibiotic choice should be guided by Gram stain and culture but initially should include aerobic and anaerobic coverage. Treatment regimens should include a penicillinase-resistant agent active against *S. aureus* and anaerobic coverage, typically with clindamycin or ticarcillin/clavulinic acid. If gram-negative bacteria are suspected or isolated, an aminoglycoside should be added.

For severely ill patients or those who fail to improve after 7–10 days of appropriate antimicrobial therapy, surgical intervention should be considered. Minimally invasive percutaneous aspiration techniques, often with CT guidance, have been used with increasing frequency. Infrequently, in rare complicated cases, thoracotomy with lobectomy and/or decortication may be necessary.

Prognosis. Overall, prognosis for children with primary pulmonary abscesses is excellent. The presence of aerobic organisms seems to be a negative prognostic indicator, particularly in those with secondary lung abscesses. Most children become asymptomatic within 7–10 days, although the fever may persist for as long as 3 wk. Radiologic abnormalities usually resolve in 1–3 mo but can persist for years.

Brook I: Lung abscesses and pleural empyema in children. *Adv Pediatr Infect Dis* 1993;8:159–76.

Emanuel S, Shulman ST: Lung abscess in infants and children. *Clin Pediatr* 1995;34:2–6.

Hoffer FA, Bloom DA, Colin AA, et al: Lung abscess versus necrotizing pneumonia: Implications for interventional therapy. *Pediatr Radiol* 1998;29:87–91.

Tan TQ, Seilheimer DK, Kaplan SL: Pediatric lung abscesses: Clinical management and outcome. *Pediatr Infect Dis J* 1995;14:51–55.

Tseng YL, Wu MH, Lin MY, et al: Surgery for lung abscess in immunocompetent and immunocompromised children. *J Pediatr Surg* 2001;36:470–73.

Chapter 393
Cystic Fibrosis *Thomas F. Boat*

Cystic fibrosis (CF) is an inherited multisystem disorder of children and adults, characterized chiefly by obstruction and infection of airways and by maldigestion and its consequences. It is the most common life-limiting recessive genetic trait among whites. A dysfunction of epithelialized surfaces is the predominant pathogenetic feature and is responsible for a broad, variable, and sometimes confusing array of presenting manifestations and complications.

CF is the major cause of severe chronic lung disease in children and is responsible for most exocrine pancreatic insufficiency during early life. It is also responsible for many cases of salt depletion, nasal polyposis, pansinusitis, rectal prolapse, pancreatitis, cholelithiasis, and insulin-dependent hyperglycemia. CF may present as failure to thrive and occasionally as cirrhosis or other forms of hepatic dysfunction. Therefore, this disorder enters into the differential diagnosis of many pediatric conditions.

Genetics. CF occurs in approximately 1/3,500 white live births and 1/17,000 black infants in the United States. The estimated incidence worldwide varies from 1/377 live births in parts of Brittany to 1/90,000 Asian infants in Hawaii. Generally, the CF gene is most prevalent among Northern and Central Europeans and in individuals who come from these areas.

CF is inherited as an autosomal recessive trait. All of the gene mutations that contribute to the CF syndrome occur at a single locus on the long arm of chromosome 7. The CF gene codes for a protein of 1,480 amino acids called the *CF transmembrane regulator* (CFTR). CFTR is expressed largely in epithelial cells of airways, the gastrointestinal tract (including pancreas and biliary system), the sweat glands, and the genitourinary system. CFTR has ion channel and regulatory functions that are perturbed variably by the different mutations. The most prevalent mutation of CFTR is the deletion of a single phenylalanine residue at amino acid 508 (ΔF508). This mutation is responsible for the high incidence of CF in northern European populations and is considerably less frequent in other populations, such as those in southern Europe and Israel. Approximately 50% of individuals with CF and Northern European ancestry are homozygous for ΔF508. The remainder of patients have an extensive array of mutations, none of which has a prevalence of more than several per cent, except in circumscribed populations. For example, the W1282X mutation occurs in 60% of the Ashkenazi Jews with CF. The relationship between genotype and phenotype is highly complex. Mutations categorized as "severe" (e.g., ΔF508) are associated almost uniformly with pancreatic insufficiency. Several mutations (e.g., 3849+10 Kb C>T) are found in patients with normal sweat chloride concentrations. Severity of lung disease and presence of liver disease cannot be predicted by genotype. This suggests a major environmental (acquired) component of organ system dysfunction or perhaps the presence of other genes that modify the CF phenotype. For example, variant alleles of the mannose-binding lectin, a key factor in systemic innate immunity, are associated with more serious lung infections and reduced survival.

Using probes for 30 of the most frequent mutations, the genotype of 80–90% of Americans with CF can be ascertained. Increasing the number of probes to 70 improves mutation ascertainment by only a few per cent. Thus, not all children with CF can be identified by DNA testing as routinely performed. In special cases, sequencing the *CFTR* gene is necessary to establish the genotype. The presence of polymorphisms in both *CFTR* genes does not always cause CF manifestations.

The high frequency of the CF gene has been hypothetically ascribed to resistance to the morbidity and mortality associated with cholera through the ages. Cultured CF intestinal epithelial cells homozygous for the ΔF508 mutation are unresponsive to the secretory effects of cholera toxin.

Pathogenesis. Four long-standing observations are of fundamental pathophysiologic importance: failure to clear mucous secretions, a paucity of water in mucous secretions, an elevated salt content of sweat and other serous secretions, and chronic infection limited to the respiratory tract. The relationships among these findings were unclear until the early 1980s when it was demonstrated that there is a greater negative potential difference across the respiratory epithelia of CF patients than across the respiratory epithelia of control subjects. Aberrant electrical properties were also demonstrated for CF sweat gland duct epithelium. Subsequent studies demonstrated that the membranes of CF epithelial cells are unable to secrete chloride ions in response to cyclic adenosine monophosphate (AMP)–mediated signals, and that, at least in the respiratory tract, excessive amounts of sodium are absorbed through these membranes (Fig. 393–1). These defects can be traced to a dysfunction of CFTR (Fig. 393–2).

After isolation of the *CFTR* gene and its characterization, it became clear that cyclic AMP-stimulated chloride conductance was a function of CFTR itself and that this function was absent in epithelial cells with many different mutations of the *CFTR* gene. CFTR mutations appear to fall into five classes, albeit with some overlap: I, defective CFTR production owing to premature transcription termination signals; II, defective CFTR processing and trafficking to the apical membrane (e.g., ΔF508); III, defective regulation of chloride channel function from mutations in CFTR phosphorylation or adenosine triphosphate–binding sites; IV, defective chloride conductance caused by missense mutations in the membrane-spanning domains of CFTR that line the channel; and V, abnormal splicing of CFTR. The importance of these

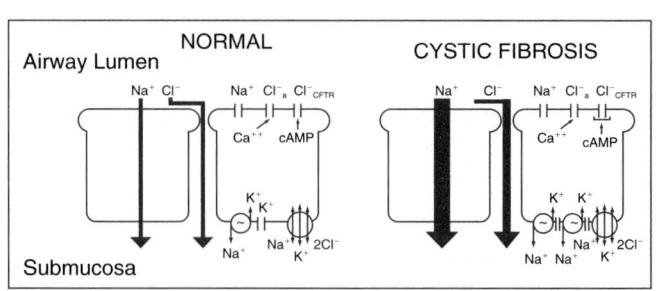

CFTR: A cAMP-Regulated Chloride Channel

FIGURE 393–1. The net ion flow across normal and cystic fibrosis (CF) airway epithelia under basal conditions *(large arrows)*. Because water follows salt movement, the predicted net flux of water would be from the airway lumen to the submucosa and would be greater across CF epithelia. The increased Na$^+$ absorption by CF cells is associated with an increased amiloride-sensitive Na$^+$ conductance across the apical (luminal) membrane and increased Na$^+$,K$^+$-ATPase sites at the basolateral membrane. The cAMP-mediated apical membrane conductance of Cl$^-$ associated with the CF transmembrane regulator (CFTR) does not function in CF epithelia, but an alternative, calcium-activated Cl$^-$ conductance is present in normal and CF cells. It is postulated that CF cells have a limited ability to secrete Cl$^-$ and absorb Na$^+$ in excessive amounts, limiting the water available to hydrate secretions and allow them to be cleared from the airways lumen. (From Knowles MR: Contemporary perspectives on the pathogenesis of cystic fibrosis. *New Insights Cystic Fibrosis* 1:1, 1993.)

functional categories is not clear, because they do not correlate with specific clinical features or their severity. Rather, clinical features correlate with the residual CFTR activity. Genotypes causing 99% loss of CFTR activity cause lung disease and pancreatic insufficiency; pancreatic function is retained with 95% loss, and 90% loss results in isolated congenital bilateral absence of the vas deferens or idiopathic chronic pancreatitis.

The postulated epithelial pathophysiology in airways involves an inability to secrete salt and secondarily to secrete water in the presence of excessive reabsorption of salt and water. The proposed outcome is insufficient water on the airway surface to form a periciliary liquid layer and hydrate secretions. Desiccated secretions become more viscous and elastic (rubbery) and are harder to clear by mucociliary and other mechanisms. Altered mucus rheology may be aggravated by low HCO$_3^-$ and a more acidic pH. These secretions are retained and obstruct airways, starting with those of the smallest caliber, the bronchioles. Airflow obstruction at the level of small airways is the earliest observable physiologic abnormality of the respiratory system.

It is plausible that similar pathophysiologic events take place in the pancreatic and biliary ducts (and in the vas deferens), leading to desiccation of proteinaceous secretions and obstruction. Because the function of sweat gland duct cells is to absorb rather than secrete chloride, salt is not retrieved from the isotonic primary sweat as it is transported to the skin surface; chloride and sodium levels consequently are elevated.

Chronic infection in CF is limited to the endobronchial spaces of the airways. The most likely explanation for infection is a sequence of events starting with failure to clear inhaled bacteria promptly and then proceeding to persistent colonization and an inflammatory response in airway walls. An alternative hypothesis, that abnormal CFTR creates an inflammatory state before first infection or amplifies the inflammatory response to initial viral infection, is based on lung lavage evidence of the presence

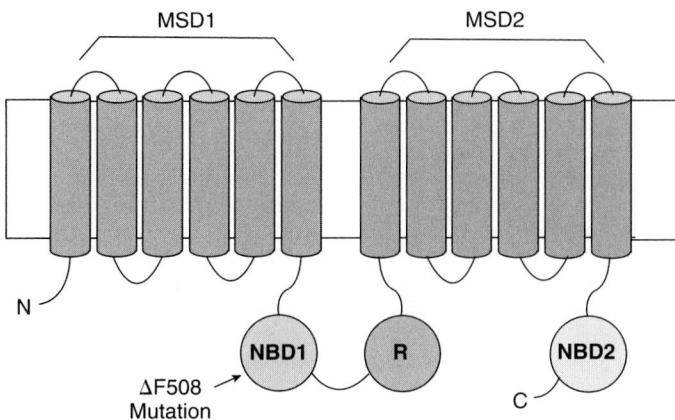

FIGURE 393–2. The predicted structure of a cystic fibrosis transmembrane regulator (CFTR) shows that the molecule is anchored in the cell membrane by two membrane-spanning domains (MSD1, MSD2). These domains form a channel through which chloride and probably water can pass. Two nucleotide-binding domains (NBD1, NBD2) interact with ATP to provide energy for CFTR functions. The R domain has many sites for phosphorylation by cAMP-dependent kinases. This domain is involved in the regulation of CFTR functions such as chloride conductance. The most common CFTR mutation, ΔF508, is localized to the NBD1 region. This region and the NBD2 site are particularly susceptible to mutation. However, mutations associated with typical manifestations of CF occur in all domains. (From Welsh MJ, Anderson MP, Rich DP, et al: Cystic fibrosis transmembrane conductance regulator. *Neuron* 8:821, 1992.)

of cytokines such as interleukin-8 and neutrophils in the absence of recovered bacteria within the first months of life. More recent evidence supports the contention that CF airway inflammation may be more exuberant but still secondary to early viral or transient bacterial infection. These events occur first in small airways, perhaps because clearance of altered secretions is more difficult from these regions. Chronic bronchiolitis and bronchitis are the initial lung manifestations, but after months to years, structural changes in airway walls produce bronchiolectasis and bronchiectasis.

The agents of airway injury include neutrophil products, such as oxidative radicals and proteases, and immune reaction products. With advanced lung disease, infection may extend to peribronchial lung parenchyma. Several inflammatory products, including proteases, are responsible for the mucus hypersecretion that is characteristic of chronic airways disease.

A finding that is not readily explained is the high prevalence of airway colonization with *Staphylococcus aureus*, *Pseudomonas aeruginosa*, and *Burkholderia cepacia*, organisms that rarely infect the lungs of other individuals. There is evidence that the CF airway epithelial cells or surface liquids provide a favorable environment for harboring these organisms. Furthermore, CF airway epithelium may be compromised in its innate defenses against the organisms, through either acquired or genetic alterations. Antimicrobial activity is diminished in CF secretions. Initially attributed to elevated salt concentrations, the effect is more likely related to hyperacidified surface liquids or other effects on innate immunity. Another puzzle is the propensity for *P. aeruginosa* to undergo mucoid transformation in the CF airways. The complex polysaccharide produced by these organisms generates a biofilm that provides a hypoxic environment and thereby protects *Pseudomonas* against antimicrobial agents.

Although functional deficits may occur in cellular immunity, mucosal immune function, and the alternate pathway for complement as lung infection progresses to an advanced stage, the immune system in CF appears to be fundamentally intact. Nutritional deficits, including fatty acid deficiency, have been implicated as predisposing factors for respiratory tract infection. The 10–15% of individuals who retain substantial exocrine pancreatic function have statistically lower sweat chloride values, delayed onset of colonization with *P. aeruginosa*, and slower deterioration of lung function. However, nutritional factors are only contributory in part because preservation of pancreatic function does not preclude development of typical lung disease.

Pathology. Striking changes are characteristically observed in the organs that secrete mucus. Eccrine sweat glands and parotid salivary glands, including ducts, are not involved pathologically despite abnormalities in the electrolyte content of their secretory product.

The earliest pathologic lesion in the *lung* is that of bronchiolitis (i.e., mucus plugging and an inflammatory response in the walls of the small airways). With time, mucus accumulation and inflammation extend to the larger airways (bronchitis). Goblet cell hyperplasia and submucosal gland hypertrophy become prominent pathologic expressions of a hypersecretory state, which is most likely a response to chronic airway infection. Organisms appear to be confined to the endobronchial space; invasive bacterial infection is not characteristic. With long-standing disease, evidence of airway destruction such as bronchiolar obliteration, bronchiolectasis, and bronchiectasis becomes prominent. Scanning electron microscopy of the airway surface appears normal, except for scattered areas of squamous cell metaplasia, although freeze-fracture studies have found alterations of tight junctions and apical membrane changes that are probably caused by chronic inflammation. Bronchiectatic cysts and emphysematous bullae or subpleural blebs are frequent with advanced lung disease, the upper lobes being most commonly involved. These enlarged air spaces may rupture and cause pneumothorax. Interstitial disease is not a prominent (common) feature, although areas of fibrosis appear eventually. True emphysema occurs but is not a general pathologic finding. Bronchial arteries are enlarged and tortuous, contributing to a propensity for hemoptysis in bronchiectatic airways. Small pulmonary arteries eventually display medial hypertrophy, which would be expected in secondary pulmonary hypertension.

The *paranasal sinuses* are uniformly filled with secretions, and the lining contains hyperplastic and hypertrophied secretory elements. Polypoid lesions within the sinuses, mucopyocele, and erosion of bone have been reported. The nasal mucosa may contain inflammatory cells, be edematous, and form large or multiple polyps, usually from a base surrounding the ostia of the maxillary and ethmoidal sinuses.

The *pancreas* is usually small, occasionally cystic, and often difficult to find at postmortem examination. The extent of involvement varies at birth. In infants, the acini and ducts are often distended and filled with eosinophilic material. In 85–90% of patients, the lesion progresses to complete or almost complete disruption of acini and replacement with fibrous tissue and fat. Infrequently, foci of calcification may be seen on radiographs of the abdomen. The islets of Langerhans contain a normal number of β cells, although they may begin to show architectural disruption by fibrous tissue during the 2nd decade of life.

The *intestinal tract* shows only minimal changes. Esophageal and duodenal glands are often distended with mucous secretions. Concretions may form in the appendiceal lumen or cecum. Crypts of the appendix and rectum may be dilated and filled with secretions.

Focal biliary cirrhosis secondary to blockage of intrahepatic bile ducts is uncommon in early life, although it is responsible for occasional cases of prolonged neonatal jaundice. This lesion becomes more prevalent and extensive with age and is found in 25% or more of patients at postmortem examination.

Infrequently, this process proceeds to symptomatic multilobular biliary cirrhosis that has a distinctive pattern of large irregular parenchymal nodules and interspersed bands of fibrous tissue. In addition, approximately 30% of patients have fatty infiltration of the liver, in some cases despite apparently adequate nutrition. At autopsy, hepatic congestion secondary to cor pulmonale is frequently observed. The gallbladder may be hypoplastic and filled with mucoid material and not infrequently contains stones. The epithelial lining often displays extensive mucous metaplasia. Atresia of the cystic duct and stenosis of the distal common bile duct have been observed.

Mucus-secreting *salivary glands* are usually enlarged and display focal plugging and dilatation of ducts.

Glands of the uterine cervix are distended with mucus, and copious amounts of mucus collect in the cervical canal. Endocervicitis may be prevalent in teenagers and young women. In more than 95% of males, the body and tail of the epididymis, the vas deferens, and the seminal vesicles are obliterated or atretic.

Generalized amyloidosis has been reported rarely (see Chapter 154).

Clinical Manifestations. Mutational heterogeneity and environmental factors appear responsible for highly variable involvement of the lung, pancreas, and other organs. A list of presenting manifestations is lengthy, although pulmonary and gastrointestinal presentations predominate (Table 393–1).

RESPIRATORY TRACT. Cough is the most constant symptom of pulmonary involvement. At first, the cough may be dry and hacking, but eventually it becomes loose and productive. In older patients, the cough is most prominent on arising in the morning or after activity. Expectorated mucus is usually purulent. Some patients remain asymptomatic for long periods or seem to have prolonged but intermittent acute respiratory infections. Others acquire a chronic cough within the first weeks of life or they repeatedly have pneumonia. Extensive bronchiolitis is attended by wheezing, which is a frequent symptom during the 1st years of life. As lung disease progresses, exercise intolerance, shortness of breath, and failure to gain weight or grow are noted. Exacerbations of lung symptoms, presumably owing to more active airways infection, eventually require hospitalization for effective treatment. Finally, cor pulmonale, respiratory failure, and death supervene. Colonization with *Burkholderia cepacia* may be associated with particularly rapid pulmonary deterioration and death.

The rate of progression of lung disease is the chief determinant of morbidity and mortality. The course of lung disease, however, is largely independent of genotype. A few mutations (e.g., R117H) may substantially or even fully spare the lungs. Male gender and exocrine pancreatic sufficiency also are associated with a slower rate of pulmonary function decline.

TABLE 393–1. Presenting Features of More Than 20,000 Cystic Fibrosis Patients in the United States

Feature	%
Acute or persistent respiratory symptoms	50.5
Failure to thrive, malnutrition	42.9
Abnormal stools	35.0
Meconium ileus, intestinal obstruction	18.8
Family history	16.8
Electrolyte, acid-base abnormality	5.4
Rectal prolapse	3.4
Nasal polyps, sinus disease	2.0
Hepatobiliary disease	0.9
Other*	1.0–2.0

Includes pseudotumor cerebri, azoospermia, acrodermatitis-like rash, vitamin deficiency states, hypoproteinemic edema, hypoprothrombinemia with bleeding, meconium plug syndrome.
Data from the Patient Registry, Cystic Fibrosis Foundation, Bethesda, MD.

However, early insults to the lungs (e.g., severe viral infections) are likely to be a major determinant of pulmonary outcome.

Early physical findings include increased anteroposterior diameter of the chest, generalized hyperresonance, scattered or localized coarse crackles, and digital clubbing. Expiratory wheezes may be heard, especially in young children. Cyanosis is a late sign. Common pulmonary complications include atelectasis, hemoptysis, pneumothorax, and cor pulmonale and usually appear beyond the 1st decade of life.

Even though radiographically the paranasal sinuses are virtually always opacified, acute sinusitis is infrequent. Nasal obstruction and rhinorrhea are common, caused by inflamed, swollen mucous membranes or, in some cases, nasal polyposis. Nasal polyps are most troublesome between 5–20 yr of age.

INTESTINAL TRACT. In 15–20% of newborn infants with CF, the ileum is completely obstructed by meconium (meconium ileus). The frequency is greater (~30%) among siblings born subsequent to a child with meconium ileus, reflecting a higher prevalence in certain genotypes. Abdominal distention, emesis, and failure to pass meconium appear within the first 24–48 hr of life (see Chapter 91.1). Abdominal radiographs (Fig. 393–3) show dilated loops of bowel with air-fluid levels and frequently a collection of granular, "ground glass" material in the lower central abdomen. Rarely, meconium peritonitis results from intrauterine rupture of the bowel wall and can be detected radiographically by the presence of peritoneal or scrotal calcifications. Meconium plug syndrome occurs with increased frequency in infants with CF but is less specific than meconium ileus for this condition. Ileal obstruction with fecal material (*distal intestinal obstruction syndrome* or *meconium ileus equivalent*) occurs in older patients, causing cramping abdominal pain and abdominal distention.

More than 85% of affected children show evidence of maldigestion from exocrine pancreatic insufficiency. Symptoms include frequent, bulky, greasy stools and failure to gain weight even when food intake appears to be large. Characteristically, stools contain readily visible droplets of fat. A protuberant abdomen, decreased muscle mass, poor growth, and delayed maturation are typical physical signs. Excessive flatus may be a problem. A number of mutations are associated with preservation of some exocrine pancreatic function, including R117H and 3849+10kbC→T. Individuals homozygous for ΔF508 virtually all have pancreatic insufficiency.

Less common gastrointestinal manifestations include intussusception, fecal impaction of the cecum with an asymptomatic right lower quadrant mass, and epigastric pain owing to duodenal inflammation. Acid or bile reflux with esophagitis symptoms is common in older children and adults. Subacute appendicitis and periappendiceal abscess have been encountered. Rectal prolapse is relatively frequent. Occasionally, hypoproteinemia with anasarca appears in malnourished infants, especially if children are fed soy-based preparations. Neurologic dysfunction (dementia, peripheral neuropathy) and hemolytic anemia may occur because of vitamin E deficiency. Deficiency of other fat-soluble vitamins is occasionally symptomatic. For example, hypoprothrombinemia owing to vitamin K deficiency may result in a bleeding diathesis. Clinical manifestations of other fat-soluble vitamin deficiencies, such as decreased bone density and night blindness, have been noted. Rickets is rare.

BILIARY TRACT. Biliary cirrhosis becomes symptomatic in only 2–3% of patients. Manifestations may include icterus, ascites, hematemesis from esophageal varices, and evidence of hypersplenism. A neonatal hepatitis-like picture and massive hepatomegaly owing to steatosis have been reported. Biliary colic secondary to cholelithiasis may occur in the 2nd decade of life. Liver disease occurs independent of genotype.

PANCREAS. In addition to exocrine pancreatic insufficiency, evidence for hyperglycemia and glycosuria including polyuria and weight loss may appear, especially after 10 yr of age when

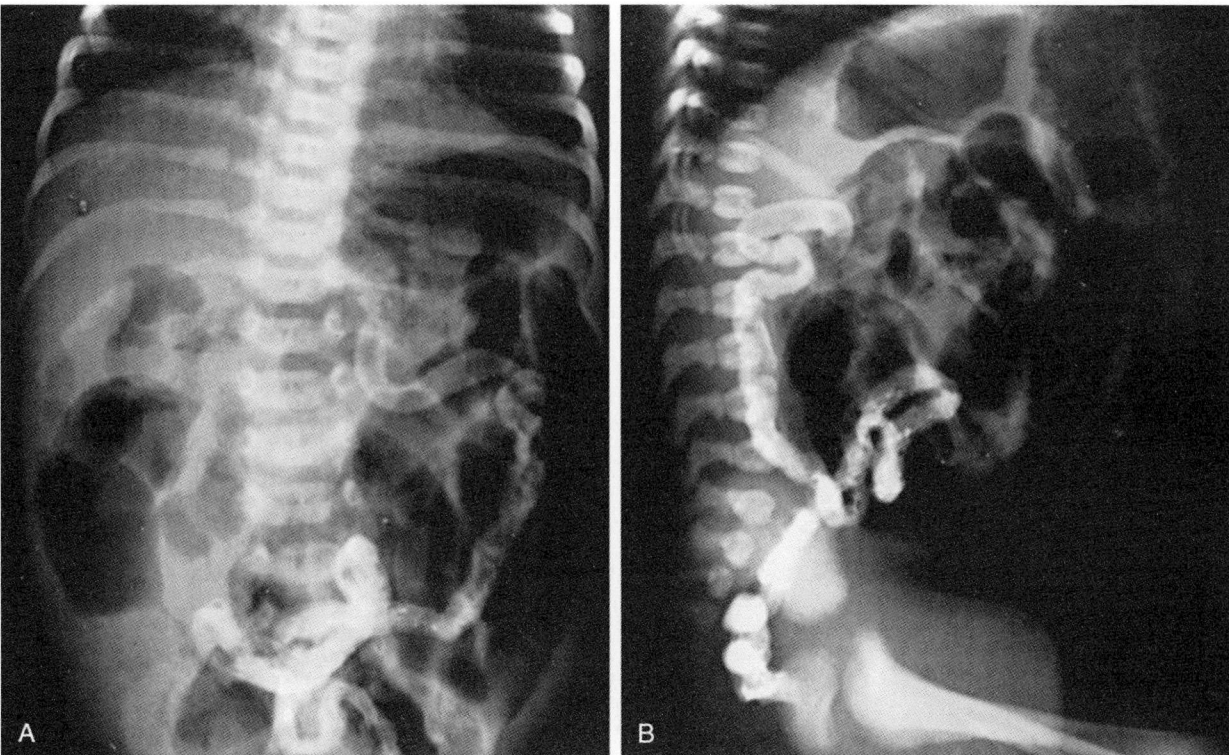

FIGURE 393–3. *A* and *B,* Contrast enema in a newborn infant with abdominal distention and failure to pass meconium. Notice the small diameter of the sigmoid and ascending colon and dilated, air-filled loops of small intestine. Several air-fluid levels in the small bowel are seen on the upright lateral view.

8% of individuals acquire diabetes. In most cases, ketoacidosis does not occur, but eye, kidney, and other vascular complications have been noted in patients living 10 yr or more after the onset of hyperglycemia. Recurrent, acute pancreatitis occurs occasionally in individuals who have residual exocrine pancreatic function.

GENITOURINARY TRACT. Sexual development is often delayed, but only by an average of 2 yr. More than 95% of males are azoospermic because of failure of development of wolffian duct structures, but sexual function is generally unimpaired. The incidence of inguinal hernia, hydrocele, and undescended testis is higher than expected. Adolescent females may experience secondary amenorrhea, especially with exacerbations of pulmonary disease. Cervicitis and accumulation of tenacious mucus in the cervical canal have been noted. The female fertility rate is diminished. Pregnancy is generally tolerated well by women with good pulmonary function but may cause a progression of pulmonary disease and even death in those with moderate or advanced lung problems.

SWEAT GLANDS. Excessive loss of salt in the sweat predisposes young children to salt depletion episodes, especially during the time of gastroenteritis and during warm weather. These children present with hypochloremic alkalosis. Frequently, parents notice salt "frosting" of the skin or a salty taste when they kiss the child. A few genotypes (e.g., 3849+10kbC→T) are associated with normal sweat chloride values.

Diagnosis and Assessment. The diagnosis of CF has been based for many years on a positive quantitative sweat test (Cl⁻ ≥ 60 mEq/L) in conjunction with one or more of the following: typical chronic obstructive pulmonary disease, documented exocrine pancreatic insufficiency, or a positive family history. New diagnostic criteria have been recommended to include additional testing procedures (Box 393–1).

BOX 393–1. Diagnostic Criteria for Cystic Fibrosis

Presence of typical clinical features (respiratory, gastrointestinal, or genitourinary)

OR

A history of CF in a sibling

OR

A positive newborn screening test

PLUS

Laboratory evidence for CFTR dysfunction:

    Two elevated sweat chloride concentrations obtained on separate days

OR

Identification of two CF mutations

OR

An abnormal nasal potential difference measurement

SWEAT TESTING. The sweat test, using pilocarpine iontophoresis to collect sweat and chemical analysis of its chloride content, remains the standard approach to diagnosis. The procedure requires care and accuracy. A 3-mA electric current is used to carry pilocarpine into the skin of the forearm and locally stimulate the sweat glands. After washing the arm with distilled water, sweat is collected on filter paper or gauze (or with a capillary tube) that has been placed on the stimulated skin and covered to prevent evaporation. After 30–60 min, the filter paper is removed, weighed, and eluted in distilled water. A chloridometer is recommended for the analysis of chloride in these samples. The amount of sweat collected should be measured and reported. For reliable results, at least 50 mg and preferably 100 mg of sweat should be collected. In infants, it may be necessary to use the upper back to obtain enough sweat. Reliable testing may be difficult in the first few weeks of life because of low sweat rates. Positive results should be confirmed;

a negative result should be repeated if suspicion of the diagnosis remains.

More than 60 mEq/L of chloride in sweat is diagnostic of CF when one or more other criteria are present. Threshold levels of 40 mEq/L for infants have been suggested. Values between 40 and 60 mEq/L suggest CF at all ages and have been reported in cases with typical involvement. In healthy adults, the sweat chloride values increase slightly, but a value of 60 mEq/L still adequately differentiates CF from other conditions. Chloride concentrations in sweat are somewhat lower in individuals who retain exocrine pancreatic function but remain within the diagnostic range. False-negative test results may be encountered in children with hypoproteinemic edema.

Non-CF conditions associated with elevated concentrations of sweat electrolytes include untreated adrenal insufficiency, ectodermal dysplasia, hereditary nephrogenic diabetes insipidus, glucose-6-phosphatase deficiency, hypothyroidism, hypoparathyroidism, familial cholestasis, pancreatitis, mucopolysaccharidoses, fucosidosis, and malnutrition. Most of these conditions can be easily distinguished from CF by clinical criteria.

OTHER DIAGNOSTIC TESTS. The finding of increased potential differences across nasal epithelium, the loss of this difference with topical amiloride application, and the absence of a voltage response to a β-adrenergic agonist have been used to confirm the diagnosis in patients with equivocal or frankly normal sweat chloride values. Failure to sweat when a combination of isoproterenol and atropine is injected into the skin has also been used to characterize CF variants.

PANCREATIC FUNCTION. Exocrine pancreatic dysfunction is clinically apparent in many patients. However, documentation is desirable if there are questions about the functional status of the pancreas. Measurement of fat balance with a 3-day stool collection or direct documentation of enzyme secretion after duodenal intubation and pancreozymin-secretin stimulation are reliable measures but are cumbersome or invasive for children and are not used routinely. Quantitation of trypsin and chymotrypsin activity in a fresh stool sample is a useful screening test but is not definitive. Measurement of immunoreactive trypsinogen in serum reliably distinguishes patients with CF, with and without pancreatic insufficiency, after 7 yr of age but not before that time. Other indirect measures of pancreatic enzyme secretion are available but have limited or unproven clinical value. Endocrine pancreatic dysfunction may be more prevalent than previously recognized. Some have advocated yearly monitoring of glycosylated hemoglobin levels after 10 yr of age. This approach is more sensitive than spot checks of blood and urine glucose levels.

RADIOLOGY. Pulmonary radiologic findings suggest the diagnosis but are not specific. Hyperinflation of lungs occurs early and may be overlooked in the absence of infiltrates or streaky densities. Bronchial thickening and plugging and ring shadows suggesting bronchiectasis usually appear first in the upper lobes. Nodular densities, patchy atelectasis, and confluent infiltrates follow. Hilar lymph nodes may be prominent. With advanced disease, impressive hyperinflation with markedly depressed diaphragms, anterior bowing of the sternum, and a narrow cardiac shadow are noted. Cyst formation, extensive bronchiectasis, dilated pulmonary artery segments, and segmental or lobar atelectasis are often apparent. Typical progression of lung disease is seen in Figure 393–4. CT of the chest can be used to detect and localize thickening of bronchial airway walls, mucus plugging, focal hyperinflation, and early bronchiectasis (Fig. 393–5); it generally is not used for routine evaluation of chest disease.

Radiographs of paranasal sinuses reveal panopacification and often failure of frontal sinus development. Fetal ultrasonography may suggest ileal obstruction with meconium early in the 2nd trimester, but this finding is not predictive of meconium ileus at birth.

PULMONARY FUNCTION. Standard pulmonary function studies are not obtained until 5–6 yr of age, by which time most patients show the typical pattern of obstructive pulmonary involvement (see Chapters 357 and 359). Decrease in the mid-maximal flow rate is an early functional change, reflecting small airway obstruction. This lesion also affects the distribution of ventilation and increases the alveolar-arterial oxygen difference. The findings of obstructive airway disease and modest responses to a bronchodilator are consistent with the diagnosis of CF at all ages. Residual volume and functional residual capacity are increased early in the course of lung disease. Restrictive changes, characterized by declining total lung capacity and vital capacity, correlate with extensive lung injury and fibrosis and are a late finding. Testing several times a year can be used to evaluate the course of the pulmonary involvement. Select CF centers are equipped to measure airflow patterns of sedated infants, but this procedure is usually done in the context of research studies. A few patients reach adolescent or adult life with normal pulmonary function and without evidence of over-inflation.

MICROBIOLOGIC STUDIES. The finding of *S. aureus* or *P. aeruginosa* on culture of the lower airways (e.g., sputum) strongly suggests a diagnosis of CF. In particular, mucoid forms of *Pseudomonas* are virtually diagnostic of CF in children. *B. cepacia* recovery also suggests CF. Increasingly, fiberoptic bronchoscopy is used to gather lower respiratory tract secretions of infants and young children who do not expectorate.

HETEROZYGOTE DETECTION AND PRENATAL DIAGNOSIS. Mutation analysis should be fully informative when testing potential carriers or a fetus provided that mutations within the family have been previously identified. Testing a spouse of a carrier with a standard panel of probes is approximately 90% sensitive. The rationale for prenatal detection of risk and termination of pregnancy is currently a matter of considerable discussion. A 1977 National Institutes of Health Consensus Conference recommendation to offer prenatal testing to all couples planning to have children as well as individuals with a family history of CF and partners of CF women has been reconsidered because of the medicolegal implications. In addition, termination of pregnancy is a less popular option because expected longevity is approximately 3 decades on average, with promise for an even better prognosis in the future.

NEWBORN SCREENING. Most newborns with CF can be identified by determination of immunoreactive trypsinogen in blood spots, coupled with confirmatory sweat or DNA testing. This screening test is at best only 95% sensitive. Although newborn diagnoses can prevent early nutritional deficiencies and improve long-term growth, there is as yet no compelling evidence that early diagnosis improves pulmonary, and therefore long-term, outcome. A number of states now screen newborns for CF, but the case for routine newborn screening remains debatable. A stronger case for screening will emerge when therapies that reverse the fundamental defect are available.

Treatment. The treatment plan should be comprehensive and linked to close monitoring and early, aggressive intervention.

GENERAL APPROACH TO CARE. Initial efforts after diagnosis should be intensive and include baseline assessment, initiation of treatment, clearing of pulmonary involvement, and education of the patient and parents. Follow-up evaluations are scheduled every 2–3 mo because many aspects of the condition require careful monitoring. An interval history and physical examination should be obtained at each visit. A sputum sample or, if that is not available, a lower pharyngeal swab taken during or after a forced cough is obtained for culture and antibiotic susceptibility studies. Even asymptomatic patients may produce sputum after forced exhalations or pharyngeal stimulation with a swab. Because irreversible loss of pulmonary function from low-grade infection can occur gradually and without acute symptoms, emphasis is placed on a thorough pulmonary history. Box 393–2 lists symptoms and signs that suggest the need for more intensive antibiotic and physical therapy. Immunoprophylaxis specifically against rubeola, pertussis, and influenza is essential. A nurse, respiratory therapist, social worker, dietitian, and psychologist should participate in the care program as needed. Considerable education and empowerment for families and older children to take responsibility for care is likely to result in the best adherence to daily care programs.

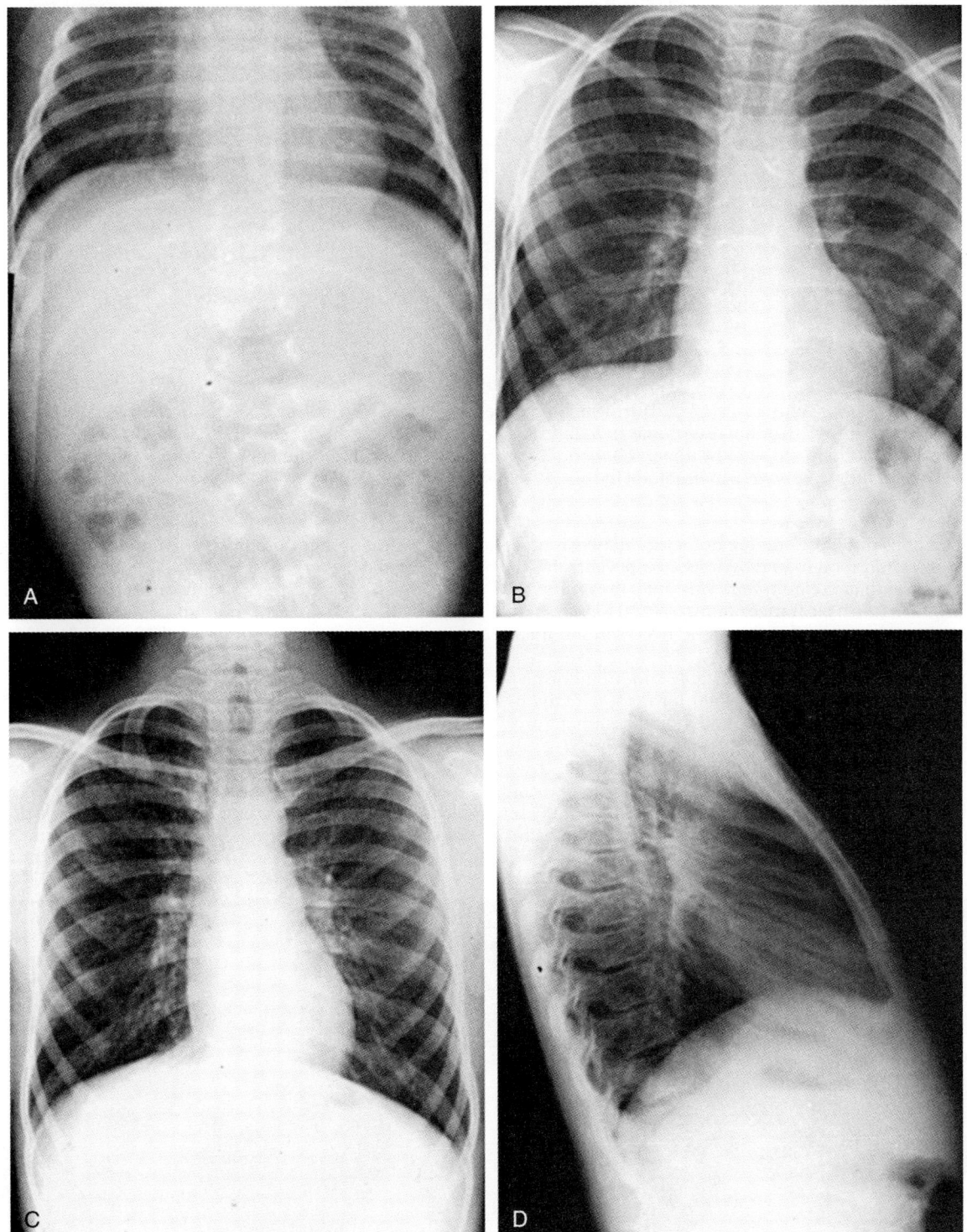

FIGURE 393–4. Roentgenographic progression of cystic fibrosis lung disease from the diagnosis in infancy to 18 yr of age. *A,* Admitted with cough and wheezing at 2 mo of age. Notice the mild increase in bronchovascular markings, especially in the upper lobe areas. *B,* At age 4 yr, cough was minimal. Bronchovascular markings were mildly increased, and there was some improvement in the upper lobes. The wheeze never recurred. *C* and *D,* At age 13 yr, there was minimal cough and occasional sputum production. The bronchovascular markings were generally further increased, with early bronchiectatic changes in the right upper lobe. The lateral view does not suggest overinflation.

Figure continued on following page

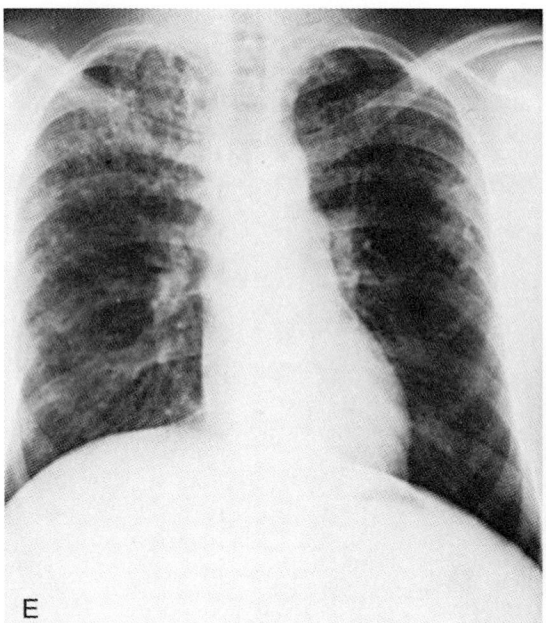
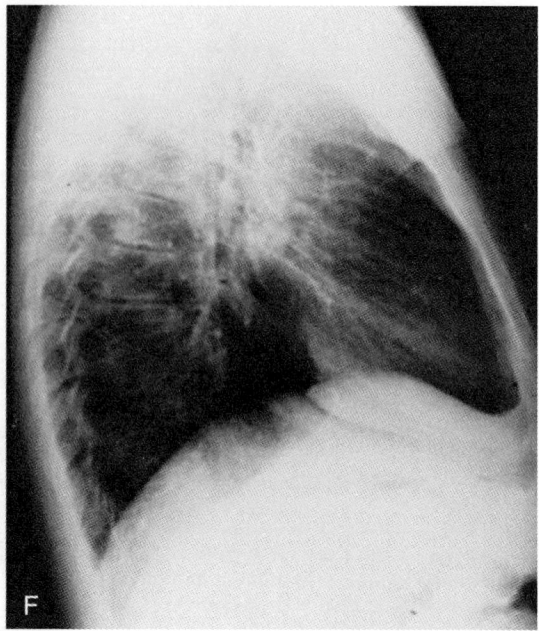

FIGURE 393–4. *Continued. E* and *F.* Age 18 yr. During adolescence, cough and sputum production increased even though outpatient antibiotic therapy was intensified. Small-volume hemoptysis, occasional paroxysms of cough, and weight loss as well as increased nodular infiltrates (especially in the right upper lobe) and hyperinflation (as seen on the lateral view) led to the first hospitalization since infancy. Height and weight were maintained in the 25th–50th percentile.

Because secretions of CF patients are not adequately hydrated, attention in early childhood to oral hydration, especially during warm weather or with acute gastroenteritis, may prevent exacerbation of problems with clearance of mucus from airways. For the same reason, intravenous therapy for dehydration should be initiated early.

The goal of therapy is to maintain a stable condition for prolonged periods. This can be accomplished for most patients by interval evaluation and adjustments of the home treatment program. However, some children have episodic acute or low-grade chronic lung infection that progresses. For these patients, 2 wk or more of intensive inhalation and physical therapy and intravenous antibiotics are indicated. Intravenous antibiotics may be required infrequently or as often as every 2–3 mo. Significant improvement in pulmonary function and the child's well-being is usually achieved.

The basic daily care program varies depending on the age of the child, the degree of pulmonary involvement, other system involvement, and the time available for therapy. The major components of this care are pulmonary and nutritional therapy. Because therapy is medication-intensive, iatrogenic problems arise frequently. Monitoring for these complications is also an important part of management (Table 393–2).

PULMONARY THERAPY. The object is to clear secretions from airways and to control infection. The effectiveness of the overall approach, including continuity of care, frequent evaluations, aggressive intervention, and an optimistic outlook, is more important than variations in the use of individual meas-

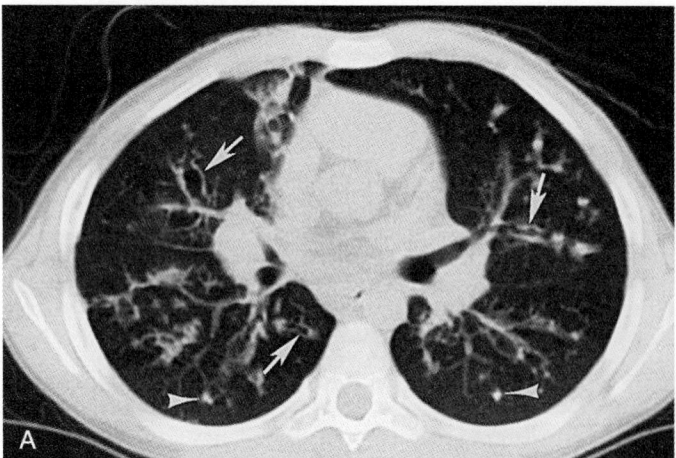
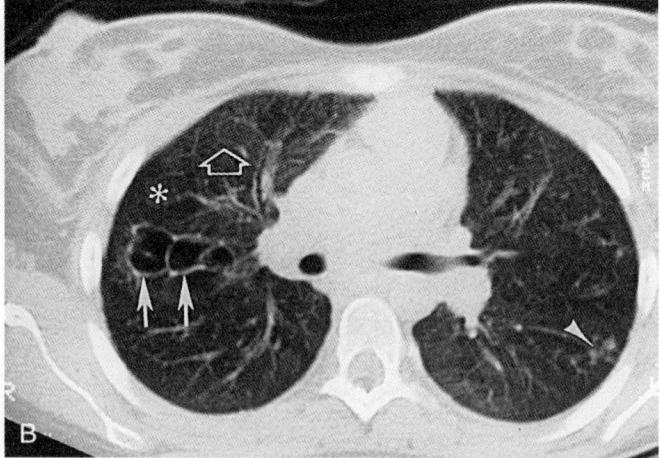

FIGURE 393–5. CT images of the chest in CF. *A,* A 12-yr-old boy with moderate lung disease. Airway and parenchymal changes are present throughout both lungs. Multiple areas of bronchiectasis *(arrows)* and mucus plugging *(arrowheads)* are seen. *B,* A 19-yr-old girl has mostly normal lung with one area of saccular bronchiectasis in the right upper lobe *(arrows)* and a focal area of peripheral mucus plugging in the right lower lobe *(arrowhead)*. Lung density is heterogeneous with areas of normal lung *(open arrow)* and areas of low attenuation reflecting segmental and subsegmental air trapping *(asterisk)*.

BOX 393-2. Symptoms and Signs Associated with Exacerbation of Pulmonary Infection in Patients with Cystic Fibrosis

SYMPTOMS
Increased frequency and duration of cough
Increased sputum production
Change in appearance of sputum
Increased shortness of breath
Decreased exercise tolerance
Decreased appetite
Feeling of increased congestion in the chest

SIGNS
Increased respiratory rate
Use of accessory muscles for breathing
Intercostal retractions
Change in results of auscultatory examination of chest
Decline in measures of pulmonary function consistent with the presence of obstructive airway disease
Fever and leukocytosis
Weight loss
New infiltrate on chest radiograph

From Ramsey B: Management of pulmonary disease in patients with cystic fibrosis. *N Engl J Med* 335:179, 1996.

ures. When a child is not doing well, every potentially useful aspect of therapy should be considered.

INHALATION THERAPY. Aerosol therapy is used to deliver medications and water to the lower respiratory tract. Some agents such as bronchodilators can be delivered by metered-dose inhaler with or without a spacer. The mainstay is intermittent delivery using a compressor that drives a hand-held nebulizer. The basic aerosol solution is 0.45–0.9% saline. In patients with reactive airways, albuterol or other β-agonists are added. Alternatively, or in addition, cromolyn sodium or inhaled corticosteroids can be administered. β-Agonists may decrease Pao_2 by increasing ventilation-perfusion mismatch, a problem if the Pao_2 is marginal.

When the airway pathogens are resistant to oral antibiotics or when the infection is difficult to control at home, aerosolized antibiotics may reduce symptoms, improve pulmonary function, and alleviate the need for hospitalization. (See Aerosolized Antibiotic Therapy.)

Human recombinant DNase (2.5 mg), given as a single daily aerosol dose, improves pulmonary function, decreases numbers of pulmonary exacerbations, and promotes a sense of well-being in patients who have moderate disease and purulent secretions. Benefit for those with normal FEV_1 values or advanced lung disease has also been documented. Improvement is sustained for 12 mo or more on continuous therapy. Another mucolytic

TABLE 393-2. Complications of Therapy for Cystic Fibrosis

Complication	Agent
Gastrointestinal bleeding	Ibuprofen
Hyperglycemia	Corticosteroids (systemic)
Growth retardation	Corticosteroids (systemic, inhaled)
Renal dysfunction	
Tubular	Aminoglycosides
Interstitial nephritis	Semisynthetic penicillins
Hearing loss, vestibular dysfunction	Aminoglycosides
Peripheral neuropathy or optic atrophy, or both	Chloramphenicol (prolonged course)
Hypomagnesemia	Aminoglycosides
Hyperuricemia, colonic stricture	Pancreatic extracts (very large doses)
Goiter	Iodine-containing expectorants
Gynecomastia	Spironolactone
Enamel hypoplasia or staining	Tetracyclines (used in first 8 yr of life)

Note: Common hypersensitivity reactions to drugs are not included.

agent, *N*-acetylcysteine, is toxic to ciliated epithelium, and repeated administration should be avoided.

CHEST PHYSICAL THERAPY. This treatment usually consists of chest percussion combined with postural drainage and derives its rationale from the idea that cough clears mucus from large airways, but chest vibrations are required to move secretions from small airways where expiratory flow rates are low. Chest physical therapy (PT) may be particularly useful for patients with CF because they accumulate secretions in small airways first, even before the onset of symptoms. Improvement of pulmonary function generally cannot be demonstrated immediately after this therapy. However, cessation of chest PT in older children with mild to moderate airflow limitation results in deterioration of lung function within 3 wk, and prompt improvement of function occurs when therapy is resumed. Chest PT is recommended one to four times a day, depending on the severity of lung dysfunction. Cough or forced expirations are encouraged after each lung segment is "drained." Hand-held or vest-type mechanical percussors may be useful for adolescents or young adults. Voluntary coughing, repeated forced expiratory maneuvers with and without positive expiratory pressure, patterned breathing, and use of a hand-held flutter device have all been suggested as additional aids to clearance of mucus. Routine aerobic exercise appears to slow the rate of decline of pulmonary function.

ANTIBIOTIC THERAPY. Antibiotics are the mainstay of therapy designed to control progression of lung infection. The goal is to reduce the intensity of endobronchial infection and to delay progressive lung damage. The usual guidelines for acute chest infections, such as fever, tachypnea, or chest pain, are often absent. Consequently, all aspects of the patient's history and examination, including anorexia, weight loss, and diminished activity, must be used to guide the frequency and duration of therapy. Antibiotic treatment varies from intermittent short courses of one antibiotic to nearly continuous treatment with one or more antibiotics. Dosages are often two to three times the amount recommended for minor infections because patients with CF have proportionately more lean body mass and higher clearance rates for many antibiotics than do other individuals. Also, it is difficult to achieve effective drug levels of many antimicrobials in respiratory tract secretions.

Oral Antibiotic Therapy. Indications include the presence of respiratory tract symptoms and identification of pathogenic organisms in respiratory tract cultures. Whenever possible, the choice of antibiotics should be guided by in vitro sensitivity testing. Common organisms include *S. aureus,* nontypable *Haemophilus influenzae,* and *P. aeruginosa. B. cepacia* is encountered with increasing frequency. The first two can be eradicated from the respiratory tract in CF, but *Pseudomonas* is more difficult to treat and rarely is eradicated outside of infancy. The usual course of therapy is 2 wk or more, and maximal doses are recommended. Useful oral antibiotics are listed in Table 393-3. Tetracycline should be avoided in children younger than 9 yr of age. The quinolones are the only broadly effective oral antibiotics for *Pseudomonas* infection, but resistance emerges rapidly. Infection with mycoplasmal or chlamydial organisms has been documented, providing a rationale for the use of macrolides on an empirical basis for flare of symptoms. Additionally, macrolides may reduce the virulence properties of *P. aeruginosa* such as biofilm production and contribute anti-inflammatory effects.

Aerosolized Antibiotic Therapy. *P. aeruginosa* and other gram-negative organisms are frequently resistant to all oral antibiotics. Aerosol delivery of antibiotics offers an option for home delivery of additional agents. Inhaled tobramycin has been studied the most extensively. When given at a dose of 300 mg twice daily on alternate months for 6 mo, *Pseudomonas* density in sputum decreases, fewer hospitalizations are required, and pulmonary function improves by 10%. Toxicity is negligible. This therapy can be recommended for increasing symptoms

TABLE 393–3. Antimicrobial Agents for Cystic Fibrosis Lung Infection

Route	Organisms	Agents	Dosage (mg/kg/24 hr)	Doses/24 hr
Oral	*Staphylococcus aureus*	Dicloxacillin	25–50	4
		Cephalexin	50	4
		Clindamycin	20	3–4
		Amoxicillin-clavulanate	40	3
	Haemophilus influenzae	Amoxicillin	50–100	3
	Pseudomonas aeruginosa	Ciprofloxacin	15–30	2–3
	Burkholderia cepacia	Trimethoprim-sulfamethoxazole	20*	2–4
	Empirical	Azithromycin	10, day 1; 5, days 2–5	1
		Erythromycin	50–100	3–4
Intravenous	*S. aureus*	Nafcillin	100–200	4–6
		Vancomycin	40	4
	P. aeruginosa	Tobramycin	8–20	1–3
		Amikacin	15–30	2–3
		Netilmicin	6–12	2–3
		Carbenicillin	400	4
		Ticarcillin	400	4
		Piperacillin	300	4
		Ticarcillin-clavulanate	400†	4
		Imipenem-cilastatin	45–90	3–4
		Ceftazidime	150	3
		Aztreonam	150	4
	B. cepacia	Chloramphenicol	50–100	4
		Meropenem	60–120	3
Aerosol		Tobramycin	300‡	2

*Quantity of trimethoprim.
†Quantity of ticarcillin.
‡In mg per dose.

or to improve long-term function in patients with moderate to severe disease. Other antimicrobials such as ticarcillin (0.5 g) and colistin (20–40 mg) have been used two to four times a day. Sensitization or resistance to inhaled antibiotics may occur, but both are surprisingly infrequent.

Intravenous Antibiotic Therapy. For the patient who has progressive or unrelenting symptoms and signs despite intensive home measures, intravenous antibiotic therapy is indicated. This therapy is usually initiated in the hospital but often is completed on an ambulatory basis. Although many patients improve within 7 days, it is usually advisable to extend the period of treatment to at least 14 days. Permanent intravenous access can be provided for long-term therapy in the hospital or at home.

Intravenous antibiotics commonly used are listed in Table 393–3. In general, treatment of *Pseudomonas* infection requires two-drug therapy. A third agent may be required for optimal coverage of *S. aureus* or other organisms. Simultaneous administration of aerosolized antimicrobial agents can increase endobronchial concentrations. The aminoglycosides have a relatively short half-life in many patients with CF. The initial parenteral dose, noted in Table 393–3, is generally given every 8 hr. After blood levels have been determined, the total daily dose should be adjusted. Peak levels of 10 mg/L are desirable, and trough levels should be kept at less than 2 mg/L to minimize the risk of ototoxicity and nephrotoxicity. Once- or twice-a-day aminoglycoside dosing may have advantages over every-8-hr dosing. Changes in therapy should be guided by culture results and by lack of improvement. If patients do not improve, heart failure, reactive airways, and infection with viruses, *Aspergillus fumigatus*, mycobacteria, or other unusual organisms should be considered. *B. cepacia* may be particularly refractory to antimicrobial therapy.

BRONCHODILATOR THERAPY. Reversible airway obstruction occurs in many children with CF, sometimes in conjunction with frank asthma or acute bronchopulmonary aspergillosis. Reversible obstruction is suggested by improvement of 15% or more in flow rates after inhalation of a bronchodilator. Treatment may include use of β-adrenergic agonists by aerosol.

Cromolyn sodium or ipratropium hydrochloride are alternative agents, but their efficacy has not been studied systematically.

ANTI-INFLAMMATORY AGENTS. Corticosteroids are useful for the treatment of allergic bronchopulmonary aspergillosis and severe reactive airway disease occasionally encountered in children with CF. Prolonged treatment of standard CF lung disease using an alternate-day regimen initially appeared to improve pulmonary function and diminish hospitalization rates. However, a 4-yr double-blind, multicenter study of this regimen for patients with mild to moderate lung disease found only modest efficacy and prohibitive side effects, including growth retardation, cataracts, and abnormalities of glucose tolerance at a dose of 2 mg/kg and growth retardation at 1 mg/kg. Inhaled corticosteroids have theoretical appeal, but there are few data concerning efficacy and safety. Ibuprofen, given chronically (dose adjusted to achieve a peak serum concentration of 50–100 μg/mL) over 4 yr, is associated with an impressive slowing of disease progression, particularly in younger patients with mild lung disease. Side effects of nonsteroidal anti-inflammatory drugs have been encountered (see Table 393–2).

ENDOSCOPY AND LAVAGE. Treatment of obstructed airways sometimes includes tracheobronchial suctioning or lavage, especially if atelectasis or mucoid impaction is present. Bronchopulmonary lavage may be performed by the instillation of saline or a mucolytic agent through a fiberoptic bronchoscope. Antibiotics (usually gentamicin or tobramycin) may also be instilled directly at lavage, transiently achieving a much higher endobronchial concentration than can be obtained by using intravenous therapy. There is no evidence for sustained benefit from repeated endoscopic or lavage procedures.

EXPECTORANTS. Systemic drugs, such as iodides and guaiphenesin, do not effectively assist with the removal of secretions from the respiratory tract.

TREATMENT OF PULMONARY COMPLICATIONS. A number of pulmonary complications require extra attention or special measures.

Atelectasis. Lobar atelectasis occurs relatively infrequently; it may be asymptomatic and noted only at the time of a routine chest radiograph. Aggressive intravenous therapy with antibiotics and increased chest PT directed at the affected lobe may be effective. If there is no improvement in 5–7 days, bronchoscopic examination of the airways may be indicated. If the atelectasis does not resolve, continued intensive home therapy is indicated, because atelectasis may resolve during a period of weeks or months. Persistent atelectasis may be asymptomatic. Lobectomy should be considered only if expansion is not achieved and the patient has progressive difficulty from fever, anorexia, and unrelenting cough (see Chapter 400).

Hemoptysis. Endobronchial bleeding usually reflects airway wall erosion secondary to infection. With increasing numbers of older patients, hemoptysis has become a relatively frequent complication. Blood streaking of sputum is particularly common. Small volume hemoptysis (<20 mL) should not trigger panic and is usually viewed as a need for intensified antimicrobial and chest PT. When the hemoptysis is persistent or increases in severity, hospital admission is indicated. Massive hemoptysis, defined as total blood loss of 250 mL or more within a 24-hr period, is rare in the first decade and occurs in less than 1% of adolescents, but it requires close monitoring and the capability to replace blood losses rapidly. Chest PT is often discontinued until 12–24 hr after the last brisk bleeding episode and is then reinstituted gradually. Patients should receive vitamin K for an abnormal prothrombin time. During brisk hemoptysis, the child and parents require a great deal of reassurance that the bleeding will stop. Blood transfusion is not indicated unless there is hypotension or the hematocrit is significantly reduced. Ticarcillin or nonsteroidal inflammatory drugs may interfere with platelet function and aggravate hemoptysis. Bronchoscopy rarely reveals the site of bleeding. Lobectomy is to be avoided, if possible, because functioning lung should be preserved. Bronchial artery embolization can be useful to control persistent, significant hemoptysis.

Pneumothorax. Pneumothorax (also see Chapter 403) is encountered in less than 1% of children and teenagers, but it is more frequently encountered in older patients and may be life-threatening. The episode may be asymptomatic but is often attended by chest and shoulder pain, shortness of breath, or hemoptysis. An open thoracotomy through a small incision with plication of blebs, apical pleural stripping, and basal pleural abrasion is recommended after the first occurrence and within 24 hr of the diagnosis. This procedure is well tolerated even in cases of advanced lung disease. Intravenous antibiotics are begun on admission. The thoracotomy tube is removed as soon as possible, usually on the 2nd or 3rd postoperative day. The patient can then be mobilized and full postural drainage therapy resumed. Rarely, bilateral simultaneous pneumothorax is encountered; in this case, control of the air leak must be achieved immediately, at least on one side.

Allergic Aspergillosis. This complication occurs in 5–10% of patients and may present as wheezing, increased cough, shortness of breath, or marked hyperinflation (see Chapters 218 and 388). In some patients there are new, focal infiltrates on the chest radiograph. The presence of rust-colored sputum, the recovery of *Aspergillus* organisms from the sputum, the demonstration of serum precipitating and specific IgE and IgG antibodies against *A. fumigatus,* or the presence of eosinophils in a fresh sputum sample support the diagnosis. The serum IgE level is usually high. Treatment is directed at controlling the inflammatory reaction with corticosteroids and preventing central bronchiectasis. For refractory cases, oral itraconazole may be required.

Nontuberculous Mycobacteria (NTM) Infection. Injured airways with poor clearance my be colonized by *Mycobacterium avium-complex,* but also *M. abscessus* and *M. kansasii.* Distinguishing endobronchial colonization (frequent) from invasive infection (infrequent) is challenging. Persistent fevers coupled with acid-fast organisms on sputum smear suggest infection. Treatment is prolonged and requires multiple

antimicrobial agents. Symptoms may improve, but NTM is usually not cleared from the lungs.

Bone and Joint Complications. Hypertrophic osteoarthropathy causes elevation of the periosteum over the distal portions of long bones and bone pain, overlying edema, and joint effusions. Acetaminophen or ibuprofen may provide relief. Control of lung infection usually reduces symptoms. Intermittent arthropathy unrelated to other rheumatologic disorders occurs occasionally, has no recognized pathogenesis, and usually responds to nonsteroidal anti-inflammatory agents. Rib fractures from vigorous coughing require pain management. These and other fractures may stem from diminished bone mineralization, the result of reduced vitamin D absorption, corticosteroid therapy, and perhaps other factors.

Acute Respiratory Failure. Acute respiratory failure (see Chapters 57.3 and 357.1) in patients with mild to moderate lung disease rarely occurs and is usually the result of a severe viral or other infectious illness. Because patients with this complication can regain their previous status, intensive therapy is indicated. In addition to aerosol, postural drainage, and intravenous antibiotic treatment, oxygen is required to raise the arterial Po_2 to greater than 50 mm Hg ($Sao_2 \geq 85$). An increasing Pco_2 may require ventilatory assistance. Endotracheal or bronchoscopic suction may be necessary and can be repeated daily. Right-sided heart failure may occur and should be treated vigorously. Recovery is often slow. Intensive intravenous antibiotic therapy and postural drainage should be continued for 1–2 wk after the patient has regained baseline status.

Chronic Respiratory Failure. Patients acquire chronic respiratory failure after prolonged deterioration of lung function. Although this can occur at any age, it is seen most frequently in adult patients. Because a long-standing Pao_2 less than 50 mm Hg promotes the development of right-sided heart failure, patients usually benefit from low-flow oxygen to raise arterial Po_2 to 55 mm Hg or greater. Increasing hypercapnia may prevent the use of optimal Fio_2. Most patients improve somewhat with intensive antibiotic and pulmonary therapy measures and can be discharged from the hospital. Low-flow oxygen therapy at home is needed, especially with sleep. Nocturnal noninvasive ventilatory support, if tolerated, can improve ventilation. These patients almost always display cor pulmonale and should be maintained on a reduced salt intake and diuretics. Caution should be exercised to avoid alkalosis that results from diuretic-induced bicarbonate retention. Chronic pain (headache, chest pain, abdominal pain, and limb pain) is frequent at the end of life and responds to judicious use of analgesics, including opioids.

Lung transplantation is an option for end-stage lung disease (see Chapter 435.2). Criteria for referral include an FEV_1 less than 30% predicted. At best, 50% of patients are now surviving 5 yr or more, and lung function as well as quality of life generally improve remarkably. Because of bronchiolitis obliterans and other complications, transplanted lungs cannot be expected to function for the lifetime of a recipient. The demand for donor lungs exceeds the supply and waiting lists as well as duration of waits continue to grow.

Heart Failure. Some patients experience reversible right-sided heart failure (see Chapters 357.1 and 434) as the result of an acute event such as a viral infection or pneumothorax. Individuals with long-standing, advanced pulmonary disease, especially those with severe hypoxemia ($Pao_2 < 50$ mm Hg), often acquire chronic right-sided heart failure. The mechanisms include hypoxemic pulmonary arterial constriction and loss of the pulmonary vascular bed. Pulmonary artery wall changes contribute to increased vascular resistance with time. Evidence for concomitant left ventricular dysfunction is often found. Cyanosis, increased shortness of breath, increased liver size with a tender margin, ankle edema, jugular venous distention, an unusual weight gain, increased heart size seen on chest radiograph, or evidence for right-sided heart enlargement seen on electrocardiogram or echocardiogram help to confirm the diagnosis. Furosemide (1 mg/kg administered intravenously)-induced diuresis confirms the suspicion of fluid retention. Repeated doses are often required at 24–48 hr intervals to reduce fluid accumulation and accompanying symptoms. Concomitant use of spironolactone may protect against potassium depletion and facilitate long-term diuresis. Hypochloremic alkalosis complicates the chronic use of loop diuretics. Digitalis is not effective in pure right-sided failure, but it may be useful when there is an associated left-sided dysfunction. The arterial Po_2 should be maintained at greater than 50 mm Hg if at all possible. Intensive pulmonary therapy including intravenous antibiotics is most important. Initially, the salt intake should be limited to 2 g sodium/24 hr. Volume overload and antibiotics with high sodium content should be avoided. No clear-cut long-term benefit from pulmonary vasodilators has been demonstrated. In the past, heart failure usually meant death within several months. However, the prognosis has been improving, and a number of patients survive for 5 yr or more after the appearance of heart failure. Lung transplantation is the best option for reversal (see Chapter 435.2).

NUTRITIONAL THERAPY. Up to 90% of patients have complete loss of exocrine pancreatic function and inadequate digestion of fats and proteins. They require diet adjustment, pancreatic enzyme replacement, and supplementary vitamins.

Diet. Many infants at the time of diagnosis have nutritional deficits. Young infants who present with wheezy breathing and are fed soy protein formulas do not use this protein well and may acquire hypoproteinemia with anasarca. Infants do not routinely need formulas containing predigested protein and medium-chain triglycerides. A low-fat, high-protein, high-calorie diet was generally recommended in the past for older children. Some children on this diet are deficient in essential fatty acids. With the advent of improved pancreatic enzyme products, normal amounts of fat in the diet are usually tolerated and preferred. Not infrequently, parent-child interactions at feeding time are maladaptive, and behavioral interventions can improve caloric intake.

Most individuals have a higher than normal caloric need because of increased work of breathing and perhaps because of increased metabolic activity related to the basic defect. When anorexia of chronic infection supervenes, weight loss occurs. Encouragement to eat high-calorie foods may be useful, but weight gain generally is not realized unless lung infection is controlled. With advanced lung disease, weight stabilization or gain has been achieved by nocturnal feeding via nasogastric tube or percutaneous enterostomy or by intravenous hyperalimentation. Long-term benefits of these interventions for lung function, quality of life, and psychologic well-being are less clearly substantiated.

Pancreatic Enzyme Replacement. Extracts of animal pancreas given with ingested food reduce but do not fully correct stool fat and nitrogen losses. Enzyme dosage and product should be individualized for each patient. Enteric-coated, pH-sensitive enzyme microspheres are most often prescribed. Several strengths up to 20,000 IU of lipase/capsule are available. Administration of large doses has been linked to colonic strictures requiring surgery. Consequently, enzyme replacement should not exceed 2,500 lipase units/kg/meal. One to three capsules/meal is sufficient for most patients; infants need 2000–4000 lipase units per feeding mixed with applesauce. Snacks should be covered. The microsphere preparations usually are sufficiently effective to permit a liberal diet, which may include homogenized milk. Although children with CF display bile salt malabsorption, enzyme preparations containing bile salts are infrequently needed. The dose of enzymes required usually increases with age, but some teenagers and young adults may later have a decrease in their requirement.

Vitamin and Mineral Supplements. Because pancreatic insufficiency results in malabsorption of fat-soluble vitamins (A, D, E, and K), vitamin supplementation is recommended. Capsules containing amounts adequate to prevent deficiency of all four vitamins for CF patients are now available. They should be taken daily. Replacement doses may be required when low serum levels are documented or the patient is symptomatic. Infants with zinc deficiency and rash have been reported. In addition, attention should be paid to iron status; in one study almost one third of children with CF had a low serum ferritin concentration.

TREATMENT OF INTESTINAL COMPLICATIONS

Meconium Ileus. When meconium ileus (see Chapter 91.1) is suggested, a nasogastric tube is placed for suction and the infant is hydrated. In some cases diatrizoate (Gastrografin) enemas with reflux of contrast material into the ileum have resulted in the passage of a meconium plug and clearing of the obstruction. Use of this hypertonic solution requires careful correction of water losses into the bowel. Children in whom this procedure fails require operative intervention. Children who are successfully treated generally have a prognosis similar to that of other patients. Infants with meconium ileus should be treated as having CF until adequate sweat testing can be carried out.

Distal Intestinal Obstruction Syndrome (Meconium Ileus Equivalent) and Other Causes of Abdominal Symptoms. Despite appropriate pancreatic enzyme replacement, 2–5% of patients accumulate fecal material in the terminal portion of the ileum and in the cecum, which may result in partial or complete obstruction. For intermittent symptoms, pancreatic enzyme replacement should be continued or even increased and laxatives or stool softeners (milk of magnesia, docusate sodium [Colace], mineral oil) given. Increased fluid intake is also recommended. Failure to relieve symptoms signals the need for large-volume bowel lavage with a balanced salt solution containing polyethylene glycol taken by mouth or by nasogastric tube. When there is complete obstruction, a diatrizoate enema, accompanied by large amounts of intravenous fluids, can be therapeutic. Intussusception and volvulus must also be considered in the differential diagnosis. Intussusception, usually ileocolic, occurs at any age and often follows a 1–2 day history of "constipation." It can often be diagnosed and reduced by a diatrizoate enema. If a nonreducible intussusception or a volvulus is present, laparotomy is required. Repeated episodes of intussusception may be an indication for cecectomy.

Chronic appendicitis with or without periappendiceal abscess may present with recurrent or persistent abdominal pain, raising the question of need for a laparotomy. A lack of acid buffering in the duodenum appears to promote duodenitis and ulcer formation in some children. Bile reflux is seen in older patients (see following section). Other reasons for surgical procedures include carcinoma of the colon or biliary tract and sclerosing colonopathy.

Gastroesophageal Reflux. Because several factors raise intra-abdominal pressure, including cough and obstructed airways, pathologic gastroesophageal reflux is not uncommon and may exacerbate lung disease secondary to reflex wheezing and repeated aspiration. Dietary, positional, and medication therapy should be considered. Cholinergic agonists are contraindicated because they trigger mucus secretion and progressive respiratory difficulty. Reduction of stomach acid secretion can help, with proton pump inhibitors being the most effective agents. Fundoplication is a procedure of last resort.

Rectal Prolapse. This occurs frequently in infants with CF and less commonly in older children. It is usually related to steatorrhea, malnutrition, and repetitive cough. The prolapsed rectum can usually be replaced manually by continuous gentle pressure with the patient in the knee-chest position. Sedation may be helpful. To prevent an immediate recurrence, the buttocks can be taped closed. Adequate pancreatic enzyme replacement, decreased fat and roughage in the diet, and control of pulmonary infection result in improvement. Occasionally, a patient may continue to have rectal prolapse and require surgery.

Liver Disease. Liver function abnormalities associated with biliary cirrhosis can be improved by treatment with ursodeoxycholic acid. The ability of bile acids to prevent progression of cirrhosis has not been clearly documented. Portal hypertension with esophageal varices, hypersplenism, or ascites occurs in 2% or fewer of children with CF (see Chapter 348). The acute management of bleeding esophageal varices includes nasogastric suction and cold saline lavage. Sclerotherapy is recommended after an initial hemorrhage. In the past, significant bleeding has also been treated successfully with portosystemic shunting. Splenorenal anastomosis has been the most effective. Pronounced hypersplenism may require splenectomy. The management of ascites is discussed in Chapter 351.

Obstructive jaundice in newborns with CF requires no specific therapy. Hepatomegaly with steatosis requires careful attention to nutrition and may respond to carnitine repletion. Rarely, biliary cirrhosis proceeds to hepatocellular failure, which should be treated as in other patients with hepatic failure (see Chapters 345 and 348). End-stage liver disease is an indication for liver transplantation in children with CF, especially if pulmonary function is good.

Pancreatitis. Pancreatitis may be precipitated by fatty meals, alcohol ingestion, or tetracycline therapy. Serum amylase and lipase levels may remain elevated for long periods. Treatment is discussed in Chapter 332.

Hyperglycemia. Onset occurs most frequently after the 1st decade. Eight percent of 13–18 yr olds and approximately 20% of young adults are treated for hyperglycemia. Prevalence is significantly higher in females and in $\Delta F508$ homozygotes. Ketoacidosis is rarely encountered. The pathogenesis includes both impaired insulin secretion and insulin resistance. Glucose intolerance without urine glucose losses is usually not treated; glycosylated hemoglobin levels should be followed at least annually. With persistent glycosuria and symptoms, insulin treatment should be instituted. Oral hypoglycemic agents, with or without drugs that reduce insulin resistance, may be effective. Exocrine pancreatic insufficiency and malabsorption make strict dietary control of hyperglycemia difficult. Corticosteroid therapy should be avoided. The development of significant hyperglycemia favors acquisition of *P. aeruginosa* and *B. cepacia* in the airways and adversely affects pulmonary function. Thus, careful control of blood sugar is an important goal.

OTHER THERAPY

Nasal Polyps. Nasal polyps (see Chapter 363) occur in 15–20% of patients with CF and are most prevalent in the 2nd decade of life. Local corticosteroids and nasal decongestants occasionally provide some relief. When the polyps completely obstruct the nasal airway, rhinorrhea becomes constant, or widening of the nasal bridge is noticed, surgical removal is indicated; polyps may recur promptly or following a symptom-free interval of months to years. Polyps inexplicably stop developing in many adults.

Salt Depletion. Sweat salt losses can be high, especially in warm arid climates. Children should have free access to salt, and precautions against overdressing infants should be observed. Regimented salt supplements are no longer prescribed. Hypochloremic alkalosis should be suspected in any infant who has had symptoms of gastroenteritis, and prompt fluid and electrolyte therapy should be instituted as needed.

Growth and Maturation. Delayed growth should be vigorously addressed by enhancing nutrition and treating lung disease more vigorously. The risk-benefit ratio of growth hormone or anabolic steroids does not support their widespread use for undersized children with CF. Delayed sexual maturation, often associated with short stature, occurs fairly frequently. Although many have severe pulmonary infection or poor nutrition, delayed

puberty also occurs in patients with otherwise mild disease and is not well explained. Adolescents with CF should receive specific counseling through their developing years concerning sexual maturation and reproductive potential.

Surgery. Minor surgical procedures, including dental work, should be performed under local anesthesia if possible. Patients with good or excellent pulmonary status can tolerate general anesthesia without any intensive pulmonary measures before the surgery. Those with moderate or severe pulmonary infection usually do better with a 1–2 wk course of intensive antibiotic treatment before surgery. If this is impossible, prompt intravenous antibiotic therapy is indicated once it is recognized that major surgery is required. The total time of anesthesia should be kept to a minimum. After induction, tracheal suctioning is useful and should be repeated at least at the end of the operation. Patients with severe disease require monitoring of their blood gases and may require ventilatory assistance in the immediate postoperative period.

After major surgery, cough should be encouraged and postural drainage treatments should be reinstituted as soon as possible, usually within 24 hr. Adequate analgesia is important if early effective therapy is to be achieved. For those with significant pulmonary involvement, intravenous antibiotics are continued for 7–14 postoperative days. Early ambulation and intermittent deep breathing are important; an incentive spirometer can also be helpful. After open thoracotomy for treatment of pneumothorax or lobectomy, the chest tube is the greatest single obstacle to effective pulmonary therapy and should be removed as soon as possible so that full postural drainage therapy can resume.

NEW THERAPIES. Several innovative therapies are under investigation. Approaches include pharmacologic stimulation of alternative chloride transport mechanisms or upregulation of mutated *CFTR*, and lung gene therapy. The lung has proved to be particularly resistant to transfer and expression of the *CFTR* gene. Earlier and more effective control of airway infection and inflammation is another experimental therapeutic goal. The use of megestrol acetate for treating malnutrition is also under study.

Prognosis. CF remains a life-limiting disorder, although survival has improved dramatically during the past 30–40 yr. Infants with severe lung disease occasionally succumb, but most children survive this difficult period and are relatively healthy into adolescence or adulthood. However, the slow progression of lung disease eventually reaches disabling proportions. Life table data now indicate a median cumulative survival of 32 yr. Male survival is somewhat better than female survival for reasons that are not readily apparent. Children in socioeconomically disadvantaged families have, on average, a much poorer prognosis.

For the most part, children with CF have good school attendance records and do not need to be restricted in their activities. A high percentage eventually attend and graduate from college. Most find satisfactory employment, and an increasing number marry. Transitioning care from pediatric to adult care centers by 18–21 years of age is an important objective and requires a thoughtful, supportive approach.

With increasing life span, a new set of psychosocial considerations has emerged, including dependence-independence issues, self-care, peer relationships, sexuality, sterility, substance abuse, educational and vocational planning, financial burdens, and anxiety concerning health and prognosis. Many of these issues are best addressed in an anticipatory fashion, prior to the onset of psychosocial dysfunction. With appropriate medical and psychosocial support, children and adolescents with CF generally cope well. Achievement of an independent and productive adulthood is a realistic goal for many.

The CF Genotype-Phenotype Consortium: Correlation between genotype and phenotype in patients with cystic fibrosis. *N Engl J Med* 1993;329:1308.
Coakley RD: Regulation of airway surface liquid pH in cystic fibrosis. *Pediatr Pulmonol* 2001;22:120 (supplement).

Cohen JA, Friedman PG, Noone MR, et al: Relations between mutations of the cystic fibrosis gene and idiopathic pancreatitis. *N Engl J Med* 1998;339:653.

Corey M, Edwards L, Levison H, et al: Longitudinal analysis of pulmonary function decline in patients with cystic fibrosis. *J Pediatr* 1997;131:809.

Eubanks V, Koppersmith N, Wooldridge N, et al: Effects of megestrol acetate on weight gain, body composition, and pulmonary function in patients with cystic fibrosis. *J Pediatr* 2002;140:439–44.

Fitzsimmons SC, Burkhart GA, Borowitz D, et al: High-dose pancreatic-enzyme supplements and fibrosing colonopathy in children with cystic fibrosis. *N Engl J Med* 1997;336:1283.

Fuchs JR, Borowitz DS, Christiansen PH, et al: Effect of aerosolized recombinant human DNase on exacerbations of respiratory symptoms and on pulmonary function in patients with cystic fibrosis. *N Engl J Med* 1994;331:637.

Knowles M, Gatzy J, Boucher R: Increased bioelectric potential difference across respiratory epithelia in cystic fibrosis. *N Engl J Med* 1981;305:1489.

Konstan M, Byard P, Hoppel C, et al: Effect of high-dose ibuprofen in patients with cystic fibrosis. *N Engl J Med* 1995;332:848.

Lemna WK, Feldman FL, Kerem B, et al: Mutation analysis for heterozygote detection and the prenatal diagnosis of cystic fibrosis. *N Engl J Med* 1990;322:291.

Lion RG, Adler FR, Cahill BC, et al: Survival effect of lung transplantation among patients with cystic fibrosis. *JAMA* 2001;286:2683–89.

Matsui H, Grubb BR, Tarran R, et al: Evidence for periciliary liquid layer depletion, not abnormal ion composition in the pathogenesis of cystic fibrosis airway disease. *Cell* 1998;95:1005.

Moran A, Hardin D, Rodman D, et al: Diagnosis, screening and management of cystic fibrosis related diabetes mellitus. A consensus conference report. *Diabetes Res Clin Pract* 1999;45:61.

Ramsey B: Management of pulmonary disease in patients with cystic fibrosis. *N Engl J Med* 1996;335:179.

Ramsey BW, Pepe MS, Quan JM, et al: Intermittent administration of inhaled tobramycin in patients with cystic fibrosis. *N Engl J Med* 1999;340:23.

Rosenstein BJ, Cutting GR: The diagnosis of cystic fibrosis: A consensus statement. *J Pediatr* 1998;132:589.

Sun L, Jiang RZ, Steinbach S, et al: The emergence of a highly transmissible lineage of *Burkholderia cepacia* causing CF centre epidemics. *Nat Med* 1995;1:661.

Zemel Bs, Jawad AF, Fitzsimmons S, et al: Longitudinal relationship among growth, nutritional status and pulmonary function in children with cystic fibrosis. *J Pediatr* 2000;137:374.

Chapter 394
Primary Ciliary Dyskinesia (Immotile Cilia Syndrome)
Gabriel G. Haddad

The group of respiratory disorders making up primary ciliary dyskinesia (PCD) have in common the malfunction of airway cilia. The ciliary abnormality is a result of various inherited primary structural defects in the cilia that lead to repeated and chronic lung infections. However, the ciliary malfunction in these diseases is *not* a result of acquired repeated pulmonary infections.

Characteristics of Cilia

LOCATION AND STRUCTURE. Airway cilia are located on epithelial surfaces in almost a ubiquitous fashion. They are present in the nose, sinuses, ears, and airways. They are also present in places other than the respiratory epithelium, such as in the fallopian tubes and in sperm. The density of cilia varies, with the majority of cells (50–80%) in the large airways having cilia, far fewer cells in the lower airways having cilia, and no cells in air sacs and alveoli having cilia. The frequency of ciliary beating, or *beatquency,* is 1–20 Hz, with the higher beatquency occurring in the larger airways, correlating with the mucus velocity in various parts of the tracheobronchial tree.

Cilia are finger-like structures that extend from the surface of cells into the lumen of airways. They have a diameter of 0.25 μm and a length of 306 μm. Each cell usually has about 200 cilia on its surface. Each cilia has a trunk, a basal body (where the cilia attaches to the cell), and a crown, which is a specialized struc-ture presumed to be important in cilia attachment to mucus. The trunk is made of an outer cell membrane and axonemes or cytoskeletal protein structures. The latter form a circular array of nine microtubules in pairs with an additional central pair. Each peripheral pair can attach to the other via bridges or dynein arms. Spokes are also cytoskeletal proteins that join peripheral and central microtubules.

FUNCTION. Cilia beat and move by a sliding motion of microtubules. At the outset of the beating cycle, they bend at the base and move backward, perpendicular to the surface. Subsequently, they extend ("slide") as they are rotating in a forward motion. These bending and rotating movements, which are clockwise, three-dimensional rotations, are made possible by adenosine triphosphate hydrolysis and the dynein arms, which are adenosine triphosphatases. When visualized under microscopy, airway cilia are seen to coordinate their activity regionally, and waves of ciliary movements (many cilia together) occur. How this is coordinated is not well understood.

The main function of cilia is to transport, through its beating movements, mucus toward the mouth. The effectiveness of this function depends on the beatquency, the composition and thickness of the periciliary fluid and mucus layer above it, and the coordination of ciliary movements. In addition, there are a number of neurochemicals that modulate ciliary beating by increasing beatquency, such as β-adrenergic compounds, acetylcholine, bradykinins, and serotonin. Alternatively, lowering airway humidity significantly lowers the frequency of ciliary beating. In addition, increasing bacterial loads decreases its beatquency.

Pathology. The structural abnormalities of these disorders can be seen with electron microscopy. Defects in both inner and outer dynein arms, radial spoke microtubular assembly, and central core cytoskeletal proteins have been described. It is estimated that there are more than 200 polypeptides in the ciliary structure, and primary ciliary dyskinesia is most likely based on the absence of one or several ciliary cytoskeletal proteins. All these structural defects result in ciliary malfunction characterized by either abnormal beating or immotility of cilia and defective mucociliary clearance of airway secretions. The most likely pathogenic sequence is airway mucus retention and failure to clear pathogenic organisms, followed by chronic or frequently recurring respiratory tract infections and, ultimately, injury to airway walls.

Genetics. PCD occurs in about 1/20,000 whites and has been reported in Japanese patients. It is probably the 3rd most common form of inherited chronic airway disease of white children, following cystic fibrosis (CF) and genetic immunodeficiency states. The inheritance pattern of PCD has not been established. An association between ciliary dyskinesia and hydrocephalus and mental retardation in four male siblings in a Jordanian family has been reported that might be caused by a mutation that affects pulmonary toilet and cerebrospinal fluid movement.

DNAH5 is a dynein heavy-chain gene localized on chromosome 5p. The cilia inner arm dynein heavy-chain gene is important in reducing the frequency of beating, although there is no gross morphologic abnormality in the cilia. This same gene is also critical for the movement of sperm from the uterus into the oviduct of the mouse. Furthermore, mutations in *DNAH5* have been found in patients with PCD. Mutations of this gene also have been described in patients exhibiting randomization of organ left-right asymmetry. It is hypothesized that normal rotation of viscera depends on the motion of ciliated intestinal cells early in development. The absence of ciliary motility allows random rotation; a dynein defect causes left-right asymmetry in the inversus viscerum (iv/iv) mouse model.

Clinical Manifestations. About 50% of patients with PCD have Kartagener syndrome: situs inversus, chronic sinusitis and otitis, and airway disease leading to bronchiectasis. However, only about 25% of patients with situs inversus also have PCD. Situs inversus does not establish or exclude the presence of PCD.

The course is variable. Individuals with PCD may have respiratory distress during the newborn period or may survive to adulthood without overt chronic sinusitis and airway disease symptoms. However, in one study of PCD, 100% of children had productive cough, sinusitis, and otitis. A feature that is helpful in differentiating PCD from CF is repeated bouts of acute otitis media or chronic serous otitis. Children diagnosed after several years of life often have been treated with tympanostomy tubes; conductive hearing loss is common. Nasal polyps or clubbing is present in about 20% of patients. Many children with PCD experience frequent wheezing and may have an initial diagnosis of asthma. The hallmark symptom is a chronic, often loose or productive, cough. Pneumonia may supervene, and lower respiratory tract disease can progress to weight loss, diminished exercise tolerance, and bronchiectasis. Respiratory failure in childhood is uncommon, as are lung complications such as pneumothorax and hemoptysis. Lobar atelectasis occurs frequently. Males are frequently infertile and display absent or poor sperm motility.

Diagnosis. PCD should be suspected in children with chronic or recurring upper and lower respiratory tract symptoms, especially in the presence of substantial middle ear disease. Radiographic or CT imaging shows involvement of the paranasal sinuses. Chest radiographs may demonstrate overinflation, bronchial wall thickening, and peribronchial infiltrates. Often, atelectasis and consolidation are present. Bronchiectasis is best detected by CT scanning (see Chapter 391). The presence of a right-sided heart in a child with chronic respiratory tract symptoms is virtually diagnostic, but this configuration occurs in only 50% of these patients. Pulmonary function testing of older children yields a typical obstructive pattern.

Mucociliary clearance can be assessed in cooperative children by ascertaining the time to taste perception of a saccharin particle placed on the inferior nasal turbinate. Scrapings or brushings of nasal mucosa can be examined directly by light or, preferably, by phase-contrast microscopy for evidence of motility. In most PCD tissue specimens, little or no ciliary motion is seen. However, because substantial motility has been documented in scrapings of several individuals with absent dynein arms, light microscopic examination of living tissue can be used as a screening tool only. The gold standard is quantitative documentation of abnormal structural elements, such as missing dynein arms or random orientation of cilia in nasal or bronchial biopsies or scrapings on electron microscopic examination. Concordance of ultrastructural abnormalities in cilia and sperm is not complete. To avoid acquired ciliary changes, mucosal specimens should not be obtained until 2 wk after an acute respiratory tract infection. Ultrastructural evaluation should be reserved for highly suspicious cases. However, some structural abnormalities are also observed after injury to ciliated epithelial cells by viral infection or sulfur dioxide exposure. Therefore, definitive evidence that any structural alteration represents a discrete form of PCD awaits the identification of specific gene mutations.

Treatment. Therapy is symptomatic. Cough should be encouraged. Chest physiotherapy assists the clearance of mucus. Antibiotics should be prescribed for evidence of infection of sinuses or lower airways. The choice of antibiotics is best dictated by identification and sensitivity testing of pathogenic organisms, often pneumococcus or untypable *Haemophilus influenzae*. Oral antibiotic administration is usually effective. Bronchodilators can be used for symptomatic wheezing or documentation of reversible airway obstruction. Children should be examined several times each year and followed by periodic chest radiographs and serial pulmonary function testing. Sinus and middle ear symptoms refractory to medical therapy deserve

consultation with an otolaryngologist. Surgical intervention may be helpful in selected cases. Prevention of lung infection by measles, pertussis, influenza, and possibly pneumococcal vaccines is highly desirable. Additional preventive measures include avoidance of cigarette smoke and other airway irritants.

Prognosis. Progression of lung disease appears to be much slower for patients with PCD than for those with CF. With proper treatment, disabling lung disease often can be avoided for long periods. A normal life span is possible.

Afzelius BA: A human syndrome caused by immotile cilia. *Science* 1976;193:317.

Al-Shroof M, Karnik AM, Karnik AA, et al: Ciliary dyskinesia associated with hydrocephalus and mental retardation in a Jordanian family. *Mayo Clin Proc* 2001;76:1219–24.

Boat TF, Carson JL: Ciliary dysmorphology and dysfunction—primary or acquired? *N Engl J Med* 1990;323:1700.

Brueckner M: Cilia propel the embryo in the right direction. *Am J Med Genet* 2001;101:339–44.

Narayan D, Krishnan SN, Upender M, et al: Unusual inheritance of primary ciliary dyskinesia (Kartagener's syndrome). *J Med Genet* 1994;31:493.

Neesen J, Kirschner R, Ochs M, et al: Disruption of an inner arm dynein heavy chain gene results in asthenozoospermia and reduced ciliary beat frequency. *Hum Mol Genet* 2001;10:1117–28.

Olbrich H, Haffner K, Kispert A, et al: Mutations in DNAH5 cause primary ciliary dyskinesia and randomization of left-right asymmetry. *Nat Genet* 2002;30:143–44.

Pedersen H, Mygind N: Absence of axonemal arms in nasal mucosal cilia in Kartagener's syndrome. *Nature* 1976;262:494.

Rutland J, deIongh RU: Random ciliary orientation: A cause of respiratory tract disease. *N Engl J Med* 1990;323:1681.

Chapter 395
Interstitial Lung Diseases
Michelle S. Howenstine

The interstitial lung diseases (ILD) in infants and children include a group of uncommon, heterogeneous diseases that cause disruption of alveolar gas exchange and symptoms of restrictive lung disease. Knowledge regarding pediatric ILD is limited because of its rare occurrence, varied spectrum of disease, and lack of controlled clinical trials investigating the disease process and treatment measures. The pathophysiology is believed to be more complex than adult disease because the injury occurs during the process of lung growth and differentiation. In ILD, the initial injury causes damage to the alveolar epithelium and capillary endothelium. An exaggerated immune response then recruits oxidants and proteases, resulting in further damage to the lung interstitium and parenchymal units.

Classification and Pathology. The classification of ILD in children is not standardized, but it is helpful to separate diseases into those of known and unknown etiology (Box 395–1). Respiratory infections caused by adenovirus, influenza, *Chlamydia*, and *Mycoplasma pneumoniae* are usually self-limited illnesses but have been associated with prolonged and progressive lung damage, often in the form of bronchiolitis obliterans. Aspiration is a frequent cause of chronic lung disease in childhood. Children with developmental delay or neuromuscular weakness are at an increased risk for aspiration of food, saliva, or foreign matter secondary to swallowing dysfunction and/or gastroesophageal reflux. An undiagnosed tracheoesophageal fistula can also result in pulmonary complications related to aspiration of gastric contents and interstitial pneumonia. Children experiencing an exaggerated immunologic response to organic dust, molds, or bird antigens may develop hypersensitivity pneumonitis. Children with malignancies also may develop ILD related to the primary malignancy, an opportunistic infection, or secondary to chemotherapy or radiation treatment. In addition, unique forms of ILD

INTERSTITIAL LUNG DISEASES OF KNOWN ETIOLOGY

Aspiration syndromes
Chronic infection (viral, bacterial, fungal, parasitic)
   Immunocompetent host
   Immunocompromised host
Bronchopulmonary dysplasia
Hypersensitivity pneumonitis (and other environmental exposures)
Lipid storage diseases

INTERSTITIAL LUNG DISEASES OF UNKNOWN ETIOLOGY

Primary pulmonary disorders
   Usual interstitial pneumonitis (UIP)
   Desquamative pneumonitis (DIP)
   Lymphocytic interstitial pneumonitis (LIP) and related disorders
   Nonspecific interstitial pneumonitis
   Pulmonary hemosiderosis
   Pulmonary infiltrates with eosinophilia
   Bronchiolitis obliterans
   Bronchiolitis obliterans with organizing pneumonia (BOOP)
   Alveolar proteinosis
   Pulmonary vascular disorders (proliferative and congenital)
   Pulmonary lymphatic disorders
   Pulmonary microlithiasis

OTHER DISORDERS WITH PULMONARY INVOLVEMENT

Connective tissue disorders
Malignancies
Histiocytosis
Sarcoidosis
Neurocutaneous syndromes

From Fan LL: Pediatric Interstitial Lung Disease. In Schwartz MI, King TE (editors): *Interstitial Lung Disease*, 3rd ed. Toronto, BC Decker, 1998, p 103.

Persistent tachypnea of infancy (PTI)
Follicular bronchitis/bronchiolitis
Infantile pulmonary hemosiderosis
Chronic pneumonitis of infancy
Surfactant protein B deficiency
Familial desquamative interstitial pneumonitis (DIP)
Idiopathic pulmonary fibrosis of infancy

From Fan LL: Pediatric Interstitial Lung Disease. In Schwartz MI, King TE (editors): *Interstitial Lung Disease*, 3rd ed. Toronto, BC Decker, 1998, p 104.

have been described in infants presenting with chronic tachypnea, retractions, crackles, and hypoxemia (Box 395–2). The prognosis in these diseases is variable.

USUAL INTERSTITIAL PNEUMONITIS (UIP). This disorder is the most common form of ILD in affected adults but is rare in children. The pulmonary lesion is characterized by a mixed distribution of ongoing inflammation and progressive end-stage fibrosis that is patchy and heterogenous. The diagnosis is made by biopsy; there is no definitive clinical or radiologic feature.

DESQUAMATIVE INTERSTITIAL PNEUMONITIS (DIP). This disease, also dependent on biopsy diagnosis, demonstrates a uniform, homogeneous process characterized by hyperplasia of alveolar epithelial cells with an accumulation of large macrophages within the air spaces. Fibrosis is usually not seen. A familial form has been described in infants that is unusually severe and often fatal.

LYMPHOCYTIC INTERSTITIAL PNEUMONITIS (LIP). This most common form of ILD in children is a form of pulmonary lymphoproliferative disease. LIP usually develops in association with conditions of impaired immunity, such as an autoimmune disease or immunodeficiency (e.g., HIV infection). The pulmonary interstitium is invaded by a diffuse infiltrate of mature lymphocytes. Fibrosis is rare. Infection with a virus such as Ebstein-Barr virus is often a contributing factor in the development of pediatric LIP.

ACUTE INTERSTITIAL PNEUMONITIS. This entity, also known as rapidly progressive interstitial pneumonitis or Hamman-Rich syndrome, is a distinct, rapidly progressive form of ILD. On biopsy, the alveolar damage progresses from an acute exudative process to severe fibrosis. An antecedent injury is often not identified; the fatality rate is greater than 50%.

Clinical Manifestations. A detailed history is needed to assess the severity of symptoms and the possibility of an underlying systemic disease. Identification of precipitating factors such as exposure to molds or birds or a severe lower respiratory infection is important in establishing the diagnosis and instituting

avoidance measures. A positive family history especially in an affected infant is suggestive of a genetic or familial disease, such as a surfactant protein B deficiency (see Chapters 396 and 397). Tachypnea, cough, dyspnea, and exercise intolerance are present in over two thirds of patients. Symptoms are usually insidious and occur in a continuous, not episodic pattern. Tachypnea and basilar crackles are present in over one half of the patients. Retractions, failure to thrive, clubbing, and wheezing are common complaints. Cyanosis and a prominent second heart sound are suggestive of severe disease. Anemia or hemoptysis suggests a pulmonary vascular disease or pulmonary hemosiderosis. Rashes or joint complaints are consistent with an underlying connective tissue disease.

Diagnosis. A systematic approach is necessary to establish a definite diagnosis of ILD. Initially, noninvasive tests are used to determine the extent and severity of the disease. Chest radiographic abnormalities may be classified as interstitial, reticular, nodular, reticulonodular, or honeycombed. The chest film also may be normal despite significant clinical impairment and may correlate poorly with the extent of disease. High-resolution CT of the chest better defines the extent and distribution of disease and can provide specific information for selection of a biopsy site. Faster modalities such as helical, spiral, or ultra-fast CT may provide precise resolution of disease patterns in tachypneic infants.

Pulmonary function tests are important in defining the degree of restrictive lung disease and in following the response to treatment. Parallel decreases in functional residual capacity (FRC) and forced expiratory volume in 1 second (FEV_1) are noted. Total lung capacity is usually low. Diffusion of carbon monoxide (DL_{CO}) is usually normal when corrected for the decreased alveolar volume. An impaired DL_{CO} may suggest vascular disease. Bronchoalveolar lavage may provide helpful information regarding secondary infection, bleeding, or aspiration but will not determine the exact diagnosis. Transthoracic lung biopsy for histopathology is necessary for a conclusive diagnosis. Conventional thoracotomy or video-assisted thoracoscopy is used to obtain tissue from children with suspected ILD. Evaluation for possible systemic disease may also be necessary.

Treatment. Supportive care is essential and includes supplemental oxygen for hypoxia and adequate nutrition for growth failure. Antimicrobial treatment may be necessary for intercurrent infections. Some patients may be responsive to bronchodilators. Anti-inflammatory treatment with corticosteroids remains the initial treatment of choice. Controlled trials in children are lacking, and the clinical responses reported in case studies are variable. The usual dose of prednisone is 1–2 mg/kg/24 hr for 6–8 wk with tapering dictated by clinical response. Alternative, but not adequately evaluated, therapy includes hydroxychloroquine, azathioprine, cyclophosphamide, cyclosporine, methotrexate, intravenous gamma globulin, and pulsed high-dose steroids. Hydroxychloroquine treatment has been successful in some children with classic ILD, particularly those with histopathologic changes of DIP. Lung transplantation for progressive or end-stage ILD also has been successful in some infants and children. Appropriate treatment for underlying systemic disease is indicated. Preventative measures include avoidance of all inhalation irritants such as tobacco smoke and, when appropriate, molds and bird antigens. Supervised pulmonary rehabilitation programs may be helpful.

Prognosis. The overall mortality of ILD is as high as 20% in infants and children. Prognosis is variable and poor in children with pulmonary hypertension, failure to thrive, and severe fibrosis.

Atival A, Godrey S, Maayan C, et al: Chloroquine treatment of interstitial lung disease in children. *Pediatr Pulmonol* 1994;18:356–60.

Fan LL: In Schwarz MI, King TE (editors): *Interstitial Lung Disease,* 3rd ed. Toronto, BC Decker, 1998, pp 103–18.

Fan LL, Langston C: Chronic interstitial lung disease in children. *Pediatr Pulmonol* 1993;16:184–96.

Fan LL, Kozinetz CA, Wojtczak HA, et al: The diagnostic value of transbronchial, thoracoscopic and open lung biopsy in immunocompetent children with chronic interstitial lung disease. *J Pediatr* 1997;131:565–69.

Kerem E, Bentur L, England S, et al: Sequential pulmonary function measurements during infantile chronic interstitial pneumonitis. *J Pediatr* 1990;116:61–67.

Sharief N, Crawford OF, Dinwiddie R: Fibrosing alveolitis and desquamative interstitial pneumonitis. *Pediatr Pulmonol* 1994;17:359–65.

Sondheimer HM, Lum Lung MC, Brugman SM, et al: Pulmonary vascular disorders masquerading as interstitial lung disease. *Pediatr Pulmonol* 1995;20:284–88.

Chapter 396

Pulmonary Alveolar Proteinosis *Aaron Hamvas,*

Lawrence M. Nogee, and F. Sessions Cole

Pulmonary alveolar proteinosis (PAP) is a disorder characterized by the intra-alveolar accumulation of pulmonary surfactant. On histopathologic examination, distal air spaces are filled with a granular, eosinophilic material that stains positively with periodic acid–Schiff reagent and is diastase resistant. Two clinically distinct forms of PAP have been described in children: a fulminant, usually fatal form presenting shortly after birth (termed *congenital PAP*) and a gradually progressive type presenting in older infants and children and similar to that observed in adults.

Etiology and Pathophysiology. Although the mechanisms that lead to alveolar proteinosis are undefined, histologic findings suggest that they result in a disruption of pulmonary surfactant metabolism. The early onset of the neonatal form of PAP along with a positive family history of similarly affected newborn infants strongly suggests a genetic basis. For example, an inherited deficiency in surfactant protein-B (SP-B) has been described with some cases of neonatal alveolar proteinosis (see Chapter 397). In addition, several genetically engineered mice with abnormal expression of granulocyte-macrophage colony-stimulating factor (GM-CSF), interleukin-4 (IL-4), and surfactant protein-D (SP-D) exhibit expanded surfactant pools and alveolar proteinosis owing to increased secretion and/or decreased clearance of otherwise normal pulmonary surfactant from the air space.

Molecular mechanisms in addition to SP-B deficiency have also been described in humans. A deficiency in expression of the β-subunit of the GM-CSF receptor occurred in four infants with alveolar proteinosis. However, human examples that mimic genetically altered mice have not been identified. Alveolar proteinosis has also been reported in children with lysinuric protein intolerance, a rare autosomal recessive disorder caused by mutations in the cationic amino acid transport peptide SLC7A7.

These children develop vomiting, hyperammonemia, and failure to thrive. The relationship between the transport defect and the PAP is unclear.

Alveolar proteinosis also may occur in association with infection, particularly in immunocompromised individuals. However, because the same pathologic process occurs in severely immunodeficient mice raised in a pathogen-free environment, it is not clear whether this is the result of a secondary infection or the underlying immunodeficiency. Possible autoimmune mechanisms of later-onset alveolar proteinosis have been described in adults with idiopathic primary alveolar proteinosis in whom IgG1 and IgG2 autoantibody directed against GM-CSF can be detected in serum and bronchoalveolar lavage (BAL) fluid. Whether these antibodies are causative or a secondary response in this disorder is unknown. These antibodies have not been identified in infants with alveolar proteinosis.

Clinical Manifestations. The congenital form of the disorder is immediately apparent in the newborn period and rapidly leads to respiratory failure. There is no gender difference in frequency. Congenital PAP is clinically and radiographically indistinguishable from more common disorders of the newborn that lead to respiratory failure, including pneumonia, generalized bacterial infection, respiratory distress syndrome, and total anomalous pulmonary venous return with obstruction. The differential diagnosis also includes primary persistent pulmonary hypertension, meconium aspiration, and alveolar capillary dysplasia, although the radiologic findings of these disorders usually differ. The incidence of congenital PAP is unknown but thought to be low; it was listed on death certificates of 37 infants who died in the first year of life in a cohort of 1,052,554 births in Missouri between 1979 and 1992.

Alveolar proteinosis in older infants and children is also rare. Males are affected three times as often as females. There may be no identifiable etiologic factor (a primary form), or it may occur in association with malignancy or several inciting agents, including dust, chemicals, and infection, particularly in the setting of systemic immunosuppression (a secondary form). Older infants and children with PAP present with dyspnea, fatigue, cough, weight loss, chest pain, or hemoptysis. In the later stages, cyanosis and digital clubbing may be seen. Pulmonary function testing reveals a restrictive pattern, and arterial blood gases show marked hypoxemia with a chronic respiratory acidosis.

Diagnosis. Histopathologic examination of lung biopsy specimens is the gold standard for diagnosis in children. The examination of sputum or BAL fluid for surfactant components has been used diagnostically in adults, but these methods have not been validated in children. In patients with alveolar proteinosis caused by mechanisms other than SP-B deficiency, immunohistochemical staining reveals abundant quantities of alveolar and intracellular surfactant proteins A and B. Examination of peripheral blood and/or bone marrow for clonogenic stimulation of monocyte-macrophage precursors, GM-CSF receptor and ligand expression, GM-CSF binding, and anti-GM-CSF autoantibodies are available through research protocols.

Treatment. Untreated alveolar proteinosis in newborns is rapidly fatal, and no successful medical therapy has been developed. Lung transplantation is the only therapeutic option, but its use is limited by concerns about disease recurrence in the absence of a defined primary mechanism of lung injury.

Repeated bronchoalveolar lavage is a temporizing measure and in some cases is therapeutic for patients with the later-onset form of PAP. In addition, recent trials have suggested that subcutaneous administration of recombinant GM-CSF may improve pulmonary function in some adults with later-onset primary alveolar proteinosis. Although experience is limited, both these interventions have been unsuccessful for the long-term management of newborn infants.

Borsani G, Bassi MT, Sperandeo MP, et al: SLC7A7, encoding a putative permease-related protein, is mutated in patients with lysinuric protein intolerance. *Nat Genet* 1999;21:297–301.

Dirksen U, Nishinakamura R, Groneck P, et al: Human pulmonary alveolar proteinosis associated with a defect in GM-CSF/IL-3/IL-5 receptor common beta chain expression. *J Clin Invest* 1997;100:2211–17.

Mahut B, Delacourt C, Scheinmann P, et al: Pulmonary alveolar proteinosis: Experience with eight pediatric cases and a review. *Pediatrics* 1996;97:117–22.

Ikegami M, Whitsett JA, Chroneos ZC, et al: IL-4 increases surfactant and regulates metabolism in vivo. *Am J Physiol* 2000;278:175–80.

Kitamura T, Uchida K, Tanaka N, et al: Serological diagnosis of idiopathic pulmonary alveolar proteinosis. *Am J Respir Crit Care Med* 2000;162:658–62.

Seymour JF, Presneill JJ, Schoch OD, et al: Therapeutic efficacy of granulocyte-macrophage colony-stimulating factor in patients with idiopathic acquired alveolar proteinosis. *Am J Respir Crit Care Med* 2001;163:524–31.

Chapter 397

Inherited Disorders of Surfactant Protein Metabolism *Aaron Hamvas,*

Lawrence M. Nogee, and F. Sessions Cole

The pulmonary surfactant is a mixture of phospholipids and proteins synthesized, packaged, and secreted by type II pneumocytes that line the distal airways. This mixture forms a monolayer at the air-liquid interface that lowers surface tension at end-expiration of the respiratory cycle and thereby prevents atelectasis and ventilation-perfusion mismatch. Four surfactant-associated proteins have been described: surfactant proteins A and D (SP-A, SP-D) participate in host defense in the lung, whereas surfactant proteins B and C (SP-B, SP-C) contribute to the surface tension–lowering activity of the pulmonary surfactant. Two genes for SP-A and one gene for SP-D are located on human chromosome 10, whereas single genes located on human chromosomes 2 and 8, respectively, encode SP-B and SP-C. Although inherited deficiencies of SP-A or SP-D have not been identified in humans, genetically engineered mice deficient in these proteins are susceptible to viral and bacterial infections and lineages deficient in SP-D accumulate lipids and foamy macrophages in their lungs and develop emphysema and pulmonary fibrosis as they age. Inherited disorders of SP-B and SP-C have been identified in humans and are discussed in detail.

DEFICIENCY OF SURFACTANT PROTEIN B

Genetics. Over 20 loss-of-function mutations in the SP-B gene have been identified. The most common is a net 2 base-pair insertion in codon 121 (termed 121ins2) that generates a frameshift and interruption of SP-B protein translation. The insertion generates a restriction fragment polymorphism (RFLP) that is useful for diagnosis. This mutation accounts for 60–70% of the alleles found to date in patients identified with SP-B deficiency. Most other mutations have been family specific.

Pathology. Although SP-B deficiency was first described in a patient with newborn-onset alveolar proteinosis, the histology is neither specific for SP-B deficiency nor universally present in lungs of affected infants. Several SP-B–deficient patients homozygous for the 121ins2 mutation have had histologic features more typical of desquamative interstitial pneumonitis with little detectable alveolar proteinosis at the time of lung transplantation. Other findings are nonspecific and include variable degrees of interstitial fibrosis and alveolar cell hyperplasia. Ultrastructural findings include a lack of tubular myelin, disorganized lamellar bodies, and an accumulation of abnormal-

appearing multivesicular bodies, suggesting abnormal lipid packaging and secretion.

Clinical Manifestations. Infants with an inherited deficiency of SP-B present in the immediate neonatal period with respiratory failure. This autosomal recessive disorder is clinically and radiographically similar to the respiratory distress syndrome of premature infants (see Chapter 90.3) but typically affects full-term infants and is refractory to mechanical ventilation, surfactant replacement therapy, glucocorticoid administration, and extracorporeal membrane oxygenation. SP-B deficiency has been recognized in diverse racial and ethnic groups. Almost all patients have died without lung transplantation, but prolonged survival is possible in cases with a partial deficiency of SP-B. Patients heterozygous for loss-of-function mutations in the SP-B gene are clinically normal as adults and have normal pulmonary function.

Diagnosis. A rapid, definitive diagnosis can be established with analyses of DNA for known mutations in the SP-B gene, particularly the 121ins2 mutation (using RFLP analysis of polymerase chain reaction–amplified genomic DNA). The sensitivity of genetic diagnosis is limited, however, because assays are not readily available for all known mutations and disease may result from yet unidentified mutations. In families in which a mutation has been previously identified, antenatal diagnosis can be established by molecular assays of DNA from chorionic villus biopsy or amniocytes, which permits advanced planning of a therapeutic regimen. Other laboratory tests remain investigational and include analysis of tracheal effluent by enzyme-linked immunosorbent assay or Western blotting for the presence or absence of SP-B protein and for aberrantly processed precursor proSP-C peptides that have been found in SP-B–deficient human infants and animals. Definitive diagnosis can also be established by immunostaining of lung biopsy tissue for the surfactant proteins. The absence of SP-B protein and abundant expression of the aberrantly processed proSP-C peptide definitively establish a diagnosis of SP-B deficiency. Such studies require a lung biopsy in a critically ill child or may be performed on lung blocks acquired at the time of autopsy. Immunohistochemical assays for SP-B and SP-C are available on a research basis.

Treatment. Because virtually all patients with SP-B deficiency die within the first year of life, prompt recognition is critical. Conventional neonatal intensive care interventions can maintain extrapulmonary organ function for a limited time (weeks to months). Replacement therapy with commercially available surfactants is ineffective. Lung transplantation has been successful, but the pre-transplant, transplant, and post-transplant medical and surgical care is highly specialized and only available at pediatric pulmonary transplant centers. The oldest living SP-B–deficient survivors after lung transplantation were born in 1994. The relative scarcity of available infants' lungs for transplantation suggests that gene therapy may be the treatment of choice in the future. Genetic counseling is also important to convey the risks for future pregnancies and the availability of antenatal diagnosis and therapeutic options. Palliative care consultation is also helpful.

SURFACTANT PROTEIN C GENE ABNORMALITIES

Surfactant protein C (SP-C) is a very low molecular weight, extremely hydrophobic protein that, along with SP-B, enhances the surface tension–lowering properties of surfactant phospholipids. It is derived from proteolytic processing of a larger precursor protein (proSP-C). A mutation in the surfactant protein C gene has been identified in a family in which affected individuals did not have respiratory symptoms at birth but developed interstitial lung disease in infancy. The mutation was present on only one allele, consistent with an autosomal dominant inheritance pattern, and resulted in the production of an abnormal proSP-C protein, decreased amounts of normal proSP-C, and nearly absent mature SP-C. Thus it is unclear if the lung disease resulted from the lack of mature SP-C or from the presence of the abnormal proSP-C protein (which suggests a possible toxic effect from this abnormal peptide).

A preliminary report suggests that SP-C mutations may be associated with other forms of both familial and sporadic chronic lung diseases. However, the epidemiology and the extent of phenotypic and pathologic variability associated with such mutations are unknown. The association of the production of an abnormal protein within the secretory pathway of the alveolar type II cell with lung disease suggests a potential novel mechanism for the initiation of lung injury.

Cole FS, Hamvas A, Nogee LM: Genetic disorders of neonatal respiratory function. *Pediatr Res* 2001;50:157–62.

Dunbar AE, Wert SE, Hamvas A, et al: Prolonged survival in hereditary surfactant protein B (SP-B) deficiency associated with a novel splicing mutation. *Pediatr Res* 2000;48:275–82.

Hamvas A: Surfactant protein B deficiency: Insights into inherited disorders of lung cell metabolism. *Curr Prob Pediatr* 1997;27:325–45.

Nogee LM, deMello DE, Dehner LP, et al: Pulmonary surfactant protein B deficiency in congenital pulmonary alveolar proteinosis. *N Engl J Med* 1993;328:406–10.

Nogee LM, Dunbar AE III, Wert SE, et al: A mutation in the surfactant protein C gene associated with familial interstitial lung disease. *N Engl J Med* 2001;344:573–79.

Nogee LM, Garnier G, Singer L, et al: A mutation in the surfactant protein B gene responsible for fatal neonatal respiratory disease in multiple kindreds. *J Clin Invest* 1994;93:1860–63.

Nogee LM, Wert SE, Proffit SA, et al: Allelic heterogeneity in hereditary surfactant protein B (SP-B) deficiency. *Am J Respir Crit Care Med* 2000;161:973–81.

Chapter 398

Pulmonary Hemosiderosis

Dorr G. Dearborn

Bleeding in the lower respiratory tract in children is unusual but can be life threatening. During infancy and prepubertal childhood, infections, trauma, and foreign bodies are the most common causes of pulmonary hemorrhage. More extensive hemorrhage in this age range can arise from any of the remaining causes listed in Box 398–1, although the rare immune-related vascular diseases are usually limited to older children and adolescents. After a hemorrhage, macrophages convert the iron of hemoglobin into hemosiderin, hence the term *hemosiderosis*. Because it takes the macrophage 36–48 hr to form hemosiderin and large numbers of hemosiderin-laden macrophages are probably only resident in the alveoli for about 5 wk, alveolar hemosiderosis is an indicator of previous bleeding and its persistence an indication of continued bleeding. The term *pulmonary hemosiderosis* should be reserved for persistent or recurrent bleeding.

Pathophysiology and Clinical Manifestations. Pulmonary hemorrhage can be either focal or diffuse. Focal hemorrhage is usually an acute process in the conducting airways whereas diffuse hemorrhage results from abnormalities of alveolar capillaries with a continuing, sometimes exacerbating course. Notably, alveolar hemorrhage can occur without sufficient blood reaching the central airways to produce hemoptysis (see Chapter 399.2) and may not produce visible infiltrates on chest radiographs. Acute pulmonary hemorrhage that does produce alveolar infiltrates can show rapid clearing in 1–2 days, distinguishing them from infectious infiltrates. An acute hemorrhage is usually accompanied by a drop in hematocrit, an increase in

BOX 398–1. Causes of Pulmonary Hemorrhage

Infection (extensive)
   Bacterial, fungal, parasitic[*]
   Chronic with bronchiectasis[*]
Trauma
   Crush injury, suffocation, foreign body
Cardiovascular
   Increased pulmonary venous pressure
   Arteriovenous malformations
   Pulmonary emboli, infarcts
Vasculitis
   Autoimmune disorders[*]
   Immune complex disorders[*]
   Anti–glomerular basement membrane antibodies[*]
Toxic (penicillamine, cocaine)
Neoplasia (carcinoid)
Associated with antibodies to cow's milk proteins
Idiopathic

[*] Limited to school-aged children and older.

reticulocyte count, and a stool positive for occult blood. The accompanying respiratory distress, including cough, wheeze, and tachypnea, may be mild and transient or may be sufficiently severe to constitute respiratory failure, depending on the quantity of blood in the alveoli and airways. A more insidious onset may occur with only fatigue, mild dyspnea, and anemia. Diagnosis is most readily confirmed with the use of Prussian blue staining for hemosiderin within alveolar macrophages, obtained most simply by bronchoalveolar lavage (BAL) or by examination of sputum or gastric aspirates. Even overt pulmonary hemorrhage requiring ventilator support should be followed by alveolar macrophage cytology several (>5) wk after the acute hemorrhage to evaluate continued elevated hemosiderosis (>20% positive cells) denoting a chronic process. Significant alveolar hemorrhage can be ongoing and clinically undetectable except by iron stain cytology of BAL samples.

Secondary Pulmonary Hemosiderosis. Heart disease that causes a chronic increase in pulmonary venous pressure, such as mitral stenosis, can lead to intrapulmonary hemorrhage and secondary hemosiderosis. Pulmonary arteriovenous malformations can be a component of hereditary hemorrhagic telangiectasia (Osler-Weber-Rendu syndrome) but are seldom accompanied by hemoptysis and hemosiderosis in infancy and childhood. Although pulmonary embolism is not often considered in infants and children, it is a well-known complication of central venous catheters (see Chapter 399). Rarely, pulmonary hemorrhage is seen with hemolytic-uremic syndrome, anaphylactoid purpura, or thrombocytopenic purpura. It can also result from graft versus host disease and is especially a concern at the end of the early neutropenic phase after bone marrow transplant, when endogenous bacterial endotoxin from the intestine can be an inflammatory stimulant in the lung.

Vascular Diseases. The entire spectrum of the pulmonary vasculature including capillaries can be involved in vascular inflammatory disorders and, in some cases, the inflammatory lesions of the capillaries may be the only pulmonary vascular manifestation of a systemic disorder. Capillary inflammation (capillaritis) may arise from immune processes, including disorders where immune complex deposition or formation can be demonstrated (e.g., systemic lupus erythematosus and Goodpasture syndrome). The role of an immune mechanism is less clear in the necrotizing vasculitis of Wegener granulomatosis. Nephritis or other systemic manifestations are usually evident, but the initial presentation of Goodpasture syndrome (pulmonary hemosiderosis with glomerulonephritis) can be similar to idiopathic pulmonary hemosiderosis with only hemoptysis and iron-deficiency anemia. Adolescents who present with hemoptysis should be evaluated for vascular diseases, including testing for circulating anti–glomerular basement membrane antibodies and antibodies to cytoplasmic components to neutrophils (ANCA). Histopathologic confirmation by biopsy of kidney, lung, or other tissue may be necessary for definitive diagnosis.

The severity of pulmonary involvement is highly variable but can be devastating. Corticosteroid immunosuppression may need to be intensified with azathioprine or cyclophosphamide. Plasmapheresis has been used successfully during acute massive pulmonary hemorrhage in Goodpasture syndrome and microscopic angiitis.

Primary Pulmonary Hemosiderosis with Hypersensitivity to Cow's Milk (Heiner Syndrome). These patients have the typical picture of idiopathic hemosiderosis often accompanied by chronic rhinitis, recurrent otitis media, gastrointestinal symptoms, and growth retardation. The symptoms improve when cow's milk is removed from the diet and return with its re-introduction. Some patients fail to improve at all on a milk-free diet, and others without multiple milk precipitins have improved. Hypertrophied nasopharyngeal lymphoid tissue can be sufficiently obstructive to lead to secondary cor pulmonale. In general, patients with hemosiderosis and precipitins to cow's milk have a better prognosis than do those with other forms of hemosiderosis, and they may eventually lose their sensitivity to milk. Corticosteroids may be useful, at least during acute bleeding episodes.

Although the pathophysiology is not understood, some infants and children with pulmonary hemosiderosis have circulating IgG antibodies toward cow's milk proteins. Heiner originally detected these "milk precipitins" by immunodiffusion. Antibody levels against cow's milk proteins in excess of 200 g/mL may be observed.

Idiopathic Pulmonary Hemosiderosis (IPH). This rare disorder of unknown etiology has a reported yearly incidence of between 0.24 (Sweden) and 1.23 (Japan) cases per million children. Onset usually occurs in early in childhood, rarely later than early adult life. Most of the clinical manifestations are related to blood in the alveoli and to the effects of chronic blood loss.

CLINICAL MANIFESTATIONS. Symptoms are those of recurrent or chronic pulmonary disease and include cough, hemoptysis, dyspnea, wheezing, and occasional cyanosis associated with fatigue and pallor. The cough may be productive of bloody sputum, or the infant or child may simply vomit large quantities of swallowed blood. During acute attacks, which usually last 2–4 days, the child may be febrile. Digital clubbing can be present. The usual clinical features of fever, tachycardia, tachypnea, leukocytosis (including eosinophilia), respiratory distress, and abnormal radiographic findings may suggest bacterial pneumonia, but accompanying anemia and rapid clearing of the chest radiographs should suggest the correct diagnosis. In some children, the early manifestations of illness are related to chronic iron-deficiency anemia and the characteristic pulmonary symptoms do not appear until much later. Although the child may have severe pulmonary manifestations without radiographic abnormalities, seldom is the radiographic picture abnormal before pulmonary symptoms have occurred.

LABORATORY FINDINGS. The anemia is typically microcytic and hypochromic; serum iron concentration is low, and there may be elevations in bilirubin, urobilinogen, and reticulocyte count. The stool usually contains occult blood, presumably swallowed. Hemosiderin is found in alveolar macrophages obtained by BAL or biopsy and in smears of sputum or gastric aspirates. Radiographic changes range from minimal infiltrates resembling pneumonia to massive pulmonary involvement with secondary atelectasis. Hilar lymphadenopathy can occur with long-standing disease.

DIAGNOSIS. This is by the exclusion of known causes for pulmonary hemorrhage and the persistence of elevated or recurrent hemosiderosis beyond the acute 5–8 wk period after a documented pulmonary hemorrhage. Significant continued hemosiderosis is indicated by iron stain cytology on BAL samples showing more than 20% of the macrophages containing hemosiderin or an iron index greater than 50 (scoring 100 macrophages for amount of hemosiderin 0 to 3+ with a maximal score of 300). Culturing of BAL samples for bacteria, viruses, and fungi helps exclude various infectious processes producing hemosiderosis. Although not required for diagnosis, open lung biopsy demonstrates intra-alveolar hemorrhage, large numbers of hemosiderin-laden macrophages, alveolar epithelial hyperplasia, and eventually interstitial fibrosis and small artery hypertensive changes. Absence of immunoglobulin or complement deposition on the alveolar basement membrane virtually excludes immune complex–based vascular disease, and all biopsy specimens should be subjected to this test.

TREATMENT. A milk-free diet may be helpful in severe cases even if antibodies toward cow's milk proteins are at low titers. Corticosteroids (prednisone, 2–30 mg/kg/24 hr) produce remission in some patients and are of no benefit to others. Maintenance corticosteroid therapy has been used between attacks with variable results, and prolonged survival has been attributed to this therapy in uncontrolled series. More extensive immune suppression with the addition of azathioprine or cyclophosphamide may be helpful. Approximately one half of the patients die within 1–5 yr, usually from acute pulmonary hemorrhage and progressive respiratory failure.

Idiopathic Pulmonary Hemorrhage and Hemosiderosis in Infants. Acute, idiopathic pulmonary hemorrhage in young infants has been reported in clusters in Cleveland, Chicago, Milwaukee, and Detroit, and sporadic cases have occurred elsewhere in the United States. A case-control study found an association with chronic water damage in the children's homes along with growth of fungi, including *Stachybotrys chartarum*. Although the strength of this association has been questioned, exposure to toxigenic fungi has continued to be found in 90% of the cases. Aerosolized spores from this fungus are sufficiently small to be inhaled out to the distal airways and contain several classes of toxins including trichothecenes, very potent protein synthesis inhibitors, and proteinases with wide substrate specificity. Local release of these toxins and proteinases especially during rapid endothelial basement membrane formation in young infants could lead to fragile capillaries, which would be at risk for stress hemorrhage. Environmental tobacco smoke might also be a contributing factor. In Cleveland, the incidence reached 1.5 cases per thousand live births and mortality was over 30%.

Most of the infants present with acute respiratory distress and overt pulmonary hemorrhage, many requiring ventilator support and blood transfusions. Some infants presenting without frank hemoptysis but with unexplained respiratory failure were found to have pulmonary hemorrhage on tracheal intubation. The subtle presentation and prodromal symptoms of some infants suggests an acute life-threatening event (ALTE). In nasal breathing young infants, hemoptysis may present as an atraumatic epistaxis. Many of the infants have had persistent hemosiderosis continuing for 3–12 mo during which time the infants appear to be at risk for a massive stress-related hemorrhage. Other manifestations observed in some infants include neurologic problems (e.g., seizures and developmental delay), concomitant infection, and hemolysis with hemoglobinuria. Fever and leukocytosis are not usually present.

Treatment for these infants beyond the initial supportive measures has included removing them from their original fungal and smoke environment. In the Cleveland infants, this has led to a 15-fold decrease in the rebleeding frequency. In addition, high-dose corticosteroids (methylprednisolone, 1 mg/kg, intravenously q6h) have been used at the time of the acute hemorrhage followed by oral prednisone (1–2 mg/kg/24 hr) for a few weeks. Daily or every-other-day prednisone (0.5–1 mg/kg) is maintained until the iron-stained BAL cytology has returned close (iron index < 50/300) to normal (<25/300). Although the use of corticosteroids is empirical, they may be suppressing inflammation, a major component in animal studies of pulmonary stachybotryomycotoxicosis. Anecdotally, several of the deaths of infants in Cleveland occurred in infants who either did not receive corticosteroids or in whom they were discontinued early. Reticulocyte counts and frequent stool guaiac testing help guide the corticosteroid therapy and scheduling of repeat bronchoscopies.

Boat TF: Pulmonary hemorrhage and hemoptysis. In Chernick V, Boat TF (editors): *Kendig's Disorders of the Respiratory Tract in Children*, 6th ed. Philadelphia, WB Saunders, 1998, pp 623–33.

Dearborn DG, Smith PG, Dahms BB, et al: Clinical profile of thirty infants with acute pulmonary hemorrhage in Cleveland. *Pediatrics* 2002;110:627–37.

Epstein CE, Elidemir O, Colasurdo GN, et al: Time course of hemosiderin production by alveolar macrophages in a murine model. *Chest* 2001;120:2013–20.

Etzel RA, Montana E, Sorenson WG, et al: Acute pulmonary hemorrhage in infants associated with exposure to *Stachybotrys atra* and other fungi. *Arch Pediatr Adolesc Med* 1998;152:757–62.

Green RJ, Ruoss SJ, Kraft SA, et al: Pulmonary capillaritis and alveolar hemorrhage. *Chest* 1996;110:1305–16.

Heggen J, Fortenberry J, Yeager AM: Diffuse alveolar hemorrhage in pediatric hematopoietic cell transplant patients. *Pediatrics* 2002;109:965–71.

Saeed MM, Woo MS, MacLaughlin EF, et al: Prognosis in pediatric idiopathic pulmonary hemosiderosis. *Chest* 1999;116:721–25.

West JB, Mathieu-Costello O: Vulnerability of pulmonary capillaries in heart disease. *Circulation* 1995;92:622–31.

Chapter 399
Pulmonary Hemorrhage, Embolism, and Infarction

Daniel Sloniewsky and Thomas P. Green

399.1 Pulmonary Embolism and Infarction

Epidemiology. Pulmonary embolism (PE) rarely occurs in children and infants. A prospective epidemiologic study in Canada revealed an incidence of deep venous thrombosis (DVT)/PE of 5.3/10,000 in hospitalized children and 0.07/10,000 in the general pediatric population. Another retrospective autopsy study found an incidence of pediatric PE of 3.7%. Males and females are equally affected, and the highest incidences occur in children younger than 1 yr old and those 11–18 yr old. Most of the patients with PE have serious underlying disorders or precipitating factors. These include the presence of a central venous catheter, immobility, heart disease, the use of oral contraceptives, ventriculoatrial shunts, trauma, infection, dehydration, collagen vascular disease, shock, and obesity.

Children with neoplasms, particularly hematologic malignancies such as acute myeloid leukemia, also are predisposed to PE. The incidence of PE in leukemic patients who receive chemotherapy is 2.9%. The reasons for this predisposition in patients with malignancies are numerous and include the presence of central venous catheters, coagulopathy associated with the disease, and endothelial damage secondary to chemotherapy.

Hematologic disorders are also common in children with PE. Patients with sickle cell anemia may present with intrapulmonary embolism and subsequent infarction, although this is difficult to differentiate from pneumonia. Coagulation abnormalities are common in children with PE (up to 70% in one study) with the presence of antiphospholipid antibodies (particularly lupus anticoagulant) and acquired or inherited deficien-

cies in proteins C and S being the most common. Other coagulation disorders such as antithrombin III deficiency, dysfibrinogenemia, and the factor V Leiden mutation can also be seen.

Surgery is an important risk factor for emboli, and studies in adults have shown a predisposition to embolic phenomena up to a month after surgery. In children, scoliosis surgery, in particular, may predispose patients to PE.

Clinical Manifestations and Diagnosis. When suspecting a pulmonary embolism in a pediatric patient, a thorough medical and family history should be taken. Patients with a family history of coagulation defects or who have had family members die of thrombotic events when younger than 50 yr of age are at high risk. The clinical presentations of PE are varied, and no group of physical findings yields a high positive predictive value. Pleuritic chest pain, dyspnea, apprehension, and cough are the most common complaints, and tachypnea is the most common physical finding. Other potential findings include rales, increased intensity of the pulmonary component of the second heart sound, tachycardia, fever, diaphoresis, phlebitis, wheezing, and hemoptysis. Patients with severe PE can even present with hemodynamic instability, cor pulmonale, and shock.

Laboratory Findings. These may be as nonspecific as the clinical findings. Arterial blood gas tensions may reveal respiratory alkalosis or arterial hypoxemia or even be normal. An alveolar-arterial gradient, when coupled to a low $Paco_2$, is present in 98% of adult patients with PE. Other laboratory tests that may aid in the diagnosis include D-dimers (which has a specificity of 56%), a complete blood cell count (which may show an elevated white blood cell count), and a coagulation profile. If acquired or familial coagulation disorders are suspected, tests such as fibrinogen, protein C activity, free protein S antigen, antithrombin III activity, DNA analysis for the factor V Leiden mutation, tests for a lupus anticoagulant, and anticardiolipin antibody assays should be considered.

Chest radiographs are often normal in patients with PE and are more useful for excluding other conditions that may mimic PE and in helping interpret ventilation-perfusion scans. Echocardiography and electrocardiography are useful in gathering supporting data for a PE and helping rule out other diseases but have little diagnostic value. An electrocardiogram can show nonspecific ST segment changes and signs of cor pulmonale when present. Echocardiograms are useful to look at cardiac function and ventricular size.

Ventilation-perfusion imaging displays regional blood flow and ventilation defects by noninvasive means and is safe and inexpensive. However, a normal ventilation-perfusion scan does not absolutely exclude a PE and reports are interpreted as high probability, intermediate probability, low probability, very low probability, and normal. Also, the presence of any other conditions that can cause ventilation-perfusion mismatching in the lung (e.g., pneumonia, obstructive lung disease) can limit the utility of this study. In the absence of any concurrent lung disease, and with high clinical suspicion of a PE, the positive predictive value of a high probability scan is 90%.

Helical spiral CT scanning is particularly useful in patients with lung disease. However, this is dependent on the experience of the radiologist and is less useful in patients with emboli to subsegmental pulmonary vessels. Pulmonary angiography is the gold standard diagnostic test for pulmonary embolism and, although invasive and expensive, is relatively safe in patients without pulmonary hypertension or cor pulmonale.

The possibility of deep venous thrombosis should be evaluated in all patients with PE. The femoral and iliac veins and the inferior vena cava are the most common sites of DVT, although emboli can originate from any vessel. Electrical impedance plethysmography and Doppler ultrasonography are useful noninvasive tests for DVT. Venography is the gold standard in the evaluation of thrombosis and should be used in patients with high clinical suspicion of DVT but negative ultrasound or plethysmography.

Pathophysiology. The mechanisms behind many of the signs and symptoms of PE arise from ventilation and perfusion mismatches. As perfusion to affected alveolar units decreases secondary to the emboli, there is an increase in alveolar dead space and the ability to eliminate CO_2 is impaired (although hypocarbia may exist secondary to tachypnea). These ventilation-perfusion mismatches can cause hypoxemia and an increased alveolar-arterial oxygen tension gradient. These abnormalities of gas exchange as well as stimulation of lung proprioceptors are responsible for the symptoms of PE.

Increases in pulmonary vascular resistance may also occur with PE, and, as the pressure increases, right ventricular function may become impaired, leading to cor pulmonale. However, it is believed that increases in pulmonary artery pressure are not likely to be evident until the vascular bed is 60% occluded; clinically significant pulmonary hypertension and shock occur with 70–80% occlusion.

Increases in airway resistance may occur when neurohumoral mediators such as serotonin and histamine are released after platelets interact with the clots. The subsequent bronchoconstriction of the small peripheral airways can be reversed with the use of heparin.

Because of the rich vascular supply of the lung and potential for retrograde flow of oxygenated blood from pulmonary veins, pulmonary infarction is an uncommon sequelae of PE. However, it can occur when a pulmonary artery is obstructed and blood subsequently extravasates into an alveolus, whose ability to clear the blood is impaired. Consequently, patients with advanced heart disease and left ventricular failure have a higher incidence of infarction associated with PE.

Treatment. In treating patients with PE, the basic tenets of resuscitation must be applied first (see Chapter 51.1). Patients with acute respiratory failure may need endotracheal intubation and mechanical ventilation to improve gas exchange. Hemodynamic instability may require the use of fluid and inotropes, but excessive fluid may cause decompensation of an already impaired right ventricle. Some agents such as dopamine also may exacerbate pulmonary hypertension.

There are three potential approaches to therapy in patients with PE, once they have been stabilized: anticoagulation, thrombolysis, and surgical thrombectomy.

Unfractionated heparin (UFH) should be used in the initial phase of anticoagulation. Heparin, derived from bovine or porcine tissue, acts by accelerating the inhibitory action of antithrombin III on factor Xa and by inactivating thrombin. Continuous intravenous heparin should be administered at 10–25 U/kg/hr after a loading dose of 50–75 U/kg is given. The goal of anticoagulation is an activated partial thromboplastin time of one and one-half to two times the control. Low molecular weight heparin (LMWH) is an alternative to UFH that is equally effective, has a longer half-life and, so, requires only once- or twice-a-day injections, and has better understood pharmacokinetics. It is only excreted by the kidney (UFH binds to numerous plasma proteins). Warfarin (Coumadin), which suppresses vitamin K–dependent clotting factors, should be started 24–48 hr after heparin therapy is begun, because it requires 5 days to reach its full effect. Coagulation profiles need to be followed when using UFH or warfarin, whereas factor Xa levels may be followed with LMWH (although commonly no laboratory tests are followed with LMWH).

Thrombolytic agents such as urokinase, streptokinase, and recombinant tissue plasminogen activator may be useful adjuncts to heparin therapy, particularly in patients with PE and hemodynamic instability. Their utility may be hindered by the presence of antibodies to these agents, and they are contraindi-cated in patients with active bleeding, recent (<2 mo) cerebrovascular accident, or trauma.

Surgical embolectomy should be reserved for patients with persistent hemodynamic compromise from a PE, despite appropriate medical therapy. This procedure requires an open thoracotomy and has high mortality. Inferior vena cava (IVC) interruption by catheter-placed filters is indicated in patients with recurrent PE despite medical therapy or in those patients who have a contraindication to anticoagulation. Although these filters are not used commonly in children, they are relatively safe and effective.

Prognosis. In pediatric patients this depends on the degree of obstruction. Ten per cent of adult patients with acute PE die within 1 hr of the event. Of those who survive, 8% will die even with early diagnosis and therapy and 30% will die if diagnosis is delayed.

Andrew M, David M, et al: Venous thromboembolic complications (VTE) in children: First analysis of the Canadian registry of VTE. *Blood* 1994;83:1251–57.

Bonduel M, Hepner M, et al: Prothrombotic abnormalities in children with venous thromboembolism. *J Pediatr Hematol Oncol* 2000;22:66–72.

Cahn MD, Rohrer MJ, et al: Long-term follow-up of Greenfield inferior vena cava filter placement in children. *J Vasc Surg* 2001;34:820–25.

Evans DA, Wilmott RW: Pulmonary embolism in children. *Pediatr Clin North Am* 1994;41:569–84.

Huang JN, Shimamura A: Low-molecular weight heparins. *Hematol Oncol Clin North Am* 1998;12:1251–81.

Manco-Johnson MJ, Nuss R, et al: Combined thrombolytic and anticoagulant therapy for venous thrombosis in children. *J Pediatr* 2000;136:446–53.

Nuss R, Hays T, et al: Antiphospholipid antibodies and coagulation regulatory protein abnormalities in children with pulmonary emboli. *J Pediatr Hematol Oncol* 1997;19:202–207.

Uderzo C, Faccini P, et al: Pulmonary thromboembolism in childhood leukemia: 8 years' experience in a pediatric hematology center. *J Clin Oncol* 1995;13:2805–11.

399.2 Hemoptysis

Hemoptysis is the expectoration of blood or blood-tinged sputum. It is a rare presenting symptom in pediatric patients and the etiology of the bleeding can be difficult to find. Bleeding can occur from disruption of the pulmonary or bronchial vessels, although bronchial arterial bleeding tends to be more brisk secondary to the higher pressure.

Clinical Manifestations. First it must be determined if a child is truly experiencing hemoptysis, because blood from the nose or gastrointestinal tract may appear similar to bleeding from the pulmonary system. The blood in hemoptysis is generally bright red and frothy, has an alkaline pH, may contain sputum, and may be accompanied by a cough. Hematemesis is characterized by dark red blood, an acidic pH, the presence of food particles, and nausea.

The differential diagnoses for hemoptysis are listed in Box 399–1. The most common causes for bleeding are infection, tracheostomy-related problems, the presence of a foreign body, cystic fibrosis, and congenital heart disease. In order to determine the cause of bleeding, a thorough history and physical examination should be performed. For example, a history of chronic lung disease, congenital heart disease, or foreign body aspiration can lead to a faster appropriate diagnostic test. Examination of the oral cavity and nasopharynx must be performed to determine if these are the sources for bleeding.

Laboratory Findings and Diagnosis. The laboratory evaluation should include a complete blood count to determine the amount of bleeding and a coagulation profile, as well as specific tests for the presumed diagnosis. A chest film may be helpful in determining the presence of a pulmonary or cardiac process or the presence of a foreign body. Computed tomography may be used to help further delineate observations in the chest film, but it should not be used as a screening tool.

BOX 399–1. Causes of Hemoptysis in Children

Infection
  Tracheobronchitis
  Pneumonia
    Bacterial
    Tuberculous
    Fungal (e.g., aspergillosis)
    Parasitic (e.g., echinococcosis)
Tracheostomy-related
Bronchiectasis
  Cystic fibrosis
  Ciliary dyskinesia
  Immunodeficiency
Foreign body
Congenital heart disease (mainly with pulmonary vascular
  obstructive diseases)
Pulmonary arteriovenous malformations
Trauma
Alveolar hemorrhage syndromes
  Connective tissue disease/vasculitis (e.g., Goodpasture
    syndrome, Wegener granuloma)
  Primary pulmonary hemosiderosis (e.g., idiopathic, Heiner
    syndrome)
Pulmonary thromboembolism
Tumor
  Bronchial adenoma
  Metastatic

Modified from Pianosi P, Al-Sadoon H: Hemoptysis in children. *Pediatr Rev* 1996;17:344–48.

Bronchoscopy may be used as a diagnostic tool and for management. If a patient has persistent bleeding that is not copious, flexible bronchoscopy may be helpful; however, a rigid bronchoscope is necessary to remove foreign bodies and blood clots and to ventilate a patient if necessary.

Treatment. The management of hemoptysis requires a stable airway, maintenance of gas exchange, and stable hemodynamics. Bleeding more than 8 mL/kg/24 hr is considered life threatening and requires replacement of blood products. Rigid bronchoscopy may be used to apply topical vasoconstrictors such as epinephrine, oxymetazoline, or iced 0.9% saline to curtail bleeding, and balloon catheters may be used to tamponade blood vessels. If this is unsuccessful, selective bronchial artery embolization may be used if the bleeding vessel is identified. Surgical management, including segmentectomy or lobectomy, is considered if embolization fails.

Batra PS, Hollinger LD: Etiology and management of pediatric hemoptysis. *Arch Otolaryngol Head Neck Surg* 2001;127(4):377–82.

Coss-Bu JA, Sachdeva RC, et al: Hemoptysis: A 10-year retrospective study. *Pediatrics* 1997;100(3):E7.

Pianosi P, Al-Sadoon H: Hemoptysis in children. *Pediatr Rev* 1996;17(10): 344–48.

Chapter 400
Atelectasis *Ranna A. Rozenfeld*

Atelectasis, the incomplete expansion or complete collapse of air-bearing tissue, is common in infants and children. Atelectasis results from obstruction of air intake into the alveolar sacs. Segmental, lobar, or whole lung collapse is associated with the absorption of air contained in the alveoli, which are no longer ventilated.

Pathophysiology. In general, the causes of atelectasis may be divided into five groups (Table 400–1). Viral infections, specifically respiratory syncytial virus (RSV) infection in young children, can cause multiple areas of atelectasis. Massive collapse of one or both lungs is most often a postoperative complication but occasionally results from other causes, such as trauma, asthma, pneumonia, tension pneumothorax, aspiration of foreign material, paralysis, or following extubation. Massive atelectasis is usually produced by a combination of factors, including immobilization or decreased use of the diaphragm and the respiratory muscles, obstruction of the bronchial tree, and abolition of the cough reflex.

Clinical Manifestations. Symptoms vary with the cause and extent of the atelectasis. A small area is likely to be asymptomatic. When a large area of previously normal lung becomes atelectatic, especially when it does so suddenly, dyspnea accompanied by rapid shallow respirations, tachycardia, cough and often cyanosis occurs. If the obstruction is removed, the symptoms disappear rapidly. Although atelectasis can cause fever, two recent studies have shown no association between atelectasis and fever. Physical findings include limitation of chest excursion, decreased breath sound intensity, and coarse crackles. Breath sounds are decreased or absent over extensive atelectatic areas.

Massive pulmonary atelectasis usually presents with dyspnea, cyanosis, and tachycardia. An affected child is extremely anxious and, if old enough, complains of chest pain. The chest appears flat on the affected side, where decreased respiratory excursion, dullness to percussion, and feeble or absent breath sounds are also noted. Postoperatively atelectasis usually presents within 24 hr after operation but may not occur for several days.

Acute lobar collapse is a frequent occurrence in patients receiving intensive care. If undetected, it can lead to impaired gas exchange, secondary infection, and subsequent pulmonary fibrosis. Initially hypoxemia may result from ventilation perfusion mismatch. In contrast to adult patients in which the lower lobes and in particular the left lower lobe is most often involved, 90% of cases in children involve the upper lobes and 63%

TABLE 400–1. Anatomic Causes of Atelectasis

Cause	Clinical Examples
External compression on the pulmonary parenchyma	Pleural effusion, pneumothorax, intrathoracic tumors, diaphragmatic hernia
Endobronchial obstruction completely obstructing the ingress of air	Enlarged lymph node, tumor, cardiac enlargement, foreign body, mucoid plug, broncholithiasis
Intraluminal obstruction of a bronchus	Foreign body, granulomatous tissue, tumor, secretions, including mucus plugs, bronchiectasis, pulmonary abscess, asthma, chronic bronchitis, acute laryngotracheobronchitis
Intrabronchiolar obstruction	Bronchiolitis, interstitial pneumonitis, asthma
Respiratory compromise or paralysis	Neuromuscular abnormalities, osseous deformities, overly restrictive casts and surgical dressings, defective movement of the diaphragm, or restriction of respiratory effort

involve the right upper lobe. There is also a high incidence of upper lobe atelectasis and especially right upper lobe collapse in neonatal intensive care units.

Diagnosis. The diagnosis of atelectasis can usually be established by chest radiographic examination. Typical findings include volume loss and displacement of fissures. Atypical presentations include atelectasis presenting as a mass-like opacity and atelectasis in an unusual location. Lobar atelectasis may be associated with pneumothorax.

A study of asthmatic children compared chest radiographs with thorax high-resolution computerized tomography (HRCT) and found a chest radiograph abnormality rate of 44% compared with the thorax HRCT scan abnormality rate of 75%, with 38% demonstrating atelectasis on HRCT. The children with atelectasis had increased incidence of right middle lobe syndrome, acute asthma exacerbations, pneumonia, and upper airway infections.

In foreign body aspiration, atelectasis is one of the most common radiographic findings (25–42%). The site of atelectasis usually indicates the site of the foreign body. Atelectasis is more common when patients have a delay in diagnosis of greater than 2 wk duration.

Bronchoscopic examination reveals a collapsed main bronchus when the obstruction is at the tracheobronchial junction and may also disclose the nature of the obstruction.

Massive pulmonary atelectasis is generally diagnosed by chest radiograph. Typical findings include elevation of the diaphragm, narrowing of the intercostal spaces, and displacement of the mediastinal structures and heart toward the affected side (Fig. 400–1).

Treatment. Treatment depends on the cause of the collapse. If effusion or pneumothorax is responsible, the external compression must first be removed. Often vigorous efforts at cough, deep breathing, and percussion will facilitate expansion. Aspiration with sterile tracheal catheters may facilitate removal of mucus plugs. In many patients, however, early fiberoptic bronchoscopy is indicated for diagnosis and aspiration of obstructing material.

Bronchoscopic examination is immediately indicated if atelectasis is the result of a foreign body or any other bronchial obstruction that may be relieved. For bilateral atelectasis, bronchoscopic aspiration should also be performed immediately. It is also indicated when an isolated area of atelectasis persists for several weeks. If no anatomic basis for atelectasis is found and no material can be obtained by suctioning, the introduction of a small amount of saline followed by suctioning allows recovery of bronchial secretions for culture and, possibly, for cytologic examination. Frequent changes in the child's position, deep breathing, and chest physiotherapy may be beneficial. Oxygen therapy is indicated when there is dyspnea or desaturation. Intermittent positive pressure breathing and incentive spirometry have been recommended when atelectasis is unchanged.

In some conditions, such as asthma, bronchodilator and corticosteroid treatment may accelerate atelectasis clearance. Recombinant human DNase (rhDNase), which is approved only for the treatment of cystic fibrosis, has been proposed for patients without cystic fibrosis but with persistent atelectasis. This product reduces the viscosity of purulent bronchial debris. In patients with acute severe asthma, diffuse airway plugging with thick viscous secretions frequently occurs, with the resulting atelectasis often refractory to conventional therapy. rhDNase has been used in both nebulized form for nonintubated patients with acute asthma as well as intratracheally for atelectasis in intubated asthmatics, with resolution of atelectasis unresponsive to conventional asthma therapies.

Lobar atelectasis in cystic fibrosis is discussed in Chapter 393.

Atelectasis can occur in patients with neuromuscular diseases. These patients tend to have ineffective cough and difficulty expelling respiratory tract secretions, which leads to pneumonia and atelectasis. Several devices are available to assist these patients including intermittent positive pressure breathing, In-Exsufflator, and noninvasive bilevel positive pressure ventilation via nasal mask or full face mask. Patients with neuromuscular disease who have undergone surgery are at substantial risk of postoperative atelectasis and subsequent pneumonia. Migrating atelectasis in the newborn infant is a rare and unique presentation and may be secondary to neuromuscular disease.

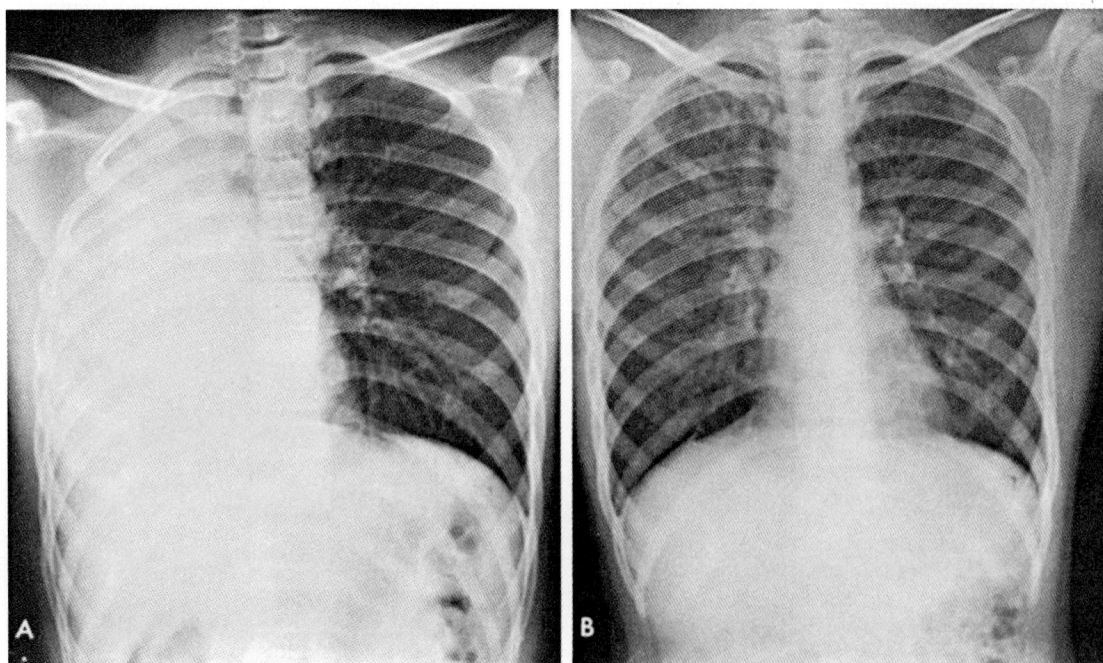

FIGURE 400–1. *A*, Massive atelectasis of the right lung. The patient has asthma. The heart and the other mediastinal structures are shifted to the right during the atelectatic phase. *B*, Comparison study after re-aeration following bronchoscopic removal of a mucus plug from the right main stem bronchus.

There is an association between the development of lobar collapse and the requirement for mechanical ventilation. Although lobar collapse is rarely a cause of long-term morbidity, its occurrence may necessitate the prolongation of mechanical ventilation or reintubation. In patients who are ventilated, positive end expiratory pressure (PEEP) or continuous positive airway pressure (CPAP) is generally indicated.

Ashizawa K, Hayashi K, Aso N, et al: Lobar atelectasis: Diagnostic pitfalls on chest radiography. *Br J Radiol* 2001;74:89–97.

Birnkrant DJ, Pope JF, Eiben RM: Management of the respiratory complications of neuromuscular diseases in the pediatric intensive care unit. *J Child Neurol* 1999;14:139–43.

Burton EM, Brick WG, Hall JD, et al: Tracheobronchial foreign body aspiration in children. *South Med J* 1996;89:195–98.

Cataneo AJM, Reibscheid SM, Ruiz RL, et al: Foreign body in the tracheobronchial tree. *Clin Pediatr* 1997;36:701–6.

Durward A, Forte V, Shemie SD: Resolution of mucus plugging and atelectasis after intratracheal rhDNase therapy in a mechanically ventilated child with refractory status asthmaticus. *Crit Care Med* 2000;28:560–62.

Engoren M: Lack of association between atelectasis and fever. *Chest* 1995;107:81–84.

Leistikow EA, Jones NE, Josephson KD, et al: Migrating atelectasis in Werdnig-Hoffmann disease: Pulmonary manifestations in two cases of spinal muscular atrophy type 1. *Pediatr Pulmonol* 1999;28:149–53.

Nuhoglu Y, Bahceciler N, Yuksel M, et al: Thorax high resolution computerized tomography findings in asthmatic children with unusual clinical manifestations. *Ann Allergy Asthma Immunol* 1999;82:311–14.

Slattery DM, Waltz DA, Denham B, et al: Bronchoscopically administered recombinant human DNase for lobar atelectasis in cystic fibrosis. *Pediatr Pulmonol* 2001;31:383–88.

Thomas K, Habibi P, Britto J, et al: Distribution and pathophysiology of acute lobar collapse in the pediatric intensive care unit. *Crit Care Med* 1999;27:1594–97.

Chapter 401
Pulmonary Tumors

Susanna A. McColley and Paul R. Haut

Primary tumors of the lung are extremely rare in children and adolescents. An accurate estimate of frequency is difficult because the literature is limited primarily to case reports, and there is a high incidence of "inflammatory pseudotumors." Metastatic lesions are the most common forms of pulmonary malignancy in children; primary processes include Wilms' tumor, osteogenic sarcoma, soft tissue sarcoma, and hepatoblastoma (see Part XXI). Bronchial adenoma and carcinoid are the most common primary tumors. Adenocarcinoma and undifferentiated histology are the most common pathologic findings in primary lung cancer; pulmonary blastoma is rarer and frequently occurs in the setting of cystic lung disease.

Pulmonary tumors may present as fever, hemoptysis, wheezing, cough, pleural effusion, chest pain, dyspnea, recurrent or persistent pneumonia, or atelectasis. Patients with symptoms or with radiographic or other laboratory findings suggesting pulmonary malignancy should be evaluated carefully for a tumor at another site before surgical excision is carried out. Isolated primary lesions and isolated metastatic lesions discovered long after the primary tumor has been removed are best treated by excision. The prognosis varies and depends on the type of tumor involved.

PULMONARY HEMANGIOMATOSIS

In this rare and ultimately fatal disease, uncontrolled vascular proliferation causes progressive dyspnea and eventually leads to death from massive hemoptysis or pulmonary hypertension. Its cause is unknown, although infection may have a role. The vascular abnormality involves the smallest (capillary size) vessels in some patients and slightly larger vessels in others. The pathologic angiogenic process may also extend into other intrathoracic tissues (e.g., mediastinum, pericardium, thymus) or the spleen. Patients usually present with hemoptysis or with right-sided heart failure secondary to pulmonary hypertension. Routine chest films are often similar to those seen in interstitial lung disease. The diagnosis is made by pulmonary angiography (which helps to preclude other forms of veno-occlusive disease) and open lung biopsy. The disease can be locally invasive but is not known to metastasize. The primary process appears to be angiogenesis. Most patients die within 1–5 yr from the onset of symptoms.

A substantial and sustained clinical improvement in a 12-yr-old boy treated with recombinant interferon-α-2a has been reported. Although some hemoptysis was still present, the patient tolerated the treatment well and was clinically stable 14 mo later.

Eggli KD, Newman B: Nodules, masses, and pseudomasses in the pediatric lung. *Radiol Clin North Am* 1993;31:651.

Epstein DM, Aronchick JM: Lung cancer in childhood. *Med Pediatr Oncol* 1989;17:510.

Faber CN, Yousem SA, Dauber JH, et al: Pulmonary capillary hemangiomatosis: A report of three cases and a review of the literature. *Am Rev Respir Dis* 1989;140:808.

Hancock BJ, Di Lorenzo M, Youssef S, et al: Childhood primary pulmonary neoplasms. *J Pediatr Surg* 1993;28:1133.

Keita O, Lagrange J-L, Michiels J-F, et al: Primary bronchogenic squamous cell carcinoma in children: Report of a case and review of the literature. *Med Pediatr Oncol* 1995;24:50.

Roviaro Gc, Varoli F, Zannini P, et al: Lung cancer in the young. *Chest* 1985;87:456.

White CW, Sondheimer HM, Crouch EC, et al: Treatment of pulmonary hemangiomatosis with recombinant interferon α-2a. *N Engl J Med* 1989;320:1197.

Chapter 402
Pleurisy *Glenna B. Winnie*

The most common cause of pleural effusion in children is bacterial pneumonia (see Chapter 389); heart failure, rheumatologic causes, and metastatic intrathoracic malignancy are the next most common causes. A variety of other diseases account for the remaining cases, including tuberculosis, lupus erythematosus, aspiration pneumonitis, uremia, pancreatitis, subdiaphragmatic abscess, and rheumatoid arthritis. Males and females are affected equally.

Inflammatory processes in the pleura are usually divided into three types: dry or plastic, serofibrinous or serosanguineous, and purulent pleurisy or empyema.

402.1 Dry or Plastic Pleurisy

Dry or plastic pleurisy may be associated with acute bacterial pulmonary infections or may develop during the course of an acute upper respiratory tract illness. The condition is also associated with tuberculosis and connective tissue diseases such as rheumatic fever.

Pathology. The process is usually limited to the visceral pleura, with small amounts of yellow serous fluid and adhesions between the pleural surfaces. In tuberculosis, the adhesions develop rapidly and the pleura is often thickened. Occasionally, fibrin deposition and adhesions may be severe enough to produce a fibrothorax that markedly inhibits the excursions of the lung.

Clinical Manifestations. Signs and symptoms are often overshadowed by the primary disease. The principal symptom is pain, which is exaggerated by deep breathing, coughing, and straining. Occasionally, pleural pain is described as a dull ache, which is less likely to vary with breathing. The pain is often localized over the chest wall and is referred to the shoulder or the back. Pain with breathing is responsible for grunting and guarding of respirations, and the child often lies on the affected side in an attempt to decrease respiratory excursions. Early in the illness, a leathery, rough, inspiratory and expiratory friction rub may be audible, but this usually disappears rapidly. Occasionally, increased dullness on percussion and decreased breath sounds are heard if the layer of exudate is thick. Pleurisy may also be asymptomatic and detected only on radiographs, showing a diffuse haziness at the pleural surface or a dense, sharply demarcated shadow. The latter finding may be indistinguishable from small amounts of pleural exudate. Chronic pleurisy is occasionally encountered with conditions such as atelectasis, pulmonary abscess, connective tissue diseases, and tuberculosis.

Differential Diagnosis. Plastic pleurisy must be distinguished from other diseases, such as epidemic pleurodynia, trauma to the rib cage (particularly fracture of a rib), lesions of the dorsal root ganglia, tumors of the spinal cord, herpes zoster, gallbladder disease, and trichinosis. Even if evidence of pleural fluid is not found on physical or radiographic examination, a pleural tap in suspected cases often results in the recovery of a small amount of exudate, which, when cultured, usually reveals the underlying bacterial cause in patients with an acute pneumonia. Patients with pleurisy and pneumonia should always be screened for tuberculosis.

Treatment. Therapy should be aimed at the underlying disease. When pneumonia is present, neither immobilization of the chest with adhesive plaster nor therapy with drugs capable of suppressing the cough reflex is indicated. If pneumonia is not present or is under good therapeutic control, strapping of the chest to restrict expansion may afford relief from pain. Analgesia with nonsteroidal anti-inflammatory agents may be helpful.

402.2 Serofibrinous Pleurisy

Serofibrinous pleurisy is most commonly associated with infections of the lung or with inflammatory conditions of the abdomen or mediastinum. Less commonly, it is found with connective tissue diseases such as lupus erythematosus, periarteritis, or rheumatic fever. On occasion, it is seen with primary or metastatic neoplasms of the lung, pleura, or mediastinum; tumors are commonly associated with a hemorrhagic pleurisy.

Clinical Manifestations. Because serofibrinous pleurisy is often preceded by the plastic type, the early signs and symptoms may be those of plastic pleurisy. As fluid accumulates, pleuritic pain may disappear and the patient may become asymptomatic if the effusion remains small, or there may be only signs and symptoms of the underlying disease. Large fluid collections may produce cough, dyspnea, retractions, tachypnea, orthopnea, or cyanosis. Physical findings depend to some degree on the amount of effusion. Dullness to flatness may be found on percussion. There is a decrease or absence of breath sounds, a diminution in tactile fremitus, a shift of the mediastinum away from the affected side, and occasionally fullness of the intercostal spaces. If the fluid is not loculated, these signs may shift with changes in position. In infants, the physical signs are less definite. Instead of decreased or absent breath sounds, bronchial breathing may be heard. If extensive pneumonia is present, crackles and rhonchi may also be audible. Friction rubs are usually detected only during the early or late plastic stage. The process is usually unilateral.

Radiographic examination shows a more or less homogeneous density obliterating the normal markings of the underlying lung. Small effusions may cause obliteration of only the costophrenic or cardiophrenic angles or a widening of the interlobar septa. Examinations should be performed with the patient

in the supine and upright positions to demonstrate a shift of the effusion with a change in position; the decubitus position may also be helpful. Ultrasonographic examinations are useful.

Differential Diagnosis. Thoracentesis should be performed when pleural fluid is present or is suggested, unless the effusion is small and the patient has a classic lobar pneumococcal pneumonia. Examination of fluid is essential to identify acute bacterial infections, and it may disclose tubercle bacilli. Thoracentesis can differentiate serofibrinous pleurisy, empyema, hydrothorax, hemothorax, and chylothorax. In hydrothorax, the fluid has a specific gravity less than 1.015, and evaluation reveals only a few mesothelial cells rather than leukocytes. Chylothorax and hemothorax usually have fluid with a distinctive appearance; differentiating serofibrinous from purulent pleurisy is impossible without microscopic examination of the fluid. The fluid of serofibrinous pleurisy is clear or slightly cloudy and contains relatively few leukocytes and, occasionally, some erythrocytes. Cytologic examination may reveal malignant cells. Protein levels greater than 3 g/dL indicate an exudate and are likely to be associated with an infectious process. Similarly, pleural fluid lactic dehydrogenase values higher than 200 IU/L suggest an exudate. Serofibrinous fluid may rapidly become purulent. A pH less than 7.20 suggests an exudate.

Course. Unless the fluid becomes purulent, it usually disappears relatively rapidly, particularly with appropriate treatment of bacterial pneumonia. It persists somewhat longer with tuberculosis and connective tissue diseases and may recur or remain for a long time with neoplasms. As the effusion is absorbed, adhesions often develop between the two layers of the pleura, but little or no functional impairment usually results. Pleural thickening may develop and is occasionally mistaken for small quantities of fluid or for persistent pulmonary infiltrates. Pleural thickening may persist for months, but the process usually disappears, leaving no residua.

Treatment. Therapy should address the underlying disease, although with large effusions, draining the fluid makes the patient more comfortable. When a diagnostic thoracentesis is performed, as much fluid as possible, up to about 1 L, should be removed for therapeutic purposes. Rapid removal of 1 L or more of pleural fluid occasionally has been associated with the ensuing development of re-expansion pulmonary edema. If the underlying disease is adequately treated, further drainage is usually unnecessary, but if sufficient fluid reaccumulates to cause respiratory embarrassment, repeated thoracentesis or chest tube drainage should be performed. In older children with parapneumonic effusion, tube thoracostomy is considered necessary if the pleural fluid pH is less than 7.20 or the pleural fluid glucose level is less than 50 mg/dL. If the fluid is clearly purulent, tube drainage is usually indicated. Systemic acidosis reduces the usefulness of pleural fluid pH measurements. Patients with pleural effusions may need analgesia, particularly after thoracentesis or insertion of a chest tube. Those with acute pneumonia often need supplemental oxygen in addition to specific antibiotic treatment.

402.3 Purulent Pleurisy (Empyema)

An accumulation of pus in the pleural spaces is most often associated with pneumonia due to *Streptococcus pneumoniae*, although *Staphylococcus aureus* is most common in developing nations and in post-traumatic empyema. The relative incidence of *Haemophilus influenzae* empyema has decreased since the introduction of Hib vaccination. Group A *Streptococcus*, gram-negative organisms, tuberculosis, fungi, and malignancy are less common causes. Empyema is most frequently encountered in infants and preschool children. It occurs in 5–10% of children with bacterial pneumonia. The disease may also be produced by rupture of a lung abscess into the pleural space, by contamination introduced from trauma or thoracic surgery or, rarely, by mediastinitis or the extension of intra-abdominal abscesses.

Pathology. Most commonly, purulent pleurisy is an extensive process consisting of a series of loculated areas involving a large portion of one or both pleural cavities. Thickening of the parietal pleura occurs. If the pus is not drained, it may dissect through the pleura into lung parenchyma, producing bronchopleural fistulas and pyopneumothorax, or into the abdominal cavity. Rarely, the pus may dissect through the chest wall (i.e., *empyema necessitatis*). Pockets of loculated pus may eventually develop into thick-walled abscess cavities or, as the exudate organizes, the lung may collapse and become surrounded by a thick, inelastic envelope (i.e., peel).

Clinical Manifestations and Diagnosis. The initial signs and symptoms are primarily those of bacterial pneumonia. Children treated inadequately or with inappropriate antibiotic agents may have an interval of a few days between the clinical pneumonia phase and the evidence of empyema. Most patients are febrile. In infants, there may be only a moderate exacerbation of respiratory distress. The older child is likely to appear more ill and have greater respiratory difficulty. Physical and radiographic findings may be identical to those described for serofibrinous pleurisy, and the two conditions are differentiated only by thoracentesis, which should always be performed when empyema is suspected. Radiographically, finding no shift of fluid with a change of position indicates a loculated empyema; this may be confirmed by ultrasonography or CT scan. The maximal amount of pus obtainable should be withdrawn by thoracentesis. The appearance of pus produced by different organisms is not distinctive; cultures must always be obtained, and Gram-stained smears should be examined for the presence of microorganisms. Blood cultures have a high yield (62% in one series), but latex agglutination may also be useful. Leukocytosis and an elevated sedimentation rate may be found.

Complications. With staphylococcal infections, bronchopleural fistulas and pyopneumothorax commonly develop. Other local complications include purulent pericarditis, pulmonary abscesses, peritonitis secondary to rupture through the diaphragm, and osteomyelitis of the ribs. Septic complications such as meningitis, arthritis, and osteomyelitis may also occur. With staphylococcal empyema, septicemia occurs infrequently; it is often encountered in *H. influenzae* and pneumococcal infections.

Treatment. If pus is obtained by thoracentesis, closed drainage should be instituted immediately and controlled by an underwater seal or continuous suction. A catheter with the largest possible internal diameter should be inserted into the site where an accumulation of pus is suspected; sometimes several tubes are required to drain loculated areas. Closed drainage is usually continued for about 1 wk, even though small amounts of material continue to drain after this time, probably in response to the presence of the tube in the pleural cavity. Chest tubes that are no longer draining should be removed.

Instillation of fibrinolytic agents into the pleural cavity to promote drainage may be beneficial, but controlled studies are needed. Antibiotics should not be instilled into the pleural cavity because they do not improve results obtained with systemic antibiotic therapy alone and are associated with local reactions. Controlling empyema by multiple aspirations of the pleural cavity rather than by closed continuous drainage should not be attempted. If the condition is diagnosed early, thoracentesis and antibiotic treatment alone can bring about complete cure.

Systemic antibiotic therapy is required; the selection of the antibiotic should be based on the in vitro sensitivities of the responsible organism. See Chapters 166, 167, and 178 for treatment of infections by *Staphylococcus, Streptococcus pneumoniae,* and *H. influenzae*, respectively. With staphylococcal infections, reso-

lution of the process is very slow, and systemic antibiotic therapy is required for 3–4 wk. Clinical response in nonstaphylococcal empyema is also slow, even with optimal treatment; little improvement may occur for as long as 2 wk. In patients with inadequately treated empyema, extensive fibrinous changes may take place over the surface of the collapsed lungs, but surgical decortication procedures are rarely indicated. In the child who remains febrile and dyspneic longer than 72 hr after initiation of therapy with intravenous antibiotics and thoracostomy tube drainage, surgical decortication via video-assisted thoracoscopic surgery or open thoracotomy may speed recovery but remains highly controversial. If pneumatoceles form, no attempt should be made to treat them surgically or by aspiration, unless they reach sufficient size to cause respiratory embarrassment or become secondarily infected. The long-term clinical prognosis for adequately treated empyema is excellent, and follow-up pulmonary function studies suggest that residual restrictive disease is uncommon, with or without surgical intervention.

Antony VB, Mohammed KA: Pathophysiology of pleural space infections. *Semin Respir Infect* 1999;14:9–17.
Givan DC, Eigen H: Common pleural effusions in children. *Clin Chest Med* 1998;19:363–71.
Lee RB: Radiologic evaluation and intervention for empyema thoracis. *Chest Surg Clin North Am* 1996;6:439–60.
Light RW, Girard WM, Jenkinson SG, et al: Parapneumonic effusions. *Am J Med* 1980;69:507–12.
Moulton JS, Benkert RE, Weisiger KH, et al: Treatment of complicated pleural fluid collections with image-guided drainage and intracavitary urokinase. *Chest* 1995;108:1252–9.
Paganini H, Guinazu JR, Hernandez C, et al: Comparative analysis of outcome and clinical features in children with pleural empyema caused by penicillin-nonsusceptible and penicillin-susceptible *Streptococcus pneumoniae. Int J Infect Dis* 2001;5:86–8.
Redding GJ, Walund L, Walund D, et al: Lung function in children following empyema. *Am J Dis Child* 1990;144:1337–42.
Subramaniam R, Joseph VT, Tan GM, et al: Experience with video-assisted thoracoscopic surgery in the management of complicated pneumonia in children. *J Pediatr Surg* 2001;36:316–9.

Chapter 403
Pneumothorax *Glenna B. Winnie*

Pneumothorax is the accumulation of extrapulmonary air within the chest. It is uncommon during childhood. Most often, pneumothorax results from leakage of air from within the lung. Air leaks can be primary or secondary and can be spontaneous, traumatic, iatrogenic, or catamenial. Pneumothorax in the neonatal period is also discussed in Chapter 90.8.

Epidemiology and Etiology. A primary spontaneous pneumothorax occurs in someone without trauma or underlying lung disease. Spontaneous pneumothorax with or without exertion (Valsalva) occurs occasionally in teenagers and young adults, most frequently in males who are tall and thin. Families have been described in which many members have had spontaneous pneumothoraces, with the onset ranging from birth to adulthood. Patients with collagen synthesis defects such as Ehlers-Danlos disease and Marfan syndrome are unusually prone to the development of pneumothorax.

A pneumothorax arising as a complication of an underlying lung disorder, but without trauma, is a secondary spontaneous pneumothorax. Pneumothorax may occur in pneumonia, usually in connection with empyema; it may also be secondary to pulmonary abscess, gangrene, infarct, rupture of a cyst or an emphysematous bleb (e.g., in asthma), or foreign bodies in the lung. In infant staphylococcal pneumonia, the incidence of pneumothorax is relatively high. It is found in about 5% of hospitalized asthmatic children and usually resolves without treatment. Pneumothorax is a serious complication in cystic fibrosis (CF) (see Chapter 393), occurring in 10–25% of patients older than 10 yr. Pneumothorax also occurs in patients with lymphoma or other malignancies.

External chest or abdominal blunt or penetrating trauma can tear a bronchus or abdominal viscus, with leakage of air into the pleural space.

Iatrogenic pneumothorax can complicate tracheotomy, subclavian line placement, thoracentesis, transbronchial biopsy, or other diagnostic or therapeutic procedures. Pneumothorax may also occur after acupuncture treatment.

Catamenial pneumothorax, an unusual condition that is by definition associated with menses, results from passage of intraabdominal air through diaphragmatic defects. When thoracotomy is performed for recurrent pneumothorax of unknown cause in a young woman, an examination of the diaphragm may be appropriate.

Pneumothorax may be associated with a serous effusion (i.e., hydropneumothorax) or a purulent effusion (i.e., pyopneumothorax). Bilateral pneumothorax is rare beyond the neonatal period but has been reported after lung transplantation and with *Mycoplasma pneumoniae* infection.

Clinical Manifestations and Diagnosis. The onset is usually abrupt, and the severity of symptoms depends on the extent of the lung collapse and on the amount of pre-existing lung disease. Pneumothorax may cause pain, dyspnea, and cyanosis. In infancy, symptoms and physical signs may be difficult to recognize. Moderate pneumothorax may cause little displacement of the intrathoracic organs and few or no symptoms. The severity of pain usually does not directly reflect the extent of the collapse.

Usually, there is respiratory distress, retractions, and markedly decreased breath sounds over the involved lung. The percussion note over the involved area is tympanitic. The larynx, trachea, and heart may be shifted toward the unaffected side. When fluid is present, there is usually a sharply limited area of tympany above a level of flatness to percussion. The presence of amphoric breathing or, when fluid is present in the pleural cavity, of gurgling sounds synchronous with respirations suggests an open fistula connecting with air-containing tissues. Confirmatory evidence is provided when the pneumothorax fills rapidly after it has been aspirated.

The diagnosis can usually be established by radiographic examination. In conditions such as CF, in which the lung is relatively noncompliant, a great deal of air can accumulate under tension without much lung collapse. The amount of air outside the lung also varies with time. A radiograph taken early shows less lung collapse than one taken later if the leak continues. Expiratory views accentuate the contrast between lung markings and the clear area of the pneumothorax. When considering the possibility of diaphragmatic hernia, a small amount of barium may be necessary to demonstrate that it is not free air but is a portion of the gastrointestinal tract that is in the thoracic cavity.

It is important to determine whether the pneumothorax is under tension (i.e., tension pneumothorax) because this condition limits expansion of the contralateral lung and may compromise venous return. It may be difficult to determine if a pneumothorax is under tension. Evidence of tension includes shift of mediastinal structures away from the side of air leak. A shift may be absent in situations in which the other hemithorax resists the shift, such as in the case of bilateral pneumothorax. When the lungs are both stiff, the unaffected lung may not collapse easily and shift may not occur. On occasion, the diagnosis of tension pneumothorax is made only on the basis of evidence of circulatory compromise or on hearing a "hiss" of rapid exit of air under tension with the insertion of the thoracostomy tube.

Differential Diagnosis. Pneumothorax must be differentiated from localized or generalized emphysema, an extensive emphysematous bleb, large pulmonary cavities or other cystic formations, diaphragmatic hernia, compensatory overexpansion with contralateral atelectasis, and gaseous distention of the stomach. In most cases, a chest radiograph differentiates among these conditions.

Treatment. Therapy varies with the extent of the collapse and the nature and severity of the underlying disease. A small or even moderate-sized pneumothorax in an otherwise normal child may resolve without specific treatment, usually within about 1 wk. A small (<5%) pneumothorax complicating asthma may also resolve spontaneously. Administering 100% oxygen may hasten resolution by increasing the nitrogen pressure gradient between the pleural air and the blood. Patients with chronic hypoxemia should be monitored closely during the administration of supplemental oxygen. Pleural pain deserves analgesic treatment. Codeine may be justified, but its respiratory depressant effect should be considered. Occasionally, morphine or meperidine is needed. If there is more than 5% collapse or if the pneumothorax is recurrent or under tension, definitive treatment is necessary. Pneumothoraces complicating CF frequently recur, and definitive treatment may be justified with the first episode, even with less than 5% collapse (see Chapter 393). Similarly, if pneumothorax complicating malignancy and its treatment does not improve rapidly with observation, chemical pleurodesis or open thoracotomy is often necessary.

Closed thoracotomy (i.e., simple insertion of a chest tube) and drainage of the trapped air through a catheter, the external opening of which is kept in a dependent position under water, is adequate to re-expand the lung in most patients. When there have been previous pneumothoraces, it may be indicated to induce the formation of strong adhesions between the lung and chest wall by a sclerosing procedure to prevent recurrence. This can be carried out by the introduction of tetracycline, talc, or silver nitrate into the pleural space (i.e., *chemical pleurodesis*). Open thoracotomy through a limited incision, with plication of blebs, closure of fistula, stripping of the pleura (usually in the apical lung where the surgeon has direct vision), and basilar pleural abrasion is also an effective treatment for recurring pneumothorax. Stripping and abrading the pleura leaves raw, inflamed surfaces that heal with sealing adhesions. Postoperative pain is comparable to chemical pleurodesis with silver nitrate, but the chest tube can usually be removed within 24–48 hr, compared with the usual 72-hr minimum for closed thoracotomy and pleurodesis. The thoracoscope has permitted a successful surgical approach to blebectomy, pleural stripping, pleural brushing, and instillation of sclerosing agents with somewhat less morbidity than occurs with traditional open thoracotomy.

Extensive pleural adhesions help to prevent recurrent pneumothorax, but they also make thoracic surgery, including lung transplantation, difficult. For conditions in which lung transplantation may be a future consideration (e.g., CF), a stepwise approach to treatment of pneumothorax has been proposed. If the patient is comfortable and the pneumothorax is small, no intervention is warranted. For a larger leak or one that does not resolve, simple thoracostomy tube drainage can be attempted. For continuing leak, or recurrence, the next step could be thoracoscopic blebectomy without pleural abrasion. Only after these steps have failed should the full aggressive pleural stripping and abrasion be undertaken. At any step during this approach, the patient and family should be given the option of the definitive procedure if they understand this may make lung transplantation difficult or impossible. It should also be kept in mind that the longer a chest tube is in place, the greater the chance of pulmonary deterioration, particularly in a patient with CF, in whom strong coughing, deep breathing, and postural drainage are important. These are all difficult to accomplish with a chest tube in place.

Treatment of the underlying pulmonary disease should begin on admission and should be continued throughout the course of treatment directed at the air leak.

Alter SJ: Spontaneous pneumothorax in infants: A 10-year review. *Pediatr Emerg Care* 1997;13:401–3.

Cook CH, Melvin WS, Groner JI, et al: A cost-effective thoracoscopic treatment strategy for pediatric spontaneous pneumothorax. *Surg Endosc* 1999;13: 1208–10.

Engdahl MS, Gershan WM: Familial spontaneous pneumothorax in neonates. *Pediatr Pulmonol* 1998;25:398–400.

Genc A, Ozcan C, Erdener A, et al: Management of pneumothorax in children. *J Cardiovasc Surg* 1998;39:849–51.

Newson TP, Parshuram CS, Berkowitz RG, et al: Tension pneumothorax secondary to grass head aspiration. *Pediatr Emerg Care* 1998;14:287–89.

Noyes BE, Orenstein DM: Treatment of pneumothorax in cystic fibrosis in the era of lung transplantation. *Chest* 1992;101:1187–88.

Roe D, Brown K: Catamenial pneumothorax heralding menarche in a 15-year-old adolescent. *Pediatr Emerg Care* 1997;13:390–91.

Chapter 404
Pneumomediastinum

Glenna B. Winnie

Pneumomediastinum usually results from alveolar rupture during acute or chronic pulmonary disease. However, a diverse group of nonrespiratory entities can also cause pneumomediastinum; in some of these, the lung is not the source of the air. For example, pneumomediastinum has been reported after dental extractions, normal menses, obstetric delivery, diabetes mellitus with ketoacidosis, acupuncture, and acute gastroenteritis. Pneumomediastinum can also result from esophageal perforation or penetrating chest trauma. Occasionally, no underlying cause is found; in an apparently normal child, the pneumomediastinum can present as chest pain associated with subcutaneous air.

After intrapulmonary alveolar rupture, air can dissect through the perivascular sheaths and other soft tissue planes toward the hilum and enter the mediastinum. Pneumomediastinum is rarely a major problem in older children because the mediastinum can be depressurized by escape of air into the neck or abdomen. In the newborn, however, the rate at which air can leave the mediastinum is limited, and pneumomediastinum can lead to dangerous cardiovascular compromise or pneumothorax (see Chapters 90.8 and 403). Acute asthma is the most common cause of pneumomediastinum in older children and teenagers. Simultaneous pneumothorax is unusual in these patients.

Clinical Manifestations. Transient stabbing pains in the chest that may radiate to the neck are the principal features of pneumomediastinum. Isolated abdominal pain and sore throat also occur. The patient may have dyspnea, but it is difficult to know if this is really a separate symptom or if it is related to the chest pain. Pneumomediastinum is difficult to detect by physical examination alone. Subcutaneous emphysema, if present, is diagnostic. Although cardiac dullness to percussion may be decreased, many of these patients' chests are chronically overinflated, and it is unlikely that the clinician can be sure of this finding. A mediastinal "crunch" is occasionally heard but is easily confused with a friction rub. On chest radiography, the cardiac border, highlighted by the mediastinal air, is more distinct than normal and, on the lateral projection, the posterior mediastinal structures are also clearly defined. Subcutaneous air, seen radiographically, confirms the pneumomediastinum.

Treatment. This is directed primarily at the underlying obstructive pulmonary disease. Analgesics are needed occasionally for chest pain. Rarely, subcutaneous emphysema can cause sufficient tracheal compression to justify tracheotomy; the tracheotomy also decompresses the mediastinum.

Chalumeau M, Le Clainche L, Sayeg N, et al: Spontaneous pneumomediastinum in children. *Pediatr Pulmonol* 2001;31:67–75.

Damore DT, Dayan PS: Medical causes of pneumomediastinum in children. *Clin Pediatr* 2001;40:87–91.

McHugh TP: Pneumomediastinum following penetrating oral trauma. *Pediatr Emerg Care* 1997;13:211–13.

Schoem SR, Choi SS, Zalzal GH: Pneumomediastinum and pneumothorax from blunt cervical trauma in children. *Laryngoscope* 1997;107:351–56.

Stack AM, Caputo GL: Pneumomediastinum in childhood asthma. *Pediatr Emerg Care* 1996;12:98–101.

Chapter 405
Hydrothorax *Glenna B. Winnie*

In hydrothorax, the fluid is noninflammatory and has a lower specific gravity (<1.015) than that of a serofibrinous exudate. It contains less protein and fewer cells and is usually associated with an accumulation of fluid in other parts of the body, such as the peritoneal cavity and the subcutaneous tissues. Hydrothorax is most often associated with cardiac, renal, or hepatic disease. It may be a manifestation of severe nutritional edema, and it rarely results from venous obstruction by neoplasms, enlarged lymph nodes, or adhesions. It may occur from a ventriculoperitoneal shunt. Hydrothorax is usually bilateral in cases of renal disease or nutritional edema; in myocardial disease, it may be bilateral, limited to the right side, or greater on the right than on the left side. The physical signs are the same as those described for serofibrinous pleurisy (see Chapter 402.2), but in hydrothorax there is more rapid shifting of the level of dullness with changes of position. Treatment is for the primary disorder; aspiration may be necessary when pressure symptoms are notable.

Kawaguchi AL, Dunn JC, Fonkalsrud EW: Management of peritoneal dialysis-induced hydrothorax in children. *Am Surgeon* 1996;62:820–24.

Xiol X, Guardiola J: Hepatic hydrothorax. *Curr Opin Pulm Med* 1998;4:239–42.

Chapter 406
Hemothorax *Glenna B. Winnie*

Extensive bleeding into the pleural cavity is rare in children but may result from erosion of a blood vessel in association with inflammatory processes such as tuberculosis and empyema. Hemothorax may complicate a variety of congenital anomalies, including sequestration, patent ductus arteriosus, and pulmonary arteriovenous malformation. It is also an occasional manifestation of intrathoracic neoplasms, blood dyscrasias, bleeding diatheses, or thrombolytic therapy. It may be the result of thoracic trauma, including surgical procedures or venous line insertion. Rupture of an aneurysm is unlikely during childhood. Hemothorax also occurs after blunt chest trauma and spontaneously in neonates and older children. A pleural hemorrhage associated with a pneumothorax is called *hemopneumothorax*.

The diagnosis of a hemothorax can be made only by thoracentesis. In every case, an effort must be made to determine and treat the cause. Surgical intervention may be required to control active bleeding, and transfusion is necessary if blood loss is excessive. Inadequate removal of blood in extensive hemothorax may lead to substantial restrictive disease secondary to organization of fibrin; fibrinolytic therapy or a decortication procedure may then be necessary.

Bagwell CE, Salzberg AM, Sonnino RE, et al: Potentially lethal complications of central venous catheter placement. *J Pediatr Surg* 2000;35:709–13.

Inci I, Ozcelik C, Nizam O, et al: Penetrating chest injuries in children: A review of 94 cases. *J Pediatr Surg* 1996;31:673–76.

Wilimas JA, Presbury G, Orenstein D, et al: Hemothorax and hemomediastinum in patients with hemophilia. *Acta Haematol* 1985;73:176–78.

Chapter 407

Chylothorax *Glenna B. Winnie*

Chylothorax results from the escape of chyle from the thoracic duct into the thoracic cavity. The incidence has increased as cardiac surgery is performed on more complex congenital abnormalities; about 50% of these cases are now operative complications resulting from rupture of the thoracic duct. Most of the remainder are associated with chest injury or with primary or metastatic intrathoracic malignancy as a result of the pressure of enlarged lymph nodes or tumor. Less common causes include lymphangiomatosis, restrictive pulmonary diseases, thrombosis of the duct or the subclavian vein, and congenital anomalies of the duct system. Chylothorax can occur in child abuse. In some patients, especially newborns, no specific cause is identified. Chylothorax is rarely bilateral and usually occurs on the left side.

Clinical Manifestations and Diagnosis. The signs and symptoms relate to the presence of fluid in the thoracic cavity. The diagnosis is established when thoracentesis demonstrates a chylous effusion, a milky fluid containing fat, protein, lymphocytes, and other constituents of chyle. In newborn infants who have not yet been fed, the fluid may be clear. A pseudochylous milky fluid has been reported in cases of serous effusion, in which the fatty material was thought to arise from degenerative changes within the fluid and not from the presence of lymph. This type of fluid may be differentiated from one containing chyle by shaking it with alkalis or ether; the fluid containing chyle tends to become clear. A more definitive test is the quantitation of fluid triglyceride, which is elevated in chylous fluid, and fluid cholesterol, which may be elevated in chronic serous effusions.

Spontaneous recovery has occurred in more than 50% of the reported cases in infants younger than 1 yr of age. Repeated aspirations may be required to relieve the symptoms of pressure. However, chyle reaccumulates quickly, and repeated thoracenteses may cause considerable loss of calories, protein, and lymphocytes. Immunodeficiencies, including hypogammaglobulinemia and abnormal cell-mediated immune responses, have been associated with repeated thoracenteses for chylothorax. Attempts to prevent these problems by intravenous infusion of pleural contents are technically difficult, dangerous, and of doubtful benefit. Despite large losses of T lymphocytes, clinical problems of infection are uncommon, but these patients should be protected from potentially dangerous viruses, including cytomegalovirus and live virus vaccines.

Treatment. Therapy should begin in most cases with a brief period of observation on a low-fat (or medium-chain triglyceride), high-protein diet. For most patients, salt restriction and diuresis are also indicated. The total caloric intake should be greater than the average requirement and, several times the daily requirements of the various vitamins, especially the fat-soluble vitamins A and D, should be added. If fluid continues to

reaccumulate over 1–2 wk, total parenteral nutrition should be instituted and, if unsuccessful, a more aggressive attempt to locate and ligate the thoracic duct may be indicated. Other therapeutic approaches include pressure control ventilation with positive end-expiratory pressure, inhalation of nitric oxide, subcutaneous octreotide, and pleuroperitoneal shunt placement.

Al-Tawil K, Ahmed G, Al-Hathal M, et al: Congenital chylothorax. *Am J Perinatol* 2000;17:121–26.

Beghetti M, La Scala G, Belli D, et al: Etiology and management of pediatric chylothorax. *J Pediatr* 2000;136:653–58.

Fishman SJ, Burrows PE, Upton J, Hendren WH: Life-threatening anomalies of the thoracic duct: Anatomic delineation dictates management. *J Pediatr Surg* 2001;36:1269–72.

Geismar SL, Tilelli JA, Campbell JB, et al: Chylothorax as a manifestation of child abuse. *Pediatr Emerg Care* 1997;13:386–89.

Chapter 408

Bronchopulmonary Dysplasia *Steven Lestrud*

Bronchopulmonary dysplasia (BPD) or *chronic lung disease due to prematurity* is discussed in detail in Chapter 90.3. This chapter focuses on the course during infancy and childhood.

Clinical Manifestations. After the neonatal course of RDS and progression of lung disease to Northway stage IV, the clinical features of BPD are varied. Whereas preterm neonates without the diagnosis of BPD may have normal pulmonary function, those requiring supplemental oxygen past 35 wk of postconceptional age have a higher incidence of lower airway obstruction and bronchodilator responsiveness and are more likely to be hospitalized during the toddler years.

Physical findings on pulmonary examination frequently include tachypnea, wheezing, or coarse crackles. Fine crackles may be present in patients prone to fluid overload. The chest wall may have an increased anteroposterior diameter, and intercostal retractions are present. Truncal motor tone is frequently increased, potentially impeding optimum chest excursion.

The most severely affected patients may require prolonged mechanical ventilation to achieve acceptable gas exchange. Infants with significant lung disease will exhibit growth failure owing to elevated energy expenditure essential to maintain increased metabolic demands. Many have baseline hypoxemia, requiring supplemental oxygen to maintain oxygen saturations above 90%; chronic respiratory insufficiency may be evident by elevated bicarbonate levels or elevated Pco_2 on blood gas analysis.

A pulmonary exacerbation is typically triggered during upper respiratory infections. During an exacerbation, the infant will exhibit increased work of breathing, tachypnea and retractions will be evident, and chest wall configuration may change with an increased anteroposterior diameter. If wheezing is a prominent baseline finding, poor air entry during an exacerbation may result in less wheezing.

Patients must be monitored for the development of cor pulmonale, especially if they require supplemental oxygen and have chronic respiratory failure. Other complicating conditions may include gastroesophageal reflux disease (GERD) and pulmonary aspiration, particularly during an exacerbation when the infants are most tachypneic and when pulmonary mechanics increase risk of GERD. For patients severely affected and those with disease out of proportion to the risk for development of chronic lung disease, other pulmonary disease may be suspected, such as asthma, cystic fibrosis, and chronic aspiration pneumonitis.

Recurrent episodes of respiratory distress may represent anatomic airway abnormalities such as subglottic stenosis and airway malacia.

Treatment. Treatment is aimed to decrease work of breathing and normalize gas exchange, allowing for optimal growth and neurodevelopment. Adequate caloric intake can be difficult for many reasons, including oral aversion, discoordinate suck and swallow, GERD, aspiration, and aspiration with GERD. In addition, disordered breathing patterns with tachypnea, frequent respiratory distress with increased work of breathing, and requirement for supplement oxygen place the infant at risk for growth failure. A high calorie intake is necessary, with ranges of 120–160 kcal/kg/day required, frequently combined with fluid restriction. To provide such high caloric intake in the compromised neonate, supplemental feedings may be considered through a nasogastric or gastrostomy tube. Careful attention is necessary to maintain fluid balance.

The administration of inhaled glucocorticoids to young children with BPD is considered, owing to the role of inflammation in the pathogenesis of this disease. A frequent finding with BPD is wheezing, particularly with onset of upper respiratory tract infections; however, a severely affected population may have chronic wheeze. The cause of the wheeze may be inflammation, bronchial smooth muscle irritation, bronchial smooth muscle hypertrophy, and airway malacia. As such, the administration of a bronchodilator is frequently undertaken to evaluate an individual's response. β-Agonists most commonly initially increase air movement and improve comfort of breathing. For patients who respond, the medication should be continued, especially during high-risk periods when triggers are present, such as an upper respiratory infection or hot humid days. Occasionally, β-agonists will worsen the air exchange; this is characteristic of infants with BPD and concomitant airway malacia. Airway malacia frequently contributes to obstructive lung disease. Bronchial smooth muscle may maintain airway caliber in the malacic airway; smooth muscle relaxation after administration of a β-agonist results in increased small airway collapse. These patients may benefit from alternative bronchodilators such as ipratropium or methylxanthines.

Gastroesophageal reflux is common and must be suspected in patients not responding to therapy and in patients with frequent exacerbations especially without clear triggers. Definitive diagnosis is necessary because these patients will be subject to prolonged promotility and antacid medications (see Chapters 304 and 387). Appropriate antireflux therapy in infants with GERD often greatly decreases respiratory complications. Gastroesophageal reflux with pulmonary aspiration or aspiration alone may present as chronic chest congestion, wheezing, and episodic hypoxic spells. Fundoplication with a gastrostomy tube is performed in patients unresponsive to medical therapy. Evaluation and treatment by a speech therapist, pediatric pulmonologist, or otolaryngologist may be necessary to decrease the risk of developing chronic lung disease associated with aspiration.

Attention must be given to prevention of respiratory viral illness. Simple measures should be encouraged, such as frequent handwashing, especially before handling the baby, and avoidance of contact with children and adults with current respiratory symptoms. Sinusitis and otitis media are frequent bacterial infections that result in an exacerbation, particularly in infants with nasogastric tubes or using nasal cannula oxygen. RSV immunoprophylaxis should be considered based on the severity of lung disease, gestational age, and current age.

In general, the *prognosis* for infants with BPD is good. Through school age, the family can expect frequent medical interactions for episodes of respiratory distress frequently triggered by simple upper respiratory tract infections and weather changes. Pulmonary function for severely affected patients will remain decreased, and exercise limitation may be present due to dyspnea. The most severely affected patients will benefit from a multidisciplinary team of caregivers, including the pediatrician, pulmonologist, speech therapist, nutritionist, and developmental specialists.

Frank L, Sosenko IRS: Undernutrition as a major contributing factor in the pathogenesis of bronchopulmonary dysplasia. *Am Rev Respir Dis* 1988;138:725–29.

Gross SJ, Iannuzzi DM, Kveselis DA, et al: Effect of preterm birth on pulmonary function at school age: A prospective controlled study. *J Pediatr* 1998;133:188–92.

Jacob SV, Coates AL, Lands LC, et al: Long-term pulmonary sequelae of severe bronchopulmonary dysplasia. *J Pediatr* 1998;133:193–200.

Prevention of Respiratory Syncytial Virus Infections: Indications for the use of palivizumab and update on the use of RSV-IGIV (RE9839). *Pediatrics* 1998;102:1211–16.

Stocker JT: Pathologic features of long-standing "healed" bronchopulmonary dysplasia. *Hum Pathol* 1986;17:943–61.

Chapter 409
Skeletal Diseases Influencing Pulmonary Function *Steven Boas*

Chest wall abnormalities can lead to restrictive pulmonary disease, impaired respiratory muscle strength, and decreased ventilatory performance in response to physical stress. Common causes of skeletal disorders affecting pulmonary function in children include kyphoscoliosis and pectus excavatum. Rarer causes include rib cage anomalies, congenital syndromes, connective tissue disorders, and neuromuscular disease and are discussed elsewhere.

409.1 Pectus Excavatum (Funnel Chest)

Pathogenesis. Midline narrowing of the thoracic cavity is usually an isolated skeletal abnormality. The cause is unknown. It may be associated with a connective tissue disorder (i.e., Marfan syndrome) or rickets, or it may be acquired.

Clinical Manifestations. The deformity is present at or shortly after birth but is usually not associated with any symptoms at that time. Over time, decreased exercise tolerance, chest pain, palpitations, recurrent respiratory infections, wheezing, stridor, and cough may be present. Because of the cosmetic nature of this deformity, many children experience significant psychological stress. Physical examination may reveal a narrowed anteroposterior diameter, rounded shoulders, kyphoscoliosis, protuberant abdomen, left shift of the cardiac impulse, and an innocent systolic murmur.

Diagnosis. Lateral chest radiograms demonstrate the depression. An electrocardiogram may show a right-axis deviation. Mitral valve prolapse, Wolff-Parkinson-White syndrome, bronchial atresia, and bronchomalacia are associated. Results of pulmonary function tests may be normal or may show a restrictive defect, if the pectus deformity is severe. Exercise testing may demonstrate either normal tolerance or limitations from underlying limited habitual activity or cardiopulmonary dysfunction. Lowered ventilatory reserves at peak exercise are common, although the clinical significance of these findings remains unclear.

Treatment. Corrective surgery is beneficial for individuals with restrictive lung disease. Although surgery itself does not reverse the lung restriction, it may halt the progression of cardiopulmonary compromise. For teenagers with exercise limitations, surgical repair may result in improved exercise tolerance. Normalization of lung perfusion scans and maximal voluntary ventilation have also been seen after surgery. Surgery is often performed for psychological or cosmetic reasons.

409.2 Pectus Carinatum and Fissuri Sterni

Pectus carinatum (pigeon breast) is an uncommon sternal deformity (⅐th the frequency of pectus excavatum) in which sternal protrusion occurs with lateral depression of the ribs. Males are affected more often than females. Three distinct subtypes (I, keel chest; II, pouter pigeon breast; III, lateral pectus carinatum) have been described with implications for surgical correction. Mitral valve disease and coarctation of the aorta are associated with this anomaly. Scoliosis may occur in these patients, with a subset of children requiring surgery. Surgery is often performed for cosmetic and psychological reasons.

Fissuri sterni congenital (sternal clefts) is a partial (more common) or total midline split in the sternum. This disorder may occur in isolation or may be associated with other congenital anomalies. Surgery is required early in life before fixation and immobility take place.

Chidambaram B, Mehta AV: Currarino-Silverman syndrome (pectus carinatum type 2 deformity) and mitral valve disease. *Chest* 1992;102:780–2.

Godfrey S: Association between pectus excavatum and segmental bronchomalacia. *J Pediatr* 1980;96:649.

Haller JA Jr, Loughlin GM: Cardiorespiratory function is significantly improved following corrective surgery for severe pectus excavatum: Proposed treatment guidelines. *J Cardiovasc Surg* 2000;41:125–30.

Haller JA Jr, Scherer LR, Turner CS, et al: Evolving management of pectus excavatum based on a single institutional experience of 664 patients. *Ann Surg* 1989;209:578–82.

Park JM, Farmer AF: Wolff-Parkinson-White syndrome in children with pectus excavatum. *J Pediatr* 1988;112:926.

Robicsek F, Cook JW, Daughetrty HK, et al: Pectus carinatum. *J Thorac Cardiovasc Surg* 1979;78:52–61.

Shamberger RC, Welch KJ, Sanders SP: Mitral valve prolapse associated with pectus excavatum. *J Pediatr* 1987;111:404.

Waters P, Welch K, Micheli LJ, et al: Scoliosis in children with pectus excavatum and pectus carinatum. *J Pediatr Orthop* 1989;9:551–56.

Xiao-Ping J, Ting-Ze H, Wen-Ying L, et al: Pulmonary function for pectus excavatum at long-term follow-up. *J Pediatr Surg* 1999;34:1787–90.

Zhao L, Feinberg MS, Gaides M, et al: Why is exercise capacity reduced in subjects with pectus excavatum? *J Pediatr* 2000;136:163–67.

409.3 Asphyxiating Thoracic Dystrophy (Thoracic-Pelvic-Phalangeal Dystrophy)

Pathogenesis. Also known as *Jeune syndrome*, this condition is an autosomal recessive disorder that results in a constricted and narrow rib cage with generalized chondrodystrophy. Other systems can be involved, including pelvic, phalangeal, and neurologic anomalies along with renal and hepatic disorders.

Clinical Manifestations. Most patients with this disorder die shortly after birth from respiratory failure, although less aggressive forms have been reported in older children. For those who survive the neonatal period, progressive respiratory failure often ensues owing to impaired lung growth, recurrent pneumonia, and atelectasis originating from the rigid chest wall.

Diagnosis. Physical examination reveals a narrowed thorax that at birth is much smaller than the head circumference. The ribs are horizontal, and these children have short extremities. Chest radiographs demonstrate a bell-shaped chest cage with short horizontal and flaring ribs and high clavicles.

Treatment. No specific treatment exists, although thoracoplasty to enlarge the chest wall and long-term mechanical ventilation have been tried with mixed results.

Prognosis. For some children, improvement in the bony abnormalities occurs with age. However, children younger than 1 yr often succumb to respiratory infection and failure. Progressive renal disease often occurs with older children. Use of vaccines for influenza and other respiratory pathogens is warranted, as is aggressive use of antibiotics for respiratory infections.

Aronson DC, Van Nierop JC, Taminiau A, et al: Homologous bone graft for expansion thoracoplasty in Jeune's asphyxiating thoracic dystrophy. *J Pediatr Surg* 1999;34:500–3.

Kajantic E, Anderson S, Kaitila I: Familial asphyxiating thoracic dysplasia: Clinical variability and impact of improved neonatal intensive care. *J Pediatr* 2001;139:130–33.

Sharoni E, Erez E, Chorev G, et al: Chest reconstruction in asphyxiating thoracic dystrophy. *J Pediatr Surg* 1998;33:1578–81.

Tahernia AC, Stamps P: "Jeune syndrome" (asphyxiating thoracic dystrophy). *Clin Pediatr* 1977;16:903–8.

Wiebicke W, Pasterkamp H: Long-term continuous positive pressure in a child with asphyxiating thoracic dystrophy. *Pediatr Pulmonol* 1988;4:54–58.

409.4 Achondroplasia

This condition is inherited as an autosomal dominant disorder that results in disordered growth (see Chapter 684). The pathogenesis is unknown.

Clinical Manifestations. Recurrent infections, cor pulmonale, and dyspnea are commonly associated with achondroplasia. There is an increased risk of obstructive sleep apnea, although the majority of patients are not affected. Hypoxemia during sleep is a common feature. Onset of restrictive lung disease can begin at a very young age. On examination, the breathing pattern is rapid and shallow with associated abdominal breathing. The anteroposterior diameter of the thorax is reduced. Special growth curves for chest circumference of patients with achondroplasia from birth to 7 yr are available. Three distinct phenotypes exist, with group 1 possessing relative adenotonsillar hypertrophy, group 2 with muscular upper airway obstruction and progressive hydrocephalus, and group 3 with upper airway obstruction without hydrocephalus. Kyphoscoliosis may develop during infancy.

Diagnosis. Pulmonary function tests reveal a reduced vital capacity that is more pronounced in males. The lungs are small but functionally normal. Chest radiographs demonstrate the decreased anteroposterior diameter along with anterior cupping of the ribs. The degree of foramen magnum involvement correlates with the degree of respiratory dysfunction.

Treatment. Treatment of sleep apnea, if present, is supportive (see Chapter 369). Physiotherapy and bracing may minimize the complications of kyphosis and of severe lordosis. Aggressive treatment of respiratory infections and scoliosis is warranted.

Prognosis. The life span is normal for most children with this condition except for the phenotypic group with hydrocephalus or with severe cervical or lumbar spinal compression.

Hunter AG, Reid CS, Pauli RM, et al: Standard curves of chest circumference in achondroplasia and the relationship of chest circumference to respiratory problems. *Am J Med Genet* 1996;62:91–7.

Mogayzel PJ Jr, Carroll JL, Loughlin GM, et al: Sleep-disordered breathing in children with achondroplasia. *J Pediatr* 1998;132:667–71.

Stokes DC, Phillips JA, Leonard Co, et al: Respiratory complications of achondroplasia. *J Pediatr* 1983;102:534–41.

Stokes DC, Wohl ME, Wise RA, et al: The lungs and airways in achondroplasia: Do little people have little lungs? *Chest* 1990;98:145–152.

Tasker RC, Dundas I, Laverty A, et al: Distinct patterns of respiratory difficulty in young children with achondroplasia: A clinical, sleep, and lung function study. *Arch Dis Child* 1998;79:99–108.

409.5 Kyphoscoliosis: Adolescent Idiopathic Scoliosis and Congenital Scoliosis

Pathogenesis. Adolescent idiopathic scoliosis (AIS) is characterized by lateral bending of the spine (see Chapter 669). It commonly affects children during their teen years and periods of rapid growth. The cause is unknown. Congenital scoliosis is uncommon, affecting girls more than boys, and is apparent within the first year of life.

Clinical Manifestations. The pulmonary manifestations of scoliosis may include chest wall restriction leading to a reduction in the total lung capacity. The angle of scoliosis deformity has been correlated with the degree of lung impairment only for those with thoracic curves. Vital capacity, FEV_1, work capacity, diffusion capacity, chest wall compliance, and Pao_2 decrease as the severity of thoracic curve increases. These findings can be seen in even mild to moderate AIS (Cobb angle < 30 degrees) but do not occur in other nonthoracic curves. Reduction in peripheral muscle function has been associated with AIS through either intrinsic mechanisms or deconditioning. Severe impairment can lead to cor pulmonale or respiratory failure and can occur before age 20 yr.

Children with severe scoliosis, especially boys, may have abnormalities of breathing during sleep, and the resultant periods of hypoxemia may contribute to the eventual development of pulmonary hypertension.

Diagnosis. Physical examination and an upright posteroanterior radiograph with subsequent measurement of the angle of curvature (Cobb technique) remain the gold standard for assessment. Curves greater than 10 degrees define the presence of scoliosis.

Treatment. Depending on the extent of the curve and the degree of skeletal maturation, treatment options include reassurance, observation, bracing, and surgery (spinal fusion). Influenza vaccine should be administered given the degree of pulmonary compromise that may co-exist. Because vital capacity is a strong predictor for the development of respiratory failure in untreated AIS, surgical goals are to diminish the scoliotic curve, maintain the correction, and prevent deterioration in pulmonary function. Abnormal vital capacity and total lung capacity, exercise intolerance, and the rate of change of these variables over time should be taken into consideration for the timing of surgical correction. Preoperative assessment of lung function may assist in predicting postsurgical pulmonary difficulties. Many patients undergoing surgical correction may be managed postoperatively without mechanical ventilation. However, even patients with mild scoliosis may have pulmonary compromise immediately after spinal fusion secondary to pain and a body cast that may restrict breathing and interfere with coughing.

Klearon C, Viviani GR, Killian KJ: Factors influencing work capacity in adolescent idiopathic thoracic scoliosis. *Am Rev Respir Dis* 1993;148:295.
Leech JA, Ernst P, Rogala EJ, et al: Cardiorespiratory status in relation to mild deformity in adolescent idiopathic scoliosis. *J Pediatr* 1985;106:143.
Mezon BL, West P, Israels J, et al: Sleep breathing abnormalities in kyphoscoliosis. *Am Rev Respir Dis* 1980;1222:617.

409.6 Congenital Rib Anomalies

Clinical Manifestations. Isolated defects of the highest and lowest ribs have minimal clinical pulmonary consequences. Missing midthoracic ribs are associated with the absence of the pectoralis muscle, and lung function can become compromised. Associated kyphoscoliosis and hemivertebrae may accompany this defect. If the rib defect is small, no significant sequelae ensue. When the 2nd to 5th ribs are absent anteriorly, lung herniation and significant abnormal respiration ensue. The lung is soft and nontender and may be easily reducible on examination. Complicating sequelae include severe lung restriction (secondary to scoliosis), cor pulmonale, and congestive heart failure. Symptoms are often minimal but can cause dyspnea. Respiratory distress is rare in infancy.

Diagnosis. Chest radiographs demonstrate the deformed and absent ribs with secondary scoliosis. Most rib abnormalities are discovered as incidental findings on a chest film.

Treatment. If symptoms are severe enough to cause clinical compromise or significant lung herniation, then homologous rib grafting can be performed. Adolescent girls may require cosmetic breast surgery.

Bronsther B, Coryllos E, Epstein B, et al: Lung hernias in children. *J Pediatr Surg* 1968;3:544.
Mehta MH, Patel RV, Mehta LV, et al: Congenital absence of ribs. *Indian Pediatr* 1992;29:1149–52.
Ricklam PP: Lung hernia secondary to congenital absence of ribs. *Arch Dis Child* 1959;34:14.

Chapter 410
Neuromuscular Diseases with Pulmonary Consequences *David Gozal*

Decreased muscle strength and endurance can affect any skeletal muscle in neuromuscular disorders including those involved in respiratory functions. Of particular concern are those muscles mediating upper airway patency, generation of cough, and lung inflation. Acute respiratory insufficiency is often one of the most prominent clinical presentations of several acute neuromuscular disorders, such as high-level spinal cord injury, poliomyelitis, Guillain-Barré syndrome, and botulism. Although much more insidious in its clinical course, development of respiratory dysfunction constitutes the leading cause of morbidity and mortality in progressive neuromuscular disorders (e.g., Duchenne muscular dystrophy, spinal muscular atrophy, congenital myotonic dystrophy, myasthenia gravis, Charcot-Marie-Tooth disease).

Clinical Manifestations. Acute respiratory distress with dyspnea, agitation, diaphoresis, and cyanosis should prompt immediate evaluation and therapy. The presence of hypoxemia is easily documented and monitored by pulse oximetry, and the severity of alveolar hypoventilation can be determined by drawing arterial or capillary blood gases. Radiographic assessment may reveal the presence of segmental or lobar atelectasis that may be difficult to differentiate from and will often coincide with a pneumonic infiltrate. In children with progressive neuromuscular disorders, decreases in total lung capacity and vital capacity are usually closely linked to the degree of muscular impairment, and the restrictive lung disease will be further accentuated by the onset and progression of kyphoscoliosis. The increased work of breathing will be further compounded by the decreased chest wall and lung compliance that result from fibrotic changes of the dystrophic chest wall muscles, shortening and stiffening of the unstretched tissues, and widespread microatelectatic changes. Despite the reduction in lung volumes, an increase in residual volume is frequently observed in patients with neuromuscular disorders and most likely reflects the disproportionate weakness of expiratory muscles. Such preferential weakness of expiratory muscles precludes, in turn, an effective expiration at lung volumes below functional residual capacity with concomitant reduction of cough and mucociliary clearance efficiency.

Because muscle weakness will reduce maximal expiratory flows, true airflow obstruction may be concealed during standard spirometric maneuvers and requires more sophisticated testing, such as the use of the forced oscillation technique for its detection. Measurement of respiratory muscle strength is an important component of the clinical evaluation of neuromuscular patients, and both maximal inspiratory and expiratory pressures will be reduced, albeit to varying degrees. The major implication of this reduction in respiratory force is the reduced capacity to develop effective clearance of secretions during cough. In the absence of competent mucociliary clearance, plugs of mucus will form and further compromise pulmonary function, especially after the onset of an otherwise benign upper respiratory tract infection. Recurrent or chronic infection and fibrosis will further accelerate the loss of functional lung parenchyma leading to hypoxemia, pulmonary hypertension, and eventually cor pulmonale.

During sleep, and particularly during rapid eye movement sleep, normally occurring decreases in central neural ventilatory output may lead to substantial aggravation of alveolar hypoventilation and hypoxemia. In addition, decreased upper airway motor tone will further promote the occurrence of upper airway obstruction. Thus, patients may complain of daytime sleepiness, fatigue, exertional dyspnea, morning headache and drowsiness, vomiting, difficulty tolerating the supine posture, and frequent need to be repositioned during the night. However, increased clinical awareness of sleep-related disturbances is needed or otherwise many of these symptoms may be misconstrued as related to the neuromuscular disorder.

Treatment. Interventions are directed at providing supportive therapy rather than curing the underlying abnormalities leading to the particular neuromuscular disease. Close surveillance through periodic history and physical examination are critical and will guide the need for further laboratory testing. Particular attention needs to be paid to the development of personality changes such as irritability, decreased attention span, and fatigue or somnolence, because these may point to the presence of sleep-associated gas exchange abnormalities and sleep fragmentation. Similarly, changes in speech and voice characteristics and the use of alae nasi and other accessory muscles during quiet breathing at rest may provide sensitive indicators of progressive muscle dysfunction and respiratory compromise. Although the frequency of periodic reevaluation needs to be individually tailored, tentative guidelines are provided in Table 410–1.

Regular administration of physical therapy, postural drainage, and a variety of manually and mechanically assisted cough maneuvers have demonstrated efficacy in the management of both acute pulmonary exacerbations as well as in long-term maintenance therapy. Parents should become proficient in the administration of such interventions. However, the role of mucolytic agents such as N-acetylcysteine or inhaled DNase remains unclear. Respiratory muscle training will improve or at least preserve muscle strength in these children and should be encouraged. Oral or intravenous antibiotic therapy should be administered early in the course of respiratory infections, and inhaled bronchodilators may alleviate any underlying bronchoconstriction. Annual administration of influenza vaccine is generally recommended and pneumococcal vaccine should be strongly considered in younger patients. The roles of theophylline or corticosteroid therapy are not established.

When respiratory insufficiency develops in the setting of neuromuscular disease, as evidenced by abnormal respiratory patterns during sleep or wakefulness, mechanical ventilatory support is needed. Tracheotomy should be avoided for as long as possible. Noninvasive mechanical ventilatory support using either nasal, oral, or face masks is the first line of treatment in both acute and chronic respiratory insufficiency. The beneficial effects of mask ventilation on lung volumes, sleep architecture, mucociliary clearance, and overall quality of life have been clearly demonstrated in patients with neuromuscular disease. Supplemental oxygen may be required to alleviate hypoxemia during either acute or chronic pulmonary insufficiency. Tracheotomy may ultimately become necessary if patients need frequent suctioning of bronchial secretions or when patients require more than 18 hr of ventilatory support a day on a long-term basis. Despite such supportive measures, most chronic neuromuscular disorders will continue to follow their progressive and irreversible course, and social and psychological assistance should be incorporated into the multidisciplinary management of the patients and their families.

Bach JR, Ishikawa Y, Kim H: Prevention of pulmonary morbidity for patients with Duchenne muscular dystrophy. *Chest* 1997;112:1024–28.

Gozal D: Pulmonary manifestations of neuromuscular disease: Focus on Duchenne muscular dystrophy and spinal muscular atrophy. *Pediatr Pulmonol* 2000;29:141–50.

Hukins CA, Hillman DR: Daytime predictors of sleep hypoventilation in Duchenne muscular dystrophy. *Am J Respir Crit Care Med* 2000;161:166–70.

Phillips ME, Smith PEM, Carroll N, et al: Nocturnal oxygenation and prognosis in Duchenne muscular dystrophy. *Am J Respir Crit Care Med* 1999;160:198–202.

Simonds AK, Ward S, Heather S, et al: Outcome of paediatric domiciliary mask ventilation in neuromuscular and skeletal disease. *Eur Respir J* 2000;16:476–81.

TABLE 410–1. Guidelines for Initial Evaluation and Follow-up of Patients with Neuromuscular Disease

Initial Evaluation	Basic Intervention/Training
History/physical examination/anthropometrics	Nutritional consultation and guidance
Lung function and maximal respiratory pressures (PFT)	Regular chest physiotherapy
Arterial blood gas analysis	Use of percussive devices
Polysomnography	Respiratory muscle training
Exercise testing (in selected cases)	Annual influenza vaccine
If vital capacity > 60% predicted or maximal respiratory pressures > 60 cm H$_2$O	Evaluate PFT every 6 mo; chest film and polysomnography yearly
If vital capacity > 60% predicted or maximal respiratory pressures > 60 cm H$_2$O	MIP/MEP every 6 mo; polysomnography every 6 mo to yearly

PFT = pulmonary function tests; MIP = maximal inspiratory pressure; MEP = maximal expiratory pressure.

Chapter 411

Extrapulmonary Diseases with Pulmonary Manifestations *Susanna A. McColley*

The embryology, anatomy, and physiology of the respiratory system lead to the occurrence of a number of respiratory symptoms that originate from extrapulmonary processes. The respiratory system adapts to metabolic demands and is exquisitely responsive to cortical input; therefore, tachypnea is common in the presence of metabolic stress such as fever, whereas dyspnea may be related to anxiety. Cough most commonly arises from upper or lower respiratory tract disorders, but it can originate from the central nervous system, as with cough tic or psychogenic cough, or it can be a prominent symptom in children with gastroesophageal reflux disease. In contrast, chest pain does not commonly arise from pulmonary processes in otherwise healthy children but more often has a neuromuscular or inflammatory etiology. Cyanosis may be caused by cardiac or hematologic disorders, and dyspnea and exercise intolerance may have a number of extrapulmonary causes. These disorders may be suspected on the basis of the history and physical examination, or they may be considered in children who have atypical findings on diagnostic studies or poor response to usual therapy. Some of the more common causes of such symptoms are listed in Table 411–1. In evaluating a child or adolescent with respiratory symptoms, it is extremely important to obtain a detailed past medical history, family history, and review of systems to evaluate the possibility of extrapulmonary origin. A comprehensive physical examination is also essential in obtaining clues to extrapulmonary disease.

Disorders of other organ systems, and many systemic diseases, may have significant respiratory system involvement. Although it is most common to encounter these complications in patients with known diagnoses, respiratory system disease is sometimes the sole or most prominent symptom at the time of presentation. For example, acute aspiration during feeding can be the presentation of neuromuscular disease in an infant who initially appears to have normal muscle tone and development. Complications may be life threatening, particularly in patients with immunocompromise. Conversely, the onset of respiratory findings may be insidious; for example, pulmonary vascular involvement in patients with systemic vasculitis may appear as an abnormality in diffusing capacity of the lung for carbon monoxide (DL_{CO}) before the onset of symptoms. Disorders that commonly have respiratory complications are listed in Table 411–2.

TABLE 411–1. **Respiratory Signs and Symptoms Originating from Outside the Respiratory Tract**

Sign Symptom	Nonrespiratory Causes	Pathophysiology	Clues to Diagnosis
Chest pain	Cardiac disease	Inflammation (pericarditis), ischemia (anomalous coronary artery, vascular disease)	Precordial pain, friction rub on examination; exertional pain, radiation to arm or neck
Chest pain	Gastroesophageal reflux disease	Esophageal inflammation and/or spasm	Heartburn, abdominal pain
Cyanosis	Congenital heart disease	Right-to-left shunt	Neonatal onset, lack of response to oxygen
Cyanosis	Methemoglobinemia	Increased levels of metHgb interfere with delivery of oxygen to tissues	Drug or toxin exposure, lack of response to oxygen
Dyspnea	Toxin exposure, drug side effect, or overdose	Variable, but often metabolic acidosis	Drug or toxin exposure confirmed by history or toxicology screen, normal SpO_2
Dyspnea	Anxiety, panic disorder	Increased respiratory drive and increased perception of respiratory efforts	Occurs during stressful situations, other symptoms of anxiety or depression
Exercise intolerance	Anemia	Inadequate oxygen deliver to tissues	Pallor, tachycardia, history of bleeding, history of inadequate diet
Exercise intolerance	Deconditioning	Self-explanatory	History of inactivity, obesity
Hemoptysis	Nasal bleeding	Posterior flow of bleeding causes appearance of pulmonary origin	History and physical examination suggest nasal source, normal chest examination, and chest radiography
Hemoptysis	Upper gastrointestinal tract bleeding	Hematemesis mimics hemoptysis	History and physical examination suggest gastrointestinal source, normal chest examination and chest radiography
Wheezing, cough, dyspnea	Congenital or acquired cardiac disease	Pulmonary overcirculation (ASD, VSD, PDA), left ventricular dysfunction	Murmur Refractory to bronchodilators Radiographic changes (prominent pulmonary vasculature, pulmonary edema)
Wheezing, cough	Gastroesophagel reflux disease	Laryngeal and bronchial response to stomach contents ?Vagally mediated bronchoconstriction	Emesis, pain, heartburn Refractory to bronchodilators

ASD = atrial septal defect; VSD = ventricular septal defect; PDA = patent ductus arteriosus.

TABLE 411–2. Disorders with Frequent Respiratory Tract Complications

Underlying Disorder	Respiratory Complications	Diagnostic Tests
Autoimmune disorders	Pulmonary vascular disease, restrictive lung disease, pleural effusion (especially lupus), upper airway disease (Wegener granulomatosis)	Spirometry, lung volume determination, oximetry, DLco, chest radiography, upper airway endoscopy and/or CT scan
Central nervous system disease (static or progressive)	Aspiration of oral or gastric contents	Chest radiography, videofluoroscopic swallowing study, esophageal pH probe, fiberoptic bronchoscopy
Immunodeficiency	Infection, bronchiectasis	Chest radiography, fiberoptic bronchoscopy, chest CT
Liver disease	Pleural effusion, hepatopulmonary syndrome	Chest radiography, assessment of orthodeoxia
Malignancy and its therapies	Infiltration, metastasis, malignant or infectious effusion, parenchymal infection, graft versus host disease (bone marrow transplant)	Chest radiography, chest CT, fiberoptic bronchoscopy, lung biopsy
Neuromuscular disease (see Part XXVII)	Hypoventilation, atelectasis, pneumonia	Spirometry, lung volume determination, respiratory muscle force measurements
Obesity	Restrictive lung disease, obstructive sleep apnea syndrome	Spirometry, lung volume determination, nocturnal polysomnography

Bowman CM: Hemoptysis. In Loughlin GM, Eigen H (editors): *Respiratory Disease in Children: Diagnosis and Management.* Baltimore, Williams & Wilkins, 1994, pp 201–5.

Loughlin GM: Chest pain. In Loughlin GM, Eigen H (editors): *Respiratory Disease in Children: Diagnosis and Management.* Baltimore, Williams & Wilkins, 1994, pp 207–14.

Methemoglobinemia. eMedicine Journal: *Medicine*, 2002.

Chapter 412

Chronic Severe Respiratory Insufficiency *Zehava Noah and*

Cynthia Budek

Infants, children, and adolescents with disorders of central control of breathing, disease of the airways, residual lung disease after severe respiratory illness, and neuromuscular disorders may develop hypercarbic and/or hypoxemic chronic respiratory failure (Chapter 357.1). In most instances it is possible to identify a primary cause for the respiratory failure; however, many children may have additional factors. Less than 1% of patients admitted to pediatric intensive care units require long-term noninvasive or invasive ventilatory assistance.

ETIOLOGIES

Obstructive Sleep Apnea. See Chapter 369.

Central Apnea and Central Hypoventilation Syndromes. Common conditions include congenital central hypoventilation syndrome (CCHS, Ondine curse); a small percentage of children with myelomeningocele, hydrocephalus, and Arnold-Chiari malformation; and survivors of brainstem tumors. Children with these disorders do not sense hypercapnia, and some of them do not sense hypoxia. Although some children may be severely bradypneic or apneic during some sleep states, the classic finding in CCHS is hypoventilation in the absence of apnea or bradypnea (see Chapter 357.2). Polysomnography confirms the diagnosis by documenting episodes of poor or absent respiratory effort and poor or absent flow during sleep.

Lung Disease. Common conditions include bronchopulmonary dysplasia (BPD) and children recuperating from adult respiratory distress syndrome (ARDS). Former premature infants recuperating from respiratory distress syndrome may develop BPD (see Chapters 90.9 and 408). When extreme, this may progress to respiratory failure.

Severe Tracheo- and/or Bronchomalacia (Airway Malacia). Conditions associated with airway malacia include tracheo-

esophageal fistula, innominate artery compression, or pulmonary artery sling after surgical repair (see Chapter 376).

Neuromuscular Weakness. Disease states resulting in neuromuscular weakness include spinal muscular atrophy (see Chapter 603.2), neurodegenerative diseases, myasthenia gravis, spinal cord injuries, and postinfectious neurologic diseases such as Guillain-Barré syndrome. In addition, children recuperating from severe illness in the intensive care unit often have neuromuscular weakness from suboptimal nutrition coupled with the devastating catabolic effects of severe illness and residual effects of sedatives, analgesics, and muscle relaxants, particularly if steroids were administered. Children with neuromuscular disease have very limited ability to increase ventilation and usually do so by increasing respiratory rate. Because of weakness, retractions may not be observed. In severe illness, some of these children respond to increased respiratory load by becoming apneic. A look of panic, changes in vital signs such as significant tachycardia or bradycardia, and cyanosis may be the only signs of respiratory failure.

EVALUATION

Children with chronic respiratory insufficiency require a thorough evaluation to determine the characteristics and severity of the condition and its effect on physical function (Chapters 357 and 370). The evaluation should include a complete physical examination, radiologic studies, pulmonary tests, nutritional evaluation, developmental assessment, and analysis of family dynamics. Most children with severe chronic respiratory insufficiency have a combination of factors contributing to their overall clinical status.

LONG-TERM MECHANICAL VENTILATION

Some children with chronic severe respiratory insufficiency will benefit from chronic ventilatory support. The goal of such support is to maintain normal oxygenation and ventilation and minimize work of breathing. Long-term ventilation in the home is a complex, physically demanding, emotionally taxing, and expensive process for the family and for society. It changes the family's way of life, priorities, and relationships. It may adversely affect marital and other relationships.

The prognosis of the disease is a critical factor in deciding to initiate long-term ventilation. The discharge process on ventilatory support should start as soon as the child is medically stable, on equipment that can be maintained in the home. Children with degenerative neuromuscular disease such as type I spinal muscular atrophy (SMA) suffer from respiratory failure very early in life, often triggered by the first respiratory illness. Although some parents decide to provide only palliative end-of-life care for the child with SMA, others choose long-term invasive or noninvasive ventilatory support. Young children with chronic lung disease and airway malacia have the potential to improve their pulmonary function and wean successfully off ventilator support if provided with adequate ventilation, good nutrition, and measures to promote development and prevent further lung injury.

Successful home discharge of a patient receiving mechanical ventilation depends on adequate resources in the community to support the family. Some hospital programs that transition children home on ventilators utilize professional nurses in the home to assist with round-the-clock care. This depends on funding as well as availability of nursing agencies in the community. Housing can be a significant barrier to home discharge because there must be adequate space for the child and caretakers; equipment and supplies; environmental safety including compliance with building and electrical codes; and home modifications for mobility, including ramping and lifts.

Funding for home care is usually a difficult issue for this population of children. If they do have private insurance, coverage for home care benefits is frequently limited. For children eligible for public aid, most states have funds available to meet the special needs of children who are ventilator dependent, although the extent of coverage varies considerably between geographic areas.

RESPIRATORY EQUIPMENT FOR HOME CARE

Modes of mechanical ventilation support are outlined in Chapter 57.4.

Noninvasive. A number of machines are available for the delivery of continuous and bilevel positive airway pressure. These machines attach to face masks and are best suited for the treatment of obstructive sleep apnea. Long-term use of these devices in small children may result in midface dysplasia. They occasionally may be used for the delivery of positive pressure through a tracheostomy for infants with tracheobronchomalacia. This type of ventilation has also been used in less severely affected patients with recurrent atelectasis, nighttime hypoventilation, or both.

Rocker Bed. A rocker bed moves in a longitudinal see-saw motion at a set rate. The child is secured to the bed with a strap. Movement of the bed promotes diaphragm movement. The bed may be an option for children with mild neuromuscular weakness, for instance when recuperating from Guillain-Barré syndrome. This device should not be placed in a home with toddlers or young children because they may get trapped in its mechanism.

Cuirass. This is a negative pressure device that resembles a turtle shell. It is designed to fit over the anterior chest and provide a tight seal. Cycled negative pressure is applied to the child's chest through a hole in the cuirass. These devices are suitable only for infants and children with mild neuromuscular weakness. A plastic bag–like device that fits snugly around the chest applies the same principle.

Iron Lung. The iron lung is a cumbersome device that applies negative pressure to the child's body. The child is placed in the iron lung cylinder with the head extending outside the device. A cuff is placed around the neck to minimize air leaks. Negative pressure is cycled within the iron lung, facilitating chest wall movement. Ventilation is disrupted when the device is opened to deliver care. This device is suitable for children with muscular weakness who require ventilation for part of the day. Its main advantage is that it does not require a tracheostomy; however, upper airway obstruction may occur, and this risk requires ongoing evaluation. A lighter version of this device is available for travel.

Diaphragmatic Pacing. Diaphragmatic pacers may be considered for children with central hypoventilation and those with high spinal cord injury. Surgically, electrodes are placed over the phrenic nerves and a receiver is placed in the subcutaneous tissue. The external pacing device is small and light with antennae secured externally over the receiver. A tracheostomy may be required if there is no coordination between the pacing of the device and the opening of the glottis. Any failure in the electrode pacing wires or the receiver requires surgical intervention.

Positive Pressure Ventilation. Ideally, a ventilator intended for home use should be lightweight and small, be able to entrain room air, preferably have continuous flow, and have a wide range of settings (pressure, volume, pressure support, and rate) that would allow ventilation from infancy to adulthood. The equipment must also be impervious to electromagnetic interference and be relatively easy to understand and troubleshoot. A variety of ventilators that can be used in the home are available, and familiarity with these devices is necessary to choose the best option for the child.

DISCHARGE PROCESS

The initial discharge process for a child going home on a ventilator is complex. A multidisciplinary, coordinated team approach is needed to develop a comprehensive plan that addresses medical, psychosocial, developmental, educational, and safety issues. The ventilated child must demonstrate medical stability that can be safely managed at home; interventions to maintain stability should be minimal before discharge. The child should be changed to a ventilator suitable for home use that allows portability as well as adequate ventilation. Medical management should also focus on weaning oxygen and ventilator parameters to settings appropriate for home care. Depending on the type of ventilation employed, a tracheostomy may be placed to promote comfort and a stable airway as soon as the decision to chronically ventilate is made.

Nutrition should be optimized to promote growth yet minimize excessive weight gain and carbon dioxide production. The nutritional requirements of a ventilated child are frequently decreased owing to supported work of breathing. The ventilated child often has problems with swallowing from dyscoordination and oral aversion secondary to intubation. Speech therapy should be introduced early to begin oromotor therapy and return of swallow. Many children require gastrostomy tube placement to replace or supplement oral intake. Evaluation and management of reflux and the risk of aspiration should also be considered because these are common problems in ventilated children. Communication devices to augment speech should be part of the planning.

Training of caregivers should be initiated early in the discharge process and be provided by nurses, respiratory care practitioners, and physical, occupational, and speech therapists. Caregivers must be trained in all aspects of care, including tracheostomy care, ventilator management, and cardiopulmonary resuscitation. Their independence in delivery of care at the bedside and while transporting the child should be emphasized. Caregivers must demonstrate their proficiency before the child is discharged.

Community agencies should be identified for provision of home support services. This may include a nursing agency to provide private duty nursing services. It is ideal to train home care nurses about the ventilator and the child's care before home discharge. An equipment vendor should be selected who can provide the ventilator equipment supplies and service. A care conference including the hospital team, funding agency, home nursing agency, equipment vendor, and family caregivers, should take place before discharge. The conference is important for coordination of last minute details and, thus, facilitate a smooth transition to home.

Providing continued support to the child and family after discharge is very important. The pediatrician in the community has a central role in providing coordination of care, well-child care, and all other medical needs, with the possible exception of ventilatory care. Equally important is the establishment of lines of communication to the medical center and the provision of timely access for advice and troubleshooting during the intervals between multidisciplinary clinic visits.

Frates RC Jr, Splaingard ML, Smith EO, et al: Outcome of home mechanical ventilation in children. *J Pediatr* 1985;106:850–56.

Hammer J: Home mechanical ventilation in children: Indications and practical aspects. *J Suisse Med* 2000;130:1894–902.

Jardine E, O'Toole M, Paton JY, et al: Current status of long term ventilation of children in the United Kingdom: Questionnaire survey. *BMJ* 1999;318:295–99.

Jardine E, Wallis C: Core guidelines for the discharge home of the child on long-term assisted ventilation in the United Kingdom. UK Working Party on Paediatric Long Term Ventilation. *Thorax* 1998;53:762–67.

Mallory GB Jr, Stillwell PC: The ventilator-dependent child: Issues in diagnosis and management. *Arch Phys Med Rehabil* 1991;72:43–55.

Nelson VS, Carroll JC, Hurvitz EA, et al: Home mechanical ventilation of children. *Dev Med Child Neurol* 1996;38:704–15.

O'Donohue WJ Jr, Giovannoni RM, Goldberg AI, et al: Long-term mechanical ventilation: Guidelines for management in the home and at alternate community sites. Report of the Ad Hoc Committee, Respiratory Care Section, American College of Chest Physicians. *Chest* 1986;90:1S–37S.

Oren J, Kelly DLH, Shannon DC: Long-term follow-up of children with congenital central hypoventilation syndrome. *Pediatrics* 1987;80:375–80.

Panitch HB, Downes JJ, Kennedy JS, et al: Guidelines for home care of children with chronic respiratory insufficiency. *Pediatr Pulmonol* 1996;21:52–56.

Quint RD, Chesterman E, Crain LS, et al: Home care for ventilator-dependent children: Psychosocial impact on the family. *Am J Dis Child* 1990;144:1238–41.

Schreiner MS, Downes JJ, Kettrick RG, et al: Chronic respiratory failure in infants with prolonged ventilator dependency. *JAMA* 1987;258:3398–404.

Splaingard ML, Frates RC Jr, Harrison GM, et al: Home positive-pressure ventilation: Twenty years' experience. *Chest* 1983;84:376–82.

The Cardiovascular System

SECTION 1 *Developmental Biology of the Cardiovascular System*

Daniel Bernstein

Chapter 413

Cardiac Development

Knowledge of the cellular and molecular mechanisms of cardiac development is necessary to understand congenital heart defects and develop strategies for prevention. Cardiac defects were grouped by common morphologic patterns: abnormalities of the outflow tracts (conotruncal lesions such as the tetralogy of Fallot and truncus arteriosus) and abnormalities of atrioventricular septation (primum atrial septal defect, complete atrioventricular canal defect). These morphologic categories may not, however, provide an understanding of the mechanisms of genetic alterations that lead to congenital heart disease.

413.1 Early Cardiac Morphogenesis

In the early presomite embryo, the first identifiable cardiac precursors are angiogenetic cell clusters arranged on both sides of the embryo's central axis; these clusters form paired cardiac tubes by 18 days of gestation. The paired tubes fuse in the midline on the ventral surface of the embryo to form the primitive heart tube by 22 days. Premyocardial cells, including epicardial cells and cells derived from the neural crest, continue their migration into the region of the heart tube. Regulation of this early phase of cardiac morphogenesis is controlled in part by the interaction of specific signaling molecules or ligands, usually expressed by one cell type, with specific receptors, usually expressed by another cell type. Positional information is conveyed to the developing cardiac mesoderm by retinoids, isoforms of vitamin A, which bind to specific nuclear receptors and regulate gene transcription. Migration of epithelial cells into the developing heart tube is directed by extracellular matrix proteins, such as fibronectin, interacting with cell surface receptors, such as the integrins. The importance of these ligands is noted clinically by the spectrum of human cardiac teratogenic effects caused by the retinoid-like drug isotretinoin.

As early as 20–22 days, before cardiac looping, the embryonic heart begins to contract and exhibit phases of the cardiac cycle that are surprisingly similar to those in a mature heart. Morphologists have identified segments of the heart tube that were believed to correspond to structures in a mature heart (Fig. 413–1): the sinus venosus and atrium (right and left atria), the primitive ventricle (left ventricle), the bulbus cordis (right ventricle), and the truncus arteriosus (aorta and pulmonary artery). This model is oversimplified, however. Only the trabecular (most heavily muscularized) portions of the left ventricular myocardium are present in the early cardiac tube; the cells that will become the inlet portion of the left ventricle migrate into

the cardiac tube at a later stage (after looping is initiated). Even later to appear are the primordial cells that give rise to the great arteries (truncus arteriosus), including cells derived from the neural crest, which are not present until after cardiac looping is complete. Chamber-specific transcription factors participate in the differentiation of the right and left ventricles. The basic helix-loop-helix transcription factor dHAND is expressed in the developing right ventricle; disruption of this gene in mice leads to hypoplasia of the right ventricle. The transcription factor eHAND is expressed in the developing left ventricle and conotruncus.

413.2 Cardiac Looping

At approximately 22–24 days, the heart tube begins to bend ventrally and toward the right (see Fig. 413–1) through unknown biomechanical forces. Looping brings the future left ventricle leftward and in continuity with the sinus venosus (future left and right atria), whereas the future right ventricle is shifted rightward and in continuity with the truncus arteriosus (future aorta and pulmonary artery). This pattern of development explains the relatively common occurrence of the cardiac anomalies double-outlet right ventricle and double-inlet left ventricle and the extreme rarity of double-outlet left ventricle and double-inlet right ventricle (see Chapter 423.5). Cardiac looping, one of the first manifestations of right-left asymmetry in the developing embryo, is critical for the successful completion of cardiac morphogenesis. When cardiac looping is abnormal, the incidence of serious cardiac malformations is high.

Potential mechanisms of cardiac looping include differential growth rates for myocytes on the convex vs the concave surface of the curve, differential rates of programmed cell death (apoptosis), and mechanical forces generated within myocardial cells via their actin cytoskeleton. The signal for this directionality may be contained in a concentration gradient between the right and left sides of the embryo by the expression of critical signaling molecules (members of the tumor growth factor-β family of peptide growth factors and signaling peptides such as *Sonic hedgehog*). In murine models of abnormal looping, one such defect resides in the dynein gene.

413.3 Cardiac Septation

When looping is complete, the external appearance of the heart is similar to that of a mature heart; internally, the structure resembles a single tube, although it now has several bulges resulting in the appearance of primitive chambers. The common atrium (comprising both the right and left atria) is connected to the primitive ventricle (future left ventricle) via the atrioventricular canal. The primitive ventricle is connected to the bulbus

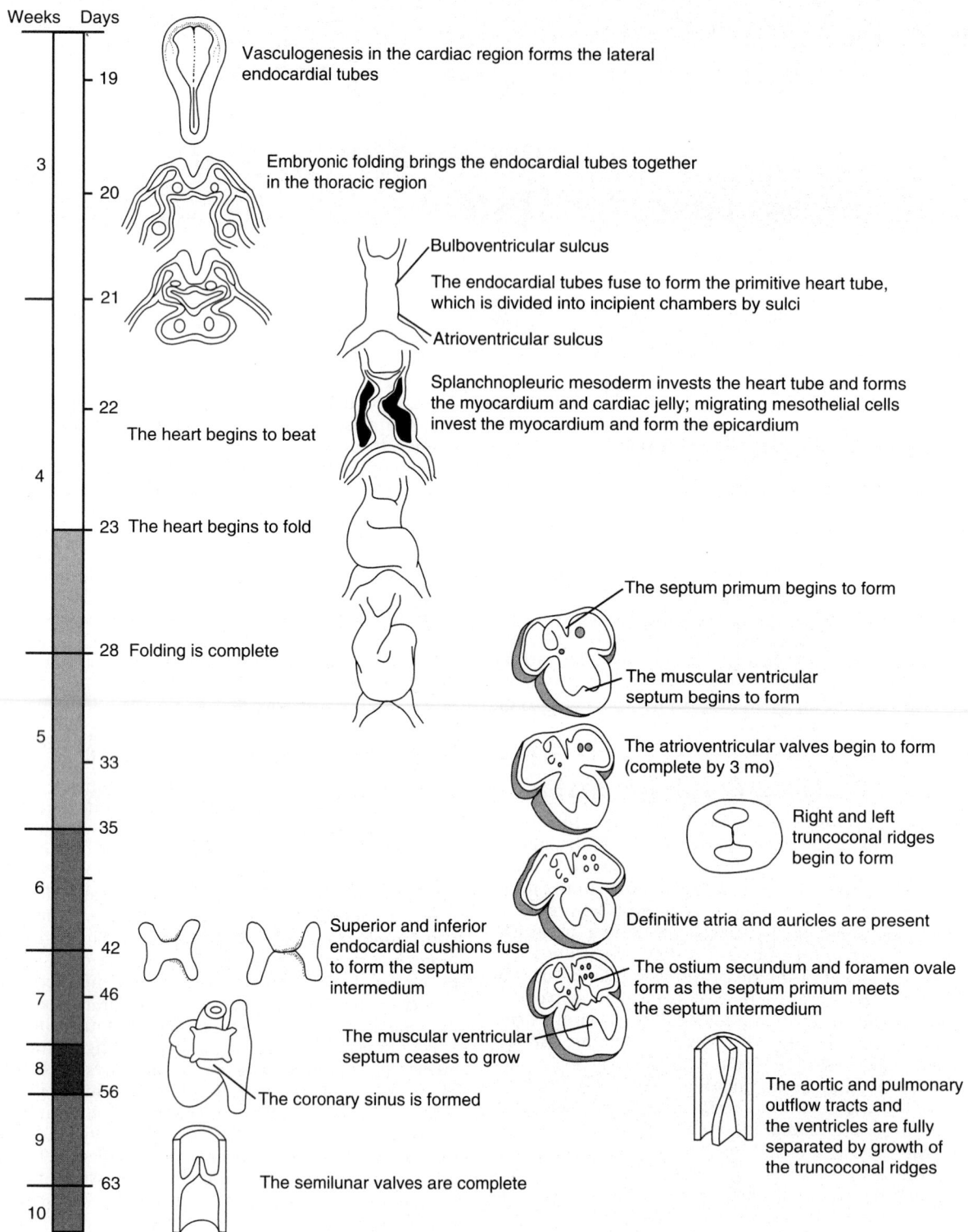

Weeks | Days

19 — Vasculogenesis in the cardiac region forms the lateral endocardial tubes

3

20 — Embryonic folding brings the endocardial tubes together in the thoracic region

21 — Bulboventricular sulcus

The endocardial tubes fuse to form the primitive heart tube, which is divided into incipient chambers by sulci

Atrioventricular sulcus

22 — Splanchnopleuric mesoderm invests the heart tube and forms the myocardium and cardiac jelly; migrating mesothelial cells invest the myocardium and form the epicardium

The heart begins to beat

4

23 — The heart begins to fold

The septum primum begins to form

28 — Folding is complete

The muscular ventricular septum begins to form

5

33 — The atrioventricular valves begin to form (complete by 3 mo)

Right and left truncoconal ridges begin to form

35 —

6

Definitive atria and auricles are present

42 — Superior and inferior endocardial cushions fuse to form the septum intermedium

7   46 —

The ostium secundum and foramen ovale form as the septum primum meets the septum intermedium

The muscular ventricular septum ceases to grow

8   56 — The coronary sinus is formed

The aortic and pulmonary outflow tracts and the ventricles are fully separated by growth of the truncoconal ridges

9

63 — The semilunar valves are complete

10

TIMELINE. FORMATION OF THE HEART.

FIGURE 413–1. Timeline of cardiac morphogenesis. (From Larsen WJ: *Essentials of Human Embryology.* New York, Churchill Livingstone, 1998.)

cordis (future right ventricle) via the bulboventricular foramen. The distal portion of the bulbus cordis is connected to the truncus arteriosus via an outlet segment (the conus).

The heart tube now consists of several layers of myocardium and a single layer of endocardium separated by cardiac jelly, an acellular extracellular matrix secreted by the myocardium.

Septation of the heart begins at approximately day 26 with the ingrowth of large tissue masses, the endocardial cushions, at both the atrioventricular and conotruncal junctions (see Fig. 413–1). These cushions consist of protrusions of cardiac jelly, which in addition to their role in development, also serve a physiologic function as primitive heart valves. Endocardial cells dedifferentiate and migrate into the cardiac jelly in the region of the endocardial cushions, eventually becoming mesenchymal cells that will form part of the atrioventricular valves.

Complete septation of the atrioventricular canal occurs with fusion of the endocardial cushions. Most of the atrioventricular valve tissue is derived from the ventricular myocardium in a process involving undermining of the ventricular walls. Because this process occurs asymmetrically, the tricuspid valve annulus sits closer to the apex of the heart than the mitral valve annulus does. Physical separation of these two valves produces the atrioventricular septum, the absence of which is the primary common defect in patients with atrioventricular canal defects (see Chapter 419.5). If the process of undermining is incomplete, one of the atrioventricular valves may not separate normally from the ventricular myocardium, a possible cause of Ebstein anomaly (see Chapter 423.7).

Septation of the atria begins at approximately 30 days with growth of the septum primum downward toward the endocardial cushions (see Fig. 413–1). The orifice that remains is the ostium primum. The endocardial cushions then fuse and, together with the completed septum primum, divide the atrioventricular canal into right and left segments. A 2nd opening appears in the posterior portion of the septum primum, the ostium secundum, and it allows a portion of the fetal venous return to the right atrium to pass across to the left atrium. Finally, the septum secundum grows downward, just to the right of the septum primum. Together with a flap of the septum primum, the ostium secundum forms the foramen ovale, through which fetal blood passes from the inferior vena cava to the left atrium (see Chapter 414).

Septation of the ventricles begins at about day 25 with protrusions of endocardium in both the inlet (primitive ventricle) and outlet (bulbus cordis) segments of the heart. The inlet protrusions fuse into the bulboventricular septum and extend posteriorly toward the inferior endocardial cushion, where they give rise to the inlet and trabecular portions of the interventricular septum. Ventricular septal defects can occur in any portion of the developing interventricular septum (see Chapter 419.6). The outlet or conotruncal septum develops from ridges of cardiac jelly, similar to the atrioventricular cushions. These ridges fuse to form a spiral septum that brings the future pulmonary artery into communication with the anterior and rightward right ventricle and the future aorta into communication with the posterior and leftward left ventricle. Differences in cell growth of the outlet septum lead to lengthening of the segment of smooth muscle beneath the pulmonary valve (conus), a process that separates the tricuspid and pulmonary valves. In contrast, disappearance of the segment beneath the aortic valve leads to fibrous continuity of the mitral and aortic valves. Defects in these processes are responsible for conotruncal and aortic arch defects (truncus arteriosus, tetralogy of Fallot, pulmonary atresia, double-outlet right ventricle, interrupted aortic arch), a group of cardiac anomalies often associated with deletions of the DiGeorge critical region of chromosome 22q11 (see Chapters 423 and 424).

413.4   Aortic Arch Development

The aortic arch, head and neck vessels, proximal pulmonary arteries, and ductus arteriosus develop from the aortic sac, arterial arches, and dorsal aortae. When the straight heart tube develops, the distal outflow portion bifurcates into the right and left 1st aortic arches, which join the paired dorsal aortae (Fig. 413–2). The dorsal aortae will fuse to form the descending aorta. The proximal aorta from the aortic valve to the left carotid artery arises from the aortic sac. The 1st and 2nd arches largely regress by about 22 days, with the 1st aortic arch giving rise to the maxillary artery and the 2nd to the stapedial and hyoid arteries. The 3rd arches participate in the formation of the innominate artery and the common and internal carotid arteries. The right 4th arch gives rise to the innominate and right subclavian arteries, and the left 4th arch participates in formation of the segment of the aortic arch between the left carotid artery and the ductus arteriosus. The 5th arch does not persist as a major structure in the mature circulation. The 6th arches join the more distal pulmonary arteries, with the right 6th arch giving rise to a portion of the proximal right pulmonary artery and the left 6th arch

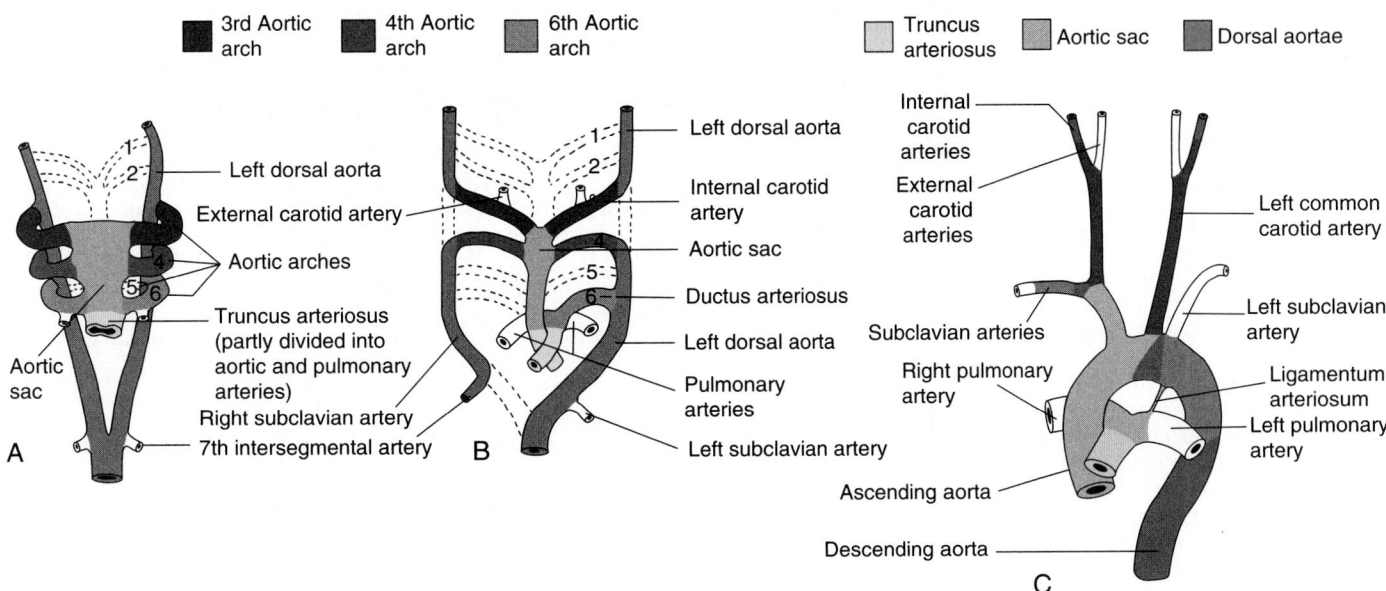

FIGURE 413–2. Schematic drawings illustrating the changes that result during transformation of the truncus arteriosus, aortic sac, aortic arches, and dorsal aortae into the adult arterial pattern. The vessels that are not shaded or colored are not derived from these structures. *A,* Aortic arches at 6 wk; by this stage the 1st two pairs of aortic arches have largely disappeared. *B,* Aortic arches at 7 wk; the parts of the dorsal aortae and aortic arches that normally disappear are indicated by *broken lines. C,* Arterial vessels of a 6-mo-old infant. (From Moore KL, Persaud TVN: *The Developing Human.* Philadelphia, WB Saunders, 1993.)

giving rise to the ductus arteriosus. The aortic arch between the ductus arteriosus and the left subclavian artery is derived from the left-sided dorsal aorta, whereas the aortic arch distal to the left subclavian artery is derived from the fused right and left dorsal aortae. Abnormalities in development of the paired aortic arches are responsible for right aortic arch, double aortic arch, and vascular rings (see Chapter 425.1).

413.5   Cardiac Differentiation

The process by which the totipotential cells of the early embryo become committed to specific cell lineages is called *differentiation*. Precardiac mesodermal cells differentiate into mature cardiac muscle cells with an appropriate complement of cardiac-specific contractile elements, regulatory proteins, receptors, and ion channels. Expression of the contractile protein myosin occurs at an early stage of cardiac development, even before fusion of the bilateral heart primordia. Differentiation in these early mesodermal cells is regulated by signals from the anterior endoderm, a process known as *induction*. Several putative early signaling molecules include fibroblast growth factor, activin, and insulin. Signaling molecules interact with receptors on the cell surface; these receptors activate 2nd messengers, which in turn activate specific *nuclear transcription factors* (GATA-4, MEF2, Nkx, bHLH, and the retinoic acid receptor family) that induce the expression of specific gene products to regulate cardiac differentiation. Some of the primary disorders of cardiac muscle, the cardiomyopathies, may be related to defects in some of these signaling molecules (see Chapter 431).

Developmental processes are chamber specific. Early in development, ventricular myocytes express both ventricular and atrial *isoforms* of several proteins, such as atrial natriuretic peptide (ANP) and myosin light chain (MLC). Mature ventricular myocytes do not express ANP and express only a ventricular-specific MLC 2v isoform, whereas mature atrial myocytes express ANP and an atrial-specific MLC 2a isoform. Heart failure (see Chapter 434, volume overload (see Chapters 419 and 421), and pressure overload hypertrophy (see Chapter 420) are associated with a recapitulation of fetal cell phenotypes in which mature myocytes re-express fetal proteins. Because different isoforms have different contractile behavior (fast vs slow activation, high vs low adenosine triphosphatase activity), expression of different isoforms may have important functional consequences.

413.6   Developmental Changes in Cardiac Function

During development, the composition of the myocardium undergoes profound changes that result in an increase in the number and size of myocytes. During prenatal life, this process involves myocyte division *(hyperplasia)*, whereas after the 1st few postnatal weeks, subsequent cardiac growth occurs by an increase in myocyte size *(hypertrophy)*. The myocytes themselves change shape from round to cylindrical, the proportion of myofibrils (which contain the contractile apparatus) increases, and the myofibrils become more regular in their orientation.

The plasma membrane (known as the *sarcolemma* in myocytes) is the location of the ion channels and transmembrane receptors that regulate the exchange of chemical information from the cell surface to the cell interior. Ion fluxes through these channels control the processes of depolarization and repolarization. Developmental changes have been described for the sodium-potassium pump, the sodium-hydrogen exchanger, and voltage-dependent calcium channels. As the myocyte matures, extensions of the sarcolemma develop toward the interior of the

cell (the t-tubule system), which dramatically increases its surface area and enhances rapid activation of the myocyte. Regulation of the membrane's α- and β-adrenergic receptors with development enhances the ability of the sympathetic nervous system to control cardiac function as the heart matures.

The *sarcoplasmic reticulum (SR)*, a series of tubules surrounding the myofibrils, controls the intracellular calcium concentration. A series of pumps regulate calcium release to the myofibrils for initiation of contraction (ryanodine-sensitive calcium channel) and calcium uptake for initiation of relaxation (adenosine triphosphate–dependent SR calcium pump). In immature hearts, this SR calcium transport system is less well developed, and such hearts consequently have an increased dependence on transport of calcium from outside the cell for contraction. In a mature heart, the majority of calcium to activate contraction comes from the SR. This developmental phenomenon may explain the sensitivity of the infant heart to sarcolemmal calcium channel blockers such as verapamil, which often results in a marked depression in contractility and cardiac arrest (see Chapter 428).

The major contractile proteins (myosin, actin, tropomyosin, and troponin) are organized into the functional unit of cardiac contraction, the sarcomere. Each has several isoforms that are expressed differentially by location (atrium vs ventricle) and by developmental stage (embryo, fetus, newborn, adult).

Changes in myocardial structure and myocyte biochemistry result in easily quantifiable differences in cardiac function with development. In isolated cardiac muscle strips, the force of contraction increases with maturation from fetus to adult. Fetal cardiac function is poorly responsive to changes in both preload (filling volume) and afterload (systemic resistance). The most effective means of increasing ventricular function in a fetus is through increasing the heart rate. After birth and with further maturation, preload and afterload play an increasing role in regulating cardiac function. The rate of cardiac relaxation is also developmentally regulated. The decreased ability of the immature SR calcium pump to remove calcium from the contractile apparatus is manifested as a decreased ability of the fetal heart to enhance relaxation in response to sympathetic stimulation. This inability of the immature myocardium to use preload effectively may partly explain the difficulty that most premature infants have in compensating for the left-to-right shunt through a patent ductus arteriosus (see Chapters 90.3 and 419.8).

Baldwin HS, Artman M: Recent advances in cardiovascular development: Promise for the future. *Cardiovasc Res* 1998;40:456–68.

Botto LD, Khoury MJ, Mulinare J, et al: Periconceptional multivitamin use and the occurrence of conotruncal heart defects: Results from a population-based, case-control study. *Pediatrics* 1996;98:911.

Bowers PN, Brueckner M, Yost HJ: The genetics of left-right development and heterotaxia. *Semin Perinatol* 1996;20:577.

Chen JN, Fishman MC: Genetics of heart development. *Trends Genet* 2000;16:383–8.

Eisenberg LM, Markwald RR: Molecular regulation of atrioventricular valvuloseptal morphogenesis. *Circ Res* 1995;77:1.

Epstein JA, Buck CA: Transcriptional regulation of cardiac development: Implications for congenital heart disease and DiGeorge syndrome. *Pediatr Res* 2000;48:717–24.

Kathiriya IS, Srivastava D: Left-right asymmetry and cardiac looping: Implications for cardiac development and congenital heart disease. *Am J Med Genet* 2000;97:271–9.

McDonald-McGinn DM, Driscoll DA, Emanuel BS, et al: Detection of a 22q11.2 deletion in cardiac patients suggests a risk for velopharyngeal incompetence. *Pediatrics* 1997;99:1.

Smith SM, Dickman ED, Power SC, Lancman J: Retinoids and their receptors in vertebrate embryogenesis. *J Nutr* 1998;128(2 Suppl):467S.

Srivastava D: HAND proteins: Molecular mediators of cardiac development and congenital heart disease. *Trends Cardiovasc Med* 1999;9:11–8.

Towbin JA, Belmont J: Molecular determinants of left and right outflow tract obstruction. *Am J Med Genet* 2000;97:297–303.

Chapter 414
The Fetal-to-Neonatal Circulatory Transition

414.1 The Fetal Circulation

The human fetal circulation and its adjustments after birth are for the most part similar to those of other large mammals, although rates of maturation differ. In the fetal circulation, the right and left ventricles exist in a parallel circuit, as opposed to the series circuit of a newborn or adult (Fig. 414–1*A*). In the fetus, the placenta provides for gas and metabolite exchange. The lungs do not provide gas exchange, and vessels in the pulmonary circulation are vasoconstricted. Three cardiovascular structures unique to the fetus are important for maintaining this parallel circulation: the ductus venosus, foramen ovale, and ductus arteriosus.

Oxygenated blood returning from the placenta flows to the fetus through the umbilical vein with a Po_2 of about 30–35 mm Hg. Approximately 50% of the umbilical venous blood enters the hepatic circulation, whereas the rest bypasses the liver and joins the inferior vena cava via the *ductus venosus,* where it partially mixes with poorly oxygenated inferior vena cava blood derived from the lower part of the fetal body. This combined lower body plus umbilical venous blood flow (Po_2 of about 26–28 mm Hg) enters the right atrium and is preferentially directed across the *foramen ovale* to the left atrium (see Fig. 414–1*B*). The blood then flows into the left ventricle and is ejected into the ascending aorta. Fetal superior vena cava blood, which is considerably less oxygenated (Po_2 of 12–14 mm Hg), enters the right atrium and preferentially traverses the tricuspid valve, rather than the foramen ovale, and flows primarily to the right ventricle.

From the right ventricle, the blood is ejected into the pulmonary artery. Because the pulmonary arterial circulation is vasoconstricted, only about 10% of right ventricular outflow enters the lungs. The major portion of this blood (which has a Po_2 of about 18–22 mm Hg) bypasses the lungs and flows through the *ductus arteriosus* into the descending aorta to perfuse the lower part of the fetal body, after which it returns to the placenta via the two umbilical arteries. Thus, the upper part of the fetal body (including the coronary and cerebral arteries and those to the upper extremities) is perfused exclusively from the left ventricle with blood that has a slightly higher Po_2 than the blood perfusing the lower part of the fetal body, which is derived mostly from the right ventricle. Only a small volume of blood from the ascending aorta (10% of fetal cardiac output) flows across the aortic isthmus to the descending aorta.

The total fetal cardiac output—the combined ventricular output of both the left and right ventricles—amounts to about 450 mL/kg/min. Approximately 65% of descending aortic blood flow returns to the placenta; the remaining 35% perfuses the fetal organs and tissues. In the sheep fetus, right ventricular output is approximately two times that of the left ventricle. In the human fetus, which has a larger percentage of blood flow going to the brain, right ventricular output is probably closer to 1.3 times left ventricular flow. Thus, during fetal life the right ventricle is not only pumping against systemic blood pressure but is also performing a greater volume of work than the left ventricle is.

414.2 The Transitional Circulation

At birth, mechanical expansion of the lungs and an increase in arterial Po_2 result in a rapid decrease in pulmonary vascular resistance. Concomitantly, removal of the low-resistance placental circulation leads to an increase in systemic vascular resistance. The output from the right ventricle now flows entirely into the pulmonary circulation, and because pulmonary vascular resistance becomes lower than systemic vascular resistance, the shunt through the ductus arteriosus reverses and becomes left to right. Over the course of several days, the high arterial Po_2 constricts the ductus arteriosus and it closes, eventually becoming the ligamentum arteriosum. The increased volume of pulmonary blood flow returning to the left atrium increases left atrial volume and pressure sufficiently to close the foramen ovale functionally, although the foramen may remain probe patent.

Removal of the placenta from the circulation also results in closure of the ductus venosus. The left ventricle is now coupled to the high-resistance systemic circulation, and its wall thickness and mass begin to increase. In contrast, the right ventricle is now coupled to the low-resistance pulmonary circulation, and its wall thickness and mass decrease slightly. The left ventricle, which in the fetus pumped blood only to the upper part of the body and brain, must now deliver the entire systemic cardiac output (approximately 350 mL/kg/min), an almost 200% increase in output. This marked increase in left ventricular performance is achieved through a combination of hormonal and metabolic signals, including an increase in the level of circulating catecholamines and the myocardial receptors (β-adrenergic) through which catecholamines have their effect.

When congenital structural cardiac defects are superimposed on these dramatic physiologic changes, they often impede this smooth transition and markedly increase the burden on the newborn myocardium. In addition, because the ductus arteriosus and foramen ovale do not close completely at birth, they may remain patent in certain congenital cardiac lesions. Patency of these fetal pathways may either provide a lifesaving pathway for blood to bypass a congenital defect (e.g., a patent ductus in pulmonary atresia or coarctation of the aorta or a foramen ovale in transposition of the great vessels) or present an additional stress to the circulation (patent ductus arteriosus in a premature infant, pathway for right-to-left shunting in infants with pulmonary hypertension). Therapeutic agents may either maintain these fetal pathways (e.g., prostaglandin E_1) or hasten their closure (indomethacin).

414.3 The Neonatal Circulation

At birth, the fetal circulation must immediately adapt to extrauterine life as gas exchange is transferred from the placenta to the lung (see Chapter 90.1). Some of these changes are virtually instantaneous with the 1st breath, whereas others develop over a period of hours or days. After an initial slight fall in systemic blood pressure, a progressive rise occurs with increasing age. The heart rate slows as a result of a baroreceptor response to an increase in systemic vascular resistance when the placental circulation is eliminated. The average central aortic pressure in a term neonate is 75/50 mm Hg.

With the onset of ventilation, pulmonary vascular resistance is markedly decreased as a consequence of both active (Po_2 related) and passive (mechanical related) vasodilation. In a normal neonate, closure of the ductus arteriosus and the fall in pulmonary vascular resistance result in a decrease in pulmonary arterial and right ventricular pressure. The major decline in pulmonary resistance from the high fetal levels to the low "adult" levels in the human infant at sea level usually occurs within the 1st 2–3 days but may be prolonged for 7 days or more. Over the 1st several weeks of life, pulmonary vascular resistance decreases even further secondary to remodeling of the pulmonary vasculature, including thinning of the vascular smooth

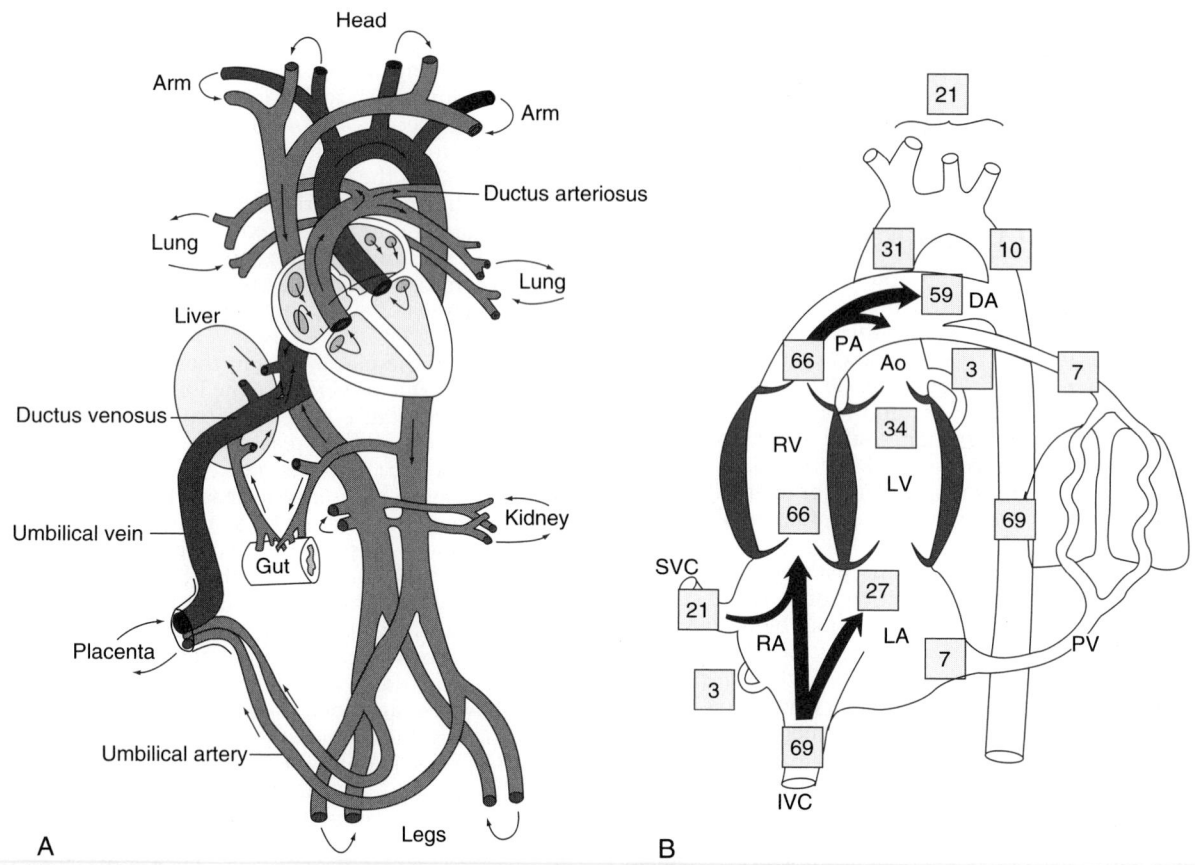

FIGURE 414–1. *A,* The human circulation before birth (partly after Dawes). *Black shading* indicates more oxygenated blood, and *arrows* indicate the direction of flow. *B,* Percentages of combined ventricular output that return to the fetal heart, that are ejected by each ventricle, and that flow through the main vascular channels. Figures are those obtained from study of late-gestation lambs. (From Rudolph AM: *Congenital Diseases of the Heart.* Chicago, Year Book, 1974.)

muscle and recruitment of new vessels. This decrease in pulmonary vascular resistance significantly influences the timing of the clinical appearance of many congenital heart lesions that are dependent on the relative systemic and pulmonary vascular resistance. For example, the left-to-right shunt through a ventricular septal defect may be minimal during the 1st wk after birth when pulmonary vascular resistance is still somewhat high. As pulmonary resistance decreases over the next week or two, the volume of the left-to-right shunt through the ventricular septal defect increases and eventually leads to symptoms of congestive heart failure.

Significant differences between the neonatal circulation and that of older infants may be summarized as follows: (1) right-to-left or left-to-right shunting may persist across the patent foramen ovale; (2) in the presence of cardiopulmonary disease, continued patency of the ductus arteriosus may allow left-to-right, right-to-left, or bidirectional shunting; (3) the neonatal pulmonary vasculature constricts more vigorously in response to hypoxemia, hypercapnia, and acidosis; (4) the wall thickness and muscle mass of the neonatal left and right ventricles are almost equal; and (5) newborn infants at rest have relatively high oxygen consumption, which is associated with relatively high cardiac output. The newborn cardiac output (about 350 mL/kg/min) falls over the 1st 2 mo of life to about 150 mL/kg/min and then more gradually to the normal adult cardiac output of about 75 mL/kg/min. The high percentage of fetal hemoglobin present in the newborn may actually interfere with delivery of oxygen to tissues in the neonate,

so increased cardiac output is needed for adequate delivery of oxygen (see Chapter 90.1).

The foramen ovale is functionally closed by the 3rd mo of life, although it is possible to pass a probe through the overlapping flaps in a large percentage of children and in 15–25% of adults. Functional closure of the ductus arteriosus is usually complete by 10–15 hr in a normal neonate, although the ductus may remain patent much longer in the presence of congenital heart disease, especially when associated with cyanosis. In premature newborn infants, an evanescent systolic murmur with late accentuation or a continuous murmur may be audible, and in the context of respiratory distress syndrome, the presence of a patent ductus arteriosus should be suspected (see Chapter 90.3).

The normal ductus arteriosus differs morphologically from the adjoining aorta and pulmonary artery in that the ductus has a significant amount of circularly arranged smooth muscle in its medial layer. During fetal life, patency of the ductus arteriosus appears to be maintained by the combined relaxant effects of low oxygen tension and endogenously produced prostaglandins, specifically prostaglandin E_2. In a full-term neonate, oxygen is the most important factor controlling ductal closure. When the Po_2 of the blood passing through the ductus reaches about 50 mm Hg, the ductal wall constricts. The effects of oxygen on ductal smooth muscle may be direct or mediated by its effects on prostaglandin synthesis. Gestational age also appears to play an important role; the ductus of a premature infant is less responsive to oxygen, even though its musculature is developed.

414.4 Persistent Pulmonary Hypertension of the Neonate (Persistence of Fetal Circulatory Pathways)

See also Chapter 90.7.

Abman SH: Abnormal vasoreactivity in the pathophysiology of persistent pulmonary hypertension of the newborn. *Pediatr Rev* 1999;20:e103–9.

Barst RJ, Gersony WM: The pharmacological treatment of patent ductus arteriosus: A review of the evidence. *Drugs* 1989;38:250.

Freed MD, Heymann MA, Lewis AB, et al: Prostaglandin E in infants with ductus arteriosus–dependent congenital heart disease. *Circulation* 1981;64:899.

Gersony WM, Peckham GH, Ellison RC, et al: Effects of indomethacin in premature infants with patent ductus arteriosus: Results of a national collaborative study. *J Pediatr* 1983;102:895.

Rudolph AM: *Congenital Diseases of the Heart: Clinical-Physiological Considerations,* 2nd ed. New York, Futura, 2001.

Rudolph AM: Distribution and regulation of blood flow in the fetal and neonatal lamb. *Circ Res* 1985;57:811.

Walsh MC, Stork EK: Persistent pulmonary hypertension of the newborn. Rational therapy based on pathophysiology. *Clin Perinatol* 2001;28:609–27.

SECTION 2 *Evaluation of the Cardiovascular System*

Daniel Bernstein

Chapter 415

History and Physical Examination

The importance of the history and physical examination cannot be overemphasized in the evaluation of infants and children with suspected cardiovascular disorders. Patients may require further laboratory evaluation and eventual treatment, or the family may be reassured that no significant problem exists. Although the ready availability of echocardiography may entice the clinician to skip these preliminary steps, an initial evaluation by a skilled cardiologist is preferred for several reasons: (1) a cardiac examination allows the cardiologist to guide the echocardiographic evaluation toward confirming or eliminating specific diagnoses, thereby increasing its accuracy; (2) because most childhood murmurs are innocent, evaluation by a pediatric cardiologist can eliminate unnecessary and expensive laboratory tests; and (3) the cardiologist's knowledge and experience are important in reassuring the patient's family and preventing unnecessary restrictions on healthy physical activity.

History. A comprehensive cardiac history starts with details of the perinatal period, including the presence of cyanosis, respiratory distress, or prematurity. Maternal complications such as gestational diabetes, medications, systemic lupus erythematosus, or substance abuse can be associated with cardiac problems. If cardiac symptoms began during infancy, the timing of the initial symptoms should be noted to provide important clues about the specific cardiac condition.

Many of the symptoms of congestive heart failure in infants and children are age specific. In infants, *feeding difficulties* are common. Inquiry should be made about the frequency of feeding and either the volume of each feeding or the time spent on each breast. An infant with heart failure often takes less volume per feeding and become dyspneic or diaphoretic while sucking. After falling asleep exhausted, the baby, inadequately fed, will awaken for the next feeding after a brief time. This cycle continues around the clock and must be carefully differentiated from colic or other feeding disorders. Additional symptoms and signs include those of *respiratory distress:* rapid breathing, nasal flaring, cyanosis, and chest retractions. In older children, heart failure may be manifested as *exercise intolerance,* difficulty keeping up with peers during sports or need for a nap after coming home from school, and poor growth. Eliciting a history of fatigue in an older child requires questions about age-specific activities, including stair climbing, walking, bicycle riding, physical education class, and competitive sports; information should be obtained regarding more severe manifestations such as orthopnea and nocturnal dyspnea.

Cyanosis at rest is often overlooked by parents; it may be mistaken for a normal individual variation in coloration. Cyanosis during crying or exercise, however, is more often noted as abnormal by observant parents. Many infants and toddlers turn "blue around the lips" when crying vigorously or during breath-holding spells; this condition must be carefully differentiated from cyanotic heart disease by inquiring about inciting factors, the length of episodes, and whether the tongue and mucous membranes also appear cyanotic. Newborns have cyanotic extremities **(acrocyanosis)** when undressed and cold, and this response to cold must be carefully differentiated from true cyanosis.

Chest pain is an unusual manifestation of cardiac disease in pediatric patients, although it is a frequent cause for referral to a pediatric cardiologist, especially in adolescents. Nonetheless, a careful history, physical examination, and if indicated, laboratory or imaging tests will assist in identifying the cause of chest pain (Box 415–1).

Cardiac disease may be a manifestation of a known congenital malformation syndrome with typical physical findings (Table 415–1) or a manifestation of a generalized disorder affecting the heart and other organ systems (Table 415–2). *Extracardiac malformations* may be noted in 20–45% of infants with congenital heart disease. Between 5 and 10% of patients have a known chromosomal abnormality; this percentage will increase as our knowledge of specific gene defects linked to congenital heart disease increases. A careful family history may also reveal early coronary artery disease or stroke (familial hypercholesterolemia or thrombophilia), generalized muscle disease (muscular dystrophy, dermatomyositis, familial or metabolic cardiomyopathy), or relatives with congenital heart disease.

General Physical Examination. After general assessment of the patient, specific attention is directed toward the presence of cyanosis, abnormalities in growth, and any evidence of respiratory distress. Evaluation of a murmur must always be performed in the context of other physical findings. Frequently, associated findings, such as the quality of the pulses or the presence of a

BOX 415–1. Differential Diagnosis of Chest Pain in Pediatric Patients

MUSCULOSKELETAL (COMMON)
Trauma (accidental, abuse)
Exercise, overuse injury (strain, bursitis)
Costochondritis (Tietze syndrome)
Herpes zoster (cutaneous)
Pleurodynia
Fibrositis
Slipping rib
Sickle cell anemia vaso-occlusive crisis
Osteomyelitis (rare)
Primary or metastatic tumor (rare)

PULMONARY (COMMON)
Pneumonia
Pleurisy
Asthma
Chronic cough
Pneumothorax
Infarction (sickle cell anemia)
Foreign body
Embolism (rare)
Pulmonary hypertension (rare)
Tumor (rare)
Bronchiectasis

GASTROINTESTINAL (LESS COMMON)
Esophagitis (gastroesophageal reflux, infectious, pill)
Esophageal foreign body
Esophageal spasm
Cholecystitis
Subdiaphragmatic abscess
Perihepatitis (Fitz-Hugh-Curtis syndrome)
Peptic ulcer disease

CARDIAC (LESS COMMON)
Pericarditis
Postpericardiotomy syndrome
Endocarditis
Cardiomyopathy
Mitral valve prolapse
Aortic or subaortic stenosis
Arrhythmias
Marfan syndrome (dissecting aortic aneurysm)
Kawasaki disease
Cocaine, sympathomimetic ingestion
Angina (familial hypercholesterolemia, anomalous coronary artery)

IDIOPATHIC (COMMON)
Anxiety, hyperventilation
Panic disorder

OTHER (LESS COMMON)
Spinal cord or nerve root compression
Breast-related pathologic condition
Castleman disease (lymph node neoplasm)

ventricular heave, provide important clues to a specific cardiac diagnosis.

Accurate measurement of *height* and *weight* and plotting on a standard growth chart are important because both cardiac failure and chronic cyanosis result in failure to thrive. Growth failure is usually manifested predominantly by poor weight gain; if length or head circumference is also affected, additional congenital malformations or metabolic disorders may be present.

Mild *cyanosis* may be too subtle for early detection, and clubbing of the fingers and toes is not usually manifested until late in the 1st yr of life, even in the presence of severe arterial oxygen desaturation. Cyanosis is best observed over the nail beds, lips, tongue, and mucous membranes. **Differential cyanosis,** manifested as blue lower extremities and pink upper extremities (usually the right arm), is seen with right-to-left shunting across a ductus arteriosus in the presence of coarctation or an interrupted aortic arch. Circumoral cyanosis or blueness around the forehead may be the result of prominent venous plexuses in

these areas rather than decreased arterial oxygen saturation. The extremities of infants often turn blue when the infant is unwrapped and cold (**acrocyanosis**), and this condition can be distinguished from central cyanosis by examination of the tongue and mucous membranes.

Heart failure in infants and children results in some degree of hepatomegaly and occasionally splenomegaly. The sites of peripheral edema are age dependent. In infants, edema is usually seen around the eyes and over the flanks, especially after first waking in the morning. Older children and teenagers manifest both periorbital edema and pedal edema. A frequent initial complaint in these older patients is that their clothes no longer fit.

The *heart rate* of newborn infants is rapid and subject to wide fluctuations (Table 415–3). The average rate ranges from 120 to 140 beats/min and may increase to 170+ beats/min during crying and activity or drop to 70–90 beats/min during sleep. As the child grows older, the average pulse rate decreases and may be as low as 40 beats/min in athletic adolescents. Persistent tachycardia (>200 beats/min in neonates, 150 beats/min in infants, or 120 beats/min in older children), bradycardia, or an irregular heartbeat other than sinus arrhythmia requires investigation to exclude pathologic arrhythmias (see Chapter 428).

Careful evaluation of the character of the pulses is an important early step in the physical diagnosis of congenital heart disease. A wide pulse pressure with bounding pulses may suggest an aortic runoff lesion such as patent ductus arteriosus, aortic insufficiency, an arterial-venous communication, or increased cardiac output secondary to anemia, anxiety, or conditions associated with increased catecholamine or thyroid hormone secretion. The presence of diminished pulses in all extremities is associated with pericardial tamponade, left ventricular outflow obstruction, or cardiomyopathy. The radial and femoral pulses should always be palpated simultaneously. Normally, the femoral pulse should be appreciated immediately before the radial pulse. In older children with coarctation of the aorta, blood flow to the descending aorta may channel through collateral vessels and result in the femoral pulse being delayed until after the radial pulse (radial-femoral delay).

Blood pressure should be measured in the arms as well as in the legs, the latter on at least one occasion to be certain that coarctation of the aorta is not overlooked. Palpation of the femoral or dorsalis pedis pulse, or both, is not reliable alone to exclude coarctation. In older children, a mercury sphygmomanometer with a cuff that covers approximately two thirds of the upper part of the arm or leg may be used for blood pressure measurement. A cuff that is too small results in falsely high readings, whereas a cuff that is too large records slightly decreased pressure. Pediatric clinical facilities should be equipped with 3, 5, 7, 12, and 18 cm cuffs to accommodate the large spectrum of pediatric patient sizes. The 1st Korotkoff sounds indicate systolic pressure. As cuff pressure is slowly decreased, the sounds usually become muffled before they disappear. Diastolic pressure may be recorded when the sounds become muffled (preferred) or when they disappear altogether; the former is usually slightly higher and the latter slightly lower than true diastolic pressure. For lower extremity blood pressure determination, the stethoscope is placed over the popliteal artery. Ordinarily, the pressure recorded in the legs with the cuff technique is about 10 mm Hg higher than that in the arms.

In infants, blood pressure can be determined by auscultation, palpation, or an oscillometric (Dinamap) device, which if used properly, provides accurate measurements in infants as well as older children.

Blood pressure varies with the age of the child and is closely related to height and weight. Significant increases occur during adolescence, and many temporary variations take place before the more stable levels of adult life are attained. Exercise, excitement, coughing, crying, and struggling may raise the systolic

TABLE 415–1. Congenital Malformation Syndromes Associated with Congenital Heart Disease

Syndrome	Features
Chromosomal Disorders	
Trisomy 21 (Down syndrome)	Endocardial cushion defect, VSD, ASD
Trisomy 21p (cat eye syndrome)	Miscellaneous, total anomalous pulmonary venous return
Trisomy 18	VSD, ASD, PDA, coarctation of aorta, bicuspid aortic or pulmonary valve
Trisomy 13	VSD, ASD, PDA, coarctation of aorta, bicuspid aortic or pulmonary valve
Trisomy 9	Miscellaneous
XXXXY	PDA, ASD
Penta X	PDA, VSD
Triploidy	VSD, ASD, PDA
XO (Turner syndrome)	Bicuspid aortic valve, coarctation of aorta
Fragile X	Mitral valve prolapse, aortic root dilatation
Duplication 3q2	Miscellaneous
Deletion 4p	VSD, PDA, aortic stenosis
Deletion 9p	Miscellaneous
Deletion 5p (cri du chat syndrome)	VSD, PDA, ASD
Deletion 10q	VSD, TOF, conotruncal lesions*
Deletion 13q	VSD
Deletion 18q	VSD
Syndrome Complexes	
CHARGE association (coloboma, heart, atresia choanae, retardation, genital and ear anomalies)	VSD, ASD, PDA, TOF, endocardial cushion defect
DiGeorge sequence, CATCH 22 (cardiac defects, abnormal facies, thymic aplasia, cleft palate, and hypocalcemia)	Aortic arch anomalies, conotruncal anomalies
Alagille syndrome (arteriohepatic dysplasia)	Peripheral pulmonic stenosis
VATER association (vertebral, anal, tracheoesophageal, radial, and renal anomalies)	VSD, TOF, ASD, PDA
FAVS (facio-auriculo-vertebral spectrum)	TOF, VSD
CHILD (congenital hemidysplasia with ichthyosiform erythroderma, limb defects)	Miscellaneous
Mulibrey nanism (muscle, liver, brain, eye)	Pericardial thickening, constrictive pericarditis
Asplenia syndrome	Complex cyanotic heart lesions with decreased pulmonary blood flow, transposition of great arteries, anomalous pulmonary venous return, dextrocardia, single ventricle, single atrioventricular valve
Polysplenia syndrome	Acyanotic lesions with increased pulmonary blood flow, azygos continuation of inferior vena cava, partial anomalous pulmonary venous return, dextrocardia, single ventricle, common atrioventricular valve
PHACE syndrome (posterior brain fossa anomalies, facial hemangiomas, arterial anomalies, cardiac anomalies and aortic coarctation, eye anomalies)	VSD, PDA, coarctation of aorta, arterial aneurysms
Teratogenic Agents	
Congenital rubella	PDA, peripheral pulmonic stenosis
Fetal hydantoin syndrome	VSD, ASD, coarctation of aorta, PDA
Fetal alcohol syndrome	ASD, VSD
Fetal valproate effects	Coarctation of aorta, hypoplastic left side of heart, aortic stenosis, pulmonary atresia, VSD
Maternal phenylketonuria	VSD, ASD, PDA, coarctation of aorta
Retinoic acid embryopathy	Conotruncal anomalies
Others	
Apert syndrome	VSD
Autosomal dominant polycystic kidney disease	Mitral valve prolapse
Carpenter syndrome	PDA
Conradi syndrome	VSD, PDA
Crouzon disease	PDA, coarctation of aorta
Cutis laxa	Pulmonary hypertension, pulmonic stenosis
de Lange syndrome	VSD
Ellis-van Creveld syndrome	Single atrium, VSD
Holt-Oram syndrome	ASD, VSD, 1st-degree heart block
Infant of diabetic mother	Hypertrophic cardiomyopathy, VSD, conotruncal anomalies
Kartagener syndrome	Dextrocardia
Meckel-Gruber syndrome	ASD, VSD
Noonan syndrome	Pulmonic stenosis, ASD, cardiomyopathy
Pallister-Hall syndrome	Endocardial cushion defect
Rubinstein-Taybi syndrome	VSD
Scimitar syndrome	Hypoplasia of right lung, anomalous pulmonary venous return to inferior vena cava
Smith-Lemli-Opitz syndrome	VSD, PDA
TAR syndrome (thrombocytopenia and absent radius)	ASD, TOF
Treacher Collins syndrome	VSD, ASD, PDA
Williams syndrome	Supravalvular aortic stenosis, peripheral pulmonic stenosis

*Conotruncal = TOF, pulmonary atresia, truncus arteriosus, transposition of great arteries.
VSD = ventricular septal defect; ASD = atrial septal defect; PDA = patent ductus arteriosus; TOF = tetralogy of Fallot.

pressure of infants and children as much as 40–50 mm Hg greater than their usual levels. Variability in blood pressure in children of approximately the same age and body build should be expected, and serial measurements should always be obtained when evaluating a patient with hypertension (Figs. 415–1 and 415–2).

Though of little use in infants, in cooperative older children, inspection of the *jugular venous pulse* wave provides information about *central venous* and right atrial pressure. The neck veins should be inspected with the patient sitting at a 90-degree angle. The external jugular vein should not be visible above the clavicles unless central venous pressure is elevated. Increased

TABLE 415–2. Cardiac Manifestations of Systemic Diseases

Systemic Disease	Cardiac Complications
Inflammatory Disorders	
Sepsis	Hypotension, myocardial dysfunction, pericardial effusion, pulmonary hypertension
Juvenile rheumatoid arthritis	Pericarditis, rarely myocarditis
Systemic lupus erythematosus	Pericarditis, Libman-Sacks endocarditis, coronary arteritis, coronary atherosclerosis (with steroids), congenital heart block
Scleroderma	Pulmonary hypertension, myocardial fibrosis, cardiomyopathy
Dermatomyositis	Cardiomyopathy, arrhythmias, heart block
Kawasaki disease	Coronary artery aneurysm and thrombosis, myocardial infarction, myocarditis, valvular insufficiency
Sarcoidosis	Granuloma, fibrosis, amyloidosis, biventricular hypertrophy, arrhythmias
Lyme disease	Arrhythmias, myocarditis
Löffler hypereosinophilic syndrome	Endomyocardial disease
Inborn Errors of Metabolism	
Refsum disease	Arrhythmia, sudden death
Hunter-Hurler syndrome	Valvular insufficiency, heart failure, hypertension
Fabry disease	Mitral insufficiency, coronary artery disease with myocardial infarction
Glycogen storage disease IIa (Pompe disease)	Short PR interval, cardiomegaly, heart failure, arrhythmias
Carnitine deficiency	Heart failure, cardiomyopathy
Gaucher disease	Pericarditis
Homocystinuria	Coronary thrombosis
Alkaptonuria	Atherosclerosis, valvular disease
Morquio-Ullrich syndrome	Aortic incompetence
Scheie syndrome	Aortic incompetence
Connective Tissue Disorders	
Arterial calcification of infancy	Calcinosis of coronary arteries, aorta
Marfan syndrome	Aortic and mitral insufficiency, dissecting aortic aneurysm, mitral valve prolapse
Congenital contractural arachnodactyly	Mitral insufficiency or prolapse
Ehlers-Danlos syndrome	Mitral valve prolapse, dilatated aortic root
Osteogenesis imperfecta	Aortic incompetence
Pseudoxanthoma elasticum	Peripheral arterial disease
Neuromuscular Disorders	
Friedreich ataxia	Cardiomyopathy
Duchenne dystrophy	Cardiomyopathy, heart failure
Tuberous sclerosis	Cardiac rhabdomyoma
Familial deafness	Occasionally arrhythmia, sudden death
Neurofibromatosis	Pulmonic stenosis, pheochromocytoma, coarctation of aorta
Riley-Day syndrome	Episodic hypertension, postural hypotension
Von Hippel-Lindau disease	Hemangiomas, pheochromocytomas
Endocrine-Metabolic Disorders	
Graves disease	Tachycardia, arrhythmias, heart failure
Hypothyroidism	Bradycardia, pericardial effusion, cardiomyopathy, low-voltage electrocardiogram
Pheochromocytoma	Hypertension, myocardial ischemia, myocardial fibrosis, cardiomyopathy
Carcinoid	Right-sided endocardial fibrosis
Hematologic Disorders	
Sickle cell anemia	High-output heart failure, cardiomyopathy, cor pulmonale
Thalassemia major	High-output heart failure, hemochromatosis
Hemochromatosis (1st or 2nd degree)	Cardiomyopathy
Others	
Appetite suppressants (fenfluramine and dexfenfluramine)	Cardiac valvulopathy, pulmonary hypertension
Cockayne syndrome	Atherosclerosis
Familial dwarfism and nevi	Cardiomyopathy
Jervell and Lange-Nielsen syndrome	Prolonged QT interval, sudden death
Kearns-Sayre syndrome	Heart block
LEOPARD syndrome (lentiginosis)	Pulmonic stenosis, prolonged QT interval
Progeria	Accelerated atherosclerosis
Rendu-Osler-Weber syndrome	Arteriovenous fistula (lung, liver, mucous membrane)
Romano-Ward syndrome	Prolonged QT interval, sudden death
Weill-Marchesani syndrome	Patent ductus arteriosus
Werner syndrome	Vascular sclerosis, cardiomyopathy

LEOPARD = multiple lentigines, electrocardiographic conduction abnormalities, ocular hypertelorism, pulmonary stenosis, abnormal genitals, retardation of growth, sensorineural deafness.

venous pressure transmitted to the internal jugular vein may appear as venous pulsations without visible distention; such pulsation is not seen in normal children reclining at an angle of 45 degrees. Because the great veins are in direct communication with the right atrium, changes in pressure and the volume of this chamber are also transmitted to the veins. The one exception occurs in superior vena cava obstruction, in which venous pulsatility is lost.

Cardiac Examination. The heart should be examined in a systematic manner starting with *inspection* and *palpation*. A **precordial bulge** to the left of the sternum with increased precordial activity suggests cardiac enlargement; such bulges can often best be appreciated by having the child lay supine with the examiner looking up from the child's feet. A **substernal thrust** indicates the presence of right ventricular enlargement, whereas an **apical heave** is noted with left ventricular hypertrophy. A **hyper-**

TABLE 415–3. **Pulse Rates at Rest**

Age	Lower Limits of Normal		Average		Upper Limits of Normal	
Newborn	70/min		125/min		190/min	
1–11 mo	80		120		160	
2 yr	80		110		130	
4 yr	80		100		120	
6 yr	75		100		115	
8 yr	70		90		110	
10 yr	70		90		110	
	Girls	*Boys*	*Girls*	*Boys*	*Girls*	*Boys*
12 yr	70	65	90	85	110	105
14 yr	65	60	85	80	105	100
16 yr	60	55	80	75	100	95
18 yr	55	50	75	70	95	90

dynamic precordium suggests a volume load such as that found with a large left-to-right shunt, although it may be normal in a thin patient. A **silent precordium** with a barely detectable apical impulse suggests pericardial effusion or severe cardiomyopathy; it may be normal in an obese patient.

The relationship of the apical impulse to the midclavicular line is also helpful in the estimation of cardiac size: the apical impulse moves laterally and inferiorly with enlargement of the left ventricle. Right-sided apical impulses signify dextrocardia, tension pneumothorax, or left-sided thoracic space-occupying lesions (e.g., diaphragmatic hernia). **Thrills** are the palpable equivalent of murmurs and correlate with the area of maximal auscultatory intensity of the murmur. It is important to palpate the suprasternal notch and neck for **aortic bruits,** which may indicate the presence of aortic stenosis or, when faint, pulmonary stenosis. Right lower sternal border and apical systolic thrills are characteristic of ventricular septal defect and mitral insufficiency, respectively. Diastolic thrills are occasionally palpable in the presence of atrioventricular valve stenosis. The timing and localization of thrills should be carefully noted.

Auscultation is an art that improves with practice. The diaphragm of the stethoscope is placed firmly on the chest for high-pitched sounds; a lightly placed bell is optimal for low-pitched sounds. The physician should initially concentrate on the characteristics of the individual heart sounds and their variation with respirations and later concentrate on murmurs. The patient should be supine, lying quietly, and breathing normally. The 1st heart sound is best heard at the apex, whereas the 2nd heart sound should be evaluated at the upper left and right sternal borders. The 1st heart sound is caused by closure of the atrioventricular valves (mitral and tricuspid); the 2nd sound is caused by closure of the semilunar valves (aortic and pulmonary; Fig. 415–3). During inspiration, the decrease in intrathoracic pressure results in increased filling of the right side of the heart, which leads to an increased right ventricular ejection time and thus delayed closure of the pulmonary valve; consequently, splitting of the 2nd heart sound increases during inspiration and decreases during expiration.

Often, the 2nd heart sound appears to be single during expiration. The presence of a normally split 2nd sound is strong evidence against the diagnosis of atrial septal defect, defects associated with pulmonary arterial hypertension, severe pulmonary valve stenosis, aortic and pulmonary atresia, and truncus arteriosus. Wide splitting is noted in atrial septal defect, pulmonary stenosis, Ebstein anomaly, total anomalous pulmonary venous return, and right bundle branch block. An accentuated pulmonic component of the 2nd sound with narrow splitting is a sign of pulmonary hypertension. A single 2nd sound occurs in pulmonary or aortic atresia or severe stenosis, truncus arteriosus, and often in transposition of the great arteries.

A 3rd heart sound is best heard with the bell at the apex in mid-diastole. A 4th sound occurring in conjunction with atrial contraction may be heard just before the 1st heart sound in late diastole. The 3rd sound may be normal in an adolescent with a relatively slow heart rate, but in a patient with the clinical signs of heart failure and tachycardia, it may be heard as a gallop rhythm and may merge with a 4th heart sound, a finding known as a *summation gallop.* A **gallop** rhythm is attributed to poor compliance of the ventricle, and exaggeration of the normal 3rd sound is associated with ventricular filling.

Ejection clicks, which are heard in early systole, may be related to dilatation of the aorta or pulmonary artery or to a mildly to moderately stenotic semilunar valve. They are heard so close to the 1st heart sound that they may be mistaken for a split 1st sound. Aortic ejection clicks are best heard at the left middle to right upper sternal border and are constant in intensity. They occur in conditions in which the aortic valve is stenotic or the aorta is dilated (tetralogy of Fallot, truncus arteriosus). Pulmonary ejection clicks, which are associated with mild to moderate pulmonary stenosis, are best heard at the left middle to upper sternal border and vary with respirations, often disappearing with inspiration. Split 1st heart sounds are usually heard best at the lower left sternal border. A midsystolic click heard at the apex, often preceding a late systolic murmur, suggests mitral valve prolapse.

Murmurs should be described according to their intensity, pitch, timing (systolic or diastolic), variation in intensity, time to peak intensity, area of maximal intensity, and radiation to other areas. Auscultation for murmurs should be carried out across the upper precordium, down the left or right sternal border, and out to the apex and left axilla. Auscultation should also always be performed in the right axilla and over the back. **Systolic murmurs** are classified as ejection, pansystolic, or late systolic according to the timing of the murmur in relation to the 1st and 2nd heart sounds. The intensity of systolic murmurs is graded from I to VI: I, barely audible; II, medium intensity; III, loud but no thrill; IV, loud with a thrill; V, very loud but still requiring positioning of the stethoscope at least partly on the chest; and VI, so loud that the murmur can be heard with the stethoscope off the chest.

Systolic ejection murmurs start a short time after a well-heard 1st heart sound, increase in intensity, peak, and then decrease in intensity; they usually end before the 2nd sound. However, in patients with severe aortic or pulmonary stenosis, the murmur may extend beyond the 1st component of the 2nd sound, thus obscuring it. *Pansystolic* or *holosystolic murmurs* begin almost simultaneously with the 1st heart sound and continue throughout systole, on occasion becoming gradually decrescendo. It is helpful to remember that after closure of the atrioventricular valves (the 1st heart sound), a brief period occurs during which ventricular pressure increases but the semilunar valves remain closed (isovolumic contraction; see Fig. 415–3). Thus, pansystolic murmurs (heard during both isovolumic contraction and the ejection phases of systole) cannot be caused by flow across the semilunar valves because these valves are closed during isovolumic contraction. Pansystolic murmurs are therefore related to blood exiting the contracting ventricle via either an abnormal opening (a ventricular septal defect) or atrioventricular (mitral or tricuspid) valve insufficiency. Systolic ejection murmurs usually imply increased flow or stenosis across one of the ventricular outflow tracts (aortic or pulmonic). In infants with rapid heart rates, it is often difficult to distinguish between ejection and pansystolic murmurs. If a clear and distinct 1st heart sound can be appreciated, the murmur is most likely ejection in nature.

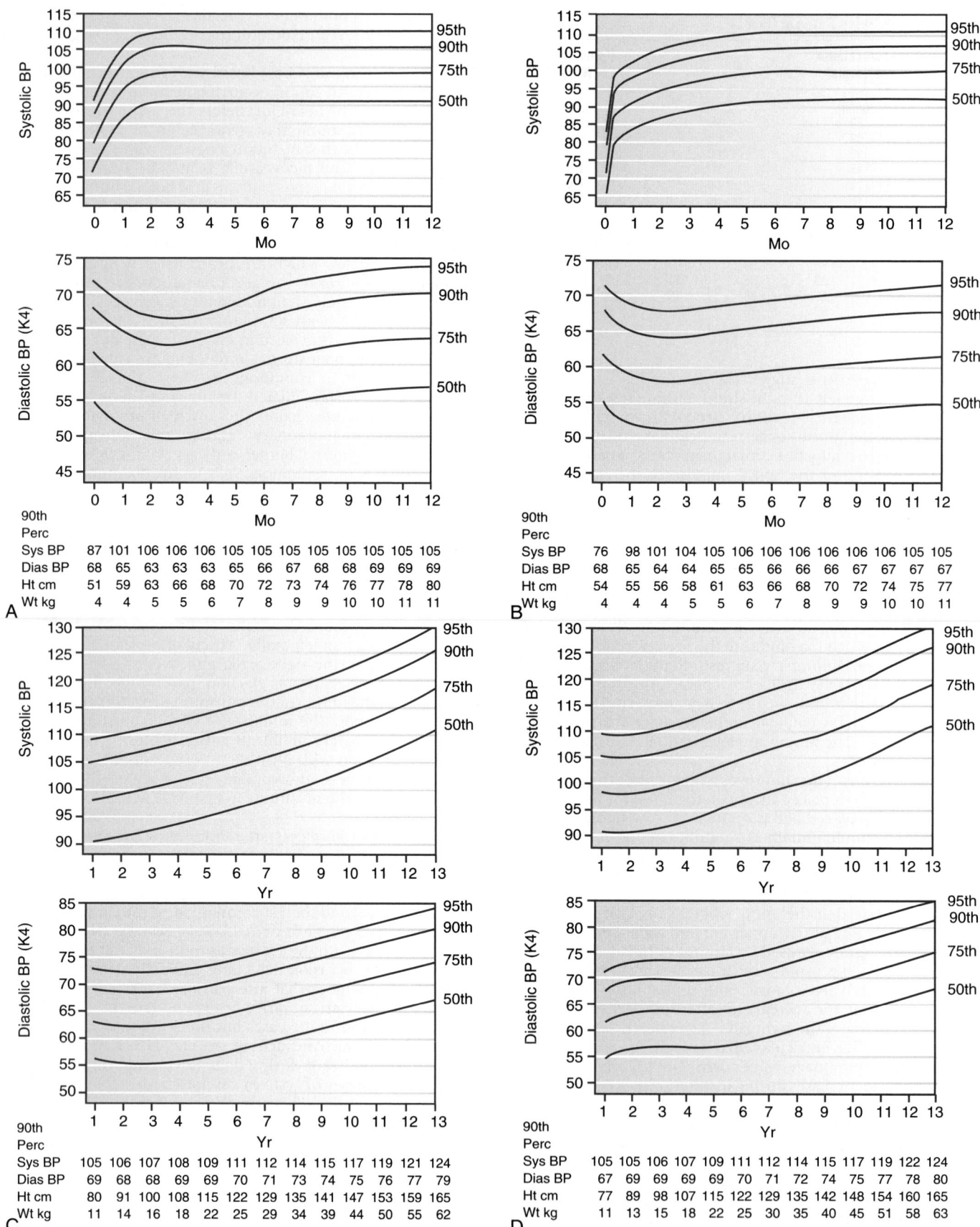

FIGURE 415–1. *A,* Age-specific percentiles of blood pressure (BP) measurements in boys from birth to 12 mo of age. *B,* Age-specific percentiles of BP measurements in girls from birth to 12 mo of age. *C,* Age-specific percentiles of BP measurements in boys 1–13 yr of age. *D,* Age-specific percentiles of BP measurements in girls 1–13 yr of age; Korotkoff phase IV (K4) used for diastolic BP. Perc = percentile; Sys = systolic; Dias = diastolic; Ht = height; Wt = weight. (From National Heart, Lung, and Blood Institute, Bethesda, MD: Report of the Second Task Force on Blood Pressure Control in Children—1987. *Pediatrics* 1987;79:1. Copyright American Academy of Pediatrics 1987.)

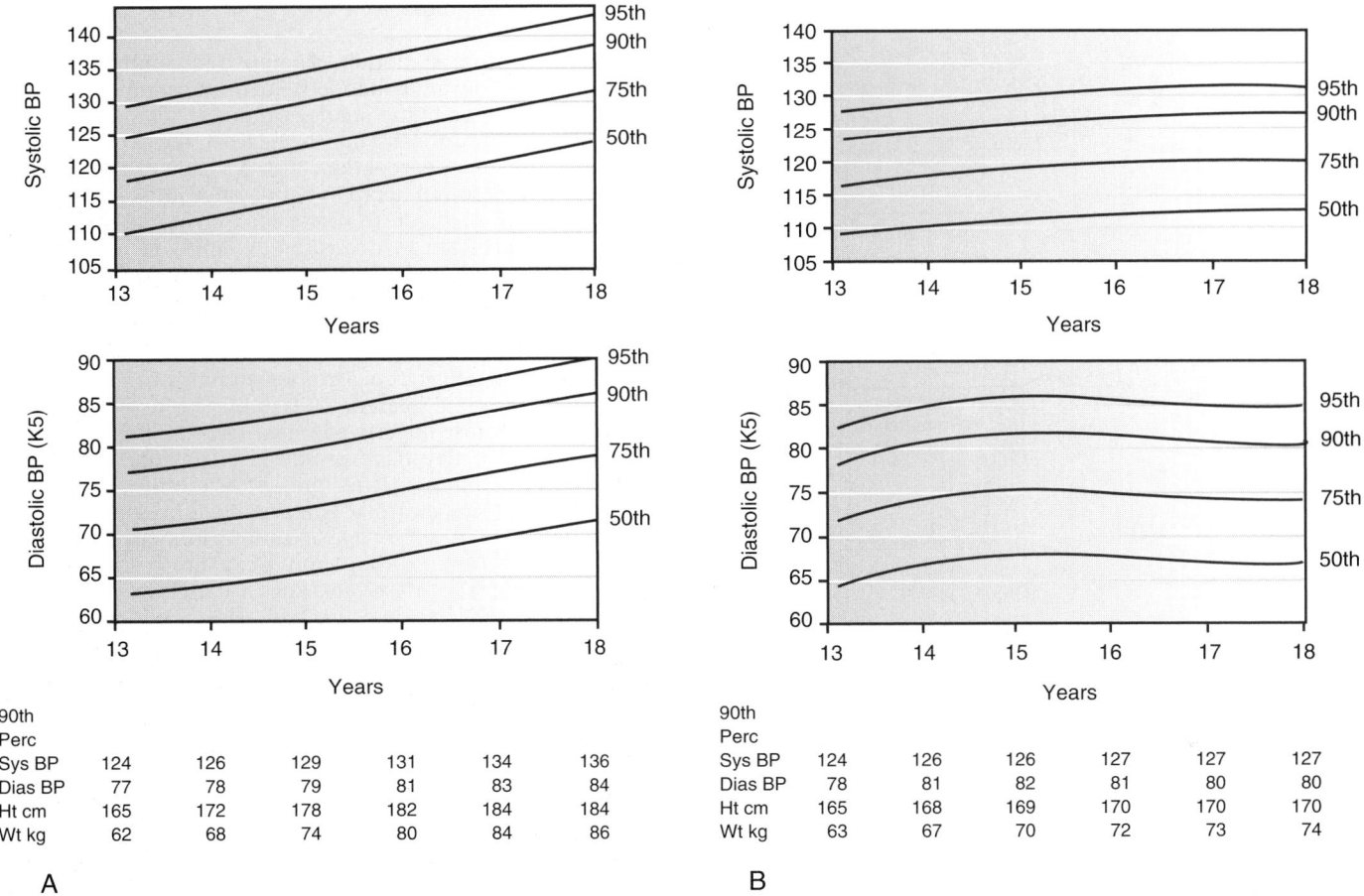

FIGURE 415–2. *A,* Age-specific percentiles of blood pressure (BP) measurements in boys 13–18 yr of age. *B,* Age-specific percentiles of BP measurements in girls 13–18 yr of age; Korotkoff phase V (K5) used for diastolic BP. Perc = percentile; Sys = systolic; Dias = diastolic; Ht = height; Wt = weight. (From Report of the second task force on blood pressure control in children—1987. Task Force on Blood Pressure Control in Children. National Heart, Lung, and Blood Institute, Bethesda, Maryland. *Pediatrics* 1987;79:1. Copyright American Academy of Pediatrics 1987.)

A **continuous murmur** is a systolic murmur that continues or "spills" into diastole and indicates continuous flow, such as in the presence of a patent ductus arteriosus or other aortopulmonary communication. This murmur should be differentiated from a **to-and-fro murmur**, which indicates that the systolic component of the murmur ends at or before the 2nd sound and the diastolic murmur begins after semilunar valve closure (e.g., aortic or pulmonary stenosis combined with insufficiency). A late systolic murmur begins well beyond the 1st heart sound and continues until the end of systole. Such murmurs may be heard after a midsystolic click in patients with mitral valve prolapse and insufficiency.

Several types of **diastolic murmurs** (graded I–IV) can be identified. A **decrescendo diastolic murmur** is a blowing murmur along the left sternal border that begins with S_2 and diminishes toward mid-diastole. When high-pitched, this murmur is associated with aortic valve insufficiency or pulmonary insufficiency related to pulmonary hypertension. When low-pitched, this murmur is associated with pulmonary valve insufficiency in the absence of pulmonary hypertension. A low-pitched decrescendo diastolic murmur is typically noted after surgical repair of the pulmonary outflow tract in defects such as tetralogy of Fallot or in patients with absent pulmonary valves. A **rumbling mid-diastolic murmur** at the left middle and lower sternal border may be due to increased blood flow across the tricuspid valve, such as occurs with an atrial septal defect or, less often, because of actual stenosis of this valve. When this

murmur is heard at the apex, it is caused by increased flow across the mitral valve, such as occurs with large left-to-right shunts at the ventricular level (ventricular septal defects), at the great vessel level (patent ductus arteriosus, aortopulmonary shunts), or with increased flow because of mitral insufficiency. When an apical diastolic rumbling murmur is longer and is accentuated at the end of diastole (presystolic), it usually indicates anatomic mitral valve stenosis.

The absence of a precordial murmur does not rule out significant congenital or acquired heart disease. Congenital heart defects, some of which are ductal dependent, may not demonstrate a murmur if the ductus arteriosus closes. These lesions include pulmonary or tricuspid valve atresia and transposition of the great arteries. Murmurs may seem insignificant in patients with severe aortic stenosis, atrial septal defects, anomalous pulmonary venous return, atrioventricular septal defects, coarctation of the aorta, or anomalous insertion of a coronary artery. Careful attention to other components of the physical examination (growth failure, cyanosis, peripheral pulses, precordial impulse, heart sounds) increases the index of suspicion of congenital heart defects in these cases. In contrast, loud murmurs may be present in the absence of structural heart disease, for example, in patients with a large noncardiac arteriovenous malformation, myocarditis, severe anemia, or hypertension.

Many murmurs are not associated with significant hemodynamic abnormalities. These murmurs are referred to as functional, normal, insignificant, or innocent (the preferred term).

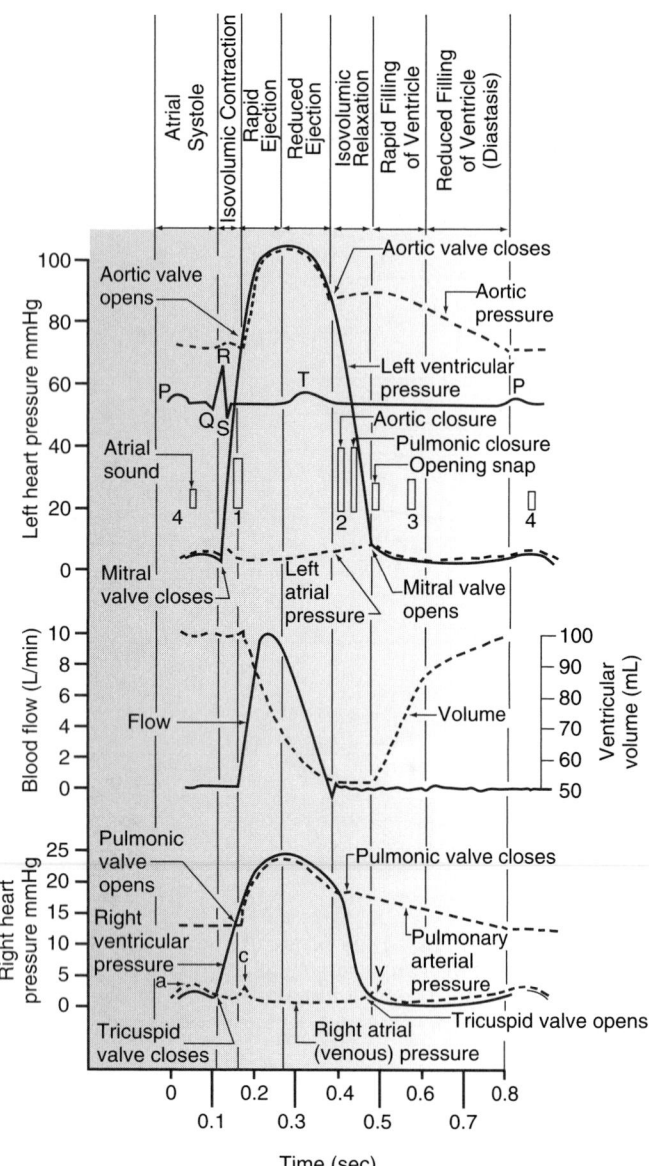

FIGURE 415–3. Idealized diagram of the temporal events of a cardiac cycle.

During routine random auscultation, more than 30% of children may have an *innocent murmur* at one time in their lives; this percentage increases when auscultation is carried out under nonbasal circumstances (high cardiac output because of fever, infection, anxiety). The most common innocent murmur is a medium-pitched, **vibratory** or **"musical,"** relatively short systolic ejection murmur, which is heard best along the left lower and midsternal border and has no significant radiation to the apex, base, or back. It is heard most frequently in children between 3 and 7 yr of age. The intensity of the murmur often changes with respiration and position and may be attenuated in the sitting or prone position. Innocent pulmonic murmurs are also common in children and adolescents and originate from normal turbulence during ejection into the pulmonary artery. They are higher pitched, blowing, brief early systolic murmurs of grade I–II in intensity and are best detected in the 2nd left parasternal space with the patient in the supine position. Features suggestive of heart disease include murmurs that are pansystolic, grade III or higher, harsh, located at the left upper sternal border, and associated

with an early or midsystolic click or an abnormal 2nd heart sound.

A **venous hum** is another example of a common innocent murmur heard during childhood. Such hums are produced by turbulence of blood in the jugular venous system; they have no pathologic significance and may be heard in the neck or anterior portion of the upper part of the chest. A venous hum consists of a soft humming sound heard in both systole and diastole; it can be exaggerated or made to disappear by varying the position of the head, or it can be decreased by lightly compressing the jugular venous system in the neck. These simple maneuvers are sufficient to differentiate a venous hum from the murmurs produced by organic cardiovascular disease, particularly a patent ductus arteriosus.

The lack of significance of an innocent murmur should be discussed with the child's parents. It is important to offer complete reassurance because lingering doubts about the importance of a cardiac murmur may have profound effects on child-rearing practices, most often in the form of overprotectiveness. An underlying fear that a cardiac abnormality is present may negatively affect a child's self-image and subtly influence personality development. The physician should explain that an innocent murmur is simply a "noise" and does not indicate the presence of a significant cardiac defect. When asked, "Will it go away?" the best response is to state that because the murmur has no meaning, it does not matter whether it "goes away" or not. Parents should be warned that the intensity of the murmur might increase during febrile illnesses. However, with growth, innocent murmurs are less well heard and often disappear completely. At times, additional studies may be indicated to rule out a congenital heart defect, but "routine" electrocardiographic, chest roentgenographic, and echocardiographic examinations should be avoided in well children with innocent murmurs.

Gutgesell HP, Barst RJ, Humes RA, et al: Common cardiovascular problems in the young: Part I. Murmurs, chest pain, syncope and irregular rhythms. *Am Fam Physician* 1997;56:1825–30.

Hohn AR, Dwyer KM, Dwyer JH: Blood pressure in youth from four ethnic groups: The Pasadena Prevention Project. *J Pediatr* 1994;125:386.

McCrindle BW, Shaffer KM, Kan JS, et al: Cardinal clinical signs in the differentiation of heart murmurs in children. *Arch Pediatr Adolesc Med* 1996;150:169.

Pelech AN: The cardiac murmur. When to refer? *Pediatr Clin North Am* 1998;45:107–2.

Rosner B, Prineas RJ, Loggie MH, et al: Blood pressure nomograms for children and adolescents, by height, sex, and age, in the United States. *J Pediatr* 1993;123:871.

Steinberger J, Moller JH, Berry JM, et al: Echocardiographic diagnosis of heart disease in apparently healthy adolescents. *Pediatrics* 2000;105:815–8.

Swenson JM, Fischer DR, Miller SA, et al: Are chest radiographs and electrocardiograms still valuable in evaluating new pediatric patients with heart murmurs or chest pain? *Pediatrics* 1997;99:1.

Talner NS, Carboni MP: Chest pain in the adolescent and young adult. *Cardiol Rev* 2000;8:49–56.

Chapter 416
Laboratory Evaluation

416.1 Radiologic Assessment

The chest roentgenogram may provide information about cardiac size and shape, pulmonary blood flow (vascularity), pulmonary edema, and associated lung and thoracic anomalies that may be associated with congenital syndromes (skeletal dysplasias, extra or deficient number of ribs, abnormal vertebrae, previous cardiac surgery). Variations are due to differences in body build, the phase of respiration or the cardiac cycle, abnormalities of the thoracic cage, position of the diaphragm, or pulmonary disease.

The most frequently used measurement of cardiac size is the maximal width of the cardiac shadow in a posteroanterior chest film taken during midinspiration. A vertical line is drawn down the middle of the sternal shadow, and perpendicular lines are drawn from the sternal line to the extreme right and left borders of the heart; the sum of the lengths of these lines is the *maximal cardiac width*. The *maximal chest width* is obtained by drawing a horizontal line between the right and left inner borders of the rib cage at the level of the top of the right diaphragm. When the maximal cardiac width is more than half the maximal chest width (**cardio-thoracic ratio** >50%), the heart is usually enlarged. Cardiac size should be evaluated only when the film is taken during inspiration with the patient in an upright position. A diagnosis of "cardiac enlargement" on expiratory or prone films is a common cause of unnecessary referrals and laboratory studies.

The cardiothoracic ratio is a less useful index of cardiac enlargement in infants than in older children because the horizontal position of the heart may increase the ratio to more than 50% in the absence of true enlargement. Furthermore, the thymus may overlap not only the base of the heart but also virtually the entire mediastinum, thus obscuring the true cardiac silhouette.

A lateral chest roentgenogram may be helpful in infants as well as in older children with pectus excavatum or other conditions that result in a narrow anteroposterior chest dimension. In these situations, the heart may appear small in the lateral view and suggest that the apparent enlargement in the posteroanterior projection was due to either the thymic image (anterior mediastinum only) or flattening of the cardiac chambers as a result of a structural chest abnormality.

In the posteroanterior view, the left border of the cardiac shadow consists of three convex shadows produced, from above downward, by the aortic knob, the main and left pulmonary arteries, and the left ventricle (Fig. 416–1). In cases of moderate to marked left atrial enlargement, the atrium may project between the pulmonary artery and the left ventricle. The outflow tract of the right ventricle does not contribute to the shadows formed by the left border of the heart. The aortic knob is not as easily seen in infants and children as in adults. However, the side of the aortic arch (left or right) can often be inferred as being opposite the side of the midline from which the air-filled trachea is visualized. This observation is important because a right-sided aortic arch is often present in cyanotic congenital heart disease, particularly the tetralogy of Fallot. Three structures contribute to the right border of the cardiac silhouette: from above downward they are the superior vena cava, the ascending aorta, and the right atrium.

Enlargement of cardiac chambers or major arteries and veins results in prominence of the areas in which these structures are normally outlined on the chest roentgenogram. In contrast, the electrocardiogram (ECG) is a more sensitive and accurate index of ventricular *hypertrophy*.

It is also important to assess the degree of *pulmonary vascularity*. Angiocardiographic studies have shown that the hilar shadows are mainly vascular. Pulmonary overcirculation is usually associated with left-to-right shunt lesions, whereas pulmonary undercirculation is associated with obstruction of the outflow tract of the right ventricle.

The esophagus is closely related to the great vessels, and a barium esophagogram can help delineate these structures in the initial evaluation of suspected vascular rings. However, echocardiographic examination best defines the morphologic features of intracardiac chambers, and CT and MRI best define extracardiac vascular morphology.

416.2 ■ Electrocardiography

DEVELOPMENTAL CHANGES

The marked changes that occur in cardiac physiology and chamber dominance during the perinatal transition (see Chapter 414) are reflected in the evolution of the ECG during

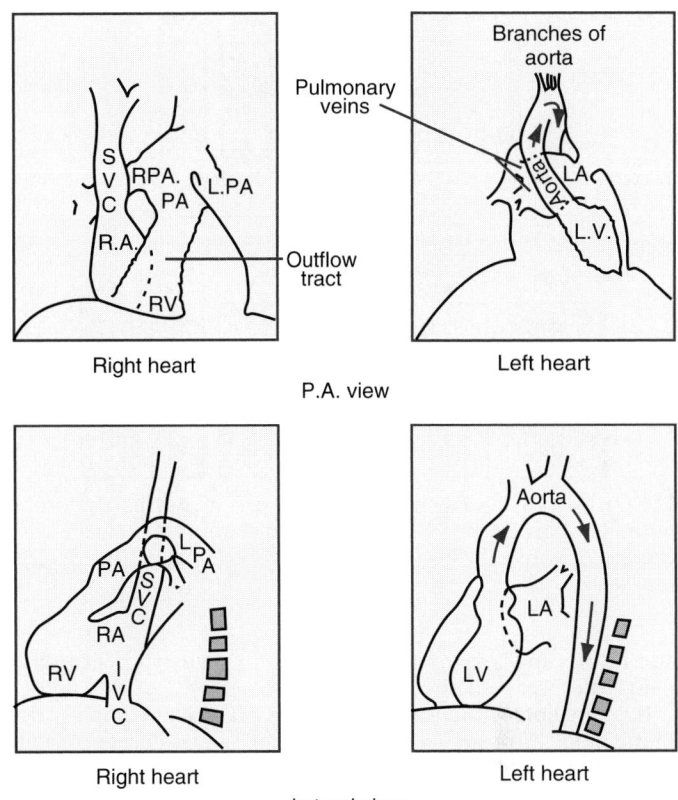

FIGURE 416–1. Idealized diagrams showing normal position of the cardiac chambers and great blood vessels. P.A. = posteroanterior; SVC = superior vena cava; RA = right atrium; RV = right ventricle; PA = pulmonary artery; RPA = right pulmonary artery; LPA = left pulmonary artery; LA = left atrium; LV = left ventricle; IVC = inferior vena cava. (Adapted and redrawn from Dotter and Steinberg: *Radiology* 1949;53:513.)

the neonatal period. Because vascular resistance in the pulmonary and systemic circulations is nearly equal in a term fetus, the intrauterine work of the heart results in an equal mass of both the right and left ventricles. After birth, systemic vascular resistance rises when the placental circulation is eliminated, and pulmonary vascular resistance falls when the lungs expand. These changes are reflected in the ECG as the right ventricular wall begins to thin.

The ECG demonstrates these anatomic and hemodynamic features principally by changes in QRS and T-wave morphologic features. It is recommended that a 13-lead ECG be performed in pediatric patients, including either lead V_3R or V_4R, which are important in the evaluation of right ventricular hypertrophy. On occasion, lead V_1 is positioned too far leftward to reflect right ventricular forces accurately. This problem is present particularly in premature infants, in whom the electrocardiographic electrode gel may produce contact among all the precordial leads.

During the 1st days of life, *right axis deviation*, large R waves, and upright T waves in the right precordial leads (V_3R or V_4R and V_1) are the norm (Fig. 416–2). As pulmonary vascular resistance decreases in the 1st few days after birth, the right precordial T waves become negative. In the great majority of instances, this change occurs within the 1st 48 hr of life. Upright T waves that persist in leads V_3R, V_4R, or V_1 beyond 1 wk of life are an abnormal finding indicating right ventricular hypertrophy or strain, even in the absence of QRS voltage criteria. The T wave in V_1 should never be positive before 6 yr of age and may remain negative into adolescence. This finding represents one of the most important, yet subtle differences between pediatric and

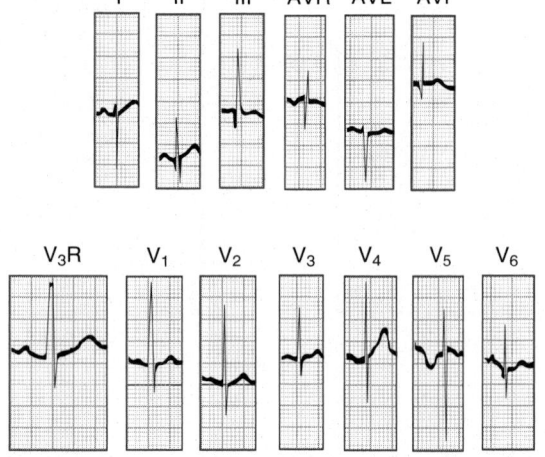

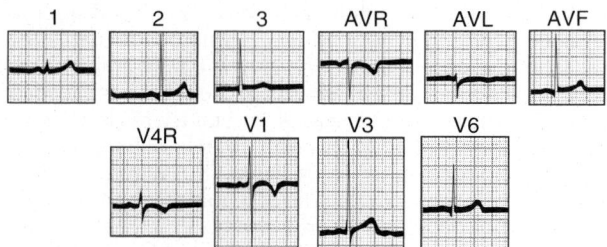

FIGURE 416–4. Electrocardiogram of a normal child. Note the relatively tall R waves and inversion of the T waves in V₄R and V₁.

FIGURE 416–2. Electrocardiogram in a normal neonate younger than 24 hr of age. Note the dominant R wave and upright T waves in leads V₃R and V₁ (V₃R paper speed = 50 mm/sec).

adult ECGs and is a common source of error when adult cardiologists interpret pediatric ECGs.

In a newborn, the mean QRS frontal-plane axis normally lies in the range of +110 to +180 degrees. The right-sided chest leads reveal a larger positive (R) than negative (S) wave and may do so for months or years because the right ventricle remains relatively thick throughout infancy. Left-sided leads (V₅ and V₆) also reflect *right-sided dominance* in the early neonatal period, when the R:S ratio in these leads may be less than 1. A dominant R wave reflecting left ventricular forces quickly becomes evident within the 1st few days of life (Fig. 416–3). Over the years, the QRS axis gradually shifts leftward, and the right ventricular forces slowly regress. Leads V₁, V₃R, and V₄R display a prominent R wave until 6 mo–8 yr of age. Most children have an R:S ratio greater than 1 in lead V₄R until they are 4 yr of age. The T waves are inverted in leads V₄R, V₁, V₂, and V₃ during infancy and may remain so into the middle of the 2nd decade of life and beyond. The processes of right ventricular thinning and left ventricular growth are best reflected in the QRS-T pattern over the right precordial leads. The diagnosis of right or left ventricular hypertrophy in a pediatric patient can be made only with an understanding of the normal developmental physiology of these chambers at various ages until adulthood is reached. As the left ventricle becomes dominant, the ECG evolves to the characteristic pattern of older children (Fig. 416–4) and adults (Fig. 416–5).

Ventricular hypertrophy may result in increased voltage in the R and S waves in the chest leads. The height of these deflections is governed by the proximity of the specific electrode to the surface of the heart; by the sequence of electrical activation through the ventricles, which can result in variable degrees of cancellation of forces; and by hypertrophy of the myocardium. Because the chest wall in infants and children, as well as in adolescents, may be relatively thin, the diagnosis of ventricular hypertrophy should not be based on voltage changes alone.

The diagnosis of pathologic right ventricular hypertrophy is difficult in the 1st wk of life because physiologic right ventricular hypertrophy is a normal finding. Serial tracings are often necessary to determine whether marked right axis deviation and potentially abnormal right precordial forces or T waves, or both, will persist beyond the neonatal period (Fig. 416–6). In contrast, an adult electrocardiographic pattern seen in a neonate suggests left ventricular enlargement (see Fig. 416–5). The exception is a premature infant, who may display a more "mature" ECG than a full-term infant (Fig. 416–7) as a result of lower pulmonary vascular resistance secondary to underdevelopment of the medial muscular layer of the pulmonary arterioles. Some premature infants display a pattern of generalized low voltage across the precordium.

The ECG should always be evaluated systematically to avoid the possibility of overlooking a minor, but important abnormality. One approach is to begin with an assessment of rate and rhythm, followed by a calculation of the mean frontal-plane QRS axis, measurements of segment intervals, assessment of voltages, and finally, assessment of ST and T-wave abnormalities.

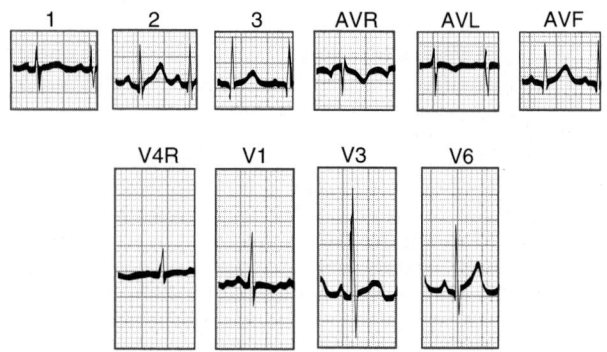

FIGURE 416–3. Electrocardiogram of a normal infant. Note the tall R and small S waves in V₄R and V₁ and the inverted T wave in these leads. A dominant R wave is also present in V₆.

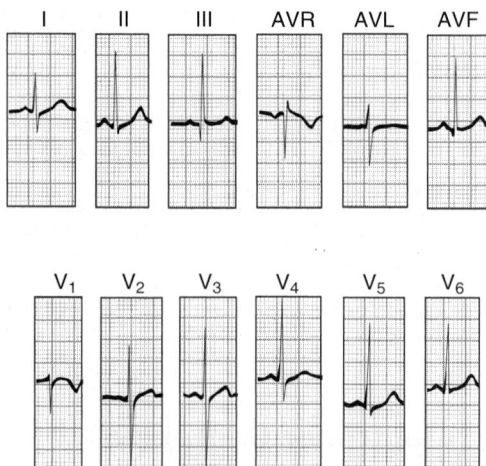

FIGURE 416–5. Normal adult electrocardiogram. Note the dominant S wave in lead V₁. This pattern in an infant would indicate the presence of left ventricular hypertrophy.

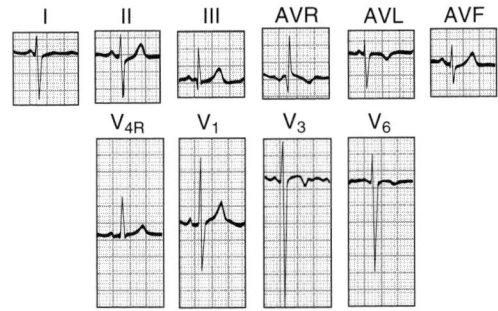

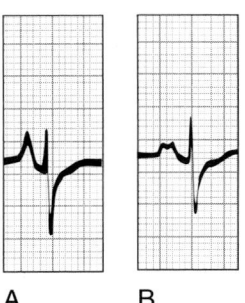

FIGURE 416–6. Electrocardiogram of an infant with right ventricular hypertrophy (tetralogy of Fallot). Note the tall R waves in the right precordium and deep S waves in V$_6$. The positive T waves in V$_4$R and V$_1$ are also characteristic of right ventricular hypertrophy.

FIGURE 416–8. Atrial enlargement. *A,* Peaked narrow P waves characteristic of right atrial enlargement. *B,* Wide bifid M-shaped P waves typical of left atrial enlargement.

RATE AND RHYTHM

A brief rhythm strip should be examined to assess whether a P wave always precedes each QRS complex. The P-wave axis should then be estimated as an indication of whether the rhythm is originating from the sinus node. If the atria are situated normally in the chest, the P wave should be upright in leads I and aVF and inverted in lead aVR. With atrial inversion (situs inversus), the P wave may be inverted in lead I. Inverted P waves in leads II and aVF are seen in nodal or junctional rhythms regardless of atrial position. The absence of P waves indicates a rhythm originating more distally in the conduction system. In this case, the morphologic features of the QRS complexes are important in differentiating a junctional (usually a narrow QRS complex) from a ventricular (usually a wide QRS complex) rhythm.

P WAVES

Tall (>2.5 mm), narrow, and spiked P waves are indicative of right atrial enlargement and are seen in congenital pulmonary stenosis, Ebstein anomaly of the tricuspid valve, tricuspid atresia, and sometimes cor pulmonale. These abnormal waves are most obvious in leads II, V$_3$R, and V$_1$ (Fig. 416–8A). Similar waves are sometimes seen in thyrotoxicosis. Broad P waves, commonly bifid and sometimes biphasic, are indicative of left atrial enlargement (see Fig. 416–8B). They are seen in some patients with large left-to-right shunts (ventricular septal defect [VSD], patent ductus arteriosus [PDA]) and with severe mitral stenosis or regurgitation. Flat P waves may be encountered in hyperkalemia.

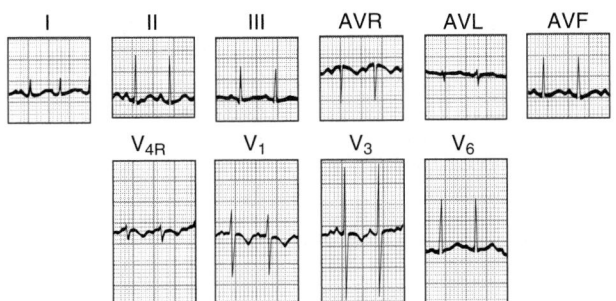

FIGURE 416–7. Electrocardiogram of a premature infant (weight 2 kg and age 5 wk at the time of the tracing). The cardiovascular system was clinically normal. Left ventricular dominance is manifested by R-wave progression across the chest, similar to tracings obtained from older children. Compare with the tracing from a normal full-term infant (Fig. 416–3).

QRS COMPLEX

Right Ventricular Hypertrophy. For the most accurate assessment of ventricular hypertrophy, pediatric ECGs should include the right precordial lead V$_3$R or V$_4$R, or both. The diagnosis of right ventricular hypertrophy depends on demonstration of the following changes (see Fig. 416–6): (1) a qR pattern in the right ventricular surface leads; (2) a positive T wave in leads V$_3$R–V$_4$R and V$_1$–V$_3$ between the ages of 6 days and 6 yr; (3) a monophasic R wave in V$_3$R, V$_4$R, or V$_1$; (4) an rsR' pattern in the right precordial leads with the 2nd R wave taller than the initial one; (5) age-corrected increased voltage of the R wave in leads V$_3$R–V$_4$R or the S wave in leads V$_6$–V$_7$, or both; (6) marked right axis deviation (>120 degrees in patients beyond the newborn period); (7) complete reversal of the normal adult precordial RS pattern; and (8) right atrial enlargement. At least two of these changes should be present to support a diagnosis of right ventricular hypertrophy.

Abnormal ventricular loading can be characterized as either systolic (as a result of obstruction of the right ventricular outflow tract, as in pulmonic stenosis) or diastolic (as a result of increased volume load, as in atrial septal defects [ASDs]). These two types of abnormal loads result in distinct electrocardiographic patterns. The *systolic overload pattern* is characterized by tall, pure R waves in the right precordial leads. In older children, the T waves in these leads are initially upright and later become inverted. In infants and children younger than 6 yr, the T waves in V$_3$R–V$_4$R and V$_1$ are abnormally upright. The *diastolic overload pattern* is characterized by an rsR' pattern (Fig. 416–9) and a slightly increased QRS duration (minor right ventricular conduction delay). Patients with mild to moderate pulmonary stenosis may also exhibit an rsR pattern in the right precordial leads.

Left Ventricular Hypertrophy. The following features indicate the presence of left ventricular hypertrophy (Fig. 416–10): (1) depression of the ST segments and inversion of the T waves in the left precordial leads (V$_5$, V$_6$, and V$_7$), known as a left ventricular strain pattern—these findings suggest the presence of a severe lesion; (2) a deep Q wave in the left precordial leads; and (3) increased voltage of the S wave in V$_3$R and V$_1$ or the R wave in V$_6$–V$_7$, or both. It is important to emphasize that evaluation of left ventricular hypertrophy should not be based on voltage criteria alone. The concepts of systolic and diastolic overload, though not always consistent, are also useful in evaluating left ventricular enlargement. Severe *systolic overload* of the left ventricle is suggested by straightening of the ST segments and inverted T waves over the left precordial leads; *diastolic overload* may result in tall R waves, a large Q wave, and normal T waves over the left precordium. Finally, an infant with an ECG that would be considered "normal" for an older child may in fact have left ventricular hypertrophy.

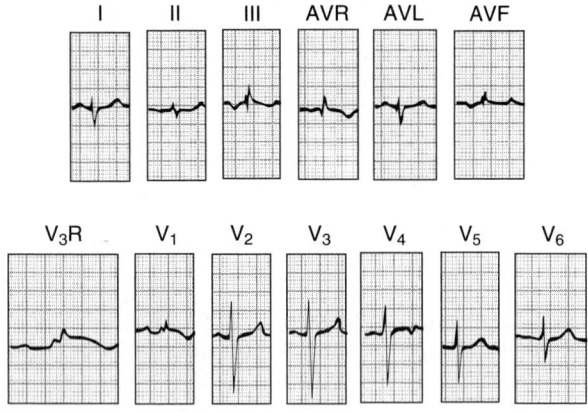

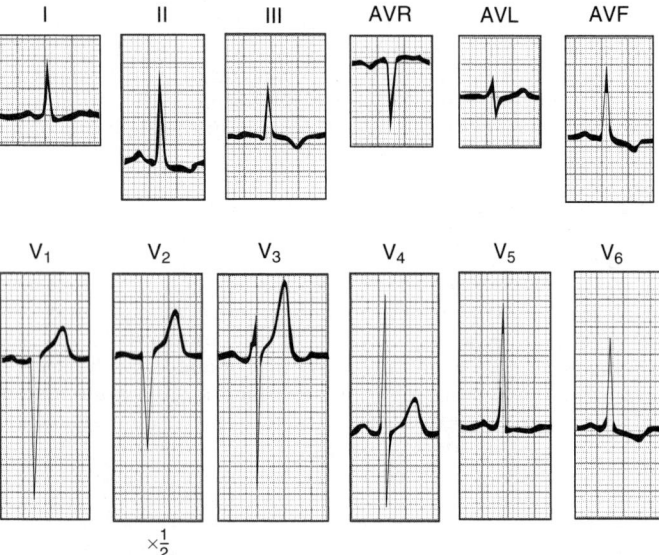

FIGURE 416–9. Electrocardiogram showing right ventricular conduction delay characterized by an rsR' pattern in V_1 and a deep S wave in V_6 (V_3R paper speed = 50 mm/sec).

Bundle Branch Block. A complete right bundle branch block may be congenital or may be acquired after surgery for congenital heart disease, especially when a right ventriculotomy has been performed as in repair of the tetralogy of Fallot. Congenital left bundle branch block is rare; this pattern is occasionally seen with cardiomyopathy. A bundle branch block pattern may be indicative of a bypass tract associated with one of the pre-excitation syndromes (see Chapter 428).

P-R AND Q-T INTERVALS

The duration of the P-R interval shortens with increasing heart rate; thus, assessment of this interval should be based on age- and rate-corrected nomograms. A long P-R interval is diagnostic of a 1st-degree heart block, the cause of which may be congenital, postoperative, inflammatory (myocarditis, pericarditis, rheumatic fever), or pharmacologic (digitalis).

The duration of the Q-T interval varies with the cardiac rate; a corrected Q-T interval (Q-Tc) can be calculated by dividing the measured Q-T interval by the square root of the preceding R-R interval. A normal Q-Tc should be less than 0.45. It is often

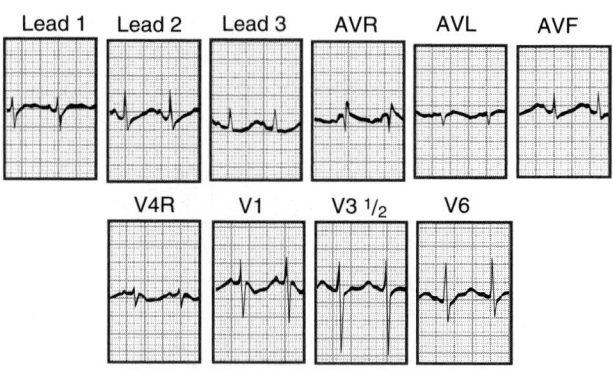

FIGURE 416–11. Electrocardiogram in hypokalemia (serum potassium, 2.7 mEq/L; serum calcium, 4.8 mEq/L at the time of the tracing). Note the prolongation of electrical systole as evidenced by a widened TU wave, as well as depression of the ST segment in V_4R, V_1, and V_6.

lengthened with hypokalemia and hypocalcemia; in the former instance, a U wave may be noted at the end of the T wave (Fig. 416–11). A congenitally prolonged Q-T interval (Fig. 416–12) may also be seen in children with one of the long Q-T syndromes. These patients are at high risk for ventricular arrhythmias, including a form of ventricular tachycardia known as *torsades de pointes*, and sudden death (see Chapter 428.6).

ST SEGMENT AND T-WAVE ABNORMALITIES

A slight elevation of the ST segment may occur in normal teenagers and is attributed to early repolarization of the heart. In pericarditis, irritation of the epicardium may cause *elevation of the ST segment* followed by abnormal T-wave inversion as healing progresses. Administration of digitalis is sometimes associated with sagging of the ST segment and abnormal inversion of the T wave.

Depression of the ST segment may also occur in any condition that produces myocardial damage or ischemia, including severe anemia, carbon monoxide poisoning, aberrant origin of the left coronary artery from the pulmonary artery, glycogen storage disease of the heart, myocardial tumors, and mucopolysaccharidoses. An aberrant origin of the left coronary artery from the pulmonary artery may lead to changes indistinguishable from those of acute myocardial infarction in adults. Similar changes may occur in patients with other rare abnormalities of the coronary arteries and in those with cardiomyopathy, even in the presence of normal coronary arteries. These patterns are often misread in young infants because of the unfamiliarity of pediatricians with this "infarct" pattern, and thus a high index of suspicion must be maintained in infants with symptoms compatible with coronary ischemia.

T-wave inversion may occur in myocarditis and pericarditis, or it may be a sign of either right or left ventricular hypertrophy and strain. Hypothyroidism may produce flat or inverted T waves in association with generalized low voltage. In hyperkalemia, the T waves are commonly of high voltage and are tent-shaped (Fig. 416–13).

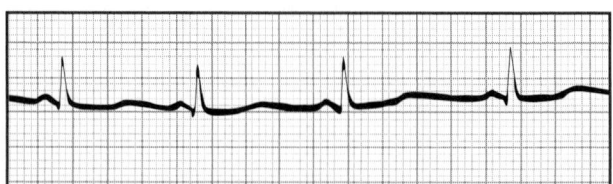

FIGURE 416–12. Prolonged Q-T interval in a patient with long Q-T syndrome.

FIGURE 416–10. Electrocardiogram showing left ventricular hypertrophy in a 12-yr-old child with aortic stenosis. Note the deep S wave in V_1–V_3 and tall R in V_5. In addition, T-wave inversion is present in leads II, III, aVF, and V_6.

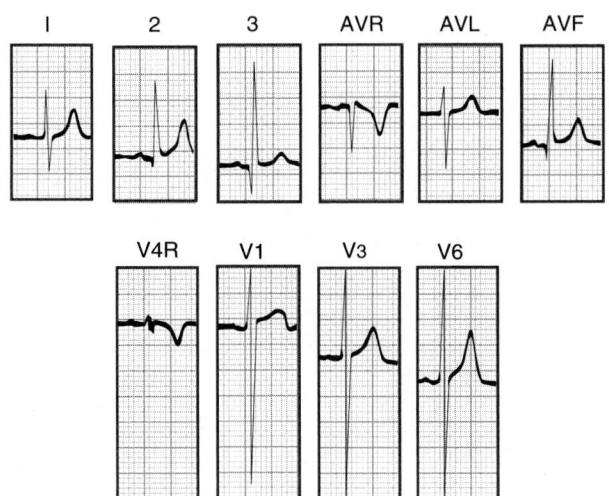

FIGURE 416–13. Electrocardiogram in hyperkalemia (serum potassium, 6.5 mEq/L; serum calcium, 5.1 mEq/L). Note the tall, tent-shaped T waves, especially in leads I, II, and V₆.

416.3 Hematologic Data

In acyanotic infants with large left-to-right shunts, the onset of heart failure often coincides with the nadir of the normal *physiologic anemia* of infancy. Increasing the hematocrit in these patients to greater than 40% can decrease shunt volume and result in an improvement in symptoms; however, this form of treatment is reserved for infants who are not otherwise surgical candidates (extremely premature infants or those with exceedingly complex congenital heart disease for whom only palliative surgery is possible). In these select infants, regular evaluation of the hematocrit and booster transfusions when appropriate may be helpful in improving growth.

Polycythemia is frequently noted in cyanotic patients with right-to-left shunts. Patients with severe polycythemia are in a delicate balance between the risks of intravascular thrombosis and a bleeding diathesis. The most frequent abnormalities include accelerated fibrinolysis, thrombocytopenia, abnormal clot retraction, hypofibrinogenemia, prolonged prothrombin time, and prolonged partial thromboplastin time. The preparation of cyanotic, polycythemic patients for elective surgery, such as dental extraction, includes evaluation and treatment of abnormal coagulation.

Because of the high viscosity of polycythemic blood (hematocrit >65%), patients with cyanotic congenital heart disease are at risk for the development of vascular thromboses, especially of cerebral veins. Dehydration increases the risk of thrombosis, and thus adequate fluid intake must be maintained during hot weather or intercurrent gastrointestinal illnesses. Diuretics should be used with caution in these patients and may need to be decreased if fluid intake is a concern. Polycythemic infants with concomitant iron deficiency are at even greater risk for cerebrovascular accidents, probably because of the decreased deformability of microcytic red blood cells. Iron therapy produces improvement, but surgical treatment of the cardiac anomaly is the best therapy.

Severely cyanotic patients should have periodic determinations of hemoglobin and hematocrit. Increasing polycythemia, often associated with headache, fatigue, dyspnea, or a combination of these conditions, is one indication for palliative or corrective surgical intervention. In cyanotic patients with inoperable conditions, phlebotomy may be required to treat individuals whose hematocrit has risen to the 65–70% level, usually when the polycythemia is associated with symptoms such as headache. This procedure is not without risk, especially in patients with an extreme elevation in pulmonary vascular resistance. Because these patients do not tolerate wide fluctuations in circulating blood volume, blood should be replaced with fresh frozen plasma or albumin. Whether routine phlebotomy should be performed in polycythemic patients who are asymptomatic is controversial.

416.4 Echocardiography

Echocardiography dramatically reduces the requirement for invasive studies such as cardiac catheterization. The echocardiographic examination can be used to evaluate cardiac structure in congenital heart lesions, estimate intracardiac pressures and gradients across stenotic valves and vessels, quantitate cardiac contractile function (both systolic and diastolic), determine the direction of flow across a defect, examine the integrity of the coronary arteries, and detect the presence of vegetations from endocarditis, as well as the presence of pericardial fluid, cardiac tumors, and chamber thrombi. Echocardiography may also be used to assist in the performance of pericardiocentesis, balloon atrial septostomy (see Chapter 424.2), and endocardial biopsy and in the placement of flow-directed pulmonary artery (Swan-Ganz) monitoring catheters. *Transesophageal echocardiography* is used to monitor ventricular function in patients during difficult surgical procedures and can provide an immediate assessment of the results of surgical repair of congenital heart lesions. *Fetal echocardiography* can detect the presence of many congenital heart lesions, often as early as 17–19 wk of gestation, and is especially valuable in evaluating fetal cardiac arrhythmias. A complete echocardiographic examination usually entails a combination of M-mode and two-dimensional imaging, as well as pulsed, continuous, and color Doppler flow studies.

M-MODE ECHOCARDIOGRAPHY

M-mode echocardiography displays a one-dimensional slice of cardiac structure varying over time. It is used mostly for the measurement of cardiac dimensions (wall thickness and chamber size) and cardiac function (fractional shortening, wall thickening). M-mode echocardiography is also useful for assessing the motion of intracardiac structures (opening and closing of valves, movement of free walls and septa) and the anatomy of valves (Fig. 416–14). The most frequently used index of cardiac function in children is *percent fractional shortening*, which is calculated as (LVED – LVES)/LVED, where LVED is left ventricular (LV) dimension at end-diastole and LVES is LV dimension at end-systole. Normal fractional shortening is 28–40%. Other M-mode indices of cardiac function include the mean velocity of fiber shortening (mean V_{CF}), systolic time intervals (LVPEP = LV pre-ejection period, LVET = LV ejection time), and isovolemic contraction time. More sophisticated indices of cardiac function can be derived noninvasively with the assistance of echocardiography (pressure-volume relationship, end-systolic wall stress-strain relationship); however, their accuracy is limited when compared with similar measurements in the catheterization laboratory.

TWO-DIMENSIONAL ECHOCARDIOGRAPHY

Two-dimensional echocardiography provides a real-time image of cardiac structures. With two-dimensional echocardiography, the contracting heart is imaged in several standard views (subxiphoid, Fig. 416–15; parasagittal, Fig. 416–16; parasternal, Fig. 416–17; and suprasternal, Fig. 416–18) that emphasize specific structures. Two-dimensional echocardiography has replaced cardiac angiography for the preoperative diagnosis of many, but not all congenital heart lesions, and it exceeds angiography in several areas, for example, in imaging the atrioventricular valves and their chordal attachments. When information from the cardiac examination is not consistent with the echocardiogram, cardiac catheterization is an important tool to confirm the

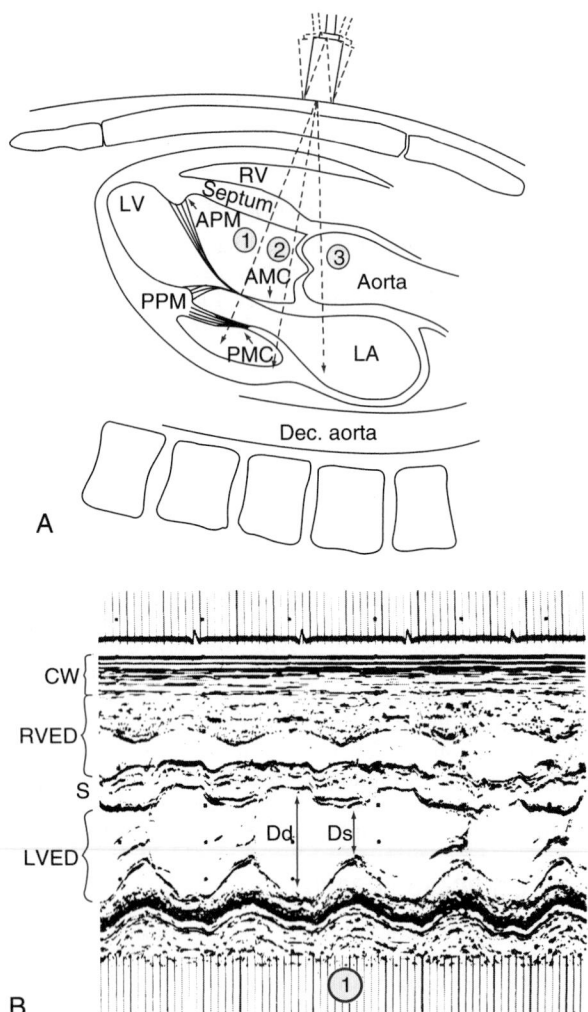

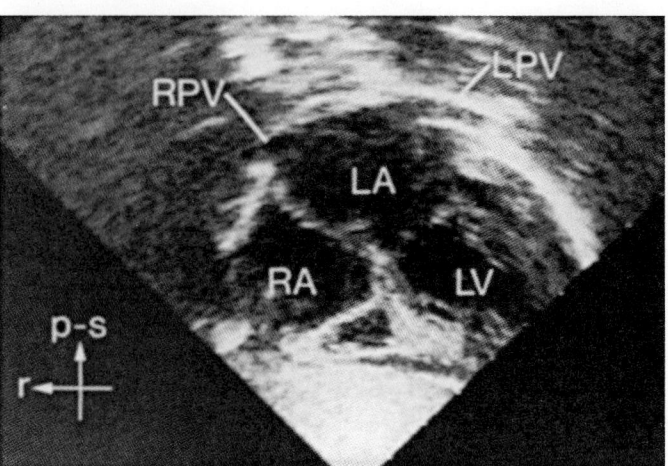

FIGURE 416–15. Subxiphoid normal echocardiographic view. The anterior angulation shows the mitral valve and the left ventricular inflow tract. Note the pulmonary veins connecting with the left atrium. LA = left atrium; LPV = left pulmonary vein; RPV = right pulmonary vein; LV = left ventricle; p-s = posterior-superior; r = right; RA = right atrium. (From Sanders SP: Echocardiography. In Long WA [editor]: *Fetal and Neonatal Cardiology*. Philadelphia, WB Saunders, 1990.)

FIGURE 416–14. M-mode echocardiogram. *A,* Diagram of a sagittal section of a heart showing the structures traversed by the echo beam as it is moved superiorly to positions (1), (2), and (3). AMC = anterior mitral cusp; APM = anterior papillary muscle; Dec. aorta = descending aorta; LA = left atrium; LV = left ventricle; PMC = posterior mitral cusp; PPM = posterior papillary muscle; RV = right ventricle. *B,* Echocardiogram from transducer position (1); this view is the best one for measuring cardiac dimensions and fractional shortening. RVED = RV dimension at end-diastole; LVED = LV dimension at end-diastole (Dd); Ds = LV dimension in systole. CW = chest wall. Fractional shortening is calculated as (LVED – LVES)/LVED.

assessment of the presence and direction of intracardiac shunts and allows identification of small or multiple left-to-right or right-to-left shunts. The severity of valvular insufficiency is also more accurately evaluated with color Doppler.

TRANSESOPHAGEAL ECHOCARDIOGRAPHY

Transesophageal echocardiography is an extremely sensitive imaging technique that produces a clearer view of smaller lesions such as vegetations in endocarditis. It is useful in visualizing posteriorly located structures such as the atria, aortic root, and atrioventricular valves. Transesophageal echocardiography has been extremely useful as an intraoperative technique for

anatomic diagnosis and evaluate the degree of physiologic derangement.

DOPPLER ECHOCARDIOGRAPHY

Doppler echocardiography displays blood flow in cardiac chambers and vascular channels based on the change in frequency imparted to a sound wave by the movement of erythrocytes. In *pulsed Doppler* and *continuous wave Doppler*, the speed and direction of blood flow in the line of the echo beam change the transducer's reference frequency. This frequency change can be translated into volumetric flow (L/min) data for estimating systemic or pulmonary blood flow and into pressure (mm Hg) data for estimating gradients across the semilunar or atrioventricular valves or across septal defects or vascular communications such as shunts (Fig. 416–19). *Color Doppler* permits highly accurate

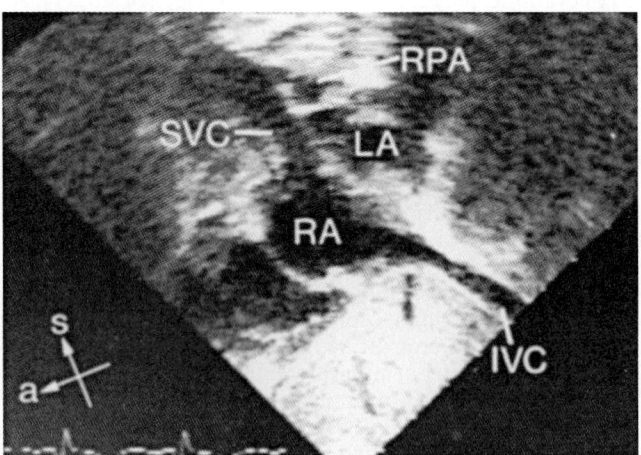

FIGURE 416–16. Right parasagittal normal echocardiographic plane view showing the junction of the inferior and superior venae cavae with the right atrium. a = anterior; IVC = inferior vena cava; LA = left atrium; RA = right atrium; RPA = right pulmonary artery; s = superior; SVC = superior vena cava. (From Sanders SP: Echocardiography. In Long WA [editor]: *Fetal and Neonatal Cardiology*. Philadelphia, WB Saunders, 1990.)

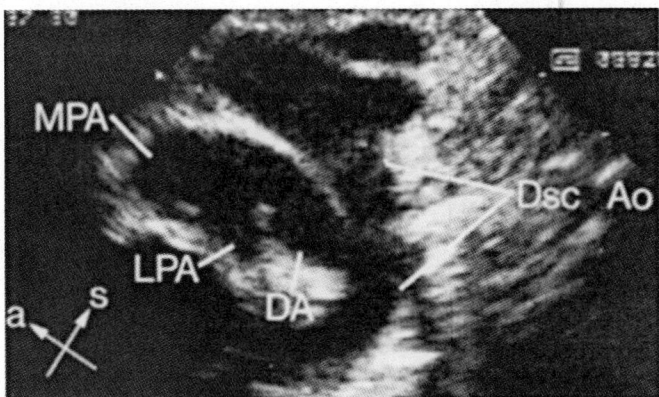

FIGURE 416–17. Normal high parasternal, parasagittal echocardiographic plane view for imaging the ductus arteriosus. a = anterior; DA = ductus arteriosus; Dsc Ao = descending aorta; LPA = left pulmonary artery; MPA = main pulmonary artery; s = superior. (From Sanders SP: Echocardiography. In Long WA [editor]: *Fetal and Neonatal Cardiology.* Philadelphia, WB Saunders, 1990.)

monitoring cardiac function during both cardiac and noncardiac surgery and for screening for residual cardiac defects after cardiopulmonary bypass. This technique has been especially helpful in evaluating the degree of residual regurgitation after repair of atrioventricular septal defects and in searching for small muscular VSDs that may have been missed during the closure of larger defects.

FETAL ECHOCARDIOGRAPHY

Fetal echocardiography can be used to evaluate cardiac structures or disturbances in cardiac rhythm. Obstetricians often detect gross abnormalities in cardiac structure on routine obstetric ultrasonography or may refer the patient because of unexplained hydrops fetalis. Fetal echocardiography may be capable of diagnosing congenital heart lesions as early as 17–19 wk of gestation; however, accuracy at this early stage is limited. Serial fetal echocardiograms have also demonstrated the importance of flow disturbance in the pathogenesis of

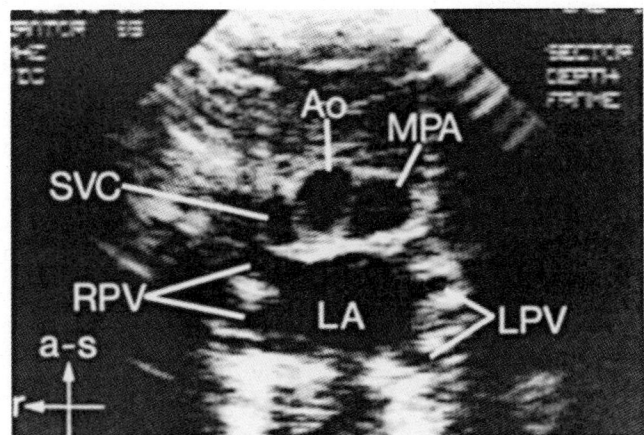

FIGURE 416–18. Suprasternal notch normal echocardiographic view showing the pulmonary veins connecting with the left atrium. Ao = aorta; a-s = anterior-superior; LA = left atrium; LPV = left pulmonary vein; MPA = main pulmonary artery; RPV = right pulmonary vein; r = right; SVC = superior vena cava. (From Sanders SP: Echocardiography. In Long WA [editor]: *Fetal and Neonatal Cardiology.* Philadelphia, WB Saunders, 1990.)

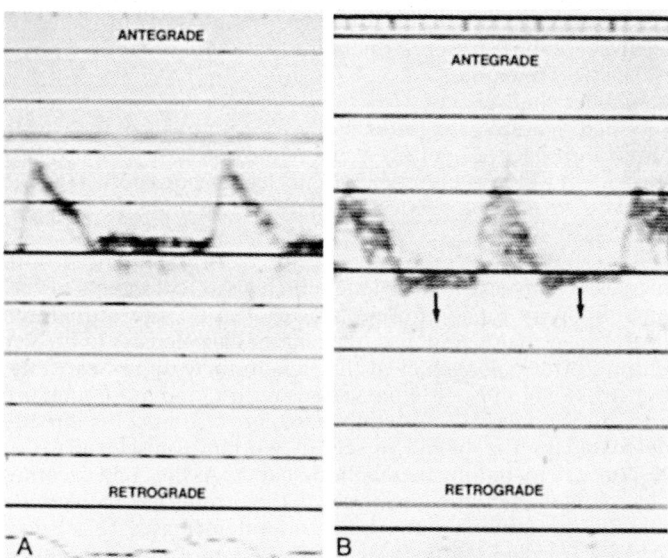

FIGURE 416–19. Patent ductus arteriosus. *A,* Doppler flow in the proximal descending aorta of a normal infant demonstrating normal antegrade systolic and diastolic flow. *B,* The Doppler flow configuration in an infant with patent ductus arteriosus reveals antegrade systolic, but retrograde diastolic flow *(arrows).*

congenital heart disease; such studies can show the intrauterine progression of a moderate lesion, such as aortic stenosis, into a more severe lesion, such as hypoplastic left heart syndrome. M-mode echocardiography can diagnose rhythm disturbances in the fetus and can determine the success of antiarrhythmic therapy administered to the mother. A screening fetal echocardiogram is recommended for patients with a previous child or 1st-degree relative with congenital heart disease, for patients who are at higher risk of having a child with cardiac disease (e.g., insulin-dependent diabetics, patients with exposure to teratogenic drugs during early pregnancy), and in any fetus in which a chromosomal abnormality is suspected or confirmed.

VENTRICULAR FUNCTION

Sophisticated M-mode and two-dimensional echocardiographic methods of assessing left ventricular systolic and diastolic function (e.g., end-systolic wall stress and dobutamine stress echocardiography) have proved useful in the serial assessment of patients at risk for the development of ventricular dysfunction. Such patients include those receiving anthracycline drugs for cancer chemotherapy, patients at risk for iron overload, and patients being monitored for rejection or coronary artery disease after heart transplantation.

416.5 Exercise Testing

The normal cardiorespiratory system adapts to the extensive demands of exercise with a several-fold increase in oxygen consumption and cardiac output. Because of the large reserve capacity for exercise, significant abnormalities in cardiovascular performance may be present without symptoms at rest or during ordinary activities. When patients are evaluated in a resting state, significant abnormalities in cardiac function may not be appreciated, or if detected, their implications for quality of life may not be recognized. Permission for children with cardiovascular disease to participate in various forms of physical activity is frequently based on totally subjective criteria. Exercise testing plays an important role in evaluating symptoms, quantitating the severity of cardiac abnormalities, and assisting in the management of these patients, including prescribing a rational physical activity schedule.

In older children, exercise studies are generally performed on a graded treadmill apparatus with timed intervals of increasing grade and speed. In younger children, exercise studies are performed on a bicycle ergometer. Many laboratories now have the capacity to measure cardiac output and pulmonary function noninvasively during exercise.

As a child grows, the capacity for work is enhanced with increased body size and skeletal muscle mass. All indices of cardiopulmonary function do not increase in a uniform manner, however. A major response to exercise is an increase in cardiac output, principally achieved through an increase in heart rate, but stroke volume, systemic venous return, and pulse pressure are also increased. Systemic vascular resistance is greatly decreased as the blood vessels in working muscle dilate in response to increasing metabolic demands. As the child becomes older and larger, the response of the heart rate to exercise remains prominent, but cardiac output increases because of growing cardiac volume capacity and hence stroke volume. Responses to dynamic exercise are not dependent solely on age. For any given body surface area, boys have a larger stroke volume than size-matched girls do. This increase is also mediated by posture. Augmentation of stroke volume with upright, dynamic exercise is facilitated by the pumping action of working muscles, which overcomes the static effect of gravity and increases systemic venous return.

Dynamic exercise testing defines not only endurance and exercise capacity but also the effect of such exercise on myocardial blood flow and cardiac rhythm. Significant ST segment depression reflects abnormalities in myocardial perfusion, for example, the subendocardial ischemia that commonly occurs during exercise in children with hypertrophied left ventricles. The exercise ECG is considered abnormal if the ST segment depression is greater than 2 mm and extends for at least 0.06 sec after the J point (onset of the ST segment) in conjunction with a horizontal-, upward-, or downward-sloping ST segment. Provocation of rhythm disturbances during an exercise study is an important method of evaluating selected patients with known or suspected rhythm disorders. The effect of pharmacologic management can also be tested in this manner.

416.6 MRI, Electron Beam CT, and Radionuclide Studies

MRI is helpful in the diagnosis and management of patients with congenital heart disease. It produces tomographic images of the heart in any projection (Fig. 416–20), with excellent contrast resolution of fat, myocardium, and lung, as well as moving blood from blood vessel walls. MRI has been particularly useful in evaluating areas that are less well visualized by echocardiography, such as distal branch pulmonary artery anatomy and anomalies in systemic and pulmonary venous return.

Magnetic resonance angiography allows the acquisition of images in several tomographic planes. Within each plane, images are obtained at different phases of the cardiac cycle. Thus, when displayed in a dynamic "cine" format, changes in wall thickening, chamber volume, and valve function can be displayed and analyzed. Blood flow velocity and blood flow volume can be approximated. Phosphorus *magnetic resonance spectroscopy* provides a means of demonstrating relative concentrations of high-energy metabolites (e.g., adenosine triphosphate, adenosine diphosphate, inorganic phosphate, and phosphocreatine) within regions of the working myocardium.

Electron beam CT (EBCT) scanning is used to perform rapid, respiration-gated cardiac imaging in children with a resolution

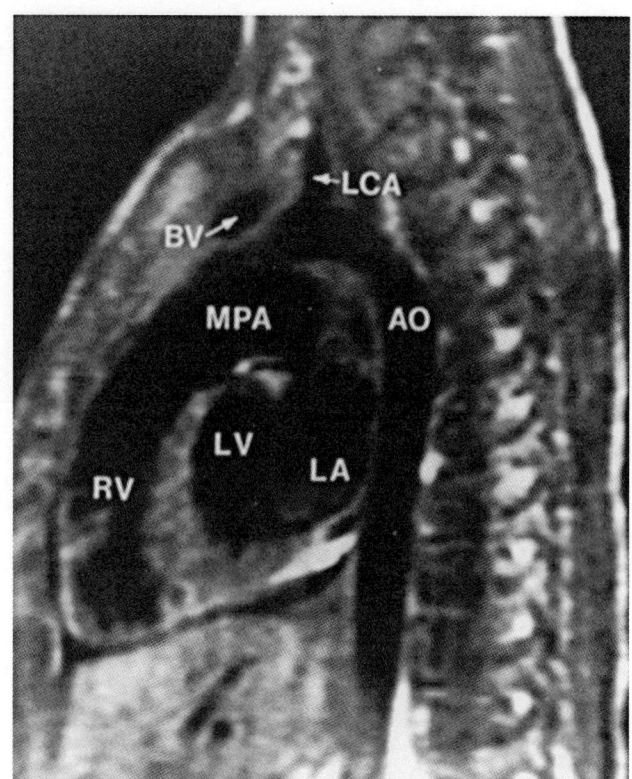

FIGURE 416–20. Sagittal normal MRI. AO = aorta; BV = brachiocephalic vein; LA = left atrium; LCA = left coronary artery; LV = left ventricle; MPA = main pulmonary artery; RV = right ventricle. (From Bisset GS III: Cardiac and great vessel anatomy. In El-Khoury GY, Bergman RA, Montgomery WJ [editors]: *Sectional Anatomy by MRI/CT.* New York, Churchill Livingstone, 1990.)

down to 0.5 mm. Three-dimensional reconstruction of EBCT images (Fig. 416–21) is especially useful in evaluating branch pulmonary arteries, anomalies in systemic and pulmonary venous return, and great vessel anomalies such as coarctation of the aorta.

Radionuclide angiography may be used to detect and quantify shunts and to analyze the distribution of blood flow to each lung. This technique is particularly useful in quantifying the volume of blood flow distribution between the two lungs in patients with abnormalities of the pulmonary vascular tree, after a shunt operation (Blalock-Taussig or Glenn), or to quantify the success of balloon angioplasty and intravascular stenting procedures. *Gated blood pool scanning* can be used to calculate hemodynamic measurements, quantify valvular regurgitation, and detect regional wall motion abnormalities. *Thallium imaging* can be performed to evaluate cardiac muscle perfusion. These methods can be used at the bedside of seriously ill children and can be performed serially, with minimal discomfort and low radiation exposure.

416.7 Cardiac Catheterization

Cardiac catheterization is an important tool in the diagnosis of congenital heart disease. During catheterization, blood samples are obtained for measuring oxygen saturation and calculating shunt volumes, pressures are measured for calculating gradients and valve areas, and contrast is injected to delineate structures. Major indications for cardiac catheterization include (1) presurgical evaluation of cardiac anatomy or shunt size, or both, in children with congenital cardiac lesions when echocardio-

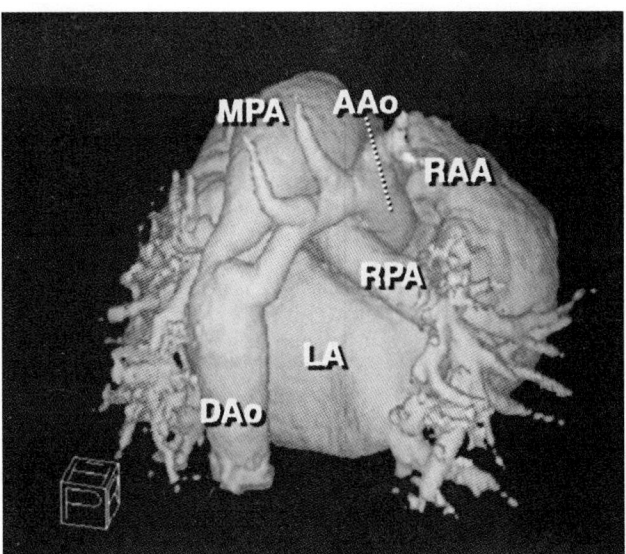

FIGURE 416–21. Three-dimensional reconstruction of electron beam CT images from a neonate with severe coarctation of the aorta. The patent ductus arteriosus can be seen toward the left leading from the main pulmonary artery to the descending aorta. The tortuous and narrow coarctated segment is just to the right of the ductus. The transverse aorta is hypoplastic as well. MPA = main pulmonary artery; AAo = ascending aorta; DAo = descending aorta; RAA = right atrial appendage; RPA = right pulmonary artery; LA = left atrium. (Image courtesy of Dr. Paul Pitlick, Stanford University, Stanford, CA.)

graphic evaluation is incomplete; (2) evaluation of pulmonary vascular resistance and its response to vasodilators or oxygen; (3) follow-up after surgical repair or palliation of complex congenital heart lesions; (4) myocardial biopsy for the diagnosis of cardiomyopathy or screening for cardiac rejection after transplantation; (5) interventional cardiac catheterization; and (6) electrophysiologic study or transcatheter ablation, or both (see Chapter 428).

Although the risks are low, cardiac catheterization involves potential complications for the patient and should not be used without an opportunity for benefit. Echocardiography, MRI, EBCT, or radionuclide studies may be used in lieu of multiple cardiac catheterizations in individual patients who require careful monitoring of their hemodynamic status. The number of postoperative catheterizations has increased with the advent of palliative surgical procedures to repair complex congenital heart lesions. Interventional cardiac catheterization has replaced surgical repair in many cases (e.g., pulmonary or aortic valve stenosis, re-coarctation of the aorta, closure of small PDAs), is competing with it in others (ASDs, muscular VSD, large PDA), and in still others is used as an adjunct to complex surgical repairs (branch pulmonary artery stenosis, closure of a fenestrated Fontan palliation [see Chapter 423.4]).

Cardiac catheterization should be performed with the patient in as close to a basal state as possible. Conscious sedation is routinely used for most of these studies; however, if general anesthesia is required, careful choice of an anesthetic agent is warranted to avoid depression of cardiovascular function and subsequent distortion of the calculations of cardiac output, pulmonary and systemic vascular resistance, and shunt ratios.

Cardiac catheterization in critically ill infants with congenital heart disease should be performed in a center where a pediatric cardiovascular surgical team is available in the event that an operation is required immediately afterward. The complication rate of cardiac catheterization and angiography is greatest in critically ill infants; they must be studied in a thermally neutral environment and treated quickly for hypothermia, hypoglycemia, acidosis, or excessive blood loss.

Catheterization usually includes both the right and left sides of the heart. The catheter is passed into the heart under fluoroscopic guidance through a percutaneous entry point in a femoral vein, although occasionally, jugular access is used. In infants and in a large number of older children, the left side of the heart can be accessed by passing the catheter across a patent foramen ovale to the left atrium and left ventricle. If the foramen is closed, the left side of the heart can also be catheterized by passing the catheter retrograde via a percutaneous entry site into the femoral artery. The catheter can be manipulated through abnormal intracardiac defects (ASDs, VSDs). Complete hemodynamics can be calculated (Box 416–1), including cardiac output, intracardiac left-to-right and right-to-left shunts, and systemic and pulmonary vascular resistance. Normal circulatory dynamics is depicted in Figure 416–22.

THERMODILUTION MEASUREMENT OF CARDIAC OUTPUT

The *thermodilution method* for measuring cardiac output is performed with a flow-directed, thermistor-tipped, pulmonary artery (Swan-Ganz) catheter. A known change in the heat content of the blood is induced at one point in the circulation (usually the right atrium or inferior vena cava), and the resultant change in temperature is detected at a point downstream (usually the pulmonary artery). The injectate is generally room tem-

---

BOX 416–1. Normal Values and Formulas for Determination of Hemodynamics in Cardiac Catheterization

1. Cardiac index: 3.0–5.0 L/min/m^2
2. Arteriovenous oxygen difference: 4.5 ± 0.7 mL/dL
3. Oxygen consumption: 140–160 mL/m^2/min
4. Arterial oxygen saturation: 94–100%
5. Pulmonary arteriolar resistance: 50–150 dyn sec cm^{-5} (1 U = 80 dynes)
6. Cardiac output (Qs) mL/min = systemic flow =

$$\frac{O_2 \text{ intake (mL/min)}}{\left\{ \begin{array}{l} O_2 \text{ content of arterial blood (mL/dL)} \\ \text{minus } O_2 \text{ content of mixed venous blood (mL/dL)} \end{array} \right.} \times 100$$

7. Cardiac index: cardiac output (L/min)/m^2 of body surface area
8. Pulmonary artery flow (Qp) =

$$\frac{O_2 \text{ intake (mL/min)}}{\left\{ \begin{array}{l} O_2 \text{ content of pulmonary venous blood (mL/dL)} \\ \text{minus } O_2 \text{ content of pulmonary arterial blood (mL/dL)} \end{array} \right.} \times 100$$

If a pulmonary venous sample is not available, it is assumed to be saturated to 95% of capacity
9. Effective pulmonary artery flow (Qep) =

$$\frac{O_2 \text{ intake (mL/min)}}{\left\{ \begin{array}{l} \text{pulmonary venous } O_2 \text{ content (100 mL/dL)} \\ \text{minus mixed venous } O_2 \text{ content (100 mL/dL)} \end{array} \right.} \times 100$$

10. Total left-to-right shunt: pulmonary artery flow minus effective pulmonary artery flow
11. Total right-to-left shunt: systemic flow minus effective pulmonary artery flow

12. Pulmonary arteriolar resistance: $Rp = \dfrac{PA - PC}{Qp}$

where R = pulmonary arteriolar resistance (resistance units)
PA = mean pulmonary artery pressure in mm Hg
PC = mean pulmonary "capillary" pressure in mm Hg
Qp = pulmonary flow in L/min/m^2

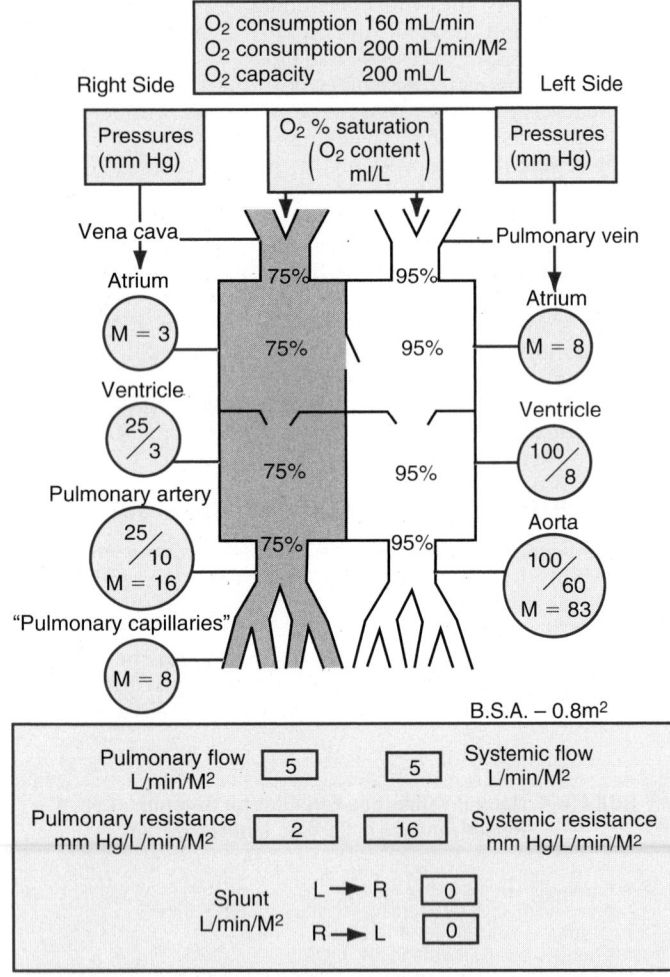

O₂ consumption 160 mL/min
O₂ consumption 200 mL/min/M²
O₂ capacity 200 mL/L

Right Side   Left Side

Pressures (mm Hg)

O₂ % saturation
(O₂ content / ml/L)

Pressures (mm Hg)

Vena cava   Pulmonary vein

Atrium   75%   95%   Atrium
M = 3   M = 8

75%   95%

Ventricle   Ventricle
25/3   100/8

Pulmonary artery   75%   95%

25/10
M = 16   Aorta
                                100/60
"Pulmonary capillaries"   75%   95%   M = 83

M = 8

B.S.A. – 0.8m²

Pulmonary flow L/min/M²	5	5	Systemic flow L/min/M²
Pulmonary resistance mm Hg/L/min/M²	2	16	Systemic resistance mm Hg/L/min/M²
Shunt L/min/M²	L → R	0	
	R → L	0	

FIGURE 416–22. Diagram of normal circulatory dynamics with pressure readings, oxygen content, and percent saturation. (Modified from Nadas AS, Fyler DC: *Pediatric Cardiology*, 3rd ed. Philadelphia, WB Saunders, 1972.)

perature saline. This method is used to measure cardiac output in the catheterization laboratory in patients without shunts. Monitoring cardiac output by the thermodilution method can also be useful in managing critically ill infants and children in an intensive care setting after cardiac surgery or in the presence of shock. In this case, a triple-lumen catheter is used for both cardiac output determination and measurement of pulmonary artery and pulmonary capillary wedge pressure.

ANGIOCARDIOGRAPHY

The major blood vessels and individual cardiac chambers may be visualized by selective angiocardiography, or the injection of contrast material into specific chambers or great vessels. This method allows identification of structural abnormalities without interference from the superimposed shadows of normal chambers. *Fluoroscopy* is used to visualize the catheter as it passes through the various heart chambers. After the cardiac catheter is properly placed in the chamber to be studied, a small amount of contrast medium is injected with a power injector, and cineangiograms are exposed at rates ranging from 15 to 90 frames/sec. *Biplane cineangiocardiography* allows detailed evaluation of specific cardiac chambers and blood vessels in two planes simultaneously with the injection of a single bolus of contrast material. This technique is standard in pediatric cardiac catheterization laboratories and allows one to minimize the vol-

ume of contrast material used, which is safer for the patient. Various angled views (e.g., left anterior oblique, cranial angulation) are used to display specific anatomic features best in individual lesions. Digital imaging is beginning to replace standard roentgenographic film for both diagnostic and archival purposes.

Rapid injection of contrast medium under pressure into the circulation is not without risk, and each injection should be carefully planned. Contrast agents consist of hypertonic solutions, with some containing organic iodides, which can cause complications, including nausea, a generalized burning sensation, central nervous system symptoms, and allergic reactions. Intramyocardial injection is generally avoided by careful placement of the catheter before injection. Hypertonicity of the contrast medium may result in transient myocardial depression and a drop in blood pressure, followed soon afterward by tachycardia, an increase in cardiac output, and a shift of interstitial fluid into the circulation. This shift can transiently increase the symptoms of heart failure in critically ill patients.

INTERVENTIONAL CATHETERIZATION

Nonsurgical treatment of certain cardiac defects is routine with interventional cardiac catheterization. Interventional techniques include balloon dilatation of stenotic valves and arteries, embolization of abnormal vascular connections, and catheter closure of both intracardiac and extracardiac defects. The procedure most often used is *balloon valvuloplasty*. A special catheter with a sausage-shaped balloon at the distal end is passed through an obstructed valve. Rapid filling of the balloon with a mixture of contrast material and saline solution results in tearing of the stenotic valve tissue, usually at the site of inappropriately fused raphe. Valvular pulmonary stenosis can be treated successfully by balloon angioplasty, and in most patients angioplasty has replaced surgical repair as the initial procedure of choice. The clinical results of this procedure are similar to those obtained by open heart surgery, but without the need for sternotomy or prolonged hospitalization. Balloon valvuloplasty for aortic stenosis has also yielded excellent results, although as with surgery, aortic stenosis often recurs as the child grows and multiple procedures may thus be required. One complication of both valvuloplasty and surgery is the creation of valvular insufficiency. This complication has more serious implications when it occurs on the aortic vs the pulmonary side of the circulation because regurgitation is less well tolerated at systemic arterial pressures.

Balloon angioplasty is the procedure of choice for patients with re-stenosis of coarctation of the aorta after earlier surgery. It is controversial whether angioplasty is the best procedure for native (unoperated) coarctation of the aorta because of reports of later aneurysm formation. The risk of angioplasty and valvuloplasty procedures on the left side of the heart is higher in younger patients, especially infants less than 1 yr of age, because of complications at the site of femoral artery catheterization. Low-profile catheters have significantly reduced, though not totally eliminated these complications. Other applications of the balloon angioplasty technique include amelioration of mitral stenosis, dilatation of surgical conduits (Mustard or Senning atrial baffles), relief of branch pulmonary artery narrowing, dilatation of venous obstructions, and the long-used balloon atrial septostomy (Rashkind procedure) for transposition of the great arteries (see Chapter 424.2).

Interventional cardiac catheterization techniques using *metal coils* have been developed for obliteration of arteriovenous shunts and pulmonary collateral vessels, which may be detrimental after surgical repair of pulmonary atresia and VSD. Coils have been used to close small and medium-sized PDAs with excellent results. In patients with branch pulmonary artery stenoses, the previously mixed results with balloon angioplasty alone have been enhanced with the use of *intravascular stents* delivered over a balloon catheter and expanded within the vessel lumen. Once placed, they can often be dilated to successively greater sizes as the patient grows. Placement of stents in small infants and children remains problematic because of problems associated with subsequent growth.

The use of catheter-introduced devices to close congenital cardiac defects has produced good results. Currently, several devices (clamshell, Helex, button) are undergoing clinical trials for closure of small to moderate-sized ASDs. Umbrella or bag devices may also be introduced to close a large PDA not amenable to coil closure. High-risk patients undergoing the Fontan operation (see Chapter 423.4) often have a small fenestration created in the baffle between the right and left sides of the circulation to serve as a "popoff valve" for high right-sided pressure in the early surgical period. Patients with these "fenestrated Fontans" are ideal candidates for subsequent closure with a catheter-delivered device. Patients with apical muscular VSDs, especially when associated with other cardiac defects, may be candidates for catheter closure with a clamshell-type device because of the higher risk of standard surgery. ASD closure devices are approved by the Food and Drug Administration for general use.

Cardiac Sounds and Phonocardiography

McNamara DG: Value and limitations of auscultation in the management of congenital heart disease. *Pediatr Clin North Am* 1990;37:93.

Mills P, Craige E: Echophonocardiography. *Prog Cardiovasc Dis* 1989;20:337.

Newburger JW, Rosenthal A, Williams RG, et al: Noninvasive tests in the initial evaluation of heart murmurs in children. *N Engl J Med* 1983;308:61.

Electrocardiogram and Vectorcardiogram

Garson A: The Electrocardiogram in Infants and Children: A Systematic Approach. Philadelphia, Lea & Febiger, 1983.

Garson A, Dick M, Fournier A, et al: The long QT syndrome in children: An international study of 287 patients. Circulation 1993;87:1866.

Lipman BF, Massey EF: Clinical Scalar Electrocardiography. Chicago, Year Book, 1984.

Marriott H: Rhythm Quizlets Self Assessment. Philadelphia, Lea & Febiger, 1987.

Schwartz PJ, Moss AJ, Vincent GM, et al: Diagnostic criteria for the long QT syndrome: An update. Circulation 1993;88:782.

Echocardiography

Allan LD: A practical approach to fetal heart scanning. *Semin Perinatol* 2000;24: 324–30.

Frommelt MA, Frommelt PC: Advances in echocardiographic diagnostic modalities for the pediatrician. *Pediatr Clin North Am* 1999;46:427–39.

Sahn DJ, Vick GW 3rd: Review of new techniques in echocardiography and magnetic resonance imaging as applied to patients with congenital heart disease. *Heart* 2001;86(Suppl 2):II41–53.

Silverman NH: *Pediatric Echocardiography*. Baltimore, Williams & Wilkins, 1993.

Stevenson JG: Role of intraoperative transesophageal echocardiography during repair of congenital cardiac defects. *Acta Paediatr Suppl* 1995;410:23–33.

Todros T: Prenatal diagnosis and management of fetal cardiovascular malformations. *Curr Opin Obstet Gynecol* 2000;12:105–9.

Van Der Velde ME, Perry SB: Transesophageal echocardiography during interventional catheterization in congenital heart disease. *Echocardiography* 1997;14: 513–28.

Exercise Testing

Braden DS, Strong WF: Cardiovascular responses to exercise in children. *Am J Dis Child* 1990;144:1255.

James FW, Blomqvist CG, Freed MD, et al: Standards for exercise testing in the pediatric age group: American Heart Association Council on Cardiovascular Disease in the Young. *Circulation* 1982;66:1377.

Nixon PA, Joswiak ML, Fricker FJ: A six-minute walk test for assessing exercise tolerance in severely ill children. *J Pediatr* 1996;129:362.

Sullivan ID: Prenatal diagnosis of structural heart disease: Does it make a difference to survival? *Heart* 2002;87:405–6.

Washington RL, van Gundy JC, Cohen C, et al: Normal aerobic and anaerobic exercise data for North American school-age children. *J Pediatr* 1988;112: 223.

Radiology, MRI, and Nuclear Medicine

Didier D, Higgins CB, Fisher MR, et al: Congenital heart disease: Gated MR imaging in 72 patients. *Radiology* 1986;158:227.

Hurwitz RA: Quantitation of aortic and mitral regurgitation in the pediatric population: Evaluation by radionuclide angiography. *Am J Cardiol* 1983;51:252.

Nienaber CA, Rehders TC, Fratz S: Detection and assessment of congenital heart disease with magnetic resonance techniques. *J Cardiovasc Magn Reson* 1999;1: 169–84.

Strife JL, Sze RW: Radiographic evaluation of the neonate with congenital heart disease. *Radiol Clin North Am* 1999;37:1093–107

Wolfson BJ: Radiologic interpretation of congenital heart disease. *Clin Perinatol* 2001;28:71–89.

Cardiac Catheterization

Allen HD, Mullins CE: Results of the Valvuloplasty and Angioplasty of Congenital Anomalies Registry. *Am J Cardiol* 1990;65:772.

Kreutzer J: Transcatheter intervention in the neonate with congenital heart disease. *Clin Perinatol* 2001;28:137–57.

McMahon CJ, El-Said HG, Grifka RG, et al: Redilation of endovascular stents in congenital heart disease: Factors implicated in the development of restenosis and neointimal proliferation. *J Am Coll Cardiol* 2001;38:521–6.

Moore JW, Ing FF, Drummond D, et al: Transcatheter closure of surgical shunts in patients with congenital heart disease. *Am J Cardiol* 2000;85:636–40.

Moore P, Lock JE: *Diagnostic and Interventional Catheterization in Congenital Heart Disease*. Boston, Kluwer, 2000.

O'Laughlin MP, Slack MC, Grifka RG, et al: Implantation and intermediate-term follow-up of stents in congenital heart disease. *Circulation* 1993;88:605.

Shaddy RE, Boucek MM, Sturtevant JE, et al: Comparison of angioplasty and surgery for unoperated coarctation of the aorta. *Circulation* 1993;87:793–9.

Simpson JM, Moore P, Teitel DF: Cardiac catheterization of low birth weight infants. *Am J Cardiol* 2001;87:1372–7.

Walsh KP: Interventional cardiology. *Arch Dis Child* 1997;76:6.

SECTION 3 *Congenital Heart Disease*

Daniel Bernstein

Chapter 417

Epidemiology and Genetic Basis of Congenital Heart Disease

Prevalence. Congenital heart disease occurs in 0.5–0.8% of live births. The incidence is higher in stillborns (3–4%), abortuses (10–25%), and premature infants (about 2% excluding patent ductus arteriosus [PDA]). This overall incidence does not include mitral valve prolapse, PDA of preterm infants, and

bicuspid aortic valves (present in 1–2% of adults). Congenital cardiac defects have a wide spectrum of severity in infants: about 2–3 in 1,000 newborn infants will be symptomatic with heart disease in the 1st yr of life. The diagnosis is established by 1 wk of age in 40–50% of patients with congenital heart disease and by 1 mo of age in 50–60% of patients. With advances in both palliative and corrective surgery in the last 20 yr, the number of children with congenital heart disease surviving to adulthood has increased dramatically. Despite these advances, congenital heart disease remains the leading cause of death in children with congenital malformations. Table 417–1 summarizes the relative frequency of the most common congenital cardiac lesions.

Most congenital defects are well tolerated in the fetus because of the parallel nature of the fetal circulation. Even the most

TABLE 417–1. Relative Frequency of Major Congenital Heart Lesions*

Lesion	% of All Lesions
Ventricular septal defect	25–30
Atrial septal defect (secundum)	6–8
Patent ductus arteriosus	6–8
Coarctation of aorta	5–7
Tetralogy of Fallot	5–7
Pulmonary valve stenosis	5–7
Aortic valve stenosis	4–7
d-Transposition of great arteries	3–5
Hypoplastic left ventricle	1–3
Hypoplastic right ventricle	1–3
Truncus arteriosus	1–2
Total anomalous pulmonary venous return	1–2
Tricuspid atresia	1–2
Single ventricle	1–2
Double-outlet right ventricle	1–2
Others	5–10

Excluding patent ductus arteriosus in preterm neonates, bicuspid aortic valve, physiologic peripheral pulmonic stenosis, and mitral valve prolapse.

severe cardiac defects (hypoplastic left heart syndrome) can usually be well compensated for by the fetal circulation. In this example, the entire fetal cardiac output would be ejected by the right ventricle via the ductus arteriosus into both the descending and ascending aortae (the latter filling in a retrograde fashion). It is only after birth when the fetal pathways (ductus arteriosus and foramen ovale) are closed that the full hemodynamic impact of an anatomic abnormality becomes apparent (see Chapter 414). One notable exception is the case of severe regurgitant lesions, most commonly of the tricuspid valve. In these lesions (Ebstein anomaly [see *Chapter 423.7*]), the parallel fetal circulation cannot compensate for the volume load imposed on the right side of the heart. In utero heart failure, often with fetal pleural and pericardial effusions, and generalized ascites (nonimmune hydrops fetalis) may occur.

Although the most significant transitions in circulation occur in the immediate perinatal period, the circulation continues to undergo changes after birth, and these later changes may also have a hemodynamic impact on cardiac lesions and their apparent incidence. As pulmonary vascular resistance falls over the 1st several weeks of life, left-to-right shunting through intracardiac defects increases and symptoms become more apparent. Thus, in patients with a ventricular septal defect (VSD), heart failure is often manifested between 1 and 3 mo of age (see Chapter 419.6). The severity of various defects can also change dramatically with growth; some VSDs may become smaller and even close as the child ages. Alternatively, stenosis of the aortic or pulmonary valve, which may be mild in the newborn period, may become worse if valve orifice growth does not keep pace with patient growth (see Chapter 420.5). The physician should always be alert for associated congenital malformations, which can adversely affect the patient's prognosis (see Table 415–2).

Etiology. The cause of most congenital heart defects is unknown, but rapid progress is being made in identifying the genetic basis of many congenital heart lesions. Most cases of congenital heart disease were thought to be multifactorial and result from a combination of genetic predisposition and environmental stimulus. A small percentage of congenital heart lesions were related to chromosomal abnormalities, in particular, trisomy 21, 13, and 18 and Turner syndrome: heart disease is found in more than 90% of patients with trisomy 18, 50% of patients with trisomy 21, and 40% of those with Turner syndrome. Other genetic factors were suspected to play a role in congenital heart disease; for example, certain types of VSDs (supracristal) are more common in Asian children. The risk of recurrence of congenital heart dis-

ease increases if a 1st-degree relative (parent or sibling) is affected.

A growing list of congenital heart lesions have been associated with specific chromosomal abnormalities, and several have even been linked to specific gene defects. Fluorescent in situ hybridization analysis allows clinicians rapid screening of suspected cases once a specific chromosomal abnormality has been identified.

A well-characterized genetic cause of congenital heart disease is the deletion of a large region of chromosome 22q11, known as the DiGeorge critical region. The estimated prevalence of 22q11 deletions is 1 in 4,000 live births. Cardiac lesions associated with 22q11 deletions are most often seen in association with either the DiGeorge syndrome or the Shprintzen (velocardiofacial) syndrome. The acronym CATCH 22 has been used to summarize the major components of these syndromes (*c*ardiac defects, *a*bnormal facies, *t*hymic aplasia, *c*left palate, and *h*ypocalcemia). The specific cardiac anomalies are conotruncal defects (tetralogy of Fallot, truncus arteriosus, double-outlet right ventricle, subarterial VSD) and branchial arch defects (coarctation of the aorta, interrupted aortic arch, right aortic arch). Congenital airway anomalies such as tracheomalacia and bronchomalacia are sometimes present. Although the risk of recurrence is extremely low in the absence of a parental 22q11 deletion, it is 50% if one of the parents carries the deletion.

Other structural heart lesions that have been associated with specific chromosomal abnormalities include familial secundum atrial septal defect associated with heart block (the transcription factor NKX2.5 on chromosome 5q35), Alagille syndrome (Jagged1 on chromosome 20p12), and Williams syndrome (elastin on chromosome 7q11). A compilation of known genetic causes of congenital heart disease is presented in Table 417–2.

The familial cardiomyopathies also require genetic evaluation. Hypertrophic cardiomyopathy is linked to missense mutations in the β-myosin heavy chain gene on chromosome 14, the cardiac troponin T gene on chromosome 1q3, α-tropomyosin on chromosome 15q2, and cardiac myosin-binding protein C on chromosome 11q11. X-linked cardiomyopathies have been linked to the dystrophin gene on Xp21, also the cause of the muscular dystrophies (see Table 417–2). The genetic basis of heritable arrhythmias, most notably the long Q-T syndromes, has been linked to mutations of genes coding for subunits of cardiac potassium and sodium channels (see Table 417–2).

Two to 4% of cases of congenital heart disease are associated with known environmental or adverse maternal conditions and teratogenic influences, including maternal diabetes mellitus, phenylketonuria, or systemic lupus erythematosus; congenital rubella syndrome; and maternal ingestion of drugs (lithium, ethanol, warfarin, thalidomide, antimetabolites, anticonvulsant agents) (see Table 415–2). Associated noncardiac malformations noted in identifiable syndromes may be seen in as many as 25% of patients with congenital heart disease (see Table 415–1).

Gender differences in the occurrence of specific cardiac lesions have been identified. Transposition of the great arteries and left-sided obstructive lesions are slightly more common in boys (approximately 65%), whereas atrial septal defect, VSD, PDA, and pulmonic stenosis are more common in girls. No racial differences in the occurrence of congenital heart lesions as a whole have been noted; for specific lesions such as transposition of the great arteries, a higher occurrence is seen in white infants.

Genetic Counseling. Parents who have a child with congenital heart disease require genetic counseling regarding the probability of a cardiac malformation occurring in subsequent children (see Chapter 72). With the exception of syndromes known to be due to mutation of a single gene, most congenital heart disease is still relegated to a multifactorial inheritance pattern, which should result in a low risk of recurrence. The

TABLE 417–2. Genetics of Congenital Heart Disease

Cardiovascular Disease	Chromosomal Location	Gene
Structural Heart Defects		
CATCH 22 (DiGeorge syndrome, velocardiofacial syndrome)	22q11	Not known
Familial ASD with heart block	5q35	Nkx2.5
Alagille syndrome (bile duct hypoplasia, right-sided cardiac lesions)	20p12	Jagged1
Holt-Oram syndrome (limb defects, ASD)	12q2	TBX5
Trisomy 21 (AV septal defect)	21q22	Not known
Familial TAPVR	4p13-q12	Not known
Noonan syndrome (PS, ASD, hypertrophic cardiomyopathy)	12q24	PTPN11
Ellis-van Creveld syndrome (polydactyly, ASD)	4p16	EVC
Char syndrome (craniofacial, limb defects; PDA)	6p12-21.1	TFAP2B
Williams syndrome (supravalvular AS, branch PS, hypercalcemia)	7q11	Elastin
Marfan syndrome (connective tissue weakness, aortic root dilatation)	15q21	Fibrillin
Familial laterality abnormalities (situs inversus, complex congenital heart disease)	Xq24-2q7	ZIC3
	1q42	Not known
	9p13-21	DNAI1
Cardiomyopathies		
Hypertrophic cardiomyopathy	14q1	ß-Myosin heavy chain
	15q2	α-Tropomyosin
	1q31	Troponin T
	19p13.2-19q13.2	Troponin I
	11p13-q13	Myosin-binding protein C
	12q23	Cardiac slow myosin regulatory light chain
	13p21	Ventricular slow myosin essential light chain
Hypertrophic cardiomyopathy with Wolf-Parkinson-White syndrome	7q3	Not known
Dilated cardiomyopathy	Xp21	Dystrophin
	Xp28	G4.5
	1q32, 1p1-1q1, 2q31, 3p22-25, 9q13-22, 10q21-23, 15q14	Not known
Arrhythmias		
Complete heart block	19q13	Not known
Long Q-T syndrome		
LQT1 (autosomal dominant)	11p15.5	KVLQT1 (K+ channel)
LQT2 (autosomal dominant)	7q35	HERG (K+ channel)
LQT3 (autosomal dominant)	3p21	SCN5A (Na+ channel)
LQT4 (autosomal dominant)	4q25-27	Not known
LQT5 (autosomal dominant)	21q22-q22	KCNE1 (K+ channel)
LQT6	21q22.1	KCNE2 (K+ channel)
Jervell and Lange-Nielsen syndrome (autosomal recessive, congenital deafness)	11p15.5	KVLQT1 (K+ channel)
Arrhythmogenic RV dysplasia	14q23-q24, 1q42-q43, 14q12-q22, 3p23, 17q21	Not known
Familial atrial fibrillation	10q22-q24	Not known
Familial ventricular fibrillation	3p21-p24	SCN5A

ASD = atrial septal defect; AV = atrioventricular; TAPVR = total anomalous pulmonary venous return; PS = pulmonic stenosis; AS = aortic stenosis; PDA = patent ductus arteriosus; RV = right ventricular.

incidence of congenital heart disease in the normal population is approximately 0.8%, and this incidence increases to 2–6% for a 2nd pregnancy after the birth of a child with congenital heart disease or if a parent is affected. This recurrence risk is highly dependent on the type of lesion in the 1st child. When two 1st-degree relatives have congenital heart disease, the risk for a subsequent child may reach 20–30%. When a 2nd child is found to have congenital heart disease, it will tend to be of a similar class as the lesion in their 1st-degree relative (e.g., conotruncal lesions, left-sided obstructive lesions, atrioventricular septation defects). The degree of severity may be variable, as is the presence of associated defects. Certain cardiac lesions, for example, left-sided obstructive lesions, may be associated with a much higher rate of recurrence because of the presence of mild and clinically silent defects in other family members, such as a bicuspid aortic valve. Consultation with a knowledgeable genetic counselor is the most reliable way of providing the family with up-to-date information regarding the risk of recurrence.

Fetal echocardiography improves the rate of detection of congenital heart lesions in high-risk patients (see Chapter 85.5). The resolution and accuracy of fetal echocardiography are not perfect, and families should be counseled that a nor-

mal fetal echocardiogram does not guarantee the absence of congenital heart disease. Congenital heart lesions may also evolve during the course of the pregnancy; for example, moderate aortic stenosis with a normal-sized left ventricle at 18 wk of gestation may evolve into aortic atresia with a hypoplastic left ventricle by 34 wk because of decreased flow through the atria, ventricle, and aorta during the latter half of gestation.

The major factor in determining whether a woman with congenital heart disease, either unoperated or operated, will be able to carry a fetus to term is the mother's cardiovascular status. In the presence of a mild congenital heart defect or after successful repair of a more severe lesion, normal childbearing is likely. However, in a woman with poor cardiac function, the increased hemodynamic burden imposed by pregnancy may result in a significantly increased risk to both the mother and fetus. The incidence of spontaneous abortion in the presence of severe congenital heart disease is high, especially when the mother is cyanotic. The maternal risk in these situations is also high. It is important to discuss various methods of birth control with young women who have repaired or palliated congenital heart lesions. Antibiotic prophylaxis against endocarditis is also indicated at the time of delivery.

Brennan P, Young ID: Congenital heart malformations: Aetiology and associations. *Semin Neonatol* 2001;6:17–25.

Donnai D, Karmiloff-Smith A: Williams syndrome; from genotype through to the cognitive phenotype. *Am J Med Genet* 2000;97:164–71.

Epstein JA, Buck CA: Transcriptional regulation of cardiac development: Implications for congenital heart disease and DiGeorge syndrome. *Pediatr Res* 2000;48:717–24.

Ferencz C, Rubin JD, McCarter RJ, et al: Congenital heart disease: Prevalence at live-birth. The Baltimore-Washington Infant Study. *Am J Epidemiol* 1985;121:31.

Fyler DC, Buckley DP, Hellenbrand WE, Cohn HE: Report of the New England Regional Infant Cardiac Program. *Pediatrics* 1980;65:376.

Gelb BD: Genetic basis of syndromes associated with congenital heart disease. *Curr Opin Cardiol* 2001;16:188–94.

Goldmuntz E: The epidemiology and genetics of congenital heart disease. *Clin Perinatol* 2001;28:1–10.

Harvey RP: NK-2 homeobox genes and heart development. *Dev Biol* 1996;178:203.

Payne RM, Johnson MC, Grant JW, et al: Toward a molecular understanding of congenital heart disease. *Circulation* 1995;91:494.

Schott JJ, Benson DW, Basson CT, et al: Congenital heart disease caused by mutations in the transcription factor NKX2-5. *Science* 1998;281:108–11.

Strauss AW, Johnson MC: The genetic basis of pediatric cardiovascular disease. *Semin Perinatol* 1996;20:564.

Whittemore R, Wells JA, Castellsague X: A second-generation study of 427 probands with congenital heart defects and their 837 children. *J Am Coll Cardiol* 1994;23:1459–67.

Wilson DI, Burn J, Scambler P, Goodship J: DiGeorge syndrome: Part of CATCH 22. *J Med Genet* 1993;30:852.

Chapter 418

Evaluation of the Infant or Child with Congenital Heart Disease

The initial evaluation for suspected congenital heart disease involves a systematic approach with three major components. First, congenital cardiac defects can be divided into two major groups based on the presence or absence of cyanosis, which can be determined by physical examination aided by pulse oximetry. Second, these two groups can be further subdivided according to whether the chest radiograph shows evidence of increased, normal, or decreased pulmonary vascular markings. Finally, the electrocardiogram can be used to determine whether right, left, or biventricular hypertrophy exists. The character of the heart sounds and the presence and character of any murmurs further narrow the differential diagnosis. The final diagnosis is then confirmed by echocardiography or cardiac catheterization, or by both.

ACYANOTIC CONGENITAL HEART LESIONS

Acyanotic congenital heart lesions can be classified according to the predominant physiologic load that they place on the heart. Although many congenital heart lesions induce more than one physiologic disturbance, it is helpful to focus on the primary load abnormality for purposes of classification. The most common lesions are those that produce a *volume load*, and the most common of these are left-to-right shunt lesions. Atrioventricular (AV) valve regurgitation and some of the cardiomyopathies are other causes of increased volume load. The second major class of lesions causes an increase in *pressure load*, most commonly secondary to ventricular outflow obstruction (e.g., pulmonic or aortic valve stenosis) or narrowing of one of the great vessels (e.g., coarctation of the aorta). The chest radiograph and electrocardiogram are useful tools for differentiating between these major classes of volume and pressure overload lesions.

Lesions Resulting in Increased Volume Load. The most common lesions in this group are those that cause left-to-right shunting (see Chapter 419): atrial septal defect, ventricular septal defect (VSD), AV septal defects (AV canal), and patent ductus arteriosus. The pathophysiologic common denominator in this group is communication between the systemic and pulmonary sides of the circulation, which results in shunting of fully oxygenated blood back into the lungs. This shunt can be quantitated by calculating the ratio of pulmonary to systemic blood flow, or Qp:Qs. Thus, a 2:1 shunt implies twice the normal pulmonary blood flow.

The direction and magnitude of the shunt across such a communication depend on the size of the defect and the relative pulmonary and systemic pressure and vascular resistance. These factors are dynamic and may change dramatically with age: intracardiac defects may grow smaller with time; pulmonary vascular resistance, which is high in the immediate newborn period, decreases to normal adult levels by several weeks of life; and chronic exposure of the pulmonary circulation to high pressure and blood flow results in a gradual increase in pulmonary vascular resistance (Eisenmenger physiology, see Chapter 426.2). Thus, a lesion such as a large VSD may be associated with little shunting and few symptoms during the initial weeks of life. When pulmonary vascular resistance declines over the next several weeks, the volume of the left-to-right shunt increases, and symptoms begin to appear.

The increased volume of blood in the lungs decreases pulmonary compliance and increases the work of breathing. Fluid leaks into the interstitial space and alveoli and causes pulmonary edema. The infant acquires the symptoms we refer to as heart failure, such as tachypnea, chest retractions, nasal flaring, and wheezing. The term *heart failure* is a misnomer, however; total left ventricular output is actually several times greater than normal, although much of this output is ineffective because it returns directly to the lungs. To maintain this high level of left ventricular output, heart rate and stroke volume are increased, mediated by an increase in sympathetic nervous system activity. The increase in circulating catecholamines, combined with the increased work of breathing, results in an elevation in total body oxygen consumption, often beyond the oxygen transport ability of the circulation. Such oxygen consumption leads to the additional symptoms of sweating, irritability, and failure to thrive. Remodeling of the heart occurs, with predominantly dilatation and a lesser degree of hypertrophy. If left untreated, pulmonary vascular resistance eventually begins to rise, and by several years of age the shunt volume will decrease and eventually reverse right to left (Eisenmenger physiology, Chapter 426.2).

Additional lesions that impose a volume load on the heart include regurgitant lesions (see Chapter 421) and the cardiomyopathies (see Chapter 431). Regurgitation through the AV valves is most commonly encountered in patients with partial or complete AV septal defects (atriseptal defects, AV canal). In these lesions, the combination of a left-to-right shunt with AV valve regurgitation increases the volume load on the heart and leads to more severe symptoms. Isolated regurgitation through the tricuspid valve is seen in Ebstein anomaly (see Chapter 423.7). Regurgitation involving one of the semilunar valves is usually also associated with stenosis; however, aortic regurgitation may be encountered in patients with a VSD directly under the aortic valve (supracristal VSD).

In contrast to left-to-right shunts, in which intrinsic cardiac muscle function is generally either normal or increased, heart muscle function is decreased in the cardiomyopathies. Cardiomyopathies may affect systolic contractility or diastolic relaxation, or both. Decreased cardiac function results in increased atrial and ventricular filling pressure, and pulmonary edema occurs secondary to increased capillary pressure. The major causes of cardiomyopathy in infants and children include viral myocarditis, metabolic disorders, and genetic defects (see Chapter 431).

Lesions Resulting in Increased Pressure Load. The pathophysiologic common denominator of these lesions is an obstruction to normal blood flow. The most frequent are obstructions to ventricular outflow: valvular pulmonic stenosis, valvular aortic stenosis, and coarctation of the aorta (see Chapter 420). Less common are obstruction to ventricular inflow: tricuspid or mitral stenosis and cor triatriatum. Ventricular outflow obstruction can occur at the valve, below the valve (e.g., double-chambered right ventricle, subaortic membrane), or above it (e.g., branch pulmonary stenosis or supravalvular aortic stenosis). Unless the obstruction is severe, cardiac output will be maintained and the clinical symptoms of heart failure will be either subtle or absent. This compensation predominantly involves an increase in cardiac wall thickness (hypertrophy), but in later stages it also involves dilatation.

The clinical picture is different when obstruction to outflow is severe, which is usually encountered in the immediate newborn period. The infant may become critically ill within several hours of birth. Severe pulmonic stenosis in the newborn period (critical pulmonic stenosis) results in signs of right-sided heart failure (hepatomegaly, peripheral edema), as well as cyanosis from right-to-left shunting across the foramen ovale. Severe aortic stenosis in the newborn period (critical aortic stenosis) is characterized by signs of left-sided heart failure (pulmonary edema, poor perfusion) and right-sided failure (hepatomegaly, peripheral edema), and it may progress rapidly to total circulatory collapse. In older children, severe pulmonic stenosis leads to symptoms of right-sided heart failure, but not to cyanosis unless a pathway persists for right-to-left shunting (e.g., patency of the foramen ovale).

Coarctation of the aorta in older children and adolescents is usually manifested as upper body hypertension and diminished pulses in the lower extremities. In the immediate newborn period, however, the occurrence of coarctation may be delayed because of the presence of a patent ductus arteriosus. In these patients, the open aortic end of the ductus may serve as a conduit for blood flow to partially bypass the obstruction. These infants then become symptomatic, often dramatically, when the ductus finally closes.

CYANOTIC CONGENITAL HEART LESIONS

This group of congenital heart lesions can also be further divided according to pathophysiology: whether pulmonary blood flow is decreased (tetralogy of Fallot, pulmonary atresia with an intact septum, tricuspid atresia, total anomalous pulmonary venous return with obstruction) or increased (transposition of the great vessels, single ventricle, truncus arteriosus, total anomalous pulmonary venous return without obstruction). The chest radiograph is a valuable tool for initial differentiation between these two categories.

Cyanotic Lesions with Decreased Pulmonary Blood Flow. These lesions must include both an obstruction to pulmonary blood flow (at the tricuspid valve or right ventricular or pulmonary valve level) and a pathway by which systemic venous blood can shunt from right to left and enter the systemic circulation (via a patent foramen ovale, atrial septal defect, or VSD). Common lesions in this group include tricuspid atresia, tetralogy of Fallot, and various forms of single ventricle with pulmonary stenosis (see Chapter 423). In these lesions, the degree of cyanosis depends on the degree of obstruction to pulmonary blood flow. If the obstruction is mild, cyanosis may be absent at rest. These patients may have hypercyanotic ("tet") spells during conditions of stress. In contrast, if the obstruction is severe, pulmonary blood flow may be dependent on patency of the ductus arteriosus. When the ductus closes during the 1st few days of life, the neonate experiences profound hypoxemia and shock.

Cyanotic Lesions with Increased Pulmonary Blood Flow. This group of lesions is not associated with obstruction to pulmonary blood flow. Cyanosis is caused by either abnormal ventricular-arterial connections or total mixing of systemic venous and pulmonary venous blood within the heart (see Chapter 424). Transposition of the great vessels is the most common of the former group of lesions. In this condition, the aorta arises from the right ventricle and the pulmonary artery arises from the left ventricle. Systemic venous blood returning to the right atrium is pumped directly back to the body, and oxygenated blood returning from the lungs to the left atrium is pumped back into the lungs. The persistence of fetal pathways (foramen ovale and ductus arteriosus) allows for a small degree of mixing in the immediate newborn period; when the ductus begins to close, these infants become extremely cyanotic.

Total mixing lesions include cardiac defects with a common atrium or ventricle, total anomalous pulmonary venous return, and truncus arteriosus (see Chapter 424). In this group, deoxygenated systemic venous blood and oxygenated pulmonary venous blood mix completely in the heart, and as a result, oxygen saturation is equal in the pulmonary artery and aorta. If pulmonary blood flow is not obstructed, these infants have a combination of cyanosis and heart failure. In contrast, if pulmonary stenosis is present, these infants have cyanosis alone, similar to patients with the tetralogy of Fallot.

Lister G, Moreau G, Moss M, Talner NS: Effect of alteration of oxygen transport on the neonate. *Semin Perinatol* 1984;8:192.

Lister G, Pitt BR: Cardiopulmonary interactions in the infant with congenital heart disease. *Clin Chest Med* 1983;4:219.

Mair DD, Ritter DG: Factors influencing systemic oxygen saturation in complete transposition of the great arteries. *Am J Cardiol* 1973;31:742.

Talner NS: The physiology of congenital heart disease. In Garson A, Bricker TJ, Fisher, DJ, Neish SR (editors): *The Science and Practice of Pediatric Cardiology.* Baltimore, Williams & Wilkins, 1998, pp 1107–1118.

Chapter 419
Acyanotic Congenital Heart Disease: The Left-to-Right Shunt Lesions

419.1 Atrial Septal Defect

Atrial septal defects (ASDs) can occur in any portion of the atrial septum (secundum, primum, or sinus venosus), depending on which embryonic septal structure has failed to develop normally (see Chapter 413). Less commonly, the atrial septum may be nearly absent, with the creation of a functional single atrium. Isolated secundum ASDs account for approximately 7% of congenital heart defects. The majority of cases of ASD are sporadic; however, autosomal dominant inheritance does occur as part of the Holt-Oram syndrome (hypoplastic or absent radii, 1st-degree heart block, ASD).

An isolated valve-incompetent patent foramen ovale (PFO) is a common echocardiographic finding during infancy. It is usually of no hemodynamic significance and is not considered an ASD; however, a PFO may play an important role if other structural heart defects are present. If another cardiac anomaly is causing increased right atrial pressure (e.g., pulmonary stenosis or atresia, tricuspid valve abnormalities, right ventricular dysfunction), venous blood may shunt across the PFO into the left atrium with resultant cyanosis. Because of the anatomic structure of the PFO, left-to-right shunting is unusual outside the immediate newborn period. In the presence of a large volume load or a hypertensive left atrium (e.g., secondary to mitral stenosis), the foramen ovale may be sufficiently dilated to result in a significant atrial left-to-right shunt. A valve-competent but probe-patent foramen ovale may be present in 15–30% of adults. An isolated PFO does not require surgical treatment, although it may be a risk for paradoxical (right to left) systemic embolization.

419.2 Ostium Secundum Defect

An ostium secundum defect in the region of the fossa ovalis is the most common form of ASD and is associated with structurally normal atrioventricular (AV) valves. Mitral valve prolapse has been described in association with this defect but is rarely an important clinical consideration. Secundum ASDs may be single or multiple (fenestrated atrial septum), and openings 2 cm or larger in diameter are common in symptomatic older children. Large defects may extend inferiorly toward the inferior vena cava and ostium of the coronary sinus, superiorly toward the superior vena cava, or posteriorly. Females outnumber males 3:1 in incidence. Partial anomalous pulmonary venous return, most commonly of the right upper pulmonary vein, may be an associated lesion.

Pathophysiology. The degree of left-to-right shunting is dependent on the size of the defect, the relative compliance of the right and left ventricles, and the relative vascular resistance in the pulmonary and systemic circulations. In large defects, a considerable shunt of oxygenated blood flows from the left to the right atrium (Fig. 419–1). This blood is added to the usual venous return to the right atrium and is pumped by the right ventricle to the lungs. With large defects, the ratio of pulmonary to systemic blood flow (Qp:Qs) is usually between 2:1 and 4:1. The paucity of symptoms in infants with ASDs is related to the structure of the right ventricle in early life when its muscular wall is thick and less compliant, thus limiting the left-to-right shunt. As the infant becomes older and pulmonary vascular resistance drops, the right ventricular wall becomes thinner and the left-to-right shunt across the ASD increases. The large blood flow through the right side of the heart results in enlargement of the right atrium and ventricle and dilatation of the pulmonary artery. The left atrium may be enlarged; however, the left ventricle and aorta are normal in size. Despite the large pulmonary blood flow, pulmonary arterial pressure is usually normal because of the absence of a high-pressure communication between the pulmonary and systemic circulations. Pulmonary vascular resistance remains low throughout childhood, although it may begin to increase in adulthood and may eventually result in reversal of the shunt and clinical cyanosis.

Clinical Manifestations. A child with an ostium secundum defect is most often asymptomatic; the lesion may be discovered inadvertently during physical examination. Even an extremely large secundum ASD rarely produces clinically evident heart failure in childhood. In younger children, subtle failure to thrive may be present; in older children, varying degrees of exercise intolerance may be noted. Often, the degree of limitation may go unnoticed by the family until after surgical repair, when the child's growth or activity level increases markedly.

The physical findings of an ASD are usually characteristic but fairly subtle and require careful examination of the heart, with special attention to the heart sounds. Examination of the chest may reveal a mild left precordial bulge. A right ventricular systolic lift is generally palpable at the left sternal border. A loud 1st heart sound and sometimes a pulmonic ejection click can be heard. In most patients, the 2nd heart sound is characteristically widely split and fixed in its splitting in all phases of respiration. Normally, the duration of right ventricular ejection varies with respiration, with inspiration increasing right ventricular volume and delaying closure of the pulmonary valve. With an ASD,

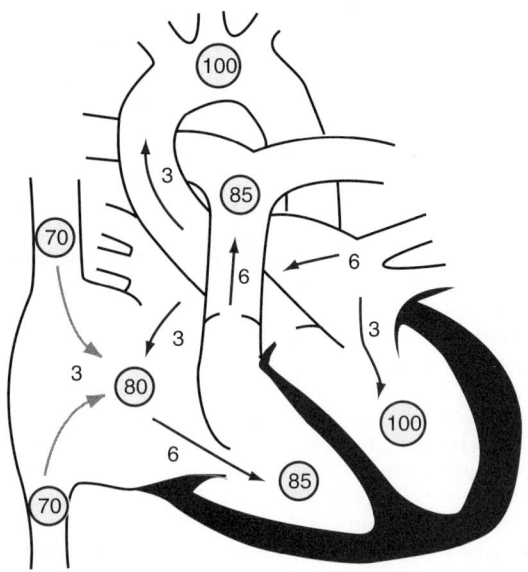

FIGURE 419–1. Physiology of atrial septal defect (ASD). Circled numbers represent oxygen saturation values. The numbers next to the arrows represent volumes of blood flow (in $L/min/m^2$). This illustration shows a hypothetical patient with a pulmonary-to-systemic blood flow ratio (Qp:Qs) of 2:1. Desaturated blood enters the right atrium from the vena cavae at a volume of 3 $L/min/m^2$ and mixes with an additional 3 L of fully saturated blood shunting left to right across the ASD; the result is an increase in oxygen saturation in the right atrium. Six liters of blood flows through the tricuspid valve and causes a mid-diastolic flow rumble. Oxygen saturation may be slightly higher in the right ventricle because of incomplete mixing at the atrial level. The full 6 L flows across the right ventricular outflow tract and causes a systolic ejection flow murmur. Six liters returns to the left atrium, with 3 L shunting left to right across the defect and 3 L crossing the mitral valve to be ejected by the left ventricle into the ascending aorta (normal cardiac output).

right ventricular diastolic volume is constantly increased and the ejection time is prolonged throughout all phases of respiration. A systolic ejection murmur is heard; it is medium pitched, without harsh qualities, seldom accompanied by a thrill, and best heard at the left middle and upper sternal border. It is produced by the increased flow across the right ventricular outflow tract into the pulmonary artery, not by low-pressure flow across the ASD. A short, rumbling mid-diastolic murmur produced by the increased volume of blood flow across the tricuspid valve is often audible at the lower left sternal border. This finding, which may be subtle and is heard best with the bell of the stethoscope, usually indicates a Qp:Qs ratio of at least 2:1.

Diagnosis. The *chest roentgenogram* shows varying degrees of enlargement of the right ventricle and atrium, depending on the size of the shunt. The pulmonary artery is large, and pulmonary vascularity is increased. These signs vary and may not be conspicuous in mild cases. Cardiac enlargement is often best appreciated on the lateral view because the right ventricle protrudes anteriorly as its volume increases. The *electrocardiogram* shows volume overload of the right ventricle; the QRS axis may be normal or exhibit right axis deviation, and a minor right ventricular conduction delay (rsR′ pattern in the right precordial leads) may be present.

The *echocardiogram* shows findings characteristic of right ventricular volume overload, including an increased right ventricular end-diastolic dimension and flattening and abnormal motion of the ventricular septum. A normal septum moves posteriorly during systole and anteriorly during diastole. With right ventricular overload and normal pulmonary vascular resistance, septal motion is reversed—that is, anterior movement in systole—or the motion may be intermediate so that the septum remains straight. The location and size of the atrial defect are readily appreciated by two-dimensional scanning, with a characteristic brightening of the echo image seen at the edge of the defect (T-artifact). The shunt is confirmed by pulsed and color flow Doppler. Patients with the classic features of a hemodynamically significant ASD on physical examination and chest radiography in whom echocardiographic identification of an isolated secundum ASD is made need not be catheterized before surgical closure, with the exception of an older patient, in whom pulmonary vascular resistance may be a concern.

If the diagnosis is suspected, shunt size cannot be reliably determined by noninvasive tests; if pulmonary vascular disease is suspected, *cardiac catheterization* confirms the presence of the defect and allows measurement of the shunt ratio and pulmonary pressure. The oxygen content of blood from the right atrium will be much higher than that from the superior vena cava. This feature is not specifically diagnostic because it may occur with partial anomalous pulmonary venous return to the right atrium, with a ventricular septal defect (VSD) in the presence of tricuspid insufficiency, with AV septal defects associated with left ventricular–to–right atrial shunts, and with aorta–to–right atrial communications (e.g., ruptured sinus of Valsalva aneurysm). Pressure in the right side of the heart is usually normal, but small to moderate pressure gradients (<25 mm Hg) may be measured across the right ventricular outflow tract because of functional stenosis related to excessive blood flow. Pulmonary vascular resistance is almost always normal. The shunt is variable and depends on the size of the defect, but it may be of considerable volume (as high as 20 L/min/m²). *Cineangiography*, performed with the catheter through the defect and in the right upper pulmonary vein, demonstrates the defect and the location of the right upper pulmonary venous drainage. Alternatively, pulmonary angiography demonstrates the defect on the levophase (return of contrast to the left side of the heart after passing through the lungs).

Prognosis and Complications. ASDs detected in term infants may close spontaneously. Secundum ASDs are well tolerated during childhood, and symptoms do not usually appear until the 3rd decade or later. Pulmonary hypertension, atrial dysrhythmias, tricuspid or mitral insufficiency, and heart failure are late manifestations; these symptoms may initially appear during the increased volume load of pregnancy. Infective endocarditis is extremely rare, and antibiotic prophylaxis for isolated secundum ASDs is not recommended. Postoperative complications such as late heart failure and atrial fibrillation are more common in patients who undergo surgery after 20 yr of age.

Secundum ASDs are usually isolated, although they may be associated with partial anomalous pulmonary venous return, pulmonary valvular stenosis, VSD, pulmonary artery branch stenosis, and persistent left superior vena cava, as well as mitral valve prolapse and insufficiency. Secundum ASDs are associated with the autosomal dominant **Holt-Oram syndrome**. The gene responsible for this syndrome, situated in the region 12q21-q22 of chromosome 12, is TBX5, a member of the T-box transcriptional family. A familial form of secundum ASD associated with AV conduction delay has been linked to mutations in the transcription factor Nkx2.5.

Treatment. Surgery or transcatheter device closure is advised for all symptomatic patients and also for asymptomatic patients with a Qp:Qs ratio of at least 2:1. The timing for elective closure is usually after the 1st yr and before entry into school. Closure carried out at open heart surgery is associated with a mortality rate of less than 1%. Repair is preferred during early childhood because surgical mortality and morbidity are significantly greater in adulthood; the long-term risk of arrhythmia is also

greater after ASD repair in adults. Atrial septal occlusion devices implanted transvenously at cardiac catheterization are approved for general use. In patients with small secundum ASDs and minimal left-to-right shunts, the consensus is that closure is not required. It is unclear at present whether the persistence of a small ASD into adulthood increases the risk for stroke enough to warrant prophylactic closure of all these defects.

The results after surgical or device closure in children with large shunts are excellent. Symptoms disappear rapidly, and physical development frequently appears enhanced. Heart size decreases to normal, and the electrocardiogram shows decreased right ventricular forces. Late arrhythmias are less frequent in patients who have had early surgical repair. Although early and mid-term results are excellent, the long-term effects of device closure are not yet known.

419.3 Sinus Venosus Atrial Septal Defect

A sinus venosus ASD is situated in the upper part of the atrial septum in close relation to the entry of the superior vena cava. Often, one or more pulmonary veins (usually from the right lung) drain anomalously into the superior vena cava. Sometimes the superior vena cava straddles the defect; in this case, some systemic venous blood enters the left atrium, but only rarely does it cause clinically evident cyanosis. The hemodynamic disturbance, clinical picture, electrocardiogram, and roentgenogram are similar to those seen in secundum ASD. The diagnosis can usually be made by two-dimensional echocardiography. If cardiac catheterization is carried out to better define venous drainage, the catheter may enter a right pulmonary vein directly from the superior vena cava. Anatomic correction generally requires the insertion of a patch to close the defect while incorporating the entry of anomalous veins into the left atrium; surgical results are generally excellent. Rarely, sinus venosus defects involve the inferior vena cava.

419.4 Partial Anomalous Pulmonary Venous Return

One or several pulmonary veins may return anomalously to the superior or inferior vena cava, the right atrium, or the coronary sinus and produce a left-to-right shunt of oxygenated blood. Partial anomalous pulmonary venous return usually involves some or all of the veins from only one lung, more often the right one. When an associated ASD is present, it is generally of the sinus venosus type (see Chapter 419.3). When a sinus venosus ASD is detected by echocardiography, one must search for associated partial anomalous pulmonary venous return. The history, physical signs, and electrocardiographic and roentgenographic findings are indistinguishable from those of an isolated ostium secundum ASD. Occasionally, an anomalous vein draining into the inferior vena cava is visible on chest radiography as a crescentic shadow of vascular density along the right border of the cardiac silhouette (*scimitar syndrome*); in these cases, an ASD is not usually present, but pulmonary sequestration and anomalous arterial supply to that lobe are common findings. Total anomalous pulmonary venous return is a cyanotic lesion and is discussed in Chapter 424.7. Echocardiography generally confirms the diagnosis. MRI and electron beam CT are also useful for defining pulmonary venous drainage. At cardiac catheterization, the presence of anomalous pulmonary veins may be demonstrated by selective pulmonary arteriography.

The prognosis is excellent, similar to that for ostium secundum ASDs. When a large left-to-right shunt is present, surgical repair is performed. The associated ASD should be closed in such a way that pulmonary venous return is directed to the left atrium. A single anomalous pulmonary vein without an atrial communication may be difficult to redirect to the left atrium; if the shunt is small, it may be left unoperated.

419.5 Atrioventricular Septal Defects (Ostium Primum and Atrioventricular Canal or Endocardial Cushion Defects)

The abnormalities encompassed by AV septal defects are grouped together because they represent a spectrum of a basic embryologic abnormality, a deficiency of the AV septum. An *ostium primum defect* is situated in the lower portion of the atrial septum and overlies the mitral and tricuspid valves. In most instances, a cleft in the anterior leaflet of the mitral valve is also noted. The tricuspid valve is usually functionally normal, although some anatomic abnormality of the septal leaflet is generally present. The ventricular septum is intact.

An *AV septal defect*, also known as an AV canal defect or an endocardial cushion defect, consists of contiguous atrial and ventricular septal defects with markedly abnormal AV valves. The severity of the valve abnormalities varies considerably; in the complete form of AV septal defect, a single AV valve is common to both ventricles and consists of an anterior and a posterior bridging leaflet related to the ventricular septum, with a lateral leaflet in each ventricle. The lesion is common in children with Down syndrome and may occasionally occur with pulmonary stenosis.

Transitional varieties of these defects also occur and include ostium primum defects with clefts in the anterior mitral and septal tricuspid valve leaflets, minor ventricular septal deficiencies, and less commonly, ostium primum defects with normal AV valves. In some patients, the atrial septum is intact, but the inlet VSD simulates that found in the full AV septal defect. These defects are also commonly associated with deformities of the AV valves.

Pathophysiology. The basic abnormality in patients with *ostium primum defects* is the combination of a left-to-right shunt across the atrial defect and mitral (or occasionally tricuspid) insufficiency. The shunt is usually moderate to large, the degree of mitral insufficiency is generally mild to moderate, and pulmonary arterial pressure is typically normal or only mildly increased. The physiology of this lesion is therefore similar to that of an ostium secundum ASD.

In *AV septal defects*, the left-to-right shunt occurs at both the atrial and ventricular levels (Fig. 419–2). Additional shunting may occur directly from the left ventricle to the right atrium because of absence of the AV septum. Pulmonary hypertension and an early tendency to increase pulmonary vascular resistance are common. AV valvular insufficiency increases the volume load on one or both ventricles. Some right-to-left shunting may also occur at both the atrial and ventricular levels and lead to mild but significant arterial desaturation. With time, progressive pulmonary vascular disease increases the right-to-left shunt so that clinical cyanosis develops (Eisenmenger physiology, see Chapter 426.2).

Clinical Manifestations. Many children with ostium primum *defects* are asymptomatic, and the anomaly is discovered during a general physical examination. In patients with moderate shunts and mild mitral insufficiency, the physical signs are similar to those of the secundum ASD, but with an additional apical murmur caused by mitral insufficiency.

A history of exercise intolerance, easy fatigability, and recurrent pneumonia may be obtained, especially in infants with large left-to-right shunts and severe mitral insufficiency. In these patients, cardiac enlargement is moderate or marked, and the precordium is hyperdynamic. Auscultatory signs produced by the left-to-right

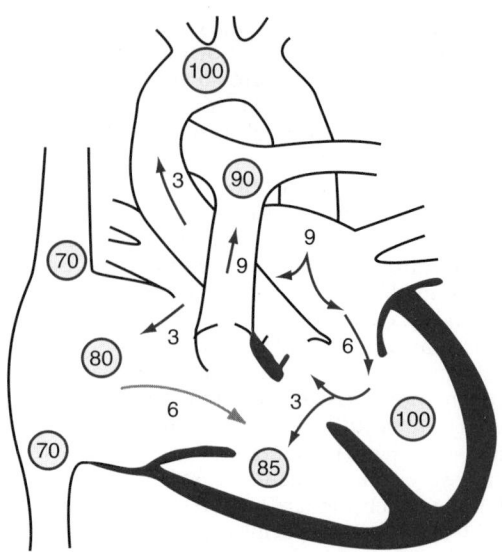

FIGURE 419–2. Physiology of atrioventricular septal defect (AVSD). Circled numbers represent oxygen saturation values. The numbers next to the arrows represent volumes of blood flow (in L/min/m^2). This illustration shows a hypothetical patient with a pulmonary-to-systemic blood flow ratio (Qp:Qs) of 3:1. Desaturated blood enters the right atrium from the vena cavae at a volume of 3 L/min/m^2 and mixes with 3 L of fully saturated blood shunting left to right across the atrial septal defect; the result is an increase in oxygen saturation in the right atrium. Six liters of blood flows through the right side of the common AV valve, joined by an additional 3 L of saturated blood shunting left to right at the ventricular level, further increasing oxygen saturation in the right ventricle. The full 9 L flows across the right ventricular outflow tract into the lungs. Nine liters returns to the left atrium, with 3 L shunting left to right across the defect and 6 L crossing the left side of the common AV valve and causing a mid-diastolic flow rumble. Three liters of this volume shunts left to right across the VSD, and 3 L is ejected into the ascending aorta (normal cardiac output).

shunt include a normal or accentuated 1st sound; wide, fixed splitting of the 2nd sound; a pulmonary systolic ejection murmur sometimes preceded by a click; and a low-pitched, mid-diastolic rumbling murmur at the lower left sternal edge or apex, or both, as a result of increased flow through the AV valves. Mitral insufficiency may be manifested by an apical harsh (occasionally very high pitched) holosystolic murmur that radiates to the left axilla.

With *complete AV septal defects*, congestive heart failure and intercurrent pulmonary infection usually appear in infancy. During these episodes, minimal cyanosis may be evident. The liver is enlarged and the infant shows signs of failure to thrive. Cardiac enlargement is moderate to marked, and a systolic thrill is frequently palpable at the lower left sternal border. A precordial bulge and lift may be present as well. The 1st heart sound is normal or accentuated. The 2nd heart sound is widely split if the pulmonary flow is massive. A low-pitched, mid-diastolic rumbling murmur is audible at the lower left sternal border, and a pulmonary systolic ejection murmur is produced by the large pulmonary flow. The harsh apical holosystolic murmur of mitral insufficiency may also be present.

Diagnosis. Chest *radiographs* of children with complete AV septal defects often show marked cardiac enlargement caused by the prominence of both ventricles and atria. The pulmonary artery is large, and pulmonary vascularity is increased.

The *electrocardiogram* in patients with a complete AV septal defect is distinctive. The principal abnormalities are (1) superior orientation of the mean frontal QRS axis with left axis deviation to the left upper or right upper quadrant, (2) counterclockwise inscription of the superiorly oriented QRS vector loop, (3) signs of biventricular hypertrophy or isolated right ventricular hypertrophy, (4) right ventricular conduction delay (RSR' pattern in leads V_3R and V_1), (5) normal or tall P waves, and (6) occasional prolongation of the P-R interval (Fig. 419–3).

The *echocardiogram* is characteristic and shows signs of right ventricular enlargement with encroachment of the mitral valve echo on the left ventricular outflow tract; the abnormally low position of the AV valves results in a "gooseneck" deformity of the left ventricular outflow tract on both echocardiography and angiography. In normal hearts, the tricuspid valve inserts slightly more toward the apex than the mitral valve does. In AV septal defects, both valves insert at the same level because of absence of the AV septum. In complete AV septal defects, the ventricular septal echo is also deficient and the common AV valve is readily appreciated (Fig. 419–4). Pulsed and color flow Doppler echocardiography will demonstrate left-to-right shunting at the atrial, ventricular, or ventricular-to-atrial levels and semiquantitate the degree of AV valve insufficiency. Echocardiography is useful for determining the insertion points of the chordae of the common AV valve and for evaluating the presence of associated lesions such as patent ductus arteriosus (PDA) or coarctation of the aorta.

Cardiac catheterization and *angiocardiography* may be required to confirm the diagnosis, although most patients can be operated on without catheterization. These studies demonstrate the magnitude of the left-to-right shunt, the severity of pulmonary hypertension, the degree of elevation of pulmonary vascular resistance, and the severity of insufficiency of the common AV valve. By oximetry, the shunt is usually demonstrable at both the atrial and ventricular levels. Arterial oxygen saturation is normal or only mildly reduced unless severe pulmonary vascular disease is present. Children with ostium primum defects generally have normal or only moderately elevated pulmonary arterial pressure. Conversely, complete AV septal defects are associated with right ventricular and pulmonary hypertension and, in older patients, with increased pulmonary vascular resistance (see Chapter 426.2).

Selective left ventriculography is extremely helpful in the diagnosis of AV septal defects. The deformity of the mitral or common AV valve and the distortion of the outflow tract of the left ventricle cause a "gooseneck"-appearing deformity of the left ventricular outflow tract. The abnormal anterior leaflet of the mitral valve is serrated, and mitral insufficiency is noted, usually with regurgitation of blood into both the left and right atria. Direct shunting of blood from the left ventricle to the right atrium may also be demonstrated.

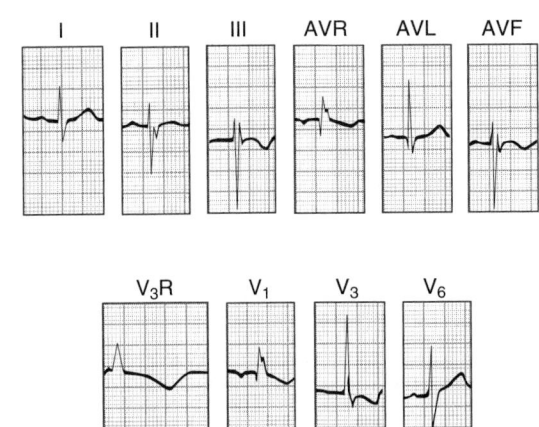

FIGURE 419–3. Electrocardiogram from a child with an atrioventricular canal. Note the QRS axis of −60 degrees and the right ventricular conduction delay with an RSR' pattern in V1 and V3R (V3R paper speed = 50 mm/sec).

Prognosis and Complications. The prognosis for complete AV septal defects depends on the magnitude of the left-to-right shunt, the degree of elevation of pulmonary vascular resistance, and the severity of AV valve insufficiency. Death from cardiac failure during infancy used to be frequent before the advent of early corrective surgery. In patients who survived without surgery, pulmonary vascular obstructive disease or, more rarely, pulmonic stenosis usually developed. Most patients with ostium primum defects and minimal AV valve involvement are asymptomatic or have only minor, nonprogressive symptoms until they reach the 3rd–4th decade of life, similar to the course of patients with secundum ASDs.

Treatment. Ostium primum defects are approached surgically from an incision in the right atrium. The cleft in the mitral valve is located through the atrial defect and is repaired by direct suture. The defect in the atrial septum is usually closed by insertion of a patch prosthesis. The surgical mortality rate for ostium primum defects is low. Surgical treatment of complete AV septal defects is more difficult, especially in infants with cardiac failure and pulmonary hypertension. Because of the risk of pulmonary vascular disease developing as early as 6–12 mo of age, surgical intervention must be performed during infancy. Correction of these defects can be accomplished in infancy, and palliation with pulmonary arterial banding is reserved for the subset of patients

FIGURE 419–4. Echocardiogram of an atrioventricular septal defect. *A*, Four-chamber view demonstrating both an interatrial and an interventricular septal defect contributing to the large central communication of this lesion (arrows). *B*, Left ventricular long-axis projection demonstrating the typical gooseneck deformity created by the anterior leaflet of the mitral valve (arrows). RA = right atrium; LA = left atrium; RVI = right ventricular inflow; LV = left ventricle; R = right; L = left; S = superior; I = inferior; Ao = aorta.

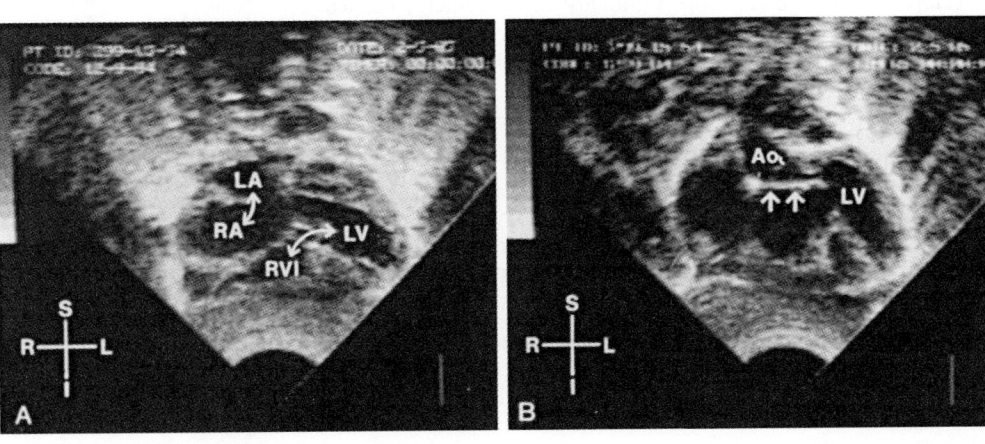

who are either too small or have other associated lesions that make early corrective surgery too risky. The atrial and ventricular defects are patched and the AV valves reconstructed. Complications include surgically induced heart block requiring placement of a permanent pacemaker, excessive narrowing of the left ventricular outflow tract requiring surgical revision, and eventual worsening of mitral regurgitation requiring replacement with a prosthetic valve.

419.6 Ventricular Septal Defect

VSD is the most common cardiac malformation and accounts for 25% of congenital heart disease. Defects may occur in any portion of the ventricular septum, but most are of the membranous type. These defects are in a posteroinferior position, anterior to the septal leaflet of the tricuspid valve. VSDs between the crista supraventricularis and the papillary muscle of the conus may be associated with pulmonary stenosis and other manifestations of the tetralogy of Fallot (see Chapter 423.1). VSDs superior to the crista supraventricularis (supracristal) are less common; they are found just beneath the pulmonary valve and may impinge on an aortic sinus and cause aortic insufficiency. VSDs in the midportion or apical region of the ventricular septum are muscular in type and may be single or multiple (Swiss cheese septum).

Pathophysiology. The physical size of the VSD is a major, but not the only determinant of the size of the left-to-right shunt. The level of pulmonary vascular resistance in relation to systemic vascular resistance also determines the shunt's magnitude. When a small communication is present (usually <0.5 cm²), the VSD is called *restrictive* and right ventricular pressure is normal. The higher pressure in the left ventricle drives the shunt left to right; the size of the defect limits the magnitude of the shunt. In large *nonrestrictive* VSDs (usually >1.0 cm²), right and left ventricular pressure is equalized. In these defects, the direction of shunting and shunt magnitude are determined by the ratio of pulmonary to systemic vascular resistance (Fig. 419–5).

After birth in patients with a large VSD, pulmonary vascular resistance may remain higher than normal, and thus the size of the left-to-right shunt may initially be limited. As pulmonary vascular resistance continues to fall in the 1st few weeks after birth because of normal involution of the media of small pulmonary arterioles, the size of the left-to-right shunt increases. Eventually, a large left-to-right shunt develops, and clinical symptoms become apparent. In most cases during early infancy, pulmonary vascular resistance is only slightly elevated, and the major contribution to pulmonary hypertension is the extremely large pulmonary blood flow. However, in some infants with a large VSD, pulmonary arteriolar medial thickness never decreases. With continued exposure of the pulmonary vascular bed to high systolic pressure and high flow, pulmonary vascular obstructive disease develops. When the ratio of pulmonary to systemic resistance approaches 1:1, the shunt becomes bidirectional, the signs of heart failure abate, and the patient becomes cyanotic (Eisenmenger physiology, see Chapter 426.2).

The magnitude of intracardiac shunts is usually described by the Qp:Qs ratio. If the left-to-right shunt is small (Qp:Qs <1.75:1), the cardiac chambers are not appreciably enlarged and the pulmonary vascular bed is probably normal. If the shunt is large (Qp:Qs >2:1), left atrial and ventricular volume overload occurs, as does right ventricular and pulmonary arterial hypertension. The main pulmonary artery, left atrium, and left ventricle are enlarged.

Clinical Manifestations. The clinical findings of patients with a VSD vary according to the size of the defect and pulmonary blood flow and pressure. *Small VSDs* with trivial left-to-right shunts and normal pulmonary arterial pressure are the most

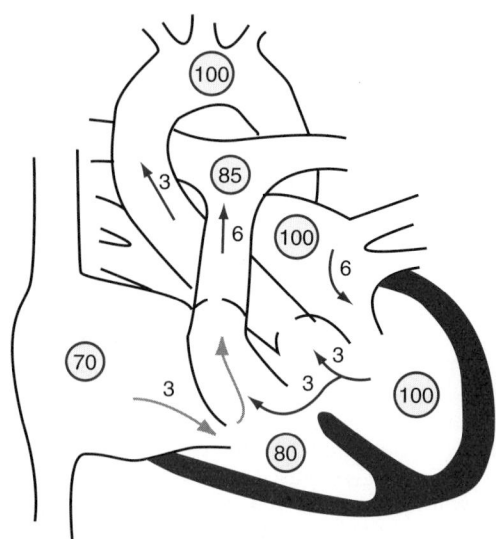

FIGURE 419–5. Physiology of a large ventricular septal defect (VSD). Circled numbers represent oxygen saturation values. The numbers next to the arrows represent volumes of blood flow (in L/min/m²). This illustration shows a hypothetical patient with a pulmonary-to-systemic blood flow ratio (Qp:Qs) of 2:1. Desaturated blood enters the right atrium from the vena cava at a volume of 3 L/min/m² and flows across the tricuspid valve. An additional 3 L of blood shunts left to right across the VSD, the result being an increase in oxygen saturation in the right ventricle. Six liters of blood is ejected into the lungs. Pulmonary arterial saturation may be further increased because of incomplete mixing at right ventricular level. Six liters returns to the left atrium, crosses the mitral valve, and causes a mid-diastolic flow rumble. Three liters of this volume shunts left to right across the VSD, and 3 L is ejected into the ascending aorta (normal cardiac output).

common. These patients are asymptomatic, and the cardiac lesion is usually found during routine physical examination. Characteristically, a loud, harsh, or blowing holosystolic murmur is present and heard best over the lower left sternal border, and it is frequently accompanied by a thrill. In a few instances the murmur ends before the 2nd sound, presumably because of closure of the defect during late systole. A short, harsh systolic murmur localized to the apex in a neonate is often a sign of a tiny muscular VSD. In the immediate neonatal period, the left-to-right shunt may be minimal because of higher right-sided pressure, and therefore the systolic murmur may not be audible during the 1st few days of life. In premature infants, the murmur may be heard early because pulmonary vascular resistance decreases more rapidly.

Large VSDs with excessive pulmonary blood flow and pulmonary hypertension are responsible for dyspnea, feeding difficulties, poor growth, profuse perspiration, recurrent pulmonary infections, and cardiac failure in early infancy. Cyanosis is usually absent, but duskiness is sometimes noted during infections or crying. Prominence of the left precordium is common, as are a palpable parasternal lift, a laterally displaced apical impulse and apical thrust, and a systolic thrill. The holosystolic murmur of a large VSD is generally less harsh than that of a small VSD and more blowing in nature because of the absence of a significant pressure gradient across the defect. It is even less likely to be audible in the newborn period. The pulmonic component of the 2nd heart sound may be increased as a result of pulmonary hypertension. The presence of a mid-diastolic, low-pitched rumble at the apex is caused by increased blood flow across the mitral valve and indicates a Qp:Qs ratio of 2:1 or greater. This murmur is best appreciated with the bell of the stethoscope.

Diagnosis. In patients with small VSDs, the *chest radiograph* is usually normal, although minimal cardiomegaly and a borderline increase in pulmonary vasculature may be observed. The *electrocardiogram* is generally normal but may suggest left ventricular hypertrophy. The presence of right ventricular hypertrophy is a warning that the defect is not small and that the patient has pulmonary hypertension or an associated lesion such as pulmonic stenosis. In large VSDs, the *chest radiograph* shows gross cardiomegaly with prominence of both ventricles, the left atrium, and the pulmonary artery. Pulmonary vascular markings are increased, and frank pulmonary edema, including pleural effusions, may be present. The *electrocardiogram* shows biventricular hypertrophy; P waves may be notched or peaked.

The *two-dimensional echocardiogram* shows the position and size of the VSD. In small defects, especially those of the muscular septum, the defect itself may be difficult to image and is visualized only by color Doppler examination. In defects of the membranous septum, a thin membrane (called a *ventricular septal aneurysm* but consisting of tricuspid valve tissue) can partially cover the defect and limit the volume of the left-to-right shunt. Echocardiography is also useful for estimating shunt size by examining the degree of volume overload of the left atrium and left ventricle; in the absence of associated lesions, the extent of their increased dimensions is a good reflection of the size of the left-to-right shunt. Pulsed Doppler examination shows whether the VSD is pressure restrictive by calculating the pressure gradient across the defect. Such calculation allows an estimation of right ventricular pressure and helps determine whether the patient is at risk for the development of early pulmonary vascular disease. In addition, the echocardiogram can be useful to determine the presence of aortic valve insufficiency or leaflet prolapse in the case of supracristal VSDs.

The hemodynamics of a VSD can also be demonstrated by *cardiac catheterization*. Catheterization is usually performed only when the size of the shunt is uncertain after a comprehensive clinical evaluation, when laboratory data do not fit well with the clinical findings, or when pulmonary vascular disease is suspected. Oximetry demonstrates increased oxygen content in the right ventricle; because some defects eject blood almost directly into the pulmonary artery (streaming), this increase is occasionally apparent only when pulmonary arterial blood is sampled. Small, restrictive VSDs are associated with normal right-sided heart pressure and pulmonary vascular resistance. Large, nonrestrictive VSDs are associated with equal or nearly equal pulmonary and systemic systolic pressure. Pulmonary blood flow may be two to four times systemic blood flow. In patients with such "hyperdynamic pulmonary hypertension," pulmonary vascular resistance is only minimally elevated because resistance is equal to pressure divided by flow. If Eisenmenger syndrome is present, pulmonary artery systolic and diastolic pressure is elevated, the degree of left-to-right shunting is minimal, and desaturation of blood in the left ventricle is encountered. The size, location, and number of ventricular defects are demonstrated by left ventriculography. Contrast medium passes across the defect or defects to opacify the right ventricle and pulmonary artery.

Prognosis and Complications. The natural course of a VSD depends to a large degree on the size of the defect. A significant number (30–50%) of small defects close spontaneously, most frequently during the 1st 2 yr of life. Small muscular VSDs are more likely to close (up to 80%) than membranous VSDs are (up to 35%). The vast majority of defects that close do so before the age of 4 yr, although spontaneous closure has been reported in adults. These VSDs often have ventricular septal aneurysms limiting the magnitude of the shunt. Most children with small defects remain asymptomatic, without evidence of an increase

in heart size, pulmonary arterial pressure, or resistance. A long-term risk is infective endocarditis. Some long-term studies of adults with unoperated small VSDs show an increased incidence of arrhythmia, subaortic stenosis, and exercise intolerance. The Council on Cardiovascular Disease in the Young of the American Heart Association states that an isolated, small, hemodynamically insignificant VSD is not an indication for surgery. The declining risk of open heart surgery has led others to suggest that all VSDs be closed electively by mid-childhood.

It is less common for moderate or large VSDs to close spontaneously, although even defects large enough to result in heart failure may become smaller and up to 8% may close completely. More commonly, infants with large defects have repeated episodes of respiratory infection and heart failure despite optimal medical management. Heart failure may be manifested in many of these infants primarily as failure to thrive. Pulmonary hypertension occurs as a result of high pulmonary blood flow. These patients are at risk for pulmonary vascular disease with time if the defect is not repaired.

Patients with VSD are also at risk for the development of aortic valve regurgitation, the greatest risk occurring in patients with supracristal VSD (see Chapter 419.7). A small number of patients with VSD have acquired infundibular pulmonary stenosis, which then protects the pulmonary circulation from the short-term effects of pulmonary overcirculation and the long-term effects of pulmonary vascular disease. In these patients, the clinical picture changes from that of a VSD with a large left-to-right shunt to a VSD with pulmonary stenosis. The shunt may diminish in size, become balanced, or even become a net right-to-left shunt (see Chapter 423). These patients must be distinguished from those in whom an Eisenmenger physiology develops (see Chapter 426.2).

Treatment. In patients with small VSDs, parents should be reassured of the relatively benign nature of the lesion, and the child should be encouraged to live a normal life, with no restrictions on physical activity. Surgical repair is currently not recommended. As protection against infective endocarditis, the integrity of primary and permanent teeth should be carefully maintained; antibiotic prophylaxis should be provided for dental visits (including cleanings), tonsillectomy, adenoidectomy, and other oropharyngeal surgical procedures, as well as for instrumentation of the genitourinary and lower intestinal tracts (see Chapter 429). These patients can be monitored by a combination of clinical examination and noninvasive laboratory tests until the VSD has closed spontaneously. The electrocardiogram is an excellent means of screening these patients for possible pulmonary hypertension or pulmonic stenosis as indicated by right ventricular hypertrophy. Echocardiography is used to screen for the development of left ventricular outflow tract pathology (subaortic membrane or aortic regurgitation) and to confirm spontaneous closure.

In infants with a large VSD, medical management has two aims: to control heart failure and prevent the development of pulmonary vascular disease. Therapeutic measures are aimed at control of the heart failure symptoms and maintenance of normal growth (see Chapter 434). If early treatment is successful, the shunt may diminish in size with spontaneous improvement, especially during the 1st yr of life. The clinician must be alert to not confuse clinical improvement caused by a decrease in defect size with clinical changes caused by the development of Eisenmenger physiology. Because surgical closure can be carried out at low risk in most infants, medical management should not be pursued in symptomatic infants after an initial unsuccessful trial. Pulmonary vascular disease can be prevented when surgery is performed within the 1st yr of life.

Indications for surgical closure of a VSD include patients at any age with large defects in whom clinical symptoms and failure to thrive cannot be controlled medically; infants between 6 and 12 mo of age with large defects associated with pulmonary hypertension, even if the symptoms are controlled by medication; and patients older than 24 mo with a Qp:Qs ratio greater than 2:1. Patients with supracristal VSD of any size are usually referred for surgery because of the high risk for aortic valve regurgitation (see Chapter 419.7). Severe pulmonary vascular disease is a contraindication to closure of a VSD.

The results of primary surgical repair are excellent, and complications leading to long-term problems (e.g., residual ventricular shunts requiring reoperation or heart block requiring a pacemaker) are rare. Pulmonary arterial palliative banding with repair in later childhood is reserved for complicated cases or very premature infants. Surgical risks are higher for defects in the muscular septum, particularly apical defects and multiple (Swiss cheese type) VSDs. These patients may require pulmonary arterial banding if symptomatic, with subsequent debanding and repair of multiple VSDs at an older age. Clamshell-type catheter occlusion devices are being tested as a means of closing apical muscular VSDs.

After obliteration of the left-to-right shunt, the hyperdynamic heart becomes quiet, cardiac size decreases toward normal (Fig. 419–6), thrills and murmurs are abolished, and pulmonary artery hypertension regresses. The patient's clinical status improves markedly. Most infants begin to thrive, and cardiac medications are no longer required. Catch-up growth occurs in most patients over the next 1–2 yr. In some instances after successful surgery, systolic ejection murmurs of low intensity may persist for months. The long-term prognosis after surgery is excellent. Patients with a small VSD and those who have undergone surgical closure without residua are considered to be at standard risk for health insurance.

419.7 Supracristal Ventricular Septal Defect with Aortic Insufficiency

A supracristal VSD is complicated by prolapse of the aortic valve into the defect and aortic insufficiency, which may eventually occur in 50–90% of patients. Although it accounts for approximately 5% of all patients with VSD, the incidence is highest in Asian children. The VSD, which may be small or moderate in size, is located anterior to and directly below the pulmonary valve in the outlet septum, superior to the crista supraventricularis. In occasional cases, aortic insufficiency is associated with VSDs located in the membranous septum. The right or, less often, the noncoronary aortic cusp prolapses into the defect and may partially or even completely occlude it. Such occlusion may limit the amount of left-to-right shunting and give the false impression that the defect is not large. Aortic insufficiency is most often not recognized until late in the 1st decade of life or beyond.

Early heart failure secondary to a large left-to-right shunt rarely occurs, but without surgery, severe aortic insufficiency and left ventricular failure may ensue. The murmur of a supracristal VSD is usually heard at the middle to upper left sternal border, as opposed to the lower left sternal border, and it is sometimes confused with that of pulmonic stenosis. The physical signs of aortic insufficiency (diastolic murmur and wide pulse pressure), when present, are added to those of the VSD. These clinical findings must be distinguished from PDA or other defects associated with aortic runoff.

The *clinical manifestations* vary widely from trivial aortic regurgitation and small left-to-right shunts in asymptomatic children to florid aortic incompetence and massive cardiomegaly in symptomatic adolescents. Closure of all supracristal ventricular VSDs at the time of diagnosis is commonly recommended to prevent the development of aortic regurgitation, even in an asymptomatic child. Patients who already have significant aortic incompetence require surgical intervention to prevent irreversible left ventricular dysfunction. Surgical options depend on the degree of damage to the valve and include valvuloplasty for mild involvement and replacement with a prosthesis or homograft or aortopulmonary translocation (see Chapter 420.5) for severe involvement.

419.8 Patent Ductus Arteriosus

During fetal life, most of the pulmonary arterial blood is shunted through the ductus arteriosus into the aorta (see

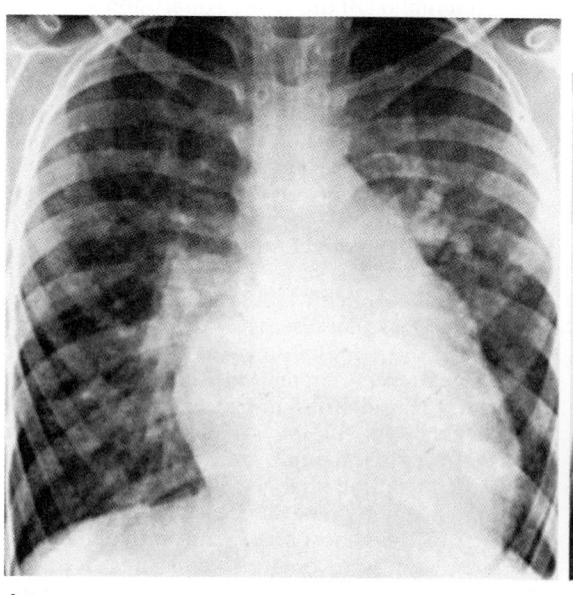 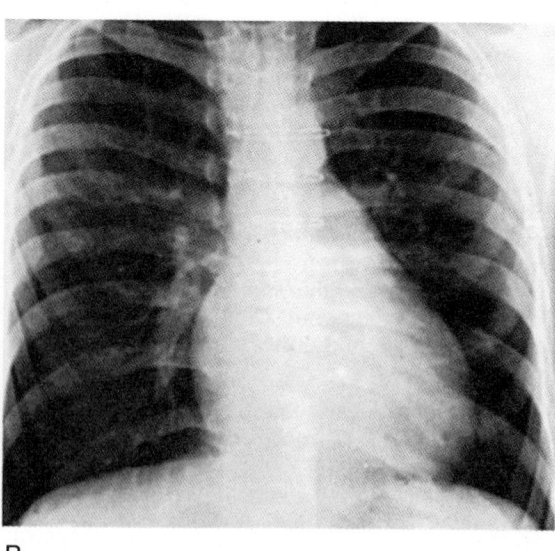

A   B

FIGURE 419–6. *A,* Preoperative roentgenogram in a patient with a ventricular septal defect with a large left-to-right shunt and pulmonary hypertension. Significant cardiomegaly, prominence of the pulmonary arterial trunk, and pulmonary overcirculation are evident. *B,* Three years after surgical closure of the defect, heart size is markedly decreased, and the pulmonary vasculature is normal.

Chapter 414). Functional closure of the ductus normally occurs soon after birth, but if the ductus remains patent when pulmonary vascular resistance falls, aortic blood is shunted into the pulmonary artery. The aortic end of the ductus is just distal to the origin of the left subclavian artery, and the ductus enters the pulmonary artery at its bifurcation. Female patients with PDA outnumber males 2:1. PDA is also associated with maternal rubella infection during early pregnancy. It is a common problem in premature infants, where it can cause severe hemodynamic derangements and several major sequelae (see Chapter 90.3).

When a term infant is found to have a PDA, the wall of the ductus is deficient in both the mucoid endothelial layer and the muscular media. In a premature infant, the PDA usually has a normal structure; patency is the result of hypoxia and immaturity. Thus, a PDA persisting beyond the 1st few weeks of life in a term infant rarely closes spontaneously or with pharmacologic intervention, whereas if early pharmacologic or surgical intervention is not required in a premature infant, spontaneous closure occurs in most instances. A PDA is seen in 10% of patients with other congenital heart lesions and often plays a critical role in providing pulmonary blood flow when the right ventricular outflow tract is stenotic or atretic (see Chapter 423) or in providing systemic blood flow in the presence of aortic coarctation or interruption (see Chapter 420).

Pathophysiology. As a result of the higher aortic pressure, blood shunts left to right through the ductus, from the aorta to the pulmonary artery. The extent of the shunt depends on the size of the ductus and on the ratio of pulmonary to systemic vascular resistance. In extreme cases, 70% of the left ventricular output may be shunted through the ductus to the pulmonary circulation. If the PDA is small, pressure within the pulmonary artery, the right ventricle, and the right atrium is normal. However, if the PDA is large, pulmonary artery pressure may be elevated to systemic levels during both systole and diastole. Patients with a large PDA are at extremely high risk for the development of pulmonary vascular disease if left unoperated. Pulse pressure is wide because of runoff of blood into the pulmonary artery during diastole.

Clinical Manifestations. A small patent ductus does not usually have any symptoms associated with it. A large PDA will result in heart failure similar to that encountered in infants with a large VSD. Retardation of physical growth may be a major manifestation in infants with large shunts.

A large PDA will result in striking physical signs attributable to the wide pulse pressure, most prominently, bounding peripheral arterial pulses. The heart is normal in size when the ductus is small but moderately or grossly enlarged in cases with a large communication. The apical impulse is prominent and, with cardiac enlargement, is heaving. A thrill, maximal in the 2nd left interspace, is often present and may radiate toward the left clavicle, down the left sternal border, or toward the apex. It is usually systolic but may also be palpated throughout the cardiac cycle. The classic continuous murmur is described as being like machinery or rolling thunder in quality. It begins soon after onset of the 1st sound, reaches maximal intensity at the end of systole, and wanes in late diastole. It may be localized to the 2nd left intercostal space or radiate down the left sternal border or to the left clavicle. When pulmonary vascular resistance is increased, the diastolic component of the murmur may be less prominent or absent. In patients with a large left-to-right shunt, a low-pitched mitral mid-diastolic murmur may be audible at the apex as a result of the increased volume of blood flow across the mitral valve.

Diagnosis. If the left-to-right shunt is small, the *electrocardiogram* is normal; if the ductus is large, left ventricular or biventricular hypertrophy is present. The diagnosis of an isolated, uncompli-

cated PDA is untenable when right ventricular hypertrophy is noted.

Radiographic studies in patients with a large PDA show a prominent pulmonary artery with increased intrapulmonary vascular markings. Cardiac size depends on the degree of left-to-right shunting; it may be normal or moderately to markedly enlarged. The chambers involved are the left atrium and ventricle. The aortic knob is normal or prominent.

The *echocardiographic* view of the cardiac chambers is normal if the ductus is small. With large shunts, left atrial and left ventricular dimensions are increased. The size of the left atrium is usually quantitated by comparison to the size of the aortic root, known as the LA:Ao ratio. Scanning from the suprasternal notch allows direct visualization of the ductus. Color and pulsed Doppler examinations demonstrate systolic or diastolic (or both) retrograde turbulent flow in the pulmonary artery and aortic retrograde flow in diastole.

The clinical pattern is sufficiently distinctive to allow an accurate diagnosis by noninvasive methods in most patients. In patients with atypical findings or when associated cardiac lesions are suspected, cardiac catheterization may be indicated. *Cardiac catheterization* demonstrates normal or increased pressure in the right ventricle and pulmonary artery, depending on the size of the ductus. The presence of oxygenated blood shunting into the pulmonary artery confirms a left-to-right shunt. The catheter may pass from the pulmonary artery through the ductus into the descending aorta. Injection of contrast medium into the ascending aorta shows opacification of the pulmonary artery from the aorta and identifies the ductus.

Other conditions can produce systolic and diastolic murmurs in the pulmonic area in the absence of cyanosis and must be differentiated. The characteristics of a venous hum are described in Chapter 415. An aorticopulmonary window defect may rarely be clinically indistinguishable from a patent ductus, although in most cases the murmur is only systolic and is loudest at the right rather than the left upper sternal border. A sinus of Valsalva aneurysm that has ruptured into the right side of the heart or pulmonary artery, coronary arteriovenous fistulas, and an aberrant left coronary artery with massive collaterals from the right coronary display dynamics similar to that of a PDA with a continuous murmur and a wide pulse pressure. Truncus arteriosus with torrential pulmonary flow also has an "aortic runoff" physiology. Pulmonary branch stenosis can be associated with systolic and diastolic murmurs, but the pulse pressure will be normal. A peripheral arteriovenous fistula also results in a wide pulse pressure, but the distinctive murmur of a PDA is not present. VSD with aortic insufficiency and combined rheumatic aortic and mitral insufficiency may be confused with a PDA, but the murmurs should be differentiated by their to-and-fro rather than continuous nature. The combination of a large VSD and a PDA results in findings more like those of an isolated VSD. Echocardiography should be able to eliminate these other diagnostic possibilities. If a PDA is suspected clinically but not visualized on echocardiography, cardiac catheterization is usually indicated.

Prognosis and Complications. Patients with a small PDA may live a normal span with few or no cardiac symptoms, but late manifestations may occur. Spontaneous closure of the ductus after infancy is extremely rare. *Cardiac failure* most often occurs in early infancy in the presence of a large ductus but may occur late in life even with a moderate-sized communication. The chronic left ventricular volume load is less well tolerated with aging.

Infective endarteritis may be seen at any age. Pulmonary or systemic emboli may occur. Rare complications include aneurysmal dilatation of the pulmonary artery or the ductus, calcification of the ductus, noninfective thrombosis of the ductus with embolization, and paradoxical emboli. Pulmonary hypertension (Eisenmenger syndrome) usually develops in patients with a large PDA who do not undergo surgical treatment (see Chapter 426.2).

Treatment. Irrespective of age, patients with PDA require surgical or catheter closure. In patients with a small PDA, the rationale for closure is prevention of bacterial endarteritis or other late complications. In patients with a moderate to large PDA, closure is accomplished to treat heart failure or prevent the development of pulmonary vascular disease, or both. Once the diagnosis of a moderate to large PDA is made, treatment should not be unduly postponed after adequate medical therapy for cardiac failure has been instituted.

Surgical closure of PDA can be accomplished by thoracoscopic techniques to minimize scarring and reduce postoperative discomfort. Because the case fatality rate with surgical treatment is considerably less than 1% and the risk without it is greater, ligation and division of the ductus are indicated in asymptomatic patients, preferably before 1 yr of age. Pulmonary hypertension is not a contraindication to surgery at any age if it can be demonstrated at cardiac catheterization that the shunt flow is still predominantly left to right and that severe pulmonary vascular disease is not present. After closure, symptoms of frank or incipient cardiac failure rapidly disappear. Infants who had failed to thrive usually have immediate improvement in physical development. The pulse and blood pressure return to normal, and the machinery-like murmur disappears. A functional systolic murmur over the pulmonary area may persist; it may represent turbulence in a persistently dilated pulmonary artery. The radiographic signs of cardiac enlargement and pulmonary overcirculation disappear over a period of several months, and the electrocardiogram becomes normal.

Transcatheter PDA closure is routinely performed in the cardiac catheterization laboratory. Small PDAs are generally closed with intravascular coils. Moderate to large PDAs may be closed with a catheter-introduced sac into which several coils are released or with an umbrella-like device.

Patent Ductus Arteriosus in Low-Birthweight Infants. See Chapter 90.3.

419.9 Aorticopulmonary Window Defect

An aorticopulmonary window defect consists of a communication between the ascending aorta and the main pulmonary artery. The presence of pulmonary and aortic valves and an intact ventricular septum distinguishes this anomaly from truncus arteriosus (see Chapter 424.8). Symptoms of heart failure appear during early infancy; occasionally, minimal cyanosis is present. The defect is usually large, and the cardiac murmur is systolic with a mid-diastolic rumble as a result of the increased blood flow across the mitral valve. In the rare instance when the communication is somewhat smaller and pulmonary hypertension is absent, the findings on examination can mimic those of a PDA (wide pulse pressure and a continuous murmur at the upper sternal borders). The electrocardiogram shows either left ventricular or biventricular hypertrophy. Radiographic studies demonstrate cardiac enlargement and prominence of the pulmonary artery and intrapulmonary vasculature. The echocardiogram shows enlarged left-sided heart chambers; the window defect can best be delineated with color flow Doppler.

Cardiac catheterization reveals a left-to-right shunt at the level of the pulmonary artery, as well as hyperkinetic pulmonary hypertension, because the defect is almost always large. Selective aortography with injection of contrast medium into the ascending aorta demonstrates the lesion, and manipulation of the catheter from the main pulmonary artery directly to the ascending aorta is also diagnostic.

An aorticopulmonary window defect is surgically corrected during infancy with cardiopulmonary bypass. If surgery is not carried out in infancy, survivors carry the risk of progressive pulmonary vascular obstructive disease, similar to that of other patients who have large intracardiac or great vessel communications.

419.10 Coronary-Arteriovenous Fistula (Coronary-Cameral Fistula)

A congenital fistula may exist between a coronary artery and an atrium, ventricle (especially the right), or pulmonary artery. Sometimes, multiple fistulas exist. Regardless of the recipient chamber, the clinical signs are similar to those of PDA, although the machinery-like murmur may be more diffuse. If the flow is substantial, the involved coronary artery may be dilated or aneurysmal. The anatomic abnormality is usually demonstrable by color flow Doppler echocardiography and, during catheterization, by injection of contrast medium into the ascending aorta. Small fistulas may be hemodynamically insignificant and may even close spontaneously. If the shunt is large, treatment consists of either transcatheter coil embolization or, for lesions not amenable to catheter intervention, surgical closure of the fistula.

419.11 Ruptured Sinus of Valsalva Aneurysm

When one of the sinuses of Valsalva of the aorta is weakened by congenital or acquired disease, an aneurysm may form and eventually rupture, usually into the right atrium or ventricle. This condition is extremely rare in childhood. The onset is usually sudden. The diagnosis should be suspected in a patient in whom symptoms of acute heart failure develop in association with a new loud to-and-fro murmur. Color Doppler echocardiography and cardiac catheterization demonstrate the left-to-right shunt at the atrial or ventricular level. Urgent surgical repair is generally required. This condition is often associated with infective endocarditis of the aortic valve.

Atrial Septal Defect

Benson DW, Silberbach GM, Kavanaugh-McHugh A, et al: Mutations in the cardiac transcription factor NKX2.5 affect diverse cardiac developmental pathways. *J Clin Invest* 1999;104:1567–73.

Boutin C, Musewe NN, Smallhorn JF, et al: Echocardiographic follow-up of atrial septal defect after catheter closure by double-umbrella device. *Circulation* 1993;88:621.

Latson LA: Per-catheter ASD closure. *Pediatr Cardiol* 1998;19:86–93.

O'Laughlin MP: Catheter closure of secundum atrial septal defects. *Tex Heart Inst J* 1997;24:287–92.

Radzik D, Davignon A, van Doesburg N, et al: Predictive factors for spontaneous closure of atrial septal defects diagnosed in the first 3 months of life. *J Am Coll Cardiol* 1993;22:851.

Rigby ML: The era of transcatheter closure of atrial septal defects. *Heart* 1999;81:227–8.

Riggs T, Sharp SE, Batton D, et al: Spontaneous closure of atrial septal defects in premature vs full term neonates. *Pediatr Cardiol* 2000;21:129–34.

Ventricular Septal Defect

Bridges ND, Perry SB, Keane JF, et al: Preoperative transcatheter closure of congenital muscular ventricular septal defects. *N Engl J Med* 1991;19:1312.

Hornberger LK, Sahn DJ, Krabill KA, et al: Elucidation of the natural history of ventricular septal defects by serial Doppler color flow mapping studies. *J Am Coll Cardiol* 1989;13:1111.

Leung MP, Beerman LB, Siewers RD, et al: Long term follow-up after aortic valvuloplasty and defect closure in ventricular septal defect with aortic regurgitation. *Am J Cardiol* 1987;60:890.

Moller JH, Patton C, Varco RL, et al: Late results (30 to 35 years) after operative closure of isolated ventricular septal defect from 1954 to 1960. *Am J Cardiol* 1991;68:1491.

Perry SB, van der Velde ME, Bridges ND, et al: Transcatheter closure of atrial and ventricular septal defects. *Herz* 1993;18:135–42.

Ramaciotti C, Keren A, Silverman NH: Importance of pseudoaneurysms of the ventricular septum in the natural history of isolated perimembranous ventricular septal defects. *Am J Cardiol* 1986;57:268.

Weidman WH, Blount SG Jr, DuShane JW, et al: Clinical course in ventricular septal defect. *Circulation* 1977;56:156.

Atrioventricular Septal Defect

Clapp SK, Perry BL, Farooki ZQ, et al: Surgical and medical results of complete atrioventricular canal: A ten-year review. *Am J Cardiol* 1987;59:454.

Drinkwater DC Jr, Laks H: Unbalanced atrioventricular septal defects. *Semin Thorac Cardiovasc Surg* 1997;9:21–5.

Marino B, Vairo U, Corno A, et al: Atrioventricular canal in Down syndrome. *Am J Dis Child* 1990;144:1120.

Murphy DJ Jr: Atrioventricular canal defects. *Curr Treat Opt Cardiovasc Med* 1999;1:323–34.

Sigfusson G, Ettedgui JA, Silverman NH, et al: Is a cleft in the anterior leaflet of an otherwise normal mitral valve an atrioventricular canal malformation? *J Am Coll Cardiol* 1995;26:508–15.

Patent Ductus Arteriosus

Bergwerff M, DeRuiter MC, Gittenberger-de Groot AC: Comparative anatomy and ontogeny of the ductus arteriosus, a vascular outsider. *Anat Embryol (Berl)* 1999;200:559–71.

Gittenberger-de Groot AC, Van Ertbruggen I, Moulaert A, et al: The ductus arteriosus in the preterm infant: Histologic and clinical observations. *J Pediatr* 1980;96:88.

Rothman A, Lucas VW, Sklansky MS, et al: Percutaneous coil occlusion of patent ductus arteriosus. *J Pediatr* 1997;130:447.

Sommer RJ, Gutierrez A, Lai WW, et al: Use of preformed nitinol snare to improve transcatheter coil delivery in occlusion of patent ductus arteriosus. *Am J Cardiol* 1994;74:836.

Coronary Arteriovenous Fistula

Velvis H, Schmidt KG, Silverman NH, et al: Diagnosis of coronary artery fistula by two-dimensional echocardiography, pulsed Doppler ultrasound, and color flow imaging. *J Am Coll Cardiol* 1989;14:968.

Chapter 420

Acyanotic Congenital Heart Disease: The Obstructive Lesions

420.1   Pulmonary Valve Stenosis with Intact Ventricular Septum

Of the various forms of right ventricular outflow obstruction with an intact ventricular septum, the most common is isolated valvular pulmonary stenosis, which accounts for 7–10% of all congenital heart defects. In this entity, the valve cusps are deformed to various degrees, and as a result the valve opens incompletely during systole. The valve may be bicuspid or tricuspid and the leaflets partially fused together with an eccentric outlet. This fusion may be so severe that only a pinhole central opening remains. If the valve is not severely thickened, it produces a domelike obstruction to right ventricular outflow during systole. Isolated infundibular stenosis, supravalvular pulmonary stenosis, and branch pulmonary artery stenosis are less commonly encountered. When pulmonary valve stenosis is the dominant lesion, a small associated ventricular septal defect (VSD) is present, and this condition is better classified as pulmonary stenosis with VSD than as tetralogy of Fallot. Pulmonary stenosis and an atrial septal defect (ASD) are occasionally seen as associated defects. The clinical and laboratory findings reflect the dominant lesion, but it is important to rule out these associated anomalies. Pulmonary stenosis as a result of valve dysplasia is the common cardiac abnormality of *Noonan syndrome* (see Chapter 70), and it is associated with a mutation in the region 12q24.1 on chromosome 12. The mechanism for pulmonic stenosis is unknown, although maldevelopment of the distal portion of the bulbus cordis and the sequelae of fetal endocarditis have been suggested as causes. Pulmonary stenosis, either of

the valve or the branch pulmonary arteries, is a common finding in patients with arteriohepatic dysplasia, also known as **Alagille syndrome**. In this syndrome and in some patients with isolated pulmonic stenosis, a mutation is present in the *Jagged1* gene.

Pathophysiology. The obstruction to outflow from the right ventricle to the pulmonary artery results in increased systolic pressure and wall stress, which eventually leads to hypertrophy of the right ventricle (Fig. 420–1). The severity of these abnormalities depends on the size of the restricted valve opening. In severe cases, right ventricular pressure may be higher than systemic arterial systolic pressure, whereas with milder obstruction, right ventricular pressure is only mildly or moderately elevated. Pulmonary artery pressure is normal or decreased. Arterial oxygen saturation will be normal even in cases of severe stenosis, unless an intracardiac communication such as a VSD or ASD is allowing blood to shunt from right to left. When severe pulmonic stenosis occurs in a neonate, markedly decreased right ventricular compliance may lead to right-to-left shunting through a patent foramen ovale, a condition termed **critical pulmonic stenosis**.

Clinical Manifestations. Patients with mild or moderate stenosis usually do not have any symptoms. Growth and development are most often normal; older infants and children appear to be well developed and healthy. If the stenosis is severe, signs of right ventricular failure such as hepatomegaly, peripheral edema, and exercise intolerance may be present. In a neonate or young infant with critical pulmonic stenosis, signs of right ventricular failure may be more prominent, and cyanosis is often present because of shunting at the foramen ovale.

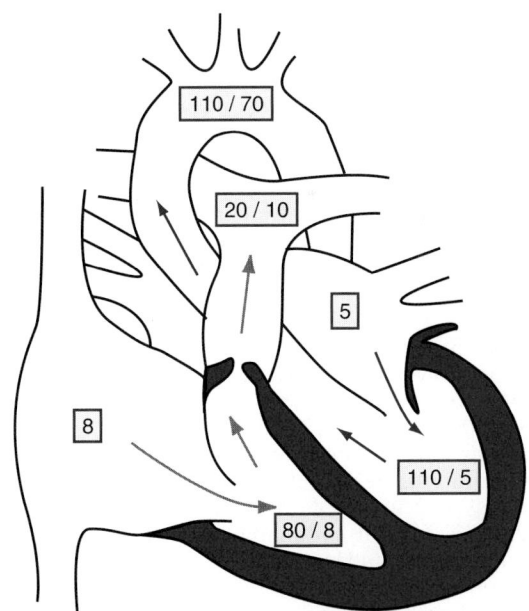

FIGURE 420–1. Physiology of valvular pulmonary stenosis. *Boxed numbers* represent pressure in mm Hg. Because of the absence of right-to-left or left-to-right shunting, blood flow through all cardiac chambers is normal at 3 L/min/m². The pulmonary-to-systemic blood flow ratio (Qp:Qs) is 1:1. Right atrial pressure is increased slightly as a result of decreased right ventricular compliance. The right ventricle is hypertrophied, and systolic and diastolic pressure is increased. The pressure gradient across the thickened pulmonary valve is 60 mm Hg. The main pulmonary artery pressure is slightly low, and poststenotic dilatation is present. Left heart pressure is normal. Unless right-to-left shunting is occurring through a foramen ovale, the patient's systemic oxygen saturation will be normal.

With **mild pulmonary stenosis**, venous pressure and pulse are normal. The heart is not enlarged, the apical impulse is normal, and the right ventricular impulse is not palpable. A sharp pulmonic ejection click immediately following the 1st heart sound is heard at the left upper sternal border during expiration. The 2nd heart sound is split, with a pulmonary component of normal intensity that may be slightly delayed. A relatively short, low- or medium-pitched systolic ejection murmur is maximally audible over the pulmonic area and radiates minimally to the lung fields bilaterally. The *electrocardiogram* is normal or characteristic of mild right ventricular hypertrophy; inversion of the T waves in the right precordial leads may be seen. The only abnormality demonstrable *radiographically* is poststenotic dilatation of the pulmonary artery. *Two-dimensional echocardiography* shows right ventricular hypertrophy and a slightly thickened and domed pulmonic valve; Doppler studies demonstrate a right ventricle–to–pulmonary artery gradient of 30 mm Hg or less.

In **moderate pulmonic stenosis,** venous pressure may be slightly elevated; in older children, a prominent *a* wave may be noted in the jugular pulse. A right ventricular lift may be palpable at the lower left sternal border. The 2nd heart sound is split, with a delayed and diminished pulmonary component. As valve motion becomes more limited with more severe degrees of stenosis, both the pulmonic ejection click and the pulmonic 2nd sound may become inaudible. With increasing degrees of stenosis, the peak of the systolic ejection murmur is prolonged later into systole, and its quality becomes louder and harsher (higher frequency). The murmur radiates more prominently to both lung fields.

The *electrocardiogram* reveals varying degrees of right ventricular hypertrophy, sometimes with a prominent spiked P wave. *Radiographically*, the heart can vary from normal size to mildly enlarged because of prominence of the right ventricle; intrapulmonary vascularity may be normal or slightly decreased. The *echocardiogram* shows a thickened pulmonic valve with restricted systolic motion. Doppler examination demonstrates a ventricular–pulmonary artery pressure gradient in the 30–60 mm Hg range. Mild tricuspid regurgitation may be present and allows Doppler confirmation of right ventricular systolic pressure.

In **severe stenosis,** mild to moderate cyanosis may be noted in those with interatrial communication. If hepatic enlargement and peripheral edema are present, they are an indication of right ventricular failure. Elevation of venous pressure is common and is caused by a large presystolic jugular "*a*" wave. The heart is moderately or greatly enlarged, and a conspicuous parasternal right ventricular lift is present and frequently extends to the midclavicular line. The pulmonary element of the 2nd sound is usually inaudible. A loud and long harsh systolic ejection murmur, frequently accompanied by a thrill, is maximally audible in the pulmonic area and may radiate widely over the entire precordium, to both lung fields, into the neck, and to the back. The peak of the murmur occurs later in systole as valve opening becomes more restricted. The murmur frequently encompasses the aortic component of the 2nd sound but is not preceded by an ejection click.

The *electrocardiogram* shows gross right ventricular hypertrophy, frequently accompanied by a tall, spiked P wave. *Radiographic studies* confirm the cardiac enlargement and prominence of the right ventricle and atrium. Prominence of the pulmonary artery segment is due to poststenotic dilatation (Fig. 420–2). Intrapulmonary vascularity is decreased. The *two-dimensional echocardiogram* shows severe deformity of the pulmonary valve and right ventricular hypertrophy. In the late stages of the disease, dysfunction of the right ventricle is seen, and the ventricle may become dilated. Doppler studies demonstrate a large gradient (>60 mm Hg) across the pulmonary valve. Tricuspid regurgitation may also be prominent. Fortunately, the classic findings of severe pulmonary stenosis in older children are rarely seen because of early intervention. Signs of critical pulmonic stenosis are usually encountered in the neonatal period.

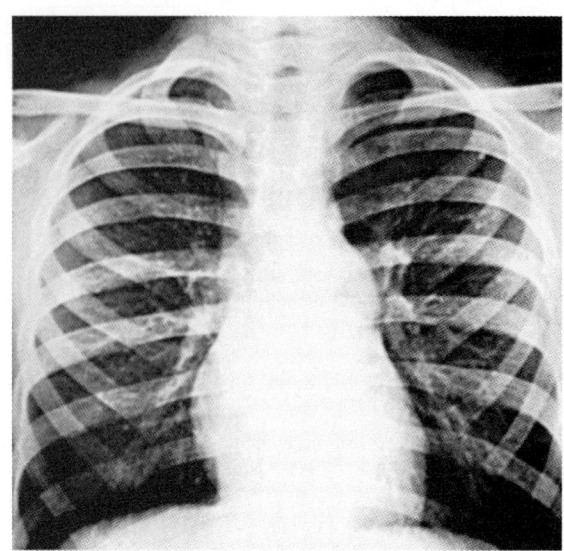

FIGURE 420–2. Roentgenogram in a patient with valvular pulmonary stenosis and a normal aortic root. The heart size is within normal limits, but poststenotic dilatation of the pulmonary artery is present.

Cardiac catheterization is not generally required for diagnostic purposes but is undertaken as part of a balloon valvuloplasty procedure. Catheterization demonstrates an abrupt pressure gradient across the pulmonary valve. Pulmonary artery pressure is either normal or low. The severity of the stenosis is based on right ventricular systolic pressure or the pressure gradient: a gradient of 10–30 mm Hg in mild cases, 30–60 mm Hg in moderate cases, and greater than 60 mm Hg or with right ventricular pressure greater than systemic pressure in severe cases. If cardiac output is low or a significant right-to-left shunt exists across the atrial septum, the pressure gradient may underestimate the degree of valve stenosis. *Selective right ventriculography* demonstrates the thickened, poorly mobile valve. In mild to moderate stenosis, doming of the valve in systole is readily seen. Flow of contrast medium through the stenotic valve in ventricular systole produces a narrow jet of dye that fills the dilated main pulmonary artery. Subvalvular hypertrophy that may intensify the obstruction may occasionally be present. The angiogram also indicates whether the ventricular septum is intact.

Prognosis and Complications. Heart failure occurs only in severe cases and most often during the 1st mo of life. The development of cyanosis from a right-to-left shunt across a foramen ovale is most often seen in infancy when the stenosis is severe. Infective endocarditis is a risk but is not common in childhood.

Children with mild stenosis can lead a normal life, but their progress should be evaluated at regular intervals. Patients who have small gradients rarely show progression and do not need intervention, but a more significant gradient is more likely to develop in children with moderate stenosis as they grow older. Worsening of obstruction may also be due to the development of secondary subvalvular muscular and fibrous tissue hypertrophy. In untreated severe stenosis, the course may abruptly worsen with the development of right ventricular dysfunction and cardiac failure. Infants with critical pulmonic stenosis require urgent catheter balloon valvuloplasty or surgical valvotomy.

Treatment. Patients with moderate or severe isolated pulmonary stenosis require relief of the obstruction. Balloon valvuloplasty is the initial treatment of choice for the majority of patients (Fig. 420–3). Patients with severely thickened pulmonic valves, especially common in those with Noonan syndrome, may require surgical intervention instead. In a neonate with critical

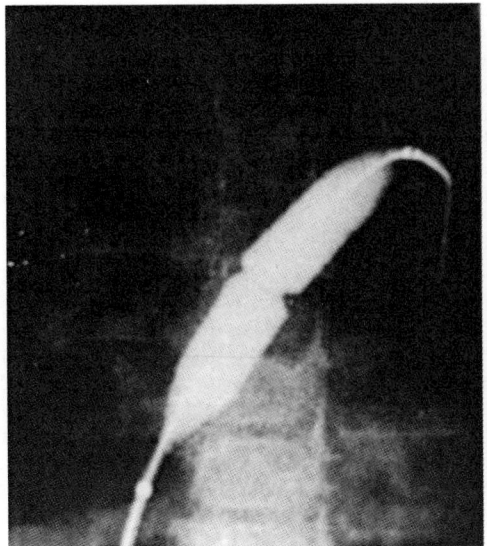
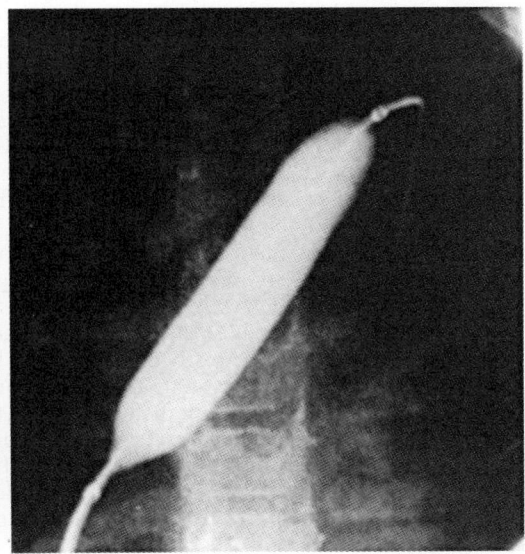

FIGURE 420–3. Balloon pulmonary valvuloplasty. *A*, Hourglass shape of the balloon at the start of inflation. *B*, Full balloon inflation. The left pulmonary artery is protected from the sharp tip of the catheter with a flexibly tipped guide wire. (From Lababidi Z: Neonatal catheter palliations. In Long WA [editor]: *Fetal and Neonatal Cardiology.* Philadelphia, WB Saunders, 1990.)

A

B

pulmonic stenosis, urgent treatment by either balloon valvuloplasty or surgical valvotomy is warranted.

Excellent results are obtained in most instances. The gradient across the pulmonary valve is markedly reduced or abolished. In the early period after balloon valvuloplasty, a small to moderate residual gradient may remain because of muscular infundibular narrowing; it nearly always resolves with time. A short, early decrescendo diastolic murmur may be heard at the mid to upper left sternal border as a result of pulmonary valvular insufficiency. The degree of insufficiency is not usually clinically significant. No difference in patient status after valvuloplasty or surgery is noted at late follow-up; recurrence is unusual after successful treatment.

420.2 Infundibular Pulmonary Stenosis and Double-Chamber Right Ventricle

Infundibular pulmonary stenosis is caused by muscular or fibrous obstruction in the outflow tract of the right ventricle. The site of obstruction may be close to the pulmonary valve or well below it; an infundibular chamber may be present between the right ventricular cavity and the pulmonary valve. In many cases, a VSD may have been present initially and later closed spontaneously. When the pulmonary valve is also stenotic, the combined defect is primarily classified as valvular stenosis with secondary infundibular hypertrophy. The *hemodynamics* and *clinical manifestations* of patients with isolated infundibular pulmonary stenosis are similar, for the most part, to those described in the discussion of isolated valvular pulmonary stenosis (see Chapter 420.1).

A common variation in right ventricular outflow obstruction below the pulmonary valve is that of a double-chambered right ventricle. In this condition, a muscular band is present in the midright ventricular region; the band divides the chamber into two parts and creates obstruction between the inlet and outlet portions. An associated VSD that may close spontaneously is often noted. Obstruction is not usually seen early in life but may progress rapidly in a similar manner to the progressive infundibular obstruction observed with the tetralogy of Fallot (see Chapter 423.1).

The *diagnosis* of isolated right ventricular infundibular stenosis or double-chambered right ventricle can be made by echocar-

diography or cardiac catheterization and angiography, or by both. The ventricular septum must be evaluated carefully to determine whether an associated VSD is present. The prognosis for untreated cases of severe right ventricular outflow obstruction is similar to that for valvular pulmonary stenosis. When the obstruction is moderate to severe, surgery is indicated. After surgery, the pressure gradient is abolished or markedly reduced and the long-term outlook is excellent.

420.3 Pulmonary Stenosis in Combination with an Intracardiac Shunt

Valvular or infundibular pulmonary stenosis, or both, may be associated with either an ASD or a VSD. In these patients, the clinical features depend on the degree of pulmonary stenosis, which determines whether the net shunt is from left to right or from right to left.

The presence of a large left-to-right shunt at the atrial or ventricular level is evidence that the pulmonary stenosis is mild. These patients have symptoms similar to those of patients with an isolated ASD or VSD. However, with increasing age, worsening of the obstruction may limit the shunt and result in a gradual improvement in symptoms. Eventually, particularly in patients with pulmonary stenosis and VSD, a further increase in obstruction may lead to right-to-left shunting and cyanosis. When a patient with a VSD has evidence of decreasing heart failure and increased right ventricular forces on the electrocardiogram, one must differentiate between the development of increasing pulmonary stenosis and the onset of pulmonary vascular disease (Eisenmenger syndrome).

These anomalies are readily repaired surgically. Defects in the atrial or ventricular septum are closed, and the pulmonary stenosis is relieved by resection of infundibular muscle or pulmonary valvotomy, or both, as indicated. Patients with a predominant right-to-left shunt have symptoms similar to those of patients with the tetralogy of Fallot (see Chapter 423.1).

420.4 Peripheral Pulmonary Stenosis

Single or multiple constrictions may occur anywhere along the major branches of the pulmonary arteries and may range from mild to severe and from localized to extensive. Frequently, these defects are associated with other types of congenital heart disease, including valvular pulmonic stenosis, tetralogy of Fallot, patent ductus arteriosus (PDA), VSD, ASD, and supravalvular aortic stenosis. A familial tendency has been recognized in some patients with peripheral pulmonic stenosis. A high incidence is found in infants with congenital rubella syndrome. The combination of supravalvular aortic stenosis with pulmonary arterial branch stenosis, idiopathic hypercalcemia of infancy, elfin facies, and mental retardation is known as Williams syndrome, a condition associated with deletion of the elastin gene in region 7q11.23 on chromosome 7.

A mild constriction has little effect on the pulmonary circulation. With multiple severe constrictions, pressure is increased in the right ventricle and in the pulmonary artery proximal to the site of obstruction. When the anomaly is isolated, the *diagnosis* is suspected by the presence of murmurs in widespread locations over the chest, either anteriorly or posteriorly. These murmurs are usually systolic but may be continuous. Most often, the physical signs are dominated by the associated anomaly, such as the tetralogy of Fallot.

In the immediate newborn period, a mild and transient form of peripheral pulmonic stenosis may be present. Physical findings are generally limited to a soft systolic ejection murmur, which can be heard over either or both lung fields. It is the absence of other physical findings of valvular pulmonic stenosis (right ventricular lift, soft pulmonic 2nd sound, systolic ejection click, murmur loudest at the upper left sternal border) that supports this diagnosis. This murmur usually disappears by 1–2 mo.

If the stenosis is severe, the electrocardiogram shows evidence of right ventricular and right atrial hypertrophy, and the *chest radiograph* shows cardiomegaly and prominence of the main pulmonary artery. Generally, the pulmonary vasculature is normal; in some cases, however, small intrapulmonary vascular shadows are seen that represent areas of poststenotic dilatation. Echocardiography is limited in its ability to visualize the distal branch pulmonary arteries. Doppler examination demonstrates the acceleration of blood flow through the stenoses and, if tricuspid regurgitation is present, allows an estimation of right ventricular systolic pressure. MRI and CT are helpful in delineating distal obstructions; if moderate to severe disease is suspected, the diagnosis is usually confirmed by *cardiac catheterization*.

Severe obstruction of the main pulmonary artery and its primary branches can be relieved during corrective surgery for associated lesions such as the tetralogy of Fallot or valvular pulmonary stenosis. If peripheral pulmonic stenosis is isolated, it may be treated by catheter balloon dilatation. When peripheral obstruction occurs distally in the intrapulmonary vessels, it is not usually amenable to surgical repair. These obstructions are often multiple and are best treated with repeat balloon angioplasty, although the rate of recurrence is high. The introduction of expandable intravascular stents, placed by catheter in the distal pulmonary arteries and then dilated with a balloon to the appropriate size, may prevent re-stenosis.

420.5 Aortic Stenosis

Pathophysiology. Congenital aortic stenosis accounts for about 5% of cardiac malformations recognized in childhood; a bicuspid aortic valve, one of the most common congenital heart lesions overall, is identified in up to 2% of adults and is usually asymptomatic in childhood. Aortic stenosis is more frequent in males (3:1). In the most common form, *valvular aortic stenosis*, the leaflets are thickened and the commissures are fused to varying degrees. Left ventricular systolic pressure is increased as a result of the obstruction to outflow. The ventricular wall hypertrophies in compensation; as its compliance decreases, end-diastolic pressure increases as well.

Subvalvular (subaortic) stenosis with a discrete fibromuscular shelf below the aortic valve is also an important form of left ventricular outflow tract obstruction. This lesion is frequently associated with other forms of congenital heart disease and may progress rapidly in severity. It is rarely diagnosed during early infancy and may develop despite previous documentation of no left ventricular outflow tract obstruction. Subvalvular aortic stenosis may become apparent after successful surgery for other congenital heart defects (e.g., coarctation of the aorta, PDA, VSD), may develop in association with mild lesions that have not been surgically repaired, or may occur as an isolated abnormality. Subvalvular aortic stenosis may also be due to a markedly hypertrophied ventricular septum, known as idiopathic hypertrophic subaortic stenosis or hypertrophic cardiomyopathy (see Chapter 431.2).

Supravalvular aortic stenosis, the least common type, may be sporadic, familial, or associated with Williams syndrome, which includes mental retardation, elfin facies (full face, broad forehead, flattened bridge of the nose, long upper lip, and rounded cheeks), and idiopathic hypercalcemia of infancy (see Chapter 70). Stenosis of other arteries, in particular, the branch pulmonary arteries, may also be present. Williams syndrome has been shown to be due to a deletion involving the elastin gene on chromosome 7q11.23.

Clinical Manifestations. Symptoms in patients with aortic stenosis depend on the severity of the obstruction. Severe aortic stenosis that occurs in early infancy is termed *critical aortic stenosis* and is associated with left ventricular failure and signs of low cardiac output. Heart failure, cardiomegaly, and pulmonary edema are severe, the pulses are weak in all extremities, and the skin may be pale or grayish. Urine output may be diminished. If cardiac output is significantly decreased, the intensity of the murmur at the right upper sternal border may be minimal. Most children with less severe forms of aortic stenosis remain asymptomatic and display normal growth and development. The murmur is usually discovered during routine physical examination. Rarely, fatigue, angina, dizziness, or syncope may develop in an older child with previously undiagnosed severe obstruction to left ventricular outflow. Sudden death has been reported with aortic stenosis but usually occurs in patients with severe left ventricular outflow obstruction in whom surgical relief has been delayed.

The physical findings are dependent on the degree of obstruction to left ventricular outflow. In mild stenosis, the pulses, heart size, and apical impulse are all normal. With increasing degrees of severity, the pulses become diminished in intensity and the heart may be enlarged, with a left ventricular apical thrust. Mild to moderate valvular aortic stenosis is usually associated with an early systolic ejection click, best heard at the apex and left sternal edge. Unlike the click in pulmonic stenosis, its intensity does not vary with respiration. Clicks are unusual in more severe aortic stenosis or in discrete subaortic stenosis. If the stenosis is severe, the 1st heart sound may be diminished because of decreased compliance of the thickened left ventricle. Normal splitting of the 2nd heart sound is present in mild to moderate obstruction. In patients with severe obstruction, the intensity of aortic valve closure is diminished, and rarely in children, the 2nd sound may be split paradoxically (becoming wider in expiration). A 4th heart sound may be audible when the obstruction is severe.

The intensity, pitch, and duration of the systolic ejection murmur are other indications of severity. Generally, the louder, harsher (higher pitch), and longer the murmur, the greater the degree of obstruction. The typical murmur is audible maximally at the right upper sternal border and radiates to the neck and the left midsternal border. It is usually accompanied by a thrill in the suprasternal notch. In patients with subvalvular aortic stenosis, the murmur may be maximal along the left sternal border or even at the apex. A soft decrescendo diastolic murmur indicative of aortic insufficiency is often present when the obstruction is subvalvular or in patients with a bicuspid aortic valve. Occasionally, an apical short mid-diastolic rumbling murmur is audible, even in the presence of a normal mitral valve; however, this murmur should always raise suspicion of associated mitral valve stenosis.

Diagnosis. The diagnosis can usually be made on the basis of the physical examination and the severity of obstruction confirmed by laboratory tests. If the pressure gradient across the aortic valve is mild, the *electrocardiogram* is likely to be normal. The electrocardiogram may occasionally be normal even with more severe obstruction, but evidence of left ventricular hypertrophy and strain (inverted T waves in the left precordial leads) is generally present if severe stenosis is long-standing. The *chest radiograph* frequently shows a prominent ascending aorta, but the aortic knob is normal. Heart size is typically normal. Valvular calcification has been noted only in older children and adults. *Echocardiography* identifies both the site and the severity of the obstruction. Two-dimensional imaging shows left ventricular hypertrophy, the thickened and domed aortic valve, the number of valve leaflets, and a subaortic or supra-aortic membrane, if present. Associated anomalies of the mitral valve or aortic arch or a VSD or PDA is present in up to 20% of cases. In the absence of left ventricular failure, the shortening fraction of the left ventricle may be increased because the ventricle is hypercontractile. In infants with critical aortic stenosis, the left ventricular shortening fraction is usually decreased and the endocardium may be bright, indicative of the development of endocardial fibrous scarring, known as **endocardial fibroelastosis**. Doppler studies show the specific site of obstruction and determine the peak and mean systolic left ventricular outflow tract gradients. When severe aortic obstruction is associated with left ventricular dysfunction, the Doppler-derived valve gradient may markedly underestimate the severity of the obstruction because of the low cardiac output.

Graded exercise testing is useful in evaluating the severity of left ventricular outflow tract obstruction in older children. As the severity of the gradient increases, working capacity decreases, systolic blood pressure fails to rise adequately, diastolic blood pressure may increase, and ST segment depression can occur. Because patients with severe aortic stenosis may deny symptoms and have normal electrocardiograms and chest roentgenograms, serial echocardiograms and graded exercise tests may be valuable in determining the timing of cardiac catheterization and surgical or balloon catheter valvuloplasty.

Left heart catheterization demonstrates the magnitude of the pressure gradient from the left ventricle to the aorta. The aortic pressure curve is abnormal if the obstruction is severe. In patients with severe obstruction and decreased left ventricular compliance, left atrial pressure is increased and pulmonary hypertension may be present. The site of obstruction is best identified by selective left ventriculography. Most infants with critical aortic stenosis do not require diagnostic cardiac catheterization but may undergo the procedure for balloon valvuloplasty. When a critically ill infant with left ventricular outflow tract obstruction undergoes cardiac catheterization, left ventricular function is often markedly decreased. As with the echocardiogram, the gradient measured across the stenotic aortic valve may underestimate the degree of obstruction because of low cardiac output. Actual measurement of cardiac output by thermodilution and calculation of the aortic valve area are helpful.

Prognosis. Neonates with critical aortic stenosis may have severe heart failure and deteriorate rapidly to a low-output shock state. Emergency surgery or balloon valvuloplasty is lifesaving, but the mortality risk is not trivial. Neonates who die of critical aortic stenosis frequently have significant left ventricular endocardial fibroelastosis.

In older infants and children with mild to moderate aortic stenosis, the prognosis is reasonably good, although disease progression over a period of 5–10 yr is common. Patients with aortic valve gradients less than 40–50 mm Hg are considered to have mild disease; those with gradients of 40–70 mm Hg have moderate disease. These patients usually respond well to treatment (either surgery or valvuloplasty), although reoperations on the aortic valve are often required later in childhood or in adult life, and many patients eventually require valve replacement. In unoperated patients with severe obstruction, sudden death is a significant risk and often occurs during or immediately after exercise. Aortic stenosis is a common cause of sudden cardiac death in the pediatric age group.

Patients with moderate to severe degrees of aortic stenosis should not participate in active competitive sports. In those with milder disease, sports participation is less severely restricted; however, patients should be encouraged to pursue less physically demanding activities. The status of each patient should be reviewed at least annually and intervention advised if progression of signs or symptoms occurs. Lifetime prophylaxis against infective endocarditis is required.

Treatment. Balloon valvuloplasty is indicated for children with moderate to severe valvular aortic stenosis to prevent progressive left ventricular dysfunction and the risk of syncope and sudden death. It is generally agreed that valvuloplasty should be advised when the peak-to-peak systolic gradient between the left ventricle and aorta exceeds 60–70 mm Hg at rest, assuming normal cardiac output, or for lesser gradients when symptoms or electrocardiographic changes are present. For more rapidly progressive subaortic obstructive lesions, a gradient of 40–50 mm Hg is considered operable. Outside the neonatal period, surgical treatment is usually reserved for valves that are not amenable to balloon therapy, generally those that are extremely thickened.

In the neonatal period, balloon valvuloplasty is made somewhat more difficult by problems of arterial access. The risk of femoral arterial complications is much higher than in older children, although low-profile balloons have reduced this risk. Both surgical and catheter approaches are used at different centers for neonatal critical aortic stenosis.

Discrete *subaortic stenosis* can be resected without damage to the aortic valve, the anterior leaflet of the mitral valve, or the conduction system. This type of obstruction is not usually amenable to catheter treatment. Relief of *supravalvular stenosis* is also achieved surgically, and the results are excellent if the area of obstruction is discrete and not associated with a hypoplastic aorta. In association with supravalvular aortic stenosis, one or both coronary arteries may be stenotic at their origins because of a thick supra-aortic fibrous ridge. For patients who have aortic stenosis in association with severe tunnel-like subaortic obstruction, the left ventricular outflow tract can be enlarged by "borrowing" space anteriorly from the right ventricular outflow tract (the *Konno procedure*).

Regardless of whether surgical or catheter treatment has been carried out, aortic insufficiency or calcification with re-stenosis is likely to occur years or even decades later and eventually require reoperation and often aortic valve replacement. When recurrence develops, it may not be associated with early symptoms. Signs of recurrent stenosis include electrocardiographic signs of left ventricular hypertrophy, an increase in the Doppler echocardiographic gradient, deterioration in echocardiographic indices of left ventricular function, and recurrence of signs or symptoms during graded treadmill exercise. Evidence of significant aortic regurgitation includes symptoms of heart failure, cardiac enlargement on roentgenogram, and left ventricular dilatation on echocardiogram. The choice of reparative procedure depends on the relative degree of stenosis and regurgitation.

When aortic valve replacement is necessary, the choice of procedure often depends on the age of the patient. Homograft valves tend to calcify more rapidly in younger children, but they do not require chronic anticoagulation. Mechanical prosthetic valves are much longer lasting, yet they require anticoagulation, which can be difficult to manage in young children. In adolescent girls who are nearing childbearing age, consideration of the teratogenic effects of warfarin may warrant the use of a homograft valve. None of these options are perfect for a younger child who requires valve replacement because neither homograft nor mechanical valves grow with the patient. An alternative operation is aortopulmonary translocation, also known as the *Ross procedure*; it involves removing the patient's own pulmonary valve and using it to replace the abnormal aortic valve. A homograft is then placed in the pulmonary position. The advantage of this procedure is the potential for growth of the translocated living "neoaortic" valve and the longer longevity of the homograft valve when placed in the lower pressure pulmonary circulation. The long-term success of this operation, especially in young children, is being investigated. Tissue-engineered replacement valves grown in the laboratory from the patient's own arterial endothelial cells are under development in animal models.

420.6 Coarctation of the Aorta

Constrictions of the aorta of varying degrees may occur at any point from the transverse arch to the iliac bifurcation, but 98% occur just below the origin of the left subclavian artery at the origin of the ductus arteriosus (juxtaductal coarctation). The anomaly occurs twice as often in males as in females. Coarctation of the aorta may be a feature of Turner syndrome (see Chapters 70 and 580.1) and is associated with a bicuspid aortic valve in more than 70% of patients. Mitral valve abnormalities (a supravalvular mitral ring or parachute mitral valve) and subaortic stenosis are potential associated lesions. When this group of left-sided obstructive lesions occurs together, they are referred to as the *Shone complex*.

Pathophysiology. Coarctation of the aorta can occur as a discrete juxtaductal obstruction or as tubular hypoplasia of the transverse aorta starting at one of the head or neck vessels and extending to the ductal area (preductal or infantile-type coarctation; Fig. 420–4). Often, both components are present. It is postulated that coarctation may be initiated in fetal life by the presence of a cardiac abnormality that results in decreased blood flow anterograde through the aortic valve (e.g., bicuspid aortic valve, VSD).

In patients with discrete juxtaductal coarctation, ascending aortic blood flows through the narrowed segment to reach the descending aorta, although left ventricular hypertension and hypertrophy result. In the 1st few days of life, the PDA may serve to widen the juxtaductal area of the aorta and provide temporary relief from the obstruction. Net left-to-right ductal shunting occurs in these acyanotic infants. With more severe juxtaductal coarctation or in the presence of transverse arch hypoplasia, right ventricular blood is ejected through the ductus to supply the descending aorta. Perfusion of the lower part of the body is then dependent on right ventricular output (see Fig. 420–4). In this situation, the femoral pulses are palpable, and differential blood pressures may not be helpful in making the diagnosis. The ductal right-to-left shunting is manifested as differential cyanosis, with the upper extremities being pink and the lower extremities blue.

Such infants may have severe pulmonary hypertension and high pulmonary vascular resistance. Signs of heart failure are prominent. Occasionally, severely hypoplastic segments of the aortic isthmus may become completely atretic and result in an **interrupted aortic arch,** with the left subclavian artery arising either proximal or distal to the interruption. Coarctation associ-

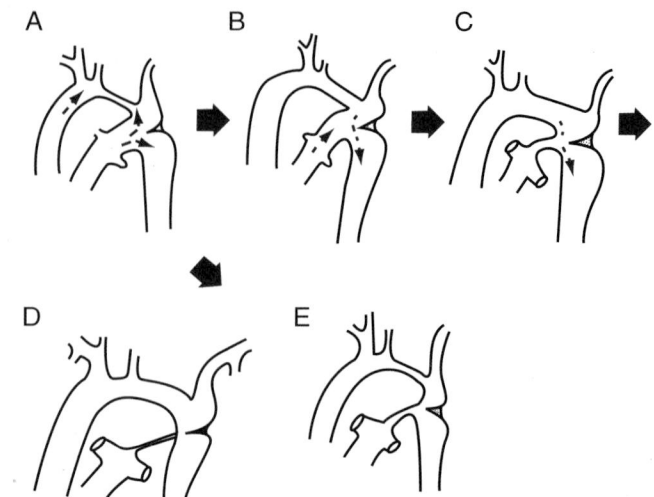

FIGURE 420–4. Metamorphosis of coarctation. *A,* Fetal prototype with no flow obstruction. *B,* Late gestation. The aortic ventricle increases its output and dilates the hypoplastic segment. Antegrade aortic flow bypasses the shelf via the ductal orifice. *C,* Neonate. Ductal constriction initiates the obstruction by removing the bypass and increasing antegrade arch flow. *D,* Mature juxtaductal stenosis. The bypass is completely obliterated, and intimal hypoplasia on the edge of the shelf is aggravating the stenosis. Collaterals develop. *E,* Persistence of the infantile-type fetal prototype. An intracardiac left-sided heart obstruction precludes an increase in antegrade aortic flow before or after birth. Both isthmus hypoplasia and a contraductal shelf are present. Lower body flow often depends on patency of the ductus. (From Gersony WM: Coarctation of the aorta. In Adams FH, Emmanouilides GC, Riemenshneider T [editors]: *Moss Heart Disease in Infants, Children, and Adolescents,* 4th ed. Baltimore, Williams & Wilkins, 1989.)

ated with arch hypoplasia was referred to as *infantile type* because its severity usually led to recognition of the condition in early infancy. *Adult type* referred to isolated juxtaductal coarctation, which if mild, was not usually recognized until later childhood. These terms have been replaced with the more accurate anatomic terms describing the location and severity of the defect.

Blood pressure is elevated in the vessels that arise proximal to the coarctation; blood pressure as well as pulse pressure is lower below the constriction. The hypertension is not due to the mechanical obstruction alone but also involves neurohumoral mechanisms. Unless operated on in infancy, coarctation of the aorta usually results in the development of an extensive collateral circulation, chiefly from branches of the subclavian, superior intercostal, and internal mammary arteries, to create channels for arterial blood to bypass the area of coarctation. The vessels contributing to the collateral circulation may become markedly enlarged and tortuous by early adulthood.

Clinical Manifestations. Coarctation of the aorta recognized after infancy is rarely associated with significant symptoms. Some children or adolescents complain about weakness or pain (or both) in the legs after exercise, but in many instances, even patients with severe coarctation are asymptomatic. Older children are frequently brought to the cardiologist's attention when they are found to be hypertensive on routine physical examination.

The classic sign of coarctation of the aorta is a disparity in pulsation and blood pressure in the arms and legs. The femoral, popliteal, posterior tibial, and dorsalis pedis pulses are weak (or absent in up to 40% of patients), in contrast to the bounding pulses of the arms and carotid vessels. The radial and femoral pulses should always be palpated simultaneously for the presence of a radial-femoral delay. Normally, the femoral pulse occurs slightly before the radial pulse. A radial-femoral delay occurs when blood flow to the descending aorta is dependent on collaterals, in which case the femoral pulse is felt after the radial pulse. In normal persons, systolic blood pressure in the legs obtained by the cuff method is 10–20 mm Hg higher than that in the arms. In coarctation of the aorta, blood pressure in the legs is lower than that in the arms; frequently, it is difficult to obtain. This differential in blood pressures is common in patients with coarctation who are older than 1 yr, about 90% of whom have systolic hypertension in an upper extremity greater than the 95th percentile for age. It is important to determine the blood pressure in each arm; a pressure higher in the right than the left arm suggests involvement of the left subclavian artery in the area of coarctation. Occasionally, the right subclavian may arise anomalously from below the area of coarctation and result in a left arm pressure that is higher than the right. With exercise, a more prominent rise in systemic blood pressure occurs, and the upper-to-lower extremity pressure gradient will increase.

The precordial impulse and heart sounds are usually normal; the presence of a systolic ejection click or thrill in the suprasternal notch suggests a bicuspid aortic valve (present in 70% of cases). A short systolic murmur is often heard along the left sternal border at the 3rd and 4th intercostal spaces. The murmur is well transmitted to the left infrascapular area and occasionally to the neck. Often, the typical murmur of mild aortic stenosis can be heard in the 3rd right intercostal space. Occasionally, more significant degrees of obstruction are noted across the aortic valve. The presence of a low-pitched mid-diastolic murmur at the apex suggests mitral valve stenosis. In older patients with well-developed collateral blood flow, systolic or continuous murmurs may be heard over the left and right sides of the chest laterally and posteriorly. In these patients, a palpable thrill can occasionally be appreciated in the intercostal spaces on the back.

Neonates or infants with more severe coarctation, usually including some degree of transverse arch hypoplasia, initially have signs of lower body hypoperfusion, acidosis, and severe heart failure. These signs may be delayed days or weeks until after closure of the ductus arteriosus. If detected before ductal closure, patients may exhibit differential cyanosis, best demonstrated by simultaneous oximetry of the upper and lower extremities. On physical examination, the heart is large, and a systolic murmur is heard along the left sternal border with a loud 2nd heart sound.

Diagnosis. Findings on *roentgenographic examination* depend on the age of the patient and on the effects of hypertension and the collateral circulation. Cardiac enlargement and pulmonary congestion are noted in infants with severe coarctation. During childhood, the findings are not striking until after the 1st decade, when the heart tends to be mildly or moderately enlarged because of left ventricular prominence. The enlarged left subclavian artery commonly produces a prominent shadow in the left superior mediastinum. Notching of the inferior border of the ribs from pressure erosion by enlarged collateral vessels is common by late childhood. In most instances, the descending aorta has an area of poststenotic dilatation.

The *electrocardiogram* is usually normal in young children but reveals evidence of left ventricular hypertrophy in older patients. Neonates and young infants display right or biventricular hypertrophy. The diagnosis can be made by careful evaluation of the pulses in all major accessible peripheral arteries and by comparative blood pressure determinations in the arms and legs. The segment of coarctation can generally be visualized by two-dimensional *echocardiography*; associated anomalies of the mitral and aortic valve can also be demonstrated. The descending aorta is hypopulsatile. Color Doppler is useful for demon-

strating the specific site of the obstruction. Pulsed and continuous wave Doppler studies determine the pressure gradient directly at the area of coarctation; in the presence of a PDA, however, the severity of the narrowing may be underestimated. *Cardiac catheterization* with selective left ventriculography and aortography is useful in certain patients with additional anomalies and as a means of visualizing collateral blood flow. In cases that are well defined by echocardiography, diagnostic catheterization is not usually required before surgery.

Prognosis and Complications. Abnormalities of the aortic valve are present in most patients. Bicuspid aortic valves are common but do not generally produce clinical signs unless the stenosis is significant. The association of a PDA and coarctation of the aorta is also common. VSDs and ASDs may be suspected by signs of a left-to-right shunt; they are exacerbated by the increased resistance to flow through the left side of the heart. Mitral valve abnormalities are also occasionally seen, as is subvalvular aortic stenosis.

Severe neurologic damage or even death may rarely occur from associated cerebrovascular disease. Subarachnoid or intracerebral hemorrhage may result from rupture of congenital aneurysms in the circle of Willis, rupture of other vessels with defective elastic and medial tissue, or rupture of normal vessels; these accidents are secondary to hypertension. Children with PHACE syndrome (*p*osterior brain fossa anomalies, facial *h*emangiomas, *a*rterial anomalies, *c*ardiac anomalies and aortic coarctation, *e*ye anomalies) may have strokes (Table 415–1). Abnormalities of the subclavian arteries may include involvement of the left subclavian artery in the area of coarctation, stenosis of the orifice of the left subclavian artery, and anomalous origin of the right subclavian artery.

Untreated, the great majority of older patients with coarctation of the aorta would succumb between the ages of 20 and 40 yr; some live well into middle life without serious disability. The common serious complications are related to systemic hypertension, which may result in premature coronary artery disease, heart failure, hypertensive encephalopathy, or intracranial hemorrhage. Heart failure may be worsened by associated anomalies. Infective endocarditis or endarteritis is a significant complication in adults. Aneurysms of the descending aorta or the enlarged collateral vessels may develop. In infants with severe coarctation, heart failure and hypoperfusion may be life threatening and require immediate medical intervention.

Treatment. In neonates with severe coarctation of the aorta, closure of the ductus often results in hypoperfusion, acidosis, and rapid deterioration. These patients should be given an infusion of prostaglandin E_1 to reopen the ductus and re-establish adequate lower extremity blood flow. Once a diagnosis has been confirmed and the patient stabilized, surgical repair should be performed. Older infants with heart failure but good perfusion should be managed with anticongestive measures to improve their clinical status before surgical intervention.

Older children with significant coarctation of the aorta should be treated relatively soon after diagnosis. Delay is unwarranted, especially after the 2nd decade of life, when the operation may be less successful because of decreased left ventricular function and degenerative changes in the aortic wall. Nevertheless, if cardiac reserve is sufficient, satisfactory repair is possible well into mid-adult life. Associated valvular lesions increase the hazards of late surgery.

The procedure of choice for isolated juxtaductal coarctation of the aorta is controversial. Surgery remains the treatment of choice, and several surgical techniques are used. The area of coarctation can be excised and a primary re-anastomosis performed. Often, the transverse aorta is splayed open and an "extended end-to-end" anastomosis performed to increase the effective cross-sectional area of the repair. The subclavian flap procedure, which involves division of the left subclavian artery and incorporation of it into the wall of the repaired coarctation, is used by some, often in the younger age group. Others favor a patch aortoplasty, in which the area of coarctation is enlarged with a roof of prosthetic material. The use of angioplasty for native coarctation remains controversial.

After surgery, a striking increase in the amplitude of pulsations in the lower extremities is noted. In the immediate postoperative course, "rebound" hypertension is common and requires medical management. This exaggerated acute hypertension gradually subsides, and in most patients, antihypertensive medications can be discontinued. Residual murmurs are common and may be due to associated cardiac anomalies, to a residual flow disturbance across the repaired area, or to collateral blood flow. Rare operative problems include spinal cord injury from aortic cross-clamping if the collaterals are poorly developed, chylothorax, diaphragm injury, and laryngeal nerve injury. If a left subclavian flap is used, the radial pulse and blood pressure in the left arm are diminished or absent. Repair of coarctation in the 2nd decade of life or beyond may be associated with a higher incidence of premature cardiovascular disease, even in the absence of residual cardiac abnormalities. Early onset of adult chronic hypertension may occur, even in patients with adequately resected coarctation.

Although re-stenosis in older patients after coarctectomy is rare, a significant number of infants operated on before 1 yr of age require revision later in childhood. All patients should be monitored carefully for the development of recoarctation and aortic aneurysm. Should recoarctation occur, balloon angioplasty is the procedure of choice. In these patients, scar tissue from previous surgery makes reoperation more difficult, yet makes balloon angioplasty safer because of the lower incidence of aneurysm formation. Relief of obstruction with this technique is usually excellent. Intravascular stents are now commonly used in many of these patients with generally excellent results.

Postcoarctectomy Syndrome. Postoperative mesenteric arteritis may be associated with acute hypertension and abdominal pain in the immediate postoperative period. The pain varies in severity and may occur in conjunction with anorexia, nausea, vomiting, leukocytosis, intestinal hemorrhage, bowel necrosis, and small bowel obstruction. Relief is usually obtained with antihypertensive drugs (nitroprusside, esmolol, captopril) and intestinal decompression; rarely, surgical exploration is required for bowel obstruction or infarction.

420.7 Coarctation with Ventricular Septal Defect

Coarctation in the presence of VSD results in both increased preload and afterload on the left ventricle, and patients with this combination of defects will be recognized either at birth or in the 1st mo of life and often have intractable cardiac failure. The magnitude of a left-to-right shunt through a VSD is dependent on the ratio of pulmonary to systemic vascular resistance. In the presence of coarctation, resistance to systemic outflow is enhanced by the obstruction, and the volume of the shunt is markedly increased. The clinical picture is that of a seriously ill infant with tachypnea, failure to thrive, and typical findings of heart failure. Often, the difference in blood pressure between the upper and lower extremities is not very marked because cardiac output may be low. Although medical management may be helpful initially, early surgical repair is necessary.

In most cases, coarctation is the major anomaly causing the severe symptoms, and resection of the coarctated segment results in striking improvement. Some repair the coarctation through a left lateral thoracotomy and at the same time place a pulmonary artery band to decrease the ventricular-level shunt.

Some do not band the pulmonary artery initially because a number of patients improve sufficiently so that further surgery is not required during early infancy. If heart failure makes it difficult to manage these infants after surgery, open repair of the VSD is then performed soon thereafter. Others routinely repair both the VSD and coarctation at the same operation through a midline sternotomy. When it is determined that a complicated VSD is present (multiple VSDs, apical muscular VSD), pulmonary arterial banding may be performed at the time of coarctation repair to avoid open heart surgery during infancy for these complex ventricular septal abnormalities.

420.8 Coarctation with Other Cardiac Anomalies and Interrupted Aortic Arch

Coarctation often occurs in infancy in association with other major cardiovascular anomalies, including hypoplastic left heart, severe mitral or aortic valve disease, transposition of the great arteries, and variations of double-outlet or single ventricle. Severe coarctation may also be associated with endocardial fibroelastosis. The clinical manifestations depend on the effects of the associated malformations, as well as on the coarctation itself.

Coarctation of the aorta associated with severe mitral and aortic valve disease may have to be treated within the context of the hypoplastic left heart syndrome (see Chapter 424.10), even if the left ventricular chamber is not severely hypoplastic. Such patients usually have a long segment of narrow transverse aortic arch with or without an isolated coarctation at the site of the ductus arteriosus. Coarctation of the aorta with transposition of the great arteries or single ventricle may be repaired alone or in combination with other palliative measures.

Complete interruption of the aortic arch is the most severe form of coarctation and is usually associated with other intracardiac pathology. Interruption may occur at any level, although it is most commonly seen between the left subclavian artery and the insertion of the ductus arteriosus. In newborns with an interrupted aortic arch, the ductus arteriosus provides the sole source of blood flow to the descending aorta, and differential oxygen saturation between the right arm (normal saturation) and the legs (decreased) can be noted. When the ductus begins to close, severe congestive heart failure, lower extremity hypoperfusion, anuria, and shock can develop in these infants. Patients with an interrupted aortic arch can be supported with prostaglandin to keep the ductus patent before surgical repair. As one of the conotruncal malformations, an interrupted aortic arch can be associated with the spectrum of lesions known as CATCH 22 (cardiac defects, abnormal facies, thymic hypoplasia, cleft palate, hypocalcemia). CATCH 22 includes patients with clinical features of the *DiGeorge syndrome* (hypocalcemia, thymic hypoplasia, mild facial anomalies) and the *Shprintzen velocardiofacial syndrome* (abnormal facies, cleft palate). Cytogenetic analysis using fluorescence in situ hybridization demonstrates deletions of a segment of chromosome 22q11 known as the DiGeorge critical region.

420.9 Congenital Mitral Stenosis

Congenital mitral stenosis is a rare anomaly that can be isolated or associated with other defects, the most common being aortic stenosis and coarctation of the aorta. The mitral valve may be funnel-shaped, with thickened leaflets and chordae tendineae that are shortened and deformed. Other mitral valve anomalies associated with stenosis include *parachute mitral valve*, caused by a single papillary muscle, and *double-orifice mitral valve*.

Symptoms usually appear within the 1st 2 yr of life. These infants are underdeveloped and generally have obvious dyspnea secondary to heart failure; cyanosis and pallor are common. In some patients whose symptoms are mainly wheezing, reactive airway disease may have been diagnosed. Heart enlargement as a result of dilatation and hypertrophy of the right ventricle and left atrium is common. Most patients have rumbling apical diastolic murmurs followed by a loud 1st sound, but the auscultatory findings may be relatively obscure. The 2nd sound is loud and split. An opening snap of the mitral valve may be present. The *electrocardiogram* reveals right ventricular hypertrophy with normal, bifid, or spiked P waves indicative of left atrial enlargement. *Roentgenograms* usually show left atrial and right ventricular enlargement and pulmonary congestion. The *echocardiogram* is characteristic and shows thickened mitral valve leaflets, a diminished E-F slope on the M-mode mitral echocardiogram, and an enlarged left atrium with a normal or small left ventricle. Two-dimensional echocardiographic examination shows a significant reduction of the mitral valve orifice in diastole. Doppler studies demonstrate a mean pressure gradient across the mitral orifice. At *cardiac catheterization*, an increase in right ventricular, pulmonary arterial, and pulmonary capillary wedge pressure can be noted. Associated anomalies such as aortic stenosis and coarctation are demonstrated. *Angiocardiography* shows delayed emptying of the left atrium and the small mitral orifice.

The prognosis for untreated patients is poor. The results of surgical treatment have been mixed; a mitral valve prosthesis is usually required, but it must be replaced as the child grows. These patients must be managed by anticoagulation with warfarin, and complications of excessive and insufficient anticoagulation are fairly common in infancy. Transcatheter balloon valvuloplasty has been used by several centers as a palliative procedure with mixed results, depending on the anatomy of the valve and the papillary muscles.

420.10 Pulmonary Venous Hypertension

A variety of lesions may give rise to chronic pulmonary venous hypertension, which when extreme may result in pulmonary arterial hypertension and right-sided heart failure. These lesions include congenital mitral stenosis, mitral insufficiency, total anomalous pulmonary venous return with obstruction, left atrial myxomas, cor triatriatum (stenosis of a common pulmonary vein), individual pulmonary vein stenosis, and supravalvular mitral rings or webs. Early symptoms can be confused with chronic pulmonary disease such as asthma because of a lack of specific cardiac findings on physical examination. Subtle signs of pulmonary hypertension may be present. The *electrocardiogram* shows right ventricular hypertrophy with spiked P waves. *Roentgenographic studies* reveal cardiac enlargement and prominence of the pulmonary veins in the hilar region, the right ventricle and atrium, and the main pulmonary artery; the left atrium is normal in size or only slightly enlarged.

The *echocardiogram* may demonstrate left atrial myxoma, cor triatriatum, or mitral valve abnormality. *Cardiac catheterization* excludes the presence of a shunt and demonstrates pulmonary hypertension with elevated pulmonary arterial wedge pressure. Left atrial pressure is normal if the lesion is at the level of the pulmonary veins, but it is elevated if the lesion is at the level of the mitral valve. Selective pulmonary arteriography usually delineates the anatomic lesion. Cor triatriatum, left atrial myxoma, and supravalvular mitral webs can all be successfully managed surgically.

The differential diagnosis includes *pulmonary veno-occlusive disease*, an idiopathic process that produces obstructive lesions in the pulmonary veins of children and young adults. The cause is uncertain. The patient is initially thought to have left-sided

heart failure on the basis of congested lungs with apparent pulmonary edema. Dyspnea, fatigue, and pleural effusions are common; cyanosis, digital clubbing, syncope, and hemoptysis are variable findings. Left atrial pressure is normal, but pulmonary arterial wedge pressure is usually elevated. A normal wedge pressure may be encountered if collaterals have formed or the wedge recording is performed in an uninvolved segment. Angiographically, the pulmonary veins return normally to the left atrium, but one or more pulmonary veins are narrowed, either focally or diffusely.

Lung biopsy demonstrates pulmonary venous and, occasionally, arterial involvement. Pulmonary veins and venules demonstrate fibrous narrowing or occlusion, and pulmonary artery thrombi may be present. Therapy is disappointing, and survival ranges from weeks to months in infants and from months to years in adults. Attempts at surgical repair, balloon dilatation, and transcatheter stenting have not significantly improved the prognosis of these patients. Combined heart-lung transplantation (see Chapter 435.2) remains the only moderately successful therapeutic option.

Pulmonary Stenosis

Benson LN, Freedom RM: Interventional cardiac catheterization. *Curr Opin Pediatr* 1989;1:106.

Crosnier C, Lykavieris P, Meunier-Rotival M, Hadchouel M: Alagille syndrome. The widening spectrum of arteriohepatic dysplasia. *Clin Liver Dis* 2000;4:765–78.

Krantz ID, Smith R, Colliton RP, et al: *Jagged 1* mutations in patients ascertained with isolated congenital heart defects. *Am J Med Gen* 1999;84:56–60.

Moller JH: Exercise responses in pulmonary stenosis. *Prog Pediatr Cardiol* 1993;2:8.

Phoon CK: Estimation of pressure gradients by auscultation: An innovative and accurate physical examination technique. *Am Heart J* 2001;141:500–6.

Aortic Stenosis

Doyle EF, Arumugham P, Lara E, et al: Sudden death in young patients with congenital aortic stenosis. *Pediatrics* 1974;53:481.

Francke U: Williams-Beuren syndrome: Genes and mechanisms. *Hum Mol Genet* 1999;8:1947–54.

Freed MD: Recreational and sports recommendations for the child with heart disease. *Pediatr Clin North Am* 1984;31:1307.

Jahangiri M, Nicholson IA, del Nido PJ, et al: Surgical management of complex and tunnel-like subaortic stenosis. *Eur J Cardiothorac Surg* 2000;17:637–42.

Laudito A, Brook MM, Suleman S, et al: The Ross procedure in children and young adults: A word of caution. *J Thorac Cardiovasc Surg* 2001;122:147–53.

Leichter DA, Sullivan I, Gersony WM: "Acquired" discrete subvalvular aortic stenosis: Natural history and hemodynamics. *J Am Coll Cardiol* 1989;14:1539.

Marino BS, Bridges ND, Paridon SM: Aortic insufficiency: Indications for surgery in children. *Semin Thorac Cardiovasc Surg Pediatr Card Surg Annu* 1998;1:147–56.

Ohye RG, Gomez CA, Ohye BJ, et al: The Ross/Konno procedure in neonates and infants: Intermediate-term survival and autograft function. *Ann Thorac Surg* 2001;72:823–30.

Pessotto R, Wells WJ, Baker CJ, et al: Midterm results of the Ross procedure. *Ann Thorac Surg* 2001;71(5 Suppl):S336–9.

Rocchini A, Beekman RH, Ben Shachar G, et al: Balloon aortic valvuloplasty: Results of the valvuloplasty and angioplasty of congenital anomalies registry. *Am J Cardiol* 1990;65:784.

Williams JCP, Barrat-Boyes BG, Lowe JB: Supravalvar aortic stenosis. *Circulation* 1961;24:1311.

Coarctation of the Aorta

Daniels SR: Repair of coarctation of the aorta and hypertension: Does age matter? *Lancet* 2001;358:89.

Hamdan MA, Maheshwari S, Fahey JT: Endovascular stents for coarctation of the aorta: Initial results and intermediate-term follow-up. *J Am Coll Cardiol* 2001;38:1518–23.

Ing FF, Starc TJ, Griffiths SP, et al: Early diagnosis of coarctation of the aorta in children: A continuing dilemma. *Pediatrics* 1996;98:378.

Metry DW, Dowd CF, Barkovich J, et al: The many faces of PHACE syndrome. *J Pediatr* 2001;139:117–23.

Rothman A: Coarctation of the aorta: An update. *Curr Probl Pediatr* 1998;28:37.

Shaddy RE, Boucek MM, Sturtevant JE, et al: Comparison of angioplasty and surgery for unoperated coarctation of the aorta. *Circulation* 1993;87:793.

Shone JD, Sellers RD, Anderson RC, et al: The developmental complex of "parachute mitral valve," supravalvar ring of left atrium, subaortic stenosis, and coarctation of the aorta. *Am J Cardiol* 1963;11:714.

Mitral Stenosis

Moore P, Adatia I, Spevak PJ, et al: Severe congenital mitral stenosis in infants. *Circulation* 1994;89:2099.

Spevak PJ, Bass JL, Ben-Shachar G, et al: Balloon angioplasty for congenital mitral stenosis. *Am J Cardiol* 1990;66:472.

Chapter 421

Acyanotic Congenital Heart Disease: Regurgitant Lesions

421.1 Pulmonary Valvular Insufficiency and Congenital Absence of the Pulmonary Valve

Pulmonary valvular insufficiency most often accompanies other cardiovascular diseases or may be secondary to severe pulmonary hypertension. Incompetence of the valve is an expected result after surgery for right ventricular outflow tract obstruction—for example, pulmonary valvotomy in patients with valvular pulmonic stenosis or valvotomy with infundibular resection in patients with the tetralogy of Fallot. Isolated congenital insufficiency of the pulmonary valve is rare. These patients are usually asymptomatic because the insufficiency is generally mild.

The prominent physical sign is a decrescendo diastolic murmur at the upper and midleft sternal border, which has a lower pitch than the murmur of aortic insufficiency because of the lower pressure involved. Roentgenograms of the chest show prominence of the main pulmonary artery and, if the insufficiency is severe, right ventricular enlargement. The electrocardiogram is normal or shows minimal right ventricular hypertrophy. Pulsed and color Doppler studies demonstrate retrograde flow from the pulmonary artery to the right ventricle during diastole. The diagnosis can be made at cardiac catheterization if necessary. Pulmonary arterial diastolic pressure is low. Selective pulmonary arteriography shows the incompetent valve, but it is difficult to evaluate in mild cases because the catheter crossing the valve usually results in some iatrogenic insufficiency during the injection. Isolated pulmonary valvular incompetence is generally well tolerated and does not require surgical treatment. When pulmonary insufficiency is severe, especially if significant tricuspid insufficiency is also present, replacement with a homograft may become necessary to preserve right ventricular function.

Congenital absence of the pulmonary valve is usually associated with a ventricular septal defect, often in the context of the tetralogy of Fallot (see Chapter 423.1). In many of these neonates, the pulmonary arteries become widely dilated and compress the bronchi, with subsequent recurrent episodes of wheezing, pulmonary collapse, and pneumonitis. The presence and degree of cyanosis are variable. Florid pulmonary valvular incompetence may not be well tolerated, and death may occur from a combination of bronchial compression, hypoxemia, and heart failure. Correction involves plication of the massively dilated pulmonary arteries, closure of the ventricular septal defect, and placement of a homograft across the right ventricular outflow tract.

421.2 Congenital Mitral Insufficiency

Congenital mitral insufficiency may be isolated but is more often associated with other anomalies, including patent ductus arteriosus, coarctation of the aorta, ventricular septal defect, corrected transposition of the great vessels, anomalous origin of the left coronary artery from the pulmonary artery, or Marfan syndrome. Mitral insufficiency is common in patients with atri-oventricular septal defects (see Chapter 419.5). Mitral insufficiency can also be seen in patients with cardiomyopathy and severe left ventricular dysfunction secondary to dilatation of the valve ring.

In isolated mitral insufficiency, the mitral valve annulus is usually dilated, the chordae tendineae are short and may insert anomalously, and the valve leaflets are deformed. When mitral insufficiency is severe enough to cause clinical symptoms, the left atrium enlarges as a result of the regurgitant flow, and the left ventricle becomes hypertrophied and dilated. Pulmonary venous pressure is increased, and the increased pressure ultimately results in pulmonary hypertension and right ventricular hypertrophy and dilatation. Mild lesions produce no symptoms; the only abnormal sign is the holosystolic murmur of mitral incompetence. Severe regurgitation results in symptoms that can appear at any age, including poor physical development, frequent respiratory infections, fatigue on exertion, and episodes of pulmonary edema or congestive heart failure. Often, a diagnosis of reactive airway disease will have been made because of the similarity in pulmonary symptoms.

The typical murmur of mitral insufficiency is a high-pitched (often referred to as a "cooing dove"), apical holosystolic murmur. If the insufficiency is moderate to severe, it is usually associated with an apical low-pitched, mid-diastolic rumbling murmur indicative of increased diastolic flow across the mitral valve. The pulmonary component of the 2nd heart sound will be accentuated in the presence of pulmonary hypertension. The *electrocardiogram* usually shows bifid P waves, signs of left ventricular hypertrophy, and sometimes signs of right ventricular hypertrophy. *Roentgenographic examination* shows enlargement of the left atrium, which at times is massive. The left ventricle is prominent, and pulmonary vascularity is normal or prominent. The *echocardiogram* demonstrates the enlarged left atrium and ventricle. Color Doppler demonstrates the extent of insufficiency, and pulsed Doppler of the pulmonary veins detects retrograde flow when mitral insufficiency is severe. *Cardiac catheterization* shows elevated left atrial pressure. Pulmonary artery hypertension of varying severity may be present. Selective left ventriculography reveals the severity of mitral regurgitation.

Mitral valvuloplasty can result in striking improvement in symptoms and heart size, but in some patients, installation of a prosthetic mechanical mitral valve may be necessary. Before surgery, associated anomalies must be identified. In children beyond 3–4 yr, it may be difficult to exclude rheumatic fever as the cause of mitral insufficiency.

421.3 Mitral Valve Prolapse

Mitral valve prolapse results from an abnormal mitral valve mechanism that causes billowing of one or both mitral leaflets, especially the posterior cusp, into the left atrium toward the end of systole. The abnormality is predominantly congenital but may not be recognized until adolescence or adulthood. Mitral valve prolapse is more common in girls and may be inherited as an autosomal dominant trait with variable expression. It is common in patients with Marfan syndrome, straight back syndrome, pectus excavatum, and scoliosis. The dominant abnormal signs are auscultatory, although occasional patients may have chest pain or palpitations. The apical murmur is late systolic and may be preceded by a click, but these signs may vary in the same patient, and at times only the click is audible. In the standing or sitting position the click may appear earlier in systole, and the murmur may be more prominent in late systole. Arrhythmias may occur and are primarily unifocal or multifocal premature ventricular contractions.

The *electrocardiogram* is usually normal but may show biphasic T waves, especially in leads II, III, aVF, and V$_6$; the T-wave abnormalities may vary at different times in the same patient. The *chest roentgenogram* is normal. The *echocardiogram* shows a characteristic posterior movement of the posterior mitral leaflet during mid or late systole or demonstrates pansystolic prolapse of both the anterior and posterior mitral leaflets. These M-mode echocardiographic findings must be interpreted cautiously because the appearance of minimal mitral prolapse may be a normal variant. Two-dimensional real-time echocardiography shows that both the free edge and the body of the mitral leaflets move posteriorly in systole toward the left atrium. The presence and severity of mitral regurgitation can be assessed by Doppler.

This lesion is not progressive in childhood, and specific therapy is not indicated. The patient may be at risk for the development of infective endocarditis. Antibiotic prophylaxis is recommended during surgery and dental procedures (see Chapter 429).

Adults (men more often than women) with mitral valve prolapse are at increased risk for cardiovascular complications (sudden death, arrhythmia, cerebrovascular accidents, progressive valve dilatation, heart failure, and endocarditis) in the presence of thickened and redundant mitral valve leaflets.

Often, confusion exists concerning the diagnosis of mitral valve prolapse. The high frequency of mild prolapse on the echocardiogram in the absence of clinical findings suggests that in these cases true *mitral valve prolapse syndrome* is not present. These patients and their parents should be reassured of this fact, and no special recommendations should be made regarding management or frequent laboratory studies. Endocarditis prophylaxis is indicated only in substantiated cases, usually those with mitral insufficiency.

421.4   Tricuspid Regurgitation

Isolated tricuspid regurgitation is generally associated with Ebstein anomaly of the tricuspid valve. Ebstein anomaly may occur either without cyanosis or with varying degrees of cyanosis, depending on the severity of the tricuspid regurgitation and the presence of an atrial-level communication (patent foramen ovale or atrial septal defect). Older children tend to have the acyanotic form, whereas if detected in the newborn period, Ebstein anomaly is usually associated with severe cyanosis (see Chapter 423.7).

Tricuspid regurgitation often accompanies right ventricular dysfunction. When the right ventricle becomes dilated because of volume overload or intrinsic myocardial disease, or both, the tricuspid annulus also enlarges, with resultant valve insufficiency. This form of regurgitation may improve if the cause of the right ventricular dilatation is corrected, or it may require surgical plication of the valve annulus. Tricuspid regurgitation is also encountered in newborns with perinatal asphyxia. The cause may be related to an increased susceptibility of the papillary muscles to ischemic damage and subsequent transient papillary muscle dysfunction.

Absent Pulmonary Valve

McDonnell BE, Raff GW, Gaynor JW, et al: Outcome after repair of tetralogy of Fallot with absent pulmonary valve. *Ann Thorac Surg* 1999;67:1391–5.

Pinsky WW: Absent pulmonary valve syndrome. In Garson A, Bricker JT, Fisher DJ, Neish SR (editors): *The Science and Practice of Pediatric Cardiology*. Baltimore, Williams & Wilkins, 1998, pp 1413–1419.

Mitral Valve Anomalies

Bouknight DP, O'Rourke RA: Current management of mitral valve prolapse. *Am Fam Physician* 2000;61:3343–50, 3353–54.

Jacobs W, Chamoun A, Stouffer GA: Mitral valve prolapse: A review of the literature. *Am J Med Sci* 2001;321:401–10.

Mitral valve prolapse and athletic competition of children and adolescents. American Academy of Pediatrics Committee on Sports Medicine and Fitness. *Pediatrics* 1995;95:789.

Chapter 422

Cyanotic Congenital Heart Disease: Evaluation of the Critically Ill Neonate with Cyanosis and Respiratory Distress

See also Chapter 90.

A severely ill neonate with cardiorespiratory distress and cyanosis is a diagnostic challenge. The clinician must perform a rapid evaluation to determine whether congenital heart disease is a cause so that potentially lifesaving measures can be instituted. The differential diagnosis of neonatal cyanosis is presented in Table 90–1.

Cardiac Disease. Congenital heart disease produces cyanosis when obstruction to right ventricular outflow causes intracardiac right-to-left shunting or when complex anatomic defects, unassociated with pulmonary stenosis, cause an admixture of pulmonary and systemic venous return in the heart. Cyanosis from pulmonary edema may also develop in patients with heart failure caused by left-to-right shunts, although the degree is usually less severe. Cyanosis may be caused by persistence of fetal pathways, for example, right-to-left shunting across the foramen ovale and ductus arteriosus in the presence of pulmonary outflow tract obstruction or persistent pulmonary hypertension of the newborn (PPHN) (see Chapter 93.7).

Differential Diagnosis. The initial evaluation of a cyanotic infant begins with observation of the breathing pattern. Weak or irregular respiration is often associated with a weak sucking reflex and a central nervous system (CNS) problem. Convulsions and general depression strongly suggest a CNS cause. An infant with primary cardiac or pulmonary disease, in contrast, displays vigorous or labored respirations with tachypnea.

The *hyperoxia test* is one method of distinguishing cyanotic congenital heart disease from pulmonary disease. Neonates with cyanotic congenital heart disease usually do not have significantly raised arterial Pao$_2$ during administration of 100% oxygen. If the Pao$_2$ rises above 150 mm Hg during 100% oxygen administration, an intracardiac shunt can usually be excluded, although the Pao$_2$ of some patients with cyanotic congenital heart lesions may be transiently increased to greater than 150 mm Hg because of intracardiac streaming patterns. The Pao$_2$ in patients with pulmonary disease generally increases significantly as ventilation-perfusion inequalities are overcome by oxygen administration. In infants with a CNS disorder, the Pao$_2$ completely normalizes during artificial ventilation. Hypoxia in many heart lesions is profound and constant, whereas in respiratory disorders and in primary hypertension of the neonate (PPHN), arterial oxygen tension is not as low and often varies with time or changes in ventilator management. Hyperventilation may improve the hypoxia in neonates with PPHN and only occasionally in those with cyanotic heart disease.

Although a significant heart murmur usually suggests a cardiac basis for the cyanosis, several of the more severe cardiac defects (transposition of the great vessels) may not initially be associated with a murmur. The chest roentgenogram may be helpful in the differentiation of pulmonary and cardiac disease; in the latter, it indicates whether pulmonary blood flow is increased, normal, or decreased.

Two-dimensional echocardiography is the definitive noninvasive test to determine the presence of congenital heart disease. The information obtained is essential in avoiding unnecessary cardiac catheterization and angiography in the absence of a cardiac defect, as well as in making a specific diagnosis. If echocardiography is not immediately available, the clinician caring for a newborn with possible cyanotic heart disease should not hesitate to start a prostaglandin infusion (for a possible ductal-dependent lesion). Because of the risk of hypoventilation associated with prostaglandins, a practitioner skilled in neonatal endotracheal intubation must be available.

Chapter 423

Cyanotic Congenital Heart Lesions: Lesions Associated with Decreased Pulmonary Blood Flow

423.1 Tetralogy of Fallot

The tetralogy of Fallot consists of (1) obstruction to right ventricular outflow (pulmonary stenosis), (2) ventricular septal defect (VSD), (3) dextroposition of the aorta with septal override, and (4) right ventricular hypertrophy (Fig. 423–1). Obstruction to pulmonary arterial blood flow is usually at both the right ventricular infundibulum (subpulmonic area) and the pulmonary valve. The main pulmonary artery is often small, and various degrees of branch pulmonary artery stenosis may be present. Complete obstruction of right ventricular outflow *(pulmonary atresia with VSD)* is classified as an extreme form of tetralogy of Fallot.

Pathophysiology. The pulmonary valve annulus may be of nearly normal size or quite small. The valve itself is often bicuspid and, occasionally, is the only site of stenosis. More commonly, the subpulmonic muscle, the crista supraventricularis, is hypertrophic, which contributes to the infundibular stenosis and results in an infundibular chamber of variable size and contour. When the right ventricular outflow tract is completely obstructed (pulmonary atresia), the anatomy of the branch pulmonary arteries is extremely variable; a main pulmonary artery segment may be in continuity with right ventricular outflow, separated by a fibrous but imperforate pulmonary valve, or the entire main pulmonary artery segment may be absent. Occasionally, the branch pulmonary arteries may be discontinuous. In these more severe cases, pulmonary blood flow may be supplied by a patent ductus arteriosus (PDA) and by *major aortopulmonary collateral arteries (MAPCAs)* arising from the aorta.

The VSD is usually nonrestrictive and large, is located just below the aortic valve, and is related to the posterior and right aortic cusps. Rarely, the VSD may be in the inlet portion of the ventricular septum (atrioventricular septal defect). The normal fibrous continuity of the mitral and aortic valves is usually maintained. The aortic arch is right sided in 20%, and the aortic root is usually large and overrides the VSD to a varying degree. When the aorta overrides the VSD more than 50% and if muscle is significantly separating the aortic valve and the mitral annulus (subaortic conus), this defect is usually classified as a form of *double-outlet right ventricle;* the pathophysiology is the same as that for tetralogy of Fallot.

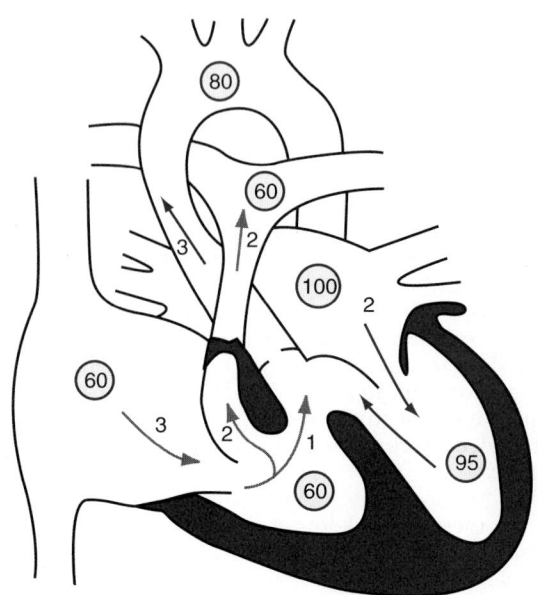

FIGURE 423–1. Physiology of the tetralogy of Fallot. *Circled numbers* represent oxygen saturation values. The numbers next to the *arrows* represent volumes of blood flow (in L/min/m²). Atrial (mixed venous) oxygen saturation is decreased because of the systemic hypoxemia. A volume of 3 L/min/m² of desaturated blood enters the right atrium and traverses the tricuspid valve. Two liters flows through the right ventricular outflow tract into the lungs, whereas 1 L shunts right to left through the ventricular septal defect (VSD) into the ascending aorta. Thus, pulmonary blood flow is two thirds normal (Qp:Qs of 0.7:1). Blood returning to the left atrium is fully saturated. Only 2 L of blood flows across the mitral valve. Oxygen saturation in the left ventricle may be slightly decreased because of right-to-left shunting across the VSD. Two liters of saturated left ventricular blood mixing with 1 L of desaturated right ventricular blood is ejected into the ascending aorta. Aortic saturation is decreased, and cardiac output is normal.

Systemic venous return to the right atrium and right ventricle is normal. When the right ventricle contracts in the presence of marked pulmonary stenosis, blood is shunted across the VSD into the aorta. Persistent arterial desaturation and cyanosis result. Pulmonary blood flow, when severely restricted by the obstruction to right ventricular outflow, may be supplemented by the bronchial collateral circulation (MAPCAs) and, in the newborn, by a PDA. Peak systolic and diastolic pressures in each ventricle are similar and at the systemic level. A large pressure gradient occurs across the obstructed right ventricular outflow tract, and pulmonary arterial pressure is normal or lower than normal. The degree of right ventricular outflow obstruction determines the timing of the onset of symptoms, the severity of cyanosis, and the degree of right ventricular hypertrophy. When obstruction to right ventricular outflow is mild to moderate and a balanced shunt is present across the VSD, the patient may not be visibly cyanotic *(acyanotic or "pink" tetralogy of Fallot).*

Clinical Manifestations. Infants with mild degrees of right ventricular outflow obstruction may initially be seen with heart failure caused by a ventricular-level left-to-right shunt. Often, cyanosis is not present at birth, but with increasing hypertrophy of the right ventricular infundibulum and patient growth, cyanosis occurs later in the 1st yr of life. It is most prominent in the mucous membranes of the lips and mouth and in the fingernails and toenails. In infants with severe degrees of right ventricular outflow obstruction, neonatal cyanosis is noted immediately. In these infants, pulmonary blood flow may be dependent on flow through the ductus arteriosus. When the ductus begins to close in the 1st few hours or days of life, severe cyanosis and circulatory collapse may occur. Older children with long-standing cyanosis who have not undergone surgery may have dusky blue skin, gray sclerae with engorged blood vessels, and marked *clubbing* of the fingers and toes. Extracardiac manifestations of long-standing cyanotic congenital heart disease are described in Chapter 427.

Dyspnea occurs on exertion. Infants and toddlers play actively for a short time and then sit or lie down. Older children may be able to walk a block or so before stopping to rest. Characteristically, children assume a *squatting* position for the relief of dyspnea caused by physical effort; the child is usually able to resume physical activity within a few minutes. These findings occur most often in patients with significant cyanosis at rest.

Paroxysmal hypercyanotic attacks (hypoxic, "blue," or "tet" spells) are a particular problem during the 1st 2 yr of life. The infant becomes hyperpneic and restless, cyanosis increases, gasping respirations ensue, and syncope may follow. The spells occur most frequently in the morning on initially awakening or after episodes of vigorous crying. Temporary disappearance or a decrease in intensity of the systolic murmur is usual as flow across the right ventricular outflow tract diminishes. The spells may last from a few minutes to a few hours but are rarely fatal. Short episodes are followed by generalized weakness and sleep. Severe spells may progress to unconsciousness and, occasionally, to convulsions or hemiparesis. The onset is usually spontaneous and unpredictable. Spells are associated with reduction of an already compromised pulmonary blood flow, which when prolonged results in severe systemic hypoxia and metabolic acidosis. Infants who are only mildly cyanotic at rest are often more prone to the development of hypoxic spells because they have not acquired the homeostatic mechanisms to tolerate rapid lowering of arterial oxygen saturation, such as polycythemia.

Depending on the frequency and severity of hypercyanotic attacks, one or more of the following procedures should be instituted in sequence: (1) placement of the infant on the abdomen in the knee-chest position while making certain that the infant's clothing is not constrictive, (2) administration of oxygen (although increasing inspired oxygen will not reverse cyanosis caused by intracardiac shunting), and (3) injection of morphine subcutaneously in a dose not in excess of 0.2 mg/kg. Calming and holding the infant in a knee-chest position may abort progression of an early spell. Premature attempts to obtain blood samples may cause further agitation and be counterproductive.

Because metabolic acidosis develops when arterial Po_2 is less than 40 mm Hg, rapid correction (within several minutes) with intravenous administration of sodium bicarbonate is necessary if the spell is unusually severe and the child shows a lack of response to the foregoing therapy. Recovery from the spell is usually rapid once the pH has returned to normal. Repeated blood pH measurements may be necessary because rapid recurrence of acidosis may ensue. For spells that are resistant to this therapy, drugs that increase systemic vascular resistance, such as intravenous methoxamine or phenylephrine, improve right ventricular outflow, decrease the right-to-left shunt, and thus improve the symptoms. β-Adrenergic blockade by the intravenous administration of propranolol (0.1 mg/kg given slowly to a maximum of 0.2 mg/kg) is also useful.

Growth and development may be delayed in patients with severe untreated tetralogy of Fallot, particularly when oxygen saturation is chronically less than 70%. Puberty may also be delayed in patients who do not undergo surgery.

The pulse is usually normal, as is venous and arterial pressure. The left anterior hemithorax may bulge anteriorly because of right ventricular hypertrophy. The heart is generally normal in size, and a *substernal right ventricular impulse* can be detected. In about half the cases, a *systolic thrill* is felt along the left sternal border in the 3rd and 4th parasternal spaces. The *systolic murmur* is usually loud and harsh; it may be transmitted widely, especially to the lungs, but is most intense at the left sternal border. The murmur is generally ejection in quality at the upper sternal border, but it may sound more holosystolic toward the lower sternal border. It may be preceded by a click. The murmur is caused by turbulence through the right ventricular outflow tract. It tends to become louder, longer, and harsher as the severity of pulmonary stenosis increases from mild to moderate; however, it can actually become less prominent with severe obstruction, especially during a hypercyanotic spell. Either the 2nd heart sound is single, or the pulmonic component is soft. Infrequently, a continuous murmur may be audible, especially if prominent collaterals are present.

Diagnosis. *Roentgenographically,* the typical configuration as seen in the anteroposterior view consists of a narrow base, concavity of the left heart border in the area usually occupied by the pulmonary artery, and normal heart size. The hypertrophied right ventricle causes the rounded apical shadow to be up-tilted so that it is situated higher above the diaphragm than normal. The cardiac silhouette has been likened to that of a boot or wooden shoe *(coeur en sabot)* (Fig. 423–2). The hilar areas and lung fields are relatively clear because of diminished pulmonary blood flow or the small size of the pulmonary arteries, or both. The aorta is usually large, and in about 20% of instances it arches to the right, which results in an indentation of the leftward-positioned air-filled tracheobronchial shadow in the anteroposterior view.

The *electrocardiogram* demonstrates right axis deviation and evidence of right ventricular hypertrophy. A dominant R wave appears in the right precordial chest leads (Rs, R, qR, qRs) or an RSR' pattern. In some cases, the only sign of right ventricular hypertrophy may initially be a positive T wave in leads V_3R and V_1. The P wave is tall and peaked or sometimes bifid (see Fig. 416–8).

Two-dimensional echocardiography establishes the diagnosis (Fig. 423–3) and provides information about the extent of aortic override of the septum, the location and degree of the right ventricular outflow tract obstruction, the size of the proximal branch pulmonary arteries, and the side of the aortic arch. The echocardiogram is also useful in determining whether a PDA is supplying a portion of the pulmonary blood flow. It may obviate the need for catheterization.

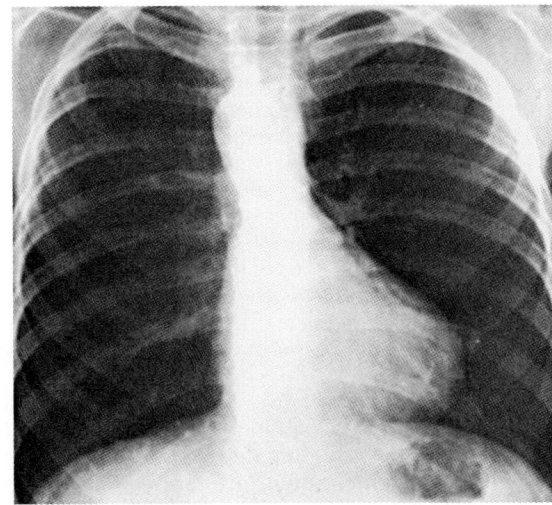

FIGURE 423–2. Roentgenogram of an 8-yr-old boy with the tetralogy of Fallot. Note the normal heart size, some elevation of the cardiac apex, concavity in the region of the main pulmonary artery, right-sided aortic arch, and diminished pulmonary vascularity.

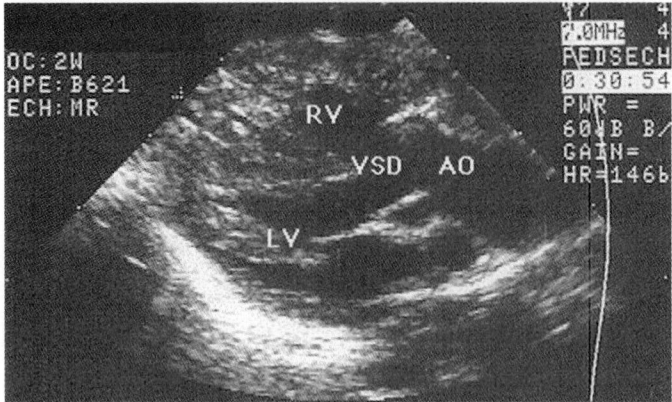

FIGURE 423–3. Echocardiogram in a patient with the tetralogy of Fallot. This short-axis, subxiphoid, two-dimensional echocardiographic projection demonstrates anterior/superior displacement of the outflow ventricular septum that resulted in stenosis of the subpulmonic right ventricular outflow tract and an associated anterior ventricular septal defect (VSD). RV = right ventricle; AO = overriding aortic valve; LV = left ventricle.

Cardiac catheterization demonstrates a systolic pressure in the right ventricle equal to systemic pressure. If the pulmonary artery is entered, the pressure is markedly decreased, although crossing the right ventricular outflow tract, especially in severe cases, may precipitate a tet spell. Pulmonary arterial pressure is usually lower than normal, in the range of 5–10 mm Hg. The level of arterial oxygen saturation depends on the magnitude of the right-to-left shunt; in "pink tets," systemic saturation may be normal, whereas in a moderately cyanotic patient at rest, it is usually 75–85%.

Selective right ventriculography best demonstrates the anatomy of the tetralogy of Fallot. Contrast medium outlines the heavily trabeculated right ventricle. The infundibular stenosis varies in length, width, contour, and distensibility (Fig. 423–4). The pulmonary valve is usually thickened, and the annulus may be small. In patients with pulmonary atresia and VSD, the anatomy of the pulmonary vessels may be extremely complex, for example, discontinuity between the right and left pulmonary arteries. Complete and accurate information regarding the anatomy of the pulmonary arteries is important when evaluating these children as surgical candidates.

Left ventriculography demonstrates the size of the left ventricle, the position of the VSD, and the overriding aorta; it also confirms mitral-aortic continuity, thereby ruling out a double-outlet right ventricle. *Aortography* or *coronary arteriography* outlines the course of the coronary arteries. In 5–10% of patients with the tetralogy of Fallot, an aberrant major coronary artery crosses over the right ventricular outflow tract; this artery must not be cut during surgical repair. Verification of normal coronary arteries is important when considering surgery in young infants who may need a patch across the pulmonary valve annulus. Echocardiography may delineate the coronary artery anatomy; angiography is reserved for cases in which questions remain.

Prognosis and Complications. Before correction, patients with the tetralogy of Fallot are susceptible to several serious complications. Fortunately, most children undergo palliation or repair in infancy, and these complications are rare. *Cerebral thromboses,* usually occurring in the cerebral veins or dural sinuses and occasionally in the cerebral arteries, are common in the presence of extreme polycythemia and dehydration. Thromboses occur most often in patients younger than 2 yr. These patients may have iron deficiency anemia, frequently with hemoglobin and hematocrit levels in the normal range. Therapy consists of ade-

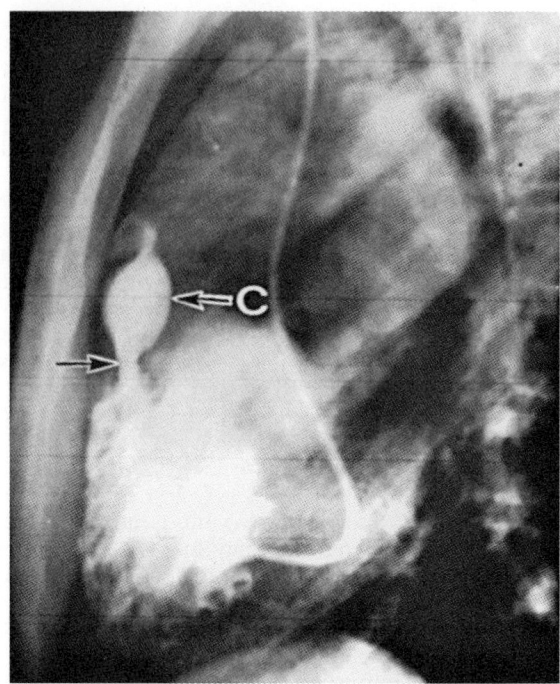

FIGURE 423–4. Lateral view of a selective right ventriculogram in a patient with the tetralogy of Fallot. The *arrow* points to an infundibular stenosis that is below the infundibular chamber (C). The narrowed pulmonary valve orifice is seen at the distal end of the infundibular chamber.

quate hydration and supportive measures. Phlebotomy and volume replacement with fresh frozen plasma are indicated in extremely polycythemic patients. Heparin is of little value and is contraindicated in patients with hemorrhagic cerebral infarction. Physical therapy should be instituted as early as possible.

Brain abscess is less common than cerebral vascular events and extremely rare when most patients are repaired at much younger ages. Patients with a brain abscess are usually older than 2 yr. The onset of the illness is often insidious and consists of low-grade fever or a gradual change in behavior, or both. Some patients have an acute onset of symptoms that may develop after a recent history of headache, nausea, and vomiting. Seizures may occur; localized neurologic signs depend on the site and size of the abscess and the presence of increased intracranial pressure. CT or MRI confirms the diagnosis. Antibiotic therapy may help keep the infection localized, but surgical drainage of the abscess is usually necessary (see Chapter 595).

Bacterial endocarditis may occur in the right ventricular infundibulum or on the pulmonic, aortic, or rarely, the tricuspid valves. Endocarditis may complicate palliative shunts or, in patients with corrective surgery, any residual pulmonic stenosis or VSD. Antibiotic prophylaxis is essential before and after dental and certain surgical procedures associated with a high incidence of bacteremia (see Chapter 429).

Heart failure is not a usual feature in patients with the tetralogy of Fallot. It may occur in a young infant with "pink" or acyanotic tetralogy of Fallot. As the degree of pulmonary obstruction worsens with age, the symptoms of heart failure resolve and eventually the patient experiences cyanosis, often by 6–12 mo of age. These patients are at increased risk for hypercyanotic spells at this time.

Associated Anomalies. An associated PDA may be present, and defects in the atrial septum are occasionally seen. A right aortic arch occurs in approximately 20% of patients with the tetralogy of Fallot, and other anomalies of the pulmonary arteries and aortic arch may also be seen. Persistence of a left superior vena cava draining into the coronary sinus may be noted. Multiple VSDs are occasionally present and must be diagnosed before corrective surgery. Tetralogy of Fallot may also occur with an atrioventricular septal defect, often associated with Down syndrome.

Congenital absence of the pulmonary valve produces a distinct syndrome that is usually marked by signs of upper airway obstruction (see Chapter 421.1). Cyanosis may be absent, mild, or moderate; the heart is large and hyperdynamic; and a loud to-and-fro murmur is present. Marked aneurysmal dilatation of the main and branch pulmonary arteries results in compression of the bronchi and produces stridulous or wheezing respirations and recurrent pneumonia. If the airway obstruction is severe, reconstruction of the trachea at the time of corrective cardiac surgery may be required to alleviate the symptoms.

Absence of a branch pulmonary artery, most often the left, should be suspected if the roentgenographic appearance of the pulmonary vasculature differs on the two sides; absence of a pulmonary artery is often associated with hypoplasia of the affected lung. It is important to recognize the absence of a pulmonary artery because occlusion of the remaining pulmonary artery during surgery seriously compromises the already reduced pulmonary blood flow.

As one of the conotruncal malformations, the tetralogy of Fallot can be associated with the spectrum of lesions known as CATCH 22 (*c*ardiac defects, *a*bnormal facies, *t*hymic hypoplasia, *c*left palate, *h*ypocalcemia). CATCH 22 includes patients with clinical features of the *DiGeorge syndrome* (hypocalcemia, thymic hypoplasia, mild facial anomalies) or the *Shprintzen velocardiofacial syndrome* (abnormal facies, cleft palate). Cytogenetic analysis using fluorescence in situ hybridization demonstrates deletions of a segment of chromosome 22q11 known as the DiGeorge critical region.

Treatment. Treatment of the tetralogy of Fallot depends on the severity of the right ventricular outflow tract obstruction. Infants with severe tetralogy require medical treatment and surgical intervention in the neonatal period. Therapy is aimed at providing an immediate increase in pulmonary blood flow to prevent the sequelae of severe hypoxia. The infant should be transported to a medical center adequately equipped to evaluate and treat neonates with congenital heart disease under optimal conditions. It is critical that oxygenation and normal body temperature be maintained during the transfer. Prolonged, severe hypoxia may lead to shock, respiratory failure, and intractable acidosis and will significantly reduce the chance of survival, even when surgically amenable lesions are present. Cold increases oxygen consumption, which places additional stress on a cyanotic infant, whose oxygen delivery is already limited. Blood glucose levels should be monitored because hypoglycemia is more likely to develop in infants with cyanotic heart disease.

Infants with marked right ventricular outflow tract obstruction may deteriorate rapidly because as the ductus arteriosus begins to close, pulmonary blood flow is further compromised. The intravenous administration of prostaglandin E$_1$ (0.05–0.20 μg/kg/min), a potent and specific relaxant of ductal smooth muscle, causes dilatation of the ductus arteriosus and usually provides adequate pulmonary blood flow until a surgical procedure can be performed. This agent should be administered intravenously as soon as cyanotic congenital heart disease is clinically suspected and continued through the preoperative period and during cardiac catheterization. Postoperatively, the infusion may be continued briefly as a pulmonary vasodilator to augment flow through a palliative shunt or through a surgical valvulotomy.

Infants with less severe right ventricular outflow tract obstruction who are stable and awaiting surgical intervention require careful observation. Prevention or prompt treatment of dehydration is important to avoid hemoconcentration and possible thrombotic episodes. Paroxysmal dyspneic attacks in infancy or early childhood may be precipitated by a relative iron deficiency; iron therapy may decrease their frequency and also improve exercise tolerance and general well-being. Red blood cell indices should be maintained in the normocytic range. Oral propranolol (0.5–1 mg/kg every 6 hr) may decrease the frequency and severity of hypercyanotic spells, but with the excellent surgery available, surgical treatment is indicated as soon as spells begin.

Infants with symptoms and severe cyanosis in the 1st mo of life have marked obstruction of the right ventricular outflow tract or pulmonary atresia. Two options are available in these infants: the first is a palliative systemic-to–pulmonary artery shunt performed to augment pulmonary artery blood flow. The rationale for this surgery, previously the only option for these patients, is to decrease the amount of hypoxia and improve linear growth, as well as augment growth of the branch pulmonary arteries. The second option is corrective open heart surgery performed in early infancy and even in the newborn period in critically ill infants. This approach has gained more widespread acceptance as excellent short- and intermediate-term results have been reported. The advantages of corrective surgery in early infancy vs a palliative shunt and correction in later infancy are still being debated. In infants with less severe cyanosis who can be maintained with good growth and absence of hypercyanotic spells, primary repair is performed electively at between 4 and 12 mo of age.

The modified *Blalock-Taussig shunt* is currently the most common aortopulmonary shunt procedure and consists of a Gore-Tex conduit anastomosed side to side from the subclavian artery to the homolateral branch of the pulmonary artery (Fig. 423–5). Sometimes the conduit is brought directly from the ascending aorta to the main pulmonary artery and is called a *central shunt*. The Blalock-Taussig operation can be successfully performed in the newborn period with shunts 3–4 mm in diameter and has also been used successfully in premature infants.

The postoperative course of patients with a successful shunt procedure is relatively uneventful. Postoperative complications may occur after a lateral thoracotomy and include chylothorax, diaphragmatic paralysis, and Horner syndrome. **Chylothorax** may require repeated thoracocentesis and, on occasion, reoperation to ligate the thoracic duct. **Diaphragmatic paralysis** from injury to the phrenic nerve may result in a more difficult postoperative course. Prolonged ventilator support and vigorous physical therapy may be required, but diaphragmatic function usually returns in 1–2 mo unless the nerve was completely divided. Surgical plication of the diaphragm may be indicated. **Horner syndrome** is usually temporary and does not require treatment. Postoperative *cardiac failure* may be caused by a large shunt; its treatment is described in Chapter 434. Vascular problems other than a diminished radial pulse and occasional long-term arm length discrepancy are rarely seen in the upper extremity supplied by the subclavian artery used for the anastomosis.

After a successful shunt procedure, cyanosis diminishes. The development of a continuous murmur over the lung fields after the operation indicates a functioning anastomosis. A good shunt murmur may not be heard until several days after surgery. The duration of symptomatic relief is variable. As the child grows, more pulmonary blood flow is needed and the shunt eventually becomes inadequate. When increasing cyanosis develops, a corrective operation should be performed if the anatomy is favorable. If not possible (e.g., because of hypoplastic branch pulmonary arteries) or if the 1st shunt lasts only a brief period in a small infant, a second aortopulmonary anastomosis may be required on the opposite side. Several groups have reported successful palliation of the tetralogy of Fallot in infants by balloon pulmonary valvuloplasty.

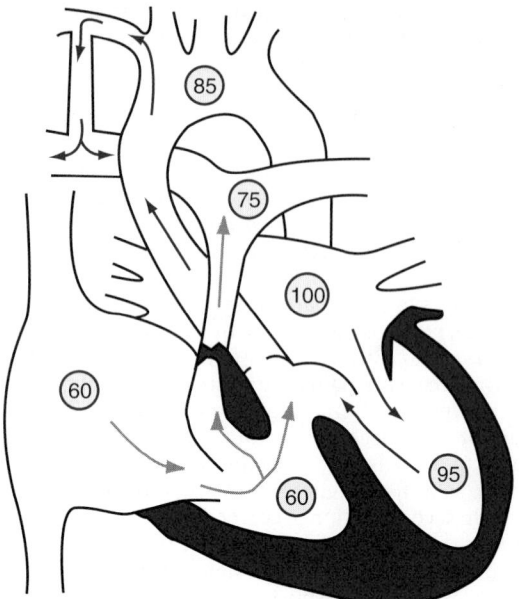

FIGURE 423–5. Physiology of a Blalock-Taussig shunt in a patient with the tetralogy of Fallot. *Circled numbers* represent oxygen saturation values. The intracardiac shunting pattern is as described for Figure 423–1. Blood shunting left to right across the shunt from the right subclavian artery to the right pulmonary artery increases total pulmonary blood flow and results in a higher oxygen saturation than would exist without the shunt (see Fig. 423–1).

Corrective surgical therapy consists of relief of the right ventricular outflow tract obstruction by removing obstructive muscle bundles and patch closure of the VSD. If the pulmonary valve is stenotic, a valvotomy is performed. If the pulmonary valve annulus is small or the valve is extremely thickened, a valvectomy may be performed, the pulmonary valve annulus split open, and a *transannular patch* placed across the pulmonary valve ring. Any previously established systemic-to-pulmonary shunt must be obliterated before full repair. The surgical risk of total correction is less than 5%. A right ventriculotomy was the standard approach; however, a transatrial-transpulmonary approach can be used to reduce the long-term risks of a ventriculotomy. Increased bleeding in the immediate postoperative period may be a complicating factor in extremely polycythemic patients.

After successful total correction, patients are generally asymptomatic and are able to lead unrestricted lives. Immediate postoperative problems include right ventricular failure, transient heart block, residual VSD with left-to-right shunting, myocardial infarction from interruption of an aberrant coronary artery, and disproportionately increased left atrial pressure because of residual bronchial collaterals. Postoperative heart failure (particularly in patients with a transannular outflow patch) requires a positive inotropic agent such as digoxin. The long-term effects of isolated, surgically induced pulmonary valvular insufficiency are unknown, but insufficiency is generally well tolerated. The majority of patients after tetralogy repair and all of those with transannular patch repairs have a to-and-fro murmur at the left sternal border, usually indicative of mild outflow obstruction and mild to moderate pulmonary insufficiency. Patients with more marked pulmonary valve insufficiency also have moderate to marked heart enlargement. Patients with a severe residual gradient across the right ventricular outflow tract may require reoperation, but mild to moderate obstruction is virtually always present and does not require re-intervention.

Follow-up of patients 5–20 yr after surgery indicates that the marked improvement in symptoms is generally maintained. Asymptomatic patients have lower than normal exercise capacity, maximal heart rate, and cardiac output. These abnormal findings are more common in patients who underwent placement of a transannular outflow tract patch and may be less frequent when surgery is performed at an early age.

Conduction disturbances can occur after surgery. The atrioventricular node and the bundle of His and its divisions are in close proximity to the VSD and may be injured during surgery. A permanent complete heart block after surgery is rare. When present, it should be treated by placement of a permanently implanted pacemaker. Even a transient complete heart block in the immediate postoperative period is rare in tetralogy patients; it may be associated with an increased incidence of late-onset complete heart block and sudden death. Right bundle branch block is quite common on the postoperative electrocardiogram. The duration of the QRS interval has been shown to predict both the presence of residual hemodynamic derangement and the long-term risk of sudden death.

A number of children have premature ventricular beats after repair of the tetralogy of Fallot. These beats are of concern in patients with residual hemodynamic abnormalities; 24-hr electrocardiographic (Holter) monitoring studies should be performed to be certain that occult short episodes of ventricular tachycardia are not occurring. Exercise studies may be useful in provoking cardiac arrhythmias that are not apparent at rest. In the presence of complex ventricular arrhythmias or severe residual hemodynamic abnormalities, prophylactic antiarrhythmic therapy is warranted. Re-repair is indicated if significant residual right ventricular outflow obstruction or severe pulmonary insufficiency is present.

423.2 Pulmonary Atresia with Ventricular Septal Defect

Pathophysiology. Pulmonary atresia with VSD is an extreme form of the tetralogy of Fallot. The pulmonary valve is atretic, rudimentary, or absent, and the pulmonary trunk is atretic or hypoplastic. The entire right ventricular output is ejected into the aorta. Pulmonary blood flow is then dependent on a PDA or on bronchial collateral vessels. The ultimate prognosis depends on the degree of development of the branch pulmonary arteries, which needs to be assessed by cardiac catheterization. If these arteries are well developed, surgical repair with a homograft conduit between the right ventricle and pulmonary arteries is feasible. If the pulmonary arteries are moderately hypoplastic, the prognosis is more guarded, and extensive reconstruction may be required. Multiple *MAPCAs* may be present and can be incorporated into the repair along with the native pulmonary arteries. If the pulmonary arteries are severely hypoplastic, heart-lung transplantation may be the only therapy (see Chapter 435.2). Pulmonary atresia with VSD is also associated with the CATCH 22 deletion and either the DiGeorge or the velocardiofacial syndrome. The association of severe tracheomalacia or bronchomalacia with these severe forms of tetralogy/pulmonary atresia may complicate postoperative recovery.

Clinical Manifestations. Patients with pulmonary atresia and VSD have findings similar to those in patients with severe tetralogy of Fallot. Cyanosis usually appears within the 1st few hours or days after birth, the prominent systolic murmur associated with the tetralogy is usually absent, the 1st heart sound is frequently followed by an ejection click caused by the enlarged aortic root, the 2nd sound is moderately loud and single, and continuous murmurs of a PDA or bronchial collateral flow may be heard over the entire precordium, both anteriorly and posteriorly. Most patients are severely cyanotic and require urgent prostaglandin

E₁ infusion and palliative surgical intervention, some patients have heart failure caused by increased pulmonary blood flow via bronchial collateral vessels (MAPCAs), and some infants have adequate pulmonary blood flow and can be managed like patients with uncomplicated tetralogy of Fallot.

Diagnosis. The chest *roentgenogram* demonstrates a small or enlarged heart (depending on the degree of pulmonary blood flow), a concavity at the position of the pulmonary arterial segment, and often the reticular pattern of bronchial collateral flow. The *electrocardiogram* shows right ventricular hypertrophy. The *echocardiogram* identifies aortic override, a thick right ventricular wall, and atresia of the pulmonary valve. Pulsed and color Doppler echocardiographic studies show an absence of forward flow through the pulmonary valve, with pulmonary blood flow being supplied by the ductus arteriosus or by MAPCAs. At cardiac catheterization, *right ventriculography* reveals a large aorta, opacified immediately by passage of contrast medium through the VSD, but with no dye entering the lungs through the right ventricular outflow tract. The pathway of pulmonary blood flow from the aorta to the lungs (ductus or collaterals) is demonstrated. Careful delineation of both native pulmonary arteries and MAPCAs by selective contrast injection is required to determine the feasibility of surgical correction.

Treatment. The surgical procedure of choice depends on whether the main pulmonary artery segment is adequate and on the size of the branch pulmonary arteries. In patients with small branch pulmonary arteries, surgical intervention is directed toward increasing pulmonary blood flow in the hope that pulmonary artery growth will be stimulated. Two options are currently considered: an aortopulmonary (*Blalock-Taussig* or central) shunt or the establishment of a connection from the right ventricle directly to the pulmonary artery, either by patch "unroofing" of the outflow tract or by implanting a homograft conduit. It is debated whether this type of bypass stimulates growth of the pulmonary arteries better than a standard shunt operation does.

To be a candidate for full repair, the pulmonary arteries must be of adequate size to accept the full volume of right ventricular output. Complete repair includes closure of the VSD and placement of a homograft conduit from the right ventricle to the pulmonary artery. At the time of reparative surgery, previous shunts are ligated. Because of proliferation of intimal tissue, conduit replacement is usually required in later life, and multiple replacements may be needed. Patients often have malformations of the primary divisions of the pulmonary arteries in the form of hypoplasia, multiple branch stenoses, absence of a pulmonary artery, and large bronchial collaterals. These vessels are difficult to surgically reconstruct. Some of these patients require repeated transcatheter balloon dilatation and eventual stenting of multiple branch pulmonary arterial stenoses.

Acquired total atresia of the right ventricular outflow tract may occur after an aortopulmonary shunt anastomosis for the tetralogy of Fallot. In this case, the systolic murmur resulting from pulmonary stenosis becomes attenuated and then disappears. The completeness of obstruction can be confirmed by echocardiography or by right ventriculography. Corrective surgery of the right ventricular outflow tract can be performed in a manner similar to that used for congenital pulmonary atresia.

423.3 Pulmonary Atresia with Intact Ventricular Septum

Pathophysiology. In pulmonary atresia with an intact ventricular septum, the pulmonary valve leaflets are completely fused to form a membrane and the right ventricular outflow tract is atretic. Because no VSD is present, no egress of blood from the right ventricle occurs. Right atrial pressure increases, and blood shunts via the foramen ovale into the left atrium, where it mixes with pulmonary venous blood and enters the left ventricle (Fig. 423–6). The combined left and right ventricular output is pumped solely by the left ventricle into the aorta. In a newborn with pulmonary atresia, the only source of pulmonary blood flow occurs via a PDA. The right ventricle is usually hypoplastic, although the degree of hypoplasia varies considerably. Patients who have a small right ventricular cavity also have a small tricuspid valve annulus, which limits right ventricular inflow. These patients may have coronary sinusoidal channels within the right ventricular wall that communicate directly with the coronary arterial circulation. The high right ventricular pressure results in desaturated blood flowing retrograde via collaterals into the coronary arteries and to the aorta. The prognosis in patients with these sinusoids is guarded. Patients with intermediate-sized or large ventricular cavities may have tricuspid insufficiency, which serves to decompress the right ventricle.

Clinical Manifestations. As the ductus arteriosus closes in the 1st hr or days of life, infants with pulmonary atresia and an intact ventricular septum become markedly cyanotic. Untreated, most patients die within the 1st wk of life. Physical examination reveals severe cyanosis and respiratory distress. The 2nd heart sound is single and loud. Often, no murmurs are audible, but sometimes a systolic or continuous murmur can be heard secondary to ductal blood flow.

Diagnosis. The *electrocardiogram* shows a frontal QRS axis between 0 and +90 degrees, the amount of leftward shift reflecting the degree of hypoplasia of the right ventricle. Tall, spiked P waves indicate right atrial enlargement. QRS voltages are consistent with left ventricular dominance or hypertrophy; right

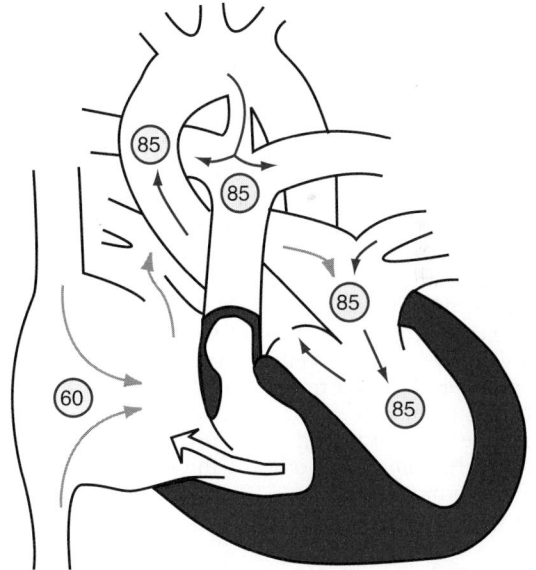

FIGURE 423–6. Physiology of pulmonary atresia with an intact ventricular septum. *Circled numbers* represent oxygen saturation values. Right atrial (mixed venous) oxygen saturation is decreased secondary to systemic hypoxemia. A small amount of the blood entering the right atrium may cross the tricuspid valve, which is often stenotic as well. The right ventricular cavity is hypertrophied and may be hypoplastic. No outlet from the right ventricle exists because of the atretic pulmonary valve; thus, any blood entering the right ventricle returns to the right atrium via tricuspid regurgitation. Most of the desaturated blood shunts right to left via the foramen ovale into the left atrium, where it mixes with fully saturated blood returning from the lungs. The only source of pulmonary blood flow is via the patent ductus arteriosus. Aortic and pulmonary arterial oxygen saturation will be identical (definition of a total mixing lesion).

ventricular forces are decreased in proportion to the decreased size of the right ventricular cavity. Most patients with small right ventricles have decreased right ventricular forces, but occasionally, patients with larger, thickened right ventricular cavities may have evidence of right ventricular hypertrophy. The chest *roentgenogram* shows decreased pulmonary vascularity, the degree depending on the size of the branch pulmonary arteries and the patency of the ductus or the size of the bronchial collaterals. The heart may be variable in size. The two-dimensional *echocardiogram* is useful in estimating right ventricular dimensions and the size of the tricuspid valve annulus, which are of prognostic value. Echocardiography can often demonstrate sinusoidal channels if they are large. *Cardiac catheterization* reveals right atrial and right ventricular hypertension. Ventriculography demonstrates the size of the right ventricular cavity, the atretic right ventricular outflow tract, the degree of tricuspid regurgitation, and the presence or absence of intramyocardial sinusoids filling the coronary vessels. Aortography shows filling of the pulmonary arteries via the PDA and is helpful in determining the size and branching patterns of the pulmonary arterial bed. The aortogram is also valuable in evaluating for coronary artery stenoses because the presence of these lesions negatively affects the prognosis.

Treatment. Infusion of prostaglandin E$_1$ is usually effective in keeping the ductus arteriosus open before intervention, thus reducing hypoxemia and acidemia before surgery. A surgical pulmonary valvotomy is carried out to relieve outflow obstruction whenever possible. To preserve adequate pulmonary blood flow, an aortopulmonary shunt is often performed during the same procedure. Some groups report success with surgical unroofing of the right ventricular outflow tract and patch grafting. Several centers report success with interventional catheterization, in which the imperforate pulmonary valve is first punctured with a wire or radiofrequency ablation catheter, followed by balloon valvuloplasty. The aim of surgery or interventional catheterization is to encourage growth of the right ventricular chamber by allowing some forward flow through the pulmonary valve while using the shunt to ensure adequate pulmonary blood flow. Later, if the tricuspid valve annulus and right ventricular chamber are of adequate size, a more extensive valvotomy is carried out and the shunt is taken down. If the right ventricular chamber remains hypoplastic, a modified Fontan procedure (see Chapter 423.4) allows blood to bypass the hypoplastic right ventricle by flowing to the pulmonary arteries directly from the venae cavae. When coronary artery stenoses are present and retrograde coronary perfusion occurs from the right ventricle via myocardial sinusoids, the prognosis may be grave because arrhythmias, coronary ischemia, and sudden death are common. Some of these infants benefit from heart transplantation.

423.4 Tricuspid Atresia

Pathophysiology. In tricuspid atresia, no outlet from the right atrium to the right ventricle is present; the entire systemic venous return enters the left side of the heart by means of the foramen ovale or an associated atrial septal defect (Fig. 423–7). Left ventricular blood usually flows into the right ventricle via a VSD. Pulmonary blood flow (and thus the degree of cyanosis) depends on the size of the VSD and the presence and severity of pulmonic stenosis. Pulmonary blood flow may be augmented by or be totally dependent on a PDA. The inflow portion of the right ventricle is always missing in these patients, but the outflow portion is of variable size. If the ventricular septum is intact, the right ventricle is completely hypoplastic and pulmonary atresia is present (see Chapter 423.3). Most patients with tricuspid atresia are recognized in the early months of life

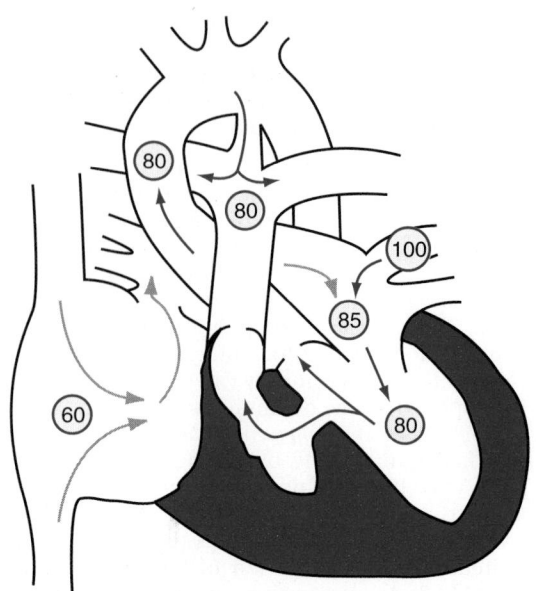

FIGURE 423–7. Physiology of tricuspid atresia with normally related great vessels. *Circled numbers* represent oxygen saturation values. Right atrial (mixed venous) oxygen saturation is decreased secondary to systemic hypoxemia. The tricuspid valve is nonpatent, and the right ventricle may manifest varying degrees of hypoplasia. The only outlet from the right atrium involves shunting right to left across an atrial septal defect or patent foramen ovale to the left atrium. There, desaturated blood mixes with saturated pulmonary venous return. Blood enters the left ventricle and is ejected either through the aorta or via a ventricular septal defect (VSD) into the right ventricle. In this example, some pulmonary blood flow is derived from the right ventricle, the rest from a patent ductus arteriosus (PDA). In patients with tricuspid atresia, the PDA may close or the VSD may grow smaller and result in a marked decrease in systemic oxygen saturation.

by decreased pulmonary blood flow and cyanosis. Less often, a large VSD in the absence of right ventricular outflow obstruction can lead to high pulmonary flow; patients have mild cyanosis and heart failure. One variant of tricuspid atresia is associated with transposition of the great arteries. In this case, left ventricular blood flows directly into the pulmonary artery, whereas systemic blood must traverse the VSD and right ventricle to reach the aorta. In these patients, pulmonary blood flow is usually massively increased and heart failure develops early. If the VSD is restrictive, aortic blood flow may be compromised.

Clinical Manifestations. Cyanosis is usually evident at birth, with the extent depending on the degree of limitation to pulmonary blood flow. An increased left ventricular impulse may be noted, in contrast to most other causes of cyanotic heart disease, in which an increased right ventricular impulse is usually present. The majority of patients have holosystolic murmurs audible along the left sternal border; the 2nd heart sound is usually single. The diagnosis is suspected in 85% of patients before 2 mo of age. In older patients, cyanosis, polycythemia, easy fatigability, exertional dyspnea, and occasional hypoxic episodes occur as a result of compromised pulmonary blood flow. Patients with tricuspid atresia are at risk for spontaneous closure of the VSD, which can occur rapidly and lead to a marked increase in cyanosis.

Diagnosis. *Roentgenographic studies* show either pulmonary undercirculation (usually in patients with normally related great vessels) or overcirculation (usually in patients with transposed great vessels). Left axis deviation and left ventricular hypertrophy are generally noted on the *electrocardiogram* (except in those with transposition of the great arteries), and these features distinguish tricuspid atresia from most other cyanotic heart lesions. The combination of cyanosis and left axis deviation is highly suggestive of tricuspid atresia. In the right precordial leads, the normally prominent R wave is replaced by an rS complex. The left precordial leads show a qR complex, followed by a normal, flat, biphasic or inverted T wave. RV_6 is normal or tall, and SV_1 is generally deep. The P waves are usually biphasic, with the initial component tall and spiked in lead II. *Two-dimensional echocardiography* reveals the presence of a fibromuscular membrane in place of a tricuspid valve, the variably small right ventricle, VSD, and the large left ventricle and aorta. The degree of obstruction at the level of the VSD or right ventricular outflow tract can be determined by direct measurement and by Doppler examination. The relationship of the great vessels (normal or transposed) can be determined. Blood flow through a patent ductus can be evaluated by color flow and pulsed Doppler examination.

Cardiac catheterization, indicated if questions remain after echocardiography, shows normal or slightly elevated right atrial pressure with a prominent "*a*" wave. If the right ventricle is entered through the VSD, the pressure may be lower than on the left because of the restrictive nature of the VSD. Right atrial angiography shows immediate opacification of the left atrium from the right atrium followed by left ventricular filling and visualization of the aorta. Absence of direct flow to the right ventricle results in an angiographic filling defect between the right atrium and the left ventricle.

Treatment. Management of patients with tricuspid atresia depends on the adequacy of pulmonary blood flow. Severely cyanotic neonates should be maintained on an infusion of prostaglandin E_1 until a surgical aortopulmonary shunt procedure can be performed to increase pulmonary blood flow. The Blalock-Taussig procedure (see Chapter 423.1) or a variation is the preferred anastomosis. Some patients with restrictive atrial-level communications also benefit from a Rashkind balloon atrial septostomy (see Chapter 424.2) or surgical septectomy.

Infants with increased pulmonary blood flow because of an unobstructed pulmonary outflow tract (most often patients with aortopulmonary transposition) require pulmonary arterial banding to decrease the symptoms of heart failure and protect the pulmonary bed from the development of pulmonary vascular disease. Infants with just adequate pulmonary blood flow who are well *balanced* between cyanosis and pulmonary overcirculation can be watched closely for the development of increasing cyanosis, which may occur as the VSD begins to get smaller and is an indication for surgery.

The next stage of palliation for patients with tricuspid atresia involves the creation of an anastomosis between the superior vena cava and the pulmonary arteries (*bidirectional Glenn shunt*; Fig. 423–8*A*). This procedure is performed after the patient has shown signs of outgrowing a previous aortopulmonary shunt, usually between 4 and 12 mo of age. The benefit of the Glenn shunt is that it reduces the volume load on the left ventricle and may lessen the chance of left ventricular dysfunction developing later in life. Some centers advocate performing the Glenn anastomosis at an even earlier age (2–4 mo); the benefit of this approach has not yet been confirmed.

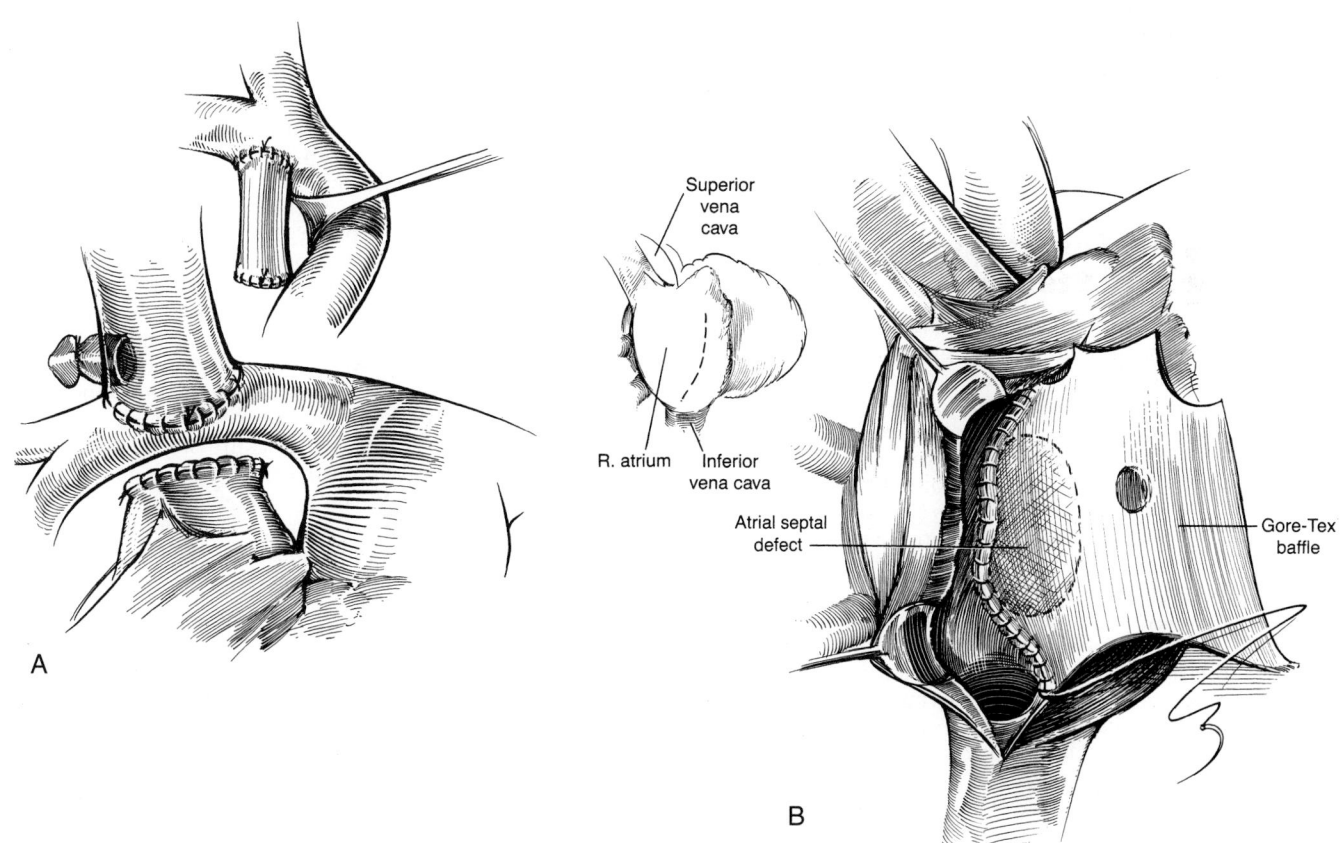

FIGURE 423–8. *A,* Bidirectional Glenn shunt showing the superior vena cava–right pulmonary anastomosis. *B,* A modified Fontan procedure (cavopulmonary isolation) is completed with placement of a baffle to convey inferior vena cava blood along the lateral wall of the right atrium to the superior vena cava orifice. A 4 mm fenestration is sometimes made on the medial aspect of the polytetrafluoroethylene baffle. (From Castaneda AR, Jonas RA, Mayer JE Jr, Hanley FL: Single-ventricle tricuspid atresia. In *Cardiac Surgery of the Neonate and Infant.* Philadelphia, WB Saunders, 1994.)

The modified Fontan operation is the preferred approach to later surgical management. It is often performed between 1.5 and 3 yr of age, usually after the patient is ambulatory. Initially, this procedure was performed by anastomosing the right atrium or atrial appendage directly to the pulmonary artery. A modification of the Fontan procedure known as a *cavopulmonary isolation procedure* involves anastomosing the inferior vena cava to the pulmonary arteries, either via a baffle that runs along the lateral wall of the right atrium (see Fig. 423–8*B*) or via a homograft or Gore-Tex tube running outside the heart. The advantage of this approach is that blood flows by a more direct route into the pulmonary arteries, thereby decreasing the possibility of right atrial dilatation and markedly reducing the incidence of postoperative pleural effusions, which were common with the earlier method. In this completed repair, desaturated blood flows from both venae cavae directly into the pulmonary arteries. Oxygenated blood returns to the left atrium, enters the left ventricle, and is ejected into the systemic circulation. The volume load is completely removed from the left ventricle, and the right-to-left shunt is abolished. Because of the reliance on passive filling of the pulmonary circulation, the Fontan procedure is contraindicated in patients with elevated pulmonary vascular resistance, in those with pulmonary artery hypoplasia, and in patients with left ventricular dysfunction. The patient must be in sinus rhythm and not have significant mitral insufficiency.

Postoperative problems after the Fontan procedure include marked elevation of systemic venous pressure, fluid retention, and pleural or pericardial effusions. Pleural effusions were a problem in 30–40% of patients, but the cavopulmonary isolation procedure reduces this risk to 5%. Late complications include baffle obstruction causing superior or inferior vena cava syndrome, vena cava or pulmonary artery thromboembolism, protein-losing enteropathy, and supraventricular arrhythmias (atrial flutter, paroxysmal atrial tachycardia), occasionally associated with sudden death. Left ventricular dysfunction may be a late occurrence, often in the teenage or young adult years. Heart transplantation is successful in patients with "failed" Fontan circuits.

423.5 Double-Outlet Right Ventricle with Pulmonary Stenosis

Both the aorta and pulmonary artery arising from the right ventricle characterize double-outlet right ventricle with pulmonary stenosis; the outlet from the left ventricle is a VSD into the right ventricle. The aortic and mitral valves are separated by a smooth muscular conus, similar to that seen under the normal pulmonary valve. The aorta may override the VSD by a variable amount but is at least 50% committed to the right ventricle. This defect may be viewed as part of a continuum with the tetralogy of Fallot, depending on the degree of aortic override. The physiology as well as the history, physical examination, electrocardiogram, and roentgenograms are similar to that in the tetralogy of Fallot (see Chapter 423.1). The two-dimensional *echocardiogram* demonstrates both great vessels arising from the right ventricle and mitral-aortic valve discontinuity. At *cardiac catheterization*, angiography shows that the aortic and pulmonary valves lie in the same horizontal plane and that the anteriorly displaced aorta arises predominantly or exclusively from the right ventricle. Surgical correction consists of creating an intraventricular tunnel so that the left ventricle ejects blood through the VSD, through the tunnel, and into the aorta. The pulmonary obstruction is relieved either with an outflow patch or with a pulmonary or aortic homograft conduit (*Rastelli operation*). In small infants, palliation with an aortopulmonary shunt provides symptomatic improvement and allows for adequate growth before corrective surgery is performed.

423.6 Transposition of the Great Arteries with Ventricular Septal Defect and Pulmonary Stenosis

This combination of anomalies may mimic the tetralogy of Fallot in its clinical features (see Chapter 423.1). However, because of the transposition, the site of obstruction is in the left as opposed to the right ventricle. The obstruction can be either valvular or subvalvular; the latter type may be dynamic, related to the interventricular septum or atrioventricular valve tissue, or acquired, as in patients with transposition and VSD after pulmonary arterial banding.

The age at which *clinical manifestations* initially appear varies from soon after birth to later infancy, depending on the degree of pulmonic stenosis. Clinical findings include cyanosis, decreased exercise tolerance, and poor physical development, similar to those described for the tetralogy of Fallot; however, the heart may be more enlarged. The pulmonary vasculature as seen on the *roentgenogram* is dependent on the degree of pulmonary obstruction, but it is often normal. The *electrocardiogram* usually shows right axis deviation, right and left ventricular hypertrophy, and sometimes tall, spiked P waves. *Echocardiography* confirms the diagnosis and is useful in sequential evaluation of the degree and progression of the left ventricular outflow tract obstruction. *Cardiac catheterization* shows that pulmonary arterial pressure is low and that oxygen saturation in the pulmonary artery exceeds that in the aorta. Selective right and left ventriculography demonstrates the origin of the aorta from the right ventricle, the origin of the pulmonary artery from the left ventricle, the VSD, and the site and severity of the pulmonary stenosis.

An infusion of prostaglandin E_1 should be started in neonates with cyanosis. The preferred surgical *treatment* in hypoxemic infants is an aortopulmonary shunt (see Chapter 423.1). When necessary, balloon atrial septostomy is performed to improve atrial-level mixing and to decompress the left atrium (see Chapter 424.2). The patient can then be monitored clinically until older, when a Rastelli operation is the preferred corrective procedure. The Rastelli procedure achieves physiologic and anatomic correction by (1) patch closure of the VSD, with left ventricular flow directed to the aorta, and (2) connection of the right ventricle to the pulmonary artery by ligating the proximal pulmonary artery and placing an extracardiac homograft conduit between the right ventricle and the distal pulmonary artery (Fig. 423–9). The conduit may eventually become stenotic or functionally restrictive with growth of the patient and require revision. Surgical correction by the Mustard operation (see Chapter 424.2) with simultaneous closure of the VSD and relief of left ventricular outflow obstruction may be an alternative when the position of the VSD is not suitable for a Rastelli operation. Patients with milder degrees of pulmonary stenosis amenable to simple valvotomy may be able to undergo complete correction with an arterial switch procedure (see Chapter 424.2).

423.7 Ebstein Anomaly of the Tricuspid Valve

Pathophysiology. Ebstein anomaly consists of downward displacement of an abnormal tricuspid valve into the right ventricle. The defect may arise from failure of the normal process by which the tricuspid valve is separated from the right ventricular myocardium (see Chapter 413). The anterior cusp of the valve retains some attachment to the valve ring, but the other leaflets are adherent to the wall of the right ventricle. The right ventricle is thus divided into two parts by the abnormal tricuspid valve: the 1st, a thin-walled *"atrialized"* portion, is contin-

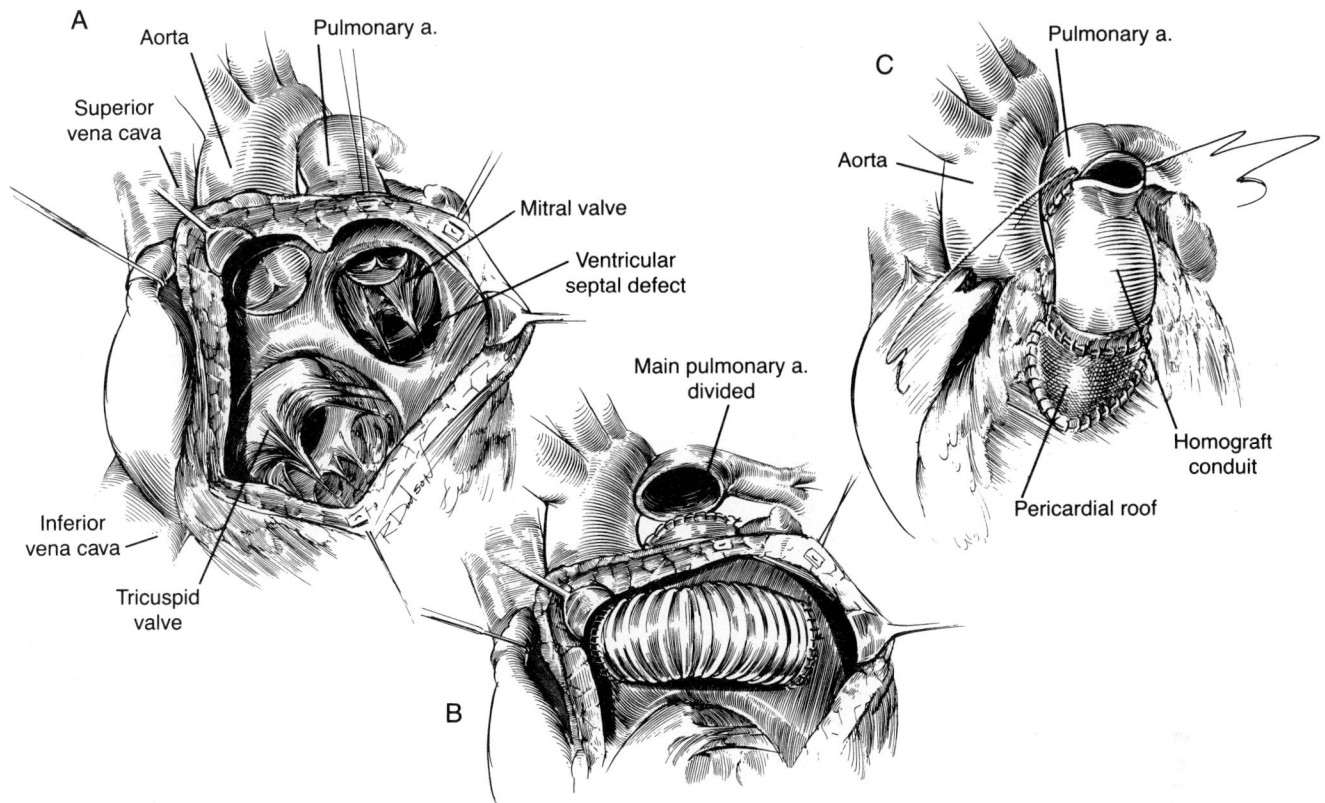

FIGURE 423–9. *A,* Taussig-Bing type of double-outlet right ventricle with subpulmonary stenosis necessitating repair by the Rastelli technique. *B,* The main pulmonary artery is divided and oversewn proximally. The pulmonary valve lies within the baffle pathway. *C,* Completion of the Rastelli repair with a right ventricle–pulmonary artery allograft conduit. (From Castaneda AR, Jonas RA, Mayer JE Jr, Hanley FL: Single-ventricle tricuspid atresia. In *Cardiac Surgery of the Neonate and Infant.* Philadelphia, WB Saunders, 1994.)

uous with the cavity of the right atrium; the 2nd, often smaller portion consists of normal ventricular myocardium. The right atrium is huge, and the tricuspid valve is generally regurgitant, although the degree is extremely variable. The effective output from the right side of the heart is decreased because of the poorly functioning small right ventricle, tricuspid valve regurgitation, and variable degrees of obstruction of the right ventricular outflow tract produced by the large, sail-like, anterior tricuspid valve leaflet. At times, right ventricular function is so compromised that it is unable to generate enough force to open the pulmonary valve in systole, thus producing "functional" pulmonary atresia. Some infants have true anatomic pulmonary atresia. The increased volume of right atrial blood shunts through the foramen ovale to the left atrium and produces cyanosis (Fig. 423–10).

Clinical Manifestations. The severity of symptoms and the degree of cyanosis are highly variable and depend on the extent of displacement of the tricuspid valve and the severity of right ventricular outflow tract obstruction. In many patients, symptoms are mild and do not occur until the teenage years or young adult life; the patient may initially have fatigue or palpitations as a result of cardiac dysrhythmias. A right-to-left shunt through the foramen ovale is responsible for cyanosis and polycythemia. Central venous pressure may be normal or increased in those with tricuspid insufficiency. On palpation, the precordium is quiet. A holosystolic murmur caused by tricuspid regurgitation is audible over most of the anterior left side of the chest. A gallop rhythm is common and often associated with multiple clicks at the lower left sternal border. A scratchy diastolic murmur may also be heard at the left sternal border. This murmur is superficial and may mimic a pericardial friction rub.

Newborn infants with severe forms of Ebstein anomaly have marked cyanosis, massive cardiomegaly, and long systolic murmurs. Death may result from cardiac failure and hypoxemia. Spontaneous improvement may occur in some neonates as pulmonary vascular resistance falls normally and improves the ability of the right ventricle to provide pulmonary blood flow. The majority are dependent on a PDA for pulmonary blood flow.

Diagnosis. The *electrocardiogram* usually shows a right bundle branch block without increased right precordial voltage, normal or tall and broad P waves, and a normal or prolonged P-R interval. Wolff-Parkinson-White syndrome (see Chapter 428) may be present; patients may have episodes of supraventricular tachycardia. On *roentgenographic examination,* heart size varies from normal to massive, box-shaped cardiomegaly caused by enlargement of the right atrium and ventricle. The pulmonary vasculature can be normal or decreased. *Echocardiography* shows the degree of displacement of the tricuspid valve leaflets, a dilated right atrium, and any right ventricular outflow tract obstruction. Pulsed and color Doppler examination demonstrates the degree of tricuspid regurgitation. In severe cases, the pulmonary valve may appear immobile and pulmonary blood flow may come solely from the ductus arteriosus. It may be difficult to distinguish true from functional pulmonary valve atresia. *Cardiac catheterization,* which is not always necessary, confirms the presence of a large right atrium, an abnormal tricuspid valve, and any right-to-left shunt at the atrial level. The risk of arrhythmia is significant during catheterization and angiographic studies.

Prognosis and Complications. The prognosis in Ebstein anomaly is extremely variable and depends on the spectrum of severity seen. The prognosis is usually poor for neonates or infants with

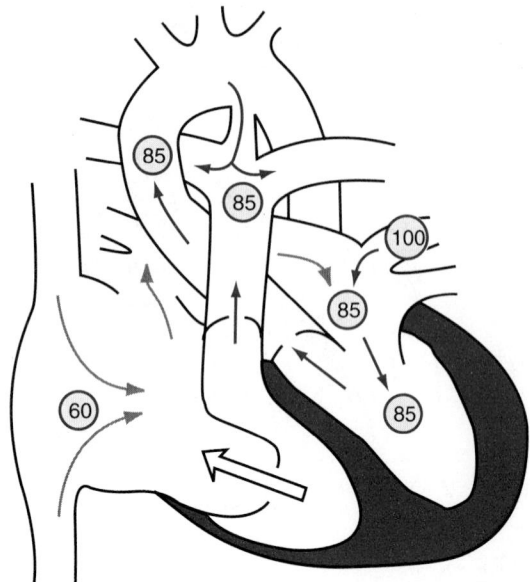

FIGURE 423–10. Physiology of Ebstein anomaly of the tricuspid valve. *Circled numbers* represent oxygen saturation values. Inferior displacement of the tricuspid valve leaflets into the right ventricle has resulted in a thin-walled, low-pressure "atrialized" segment of right ventricle. The tricuspid valve is grossly insufficient *(clear arrow)*. Right atrial blood flow is shunted right to left across an atrial septal defect or patent foramen ovale into the left atrium. Some blood may cross the right ventricular outflow tract and enter the pulmonary artery; however, in severe cases, the right ventricle may generate insufficient force to open the pulmonary valve, and "functional pulmonary atresia" results. In the left atrium, desaturated blood mixes with saturated pulmonary venous return. Blood enters the left ventricle and is ejected via the aorta. In this example, some pulmonary blood flow is derived from the right ventricle, the rest from a patent ductus arteriosus (PDA). Severe cyanosis will develop in neonates with a severe Ebstein anomaly when the PDA closes.

intractable symptoms and cyanosis. Patients with milder degrees of Ebstein anomaly usually survive well into adult life.

Treatment. Neonates with severe hypoxia who are prostaglandin dependent have been treated with an aortopulmonary shunt alone or by surgical patch closure of the tricuspid valve, atrial septectomy, and placement of an aortopulmonary shunt (*Starnes procedure*). This operation creates a functional tricuspid atresia, which can then be further repaired with first a Glenn and then a Fontan operation (see Chapter 423.4). In older children with mild or moderate disease, control of supraventricular dysrhythmias is of primary importance; surgical treatment may not be necessary until adolescence or young adulthood. In patients with severe tricuspid regurgitation, repair or replacement of the abnormal tricuspid valve along with closure of the atrial septal defect is then carried out. In some patients, a bidirectional Glenn shunt is performed, with the superior vena cava anastomosed to the pulmonary arteries. This procedure reduces the volume of blood that the dysfunctional right side of the heart has to pump, thus creating a "one-and-one-half" ventricle repair.

Tetralogy of Fallot, Pulmonary Atresia with Ventricular Septal Defect, and Double-Outlet Right Ventricle
Boudjemline Y, Fermont L, Le Bidois J, et al: Prevalence of 22q11 deletion in fetuses with conotruncal cardiac defects: A 6-year prospective study. *J Pediatr* 2001;138:520–4.
Hanley FL: Management of the congenitally abnormal right ventricular outflow tract—what is the right approach? *J Thorac Cardiovasc Surg* 2000;119:1–3.

McCaughan BC, Danielson GK, Driscoll DJ, et al: Tetralogy of Fallot with absent pulmonary valve: Early and late results of surgical treatment. *J Thorac Cardiovasc Surg* 1985;89:280.
Oku H, Shirotani H, Sunakawa A, et al: Postoperative long term results in total correction of tetralogy of Fallot: Hemodynamics and cardiac function. *Ann Thorac Surg* 1986;41:413.
Pacifico AO, Saro ME, Bargeron LM Jr, et al: Transatrial-transpulmonary repair of tetralogy of Fallot. *J Thorac Cardiovasc Surg* 1987;74:382.
Parry AJ, McElhinney DB, Kung GC, et al: Elective primary repair of acyanotic tetralogy of Fallot in early infancy: Overall outcome and impact on the pulmonary valve. *J Am Coll Cardiol* 2000;36:2279–83.
Reddy VM, McElhinney DB, Amin Z, et al: Early and intermediate outcomes after repair of pulmonary atresia with ventricular septal defect and major aortopulmonary collateral arteries: Experience with 85 patients. *Circulation* 2000;101:1826–32.
Sluysmans T, Neven B, Rubay J, et al: Early balloon dilatation of the pulmonary valve in infants with tetralogy of Fallot. Risks and benefits. *Circulation* 1995;91:1506.

Pulmonary Atresia with Intact Septum
Hanley FL, Sade RM, Blackstone EH, et al: Outcomes in neonatal pulmonary atresia with intact ventricular septum. A multiinstitutional study. *J Thorac Cardiovasc Surg* 1993;105:406.
Latson LA: Nonsurgical treatment of a neonate with pulmonary atresia and intact ventricular septum by transcatheter puncture and balloon dilatation of the atretic valve membrane. *Am J Cardiol* 1991;68:277.
L'Ecuyer TJ, Poulik JM, Vincent JA: Myocardial infarction due to coronary abnormalities in pulmonary atresia with intact ventricular septum. *Pediatr Cardiol* 2001;22:68–70.

Tricuspid Atresia
Donnelly JP, Rosenthal A, Castle VP, et al: Reversal of protein-losing enteropathy with heparin therapy in three patients with univentricular hearts and Fontan palliation. *J Pediatr* 1997;130:474.
Freedom RM, Hamilton R, Yoo SJ, et al: The Fontan procedure: Analysis of cohorts and late complications. *Cardiol Young* 2000;10:307–31.
Gelatt M, Hamilton R, McCrindle W, et al: Risk factors for atrial tachyarrhythmias after the Fontan operation. *J Am Coll Cardiol* 1994;24:1735.
Hess J: Long-term problems after cavopulmonary anastomosis: Diagnosis and management. *Thorac Cardiovasc Surg* 2001;49:98–100.
Mair DD, Puga FJ, Danielson GK: The Fontan procedure for tricuspid atresia: Early and late results of a 25-year experience with 216 patients. *J Am Coll Cardiol* 2001;1;37:933–9.
Petrossian E, Reddy VM, McElhinney DB, et al: Early results of the extracardiac conduit Fontan operation. *J Thorac Cardiovasc Surg* 1999;117:688–96.
Shirai LK, Rosenthal DN, Reitz BA, et al: Arrhythmias and thromboembolic complications after the extracardiac Fontan operation. *J Thorac Cardiovasc Surg* 1998;115:499–505.

Ebstein Anomaly
Kiziltan HT, Theodoro DA, Warnes CA, et al: Late results of bioprosthetic tricuspid valve replacement in Ebstein's anomaly. *Ann Thorac Surg* 1998;66:1539–45.
Marianeschi SM, McElhinney DB, Reddy VM, et al: Alternative approach to the repair of Ebstein's malformation: Intracardiac repair with ventricular unloading. *Ann Thorac Surg* 1998;66:1546–50.
Schreiber C, Cook A, Ho SY, et al: Morphologic spectrum of Ebstein's malformation: Revisitation relative to surgical repair. *J Thorac Cardiovasc Surg* 1999;117:148–55.
Starnes VA, Pitlick PT, Bernstein D, et al: Ebstein's anomaly appearing in the neonate. *J Thorac Cardiovasc Surg* 1991;101:1082.

Chapter 424

Cyanotic Congenital Heart Disease: Lesions Associated with Increased Pulmonary Blood Flow

424.1 d-Transposition of the Great Arteries

Transposition of the great vessels, a common cyanotic congenital anomaly, accounts for approximately 5% of all congenital heart disease. In this anomaly, the systemic veins return normally to the right atrium and the pulmonary veins return to the left atrium. The connections between the atria and ventricles are also normal *(atrioventricular concordance)*. However, the aorta arises from the right ventricle and the pulmonary artery from the left ventricle (Fig. 424–1). In normally related great vessels, the aorta is *posterior* and to the right of the pulmonary artery; in d-transposition of the great arteries (d-TGA), the aorta is *anterior* and to the right of the pulmonary artery (the "d" indicates a dextropositioned aorta). Desaturated blood returning from the body to the right side of the heart inappropriately goes right out the aorta and back to the body again, whereas oxygenated pulmonary venous blood returning to the left side of the heart is returned directly to the lungs. The systemic and pulmonary circulations consist of two parallel circuits. Survival in these newborns is provided by the foramen ovale and the ductus arteriosus, which permit some mixture of oxygenated and deoxygenated blood. About half of patients with TGA also have a ventricular septal defect (VSD), which provides for better mixing. The clinical findings and hemodynamics vary in relation to the presence or absence of associated defects. TGA is more common in infants of diabetic mothers and in males (3:1). TGA, especially when accompanied by other cardiac defects such as pulmonic stenosis or right aortic arch, can be associated with deletion of chromosome 22q11 (CATCH 22 [*c*ardiac defects, *a*bnormal facies, *t*hymic aplasia, *c*left palate, *h*ypoplasia], DiGeorge syndrome). Before the modern era of corrective or palliative surgery, mortality was greater than 90% in the 1st yr of life.

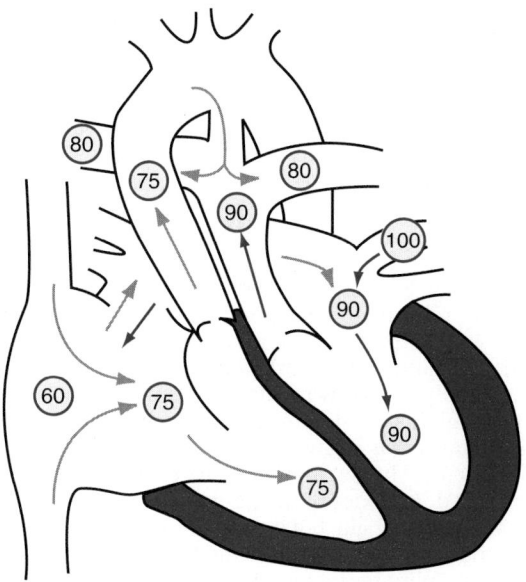

FIGURE 424–1. Physiology of d-transposition of the great arteries (d-TGA). *Circled numbers* represent oxygen saturation values. Right atrial (mixed venous) oxygen saturation is decreased secondary to systemic hypoxemia. Desaturated blood enters the right atrium, flows through the tricuspid valve into the right ventricle, and is ejected into the transposed aorta with resultant severe aortic desaturation. Fully saturated pulmonary venous blood flows into the left atrium, across the mitral valve into the left ventricle, and across the transposed pulmonary artery into the lungs. Pulmonary arterial oxygen saturation is thus increased. This lesion would not be compatible with life were it not for the ability of blood to shunt via two fetal pathways: the patent foramen ovale (PFO) and patent ductus arteriosus (PDA). Blood may shunt left to right or bidirectionally at the PFO. Because systemic vascular resistance tends to be higher than pulmonary vascular resistance, blood tends to shunt across the PDA mostly from the aorta to the pulmonary artery. As pulmonary resistance drops in the 1st few weeks of life, pulmonary blood flow will gradually increase in patients with d-TGA.

424.2   d-Transposition of the Great Arteries with Intact Ventricular Septum

d-TGA with an intact ventricular septum is also referred to as *simple TGA* or *isolated TGA*. Before birth, oxygenation of the fetus is nearly normal, but after birth, once the ductus begins to close, the minimal mixing of systemic and pulmonary blood via the patent foramen ovale is usually insufficient and severe hypoxemia ensues, generally within the 1st few days of life.

Clinical Manifestations. Cyanosis and tachypnea are most often recognized within the 1st hours or days of life. Untreated, the vast majority of these infants would not survive the neonatal period. Hypoxemia is usually severe, but heart failure is less common. This condition is a medical emergency, and only early diagnosis and appropriate intervention can avert the development of prolonged severe hypoxemia and acidosis, which lead to death. Physical findings associated with cyanosis may be nonspecific, with the exception of cyanosis itself. The precordial impulse may be normal, or a parasternal heave may be present. The 2nd heart sound is usually single and loud, although occasionally it may be split. Murmurs may be absent, or a soft systolic ejection murmur may be noted at the midleft sternal border.

Diagnosis. The *electrocardiogram* shows the normal neonatal right-sided dominant pattern. *Roentgenograms* of the chest may show mild cardiomegaly, a narrow mediastinum, and normal to increased pulmonary blood flow. In the early newborn period, the chest roentgenogram is generally normal. As pulmonary vascular resistance drops over the 1st wk or two of life, evidence of increased pulmonary blood flow is apparent. Arterial Po_2 is low and does not rise appreciably after the patient breathes 100% oxygen (*hyperoxia test*), although this finding may not be totally reliable. *Echocardiography* confirms the transposed ventricular-arterial connections. In addition, the size of the interatrial communication and the ductus arteriosus can be visualized; the degree of mixing is assessed by pulsed and color Doppler examination. The presence of left ventricular outflow tract obstruction or a VSD can also be assessed. The origins of the coronary arteries can often be imaged, although echocardiography is not as accurate as catheterization for this purpose. *Cardiac catheterization* is occasionally performed in patients for whom noninvasive imaging is diagnostically inconclusive or in patients who require emergency balloon atrial septostomy (see later). Catheterization will show right ventricular pressure to be systemic because this ventricle is supporting the systemic circulation. The blood in the left ventricle and pulmonary artery has higher oxygen saturation than that in the aorta. Depending on the age at catheterization, left ventricular and pulmonary arterial pressure can vary from systemic level to less than 50% of systemic-level pressure. *Right ventriculography* demonstrates the anterior and rightward aorta originating from the right ventricle, as well as the intact ventricular septum. Anomalous coronary arteries are noted in 10–15% of patients. *Left ventriculography* shows that the pulmonary artery arises exclusively from the left ventricle.

Treatment. When transposition is suspected, an *infusion of prostaglandin E_1* should be initiated immediately to maintain patency of the ductus arteriosus and improve oxygenation (dosage, 0.05–0.20 µg/kg/min). Because of the risk of apnea associated with prostaglandin infusion, an individual skilled in neonatal endotracheal intubation should be available. Hypothermia intensifies the metabolic acidosis resulting from hypoxemia, and thus the patient should be kept warm. Prompt correction of acidosis and hypoglycemia is essential.

Infants who remain severely hypoxic or acidotic despite prostaglandin infusion should undergo *Rashkind balloon atrial septostomy* (Fig. 424–2). A Rashkind atrial septostomy is usually

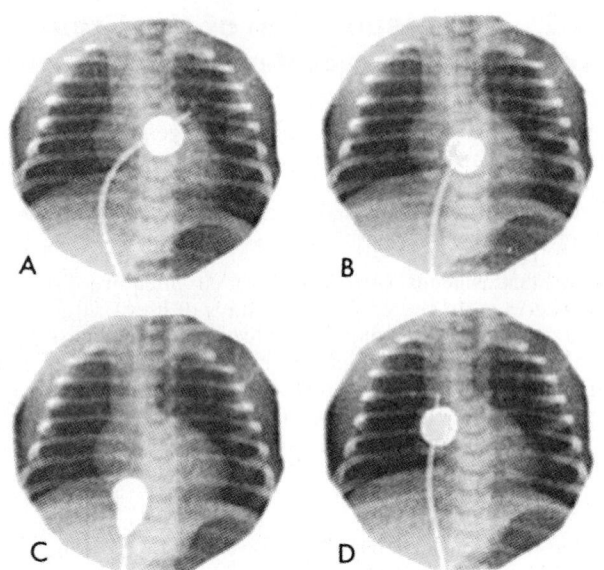

FIGURE 424–2. Rashkind balloon atrial septostomy. Four frames from a continuous cineangiogram show the creation of an atrial septal defect in a hypoxemic newborn infant with transposition of the great arteries and an intact ventricular septum. *A,* Balloon inflated in the left atrium. *B,* The catheter is jerked suddenly so that the balloon ruptures the foramen ovale. *C,* Balloon in the inferior vena cava. *D,* Catheter advanced to the right atrium to deflate the balloon. The time from *A* to *C* is less than 1 sec.

performed in all patients in whom any significant delay in surgery is necessary. At most centers, the arterial switch (Jantene) operation is performed within the 1st 2 wk of life. If the arterial switch is planned immediately, catheterization and atrial septostomy may often be avoided.

A successful Rashkind atrial septostomy should result in a rise in Pao$_2$ to 35–50 mm Hg and elimination of any pressure gradient across the atrial septum. Some patients with TGA and VSD may require balloon atrial septostomy because of poor mixing, even though the VSD is large. Others may benefit from decompression of the left atrium to alleviate the symptoms of increased pulmonary blood flow and left-sided heart failure.

The *arterial switch (Jantene) procedure* is the surgical treatment of choice for neonates with d-TGA and an intact ventricular septum and is usually performed within the 1st 2 wk of life. The reason for this urgency is that as pulmonary vascular resistance declines after birth, pressure in the left ventricle (connected to the pulmonary vascular bed) also declines. This drop in pressure results in a decrease in left ventricular mass over the 1st few weeks of life. If the arterial switch operation is attempted after left ventricular pressure has declined too far, the left ventricle will be unable to generate adequate pressure to pump blood to the systemic circulation. The operation involves dividing the aorta and pulmonary artery just above the sinuses and re-anastomosing them in their correct anatomic positions. The coronary arteries are then removed from the old aortic root along with a button of aortic wall and re-implanted in the old pulmonary root (the "neoaorta"). By using a button of great vessel tissue, the surgeon avoids having to suture directly onto the coronary artery (Fig. 424–3). Rarely, a two-stage arterial switch procedure, with initial placement of a pulmonary artery band, may be used in patients older than 3–4 wk who already have a reduction in left ventricular muscle mass and pressure.

The arterial switch procedure has a survival rate of 90–95% for uncomplicated d-TGA. It restores the normal physiologic relationships of systemic and pulmonary arterial blood flow and

eliminates the long-term complications of the atrial switch procedure (see the next paragraph).

Previous operations for d-TGA consisted of some form of *atrial switch procedure* (Mustard or Senning operation). In older infants, these procedures produced excellent early survival (about 85–90%), but significant long-term morbidity. Atrial switch procedures reverse blood flow patterns at the atrial level by the surgical creation of an intra-atrial baffle that allows systemic venous blood to be directed to the left atrium and the left ventricle and then, via the pulmonary artery, into the lungs. The same baffle also permits oxygenated pulmonary venous blood to cross over to the right atrium, right ventricle, and aorta. Atrial switch procedures involve significant atrial surgery and may result in the late development of atrial conduction disturbances, sick sinus syndrome with bradyarrhythmia and tachyarrhythmia, atrial flutter, sudden death, superior or inferior vena cava syndrome, edema, ascites, and protein-losing enteropathy. Atrial switch operations are reserved for patients who are not candidates for the arterial switch procedure (TGA and severe pulmonic stenosis).

424.3 Transposition of the Great Arteries with Ventricular Septal Defect

If the VSD associated with TGA is small, the clinical manifestations, laboratory findings, and treatment are similar to those described previously for transposition with an intact ventricular septum. A harsh systolic murmur is audible at the lower left sternal border and results from flow through the defect. Many of these small defects eventually close spontaneously and are often not addressed at the time of surgery.

When the VSD is large and not restrictive to ventricular ejection, significant mixing of oxygenated and deoxygenated blood usually occurs and *clinical manifestations* of cardiac failure are seen. The onset of cyanosis may be subtle and frequently delayed, and its intensity is variable. Cyanosis can generally be recognized within the 1st mo of life, but it may remain undiagnosed in some infants for several months. The murmur is holosystolic and generally indistinguishable from that produced by a large VSD in patients with normally related great arteries. The heart is usually significantly enlarged.

Cardiomegaly, a narrow mediastinal waist, and increased pulmonary vascularity are demonstrated on the *chest roentgenogram.* The *electrocardiogram* shows prominent P waves and isolated right ventricular hypertrophy or biventricular hypertrophy. Occasionally, dominance of the left ventricle is present. Usually, the QRS axis is to the right, but it is sometimes normal or even to the left. The diagnosis can be confirmed by *echocardiography,* and the extent of pulmonary blood flow can also be assessed by the degree of enlargement of the left atrium and ventricle. In equivocal cases, the diagnosis can be confirmed by *cardiac catheterization.* Right and left ventriculography can indicate the presence of arterial transposition and demonstrate the site and size of the VSD. Peak systolic pressure is equal in the two ventricles, the aorta, and the pulmonary artery. Left atrial pressure may be much higher than right atrial pressure, a finding indicative of a restrictive communication at the atrial level. At the time of cardiac catheterization, Rashkind balloon atrial septostomy may be performed to decompress the left atrium, even when adequate mixing is occurring at the ventricular level.

Surgical treatment is advised soon after diagnosis, usually within the 1st months of life, because heart failure and failure to thrive are difficult to manage and pulmonary vascular disease can develop unusually rapidly. Management includes digitalis and diuretics to lessen the symptoms of heart failure while awaiting surgical repair.

Patients with TGA and a VSD without pulmonic stenosis can be managed with an arterial switch procedure combined with

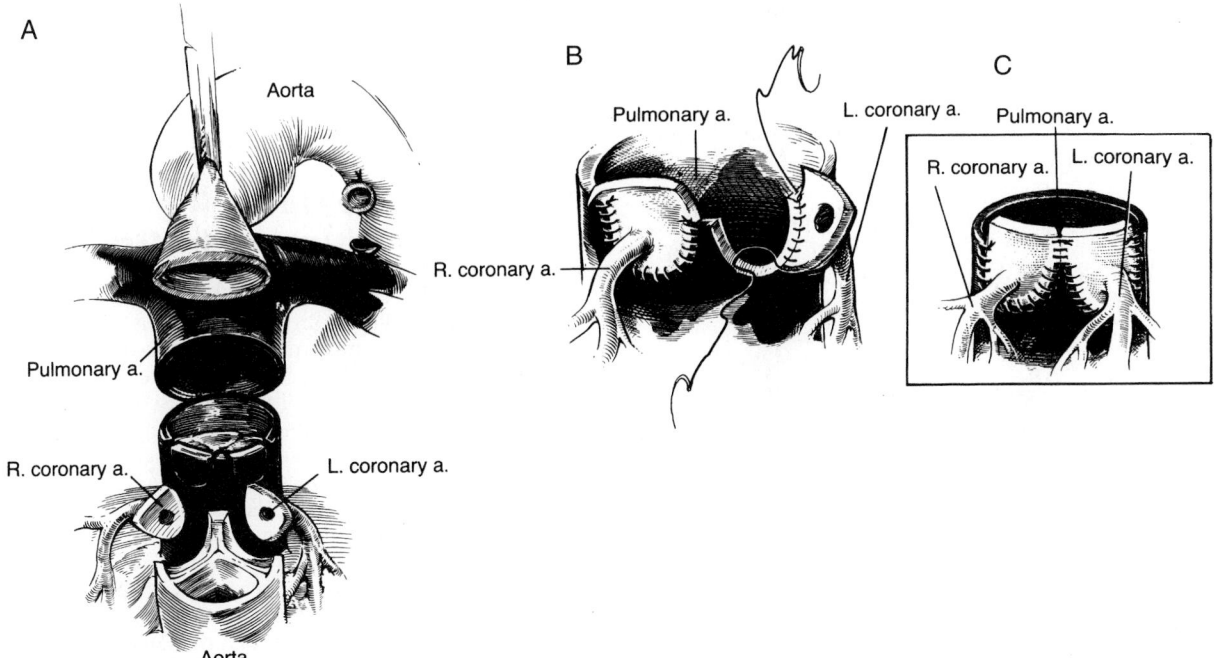

FIGURE 424–3. Method for translocating the coronary arteries in the arterial switch (Jantene) procedure. *A,* The aorta (anterior) and the pulmonary artery (posterior) have been transected to allow visualization of the left and right coronary arteries. The coronaries have been excised from their respective sinuses, including a large flap (button) of arterial wall. Equivalent segments of the wall of the pulmonary artery (which will become the neoaorta) are also removed. *B,* The aortocoronary buttons are sutured into the proximal portion of the neoaorta. With this technique all sutures are placed in the button of aortic wall rather than directly on the coronary arteries. *C,* Completed anastomosis of the left and right coronary arteries to the neoaorta. (Adapted from Castañeda AR, Jonas RA, Mayer JE Jr, Hanley FL: *Cardiac Surgery of the Neonate and Infant.* Philadelphia, WB Saunders, 1994.)

VSD closure. The arterial switch operation can be safely performed after the 1st 2 wk of life because the VSD results in equal pressure in both ventricles and prevents regression of left ventricular muscle mass.

Without treatment, the *prognosis* is poor; most patients succumb in the 1st yr of life because of heart failure, hypoxemia, and pulmonary hypertension. In the past, some survived infancy with medical therapy alone, but pulmonary vascular disease often developed. The clinical picture and treatment of these patients are similar to those described with Eisenmenger syndrome secondary to an isolated large VSD (see Chapter 426.2).

424.4 l-Transposition of the Great Arteries (Corrected Transposition)

In l-transposition, the atrioventricular relationships are discordant, with the right atrium connected to the left ventricle and the left atrium to the right ventricle *(ventricular inversion).* The great arteries are also transposed, with the aorta arising from the right ventricle and the pulmonary artery from the left. The aorta arises to the left of the pulmonary artery (hence the designation "l" for levotransposition). The aorta may be anterior to the pulmonary artery; usually, they are nearly side by side. Desaturated systemic venous blood is returned to a normally positioned right atrium, from which it passes through a bicuspid atrioventricular (mitral) valve into a right-sided ventricle that has the architecture and smooth wall morphologic features of the normal left ventricle (Fig. 424–4). Because transposition is also present, desaturated blood ejected from this left ventricle enters the transposed pulmonary artery and flows into the lungs. Oxygenated pulmonary venous blood returns to a normally

positioned left atrium, passes through a tricuspid atrioventricular valve into a left-sided ventricle, which has the trabeculated morphologic features of a normal right ventricle, and is then ejected into the transposed aorta. The double inversion of the atrioventricular and ventriculoarterial relationships results in desaturated right atrial blood reaching the lungs and oxygenated pulmonary venous blood appropriately flowing to the aorta. The circulation is physiologically "corrected." Without other defects, the hemodynamics would be nearly normal. However, in most patients, associated anomalies coexist: VSD, Ebstein-like abnormalities of the left-sided atrioventricular (tricuspid) valve, pulmonary valvular or subvalvular stenosis (or both), and atrioventricular conduction disturbances (complete heart block).

Clinical Manifestations. Symptoms and signs are widely variable and are determined by the associated lesions. If pulmonary outflow is unobstructed, the clinical signs are similar to those of an isolated VSD. If the TGA is associated with pulmonary stenosis and a VSD, the clinical signs are similar to those of tetralogy of Fallot.

Diagnosis. The *chest roentgenogram* may suggest the abnormal position of the great arteries; the ascending aorta occupies the upper left border of the cardiac silhouette and has a straight profile. In addition to atrioventricular conduction disturbances, the *electrocardiogram* may show abnormal P waves; absent Q waves in V_6; abnormally present Q waves in leads III, aVR, aVF, and V_1; and upright T waves across the precordium.

Surgical treatment of the associated anomalies, most often the VSD, is complicated by the position of the bundle of His, which can be injured at the time of surgery and result in heart block. Identification of the usual course of the bundle in corrected transposition (running superior to the defect) has been

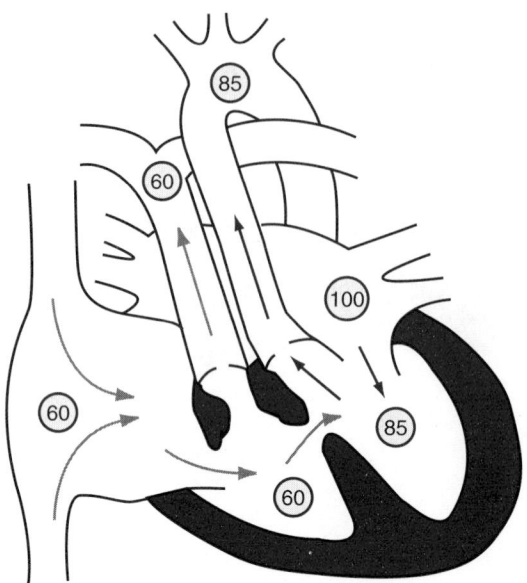

FIGURE 424–4. Physiology of l- or corrected transposition of the great arteries (l-TGA) with a ventricular septal defect and pulmonic stenosis (VSD + PS). *Circled numbers* represent oxygen saturation values. Right atrial (mixed venous) oxygen saturation is decreased secondary to systemic hypoxemia. Blood from the right atrium flows through the mitral valve into the "inverted" left ventricle. However, the left ventricle is attached to the transposed pulmonary artery. Therefore, despite the anomalies, desaturated blood still winds up in the pulmonary circulation. Saturated blood returns to the left atrium, traverses the tricuspid valve into the "inverted" right ventricle, and is pumped into the transposed aorta. This circulation would be totally "corrected" were it not for the frequent association of other congenital anomalies, in this case, VSD + PS. Because of the stenotic pulmonary valve, some left ventricular blood flow crosses the VSD and into the right ventricle and the ascending aorta, and systemic desaturation results.

accomplished by mapping of the conduction system so that the surgeon can avoid the bundle of His during open heart repair.

424.5 Double-Outlet Right Ventricle Without Pulmonary Stenosis

In double-outlet right ventricle without pulmonary stenosis, both the aorta and the pulmonary artery arise from the right ventricle. The only outlet from the left ventricle is through a VSD. The *clinical manifestations* closely simulate those of an uncomplicated VSD with a large left-to-right shunt, although mild systemic desaturation may be present because of mixing of oxygenated and deoxygenated blood in the right ventricle. The *electrocardiogram* usually shows biventricular hypertrophy. *Echocardiography* is diagnostic and shows the right ventricular origin of both great vessels and their anteroposterior relationship, as well as the position of the VSD. *Cardiac catheterization* demonstrates the proximity of the VSD to the aorta, which results in most of the left ventricular blood being ejected directly into the systemic circulation. The angiogram also confirms the lack of mitral-aortic fibrous continuity and shows the aortic valve displaced superiorly and at the same level as the pulmonary valve. It is important to differentiate this condition from a simple VSD.

Surgical correction is accomplished by creation of an intracardiac tunnel. Blood is then ejected from the left ventricle via the VSD into the aorta. Pulmonary arterial banding may be required in infancy, followed by surgical correction when the child is bigger. When associated pulmonary stenosis is present, the cyanosis is more marked and pulmonary blood flow is decreased (see Chapter 423).

424.6 Double-Outlet Right Ventricle with Transposition of the Great Arteries (Taussig-Bing Anomaly)

In double-outlet right ventricle with TGA, the VSD is located above the crista supraventricularis (subarterial VSD) and is either directly subpulmonary or related to both the pulmonary and aortic valves (doubly committed VSD). Patients experience cardiac failure early in infancy and are at risk for the development of pulmonary vascular disease and cyanosis. Cardiomegaly is usual, and a parasternal systolic ejection murmur is audible, sometimes preceded by an ejection click and loud closure of the pulmonary valve. Left-sided obstructive lesions are frequent, including coarctation of the aorta, interruption of the aortic arch, and a restrictive VSD, which obstructs left ventricular ejection. The *electrocardiogram* shows right axis deviation and right, left, or biventricular hypertrophy. The *roentgenogram* documents cardiomegaly, a large left atrium, and prominence of the pulmonary artery and pulmonary vasculature. The anatomic features of the anomaly and associated abnormalities are best demonstrated by a combination of echocardiography and selective right and left ventriculography. Palliation may be achieved by pulmonary arterial banding in infancy and surgical correction at a later age, which may be accomplished by a Rastelli procedure (see Chapter 423) or by an arterial switch procedure (see Chapter 424.2).

424.7 Total Anomalous Pulmonary Venous Return

Pathophysiology. Abnormal development of the pulmonary veins may result in either partial or complete anomalous drainage into the systemic venous circulation. Partial anomalous pulmonary venous return is usually an acyanotic lesion (see Chapter 419.4). Total anomalous pulmonary venous return (TAPVR) allows total mixing of systemic venous and pulmonary venous blood flow within the heart and thus produces cyanosis.

In TAPVR, the heart has no direct pulmonary venous connection into the left atrium. The pulmonary veins may drain *above the diaphragm* into the right atrium directly, into the coronary sinus, or into the superior vena cava via a "vertical vein," or they may drain *below the diaphragm* and join into a "descending vein" that enters into the inferior vena cava or one of its major tributaries, often via the ductus venosus. This latter form of anomalous venous drainage is most commonly associated with obstruction, usually as the ductus venosus closes soon after birth, although supracardiac anomalous veins may also become obstructed. Occasionally, the drainage may be mixed, with some veins draining above and others below the diaphragm.

All forms of TAPVR involve mixing of oxygenated and deoxygenated blood before or at the level of the right atrium. Right atrial blood either passes into the right ventricle and pulmonary artery or passes through an atrial septal defect (ASD) or patent foramen ovale into the left atrium. The right atrium and ventricle and the pulmonary artery are generally enlarged, whereas the left atrium and ventricle may be normal or small. The manifestations of TAPVR depend on the presence or absence of obstruction of the venous channels (Table 424–1). If pulmonary venous return is obstructed, severe pulmonary congestion and pulmonary hypertension develop; rapid deterioration occurs

TABLE 424–1. Anomalous Pulmonary Venous Return

% and Site of Connection	% with Severe Obstruction
Supracardiac (50)	
Left superior vena cava (40)	40
Right superior vena cava (10)	75
Cardiac (25)	
Coronary sinus (20)	10
Right atrium (5)	5
Infracardiac (20)	95–100
Mixed (5)	

without surgical intervention. Obstructed TAPVR is a pediatric cardiac surgical emergency because prostaglandin therapy may not be helpful.

Clinical Manifestations. Three major clinical patterns of TAPVR are seen. Some are manifested in the neonatal period as severe obstruction to pulmonary venous return, most prevalent in the infracardiac group (see Table 424–1). Cyanosis and severe tachypnea are prominent, but murmurs may not be present. Infants are severely ill and fail to respond to mechanical ventilation. Rapid diagnosis and surgical correction are necessary for survival. Another group is characterized by heart failure in early life, but these infants have only mild or moderate obstruction to pulmonary venous return and a large left-to-right shunt. Because pulmonary artery hypertension is present, these infants are severely ill. Systolic murmurs are audible along the left sternal border, and a gallop rhythm may be present. A continuous murmur is occasionally heard along the upper left sternal border over the pulmonary area. Cyanosis is mild. The third group of patients with TAPVR consists of those in whom pulmonary venous obstruction is not present; these patients have total mixing of systemic venous and pulmonary venous blood and a large left-to-right shunt. Pulmonary hypertension is absent, and these patients are less likely to be severely symptomatic during infancy. Clinical cyanosis is usually mild or absent.

Diagnosis. The *electrocardiogram* demonstrates right ventricular hypertrophy (usually a qR pattern in V_3R and V_1, and the P waves are frequently tall and spiked). *Roentgenograms* are

pathognomonic in older children if the anomalous pulmonary veins enter the innominate vein and persistent left superior vena cava (Fig. 424–5). A large supracardiac shadow can be seen, which together with the normal cardiac shadow forms a "snowman" appearance. This appearance is not helpful for diagnosis in early infancy because of the thymus. In most cases without obstruction, the heart is enlarged, the pulmonary artery and right ventricle are prominent, and pulmonary vascularity is increased. In neonates with marked pulmonary venous obstruction, the chest roentgenogram demonstrates a perihilar pattern of pulmonary edema and a small heart. This appearance can be confused with primary pulmonary disease. The differential diagnosis includes persistent pulmonary hypertension of the newborn, respiratory distress syndrome, pneumonia (bacterial, meconium aspiration), pulmonary lymphangiectasia, and other heart defects (hypoplastic left heart syndrome).

The *echocardiogram* demonstrates a large right ventricle and usually identifies the pattern of abnormal pulmonary venous connections. The demonstration of a vessel in the abdomen with Doppler venous flow away from the heart is pathognomonic of TAPVR below the diaphragm. Shunting occurs almost exclusively from right to left at the atrial level.

Cardiac catheterization shows that the oxygen saturation of blood in both atria, both ventricles, and the aorta is more or less similar, indicative of a *total mixing lesion*. An increase in systemic venous saturation occurs at the site of entry of the abnormal pulmonary venous channel. In older patients, pulmonary arterial and right ventricular pressure may be only moderately elevated, but in infants with pulmonary venous obstruction, pulmonary hypertension is usual. *Selective pulmonary arteriography* shows the anatomy of the pulmonary veins and their point of entry into the systemic venous circulation. MRI and CT may be alternative methods of confirming the diagnosis.

Treatment. Surgical correction of TAPVR is indicated during infancy. Before surgery, infants may be stabilized with prostaglandin E_1 to dilate the ductus venosus and the ductus arteriosus. Some may require balloon atrial septostomy, but it is of little or no benefit in the presence of pulmonary venous obstruction. Surgically, the common pulmonary venous trunk is anastomosed directly to the left atrium, the ASD is closed, and the

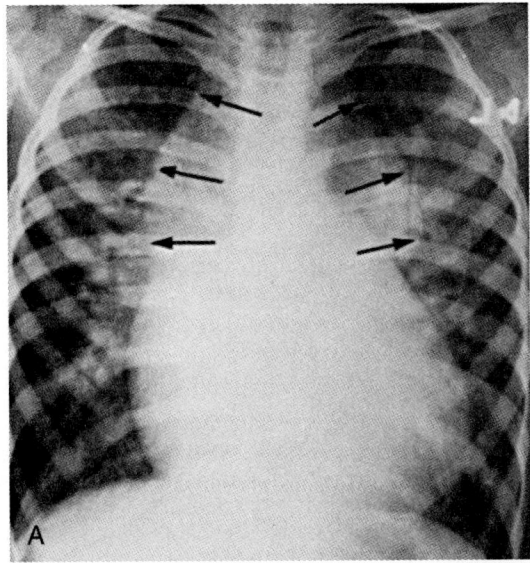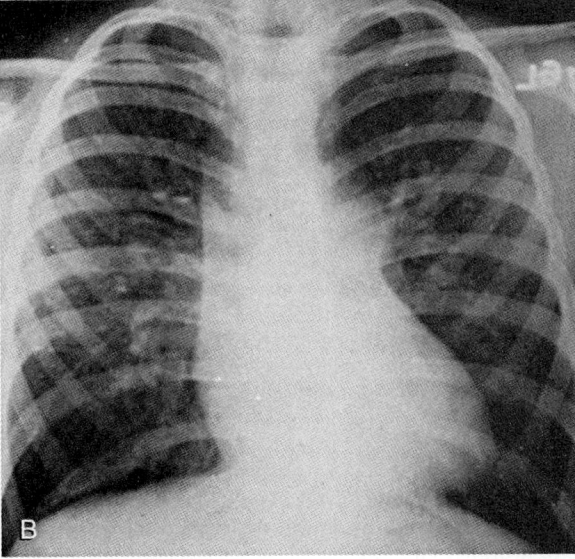

FIGURE 424–5. Roentgenograms of total anomalous pulmonary venous return to the left superior vena cava. *A*, Preoperative image. *Arrows* point to the supracardiac shadow, which produces the snowman or figure 8 configuration. Cardiomegaly and increased pulmonary vascularity are evident. *B*, Postoperative image showing a decrease in the size of the heart and the supracardiac shadow.

connection to the systemic venous circuit is interrupted. Results have been generally good, even for critically ill neonates. If post-operative hemodynamics are normal, the prognosis is excellent. The postoperative period may be complicated by pulmonary vascular hypertensive crises. In some patients, especially those in whom the diagnosis was delayed, persistent pulmonary hypertension may occur, and the long-term prognosis in these patients is poor. Inhaled nitric oxide or extracorporeal membrane oxygenation may be necessary. Long-term complications include re-stenosis of the pulmonary venous channel–to–left atrial communication. In patients with stenosis or hypoplasia of the individual pulmonary veins, the prognosis is poor.

424.8 Truncus Arteriosus

Pathophysiology. In truncus arteriosus, a single arterial trunk (truncus arteriosus) arises from the heart and supplies the systemic, pulmonary, and coronary circulations. A VSD is always present, with the truncus overriding the defect and receiving blood from both the right and left ventricles (Fig. 424–6). The number of truncal valve cusps varies from two to as many as six. The pulmonary arteries may arise together from the posterior left side of the persistent truncus arteriosus and then divide into left and right pulmonary arteries (type I truncus arteriosus). In types II and III truncus arteriosus, no main pulmonary artery is present, and the right and left pulmonary arteries arise from separate orifices in the posterior (type II) or lateral (type III) aspects of the truncus arteriosus. Type IV truncus has no identifiable connection between the heart and pulmonary arteries, and pulmonary blood flow is derived from *major aortopulmonary*

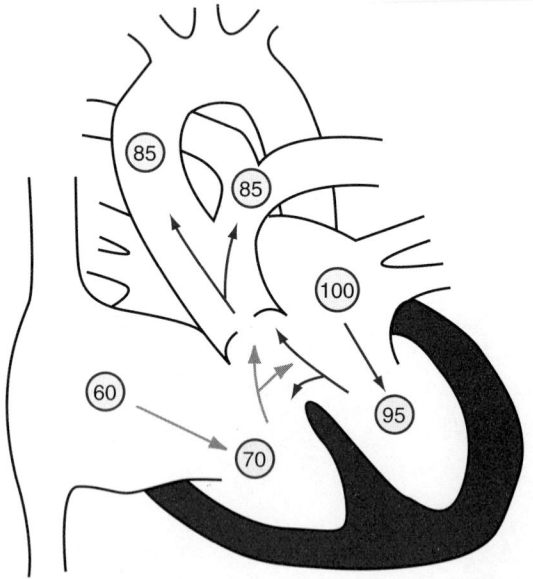

FIGURE 424–6. Physiology of truncus arteriosus. *Circled numbers* represent oxygen saturation values. Right atrial (mixed venous) oxygen saturation is decreased secondary to systemic hypoxemia. Desaturated blood enters the right atrium, flows through the tricuspid valve into the right ventricle, and is ejected into the truncus. Saturated blood returning from the left atrium enters the left ventricle and is also ejected into the truncus. The common aortopulmonary trunk gives rise to the ascending aorta and to the main or branch pulmonary arteries. Oxygen saturation in the aorta and pulmonary arteries is usually the same (definition of a total mixing lesion). As pulmonary vascular resistance decreases over the 1st few weeks of life, pulmonary blood flow increases dramatically and mild cyanosis and congestive heart failure result.

collateral arteries arising from the transverse or descending aorta; this form has also been called *pseudotruncus* but is essentially a form of pulmonary atresia with a VSD (see Chapter 423.2).

Both ventricles are at systemic pressure and both eject blood into the truncus. When pulmonary vascular resistance is relatively high immediately after birth, pulmonary blood flow may be normal; as pulmonary resistance drops over the 1st mo of life, blood flow to the lungs is greatly increased and heart failure ensues. Truncus arteriosus is a *total mixing lesion* with total admixture of pulmonary and systemic venous return. Because of the large volume of pulmonary blood flow, clinical cyanosis is usually minimal. If the lesion is left untreated, pulmonary resistance eventually increases, pulmonary blood flow decreases, and cyanosis becomes more apparent (Eisenmenger physiology; see Chapter 426.2). The truncal valve is occasionally incompetent, which significantly complicates medical and surgical management.

Clinical Manifestations. The clinical signs of truncus arteriosus vary with age and depend on the level of pulmonary vascular resistance. In the immediate newborn period, signs of heart failure are usually absent; a murmur and minimal cyanosis are the initial signs. In most older infants, pulmonary blood flow is torrential and the clinical picture is dominated by heart failure. Cyanosis is minimal. Runoff of blood from the truncus to the pulmonary circulation may result in a wide pulse pressure and bounding pulses. These findings may be further exaggerated if truncal valve insufficiency is present. The heart is usually enlarged, and the precordium is hyperdynamic. The 2nd heart sound is loud and single. A systolic ejection murmur, sometimes accompanied by a thrill, is generally audible along the left sternal border. The murmur is frequently preceded by an early systolic ejection click. In the presence of truncal valve insufficiency, a high-pitched early diastolic decrescendo murmur is heard at the midleft sternal border. An apical mid-diastolic rumbling murmur caused by increased flow through the mitral valve is audible with the bell of the stethoscope. In older children with restricted pulmonary blood flow secondary to pulmonary vascular obstructive disease, progressive cyanosis, polycythemia, and clubbing develop. Truncus arteriosus may be associated with DiGeorge syndrome (Chapter 115.1).

Diagnosis. The *electrocardiogram* shows right, left, or combined ventricular hypertrophy. The *chest roentgenogram* also shows considerable variation. The cardiac enlargement is due to prominence of both ventricles. The truncus may produce a prominent shadow that follows the normal course of the ascending aorta and aortic knob; the aortic arch is to the right in 50% of patients. Sometimes a high bulge left of the aortic knob is produced by the main or left pulmonary artery. Pulmonary vascularity is increased . after the 1st few weeks of life. *Echocardiography* demonstrates the large truncal artery overriding the VSD and the pattern of origin of the branch pulmonary arteries. Associated anomalies such as an interrupted aortic arch may be noted. Pulsed and color Doppler studies are used to evaluate truncal valve regurgitation. If required, *cardiac catheterization* shows a left-to-right shunt at the ventricular level, with right-to-left shunting into the truncus. Systolic pressure in both ventricles and the truncus is similar. Angiography reveals the large truncus arteriosus and more precisely defines the origin of the pulmonary arteries.

Prognosis and Complications. Without surgery, many of these patients succumb during infancy or by the 1st or 2nd yr of life. If pulmonary blood flow is restricted by the development of pulmonary vascular disease, the patient may survive into early adulthood. Starting in the late 1970s, surgical results have been very good, and many patients with repaired truncus are entering young adulthood. As a conotruncal lesion, truncus arteriosus is often associated with a deletion of chromosome 22q11 (CATCH

22, DiGeorge syndrome) and associated endocrine, immunologic, facial, and pulmonary abnormalities.

Treatment. In the 1st few weeks of life, many of these infants can be managed with anticongestive medications; however, as pulmonary vascular resistance falls, heart failure symptoms worsen and surgery is indicated, usually in the 1st few weeks of life. Delay of surgery much beyond 4–8 wk may increase the likelihood of pulmonary vascular disease; some centers advocate neonatal repair at the time of diagnosis. At surgery, the VSD is closed, the pulmonary arteries are separated from the truncus, and continuity is established between the right ventricle and the pulmonary arteries with a homograft conduit (Rastelli repair). Immediate surgical results are excellent, but after repair the conduit must be replaced, often several times, as the child grows. In older patients who already have pulmonary vascular obstruction, routine surgical treatment is contraindicated and heart-lung transplantation is the only option.

424.9 Single Ventricle (Double-Inlet Ventricle, Univentricular Heart)

Pathophysiology. With a single ventricle, both atria empty through a common atrioventricular valve or via two separate valves into a single ventricular chamber, with *total mixing* of systemic and pulmonary venous return. This chamber may have left, right, or indeterminate ventricular anatomic characteristics. The aorta and pulmonary artery both arise from this single chamber, although one of the great vessels may originate from a rudimentary outflow chamber. The aorta may be posterior, anterior *(malposition)*, or side by side with the pulmonary artery and either to the right or to the left. Pulmonary stenosis or atresia is common.

Clinical Manifestations. The clinical picture is variable and depends on the associated intracardiac anomalies. If pulmonary outflow is obstructed, the findings may be similar to those of tetralogy of Fallot: marked cyanosis without heart failure. If pulmonary outflow is unobstructed, the findings are similar to those of transposition with VSD: minimal cyanosis with marked heart failure.

In patients with pulmonary stenosis, cyanosis is present in infancy and increases in intensity during childhood, when clubbing and polycythemia appear. Dyspnea and fatigue are frequent, cardiomegaly is mild or moderate, a left parasternal lift is palpable, and a systolic thrill is common. The systolic ejection murmur is usually loud; an ejection click may be audible, and the 2nd heart sound is single and loud.

Patients with unobstructed pulmonary outflow have torrential pulmonary blood flow and are initially seen in early infancy with tachypnea, dyspnea, failure to thrive, and recurrent pulmonary infections. Cyanosis is only mild or moderate. Cardiomegaly is generally marked, and a left parasternal lift is palpable. The systolic ejection murmur is not usually intense, and the 2nd heart sound is loud and closely split. A 3rd heart sound is common and may be followed by a short mid-diastolic rumbling murmur caused by increased flow through the atrioventricular valves. The eventual development of pulmonary vascular disease reduces pulmonary blood flow so that the cyanosis increases and signs of cardiac failure appear to improve (Eisenmenger physiology; see Chapter 426.2).

Diagnosis. Findings on the *electrocardiogram* are nonspecific. P waves are normal, spiked, or bifid. The precordial lead pattern suggests right ventricular hypertrophy, combined ventricular hypertrophy, or sometimes left ventricular dominance. The initial QRS forces are usually to the left and anterior. *Roentgenographic examination* confirms the degree of cardiomegaly. If present, a rudimentary outflow chamber may produce a bulge on the upper left border of the cardiac silhouette in the posteroanterior projection. In the absence of pulmonary stenosis, pulmonary vasculature is increased, whereas in the presence of pulmonary stenosis, pulmonary vasculature is diminished. Absence or near absence of the ventricular septum is the principal *echocardiographic* sign. The echocardiogram can usually determine whether the single ventricle has right, left, or mixed morphologic features. The presence of a rudimentary outflow chamber under one of the great vessels can be identified, and pulsed Doppler can be used to determine whether flow through this communication *(bulboventricular foramen)* is obstructed.

If *cardiac catheterization* is performed, arterial oxygen saturation is seen to be decreased in the presence of severe pulmonary stenosis or obstructive pulmonary hypertension, but it may be near normal when pulmonary blood flow is unimpeded. The pressure in the ventricular chamber is at systemic level; a gradient may be demonstrated across the entrance to a rudimentary outflow chamber. Pressure measurements and angiography demonstrate whether pulmonary stenosis is present. Severe pulmonary hypertension may be demonstrated in older patients in the absence of pulmonary stenosis.

Prognosis and Complications. Unoperated, some patients succumb during infancy from heart failure. Others may survive to adolescence and early adult life but finally succumb to the effects of chronic hypoxemia or, in the absence of pulmonary stenosis, to the effects of pulmonary vascular disease. Patients with moderate pulmonary stenosis have the best prognosis because pulmonary blood flow, though restricted, is still adequate.

Treatment. If pulmonary stenosis is severe, an aortopulmonary shunt is indicated. If pulmonary blood flow is unrestricted, pulmonary arterial banding is used to control heart failure and prevent progressive pulmonary vascular disease. The *Glenn shunt* followed by a modified *Fontan* operation (cavopulmonary isolation procedure, see Chapter 423.4) is the ultimate treatment of choice. If subaortic stenosis is present because of a restrictive connection to a rudimentary outflow chamber, surgical relief can be provided by anastomosing the proximal pulmonary artery to the side of the ascending aorta *(Damus-Stansyl-Kaye operation)*.

424.10 Hypoplastic Left Heart Syndrome

Pathophysiology. The term *hypoplastic left heart* is used to describe a related group of anomalies that include underdevelopment of the left side of the heart (e.g., atresia of the aortic or mitral orifice) and hypoplasia of the ascending aorta. The left ventricle may be small and nonfunctional or totally atretic; the right ventricle maintains both the pulmonary and systemic circulation (Fig. 424–7). Pulmonary venous blood passes through an atrial defect or dilated foramen ovale from the left to the right side of the heart, where it mixes with systemic venous blood *(total mixing lesion)*. When the ventricular septum is intact, which is usually the case, all the right ventricular blood is ejected into the main pulmonary artery; the descending aorta is supplied via the ductus arteriosus, with flow from the ductus also filling the ascending aorta and coronary arteries in a retrograde fashion. In the presence of a VSD and a patent but small aortic orifice, right ventricular blood is ejected into the small left ventricle and ascending aorta, as well as the pulmonary artery. The major hemodynamic abnormalities are inadequate maintenance of the systemic circulation and, depending on the size of the atrial-level communication, either pulmonary venous hypertension (restrictive foramen ovale) or pulmonary overcirculation (moderate or large ASD).

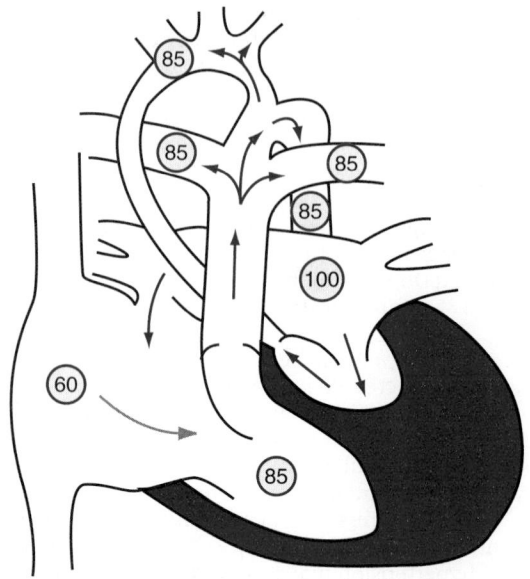

FIGURE 424–7. Physiology of hypoplastic left heart syndrome (HLHS). *Circled numbers* represent oxygen saturation values. HLHS is not a single lesion but a constellation of different degrees of hypoplasia of the left-sided heart structures. This drawing shows a patent mitral valve, a small left ventricular cavity, and a diminutive ascending aorta. Right atrial (mixed venous) oxygen saturation is decreased secondary to systemic hypoxemia. Desaturated blood enters the right atrium, flows through the tricuspid valve into the right ventricle, and is ejected into the pulmonary artery. Because of the markedly decreased left ventricular compliance, most of the pulmonary venous blood returning to the left atrium shunts left to right at the atrial level. A small amount of left atrial blood will cross the mitral valve and be ejected into the tiny ascending aorta. The right ventricular oxygen saturation represents a mixing of desaturated systemic venous blood and saturated pulmonary venous blood. Pulmonary artery blood flows into the pulmonary arteries as well as right to left across the patent ductus arteriosus (PDA) into the aorta. Ductal blood flows prograde to the descending aorta as well as retrograde to the ascending aorta, where it supplies the head and neck vessels in addition to the coronary arteries (which arise off the small ascending aorta). Closure of the PDA results in profound hypoxia and circulatory collapse.

Clinical Manifestations. Although cyanosis may not always be obvious in the 1st 48 hr of life, a grayish blue color of the skin is soon apparent and denotes a mix of cyanosis and hypoperfusion. The condition is diagnosed in most infants in the 1st few hours or days of life. If the ductus arteriosus partially closes, signs of systemic hypoperfusion and shock predominate. Signs of heart failure usually appear within the 1st few days or weeks of life and include dyspnea, hepatomegaly, and low cardiac output. The peripheral pulses may be weak or absent. Cardiac enlargement is usual, with a palpable right ventricular parasternal lift. A nondescript systolic murmur is generally audible. Extracardiac anomalies, particularly of the kidneys and central nervous system, may be present.

Diagnosis. On the *chest roentgenogram*, the heart is variable in size in the 1st days of life, but cardiomegaly develops rapidly and is associated with increased pulmonary vascularity. The initial *electrocardiogram* may show only the normal right ventricular dominance with poor ventricular voltage, but later, P waves become prominent and right ventricular hypertrophy is usual. The *echocardiogram* is diagnostic and demonstrates

absence or hypoplasia of the mitral valve and aortic root, a variably small left atrium and left ventricle, and a large right atrium and right ventricle. The size of the atrial communication by which pulmonary venous blood leaves the left atrium can be assessed directly and by pulsed and color flow Doppler studies. Suprasternal notch views identify the small ascending aorta and transverse aortic arch and may also show a discrete coarctation of the aorta in the juxtaductal area. Doppler echocardiography demonstrates the absence of anterograde flow in the ascending aorta and retrograde flow via the ductus arteriosus. These findings are so characteristic that the diagnosis of hypoplastic left heart syndrome can usually be made without any need for *cardiac catheterization*. If catheterization is necessary, the hypoplastic ascending aorta can be demonstrated by angiography.

Prognosis and Complications. Patients most often succumb during the 1st months of life, usually during the 1st wk or two. Occasionally, unoperated patients may live for months or rarely years. One third of infants with hypoplastic left heart syndrome have evidence of either a major or minor central nervous system abnormality. Other dysmorphic features may be found in up to 40% of patients. Thus, careful preoperative evaluation (genetic, neurologic, and ophthalmologic) should be performed in patients being considered for either standard surgical therapy or cardiac transplantation.

Treatment. Surgical therapy for hypoplastic left heart syndrome has been associated with survival rates of 80–90% for the first-stage Norwood operation in many centers. Management options include palliation (the Norwood procedure; Fig. 424–8), heart transplantation, and in very few patients, supportive expectant care. Considerable controversy has arisen regarding which of the two surgical options is optimal, as well as concern over whether a "do nothing" option should be offered to parents given the good surgical results.

If a **Norwood procedure** is to be performed, preoperative medical management includes correction of acidosis and hypoglycemia, maintenance of ductus arteriosus patency with prostaglandin E_1 to support systemic blood flow, and prevention of hypothermia. Preoperative management should avoid excessive pulmonary blood flow; often, patients are managed on room air or with a F_{IO_2} of 18% with nitrogen gas blended into the oxygen source. Balloon dilatation of the atrial septum may be indicated if surgery is delayed.

The Norwood procedure is usually performed in three stages. The first stage (see Fig. 424–8) includes an atrial septectomy and transection and ligation of the distal main pulmonary artery; the proximal pulmonary artery is then connected to the transversely opened hypoplastic aortic arch to form a neoaorta, and the coarcted segment of the aorta is repaired. A synthetic aortopulmonary shunt connects the aorta to the main pulmonary artery to provide controlled pulmonary blood flow. The operative risk for the first-stage Norwood procedure is high and varies greatly among centers, although the best reported results demonstrate a better than 85–90% survival rate.

The second stage consists of a Glenn anastomosis to connect the superior vena cava to the pulmonary arteries (see Chapter 423.4), followed by a modified Fontan procedure (cavopulmonary isolation) to connect the inferior vena cava to the pulmonary arteries via either an intra-atrial or external baffle. After the third stage, all systemic venous return enters the pulmonary circulation directly. Pulmonary venous flow enters the left atrium and is directed across the atrial septum to the tricuspid valve and subsequently to the right (now the systemic) ventricle. Blood leaves the right ventricle via the neoaorta, which supplies the systemic circulation. The old aortic root now attached to the neoaorta provides coronary blood flow. The risks associated with stages II and III are considerably less than those of

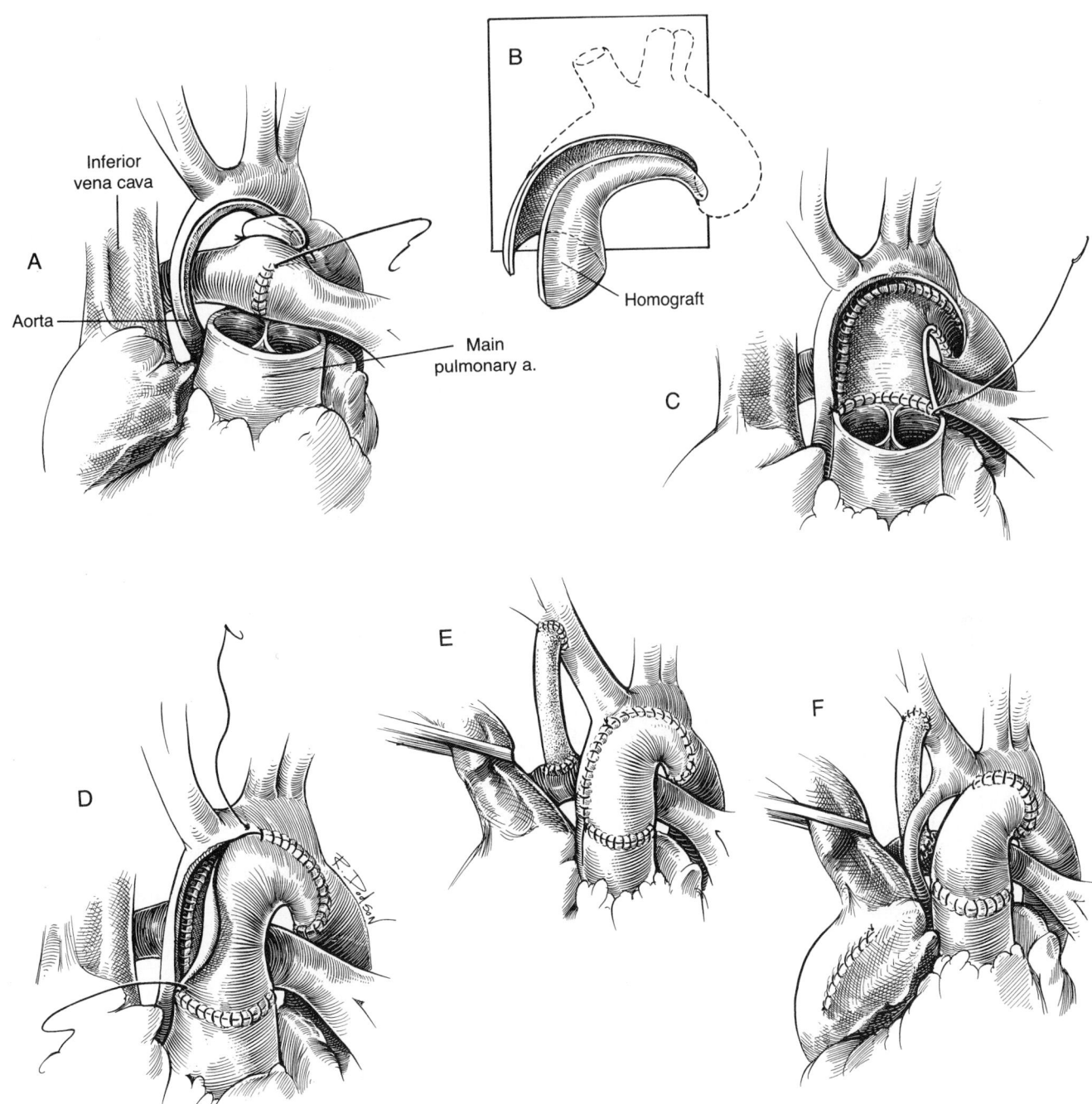

FIGURE 424–8. Current technique for first-stage palliation of hypoplastic left heart syndrome. *A,* Incisions used for the procedure incorporate a cuff of arterial wall allograft. The distal divided main pulmonary artery may be closed by direct suture or with a patch. *B,* Dimensions of the cuff of the arterial wall allograft. *C,* The arterial wall allograft is used to supplement the anastomosis between the proximal divided main pulmonary artery and the ascending aorta, aortic arch, and proximal descending aorta. *D* and *E,* The procedure is completed by an atrial septectomy and a 3.5 mm modified right Blalock shunt. *F,* When the ascending aorta is particularly small, an alternative procedure involves placement of a complete tube of arterial allograft. The tiny ascending aorta may be left in situ, as indicated, or implanted into the side of the neoaorta. (From Castañeda AR, Jonas RA, Mayer JE Jr, Hanley FL: Single-ventricle tricuspid atresia. In *Cardiac Surgery of the Neonate and Infant.* Philadelphia, WB Saunders, 1994.)

stage I; the long-term results of the Norwood procedure remain to be demonstrated.

An alternative therapy is *cardiac transplantation,* either in the immediate neonatal period, thereby obviating stage I of the Norwood procedure, or after a successful stage I Norwood procedure is performed as a bridge to transplantation. After transplantation, patients usually have normal cardiac function and no symptoms of heart failure; however, these patients have the chronic risk of organ rejection and lifelong immunosuppressive therapy (see Chapter 435.1). The combination of donor shortage and good results with the Norwood procedure has caused many centers to stop recommending transplantation except when associated lesions make the Norwood operation an exceptionally high-risk procedure.

424.11 Abnormal Positions of the Heart and the Heterotaxy Syndromes (Asplenia, Polysplenia)

Classification and diagnosis of abnormal cardiac position are best performed via a segmental approach, with the position of the viscera and atria first identified, then the ventricles, followed by the great vessels. Determination of *visceroatrial situs* can be made by roentgenographic demonstration of the position of the abdominal organs and the tracheal bifurcation for recognition of the right and left bronchi and by *echocardiography*. The atrial situs is related to the situs of the viscera and lungs. In **situs solitus**, the viscera are in their normal positions (stomach and spleen on the left, liver on the right), the three-lobed right lung is on the right, and the two-lobed left lung on the left; the right atrium is on the right, whereas the left atrium is on the left. When the abdominal organs and lungs are reversed, an arrangement known as **situs inversus**, the left atrium is on the right and the right atrium on the left. If the visceroatrial situs cannot be readily determined, a condition known as **situs indeterminus** or **heterotaxia** exists. The two major variations are (1) **asplenia syndrome** (right isomerism or bilateral right-sidedness), which is associated with a centrally located liver, absent spleen, and two morphologic right lungs, and (2) **polysplenia syndrome** (left isomerism or bilateral left-sidedness), which is associated with multiple small spleens, absence of the intrahepatic portion of the inferior vena cava, and bilateral left lung morphology (i.e., in both lungs). The heterotaxia syndromes are usually associated with severe congenital heart lesions: ASD, VSD, atrioventricular septal defect, pulmonary stenosis or atresia, and anomalous systemic venous or pulmonary venous return (Table 424–2).

The next segment is *localization of the ventricles,* which depends on the direction of development of the embryonic cardiac loop. Initial protrusion of the loop to the right (**d-loop**) carries the future right ventricle to the right, whereas the left ventricle remains on the left. With situs solitus, this arrangement yields normal atrioventricular connections (right atrium connecting to the right ventricle, left atrium to the left ventricle). Protrusion of the loop to the left (**l-loop**) carries the future right ventricle to the left and the left ventricle to the right. In this case, in the presence of situs solitus, the right atrium connects with the left ventricle and the left atrium with the right ventricle (**ventricular inversion**).

The final segment is that of the *great vessels.* With each type of cardiac loop, the ventricular-arterial relationships may be regarded as either normal (right ventricle to the pulmonary artery, left ventricle to the aorta) or transposed (right ventricle to the aorta, left ventricle to the pulmonary artery). A further classification can be based on the position of the aorta (normally to the right and posterior) relative to the pulmonary artery. In transposition, the aorta is usually anterior and either to the right of the pulmonary artery (**d-transposition**) or to the left (**l-transposition**). These segmental relationships can be determined by *echocardiographic* and *angiographic* studies demonstrating both atrioventricular and ventriculoarterial relationships. The clinical manifestations of these syndromes of abnormal cardiac position are determined primarily by their associated cardiovascular anomalies.

Dextrocardia occurs when the heart is in the right side of the chest; **levocardia** (the normal situation) is present when the heart is in the left side of the chest. *Dextrocardia without associated situs inversus* and *levocardia in the presence of situs inversus* are most often complicated by severe malformations that include various combinations of single ventricle, arterial transposition, pulmonary stenosis, ASDs and VSDs, atrioventricular septal defect, anomalous pulmonary venous return, tricuspid atresia, and pulmonary arterial hypoplasia or atresia. Surveys of older children and adults indicate that dextrocardia with situs inversus and normally related great arteries (so-called *mirror-image dextrocardia*) is often associated with a functionally normal heart, although congenital heart disease of a less severe nature is common.

Anatomic or functional abnormalities of the lungs, diaphragm, and thoracic cage may result in displacement of the heart to the right (**dextroposition**). However, in this case the *cardiac apex* is pointed normally to the left. This anatomic position is less often associated with congenital heart lesions, although hypoplasia of a lung may be accompanied by anomalous pulmonary venous return from that lung (scimitar syndrome).

The *electrocardiogram* is difficult to interpret in the presence of lesions with discordant atrial, ventricular, and great vessel anatomy. Diagnosis usually requires detailed *echocardiographic* and *cardiac catheterization* studies. The prognosis and treatment of patients with one of the cardiac positional anomalies are determined by the underlying defects. Asplenia increases the

TABLE 424–2. Comparison of Cardiosplenic Heterotaxy Syndromes

Feature	Asplenia (Right Isomerism)	Polysplenia (Left Isomerism)
Spleen	Absent	Multiple
Sidedness (isomerism)	Bilateral right	Bilateral left
Lungs	Bilateral trilobar with eparterial bronchi	Bilateral bilobar with hyparterial bronchi
Sex	Male (65%)	Female ≥ male
Right-sided stomach	Yes	Less common
Symmetric liver	Yes	Yes
Partial intestinal rotation	Yes	Yes
Dextrocardia (%)	30–40	30–40
Pulmonary blood flow	Decreased (usually)	Increased (usually)
Severe cyanosis	Yes	No
Transposition of great arteries (%)	60–75	15
Total anomalous pulmonary venous return (%)	70–80	Rare
Common atrioventricular valve (%)	80–90	20–40
Single ventricle (%)	40–50	10–15
Absent inferior vena cava with azygos continuation	No	Characteristic
Bilateral superior vena cava	Yes	Yes
Other common defects	PA, PS	Partial anomalous pulmonary venous return, ventricular septal defect, double-outlet right ventricle
Risk of sepsis	Yes	No
Howell-Jolly and Heinz bodies, pitted erythrocytes	Yes	No
Absent gallbladder; biliary atresia	No	Yes
Mortality	High	Moderately high if symptomatic

PA = pulmonary atresia; PS = pulmonary stenosis.

risk of serious infections such as bacterial sepsis and thus requires daily antibiotic prophylaxis. The risk of sudden death from arrhythmias after palliative surgery is also increased.

Transposition of the Great Arteries

Dearani JA, Danielson GK, Puga FJ, et al: Late results of the Rastelli operation for transposition of the great arteries. *Semin Thorac Cardiovasc Surg Pediatr Card Surg Annu* 2001;4:3–15.

Dunbar-Masterson C, Wypij D, Bellinger DC, et al: General health status of children with D-transposition of the great arteries after the arterial switch operation. *Circulation* 2001;104(12 Suppl 1):I138–42.

Hayes CJ, Gersony WM: Arrhythmias after the Mustard operation for transposition of the great arteries: A long-term study. *J Am Coll Cardiol* 1986;7:133.

Losay J, Touchot A, Serraf A, et al: Late outcome after arterial switch operation for transposition of the great arteries. *Circulation* 2001;104(12 Suppl 1):I121–6.

Pretre R, Tamisier D, Bonhoeffer P, et al: Results of the arterial switch operation in neonates with transposed great arteries. *Lancet* 2001;357:1826–30.

Wetter J, Belli E, Sinzobahamvya N, et al: Transposition of the great arteries associated with ventricular septal defect: Surgical results and long-term outcome. *Eur J Cardiothorac Surg* 2001;20:816–23.

Truncus Arteriosus

Reddy VM, Hanley F: Late results of repair of truncus arteriosus. *Semin Thorac Cardiovasc Surg Pediatr Card Surg Annu* 1998;1:139–46.

Reddy VM, McElhinney DB, Sagrado T, et al: Results of 102 cases of complete repair of congenital heart defects in patients weighing 700 to 2500 grams. *J Thorac Cardiovasc Surg* 1999;117:324–31.

Thompson LD, McElhinney DB, Reddy M, et al: Neonatal repair of truncus arteriosus: Continuing improvement in outcomes. *Ann Thorac Surg* 2001;72:391–5.

Wilson DI, Burn J, Scambler P, et al: DiGeorge syndrome: Part of CATCH 22. *J Med Genet* 1993;30:852.

Total Anomalous Pulmonary Venous Return

Choe YH, Lee HJ, Kim HS, et al: MRI of total anomalous pulmonary venous connections. *J Comput Assist Tomogr* 1994;18:243.

Duff DG, Nihill MR, McNamara DG: Infradiaphragmatic total anomalous pulmonary venous return. Review of clinical and pathological findings and results of operation in 28 cases. *Br Heart J* 1977;39:619.

Huhta J, Gutgesell HP, Nihill MR: Cross sectional echocardiographic diagnosis of total anomalous pulmonary venous connection. *Br Heart J* 1985;53:525.

Hypoplastic Left Heart Syndrome

Bove EL: Current status of staged reconstruction for hypoplastic left heart syndrome. *Pediatr Cardiol* 1998;19:308–15.

Chiavarelli M, Gundry SR, Razzouk AJ, et al: Cardiac transplantation for infants with hypoplastic left heart syndrome. *JAMA* 1993;270:2944.

Daebritz SH, Nollert GD, Zurakowski D, et al: Results of Norwood stage I operation: Comparison of hypoplastic left heart syndrome with other malformations. *J Thorac Cardiovasc Surg* 2000;119:358–67.

Forbess JM, Visconti KJ, Bellinger DC, et al: Neurodevelopmental outcomes in children after the Fontan operation. *Circulation* 2001;104(12 Suppl 1):I127–32.

Starnes VA, Griffin ML, Pitlick PT, et al: Current approach to hypoplastic left heart syndrome: Palliation, transplantation or both? *J Thorac Cardiovasc Surg* 1992;104:189.

Dextrocardia and Levocardia

Britz-Cunningham SH, Shah MM, Zuppan CW, et al: Mutation of the connexin 43 gap-junction gene in patients with heart malformations and defects of laterality. *N Engl J Med* 1995;332:1323.

Rose V, Izukawa T, Moes CAF: Syndromes of asplenia and polysplenia: A review of cardiac and non-cardiac malformations in 60 cases with special reference to diagnosis and prognosis. *Br Heart J* 1975;37:840.

Wa MH, Wang JK, Lue HC: Sudden death in patients with right isomerism (asplenism) after palliation. *J Pediatr* 2002;140:93–6.

Chapter 425

Other Congenital Heart and Vascular Malformations

425.1 Anomalies of the Aortic Arch

Right Aortic Arch. In this abnormality, the aorta curves to the right and, if it descends on the right side of the vertebral column, is usually associated with other cardiac malformations. It is found in 20% of cases of tetralogy of Fallot and is common in truncus arteriosus. A right aortic arch without other cardiac anomalies is not associated with symptoms. It can often be visu-

alized on the chest roentgenogram. The trachea is deviated to the left of the midline rather than to the right, as in the presence of a normal left arch. On a barium esophagogram, the esophagus is indented on its right border at the level of the aortic arch.

Vascular Rings. Congenital abnormalities of the aortic arch and its major branches result in the formation of vascular rings around the trachea and esophagus with varying degrees of compression. Common anomalies include (1) double aortic arch (Fig. 425–1A), (2) right aortic arch with a left ligamentum arteriosum, (3) anomalous innominate artery arising further to the left on the arch than usual, (4) anomalous left carotid artery arising further to the right than usual and passing anterior to the trachea, and (5) anomalous left pulmonary artery (vascular sling). In the latter anomaly, the abnormal vessel arises from an elongated main pulmonary artery or from the right pulmonary artery. It courses between and compresses the trachea and the esophagus. Associated congenital heart disease may be present in 5–50% of patients, depending on the vascular anomaly.

Clinical Manifestations. If the vascular ring produces compression of the trachea and esophagus, symptoms are frequently present during infancy. Chronic wheezing is exacerbated by crying, feeding, and flexion of the neck. Extension of the neck tends to relieve the noisy respiration. Vomiting is frequent. Affected infants may have a brassy cough, pneumonia, or sudden death from aspiration.

Diagnosis. Roentgenographic examination of the barium-filled esophagus (Fig. 425–2) and aortography identify the anomaly. An aberrant right subclavian artery is commonly seen but does not cause compression of the trachea. The diagnosis is confirmed by two-dimensional echocardiography, MRI, CT, or angiography during cardiac catheterization. Bronchoscopy may be used to determine the extent of airway narrowing.

Treatment. Surgery is advised for symptomatic patients who have roentgenographic evidence of tracheal compression. The anterior vessel is usually divided in patients with a double aortic arch (see Fig. 425–1B). Compression produced by a right aortic arch and left ligamentum arteriosum is relieved by division of the latter. Anomalous innominate or carotid arteries cannot be divided; the tracheal compression is usually relieved by attaching the adventitia of these vessels to the sternum. An anomalous left pulmonary artery is corrected during cardiopulmonary bypass by division at its origin and re-anastomosis to the main pulmonary artery after it has been brought in front of the trachea. Severe tracheomalacia may be present and require reconstruction of the trachea as well.

425.2 Anomalous Origin of the Coronary Arteries

ANOMALOUS ORIGIN OF THE LEFT CORONARY ARTERY FROM THE PULMONARY ARTERY

In anomalous origin of the left coronary artery from the pulmonary artery, the blood supply to the left ventricular myocardium is severely compromised. Soon after birth, as pulmonary arterial pressure falls, perfusion pressure to the left coronary artery becomes inadequate; myocardial ischemia, infarction, and fibrosis result. In some cases, interarterial collateral anastomoses develop between the right and left coronary arteries. Blood flow in the left coronary artery is then reversed, and it empties into the pulmonary artery, a condition known as the "myocardial steal" syndrome. The left ventricle becomes dilated, and performance is decreased. Mitral insufficiency is a frequent complication secondary to a dilated valve ring or infarction of a papillary muscle. Localized aneurysms may also

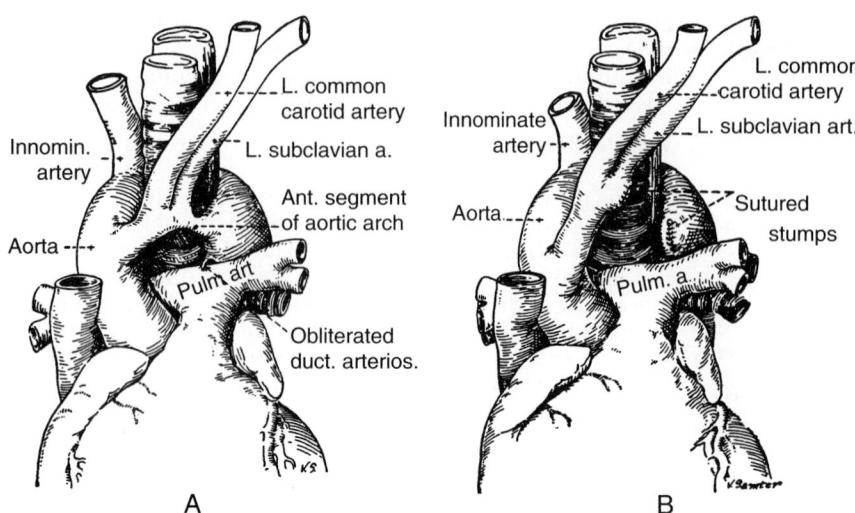

FIGURE 425–1. Double aortic arch. *A*, Small anterior segment of the double aortic arch (most common type). *B*, Operative procedure for release of the vascular ring.

develop in the left ventricular free wall. Occasional patients have adequate myocardial blood flow during childhood and, later in life, a continuous murmur and a small left-to-right shunt via the dilated coronary system (aorta to right coronary to left coronary to pulmonary artery).

Clinical Manifestations. Evidence of heart failure becomes apparent within the 1st few months of life, and it is often precipitated by respiratory infection. Recurrent attacks of discomfort, restlessness, irritability, sweating, dyspnea, and pallor with or without mild cyanosis occur and probably represent angina pectoris. Cardiac enlargement is moderate to massive. A gallop rhythm is common. If a gallop is present, murmurs may be of the nonspecific, ejection type or may be holosystolic and due to mitral insufficiency. Older patients with abundant intercoronary anastomoses may have continuous murmurs and minimal left ventricular dysfunction. During adolescence, they may experience angina during exercise. Rare patients with an anomalous right coronary artery may also have such clinical findings.

Diagnosis. *Roentgenographic examination* confirms the cardiomegaly. The *electrocardiogram* resembles the pattern described in lateral wall myocardial infarction in adults. A QR pattern followed by inverted T waves is seen in leads I and aVL. The left ventricular surface leads (V_5 and V_6) may also show deep Q waves and exhibit elevated ST segments and inverted T waves (Fig. 425–3). In older patients, an exercise study may be helpful as ST-T wave changes or symptoms occur. *Two-dimensional echocardiography* may suggest the diagnosis; echocardiography is not always reliable in diagnosing this condition. On two-dimensional imaging alone, the left coronary artery can appear as though it were arising from the aorta. Color Doppler ultrasound examination has improved the accuracy of diagnosis of this lesion and may demonstrate retrograde flow in the left coronary artery. *Cardiac catheterization* is diagnostic; *aortography* shows immediate opacification of the right coronary artery only. This vessel is large and tortuous. After filling of the intercoronary anastomoses, the left coronary artery is opacified, and contrast can be seen to enter the pulmonary artery. Pulmonary arteriography may also opacify the origin of the anomalous left coronary artery. Selective left ventriculography usually demonstrates a dilated left ventricle that empties poorly.

Treatment and Prognosis. Untreated, death often occurs from heart failure within the 1st 6 mo. Those who survive generally have abundant intercoronary collateral anastomoses. Medical management includes standard therapy for heart failure

(diuretics, digoxin, captopril) and for controlling ischemia (nitrates, β-blocking agents).

Surgical treatment consists of detaching the anomalous coronary artery from the pulmonary artery and anastomosing it to the aorta to establish normal myocardial perfusion. A seriously ill infant with a tiny left coronary artery may present a difficult technical problem. Ligation of the anomalous left coronary artery at its origin was once performed to prevent runoff from the coronary circuit and possibly to increase myocardial perfusion by the collateral circulation. This operation may occasionally be required. In patients who have already sustained a significant myocardial infarction, cardiac transplantation is another option.

ANOMALOUS ORIGIN OF THE RIGHT CORONARY ARTERY FROM THE PULMONARY ARTERY

Anomalous origin of the right coronary artery from the pulmonary artery is rarely manifested in infancy or early childhood. The left coronary artery is enlarged, whereas the right is thin walled and mildly enlarged. In early infancy, perfusion of the right coronary artery is from the pulmonary artery, whereas later, perfusion is from collaterals of the left coronary vessels. Angina and sudden death can occur in adolescence or adulthood. When recognized, this anomaly should be repaired by re-anastomosis of the right coronary artery to the aorta.

ECTOPIC ORIGIN OF THE CORONARY ARTERY FROM THE AORTA WITH ABERRANT PROXIMAL COURSE

In ectopic origin of the coronary artery from the aorta with an aberrant proximal course, the aberrant artery may be a left, right, or major branch coronary artery. The site of origin may be the wrong sinus of Valsalva or a proximal coronary artery. The ostium may be hypoplastic, slitlike, or of normal caliber. The aberrant vessel may pass anteriorly, posteriorly, or between the aorta and right ventricular outflow tract; it may tunnel in the conal or interventricular septal tissue. Obstruction resulting from hypoplasia of the ostia, tunneling between the aorta and right ventricular outflow tract or interventricular septum, and acute angulation produces focal myocardial fibrosis or myocardial infarction. Unobstructed vessels produce no symptoms. Patients with this extremely rare abnormality are often initially seen with severe myocardial infarction, ventricular arrhythmias, angina pectoris, or syncope; sudden death may occur in young adult or adolescent athletes.

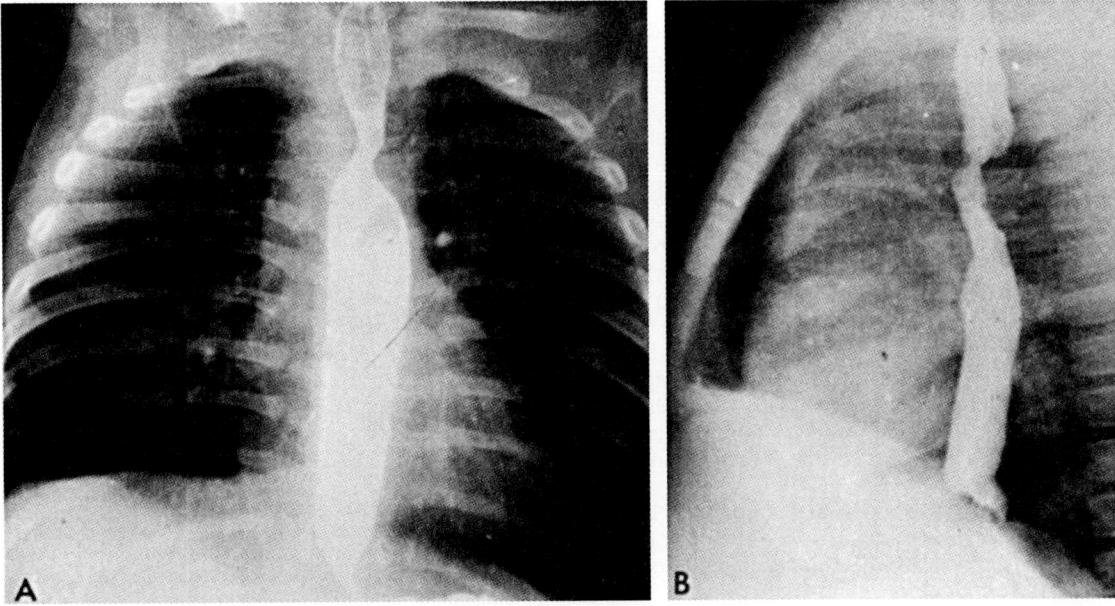

FIGURE 425–2. Double aortic arch in an infant aged 5 mo. *A*, Anteroposterior view. The barium-filled esophagus is constricted on both sides. *B*, Lateral view. The esophagus is displaced forward. The anterior arch was the smaller and was divided at surgery.

Diagnosis should include an electrocardiogram, stress testing, two-dimensional echocardiography, and cardiac catheterization with selective coronary angiography.

Treatment is indicated for obstructed vessels and consists of aortoplasty with re-anastomosis of the aberrant vessel or, occasionally, coronary artery bypass grafting.

425.3 Pulmonary Arteriovenous Fistula

Fistulous vascular communications in the lungs may be large and localized or multiple, scattered, and small. The most common form of this unusual condition is the **Osler-Weber-Rendu syndrome** (hereditary hemorrhagic telangiectasia type I), which is also associated with angiomas of the nasal and buccal mucous membranes, gastrointestinal tract, or liver. This syndrome is caused by mutations in the endoglin gene, a cell surface component of the transforming growth factor-β receptor complex. The usual communication is between the pulmonary artery and pulmonary vein; direct communication between the pulmonary artery and left atrium is extremely rare. Desaturated blood in the pulmonary artery is shunted through the fistula into the pulmonary vein, thus bypassing the lungs, and then enters the left side of the heart; this aberrant direction of flow results in systemic arterial desaturation and, sometimes, clinical cyanosis. The shunt across the fistula is at low pressure and resistance, so pulmonary arterial pressure is normal; cardiomegaly and heart failure are not present.

The *clinical manifestations* depend on the magnitude of the shunt. Large fistulas are associated with dyspnea, cyanosis, clubbing, a continuous murmur, and polycythemia. Hemoptysis is

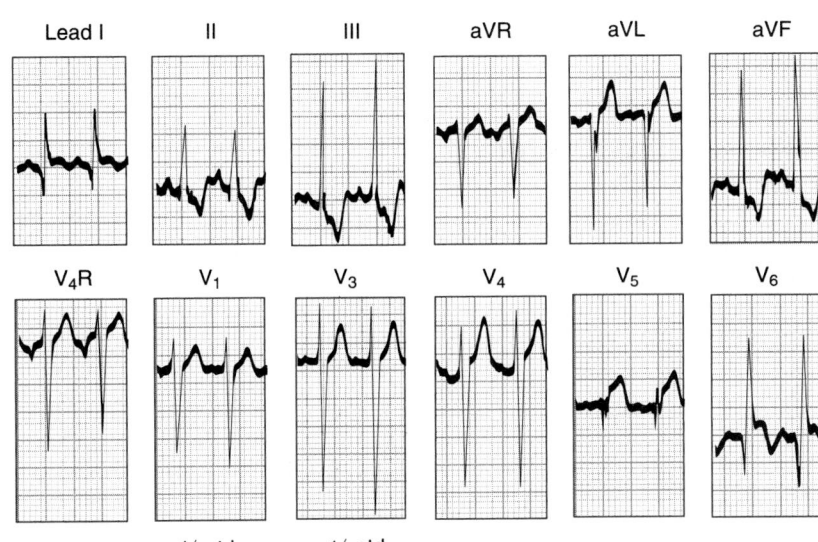

FIGURE 425–3. Electrocardiogram of a 3-mo-old child with anomalous origin of the left coronary artery from the pulmonary artery. Lateral myocardial infarction is present as evidenced by abnormally large and wide Q waves in leads I, V_5, and V_6; an elevated ST segment in V_5 and V_6; and inversion of TV_6.

rare, but when it occurs, it may be massive. Features of the Osler-Weber-Rendu syndrome are seen in about 50% of patients (or other family members) and include recurrent epistaxis and gastrointestinal tract bleeding. Transitory dizziness, diplopia, aphasia, motor weakness, or convulsions may result from cerebral thrombosis, abscess, or paradoxical emboli. Soft systolic or continuous murmurs may be audible over the site of the fistula. The electrocardiogram is normal. Roentgenographic examination of the chest may show opacities produced by large fistulas; multiple small fistulas may be visualized by fluoroscopy (as abnormal pulsations), MRI, or CT. Selective pulmonary arteriography demonstrates the site, extent, and distribution of the fistulas.

Treatment consisting of excision of solitary or localized lesions by lobectomy or wedge resection results in complete disappearance of symptoms. In most instances, fistulas are so widespread that surgery is not possible. Direct communication between the pulmonary artery and the left atrium, if present, can be obliterated by division and suture.

Patients who have undergone a *Glenn cavopulmonary anastomosis* for cyanotic congenital heart disease are also at risk for the development of pulmonary arteriovenous malformations. In these patients the arteriovenous malformations are usually multiple and the risk increases over time after the Glenn procedure. These malformations rarely occur after the heart disease is fully palliated by completion of the Fontan operation. The pulmonary circulation may require an unknown hepatic factor to suppress the development of arteriovenous malformations. The hallmark of the development of these malformations is a decrease in the patient's oxygen saturation. The diagnosis can often be made with contrast echocardiography; cardiac catheterization is the definitive test. Completion of the Fontan circuit so that inferior vena cava blood flow is routed through the lungs results in improvement or resolution of the malformations.

425.4 Ectopia Cordis

In the most common thoracic form of ectopia cordis, the sternum is split and the heart protrudes outside the chest. In other forms, the heart protrudes through the diaphragm into the abdominal cavity or may be situated in the neck. Associated intracardiac anomalies are common. Death occurs in the 1st days of life in most, usually from infection, cardiac failure, or hypoxemia. Surgical therapy for neonates without overwhelmingly severe cardiac anomalies consists of covering the heart with skin without compromising venous return or ventricular ejection. Palliation of associated defects is also often necessary. Occasional patients with the abdominal type have survived to adulthood.

425.5 Diverticulum of the Left Ventricle

In this rare anomaly, a diverticulum of the left ventricle protrudes into the epigastrium. The lesion may be isolated or associated with complex cardiovascular anomalies. A pulsating mass is visible and palpable in the epigastrium. Systolic or systolic-diastolic murmurs produced by blood flow into and out of the diverticulum may be audible over the lower part of the sternum and the mass. The *electrocardiogram* shows a pattern of complete or incomplete left bundle branch block. *Roentgenograms* of the chest may or may not show the mass. Associated abnormalities include defects of the sternum, abdominal wall, diaphragm, and pericardium. Surgical treatment of the diverticulum and associated cardiac defects can be performed in selected cases. Occasionally, a diverticulum may be small and not associated with clinical signs

or symptoms. These small diverticula are diagnosed at the time of echocardiographic examination for other indications.

Vascular Rings

Azarow KS, Pearl RH, Hoffman MA, et al: Vascular ring: Does magnetic resonance imaging replace angiography? *Ann Thorac Surg* 1992;53:882.
Bertrand J-M, Chartrand C, Lamarre A, et al: Vascular ring: Clinical and physiological assessment of pulmonary function following surgical correction. *Pediatr Pulmonol* 1986;2:378.
Murdison KA, Andrews BA, Chin AJ: Ultrasonographic display of complex vascular rings. *J Am Coll Cardiol* 1990;15:1645.
van Son JA, Julsrud PR, Hagler DJ, et al: Imaging strategies for vascular rings. *Ann Thorac Surg* 1994;57:604–10.

Anomalous Coronary Artery

Chang RR, Allada V: Electrocardiographic and echocardiographic features that distinguish anomalous origin of the left coronary artery from pulmonary artery from idiopathic dilated cardiomyopathy. *Pediatr Cardiol* 2001;22:3–10.
Frommelt PC, Berger S, Pelech AN, et al: Prospective identification of anomalous origin of left coronary artery from the right sinus of Valsalva using transthoracic echocardiography: Importance of color Doppler flow mapping. *Pediatr Cardiol* 2001;22:327–32.
Johnsrude CL, Perry JC, Cecchin F, et al: Differentiating anomalous left main coronary artery originating from the pulmonary artery in infants from myocarditis and dilated cardiomyopathy by electrocardiogram. *Am J Cardiol* 1995;75:71.
Schmidt KG, Cooper MJ, Silverman NH, et al: Pulmonary artery origin of the left coronary artery: Diagnosis by two-dimensional echocardiography, pulsed Doppler ultrasound and color flow mapping. *J Am Coll Cardiol* 1988;11:396.

Pulmonary Arteriovenous Fistulas

Feinstein JA, Moore P, Rosenthal DN, et al: Comparison of contrast echocardiography versus cardiac catheterization for detection of pulmonary arteriovenous malformations. *Am J Cardiol* 2002;89:281–5.
Marchuk DA: Genetic abnormalities in hereditary hemorrhagic telangiectasia. *Curr Opin Hematol* 1998;5:332–8.
Srivastava D, Preminger T, Lock JE, et al: Hepatic venous blood and the development of pulmonary arteriovenous malformations in congenital heart disease. *Circulation* 1995;92:1217–22.

Chapter 426
Pulmonary Hypertension

426.1 Primary Pulmonary Hypertension

Pathophysiology. Primary pulmonary hypertension is characterized by pulmonary vascular obstructive disease and right-sided heart failure. It occurs at any age, although in pediatric patients the diagnosis is initially made in the teenage years. In older patients, females outnumber males 1.7:1; in younger patients, both genders are represented equally. Some patients have evidence of either an immunologic disorder or a hypercoagulable state. Mutations in the gene for bone morphogenetic protein receptor-II (a member of the transforming growth factor-β receptor family) have been identified in patients with autosomal dominant familial primary pulmonary hypertension (known as *PPH1*). This genetic variant demonstrates anticipation and a female preponderance. Up to 25% of patients may have a mutation in this gene. Angiopoietin-1, an angiogenic factor, and its receptor are overexpressed in patients. Angiopoietin-1 inhibits expression of bone morphogenetic protein receptors. Diet pills, particularly fenfluramine, have also been implicated. Pulmonary hypertension is associated with precapillary obstruction of the pulmonary vascular bed as a result of hyperplasia of the muscular and elastic tissues and a thickened intima of the small pulmonary arteries and arterioles. Atherosclerotic changes may be found in the larger pulmonary arteries. In children, veno-occlusive disease may account for some cases of primary pulmonary hypertension. For the diagnosis other causes of elevated pulmonary pressure must be eliminated (chronic pulmonary parenchymal disease, persistent obstruction of the upper airway, congenital cardiac malformations, recurrent pulmonary emboli, alveolar capillary dysplasia, liver disease, autoimmune disease, and moyamoya disease). Pulmonary hypertension places an afterload burden on the right ventricle, which results in right ventricular hypertrophy. Dilatation of the pulmonary artery is present, and pulmonary valve insufficiency may occur. In the later stages of the disease, the right ventricle dilates, tricuspid insufficiency develops, and cardiac output is decreased. Arrhythmias, syncope, and sudden death are common.

Clinical Manifestations. The predominant symptoms include exercise intolerance and fatigability; occasionally, precordial chest pain, dizziness, syncope, or headaches are noted. Peripheral cyanosis may be present, especially in patients with a patent foramen ovale through which blood can shunt from right to left; in the late stages of disease, patients may have cold extremities and a gray appearance associated with low cardiac output. Arterial oxygen saturation is usually normal. If right-sided heart failure has supervened, jugular venous pressure is elevated, and hepatomegaly and edema are present. Jugular venous "*a*" waves are present, and in those with functional tricuspid insufficiency, a conspicuous jugular "*cv*" wave and systolic hepatic pulsations are manifested. The heart is moderately enlarged, and a right ventricular heave can be noted. The 1st heart sound is often followed by an ejection click emanating from the dilated pulmonary artery. The 2nd heart sound is narrowly split, loud, and sometimes booming in quality; it is frequently palpable at the upper left sternal border. A presystolic gallop rhythm may be audible at the lower left sternal border. The systolic murmur is soft and short and is sometimes followed by a blowing decrescendo diastolic murmur caused by pulmonary insufficiency. In later stages, a holosystolic murmur of tricuspid insufficiency is appreciated at the lower left sternal border.

Diagnosis. *Chest roentgenograms* reveal a prominent pulmonary artery and right ventricle (Fig. 426–1). The pulmonary vascularity in the hilar areas may be prominent, in contrast to the peripheral lung fields, in which pulmonary markings are decreased. The *electrocardiogram* shows right ventricular hypertrophy, often with spiked P waves.

At *cardiac catheterization* this condition must be differentiated from **Eisenmenger syndrome** (see Chapter 426.2), which is associated with a communication between the left and right sides of the heart or great arteries, as well as from left-sided obstructive lesions (pulmonary venous stenosis, mitral stenosis) that result in pulmonary venous hypertension (see Chapter 420). The presence of pulmonary artery hypertension with a normal pulmonary capillary wedge pressure is diagnostic of primary pulmonary hypertension. If the wedge pressure is elevated and left ventricular end-diastolic pressure is normal, obstruction at the level of the pulmonary veins, left atrium, or mitral valve should be suspected. The risks associated with cardiac catheterization may be high in severely ill patients with primary pulmonary hypertension.

Prognosis and Treatment. Primary pulmonary hypertension is progressive, and no cure is currently available. Some success has been reported with oral calcium channel blocking agents such as nifedipine in children who demonstrate pulmonary vasoreactivity when these agents are administered during catheterization. Continuous intravenous infusion of prostacyclin (prostaglandin I_2) provides relief as long as the infusion is continued. Continuous administration of nitric oxide via nasal cannula, nebulized forms of prostacyclin, and orally administered pulmonary vasodilators (bosentan, an antagonist of endothelin receptors; or sildenafil, a phosphodiesterase type 5 inhibitor and generator of nitric oxide) are all being investigated. Anticoagulation may be of value in patients with previous pulmonary thromboemboli, and some of these patients will respond to balloon angioplasty of narrowed pulmonary artery

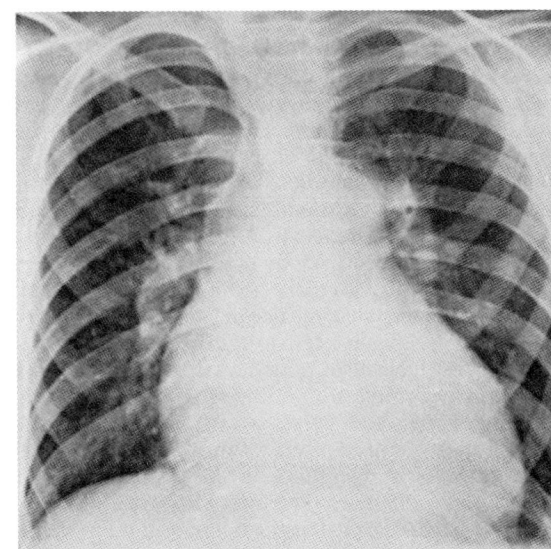

FIGURE 426–1. Roentgenogram in primary pulmonary hypertension. Note the moderate cardiac enlargement, dilatation of the pulmonary artery, and relative pulmonary undervascularity in the outer two thirds of the lung fields.

segments. Despite many advances, definitive therapy is still heart-lung or lung transplantation (see Chapter 435). In patients with severe pulmonary hypertension and low cardiac output, the terminal event is often sudden and related to a lethal arrhythmia. Patients with primary pulmonary hypertension diagnosed in infancy often have rapid progression and high mortality.

426.2 Pulmonary Vascular Disease (Eisenmenger Syndrome)

Pathophysiology. The term *Eisenmenger syndrome* refers to patients with a ventricular septal defect in which blood is shunted partially or totally from right to left as a result of the development of pulmonary vascular disease. This physiologic abnormality can also occur with atrial septal defect, atrioventricular septal defect, patent ductus arteriosus, or any other communication between the aorta and pulmonary artery. Pulmonary vascular disease with an isolated atrial septal defect is less common and does not occur until late in adulthood.

In Eisenmenger syndrome, pulmonary vascular resistance after birth either remains high or, after having decreased during early infancy, rises thereafter because of increased shear stress on pulmonary arterioles. Factors playing a role in the rapidity of development of pulmonary vascular disease include increased pulmonary arterial pressure, increased pulmonary blood flow, and the presence of hypoxia or hypercapnia. Early in the course of disease, pulmonary hypertension (elevated pressure in the pulmonary arteries) is the result of markedly increased pulmonary blood flow (*hyperkinetic pulmonary hypertension*). This form of pulmonary hypertension decreases with the administration of pulmonary vasodilators or oxygen, or both. With the development of Eisenmenger syndrome, pulmonary hypertension is the result of *pulmonary vascular disease* (obstructive pathologic changes in the pulmonary vessels). This form of pulmonary hypertension is usually only minimally responsive to pulmonary vasodilators or oxygen or not at all.

Pathology and Pathophysiology. The pathologic changes of Eisenmenger syndrome occur in the small pulmonary arterioles and muscular arteries (<300 mm) and are graded on the basis of histologic characteristics (Heath-Edwards classification): grade I changes involve medial hypertrophy alone, grade II consists of medial hypertrophy and intimal hyperplasia, grade III involves near obliteration of the vessel lumen, grade IV includes arterial dilatation, and grades V and VI include plexiform lesions, angiomatoid formation, and fibrinoid necrosis. Grades IV–VI indicate irreversible pulmonary vascular obstructive disease. Eisenmenger physiology is defined by an absolute elevation in pulmonary arterial resistance to greater than 12 Wood units (resistance units indexed to body surface area) or by a ratio of pulmonary to systemic vascular resistance of 1.0 or higher.

Pulmonary vascular disease occurs more rapidly in patients with trisomy 21 who have left-to-right shunts. It also complicates the natural history of patients with elevated pulmonary venous pressure secondary to mitral stenosis or left ventricular dysfunction, any patient with transmission of systemic pressure to the pulmonary circulation via a shunt at the interventricular or great vessel level, and patients chronically exposed to low Po_2 (because of high altitude). Patients with cyanotic congenital heart lesions associated with unrestricted pulmonary blood flow are at particularly high risk.

Clinical Manifestations. Symptoms do not usually develop until the 2nd or 3rd decade of life, although a more fulminant course may occur. Many patients survive for decades with minimal symptoms. Intracardiac or extracardiac communications that would normally shunt from left to right are converted to right-to-left shunting as pulmonary vascular resistance exceeds systemic vascular resistance. Cyanosis becomes apparent, and dyspnea, fatigue, and a tendency toward dysrhythmias begin to occur. In the late stages of the disease, heart failure, chest pain, headaches, syncope, and hemoptysis may be seen. Physical examination reveals a right ventricular heave and a narrowly split 2nd heart sound with a loud pulmonic component. Palpable pulmonary artery pulsation may be present at the left upper sternal border. A holosystolic murmur of tricuspid regurgitation may be audible along the left sternal border. An early decrescendo diastolic murmur of pulmonary insufficiency may also be heard along the left sternal border. The degree of cyanosis depends on the stage of the disease.

Diagnosis. Cyanotic patients have various degrees of polycythemia that depend on the severity and duration of hypoxia. Roentgenographically, the heart varies in size from normal to greatly enlarged; the latter usually occurs late in the course of the disease. The main pulmonary artery is generally prominent, similar to primary pulmonary hypertension (see Fig. 426–1).

The pulmonary vessels are enlarged in the hilar areas and taper rapidly in caliber in the peripheral branches. The right ventricle and atrium are prominent. The electrocardiogram shows marked right ventricular hypertrophy. The P wave may be tall and spiked.

The echocardiogram shows a thick-walled right ventricle and demonstrates the underlying congenital heart lesion. Two-dimensional echocardiography assists in eliminating from consideration lesions such as obstructed pulmonary veins, a supramitral membrane, and mitral stenosis. The pulmonary valve echocardiogram shows a characteristic early midsystolic closure, the "W sign." Doppler studies demonstrate the direction of the shunt and the presence of a typical hypertension waveform in the main pulmonary artery. Tricuspid and pulmonary regurgitation can be used in the Doppler examination to estimate pulmonary arterial pressure.

Cardiac catheterization usually shows a bidirectional shunt at the site of the defect. Systolic pressure is generally equal in the systemic and pulmonary circulations. Pulmonary capillary wedge pressure is normal unless a left-sided heart obstructive lesion or left ventricular failure is the cause of the pulmonary artery hypertension. Arterial oxygen saturation is decreased because of the magnitude of the right-to-left shunt. The response to vasodilator therapy (oxygen, nitroprusside, calcium channel blockers, prostacyclin, nitric oxide) may identify patients with hyperdynamic pulmonary hypertension. Selective angiocardiography can locate the site of the shunt, but these studies are usually avoided in such patients because of increased risk and the accuracy of echocardiography. Selective pulmonary artery injections may be necessary if pulmonary venous obstruction is suspected because of high wedge pressure and low left ventricular end-diastolic pressure.

Treatment. The best management for patients who are at risk for the development of late pulmonary vascular disease is prevention by early surgical elimination of large intracardiac or great vessel communications during infancy. Some patients may be missed because they have not shown early clinical manifestations. Pulmonary vascular resistance never decreases substantially at birth in some of these infants, and therefore they never acquire enough left-to-right shunting to become clinically apparent. Such delayed recognition is a particular risk in patients with congenital heart disease who live at high altitude. It is also a risk in infants with trisomy 21, who have a propensity for earlier development of pulmonary vascular disease. Because of the high incidence of congenital heart disease associated with trisomy 21, many physicians recommend routine

---

TABLE 426–1. Extracardiac Complications of Cyanotic Congenital Heart Disease and Eisenmenger Physiology

Problem	Etiology	Therapy
Polycythemia	Persistent hypoxia	Phlebotomy
Relative anemia	Nutritional deficiency	Iron replacement
CNS abscess	Right-to-left shunting	Antibiotics, drainage
CNS thromboembolic stroke	Right-to-left shunting or polycythemia	Phlebotomy
Low-grade DIC, thrombocytopenia	Polycythemia	None for DIC unless bleeding, then phlebotomy
Hemoptysis	Pulmonary infarct, thrombosis, or rupture of pulmonary artery plexiform lesion	Embolization
Gum disease	Polycythemia, gingivitis, bleeding	Dental hygiene
Gout	Polycythemia, diuretic agent	Allopurinol
Arthritis, clubbing	Hypoxic arthropathy	None
Pregnancy complications: abortion, fetal growth retardation, prematurity, maternal illness	Poor placental perfusion, poor ability to increase cardiac output	Bed rest, pregnancy prevention counseling
Infections	Associated asplenia, DiGeorge syndrome, endocarditis	Antibiotics
	Fatal RSV pneumonia with pulmonary hypertension	Ribavirin; RSV immunoglobulin (prevention)
Failure to thrive	Increased oxygen consumption, decreased nutrient intake	Treat heart failure; correct defect early; increase caloric intake
Psychosocial adjustment	Limited activity, cyanotic appearance, chronic disease, multiple hospitalizations	Counseling

CNS = central nervous system; DIC = disseminated intravascular coagulation; RSV = respiratory syncytial virus.

echocardiography at the time of initial diagnosis, even in the absence of other clinical findings.

Medical treatment of Eisenmenger syndrome is entirely symptomatic (Table 426–1). Older children and adolescents with symptomatic polycythemia may be improved by cautious, repeated phlebotomies with volume replacement. Clinical trials in adults have described short-term benefits from chronic calcium channel blocker or prostacyclin therapy, but experience with these agents in children is minimal. Combined heart-lung or bilateral lung transplantation is the only surgical option for many of these patients (see Chapter 435).

Barst RJ: Medical therapy of pulmonary hypertension. An overview of treatment and goals. *Clin Chest Med* 2001;22:509–15.

Channick RN, Simonneuar G, Sitbon IM, et al: Effects of the dual endothelin-receptor antagonist bosentan in patients with pulmonary hypertension: A randomized placebo-controlled study. *Lancet* 2001;358:1119–23.

Du L, Sullivan CC, Chu D, et al: Signaling molecules in nonfamilial pulmonary hypertension. *N Engl J Med* 2003;348:500–9.

Ghofrani HA, Wiedemann R, Rose F, et al: Sildenafil for a treatment of lung fibrosis and pulmonary hypertension: A randomized controlled trial. *Lancet* 2002;360:895–900.

Feinstein JA, Goldhaber SZ, Lock JE, et al: Balloon pulmonary angioplasty for treatment of chronic thromboembolic pulmonary hypertension. *Circulation* 2001;103:10–3.

Gammie JS, Keenan RJ, Pham SM, et al: Single- versus double-lung transplantation for pulmonary hypertension. *J Thorac Cardiovasc Surg* 1998;115:397.

McCann UD, Seiden LS, Rubin LJ, et al: Brain serotonin neurotoxicity and primary pulmonary hypertension from fenfluramine and dexfenfluramine. A systemic review of the evidence. *JAMA* 1997;278:666.

McLaughlin VV, Shillington A, Rich S: Survival in primary pulmonary hypertension. The impact of epoprostenol therapy. *Circulation* 2002;106:1477–82.

Mikhail G, Gibbs J, Richardson M, et al: An evaluation of nebulized prostacyclin in patients with primary and secondary pulmonary hypertension. *Eur Heart J* 1997;18:1499.

Newman JH, Wheeler L, Lane KB, et al: Mutation in the gene for bone morphogenetic protein receptor II as a cause of primary pulmonary hypertension in a large kindred. *N Engl J Med* 2001;345:319–24.

Sandoval J, Bauerle O, Gomez A, et al: Primary pulmonary hypertension in children: Clinical characterization and survival. *J Am Coll Cardiol* 1995;25:466.

Chapter 427
General Principles of Treatment of Congenital Heart Disease

Most patients who have mild congenital heart disease require no treatment. The parents and child should be made aware that a normal life is expected and that no restriction of the child's activities is necessary. Overprotective parents may use the presence of a mild congenital heart lesion or even a functional heart murmur as a means to exert excessive control over their child's activities. Although fears may not be expressed overtly, the child may become anxious regarding early death or debilitation, especially when an adult member of the family acquires symptomatic heart disease. The family may have an unexpressed fear of sudden death, and the rarity of this manifestation should be emphasized in discussions directed at improving their understanding of the child's congenital heart defect. The difference between congenital heart disease and degenerative coronary disease in adults should be emphasized. General health maintenance, including a well-balanced, "heart-healthy" diet, aerobic exercise, and avoidance of smoking, should be encouraged.

Even patients with moderate to severe heart disease need not be markedly restricted in physical activity. Physical education should be modified appropriately to the child's capacity to participate. The extent of such modification can generally be determined best by exercise testing. Competitive sports for most of

these patients should be discouraged. Patients with severe heart disease and decreased exercise tolerance usually tend to limit their own activities. Dyspnea, headache, and fatigability in cyanotic patients may be a sign of increasing hypoxemia and may require some limitation of activity in those for whom specific medical or surgical treatment is not available. Routine immunizations should be given, with the inclusion of influenza vaccine; patients who might be considered candidates for heart or heart-lung transplantation should not receive live-virus vaccinations just before transplantation.

Bacterial infections should be treated vigorously, but the presence of congenital heart disease is not an appropriate reason to use antibiotics indiscriminately. Prophylaxis against infective endocarditis should be carried out during dental procedures, during instrumentation of the urinary tract, and before lower gastrointestinal tract manipulation (see Table 429–2).

Cyanotic patients need to be monitored for a multitude of noncardiac manifestations of oxygen deficiency (Table 427–1). Treatment of iron deficiency anemia is important in cyanotic patients who show improved exercise tolerance and general well-being with adequate hemoglobin levels. These patients should also be carefully observed for excessive polycythemia. Cyanotic patients should avoid situations in which dehydration may occur, which leads to increased viscosity and increases the risk of stroke. Diuretics may need to be decreased or temporarily discontinued during episodes of acute gastroenteritis. High altitudes and sudden changes in the thermal environment should also be avoided. Phlebotomy with volume replacement should be carried out in symptomatic patients with severe polycythemia (hematocrit >65%); the use of routine phlebotomy in the absence of symptoms is controversial. Patients with severe congenital heart disease or a history of rhythm disturbance should be carefully monitored during anesthesia for even routine surgical procedures. Women with nonrepaired severe congenital heart disease should be counseled on the risks associated with childbearing and on the use of contraceptives and tubal ligation. Pregnancy may be extremely dangerous for patients with chronic cyanosis or pulmonary artery hypertension, or both. Women with mild to moderate heart disease and many of those who have had corrective surgery can have normal pregnancies.

Postoperative Management. After successful open heart surgery, the severity of the congenital heart defect, the age and condition (nutritional status) of the patient before surgery, the events in the operating room, and the quality of the postoperative care influence the patient's course. Intraoperative factors that influence survival and that should be noted when a patient returns from the operating room include the duration of cardiopulmonary bypass, the duration of aortic cross-clamping (the time during which the heart is not being perfused), and the duration of profound hypothermia (generally used in infants: the period during which the entire body is not being perfused).

Immediate postoperative care should be provided in an intensive care unit staffed by a team of physicians, nurses, and technicians experienced with the unique problems encountered after open heart surgery. Preparation for postoperative monitoring begins in the operating room, where the anesthesiologist or surgeon places an arterial catheter to allow direct arterial pressure measurements and arterial sampling for blood gas determination. A central venous catheter is also placed for measuring central venous pressure and for infusions of cardioactive medications. In more complex cases, left atrial or pulmonary artery catheters may be inserted directly into these cardiac structures and used for pressure monitoring purposes. Flow-directed thermodilution monitoring (Swan-Ganz) catheters are sometimes used for monitoring pulmonary capillary wedge pressure and the cardiac index. Temporary pacing wires are placed on the atrium or ventricle, or both, in case temporary heart block

TABLE 427–1. Systems Approach to Postoperative Care Following Surgery for Congenital Heart Disease

System and Problem	Etiology	Treatment or Prevention
Nervous System		
Coma	Global ischemia	Monitor and treat increased intracranial pressure
	Prolonged anesthetic effect	Reverse anesthesia
	Hypoglycemia	Glucose
Focal lesions	Emboli (air, thrombi)	
Seizures	Metabolic (hyponatremia, hypoglycemia), ischemic, embolic disturbances	Phenytoin, correct metabolic disturbances
Diaphragm paralysis	Phrenic nerve injury	Respiratory care
Vocal cord paralysis	Traction on recurrent laryngeal nerve	Respiratory care
Horner syndrome	Dissection of subclavian artery with sympathetic chain injury	None
Paraplegia	Postcoarctation repair with spinal artery ischemia	Avoid ischemia
Pain	Surgical trauma	Fentanyl, morphine
Anxiety	Stress	Midazolam (Versed), diazepam (Valium)
Respiratory System		
ARDS postpump syndrome	Unknown; possible release of vasoactive substances by cardiopulmonary bypass	PEEP, mechanical ventilation, oxygen
Pulmonary edema	Heart failure, left-sided obstructions, fluid overload	Diuresis, PEEP, mechanical ventilation, inotropic agents
Pleural effusions	Hemothorax	Thoracocentesis
	Early serous effusion	Thoracocentesis
	Delayed postpericardiotomy syndrome	Anti-inflammatory agents
Chylothorax	Injury to thoracic duct	NPO or medium-chain triglyceride diet
		Rarely surgical ligation of thoracic duct
Atelectasis	Hypoventilation, poor cough	Chest physiotherapy, PEEP
Pneumonia	Aspiration, nosocomial, bacteremia	Identify bacterial-viral (respiratory syncytial virus) cause; specific antimicrobial therapy
Pulmonary hypertension	Repair of TAPVR, Norwood 1st stage, trisomy 21; prior preoperative pulmonary hypertension	Hyperventilation, hyperoxia, nitroprusside, prostaglandins, nitric oxide, ECMO
Stridor	Vocal cord edema, paralysis	Steroids, rarely tracheotomy
Cardiovascular System		
Bradycardia, sick sinus syndrome, atrioventricular block	Injury to interatrial or interventricular conduction system	Atropine, isoproterenol, pacemaker
Right bundle branch block	Right ventriculotomy	Atrial approach to ventricular septal defect repair or tetralogy of Fallot
Tachyarrhythmias	Supraventricular, junctional tachycardia	Antiarrhythmic agents
	Ventricular tachycardia	Defibrillation, antiarrhythmic agents
Poor cardiac output	Cardiogenic—right ventriculotomy or cardiac "stun" (prolonged pump and cross-clamp time) or infarction	Inotropic agents, support preload, reduce afterload, LVAD, ECMO
	Hypocalcemia	Calcium
	Hypovolemia	Support preload with fluids
Pericardial tamponade	Pericardial effusion, acute hemorrhage	Pericardiocentesis
	Serous postpericardiotomy syndrome	Anti-inflammatory agents
Hypertension	Stress or pain	Analgesia
	Postcoarctectomy syndrome	Nitroprusside
Mesenteric arteritis	Postcoarctectomy syndrome	NPO, nitroprusside
Renal-Metabolic System		
Prerenal oliguria	Hypovolemia	Fluid administration
	Poor cardiac output	Inotropic agents
Renal failure	Hypotension, prolonged pump–cross-clamp time, acute tubular necrosis	Improve blood pressure, diuretics, dialysis
Edema	Fluid resuscitation, capillary leak, poor cardiac output, elevated systemic venous pressure	Diuresis, inotropic agents
Hyponatremia	Dilutional, SIADH	Fluid restriction
	Diuretics	Fluid restriction
Hyperglycemia	Hypothermia, inhibition of insulin	None needed (usually), insulin
Hypoglycemia	Rebound following hyperglycemia, hepatic failure	Glucose infusion
Hematologic System		
Hemorrhage	Abnormal PT, PTT, thrombocytopenia	Correct coagulopathy
	Surgical leak	Reoperation, suture
Shunt thrombosis	Poor cardiac output, hypovolemia	Fluids, heparin, reoperation
Anemia (usually reflecting reduced blood volume)	Hemorrhage, hemolysis	Transfuse packed red blood cells
Graft-vs-host disease	Infusion of viable leukocytes to patients with DiGeorge syndrome	Irradiate blood products
Infectious Diseases		
Wound infection (cutaneous, costochondral, sternotomy, mediastinitis, vascular lines, chest tubes)	Contamination in operating room	Antibiotics
Endocarditis	*Staphylococcus epidermidis, Corynebacterium*, contamination in operating room	Antibiotics
Cystitis, pyelonephritis	Contamination of indwelling urinary catheter	Antibiotics, remove catheter
Hepatitis	Blood-borne: cytomegalovirus, Epstein-Barr virus, hepatitis B and C viruses	Screen blood products

TABLE 427–1. **Systems Approach to Postoperative Care Following Surgery for Congenital Heart Disease** *Continued*

System and Problem	Etiology	Treatment or Prevention
Postperfusion syndrome (fever, hepatosplenomegaly, atypical lymphocytes, lymphadenopathy, transient rash)	Cytomegalovirus, Epstein-Barr virus	Screen blood products
Psychosocial Conditions		
Anxiety, separation	Age related, fears, etc.	Preparedness (videotape, play acting); parent visitation, sedation

ARDS = acute respiratory distress syndrome; PEEP = positive end-expiratory pressure; NPO = nothing per os (by mouth); TAPVR = total anomalous pulmonary venous return; ECMO = extracorporeal membrane oxygenation; LVAD = left ventricular assist device; SIADH = syndrome of inappropriate antidiuretic hormone; PT = prothrombin time; PTT = partial thromboplastin time.

occurs. Transcutaneous oximetry provides for continuous monitoring of arterial oxygen saturation.

Functional failure of one organ system may cause profound physiologic and biochemical changes in another (see Table 427–1). Respiratory insufficiency, for example, leads to hypoxia, acidosis, and hypercapnia, which in turn compromises cardiac, vascular, and renal function. The latter problems cannot be managed successfully until adequate ventilation is re-established. Thus, it is essential that the primary source of each postoperative problem be identified and treated.

Respiratory failure is a major postoperative complication encountered after open heart surgery. Cardiopulmonary bypass carried out in the presence of pulmonary congestion results in decreased lung compliance, copious tracheal and bronchial secretions, atelectasis, and increased breathing effort. Because fatigue and subsequently hypoventilation and acidosis may rapidly ensue, mechanical positive pressure endotracheal ventilation may be continued after open heart surgery for a minimum of several hours in relatively stable patients and for up to 2–3 days or longer in severely ill patients, especially infants. Patients with certain congenital heart lesions may also have airway abnormalities that could make extubation more difficult.

The electrocardiogram should be monitored continuously during the postoperative period. A change in heart rate may be the 1st indication of a serious complication such as hemorrhage, hypothermia, hypoventilation, or heart failure. *Cardiac rhythm disorders* must be diagnosed quickly because a prolonged untreated arrhythmia may add a severe hemodynamic burden to the heart in the critical early postoperative period (see Chapter 428). Injury to the heart's conduction system during surgery can result in postoperative *complete heart block*. This complication is usually temporary and is treated with surgically placed pacing wires that can later be removed. Occasionally, complete heart block is permanent. If heart block persists beyond 10–14 days postoperatively, insertion of a permanent pacemaker is required. Tachyarrhythmias are a more common problem in postoperative patients. Junctional ectopic tachycardia can be a particularly troublesome rhythm to manage (see Chapter 428).

Heart failure with poor cardiac output (see Table 427–1) after cardiac surgery may be secondary to respiratory failure, serious arrhythmias, myocardial injury, blood loss, hypervolemia or hypovolemia, or a significant residual hemodynamic abnormality. Treatment specific to the cause should be instituted. Catecholamines, phosphodiesterase inhibitors, digoxin, nitroprusside and other afterload-reducing agents, and diuretics are the cardioactive agents most often used in patients with myocardial dysfunction in the early postoperative period (see Chapter 434). Postoperative pulmonary hypertension can be managed with inhaled nitric oxide. In patients who are unresponsive to standard pharmacologic treatment, various ventricular assist devices are available, depending on the patient's size. If pulmonary function is adequate, an intra-aortic balloon counterpulsation pump or an external or implantable left ventricular assist

device may be used. If pulmonary function is inadequate, extracorporeal membrane oxygenation may be used. These extraordinary measures are helpful in maintaining the circulation until cardiac function improves, usually within 2–3 days. They have also been used with some success as a bridge to transplantation in patients with severe nonremitting postoperative cardiac failure.

Acidosis secondary to low cardiac output, renal failure, or hypovolemia must be prevented or promptly corrected. An arterial pH less than 7.3 may result in a decrease in cardiac output with an increase in lactic acid production and may be the forerunner of a series of arrhythmias or cardiac arrest.

Kidney function may be compromised by congestive heart failure and further impaired by prolonged cardiopulmonary bypass (see Table 427–1). Blood and fluid replacement, cardiac inotropic agents, and sometimes vasodilators will usually re-establish normal urine flow in patients with hypovolemia or cardiac failure. Dopamine is a useful inotropic agent because it also increases renal blood flow directly. Renal failure secondary to tubular injury may require temporary peritoneal dialysis or hemofiltration.

Neurologic abnormalities can develop after cardiopulmonary bypass, especially in the neonatal period. Seizures may occur when the patient awakens from sedation and can usually be controlled with phenytoin (Dilantin) or phenobarbital. In the absence of other neurologic signs, isolated seizures in the immediate postoperative period usually carry a good prognosis. Thromboembolism and stroke are rare, but serious complications of open heart surgery. Over the long term, both subtle and more substantial learning disabilities may develop. Patients who have undergone surgery entailing the use of cardiopulmonary bypass, especially in the newborn period, should be watched carefully during their early school years for signs of learning disabilities, which are often amenable to early remedial intervention.

The *postpericardiotomy syndrome* may occur toward the end of the 1st postoperative week or may sometimes be delayed until weeks or months after surgery. This febrile illness is characterized by fever, decreased appetite, listlessness, nausea, and vomiting. Chest pain is not always present, so a high index of suspicion should be maintained in any recently postoperative patient. Echocardiography is diagnostic. In most instances the postpericardiotomy syndrome is self-limited; however, when pericardial fluid accumulates rapidly, the potential danger of cardiac tamponade should be recognized (see Chapter 432). Rarely, arrhythmias may also occur. Symptomatic patients usually respond to salicylates or indomethacin and bed rest. Occasionally, steroid therapy or pericardiocentesis is required. A prolonged illness or late recurrences are less usual.

Hemolysis of mechanical origin is seen rarely after repair of certain cardiac defects, for example, atrioventricular septal defects, or after the insertion of a mechanical prosthetic valve. It is due to unusual turbulence of blood at increased pressure. Reoperation may be necessary in rare patients with severe and progressive hemolysis who require frequent blood transfusions, but in most instances the problem slowly regresses.

Infection is another potential postoperative problem. Patients usually receive a broad-spectrum antibiotic for the initial postoperative period. Potential sites of infection include the lungs (generally related to postoperative atelectasis), the subcutaneous tissues at the incision site, the sternum, and the urinary tract (especially after an indwelling catheter has been in place). Sepsis with infective endocarditis is an infrequent complication but can be difficult to manage (see Chapter 429).

Dunbar-Masterson C, Wypij D, Bellinger DC, et al: General health status of children with D-transposition of the great arteries after the arterial switch operation. *Circulation* 2001;104(12 Suppl 1):I138–42.

Galioto FM: Physical activity for children with cardiac disease. In Garson A, Bricker JT, Fisher DJ, Neish SR (editors): *The Science and Practice of Pediatric Cardiology*. Baltimore, Williams & Wilkins, 1998, pp 2585–92.

Leitch CA, Karn CA, Ensing GJ, et al: Energy expenditure after surgical repair in children with cyanotic congenital heart disease. *J Pediatr* 2000;137:381–5.

Limperopoulos C, Majnemer A, Shevell MI, et al: Predictors of developmental disabilities after open heart surgery in young children with congenital heart defects. *J Pediatr* 2002;141:51–8.

Limperopoulos C, Majnemer A, Shevell MI, et al: Functional limitations in young children with congenital heart defects after cardiac surgery. *Pediatrics* 2001;108;1325–31.

Mehta U, Laks H, Sadeghi A, et al: Extracorporeal membrane oxygenation for cardiac support in pediatric patients. *Am Surg* 2000;66:879–86.

Todd JL, Todd NW: Conotruncal cardiac anomalies and otitis media. *J Pediatr* 1997;131:215.

Visconti KJ, Bichell DP, Jonas RA, et al: Developmental outcome after surgical versus interventional closure of secundum atrial septal defect in children. *Circulation* 1999;100(19 Suppl):II145–50.

Wernovsky G, Stiles KM, Gauvreau K, et al: Cognitive development after the Fontan operation. *Circulation* 2000;102:883–9.

SECTION 4 *Cardiac Arrhythmias*

Anne Dubin

Chapter 428

Disturbances of Rate and Rhythm of the Heart

Pediatric arrhythmias may be transient or permanent, congenital (in a structurally normal or abnormal heart) or acquired (rheumatic fever, myocarditis), or caused by a toxin (diphtheria), cocaine, or theophylline or by proarrhythmic or antiarrhythmic drugs. Arrhythmias may be a sequela of surgical correction of congenital heart disease or a result of congenital metabolic disorders of mitochondria or fetal inflammation as in systemic lupus erythematosus (SLE). The major risk of any arrhythmia is either severe tachycardia or bradycardia leading to decreased cardiac output or degeneration into a more critical arrhythmia such as ventricular fibrillation. These complications may lead to syncope, which itself can be dangerous under certain circumstances (e.g., swimming, driving), or to sudden death. When a patient has an arrhythmia, it is vital to determine whether the particular rhythm is prone to deteriorate into a life-threatening tachyarrhythmia or bradyarrhythmia. Some rhythm abnormalities, such as single premature atrial and ventricular beats, are common in children without heart disease and in the great majority of instances do not pose a risk to the patient.

A number of powerful pharmacologic agents are available for treating dysrhythmias in adults, but many have not been studied extensively in children. Problems with frequency of administration, compliance, side effects, drug interactions, and variable responses remain, and selection of an appropriate agent involves empiricism. Fortunately, the majority of rhythm disturbances in children can be reliably controlled with a single agent (Table 428–1). Transcatheter radiofrequency ablation is used not only for resistant tachyarrhythmias but also for elective definitive treatment of arrhythmias. For patients with bradyarrhythmias, implantable pacemakers are small enough for use in premature infants. Implantable cardioverter-defibrillators (ICDs) are available for use in high-risk patients with malignant ventricular arrhythmias and an increased risk of sudden death.

428.1 Sinus Arrhythmias and Extrasystoles

Sinus arrhythmia represents a normal physiologic variation in impulse discharges from the sinus node related to respirations. The heart rate slows during expiration and accelerates during inspiration. Occasionally, if the sinus rate becomes slow enough, an escape beat arises from the atrioventricular (AV) junction region (Fig. 428–1). Irregularities in sinus rhythm are commonly seen in premature infants, especially bradycardia associated with periodic apnea. Sinus arrhythmia is exaggerated during febrile illnesses and by drugs that increase vagal tone, such as digitalis; it is usually abolished by exercise.

Sinus bradycardia is due to slow discharge of impulses from the sinus node. A sinus rate less than 90 beats/min in neonates and less than 60 beats/min thereafter is considered to be sinus bradycardia. It is commonly seen in athletes; in healthy individuals it is without significance. Sinus bradycardia may occur in systemic disease, for example, myxedema, and it resolves when the disorder is under control. Sinus bradycardia must be differentiated from sinoatrial and AV block. Children with sinus bradycardia are able to increase their heart rate with exercise to much higher than 100 beats/min, whereas patients with AV block are usually unable to do so. Low-birthweight infants display great variation in sinus rate. Sinus bradycardia is common in these infants and may be associated with junctional escape beats. Premature atrial contractions are also frequent. These rhythm changes, especially bradycardia, appear more commonly during sleep and are not associated with symptoms. No therapy is usually necessary.

Wandering atrial pacemaker (Fig. 428–2) is defined as an intermittent shift in the pacemaker of the heart from the sinus node to another part of the atrium. It is not uncommon in childhood and usually represents a normal variant, but it may also be seen in patients with central nervous system disturbances, for example, subarachnoid hemorrhage.

Extrasystoles are produced by the discharge of an ectopic focus that may be situated anywhere in atrial, junctional, or ventricular tissue. Usually, isolated extrasystoles are of no clinical or prognostic significance. Under certain circumstances, however, premature beats may be due to organic heart disease (inflammatory, ischemic, fibrotic, and so on) or to drug toxicity, especially from digitalis.

TABLE 428–1. Antiarrhythmic Drugs Commonly Used in Pediatric Patients, by Class

Drug	Indications	Oral Administration — Maintenance Dose	Oral Administration — Maximal Maintenance Dose	Intravenous Administration* — Loading Dose	Intravenous Administration* — Maximal Dose	Comments	Side Effects	Drug Interactions	Proarrhythmias	Drug Level
Class IA: Inhibit Na+ Fast Channel, Prolong Repolarization										
Quinidine sulfate	SVT,[†] atrial fibrillation, atrial flutter, VPC Digoxin, verapamil, or propranolol must be given first to prevent 1:1 conduction and fast ventricular rate in atrial flutter	20–60 mg/kg/24 hr q6h	2.4 g/24 hr	—	—	—	Nausea, vomiting, diarrhea, fever, cinchonism, QRS and QT prolongation, AV node block, asystole, syncope, thrombocytopenia, hemolytic anemia, SLE, blurred vision, convulsions, allergic reactions, exacerbation of periodic paralysis	Enhances digoxin effects may ↑ PTT when administered with Warfarin	Yes, torsades de pointes	2–7 µg/mL
Quinidine gluconate	Digoxin, verapamil, or propranolol must be given first to prevent 1:1 conduction and fast ventricular rate in atrial flutter	20–60 mg/kg/ 24 hr q8–12h	2.0 g/24 hr	—	—	Oral test dose, 2 mg/kg	Same as above	Same as above	Same as above	Same as above
Procainamide	SVT,[†] atrial fibrillation, atrial flutter, VPC, ventricular tachycardia[‡]	15–50 mg/kg/ 24 hr q4h or q6h[§]	4.0 g/24 hr	3–6 mg/kg over 5 min; repeat to 15 mg/kg/ load	20 mg/min to 1.0 g	Intravenous maintenance, 20–80 µg/ kg/min	P-R, QRS, Q-T interval prolongation, anorexia, nausea, vomiting, rash, fever, agranulocytosis, thrombocytopenia, Coombs-positive hemolytic anemia, SLE, hypotension, exacerbation of periodic paralysis	Toxicity increased by amiodarone, cimetidine	Yes, torsades de pointes	4–10 µg/mL
Disopyramide	SVT,[†] atrial fibrillation, atrial flutter, VPC	<2 yr: 20–30 mg/kg/24 hr divided q6h or q12 h for long acting form 2–10 yr: 9–24 mg/ kg/24 hr divided q6h or q12h for long acting form ≥11 yr: 5–13 mg/kg/24 hr divided q6h or q12h for long acting form	1.2 g/24 hr	—	—	—	Anticholinergic effects, urinary retention, blurred vision, dry mouth, QT and QRS prolongation, hepatic toxicity, negative inotropic effects, agranulocytosis, psychosis, hypoglycemia	—	Yes, torsades de pointes	2–5 µg/mL

Table continued on following page

TABLE 428–1. Antiarrhythmic Drugs Commonly Used in Pediatric Patients, by Class *Continued*

Drug	Indications	Oral Administration — Maintenance Dose	Oral Administration — Maximal Maintenance Dose	Intravenous Administration* — Loading Dose	Intravenous Administration* — Maximal Dose	Comments	Side Effects	Drug Interactions	Proarrhythmias	Drug Level
Class IB: Inhibit Na⁺ Fast Channel, Shorten Repolarization										
Lidocaine (class IB)	VPC, ventricular tachycardia,‡ ventricular fibrillation‖	—	—	1 mg/kg; repeat q5 min 2 times	50–75 mg	IV maintenance, 20–50 µg/kg/min	CNS effects, confusion, convulsions, high-degree AV block, asystole, coma, paresthesias, respiratory failure	Propranolol, cimetidine, tocainide increase toxicity	No	1–5 µg/mL
Mexiletene	VT, VPCs, ?long QT	6–15 mg/kg/24 hr, divided q24hr	—	—	—		GI upset, skin rash, neurologic	Cimetidine	No	—
Phenytoin (class IB)	Digoxin-induced arrhythmias with heart block	3–6 mg/kg/24 hr q12h	600 mg	10–15 mg/kg over 1 hr	20 mg/min to 1.0 g		Rash, gingival hyperplasia, ataxia, lethargy, vertigo, tremor, macrocytic anemia, bradycardia with rapid push	Amiodarone, oral anticoagulants, cimetidine, nifedipine, disopyramide increase toxicity Phenytoin decreases effect of quinidine, mexiletine, furosemide, disopyramide	No	10–20 µg/mL
Class II: β-Blockers										
Propranolol	SVT,† PVCs, LQTS	1–4 mg/kg/24 hr q6h	16 mg/kg/24 hr or 60 mg/24 hr	0.1–0.15 mg/kg over 5 min	1 mg/min to 10 mg	Long-acting β-blocking agents (nadolol, atenolol) are preferred for long-term therapy (less frequent administration and fewer CNS side effects); caution with IV administration—significant hypotension	Bradycardia, loss of concentration or memory, bronchospasm, hypoglycemia, hypotension, heart block, CHF	Use with disopyramide or verapamil exacerbates or precipitates CHF	No	—
Class III: Prolong Repolarization										
Amiodarone	Drug-resistant SVT, JET (congenital or postoperative), VT	Loading dose: 10 mg/kg/24 hr in 1–2 divided doses for 4–14 days; reduce to 5 mg/kg/24 hr for several weeks; if no recurrence,	Adult doses: loading = 800–1600 mg/24 hr for 2 wk, then 600–800 mg/24 hr for 1 mo, then 400 mg/24 hr	Loading dose: 2.5–5 mg/kg over 30–60 min, may repeat 3 times; then 2–10 mg/kg/24h q24h		Contraindicated in severe sinus node disease or in AV block without pacemaker	Hypothyroidism or hyperthyroidism, elevated triglycerides, hepatic toxicity, pulmonary fibrosis	Digoxin (increases levels), flecainide, procainamide, quinidine, warfarin, phenytoin	Torsades de pointes, bradycardia	0.5–2.5 mg/L

Class IV: Miscellaneous

reduce to 2.5 mg/kg/24 hr; may be given for 5 of 7 days/wk

Drug	Indication	Dose (PO)	Maximum dose (PO)	Dose (IV)	Maximum dose (IV)	Side effects	Drug interactions	Proarrhythmic effect	Therapeutic level
Digoxin (digitalis glycoside)	SVT† (non-WPW), atrial flutter, atrial fibrillation	10 µg/kg/24 hr q12h	0.5 mg	PO total loading dose: Premature: 20 µg/kg; Term newborn: 30 µg/kg; >6-mo-old infant: 40 µg/kg; Give 1/2 total dose followed by 1/4 q8–12h ×2; IV dose = 3/4 PO dose	0.5 mg	APC, VPC, bradycardia, nausea, vomiting, anorexia; prolongs P-R interval	Quinidine, amiodarone, verapamil increase digoxin levels; Diuretic, amphotericin-induced hypokalemia increases digoxin arrhythmia	Induces APC, VPC, accelerated AV junctional tachycardia	1–2 ng/mL (>6 mo old); 1.5–3 ng/mL (<6 mo old)
Verapamil (Ca²⁺ channel blocker)	SVT†	2–7 mg/kg/24 hr q8h	480 mg	0.1–0.2 mg/kg q20min 2 times (have IV CaCl₂ ready)	5–10 mg	Bradycardia, asystole, high-degree AV block, P-R prolongation, hypotension, CHF; Not for use in infants; Contraindicated in VT, severe CHF, and atrial fibrillation with WPW	Use with β-blocking agent or disopyramide exacerbates or precipitates CHF; increases digoxin levels and toxicity	No, but may increase AV block	—
Adenosine (purinergic agonist)	SVT†	—	—	50–300 µg/kg; begin with 50 µg/kg and increase by 50–100 µg/kg/dose if no effect; 6–12 mg in adolescents	Must be given as rapid IV (not arterial) push, repeat at higher dose if no effect	Because of short half-life, adverse effects (chest pain, dyspnea, facial flushing) last <1 min; may see transient bradycardia, rarely transient asystole, VPC	May be less effective in patients receiving theophylline; increased heart block with carbamazepine	—	—

*IV administration of antiarrhythmic drugs should always be at a slow rate, with constant monitoring of blood pressure and an electrocardiogram, particularly in patients with compromised cardiac, renal, or hepatic function. The dose must be modified in patients with abnormal renal or hepatic function. The exception is adenosine, which must be given by rapid IV push, usually followed by a saline flush. It is generally ineffective if given intra-arterially.

†Vagotonic maneuvers (placing the face in iced saline or an ice bag over the face) may be attempted first. If the patient is severely compromised and critically ill, synchronized DC cardioversion is the treatment of choice for SVT, atrial flutter, and atrial fibrillation.

‡Cardioversion is the treatment of choice for sustained VT with significant hemodynamic compromise. Some cardiologists try a chest thump or IV lidocaine, or both. If heart block is present, a temporary ventricular pacemaker may be needed.

§Sustained-release preparations available for clinical use.

‖Defibrillation is the treatment of choice.

SVT = supraventricular tachycardia; VPC = ventricular premature contraction; AV = atrioventricular; SLE = systemic lupus erythematosus–like illness, antinuclear antibody positive; CNS = central nervous system; PVCs = premature ventricular complexes; LQTS = long QT syndrome; CHF = congestive heart failure; JET = junctional ectopic tachycardia; VT = ventricular tachycardia; WPW = Wolff-Parkinson-White (pre-excitation) syndrome; IV = intravenous; PO = oral; APC = atrial premature contraction.

Lead 2

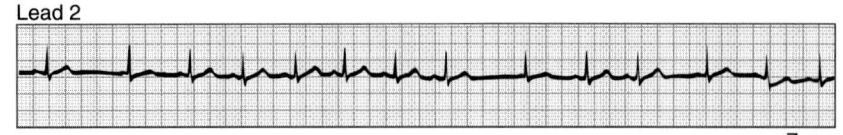

7 yrs.

FIGURE 428–1. Sinus arrhythmia with a junctional escape beat. Note the variation in P-P interval with little change in P morphology or P-R interval. When the sinus rate is slow enough, the atrioventricular junction takes over and produces escape beats. This rhythm is normal.

Lead 2

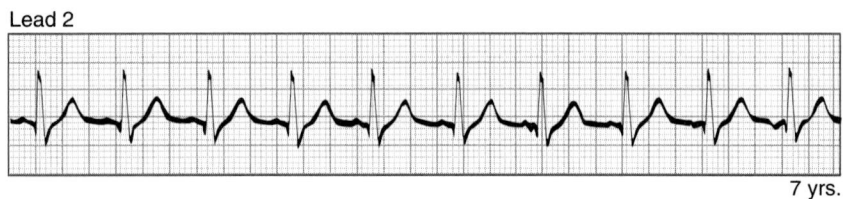

7 yrs.

FIGURE 428–2. Wandering atrial pacemaker. Note the change in P-wave configuration in the 7th, 9th, and 10th beats. The 7th P wave may represent a fusion between the sinus P and the ectopic atrial pacemaker seen in the 10th beat.

Premature atrial complexes are common in childhood, even in the absence of cardiac disease. Depending on the degree of prematurity of the beat (coupling interval) and the preceding R-R interval (cycle length), premature atrial complexes may result in a normal, a prolonged (*aberrancy*), or an absent (*blocked premature atrial complex*) QRS complex. The last occurs when the premature impulse is conducted to the ventricle while the specialized ventricular conducting system is partially refractory (Fig. 428–3). Atrial extrasystoles must be distinguished from premature ventricular complexes (PVCs). Careful scrutiny of the electrocardiogram for a premature P wave preceding the QRS that has a different contour from that of the other sinus P waves is essential for diagnosis. Atrial premature complexes often reset the sinus node pacemaker (lack of a compensatory pause), but this feature is not regarded as a reliable means of differentiating atrial from ventricular premature complexes.

PVCs may arise in any region of the ventricles. They are characterized by premature, widened, bizarre QRS complexes that are not preceded by a P wave (Fig. 428–4). When all premature beats have identical contours, they are classified as unifocal in origin. When PVCs vary in contour, they are designated as multifocal. Ventricular extrasystoles are often, but not always followed by a compensatory pause. The presence of fusion beats, that is, complexes with morphologic features that are intermediate between those of normal sinus beats and those of PVCs, is a clue to the ventricular origin of the extrasystole. Extrasystoles produce a smaller stroke and pulse volume than normal and, if quite premature, may not be audible with a stethoscope or palpable at the radial pulse. When frequent, extrasystoles may assume a definite rhythm, for example, alternating with normal beats (**bigeminy**) or occurring after two normal beats (**trigeminy**). Most patients are unaware of single premature ventricular contractions, although some may be aware of a "skipped beat" over the precordium. This sensation is due to the increased stroke volume of the normal beat following a compensatory pause. Anxiety, a febrile illness, or ingestion of

Lead 2   17 yrs.

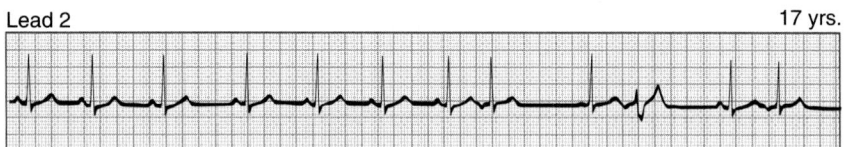

FIGURE 428–3. Premature atrial contraction (PAC). QRS complexes—the 8th, 10th, and final—in this strip are preceded by a P wave that is inverted, indicative of an ectopic origin of atrial depolarization. Note that the 8th and final QRS complexes resemble those of sinus origin whereas the 10th is aberrantly conducted. This shift in origin is a function of the preceding cycle length, which influences the refractory period of the bundle branches. The fact that the pause after the PAC is longer than two P-P intervals implies that the premature atrial depolarization has invaded and discharged the sinus node and then reset it so that it fires later.

Lead 2   15 yrs.

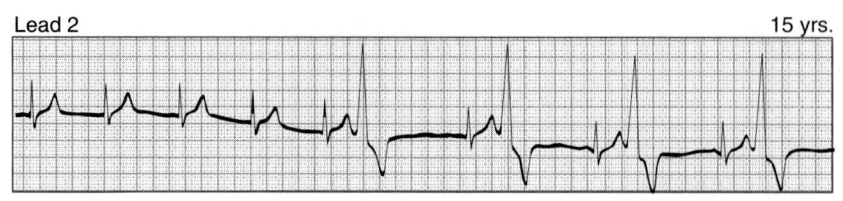

FIGURE 428–4. Premature ventricular contractions (PVCs) induced by hyperventilation. Note that the premature beat is wide and has a completely different morphology from that of the sinus beat. The fact that the premature beat is not preceded by a P wave and the pause following it is fully compensatory (i.e., the P-P interval containing the PVC equals two sinus cycles) indicates that the sinus mechanism has not been disturbed by the premature beats.

various drugs or stimulants may cause premature ventricular beats.

It is important to distinguish PVCs that are benign from those that are likely to degenerate into more severe dysrhythmias. The former usually disappear during the tachycardia of exercise. If they persist or become more frequent during exercise, the arrhythmia may have greater significance. The following criteria are indications for further investigation of PVCs that could require suppressive therapy: (1) two or more ventricular premature beats in a row, (2) multifocal origin, (3) increased ventricular ectopic activity with exercise, (4) R on T phenomenon (premature ventricular depolarization occurs on the T wave of the preceding beat), and (5) presence of underlying heart disease. The basis of therapy for benign PVCs is reassurance that the arrhythmia is not life threatening. Malignant PVCs are usually secondary to another medical problem, for example, electrolyte imbalance, hypoxia, drug toxicity, cardiac injury, or an intraventricular catheter. Successful treatment includes correction of the underlying abnormality. An intravenous lidocaine bolus and drip is the 1st line of therapy, with more powerful drugs such as amiodarone reserved for refractory cases or for patients with hemodynamic compromise. The choice of a maintenance oral antiarrhythmic agent is determined empirically or during an electrophysiologic study in the catheterization laboratory.

428.2 Supraventricular Tachycardia

Supraventricular tachycardias (SVTs) involve components of the conduction system within or above the bundle of His and can be divided into three major categories: *re-entrant tachycardias using an accessory pathway*, *re-entrant tachycardias without an accessory pathway*, and *ectopic or automatic tachycardias*. Re-entry using an accessory pathway is the most common mechanism of SVT in infants, with an increasing incidence of AV nodal re-entry noted in childhood. The tachycardia is initiated by a premature atrial beat that is most often conducted to the ventricle through the normal AV nodal pathway (*orthodromic conduction*). The ventricular response finds the AV nodal pathway refractory, but the bypass tract, readily able to conduct in a retrograde fashion, returns to the atrium as an echo beat, which in turn transmits back to the ventricle, and so on (Fig. 428–5). Atrial and junctional ectopic tachycardias are more commonly associated with abnormal hearts (e.g., cardiomyopathy) or with postoperative congenital heart disease.

Clinical Manifestations. Re-entrant SVT is characterized by an abrupt onset and cessation; it may be precipitated by an acute infection and usually occurs when the patient is at rest. Attacks may last only a few seconds or may persist for hours. The heart rate usually exceeds 180 beats/min and may occasionally be as rapid as 300 beats/min (Fig. 428–6). The only complaint may be awareness of the rapid heart rate. Many children tolerate these episodes extremely well, and it is unlikely that short paroxysms are a danger to life. If the rate is exceptionally rapid or if the attack is prolonged, precordial discomfort and heart failure may supervene. SVT may occur in the presence of unoperated congenital heart disease (Ebstein anomaly). In children, SVT may be precipitated by exposure to the sympathomimetic amines contained in over-the-counter decongestants.

In *young infants*, the diagnosis may be more obscure because of the inability to communicate their symptoms. The heart rate at this age is normally rapid, and even in the absence of tachyarrhythmia it increases greatly with crying. Infants with SVT are often initially seen in heart failure because the tachycardia goes unrecognized for a long time. The heart rate during paroxysms is frequently in the range of 200–300 beats/min. If the attack lasts 6–24 hr or more with an extremely fast heart rate, the infant may become acutely ill, have an ashen color, and be restless and irritable. Tachypnea and hepatomegaly are the prominent signs of cardiac failure, and fever and leukocytosis may be present. When tachycardia occurs in the fetus, it can cause severe heart failure and hydrops fetalis.

In *neonates*, SVT is usually manifested as a narrow QRS complex (<0.08 sec). The P wave is visible on a standard electrocardiogram in only 50–60% of neonates with SVT, but it is detectable with a transesophageal lead in most patients. Differentiation from sinus tachycardia may be difficult; if the rate is greater than 230 beats/min with an abnormal P-wave axis (a normal P wave is positive in leads I and aVF), SVT is more likely. The heart rate in SVT also tends to be unvarying, whereas in sinus tachycardia the heart rate varies with changes in vagal and sympathetic tone. Differentiation from ventricular tachycardia is critical because digoxin can precipitate ventricular fibrillation in patients with ventricular tachycardia. The absence of ventricular-to-atrial conduction (and thus only intermittent p waves), the presence of fusion beats, and wide QRS complexes that are dissimilar to the QRS complex during sinus rhythm are diagnostic of ventricular tachycardia.

AV re-entrant tachycardia uses a bypass tract that may either be able to conduct antegrade (Wolff-Parkinson-White [WPW]

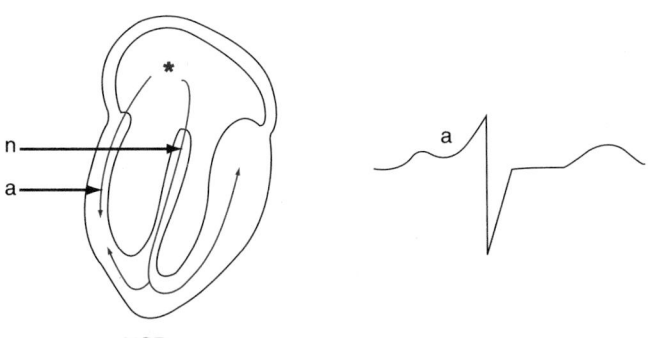

FIGURE 428–5. Schematic representation of the heart with a right-sided anomalous pathway. The *asterisk* indicates initiation of the sinus beat. The *arrows* indicate the direction and spread of excitation. The electrocardiographic complex shown represents a fusion beat that combines activation over the normal (n) and accessory (a) pathways. The latter inscribes the delta wave. NSR = normal sinus rhythm.

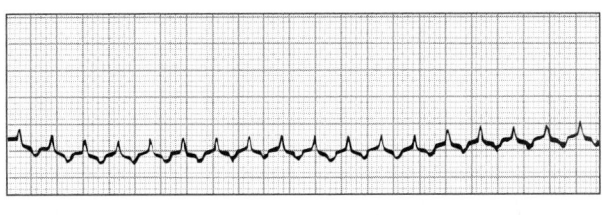
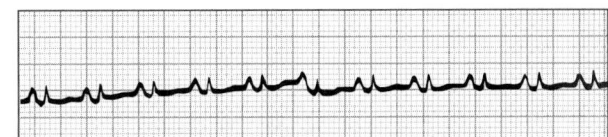

FIGURE 428–6. The *upper tracing* shows paroxysmal supraventricular or atrial tachycardia with a ventricular rate of 230/min. The *lower tracing* shows sinus rhythm after DC cardioversion. Note that during the tachycardia the T wave is deformed by an inverted, presumably retrograde P wave. The QRS morphology is unchanged during the tachycardia. The low voltage is due to peripheral edema in a 1-day-old infant who had intrauterine tachycardia and hydrops fetalis.

syndrome) or remain concealed. Patients with WPW syndrome have a small, but real risk of sudden death. If the accessory pathway rapidly conducts in antegrade fashion, the patient is at risk for atrial fibrillation begetting ventricular fibrillation. Risk stratification, including 24 hr Holter monitoring and exercise study, can help differentiate patients at higher risk for sudden death from WPW. Concurrently, any patient with syncope and WPW syndrome should have an electrophysiology study performed.

The typical electrocardiographic features of the **Wolff-Parkinson-White** *syndrome* are usually seen when the patient is not having the tachycardia. These features include a short P-R interval and slow upstroke of the QRS (delta wave) (Fig. 428–7). Though most often present in patients with a normal heart, this syndrome may also be associated with Ebstein anomaly and other congenital heart lesions. The anatomic substrates included in the re-entrant circuit are the AV node and an accessory pre-excitation pathway consisting of a muscular bridge connecting atrium to ventricle on either the right or the left side of the AV ring (see Fig. 428–5). During sinus rhythm, the impulse is carried over both the AV node and the accessory pathway; it produces some degree of fusion of the two depolarization fronts that results in an abnormal QRS. During tachycardia, an impulse is usually carried in anterograde fashion through the AV node (*orthodromic conduction*), which results in a normal QRS complex, and in retrograde fashion through the accessory pathway to the atrium, thereby perpetuating the tachycardia. In these cases, only after cessation of the tachycardia are the typical features of WPW syndrome recognized (see Fig. 428–7). When rapid anterograde conduction occurs through the pre-excitation pathway during tachycardia and the retrograde re-entry pathway to the atrium is via the AV node (*antidromic conduction)*, the tachycardiac complexes are wide and the potential for more serious arrhythmias (i.e., ventricular fibrillation) is greater, especially if atrial fibrillation occurs.

AV nodal re-entrant tachycardia involves the use of two pathways within the AV node. This arrhythmia is more commonly seen in adolescence. It is one of the few SVTs that is frequently associated with syncope. This arrhythmia is usually amenable to antiarrhythmic therapy, such as digoxin or propranolol, or to radiofrequency ablation therapy.

Treatment. Vagal stimulation by submersion of the face in iced saline (in older children) or by placing an ice bag over the face (in infants) may abort the attack. To abolish the paroxysm, older children may be taught **vagotonic maneuvers** such as the Valsalva maneuver, straining, breath holding, drinking ice water, or adopting a particular posture. When these measures fail, several pharmacologic alternatives are available (see Table 428–1). In stable patients, adenosine by rapid intravenous push is the treatment of choice because of its rapid onset of action and minimal effects on cardiac contractility. Other drugs that have been used for initial treatment of SVT include infusions of phenylephrine (Neo-Synephrine) or edrophonium (Tensilon), which increase vagal tone through the baroreflex, as well as the antiarrhythmic agents quinidine, procainamide, and propranolol. Calcium channel blockers such as verapamil have also been used in the initial treatment of SVT in older children. Verapamil may reduce cardiac output and produce hypotension and cardiac arrest in infants younger than 1 yr; it is therefore contraindicated in this age group. In urgent situations when symptoms of severe heart failure have already occurred, **synchronized DC cardioversion** (0.5–2 W-sec/kg) is recommended as the initial management (Chapter 57.1).

Once the patient has been converted to sinus rhythm, a longer acting agent is selected for maintenance therapy. In patients without an antegrade accessory pathway, digoxin or propranolol is the mainstay of therapy. In children with evidence of pre-excitation (e.g., WPW syndrome), digoxin or calcium channel blockers may increase the rate of anterograde conduction of impulses through the bypass tract and should be avoided. These patients are usually managed in the long term with propranolol. In patients with resistant tachycardias, procainamide, quinidine, flecainide, propafenone, sotalol, and amiodarone have all been used. It should be recognized that most antiarrhythmic agents could have proarrhythmic and negative inotropic effects. Flecainide in particular should be limited to use in patients with otherwise normal hearts.

If cardiac failure occurs because of prolonged tachycardia in an infant with a normal heart, cardiac function usually returns to normal after sinus rhythm is re-instituted, although it may take days to weeks. Infants with SVT diagnosed within the 1st 3–4 mo of life have a lower incidence of recurrence than do those in whom it is initially diagnosed at a later age. These patients have a 40% chance of resolution and are usually treated for a minimum of 1 yr after diagnosis, after which the antiarrhythmic agents can be tapered and the patient watched for signs of recurrence.

Twenty-four hour electrocardiographic (Holter) recordings are useful in monitoring the course of therapy and in detecting brief runs of asymptomatic tachycardia. A brief assessment of arrhythmia control can be made at the bedside with *transesophageal pacing*. More detailed *electrophysiologic studies* performed in the cardiac catheterization laboratory are often indicated in patients with refractory SVTs. During an electrophysiologic study, multiple electrode catheters are placed in different locations in the heart. By comparing the timing of premature beats in different leads, the location of an ectopic focus or bypass tract can be identified. The tachyarrhythmia can be induced by pacing, and different pharmacologic agents can be tested for their ability to inhibit the arrhythmia. These studies are necessary prerequisites to radiofrequency ablation.

Radiofrequency ablation of an accessory pathway is another treatment option commonly used in patients with re-entrant rhythms. It is often used electively in older children and teenagers, as well as for patients in whom multiple agents are required or drug side effects are intolerable or when arrhythmia control is poor. The overall initial success rate ranges from approximately 80 to 95%, depending on the location of the bypass tract or tracts. Surgical ablation of bypass tracts can also be successful in selected patients.

Atrial ectopic tachycardia is an uncommon tachycardia in childhood. It is characterized by a variable rate (seldom greater than 200 beats/min), identifiable P waves with an abnormal axis, and chronicity in either a sustained or intermittent tachycardia.

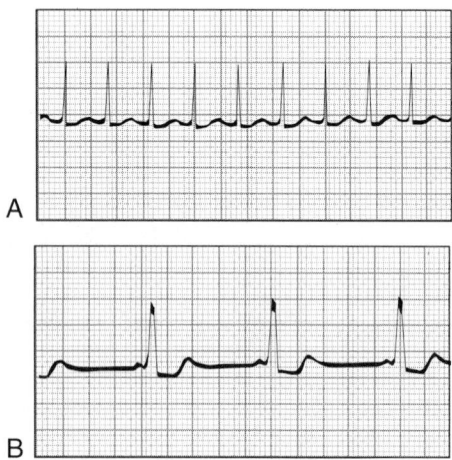

FIGURE 428–7. *A,* Supraventricular tachycardia in a child with Wolff-Parkinson-White (WPW) syndrome. Note the normal QRS complexes during the tachycardia. *B,* Later, the typical features of WPW syndrome are apparent (short P-R interval, delta wave, and wide QRS).

This form of atrial tachycardia has a single automatic focus rather than the more usual re-entry mechanism. Identification of this mechanism is aided by monitoring the electrocardiogram while initiating vagal or pharmacologic therapy. Re-entry tachycardias "break" suddenly, whereas automatic tachycardias gradually slow down and then gradually speed up again. Atrial ectopic tachycardias are usually more difficult to control pharmacologically than the more common re-entrant tachycardias are. If pharmacologic therapy with a single agent is unsuccessful, catheter ablation is suggested and has a greater than 90% success rate.

Chaotic or multifocal atrial tachycardia is characterized by three or more ectopic P waves with three or more different ectopic P-P cycles, frequent blocked P waves, and varying P-R intervals of conducted beats. This arrhythmia occurs most often in infants younger than 1 yr, usually without cardiac disease, although some evidence suggests an association with viral myocarditis. Drug treatment may not be effective, and multiple agents are often required. Fortunately, when this arrhythmia occurs in infancy, it usually terminates spontaneously by 3 yr of age.

Accelerated junctional ectopic tachycardia (JET) is an automatic (non–re-entry) arrhythmia in which the junctional rate exceeds that of the sinus node and AV dissociation results. This arrhythmia is most often recognized in the early postoperative period after cardiac surgery and may be extremely difficult to control. Reduction of the infusion rate of catecholamines and control of fever are important adjuncts to management. JET in these patients often disappears spontaneously without specific treatment; JET in the absence of surgery carries a more guarded prognosis. Junctional tachycardia may also be a sign of digitalis intoxication; when intoxication occurs, the drug should be discontinued. Intravenous amiodarone is effective in the treatment of postoperative JET. Patients who require chronic therapy may respond to amiodarone or sotalol.

Atrial flutter, also known as *intra-atrial re-entrant tachycardia*, is a regular or regularly irregular tachycardia characterized by atrial activity at a rate of 250–400 beats/min. These contractions are thought to be due to a re-entrant or circus rhythm originating in the atria and involving a micro–re-entrant loop within the atrial tissue and some form of anatomic obstacle that creates a discontinuity in conduction (fibrosis, surgical suture site, valve annulus). Because the AV node cannot transmit such rapid impulses, some degree of AV block is virtually always present, and the ventricles respond to every 2nd–4th atrial beat. Occasionally, the response is variable and the rhythm appears irregular.

In older children, atrial flutter usually occurs in the setting of congenital heart disease; however, neonates with atrial flutter frequently have normal hearts. Atrial flutter may occur during acute infectious illnesses but is most often seen in patients with large stretched atria, such as those associated with long-standing mitral or tricuspid insufficiency, tricuspid atresia, Ebstein anomaly, or rheumatic mitral stenosis. Atrial flutter can also occur after palliative or corrective intra-atrial surgery. Uncontrolled atrial flutter may precipitate heart failure. Vagal maneuvers (such as carotid sinus pressure or iced saline submersion) or adenosine generally produce a temporary slowing of the heart rate. The diagnosis is confirmed by electrocardiography, which demonstrates the rapid and regular atrial saw-toothed flutter waves. Atrial flutter usually converts immediately to sinus rhythm by synchronized DC cardioversion, which is most often the treatment of choice. Patients with chronic atrial flutter in the setting of congenital heart disease may be at increased risk for thromboembolism and stroke and should thus undergo anticoagulation before elective cardioversion. Digitalis slows the ventricular response in atrial flutter by prolonging conduction time through the AV node. After digitalization, a type I agent such as quinidine or procainamide is usually needed to maintain adequate control. Type III agents such as amiodarone and sotalol have shown promise and may be useful in patients refractory to type I agents. Other modalities, including radiofrequency and surgical ablation, have been used in older patients with congenital heart disease with moderate success. Neonates with normal hearts who respond to digoxin may be treated for 6–12 mo, after which the medication can often be discontinued.

Atrial fibrillation is much less common in children and rare in infants. The atrial excitation is chaotic and more rapid (300–700 beats/min) and produces an irregularly irregular ventricular response and pulse (Fig. 428–8). This rhythm disorder is most often the result of a chronically stretched atrial myocardium. Atrial fibrillation occurs most frequently in older children with rheumatic mitral valve disease. It is also seen rarely as a complication of intra-atrial surgery, in patients with left atrial enlargement secondary to left AV valve insufficiency, in conditions producing atrial flutter, and in patients with WPW syndrome. Thyrotoxicosis, pulmonary emboli, and pericarditis should be suspected in a previously normal older child or adolescent with atrial fibrillation. Atrial fibrillation may be familial. The best initial treatment is digitalization, which restores the ventricular rate to normal, although the atrial fibrillation usually persists. Digoxin is not given if WPW syndrome is present. Normal sinus rhythm may then be restored with a type I agent such as quinidine or procainamide or by DC cardioversion. Patients with chronic atrial fibrillation are at risk for the development of thromboemboli and stroke and should undergo anticoagulation with warfarin. Patients being treated by elective cardioversion should also undergo anticoagulation.

428.3 Ventricular Tachyarrhythmias

Ventricular tachycardia (VT) is less common than SVT in pediatric patients. VT is defined as at least three PVCs at greater than 120 beats/min. It may be paroxysmal or incessant. VT may be associated with myocarditis, anomalous origin of a coronary artery, arrhythmogenic right ventricular dysplasia, mitral valve prolapse, primary cardiac tumors, cardiomyopathy, prolonged Q-T interval of either congenital or acquired (proarrhythmic drugs) cause, WPW syndrome, or drugs (cocaine, amphetamines); it may develop many years after intraventricular surgery (tetralogy of Fallot, ventricular septal defect) or occur without obvious organic heart disease. VT must be distinguished from SVT with aberrancy or rapid conduction over an accessory pathway (Table 428–2). The presence of capture and fusion

FIGURE 428–8. Atrial fibrillation, characterized by the absence of P waves; presence of fibrillatory waves, which are grossly irregular, rapid undulations; and an irregular ventricular response. Fibrillatory waves may not be visible in all leads and should be carefully sought in every tracing with irregular R-R intervals. (The coexisting qR in V_1 is diagnostic of right ventricular hypertrophy in this patient with Eisenmenger syndrome.)

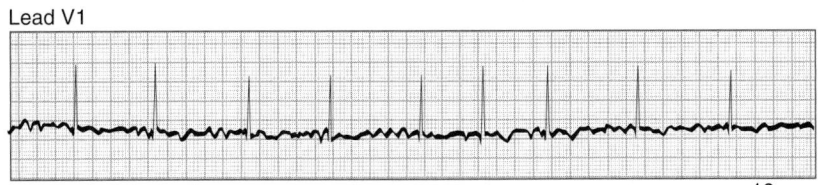

Lead V1

16 yrs.

TABLE 428–2. Diagnosis of Tachyarrhythmias

	Electrocardiographic Findings			
	Heart Rate (Beats/min)	*P Wave*	*QRS Duration*	*Regularity*
Sinus tachycardia	<225	Always present Normal axis	Normal	Rate varies with respiration
Atrial tachycardia	180–320	Present—50% Superior axis common	Normal or prolonged (RBBB pattern)	Regular
Atrial fibrillation	120–180	Fibrillatory waves	Normal or prolonged (RBBB pattern)	Irregularly irregular
Atrial flutter	Atrial: 250–400 Ventricular response variable: 100–320	Saw-toothed flutter waves	Normal or prolonged (RBBB pattern)	Regular ventricular response (e.g., 2:1, 3:1, 3:2, and so on)
Ventricular tachycardia	120–240	Absent or atrioventricular dissociation	Usually prolonged	Slightly irregular

RBBB = right bundle branch block.

beats helps confirm the diagnosis. Although some children tolerate rapid ventricular rates for many hours, this arrhythmia should be promptly treated because hypotension and degeneration into ventricular fibrillation may result. For patients who are hemodynamically stable, intravenous lidocaine is the initial drug of choice. If treatment is to be successful, it is critical to search for and correct any underlying abnormalities such as electrolyte imbalance, hypoxia, or drug toxicity. Alternative drugs include amiodarone, procainamide, and propranolol (see Table 428–1). Amiodarone is quite useful during cardiac arrest (Chapter 57.1). Overdrive ventricular pacing may also be effective, although it may occasionally cause the arrhythmia to deteriorate into ventricular fibrillation. In the neonatal period, ventricular tachycardia may be associated with an anomalous left coronary artery (see Chapter 425.2) or a myocardial tumor.

Unless a clearly reversible cause is identified, electrophysiologic study is usually indicated for patients in whom VT has developed.

Ventricular fibrillation is a chaotic dysrhythmia that results in death unless an effective ventricular beat is rapidly re-established. A thump on the chest sometimes restores sinus rhythm. Usually, external cardiac massage with artificial ventilation and DC defibrillation is necessary. If defibrillation is ineffective or fibrillation recurs, amiodarone may be given intravenously and defibrillation repeated. After recovery from ventricular fibrillation, a search should be made for the underlying cause. The Q-T interval should be measured to rule out long Q-T syndrome (LQTS). Electrophysiologic study is usually indicated for patients in whom ventricular fibrillation has developed unless a clearly reversible cause is identified. If WPW syndrome is noted, ablation should be performed. For patients in whom no correctable abnormality can be found, an ICD should be strongly considered because of the high risk of sudden death.

428.4 Long Q-T Syndrome

A particularly malignant form of ventricular arrhythmia called *torsades de pointes* occurs in patients with LQTS; it is a cause of syncope and sudden death and may be associated with sudden infant death syndrome or drowning. About 50% of cases are familial: **Romano-Ward syndrome** (RWS) is a common form of LQTS that exhibits autosomal dominant transmission with low penetrance, but some cases are autosomal recessive; **Jervell-Lange-Nielsen syndrome** (JLNS) is an uncommon form of LQTS, has autosomal recessive transmission, and may be associated with congenital deafness. The remainder of cases are sporadic. Genetic studies have identified mutations in cardiac potassium and sodium channels. In LQT1, a form of RWS, the gene is on chromosome 11p15.5 and encodes a potassium

channel (KVLQT1). *LQT2* gene is on chromosome 7q35-36, which encodes HERG (human ether a go-go related gene), a potassium channel. *LQT3* is a defect on chromosome 3p21-24 and encodes a sodium channel (SCN5A). The cause of *LQT4* is unknown. *LQT5* is a mutation on chromosome 21q22.1 and encodes a regulator (minK) of potassium channels. *LQT6* is on chromosome 21q22.1 and is a minK-related peptide. At least one form of JLNS is due to homozygous mutations of *KVLQT1*, whereas the heterozygous state is manifested as RWJ. Genotype may predict clinical manifestations; for example, LQT1 events are stress induced whereas events in LQT3 occur during sleep. LQT2 events have an intermediate pattern. LQT3 has the highest probability for sudden death, followed by LQT2 and then LQT1. Drugs may prolong the Q-T interval directly (terfenadine, astemizole) or more often when drugs such as erythromycin or ketoconazole inhibit their metabolism.

The clinical manifestation of LQTS in children is most often a syncopal episode often brought on by exercise, fright, or a sudden startle; some events occur during sleep. Patients can initially be seen with seizures, presyncope, and palpitations, and about 10% are initially in cardiac arrest. The diagnosis is based on electrocardiographic and clinical criteria. Not all patients with long Q-T intervals have LQTS, and rare patients with normal Q-T intervals on a resting electrocardiogram may have LQTS. A heart rate–corrected Q-T interval of greater than 0.47 sec is highly indicative, whereas a Q-T interval of greater than 0.44 sec is suggestive. Other features include notched T waves, T wave alternans, a low heart rate for age, a history of syncope (especially with stress), and a familial history of either LQTS or unexplained sudden death. Twenty-four hour Holter monitoring and exercise testing are adjuncts to the diagnosis.

Treatment of LQTS includes the use of β-blocking agents at doses that blunt the heart rate response to exercise. Some patients may require a pacemaker because of drug-induced profound bradycardia. In patients with continued syncope despite treatment and for those who have experienced cardiac arrest, many authorities recommend an ICD.

428.5 Bradyarrhythmias

Sinus arrest and *sinoatrial block* may cause a sudden pause in the heartbeat. The former is presumably caused by failure of impulse formation within the sinus node and the latter by a block between the sinus impulse and the surrounding atrium. These arrhythmias are rare in childhood except as manifestations of digitalis intoxication or in patients who have had extensive atrial surgery.

AV block may be divided into three forms. In **1st-degree block**, the P-R interval is prolonged, but all the atrial impulses are conducted to the ventricle. In **2nd-degree block**, some impulses are not conducted to the ventricle. In one variant of *2nd-degree block* known as the **Wenckebach type** (also called *Mobitz type I*), the P-P interval remains constant and the P-R interval increases progressively until a P wave is not conducted. In the cycle following the dropped beat, the P-R interval is again shorter (Fig. 428–9). In *Mobitz type II*, occasional atrial beats are not conducted to the ventricle; this conduction defect has more potential to cause syncope and may be progressive. In **3rd-degree block** (complete heart block), no impulses from the atria reach the ventricles.

Congenital complete AV block in children is most often caused by autoimmune injury of the fetal conduction system by maternally derived IgG antibodies (anti-SSA/Ro, anti-SSB/La) in a mother with overt or, more often, asymptomatic SLE. Rheumatoid arthritis, dermatomyositis, or Sjögren syndrome is rarely the primary autoimmune process. Autoimmune disease accounts for 60–70% of all cases of congenital complete heart block and about 80% of cases in which the heart is structurally normal. Complete heart block is also seen in patients with complex congenital heart disease, abnormal embryonic development of the conduction system, myocardial tumors, myocarditis, myocardial abscess secondary to endocarditis, LQTS, postsurgical repair of congenital heart disease involving the ventricular septum, and Kearns-Sayre syndrome. The incidence of congenital complete heart block is 1 in 20,000–25,000 live births; a high fetal wastage rate may cause an underestimation of its true incidence, however. In some infants of mothers with SLE, complete heart block is not present at birth but develops within the 1st 3–6 mo after birth. Steroids may be helpful in preventing the development of complete heart block. The arrhythmia is occasionally suspected in the fetus and may produce hydrops fetalis. The dissociation between atrial and ventricular contractions can be diagnosed by fetal echocardiography. Infants with associated congenital heart disease who experience heart failure in the 1st wk of life are at greatest risk for serious illness.

In older children with otherwise normal hearts, the condition is commonly asymptomatic, although syncope may occur. Older infants may have night terrors, tiredness with frequent naps, and irritability. The peripheral pulse is prominent as a result of the compensatory large ventricular stroke volume and peripheral vasodilation; systolic blood pressure is elevated. Jugular venous pulsations occur irregularly and may be large when the atrium contracts against a closed tricuspid valve (cannon wave). Exercise and atropine may produce an acceleration of 10–20 beats/min or more. Systolic murmurs are frequently audible along the left sternal border, and apical mid-diastolic murmurs are not unusual. Heart block results in enlargement of the heart on the basis of increased diastolic ventricular filling.

The *diagnosis* is confirmed by electrocardiography; the P waves and QRS complexes have no constant relationship (Fig. 428–10).

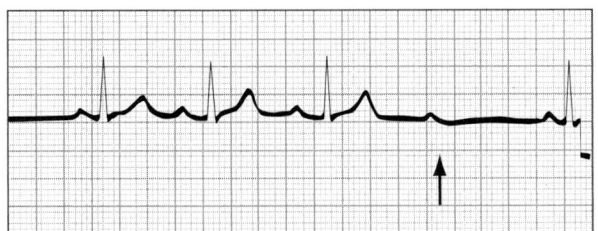

FIGURE 428–9. Wenckebach phenomenon (Mobitz I). The P-R interval gradually lengthens until the 4th P wave in the cycle is not conducted to the ventricle (*arrow*). The ensuing P-R interval is once again normal.

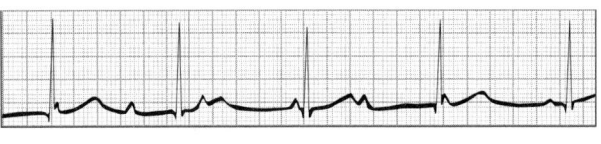

Lead II

FIGURE 428–10. Complete atrioventricular (AV) block. The ventricular rate is regular at 53/min. The atrial rate varied from 65 to 95/min. The QRS morphology is normal, which is usual in congenital AV block.

The QRS duration may be prolonged, or it may be normal if the heartbeat is initiated high in the bundle of His.

The *prognosis* for congenital complete heart block is usually favorable; patients who have been observed to the age of 30–40 yr have lived normal, active lives. Some patients have episodes of dizziness with or without syncope (**Stokes-Adams attacks**); this symptom requires the implantation of a permanent cardiac pacemaker. Pacemaker implantation should be considered for patients in whom symptoms develop, such as progressive cardiac enlargement, prolonged pauses, or awake heart rates of 40 beats/min or less.

Cardiac pacing is required in neonates with ventricular rates of 50 beats/min or less who show evidence of hydrops or experience heart failure after birth. Isoproterenol, atropine, or epinephrine may be used to try to increase the heart rate temporarily until pacemaker placement can be arranged. Patients with complete heart block and congenital heart disease should also receive a pacemaker. Transthoracic epicardial pacemaker implants have traditionally been used in infants; transvenous placement of pacemaker leads is available for older infants and young children.

Postsurgical complete AV block can occur after any open heart procedure requiring suturing near the AV valves or crest of the ventricular septum. Because postoperative heart block may be transient, the patient should be maintained with temporary pacing wires inserted at the time of surgery until at least 10–14 days, after which it is much less likely that sinus rhythm will return.

428.6 Sick Sinus Syndrome

Sick sinus syndrome is the result of abnormalities in the sinus node or atrial conduction pathways, or both. This syndrome may occur in the absence of congenital heart disease and has been reported in siblings, but it is most commonly seen after surgical correction of congenital heart defects, especially the atrial switch (Mustard or Senning) operation for transposition of the great arteries. *Clinical manifestations* depend on the heart rate. Most patients remain asymptomatic without treatment, but dizziness and syncope can occur during periods of marked sinus slowing with failure of junctional escape (Fig. 428–11). SVT may alternate with bradycardia (*bradycardia-tachycardia syndrome*) and cause palpitations, exercise intolerance, or dizziness. Treatment must be individualized. Drug therapy to control tachyarrhythmias (e.g., propranolol, quinidine, procainamide) may suppress sinus and AV node function to such a degree that symptomatic bradycardia may be produced. Therefore, insertion of a demand ventricular pacemaker in conjunction with drug therapy is usually necessary for symptomatic patients.

428.7 Sudden Death

Sudden death other than sudden infant death syndrome (see Chapter 360) is rare in children younger than 18 yr. Potential causes are noted in Box 428–1. Competitive high-school sports

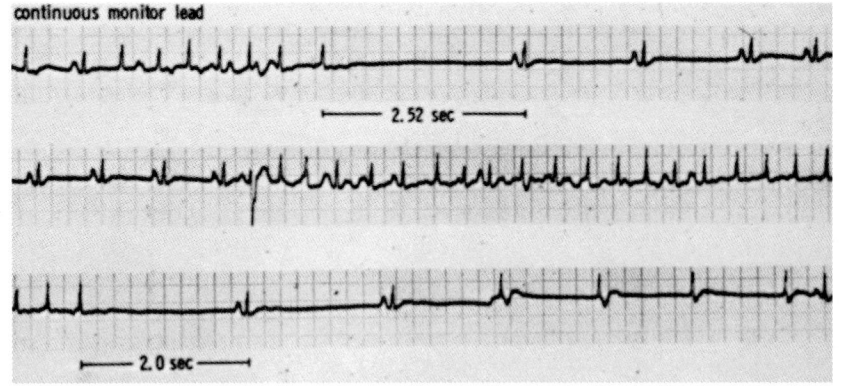

continuous monitor lead

|— 2.52 sec —|

|— 2.0 sec —|

FIGURE 428–11. Sick sinus syndrome with bradytachycardia. Note the bursts of supraventricular tachycardia, probably multifocal in origin, followed by long periods of sinus arrest and by sinus bradycardia.

(basketball, football) are high-risk environmental factors. Approximately 65% of sudden deaths are due to heart-related problems in patients with normal or congenitally (corrected, palliated, or unoperated) abnormal hearts. Symptoms may be absent before the event but, if present, include syncope, chest pain, dyspnea, and palpitations. Patients may have a family his-

---

BOX 428–1. Potential Causes of Sudden Death in Infants, Children, and Adolescents

SIDS AND SIDS "MIMICS"
SIDS
Long Q-T syndromes
Inborn errors of metabolism
Child abuse
Myocarditis
Duct-dependent congenital heart disease

CORRECTED OR UNOPERATED CONGENITAL HEART DISEASE
Aortic stenosis
Tetralogy of Fallot
Transposition of great vessels (postoperative atrial switch)
Mitral valve prolapse
Hypoplastic left heart syndrome
Eisenmenger syndrome

CORONARY ARTERIAL DISEASE
Anomalous origin
Anomalous tract
Kawasaki disease
Periarteritis
Arterial dissection
Marfan syndrome
Myocardial infarction

MYOCARDIAL DISEASE
Myocarditis
Hypertrophic cardiomyopathy
Dilated cardiomyopathy
Arrhythmogenic right ventricular dysplasia

CONDUCTION SYSTEM ABNORMALITY/ARRHYTHMIA
Long Q-T syndromes
Proarrhythmic drugs
Pre-excitation syndromes
Heart block
Commotio cordis
Idiopathic ventricular fibrillation
Heart tumor

MISCELLANEOUS
Pulmonary hypertension
Pulmonary embolism
Heat stroke
Cocaine
Anorexia nervosa
Electrolyte disturbances

SIDS = sudden infant death syndrome.

---

tory (dilated or hypertrophic cardiomyopathy, long Q-T interval, right ventricular dysplasia, mitral valve prolapse, Marfan syndrome) of heart disease or sudden death. Death often follows exertion or exercise.

Commotio cordis is a nearly universally fatal condition that follows blunt nonpenetrating trauma to the chest (e.g., from a baseball or hockey puck). Occasionally innocent-appearing chest blows while at home or at a playground may be fatal. Patients experience immediate ventricular fibrillation in the absence of identifiable cardiac trauma (contusion, hematoma, lacerated coronary artery). Death results from ventricular fibrillation that is unresponsive to all resuscitative efforts in 85–90% of children.

Prevention of Sudden Death. Many of the more common causes of sudden death in children and adolescents can be identified from the patient's history (prodromal symptoms), the family history, and physical examination.

Avoiding high-risk behavior (cocaine, anorexia nervosa) and knowledge of drug side effects (tricyclic antidepressants) or drug interactions (terfenadine [Seldane]-erythromycin) is critical. Chest-protecting equipment and softer baseballs may prevent *commotio cordis*. Prompt cardiopulmonary resuscitation *and* rapid defibrillation by an automatic external defibrillator or by an emergency medical services rescue team improves survival.

In patients with known risk factors for sudden death, ICD therapy may be used as a protective measure.

Ackerman MJ, Tester DJ, Porter CJ, et al: Molecular diagnosis of the inherited long-QT syndrome in a woman who dies after near-drowning. *N Engl J Med* 1999;341:1121–5.

Benson DW Jr, Smith WM, Dunnigan A, et al: Mechanisms of regular, wide QRS tachycardia in infants and children. *Am J Cardiol* 1982;49:1778.

Blaufox AD, Felix GL, Saul JP, et al: Radiofrequency catheter ablation in infants ≤18 months old. *Circulation* 2001;104:2803–8.

Brugada R, Tapscott T, Czernuszewicz GZ, et al: Identification of a genetic locus for familial atrial fibrillation. *N Engl J Med* 1997;336:905.

Case C, Crawford F, Gillette P: Surgical treatment of dysrhythmias. *Pediatr Clin North Am* 1990;37:79.

Cecchin F, Jorgenson DB, Berul CI, et al: Is arrhythmia detection by automatic external defibrillator accurate for children? *Circulation* 2001;103:2483–8.

Dungan WT, Garson A Jr, Gillette PC: Arrhythmogenic right ventricular dysplasia: A cause of ventricular tachycardia in children with apparently normal hearts. *Am Heart J* 1981;102:745.

Dunnigan A, Benson DW Jr, Banditt DG: Atrial flutter in infancy: Diagnosis, clinical features, and treatment. *Pediatrics* 1985;75:725.

Eronen M, Siren MK, Ekblad H, et al: Short- and long-term outcome of children with congenital complete heart block diagnosed in utero as a newborn. *Pediatrics* 2000;106:86–91.

Esberger D, Jones S, Morris F, et al: Junctional tachycardias. *Br Med J* 2002;324:662–665.

Etheridge SP, Judd VE: Supraventricular tachycardia in infancy. *Arch Pediatr Adolesc Med* 1999;153:267–71.

Fenrich AL, Perry JC, Friedman RA: Flecainide and amiodarone: Combined therapy for refractory tachyarrhythmias in infancy. *J Am Coll Cardiol* 1995;25:1195.

Goodacre S, McLeod K: Paediatric electrocardiography. *Br Med J* 2002;324:1382–5.

Goodwin JF: Sudden cardiac death in the young. *Br Med J* 1997;314:843.

Gow R: Ventricular arrhythmias in infants and children. *Curr Opin Pediatr* 1990;2:963.

Josephson ME: Antiarrhythmic agents and the danger of proarrhythmic events. *Ann Intern Med* 1989;111:101.

Kirk CR, Gibbs JL, Thomas R: Cardiovascular collapse after verapamil in supraventricular tachycardia. *Arch Dis Child* 1987;62:1265.

Kugler JD, Danford DA: Management of infants, children, and adolescents with paroxysmal supraventricular tachycardia. *J Pediatr* 1996;129:324.

Kugler JD, Danford DA, Deal BJ, et al: Radiofrequency catheter ablation for tachyarrhythmias in children and adolescents. *N Engl J Med* 1994;330:1481.

Kusumoto FM, Goldschlager N: Device therapy for cardiac arrhythmias. *JAMA* 2002;287:1848–52.

Liberthson RR: Sudden death from cardiac causes in children and young adults. *N Engl J Med* 1996;334:1039.

Link MS, Wang PJ, Pandian NG, et al: An experimental model of sudden death due to low-energy chest-wall impact (commotio cordis). *N Engl J Med* 1998;338:1805.

Maron BJ, Gohman TE, Kyle SB, et al: Clinical profile and spectrum of commotio cordis. *JAMA* 2002;287:1142–6.

Maron BJ, Shirani J, Poliac LC, et al: Sudden death in young competitive athletes. *JAMA* 1996;276:199.

Miller MD, Porter CJ, Ackerman MJ: Diagnostic accuracy of screening electrocardiograms in long QT syndrome I. *Pediatrics* 2001;108:8–12.

Narayan SM, Cain ME, Smith JM: Atrial fibrillation. *Lancet* 1997;350:943.

Ommen SR, Odell JA, Stanton MS: Atrial arrhythmias after cardiothoracic surgery. *N Engl J Med* 1997;336:1429.

Perry JC, Garson A Jr: Supraventricular tachycardia due to Wolff-Parkinson-White syndrome in children: Early disappearance and late recurrence. *J Am Coll Cardiol* 1990;16:1215.

Priori SG, Napolitano C, Schwartz PJ: Low penetrance in the long-QT syndrome: Clinical impact. *Circulation* 1999;102:529.

Ralston MA, Knilans TK, Hannon DW, et al: Use of adenosine for diagnosis and treatment of tachyarrhythmias in pediatric patients. *J Pediatr* 1994;124:139.

Rankin AC: Non-sedating antihistamines and cardiac arrhythmia. *Lancet* 1997;350:1115.

Risser WL, Anderson SJ, Bolduc SP, et al: Cardiac dysrhythmias and sports. *Pediatrics* 1995;95:786.

Splawski I, Timothy KW, Vincent GM, et al: Molecular basis of the long-QT syndrome associated with deafness. *N Engl J Med* 1997;336:1562.

Tan HL, Hou CJY, Lauer MR, et al: Electrophysiologic mechanisms of the long QT interval syndromes and torsades de pointes. *Ann Intern Med* 1995;122:701.

Tanel RE, Walsh EP, Triedman JK, et al: Five-year experience with radiofrequency catheter ablation: Implications for management of arrhythmias in pediatric and young adult patients. *J Pediatr* 1997;131:878.

Tchou PJ, Kadri N, Anderson J, et al: Automatic implantable cardioverter defibrillators and survival of patients with left ventricular dysfunction and malignant ventricular arrhythmias. *Ann Intern Med* 1988;109:529.

Towbin JA, Wang Z, Li H: Genotype and severity of long QT syndrome. *Arch Pathol Lab Med* 2001;125:116–21.

Van Hare GF: Indications for radiofrequency ablation in the pediatric population. *J Cardiovasc Electrophysiol* 1997;8:952.

Wellens HJJ, Brugada P, Penn OC: The management of preexcitation syndromes. *JAMA* 1987;257:2325.

Zimetbaum P, Josephson ME: Evaluation of patients with palpitations. *N Engl J Med* 1998;338:1369.

SECTION 5 *Acquired Heart Disease*

Daniel Bernstein

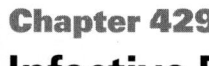

Chapter 429
Infective Endocarditis

Infective endocarditis includes acute and subacute bacterial endocarditis, as well as nonbacterial endocarditis caused by viruses, fungi, and other microbiologic agents. It is a significant cause of morbidity and mortality in children and adolescents despite advances in the management and prophylaxis of the disease with antimicrobial agents. The inability to eradicate infective endocarditis by prevention or early treatment stems from several factors: the nature of the infecting organism has changed; physicians, dentists, and the public are not sufficiently aware of the threat of infective endocarditis and the preventive measures available; diagnosis may be difficult when delayed; and special risk groups have emerged, including an increasing number of intravenous drug users, survivors of cardiac surgery, patients taking immunosuppressant medications, and patients who require chronic intravascular catheters. In addition, many patients get endocarditis on what was thought to be a previously healthy native valve. Furthermore, endocarditis from oral flora may occur without a preceding dental procedure.

Etiology. Viridans-type streptococci (α-hemolytic streptococci) and *Staphylococcus aureus* are the leading causative agents responsible for endocarditis in pediatric patients. Other organisms cause endocarditis less frequently, and in approximately 6% of cases, blood cultures are negative for any organisms (Box 429–1). No relationship exists between the infecting organism and the type of congenital defect, the duration of illness, or the age of the child. Staphylococcal endocarditis is more common in patients with no underlying heart disease; viridans group streptococcal infection is more common after dental procedures, group D enterococci are seen more often after lower bowel or genitourinary manipulation, *Pseudomonas aeruginosa* or *Serratia marcescens* is seen more frequently in intravenous drug users, and fungal organisms are encountered after open heart surgery. Coagulase-negative staphylococci are common in the presence of an indwelling central venous catheter.

Epidemiology. Infective endocarditis is often a complication of congenital or rheumatic heart disease but can also occur in children without any abnormal valves or cardiac malformations. In developed countries, congenital heart disease is the overwhelming predisposing factor. Endocarditis is rare in infancy; in this age group it usually follows open heart surgery or is associated with a central venous line.

Patients with congenital heart lesions in which blood is ejected at high velocity through a hole or stenotic orifice are most susceptible to endocarditis. Vegetations usually form at the site of the endocardial or intimal erosion that results from the turbulent flow. Children with ventricular septal defects (VSDs), left-sided valvular disease, and systemic-pulmonary arterial communications (including palliative shunts) are at highest risk. Tetralogy of Fallot, VSD, aortic stenosis, patent ductus arteriosus, transposition of the great arteries, and Blalock-Taussig shunts are the most frequent structural lesions associated with endocarditis. In older patients, congenital bicuspid aortic valves and mitral valve prolapse pose additional risks for endocarditis. Surgical correction of congenital heart disease may reduce, but does not eliminate the risk of endocarditis, with the exception of repair of a simple atrial septal defect or patent ductus arteriosus. Children who have undergone valve replacement or valved conduit repair are at particularly high risk.

BOX 429–1. Bacterial Agents in Pediatric Infective Endocarditis

COMMON: NATIVE VALVE OR OTHER CARDIAC LESIONS

Viridans group streptococci (*S. mutans, S. sanguis, S. mitis*)
Staphylococcus aureus
Group D streptococcus (enterococcus) (*S. bovis, S. faecalis*)

UNCOMMON: NATIVE VALVE OR OTHER CARDIAC LESIONS

Streptococcus pneumoniae
Haemophilus influenzae
Coagulase-negative staphylococci
Coxiella burnetii (Q fever)*
Neisseria gonorrhoeae
*Brucella**
*Chlamydia psittacli**
*Chlamydia trachomatis**
*Chlamydia pneumoniae**
*Legionella**
*Bartonella**
HACEK group[†]
*Streptobacillus moniliformis**
*Pasteurella multocida**
Campylobacter fetus
Culture negative (6% of cases)

PROSTHETIC VALVE

Staphylococcus epidermidis
Staphylococcus aureus
Viridans group streptococcus
Pseudomonas aeruginosa
Serratia marcescens
Diphtheroids
Legionella species*
HACEK group[†]
Fungi[‡]

---

*These fastidious bacteria plus some fungi may produce culture-negative endocarditis. Detection may require special media, incubation for more than 7 days, or serologic tests.
[†]The HACEK group includes *Haemophilus* species (*H. paraphrophilus, H. parainfluenzae, H. aphrophilus*), *Actinobacillus actinomycetemcomitans, Cardiobacterium hominis, Eikenella corrodens,* and *Kingella* species.
[‡]*Candida* species, *Aspergillus* species, *Pseudallescheria boydii, Histoplasma capsulatum.*

BOX 429–2. Manifestations of Infective Endocarditis

HISTORY

Prior congenital or rheumatic heart disease
Preceding dental, urinary tract, or intestinal procedure
Intravenous drug use
Central venous catheter
Prosthetic heart valve

SYMPTOMS

Fever
Chills
Chest and abdominal pain
Arthralgia, myalgia
Dyspnea
Malaise
Night sweats
Weight loss
CNS manifestations (stroke, seizures, headache)

SIGNS

Elevated temperature
Tachycardia
Embolic phenomena (Roth spots, petechiae, splinter nail bed
   hemorrhages, Osler nodes, CNS or ocular lesions)
Janeway lesions
New or changing murmur
Splenomegaly
Arthritis
Heart failure
Arrhythmias
Metastatic infection (arthritis, meningitis, mycotic arterial aneurysm,
   pericarditis, abscesses, septic pulmonary emboli)
Clubbing

LABORATORY

Positive blood culture
Elevated erythrocyte sedimentation rate; may be low with heart or
   renal failure
Elevated C-reactive protein
Anemia
Leukocytosis
Immune complexes
Hypergammaglobulinemia
Hypocomplementemia
Cryoglobulinemia
Rheumatoid factor
Hematuria
Renal failure: azotemia, high creatinine (glomerulonephritis)
Chest radiograph: bilateral infiltrates, nodules, pleural effusions
Echocardiographic evidence of valve vegetations, prosthetic valve
   dysfunction or leak, myocardial abscess, new-onset valve
   insufficiency

CNS = central nervous system.

In approximately 30% of patients with infective endocarditis, a predisposing factor is recognized. A surgical or dental procedure can be implicated in approximately 65% of cases in which the potential source of bacteremia is identified. Poor dental hygiene in children with cyanotic heart disease results in a greater risk for endocarditis. The occurrence of endocarditis directly after heart surgery is relatively low, but it is frequently an antecedent event.

Clinical Manifestations (Box 429–2). Early manifestations are usually mild, especially when viridans group streptococci are the infecting organisms. Prolonged fever without other manifestations (except occasionally weight loss) that persists for as long as several months may be the only symptom. Alternatively, the onset may be acute and severe, with high, intermittent fever and prostration. Usually, the onset and course vary between these two extremes. The symptoms are often nonspecific and consist of low-grade fever with afternoon elevations, fatigue, myalgia, arthralgia, headache, and at times, chills, nausea, and vomiting. New or changing heart murmurs are common, particularly with associated heart failure. Splenomegaly and petechiae are relatively common. Serious neurologic complications such as embolic strokes, cerebral abscesses, mycotic aneurysms, and hemorrhage are most often associated with staphylococcal disease and may be late manifestations. Meningismus, increased intracranial pressure, altered sensorium, and focal neurologic signs are manifestations of these complications. Myocardial abscesses may

occur with staphylococcal disease and may rupture into the pericardium and produce purulent pericarditis. Pulmonary and other systemic emboli are infrequent, except with fungal disease. Many of the classic skin findings develop late in the course of the disease; they are seldom seen in appropriately treated patients. Such manifestations include *Osler nodes* (tender, pea-sized intradermal nodules in the pads of the fingers and toes), *Janeway lesions* (painless small erythematous or hemorrhagic lesions on the palms and soles), and *splinter hemorrhages* (linear lesions beneath the nails). These lesions may represent vasculitis produced by circulating antigen-antibody complexes.

Identification of infective endocarditis is most often based on a high index of suspicion during evaluation of an infection in a child with an underlying contributory factor.

Diagnosis. The critical information for appropriate treatment of infective endocarditis is obtained from blood cultures. All other laboratory data are secondary in importance (see Box 429–2). Blood specimens for culture should be obtained as promptly as possible, even if the child feels well and has no other physical findings. Three to five separate blood collections should be obtained after careful preparation of the phlebotomy site. Contamination presents a special problem inasmuch as bacteria found on the skin may themselves cause infective endocarditis. The timing of collections is not important because bacteremia can be expected to be relatively constant. In 90% of cases of endocarditis, the causative agent is recovered from the 1st two blood cultures. The laboratory should be notified that endocarditis is suspected so that if necessary, the blood can be cultured on enriched media for longer than usual (>7 days) to detect nutritionally deficient and fastidious bacteria or fungi. Antimicrobial pretreatment of the patient reduces the yield of blood cultures to 50–60%. The microbiology laboratory should be notified if the patient has received antibiotics so that more sophisticated methods can be used to recover the offending agent. Other specimens that may be cultured include scrapings from cutaneous lesions, urine, synovial fluid, abscesses, and in the presence of manifestations of meningitis, cerebrospinal fluid. Serologic diagnosis is necessary in patients with unusual or fastidious microorganisms (see Box 429–1).

The index of suspicion should be high when evaluating infection in a child with an underlying contributing factor. The combination of M-mode, two-dimensional, and transesophageal echocardiography enhances the ability to diagnose endocarditis. M-mode echocardiography can detect valvular vegetations larger than 2–3 mm. Two-dimensional echocardiography can identify the size, shape, location, and mobility of the lesion; when combined with Doppler studies, the presence of valve dysfunction (regurgitation, obstruction) can be determined and its effect on left ventricular performance quantified. Echocardiography may also be helpful in predicting embolic complications given that lesions greater than 1 cm and fungating masses are at greatest risk for embolization. The absence of vegetations does not exclude endocarditis, and vegetations are often not visualized in the early phases of the disease or in patients with complex congenital heart lesions.

The Duke criteria help in the diagnosis of endocarditis. Major criteria include (1) positive blood cultures (two separate cultures for a usual pathogen, two or more for less typical pathogens) and (2) evidence of endocarditis on echocardiography (intracardiac mass on a valve or other site, regurgitant flow near a prosthesis, abscess, partial dehiscence of prosthetic valves, or new valve regurgitant flow). Minor criteria include predisposing conditions, fever, embolic-vascular signs, immune complex phenomena (glomerulonephritis, arthritis, rheumatoid factor, Osler nodes, Roth spots), a single positive blood culture or serologic evidence of infection, and echocardiographic signs not meeting the major criteria. Two major criteria, one major and three minor, or five minor criteria suggest definite endocarditis.

Prognosis and Complications. In the pre-antibiotic era, infective endocarditis was a fatal disease. Despite the use of antibiotic agents, mortality remains at 20–25%. Serious morbidity occurs in 50–60% of children with documented infective endocarditis; the most common is heart failure caused by vegetations involving the aortic or mitral valve. Myocardial abscesses and toxic myocarditis may also lead to heart failure without characteristic changes in auscultatory findings. Systemic emboli, often with central nervous system manifestations, are a major threat. Pulmonary emboli may occur in children with VSD or the tetralogy of Fallot, although massive life-threatening pulmonary embolization is rare. Other complications include mycotic aneurysms, rupture of a sinus of Valsalva, obstruction of a valve secondary to large vegetations, acquired VSD, and heart block as a result of involvement (abscess) of the conduction system. Additional complications include meningitis, osteomyelitis, arthritis, renal abscess, and immune complex–mediated glomerulonephritis.

Treatment. Antibiotic therapy should be instituted immediately once a definitive diagnosis is made. When virulent organisms are responsible, small delays may result in progressive endocardial damage and are associated with a greater likelihood of severe complications. The choice of antibiotics, method of administration, and length of treatment are outlined in Table 429–1. High serum bactericidal levels must be maintained long enough to eradicate organisms that are growing in relatively inaccessible avascular vegetations. Between 5 and 20 times the minimal in vitro inhibiting concentration must be produced at the site of infection to destroy bacteria growing at the core of these lesions. Several weeks is required for a vegetation to organize completely; therapy must be continued through this period so that recrudescence can be avoided. A total of 4–6 wk of treatment is recommended, with serumcidal levels by tube dilution of at least 1:8 after a dose of antibiotic. Depending on the clinical and laboratory responses, antibiotic therapy may require modification, and in some instances more prolonged treatment is required. With highly sensitive viridans group streptococcal infections, shortened regimens that include oral penicillin for some portion have been recommended. In nonstaphylococcal disease, bacteremia usually resolves in 24–48 hr, whereas fever resolves in 5–6 days with appropriate antibiotic therapy. Resolution with staphylococcal disease takes longer.

Digitalis, salt restriction, and diuretic therapy should be used for the treatment of heart failure. Surgical intervention for infective endocarditis is indicated for severe aortic or mitral valve involvement with intractable heart failure. Rarely, a mycotic aneurysm, rupture of an aortic sinus, or dehiscence of an intracardiac patch requires an emergency operation. Other surgical indications include failure to sterilize the blood despite adequate antibiotic levels, myocardial abscess, recurrent emboli, and increasing size of vegetations while receiving therapy. Although antibiotic therapy should be administered for as long as possible before surgical intervention, active infection is not a contraindication if the patient is critically ill as a result of severe hemodynamic deterioration from infective endocarditis. Removal of vegetations and, in some instances, valve replacement may be lifesaving, and sustained antibiotic administration will most often prevent re-infection. Replacement of infected prosthetic valves carries a higher risk.

Fungal endocarditis is difficult to manage and has a poor prognosis regardless of treatment. It has been encountered after cardiac surgery, especially in severely debilitated or immunosuppressed patients. The drugs of choice are amphotericin B and 5-fluorocytosine. Surgery to excise infected tissue is occasionally attempted, though often with limited success.

Prevention. Antimicrobial prophylaxis before various procedures, including dental cleaning and other forms of dental manipulation, reduces the incidence of infective endocarditis in susceptible patients (Tables 429–2 and 429–3). Continuing education regarding prophylaxis is important, especially in teenagers and young adults, who often have poor knowledge of their own congenital heart lesion. Proper general dental care and oral hygiene are most important in decreasing the risk of infective endocarditis in susceptible individuals. Vigorous treatment of sepsis and local infections and careful asepsis during heart surgery and catheterization reduce the incidence of infective endocarditis.

TABLE 429–1. Treatment of Infective Endocarditis

Etiologic Agent	Drug	Dose	Route	Duration of Therapy (wk)
Streptococcus viridans, Streptococcus bovis (minimal inhibitory concentration [MIC] ≤0.1 µg/mL)	(1) Penicillin G *or*	200,000–300,000 U/kg/24 hr q4h, not to exceed 20 million U/24 hr	IV	4–6
	(2) Penicillin G	As above No. 1	IV	2–4
	plus gentamicin	3–7.5 mg/kg/24 hr q8h, not to exceed 240 mg/24 hr	IV	2
S. viridans, S. bovis (MIC ≥0.1 µg/mL)	(3) Penicillin G	As above No. 2	IV	4–6
	plus gentamicin	As above No. 2	IV	2
S. viridans or enterococci (*S. bovis* or *Streptococcus faecalis*) (MIC >0.5 µg/mL)	(4) Penicillin G *or*	As above No. 2	IV	4–6
	Ampicillin	300 mg/kg 24 hr q4–6h, not to exceed 12 g/24 hr	IV	4–6
	plus gentamicin	As above No. 2	IV	4–6
S. viridans, S. bovis* (penicillin allergy†)	(5) Vancomycin plus	40–60 mg/kg/24 hr q8–12h, not to exceed 2 g/24 hr	IV	4–6
	(6) Gentamicin if resistant*	As above No. 2	IV	4–6
Staphylococcus aureus	(7) Nafcillin *or*	200 mg/kg/24 hr q4–6h, not to exceed 12 g/24 hr	IV	6–8
	Oxacillin	As above No. 2		
	plus optional gentamicin		IV	1–2
S. aureus (methicillin resistant) (penicillin allergy)	(8) Vancomycin	As above No. 5	IV	6–8
	plus optional trimethoprim-sulfamethoxazole	12 mg/kg/24 hr trimethoprim q8h, not to exceed 1 g/24 hr	IV, PO	4–8
S. aureus (with prosthetic device, methicillin sensitive)‡	(9) Nafcillin	As above No. 7	IV	6–8
	plus gentamicin	As above No. 2	IV	2
	plus optional rifampin	10–20 mg/kg/24 hr q12h, not to exceed 600 mg/24 hr	PO	≥6
S. aureus (with prosthetic device, methicillin resistant)	(10) Vancomycin	As above No. 5	IV	6–8
	plus gentamicin	As above No. 9	IV	2
	plus optional rifampin	As above No. 9	PO	≥6
Staphylococcus epidermidis	(11) Vancomycin	As above No. 5	IV	6–8
	plus optional rifampin	As above No. 9	PO	6–8
Haemophilus species	(12) Ampicillin	As above No. 4	IV	4–6
	plus optional gentamicin	As above No. 2	IV	2–4
Unknown				
Postoperative	(13) Vancomycin	As above No. 5	IV	6–8
	plus gentamicin	As above No. 2	IV	2–4
Nonoperative	(14) Nafcillin *or*	As above No. 7	IV	6–8
	Vancomycin	As above No. 5	IV	6–8
	plus gentamicin	As above No. 2	IV	2–4
	plus optional ampicillin	As above No. 4	IV	6–8

*Add gentamicin for relatively resistant organisms. Monitor vancomycin peaks 1 hr after infusion (30–45 µg/mL). Adjust the dose according to vancomycin levels.
†Desensitization should be considered for patients who are allergic to penicillin. Cephalosporins are not recommended.
‡May require valve (device) replacement.
IV = intravenous; PO = oral.

TABLE 429–2. Recommendations of the American Heart Association for Prophylaxis Against Bacterial Endocarditis

Dental and Oral Procedures or Surgery of the Upper Respiratory Tract or Esophagus		Gastrointestinal and Genitourinary Tract Surgery and Instrumentation	
For most patients	Oral amoxicillin Adults, 2.0 g, children, 50 mg/kg 1 hr before procedure	High-risk patients	IM or IV ampicillin Adults, 2.0 g, children, 50 mg/kg *plus*
For patients unable to take oral medication	IM or IV ampicillin Adults, 2.0 g, children, 50 mg/kg given within 30 min before procedure		IM or IV gentamicin 1.5 mg/kg (maximal dose, 120 mg) given within 30 min before procedure *plus 6 hr later*
Ampicillin- and amoxicillin-allergic patients	Oral clindamycin Adults, 600 mg, children, 20 mg/kg 1 hr before procedure *or*		IM or IV ampicillin or oral amoxicillin Adults, 1 g, children, 25 mg/kg
	Oral cephalexin* or cefadroxil* Adults, 2.0 g, children, 50 mg/kg 1 hr before procedure *or*	High-risk patients allergic to ampicillin and amoxicillin	IV vancomycin Adults, 1.0 g, children, 20 mg/kg given over 1–2 hr *plus* IM or IV gentamicin
	Oral azithromycin *or* clarithromycin Adults, 500 mg, children, 15 mg/kg 1 hr before procedure		1.5 mg/kg (maximal dose, 120 mg); complete injection/infusion within 30 min before starting procedure
Ampicillin- and amoxicillin-allergic patients unable to take oral medications	IV clindamycin Adults, 600 mg, children, 20 mg/kg given within 30 min before procedure *or*	Moderate-risk patients	Oral amoxicillin Adults, 2.0 g, children, 50 mg/kg 1 hr before procedure *or*
	IV cefazolin		IM or IV ampicillin Adults, 2.0 g, children, 50 mg/kg given within 30 min before procedure

TABLE 429–2. Recommendations of the American Heart Association for Prophylaxis Against Bacterial Endocarditis *Continued*

Dental and Oral Procedures or Surgery of the Upper Respiratory Tract or Esophagus	Gastrointestinal and Genitourinary Tract Surgery and Instrumentation	
Adults, 1.0 g, children, 25 mg/kg given within 30 min before procedure	Moderate-risk patients who are allergic to ampicillin and amoxicillin	IV vancomycin Adults, 1.0 g, children, 20 mg/kg given over 1–2 hr; complete infusion within 30 min of starting procedure

*Cephalosporins should not be used in patients with an immediate-type hypersensitivity reaction to penicillins.

High-risk patients: *prosthetic heart valves (including homografts), previous endocarditis, complex cyanotic congenital heart disease (e.g., transposition of great vessels, tetralogy of Fallot, single ventricle), systemic-to-pulmonary artery shunts or conduits.*

Moderate-risk patients: *most other congenital heart diseases (other than those specifically listed previously or further on), acquired valve dysfunction (e.g., rheumatic heart disease), hypertrophic cardiomyopathy.*

Negligible-risk patients (prophylaxis not recommended): *isolated secundum ASD; surgical repair of ASD, VSD, or PDA (without residua and beyond 6 mo after repair); previous coronary artery bypass surgery; functional heart murmurs; previous Kawasaki disease or rheumatic fever without valve dysfunction; cardiac pacemakers; implantable defibrillators.*

The risk for mitral valve prolapse is controversial. The latest American Heart Association recommendations categorize mitral valve prolapse with regurgitation or thickened leaflets, or both, as a moderate risk; mitral valve prolapse without regurgitation is categorized as negligible risk (for further details see the reference).

IM = intramuscularly; IV = intravenously; ASD = atrial septal defect; VSD = ventricular septal defect; PDA = patent ductus arteriosus.

Adapted from Dajani AS, Taubert KA, Wilson W, et al: Prevention of bacterial endocarditis. Recommendations by the American Heart Association. JAMA 1997; 277:1794.

TABLE 429–3. Procedures and Endocarditis Prophylaxis

Endocarditis Prophylaxis Recommended*	Endocarditis Prophylaxis Not Recommended

Dental

Tooth extractions
Periodontal procedures, including surgery, scaling and root planing, probing, and recall maintenance
Dental implant placement and re-implantation of avulsed teeth
Endodontic (root canal) instrumentation or surgery only beyond the apex
Subgingival placement of antibiotic fibers or strips
Initial placement of orthodontic bands but not brackets
Intraligamentary local anesthesia injections
Prophylactic cleaning of teeth or implants when bleeding is anticipated

Respiratory Tract

Tonsillectomy or adenoidectomy, or both
Surgical operations that involve respiratory mucosa
Bronchoscopy with a rigid bronchoscope

Gastrointestinal Tract[†]

Sclerotherapy for esophageal varices
Esophageal stricture dilatation
Endoscopic retrograde cholangiography with biliary obstruction
Biliary tract surgery
Surgical operations that involve intestinal mucosa

Genitourinary Tract

Cystoscopy

Dental

Restorative dentistry[‡] (operative and prosthodontic) with or without retraction cord[§]
Local anesthesia injections (non-intraligamentary)
Intracanal endodontic treatment, after placement and buildup
Placement of rubber dams
Postoperative suture removal
Placement of removable prosthodontic or orthodontic appliances
Taking of oral impressions
Fluoride treatments
Taking of oral radiographs
Orthodontic appliance adjustment
Shedding of primary teeth

Respiratory Tract

Endotracheal intubation
Bronchoscopy with a flexible bronchoscope, with or without biopsy[§]
Tympanostomy tube insertion

Gastrointestinal Tract

Transesophageal echocardiography[§]
Endoscopy with or without gastrointestinal biopsy[§]

Genitourinary Tract

Vaginal delivery[§]
Cesarean section
In uninfected tissue:
    Urethral catheterization
    Uterine dilatation and curettage
    Therapeutic abortion
    Sterilization procedures
    Insertion or removal of intrauterine devices

Other

Cardiac catheterization, including balloon angioplasty
Implanted cardiac pacemakers, implanted defibrillators, and coronary stents
Incision or biopsy of surgically scrubbed skin
Circumcision

---

*Prophylaxis is recommended for patients with high- or moderate-risk heart conditions.
[†]Prophylaxis is recommended for high-risk patients; optional for medium-risk patients.
[‡]Includes restoration of decayed teeth (filling cavities) and replacement of missing teeth.
[§]Prophylaxis is optional for high-risk patients.

Bayer AS, Bolger AF, Taubert KA, et al: Diagnosis and management of infective endocarditis and its complications. *Circulation* 1998;98:2936–48.

Bouza E, Menasalvas A, Munoz P, et al: Infective endocarditis—a prospective study at the end of the twentieth century. *Medicine (Baltimore)* 2001;80:298–307.

Dajani AS, Taubert KA, Wilson W, et al: Prevention of bacterial endocarditis. Recommendations by the American Heart Association. *JAMA* 1997; 277:1794.

Ellis ME, Al-Abdely H, Sandridge A, et al: Fungal endocarditis: Evidence in the world literature, 1965–1995. *Clin Infect Dis* 2001;32:50–62.

Ferrieri P, Gewitz MH, Berger M, et al: Unique features of infective endocarditis in childhood. *Pediatrics* 2002;109:931–43.

Gonzalez-Juanatey C, Gonzalez-Gay M, Llorca J, et al: Rheumatic manifestations of infective endocarditis in non-addicts. A 12-year study. *Medicine (Baltimore)* 2001;80:9–19.

Hoen B, Alla F, Selton-Suty C, et al: Changing profile of infective endocarditis. Results of a 1-year survey in France. *JAMA* 2002;288:75–80.

Martin JM, Neches WH, Wald ER: Infective endocarditis: 35 years of experience at a children's hospital. *Infect Dis* 1997;24:669.

Milazzo AS Jr, Li JS: Bacterial endocarditis in infants and children. *Pediatr Infect Dis J* 2001;20:799–801.

Morris CD, Reller MD, Menashe VD: Thirty-year incidence of infective endocarditis after surgery for congenital heart disease. *JAMA* 1998;279:599.

Chapter 430
Rheumatic Heart Disease

Rheumatic involvement of the valves and endocardium is the most important manifestation of rheumatic fever (see Chapter 147). The valvular lesions begin as small verrucae composed of fibrin and blood cells along the borders of one or more of the heart valves. The mitral valve is affected most often, followed in frequency by the aortic valve; right-sided heart manifestations are rare. As the inflammation subsides, the verrucae tend to disappear and leave scar tissue. With repeated attacks of rheumatic fever, new verrucae form near the previous ones, and the mural endocardium and chordae tendineae become involved.

PATTERNS OF VALVULAR DISEASE

Mitral Insufficiency

Pathophysiology. Mitral insufficiency is the result of structural changes that usually include some loss of valvular substance and shortening and thickening of the chordae tendineae. During acute rheumatic fever with severe cardiac involvement, heart failure is caused by a combination of mitral insufficiency coupled with inflammatory disease of the pericardium, myocardium, endocardium, and epicardium. Because of the high volume load and inflammatory process, the left ventricle becomes enlarged. The left atrium dilates as blood regurgitates into this chamber. Increased left atrial pressure results in pulmonary congestion and symptoms of left-sided heart failure. Spontaneous improvement usually occurs with time, even in patients in whom mitral insufficiency is severe at the onset. The resultant chronic lesion is most often mild or moderate in severity, and the patient is asymptomatic. More than half of patients with acute mitral insufficiency no longer have the mitral murmur 1 yr later. In patients with severe chronic mitral insufficiency, pulmonary arterial pressure becomes elevated, the right ventricle and atrium become enlarged, and right-sided heart failure subsequently develops.

Clinical Manifestations. The physical signs of mitral insufficiency depend on its severity. With mild disease, signs of heart failure are not present, the precordium is quiet, and auscultation reveals a high-pitched holosystolic murmur at the apex that radiates to the axilla. With severe mitral insufficiency, signs of chronic heart failure may be noted. The heart is enlarged, with a heaving apical left ventricular impulse and often an apical systolic thrill. The 2nd heart sound may be accentuated if pulmonary hypertension is present. A 3rd heart sound is generally prominent. A holosystolic murmur is heard at the apex with radiation to the axilla. A short mid-diastolic rumbling murmur is caused by increased blood flow across the mitral valve as a result of the insufficiency. Auscultation of a diastolic murmur does not necessarily mean that mitral stenosis is present. The latter lesion takes many years to develop and is characterized by a diastolic murmur of greater length with presystolic accentuation.

The electrocardiogram and roentgenograms are normal if the lesion is mild. With more severe insufficiency, the *electrocardiogram* shows prominent bifid P waves, signs of left ventricular hypertrophy, and associated right ventricular hypertrophy if pulmonary hypertension is present. *Roentgenographically*, prominence of the left atrium and ventricle can be seen. Congestion of perihilar vessels, a sign of pulmonary venous hypertension, may also be evident. Calcification of the mitral valve is rare in children. *Echocardiography* shows enlargement of the left atrium and ventricle, and Doppler studies demonstrate the severity of the mitral regurgitation. *Heart catheterization* and left ventriculography are considered only if diagnostic questions are not totally resolved by noninvasive assessment. The degree of opacification of the left atrium during left ventriculography is used as a qualitative assessment of the severity of mitral insufficiency.

Complications. Severe mitral insufficiency may result in cardiac failure that may be precipitated by progression of the rheumatic process, the onset of atrial fibrillation, or infective endocarditis. The effects of chronic mitral insufficiency may become manifested after many years and include right ventricular failure and atrial and ventricular arrhythmias.

Treatment. In patients with mild mitral insufficiency, prophylaxis against recurrences of rheumatic fever is all that is required. Treatment of complicating heart failure (see Chapter 434), arrhythmias (see Chapter 428), and infective endocarditis (see Chapter 429) is described elsewhere. Afterload-reducing agents (captopril, hydralazine) may reduce the regurgitant volume and preserve left ventricular function. Surgical treatment is indicated for patients who despite adequate medical therapy have recurrent episodes of heart failure, dyspnea with moderate activity, and progressive cardiomegaly, often with pulmonary hypertension. Although annuloplasty provides good results in some children and adolescents, valve replacement may be required. Prophylaxis against bacterial endocarditis is warranted in these patients for dental or other surgical procedures. The routine antibiotics taken by these patients for rheumatic fever prophylaxis are insufficient to prevent endocarditis.

Mitral Stenosis

Pathophysiology. Mitral stenosis of rheumatic origin results from fibrosis of the mitral ring, commissural adhesions, and contracture of the valve leaflets, chordae, and papillary muscles over time. It takes 10 yr or more for the lesion to become fully established, although the process may occasionally be accelerated. Rheumatic mitral stenosis is seldom encountered before adolescence and is not usually recognized until adult life. Significant mitral stenosis results in increased pressure and enlargement and hypertrophy of the left atrium, pulmonary venous hypertension, increased pulmonary vascular resistance, and pulmonary hypertension. Right ventricular and atrial dilatation and hypertrophy ensue and are followed by right-sided heart failure.

Clinical Manifestations. Generally, the correlation between symptoms and the severity of obstruction is good. Patients with mild lesions are asymptomatic. More severe degrees of obstruction are associated with exercise intolerance and dyspnea. Critical lesions can result in orthopnea, paroxysmal nocturnal dyspnea, and overt pulmonary edema, as well as atrial arrhythmias. When pulmonary hypertension has developed, right ventricular dilatation may result in functional tricuspid insufficiency, hepatomegaly, ascites, and edema. Hemoptysis caused by rupture of bronchial or pleurohilar veins and, occasionally, by pulmonary infarction may occur.

Jugular venous pressure is increased in severe disease with heart failure, tricuspid valve disease, or severe pulmonary hypertension. In mild disease, heart size is normal; however, moderate cardiomegaly is usual with severe mitral stenosis. Cardiac enlargement can be massive when atrial fibrillation and heart failure supervene. A parasternal right ventricular lift is palpable when pulmonary pressure is high. The principal auscultatory findings are a loud 1st heart sound, an opening snap of the mitral valve, and a long, low-pitched, rumbling mitral diastolic murmur with presystolic accentuation at the apex. The mitral diastolic murmur may be virtually absent in patients who are in heart failure. A holosystolic murmur secondary to tricuspid insufficiency may be audible. In the presence of pulmonary hypertension, the pulmonic component of the 2nd heart sound is accentuated. An early diastolic murmur may be caused by associated aortic insufficiency or secondary pulmonary valvular insufficiency.

Electrocardiograms and *roentgenograms* are normal if the lesion is mild; as the severity increases, prominent and notched P waves and varying degrees of right ventricular hypertrophy become evident. Atrial fibrillation is a common late manifestation. Moderate or severe lesions are associated with roentgenographic signs of left atrial enlargement and prominence of the pulmonary artery and right-sided heart chambers; calcifications may be noted in the region of the mitral valve. Severe obstruction is associated with a redistribution of pulmonary blood flow so that the apices of the lung have greater perfusion (the reverse of normal). *Echocardiography* shows distinct narrowing of the mitral orifice during diastole and left atrial enlargement, and Doppler can estimate the transmitral pressure gradient. *Cardiac catheterization* quantitates the diastolic gradient across the mitral valve and the degree of elevation of pulmonary arterial pressure.

Treatment. Intervention is indicated in patients with clinical signs and hemodynamic evidence of severe obstruction but before the severe manifestations outlined earlier. Surgical valvotomy or balloon catheter mitral valvuloplasty generally yields good results; valve replacement is avoided unless absolutely necessary. Balloon valvuloplasty is indicated for symptomatic, stenotic, pliable, noncalcified valves of patients without atrial arrhythmias or thrombi.

Aortic Insufficiency

In chronic rheumatic aortic insufficiency, sclerosis of the aortic valve results in distortion and retraction of the cusps. Regurgitation of blood leads to volume overload with dilatation and hypertrophy of the left ventricle. Combined mitral and aortic insufficiency is more common than aortic involvement alone.

Clinical Manifestations. Symptoms are unusual except in severe aortic insufficiency. The large stroke volume and forceful left ventricular contractions may result in palpitations. Excessive sweating and heat intolerance are related to vasodilation. Dyspnea on exertion can progress to orthopnea and pulmonary edema; angina may be precipitated by heavy exercise. Nocturnal attacks with sweating, tachycardia, chest pain, and hypertension may occur.

The pulse pressure is wide with bounding peripheral pulses. Systolic blood pressure is elevated, and diastolic pressure is lowered. In severe aortic insufficiency, the heart is enlarged, with a left ventricular apical heave. A diastolic thrill may be present. The typical murmur begins immediately with the 2nd heart sound and continues until late in diastole. The murmur is heard over the upper and midleft sternal border with radiation to the apex and the aortic area. Characteristically, it has a high-pitched blowing quality and is easily audible in full expiration with the diaphragm of the stethoscope placed firmly on the chest and the patient leaning forward. A systolic ejection murmur is frequent because of the increased stroke volume. An apical presystolic murmur (Austin Flint murmur) resembling that of mitral stenosis is sometimes heard and is a result of the large regurgitant aortic flow in diastole that prevents the mitral valve from opening fully.

Roentgenograms show enlargement of the left ventricle and aorta. The *electrocardiogram* may be normal, but in advanced cases it reveals signs of left ventricular hypertrophy and strain with prominent P waves. The *echocardiogram* shows a large left ventricle and diastolic mitral valve flutter or oscillation caused by regurgitant flow hitting the valve leaflets. Doppler studies demonstrate the degree of aortic runoff into the left ventricle. *Cardiac catheterization* is necessary only when the echocardiographic data are equivocal.

Prognosis and Treatment. Mild and moderate lesions are well tolerated. Many adolescents with severe regurgitation are symptom free and tolerate advanced lesions into the 3rd–4th decades. Unlike mitral insufficiency, aortic insufficiency does not regress. Patients with combined lesions during the episode of acute rheumatic fever may have only aortic involvement 1–2 yr later. Treatment consists of afterload reducers (e.g., captopril, hydralazine) and prophylaxis against recurrence of acute rheumatic fever and the development of infective endocarditis. Surgical intervention (valve replacement) should be carried out well in advance of the onset of heart failure, pulmonary edema, or angina, when signs of decreasing myocardial performance become evident as manifested by increasing left ventricular dimensions on the echocardiogram. Surgery is considered when early symptoms are present, ST-T wave changes are seen on the electrocardiogram, or evidence of decreasing left ventricular ejection fraction is noted.

Tricuspid Valve Disease

Primary tricuspid involvement is rare after rheumatic fever. *Tricuspid insufficiency* is more common secondary to right ventricular dilatation resulting from unrepaired left-sided lesions. The signs produced by tricuspid insufficiency include prominent pulsations of the jugular veins, systolic pulsations of the liver, and a blowing holosystolic murmur at the lower left sternal border that increases in intensity during inspiration. Concomitant signs of mitral or aortic valve disease, with or without atrial fibrillation, are frequent. Signs of tricuspid insufficiency decrease or disappear when heart failure produced by the left-sided lesions is successfully treated. Tricuspid valvuloplasty may be required in rare cases.

Pulmonary Valve Disease

Pulmonary insufficiency usually occurs on a functional basis secondary to pulmonary hypertension and is a late finding with severe mitral stenosis. The murmur (Graham Steell murmur) is similar to that of aortic insufficiency, but peripheral arterial signs (bounding pulses) are absent. The correct diagnosis is confirmed by two-dimensional echocardiography and Doppler studies.

Figueroa FE, Fernandez MS, Valdes P, et al: Prospective comparison of clinical and echocardiographic diagnosis of rheumatic carditis: Long term follow up of patients with subclinical disease. *Heart* 2001;85:407–10.

Griffiths SP, Gersony WM: Acute rheumatic fever in New York City (1969 to 1988): A comparative study of two decades. *J Pediatr* 1990;116:882.

Holmes DR, Nishimura RA, Reeder GS: Aortic and mitral balloon valvuloplasty: Emergence of a new percutaneous technique. *Int J Cardiol* 1987;16:227.

Narula J, Chandrasekhar Y, Rahimtoola S: Diagnosis of active rheumatic carditis. *Circulation* 1999;100:1576–81.

Stollerman GH: Rheumatic fever in the 21st century. *Clin Infect Dis* 2001;33:806–14.

Westlake RM, Graham TP, Edwards KM: An outbreak of acute rheumatic fever in Tennessee. *Pediatr Infect Dis J* 1990;9:97.

SECTION 6 *Diseases of the Myocardium and Pericardium*

Daniel Bernstein

Chapter 431
Diseases of the Myocardium

In children, myocardial function is relatively unimpaired early in the course of the majority of congenital heart lesions. In some congenital lesions (left-to-right shunts), the myocardium may even be functioning at a supranormal level (high-output state). Children with unoperated congenital heart disease, long-standing volume, pressure overload, or chronic hypoxia may eventually experience myocardial dysfunction. In most children with diseases of the myocardium, causes other than congenital heart disease are predominant (Table 431–1).

Cardiomyopathies were divided into primary or idiopathic (those with unknown cause) and secondary (those resulting from infections, endocrine disorders, metabolic and nutritional diseases, neuromuscular diseases, blood diseases, and tumors). Molecular biology has identified specific causes in many patients who were classified as "idiopathic." In some, specific gene defects have been identified; in others, polymerase chain reaction (PCR) has detected evidence of a viral genome, thus suggesting previous or chronic viral myocarditis. A useful scheme for classifying cardiomyopathies is based on the predominant structural and functional abnormalities: *dilated cardiomyopathy, hypertrophic cardiomyopathy,* and *restrictive cardiomyopathy* (Table 431–2). The prevalence of cardiomyopathy in the newborn period is 10/100,000 live births, whereas for all children the prevalence is 36/100,000 for dilated cardiomyopathy and 2/100,000 for hypertrophic and restrictive cardiomyopathy.

431.1 Dilated Cardiomyopathy

Pathophysiology. Dilated cardiomyopathy is characterized by cardiomegaly secondary to extensive dilatation of the ventricles, most prominently the left. Varying degrees of ventricular hypertrophy are also present. The cause in the vast majority of pediatric cases is still unknown *(idiopathic dilated cardiomyopathy)* but may have a genetic basis; a remote history of viral illness in many patients suggests that the disease may be a sequela of a previous myocarditis. Active myocarditis is identified in 2–15% of patients. In as many as 20% of cases, the disease is recognized as familial, with autosomal dominant, autosomal recessive, X-linked, and mitochondrial inheritance patterns (see Table 431–2). Potential gene loci for the autosomal dominant form include chromosome 1p1-1q1 and chromosome 3p25. For the X-linked form, the Xp21 region containing the dystrophin gene is implicated. Mitochondrial myopathies may be due to mutations of either nuclear DNA (in which inheritance will follow mendelian genetic patterns) or mitochondrial DNA (which is inherited solely from the mother). Mitochondrial abnormalities leading to dilated cardiomyopathy involve enzymes of the electron transport chain (nuclear DNA) or enzymes of fatty acid oxidation (mitochondrial DNA). Patients with dilated cardiomyopathy may have infectious causes other than viral infection, including endocrine disorders such as hypothyroidism, metabolic disorders such as storage disease, nutritional deficiency, exposure to cardiotoxic agents such as doxorubicin, systemic disorders such as connective tissue disease, and familial muscular or neuromuscular disorders such as the muscular dystrophies. Specific cardiac causes include congenital and acquired abnormalities of the coronary arteries, tachyarrhythmias, and familial hypercholesterolemia.

Myocardial biopsy early in the disease process may be useful; a specific cause is rarely found when biopsy samples are obtained after long-standing disease, in which case the histologic findings consist mainly of areas of fibrosis and compensatory hypertrophy. A viral origin of many of these "idiopathic" cases may be detected with PCR. A complete family history is important, and unless a viral diagnosis is confirmed, first-degree family members should be screened for subclinical cardiomyopathy by echocardiography. DNA studies on both affected and nonaffected family members may help determine the specific gene defect. In several states, neonatal screening is becoming available for some of the mitochondrial disorders of fatty acid oxidation.

Clinical Manifestations. All age groups may be affected. Usually, the onset is insidious, but sometimes symptoms of heart failure occur suddenly. Irritability, anorexia, abdominal pain, cough from pulmonary congestion, and dyspnea with exertion are common. Infants and younger children tend to have respiratory symptoms and failure to thrive, whereas older children and adolescents often initially have primarily abdominal complaints such as nausea and anorexia. Although the typical sign of pulmonary edema is the presence of rales, younger infants can exhibit wheezing. When the disease is fully established, the skin is cool and pale, the arterial pulse is decreased, pulse pressure is narrow, and tachycardia is present. Jugular venous pressure is increased, and hepatomegaly and edema are common. The heart is enlarged, and holosystolic murmurs of mitral and tricuspid insufficiency may be present. A summation gallop rhythm is usually audible.

Diagnosis. The *electrocardiogram* shows a combination of atrial enlargement, varying degrees of left or right ventricular hypertrophy, and nonspecific T-wave abnormalities. The *roentgenogram* confirms the cardiomegaly. Pulmonary congestion and pleural effusions may also be present. Often, the initial diagnosis of dilated cardiomyopathy is suspected when a chest roentgenogram is performed to evaluate a suspected pneumonia. The *echocardiogram* shows dilatation of the left atrium and ventricle and poor contractility. The right ventricle may also be affected. Doppler studies show decreased flow velocity through the aortic valve and mitral regurgitation. In long-standing cases, evidence of pulmonary hypertension may exist.

Prognosis and Management. The course of the disease is usually progressively downhill, although some patients may remain stable for years. Vigorous treatment of heart failure (see Chapter 434) may result in temporary remission, but relapses are common, and in time patients tend to become resistant to therapy. Once this point is reached, the prognosis for survival beyond a year is poor. Serious complications include ventricular arrhythmias leading to syncope and sudden death, as well as pulmonary or systemic emboli from intracardiac thrombi. Patients with severely depressed myocardial function should be monitored closely for arrhythmias and, if present, treated aggressively with

TABLE 431–1. Etiology of Myocardial Disease

Familial-Hereditary

Mitochondrial myopathy syndromes*
Hypertrophic cardiomyopathy*
Duchenne muscular dystrophy*
Other muscular dystrophies (Becker, limb girdle)
Myotonic dystrophy
Kearns-Sayre syndrome (progressive external ophthalmoplegia)
Friedreich ataxia
Hemochromatosis
Fabry disease
Primary endocardial fibroelastosis
Idiopathic dilated cardiomyopathy (familial, enteroviral, autoimmune)
Arrhythmogenic right ventricular dysplasia (familial and nonfamilial)

Infection

Virus: coxsackievirus A and B,* adenovirus,* HIV, echovirus, rubella, varicella,
 influenza, mumps, Epstein-Barr, measles, poliomyelitis
Rickettsiae: psittacosis, *Coxiella*, Rocky Mountain spotted fever
Bacteria: diphtheria, *Mycoplasma*, meningococcus, leptospirosis, Lyme disease,
 typhoid fever, tuberculosis, *Streptococcus*, listeriosis
Parasites: Chagas disease, toxoplasmosis, *Loa loa, Toxocara canis*, schistosomiasis,
 cysticercosis, *Echinococcus*, trichinosis
Fungi: histoplasmosis, coccidioidomycosis, actinomycosis

Metabolic, Nutritional, Endocrine

Pompe disease
Carnitine deficiency syndromes*
Mucopolysaccharidosis
Beriberi (thiamine deficiency)
Keshan disease (selenium deficiency)
Kwashiorkor
Hyperthyroidism
Carcinoid
Pheochromocytoma
Hypercholesterolemia
Infant of diabetic mother*
Sphingolipidoses
3-Methylglutaconic acidura type II

Connective Tissue–Granulomatous Disease—Infiltrative

Systemic lupus erythematosus (SLE)
Infant of mother with SLE
Scleroderma
Churg-Strauss vasculitis
Rheumatoid arthritis
Rheumatic fever
Sarcoidosis
Amyloidosis
Dermatomyositis
Periarteritis nodosa
Leukemia

Drugs-Toxins

Doxorubicin (Adriamycin)*
Cyclophosphamide
Chloroquine
Ipecac (emetine)
Iron overload (hemosiderosis)
Sulfonamides
Mesalezine
Chloramphenicol
Hypersensitivity reaction
Alcohol
Irradiation
Herbal remedy (blue cohosh)

Coronary Arteries

Kawasaki disease*
Medial necrosis
Anomalous left coronary artery

Other

Anemia*
Sickle cell anemia (sickling)*
Hypereosinophilic syndrome (Löffler syndrome)
Endomyocardial fibrosis
Ischemia-hypoxia
Peripartum cardiomyopathy
Uhl right ventricular anomaly
Histiocytoid (oncocytic, lipidotic) cardiomyopathy
Acute eosinophilic necrotizing myocarditis
Restrictive cardiomyopathy
Chronic tachyarrhythmias

Relatively common etiology of myocarditis-cardiomyopathy.

antiarrhythmic agents or an implantable cardioverter-defibrillator (ICD). They should also receive systemic anticoagulation with warfarin. The use of β-adrenergic blocking agents such as metoprolol and carvedilol in adults with cardiomyopathy has resulted in improvement in exercise capacity and a reduction in hospitalization and mortality. The initial experience with these drugs in children is encouraging. A trial of oral carnitine is worthwhile. When medical therapy fails, heart transplantation has been effective in infants and children with dilated cardiomyopathy (see Chapter 435). Because of the scarcity of pediatric donor organs, patients with cardiomyopathy should be referred to a pediatric heart transplant center for an initial evaluation early in the course of their disease.

Neuromuscular Diseases. Heart disease is common in patients with *Friedreich ataxia* (see Chapter 590.1), which chiefly affects the left ventricle and results in a dilated or restrictive cardiomyopathy. In some patients, exercise intolerance, chest pain, and heart failure have been the initial symptoms. Arrhythmias may also occur and consist of atrial tachycardia, fibrillation, or extrasystoles. In *Duchenne muscular dystrophy* (see Chapter 600.1), 50% of children have postmortem evidence of myocardial involvement similar to that of the striated muscle. Most often the cardiac symptoms are overshadowed by peripheral muscular and pulmonary complications, although separating disability caused by cardiac failure from that caused by periph-

eral muscle or pulmonary complications can be difficult. The electrocardiogram may reveal tachycardia, abnormalities in P waves, a short P-R interval, and abnormal Q and T waves. Minimal evidence of right or left ventricular hypertrophy may also be noted. In the less severe forms of muscular dystrophy, for example, *Becker dystrophy*, cardiac involvement may be more prominent and the primary cause of exercise intolerance and respiratory symptoms. Other X chromosome–linked dilated cardiomyopathies have been described without associated skeletal muscle involvement. Some limited experience with heart transplantation exists in patients with the milder Becker dystrophy.

Kawasaki Disease (see Chapter 156). The arteritis associated with Kawasaki disease initially involves small arterioles, but in the 2nd and 3rd wk of illness, medium-sized arteries become inflamed and aneurysmal dilatation of the coronary arteries may occur. During the healing phase, areas of both coronary dilatation and stenosis may result and can lead to myocardial infarction and death. Myocarditis is a less common sequela of Kawasaki disease but, when present, is manifested as heart failure early in the course.

Autoimmune Diseases. *Rheumatic carditis* is described in Chapters 147 and 430. The cardiovascular manifestations of juvenile rheumatoid arthritis, systemic lupus erythematosus, periarteritis nodosa, dermatomyositis, and scleroderma are described in Part XV.

TABLE 431–2. Cardiomyopathies

	Dilated	Hypertrophic	Arrhythmogenic Right Ventricular	Restrictive
Prevalence	50/100,000	1/500	Unknown	Unknown
Familial	30% AD, AR, X-L, Mt	50% AD	30% AD, rare AR (Naxos disease)	Unknown
Genes	Dystrophin	2 myosin heavy chain	Plakoglobin	None identified
	Tafazzin	Troponin T or I	Desmoplakin	
	Troponin T	K tropomycin	Ryanodine receptor	
	Sarcoglycans	Myosin-binding protein C		
	Actin	α-Actin		
	Myosin heavy chain	Myosin light chain 1 or 2		
	Lamin A/C	Titin		
	Desmin			
	Tropomyosin			
	tRNA-Lys			
	Vinculin			
Sudden death	Yes	Depends on gene 0.7–11%/yr with exercise	Yes	1.5%/yr
Arrhythmias	Atrial, ventricular, and conduction disturbances	Atrial and ventricular	Ventricular and conduction disturbances	Atrial fibrillation
Ventricular function	Systolic and diastolic dysfunction	Diastolic dysfunction Dynamic systolic outflow obstruction	Normal to reduced systolic Reduced diastolic	Severely reduced diastolic
Diagnosis	Dilated left ventricular cavity with normal to thin wall thickness	Asymmetric left ventricular hypertrophy	Right ventricular fibrofatty replacement on biopsy, right ventricular dilatation	Normal or reduced ventricles, cavity size, and thickness Biatrial enlargement
Management	ACE inhibitors Spironolactone, β$_2$-Blocking agents Carnitine ICD Transplantation	Propranolol Pacemaker ICD Surgery: septal myotomymyectomy Transplantation	β$_2$-Blocking agents, Class III antiarrhythmic agents Catheter ablation ICD Transplantation	Antiarrhythmic agents Support diastolic dysfunction ICD Transplantation

AD = autosomal dominant inheritance; AR = autosomal recessive inheritance; X-L = X-linked inheritance; Mt = mitochondrial inheritance; ACE = angiotensin-converting enzyme; ICD = implantable cardiac defibrillator.

Endocrine Disorders. Hyperthyroidism (see Chapter 562) produces tachycardia, vasodilation, a wide pulse pressure, cardiac enlargement, and occasionally, atrial fibrillation. Hypothyroidism can produce cardiac dysfunction in adults but seldom produces gross cardiac involvement in children. The electrocardiogram is characterized by bradycardia, low voltage of all complexes (especially the P and T waves), left axis deviation, and prolonged electrical systole. These signs usually disappear within 1 mo after initiation of adequate thyroid therapy. Diabetic cardiomyopathy is rare in children; however, infants of diabetic mothers can experience cardiac hypertrophy and dilatation. Cardiomyopathy may be caused by chronic exposure to elevated catecholamines in patients with pheochromocytoma.

Metabolic and Nutritional Diseases. Among the vitamin deficiency diseases, *beriberi* (see Chapter 44.2) causes the most conspicuous cardiac damage. In patients with malnutrition such as kwashiorkor, the deficiencies are often multiple, and it may be difficult to separate the cardiac lesion of one nutritional disease from that of another (see Chapters 42.1 and 42.2). Other nutritional and metabolic causes of cardiac dysfunction include selenium (see Chapter 41.6) and taurine deficiency and carnitine deficiency (Chapter 75.1). In children suffering from malabsorption because of their primary illness, for example, epidermolysis bullosa, nutritional cardiomyopathies may develop as well.

Hematologic Diseases. In infants and children, severe anemia may be associated with cardiac involvement. Although cardiac output increases when the hemoglobin content is less than about 7 g/dL, significant cardiac enlargement occurs with an extreme reduction in hemoglobin (3–4 g or less). The heart rate is rapid, pulse pressure is widened, and venous pressure is increased. A systolic flow murmur at the apex or along the left sternal border is usual; diastolic murmurs may occur in the same areas, and a gallop rhythm is also common. Electrocardiographic changes include depressed ST segments and flat T waves. In patients with congenital heart lesions, anemia can place extra stress on the heart's ability to maintain adequate oxygen delivery and can result in considerable worsening of heart failure symptoms. *Treatment* is directed toward the cause of the anemia. If blood transfusions are indicated in the presence of cardiomegaly or heart failure, only small volumes (5 mL/kg) of packed red blood cells should be administered at any one time and followed by a dose of diuretic (see Chapter 462). Sometimes, exchange transfusion may be prudent to avoid an acute increase in blood volume.

Disorders of the Coronary Arteries. Anomalous origin of the left coronary artery from the pulmonary artery is one of the major causes of myocardial ischemia in infants (see Chapter 425.2). Anomalous origin of one of the coronaries from the aorta may result in its course running between the aorta and pulmonary artery ("suicide coronary") and lead to myocardial ischemia and infarction with exercise. Coronary calcinosis is a rare disorder in infants and children in which the coronary arteries are tortuous and calcareous. Other blood vessels may be similarly involved. The onset of cardiac failure is sudden; death usually occurs in infancy. Rare coronary artery malformations include coronary ostial stenosis and coronary artery stenosis in the setting of supravalvular aortic stenosis (see Chapter 420.5). Patients with homozygous familial hypercholesterolemia may have a propensity for coronary atherosclerosis at an early age. Patients who have undergone heart transplantation are at risk for the development of graft coronary artery disease (see Chapter 435).

Doxorubicin (Adriamycin) Cardiotoxicity. This chemotherapeutic agent can cause acute myocarditis but more often results in chronic dilated cardiomyopathy. The most common manifestation is a severe, chronic, dose-dependent cardiomyopathy, which occurs in about 30% of patients when the total cumulative dose exceeds 550 mg/m² but may be seen occasionally in patients after doses as low as 200 mg/m². One study has shown abnormalities in the echocardiographic indices of left ventricular function (wall stress) in as many as 65% of children receiving doses larger than 220 mg/m². When radiation therapy is combined with doxorubicin, the risk of cardiac damage is even greater.

Cardiomyopathy may become manifested months or even years after doxorubicin treatment. Cardiomegaly is principally due to left ventricular and left atrial enlargement. T-wave flattening or inversion is nonspecific evidence of cardiac involvement. Acute electrocardiographic changes, including a long Q-T interval, may be present in 40% of patients immediately after a single dose. Early changes in cardiac function, even in the absence of symptoms, may be detected by serial echocardiograms or radionuclide (MUGA [multigated acquisition]) scans, but no method is totally able to predict which patients are at risk. The child's condition may remain clinically stable for many years, even with decreased fractional shortening. Once symptoms of heart failure develop, the case fatality rate is as high as 30–50%. Cardiac transplantation has been used with success in these patients (see Chapter 435).

Acute myocarditis is less common and typically occurs during the course of administration of the drug. It is frequently reversible, and the long-term prognosis may be somewhat better. Supportive treatment consists of anticongestive medications such as digoxin, diuretics, and afterload-reducing agents.

Ipecac Cardiac Toxicity. Cardiac toxicity can occur with chronic intentional ipecac abuse secondary to anorexia nervosa or bulimia nervosa. Manifestations include chest pain, tachycardia, dyspnea, hypotension, arrhythmias, flattening and inversion of T waves, ST segment abnormalities, prolongation of the Q-T and P-R intervals, cardiac failure, and potentially death. Differentiating the cardiac abnormalities caused by ipecac from those of chronic starvation, abnormal diets, and electrolyte abnormalities may be difficult.

431.2 Hypertrophic Cardiomyopathy

Pathophysiology. Hypertrophic cardiomyopathies in children may be secondary to obstructive congenital heart disease (critical aortic stenosis, coarctation of the aorta) or to an inborn error of metabolism (glycogen storage disease or mucopolysaccharidosis), or it may be idiopathic. This latter condition is known variably as *hypertrophic cardiomyopathy, hypertrophic obstructive cardiomyopathy, idiopathic hypertrophic subaortic stenosis,* or *asymmetric septal hypertrophy,* although subaortic obstruction is present in only about 25% of cases. Massive ventricular hypertrophy with principal involvement of the ventricular septum characterizes the disease, but all portions of the left ventricle and sometimes the right ventricle can be affected. Varying degrees of myocardial fibrosis are also present. The mitral valve is displaced anteriorly by hypertrophy of the papillary muscles, and the left ventricular cavity is distorted by the massive generalized hypertrophy. Microscopically, patchy areas of abnormally thick and short muscle fibers are arranged in circular collections and interspersed among normal as well as hypertrophied muscle fibers. Electron microscopy shows a disarray of myofibrils and myofilaments.

The hypertrophic and fibrosed muscle has decreased distensibility (compliance), so resistance to left ventricular filling occurs; systolic pumping function remains intact (or may even be hyperdynamic) until late in the course of the disease. Obstruction to left ventricular outflow develops in 25% of patients because of apposition of the abnormally placed anterior mitral leaflet against the hypertrophied septum. Varying degrees of mitral valve insufficiency are also common.

Epidemiology. Hypertrophic cardiomyopathy is most often inherited in an autosomal dominant pattern with wide variability in penetrance. Manifestations can begin at any age. Siblings of the proband may not be affected as children but may show evidence of the disease as they reach adolescence and adulthood. Mutations of the cardiac β-myosin heavy-chain gene on chromosome 14 are responsible for 30–40% of cases of familial hypertrophic cardiomyopathy (see Table 431–2). Other mutations include the cardiac troponin T gene on chromosome 1q3, α-tropomyosin on chromosome 15q2, and cardiac myosin-binding protein C on chromosome 11q11. Genetic testing may eventually make it possible to predict which patients are more likely to suffer from arrhythmias and sudden death. Other gene alterations associated with hypertrophic cardiomyopathy include those of the mitochondrial respiratory chain enzymes, which give rise to a maternal pattern of inheritance.

In childhood, hypertrophic cardiomyopathy may be somewhat different from the disease in adults in that children have a greater tendency for the development of left and right ventricular outflow obstruction. The left ventricular wall may be diffusely thickened, as opposed to only the septal portion being thickened.

Clinical Manifestations. Many children are asymptomatic, and about 50% of cases are first evaluated because of a heart murmur or because another family member has come to medical attention. In others, the clinical pattern is dominated by weakness, fatigue, dyspnea on effort, palpitations, angina pectoris, dizziness, and syncope. Even asymptomatic children have a risk of sudden death. The pulse can be brisk because of the early systolic ejection of blood from the ventricle. A prominent left ventricular lift and double apical impulse may be noted. The 1st and 2nd heart sounds are usually normal. The rarity of systolic ejection clicks helps differentiate hypertrophic obstructive cardiomyopathy from valvular aortic stenosis. The systolic murmur is ejection in type and of medium intensity; it is heard maximally at the left sternal edge and apex. The murmur may increase shortly after exercise is discontinued, during the Valsalva maneuver, or on assumption of the erect position.

Diagnosis. The *electrocardiogram* shows left ventricular hypertrophy with or without ST segment depression and T-wave inversion. Signs of the Wolff-Parkinson-White syndrome and other intraventricular conduction defects may be present. *Roentgenograms* demonstrate mild cardiomegaly with prominence of the left ventricle. The *echocardiogram* shows left ventricular hypertrophy predominantly affecting the interventricular septum, although concentric hypertrophy, systolic anterior motion of the anterior leaflet of the mitral valve, and premature closure of the aortic valve are also seen. Doppler studies demonstrate the presence of a left ventricular outflow tract gradient, which usually occurs in mid to late systole, when the muscular obstruction to outflow is maximal.

Echocardiography has largely replaced *cardiac catheterization* for initial diagnosis, although catheterization is useful in assessing a patient's candidacy for surgery. Many patients who do not have a left ventricular outflow tract gradient at rest may acquire a significant gradient after the administration of isoproterenol, amyl nitrite, or nitroglycerin. Left ventriculography shows encroachment on the left ventricular cavity by the hypertrophied muscle, especially by the interventricular septum. Midsystolic cavity obliteration occurs in more severe cases. Mitral insufficiency is common. A discrete subaortic obstruction with secondary muscular hypertrophy should be ruled out because surgical management of discrete subaortic stenosis is much more effective (see Chapter 420.5). The *prognosis* of hypertrophic cardiomyopathy in an individual patient is unpredictable. Asymptomatic patients may remain stable for years. Some patients progress to chronic heart failure, whereas others are at risk for sudden death from arrhythmia. The clinical course of other affected family members may be of some use in stratifying risk in an affected child.

Treatment. No standardized therapy has been established. Competitive sports and strenuous physical activity should be prohibited because most sudden deaths occur during or immediately after vigorous physical exertion. Digitalis or aggressive diuresis is contraindicated in most patients. Infusion of isoproterenol or other inotropic agents should also be avoided other than for diagnostic purposes in the controlled environment of the catheterization laboratory. β-Adrenergic blocking agents (propranolol) and calcium channel blocking agents (verapamil, nifedipine) have been used with some success in decreasing the degree of outflow obstruction and slowing the development of hypertrophy; these drugs do not necessarily affect the long-term prognosis and do not reduce the incidence of sudden death. Calcium channel blockers should not be used during infancy because of the increased risk of cardiovascular collapse. Patients with arrhythmias should be treated aggressively with either pharmacologic agents or an ICD. A pacemaker has been used to alter septal depolarization in some patients, although this modality is less effective in reducing the gradient and may be reserved for patients who are high surgical risks. Surgery involving ventricular septal myotomy has been successfully accomplished in some patients, especially in those with disabling angina or syncope associated with left ventricular outflow tract obstruction (resting or provoked gradient of ≥50 mm Hg). Although surgical reduction of the outflow tract gradient may improve symptoms, it does not reduce the risk of sudden death. Mitral valve replacement may be needed if the obstruction cannot be alleviated.

Hypertrophic Cardiomyopathy in Infants of Diabetic Mothers. In *infants of diabetic mothers,* a transient form of hypertrophic cardiomyopathy may be encountered with or without left ventricular outflow tract obstruction. The increased left ventricular mass usually regresses within several months (Chapter 96.1).

Corticosteroids in Premature Infants. Premature infants who are receiving *corticosteroids* for chronic lung disease may also experience transient hypertrophic cardiomyopathy, which usually resolves rapidly with cessation of steroid therapy.

Glycogen Storage Disease. Cardiac as well as skeletal muscles are affected in the generalized form of glycogen storage disease known as type II or *Pompe disease* (see Chapter 76.1). The cardiomegaly is massive, but murmurs are insignificant. Pulmonary atelectasis with secondary infection is common and related to compression by the enlarged heart. The *electrocardiogram* is characteristic and shows prominent P waves, a short P-R interval, massive QRS voltage, signs of isolated left or biventricular hypertrophy, and intraventricular conduction delays. *Roentgenograms* confirm the striking cardiomegaly with prominence of the left ventricle. The echocardiogram shows severe ventricular hypertrophy. The prognosis is poor. Recombinant enzyme therapy holds some promise to improve the outcome.

431.3 Restrictive Cardiomyopathy

Poor ventricular compliance is the major abnormality in restrictive cardiomyopathies, and inadequate filling of the ventricular cavities occurs during diastole and results in *clinical manifestations* that closely simulate those of constrictive pericarditis (see Chapter 432.1). In its full-blown form, restrictive cardiomyopathy results in dyspnea, edema, ascites, hepatomegaly, increased venous pressure, and pulmonary congestion. The heart is mildly or moderately enlarged, and murmurs are nonspecific. The electrocardiogram shows very prominent P waves, often normal QRS voltage, ST segment depression, and T-wave inversion. Roentgenographic examination shows mild to moderate cardiomegaly. The echocardiogram shows markedly enlarged atria and small to normal-sized ventricles with often preserved systolic function but highly abnormal filling characteristics by Doppler echocardiography. *Differential diagnosis* from constrictive pericarditis is critical, though difficult, because the latter can be treated surgically. Restrictive cardiomyopathy may be idiopathic, or it may be associated with a systemic disease such as scleroderma, amyloidosis, or sarcoidosis; an inborn error of metabolism (mucopolysaccharidosis); hypereosinophilic syndrome; malignancies; or radiation therapy. It may also result from a congenital abnormality such as isolated noncompaction of the left ventricular myocardium. The *prognosis* for restrictive cardiomyopathy is generally poor, and clinical deterioration can be rapid. Treatment is directed toward relief of heart failure, although these patients may show a poor response to standard heart failure management (see Chapter 434); calcium channel blocking agents have been used by some in an effort to increase diastolic compliance. Antiarrhythmic agents are used as required, and anticoagulation with warfarin is indicated for lesions with an increased risk of mural thrombosis and stroke. Cardiac transplantation has been used effectively in some of these patients as long as multiple organ involvement from systemic disease is not present. Referral to a transplant center should be considered as soon as a diagnosis of restrictive cardiomyopathy is made.

Löffler Hypereosinophilic Syndrome. This disorder produces severe multisystem dysfunction (skin, lungs, nervous system, liver), and the predominant cause of death is restrictive cardiomyopathy with endocardial fibrosis of the mitral and tricuspid valves and the right and left ventricles. The subsequent formation of endocardial thrombi results in embolization. Löffler syndrome should be distinguished from nonrestrictive, nonfibrotic acute *eosinophilic necrotizing myocarditis,* an acute rapidly fatal illness, and from *hypersensitivity myocarditis* (characterized by fever, rash, tachycardia, eosinophilia, drug allergy, and arrhythmias). Steroids and cytotoxic agents may be beneficial in the hypereosinophilic syndromes. Anticoagulant therapy may reduce the incidence of thromboembolism.

Mucopolysaccharidosis. In this disorder, most commonly *Hurler syndrome,* mucopolysaccharides accumulate in many organs, including the heart and great vessels (see Chapter 77). The most pronounced lesions are found in the valves and coronary arteries, but abnormalities in the pericardium and aorta are not uncommon. The heart may be moderately enlarged, with electrocardiographic signs of left ventricular hypertrophy. Cardiac murmurs may result from insufficiency and stenosis of the mitral and aortic valves. Sometimes the pulmonary and tricuspid valves are also involved. Coronary arterial disease may result in angina, which perhaps explains the frequent occurrence of sudden death. The prognosis is poor.

Isolated Noncompaction of the Left Ventricle. This cardiomyopathy of unknown cause results in elements of both left ventricular restriction and dilatation. The condition may be diagnosed at any age, from infancy to young adulthood, and the severity of congestive heart failure varies. The echocardiogram is diagnostic and shows a specific pattern of left ventricular hypertrophy with deep muscular crypts. Patients may be at risk for ventricular arrhythmias and sudden death, as well as mural thromboses and stroke. Although some patients may remain stable for years, others may deteriorate rapidly. Cardiac transplantation has been used successfully in this group of patients.

431.4 Myocarditis

Myocarditis refers to inflammation, necrosis, or myocytolysis and may be caused by many infectious, connective tissue, granulomatous, toxic, or idiopathic processes affecting the myocardium with or without associated systemic manifestations of the disease process or involvement of the endocardium or pericardium (see Table 431–1). Coronary pathology is uniformly absent. The most common manifestation is heart failure, although arrhythmias and sudden death may be the 1st detectable signs. Viral infections are the most common cause.

Etiology and Epidemiology. The true incidence of viral myocarditis in children is unknown because many mild cases go undetected. Viral myocarditis is typically a sporadic, but occasionally an epidemic illness. Its manifestations are to some degree age dependent: in early infancy, viral myocarditis often occurs as an acute, fulminant disease; in toddlers and young children, it occurs as an acute, but less fulminant myopericarditis; and in older children and adolescents, it is often asymptomatic and comes to clinical attention primarily as a precursor to idiopathic dilated cardiomyopathy. The most common causative agents are coxsackievirus B and adenovirus, although many known viral agents have been implicated.

Pathophysiology. Acute viral myocarditis may produce a fulminant inflammatory process characterized by cellular infiltrates, cell degeneration and necrosis, and subsequent fibrosis. Viral myocarditis may also become a chronic process with persistence of viral RNA or DNA (but not infectious virus particles) in the myocardium. Chronic inflammation is then perpetuated by the host immune response, which includes T lymphocytes activated against viral-host antigenic alterations. Such cytotoxic lymphocytes and natural killer cells, together with persistent and possibly defective viral replication, may impair myocyte function without obvious cytolysis. Alternatively, the persistent viral infection may alter the expression of major histocompatibility complex antigens, with resultant exposure of neoantigens to the immune system. In addition, some viral proteins may share antigenic epitopes with host cells, which results in autoimmune damage to the antigenically related myocyte. Cytokines such as tumor necrosis factor-α and interleukin 1 may be released and participate in initiation of the altered immune response. The net final result of chronic viral-associated inflammation is often dilated cardiomyopathy.

Clinical Manifestations. Signs and symptoms depend on the patient's age and the acute or chronic nature of the infection. A *neonate* may initially have fever, severe heart failure, respiratory distress, cyanosis, distant heart sounds, weak pulses, tachycardia out of proportion to the fever, mitral insufficiency caused by dilatation of the valve annulus, a gallop rhythm, acidosis, and shock. Evidence of viral hepatitis, aseptic meningitis, and an associated rash may be present. In the most fulminant form, death may occur within 1–7 days of the onset of symptoms. The chest roentgenogram demonstrates an enormously enlarged heart and pulmonary edema; the electrocardiogram reveals sinus tachycardia, reduced QRS complex voltage, and ST segment and T-wave abnormalities. Arrhythmias may be the first clinical manifestation and, in the presence of fever and a large heart, strongly suggest acute myocarditis.

An *older patient* with acute myocarditis may also initially be seen with acute congestive heart failure; however, more commonly, patients have a gradual onset of congestive heart failure or a sudden onset of ventricular arrhythmias. In these patients, the acute infectious phase has usually passed and an idiopathic dilated cardiomyopathy is present (see Chapter 431.1).

Diagnosis. The sedimentation rate and heart enzymes (creatine phosphokinase, lactate dehydrogenase) may be elevated in acute or chronic myocarditis. If positive, serum viral titers are helpful; negative titers do not eliminate the diagnosis. Paired studies involving PCR of ventricular biopsy and serum samples have shown viral genome routinely present in cardiac samples yet absent in peripheral blood. *Echocardiography* demonstrates poor ventricular function and often a pericardial effusion, mitral valve regurgitation, and the absence of coronary artery or other congenital heart lesions. Myocarditis can be confirmed by endomyocardial biopsy. Biopsy is performed during cardiac catheterization and can also be used to detect other causes of

cardiomyopathy (storage disease, mitochondrial defects). PCR can identify specific viral RNA or DNA.

Differential Diagnosis. The predominant diseases mimicking acute myocarditis include carnitine deficiency, hereditary mitochondrial defects, idiopathic dilated cardiomyopathy, pericarditis, fibroelastosis of the endocardium, and anomalous origin of the left coronary artery (see Table 431–1).

Treatment. The approach to treating acute myocarditis involves supportive measures for severe congestive heart failure (see Chapter 434). Dopamine or epinephrine may be helpful in those with poor cardiac output and systemic hypotension. However, all inotropic agents, including digoxin, should be used with caution because patients with myocarditis may be more susceptible to the arrhythmogenic properties of these agents. Digoxin is often started at half the normal dosage. Pericardiocentesis should be performed in patients with evidence of cardiac tamponade, and culture of pericardial fluid may yield the offending viral agent. Arrhythmias should be treated aggressively and may require the use of intravenous amiodarone to achieve adequate control. For infants and children in cardiogenic shock, extracorporeal membrane oxygenation may be indicated. In larger children and adolescents, implantation of a left ventricular assist device has been performed, usually as a bridge to heart transplantation, which is the treatment of choice in those with refractory heart failure (see Chapter 435). The role of corticosteroids in the treatment of acute viral myocarditis is controversial. In a small series of pediatric patients, treatment with prednisone (2 mg/kg daily, tapered to 0.3 mg/kg daily over a period of 3 mo) was effective in reducing myocardial inflammation and improving cardiac function. Relapse was noted to occur when immunosuppression was discontinued. Trials in adult patients have shown mixed results. Specific antiviral therapy for enterovirus (pleconaril) or Epstein-Barr virus (acyclovir) may be effective.

Prognosis. The outcome of symptomatic neonates with acute viral myocarditis has been poor, but pleconaril therapy has been quite effective in those infected with enteroviruses. Patients with lesser symptoms have a better prognosis, and complete resolution has been described. The outcome of older patients with chronic dilated cardiomyopathy associated with previous viral infection is also poor without therapy. These patients continue to have dilatation, fibrosis, and deteriorating cardiac function. Spontaneous resolution has occurred in various adult studies in 10–50% of patients. However, as many as 50% of untreated older patients die within 2 yr of diagnosis and 80% within 8 yr without heart transplantation.

431.5 Nonviral Causes of Myocarditis

Bacterial Infections. In *diphtheria* (see Chapter 172), the toxin of the bacillus may produce peripheral circulatory failure or toxic myocarditis within the 1st 2 wk of the disease. In addition to therapy for diphtheria, treatment of cardiogenic shock is essential. Diphtheritic toxic myocarditis is characterized by the development of atrioventricular block, bundle branch block, or extrasystoles. Heart failure occurs later and is associated with cardiac enlargement and a gallop rhythm. In addition to the arrhythmia, the electrocardiogram shows ST segment depression and T-wave inversion in most leads. The immediate prognosis is grave (about 50% mortality). Treatment includes strict bed rest until all signs of myocarditis have disappeared, as well as management of arrhythmias, including cardiac pacing. Digitalis is reserved for patients with frank congestive heart failure, but this drug must be used with care because of the possibility of increased myocardial sensitivity.

In many *systemic bacterial infections*, circulatory involvement is manifested as peripheral circulatory collapse or toxic myocarditis. Toxic myocarditis, as evidenced by tachycardia, a gallop rhythm, and cardiac enlargement, may complicate pneumonia, infective endocarditis, and septicemia. A myocardial depressant factor may produce an acute toxic cardiomyopathy. The prognosis depends on the ability to control the primary infection.

Rickettsial Diseases. *Rocky Mountain spotted fever* (see Chapter 210.1) may be complicated by hypotension and peripheral vascular collapse. This complication has been attributed to the general vasculitis characteristic of the disease, but acute myocarditis may be a contributing factor.

Parasitic and Fungal Infections. Lesions in the myocardium have been described in association with *histoplasmosis, coccidioidomycosis, toxoplasmosis,* and *trichinosis*. In these conditions, the cardiac lesion seldom produces clinical signs of myocarditis. *Actinomycosis* may involve the pericardium and myocardium by direct contiguity to a pulmonary abscess. *Hydatid cysts* of the pericardium may be found on routine roentgenograms of the chest and usually produce symptoms only when they rupture. *Schistosomiasis* may result in pulmonary hypertension and cor pulmonale. *Cruz trypanosomiasis* (Chagas disease) may produce either acute or subacute myocarditis and can lead to sudden death.

431.6 Endocardial Fibroelastosis

Endocardial fibroelastosis (EFE) has been called *fetal endocarditis, endocardial fibrosis, prenatal fibroelastosis, elastic tissue hyperplasia,* and *endocardial sclerosis*. In *primary* EFE, no apparent predisposing valvular lesion or other congenital heart abnormality can be found. In *secondary* EFE, severe congenital heart disease of the left-sided obstructive type (e.g., aortic stenosis or atresia, forms of hypoplastic left heart syndrome, or severe coarctation of the aorta) is present. In *secondary* EFE, the ventricular cavity is often contracted, whereas with primary disease, a dilated left ventricular chamber is seen, usually during infancy. However, in young adults, a contracted form of primary EFE has been observed. No cause for primary EFE has been firmly established, although an association with mumps infection has been implied through analysis of affected myocardial specimens by PCR.

Pathologically, a white, opaque fibroelastic thickening of the endocardium is present, usually in the left ventricle, and it frequently obscures the trabeculation of the inner surfaces of the cardiac chamber. The lesion may spread to involve the valves. Microscopically, the lesion consists of fibroelastic thickening of the endocardium and may result in subendocardial degeneration or necrosis of muscle with vacuolation of muscle fibers. The involved valve leaflets are characterized by myxomatous proliferation with an increase in collagenous elements.

The *clinical manifestations* are variable. Infants, usually those younger than 6 mo who had apparently been in good health, experience severe congestive heart failure, often precipitated by a respiratory infection. Affected infants may manifest dyspnea, cough, anorexia, hepatomegaly, edema, failure to thrive, and recurrent pulmonary infections. Chronic heart failure can be controlled for some time by digitalis and diuretics; however, most patients eventually succumb. Infants in whom valvular lesions or associated congenital cardiovascular defects are predominant usually expire in the 1st mo of life. *Roentgenograms* confirm significant cardiac enlargement (Fig. 431–1). The electrocardiogram is abnormal, with changes indicative of left atrial and left ventricular hypertrophy with strain. The echocardiogram shows a bright-appearing endocardial surface and a dilated, poorly functioning left ventricle.

Treatment is directed toward alleviation of congestive heart failure and prevention of intercurrent infections. End-stage EFE, with signs of heart failure despite maximal medical treatment, is an indication for heart transplantation (see Chapter 435).

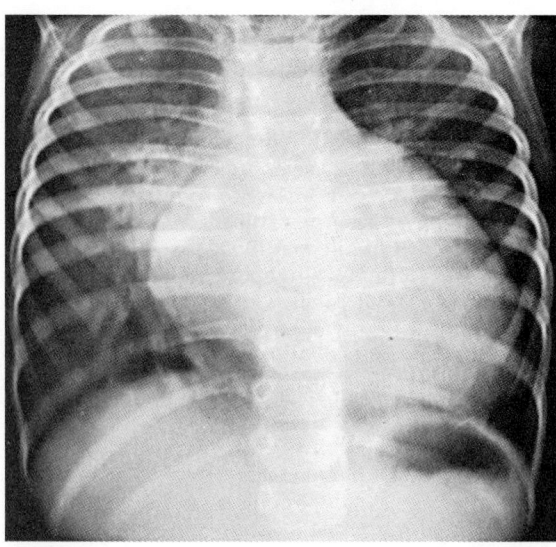

FIGURE 431–1. Roentgenogram of a 7-mo-old girl with endocardial fibroelastosis. Note the enlargement of the heart, without a distinctive contour and clear lung fields.

Dilated Cardiomyopathy
Barbaro G, Lipshultz SE: Pathogenesis of HIV-associated cardiomyopathy. *Ann N Y Acad Sci* 2001;946:57–81.
Brown CA, O'Connell JB: Myocarditis and idiopathic dilated cardiomyopathy. *Am J Med* 1995;99:309.
Burch M, Runciman M: Dilated cardiomyopathy. *Arch Dis Child* 1996;74:479.
Dubin AM, Rosenthal DN, Chin C, Bernstein D: QT dispersion predicts ventricular arrhythmia in pediatric cardiomyopathy patients referred for heart transplantation. *J Heart Lung Transplant* 1999;18:781–5.
Lipshultz SE, Colan SD, Gelber RD, et al: Late cardiac effects of doxorubicin therapy for acute lymphoblastic leukemia in childhood. N Engl J Med 1991;324:808.
Schonberger J, Seidman CE: Many roads lead to a broken heart: The genetics of dilated cardiomyopathy. *Am J Hum Genet* 2001;69:249–60.
Seidman JG, Seidman C: The genetic basis for cardiomyopathy: From mutation identification to mechanistic paradigms. *Cell* 2001;23:104:557–67.
Shaw T, Elliott P, McKenna WJ: Dilated cardiomyopathy: A genetically heterogeneous disease. *Lancet* 2002;360:654–5.
Towbin JA, Bowles NE: Genetic abnormalities responsible for dilated cardiomyopathy. *Curr Cardiol Rep* 2000;2:475–80.
Towbin JA, Lipshultz SE: Genetics of neonatal cardiomyopathy. *Curr Opin Cardiol* 1999;14:250–62.

Hypertrophic Cardiomyopathy
Maron BJ: Hypertrophic cardiomyopathy. *JAMA* 2002;287:1308–20.
Niimura H, Bachinski LL, Sangwatanaroj S, et al: Mutations in the gene for cardiac myosin-binding protein C and late-onset familial hypertrophic cardiomyopathy. *N Engl J Med* 1998;338:1248.
Roberts R, Sigwart U: New concepts in hypertrophic cardiomyopathies, part I. *Circulation* 2001;104:2113–6.
Roberts R, Sigwart U: New concepts in hypertrophic cardiomyopathies, part II. *Circulation* 2001;104:2249–52.
Spirito P, Seidman CE, McKenna WJ, Maron BJ: The management of hypertrophic cardiomyopathy. *N Engl J Med* 1997;336:775.
Towbin JA: Molecular genetics of hypertrophic cardiomyopathy. *Curr Cardiol Rep* 2000;2:134–40.
Watkins H, McKenna WJ, Thierfelder L, et al: Mutations in the genes for cardiac troponin T and alpha-tropomyosin in hypertrophic cardiomyopathy. *N Engl J Med* 1995;332:1058.

Restrictive Cardiomyopathy
Cetta F, O'Leary PW, Seward JB, Driscoll DJ: Idiopathic restrictive cardiomyopathy in childhood: Diagnostic features and clinical course. *Mayo Clin Proc* 1995;70:634.
Chen SC, Balfour IC, Jureidini S: Clinical spectrum of restrictive cardiomyopathy in children. *J Heart Lung Transplant* 2001;20:90–2.
Denfield SW, Rosenthal G, Gajarski RJ, et al: Restrictive cardiomyopathies in childhood. *Tex Heart J* 1997;24:38.
Kushwaha SS, Fallon JT, Fuster V: Restrictive cardiomyopathy. *N Engl J Med* 1997;336:267.

Myocarditis
Batra AS, Lewis AB: Acute myocarditis. *Curr Opin Pediatr* 2001;13:234–9.
Bowles NE, Towbin JA: Molecular aspects of myocarditis. *Curr Opin Cardiol* 1998;13:179–84.
Feldman AM, McNamara D: Myocarditis. *N Engl J Med* 2000;343:1388–98.

Hrobon P, Kuntz KM, Hare JM: Should endomyocardial biopsy be performed for detection of myocarditis? A decision analytic approach. *J Heart Lung Transplant* 1998;17:479–86.

Kleinert S, Weintraub RG, Wilkinson JL, Chow CW: Myocarditis in children with dilated cardiomyopathy: Incidence and outcome after dual therapy immuno-suppression. *J Heart Lung Transplant* 1997;16:1248–54.

Levi D, Alejos J: Diagnosis and treatment of pediatric viral myocarditis. *Curr Opin Cardiol* 2001;16:77–83.

Liu PP, Mason JW: Advances in the understanding of myocarditis. *Circulation* 2001;104:1076–82.

Mason JW: Immunopathogenesis and treatment of myocarditis: The United States Myocarditis Treatment Trial. *J Card Fail* 1996;2(4 Suppl):173–7.

Chapter 432
Diseases of the Pericardium

Major diseases that involve the pericardium are noted in Box 432–1. In some diseases, pericardial involvement is one manifestation of a generalized illness; prominence of the pericardial component varies with the disease.

Pathophysiology. Pericardial inflammation results in an accumulation of fluid in the pericardial space. The fluid varies according to the cause of the pericarditis and may be serous, fibrinous, purulent, or hemorrhagic. **Cardiac tamponade** occurs when the amount of pericardial fluid reaches a level that compromises cardiac function. In a healthy child, 10–15 mL of fluid is normally found in the pericardial space, whereas in an adolescent with pericarditis, fluid in excess of 1,000 mL may accumulate. For every small increment of fluid, pericardial pressure rises slowly; once a critical level is reached, pressure rises rapidly and culminates in severe cardiac compression. Inhibition of ventricular filling during diastole, elevated systemic and pulmonary venous pressure, and if untreated, eventual compromised cardiac output and shock occur.

Clinical Manifestations. The 1st symptom of pericardial disease is often precordial pain. The major complaint is a sharp, stabbing sensation over the precordium and often the left shoulder and back; the pain may be exaggerated by lying supine and relieved by sitting, especially leaning forward. Because of the absence of sensory innervation of the pericardium, the pain is probably referred pain from diaphragmatic and pleural irritation. Cough, dyspnea, abdominal pain, vomiting, and fever may also occur. The presence of symptoms or signs associated with other organs depends on the cause of the pericarditis.

Many of the findings on physical examination are related to the degree of fluid accumulation in the pericardial sac. The presence of a friction rub is helpful but is a variable sign in acute pericarditis; it usually becomes apparent when the effusion is small. When the effusion is larger, muffled heart sounds may be the only auscultatory finding. Narrow pulses, tachycardia, neck vein distention, and increased **pulsus paradoxus** suggest significant fluid accumulation.

Pulsus paradoxus is caused by the normal slight decrease in systolic arterial pressure during inspiration. With cardiac tamponade, this normal phenomenon is exaggerated, probably because of decreased filling of the left side of the heart with the inspiratory phase of respiration. The degree of pulsus paradoxus is determined with a mercury manometer. The patient is told to breathe normally without exaggeration. By allowing the manometer to fall slowly, the 1st Korotkoff sound will initially be heard intermittently (varying with respirations). This 1st point is noted, and the manometer is then allowed to fall until the 1st Korotkoff sound is heard continuously. The difference between these two systolic pressures is the pulsus paradoxus. A pulsus paradoxus greater than 20 mm Hg in a child with pericarditis is an indicator of the presence of cardiac tamponade; a

---

BOX 432–1. Etiology of Pericardial Disease

CONGENITAL ANOMALIES
Absence (partial, complete)
Cysts
Mulibrey nanism (*muscle*, *liver*, *brain*, *eye*) with congenital pericardial thickening and constriction

INFECTIOUS
Viral (coxsackievirus B, Epstein-Barr virus influenza, adenovirus)
Bacterial (*Streptococcus, Pneumococcus, Staphylococcus, Meningococcus, Mycoplasma*, tularemia)
Immune complex (*Meningococcus, Haemophilus influenzae*)
Tuberculosis
Fungal (histoplasmosis, actinomycosis)
Parasitic (toxoplasmosis, echinococcosis)

CONNECTIVE TISSUE DISEASES
Rheumatoid arthritis
Rheumatic fever
Systemic lupus erythematosus
Systemic sclerosis
Sarcoidosis

METABOLIC-ENDOCRINE
Uremia
Hypothyroidism
Chylopericardium

HEMATOLOGY-ONCOLOGY
Bleeding diathesis
Malignancy (primary, metastatic)
Radiotherapy-induced

OTHER
Trauma (penetrating or blunt injury)
Iatrogenic (catheter related)
Postpericardiotomy (cardiac surgery)
Aortic dissection
Idiopathic
Familial Mediterranean fever

10–20 mm Hg change is equivocal. Increased pulsus paradoxus may also be seen in patients with severe dyspnea of any cause, in patients with pulmonary disease (emphysema or asthma), in obese individuals, or in patients being ventilated with a positive pressure respirator. In these patients, the paradoxical pulse is due to a marked increase in intrathoracic pressure. The cause of a paradoxical pulse in a child maintained on a ventilator after heart surgery may therefore be difficult to assess.

Diagnosis. The specific findings depend on the underlying disease. The effects of pericarditis on the *electrocardiogram* are multiple. Low voltage of the QRS complexes results from a damping effect of pericardial fluid. Pressure on the myocardium by fluid or exudate produces a current of injury that results in mild elevation of ST segments. Generalized T-wave inversion occurs as a consequence of associated myocardial inflammation. The ST segment and T-wave changes with pericarditis are more generalized than those seen with myocardial infarction, and the ST segment elevations tend to precede the T-wave changes. *Electrical alternans* may be present and is demonstrated by a variable QRS complex amplitude. An interval when the electrocardiogram is in a transitional phase and appears to be normal may occur during the acute phase of the illness before diagnosis. In some instances, clear-cut abnormalities are never identified.

A relatively large pericardial effusion must be present to cause an enlarged cardiac shadow with the usual "water bottle" configuration on a *chest roentgenogram* (Fig. 432–1). In most instances, the lung fields are clear. With constrictive pericardial disease, the heart is relatively small and calcification may be present.

The *echocardiogram* is the most sensitive technique for evaluating the size and progression of pericardial effusions. Normally, the pericardium is closely adherent to the epicardium, and the two layers can only be narrowly separated by the ultrasound beam. In patients with pericardial effusion, a clear, echo-free space is recorded between the epicardium and pericardium. A posterior effusion is recorded behind the left ventricular epicardium and ends at the junction of the left ventricle and left atrium. An anterior effusion will be recorded between the chest wall and the anterior right ventricular wall. The presence of both anterior and posterior effusion generally indicates a large collection of fluid. Flattening of septal motion and collapse of right ventricular outflow during diastole are signs of pericardial tamponade.

Differential Diagnosis

VIRAL AND ACUTE BENIGN PERICARDITIS. These entities are considered synonymous because most episodes of acute benign pericarditis follow or coincide with viral illness. Viruses recognized to cause pericarditis include coxsackievirus B, influenza, echovirus, and adenovirus. The pathogenesis is unclear but may be related to a hypersensitivity reaction to the viral disease. Pericardial inflammation is not necessarily the precursor of a generalized inflammatory process. Most cases are mild, and recovery occurs within several weeks. Only symptomatic treatment is indicated, usually with nonsteroidal anti-inflammatory agents such as indomethacin. In rare instances, the patient is severely ill, and cardiac tamponade may ensue. In addition, in some patients a chronic relapsing illness occurs. Differential diagnosis between these patients and those with collagen vascular disease may be difficult. The latter patients respond dramatically to corticosteroids or nonsteroidal anti-inflammatory agents; milder forms may be controlled with aspirin. The clinical course may vary from months to 1–2 yr, during which time patients are dependent on drug therapy for suppression of the pericarditis. Ultimately, these patients improve, and the prognosis is good.

The clinical differential diagnosis between acute pericarditis and myocarditis may be difficult; usually, each includes a component of the other. Management of these conditions is quite different: anti-inflammatory treatment and urgent response to cardiac tamponade are appropriate in the former, whereas therapy for heart failure is required in the latter. The echocardiogram can demonstrate the size of the pericardial effusion and also indicate the presence of myocardial dysfunction.

PURULENT PERICARDITIS. This condition is most often associated with bacterial infections such as pneumonia, epiglottitis, meningitis, or osteomyelitis. Generally, signs and symptoms of the primary infection are present. Once the purulent process is established, if untreated, the course is ful-minant and terminated by acute cardiac tamponade and death. Open pericardial drainage is required along with appropriate intravenous antibiotics. Although closed pericardial aspiration provides a sample of the exudate for diagnostic purposes and may be lifesaving in the face of severe cardiac compression, without open drainage and removal of adhesions, tamponade almost invariably recurs. Open pericardial drainage has significantly increased survival. Rarely, with infections that are identified extremely early and with pericardial fluid that is more of a transudate than an exudate, multiple pericardial taps with placement of a drain and antibiotic therapy have been successful. The most common organisms implicated in purulent pericarditis are *Staphylococcus aureus*, *Haemophilus influenzae* type b, and *Neisseria meningitidis*. (For antimicrobial treatment, see Chapters 166, 178, and 176, respectively.) *Tuberculous pericarditis* rarely occurs in children. Extensive treatment with antituberculous chemotherapy is required (see Chapter 197). *Immune complex–mediated pericarditis* (sterile) may occur 5–7 days after the initiation of therapy for severe systemic or meningeal infection with meningococcus or *H. influenzae* type b. Therapy includes anti-inflammatory agents and pericardiocentesis if tamponade develops.

ACUTE RHEUMATIC FEVER. Pericarditis occurs in acute rheumatic fever as a component of pancarditis (see Chapters 147.1 and 430). It is associated with acute valvulitis. Pericarditis and other manifestations of acute rheumatic pancarditis respond to therapy with steroids. Cardiac tamponade is extremely rare.

JUVENILE RHEUMATOID ARTHRITIS. Pericarditis is a common manifestation of juvenile rheumatoid arthritis (see Chapter 145). Rarely, it may be the only manifestation and precede the onset of arthritis by months or even years. Differentiation of rheumatoid pericarditis from that seen with other collagen vascular disease, particularly lupus erythematosus, may be difficult. Treatment consists of steroids or salicylates, which may be needed on a long-term basis.

UREMIA. Uremic pericarditis occurs only in the presence of prolonged severe renal failure and results from chemical irritation of the pericardium secondary to the metabolic abnormalities. It may culminate in cardiac tamponade or cause recurrent hypotension during hemodialysis. If adequate relief of uremic pericarditis does not occur with hemodialysis, pericardiectomy is recommended.

NEOPLASTIC DISEASE. Neoplastic pericardial effusion is seen in patients with Hodgkin disease, lymphosarcoma, and leukemia, and it results from direct neoplastic invasion of the

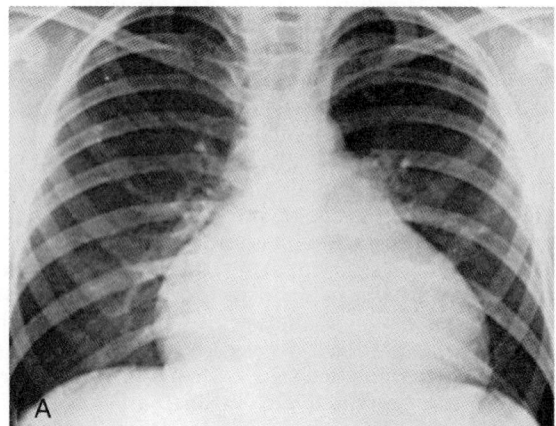
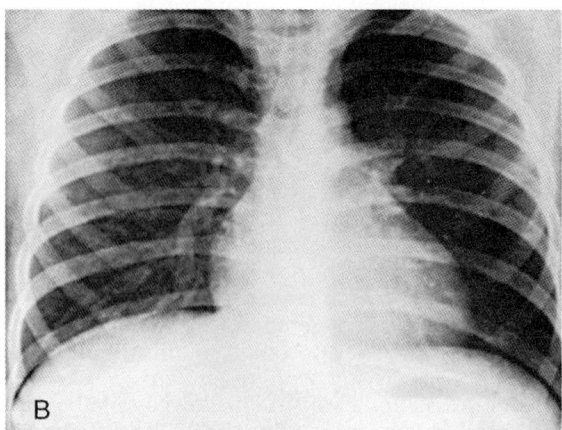

FIGURE 432–1. Roentgenograms in acute nonspecific pericarditis. *A,* Increase in cardiopericardial shadow caused by pericardial effusion. *B,* One month later after complete recovery.

pericardium. Cardiac tamponade may occur late in the course of the illness. Rarely, pericardial infiltration is the initial manifestation of neoplastic disease. Patients with malignancy may also acquire pericarditis as a result of radiation therapy to the mediastinum.

POSTPERICARDIOTOMY SYNDROME (Chapter 427). Pericardial effusions may be seen 1–2 wk or longer after open heart surgery and in some echocardiographic series are diagnosed in 15–23% of postoperative patients. The syndrome is a nonspecific hypersensitivity reaction to trauma to the pericardium and the epicardial surface of the heart. High titers of antiheart antibodies have been reported to correlate with clinical signs of the syndrome. Patients may initially have low-grade fever, lethargy, loss of appetite, or abdominal pain. Precordial or pleural chest pain may or may not be present. A high index of suspicion should accompany any acute illness in a child within the 1st 4–6 weeks after cardiac surgery. In most children, the syndrome responds well to therapy with aspirin or other nonsteroidal anti-inflammatory agents. Corticosteroids may be needed for more severe cases, and progression to tamponade can occur if untreated. Treatment is maintained for 1–3 mo, but recurrences may be seen as long as 1 yr postoperatively and require re-institution of therapy.

432.1 Constrictive Pericarditis

In most instances, constriction occurs months or years after the initial pericarditis, but it may occasionally be an acute, rapidly progressive process. Constrictive pericarditis most often occurs without an immediately preceding illness or generalized systemic disease.

Clinical manifestations occur as a result of impaired diastolic ventricular filling, compromised myocardial contractility, and resultant depression of cardiac function. Hepatomegaly and ascites may be out of proportion to the other signs and symptoms and thus suggest chronic liver disease. Liver function studies are only mildly abnormal; careful physical examination reveals other subtle findings of constriction, including neck vein distention, narrow pulses, quiet precordium, distant heart sounds, a faint pericardial friction rub, and increased pulsus paradoxus. Typical findings become apparent gradually and may be overlooked. The auscultatory presence of an early pericardial knock and the appearance of calcification of the pericardium on chest roentgenograms are the more obvious manifestations. Protein-losing enteropathy with hypoproteinemia and lymphopenia may be seen in association with severe constriction.

Constrictive pericarditis may be difficult to distinguish from chronic restrictive cardiomyopathy (see Chapter 431.3). Impaired myocardial function occurs with both conditions. The myocardial disease of constrictive pericarditis is usually reversible with pericardiectomy. At times, a definite diagnosis can be made only by exploratory thoracotomy and direct examination of the pericardium.

Radical pericardiectomy with decortication of the pericardium over a wide area of the heart, including the systemic and pulmonary veins, is the only effective treatment of constrictive pericarditis. In most patients, surgical intervention elicits a rapid response characterized by increased cardiac output and prompt diuresis. The long-term prognosis is usually excellent.

Fowler NO: Cardiac tamponade: A clinical or an echocardiographic diagnosis? *Circulation* 1993;87:1738.

Gersony WM, Hordof AH: Infective endocarditis and diseases of the pericardium. *Pediatr Clin North Am* 1978;25:831.

Hara KS, Ballard DJ, Ilstrup DM, et al: Rheumatoid pericarditis: Clinical features and survival. *Medicine (Baltimore)* 1990;69:81.

Nishimura RA, Connolly DC, Parkin TW, et al: Constrictive pericarditis: Assessment of current diagnostic procedures. *Mayo Clin Proc* 1985;60:397.

Sinzobahamvya N, Ikeogu MO: Purulent pericarditis. *Arch Dis Child* 1987;62:696.

Chapter 433
Tumors of the Heart

Primary tumors of the heart are rare in infancy and childhood and are most often benign. Clinical manifestations depend primarily on the location of the tumor and, to a lesser extent, on the histologic type.

The most common benign cardiac tumors in children are rhabdomyomas, fibromas, and myxomas. *Rhabdomyomas* occur as single or, usually, multiple nodules embedded in chamber walls. They often remain clinically unimportant and regress with age, but they may cause mechanical obstruction, heart failure, or arrhythmias. They may be familial and are often found in association with **tuberous sclerosis**. Most rhabdomyomas are seen in infants younger than 1 yr. Incessant ventricular tachycardia in a child younger than 2 yr should raise suspicion of a small endocardial or epicardial *rhabdomyoma* or *Purkinje cell tumor*. *Fibromas* are usually solitary, nonencapsulated nodules located in the ventricles; they can be massive. Treatment of rhabdomyomas and fibromas depends on their location and size. Small asymptomatic tumors in the myocardial wall or ventricular septum may be observed for growth or regression. Rhabdomyomas associated with tuberous sclerosis often resolve as the child grows older. Large tumors that show signs of obstructing blood flow and those producing ventricular arrhythmias should be removed. Large and diffuse tumors may interfere with cardiac performance. Removal of large lesions is often difficult because insufficient normal myocardium may remain. Heart transplantation may be the only recourse for patients with extensive tumors.

Myxomas develop in intracavitary locations, most frequently in the left atrium (75%) and most often in females (75%). These tumors are solid, smooth, pedunculated masses (1–8 cm) that attach to the interatrial septum, protrude into the atrial chamber, and by their position relative to the mitral or tricuspid valve, cause intermittent obstruction and a clinical picture consistent with stenosis (syncope, heart failure, atrial fibrillation). A myxoma should be considered in patients with fainting spells, a positional character (supine vs erect) of the murmur, or evidence of systemic or pulmonary embolization. Atrial myxomas can also cause fever, malaise, arthralgias, and systemic emboli mimicking endocarditis, rheumatic fever, or systemic lupus erythematosus. Laboratory features include a high sedimentation rate, hematuria, and echocardiographic evidence of the tumor. Atrial myxomas may be associated with multiple pigmented skin lesions (lentiginosis), myxoid fibroadenomas of the breast, cutaneous myxomas, and adrenal pigmented nodules. Some are associated with various cutaneous and connective tissue lesions and testicular tumors or pituitary adenomas (Carney syndrome). Treatment consists of surgical excision, which must include the entire base of the tumor to prevent recurrence.

Other benign tumors include *papillomas*, which are attached to valve leaflets and may occur in neonates; *lipomas*, which are situated in ventricular walls; and *mesotheliomas*, which may involve the atrioventricular node and cause abnormalities in electrical conduction, including complete heart block.

Primary malignant cardiac tumors in children are almost exclusively *sarcomas*. These tumors are usually located in the right side of the heart, atrial septum, right atrial wall, or root of the pulmonary artery. They may extend either into the adjacent chamber and cause obstruction to blood flow or into the pericardial cavity and produce effusion or tamponade. The heart may also be involved in metastatic dissemination of a noncardiac malignancy, such as leukemia or lymphoma, or in Wilms tumor by direct extension of the tumor into the right atrium via the inferior vena cava. Physical examination may reflect the location and size of the tumor if it interferes with blood flow. Conduction system involvement can be assessed by electrocardiography. Two-dimensional echocardiography is diagnostic and allows excellent visualization of the location and extent of the tumor. Doppler studies evaluate the extent of blood flow obstruction caused by the tumor. Cardiac catheterization may provide further information about the anatomy of the tumor and its hemodynamic effects. When indicated, surgical intervention is directed toward complete removal of the tumor, relief of obstruction, and control of any arrhythmias. The long-term outcome depends on the type of tumor, the completeness of surgical removal, and postsurgical integrity of the normal heart structures and myocardium. For tumors that are unresectable because of an inability to separate them from normal heart tissue, heart transplantation is an effective treatment.

Bini RM, Westaby S, Bargeron LM, et al: Investigation and management of primary cardiac tumors in infants and children. *J Am Coll Cardiol* 1983;2:351.
Birnbaum S, McGahan JP, Janos GG, et al: Fetal tachycardia and intramyocardial tumors. *J Am Coll Cardiol* 1985;6:1358.
Garson A Jr, Gillette PC, Titus JL, et al: Surgical treatment of ventricular tachycardia in infants. *N Engl J Med* 1984;310:1443.
Shapiro LM: Cardiac tumours: Diagnosis and management. *Heart* 2001;85:218–22.
Stratakis CA, Kirschner LS, Carney JA: Clinical and molecular features of the Carney complex: Diagnostic criteria and recommendations for patient evaluation. *J Clin Endocrinol Metab* 2001;86:4041–6.

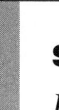

SECTION 7 *Cardiac Therapeutics*

Daniel Bernstein

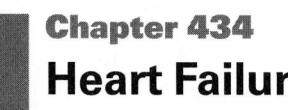

Chapter 434
Heart Failure

Heart failure occurs when the heart cannot deliver adequate cardiac output to meet the metabolic needs of the body. In the early stages of heart failure, various compensatory mechanisms are evoked to maintain normal metabolic function. When these mechanisms become ineffective, increasingly severe clinical manifestations result (Chapter 57.2).

Pathophysiology. The heart can be viewed as a pump with an output proportional to its filling volume and inversely proportional to the resistance against which it pumps. As ventricular end-diastolic volume increases, a healthy heart increases cardiac output until a maximum is reached and cardiac output can no longer be augmented (the Frank-Starling principle; Fig. 434–1). The increased stroke volume obtained in this manner is due to stretching of myocardial fibers, but it also results in increased wall tension, which elevates myocardial oxygen consumption. Hearts working under various types of stress function along different Frank-Starling curves. Cardiac muscle with compromised intrinsic contractility requires a greater degree of dilatation to produce increased stroke volume and does not achieve the same maximal cardiac output as normal myocardium does. If a cardiac chamber is already dilated because of a lesion causing increased preload (e.g., a left-to-right shunt or valvular insufficiency), there is little room for further dilatation and augmentation of cardiac output. The presence of lesions that result in increased afterload to the ventricle (aortic or pulmonic stenosis, coarctation of the aorta) decreases cardiac performance, thereby resulting in a depressed Frank-Starling relationship. The ability of an immature heart to increase cardiac output in response to increased preload is less than that of a mature heart. Premature infants are more compromised by a left-to-right shunt than full-term infants are.

Systemic oxygen transport is calculated as the product of cardiac output and systemic oxygen content. Cardiac output can be calculated as the product of heart rate and stroke volume. The primary determinants of stroke volume are the *afterload* (pressure work), *preload* (volume work), and *contractility* (intrinsic myocardial function). Abnormalities in heart rate can also compromise cardiac output and produce both bradyarrhythmias and tachyarrhythmias; the latter shorten the diastolic time interval for ventricular filling. Alterations in the oxygen-carrying capacity of blood (e.g., anemia or hypoxemia) also lead to a decrease in systemic oxygen transport and, if compensatory mechanisms are inadequate, can result in decreased delivery of substrate to tissues.

In some cases of heart failure, cardiac output is normal or increased, yet because of decreased systemic oxygen content (secondary to anemia) or increased oxygen demands (secondary to hyperventilation, hyperthyroidism, or hypermetabolism), an inadequate amount of oxygen is delivered to meet the body's needs. This condition, **high-output failure**, results in the development of signs and symptoms of heart failure when there is no basic abnormality in myocardial function and cardiac output is greater than normal. It is also seen with large systemic

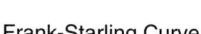

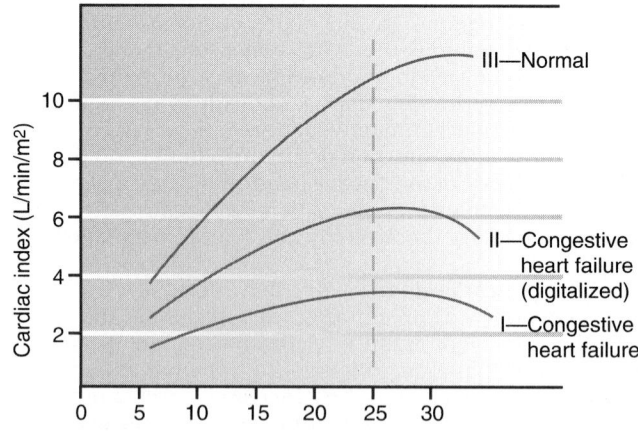

FIGURE 434–1. The Frank-Starling relationship. As left ventricular end-diastolic pressure (LVED) increases, the cardiac index increases, even in the presence of congestive heart failure, until a critical level of LVED is reached. Adding an inotropic agent (digoxin) shifts the curve from I and II. (From Gersony WM, Steep CN: In Dickerman JD, Lucey JF [editors]: *Smith's The Critically Ill Child: Diagnosis and Medical Management*, 3rd ed. Philadelphia, WB Saunders, 1984.)

arteriovenous fistulas. These conditions reduce peripheral vascular resistance and cardiac afterload and increase myocardial contractility. Heart "failure" results when the demand for cardiac output exceeds the ability of the heart to respond. Chronic severe high-output failure may eventually result in a decrease in myocardial performance as the metabolic requirements of the myocardium are not met.

One major compensatory mechanism for increasing cardiac output is an increase in sympathetic tone secondary to increased adrenal secretion of circulating epinephrine and increased neural release of norepinephrine. The initial beneficial effects of sympathetic stimulation include an increase in heart rate and myocardial contractility; both serve to increase cardiac output. Because of localized vasoconstriction, blood flow may be redistributed from the cutaneous, visceral, and renal beds to the heart and brain. Prolonged increases in sympathetic stimulation can have deleterious effects as well, including hypermetabolism, increased afterload, arrhythmogenesis, increased myocardial oxygen requirements, and direct myocardial toxicity. Peripheral vasoconstriction can result in decreased renal, hepatic, and gastrointestinal tract function.

Clinical Manifestations. The clinical manifestations depend on the degree of cardiac reserve under various conditions. A critically ill infant or child who has exhausted the compensatory mechanisms to the point that cardiac output is no longer sufficient to meet the basal metabolic needs of the body is symptomatic at rest. Other patients may be comfortable when quiet but are incapable of increasing cardiac output in response to even mild activity without experiencing significant symptoms. Conversely, it may take rather vigorous exercise to compromise cardiac function in children who have less severe heart disease. A thorough history is extremely important in making the diagnosis of heart failure and in evaluating the possible causes. Parents who observe their infant on a daily basis may not recognize subtle changes that have occurred over the course of days or weeks. Cyanosis may be considered merely "a deep coloring" and not be recognized as an abnormal finding. The history of a young infant should also focus on feeding (see Chapter 415). An infant with heart failure often takes less volume per feeding, becomes dyspneic while sucking, and may perspire profusely. Eliciting a history of fatigue in an older child requires specific questions about activity.

In children, the signs and symptoms of heart failure are often similar to those in adults and include fatigue, effort intolerance, anorexia, abdominal pain, dyspnea, and cough. However, older children and adolescents may have primarily abdominal symptoms and a surprising lack of respiratory complaints. The elevation in systemic venous pressure may be gauged by clinical assessment of jugular venous pressure and liver enlargement. Orthopnea and basilar rales are variably present; edema is usually discernible in dependent portions of the body, or anasarca may be present. Cardiomegaly is invariably noted. A gallop rhythm is common; when ventricular dilatation is advanced, the holosystolic murmur of mitral or tricuspid valve regurgitation may be heard.

In infants, heart failure may be difficult to identify. Prominent manifestations include tachypnea, feeding difficulties, poor weight gain, excessive perspiration, irritability, weak cry, and noisy, labored respirations with intercostal and subcostal retractions, as well as flaring of the alae nasi. The signs of cardiac-induced pulmonary congestion may be indistinguishable from those of bronchiolitis; wheezing is prominent. Pneumonitis with or without atelectasis is common, especially in the right middle and lower lobes; it is due to bronchial compression by the enlarged heart. Hepatomegaly usually occurs, and cardiomegaly is invariably present. In spite of pronounced tachycardia, a gallop rhythm can frequently be recognized. The other auscultatory signs are those produced by the underlying cardiac lesion. Clinical assessment of jugular venous pressure in infants

may be difficult because of the shortness of the neck and the difficulty of observing a relaxed state. Edema may be generalized and usually involves the eyelids as well as the sacrum and less often the legs and feet. The differential diagnosis is age dependent (Box 434–1).

Diagnosis. *Roentgenograms of the chest* show cardiac enlargement. Pulmonary vascularity is variable and depends on the cause of the heart failure. Infants and children with large left-to-right shunts have exaggeration of the pulmonary arterial vessels to the periphery of the lung fields, whereas patients with cardiomyopathy may have a relatively normal pulmonary vascular bed early in the course of disease. Fluffy perihilar pulmonary markings suggestive of venous congestion and acute pulmonary edema are seen only with more severe degrees of heart failure. Cardiac enlargement is often noted as an unexpected finding on a chest roentgenogram performed to evaluate for a possible pulmonary infection or asthma.

Chamber hypertrophy noted by *electrocardiography* may be helpful in assessing the cause of heart failure but does not establish the diagnosis. In cardiomyopathies, left or right ventricular ischemic changes may correlate well with clinical and other noninvasive parameters of ventricular function. Low-voltage QRS morphologic characteristics with ST-T wave abnormalities may also suggest myocardial inflammatory disease but can be seen with pericarditis as well. The electrocardiogram is the best tool for evaluating rhythm disorders as a potential cause of heart failure.

Echocardiographic techniques are useful in assessing ventricular function. The most commonly used parameter is fractional

---

BOX 434–1. Etiology of Heart Failure

FETAL

Severe anemia (hemolysis, fetal-maternal transfusion, parvovirus B19–induced anemia, hypoplastic anemia)
Supraventricular tachycardia
Ventricular tachycardia
Complete heart block

PREMATURE NEONATE

Fluid overload
Patent ductus arteriosus
Ventricular septal defect
Cor pulmonale (bronchopulmonary dysplasia)
Hypertension

FULL-TERM NEONATE

Asphyxial cardiomyopathy
Arteriovenous malformation (vein of Galen, hepatic)
Left-sided obstructive lesions (coarctation of aorta, hypoplastic left heart syndrome)
Large mixing cardiac defects (single ventricle, truncus arteriosus)
Viral myocarditis

INFANT-TODDLER

Left-to-right cardiac shunts (ventricular septal defect)
Hemangioma (arteriovenous malformation)
Anomalous left coronary artery
Metabolic cardiomyopathy
Acute hypertension (hemolytic-uremic syndrome)
Supraventricular tachycardia
Kawasaki disease
Viral myocarditis

CHILD-ADOLESCENT

Rheumatic fever
Acute hypertension (glomerulonephritis)
Viral myocarditis
Thyrotoxicosis
Hemochromatosis-hemosiderosis
Cancer therapy (radiation, doxorubicin)
Sickle cell anemia
Endocarditis
Cor pulmonale (cystic fibrosis)
Cardiomyopathy (hypertrophic, dilated)

shortening, determined as the difference between end-systolic and end-diastolic diameter divided by end-diastolic diameter. Normal fractional shortening is between 28 and 40%, whereas a normal ejection fraction (which measures volume) is 55–65% as measured by angiography. The pre-ejection:ejection period ratio measured by M-mode echocardiography should be less than 40%. A long pre-ejection time with a short ejection time usually denotes myocardial failure. Doppler studies can be used to calculate cardiac output. *Arterial oxygen levels* may be decreased when ventilation-perfusion inequalities occur secondary to pulmonary edema. When heart failure is severe, respiratory or metabolic *acidosis*, or both, may be present. Infants with heart failure often display *hyponatremia* as a result of renal water retention. Total body sodium may actually be increased. Chronic diuretic treatment can decrease serum sodium levels further.

Measurement of B-type natriuretic peptide, a cardiac neurohormone released in response to increased ventricular wall tension, is elevated in adult patients whose dyspnea is due to congestive heart failure. Rapid measurement may be helpful in distinguishing heart failure from other causes of dyspnea.

Treatment. The underlying cause of cardiac failure must be removed or alleviated if possible. If the cause is a congenital cardiac anomaly amenable to surgery, medical treatment is indicated to prepare the patient for surgery and in the immediate postoperative period while the heart is recovering from the effects of cardiopulmonary bypass. If the cause is cardiomyopathy, medical management provides temporary relief from symptoms and allows the patient to recover if the insult is reversible (e.g., myocarditis) or provides time to wait for a heart donor if heart transplantation is indicated.

GENERAL MEASURES. Strict bed rest is rarely necessary except in extreme cases, but it is important that the child rest often and sleep adequately. Most older patients feel better sleeping in a semi-upright position. For infants with heart failure, an infant chair may be advisable. After patients begin to respond to treatment, restrictions on activities can often be modified within the context of the specific diagnosis and the patient's ability. Competitive and strenuous sports activities are usually contraindicated. For patients with severe pulmonary edema, positive pressure ventilation may be required along with other drug therapy. β-Adrenergic agonists such as dopamine, epinephrine, and dobutamine, along with phosphodiesterase inhibitors and afterload-reducing agents (e.g., nitroprusside, captopril), may be required in an intensive care setting.

DIET. Infants with heart failure may fail to thrive because of increased metabolic requirements and decreased caloric intake. Increasing daily calories is an important aspect of their management. Increasing the number of calories per ounce of infant formula (or supplementing breast-feeding) may be beneficial. Many infants do not tolerate an increase beyond 24 calories/oz because of diarrhea or because these formulas provide too large a solute load for compromised kidneys.

Severely ill infants may lack sufficient strength for effective sucking because of extreme fatigue, rapid respirations, and generalized weakness. In these circumstances, nasogastric feedings may be helpful. In many children with cardiac enlargement, gastroesophageal reflux is a major problem. The use of continuous drip nasogastric feedings at night, administered by pump, may improve caloric intake while decreasing problems with reflux. Occasionally, medical or surgical intervention to correct reflux is necessary (Nissen fundoplication). Continued malnutrition may be an important factor in the decision to undertake earlier surgical intervention in patients who have an operable congenital heart lesion.

The use of low sodium formulas in the routine management of infants with heart failure is not recommended because these preparations are often poorly tolerated and may exacerbate diuretic-induced hyponatremia. Human breast milk is the ideal low sodium nutritional source. The use of more potent diuretic agents allows more palatable standard formulas to be used for nutrition while controlling salt and water balance by chronic diuretic administration. Most older children can be managed with "no added salt" diets and abstinence from foods containing large amounts of sodium. A strict, extremely low sodium diet is rarely required.

DIGITALIS. Digoxin is the digitalis glycoside used most often in pediatric patients. Its half-life of 36 hr is long enough to allow daily or twice-daily administration and short enough to limit toxic effects from overdosage. It is absorbed well by the gastrointestinal tract (60–85%), even in infants. Absorption is greater with the elixir than with tablets. An initial effect can be seen as early as 30 min after administration, and the peak effect for oral digoxin occurs at approximately 2–6 hr. When the drug is administered intravenously, the initial effect is seen in 15–30 min, and the peak effect occurs at 1–4 hr. The drug crosses the placenta, and therefore a fetus with heart failure (secondary to arrhythmia) can be treated by administering digoxin to the mother. The kidney eliminates digoxin, so dosing must be adjusted according to the patient's renal function. The rate of excretion is proportional to the glomerular filtration rate. After intravenous administration, 50–70% is excreted unchanged in the urine. The half-life of digoxin may be up to 6 days in patients with anuria because slower hepatic excretion pathways are used in these patients.

Rapid digitalization of infants and children in heart failure may be carried out intravenously. The dose depends on the patient's age (Table 434–1). The recommended schedule is to give half the total digitalizing dose immediately and the succeeding two one-quarter doses at 12 hr intervals later. The electrocardiogram must be closely monitored and rhythm strips obtained before each of the three digitalizing doses. Digoxin should be discontinued if a new rhythm disturbance is noted. Prolongation of the P-R interval is not necessarily an indication to withhold digitalis, but a delay in administering the next dose or a reduction in the dosage should be considered, depending on the patient's clinical status. Serum digoxin determination is helpful when digitalis toxicity is suspected, although it may be less reliable in infants. ST segment or T-wave changes are commonly noted with digitalis administration and should not affect the digitalization regimen. Baseline serum electrolyte levels should be measured before and after digitalization. Hypokalemia and hypercalcemia exacerbate digitalis toxicity. Because hypokalemia is relatively common in patients receiving diuretics, potassium levels should be monitored closely in those receiving a potassium-wasting diuretic (e.g., furosemide) in combination with digitalis.

Maintenance digitalis therapy is started approximately 12 hr after full digitalization. The daily dosage is divided in two and given at 12 hr intervals for more consistent blood levels and more flexibility in case of toxicity. The dosage is one quarter of the total digitalizing dose. For patients who are initially given digitalis intravenously, maintenance digoxin can be given orally once oral feedings are tolerated. Because absorption from the gastrointestinal tract is less certain, the oral maintenance dose is usually 20–25% higher than when digoxin is used parenterally (see Table 448–1). The normal daily dose of digoxin for older children (>5 yr of age) calculated by body weight should not exceed the usual adult dose of 0.2–0.5 mg/24 hr.

Patients who are not critically ill may be given digitalis initially by the oral route, and in most instances digitalization is completed within 24 hr. When slow digitalization is desirable, for example, in the immediate postoperative period, initiation of a maintenance digoxin schedule without a previous loading dose achieves full digitalization in 7–10 days. Often, it can be carried out on an outpatient basis.

Measurement of *serum digoxin levels* is useful under several circumstances: (1) when an unknown amount of digoxin has been

TABLE 434–1. Dosage of Drugs Commonly Used for the Treatment of Congestive Heart Failure

Drug	Dosage
Digoxin	Premature: 20 µg/kg
Digitalization PO (1/2 initially, followed by 1/4 q8–12h 12 × 2)	Full-term neonate (up to 1 mo): 20–30 µg/kg Infant or child: 25–40 µg/kg Adolescent or adult: 0.5–1 mg in divided doses IV dose is 75% of PO dose
Digoxin maintenance	5–10 µg/kg/day, divided q12h Trough serum level: 1.5–3.0 ng/mL < 6 mo old; 1–2 ng/mL >6 mo old IV dose is 75% of PO dose
Furosemide (Lasix)	
IV	1–2 mg/dose prn
PO	1–4 mg/kg/day, divided qd–qid
Bumetanide (Bumex)	
IV	0.01–0.1 mg/kg/dose
PO	0.05–0.1 mg/kg/day, divided q6–8h
Chlorothiazide (Diuril) PO	20–50 mg/kg/day, divided bid or tid
Spironolactone (Aldactone) PO	1–3 mg/kg/day, divided bid or tid
β-Adrenergic agonists IV	
Dobutamine	2–20 µg/kg/min
Dopamine	2–30 µg/kg/min
Isoproterenol	0.01–0.5 µg/kg/min
Epinephrine	0.05–1.0 µg/kg/min
Norepinephrine	0.1–2.0 µg/kg/min
Phosphodiesterase inhibitors IV	
Amrinone	3–10 µg/kg/min
Milrinone	0.25–1.0 µg/kg/min
Afterload-reducing agents	
Captopril (Capoten) PO	
Infants	0.1–0.5 mg/kg/dose q8–12h (maximum, 4 mg/kg/day) Prematures: start at 0.01 mg/kg/dose
Children	0.1–2 mg/kg/day q8–12h (adult dose is 6.25–25 mg/dose)
Enalapril (Vasotec) PO	0.08–0.5 mg/kg/dose q12–24h (maximum, 1 mg/kg/day)
Hydralazine (Apresoline) PO	
IV or IM	0.1–0.5 mg/kg/dose (maximum, 20 mg)
PO	0.25–1.0 mg/kg/dose q6–8h (maximum, 200 mg/day)
Nitroglycerin	0.25–5 µg/kg/min
Nitroprusside (Nipride) IV	0.5–8 µg/kg/min
Prazosin	0.005–0.05 mg/kg/dose q6–8h (maximum, 0.1 mg/kg/dose)
Carvedilol	Test dose, 0.08–0.09 mg/kg 0.18 mg/kg/day bid increased to 0.4–0.7 mg/kg/day bid over 8–12 wk PO; adult maximal dose, 50 mg/day

Note: Pediatric doses based on weight should not exceed adult doses. Because recommendations may change, these doses should always be double checked. Doses may also need to be modified in any patient with renal or hepatic dysfunction.

PO = by mouth; IV = intravenously; prn = as necessary; qd = every day; qid = three times per day; bid = twice daily.

administered or ingested accidentally, (2) when renal function is impaired or if drug interactions are possible, (3) when questions regarding compliance are raised, and (4) when a toxic response is suspected. Blood is usually drawn immediately before a dose but at minimum 4 hr after the last dose to ensure that tissue-plasma equilibration has occurred. An appropriate blood level is approximately 2–4 ng/mL in infants and 1–2 ng/mL in older children. Exceeding these levels does not generally add to the management of heart failure significantly and only increases the risk of toxicity. In suspected toxicity, elevated serum digoxin levels are not in themselves diagnostic of toxicity but must be interpreted as an adjunct to other clinical and electrocardiographic findings (rhythm and conduction disturbances). Nausea and vomiting are less frequent in pediatric patients. Hypokalemia, hypomagnesemia, hypercalcemia, cardiac inflammation secondary to myocarditis, and prematurity may all potentiate digitalis toxicity. A cardiac arrhythmia that develops in a child who is taking digitalis may also be related to the primary cardiac disease rather than the drug. Any form of arrhythmia occurring after the institution of digitalis therapy must be considered to be drug related until proved otherwise. Succeeding doses should be withheld until the issue is resolved.

DIURETICS. These agents interfere with reabsorption of water and sodium by the kidneys, which results in a reduction in circulating blood volume and thereby reduces pulmonary fluid overload and ventricular filling pressure. Diuretics are most often used in conjunction with digitalis therapy in patients with severe congestive heart failure.

Furosemide is the most commonly used diuretic in patients with heart failure. It inhibits the reabsorption of sodium and chloride in the distal tubules and the loop of Henle. Patients requiring acute diuresis should be given intravenous or intramuscular furosemide at an initial dose of 1–2 mg/kg, which usually results in rapid diuresis and prompt improvement in clinical status, particularly if symptoms of pulmonary congestion are present. Chronic furosemide therapy is then prescribed at a dose of 1–4 mg/kg/24 hr given between one and four times a day. Careful monitoring of electrolytes is necessary with long-term furosemide therapy because of the potential for significant loss of potassium. Potassium chloride supplementation is usually required unless the potassium-sparing diuretic spironolactone is given concomitantly. When furosemide is administered every other day, dietary potassium supplementation may be adequate to maintain normal serum potassium levels. Chronic administration of furosemide may cause contraction of the extracellular fluid compartment and result in "contraction alkalosis" (see Chapter 48.8). Diuretic-induced hyponatremia may become difficult to manage in patients with severe heart failure.

Spironolactone is an inhibitor of aldosterone and enhances potassium retention, often eliminating the need for oral potassium supplementation, which is frequently poorly tolerated. This drug is usually given orally in two to three divided doses of 2–3 mg/kg/24 hr. Combinations of spironolactone and chlorothiazide are commonly used for convenience. Adult patients have shown improved survival when this aldosterone inhibitor is included in the diuretic regimen.

Chlorothiazide is used occasionally for diuresis in children with less severe chronic heart failure. It is less immediate in action and less potent than furosemide, and it affects the reabsorption of electrolytes in the renal tubules only. The usual dose is 20–40 mg/kg/24 hr in divided doses. Potassium supplementation is often required if this agent is used alone.

AFTERLOAD-REDUCING AGENTS AND ACE INHIBITORS. This group of drugs reduces ventricular afterload by decreasing peripheral vascular resistance and thereby improving myocardial performance. Some of these agents also decrease systemic venous tone, which significantly reduces preload. Afterload reducers are especially useful in children with heart failure secondary to cardiomyopathy and in patients with severe mitral or aortic insufficiency. They may also be effective in patients with heart failure caused by left-to-right shunts. They are not generally used in the presence of stenotic lesions of the left ventricular outflow tract. Angiotensin-converting enzyme (ACE) inhibitors may have additional beneficial effects on cardiac remodeling independent of their influence on afterload. In adult patients with dilated cardiomyopathy, the addition of an ACE inhibitor to standard medical therapy reduces both morbidity and mortality. Afterload-reducing agents and ACE inhibitors are most often used in conjunction with other anticongestive drugs such as digoxin and diuretics.

Intravenously administered agents such as *nitroprusside* should be administered only in an intensive care setting and for as short a time as possible. Nitroprusside's short intravenous half-life makes it ideal for titrating the dose in critically ill patients. Peripheral arterial vasodilation and afterload reduction are the major effects, but venodilation causing a decrease in venous return to the heart may also be beneficial. Blood pressure must be continuously monitored because sudden hypotension can occur. Nitroprusside is contraindicated in patients with pre-existing hypotension. As the drug is metabolized, small amounts of circulating cyanide are produced and detoxified in the liver to thiocyanate, which is excreted in urine. When high doses of nitroprusside are administered for several days, toxic symptoms related to thiocyanate poisoning may occur (fatigue, nausea, disorientation, acidosis, and muscular spasm). If nitroprusside use is prolonged, blood thiocyanate levels should be monitored; values greater than 10 g/dL are consistent with clinical symptoms of toxicity. Phosphodiesterase inhibitors (see later) are also excellent afterload-reducing agents.

The orally active ACE inhibitor *captopril* produces arterial dilatation by blocking the production of angiotensin II, thereby resulting in significant afterload reduction. Venodilation and consequent preload reduction have also been reported. In addition, this agent interferes with aldosterone production and therefore also helps control salt and water retention. ACE inhibitors have additional beneficial effects on cardiac structure and function that may be independent of their effect on afterload. The oral dose is 0.3–6 mg/kg/24 hr given in two to three divided doses. Adverse reactions to captopril include hypotension and its sequelae (e.g., syncope, weakness, and dizziness). A maculopapular pruritic rash is encountered in 5–8% of patients, but the drug may be continued because the rash often disappears spontaneously with time. Neutropenia, renal toxicity, and chronic cough also occur. *Enalapril* is a longer acting ACE inhibitor that can be taken once or twice daily. Angiotensin II receptor blocking drugs have recently been introduced into management protocols for adults with heart failure; however, data on these agents in children are limited.

Intravenous nesiritide is a recombinant human brain (B-type) natriuretic peptide that has venous, arterial, and coronary vasodilatory effects. B-type natriuretic peptide is normally released by the failing ventricular myocardium. Exogenous infusion of nesiritide in adults with decompensated heart failure improves hemodynamic function and the clinical manifestations of heart failure.

α- AND β-ADRENERGIC AGONISTS. These drugs are usually administered in an intensive care setting, where the dose can be carefully titrated to hemodynamic response. Continuous determinations of arterial blood pressure and heart rate are performed; measuring cardiac output at the bedside with a pulmonary thermodilution (Swan-Ganz) catheter may also be helpful in assessing drug efficacy. Though extremely efficacious in the acute intensive care setting, some evidence indicates that long-term administration of adrenergic agonists may in certain cases increase morbidity and mortality in patients with heart failure.

Dopamine is a predominantly ß-adrenergic receptor agonist, but it has α-adrenergic effects at higher doses. Dopamine has less chronotropic and arrhythmogenic effect than the pure β-agonist isoproterenol does. In addition, it results in selective renal vasodilation because of its interaction with renal dopamine receptors, which is particularly useful in patients with the compromised kidney function that is often associated with low cardiac output. At a dose of 2–10 μg/kg/min, dopamine results in increased contractility with little peripheral vasoconstrictive effect. However, if the dose is increased beyond 15 μg/kg/min, its peripheral α-adrenergic effects may result in vasoconstriction.

Dobutamine, a derivative of dopamine, is useful in treating low cardiac output. It causes direct inotropic effects with a moderate reduction in peripheral vascular resistance. Dobutamine can be used as an adjunct to dopamine therapy to avoid the vasoconstrictive effects of high-dose dopamine. Dobutamine is also less likely to cause cardiac rhythm disturbances than isoproterenol is. The usual dose is 2–20 μg/kg/min.

Isoproterenol is a pure β-adrenergic agonist that has a marked chronotropic effect; it is most effective in patients with slow heart rates and should be used with caution in those who already have significant tachycardia. Children receiving isoproterenol must be carefully monitored for arrhythmias.

Epinephrine is a mixed α- and β-adrenergic receptor agonist that is usually reserved for patients with cardiogenic shock and low arterial blood pressure. Although epinephrine can raise blood pressure effectively, it also increases systemic vascular resistance and therefore increases the afterload against which the heart has to work.

PHOSPHODIESTERASE INHIBITORS. *Milrinone* is useful in treating patients with low cardiac output who are refractory to standard therapy. It works by inhibition of phosphodiesterase, which prevents the degradation of intracellular cyclic adenosine monophosphate. Milrinone has both positive inotropic effects on the heart and significant peripheral vasodilatory effects and has generally been used as an adjunct to dopamine or dobutamine therapy in the intensive care unit. It is given by intravenous infusion at 0.25–1 μg/kg/min, sometimes with an initial loading dose of 50 μg/kg. A major side effect is hypotension secondary to peripheral vasodilation, especially when a loading dose is used. The hypotension can generally be managed by the administration of intravenous fluids to restore adequate intravascular volume. *Amrinone*, another phosphodiesterase inhibitor, can cause thrombocytopenia; the severity appears to be related to both the rate of infusion and the duration of therapy. It is reversible when use of the drug is discontinued.

CHRONIC TREATMENT WITH β BLOCKERS. Studies in children and adults with dilated cardiomyopathy show that β-adrenergic blocking agents, introduced gradually as part of a comprehensive heart failure treatment program, improve exercise tolerance, decrease hospitalizations, and reduce overall mortality. The agents most often used are metoprolol, a β₁-adrenergic receptor selective antagonist, and carvedilol, an agent with both α- and β-adrenergic receptor blocking as well as free radical scavenging effects. β blockers are used for the chronic treatment of patients with heart failure and should not be administered when patients are still in the acute phase of heart failure (i.e., in the intensive care unit and receiving intravenous adrenergic agonist infusions). Preliminary noncontrolled studies in children show that β blockers are well tolerated and appear to be efficacious; a multicenter controlled trial of carvedilol in pediatric patients is currently in progress.

434.1 Cardiogenic Shock (see also Chapter 57.2)

Cardiogenic shock may occur as a complication of (1) severe cardiac dysfunction before or after cardiac surgery, (2) septicemia, (3) severe burns, (4) anaphylaxis, (5) cardiomyopathy, (6) myocarditis, (7) myocardial infarction or stunning, and (8) acute central nervous system disorders. It is characterized by low cardiac output and hypotension and therefore results in inadequate tissue perfusion.

Treatment is aimed at re-institution of adequate cardiac output and peripheral perfusion to prevent the untoward effects of prolonged ischemia on vital organs, as well as management of the underlying cause. Under physiologic conditions, cardiac output is increased as a result of sympathetic discharge, which increases the heart rate. However, in the presence of cardiogenic shock with marked tachycardia, the heart rate will not increase further, and cardiac output may be reduced because of decreased diastolic filling time. Cardiac output must be increased by increasing stroke volume. If the rate of fluid administration is increased, central venous pressure and ventricular filling pressure (preload) increase, and the Frank-Starling mechanism results in increased stroke volume. Optimal filling pressure is variable and depends on a number of extracardiac factors, including ventilatory support with high positive end-expiratory

TABLE 434–2. Treatment of Cardiogenic Shock*

	Determinants of Stroke Volume		
	Preload	*Contractility*	*Afterload*
Parameters measured	CVP, PCWP, LAP, cardiac chamber size on echocardiography	CO, BP, fractional shortening on echocardiography, MV O₂ saturation	BP, peripheral perfusion, SVR
Abnormal physiologic manifestations	Low CVP, PCWP, or LAP ↓ CO ↓ BP	High CVP, PCWP, or LAP; low MV O₂ saturation ↓ CO ↓ BP	High CVP, PCWP, LAP, or SVR ↓ CO → or ↑ BP
Treatment to improve cardiac output	Volume expansion, crystalloid, colloid, blood	β-Adrenergic agonists, phosphodiesterase inhibitors	Afterload-reducing agents: captopril, enalapril, lisinopril

The goal is to improve peripheral perfusion by increasing cardiac output: cardiac output = heart rate × stroke volume.
CVP = central venous pressure; PCWP = pulmonary capillary wedge pressure; LAP = left atrial pressure (measured with an indwelling LA line); CO = cardiac output (measured with a thermodilation catheter); BP = blood pressure; SVR = systemic vascular resistance (calculated from CO and mean BP); MV O₂ saturation = mixed venous oxygen saturation (measured with a central venous catheter); ↓ = decreased; → = normal; ↑ = increased.

pressure, peak inspiratory pressure, and intra-abdominal pressure. The increased pressure necessary to fill a relatively noncompliant ventricle should also be considered, particularly after open heart surgery. If carefully administered incremental fluid administration does not result in improved cardiac output, abnormal myocardial contractility or an abnormally high afterload, or both, must be implicated as the cause of the low cardiac output.

Myocardial contractility improves when treatment of the basic cause of shock is instituted, hypoxia is eliminated, and acidosis is corrected. However, dopamine, epinephrine, and dobutamine improve cardiac contractility, increase the heart rate, and ultimately increase cardiac output.

The use of cardiac glycosides to treat acute low cardiac output states should be avoided. Digoxin has a slower effect than catecholamines do, even with intravenous administration. In addition, adverse effects may result from larger doses, and toxicity is less predictable and depends on myocardial and serum potassium and calcium levels. It is common for patients in cardiovascular shock to have compromised renal perfusion, so administration of digoxin may result in high persistent blood levels because it is excreted by the kidneys. When digoxin is required for these patients, a lower and less frequent dosage should be used, and serum digoxin levels must be monitored frequently.

Patients in cardiogenic shock may have a marked increase in systemic vascular resistance resulting in high afterload and poor peripheral perfusion. If the increased systemic vascular resistance is persistent and the administration of positive inotropic agents alone does not improve tissue perfusion, the use of afterload-reducing agents may be appropriate, for example, nitroprusside or milrinone in combination with dopamine. In these patients, the use of a pulmonary thermodilution catheter to measure the cardiac index and to calculate systemic vascular resistance can be indispensable in guiding therapeutic decisions.

Sequential evaluation and management of cardiovascular shock are mandatory (see Chapter 57.2). Table 434–2 outlines the general *treatment principles* for acute cardiac circulatory failure under most circumstances. Treatment of infants and children with low cardiac output after cardiac surgery depends on the nature of the operative procedure and the patient's status after surgery (see Chapter 427).

Patients with deteriorating cardiogenic shock may benefit from a left ventricular assist device (LVAD). These devices have been used successfully in children and adolescents as a bridge to cardiac transplantation. In some cases, both right and left ventricular assist is necessary (BiVAD). Once implanted, assist devices allow patients to recover sufficiently to be extubated, become ambulatory, and often leave the intensive care setting while awaiting transplantation. Patients with reversible ventricular failure, for example, those in the immediate postoperative

state or those with acute myocarditis, may also benefit from extracorporeal membrane oxygenation (ECMO).

Bruns LA, Chrisant MK, Lamour JM, et al: Carvedilol as therapy in pediatric heart failure: An initial multicenter experience. *J Pediatr* 2001;138:505–11.
Clark BJ 3rd: Treatment of heart failure in infants and children. *Heart Dis* 2000;2:354–61.
Colucci WS, Elkayam U, Horton DP, et al: Intravenous nesiritide, a natriuretic peptide, in the treatment of decompensated congestive heart failure. *N Engl J Med* 2000;343:246–53.
Cowie MR, Zaphiriou A: Management of chronic heart failure. *Br Med J* 2002;325:422–5.
HFSA guidelines for management of patients with heart failure caused by left ventricular systolic dysfunction—pharmacological approaches. Heart Failure Society of America. *Pharmacotherapy* 2000;20:495–522.
Hunt SA, Baker DW, Chin MH, et al: ACC/AHA guidelines for the evaluation and management of chronic heart failure in the adult: Executive summary. A report of the American College of Cardiology/American Heart Association Task Force on Practice Guidelines (Committee to Revise the 1995 Guidelines for the Evaluation and Management of Heart Failure) developed in collaboration with the International Society for Heart and Lung Transplantation endorsed by the Heart Failure Society of America (1). *J Heart Lung Transplant* 2002;21:189–203.
Intravenous nesiritide vs nitroglycerin for treatment of decompensated congestive heart failure: A randomized controlled trial. *JAMA* 2002;287:1531–40.
Kay JD, Colan SD, Graham TP Jr: Congestive heart failure in pediatric patients. *Am Heart J* 2001;142:923–8.
Laer S, Mir TS, Behn F, et al: Carvedilol therapy in pediatric patients with congestive heart failure: A study investigating clinical and pharmacokinetic parameters. *Am Heart J* 2002;143:916–22.
Maisel AS, Krishnaswamy P, Nowak RM, et al: Rapid measurement of B-type natriuretic peptide in the emergency diagnosis of heart failure. *N Engl J Med* 2002;347:161–6.
Nohria A, Lewis E, Stevenson LW: Medical management of advanced heart failure. *JAMA* 2002;287:628–40.
Shaddy RE: Optimizing treatment for chronic congestive heart failure in children. *Crit Care Med* 2001;29(Suppl):237–40.
Weber KT: Aldosterone in congestive heart failure. *N Engl J Med* 2001;345:1689–97.

Chapter 435
Pediatric Heart and Heart-Lung Transplantation

435.1 Pediatric Heart Transplantation

As of 1999, over 4600 heart transplants had been performed on children at 226 centers worldwide. Survival rates in children compare favorably with those in adults: 78% at 1 yr and 68% at 5 yr (Fig. 435–1). Nearly 60% of patients are alive at 10 yr. As new therapeutic regimens are introduced, the long-term outlook for pediatric heart transplant recipients continues to improve. A small, but growing number of children are surpassing 15- and 20-yr survival.

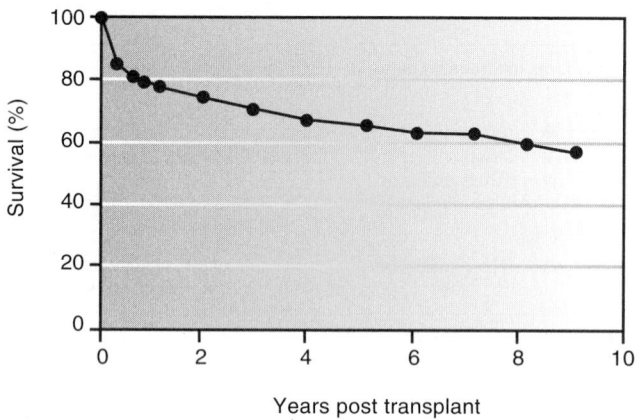

FIGURE 435–1. Survival after pediatric heart transplantation. (Data based on over 4500 patients worldwide who received heart transplants from 1982 through 1999 as listed with the Registry of the International Society for Heart and Lung Transplantation.)

Indications. Heart transplantation is performed in infants and children with end-stage cardiomyopathy who have become refractory to medical therapy and in patients with some forms of complex congenital heart disease (e.g., hypoplastic left heart syndrome) for whom standard surgical procedures are extremely high risk. Cardiomyopathies account for over 50% of heart transplants in pediatric patients older than 1 yr, although the percentage of patients with congenital lesions (approximately 25%) is gradually increasing. In infants younger than 1 yr, congenital heart lesions represent 75% of transplants. Heart transplantation is performed in children who have previously undergone conventional surgery for congenital heart disease and in whom myocardial dysfunction later develops.

Recipient and Donor Selection. Potential heart transplant recipients must be free of serious noncardiac medical problems such as neurologic disease, systemic infection, severe hepatic or renal disease, or severe malnutrition. Many children with ventricular dysfunction may have pulmonary hypertension and even pulmonary vascular disease, which would preclude heart transplantation. For this reason, pulmonary vascular resistance is measured at cardiac catheterization, both at rest and in response to vasodilators. Patients with fixed elevated pulmonary vascular resistance (>6–8 Wood units) are at higher risk for heart transplantation and may be considered candidates for heart-lung transplantation (see Chapter 435.2). A comprehensive social services consultation is an important component of the recipient evaluation. Because of the complex post-transplantation medical regimen, the family must have a history of compliance. Detailed informed consent must be obtained.

Donor shortage is a serious problem for both adults and children. At the national registry of transplant recipients in the United States (UNOS—the United Network for Organ Sharing), allografts are matched by ABO blood group and body weight. HLA matching is not currently feasible for heart transplantation; however, with modern immunosuppression, it may offer only minimal advantage. ABO matching may not be needed for infants. Physicians caring for a patient who may be a potential donor should contact the organ donor coordinator at a transplanting institution, who can best judge the appropriateness of organ donation and has experience in interacting with donor families. Contraindications to *organ donation* include prolonged cardiac arrest with moderate to severe cardiac dysfunction, ongoing systemic illness or infection, and pre-existing severe cardiac disease. A history of resuscitation alone or reparable congenital heart disease is not an automatic exclusion for dona-

tion. Non–heart-beating donors may provide additional hearts for those on the long waiting list.

The decision of when to place a patient on the transplant waiting list is based on many factors, including extremely poor ventricular function (left ventricular fractional shortening <10%; normal is 28–40%), poor response to medical anticongestive therapy, multiple hospitalizations for heart failure, arrhythmia, progressive deterioration in renal or hepatic function, early stages of pulmonary vascular disease, and poor nutritional status. In patients awaiting transplantation, those with poor left ventricular function (fractional shortening <15%) are usually started on a regimen of warfarin to reduce the risk of mural thrombosis and thromboembolism. Patients with cardiogenic shock unresponsive to standard pharmacologic treatment may be candidates for placement of left ventricular (LVAD) or biventricular (BiVAD) assist devices, which can stabilize hemodynamics and serve as a bridge to transplantation.

Perioperative Management. In the classic operation, both donor and recipient hearts are excised so that the posterior portions of the atria containing the venae cavae and pulmonary veins are left intact. The aorta and pulmonary artery are divided above the level of the semilunar valves. The anterior portion of the donor's atria is then connected to the remaining posterior portion of the recipient's atria, thereby avoiding the need for delicate suturing of the venae cavae or pulmonary veins. The donor and recipient great vessels are connected via end-to-end anastomoses. A bicaval anastomosis may be used, with the donor right atrium left intact; the left atrial connection is still performed as in the classic procedure.

In the immediate postoperative period, immunosuppression is most commonly achieved with a triple-drug regimen. One protocol calls for cyclosporine, 2–10 mg/kg/24 hr; azathioprine, 2 mg/kg/24 hr; and prednisone, started at 0.6–1.0 mg/kg/24 hr and tapered to 0.2 mg/kg/24 hr over the 1st 6–12 wk, although in children, a wide range of cyclosporine doses are required to achieve therapeutic serum levels. In many centers, an antilymphocyte preparation is added in the 1st wk, either antithymocyte globulin, monoclonal murine antihuman T-lymphocyte antibody (OKT3), or one of the humanized anti–interleukin 2 receptor antibodies. In children who do not experience significant graft rejection, steroids can be tapered to an alternate-day regimen after the 1st 6–12 mo; in many patients, steroids can be totally eliminated. In some centers, steroids are not routinely included as part of maintenance immunosuppression but are added later for the treatment of acute rejection episodes. Some centers prefer tacrolimus (FK506, Prograf) as part of the initial regimen instead of cyclosporine. Agents such as mycophenolate mofetil (CellCept) and rapamycin have gained increased use as a substitute for azathioprine.

Most pediatric heart transplant recipients can be extubated within the 1st 48 hr after transplantation and are out of bed within 3–4 days. These patients are often discharged within the 1st 2 wk after transplantation. In patients with pre-existing high-risk factors, postoperative care is considerably prolonged.

Diagnosis and Management of Acute Graft Rejection. Post-transplantation management consists of adjusting medications to maintain a balance between the risk of rejection and the side effects of over-immunosuppression. Along with infection, acute graft rejection is a leading cause of death in adult and pediatric heart transplant recipients. The incidence of acute rejection is greatest within the 1st 3 mo after transplantation and decreases considerably thereafter. Most pediatric patients experience at least one episode of acute rejection within the 1st 2 yr after transplantation, usually at the time of weaning of one of their immunosuppressive medications. Because the symptoms of rejection can mimic many routine pediatric illnesses (e.g., gastroenteritis), the transplant center should be notified any time that a heart transplant recipient is seen in the office or emergency room for acute illness.

Clinical manifestations of acute rejection may include fatigue, fluid retention, fever, diaphoresis, abdominal symptoms, and a gallop rhythm. The *electrocardiogram* may show reduced voltage, atrial or ventricular arrhythmias, or heart block. *Roentgenographic* examination may show an enlarged heart, effusions, or pulmonary edema. Cyclosporine modifies the clinical course of rejection; most rejection episodes occur without any detectable clinical symptoms. On *echocardiography*, indices of systolic left ventricular function usually do not deteriorate until rejection is severe. Techniques to evaluate wall thickening and left ventricular diastolic function have not fulfilled their promise as predictors of early rejection. Most transplant centers do not rely on echocardiography alone in rejection surveillance.

Myocardial biopsy is the most reliable method of monitoring patients for rejection. Biopsy specimens are taken from the right ventricular side of the interventricular septum and can be harvested relatively safely in small infants and children. In older children, myocardial biopsies may be performed as often as every 1–4 wk during the 1st 3–6 mo after transplantation. The frequency is then reduced to two or four biopsies per year unless the patient has an episode of rejection. In infants, surveillance biopsies are usually performed less often and may be as infrequent as once or twice per year. Children may have clinically unsuspected rejection episodes even 5–10 yr after transplantation; most pediatric transplant centers continue routine surveillance biopsies, albeit at less frequent intervals (every 6–12 mo).

Criteria for grading cardiac rejection are based on a system developed by the International Society for Heart and Lung Transplantation (ISHLT); these criteria take into account the degree of cellular infiltration and whether myocyte necrosis is present. ISHLT rejection grades 1A, 1B, and 2 are usually mild enough to not warrant immediate treatment, and more than 50% of these episodes may resolve spontaneously. A repeat biopsy specimen is usually obtained within several weeks. For patients with ISHLT grade 3A rejection, treatment is instituted with either intravenous methylprednisolone or a "bump and taper" of oral prednisone. Asymptomatic patients more than 3 mo post-transplant and with normal echocardiograms are often treated as outpatients. For grades 3B or 4, especially with hemodynamic instability, patients are admitted to the hospital for intravenous steroid therapy. For rejection episodes resistant to steroid therapy, additional therapeutic regimens include a repeat course of an antilymphocyte preparation (OKT3 or antithymocyte globulin), methotrexate, or total lymphoid irradiation. Patients with repeated episodes of rejection may also benefit from being switched from cyclosporine to tacrolimus (or vice versa) and from azathioprine to mycophenolate therapy. Rare patients with refractory rejection require retransplantation.

Complications of Immunosuppression

INFECTION. Infection is one of the two leading causes of death in pediatric transplant patients (Fig. 435–2). The incidence of infection is greatest in the 1st 3 mo after transplantation when immunosuppressive doses are highest. Viral infections are the most common, especially cytomegalovirus, which accounts for as many as 25% of infectious episodes. Cytomegalovirus infection may occur as a primary infection in patients without previous exposure to the virus or as a reactivation. Severe cytomegalovirus infection can be disseminated or associated with pneumonitis and may provoke an episode of acute graft rejection or graft coronary disease (see later). Many centers use intravenous ganciclovir or cytomegalovirus immune globulin (CytoGam), or both, as prophylaxis in any patient receiving a heart from a donor who is positive for cytomegalovirus or in any recipient who has serologic evidence of previous cytomegalovirus disease. Polymerase chain reaction has markedly improved the ability to diagnose

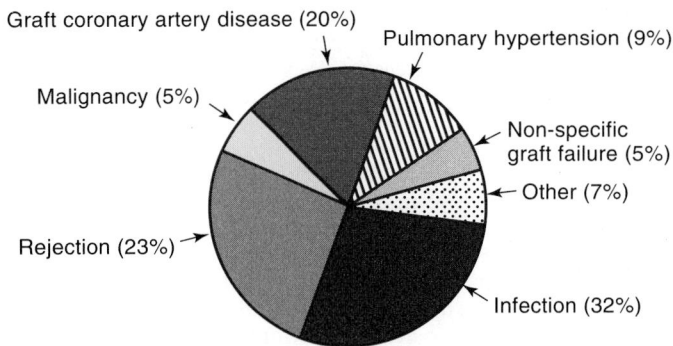

FIGURE 435–2. Major causes of death after pediatric heart transplantation. (Data from Stanford University.)

cytomegalovirus infection and to serially monitor the efficacy of therapy. Oral preparations of ganciclovir are available for chronic therapy. Adenovirus infection may be associated with graft loss.

Most normal childhood viral illnesses are well tolerated and do not usually require special treatment. Otitis media and routine upper respiratory tract infections can be treated in the outpatient setting, although fever or symptoms that last beyond the usual course require further investigation. Gastroenteritis, especially with vomiting, can result in markedly reduced absorption of immunosuppressive medications and provoke a rejection episode. In this setting, drug levels should be closely monitored and the use of intravenous medications considered. Varicella exposure is treated with varicella immune globulin, and if the patient acquires clinical varicella infection, treatment with intravenous acyclovir attenuates the illness.

Bacterial infections are the next most frequent, with the lung being the most common site of infection (35%), followed by the blood, urinary tract, and less commonly, the sternotomy site. Other sources of post-transplantation infection include fungi (14%) and protozoa (6%). The incidence of serious infection is lower in children who can be managed without steroids.

GROWTH RETARDATION. Patients requiring chronic steroid administration usually have decreased linear growth. Alternate-day steroid regimens generally result in improved linear growth. In patients who experience rejection when steroids are weaned, other immunosuppressants (methotrexate, total lymphoid irradiation) have shown promise as steroid-sparing agents. In children surviving longer than 5 yr after transplantation, growth is normal in 75%.

HYPERTENSION. Hypertension is common in patients treated with cyclosporine. It is due to a combination of plasma volume expansion and defective renal sodium excretion. Corticosteroids usually potentiate cyclosporine-induced hypertension. Patients are typically managed with a combination of a diuretic and a vasodilator. Agents that work via calcium channel blockade have the additional advantage of possibly attenuating graft coronary disease (see later). The incidence of hypertension may be slightly lower in patients treated with tacrolimus.

RENAL FUNCTION. Chronic administration of cyclosporine or tacrolimus can lead to a tubulointerstitial nephropathy in adults, but severe renal dysfunction is rare in children. Most pediatric patients gradually have an increase in serum creatinine during the 1st yr after transplantation; if renal dysfunction occurs, it usually responds to a decrease in cyclosporine dosage. Long-term patients rarely require renal transplantation.

NEUROLOGIC COMPLICATIONS. Neurologic side effects of cyclosporine and tacrolimus include tremor, myalgias, paresthesias, and rarely, seizures. These complications can be treated with reduced doses of medication and occasionally with oral magnesium supplementation. Intracranial infections pose a significant risk, especially because some of the more frequent signs (nuchal rigidity) may be absent in immunosuppressed patients. The most common organisms are *Aspergillus, Cryptococcus neoformans,* and *Listeria monocytogenes.* Aseptic meningitis can be seen days or weeks after OKT3 administration and is usually self-limited.

TUMORS. One of the serious complications limiting long-term survival in pediatric heart transplant patients is the risk of neoplastic disease. The most common is post-transplant lymphoproliferative disease (PTLD), a condition associated with Epstein-Barr virus. PTLD usually responds to a reduction in immunosuppression and acyclovir and only occasionally requires chemotherapy. Monoclonal antibodies directed against the CD20 antigen on activated lymphocytes show promise against PTLD. An increased risk of skin cancer requires that children use appropriate precautions when exposed to sunlight.

CHRONIC REJECTION. Graft coronary artery disease (CAD) is a manifestation of chronic graft rejection that occurs in 10–20% of children. The cause is still unclear, although it is thought to be a form of immunologically mediated vessel injury. Hypercholesterolemia and hyperglycemia increase the risk of this disease. Unlike native coronary atherosclerosis, graft CAD is a diffuse process with a high degree of distal vessel involvement. Because the transplanted heart has been denervated, patients do not experience symptoms such as angina pectoris during ischemic episodes, and the initial manifestation may be cardiovascular collapse or sudden death. Most centers perform coronary angiography annually to screen for coronary abnormalities; some also perform coronary intravascular ultrasound. Several reports have suggested that dobutamine stress echocardiography is useful as a screening tool. Standard coronary artery bypass procedures are not usually helpful because of the diffuse nature of the process, although transcatheter stenting is sometimes effective for isolated lesions. For severe cases, repeat heart transplantation has been the only effective treatment. Calcium channel blockers such as diltiazem have been shown to either prevent or delay the onset of graft coronary disease in adult transplant patients. One class of cholesterol-lowering agents, the HMG-CoA (3-hydroxy-3-methyl–coenzyme A) reductase inhibitors (pravastatin, atorvastatin), may be effective in reducing the risk of both graft CAD and rejection.

OTHER COMPLICATIONS. Corticosteroids usually result in cushingoid facies, steroid acne, and striae. Cyclosporine can cause a subtle change in facial features such as hypertrichosis and gingival hyperplasia. These cosmetic features can be particularly disturbing to adolescents and may be the motivation for noncompliance. Many of these complications are dose related and improve as immunosuppressive medications are weaned. Osteoporosis and aseptic necrosis are additional reasons for reducing the steroid dosage as soon as possible. Diabetes and pancreatitis are rare, but serious complications.

REHABILITATION. Despite the potential risks of immunosuppression, the prospect for rehabilitation in pediatric heart transplant recipients is excellent. Almost 95% of pediatric heart transplant recipients have no functional limitations in their daily lives. At 2 yr follow-up, almost 70% of patients do not require rehospitalization for transplant-related problems.

Pediatric heart transplant recipients can attend daycare or school and participate in noncontact competitive sports and other age-appropriate activities. Standardized measurements of ventricular function are close to normal. Because the transplanted heart is denervated, the increase in heart rate and cardiac output during exercise is slower in transplant recipients, and maximal heart rate and cardiac output responses are mildly attenuated. These subtle abnormalities are rarely noticeable by the patient.

Growth of the transplanted heart is excellent, although a mild degree of ventricular and septal hypertrophy is commonly seen, even years after transplantation. The sites of atrial and great vessel anastomoses grow without the development of obstruction.

However, in neonates who undergo transplantation for hypoplastic left heart syndrome, juxtaductal aortic coarctation may recur.

As assessed by standardized psychologic testing, the psychologic adjustment to heart transplantation in children is usually good. A problem sometimes occurs with noncompliance once patients reach adolescence, and life-threatening rejection may result. Early intervention by social services counselors may be able to reduce this risk.

435.2 Heart-Lung and Lung Transplantation

More than 400 heart-lung and over 580 lung (single or double) transplants have been performed in children at approximately 60 institutions worldwide. Primary indications for heart-lung transplantation include complex congenital heart disease with pulmonary hypoplasia or Eisenmenger syndrome, primary pulmonary hypertension, congenital lung abnormalities, α_1-antitrypsin deficiency, and end-stage parenchymal lung disease (bronchopulmonary dysplasia, chronic lung disease, interstitial fibrosis, and cystic fibrosis). Many of these patients with normal hearts may also be candidates for single- or double-lung transplantation if right ventricular function is preserved. In some patients with Eisenmenger physiology, double-lung transplantation can be performed in combination with repair of intracardiac defects. Patients with cystic fibrosis are not candidates for single-lung grafts because of the risk of infection from the diseased contralateral lung. Patients are selected according to many of the same criteria as for heart transplant recipients (see Chapter 435.1).

Post-transplant immunosuppression is achieved with a triple-drug regimen, similar to that used for heart transplantation; many groups avoid steroids during the early postoperative period to promote better airway healing. Unlike patients with isolated heart transplants, few patients with lung transplants can be weaned off steroids. Prophylaxis against infection is achieved with trimethoprim-sulfamethoxazole or aerosolized pentamidine. Ganciclovir and cytomegalovirus immune globulin prophylaxis are used as in heart transplant recipients (see Chapter 435.1).

Pulmonary rejection is common in heart-lung transplant recipients, whereas heart rejection is encountered less often than in patients with isolated heart transplants. Symptoms of lung rejection may include fever and fatigue, although many episodes are minimally symptomatic. Surveillance for rejection is performed by monitoring pulmonary function (forced vital capacity; forced expiratory volume in 1 sec [FEV_1]; forced expiratory flow, midexpiratory phase [$FEF_{25-75\%}$]), systemic arterial oxygen tension, and chest roentgenograms and by serial transbronchial biopsy. Routine biopsies are performed frequently in the 1st 3 mo and then quarterly thereafter. Because of technical limitations, biopsies are not performed in infants, who are monitored by clinical criteria alone.

Actuarial *survival* rates after heart-lung or lung transplantation in children are currently 75% at 1 yr and 45% at 5 yr; improved patient selection and postoperative management are continually improving these survival statistics. As in isolated heart transplantation, infection remains the leading cause of early death and accounts for nearly 50% of all mortality in the 1st yr after transplantation. Other causes of early morbidity and mortality include tracheal complications, pulmonary venous obstruction, donor lung dysfunction, bleeding, and acute rejection. *Obliterative bronchiolitis* (OB), a form of chronic rejection, remains a major limitation to long-term survival in a significant number of patients. OB develops in 10–50% of long-term survivors of lung transplantation. Increasing immunosuppression has markedly reduced the incidence of OB. Additional late complications include the development of airway stenosis, accelerated graft CAD (though less common than in isolated heart transplantation), and other side effects of chronic immunosuppression (see Chapters 128 and 129).

Postoperative indices of *cardiopulmonary function* and exercise capacity show significant improvement. More than 95% of patients are without activity limitations at 2 yr follow-up. Problems of donor availability are even more severe with lung transplantation. Living related lung transplantation, in which a lobe from a parent is transplanted into a child, may partially alleviate this problem.

Heart Transplantation

Bernstein D, Baum D, Berry G, et al: Neoplastic disorders after pediatric heart transplantation. *Circulation* 1993;88:230.

Boucek MM, Faro A, Novick RJ, et al: The Registry of the International Society for Heart and Lung Transplantation: Fourth Official Pediatric Report—2000. *J Heart Lung Transplant* 2001;20:39–52.

Canter C, Naftel D, Caldwell R, et al: Survival and risk factors for death after cardiac transplantation in infants. A multi-institutional study. The Pediatric Heart Transplant Study. *Circulation* 1997;96:227.

Elliott MJ, Mallory G Jr, Khagani A: Transplantation from non–heart-beating donors. *Lancet* 2001;357:819.

Gao SZ, Schroeder JS, Alderman EL, et al: Clinical and laboratory correlates of accelerated coronary artery disease in the cardiac transplant patient. *Circulation* 1987;76:56.

Hornung TS, de Goede C, O'Brien C, et al: Renal function after pediatric cardiac transplantation: The effect of early cyclosporin dosage. *Pediatrics* 2001;107:1346–50.

Hotson JR, Enzmann DR: Neurologic complications of cardiac transplantation. *Neurol Clin* 1988;6:346.

Pahl E, Zales VR, Fricker FJ, Addonizio LJ: Posttransplant coronary artery disease in children. A multicenter national survey. *Circulation* 1994;90:II56.

Ringewald JM, Gidding SS, Crawford SE, et al: Nonadherence is associated with late rejection in pediatric heart transplant recipients. *J Pediatr* 2001;139:75–8.

Schowengerdt KO, Naftel DC, Seib PM, et al: Infection after pediatric heart transplantation: Results of a multi-institutional study. The Pediatric Heart Transplant Study Group. *J Heart Lung Transplant* 1997;16:1207.

Schroeder JS, Gao SZ, Alderman EL: A preliminary study of diltiazem in the prevention of coronary artery disease in heart transplant recipients. *N Engl J Med* 1993;3:164.

Shaddy RE, Naftel DC, Kirklin JK, et al: Outcome of cardiac transplantation in children. Survival in a contemporary multi-institutional experience. Pediatric Heart Transplant Study. *Circulation* 1996;94(9 Suppl):II69.

Shirali GS, Ni J, Chinnock RE, et al: Association of viral genome with graft loss in children after cardiac transplantation. *N Engl J Med* 2001;344:1498–1503.

Sigfusson G, Fricker FJ, Bernstein D, et al: Long term survivors of pediatric heart transplantation: A multicenter report of 68 children who have survived greater than five years. *J Pediatr* 1997;130:862.

Webber SA: Immunology of pediatric heart transplantation: A clinical update. *Semin Thorac Cardiovasc Surg Pediatr Card Surg Annu* 2001;4:158–84.

West LJ, Pollock-Barziv SM, Dipchand AI, et al: ABO-incompatible heart transplantation in infants. *N Engl J Med* 2001;344:793–800.

Lung Transplantation

Conte JV, Robbins RC, Reichenspurner H, et al: Pediatric heart-lung transplantation: Intermediate-term results. *J Heart Lung Transplant* 1996;15:692.

Mendeloff EN, Huddleston CB, Mallory GB: Pediatric and adult lung transplantation for cystic fibrosis. *J Thorac Cardiovasc Surg* 1998;115:404.

Spray TL, Mallory GB, Canter CE, et al: Pediatric lung transplantation for pulmonary hypertension and congenital heart disease. *Ann Thorac Surg* 1992;54:216.

Starnes VA, Oyer PE, Bernstein D, et al: Heart, heart-lung, and lung transplantation in the first year of life. *Ann Thorac Surg* 1992;53:306.

Sweet SC, Spray TL, Huddleston CB, et al: Pediatric lung transplantation at St. Louis Children's Hospital, 1990–1995. *Am J Respir Crit Care Med* 1997;155:1027.

Theodore J, Starnes VA, Lewiston NJ: Obliterative bronchiolitis. *Clin Chest Med* 1990;11:309.

Watson TJ, Starnes VA: Pediatric lobar lung transplantation. *Semin Thorac Cardiovasc Surg* 1996;8:313.

SECTION 8 *Diseases of the Peripheral Vascular System*

Daniel Bernstein

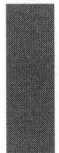

Chapter 436
Disease of the Blood Vessels (Aneurysms and Fistulas)

436.1 Kawasaki Disease

(see also Chapters 156 and 431.5)

Aneurysms of the coronary or systemic arteries may complicate Kawasaki disease and are the leading cause of morbidity in this disease (Fig. 436–1). Other than in Kawasaki disease, aneurysms are not common in children and occur most frequently in the aorta in association with coarctation of the aorta, patent ductus arteriosus, and Marfan syndrome and in intracranial vessels (see Chapter 593). They may also occur secondary to an infected embolus; infection contiguous to a blood vessel; trauma; congenital abnormalities of vessel structure, especially the medial wall; and arteritis, for example, polyarteritis nodosa and Takayasu arteritis (see Chapter 157).

436.2 Arteriovenous Fistulas

Arteriovenous fistulas may be limited to small cavernous hemangiomas or may be extensive (see Chapters 497 and 640). The most common sites in infants and children are within the cranium, in the liver, in the lung, in the extremities, and in vessels in or near the thoracic wall. These fistulas, though usually congenital, may follow trauma or be a manifestation of hereditary hemorrhagic telangiectasia (Osler-Weber-Rendu disease). Femoral arteriovenous fistulas are a rare complication of percutaneous femoral catheterization.

Clinical Manifestations. Clinical symptoms occur only in association with large arteriovenous communications when arterial blood flows into a low-pressure venous system; local venous pressure is increased, and arterial flow distal to the fistula is decreased. Systemic arterial resistance falls because of the runoff of blood through the fistula. Compensatory mechanisms include tachycardia and increased stroke volume so that cardiac output rises. Total blood volume is also increased. In large fistulas, left ventricular dilatation, a widened pulse pressure, and heart failure occur. Injection of contrast material into an artery proximal to the fistula confirms the diagnosis.

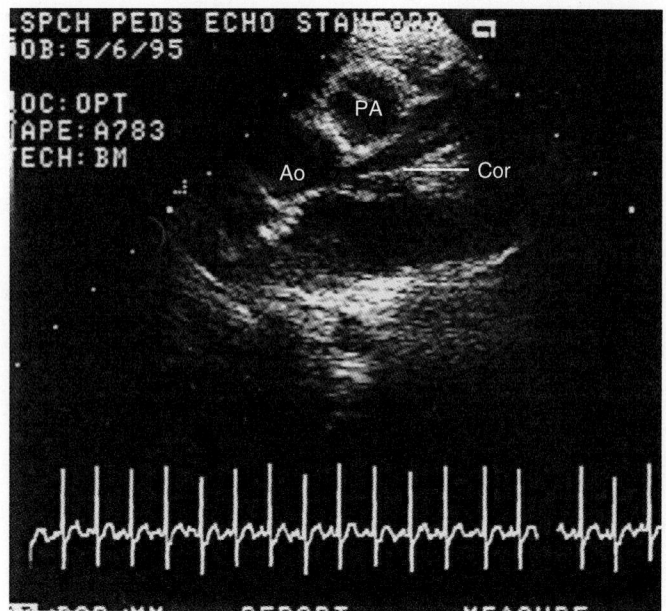

FIGURE 436–1. Two-dimensional echocardiogram showing giant coronary artery aneurysms in a patient with Kawasaki disease. PA = pulmonary artery; Ao = aorta; Cor = coronary artery

Large *intracranial arteriovenous fistulas* most often occur in newborn infants in association with a *vein of Galen malformation*. The large intracranial left-to-right shunt results in heart failure secondary to the demand for high cardiac output. Patients with smaller communications may not have cardiovascular manifestations but may later be disposed to hydrocephalus (see Chapter 585.11) or seizure disorders. A newborn infant with a large symptomatic intracranial arteriovenous fistula has a grave prognosis; some survive with medical management but are subject to later complications caused by the intracranial mass. The diagnosis can often be made by auscultation of a continuous murmur over the cranium. Older children with more diffuse intracranial arteriovenous malformations may be recognized on the basis of intracranial calcification and high cardiac output without cardiac failure.

Hepatic arteriovenous fistulas may be generalized or localized in the liver and may be hemangioendotheliomas or cavernous hemangiomas. The fistula may be located between the hepatic artery and the ductus venosus or portal vein. Congenital hemorrhagic telangiectasia may also be present. Large arteriovenous fistulas are associated with increased cardiac output and heart failure. Hepatomegaly is usual, and systolic or continuous murmurs may be audible over the liver.

Peripheral arteriovenous fistulas generally involve the extremities and are associated with disfigurement, swelling of the extremity, and visible hemangiomas. Some are located in areas that result in upper airway obstruction. Because only a small minority result in large arterial runoff, cardiac failure is uncommon.

Treatment. Medical management of heart failure is initially helpful in neonates with these conditions; with time, the size of the shunt may diminish and symptoms spontaneously regress. Hemangiomas of the liver often eventually disappear completely. Large liver hemangiomas have been treated with steroids, ε-aminocaproic acid, interferon, local compression, embolization, or local irradiation; the beneficial effects of these management options are not firmly established because individual patients display marked variation in clinical course without treatment. *Catheter embolization* is rapidly becoming the treatment of choice for many patients with a symptomatic arteriovenous fistula. Embolic agents that have been used include detachable balloons, steel (Gianturco) coils, and liquid tissue adhesives (cyanoacrylate). Often, multiple procedures are necessary before flow is significantly reduced. *Surgical removal* of a large fistula may be attempted in patients with severe cardiac failure and lack of improvement with medical treatment. Surgical treatment may be contraindicated or unsuccessful when the lesion is extensive and diffuse or is located in a position where adjoining tissue may be injured during the surgery or related procedures.

Fong LV, Lee SH, Salmon AP: Diagnosis of cerebral arteriovenous malformations by colour Doppler examination. *Eur Heart J* 1992;13:415.

Ford EG, Stanley P, Tolo V, et al: Peripheral congenital arteriovenous fistulae: Observe, operate, or obturate? *J Pediatr Surg* 1992;27:714.

Friedman DM, Verma R, Madrid M, et al: Recent improvement in outcome using transcatheter embolization techniques for neonatal aneurysmal malformations of the vein of Galen. *Pediatrics* 1993;91:583.

Grifka RG, Mullins CE, Gianturco C, et al: New Gianturco-Grifka vascular occlusion device. Initial studies in a canine model. *Circulation* 1995;91:1840.

Chapter 437
Systemic Hypertension

Systemic hypertension occurs commonly in adults and if untreated is a major risk factor for myocardial infarction, stroke, and renal failure. The prevalence of hypertension increases with age: 15% in young adults to 60% in individuals older than 65 yr. In infants and younger children, systemic hypertension is uncommon, but when present, it is usually indicative of an underlying disease process *(secondary hypertension)*. Adolescents may acquire *primary or essential hypertension* (with no underlying cause); the hypertension may track into adulthood. To increase early detection of hypertension, accurate blood pressure measurements should be part of the routine annual physical examination of all children 3 yr or older. A complete family history of hypertension should be elicited.

Accurate measurement of blood pressure requires careful attention to the comfort of the patient and is highly dependent on proper use of the equipment, whether it be a simple sphygmomanometer or a state-of-the-art automated device. Obtaining an accurate blood pressure measurement in infants is often the most difficult and time-consuming part of the physical examination. Patients of any age have some level of anxiety associated with measurement of blood pressure that may lead to a false diagnosis of hypertension. Blood pressure can be measured with the patient either seated or supine; infants may be held in the lap of a parent. Subsequent measurements taken for comparison should be obtained with the patient in the same position. Careful attention to cuff size is necessary to avoid overdiagnosis. A wide variety of bladder sizes should be available in any medical office where children are routinely cared for. The cuff should completely encircle the upper part of the arm to ensure uniform compression; the inflatable bladder should cover at least two thirds of the upper arm length and three quarters of its circumference. A cuff that is too short or narrow artificially increases blood pressure readings. Blood pressure should be obtained in all four extremities to detect coarctation of the aorta (see Chapter 420.6).

Systolic pressure is indicated by appearance of the 1st Korotkoff sound. True diastolic pressure probably lies between the muffling and the disappearance of Korotkoff sounds; muffling may be difficult to appreciate in smaller children. Palpation is useful for rapid assessment of systolic blood pressure, although the palpated pressure is generally about 10 mm Hg less than that obtained via auscultation. Doppler is an extremely accurate method of measuring systolic blood pressure; it is less so for diastolic pressure. Oscillometric techniques are used frequently in infants and young children, but they are susceptible to artifacts and are best for measuring mean blood pressure.

Blood pressure increases gradually with age; therefore, standard nomograms are necessary for interpretation of blood pressure values (see Figs. 415–1 and 415–2). If mild hypertension is found, it is imperative that the measurement be repeated twice more over a period of 6 wk. Anxiety usually decreases as the patient becomes more comfortable with the procedure; thus, repeated measurements are necessary to avoid inappropriately labeling a patient as hypertensive. Blood pressure that is consistently above the 95th percentile for age requires further evaluation. Ambulatory blood pressure monitoring may be especially useful in adolescents who have borderline hypertension in the office setting.

Etiology and Pathophysiology. Blood pressure is the product of cardiac output and peripheral vascular resistance. An increase in either cardiac output or peripheral resistance results in an increase in blood pressure; if one of these factors increases while the other decreases, blood pressure may not increase. When hypertension is the result of another disease process, it is referred to as *secondary hypertension*. When no identifiable cause can be found, it is referred to as *primary* or *essential hypertension*. Many factors, including heredity, diet, stress, and obesity, may play a role in the development of essential hypertension.

Secondary hypertension is most common in infants and younger children. Many childhood diseases may be responsible for both acute and chronic elevation of blood pressure (Boxes 437–1 and 437–2). The most likely cause varies with age. Hypertension in the newborn is most often associated with umbilical artery catheterization and renal artery thrombosis. Hypertension during early childhood may be due to renal disease, coarctation of the aorta, endocrine disorders, or medications. In adolescents, essential hypertension becomes increasingly common. The severity of hypertension is also helpful in distinguishing secondary from primary hypertension; in general, children and adolescents with essential hypertension have blood pressure values at or only slightly above the 95th percentile for age.

Renal and renovascular hypertension accounts for the majority of children with secondary hypertension. A history of urinary tract infection is present in 25–50% of these patients and is often related to an obstructive lesion of the urinary tract. Renovascular hypertension may be associated with sodium retention and increased renin secretion. Other renal parenchymal lesions associated with hypertension are detailed in Boxes 437–1 and 437–2. The reduced glomerular filtration rate in patients with nephritis results in salt and water retention, whereas mass lesions (cysts, solid tumors, hematoma) may impair renal perfusion and stimulate renin production by the juxtaglomerular apparatus. Both Wilms tumor and juxtaglomerular cell tumor (hemangiopericytoma) may secrete renin or other pressors without feedback control.

Lesions such as renal artery stenosis cause hypertension through stimulation of the *renin-angiotensin-aldosterone system*. Renin is a proteolytic enzyme secreted by juxtaglomerular cells that converts angiotensinogen to angiotensin I. Renin secretion is affected by afferent arteriolar perfusion pressure in the kidney, sodium concentration in plasma and tubular urine, sympathetic nervous system activation, and other factors such as prostaglandins, potassium intake, and atrial natriuretic peptides. Angiotensin I possesses little physiologic activity and is rapidly converted to angiotensin II by angiotensin-converting enzyme (ACE). This enzyme is also responsible for the metabolic degradation of vasodilating kinins. Angiotensin II is a potent vasoconstrictor and also stimulates aldosterone secretion, which leads to salt and water retention.

Several *endocrinopathies* are associated with hypertension, usually those involving the thyroid, parathyroid, and adrenal

---

BOX 437–1. Conditions Associated with Transient or Intermittent Hypertension in Children

RENAL
Acute postinfectious glomerulonephritis
Anaphylactoid (Henoch-Schönlein) purpura with nephritis
Hemolytic-uremic syndrome
Acute tubular necrosis
After renal transplantation (immediately and during episodes of rejection)
After blood transfusion in patients with azotemia
Hypervolemia
After surgical procedures on the genitourinary tract
Pyelonephritis
Renal trauma
Leukemic infiltration of the kidney
Obstructive uropathy associated with Crohn disease

DRUGS AND POISONS
Cocaine
Oral contraceptives
Sympathomimetic agents
Amphetamines
Phencyclidine
Corticosteroids and adrenocorticotropic hormone
Cyclosporine or sirolimus treatment post-transplantation
Licorice (glycyrrhizic acid)
Lead, mercury, cadmium, thallium
Antihypertensive withdrawal (clonidine, methyldopa, propranolol)
Vitamin D intoxication

CENTRAL AND AUTONOMIC NERVOUS SYSTEM
Increased intracranial pressure
Guillain-Barré syndrome
Burns
Familial dysautonomia
Stevens-Johnson syndrome
Posterior fossa lesions
Porphyria
Poliomyelitis
Encephalitis

MISCELLANEOUS
Preeclampsia
Fractures of long bones
Hypercalcemia
After coarctation repair
White cell transfusion
Extracorporeal membrane oxygenation
Chronic upper airway obstruction

---

glands. Systemic hypertension and tachycardia are common in hyperthyroidism; however, diastolic pressure is not usually elevated. Hypercalcemia, whether secondary to hyperparathyroidism or other causes, often results in mild elevation in blood pressure because of an increase in vascular tone. Adrenocortical disorders (aldosterone-secreting tumors, congenital adrenal hyperplasia, Cushing syndrome) may produce hypertension in patients with increased mineralocorticoid secretion. **Pheochromocytomas** are catecholamine-secreting tumors that give rise to hypertension because of the cardiac and peripheral vascular effects of epinephrine and norepinephrine. Children with pheochromocytoma usually have sustained rather than intermittent hypertension (see Chapter 574). Pheochromocytoma develops in approximately 5% of patients with neurofibromatosis. Altered sympathetic tone can be responsible for acute or intermittent elevation of blood pressure in children with Guillain-Barré syndrome, poliomyelitis, burns, and Stevens-Johnson syndrome. Sympathetic outflow from the central nervous system is also affected by intracranial lesions.

In adolescents, a number of *drugs of abuse, therapeutic agents*, and *toxins* may cause hypertension. Cocaine may provoke a rapid increase in blood pressure and can result in seizures or intracranial hemorrhage. Phencyclidine causes transient hypertension that may become persistent in chronic abusers. Tobacco

BOX 437–2. Conditions Associated with Chronic Hypertension in Children

RENAL
Chronic pyelonephritis
Chronic glomerulonephritis
Hydronephrosis
Congenital dysplastic kidney
Multicystic kidney
Solitary renal cyst
Vesicoureteral reflux nephropathy
Segmental hypoplasia (Ask-Upmark kidney)
Ureteral obstruction
Renal tumors
Renal trauma
Rejection damage following transplantation
Postirradiation damage
Systemic lupus erythematosus (other connective tissue diseases)

VASCULAR
Coarctation of thoracic or abdominal aorta
Renal artery lesions (stenosis, fibromuscular dysplasia, thrombosis, aneurysm)
Umbilical artery catheterization with thrombus formation
Neurofibromatosis (intrinsic or extrinsic narrowing of vascular lumen)
Renal vein thrombosis
Vasculitis
Arteriovenous shunt
Williams-Beuren syndrome
Moyamoya disease

ENDOCRINE
Hyperthyroidism
Hyperparathyroidism
Congenital adrenal hyperplasia (11 β-hydroxylase and 17-hydroxylase defect)
Cushing syndrome
Primary aldosteronism
Dexamethasone-suppressible hyperaldosteronism
Pheochromocytoma
Other neural crest tumors (neuroblastoma, ganglioneuroblastoma, ganglioneuroma)
Diabetic nephropathy
Liddle syndrome

CENTRAL NERVOUS SYSTEM
Intracranial mass
Hemorrhage
Residual following brain injury
Quadriplegia

ESSENTIAL HYPERTENSION
Low renin
Normal renin
High renin

use may also increase blood pressure. Sympathomimetic agents used as nasal decongestants, appetite suppressants, and stimulants for attention deficit disorder produce peripheral vasoconstriction and varying degrees of cardiac stimulation. Individuals vary in their susceptibility to these effects. Oral contraceptives should be suspected as a cause of hypertension in adolescent girls, although the incidence is low with the use of low-estrogen preparations. Immunosuppressant agents such as cyclosporine and tacrolimus cause hypertension in organ transplant recipients, and the effect is exacerbated by the co-administration of steroids. Blood pressure may be elevated in patients with poisoning by a heavy metal.

Essential hypertension is the most common form of hypertension in adults, and it is recognized more often in adolescents than in younger children. It is often accompanied by a strong family history. The cause of essential hypertension is likely to be multifactorial; however, obesity, genetic alterations in calcium and sodium transport, vascular smooth muscle reactivity, the renin-angiotensin system, and insulin sensitivity have been implicated in this disorder. Normotensive children of hypertensive parents may show abnormal physiologic responses that are similar to those of their parents. When subjected to stress or competitive tasks, the offspring of hypertensive adults, as a group, respond with greater increases in heart rate and blood pressure than do children of normotensive parents. Similarly, some children of hypertensive parents may excrete higher levels of urinary catecholamine metabolites or may respond to sodium loading with greater weight gain and increases in blood pressure than do those without a family history of hypertension. The abnormal responses in children with affected parents tend to be greater in the black population than in white individuals. Erythrocyte sodium transport, the free calcium concentration in platelets and leukocytes, urine kallikrein excretion, and sympathetic nervous system receptors have been investigated as other possible markers for the subsequent development of hypertension.

Categorization of essential hypertension according to the level of plasma renin activity (high, normal, low) has been useful in understanding the pathophysiology and in developing treatment regimens for adults; similar large studies have not been conducted in adolescents with primary hypertension. A large number of adult patients with essential hypertension appear to be especially sensitive to salt intake. The mechanism of salt sensitivity is not clear and may involve the chloride ion rather than sodium. A subgroup of salt-sensitive individuals appear to have impaired ability for urinary excretion of a sodium load. Atrial natriuretic peptides stimulate sodium excretion by the kidneys; their role in maintenance of normal blood pressure and development of hypertension is being investigated.

Tracking of blood pressure is the process by which individuals over time maintain their relative ranking of blood pressure with respect to their peers. Children and young adolescents with blood pressure greater than the 90th percentile for age have a threefold greater likelihood of becoming adults with hypertension than do children with blood pressure at the 50th percentile. Adolescents with essential hypertension may progress from high cardiac output and normal systemic vascular resistance to the adult pattern of normal cardiac output with elevated systemic vascular resistance. Racial differences have been noted: black adults with hypertension have greater elevations in peripheral resistance, whereas hypertensive white adults predominantly show an increase in cardiac output.

Clinical Manifestations. Children and adolescents with essential hypertension are usually asymptomatic; the blood pressure elevation is usually mild and is detected during a routine examination or evaluation before athletic participation. These children may have mild to moderate obesity.

Children with secondary hypertension can have blood pressure elevations ranging from mild to severe. Unless the pressure has been sustained or is rising rapidly, hypertension does not usually produce symptoms. Therefore, clinical manifestations of the underlying disease, such as growth failure in children with chronic renal disease, are the most frequent reasons for detecting the hypertension. With substantial hypertension, however, headache, dizziness, epistaxis, anorexia, visual changes, and seizures may occur. Hypertensive encephalopathy is suggested by the presence of vomiting, temperature elevation, ataxia, stupor, and seizures. Regardless of the cause, end-organ (cardiac and renal) dysfunction occurs in the face of marked hypertension.

Young children and infants with unexplained heart failure or seizures should have their blood pressure measured. Such patients often cannot communicate symptoms such as headache, and their behavior may not be considered abnormal until the complications of hypertension are present. After blood pressure has been lowered, parents of hypertensive infants often comment in retrospect that their child had been increasingly irritable before the hypertension was recognized.

Diagnosis. The diagnosis of essential hypertension is suggested by the patient's age (usually adolescent), level of blood pressure elevation (usually mild), weight (mild to moderate obesity), positive family history, and the paucity of signs and symptoms of underlying disease. It is uncommon to make this diagnosis in children younger than 10 yr. Obesity is associated with essential hypertension, but except for disorders of the adrenal cortex, patients with secondary hypertension are rarely obese. Heredity is also a strong determinant of blood pressure; therefore, an adolescent with mild elevation of pressure and a strong family history of essential hypertension is less likely to have an underlying disease. Adolescents suspected of having essential hypertension require regular measurement of blood pressure to determine the course of the elevation over time. If blood pressure continues to rise over several weeks or months of observation, additional diagnostic studies to eliminate secondary hypertension are indicated.

The diagnosis of secondary hypertension is also suggested by the patient's age (younger), level of blood pressure elevation (varying from mild to extreme), and presence of symptoms. The history may include intermittent febrile illnesses, which might suggest recurring infection of the urinary tract (reflux nephropathy). A family history of renal disease or premature cardiovascular disease should be elicited. Careful measurement of height and weight are important because they are often less than normal in children with chronic disease. Physical examination should determine the presence of flank masses or abdominal bruits. Examination should always include palpation of pulses in all extremities and blood pressure in both arms and one leg to evaluate for possible coarctation of the aorta. Systolic blood pressure in the lower limbs of children should be 10–20 mm Hg higher than that in the upper limbs. Screening tests should include a complete blood count, urinalysis, and determination of serum electrolyte, blood urea nitrogen, serum creatinine, calcium, and uric acid levels. Urine culture should be performed even if the sediment is unremarkable. A lipid panel is indicated if the family history is suggestive or if primary hypertension is suspected. Echocardiography is helpful in assessing the chronicity of the hypertension, which if long-standing, should lead to left ventricular hypertrophy.

Renal imaging is discussed in Chapters 529–533. Renal ultrasonography provides a comparison of kidney size and a view of the anatomy of the collecting system. A radionuclide scan is helpful in distinguishing variation in perfusion or scarring of the two kidneys. Renal Doppler ultrasonography and angiography can demonstrate lesions in the main arteries or in the segmental branches; if angiography is performed, venous blood samples should be collected from both renal veins and the inferior vena cava for assay of plasma renin activity. Doppler ultrasonography may demonstrate abnormal arterial and venous blood flow.

Peripheral plasma renin activity is a useful screening test for both renovascular and renal parenchymal disease. Normal values gradually decrease with age and vary among laboratories. A suppressed value suggests excess mineralocorticoid effect, and an elevated value is associated with renal or renovascular involvement. Urinary catecholamines should be measured as well as plasma and urinary steroids. One approach to an adolescent with hypertension is summarized in Figure 437–1. A pregnancy test may be useful in a sexually active female who is noted to be hypertensive (preeclampsia).

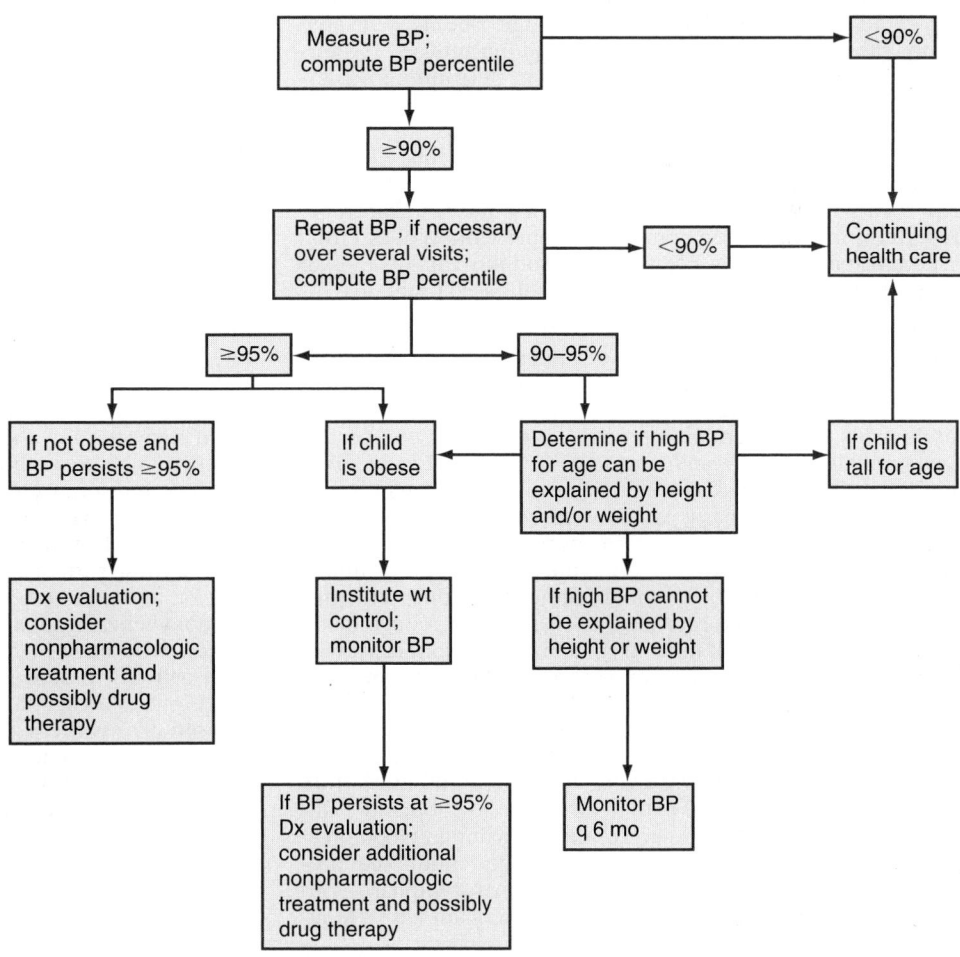

FIGURE 437–1. Algorithm for identifying children with high blood pressure (BP). Note that whenever BP measurement is stipulated, the average of at least two measurements should be used. (From Report of the second task force on blood pressure control in children—1987. Task Force on Blood Pressure Control in children. National Heart, Lung, and Blood Institute, Bethesda, Maryland. *Pediatrics* 1987;79:1. Copyright American Academy of Pediatrics 1987.)

Course and Prognosis. The natural history of essential hypertension that is initially detected during childhood or adolescence is under investigation in several large long-term population studies. Many of these children continue to have essential hypertension as adults, although the correlation is not perfect. In adults with essential hypertension, drug therapy has been shown to be beneficial in reducing the incidence of congestive heart failure, renal failure, and stroke.

The prognosis of a child with secondary hypertension is primarily determined by the nature of the underlying disease and its responsiveness to specific therapy. Survival in patients with underlying chronic renal disease is determined by the patient's response to dialysis and the success of renal transplantation. In patients with renovascular disease, the degree of elevation in renal vein renin activity may help predict response to therapy. A discrepancy in renin secretion between the two kidneys of more than 1.5:1 suggests that the kidney producing the higher level is primarily responsible for the hypertension. In this case, surgical correction yields a high probability of marked improvement or resolution of the hypertension. The prognosis after surgical repair of coarctation of the aorta is variable and partly dependent on the age at which the correction is performed. Most patients operated on during infancy and childhood establish normal systemic blood pressure after surgery unless the coarctation recurs; patients in whom the diagnosis is made during adolescence, however, are at risk for persistently elevated pressure. The long-term outcome is favorable for neonates who experience hypertension as a complication of umbilical artery catheterization. Few of these infants require therapy beyond 12 mo of age, and most show marked improvement in renal perfusion.

Prevention. Prevention of high blood pressure may be viewed as part of the prevention of cardiovascular disease and stroke, the leading cause of death in adults in the United States. Other risk factors for cardiovascular disease include obesity, elevated serum cholesterol levels, high dietary sodium intake, a sedentary lifestyle, and alcohol and tobacco use. Beginning in childhood and continuing through adolescence, it is especially important to discourage cigarette smoking because of the pulmonary and cardiovascular consequences. The increase in arterial wall rigidity and blood viscosity that is associated with exposure to the components of tobacco may cause or exacerbate hypertension. Population approaches to prevention of essential hypertension include a reduction in sodium intake and an increase in physical activity through school-based programs.

Treatment. The goal of therapy for hypertension should be to reduce blood pressure below the 95th percentile for age. Both nonpharmacologic and pharmacologic approaches to treatment are useful in managing children with elevated blood pressure. Adolescents with essential hypertension are usually best managed initially with *nonpharmacologic* therapy. Intervention should focus on the risk factors that were cited as important in prevention. Because many patients with mild elevation of pressure are obese, weight reduction may result in a 5–10 mm Hg reduction in systolic pressure. A reduction in sodium intake often lowers pressure by a similar amount. A consistent program of aerobic exercise has also been noted to reduce blood pressure in patients with mild essential hypertension. In view of these benefits and the undesirable effects of many antihypertensive drugs, a well-supervised program of nonpharmacologic therapy should be enthusiastically prescribed for most young patients with essential hypertension. Adolescents should be counseled about the adverse effects of tobacco and alcohol on blood pressure. When the patient is unable to cooperate with the nonpharmacologic approach or the reduction in blood pressure is insufficient, antihypertensive agents should be prescribed. However, adolescents who are poorly compliant with changes in lifestyle are also unlikely to be compliant with a long-term drug regimen.

For many children with secondary hypertension and for selected patients with essential hypertension, *pharmacologic* therapy is required. A number of antihypertensive drugs are available for both hypertensive emergencies and chronic therapy (Table 437–1). In response to a *hypertensive crisis*, it is important to select an agent with a rapid and predictable onset of action and to monitor blood pressure carefully as it is being reduced. Because hypertensive encephalopathy is a possible complication of hypertensive emergencies, antihypertensive agents with minimal central nervous system side effects should be chosen to avoid confusion between symptoms of disease and adverse effects of the drug. Intravenous administration is often preferred so that the fall in blood pressure can be carefully titrated. Because too rapid a reduction in blood pressure may interfere with adequate organ perfusion, a stepwise reduction in pressure should be planned. In general, the pressure should be reduced by about one third of the total planned reduction during the 1st 6 hr and the remaining amount over the following 48–72 hr.

In most *hypertensive emergencies*, the drugs of choice are intravenous labetalol or nitroprusside or sublingual nifedipine. Labetalol blocks both α- and β-adrenergic receptors; with a single dose followed by continuous infusion, controlled reduction of blood pressure can be achieved. Similar control is possible with an infusion of nitroprusside. Nifedipine has a rapid onset of action, but its short duration of action must be anticipated. Because nifedipine is available only as a liquid within a capsule, administration to younger children has presented some difficulty. Although the drug has often been placed in the sublingual space to achieve rapid absorption, gastrointestinal absorption is also sufficiently rapid to be effective in a hypertensive crisis. Intravenous hydralazine and diazoxide, when given at intervals, are alternative agents for the management of acute hypertensive crises, but such an approach may not provide the desired gradual reduction in blood pressure. Most children with hypertensive crisis have chronic or acute renal disease; in these patients, management of blood pressure also requires careful attention to fluid balance, as well as diuresis. Intravenous furosemide is usually effective, even though glomerular filtration may be impaired.

In selecting a drug regimen for *long-term use*, an understanding of the underlying pathophysiology is helpful. Drugs with different sites and mechanisms of action are available so that therapy can be tailored to the specific pathologic condition. For example, excessive activity of the renin-angiotensin-aldosterone system may be treated effectively with a β-blocking drug (e.g., propranolol) for suppression of renin secretion, an ACE inhibitor (e.g., captopril), or rarely, an aldosterone antagonist (e.g., spironolactone). ACE inhibitors are useful, not only in patients with high-renin hypertension that is secondary to renovascular or renal parenchymal disease but also in patients with high-renin essential hypertension. Excess angiotensin production is the probable cause of most hypertension in neonates after partial occlusion of a renal vessel by thrombus. Captopril is an effective agent in most of these patients, but it must be used with careful attention to renal function. α-Adrenergic blocking agents (phentolamine, phenoxybenzamine) are beneficial in patients with neural crest tumors who have high circulating levels of catecholamines. In such patients, β-blocking drugs are also needed to control the heart rate, or an agent with dual blocking action (labetalol) may be used. Sympathetic blockade with labetalol is likewise efficacious in patients who experience marked stimulation of the cardiovascular system from high doses of cocaine.

Young patients with essential hypertension who require drug therapy may be treated initially with a diuretic or a β-blocking agent. Patients with volume-dependent hypertension usually have an adequate response to diuretics; those with high-renin, high cardiac output physiology respond best to β blockers. If the pressure is not lowered adequately, a calcium channel blocker

TABLE 437–1. Antihypertensive Drugs

Drug	Mechanism of Action	Dosage Range	Route	Duration	Side Effects
Arterial Vasodilators					
Hydralazine	Relax arteriolar smooth muscle	0.1–0.4 mg/kg/dose 0.25–1 mg/kg/dose and increase to max of 200 mg/24 hr	IV PO	2–4 hr 6–8 hr	Tachycardia, nausea Drug-induced lupus
Diazoxide	Relax smooth muscle	1–3 mg/kg/dose, max of 150 mg	IV	6–24 hr	Tachycardia, hypotension, hyperglycemia
Nitroprusside	Dilatation of arterioles and venules	0.5–8.0 μg/kg/min	IV	With infusion	Thiocyanate production, rarely hypothyroidism
Minoxidil	Arteriolar dilatation	0.1–0.2 mg/kg/24 hr, max of 50 mg/24 hr	PO	12–24 hr	Hypertrichosis, fluid retention
Adrenergic Blockers					
Phentolamine	α-Receptor blockade	0.05–0.1 mg/kg/dose, max of 5 mg	IV	1–2 hr	Reflex tachycardia
Phenoxybenzamine	α-Receptor blockade	0.2–1.2 mg/kg/24 hr, max single dose of 10 mg	PO	6–12 hr	Tachycardia may progress to arrhythmia
Prazosin	α-Receptor blockade	0.005–0.1 mg/kg/dose	PO	6–12 hr	First dose, orthostatic hypotension
Propranolol	β-Receptor blockade	0.01–0.1 mg/kg/dose	IV slow push	6–8 hr	Bronchospasm, bradycardia, vivid dreams
	Reduces renin release	0.5–6.0 mg/kg/24 hr, max of 16 mg/kg/24 hr or 60 mg/24 hr	PO		
Labetalol	α and β blockade	0.2–1.0 mg/kg/dose, max of 20 mg dose 0.25–2.0 mg/kg/hr 1–3 mg/kg/24 hr	IV bolus IV continuous PO	With infusion 6–12 hr	Orthostasis, dizziness, bronchospasm
Clonidine	CNS α₂-agonist	0.005–0.025 mg/kg/24 hr initially, max of 0.9 mg/24 hr	PO	6–12 hr	Sedation, constipation, rebound withdrawal, hypertension
Renin-Angiotensin Inhibitors					
Captopril	ACE inhibition	Neonates <2 mo: 0.05–0.1 mg/kg/dose up to 0.5 mg/kg/dose	PO	6–24 hr	Proteinuria, neutropenia, rash, dysgeusia, chronic cough
		Infants and children: 0.15–0.5 mg/kg/dose up to 6 mg/kg/24 hr	PO	8–12 hr	
		Older children and adolescents: 6.25–12.5 mg/dose up to 450 mg/24 hr	PO	8–12 hr	
Enalaprilat	ACE inhibition	Children: 0.005–0.010 mg/kg/dose Adults: 0.625–1.25 mg/dose	IV over 5 min	8–24 hr	Transient hypotension
Enalapril	ACE inhibition	Children: 0.2–1 mg/kg/24 hr Adolescents: 2.5–5 mg/24 hr up to 40 mg/24 hr	PO	12–24 hr	Hypotension
Calcium Channel Blockers					
Nifedipine	Calcium channel blocker	Children: 0.25–0.5 mg/kg/dose, max of 10 mg/dose and 1–2 mg/kg/24 hr Adolescents: 10–30 mg (capsules) 30–120 mg qd (sustained release)	PO, SL PO PO	Repeat q 4–6h 6–8 hr 24 hr	Facial flushing, tachycardia
Diuretic Agents					
Hydrochlorothiazide	Diuresis	1–2 mg/kg/24 hr, max of 100 mg/24 hr	PO	12–24 hr	Hypokalemia, hyperuricemia, hypercalcemia
Furosemide	Diuresis	1 mg/kg/dose 1–2 mg/kg/dose up to 6 mg/kg/24 hr	IV PO	4–6 hr 6–12 hr	Hypokalemia, alkalosis
Bumetanide	Diuresis	0.015–0.1 mg/kg/dose, max of 10 mg/24 hr	PO	6–24 hr	Hypokalemia, hyperglycemia, hyperuricemia

Note: Pediatric doses based on weight should not exceed adult doses. Because recommendations may change, these doses should always be double-checked. Doses may also need to be modified in any patient with renal or hepatic dysfunction.

ACE = angiotensin = converting enzyme; SL = sublingual.

may be added to the diuretic, and an ACE inhibitor may replace the β blocker. Chronic use of diuretics may result in elevation of serum lipids, which may increase the risk of ischemic heart disease in adults with hypertension. Long-term investigations of this side effect in children are not available. β-Blocking agents have also been associated with changes in serum lipids, and some studies suggest a mild reduction in exercise tolerance in patients treated with propranolol. Patients with reactive airway disease are not able to tolerate a β-blocking agent.

Because of these side effects, ACE inhibitors and calcium channel blockers may be considered for initial therapy in an adolescent with significant hypertension. Although captopril has been used more often in the pediatric and adolescent populations, newer ACE inhibitors such as enalapril have a longer duration of action and require less frequent administration.

In patients with long-standing or poorly controlled hypertension, the underlying pathophysiology is often complex. Such patients frequently require trials of combinations of antihypertensive agents to gain control of markedly elevated or labile pressure. The basic principle of combination antihypertensive therapy is the co-administration of drugs with different sites or mechanisms of action. Because compliance may become a problem, the drug regimen should be as simple as possible and should take advantage of longer acting agents that can be administered once or twice daily, when available. Drug calendars, parental supervision, and close patient-physician communication also help ensure compliance.

In patients with renal artery stenosis secondary to fibromuscular dysplasia, percutaneous balloon angioplasty may cure as many as 50%. Angioplasty is not successful for renal artery stenosis because of atherosclerotic plaques. If angioplasty is unsuccessful, placement of an intravascular stent or surgery may be indicated.

Athletic participation by children and adolescents who have systemic hypertension. American Academy of Pediatrics Committee on Sports Medicine and Fitness. *Pediatrics* 1997;99:637.

Bartosh SM, Aronson AJ: Childhood hypertension. An update on etiology, diagnosis, and treatment. *Pediatr Clin North Am* 1999;46:235–52.

Blaszak RT, Savage JA, Ellis EN: The use of short-acting nifedipine in pediatric patients with hypertension. *J Pediatr* 2001;139:34–7.

Choi Y, Kang BC, Kim KJ, et al: Renovascular hypertension in children with moyamoya disease. *J Pediatr* 1997;131:258.

Drugs for hypertension. *Med Lett* 2001;43:17–22.

Egger DW, Deming DD, Hamada N, et al: Evaluation of the safety of short-acting nifedipine in children with hypertension. *Pediart Nephrol* 2002;17:35–40.

Flynn JT: What's new in pediatric hypertension? *Curr Hypertens Rep* 2001;3:503–10.

Flynn JT, Pasko DA: Calcium channel blockers: Pharmacology and place in therapy of pediatric hypertension. *Pediatr Nephrol* 2000;15:302–16.

Harshfield GA, Alpert BS, Pullman DA, et al: Ambulatory blood pressure readings in children and adults. *Pediatrics* 1994;94:180.

Kay JD, Sinaiko AR, Daniels SR: Pediatric hypertension. *Am Heart J* 2001;142:422–32.

Sinaiko AR: Hypertension in children. *N Engl J Med* 1996;335:1968.

Tyagi S, Kaul UA, Satsangi DK, et al: Percutaneous transluminal angioplasty for renovascular hypertension in children: Initial and long-term results. *Pediatrics* 1997;99:44.

Update on the 1987 task force report on high blood pressure in children and adolescents: A working group report from the National High Blood Pressure Education Program. National High Blood Pressure Education Program Working Group on Hypertension Control in Children and Adolescents. *Pediatrics* 1996;98:649.

Weir MR: Impact of age, race, and obesity on hypertensive mechanisms and therapy. *Am J Med* 1991;90(Suppl):3.

Wolfish NM, Delbrouck NF, Shanon A, et al: Prevalence of hypertension in children with primary vesicoureteral reflux. *J Pediatr* 1993;123:559.

Diseases of the Blood

SECTION 1 *The Hematopoietic System*

Chapter 438

Development of the Hematopoietic System

Robin K. Ohls and Robert D. Christensen

Hematopoietic regulation in the human fetus differs markedly from that in the adult. In the adult, homeostatic maintenance is a prime function of hematopoietic regulation, whereas in the embryo and fetus, constant changes characterize all phases of hematopoiesis. During developmental erythropoiesis, the constant growth of the fetus and the resultant need to increase the red cell mass necessitates an extraordinary erythropoietic effort. In addition, the relatively low oxygen tensions but high metabolic rates of fetal tissues demand a system of oxygen delivery unique from that present in adults. During developmental granulopoiesis, the sterile intra-amniotic environment results in a low demand for neutrophils and obviates the need for maintenance of a large neutrophil reserve. Knowledge of developmental hematopoietic regulation aids the clinician in interpretation of postnatal hematologic data and results in greater appreciation for the erythropoietic and granulocytopoietic capacities and limitations of prematurely delivered neonates.

Developmental hematopoiesis occurs in three anatomic stages: mesoblastic, hepatic, and myeloid. Mesoblastic hematopoiesis occurs in extraembryonic structures, principally in the yolk sac, and begins between the 10th and 14th days of gestation. By 6–8 wk of gestation the liver replaces the yolk sac as the primary site of blood cell production, and by 10–12 wk extraembryonic hematopoiesis has essentially ceased. Hematopoiesis occurs in the liver throughout the remainder of gestation, although production begins to diminish during the second trimester as bone marrow hematopoiesis increases. The liver, however, remains the predominant hematopoietic organ through weeks 20–24 of gestation.

Each hematopoietic organ houses distinct hematopoietic populations. For example, at 18–20 wk of gestation over 85% of the cells in the fetal liver are erythroid and virtually no neutrophils are present. In contrast, at this same time, less than 40% of the cells within the bone marrow are erythroid and up to 15% are neutrophils. Moreover, the subpopulations of leukocytes present in the liver and marrow differ with gestation. Macrophages precede the presence of granulocytes in both the liver and marrow, and the ratio of macrophages to granulocytes decreases with increasing gestation. Thus, not only does the anatomic site of hematopoiesis change during gestation, but the populations of cells generated at those sites are also distinct. The mechanisms responsible for the changing anatomic sites of hematopoiesis and for the differences in blood cells produced in the yolk sac, liver, and marrow have not been determined. Regardless of gestational age or anatomic location, production of all

hematopoietic tissues begins with pluripotent stem cells that are capable of both self-renewal and of clonal maturation into all blood cell lineages. Progenitor cells differentiate under the influence of hematopoietic growth factors (Table 438–1) produced by the fetus.

Erythroid and granulocytic blood cell indices change during gestation and continue to change through the first year of life. Circulating erythrocyte and granulocyte concentrations gradually increase during the second and third trimesters (Table 438–2). In parallel with increasing erythrocyte concentrations, hematocrits increase from 30–40% during the second trimester and continue to increase to term values over the latter part of the third trimester. Term hematocrits range from 50–63% (with variability due to delayed clamping of the umbilical cord and the sampling site). Unlike the blood concentrations of erythrocytes and neutrophils, platelet concentrations remain constant from 18 wk of gestation through term, with a range of 150,000–450,000/μL.

Mean cell volumes generally are inversely proportional to gestation and to the life span of the cell. The mean cell volume (MCV) of erythrocytes is more than 180 fL in the embryo, falls to around 130 by mid gestation, then decreases to 115 fL by 40 wk of gestation (see Table 438–2). Mean platelet volumes (MPV) range from 10–12 fL at birth and can sometimes be helpful in determining whether diminished platelet counts are primarily caused by decreased production (small MPV) or increased destruction (normal to large MPV).

Granulocytopoiesis. The process whereby hematopoiesis moves from the yolk sac to the liver to the marrow is not a simple transfer in location, because the type of cells produced at each anatomic site is unique. For instance, the human yolk sac does not engage in neutrophil production. Also, the human fetal liver produces few, if any, neutrophils. Those few neutrophils seen in human fetal liver are not arranged in hematopoietic islands like the developing hepatic erythroblasts but are widely separated, generally near vessels, suggesting they were made elsewhere and carried to the liver by the circulation. Similarly, no neutrophil production occurs in the human fetal spleen. The neutrophils seen within the spleen are mostly mature and evenly dispersed, suggesting that, like the neutrophils in the fetal liver, they were produced elsewhere and carried to that site by the circulation.

Neutrophils are first observed in the human fetus about 5 wk post conception as small clusters of cells around the aorta. These cells contain myeloperoxidase, and they mature into cells with segmented nuclei, but other similarities between them and the neutrophils of adults have not been reported. The fetal bone marrow space begins to develop around the eighth week post conception. From 8–10 wk the bone marrow space enlarges, but no neutrophils are apparent in this space until 10.5 wk. These first marrow neutrophils have round nuclei, contain myeloperoxidase, and express cell surface characteristics of myeloblasts and promyelocytes. From 14 wk through term the

TABLE 438–1. Characteristics of Hematopoietic Growth Factors

Growth Factors	Molecular Mass (kd)	Chromosomal Location	Principal Target Cell
Erythropoietin	30–39	7q11-22	CFU-E, fetal BFU-E
Colony-Stimulating Factors			
G-CSF	18–22	17q11.2-21	CFU-G, CFU-MIX, mature neutrophil
GM-CSF	18–30	5q23-31	CFU-MIX, CFU-GM, BFU-E, monocyte, mature neutrophil
M-CSF	45–70 Dimer of 2 subunits	5q33.1	CFU-M, macrophage
SCF	36	12	CFU-MIX, BFU-E, CFU-GM, mast cell
Interleukins			
IL-1	17	Alpha 2q13 Beta 2q13-21	Hepatocyte, macrophage, lymphocyte
IL-2	15–20	4q26-27	T cell, cytotoxic lymphocyte
IL-3	14–30	5q23-31	CFU-MIX, CFU-Meg, CFU-GM, BFU-E, macrophage
IL-4	16–20	5q23-31	T cell, B cell
IL-5	46 Dimer of 2 subunits	5q23-31	CFU-Eo, B cell
IL-6	19–26	7p21-24	CFU-MIX, CFU-GM, BFU-E, monocyte, B cell, T cell, cytotoxic lymphocyte
IL-7	35	8q12-13	B cell
IL-8	8–10	4	Neutrophil, endothelial cell, T cell
IL-9	16	5q31-32	BFU-E, CFU-MIX
IL-10	18.7	1	Macrophage, lymphocyte
IL-11	23	19q13	CFU-Meg, B cell, keratinocyte
IL-12	70-75 Dimer of subunits p35/p40	3 (p35) and 11 (p40)	T cells, NK cells, macrophages
IL-13	9	5q23-31	Pre-B lymphocyte, macrophage
IL-14	53	5q31	B cells
IL-15	14–15	4q25-35	B cells, T cells
IL-16	12–14		T cell
IL-17	20–30	2q31	Marrow stromal cells
IL-18	24	9p13	CD4+ T cells, NK cells
IL-21			T cells
IL-23	Dimer of subunits p19/IL-12p40		CD4+ T cells
Thrombopoietin	35–38	3q27-28	Megakaryocyte progenitor, megakaryocyte

G-CSF = granulocyte colony-stimulating factor; GM-CSF = granulocyte-macrophage colony-stimulating factor; M-CSF = macrophage colony-stimulating factor; SCF = stem cell factor.

TABLE 438–2. Blood Cell Indices During Gestation and at Birth

Week of Gestation	Total WBC Counts* ($\times 10^9$/L)	Corrected WBC Counts ($\times 10^9$/L)	Platelets ($\times 10^9$/L)	RBC ($\times 10^9$/L)	Hb (g/dL)	Hct (%)	MCV (fL)
18–21 (n = 760)	4.68 ± 2.96	2.57 ± 0.42	234 ± 57	2.85 ± 0.36	11.69 ± 1.27	37.3 ± 4.3	131.1 ± 11.0
22–25 (n = 1,200)	4.72 ± 2.84	3.73 ± 2.17	247 ± 59	3.09 ± 0.34	12.2 ± 1.6	38.6 ± 3.9	125.1 ± 7.8
26–29 (n = 460)	5.16 ± 2.53	4.08 ± 0.84	242 ± 69	3.46 ± 0.41	12.91 ± 1.38	40.9 ± 4.4	118.5 ± 8.0
> 30 (n = 440)	7.71 ± 4.99	6.40 ± 2.99	232 ± 87	3.82 ± 0.64	13.64 ± 2.21	43.6 ± 7.2	114.4 ± 9.3
Term		18.1 (9.0–30.0)	290 ± 100	4.70 ± 0.40	16.5 ± 1.5	51.0 ± 4.5	108 ± 5.0

*Including normoblasts.
RBC = red blood cells; Hb = hemoglobin; Hct = hematocrit.
Adapted from Forester F, Daffos F, Catherine N, et al: Developmental hematopoiesis in normal human fetal blood. Blood 1991; 77:2361.

most common cell type found in the fetal bone marrow space is the neutrophil.

In children and adults neutrophils and macrophages originate from a common progenitor cell. It is not clear whether this is the case in the fetus, because neutrophils and macrophages appear at different times and in different anatomic locations. Macrophages first appear in the yolk sac, liver, lung, and brain, before the bone marrow cavity is formed.

The mechanisms regulating fetal granulocyte production have not been well defined. Granulocyte colony-stimulating factor (G-CSF) and macrophage colony-stimulating factor (M-CSF) are likely to be involved, as they are in adults, because both are expressed in the developing fetal bone as early as 6 wk post conception and both are expressed in the fetal liver as early as 8 wk. Granulocyte-macrophage colony-stimulating factor (GM-CSF) and stem cell factor (SCF) are also distributed widely in human fetal tissues. However, no changes in mRNA expression of any of these factors, or of their specific receptors, or in

the concentrations of proteins (as judged by immunohistochemical staining) appear to be the signal for fetal production of neutrophils or macrophages. The precise signals have not yet been identified.

Few neutrophils are found in the circulation until the third trimester. Forester and Daffos observed a mean circulating neutrophil count of 190/mm^3 (range, 0–490/mm^3, mode concentration of zero) in fetuses of 20 wk gestation. Although mature neutrophils are scarce, progenitor cells, with the capacity to generate neutrophil clones, are relatively abundant in fetal blood. When these fetal progenitor cells are cultured in vitro in the presence of recombinant G-CSF they undergo maturation into large colonies of neutrophils. The physiologic role of G-CSF includes upregulation of neutrophil production, and this appears to be the case for the fetus and neonate as well as for adults. Thus, the low quantities of circulating and storage neutrophils in the mid-trimester human fetus may be due in part to low production of G-CSF. Monocytes isolated from the blood of adults produce G-CSF when stimulated with a variety of inflammatory mediators such as bacterial lipopolysaccharide (LPS) or interleukin-1 (IL-1). In contrast, monocytes isolated from the umbilical cord blood of preterm infants, and from the liver and bone marrow of aborted fetuses up to 24 wk gestation, generate only small quantities (10–100 times less per cell) of G-CSF protein and mRNA after LPS or IL-1 stimulation. Despite this low capacity to generate G-CSF, G-CSF receptors on the surface of neutrophils of newborn infants are equal in number and affinity to those on adult neutrophils.

In the fetus, the actions of G-CSF, M-CSF, GM-CSF, and SCF are not limited to hematopoiesis. Receptors for each of these factors are located in distinct areas of the fetal central nervous system and gastrointestinal tract, where their patterns of expression change with development. Important developmental roles exist for these factors beyond those known for hematopoiesis.

Thrombopoiesis. The marrow megakaryocyte compartment can be conceptualized as consisting of two pools of cells: *megakaryocyte progenitors* and *megakaryocytes*. The megakaryocyte progenitor pool can be identified by two methods: a culture system, in which the progenitors are identified by their ability to form colonies of megakaryocytes, and immunologic staining methods, which allow characterization on the basis of the specific antigens. Megakaryocytes are identified by their morphologic characteristics, as they undergo endoreduplication that results in large cells with polyploid nuclei.

Megakaryocyte progenitors can be subcategorized into two populations: burst-forming unit-megakaryocytes (BFU-MK), which are primitive megakaryocyte progenitors, and colony-forming unit-megakaryocytes (CFU-MK), which are more differentiated cells. BFU-MK produce large multifocal colonies containing 50 or more megakaryocytes, whereas CFU-MK generate smaller (3–50 cells/colony) unifocal colonies. BFU-MK express CD34 but not HLA-DR, whereas CFU-MK express CD34 and HLA-DR. The colonies generated by BFU-MK of fetal origin contain significantly more megakaryocytes than do those of adult origin and on that basis are thought to represent somewhat more primitive cells.

Megakaryocytes, unlike megakaryocyte progenitors, do not have the capacity to generate clones. Rather, they undergo maturation, progressing from small mononuclear cells to large polyploid cells. The modal megakaryocyte ploidy in normal adult marrow is 16N. In the fetus and neonate, modal ploidy is lower and megakaryocyte size is smaller. However, umbilical cord blood has a higher concentration of megakaryocytes than does adult blood. Large megakaryocytes generate more platelets than do small megakaryocytes; thus, it is assumed that megakaryocytes of neonates produce fewer platelets than do their adult counterparts.

The processes of platelet production and release from megakaryocytes are not well understood. It has been speculated that small buds, proplatelets, are formed on marrow megakaryocytes and that these are released from the marrow as platelets. An alternate possibility is that platelets are principally released from megakaryocytes in the lungs, as a consequence of shear forces. That theory is supported by the observation that megakaryocytes are abundant in the lungs.

Thrombopoietin (TPO) is the physiologic regulator of platelet production and acts as a potent stimulator of all stages of megakaryocyte growth and development. The gene that encodes TPO is located on the long arm of human chromosome 3, and TPO-mRNA is expressed primarily in liver and kidney and, to a lesser extent, in bone marrow stroma. TPO is a primary, but not exclusive, regulator of platelet production. TPO also stimulates the proliferation and survival of not only megakaryotic progenitors but also erythroid, myeloid, and multipotential progenitors. Phase I/II human trials have demonstrated that rTPO acts as a stimulator of platelet production in nonthrombocytopenic adults and in patients with chemotherapy-induced thrombocytopenia. Recombinant TPO clearly supports the growth of megakaryocytic colonies of neonates and children. Progenitors of preterm neonates are more sensitive to rTPO than are progenitors of term neonates. However, nothing is known about the benefits and risks of rTPO administration in neonates and children.

Erythropoiesis. Erythropoiesis in utero is controlled by erythroid growth factors produced solely by the fetus. Erythropoietin (EPO) does not cross the placenta in humans; therefore, stimulation of maternal EPO production does not result in stimulation of fetal red cell production. Moreover, suppression of maternal erythropoiesis by hypertransfusion does not suppress fetal erythropoiesis.

It is unclear whether the same mechanism of erythropoietic regulation defining adult erythropoiesis exists in the fetus or in the infant born prematurely. The production of red blood cells is governed by a variety of growth factors produced by a variety of accessory cells such as macrophages, lymphocytes, and stromal cells. These cells and cell products make up the erythropoietic microenvironment and stimulate maturation, growth, and differentiation at various stages of red blood cell production. Of all the factors stimulating erythropoiesis, none plays a more important regulatory role than EPO. EPO is a 30–39 kd glycoprotein that binds to specific receptors on the surface of erythroid precursors and stimulates their differentiation and clonal maturation into mature erythrocytes. The regulation of EPO gene expression involves an oxygen-sensing mechanism, and both hypoxia and anemia stimulate erythropoiesis by stimulating mRNA transcription and EPO production. EPO mRNA production is regulated by *cis*-acting elements in the promoter and 3' enhancer regions that are responsive to hypoxia. Two factors, hepatic nuclear factor 4 (HNF-4) and hypoxic inducible factor (HIF-1), exhibit transcriptional activation for EPO and other hypoxia-inducible genes. HNF-4 has been shown to bind specifically to the EPO promoter and enhancer regions of the gene and is expressed in kidney, liver, and Hep3B cells. HIF-1 is a basic helix-loop-helix transcription factor composed of HIF-1α and HIF-1β subunits that bind to *cis*-acting hypoxia-response elements and induce EPO transcription. HIF-1 is expressed in many cells and is involved in upregulation of a variety of hypoxically regulated proteins. HIF-1α appears to be constitutively expressed and rapidly degraded under normoxic conditions. HIF-1 regulation occurs through DNA binding and protein stabilization. RNA stability may be dependent on the ubiquitin proteasome degradation system; inhibition of this system leads to increased HIF-1 and increased EPO, even under normoxic conditions. In mouse models exposed to hypoxia, HIF-1α mRNA concentrations do not change significantly. It is unknown whether HIF-1α operates in the same fashion in the fetus. Moreover, the development of these transcription activating factors in the fetus and premature infant remains to be determined. There is some evidence that HIF-1 is present to varying degrees during fetal development.

The fetal liver produces EPO during the first and second trimesters, principally by cells of monocyte/macrophage origin. At some time during the third trimester and the first few weeks of life, the anatomic site of EPO production shifts from the liver to the kidney. The specific stimulus for the shift of EPO production from liver to kidney is unknown but might involve the significant changes in arterial oxygen tension that occur at birth. In animal models, the sensitivity of the hepatic hypoxia-sensing mechanism appears decreased compared with renal sensitivity. The liver also appears to require more prolonged hypoxia to achieve an EPO response. Although EPO mRNA and protein can be found in the human fetal kidney, it is not known whether this production is biologically relevant. However, it appears that renal production of EPO is not essential for normal fetal erythropoiesis, as evidenced by the normal serum EPO concentrations and normal hematocrits of anephric fetuses.

Studies of bone marrow cells in tissue culture have added to our understanding of how erythroid precursors respond to growth factors. When bone marrow cells are placed in semi-solid media culture systems for 5–7 days, the EPO-sensitive precursors, termed colony-forming units–erythroid (CFU-E) clonally mature into clusters containing 30–100 normoblasts. Erythroid-specific progenitors that are less well differentiated than CFU-E, hence more primitive cells, are termed burst-forming units–erythroid (BFU-E). Twelve to 14 days after these cells are placed in culture, BFU-E develop into large clusters of normoblasts, each containing 200–10,000 cells. BFU-E from human fetuses respond in a slightly different fashion than BFU-E isolated from adults. Specifically, BFU-E of fetal origin generally develop into erythroid clones more rapidly and generally develop substantially more normoblasts than do BFU-E of adult origin. Moreover, BFU-E from adult bone marrow require a combination of EPO plus another factor such as IL-3 or GM-CSF to clonally mature, whereas many fetal BFU-E mature in the presence of EPO alone.

Hemoglobin. The combustion essential to life requires that tissues receive a constant supply of oxygen. The evolutionary development of oxygen-carrying proteins, the hemoglobins, increased the ability of blood to transport oxygen. Furthermore, the combination of oxygen with hemoglobin and its dissociation from it are accomplished without expenditure of metabolic energy.

Hemoglobin is a complex protein consisting of iron-containing heme groups and the protein moiety globin. A dynamic interaction between heme and globin gives hemoglobin its unique properties in the reversible transport of oxygen. The hemoglobin molecule is a tetramer made up of two pairs of polypeptide chains, each chain having a heme group attached. The polypeptide chains of various hemoglobins are of chemically different types. The major hemoglobin of a normal adult (Hb A) is made up of one pair of alpha (α) and one pair of beta (β) polypeptide chains and represented as $\alpha_2\beta_2$. The major hemoglobin in the fetus (Hb F) is represented by $\alpha_2\gamma_2$.

The various globin chains differ in both the number and sequence of amino acids, and their synthesis is directed by separate genes (Fig. 438–1). Two sets of genes for the α chains are located on human chromosome 16. Two pairs of alleles provide the genetic information for the structure of the α chain. β, γ, δ genes are closely linked on chromosome 11.

Within the RBCs of an embryo, fetus, child, and adult, six different hemoglobins may normally be detected: the embryonic hemoglobins, Gower-1, Gower-2, and Portland; the fetal hemoglobin, Hb F; and the adult hemoglobins, Hb A and Hb A_2. The electrophoretic mobilities of hemoglobins vary with their chemical structures. The time of appearance and quantitative relationships among the hemoglobins are determined by complex developmental processes (Fig. 438–2).

Embryonic Hemoglobins. The blood of early human embryos contains two slowly migrating hemoglobins, Gower-1 and Gower-2, and Hb Portland, which has Hb F–like mobility. The zeta (ζ) chains of Hb Portland and Gower-1 are structurally quite similar to α chains. Both Gower hemoglobins contain a unique type of polypeptide chain, the epsilon (ϵ) chain. Hb Gower-1 has the structure $\zeta_2\epsilon_2$, and Gower-2, $\alpha_2\epsilon_2$. Hb Portland has the structure $\zeta_2\gamma_2$. In embryos of 4–8 wk gestation, the Gower hemoglobins predominate, but by the 3rd mo they have disappeared.

Fetal Hemoglobin. Hb F contains γ polypeptide chains in place of the β chains of Hb A. Its resistance to denaturation by strong alkali is the basis for determining the presence of fetal RBCs in the maternal circulation (the Kleihauer-Betke test). After the

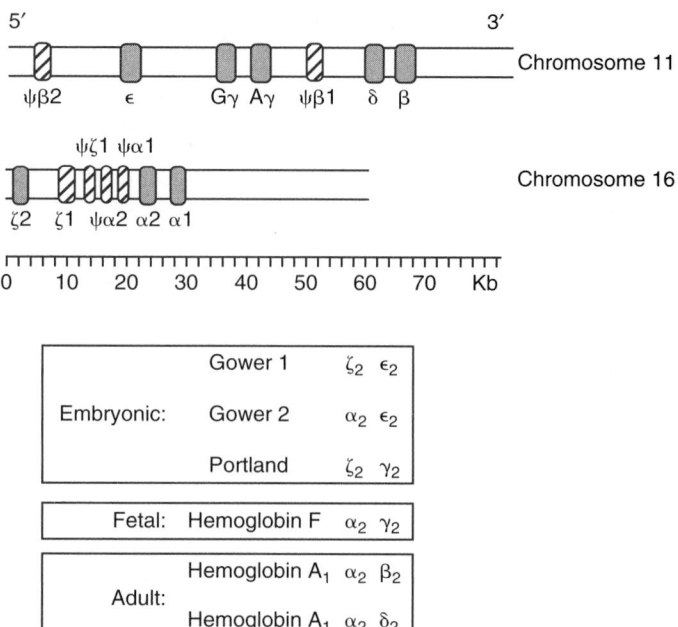

FIGURE 438–1. Organization of the globin genes. The bottom line reflects the scale in kilobases. Transcription of mRNA takes place from the 5′ to the 3′ end. The upper segment represents the beta-like globin genes on chromosome 11, and the lower segment the alpha-like genes on chromosome 16. Regions of the gene that code for primary globin proteins are shown as shaded segments, and regions that code for pseudogenes ("ψ," nonexpressed remnants) are shown as hatched segments. The composition of embryonic, fetal, and adult hemoglobins is listed. α = alpha; β = beta; γ = gamma; δ = delta; ϵ = epsilon; ζ = zeta.

8th gestational wk, Hb F is the predominant hemoglobin; at 24 wk gestation it constitutes 90% of the total hemoglobin. During the 3rd trimester, a gradual decline occurs, so that at birth Hb F averages 70% of the total. Synthesis of Hb F decreases rapidly postnatally, and by 6–12 mo of age only a trace is present. Less than 2.0% can be detected by alkali denaturation in older children and adults. Hb F is heterogeneous because of two types of γ chains, whose synthesis is directed by two sets of genes. The chains differ at position 136 in the presence of either a glycine (Gγ) or an alanine (Aγ) residue. In newborns, the relative proportion or ratio of Gγ to Aγ chain is 3:1.

Adult Hemoglobins. Some Hb A ($\alpha_2\beta_2$) can be detected in even the smallest embryos. Accordingly, it is possible as early as 16–20 wk gestation to make a prenatal diagnosis of major β-chain hemoglobinopathies, such as thalassemia major. Prenatal diagnosis is based on techniques that examine the rates of synthesis of β chains or the structure of newly synthesized β chains. Earlier diagnosis is possible using molecular biology techniques and sampling of chorionic villus tissue or amniotic fluid if DNA structural defects are a cause of the hemoglobinopathies. Similarly, gene deletion disorders such as the α-thalassemias are detectable by the same method.

By the 24th wk of gestation, 5–10% of Hb A is present. A steady increase follows, so that at term, Hb A averages 30%. By 6–12 mo of age, the normal Hb A pattern appears. The minor Hb A component Hb A_2 contains delta (δ) chains and has the structure $\alpha_2\delta_2$. It is seen only when significant amounts of Hb A are also present. At birth, less than 1.0% of Hb A_2 is seen, but by 12 mo of age the normal level of 2.0–3.4% is attained. Throughout life, the normal ratio of Hb A to A_2 is about 30:1.

Normal Relationships Among the Hemoglobins. During fetal life and early childhood, the rates of synthesis of γ and β chains and the

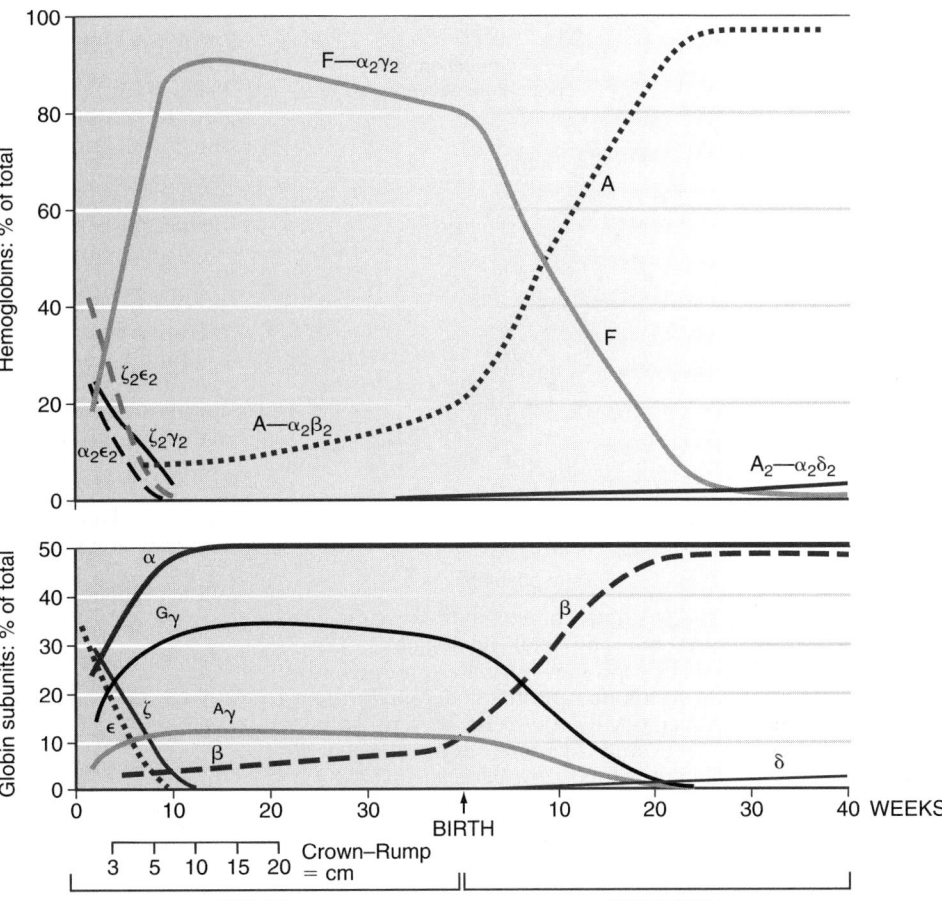

FIGURE 438–2. Changes in hemoglobin tetramers (*top*) and in globin subunits (*bottom*) during human development from embryo to early infancy. (From Polin RA, Fox WW: Fetal and Neonatal Physiology, 2nd ed. Philadelphia, WB Saunders, 1998, p 1769.)

amounts of Hb A and Hb F are inversely related. This relationship has been attributed to a "switch mechanism" similar to genetic regulatory mechanisms in bacteria, but the genetic, biologic, and developmental processes that direct a switchover from predominantly γ-chain synthesis in utero to predominantly β-chain synthesis after birth are unclear. It is not certain whether the mechanisms involve selective genetic inhibition or facilitation. The increase in the α_1/α_2 globin ratio occurring after 36 wk gestation corresponds with a rapid decline in γ-globin synthesis, suggesting that these changes could be regulated by a coordinated molecular mechanism. Differential selection and amplified production of RBC precursors derived from BFU-E result in considerable Hb F production. This may be the basis for the increased levels of Hb F that occur in many hypoproliferative or hemolytic anemias. Alternative explanations involve more basic genetic regulators in the DNA sequences that flank the hemoglobin gene complexes.

Alterations of the Hemoglobins by Disease. Because hemoglobins containing ε chains are normally present only very early in intrauterine life, they are largely of theoretical interest. Small amounts of the Gower hemoglobins have been detectable in a few newborns with 13/15-trisomy. Increased levels of Hb Portland have been found in cord blood of stillborn infants with homozygous α-thalassemia.

Hb F levels may be influenced by various factors. Because the Hb F level is elevated during the 1st year of life, knowledge of its normal decline is important (Fig. 438–3). In persons heterozygous for β-thalassemia (β-thalassemia trait), postpartum decrease of Hb F is retarded; about 50% of such persons have elevated levels of Hb F (>2.0%) in later life. In homozygous thalassemia (Cooley anemia) and in hereditary persistence of Hb F, large amounts of Hb F are characteristically found. In patients with major β-chain hemoglobinopathies (e.g., Hb SS, SC), Hb F is usually increased, particularly during childhood. Preterm infants treated with human recombinant EPO may increase Hb F production during active erythropoiesis. Finally, moderate elevations of Hb F may occur in many diseases accompanied by hematologic stress, such as hemolytic anemias, leukemia, and aplastic anemia, because of a minor population of RBCs that contains increased amounts of Hb F. Tetramers of γ chains (γ_4 or Hb Barts) or β chains (β_4, Hb H) may be found in α-thalassemia syndromes.

The normal adult level of Hb A_2 (2.0–3.4%) is seldom altered. Levels of Hb A_2 exceeding 3.4% are found in most persons with the β-thalassemia trait and in those with megaloblastic anemias secondary to vitamin B_{12} and folic acid deficiency. Decreased HbA_2 levels are found in those with iron-deficiency anemia and α-thalassemia.

Metabolism of the RBC. The nucleated RBCs in bone marrow participate in various metabolic functions, including active protein synthesis. After extrusion of the nucleus, much of this metabolic ability is lost, including the ability to synthesize proteins. Loss of the nucleus makes the RBC a better vessel for oxygen transport, but it imposes on the RBC a finite life span, because the cell cannot replace or repair its vital enzymatic proteins. Mature RBCs contain more than 40 enzymes. Many of these are essential for cellular viability, but genetically determined deficiencies of others, such as catalase, do not interfere with normal survival.

Mature RBCs are not metabolically inert. They have no mitochondria, however, and adenosine triphosphate (ATP) generation cannot occur by oxidative phosphorylation in Krebs' cycle reactions. Rather, glucose is taken up and lactic acid produced mostly by anaerobic glycolysis (Embden-Meyerhof pathway);

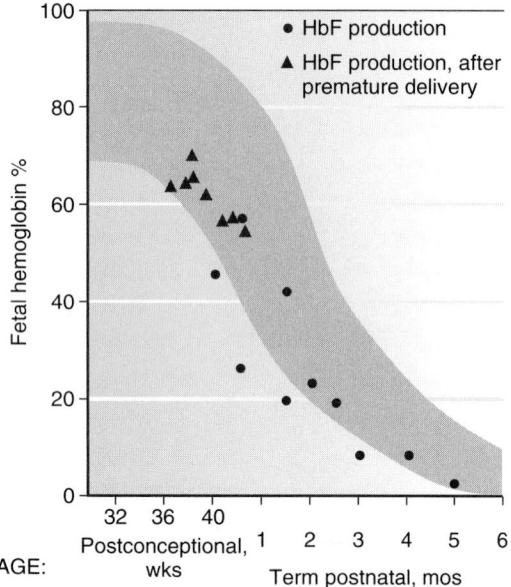

FIGURE 438–3. Pre- and postnatal changes in the percentage of total hemoglobin represented by fetal hemoglobin (Hb F) *(shaded area)*. The triangles represent postnatal production by reticulocytes in premature infants, and the dots represent cord blood and postnatal reticulocyte production in term infants. (From Brown MS: Fetal and neonatal erythropoiesis. In Stockman JA, Pochedly C [editors]: *Developmental and Neonatal Hematology.* New York, Raven Press, 1988.)

about 10% of glucose is metabolized oxidatively through the pentose phosphate pathway. At least five functions for ATP generated by glucose metabolism are essential to normal cell viability:

1. Maintenance of electrolyte gradients. The principal intracellular cation of RBCs is potassium, whereas that in plasma is sodium. Reversal of the constant tendency for sodium to enter the RBCs and concomitantly for potassium to leak out, with preservation of normal ionic gradients, is accomplished by an energy (ATP)-dependent membrane mechanism, the cation pump. When the cation pump fails, sodium and water enter the RBCs, causing them to swell and ultimately to hemolyze. Energy is also used to maintain low intracellular levels of calcium ion.

2. Initiation of energy production. ATP is required for the initial reaction of glycolysis involving phosphorylation of glucose to glucose-6-phosphate.

3. Maintenance of RBC membrane and shape. Energy is required to maintain the complex phospholipid structure of the RBC membrane. Maintenance of the biconcave shape is probably also energy dependent.

4. Maintenance of heme iron in the reduced (ferrous) form. Oxidative potentials within the RBC may cause oxidation of the iron of hemoglobin. Hemoglobin containing ferric iron (methemoglobin) is ineffective in oxygen transport. Moreover, if peroxides and other oxidant substances are not inactivated, hemoglobin may be denatured and precipitated. Cells containing such denatured hemoglobin (Heinz bodies) are rapidly removed from the circulation. Protection of RBCs from the effects of oxidation ultimately depends on NADPH and NADH. These compounds are continually regenerated by activities of the glycolytic pathway and pentose shunt. In many genetically determined deficiencies of glycolytic and pentose pathway enzymes, hemolytic states occur because the energy necessary to perform these vital functions cannot be generated.

5. Maintenance of the levels of organic phosphates such as 2,3-diphosphoglycerate and ATP within the RBCs. These com-

pounds interact with hemoglobin and have profound effects on oxygen affinity.

Red Cell Life Span. The differences in physical properties of RBCs derived from term and preterm infants may in part account for the decreased life span of neonatal RBCs within the circulation. The average life span for a neonatal RBC is 60–90 days, approximately one half to two thirds that of an adult RBC. When neonatal RBCs are transfused into adults, they exhibit a shortened life span, owing to alterations intrinsic to the neonatal RBC. In contrast, cells transfused from adult donors appear to survive normally in newborns. With increasing degrees of prematurity, remarkably shorter red cell life spans (35 to 50 days) are found. The shortened red cell life span of the preterm and term neonate may be explained by some of the characteristics specific to newborn cells: a rapid decline in intracellular enzyme activity and ATP, loss of membrane surface area by internalization of membrane lipids, decreased levels of intracellular carnitine, increased susceptibility of membrane lipids and protein to peroxidation, and increased mechanical fragility due to increased membrane deformability.

Athens JW: Granulocytes—Neutrophils. In Lee RG, Bithell TD, Forester J, Athens JW, Leukins JN (editors): *Wintrobe's Clinical Hematology.* Philadelphia, Lea & Febiger, 1993, vol 9, pp 236–39.

Cairo MS: Therapeutic implications for dysregulated colony-stimulating factor expression in neonates. *Blood* 1993;82:2269.

Calhoun DA, Christensen RD: Human developmental biology of granulocyte colony-stimulating factor. *Clin Perinatol* 2000;27:559.

Carbonell F, Calvo W, Fliedner TM: Cellular composition of human fetal bone marrow. *Acta Anat* 1982;113:371.

Dame C, Juul S: The switch from fetal to adult erythropoiesis. *Clin Perinatol* 2000;27:507.

Forester F, Daffos F: Hematological values of 163 normal fetuses between 18 and 30 weeks of gestation. *Pediatr Res* 1985;20:342.

Goldberg MA, Dunning SP, Bunn HF: Regulation of the erythropoietin gene: Evidence that the oxygen sensor is a heme protein. *Science* 1988;242:524.

Kaushansky K: Thrombopoietin and hematopoietic stem cell development. *Ann N Y Acad Sci* 1999;30:314.

Keleman E, Janossa M: Macrophages are the first differentiated blood cells formed in human embryonic liver. *Exp Hematol* 1980;8:996.

Metcalf D: Hematopoietic regulators: Redundance or subtlety? *Blood* 1993;82:3515.

Nathan DG: Regulation of hematopoiesis. *Pediatr Res* 1990;27:423.

Ohls RK, Li Y, Abdel-Mageed A, et al: Neutrophil pool sizes and granulocyte colony-stimulating factor production in human mid-trimester fetuses. *Pediatr Res* 1995;37:806.

Oski FA: The erythrocyte and its disorders. In Nathan DG, Oski FA (editors): *Hematology of Infancy and Childhood.* Philadelphia, WB Saunders, 1993, vol 4, pp 18–43.

Roberts IA, Murray NA: Neonatal thrombocytopenia: New insights into pathogenesis and implications for clinical management. *Curr Opin Pediatr* 2001;131:16.

Schibler KR, Li Y, Ohls RK, et al: Possible mechanisms accounting for the growth factor independence of hematopoietic progenitors from umbilical cord blood. *Blood* 1994;84:3679.

Slayton WB: Development of the immune system in the human fetus. In Christensen RD (editor): *Hematologic Problems of the Neonate.* Philadelphia, WB Saunders, 2000, pp 21–42.

Sola MC, Dame C, Christensen RD: Toward a rational use of recombinant thrombopoietin in the neonatal intensive care unit. *J Pediatr Hematol Oncol* 2001;23:179.

Chapter 439
The Anemias *Bertil Glader*

Anemia is defined as a reduction of the red blood cell (RBC) volume or hemoglobin concentration below the range of values occurring in healthy persons. Table 439–1 lists the means and ranges for hemoglobin and hematocrit values by age groups of well-nourished children. There may be racial differences in hemoglobin levels. Black children have levels about 0.5 g/dL lower than those of white and Asian children of comparable age

TABLE 439–1. Hematologic Values During Infancy and Childhood

Age	Hemoglobin (g/dL) Mean	Hemoglobin (g/dL) Range	Hematocrit (%) Mean	Hematocrit (%) Range	Reticulocytes (%) Mean	MCV (fL) Lowest	Leukocytes (WBC/mm³) Mean	Leukocytes (WBC/mm³) Range	Neutrophils (%) Mean	Neutrophils (%) Range	Lymphocytes (%) Mean*	Eosinophils (%) Mean	Monocytes (%) Mean
Cord blood	16.8	13.7–20.1	55	45–65	5.0	110	18,000	(9,000–30,000)	61	(40–80)	31	2	6
2 wk	16.5	13.0–20.0	50	42–66	1.0		12,000	(5,000–21,000)	40		63	3	9
3 mo	12.0	9.5–14.5	36	31–41	1.0		12,000	(6,000–18,000)	30		48	2	5
6 mo–6 yr	12.0	10.5–14.0	37	33–42	1.0	70–74	10,000	(6,000–15,000)	45		48	2	5
7–12 yr	13.0	11.0–16.0	38	34–40	1.0	76–80	8,000	(4,500–13,500)	55		38	2	5
Adult													
Female	14	12.0–16.0	42	37–47	1.6	80	7,500	(5,000–10,000)	55	(35–70)	35	3	7
Male	16	14.0–18.0	47	42–52		80							

*Relatively wide range.
fL = femtoliters; MCV = mean corpuscular volume; WBC = white blood cells.

and socioeconomic status, possibly, in part, because of the high incidence of α-thalassemia in blacks.

Although a reduction in the amount of circulating hemoglobin decreases the oxygen-carrying capacity of the blood, few clinical disturbances occur until the hemoglobin level falls below 7–8 g/dL. Below this level, pallor becomes evident in the skin and mucous membranes. Physiologic adjustments to anemia include increased cardiac output, increased oxygen extraction (increased arteriovenous oxygen difference), and a shunting of blood flow toward vital organs and tissues. In addition, the concentration of 2,3-diphosphoglycerate (2,3-DPG) increases within the RBC. The resultant "shift to the right" of the oxygen dissociation curve, reducing the affinity of hemoglobin for oxygen, results in more complete transfer of oxygen to the tissues. The same shift in the oxygen dissociation curve may also occur at high altitude. When moderately severe anemia develops slowly, surprisingly few symptoms or objective findings may be evident. However, weakness, tachypnea, shortness of breath on exertion, tachycardia, cardiac dilatation, and congestive heart failure ultimately result from increasingly severe anemia, regardless of its cause.

When oxygen delivery by RBCs to tissues is decreased, various mechanisms, including expanded cardiac output, increased production of 2,3-DPG in RBCs, and higher levels of erythropoietin (EPO), help the body compensate for the deficiency. RBC production by the bone marrow in response to EPO may expand severalfold and thereby compensate for mild to moderate reductions in RBC life span. However, in some anemias, the bone marrow loses its usual capacity for sustained production and expansion of the RBC mass; and, in these instances, absolute reticulocyte numbers in the peripheral blood are decreased. If the normal reticulocyte percentage of total RBCs during most of childhood is about 1.0% and the expected RBC count is approximately $4.0 \times 10^6/mm^3$, then the normal absolute reticulocyte number should be about 40,000/mm³. In the presence of anemia, EPO production and the absolute number of reticulocytes should rise. A normal or low absolute number or percentage of reticulocytes in response to anemia indicates relative bone marrow failure or ineffective erythropoiesis (e.g., megaloblastic anemia, thalassemia). Measurement of the serum transferrin receptor (TfR) level or examination of the bone marrow distinguishes between these possibilities, because TfR is elevated in ineffective erythropoiesis (or in iron deficiency) and is decreased in marrow RBC hypoproliferation.

Anemia is not a specific entity but results from many underlying pathologic processes. RBC size changes with age; and before an anemia can be specifically characterized with respect to RBC size, normal developmental changes in the mean corpuscular volume (MCV) should be understood (see Table 439–1). It is important that pediatricians recognize the MCV variations in

childhood because many laboratories use only adult normal values, which differ considerably. For every child with significant anemia, it is essential also to review the appearance of RBCs on a peripheral blood smear (Fig. 439–1). Specific morphologic features may point to the underlying diagnosis. In addition, the presence of polychromatophilia, which generally correlates the degree of reticulocytosis, indicates that the marrow is able to respond to RBC loss or destruction.

A useful approach to assessing the common causes of anemia in children is summarized next and in Box 439–1.

Is anemia associated with other hematologic abnormalities? The presence of thrombocytopenia, abnormalities in white blood cell numbers, or the presence of abnormal leukocytes often indicates bone marrow failure caused by aplastic anemia, leukemia, or other malignant marrow disease. These disorders can be differentiated by careful review of screening hematologic studies and close attention to the medical history and physical examination.

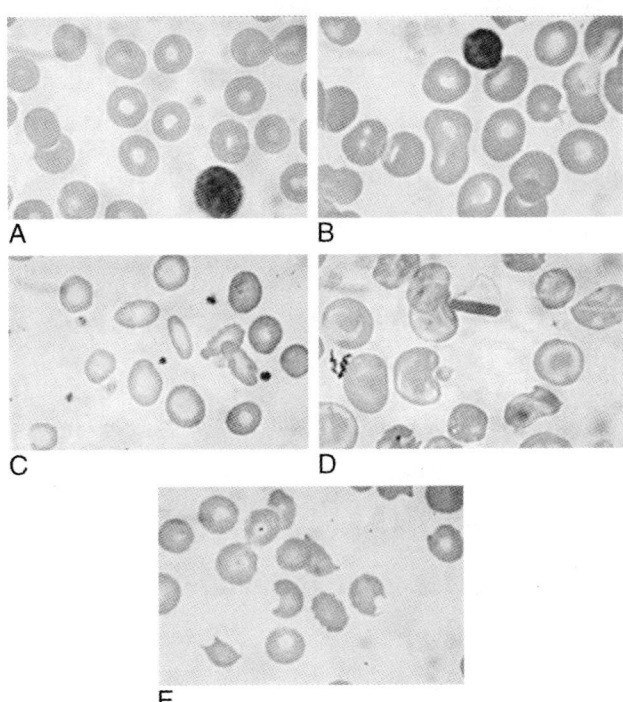

FIGURE 439–1. Morphologic abnormalities of the red blood cell. A, normal. B, Macrocytes (folic acid or vitamin B_{12} deficiency). C, Hypochromic microcytes (iron deficiency). D, Target cells (Hb CC disease). E, Schizocytes (hemolytic-uremic syndrome). (Courtesy Dr. E. Schwartz.) See also color plates.

BOX 439–1. Approach to Common Causes of Anemia in Children

Is anemia associated with other hematologic abnormalities?
  If yes, consider
  Aplastic anemia
  Leukemia
  Other bone marrow replacement disorders
Is anemia associated with reticulocytosis?
  If yes, usually a consequence of bleeding or ongoing hemolysis
Is there associated hyperbilirubinemia or increased serum lactate dehydrogenase
  If yes, usually due to hemolysis
  Review of peripheral blood smear
  Spherocytes (hereditary spherocytosis, autoimmune hemolytic anemia, Wilson disease)
  Sickle forms (sickle cell disease, sickle-β-thalassemia)
  Target cells (hemoglobin SC disease)
  Hypochromic RBC, nucleated RBC (homozygous β-thalassemia, Hgb E-β-thalassemia)
  Microangiopathy (hemolytic-uremic syndrome, thrombotic thrombocytopenia)
  Bite cells/blister cells (G6PD deficiency)
Is anemia associated with a lower than appropriate reticulocyte response?
  If yes, assess red blood cell size
Are red blood cells microcytic?
  If yes, usually due to defect in hemoglobin synthesis
  Iron deficiency
  α or β-Thalassemia trait
  Hemoglobin E disorders (AE, EE)
  Lead poisons
Are red blood cells macrocytic?
  If yes, is there neutrophil hypersegmentation (megaloblastic changes)?
  If yes, consider
  Folate deficiency, vitamin B12 deficiency, inborn errors of metabolism
  If no, consider
  Diamond-Blackfan anemia
  Congenital dyserythropoietic anemia
  Pearson syndrome
Are red blood cells normocytic?
  If yes, consider
  Anemia of chronic disease usually (associated comorbid conditions)
  Anemia of renal disease (renal failure)
  Transient erythroblastopenia of childhood
  Anemia associated with hypothyroidism

Is anemia associated with reticulocytosis? In anemic children with an appropriate reticulocyte response, the cause usually is a consequence of bleeding or ongoing hemolysis. The most characteristic feature of hemolysis is reticulocytosis with indirect hyperbilirubinemia and often increased serum lactate dehydrogenase as indicators of accelerated erythrocyte destruction. Review of the peripheral blood smear to identify abnormal RBC morphology (e.g., spherocytes, sickle forms, microangiopathy) often is helpful in ascertaining the cause of hemolysis.

Is anemia associated with reticulocytopenia? Anemia in children with a less than appropriate reticulocyte response reflects an impairment of normal erythropoiesis, and it is in this group that analysis of red blood cell size (MCV) is particularly useful.

Are red blood cells microcytic? Almost all children in this category have defects in hemoglobin synthesis from either iron deficiency, thalassemia trait, hemoglobin E disorders, or hemoglobin C. Thalassemia trait disorders and other hemoglobinopathies are considered in patients of Mediterranean, Near Eastern, African, or Asian background. A distinguishing feature of thalassemia trait conditions and hemoglobin E is that the RBC count often is elevated above normal despite the presence of a mild anemia and microcytosis; this is in marked contrast to iron deficiency, in which the RBC count decreases along with the reduced hemoglobin and MCV.

Are red blood cells macrocytic? The anemia in these children is sometimes megaloblastic, a result of impaired DNA synthesis and nuclear development, and the formation of other blood cells is also affected. The peripheral blood smear in megaloblastic anemias contains large macrovalocytes, and frequently there is nuclear hypersegmentation of the neutrophils. The varied major causes of megaloblastic anemia include folate deficiency, Vitamin B_{12} deficiency, and rare inborn errors of metabolism. However, not all macrocytic anemias are megaloblastic, and one such important condition in children is Diamond-Blackfan anemia.

Are red blood cells normocytic? Normocytic anemia, low reticulocyte count, and normal bilirubin levels characterize a large number of anemias. The anemia of chronic disease usually is normocytic, although rarely it may be slightly microcytic. In these cases there usually is clinical evidence of associated inflammatory disease or chronic illness. The anemia of renal failure is normocytic and is caused by reduced erythropoietin production. Invariably, there is clinical and laboratory evidence of significant renal disease. The most common cause of acquired pure red cell aplasia seen in pediatrics is transient erythroblastopenia of childhood, a normocytic anemia.

SECTION 2 *Anemias of Inadequate Production*

Bertil Glader

Chapter 440

Congenital Hypoplastic Anemia (Diamond-Blackfan Anemia)

This rare condition usually becomes symptomatic in early infancy, often with pallor in the neonatal period, but occasionally may first be noted later in childhood. Over 90% of cases are recognized in the 1st year of life, and the average age of diagnosis is 3 mo. The most characteristic hematologic features are macrocytic anemia, reticulocytopenia, and a deficiency or absence of red blood cell (RBC) precursors in an otherwise normally cellular bone marrow.

Etiology. The majority of cases are sporadic, although dominant or recessive patterns of inheritance are indicated by familial occurrence in about 15% of patients. The primary defects are in the erythroid progenitor cells, where there is an intrinsic defect that results in increased apoptosis (programmed cell death). High levels of erythropoietin (EPO) are present in serum and urine, although a search for mutations in the EPO receptor gene has been negative. In about 25% of sporadic and inherited cases there are mutations in a gene *(DBA1)* for a ribosomal protein S19, mapped to chromosome 19q13. A second gene for Diamond-Blackfan anemia has been linked to chromosome 8p, and most likely other genetic abnormalities will be identified. A unifying etiology for this disorder and the significance of these genetic alterations is being defined.

Clinical Manifestations. Although hematopoiesis is generally adequate in fetal life, some affected infants appear pale in the first days after birth; rarely, hydrops fetalis occurs. Profound anemia usually becomes evident by 2–6 mo of age, occasionally somewhat later. Over 50% of affected children have congenital anomalies, including short stature, craniofacial deformities, or defects of the upper extremities, including triphalangeal thumbs. The abnormalities are diverse, with no specific pattern emerging in the majority of those affected.

Laboratory Findings. The RBCs are almost always macrocytic for age, but there is no hypersegmentation of neutrophils or other peripheral blood characteristics of megaloblastic anemia. Folic acid and vitamin B_{12} levels are normal. Chemical evaluation of RBCs reveals an enzyme pattern similar to a "fetal" RBC population, and there is also elevated fetal hemoglobin (Hb F) and increased expression of "i" antigen. Erythrocyte adenosine deaminase (ADA) activity is increased in most patients with this disorder, a finding that helps distinguish congenital RBC aplasia from acquired transient erythroblastopenia of childhood (see Chapter 442). Also, because elevated ADA activity is not a fetal RBC feature, measurement of this enzyme is helpful in diagnosing Diamond-Blackfan anemia in very young infants. Thrombocytosis or thrombocytopenia and occasionally neutropenia may also be present initially. Reticulocytes are characteristically very low despite severe anemia. RBC precursors in the marrow are markedly reduced in most patients, but other marrow elements are usually normal. Serum iron levels are elevated. Bone marrow chromosome studies are normal and, unlike in Fanconi anemia, there is no increase in chromosomal breaks when lymphocytes are stressed with alkylating agents.

Differential Diagnosis. Congenital hypoplastic anemia must be differentiated from other anemias with low reticulocyte counts. The anemia of hemolytic disease of the newborn can have a protracted course and, on occasion, be associated with markedly reduced erythropoiesis. This usually terminates spontaneously at 5–8 wk of age. Aplastic anemic crises characterized by reticulocytopenia and by decreased numbers of RBC precursors, frequently caused by parvovirus B19 infections, may complicate various types of chronic hemolytic disease, but usually after the first several months of life (see Chapter 442). Infection with parvovirus B19 in utero may also cause pure RBC aplasia in infancy, even with hydrops fetalis at birth. The absence of parvovirus B19 detected by polymerase chain reaction (PCR) is now considered an essential feature in establishing the diagnosis of Diamond-Blackfan anemia in young infants. The syndrome of transient erythroblastopenia of childhood (see Chapter 442) may be differentiated from Diamond- Blackfan syndrome by its relatively late onset (although it may occasionally develop in infants younger than 6 mo). In very young infants whose RBCs have many fetal features, a determination of elevated erythrocyte ADA activity is particularly useful because this increased enzyme activity is not a characteristic of fetal RBCs.

Treatment. Corticosteroid therapy is beneficial in three fourths of patients who respond initially. The mechanism of its effect is unknown. Prednisone in three divided doses totaling 2 mg/kg/24 hr is used as an initial trial. An increase in RBC precursors appears in bone marrow 1–3 wk after therapy is begun, and this is followed by peripheral reticulocytosis. The hemoglobin may reach normal levels in 4–6 wk, although there is much variability in the rate of response. Once the hemoglobin concentration is clearly increasing, the dose of corticosteroid may be reduced gradually by tapering divided doses and then by eliminating all except a single, lowest effective daily dose. This dose should then be doubled, used on alternate days, and tapered still

further while maintaining the hemoglobin level at 9 g/dL or above. In some patients, very small amounts of prednisone, as low as 2.5 mg twice a week, may be sufficient to sustain adequate erythropoiesis. Overall, 60% of children with Diamond-Blackfan anemia initially started on steroids stop taking the drug. This occurs because of unacceptable steroid side effects or evolution of steroid refractoriness at acceptable steroid doses, or, occasionally, there is spontaneous remission of anemia.

In patients who do not respond to corticosteroid therapy, transfusions at intervals of 4–8 wk are necessary to sustain normal growth and activities. Chelation therapy for iron overload with deferoxamine administered subcutaneously through a portable pump should be started when excess iron accumulation is reflected by serum ferritin levels exceeding 1,500 mg/dL, but preferably after 5 yr of age, because the medication may interfere with normal growth. An oral iron chelator, deferiprone (L1), is in clinical trials and may be almost as effective as deferoxamine; however, there is some controversy related to possible hepatic toxicity. The drug is licensed for use in Canada, the United Kingdom, and India but not in the United States. Other therapies, including androgens, cyclosporine, cyclophosphamide, antithymocyte globulin (ATG), high-dose intravenous immunoglobulin, high-dose methylprednisolone, EPO, and interleukin-3 have not had a consistent beneficial effect and may have a high incidence of side effects. Splenectomy may decrease the need for transfusion if hypersplenism or isoimmunization develops. Stem cell transplantation from a related histocompatible donor has a role in children who do not respond to corticosteroids and who have demonstrated a several-year need for RBC transfusions. The survival results for matched-related donors have been very encouraging, but the responses have been much inferior with the use of partially mismatched siblings or matched unrelated donors.

Prognosis. Median survival is probably more than 40 yr of age, although definitive data are lacking. The outlook is best in those who respond to corticosteroid therapy. About half of patients are long-term responders. In the others, survival depends on transfusions. Some children in each group may eventually have spontaneous remissions (about 20%), and most of these remissions occur in the first decade. In children who are regularly transfused, total body iron increases and hemosiderosis ensues. The liver and spleen may enlarge, and secondary hypersplenism with leukopenia and thrombocytopenia can occur. The complications of chronic transfusions in Diamond-Blackfan anemia are similar to those in β-thalassemia major, and prevention and treatment of iron overload should be equally aggressive in both groups of transfused patients (see Chapter 454). Diamond-Blackfan anemia may be a premalignant syndrome, with acute leukemia (usually myeloid) and myelodysplasia occurring in a small fraction (less than 5%) of patients. Solid tumor malignancies also have been reported, in particular osteosarcoma. Other significant causes of death include complications associated with stem cell transplantation, steroid therapy (opportunistic infections), and iron overload.

Chapter 441
Pearson Marrow-Pancreas Syndrome

This form of congenital hypoplastic anemia may be initially confused with Diamond-Blackfan syndrome or transient erythroblastopenia of childhood. The marrow failure usually appears in the neonatal period and is characterized by a macrocytic anemia and, occasionally, neutropenia and thrombocytopenia. The level of hemoglobin F is elevated. There are vacuolated erythroblasts and myeloblasts in the marrow. This disorder is considered a unique variant of congenital sideroblastic anemia because the marrow also contains ringed sideroblasts. Other clinical features are failure to thrive, pancreatic fibrosis with insulin-dependent diabetes and exocrine pancreatic deficiency, muscle and neurologic impairment, and, frequently, early death. This multiorgan disorder is caused by mitochondrial DNA deletions, with heterogeneity in different tissues and between patients. The heterogeneity accounts for the variable clinical picture, and a change in proportions of mtDNA types in tissues over time may result in spontaneous improvement of red blood cell hypoproliferation. Therapy includes transfusions of red blood cells as needed. Filgrastim (granulocyte colony-stimulating factor) may reverse episodes of severe neutropenia.

Chapter 442
Acquired Pure Red Blood Cell Anemias

Transient Erythroblastopenia of Childhood (TEC). This is the most common acquired red cell aplasia occurring in children, and it is more common than congenital hypoplastic anemia. This syndrome of severe, transient hypoplastic anemia occurs mainly in previously healthy children between 6 mo and 3 yr of age, with most older than 12 mo at onset. The cause of this decrease in red blood cell (RBC) production is a transient immunologic suppression of erythropoiesis. It frequently follows a viral illness, although a specific virus has not been identified. Parvovirus B19 infections, which may cause hypoplasia in children with chronic hemolytic anemia (see Chapter 461), are not responsible for TEC. Reticulocytes and bone marrow erythroid precursors are markedly decreased, although examination of the bone marrow rarely is needed to make the diagnosis. Some degree of neutropenia may occur in up to 20% of cases while platelet numbers are normal or elevated. Just as is the case in iron-deficiency anemia and other RBC hypoplasias, thrombocytosis presumably is caused by increased erythropoietin, which is known to have some homology with thrombopoietin. Mean corpuscular volume (MCV) is characteristically normal for age, and fetal hemoglobin (Hb F) levels are normal before the recovery phase. RBC adenosine deaminase (ADA) levels are normal in this disorder, whereas they are elevated in a majority of children with congenital hypoplastic anemia. Differentiation from the latter disease sometimes may be difficult, but differences in age at onset and in age-related MCV, Hb F, and ADA usually are helpful. The peak occurrence of TEC coincides with that of iron-deficiency anemia in infants receiving milk as their main caloric source; however, differences in MCV clearly distinguish these two disorders.

Virtually all children recover within 1–2 mo. RBC transfusions may be necessary for severe anemia in the absence of signs of early recovery. The anemia develops slowly, and marked symptoms usually develop only with severe anemia. Corticosteroid therapy is of no value in this disorder. Any child with presumed TEC who requires more than one transfusion should be re-evaluated for another possible diagnosis. In rare instances a prolonged case of apparent TEC may be caused by parvovirus-induced RBC aplasia occurring in children with congenital or acquired immunodeficiencies.

Red Cell Aplasia Associated with Chronic Hemolysis. Parvovirus B19 is the best documented viral cause of RBC aplasia; it is the cause of fifth disease or erythema infectiosum (see Chapter 230). The virus is particularly infective and cytotoxic for erythroid progenitor cells in the marrow, interacting specifically with the RBC P antigen as a receptor. Characteristic nuclear inclusions in erythroblasts and giant pronormoblasts can be seen with light microscopy of bone marrow. Hemophagocytosis may also be seen in the marrow, perhaps accounting for the occasional granulocytopenia and thrombocytopenia. Because infection with this virus is usually transient, with recovery occurring in less than 2 wk, anemia is not present or not noticed in otherwise normal children, in whom the life span of peripheral RBCs is 110–120 days. However, in patients with hemolysis, such as that caused by hereditary spherocytosis or sickle cell disease, in whom RBC life span is much shorter, a brief cessation of erythropoiesis from parvovirus infection may cause severe anemia, the "aplastic crisis" occurring in these diseases. Recovery from moderate to severe anemia is usually spontaneous, heralded by a wave of nucleated RBCs and subsequent reticulocytosis in the peripheral blood. An RBC transfusion occasionally is necessary for marked symptoms caused by anemia. In children with chronic hemolysis this "aplastic crisis" from parvovirus usually occurs only once.

Red Cell Aplasia Associated with Immunodeficiency. Rarely, persistence of parvovirus infection may occur in patients unable to mount an adequate antibody response to the virus, as in children with congenital immunodeficiency diseases, those being treated with immunosuppressive agents, and those with AIDS. The resultant pure RBC aplasia may be severe and affected children are often thought to have TEC. This type of RBC aplasia differs from TEC in that there is no spontaneous recovery and more than one transfusion needs to be given. The diagnosis of parvovirus infection is made by detecting viral particles (by polymerase chain reaction) because the usual serologic responses are impaired in these immunodeficient children. The viral infection in these chronically infected patients may be treated with high doses of intravenous immunoglobulin (IVIG), which contains neutralizing antibody to parvovirus.

Red Cell Aplasia with Miscarriage and Hydrops Fetalis. Different clinical manifestations of infection with this virus and destruction of erythroid precursors occur with infections in utero, in which there is increased fetal wastage in the first and second trimesters, and infants may be born with hydrops fetalis and viremia. The presence of persistent congenital parvovirus infection needs to be detected by examination of bone marrow DNA because immunologic tolerance to the virus may prevent the usual development of specific antibodies.

Other Red Cell Aplasias in Children. Adult types of red cell aplasia are usually chronic antibody mediated and frequently associated with disorders such as chronic lymphocytic leukemia, lymphoma, thymoma, and systemic lupus erythematosus. This chronic antibody–mediated type of RBC aplasia is extremely rare in childhood. Certain drugs such as chloramphenicol also can inhibit erythropoiesis in a dose-dependent manner. Reticulocytopenia, erythroid hypoplasia, and vacuolated pronormoblasts in the marrow are reversible effects of this drug; and these effects are distinct from the idiosyncratic and rare development of severe aplastic anemia in recipients of chloramphenicol.

Chapter 443
Anemia of Chronic Disorders (ACD) and Renal Disease

Anemia complicates a number of chronic systemic diseases associated with infection, inflammation, or tissue breakdown. Examples include chronic pyogenic infections, such as bronchiectasis and osteomyelitis, and chronic inflammatory processes, such as rheumatoid arthritis, systemic lupus erythematosus, and ulcerative colitis. Despite diverse underlying causes, the erythroid abnormalities are similar, although incompletely understood. The red blood cell (RBC) life span is mildly decreased, but this increased hemolysis is not the major problem. More importantly, there is a relative failure of bone marrow to respond adequately to the anemia. This impaired erythropoietic response is believed to be related to three factors. First, iron is trapped in the macrophages and is unavailable for hemoglobin synthesis. Second, despite slightly increased erythropoietin (EPO) levels the morphologically appearing normal marrow is unable to increase erythropoiesis. Third, although EPO production is slightly increased, this elevation is inadequate for the degree of anemia. A unifying explanation for the abnormal findings in this type of anemia is not available. One hypothesis is that the underlying medical conditions cause the release of interleukin-1 (IL-1) and tumor necrosis factor (TNF), and, subsequently, these cytokines lead to the production of interferon-beta (IFN-β) and interferon-gamma (IFN-γ). This hypothesis is supported by the observation that IFN-β and IFN-γ given to experimental animals causes a disorder similar to the anemia of chronic disease. The specific stimulant of increased TNF and IL-1 production in these patients has not been identified.

The anemia seen in chronic renal disease shares some features with the anemia of chronic disease, such as a mild degree of hemolysis. However, the major component of this anemia is decreased EPO production owing to damage of the renal cells producing this cytokine.

Clinical Manifestations. Although the important symptoms and signs are those of the underlying disease, the quality of life may be affected by the mild to moderate anemia that is present.

Laboratory Findings. Hemoglobin concentrations are usually 6–9 g/dL. The anemia is usually normochromic and normocytic, although occasionally some patients may have modest hypochromia and microcytosis. Absolute reticulocyte counts are normal or low, and leukocytosis is common. The serum iron level is low, without the increase in total iron-binding capacity (serum transferrin) that occurs in iron deficiency. This pattern of low serum iron and low to normal iron-binding protein (serum transferrin) is a regular and valuable diagnostic feature. The serum ferritin level may be elevated. The bone marrow has normal cellularity; the RBC precursors are low to adequate, marrow hemosiderin may be increased, and granulocytic hyperplasia may be present. A frequent clinical challenge is to identify concomitant iron deficiency in patients with an inflammatory disease. Measurement of the TfR/ferritin ratio may be useful, because it is elevated when iron deficiency is present (see Chapter 439). A trial of iron therapy also may help resolve the issue, although there may be no response when inflammation caused by the primary disease persists.

Treatment and Prognosis. Because these anemias are secondary to other disease processes, they do not respond to iron or hematinics unless there is concomitant deficiency. Transfusions raise the hemoglobin concentration temporarily, but they are rarely indicated. If the underlying systemic disease can be controlled, the anemia will resolve. Recombinant human EPO can increase the hemoglobin level and improve activity and the sense of well-being in patients with cancer and end-stage renal failure and in those with anemia of chronic inflammation. Treatment with iron is usually necessary for an optimal EPO effect.

Chapter 444
Congenital Dyserythropoietic Anemias (CDA)

These are a class of hemolytic disorders characterized by unique morphologic abnormalities in marrow erythroblasts (multinuclearity, abnormal nuclear fragments, and intrachromatin bridges between cells). Glycosylation of membrane proteins is impaired, and there also is an accumulation of red blood cell (RBC) glycolipids. The cause of both of these abnormalities is thought to be a deficiency of N-acetyl-glucosaminyltransferase II, an RBC enzyme responsible for membrane protein glycosylation. Clinically, these disorders are characterized by variable degrees of anemia despite the fact that there is increased marrow erythroid activity (i.e., ineffective erythropoiesis). CDA has been reported in newborn infants with hydrops fetalis. Three major types of CDA (types I, II, and III) have been defined.

Type I CDA is a rare autosomal recessive disorder in which the onset of macrocytic anemia and/or jaundice may be noted at any age, although the majority of cases are first recognized in the neonatal period. The reticulocyte count is less than expected for the degree of anemia. White blood cells and platelets are normal. Indirect bilirubin levels are slightly elevated, haptoglobin levels are low, and transferrin is saturated with iron (serum iron level approximates the total iron-binding capacity concentration). The marrow exhibits erythroid hyperplasia, shown by megaloblastic erythroblasts in the absence of vitamin B$_{12}$ or folate deficiency. A small number of erythroblasts manifest dyserythropoietic features with interchromatin bridges between cells. *Treatment* of this disorder has been unsuccessful with the usual hematinics (vitamins and steroids), but some improvement has been achieved with interferon alfa. Although splenomegaly is common, splenectomy is not helpful. The most important long-term complication is hemosiderosis caused by increased intestinal absorption of iron and ineffective erythropoiesis. The gene for CDA type I has been mapped to chromosome 15q15.1.

Type II CDA is an autosomal recessive disorder, and it is the most common variant of CDA. The gene for CDA II has been mapped to chromosome 20q11.2. The clinical and laboratory features are similar to those seen in type I CDA; however, the magnitude of anemia usually is greater. Many more late marrow erythroblasts (up to 50%) may be abnormal, as manifested by binuclearity, multinuclearity, and abnormal lobulation. The pathognomonic findings in CDA type II are that the patient's RBCs are lysed by acidified serum. The combination of erythroblast multinuclearity and the sensitivity of circulating RBC to lysis by acidified normal serum is the reason that type II CDA is known by the acronym HEMPAS (*h*ereditary *e*rythroblastic *m*ultinuclearity with a *p*ositive *a*cidified *s*erum test). Patients with severe anemia require blood transfusions. Iron overload occurs from both transfusions and increased intestinal absorption (even in untransfused patients), and in select patients iron chelation therapy should be considered.

Type III CDA, the least common type of CDA, is a mild-to-moderate macrocytic anemia. Transfusions usually are not required. In contrast to CDA types I and II, this disorder is inherited as an autosomal dominant defect. A characteristic bone marrow feature is erythroid hyperplasia, with many multinucleated erythroblasts containing up to 12 nuclei. The gene for type III CDA has been mapped to chromosome 15q21.

Chapter 445
Physiologic Anemia of Infancy

Normal newborn infants have higher hemoglobin and hematocrit levels with larger red blood cells (RBCs) than older children and adults. Within the first week of life, a progressive decline in hemoglobin level begins and persists for 6–8 wk. The result of this decline is generally referred to as **physiologic anemia of infancy**. Several factors are operative. With the onset of respirations at birth, considerably more oxygen is available for binding to hemoglobin and the hemoglobin-oxygen saturation increases from 50–95% or more. Furthermore, the normal developmental switch from fetal to adult hemoglobin synthesis actively replaces high oxygen affinity fetal hemoglobin with lower oxygen affinity adult hemoglobin, which can deliver a greater fraction of hemoglobin-bound oxygen to the tissues. Therefore, immediately after birth the increase in blood oxygen content and tissue oxygen delivery downregulates erythropoietin (EPO) production and, as a consequence, erythropoiesis is suppressed. In the absence of erythropoiesis, hemoglobin levels decrease because there is no replacement of aged RBCs as they are normally removed from the circulation. Iron from degraded RBCs is stored for future hemoglobin synthesis. The hemoglobin concentration continues to decrease until tissue oxygen needs are greater than oxygen delivery. Normally, this point is reached between 8–12 wk of age when the hemoglobin concentration is 9–11 g/dL. As hypoxia is detected by renal or hepatic oxygen sensors, EPO production increases and erythropoiesis resumes. The iron previously stored in reticuloendothelial tissues can then be used for hemoglobin synthesis. The supply of stored iron is sufficient for hemoglobin synthesis, even in the absence of dietary iron intake, until approximately 20 wk of age. This "anemia" should be viewed as a physiologic adaptation to extrauterine life, reflecting the excess capability for oxygen delivery relative to tissue oxygen requirements. There is no hematologic problem, and no therapy is required.

Premature infants also develop a physiologic anemia. The same factors are operative as in term infants, but they are exaggerated. The decline in hemoglobin level is both more extreme and more rapid. Minimal hemoglobin levels of 7–9 g/dL commonly occur by 3–6 wk of age, and in very small premature infants levels may be even lower (see Chapter 86). The cause of this anemia is multifaceted. An important component in the first few weeks of life is blood loss as a result of sampling for the many laboratory tests necessary to stabilize the clinical status of these infants, particularly those with cardiorespiratory problems. The erythropoietic response to anemia is also suboptimal, a significant problem because demands on erythropoiesis are heightened by the short survival of the RBCs of premature infants (40–60 days instead of 120 days as in adults) and the rapid expansion of the RBC mass that accompanies growth. The basis for suboptimal erythropoiesis in prematurity appears to be inadequate synthesis of EPO in response to hypoxia. Because the liver is the predominant source of EPO during fetal life, it has been proposed that relative insensitivity of the hepatic oxygen sensor to hypoxia explains the blunted EPO response seen in premature infants. The spontaneous resolution of the anemia that occurs by approximately 40 wk gestational age is in keeping with a developmental switch from the relatively insensitive hepatic oxygen sensor to the renal oxygen sensor, which is exquisitely sensitive to hypoxia, because by this time the predominant site of EPO synthesis has shifted to the kidneys.

The magnitude of the physiologic anemia of infancy can be modified by other ongoing processes. For example, a late hyporegenerative anemia, with absence of reticulocytes, may occur in infants with mild hemolytic disease of the newborn, requiring only phototherapy to effectively decrease the bilirubin concentration. The persistence of maternally derived anti-RBC antibodies in the infant's circulation can lead to a low-grade hemolytic anemia for several weeks, and this may present as an exaggeration of the physiologic anemia of infancy. In part, it also might reflect an impaired EPO response. Another observation is the lower than expected hemoglobin at the "physiologic" nadir seen in infants after intrauterine or neonatal RBC transfusions. When premature infants are transfused with adult blood containing Hb A, the shift of the oxygen dissociation curve as a result of the presence of Hb A facilitates delivery of oxygen to the tissues. Accordingly, the definition of anemia and the need for transfusion in premature infants must be based not only on hemoglobin level but also on oxygen requirements and the ability of an infant's circulating hemoglobin to release oxygen.

Dietary factors may also aggravate physiologic anemia. Deficiency of folic acid superimposed on the physiologic process may result in more severe anemia. Vitamin E deficiency and therapy do not appear to have a role in anemia of prematurity, despite early suggestions to the contrary. A controlled and blinded study of oral vitamin E administration (25 IU/dL-α-tocopherol, colloidal aqueous solution) to infants weighing less than 1,500 g showed no difference in hemoglobin levels, reticulocytes, RBC morphology, or platelet counts. Breast milk and modern formulas appear to provide adequate vitamin E. Oral vitamin C supplementation (50 mg/24 hr) does not cause hemolysis in premature infants. Supplemental iron starting at approximately 4 mg/kg/24 hr for preterm babies 4–8 wk old and by 4 mo in full-term infants should not cause significant hemolysis due to oxidation.

Unless perinatal blood loss has been significant, iron deficiency should not be considered as a cause of anemia in term infants in the first 4 mo of life. Assuming an infant is born with adequate iron stores, dietary iron deficiency cannot be a cause of anemia until these iron stores have been exhausted. In the absence of blood loss, this does not occur until the birthweight has approximately doubled.

Treatment. Physiologic anemia requires no therapy other than ensuring that the diet of the infant contains essential nutrients for normal hematopoiesis, especially folic acid and iron. Premature infants who are feeding well and growing normally rarely need transfusion unless iatrogenic blood loss has been significant. In otherwise healthy premature infants, hemoglobin levels as low as 6.5 g/dL are usually well tolerated. However, the optimal level of hematocrit for premature infants is not settled (see Chapter 462). Assessment of the overall clinical condition, including growth rate, and monitoring of hematocrit are the best guides to transfusion of RBCs. RBC transfusions do not appear to affect the course of apneic spells and bradycardia. When transfusions are necessary, a volume of RBCs of 10–15 mL/kg is recommended. The number of donors for an infant should be minimized. In early preterm infants (<1,250 g), the half-life of transfused RBCs is about 30 days.

Anemia in very-low-birthweight preterm infants may be related to a relative deficiency of EPO, and clinical trials indicate that premature infants who do not have severe illnesses and are treated with recombinant human EPO (rHuEPO) and iron during the first 6 wk of life require fewer transfusions. The optimal timing for initiation of rHuEPO therapy and the optimal dose have yet to be determined. To achieve the best results, supplemental oral iron at a dose of at least 4–6 mg/kg/day needs to be administered. It may be possible to use parenteral iron supplements, particularly in young very-low-birthweight infants who are not able to take oral iron to reduce the need for transfusions. The cost of rHuEPO treatment currently is higher than that of RBC transfusion; however, EPO treatment may have a significant role to play in the management of infants whose parents refuse to allow blood transfusions on religious grounds.

Chapter 446
Megaloblastic Anemias

Megaloblastic anemias have in common certain abnormalities of red blood cell (RBC) morphology and maturation. The RBCs at every stage of development are larger than normal and have an open, finely dispersed nuclear chromatin and an asynchrony between the maturation of nucleus and cytoplasm, with the delay in nuclear progression being more evident with further cell divisions. Giant metamyelocytes and bands are also present in the marrow. All megaloblastic anemias are characterized by ineffective erythropoiesis, a kinetic term that describes active erythropoiesis with premature death of cells, a decreased output of RBC from the marrow, and, consequently, anemia. In the peripheral blood, RBCs are large (increased mean corpuscular volume [MCV]) and frequently oval. Another characteristic is the presence of hypersegmented neutrophils (many neutrophils with more than four to five lobes). Almost all cases of childhood megaloblastic anemia result from a deficiency of folic acid or vitamin B_{12}; rarely, they are caused by inborn errors of metabolism. Both vitamin B_{12} and folate are cofactors required in the synthesis of nucleoproteins, and deficiencies result in defective synthesis of DNA and, to a lesser extent, RNA and protein. Megaloblastic anemias resulting from malnutrition are relatively uncommon in the United States but important worldwide (see Chapters 4 and 42).

446.1 Folic Acid Deficiency

Folates are abundant in many foods, including green vegetables, fruits, and animal organs (liver, kidney). Folates are heat labile and water soluble, and consequently boiling or heating folate sources will lead to decreased amounts of vitamin. Naturally occurring folates are in a polyglutamated form and are absorbed less efficiently than the monoglutamate species (folic acid). Folate conjugase activity in the intestinal brush border aids the conversion of polyglutamates to the monoglutamate and thereby enhances absorption. Folic acid is absorbed throughout the small intestine, and there is an active enterohepatic circulation. Much of the folate in plasma is loosely bound to albumin. Folic acid is not biologically active. It is reduced by dihydrofolate reductase to tetrahydrofolate, which is transported into tissue cells and polyglutamated. Body stores of folate are limited, and megaloblastic anemia occurs after 2–3 mo on a folate-free diet.

Clinical Manifestations. Mild megaloblastic anemia has been reported in very-low-birthweight infants, and routine folic acid supplementation is advised. Megaloblastic anemia has its peak incidence at 4–7 mo of age, somewhat earlier than iron deficiency anemia, although the two may be present concomitantly in infants with poor nutrition. Besides having the usual clinical features of anemia, affected infants with folate deficiency are irritable, fail to gain weight adequately, and have chronic diarrhea.

Hemorrhages from thrombocytopenia occur in advanced cases. In older children with folate deficiency the signs and symptoms are related to anemia and to any underlying pathologic process responsible for the vitamin deficiency. Folic acid deficiency may accompany kwashiorkor, marasmus, or sprue.

Etiology. Folic acid deficiency can occur as a consequence of inadequate folate intake, decreased folate absorption, or acquired and congenital disorders of folate metabolism.

INADEQUATE FOLATE INTAKE. Anemia due to decreased folate intake usually becomes manifest under clinical conditions where there are increased vitamin requirements (pregnancy, growth in infancy, chronic hemolysis). The normal infant daily requirement is 25–35 μg/day. The requirements on a weight basis are higher in children than adults, owing to the increased needs of growth. Human breast milk, pasteurized cow's milk, and infant formulas provide adequate amounts of folic acid. Goat's milk is deficient; folic acid supplementation must be given when it is the main food. Unless supplemented, powdered milk may also be a poor source of folic acid.

Folate requirements increase markedly during pregnancy, in part to meet fetal needs. Decreases in serum and RBC folate levels occur in as many as 25% of pregnant women at term and may be aggravated by infection. Folate supplementation of at least 400 μg/day is recommended from the start of pregnancy to prevent neural tube defects and to meet growth needs. Mothers with folate deficiency may have infants with normal folate stores, owing to selective transfer of folate to the fetus via placental folate receptors.

DECREASED FOLATE ABSORPTION. Malabsorption due to chronic diarrheal states or diffuse inflammatory disease can lead to folate deficiency. Megaloblastic anemia due to folic acid deficiency occurs in celiac disease, chronic infectious enteritis, and in association with enteroenteric fistulas. With both inflammatory bowel disease and diarrhea some of the decreased folate absorption may be caused by impaired folate conjugase. Chronic diarrhea also interferes with the enterohepatic circulation of folate, thereby enhancing folate losses because of rapid intestinal passage. Previous intestinal surgery also can be a cause of decreased folate absorption.

Certain anticonvulsant drugs (e.g., phenytoin, primidone, phenobarbital) can impair absorption of folic acid, and many treated patients have low serum levels of folic acid. Frank megaloblastic anemia is rare, however, and responds to folic acid therapy even if administration of the offending drug is continued.

CONGENITAL ABNORMALITIES IN FOLATE METABOLISM. Megaloblastic anemia resulting from congenital dihydrofolate reductase deficiency has been reported in several patients who were unable to form biologically active tetrahydrofolate and who developed severe megaloblastic anemia in early infancy. These patients were successfully treated with large doses of folic acid or folinic acid. Deficiency of methylene tetrahydrofolate reductase has been described in some patients with homocystinuria without hematologic abnormalities.

DRUG-INDUCED ABNORMALITIES IN FOLATE METABOLISM. A number of drugs have anti–folic acid activity as their primary pharmacologic effect and regularly produce megaloblastic anemia. Methotrexate binds to dihydrofolate reductase and prevents formation of tetrahydrofolate, the active form. Pyrimethamine, used in the therapy of toxoplasmosis, and trimethoprim, used for treatment of various infections, may induce folic acid deficiency and, occasionally, megaloblastic anemia. Therapy with folinic acid (5-formyltetrahydrofolate) is usually beneficial.

Laboratory Findings. The anemia is macrocytic (mean corpuscular volume > 100 fL). Variations in RBC shape and size are common (see Fig. 439–1B). The reticulocyte count is low, and nucleated RBCs demonstrating megaloblastic morphology are often seen in the blood. Neutropenia and thrombocytopenia may be present, particularly in patients with long-standing deficiencies. The neutrophils are large, some with hypersegmented nuclei. Normal serum folic acid levels are 5–20 ng/mL; with deficiency, levels are less than 3 ng/mL. Levels of RBC folate are a better indicator of chronic deficiency. The normal RBC folate level is 150–600 ng/mL of packed cells. Levels of iron and vitamin B$_{12}$ in serum are usually normal or elevated. Serum activity of lactate dehydrogenase (LDH) is markedly elevated. The bone marrow is hypercellular because of erythroid hyperplasia. Megaloblastic changes are prominent, although some normal RBC precursors may also be found. Large, abnormal neutrophilic forms (giant metamyelocytes) with cytoplasmic vacuolation are seen, as well as hypersegmentation of the nuclei of megakaryocytes.

Treatment. When the diagnosis of folate deficiency is established, folic acid may be administered orally or parenterally in a dose of 0.5–1 mg/day. If the specific diagnosis is in doubt, smaller doses of folate (0.1 mg/day) may be used for a week as a diagnostic test, because a hematologic response can be expected within 72 hr. Larger doses of folate (greater than 0.1 mg) can correct the anemia of vitamin B$_{12}$ deficiency but may aggravate any associated neurologic abnormalities. In most medical settings in developed countries, this therapeutic trial to distinguish the different causes of megaloblastic anemia rarely is necessary because vitamin B$_{12}$ and folate blood levels usually are readily available. Transfusions are indicated only when the anemia is severe or the child is very ill. Folic acid therapy (0.5–1.0 mg/day) should be continued for 3–4 wk until a definite hematologic response has occurred. Maintenance therapy with a multivitamin (containing 0.2 mg folate) is adequate.

446.2 Vitamin B$_{12}$ (Cobalamin) Deficiency

Vitamin B$_{12}$ is derived from cobalamin in food (mainly animal sources) secondary to production by microorganisms. Humans cannot synthesize vitamin B$_{12}$. The cobalamins are released in the acidity of the stomach and combine there with R proteins and intrinsic factor (IF), traverse the duodenum, where pancreatic proteases break down the R proteins, and are absorbed in the distal ileum via specific receptors for IF-cobalamin. In addition, some vitamin B$_{12}$ from large doses may diffuse through mucosa in the intestine and mouth. In the plasma, cobalamin binds to a transport protein, transcobalamin II (TC-II), which carries the vitamin B$_{12}$ to the liver, bone marrow, and other tissue storage sites. TC-II enters cells by receptor-mediated endocytosis, and cobalamin is converted to active forms (methylcobalamin and adenosylcobalamin) important in the transfer of methyl groups and DNA synthesis. Plasma also contains two other vitamin B$_{12}$–binding proteins, transcobalamin I and III (TC-I and TC-III). These latter two forms of transcobalamin have no specific transport role but are known to reflect vitamin B$_{12}$ tissue stores. In fact, almost all vitamin B$_{12}$ in plasma is bound to TC-I and TC-III and thus the measurement of serum B$_{12}$ concentration reflects the storage of this vitamin. In contrast to folate stores, older children and adults have sufficient vitamin B$_{12}$ stores to last 3–5 yr. However, in young infants born to mothers with low vitamin B$_{12}$ stores, clinical signs of cobalamin deficiency can become apparent in the first 4–5 mo of life.

Etiology. Vitamin B$_{12}$ deficiency may result from inadequate dietary intake of vitamin, lack of IF secretion by the stomach, impaired intestinal absorption of IF-cobalamin, or absence of vitamin B$_{12}$ transport protein.

INADEQUATE VITAMIN B$_{12}$ INTAKE. Because vitamin B$_{12}$ is present in many foods, dietary deficiency is rare. It may occur in cases of extreme dietary restriction (strict vegetarians or vegans) in which no animal products are consumed. Vitamin B$_{12}$ deficiency is not common in kwashiorkor or infantile marasmus. In children, megaloblastic anemia from inadequate intake of vitamin B$_{12}$ occurs in breast-fed infants whose mothers are vegans or themselves have pernicious anemia. Maternal pernicious anemia may be manifest by reduced serum vitamin B$_{12}$ with or without macrocytic anemia in the mother. This cause of childhood megaloblastic anemia often appears in the first year of life.

LACK OF INTRINSIC FACTOR. *Congenital pernicious anemia* is a rare autosomal recessive disorder due to an inability to secrete gastric IF or secretion of functionally abnormal IF. It differs from the typical disease in adults in that the stomach secretes acid normally and is histologically normal. There are no antibodies to parietal cells and no associated endocrine disorders. The symptoms of juvenile pernicious anemia become prominent at around 1 yr of age. This interval is consistent with exhaustion of the stores of vitamin B$_{12}$ acquired in utero. As the anemia becomes severe, weakness, irritability, anorexia, and listlessness occur. The tongue is smooth, red, and painful. Neurologic manifestations include ataxia, paresthesias, hyporeflexia, Babinski responses, and clonus. *Juvenile pernicious anemia* is another rare disorder occurring in older children. It is an immunologic disorder akin to adult-type pernicious anemia. There may be atrophy of the gastric mucosa, achlorhydria, and antibodies in serum against IF and parietal cells. These children may have additional immunologic abnormalities, cutaneous candidiasis, hypoparathyroidism, and other endocrine deficiencies. An abnormal Schilling result is corrected by addition of exogenous IF. Parenteral vitamin B$_{12}$ should be administered regularly to these patients. *Gastric surgery* can lead to intrinsic factor deficiency, and susceptible individuals need lifelong parenteral vitamin B$_{12}$ supplementation.

IMPAIRED VITAMIN B$_{12}$ ABSORPTION. Patients with inflammatory diseases such as regional enteritis or neonatal necrotizing enterocolitis may have impaired absorption of vitamin B$_{12}$. When the terminal ileum has been surgically removed, lifelong parenteral administration should be used if there is evidence that vitamin B$_{12}$ is not absorbed. An overgrowth of intestinal bacteria within diverticula or duplications of the small intestine may cause vitamin B$_{12}$ deficiency by consumption of or competition for the vitamin or by splitting of its complex with IF. In these cases, hematologic response may follow appropriate antibiotic therapy. Similar mechanisms may operate when the fish tapeworm *Diphyllobothrium latum* infests the upper small intestine. When megaloblastic anemia occurs in these situations, the serum vitamin B$_{12}$ level is low, the gastric juice contains intrinsic factor, and the abnormal Schilling test result is not corrected by addition of exogenous IF.

Rare cases have been reported of familial occurrence of absence or defect of the receptor for IF-B$_{12}$ in the terminal ileum, in some instances associated with proteinuria *(Imerslund-Grasbeck syndrome)*. Decreased receptor activity may be detected in the urine of affected patients by a radioisotope binding assay. Histology of the stomach is normal, and IF and acid are present in gastric secretions. This autosomal recessive disorder is caused by defects in the *CUBN* gene on chromosome 10p12.1, resulting in decreased expression of the IF-B$_{12}$ receptor cubilin. Parenteral treatment with vitamin B$_{12}$ monthly corrects the deficiency.

ABSENCE OF VITAMIN B$_{12}$ TRANSPORT PROTEIN. Transcobalamin II (TC-II) deficiency is a rare cause of megaloblastic anemia due to decreased utilization of cobalamin. TC-II is the principal physiologic transport vehicle for vitamin B$_{12}$. The role of TC-II in B$_{12}$ transport is similar to that of transferrin (Tf) for iron; specific receptors for TC-II and Tf exist on cells needing vitamin B$_{12}$ or iron. A congenital deficiency is inherited as an autosomal recessive condition, with failure to absorb and transport vitamin B_{12}. Most patients lack TC-II, but some have functionally defective forms. Serum vitamin B_{12} levels are normal because the storage forms of cobalamin, TC-I and TC-III, are not affected. This disorder usually manifests in the first weeks of life. Characteristically, there is failure to thrive, diarrhea, vomiting, glossitis, neurologic abnormalities, and megaloblastic anemia. The diagnosis of this disorder is suggested by the presence of severe megaloblastic anemia with normal serum vitamin B_{12} and folate levels and no evidence of any other inborn errors of metabolism. The diagnosis is made by specific tests for TC-II. The serum vitamin B_{12} levels must be kept high to utilize cobalamin. Hence, the therapy for this disorder is large parenteral doses of vitamin B_{12} given twice a week for life. These frequent and large doses of cobalamin appear to overcome the transport deficiency. Most children with this disorder die if treatment is not provided in infancy.

Clinical Manifestations. Children with cobalamin deficiency often present with nonspecific manifestations such as weakness, fatigue, failure to thrive, or irritability. Other common findings include pallor, glossitis, vomiting, diarrhea, and icterus. Neurologic symptoms also occur, and these include paresthesias, sensory deficits, hypotonia, seizures, developmental delay, developmental regression, and neuropsychiatric changes. Neurologic problems from vitamin B_{12} deficiency can occur in the absence of any hematologic abnormalities.

Laboratory Findings. The hematologic manifestations of folate and cobalamin deficiency are identical. The anemia resulting from cobalamin deficiency is macrocytic, with prominent macroovalocytosis of the RBCs (see Fig. 439–1B). The neutrophils may be large and hypersegmented. In advanced cases, neutropenia and thrombocytopenia, simulating aplastic anemia or leukemia, occur. Serum vitamin B_{12} levels are less than 100 pg/mL. Concentrations of serum iron and serum folic acid are normal or elevated. Serum LDH activity is markedly increased, a reflection of the ineffective erythropoiesis. Moderate elevations (2–3 mg/dL) of serum bilirubin levels also may be found. Excessive excretion of methylmalonic acid in the urine (normal amount, 0–3.5 mg/24 hr) is a reliable and sensitive index of vitamin B_{12} deficiency.

Diagnosis. The specific cause of vitamin B_{12} often is apparent from the clinical history. In cases where there is a reasonable explanation for decreased vitamin B_{12} absorption (previous gastric or ileal surgery) it may be reasonable to start appropriate therapy without further evaluation. In very young children in whom dietary insufficiency may be a factor, evaluation of the mother for anemia and serum vitamin B_{12} often is rewarding. If there is no obvious cause for decreased serum vitamin B_{12}, absorption of vitamin B_{12} is usually assessed by the **Schilling test.** When a normal person ingests a small amount of vitamin B_{12} into which ^{57}Co has been incorporated, the radioactive vitamin combines with the IF in stomach secretions and passes to the terminal ileum, where absorption occurs. Because the absorbed vitamin is bound to TC-II and incorporated into tissues, little or none is normally excreted in the urine. If a large dose (1 mg) of nonradioactive vitamin B_{12} is injected parenterally after 2 hr ("flushing dose"), 10–30% of the previously absorbed radioactive vitamin appears in the urine in 24 hr. Children with pernicious anemia usually excrete 2% or less under these conditions. To confirm that absence of IF is the basis of the vitamin B_{12} malabsorption, 30 mg of IF is given with a second dose of radioactive vitamin B_{12}. Normal amounts of radioactive vitamin should now be absorbed and flushed out in the urine. On the other hand, when vitamin B_{12} malabsorption results from absence of ileal receptor sites or other intestinal causes, no improvement in absorption occurs with IF. The

Schilling test result remains abnormal in patients with pernicious anemia, even when therapy has completely reversed the hematologic and neurologic manifestations of the disease.

Treatment. A prompt hematologic response follows parenteral administration of vitamin B_{12} (1 mg), usually with reticulocytosis in 2–4 days, unless there is concurrent inflammatory disease. The physiologic requirement for vitamin B_{12} is 1–5 µg/day, and hematologic responses have been observed with these small doses, indicating that administration of a minidose may be used as a therapeutic test when the diagnosis of vitamin B_{12} deficiency is in doubt. If there is evidence of neurologic involvement, 1 mg should be injected intramuscularly daily for at least 2 wk. Maintenance therapy is necessary throughout a patient's life; monthly intramuscular administration of 1 mg of vitamin B_{12} is sufficient. Oral therapy may succeed because of mucosal diffusion with high doses, but it is not generally advisable, owing to uncertainty of absorption.

446.3 Other Rare Megaloblastic Anemias

Oroticaciduria is a rare autosomal recessive disorder that usually appears in the first year of life and is characterized by growth failure, developmental retardation, megaloblastic anemia, and increased urinary excretion of orotic acid (see Chapter 78). This defect, the most common metabolic error in the de novo synthesis of pyrimidines, therefore affects nucleic acid synthesis. The usual form of hereditary orotic aciduria is caused by a deficiency (in all body tissues) of both orotic phosphoribosyl transferase (OPT) and orotidine-5-phosphate decarboxylase (ODC), two sequential enzymatic steps in pyrimidine nucleotide synthesis. The diagnosis of this disorder is suggested by the presence of severe megaloblastic anemia with normal serum B_{12} and folate levels and no evidence of TC-II deficiency. A presumptive diagnosis is made by finding increased urinary orotic acid. Confirmation of the diagnosis, however, requires assay of the transferase and decarboxylase enzymes in the patient's erythrocytes. Physical and mental retardation are frequently present. The anemia is refractory to vitamin B_{12} or folic acid but responds promptly to administration of the pyrimidine uridine (100–150 µg/kg/24 hr). Megaloblastic anemia can also occur in the *Lesch-Nyhan syndrome*, in which regeneration of purine nucleotides is blocked (see Chapter 78).

Thiamine-responsive megaloblastic anemia (TRMA) is a syndrome characterized by megaloblastic anemia, sensorineural deafness, diabetes mellitus, and, occasionally, cardiomyopathy and optic nerve atrophy. It previously had been observed that the megaloblastic anemia in some patients responded to high doses of thiamine. It now is known that the defect in this disorder is due to an abnormality in a thiamine transport gene located on chromosome 1. This is an autosomal recessive disorder presenting in childhood and occurring in several ethnically distinct populations.

Deficiency of adenosylcobalamin and methylcobalamin along with megaloblastic anemia has been encountered in a few children with inability to convert cobalamin to its biologically active metabolites. These disorders are characterized by neurologic abnormalities and either methylmalonic aciduria, homocystinuria, or both. Abnormalities are usually noted in the early weeks of life and include failure to thrive, lethargy, hypotonia, macrocytosis with megaloblastic bone marrow changes and anemia or pancytopenia, and hepatic dysfunction. The megaloblastic changes may reverse and other symptoms may improve with hydroxycobalamin treatment, 1 mg/24 hr IM initially, gradually changed to a dose two to three times per week, then once a month.

Chapter 447
Iron-Deficiency Anemia

Anemia resulting from lack of sufficient iron for synthesis of hemoglobin is the most common hematologic disease of infancy and childhood. Its frequency is related to certain basic aspects of iron metabolism and nutrition. The body of a newborn infant contains about 0.5 g of iron, whereas the adult content is estimated at 5 g. To make up for this discrepancy, an average of 0.8 mg of iron must be absorbed each day during the first 15 yr of life. In addition to this growth requirement, a small amount is necessary to balance normal losses of iron by shedding of cells. Accordingly, to maintain positive iron balance in childhood, about 1 mg of iron must be absorbed each day.

Iron is absorbed in the proximal small intestine, mediated in part by a variety of duodenal proteins. Because absorption of dietary iron is assumed to be about 10%, a diet containing 8–10 mg of iron daily is necessary for optimal nutrition. Iron is absorbed two to three times more efficiently from human milk than from cow's milk, perhaps partly because of differences in calcium content. Breast-fed infants may, therefore, require less iron from other foods. During the first years of life, because relatively small quantities of iron-rich foods are eaten, it is often difficult to attain sufficient iron. For this reason, the diet should include such foods as infant cereals or formulas that have been fortified with iron; both of these are very effective in preventing iron deficiency. Formulas with 7–12 mg Fe/L for full-term infants and premature infant formulas with 15 mg/L for infants less than 1,800 g at birth are effective. Infants breast-fed exclusively should receive iron supplementation from 4 mo of age. At best, an infant is in a precarious situation with respect to iron. Should the diet become inadequate or external blood loss occur, anemia ensues rapidly.

Adolescents are also susceptible to iron deficiency because of high requirements due to the growth spurt, dietary deficiencies, and menstrual blood loss. In the United States, about 9% of 1–2 yr-old children are iron deficient; 3% have anemia. Of adolescent girls, 9% are iron deficient and 2% have anemia. In boys, a 50% decrease in stored iron occurs as puberty progresses.

Etiology. Low birthweight and unusual perinatal hemorrhage are associated with decreases in neonatal hemoglobin mass and stores of iron. As the high hemoglobin concentration of the newborn infant falls during the first 2–3 mo of life, considerable iron is reclaimed and stored. These reclaimed stores are usually sufficient for blood formation in the first 6–9 mo of life in term infants. In low-birthweight infants or those with perinatal blood loss, stored iron may be depleted earlier and dietary sources become of paramount importance. In term infants, anemia caused solely by inadequate dietary iron is unusual before 6 mo and usually occurs at 9–24 mo of age. Thereafter, it is relatively infrequent. The usual dietary pattern observed in infants with iron-deficiency anemia is consumption of large amounts of cow's milk and of foods not supplemented with iron.

Blood loss must be considered a possible cause in every case of iron-deficiency anemia, particularly in older children. Chronic iron-deficiency anemia from occult bleeding may be caused by a lesion of the gastrointestinal tract, such as a peptic ulcer, Meckel diverticulum, polyp, or hemangioma, or by inflammatory bowel disease. In some geographic areas, hookworm infestation is an important cause of iron deficiency. Pulmonary hemosiderosis may be associated with unrecognized bleeding in the lungs and recurrent iron deficiency after treatment with iron. Chronic diarrhea in early childhood may be associated with considerable unrecognized blood loss. Some infants with severe iron deficiency in the United States have chronic intestinal blood loss induced by exposure to a heat-labile protein in whole cow's milk. Loss of blood in the stools each day can be prevented either by reducing the quantity of whole cow's milk to 1 pint/24 hr or less, by using heated or evaporated milk, or by feeding a milk substitute. This gastrointestinal reaction is not related to enzymatic abnormalities in the mucosa, such as lactase deficiency, or to typical "milk allergy." Involved infants characteristically develop anemia that is more severe and occurs earlier than would be expected simply from an inadequate intake of iron.

Histologic abnormalities of the mucosa of the gastrointestinal tract, such as blunting of the villi, are present in advanced iron-deficiency anemia and may cause leakage of blood and decreased absorption of iron, further compounding the problem.

Intense exercise conditioning, as occurs in competitive athletics in high school, may result in iron depletion in girls; this occurs less commonly in boys.

Clinical Manifestations. Pallor is the most important sign of iron deficiency. In mild to moderate iron deficiency (hemoglobin levels of 6–10 g/dL), compensatory mechanisms, including increased levels of 2,3-diphosphoglycerate (2,3-DPG) and a shift of the oxygen dissociation curve, may be so effective that few symptoms of anemia are noted, although affected children may be irritable. Pagophagia, the desire to ingest unusual substances such as ice or dirt, may be present. In some children, ingestion of lead-containing substances may lead to concomitant plumbism. When the hemoglobin level falls below 5 g/dL, irritability and anorexia are prominent. Tachycardia and cardiac dilation occur, and systolic murmurs are often present.

Children with iron deficiency anemia may be obese or may be underweight, with other evidence of poor nutrition. The irritability and anorexia characteristic of advanced cases may reflect deficiency in tissue iron, because with iron therapy striking improvement in behavior frequently occurs before significant hematologic improvement is noted.

Iron deficiency may have effects on neurologic and intellectual function. A number of reports suggest that iron-deficiency anemia, and even iron deficiency without significant anemia, affects attention span, alertness, and learning of both infants and adolescents. In a controlled trial, adolescent girls with serum ferritin levels of 12 ng/L or less but without anemia had improved verbal learning and memory after taking iron for 8 wk.

Some of the clinical manifestations may be related to the role of iron in certain enzymatic reactions. Monoamine oxidase (MAO), an iron-dependent enzyme, has a crucial role in neurochemical reactions in the central nervous system. Iron deficiency produces decreases in the activities of enzymes such as catalase and cytochromes. Catalase and peroxidase contain iron, but their biologic essentiality is not well established. Administration of iron may decrease the frequency of breath-holding spells, suggesting a role for iron deficiency or anemia.

Laboratory Findings. In progressive iron deficiency, a sequence of biochemical and hematologic events occurs. First, the tissue iron stores represented by bone marrow hemosiderin disappear. The level of serum ferritin, an iron-storage protein, provides a relatively accurate estimate of body iron stores in the absence of inflammatory disease. Normal ranges are age dependent, and decreased levels accompany iron deficiency. Next, serum iron level decreases (also age dependent), the iron-binding capacity of the serum (serum transferrin) increases, and the percent saturation (transferrin saturation) falls below normal. When the availability of iron becomes rate limiting for hemoglobin synthesis, free erythrocyte protoporphyrins (FEP) accumulates.

As the deficiency progresses, the red blood cells (RBCs) become smaller than normal and their hemoglobin content decreases. The morphologic characteristics of RBCs are best quantified by the determination of mean corpuscular hemoglobin

(MCH) and mean corpuscular volume (MCV). Developmental changes in MCV require the use of age-related standards for diagnosis of microcytosis (see Table 439–1). With increasing deficiency, the RBCs become deformed and misshapen and present characteristic microcytosis, hypochromia, poikilocytosis, and increased RBC distribution width (RDW) (see Fig. 439–1*C*). The reticulocyte percentage may be normal or moderately elevated, but absolute reticulocyte counts indicate an insufficient response to anemia. Nucleated RBCs occasionally are seen in the peripheral blood if the anemia is severe. White blood cell counts are normal. Sometimes there is a striking thrombocytosis (600,000–1 million/mm^3). Just as in the case of transient erythroblastopenia of childhood, thrombocytosis presumably is caused by increased erythropoietin, which is known to have some structural homology with thrombopoietin. However, it should also be noted that very severe iron-deficiency anemia occasionally may be associated with thrombocytopenia, and this can confuse the diagnosis with other bone marrow failure disorders. The bone marrow is hypercellular, with erythroid hyperplasia. The normoblasts may have scanty, fragmented cytoplasm with poor hemoglobination. Leukocytes and megakaryocytes are normal. There is no stainable iron in marrow reticulum cells. In about a third of cases, occult blood can be detected in the stools.

Differential Diagnosis. Iron deficiency must be differentiated from other hypochromic microcytic anemias. The most common scenario is the need to distinguish iron deficiency from α– and β–thalassemia trait and other hemoglobinopathies, particularly those related to hemoglobin E (see Chapter 454). A simple distinguishing feature of the latter conditions is that the RBC count often is elevated above normal despite the presence of a mild anemia and microcytosis; and this is in marked contrast to iron deficiency in which the RBC count decreases along with the reduced hemoglobin and MCV. Another difference between α– and β–thalassemia trait and iron deficiency is that the RDW is elevated in iron deficiency.

β-Thalassemia trait occurs in people from the Mediterranean area, Africa, and Asia. It is a mild microcytic anemia characterized by elevated levels of hemoglobin A$_2$ and/or increased fetal hemoglobin concentration; serum iron, total iron-binding capacity (transferrin), and ferritin are normal; and no abnormal hemoglobin is seen on electrophoresis. *Homozygous β-thalassemia (or thalassemia major)*, with its pronounced erythroblastosis and severe hemolytic component, should present no diagnostic confusion.

α-Thalassemia trait occurs in blacks, Chinese, and Southeast Asians. This mild microcytic disorder is caused by a deletion of two of four genes that regulate α-globin production. In the usual clinical setting the diagnosis of α-thalassemia trait can be assumed when a patient with a familial hypochromic microcytic anemia has normal results of iron studies (including ferritin), normal levels of Hb A2 and Hb F, and a normal hemoglobin electrophoresis. It is a diagnosis of exclusion except in the newborn period when infants with α-thalassemia trait have 3–10% hemoglobin Barts (γ$_4$) (see Chapter 454). A specific diagnosis for α-thalassemia disorders is possible using molecular diagnostic strategies, which are also important for prenatal diagnosis.

Hb H disease, another form of α-thalassemia results from deletion of three of the four α-globin genes. It also is characterized by hypochromia and microcytosis, but in addition there is a mild hemolytic component from instability of the β-chain tetramers (Hb H) resulting from a deficiency of α-globin chains. Beyond infancy, Hb H is readily identified by hemoglobin electrophoresis. During the newborn period, the moderately severe α-globin deficiency allows for the accumulation of more γ chains and the concentration of hemoglobin Barts is over 20%.

The *anemia of chronic disease (ACD)* and infection is usually normocytic, although occasionally it may be slightly microcytic. In contrast to iron-deficiency anemia, in these inflammatory conditions both the serum iron level and iron-binding capacity (transferrin) are reduced and serum ferritin levels are normal or elevated. The serum transferrin receptor (TfR) level is useful in the distinction between iron-deficiency anemia and anemia of chronic disease because it is not affected by inflammation. The concentration of TfR is elevated in iron deficiency and is within the normal range in anemia of chronic disease. An elevation of the TfR/log ferritin ratio is especially sensitive in detecting iron-deficiency anemia.

Lead poisoning and iron-deficiency anemia both are associated with elevations of FEP. In cases of lead poisoning associated with iron deficiency, the RBCs are morphologically similar but coarse basophilic stippling of the RBCs is frequently prominent. Elevations of blood lead, FEP, and urinary coproporphyrin levels are seen (see Chapter 703).

Treatment. The regular response of iron-deficiency anemia to adequate amounts of iron is an important diagnostic and therapeutic feature. Oral administration of simple ferrous salts (sulfate, gluconate, fumarate) provides inexpensive and satisfactory therapy. No evidence shows that addition of any trace metal, vitamin, or other hematinic substance significantly increases the response to simple ferrous salts. The therapeutic dose should be calculated in terms of elemental iron; ferrous sulfate is 20% elemental iron by weight. A daily total of 4–6 mg/kg of elemental iron in three divided doses provides an optimal amount of iron for the stimulated bone marrow to use. Intolerance to oral iron is uncommon in young children, although older children and adolescents sometimes have gastrointestinal complaints. A parenteral iron preparation (iron dextran) is an effective form of iron and is usually safe when given in a properly calculated dose, but the response to parenteral iron is no more rapid or complete than that obtained with proper oral administration of iron, unless malabsorption is a factor.

While adequate iron medication is given, the family must be educated about the patient's diet, and the consumption of milk should be limited to a reasonable quantity, preferably 500 mL (1 pint)/24 hr or less. This reduction has a dual effect: The amount of iron-rich foods is increased, and blood loss from intolerance to cow's milk proteins is reduced. When the re-education of child and parent is not successful, parenteral iron medication may be indicated. Iron deficiency can be prevented in high-risk populations by providing iron-fortified formula or cereals during infancy.

Within 72–96 hr after administration of iron to an anemic child, peripheral reticulocytosis is noted (Table 447–1). The height of this response is inversely proportional to the severity of the anemia. Reticulocytosis is followed by a rise in the hemoglobin level, which may increase as much as 0.5 g/dL/24 hr. Iron medication should be continued for 8 wk after blood values are normal. Failures of iron therapy occur when a child does not receive the prescribed medication, when iron is given in a form that is poorly absorbed, or when there is continuing unrecognized blood loss, such as intestinal or pulmonary loss, or loss with menstrual periods. An incorrect original diagnosis of nutritional iron deficiency may be revealed by therapeutic failure of iron medication.

Because a rapid hematologic response can be confidently predicted in typical iron deficiency, blood transfusion is indicated only when the anemia is very severe or when superimposed infection may interfere with the response. It is not necessary to attempt rapid correction of severe anemia by transfusion; the procedure may be dangerous because of associated hypervolemia and cardiac dilatation. Packed or sedimented RBCs should be administered slowly in an amount sufficient to raise the hemoglobin to a safe level at which the response to iron therapy can be awaited. In general, severely anemic children with hemoglobin values less than 4 g/dL should be given only

TABLE 447–1. Responses to Iron Therapy in Iron-Deficiency Anemia

Time After Iron Administration	Response
12–24 hr	Replacement of intracellular iron enzymes; subjective improvement; decreased irritability; increased appetite
36–48 hr	Initial bone marrow response; erythroid hyperplasia
48–72 hr	Reticulocytosis, peaking at 5–7 days
4–30 days	Increase in hemoglobin level
1–3 mo	Repletion of stores

2–3 mL/kg of packed cells at any one time (furosemide may also be administered as a diuretic). If there is evidence of frank congestive heart failure, a modified exchange transfusion using fresh-packed RBCs should be considered, although diuretics followed by slow infusion of packed RBCs may suffice.

Chapter 448
Other Microcytic Anemias

Sideroblastic Anemias. Sideroblastic anemias result from acquired and hereditary disorders of heme synthesis. The anemias are characterized by hypochromic microcytic red blood cells (RBCs) mixed with normal RBCs, thus giving an overall picture of a dimorphic population of erythrocytes, and the complete blood cell count indicates an extremely high RBC distribution width (RDW). The serum iron concentration usually is elevated, and the transferrin saturation of iron is increased. In all cases of sideroblastic anemia, regardless of the specific cause, impaired heme synthesis leads to retention of iron within the mitochondria. Morphologically, this is seen in marrow nucleated RBCs with iron granules (i.e., aggregates of iron in mitochondria) that have a perinuclear distribution. These unusual cells, known as ringed sideroblasts, are found only in pathologic states and are distinct from the sideroblasts in the marrows of normal subjects (i.e., RBC precursors that contain diffused cytoplasmic ferritin granules). Sideroblastic anemias most commonly occur in adulthood, and these acquired disorders can be idiopathic or secondary to drugs, alcohol, or myelodysplastic disorders. A few sideroblastic anemias are seen in children.

CONGENITAL SIDEROBLASTIC ANEMIA. This rare sideroblastic anemia usually conforms to an X-linked pattern of inheritance, and it usually occurs in males, although skewed lyonization has resulted in affected females. Autosomal dominant and sporadic cases also occur. Hereditary sideroblastic anemias result from abnormalities of the erythrocytic isozyme for 5-aminolevulinic acid synthetase (ALAS), the rate-limiting enzyme reaction in heme synthesis. An important cofactor for ALAS is pyridoxal phosphate. The gene for the erythrocyte-specific ALAS (ALAS2) is located on the X chromosome, and over 20 different missense mutations have been identified. Several of these mutations occur near the binding site for pyridoxal phosphate.

Severe anemias are recognized in infancy or early childhood whereas milder cases may not become apparent until early adulthood or later. Clinical findings include pallor, icterus, and moderate splenomegaly and/or hepatomegaly. The severity of the anemia varies such that some patients require no therapy while others need regular RBC transfusions. A subset of patients with hereditary sideroblastic anemia manifest a hematologic response to pharmacologic doses of pyridoxine. Iron overload as manifested by elevated serum ferritin, elevated serum iron, and increased transferrin saturation is a major complication of this disorder. In some cases in which there is little or no anemia there still may be clinical evidence of iron overload (e.g., diabetes mellitus, liver dysfunction). Stem cell transplantation has been utilized for affected children who were RBC transfusion dependent.

A unique variant of congenital sideroblastic anemia is **Pearson's syndrome**, characterized by the early onset of transfusion-dependent anemia, neutropenia, and thrombocytopenia. In addition to the usual marrow abnormalities of sideroblastic anemia, these children also have vacuolization of RBC and myeloid precursors. In contrast to other sideroblastic anemias that are microcytic, this is a macrocytic anemia and, for this reason, it often is sometimes confused with Diamond-Blackfan anemia (see Chapter 440).

Lead Poisoning. See Chapter 703.

Rare Types of Hypochromic Microcytic Anemia. Isolated cases of hypochromic microcytic anemia with other abnormalities of iron metabolism are known; some patients have had defects in iron mobilization or reutilization. *Congenital absence of iron-binding protein* (atransferrinemia) is a very rare disorder associated with severe hypochromic anemia despite iron overload and requires infusions of apo-transferrin and iron chelation therapy, although the latter may be avoided if the transferrin infusions are started early. Iron is absorbed normally and is deposited in the visceral organs rather than in bone marrow.

Several patients have had refractory hypochromic anemia associated with lymphatic tumors or lymphoid hyperplasia. Correction of the anemia followed removal of the abnormal lymphatic tissue in these patients. (See also Chapters 481 and 498.)

General

Greer JP, Foerster J, Lukens J, et al: *Wintrobe's Clinical Hematology,* 11th ed. Baltimore, Williams & Wilkins, in press.

Hoffman R, Benz EJ, Shattil SJ, et al: *Basic Principles and Practice,* 3rd ed. New York, Churchill Livingstone, 2000.

Nathan DG, Orkin SH: *Nathan and Oski's Hematology of Infancy and Childhood,* 5th ed. Philadelphia, WB Saunders, 2002.

Rimoin DL, Connor JM, Pyeritz RE, et al: *Emery and Rimoin's Principles and Practice of Medical Genetics,* 4th ed. London, Churchill Livingstone, 2002.

Pure RBC Anemias

Cherrick I, Karayalcin G, Lanzkowsky P: Transient erythroblastopenia of childhood. *Am J Pediatr Hematol Oncol* 1994;16:320.

Costa LD, Willig TN, Fixler J, et al: Diamond-Blackfan anemia. *Curr Opin Pediatr* 2001;13:10.

Delaunay J, Iolascon A: The congenital dyserythropoietic anaemias. *Baillieres Clin Haematol* 1999;12:691.

Freedman MH: Diamond-Blackfan anaemia. *Baillieres Clin Haematol* 2000;13:391.

Gustavsson P, Willig TN, van Haeringen A, et al: Diamond-Blackfan anaemia: Genetic homogeneity for a gene on chromosome 19q13 restricted to 1.8 Mb. *Nat Genet* 1997;16:368.

Vlachos A, Klein GW, Lipton JM: The Diamond Blackfan anemia registry: Tool for investigating the epidemiology and biology of Diamond-Blackfan anemia. *J Pediatr Hematol Oncol* 2001;23:377.

Willig TN, Niemeyer CM, Leblanc T, et al: Identification of new prognosis factors from the clinical and epidemiologic analysis of a registry of 229 Diamond-Blackfan anemia patients. *Pediatr Res* 1999;46:553.

Anemia of Chronic Disease

Cazzola M, Ponchio L, de Benedetti F, et al: Defective iron supply for erythropoiesis and adequate endogenous erythropoietin production in the anemia associated with systemic-onset juvenile chronic arthritis. *Blood* 1996;87:4824.

Means RT, Krantz SB: Progress in understanding the pathogenesis of the anemia of chronic disease. *Blood* 1992;80:1639.

Physiologic Anemia of Infancy

Bednarek FJ, Weisberger S, Richardson DK, et al: Variations in blood transfusions among newborn intensive care units. *J Pediatr* 1998;133:601.

Fain J, Hilsenrath P, Widness JA, et al: A cost analysis comparing erythropoietin and red cell transfusions in the treatment of anemia of prematurity. *Transfusion* 1995;35:936.

Meyer MP, Haworth C, Meyer JH: A comparison of oral and intravenous iron supplementation in preterm infants receiving recombinant erythropoietin. *J Pediatr* 1996;129:258.

Ohls RK: The use of erythropoietin in neonates. *Clin Perinatol* 2000;27:681.

Megaloblastic Anemias

Monagle PT, Tauro GP: Infantile megaloblastosis secondary to maternal vitamin B$_{12}$ deficiency. *Clin Lab Haematol* 1997;19:23.

Rasmussen SA, Fernhoff PM, Scanlon KS: Vitamin B$_{12}$ deficiency in children and adolescents. *J Pediatr* 2001;138:10.

Rosenblatt DS, Whitehead VM: Cobalamin and folate deficiency: Acquired and hereditary disorders in children. *Semin Hematol* 1999;36:19.

Xu D, Kozyraki R, Newman TC, et al: Genetic evidence of an accessory activity required specifically for cubilin brush-border expression and intrinsic factor-cobalamin absorption. *Blood* 1999;94:3604.

Microcytic Anemia

Andrews N: Disorders of iron metabolism. *N Engl J Med* 1999;341:1986.

Ayas M, Al-Jefri A, Mustafa MM, et al: Congenital sideroblastic anaemia successfully treated using allogeneic stem cell transplantation. *Br J Haematol* 2001;113:938.

Booth IW, Aukett MA: Iron deficiency anaemia in infancy and early childhood. *Arch Dis Child* 1997;76:549.

Bottomley SS: Sideroblastic anemias. In Lee GR, et al (editors): *Wintrobe's Clinical Haematology*, 10th ed. Baltimore, Williams & Wilkins, 1999, pp 1022-45.

Bruner AB, Joffe A, Duggan AK, et al: Randomised study of cognitive effects of iron supplementation in non-anaemic iron-deficient adolescent girls. *Lancet* 1996;348:992.

Centers for Disease Control and Prevention: Recommendations to prevent and control iron deficiency in the United States. *MMWR Morb Mortal Wkly Rep* 1998;47:1.

Fleming MD, Trenor CC III, Su MA, et al: Microcytic anaemia mice have a mutation in *Nramp2*, a candidate iron transporter gene. *Nat Genet* 1997;16:383.

Looker AC, Dallman PR, Caroll MD, et al: Prevalence of iron deficiency in the United States. *JAMA* 1997;277:973.

Lozoff B, Jimenez E, Hagen J, et al: Poorer behavioral and developmental outcome more than 10 years after treatment for iron deficiency in infancy. *Pediatrics* 2000;105:1.

Lozoff B, Wolf AW, Jimenez E: Iron-deficiency anemia and infant development: Effects of extended oral iron therapy. *J Pediatr* 1996;129:382.

Pearson HA: The naming of a syndrome. *J Pediatr Hematol Oncol* 1997;19:271.

Punnonen K, Irjala K, Rajamaki A: Serum transferrin receptor and its ratio to serum ferritin in the diagnosis of iron deficiency. *Blood* 1997;89:1052.

Walter T, Pino P, Pizarro F, et al: Prevention of iron-deficiency anemia: Comparison of high- and low-iron formulas in healthy infants after 6 months of life. *J Pediatr* 1998;132:635.

SECTION 3 *Hemolytic Anemias*

Chapter 449

Definitions and Classification of Hemolytic Anemias *George B. Segel*

Hemolysis is defined as the premature destruction of red blood cells (RBCs). If the rate of destruction exceeds the capacity of the marrow to produce RBCs, anemia results. Normal RBC survival time is 110–120 days (half-life, 55–60 days), and approximately 1% of RBCs (the senescent ones) are removed each day and replaced by the marrow to maintain the RBC count. During hemolysis, RBC survival is shortened and increased marrow activity results in a heightened reticulocyte percentage and number. Hemolysis should be suspected as a cause of anemia if an elevated reticulocyte count is present. The reticulocyte count also may be elevated as a response to acute blood loss or for a short period after replacement therapy for iron, vitamin B$_{12}$, or folate deficiencies. The marrow can increase its output two- to threefold acutely, with a maximum of six- to eightfold if hemolysis is of long standing. The reticulocyte percentage can be corrected to measure the magnitude of the marrow production in response to hemolysis as follows:

$$\text{Reticulocyte index} = \text{reticulocyte } \% \times \frac{\text{observed hematocrit}}{\text{normal hematocrit}} \times \frac{1}{\mu}$$

where μ is a maturation factor related to the severity of the anemia (Fig. 449–1). The normal reticulocyte index is 1.0.

As anemia becomes more severe, there is more erythropoietin stimulation of erythropoiesis, and *reticulocytes* are released from the marrow earlier, spending more than 1 day as reticulocytes in the blood. In terms of measuring the marrow response, it is inappropriate to count reticulocytes produced yesterday in today's calculation of the reticulocyte index. The maturation factor, μ, provides this correction (see Fig. 449–1). The usual marrow response in a chronic hemolytic anemia is reflected by a

MATURATION TIME - DAYS

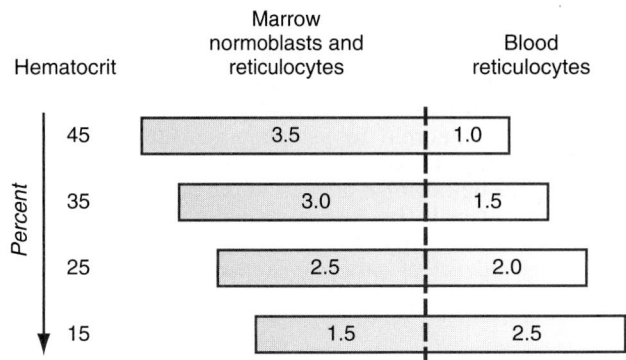

FIGURE 449–1. Number of days for maturation of reticulocytes in the marrow and blood. The duration of maturation as blood reticulocytes is taken as μ. (Modified from Hillman RS, Finch CA: *Red Cell Manual*. Philadelphia, FA Davis, 1983.)

reticulocyte index of 3–4, with a maximum of 6–8 corresponding to maximal marrow output.

The *erythroid hyperplasia* resulting from chronic hemolytic anemia in children, especially thalassemia, may be so extensive that the medullary spaces expand at the expense of the cortical bone. These changes may be evident on physical examination or on radiographs of the skull and long bones (see Fig. 454–3). A propensity to fracture long bones can also occur.

Direct assessment of the severity of hemolysis requires measurement of the RBC survival time using RBCs tagged with the radioisotope Na$_2$^{51}CrO$_4$. The normal value for the ^{51}Cr half-life is 25–35 days. This value is less than the expected half-life of 55–60 days because of the elution of ^{51}Cr from the labeled RBCs at the rate of about 1% per day.

Several other plasma, urinary, or fecal chemical alterations reflect the presence of hemolysis. The exaggerated *degradation of hemoglobin* results in increased biliary excretion of heme pigment derivatives and increased fecal urobilinogen (Fig. 449–2). Gallstones composed of calcium bilirubinate may be formed in children with chronic hemolysis as young as 4 yr of age.

RED CELL DESTRUCTION

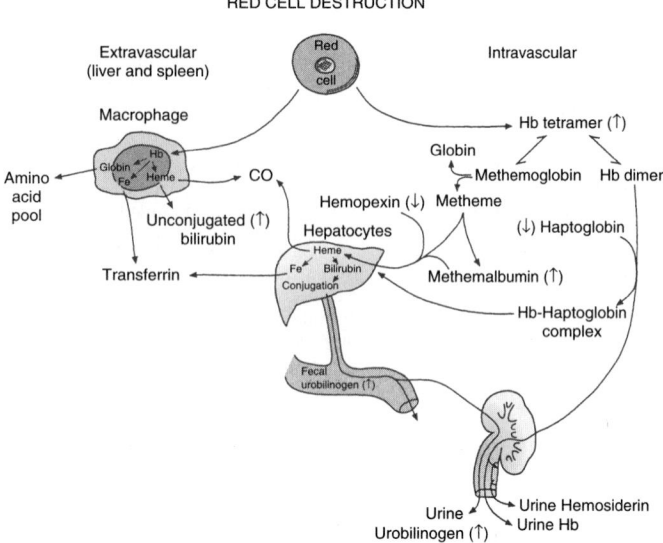

FIGURE 449–2. Red cell destruction and the catabolism of hemoglobin (Hb) based on the description by Hillman and Finch. (From Hillman RS, Finch CA: *Red Cell Manual*. Philadelphia, FA Davis, 1983.)

Elevations of serum unconjugated bilirubin also may accompany hemolysis.

Three heme-binding proteins in the plasma are altered during hemolysis (see Fig. 449–2). Hemoglobin binds to haptoglobin and hemopexin, both of which are cleared more rapidly as conjugates and their plasma concentration is decreased. Oxidized heme binds to albumin to form methemalbumin, which is increased. When the capacity of these binding molecules is exceeded, free hemoglobin appears in the plasma, and the pink color can be seen if the RBCs are sedimented in a capillary hematocrit tube. If present, free hemoglobin in the plasma is prima facie evidence of intravascular hemolysis. Free hemoglobin dissociates into dimers and is filtered by the kidneys. When

the tubular reabsorptive capacity of the kidneys for hemoglobin is exceeded, free hemoglobin appears in the urine. Even in the absence of hemoglobinuria, iron loss may result from reabsorbed hemoglobin and the shedding of renal epithelial cells in which the iron from hemoglobin is stored as hemosiderin. This may lead to secondary iron deficiency during chronic intravascular hemolysis. When hemoglobin is degraded, an α-methene bridge is broken in the cyclic tetrapyrrole of the heme moiety, with release of carbon monoxide (CO) (see Fig. 449–2). The amount of CO in the blood or expired air provides a dynamic measure of the hemolytic rate. End-tidal CO is used as a research tool but is not used in clinical laboratories to measure hemolysis.

The hematocrit during hemolysis is dependent on the severity of the hemolysis and on the marrow response in producing RBCs. The shortened RBC life span and heightened RBC production result in a marked susceptibility to *aplastic* or *hypoplastic crises*, characterized by erythroid marrow failure and reticulocytopenia, accompanied by a rapid further reduction in hemoglobin and hematocrit to extremely low levels. The most common cause of aplastic crises is parvovirus B19, which is erythrocytotropic in marrow culture in vitro (see Chapters 230 and 454). Aplastic crises may produce a precipitous and life-threatening decline in the hematocrit, which usually lasts 10–14 days. Such transient erythroid marrow failure has only a mild effect on persons with a normal RBC life span but has a proportionately greater effect as the RBC life span is shortened by hemolysis. A second infection with parvovirus is uncommon, but other infections may compromise the erythroid marrow output, resulting in various degrees of hypoplasia or hypoplastic crises.

The hemolytic anemias may be classified as either (1) cellular, resulting from intrinsic abnormalities of the membrane, enzymes, or hemoglobin; or (2) extracellular, resulting from antibodies, mechanical factors, or plasma factors. Most of the cellular defects are inherited (paroxysmal nocturnal hemoglobinuria is acquired), and most of the extracellular defects are acquired (abetalipoproteinemia with acanthocytosis is inherited). Table 449–1 shows the most common hemolytic anemias, their underlying defects, the diagnostic laboratory tests, and the current recommendations for treatment.

TABLE 449–1. Hemolytic Anemias and Their Treatment

Diagnosis	Defect	Laboratory Tests	Treatment
Cellular Defects			
Membrane Defects			
Hereditary spherocytosis	Cytoskeletal protein defects Frequently involve vertical interactions of spectrin ankyrin, protein 3	Spherocytes on blood film Negative Coombs test eliminates immune hemolysis Increased incubated osmotic fragility Abnormal cytoskeletal protein analysis	If Hb > 10 g/dL and retic < 10%–none If severe anemia, poor growth, aplastic crises and age < 2 yr–transfusion If Hb < 10 g/dL and retic > 10% or massive spleen-splenectomy, preferably > age 6 yr but earlier if necessary Folic acid, 1 mg qd
Hereditary elliptocytosis	Cytoskeletal protein defects Frequently involve horizontal interactions of spectrin, protein 4.1, glycophorin C	Elliptocytes on blood film RBCs mildly heat sensitive Abnormal cytoskeletal protein analysis	Mild types–no treatment Chronic hemolysis—transfusion and splenectomy as recommended for spherocytosis (above) Folic acid, 1 mg qd
Hereditary pyropoikilocytosis	Cytoskeletal protein defects Homozygous or double heterozygous abnormality in horizontal interactions of α spectrin	Extreme variation in RBC size and shape on blood film Thermal sensitivity-fragmentation at 45°C for 15 min	Transfusion and splenectomy as recommended for spherocytosis (above) Folic acid 1 mg qd
Hereditary stomatocytosis	Cytoskeletal protein defects Decreased protein 7.2b (one subset) Abnormal RBC cation and water content	Stomatocytes on blood film	Splenectomy should be avoided (see text) Folic acid 1 mg qd

Continued

TABLE 449–1. Hemolytic Anemias and Their Treatment *Continued*

Diagnosis	Defect	Laboratory Tests	Treatment
Paroxysmal nocturnal hemoglobinuria	Primary acquired marrow disorder RBCs unusually sensitive to complement-mediated lysis	Ham's test, sucrosis lysis test Marrow aspirate and biopsy to assess cellularity Decreased decay accelerating factor Decreased WBC, CD55, and CD59 or decreased RBC CD59 by flow cytometry	Folic acid 1 mg qd Mild cytopenias—no treatment Chronic hemolysis and other cytopenias—prednisone, 60 mg qd initially, then taper if possible; chronic 15–40 mg qod Iron for secondary iron deficiency Androgens—fluoxymesterone, danazol Anticoagulation Marrow transplant for pancytopenia
Enzyme Deficiencies			
Pyruvate kinase deficiency	Decreased or abnormal enzyme	PK assay—decreased V̇max or rarely high Km variant	If severe anemia with symptoms, poor growth and age < 2 yr—transfusion Splenectomy > age 6 yr but earlier if necessary Folic acid, 1 mg qd
G6PD deficiency	A type: age-labile enzyme Mediterranean type: no enzyme activity in circulating RBCs	Glucose-6-phosphate dehydrogenase	Avoid oxidant stress to RBCs Transfusion if acute anemia is symptomatic
Hemoglobin Abnormalities (For discussion of hemoglobinopathies, see sections on these topics)			
Extracellular Defects			
Autoimmune			
Autoimmune hemolytic anemia "Warm" antibody	Alteration in membrane surface antigen (Rh) or abnormal response of B lymphocytes, causing autoantibody formation	Spherocytes on blood film Positive direct Coombs test to IgG "warm" antibody directed against RBCs Positive indirect Coombs test and antibody detectable in plasma Thermal amplitude 35–40°C Some complement (C3b) may be detected on RBCs Tests for underlying disease	If Hb > 10 g/dL + retic <10%—none Severe anemia may require transfusion Prednisone, 2 mg/kg/24 hr IVIG Danazol Splenectomy Immunosuppressives Folic acid 1 mg/24 hr if chronic
"Cold" antibody	"Cold" or IgM autoantibody directed against I/i antigen system	Agglutination or rouleaux on blood film Positive direct Coombs test to complement (C3b) Tests for underlying disease Serology for infectious mononucleosis; anti-i present Serology for *Mycoplasma pneumoniae*; anti-I present	If Hb >10 g/dL + retic <10%—none Severe anemia may require transfusion Avoid exposure to cold If severe: immunosuppressives and plasmapheresis Prednisone—*less* effective Splenectomy—*not* useful Folic acid, 1 mg/24 hr if chronic
Fragmentation Hemolysis			
DIC, TTP, HUS	Direct damage to RBC membrane	Fragments on blood film	Treat underlying condition Transfusion: but transfused cells also will have shortened life span
Extracorporeal membrane oxygenation	Direct damage to RBC membrane	Fragments on blood film	Supportive Transfusion until ECMO discontinued
Prosthetic heart valve	Direct damage to RBC membrane	Fragments on blood film	Folic acid, 1 mg/24 hr Iron for secondary iron deficiency
Burns—thermal injury	Direct damage to RBC membrane	Spherocytes on blood film	Supportive Transfusion
Hypersplenism	Effects of sequestration, ↓ pH, lipases and other enzymes, and macrophages on RBCs	Thrombocytopenia and neutropenia	Treat underlying condition—cytopenias usually mild Splenectomy if complicating other anemia (e.g., thalassemia major) Folic acid, 1 mg/24 hr
Plasma Factors			
Liver disease	Alteration in plasma cholesterol and phospholipids	Target cells or spiculated RBCs on blood film Abnormal liver function tests	Treat underlying condition Transfusion: but transfused cells also will have shortened life span Folic acid, 1 mg/24 hr
Abetalipoproteinemia	Absence of apolipoprotein β Vitamin E deficiency and heightened sensitivity to oxidative damage	Acanthocytes on blood film Absent chylomicrons, VLDL and LDL	Vitamin E (A, K, and D) Folic acid, 1 mg/24 hr Dietary restriction of triglycerides
Infections	Toxic effects on RBCs	Associated symptoms and signs Cultures	Antibiotics Supportive
Wilson disease	Effect of copper on RBC membrane, usually self-limited	Spherocytes on blood film Copper, ceruloplasmin Penicillamine challenge and urine copper excretion	Penicillamine Supportive Transfusion if acute anemia is symptomatic

ECMO = extracorporeal membrane oxygenation; retic = reticulocyte count; DIC = disseminated intravascular coagulation; TTP = thrombotic thrombocytopenic purpura; HUS = hemolytic-uremic syndrome; VLDL = very low density lipoproteins; LDL = low density lipoproteins; IVIG = intravenous immunoglobin; RBC = red blood cell; Hb = hemoglobin.
Modified from Asselin BL, Segel GB: In Rakel R (editor): Conn's Current Therapy. Philadelphia, WB Saunders, 1994, pp 338–9.

Chapter 450
Hereditary Spherocytosis

George B. Segel

Hereditary spherocytosis is a common cause of hemolysis and hemolytic anemia, with a prevalence of approximately 1/5,000 in people of Northern European extraction. It is the most common familial and congenital abnormality of the red blood cell (RBC) membrane. Affected individuals may be asymptomatic without anemia and with minimal hemolysis or may have a severe hemolytic anemia. Hereditary spherocytosis has been described in most ethnic groups but is most common among persons of Northern European origin.

Etiology. Hereditary spherocytosis usually is transmitted as an autosomal dominant and, less frequently, as an autosomal recessive disorder. As many as 25% of patients have no previous family history. Of these patients, most represent new mutations, and a few result from recessive inheritance or represent nonpaternity. The most common molecular defects are abnormalities of spectrin or ankyrin, which are major components of the cytoskeleton responsible for RBC shape. A recessive defect has been described in α-spectrin; dominant defects, in β-spectrin and in protein 3; and dominant and recessive defects, in ankyrin. A deficiency in spectrin, protein 3, or ankyrin results in uncoupling in the "vertical" interactions of the lipid bilayer skeleton

and the loss of membrane microvesicles (Fig. 450–1). The loss of membrane surface area without a proportional loss of volume causes sphering of the RBCs and an associated increase in cation permeability, cation transport, adenosine triphosphate utilization, and glycolysis. The decreased deformability of the spherocytic RBCs impairs cell passage from the splenic cords to the splenic sinuses, and the spherocytic RBCs are destroyed prematurely in the spleen. Splenectomy markedly improves the RBC life span and cures the anemia.

Clinical Manifestations. Hereditary spherocytosis may be a cause of hemolytic disease in the newborn and may present as anemia and hyperbilirubinemia sufficiently severe to require phototherapy or exchange transfusions. The severity in infants and children is variable. Some children remain asymptomatic into adulthood, but others may have severe anemia with pallor, jaundice, fatigue, and exercise intolerance. Severe cases may be marked by expansion of the diploë of the skull and the medullary region of other bones, but to a lesser extent than in thalassemia major. After infancy, the spleen is usually enlarged, and pigmentary (bilirubin) gallstones may form as early as age 4–5 yr. At least 50% of unsplenectomized patients ultimately form gallstones, although for the most part they remain asymptomatic. Because of the high RBC turnover and heightened erythroid marrow activity, children with hereditary spherocytosis are susceptible to aplastic crisis, primarily as a result of parvovirus infection, and to hypoplastic crises associated with various other infections. Such erythroid marrow failure may result rapidly in profound anemia (hematocrit

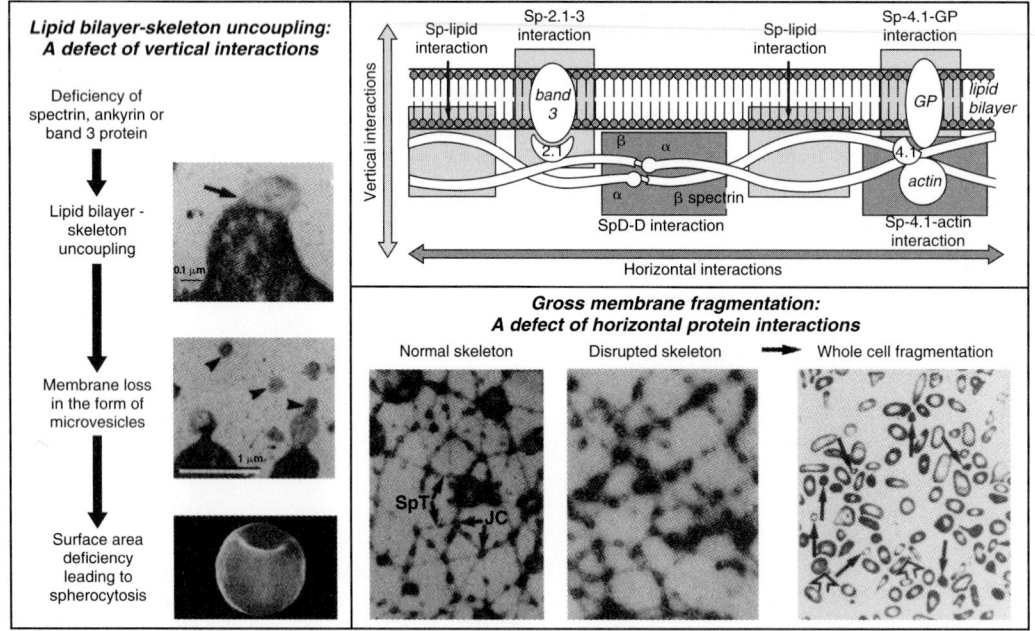

FIGURE 450–1. Vertical and horizontal interactions of membrane proteins and the pathobiology of the red cell lesion in hereditary spherocytosis (HS) and hereditary elliptocytosis/hereditary pyropoikilocytosis (HE/HPP). *Left,* A defect of vertical or transverse interactions as exemplified by the red cell membrane lesion in HS. Partial deficiencies of spectrin, ankyrin (band 2.1), or band 3 protein lead to uncoupling of the membrane lipid bilayer from the underlying skeleton *(arrow)* followed by a formation of spectrin-free microvesicles of 0.2–0.5 μm in diameter *(arrowheads).* These vesicles can be visualized by transmission electron microscopy, but they are not seen during examination of blood films. The subsequent loss of cell surface and a decrease in the surface/volume ratio leads to spherocytosis. *Right,* Defect of horizontal or parallel interactions of skeletal proteins as exemplified by the membrane lesion in hemolytic forms of HE associated with a defect of spectrin heterodimer self-association. The molecular lesion involving a weakened self-association of spectrin heterodimers to tetramers represents a horizontal defect of the stress-supporting protein interactions. It leads to a disruption of the membrane skeletal lattice and, consequently, whole cell destabilization followed by red cell fragmentation and poikilocytosis. Such fragments are readily seen on stained blood films. (Modified from Palek J, Jarolim P: Clinical expression and laboratory detection of red blood cell membrane protein mutations. *Semin Hematol* 1993;30:249.)

<10%), high-output heart failure, hypoxia, cardiovascular collapse, and death.

Laboratory Findings. Evidence for hemolysis includes reticulocytosis and indirect hyperbilirubinemia. The hemoglobin level usually is 6–10 g/dL, but it can be in the normal range. The reticulocyte percentage often is heightened to 6–20%, with a mean of approximately 10%. The mean corpuscular volume is normal, whereas the mean corpuscular hemoglobin concentration often is increased (36–38 g/dL RBCs). The RBCs on the blood film vary in size and include polychromatophilic reticulocytes and spherocytes (Fig. 450–2A). The spherocytes are smaller in diameter and on the blood film are hyperchromic as a result of the high hemoglobin concentration. The central pallor is less conspicuous than in normal cells. Spherocytes may be the predominant cell or may be relatively sparse, depending on severity of the disease, but they usually account for more than 15–20% of the cells when hemolytic anemia is present. Erythroid hyperplasia is evident in the marrow aspirate or biopsy. The marrow expansion may be evident on routine roentgenographic examination. Other evidence of hemolysis may include decreased haptoglobin and the presence of gallstones by ultrasonography.

The *diagnosis* of hereditary spherocytosis usually is established clinically from the blood film, showing many spherocytes and reticulocytes, from the family history, and from splenomegaly. The presence of spherocytes in the blood can be confirmed with an osmotic fragility test. The RBCs are incubated in progressive dilutions of an iso-osmotic buffered salt solution. Exposure to hypotonic saline causes RBCs to swell, and the spherocytes lyse more readily than biconcave cells in hypotonic solutions. This feature is accentuated by depriving the cells of glucose overnight at 37°C, a so-called incubated osmotic fragility test.

As a research tool, the specific protein abnormality can be established in 80% of these patients by RBC membrane protein analysis using gel electrophoresis and densitometric quantitation. The protein abnormalities are more evident in patients who have had a splenectomy. Studies to define the underlying defects in the cytoskeleton may require assessment of protein synthesis, stability, assembly, and binding to the other membrane proteins. Molecular diagnosis also is possible. Most patients have family-specific private mutations that can be detected by DNA analysis. De novo mutations in the β-spectrin and ankyrin genes have been described in 50% of patients with unaffected parents.

Differential Diagnosis. The major alternative considerations when large numbers of spherocytes are seen on the blood film are isoimmune or autoimmune hemolysis. Isoimmune hemolytic disease of the newborn, particularly due to ABO incompatibility, mimics hereditary spherocytosis. The detection of antibody on an infant's RBCs using a direct antiglobulin (Coombs) test should establish the diagnosis of immune hemolysis. Autoimmune hemolytic anemias also are characterized by spherocytes, and there may be evidence of a previously normal hemoglobin, hematocrit, and reticulocyte count. Rare causes of spherocytosis include thermal injury, clostridial septicemia with exotoxemia, and Wilson disease, each of which may present as a transient hemolytic anemia (see Table 449–1).

Treatment. Because the spherocytes in hereditary spherocytosis are destroyed almost exclusively in the spleen, splenectomy eliminates most of the hemolysis associated with this disorder. After splenectomy, osmotic fragility often improves because of diminished splenic conditioning and less RBC membrane loss, and the anemia, reticulocytosis, and hyperbilirubinemia resolve. Whether all patients with hereditary spherocytosis should undergo splenectomy is controversial. Some hematologists do not recommend splenectomy for those patients whose hemoglobin values exceed 10 g/dL and whose reticulocyte percentage is less than 10. Folic acid, 1 mg/24 hr, should be administered to prevent secondary folic acid deficiency. For patients with more severe anemia and reticulocytosis or those with hypoplastic or aplastic crises, poor growth, or cardiomegaly, splenectomy is recommended after age 5–6 yr to avoid the heightened risk of postsplenectomy sepsis in younger children. The introduction of laparoscopic splenectomy decreases the length of hospital stay and has replaced open splenectomy for many patients. Vaccines for encapsulated organisms such as pneumococcus, meningococcus, and *Haemophilus influenzae* type b should be administered before splenectomy, and oral prophylactic penicillin V (age <5 yr: 125 mg twice daily; age ≥5 yr through adulthood: 250 mg twice daily) administered thereafter. Postsplenectomy thrombocytosis is commonly observed but needs no treatment and usually resolves spontaneously. Partial splenectomy also may be useful in children younger than age 5 yr and can provide some increase in hemoglobin and reduction in the reticulocyte count, with potential maintenance of splenic phagocytic and immune function.

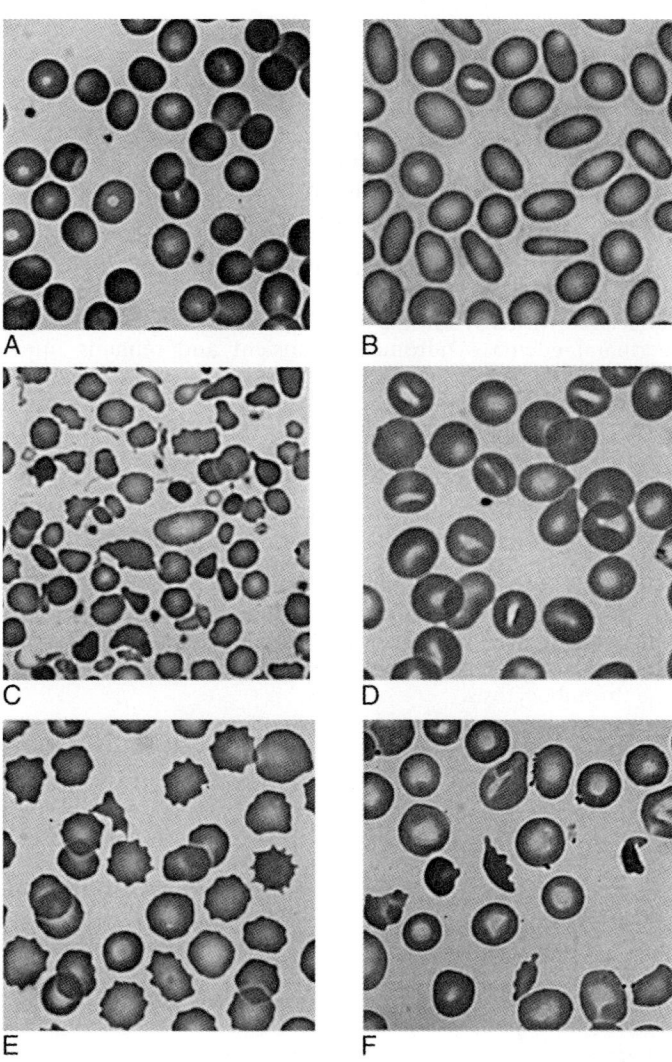

FIGURE 450–2. Morphology of abnormal red cells. *A,* Hereditary spherocytosis; *B,* hereditary elliptocytosis; *C,* hereditary pyropoikilocytosis; *D,* hereditary stomatocytosis; *E,* acanthocytosis; *F,* fragmentation hemolysis. See also color plates.

Chapter 451
Hereditary Elliptocytosis
George B. Segel

Hereditary elliptocytosis is an uncommon disorder that varies markedly in severity. Mild hereditary elliptocytosis produces no symptoms, but more severe varieties may result in neonatal poikilocytosis (shape variation) and hemolysis, chronic or sporadic hemolytic anemias, or hereditary pyropoikilocytosis (HPP), which is a severe disorder with microspherocytosis and poikilocytosis. Although hereditary elliptocytosis is rare in Western populations, it is more commonly found in West Africa, where the abnormalities (spectrin mutations) may provide resistance to malarial infection.

Etiology. Hereditary elliptocytosis is inherited as a dominant disorder. In the rare instances when two abnormal alleles are inherited (HPP), the patient exhibits a particularly severe hemolytic anemia. Various molecular defects have been described in hereditary elliptocytosis; these produce abnormalities of α- and β-spectrin and defective spectrin heterodimer self-association (see Fig. 450–1). Such defects in the horizontal protein interactions result in gross membrane fragmentation, particularly in homozygous HPP. Less commonly, mutations in protein 4.1 and glycophorin C may produce elliptocytosis.

Clinical Manifestations. Elliptocytosis may be noted as an incidental finding on a blood film examination and may not be associated with clinically significant hemolysis (see Fig. 450–2B). The diagnosis of hereditary elliptocytosis is established by the findings on the blood film, the autosomal dominant inheritance pattern, and the absence of other causes of elliptocytosis, such as deficiencies of iron, folic acid, or vitamin B_{12}. Hemolytic elliptocytosis may produce neonatal jaundice, even though characteristic elliptocytosis may not be evident at that time. The blood of the affected newborn may show bizarre poikilocytes and pyknocytes. The usual features of a chronic hemolytic process with elliptocytosis are manifested later as anemia, jaundice, splenomegaly, and osseous changes. Cholelithiasis may occur in later childhood, and aplastic crises have been reported. The most severe form is HPP, which is characterized by extreme microcytosis (mean corpuscular volume 50–60 fL/cell), extraordinary variation in the cell size and shape, and primarily microspherocytic rather than elliptocytic cells (see Fig. 450–2C). These patients inherit a mutant spectrin from one parent, who has mild or no elliptocytosis, and a partial spectrin deficiency from the other parent, who is hematologically normal.

Ovalocytes, in contrast to elliptocytes, are less elongated and may reflect a condition termed *Southeast Asian ovalocytosis* (SAO). SAO is associated with an abnormal protein 3, which functions as an anion exchanger. This disorder may produce augmented neonatal hyperbilirubinemia but causes little hemolysis later and may offer protection against *Plasmodium falciparum* malaria. This anion exchanger also is expressed in renal tubular cells and may cause distal renal tubular acidosis in association with SAO.

Laboratory Findings. The blood film is the most important test to establish hereditary elliptocytosis (see Fig. 450–2B). The red blood cells (RBCs) show various degrees of elongation and may actually be rod shaped. In hereditary elliptocytosis, other abnormal RBC shapes may be present, depending on the severity of hemolysis. They include microcytes, spherocytes, and other poikilocytes. The reticulocyte percentage reflects the severity of hemolysis, and erythroid hyperplasia and indirect hyperbilirubinemia may be present. Increased thermal instability is characteristic of HPP, hence its name. The abnormal spectrin denatures and the cells lyse at 45–46°C instead of the usual 49–50°C. The specific protein abnormality can be established by protein separation and analysis techniques. Molecular defects currently are defined only in research laboratories.

Treatment. If hereditary elliptocytosis represents a morphologic abnormality on the blood film without evident hemolysis, no treatment is necessary. Patients with chronic hemolysis should receive folic acid, 1 mg/24 hr, to prevent secondary folic acid deficiency. Splenectomy decreases the hemolysis and should be considered if the hemoglobin is less than 10 g/dL and the reticulocyte count is greater than 10%. The RBCs on the blood film may be more abnormal after splenectomy even though hemoglobin increases and the reticulocytes decrease. The hematologic features of SAO do not require treatment beyond the newborn period.

Chapter 452
Hereditary Stomatocytosis
George B. Segel

Hereditary stomatocytosis is a rare condition in which the red blood cells (RBCs) are cup shaped. On stained blood film, they present a mouthlike slit in place of the usual circular area of central pallor (see Fig. 450–2D). Acquired stomatocytosis may be seen in several conditions, especially liver disease. Hereditary stomatocytosis is associated with increased RBC membrane permeability to Na+ and K+ and alterations in RBC hydration status. Dehydrated hereditary stomatocytosis is the most common type, but it is heterogeneous and sometimes is associated with pseudohyperkalemia from heightened RBC K+ leak, particularly when the blood is cooled to room temperature, or it may be associated with a syndrome of perinatal edema and ascites. The perinatal edema syndrome is transient and remains unexplained. The hydrocytic or overhydrated variety is associated with abnormalities within the region of protein 7.2, or "stomatin," which has been mapped to chromosome 9. A defective transcription promoter results in stomatin reduction, which may impair regulation of cation transport. Hemolytic anemia may be associated with hereditary stomatocytosis, but splenectomy is not a recommended treatment. Persistent symptomatic thrombocytosis may follow splenectomy if the hemolysis is not eliminated or markedly decreased. Patients have developed a life-threatening tendency toward in situ thrombosis after splenectomy in association with the abnormal adherence of the stomatocytic RBC to vascular endothelium in conjunction with the thrombocytosis.

Chapter 453
Other Membrane Defects
George B. Segel

PAROXYSMAL NOCTURNAL HEMOGLOBINURIA

Etiology. Paroxysmal nocturnal hemoglobinuria (PNH) reflects an abnormality of marrow stem cells that affects many blood cell lines. The disease is not inherited; it is an acquired disorder of hematopoiesis characterized by a defect in proteins of the cell membrane that renders the red blood cells (RBCs) (and other cells) susceptible to damage by serum complement. The deficient membrane-associated proteins include decay-accelerating factor, the C8 binding protein, and other proteins that normally impede complement lysis at various steps. The underlying defect involves the glycolipid anchor that maintains these proteins on the cell surface. Various mutations in the *PIGA* gene involved in glycosylphosphatidylinositol biosynthesis have been identified in patients with PNH. More than one *PIGA* mutation often occurs in an individual patient, suggesting multiclonality. Furthermore, glycosylphosphatidylinositol-deficient cells are found at low frequency in normal persons. This suggests that injury to the normal marrow stem cells provides a selective advantage to the PNH clones in the genesis of this disease.

Clinical Manifestations. PNH is a rare disorder, particularly in children, but 26 patients with a mean age of 13 yr (0.8–21.4 yr) were diagnosed at Duke University Medical Center between 1966 and 1991. Approximately 60% of these patients presented with marrow failure, and the remainder had either intermittent or chronic anemia, often with prominent intravascular hemolysis. Nocturnal and morning hemoglobinuria is a classic finding in adults if hemolysis is worse during sleep. However, chronic hemolysis is more common in PNH despite its name. In addition to chronic hemolysis, thrombocytopenia and leukopenia are often characteristic. Thrombosis and thromboembolic phenomena are serious complications that may be related to altered glycoproteins on the platelet surface and resultant platelet activation. Abdominal, back, and head pain may be prominent complaints. Hypoplastic or aplastic pancytopenia may precede or follow the onset of PNH, and rarely PNH progresses to acute myelogenous leukemia. The mortality in PNH is related primarily to the development of aplastic anemia or thrombotic complications. The predicted survival for children is 80% for 5 yr, 60% for 10 yr, and 28% for 20 yr.

Laboratory Findings. The diagnosis of PNH was established classically by a positive result in either the acidified serum hemolysis (Ham) test or the sucrose lysis test, which activate the alternative and classic pathways of complement lysis, respectively. Hemosiderinuria is common and reflects the chronic intravascular hemolysis. Markedly reduced levels of RBC acetylcholinesterase activity and reduced levels of decay-accelerating factor also are found. Flow cytometry now is the best diagnostic test for PNH. With the use of anti-CD59 for RBCs and anti-CD55 and anti-CD59 for granulocytes, flow cytometry is more sensitive than the classic RBC lysis tests in detecting the reduced glycolipid-bound membrane proteins. Newer reagents, such as fluorescent aerolysin, may heighten the sensitivity of detection by binding selectively to glycosylphosphatidylinositol anchors.

Treatment. Splenectomy is not indicated. Glucocorticoids such as prednisone (2 mg/kg/24 hr) have been used to treat acute hemolytic episodes, and their dosage should be tapered as soon as the hemolysis abates. Prolonged anticoagulation therapy may be of benefit when thromboses occur, and heparin and low molecular heparin may inhibit complement-mediated hemolysis. Because of chronic loss of iron as hemosiderin in the urine, iron therapy may be necessary. Androgens, such as fluoxymesterone (Halotestin) and danazol, antithymocyte globulin, cyclosporine, and growth factors, such as erythropoietin and granulocyte colony-stimulating factor, have been used to treat marrow failure. Bone marrow transplantation has been successful in treating some cases, and nonmyeloablative transplantation may reduce transplant-related mortality and morbidity. Retroviral gene transfer of *PIGA* restores the glycolipid anchor in cultured cells and may be the basis for future gene therapy.

ACANTHOCYTOSIS

Acanthocytosis is characterized by RBCs with irregular circumferential pointed projections (see Fig. 450–2E). This morphologic finding is seen with alterations in the cholesterol/phospholipid ratio in some patients with liver disease and in congenital abetalipoproteinemia associated with malabsorption, neuromuscular abnormalities, and retinitis pigmentosa (see Chapters 75.3 and 320.12). It also is associated with the rare X-linked *McLeod syndrome*: absence of the Kx (Kell) antigen, late-onset myopathy, neurologic abnormalities such as chorea, splenomegaly, and hemolysis with acanthocytosis.

Hereditary Spherocytosis and Other Membrane Proteins
Bader-Meunier B, Gauthier F, Archambaud F, et al: Long-term evaluation of the beneficial effect of subtotal splenectomy for management of hereditary spherocytosis. *Blood* 2001;97:399–403.
Bolton-Maggs PH: The diagnosis and management of hereditary spherocytosis. *Baillieres Best Pract Res Clin Haematol* 2000;13:327–42.
Carella M, Stewart GW, Ajetunmobi JF, et al: Genetic heterogeneity of hereditary stomatocytosis. *Haematologica* 1999;84:862–3.
Delaunay J, Stewart G, Iolascon A: Hereditary dehydrated and overhydrated stomatocytosis: Recent advances. *Curr Opin Hematol* 1999;6:110–4.
Delhommeau F, Cynober T, Schischmanoff PO, et al: Natural history of hereditary spherocytosis during the first year of life. *Blood* 2000;95:393–7.
Gallagher PG, Forget BG: Structure, organization and expression of the human band 7.2b gene, a candidate gene for hereditary hydrocytosis. *J Biol Chem* 1995;270:26358.
Minkes RK, Lagzdins M, Langer JC, et al: Laparoscopic versus open splenectomy in children. *J Pediatr Surg* 2000;35:699–700.
Miragha del Guidice E, Francese M, Nobili B, et al: High frequency of de novo mutations in ankyrin gene *(ANK1)* in children with hereditary spherocytosis. *J Pediatr* 1998;132:117.
Stewart GW, Amess JA, Eber SW, et al: Thromboembolic disease after splenectomy for hereditary stomatocytosis. *Br J Haematol* 1996;93:303.
Tse WT, Lux SE: Red blood cell membrane disorders. *Br J Haematol* 1999;104:2–13.
Vasuvattakul S, Yenchitsomanus PT, Vachuanichsanong P, et al: Autosomal recessive distal renal tubular acidosis associated with Southeast Asian ovalocytosis. *Kidney Int* 1999;56:1674–82.

Paroxysmal Nocturnal Hemoglobinuria
Hall SE, Rosse WF: The use of monoclonal antibodies and flow cytometry in the diagnosis of paroxysmal nocturnal hemoglobinuria. *Blood* 1996;87:5332.
Hillmen P, Lewis SM, Bessler M, et al: Natural history of paroxysmal nocturnal hemoglobinuria. *N Engl J Med* 1995;333:1253.
Rosse WF: New insights into paroxysmal nocturnal hemoglobinuria. *Curr Opin Hematol* 2001;8:61.
Suenaga K, Kanda Y, Niiya H, et al: Successful application of nonmyeloablative transplantation for paroxysmal nocturnal hemoglobinuria. *Exp Hematol* 2001;29:639–42.
Ware RE, Hall SE, Rosse WF: Paroxysmal nocturnal hemoglobinuria with onset in childhood and adolescence. *N Engl J Med* 1991;325:991.

Chapter 454

Hemoglobin Disorders

Keith Quirolo and Elliott Vichinsky

Point mutations and deletions in the hemoglobin genes result in structural changes in the hemoglobin molecule leading to a change in function. The globin genes are found in clusters on chromosomes 11 (β globins) and 16 (α globins) as at least six conserved, duplicated genes. Their control is complex, including an upstream locus control region as well as an X-linked control site. It is likely that fetal and adult non-α genes are present in a single cluster. The order of the genes on the chromosomes follows ontogeny. The α- and β-gene clusters are translated and the globin molecules combine to form the embryonic hemoglobins: Gower-1 ($\zeta_2\epsilon_2$), Gower-2 ($\alpha_2\epsilon_2$), and Portland ($\zeta_2\gamma_2$). Embryonic hemoglobins are not found in the circulation after 8 wk of gestational age, and by 9 wk gestational age the major hemoglobin is Hb F ($\alpha_2\gamma_2$). In the normal individual, Hb A ($\alpha_2\beta_2$) appears in the first month of gestation but does not become the dominant hemoglobin until after birth. Hb A$_2$ ($\alpha_2\delta_2$) appears shortly before birth and remains at a low level throughout adult life. (Also see Chapter 438.)

Hemoglobin disorders can be functionally classified as noted in Table 454–1. The functionality of the altered hemoglobin can

TABLE 454–1. Functional Classification of Hemoglobins

Functional Abnormality of Hemoglobin	Location of Substitution	Clinical Abnormality	Example Hemoglobin
None	Surface	None	G Philadelphia
Aggregation	Surface	Hemolytic anemia	S
Unstable	Internal	Hemolytic anemia	Köln
Increased O_2 affinity	$\alpha_1\beta_2$ Contact or βC terminal	Erythrocytosis	Chesapeake
Decreased O_2 affinity	Near heme $\alpha_1\beta_2$ contact	Cyanosis	Kansas
Methemoglobinemia	Proximal or distal histidine	Cyanosis	M
α-Thalassemia	Variable	Hemolytic anemia	Constant Spring
β-Thalassemia	Variable	Hemolytic anemia	Lepore

be predicted to some degree by the site of the mutation. Those in the heme pocket region will affect oxygen affinity, and those in the periphery will affect the behavior of the hemoglobin, as can be seen in the table. Some hematologists refer to qualitative (structural abnormalities, i.e., sickle hemoglobins) and quantitative (hemoglobin production, i.e., thalassemias, hemolytic anemias) abnormalities to be more concise.

THE HEMOGLOBINOPATHIES

There are approximately 700 variant hemoglobins; the majority are the result of point mutations (634), and the rest are two amino acid substitutions, deletions or insertions, extended chains, and fusions. The majority of these hemoglobin variants are extremely rare. Those variants that are caused by the evolutionary pressures of malaria are the most prevalent worldwide and are a major public health challenge owing to improvements in health care leading to a much longer life expectancy for affected individuals. The diagnosis of the common inherited hemoglobinopathies can be made by newborn screening programs, which should improve access to appropriate medical care.

454.1 Sickle Cell Disease

Epidemiology. Sickle cell disease has been recognized in the malarial areas of the world for millennia but has only been recognized by the western scientific community since the description of "sickled" red cells in 1910 by Herrick. In malarial areas there is a selective advantage to the heterozygote (Hb AS), although the actual mechanism of this advantage is not known. Individuals with sickle cell trait have lower levels of *Plasmodium falciparum* parasitemia, higher hemoglobin counts, and less severe reinfections than individuals with homozygous Hb A. In these areas there are confounding factors that influence resistance to malaria, including the Duffy chemokine receptor, glucose-6-phosphate dehydrogenase, and HLA-B53 and HLA-DRB1*1302. Sickle cell disease occurs in endemic malarial areas, including North Africa, Italy, Greece, Central India, and most predominantly in sub-Saharan Africa. Because of the slave trade, sickle cell disease is also common in North, Central, and South America as well as the Caribbean. Sickle cell disease is most common in individuals of African descent but is seen in Hispanics, Arabians, Indians, and whites. In the United States the incidence is 1 in 625 live births to African-Americans. The severity of sickle cell disease is somewhat influenced by haplotypes specific to areas of origin of the Hb S mutation: Senegal, Benin, Bantu, and Asian.

Pathophysiology. Hb S is the result of a single base-pair change, thymine for adenine, at the sixth codon of the β gene. This change encodes valine instead of glutamine in the sixth position on the β-globin molecule. The charge at this site is altered and allows for polymerization of hemoglobin under conditions of hypoxia. Acidosis, hemoglobin concentration, and the combination of Hb S with other hemoglobins affect the ability of Hb S to polymerize. Oxygen affinity is affected by 2,3-diphosphoglycerate (2,3-DPG) and pH; an increase in 2,3-DPG and a decrease in pH increase polymerization. Hemoglobin concentration has a lesser effect, a higher concentration leading to increased polymerization. The effect of other hemoglobins depends on the extent of their homology with Hb S; in descending order of ability to copolymerize are hemoglobins S, C, D, O Arab, A, J, and F. Based on the effect of other hemoglobins, intracellular pH, and mean corpuscular hemoglobin concentration on polymerization, new therapies for sickle cell disease can be hypothesized. Because of the disruption of the red cell membrane, the increased adhesiveness of sickle reticulocytes, and the increased leukocyte count there is a thrombotic coagulopathy associated with sickle cell anemia that contributes to the severity of the disease.

Sickle Cell Anemia (Homozygous Hemoglobin S or S β^0-thalassemia)

Children who have only hemoglobin S usually have a lifetime of severe intermittent illness, with painful vaso-occlusive episodes and eventually the sequelae of complications of their sickle cell disease (Table 454–2). A few children will have a less severe course, owing to higher levels of Hb F.

Clinical Manifestations. Affected newborns seldom exhibit clinical features of sickle cell disease; hemolytic anemia gradually develops over the first 2–4 mo, paralleling the replacement of much of the fetal hemoglobin by Hb S. Other clinical manifestations are uncommon before 5–6 mo of age. However, infants with sickle cell anemia have abnormal immune function and by about 6 mo of age many will have functional asplenia, making bacterial sepsis the greatest risk for morbidity and mortality. By the age of 5 yr, 95% of children with sickle cell anemia will have functional asplenia. Acute sickle dactylitis, presenting as the *hand-foot syndrome*, is frequently the first overt evidence that sickle cell disease is present in an infant. Dactylitis in infants requires medical attention for hydration and pain management. Its associated findings include painful, usually symmetric, swelling of the hands and feet. The underlying abnormality is ischemic necrosis of the small bones, believed to be caused by a choking off of the blood supply as a result of the rapidly expanding bone marrow. Roentgenograms are not informative in the acute phase of dactylitis but later show evidence of extensive bony destruction and repair (Fig. 454–1). Predictors of a severe course of sickle cell disease are anemia, painful episodes, and dactylitis before the age of 24 mo.

TABLE 454–2. Complications of Sickle Cell Disease

Complication	Hemoglobin SS*	Hemoglobin δβ⁰-Thalassemia	Hemoglobin SC	Hemoglobin δβ⁺-Thalassemia
Infection	++++	++++	+++	+
Acute chest	++++	++++	++++	++
Splenic sequestration	++++	++++	++	0
Severe anemia	++++	++++	+++	+
Stroke	++++	++++	++	0
Priapism	++++	++++	++++	++
Renal disease	++++	++++	+++	+
Skin ulcers	++++	++++	+	0
Avascular necrosis	++++	+++++	+++	+
Retinopathy	++	++	++++	+

Hemoglobin SO Arab and hemoglobin D have equivalent severity.

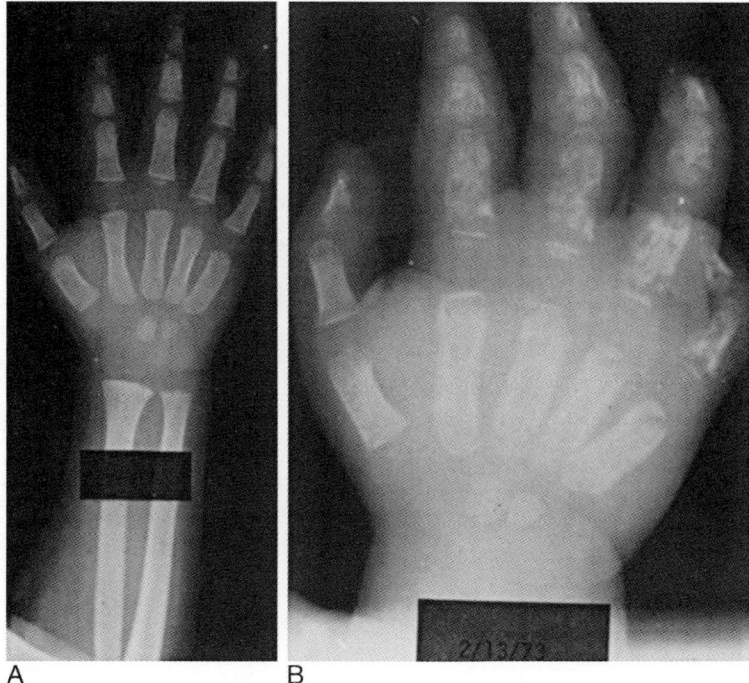

FIGURE 454–1. Roentgenograms of an infant with sickle cell anemia and acute dactylitis. *A,* The bones appear normal at the onset of the episode. *B,* Destructive changes and periosteal reaction are evident 2 wk later.

A   B

Acute painful episodes represent the most frequent and prominent manifestation of sickle cell disease. Most patients experience some pain on a nearly daily basis. Episodes of severe pain that require hospitalization and parenteral analgesic administration average about one per year in children with Hb SS, but this interval varies considerably. Some patients never experience severe pain, and others require hospital admission with such frequency that they become seriously disabled. In young children, pain often involves the extremities; in older patients, pain in the head, chest, abdomen, and back occurs more commonly. In an individual patient, pain tends to recur in a limited number of sites. Intercurrent illnesses accompanied by fever, hypoxia, and acidosis, all of which promote the deoxygenation of Hb S, may precipitate sickle pain episodes, but acute pain also develops frequently without an apparent antecedent event. Sickle-related abdominal pain may mimic that of an acute surgical condition.

More extensive vaso-occlusive events in children can produce gross ischemic damage. Acute pain episodes may progress to infarction of bone marrow or bone. Splenic infarcts are common in children, causing pain and contributing to the process of "autosplenectomy." Pulmonary infarction, often occurring in association with pneumonitis or microscopic fat emboli (from bone marrow infarction), may produce the severe clinical picture of *acute chest syndrome*. Strokes caused by cerebrovascular occlusion are among the most catastrophic acute events and are a frequent cause of hemiplegia. As many as 10% of children with sickle cell anemia, mainly preadolescent and older patients, exhibit sequelae of cerebrovascular occlusion. Findings of increased blood flow velocity by transcranial Doppler studies may be predictive of increased risk of stroke in these patients, and this may help to identify children who will benefit from preventive therapy. Ischemic damage may also affect the myocardium, liver, and kidneys. Renal function is progressively impaired by diffuse glomerular and tubular fibrosis, and hyposthenuria accompanied by polyuria is a characteristic finding in patients older than 5 yr. Renal papillary necrosis and nephrotic syndrome also develop occasionally. *Priapism* is a relatively frequent complication that results from the pooling of blood in the corpora cavernosa, causing obstruction of the venous outflow.

In the first 5 yr of life common complications of sickle cell disease include bacterial sepsis, splenic or hepatic sequestration, acute chest syndrome, parvovirus B19 infection, and vaso-occlusive episodes. Occasionally, children will have priapism, stroke, and chronic splenic sequestration with severe chronic anemia (Fig. 454–2A). Urinary tract infections are more

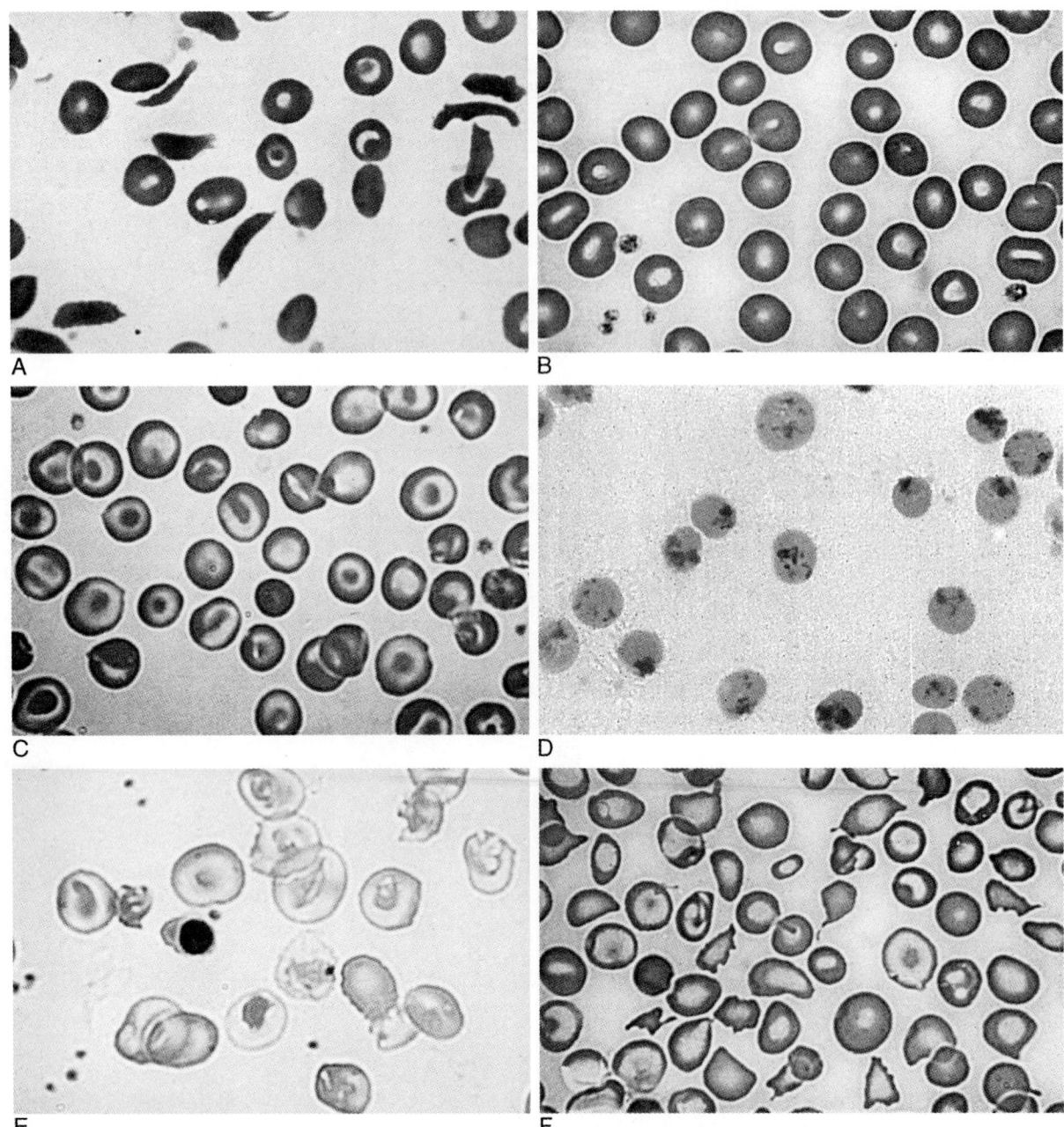

FIGURE 454–2. Red blood cell (RBC) morphology associated with hemoglobin disorders. *A*, Sickle cell anemia (Hb SS): target cells and fixed (irreversibly sickled) cells. *B*, Sickle cell trait (Hb AS): normal RBC morphology. *C*, Hemoglobin CC: target cells and occasional spherocytes. *D*, Congenital Heinz body anemia (unstable hemoglobin): RBCs stained with supravital stain (brilliant cresyl blue) reveal intracellular inclusions. *E*, Homozygous B^0-thalassemia: severe hypochromia with deformed RBCs and normoblasts. *F*, Hemoglobin H disease (α-thalassemia): anisopoikilocytosis with target cells. (Courtesy of Dr. John Bolles, The ASH Collection, University of Washington, Seattle.)

common and can lead to bacteremia. Viral pneumonia and reactive airways disease can rapidly become acute chest syndrome. Acute splenic sequestration has a peak incidence between 6 mo and 3 yr and can be rapid in onset and lead to death. The most common cause of mortality is sepsis and acute chest syndrome.

Young children with Hb SS may have splenic enlargement associated with their hemolytic disease, with progression to the syndrome of *hypersplenism* accompanied by worsening anemia and sometimes thrombocytopenia. *Acute splenic sequestration* is a distinct and episodic event that occurs in infants and young children with sickle cell anemia, often following an acute febrile illness. For unknown reasons, large amounts of blood become acutely pooled in the spleen, which becomes massively enlarged, and signs of circulatory collapse rapidly develop. Blood transfusions in the acute phase may be lifesaving. Altered splenic function in young children with sickle cell disease is a significant factor leading to their increased susceptibility to meningitis, sepsis, and other serious infections, mainly caused by pneumococci and *Haemophilus influenzae*. In the absence of specific antibody to the polysaccharide capsular antigens of these organisms, splenic activity is essential for removing these bacteria when they invade the blood. Despite frequent enlargement of the spleen in young patients with Hb SS, its phagocytic and reticuloendothelial functions have been shown to be markedly reduced. As an additional risk factor, children with sickle cell disease have also been shown to have deficient levels of serum opsonins, of the alternate complement pathway, against pneumococci. Children with sickle cell disease also have increased susceptibility to *Salmonella* osteomyelitis (partly because of bone necrosis).

As children become older they more frequently develop other complications of sickle cell anemia. Stroke is more common after the age of 5 yr, with the peak being between 6 and 9 yr. Children often begin to have more frequent vaso-occlusive episodes from 5–10 yr of age, and the episodes sometimes become more severe. Some children develop avascular necrosis of the hips; others develop cholelithiasis requiring cholecystectomy. *Salmonella* osteomyelitis may occur. With matriculation to school, affected children are exposed to more infectious agents, including parvovirus, which can cause a severe anemia characterized by the absence of reticulocytes during the anemic phase; blood transfusion is frequently required. Enuresis is a common sequela of sickle renal disease. Children with sickle cell anemia may develop school problems because of frequent absence; they begin to have fears related to their sickle cell disease and often fear death from their disease. There is growing evidence that there may be subtle, sickle cell–related brain injury in young children with sickle cell disease, with 25–30% of children suffering occult strokes.

Adolescents begin to develop some of the chronic changes of sickle cell disease. These children are still at risk for all of the complications of younger children. In addition, there is an increased incidence of urinary tract infection with bacteremia in young women and severe priapism in young men, leading to impotence. Frequent episodes of acute chest syndrome in early childhood may subsequently manifest as pulmonary hypertension. Hip pain in this age group may be the harbinger of avascular necrosis. Skin ulcers may also develop in adolescence and pose a chronic problem. Proteinuria is the first indication of sickle nephropathy; over 12% of adolescents will develop chronic renal disease. Retinopathy may develop in 3% of patients with sickle cell anemia but in 30% of those with Hb SC disease. Hyphema is a medical emergency in sickle cell disease. Stroke is still a risk in these young men and women.

Development must be monitored closely. By mid childhood most patients are underweight. Some adolescents have marked pubertal delay, although the majority of adolescents eventually develop normally. Zinc deficiency, which is prevalent in children with sickle cell disease, may contribute to their poor growth and delayed maturation. Coping can be extremely problematic for those adolescents who have had frequent hospitalizations, more than one chronic complication of sickle cell disease, or poor social support systems.

In common with patients having other forms of chronic hemolytic anemia, children with Hb SS are at risk of developing a rapid, potentially life-threatening decrease in their hemoglobin level (aplastic episodes) in association with parvovirus B19 infection (see Chapter 230). Cardiomegaly is invariably present in older children, often caused partly by sickle cell–related cardiomyopathy. Increased iron absorption contributes to parenchymal damage of the liver, pancreas, and heart. Symptomatic gallstone formation is common in adolescent and older patients, occasionally occurring in children as young as 5 yr.

Laboratory Findings. Sickle cell disease should be suspected in all patients who have the clinical manifestations of sickle cell disease regardless of their ethnic origin (see Table 454–2). A complete blood cell count usually reveals an increased reticulocyte count (5–15%), upper limit of normal or greater leukocyte count (12,000–20,000/mm^3), normal mean corpuscular volume (MCV) (unless a thalassemic hemoglobin is present), mild to moderate anemia (5–9 g/dL), normal to increased platelet count, and a normal differential (or predominance of neutrophils); if severe anemia is present, nucleated red cells can be found. A diagnosis of sickle cell disease can be suspected by examination of the blood smear (see Fig. 454–2A) for target cells, poikilocytes, hypochromasia, sickle red cells, nucleated RBCs, and Howell-Jolly bodies and confirmed by hemoglobin electrophoresis or high-pressure liquid chromatography (HPLC). Bone marrow is markedly hyperplastic with erythroid predominance. If variant hemoglobins are present, only minor changes in the blood cell count may occur, and other diagnostic studies should be used for identification.

Radiologic studies may reveal characteristic bony findings of sickle cell disease in the vertebral bodies, mild expansion of the marrow cavities, osteoporosis, and possibly sclerosis of the long bones and femoral heads. Renal concentrating capacity is usually decreased.

Diagnosis. In the United States, sickle cell disease is diagnosed in most states at birth through newborn screening programs (Table 454–3). These programs use hemoglobin electrophoresis or HPLC to define abnormal hemoglobins. Confirmatory studies for Hb S or variants are performed after birth. Newborn infants who have HbFS on screening could also have Sδβ^0-thalassemia or S-hereditary persistence of fetal hemoglobin (HPFH); some hemoglobin variants need to be defined by further diagnostic studies. Prenatal diagnosis is also possible for parents who both have sickle cell trait. Most African-Americans of reproductive age do not know their trait status; this is problematic because 1 of 14 African-Americans carries the trait. Hispanics and other peoples almost never know they are heterozygous for Hb S, Hb C, or thalassemia trait.

Differential Diagnosis. The various clinical manifestations of sickle cell disease, including limb pain, heart murmurs, hepatosplenomegaly, and anemia, may suggest a number of other diagnoses, including rheumatic fever or rheumatoid arthritis, osteomyelitis, and leukemia. In patients who have an Hb SS electrophoresis pattern and concomitant microcytosis (MCV < 78 fL), possibilities that require consideration include iron deficiency or a combination of Hb S with α- or β^0-thalassemia.

Treatment. Treatment in sickle cell disease is directed toward the *prevention* of complications and optimization of health and healthy coping strategies. All children who have sickle cell disease should be immunized with the conjugate pneumococcal vaccine and all other routine vaccines of childhood. At the age of 2 mo all children should begin penicillin prophylaxis with 125 mg twice daily. It is extremely important that the physicians and the caretakers of these children understand the risks to children with this disease. Caretakers need to be taught how to take a reliable temperature, assess illness, palpate their child's spleen, and recognize the symptoms of anemia and stroke. Adequate medical care should be available and reliable. At the age of 3 yr the penicillin dose is increased to 250 mg twice a day. There is some controversy as to when to discontinue penicillin prophylaxis; some physicians discontinue this medication at 5 yr age,

TABLE 454–3. Newborn Screening for Hemoglobinopathy

Hemoglobin Electrophoresis	Hemoglobinopathy
FA	Normal
FAS	Sickle cell trait
FSA	δβ$^+$-Thalassemia
FS	Sickle cell anemia or Sβ^0-thalassemia
FSC	SC disease
FSV	S variant (D, O Arab, other)
F	β^0-Thalassemia
E	EE, Eβ^0-Thalassemia
FABart's	α-Thalassemia

others later. Because of the thrombotic nature of the sickle hemoglobins and the high red cell turnover, folate supplementation is recommended as well.

Although there have been reports of outpatient management of *febrile infants* older than the age of 6 mo, this approach is not recommended. After the age of 18 to 24 mo, outpatient treatment may be considered if the treating physician knows the patients well, there is the ability to return to the hospital for follow-up, and the treating physician and parent believe the child is well enough for outpatient management of a febrile illness. In this situation, a thorough examination be performed; a blood cell count, blood culture, urine culture, and chest radiograph obtained; and ceftriaxone administered. Children with any physical findings, high fever or previous episodes of sepsis, or splenectomy should be hospitalized.

Treatment of *pain* in children with sickle cell disease requires patience and attention to detail (also see Chapters 38 and 66). Children may begin having painful episodes at a young age, and their caretakers must be taught how to treat this symptom and when to seek medical assistance. Limited amounts of opiate medication should be prescribed (usually acetaminophen with codeine) to avoid masking disease with opiates and to ensure that the child will be evaluated if a painful event is long lasting. Day treatment center care may avoid hospitalization, which is frequently necessary. Children older than the age of 7–10 yr may be able to use a patient-controlled analgesia (PCA) pump. A nonsteroidal anti-inflammatory drug and opiate medication should be instituted together. The opiate medication should be weaned after 3–4 days in most cases. Patients may have withdrawal symptoms if opiates are abruptly withdrawn. A cause should be sought for pain symptoms, and patients should be monitored for other complications of sickle cell disease and treated expectantly.

Blood transfusion is indicated for acute chest syndrome, stroke, stroke prevention, severe anemia, and splenic sequestration and before general surgery. In some patients, transfusion may be instituted for chronic pain syndromes, if accompanied by psychotherapy to enhance coping strategy. Blood transfusions usually do not reverse ischemic damage but do prevent most of the manifestations of sickle cell disease. Even while on chronic transfusion therapy children can still have transient cerebral ischemia as well as avascular necrosis of the hips and shoulders.

Children who have Hb SS or Sβ⁰-thalassemia have the highest risk of stroke and should be monitored for risk of stroke with transcranial Doppler (TCD) as recommended by the STOP study. This should be done at a sickle cell center under the direction of a physician familiar with sickle cell disease, transfusion therapy, and monitoring for stroke and complications of transfusion. Increased blood flow velocity in the cerebral arteries (> 200 cm/sec) diagnosed by TCD is an indication for initiation of transfusions to maintain Hb S below 30%. All children who have sickle cell disease should have a red cell phenotype determination in infancy and receive partially phenotypically matched (for C, E, and Kell at least), leukocyte-depleted red cell products.

Drug therapy with hydroxyurea has successfully elevated fetal hemoglobin levels and reduced morbidity in adults with sickle cell anemia. There have been several encouraging studies of hydroxyurea therapy in children. One study did not detect adverse effects on height, weight gain, or pubertal development. However, there are no large, randomized studies of efficacy and long-term safety when hydroxyurea is used in children. Children with sickle cell complications (see Table 454–2) are usually begun on hydroxyurea at 15 mg/kg/24 hr, and, if tolerated, the dose is gradually increased to a maximum of less than 30 mg/kg/24 hr. Complete blood cell counts, liver function tests, and fetal hemoglobin levels are monitored at least monthly as long as patients are on this medication. An increase in MCV of over 100 fL/dL, a decrease in the leukocyte count to low normal, and an increase in fetal hemoglobin is an indication

of compliance and of efficacy. The increase in fetal hemoglobin is variable but is usually between 10–25%. The fetal hemoglobin is not uniformly distributed in the red cells but appears in clones of F cells. There is a reduction in severity of disease in children who have only moderate increases in fetal hemoglobin. Other medical therapies are now in clinical trials.

Bone marrow transplantation is the only cure for sickle cell disease, but it is only an option for children younger than 16 yr of age who have an HLA-matched sibling. An initial problem of increased neurologic complications during transplantation has been minimized by improved transplantation regimens. There is a 5% mortality rate. An innovative method of transplant referred to as a nonmyeloablative regimen has been used in a few patients. This technique induces a stable stem cell chimera with phenotypic overexpression of the healthy graft resulting in an asymptomatic patient. This regimen does not cause the significant myelosuppression or immune deficiency observed in full transplant protocols. Long-term stability of the chimera graft needs to be proven before this technique is accepted.

Other experimental treatments are aimed at increasing intracellular hydration, decreasing red cell adhesion, lowering blood viscosity, elevating nitric oxide levels, and decreasing thrombosis. Combination therapy of different treatment modalities appears likely in the future.

Other Sickle Cell Syndromes. The most commonly occurring sickle syndromes besides Hb SS are Hb SC and Sβ⁰-thalassemia and Sβ⁺-thalassemia. The other syndromes—SD, SO, Arab, and other variants—are much less common. Sβ⁰-thalassemia is a severe sickle cell anemia. Hb SC does not polymerize like Hb SS, but the presence of crystals of Hb C interact with the membrane ion transport dehydrating the cell, inducing sickling. Children who have Hb SC disease can experience the same symptoms and complications as those with severe Hb SS disease, but the frequency is less. These children have an increased hemoglobin concentration and better growth. However, they have more fat in their bone marrow, and this can lead to more severe acute chest syndrome and organ failure caused by fat emboli from bone necrosis. There is also an increased incidence of retinopathy and chronic hypersplenism. Despite a well-developed appearance, these children may develop all the chronic complications of sickle cell disease. Sβ⁺-thalassemia is a less severe form of sickle cell disease with a much lower frequency of the severe manifestations.

454.2 Sickle Cell Trait (Hemoglobin AS)

The prevalence of sickle cell trait varies throughout the world; in the United States the incidence is 7–10% of African-Americans. The incidence of Hb S in most individuals with hemoglobin AS on electrophoresis is 35–45%; this is influenced by α-thalassemia, which is common in this population. Individuals with α-thalassemia have a two-gene deletion resulting in an Hb S of 25–30%. The life span of people with this trait is normal, and serious complications are very rare. The complete blood cell count is within the normal range (see Fig. 454–2B). Hemoglobin electrophoresis is diagnostic.

Complications of sickle cell trait include sudden death during rigorous exercise, splenic infarcts at high altitude, hematuria, hyposthenuria, bacteriuria, and intraocular bleeding leading to blindness. A rare cancer, renal medullary carcinoma, is also associated with sickle cell trait. Most of these complications have been not adequately studied, making counseling difficult. In general, children with sickle cell trait should not have any restrictions on activities. The most importance risk is to future progeny, and the pediatrician should offer counseling to at-risk individuals and families.

454.3 Other Hemoglobinopathies

Hemoglobin C. The mutation for Hb C is at the same site as Hb S, with lysine instead of valine substituted for glutamine. In the United States, Hb AC occurs in 1:50 and Hb CC occurs in 1:5,000 African-Americans. Hb AC is asymptomatic. Hb CC may result in a mild anemia, splenomegaly, and cholelithiasis; rare cases of spontaneous splenic rupture have been reported. Sickling does not occur. This condition is usually diagnosed through newborn screening programs. Hb C crystallizes, disrupting the red cell membrane (see Fig. 454–2C).

Hemoglobin E ($\alpha_2\beta_2^{26Glu-Lys}$). This is the second most common globin mutation worldwide. The hemoglobin mutation activates a cryptic splice site, and the mRNA is less efficiently processed. There are two other hemoglobins with a similar RNA processing defect: hemoglobins Knossos and Malay; these are sometimes called thalassemic hemoglobinopathies, owing to the ineffective erythropoiesis that results from the hemoglobin mutation. Heterozygotes are asymptomatic and homozygotes have a mild microcytic anemia. The phenotype is altered with co-inheritance of α-thalassemia.

Hemoglobin D. There are 16 variants of Hb D; only one, D-Punjab (Los Angeles), in combination with Hb S produces symptoms of sickle cell disease. This rare hemoglobin is seen in 1–3% of Western Indians and in some Europeans with a tie to India. Heterozygous D is clinically silent. Homozygous D produces a mild to moderate anemia with splenomegaly.

454.4 Unstable Hemoglobin Disorders

About 200 rare unstable hemoglobins have been identified; the most common is Hb Köln. Most individuals seem to have de novo mutations rather than inherited hemoglobin disorders. The most studied are those whose mutation causes unstable heme binding that eventually leads to the denaturation of the hemoglobin molecule. The denatured hemoglobin can be visualized during severe hemolysis or after splenectomy as Heinz bodies. Unlike the Heinz bodies seen after toxic exposure, in unstable hemoglobins Heinz bodies are present in reticulocytes and older red cells (see Fig. 454–2D). Heterozygotes are asymptomatic.

Homozygous children can present in early childhood with anemia and splenomegaly or with unexplained hemolytic anemia. Hemolysis is increased with febrile illness and, with some unstable hemoglobins, the ingestion of oxidant medications (similar to glucose-6-phosphate dehydrogenase). If the spleen is functional, the smear may appear almost normal or have only hypochromasia and basophilic stippling. A diagnosis may be made by demonstrating Heinz bodies, hemoglobin instability, or an abnormal electrophoresis (although some unstable hemoglobins have normal mobility).

Treatment is supportive. Transfusion may be required during hemolytic episodes in severe cases. Oxidative drugs should be avoided, and folate supplementation provided. Splenectomy has been performed, but the complications of splenectomy, including bacterial sepsis and the possibility of developing pulmonary hypertension, should be considered before this therapy.

454.5 Abnormal Hemoglobins with Increased Oxygen Affinity

Over 110 high-affinity hemoglobins have been characterized. These mutations affect the state of configuration of hemoglobin during oxygenation and deoxygenation. Hemoglobin changes structure when in the oxygenated versus the deoxygenated state. The deoxygenated state is termed the T (tense) state and is stabilized by 2,3-DPG. When fully oxygenated, hemoglobin assumes the R (relaxed) state. The exact molecular interactions between these two states are not known. The high-affinity hemoglobins contain mutations that either stabilize the R form or destabilize the T form. The interactions between these two forms are complex, and the mechanisms of the mutations are not known. In most cases the hemoglobins can be identified by hemoglobin electrophoresis; about 20% must be characterized under controlled conditions of measurements of the P_{50}, which will be 9–21 mm Hg (normal: 23–29 mm Hg). Because of a decrease in the P_{50} most of these hemoglobins cause an erythrocytosis of 17 to 20 g/dL of hemoglobin. Levels of erythropoietin and 2,3-DPG are normal. Patients are usually asymptomatic, and do not need phlebotomy. If phlebotomy is performed, oxygen delivery could be problematic owing to a lowered hemoglobin.

454.6 Abnormal Hemoglobins Causing Cyanosis

These hemoglobin variants are rare. The major group is the M hemoglobins, of which there are seven. Hemoglobin M variants have mutations in either the α or the β chain, all in the heme pocket of the hemoglobin molecule. Six of the 7 have a tyrosine residue that covalently bonds with the heme iron, stabilizing it in the oxidized form. These unstable hemoglobins lead to a hemolytic anemia, most pronounced in the β forms. Clinically, these children are cyanotic from birth without other signs or symptoms of disease if the tyrosine is on the α chain (Hb M Boston, M Iwate). Infants with β-chain mutations become cyanotic later in infancy owing to the fetal hemoglobin switch (Hb M Saskatoon, Hyde Park, Milwaukee). The abnormal hemoglobins are autosomal dominant and diagnosed by hemoglobin electrophoresis using special techniques and HPLC. There is no treatment; children with the β form should avoid oxidant drugs.

Low affinity hemoglobins have less cyanosis than the M hemoglobins. The amino acid substitutions destabilize the oxyhemoglobin and lead to decreased oxygen saturation. The best characterized are Hb Kansas and Hb Beth Israel.

454.7 Hereditary Methemoglobinemia

The iron in hemoglobin is normally in the ferrous state (Fe^{2+}), which is essential for its oxygen-transporting function. Under physiologic conditions there is a slow, constant loss of electrons to released oxygen and the ferric (Fe^{3+}) form combines with water, producing methemoglobin (MHg). The predominant intracellular mechanism for the reduction of MHg is cytochrome 5b. This mechanism is over a hundredfold more efficient than the production of MHg, and only 1% of hemoglobin is in the ferric state normally.

MHg may be increased in the red cell owing to exposure to toxic substances or to absence of reductive pathways (NADH-cytochrome b5 reductase deficiency). Toxic methemoglobinemia is much more common than hereditary methemoglobinemia. Infants are particularly vulnerable to hemoglobin oxidation because they have 50% the level of cytochrome b5 reductase that adults do, fetal hemoglobin is more susceptible to oxidation than hemoglobin A, and the more alkaline infant gastrointestinal tract may promote the growth of nitrite producing gram-negative bacteria. When MHg levels are greater than 1.5 g/24 hr, cyanosis is visible (15% MHb); a level of 70% MHg is lethal. The level is usually reported as a percent of normal hemoglobin, and the toxic level is lower at a lower hemoglobin level. Methemoglobinemia has been described in infants who ingested foods and water high in nitrates, who were exposed to aniline teething gels or other chemicals, and in some infants with severe gastroenteritis and acidosis. Methemoglobin may color the blood brown.

Hereditary Methemoglobinemia with Deficiency of NADH Cytochrome b5 Reductase. These rare disorders are classified as four types. In type I (most common) the deficiency of NADH cytochrome b5 activity is deficient only in the red cells. In type II, the enzyme deficiency is present in all tissues and is characterized in infancy by encephalopathy, mental retardation, spasticity, microcephaly, and growth retardation. In type III, the deficiency occurs in leukocytes, platelets, and red cells; and in type IV there is deficiency of only red cell cytochrome b5.

Clinically, cyanosis may vary in intensity with season and diet. The time at onset of cyanosis also varies; in some patients it appears at birth, in others as late as adolescence. Although as much as 50% of the total circulating hemoglobin may be in the form of nonfunctional methemoglobin, little or no cardiorespiratory distress occurs in these patients, except on exertion.

Daily oral *treatment* with ascorbic acid (200–500 mg/day in divided doses) gradually reduces the methemoglobin to about 10% of the total pigment and alleviates the cyanosis as long as therapy is continued. Chronic high doses of ascorbic acid have been associated with hyperoxaluria and renal stone formation. Ascorbic acid should not be used for treatment of toxic methemoglobinemia. Methylene blue given intravenously (1–2 mg/kg initially) is used to treat toxic methemoglobinemia. An oral dose can be administered (3–5 mg/kg/24 hr) as maintenance therapy. Methylene blue should not be used in patients with glucose-6-dehydrogenase deficiency; it is ineffective and can cause severe oxidant hemolysis.

454.8 Syndromes of Hereditary Persistence of Fetal Hemoglobin (HPFH)

These syndromes are a form of thalassemia; a mutation is associated with a decrease in the production of either or both β and δ globins. There is an imbalance in the α:non-α synthetic ratio (see Chapter 454.9) characteristic of thalassemia. Over 20 variants of HPFH have been described. They are deletional, δβ⁰ (Black, Ghanaian, Italian), nondeletional (Tunisian, Japanese, Australian), linked to the β-globin-gene cluster (British, Italian-Chinese, Black), or unlinked to the β-globin-gene cluster (Atlanta, Czech, Seattle). The δβ⁰ forms have deletions of the entire δ- and β-gene sequences, the most common in the United States being the Black (HPFH 1) variant. Because the δ and β genes have been deleted there is production only of γ globin and formation of Hb F. In the homozygous form there are no manifestations of thalassemia. There is only Hb F with very mild anemia and slight microcytosis. When inherited with other variant hemoglobins, Hb F is elevated in the 20–30% range; when inherited with Hb S, there is an amelioration of sickle hemoglobinopathy with some mild manifestations. Avascular necrosis of the hips has been reported in Hb SS disease with HPFH.

454.9 Thalassemia Syndromes

The thalassemias are the most common genetic disorder on a worldwide basis. The selective pressures that have made the thalassemias so common are not known but are assumed to relate to the geographic distribution of malaria. Children with thalassemia have a shorter red cell life, fetal hemoglobin in their red cells until an older age than normal, and red cells that are more sensitive to oxidative stress.

Epidemiology. Although there are more than 200 mutations for β-thalassemia, most are rare. About 20 common alleles constitute 80% of the known thalassemias worldwide; 3% of the world's population carry genes for β-thalassemia, and in Southeast Asia 5–10% of the population carry genes for α-thalassemia. In a particular area there are fewer common alleles.

Pathophysiology. Mutations in β-thalassemia involve globin gene deletions, promoter region mutations, termination mutations, splice site mutations, and other rare mutations. There are relatively few α-thalassemia mutations; most are deletions. Selected features of the thalassemias can be seen in Table 454–4. The key feature is the fact that there is a globin chain imbalance. In the bone marrow the thalassemic mutations disrupt the maturation of the red cell, resulting in ineffective erythropoiesis; the marrow is hyperactive, but there are relatively few reticulocytes and severe anemia. In β-thalassemias there is an excess of α-globin chains relative to β- and γ-globin chains; α-globin tetramers (α_4) are formed, and these inclusions interact with the red cell membrane and shorten red cell survival, leading to anemia and increased erythroid production. The γ-globin chains are produced in normal amounts, leading to an elevated Hb F ($\alpha_2\gamma_2$). The δ-globin chains are also produced in normal amounts, leading to an elevated Hb A$_2$ ($\alpha_2\delta_2$) in β-thalassemia. In α-thalassemia there are relatively fewer α-globin chains and an excess of β- and γ-globin chains. These excess chains form Bart's hemoglobin (γ_4) in fetal life and Hb H (β_4) after birth. These abnormal tetramers are not as lethal but lead to extravascular hemolysis.

Homozygous β⁰-Thalassemia (Thalassemia Major, Cooley's Anemia)

Clinical Manifestations. These children usually become symptomatic from progressive hemolytic anemia with profound weakness and cardiac decompensation during the second 6 mo of life if not treated. Depending on the mutation and degree of fetal hemoglobin production, transfusions in thalassemia major are necessary in the second month of life or the second year of life but rarely later. The decision to transfuse depends on the child's ability to compensate for the degree of anemia. Most infants and children have cardiac decompensation at hemoglobins of 4 g/dL or less. Generally, fatigue, poor appetite, and lethargy are late findings of severe anemia in an infant or child. These were common before transfusions were standard therapy. The classic presentation of children with severe thalassemic facies, pathologic fractures, marked hepatosplenomegaly, and cachexia is still seen in some developing countries. The spleen may become so enlarged that it causes mechanical discomfort and secondary hypersplenism. These are features of ineffective erythropoiesis (Fig. 454–3): expanded medullary spaces (with massive expansion of the marrow of the face and skull), extramedullary hematopoiesis, and a huge caloric need. The hepatosplenomegaly may interfere with nutritional support. Pallor, hemosiderosis, and jaundice may combine to produce a greenish brown complexion. Because of the anemia there is also an increase in iron absorption, with toxicity leading to further complications, if the child survives long enough to develop them. Many of these features became less severe and infrequent with transfusion therapy, but transfusional hemosiderosis is a consequent complication. Many of the complications of thalassemia seen in developed countries today are the result of iron overload: in the liver, fibrosis and cirrhosis; in the beta cells of the pancreas, diabetes mellitus; in the pituitary, testis, and ovaries, growth retardation and hypogonadotropic hypogonadism; in the parathyroid, hypocalcemia and osteoporosis; and in the heart, arrhythmias, myocarditis, and intractable cardiac failure. Most, if not all, of these complications can be avoided by the consistent use of an iron chelator. However, chelation therapy also has associated complications.

Laboratory Findings. The infant is born only with Hb F or, in some cases, Hb F and Hb E (heterozygosity for β⁰-thalassemia). Eventually in β⁰-thalassemia there is severe anemia, few reticulocytes, numerous nucleated red cells, and microcytosis with almost no normal-appearing red cells on the smear (see Fig. 454–2E). The hemoglobin level falls progressively to lower than

TABLE 454–4. The Thalassemias

Thalassemia	Globin Genotype	Features	Expression	Hemoglobin Electrophoresis
α-Thalassemia				
1 gene deletion	$-\alpha/\alpha,\alpha$	Normal	Normal	Newborn: Bart's 1–2%
2 gene deletion trait	$-\alpha/-,\alpha$ $-,-/\alpha,\alpha$	Microcytosis, mild hypochromasia	Normal, mild anemia	Newborn: Bart's 5–10%
3 gene deletion hemoglobin H	$-,-/-,\alpha$	Microcytosis, hypochromic	Mild anemia, transfusions not required	Newborn: Bart's 20–30%
2 gene deletion + Constant Spring	$-,-/\alpha,\alpha^{Constant\ Spring}$	Microcytosis, hypochromic	Moderate to severe anemia, transfusion, splenectomy.	2–3% Constant Spring, 10–15% hemoglobin H
4 gene deletion	$-,-/-,-$	Anisocytosis, poikilocytosis	Hydrops fetalis	Newborn: 89–90% Bart's with Gower 1 and 2 and Portland
Nondeletional	$\alpha,\alpha/\alpha,\alpha^{variant}$	Microcytosis, mild anemia	Normal	1–2% variant hemoglobin
β-Thalassemia				
β0 or β+ heterozygote: trait	$\beta^0/A,\beta^+/A$	Variable microcytosis	Normal	Elevated A_2, variable elevation of F
β0-Thalassemia	$\beta^0/\beta^0, \beta^+/\beta^0, E/\beta^0$	Microcytosis, nucleated RCB	Transfusion dependent	F 98% and A_2 2%, E 30–40%
β+-Thalassemia severe	β^+/β^+	Microcytosis nucleated RBC	Transfusion dependent/thalassemia intermedia	F 70–95%, A_2 2%, trace A
Silent	β^+/A	Microcytosis	Normal with only microcytosis	A_2 3.3–3.5%
	β^+/β^+	Hypochromic, microcytosis	Mild to moderate anemia	A_2 2–5%, F 10–30%
Dominant (rare)	B^0/A	Microcytosis, abnormal RBCs	Moderately severe anemia, splenomegaly	Elevated F and A_2
δ-Thalassemia	A/A	Normal	Normal	A_2 absent
(δβ)0-Thalassemia	$(\delta\beta)^0/A$	Hypochromic	Mild anemia	F 5–20%
(δβ)+-Thalassemia Lepore	β^{Lepore}/A	Microcytosis	Mild anemia	Lepore 8–20%
Lepore	$\beta^{Lepore}/\beta^{Lepore}$	Microcytic, hypochromic	Thalassemia intermedia	F 80%, Lepore 20%
γδβ-Thalassemia	$(\gamma^A\delta\beta)^0/A$	Microcytosis, microcytic, hypochromic	Moderate anemia. Splenomegaly. Homozygote: thalassemia intermedia	Decreased F and A2 compared with δβ-thalassemia
γ-Thalassemia	$(\gamma^A\gamma\beta^0)/A$	Microcytosis	Insignificant unless homozygote	Decreased F
Hereditary Persistence of Fetal Hemoglobin				
Deletional	A/A	Microcytic	Mild anemia	F 100% homozygotes
Nondeletional	A/A	Normal	Normal	F 20–40%

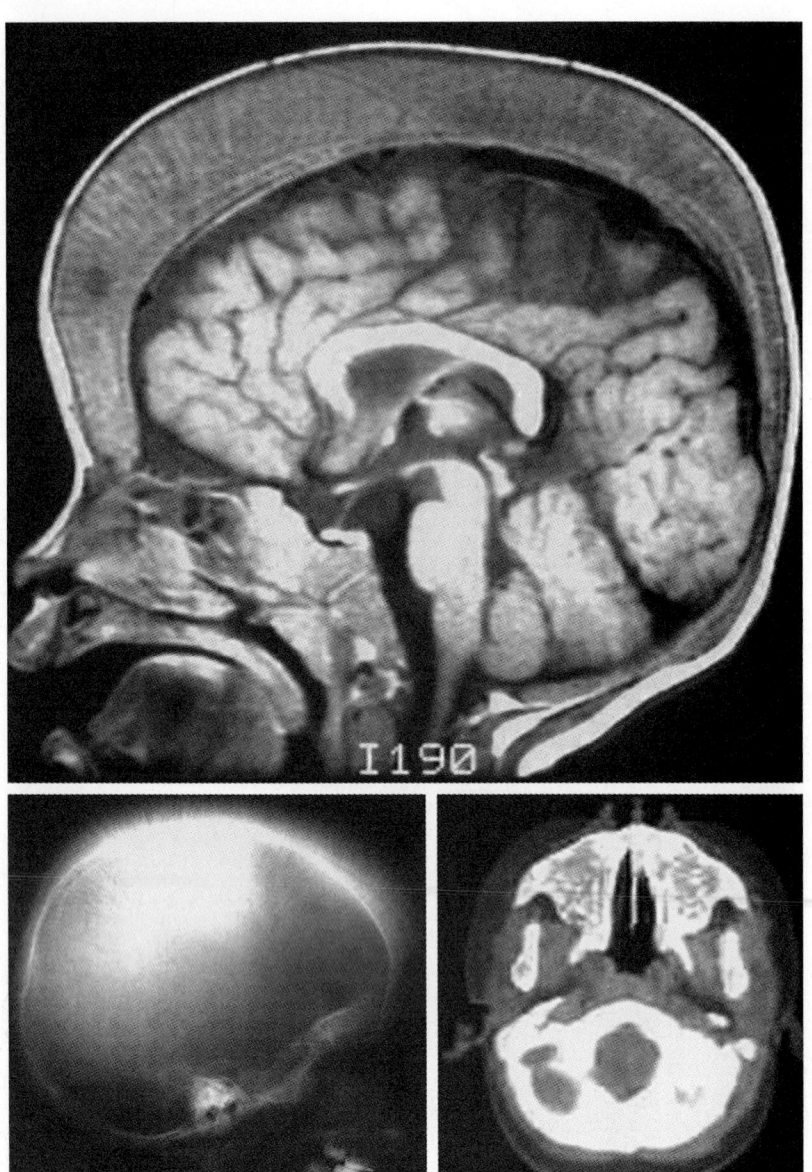

FIGURE 454–3. Ineffective erythropoiesis in untransfused 3-year-old patient with thalassemia major. Massive widening of the diploic spaces of the skull on MRI, radiographic appearance of trabeculae seen on plain radiograph, and obliteration of the maxillary sinuses with hematopoietic tissue as seen on computed tomography.

5 g/dL unless transfusions are given. The unconjugated serum bilirubin level is usually elevated, but other chemistries may be normal at an early stage. Even if untransfused, eventually there is iron accumulation with an elevated serum ferritin and saturation of the transferrin. Bone marrow hyperplasia can be seen on radiographs (see Fig. 454–3).

Treatment. Before initiating chronic transfusions, the diagnosis of β^0-thalassemia should be confirmed and the parents counseled concerning this life-long therapy. Beginning transfusion and chelation therapy are difficult challenges for parents to face early in their child's life. Before beginning transfusion therapy, a red cell phenotype is obtained; blood products that are leukoreduced and phenotypically matched for the Rh and Kell antigens are required for transfusion. If there is the possibility of a bone marrow transplant, the blood should be negative for cytomegalovirus and irradiated. Transfusion therapy promotes general health and well-being and avoids the consequences of ineffective erythropoiesis. Iron overload is inevitable, and "hyper"-transfusion should be avoided. A post-transfusion hemoglobin level of

9.5 g/dL is the goal. Banked blood in developed countries is generally safe. Designated donors are not encouraged; some blood centers have "partner" programs, pairing donors and recipients, which decreases the exposure to multiple red cell antigens. As a child grows, more donors will be needed.

Transfusional hemosiderosis causes many of the complications of thalassemia major. Assessment of iron overloading is best achieved by liver biopsy, supplemented by ferritometry and the measurement of serum ferritin. Liver biopsy is the only method that is reproducible and should be available in centers caring for thalassemic patients. There are few available ferritometers. Ferritin can only provide an assessment of the trend of the iron status for a particular patient.

Transfusional hemosiderosis can be prevented by the use of deferoxamine (Desferal). Deferoxamine chelates iron and some other divalent cations, allowing their excretion in the urine and the stool. If used appropriately, a negative iron balance can be achieved. Deferoxamine is given subcutaneously over 10–12 hr, 5–6 days a week. It should be used cautiously in young children. The side effects include ototoxicity with high-frequency hearing loss, retinal changes, and bone dysplasia with truncal shortening. Oral iron chelators (deferiprone: L-1) have not been as effective as deferoxamine and there is a concern about their causing neutropenia, arthritis, and hepatic fibrosis. Other iron chelators are being studied for oral and subcutaneous use.

Splenectomy may be indicated for patients with thalassemia intermedia who have a falling steady-state hemoglobin and for transfused patients with a rising transfusion requirement. However, splenectomy may have serious infectious consequences. Because of the increased risk of infection after splenectomy, all patients should be fully immunized against encapsulated bacteria before splenectomy, and they subsequently should be on long-term penicillin prophylaxis. Preliminary evidence that splenectomy may lead to pulmonary hypertension has led to anticoagulation being considered for some splenectomized patients.

Bone marrow transplantation has successfully cured over a thousand patients who have thalassemia major. Most success has been in children younger than 15 yr of age without iron overload and hepatomegaly who have HLA-matched siblings. All children who have an HLA-matched sibling should be offered the option of bone marrow transplantation.

Other β-Thalassemia Syndromes

The β-thalassemia syndromes are broken into six groups: β-thalassemias, δβ-thalassemias, γ-thalassemias, δ-thalassemias, εγδβ-thalassemias, and the HPFH syndrome (see Chapter 454.8). Most of these thalassemias are relatively rare, some being found only in family groups. The β-thalassemias can also be classified clinically as thalassemia trait, minima, minor, intermediate, and major, reflecting the degree of anemia. The genetic classification does not necessarily define the phenotype, and the degree of anemia does not always predict the genetic classification.

Thalassemia intermedia can be any combination of β-thalassemia mutations (β^0/β^+, $\beta^0/\beta^{variant}$, E/β^0), which will lead to a phenotype of microcytic anemia with hemoglobin of about 7 g/dL. There is controversy about whether to transfuse these children. They will certainly develop a degree of medullary hyperplasia, nutritional hemosiderosis perhaps requiring chelation, splenomegaly, and other complications of thalassemia and iron overload. Extramedullary hematopoiesis can occur in the vertebral canal, compressing the spinal cord and causing neurologic symptoms; the latter is a medical emergency requiring immediate local radiation therapy to halt erythropoiesis. Transfusion will alleviate the thalassemic manifestations and hasten the need for chelation. A splenectomy puts the child at risk for infection and pulmonary hypertension.

The thalassemias classified as *minima* and *minor* are usually heterozygotes (β^0/β, β^+/β^+) having a phenotype more severe than trait but not as severe as intermedia. These children should be investigated for their genotype and monitored for iron accumulation. The β-thalassemias are influenced by the presence of α-thalassemia: α-thalassemia trait leading to less severe anemia and duplicated α genes ($\alpha\alpha\alpha/\alpha\alpha$) leading to more severe thalassemia. Frequently, individuals who are in these groups require transfusions in adolescence or adulthood; some may be candidates for chemotherapy such as hydroxyurea.

Thalassemia trait is frequently misdiagnosed as iron deficiency in children because the two are similar hematologically and iron deficiency is much more prevalent. A short course of iron and re-evaluation is all that is required to separate those children who will need further evaluation. Children who have β-thalassemia trait will have a persistent red cell distribution width, and on hemoglobin electrophoresis they will have an elevated Hb F and diagnostically elevated Hb A_2. There are "silent" forms

of thalassemia trait, and if the family history is suggestive, further studies may be indicated.

α-Thalassemia

The same evolutionary pressures that produced the β-thalassemia and sickle hemoglobinopathies produced α-thalassemia. Infants are identified in the newborn period by the increased production of Bart's hemoglobin (γ_4) during fetal life and its presence at birth. Although these thalassemias occur in all malarious areas, they are most common in Southeast Asia. Deletion mutations are common in the α-thalassemias and rare in β-thalassemia. The variety of phenotypes seen in β-thalassemia are lacking in α-thalassemia. There are four α-globin genes and four deletional α-thalassemia phenotypes. There are five common α^0-thalassemia mutations, $^{-FIL}$, $^{-MED}$, $^{-THAI}$, $^{-SEA}$, and $^{-(\alpha)20.5}$ deletions, and two α^+-thalassemia mutations, $-\alpha^{3.7}$ and $-\alpha^{4.2}$. They can be identified by polymerase chain reaction analysis. Most of these deletions, with the exception of the SEA deletion, common in Southeast Asia, include the ζ-globin gene and are not compatible with life in the homozygous state. In addition to these deletional mutations there are also nondeletional α-globin gene mutations, the most common being Constant Spring ($\alpha^{CS}\alpha$); these mutations cause a more severe anemia and clinical course than the deletional mutations.

The deletion of one α-globin gene (silent trait) is not identifiable hematologically; individuals with this deletion are usually diagnosed after the birth of a child with a two gene deletion or Hb H (β_4). This deletion is common in African-Americans.

The deletion of two α-globin genes results in α-thalassemia trait. The globin genes can be lost in trans, $-\alpha/-\alpha$ or cist, such as $\alpha,\alpha/^{-SEA}$. The cist or α^0 mutations combined with other mutations can lead to Hb H or α-thalassemia major. The α-thalassemia traits present as a microcytic anemia that can be mistaken for iron-deficiency anemia (see Fig. 454–2F). The hemoglobin electrophoresis is normal. The diagnosis of iron deficiency must be eliminated and the diagnosis presumed or confirmed by DNA testing.

The deletion of three α-globin genes leads to the diagnosis of **Hb H disease**. This form of α-thalassemia is significant for a marked microcytosis and anemia; it is identified by hemoglobin electrophoresis. Although there have been few studies of this hemoglobinopathy, it is generally asymptomatic with a moderate anemia and mild splenomegaly, and, occasionally, scleral icterus or cholelithiasis is present. Although brilliant cresyl blue can stain Hb H, it is rarely used for diagnosis. Transfusion is not usually necessary for treatment of the anemia.

The deletion of all four α-globin genes causes profound anemia during fetal life, resulting in hydrops fetalis; the ζ-globin gene must be present for fetal survival. There are no normal hemoglobins present at birth (primarily Bart's, with hemoglobins Gower 1, Gower 2, and Portland). If the fetus survives, immediate exchange transfusion is indicated. These infants with α-thalassemia major are transfusion dependent. There have been at least two successful bone marrow transplants that cured this disease.

The presence of *a nondeletional α-globin mutation* with a two-gene deletion results in a more severe anemia, increased hepatosplenomegaly, increased jaundice, and a much more severe clinical course than Hb H disease. Hb H Constant Spring is the most common form ($-\alpha/\alpha,\alpha^{CS}$).

Treatment of the α-thalassemia deletion syndromes consists of folate supplementation, possible splenectomy (with the attendant risks), intermittent transfusion during severe anemia for the nondeletion Hb H diseases, and chronic transfusion therapy or bone marrow transplant for survivors of hydrops fetalis. These children also should not be exposed to oxidant medications.

Iron Overload Disorders

The disorders leading to iron overload are not disorders of hemoglobin. **Hereditary hemochromatosis** (HH) is a disorder of iron absorption leading to toxicity in the fourth to fifth decades of life. Iron absorption is primarily in the liver, heart, and pancreas leading to hepatic cirrhosis and liver failure. It has a prevalence of 1:250 in white Northern Europeans. There are two alleles of the *HFE* gene: 845 G→A (C282Y) and 187 C→G (H63D). These alleles have been associated with hereditary hemtochomatosis. Expression of the C282Y gene is homozygous in 84–100% of individuals with HH (type 1). A second mutation, H63D, is found in combination with C282Y in 2–7% of HH. There are individuals with HH who have neither mutation (type 3). Diagnosis can be made by evaluation of transferrin saturation and ferritin. Treatment is phlebotomy.

There are three pediatric forms of iron overload. Juvenile hemochromatosis (type 2), atransferrinemia/hypotransferrinemia, and neonatal hemochromatosis. **Juvenile hemochromatosis** differs from HH in that the iron loading is primarily in the heart and endocrine system with associated morbidity (i.e., cardiac arrhythmias and failure, diabetes mellitus). Without phlebotomy, death occurs in the third decade. There is no genetic determinant. Infants born with **atransferrinemia** have a disorder similar to HH but also have anemia owing to the lack of transferrin. **Neonatal hemochromatosis** is a rare disease that presents as hepatic iron overload leading to liver dysfunction and failure in the neonatal period. It is sometimes associated with neonatal giant cell hepatitis.

Hemoglobin Disorders

Arcasoy MO, Gallagher PG: Molecular diagnosis of hemoglobinopathies and other red blood cell disorders. *Semin Hematol* 1999;36:328–9.

Weatherall D, Clegg J (editors): *The Thalassemia Syndromes*, 4th ed. Oxford, Blackwell Science, 2001.

Sickle Cell Disease

Adams RJ: Stroke prevention and treatment in sickle cell disease. *Arch Neurol* 2001;58:565–8.

Adams RJ, McKie VC, Hsu L, et al: Prevention of a first stroke by transfusions in children with sickle cell anemia and abnormal results on transcranial Doppler ultrasonography. *N Engl J Med* 1998;339:5–11.

Bunn HF: Pathogenesis and treatment of sickle cell disease. *N Engl J Med* 1997;337:762–9.

Gladwin MT, Schechter AN: Nitric oxide therapy in sickle cell disease. *Semin Hematol* 2001;38:333–42.

Hoppe C, Vichinsky E, Quirolo K, et al: Use of hydroxyurea in children ages 2 to 5 years with sickle cell disease. *J Pediatr Hematol Oncol* 2000;22:330–4.

Hoppe CC, Walters MC: Bone marrow transplantation in sickle cell anemia. *Curr Opin Oncol* 2001;13:85–90.

Kinney TR, Sleeper LA, Wang WC, et al: Silent cerebral infarcts in sickle cell anemia: A risk factor analysis. The Cooperative Study of Sickle Cell Disease. *Pediatrics* 1999;103:640–5.

Kinney TR, Helms RW, O'Branski EE, et al: Safety of hydroxyurea in children with sickle cell anemia: Results of the HUG-KIDS study, a phase I/II trial. Pediatric Hydroxyurea Group. *Blood* 1999;94:1550–4.

Knight-Madden J, Serjeant GR: Invasive pneumococcal disease in homozygous sickle cell disease: Jamaican experience 1973–1997. *J Pediatr* 2001;138:65–70.

Koumbourlis AC, Zar HJ, Hurlet-Jensen A, et al: Prevalence and reversibility of lower airway obstruction in children with sickle cell disease. *J Pediatr* 2001;138:188–92.

Miller MK, Zimmerman SA, Schultz WH, et al: Hydroxyurea therapy for pediatric patients with hemoglobin SC disease. *J Pediatr Hematol Oncol* 2001;23:306–8.

Miller ST, Sleeper LA, Pegelow CH, et al: Prediction of adverse outcomes in children with sickle cell disease. *N Engl J Med* 2000;342:83–9.

Miller ST, Wright E, Abboud M, et al: Impact of chronic transfusion on incidence of pain and acute chest syndrome during the Stroke Prevention Trial (STOP) in sickle cell anemia. *J Pediatr* 2001;139:785–9.

Milner PF, Kraus AP, Sebes JI, et al: Sickle cell disease as a cause of osteonecrosis of the femoral head. *N Engl J Med* 1991;325:1476–81.

Morris CR, Kuypers FA, Larkin S, et al: Patterns of arginine and nitric oxide in patients with sickle cell disease with vaso-occlusive crisis and acute chest syndrome. *J Pediatr Hematol Oncol* 2000;22:515–20.

Olivieri NF: Progression of iron overload in sickle cell disease. *Semin Hematol* 2001;38(1 Suppl 1):57–62.

Steen RG, Helton KJ, Horwitz EM, et al: Improved cerebrovascular patency following therapy in patients with sickle cell disease: Initial results in 4 patients who received HLA-identical hematopoietic stem cell allografts. *Ann Neurol* 2001;49:222–9.

Vernacchio L, Neufeld EJ, MacDonald K, et al: Combined schedule of 7-valent pneumococcal conjugate vaccine followed by 23-valent pneumococcal vaccine in children and young adults with sickle cell disease. *J Pediatr* 1998;133:275–8.

Vichinsky EP, Haberkern CM, Neumayr L, et al: A comparison of conservative and aggressive transfusion regimens in the perioperative management of sickle cell disease. The Preoperative Transfusion in Sickle Cell Disease Study Group. *N Engl J Med* 1995;333:206–13.

Vichinsky EP, Neumayr LD, Earles AN, et al: Causes and outcomes of the acute chest syndrome in sickle cell disease. National Acute Chest Syndrome Study Group. *N Engl J Med* 2000;342:1855–65.

Walker TM, Hambleton IR, Serjeant GR: Gallstones in sickle cell disease: Observations from The Jamaican Cohort study. *J Pediatr* 2000;136:80–5.

Walters MC, Patience M, Leisenring W, et al: Bone marrow transplantation for sickle cell disease. *N Engl J Med* 1996;335:369–76.

Wang W, Enos L, Gallagher D, et al: Neuropsychologic performance in school-aged children with sickle cell disease: A report from the Cooperative Study of Sickle Cell Disease. *J Pediatr* 2001;139:391–7.

Wang W, Holms RW, Lynn HS, et al: Effect of hydroxyurea on growth in children with sickle cell anemia: Results of the HUG-KIDS study. *J Pediatr* 2002;140:225–9.

Ware RE, Eggleston B, Redding-Lallinger R, et al: Predictors of fetal hemoglobin response in children with sickle cell anemia receiving hydroxyurea therapy. *Blood* 2002;99:10–14.

Wigfall DR, Ware RE, Burchinal MR, et al: Prevalence and clinical correlates of glomerulopathy in children with sickle cell disease. *J Pediatr* 2000;136:749–53.

Methemoglobinemia

Rehman HU: Methemoglobinemia. *West J Med* 2001;175:193–6.

Sanchez-Echaniz J, Benito-Fernandez J, Mintegui-Raso S: Methemoglobinemia and consumption of vegetables in infants. *Pediatrics* 2001;107:1024–8.

Thalassemia

Aessopos A, Tsironi M, Vassiliadis I, et al: Exercise-induced myocardial perfusion abnormalities in sickle beta-thalassemia: Tc-99m tetrofosmin gated SPECT imaging study. *Am J Med* 2001;111:355–60.

Berkovitch M, Bistritzer T, Milone SD, et al: Iron deposition in the anterior pituitary in homozygous beta-thalassemia: MRI evaluation and correlation with gonadal function. *J Pediatr Endocrinol Metab* 2000;13:179–84.

Chen FE, Ooi C, Ha SY, et al: Genetic and clinical features of hemoglobin H disease in Chinese patients. *N Engl J Med* 2000;343:544–50.

Chern JP, Lin KH, Lu MY, et al: Abnormal glucose tolerance in transfusion-dependent beta-thalassemic patients. *Diabetes Care* 2001;24:850–4.

Chik KW, Shing MM, Li CK, et al: Treatment of hemoglobin Bart's hydrops with bone marrow transplantation. *J Pediatr* 1998;132:1039–42.

Eldor A, Rachmilewitz EA: The hypercoagulable state in thalassemia. *Blood* 2002;99:36–43.

Gulati R, Bhatia V, Agarwal SS: Early onset of endocrine abnormalities in beta-thalassemia major in a developing country. *J Pediatr Endocrinol Metab* 2000;13:651–6.

Hahalis G, Manolis AS, Gerasimidou I, et al: Right ventricular diastolic function in beta-thalassemia major: Echocardiographic and clinical correlates. *Am Heart J* 2001;141:428–34.

Kattamis AC, Antoniadis M, Manoli I, et al: Endocrine problems in ex-thalassemic patients. *Transfus Sci* 2000;23:251–2.

Jensen CE, Tuck SM, Agnew JE, et al: High prevalence of low bone mass in thalassaemia major. *Br J Haematol* 1998;103:911–5.

Olivieri NF: The beta-thalassemias. *N Engl J Med* 1999;341:99–109.

Olivieri NF, Brittenham GM: Iron-chelating therapy and the treatment of thalassemia. *Blood* 1997;89:739–61.

Telfer PT, Prescott E, Holden S, et al: Hepatic iron concentration combined with long-term monitoring of serum ferritin to predict complications of iron overload in thalassaemia major. *Br J Haematol* 2000;110:971–7.

Theodoridis C, Ladis V, Papatheodorou A, et al: Growth and management of short stature in thalassaemia major. *J Pediatr Endocrinol Metab* 1998;11(Suppl 3):835–44.

Weatherall DJ: Introduction to the problem of hemoglobin E-beta thalassemia. *J Pediatr Hematol Oncol* 2000;22:551.

Winichagoon P, Fucharoen S, Chen P, et al: Genetic factors affecting clinical severity in beta-thalassemia syndromes. *J Pediatr Hematol Oncol* 2000;22:573–80.

Wonke B: Clinical management of beta-thalassemia major. *Semin Hematol* 2001;38:350–9.

Iron Overload Disorders

Andrews NC: Inherited iron overload disorders. *Curr Opin Pediatr* 2000;12:596–602.

McCullen MA, Crawford DH, Hickman PE: Screening for hemochromatosis. *Clin Chim Acta* 2002;315(1–2):169–86.

Murray KF, Kowdley KV: Neonatal hemochromatosis. *Pediatrics* 2001;108:960–4.

Roy CN, Andrews NC: Recent advances in disorders of iron metabolism: Mutations, mechanisms and modifiers. *Hum Mol Genet* 2001;10:2181–6.

Sanchez AM, Schreiber GB, Bethel J, et al: Prevalence, donation practices, and risk assessment of blood donors with hemochromatosis. *JAMA* 2001;286:1475–81.

Vohra P, Haller C, Emre S, et al: Neonatal hemochromatosis: The importance of early recognition of liver failure. *J Pediatr* 2000;136:537–41.

Enzymatic Defects *George B. Segel*

DEFICIENCIES OF ENZYMES OF THE GLYCOLYTIC PATHWAY

Various red blood cell (RBC) enzymatic defects produce hemolytic anemias, characterized by a lack of spherocytes and few distinguishing features on the blood film. Deficiencies of most of the enzymes in both the anaerobic Embden-Meyerhof pathway and the oxidative hexose monophosphate (pentose) shunt have been described (Fig. 455–1). The most common glycolytic enzyme defect as a cause of hemolytic anemia is pyruvate kinase (PK) deficiency, although it is a rare disorder, with only 300–400 cases reported.

455.1 Pyruvate Kinase (PK) Deficiency

A congenital hemolytic anemia occurs in persons homozygous for an autosomal recessive gene that causes either a marked reduction in RBC PK or production of an abnormal enzyme with decreased activity. Generation of adenosine triphosphate (ATP) within RBCs is impaired, and low levels of ATP, pyruvate, and the oxidized form of nicotinamide-adenine dinucleotide (NAD$^+$) are found (see Fig. 455–1). The concentration of 2,3-diphosphoglycerate (2,3-DPG) is increased, and this increase is beneficial in facilitating oxygen release from hemoglobin but detrimental in inhibiting hexokinase as well as enzymes of the hexose monophosphate shunt. In addition, an unexplained decrease occurs in the sum of the adenine (ATP, adenosine diphosphate [ADP], and adenosine monophosphate [AMP]) and pyridine (NAD$^+$ and NADH) nucleotides, and this further impairs glycolysis. As a consequence of decreased ATP, RBCs cannot maintain the potassium and water content; the cells become rigid, and the RBC life span is considerably reduced.

Etiology. There are two mammalian PK genes, but only the *PKLR* gene is expressed in red cells. The human *PKLR* gene has been mapped to chromosome 1q21, and 133 mutations are reported in this structural gene, which codes for a protein with 574 amino acids and forms a functional tetramer. Most affected patients are compound heterozygotes for two different PK gene defects. The many possible combinations likely account for the variability in clinical severity.

Clinical Manifestations and Laboratory Findings. The clinical manifestations vary from a severe neonatal hemolytic anemia to mild, well-compensated hemolysis noted first in adulthood. Severe jaundice and anemia may occur in the neonatal period, and kernicterus has been reported. The hemolysis in older children and adults varies in severity, with hemoglobin values from 8–12 g/dL associated with some pallor, jaundice, and splenomegaly. These patients usually do not require transfusion. A severe form of the disease has a relatively high incidence among the Amish of the midwestern United States.

Polychromatophilia and mild macrocytosis reflect the elevated reticulocyte count. Spherocytes are uncommon, but a few spiculated pyknocytes usually are found. Nonincubated osmotic fragility is normal. Autohemolysis is moderately or markedly increased, but the addition of glucose does not regularly correct the abnormality as it does in hereditary spherocytosis.

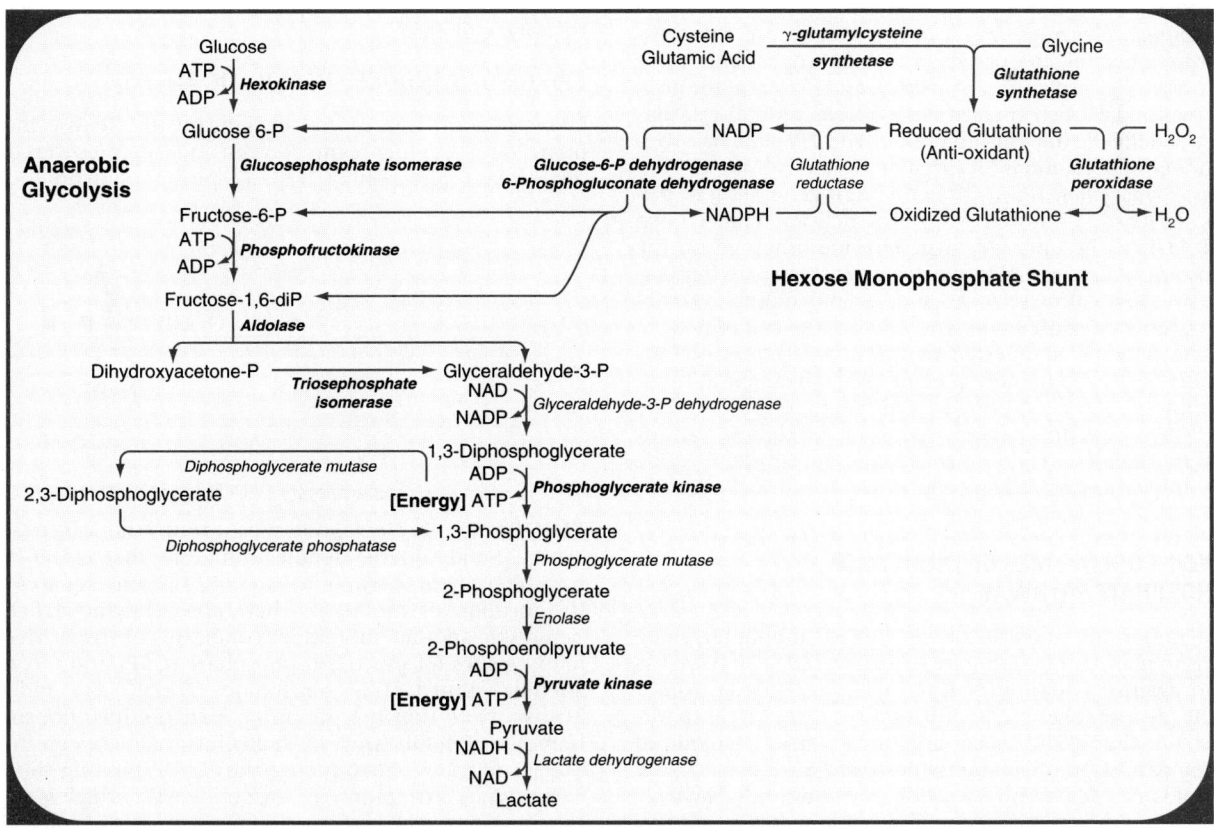

FIGURE 455–1. Red cell metabolism. Glycolysis and the hexose monophosphate pathway. The enzyme deficiencies clearly associated with hemolysis are shown in bold type.

Diagnosis relies on demonstration of a marked reduction of PK activity or an increase in the Michaelis-Menten dissociation constant (Km) for its substrate, phosphoenolpyruvate, in the RBCs. Other RBC enzyme activities are normal, or elevated reflecting the reticulocytosis. No abnormalities of hemoglobin are noted. The white cells have normal PK activity and must be rigorously excluded from hemolysates used to measure PK activity. Heterozygous carriers usually have moderately reduced levels of PK activity.

Treatment. Exchange transfusions may be indicated for hyperbilirubinemia in newborns. Transfusions of packed RBCs are necessary for severe anemia or for aplastic crises. If the anemia is consistently severe or if frequent transfusions are required, splenectomy should be performed after 5–6 yr of age. Although not curative, the operation may be followed by higher hemoglobin levels and by strikingly high (30–60%) reticulocyte counts. Deaths resulting from overwhelming pneumococcal sepsis have followed splenectomy; thus, immunization with vaccines for encapsulated organisms should be given before splenectomy and prophylactic penicillin should be administered after splenectomy.

455.2 Other Glycolytic Enzyme Deficiencies

Chronic nonspherocytic hemolytic anemias of varying severity have been associated with deficiencies of other enzymes in the glycolytic pathway, including hexokinase, glucose phosphate isomerase, and aldolase, which are inherited as autosomal recessive disorders. *Phosphofructokinase (PFK) deficiency* occurs primarily in Ashkenazi Jews in the United States and results in hemolysis associated with a myopathy classified as glycogen storage disease type VII (see Chapter 76.1). Clinically, a hemolytic anemia is complicated by muscle weakness, exercise intolerance, cramps, and possibly myoglobinuria. Enzyme assays for PFK are low in RBCs and muscle.

Triose phosphate isomerase (TPI) deficiency is an autosomal recessive disorder affecting many systems. Affected patients have hemolytic anemia, cardiac abnormalities, and lower motor neuron and pyramidal tract impairment without mental retardation. They usually die in early childhood. The *TPI* gene has been cloned and sequenced and is localized on chromosome 12.

Phosphoglycerate kinase (PGK) is the first ATP-generating step in glycolysis. At least 23 kindreds with PGK deficiency have been described. PGK is the only glycolytic enzyme inherited on the X chromosome. Affected males may have progressive extrapyramidal disease, myopathy, seizures, and variable mental retardation in conjunction with hemolytic anemia. In a report from Tokyo, nine patients manifested neural/myopathic symptoms with hemolysis; six had hemolysis alone, seven had neural/myopathic symptoms alone, and one person had no symptoms. The gene for PGK is particularly large, spanning 23 kb, and various genetic abnormalities including nucleotide substitutions, gene deletions, missense and splicing mutations result in PGK deficiency.

DEFICIENCIES OF ENZYMES OF THE HEXOSE MONOPHOSPHATE PATHWAY

The most important function of the hexose monophosphate pathway is to maintain glutathione in its reduced state (GSH) as protection against oxidation of RBCs (see Fig. 455–1). About 10% of the glucose taken up by RBCs passes through this pathway to provide the NADPH necessary for conversion of oxidized glutathione (GSSG) to GSH. Maintenance of GSH is essential for the physiologic inactivation of oxidant compounds, such as hydrogen peroxide, that accumulate within RBCs. If glutathione, or any compound or enzyme necessary for maintaining it in the reduced state, is decreased, the SH groups of the

RBC membrane are oxidized and the hemoglobin becomes denatured and may precipitate into RBC inclusions called *Heinz bodies*. Once Heinz bodies have formed, an acute hemolytic process results from damage to the RBC membrane by the precipitated hemoglobin, the oxidant agent, and the action of the spleen. The damaged RBCs then are rapidly removed from the circulation.

455.3 Glucose-6-Phosphate Dehydrogenase (G6PD) and Related Deficiencies

G6PD deficiency is the most important disease of the hexose monophosphate pathway and is responsible for two clinical syndromes, an episodic hemolytic anemia induced by infections, certain drugs, or, rarely, fava beans and a spontaneous chronic nonspherocytic hemolytic anemia. This X-linked enzyme deficiency affects more than 200 million people worldwide, and it represents an example of "balanced polymorphism" in which there is an evolutionary advantage of resistance to falciparum malaria in heterozygous females that outweighs the small negative effect of affected hemizygous males.

The deficiency is caused by inheritance of any of a large number of abnormal alleles of the gene responsible for the synthesis of the G6PD molecule. The *G6PD* gene has been cloned and sequenced, and at least 90 mutations have been identified. Some of these mutations that cause episodic versus chronic hemolysis are shown in Figure 455–2. Milder disease is associated with mutations near the amino terminus of the G6PD molecule, and chronic nonspherocytic hemolytic anemia with mutations clustered near the carboxyl terminus. The normal enzyme found in most populations is designated G6PD B+. A normal variant designated G6PD A+ is common in the African-American population. More than 100 distinct enzyme variants of G6PD are associated with a wide spectrum of hemolytic disease.

EPISODIC OR INDUCED HEMOLYTIC ANEMIA

Etiology. G6PD is a central enzyme in the hexose monophosphate shunt of glucose metabolism and catalyzes the conversion of glucose-6-phosphate (G6P) to 6-phosphogluconic acid (6PG).

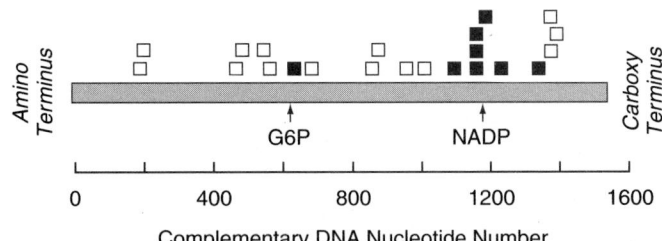

FIGURE 455–2. Nucleotide substitutions that cause G6PD deficiency. Solid squares denote mutations that cause hereditary nonspherocytic hemolytic anemia. Open squares indicate the location of mutations that cause enzyme deficiency but hemolytic anemia only under conditions of stress. The putative binding sites for glucose-6-phosphate (G6P) and nicotinamide-adenine dinucleotide phosphate (NADP) are indicated by arrows. Note that the mutations that produce nonspherocytic hemolytic anemia are almost all clustered between nucleotides 1089 and 1361, surrounding the NADP-binding domain. The exception is a mutation at nucleotide 637, which is adjacent to the putative G-6-P binding domain at nucleotide 605. (Modified from Beutler E: Glucose-6-phosphate deficiency. N Engl J Med 1991;324:169.)

NADPH is produced in this process and is necessary to maintain glutathione in the reduced state, that is, GSSG→GSH. Glutathione is present in the red cell in millimolar amounts and acts to neutralize agents that potentially oxidize either hemoglobin or components of the red cell membrane. If reduced glutathione cannot be sustained to remove oxygen radicals generated by oxidant drugs, the hemoglobin precipitates forming Heinz bodies, and the red cell membrane is critically damaged. The precipitation of hemoglobin and damage to the membrane result in premature red cell destruction or hemolysis.

Synthesis of RBC G6PD is determined by a gene on the X chromosome. Diseases involving this enzyme therefore occur more frequently in males than in females. About 13% of male African-Americans have a mutant enzyme (G6PD A⁻) that results in a deficiency of RBC G6PD activity to 5–15% or less of normal. Italians, Greeks, and other Mediterranean, Middle Eastern, African, and Asian ethnic groups also have a high incidence, ranging from 5–40%, of a variant designated G6PD B⁻ (G6PD Mediterranean). In these variants, the G6PD activity of homozygous females or hemizygous males is less than 5% of normal. Heterozygous females have an intermediate enzymatic activity and, as an example of random X chromosome inactivation (Lyon hypothesis), have two populations of RBCs: One is normal, and the other is deficient in G6PD activity. Most heterozygous females do not have clinical hemolysis after exposure to oxidant drugs. Rarely, the majority of the RBCs are G6PD deficient in heterozygous females because of random inactivation of the normal X chromosome.

Considerable variation in the defect among various racial groups is noted. For example, the defect in Americans of African descent is less severe than in affected Americans of European descent. In Americans of African descent, the electrophoretically distinct enzyme variant is unstable in vivo, and its activity is decreased primarily in the older RBCs in the circulation. The enzyme activity of RBCs containing the variant enzyme (G6PD B⁻) in Americans of European descent is very low, often less than 1% of normal in the entire RBC population. A third common mutant enzyme with markedly reduced activity (G6PD Canton) occurs in about 5% of the Chinese population. A large number of other rare enzyme variants have been associated with drug-induced hemolysis.

Clinical Manifestations. In the usual pattern of G6PD deficiency, symptoms develop 24–48 hr after a patient has ingested a substance that has oxidant properties. Drugs that have these properties include aspirin, sulfonamides, and antimalarials such as primaquine (Box 455–1). In some patients, ingestion of fava beans, a Mediterranean dietary staple, may also produce an acute and severe hemolytic syndrome called *favism*. This results from oxidative products derived from two glucosidic compounds, vicine and convicine, which are hydrolyzed to divicine and isouramil, ultimately producing hydrogen peroxide and other reactive oxygen products.

The degree of hemolysis varies with the inciting agent, the amount ingested, and the severity of the enzyme deficiency in the patient. In severe cases, hemoglobinuria and jaundice result, and the hemoglobin concentration may fall precipitously and be life threatening. In the A⁻ variety (Americans of African descent), the stability of the folded protein dimer is impaired, and this defect is accentuated as RBCs age. Thus, some spontaneous recovery of the hemolysis may be observed even if administration of the drug is continued. This recovery is a result of the age-labile enzyme, which is abundant and more stable in younger RBCs. The associated reticulocytosis produces a compensated hemolytic process. Infection also may result in hemolysis, and significant but insidious hemolysis may occur in patients hospitalized for other illnesses even when no exposure to drugs can be documented. In A⁻ G6PD deficiency, spontaneous hemolysis

---

BOX 455–1. Agents Precipitating Hemolysis in Glucose-6-Phosphate Dehydrogenase Deficiency

MEDICATIONS

Antibacterials
Sulfonamides
Trimethoprim-sulfamethoxazole
Nalidixic acid
Chloramphenicol
Nitrofurantoin

Antimalarials
Primaquine
Pamaquine
Chloroquine
Quinacrine

Others
Phenacetin
Vitamin K analogs
Methylene blue
Probenecid
Acetylsalicylic acid
Phenazopyridine

CHEMICALS
Phenylhydrazine
Benzene
Naphthalene

ILLNESS
Diabetic acidosis
Hepatitis

Reproduced from Asselin BL, Segel GB. In Rakel R (editor): *Conn's Current Therapy*. Philadelphia, WB Saunders, 1994, p 341.

---

may occur in premature but not term infants. In Greek and Chinese newborns with the G6PD B⁻ and Canton varieties, the deficiency of G6PD is an important cause of hyperbilirubinemia and potential kernicterus. In a group of Sephardic Jewish female newborn heterozygotes, there was heightened hyperbilirubinemia particularly if the variant promoter (UGT1A1) seen in Gilbert's syndrome was present. When a pregnant woman ingests oxidant drugs, they may be transmitted to her G6PD-deficient fetus, and hemolytic anemia and jaundice may be apparent at birth.

Laboratory Findings. The onset of acute hemolysis results in a precipitous fall in hemoglobin and hematocrit. If the episode is severe, the hemoglobin-binding proteins such as haptoglobin are saturated, and free hemoglobin may appear in the plasma and subsequently in the urine (see Fig. 449–2). Unstained or supravital preparations of RBCs reveal Heinz bodies (precipitated hemoglobin), which are not visible on the Wright-stained blood film. Because cells containing these inclusions are rapidly removed from the circulation, they are not seen after the first 3–4 days of illness. The blood film reveals a few fragmented cells and polychromatophilic cells (bluish, large RBCs), representing the reticulocytosis, which often is substantial (5–15%).

Diagnosis. The diagnosis depends on direct or indirect demonstration of reduced G6PD activity in RBCs. By direct measurement, enzyme activity in affected persons is 10% of normal or less, and the reduction of enzyme is more extreme in Americans of European descent and Asians than in Americans of African descent. Satisfactory screening tests are based on decoloration of methylene blue, on the reduction of methemoglobin, or on the fluorescence of NADPH. Immediately after a hemolytic episode, reticulocytes and young RBCs predominate. These young cells have significantly higher enzyme activity than do older cells in the A⁻ variety. Testing may therefore have to be deferred for a few weeks before a diagnostically low level of enzyme can be shown. The diagnosis can be suspected when the G6PD activity is within the low normal range in the presence of a high reticulocyte count. G6PD variants also can be detected by electrophoretic analysis.

Prevention and Treatment. Prevention of hemolysis constitutes the most important therapeutic measure. When possible, males belonging to ethnic groups with a significant incidence of G6PD deficiency (e.g., Greeks, southern Italians, Sephardic Jews, Filipinos, southern Chinese, Americans of African descent, and Thais) should be tested for the defect before known oxidant drugs are given. The usual doses of aspirin and trimethoprim sulfamethoxazole do not cause clinically relevant hemolysis in the A⁻ variety. However, aspirin administered in doses used for acute rheumatic fever (60–100 mg/kg/24 hr) may produce a severe hemolytic episode. When hemolysis has occurred, supportive therapy may require blood transfusions, although recovery is the rule when the oxidant agent is removed.

CHRONIC HEMOLYTIC ANEMIAS ASSOCIATED WITH DEFICIENCIES OF G6PD OR RELATED FACTORS

Chronic nonspherocytic hemolytic anemia has been associated with profound deficiency of G6PD caused by enzyme variants, particularly those defective in quantity, activity, or stability. The gene defects leading to chronic hemolysis are located primarily in the region of the NADP binding site near the carboxyl terminus of the protein (see Fig. 455–2). These include the Loma Linda, Tomah, Iowa, Beverly Hills, Nashville, Riverside, Santiago de Cuba, and Andalus variants. Persons with G6PD B⁻ (Mediterranean) enzyme deficiency occasionally have chronic hemolysis, and the hemolytic process may worsen after ingestion of oxidant drugs. Splenectomy is of little value in these types of chronic hemolysis.

Other enzyme defects may impair the regeneration of GSH as an oxidant "sump" (see Fig. 455–1). A mild, chronic nonspherocytic anemia has been reported in association with decreased RBC GSH, resulting from γ-glutamylcysteine synthetase or glutathione synthetase deficiencies. 6-Phosphogluconate dehydrogenase deficiency has been associated primarily with drug-induced hemolysis, and hemolysis with hyperbilirubinemia has been related to a deficiency of glutathione peroxidase in newborn infants.

Chapter 456

Hemolytic Anemias Resulting from Extracellular Factors *George B. Segel*

AUTOIMMUNE HEMOLYTIC ANEMIAS

A number of extrinsic agents and disorders may lead to premature destruction of red blood cells (RBCs) (see Table 449–1). Among the most clearly defined are antibodies associated with immune hemolytic anemias. The hallmark of this group of diseases is a positive direct antiglobulin (Coombs) test, which detects a coating of immunoglobulin or components of complement on the RBC surface. The most important immune hemolytic disorder in pediatric practice is hemolytic disease of the newborn (erythroblastosis fetalis), caused by transplacental transfer of maternal antibody active against the RBCs of the fetus, that is, isoimmune hemolytic anemia (see Chapter 92.2). Various other immune hemolytic anemias are autoimmune

(Box 456–1) and may be idiopathic or related to various infections (Epstein-Barr virus, rarely HIV, cytomegalovirus, and *Mycoplasma*), immunologic diseases (systemic lupus erythematosus [SLE], rheumatoid arthritis), immunodeficiency diseases (agammaglobulinemia and dysgammaglobulinemias), neoplasms (lymphoma, leukemia, and Hodgkin's disease), or drugs (methyldopa, levodopa). Other drugs (penicillins, cephalosporins) cause immune hemolysis that is not autoimmune. The antibodies are "drug dependent" and usually (although not always) have no "specificity" for RBC membrane antigens.

AUTOIMMUNE HEMOLYTIC ANEMIAS ASSOCIATED WITH "WARM" ANTIBODIES

Etiology. In the autoimmune hemolytic anemias, abnormal antibodies are directed against RBCs but the pathogenetic mechanisms are uncertain. The autoantibody may be produced as an inappropriate immune response to an RBC antigen or to another antigenic epitope similar to an RBC antigen. Alternatively, an infectious agent may in some way alter the RBC membrane so that it becomes "foreign" or antigenic to the host. The antibodies usually react to epitopes (antigens) that are "public" or common to all human RBC such as Rh proteins.

In most instances of warm antibody hemolysis, no underlying cause can be found, and it is called *primary* or *idiopathic* (see Box 456–1). If the autoimmune hemolysis is associated with an underlying disease such as a lymphoproliferative disorder, SLE, or immunodeficiency, it is called *secondary*. In as many as 20% of cases of immune hemolysis, drugs may be implicated.

Drugs (e.g., penicillin or sometimes cephalosporins) that cause hemolysis via the "hapten" mechanism (immune but not autoimmune) bind tightly to the RBC membrane (see Box 456–1). Antibodies to the drug, either newly or previously formed, bind to the drug molecules on RBCs, mediating their destruction in the spleen. In other cases, certain drugs, such as quinine and quinidine, do not bind to RBCs but rather form part of a "ternary complex," consisting of the drug, an RBC membrane

---

BOX 456–1. Diseases Characterized by Immune-Mediated Red Blood Cell Destruction

AUTOIMMUNE HEMOLYTIC ANEMIA DUE TO WARM REACTIVE AUTOANTIBODIES
Primary (idiopathic)
Secondary
    Lymphoproliferative disorders
    Connective tissue disorders (especially systemic lupus erythematosus)
    Nonlymphoid neoplasms (e.g., ovarian tumors)
    Chronic inflammatory diseases (e.g., ulcerative colitis)
 	
AUTOIMMUNE HEMOLYTIC ANEMIA DUE TO COLD REACTIVE AUTOANTIBODIES (CRYOPATHIC HEMOLYTIC SYNDROMES)
Primary (idiopathic) cold agglutinin disease
Secondary cold agglutinin disease
    Lymphoproliferative disorders
    Infections (*Mycoplasma pneumoniae*, Epstein-Barr virus)
Paroxysmal cold hemoglobinuria
    Primary (idiopathic)
    Congenital or tertiary syphilis
    Viral syndromes (most common)
 	
DRUG-INDUCED IMMUNE HEMOLYTIC ANEMIA
Hapten/drug adsorption (e.g., penicillin)
Ternary (immune) complex (e.g., quinine or quinidine)
True autoantibody induction (e.g., methyldopa)

Modified from Packman CH: Autoimmune hemolytic anemias. In Rakel R (editor): *Conn's Current Therapy.* Philadelphia, WB Saunders, 1995, p 305.

antigen, and an antibody that recognizes both (see Box 456–1). Methyldopa and sometimes cephalosporins may by unknown mechanisms incite true autoantibodies to RBC membrane antigens, so that the presence of the drug is not required to cause hemolysis.

Clinical Manifestations. Autoimmune hemolytic anemias may occur in either of two general clinical patterns. The first, an acute transient type lasting 3–6 mo and occurring predominantly in children ages 2–12 yr, accounts for 70–80% of patients. It is frequently preceded by an infection, usually respiratory. The onset may be acute, with prostration, pallor, jaundice, pyrexia, and hemoglobinuria, or may be more gradual in onset, with primarily fatigue and pallor. The spleen is usually enlarged and is the primary site for destruction of IgG-coated RBCs. Underlying systemic disorders are unusual in this group. A consistent response to glucocorticoid therapy, low mortality, and full recovery are characteristic of the acute form. The other clinical pattern involves a prolonged and chronic course, which is more frequent in infants and in children older than 12 yr. Hemolysis may continue for many months or years. Abnormalities involving other blood elements are common, and the response to glucocorticoids is variable and inconsistent. Mortality is about 10%, often attributable to an underlying systemic disease.

Laboratory Findings. In many cases, the anemia is profound, with hemoglobin levels less than 6 g/dL. Considerable spherocytosis and polychromasia are present. More than 50% of the circulating RBCs may be reticulocytes, and nucleated RBCs usually are present. In some cases, a low reticulocyte count may be present, particularly early in the episode. Leukocytosis is common. The platelet count is usually normal, but immune thrombocytopenic purpura is an occasional concomitant (*Evans syndrome*). The prognosis for patients with Evans syndrome is poor, because many develop chronic disease, including some with SLE.

Results of the direct antiglobulin test are strongly positive, and free antibody can sometimes be demonstrated in the serum (indirect Coombs test). These antibodies are active between 35°C and 40°C ("warm" antibodies) and most often belong to the immunoglobulin G (IgG) class. They do not require complement for activity and usually do not produce agglutination in vitro; they are "incomplete." Antibodies from the serum and those eluted from the RBCs react with RBCs of many persons, in addition to those of the patient. They often have been regarded as nonspecific panagglutinins, but careful studies have revealed specificity for RBC antigens of the Rh system in 70% (~50% adults) of patients. Complement, particularly C3b, may be detected on the RBCs in conjunction with IgG. The Coombs test result is occasionally negative because of the limited sensitivity of the Coombs reaction. A minimum of 260–500 molecules of IgG per cell is necessary on the RBC membrane to produce a positive reaction. Special tests are required to detect the antibody in cases of "Coombs-negative" autoimmune hemolytic anemia.

Treatment. Transfusions usually are only of transient benefit but may be required initially because of the severity of the anemia until the effect of other treatment is observed. It may be extremely difficult to find compatible blood; blood in which the RBCs give the least positive in vitro reaction by Coombs technique should be chosen. It is sometimes necessary to give blood that is "incompatible" as judged by cross matching. Failure to transfuse a profoundly anemic infant or child may lead to serious morbidity and even death.

Those patients with mild disease and compensated hemolysis may not require any treatment. If the hemolysis is severe and results in significant anemia or symptoms, treatment with glucocorticoids is initiated. Glucocorticoids decrease the rate of hemolysis by blocking macrophage function, decreasing the production of the autoantibody, and perhaps by enhancing the elution of antibody from the RBCs. Prednisone or its equivalent is administered in a dose of 2 mg/kg/24 hr. In some patients with severe hemolysis, doses up to 6 mg/kg/24 hr of prednisone may be required to reduce the rate of hemolysis. Treatment should be continued until the rate of hemolysis decreases, and then the dose is gradually reduced. If relapse occurs, resumption of full dosage may be necessary. The disease tends to remit spontaneously within a few weeks or months. The Coombs test result may remain positive, even after hemolysis has subsided. When hemolytic anemia remains severe despite glucocorticoid therapy, or if very large doses are necessary to maintain a reasonable hemoglobin level, intravenous immunoglobulin and danazol may be tried. Splenectomy may be beneficial but is complicated by a heightened risk of infection with encapsulated organisms, particularly in patients younger than 2 yr. Prophylaxis is indicated with appropriate vaccines (pneumococcal, meningococcal, and *Haemophilus influenzae* type b) before splenectomy and with oral penicillin after splenectomy. Immunosuppressive agents including new treatments such as rituximab that target β-lymphocytes, the source of antibody production, may prove useful in chronic cases refractory to conventional therapy. Various plasmapheresis techniques may be used in refractory cases but generally are not helpful.

Course and Prognosis. The acute variety of idiopathic autoimmune hemolytic disease in childhood varies in severity but is self-limited, and mortality from untreatable anemia is rare. Approximately 30% of patients develop chronic hemolysis, often associated with an underlying disease, such as SLE, lymphoma, or leukemia. Mortality in the chronic cases depends on the primary disorder.

AUTOIMMUNE HEMOLYTIC ANEMIAS ASSOCIATED WITH "COLD" ANTIBODIES

RBC antibodies that are more active at low temperatures and agglutinate RBCs at temperatures below 37°C have been called "cold" antibodies. They are primarily of the IgM class and require complement for activity. The range of temperature associated with RBC agglutination is called the *thermal amplitude*. A higher thermal amplitude results in hemolysis with less severe exposure to a cold environment. High antibody titers are associated with high thermal amplitude.

Cold Agglutinin Disease. Cold antibodies usually have specificity for the oligosaccharide antigens of the I/i system. They may occur in primary or idiopathic cold agglutinin disease, secondary to infections such as those from *Mycoplasma pneumoniae* and Epstein-Barr virus or secondary to lymphoproliferative disorders. After *M. pneumoniae* infection, the anti-I levels may increase considerably, and, occasionally, enormous increases may occur to titers of 1:30,000 or greater. The antibody has specificity for the I antigen and, thus, reacts poorly with human cord red blood cells, which possess the i antigen but exhibit low levels of I. Patients with infectious mononucleosis occasionally develop cold agglutinin disease, and the antibodies in these patients often have anti-i specificity. Spontaneous RBC agglutination is observed in the cold, and RBC aggregates are seen on the blood film. The mean corpuscular volume may be spuriously elevated because of cell agglutination. The severity of the hemolysis is related to the thermal amplitude of the antibody, which itself is partly dependent on the IgM antibody titer.

When very high titers of cold antibodies are present and active near body temperature, severe intravascular hemolysis with hemoglobinemia and hemoglobinuria may occur and be heightened on a patient's exposure to cold. Each IgM molecule has the potential to activate a C1 molecule so that large amounts of complement are found on the RBCs in cold agglutinin disease. These sensitized RBCs may undergo intravascular complement lysis or be destroyed in both the liver and spleen.

Cold agglutinin disease is less common in children than in adults, and it more frequently results in an acute, self-limited episode of hemolysis. Glucocorticoids are much less effective in cold agglutinin disease than in disease with warm antibodies. Patients should avoid exposure to cold and should be treated for any underlying disease. In the infrequent patients with severe hemolytic disease, the treatment includes immunosuppression and plasmapheresis. There are several reports of successful treatment of cold agglutinin disease with the monoclonal antibody rituximab that effectively depletes β-lymphocytes. Splenectomy is not useful in cold agglutinin disease.

Paroxysmal Cold Hemoglobinuria. This form of hemolytic anemia is mediated by the Donath-Landsteiner hemolysin, which is an IgG cold-reactive autoantibody with anti-P specificity. This antibody fixes large amounts of complement in the cold, and the RBCs lyse as the temperature is increased. Most reported cases are self-limited and usually are associated with nonspecific viral infections. They are now rarely found in association with congenital or acquired syphilis. This disorder may account for 30% of immune hemolytic episodes among children. Treatment includes transfusions for severe anemia and avoidance of cold ambient temperatures.

Chapter 457
Hemolytic Anemias Secondary to Other Extracellular Factors (See Table 449-1)

George B. Segel

Fragmentation Hemolysis. Red blood cell (RBC) destruction occurs in this group of diseases because of mechanical injury as the cells traverse a damaged vascular bed. This may be microvascular when RBCs are sheared by fibrin in the capillaries during intravascular coagulation or when renovascular disease accompanies the hemolytic-uremic syndrome (see Chapter 510) or thrombotic thrombocytopenic purpura. Larger vessels may be involved in the Kasabach-Merritt syndrome (giant hemangioma and thrombocytopenia) or when a replacement heart valve is poorly epithelialized. The blood film shows many "schistocytes" or fragmented cells as well as polychromatophilia, reflecting the reticulocytosis (see Fig. 450–2F). Secondary iron deficiency may complicate the intravascular hemolysis because of urinary hemoglobin and hemosiderin iron loss (see Fig. 449–2). Treatment should be directed toward the underlying condition, and the prognosis depends on the effectiveness of this treatment. The benefit from transfusion is transient because the transfused cells are destroyed as quickly as those produced by the patient.

Thermal Injury. Extensive burns may directly damage the RBCs and result in hemolysis that results in the formation of spherocytes. Blood loss and marrow suppression may contribute to anemia and require blood transfusion. Erythropoietin (EPO) has been used as treatment for diminished RBC production.

Renal Disease. The anemia of uremia is multifactorial in origin. EPO production may be decreased and the marrow suppressed by toxic metabolites. Furthermore, the RBC life span often is shortened owing to retention of metabolites and organic acidemia. The use of EPO in chronic renal disease has markedly decreased the need for blood transfusion.

Liver Disease. Change in the ratio of cholesterol to phospholipids in the plasma may result in changes in the composition of the RBC membrane and shortening of the RBC life span. Some patients with liver disease have many target RBCs on the blood film, whereas others have a preponderance of spiculated cells.

Toxins and Venoms. Bacterial sepsis due to *Haemophilus influenzae*, staphylococci, and streptococci may be complicated by accompanying hemolysis. A particularly severe hemolytic anemia has been observed in clostridial infections and results from a hemolytic clostridial toxin. Large numbers of spherocytes may be seen on the blood film in this condition. Spherocytic hemolysis also may be noted after bites by various snakes, including cobras, vipers, and rattlesnakes, which have phospholipases in their venom. Large numbers of bites by insects such as bees, wasps, and yellow jackets also may cause spherocytic hemolysis by a similar mechanism (see Chapter 708).

Wilson Disease. An acute and self-limited episode of hemolytic anemia may precede by years the onset of hepatic or neurologic symptoms in Wilson disease. This appears to result from the toxic effects of free copper on the RBC membrane. The blood film often (but not always) shows large numbers of spherocytes, and the Coombs test result is negative. Because early diagnosis of Wilson disease permits prophylactic treatment with penicillamine and prevention of hepatic and neurologic disease, correct assessment of this rare type of hemolysis is most important.

Enzymatic Defects of Red Cells
Beutler E: Glucose-6-phosphate dehydrogenase deficiency. *N Engl J Med* 1994;324:169.
Fujii H, Miwa S: Other erythrocyte enzyme deficiencies associated with non-haematological symptoms: Phosphoglycerate kinase and phosphofructokinase deficiency. *Baillieres Best Pract Res Clin Haematol* 2000;13:141–8.
Kaplan M, Muraca M, Hammerman C, et al: Bilirubin conjugation, reflected by conjugated bilirubin fractions, in glucose-6-phosphate dehydrogenase-deficient neonates: A determining factor in the pathogenesis of hyperbilirubinemia. *Pediatrics* 1998;102:E37.
Kaplan M, Beutler E, Vreman HJ, et al: Neonatal hyperbilirubinemia in glucose-6-phosphate dehydrogenase–deficient heterozygotes. *Pediatrics* 1999; 104:68–74.
Martinov MV, Plotnikov AG, Vitvitsky VM, et al: Deficiencies of glycolytic enzymes as a possible cause of hemolytic anemia. *Biochim Biophys Acta* 2000;1474:75–87.
McMullin MF: The molecular basis of disorders of red cell enzymes. *J Clin Pathol* 1999;52:241.
Zanella A, Bianchi P: Red cell pyruvate kinase deficiency: From genetics. *Baillieres Best Pract Res Clin Haematol* 2000;13:57–81.

Autoimmune Hemolytic Anemia
Buchanan GR, Boxer LA, Nathan DG: The acute and transient nature of idiopathic immune hemolytic anemia in childhood. *J Pediatr* 1976;88:780.
Flores G, Cunningham-Rundles C, Newland AC, et al: Efficacy of intravenous immunoglobulin in the treatment of autoimmune hemolytic anemia: Results in 73 patients. *Am J Hematol* 1993;44:237.
Packman CH: Acquired hemolytic anemia due to warm-reacting autoantibodies. In Beutler E, Lichtman MA, Coller BS, Kipps TC, Seligsohn U (editors): *Williams Hematology*, 6th ed. New York, McGraw-Hill, 2001, pp 639-48.
Packman CH: Cryopathic hemolytic syndromes. In Beutler E, Lichtman MA, Coller BS, Kipps TC, Seligsohn U (editors): *Williams Hematology*, 6th ed. New York, McGraw-Hill, 2001, pp 649–57.
Sparling TM, Andricevic M, Wass H: Remission of cold hemagglutinin disease induced by rituximab therapy. *Can Med Assoc J* 2001;164:1405.

SECTION 4 *Polycythemia (Erythrocytosis)*
Bruce M. Camitta

Chapter 458
Primary Polycythemia (Polycythemia Rubra Vera)

Polycythemia exists when the red blood cell (RBC) count, the hemoglobin level, and the total RBC volume all exceed the upper limits of normal. In postpubertal individuals, a red cell mass greater than 25%, above the mean normal value (based on body surface area), or a hematocrit greater than 60 (males) or 56 (females) indicate an absolute erythrocytosis. True polycythemia is characterized by increases of both the RBC and total blood volumes. A decrease in plasma volume, such as occurs in acute dehydration and burns, may result in a high hemoglobin value. However, these situations are more accurately designated hemoconcentration because the RBC mass is not increased and normalization of the plasma volume restores the hemoglobin to normal levels.

Polycythemia vera, a myeloproliferative disorder, has been reported in only a few children. Its pathogenesis is not known. The erythropoietin receptor is normal, and in vitro cultures of erythroid precursors of affected persons do not require added erythropoietin to stimulate growth. Serum erythropoietin levels are normal or low. Diagnostic criteria are listed in Box 458–1. Phlebotomy and antiplatelet agents (aspirin) reduce the risks of thrombosis and abnormal bleeding. If these are unsuccessful, antiproliferative treatments (hydroxyurea, anagrelide, interferon-α) may be helpful. The risk of transformation of the disease into myelofibrosis or acute leukemia has diminished with discontinuation of the use of alkylating agents and radioactive phosphorus. Prolonged survival is not unusual.

BOX 458–1. Diagnosis of Polycythemia Vera

MAJOR CRITERIA

1. Increased red cell mass (see text)
2. Absent causes of secondary polycythemia
3. Palpable splenomegaly
4. Abnormal bone marrow karyotype (acquired)

MINOR CRITERIA

a. Platelets > 400 × 10⁹/L
b. Neutrophils > 400 × 10⁹/L
c. Splenomegaly by scanning
d. Erythropoietin-independent red cell precursor growth or reduced serum erythropoietin

DIAGNOSIS

1 + 2 and 3 or 4
1 + 2 and 2 minor criteria

Butcher C, D'Andrea RJ: Molecular aspects of polycythemia vera. *Int J Mol Med* 2000;6:243–52.
Gilbert HS: Current management in polycythemia vera. *Semin Hematol* 2001;38:25–8.
Pearson TC: Evaluation of diagnostic criteria in polycythemia vera. *Int J Mol Med* 2000;6:21–4.

Chapter 459
Secondary Polycythemia

The differential diagnosis of secondary polycythemia is shown in Box 459–1. Polycythemia may be present in any clinical situation associated with chronic arterial oxygen desaturation. *Cardiovascular defects involving right-to-left shunts* and *pulmonary diseases interfering with proper oxygenation* are the most common causes of hypoxic polycythemia. Clinical findings usually include cyanosis, hyperemia of the sclerae and mucous membranes, and clubbing of the fingers. As the hematocrit rises above 65%, clinical manifestations of hyperviscosity, such as headache and hypertension, may require phlebotomy (see also Chapter 92.3). On the other hand, the increased demand for red blood cell (RBC) production may cause iron deficiency. Iron-deficient RBCs are more rigid, further increasing the risk of intracranial thrombosis in these patients. Because microcytosis may occur only as a late manifestation of iron deficiency in children with hypoxic polycythemia, routine periodic assessment of iron status, with treatment of iron deficiency, should be performed in these children. Living at *high altitudes* also causes hypoxic polycythemia; the hemoglobin level increases about 4% for each rise of 1,000 m in altitude. *Partial obstruction of a renal artery* rarely results in polycythemia.

BOX 459–1. Differential Diagnosis of Polycythemia

POLYCYTHEMIA VERA

SECONDARY

Neonatal
  Normal intrauterine environment
  Twin-twin or maternal-fetal hemorrhage
  Infants of diabetic mothers
  Intrauterine growth retardation
  Trisomies 13, 18, or 21
  Adrenal hyperplasia
  Thyrotoxicosis
Hypoxia
  Altitude
  Cardiac disease
  Lung disease
  Central hypoventilation
Hemoglobinopathy
  High oxygen affinity variants
  Methemoglobin reductase deficiency
  Chronic carbon monoxide exposure
Metabolic
  2,3-DPG deficiency
Hormonal
  Malignant tumors
    Renal, hepatic, adrenal, cerebellar, other
  Renal disease
    Cysts, hydronephrosis
  Adrenal disease
    Virilizing hyperplasia, Cushing syndrome
  Anabolic steroid therapy
Familial

SPURIOUS (PLASMA VOLUME DECREASE)

BOX 459–2. Sequential Evaluation of Polycythemia

1. Complete blood cell count including differential white blood cell count
2. Rule out plasma volume decrease
3. Diagnose secondary polycythemia vera
   Arterial oxygen saturation
   Carboxyhemoglobin
   Renal ultrasonography
   Abdominal/cranial computed tomography
4. Special studies for polycythemia vera
   Leukocyte alkaline phosphatase
   B_{12}/B_{12} binding capacity
   Erythropoietin level
   Red blood cell colony formation

More subtle forms of hypoxia may also cause polycythemia. *Congenital methemoglobinemia* resulting from a deficiency of cytochrome b5 reductase may cause cyanosis and polycythemia (see Chapter 454.7). This condition is transmitted as an autosomal recessive trait. Most affected individuals are asymptomatic. Neurologic abnormalities may be present in patients whose enzyme deficit is not limited to hematopoietic cells. Dominantly transmitted polycythemia is caused by hemoglobins that have increased oxygen affinity. Cyanosis may occur in the presence of as little as 1.5 g/dL of methemoglobin but is uncommon in other hemoglobin variants unless hyperviscosity results in localized hypoxemia (see Chapter 92.3).

Polycythemia has also been associated with benign and malignant *tumors* that secrete erythropoietin. Exogenous or endogenous excess of *anabolic steroids* also may cause polycythemia. Polycythemias have been transmitted as dominant or recessive conditions. In about 10% of these families, there is an abnormality of the erythropoietin receptor.

Sequential studies to evaluate polycythemia are outlined in Box 459–2. For mild disease, observation is sufficient. When the hematocrit exceeds 65–70% (hemoglobin > 23 g/dL), blood viscosity markedly increases. Periodic phlebotomies may prevent or decrease symptoms. Apheresed blood should be replaced with plasma or saline to prevent hypovolemia in patients accustomed to a chronically elevated total blood volume.

Prchal JT: Pathogenetic mechanisms of polycythemia vera and congenital polycythemia disorders. *Semin Hematol* 2001;38:10.

SECTION 5 *The Pancytopenias*

Pancytopenia can result from a failure of production of hematopoietic progenitors, their destruction, or replacement of the bone marrow by tumor or fibrosis. Although selective cytopenias are important clinical entities (see Chapters 121.1, 440–444, and 476), pancytopenia is a loss of all marrow elements. The clinical consequences include anemia, neutropenia, and thrombocytopenia and, depending on the degree and duration of their impairment, can lead to serious illness and death. Pancytopenia can be constitutional, arising as a consequence of an inherited genetic defect affecting hematopoietic progenitors, or can be acquired as a consequence of either direct destruction of progenitors, immune-mediated damage to either hematopoietic progenitors or their nurturing microenvironment, or suppression of or crowding out of progenitors by tumor cells or fibrosis. In this section, the constitutional and acquired pancytopenias are considered separately. Because the principles of supportive care are generally independent of the etiology of the pancytopenia, they are presented in Chapters 462–466.

Chapter 460
The Constitutional Pancytopenias

Alan D. D'Andrea

Etiology. Although Fanconi anemia is the best-recognized constitutional pancytopenia, a number of other infrequent genetic disorders have also been implicated. These genetic syndromes (Table 460–1) include various modes of inheritance and may be associated with a number of congenital abnormalities, especially of the bones, kidneys, and heart. Because the hematologic manifestations of the congenital pancytopenias may not become manifested until the first years to even decades of life, a genetic predisposition to bone marrow failure should be considered in all cases of aplastic anemia in children (see later). These disorders can be autosomal recessive (e.g., Fanconi anemia, dyskeratosis congenita), X linked, or autosomal dominant (e.g., dyskeratosis congenita). Several of these genetic disorders may present initially with a single cytopenia and subsequently progress to pancytopenia (e.g., Shwachman-Diamond syndrome, amegakary-ocytic thrombocytopenia, reticular dysgenesis). In addition, a number of inheritable familial marrow dysfunction syndromes have been associated with pancytopenia (which can also be autosomal recessive, autosomal dominant, or X linked), and aplastic anemia also occurs in association with other genetic disorders (e.g., Down, Dubowitz, and Seckel syndromes). Thus, pancytopenia can be either the primary disease manifestation or can emerge as a rare complication during the course of another illness. Because of the chromosomal fragility or defective repair mechanisms that may be associated, several of these disorders can also be complicated by cancer or other organ dysfunction(s). In addition, if such patients are treated for a malignancy with radiation or chemotherapy, they may experience excessive toxicity owing to their underlying defect.

Epidemiology. Although the true incidence of these disorders is unknown, the constitutional pancytopenias are rare. The most common disorder is Fanconi anemia, of which approximately 1,000 cases have been described, in contrast to only about 45 cases of amegakaryocytic thrombocytopenia. Depending on geography, the heterozygote frequency of Fanconi anemia ranges from 1/100 to 1/300. The familial aplastic anemias are much less common.

Pathology and Pathogenesis. One of the hallmarks of Fanconi anemia is evidence of spontaneous or clastogen-induced

TABLE 460–1. Inherited Bone Marrow Failure Syndromes

Feature	Fanconi Anemia	Dyskeratosis Congenita	Shwachman-Diamond Syndrome	Amegakaryocytic Thrombocytopenia
Cases reported	1,000	225	200	45
Male/female	1.3	4.3	1.7	1.6
Genetics	Autosomal recessive	X linked; autosomal recessive, dominant	Autosomal recessive	X linked, or autosomal recessive
Physical abnormalities (%)	80	100	40	60
Hand/arm anomalies (%)	48	15	<2	0
Median age (yr) at diagnosis of initial hematologic disease	7.5	16	4 mo	<1 wk
First hematologic manifestation	Pancytopenia	Pancytopenia	Neutropenia	Thrombocytopenia
Bone marrow	Aplastic	Aplastic	Hypocellular or myeloid arrest	Absent or small megakaryocytes
Aplastic anemia (%)	>95	50	20	45
Leukemia (%)	12	0.4	5	5
Liver disease (%)	4	0	0	0
Cancer	5	10	0	0
Hb F	Increased	Increased	Increased	Increased
Chromosomes	Breaks increased with clastogens	Bleomycin sensitive	Normal	Normal
Spontaneous remissions	Very rare	None	Rare	BMT
Treatment, responses	BMT, androgens, 50%, transient	Androgens, 50%, transient	G-CSF, BMT, 80%	None
Prognosis	Poor	Poor	Fair	Poor
Prenatal diagnosis	Chromosome breaks, FAC	Xq28 RFLP	Neutropenia	Thrombocytopenia
Predicted median survival age (yr)	30	33	35	3

RFLP = restriction fragment length polymorphism; BMT = bone marrow transplantation; G-CSF = granulocyte colony-stimulating factor; FAC = Franconi anemia gene, complementation group C.

Modified from Alter BP, Young NS: The bone marrow failure syndromes. In Nathan DG, Orkin FA (editors): Nathan and Oski's Hematology of Infancy and Children, 5th ed. Philadelphia, WB Saunders, 1998.

chromosome breaks. Lymphoid, hematopoietic (including progenitors), and fibroblast cells from patients with Fanconi anemia demonstrate a number of cytogenetic abnormalities, including defective DNA repair, increased susceptibility of hematopoietic cells to oxidant stress, and decreased cell survival. Eight genetic complementation groups of Fanconi anemia have been identified (FA subtypes A, B, C, D1, D2, E, F, and G). Six of the corresponding FA genes have been cloned, and the six encoded FA proteins interact in a common biochemical pathway regulating DNA repair. It is likely that the absence of these gene products contributes directly to the poor growth of hematopoietic progenitor cells and the heightened risk of malignancies. Depressed levels of granulocyte-macrophage colony-stimulating factor (GM-CSF), stem cell factor, and interleukin-6 (IL-6) also have been observed in children with Fanconi syndrome, suggesting that an abnormal cytokine network contributes to the pathogenesis of the bone marrow failure in these patients. Increased cellular sensitivity to interferon-γ may account, at least in part, for the pancytopenia of Fanconi anemia.

Chromosome breakage has also been observed in approximately 10% of patients with dyskeratosis congenita, and decreased hematopoietic cytokines have been found in some patients with the Shwachman-Diamond syndrome. However, the pathogenesis of these disorders and that of the familial marrow dysfunction syndromes remains poorly defined. Two of the human disease genes corresponding to dyskeratosis congenita have been cloned.

Clinical Manifestations. Various physical abnormalities accompany most of the congenital pancytopenias, particularly Fanconi anemia and dyskeratosis congenita. Patients having Fanconi anemia have hyperpigmentation and café-au-lait spots, skeletal abnormalities (especially absent or hypoplastic thumbs), short stature, and a wide array of integumentary and organ abnormalities. *Dyskeratosis congenita* is also very commonly associated with

hyperpigmentation as well as nail dystrophy of both the hands and feet, leukoplakia, and a number of ocular abnormalities, including epiphora, blepharitis, and cataracts. The relative frequencies of these abnormalities are compared in Table 460–1. Fourteen to 25% of patients with the cytogenetic abnormalities of Fanconi anemia lack the major physical stigmas of Fanconi syndrome and have been designated as having the Estren-Damashek subtype. Such patients may present with isolated bone marrow failure or a new malignancy, in the absence of other manifestations of a genetic syndrome. A diversity of cutaneous, skeletal, growth, and organ abnormalities can also be found in 30–40% of the other congenital and familial pancytopenias, although they do not follow any uniform pattern.

Laboratory Findings. Depending on the specific disorder, thrombocytopenia, leukopenia, lymphopenia, or anemia generally precedes the onset of pancytopenia. Further, hematologic abnormalities may precede or follow elucidation of other physical defects. As noted earlier, chromosomal breaks occur in most patients with Fanconi anemia compared with 10% of those with dyskeratosis congenita. Children with Fanconi anemia and dyskeratosis congenita generally have macrocytosis as well as mild poikilocytosis and anisocytosis, and their red blood cells (RBCs) contain higher levels of i antigen and hemoglobin F than are found in acquired aplasia. The age at onset of hematologic abnormalities ranges from infancy to adolescence. Once peripheral pancytopenia is evident, bone marrow examination generally confirms a hypoplastic or aplastic state comparable to that in acquired aplastic anemias.

Additional laboratory examination should include skeletal radiographs as well as examination of the genitourinary tract and, depending on the diagnosis, more detailed examination of the eyes, gastrointestinal tract, heart, teeth, and gonads (in males).

Diagnosis. The presence of characteristic skeletal and cutaneous abnormalities coupled with short stature should suggest the diagnosis of congenital pancytopenia even in the absence of hematologic problems. In contrast, when a child presents with evidence of bone marrow failure, a genetic or familial defect should always be considered and evaluated by cytogenetic examination, including chromosomal breakage studies. This is particularly important because approximately 20% of individuals with congenital pancytopenias may occasionally not have any of the physical abnormalities that are considered characteristic of these syndromes (see Table 460–1).

Complications. The major complications related to the congenital pancytopenias include the consequences of bone marrow failure, a heightened risk for leukemia and other cancers, and organ complications that are specific to the primary defect (e.g., liver problems in Fanconi syndrome, malabsorption in Shwachman-Diamond syndrome). Because Fanconi anemia has eight distinct subtypes (see earlier), knowledge of a patient's specific subtype or specific mutation may allow a more accurate prediction of the clinical course and the need for early therapy. Infection and bleeding represent the major hematologic manifestations leading to life-threatening complications (see Chapter 462). Depending on their degree and duration, the hematologic abnormalities may respond to supportive care initially, but when pancytopenia ensues (depending on the syndrome, this occurs in 20–90% of patients), more aggressive therapies are required. As more knowledge is gained about the molecular and cellular pathogenesis of these syndromes, it may be possible to delay some of the hematologic complications (see Treatment).

Treatment. The traditional backbone of therapy for patients with congenital anemias has been steroids and androgens (especially oxymetholone or nandrolone), alone or in combination. Although 50–75% of patients show some evidence of improvement with androgens, relapse is common and complications (especially hepatic tumors or obstructive liver disease) occur. Improvements in RBCs generally precede those in white blood cells, and it may take months to achieve a maximum benefit. These therapies have been shown to prolong life by approximately 2 yr and hence can only be considered palliative.

The only "curative" therapy to date has been bone marrow transplantation. However, patients with congenital pancytopenias also have an increased predisposition to malignancy, and the preparative regimens generally used during bone marrow transplantation can adversely affect this susceptibility. Accordingly, lower doses of alkylating agents in the preparative regimens are appropriate. Furthermore, most patients with Fanconi anemia do not have histocompatible donors. Transplantation from unmatched donors results in considerable morbidity, owing to the increased intensity of graft versus host disease in these children. Encouraging results have been reported when GM-CSF was administered subcutaneously to children with Fanconi anemia and pancytopenia. A significant increase in the neutrophil count was observed in six of seven patients who were treated at the Children's Hospital (Boston), and this was sustained for more than a year without any evidence of leukemia. More transient responses have been observed with granulocyte colony-stimulating factor (G-CSF). Additional follow-up is important, and it is possible that treatment of these patients with multiple cytokines (erythropoietin, IL-3, IL-6) may offer additional benefits. Ultimately, the best hope for these children will emerge from an understanding of the molecular defects that produce the syndromes; once these are identified, gene therapy may become a feasible consideration.

Prognosis. When marrow failure develops, the prognosis is guarded. Although bone marrow transplantation and hematopoietic growth factor reconstitution offer some hope, neither overcomes the risks for subsequent cancer or other organ complications.

Genetic Counseling. Once an index case has been identified, genetic counseling is important and must be oriented to the patterns of inheritance and the prospect for prenatal diagnosis. Based on the presence of cytogenetic and chromosomal breakage or, in the case of amegakaryocytic thrombocytopenia, fetal blood platelet counts, a diagnosis can be suspected or confirmed.

Alter BP: Fanconi's anemia and malignancies. *Am J Hematol* 1996;53:99–110.

Alter BP, D'Andrea AD: Inherited bone marrow failure syndromes. In Handin RL, Lux SE, Stossel TP (editors): *Blood: Principles and Practice of Hematology*, 2nd ed. Philadelphia, Lippincott Williams & Wilkins, in press.

Grompe M, D'Andrea AD: Fanconi anemia and DNA repair. *Hum Mol Genet* 2001;10:2253–9.

Heiss NS, Knight SW, Vulliamy TJ, et al: X-linked dyskeratosis congenita is caused by mutations in a highly conserved gene with putative nucleolar functions. *Nat Genet* 1998;19:32–8.

Jonje H, Patel KJ: The emerging genetic and molecular basis of Fanconi anemia. *Nat Rev Genet* 2001;2:446–59.

Vulliamy T, Marrone A, Goldman F, et al: The RNA component of telomerase is mutated in autosomal dominant dyskeratosis congenita. *Nature* 2001;413:432–5.

Chapter 461
The Acquired Pancytopenias

Jeffrey D. Hord

Etiology and Epidemiology. Various drugs, chemicals, toxins, infectious agents, radiation, or immune disorders can result in pancytopenia, by either direct destruction of hematopoietic progenitors, disruption of the marrow microenvironment, or immune-mediated suppression of marrow elements (Box 461–1). Whenever a child presents with pancytopenia, a careful history of exposure to known risk factors should be obtained. The possibility of a genetic predisposition to bone marrow failure should always be considered, even in the absence of the classic associated physical findings (see Chapter 460). A specific cause cannot be identified in most cases of acquired marrow failure in childhood, and these cases are termed "idiopathic." The overall incidence of acquired aplastic anemia is relatively low, with an approximate incidence in both children and adults, in the United States and Europe, of 2–6 cases per million per year.

Severe bone marrow suppression can develop after exposure to many different drugs and chemicals, including certain chemotherapeutic agents, insecticides, antibiotics, anticonvulsants, nonsteroidal anti-inflammatory agents, antihistamines, sedatives, and metals. Some of the most notable agents are benzene, chloramphenicol, and gold. The severity and duration of the pancytopenia is dependent on the extent of exposure to these agents. A genetic predisposition may exist and may increase the likelihood of pancytopenia after exposure.

A number of viruses can either directly or indirectly result in bone marrow failure. Parvovirus B19 is classically associated with isolated red cell aplasia, but in patients with sickle cell disease or immunodeficiencies it can result in transient pancytopenia (see Chapters 230 and 454). Prolonged pancytopenia can occur after infections with many of the hepatitis viruses, herpesviruses, Epstein-Barr virus (EBV), and cytomegalovirus (CMV). HIV has also been associated with a number of hematologic abnormalities, including anemia, neutropenia, thrombocytopenia, and pancytopenia.

Patients with evidence of bone marrow failure should also be evaluated for paroxysmal nocturnal hemoglobinuria (PNH) and collagen vascular diseases, although these are uncommon causes of pancytopenia in childhood. Pancytopenia without

BOX 461-1. Etiology of Acquired Aplastic Anemia

RADIATION

DRUGS AND CHEMICALS
Predictable: chemotherapy, benzene
Idiosyncratic: chloramphenicol, antiepileptics, gold

VIRUSES
Cytomegalovirus
Epstein-Barr
Hepatitis B
Hepatitis C
Hepatitis non–A,B,C
Human immunodeficiency (HIV)

IMMUNE DISEASES
Eosinophilic fasciitis
Hypoimmunoglobulinemia
Thymoma

PREGNANCY

PAROXYSMAL NOCTURNAL HEMOGLOBINURIA

MARROW REPLACEMENT
Leukemia
Myelodysplasia
Myelofibrosis

peripheral blasts may be caused by bone marrow replacement by leukemic blasts or neuroblastoma cells.

Pathology and Pathogenesis. The hallmark of aplastic anemia is peripheral pancytopenia coupled with hypoplastic or aplastic bone marrow. The severity of the clinical course is related to the degree of myelosuppression. Severe aplastic anemia is defined as a condition in which two or more cell components have become seriously compromised (i.e., an absolute neutrophil count $< 500/mm^3$, a platelet count $< 20,000/mm^3$, a reticulocyte count $< 1\%$ after correction for the hematocrit) in a patient whose bone marrow biopsy material is moderately or severely hypocellular. Bone marrow failure can result from various causes and mechanisms. For example, it may be a consequence of a direct cytotoxic effect on hematopoietic stem cells from a drug or chemical or may result from either cell-mediated or antibody-dependent cytotoxicity. There is evidence that many cases of aplastic anemia are caused by an immune-mediated process with increased circulating activated T lymphocytes producing cytokines (e.g., interferon-γ) that suppress hematopoiesis. Abnormalities of the supporting microenvironment or a loss of critical hematopoietic growth factors can contribute to the marrow failure.

Clinical Manifestations, Laboratory Findings, and Differential Diagnosis. Acquired pancytopenia is usually characterized by anemia, leukopenia, and thrombocytopenia, in the setting of elevated serum cytokine levels. The pancytopenia results in increased risks of fatigue, cardiac failure, infection, and bleeding. Other treatable disorders, such as cancer, collagen vascular disorders, PNH, or infections that may respond to specific therapies (e.g., intravenous immune globulin for parvovirus) should be considered in the differential diagnosis. Careful examination of the peripheral blood smear for RBC, leukocyte, and platelet morphology is important. A reticulocyte count should be performed to assess erythropoietic activity. In children, the possibility of a congenital pancytopenia must always be considered and chromosomal breakage analysis should be performed to evaluate for Fanconi anemia. The presence of fetal hemoglobin suggests a congenital pancytopenia but is not diagnostic. To assess for the possibility of PNH, flow cytometric analysis of erythrocytes for CD48 and CD59 is the most sensitive test. Bone marrow examination should include both aspiration and a biopsy, and the marrow should be carefully evaluated for morphology, cellularity, and cytogenetics.

Complications. The major complications of severe pancytopenia are predominantly related to the risk of life-threatening bleeding from prolonged thrombocytopenia or to infection secondary to protracted neutropenia. Patients with protracted neutropenia due to bone marrow failure are at risk not only for serious bacterial infections but also for invasive mycoses. The general principles of supportive care that have evolved from the treatment of cancer patients with chemotherapy-related myelosuppression should be fully extended to the care of patients with acquired pancytopenias (see Chapter 164).

Treatment. The treatment of children with acquired pancytopenia requires comprehensive supportive care coupled with an attempt to treat the underlying marrow failure. For patients with a human leukocyte antigen (HLA)–identical sibling marrow donor, allogeneic bone marrow transplantation offers a 90% chance of long-term survival. The risks associated with this approach include the immediate complications of the transplantation, graft failure, graft versus host disease, and the risk of secondary cancers (see Chapters 125 and 129). The life-threatening problem of graft failure has diminished with the incorporation of antithymocyte globulin (ATG) and cyclophosphamide into the transplant conditioning regimen. Only one of five patients has an HLA-matched sibling donor so allogeneic bone marrow transplant is not an option for the majority of patients.

For those without a sibling donor, the major form of therapy is immunosuppression with ATG and cyclosporine combined with a hematopoietic colony-stimulating factor (e.g., granulocyte colony-stimulating factor, granulocyte-macrophage colony-stimulating factor). Response to this combination therapy is in the range of 60–80%, but a few responders will relapse. There is an increased risk of developing clonal bone marrow diseases such as leukemia, myelodysplasia, or PNH after immunosuppression. The risk for developing clonal disease after immunosuppression has been estimated as high as 40%. For those who fail to respond to immunosuppression or relapse after immunosuppression, matched unrelated donor bone marrow transplantation and high-dose cyclophosphamide remain treatment options. Other therapies that have been used in the past with inconsistent results include androgens, corticosteroids, and plasmapheresis. Alternative marrow transplants continue to be studied as a therapeutic intervention in refractory aplastic anemia.

Prognosis. Spontaneous recovery rarely occurs. Severe pancytopenia left untreated has an overall mortality rate of approximately 50% within 6 mo of diagnosis and more than 75% overall, with infection and hemorrhage the major causes of morbidity and mortality. Fortunately, the majority of children with acquired severe aplastic anemia will respond to allogeneic marrow transplantation or immunosuppression/cytokine, leaving them with normal or near-normal blood cell counts. For those who fail to respond to front-line therapy, prognosis remains poor.

PANCYTOPENIA CAUSED BY MARROW REPLACEMENT

Processes that either infiltrate or replace the bone marrow can present as acquired pancytopenia. This can occur either before or during malignancy (classically, neuroblastoma or leukemia) or as a consequence of myelofibrosis, myelodysplasia, or osteoporosis. Although uncommon, evidence of a hypoplastic anemia can precede, generally by months, the onset of acute leukemia. This is important to appreciate in evaluating and monitoring children who present with what appears to be an acquired aplastic anemia. Morphologic examination of the peripheral blood and the bone marrow as well as marrow cytogenetic studies are critically important in making the diagnoses of leukemia, myelofibrosis, and myelodysplasia.

Myelodysplasia (MDS) in children is very rare but the clinical course is more aggressive than the same category of MDS in adults. About one half of the children with reported cases of MDS have had clonal abnormalities involving chromosome 7 (usually monosomy 7). The transition time from pediatric MDS to acute leukemia is relatively short at 14 to 26 mo, so aggressive treatment such as bone marrow transplantation (BMT) must be considered shortly after diagnosis. With conventional chemotherapy there is a 20–25% long-term survival, but with allogeneic BMT the survival increases to about 50%. One exception may be MDS/acute myelocytic leukemia in children with Down syndrome because this disease in this specific population is very responsive to conventional chemotherapy, with long-term survival rates of greater than 80%.

Alter BP, Young NS: In Nathan DG, Orkin SH (editors): *Hematology of Infancy and Childhood*, 5th ed. Philadelphia, WB Saunders, 1998, pp 237–335.

Bacigalupo A, Bruno B, Saracco P, et al: Antilymphocyte globulin, cyclosporine, prednisolone, and granulocyte colony stimulating factor for severe aplastic anemia: An update of the GITMO/EBMT on 100 patients. *Blood* 2000; 95:1931–4.

Brodsky RA, Sensenbrenner LL, Jones RJ: Complete remission in severe aplastic anemia after high-dose cyclophosphamide without bone marrow transplantation. *Blood* 1996;87:491–4.

Socie G, Rosenfeld S, Frickhofen N, et al: Late clonal diseases of treated aplastic anemia. *Semin Hematol* 2000;37:91–101.

Tisdale JF, Dunn DE, Geller N, et al: High-dose cyclophosphamide in severe aplastic anaemia: A randomised trial. *Lancet* 2000;356:1554–9.

Young NS: *Bone Marrow Failure Syndromes*. Philadelphia, WB Saunders, 2000.

Young NS, Alter BP: *Aplastic Anemia Acquired and Inherited*. Philadelphia, WB Saunders, 1994.

SECTION 6 *Risks of Blood Component Transfusions*

Ronald G. Strauss

Blood component and derivative transfusions frequently are lifesaving. Intensive care of premature neonates and modern therapy for many children with cancer, hematologic disorders, and transplant recipients would be impossible without them. However, transfusions are not without risks and should be given only when true benefits are likely (e.g., to correct a deficiency or dysfunction of a blood element causing a clinically significant problem). The principles of transfusion support for children and adolescents are similar to those for adults, but infants have special needs. Accordingly, each of these two age groups is discussed separately within each section. Many of the transfusion guidelines presented are based on those formulated by the Pediatric Hemotherapy Committee of the American Association of Blood Banks, but they must be adapted to fit local standards of practice. In particular, terms expressed on the tables, such as "severe" and "symptomatic," must be defined by local physicians.

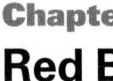

Chapter 462
Red Blood Cell Transfusions and Erythropoietin Therapy

Red blood cells (RBCs) are transfused to increase the oxygen-carrying capacity of the blood and, in turn, to maintain satisfactory tissue oxygenation. Guidelines for RBC transfusions in children and adolescents are similar to those for adults (Box 462–1). However, transfusions may be given more stringently to children because normal hemoglobin levels are lower in healthy children than in adults and, except in defined circumstances, children do not have the underlying cardiorespiratory and vascular diseases that develop with aging in adults. Thus, children should be better able to compensate for RBC loss. In the perioperative period, for example, it is unnecessary for most children to maintain hemoglobin levels of 80 g/L or greater, a level frequently desired for adults. There should be a compelling reason for any postoperative RBC transfusion because most children (without continued bleeding) can quickly restore their RBC mass with iron therapy. As is true for adults, the most important measures in the treatments of acute hemorrhage are, first, to control the hemorrhage and to restore tissue with crystalloid and/or colloid solutions. Then, if the estimated blood loss is greater than 25% of the circulating blood volume (i.e., >17 mL/kg) and the patient's condition remains unstable, RBC transfusions may be indicated. In acutely ill children with severe pulmonary disease requiring assisted ventilation, it is common practice to maintain the hemoglobin level close to the normal range. Although this recommendation seems logical, its efficacy has not been documented by controlled scientific studies.

With chronic anemias, the decision to transfuse RBCs should not be based solely on blood hemoglobin levels because children compensate well and may be asymptomatic despite very low hemoglobin levels. Patients with iron-deficiency anemia, for example, often are treated successfully with oral iron alone, even at hemoglobin levels below 50 g/L. Factors other than hemoglobin concentration to be considered in the decision to transfuse RBCs include (1) the patient's symptoms, signs, and functional capacities; (2) the presence of cardiorespiratory, vascular, and central nervous system disease; (3) the cause and anticipated course of the anemia; and (4) alternative therapies such as recombinant human erythropoietin (EPO) therapy, which is known to reduce RBC transfusions and to improve the overall condition of children with chronic renal insufficiency (see Chapter 527.2). In anemias likely to be permanent, one must also balance the detrimental effects of anemia on growth and development versus the potential toxicity of repeated transfusions. RBC transfusions for disorders such as sickle cell anemia and thalassemia are discussed in Chapters 454.1 and 454.9.

For *neonates*, clearly established indications for RBC transfusions, based on controlled scientific studies, do not exist. Generally, RBCs are given to maintain a hemoglobin value believed to be most desirable for each neonate's clinical status (see Box 462–1). This clinical approach is imprecise, but more physiologic indications, such as RBC mass, available oxygen, and measurements of oxygen delivery and tissue extraction are too cumbersome for clinical practice. Because definitive data are limited, it is important that the pediatricians critically evaluate the need for neonatal RBC transfusions in light of the pathophysiology involved.

BOX 462–1. Guidelines for Pediatric RBC Transfusions

CHILDREN AND ADOLESCENTS

Acute loss > 25% circulating blood volume
Hemoglobin < 8.0 g/dL* in perioperative period
Hemoglobin < 13.0 g/dL and *severe* cardiopulmonary disease
Hemoglobin < 8.0 g/dL and *symptomatic* chronic anemia
Hemoglobin < 8.0 g/dL and *marrow failure*

INFANTS WITHIN FIRST 4 MO OF LIFE

Hemoglobin < 13.0 g/dL and *severe* pulmonary disease
Hemoglobin < 10.0 g/dL and *moderate* pulmonary disease
Hemoglobin < 13.0 g/dL and *severe* cardiac disease
Hemoglobin < 10.0 g/dL and major surgery
Hemoglobin < 8.0 g/dL and *symptomatic* anemia

---

*Hematocrit estimated by Hb g/dL × 3.
Words in *italics* must be defined for local transfusion guidelines.

During the first weeks of life, all neonates experience a decline in circulating RBC mass caused both by physiologic factors and, in sick premature infants, by phlebotomy blood losses. In healthy term infants, the nadir hemoglobin value rarely falls below 9 g/dL at an age of 10–12 wk. This "physiologic" drop in RBCs does not require transfusions. In contrast, the decline occurs earlier and is more pronounced in premature infants, even in those without complicating illnesses, in whom the mean hemoglobin concentration falls to approximately 8 g/dL in infants of 1.0–1.5 kg birthweight and to 7 g/dL in infants weighing less than 1.0 kg. Most infants with birthweight of less than 1.0 kg need RBC transfusions. A key reason the nadir hemoglobin values of premature infants are lower than those of term infants is the former group's relatively diminished EPO output in response to anemia (see Chapters 92.1 and 438). The mechanisms responsible for low plasma EPO levels are only partially defined. One factor is reliance of preterm infants on the liver as the primary site of EPO production during the first weeks of life. This is important because the liver is less responsive than kidneys to anemia and tissue hypoxia. Thus, preterm infants exhibit a sluggish EPO response to falling hematocrit values. Low plasma EPO levels provide a rationale to use recombinant EPO in the treatment of the anemia of prematurity. Unquestionably, proper doses of EPO and iron effectively stimulate neonatal erythropoiesis. However, the efficacy of EPO therapy to substantially diminish the need for RBC transfusions has not been convincingly demonstrated—particularly, for sick, extremely premature neonates—and recombinant EPO has not been widely accepted as treatment for the anemia of prematurity (see Chapter 92.1).

Despite the promise of EPO therapy, many low-birthweight preterm infants need RBC transfusions (see Box 462–1). In neonatal patients with severe respiratory disease, defined as those requiring relatively large quantities of oxygen and ventilator support, it is customary to maintain the blood hemoglobin above 130 g/L (hematocrit > 40%). Proponents believe that transfused RBCs containing adult hemoglobin, with their superior interaction with 2,3-diphosphoglycerate (2,3-DPG), leading to better oxygen offloading than that of fetal hemoglobin, are likely to provide optimal oxygen delivery throughout the period of diminished pulmonary function. Although this practice is widely recommended, little evidence is available to establish its efficacy or to define its optimal use (i.e., the best hemoglobin level for each degree of pulmonary dysfunction). It seems logical to presume that infants with less severe cardiopulmonary disease require less vigorous support, hence, the lower hemoglobin level suggested for those with only moderate disease. Consistent with the rationale for oxygen delivery in neonates with severe respiratory disease, it seems logical to maintain the hemoglobin value above 130 g/L (hematocrit > 40%) in neonates with

severe cardiac disease leading to either cyanosis or congestive heart failure.

The optimal hemoglobin level for neonates facing *major surgery* has not been established by definitive studies. However, it seems reasonable to maintain the hemoglobin above 100 g/dL (hematocrit > 30%) because of limited ability of a neonate's heart, lungs, and vasculature to compensate for anemia; the inferior offloading of oxygen because of the diminished interaction between fetal hemoglobin and 2,3-DPG; and the developmental impairment of neonatal renal, hepatic, and neurologic function. This transfusion guideline must be applied with flexibility to individual infants facing different kinds of surgery.

Stable neonates do not require RBC transfusion unless they exhibit clinical problems attributable to anemia. Proponents of RBC transfusions for symptomatic anemia believe that the low RBC mass contributes to tachypnea, dyspnea, apnea, tachycardia, bradycardia, feeding difficulties, and lethargy and that these problems can be alleviated by transfusing RBCs. However, it is important to remember that the anemia is only one of several possible causes of these problems, and RBC transfusions should only be given when clinical problems seem to be manifestations of anemia (i.e., not otherwise explained).

The RBC product of choice for children and adolescents is the standard suspension of RBCs separated from whole blood by centrifugation and resuspended in an anticoagulant/preservative storage solution at a hematocrit value of about 60%. The usual dose is 10–15 mL/kg, but transfusion volumes vary greatly depending on clinical circumstances (e.g., continued vs. arrested bleeding, hemolysis). For neonates, many centers transfuse the same RBC product as selected for older children, whereas others prefer a packed RBC concentrate (hematocrit of 70–90%). Either is infused slowly (2–4 hr) at a dose of about 15 mL/kg. Because of the small quantity of extracellular fluid given at these relatively high hematocrit values and the slow rate of transfusion, the type of RBC anticoagulant/preservative solution used does not pose risks for premature infants. Packing RBCs by centrifugation at the time the aliquot is issued for transfusion ensures a consistent RBC dose is infused with each transfusion.

The traditional use of relatively fresh RBCs (< 7 days of storage) has been halted in many centers in favor of diminishing donor exposure by using a single unit of RBCs to obtain aliquots for transfusing each infant, regardless of the duration of RBC storage. Neonatologists who insist on transfusing only fresh RBCs generally are fearful of the rise in plasma potassium (K^+) level that occurs in RBC units during extended storage. After 42 days of storage, plasma K^+ levels are $\simeq$ 50 mEq/L (0.05 mEq/mL), a value that at first glance seems alarmingly high. However, the actual dose of K^+ transfused in the extracellular fluid is tiny. An infant weighing 1.0 kg, given a 15 mL/kg transfusion of packed RBCs (hematocrit 80%), will receive 3 mL of extracellular fluid that contains only 0.15 mEq of K^+, and it will be transfused slowly. However, the safety of stored RBCs may not apply to large-volume (>25 mL/kg) transfusions infused rapidly, in which greater doses of K^+ may be harmful.

Chapter 463
Platelet Transfusions

Guidelines for platelet (PLT) support of *children and adolescents* with quantitative and qualitative PLT disorders are similar to those for adults (Box 463–1), in which the risk of life-threatening bleeding after injury or occurring spontaneously can be related to the severity of thrombocytopenia. PLT transfusions should be given to patients with PLT counts less than 50×10^9/L when they are bleeding or are scheduled for an invasive procedure. Studies of patients with thrombocytopenia resulting from bone marrow failure indicate that spontaneous bleeding increases markedly when PLT levels fall below 20×10^9/L, if serious complications (e.g., infection, organ failure, clotting abnormalities, or anemia) are present. In this setting, prophylactic PLT transfusions are given to maintain a PLT count above 20×10^9/L. This threshold has been challenged by several studies of adult patients, and a lower PLT transfusion trigger of $5–10 \times 10^9$/L is recommended for stable patients. However, in practice, severe thrombocytopenia commonly occurs in association with the complications of fever, antimicrobial therapy, active bleeding, need for an invasive procedure, disseminated intravascular coagulation, and other severe clotting abnormalities—situations in which PLT transfusions are given to maintain relatively high PLT counts.

Qualitative PLT disorders may be inherited or acquired (e.g., in advanced hepatic or renal insufficiency or after cardiopulmonary bypass). In such patients, PLT transfusions are justified only if significant bleeding occurs. Because inherited PLT dysfunction is long term and repeated transfusions may lead to alloimmunization and refractoriness, prophylactic PLT transfusions are rarely justified, unless an invasive procedure is planned. In these cases, a bleeding time of greater than twice the upper limit of laboratory normal may be taken as diagnostic evidence that PLT dysfunction exists, but the bleeding time is poorly predictive of hemorrhagic risk or the need to transfuse PLTs. Alternative therapies, particularly desmopressin acetate, should be considered to avoid PLT transfusions.

In *neonates*, hemostasis is quantitatively and qualitatively different from that of older children, and the potential exists for either serious hemorrhage or thrombosis. About 25% of neonates treated in intensive care units exhibit blood PLT counts less than 150×10^9/L at some time during admission. Multiple pathogenetic mechanisms are involved in these sick neonates, the predominant ones being accelerated PLT destruction plus diminished PLT production, as evidenced by decreased numbers of megakaryocyte progenitors and relatively low levels of thrombopoietin in thrombocytopenic neonates, when compared with thrombocytopenic children and adults.

Blood PLT counts less than 100×10^9/L pose significant clinical risks for premature neonates. In one study, infants with birthweight less than 1.5 kg and a blood PLT count less than 100×10^9/L were compared with nonthrombocytopenic infants of similar birthweight. The bleeding time was prolonged at PLT counts less than 100×10^9/L, PLT dysfunction was suggested by bleeding times that were disproportionately long for the degree of thrombocytopenia, and hemorrhage was greater in thrombocytopenic infants. Of particular importance, the incidence of intracranial hemorrhage in thrombocytopenic infants with birthweights less than 1.5 kg was 78% versus 48% for nonthrombocytopenic infants of similar size. Moreover, the extent of hemorrhage and neurologic morbidity was greater in the thrombocytopenic group. However, in a randomized trial, transfusing PLTs prophylactically whenever the PLT count fell below 150×10^9/L to maintain the average PLT count above 200×10^9/L versus transfusing PLTs only when the PLT count fell below 50×10^9/L to maintain the average PLT count at about 100×10^9/L did not diminish the incidence of intracranial hemorrhage (28% vs 26%). Thus, there is no documented benefit to transfusing PLTs for mild thrombocytopenia (i.e., PLT counts < 150 but > 100×10^9/L). Although basic questions about the relative risks of different degrees of thrombocytopenia in various clinical settings are only partially answered, guidelines acceptable to many neonatologists are listed in Box 463–1.

The ideal goal of most PLT transfusions is to raise the PLT count to greater than 50×10^9/L, and that for neonates to greater than 100×10^9/L. This can be achieved consistently in children weighing up to 30 kg by infusing 10 mL/kg of standard (unmodified) PLT concentrates, obtained either from whole

---

BOX 463–1. Guidelines for Pediatric Platelet Transfusions

CHILDREN AND ADOLESCENTS

PLTs < 50×10^9/L and bleeding
PLTs < 50×10^9/L and *invasive* procedure
PLTs < 20×10^9/L and *marrow failure* with hemorrhagic risk factors
PLTs < 10×10^9/L and *marrow failure* without hemorrhagic risk factors
PLTs at any count, but with PLT dysfunction plus bleeding or invasive procedure

INFANTS WITHIN FIRST 4 MO OF LIFE

PLTs < 100×10^9/L and bleeding
PLTs < 50×10^9/L and *invasive* procedure
PLTs < 20×10^9/L and *clinical stable*
PLTs < 100×10^9/L and *clinically unstable*
PLTs at any count, but with PLT dysfunction plus bleeding or invasive procedure

---

PLTs = platelets.
Words in *italics* must be defined for local transfusion guidelines.

---

blood units or by plateletpheresis. For larger children, the appropriate dose is four to six pooled whole blood–derived PLT units or one apheresis unit. PLT concentrates should be transfused as rapidly as the patient's overall condition permits, certainly within 2 hr. Patients requiring repeated PLT transfusions should receive leukocyte-reduced blood products, including PLT concentrates, to diminish alloimmunization and PLT-refractoriness and to reduce the risk of transfusion-transmitted cytomegalovirus infections.

Routinely reducing the volume of platelet concentrates for infants and small children by additional centrifugation steps is both unnecessary and unwise. Transfusion of 10 mL/kg of an unmodified PLT concentrate is adequate because it adds 10×10^9 PLTs to 70 mL of blood (the blood volume of a 1-kg neonate), a number calculated to increase the PLT count by 100×10^9/L. This calculated increment is consistent with the actual increment reported in clinical studies. Moreover, 10 mL/kg is not an excessive transfusion volume, providing the intake of other intravenous fluids, medications, and nutrients is monitored and adjusted. It is important to minimize repeated transfusion of group O PLTs to group A or B recipients because passive anti-A or anti-B in group O plasma can lead to hemolysis. Although proven methods exist to reduce the volume of PLT concentrates when truly warranted (i.e., many transfusions anticipated, in which the quantity of passive anti-A or anti-B might lead to hemolysis, or failure of 10 mL/kg of unmodified PLT concentrate to increase the PLT count), additional processing should be performed with great care because of probable PLT loss, clumping, and dysfunction caused by the additional handling—all of which could diminish the efficacy and increase the toxicity of PLT transfusions.

Chapter 464
Neutrophil (Granulocyte) Transfusions

Guidelines for granulocyte transfusions (GTX) are listed in Box 464–1. Although GTX have been used sparingly in the past, the ability to collect markedly higher numbers of neutrophils from donors stimulated with recombinant granulocyte colony-stimulating factor (G-CSF) has led to renewed interest, particularly for marrow or peripheral blood progenitor cell transplantation. GTX should be reconsidered at institutions where neutropenic patients continue to die of progressive bacterial and fungal infections despite the optimal use of antimicrobial agents and recombinant myeloid growth factors.

The role of GTX added to antibiotics for patients with severe neutropenia ($<0.5 \times 10^9$/L) due to bone marrow failure is similar for both adults and children. Infected neutropenic patients usually respond to antibiotics alone, provided bone marrow function recovers early during the infection. Because children with newly diagnosed leukemia respond rapidly to induction chemotherapy, only rarely are they candidates for GTX. In contrast, infected children with sustained bone marrow failure (i.e., malignant neoplasms resistant to treatment, aplastic anemia, and hematopoietic progenitor cell transplant recipients) may benefit when GTX are added to antibiotics. The use of GTX for bacterial sepsis unresponsive to antibiotics in patients with severe neutropenia ($<0.5 \times 10^9$/L) is supported by most of the controlled studies (see Chapter 164).

Children with qualitative neutrophil defects (neutrophil dysfunction) usually have adequate numbers of blood neutrophils but are susceptible to serious infections because their cells kill pathogenic microorganisms inefficiently. Neutrophil dysfunction syndromes are rare, and no definitive studies have established the efficacy of GTX. However, several patients with progressive life-threatening infections have improved strikingly with the addition of GTX to antimicrobial therapy. These disorders are chronic, and because of the risk of inducing alloimmunization, GTX are recommended only when infections are clearly unresponsive to antimicrobial drugs.

Neonates are unusually susceptible to severe bacterial infections, and a number of defects of neonatal body defenses may be contributing factors (see Chapter 98). These abnormalities are accentuated in sick premature neonates, and it is logical to consider GTX. Neonates exhibiting fulminant sepsis, relative neutropenia ($<3.0 \times 10^9$/L during the first week of life; $<1.0 \times 10^9$/L thereafter), and a severely diminished neutrophil marrow storage pool ($<10\%$ of nucleated marrow cells being postmitotic neutrophils) are at particularly great risk of dying if only treated with antibiotics. Although some studies have shown a significant benefit from GTX, they are rarely used. Instead, some neonatologists consider alternative therapies including intravenous immunoglobulin (IVIG) and recombinant myeloid growth factors (G-CSF or granulocyte-macrophage colony-stimulating factor [GM-CSF]). Results of studies evaluating IVIG have been mixed, but a meta-analysis found significant benefit for neonates with proven sepsis. Current data are insufficient to determine whether recombinant myeloid growth factors have a role in treating these neonates, although both G-CSF and GM-CSF have been demonstrated to enhance myelopoiesis and to increase neutrophil blood counts in infants. Importantly, G-CSF clearly is efficacious for the treatment of several types of severe congenital neutropenia.

Once the decision to provide GTX has been made, an adequate dose of fresh leukapheresis cells must be transfused. Neonates and infants weighing less than 10 kg should receive

---

BOX 464–1. Guidelines for Pediatric Granulocyte Transfusions

CHILDREN AND ADOLESCENTS

Neutrophils $< 0.5 \times 10^9$/L and bacterial infection *unresponsive* to appropriate antimicrobial therapy

Qualitative neutrophil defect and infection (bacterial or fungal) *unresponsive* to appropriate antimicrobial therapy

INFANTS WITHIN FIRST 4 MO OF LIFE

Neutrophils $< 3.0 \times 10^9$/L (1st wk of life) or $< 1.0 \times 10^9$/L (thereafter) and *fulminant* bacterial infection

---

Words in *italics* must be defined for local transfusion guidelines.

$1-2 \times 10^9$/kg neutrophils per GTX. Larger infants and children should receive a total dose of at least 1×10^{10} neutrophils per each GTX; the preferred dose for adolescents is $5-8 \times 10^{10}$ per GTX—a dose requiring donors to be stimulated with G-CSF. GTX should be given daily until either the infection resolves or the blood neutrophil count exceeds 1.0×10^9/L for a few days.

Chapter 465
Fresh Frozen Plasma Transfusions

Guidelines for fresh frozen plasma (FFP) transfusions in children (Box 465–1) are similar to those for adults. FFP is transfused to replace clinically significant deficiencies of plasma proteins for which more highly purified concentrates are not available. Requirements for FFP vary with the specific factor being replaced, but a starting dose of 15 mL/kg is usually satisfactory. Transfusion of FFP is efficacious for the treatment of deficiencies of clotting factors II, V, X, and XI. Factor XIII and fibrinogen deficiencies are treated with cryoprecipitate. Transfusion of FFP is no longer recommended for treatment of patients with severe hemophilia A or B or for factor VII deficiency because safer factor VIII, IX, and VII concentrates are available. Moreover, mild to moderate hemophilia A and certain types of von Willebrand's disease can be treated with desmopressin (see Chapter 469). An important use of FFP, albeit rare in children, is for rapid reversal of warfarin effects in patients who are actively bleeding or who require emergency surgery (i.e., in whom functional deficiencies of factors II, VII, IX, and X cannot be rapidly reversed by vitamin K). Results of screening coagulation tests (prothrombin, activated partial thromboplastin, and thrombin times) should not be assumed, by themselves, to reflect the integrity of the coagulation system. To justify FFP transfusions, coagulation test results must be related to the clinical condition of the patient. Transfusion of FFP in patients with chronic liver disease and prolonged clotting times is not recommended unless bleeding is present or an invasive procedure is planned.

Although its major benefit has been in the treatment of bleeding associated with clotting factor deficiencies, FFP also contains several anticoagulant proteins (antithrombin III, protein C, and protein S), whose deficiencies have been associated with thrombosis. In selected situations, FFP may be appropriate as replacement therapy—along with anticoagulant treatment—in patients with these disorders. However, when available, purified concentrates are preferred. Other indications for FFP include replacement fluid during plasma exchange in patients with thrombotic thrombocytopenic purpura or other disorders for which FFP is likely to be beneficial (e.g., plasma exchange in a patient with bleeding and a severe coagulopathy). FFP is not indicated for correction of hypovolemia or as immunoglobulin replacement therapy, because safer alternatives exist (e.g., albumin solutions and intravenous immunoglobulin, respectively).

In *neonates*, FFP transfusions merit special considerations. Clotting times are prolonged, owing to developmental deficiency of clotting proteins, and FFP should be transfused only after reference to normal values expected for the birthweight and age of the infant in question. The indications for FFP in neonates include (1) reconstitution of red blood cell (RBC) concentrates to simulate whole blood for use in massive transfusions (e.g., exchange transfusion or cardiovascular surgery), (2) hemorrhage secondary to vitamin K deficiency, (3) disseminated intravascular coagulation with bleeding, and (4) bleeding in congenital coagulation factor deficiency when more specific treatment is either unavailable or inappropriate. The use of prophylactic FFP transfusions to prevent intraventricular hemorrhage in premature infants is not recommended. FFP should not be used as a suspending agent to adjust the hematocrit values of RBC concentrates before small-volume RBC transfusions to neonates because it offers no apparent medical benefit over the use of sterile solutions for this purpose. Similarly, the use of FFP in partial exchange transfusion for the treatment of neonatal hyperviscosity syndrome is unnecessary because safer colloid solutions are available.

When treating bleeding infants, cryoprecipitate is often considered because of its small infusion volume. However, cryoprecipitate contains only fibrinogen and factors VIII and XIII. Thus, it is not effective for treating the usual clinical situation in bleeding infants of multiple clotting factor deficiencies despite the convenience of a small infusion volume. In preliminary studies, infusions of very small volumes of recombinant activated factor VII have been life saving with hemorrhage due to several mechanisms.

Chapter 466
Risks of Blood Transfusions

Although the risks of allogeneic blood transfusions are extraordinarily low, transfusions must be given judiciously. Actual infectious disease risks are too low to be known accurately, but taking nucleic amplification testing and all other donor screening activities into account, a current estimate for risk of transfusion-associated HIV is 1/1 million donor exposures, with estimates ranging from 1/800,000 to 1/2 million donor exposures. Similarly, the risk of viral hepatitis C is 1/1 million donor exposures. Transfusion-associated cytomegalovirus can be nearly eliminated by transfusing leukocyte-reduced cellular blood products or by selecting blood from donors seronegative for antibody to cytomegalovirus. Additional infectious risks include other types of hepatitis and retroviruses, syphilis, parvovirus B19, Epstein-Barr virus, and Chagas disease.

Transfusion-associated risks of a noninfectious nature that may occur include fluid overload, graft versus host disease, electrolyte and acid-base imbalances, iron overload, increased susceptibility to oxidant damage, exposure to plasticizers, hemolysis when T-antigen activation of red blood cells (RBCs) has occurred, immunosuppression, and alloimmunization. Curiously, alloimmunization to RBC and leukocyte antigens seems to be very uncommon in infants. Some adverse effects are seen only in massive transfusion settings such as exchange transfusions, when relatively large quantities of blood are needed, and are rare with the small-volume transfusions usually given.

Premature infants are known to have immune dysfunction, but their relative risk of post-transfusion graft versus host disease is controversial. The postnatal age of the infant, the number of immunocompetent lymphocytes in the transfusion product, the degree of human leukocyte antigen (HLA) compatibility between donor and recipient, and other poorly described phenomena determine which infants are truly at risk. Regardless, many centers caring for preterm infants transfuse exclusively gamma-irradiated cellular products. Directed donations with blood drawn from blood relatives should always be irradiated because of the risk of engraftment with transfused HLA homozygous haploidentical lymphocytes. Cellular blood products given as intrauterine and exchange transfusions are gamma irradiated, as are transfusions for patients with severe congenital immunodeficiency disorders and recipients of hematopoietic progenitor cell transplants. Other groups potentially at risk, but for whom no conclusive data are available, are patients given T-cell antibody therapy (antithymocyte globulin or OKT3), organ allografts, immunosuppressive drug regimens, and patients infected with HIV.

Current practice uses gamma irradiation from a cesium, cobalt, or linear acceleration source at doses ranging from 2,500–5,000 cGy; a minimum dose of 2,500 cGy is required. All cellular blood components should be irradiated, but frozen "acellular" products such as plasma and cryoprecipitate do not require it. Leukocyte reduction cannot be substituted for gamma irradiation to prevent graft versus host disease.

Andrew M, Castle V, Saigal S, et al: Clinical impact of neonatal thrombocytopenia. *J Pediatr* 1987;110:457.

Andrew M, Vegh P, Caco C, et al: A randomized, controlled trial of platelet transfusions in thrombocytopenic premature infants. *J Pediatr* 1993;123:285.

Blanchette VS, Hume HA, Levy GJ, et al: Guidelines for auditing pediatric blood transfusion practices. *Am J Dis Child* 1991;145:787.

College of American Pathologists Task Force: Practice parameter for the use of fresh-frozen plasma, cryoprecipitate, and platelets. *JAMA* 1994;271:777.

Del Vecchio A, Sola MC, Theriaque DW, et al: Platelet transfusions in the neonatal intensive care unit: Factors predicting which patients will require multiple transfusions. *Transfusion* 2001;41:803.

Strauss RG: Current status of granulocyte transfusions to treat neonatal sepsis. *J Clin Apheresis* 1989;5:25

Strauss RG: Transfusion approach to the anemia of prematurity. *NeoReviews* 2000;1:e74.

Strauss RG: Data-driven blood banking practices for neonatal red blood cell transfusions. *Transfusion* 2000;40:1528.

Vamvakas EC, Strauss RG: Meta-analysis of controlled clinical trials studying the efficacy of recombinant human erythropoietin in reducing blood transfusions in the anemia of prematurity. *Transfusion* 2001;41:406.

SECTION 7 *Hemorrhagic and Thrombotic Diseases*

Robert R. Montgomery and J. Paul Scott

When blood vessels are injured, hemostasis maintains vascular integrity or causes blood flow to cease through the injured vessel. If clotting is impaired, hemorrhage occurs. If clotting is excessive, thrombosis and its complications occur. The hemostatic response needs to be rapid and regulated. Trivial trauma should not trigger a systemic reaction but must initiate a rapid, localized response. Once clotting begins, anticoagulants must confine the clotting process to the site of injury to prevent extensive thrombosis. The clot must then be physiologically lysed to re-establish blood vessel patency. These hemostatic mechanisms are very complex and involve local reactions of the blood vessel, the multiple activities of the platelet, the interaction of specific coagulation factors both with each other and with platelets, the regulation of clotting by anticoagulant factors and their inhibitors, and the factors that initiate and regulate the fibrinolytic process.

The vascular endothelium is the primary barrier against hemorrhage. When small vessels are transected, active vasoconstriction minimizes the local hemorrhage even without activation of clotting. Platelets are essential for the control of hemorrhage from small blood vessels. More extensive injury (involvement of large blood vessels) requires the participation and coordination of the full hemostatic process to provide a firm, stable, fibrin clot. The extent of this clotting is localized by the anticoagulation system; the removal of the clot requires appropriate fibrinolysis.

Isolated deficiencies of individual anticoagulants (clotting factor inhibitors) predispose the patient to excessive thrombosis. In acquired hemostatic disorders, there are frequently multiple problems with homeostasis that perturb and dysregulate hemostasis. As an example, a primary illness (sepsis) and its secondary effects (shock, acidosis) activate coagulation and fibrinolysis and impair the host's ability to restore normal hemostatic function. In disseminated intravascular coagulation (DIC), procoagulant clotting factors and anticoagulant proteins are consumed, leaving the hemostatic system unbalanced and prone to bleeding or clotting. Similarly, newborn infants or patients with severe liver disease have synthetic deficiencies of both procoagulant and anticoagulant proteins. Such dysregulation causes the patient to be predisposed to both hemorrhage and thrombosis with mild or moderate triggers that result in major alterations in the hemostatic process.

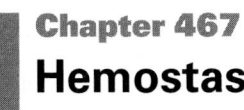

Chapter 467

Hemostasis

467.1 Hemostatic Mechanism

The classic hemostatic mechanism includes the vascular response, platelet adhesion, platelet aggregation, clot formation, clot stabilization, limitation of clotting to the site of injury by regulatory anticoagulants, and re-establishment of vascular patency through fibrinolysis and vascular healing. The laboratory evaluation of this mechanism requires the isolated study of this response as a series of independent events; however, in vivo, these events are tightly integrated. For example, fibrinogen serves as the ligand between platelets during platelet aggregation and also serves as the substrate for thrombin that forms the fibrin clot. von Willebrand factor (VWF) provides another example of a single protein with multiple functions. It circulates in a complex with factor VIII, with VWF serving as the adhesive ligand for platelet adhesion and factor VIII serving as one of the major regulating cofactors controlling clotting. The hemostatic mechanism is further complicated in that in vivo the interactions may utilize different pathways from those studied in clinical laboratory testing. In vitro clotting is characterized by using the activated partial thromboplastin time (PTT) and the prothrombin time (PT). The PT measures the clotting process through the addition of tissue factor, which, together with factor VII, activates factor X (Fig. 467–1). In vivo, factor VIIa activates factor X and factor IX, but as routinely studied in the clinical laboratory, the pathway through which factor VIIa activates factor IX is not evaluated. If the tissue factor/factor VIIa complex activated only factor X, it would be difficult to explain why the most severe bleeding disorders are factor VIII (hemophilia A) and factor IX (hemophilia B) deficiency. Nevertheless, the mechanisms studied by the PTT and the PT permit us to evaluate clotting factor deficiencies even though these pathways may not be the same as those occurring physiologically.

After vascular injury, vasoconstriction occurs and flowing blood is subjected to exposure to the subendothelial matrix (Fig. 467–2). VWF in flowing blood contacts the subendothelial matrix proteins, changes conformation, and provides the glue to which the platelet VWF receptor binds. After adherence, platelets become activated and release storage granules containing adenosine diphosphate (ADP), thromboxane A_2, and other stored proteins. These result in the aggregation and recruitment of other platelets to the platelet plug. Aggregation involves the interaction of specific receptors on the platelet surface with plasma hemostatic proteins, primarily fibrinogen. During the process of platelet activation, internalized platelet phospholipids (primarily phosphatidylserine) become externalized and interact at two specific, rate-limiting steps in the clotting process—those involving the cofactors factor VIII (X-ase complex) and factor V (prothrombinase complex). Vascular injury also releases tissue factor and alters the vascular surface that initiates the clotting cascade and results in the generation of the fibrin clot. The stable fibrin-platelet plug is ultimately formed through clot retraction and cross linking of the fibrin clot by factor XIII.

Examination of the interaction of clotting factors shown in Figure 467–1 discloses what has been termed the *waterfall cascade*. Inactive clotting factors denoted by roman numerals become activated. The activated clotting factor then initiates the activation of the next sequential clotting factor in a systematic manner. This results in the amplification of the process to give a burst of clotting where it is physiologically needed. In vivo, autocatalysis of factor VII generates small amounts of factor VII continuously so the system is always poised to act. Clotting is held in check by the coagulation inhibitory proteins. The release of tissue factor at the site of vascular injury generates an over thousandfold increase in factor VIIa generation. Activated platelets at the site of injury provide the membrane surface upon which the activated clotting factor, its substrate (next in the waterfall), and its cofactor all localize in close proximity to maximize the efficiency of the reactions and provide a burst of clotting where it is needed. Once generated, thrombin amplifies these reactions by providing a positive feedback loop by activating additional molecules of factors XI, VIII, and V as well as aggregating additional platelets.

In the clinical laboratory, factor XII is activated using a surface (silica or glass) or a contact activator, such as ellagic acid. Factor VII is activated and interacts with tissue factor through a similar cascade. The former is the pathway measured by the PTT and the latter that measured by the PT. This process is accelerated by the interaction with phospholipid and calcium at the steps involving factor VIII and factor V. Deficiencies of clotting factors

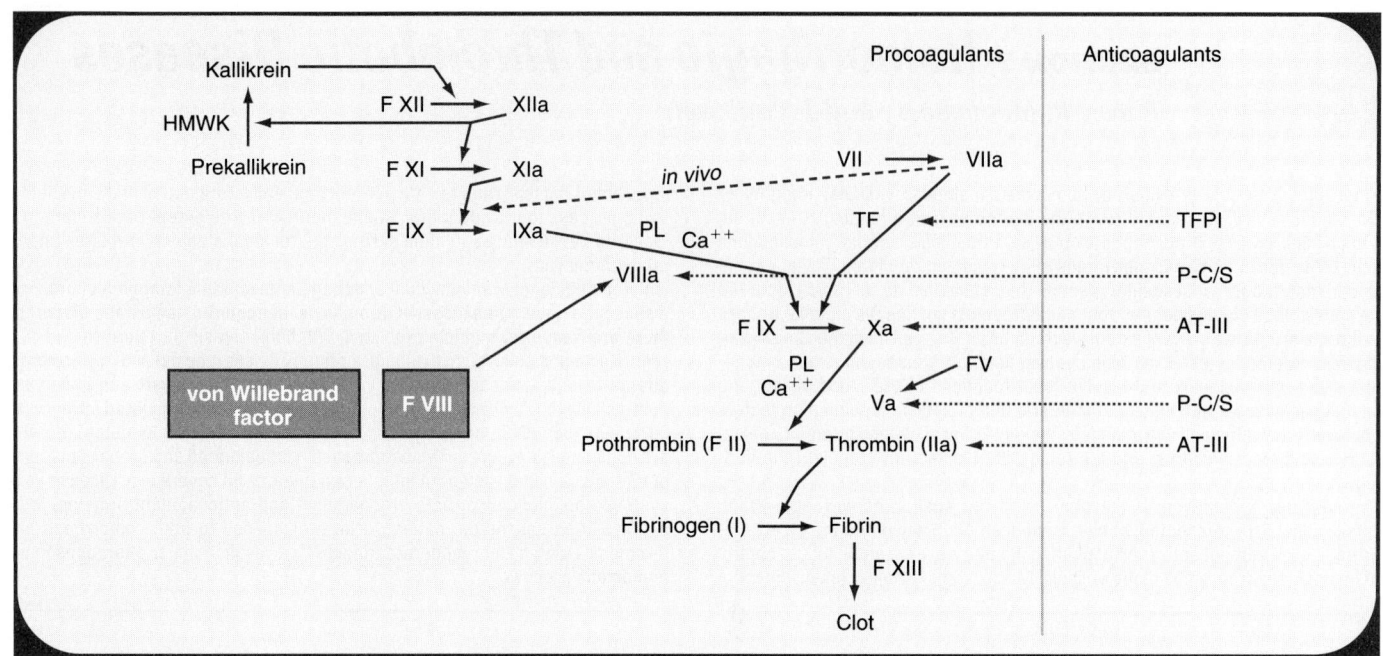

FIGURE 467–1. Clotting cascade with sequential activation and amplification of clot formation. Many of the factors are activated by the clotting factor above them in the cascade. The activated factors are designated by the addition of an "a." *Right side,* The major anticoagulants and the sites that they regulate (TFPI regulates TF and VIIa; protein C and S regulate factors VIII and V; and AT-III regulates Xa and thrombin [Xa]). The dotted line illustrates that in vivo TF and VIIa activate both IX and X, but in vitro we measure only the activation of factor X. Unactivated factor VIII, when bound to its carrier protein, von Willebrand factor, is protected from protein C inactivation. When thrombin or Xa activates factor VII, it becomes unbound to von Willebrand factor, where it can participate with IXa in the activation of factor X in the presence of phospholipid and calcium. Factor XIII cross links the fibrin clot and thereby makes it more stable. HMWK = high molecular weight kininogen; PL = phospholipid; Ca^{++} = calcium; TF = tissue factor; TFPI = tissue factor pathway inhibitor; P-C/S = protein C and protein S; AT-III = antithrombin III.

result in either isolated prolongation of the PTT or PT or an alteration in both. This is useful in determining hereditary clotting factor deficiencies; in acquired hemostatic disorders encountered in clinical practice, however, more than one clotting factor is frequently deficient so that the relative prolongation of the PTT and PT must be assessed.

Because clotting factors were named in the order of discovery they do not necessarily reflect the sequential order of activation (Table 467–1). In fact, factors III, IV, and VI were not subsequently found to be independent proteins, and thus these terms are no longer used. The dual mechanisms of activating clotting have been termed the *intrinsic* (surface activation) and *extrinsic* (tissue factor–mediated) pathways. The intrinsic pathway involves the initial activation of factor XII, which is accelerated by two other plasma proteins, prekallikrein and high molecular weight kininogen. Activated factor XII (XIIa), in turn, activates XI to XIa, which then catalyzes IX to IXa. On the platelet phospholipid surface, factor IXa complexes with factor VIII and calcium to activate factor X (the "tenase" complex). The extrinsic system is measured by the prothrombin time. Addition of tissue factor causes a burst of factor VIIa generation. The tissue factor/factor VIIa complex activates factor X. This is the in vitro pathway, but in vivo the complex between tissue factor and factor VIIa triggers activation of factor IX. Whether factor X is activated by the intrinsic or the extrinsic pathway, Xa is generated. On the platelet phospholipid surface, Xa complexes with factor V and calcium (the "prothrombinase" complex) to activate prothrombin to thrombin (also referred to as IIa). Once thrombin is generated, fibrinogen is converted to a fibrin clot. This loose fibrin clot is then cross-linked by factor XIII (transglutaminase). Figure 467–1 is oversimplified because Xa can activate both factor VIII and factor V, and thrombin can activate factor V, factor VIII, factor XI, and platelets. After

thrombin activates the procoagulant system, thrombin binds to thrombomodulin on the intact endothelial cell surface, where it activates the anticoagulant system. Thrombomodulin-bound thrombin is no longer a procoagulant but acts as an anticoagulant by activating protein C. Activated protein C inactivates factor V and factor VIII, which, in turn, limit further thrombin generation. Thus, when thrombin encounters intact healthy endothelium, it now functions to activate the anticoagulant mechanism and limit clotting.

Virtually all procoagulant proteins are balanced by an anticoagulant protein that regulates or inhibits procoagulant function. There are four clinically important, naturally occurring anticoagulants that regulate the extension of the clotting process. These include antithrombin III (AT III), protein C, protein S, and tissue factor pathway inhibitor (TFPI). The primary action of antithrombin III is to regulate factor Xa and thrombin. It may also serve to regulate IXa, XIa, and XIIa, but this activity is less important. Protein C, in the presence of thrombin bound to thrombomodulin, becomes activated protein C (APC). In the presence of the cofactor protein S, activated protein C proteolyses and inactivates activated factor V and activated factor VIII. The final inhibitor is TFPI, which quickly shuts down the activation of factor X by factor VII and tissue factor and shifts the activation site of tissue factor and factor VII to that of factor IX (see Figs. 467–1 and 467–2).

Once a stable fibrin-platelet plug is formed, the fibrinolytic system limits its extension and also lyses the clot (fibrinolysis) to re-establish vascular integrity. Plasmin, generated from plasminogen by either urokinase-like or tissue-type plasminogen activator, degrades the fibrin clot. In the process of dissolving the fibrin clot, fibrin degradation products are produced. This pathway is regulated by plasminogen activator inhibitors (PAI-1) and α_2-antiplasmin.

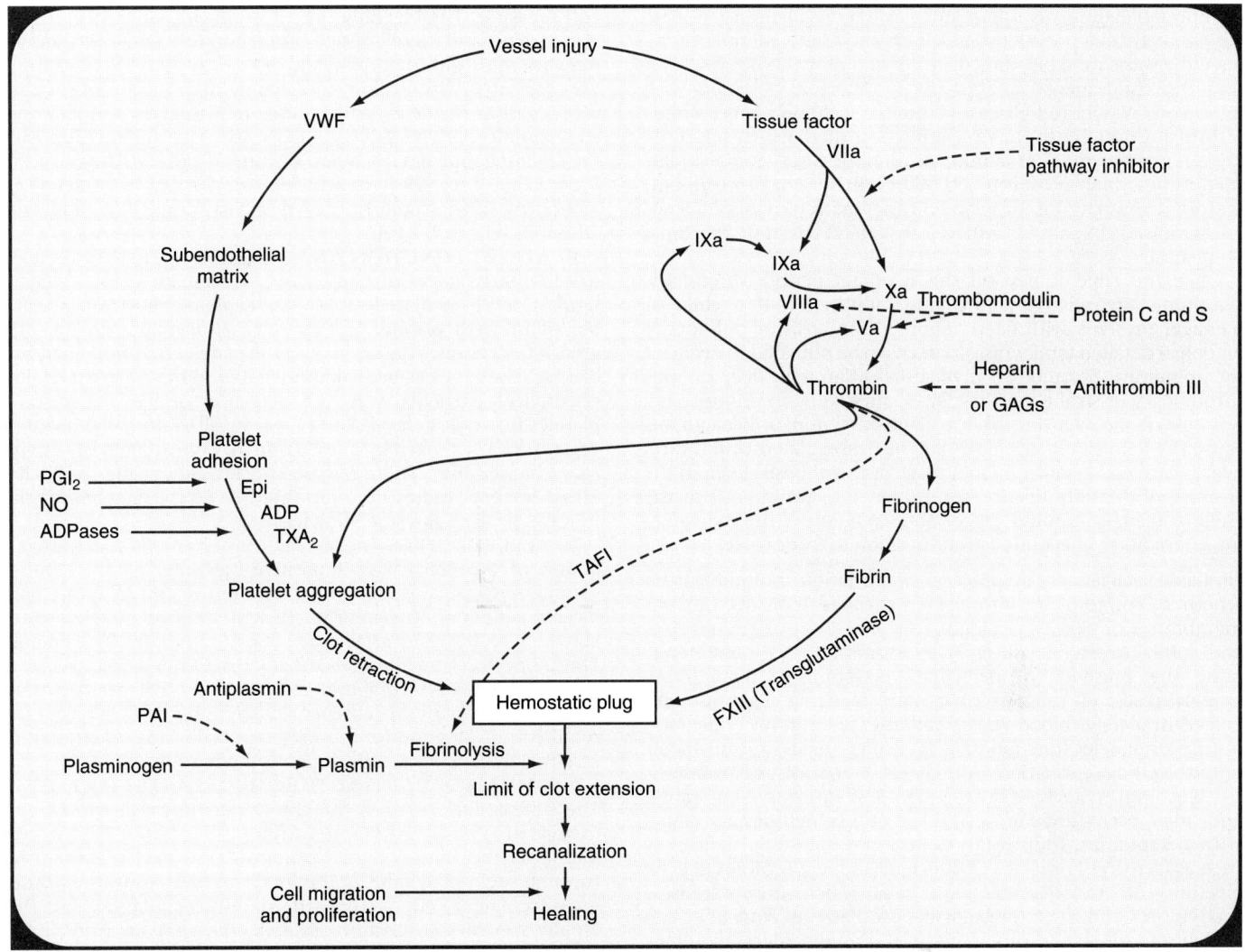

FIGURE 467–2. Diagrammatic representation of the hemostatic mechanism. PGI_2 = prostacyclin; NO = nitric oxide; ADP = adenosine diphosphate; Epi = epinephrine; TXA_2 = thromboxane A_2; PAI = plasminogen activator inhibitor; GAGs = glycosaminoglycans; TAFI = thrombin activated fibrinolytic inhibitor.

TABLE 467–1. The Coagulation Factors

Clotting Factors	Synonym	Disorder
I	Fibrinogen	Congenital deficiency (afibrinogenemia) and dysfunction (dysfibrinogenemia)
II	Prothrombin	Congenital deficiency or dysfunction
V	Labile factor, proaccelerin	Congenital deficiency (parahemophilia)
VII	Stable factor or proconvertin	Congenital deficiency
VIII	Antihemophilic factor (AHF)	Congenital deficiency is hemophilia A (classic hemophilia)
IX	Christmas factor	Congenital deficiency is hemophilia B
X	Stuart-Prower factor	Congenital deficiency
XI	Plasma thromboplastin antecedent	Congenital deficiency, sometimes referred to as hemophilia C
XII	Hageman factor	Congenital deficiency is not associated with clinical symptoms
XIII	Fibrin-stabilizing factor	Congenital deficiency

467.2 The Clinical and Laboratory Evaluation

History. For most hemostatic disorders, whether they be hemorrhagic or thrombotic, the clinical history provides the most useful information. For a hemorrhagic condition the history should determine the site or sites of bleeding, the severity and duration of hemorrhage, and the age at symptom onset. Was the bleeding spontaneous or after trauma? Was there a previous personal or family history of similar problems? One should determine if symptoms correlate with the degree of injury or trauma. Does bruising occur spontaneously? Are there lumps with bruises for which there is minimal trauma? If there has been previous surgery or significant dental procedures, was there any increased bleeding? If a child or adolescent has had surgery to mucosal surfaces, such as a tonsillectomy or major dental extractions, the absence of bleeding usually rules out a hereditary bleeding disorder. Delayed or slow healing of superficial injuries may suggest a hereditary bleeding disorder. In postpubertal females, it is important to take a careful menstrual history. Because some common bleeding disorders such as von Willebrand disease have a fairly high prevalence, mothers and family members may have the same mild bleeding disorder and may not be cognizant that the child menstrual history is abnormal. Women with mild von Willebrand disease who have a moderate history of bruising frequently have a reduction of that bruising during pregnancy or after administration of birth control pills. Medications such as aspirin and other nonsteroidal anti-inflammatory drugs may inhibit platelet function and increase bleeding symptoms in patients with a low platelet count or abnormal hemostasis.

Once the child is beyond the neonatal period, thrombotic symptoms are relatively rare until adulthood. If a child or teenager presents with deep venous thrombosis or pulmonary emboli, a detailed family history needs to be obtained to evaluate for premature thrombosis, myocardial infarction, deep venous thrombosis, or stroke in other family members. In the neonate, physiologic deficiencies of procoagulants and anticoagulants cause the hemostatic mechanism to be dysregulated, and clinical events can lead to either hemorrhage or thrombosis. Even in the absence of a family history, the presence of thrombosis in the child or teenager should trigger an evaluation of the individual for a hereditary or acquired predisposition to thrombosis.

Physical Examination. The physical examination should focus on whether symptoms are primarily associated with the mucous membranes or skin (mucocutaneous bleeding) or the muscles and joints (deep bleeding). The examination should determine the presence of petechiae, ecchymoses, hematomas, hemarthroses, or mucous membrane bleeding. Patients with defects in platelet/blood vessel wall interaction (von Willebrand disease or platelet function defects) usually have mucous membrane bleeding (epistaxis, menorrhagia, hematuria, gastrointestinal bleeding); petechiae on the skin and mucous membranes; and small, ecchymotic lesions of the skin sometimes associated with hematomas. Individuals with a clotting factor deficiency such as factor VIII or factor IX deficiency have symptoms of deep bleeding into muscles and joints with much more extensive ecchymoses and hematoma formation. Patients with mild von Willebrand disease or other mild bleeding disorders may have no abnormal findings on physical examination.

Patients at risk for thrombotic disorders should be evaluated for swollen, warm, tender extremities or internal organs (venous thrombosis), unexplained dyspnea or persistent pneumonia especially in the absence of fever (pulmonary emboli), as well as varicosities and postphlebitic changes. Arterial thrombi usually cause an acute, dramatic impairment of organ function: stroke, myocardial infarction, and a painful white, cold extremity.

Laboratory Tests. Patients who have a positive bleeding history or who are actively hemorrhaging should have a platelet count, bleeding time, PTT, and PT. If the results are normal, a thrombin time and VWF testing should be considered. In individuals with abnormal screening tests, further specific factor work-up should be undertaken. In a patient with an abnormal bleeding history and a positive family history, normal screening tests should not preclude further laboratory evaluation.

There are no effective routine screening tests for hereditary thrombotic disorders. If the family history is positive or the clinical thrombosis is unexplained, specific anticoagulant assays should be undertaken. Thrombosis is rare in children, and, when present, the possibility of a hereditary predisposition must be considered and evaluated in the laboratory.

BLEEDING TIME. The bleeding time assesses the function of platelets and their interaction with the vascular wall. Disposable standardized devices have been developed that control the length and depth of the skin incision. A blood pressure cuff is applied to the upper arm and inflated to 40 mm Hg for children and adults. In term newborns and younger children a modified device has been developed and used with a lower blood pressure

cuff pressure. The bleeding time is a difficult laboratory test to standardize, and there is much interlaboratory and interindividual variation. Although platelet counts less than 100,000/mm^3 are associated with prolonged bleeding times, disproportionate prolongation of the bleeding times may suggest a qualitative platelet defect or von Willebrand disease. After the incision with the bleeding time device, blood is blotted from the margin of the incision at 30 sec intervals until bleeding ceases. Although each laboratory must establish its own normal range, bleeding usually stops within 4–8 min.

PLATELET FUNCTION ANALYZER. In an attempt to measure the early stages of hemostasis to evaluate shear, collagen binding, VWF-mediated adhesion, and platelet function, a number of in vitro platelet analyzers have been developed. The greatest experience has been with the platelet function analyzer, or PFA. The PFA has been demonstrated to have a great deal of sensitivity—particularly in the detection of VWD and some platelet function defects. The PFA is sensitive to VWD in those variants characterized by a reduction in VWF antigen or activity (see Chapter 469). There remain concerns about the specificity. Thus, further studies are warranted to establish whether the PFA can be used as a screening tool.

PLATELET COUNT. The platelet count is essential in the evaluation of the child with a positive bleeding history because thrombocytopenia is the most common acquired cause of a bleeding diathesis in children. Patients with a platelet count above 50,000/mm^3 rarely have significant clinical bleeding. Thrombocytosis in children is usually reactive and not associated with bleeding or thrombotic complications. Persistent, severe thrombocytosis in the absence of an underlying illness may require an evaluation for the very rare pediatric presentation of essential thrombocythemia or polycythemia vera.

"ACTIVATED" PARTIAL THROMBOPLASTIN TIME (PTT). The PTT as performed in the clinical laboratory is actually an "activated" PTT (or APTT); most refer to it as the PTT. This test measures the initiation of clotting at the level of factor XII through sequential steps to the final clot end-point. It does not measure factor VII, factor XIII, or anticoagulants. The PTT employs a contact activator (silica, kaolin, or ellagic acid) in the presence of calcium and phospholipid. Because of different reagents and laboratory instruments the normal range for the PTT varies between one hospital laboratory and another. Normal ranges are much more variable from laboratory to laboratory than with the PT.

PROTHROMBIN TIME (PT). The PT measures the extrinsic clotting system after the activation of clotting by tissue factor (thromboplastin) in the presence of calcium. It is not prolonged with deficiencies of factors VIII, IX, XI, or XII. In most laboratories the normal PT ranges between 10–13 sec. The PT has been standardized using the International Normalized Ratio (INR) so that values can be compared from one laboratory or instrument to another. The INR is used to determine similar degrees of anticoagulation with warfarin (Coumadin)–like medications.

THROMBIN TIME. The thrombin time measures the final step of the clotting cascade in which fibrinogen is converted to fibrin. The normal thrombin time varies between laboratories but is usually between 11–15 sec. Prolongation of the thrombin time occurs with reduced fibrinogen levels (hypofibrinogenemia or afibrinogenemia), with dysfunctional fibrinogen (dysfibrinogenemia), or by substances that interfere with fibrin polymerization, such as heparin or fibrin split products. If heparin contamination is a potential cause for a long thrombin time, a reptilase time is usually ordered.

REPTILASE TIME. The reptilase time uses a snake venom to clot fibrinogen. Unlike the thrombin time, the reptilase time is not sensitive to heparin and is prolonged only by reduced or dysfunctional fibrinogen and fibrin split products. Therefore, if the thrombin time is prolonged but the reptilase time is normal, the prolonged thrombin time is due to heparin and does not

TABLE 467–2. Reference Values for Coagulation Tests in Healthy Children*

Tests	28–31 Wk Gestation	30–36 Wk Gestation	Full Term	1–5 Yr	6–10 Yr	11–18 Yr	Adult
Screening Tests							
PT (sec)	15.4 (14.6–16.9)	13.0 (10.6–16.2)	13.0 (10.1–15.9)	11 (10.6–11.4)	11.1 (10.1–12.0)	11.2 (10.2–12.0)	12 (11.0–14.0)
APTT (sec)	108 (80–168)	53.6 (27.5–79.4)‡§	42.9 (31.3–54.3)‡	30 (24–36)	31 (26–36)	32 (26–37)‡	33 (27–40)
BT (min)	—	—	—	6 (2.5–10)‡	7 (2.5–13)‡	5 (3–8)‡	4 (1–7)
Procoagulants							
Fibrinogen	256 (160–550)	243 (150–373)‡§	283 (167–399)	276 (170–405)	279 (157–40)	30 (154–448)	278 (156–40)
II	31 (19–54)	45 (20–77)‡	48 (26–70)‡	94 (71–116)‡	88 (67–107)‡	83 (61–104)‡	108 (70–146)
V	65 (43–80)	88 (41–144)§	72 (34–108)‡	103 (79–127)	90 (63–116)‡	77 (55–99)‡	106 (62–150)
VII	37 (24–76)	67 (21–113)‡	66 (28–104)‡	82 (55–116)‡	86 (52–120)‡	83 (58–115)‡	105 (67–143)
VII procoagulant	79 (37–126)	111 (5–213)	100 (50–178)	90 (59–142)	95 (58–132)	92 (53–131)	99 (50–149)
vWF	141 (83–223)	136 (78–210)	153 (50–287)	82 (60–120)	95 (44–144)	100 (46–153)	92 (50–158)
IX	18 (17–20)	35 (19–65)§‡	53 (15–91)†‡	73 (47–104)‡	75 (63–89)‡	82 (59–122)‡	109 (55–163)
X	36 (25–64)	41 (11–71)‡	40 (12–68)‡	88 (58–116)‡	75 (55–101)‡	79 (50–117)	106 (70–152)
XI	23 (11–33)	30 (08–52)‡§	38 ± (40–66)‡	30 (08–52)‡	38 (10–66)	74 (50–97)‡	97 (56–150)
XII	25 (05–35)	38 (10–66)‡§	53 (13–93)‡	93 (64–129)	92 (60–140)	81 (34–137)‡	108 (52–164)
PK	26 (15–32)	33 (09–89)‡	37 (18–69)‡	95 (65–130)	99 (66–131)	99 (53–145)	112 (62–162)
HMWK	32 (19–52)	49 (09–89)‡	54 (06–102)‡	98 (64–132)	93 (60–130)	91 (63–119)	92 (50–136)
XIIIa‖	—	70 (32–108)‡	79 (27–131)‡	108 (72–143)	109 (65–151)	99 (57–140)	105 (55–155)
XIIIb‖	—	81 (35–127)‡	76 (30–122)‡	113 (69–156)‡	116 (77–154)‡	102 (60–143)	98 (057–137)
Anticoagulants							
ATIII	28 (20–38)	38 (14–62)‡§	63 (39–87)‡	111 (82–139)	111 (90–131)‡	106 (77–132)	100 (74–126)
Protein C	—	28 (12–44)‡§	35 (17–53)‡	66 (40–92)‡	69 (45–93)‡	83 (55–111)‡	96 (64–128)
Protein S							
Total (U/mL)	—	26 (14–38)‡§	36 (12–60)‡	86 (54–118)	78 (41–114)	72 (52–92)	81 (61–113)
Free (U/mL)	—	—	—	45 (21–69)	42 (22–62)	38 (26–55)	45 (27–061)
Plasminogen (U/mL)	—	170 (112–248)‖	195 (125–265)‖	98 (78–118)	92 (75–108)	86 (68–103)	99 (77–122)
TPA (ng/mL)	—	8.48 (3.00–16.70)	9.6 (5.0–18.9)	2.15 (1.0–4.5)‡	2.42 (1.0–5.0)‡	2.16 (1.0–4.0)‡	1.02 (.68–1.36)
a_2AP (U/mL)	—	78 (40–116)	85 (55–115)	105 (93–117)	99 (89–110)	98 (78–118)	102 (68–136)
PAI-1	—	5.4 (0.0–12.2)‡	6.4 (2.0–15.1)	5.42 (1.0–10.0)	6.79 (2.0–12.0)‡	6.07 (2.0–10.0)‡	3.60 (0–11.0)

*All factors except fibrinogen are presented as units/mL (fibrinogen in mg/mL), where pooled normal plasma contains 1 unit/mL. All data are expressed as the mean followed by the upper and lower boundaries encompassing 95% of the normal population.

†Levels for 19–27 wk and 28–31 wk are from multiple sources and cannot be analyzed statistically.

‡Values are significantly different from those of adults.

§Values are significantly different from those of full-term infants.

‖Value given as CTA units/mL.

PT = prothrombin time; INR = international normalized ratio; APTT = activated partial thromboplastin time; VIII = factor VIII procoagulant activity; vWf = von Willebrand factor; PK = prekallikrein; HMWK = high molecular weight kininogen.

Data from Andrew M, Paes B, Johnston M: Development of the hemostatic system in the neonate and young infant. Am J Pediatr Hematol Oncol 1990; 12:95; and Andrew M, Vegh P, Johnston M, et al: Maturation of the hemostatic system during childhood. Blood 1992; 80:1998.

indicate the presence of fibrin split products or reduced concentration or function of fibrinogen.

MIXING STUDIES. If there is an unexplained prolongation of the PT, PTT, or thrombin time, a mixing study is usually performed. Normal plasma is added to the patient's plasma, and the PTT or PT is repeated. Correction of the PT or PTT by 1:1 mixing with normal plasma suggests the deficiencies of a clotting factor, since a 50% level of individual clotting proteins is sufficient to produce a normal PT or PTT. If the clotting time is not corrected or only partially corrected, an inhibitor is usually present. In the inpatient setting, the most common cause of this finding is heparin contamination of the sample. The presence of heparin in the sample can be ruled in or out using the thrombin time and reptilase time as noted earlier. If the mixing study does not correct or becomes more prolonged and the patient has clinical bleeding, an inhibitor (antibody directed against) of a specific clotting factor, most commonly factor VIII, or IX or XI, may be present. If the patient has no bleeding symptoms and both the PTT and the mixing study are prolonged, a lupus-like anticoagulant (see Chapter 474) is often present. These patients usually have a long PTT, do not bleed, and may have a clinical predisposition to excessive clotting.

CLOTTING FACTOR ASSAYS. Each of the clotting factors can be measured in the clinical laboratory using individual factor-deficient plasmas. For most clotting factors, their activity is measured against a pooled normal plasma or standard where 100% activity is expressed as 100 U/dL. In general, severe deficiency of factor VIII or factor IX is less than 1 U/dL of normal plasma (< 1% of normal), moderate deficiency between 1–5 U/dL of normal, and mild deficiencies greater than 5 U/dL but below the normal range. For most clotting factors the normal range is between 50–150 U/dL (50–150%).

In patients with hemophilia A or hemophilia B, inhibitors of factor VIII or factor IX may develop after exposure to replacement therapy. To quantitate the amount of inhibitor present, the standardized clinical assay of these clotting inhibitors is termed the *Bethesda assay*. One Bethesda unit is defined as the amount that will inhibit 50% of the clotting factor in normal plasma.

PLATELET AGGREGATION. When a qualitative platelet function defect is suspected, platelet aggregation testing is usually ordered. Platelet-rich plasma from the patient is activated with one of a series of agonists (ADP, epinephrine, collagen, thrombin or thrombin-receptor peptide, and ristocetin). Repeat testing or testing of other symptomatic family members can help determine the hereditary nature of the defect. Many medications, especially aspirin, other nonsteroidal anti-inflammatory drugs, and valproic acid alter platelet function testing. Some platelet aggregometers measure specific ADP release from the plates, as reflected in generating luminescence (lumiaggregometer) and are more sensitive in detecting abnormalities of the platelet release reaction from storage granules.

TESTING FOR THROMBOTIC PREDISPOSITION. Hereditary predisposition to thrombosis is associated with a reduction of anticoagulant function (protein C, protein S, AT-III); presence of a factor V molecule that is resistant to inactivation by protein C (factor V Leiden); elevated procoagulants (a mutation of the prothrombin gene); or deficiency of fibrinolysis (plasminogen deficiency). If warranted by the clinical severity and history of thrombosis, specific tests of the natural anticoagulants are ordered. Whereas both immunologic and functional tests are usually available, the functional assay of protein C, protein S, and antithrombin III is more clinically useful.

Factor V Leiden is a common mutation in factor V that is associated with significant risk of thrombosis. A point mutation in the factor V molecule prevents the inactivation of activated factor V by protein C and, thereby, the persistence of activated factor V. This defect has also been termed *APC resistance* and is easily diagnosed by DNA testing.

The *prothrombin gene mutation (G20210A)* is a mutation in the noncoding portion of the prothrombin gene with a G at position 20210 being replaced by an A. This mutation increases the amount of prothrombin mRNA, is associated with elevated levels of prothrombin, and causes a thrombotic predisposition. This abnormality is easily identified using molecular (DNA) diagnostic testing.

ELEVATED HOMOCYSTEINE. Homocysteine levels may be increased as a result of genetic mutations causing homocystinuria. Such patients have a predisposition to both arterial and venous thrombosis as well as an increase in arteriosclerosis.

TESTS OF THE FIBRINOLYTIC SYSTEM. The euglobulin clot lysis time (ELT) is used to assess a reduction of fibrinolysis. More specific tests are available in most laboratories to determine the levels of plasminogen, plasminogen activator, and inhibitors of fibrinolysis. An increase in fibrinolysis may be associated with hemorrhagic symptoms, and a delay in fibrinolysis is associated with thrombosis.

Developmental Hemostasis. The normal newborn infant has a reduced level of most procoagulants and anticoagulants. Table 467–2 lists the levels of hemostatic proteins in the newborn and older children. In general, there is a more marked abnormality in the preterm infant. While major differences exist in the normal ranges for newborn and preterm infants, these ranges vary greatly between laboratories. During gestation there is progressive maturation and increase of the clotting factors synthesized by the liver. The extremely premature infant will have a prolonged PTT and PT as well as a marked reduction in anticoagulant proteins (proteins C, S, and AT III). Note that fibrinogen, factor V, factor VIII, VWF, and platelets are near-normal throughout the later stages of gestation (see Chapter 92.4). Because protein C and protein S are physiologically reduced, the normal factor V and factor VIII are not balanced with their regulatory proteins. In contrast, the physiologic deficiency of vitamin K–dependent procoagulant proteins (factors II, VII, IX, and X) is partially balanced by the physiologic reduction of AT III. The net effect is that newborns (especially premature infants) are at increased risk for bleeding and clotting complications or both.

Andrew M: The relevance of developmental hemostasis to hemorrhagic disorders of newborns. *Semin Perinatol* 1997;21:70–85.

Andrew M, Booker L: Hemostatic disorders in newborns. In Polin RA, Fox WW (editors): *Fetal and Neonatal Physiology*, 2nd ed. Philadelphia, WB Saunders, 1998, p 1368.

Andrew M, Montgomery RR: Acquired disorders of hemostasis. In Nathan DG, Orkin SH (editors): *Hematology of Infancy and Childhood*, 5th ed. Philadelphia, WB Saunders, 1998, pp 1677–1717.

Esmon CT: Blood coagulation. In Nathan DG, Orkin SH (editors): *Nathan and Oski's Hematology of Infancy and Childhood*, 5th ed. Philadelphia, WB Saunders, 1998.

Handin RI: Blood platelets and the vessel wall. In Nathan DG, Orkin SH (editors): *Hematology of Infancy and Childhood*, 5th ed. Philadelphia, WB Saunders, 1998, pp 1511–29.

Hathaway WE, Goodnight SH Jr: *Disorders of Hemostasis and Thrombosis: A Clinical Guide*. New York, McGraw-Hill, 1993.

Lusher JM: Approach to the bleeding patient. In Nathan DG, Orkin SH (editors): *Hematology of Infancy and Childhood*, 5th ed. Philadelphia, WB Saunders, 1998, pp 1574–84.

Montgomery RR, Scott JP: Hemostasis: Diseases of the fluid phase. In Nathan DG, Orkin SH (editors): *Hematology of Infancy and Childhood*, 4th ed. Philadelphia, WB Saunders, 1993, pp 1605–50.

Scott JP: Bleeding and thrombosis. In Kliegman R, Super, Lye P (editors): *Practical Strategies in Pediatric Diagnosis and Therapy*, 2nd ed. Philadelphia, WB Saunders, 2002, pp 240–47.

Stuart MF, Graeber JE: Normal hemostasis in the fetus and newborn: Vessels and platelets. In Polin RA, Fox WW (editors): *Fetal and Neonatal Physiology*, 2nd ed. Philadelphia, WB Saunders, 1998, p 1834.

Hereditary Clotting Factor Deficiencies (Bleeding Disorders)

Hemophilia A (factor VIII deficiency) and hemophilia B (factor IX deficiency) are the most common and serious congenital coagulation factor deficiencies. The clinical findings in hemophilia A and B are virtually identical. Hemophilia C refers to the bleeding disorder associated with reduced levels of factor XI and is discussed separately in Chapter 468.2. The contact factors (factor XII, high molecular weight kininogen, and prekallikrein), which are associated with significant prolongation of the activated partial thromboplastin time (APTT) but are not associated with hemorrhage, are discussed in Chapter 468.3. Other coagulation factor deficiencies that are less common are briefly discussed in subsequent subchapters.

468.1 Factor VIII or Factor IX Deficiency (Hemophilia A or B)

Factor VIII and factor IX deficiencies are the most common severe inherited bleeding disorders. Hemophilia has been recognized as a clinical entity since Biblical times; Talmudic writings permitted the avoidance of circumcision when there was a repeated history of death from circumcisional bleeding in male siblings. Whole blood or plasma was used during the mid-20th century for treatment of hemophilia. The "concentrate" era of treatment began in 1964 with the discovery that cryoprecipitate, a fraction of plasma that contained factor VIII, could be used to treat hemophilia A. Shortly thereafter, concentrates for both factor VIII and factor IX were commercially developed. In 1985 the genes for both factor VIII and factor IX were cloned. Subsequently, recombinant factor VIII and factor IX concentrates were developed to treat patients with hemophilia and thereby avoid the infectious risk of plasma-derived transfusion-transmitted diseases.

Pathophysiology. Factor VIII and factor IX participate in a complex required for the activation of factor X. Together with phospholipid and calcium, they form the "tenase," or factor X–activating, complex. Figure 467–1 illustrates the clotting process as it occurs in the test tube, with factor X being activated by either the complex of factor VIII and factor IX or the complex of tissue factor and factor VII. In vivo factor VII and tissue factor can also activate factor IX. This may be one reason that deficiencies of factor VIII and factor IX are the severest bleeding disorders. In the laboratory, however, the prothrombin time (PT) measures the activation of factor X by factor VII and is therefore normal in patients with factor VIII or factor IX deficiency.

After injury, the initial hemostatic event is the formation of the platelet plug together with the generation of the fibrin clot that prevents further hemorrhage. In hemophilia A or hemophilia B, clot formation is delayed and is not robust. Thus, patients with hemophilia do not bleed more rapidly. There is, instead, a slowing of the rate of clot formation. When untreated bleeding occurs in a closed space such as a joint, cessation of bleeding may be the result of tamponade. With open wounds, in which tamponade cannot occur, profuse bleeding may result in significant blood loss. The clot that is formed may be friable, and rebleeding occurs during the physiologic lysis of clots or with minimal new trauma.

Clinical Manifestations. Neither factor VIII nor factor IX crosses the placenta; thus, bleeding symptoms may be present from birth or occur in the fetus. Occasionally, neonates with hemo-philia may sustain intracranial hemorrhage. Surprisingly, only about 30% of affected male infants with hemophilia bleed with circumcision. Thus, if the family history does not alert the physician to be suspicious for its presence, hemophilia may go undiagnosed in the newborn. It is only when a child begins to crawl and walk that mobility causes the initiation of easy bruising, intramuscular hematomas, and hemarthroses. Bleeding from minor traumatic lacerations of the mouth may persist for hours or days and may cause the parents to seek medical evaluation. Even in patients with severe hemophilia, only 90% have evidence of increased bleeding by 1 yr of age. Although bleeding may occur in any area of the body, the hallmark of hemophilia is the hemarthrosis. Bleeding into joints may be induced by minor trauma; nonetheless, many hemarthroses are spontaneous. The earliest joint hemorrhages appear most commonly in the ankle, because of the lack of stability of this joint as the toddler assumes an upright posture. In the older child and adolescent, hemarthroses of the knees and elbows are the most debilitating. Whereas the child's early joint hemorrhages are recognized only after major swelling and fluid accumulation in the joint space, older children are frequently able to recognize bleeding earlier than the physician. Patients with severe hemophilia often develop a "target" joint where repetitive episodes of bleeding occur. Recurrent bleeding may then become spontaneous because of the underlying pathologic changes to the joint.

Although most muscular hemorrhages are clinically evident owing to localized pain or swelling, bleeding into the iliopsoas muscle requires specific mention. Patients may lose large volumes of blood into the iliopsoas muscle and verge on hypovolemic shock with only a vague area of referred pain in the groin. The diagnosis is made clinically by the inability to extend the hip but demands confirmation with ultrasonography or CT scan together with aggressive replacement therapy.

Life-threatening bleeding in the hemophilic patient is caused by bleeding into vital structures (central nervous system, upper airway) or by exsanguination (external, gastrointestinal, or iliopsoas hemorrhage). Prompt treatment with clotting factor concentrate for these life-threatening hemorrhages is imperative. If head trauma is of sufficient concern so as to suggest radiologic evaluation, factor replacement should precede radiologic evaluation. Life-threatening hemorrhages require replacement therapy to achieve a level equal to that of normal plasma (100 U/dL or 100%).

Patients with mild hemophilia who have factor VIII or IX levels greater than 5 U/dL usually do not have spontaneous hemorrhages. These individuals may experience prolonged bleeding after dental work, surgery, or injuries from moderate trauma.

Laboratory Findings. The laboratory screening test that is affected by a reduced level of factor VIII or factor IX is the APTT. In severe hemophilia, this APTT is usually two to three times the upper limits of normal. The other screening tests of the hemostatic mechanism (platelet count, bleeding time, prothrombin time, and thrombin time) are normal. Unless the patient has an inhibitor to factor VIII, the mixing of normal plasma with patient plasma results in correction of the PTT. The specific assay for factor VIII and factor IX will confirm the diagnosis of hemophilia. If correction does not occur on mixing, an inhibitor may be present. In 14–25% of patients who receive infusions of factor VIII or factor IX, a factor-specific antibody may develop. These antibodies are directed against the active clotting site and are termed *inhibitors*. In such patients the quantitative Bethesda assay for inhibitor should be performed.

Genetics and Classification. Hemophilia occurs in approximately 1:5,000 males, with 85% having factor VIII deficiency and 10–15% having factor IX deficiency. Hemophilia shows no apparent racial predilection, appearing in all ethnic groups. The severity of hemophilia is classified on the basis of the patient's baseline level of factor VIII or factor IX because factor levels usually correlate with the severity of the bleeding symptoms. By convention, 1 unit (U) of each factor is defined as the amount found in 1 mL of normal plasma, thus 100 mL of normal plasma has 100 U/dL (100% activity) of each factor. Severe hemophilia is characterized by having less than 1.0 U/dL (<1%) of the specific clotting factor, and bleeding is often spontaneous. Patients with moderate hemophilia have 1–5 U/dL and require mild trauma to induce bleeding. Individuals with mild hemophilia have levels greater than 5 U/dL, may go many years before the condition is diagnosed, and frequently require significant trauma to cause bleeding. The hemostatic level for factor VIII is more than 30–40 U/dL, and for factor IX it is more than 25–30 U/dL.

The genes for both factor VIII and factor IX are carried near the terminus of the long arm of the X chromosome and are therefore X-linked traits. The majority of patients have reduction in the amount of clotting factor protein; however, 5–10% of hemophilia A and 40–50% of hemophilia B patients make a dysfunctional protein. One specific genetic mutation in hemophilia A warrants further discussion. Forty-five to 50% of patients with severe hemophilia A have the same mutation, in which there is an internal inversion within the factor VIII gene that results in no protein being produced. This mutation can be detected in the blood of patients or carriers and in the amniotic fluid by molecular techniques. Because of the multiple genetic causes of either factor VIII or factor IX deficiency, however, most patients are classified based on the amount of factor VIII or factor IX clotting activity. In the newborn, factor VIII levels may be artificially elevated because of the acute-phase response elicited by the birth process. This may cause a mildly affected patient to have normal or near-normal levels of factor VIII. Patients with severe hemophilia will not have detectable levels. In contrast, factor IX levels are physiologically low in the newborn. If severe hemophilia is present in the family, an undetectable level of factor IX is diagnostic of severe hemophilia B. Sometimes with mild factor IX deficiency, the presence of hemophilia can be confirmed only after several weeks of life.

Some female carriers of hemophilia A or hemophilia B will have sufficient reduction of their factor VIII or factor IX through lionization of the X chromosome to produce mild bleeding disorders in carriers. Factor VIII or factor IX levels should be determined in all known carriers to assess the need for treatment in the event of surgery or clinical bleeding.

Because factor VIII is carried in plasma by von Willebrand factor (VWF), the ratio of factor VIII to VWF is sometimes used to diagnose carriers of hemophilia. When possible, specific genetic mutations should be identified in the propositus and used to test other family members at risk for either having hemophilia or being carriers.

Treatment. The prevention of trauma is important to the care of the child with hemophilia, but hemorrhages may occur in the absence of trauma. Early psychosocial intervention helps the family achieve a balance between overprotection and permissiveness. Aspirin and other nonsteroidal anti-inflammatory drugs that affect platelet function should be avoided by patients with hemophilia. Although recombinant products may avoid exposure to transfusion-transmitted diseases, the infant should be immunized against hepatitis B virus in the neonatal period in case plasma-derived products are used with future hemorrhages. Patients should be periodically screened for hepatitis and abnormalities in liver function. Calculation of the dose of recombinant factor VIII (FVIII) or recombinant factor IX (FIX) is as follows:

$$\text{Dose of FVIII (units, U)} = \begin{pmatrix} \text{U/dL (\%) desired} \\ \text{rise in plasma FVIII} \end{pmatrix} \times \text{Body Weight (kg)} \times 0.5^*$$

---

* B-domain deleted recombinant factor VIII (Refacto) may require special assays to determine plasma level—chromogenic assay or referencing versus a Refacto Standard.

$$\text{Dose of FIX (units, U)} = \begin{pmatrix} \text{U/dL (\%) desired} \\ \text{rise in plasma FIX} \end{pmatrix} \times \text{Body Weight (kg)} \times 1.4^{\dagger}$$

REPLACEMENT THERAPY. When bleeding occurs, levels of factor VIII or IX must be raised to hemostatic levels (35–40 U/dL) or for life-threatening or major hemorrhages to 100 U/dL (100%). Table 468–1 summarizes the treatment of some common types of hemorrhage in a patient with hemophilia.

With the availability of recombinant replacement products, prophylaxis has been recommended for many young children with severe hemophilia to prevent spontaneous bleeding and early joint deformities. The results of prophylaxis have been impressive in the prevention of chronic joint disease. If patients develop target joints, "secondary" prophylaxis is often initiated.

With mild factor VIII hemophilia, the patient's endogenously produced factor VIII can be released by the administration of desmopressin acetate. In patients with moderate or severe factor VIII deficiency, the stored levels of factor VIII in the body are inadequate, and desmopressin treatment is ineffective. On the other hand, exposing the patient with mild hemophilia to transfusion-transmitted diseases or the cost of recombinant products warrants the use of desmopressin if it is effective. Stimate, a concentrated intranasal form of desmopressin acetate, can also be used to treat patients with mild hemophilia A. The Stimate dose is 150 µg (one puff) for children weighing less than 50 kg and 300 µg (two puffs) for children and young adults weighing more than 50 kg. Most centers administer a trial of desmopressin to determine the level of factor VIII achieved after its infusion. Desmopressin is not effective in the treatment of factor IX–deficient hemophilia.

Prophylaxis. Many patients are now placed on lifelong prophylaxis programs to prevent spontaneous joint bleeding. Usually, such programs are initiated with the first joint hemorrhage. Young children often require the insertion of a central catheter to ensure venous access. Such programs, although expensive, are highly effective at preventing or greatly modulating the degree of joint pathology. Treatment is usually provided every 2–3 days to maintain a measurable plasma level of clotting factor (1–2 U/dL) when assayed just before the next infusion (trough level). Because gene therapy may be available within the lifetime of pediatric patients, keeping joints normal through prophylaxis is a logical priority. If moderate arthropathy develops, prevention of future bleeding will require higher plasma levels of clotting factors and the individual will be less amenable to gene therapy. In the older child who is not placed on primary prophylaxis, secondary prophylaxis is sometimes initiated if a target joint develops.

Chronic Complications. The long-term complications of hemophilia A and B include chronic joint destruction, the risk of transfusion-transmitted infectious diseases, and the development of an inhibitor to either factor VIII or factor IX. Although the aggressive or prophylactic approach to treatment has reduced the problems of chronic arthropathy, these problems have not been eliminated. Furthermore, whereas transfusion-transmitted diseases are minimized or negated by using highly purified or recombinant products, many older patients have been exposed to plasma-derived products. As a result, transfusion-transmitted diseases, including HIV infection and hepatitis C or B, may be the major long-term cause of morbidity and mortality in older adolescents and adults with hemophilia. The incidence of inhibitors appears similar in patients using either recombinant or plasma-derived products for factor VIII replacement. Highly purified factor IX or recombinant factor IX seems to increase the incidence of factor IX inhibitors, and some may induce anaphy-

---

† Correction factor is 1.0 for plasma-derived factor IX.

TABLE 468–1. Treatment of Hemophilia

Type of Hemorrhage	Hemophilia A	Hemophilia B
Hemarthrosis*	20–40 U/kg factor VIII concentrate†; 15 U/kg if treated early. Repeat the dose daily until joint function is normal or back to baseline. Consider additional treatment every other day for 7–10 days. Consider prophylaxis.	40 U/kg factor IX concentrate‖; 30 U/kg if treated early. Repeat the dose daily until joint function is normal or back to baseline. Consider additional treatment every other day for 7–10 days. Consider prophylaxis.
Muscle or significant subcutaneous hematoma	20 U/kg factor VIII concentrate; may need every-other-day treatment until resolved	40 U/kg factor IX concentrate‖; may need treatment every 2–3 days until resolved
Mouth, deciduous tooth, or tooth extraction	20 U/kg factor VIII concentrate; antifibrinolytic therapy; remove loose deciduous tooth	40 U/kg factor IX concentrate‖; antifibrinolytic therapy‡; remove loose deciduous tooth
Epistaxis	Apply pressure for 15–20 min; pack with petrolatum gauze; antifibrinolytic therapy; 20 U/kg factor VIII concentrate if above fails	Apply pressure for 15–20 min; pack with petrolatum gauze; antifibrinolytic therapy; 30 U/kg factor IX concentrate‖ if above fails
Major surgery, life-threatening hemorrhage (e.g., central nervous system, gastrointestinal, airway)	50–75 U/kg factor VIII concentrate, then initiate continuous infusion of 2–4 U/kg/hr to maintain factor VIII >100 U/dL for 24 hr, then give 2–3 U/kg/hr continuously for 5–7 days to maintain the level > 50 U/dL and an additional 5–7 days at a level > 30 U/dL.	120 U/kg factor IX concentrate‖, then 50–60 U/kg every 12–24 hr to maintain factor IX > 40 U/dL for 5–7 days, and then > 30 U/dL for 5 days
Iliopsoas hemorrhage	50 U/kg factor VIII concentrate, then 25 U/kg every 12 hr until asymptomatic, then 20 U/kg every other day for total 10–14 days§	120 U/kg factor IX concentrate‖; then 50–60 U/kg every 12–24 hr to maintain factor IX > 40 U/dL until asymptomatic, then 40–50 U every other day for total 10–14 days§¶
Hematuria	Bed rest; 1½ × maintenance fluids; if not controlled in 1–2 days, 20 U/kg factor VIII concentrate; if not controlled, give prednisone (unless HIV-infected)	Bed rest: 1½ × maintenance fluids; if not controlled in 1–2 days, 40 units/kg factor IX concentrate‖; if not controlled, give prednisone (unless HIV-infected)
Prophylaxis	20 U/kg factor VIII concentrate every other day to achieve trough level ≥ 1%.	30 U/kg factor IX concentrate‖ every 2–3 days to achieve trough level ≥ 1%

*For hip hemarthrosis, orthopedic evaluation for possible aspiration is advisable to prevent avascular necrosis of the femoral head.
†For mild or moderate hemophilia, desmopressin, 0.3 μg/kg, should be used instead of factor VIII concentrate, if patient is known to respond with a hemostatic level of factor VIII; if repeated doses are given, monitor factor VIII levels for tachyphylaxis.
‡Do not give antifibrinolytic therapy until 4–6 hr after a dose of prothrombin complex concentrate.
§Repeat radiologic assessment should be performed before discontinuation of therapy.
‖Stated doses apply for recombinant factor IX concentrate; for plasma-derived factor IX concentrate, use 70% of stated dose.
¶If repeated doses of factor IX concentrate are required, use highly purified, specific factor IX concentrate.

Adapted from Montgomery RR, Gill JC, Scott JP: Hemophilia and von Willebrand disease. In Nathan DG, Orkin SH (editors): Nathan and Oski's Hematology of Infancy and Childhood, 5th ed. Philadelphia, WB Saunders, 1998.

laxis. Factor IX immune tolerance induction has also resulted in nephrotic syndrome in some patients.

Historically, chronic arthropathy is the major long-term disability of hemophilia. The natural history of untreated hemophilia is one of cyclical recurrent hemorrhages into specific joints, including hemorrhages into the same or "target" joint. After joint hemorrhage, proteolytic enzymes are released by white blood cells into the joint space and heme iron induces macrophage proliferation—all of which contributes to inflammation in the synovium. The synovium thickens and develops frond-like projections into the joint that are susceptible to being pinched and may induce further hemorrhage. The cartilaginous surface becomes eroded and ultimately may even expose raw bone, leaving the joint susceptible to articular fusion. When the first hemorrhages occur in a child's joints, the joint has not been previously damaged. The synovium is therefore elastic and can accommodate a large amount of blood. Frequently, the swelling is much greater than the pain. In contrast, the older patient with advanced arthropathy may have such a scarred joint that there is little space for accommodating blood. In these patients the pain is much greater than the degree of swelling. Once a target joint is seen to be developing, the patient is usually placed on short- or long-term prophylaxis to prevent progression of the arthropathy and to reduce inflammation.

Whereas infection from transfusion-transmitted diseases has been dramatically reduced by using plasma-derived products that are heat treated, immuno-purified, and chemically treated, most hemophilia centers recommend the use of recombinant products, because they are free from known human transmitted viruses. Although some of these products have been produced or even reformulated in human albumin, the risk of viral infection is theoretical. Recombinant products are being developed that contain no human or other animal protein. Although HIV infection devastated the adult hemophilic population, alteration in manufacturing practices in the early to mid 1980s has eliminated this risk. However, many adults remain with HIV infection. The experience with this "epidemic" requires that great vigilance be exercised to prevent similar unexpected infections in the future. Chronic hepatitis C and even hepatitis B remain as problems for many older patients with hemophilia, but the use of recombinant products has virtually eliminated this risk in younger patients. Parvovirus and hepatitis A are nonenveloped viruses that may escape solvent detergent treatment and heat treatment. Thus, plasma-derived products may continue to transmit these infectious agents. The potential for Creutzfeldt-Jakob disease to be transmitted through blood remains controversial but unsubstantiated.

Infusion of the deficient clotting factor may initiate an immune response in patients with either factor VIII or factor IX deficiency. Inhibitors are antibodies directed against factor VIII or factor IX that block the clotting activity. Failure of a bleeding episode to respond to appropriate replacement therapy is the usual first sign of an inhibitor. Less often they are identified during routine follow-up testing. Inhibitors develop in approximately 25% of patients with hemophilia A; the percentage is somewhat lower in patients with hemophilia B, many of whom make an inactive dysfunctional protein that renders them less susceptible to an immune response. Many patients who develop an inhibitor lose this inhibitor with continued regular infusions. Others develop a higher titer with subsequent infusions and may need to go through desensitization programs, in which high doses of factor VIII or factor IX are infused in an attempt to saturate the antibody and to permit the body to develop tolerance. If desensitization fails, bleeding episodes are treated with either activated prothrombin complex concentrates or recombinant factor VIIa. The use of these products bypasses the inhibitor in many instances but may increase the risk for thrombosis. Patients with inhibitors require referral to a hospital that cares for many such patients and has a comprehensive hemophilia program.

Comprehensive Care. Hemophilia patients today are best managed through comprehensive hemophilia care centers. Such centers are dedicated to patient and family education as well as prevention and/or treatment of the complications of hemophilia including chronic joint disease and inhibitor development as well as infectious complications such as hepatitis C and HIV. Such centers involve a team of physicians, nurses, orthopedists, physical therapists, and psychosocial workers among others.

468.2 Factor XI Deficiency (Hemophilia C)

Factor XI deficiency is an autosomal deficiency associated with mild to moderate bleeding symptoms. It is frequently encountered in Ashkenazi Jews but has been found in many other ethnic groups. In Israel, 1–3/1,000 are homozygous for this deficiency. Sephardic Jews are rarely affected.

Although the condition is referred to as hemophilia C, the bleeding tendency is not as severe as in factor VIII or factor IX deficiency. The bleeding associated with factor XI deficiency is not correlated with the amount of factor XI. Some patients with severe deficiency may have minimal or no symptoms at the time of major surgery. Unless the patient previously had surgery without bleeding, replacement therapy should be considered and given preoperatively depending on the nature of the surgical procedure. There is no licensed concentrate of factor XI available in the United States; therefore, the physician must use fresh frozen plasma (FFP) or enroll the patient in a clinical trial of factor XI concentrate.

Minor surgeries can be controlled with local pressure; dental extractions can be monitored closely and the patient treated only if hemorrhage occurs. In a patient with homozygous deficiency of factor XI, the PTT is often longer than it is in patients with either severe factor VIII or factor IX deficiency. The paradox of fewer clinical symptoms with a longer PTT is surprising, but this is the result of factor VIIa being able to activate factor IX in vivo. The deficiency of factor XI can be confirmed by specific factor XI assays. Plasma infusions of 1 U/kg usually increase the plasma concentration by 2 U/dL. Thus, the infusion of 10–15 mL of plasma/kg will result in a plasma level of 20–30 U/dL (20–30%), a level usually sufficient to control moderate hemorrhage. Frequent infusions of plasma would be necessary to achieve higher levels of factor XI. Because the factor XI half-life is usually 48 hr or greater, maintaining adequate levels of factor XI is not usually difficult.

Chronic joint bleeding is rarely a problem, and, for most patients, factor XI deficiency is a concern only at the time of major surgery unless there is a second underlying hemostatic defect (e.g., von Willebrand disease).

468.3 Deficiencies of the Contact Factors (Nonbleeding Disorders)

Deficiencies of factor VIII, factor IX, and factor XI all cause isolated prolongation of the PTT. Deficiencies of the contact factors also prolong the PTT but are not causes of clinical bleeding. These factors include factor XII, prekallikrein, and high molecular weight kininogen. Because these contact factors function at the step of initiation of the intrinsic clotting system, the PTT is markedly prolonged when these factors are absent. Thus, one encounters the paradoxical situation in which there is an extremely prolonged PTT but no evidence of clinical bleeding. It is important that these individuals be well informed about the meaning of their clotting factor deficiency, since they do not need treatment even if major surgery is undertaken. On rare occasions, factor XII deficiency is associated with von Willebrand disease and has been termed von Willebrand San Diego. Thus, if a patient with low factor XII level is identified who has bleeding symptoms, it is advisable to carry out screening for von Willebrand disease.

468.4 Factor VII Deficiency

Factor VII deficiency is a rare bleeding disorder that is usually detected only in the homozygous state. Individuals with this deficiency may have spontaneous intracranial hemorrhage and frequent mucocutaneous bleeding. Such patients will have a markedly prolonged PT but a normal PTT. Factor VII assays demonstrate a marked reduction of factor VII. Because the plasma half-life of factor VII is 2–4 hr, therapy with FFP is difficult and often complicated by fluid overload. A commercial concentrate of recombinant factor VIIa is now available for treating factor VIII or factor IX inhibitor patients, but this concentrate may be useful in treating patients with factor VII deficiency as well. Clinical trials are currently evaluating this approach.

Deficiencies in the Factors of the Common Pathway (X, V, II, I) Causing Prolongation of Both the PT and the PTT

468.5 Factor X Deficiency

This is a rare autosomal disorder that results in mucocutaneous and post-traumatic bleeding. This deficiency is the result of either a quantitative deficiency or a dysfunctional molecule. A reduced factor X level is associated with a prolongation of both the PT and the PTT. In patients with hereditary deficiency of factor X, factor X levels can be increased using either FFP or prothrombin complex concentrate. The half-life of factor X is approximately 30 hr, and its volume of distribution is similar to factor IX. Thus, 1 U/kg will increase the plasma level of factor X 1 U/dL (1%).

Although rarely a problem in pediatric patients, systemic amyloidosis may be associated with factor X deficiency owing to the adsorption of factor X on the amyloid protein. In the setting of amyloidosis, transfusion therapy is often not successful because of the rapid clearance of factor X.

468.6 Prothrombin (Factor II) Deficiency

This deficiency is caused either by a markedly reduced prothrombin level (hypoprothrombinemia) or by a functionally abnormal prothrombin (dysprothrombinemia). Laboratory testing in homozygous patients demonstrates a prolonged PT and PTT. Factor II or prothrombin assays demonstrate the markedly reduced prothrombin level. Treatment can be achieved using either prothrombin complex concentrates or FFP. In prothrombin deficiency, FFP is useful, because the half-life of prothrombin is 3.5 days. Administration of 1 U/kg of prothrombin will increase the plasma concentration by 1 U/dL (1%).

468.7 Factor V Deficiency

The deficiency of factor V, also known as labile factor, is an autosomal recessive, mild to moderate bleeding disorder that has also been termed *parahemophilia*. Hemarthroses occur rarely; mucocutaneous bleeding and hematomas are the most common symptoms. Severe menorrhagia is a frequent symptom in women. Laboratory evaluation demonstrates a prolonged PTT and PT. Specific assays for factor V demonstrate a reduction in factor V levels. FFP is the only currently available therapeutic product that contains factor V. Factor V is lost rapidly from FFP. It is therefore important to use FFP that is less than 2 mo old.

Infusing 10 mL/kg of FFP every 12 hr can treat patients with severe factor V deficiency. Rarely, one encounters the patient with a negative family history of bleeding who has an acquired antibody to factor V. Often, these patients do not bleed because the factor V in platelets prevents excessive bleeding.

468.8 Combined Deficiency of Factors V and VIII

Combined deficiency of factor V and factor VIII has been demonstrated to be secondary to the absence of an intracellular transport protein, ERGIC-53, that is responsible for transporting factor V and factor VIII from the endoplasmic reticulum to the Golgi compartments. ERGIC-53 is encoded on chromosome 18. The deficiency of factor VIII and factor V is not related to defective genes for those proteins but is secondary to a deficiency of a transport protein. This explains the paradoxical deficiency of two factors, one encoded on chromosome 1 and the other on the X chromosome.

468.9 Fibrinogen Deficiency

Congenital afibrinogenemia is a rare autosomal recessive disorder in which there is an absence of fibrinogen. These patients do not bleed as frequently as hemophilia patients and rarely have hemarthroses. Affected patients may present in the neonatal period with gastrointestinal hemorrhage or hematomas after vaginal delivery. In addition to marked prolongation of the PTT and PT, the thrombin time is prolonged. In the absence of a consumptive coagulopathy, an unmeasurable fibrinogen level is diagnostic. In addition to the quantitative deficiency of fibrinogen, a number of dysfunctional fibrinogens have been reported (dysfibrinogenemia). Currently, no fibrinogen concentrates are commercially available. Because the plasma half-life of fibrinogen is between 2 and 4 days, treatment with either FFP or cryoprecipitate is effective. The hemostatic level of fibrinogen is above 60 mg/dL. Each bag of cryoprecipitate contains 100–150 mg of fibrinogen. Some clinical assays for fibrinogen are inhibited by high doses of heparin. Thus, a markedly prolonged thrombin time when associated with a low fibrinogen level should be evaluated with a reptilase time. A prolonged reptilase time confirms that functional levels of fibrinogen are low and that heparin is not present.

468.10 Factor XIII Deficiency (Fibrin-Stabilizing Factor or Transglutaminase Deficiency)

Because factor XIII is responsible for the cross linking of fibrin or the stabilization of fibrin clot, symptoms of delayed hemorrhage are secondary to instability of the clot. Typically, patients will have trauma one day and then develop a bruise or hematoma on the following day. Clinical symptoms include mild bruising, delayed separation of the umbilical stump beyond 4 wk, poor wound healing, and, in women, recurrent spontaneous abortions. The usual screening tests for hemostasis are normal in patients with factor XIII deficiency. Screening tests for factor XIII deficiency are based on the observation that there is an increased solubility of the clot because of the failure of cross linking. The normal clot remains insoluble in the presence of 5 M urea, whereas the clot formed from a patient with factor XIII deficiency dissolves. More specific assays for factor XIII are immunologic. Because the half-life of factor XIII is 5–7 days and the hemostatic level is 2–3 U/dL, infusion of FFP or cryoprecipitate will correct the deficiency in these patients. Plasma contains 1 U/dL, and cryoprecipitate contains 75 U/bag. In patients with significant bleeding symptoms, prophylaxis can be achieved with infusion of cryoprecipitate every 3–4 wk.

468.11 Antiplasmin or Plasminogen Activator Inhibitor (PAI) Deficiency

Deficiency of either of these two antifibrinolytic proteins results in increased plasmin generation and the premature lysis of fibrin clots. Patients have mucocutaneous bleeding but rarely have joint hemorrhages. Because the usual hemostatic tests are normal, further work-up of a patient with a positive bleeding history should include the euglobulin clot lysis time that measures fibrinolytic activity and is shortened in the presence of these deficiencies. Specific assays for α_2-antiplasmin and PAI are available. Treatment can be accomplished using FFP.

Andrew ME, Montgomery RR: Acquired disorders of hemostasis. In Nathan DG, Orkin SH (editors): *Nathan and Oski's Hematology of Infancy and Childhood*, 5th ed. Philadelphia, WB Saunders, 1998.

Bauer KA: Rare hereditary coagulation factor abnormalities. In Nathan DG, Orkin SH (editors): *Hematology of Infancy and Childhood*, 5th ed. Philadelphia, WB Saunders, 1998, pp 1660–75.

Funk M, Schmidt H, Escuriola-Ettingshausen C, et al: Radiological and orthopedic score in pediatric hemophilic patients with early and late prophylaxis. *Ann Hematol* 1998;77:171–4.

Hedner U: Recombinant factor VIIa (Novoseven) as a hemostatic agent. *Semin Hematol* 2001;38(4 Suppl 12):43–7.

Ljung RC: Prophylactic infusion regimens in the management of hemophilia. *Thromb Haemost* 1999;82:525–30.

Mannucci PM: Desmopressin (DDAVP) in the treatment of bleeding disorders: The first 20 years. *Blood* 1997;90:2515–21.

Mannucci PM, Tuddenham EG: The hemophilias—from royal genes to gene therapy. *N Engl J Med* 2001;344:1773–79.

Menitove JE, Gill JC, Montgomery RR: Preparation and clinical use of plasma and plasma fractions. In *Hematology*, 5th ed. New York, McGraw-Hill, 1994.

Montgomery RR, Gill JC, Scott JP: Hemophilia and von Willebrand disease. In Nathan DG, Orkin SH (editors): *Hematology of Infancy and Childhood*, 5th ed. Philadelphia, WB Saunders, 1998, pp 1631–59.

Chapter 469

von Willebrand Disease

von Willebrand disease (VWD) is the most common hereditary bleeding disorder, with some reports suggesting that it is present in 1–2% of the general population. VWD is inherited autosomally, but most centers report more women than men affected. Because menorrhagia is a major symptom, it may cause more women to seek diagnosis. VWD is classified on the basis of whether the protein is quantitatively reduced but not absent (type 1), qualitatively abnormal (type 2), or absent (type 3) (Fig. 469–1). Mutations in different loci that code for different functional domains of the VWF protein cause the different variants of VWD.

Pathophysiology. von Willebrand factor (VWF) is a large multimeric glycoprotein that is synthesized in megakaryocytes and endothelial cells and stored in α-granules and Weibel-Palade bodies, respectively. The highest molecular weight multimers of VWF are responsible for the normal interaction of VWF with the subendothelial matrix and platelets. During normal hemostasis, VWF adheres to the subendothelial matrix after vascular damage. When VWF binds to the subendothelial matrix, the conformation of VWF is changed so that it causes platelets to adhere to VWF through their glycoprotein IB (GPIb) receptor. These platelets are then activated, causing the recruitment of additional platelets and exposing phosphatidylserine, which is an important regulatory step for factor V– and factor VIII–dependent steps in the clotting cascade. VWF also serves as the carrier protein for plasma factor VIII. A severe deficiency of VWF may cause a secondary deficiency in factor VIII, even though the gene for factor VIII is normal. This is the cause of autosomal deficiency of factor VIII, now known to be a molecular abnormality of VWF and termed type 2N VWD.

Clinical Manifestations. Patients with VWD usually have symptoms of mucocutaneous hemorrhage, including excessive bruising, epistaxis, menorrhagia, and postoperative hemorrhage, particularly after mucosal surgery such as tonsillectomy or wisdom tooth extraction. Because a teenager's menstrual history is usually put in the context of other family members, excessive menstrual bleeding is not always recognized as being abnormal, because others in the family may be affected with the same disorder. If a menstruating female presents with iron deficiency, a detailed history of bruising and other bleeding should be elicited and further hemostatic evaluation undertaken. The American College of Obstetrics and Gynecology recommends VWD testing on all teenage females with menorrhagia before initiating hormonal therapy or oral contraceptives.

Because VWF is an acute-phase protein, stress will increase its level. Thus, patients may not bleed with procedures that incur major stress, such as appendectomy and childbirth, but may bleed excessively at the time of cosmetic or mucosal surgery. Bruising symptoms may diminish during pregnancy, because the VWF levels may double or triple during pregnancy. Rarely, patients with VWD may have gastrointestinal telangiectasia. This combination results in major bleeding and accounts for numerous hospital admissions for patients with severe disease. In patients with type 3 or homozygous VWD, bleeding symptoms are much more profound. These patients are usually diagnosed early in life and may have severe epistaxis or menorrhagia that results in major blood loss and possibly shock. Rarely, patients with severe type 3 VWD have joint hemorrhages or spontaneous central nervous system hemorrhages.

Laboratory Findings. Patients with VWD were said to have a long bleeding time and a long PTT. Nevertheless, these tests are frequently normal in patients with type 1 VWD. Therefore, normal screening tests do not preclude the diagnosis of VWD. If the history is suggestive of a bleeding disorder, VWD testing must be undertaken, including a quantitative assay for VWF antigen, VWF activity (ristocetin cofactor activity, or VWF:RCo), plasma factor VIII activity, determination of VWF structure (VWF multimers), and a platelet count. While the platelet count is usually normal in most patients, those with type 2B disease or platelet type (pseudo-VWD) may have lifelong thrombocytopenia. Figure 469–1 lists the variants of VWD and summarizes their laboratory findings.

Genetics. Chromosome 12 contains the gene for VWF. Each of the type 2 variants listed in Figure 469–1 has specific areas of the molecule affected. The phenotype can guide the genetic diagnosis of the specific mutation. Clinical genetic testing for VWD variants is only available in a few referral laboratories.

Treatment. Treatment of VWD is directed toward increasing the plasma level of VWF and factor VIII. Because the gene for factor VIII is normal in patients with VWD, elevating the plasma concentration of VWF will permit the normal recovery and survival of the endogenously produced factor VIII. The most common form of VWD is type 1. In these patients the synthetic drug desmopressin (DDAVP) induces the release of VWF from the endothelial cells. In some patients with type 2 variants, desmopressin may be similarly effective, but in other circumstances the released VWF is dysfunctional. Patients with VWD may fail to respond adequately to desmopressin because they release an abnormal VWF molecule (most type 2 variants), because they have type 3 disease in which there is no VWF to be released, or because they have accelerated clearance of released VWF. A small subset of children and adults, especially infants, fail to release VWF in response to DDAVP. In these circumstances replacement therapy must be used. Current replacement therapy uses plasma-derived VWF containing concentrates that also contain factor VIII. VWF distributes only to the intravascular space, because it is so large. During plasma fractionation, VWF multimers are altered to a variable extent. Therefore, 1 U/kg will

von Willebrand Disease Variants									
	Normal	**Type I**	**Type 3**	**Type 2A**	**Type 2B**	**Type 2N**	**Type 2M**	**PT-VWD**	**BSS**
VWF:Ag	N	↓	Absent	↓	↓	N or ↓	↓ or N	↓	N
VFW:RCo	N	↓	Absent	↓↓↓	↓	N or ↓	↓↓↓	↓	N
FVIII	N	↓ or N	1–3%	N or ↓	No or ↓	↓↓	N	N	N
RIPA	N	Often normal	Absent	↓	Often normal	N	↓	N	Absent
LD-RIPA	Absent	Absent	Absent	Absent	↑↑↑	Absent	Absent	↑↑↑	Absent
PFA	N	↑	↑↑↑	↑	↑	N	↑	↑	↑↑↑
BT	N	N or ↑	↑↑↑	↑	↑	N	↑	↑	↑↑↑
Platelet count	N	N	N	N	↓	N	N	↓	↓
Usual Tx		DDAVP VWF conc	VWF conc	VWF conc (DDAVP)	VWF conc	VWF conc (DDAVP)	VWF conc	Platelets	Platelets
Response to DDAVP		Good	None	Poor	Decreases platelets	Poor	Poor	Decreases platelets	None or modest
Response to VWF conc		Good	Good	Good	Good	Good	Good	Decreases platelets	No response
Frequency in general population		1–2%	Very rare 1:250,000	Rare	Rare	Rare	Rare	Rare	Rare
VWF multimers	N	N but ↓	Absent / Absent	Abnormal	Abnormal	N but ↓	N but ↓	Abnormal	Normal

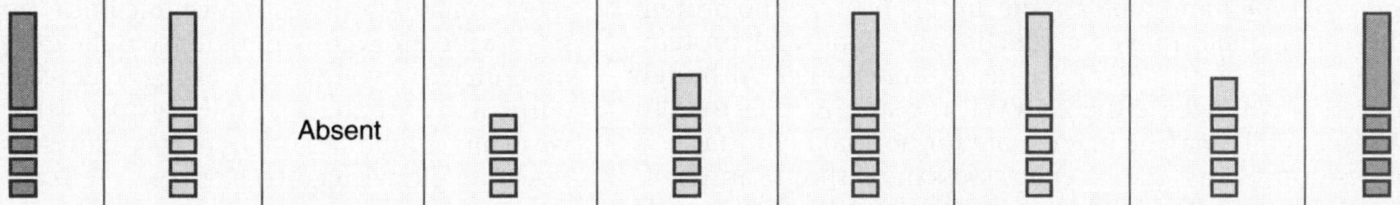

FIGURE 469–1. Common variants of VWD and other related disorders. Laboratory testing is listed on the left and the results most commonly identified in patients with these conditions are shown. N is normal, ↑ is degree of increase, and ↓ is degree of decrease. A graph representing VWF multimers is shown at the bottom of each column. A lighter shade of color illustrates a reduction in staining intensity, and figure length represents the relative size of the multimers. PT-VWD = platelet-type pseudo VWD; BSS = Bernard Soulier syndrome; FVIII = factor VIII; VWF:Ag = von Willebrand antigen; VWF:RCo = ristocetin cofactor activity; BT = bleeding time; PFA = platelet function analyzer; VWF conc = VWF concentrate; Tx = treatment.

increase the plasma level by 1.5 U/dL (1.5%). The plasma half-life of both factor VIII and VWF is 12 hr, but the alteration of VWF during fractionation results in half-lives of 8–10 hours when infusing concentrates. Purified VWF concentrates or recombinant VWF concentrates (containing no factor VIII) may become available in the near future. These will be useful in presurgical management or in prophylaxis. When used for acute bleeding, however, these VWF concentrates may need to be supplemented by an infusion of recombinant factor VIII for the first infusion. Both VWF and factor VIII are required for normal hemostasis. If only VWF is replaced, the endogenous correction of the factor VIII level takes 12–24 hr. Dental extractions and sometimes nose-

bleeds can be managed with both desmopressin and an antifibri-nolytic agent such as ε-aminocaproic acid (Amicar).

VWD VARIANTS

Type 1 VWD is the most common form and accounts for 85% of cases. Bleeding symptoms include epistaxis, bruising, and menorrhagia. If bleeding is excessive, desmopressin administration at a dose of 0.3 μg/kg given intravenously will increase the level of VWF and factor VIII by three- to fivefold. Intranasal desmo-pressin (Stimate) is particularly helpful for the outpatient treat-ment of bleeding episodes. The dose of Stimate is 150 μg (one puff) for children weighing less than 50 kg and 300 µg (two puffs) for those weighing more than 50 kg.

Type 2A VWD is caused by the abnormal proteolysis of VWF, with only the smallest VWF multimers being present. This results in a reduction in VWF antigen with a much greater reduction in VWF activity. Although desmopressin is safe in these patients, it is not always effective, because normal multimers are not maintained in plasma. Significant bleeding should be treated with VWF replacement therapy.

Type 2B VWD may be caused by one of several mutations resulting in "hyperactive" VWF. The abnormal VWF binds spontaneously to platelets with resulting rapid clearance of VWF and platelets. The larger molecular weight multimers of VWF are preferentially cleared from the circulation, and moderate to severe thrombocytopenia is common. The laboratory diagnosis is based on demonstration that the "hyperactive" 2B VWF binds to platelets and agglutinates them at low concentrations of ristocetin, a concentration that would not agglutinate normal platelets. If one administers desmopressin to these patients, the abnormal "hyperactive" 2B VWF would be released and more profound thrombocytopenia might occur. These patients usually respond to the infusion of VWF.

Type 2M VWD is caused by mutations that result in the reduction of the platelet-binding function of VWF. The binding of this protein to factor VIII is normal, so that the factor VIII levels will be equal to the VWF levels, but the platelet-dependent interaction of VWF is reduced significantly. Desmopressin will increase VWF and factor VIII levels, but the released type 2M VWF may not have sufficient activity to cause cessation of bleeding. Thus, VWF replacement therapy may need to be employed.

Type 2N VWD is caused by the reduction of factor VIII binding by VWF. This disorder has also been termed *autosomal hemophilia*. With this variant, platelet interaction with VWF is normal but the 2N VWF binds weakly (or not at all) to factor VIII, resulting in rapid clearance of factor VIII that is weakly complexed to VWF. Thus, the factor VIII level is reduced much more than the VWF levels. Commonly, patients who have symptomatic bleeding are compound heterozygotes who have inherited a gene for type 1 VWD from one parent and one for type 2N VWD from the other. Rarely, 2N mutations are inherited from both parents and the VWF levels are normal. In the patient who is compound heterozygous of type 1 and type 2N, the one allele makes no protein and the other allele makes a functionally abnormal protein, resulting in all of the VWF being dysfunctional. Although desmopressin will release the 2N VWF, the sustained factor VIII levels occasionally may be inadequate for normal hemostasis. A trial of desmopressin is indicated to assess the response and half-life of VWF and factor VIII after infusion. VWF replacement therapy is usually effective.

Platelet type (pseudo-) VWD is actually an abnormality of the GPIb receptor on platelets. This can be considered the converse abnormality of type 2B, in that the GPIb receptor on platelets is hyperfunctional and binds plasma VWF spontaneously. This results in thrombocytopenia and a loss of high molecular weight VWF multimers that are indistinguishable from those seen in type 2B VWD. Specific testing, however, will demonstrate that this is a platelet abnormality rather than a plasma abnormality.

Type 3 VWD is the homozygous or compound heterozygous inheritance of VWF deficiency. Patients exhibit undetectable plasma levels of VWF and only low, but measurable, levels of factor VIII. These patients will have major hemorrhage but only rarely have joint hemorrhages. This severe, very rare form occurs in approximately 1:500,000 individuals. Intracranial hemorrhage, major epistaxis, and menorrhagia in women are the major features. Bleeding episodes require treatment with VWF-containing concentrates. Desmopressin is not effective.

Ginsburg D, Konkle BA, Gill JC, et al: Molecular basis of human von Willebrand disease: Analysis of von Willebrand factor mRNA. *Proc Natl Acad Sci USA* 1989;86:3723.

Hillery CA, Mancuso DJ, Sadler JE, et al: Type 2M von Willebrand disease: F606I and I662F, mutations in the glycoprotein Ib binding domain selectively impair ristocetin, but not botrocetin-mediated binding of von Willebrand factor to platelets. *Blood* 1998;91:1011.

Kroner PA, Kluesendorf KL, Montgomery RR: Expressed full-length von Willebrand factor containing missense mutations linked to type IIb von Willebrand's disease shows enhanced binding to platelets. *Blood* 1991;79:2048.

Kroner PA, Friedman KD, Fahs SA, et al: Abnormal binding of factor VIII is linked with the substitution of Gln for Arg91 in von Willebrand factor in a variant form on von Willebrand disease. *J Biol Chem* 1991;266:10146.

Mannucci PM: Desmopressin (DDAVP) in the treatment of bleeding disorders: The first 20 years. *Blood* 1997;90:2515–21.

Montgomery RR, Gill JC, Scott JP: Hemophilia and von Willebrand disease. In Nathan DG, Orkin SH (editors): *Hematology of Infancy and Childhood*, 5th ed. Philadelphia, WB Saunders, 1998, pp 1631–59.

Montgomery RR, Coller BS: von Willebrand disease. In Colman RW, Hirsh J, Marder VJ, Salzman E (editors): *Hemostasis and Thrombosis, Basic Principles and Clinical Practice*. Philadelphia, JB Lippincott, 1994, pp 134–68.

Scott JP, Montgomery RR: Therapy of von Willebrand disease. *Semin Thromb Hemost* 1993;19:37.

Werner EJ: von Willebrand disease in children and adolescents. *Pediatr Clin North Am* 1996;43:683–707.

White GC, Montgomery RR: Clinical aspects and therapy of von Willebrand disease. In *Hematology: Basic Principles and Practice*, 3rd ed. New York, Churchill Livingstone, 1999.

Chapter 470

Hereditary Predisposition to Thrombosis

Thromboses in children are frequently caused by a hereditary or acquired prothrombotic state. Over the past 20 years a large number of hereditary causes of thrombosis have been identified. The newborn infant because of the physiologic deficiency of various regulatory proteins is particularly predisposed to both hemorrhage and thrombosis. The more premature the infant, the greater the deficiency. The sick newborn infant is particularly at risk since interventions to provide support often include placement of large indwelling catheters into major veins or arteries. Those with hereditary deficiencies of anticoagulants may have major symptoms. After the neonatal period, young children seem to have some resistance to clinical thrombosis even if they have a heterozygous hereditary deficiency of an anticoagulant protein. However, when clotting is identified in the young child, particularly when the family history is abnormal, a thrombotic work-up should be initiated. In children and teenagers, thromboses are often triggered by major medical or surgical challenges.

Pathophysiology and Clinical Manifestations The predominant anticoagulants are illustrated in Figures 467–1 and 467–2. A hereditary predisposition to thrombosis can be caused by deficiencies of the regulatory proteins: protein C, protein S, antithrombin III, and plasminogen; synthesis of a procoagulant protein unable to be inhibited by its regulatory protein, *factor V Leiden;* elevated levels of procoagulant protein, *prothrombin mutation (G20210A);* and elevated levels of a toxic organic acid, homocystinuria.

The hereditary mutation of factor V, termed *factor V Leiden*, results in a factor V molecule that, when activated, is not subsequently inactivated by activated protein C. This leaves the patient with unregulated "active" factor V and so-called resistance to activated protein C. Individuals with the *prothrombin mutation (G20210A)* have a mutation in the 3'-untranslated end of the mRNA for prothrombin that results in increased levels of prothrombin synthesis. Children with these hereditary mutations have an increased frequency of venous thrombosis. Young women are at increased risk of venous thrombosis during pregnancy or while receiving oral contraceptive agents. There is also an increased risk of recurrent abortions. If one evaluates young adults with thrombosis, factor V Leiden and the prothrombin mutation (G20210A) are the most common associated abnormalities.

While patients with heterozygous deficiencies may be predisposed to thrombosis, those with *homozygous protein C deficiency* have fatal purpura fulminans in the neonatal period if untreated. Such infants were probably overlooked in the past because the symptoms were thought to be secondary to sepsis and disseminated intravascular coagulation. Because the newborn is physiologically deficient in protein C, its absence is difficult to determine except in a laboratory that has established normal ranges for neonates and preterm infants. If an individual has undetectable levels of protein C, this is most likely a hereditary disorder. The physiologic deficiency of protein C in the newborn coupled with true sepsis may also lead to nearly undetectable levels of protein C.

Laboratory Findings. There are no screening tests for hereditary deficiencies of anticoagulants such as protein C, protein S, antithrombin III, or factor V Leiden and prothrombin 20210; thus, specific testing is required. A careful family history may reveal thromboembolic diseases in family members at a young age, but the absence of a positive history does not rule out a hereditary predisposition to thrombosis. If hereditary deficiency of anticoagulant or regulatory proteins is suspected, specific assays should be undertaken. Techniques that quantitate the amount and function of antithrombin III, protein C, and free protein S are well established. Genetic DNA testing for factor V Leiden and the prothrombin mutation (G20210A) are more sensitive and specific than clotting-based tests.

Treatment. Homozygous deficiency of protein C presents with purpura fulminans in the first few hours of life. A recombinant activated protein C concentrate has been licensed for adult sepsis, but it has not been licensed for treating hereditary deficiency. Fresh frozen plasma (FFP) is the only immediately available source of protein C. Amelioration of symptoms usually requires 10–15 mL/kg of FFP every 8–12 hr. Clinical trials are in progress using a plasma protein C concentrate, which eliminates the need for large amounts of FFP. After the infant's symptoms are reduced, the amount of FFP or protein C concentrate is adjusted and monitored by frequent protein C levels. When the infant is beyond the neonatal period, high-dose warfarin (to achieve an INR of 4–5) may prevent most of the thrombotic problems, but acute intermittent thromboses require additional FFP or protein C concentrate (see also Chapter 471). Thromboses associated with a hereditary predisposition to clotting should be treated with anticoagulants as outlined in Chapter 471. Replacement therapy is usually not indicated. Individuals with homocystinuria should receive anticoagulation as well as management of their primary disease (see Chapter 74.3).

Andrew M, Montgomery RR: Acquired disorders of hemostasis. In Nathan DG, Orkin SH (editors): *Nathan and Oski's Hematology of Infancy and Childhood,* 5th ed. Philadelphia, WB Saunders, 1998, pp 1677–1717.

David M, Andrew M: Venous thromboembolic complications in children. *J Pediatr* 1993;123:337.

Esmon CT: Blood coagulation. In Nathan DG, Orkin SH (editors): *Hematology of Infancy and Childhood,* 5th ed. Philadelphia, WB Saunders, 1998, pp 1531–1556.

Seligsohn U, Lubetsky A: Genetic susceptibility to venous thrombosis. *N Engl J Med* 2001;344:1222.

Chapter 471
Acquired Thrombotic Disorders

The occlusion of a blood vessel with a platelet plug or fibrin clot may occur in vessels of any size. A large number of systemic disorders are associated with occlusion of arterial or venous vessels of diverse caliber, including vasculitic diseases like systemic lupus erythematosus and Kawasaki disease, metabolic defects like homocystinuria, and red cell disorders like sickle cell anemia and polycythemia. Activation of clotting as a complication of disseminated intravascular coagulation (DIC) can cause microvascular and macrovascular thrombosis. Medical interventions themselves can predispose to thrombosis, such as when sick newborns have indwelling catheters placed in major vessels or when children with acute lymphoblastic leukemia receive the chemotherapeutic agent L-asparaginase that depletes anticoagulant proteins. Mechanism(s) leading to thrombosis, in addition to vessel injury, include one or all of the following: abnormal platelet adhesiveness-aggregation, an activated coagulation mechanism, a defective/deficient anticoagulant system, a dysfunctional fibrinolytic mechanism, and reduced blood flow. Arterial thrombosis appears to depend on vascular injury and platelet activation under high shear, whereas venous thrombosis generally occurs in low-flow (low-shear) conditions associated with activation of the coagulation mechanism or with an impaired inhibitor-fibrinolytic system.

The *clinical manifestations* reflect organ or tissue injury resulting from a severe reduction in blood perfusion or distention from occlusion of venous outflow. In general, vascular occlusive events in children have an acute or sudden onset. The diagnosis is made noninvasively by Doppler ultrasonography or MRI or by contrast angiography. Routine coagulation screening studies are rarely helpful in diagnosing a thromboembolic event. Studies in adults have suggested that quantitative assays of the D-dimer (formed when cross-linked fibrin is proteolysed by plasmin) are a sensitive screening tool for deep venous thrombosis (DVT) and especially for pulmonary emboli. In acute DIC, screening tests are strikingly abnormal, characterized by thrombocytopenia, hypofibrinogenemia, prolongation of the PT and PTT, and elevated D-dimers (see Chapter 475).

Acquired thrombotic and embolic events are uncommon in otherwise healthy children. Nevertheless, there are increasing reports of thromboembolism in newborns and in patients with specific diseases (Box 471–1). Arterial events usually present as stroke (at any age), a cold and pulseless lower extremity with or without renal involvement (aortic thrombosis in the newborn), and, rarely, myocardial infarction, although any organ can be affected. Venous events usually present as DVT with or without phlebitis, pulmonary embolism, and renal vein thrombosis.

The *lupus anticoagulant* causes a prolongation of the PTT that fails to correct on 1:1 mixing with normal plasma. The antibody is directed against the phospholipid used as a reagent in the PTT. The activated partial thromboplastin time (PTT or APTT) may be prolonged, but specific assays are needed to confirm the antiphospholipid antibody. Although the PTT is prolonged, the patient with an isolated lupus anticoagulant is not at increased risk of bleeding. Paradoxically, 5–20% of such individuals may develop arterial or venous thromboses. The lupus anticoagulant, either alone or as a component of the **antiphospholipid syndrome,** may be primary (idiopathic) or associated with systemic lupus erythematosus, infections, especially HIV, drug reactions, or other autoimmune diseases. Associated features include *livedo reticularis,* thrombocytopenia, recurrent fetal loss, and thrombosis (arterial or venous or both). Some children may develop an evanescent lupus anticoagulant after a viral illness. Treatment of thromboses includes warfarin with or without aspirin.

Venous Thrombosis and Thrombophlebitis. Superficial thrombophlebitis is treated by anti-inflammatory drugs (nonsteroidal anti-inflammatory agents), heat compresses, rest, and elevation of the affected part. Patients with DVT or thrombophlebitis are treated with anticoagulation and sometimes with thrombolytic agents. Heparin anticoagulation should be used in a full dose for

BOX 471–1. Causes of Disseminated Intravascular Coagulation

INFECTIOUS

Meningococcemia (purpura fulminans)
Other gram-negative bacteria (*Haemophilus, Salmonella, Escherichia coli*)
Gram-positive bacteria (group B streptococci, staphylococci)
Rickettsia (Rocky Mountain spotted fever)
Virus (cytomegalovirus, herpes simplex, hemorrhagic fevers)
Malaria
Fungus

TISSUE INJURY

Central nervous system trauma (massive head injury)
Multiple fractures with fat emboli
Crush injury
Profound shock or asphyxia
Hypothermia or hyperthermia
Massive burns

MALIGNANCY

Acute promyelocytic leukemia
Acute monoblastic or myelocytic leukemia
Widespread malignancies (neuroblastoma)

VENOM OR TOXIN

Snake bites
Insect bites

MICROANGIOPATHIC DISORDERS

"Severe" thrombotic thrombocytopenic purpura or hemolytic-uremic syndrome
Giant hemangioma (Kasabach-Merritt syndrome)

GASTROINTESTINAL DISORDERS

Fulminant hepatitis
Severe inflammatory bowel disease
Reye syndrome

HEREDITARY THROMBOTIC DISORDERS

Antithrombin III deficiency
Homozygous protein C deficiency

NEWBORN

Maternal toxemia
Group B streptococcal infections
Abruptio placentae
Severe respiratory distress syndrome
Necrotizing enterocolitis
Congenital viral disease (cytomegalovirus, herpes simplex)
Erythroblastosis fetalis

MISCELLANEOUS

Severe acute graft rejection
Acute hemolytic transfusion reaction
Severe collagen-vascular disease
Kawasaki disease
Heparin-induced thrombosis
Infusion of "activated" prothrombin complex concentrates
Hyperpyrexia/encephalopathy, hemorrhagic shock syndrome

Modified from Montgomery RR, Scott IP. Hemostasis: Diseases of the fluid phase. In Nathan DG, Oski FA (editors): *Hematology of Infancy and Childhood,* 4th ed. Vol 2. Philadelphia, WB Saunders, 1993.

3–5 days, with warfarin added for an additional 6 mo in those patients with proximal (above the knee) venous thrombosis. Patients with calf vein thrombosis may not require treatment. Experience with thrombolytic therapy in children is limited, but its efficacy is probably similar to that seen in adults. At this time, use of thrombolytic therapy should probably be limited to life- or limb-threatening situations.

Pulmonary Embolism. The patient with acute pulmonary embolism (PE) can be treated with heparin or thrombolytic drugs. Thrombolytic therapy in adults produces a more rapid clinical improvement than heparin therapy, but the overall survival and long-term pulmonary function abnormalities appear to be the same in both treatment groups. Rarely, embolectomy is used when there is a large embolism and no benefit from thrombolytic or anticoagulant therapy.

Arterial Thrombosis. Fibrinolytic therapy with either recombinant tPA (rTPA) or urokinase followed by heparin anticoagulation has been used successfully to treat acute arterial thromboses. Rarely, surgical removal of the clot is performed if lytic therapy is not successful or if the thrombosis affects a major organ or limb. Thrombolytic therapy cannot be employed if there has been recent surgery or central nervous system thrombosis/hemorrhage.

Stroke. Arterial occlusion in the brain occurs when there is a vascular injury or anomaly or embolization from the heart; often these strokes are idiopathic. The most common cause of stroke in children is sickle cell disease. Venous thrombosis of cerebral vessels can be seen in those with cyanotic heart disease, inflammatory/infectious lesions of the brain or surrounding tissues, hyperviscosity states, or congenital thrombophilia. The therapeutic approach is directed toward the cause of the occlusion. Anticoagulation and/or platelet inhibitor drugs may be used. The presence of a hemorrhagic infarct is a contraindication to anticoagulant therapy. It is not known whether thrombolytic therapy is effective or safe in children with non-hemorrhagic strokes; but if used, it should only be used in patients with less than 3 hr of symptoms. Heparin therapy may improve the outcome of stroke in adults, although this is controversial.

471.1 Anticoagulant and Thrombolytic Therapy

Standard Unfractionated Heparin. Heparin enhances the rate by which antithrombin III neutralizes the activities of several of the activated clotting proteins, especially factor Xa and thrombin. The average half-life of intravenously administered heparin is about 60 min in adults and can be as short as 30 min in the newborn. Heparin does not cross the placenta. The half-life of heparin is dose dependent; the higher the dose, the longer the circulating half-life. In thrombotic disease the half-life may be shorter than normal in patients with significant thromboembolism (e.g., pulmonary embolism) and longer than normal in patients with cirrhosis and uremia.

Anticoagulation with heparin is contraindicated in the following circumstances: a pre-existing coagulation defect or bleeding abnormality; a recent central nervous system hemorrhage; bleeding from inaccessible sites; malignant hypertension; bacterial endocarditis; recent surgery of the eye, brain, or spinal cord; and current administration of regional or lumbar block anesthesia. Despite these precautions, the frequency of bleeding in patients given heparin anticoagulation is 0.2–1%.

Heparin can be given as an intravenous or subcutaneous injection. It should not be given as an intramuscular injection. Although heparin can be administered by intermittent bolus injections of 75–100 U/kg every 4 hr, continuous administration is associated with a lower risk of secondary hemorrhage. The current recommendation for continuous heparin is to give a bolus injection of 75 U/kg, followed by a continuous infusion of 28 U/kg/hr in infants younger than 1 yr of age or 20 U/kg/hr in children older than 1 yr. The goal is a PTT between 60 and 85 sec, which should correlate with a heparin level of 0.35–0.7 anti–factor Xa U/mL. If the PTT is less than 60 sec, increase the heparin dose rate by 10%. If it is less than 50 sec, re-administer a bolus of 50 U/kg and then increase the dose rate by 10%. If the PTT is more than 90 sec, stop the heparin dose for 30 min and then decrease the dose rate by 10%. If the dose must be adjusted, repeat the PTT in 4 hr. Once a stable therapeutic level has been reached, recheck the PTT daily. In newborns with low clotting factors, in patients with a lupus inhibitor, or in patients with elevated factor VIII (stress or surgery), the PTT may not reflect the correct degree of anticoagulation, and specific heparin levels should be performed so that the heparin level is 0.35–0.70 U/mL by anti–factor Xa assay or 0.2–0.4 U/mL by protamine sulfate assay.

Heparin can be neutralized immediately by using protamine sulfate. Because of the rapid clearance rate of heparin, however, most patients can be treated by stopping the infusion. One milligram of protamine sulfate neutralizes between 90 and 110 U of heparin. Because heparin has a rapid in vivo metabolic decay, only half the total dose of protamine should be administered. A clotting test is performed to determine whether adequate neutralization has occurred; if not, the additional protamine can be given. Protamine itself is an anticoagulant; thus, if too much is given the clotting time may be prolonged. Although excess protamine has an anticoagulant effect, it rarely (if ever) is a cause of clinical bleeding. Once heparin is neutralized, the patient is returned to the original "prothrombotic" state.

LOW MOLECULAR WEIGHT HEPARIN. Low molecular weight (LMW) heparin is an effective, convenient alternative to standard heparin therapy. Several heparins and heparinoids are undergoing clinical trials. The majority of the pediatric experience is with enoxaparin. Adult patients receiving LMW heparin rarely need to have heparin levels monitored, but in pediatric patients there is more diversity of response. Thus, monitoring should be performed to be sure that a therapeutic level is achieved. To treat a thrombus in older children, 1 mg/kg of enoxaparin every 12 hr subcutaneously is usually effective. In newborn and young infants, the dose is 1.6 mg/kg every 12 hr to achieve a therapeutic level. The PTT cannot be used to monitor LMW heparin; a specific assay for LMW heparin level should be used. The therapeutic level is more than 0.6 U/mL at 3 hr after injection. Prophylaxis is achieved with doses of 0.5 mg/kg every 12 hr subcutaneously. Prophylaxis levels demonstrate an anti-Xa assay of more than 0.3 U. Once a therapeutic range is achieved, routine monitoring is not required or required only infrequently.

Warfarin. The coumarin derivatives are oral anticoagulant drugs that act by decreasing the functional levels of the vitamin K–dependent coagulation factors: II, VII, IX, and X. In addition, protein C and protein S (the vitamin K–dependent anticoagulants) are reduced. These drugs inhibit vitamin K–dependent carboxylation of the precursor coagulation proteins. Warfarin probably acts by competitively inhibiting vitamin K metabolism. After the administration of warfarin, the levels of factors II, VII, IX, and X decrease gradually, according to their respective plasma half-life. Because factor VII has the shortest half-life, its level is the first to decrease, followed by factors IX and X, and finally factor II. It generally takes 4–5 days to reduce levels of all four coagulation factors consistent with effective anticoagulation.

The prothrombin time (PT) is the clotting test used to assess warfarin anticoagulation. Current recommendations are based on the International Normalized Ratio (INR), which permits comparison of PTs using a wide variety of reagents or instrument. The INR for standard treatment of thrombosis is 2.0–3.0. For mechanical heart valves, treatment of homozygous protein C deficiency, and DVT associated with the lupus anticoagulant, the INR should be between 3.0–4.0.

The starting dose of warfarin in children is 0.2 mg/kg/24 hr orally. After 48 hr the dose is adjusted based on the INR. If the INR is 1.1–1.4, increase the dose by 20%; if it is 1.5–1.9, increase by 10%. If the INR is 3.2–3.5, decrease the dose by 20%. If the INR is more than 3.5, hold the dose until the INR is less than 3.5, then restart at 20% less than the previous dose. If the INR is 2.0–3.0, continue the same dose.

The most serious side effect of warfarin is hemorrhage. This is often related to changes in the dose or metabolism of the drug. The addition or removal of certain drugs in the patient's ther-

apeutic regimen can have significant effects on oral anticoagulation. For example, warfarin's effect can be enhanced by the administration of antibiotics, salicylates, anabolic steroids, chloral hydrate, laxatives, allopurinol, vitamin E, and methylphenidate HCl; its effect can be diminished by barbiturates, vitamin K, oral contraceptives, phenytoin, and others. Warfarin-induced bleeding is treated by discontinuation of the drug and the oral administration of vitamin K. Generally, the amount of vitamin K given is equal to the amount of the daily warfarin dose. Vitamin K can be administered orally, subcutaneously, or intravenously (not intramuscularly) but the parenteral forms have a much longer half-life and may overshoot the correction. Correction of the coagulopathy begins within 6–8 hr and should be complete in 24–48 hr. If the patient is having a significant or life-threatening hemorrhage, fresh frozen plasma (15 mL/kg) should be given at the same time as the vitamin K is administered.

Coumarin anticoagulants are contraindicated in essentially the same circumstances as those for heparin therapy. The oral anticoagulants are teratogenic, cross the placenta, and should not be given during pregnancy—particularly during the first trimester. Although breast milk contains warfarin, the quantity is insignificant and the drug can be used to treat the lactating mother.

Thrombolytic Therapy. Thrombolytic agents such as streptokinase, urokinase, and tissue-type plasminogen activator (rTPA) activate plasminogen to lyse blood clots by enzymatic digestion. Urokinase and rTPA act as direct activators, whereas streptokinase acts by binding to plasminogen, and the streptokinase-plasminogen complex becomes the plasminogen activator. For this therapy to be effective, the patient should have a relatively fresh clot (<3–5 days old), the clot must be accessible to the lytic agent, and there must be an adequate amount of plasminogen. Once plasmin has been formed, it lyses fibrin. The plasmin generated by urokinase and streptokinase can produce a systemic hyperfibrinolytic state; when this occurs, the plasmin can degrade other plasma proteins, including fibrinogen, and factors V and VIII, resulting in a hemorrhagic disorder. rTPA is relatively more fibrin specific than urokinase; it serves as an activator within or on a fibrin clot. Clinical trials with rTPA suggest that a systemic hyperfibrinolytic state is rarely produced. The initial dose of rTPA is 0.1 mg/kg/hr with therapeutic effect determined by an increase in concentration of D-dimers or fibrin degradation products (FDP). With urokinase, a loading dose of 4400 U/kg is administered and then followed by 4400 U/kg/hr with therapeutic effectiveness monitored by a moderate drop in fibrinogen and the presence of detectable D-dimers. Higher doses or more prolonged courses of thrombolytic therapy are likely associated with an increased risk of bleeding complications.

Thrombolytic therapy has been reported to be beneficial in those with pulmonary embolism, DVT, certain arterial occlusive events, and occluded vascular access catheters. However, there are no controlled trials on its use in the pediatric group.

Andrew M, Michelson AD, Bovill E, et al: Guidelines for antithrombotic therapy in pediatric patients. *J Pediatr* 1998;132:575–8.

Andrew M, Montgomery RR: Acquired disorders of hemostasis. In Nathan DG, Orkin SH (editors): *Nathan and Oski's Hematology of Infancy and Childhood*, 5th ed. Philadelphia, WB Saunders, 1998, pp 1677–1717.

Andrew M, Vegh P, Johnston M, et al: Maturation of the hemostatic system during childhood. *Blood* 1992;80:1998.

Dix D, Andrew M, Marzinotto V, et al: The use of low molecular weight heparin in pediatric patients: A prospective cohort study. *J Pediatr* 2000;136:439-45.

Hathaway WE, Bonnar J: *Hemostatic Disorders of the Pregnant Woman and Newborn Infant*. New York, Elsevier Science, 1987.

Manco-Johnson MJ: Disorders of hemostasis in childhood: Risk factors for venous thromboembolism. *Thromb Haemost* 1997;78:710-14.

Wells PS, Anderson DR, Rodger M, et al: Excluding pulmonary embolism at the bedside without diagnostic imaging: Management of patients with suspected pulmonary embolism presenting to the emergency department by using a simple clinical model and D-dimer. *Ann Intern Med* 2001;135:98-107.

Chapter 472
Postneonatal Vitamin K Deficiency

Although "late" hemorrhagic disease has been reported in breast-fed children, vitamin K deficiency occurring after the neonatal period is usually secondary to a lack of oral intake of vitamin K, alterations in the gut flora due to the long-term use of broad-spectrum antibiotics, or malabsorption of vitamin K (see also Chapter 92). Intestinal malabsorption of fats may accompany cystic fibrosis or biliary atresia and result in a deficiency of fat-soluble, dietary vitamin K with a reduced synthesis of the vitamin K–dependent clotting factors (factors II, VII, IX, X, protein C, and protein S). Prophylactic administration of water-soluble vitamin K orally is indicated in these cholestatic situations (2–3 mg/24 hr for children and 5–10 mg/24 hr for adolescents and adults) or vitamin K, 1–2 mg, may be administered intravenously. In patients with advanced cirrhosis, synthesis of many of the clotting factors may be reduced because of hepatocellular damage. In these patients, vitamin K may be ineffective. The anticoagulant properties of warfarin (Coumadin) and related anticoagulants depend on interference with vitamin K with a concomitant reduction of factors II, VII, IX, and X. Rat poison (superwarfarin) produces a similar deficiency; vitamin K is a specific antidote.

Andrew M, Montgomery RR: Acquired disorders of hemostasis. In Nathan DG, Orkin SH (editors): *Hematology of Infancy and Childhood,* 5th ed. Philadelphia, WB Saunders, 1998, pp 1677–1717.

Chapter 473
Liver Disease

Since all the clotting factors are produced exclusively in the liver except factor VIII, coagulation abnormalities are very common in patients with severe liver disease. Only 15% of such patients, however, have significant clinical bleeding states. The severity of the coagulation abnormality appears to be directly proportional to the extent of hepatocellular damage. The most common mechanism causing the defect is decreased synthesis of the coagulation factors. Severe liver disease characteristically has normal to increased (not reduced) levels of factor VIII activity in plasma. In some instances, disseminated intravascular coagulation (DIC) or hyperfibrinolysis may complicate liver diseases, making the laboratory differentiation of severe liver disease from DIC difficult.

The treatment of the coagulopathy of liver disease consists of replacement with fresh frozen plasma (FFP) or cryoprecipitate. FFP (10–15 mL/kg) contains all clotting factors, but replacement of fibrinogen may require cryoprecipitate. For severe hypofibrinogenemia, cryoprecipitate is recommended to replace fibrinogen at a dose of 1 bag/5 kg body weight. Because a reduction in the vitamin K-dependent coagulation factors is common in those with acute and chronic liver disease, vitamin K therapy can be given as a trial. The vitamin K can be given orally, subcutaneously, or intravenously (not intramuscularly) in a dose of 1 mg/24 hr for infants, 2–3 mg for children, and 5–10 mg for adolescents and adults. An inability to correct the coagulopathy indicates that the coagulopathy may be caused by a reduction in one or more of the non-vitamin K dependent proteins or because the liver is severely impaired and cannot produce the precursor vitamin K proteins.

Frequently, severe liver disease is associated with moderate prolongation of the bleeding time that is not corrected by either vitamin K or plasma replacement. DDAVP (0.3 μg/kg IV) has been found to be effective in shortening the bleeding time and has been used effectively to augment hemostasis prior to liver biopsy.

Andrew M, Montgomery RR: Acquired disorders of hemostasis. In Nathan DG, Orkin SH (editors): *Hematology of Infancy and Childhood*, 5th ed. Philadelphia, WB Saunders, 1998, pp 1677–717.

Chapter 474
Acquired Inhibitors of Coagulation

Acquired circulating anticoagulants (inhibitors) are antibodies that react or cross react with clotting proteins and cause screening tests such as the partial thromboplastin time and prothrombin time to be prolonged. Many of these anticoagulants are autoantibodies that react with phospholipid and thereby interfere with clotting in vitro but not in vivo. These antibodies have been referred to as the lupus anticoagulant (see also Chapter 471). These circulating anticoagulants are uncommon in otherwise normal children. They are found in patients with systemic lupus erythematosus (SLE) or lymphomas or in those with penicillin or other drug reactions. They are a subset of antibodies found as a component of the *antiphospholipid syndrome.* Spontaneous inhibitors have been reported in children after incidental viral infections. Paradoxically, the lupus anticoagulant is rarely associated with bleeding symptoms but is associated with a predisposition to thrombosis. The mechanism(s) for the prothrombotic tendency associated with the lupus anticoagulant is likely multifactorial as these antibodies are heterogeneous in character.

Clinical Manifestations. Bleeding symptoms in a patient with the lupus anticoagulant may be caused by thrombocytopenia, as a manifestation of the antiphospholipid syndrome or lupus itself, or rarely by a specific autoantibody against prothrombin (factor II). This antibody does not inactivate prothrombin but causes accelerated clearance of prothrombin, resulting in low levels of prothrombin.

Rarely, antibodies may arise spontaneously against a specific clotting factor, such as factor VIII or von Willebrand factor, similar to those seen more frequently in elderly patients. These patients are prone to excessive hemorrhage and may require specific treatment. In patients with a hereditary deficiency of a clotting factor (factor VIII or factor IX), antibodies may develop after exposure to transfused factor concentrates. These hemophilic inhibitory antibodies are discussed in Chapter 468.

Laboratory Findings. Inhibitors against specific coagulation factors usually affect factors VIII, IX, and XI or, rarely, prothrombin. The PTT or the PT may be prolonged and is not corrected in vitro with the addition of normal plasma, unless the antibody is a noninhibitory antibody that promotes rapid clearance of the protein. Specific factor assays determine which factor is involved.

The most common inhibitor is the "lupus anticoagulant" that is found in patients with SLE, other collagen-vascular diseases, or sometimes after common viral infections, including HIV. The lupus anticoagulant produces a prolonged PTT and, if severe, a prolonged PT. The addition of normal, platelet-poor plasma in a 1:1 ratio with the test plasma does not correct the abnormal tests, but the addition of platelets neutralizes the anticoagulant.

More specific assays are necessary to confirm the presence of the lupus anticoagulant.

Treatment. Management of the patient with an inhibitor against a specific coagulation factor is the same as for the hemophilia patient who develops an alloantibody against factor VIII or IX. Infusions of a prothrombin complex concentrate, activated prothrombin complex concentrate (FEIBA or Autoplex), porcine factor VIII, or recombinant factor VIIa concentrate may be needed to control significant bleeding. Spontaneous inhibitors that arise after a viral infection tend to disappear within a few weeks to months. Inhibitors seen with an underlying disease often disappear when the primary disease is treated. The lupus anticoagulant will often disappear after appropriate treatment of SLE. Thrombotic complications of the lupus anticoagulant should be treated with anticoagulants similar to other thrombotic events. Monitoring anticoagulant treatment may be complicated by the lupus anticoagulant and may require specific assays such as a heparin assay rather than the PTT or a factor X level rather than a PT. Maintenance of an International Normalized Ratio of 3–4, higher than for other patients with deep venous thrombosis, is recommended when thrombosis occurs with lupus inhibitors.

Andrew M, Montgomery RR: Acquired disorders of hemostasis. In Nathan DC, Orkin SH (editors): *Hematology of Infancy and Childhood,* 5th ed. Philadelphia, WB Saunders, 1998, pp 1677–1717.

Bernini JC, Buchanan GR, Ashcroft J: Hypoprothrombinemia and severe hemorrhage associated with lupus anticoagulant. *J Pediatr* 1993;123:937.

Levine JS, Branch DW, Rauch J: The antiphospholipid syndrome. *N Engl J Med* 2002;346:752–63.

Manco-Johnson MJ: Antiphospholipid antibodies in children. *Semin Thromb Hemost* 1998;24:591–8.

Chapter 475

Disseminated Intravascular Coagulation (Consumptive Coagulopathy)

Consumption coagulopathy refers to a heterogeneous group of conditions, including disseminated intravascular coagulation (DIC), that result in consumption of clotting factors, platelets, and anticoagulant proteins. Consequences of this process include widespread intravascular deposition of fibrin leading to tissue ischemia and necrosis, a generalized hemorrhagic state, and hemolytic anemia.

Etiology. A number of life-threatening pathologic processes, including hypoxia, acidosis, tissue necrosis, shock, and endothelial damage, may trigger DIC. Accordingly, it is not surprising that a large number of conditions have been reported to be associated with DIC, including septic shock (especially meningococcemia), incompatible blood transfusions, rickettsial infections, snakebite, purpura fulminans, giant hemangioma, and malignancies, especially acute promyelocytic leukemia. Although the clinical symptoms are primarily hemorrhagic, the initiating event is usually excessive activation of clotting that consumes both the physiologic anticoagulants (protein C, protein S, antithrombin III) and procoagulants, resulting in a deficiency of factor VIII, factor V, prothrombin, fibrinogen, and platelets. Commonly, the clinical result of this sequence of events is hemorrhage. The hemostatic dysregulation may also result in thrombotic susceptibility in the skin, kidneys, and other organs.

Clinical Manifestations. Most frequently, DIC accompanies a severe systemic disease process. Bleeding frequently first occurs from sites of venipuncture or surgical incision. The skin may show petechiae and ecchymoses. Tissue necrosis may involve many organs and can be most spectacularly seen as infarction of large areas of skin, subcutaneous tissue, or kidneys. Anemia caused by hemolysis may develop rapidly owing to microangiopathic hemolytic anemia.

Laboratory Findings. There is no well-defined sequence of events. Certain coagulation factors (II, V, VIII, and fibrinogen) and platelets may be consumed by the ongoing intravascular clotting process, with resultant prolongation of the prothrombin, partial thromboplastin, and thrombin times. Platelet counts may be profoundly depressed. The blood smear may contain fragmented, burr, and helmet-shaped red blood cells (schistocytes). In addition, because the fibrinolytic mechanism is activated, fibrinogen degradation products (FDPs, D-dimers) appear in the blood. The D-dimer is formed by fibrinolysis of a cross-linked fibrin clot. The D-dimer assay is equally sensitive and more specific for activation of coagulation and fibrinolysis than the FDP test.

Treatment. The first two steps in the treatment of DIC are the critical ones: (1) treat the trigger that caused the DIC and (2) restore normal homeostasis by correcting the shock, acidosis, and hypoxia that usually complicate the DIC. If the underlying problem can be controlled, bleeding quickly ceases, and there is improvement of the abnormal laboratory findings. Blood components are used for replacement therapy in patients who have hemorrhage. This may consist of platelet infusions (for thrombocytopenia), cryoprecipitate (for hypofibrinogenemia), and/or fresh frozen plasma (for replacement of other coagulation factors and natural inhibitors).

In DIC associated with sepsis, a recent controlled trial of activated protein C (APC) in adults with sepsis demonstrated a statistically significant survival advantage for those treated with APC. Studies of APC in purpura fulminans in adults and children also suggest that APC helps reverse or ameliorate the process.

Heparin has been found occasionally to be effective in children with DIC associated with purpura fulminans and acute promyelocytic leukemia. Continuous heparin at a dose of 5–10 U/kg/hr without a loading dose may be used for those with acute promyelocytic leukemia. Heparin is not indicated and has been reported to be ineffective in septic shock, snake envenomation, heat stroke, massive head injury, and incompatible blood transfusion reaction, unless there is clear evidence of vascular thrombosis. Patients who develop vascular thrombosis due to DIC should be treated as outlined in Chapter 471.1 with careful attention to replacement therapy to maintain an adequate platelet count. Some individuals with DIC appear to have incipient ischemia with poorly perfused extremities. When this occurs, the DIC may be treated with heparin to prevent ongoing consumption of factors and progression of thromboses. Because administering heparin to patients with a deficiency of both clotting factors and platelets may result in profound hemorrhage, the heparin is usually started together with clotting factor and platelet replacement. Heparin is usually administered continuously, starting with a low dose of 5–10 U/kg/hr. The duration and effectiveness of heparin therapy can be judged by serial measurements of the platelet count, fibrinogen level, and D-dimer assay.

Andrew M, Montgomery RR: Acquired disorders of hemostasis. In Nathan DG, Orkin SH (editors): *Hematology of Infancy and Childhood,* 5th ed. Philadelphia, WB Saunders, 1998, pp 1677–1717.

Bernard GR, Vincent JL, Laterre PF, et al: Efficacy and safety of recombinant human activated protein C for severe sepsis. *N Engl J Med* 2001;344:699–709.

Hathaway WE, Bonnar J: *Hemostatic Disorders of the Pregnant Woman and Newborn Infant.* New York, Elsevier, 1987.

Levi M, Ten Cate H: Disseminated intravascular coagulation. *N Engl J Med* 1999;341:586–92.

Chapter 476
Platelet and Blood Vessel Disorders

Megakaryopoiesis. Platelets are non-nucleated cellular fragments produced by megakaryocytes within the bone marrow and other tissues. Megakaryocytes are large polyploid cells. When the megakaryocyte approaches maturity, budding of the cytoplasm occurs and large numbers of platelets are liberated. Platelets circulate with a life span of 10 to 14 days. Thrombopoietin (TPO) is the major hormone that controls platelet production. Levels of TPO appear to correlate inversely with platelet number and with megakaryocyte mass. Thus, levels of TPO are highest in thrombocytopenic states associated with decreased marrow megakaryopoiesis and may be variable in states of increased platelet production.

The platelet plays multiple hemostatic roles. The platelet surface possesses a number of important receptors for adhesive proteins, including von Willebrand factor (VWF) and fibrinogen as well as receptors for agonists that trigger platelet aggregation, such as thrombin, collagen, and adenosine diphosphate (ADP). After injury to the blood vessel wall, subendothelial collagen binds VWF. VWF undergoes a conformational change that induces binding of the platelet glycoprotein Ib complex (the VWF receptor). This process is called platelet adhesion. Platelets then undergo activation. During the process of activation, the platelets generate thromboxane A_2 from arachidonic acid via the enzyme cyclooxygenase. After activation they release agonists such as ADP, adenosine triphosphate (ATP), Ca^{2+}, serotonin, and coagulation factors into the surrounding milieu. Circulating fibrinogen binds to its receptor on the activated platelets, the GPIIb-IIIa complex, linking platelets together in a process called aggregation. This series of events forms a hemostatic plug at the site of vascular injury. The serotonin and histamine liberated during activation increase local vasoconstriction. In addition to acting in concert with the vessel wall to form the platelet plug, the platelet provides the catalytic surface on which coagulation factors assemble and eventually generate thrombin through a sequential series of enzymatic cleavages. Last, the platelet contractile apparatus mediates clot retraction.

Thrombocytopenia. The normal platelet count is 150 to 450 × 10^9/L. Thrombocytopenia refers to a reduction in platelet count below 150 × 10^9/L. Causes of thrombocytopenia include (1) decreased production on either a congenital or an acquired basis, (2) sequestration of the platelets within an enlarged spleen or other organ, and (3) increased destruction of normally synthesized platelets either on an immune or a nonimmune basis. See also Chapters 460, 461, and 475.

476.1 Idiopathic Thrombocytopenic Purpura

The most common cause for acute onset of thrombocytopenia in an otherwise well child is (autoimmune) idiopathic thrombocytopenic purpura (ITP).

Etiology. One to 4 wk after exposure to a common viral infection, a small number of children develop an autoantibody directed against the platelet surface. The exact antigenic target for most such antibodies in acute ITP remains undetermined. After binding of the antibody to the platelet surface, circulating antibody-coated platelets are recognized by the Fc receptor on the splenic macrophages, ingested, and destroyed. A preceding history of a viral illness is described in 50–65% of cases of childhood ITP. The

reason why some children respond to a common infection with an autoimmune disease remains unknown. Virtually every common infectious virus has been described in association with ITP, including Epstein-Barr (EBV) and HIV. EBV-related ITP is usually of short duration and follows the course of infectious mononucleosis. HIV-associated ITP is usually chronic.

Clinical Manifestations. The classic presentation of ITP is that of a previously healthy 1–4 yr old child who has the sudden onset of generalized petechiae and purpura. The parents often state that the child was fine yesterday and now is covered with bruises and purple dots. Often there is bleeding from the gums and mucous membrane, particularly with profound thrombocytopenia (platelet count < 10 × 10^9/L). There is a history of a preceding viral infection 1 to 4 wk before onset of the thrombocytopenia. The physical examination is normal other than the finding of petechiae and purpura. Splenomegaly is rare. The presence of abnormal findings such as hepatosplenomegaly or remarkable lymphadenopathy suggests other diagnoses. When the onset is insidious, especially in an adolescent, the possibility of chronic ITP or that thrombocytopenia is a manifestation of a systemic illness such as systemic lupus erythematosus (SLE) is more likely.

In 70–80% of children who present with acute ITP, spontaneous resolution of their ITP will occur within 6 mo. Therapy does not appear to affect the natural history of the illness. Less than 1% of cases develop intracranial hemorrhage. Nevertheless, the objective of early therapy is to raise the platelet count to more than 20 × 10^9/L and prevent the rare development of intracranial hemorrhage. Ten to 20 percent of children who present with acute ITP go on to develop chronic ITP.

Laboratory Findings. Severe thrombocytopenia (platelet count < 20 × 10^9/L) is common, and platelet size is normal or increased, reflective of increased platelet turnover. In acute ITP, the hemoglobin value, white blood cell (WBC) count, and differential count should be normal. The hemoglobin may be decreased if there have been profuse nosebleeds or menorrhagia. The bone marrow examination, when done, reveals normal granulocytic and erythrocytic series with characteristically normal or increased numbers of megakaryocytes. Some of the megakaryocytes may appear to be immature and are reflective of increased platelet turnover. Indications for a bone marrow aspiration include an abnormal WBC count or differential or unexplained anemia as well as findings suggestive of bone marrow disease on history and physical examination. Other laboratory tests should be done as indicated by history and physical examination. An antinuclear antibody (ANA) test is more often positive in adolescents with ITP than in younger children and may indicate a higher likelihood of eventual chronic ITP. HIV studies should be done in at-risk populations, especially sexually active teens. Platelet antibody testing is seldom useful in acute ITP. A Coombs test should be done if there is unexplained anemia to rule out Evans syndrome (autoimmune hemolytic anemia and thrombocytopenia).

Differential Diagnosis. The well-appearing child with moderate to severe thrombocytopenia and otherwise normal complete blood cell count (CBC) has a limited differential diagnosis that includes exposure to medication that induces drug-dependent antibodies, splenic sequestration due to previously unappreciated portal hypertension, and, rarely, early aplastic processes such as Fanconi anemia. Other than congenital syndromes such as amegakaryocytic thrombocytopenia and thrombocytopenia–absent radius syndrome, most marrow processes that interfere with platelet production will also cause abnormal synthesis of red blood cells and leukocytes and therefore will manifest abnormalities in the CBC. Disorders that cause increased platelet destruction on a nonimmune basis are usually serious systemic illnesses with obvious clinical findings (hemolytic-uremic syndrome, disseminated intravascular coagulation). Isolated enlargement of the spleen suggests the potential for hypersplenism owing to either liver disease or portal vein thrombosis. Autoimmune thrombocytopenia may be an initial manifestation of SLE, HIV infection, or rarely, lymphoma. Wiskott-Aldrich syndrome must be considered in young males found to have low platelet counts, particularly if there is a history of eczema and recurrent infections.

Treatment. There are no data that treatment affects either short- or long-term clinical outcome of ITP. When compared with untreated controls, treatment appears to be capable of inducing a more rapid rise in platelet count to the theoretically safe level of more than 20×10^9/L. Antiplatelet antibodies will bind to transfused platelets as well as they do to autologous platelets. Thus, platelet transfusion in ITP is usually contraindicated unless life-threatening bleeding is present. Initial treatment options for ITP include the following:

1. *Intravenous immunoglobulin* (IVIG). IVIG in a dose of 0.8–1 g/kg/day × 1–2 days, induces a rapid rise in platelet count (usually >20×10^9/L) in 95% of patients within 48 hr. IVIG therapy is both expensive and time-consuming to administer. Additionally, there is a high frequency of headaches and vomiting suggestive of aseptic meningitis after IVIG infusions.

2. *Prednisone.* Corticosteroid therapy has been used for many years to treat acute and chronic ITP in adults and children. Doses of 1–4 mg/kg/24 hr of prednisone appear to induce a more rapid rise in platelet counts than in untreated patients with ITP. Whether a bone marrow examination should be performed to rule out other causes for thrombocytopenia, especially acute lymphoblastic leukemia, before institution of prednisone therapy in acute ITP is controversial. Corticosteroid therapy is usually continued for 2–3 wk or until a rise in platelet count above 20,000 has been achieved with a rapid taper to avoid the long-term side effects of corticosteroid therapy, especially growth failure, diabetes mellitus, and osteoporosis.

3. *IV Anti-D Therapy.* The role of IV anti-D in initial therapy of acute ITP is under investigation. When given to Rh-positive individuals, IV anti-D induces a mild hemolytic anemia. RBC-antibody complexes bind to macrophage Fc receptors and interfere with platelet destruction, thereby causing a rise in platelet count. This increase appears to be somewhat slower than after IVIG. Whether this is a biologically relevant delay remains unclear, because 80–85% of patients receiving anti-D in a dose of 50 μg/kg have demonstrated a rise in platelet count to levels above 20×10^9/L within 2 days.

Each of these medications may be used to treat exacerbations of ITP, which commonly occur several weeks after an initial course of therapy.

At the present time, there is no consensus regarding the management of acute ITP. Treatment guidelines have been published by the American Society of Hematology for adults with ITP, but there is significant disagreement within the field. Intracranial hemorrhage remains rare, and there are no data that treatment actually reduces the incidence of intracranial hemorrhage in ITP because of the rarity of the event.

The role of splenectomy in ITP should be reserved for one of two circumstances. The older child (≥4 yr) with severe ITP that has lasted longer than 1 yr (chronic ITP) and whose symptoms are not easily controlled with therapy is a candidate for splenectomy. Splenectomy must also be considered when life-threatening hemorrhage (intracranial hemorrhage) complicates acute ITP if the platelet count cannot rapidly be corrected with transfusion of platelets and administration of IVIG and corticosteroids. Splenectomy is associated with a lifelong risk of overwhelming post-splenectomy infection caused by encapsulated organisms.

Chronic ITP. Those 10–20% of patients who present with acute ITP and who have persistent thrombocytopenia for more than 6 mo have chronic ITP. At that time a careful re-evaluation for associated disorders should be performed, especially for autoimmune disease such as SLE and chronic infectious disorders such as HIV as well as nonimmune causes of chronic thrombocytopenia such as type 2B von Willebrand disease, X-linked thrombocytopenia, and Wiskott-Aldrich syndrome. Therapy should be aimed at controlling symptoms and preventing serious bleeding. In ITP the spleen is the primary site of antiplatelet antibody synthesis as well as the primary site of platelet destruction. Splenectomy is successful in inducing a complete remission in 64–88% of children with chronic ITP. This must be balanced against the lifelong risk of overwhelming post-splenectomy infection. This decision is often affected by lifestyle issues as well as the ease with which the child can be managed using medical therapy such as IVIG, corticosteroids, or IV anti-D. Before splenectomy the child should receive pneumococcal vaccine, and after splenectomy he or she should receive penicillin prophylaxis for a number of years. Whether penicillin prophylaxis should be lifelong is controversial.

476.2 Drug-Induced Thrombocytopenia

A number of drugs are associated with immune thrombocytopenia as the result of either an immune process or a megakaryocyte injury. Some common drugs used in pediatrics that cause thrombocytopenia include valproic acid, phenytoin, sulfonamides, and trimethoprim-sulfamethoxazole. Heparin-induced thrombocytopenia (and rarely thrombosis) is seldom seen in pediatrics but occurs when, after exposure to heparin, the patient develops an antibody directed against the heparin/ platelet factor IV complex.

476.3 Nonimmune Platelet Destruction

The syndromes of DIC, hemolytic-uremic syndrome, and thrombotic thrombocytopenic purpura share the hematologic picture of a *thrombotic microangiopathy* in which there is red cell destruction and a consumptive thrombocytopenia caused by platelet and fibrin deposition in the microvasculature. The microangiopathic hemolytic anemia is characterized by the presence of RBC fragments, including helmet cells, schistocytes, spherocytes, and burr cells.

476.4 Hemolytic-Uremic Syndrome (HUS) (see also Chapter 510)

This acute disease of infancy and early childhood usually follows an episode of acute gastroenteritis, often triggered by *Escherichia coli* 0157:H7. Shortly thereafter, signs and symptoms of hemolytic anemia, thrombocytopenia, and acute renal failure ensue. Sometimes neurologic symptoms are associated with these findings. *E. coli* 0157:H7 produces a specific toxin (verotoxin) that binds to and damages renal endothelial cells preferentially.

The hemolytic anemia is characterized by abnormal red cell morphology with the presence of helmet cells, spherocytes, schistocytes, burr cells, and other distorted forms. Thrombocytopenia despite normal numbers of megakaryocytes in the marrow indicates excessive platelet destruction. Tests for DIC are usually normal except for elevated fibrin(ogen) degradation products. Evaluation of the urine shows the presence of protein, red blood cells, and casts. The presence of anuria and severe azotemia indicates grave renal damage. Treatment of most cases of hemolytic-uremic syndrome involves institution of careful fluid management and prompt appropriate dialysis. Treatment using plasmapheresis is usually reserved for patients with hemolytic-uremic syndrome associated with major neurologic complications.

476.5 Thrombotic Thrombocytopenic Purpura (TTP)

This rare pentad of fever, microangiopathic hemolytic anemia, thrombocytopenia, abnormal renal function, and CNS changes is clinically similar to hemolytic-uremic syndrome, although TTP usually presents in adults and occasionally in adolescents. Microvascular thrombi within the central nervous system cause subtle, shifting neurologic signs that vary from changes in affect and orientation to aphasia, blindness, and convulsions. Prompt recognition of this disorder is critical. Laboratory findings demonstrate a microangiopathic hemolytic anemia characterized by abnormal red cell morphology with schistocytes, spherocytes, helmet cells, and an elevated reticulocyte count in association with thrombocytopenia. Coagulation studies are usually nondiagnostic. The treatment of TTP is plasmapheresis (plasma exchange), which is effective in 80–95% of cases. Corticosteroids and splenectomy are reserved for refractory cases.

The majority of cases of TTP are caused by an acquired deficiency of a metalloproteinase responsible for cleaving the high molecular weight multimers of VWF, which appear to play a pivotal role in the evolution of the thrombotic microangiopathy. In contrast, levels of the metalloproteinase in HUS are usually normal. A congenital deficiency of the metalloproteinase causes rare familial cases of TTP.

476.6 Kasabach-Merritt Syndrome (see

also Chapter 640)

The association of a giant hemangioma with localized intravascular coagulation causing thrombocytopenia and hypofibrinogenemia is called the Kasabach-Merritt syndrome. In most patients the site of the hemangioma is obvious, but retroperitoneal and intra-abdominal hemangiomas may require body imaging for detection. Inside the hemangioma there is platelet trapping and activation of coagulation with fibrinogen consumption and generation of fibrin(ogen) degradation products. Arteriovenous malformation within the lesions can cause heart failure. Some authors contend that Kasabach-Merritt syndrome is really a kaposiform hemangioendothelioma rather than a simple hemangioma. The peripheral blood smear shows microangiopathic changes. Multiple modalities have been used to treat Kasabach-Merritt syndrome, including surgical excision (if possible), laser photocoagulation, corticosteroids in high doses, local x-ray therapy, and antiangiogenic agents such as interferon α_2. Over time most patients who present in infancy have regression of the hemangioma. Treatment of the associated coagulopathy may benefit from a trial of antifibrinolytic therapy with ε-aminocaproic acid (Amicar).

476.7 Sequestration

Individuals with massive splenomegaly develop thrombocytopenia, since the spleen acts as a sponge for platelets and sequesters large numbers. Most such patients will also have mild leukopenia and anemia on the CBC. Individuals who have thrombocytopenia caused by splenic sequestration should undergo a work-up to diagnose the etiology of splenomegaly, including infectious, infiltrative, neoplastic, obstructive, and hemolytic causes.

476.8 Congenital Thrombocytopenic Syndromes

Congenital amegakaryocytic thrombocytopenia is caused by a rare defect in hematopoiesis that usually manifests within the first few days to weeks of life, when the child presents with petechiae and purpura caused by profound thrombocytopenia. Other than skin and mucous membrane findings, the physical examination is normal. Examination of the bone marrow shows an absence of megakaryocytes. These patients often progress to marrow failure (aplasia) over time. Bone marrow transplantation is curative.

Thrombocytopenia–absent radius (TAR) syndrome consists of thrombocytopenia that presents in early infancy with radial anomalies of variable severity from mild changes to marked limb shortening. In many such individuals there are also other skeletal abnormalities of the lower extremities. Intolerance to formula may complicate management by triggering gastrointestinal bleeding. The thrombocytopenia of TAR syndrome frequently remits over the first few years of life. The molecular basis for amegakaryocytic thrombocytopenia and TAR syndrome is undefined at present.

The *Wiskott-Aldrich syndrome (WAS)* is characterized by thrombocytopenia with tiny platelets, eczema, and recurrent infections due to immune deficiency (see Chapter 116.11). WAS is inherited as an X-linked disorder, and the gene for WAS has been sequenced. The WAS protein appears to play an integral role in regulating the cytoskeletal architecture of both platelets and T lymphocytes in response to receptor-mediated cell signaling. The WAS protein is common to all cells of hematopoietic lineage. Molecular analysis of families with *X-linked thrombocytopenia* has shown that many members have a point mutation within the WAS gene, whereas individuals with the full manifestation of WAS have large gene deletions. Examination of the bone marrow in WAS shows the normal number of megakaryocytes, although the megakaryocytes may have bizarre morphology. Transfused platelets have a normal life span. Splenectomy often corrects the thrombocytopenia, suggesting that the platelets formed in WAS have accelerated destruction. After splenectomy, these patients are at increased risk of overwhelming infection and require lifelong antibiotic prophylaxis against encapsulated organisms. About 5% of WAS patients develop lymphoreticular malignancies. Successful bone marrow transplantation cures WAS.

476.9 Neonatal Thrombocytopenia (see

also Chapter 92.4)

Thrombocytopenia in the newborn rarely is indicative of a primary disorder of megakaryopoiesis but more often is the result of either systemic illness or transfer of maternal antibodies directed against fetal platelets.

Thrombocytopenia may occur in various fetal and neonatal infections and be responsible for severe spontaneous bleeding. Neonatal thrombocytopenia often occurs in association with congenital viral infections, especially rubella and CMV; protozoal infections such as toxoplasmosis; syphilis; and bacterial infections, especially those caused by gram-negative bacilli. The constellation of marked thrombocytopenia and abnormal abdominal findings is common in necrotizing enterocolitis and other causes of necrotic bowel. The presence of thrombocytopenia in an ill child requires a prompt search for viral and bacterial pathogens.

Antibody-mediated thrombocytopenia in the newborn occurs because of transplacental transfer of maternal antibodies directed against fetal platelets. **Neonatal alloimmune thrombocytopenic purpura (NATP)** is caused by the development of maternal antibodies against antigens present on fetal platelets that are shared with the father and recognized as foreign by the maternal immune system. This is the platelet equivalent of Rh disease of the newborn (see Chapter 92.2). The incidence of NATP is 1 in 4,000–5,000 live births. The *clinical manifestations* of NATP are those of an apparently well child who, within the first few days after delivery, develops generalized petechiae and purpura. Laboratory studies show a normal maternal platelet count, yet moderate to severe thrombocytopenia in the newborn. Detailed historical review should show no evidence of maternal thrombocytopenia in the past. Up to 30% of infants with severe NATP may develop intracranial hemorrhage, either prenatally or in the perinatal period. Unlike Rh disease, first pregnancies may develop severe thrombocytopenia, and subsequent pregnancies may be more severely affected than the first.

The *diagnosis* of NATP is made by checking for the presence of maternal alloantibodies directed against the father's platelets. Specific studies can be done to identify the target alloantigen. The most common cause is incompatibility for P1^{A1}. Specific DNA sequence polymorphisms have been identified that permit informative prenatal testing to identify at-risk pregnancies. The differential diagnosis of NATP includes transplacental transfer of maternal antiplatelet autoantibodies (maternal ITP) and, more commonly, viral or bacterial infection.

Treatment for NATP is the administration of intravenous immunoglobulin (IVIG) prenatally to the mother. Therapy usually begins in the second trimester and is continued throughout the pregnancy. Fetal platelet counts can be monitored by percutaneous umbilical blood sampling (PUBS). Delivery should be performed by cesarean section. After delivery, if severe thrombocytopenia persists, transfusion of one unit of phenotypically matched platelets (washed maternal platelets) will cause a rise in platelet counts to provide effective hemostasis. After there has been one affected child, genetic counseling is critical to inform the parents of the high risk of thrombocytopenia in subsequent pregnancies.

Children born to mothers with ITP (maternal ITP) appear to have a lower risk of serious hemorrhage than infants born with NATP, although severe thrombocytopenia occurs. The mother's preexisting platelet count may have some predictive value, in that severe maternal thrombocytopenia before delivery appears to predict a higher risk of fetal thrombocytopenia. Nevertheless, in mothers who have had splenectomy for ITP, the maternal platelet count may be normal and is not predictive of fetal thrombocytopenia.

Treatment includes prenatal administration of corticosteroids to the mother and administration of IVIG and sometimes corticosteroids to the infant after delivery. The thrombocytopenia in an infant, whether due to NATP or maternal ITP, usually resolves within 2 to 4 mo after delivery. The highest risk period remains in the immediate perinatal period.

476.10 Thrombocytopenia Due to Acquired Disorders Causing Decreased Production

Disorders of the bone marrow that inhibit megakaryopoiesis usually affect red cell and white cell production. Infiltrative disorders, including malignancies such as acute lymphocytic leukemia, histiocytosis, lymphomas, and storage disease, usually cause either abnormalities on physical examination (lymphadenopathy, hepatosplenomegaly, masses) or abnormalities of the WBC count, or anemia. Aplastic processes may present as isolated thrombocytopenia, although there are usually clues on the CBC (leukopenia, neutropenia, anemia, or macrocytosis). Children with constitutional aplastic anemia (Fanconi anemia) often have abnormalities on examination, including radial anomalies, other skeletal anomalies, short stature, microcephaly, and hyperpigmentation. A bone marrow examination should be done when thrombocytopenia is associated with abnormalities found on physical examination or on examination of the other blood cell lines.

476.11 Platelet Function Disorders

The bleeding time is the only commonly available test to screen for abnormal platelet function. The bleeding time measures indirectly the platelet count, platelet function, and interaction of platelets with the blood vessel wall. Unfortunately, the bleeding time is dependent on a number of other factors, including the skill of the technician and the cooperation of the patient. Therefore, its predictive value is often problematic. A normal bleeding time does not rule out a mild platelet function defect in a clinically symptomatic individual. The Platelet Function Analyzer (PFA) is being evaluated as a screening tool for platelet function disorders (see Chapter 467.2) and may supplant the bleeding time as a screening test in the future. Platelet function in the clinical laboratory is currently measured using platelet aggregometry. In the aggregometer, agonists such as collagen, ADP, ristocetin, arachidonic acid, and thrombin are added to platelet-rich plasma, and the clumping of platelets over time is measured by an automated machine. At the same time, other instruments measure the release of granular contents such as ATP from the platelets after activation. In this manner, the ability of platelets to aggregate and their metabolic activity can be assessed simultaneously. Mild disorders can frequently be managed with desmopressin (see hemophilia and von Willebrand disease treatment), but severe or life-threatening bleeding may require platelet transfusions. Because transfused platelets must compete with the patient's abnormal platelets, the clinical response to transfusion may be less than that seen with thrombocytopenia due to decreased production.

476.12 Acquired Disorders of Platelet Function

A number of systemic illnesses are associated with platelet dysfunction, most commonly liver disease, kidney disease (uremia), and those disorders that trigger increased amounts of fibrin degradation products. These disorders frequently cause a prolonged bleeding time and are often associated with other abnormalities of the coagulation mechanism. The most important element of management is to treat the primary illness. If treatment of the primary process is not feasible, infusions of desmopressin have been helpful in augmenting hemostasis and correcting the bleeding time. In some patients, transfusions of platelets and/or cryoprecipitate have also been helpful in improving hemostasis.

Many drugs alter platelet function. The most commonly used drug in adults that alters platelet function is acetylsalicylic acid (aspirin). Aspirin irreversibly acetylates the enzyme cyclooxygenase, which is critical in the formation of thromboxane A$_2$. Aspirin usually causes moderate platelet dysfunction, which becomes more prominent if there is some other abnormality of the hemostatic mechanism. Other commonly used drugs that affect platelet function include other nonsteroidal anti-inflammatory drugs, valproic acid, and high-dose penicillin. Therefore, when evaluating a patient for a possible platelet dysfunction, it is critically important to exclude the presence of other exogenous agents and to study the patient, if possible, off all medications for 2 wk.

476.13 Congenital Abnormalities of Platelet Function

Severe platelet function defects usually present with petechiae and purpura shortly after birth, especially after vaginal delivery. Defects in the VWF receptor, the glycoprotein Ib (GPIb) complex, or the fibrinogen receptor, the glycoprotein IIb-IIIa (GPIIb-IIIa) complex, cause severe congenital platelet dysfunction.

Bernard-Soulier syndrome, a congenital bleeding disorder, is characterized by thrombocytopenia with giant platelets and a markedly prolonged bleeding time (>20 minutes). Platelet aggregation tests show absent ristocetin-induced platelet aggregation but normal aggregation to all other agonists. Studies of VWF are normal. Ristocetin induces the binding of VWF to platelets. The cause for this severe platelet dysfunction is the absence or severe deficiency of the VWF receptor (GPIb complex) on the platelet membrane. This complex interacts with the platelet cytoskeleton; the defect in this interaction is thought to be the cause for the large platelet size. Bernard-Soulier syndrome is inherited as an autosomal recessive disorder.

Glanzmann thrombasthenia is a congenital disorder associated with severe platelet dysfunction that yields a prolonged bleeding time and a normal platelet count. The platelet morphology and size are normal on the peripheral blood smear. The bleeding time is markedly prolonged. Aggregation studies show abnormality of aggregation with all agonists used except ristocetin, because ristocetin agglutinates platelets and does not require a metabolically active platelet. This disorder is caused by deficiency of the platelet fibrinogen receptor, GPIIb-IIIa, an integrin complex on the platelet surface that undergoes conformational changes when platelets are activated. Fibrinogen binds to this complex and causes platelets to aggregate. This disorder is inherited in an autosomal recessive manner.

Hereditary deficiency of platelet storage granules occurs in two well-characterized but rare syndromes that involve deficiency of intracytoplasmic granules. **Dense body deficiency** is characterized by the absence of the granules that contain ADP, ATP, Ca^{2+}, and serotonin. This disorder is diagnosed by absent release of ATP on platelet aggregation studies and ideally characterized by electron microscopic studies. **Gray platelet syndrome** is caused by the absence of platelet α granules resulting in platelets that appear gray on Wright stain of peripheral blood. This rare syndrome has absent aggregation and release with most agonists other than thrombin and ristocetin. Electron microscopic studies are diagnostic.

Other Hereditary Disorders of Platelet Function. Abnormalities in the pathways of platelet activation and release of granular contents cause a heterogeneous group of platelet function defects that are usually manifested as increased bruising, epistaxis, and/or menorrhagia. Symptoms may be subtle and are often made more obvious by high-risk surgery, such as tonsillectomy/adenoidectomy, or by administration of nonsteroidal antiinflammatory drugs. In the laboratory, the bleeding time is variable, although it is frequently but not always prolonged. Platelet aggregation studies show deficient aggregation with one or two agonists and/or abnormal release of granular contents.

Formation of thromboxane from arachidonic acid after activation of phospholipase is critical to normal platelet function. Deficiency or dysfunction of enzymes such as cyclooxygenase and thromboxane synthase, which metabolize arachidonic acid, causes abnormal platelet function. In the aggregometer, platelets from such patients fail to aggregate in response to arachidonic acid.

The most common platelet function defects are those characterized by a variable bleeding time and abnormal aggregation with one or two agonists, usually ADP and/or collagen. These patients have normal aggregation with thrombin. Some of these individuals have only decreased release of ATP from intracytoplasmic granules. This selective release defect is a common cause of a mild platelet function defect.

Treatment of Platelet Function Defects. Successful treatment depends on the severity of the diagnosis and of the hemorrhagic event. In all but the severe platelet function defects, desmopressin, 0.3 μg/kg IV, may be used for mild to moderate bleeding episodes. In addition to its effect on stimulating levels of VWF and factor VIII, desmopressin corrects the bleeding time and provides normal hemostasis in many individuals with mild to moderate platelet function defects. For individuals with Bernard-Soulier

syndrome or Glanzmann thrombasthenia, platelet transfusions, 1 U/5–10 kg, will correct the defect in hemostasis and may be life-saving. Both alloantibodies and anti-HLA antibodies that may develop after numerous platelet transfusions may limit the effectiveness of platelet transfusion therapy. In such patients, the use of recombinant factor VIIa has been effective and is undergoing clinical trials. In both conditions, stem cell transplants would be expected to be curative. Because the first hemostatic event involves the GPIb receptor, partial stem cell reconstitution may be successful in Bernard-Soulier syndrome patients because the normal platelets would be those that preferentially adhere.

476.14 ■ Disorders of the Blood Vessels

Henoch-Schönlein Purpura (HSP). This syndrome is characterized by the sudden development of a purpuric rash, arthritis, abdominal pain, and renal involvement (see Chapter 157.1). The characteristic rash, consisting of petechiae and often palpable purpura, usually involves the lower extremities and buttocks. Coagulation studies are normal. The pathologic lesions in the skin, intestines, and synovium are a *leukocytoclastic angiitis*—inflammatory damage to the endothelium of the capillary and postcapillary venules mediated by WBCs and macrophages. The trigger for HSP is unknown. In the kidney the lesion is focal glomerulonephritis with deposition of IgA. Coagulation studies and the platelet count are normal in HSP.

Ehlers-Danlos Syndrome. This disorder of collagen structure causes easy bruising and poor wound healing (see Chapter 649). Suggestive findings on physical examination include soft, velvety skin that is hyperelastic and lax joints that are easily subluxed. More than 10 variants of Ehlers-Danlos syndrome have been described. The most serious forms have been associated with sudden rupture of visceral organs. Coagulation screening tests are usually normal, other than the bleeding time, which may be mildly prolonged. Platelet aggregation studies are either normal or mildly abnormal with deficient aggregation to collagen.

Acquired Disorders. Scurvy, chronic corticosteroid therapy, and severe malnutrition are associated with "weakening" of the collagen matrix that supports the blood vessels and therefore are associated with easy bruising and, particularly in the case of scurvy, bleeding gums and loosening of the teeth. Lesions of the skin that initially look like petechiae and purpura may be seen in vasculitic syndromes such as SLE.

Athreya B: Vasculitis in children. *Pediatr Clin North Am* 1995;42:1239.

Beardsley DS, Nathan DG: Platelet abnormalities in infancy and childhood. In Nathan DG, Orkin SH (editors): *Hematology of Infancy and Childhood*, 5th ed. Philadelphia, WB Saunders, 1998, pp 1585–1630.

Beighton P, De Paepe A, Steinmann B, et al: Ehlers-Danlos syndromes: Revised nosology. *Am J Med Genet* 1998;77:31.

Blanchette V, Imbach P, Andrew M, et al: Randomised trial of intravenous immunoglobulin G, intravenous anti-D, and oral prednisone in childhood acute immune thrombocytopenic purpura. *Lancet* 1994;344:703.

Brickell PM, Katz DR, Thrasher AJ: Wiskott-Aldrich syndrome: Current research concepts. *Br J Haematol* 1998;101:603.

Bussel JB, Zabusky MR, Berkowitz RL, et al: Fetal alloimmune thrombocytopenia. *N Engl J Med* 1997;337:22.

Drolet BA, Esterly NB, Frieden IJ: Hemangiomas in children. *N Engl J Med* 1999;341:173–81.

George JN, Woolf SH, Raskob GE, et al: Idiopathic thrombocytopenic purpura: A practice guideline developed by explicit methods for The American Society of Hematology. *Blood* 1996;88:3.

Lilleyman JS: Intracranial haemorrhage in idiopathic thrombocytopenic purpura. *Arch Dis Child* 1994;71:251.

Levy GG, Nichols WC, Lian EC, et al: Mutations in a member of the ADAMTS gene family cause thrombotic thrombocytopenic purpura. *Nature* 2001;413:488–94.

Sarkar M, Mulliken JB, Kozakewich HP, et al: Thrombocytopenic coagulopathy (Kasabach-Merritt phenomenon) is associated with kaposiform hemangioendothelioma and not with common infantile hemangioma. *Plast Reconstr Surg* 1997;100:1377.

Sutor AH: Thrombocytosis in childhood. *Semin Thromb Hemost* 1995;21:330.

SECTION 8 *The Spleen*
James French and Bruce M. Camitta

Chapter 477
Anatomy and Function of the Spleen

Anatomy. The splenic precursor is recognizable by the 5th wk of gestation. At birth, the spleen weighs approximately 11 g. Thereafter, it enlarges until puberty, reaching an average weight of 135 g before diminishing in size during adulthood. The major splenic components are a lymphoid compartment (white pulp) and a filtering system (red pulp). The white pulp consists of peri-arterial lymphatic sheaths of T cells with embedded germinal centers containing B cells. The red pulp has a skeleton of fixed reticular cells, mobile macrophages, partially collapsed endothelial passages (cords of Billroth), and splenic sinuses. A marginal zone rich in dendritic (antigen-presenting) cells separates the red pulp from the white. The splenic capsule contains smooth muscle and contracts in response to epinephrine. Approximately 10% of the blood delivered to the spleen flows rapidly through a closed vascular network. The other 90% flows more slowly through an open system (the splenic cords) where it is filtered through 1–5 μm slits before entering the splenic sinuses.

Function. Unique anatomy and blood flow enable the spleen to perform reservoir, filtering, and immunologic functions more effectively. The spleen receives 5–6% of the cardiac output but normally contains only 25 mL of blood. It can retain much more when it enlarges. Hematopoiesis is a major splenic function from 3–6 mo of fetal life but then disappears. Splenic blood formation can be resumed in patients with myelofibrosis or severe hemolytic anemia. Factor VIII and platelets are stored in the spleen and can be released by stress or an epinephrine injection. Thrombocytosis and leukocytosis occur with loss of the splenic reservoir function. The high platelet counts do not appear to be associated with an increased risk of thrombosis in children.

Slow blood flow past macrophages and through small openings in the sinus walls facilitates the filtering functions of the spleen. Excess membrane is removed from young red blood cells (RBCs); loss of this function is characterized by target cells, poikilocytosis, and decreased osmotic fragility. The spleen is the primary site for destruction of old RBCs; this function is assumed by other reticuloendothelial cells after splenectomy. The spleen also removes damaged and abnormal cells such as spherocytes and antibody-coated RBCs. Intracytoplasmic inclusions may be removed from RBCs without cell lysis. Functional or anatomic hyposplenia is characterized by continued circulation of cells containing nuclear remnants (Howell-Jolly bodies), denatured hemoglobin (Heinz bodies), and other debris in the RBC. The latter may appear as "pits" on indirect microscopy. The spleen may be an important site of antibody production in immune thrombocytopenia.

Immunoglobulin, properdin, and tuftsin are produced in the spleen. The spleen has a minor role in antibody responses to intramuscularly or subcutaneously injected antigens but is required for early antibody production after exposure to intravenous antigens. Thus, young (nonimmune) or hyposplenic individuals are at increased risk for sepsis caused by pneumococci and other encapsulated bacteria. The spleen can also use phagocytosis to trap and destroy intracellular parasites. The spleen may be an important site of antibody production in immune thrombocytopenic purpura.

Chadburn A: The spleen: Anatomy and anatomical function. *Semin Hematol* 2000;37 (Suppl 1):13–21.
Steininger B, Barth P: Microanatomy and function of the spleen. *Adv Anat Embryol Cell Biol* 2000;151:1–101.

Chapter 478
Splenomegaly

Clinical Manifestations. A soft, thin spleen may be palpable in 15% of neonates, 10% of normal children, and 5% of adolescents. However, in most individuals, the spleen must be two to three times its normal size before it is palpable. The spleen is best examined in a supine patient by palpating across the abdomen toward the left costal margin from below as the patient inspires deeply. One should remember that an enlarged spleen may descend into the pelvis; thus, when splenomegaly is suspected, the abdominal examination should begin at a lower starting point. Superficial abdominal venous distention may be present when splenomegaly is a result of portal hypertension. Radiologic detection or confirmation of splenic enlargement is done with ultrasonography, CT, or a technetium-99m sulfur colloid scan. The latter also assesses splenic function.

Differential Diagnosis. Specific causes of splenomegaly are listed in Box 478–1. Unique problems are discussed next.

Pseudosplenomegaly. Abnormally elongated mesenteric connections may produce a wandering or ptotic spleen. An enlarged left lobe of the liver, a left upper quadrant mass, or a splenic hematoma may be mistaken for splenomegaly. Splenic cysts may contribute to splenomegaly or mimic it; these may be congenital (epidermoid) or acquired (pseudocyst) after trauma or infarction. Cysts are usually asymptomatic and are found on radiologic evaluation. Splenosis after splenic rupture or an accessory spleen (present in 10% of normal individuals) may also mimic splenomegaly; most, however, are not palpable. The syndrome of *congenital polysplenism* includes cardiac defects, left-sided organ anomalies, bilobed lungs, biliary atresia, and pseudosplenomegaly (see Chapter 424.11)

Hypersplenism. Hypersplenism is characterized by increased splenic function (sequestration or destruction of circulating cells), which results in peripheral blood cytopenias, increased bone marrow activity, and splenomegaly. It is usually secondary to another disease and may be cured by treatment of the underlying condition or, if absolutely necessary, moderated by splenectomy.

Congestive Splenomegaly (Banti's Syndrome). Splenomegaly may result from obstruction in the hepatic, portal, or splenic veins. Wilson disease, galactosemia, biliary atresia, and α-antitrypsin deficiency result in hepatic inflammation, fibrosis, and vascular obstruction. Congenital abnormalities of the portal or splenic veins may cause vascular obstruction. Septic omphalitis or umbilical venous catheterization in neonates may also result in secondary obliteration of these vessels. Splenic venous flow may be obstructed by masses of sickled erythrocytes. When the spleen is the site of vascular obstruction, splenectomy cures hypersplenism. However, the obstruction usually is in the hepatic or portal systems, and portocaval shunting may be more helpful, because both portal hypertension and thrombocytopenia contribute to variceal bleeding.

■ **BOX 478–1. Common Causes of Splenomegaly**

INFECTION

Bacterial: Typhoid fever, endocarditis, septicemia, abscess

Viral: Epstein-Barr, cytomegalovirus, and others

Protozoal: Malaria, toxoplasmosis

HEMATOLOGIC PROCESSES

Hemolytic anemia: Congenital, acquired

Extramedullary hematopoiesis: Thalassemia, osteopetrosis, myelofibrosis

NEOPLASMS

Malignant: Leukemia, lymphoma, histiocytoses, metastatic tumors

Benign: Hemangioma, hamartoma

METABOLIC DISEASES

Lipidoses: Niemann-Pick, Gaucher diseases

Mucopolysaccharidosis infiltration: Histiocytosis

CONGESTION

Cirrhosis or hepatic fibrosis

Hepatic portal or splenic vein obstruction

Congestive heart failure

CYSTS

Congenital (true cysts)

Acquired (pseudocysts)

MISCELLANEOUS

Lupus erythematosus, sarcoidosis, rheumatoid arthritis

Grover SA, Barkun AN, Sackett DL: Does this patient have splenomegaly? *JAMA* 1993;270:2218–21.

Chapter 479
Hyposplenism, Splenic Trauma, and Splenectomy

Congenital absence of the spleen is associated with complex cyanotic heart defects, dextrocardia, bilateral trilobed lungs, and heterotopic abdominal organs (Ivemark's syndrome; see Chapter 424.11). Splenic function is usually normal in children with congenital polysplenia. *Functional hyposplenism* may occur in normal neonates, especially premature infants. Children with sickle cell hemoglobinopathies may develop splenic hypofunction as early as 6 mo of age. Initially, this is caused by vascular obstruction, which can be reversed with red blood cell (RBC) transfusions. The spleen eventually autoinfarcts, resulting in a fibrotic, permanently nonfunctioning spleen. Functional hyposplenism may also occur in malaria, after irradiation to the left upper quadrant, and when the reticuloendothelial function of the spleen is overwhelmed (as in severe hemolytic anemias or metabolic storage diseases). Splenic hypofunction has been reported occasionally in patients with vasculitides, nephritis, inflammatory bowel disease, coeliac disease, Pearson syndrome, Fanconi anemia, and graft versus host disease. Splenic hypofunction is characterized by RBC inclusions in peripheral blood smears, "pits" on interference microscopy, and poor uptake of technetium on spleen scan. Patients with functional hyposplenism or asplenia are at increased risk of sepsis from encapsulated organisms.

Trauma. Injury to the spleen may occur with left flank or abdominal trauma. Small splenic capsular tears may cause abdominal or referred left shoulder pain as a result of peritoneal irritation by blood. Larger tears result in more severe blood loss with similar pain and signs of hypovolemia. Previously enlarged spleens (as in infectious mononucleosis) are more likely to rupture with minor trauma.

Treatment of a small capsular injury should include careful observation with attention to changes in vital signs or abdominal findings, serial hemoglobin determinations, and the availability of prompt surgical intervention should a patient's condition deteriorate. RBC transfusion requirements should be minimal (<25 mL/kg/48 hr). These patients are usually hospitalized 10–14 days and have their activities restricted for months. A laparotomy with or without splenectomy is indicated for more marked abdominal bleeding, for clinical instability or deterioration, or when other organ damage is suspected. Partial splenectomy and splenic repairs should be substituted for total splenectomy when feasible.

Splenectomy. Because of the risk of postoperative sepsis, splenectomy should be limited to specific indications. These include splenic rupture, anatomic defects, severe hemolytic anemias, immune cytopenias, metabolic storage diseases, secondary hypersplenism, and (rarely) surgical indications, including exposure of the left upper quadrant. The major long-term risk of splenectomy is sudden overwhelming infection (sepsis or meningitis). This risk is especially high in children younger than 5 yr at the time of surgery. The risk of sepsis is less after splenectomies performed for trauma, RBC membrane defects, and immune thrombocytopenia (2–4%) than when there is pre-existing immune deficiency (Wiskott-Aldrich syndrome, Hodgkin disease) or reticuloendothelial blockade (storage diseases, severe hemolytic anemias) (8–30%). Laparoscopic splenectomy has decreased morbidity and hospitalization time after splenectomy.

Encapsulated bacteria such as *Streptococcus pneumoniae* (>60% of cases), *Haemophilus influenzae,* and *Neisseria meningitides* account for more than 80% of post-splenectomy sepsis. Because the spleen is responsible for filtering the blood and early antibody responses, sepsis (with or without meningitis) can progress rapidly, leading to death within 12–24 hr of onset. Febrile splenectomized patients should be treated promptly with antibiotics. This should be initiated at home if access to definitive medical care will be delayed. A broad-spectrum cephalosporin (cefotaxime: 50 mg/kg q 8 hr) or vancomycin (10 mg/kg q 6 hr) to cover penicillin-resistant pneumococci is recommended until specific antibiotic susceptibility is known. Splenectomized patients are also at increased risk for contracting protozoal infections such as malaria and babesiosis.

Preoperative, intraoperative, and postoperative management may decrease the risk of post-splenectomy infection. It is important to be certain of the need for splenectomy and, if possible, to postpone the operation until the patient is 5 yr of age or older. Vaccination with pneumococcal, *H. influenzae,* and meningococcal vaccines before splenectomy may be helpful to reduce post-splenectomy sepsis. However, vaccine efficacy is lower in children younger than 2 yr and in immune-suppressed patients. In trauma cases, splenic repair or partial splenectomy should be considered in an attempt to preserve splenic function. Partial splenectomy or partial splenic embolization may be sufficient to ameliorate some forms of hemolytic anemia. Up to 50% of children whose spleen is removed for trauma have spontaneous splenosis; surgical splenosis (distributing small pieces of spleen throughout the abdomen) has been suggested as a way to decrease the risk of sepsis in patients whose splenectomy is necessitated by trauma. However, in both of these settings, the splenic tissue that regrows frequently has inadequate function. Prophylaxis with oral penicillin V (125 mg twice daily for children younger than 5 yr; 250 mg twice daily for children 5 yr or older) should be given for at least 2 yr after splenectomy (to at least 6 yr of age). Prophylaxis may be continued into adulthood for higher-risk patients. Penicillin reduces the risk of pneumococcal sepsis in patients with hemoglobin SS, but other populations have not been well studied. Although the greatest risk is in the immediate postoperative period, reports of deaths occurring many years after splenectomy suggest that the risk (and need for prophylaxis) may be lifelong. Other postoperative measures include patient and family education, wearing a medical information bracelet, and prompt evaluation and treatment of fevers.

Bader-Meunier B, Gauthier F, Archambaud F, et al: Long-term evaluation of the beneficial effect of subtotal splenectomy for management of hereditary spherocytosis. *Blood* 2001;97:399–403.

Hansen K, Singer DB: Asplenic-hyposplenic overwhelming sepsis: Postsplenectomy sepsis revisited. *Pediatr Dev Pathol* 2001;4:105–21.

Pachter HL, Grau J: The current status of splenic preservation. *Adv Surg* 2000;34:137–74.

Stylianos S: Evidence-based guidelines for resource utilization in children with isolated spleen or liver injury. *J Pediatr Surg* 2000;35:164–9.

Working Party for the British Committee for Standards in Haematology, Clinical Haematology Task Force: Guidelines for the prevention and treatment of infection in patients with an absent or dysfunctional spleen. *BMJ* 1996;312:430–4.

SECTION 9 *The Lymphatic System*
Bruce M. Camitta

Chapter 480
Anatomy and Function of the Lymphatic System

The lymphatic system includes circulating lymphocytes, lymphatic vessels, lymph nodes, spleen, tonsils, adenoids, Peyer patches, and thymus. Lymph, an ultrafiltrate of blood, is collected by lymphatic capillaries that are present in all organs except the brain and the heart. These join to form progressively larger vessels that drain regions of the body. During their course, the lymphatic vessels carry lymph to the lymph nodes. In the nodes, lymph is filtered through sinuses where particulate matter and infectious organisms are phagocytosed, processed, and presented as antigens to surrounding lymphocytes. This results in stimulation of antibody production, T-cell responses, and cytokine secretion (see Chapter 113).

Lymph composition can vary with the site of lymph drainage. It is usually clear, but drainage of lymph from the intestinal tract may be milky (chylous) because of the presence of fats. The protein content is intermediate between an exudate and a transudate. The protein level may be increased with inflammation or in lymph from the liver or intestines. Lymph also contains variable numbers of lymphocytes.

Chapter 481
Abnormalities of Lymphatic Vessels

Abnormalities of the lymph vessels may be congenital or acquired. Signs and symptoms may result from increased lymphatic tissue mass or from leakage of lymph. *Lymphangiectasia* is a dilation of the lymphatics. Pulmonary lymphangiectasia causes respiratory distress (see Chapter 383). Involvement of the intestinal lymphatics causes hypoproteinemia and lymphocytopenia secondary to loss of lymph into the intestines (see Chapter 320.10). *Lymphangioma* (cystic hygroma) is a mass of dilated lymphatics. Some of these lesions also have a hemangiomatous component (see Chapter 497). Because surgical treatment is complicated by a high incidence of recurrence, intralesional sclerosing with OK-432, a streptococcal derivative, has been used in selected patients. *Lymphatic dysplasia* may cause multisystem problems. These include lymphedema, chylous ascites, chylothorax, and lymphangiomas of bone, lung, or other locations.

Lymphedema is caused by obstruction of lymph flow. Congenital lymphedema may be found in Turner syndrome, Noonan syndrome, and the autosomal dominantly inherited Milroy disease. *Lymphedema praecox* causes progressive lower extremity edema, usually in females (10–25 yr old). Lymphedema has also been found in association with intestinal lymphangiectasia, cerebrovascular malformation, ptosis, yellow dystrophic nails, distichiasis, and cholestasis. Acquired obstruction of the lymphatics can result from tumor, postirradiation fibrosis, filariasis, and postinflammatory scarring. Injury to the major lymphatic vessel can cause collection of lymph fluid in the abdomen (chylous ascites) and chest (chylothorax).

Lymphangitis is an inflammation of the lymphatics draining an area of infection. On examination, tender red streaks extend proximally from the infected site. Regional nodes may also be enlarged and tender. *Staphylococcus aureus* and group A streptococci are the most frequent pathogens.

Gallagher PG, Mahoney MJ, Gosche JR: Cystic hygroma in the fetus and newborn. *Semin Perinatol* 1999;23:341–56.

Luzatto C, Midrio P, Tchaprassi Z, et al: Sclerosing treatment of lymphangiomas with OK-432. *Arch Dis Child* 2000;82:316–8.

Mulliken JB, Fishman SJ, Burrows PE: Vascular anomalies. *Curr Pediatr Surg* 2000;37:527–84.

Orvidan LJ, Kasperbauer JL: Pediatric lymphangioma of the head and neck. *Ann Otol Rhinol Laryngol* 2000;109:411–21.

Chapter 482
Lymphadenopathy

Most lymph nodes are not palpable in the newborn infant. With antigenic exposure, lymphoid tissue increases in volume so that cervical, axillary, and inguinal nodes are often palpable during childhood. They are not considered enlarged until their diameter exceeds 1 cm for cervical or axillary nodes and 1.5 cm for inguinal nodes. Other lymph nodes usually are not palpable or visualized with plain radiographs.

Lymph node enlargement is caused by proliferation of normal lymphoid elements or to infiltration by malignant or phagocytic cells. In most patients, a careful history and a complete physical examination suggest the proper diagnosis (Box 482–1). Nonlymphoid masses (cervical rib, thyroglossal cyst, branchial sinus or cystic hygroma, goiter, sternomastoid muscle tumor, neurofibroma) occur frequently in the neck and less often in other areas. Acutely infected nodes are usually tender. There may also be erythema and warmth of the overlying skin. Fluctuance suggests abscess formation. Tuberculous nodes may be matted. With chronic infection, most of the just described signs are not

■ **BOX 482–1. Evaluation of Possible Adenopathy**

1. Is the swelling a lymph node?
2. Is the node enlarged?
3. What are the characteristics of the node?
4. Is the adenopathy local or generalized?

present. Tumor-bearing nodes are usually firm and nontender and may be matted or fixed to the skin or underlying structures.

Generalized adenopathy (enlargement of more than two non-contiguous node regions) is caused by systemic disease (Box 482–2) and is often accompanied by abnormal physical findings in other systems. In contrast, localized adenopathy is most frequently the result of infection in the involved node and/or its drainage area (Boxes 482–3 and 482–4).

Regional lymphadenitis, as a result of infectious agents other than bacteria, may be characterized by atypical anatomic areas, a prolonged course, a draining sinus, lack of prior pyogenic infection, and unusual clues in the history (cat scratches, tuberculosis exposure, venereal disease).

A firm fixed node should always raise the question of malignancy, regardless of the presence or absence of systemic symptoms or other abnormal physical findings.

Evaluation and treatment of lymphadenopathy is guided by the probable etiologic factor, as determined from the history and physical examination. For example, many patients with cervical adenopathy have a history of viral infection and need no intervention. If a bacterial infection is suspected, antibiotic treatment covering at least streptococci and staphylococci is indicated. Surgical drainage is required if an abscess forms. The size of involved nodes should be documented before treatment. Failure to decrease in size within 10–14 days suggests the need for further evaluation. This may include complete blood cell count with differential; Epstein-Barr virus, cytomegalovirus, *Toxoplasma*, and cat-scratch disease titers; antistreptolysin O or anti-DNAase serologic tests; tuberculin skin test; and chest radiograph. If these are not diagnostic, consultation with infectious disease or oncology specialists may be helpful. Biopsy should be considered if there is persistent or unexplained fever, weight loss, night sweats, hard nodes, or fixation of the nodes to surrounding tissues. Biopsy may also be indicated if there is an increase in size over baseline in 2 wk, no decrease in size in 4–6 wk, no regression to "normal" in 8–12 wk, or the development of new signs and symptoms.

■ **BOX 482–2. Common Causes of Generalized Lymphadenopathy**

AUTOIMMUNE DISEASES
Dermatomyositis, lupus erythematosus, rheumatoid arthritis

DRUG REACTIONS

INFECTIONS
Cytomegalovirus, histoplasmosis, HIV, HTLV, mononucleosis, rubella, rubeola, toxoplasmosis, varicella, tuberculosis

LIPID STORAGE DISEASES
Gaucher disease, Niemann-Pick disease

MALIGNANCIES
Primary: histiocytic disorders, Hodgkin disease, lymphoproliferative disease (PTLPD), non-Hodgkin lymphoma, post transplant lymphoproliferation
Metastatic: leukemia, neuroblastoma, rhabdomyosarcoma

OTHER
Castleman disease, sarcoidosis, serum sickness

■ **BOX 482–3. Drainage Areas of Regional Nodes**

ABDOMINAL AND PELVIC
Abdomen, lower extremity, pelvic organs

AXILLARY
Arm, breast, chest wall, hand, upper and lateral abdominal wall

CERVICAL
External ear, larynx, parotid, superficial tissues of the head and neck, thyroid, tongue, trachea

EPITROCHLEAR
Forearm, hand

ILIAC
Bladder, lower abdomen, part of the genitalia, urethra

INGUINAL
Gluteal region, lower anal canal, lower extremity, perineum, scrotum and penis in males, skin of the lower abdomen, vulva and vagina in females

MEDIASTINAL
Thoracic viscera

OCCIPITAL
Posterior scalp

POPLITEAL
Knee joint, skin of the lateral lower leg and foot

PREAURICULAR
Cheek, conjunctivas, eyelid, temporal scalp

SUBMAXILLARY/SUBMENTAL
Buccal mucosa, gums, teeth, tongue

SUPRACLAVICULAR
Abdomen, arms, head, lungs, mediastinum, neck, superficial thorax
Left supraclavicular adenopathy is usually due to an intra-abdominal problem.
Right supraclavicular adenopathy is usually due to an intrathoracic problem.

■ **BOX 482–4. Common Causes of Regional Node Enlargement**

ABDOMINAL
Malignancies, mesenteric adenitis

AXILLARY
Cat-scratch disease, infections of the arm/chest wall, malignancies

CERVICAL
Kawasaki disease, malignancies, mononucleosis, sinus histiocytosis (Rosai-Dorfman disease), streptococcal/staphylococcal adenitis or tonsillitis, toxoplasmosis

ILIOINGUINAL
Infections of the leg, groin

MEDIASTINAL
Coccidioidomycosis, histoplasmosis, malignancies, sarcoidosis (T-cell lymphoma/leukemia, teratoma, thymoma, other), tuberculosis

OCCIPITAL
Roseola, rubella, scalp infections

PERIAURICULAR
Cat-scratch disease, eye infections

SUBMAXILLARY
Histoplasmosis, Hodgkin or non-Hodgkin lymphoma, tuberculosis

Haberman TM, Steensma DP: Lymphadenopathy. *Mayo Clin Proc* 2000;75:723–32.
Kelly CS, Kelly RE Jr: Lymphadenopathy in children. *Pediatr Clin North Am* 1998;45:875–88.

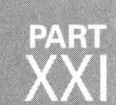

PART XXI Cancer and Benign Tumors

Chapter 483

Epidemiology of Childhood and Adolescent Cancer

James G. Gurney and Melissa L. Bondy

Only about 1% of new cancer cases in the United States occur in children age 19 yr or younger (~12,400 cases/yr), yet children dying of cancer lose an average of 69.5 yr of life, a span far exceeding the average loss from any adult cancer. Despite impressively improved 5-yr survival probabilities for children diagnosed with cancer, from 56% in 1974 to over 75% in 2000, malignant neoplasms remain the second leading death cause (10.6% of all deaths) among 1–14 yr olds in the United States. Although most pediatric cancer patients survive their disease and the associated treatment, the long-term consequences of cure, the **late adverse effects**, are only now becoming a focus of clinical research. The number of children alive today who either have or had a malignancy is difficult to determine. Prevalence estimates from the National Cancer Institute for U.S. children age 19 yr or younger range from 90,000–174,000.

Pediatric cancers differ markedly from adult malignancies in their prognosis and their distribution by histology and tumor site. Acute lymphoblastic leukemia, brain cancers, lymphomas, and sarcomas of soft tissue and bone predominate in children and adolescents (Table 483–1). In adults, in contrast, epithelial tumors of organs such as lung, colon, breast, and prostate are most common. Unlike incidence patterns in adults where cancer rates tend to rapidly increase with increasing age, relatively wide age variability exists during development, with two peaks, in early childhood and in adolescence (Fig. 483–1). During the 1st yr of life, **embryonal tumors** such as neuroblastoma, Wilms' tumor (nephroblastoma), retinoblastoma, rhabdomyosarcoma, and medulloblastoma are most common (Fig. 483–2). These tumors, which are likely congenital, occur far less often among older children, whose developmental processes and cell differentiation have slowed considerably, and are extremely unusual in adults. Embryonal tumors combine with acute leukemias, non-Hodgkin lymphomas, and gliomas, which together peak in incidence from 2–5 yr of age, for the highest cancer incidence during childhood and adolescence other than in infancy. As children age, especially after they pass puberty, bone malignancies, Hodgkin disease, **gonadal germ cell malignancies** (testicular and ovarian carcinomas), and various carcinomas such as thyroid cancer and malignant melanoma increase in incidence. It appears that adolescence is a transitional period between the common early childhood malignancies and characteristic carcinomas of adulthood.

Pediatric oncologists face unique challenges because treatment with radiation, surgery, and chemotherapy may adversely affect growth and development and may cause serious long-term medical and psychosocial effects. Given the relative rarity of specific types of childhood cancer and the sophisticated technology and expertise required for diagnosis, treatment, and monitoring of late effects, all children with cancer should be treated on standardized clinical protocols in clinical research settings whenever possible.

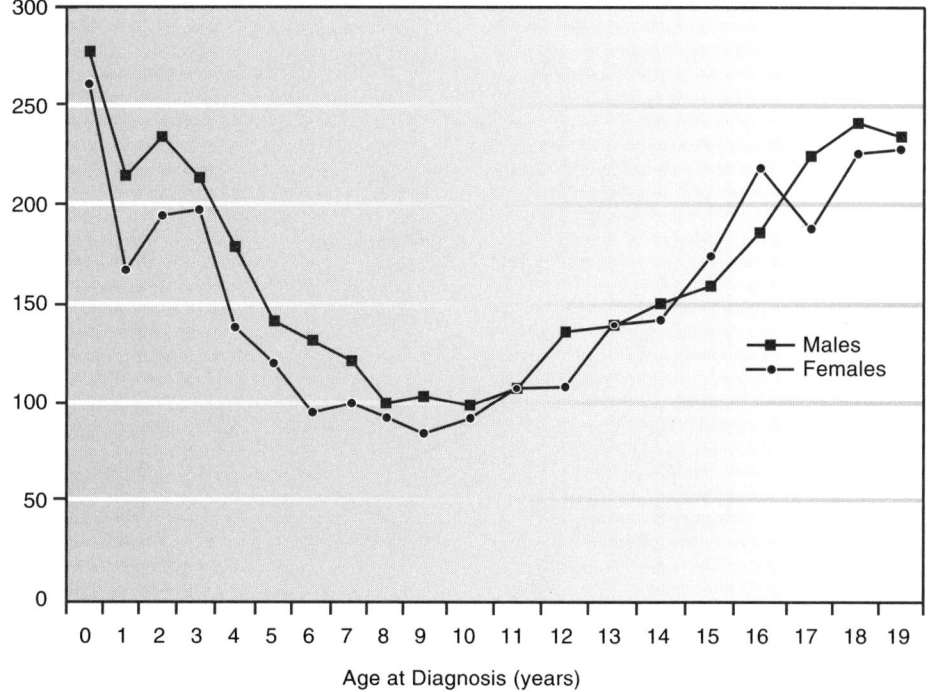

FIGURE 483–1. Age- and sex-specific cancer incidence rates per million children in the United States. (From Ries LAG, Smith MA, Gurney JG, et al (editors): *Cancer Incidence and Survival Among Children and Adolescents: United States SEER Program 1975–1995.* Bethesda, MD, National Cancer Institute, SEER Program, 1999. http://seer.cancer.gov/publications/childhood/

TABLE 483–1. Rates of Malignant Neoplasms by Age Among U.S. Children

	Average Age-Adjusted Annual Incidence Rates per Million Children, 1975–1998						5-yr Survival Percentage, ≤19 yr of Age at Diagnosis, 1985–1997
	≤14 y	≤19 y	≤4 y	5–9 y	10–14 y	15–19 y	
All malignancies combined	136.4	151.4	193.7	107.9	116.5	197.1	75.2
Leukemias	40.6	36.2	67.6	34.8	24.0	22.6	69.6
Acute lymphoblastic	31.6	26.6	54.8	28.0	15.8	11.4	78.6
Acute myeloid	4.3	4.7	5.2	3.4	4.2	6.0	40.8
Brain and central nervous system	28.7	26.3	32.7	30.3	23.9	19.2	67.2
Astrocytoma	14.3	13.7	13.4	15.3	14.0	12.1	76.4
PNET/medulloblastoma	6.1	5.1	8.1	6.8	3.8	1.8	57.3
Ependymoma	2.6	2.2	5.2	1.5	1.4	0.9	58.7
Lymphomas	15.4	24.4	6.9	13.3	24.3	51.7	83.9
Hodgkin	6.4	13.9	0.5	4.2	13.3	36.8	92.2
Non-Hodgkin	5.4	7.0	3.5	5.4	7.1	11.8	73.4
Bone	6.8	8.8	1.2	5.0	13.1	15.0	65.1
Osteosarcoma	3.7	4.8	0.5	2.4	7.5	8.3	65.3
Ewing sarcoma	2.5	3.1	0.6	2.3	4.3	4.8	58.7
Soft tissue sarcomas	9.7	11.0	10.2	8.5	10.3	15.0	70.9
Rhabdomyosarcomas	4.7	4.4	6.5	4.8	3.1	3.5	65.1
Germ cell	4.7	10.3	6.1	2.2	6.1	27.3	88.6
Carcinomas	5.3	14.2	1.6	2.9	10.7	41.3	89.0
Hepatic	1.8	1.6	4.5	0.6	0.6	0.9	54.4
Sympathetic nervous system	10.3	8.0	29.7	3.2	1.1	1.1	66.1
Retinoblastoma	3.8	2.8	11.9	0.6	0.1	0.0	93.9
Renal	8.3	6.5	19.2	6.1	1.3	1.2	89.9

PNET = primitive neuroectodermal tumor. From Ries LAG, Eisner MP, Kosary CI, et al (editors): SEER Cancer Statistics Review, 1973–1998. Bethesda MD, National Cancer Institute, 2001; http://seer.cancer.gov/childhood/

Promoting such treatment, the Children's Oncology Group facilitates clinical, biologic, and epidemiologic research in 238 affiliated institutions in North America. These centers have the required facilities and expertise and are committed to learning more about and defining the optimal treatment of pediatric malignancy through participation in national clinical trials. Such coordinated treatment efforts have substantially increased survival for many children with cancer. The continuing poor prognosis, however, for specific malignancies such as acute myeloid leukemia, high-risk neuroblastoma, and many brain cancers demands continuing concerted and coordinated clinical research efforts. So, too, does the need for clinical and epidemiologic research on the late effects of therapy.

RISK FACTORS

Childhood neoplasms comprise a diverse array of malignant (cancers) and nonmalignant tumors arising from disorders of genetic processes involved in control of cellular growth and development. Although a number of genetic conditions are associated with elevated risks for childhood cancer, such conditions are believed to account for less than 5% of all occurrences. The most notable genetic conditions that impart childhood cancer susceptibility are neurofibromatosis types 1 and 2, Down syndrome, Beckwith-Wiedemann syndrome, tuberous sclerosis, von Hippel-Lindau disease, xeroderma pigmentosum, ataxia-telangiectasia, nevus basal cell carcinoma syndrome, and Li-Fraumeni (*P53*) syndrome.

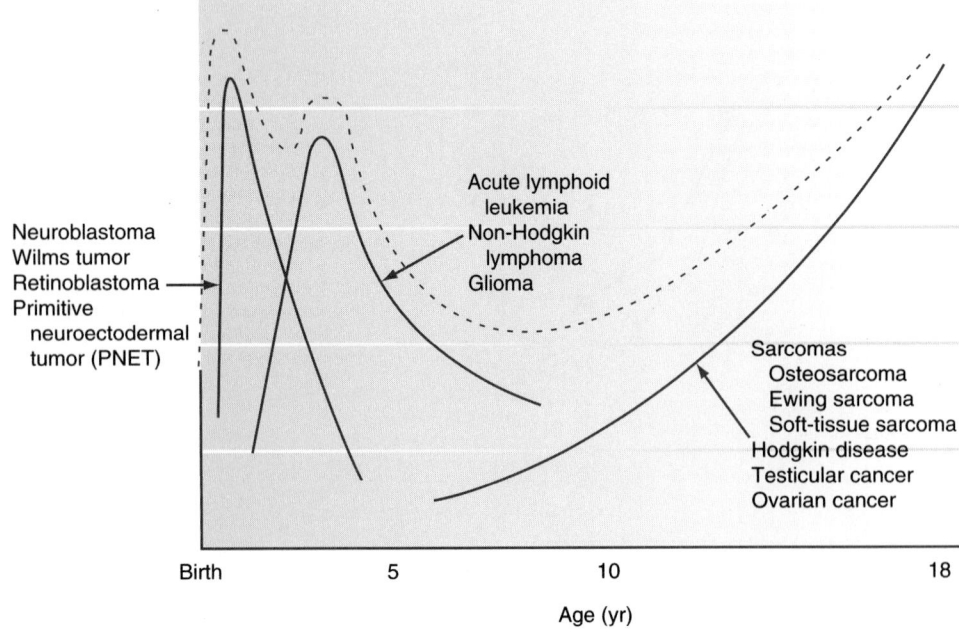

FIGURE 483–2. Incidence of the most common types of cancer in children by age. The cumulative incidence is shown as a dashed line. (Courtesy of Archie Bleyer, MD.)

TABLE 483–2. Known Risk Factors for Selected Pediatric Cancers

Cancer Type	Risk Factor	Comments
Acute lymphoid leukemia	Ionizing radiation	Although primarily of historical significance, prenatal diagnostic x-ray exposure increases risk. Therapeutic irradiation for cancer treatment also increases risk.
	Race	White children have a 2-fold higher rate than black children in the United States.
	Genetic conditions	Down syndrome is associated with an estimated 10- to 20-fold increased risk. Neurofibromatosis type 1, Bloom's syndrome, ataxia-telangiectasia, and Langerhans cell histiocytosis, among others, are associated with an elevated risk.
Acute myeloid leukemias	Chemotherapeutic agents	Alkylating agents and epipodophyllotoxins increase risk.
	Genetic conditions	Down syndrome and neurofibromatosis type 1 are strongly associated. Familial monosomy 7 and several other genetic syndromes are also associated with increased risk.
Brain cancers	Therapeutic ionizing radiation to the head	With the exception of cancer radiotherapy, higher risk from radiation treatment is essentially of historical importance.
	Genetic conditions	Neurofibromatosis type 1 is strongly associated with optic gliomas, and, to a lesser extent, with other CNS tumors. Tuberous sclerosis and several other genetic syndromes are associated with increased risk.
Hodgkin disease	Family history	Monozygotic twins and siblings of cases are at increased risk.
	Infections	Epstein-Barr virus is associated with increased risk.
Non-Hodgkin lymphoma	Immunodeficiency	Acquired and congenital immunodeficiency disorders, and immunosuppressive therapy, increase risk.
	Infections	Epstein-Barr virus is associated with Burkitt lymphoma in Africa.
Osteosarcoma	Ionizing radiation	Cancer radiotherapy and high radium exposure increase risk.
	Chemotherapy	Alkylating agents increase risk.
	Genetic conditions	Increased risk is apparent with Li-Fraumeni syndrome and hereditary retinoblastoma.
Ewing sarcoma	Race	White children have about a 9-fold higher incidence rate than black children in the United States.
Neuroblastoma		No established risk factors.
Retinoblastoma		No established nonhereditary risk factors.
Wilms tumor	Congenital anomalies	Aniridia, Beckwith-Wiedemann syndrome, and other congenital and genetic conditions are associated with increased risk.
	Race	Asian children reportedly have about half the rates of white and black children.
Rhabdomyosarcoma	Congenital anomalies and genetic conditions	Li-Fraumeni syndrome and neurofibromatosis type 1 are believed to be associated with increased risk. There is some concordance with major birth defects.
Hepatoblastoma	Genetic conditions	Beckwith-Wiedemann syndrome, hemihypertrophy, Gardner syndrome, and family history of adenomatous polyposis are associated with increased risk.
Malignant germ cell tumors	Cryptorchidism	Cryptorchidism is a risk factor for testicular germ cell tumors.

From Gurney JG, Bondy ML: Epidemiologic research methods and childhood cancer. In Pizzo PA, Poplack DG (editors): Principles and Practice of Pediatric Oncology, *4th ed. Philadelphia, Lippincott Williams & Wilkins, 2001, pp 13–20.*

Because of the relatively minor role of directly heritable conditions, research efforts in cancer epidemiology are moving to the exploration of potential interactions between genetic susceptibility traits and environmental exposures, but very few established environmental causes of childhood cancer are known (Table 483–2). Risk factors for the major pediatric cancers such as ionizing radiation exposure and several chemotherapeutic agents explain very few cases overall. Among environmental exposures studied, but currently without convincing evidence for a causal role, are non-ionizing power frequency electromagnetic fields, pesticides, parental occupational chemical exposures, dietary factors, and environmental cigarette smoke. Pediatric cancers have been associated with some viruses whose etiologic importance remains unclear, such as the polyomaviruses (BK, JC, and SV 40) that have been associated with brain cancer, and Epstein-Barr virus with non-Hodgkin lymphoma. The connection, also, of transplacental fetal exposures to pediatric cancer is largely unestablished in humans, with the exception of maternal diethylstilbestrol intake during pregnancy and subsequent vaginal cancer in adolescent female offspring. In notable contrast to adult epithelial tumors, a very low fraction of pediatric cancers, at least based on current evidence, appears to be explainable from known environmental exposures.

Ahlbom A, Cardis E, Green A, et al: Review of the epidemiologic literature on EMF and Health. ICNIRP (International Commission for Non-Ionizing Radiation Protection) Standing Committee on Epidemiology. *Environ Health Perspect* 2001;109(Suppl 6):911–33.

Gurney JG, Smith MA, Olshan AF, et al: Clues to the etiology of childhood brain cancer: *N*-nitroso compounds, polyomaviruses and other factors of interest. *Cancer Invest* 2001;19:640–50.

Gurney JG, Bondy ML: Epidemiologic research methods and childhood cancer. In Pizzo PA, Poplack DG (editors): *Principles and Practice of Pediatric Oncology.* Philadelphia, Lippincott Williams & Wilkins, 2002, pp 13–20.

Little J: *Epidemiology of Childhood Cancer.* Lyon, International Agency for Research on Cancer, 1999.

Look AT, Kirsch IR: Molecular basis of childhood cancer. In Pizzo PA, Poplack DG (editors): *Principles and Practice of Pediatric Oncology,* 4th ed. Philadelphia, Lippincott Williams & Wilkins, 2001, pp 45–87.

Neglia JP, Friedman DL, Yasui Y, et al: Second malignant neoplasms in five-year survivors of childhood cancer: Childhood Cancer Survivor Study. *J Natl Cancer Inst* 2001;93:618–29.

Plon SE, Malkin D: Childhood cancer and heredity. In Pizzo PA, Poplack DG (editors): *Principles and Practice of Pediatric Oncology,* 4th ed. Philadelphia, Lippincott Williams & Wilkins, 2001, pp 21–44.

Ries LAG, Smith MA, Gurney JG, et al (editors): *Cancer Incidence and Survival Among Children and Adolescents: United States SEER Program 1975–1995.* Bethesda, MD, National Cancer Institute, SEER Program, 1999.

Chapter 484

Molecular and Cellular Biology of Cancer *Laura L. Worth*

Cancer is a complex of diseases arising from alterations that can occur in a wide variety of genes. Alterations in normal cellular processes such as signal transduction, cell cycle control, DNA repair, cellular growth and differentiation, translational regulation, senescence, and apoptosis (programmed cell death) can result in a malignant phenotype.

GENES INVOLVED IN ONCOGENESIS

Two major classes of genes have been implicated in the development of cancer: oncogenes and tumor suppressor genes. **Proto-oncogenes** are cellular genes that are important for normal cellular function and code for various proteins, including transcriptional factors, growth factors, and growth factor receptors.

These proteins are vital components in the network of signal transduction that regulate cell growth, division, and differentiation. Proto-oncogenes can be altered to form **oncogenes**, genes that when translated can result in the malignant transformation of a cell.

The three main mechanisms by which proto-oncogenes can be activated include amplification, point mutations, and translocation (Table 484–1). *MYC*, which codes for a protein that regulates transcription, is an example of a proto-oncogene that is activated by amplification. Patients with neuroblastoma in which the *MYC* gene is amplified 10–300 fold have a poorer outcome. Point mutations can also activate proto-oncogenes. The *NRAS* proto-oncogene codes for a guanine nucleotide-binding protein with guanosine triphosphatase activity that is important in signal transduction and is mutated in 25–30% of acute nonmyelogenous leukemias, resulting in a constitutively active protein. The RET protein is a transmembrane tyrosine kinase receptor that is important in signal transduction. A point mutation in the *RET* gene results in the constitutive activation of a tyrosine kinase, as found in multiple neoplasia syndromes and familial thyroid carcinoma. The third mechanism by which proto-oncogenes become activated is chromosomal translocation. In some leukemias and lymphomas, transcription factor controlling sequences are relocated in front of T-cell receptors or immunoglobulin genes, resulting in unregulated transcription of the genes and leukemogenesis. Chromosomal translocations can also result in **fusion genes;** transcription of the fusion gene can result in the production of a chimeric protein with new and potentially oncogenic activity. Examples of cancers associated with fusion genes include the childhood solid tumors such as Ewing sarcoma [t(11;22)] and alveolar rhabdomyosarcoma [t(2;13) or t(1;13)]. The translocations result in novel proteins that are useful as diagnostic markers. The best described translocation in leukemia is the **Philadelphia chromosome t(9;22)**, which results in the BCR/ABL protein found in chronic myelogenous leukemia. This translocation results in a tyrosine kinase protein that is constitutively activated. In addition, the protein is localized to the cytoplasm instead of the nucleus, exposing the kinase to a new spectrum of substrates.

Alteration in the regulation of tumor suppressor genes is another mechanism involved in oncogenesis. Tumor suppressor genes are important regulators of cellular growth and programmed cell death or apoptosis. They have been called recessive oncogenes because the inactivation of both alleles of a tumor suppressor gene is required for expression of a malignant phenotype.

Knudson's **"two-hit" model of cancer development** was based on the observation of the behavior of the tumor suppressor gene *RB*. In sporadic cases of retinoblastoma, both alleles of the *RB* gene must be inactivated. However, in familial cases, children inherit an inactivated allele from one parent and consequently require the inactivation of the only remaining normal allele. This helps explain why familial cases of retinoblastoma

present earlier in childhood than do sporadic cases, because only one "hit" is required.

Another major tumor suppressor protein is p53, which is known as the "guardian of the genome" because it detects the presence of chromosomal damage and prevents the cell from dividing until repairs have been made. In the presence of damage beyond repair, p53 initiates apoptosis and the cell dies. More than 50% of all tumors have abnormal p53 proteins. Mutations in the *P53* gene are important in many cancers, including breast, colorectal, lung, esophageal, stomach, ovarian, and prostatic carcinomas as well as gliomas, sarcomas, and some leukemias.

SYNDROMES PREDISPOSING TO CANCER

Several syndromes are associated with an increased risk of developing malignancies, which can be characterized by different mechanisms (Table 484–2). One mechanism involves the inactivation of tumor suppressor genes, such as *RB* in familial retinoblastoma. Interestingly, patients with retinoblastoma in which one of the alleles is inactivated throughout all of the patient's cells are at very high risk for developing osteosarcoma. A familial syndrome, Li-Fraumeni syndrome, in which one mutant *P53* allele is inherited, has also been described in which patients can develop sarcomas, leukemias, and cancers of the breast, bone, lung, and brain. Neurofibromatosis is a condition characterized by the proliferation of cells of neural crest origin, leading to neurofibromas. These patients are at a higher risk of developing malignant schwannomas and pheochromocytomas. Neurofibromatosis is often inherited in an autosomal dominant fashion, although 50% of the cases present without a family history and occur secondary to the high rate of spontaneous mutations of the *NF1* gene.

A second mechanism responsible for inherited predisposition to develop cancer involves defects in DNA repair. Syndromes associated with an excessive number of broken chromosomes due to repair defects include Bloom syndrome (short stature, photosensitive telangiectatic erythema), ataxia-telangiectasia (childhood ataxia with progressive neuromotor degeneration), and Fanconi anemia (short stature, skeletal and renal anomalies, pancytopenia). Because of the decreased ability to repair chromosomal defects, cells accumulate abnormal DNA that results in significantly increased rates of cancer, especially leukemia. Xeroderma pigmentosum likewise increases the risk of skin cancer, owing to defects in repair of DNA damaged by ultraviolet light. These disorders display an autosomal recessive pattern.

A third category of inherited cancer predisposition is characterized by defects in immune surveillance. This group includes patients with Wiskott-Aldrich syndrome, severe combined immunodeficiency, common variable immunodeficiency, and the X-linked lymphoproliferative syndrome. The most common types of malignancy in these patients are lymphoma and leukemia. Cure rates for immunodeficient children with cancer are much poorer than for immunocompetent children with sim-

TABLE 484–1. Oncogene Activation in Pediatric Tumors

Mechanism	Chromosome	Genes	Protein Function	Tumor
Chromosomal translocation	t(9;22)	BCR-ABL	Chimeric tyrosine kinase	CML, ALL
	t(1;19)	E2A-PBX1	Chimeric transcription factor	Pre-B ALL
	t(14;18)	CMYC	Transcription factor	Burkitt lymphoma
	t(15;17)	APL-RARα	Chimeric transcription factor	APL
Gene amplification	Amplicon	NMYC	Transcription factor	Neuroblastoma
	Amplicon	EGFR	Growth factor receptor, tyrosine kinase	Glioblastoma
Point mutation	1p	NRAS	GTPase	AML
	10q	RET	Tyrosine kinase	MEN2

ALL = acute lymphocytic anemia; AML = acute myelocytic leukemia; APL = acute promyelocytic leukemia; CML = chronic myelocytic leukemia; MEN2 = multiple endocrine neoplasia type 2.

TABLE 484–2. Familial or Genetic Susceptibility to Malignancy

Disorder	Tumor/Cancer	Comment
Chromosomal Syndromes		
Chromosome 11p—(deletion) with sporadic aniridia	Wilms tumor	Associated with genitourinary anomalies, mental retardation, *WT1* gene
Chromosome 13q—(deletion)	Retinoblastoma, sarcoma	Associated with mental retardation, skeletal malformations: autosomal dominant (bilateral) or sporadic new mutation, *RB1* gene
Trisomy 21	Lymphocytic or nonlymphocytic leukemia	Risk is 15 times normal
Klinefelter syndrome (47, XXY)	Breast cancer, extragonadal germ cell tumors	
Gonadal dysgenesis XO/XY	Gonadoblastoma	Gonads must be removed; 25% chance of gonadal malignancy
Trisomy 8	Preleukemia	
Noonan syndrome	Schwannoma, myelodysplasia	
Monosomy 5 or 7	Myelodysplastic syndromes	Recurrent infections may precede neoplasia
DNA Fragility		
Xeroderma pigmentosum	Basal, squamous cell skin cancers	Autosomal recessive; failure to repair solar-damaged DNA
Fanconi anemia	Leukemia	Autosomal recessive; 10% risk for acute myelogenous leukemia; chromosome fragility, positive diepoxybutane test result
Bloom syndrome	Leukemia, lymphoma	Autosomal recessive; chromosome fragility; high risk for malignancy
Ataxia-telangiectasia	Lymphoma, leukemia	Autosomal recessive; sensitive to x-radiation, radiomimetic drugs; chromosome fragility
Dysplastic nevus syndrome	Melanoma	Autosomal dominant
Immunodeficiency Syndromes		
Wiskott-Aldrich syndrome	Lymphoma, leukemia	Immunodeficiency; X-linked recessive
X-linked immunodeficiency (Duncan syndrome)	Lymphoma	Epstein-Barr virus is inciting agent
X-linked agammaglobulinemia	Lymphoma, leukemia	Immunodeficiency
Severe combined immunodeficiency	Leukemia, lymphoma	Immunodeficiency; X-linked recessive
Others		
Neurofibromatosis 1	Neurofibroma, optic glioma, acoustic neuroma, astrocytoma, meningioma, pheochromocytoma, sarcoma	Autosomal dominant; *NF1* gene
Neurofibromatosis 2	Bilateral acoustic neuromas, meningioma	Autosomal dominant; *NF2* gene
Tuberous sclerosis	Fibroangiomatous nevi, myocardial rhabdomyoma	Autosomal dominant
Hemochromatosis	Hepatoma	Cirrhosis; autosomal dominant/recessive
Retinoblastoma	Sarcoma	Increased risk of secondary malignancy 10–20 yr later, *RB1* gene
Glycogen storage disease I	Hepatic adenoma	Usually with cirrhosis, autosomal recessive
Familial adenomatous polyposis coli	Adenocarcinoma of colon	Autosomal dominant, *APC* gene
Gardner syndrome	Adenocarcinoma of colon; skull and soft tissue tumors	Autosomal dominant, *APC* gene
Peutz-Jeghers syndrome	Gastrointestinal carcinoma, ovarian neoplasia	Autosomal dominant
Hemihypertrophy ± Beckwith's syndrome	Wilms tumor, hepatoblastoma, adrenal carcinoma	25% develop tumor, most in first 5 yr of life
Tyrosinemia, galactosemia	Hepatic carcinoma	Nodular cirrhosis; autosomal recessive
Multiple endocrine neoplasia syndrome, type I (Werner syndrome)	Parathyroid adenoma, pancreatic islet tumor, pituitary adenoma carcinoid	Autosomal dominant; Zollinger-Ellison syndrome
Multiple endocrine neoplasia syndrome, type II (Sipple syndrome)	Medullary carcinoma of the thyroid, hyperparathyroidism, pheochromocytoma	Autosomal dominant; monitor calcitonin and calcium levels
Multiple endocrine neoplasia, type III (multiple mucosal neuroma syndrome)	Mucosal neuroma, pheochromocytoma, medullary thyroid carcinoma; Marfan habitus; neuropathy	Autosomal dominant
Rendu-Osler-Weber syndrome	Angioma	Autosomal dominant
von Hippel-Lindau disease	Hemangioblastoma of the cerebellum and retina, pheochromocytoma, renal cancer	Autosomal dominant, mutation of tumor-suppressor gene, *VHL* gene
Cancer family syndrome	Colonic, uterine carcinoma	Autosomal dominant
Li-Fraumeni syndrome	Bone, soft tissue sarcoma, breast	Mutation of *P53* tumor-suppressor gene, autosomal dominant
BRCA1 and 2	Breast, ovarian	DNA repair defect

From Behrman R, Kliegman R (eds): Nelson Essentials of Pediatrics, 2nd ed. Philadelphia, WB Saunders, 1994.

ilar malignancies, suggesting a role for the immune system in cancer treatment as well as in cancer prevention.

OTHER FACTORS ASSOCIATED WITH ONCOGENESIS

Viruses. Several viruses have been implicated in the pathogenesis of malignancy. The association of the Epstein-Barr virus (EBV) with Burkitt lymphoma and nasopharyngeal carcinoma was identified more than 30 yr ago, but EBV infection alone is not sufficient for malignant transformation. EBV is also associated with mixed cellularity and lymphocyte-depleted Hodgkin disease as well as some T-cell lymphomas, which is particularly intriguing because EBV normally does not infect T lymphocytes. The most conclusive evidence for a role of EBV in lymphogenesis is the direct causal role of EBV for B-cell lymphoproliferative disease in immunocompromised persons, especially those with AIDS.

As is the case with adults, children who are chronically infected with hepatitis B (HBsAg-positive) have a greater than 200-fold risk of developing hepatocellular carcinoma. In adults, the latency period between viral infection and the development of hepatocellular carcinoma approaches 20 yr. However, in children who acquire the viral infection through perinatal transmission, the latency period can be as short as 6–7 yr. The additional factors that are required for malignant transformation of the virally infected hepatocytes are not clear. Hepatitis C virus infection is also a risk factor for hepatocellular carcinoma and is also associated with splenic lymphoma.

Nearly all cervical carcinomas contain human papillomaviruses (HPV). High-risk papillomaviruses include types 16 and 18 but also 31, 33, 35, 45, and 56, which are also most commonly found in women without lesions. The low-risk papillomaviruses, including types 6 and 11 that are most commonly found in genital warts, are almost never associated with malignancies. Like other virus-associated cancers, the presence of HPV alone is not sufficient to cause malignant transformation. The mechanism by which HPV 19 induces malignant transformation is thought to involve *P53* and *RB* tumor suppressor genes, which regulate the cell cycle by acting as gatekeepers of the G1/S and G2/M checkpoints. By interfering with these proteins, HPV alters the regulation of cell growth.

Human herpesvirus 8 (HHV8) is associated with Kaposi sarcoma, primary effusion B-cell lymphoma, and the plasma cell variant of Castleman disease, all of which occur primarily in persons with AIDS. Human T-cell leukemia virus type 1 (HTLV-1) is associated with adult T-cell leukemia and lymphoma.

Genomic Imprinting. The development of cancer has also been linked to genomic imprinting, which is the selective inactivation of one of two alleles of a certain gene. The inactivated gene is determined by whether the gene is inherited from the mother or father. For example, normally the maternal *IGF2* (insulin-like growth factor receptor 2) gene is inactivated. The inactivation is thought to be secondary to methylation of specific CpG sequences upstream of the IGF2 promoter, which interferes with the transcription of the *IGF2* gene. In some Wilms tumors, there is loss of methylation in the upstream area of the maternal gene, which, in turn, allows transcript expression of the maternal *IGF2* gene. At the same time the *H19* gene (whose function is not yet clear), a previously actively transcribed maternal gene, is silenced by methylation. Beckwith-Weidemann syndrome, an overgrowth syndrome characterized by macrosomia, macroglossia, hemihypertrophy, omphalocele, and renal anomalies, is associated with an increased risk of Wilms tumor, hepatoblastoma, rhabdomyosarcoma, neuroblastoma, and adrenal cortical carcinoma. The increased risk in developing cancer is associated with changes in the methylation pattern of genes on the 11p15 chromosome.

Telomerase. Telomeres are a series of tens to thousands of TTAGGG repeats at the ends of chromosomes that are important for stabilizing the chromosomal ends and limiting breakage,

translocation, and loss of DNA maternal. With DNA replication there is a progressive shortening of telomere length, which is a hallmark of cellular aging and may be a senescence signal. In some instances, telomerase, which is an enzyme that adds telomeres to the ends of chromosomes, becomes active. The addition of telomeres occurs in immortalized cell lines and most tumor types and, as a consequence, these cells may have a survival advantage allowing them to undergo additional cell divisions. Therapy aimed at inhibition of telomerase activity may result in cell death.

Butel JS: Viral carcinogenesis: Revelation of molecular mechanisms and etiology of human disease. *Carcinogenesis* 2000;21:405–26.
Helder MN, Wisman GB, van der Zee GJ: Telomerase and telomeres: From basic science to cancer treatment. *Cancer Invest* 2002;20:82–101.
Momparler RL, Boverzis V: DNA methylation and cancer. *J Cell Physiol* 2000;183: 145–54.

Chapter 485
Principles of Diagnosis
Archie Bleyer

Symptoms and physical findings are important in the recognition of malignant diseases and life-threatening benign tumors in children and adolescents. In addition to the classic manifestations, any persistent, unexplained symptom or sign should be evaluated as potentially emanating from a cancerous or precancerous condition. As part of the diagnostic evaluation, the pediatrician and pediatric oncologist must convey the diagnosis to the patient and family in a sensitive and informative manner.

SIGNS AND SYMPTOMS

In contrast to the classic warning signs of cancer in adults, there is no established set of similar symptoms and signs of cancer in children, although the most frequent cancers in children suggest 10 signs and symptoms that are helpful for early recognition (Box 485–1). This lack of explicit criteria is caused by multiple factors. The symptoms and signs of cancer are more variable and nonspecific in children. Most childhood cancers originate from deeper structures in the body, from the parenchyma or organs rather than from epithelial layers that compose the skin and that line the ducts and glands of organs. In children, metastases are present at diagnosis in approximately 80% of cases, whereas only about 20% of adults have evidence of metastases at diagnosis. In children, therefore, the presenting symptoms or signs are more likely to be caused by metastases than by the primary tumor. Thus, the signs of cancer in children are frequently attributed to other causes before the malignancy is recognized. There are several additional but less common signs and symptoms of cancer in children (Box 485–2).

Diffuse enlargement of the pons is a radiographic finding, usually on MRI, which is nearly always indicative of malignant disease and may be considered pathognomonic (Fig. 485–1). Diffuse, not local, enlargement of the pons is regarded as astrocytoma and treated accordingly without tissue biopsy, in part because or the risk and difficulty of procedure on this part of the brain. The hematopoietic sign of more than one abnormal hematopoietic lineage is primarily a laboratory observation in which more than one of the three blood cell lineages (leukocytes, erythrocytes, and platelets) are affected. Related signs may also be apparent on physical examination. A white pupillary reflex (Fig. 485–2), instead of the usual red reflection from incident light, is almost pathognomonic for retinoblastoma, although astrocytic hamartoma, Coats disease, and posterior persistent hyperplastic vitreous (PPHV) may mimic this finding.

BOX 485–1. The Most Frequent Signs and Symptoms of Cancer in Children and Adults

ADULTS
(American Cancer Society, 1950s)
Change in bowel or bladder habits
Blood in stool
Lump in breast or elsewhere
Hoarseness or nagging cough
Difficulty in swallowing
Sore that will not heal
Change in wart or mole

CHILDREN
(University of Texas M.D. Anderson Cancer Center)
Abdominal mass
Persistent lymphadenopathy
More than one abnormal hematopoietic lineage
Specific neurologic deficit
Increased intracranial pressure
Diffuse enlargement of pons
Proptosis
White pupillary reflex
Unilateral knee or shoulder pain or swelling
Vaginal bleeding or mass

Physical Examination. The physical examination should focus on the tissues and organ systems that are most likely to be affected by cancer in children (Table 485–1). Accordingly, paying particular attention to blood, brain, belly, and bone—the

BOX 485–2. Uncommon Signs and Symptoms of Cancer in Children

DIRECTLY RELATED TO TUMOR
Superior vena cava syndrome
Subcutaneous nodules
Leukemoid reaction
Myasthenia gravis
Heterochromia

NOT DIRECTLY RELATED TO TUMOR GROWTH
Chronic diarrhea
Polymyoclonus-opsoclonus
Failure to thrive
Cushing syndrome
Pseudomuscular dystrophy

Modified from Vietti TJ, Steuber CP: Clinical assessment and differential diagnosis of the child with suspected cancer. In Pizzo PA, Poplack DG (editors): *Principles and Practice of Pediatric Oncology*, 4th ed. Philadelphia, Lippincott Williams & Wilkins, 2002, pp 149–59.

4 Bs—is helpful in eliciting evidence of malignancy by physical examination.

Abnormalities of the hematopoietic system are manifested as (1) pallor, which indicates anemia; (2) bleeding from orifices, petechiae, purpura, and ecchymosis, which indicate thrombocytopenia and disseminated intravascular coagulation; (3) cellulitis and other infection, which indicate leukopenia; (4) skin nodules, which indicate leukocytosis; and (5) other abnormalities of the formed elements of the blood. Abnormalities of the lymphatic system include lymphadenopathy (Fig. 485–3), superior vena cava syndrome, or respiratory distress when the patient is in a supine position resulting from upper anterior mediastinal mass or thymic enlargement (Fig. 485–4). Enlargement of the cervical lymph nodes is common in children with infection and in patients with lymphoma. Persistent or progressive enlargement of lymph nodes, often painless, is suggestive of lymphoma and indicates the need for biopsy.

Abnormalities of the central nervous system that indicate cancer include decreased level of consciousness, paresis of the sixth nerve, and increased intracranial pressure, which may be diagnosed by the presence of papilledema (Fig. 485–5). Any focal neurologic deficit in the motor or sensory system, especially a decrease in cranial nerve function, should prompt further investigation for malignancy.

Abnormalities of the embryonal system are usually apparent on physical examination as organomegaly or an abdominal mass. However, an unexplained mass in any area of the body should be considered malignant until proven otherwise. Retinoblastoma is, of course, usually manifest as a white pupillary reflex (see Fig. 485–2). In neonates, "blueberry muffin" spots on the skin may be neuroblastoma. A sacrococcygeal mass is usually a teratoma that may undergo malignant transformation if it is not removed.

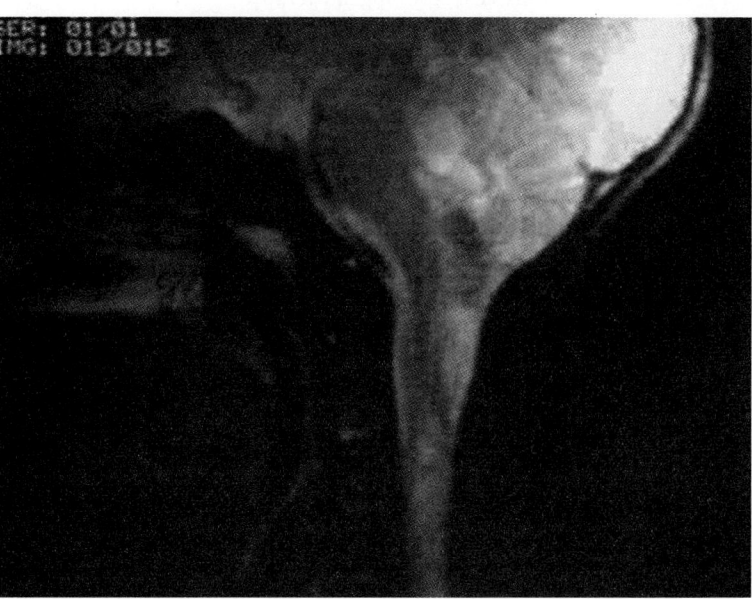

FIGURE 485–1. Brain stem tumor apparent on MRI. (From Sinniah D, D'Angio GJ, Chatten J, et al: *Atlas of Pediatric Oncology*. London, Arnold, 1996.)

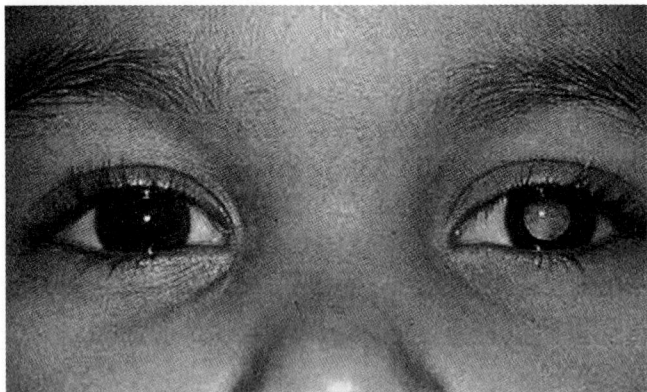

FIGURE 485–2. White pupillary reflex. (From Sinniah D, D'Angio GJ, Chatten J, et al: *Atlas of Pediatric Oncology.* London, Arnold, 1996.)

Age-Related Manifestations. Because the types of cancer in children occur at specific ages, the physician should tailor the history and physical examination based on the age of the child. The embryonal tumors, including neuroblastoma, usually occur during the first 2 yr of life (see Fig. 483–2). From 2–5 yr of age, acute lymphoblastic leukemias, non-Hodgkin's lymphoma, and gliomas peak in incidence. During adolescence, bone tumors, Hodgkin disease, and the gonadal and connective tissue tumors predominate. Hence, for infants and toddlers, special attention should be paid to the possibility of embryonal and intra-abdominal tumors (i.e., Wilms tumor, retinoblastoma, teratoma, neuroblastoma, and liver tumors). Preschool-aged and early school-aged children showing compatible signs and symptoms should be specifically evaluated for leukemia, lymphoma, and brain tumors. Adolescents require assessment for sarcomas and genital or gonadal malignancies, as well as for Hodgkin disease.

IMPORTANCE OF EARLY DETECTION

Because most of childhood cancers are curable, early detection is paramount. In addition, there are several types of cancer for which less therapy is indicated for early-stage disease than for advanced disease. Indeed, early detection often minimizes the amount and duration of treatment required for cure and may therefore not only lead to a higher potential for cure but also spare the patient intensive or prolonged therapy.

The prognosis of malignancy in children depends primarily on tumor type, extent of disease at diagnosis, and rapidity of response to treatment. Early diagnosis helps to ensure that appropriate therapy is given in a timely fashion and, hence, optimizes the chances of cure. Because most physicians in general practice rarely encounter children with cancer, they should investigate the possibility of malignancy when they encounter an atypical course of a common childhood condition.

Delayed diagnosis is particularly likely in certain clinical situations. The cardinal symptom of both osteosarcoma and Ewing sarcoma is localized and usually persistent pain. Because these

TABLE 485–1. Organ Systems and Tissues of the Most Common Cancers in Children

Type of Cancer	Proportion of All Cancers (%)
Lymphohematopoietic	44
Nervous system	29
Embryonal	12
Connective tissue	10

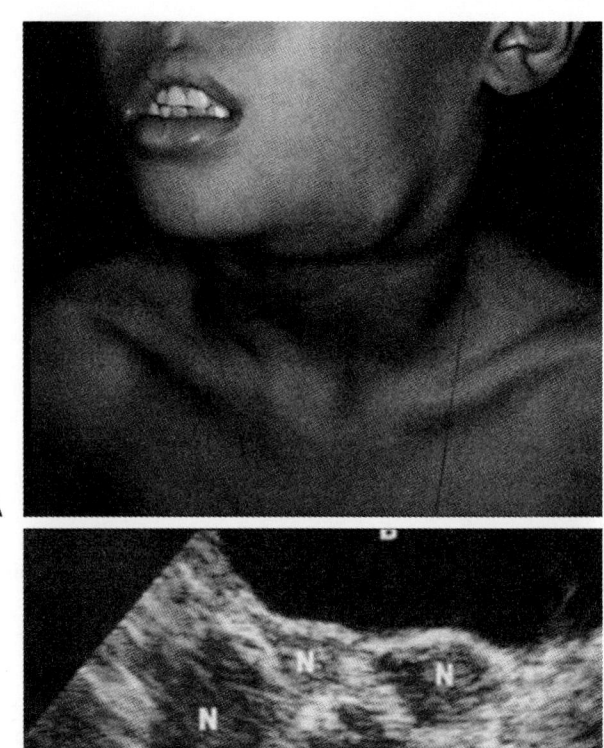

FIGURE 485–3. *A,* Cervical lymphadenopathy. *B,* Manifestations on ultrasonography. N = abnormally enlarged lymph nodes. (From Sinniah D, D'Angio GJ, Chatten J, et al: *Atlas of Pediatric Oncology.* London, Arnold, 1996.)

tumors occur during the 2nd decade of life, a time of increased physical activity, patients often associate the pain with an episode of trauma. Prompt radiologic evaluation can help confirm the diagnosis. Tumors of the nasopharynx or middle ear may mimic infection. Prolonged unexplained ear pain, nasal discharge, retropharyngeal swelling, and trismus should be investigated as possible signs of malignancy.

Early symptoms of leukemia may be limited to low-grade fever or bone and joint pain. Blood counts, with particular attention to the presence of normocytic anemia or mild thrombocytopenia, may indicate the need for bone marrow examination, even when leukemic blast cells are not seen in the peripheral blood smear. Malignancy can also occur in neonates and should be considered in children with masses in any area or with "blueberry muffin" spots on their skin; the latter sign indicates neuroblastoma.

STAGING

When a patient is suspected to have a malignant neoplasm, the immediate goal is to determine its type and extent. A tentative diagnosis can often be established on the basis of the patient's age, presenting symptoms, and the location of a suspected mass. A thorough search for metastatic disease usually precedes biopsy of a suspicious lesion. The surgeon can make a more informed choice between an attempt at complete resection and a more limited procedure when the presence or likelihood of disseminated disease is known. The appropriate preoperative studies depend on the tentative diagnosis. Several noninvasive techniques (e.g., CT and MRI) are useful in evaluating patients

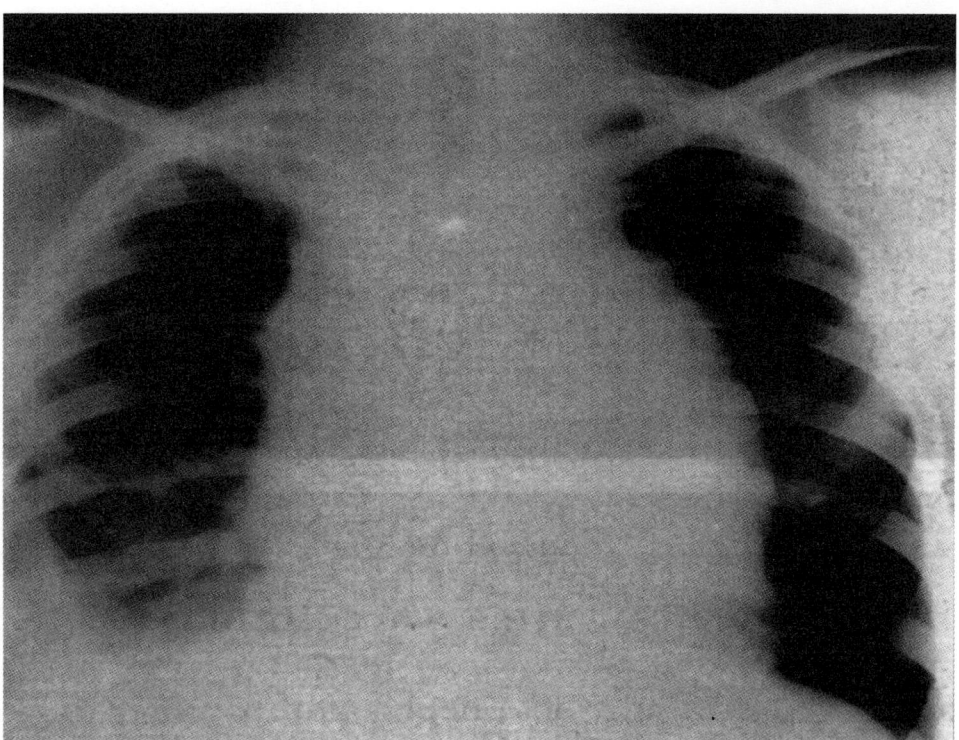

FIGURE 485–4. Anterior upper mediastinal mass due to non-Hodgkin lymphoma. (From Sinniah D, D'Angio GJ, Chatten J, et al: *Atlas of Pediatric Oncology*. London, Arnold, 1996.)

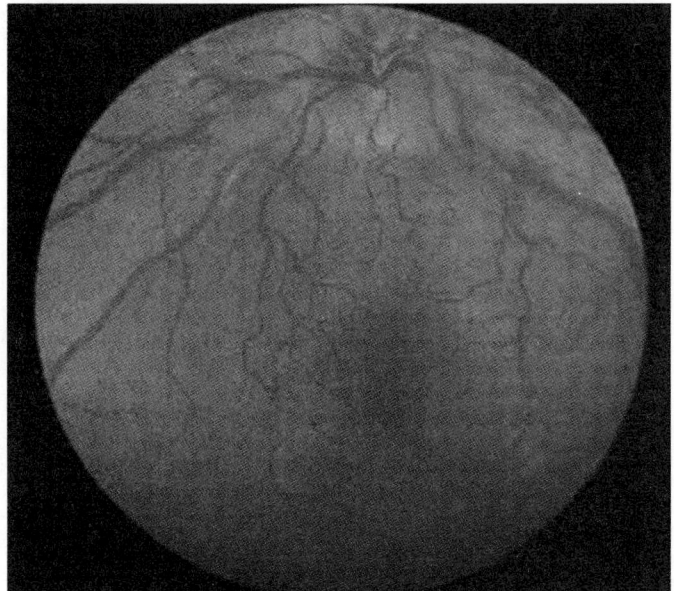

FIGURE 485–5. Papilledema. (From Sinniah D, D'Angio GJ, Chatten J, et al: *Atlas of Pediatric Oncology*. London, Arnold, 1996.)

for the presence of metastatic lesions; also, bone marrow aspiration, biopsy, or both may be needed. These studies are also used in assessing the disease stage, information that is critical in determining the prognosis and developing a treatment plan.

HISTOPATHOLOGY

Central to the diagnosis of any tumor is histologic examination of specimens. The initial specimen of tumor tissue should be obtained under conditions that allow for a full range of pathologic studies. In some cases, such as suspected lymphomas, fresh tissue may be required for special studies. Some of these studies

are time consuming; thus, it is often impossible to discuss the specific diagnosis with the patient's family immediately after surgery.

In many cases, the diagnosis can be ascertained by means of a fine-needle biopsy, thus eliminating the need for an incision or major operation. However, a diagnosis based on the results of a fine-needle biopsy requires the availability of an experienced radiologist and an experienced cytologist and usually can be performed only at major medical centers. Similarly, minimally invasive surgery utilizing endoscopic techniques is commonly performed in patients with abdominal and thoracic masses. At the time of biopsy, excision, or exploration the surgeon must search carefully for evidence of regional dissemination to lymph node groups or to adjacent organs. If total resection is attempted, the pathologist must carefully examine the margins for microscopic residual tumor because this information is needed for determining subsequent treatment.

Explaining the Diagnostic Evaluation to Pediatric Patients and Their Families. The diagnostic and treatment plan must be carefully explained to parents and, if old enough to understand, to the patient. An honest discussion of the facts is the best policy. Children should be told all information that they can understand and would find useful or that they express a desire or wish to know. Effects of treatment, such as the possible need to amputate a limb, loss of hair during chemotherapy, and possible temporary or permanent functional impairment must be anticipated and fully discussed. The possibility and probability of death from cancer should be covered in an age-appropriate manner. It is usually necessary to repeat explanations several times before distraught family members fully and uniformly understand what is being communicated. Throughout treatment, parents, patients, siblings, and medical staff will need help in expressing feelings of anxiety, depression, guilt, and anger. Experienced professionals, including pediatric social workers, child psychologists and psychiatrists, child life specialists, and schoolteachers with special expertise in managing students with cancer should be called on by the pediatrician, pediatric oncologist, and nurses to assist when needed.

Sinniah D, D'Angio GJ, Chatten J, et al: *Atlas of Pediatric Oncology.* London, Arnold, 1996.

Triche TJ: Pathology and molecular diagnosis of pediatric malignancies. In Pizzo PA, Poplack DG (editors): *Principles and Practice of Pediatric Oncology,* 3rd ed. Philadelphia, Lippincott-Raven, 1997.

Vietti TJ, Steuber CP: Clinical assessment and differential diagnosis of the child with suspected cancer. In Pizzo PA, Poplack DG (editors): *Principles and Practice of Pediatric Oncology,* 3rd ed. Philadelphia, Lippincott Williams & Wilkins, 2002, pp 149–59.

Chapter 486
Principles of Treatment

Archie Bleyer

Treatment of children with cancer is one of the most complex endeavors in practice of pediatrics. It begins with an absolute requirement for the correct diagnosis (including subtype), proceeds through accurate and thorough staging of the extent of disease and determination of prognostic subgroup, provides appropriate multidisciplinary and usually multimodal therapy, and assiduously evaluates the possibilities of recurrent disease and of adverse late effects of the disease and the therapies rendered. Throughout treatment, every child with cancer should have the benefit of the expertise of specialized teams of providers of pediatric cancer care, including pediatric oncologists, pathologists, radiologists, surgeons, radiotherapists, nurses, and various support staff including nutritionists, social workers, psychologists, pharmacists, and other medical specialists.

The best chance for cure of cancer is during the initial course of treatment; the cure rates for patients with recurrent disease are much lower than those for patients with primary disease. All patients with cancer should be referred to an appropriate specialized center as soon as possible when the diagnosis of cancer is suspected. All such centers in North American are identified on the Children's Oncology Group Website (www.childrensoncology group.org) and on the National Cancer Institute cancer trials website (www.cancernet.nci.nih.gov). The remarkable increases in cure rates for childhood malignancies over the past 30 yr would not have occurred without the collective participation of patients and their physicians in clinical research programs at these centers. In the United States, the national organization of cancer clinical trials cooperative groups has been associated with a more than 80% reduction in the incidence of mortality due to cancer among children younger than 15 yr of age despite an overall increase in cancer incidence during this interval (Fig. 486–1). This remarkable achievement represents the effects of an effective multimodal, multi-institutional, multidisciplinary collaboration.

DIAGNOSIS AND STAGING

Accurate diagnosis and staging of the extent of disease is imperative, especially for children, whose cure rates are so high. Accuracy also is essential, not only because the nature of therapy depends strongly on the type of cancer but also because better and worse prognostic subgroups, based on stage of disease, have been established for most cancers that occur in children. Accordingly, children with a better prognosis are treated with less intensive therapy, including lower doses of chemotherapy or radiotherapy, a shorter duration of treatment, or elimination of at least one treatment modality (e.g., radiotherapy, chemotherapy, or surgery). Accurate staging thus avoids the occurrence of excessive acute adverse effects and long-term complications of therapy in patients whose prognosis indicates

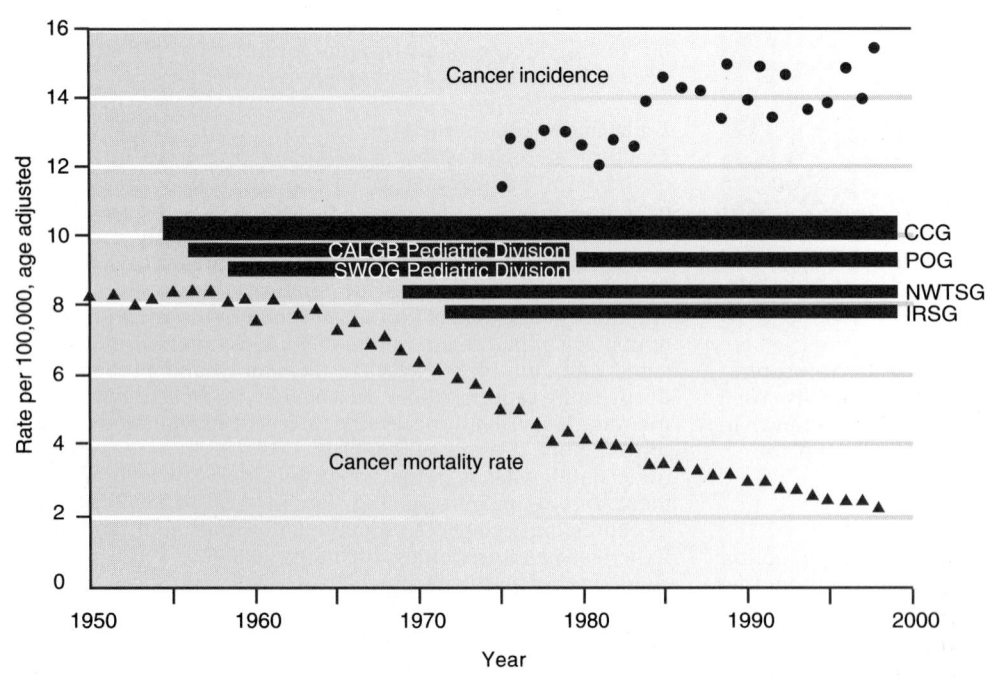

FIGURE 486–1. Reduction in the U.S. national cancer mortality rate among children younger than age 15 yr as a direct consequence of the National Cooperative Group Program sponsored by the National Cancer Institute. *Horizontal bars* indicate the duration of the existence of the national pediatric cancer cooperative groups, beginning with the Children's Cancer Group (CCG) in 1955. Other groups are the Pediatric Oncology Group (POG), which was derived from the Pediatric Divisions of the Southwest Oncology Group (SWOG) and the Cancer and Acute Leukemia Group B (CALGB), the National Wilms' Tumor Study Group (NWTSG), and the Intergroup Rhabdomyosarcoma Study Group (IRSG). *Solid triangles* represent the annual national mortality rate before age 15, and *solid circles* indicate the national cancer incidence rate before age 15 yr from the Surveillance, Epidemiology and End-Results (SEER) program of the National Cancer Institute. (Incidence and mortality data from Ries LAG, Eisner MP, Kosary CL, et al [editors]: *SEER Cancer Statistics Review, 1973–1999.* Bethesda, MD, National Cancer Institute, 2002. http://seer.cancer.gov/csr/1973_1999/)

that less therapy is required for cure. Overtreatment of patients with a more favorable prognosis is a definite risk if the patient is not referred to a cancer treatment center for management of adverse effects of such treatment. Conversely, undertreatment is also a clear risk if the diagnosis and stage are not correct, with the result being a compromise of an otherwise high potential for cure.

Diagnostic imaging is a critical phase of evaluation in most children with solid tumors (i.e., cancers other than leukemia). In the evaluation of children with cancer, MRI, CT, ultrasonography, scintigraphy (nuclear medicine scans), positron emission tomography, and spectroscopy, as appropriate, all serve a clear purpose, not only before treatment to determine the extent of disease and the appropriate therapy but also during follow-up to determine whether the therapy was effective. In addition, rapidity and completeness of response to treatment of an increasing number of malignant diseases in children are being evaluated and imaging techniques are used to quantify the magnitude of the response and to guide appropriate changes in the therapy if it is not adequate. Competence in the sedation of children for diagnostic imaging is also critical.

Expertise in pathology and laboratory medicine provides critical diagnostic support and guides therapy in most children with cancer. Fine-needle aspiration cytology avoids the need for open biopsies of masses in most locations of the body and can be performed in pediatric centers with appropriate expertise in diagnostic imaging, cytology, analgesia, and local anesthesia. Sentinel node mapping is increasingly being applied in the staging of children's cancers. The adequacy of surgery by evaluation of frozen sections of the surgical margins for tumor cells is essential in many tumor operations.

MULTIMODAL, MULTIDISCIPLINARY APPROACH

Many pediatric subspecialties are required to evaluate, treat, and manage children with cancer, including provision of primary modalities and multiple supportive care services (Fig. 486–2). Among the primary treatment modalities, more than two modalities are frequently used, with chemotherapy being the most widely used, followed, in order of use, by surgery, radiotherapy, and biologic agent therapy (Fig. 486–3).

The leukemias that occur in childhood are generally managed with chemotherapy alone, with a minor proportion of patients receiving cranial or craniospinal radiotherapy for prevention or treatment of overt central nervous system leukemia. Most children with non-Hodgkin lymphoma also are treated with chemotherapy alone. Exceptions include bulky nonlymphoblastic non-Hodgkin tumors, for which radiotherapy is often benefi-cial, and resectable primary Burkitt tumor in the abdomen, for which surgery is usually therapeutic. Localized therapy with surgery or irradiation or both is an important component of treatment of most solid tumors, including Hodgkin disease, but systemic multiagent chemotherapy is usually necessary because tumor dissemination is generally present even if undetectable. Chemotherapy alone is usually insufficient to eradicate gross residual tumors. Hence, children with malignant tumors not infrequently require treatment with all three modalities (see Fig. 486–3). Unfortunately, most treatments effective in children with cancer have a narrow therapeutic index (i.e., a low ratio of efficacy to toxicity). The acute and chronic adverse effects of these treatments can be minimized but not entirely avoided.

Over the past 10 yr, biologic agent therapy has become an important modality in a few childhood cancers (see Fig. 486–3). This type of treatment generally refers to immunotherapy, biologic response modifiers, or endogenously occurring molecules that in supraphysiologic doses have therapeutic effects. Examples are retinoic acid therapy in acute progranulocytic leukemia, monoclonal antibody therapy for certain non-Hodgkin lymphomas, imatinib mesylate for chronic myelogenous and Philadelphia chromosome–positive leukemias, and radioactive meta-iodobenzylguanidine (MIBG) therapy for neuroblastoma.

Chemotherapy is more widely used in children than in adults because children better tolerate the acute adverse effects and, in general, have malignant diseases that are more responsive to chemotherapy than are malignant diseases of adults. In general, radiotherapy is used sparingly in children because they are more vulnerable than adults to its late adverse effects.

Whenever possible, treatment is given on an outpatient basis. Children should remain living at home and in school as much as possible throughout treatment. Increasingly, pediatric cancer therapies are being administered to ambulatory patients, with the advent of such innovations as programmable infusion pumps, oral chemotherapeutic regimens, early discharge from hospital with intensive outpatient supportive care, and home health care services. Some patients miss a considerable amount of school in the 1st year after diagnosis owing to the intensity of therapy or its adverse effects and to the ensuing complications of the disease or therapy. Tutoring should be encouraged so that children do not fall behind in their schooling; counseling should be provided as appropriate. In-hospital school services should be provided for those patients who must spend much of their time as inpatients receiving therapy for disease or for managing adverse effects.

Development of selective, highly effective therapy for cancer both in children and in adults is generally hindered by a lack of understanding of the molecular mechanisms that underlie malig-

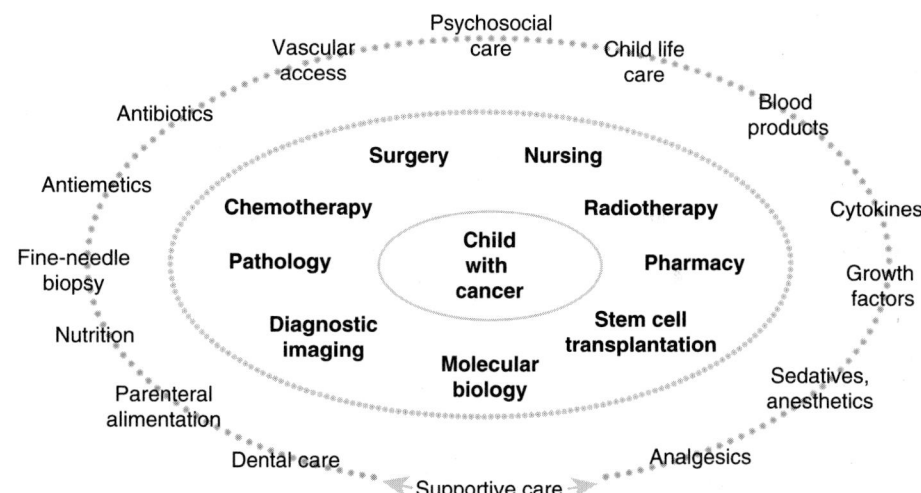

FIGURE 486–2. Multidisciplinary care of children with cancer. *Inner circle* designates primary modalities, and *outer ring* identifies supportive care elements to which all children with cancer have access.

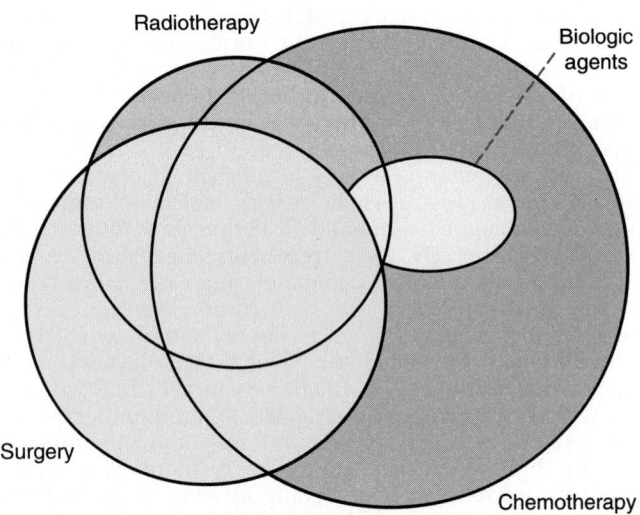

FIGURE 486–3. The primary modalities of therapy used in the treatment of children with cancer. The relative sizes of the circles reflect the approximate proportion of the overall role in the management of pediatric cancer.

nant transformation. Also, de novo or acquired resistance to chemotherapy and radiotherapy remains an obstacle. Dramatic advances in the discipline have reduced the empiricism of therapy for cancer, but much remains unknown.

CHEMOTHERAPY

The most widely used modality in pediatric cancer therapy is chemotherapy (see Fig. 486–3). Moreover, therapy nearly always involves combinations of drugs, such as VAC (vincristine, doxorubicin [Adriamycin] or dactinomycin [Actinomycin D], and cyclophosphamide) and CHOP (cyclophosphamide, doxorubicin [Adriamycin], vincristine [Oncovin], and prednisone). Historically, sequential single-drug therapy rarely resulted in complete responses, and partial responses generally were infrequent and transient and grew progressively shorter in duration with each drug used. Combination chemotherapy became the standard when combinations of drugs with different mechanisms of action and nonoverlapping toxicities (e.g., POMP [mercaptopurine, vincristine (Oncovin), methotrexate, and prednisone], VAMP [vincristine, doxorubicin (Adriamycin), methotrexate, and prednisone], and MOPP [nitrogen mustard, vincristine (Oncovin), prednisone, and procarbazine] were first demonstrated to be effective in childhood leukemia. Most of the cytotoxic drugs for childhood cancer are selected from several classes of agents, including alkylating agents, antimetabolites, antibiotics, hormones, plant alkaloids, and topoisomerase inhibitors (Tables 486–1 and 486–2). The increased metabolic and cell cycle activity of malignant cells makes them more susceptible to the cytotoxic effects of these types of agents.

Because most antineoplastic agents are cell cycle dependent, their adverse effects are generally related to the proliferation kinetics of individual cell populations (Table 486–3). Most susceptible are those tissues or organs with high rates of cell turnover: bone marrow, oral and intestinal mucosa, epidermis,

---

TABLE 486–1. Antineoplastic Agents Used in Pediatric Solid Tumors

Agent	Type of Tumor								
	Brain Tumors	Neuro-blastoma	Wilms Tumor	Osteo-sarcoma	Ewing Sarcoma	Rhabdomyo-sarcoma	Retino-blastoma	Hepato-blastoma	Testicular Carcinoma
Antimetabolites									
Methotrexate–high dose	+	–	–	+	–	–	–	–	–
Cytarabine	±	–	–	–	–	–	–	–	–
Fluorouracil	–	–	–	–	–	–	–	+	–
Alkylating agents									
Cyclophosphamide	+	+	+	+	+	+	+	+	+
Ifosfamide	+	±	+	+	+	+	+	+	+
Nitrogen mustard	+	–	–	–	+	–	–	–	–
Chlorambucil	–	–	–	–	+	–	–	–	–
Melphalan*	+	+	+	+	+	+	+	+	–
Busulfan*	+	–	–	–	–	+	–	+	–
Triethylenethiophosphoramide (thioTEPA)*	+	+	+	+	+	+	+	+	–
Antitumor Antibiotics									
Doxorubicin (Adriamycin)	–	+	+	+	+	+	+	+	+
Daunomycin	–	±	+	–	+	+	–	–	–
Dactinomycin (Actinomycin D)	–	–	+	±	+	+	+	+	+
Bleomycin	–	–	–	–	–	–	–	–	+
Vinca Alkaloids									
Vincristine	+	+	+	–	+	+	+	–	+
Vinblastine	–	–	–	–	–	–	–	–	+
Vinorelbine	–	–	–	–	+	+	–	–	–
Miscellaneous agents									
Corticosteroids	+	–	–	–	–	–	–	–	–
Lomustine (CCNU)	+	–	–	–	–	–	–	–	–
Dacarbazine (DTIC)	+	+	–	±	+	+	–	–	–
Procarbazine	+	–	–	–	–	–	–	–	–
Cisplatin	+	+	+	+	–	±	+	+	+
Carboplatin	+	+	±	–	–	–	±	+	+
Hydroxyurea	+	–	–	–	–	–	–	–	–
Etoposide (VP-16)	+	+	–	–	+	+	+	–	+

Includes high–dose chemotherapy with hematopoietic stem cell rescue.
+ = commonly used; – = not used or rarely used; ± = occasionally used as second-line or substitute agent.

TABLE 486–2. Antineoplastic Agents Used in Pediatric Leukemias and Lymphomas

Agent	Leukemias						Lymphomas			
	ALL pre-B	ALL T-cell	ALL B-cell	AML	APL	CML	Lympho-blastic	B-cell Burkitt	Large Cell	Hodgkin Disease
Antimetabolites										
Methotrexate—low dose	+	+	+	±	–	–	±	+	±	–
Methotrexate—high dose	+	+	+	±	–	–	+	+	+	+
Mercaptopurine	+	+	+	±	–	–	±	±	±	–
Cytarabine	+	+	+	+	–	–	+	+	+	+
Thioguanine	+	+	+	+	–	–	+	–	+	–
5-Azacytidine	–	–	–	+	–	–	–	–	–	–
Alkylating agents										
Cyclophosphamide	+	+	+	+	–	–	+	+	+	+
Ifosfamide	±	±	±	–	–	–	±	±	±	+
Nitrogen mustard	–	–	–	–	–	–	–	–	±	+
Chlorambucil	–	–	–	–	–	–	–	–	–	+
Melphalan*	+	+	+	+	+	+	+	+	+	+
Busulfan*	+	+	+	+	+	+	+	+	+	+
ThioTEPA*	+	+	+	+	+	+	+	+	+	+
Antitumor Antibiotics										
Doxorubicin (Adriamycin)	+	+	+	+	–	–	+	±	+	+
Daunomycin	+	+	+	+	–	–	+	+	+	+
Idarubicin	+	+	–	+	–	–	–	–	–	–
Dactinomycin (Actinomycin D)	–	–	–	–	–	–	–	–	–	–
Bleomycin	–	–	–	–	–	–	–	–	±	+
Vinca Alkaloids										
Vincristine	+	+	+	+	–	–	+	+	+	+
Vinblastine	–	–	–	–	–	–	±	±	+	+
Miscellaneous Agents										
Corticosteroid	+	+	+	+	–	±	+	+	+	+
Retinoic acid	–	–	–	–	+	–	–	–	–	–
Interferon-a	–	–	–	–	–	+	–	–	–	–
Lomustine (CCNU)	–	–	–	–	–	–	±	–	–	+
Dacarbazine (DTIC)	–	–	–	–	–	–	–	–	–	+
Procarbazine	–	–	–	–	–	–	±	–	–	+
L-Asparaginase	+	+	+	+	–	–	+	±	–	–
Cisplatin	–	–	–	+	–	–	–	–	–	±
Carboplatin	–	–	–	+	–	–	–	–	–	–
Hydroxyurea	–	–	–	–	–	+	–	–	–	–
Etoposide (VP-16)	+	+	±	+	–	–	+	±	+	+

*Includes high-dose chemotherapy with hematopoietic stem cell rescue.

+ = commonly used; – = not used or rarely used; ± = occasionally used as second-line or substitute agent; ALL = acute lymphoblastic leukemia; AML = acute myelogenous leukemia; APL = acute progranulocytic leukemia; CML = chronic myelogenous leukemia.

liver, and spermatogonia. The most common acute adverse effects are myelosuppression (with neutropenia and thrombocytopenia being the most problematic), immunosuppression, nausea and vomiting, hepatic dysfunction, upper and lower gastrointestinal mucositis, dermatitis, and alopecia. Fortunately, the tissues affected also recover relatively quickly such that the acute adverse effects are nearly always reversible. Life-threatening effects of many chemotherapy agents include severe neutropenia with infection, fungemia or fungal pneumonia due to immunosuppression, and septicemia, which is frequently contributed to by indwelling intravascular devices. Cardiomyopathy caused by anthracyclines (doxorubicin and daunorubicin) and renal failure from platinum-containing agents may also be life threatening and frequently disabling.

Least susceptible to chemotherapy and radiotherapy are cells that do not replicate or that replicate slowly, such as neurons, muscle cells, connective tissue, and bone. However, children are not exempt from toxicities of these tissues, probably because they are still undergoing proliferation, albeit at a slower pace than other tissues, during growth and growth spurts. Certain chemotherapeutic agents are particularly toxic to these tissues, and more so in adults than children; for instance, children are spared the neurotoxic effects of vin-cristine and methotrexate and the cardiotoxic effect of anthracyclines that occur in adults.

Children can in many ways physically endure the acute adverse effects of chemotherapy better than can adults. The maximum tolerated dose in children, when expressed on the basis of body surface area or body weight, is commonly greater than that in adults. A comparison of anticancer drugs tested in phase I trials in both adult and pediatric patients showed that the maximum tolerated dose in children was greater than that in adults for 70% of the agents, equal to that in adults for 15% of the agents, and less than the adult dose for only 15% of the agents. For all the drugs that were compared, the mean pediatric maximum tolerated dose was greater than the adult mean.

Newer treatment approaches that have not reached general clinical application in children are specific tumor-directed therapies such as tumor antigen–specific monoclonal antibodies, tumor vaccines, antisense DNA and RNA transcripts, and antiangiogenic agents.

SURGERY

Superb pediatric surgical and anesthesia services are indispensable for children with cancer. The pediatric surgeon's role varies depending on the type of tumor. In children with solid tumors,

TABLE 486–3. Adverse Effects of Various Chemotherapeutic Agents

Drug	Common Adverse Effects	Uncommon Adverse Effects
Antimetabolites		
Methotrexate	Myelosuppression, mucositis, hepatitis, dermatitis	Neurotoxicity, osteoporosis, pneumonitis, cirrhosis
Cytarabine (Ara-C)	Myelosuppression, nausea and vomiting	Mucositis, hepatitis, neurotoxicity with intrathecal administration
6-Thioguanine	Myelosuppression	Nausea and vomiting
6-Mercaptopurine	Myelosuppression, nausea and vomiting, abdominal pain, hepatitis	Mucositis
5-Azacytidine	Nausea and vomiting, myelosuppression	Hepatitis
5-Fluorouracil	Myelosuppression, anorexia, nausea and vomiting, mucositis	Dermatitis, alopecia, hyperpigmentation, cerebellar ataxia
Alkylating Agents		
Cyclophosphamide, ifosfamide	Myelosuppression, hemorrhagic cystitis, nausea and vomiting, alopecia	Mucositis, hyperpigmentation, hypo-osmolarity, infertility
Mechlorethamine (nitrogen mustard)	Nausea and vomiting, myelosuppression	Mucositis, alopecia
Chlorambucil	Myelosuppression	Nausea and vomiting, hepatitis
Melphalan	Myelosuppression	Anorexia, nausea and vomiting
Busulfan	Myelosuppression	Nausea and vomiting, alopecia, hyperpigmentation, pneumonitis
Antibiotics		
Doxorubicin, daunorubicin, idarubicin	Myelosuppression, nausea and vomiting, alopecia, mucositis	Cardiomyopathy
Dactinomycin (Actinomycin D)	Myelosuppression, nausea and vomiting, mucositis, alopecia	Dermatitis, hyperpigmentation, radiation recall
Bleomycin	Nausea and vomiting, dermatitis, hyperpigmentation, alopecia	Pulmonary fibrosis, mucositis, hypersensitivity reactions
Vinca Alkaloids		
Vincristine	Peripheral neuropathy, jaw pain, constipation, alopecia	Obstipation, cranial nerve palsies, seizures, myelosuppression, hemolysis, hypo-osmolarity
Vinblastine	Myelosuppression, nausea and vomiting, mucositis	Peripheral neuropathy, alopecia
Miscellaneous Agents		
Corticosteroids	Cushing's syndrome, diabetes, hypertension, growth delay	Hypokalemia, myopathy, osteoporosis, psychosis, adrenal insufficiency
Lomustine/carmustine (CCNU/BCNU)	Nausea and vomiting, delayed immunosuppression, myelosuppression	Hepatitis, stomatitis
Dacarbazine (DTIC)	Myelosuppression, nausea and vomiting, stomatitis	Hepatitis, alopecia
Procarbazine	Nausea and vomiting, myelosuppression, lethargy, dermatitis	Stomatitis, peripheral neuropathy, seizures, myopathy/myalgias
L-Asparaginase	Hypersensitivity reactions, coagulopathy, hyperglycemia, hepatic dysfunction	Encephalopathy, pancreatitis, abdominal pain
Cisplatin	Nausea and vomiting, nephrotoxicity, ototoxicity	Myelosuppression, seizures, peripheral and autonomic neuropathy
Hydroxyurea	Myelosuppression	Nausea and vomiting, mucositis, dermatitis, alopecia
Etoposide (VP-16)	Myelosuppression, nausea and vomiting	Hypersensitivity reactions, hypotension

complete resection with documented evidence of negative margins is often required for cure or long-term control. Considerable prolongation of life nearly always depends on whether the tumor is resectable and on the actual extent of resection.

With the exception of brainstem tumors and retinoblastoma, all solid tumors in children require a tissue diagnosis; therefore, biopsy of the suspected neoplasm is paramount. Staging with sentinel node biopsies has become a standard of care for several pediatric malignancies. Surgical expertise is essential for implantation of vascular access devices and removal and replacement of such devices when infection or thrombosis supervenes (see Chapter 165).

Increasingly, minimally invasive endoscopic surgical techniques are being used when indicated and, if the patient's condition permits, for biopsy and resection of tumor, direct ascertainment of residual disease and assessment of response, lysis of adhesions, and splenectomy.

RADIOTHERAPY

Radiotherapy is used sparingly in children, who are more susceptible than are adults to the adverse delayed effects of ionizing radiation. With more focused beams, such as conformal radiotherapy (a technology in which the beam conforms to the shape of the tumor and thus maximizes the amount of normal tissue spared) and better sedation and immobilization techniques, radiotherapy is becoming more frequently applied in children. Acute adverse effects from radiotherapy are less severe than those from chemotherapy and depend entirely on which part of the body is irradiated and the means of administration. Dermatitis is the most common general adverse effect, because skin is always in the treatment field. Nausea and diarrhea are common subacute adverse effects with abdominal radiotherapy. Mucositis nearly always occurs to some extent whenever oral or intestinal mucosa is in the treatment volume. Somnolence is common with cranial irradiation. Alopecia occurs where hair is in the radiation port.

Most radiotherapy schedules require treatment 5 days/wk for 4–7 wk, depending on the dose needed to control the tumor and on the amount and nature of normal tissue in the field. Most adverse effects are not noted until the second half of the course of irradiation. Late effects may occur months to years after radiotherapy and usually are dose-limiting manifestations. The type of delayed toxicity also depends on the site of irradiation. Examples are impaired growth resulting from cranial or vertebral irradiation, endocrine dysfunction from midbrain irradiation, pulmonary or cardiac insufficiency from chest irradiation, strictures and adhesions from abdominal irradiation, and infertility from pelvic irradiation.

ACUTE ADVERSE EFFECTS AND SUPPORTIVE CARE

Adverse treatment effects that occur early in therapy include metabolic disorders, bone marrow suppression, and immunosuppression. Patients with a large tumor burden may have had substantial breakdown of tumor cells, which, in some cases, causes renal function impairment, owing to tubular precipitates of uric acid crystals. This effect occurs most often in patients with leukemia and lymphoma (particularly Burkitt lymphoma) but also can occur in cases of large solid tumors (e.g., hepatoblastoma, germ cell tumors, and neuroblastoma). Before therapy is initiated, the serum levels of uric acid and creatinine should be measured and adequate hydration ensured; allopurinol (a xanthine oxidase inhibitor) can be given, if necessary, to lower uric acid levels to within the normal range. In the metabolic **tumor lysis syndrome,** phosphates and potassium are released into the circulation in large quantities as cells are lysed by treatment. Symptomatic hyperkalemia and hyperphosphatemia with subsequent hypocalcemia may develop in the setting of inadequate renal function.

Virtually all chemotherapy regimens can produce myelosuppression, as can tumors that invade and replace bone marrow. Anemia can be corrected by transfusions of packed erythrocytes, and thrombocytopenia, by platelet infusions. Patients receiving immunosuppressive therapy should receive irradiated blood products to prevent graft versus host disease. Granulocytopenia (granulocyte counts < 500/mm^3) poses a risk of life-threatening infection. Febrile granulocytopenic patients should be hospitalized and treated with empirical broad-spectrum intravenous antimicrobial therapy pending the results of appropriate cultures of blood, urine, or any obvious sites of infection (see Chapter 164). Treatment is continued until fever resolves and the granulocyte count rises. If fever persists more than 1 wk while the patient is receiving broad-spectrum antibiotics, the possibility of fungal infection must be considered. Fungal infections caused by *Candida* and *Aspergillus* are common in immunosuppressed patients. Opportunistic organisms such as *Pneumocystis carinii* can produce fatal pneumonia. Prophylactic treatment with trimethoprim/sulfamethoxazole is given when severe or prolonged immunosuppression is anticipated.

Viruses of low pathogenicity can produce serious disease in the setting of immunosuppression caused by malignancy or its treatment. Patients should not be given live virus vaccines. Children who are receiving chemotherapy and who are exposed to chickenpox should receive varicella-zoster immunoglobulin and, if clinical disease develops, should be hospitalized and treated with intravenous acyclovir.

Adequate pain management is critical. The World Health Organization (WHO) guidelines are particularly useful in the management of pain associated with cancer and cancer therapy (see Chapter 66).

It is common for patients undergoing cancer therapy to lose more than 10% of body weight. Patients sometimes reduce their food intake because of temporary, treatment-associated nausea, stomatitis, and vomiting. Appetite loss is not a cause for alarm. Malnutrition is a particular risk in patients receiving radiotherapy involving the abdomen or the head and neck, intensive chemotherapy, or total body irradiation and high-dose chemotherapy before marrow transplantation. If oral supplementation proves inadequate, such patients may require enteral tube feedings or parenteral hyperalimentation.

CHRONIC ADVERSE EFFECTS AND DELAYED SEQUELAE

Injury to tissues with low repair potential often results in long-lasting or permanent deficit. For example, anthracycline-induced cardiomyopathy usually produces refractory cardiac dysfunction, and the leukoencephalopathy caused by intrathecal methotrexate and by central nervous system radiotherapy is frequently only partially reversible.

Late consequences of therapy can cause substantial morbidity (Table 486–4). Successful surgical resection may result in loss of important functional structures. Irradiation can produce irreversible organ damage, with symptoms and functional limitations depending on the organ involved and the severity of the damage. Many radiotherapy-related problems do not become obvious until the patient is fully grown, such as asymmetry between irradiated and nonirradiated areas or extremities. Irradiation of fields that include endocrine organs can cause hypothyroidism, pituitary dysfunction, or infertility. In suffi-

TABLE 486–4. Long-Term Sequelae of Cancer Therapy

Sequela	Causative Treatment
Second cancers	Genetic predisposition, irradiation, alkylating agents
Sepsis	Splenectomy
Hepatotoxicity	Methotrexate, 6-mercaptopurine, irradiation
Amputation	Surgery for osteogenic sarcoma
Scoliosis	Irradiation, surgery
Osteonecrosis (hip)	Corticosteroids, methotrexate
Pulmonary dysfunction (interstitial fibrosis)	Irradiation, bleomycin, busulfan, nitrosourea
Cardiomyopathy	Doxorubicin, daunomycin, irradiation
Leukoencephalopathy	Cranial irradiation, methotrexate
Impaired cognition or intelligence	Cranial irradiation, methotrexate
Infertility	Alkylating agents, irradiation
Pituitary dysfunction	Cranial irradiation
Cataracts	Corticosteroids, cranial irradiation
Hypothyroidism	Neck irradiation

cient doses, cranial irradiation can produce neurologic dysfunction and spinal irradiation can produce growth retardation.

Chemotherapy also carries the risk of long-lasting organ damage. Of particular concern are leukoencephalopathy after high-dose methotrexate therapy; infertility in male patients treated with alkylating agents (e.g., cyclophosphamide); myocardial damage caused by anthracyclines; pulmonary fibrosis caused by bleomycin; pancreatitis caused by asparaginase; renal dysfunction due to ifosfamide, nitrosourea, or platinum agent; and hearing loss from cisplatin. Development of these sequelae may be dose related and is usually irreversible. Appropriate baseline and intermittent testing should be performed before these drugs are administered to ensure that there is no pre-existing damage to the organs likely to be affected and to permit monitoring of the effects of treatment-induced changes.

Perhaps the most serious late effect is the occurrence of second cancers in patients successfully cured of a first malignancy. The risk appears to be cumulative, increasing by about 0.5% per year, resulting in approximately a 12% incidence at 25 years after treatment. Patients who have been treated for childhood cancer should be examined annually, with particular attention to possible late effects of therapy, including second malignancies.

PALLIATIVE CARE

At all stages of caring for children with cancer, principles of palliative care should be applied to relieve pain and suffering and to provide comfort (see Chapter 38). Pain is a serious cause of suffering among patients with cancer and may be the result of organ obstruction or compression or bone metastasis or may be neuropathic. Pain should be managed in a stepwise manner, as recommended by the WHO, in accordance with the principles of selecting the appropriate analgesic, prescribing the appropriate dosage, administering the drug by the appropriate route, and choosing an appropriate dosing schedule to prevent persistent pain and to relieve breakthrough pain (see Chapter 66). In addition, the dosage should be aggressively titrated while attempts are made to prevent, anticipate, and manage side effects. Adjuvant drugs and sequential trials of analgesic drugs should be considered.

The goals in the care of dying patients are to avoid distress for the patient, family, and caregivers; to provide care consistent with the patient's and family's wishes; and to comply with and advocate for clinical, cultural, and ethical standards.

Andrassy RJ: *Pediatric Surgical Oncology*. Philadelphia, WB Saunders, 1998.
Andrassy RJ, Chwals WJ: Nutritional support of the pediatric oncology patient. *Nutrition* 1998;14:124–9.
Bernstein ML, Reaman GH, Hirschfeld S: Developmental therapeutics in childhood cancer. A perspective from the children's oncology group and the US Food and Drug Administration. *Hematol Oncol Clin North Am* 2001;1:631–55.

Blatt J, Dreyer ZE, Bleyer A: Late effects of childhood cancer and its treatment. In Pizzo PA, Poplack DG (editors): *Principles and Practice of Pediatric Oncology*, 4th ed. Philadelphia, Lippincott Williams & Wilkins, 2002, pp 1431–61.

Bleyer WA: Principles of cancer chemotherapy in children. *Cancer Bull* 1992;44: 461–9.

Bleyer WA: The past and future of cancer in the young. *Pediatr Dent* 1995;17:285–90.

Coppes M, Tubergen DG, Arceci RJ: Pediatric oncology in the 21st century: I and II. *Hematol Oncol Clin North Am* 2001;15:631–910.

Neville HL, Andrassy RJ, Lally KP, et al: Lymphatic mapping with sentinel node biopsy in pediatric patients. *J Pediatr Surg* 2000;35:961–4.

Steen RG, Mirro J Jr: *Childhood Cancer: A Handbook from St. Jude Children's Research Hospital*. Cambridge, MA, Perseus, 2000.

Weitman S, Kamen BA: Cancer chemotherapy and pharmacology in children. In Shilsky R, Milano G, Ratain M (editors): *Principles of Cancer Drug Pharmacology*. New York, Marcel Dekker, 1996.

Chapter 487

The Leukemias

David G. Tubergen and Archie Bleyer

The leukemias are the most common malignant neoplasms in childhood, accounting for about 41% of all malignancies that occur in children younger than 15 yr of age. In 2000, approximately 3,600 children were diagnosed with leukemia in the United States, for an annual incidence of 4.1 new cases per 100,000 children younger than 15 yr of age. Acute lymphoblastic leukemia (ALL) accounts for about 77% of cases of childhood leukemia, acute myelogenous leukemia (AML) for about 11%, chronic myelogenous leukemia (CML) for 2–3%, and juvenile chronic myelogenous leukemia (JCML) for 1–2%. The remaining 7–9% of cases include a variety of acute and chronic leukemias that do not fit classic definitions for ALL, AML, CML, or JCML.

The leukemias may be defined as a group of malignant diseases in which genetic abnormalities in a hematopoietic cell give rise to a clonal proliferation of cells. The progeny of these cells have a growth advantage over normal cellular elements owing to an increased rate of proliferation, a decreased rate of spontaneous apoptosis, or both. The result is a disruption of normal marrow function and, ultimately, marrow failure. The clinical features, laboratory findings, and responses to therapy vary depending on the type of leukemia.

487.1 Acute Lymphoblastic Leukemia

Childhood ALL was the first disseminated cancer shown to be curable and as such has represented the model malignancy for the principles of cancer diagnosis, prognosis, and treatment. It is actually a heterogeneous group of malignancies with a number of distinctive genetic abnormalities that result in varying clinical behaviors and responses to therapy.

Epidemiology. Approximately 2,800 children are diagnosed with ALL in the United States annually. It has a striking peak incidence between 2–6 yr of age and occurs slightly more frequently in boys than in girls. This peak age incidence was apparent decades ago in white populations in advanced socioeconomic countries, but more recently has also been confirmed in the black population of the United States. The disease is more common in children with certain chromosomal abnormalities such as Down syndrome, Bloom syndrome, ataxia-telangiectasia, and Fanconi syndrome. Among identical twins, the risk to the second twin if one develops leukemia is greater than that in the general population. The risk may be as high as 100% if the first twin is diagnosed during the first year of life and the twins shared the same (monochorionic) placenta. If the first twin

develops ALL by 5–7 yr of age, the risk to the second twin is at least twice that in the general population, regardless of zygosity.

Etiology. In virtually all cases, the etiology of ALL is unknown, although several genetic and environmental factors are associated with childhood leukemia (Box 487–1). Exposure to medical diagnostic radiation both in utero and in childhood has been associated with an increased incidence of ALL. In addition, published descriptions and investigations of geographic clusters of cases have raised concern that environmental factors may increase the incidence of ALL. Thus far, no such factors other than radiation have been identified, except for an association between B-cell ALL and Epstein-Barr viral infections in certain developing countries.

Pathogenesis. The classification of ALL depends on characterizing the malignant cells in the bone marrow to determine the morphology, phenotypic characteristics as measured by cell membrane markers, and cytogenetic and molecular genetic features. Morphology alone is usually adequate to establish a diagnosis, but the other studies are essential for disease classification, which may have a major influence on both the prognosis and the choice of appropriate therapy. In terms of clinical significance, the most important distinguishing morphologic feature is the French-American-British (FAB) L3 subtype, which is evidence of a mature B-cell leukemia. The L3 type, also known as Burkitt leukemia, is one of the most rapidly growing cancers in humans and requires a different therapeutic approach. Phenotypically, surface markers show that about 85% of cases of ALL are derived from progenitors of B cells, about 15% are derived from T cells, and about 1% are derived from B cells. A small percentage of children diagnosed with leukemia have a disease characterized by surface markers of both lymphoid and myeloid derivation.

Chromosomal abnormalities are found in most patients with ALL (Table 487–1). The abnormalities, which may be related to chromosomal number, translocations, or deletions, provide important prognostic information. Specific chromosomal findings, such as the t(9;22) translocation, suggest a need for additional, molecular genetic studies. The polymerase chain reaction and fluorescence in situ hybridization techniques, for example, offer the ability to pinpoint molecular genetic abnormalities and to detect small numbers of malignant cells during follow-up; however, the clinical utility of these findings has yet to be firmly established.

Clinical Manifestations. The initial presentation of ALL is usually nonspecific and relatively brief. Anorexia, fatigue, and irritability are often present, as is an intermittent, low-grade fever. Bone or joint pain, particularly in the lower extremities, may be present. Patients often have a history of an upper respiratory tract infection in the proceeding 1–2 mo. Less commonly, symptoms

---

BOX 487–1. Factors Predisposing to Childhood Leukemia

GENETIC CONDITIONS	ENVIRONMENTAL FACTORS
Down syndrome	Ionizing radiation
Fanconi syndrome	Drugs
Bloom syndrome	Alkylating agents
Diamond-Blackfan anemia	Nitrosourea
Schwachman syndrome	Epipodophyllotoxin
Klinefelter syndrome	Benzene exposure
Turner syndrome	Advanced maternal age
Neurofibromatosis	
Ataxia-telangiectasia	
Severe combined immune deficiency	
Paroxysmal nocturnal hemoglobinuria	
Li-Fraumeni syndrome	

TABLE 487–1. Common Chromosomal Abnormalities in the Acute Leukemias of Childhood

Disease, Subtype	Chromosomal Abnormality	Influence on Prognosis
ALL, pre-B	Trisomy 4 and 10	Favorable
	t(12;21)	
ALL, pre-B	t(4;11)	Unfavorable
ALL, pre-B	t(9;22)	Unfavorable
ALL, B-cell	t(8;14)	None
ALL (general)	Hyperdiploidy	Favorable
ALL (general)	Hypodiploidy	Unfavorable
AML, M1*	t(8;21)	Favorable
AML, M4*	inv(16)	Favorable
AML, M3*	t(15;17)	Favorable
AML (general)	del(7)	Unfavorable
AML, infant	t(4;11)	Unfavorable

Per the French-American-British classification of acute myelogenous leukemia (see Table 487–2).
ALL = acute lymphoblastic leukemia; AML = acute myelogenous leukemia.

may be of several months' duration, may be predominantly localized to the bones or joints, and may include joint swelling. As the disease progresses, signs and symptoms of bone marrow failure become more obvious with the occurrence of pallor, fatigue, bruising, or epistaxis, as well as fever, which may be caused by infection.

On physical examination, findings of pallor, listlessness, purpuric and petechial skin lesions, or mucous membrane hemorrhage may reflect bone marrow failure. The proliferative nature of the disease may be manifested as lymphadenopathy, splenomegaly, or, less commonly, hepatomegaly. In patients with bone or joint pain, there may be exquisite tenderness on bone palpation or objective evidence of joint swelling and effusion. Rarely, patients show signs of increased intracranial pressure that indicate leukemic involvement of the central nervous system (CNS). These include papilledema (see Fig. 485–5), retinal hemorrhages, and cranial nerve palsies. Respiratory distress is usually related to anemia but may occur in patients with an obstructive airway problem, owing to a large mediastinal mass of lymphoblasts. This problem is most typically seen in adolescent boys with T-cell ALL.

Diagnosis. The diagnosis of ALL is strongly suggested by peripheral blood findings indicative of bone marrow failure. Anemia and thrombocytopenia are seen in most patients. Leukemic cells are often not observed in the peripheral blood in routine laboratory examinations. Most patients with ALL present with total leukocyte counts of less than 10,000/µL. In such cases, the leukemic cells are often initially reported to be atypical lymphocytes, and it is only with further evaluation that the cells are found to be part of a malignant clone. When the results of an analysis of peripheral blood suggest the possibility of leukemia, a bone marrow examination should be done promptly to establish the diagnosis. Bone marrow aspiration alone is usually sufficient, but sometimes a bone marrow biopsy is needed to provide adequate tissue for study or to exclude other possible causes of bone marrow failure.

ALL is diagnosed by a bone marrow evaluation that demonstrates more than 25% of the bone marrow cells as a homogeneous population of lymphoblasts. Staging of ALL is partly based on a cerebrospinal fluid (CSF) examination. If lymphoblasts are found and the CSF leukocyte count is elevated, overt CNS (or meningeal) leukemia is present; a worse stage is implied and additional CNS and systemic therapies are indicated. The staging lumbar puncture may be performed in conjunction with the first dose of intrathecal chemotherapy if the diagnosis of leukemia has been previously established from bone marrow evaluation.

DIFFERENTIAL DIAGNOSIS. Acute lymphoblastic leukemia must be differentiated from acute myelogenous leukemia (AML); other malignant diseases that may invade the bone marrow and cause marrow failure such as neuroblastoma, rhabdomyosarcoma, Ewing's sarcoma, and retinoblastoma; and causes of primary bone marrow failure, such as aplastic anemia (either congenital or acquired) and myelofibrosis. Failure of a single cell line, as in transient erythroblastic anemia, immune thrombocytopenia, and congenital or acquired neutropenia, sometimes produces a clinical picture that is difficult to distinguish from ALL and that may require bone marrow examination. A high index of suspicion is required to differentiate ALL from infectious mononucleosis in patients with acute onset of fever and lymphadenopathy and from rheumatoid arthritis in patients with fever and joint swelling. These presentations also may require bone marrow examination.

Treatment. The single most important prognostic factor in ALL is the treatment: without effective therapy the disease is fatal. The survival rates of children with ALL over the past 40 yr have improved as the results of clinical trials have improved the therapies and outcomes (Fig. 487–1).

The choice of treatment of ALL is based on the estimated clinical risk of relapse in the patient, which varies widely among the subtypes of ALL. Three of the most important predictive factors are the age of the patient at the time of diagnosis, the initial leukocyte count, and the speed of response to treatment (i.e., how rapidly the blast cells can be cleared from the marrow or peripheral blood). Different study groups use various factors to define risk, but a patient between 1–10 yr of age and with a leukocyte count of less than 50,000/µL is widely used to define average

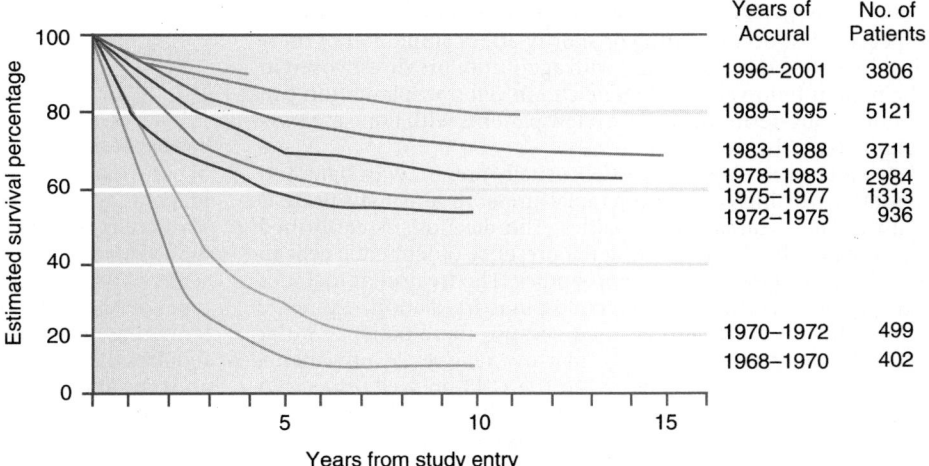

FIGURE 487–1. Survival rates of children with acute lymphoblastic leukemia treated on sequential Children's Cancer Group (COG) clinical trials over 30 yr. (Data provided by H. N. Sather.)

Years of Accural	No. of Patients
1996–2001	3806
1989–1995	5121
1983–1988	3711
1978–1983	2984
1975–1977	1313
1972–1975	936
1970–1972	499
1968–1970	402

risk. Patients considered to be at higher risk are children who are older than 10 yr of age or who have an initial leukocyte count of more than 50,000/μL. Recent trials have shown that the outcome for patients at higher risk can be improved by administration of more intensive therapy despite the greater toxicity of such therapy. Infants with ALL, along with patients who present with specific chromosomal abnormalities such as t(9;22) or t(4;11), have an even higher risk of relapse despite intensive therapy. Clinical trials have also demonstrated that the prognosis for patients with a slower response to initial therapy may be improved by therapy that is more intensive than the therapy considered necessary for patients who respond more rapidly.

Most children with ALL are treated on clinical trials conducted by national or international cooperative groups. In general, the initial therapy is designed to eradicate the leukemic cells from the bone marrow and is known as **remission induction.** During this phase, therapy is usually given for 4 wk and consists of vincristine weekly, a corticosteroid such as dexamethasone or prednisone, and either repeated doses of native L-asparaginase or a single dose of a long-acting asparaginase preparation. Intrathecal cytarabine or methotrexate, or both, may also be given. Patients at higher risk also receive daunomycin at weekly intervals. With this approach, 98% of patients are in remission, as defined by less than 5% blasts in the marrow and a return of neutrophil and platelet counts to near-normal levels after 4–5 wk of treatment. Intrathecal chemotherapy is usually given at the time of diagnosis and once more during induction.

The second phase of treatment focuses on **CNS therapy** in an effort to prevent later CNS relapses. Intrathecal chemotherapy is given repeatedly by lumbar puncture in conjunction with intensive systemic chemotherapy. The likelihood of later CNS relapse is thereby reduced to less than 5%. A small proportion of patients with features that predict a high risk of CNS relapse receive irradiation to the brain and spinal cord. This includes those patients who have lymphoblasts in the CSF and an elevated CSF leukocyte count at the time of diagnosis.

After remission induction, many regimens provide 14–28 wk of multiagent therapy, with the drugs and schedules used varying depending on the risk group of the patient. Finally, patients are given daily mercaptopurine and weekly methotrexate, usually with intermittent doses of vincristine and a corticosteroid. This period, known as the **maintenance phase** of therapy, lasts for 2–3 yr, depending on the protocol used. A small number of patients with particularly poor prognostic features, principally those with the t(9;22) translocation known as the Philadelphia chromosome, may undergo bone marrow transplantation during the first remission. In ALL, this chromosome is similar but not identical to the Philadelphia chromosome of chronic myelogenous leukemia (CML).

The major impediment to a successful outcome is relapse of the disease. Relapse occurs in the bone marrow in 15–20% of patients with ALL and carries the most serious implications, especially if it occurs during or shortly after completion of therapy. Intensive chemotherapy with agents not previously used in the patient followed by allogeneic stem cell transplantation can result in long-term survival for a few patients with bone marrow relapse (see Chapter 125).

Patients with relapse in the CNS usually present with signs and symptoms of increased intracranial pressure and may present with isolated cranial nerve palsies. The diagnosis is confirmed most readily by demonstrating the presence of leukemic cells in the CSF and, rarely, by imaging studies. The treatment includes intrathecal medication and craniospinal irradiation. Systemic chemotherapy must also be used because these patients are at high risk for subsequent bone marrow relapse. Most patients with leukemic relapse confined to the CNS do well, especially those in whom the CNS relapse occurs after chemotherapy has been completed or during the latter phase of chemotherapy.

Testicular relapse occurs in 1–2% of boys with ALL, usually after completion of therapy. Such relapse presents as painless swelling of one or both testes. The diagnosis is confirmed by biopsy of the affected testis. Treatment includes systemic chemotherapy and local irradiation. A high proportion of boys with a testicular relapse can be successfully re-treated, and the survival rate of these patients is good.

SUPPORTIVE CARE. Close attention to the medical supportive care needs of the patients is essential in successfully administering aggressive chemotherapeutic programs. Patients with a large tumor burden are prone to tumor lysis syndrome as therapy is initiated. Chemotherapy often produces severe myelosuppression, which may require erythrocyte and platelet transfusion and which always requires a high index of suspicion and aggressive empirical antimicrobial therapy for sepsis in febrile children with neutropenia. Patients need to receive prophylactic treatment of *Pneumocystis carinii* pneumonia during chemotherapy and for several months after completing treatment.

The success of therapy has changed ALL from an acute disease with a high mortality rate to a chronic disease. However, such chronic treatment can incur substantial academic, developmental, and psychosocial costs for children with ALL and considerable financial costs and stress for their families. Because of the intensity of therapy, long-term and acute toxicity effects may occur. An array of cancer care professionals with training and experience in addressing the myriad of problems that may arise is essential to minimize the complications and achieve an optimal outcome.

Prognosis. Most children with ALL can now be expected to have long-term survival, with the rate greater than 80% after 5 yr (see Fig. 487–1). The most important prognostic factor is the choice of appropriate risk-directed therapy, with the type of treatment chosen according to the type of ALL, the stage of disease, the age of the patient, and the rate of response to initial therapy. Characteristics generally believed to adversely affect outcome include an age younger than 1 yr or older than 10 yr at diagnosis, a leukocyte count of more than 100,000/μL at diagnosis, or a slow response to initial therapy. Chromosomal abnormalities, including hypodiploidy, the Philadelphia chromosome, and t(4;11), portend a poorer outcome. More favorable characteristics include a rapid response to therapy, hyperdiploidy, and rearrangements of the *TEL/AML1* genes.

487.2 Acute Myelogenous Leukemia

Epidemiology. AML comprises 11% of the cases of leukemia in childhood in the United States, with approximately 380 children diagnosed with AML annually. One subtype, acute promyelocytic leukemia (APL), is more common in certain other regions of the world, but incidence of the other types is generally uniform. Several chromosomal abnormalities associated with AML are identified, but no predisposing genetic or environmental factors can be identified in most patients (see Table 487–1).

Pathogenesis. The characteristic feature of AML is more than 30% of bone marrow cells on bone marrow aspiration or biopsy touch preparations that constitute a rather homogeneous population of blasts cells with features similar to those that characterize early differentiation states of the myeloid-monocyte-megakaryocyte series of blood cells. The most common classification of the subtypes of AML is the FAB system (Table 487–2). Although this system is based on morphologic criteria alone, current practice also requires the use of flow cytometry for identification of cell surface antigens and of chromosomal and molecular genetic techniques for additional diagnostic precision and also to aid the choice of therapy.

TABLE 487–2. French-American-British (FAB) Classification of Acute Myelogenous Leukemia

Subtype	Common Name
M1	Acute myeloblastic leukemia without maturation
M2	Acute myeloblastic leukemia with maturation
M3	Acute promyeloblastic leukemia
M4	Acute myelomonocytic leukemia
M5	Acute monocytic leukemia
M6	Erythroleukemia
M7	Acute megakaryocytic leukemia

Clinical Manifestations. The production of symptoms and signs of AML, as in ALL, is due to replacement of bone marrow by malignant cells and to secondary bone marrow failure. Thus, patients with AML may present with any or all of the findings associated with marrow failure in ALL. In addition, patients with AML present with signs and symptoms that infrequently occur with ALL, including subcutaneous nodules or "blueberry muffin" lesions, infiltration of the gingiva, signs and laboratory findings of disseminated intravascular coagulation (especially indicative of acute promyelocytic leukemia), and discrete masses, known as **chloromas** or **granulocytic sarcomas.** These masses may occur in the absence of apparent bone marrow involvement and are typically associated with the M2 subcategory of AML with a t(8;21) translocation.

Diagnosis. Analysis of bone marrow aspiration and biopsy specimens of patients with AML typically reveals the features of a hypercellular marrow consisting of a rather monotonous pattern of cells with features that permit FAB subclassification of disease. Special stains assist in identification of myeloperoxidase-containing cells, thus confirming both the myelogenous origin of the leukemia and the diagnosis. Some chromosomal abnormalities and molecular genetic markers are characteristic of specific subtypes of disease (see Box 487–1).

Treatment. Aggressive multiagent chemotherapy is successful in inducing remission in about 80% of patients. Up to 10% of patients die of either infection or bleeding before a remission can be achieved. Matched-sibling bone marrow or stem cell transplantation after remission has been shown to achieve long-term disease-free survival in 60–70% of patients. Continued chemotherapy for patients who do not have a matched donor is less effective than marrow transplantation but nevertheless is curative in some patients.

Acute promyelocytic leukemia, characterized by a gene rearrangement involving the retinoic acid receptor, is very responsive to retinoic acid combined with anthracyclines. The success of this therapy makes marrow transplantation in first remission unnecessary for patients with this disease.

The supportive care needs of patients with AML are basically the same as those given for ALL. The very intensive therapy required in AML produces prolonged bone marrow suppression with a very high incidence of serious infections.

487.3 Down Syndrome and Acute Leukemia and Myeloproliferation

Acute leukemia occurs about 14 times more frequently in children with Down syndrome than in the general population. The ratio of ALL to AML in patients with Down syndrome is the same as that in the general population. In Down children with ALL, the expected outcome of treatment is the same as that for other children. However, patients with Down syndrome demonstrate a remarkable sensitivity to methotrexate and other antimetabolites, which can result in substantial toxicity if stan-

dard doses are administered. In AML, however, patients with Down syndrome have much better outcomes, with a greater than 80% long-term survival rate, than does the non-Down syndrome population. After induction therapy, these patients require less intensive therapy to achieve the better results.

Neonates with Down syndrome are prone to develop a transient leukemia or myeloproliferative syndrome characterized by high leukocyte counts, blast cells in the peripheral blood, and associated anemia, thrombocytopenia, and hepatosplenomegaly. These features usually resolve within days to a few weeks after onset. Although these neonates may require temporary transfusion support, they do not require chemotherapy. However, patients who have Down syndrome and who develop this transient leukemia or myeloproliferative syndrome require close follow-up because 20–30% will develop typical leukemia within the first few years of life.

487.4 Chronic Myelogenous Leukemia

CML is a clonal disorder of the hematopoietic tissue that accounts for 2–3% of all cases of childhood leukemia. About 99% of the cases are characterized by a specific translocation, t(9;22)(q34;q11), known as the **Philadelphia chromosome.** The disease has been associated with exposure to ionizing radiation but very few children with CML have a history of such exposure. The disease is characterized clinically by an initial chronic phase in which the malignant clone produces an elevated leukocyte count with a predominance of mature forms but with increased numbers of immature granulocytes. The spleen is often greatly enlarged, often resulting in pain in the left upper quadrant of the abdomen. In addition to leukocytosis, the blood counts may reveal mild anemia and thrombocytosis.

Typically, the chronic phase terminates 3–4 yr after onset when the CML moves into the accelerated or "blast crisis" phase. At this point, the blood counts rise dramatically and cannot be controlled with drugs such as hydroxyurea. Additional manifestations may occur, including hyperuricemia and neurologic symptoms, which are related to increased blood viscosity with decreased CNS perfusion.

The presenting symptoms of CML are entirely nonspecific and may include fever, fatigue, weight loss, and anorexia. Splenomegaly may also be present. The diagnosis is suggested by increased numbers of myeloid cells with differentiation to mature forms in the peripheral blood and bone marrow and is confirmed by cytogenetic studies that demonstrate the presence of the characteristic Philadelphia chromosome. Molecular techniques usually demonstrate the *BCR-ABL* gene rearrangement. The translocation, although characteristic of CML, is also found in a small percentage of patients with ALL or AML.

The signs and symptoms of CML in the chronic phase can be controlled with hydroxyurea, which will gradually return the leukocyte count to normal. However, this treatment is not definitive and does not eliminate the abnormal clone or prevent progression of the disease. Therapy with interferon-α produces hematologic remission in up to 70% of patients and cytogenetic remission in about 20% of patients. Combination chemotherapy has been successful in achieving remission in a small proportion of patients with CML; however, the optimum therapy is allogeneic bone marrow or stem cell transplantation from an HLA-matched sibling, which is curative in up to 80% of children.

Exciting results have recently been reported with imatinib mesylate, an agent designed specifically to inhibit the *BCR-ABL* tyrosine kinase. Although this drug is very effective in adult patients, trials in children are just beginning. It is hoped that this agent will usher in a new era of therapy for CML by specifically targeting the genetic abnormality of the malignant clone of cells.

487.5 Juvenile Chronic Myelogenous Leukemia

Juvenile chronic myelogenous leukemia (JCML), also known as juvenile myelomonocytic leukemia, is a clonal proliferation of hematopoietic stem cells that typically affects children younger than 2 yr of age. Patients with this disease do not have the Philadelphia chromosome that is characteristic of CML. Patients with JCML present with rashes, lymphadenopathy, and splenomegaly. Analysis of the peripheral blood often shows an elevated leukocyte count and may also show thrombocytopenia and the presence of erythroblasts. The bone marrow shows a myelodysplastic pattern, with blasts accounting for less than 30% of cells. No distinctive cytogenetic abnormalities are seen. JCML is rare constituting less than 2% of all cases of childhood leukemia. Therapeutic reports are largely anecdotal. Patients with neurofibromatosis have a predilection for this type of leukemia. Stem cell transplantation offers the best opportunity for cure, but much less so than for classic CML.

487.6 Infant Leukemia

Only about 2% of cases of leukemia during childhood occur before the age of 1 yr. Several unique biologic features and a particularly poor prognosis are characteristic of ALL during infancy. More than two thirds of the cases demonstrate rearrangements of the *MLL* gene, classically a translocation involving the q23 band of chromosome 11, and it is this subset of patients that largely accounts for the very high relapse rate. These patients often present with hyperleukocytosis and extensive tissue invasion, including CNS disease. Subcutaneous nodules **(leukemia cutis)** and tachypnea due to diffuse pulmonary infiltration by leukemic cells are more frequently observed in infants than in older children. The leukemic cell morphology is usually that of large irregular lymphoblasts (FAB L2) with a phenotype negative for the CD10 (cALLa) marker.

Very intensive chemotherapy programs including stem cell transplantation are being explored in infants with rearrangement of *MLL* in band 11q23, but none has yet proved satisfactory. Infants with leukemia who lack the 11q23 rearrangements have a prognosis similar to that of older children with ALL. Infants with AML often present with CNS or skin involvement and have the FAB M4 subtype, which is commonly known as **acute myelomonocytic leukemia.** The treatment may be the same as that for older children with AML. Meticulous supportive care is necessary because of the young age and aggressive therapy needed in these patients.

General
Fisher DE: Pathways of apoptosis and the modulation of cell death. *Hematol Oncol Clin North Am* 2001;15:931–56.
Reynolds CP, Lemons RS: Retinoid therapy of childhood cancer. *Hematol Oncol Clin North Am* 2001;15:867–910.
Ries LAG, Eisner MP, Kosary CL, et al (editors): *SEER Cancer Statistics Review, 1973–1999.* Bethesda, MD, National Cancer Institute, 2002. http://seer.cancer.gov/csr/1973_1999/
Rubnitz JE, Look AT: Molecular genetics of childhood leukemias. *J Pediatr Hemat Oncol* 1998;20:1–11.

Acute Lymphoblastic Leukemia
Arico M, Valsecchi MG, Camitta B, et al: Outcome of treatment in children with Philadelphia chromosome–positive acute lymphoblastic leukemia. *N Engl J Med* 2000;342:998–1006.
Bleyer WA: Acute lymphoblastic leukemia. In Herzog CE, Pratt CB (editors): *Therapy of Cancer in Children.* New York, Clinical Insights 2000, pp 8–10.
Chessels JM: The management of high risk lymphoblastic leukemia in children. *Br J Hematol* 2000;108:204–16.
Coustan-Smith E, Sancho J, Hancock ML, et al: Clinical importance of minimal residual disease in childhood acute lymphoblastic leukemia. *Blood* 2000;96:2691–96.
Gaynon PS, Trigg ME, Heerema NA, et al: Children's Cancer Group trials in acute lymphoblastic leukemia 1983–1995. *Leukemia* 2000;14:2223–33.
Pui CH, Evans WE: Acute lymphoblastic leukemia. *N Engl J Med* 1998;339:605–14.

Roberts WM, Estrov Z, Ouspenskaia MV, et al: Measurement of residual leukemia during remission in childhood acute lymphoblastic leukemia. *N Engl J Med* 1997;336:317–23.
Schrappe M, Reiter A, Ludwig WD, et al: Improved outcome in childhood acute lymphoblastic leukemia despite reduced use of anthracyclines and cranial radiotherapy: Results of trial ALL-BFM 90. *Blood* 2000;95:3310–22.
Zipf TF, Berg SL, Roberts WM, et al: Childhood leukemias. In Abeloff MD, Armitage JO, Lichter AS, et al (editors): *Clinical Oncology*, 2nd ed. New York, Churchill Livingstone, 2000, pp 2402–34.

Acute and Chronic Myelogenous Leukemia
Druker BJ, Talpaz M, Resta DJ, et al: Efficacy and safety of a specific inhibitor of the BCR-ABL tyrosine kinase in chronic myeloid leukemia. *N Engl J Med* 2001;344:1031–37.
Fenaux P, Chomienne C, Degos J: All-*trans* retinoic acid and chemotherapy in the treatment of acute promyelocytic leukemia. *Semin Hematol* 2001;38:13–25.
Perentesis JP, Sievers EL: Targeted therapies for high-risk acute myeloid leukemia. *Hematol Oncol Clin North Am* 2001;15:677–701.
Powell BL: Acute progranulocytic leukemia. *Curr Opin Oncol* 2001;13:8–13.
Smith FO, Sanders JE: Juvenile myelomonocytic leukemia: What we don't know. *J Pediatr Hemat Oncol* 1999;21:461–63.
Sande LE, Arcecci RJ, Lampkin BC: Congenital and neonatal leukemia. *Semin Perinatol* 1999;23:274–85.
Woods WG, Neudorf S, Gold S, et al: A comparison of allogeneic bone marrow transplantation, autologous bone marrow transplantation, and aggressive chemotherapy in children with acute myeloid leukemia in first remission: A report from the Children's Cancer Group. *Blood* 2001;97:56–62.
Zipf TF, Berg SL, Roberts WM, et al: Childhood leukemias. In Abeloff MD, Armitage JO, Lichter AS, et al (editors): *Clinical Oncology*, 2nd ed. New York, Churchill Livingstone, 2000, pp 2402–34.

Chapter 488

Lymphoma *Gerald S. Gilchrist*

Lymphoma is the third most common cancer in children in the United States, with an annual incidence of 13–14 per million children. The two broad categories of lymphoma, Hodgkin disease and non-Hodgkin lymphoma (NHL), have such different clinical manifestations and treatments that they are considered separately.

488.1 Hodgkin Disease

Epidemiology. In the United States, Hodgkin disease accounts for about 5% of cancers in persons younger than 15 yr of age and for about 15% in persons 15–19 yr of age, with an incidence ratio among blacks and whites of 1.6. In industrialized countries the highest rate is in adolescents and young adults, in contrast to developing countries, where the highest rate is in younger children.

Three forms of Hodgkin disease have been identified in epidemiologic studies: a childhood form ($\leq$ 14 yr of age), a young adult form (15–34 yr of age), and an older adult form (55–74 yr of age). The epidemiologic similarities of Hodgkin disease in young adults to paralytic polio in the pre-vaccine era suggest an infectious cause. The role of Epstein-Barr virus (EBV) is supported by serologic studies and the frequent presence of EBV genome in biopsy material. Males predominate in patients younger than 10 yr of age at diagnosis, with roughly equal gender incidence in adolescence. Pre-existing immunodeficiency, either congenital or acquired, increases the risk of developing Hodgkin disease. A genetic predisposition or a common exposure to the same etiologic agent could account for an apparent increased risk in twins and first-degree relatives ranging from 3- to 7-fold.

Pathogenesis. The **Reed-Sternberg cell,** a large cell (15–45 μm in diameter) with multiple or multilobulated nuclei, is considered the hallmark of Hodgkin disease, although similar cells are seen in infectious mononucleosis, NHL, and other conditions. There is now general agreement that the Reed-Sternberg cell arises from germinal center B-cells in most cases. An infiltrate of apparently normal lymphocytes, plasma cells, and eosinophils surround the Reed-Sternberg cell and varies with the histologic subtype. Other features that distinguish the histologic subtypes include various degrees of fibrosis and the presence of collagen bands, necrosis, or malignant reticular cells. The four major histologic subtypes are **lymphocyte predominant, nodular sclerosing, mixed cellularity, and lymphocyte depleted.** More recently, additional immunohistochemically identifiable subtypes have been described but their prognostic or therapeutic significance is not yet apparent in pediatric patients. Most cases previously classified as lymphocyte depleted are now considered to represent high-grade non-Hodgkin lymphoma. Since the advent of curative therapy, the prognostic significance of histologic subtype has been virtually eliminated.

Hodgkin disease appears to arise in lymphoid tissue and spreads to adjacent lymph node areas in a relatively orderly fashion. Hematogenous spread also occurs, leading to involvement of the liver, spleen, bone, bone marrow, or brain, and is usually associated with systemic symptoms. Levels of various cytokines have been shown to be elevated in patient sera or are produced by cultured cell lines or Hodgkin disease tissue. They may well be responsible for the systemic symptoms of fever and night sweats (interleukin 1 or 2) and weight loss (tissue necrosis factor [TNF]), in addition to influencing the proliferation of Reed-Sternberg cells and inducing immunosuppression (transforming growth factor-β)

Various degrees of cellular immune impairment can be identified in the majority of newly diagnosed cases of Hodgkin disease. The severity of the immune defect varies with the extent of disease and persists even after successful curative therapy. Whether it predisposes to the disease or results from it is unknown.

Clinical Manifestations. Painless, firm, cervical, or supraclavicular lymphadenopathy is the most common presenting sign. Inguinal or axillary lymphadenopathy sites are uncommon areas of presentation. An anterior mediastinal mass is often present and can rapidly disappear with therapy (Fig. 488–1). Clinically detectable hepatosplenomegaly is rarely encountered. Depending on the extent and location of nodal and extranodal disease, patients might present with symptoms and signs of airway obstruction, pleural or pericardial effusion, hepatocellular dysfunction, or bone marrow infiltration (anemia, neutropenia, or thrombocytopenia). Nephrotic syndrome is a rare but recognized presenting manifestation of Hodgkin disease.

Systemic symptoms considered important in staging are unexplained fever, weight loss, or drenching night sweats. Less common and not considered of prognostic significance are symptoms of pruritus, lethargy, anorexia, or pain that worsens after ingestion of alcohol.

Because of the impaired cellular immunity, concomitant tuberculous or fungal infections may complicate Hodgkin disease and predispose to complications during immunosuppressive therapy. In the pre-vaccine era varicella-zoster infections occurred at some time during the course of the disease in about 30% of cases.

Diagnosis. Any patient with persistent, unexplained lymphadenopathy unassociated with an obvious underlying inflammatory or infectious process should have a chest radiograph to identify the presence of a mediastinal mass before undergoing node biopsy. Unless signs or symptoms dictate otherwise, additional laboratory studies can be delayed until the biopsy results are available. Patients with persistently enlarged lymph nodes, even after serologically proven infectious mononucleosis, should also be considered for biopsy.

Formal excisional biopsy is preferred over needle biopsy to ensure that adequate tissue is obtained, both for light microscopy and for appropriate immunocytochemical and molecular studies, culture, and cytogenetic analysis if routine studies fail to provide a firm diagnosis. Hodgkin disease is rarely diagnosed with certainty on frozen section. Ideally, a portion of the biopsy specimen should be frozen and stored to allow for additional studies.

Once the diagnosis of Hodgkin disease is established, extent of disease (i.e., stage) should be determined. These studies should provide all the information needed to clinically stage the disease based on the Ann Arbor classification (Boxes 488–1 and 488–2). A complete blood cell count (CBC) identifies abnormalities that might suggest marrow involvement. Erythrocyte sedimentation rate (ESR), serum copper determination, and serum ferritin levels are of some prognostic significance and, if abnormal at diagnosis, serve as a baseline to evaluate the effects of treatment. Liver function tests, although not particularly sensitive to the

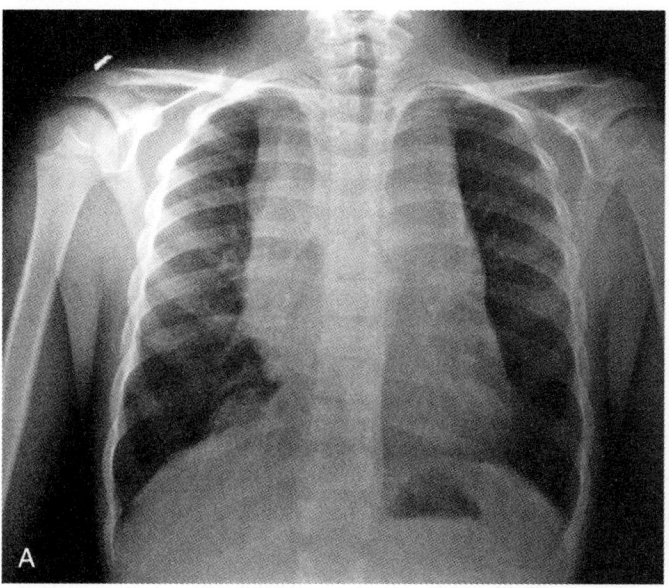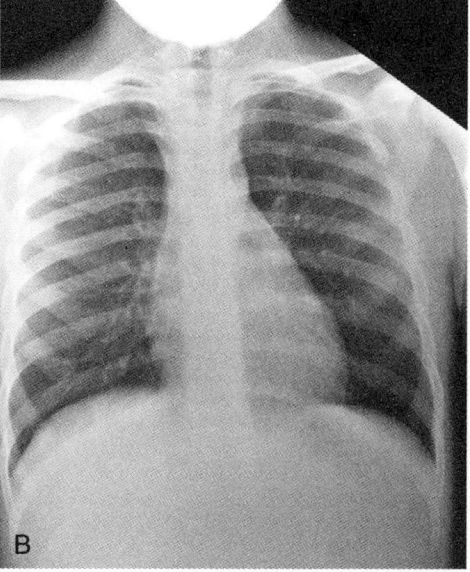

FIGURE 488–1. *A,* Anterior mediastinal mass in a patient with Hodgkin disease before therapy. *B,* Complete disappearance of mediastinal mass in the same patient after 2 mo of chemotherapy.

STAGE I
Involvement of a single lymph node region or of a single extralymphatic organ or site

STAGE II
Involvement of two or more lymphoid regions on the same side of the diaphragm; or localized involvement of an extralymphatic organ or site and of one or more lymph node regions on the same side of the diaphragm

STAGE III
Involvement of lymph node regions on both sides of the diaphragm, which may be accompanied by localized involvement of an extralymphatic organ or site or by splenic involvement

STAGE IV
Diffuse or disseminated involvement of one or more extralymphatic organs or tissues, with or without associated lymph node enlargement

*Stages are further categorized as:

A or B, based on the absence or presence, respectively, of systemic symptoms of fever and/or weight loss

Bulky disease, based on mediastinal mass larger than one third thoracic diameter; lymph node masses ≥10 cm in diameter and/or four or more nodal regions involved

From Lister TA, Crowther D, Sutcliffe SB, et al: Report of a committee convened to discuss the evaluation and staging of patients with Hodgkin's disease: Cotswolds meeting. *J Clin Oncol* 1989;7:1630–36.

presence of liver involvement, can influence treatment and treatment complications. A chest radiograph is particularly important for measuring the size of the mediastinal mass in relation to the maximal diameter of the thorax. Chest CT more clearly defines the extent of a mediastinal mass if present and identifies hilar nodes and pulmonary parenchymal involvement, which may not be evident on chest radiographs. Abdominal CT or MRI can identify gross subdiaphragmatic involvement of nodes together with enlargement and defects in the liver and spleen. Gallium-67 scan is particularly helpful in identifying areas of increased uptake, which can then be re-evaluated at the end of treatment, especially in patients with mediastinal masses that do not completely resolve on chest radiographs or CT. Lymphangiography, although unique in its ability to demonstrate intrinsic abnormalities in lymph nodes, is not without risk, is very labor intensive and uncomfortable, and fails to visualize upper para-aortic nodes. It is rarely performed in pediatric practice, where systemic therapy has become the cornerstone of treatment and would be expected to eliminate relatively small foci of disease.

Staging is based on involvement of lymph node regions (see Box 488–1). Surgical staging is no longer routinely performed and

BOX 488–2. Studies Necessary for Clinical Staging of Hodgkin Disease

Measurement of palpable lymph nodes, liver, and spleen
Complete blood cell count
Erythrocyte sedimentation rate, serum ferritin, serum copper
Liver function tests
Chest radiograph with measurement of mediastinal ratio
Chest CT with contrast medium enhancement
Neck CT if high cervical nodes palpable
Abdominal CT or MRI
Gallium scan
Bone marrow biopsy with advanced disease or "B" symptoms
Bone scan with elevated serum alkaline phosphatase level and/or bone pain

should be considered only if findings will significantly influence therapy. Bone marrow biopsy is necessary in only those patients with advanced (stage III or IV) disease or with "B" symptoms.

Treatment. Because of concern about late effects, treatment of children in North America and Europe has evolved from primary treatment with extended-field radiation therapy to use of multiagent chemotherapy as the cornerstone of treatment, supplemented in selected cases by relatively low-dose involved-field irradiation (2,000–2,500 cGy). Treatment is largely determined by disease stage, patient's age at diagnosis, the presence or absence of "B" symptoms, and the presence of hilar lymphadenopathy and/or bulky nodal disease. Although there is not yet general agreement on their definitions, three risk groups have been identified. Favorable presentations include stages I and IIA. Intermediate presentations include stages I, IIB (with symptoms, bulky disease, or hilar lymphadenopathy), and stage IIIA. Unfavorable presentations include stages IIIB and IV.

FAVORABLE AND INTERMEDIATE PRESENTATIONS. Cure rates with radiation alone (3,500–4,500 cGy) in surgically staged localized disease range from 40–80%, and the overwhelming majority of those who suffer relapse can be salvaged with a combination of multiagent chemotherapy or additional irradiation or both, resulting in cure rates of more than 90%. Unfortunately, this approach produces growth retardation in skeletally immature children and is associated with significant long-term morbidity, including thyroid failure, cardiac and pulmonary dysfunction, and an increased risk of breast cancer. For these reasons, many centers treating children and adolescents use combined modality therapy or even chemotherapy alone.

The chemotherapy regimens in current use are based on **MOPP** (nitrogen mustard [Mustargen], vincristine [Oncovin], procarbazine, and prednisone), or **ABVD** (doxorubicin [Adriamycin], bleomycin, vinblastine, and dacarbazine), or variations and/or combinations of the two together with additional active agents such as etoposide and methotrexate. As originally conceived, a minimum of six cycles of chemotherapy was given with significant cumulative toxicity, including second malignancies, sterility, and cardiac and pulmonary dysfunction. The long-term toxicity is determined by the total dose of the agents. Newly developed "risk-adapted" programs are based on staging criteria as well as rapidity of response to initial chemotherapy. Their aim is to reduce total drug doses and treatment duration and even eliminate radiation therapy.

UNFAVORABLE PRESENTATIONS. Chemotherapy, based on the same regimens used in early stage disease, is considered the primary treatment for patients with advanced disease, but the role of radiation is still under study. Because the cure rate with conventional drug combinations, with or without radiation therapy, is only 60–70%, newer and more aggressive regimens have been developed and are now in clinical trials.

RELAPSE. Patients who suffer relapse after initial treatment with radiation alone or after an initial remission of more than 12 mo after chemotherapy alone or combined modality therapy usually respond to additional chemotherapy or radiation or both. Those who never achieve remission or who suffer relapse after an initial remission of less than 12 mo after chemotherapy or combined modality therapy have a poorer prognosis and are candidates for myeloablative chemotherapy and autologous stem cell or bone marrow rescue.

Prognosis. Most treatment programs result in disease-free survival rates of more than 60%, with overall cure rates greater than 90% in those with early stage disease and more than 70% in more advanced cases. All newly diagnosed cases in children and adolescents should be treated with curative intent; this is consistently and effectively achieved with combined modality therapy. The choice of regimen is then selected on the basis of risk category and observed or anticipated long-term complications. Elimination of routine staging laparotomy and splenectomy avoids concerns about surgical morbidity and postsplenectomy infections.

488.2 Non-Hodgkin Lymphoma

Non-Hodgkin lymphoma (NHL) results from malignant clonal proliferation of lymphocytes of T-, B-, or indeterminate cell origin. In the United States, NHL occurs with an annual incidence of 10.5 per million white and 7.3 per million black children younger than 20 yr of age. In equatorial Africa, 50% of childhood cancers are lymphomas, a result of the very high incidence of Burkitt lymphoma and possibly related to the immunosuppressive effects of malaria. Unlike that of Hodgkin disease, the incidence of NHL increases steadily throughout life. In some situations there is overlap with acute lymphoblastic or B-cell leukemia. Patients with lymphoblastic NHL and more than 25% lymphoblasts in the bone marrow are arbitrarily classified and treated as if they had acute lymphoblastic leukemia, whereas patients with B-cell ALL are treated similarly to patients with Burkitt lymphoma even if no extramedullary disease is present.

Pathogenesis. EBV infection has a major role in the pathogenesis of Burkitt lymphoma. The EBV genome is present in tumor cells in 95% of "endemic" cases in equatorial Africa compared with 15% in "sporadic" cases in the United States. How EBV contributes to the pathogenesis of Burkitt lymphoma remains unclear. Congenital or acquired immunodeficiency also predisposes to the development of NHL. Epidemiologic studies have also implicated pesticide exposure as a possible risk factor.

Although elaborate classifications of NHL have been developed, they have little application to the pediatric disease. Most cases of NHL in children are high-grade, diffuse neoplasms. Three histologic subtypes are recognized: **lymphoblastic,** usually of T-cell origin; **small noncleaved cell lymphoma (SNCCL),** with Burkitt and non-Burkitt subtypes and of B-cell origin; and **large cell lymphoma (LCL),** with diffuse and anaplastic subtypes and of T-, B-, or indeterminate cell origin. The diagnosis and classification of childhood NHL requires considerable hematopathologic expertise and adequate diagnostic tissue, both fresh and frozen.

Different chromosomal translocations are specific for some histologic subtypes and involve various proto-oncogenes, resulting in malignant transformation through a variety of mechanisms. In SNCCL (Burkitt type), one of three chromosomal translocations [t(8;14), t(8;22), t(2;8)] results in approximation of the *MYC* proto-oncogene on chromosome 8 to a regulatory region of one of the immunoglobulin chain genes, resulting in dysregulation of *MYC*; in anaplastic LCL, fusion of the *NPM* gene on chromosome 5 with the *ALK* gene on chromosome 2 leads to formation of a chimeric protein that can influence cell growth and proliferation.

Clinical Manifestations. Presenting signs and symptoms vary with disease site and extent, and these in turn differ with histologic subtype.

Lymphoblastic NHL often presents as an intrathoracic tumor, usually a mediastinal mass, and is associated with dyspnea, chest pain, dysphagia, pleural effusion, and superior vena cava syndrome. Cervical or axillary lymphadenopathy is present in up to 80% of patients at diagnosis. Primary involvement of bone, bone marrow, testis, or skin is not uncommon. The central nervous system (CNS) may also be involved.

SNCCL presents as an abdominal tumor in 80% of U.S. cases in patients with abdominal pain or distention, bowel obstruction, change in bowel habits, intestinal bleeding, or, rarely, intestinal perforation. Other sites include CNS, bone marrow, and peripheral lymph nodes. Jaw involvement occurs in less

than 20% of U.S. cases, compared with 70% of younger patients in equatorial Africa.

LCL occurs in many sites, including the abdomen and mediastinum. Extramedullary sites include skin, bone, and soft tissues. CNS involvement is rare, in contrast to SNCCL and lymphoblastic NHL.

Diagnosis. Prompt tissue diagnosis and staging is important because of the rapid growth rate of lymphomas, especially SNCCL. To ensure adequate tissue for accurate diagnosis and subtyping, multiple needle biopsy specimens or a large wedge of tumor should be obtained. Several studies are necessary to accurately stage the disease and provide baseline measurements of organ function before treatment is instituted (Box 488–3). In cases with airway compromise, potential for anesthetic complications, and no easily accessible tissue to sample, empirical therapy may be started using corticosteroids.

The St. Jude staging system defines tumor extent, which is important for designing treatment (Box 488–4). Stage I applies to localized disease, stage II to regional disease (except for mediastinal tumors, which are designated stage III), stage III to extensive disease, and stage IV to disseminated (CNS and/or bone marrow) disease. Elevated levels of serum lactic dehydrogenase (>500 U/L) correlate with tumor mass and have proved useful for stratifying therapy intensity.

LABORATORY FINDINGS. Laboratory findings vary, depending on sites or organs involved. Elevated serum uric acid levels and other features of tumor lysis syndrome often compli-

---

BOX 488–3. Pretreatment Studies for Staging Pediatric Non-Hodgkin Lymphoma

Complete blood cell count
Serum electrolytes, uric acid, lactate dehydrogenase, creatinine, calcium, phosphorus
Liver function tests
Chest radiograph and chest CT if abnormal
Abdominal and pelvic ultrasonography and/or CT
Gallium scan and/or bone scan
Bilateral bone marrow aspirate and biopsy
Cerebrospinal fluid cytology

BOX 488–4. St. Jude Staging System for Childhood Non-Hodgkin Lymphoma

STAGE I

A single tumor (extranodal) or single anatomic area (nodal), with the exclusion of mediastinum or abdomen.

STAGE II

A single tumor (extranodal) with regional node involvement.
Two or more nodal areas on the same side of the diaphragm.
Two single (extranodal) tumors with or without regional node involvement on the same side of the diaphragm.
A primary gastrointestinal tract tumor, usually in the ileocecal area, with or without involvement of associated mesenteric nodes only, which must be grossly (>90%) resected.

STAGE III

Two single tumors (extranodal) on opposite sides of the diaphragm.
Two or more nodal areas above and below the diaphragm.
Any primary intrathoracic tumor (mediastinal, pleural, or thymic).
Any extensive primary intra-abdominal disease.

STAGE IV

Any of the above, with initial involvement of central nervous system and/or bone marrow at time of diagnosis.

From Murphy SB: Classification, staging and end results of treatment of childhood non-Hodgkin's lymphomas: Dissimilarities from lymphomas in adults. *Semin Oncol* 1980;7:332–99.

cate the presentation of SNCCL. Elevated serum level of lactate dehydrogenase is a measure of tumor burden and may occur with any NHL subtype. A normal CBC does not preclude marrow involvement. CT or MRI of the chest or abdomen or both provides key information on disease extent. Surgical staging is not necessary.

Treatment and Prognosis. Surgical excision of localized intra-abdominal tumors often precedes the diagnosis of NHL and should always be attempted, if feasible. In this and other situations, multiagent chemotherapy is the primary treatment. Tumor lysis syndrome (i.e., high serum potassium, uric acid, and high phosphorus with low calcium levels) frequently complicates initial treatment of disseminated disease. Appropriate hydration with addition of sodium bicarbonate to produce dilute alkaline urine, administration of allopurinol, and correction of electrolyte abnormalities are essential to minimize this life-threatening complication.

In contrast to HD, second malignancies and infertility have not been major problems in long-term survivors of NHL.

EARLY-STAGE NHL. Unlike HD, NHL is considered a disseminated disease from the time of diagnosis. Even patients with apparently localized and resected disease require chemotherapy. Patients with stage I/II NHL, irrespective of histologic subgroup, are effectively treated with six cycles of **COMP** (cyclophosphamide, vincristine [Oncovin], methotrexate, and prednisone) or three cycles of **COPA** (substituting doxorubicin for methotrexate) followed by 6 mo of mercaptopurine and methotrexate or, in the case of T-cell lymphoblastic NHL, an acute lymphoblastic leukemia–like regimen. About 90% of cases are cured with these regimens. The emphasis now is on decreasing morbidity of therapy for these children while maintaining the high cure rate.

ADVANCED-STAGE NHL. Patients with stage III/IV NHL are best treated with therapy based on the histologic subtype.

Lymphoblastic lymphoma is treated with intensive chemotherapy regimens, generally of 2 yr duration and consisting of multiple chemotherapeutic agents given in cycles or a regimen based on those used for high-risk acute lymphoblastic leukemia. Cranial radiation, intrathecal chemotherapy, and/or high-dose methotrexate are important for prevention of CNS disease. Early relapses require cytoablative chemotherapy, followed by allogeneic bone marrow transplantation, if possible.

SNCCL is treated with relatively short-duration (3–6 mo) intensive chemotherapy regimens, including an alkylating agent (usually cyclophosphamide) coupled with other active systemic agents (vincristine, prednisone, methotrexate, cytarabine, etoposide, and/or doxorubicin) and intrathecal therapy, which produces survival rates of more than 90% in localized and 70–80% in those with disseminated disease. If relapse occurs, it becomes evident in the 1st yr after diagnosis and is often rapidly progressive and relatively resistant to additional therapy, especially in patients with stage IV disease.

LCL is treated with intensive multiagent chemotherapy regimens similar to those used for lymphoblastic lymphoma, which have produced long-term survival rates of 50–70% in those of T-cell origin. For B cell–derived LCL, short, intensive regimens as outlined earlier for SNCLL have produced 6-yr event-free survival as high as 95%.

Hodgkin Disease
Flavell KJ, Murray PG: Hodgkin's disease and the Epstein-Barr virus. *Mol Pathol* 2000;53:262–9.
Hudson MM, Donaldson SS: Hodgkin's disease. In Pizzo PA, Poplack DG (editors): *Principles and Practice of Pediatric Oncology*, 4th ed. Philadelphia, Lippincott, Williams and Wilkins 2002, pp 637–60.
Hudson MM, Donaldson SS: Treatment of pediatric Hodgkin's disease. *Semin Hematol* 1999;36:313–23.

Non-Hodgkin Lymphoma
Biggar RJ, Frisch M, Goedert JJ: Risk of cancer in children with AIDS. *JAMA* 2000;284:205–9.

Buckley JD, Meadows AT, Kadin ME: Pesticide exposures in children with non-Hodgkin lymphoma. *Cancer* 2000;89:2315–21.
McGrath IT: Malignant non-Hodgkin's lymphoma in children. In Pizzo PA, Poplack DG (editors): *Principles and Practice of Pediatric Oncology*, 4th ed. Philadelphia, Lippincott Williams and Wilkins, 2002, pp 661–706.
Pinkerton CR: The continuing challenge of treatment for non-Hodgkin's lymphoma in children. *Br J Haematol* 1999;107:220–34.
Reiter A, Schrappe M, Tiemann M, et al: Improved treatment results in childhood B-cell neoplasms with tailored intensification of therapy: A report of the Berlin-Frankfurt-Munster Group Trial NHL-BFM 90. *Blood* 1999;94:3294–306.

Chapter 489
Brain Tumors in Childhood
John F. Kuttesch, Jr. and Joann L. Ater

Primary central nervous system (CNS) tumors are a heterogeneous group of diseases that collectively are the second most frequent malignancy in childhood and adolescence. Mortality among this group approaches 45%. In addition, these patients have the highest morbidity, primarily neurologic, of all childhood malignancies. However, outcomes have improved over time, owing to innovations in neurosurgery and radiation therapy as well as to identification of chemotherapy as a therapeutic modality. The treatment approach for these tumors is multimodal. Surgery with complete resection, if feasible, is the foundation of this approach. Based on the diagnosis, patient age, and other factors, radiation therapy and/or chemotherapy are used.

Epidemiology. Approximately 2,200 primary brain tumors are diagnosed each year in children and adolescents, with an overall annual incidence of 28 cases/per million children. There is a higher incidence of CNS tumors in infants and young children up to 7 yr of age (~36 cases/million children annually) compared with older children and adolescents (~21 cases/million children annually) (Fig. 489–1).

Pathogenesis. Among the more than 100 histologic categories and subtypes of primary brain tumors described in the World Health Organization (WHO) classification of tumors of the CNS and meninges, 5 categories (juvenile pilocytic astrocytoma, medulloblastoma/primitive neuroectodermal tumor [PNET], diffuse astrocytomas, ependymoma, and craniopharyngioma) constitute 80% of all pediatric brain tumors (Table 489–1).

In a survey of children with sampled brain tumors, the Childhood Brain Tumor Consortium reported a slight predominance of infratentorial tumor location (43.2%), followed by the supratentorial location (40.9%), spinal cord (4.9%), and multiple sites (11%). There are age-related differences in primary location of tumor (Fig. 489–2). Within the 1st year of life, supratentorial tumors predominate and include, most commonly, choroid plexus complex tumors and teratomas. From 1–10 yr of age, infratentorial tumors predominate, owing to the high incidence of juvenile pilocytic astrocytoma and medulloblastoma. After 10 yr of age, once again, supratentorial tumors predominate, with the diffuse astrocytomas most common. Tumors of the optic pathway and hypothalamus region, the brainstem, and pineal-midbrain region occur with a greater incidence in children and adolescents than in adults.

There is little understanding of the etiology of pediatric brain tumors. A male predominance is noted in the incidence of medulloblastoma and ependymoma. Familial and hereditary syndromes associated with increased incidence of brain tumors account for approximately 5% of cases (Table 489–2). Cranial exposure to ionizing radiation is also associated with an increased incidence of brain tumors. Additionally, there are sporadic reports of brain tumors within families without evidence of a heritable syndrome. The molecular events associated with

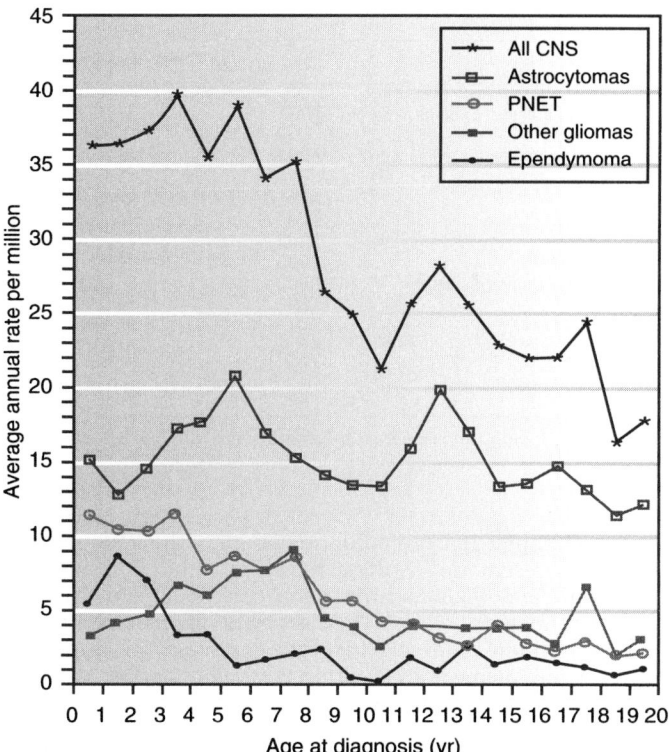

FIGURE 489–1. Age-specific incidence rates of malignant brain tumors of childhood from SEER 1986–1994. (From Gurney JC, Smith MA, Bunin GR: *National Cancer Institute SEER Program.* NIH publication No. 99-4649, 1999, pp 51–63.)

tumorigenesis of pediatric brain tumors are not known; however, our understanding of the molecular biology of these diseases is expanding.

Clinical Manifestations. The clinical presentation of patients with brain tumors depends on the tumor location, tumor type, and the age of the child. Signs and symptoms are related to the tumor causing obstruction of cerebrospinal fluid (CSF) drainage paths, leading to increased intracranial pressure (ICP) and/or

TABLE 489–1. Distribution of Childhood Brain Tumors Based on Histology

Histology	Distribution (% of total)
Medulloblastoma/PNET	20
Juvenile pilocytic astrocytoma	20
Low-grade astrocytoma	15
High-grade astrocytoma	7
Ependymoma	7
Craniopharyngioma	7
Unclassified primary tumors	7
Choroid plexus tumors, germ cell tumors, oligodendroglioma, meningioma, mixed tumors, pineal parenchymal tumors	1–2 (each histologic group)

Adapted from Fuller GN: Central nervous system tumors. In Parham DM (editor): Pediatric Neoplasia: Morphology and Biology. Philadelphia, Lippincott-Raven, 1996, pp 153–204.

causing focal brain dysfunction. Subtle changes in personality, mentation, and/or speech may precede these classic signs and symptoms of brain tumors. In young children the diagnosis of a brain tumor may be delayed because their symptoms are similar to those of more common illnesses, such as gastrointestinal disorders. Infants with open cranial sutures may present with the common signs of increased ICP (vomiting, lethargy, and irritability) as well as macrocephaly. The classic triad of headache, nausea and/or vomiting, and papilledema is associated with midline or infratentorial tumors. Disorders of equilibrium, gait, and coordination occur with infratentorial tumors. Torticollis may result in patients with cerebellar tonsil herniation. Blurred vision, diplopia, and nystagmus are also associated with infratentorial tumors. Brainstem region tumors may be associated with gaze palsy, cranial nerve palsies, and upper motor neuron deficits (hemiparesis, hyperreflexia, and clonus). Supratentorial tumors are more commonly associated with focal disorders such as motor weaknesses, sensory changes, speech disorders, seizures, and reflex abnormalities. Infants with supratentorial tumors may present with hand preference. Optic pathway tumors present with visual disturbances such as decreased visual acuity, Marcus Gunn pupil (afferent papillary defect), nystagmus, and/or visual field defects. Suprasellar region tumors and third ventricular region tumors may present initially with neuroendocrine deficits such as diabetes insipidus and hypothyroidism. **The diencephalic syndrome,** a classic presentation of failure to

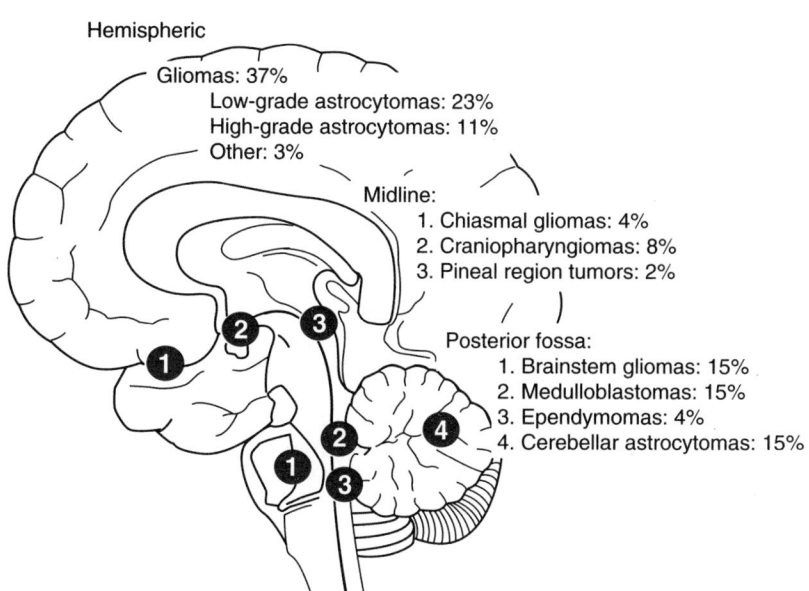

FIGURE 489–2. Childhood brain tumors occur at any location within the central nervous system. The relative frequency of brain tumor histologic types and the anatomic distribution are shown. (From Albright AL: Pediatric brain tumors. *CA Cancer J Clin* 1993;43:272–88.)

TABLE 489–2. Familial Syndromes Associated with Pediatric Brain Tumors

Syndrome	CNS Manifestations	Chromosome	Gene
Neurofibromatosis 1 (autosomal dominant)	Optic pathway gliomas, astrocytoma, malignant peripheral nerve sheath tumors (MPNST), neurofibromas	17q11	NF1
Neurofibromatosis 2 (autosomal dominant)	Vestibular schwannomas, meningiomas, spinal cord ependymoma, spinal cord astrocytoma, hamartomas	22q12	NF2
von Hippel-Lindau (autosomal dominant)	Hemangioblastoma	3p25–26	VHL
Tuberous sclerosis (autosomal dominant)	Subependymal giant cell astrocytoma, cortical tubers	9q34	TSC1
		16q13	TSC2
Li-Fraumeni (autosomal dominant)	Astrocytoma, PNET	17q13	TP53
Cowden (autosomal dominant)	Dysplastic gangliocytoma of the cerebellum (Lhermitte-Duclos disease)	10q23	PTEN
Turcot (autosomal dominant)	Medulloblastoma	5q21	APC
	Glioblastoma	3p21	hMLH1
		7p22	hPSM2
Nevoid basal cell carcinoma (autosomal dominant)	Medulloblastoma	9q31	PTCH

Modified from Kleihues P, Cavenee WK: World Health Organization Classification of Tumors: Pathology and Genetics of Tumors of the Nervous System. *Lyon, IARC Press, 2000.*

thrive, emaciation, increased appetite, and euphoric affect, occurs in infants with tumors in these regions. **Parinaud syndrome,** a classic presentation of pineal region tumors, is manifested by (1) paresis of upward gaze, (2) pupillary dilatation reactive to accommodation but not to light, (3) nystagmus to convergence or retraction, and (4) eyelid retraction. Spinal cord tumors and spinal cord dissemination of brain tumors may manifest as long nerve tract motor and/or sensory deficits, bowel and bladder deficits, and back or radicular pain. Patients with meningeal metastatic disease from brain tumors or leukemia may present with signs and symptoms similar to those of patients with infratentorial tumors.

Diagnosis. The evaluation of a patient suspected to have a brain tumor is an emergency. Initial evaluation should include a complete history, physical examination, and neurologic assessment with neuroimaging. For primary brain tumors, MRI is the neuroimaging standard. Tumors in the pituitary/suprasellar region, optic path, and infratentorium are better delineated with MRI than with CT. Patients with tumors of the midline and the pituitary/suprasellar/optic chiasmal region should undergo evaluation for neuroendocrine dysfunction. Formal ophthalmologic examination is beneficial in patients with optic path region tumors to document impact of the disease on oculomotor function, visual acuity, and fields of vision. The suprasellar region and pineal region are preferential sites for germ cell tumors. Both serum and CSF measurements of β-human chorionic gonadotropin and α-fetoprotein can assist in the diagnosis of germ cell tumors. In tumors with the propensity of spreading to the leptomeninges such as medulloblastoma/PNET, ependymoma, and germ cell tumors, lumbar puncture and cytologic analysis of the CSF is indicated; however, lumbar puncture is contraindicated in individuals with newly diagnosed hydrocephalus secondary to CSF flow obstruction or in individuals with infratentorial tumors. Lumbar puncture in these individuals may lead to brain herniation, resulting in neurologic compromise and death.

ASTROCYTOMAS. Astrocytomas are the most common pediatric brain tumors and comprise a heterogeneous group of tumors accounting for approximately 40% of cases. These tumors occur throughout the CNS.

Low-grade astrocytomas (LGAs) are the predominant group of astrocytomas in childhood and are characterized by their indolent clinical course. The two most common types of LGAs are the pilocytic astrocytomas and the fibrillary infiltrating astrocytomas. **Juvenile pilocytic astrocytoma (JPA)** is the most common astrocytoma in children, comprising 20% of all brain tumors. Based on clinicopathologic features using the WHO Classification System, JPA is classified as a WHO grade I

tumor. Although JPA can occur anywhere in the CNS, the classic site of presentation is the cerebellum. Other common sites include the hypothalamic/third ventricular region and the optic nerve and chiasmal region. The classic but not exclusive neuroradiologic findings of JPA are the presence of a contrast medium–enhancing nodule within the wall of a cystic mass (Fig. 489–3). The microscopy findings exhibit a biphasic appearance of bundles of compact fibrillary tissue interspersed with loose microcystic, spongy areas. The presence of **Rosenthal fibers,** condensed masses of glial filaments occurring in the compact areas, helps to establish the diagnosis. JPA has a low metastatic potential and is rarely invasive. A small proportion of these tumors can progress and develop leptomeningeal spread, particularly tumors occurring in the optic path region. JPA very rarely undergoes malignant transformation to a more aggressive tumor. JPA of the optic nerve and chiasmal region is a relatively common finding in patients with neurofibromatosis type 1 (15% incidence). Unlike diffuse fibrillary astrocytomas, there are no characteristic cytogenetic abnormalities in JPA nor are there any known molecular abnormalities. Other tumors occurring in the pediatric age group with similar clinicopathologic characteristics as JPA include pleomorphic xanthoastrocytoma, desmoplastic cerebral astrocytoma of infancy, and subependymal giant cell astrocytoma. The fibrillary astrocytomas are a group of tumors characterized by a pattern of diffuse infiltration of tumor cells among normal neural tissue and a potential for anaplastic progression. Based on their clinicopathologic characteristics, they are grouped as low-grade astrocytomas (WHO grade II), malignant astrocytomas (anaplastic astrocytoma [AA, WHO grade III], and glioblastoma multiforme (GBM, WHO grade IV). Of this group the fibrillary LGA is the second most common astrocytoma in children, accounting for 15% of brain tumors. Histologically, these low-grade tumors demonstrate increased cellularity compared with normal brain parenchyma, with few mitotic figures, nuclear pleomorphism, and microcysts. The characteristic MRI finding is the lack of enhancement after contrast agent infusion. Molecular genetic abnormalities found among low-grade diffuse infiltrating astrocytomas include mutations of *TP53* and overexpression of platelet-derived growth factor α-chain and platelet-derived growth factor receptor-α. These tumors have the potential to evolve into malignant astrocytomas, a development that is associated with cumulative acquisition of multiple molecular abnormalities.

The clinical management of LGAs focuses on a multimodal approach incorporating surgery, radiation therapy, and/or chemotherapy. Outcome among patients with JPA is better than outcome among those with fibrillary LGAs. Surgery is the primary therapeutic modality for LGAs. After complete surgical

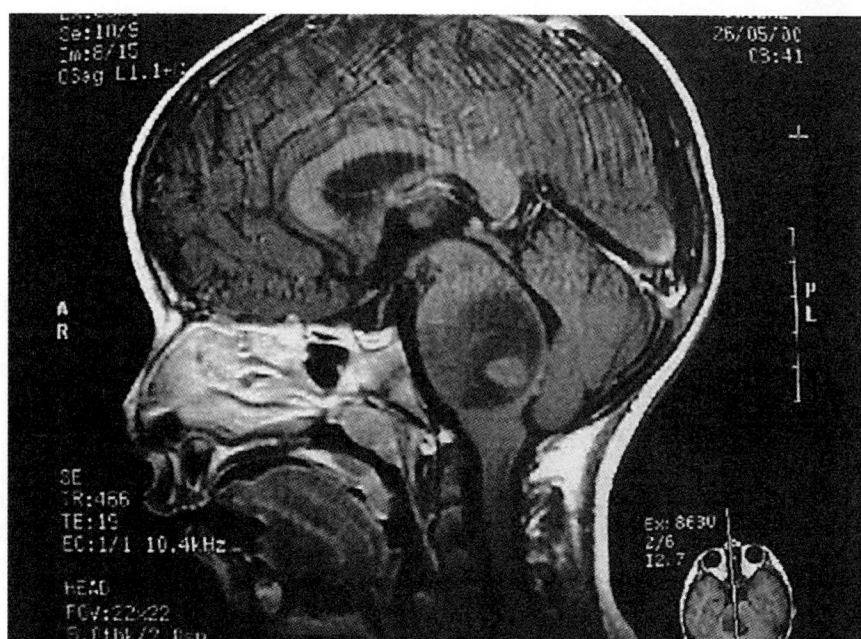

FIGURE 489–3. T1 weighted sequence post gadolinium MR (axial image) in a 4-yr-old boy presenting with headaches, nausea and vomiting, and ataxia who was found to have a juvenile pilocytic astrocytoma. (Adapted from Fuller GN: Central nervous system tumors. In Parham DM [editor]: *Pediatric Neoplasia: Morphology and Biology.* Philadelphia, Lippincott–Raven, 1996, pp 153–204.)

resection the overall survival approaches 80–100%. In patients with partial resection (<90% resection), overall survival varies from 50–95% depending on the anatomic location of the tumor. In those patients with partial resection and stable neurologic status, the current approach is to follow the patient closely by examination and imaging. With evidence of progression, surgical re-resection should be considered. In those patients in whom second surgery was less than complete or not feasible, radiation therapy is of benefit. Radiation therapy is given to the tumor bed at a total cumulative dose ranging from 50–55 Gy given at a daily schedule over 6 wk. Historically, patients with deep midline tumors were treated empirically without surgery or biopsy using radiation therapy, with variable survival rates from 33–75%. However, modern surgical techniques and innovative radiation therapy methodology may positively impact on the survival and clinical outcome of these patients. The role of chemotherapy in management of LGAs is evolving. Because of the concerns for young children of the morbidity from radiation therapy, several chemotherapy approaches have been evaluated, especially in children younger than 5 yr of age. Complete response to chemotherapy is low; however, these approaches have yielded prolonged disease control in 70–100% of patients. Patients with midline tumors as in the hypothalamic/optic chiasmatic region have tended to do less well. Taken together, the chemotherapy approaches have permitted delay and, potentially, avoidance of radiation therapy. Currently, in a national trial investigators are comparing the effectiveness and tolerance between a carboplatin-based chemotherapy schedule and a lomustine (CCNU)-based schedule in children younger than 10 yr of age with a progressive LGA. Observation is the primary approach in clinical management of selective patients with LGAs that are biologically indolent. One group includes patients with neurofibromatosis 1 who may develop an LGA of the optic chiasm/optic pathway or brainstem that is found incidentally. Another group is patients with midbrain astrocytomas who have resolution of clinical symptoms after ventricular shunting and do not require further intervention.

Malignant astrocytomas are much less common in children and adolescents than in adults, accounting for 7–10% of all childhood tumors. Among this group, **anaplastic astrocytoma** (WHO grade III) is more common than **glioblastoma multiforme** (WHO grade IV). The histopathology of anaplastic astrocytomas demonstrates increased cellularity compared with low-grade diffuse astrocytomas, cellular and nuclear atypia, presence of mitoses, and, variably, microvascular proliferation. Characteristic histopathology findings in glioblastoma multiforme include dense cellularity, high mitotic index, microvascular proliferation, and foci of tumor necrosis. There is limited information regarding the molecular abnormalities in malignant astrocytomas of children. Overexpression of P53 in malignant astrocytomas of children is an adverse prognostic factor. The frequency of mutations in *TP53* in childhood malignant astrocytomas is similar to that noted in adults; however, the frequency of such mutations in malignant astrocytomas of children younger than 3 yr of age is lower. These observations suggest differing mechanisms of oncogenesis between young children (<3 yr old) and older children. As in adults, optimal therapeutic approaches for malignant astrocytomas have yet to be defined. The "standard therapy" continues to be surgical resection followed by involved-field radiation therapy, although patient outcome is poor.

Oligodendrogliomas are uncommon tumors of childhood. These infiltrating tumors occur predominately in the cerebral cortex and originate in the white matter. In childhood, oligodendroglioma, a well-differentiated neoplasm, predominates. Histologically, oligodendrogliomas are composed of rounded cells with little cytoplasm and the presence of microcalcifications. Observation of a calcified cortical mass on CT in a patient presenting with a seizure is suggestive of oligodendroglioma. Treatment approaches are similar to those for infiltrating astrocytomas.

MIXED GLIOMAS. Mixed gliomas are composed of two or more distinct glial cell types (astrocytoma, oligodendroglioma, and/or ependymoma) and occur uncommonly in pediatric patients.

EPENDYMAL TUMORS. Ependymal tumors are derived from the ependymal lining of the ventricular system. Ependymoma (WHO grade II) is the most common of these neoplasms, occurring predominately in childhood and accounting for 10% of childhood tumors. Approximately 70% of ependymomas in childhood occur in the posterior fossa. The mean age of patients is 6 yr, with approximately 30% of cases occurring in children younger than 3 yr of age. The incidence of leptomeningeal spread approaches 10% overall. Clinical presentation is dependent on the anatomic location of the tumor. MRI demonstrates a well-circumscribed tumor with variable and complex patterns of gadolinium enhancement with or without cystic structures. These tumors generally are noninvasive, extending into the ventricular lumen and/or displacing normal structures. Histologic characteristics of these tumors include perivascular pseudorosettes, ependymal rosettes, monomorphic nuclear morphology, and occasional nonpalisading foci of necrosis. Surgery is the primary treatment modality, with extent of surgical resection a major prognostic factor. Two other major prognostic factors are age, with younger children having poorer outcomes, and tumor location, with localization in the posterior fossa that is often seen in young children associated with poorer outcomes. Surgery alone is rarely curative. Multimodal therapy incorporating radiation with surgery has resulted in long-term survival in approximately 40% of patients after gross total resection. Recurrence is predominately local. Ependymoma is sensitive to a spectrum of chemotherapeutic agents; however, the role of chemotherapy in multimodal therapy of ependymoma is still unclear. Several limited trials have shown no benefit to the use of high-dose chemotherapy with peripheral blood stem cell rescue in ependymoma. Current investigations are directed toward identification of optimal radiation dose, surgical questions addressing the use of second-look procedures after chemotherapy, and further evaluation of classic as well as novel chemotherapeutic agents. There are no characteristic cytogenetic or molecular genetic alterations in ependymoma. However, preliminary studies suggest that there are genetically distinct subtypes, exemplified by an association between alterations in the *NF2* gene and spinal ependymoma. **Anaplastic ependymoma** (WHO grade III) is much less common in childhood, and these tumors are characterized by a high mitotic index and histologic features of microvascular proliferation and pseudopalisading necrosis. **Myxopapillary ependymoma** (WHO grade I) is a slow-growing tumor arising from the filum terminale and conus medullaris.

CHOROID PLEXUS TUMORS. Choroid plexus tumors account for 2–4% of childhood CNS tumors. They are the most frequent CNS tumor in children younger than 1 yr of age and account for 10–20% of CNS tumors occurring in infancy. These tumors are intraventricular papillary neoplasms arising from choroid plexus epithelium. Children present with signs and symptoms of increased ICP. Infants may present with macrocephaly and focal neurologic deficits. In children, these tumors occur predominately supratentorially in the lateral ventricles. **Choroid plexus papilloma** (WHO grade I), the most common of this group, is a well-circumscribed lesion by neuroimaging and closely resembles normal choroid plexus histologically. **Choroid plexus carcinoma** (WHO grade III) is a malignant tumor with metastatic potential to seed into the CSF pathways. This malignancy has histologic characteristics of nuclear pleomorphism, high mitotic index, and increased cell density. Immunopositivity for transthyretin (prealbumin) is useful in confirming the diagnosis of these tumors. These tumors are associated with the Li-Fraumeni syndrome. Simian virus 40 (SV40) may play an etiologic role in choroid plexus tumors. After complete surgical resection, outcome for choroid plexus papilloma approaches 100% whereas outcome for choroid plexus carcinoma approaches 20–40%. Reports suggest that radiation therapy and/or chemotherapy may lead to better disease control for choroid plexus carcinoma.

EMBRYONAL TUMORS. Embryonal tumors or **primitive neuroectodermal tumors (PNET)** are the most common group of malignant CNS tumors of childhood, accounting for 20–25% of pediatric CNS tumors. These tumors have the potential to metastasize to the neuraxis. This group includes medulloblastoma, supratentorial PNET, ependymoblastoma, medulloepithelioblastoma, and atypical teratoid/rhabdoid tumor (ATRT). These tumors are histologically classified as WHO grade IV tumors.

Medulloblastoma, accounting for 90% of embryonal tumors, is a cerebellar tumor occurring predominately in males and at a median age of 5–7 yr. The majority of tumors occur in the midline cerebellar vermis; however, older patients may present with tumors in the cerebellar hemisphere. CT demonstrates a solid, homogeneous, contrast medium–enhancing mass in the posterior fossa causing 4th ventricular obstruction and hydrocephalus. MRI shows similar characteristics. Up to 30% of patients present with neuroimaging evidence of leptomeningeal spread. Among a variety of diverse histologic patterns of this tumor, the most common is a monomorphic sheet of undifferentiated cells classically noted as small, blue, round cells. Neuronal differentiation is more common among these tumors and histologically characterized by the presence of Homer Wright rosettes and by immunopositivity for synaptophysin. Patients present with signs and symptoms of increased intracranial pressure (headache, nausea, vomiting, mental status changes, and hypertension) and cerebellar dysfunction (ataxia, poor balance, dysmetria). Standard clinical staging evaluation includes MRI of brain and spine, both preoperatively and postoperatively, as well as lumbar punctures. The Chang staging system, originally based on surgical information, has been modified to incorporate information from neuroimaging to identify risk categories. Clinical features that have consistently demonstrated prognostic significance include age at diagnosis, extent of disease, and extent of surgical resection. Younger patients (<4 yr of age) have poor outcome that is partly caused by a higher incidence of disseminated disease on presentation and past therapeutic approaches that have used less intense therapies. Patients with disseminated disease at diagnosis (M > 0), including positive CSF cytology alone (M1), have a markedly worse outcome than those patients with no dissemination (M0). Similarly, patients with gross residual disease after surgery have worse outcomes compared with those who had gross total resection of their disease.

Multimodal treatment approach is pursued in medulloblastoma, with surgery being the cornerstone of treatment. Medulloblastoma is both a chemotherapy-sensitive and irradiation-sensitive disease. Historically, surgery alone was ineffective. In the 1940s radiation therapy was found to be effective, improving overall outcome to a 30% survival rate. With technologic advances in neurosurgery, neuroradiology, and radiation therapy, as well as identification of chemotherapy as an effective modality, overall outcome among all patients approaches 60–70%. Standard radiation treatment in medulloblastoma incorporates craniospinal radiation at a total cumulative dose of 30–36 Gy with a cumulative dose of 50–55 Gy to the tumor bed. Craniospinal radiation at this dose in very young children (those < 4 years) results in severe late neurologic sequelae, including microcephaly, learning disabilities, mental retardation, neuroendocrine dysfunction (growth failure, hypothyroidism, hypogonadism, and absent/delayed puberty), and/or second malignancies. Similarly, in older children, late sequelae, such as learning disabilities, neuroendocrine dysfunction, and/or second malignancies, can occur. These observations have resulted in stratification of treatment approaches into three strata: (1) patients younger than 4 yr of age; (2) standard risk patients age 4 yr and older with surgical total resection and no disease dissemination (M0); and (3) high-risk patients age 4 yr and older with disease dissemination (M > 0) and/or bulky residual disease after surgery.

Cytogenetic and molecular genetic studies have demonstrated multiple abnormalities in medulloblastoma. The most common cytogenetic abnormality involves chromosome 17p deletions. Molecular studies have identified these lesions as the most common molecular defect in medulloblastoma, occurring in 30–40% of all cases. These deletions are not associated with *TP53* mutations. In 10–20% of medulloblastoma cases, genetic material losses are noted on chromosomes 1q and 10p. In approximately 10% of cases, abnormalities of 9p have been detected. Molecular lesions in this region are associated with inactivation of the human homologue of the hedgehog/patched signaling pathway and are implicated in the nevoid basal cell carcinoma syndrome. The finding of mutations in the *APC* gene and β-catenin gene suggests the involvement of the Wnt pathway in the pathogenesis of medulloblastoma. Increased *PAX5* and *PAX6* gene expression in medulloblastoma suggests that abnormalities in neural transcription factors may play a role in early tumorigenesis of these tumors. Most recently, high expression of neurotrophin receptor TrkC and low expression of the oncogene *MYC* have been demonstrated to be associated with favorable outcome and appear to be strong independent prognostic factors. Further analysis has shown that the cohort of patients with tumors with high expression of TrkC and low expression of *MYC* have very favorable outcomes independent of clinical prognostic factors. With the evolution of gene array technology, recent preliminary studies have identified clusters of genes/gene expression that appear to be associated with metastatic medulloblastoma and outcome. Using gene micro array technology and the development of proteomic technology will, it is hoped, offer insight into the molecular events associated with medulloblastoma tumorigenesis. Additionally, information obtained may lead to novel molecularly targeted approaches in this disease.

Supratentorial primitive neuroectodermal tumors (SPENT) account for 2–3% of childhood brain tumors primarily in children within the 1st decade of life. These tumors are similar histologically to medulloblastoma and composed of undifferentiated or poorly differentiated neuroepithelial cells. Historically, patients with SPNET have had poorer outcomes than those with medulloblastoma after combined modality therapy. In current clinical trials, children with these tumors are considered among the high-risk group and received dose-intense therapy with craniospinal radiation therapy.

Atypical teratoid/rhabdoid tumor (ATRT) is a very aggressive embryonal malignancy that occurs predominantly in children younger than 5 yr of age and can occur at any location in the neuraxis. The histology demonstrates a heterogeneous pattern of cells, including rhabdoid cells that express epithelial membrane antigen and neurofilament antigen. The characteristic cytogenetic pattern is partial or complete deletion of chromosome 22q that has been associated with mutation in the *INI1* gene. The relationship between this mutation and tumorigenesis is unclear. Outcome after combined modality therapy with intensive chemotherapy is very poor.

Ependymoblastoma and **medullomyoblastoma** are rare, highly malignant embryonal tumors of early childhood and infancy.

PINEAL PARENCHYMAL TUMORS. The pineal parenchymal tumors are the second most common malignancies after germ cell tumors that occur in the pineal region. These include pineoblastoma, occurring predominantly in childhood, pineocytoma, and the mixed pineal parenchymal tumors. Therapeutic approach in this group of diseases is multimodal. In the past there was significant concern owing to the location of these masses and the potential complications of surgical intervention. With recent developments in neurosurgical technique and surgical technology, the morbidity and mortality associated with these approaches have markedly decreased. Stereotactic biopsy of these tumors may be adequate to establish diagnosis; however, consideration should be pursued for total resection of the lesion before institution of additional therapy. Pineoblastoma is the more malignant variant and is considered a subgroup of PNETs of childhood. Chemotherapy regimens incorporate cisplatin, cyclophosphamide (Cytoxan), etoposide (VP-16), and vincristine and/or lomustine. Data have shown that survival outcome of pineal region PNETs with combined modality therapy of chemotherapy and radiation approaches 70% at 5 yr, similar to that noted for medulloblastoma. Pineocytoma is a disease that is generally approached with surgical resection.

NEURONAL/MIXED NEURONAL-GLIAL TUMORS. These tumors are a heterogeneous group of tumors that are slow growing and of low malignant progression. They are associated with favorable outcome after surgical resection. They are categorized as WHO grade I or WHO grade II tumors. The diseases within this category include ganglioglioma, dysembryoplastic neuroepithelial tumor, desmoplastic infantile astrocytoma, and desmoplastic infantile ganglioglioma.

CRANIOPHARYNGIOMA. Craniopharyngioma (WHO grade I) is a common tumor of childhood, accounting for 7–10% of all childhood tumors. The adamantinomatous variant of craniopharyngioma predominates in childhood. These tumors are solid with cystic components and occur within the suprasellar region. These tumors are minimally invasive, adhere to adjacent brain parenchyma, and engulf normal brain structures. MRI demonstrates the solid tumor with cystic structures containing fluid of intermediate density. CT may show calcifications associated with the solid and cystic wall components. Surgery is the primary treatment modality, with gross total resection curative in small lesions. Controversy exists in the relative roles of surgery and radiation therapy in large, complex tumors. There is significant morbidity (panhypopituitarism, growth failure, visual loss) associated with these tumors and their therapy owing to the anatomic location. No role has been identified for chemotherapy in craniopharyngioma.

MENINGEAL TUMORS. Meningiomas are uncommon tumors of childhood. These tumors arise from the arachnoid layer of the meninges and are generally very slow growing. Among children, a large proportion of these tumors can be associated with either a genetic disposition such as neurofibromatosis 2 or basal cell nevus syndrome or prior radiation exposure (secondary malignancy).

GERM CELL TUMORS. Germ cell tumors of the CNS are a heterogeneous group of tumors that are primarily tumors of childhood arising predominantly in midline structures of the pineal and suprasellar regions. They account for 1–2% of pediatric brain tumors. The peak incidence of these tumors is 10–12 yr of age. Overall, there is a male preponderance, although there is a female preponderance for suprasellar tumors. These tumors can occur multifocally in 5–10% of cases. This group of tumors is much more prevalent in Asian populations than European populations. As in peripheral germ cell tumors, the analysis of protein markers, α-fetoprotein, and β-human chorionic gonadotropin may be useful in establishing the diagnosis and monitoring treatment response. Surgical biopsy is recommended to establish the diagnosis; however, nongerminomatous germ cell tumors may be diagnosed based on protein marker elevations. Therapeutic approaches to germinomas and mixed germ cell tumors are different. The survival proportion among patients with pure germinoma exceeds 90%. The postsurgical treatment of pure germinomas is somewhat controversial in defining the relative roles of chemotherapy and radiation therapy. Excellent outcomes are reported in patients who have received local field doses of radiation of more than 40 Gy and craniospinal radiotherapy. Similarly, groups have reported excellent outcomes when chemotherapy has been incorporated in regimens that utilize reduced doses of radiation therapy (24 Gy to the local field alone). More recently, clinical trials have investigated the use of chemotherapy alone after surgery in pure germinomas. The therapeutic approach in nongerminomatous germ cell tumors is more aggressive, combining more intense chemotherapy regimens with craniospinal radiation therapy. Survival rates among these tumors are markedly less than noted in germinoma, ranging from 40–70% at 5 yr. Recent trials have shown benefit using high doses of chemotherapy with blood stem cell rescue. If confirmed in larger studies, future approaches may test the use of high doses of chemotherapy with dose-reduced radiation therapy.

TUMORS OF THE BRAINSTEM. Tumors of the brainstem comprise 10–15% of childhood primary CNS tumors. This is a heterogeneous group of tumors. Outcome is associated with tumor location, imaging characteristics, and clinical status of the patient. Patients with these tumors may present with motor weakness, cranial nerve deficits, cerebellar deficits, and/or signs of increased intracranial pressure. Based on MR evaluation and clinical findings, tumors of the brainstem can be classified into four types: (1) focal, 5–10% of patients; (2) dorsally exophytic, 5–10% of patients; (3) cervicomedullary, 5–10% of patients; and (4) diffuse intrinsic tumors, 70–85% of patients. Surgical resection is the primary treatment approach for focal and dorsally exophytic tumors leading to a favorable outcome. Histologically, these two groups are generally low-grade gliomas. Cervicomedullary tumors, owing to their location, may not be amenable to surgical resection but are radiotherapy sensitive. Diffuse intrinsic tumors, characterized by the diffuse infiltrating pontine glioma, are associated with very poor outcome independent of histologic diagnosis (Fig. 489–4). These tumors are not amenable to surgical resection. Biopsy in children with MR findings of a diffuse intrinsic tumor is controversial and is not recommended unless there is suspicion of another diagnosis, such as infection, demyelination, vascular malformation, multiple sclerosis, or metastatic tumors. These diagnoses are much more common in adults. The standard approach for treatment in diffuse infiltrating pontine gliomas has been radiation therapy; however, median survival associated with this treatment is 12 mo, at best. Use of chemotherapy, including high-dose chemotherapy with blood stem cell rescue, has not been of survival benefit in this group of patients. Current approaches include evaluation of investigational agents alone or in combination with radiation therapy, similar to approaches being pursued in patients with malignant gliomas.

METASTATIC TUMORS. Metastatic spread of other childhood malignancies to the brain is uncommon. Childhood acute lymphoblastic leukemia and non-Hodgkin lymphoma can spread to the leptomeninges, causing symptoms of communicating hydrocephalus. Chloromas, which are collections of myeloid leukemia cells, can occur throughout the neuraxis. Rarely, brain parenchymal metastases occur from lymphoma, neuroblastoma, rhabdomyosarcoma, Ewing sarcoma, osteosarcoma, and clear cell sarcoma of the kidney. Therapeutic approaches are based on the specific histologic diagnosis and may incorporate radiation therapy, intrathecal administration of chemotherapy, and/or systemic administration of chemotherapy. Medulloblastoma is the most common childhood brain tumor to metastasize extraneuronally. Less commonly, extraneuronal metastases from malignant glioma, PNET, and ependymoma can occur. Ventriculoperitoneal shunts have been known to allow extraneural metastases, primarily within peritoneal cavity but also systemically.

Complications and Long-Term Management. Data from the National Cancer Institute SEER Program indicate that more than 70% of patients with childhood brain tumors will be long-term survivors. At least one half of these survivors will experience chronic problems as a direct result of their tumor and treatment. These include chronic neurologic deficits such as focal motor and sensory abnormalities, seizure disorders, neurocognitive deficits (developmental delays, learning disabilities), and neuroendocrine deficiencies (hypothyroidism, growth failure, delayed or absent puberty). Additionally, these patients are at significant risk of secondary malignancies. The impact of these chronic complications in these survivors of childhood brain tumors on their quality of life is only now being to be appreciated.

Future Directions. Efforts will continue to define more specific and selective chemotherapeutic agents and to refine the use of radiation therapy. Technologic advances have made feasible extensive laboratory studies of genomics and, soon, proteomics in childhood malignancies. A major effort is being directed to understand the molecular biology of tumorigenesis, cellular proliferation and survival, and metastasis in childhood brain tumors. The underlying mechanisms of these processes may be different among primary childhood malignancies compared with malignancies of adulthood. National and international collaborative research efforts are ongoing to elucidate the molecular events associated with these processes. The ultimate goal is translation of this information to define molecular targets for the development of novel therapeutic approaches in these diseases.

Barkovich AJ, Krischer J, Kun LE, et al: Brain stem gliomas: A classification based on magnetic resonance imaging. *Pediatr Neurosurg* 1990–91;16:73–83.

Biegel JA: Cytogenetics and molecular genetics of childhood brain tumors. *Neurooncol* 1999;1:139–51.

Bouffet E, Foreman N: Chemotherapy for intracranial ependymomas. *Childs Nerv Syst* 1999;15:563–70.

Burger PC, Scheithauer BW: *Atlas of Pathology: Tumors of the Central Nervous System*, third series. Washington, DC, Armed Forces Institute of Pathology, 1994.

Freeman CR, Perilongo G: Chemotherapy for brain stem gliomas. *Childs Nerv Syst* 1999;15:545–53.

Fuller GN: Central nervous system tumors. In Parham DM (editor): *Pediatric Neoplasia: Morphology and Biology*. Philadelphia, Lippincott-Raven, 1996, pp 153–204.

Gajjar A, Kuhl J, Epelman S, et al: Chemotherapy for medulloblastoma. *Childs Nerv Syst* 1999;15:554–62.

Grotzer MA, Hogarty MD, Janss AJ, et al: *MYC* messenger RNA expression predicts survival outcome in childhood primitive neuroectodermal tumor/medulloblastoma. *Clin Cancer Res* 2001;7:2425–33.

Grotzer MA, Janss AJ, Fung K-M, et al: TrkC expression predicts good clinical outcome in primitive neuroectodermal brain tumors. *J Clin Oncol* 2000;18:1027–35.

Gurney JC, Smith MA, Bunin GR: In Reis LAG, Smith MA, Gurney JC, et al (editors): *Cancer Survival and Incidence Among Children and Adolescents: United States SEER Program 1975–1995*. Bethesda, MD, National Cancer Institute SEER Program. NIH publication No. 99-4649, 1999, pp 51–63.

Kleihues P, Cavenee WK: *World Health Organization Classification of Tumours: Pathology and Genetics of Tumours of the Nervous System*. Lyon, IARC Press, 2000.

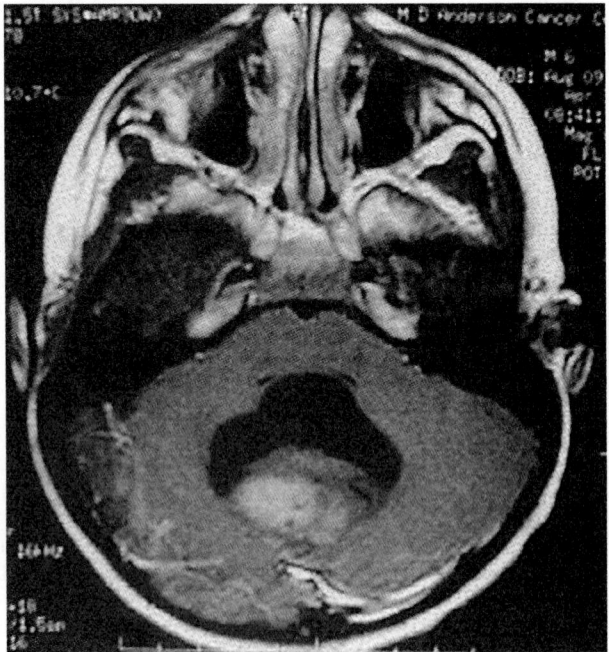

FIGURE 489–4. T1 weighted sequence post-gadolinium MRI (sagittal image) of a pontine diffuse infiltrating glioma in a 10-yr-old girl presenting with headache, cranial nerve palsies, and left-sided weakness. (Modified from Kleihues P, Cavenee WK: *World Health Organization Classification of Tumors: Pathology and Genetics of Tumors of the Nervous System*. Lyon, IARC Press, 2000.)

Packer RJ, Cohen BH, Coney K: Intracranial germ cell tumors. *Oncologist* 2000;5:312–20.

Packer RJ, Goldwein J, Nicholson HS, et al: Treatment of children with medulloblastoma with reduced-dose craniospinal radiation therapy and adjuvant chemotherapy: A Children's Cancer Group Study. *J Clin Oncol* 1999;17:2127–36.

Pollack IF, Boyett JM, Finlay JL: Chemotherapy for high grade gliomas of childhood. *Childs Nerv Syst* 1999;15:529–44.

Pollack IF, Finkelstein SD, Woods J, et al: Expression of p53 and prognosis in children with malignant gliomas. *N Engl J Med* 2002;346:420–26.

Pomeroy SL, Tamayo P, Gaasenbeek M, et al: Prediction of central nervous system embryonal tumor outcome based on gene expression. *Nature* 2002;415:436–42.

Reddy AT, Packer RJ: Chemotherapy for low grade gliomas. *Childs Nerv Syst* 1999;15:506–13.

Stiller CA, Bunch KJ, Lewis IJ: Ethnic group and survival from childhood cancer: Report from the UK Children's Cancer Study Group. *Br J Cancer* 2000; 82:1339–43.

Strother DR, Pollac IF, Fisher PG, et al: Tumors of the central nervous system. In Pizzo PA, Poplack DG (editors): *Principles and Practices of Pediatric Oncology*, 4th ed. Philadelphia, Lippincott Williams & Wilkins, 2002;751–824.

Chapter 490

Neuroblastoma *Joann L. Ater*

Epidemiology. Neuroblastoma (NB) is an embryonal cancer of the peripheral sympathetic nervous system. It is the third most common pediatric cancer, accounting for about 8% of childhood malignancies. About 500 new cases are diagnosed each year in the United States. NB is the most frequently diagnosed neoplasm in infants, accounting for 28–39% of neonatal malignancies. The median age at diagnosis is 2 yr; 90% of cases are diagnosed before 5 yr of age. The incidence is slightly higher in males and in whites.

Pathogenesis. NB includes a spectrum of tumors with variable degrees of neural differentiation, ranging from undifferentiated small round cells (neuroblastoma) to tumors containing mature ganglion cells (ganglioneuroblastoma or ganglioneuroma). The tumors may resemble other small round cell tumors, such as rhabdomyosarcoma, Ewing sarcoma, and non-Hodgkin lymphoma.

The prognosis varies with the histologic definition of tissue pattern (Shimada classification). A favorable prognosis NB subtype is based on the amount of stroma, degree of tumor cell differentiation, and number of tumor cell mitoses.

The genetic event that initially triggers formation of NB is not known. The pathogenesis is likely to be related to a succession of mutational events, prenatally and perinatally, that may be caused by environmental and genetic factors. Increased incidence of NB is associated with some maternal and paternal occupational chemical exposures, work in farming, and work related to electronics. Familial NB is found in 1–2% of cases. Genetic characteristics of NB that are of prognostic importance and currently used along with clinical factors to determine treatment include amplification of the *MYCN* (N-*myc*) proto-oncogene and hyperdiploidy of tumor cell DNA content (Table 490–1). Amplification of *MYCN* has prognostic importance independent of stage and age and is strongly associated with advanced tumor stage and poor outcome. Hyperdiploidy confers better prognosis if the child is younger than 1 yr of age at diagnosis. Genetic abnormalities, including loss of heterozygosity (LOH) of 1p, 11q, and 14q, and gain of 17q, are found commonly in NB tumor tissue. In addition, other biologic factors that correlate with prognosis include the level of nerve growth factor receptor (Trk-A) expression, multidrug-resistance–associated protein, and telomerase activity. These factors are under investigation in clinical trials to determine if they can be used to further refine risk-based therapy, to reduce therapy for patients predicted to fare well with minimal therapy and intensify therapy for those predicted to be at high risk of relapse.

Clinical Manifestations. NB may develop at any site of sympathetic nervous system tissue. The signs and symptoms of NB reflect the tumor site and extent of disease. Most cases of NB arise in the abdomen, either in the adrenal gland or in retroperitoneal sympathetic ganglia. Usually a firm, nodular mass is palpable in the flank or midline that is causing abdominal discomfort. On plain radiography or CT the mass often contains calcification and hemorrhage. Wilms tumor, another common flank mass in a young child, usually does not calcify. NB originates from cervical, thoracic, or pelvic ganglia in 30% of cases. Metastatic disease can be associated with myriad signs and symptoms, including fever, irritability, failure to thrive, bone pain, bluish subcutaneous nodules, orbital proptosis, and periorbital ecchymoses (Fig. 490–1). The most common sites of metastasis are the long bones and skull, bone marrow, liver, lymph nodes, and skin. Lung metastases are rare, occurring in less than 3% of cases. Prenatal diagnosis of NB is, at times, possible on maternal ultrasound scans.

Less commonly, children present first with neurologic signs and symptoms. Location in the superior cervical ganglion can result in Horner syndrome. Paraspinal NB can invade the neural foramina, producing symptoms of spinal cord and nerve root compression. Finally, NB can present as a paraneoplastic syndrome of autoimmune origin manifesting as ataxia or **opsomyoclonus** ("dancing eyes and dancing feet"). In such cases, the primary tumor is in the chest or abdomen, and the brain is negative for tumor. Some tumors produce catecholamines that can cause increased sweating and hypertension, and some release vasoactive intestinal peptide, causing a secretory diarrhea. Children younger than 1 yr of age can also present with a unique stage, 4S, that often includes subcutaneous tumor nodules, massive liver involvement, and a small primary tumor without bone involvement.

TABLE 490–1. Neuroblastoma Risk Groups

Risk Group	Survival	INSS Stage	Age	*MYCN* Status	Shimada Histology	DNA Ploidy
Low	90–100%	1	All	Any	Any	Any
		2	<1 yr	Any	Any	Any
		2	>1 yr	Any	Favorable	
		4S	<1 yr	<10 copies	Favorable	Hyperdiploid
Average	75–98%	3	>1 yr	<10 copies	Favorable	
		3 and 4	<1 yr	<10 copies	Any	Any
		4S	<1 yr	<10 copies	Unfavorable	Any
		4S	<1 yr	<10 copies	Any	Diploid
High	20–60%	2	>1 yr	Any	Unfavorable	
		3	All	>10 copies	Any	
		4	<1 yr	>10 copies	Any	Any
		4	>1 yr	Any	Any	

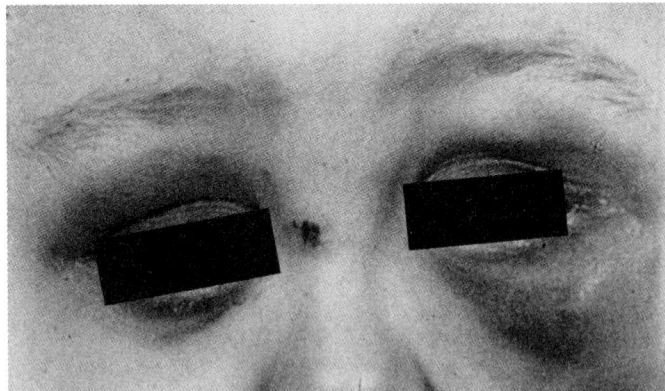

FIGURE 490–1. Periorbital metastases of neuroblastoma, with proptosis and ecchymoses.

Diagnosis. NB is generally discovered as a mass or multiple masses on plain radiographs, CT, or MRI (Fig. 490–2). Tumor markers, including elevated homovanillic acid (HVA) and vanillylmandelic acid (VMA) in urine, are elevated in 95% of cases and help to confirm the diagnosis. A pathologic diagnosis is established from tumor tissue obtained by biopsy. NB can be diagnosed in a typical presentation without a primary tumor biopsy if the patient has neuroblasts observed in bone marrow (Fig. 490–3) and elevated VMA or HVA in the urine.

Evaluation for metastatic disease should include bone scan to detect cortical bone involvement and bone marrow aspirates and biopsies to detect marrow disease. The clinical extent of disease and age, together with cytogenetic and molecular markers performed on the tumor tissue, are used to estimate the prognosis and for determination of risk-directed therapy. Although several staging systems have been used, the International Neuroblastoma Staging System (INSS) is universally used. In the INSS, stage 1 includes tumors confined to the organ or structure of origin. Stage 2 tumors extend beyond the structure of origin but not across the midline, with (stage 2B) or without (stage 2A) ipsilateral lymph node involvement. Stage 3 tumors extend beyond the midline, with or without bilateral lymph node involvement. Stage 4 tumors are disseminated to distant sites (e.g., bone, bone marrow, liver, distant lymph nodes, other organs). Stage 4S refers to children younger than 1 yr of age with dissemination to liver, skin, or bone marrow without bone involvement and with a primary tumor that would otherwise be stage 1 or 2.

Treatment. The most important clinical and biologic prognostic factors currently used to determine treatment are the age of the patient at diagnosis, stage, *MYCN* status, Shimada histology, and ploidy for infants (see Table 490–1). The prognoses shown are the best published survival rates with recently published therapies (see references). Treatment of low-risk NB is usually surgery for stages 1 and 2 and observation for stage 4S. Even in stage 2 with small amounts of residual tumor, the cure rate is over 90% without further therapy. Furthermore, treatment with chemotherapy or radiation for the rare child with local recurrence can still be curative. Children with spinal cord compression at diagnosis may also require urgent therapy with chemotherapy, surgery, or radiation to avoid neurologic damage. Stage 4S also has a favorable prognosis, with nearly 100% survival with supportive care only, because the tumor regresses spontaneously. Chemotherapy or resection of the primary tumor does not improve survival. Infants younger than 2 months old with stage 4S are at more risk if they have massive liver involvement and respiratory compromise. In such infants, low-dose cyclophosphamide or very low-dose hepatic radiation may be recommended to alleviate symptoms. For

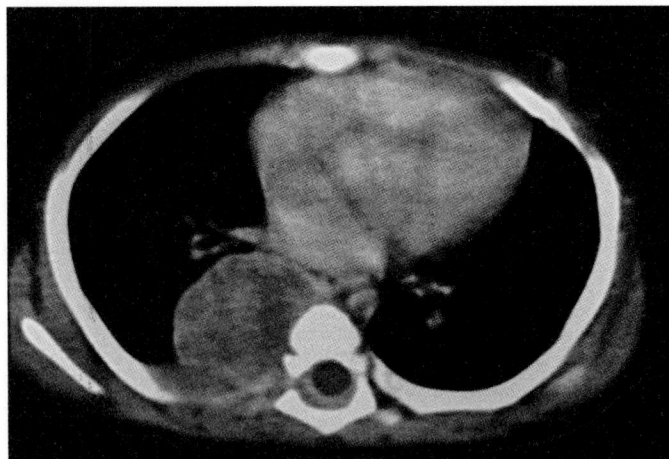

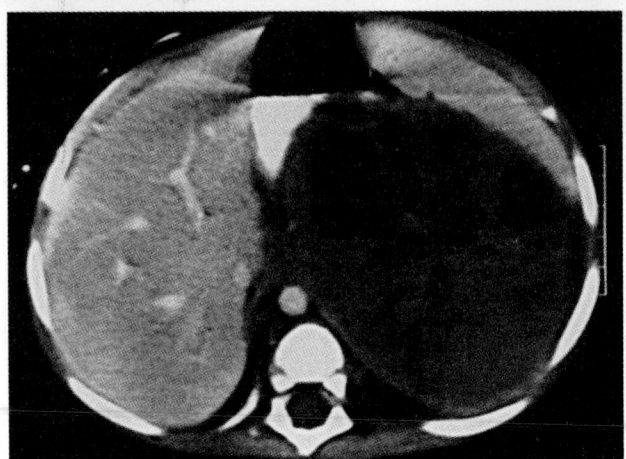

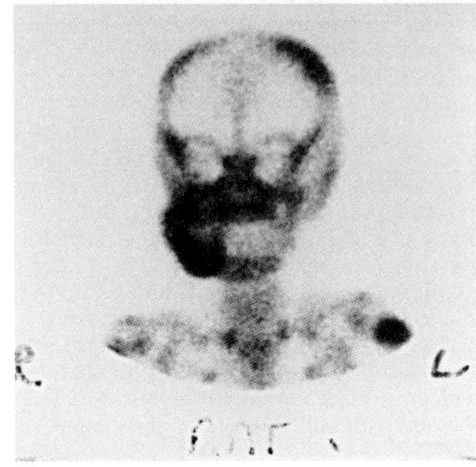

FIGURE 490–2. *Top,* CT of a thoracic neuroblastoma with intraspinal extension at diagnosis. *Middle,* CT of adrenal primary with extensive lymph node involvement. *Bottom,* Bone scintigraphy with technetium diphosphonate demonstrating diffuse skeletal involvement.

children with stage 4S NB who require treatment for symptoms, the survival rate is 81%.

Treatment of intermediate-risk NB includes surgery, chemotherapy, and, in some cases, radiation. The chemotherapy usually includes moderate doses of cisplatin or carboplatin, cyclophosphamide, etoposide, and doxorubicin given for several months. Radiotherapy is utilized for incomplete response of the tumor to chemotherapy. Children with stage 3 and infants

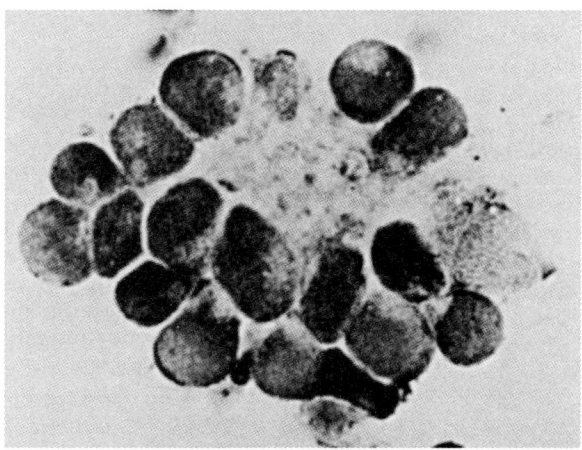

FIGURE 490–3. Neuroblastoma cells aspirated from the bone marrow. Clumps of cells often contain three or more cells with or without evidence of rosette formation. Rosettes of cells surrounding an inner mass of fibrillary material are characteristic of neuroblastoma.

younger than 12 mo of age with stage 4 and favorable characteristics have an excellent prognosis of more than 90% survival with this moderate treatment. In this intermediate-risk group, obtaining adequate diagnostic material for determination of Shimada pathologic classification system and for *MYCN* amplification is critical so that children with unfavorable characteristics can receive more aggressive treatment and those with favorable features can be spared excessive toxic therapy.

Treatment of high-risk NB (see Table 490–1) is usually induction chemotherapy followed by high-dose chemotherapy and autologous bone marrow or stem cell transplantation (BMT). A randomized study performed nationally showed significantly improved survival with BMT compared with chemotherapy without BMT. The addition of *cis*-retinoic acid after BMT for 1 yr further improved the 5-yr event-free survival to 50% compared with 20% for those treated with chemotherapy without BMT or *cis*-retinoic acid. However, better therapy is needed for the majority of patients with high-risk NB. New therapies currently under investigation include new chemotherapeutic agents, high-dose chemotherapy with multiple stem cell rescues, monoclonal antibodies combined with growth factors, and antitumor vaccines. It is also hoped that biologic studies of NB will eventually lead to new genetic targets for therapy.

De Roos AJ, Olshan AF, Teschke K, et al: Parental occupational exposures to chemicals and incidence of neuroblastoma in offspring. *Am J Epidemiol* 2001;154:106–14.

Maris JM, Matthay KK: Molecular biology of neuroblastoma. *J Clin Oncol* 1999;17:2264–79.

Matthay KK, Villablanca JG, Seeger RC, et al: Treatment of high-risk neuroblastoma with intensive chemotherapy, radiotherapy, autologous bone marrow transplantation, and 13-*cis*-retinoic acid. *N Engl J Med* 1999;341:1165–73.

Moppett J, Haddadin I, Foot ABM: Neonatal neuroblastoma. *Arch Dis Fetal Neonatal Ed* 1999;81:F134–37.

Nickerson HJ, Matthay KK, Seeger RC, et al: Favorable biology and outcome of stage IV-S neuroblastoma with supportive care or minimal therapy: A Children's Cancer Group study. *J Clin Oncol* 2000;18:477–86.

Perez CA, Matthay KK, Atkinson JB, et al: Biological variables in the outcome of stages I and II neuroblastoma treated with surgery as primary therapy: A Children's Cancer Group study. *J Clin Oncol* 2000;18:18–26.

Rudnick E, Khakoo Y, Antunes NL, et al: Opsoclonus-myoclonus-ataxia syndrome in neuroblastoma: Clinical outcome and antineuronal antibodies: A report from the Children's Cancer Group Study. *Med Pediatr Oncol* 2001;36:612–22.

Schmidt ML, Lukens JN, Seeger RC, et al: Biologic factors determine prognosis in infants with stage IV neuroblastoma: A prospective Children's Cancer Group Study. *J Clin Oncol* 2000;18:1260–68.

Chapter 491
Neoplasms of the Kidney
Norman Jaffe and Vicki Huff

WILMS TUMOR

Epidemiology. Wilms tumor, also designated **nephroblastoma,** is a complex mixed embryonal neoplasm of the kidney composed of three elements: blastema, epithelia, and stroma. The incidence is approximately 8 cases/million children younger than 15 yr of age. It usually occurs in children between 2–5 yr of age, although it has also been encountered in neonates, adolescents, and adults. It comprises approximately 6% of pediatric cancers and is the second most common malignant abdominal tumor in childhood. It may arise in one or both kidneys; the incidence of bilateral Wilms tumor is 7%. It may be associated with hemihypertrophy, aniridia, and other congenital anomalies, usually of the genitourinary tract. It has also been described in association with a variety of syndromes.

Pathogenesis. The majority of Wilms tumors cases are sporadic, although 1–2% of patients have a family history. Familial predisposition to Wilms tumor is inherited in an autosomal dominant manner. Familial cases are associated with a decreased age at diagnosis and an increased frequency of bilateral disease, although these features are not observed in all families. Congenital anomalies are absent in most families.

One Wilms tumor gene, *WT1*, located at 11p13, has been isolated. *WT1* encodes a zinc finger transcription factor that is critical for normal kidney development. Roughly 20% of all Wilms tumors carry *WT1* mutations, and most of these mutations are tumor specific. Wilms tumor patients with associated congenital anomalies frequently carry germline *WT1* mutations. Familial predisposition to Wilms tumor is usually not associated with *WT1* alterations; familial predisposition genes have been localized to 19q13 and 17q.

Histologically, two broad categories have been recognized: favorable and unfavorable. The favorable type is considered to be the "conventional" form and usually carries a good prognosis. It is characterized by blastema, epithelia, and stromal elements devoid of ectopia or anaplasia. Small amounts of sarcomatous elements in the stroma in an otherwise favorable type apparently do not adversely influence the prognosis. The unfavorable subtype is characterized by marked enlargement of the nuclei, hyperchromatism of the enlarged nuclei, and multipolar mitotic figures. Areas of anaplasia may be focal or diffuse and predict probable high rates of tumor relapse and death. It tends to occur in older, nonwhite patients. Clear cell sarcoma is a subtype of the unfavorable form and usually metastasizes to bone. Rhabdoid tumor, which may metastasize to the brain, is no longer classified as a subtype of Wilms tumor.

Nodal or other potential metastatic sites are usually the most fruitful areas to identify anaplasia, which is extremely uncommon in children younger than 2 yr of age. A high index of suspicion and more thorough sampling of techniques are appropriate if anaplasia is detected, particularly in older children. The phenomenon is generally not found once chemotherapy has been administered. Anaplasia related to skeletal muscle cells does not appear to be associated with an increased incidence of relapse.

Recent studies have shown a remarkable correlation among the DNA content in the cells of Wilms tumor, histologic subtype, and treatment outcome. Stem lines of both the primary tumor and metastases are in the diploid and low aneuploid (hyperdiploid) range. Tumors with hyperdiploid content are also characteristic of the anaplastic (unfavorable) varieties and have enormous complex translocations. They respond poorly to chemotherapy.

CONGENITAL ABNORMALITIES. Several syndromes, congenital abnormalities, and chromosomal aberrations are commonly reported in Wilms tumor (Tables 491–1 and 491–2). **WAGR syndrome** comprises Wilms tumor, aniridia, genitourinary abnormalities, and mental retardation. Patients with this syndrome have a constitutional deletion of chromosome 11p13 where both the Wilms tumor gene, *WT1*, and the aniridia gene, *PAX6*, are located. **Denys-Drash syndrome** comprises male pseudohermaphrodism, early-onset renal failure characterized by mesangial sclerosis, and an increased risk of Wilms tumor. Patients with this syndrome typically carry a point mutation within the *WT1* gene. The **Beckwith-Wiedemann syndrome** is characterized by hemihypertrophy, macroglossia, and visceromegaly, with a risk of developing Wilms tumor of 3–5%. A variety of 11p15.5 abnormalities have been reported in patients with this syndrome, and it is postulated that a second Wilms tumor gene, *WT2*, is located in this region. Other syndromes or conditions with an increased risk of Wilms tumor include hemihypertrophy, aniridia, genitourinary anomalies, Pearlman syndrome, Sotos syndrome, neurofibromatosis (von Recklinghausen disease), and von Willebrand disease. The most common genitourinary anomalies associated with Wilms tumor are hypoplasia, fusion and ectopia of the kidney, duplications of the collecting systems, hypospadias, and cryptorchidism.

Clinical Manifestations. Wilms tumor usually presents as an abdominal mass. It is generally discovered fortuitously, and it is not uncommon for it to be brought to the mother's attention while bathing the infant. It may also be identified during a well-child clinical examination. Renal masses of this type are usually smooth and firm and occasionally may cross the midline. They vary in size. Some patients may present with abdominal pain and vomiting and, infrequently, hematuria. Hypertension has also been described and is probably due to renal ischemia. Occasionally, rapid abdominal enlargement and anemia may occur owing to bleeding into the renal parenchyma or pelvis. Hematuria has been reported in 12–25% of patients.

Diagnosis. Any abdominal mass in a child must be considered malignant until diagnostic imaging and laboratory findings define its true nature. If there is any doubt, biopsy or excision and histologic verification is the final arbiter. Wilms tumor must be differentiated from a variety of malignant abdominal and pelvic tumors (Table 491–3). Once an abdominal mass is discovered, a complete physical examination should be performed followed by a complete blood cell count, liver and kidney function studies, and a search for specific tumor markers secreted by the suspected tumor. Imaging studies include a flat plate of the abdomen, ultrasonography, and CT and/or MRI.

CT scan permits confirmation of the intrarenal origin of the mass. It may also provide information on the extent of tumor, involvement of the inferior vena cava, and integrity of the contralateral kidney. Tumors enhance slightly after injection of contrast medium, which is useful to determine the function of the uninvolved kidney in the event that nephrectomy is required. MRI may also help define the extent of tumor. Ultrasonography may also contribute to identification of the tumor and integrity of the inferior vena cava. Occasionally, angiography may be requested to plan the surgical procedure. Bone scans are obtained for clear cell sarcoma of the kidney and MRI or CT of the brain in a malignant rhabdoid tumor.

Radiographic examination of the chest is required to determine the presence of pulmonary metastases. Pulmonary metastases from Wilms tumor can generally be identified on conventional radiograph; therefore, CT scans of the lungs are not routinely obtained. Occasionally, a CT scan demonstrates isolated nodules in patients with normal chest radiographs; the true nature of these nodules is uncertain.

STAGING. The staging system frequently utilized was developed by the National Wilms Tumor Study Group (Table 491–4) and correlates with prognosis (Table 491–5). Stage I Wilms tumor is confined to the kidney and, by definition, is completely excised with the capsular surface intact. Stage II Wilms tumor is also confined to the kidney, although the capsule is penetrated or tumor is present in the perirenal soft tissue. Stage III Wilms tumor has postsurgical residual nonhematogenous extension present. Spread is confined to the abdomen and may involve the perirenal bed, draining lymph nodes, or the surrounding tissue and organs by contiguity. Stage IV Wilms tumor is characterized by hematogenous metastases. The metastases generally involve the lungs and occasionally the liver. Stage V Wilms tumor is designated by bilateral renal involvement.

Treatment. Surgical extirpation of the tumor should be performed. The patency of the inferior vena cava should be established before the resection; if it is not patent, preoperative chemotherapy should be administered. During the operation the contralateral kidney should be examined to exclude bilateral Wilms tumor. The liver should be inspected for possible metas-

TABLE 491–1. Syndromes Associated with Wilms Tumor and Their Clinical and Genetic Characteristics

Syndrome	Clinical Characteristics	Chromosome or other abnormalities
WAGR	Aniridia, genitourinary abnormalities, mental retardation	Del 11p13 (*WT1* & *PAX6* loci)
Denys-Drash	Early-onset renal failure with renal mesangial sclerosis, male pseudohermaphrodism, increase risk of Wilms tumor	*WT1* mutations
Beckwith-Wiedemann	Organomegaly (liver, kidney, adrenal, pancreas), macroglossia omphalocele, hemihypertrophy	Uniparental paternal disomy, duplication 11p15.5, loss of imprinting, mutation of p57KIP57 have been described. Del 11p15.5 (*WT2* locus) May also involve *IGF2* and/or *H19* genes

TABLE 491–2. Genetic Alterations Observed in Wilms Tumors

Gene	Wilms Tumor Characteristic	Frequency	Type of Alteration
WT1	Unselected	~20%	Deletions, truncating mutations, missense mutations in zinc finger–encoding exons
β-Catenin	Unselected	~15%	Missense mutations or deletions affecting protein phosphorylation sites
	Tumors with *WT1* mutations (~20% of total)	~50%	
P53	Anaplastic histology (~5% of total)	~80%	Missense and truncating mutations

TABLE 491-3. Differential Diagnosis of Abdominal and Pelvic Tumors in Infants and Children

Tumor	Age	Clinical Signs	Laboratory Findings
Wilms tumor	Preschool	Unilateral flank mass, aniridia, hemihypertrophy	Hematuria; bone scintigraphy (clear cell sarcoma)
Neuroblastoma	Preschool	Gastrointestinal/ genitourinary obstruction, raccoon eyes, myoclonus-opsoclonus, diarrhea, skin nodules (infants)	Increased VMA; increased HVA; increased ferritin; stippled calcification in mass. Bone marrow +
Non-Hodgkin lymphoma	>1 yr	Intussusception in >2-yr-old child	Increased urate; bone marrow +
Rhabdomyosarcoma	All	Gastrointestinal/genitourinary obstruction, sarcoma botryoides, vaginal bleeding, paratesticular mass	
Germ cell/teratoma	Preschool, teens	Girls: abdominal pain, vaginal bleeding	Increased hCG;
		Boys: testicular mass, new onset "hydrocele" Sacrococcygeal mass/dimple	Increased AFP
Hepatoblastoma	Birth–3 yr	Large, firm liver	Increased AFP
Hepatoma	School age, teens	Large, firm liver; hepatitis B, cirrhosis	Increased AFP

VMA = vanillylmandelic acid; HMA = homovanillic acid; hCG = human chorionic gonadotropin; AFP = α-fetoprotein.

TABLE 491-4. Staging System Developed by the Third National Wilms Tumor Study Group

Stage I	Tumor limited to kidney and is completely excised. Capsular surface intact; no tumor rupture; no residual tumor apparent beyond margins of excision
Stage II	Tumor extends beyond kidney but is completely excised. Regional extension of tumor; vessel infiltration; tumor biopsied or local spillage of tumor confined to the flank. No residual tumor apparent at or beyond margins of excision
Stage III	Residual nonhematogenous tumor confined to the abdomen. Lymph node involvement of hilus, periaortic chains, or beyond; diffuse peritoneal contamination by tumor spillage; peritoneal implants of tumor; tumor extends beyond surgical margins microscopically or macroscopically; tumor not completely removable because of local infiltration into vital structures
Stage IV	Deposits beyond stage III (e.g., lung, liver, bone, brain)
Stage V	Bilateral renal involvement at diagnosis

tases, although CT, MRI, or ultrasonography may have identified metastases preoperatively. The retroperitoneal lymph nodes should be examined and suspicious nodes sampled for tumor involvement. Every attempt should be made to avoid spillage of tumor.

Most centers utilize chemotherapy guidelines provided by the National Wilms Tumor Study Group. For stage I and II, favorable histology tumors, vincristine and dactinomycin are administered. For stage III, favorable histology, vincristine, dactinomycin, and doxorubicin are administered. Radiation therapy is also administered to the tumor bed. In stage IV, favorable histology, vincristine, dactinomycin, and doxorubicin are administered. In addition, radiation therapy is administered to the sites of known disease, particularly the lungs. If tumor in the liver is present, surgical resection as opposed to radiation therapy may be considered. Resistant tumors that fail to respond to chemotherapy and radiation, or tumors that recur, may be considered for surgical resection and alternate (investigational) chemotherapy.

In the unfavorable histology subtype, vincristine, dactinomycin, doxorubicin, and cyclophosphamide are administered. Treatment is more aggressive and usually incorporates radiation therapy to the tumor bed and sites of established metastases. Clear cell sarcoma of bone has responded to a combination of cisplatin, doxorubicin, and radiation therapy. Additional therapy with cyclophosphamide or ifosfamide may also be considered.

INOPERABLE WILMS TUMOR. Chemotherapy is administered for all Wilms tumors that appear inoperable. In these circumstances the diagnosis is usually established by percutaneous needle biopsy. The selection of chemotherapy is dictated by histologic criteria: for favorable histologic subtypes, vincristine and dactinomycin are utilized for stages I and II and vincristine, dactinomycin, and doxorubicin for stages III and IV. Tumors of the unfavorable variety are treated with vincristine, dactinomycin, doxorubicin, and cyclophosphamide. In most instances a reduction in tumor size will be obtained. The prognosis for inoperable tumors treated with chemotherapy, surgery, and, if required, radiation therapy is generally favorable, with survival rates of more than 50%.

BILATERAL WILMS TUMOR. Chemotherapy for bilateral Wilms tumor is identical to that employed for inoperable tumors and is utilized to render the tumor amenable to surgical extirpation. This may comprise unilateral nephrectomy and contralateral partial nephrectomy or bilateral partial nephrectomies. These maneuvers permit ablation of viable neoplasm and conservation of renal tissue. Surgical procedures are dictated by the extent of tumor and response to chemotherapy. Postoperatively, chemotherapy and, not infrequently, radiation therapy are administered. Occasionally, preoperative radiation is also utilized. These therapeutic strategies have yielded survival rates of 60–85%.

SALVAGE CHEMOTHERAPY. Patients may relapse during or after treatment with conventional therapy. Such patients, particularly those with favorable hematology, can often be salvaged with alternate treatment. In these circumstances, combination chemotherapy with vincristine, doxorubicin (Adriamycin), cyclophosphamide, and dactinomycin (Actinomycin D) (VACA) or ifosfamide, carboplatin, and etoposide (ICE) may be attempted. High-dose chemotherapy with bone marrow rescue has also been employed. A multidisciplinary strategy with surgery, radiation therapy, and chemotherapy will generally yield the best result.

Prognosis. Major prognostic factors are tumor size, stage, and histology (see Table 491–5). The prognosis is worse in patients with a larger tumor (>500 g), advanced stage (III and IV), and unfavorable histologic subtype. Nonetheless, Wilms tumor

TABLE 491–5. Wilms Tumor: Survival by Histology and Stage

Histology/Stage	Survival 2 Yr (%)	Survival 4 Yr (%)
Favorable I	98	97
Favorable II	96	94
Favorable III	91	88
Favorable IV	88	82
Anaplastic I	89	89
Anaplastic II–IV	56	54

Modified from Wilms' tumor: Status report, 1990. By the National Wilms' Tumor Study Committee. J Clin Oncol *1991;9:877–87.*

constitutes a paradigm of successful multidisciplinary treatment; more than 60% of patients with all stages generally survive. Stages I through III have a cure rate varying from 88–98%.

OTHER KIDNEY TUMORS IN CHILDREN

Congenital Mesoblastic Nephroma. This is a unique congenital neoplasm of the infant kidney that rarely metastasizes. It occurs more often in males and has been noted to produce renin. The tumor is a massive, firm, infiltrative, solitary renal mass. Grossly and microscopically it resembles a leiomyoma or a low-grade leiomyosarcoma with trapped nephrons. Microscopy reveals fibroblast or myofibroblast cells. The tumor accounts for the majority of congenital renal tumors. Most cases are considered benign, and there is division of opinion regarding the utility of chemotherapy. One report noted that vincristine and dactinomycin administered as adjuvant therapy did not prevent metastases. In another report, metastatic disease apparently responded to vincristine, doxorubicin, and cyclophosphamide.

Nephroblastomatosis. Nephroblastomatosis generally refers to the abnormal persistence of embryonal renal tissue that may be associated with the development of Wilms tumor. It has been suggested that a brief course of relatively nontoxic chemotherapy (vincristine and dactinomycin) may be beneficial by reducing the large volume of the kidneys. Persistent nodule renal blastema and associated nephroblastic abnormalities appear to remain in the kidneys of many, if not all, treated patients despite the reduction in renal volume. The favorable survival and response rate of bilateral Wilms tumor suggests a strong relationship of the latter to the nodular renal blastema nephroblastomatosis complex. Nephrogenic nests detected in one kidney should prompt a careful evaluation of the contralateral kidney. Radiographic follow-up with CT may also be indicated. Whether chemotherapy can reduce the incidence of development of subsequent Wilms tumor is unknown.

Multicystic Nephroblastoma. Tumors of the kidney may occasionally contain cysts, some of which may be linked to Wilms tumor. There is a melange of diagnostic terms applied to such tumors, including cystic partially differentiated nephroblastoma (CPDN), polycystic nephroblastoma, and multilocular nephroma. The majority of the reported cases of multicystic nephroblastoma occur in patients younger than 1 yr of age. When confronted with this type of tumor biology, a benign process may be considered to be present. However, if there is definite evidence of Wilms tumor, treatment with chemotherapy is justified.

Renal Cell Carcinoma. The tumor is rare in the first decades of life, but it has occasionally been reported in children and teenagers. It usually presents as an abdominal mass and/or hematuria. Complete resection may achieve cure. Occasionally, adjuvant treatment with interferon and 5-fluorouracil has been recommended.

Bracken RB, Sutow WW, Jaffe N, et al: Preoperative chemotherapy for Wilms tumor. *Urology* 1982;19:55–60.
Brodeur AE, Brodeur GM: Abdominal masses in children: Neuroblastoma, Wilms' tumor, and other considerations. *Pediatr Rev* 1991;12:196–207.

Green DM, Breslow NE, Beckwith JB, et al: Effect of duration of treatment on treatment outcome and cost of treatment for Wilms' tumor: A report from the National Wilms' Tumor Study Group. *J Clin Oncol* 1998;16:3744–51.
Huff V: Wilms' tumor genetics. *Am J Med Genet* 1998;79:260–67.
National Wilms' Tumor Study Committee: Wilms' tumor: Status report, 1990. *J Clin Oncol* 1991;9:877–87.
Paulino AC: Current issues in the diagnosis and management of Wilms' tumor. *Oncology* 1996;10:1553–71.

Chapter 492
Soft Tissue Sarcomas
Carola A. S. Arndt

Soft tissue sarcomas occur with an annual incidence of 8.4 cases/million white children younger than 15 yr of age. The incidence in black children is 50% of that in white children. Rhabdomyosarcoma accounts for more than half of soft tissue sarcomas. The prognosis most strongly correlates with extent of disease at diagnosis, primary tumor site, and type of treatment.

RHABDOMYOSARCOMA

Epidemiology. The most common pediatric soft tissue sarcoma, rhabdomyosarcoma, accounts for 5–8% of childhood cancers. These tumors occur at virtually any anatomic site but are most often found in the head and neck (40%), genitourinary tract (20%), extremities (20%), and trunk (10%); retroperitoneal and other sites account for the remainder of primary sites. The primary anatomic site is related to both age and tumor histology. Extremity lesions are more likely to occur in older children and to have alveolar histology. Rhabdomyosarcoma occurs with increased frequency in patients with neurofibromatosis and has been associated with maternal breast cancer in the Li-Fraumeni syndrome, suggesting a genetic influence.

Pathogenesis. Rhabdomyosarcoma is thought to arise from the same embryonic mesenchyme as striated skeletal muscle. On the basis of light microscopic appearance, it belongs to the group of small round cell tumors that includes Ewing sarcoma, neuroblastoma, and non-Hodgkin lymphoma. Definitive diagnosis of a pathologic specimen may require immunohistochemical studies using antibodies to skeletal muscle (e.g., desmin, muscle-specific actin, and Myo-D) and electron microscopy.

Determination of the specific histologic subtype is important in treatment planning and assessment of prognosis. There are four recognized histologic subtypes. The **embryonal type** accounts for about 60% of all cases and has an intermediate prognosis. The **botryoid type**, a variant of the embryonal form in which tumor cells and an edematous stroma project into a body cavity like a bunch of grapes, accounts for 6% of cases and is most often found in the vagina, uterus, bladder, nasopharynx, and middle ear. **Alveolar tumors**, which account for about 15% of cases, are often characterized by 2;13 or 1;13 chromosomal translocations. The tumor cells tend to grow in cores that often have cleftlike spaces resembling alveoli. Alveolar tumors occur most often in the trunk and extremities and carry the poorest prognosis. The **pleomorphic type (adult form)** is rare in childhood (1% of cases). About 20% of retinoblastomas are considered to be **undifferentiated sarcomas**.

Clinical Manifestations. The most common presenting feature is a mass that may or may not be painful. Symptoms are caused by displacement or obstruction of normal structures. Origin in the nasopharynx may be associated with nasal congestion, mouth breathing, epistaxis, and difficulty with swallowing and chewing. Regional extension into the cranium can produce cranial nerve paralysis, blindness, and signs of increased intracranial pressure with headache and vomiting. When the tumor develops in the face or cheek, there may be swelling, pain, trismus, and, as extension occurs, paralysis of cranial nerves. Tumors in the neck can produce progressive swelling with neurologic symptoms after regional extension. Orbital primary tumors are usually diagnosed early in their course because of associated proptosis, periorbital edema, ptosis, change in visual acuity, and local pain. When the tumor arises in the middle ear, the most common early signs are pain, hearing loss, chronic otorrhea, or a mass in the ear canal; extensions of tumor produce cranial nerve paralysis and signs of an intracranial mass on the involved side. An unremitting croupy cough and progressive stridor can accompany rhabdomyosarcoma of the larynx. Because most of these signs and symptoms are also associated with common childhood conditions, clinicians must be alert to the possibility of tumor.

Rhabdomyosarcoma of the trunk or extremities is often first noticed after trauma and may be regarded initially as a hematoma. When the swelling does not resolve or increases, malignancy should be suspected. Involvement of the genitourinary tract can produce hematuria, obstruction of the lower urinary tract, recurrent urinary tract infections, incontinence, or a mass detectable on abdominal or rectal examination. Paratesticular tumors usually present as a painless, rapidly growing mass in the scrotum. Vaginal rhabdomyosarcoma may present as a grapelike mass of tumor tissue bulging through the vaginal orifice **(sarcoma botryoides)** and can cause urinary tract or large bowel symptoms. Vaginal bleeding or obstruction of the urethra or rectum may occur. Similar findings can be noted with uterine primaries.

Tumors in any location may disseminate early, with presenting symptoms of pain or respiratory distress associated with pulmonary metastases. Extensive bone involvement can produce symptomatic hypercalcemia. In such cases, it may be difficult to identify the primary lesion.

Diagnosis. Early diagnosis of rhabdomyosarcoma requires a high index of suspicion. The microscopic appearance is that of a small round blue cell tumor. Neuroblastoma, lymphoma, and Ewing sarcoma are also small round blue cell tumors. The differential diagnosis depends on the site of presentation. Definitive diagnosis is established by biopsy, microscopic appearance, and immunohistochemical stains. A lesion in an extremity may be thought to be a hematoma or hemangioma, an orbital lesion resulting in proptosis may be treated as an orbital cellulitis, or

bladder obstructive symptoms may be missed. Paratesticular lesions may be ignored for a long time by adolescents. Unfortunately, several months often elapse between the initial symptoms and biopsy. Diagnostic procedures are determined mainly by the area of involvement. MRI or CT is necessary for evaluation of the primary tumor site. With signs and symptoms in the head and neck area, radiographs should be examined for evidence of a tumor mass and for indications of bony erosion. CT scans should be performed to identify intracranial extension and may also reveal bony involvement at the base of the skull; this may be difficult to visualize. For abdominal and pelvic tumors, ultrasound examination and CT with oral and intravenous contrast media or MRI can help delineate the tumor. Figure 492–1 shows a CT scan of the pelvis in a child with a bladder rhabdomyosarcoma. A radionuclide bone scan, chest CT scan, and bilateral bone marrow aspirate and biopsy should be performed to evaluate the patient for the presence of metastatic disease. The results of these studies are used to plan treatment. The most essential element of the diagnostic workup is examination of tumor tissue, which includes the use of special histochemical stains and immunostains. Lymph nodes should be sampled also for presence of disease spread, especially in extremity tumors.

Treatment. Patients with completely resected tumors have the best prognosis. Unfortunately, most rhabdomyosarcomas are not completely resectable. At the initial surgery, tumor margins should be carefully defined and an appropriate search for regional or metastatic disease (e.g., to regional lymph nodes or adjacent structures) should be completed even if the procedure is limited to biopsy. Treatment is based on the primary tumor location and disease stage ("clinical group"). Most patients are given preoperative chemotherapy in an attempt to reduce the extent of surgery required and to preserve vital organs, particularly in the genitourinary tract. For patients with group I tumors, complete local excision is followed by chemotherapy to reduce the likelihood of subsequent metastatic disease. For patients with group II tumors (microscopic residual tumor), surgery is followed by local irradiation and systemic multiagent chemotherapy. Patients with group III tumors (gross residual tumor) receive initial systemic multiagent chemotherapy, followed by irradiation and surgery if possible. Children with metastatic (group IV) rhabdomyosarcoma are treated principally with systemic chemotherapy and irradiation. Standard chemotherapeutic agents include vincristine, dactinomycin,

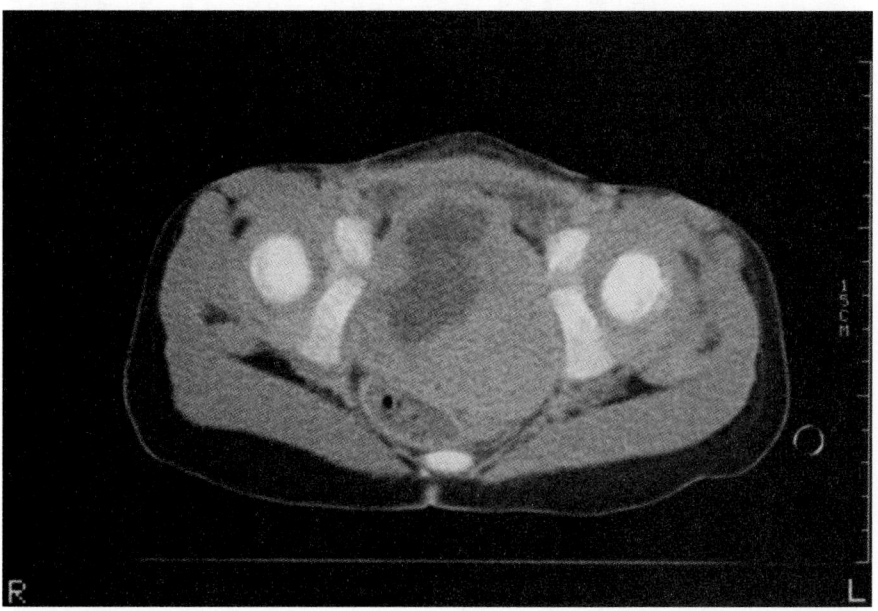

FIGURE 492–1. CT scan of pelvis in a patient with an embryonal rhabdomyosarcoma of the bladder.

TABLE 492–1. Features of Most Common Types of Nonrhabdomyocarcoma Soft Tissue Sarcomas

Tissue Type	Tumor	Natural History and Biology
Adipose	Liposarcoma	A very rare tumor. Usually arises in the extremities or retroperitoneum; associated with a nonrandom translocation, t(12;16) (q13;p11). Tends to be locally invasive and rarely metastasizes; wide local excision is the treatment of choice. The role of radiation therapy and chemotherapy in treating gross residual or metastatic disease is not established.
Fibrous	Fibrosarcoma	Most common soft tissue sarcoma in children younger than 1 yr. Congenital fibrosarcoma is a low-grade malignancy that commonly arises in the extremities or trunk and rarely metastasizes. Surgical excision is treatment of choice; dramatic responses to preoperative chemotherapy may occur. In children older than 4 yr, the natural history is similar to that in adults (a 5-yr survival rate of 60%); wide surgical excision and preoperative chemotherapy are commonly used.
	Malignant fibrous histiocytoma	Most commonly arises in the trunk and extremities, deep in the subcutaneous layer. Histologically subdivided into storiform, giant cell, myxoid, and angiomatoid variants. The angiomatoid type tends to affect younger patients and is curable with surgical resection alone. Wide surgical excision is the treatment of choice. Chemotherapy has produced objective tumor regressions.
Vascular	Hemangiopericytoma	Often arises in the lower extremities or retroperitoneum; may present with hypoglycemia and hypophosphatemic rickets. Both benign and malignant histology. Nonrandom translocations t(12;19) (q13;q13) and t(13;22) (q22;q11) have been described. Complete surgical excision is the treatment of choice. Chemotherapy and radiotherapy may produce responses.
	Angiosarcoma	Rare in children; 33% arise in skin, 25% in soft tissue, and 25% in liver, breast, or bone. Associated with chronic lymphedema and exposure to vinyl chloride in adults. Survival rate is poor (12% at 5 yr) despite some responses to chemotherapy/radiotherapy.
	Hemangioendothelioma	Can occur in soft tissue, liver, and lung. Localized lesions have a favorable outcome; lesions in lung and liver are often multifocal and have a poor prognosis.
Peripheral nerves	Neurofibrosarcoma	Also known as the malignant peripheral nerve sheath tumor. Develops in up to 16% of patients with NF1; almost 50% occur in patients with NF1. Deletions of chromosome 22q11–q13 or 17q11 and p53 mutations have been reported. Commonly arises in trunk and extremities and is usually locally invasive. Complete surgical excision is necessary for survival; response to chemotherapy is suboptimal.
Synovium	Synovial sarcoma	The most common NRSTS in some series. Often presenting in the 3rd decade, but 33% of patients are younger than 20 yr. Typically arises around the knee or thigh and is characterized by a nonrandom translocation t(X;18) (p11;q11). Wide surgical excision is necessary. Radiotherapy is effective in microscopic residual disease, and ifosfamide-based therapy is active in advanced disease.
Unknown	Alveolar soft part sarcoma	Slow-growing tumor; tends to recur or metastasize to lung and brain years after diagnosis. Often arises in the extremities and head and neck. A myogenic origin has been proposed. Resection of primary and metastatic sites, when possible, is recommended.
Smooth muscle	Leiomyosarcoma	Often arises in the gastrointestinal tract and may be associated with a t(12;14) (q14;q23) translocation. Associated with Epstein-Barr virus in immunodeficiency syndromes (including AIDS). Complete surgical excision is the treatment of choice.

NF = Neurofibromatosis; NRSTS = nonrhabdomyosarcoma soft tissue sarcoma.

and cyclophosphamide. Topotecan is being evaluated in therapeutic trials.

Prognosis. Among patients with resectable tumor, 80–90% have prolonged, disease-free survival. Unresectable tumor localized to certain "favorable" sites (e.g., the orbit) also has a high likelihood of cure. About 70% of patients with incompletely resected tumor also achieve long-term disease-free survival. Patients with disseminated disease have a poor prognosis; only about half achieve remission, and fewer than half of these are cured. Older children have a poorer prognosis than younger ones. For all patients, surveillance for late effects of cancer treatment, such as impaired bone growth due to radiation, sterility from cyclophosphamide, and second malignancies, is important.

OTHER SOFT TISSUE SARCOMAS

The nonrhabdomyosarcoma soft tissue sarcomas (NRSTS) constitute a heterogeneous group of tumors that account for 3% of all childhood malignancies. Because they are relatively rare in children, much of the information about their natural history and treatment has been derived from studies of adult patients. In children, the median age at diagnosis is 12 yr of age and males predominate (male:female ratio 2.3:1). The most common histologic types are synovial sarcoma (42%), fibrosarcoma (13%), malignant fibrous histiocytoma (12%), and neurogenic tumors (10%). Table 492–1 describes the clinical features, treatment, and prognosis of the most common NRSTS. These tumors commonly arise in the trunk or lower extremities. Tumor size, stage (clinical group), invasiveness, and histologic grade correlate with survival.

Surgery remains the mainstay of therapy, but a careful search for lung and bone metastases should be undertaken before surgical excision. Lymph node spread is rare, and routine dissection is not recommended. Chemotherapy and radiotherapy should be considered for large, high-grade, and unresectable tumors. The role of chemotherapy in nonrhabdomyosarcomatous tumors is not as well defined as in rhabdomyosarcoma. Patients with unresectable or metastatic disease are treated with multi-agent chemotherapy in addition to radiation and/or surgery.

Arndt CAS, Crist WM: Medical progress: Common musculoskeletal tumors of childhood and adolescence. *N Engl J Med* 1999;341:342–52.

Baker KS, Anderson JR, Lind MP, et al: Benefit of intensified therapy for patients with local or regional embryonal rhabdomyosarcoma: Results from the Intergroup Rhabdomyosarcoma Study IV. *J Clin Oncol* 2000;18:2427–34.

Crist WM, Anderson JR, Meza JL, et al: Intergroup rhabdomyosarcoma study: IV. Results for patients with nonmetastatic disease. *J Clin Oncol* 2001;19:3091–102.

Palumbo JS, Zwerdling J: Soft tissue sarcomas of infancy. *Semin Perinatol* 1999;23:299–309.

Spunt SL, Poquette CA, Hurt YS, et al: Prognostic factors for children and adolescents with surgically resected nonrhabdomyosarcoma soft tissue sarcoma: An analysis of 121 patients treated at St. Jude Children's Research Hospital. *J Clin Oncol* 1999;17:3697–705.

Chapter 493
Neoplasms of Bone
Carola A. S. Arndt

493.1 Malignant Tumors of Bone

The annual incidence of malignant bone tumors in the United States is approximately 7 cases/million white children younger than 15 yr of age, with a slightly lower incidence in black children. Osteosarcoma is the most common primary malignant bone tumor in children and adolescents, followed by Ewing sarcoma (Table 493–1 and Fig. 493–1). In children younger than 10 yr of age, Ewing sarcoma is more common than osteosarcoma. Both tumor types occur most frequently in the 2nd decade of life.

OSTEOSARCOMA

Epidemiology. The annual incidence of osteosarcoma in the United States is 5.6 cases/million children younger than 15 yr of age. The highest risk period for development of osteosarcoma is during the adolescent growth spurt, which suggests an association between rapid bone growth and malignant transformation. Patients with osteosarcoma are taller than their peers of similar age.

Pathogenesis. Although the cause of osteosarcoma is unknown, certain genetic or acquired conditions predispose patients to development of osteosarcoma. Patients with hereditary retinoblastoma have a significantly increased risk of developing osteosarcoma. The sites of osteosarcoma in these patients were initially thought to be in previously irradiated areas; however, they have since been shown to arise in sites far from the radiation field. Predisposition to development of osteosarcoma in these patients is thought to be related to loss of heterozygosity of the *RB* gene. Osteosarcoma also occurs in the **Li-Fraumeni syndrome**, which is a familial cancer syndrome associated with germline mutations of the *TP53* gene. Kindreds with Li-Fraumeni syndrome have a spectrum of malignancies in 1st-degree relatives, including carcinoma of the breast, soft tissue sarcomas, brain tumors, leukemia, adrenal cortical carcinoma, and other malignancies. **Rothmund-Thomson syndrome** is a rare syndrome associated with short stature, skin telangiectasia, small hands and feet, hypoplastic or absent thumbs, and a high risk of osteosarcoma. Osteosarcoma can also be induced by irradiation for Ewing sarcoma, craniospinal irradiation for brain tumors, or high-dose irradiation for other malignancies. Other benign conditions that can be associated with malignant

TABLE 493–1. Comparison of Features of Osteosarcoma and the Ewing Family of Tumors

Feature	Osteosarcoma	Ewing Family of Tumors
Age	Second decade	Second decade
Race	All races	Primarily whites
Sex (M:F)	1.5:1	1.5:1
Cell	Spindle cell–producing osteoid	Undifferentiated small round cell, probably of neural origin
Predisposition	Retinoblastoma, Li-Fraumeni syndrome, Paget's disease, radiotherapy	None known
Site	Metaphyses of long bones	Diaphyses of long bones, flat bones
Presentation	Local pain and swelling; often history of injury	Local pain and swelling; fever
Radiographic findings	Sclerotic destruction (less commonly lytic); sunburst pattern	Primarily lytic, multilaminar periosteal reaction ("onion skinning")
Differential diagnosis	Ewing's sarcoma, osteomyelitis	Osteomyelitis, eosinophilic granuloma, lymphoma, neuroblastoma, rhabdomyosarcoma
Metastasis	Lungs, bones	Lung, bones
Treatment	Chemotherapy Ablative surgery of primary tumor	Chemotherapy Radiotherapy and/or surgery of primary tumor
Outcome	Without metastases: 70% cured; with metastases at diagnosis, ≤20% survival	Without metastases: 60% cured; with metastases at diagnosis, 20–30% survival

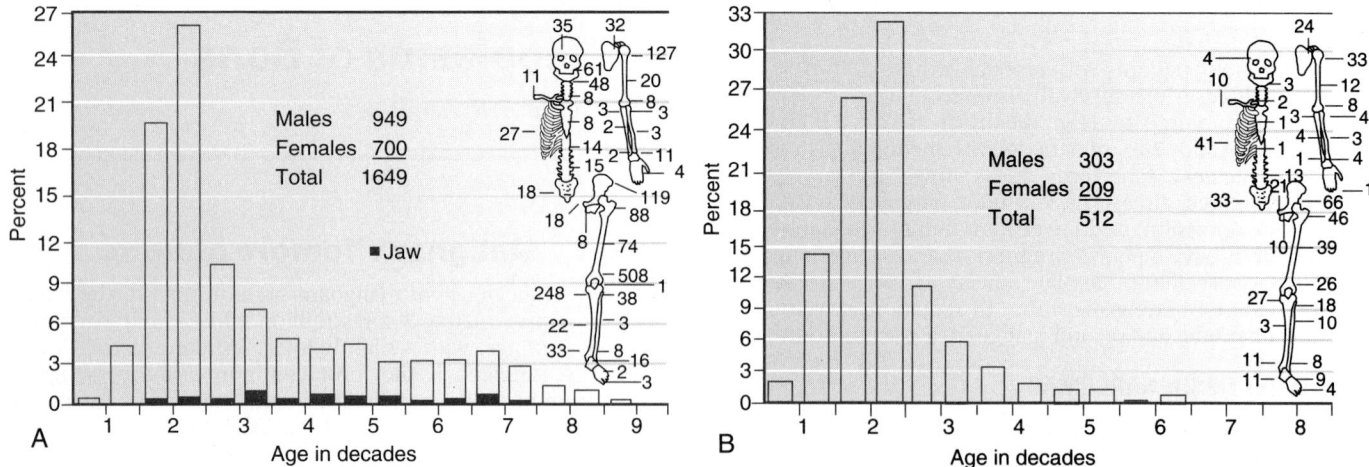

FIGURE 493–1. *A,* Age and skeletal distribution of 1,649 cases of osteosarcoma in the Mayo Clinic files. *B,* Age and skeletal distribution of 512 cases of Ewing sarcoma in the Mayo Clinic files. (From Unni KK [editor]: *Dahlin's Bone Tumors: General Aspects and Data on 11,087 Cases,* 5th ed. Philadelphia, Lippincott-Raven, 1996. Reprinted by permission of the Mayo Foundation.)

transformation to osteosarcoma include Paget disease, enchondromatosis, multiple hereditary exostoses, and fibrous dysplasia.

The pathologic diagnosis of osteosarcoma is made by demonstration of a highly malignant, pleomorphic, spindle cell neoplasm associated with the formation of malignant osteoid and bone. There are four pathologic subtypes of conventional high-grade osteosarcoma: osteoblastic, fibroblastic, chondroblastic, and telangiectatic. No significant differences in outcome are associated with the various subtypes, although the chondroblastic component of that subtype may not respond as well to chemotherapy. The role of various genes in prognosis such as drug resistance–related genes, tumor suppressor genes, and genes related to apoptosis is being evaluated.

Telangiectatic osteosarcoma may be confused with aneurysmal bone cyst because of its lytic appearance radiographically. High-grade osteosarcoma typically arises in the diaphyseal region of long bones and invades the medullary cavity. It may also be associated with a soft tissue mass. Two variants of osteosarcoma, parosteal and periosteal osteosarcoma, should be distinguished from conventional osteosarcoma because of their characteristic clinical features. **Parosteal osteosarcoma** is a low-grade, well-differentiated tumor that does not invade the medullary cavity and is most commonly found in the posterior aspect of the distal femur. Surgical resection alone is often curative in this lesion, which has a low propensity for metastatic spread. **Periosteal osteosarcoma** is a rare variant, which arises on the surface of the bone but has a higher rate of metastatic spread than the parosteal type and an intermediate prognosis.

Clinical Manifestations. Pain and swelling are the most common presenting manifestations of osteosarcoma. Because these tumors occur most frequently in active adolescents, initial complaints may be attributed to a sports injury or sprain; any bone or joint pain not responding to conservative therapy within a reasonable amount of time should be investigated thoroughly. Additional clinical findings may include limitation of motion, joint effusion, tenderness, and warmth. Results of routine laboratory tests, such as a complete blood cell count and chemistry panel, are usually normal, although alkaline phosphatase or lactic dehydrogenase levels may be elevated.

Diagnosis. The diagnosis of a bone tumor should be suspected in a patient who presents with deep bone pain, often causing nighttime awakening, a palpable mass, and a radiograph demonstrating a lesion. The lesion may be mixed lytic and blastic in appearance, but new bone formation is usually visible. The

classic radiographic appearance of osteosarcoma is the **sunburst** pattern (Fig. 493–2). When osteosarcoma is suspected, the patient should be referred to a center with experience in managing bone tumors. The biopsy should be performed by the surgeon who will ultimately perform the definitive surgery so that the incisional biopsy site can be placed in a manner that will not compromise the ultimate limb salvage procedure. Tissue is usually obtained for molecular and biologic studies at the time of the initial biopsy. Before biopsy, MRI of the primary lesion and the entire bone should be performed to evaluate the tumor for its proximity to nerves and blood vessels and soft tissue and joint extension as well as for skip lesions. The metastatic work-up should be performed before biopsy and includes CT of the chest and radionuclide bone scan to evaluate for lung and bone metastases, respectively. The differential diagnosis of a lytic bone lesion includes histiocytosis, Ewing sarcoma, lymphoma, and bone cyst.

Treatment. The survival of children with nonmetastatic osteosarcoma was only 20% at 5 yr with surgery alone. It is well established that with chemotherapy and surgery, the 5-yr disease-free survival rate of patients with nonmetastatic extremity osteosarcoma is 65–75%. Complete surgical resection of the tumor is important for cure. The current approach is to treat patients with preoperative chemotherapy in an attempt to facilitate limb salvage operations and to immediately treat micrometastatic disease. Up to 80% of patients are able to undergo limb salvage operations after initial chemotherapy. Some institutions use intra-arterial chemotherapy to infuse chemotherapy directly into an artery feeding the tumor, although this has not been proved to be better than conventional intravenous chemotherapy. It is important to resume chemotherapy as soon as possible after surgery. Lung metastases present at diagnosis should be resected by thoracostomies at some time during the course of treatment. Active agents currently in use in multidrug chemotherapy regimens for conventional osteosarcoma include doxorubicin, cisplatin, methotrexate, and ifosfamide. Current national treatment protocols are investigating dose intensification of various agents for patients who have a poor histologic response at time of surgery. After limb salvage surgery, intensive rehabilitation and physical therapy is necessary to ensure maximal functional outcome. For patients who require amputation, early prosthetic fitting and gait training is essential to enable them to resume as normal activities as possible. Before definitive surgery, patients with tumors on weight-bearing bones should be instructed to use

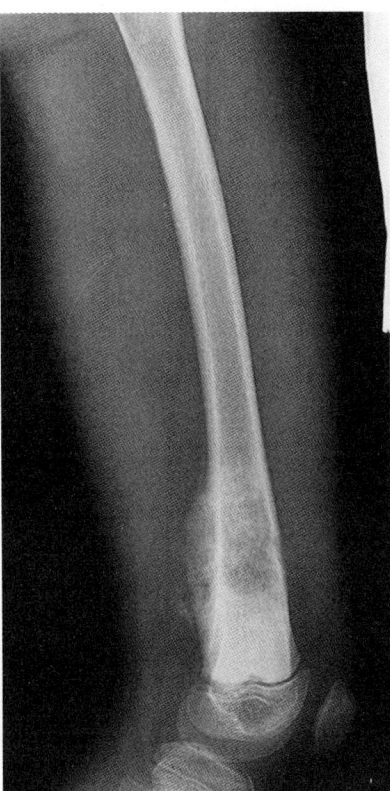

FIGURE 493–2. Radiograph of an osteosarcoma of the femur with typical "sunburst" appearance of bone formation.

crutches to avoid stressing the weakened bone and causing a pathologic fracture. The role of chemotherapy in parosteal and periosteal osteosarcoma is not well defined.

Prognosis. Surgical resection alone is curative only for patients with parosteal osteosarcoma. Conventional osteosarcoma requires multiagent chemotherapy. Up to 75% of patients with nonmetastatic extremity osteosarcoma are cured with current multiagent treatment protocols. Patients with pelvic tumors do not have as favorable a prognosis as those with extremity primaries. From 20–30% of patients who have limited numbers of pulmonary metastases can also be cured with aggressive chemotherapy and resection of lung nodules. Patients with bone metastases and those with widespread lung metastases have an extremely poor prognosis. Long-term follow-up of patients with osteosarcoma is important to monitor for late effects of chemotherapy such as cardiotoxicity from anthracycline. Patients who develop late isolated lung metastases may be cured with surgical resection alone.

EWING SARCOMA

Epidemiology. The incidence of Ewing sarcoma is 2.1 cases/million children in the United States. It is extremely rare among black children. Ewing sarcoma, an undifferentiated sarcoma of bone, may also arise from soft tissue. The term **Ewing sarcoma family of tumors** refers to a group of small round cell undifferentiated tumors thought to be of neural crest origin that generally carry the same chromosomal translocation. This family of tumors includes Ewing sarcoma of bone and soft tissue and **peripheral primitive neuroectodermal tumor (PPNET).** Treatment protocols for these tumors are the same whether the tumors arise in bone or soft tissue. Anatomic sites of primary tumors arising in bone are evenly distributed between the extremities and the central axis (pelvis, spine, and chest wall). Primary tumors arising in the chest wall are often referred to as **Askin tumors.**

Pathogenesis. Immunohistochemical staining assists in the diagnosis of Ewing sarcoma to differentiate it from other small, blue, round cell tumors such as lymphoma, rhabdomyosarcoma, and neuroblastoma. Histochemical stains may react positively with certain neural markers on tumor cells (neuron-specific enolase and S-100), especially in PPNET. Reactivity with muscle markers (e.g., desmin, actin) is absent. Additionally, the cell surface glycoprotein MIC-2 is usually positive. A specific chromosomal translocation, t(11;22), or a variant thereof is found in most of the Ewing sarcoma family of tumors. Analysis for the translocation by routine cytogenetics or polymerase chain reaction analysis for the chimeric fusion gene products EWS/FLI1 or EWS/ERG can be helpful in confirming the diagnosis in very undifferentiated tumors.

Clinical Manifestations. Symptoms of Ewing sarcoma are similar to those of osteosarcoma. Pain, swelling, limitation of motion, and tenderness over the involved bone or soft tissue are common presenting symptoms. In the case of huge chest wall primary tumors, patients may present with respiratory distress. Patients with paraspinal or vertebral primary tumors may present with symptoms of cord compression. Ewing sarcoma is often associated with systemic manifestations such as fever or weight loss; patients may have undergone treatment for a presumptive diagnosis of osteomyelitis. Patients may also have a delay in diagnosis when their pain or swelling is attributed to a sports injury.

Diagnosis. The diagnosis of Ewing sarcoma should be suspected in a patient who presents with pain and swelling, with or without systemic symptoms, and with a radiographic appearance of a primarily lytic bone lesion with periosteal reaction, the characteristic **onion-skinning** (Fig. 493–3). A large associated soft tissue mass is often visualized on MRI or CT (Fig. 493–4). The differential diagnosis includes osteosarcoma, osteomyelitis, Langerhans cell histiocytosis, primary lymphoma of bone, metastatic neuroblastoma, or rhabdomyosarcoma in the case of a pure soft tissue lesion. Patients should be referred to a center with experience in managing bone tumors for evaluation and biopsy. Thorough evaluation for metastatic disease includes CT of the chest, radionuclide bone scan, and bone marrow aspirate and biopsy specimens from at least two sites. MRI of the tumor and the entire length of involved bone should be performed to determine the exact extension of the soft tissue and bony mass and the proximity of tumor to neurovascular structures. Biopsy should be performed preferably by the surgeon who will perform the ultimate surgical procedure to avoid compromising an ultimate potential for limb salvage by a poorly planned biopsy incision. CT-guided biopsy of the lesion often provides diagnostic tissue. It is important to obtain adequate tissue for special stains, cytogenetics, and molecular studies.

Treatment. Ewing sarcoma family of tumors are best managed with a comprehensive multidisciplinary approach incorporating the surgeon, chemotherapist, and radiation oncologist in planning therapy. Multiagent chemotherapy is important because it can rapidly shrink the tumor and is generally given before attempting local control. The addition of ifosfamide and etoposide to the standard agents of vincristine, doxorubicin, and cyclophosphamide improves the outcome of nonmetastatic Ewing sarcoma. Chemotherapy usually causes dramatic shrinkage of the soft tissue mass and rapid significant pain relief. Recent randomized studies of chemotherapy in Ewing sarcoma are evaluating the role of dose intensity in treatment. Ewing sarcoma is considered a radiosensitive tumor, and local control may be achieved with radiation or surgery. Radiation therapy is associated with a risk of radiation-induced second malignancies, especially osteosarcoma, as well as failure of bone growth in skeletally immature patients. Many centers prefer surgical resection if possible to achieve local control. It is important to

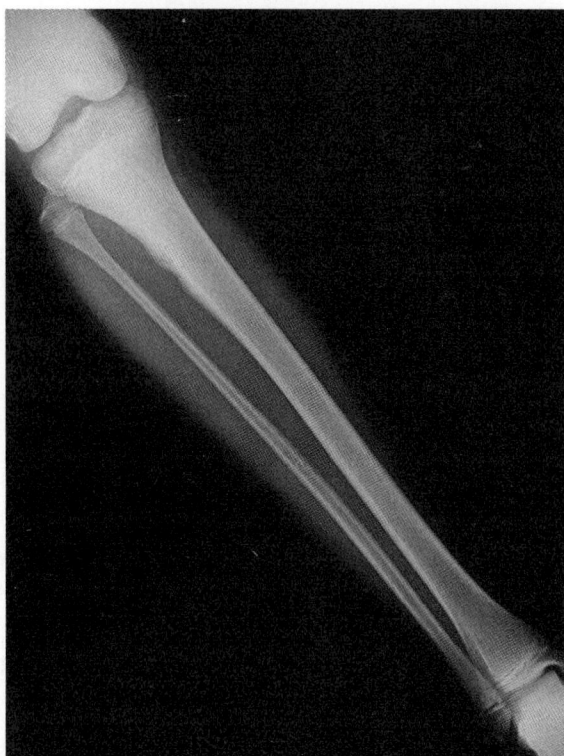

FIGURE 493–3. Radiograph of tibial Ewing sarcoma showing periosteal elevation or "onion-skinning."

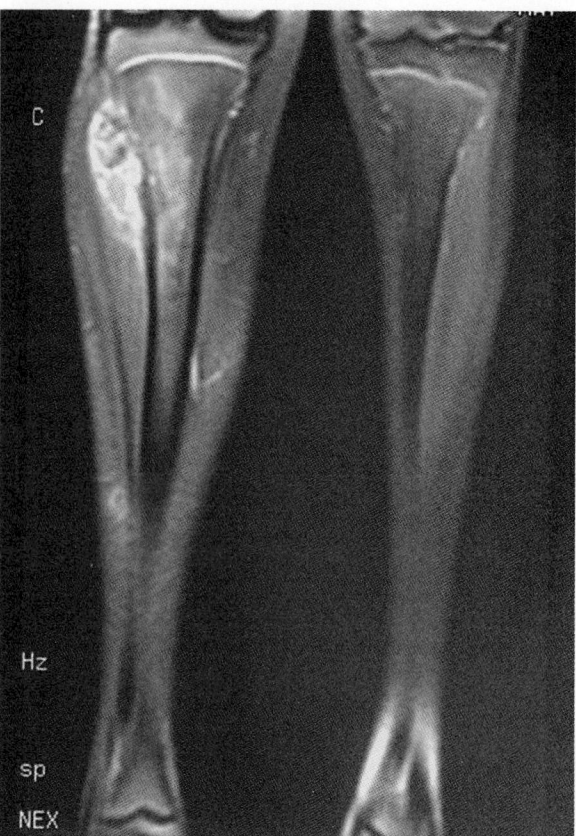

FIGURE 493–4. Magnetic resonance image (MRI) of tibial Ewing sarcoma showing a large associated soft tissue mass.

provide patients with crutches if the tumor is in a weight-bearing bone to avoid a pathologic fracture before definitive local control. Chemotherapy should be resumed as soon as possible after surgery.

Prognosis. Patients with small, nonmetastatic, distally located extremity tumors have the best prognosis. Such patients enjoy up to a 75% cure rate. The type of chromosomal translocation may be related to prognosis. Patients with pelvic tumors have, until recently, had a much worse outcome. Patients with metastatic disease at diagnosis, especially bone or bone marrow metastases, have a poor prognosis, with fewer than 30% surviving long term. New approaches, such as very intensive chemotherapy with peripheral blood stem cell rescue, are being investigated in these patients.

Long-term follow-up of patients with Ewing sarcoma is important because of the potential for late effects of treatment such as anthracycline cardiotoxicity, second malignancies, especially in the radiation field, and late relapses even 10 yr after initial diagnosis.

493.2 Benign Tumors and Tumor-like Processes of Bone

Benign bone lesions in children are common in comparison with the relatively rare malignant neoplasms of bone and present diagnostic challenges (see Table 493–1). Some, although histologically benign, can be life threatening. No single history element or diagnostic test is sufficient to rule out malignancies or suggest non-neoplastic conditions. A broad range of diagnostic possibilities must be considered when confronted with an unknown bone lesion. Benign lesions may be painless or painful, especially if a pathologic fracture is impending. Night pain that awakens a child is suggestive of malignancy; relief of such pain with aspirin is common with benign lesions such as

osteoid osteomas. Rapidly enlarging lesions are usually associated with malignancy, but several benign lesions, such as aneurysmal bone cysts, may enlarge faster than most malignancies. Several conditions, such as osteomyelitis, may simulate the appearance of benign bone tumors.

Many benign bone tumors are diagnosed incidentally or after pathologic fracture. Management of these fractures is similar to that of nonpathologic fractures in the same location. It is unusual for benign bone tumors to interfere with fracture healing. Likewise, the fractures rarely result in changes or healing of these tumors, which are usually treated after the fracture has healed.

Radiographs of any suspected bone lesion should always be obtained in two planes. Additional studies may be necessary to help arrive at the correct diagnosis and to guide treatment. Despite the benign nature of these lesions, many require intervention.

Osteochondroma (exostosis) is one of the most common benign bone tumors in children. Many are completely asymptomatic and unrecognized. The true incidence of this lesion is therefore unknown. Most osteochondromas develop in childhood, arising from the metaphysis of long bones, particularly the distal femur, proximal humerus, and proximal tibia. The lesion enlarges with the child until skeletal maturity. Most are discovered from 5–15 yr of age when the child or parent notices a bony, nonpainful mass. Some are discovered when irritated by pressure during athletic or other activities. Osteochondromas appear radiographically as stalks or broad-based projections from the surface of the bone, usually in a direction away from the adjacent joint. Invariably, the lesion is radiographically smaller than suggested by palpation because the cartilage "cap" covering the lesion is not seen. This cartilage cap may be up to 1 cm thick. Both the cortex of the bone and the marrow space of the involved bone are continuous with the lesion. Malignant degeneration to a chondrosarcoma is rare in children but may occur in as many as 1% of adults. Routine removal is not performed unless the lesion is large enough to cause symptoms or if rapid growth occurs. **Multiple hereditary exostoses** is a related but rare condition characterized by the presence of multiple osteochondromas. Severely involved children may have short stature, limb-length inequality, premature partial physeal arrests, and deformity of both the upper and lower extremities. These individuals need to be monitored carefully during growth.

Enchondroma is a benign lesion of hyaline cartilage occurring centrally in the bone. The majority are asymptomatic and occur in the hands. Most are discovered incidentally, although pathologic fractures often lead to the diagnosis. Radiographically, the lesions occupy the medullary canal, are radiolucent, and are sharply marginated. Punctate or stippled calcification may be present within the lesion, but this is much more common in adults than children. The vast majority of enchondromas are solitary. Most can be observed, with curettage and bone grafting reserved for those lesions that are symptomatic or large enough to weaken the bone structurally. Multifocal involvement is referred to as **Ollier disease** and may result in bony dysplasia, short stature, limb-length inequality, and joint deformity. Surgery may be necessary to correct or prevent such deformities. When multiple enchondromas are associated with angiomas of the soft tissue, the condition is referred to as **Maffucci syndrome**. A high rate of malignant transformation has been reported in both of these multifocal conditions.

Chondroblastoma is a rare lesion usually found in the epiphysis of long bones. Most patients present in the 2nd decade with complaints of mild to moderate pain in the adjacent joint. Common sites include the hip, shoulder, and knee. Muscle atrophy and local tenderness may be the only clinical findings. The lesion appears radiographically as a sharply marginated radiolucency within the epiphysis or apophysis, occasionally with metaphyseal extension across the physis. Proximity to the joint may cause deformity of the subchondral bone, an effusion, or erosion into the joint. Recognition is important because most lesions can be cured with curettage and bone grafting before joint destruction occurs.

Chondromyxoid fibroma is an uncommon benign bone tumor in children. This metaphyseal lesion usually causes pain and local tenderness. The lesion may occasionally be asymptomatic. Chondromyxoid fibroma appears radiographically as an eccentric, lobular, metaphyseal radiolucency with sharp, sclerotic, and scalloped margins. The lower extremity is most often involved. Treatment usually consists of curettage and bone grafting or en bloc resection.

Osteoid osteoma is a small benign bone tumor; most of these tumors are diagnosed between 5–20 yr of age. The clinical pattern is characteristic, consisting of unremitting and gradually increasing pain that is often worst at night and relieved by aspirin. Males are affected more often than females. Any bone can be involved, but the most common sites are the proximal femur and tibia. Vertebral lesions may cause scoliosis or symptoms that mimic a neurologic disorder. Examination may reveal a limp, atrophy, and weakness when the lower extremity is involved. Palpation and range of motion do not alter the discomfort. Radiographs are distinctive, showing a round or oval metaphyseal or diaphyseal lucency (0.5–1.0 cm diameter) surrounded by sclerotic bone. The central lucency, or nidus, shows intense uptake on bone scan. About 25% of osteoid osteomas are not visualized on plain radiographs but can be identified with CT. Because of the small size of the lesion and the location adjacent to thick cortical bone, MRI is poor at detecting osteoid osteomas. Treatment is directed at removing the lesion. This may involve en bloc excision, curettage, or percutaneous CT-guided ablation of the nidus. Patients with mild pain may be treated with salicylates. Some lesions spontaneously resolve after skeletal maturity.

Osteoblastoma is a locally destructive, progressively growing lesion of bone with a predilection for the vertebrae, although almost any bone may be involved. Most patients note the insidious onset of dull aching pain, which may be present for months before they seek medical attention. Spinal lesions may cause neurologic symptoms or deficits. The radiographic appearance is variable and less distinctive than that of other benign bone tumors. About 25% show features suggesting a malignant neoplasm, making biopsy necessary in many cases. Expansile spinal lesions often involve the posterior elements. Treatment involves curettage and bone grafting or en bloc excision, taking care to preserve nerve roots when treating spinal lesions. Surgical stabilization of the spine may be necessary.

Fibromas (nonossifying fibroma, fibrous cortical defect, metaphyseal fibrous defect) are fibrous lesions of bone that occur in 40% of children older than 2 yr of age. They likely represent a defect in ossification rather than a neoplasm. As such, these lesions are usually asymptomatic. Most are discovered incidentally when radiographs are taken for other reasons, usually to rule out a fracture after trauma. Occasional pathologic fractures can occur through rare large lesions. Physical examination is usually unrevealing. Radiographs show a sharply marginated eccentric lucency in the metaphyseal cortex. Lesions may be multilocular and expansile, with extension from the cortex into the medullary bone. The long axis of the lesion is parallel with that of the bone. Approximately 50% are bilateral or multiple. Because of the characteristic radiographic appearance, most lesions do not require biopsy or treatment. Spontaneous regression can be expected after skeletal maturity. Curettage and bone grafting may be recommended for lesions occupying more than 50% of the bone diameter because of the risk of a pathologic fracture.

Unicameral bone cysts can occur at any age in childhood but are rare before 3 yr of age and after skeletal maturity. The cause of these fluid-filled lesions is unknown. Some resolve spontaneously after skeletal maturity. Most are asymptomatic until diagnosis, which usually follows a pathologic fracture. Such fractures may occur with relatively minor trauma, such as with throwing or catching a ball. Unicameral bone cysts appear radiographically as solitary, centrally located lesions within the medullary portion of the bone. These cysts are most common in the proximal humerus or femur. They often extend to (but not through) the physis and are sharply marginated. Thinning and expansion of the cortex occurs but does not exceed the width of the adjacent physis. Treatment involves allowing the pathologic fracture to heal, followed by aspiration and injection with methylprednisolone or bone marrow. Repeat injections, curettage, and bone grafting are occasionally necessary to treat recurrent lesions.

Aneurysmal bone cyst is a reactive lesion of bone seen during the 1st and 2nd decades of life. The lesion is characterized by cavernous spaces filled with blood and solid aggregates of tissue. Although the femur, tibia, and spine are most commonly involved, this progressively growing, expansile lesion develops in any bone. Pain and swelling are common. Spinal involvement may lead to cord or nerve root compression and associated neurologic symptoms, including paralysis. Radiographs show eccentric lytic destruction and expansion of the metaphysis surrounded by a thin sclerotic rim of bone. Posterior elements of the spine are more commonly involved than the vertebral body. Unlike most other benign bone tumors, which are usually confined to a single bone, aneurysmal bone cysts may involve adjacent vertebrae. Rapid growth is characteristic and may lead to confusion with malignant neoplasms. Treatment consists of curettage and bone grafting or excision. Spinal lesions may require stabilization after excision. As with other benign tumors, attempts are made to preserve nerve roots and other vital structures. Recurrence after surgical treatment occurs in 20–30%, is more common in younger than older children, and usually occurs in the first 1–2 yr after treatment.

Fibrous dysplasia is a developmental abnormality characterized by fibrous replacement of cancellous bone. Lesions may be solitary or multifocal (polyostotic), relatively stable, or progressively more severe. Most children are asymptomatic, although those with skull involvement may have swelling or exophthalmos. Pain and limp are characteristic of proximal femoral involvement. Limb-length discrepancy, bowing of the tibia or femur, and pathologic fractures may be presenting complaints. The triad of polyostotic disease, precocious puberty, and cutaneous pigmentation is known as **Albright syndrome.** Radiographic features of fibrous dysplasia include a lytic or ground-glass expansile lesion of the metaphysis or diaphysis. The lesion is sharply marginated and often surrounded by a thick rim of sclerotic bone. Bowing, especially of the proximal femur, may be present. Treatment usually involves observation. Surgery is indicated for patients with progressive deformity, pain, or impending pathologic fractures. Bone grafting is not as successful in the treatment of fibrous dysplasia as with other benign tumors because the lesion often recurs within the grafted bone. Reconstructive surgical techniques are often necessary to provide stability.

Osteofibrous dysplasia is a lesion that affects children 1–10 yr old. This lesion usually involves the tibia. It is clinically, radiographically, and histologically distinct from fibrous dysplasia. Most children present with anterior swelling or enlargement of the leg, and most have no pain unless there is an associated pathologic fracture. Progression is unlikely after 10 yr of age. Radiographs show solitary or multiple lucent, cortical, diaphyseal lesions surrounded by sclerosis. Anterior bowing of the tibia is often present. The radiographic appearance closely resembles that of adamantinoma, a malignant neoplasm, making biopsy more common than with other benign bone tumors. Treatment involves observation. Some lesions heal spontaneously. Excision and bone grafting should be delayed after age 10 yr because of a high recurrence rate after this age. Pathologic fractures heal with immobilization.

Eosinophilic granuloma is a monostotic or polyostotic disease with no extraskeletal involvement. This latter finding distinguishes eosinophilic granuloma from the other forms of Langerhans cell histiocytosis (Hand-Schüller-Christian or Letterer-Siwe variants), which may have a less favorable prognosis (see Chapter 499). Eosinophilic granuloma usually occurs during the first 3 decades of life and is most common in boys 5–10 yr of age. The skull is most commonly affected, but any bone may be involved. Patients usually present with local pain and swelling. There is often marked tenderness and warmth in the area of the involved bone. Spinal lesions may cause pain, stiffness, and occasional neurologic symptoms. The radiographic appearance of the skeletal lesions is similar in all forms of Langerhans cell histiocytosis but is variable enough to mimic many other benign and malignant lesions of bone. The radiolucent lesions have well-defined or irregular margins with expansion of the involved bone and periosteal new bone formation. Spine involvement may cause uniform compression or flattening of the vertebral body. A skeletal survey is warranted because polyostotic involvement and the typical skull lesions strongly suggest the diagnosis of eosinophilic granuloma. Biopsy is often necessary to confirm the diagnosis because of the broad radiographic differential diagnosis. Treatment includes curettage and bone grafting, low-dose radiation therapy, or steroid injection. Observation for symptomatic lesions is reasonable because most osseous lesions heal spontaneously and do not recur. Children with bone lesions should be evaluated for visceral involvement because treatment of Hand-Schüller-Christian disease and Letterer-Siwe disease is more complex and often systemic.

Arndt CAS, Crist WM: Common musculoskeletal tumors of childhood and adolescence. *N Engl J Med* 1999;341:342–52.

Campanacci M, Capanna R, Picci P: Unicameral and aneurysmal bone cysts. *Clin Orthop* 1986;204:25–36.

Campanacci M, Laus M: Osteofibrous dysplasia of the tibia and fibula. *J Bone Joint Surg Am* 1981;63:367–75.

Dahlin DC, Ivins JC: Benign chondroblastoma: A study of 125 cases. *Cancer* 1972;30:401–13.

De Alava E, Gerald WL: Molecular biology of the Ewing's sarcoma/primitive neuroectodermal tumor family. *J Clin Oncol* 2000;18:204–13.

Ferguson WS, Goorin AM: Current treatment of osteosarcoma. *Cancer Invest* 2001;19:292–315.

Freiberg AA, Loder RT, Heidelberger KT: Aneurysmal bone cysts in young children. *J Pediatr Orthop* 1994;14:86–91.

Ginsberg JP, Woo SY, Johnson ME, et al: Ewing's sarcoma family of tumors. In Pizzo PA, Poplack DG (editors): *Principles and Practice of Pediatric Oncology,* 4th ed. Philadelphia, Lippincott Williams & Wilkins, 2002, pp 973–1016.

Kneisl JS, Simon MA: Medical management compared with operative treatment for osteoid osteoma. *J Bone Joint Surg Am* 1992;74:179–85.

Schmale GA, Conrad EU III, Raskind WH: The natural history of hereditary multiple exostoses. *J Bone Joint Surg Am* 1994;76:986–92.

Chapter 494

Retinoblastoma *Cynthia E. Herzog*

Epidemiology. Retinoblastoma occurs at a rate of 3.7 cases/million in the United States, with no racial or gender predilection. Overall, about 60% of cases are unilateral and nonhereditary, 15% unilateral and hereditary, and 25% bilateral and hereditary. Bilateral involvement is found in 42% of those presenting when younger than 1 yr of age but in only 21% of those presenting during 1 yr of age and is even less common at older ages of presentation.

The hereditary form is associated with a germline defect in the retinoblastoma gene *(RB1)* located on the long arm of chromosome 13. *RB1* encodes a tumor suppressor protein. Familial cases are generally multifocal and bilateral, whereas nonfamilial cases tend to have unilateral, unifocal involvement. According to the "two-hit" model, two mutational events are required for tumor development. In the heritable form, one mutated *RB* gene is inherited through the germ line and a second mutation occurs subsequently in the somatic retinal cell. In the noninherited form, both mutations occur in retinal cells.

Pathogenesis. The histology of retinoblastoma is a small, round, blue cell tumor with rosette formation. It may arise in any of the nucleated layers of the retina and exhibits various degrees of differentiation; it tends to outgrow its blood supply, resulting in necrosis and calcification.

Endophytic tumors arise from the inner surface of the retina, grow into the vitreous, and tend to seed to other areas of the retina. **Exophytic tumors** grow from the outer retinal layer and may produce retinal detachment. Hematogenous or lymphatic spread to more distant sites can occur with extension to the choroid or along the optic nerve beyond the lamina cribrosa.

Clinical Manifestations. Only about 10% of retinoblastomas are detected by routine ophthalmologic screening in the context of a positive family history. Retinoblastoma classically presents with **leukocoria,** a white pupillary reflex (Fig. 494–1). This abnormality is often first noticed when a red reflex is not present at routine newborn or well-child examination or in a flash photograph of the child. Strabismus is commonly the initial presenting complaint. Orbital inflammation, hyphema, or pupil irregularity occurs with advancing disease. Pain is usually a feature if secondary glaucoma is present.

Diagnosis. The diagnosis does not require a biopsy but is established by characteristic ophthalmologic findings. Evaluation generally requires an examination under general anesthesia by

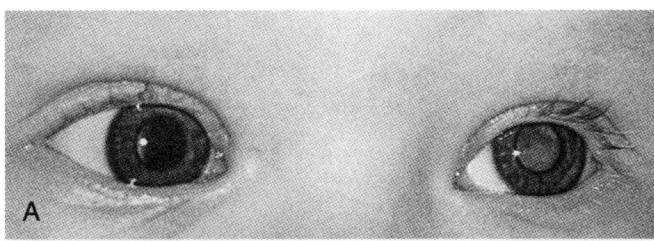

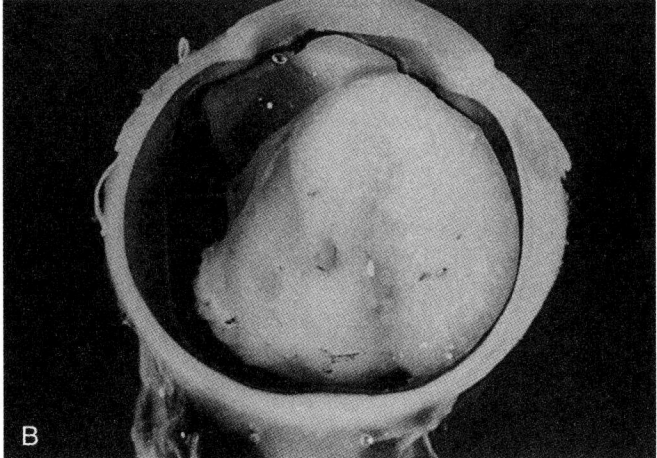

FIGURE 494–1. *A,* Leukocoria noted in the left eye of a child presenting with retinoblastoma. *B,* A large white tumor mass noted within the posterior chamber of the enucleated eye. (From Shields JA, Shields CL: Current management of retinoblastoma. *Mayo Clin Proc* 1994;69:50–6.)

an ophthalmologist to obtain a complete visualization of both eyes, which also facilitates photographing and mapping of the tumors. Retinal detachment or vitreous hemorrhage can complicate the evaluation.

Orbital ultrasonography and CT or MRI are used to evaluate the extent of intraocular disease and extraocular spread. Occasionally, a pineal area tumor will be detected, a phenomenon known as **trilateral retinoblastoma.** MRI allows for better evaluation of optic nerve involvement. Bone scan, cerebrospinal fluid evaluation, and bone marrow evaluation are necessary only if indicated by other clinical, laboratory, or imaging studies.

The differential diagnosis includes hyperplastic primary vitreous, Coats disease, cataract, visceral larva migrans, choroidal coloboma, and retinopathy of prematurity.

Treatment. The treatment is determined by the size and location of the tumor, with the primary goal being cure and a secondary goal of preserving vision. As newer modalities for local control of intraocular tumor and more effective systemic chemotherapy have been developed, primary enucleation is less frequently undertaken routinely.

Most unilateral disease presents as a large tumor. Enucleation is undertaken if there is no potential for useful vision. In bilateral disease the traditional approach involves enucleation of the more severely affected eye and irradiation of the remaining eye in hope of salvaging some useful vision. With the availability of effective chemotherapy, an attempt can be made to salvage both eyes with some degree of functional vision. If feasible, small tumors can be treated with laser photocoagulation or cryotherapy with careful follow-up for evidence of recurrence or new tumor growth. Larger tumors often respond to multiagent chemotherapy, including carboplatin, vincristine, and etoposide, thus facilitating successful focal therapy. If this approach fails, external-beam irradiation or brachytherapy should be con-

sidered, although this approach may result in significant orbital deformity and increased incidence of second malignancies in patients with germ line mutations. Enucleation may be required for nonresponsive or recurrent tumors.

Prognosis. Close to 95% of retinoblastomas are cured in the United States, where extraocular extension is rarely seen. Current efforts using chemotherapy in combination with local therapy are focused on trying to preserve useful vision and avoidance of irradiation or enucleation. Routine ophthalmologic examinations should continue until about 6 yr of age to detect new lesions. The prognosis for patients with metastases is poor.

Children with germ line *RB1* mutations are at significant risk for development of second malignancies, primarily osteosarcoma. This risk is further increased by the use of radiation therapy. Other radiation-related complications include cataracts, orbital growth deformities, lacrimal dysfunction, and late retinal vascular injury.

DiCiommo D, Gallie BL, Bremner R: Retinoblastoma: The disease, gene and protein provide critical leads to understand cancer. *Semin Cancer Biol* 2000;10:255–69.
Finger PT, Czechonska G, Demirci H, et al: Chemotherapy for retinoblastoma: A current topic. *Drugs* 1999;58:983–96.
Friedman DL, Himelstein B, Shields CL, et al: Chemoreduction and local ophthalmic therapy for intraocular retinoblastoma. *J Clin Oncol* 2000;18:12–7.

Chapter 495
Gonadal and Germ Cell Neoplasms

Cynthia E. Herzog

Epidemiology. Malignant germ cell tumors (GCTs) and gonadal tumors occur with an incidence of 12 cases/million in persons younger than 20 yr of age. Most malignant tumors of the gonads in children are GCTs. The incidence varies according to age and sex of the patient. Sacrococcygeal tumors occur predominantly in female infants. Testicular GCTs occur predominantly before age 4 yr and after puberty. Testicular GCTs occur with much greater frequency in whites than in blacks, whereas ovarian tumors have a slight predominance in blacks. Undescended testes are associated with an increased risk of testicular cancer.

Pathogenesis. The GCTs and non-GCTs arise from primordial germ cells and coelomic epithelium, respectively. GCTs may contain benign and malignant elements in different areas of the tumor; extensive sectioning is essential to make the correct diagnosis. There are many histologically distinct subtypes of GCTs, including teratomas (mature and immature), endodermal sinus tumor, and embryonal carcinoma (Fig. 495–1). Non-GCTs of the ovary include epithelial (serous and mucinous) and sex cord/stromal tumors; testicular tumors include sex cord/stromal tumors (e.g., Leydig cell, Sertoli cell).

Clinical Manifestations and Diagnosis. The clinical presentation of germ cell neoplasms depends on location. Ovarian tumors are often quite large before diagnosis. Extragonadal GCTs occur in the midline, including the suprasellar region, pineal region, neck, mediastinum, and retroperitoneal and sacrococcygeal areas. Symptoms relate to mass effect, but the intracranial GCTs often present with anterior and posterior pituitary deficits.

α-Fetoprotein (AFP) level is elevated in endodermal sinus tumors and may have minimally elevated levels in teratomas. Infants have elevated levels of AFP that reach adult normal by about 8 mo; therefore, high AFP levels must be interpreted with

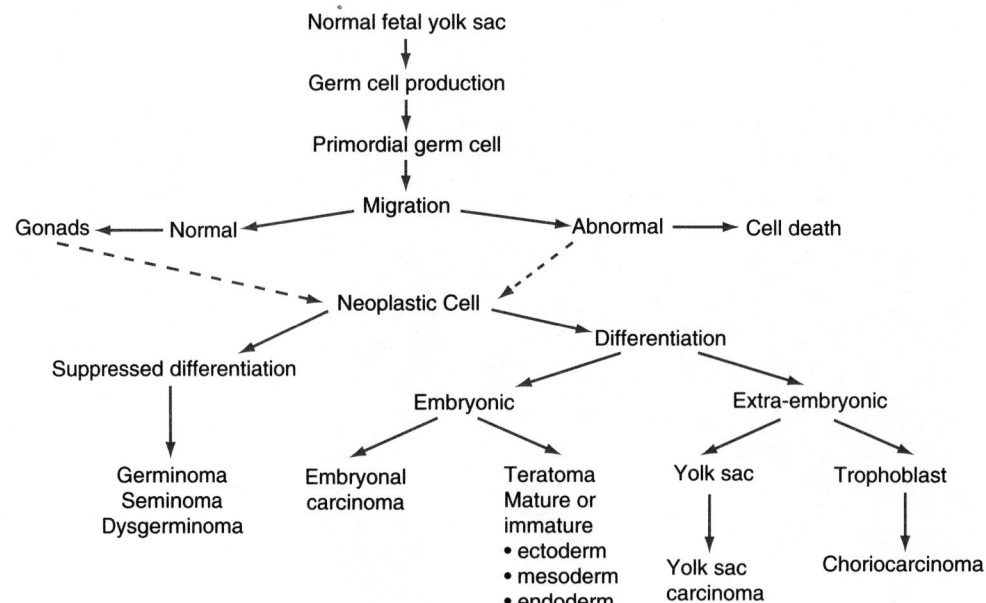

FIGURE 495–1. Tumors of germ cell origin. (Adapted from Pierce GB, Abell MR: Embryonal carcinoma of the testis. *Pathol Annu* 1970;5:27–60.)

caution in this age group. Elevation of the β subunit of human chorionic gonadotropin (β-hCG) is seen in choriocarcinoma and germinomas. Lactate dehydrogenase (LDH), although nonspecific, is sometimes a useful marker. If elevated, these markers provide important confirmation of the diagnosis and serve as a means to monitor the patient for tumor response and recurrence. Both serum and cerebrospinal fluid should be assayed for these markers in the case of intracranial lesions.

Diagnosis begins with physical examination and imaging studies, including plain radiographs of the chest and ultrasonography of the abdomen. CT or MRI can further delineate the primary tumor. If germ cell malignancy is strongly suggested, preoperative staging with CT of the chest and bone scan is appropriate. Primary surgical resection is indicated for tumors deemed resectable. The exception is intracranial lesions; in this site, the diagnosis can be made with imaging and AFP or β-hCG determinations. For intracranial lesions, primary therapy comprises irradiation and chemotherapy.

Gonadoblastoma frequently occurs in patients with gonadal dysgenesis and a Y chromosome. This syndrome is characterized by failure to fully masculinize the external genitalia. If this syndrome is diagnosed, imaging with ultrasonography or CT of the gonad is performed, and surgical resection of the tumor is generally curative. Prophylactic resection of dysgenetic gonads at the time of diagnosis is recommended because gonadoblastomas, some of which contain malignant germ cell tumor elements, frequently develop. Gonadoblastomas may produce abnormal amounts of estrogen.

Teratomas occur in many locations, presenting as masses. They are not associated with elevated markers unless malignancy is present. The sacrococcygeal region is the most frequent tumor site of teratomas. Sacrococcygeal teratomas occur most commonly in infants and may be diagnosed in utero, or at birth, with the majority arising in females. The frequency of malignancy in this location varies from less than 10% when younger than 2 mo of age to more than 50% when older than 4 mo of age.

Germinomas occur intracranially, in the mediastinum, and in the gonads. In the ovary, they are called **dysgerminomas;** in the testis, **seminomas.** They are usually tumor marker negative despite being malignant. **Endodermal sinus or yolk sac tumor** and **choriocarcinoma** appear highly malignant by his-

tologic criteria. Both occur at gonadal and extragonadal sites. **Embryonal carcinoma** most often occurs in the testes.

Non–germ cell gonadal tumors are very uncommon in pediatrics and occur predominantly in the ovary. **Epithelial carcinomas** (usually an adult tumor), **Sertoli-Leydig cell tumors,** and **granulosa cell tumors** may occur in children. Both of the latter tumors produce hormones that can cause virilization or feminization or precocious puberty, depending on pubertal stage and the balance between Sertoli (estrogen production) and Leydig cells (androgen production). Diagnostic evaluation usually focuses on the chief complaint of inappropriate sex steroid effect and includes hormone measurements, which reflect gonadotropin-independent sex steroid production. Appropriate imaging, to rule out a functioning gonadal tumor, is also performed. Surgery is usually curative. Effective therapy for nonresectable disease has not been found.

Treatment. Complete surgical excision of the tumor is generally indicated, except for patients with central nervous system (CNS) primary tumors. For testicular tumors, an inguinal approach is indicated. When complete excision cannot be accomplished, preoperative chemotherapy is indicated, with second-look surgery. For teratomas, both mature and immature, and completely resected malignant tumors, surgery alone is the treatment. Cisplatin-based chemotherapy regimens are generally curative in GCTs that cannot be completely resected, even if metastases are present. Except for GCTs of the CNS, irradiation is limited to those tumors that are not amenable to complete excision and are refractory to chemotherapy.

Prognosis. The overall cure rate for children with GCTs is more than 80%. There is little impact of histology or site on prognosis, although nonresected extragonadal GCTs have a slightly worse prognosis.

Gobel U, Schneider DT, Calaminus G, et al: Germ-cell tumors in childhood and adolescence. GPOH MAKEI and the MAHO study groups. *Ann Oncol* 2000;11:263–71.

Mann JR, Raafat F, Robinson K, et al: The United Kingdom Children's Cancer Study Group's second germ cell tumor study: Carboplatin, etoposide, and bleomycin are effective treatment for children with malignant extracranial germ cell tumors, with acceptable toxicity. *J Clin Oncol* 2000;18:3809–18.

Rescorla FJ: Pediatric germ cell tumors. *Semin Surg Oncol* 1999;16:144–58.

Neoplasms of the Liver

Cynthia E. Herzog

Hepatic tumors are rare in children. Primary tumors of the liver account for approximately 1% of malignancies in children, with an annual incidence of 1.6 cases/million children in the United States. From 50–60% of hepatic tumors in children are malignant, with more than 65% of these malignancies being hepatoblastomas and most of the remainder hepatocellular carcinomas. Rare hepatic malignancies include angiosarcoma, malignant germ cell tumor, rhabdomyosarcoma of the liver, and undifferentiated sarcoma. More common childhood malignancies such as neuroblastoma and lymphoma can metastasize to the liver. Benign liver tumors, which usually present within the first 6 mo of life, include hemangiomas, hamartomas, and hemangioendotheliomas.

HEPATOBLASTOMA

Epidemiology. Hepatoblastoma occurs predominantly in children younger than 3 yr of age. The etiology is unknown. Hepatoblastomas are associated with familial adenomatous polyposis; alterations in the antigen-presenting cell (APC)/β-catenin pathway have been found in a majority of tumors evaluated. Hepatoblastoma is also associated with Beckwith-Wiedemann syndrome, which can show a similar loss of genomic imprinting of the insulin-like growth factor-2 gene. Low birthweight is associated with increased incidence of hepatoblastoma, with the risk increasing as birthweight decreases.

Pathogenesis. Hepatoblastoma can be epithelial type, containing fetal or embryonal malignant cells (either as a mixture or as pure elements), or the mixed type, containing mesenchymal and epithelial elements. Pure fetal histology predicts a more favorable outcome.

Clinical Manifestations. Hepatoblastoma generally presents as a large, asymptomatic abdominal mass. It arises from the right lobe three times more often than the left and is usually unifocal. As the disease progresses, weight loss, anorexia, vomiting, and abdominal pain may ensue. Metastatic spread of hepatoblastoma most commonly involves regional lymph nodes and the lungs.

A valuable serum tumor marker, α-fetoprotein (AFP), is used in the diagnosis and monitoring of hepatic tumors. AFP level is elevated in almost all hepatoblastomas. Bilirubin and liver enzymes are usually normal. Anemia is common, and thrombocytosis occurs in about a third of patients. Hepatitis B and C serology should be obtained but are usually negative in hepatoblastoma.

Diagnostic imaging should include plain radiographs and ultrasonography of the abdomen to characterize the hepatic mass. Ultrasonography can differentiate malignant hepatic masses from benign vascular lesions. Either CT or MRI is an accurate method of defining the extent of intrahepatic tumor involvement and the potential for surgical resection. Evaluation for metastatic disease should include CT of the chest and bone scan.

Treatment. In general, the cure of malignant hepatic tumors in children depends on complete resection of the primary tumor. As much as 85% of the liver can be resected, with hepatic regeneration noted within 3–4 mo after surgery. Cisplatin in combination with vincristine and 5-fluorouracil or doxorubicin is effective treatment for hepatoblastoma and increases the chances of cure after complete surgical resection. In low-stage tumors, survival rates more than 90% can be achieved with multimodal treatment, including surgery and adjuvant chemotherapy. With tumors unresectable at diagnosis, survival rates of approximately 60% can be obtained. Metastatic disease further reduces survival, but complete regression of disease can often be obtained with chemotherapy and surgical resection of the primary tumor and isolated pulmonary metastatic disease, resulting in survival rates of about 25%.

HEPATOCELLULAR CARCINOMA

Epidemiology. Hepatocellular carcinoma occurs mostly in adolescents and is often associated with hepatitis B or C infection. It is more common in East Asia and other areas where hepatitis B is endemic. In these areas it also tends to occur in a bimodal pattern, with the younger age peak overlapping the age of hepatoblastoma presentation. It also occurs in the chronic form of hereditary tyrosinemia, glycogen storage disease, α₁-antitrypsin deficiency, and biliary cirrhosis.

Pathogenesis. Hepatocellular carcinoma generally presents as a multicentric, invasive tumor consisting of large pleomorphic cells with a lack of underlying cirrhosis. The fibrolamellar variant of hepatocellular carcinoma has a somewhat better prognosis.

Clinical Manifestations. Hepatocellular carcinoma generally presents as a hepatic mass, abdominal distention, and symptoms of anorexia, weight loss, and abdominal pain. Hepatocellular carcinoma can present as an acute abdominal crisis with rupture of the tumor and hemoperitoneum. AFP level is elevated in approximately 60% of children with hepatocellular carcinoma. Evidence of hepatitis B and C infection is usually found in areas where it is endemic, but not in Western countries or with the fibrolamellar type. Bilirubin is usually normal, but liver enzymes may be abnormal.

Diagnostic imaging should include plain radiographs and ultrasonography of the abdomen to characterize the hepatic mass. Ultrasonography can differentiate malignant hepatic masses from benign vascular lesions. Either CT or MRI is an accurate method of defining the extent of intrahepatic tumor involvement and the potential for surgical resection. Evaluation for metastatic disease should include CT of the chest and bone scan.

Treatment. Because of the multicentric origin of hepatocellular carcinoma, complete resection of this tumor is accomplished in only 30–40% of cases. Even with complete surgical resection, only 30% of children are long-term survivors. Chemotherapy, including cisplatin, doxorubicin, etoposide, and 5-fluorouracil, has shown some activity against this tumor, but improved long-term outcome has been difficult to achieve. Other techniques such as chemoembolization and liver transplantation are under study as therapy for hepatocellular carcinomas.

Herzog CE, Andrassy RJ, Eftekhari F: Childhood cancers: Hepatoblastoma. *Oncologist* 2000;5:445–53.

Ortega JA, Douglass EC, Feusner JH, et al: Randomized comparison of cisplatin/vincristine/fluorouracil and cisplatin/continuous infusion doxorubicin for treatment of pediatric hepatoblastoma: A report from the Children's Cancer Group and the Pediatric Oncology Group. *J Clin Oncol* 2000;18:2665–75.

Pritchard J, Brown J, Shafford E, et al: Cisplatin, doxorubicin, and delayed surgery for childhood hepatoblastoma: A successful approach: Results of the first prospective study of the International Society of Pediatric Oncology. *J Clin Oncol* 2000;18:3819–28.

Stocker JT: Hepatic tumors in children. *Clin Liver Dis* 2001;5:259–81.

Stringer MD: Liver tumors. *Semin Pediatr Surg* 2000;9:196–208.

Chapter 497

Benign Vascular Tumors

Cynthia E. Herzog

HEMANGIOMAS

Hemangiomas are the most common benign tumors of infancy and occur in about 10% of term infants. The risk of hemangioma is 3 times higher in females than males. The risk is doubled in premature infants and 10 times higher in offspring of women who had chorionic villus sampling. Although hemangiomas can be present at birth, they usually arise shortly after birth and grow rapidly during the first year of life, with slowing of growth in the next 5 yr and involution by 10–15 yr of age.

Clinical Manifestations. More than half of these tumors are located in the head and neck region. The majority are solitary lesions, but the presence of more than one cutaneous lesion increases the likelihood of visceral hemangiomas. The liver is the primary site of visceral involvement; other involved organs include the brain, intestines, and lung. Most hemangiomas require no therapy, but approximately 10% of hemangiomas cause significant impairment and 1% are life threatening because of their location. Hemangiomas around the airway can cause airway obstruction, and those around the eyes can result in loss of vision. Ulceration is a frequent complication and can lead to secondary infection. Large hepatic hemangiomas or hemangioendotheliomas may result in hepatomegaly, anemia, thrombocytopenia, and high-output heart failure.

Kasabach-Merritt syndrome is characterized by rapidly enlarging lesion, thrombocytopenia, microangiopathic hemolytic anemia, and coagulopathy as a result of platelet and red blood cell trapping and activation of the clotting system within the vasculature of the hemangioma. This syndrome has now been shown to be associated with kaposiform hemangioendotheliomas or tufted hemangiomas.

Cutaneous lesions can usually be diagnosed by typical appearance and rapid proliferation. Deep lesions may require imaging studies to help differentiate from a lymphangioma. The presence of a midline hemangioma in the lumbosacral area indicates the need for an MRI for underlying asymptomatic neurologic abnormalities. Location may also dictate the need for an ophthalmologic or surgical consultation. A scan of the liver should be performed if multiple cutaneous lesions are present.

Treatment. Most require no specific therapy and only parental reassurance. For those hemangiomas that are life threatening or that threaten vital functions such as eyesight, treatment is warranted. Prednisone (1–3 mg/kg/24 hr PO) is typically the initial therapy. Occasionally, higher doses are used. Approximately 30% of hemangiomas respond dramatically to corticosteroids and begin to regress within 1 wk; 40% stabilize or show minimal response; and the remainder do not respond. Interferon-α (1–3 MU/m^2/24 hr) has also been used as initial therapy and in those that do not respond to corticosteroid therapy. Although response rates of up to 70% have been reported, the risk of neurologic adverse effects in 10–20% indicates the need for caution in using interferon-α. Laser therapy has been used in some situations.

Treatment of patients with Kasabach-Merritt syndrome usually consists of supportive care while also beginning therapy with corticosteroids or interferon-α. Heparin therapy is contraindicated, and platelet transfusions should be avoided in the absence of life-threatening hemorrhage because they may exacerbate the bleeding. The use of aminocaproic acid or tranexamic acid may be beneficial. Failure to respond to therapy warrants the use of less conventional treatments, such as irradiation, embolization, or surgical resection.

Dinehart SM, Kincannon J, Geronemus R: Hemangiomas: Evaluation and treatment. *Dermatol Surg* 2001;27:475–85.
Donnelly LF, Adams DM, Bisset GS III: Vascular malformations and hemangiomas: A practical approach in a multidisciplinary clinic. *Am J Radiol* 2000;174:597–608.
Drolet BA, Esterly NB, Frieden IJ: Hemangiomas in children. *N Engl J Med* 1999;341:173–81.
Greinwald JH Jr, Burke DK, Bonthius DJ, et al: An update on the treatment of hemangiomas in children with interferon alfa-2a. *Arch Otolaryngol Head Neck Surg* 1999;125:21–27.

LYMPHANGIOMAS AND CYSTIC HYGROMAS

Lymphatic malformations, including lymphangiomas and cystic hygromas, which arise in the embryonic lymph sac, are the second most common benign vascular tumors in children. About half are located in the head and neck area. Approximately 50% are present at birth, with most presenting by 2 yr of age. There is no gender predisposition. Spontaneous regression has been reported but is not typical.

Lymphatic malformations present as soft, painless masses that transilluminate if superficial. Intrathoracic lymphatic malformation can present as symptoms related to a mediastinal mass or pericardial or pleural effusion. Rapid enlargement can occur with infection or hemorrhage. Localized lesions may be surgically resected, but this can be difficult, owing to their infiltrative nature. Recurrence is common with incompletely resected lesions. Aspiration can provide temporary relief in an emergency, such as in the presence of dyspnea, but reaccumulation will occur. Treatment by injection of sclerosing agents and laser therapy has also been used. Systemic therapy with interferon has also been reported.

Alqahtani A, Nguyen LT, Flageole H, et al: 25 Years' experience with lymphangiomas in children. *J Pediatr Surg* 1999;34:1164–68.

Chapter 498

Rare Tumors *Cynthia E. Herzog*

THYROID TUMORS

The incidence of thyroid cancer in patients younger than 20 yr of age is 4.9 cases/million in the United States. Most thyroid cancer in this age group occurs in the adolescent female. Thyroid cancer occurrence is about 4 times greater in females than males and 2.5 times more common in whites than blacks. The greatest risk factor for thyroid cancer is radiation exposure, especially from head and neck irradiation. Thyroid cancer accounts for about 10% of second malignancies among cancer survivors, especially survivors of Hodgkin lymphoma. This is due to treatment not only with radiation but also with alkylating agents. The vast majority are differentiated carcinomas (papillary or follicular). However, medullary thyroid carcinoma (MTC) may occur in familial cases, especially with multiple endocrine neoplasia (MEN type 2). MEN type 2b is associated with onset of MTC at a very early age. Other findings of MEN 2b include mucosal neuromas and marfanoid habitus. MEN type 2 is associated with mutations in the *RET* proto-oncogene, whereas genetic translocations involving *RET* are found in about half of the pediatric thyroid cancers with differentiated histology.

Patients present with a thyroid mass and/or cervical lymphadenopathy; symptoms related to abnormal hormone levels are rare. About 20% of thyroid nodules in young children are malignant, compared with about 10% in adolescents and adults. Fine-needle aspiration (FNA) is commonly used to assess thyroid nodules in adults, but the use of FNA in the pediatric population has not been firmly established, especially in preadolescent patients; surgical resection of nodules is recommended for these patients. Evaluation should include determination of thyroid hormone levels, thyroid scan, chest radiography, and CT of the chest. Total thyroidectomy for disease confined to one lobe remains controversial in pediatrics owing to good prognosis and the risk of complications such as hypoparathyroidism. With more extensive disease, or radiation-related cancer, total thyroidectomy is indicated, with lymph node dissection if cervical nodes are involved. Treatment with iodine-131 is then used to eradicate residual disease and treat pulmonary metastases, which occur in 6–10% of cases. Pulmonary metastases are best detected with radioiodine after resection of bulk disease.

Skinner MA: Cancer of the thyroid gland in infants and children. *Semin Pediatr Surg* 2001;10:119–26.

MELANOMA

The incidence of melanoma in persons younger than 20 yr of age is 4.2 cases/million in the United States, with almost all of these cases occurring in adolescents. Incident rates of melanoma in younger age groups have remained stable in the United States, but the incidence is rapidly increasing in adults. Although sun exposure is a well-known risk factor for melanoma in adults, its role in pediatric melanoma is less clear. Pediatricians should counsel patients regarding avoidance of sun exposure to decrease the risk of later development of melanoma. Patients with fair skin and a family history of melanoma are at particularly high risk. Known risk factors in pediatrics are giant hairy nevus (>20 cm), dysplastic nevus syndrome, and xeroderma pigmentosum.

Findings of a rapidly enlarging nevus that is dark or has changed colors, has irregular borders, or bleeds easily should raise a concern of melanoma. Diagnosis is based on pathology. However, extra care must be taken in the diagnosis of melanoma in children because the distinction from other lesions, particularly Spitz nevus, can be difficult.

Treatment recommendations are based on adult data. The primary treatment is local excision with lymph node mapping and biopsy for all but the most superficial melanomas. If the sentinel node is positive, a formal lymph node dissection is recommended. Chemotherapy in combination with biologic agents and vaccine therapy has been used for treatment of distant metastases. Whether the outcome is better for children than adults is unclear.

Chamlin SL, Williams ML: Pigmented lesions in adolescents. *Adolesc Med* 2001;12:195–212.

Gibbs P, Moore A, Robinson W, et al: Pediatric melanoma: Are recent advances in the management of adult melanoma relevant to the pediatric population? *J Pediatr Hematol Oncol* 2000;22:428–32.

NASOPHARYNGEAL CARCINOMA

Nasopharyngeal carcinoma is rare in the pediatric population, but is one of the most common nasopharyngeal tumors to occur in pediatric patients. In adults it occurs with highest incidence in South China, but it also has a high incidence among Eskimos and in North Africa and Northeast India. In China, it is rare in the pediatric population, but in other populations a substantial proportion of cases occur in the pediatric age group, primarily in adolescents. It occurs in males twice as often as in females. In the pediatric population the tumors are more commonly of undifferentiated histology and associated with Epstein-Barr virus.

Most pediatric patients present with advanced locoregional disease manifest by cervical lymphadenopathy. Epistaxis, trismus, and cranial nerve deficits may also be present. The diagnosis is established from biopsy of the nasopharynx or cervical lymph nodes. In most cases the lactate dehydrogenase level is elevated, but this finding is nonspecific. Evaluation of the head and neck with CT or MRI is performed to determine the extent of locoregional disease. Chest radiography, CT, bone scan, and liver scan are used to evaluate for metastatic disease.

Treatment is a combination of chemotherapy and irradiation. Cisplatin-based chemotherapy is given before or concurrent with irradiation. The outcome depends on the extent of disease; those with distant metastases have a very poor prognosis. Late effects as a result of radiation therapy are common, including hormonal dysfunction, dental caries, fibrosis, and second malignancies.

McDermott AL, Dutt SN, Watkinson JC: The aetiology of nasopharyngeal carcinoma. *Clin Otolaryngol Allied Sci* 2001;26:82–92.

Sahraoui S, Acharki A, Benider A, et al: Nasopharyngeal carcinoma in children under 15 years of age: A retrospective review of 65 patients. *Ann Oncol* 1999;10:1499–502.

ADENOCARCINOMA OF THE COLON AND RECTUM

Colorectal carcinoma rarely presents in the pediatric population. There is a male predominance, as compared with a female predominance in adults. Even in patients with predisposing conditions, such as familial adenomatous polyposis and Peutz-Jeghers syndrome, cancer usually does not present until adulthood, although screening should begin during childhood or adolescence. Presenting symptoms include bloody stools or melena, abdominal pain, weight loss, and changes in bowel pattern. Signs are often vague, often resulting in a delay in diagnosis and advanced disease. The histologic subtype differs from that seen in adults, with the majority of pediatric tumors being mucinous. Treatment consists of surgical resection when possible, with chemotherapy for unresectable tumors. Irradiation is useful in the treatment of rectal carcinomas.

ADRENOCORTICAL CARCINOMA

Adrenocortical carcinoma is rare but is associated with the Li-Fraumeni and Beckwith-Wiedemann syndromes. It may occur at any age during childhood but is more common during the first few years of life. In Brazil, there is a 10-fold higher frequency of childhood adrenocortical carcinoma, with a female predominance. Patients typically present with endocrine symptoms of Cushing syndrome or virilization. Most tumors are secretory, producing androgens, glucocorticoids, or estrogens. Prognosis depends on tumor size, extent of tumor, and resectability. Although responses are seen to mitotane- and cisplatin-based chemotherapy, the prognosis is poor for unresectable or metastatic disease.

Teinturier C, Pauchard MS, Brugières L, et al: Clinical and prognostic aspects of adrenocortical neoplasms in childhood. *Med Pediatr Oncol* 1999;32:106–11.

Chapter 499

Histiocytosis Syndromes of Childhood *Stephan Ladisch*

The childhood histiocytoses constitute a diverse group of disorders, which, although rare in occurrence, may be severe in their clinical expression. These disorders are grouped together because they have in common a prominent proliferation or accumulation of cells of the monocyte-macrophage system of bone marrow origin. Although these disorders are sometimes difficult to distinguish clinically, accurate diagnosis is nevertheless essential for facilitating progress in treatment. To this end, a systematic classification of the childhood histiocytoses has been developed (Table 499–1). This diagnostic classification rests on

TABLE 499–1. Classification of the Childhood Histiocytoses

	Diseases	Cellular Characteristics of the Lesions	Treatment
Class I	Langerhans cell histiocytosis	Langerhans cells (CD1a positive) with Birbeck granules	Local therapy for isolated lesions; chemotherapy for disseminated disease
Class II	Familial erythrophagocytic lymphohistiocytosis	Morphologically normal reactive macrophages with prominent erythrophagocytosis	Chemotherapy; allogeneic bone marrow transplantation
	Infection-associated hemophagocytic syndrome		
Class III	Malignant histiocytosis	Neoplastic proliferation of cells with characteristics of monocytes/macrophages or their precursors	Antineoplastic chemotherapy, including anthracyclines
	Acute monocytic leukemia		

histopathologic findings; thus, a thorough, comprehensive evaluation of a biopsy specimen obtained at the time of diagnosis is essential. This evaluation includes studies (electron microscopy, immunostaining) that may require special sample processing.

Classification and Pathology. Three classes of childhood histiocytosis are recognized, based on histopathologic findings. The most well-known childhood histiocytosis, previously known as **histiocytosis X,** constitutes class I and includes the clinical entities of eosinophilic granuloma (see Chapter 493), **Hand-Schüller-Christian disease,** and **Letterer-Siwe disease.** The name **Langerhan cell histiocytosis** (LCH) has been applied to the class I histiocytoses. The normal Langerhans cell is an antigen-presenting cell (APC) of the skin. The hallmark of LCH in all forms is the presence of a clonal proliferation of cells of the monocyte lineage containing the characteristic electron microscopic findings of a Langerhans cell. This is the **Birbeck granule,** a tennis racket–shaped bilamellar granule, which when seen in the cytoplasm of lesional cells in LCH is diagnostic of the disease. Alternatively, the definitive diagnosis of LCH can be made by demonstrating CD1a positivity of lesional cells. The lesions may contain various proportions of these Langerhans granule–containing cells, lymphocytes, granulocytes, monocytes, and eosinophils.

In contrast to a prominence of an APC (the Langerhans cell) in the class I histiocytoses, the class II histiocytoses are characterized by accumulation of antigen-processing cells (i.e., macrophages). With the characteristic morphology of normal macrophages by light microscopy, these phagocytic cells lack the two markers (Birbeck granules and CD1a positivity) characteristic of the cells found in LCH. The two major diseases among the class II histiocytoses have indistinguishable pathologic findings. One is **familial erythrophagocytic lymphohistiocytosis** (FEL), which is the only inherited form of histiocytosis and is

autosomal recessive. Most recently, several specific gene mutations underlying FEL have been discovered. The other is the **infection-associated hemophagocytic syndrome** (IAHS). Both diseases are characterized by disseminated lesions that involve many organ systems. The lesions are characterized by infiltration of the involved organ with activated phagocytic macrophages and lymphocytes, and the diseases are grouped together under the term **hemophagocytic lymphohistiocytosis** (HLH).

The mixed cellular lesions of both the class I and class II histiocytoses suggest that these may be disorders of immune regulation, resulting from either an unusual and unidentified antigenic stimulation or an abnormal and somehow defective cellular immune response. In fact, the genetic defect in some cases of FEL has been identified as a defect in perforin, the effector molecule of cytotoxic lymphocytes whose function has been found to be inhibited in FEL. In contrast, the class III histiocytoses are unequivocal malignancies of cells of monocyte-macrophage lineage. By this definition, acute monocytic leukemia and true malignant histiocytosis are included among the class III histiocytoses (see Chapter 487). The existence of neoplasms of Langerhans cells is controversial. Some cases of LCH demonstrate clonality.

CLASS I HISTIOCYTOSES

Clinical Manifestations. LCH has an extremely variable presentation. The skeleton is involved in 80% of patients and may be the only affected site, especially in children older than 5 yr of age. Bone lesions may be single or numerous and are seen most commonly in the skull (Fig. 499–1). They may be asymptomatic or associated with pain and local swelling. Involvement of the spine may result in collapse of the vertebral body, which can be seen radiographically, and may cause secondary compression of

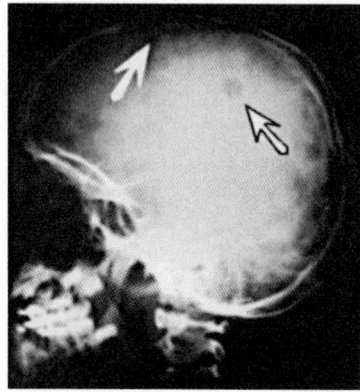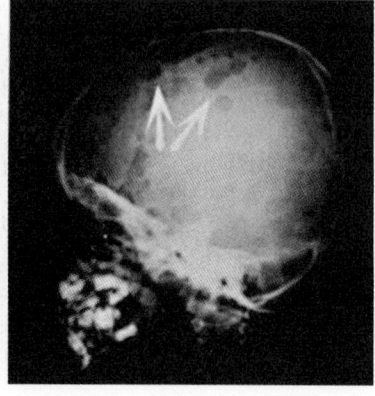

FIGURE 499–1. Two skull radiographs from patients with LCH. *Left,* The patient was older than 2 yr of age and had involvement limited to isolated bone lesions *(arrows).* She had a good recovery. *Right,* The patient was younger than 2 yr of age and had extensive bone disease *(arrows),* febrile course, anemia, severe skin eruption, generalized lymphadenopathy, hepatosplenomegaly, pulmonary infiltrates, and a fatal outcome despite antitumor chemotherapy. These patients represent opposite ends of the clinical spectrum of LCH.

the spinal cord. In flat and long bones, osteolytic lesions with sharp borders occur and no evidence exists of reactive new bone formation (until the lesions begin to heal). Lesions that involve weight-bearing long bones may result in pathologic fractures. Chronically draining, infected ears are commonly associated with destruction in the mastoid area. Bone destruction in the mandible and maxilla may result in teeth that, on radiographs, appear to be free floating. With response to therapy, healing may be complete.

Skin involvement occurs in about 50% of patients at some time during their course (usually, a seborrheic dermatitis of the scalp or diaper region). The lesions may spread to involve the back, palms, and soles. The exanthem may be petechial or hemorrhagic, even in the absence of thrombocytopenia. Localized or disseminated lymphadenopathy is present in approximately 33% of patients. Hepatosplenomegaly occurs in approximately 20% of patients. Various degrees of hepatic malfunction may occur, including jaundice and ascites.

Exophthalmos, when present, is often bilateral and is caused by retro-orbital accumulation of granulomatous tissue. Gingival mucous membranes may be involved with infiltrative lesions that appear superficially like candidiasis. In 10–15% of patients, pulmonary infiltrates are found on radiography. The lesions may vary from diffuse fibrosis and disseminated nodular infiltrates to diffuse cystic changes. Rarely, pneumothorax may be a complication. If the lungs are severely involved, tachypnea and progressive respiratory failure may result.

Pituitary dysfunction or hypothalamic involvement may result in growth retardation. In addition, patients may have diabetes insipidus; patients suspected of having LCH should demonstrate the ability to concentrate their urine before going to the operating room for a biopsy. Rarely, panhypopituitarism may occur. Primary hypothyroidism due to thyroid gland infiltration may also occur.

Patients who are affected more severely may have systemic manifestations, including fever, weight loss, malaise, irritability, and failure to thrive. Bone marrow involvement may cause anemia and thrombocytopenia. Two uncommon but serious and unusual manifestations of LCH are hepatic involvement (leading to cirrhosis) and a peculiar central nervous system (CNS) involvement characterized by ataxia, dysarthria, and other neurologic symptoms. Associated with multisystem disease, hepatic involvement is frequently already present at the time of diagnosis. In contrast, the CNS involvement, which is progressive, histopathologically characterized by gliosis, and for which no treatment is known, may be observed only many years after the initial diagnosis of LCH, which may have consisted only of mild bone disease. Striking is that neither of these manifestations evidence Langerhans cells or Birbeck granules.

After tissue biopsy, which is diagnostic and easiest to perform on skin or bone lesions, a thorough clinical and laboratory evaluation should be undertaken. This should include a series of studies in all patients (complete blood cell count, liver function tests, coagulation studies, skeletal survey, chest radiograph, and measurement of urine osmolality). In addition, detailed evaluation of any organ system that has been shown to be involved by physical examination or by these studies should be performed to establish the extent of disease before initiation of treatment.

Treatment and Prognosis. The clinical course of single-system disease (usually, bone, lymph node, or skin) is generally benign, with a high chance of spontaneous remission. Therefore, treatment should be minimal and should be directed at arresting the progression of a lesion (e.g., a bone lesion) that could result in permanent damage before it resolves spontaneously. Curettage or low-dose local radiation therapy (5–6 Gy) may accomplish this goal. Multisystem disease, in contrast, should be treated with systemic multiagent chemotherapy. Several different regimens have been proposed, but a central element is the inclusion

of either vinblastine or etoposide, which have been found to be very effective in treating LCH. Based on the most recent findings, treatment of multisystem LCH includes therapy with multiple agents, designed to reduce reactivation of disease and long-term consequence. The response rate to therapy, contrary to previous opinion, may be high, especially if the diagnosis is accurately and expeditiously ascertained. Experimental therapies, suggested only for unresponsive disease (frequently very young children with multisystem disease who have not responded to initial treatment), include immunosuppressive therapy with cyclosporine/antithymocyte globulin and possibly certain new agents and modalities, such as 2-chlorodeoxyadenosine and stem cell transplantation. Current treatment approaches and experimental protocols for both class I and class II histiocytoses can be obtained at *www.histio.org/society*, the website for the Histiocyte Society.

CLASS II HISTIOCYTOSES

Clinical Manifestations. The major forms of class II histiocytosis, FEL and IAHS, have a remarkably similar presentation, consisting of a generalized disease process, most often with fever, weight loss, and irritability. FEL is also characterized by severe immunodeficiency. Children with FEL are always younger than 4 yr of age; children with IAHS may present at an older age. Physical examination frequently reveals hepatosplenomegaly and symptoms of CNS involvement (with an aseptic meningitis, the cerebrospinal fluid cells are the same phagocytic macrophages as found in the peripheral blood or bone marrow). As in the class I histiocytoses, the diagnosis rests on the pathologic findings. Associated laboratory findings in both forms of class II histiocytosis include hyperlipidemia, hypofibrinogenemia, elevated levels of hepatic enzymes, extremely elevated levels of circulating soluble interleukin-2 receptors released by the activated lymphocytes, and sometimes cytopenias. No absolute clinical or laboratory distinction can be made between FEL and IAHS. Without a genetic marker for FEL at present, the distinction can definitively be made only by a positive family history for other affected children.

Treatment and Prognosis. The diagnostic distinction between FEL and IAHS can sometimes be based on the acute onset of IAHS in the presence of a documented infection. In this case, treatment of the underlying infection, coupled with supportive care, is critical. If the diagnosis is made in a setting of iatrogenic immunodeficiency, immunosuppressive treatment should be withdrawn and supportive care should be instituted along with specific therapy for underlying infection. When FEL is diagnosed or suspected and when an infection cannot be documented, therapy currently includes etoposide and immunosuppressive therapy. Nevertheless, even with chemotherapy, FEL remains uniformly fatal. However, allogeneic bone marrow transplantation may be effective in curing a significant fraction of patients with FEL and provides hope for the outcome of this disease.

In contrast, in IAHS, when an infection can be documented and effectively treated, the prognosis is good without any other specific treatment. When a treatable infection cannot be documented (as is the case in most patients presumed to have IAHS), the prognosis is as poor as that of FEL; and an identical chemotherapeutic approach, including etoposide, is recommended. It is theorized that, by its cytotoxic effect on macrophages, etoposide interrupts cytokine production, the hemophagocytic process, and the accumulation of macrophages, all of which may contribute to the pathogenesis of IAHS. A broad spectrum of infectious agents, viruses (e.g., cytomegalovirus, Epstein-Barr virus, human herpesvirus 6), fungi, protozoa, and bacteria may trigger IAHS, usually in the setting of immunodeficiency. A thorough evaluation for infection should be undertaken in immunodeficient patients with hemophagocytosis. Rarely, the same syndrome may be identified in conjunction with a neoplasm (e.g., leukemia); in this case, treatment of the underlying disease causes resolution of the hemophagocytosis. In some patients, interferon and intravenous immunoglobulin have been effective.

CLASS III HISTIOCYTOSES

By this definition, acute monocytic leukemia and true malignant histiocytosis are included among the class III histiocytoses (see Chapter 487).

Arico M, Danesino C, Pende D, et al: Pathogenesis of haemophagocytic lymphohistiocytosis. *Br J Haematol* 2001;114:761–9.

Arico M, Imashuku S, Clementi R, et al: Hemophagocytic lymphohistiocytosis due to germline mutations in *SH2D1A*, the X-linked lymphoproliferative disease gene. *Blood* 2001;97:1131–3.

Broadbent V, Gadner, H: Current therapy for Langerhans cell histiocytosis. *Hematol Oncol Clin North Am* 1998;12:327–8.

Durken M, Finckenstein FG, Janka GE: Bone marrow transplantation in hemophagocytic lymphohistiocytosis. *Leuk Lymphoma* 2001;41:89–95.

Filipovich AH: Hemophagocytic lymphohistiocytosis: A lethal disorder of immune regulation. *J Pediatr* 1997;130:337–8.

Gadner H, Grois N, Arico M, et al: A randomized trial of treatment for multisystem Langerhans' cell histiocytosis. *J Pediatr* 2001;138:728–34.

Henter, JI, Arico M, Egeler RM, et al: HLH-94: A treatment protocol for hemophagocytic lymphohistiocytosis. HLH Study Group of the Histiocyte Society. *Med Pediatr Oncol* 1997;28:342–7.

Lahey ME: Histiocytosis X: An analysis of prognostic factors. *J Pediatr* 1975;87:184–9.

Kogawa K, Lee SM, Villanueva J, et al: Perforin expression in cytotoxic lymphocytes from patients with hemophagocytic lymphohistiocytosis and their family members. *Blood* 2002;99:61–6.

Stepp SE, Dufourcq-Lagelouse R, Le Deist F, et al: Perforin gene defects in familial hemophagocytic lymphohistiocytosis. *Science* 1999;286:1957–9.

Writing Group of the Histiocyte Society: Histiocytosis syndromes in childhood. *Lancet* 1987;208–9.

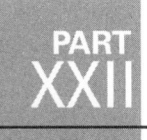

PART XXII Nephrology

SECTION 1 *Glomerular Disease*

Ira D. Davis and Ellis D. Avner

Chapter 500

Introduction to Glomerular Diseases

500.1 Anatomy of the Glomerulus

The kidneys lie in the retroperitoneal space slightly above the level of the umbilicus. They range in length and weight, respectively, from approximately 6 cm and 24 g in a full-term newborn to 12 cm or more and 150 g in an adult. The kidney (Fig. 500–1) has an outer layer, the cortex, which contains the glomeruli, proximal and distal convoluted tubules, and collecting ducts, and an inner layer, the medulla, which contains the straight portions of the tubules, the loops of Henle, the vasa recta, and the terminal collecting ducts (Fig. 500–2).

The blood supply to each kidney usually consists of a main renal artery that arises from the aorta; multiple renal arteries may occur. The main artery divides into segmental branches within the medulla and these into interlobar arteries that pass through the medulla to the junction of the cortex and medulla. At this point, the interlobar arteries branch to form the arcuate arteries, which run parallel to the surface of the kidney. Interlobular arteries originate from the arcuate arteries and give rise to the afferent arterioles of the glomeruli. Specialized muscle cells in the wall of the afferent arteriole and the macula densa within the distal tubule next to the glomerulus form the juxtaglomerular apparatus that controls the secretion of renin. The afferent arteriole divides into the glomerular capillary network, which then merges into the efferent arteriole (Fig. 500–3). The efferent arterioles of glomeruli next to the medulla (juxtamedullary glomeruli) are larger than those in the outer cortex and provide the blood supply (vasa recta) to the tubules and medulla.

Each kidney contains approximately 1 million nephrons (glomeruli and associated tubules). In humans, formation of nephrons is complete at birth, but functional maturation with tubular growth and elongation continues during the first decade of life. Because new nephrons cannot be formed after birth, progressive loss of nephrons may lead to renal insufficiency.

The glomerular network of specialized capillaries serves as the filtering mechanism of the kidney. The glomerular capillaries are lined by endothelial cells (Fig. 500–4) having very thin cytoplasm that contains many holes (fenestrations). The glomerular basement membrane (GBM) forms a continuous layer between the endothelial and mesangial cells on one side and the epithelial cells on the other. The membrane has three layers: (1) a central electron-dense lamina densa; (2) the lamina rara interna, which lies between the lamina densa and the endothelial cells;

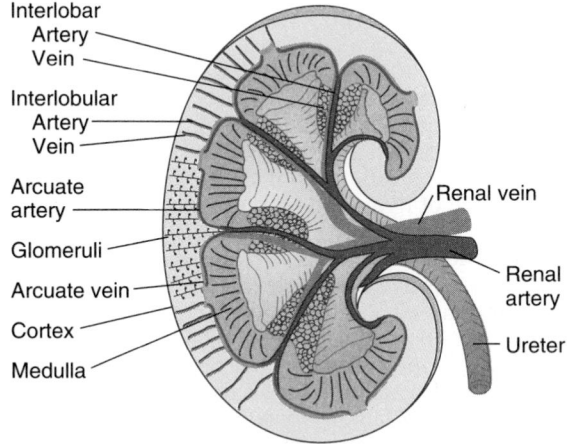

FIGURE 500–1. Gross morphology of the renal circulation. (From Pitts RF: *Physiology of the Kidney and Body Fluids*, 3rd ed. Chicago, Year Book Medical Publishers, 1974.)

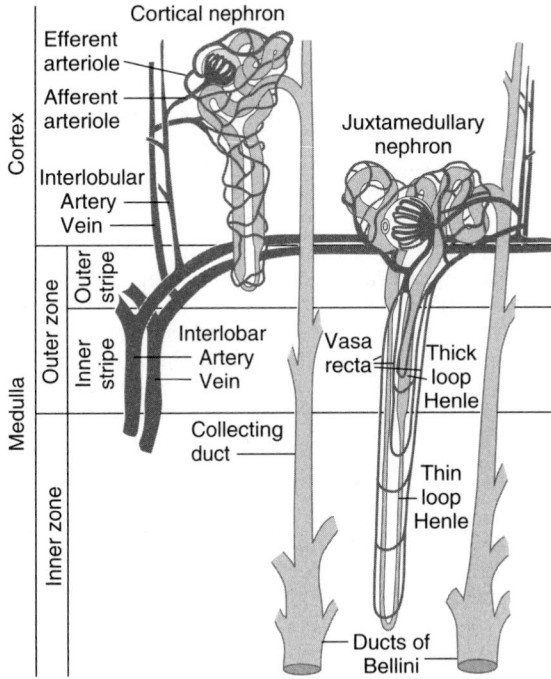

FIGURE 500–2. Comparison of the blood supplies of cortical and juxtamedullary nephrons. (From Pitts RF: *Physiology of the Kidney and Body Fluids*, 3rd ed. Chicago, Year Book Medical Publishers, 1974.)

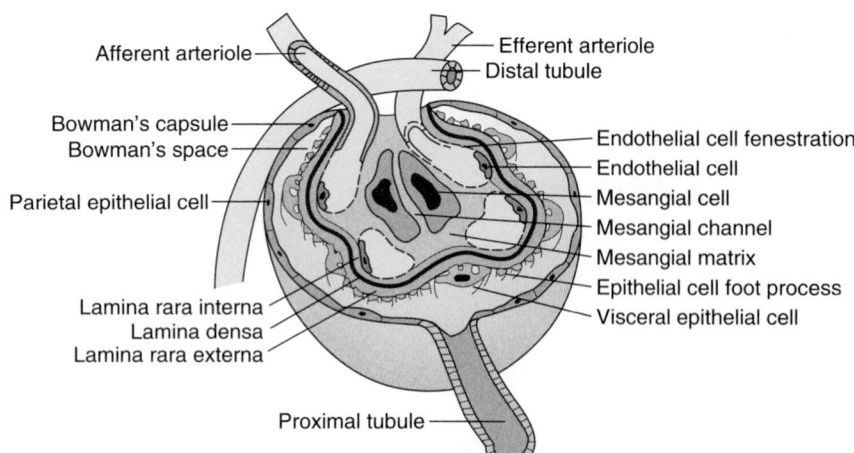

FIGURE 500–3. Schematic depiction of the glomerulus and surrounding structures.

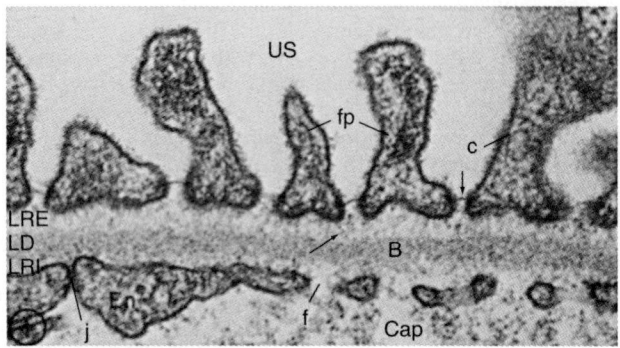

FIGURE 500–4. Electron micrograph of the normal glomerular capillary (Cap) wall demonstrating the endothelium (En) with its fenestrations (f), the glomerular basement membrane (B) with its central dense layer, the lamina densa (LD) and adjoining lamina rara interna (LRI) and externa (LRE; *long arrow*) and the epithelial cell foot processes (fp) with their thick cell coat (c). The glomerular filtrate passes through the endothelial fenestrae, crosses the basement membrane, and passes through the filtration slits *(short arrow)* between the epithelial cell foot processes to reach the urinary space (US). (×60,000.) J is the junction between two endothelial cells. (From Farquhar MG, Kanwar YS: Functional organization of the glomerulus: State of the science in 1979. In Cummings NB, Michael AF, Wilson CB [editors]: *Immune Mechanisms in Renal Disease.* New York, Plenum, 1982. Reprinted by permission.)

and (3) the lamina rara externa, which lies between the lamina densa and the epithelial cells. The visceral epithelial cells cover the capillary and project cytoplasmic "foot processes," which attach to the lamina rara externa. Between the foot processes are spaces or filtration slits. The mesangium (mesangial cells and matrix) lies between the glomerular capillaries on the endothelial cell side of the GBM and forms the medial part of the capillary wall. The mesangium may serve as a supporting structure for the glomerular capillaries and probably has a role in the regulation of glomerular blood flow and filtration and in the removal of macromolecules (such as immune complexes) from the glomerulus, either through intracellular phagocytosis or by transport through intercellular channels to the juxtaglomerular region. Bowman capsule, which surrounds the glomerulus, is composed of (1) a basement membrane, which is continuous with the basement membranes of the glomerular capillaries and the proximal tubules, and (2) the parietal epithelial cells, which are continuous with the visceral epithelial cells.

Price CP, Finney H: Developments in assessment of glomerular filtration rate. *Clin Chim Acta* 2000;297:55–66.

500.2 Glomerular Filtration

As the blood passes through the glomerular capillaries, the plasma is filtered through the glomerular capillary walls. The ultrafiltrate, which is cell free, contains all the substances in the plasma (electrolytes, glucose, phosphate, urea, creatinine, peptides, low molecular weight proteins) except proteins (like albumin and the globulins) having a molecular weight of 68,000 or more. The filtrate is collected in Bowman space and enters the tubules, where its composition is modified by solute and fluid secretion and absorption in accordance with tightly regulated homeostatic mechanisms until it leaves the kidney as urine.

Glomerular filtration is the net result of opposing forces across the capillary wall. The force for ultrafiltration (glomerular capillary hydrostatic pressure) stems from the systemic arterial pressure, as modified by the tone of the afferent and efferent arterioles. The major force opposing ultrafiltration is the glomerular capillary oncotic pressure, which is created by the gradient between the high concentration of plasma proteins within the capillary and the almost protein-free ultrafiltrate in Bowman space. Filtration may be modified by the rate of glomerular plasma flow, the hydrostatic pressure within Bowman space, and the permeability of the glomerular capillary wall.

Although glomerular filtration begins around the 9th wk of fetal life, kidney function is not necessary for normal intrauterine homeostasis because the placenta serves as the major excretory organ. After birth, the glomerular filtration rate (GFR) increases until growth ceases toward the end of the 2nd decade of life. To facilitate the comparison of the GFRs of children and adults, GFR is standardized to the surface area (1.73 m^2) of a 70-kg adult. Even after correction for surface area, the GFR of a child does not approximate adult values until the 3rd yr of life (Fig. 500–5).

The GFR may be estimated by measurement of the serum creatinine level (Fig. 500–6). Creatinine is derived from muscle metabolism. Its production is relatively constant, and its excretion is primarily through glomerular filtration, although tubular secretion may become important in renal insufficiency. In contrast to the concentration of blood urea nitrogen, which is affected by state of hydration and nitrogen balance, the serum creatinine level is primarily influenced by the level of glomerular function. The serum creatinine is of value only in estimating the GFR in the steady state. For example, a patient may have a normal creatinine level without effective renal function very shortly after the onset of acute renal failure with anuria. In this clinical setting, serum creatinine may be an insensitive measure of decreased renal function, because its level does not rise above normal until the GFR falls by 30–40%.

The precise measurement of the GFR is accomplished by quantitating the "clearance" of a substance that is freely filtered across the capillary wall and that is neither reabsorbed nor secreted by the tubules. The clearance (C_s) of such a substance is

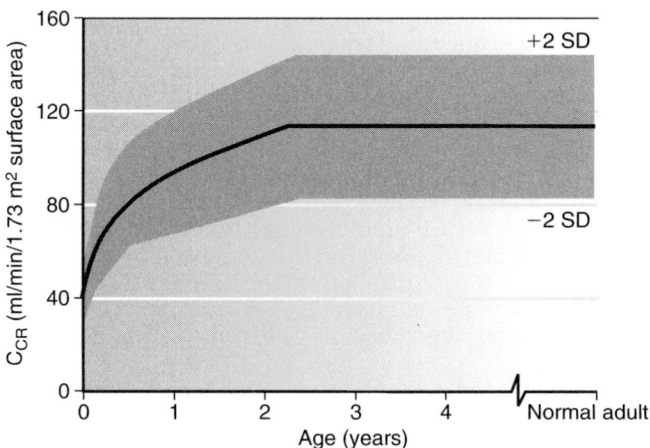

FIGURE 500–5. Changes in the normal value of the glomerular filtration rate, as measured by the creatinine clearance (C_{CR}), when standardized to mL/min/1.73 m^2 of body surface area. The *solid line* depicts the mean value, and the *shaded area* includes two standard deviations. (Reprinted by permission of the publishers from McCrory W: *Developmental Nephrology.* Cambridge, MA, Harvard University Press. Copyright © 1972 by the President and Fellows of Harvard College.)

that volume of plasma that, when completely "cleared" of the contained substance, would yield a quantity of that substance equal to that excreted in the urine over a specified time. The clearance is represented by the following formula:

$$C_s \text{ (mL/min)} = U_s \text{ (mg/mL)} \times V \text{ (mL/min)}/P_s \text{ (mg/mL)}$$

where C_s equals the clearance of substance s, U_s reflects the urinary concentration of s, V represents the urinary flow rate, and P_s equals the plasma concentration of s. To correct the clearance for body surface area, the formula is

$$\text{Corrected clearance} = C_s \text{ (mL/min)} \times \frac{1.73}{\text{patient's surface area (m}^2)}$$

The GFR is optimally measured by the clearance of inulin, a fructose polymer having a molecular weight of approximately 5,000. Because the inulin clearance technique is cumbersome, the GFR is commonly estimated by the clearance of endogenous creatinine. When the GFR is relatively normal, the creatinine clearance closely approximates the inulin clearance. As the GFR declines, an increasing proportion of the total creatinine in the urine is secreted by tubules, resulting in a creatinine clearance that progressively overestimates the actual GFR. Therefore, changes in renal function should be monitored by serum creatinine concentration when the serum creatinine level exceeds 2.0 mg/dL (180 μmol/L).

The absence of plasma proteins larger than the size of albumin from the glomerular filtrate confirms the effectiveness of the glomerular capillary wall as a filtration barrier. Major factors restricting the filtration of these and other macromolecules include their size and their ionic charge.

Clearance studies of macromolecules in animals have shown no restriction to the filtration of molecules up to the size of inulin. As size increases farther, filtration diminishes progressively, approaching zero for substances the size of albumin. Morphologic studies suggest that the size-selective filtration barrier resides within the GBM.

The endothelial cell, basement membrane, and epithelial cell of the glomerular capillary wall possess strong negative ionic charges. These anionic charges are a consequence of two negatively charged moieties: proteoglycans (heparan sulfate) and glycoproteins containing sialic acid. Proteins in the blood have a relatively low isoelectric point and carry a net negative charge. Consequently, they are repelled by the negatively charged sites in the glomerular capillary wall, thus restricting filtration.

Arant BS Jr: Postnatal development of renal function during the first year of life. *Pediatr Nephrol* 1987;1:308.

Price CP, Finney H: Developments in assessment of glomerular filtration rate. *Clin Chim Acta* 2000;297:55–66.

Schwartz GJ, Haycock GB, Spitzer A: Plasma creatinine and urea concentration in children: Normal values for age and sex. *J Pediatr* 1976;88:828–37.

Yared A, Ichikawa I: In Barratt TM, Avner ED, Harmon WE (editors): *Pediatric Nephrology,* 4th ed. Baltimore, Lippincott, Williams, & Wilkins, 2000, pp 39–58.

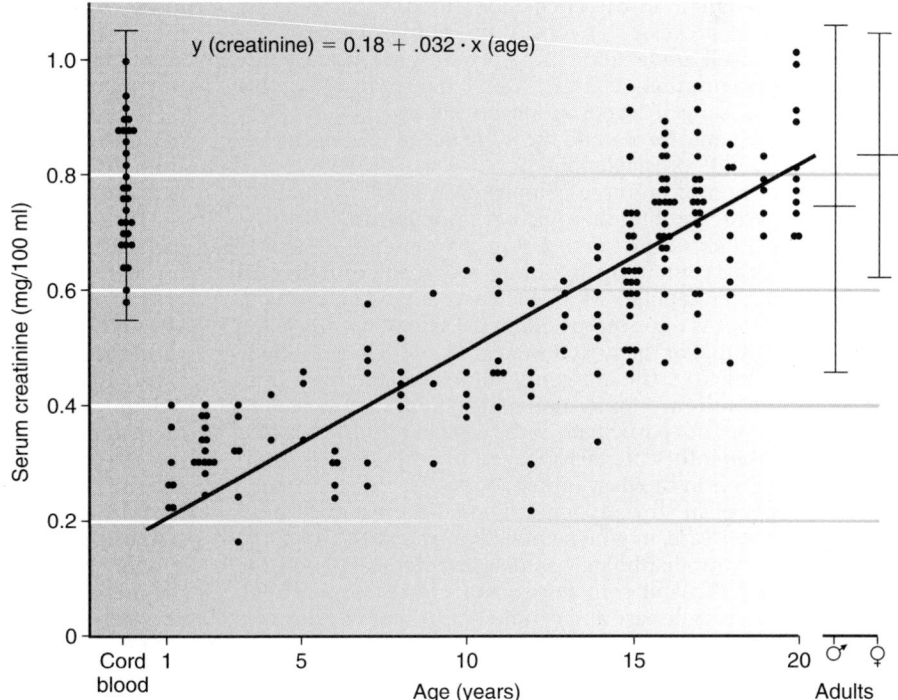

FIGURE 500–6. The serum creatinine in relation to age. (Reprinted by permission of the publishers from McCrory W: *Developmental Nephrology.* Cambridge, MA, Harvard University Press. Copyright © 1972 by the President and Fellows of Harvard College.)

500.3 Glomerular Diseases

Pathogenesis. Glomerular injury may be a result of genetic, immunologic, or coagulation disorders. Genetic disorders of the glomerulus result from (1) mutations in the exons of DNA encoding transcriptional units that undergo translation in the ribosomes forming proteins located within the glomerulus, interstitium, or tubular epithelium; (2) mutations in the regulatory genes controlling DNA transcription; (3) abnormal posttranscriptional modification of RNA transcripts; or (4) abnormal post-translational modification of proteins. Immunologic injury is the most common cause and results in *glomerulonephritis*, which is both a generic term for several diseases and a histopathologic term signifying inflammation of the glomerular capillaries. Evidence that glomerulonephritis is caused by immunologic injury includes (1) morphologic and immunopathologic similarities to experimental immune-mediated glomerulonephritis; (2) the demonstration of immune reactants (immunoglobulin and complement components) in glomeruli; and (3) abnormalities in serum complement and the finding of autoantibodies (e.g., anti-GBM) in some of these diseases. There appear to be two major mechanisms of immunologic injury: (1) localization of circulating antigen-antibody immune complexes and (2) interaction of antibody with local antigen in situ. In the latter circumstance, the antigen may be a normal component of the glomerulus (e.g., the noncollagenous domain [NC-1] of type IV collagen, which is the putative antigen in human anti-GBM nephritis) or an antigen that has been deposited in the glomerulus.

In immune complex–mediated diseases, antibody is produced against and combines with a circulating antigen that is usually unrelated to the kidney. The immune complexes accumulate in glomeruli and activate the complement system, leading to immune injury. Experimental studies suggest that the complexes are formed in the circulation and deposited in the kidney. Acute serum sickness in rabbits is produced by a single intravenous injection of bovine albumin. Within 1 wk after injection, a rabbit produces antibody against bovine albumin, while the antigen remains in the blood in high concentration. As antibody enters the circulation, it forms immune complexes with antigen. Although the amount of antigen in the circulation exceeds that of antibody (antigen excess), the complexes formed are small, remain soluble in the circulation, and are deposited in glomeruli. The processes involved in glomerular localization are not well understood but include attributes of the complex (concentration, charge, size), characteristics of the glomerulus (mesangial trapping, negatively charged capillary wall), hydrodynamic forces, and the influence of various mediators (angiotensin II, prostaglandins).

With deposition of immune complexes in glomeruli, rabbits develop an acute proliferative glomerulonephritis. Immunofluorescence microscopy demonstrates granular ("lumpy-bumpy") deposits containing immunoglobulin and complement in the glomerular capillary wall. Electron microscopic studies show these deposits to be on the epithelial side of the GBM and in the mesangium. For the next few days, as additional antibody enters the circulation, the antigen is ultimately removed from the circulation and the glomerulonephritis subsides. In rabbits, complement does not participate in the capillary injury, which is largely related to influx of macrophages. In other models, complement has a role in capillary injury.

An example of in situ antigen-antibody interaction is anti-GBM antibody disease, in which antibody reacts with antigen(s) of the GBM. Immunopathologic studies reveal linear deposition of immunoglobulin and complement on the GBM, similar to that in Goodpasture disease and certain types of rapidly progressive glomerulonephritis.

The inflammatory reaction that follows immunologic injury results from activation of one or more mediator pathways. The most important of these is the complement system, which has two initiating sequences: (1) the classic pathway, which is activated by antigen-antibody immune complexes, and (2) the alternative or properdin pathway, which is activated by polysaccharides and endotoxin. These pathways converge at C3; from that point on, the same sequence leads to lysis of cell membranes (see Fig. 123–1). The major noxious products of complement activation are produced after activation of C3 and include anaphylatoxin (which stimulates contractile proteins within vascular walls and increases vascular permeability) and chemotactic factors (C5a) that direct neutrophils and perhaps macrophages to the site of complement activation, where the cells release substances that damage vascular cells and basement membranes.

The coagulation system may be activated directly, after endothelial cell injury, which bares the thrombogenic subendothelial layer (initiating the coagulation cascade), or indirectly, after complement activation. Fibrin deposits may occur within glomerular capillaries or within Bowman space in crescents. Activation of the coagulation process may activate the kinin system, which also produces chemotactic and anaphylatoxin-like factors.

Pathology. The glomerulus may be injured by several mechanisms but has only a limited number of histopathologic responses; accordingly, different disease states may produce similar microscopic changes.

Proliferation of glomerular cells occurs in most forms of glomerulonephritis and may be generalized, involving all glomeruli, or focal, involving only some glomeruli while sparing others. Within a single glomerulus, proliferation may be diffuse, involving all parts of the glomerulus, or segmental, involving only some areas but not others. Proliferation commonly involves the endothelial and mesangial cells and is frequently associated with an increase in the mesangial matrix. Mesangial proliferation may result from immune complex deposition within the mesangium. The resultant increase in cell size and number, and in mesangial matrix, may increase glomerular size and narrow the lumens of glomerular capillaries, leading to renal insufficiency.

Crescent formation in Bowman space (capsule) is a result of proliferation of parietal epithelial cells. Crescents develop in several forms of glomerulonephritis (termed *rapidly progressive*) and are thought to be a response to fibrin deposited in Bowman space. New crescents contain fibrin, the proliferating epithelial cells of Bowman space, basement membrane–like material produced by these cells, and macrophages that may have a role in the genesis of glomerular injury. In days to weeks, the crescent is invaded by connective tissue (fibroepithelial crescent); this generally results in glomerular obsolescence. Crescent formation is frequently associated with glomerular cell death. The necrotic glomerulus has a characteristic eosinophilic appearance and usually contains nuclear remnants. Crescent formation is usually associated with generalized proliferation of the mesangial cells and with either immune complex or anti-GBM antibody deposition in the glomerular capillary wall.

In addition to proliferation, certain forms of acute glomerulonephritis show glomerular *exudation of blood cells*, including neutrophils, eosinophils, basophils, and mononuclear cells. The thickened appearance of GBM may result from a true *increase in the width of the membrane* (as seen in membranous glomerulopathy), from massive deposition of immune complexes that have staining characteristics similar to the membrane (as seen in systemic lupus erythematosus), or from the interposition of mesangial cells and matrix into the subendothelial space between the endothelial cells and the membrane. The latter may give the basement membrane a split appearance, as seen in type I membranoproliferative glomerulonephritis and other diseases.

Sclerosis refers to the presence of scar tissue within the glomerulus. Occasionally, pathologists use this term to refer to an increase in mesangial matrix.

Tubulointerstitial fibrosis is present in all patients with glomerular disease who develop progressive renal injury. This fibrosis is initiated by injury to the renal tubules resulting in mononuclear cell infiltrates that release soluble factors that have fibrosis-promoting effects. Additionally, matrix proteins of the renal interstitium begin to accumulate, leading to eventual destruction of renal tubules and peritubular capillaries.

SECTION 2 *Conditions Particularly Associated with Hematuria*

Ira D. Davis and Ellis D. Avner

Chapter 501
Clinical Evaluation of the Child with Hematuria

Hematuria is defined as the presence of at least five red blood cells (RBCs) in the urine and occurs with a prevalence of 0.5–2.0% among school-aged children. Quantitative studies demonstrate that the normal child aged 4–12 yr excretes more than 100,000 RBCs per 12-hr period and that this increases with fever and/or exercise. In the clinical setting, qualitative estimates are provided by a urinary "dipstick" that uses a peroxidase-like chemical reaction between hemoglobin (or myoglobin) and a chemical indicator compound impregnated on the dipstick. Chemstrip (Boehringer Mannheim), a common commercially available dipstick, is capable of detecting 3–10 RBCs per microliter of unspun urine with significant hematuria suggested by the presence of more than 50 RBCs/μL. False-negative results may occur in the presence of formalin (used as a urine preservative) or high urinary concentrations of ascorbic acid. False-positive results may be seen in the presence of menstrual blood, alkaline urine with a pH greater than 9, or contamination with oxidizing agents used to clean the perineum before obtaining a specimen. Microscopic analysis of 10–15 mL of fresh centrifuged urine is essential in confirming the diagnosis of hematuria suggested by a positive dipstick. Screening urinalyses should be obtained during well child care visits at 5 yr and once during the second decade of life (see Chapter 5).

Red urine *without RBCs* is seen in a number of conditions (Box 501–1). Heme-positive urine without RBCs is caused by the presence of either hemoglobin or myoglobin. *Hemoglobinuria* without hematuria may occur in the presence of hemolytic anemia. *Myoglobinuria* without hematuria occurs in the presence of rhabdomyolysis syndrome resulting from skeletal muscle injury and is generally associated with a fivefold increase in the plasma concentration of creatine kinase. *Rhabdomyolysis* may occur secondary to viral disease, crush injury, severe electrolyte abnormalities (i.e., hypernatremia, hypophosphatemia), hypotension, disseminated intravascular coagulation, and prolonged seizures. Heme-negative urine may appear red, cola colored, or burgundy, owing to ingestion of various drugs or food dyes, whereas dark brown (or black) urine may result from various urinary metabolites.

Evaluation of the child with hematuria begins with a careful history, physical examination, and urinalysis. This information is used to determine the level of hematuria (i.e., upper vs. lower urinary tract) and to determine the urgency of the evaluation

BOX 501–1. Imposters of Hematuria

HEME-POSITIVE
Hemoglobin
Myoglobin

HEME-NEGATIVE

Drugs
Chloroquine
Deferoxamine
Ibuprofen
Iron sorbitol
Metronidazole
Nitrofurantoin
Phenazopyridine (Pyridium)
Phenolphthalein
Phenothiazines
Rifampin
Salicylates
Sulfasalazine

Dyes (vegetable/fruit): beets, blackberries, food coloring

Metabolites
Homogentisic acid
Melanin
Methemoglobin
Porphyrin
Tyrosinosis
Urates

based on the symptomatology. In addition, special consideration needs to be given to family history, identification of anatomic abnormalities/malformation syndromes, and presence of gross hematuria.

Causes of hematuria are listed in Box 501–2. Upper urinary tract sources of hematuria originate within the nephron (i.e., glomerulus, convoluted/collecting tubules and interstitium). Lower urinary tract sources of hematuria originate from the pelvocalyceal system, ureter, bladder, or urethra. Hematuria from within the glomerulus is frequently associated with brown, cola-colored, or burgundy urine, proteinuria exceeding 100 mg/dL via dipstick, red blood cell casts, and deformed urinary RBCs. Hematuria originating within the convoluted or collecting tubules may be associated with the presence of leukocyte or renal tubular epithelial cell casts. On the other hand, lower urinary tract sources of hematuria may be associated with gross hematuria, terminal hematuria (i.e., onset of gross hematuria occurs at the end of the urine stream), blood clots, normal urinary RBC morphology, and minimal proteinuria on dipstick (i.e. <100 mg/dL).

Patients with hematuria may present with a number of symptoms suggestive of specific disorders. Tea or cola-colored urine,

BOX 501–2. Causes of Hematuria in Children

GLOMERULAR HEMATURIA

Isolated Renal Disease

IgA nephropathy (i.e., Berger disease)
Alport syndrome (hereditary nephritis)
Thin glomerular basement membrane nephropathy
Postinfectious GN* (i.e., poststreptococcal GN)
Membranous nephropathy
Membranoproliferative GN
Focal segmental glomerulosclerosis
Anti–glomerular basement membrane disease

Multisystem Disease

Systemic lupus erythematosus nephritis*
Henoch-Schönlein purpura nephritis
Wegener granulomatosis
Polyarteritis nodosa
Goodpasture syndrome
Hemolytic-uremic syndrome
Sickle cell glomerulopathy
HIV nephropathy

EXTRAGLOMERULAR HEMATURIA

Upper Urinary Tract
Tubulointerstitial
  Pyelonephritis
  Interstitial nephritis
  Acute tubular necrosis
  Papillary necrosis
  Nephrocalcinosis
Vascular
  Arterial/venous thrombosis
  Malformations (aneurysms, hemangiomas)
  Nutcracker syndrome
Crystalluria
  Calcium
  Oxalate
  Uric acid
Hemoglobinopathy (sickle cell trait/disease, SC hemoglobin)
Anatomic
  Hydronephrosis
  Cystic kidney disease
    Polycystic kidney disease
    Multicystic dysplasia
  Tumor (Wilms, rhabdomyosarcoma, angiomyolipoma)
  Trauma

Lower Urinary Tract
Inflammation (infectious and noninfectious)
  Cystitis
  Urethritis
Urolithiasis
Trauma
Coagulopathy
Heavy exercise
Munchausen/Munchausen-by-proxy syndrome

---

*Denotes glomerulonephritides presenting with hypocomplementemia.
GN = glomerulonephritis

Finally, patients with a history of trauma require immediate evaluation. Child abuse must always be suspected in the child presenting with unexplained bruising and hematuria.

A careful family history is crucial in the initial assessment of the child with hematuria in view of numerous genetic causes of renal disorders. Hereditary glomerular diseases include hereditary nephritis (Alport syndrome), thin glomerular basement membrane disease, SLE nephritis, and IgA nephropathy (Berger disease). Other renal disorders with a hereditary component include polycystic kidney disease, urolithiasis, and sickle cell disease/trait.

Physical examination is critical in assessing the cause of hematuria. Hypertension, body edema, hepatosplenomegaly, or signs of congestive heart failure suggest acute glomerulonephritis. Several malformation syndromes are associated with renal disease including VATER (*v*ertebral body anomalies, *a*nal atresia, *t*racheo-*e*sophageal fistula and *r*enal dysplasia) syndrome. Abdominal masses may be caused by posterior urethral valves, ureteropelvic junction obstruction, polycystic kidney disease, or Wilms tumor. Hematuria seen in patients with neurologic or cutaneous abnormalities may be the result of renal cystic disease or tumors associated with several syndromes, including tuberous sclerosis, von Hippel-Lindau syndrome, and Zellweger (cerebrohepatorenal) syndrome. Finally, anatomic abnormalities of the external genitals may be associated with renal disease.

Patients with gross hematuria present additional challenges because of the associated parental anxiety. This entity must be distinguished from *urethrorrhagia,* which refers to urethral bleeding (in the absence of urine) associated with dysuria and blood spots on underwear after voiding. This condition, which often occurs in prepubertal boys at intervals several months apart over a period of many years, has a benign self-limited course. Common causes of gross hematuria are listed in Box 501–3. The most common cause of gross hematuria is either documented or suspected urinary tract infections. Less than 10% of patients have evidence of glomerulonephritis. Recurrent episodes of gross hematuria suggest IgA nephropathy, Alport syndrome, thin glomerular basement membrane disease, hypercalciuria, or urolithiasis.

A general approach to the laboratory and radiologic evaluation of the patient with glomerular or extraglomerular hematuria is outlined in Figure 501–1. Asymptomatic patients with isolated microscopic hematuria should not undergo diagnostic evaluation until at least two additional urine specimens collected over a 1–2 wk period demonstrate an abnormal number of RBCs. This will reduce the number of unnecessary evaluations by tenfold to a hundredfold.

The child with persistent asymptomatic isolated microscopic hematuria of greater than 2 wk duration poses a dilemma as to the extent to which one should pursue diagnostic evaluation. It is recommended that the initial evaluation of these children includes a urine culture followed by a spot urine for calcium and creatinine

facial/body edema, hypertension, and oliguria suggest the acute nephritic syndrome. Diseases commonly presenting as acute nephritic syndrome include postinfectious glomerulonephritis, IgA nephropathy, membranoproliferative glomerulonephritis, Henoch-Schönlein purpura nephritis (HSP), systemic lupus erythematosus (SLE) nephritis, Wegener granulomatosis, microscopic polyarteritis nodosa, Goodpasture syndrome, and hemolytic-uremic syndrome. A history of recent upper respiratory, skin, or gastrointestinal infection suggests acute glomerulonephritis, hemolytic-uremic syndrome, or HSP. Rash and joint complaints point toward HSP or SLE. Frequency, dysuria, and unexplained fevers suggest a urinary tract infection whereas renal colic suggests nephrolithiasis. A flank mass may signal hydronephrosis, cystic disease, renal vein thrombosis, or tumor. Hematuria associated with headache, visual changes, epistaxis, or congestive heart failure suggests significant hypertension.

BOX 501–3. Common Causes of Gross Hematuria

Urinary tract infection
Meatal stenosis
Perineal irritation
Trauma
Urolithiasis/hypercalciuria
Coagulopathy
Tumor
Glomerular
  IgA nephropathy
  Alport syndrome (hereditary nephritis)
  Thin glomerular basement membrane disease
  Postinfectious glomerulonephritis
  Henoch-Schönlein purpura nephritis
  Systemic lupus erythematosus nephritis

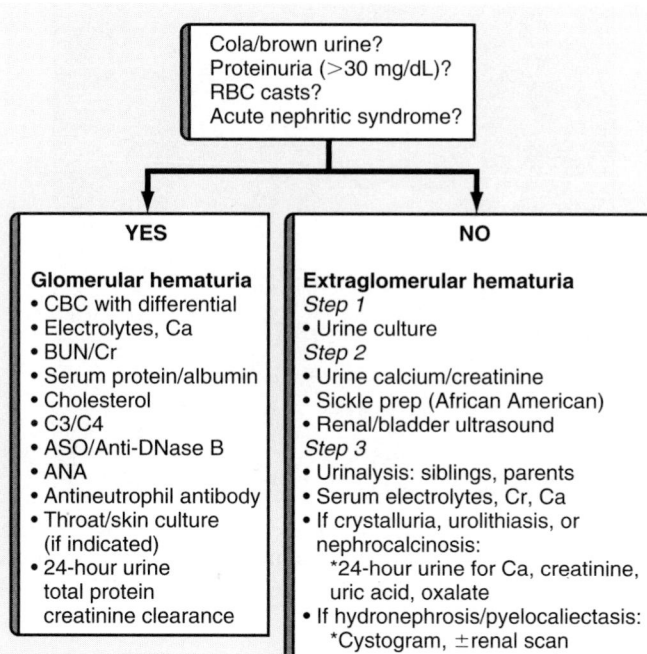

Cola/brown urine?
Proteinuria (>30 mg/dL)?
RBC casts?
Acute nephritic syndrome?

YES

Glomerular hematuria
• CBC with differential
• Electrolytes, Ca
• BUN/Cr
• Serum protein/albumin
• Cholesterol
• C3/C4
• ASO/Anti-DNase B
• ANA
• Antineutrophil antibody
• Throat/skin culture
  (if indicated)
• 24-hour urine
  total protein
  creatinine clearance

NO

Extraglomerular hematuria
Step 1
• Urine culture
Step 2
• Urine calcium/creatinine
• Sickle prep (African American)
• Renal/bladder ultrasound
Step 3
• Urinalysis: siblings, parents
• Serum electrolytes, Cr, Ca
• If crystalluria, urolithiasis, or
  nephrocalcinosis:
    *24-hour urine for Ca, creatinine,
    uric acid, oxalate
• If hydronephrosis/pyelocaliectasis:
    *Cystogram, ±renal scan

FIGURE 501–1. Algorithm of general approach to the laboratory and radiologic evaluation of the patient with glomerular or extraglomerular hematuria. CBC = complete blood cell count; BUN = blood urea nitrogen; C3/C4 = complement; ASO = antistreptolysin O; ANA = antinuclear antibody; Cr = creatinine.

concentration in culture-negative patients. In African-American patients, a sickle cell screen should be included. Renal and bladder ultrasonography should be considered to rule out structural lesions such as tumor, cystic disease, hydronephrosis, or urolithiasis. Ultrasonography of the urinary tract is most informative in patients presenting with gross hematuria, abdominal pain, flank pain, or trauma. If these initial studies are normal, assessment of serum creatinine and electrolytes is recommended.

The finding of certain hematologic abnormalities may narrow the differential diagnosis. Anemia in this setting may be caused by (1) intravascular dilution secondary to hypervolemia associated with acute renal failure; (2) decreased RBC production in chronic renal failure; (3) hemolysis from hemolytic-uremic syndrome or SLE; and (4) blood loss from pulmonary hemorrhage as seen in Goodpasture syndrome or melena in patients with Henoch-Schönlein purpura or hemolytic-uremic syndrome. Inspection of the peripheral blood smear may reveal a microangiopathic process as seen in the hemolytic-uremic syndrome, renal vein thrombosis, vasculitis, and SLE. In the latter, the presence of autoantibodies may result in a positive Coombs test, the presence of antinuclear antibody, leukopenia, and multisystem disease. Thrombocytopenia may result from decreased platelet production (malignancies) or increased platelet consumption (SLE, idiopathic thrombocytopenic purpura, hemolytic-uremic syndrome, renal vein thrombosis). Although urinary RBC morphology may be normal with lower tract bleeding and dysmorphic from glomerular bleeding, cell morphology does not reliably correlate with the site of hematuria. The best screening test for a bleeding diathesis is a thorough history. Coagulation studies are not routinely obtained unless personal or family history suggests a bleeding tendency.

A voiding cystourethrogram is only required in patients with a urinary tract infection, renal scarring, hydroureter, or pyelocaliectasis. Cystoscopy, an unnecessary and costly procedure in patients with hematuria that carries the associated risks of anesthesia, should be reserved for the evaluation of the rare child

with a bladder mass noted on ultrasound, urethral abnormalities caused by trauma, posterior urethral valves, or tumor. Unilateral gross hematuria identified by cystoscopy is rarely encountered in the pediatric patient.

Referral to a pediatric nephrologist is recommended for patients with nephritis (i.e., glomerulonephritis and tubulointerstitial nephritis), hypertension, renal insufficiency, urolithiasis/nephrocalcinosis, or a family history of renal disease such as polycystic kidney disease or hereditary nephritis. Renal biopsy is indicated for children with persistent microscopic hematuria or recurrent gross hematuria associated with decreased renal function, proteinuria, or hypertension.

Children with persistent asymptomatic isolated hematuria and a normal evaluation should have their serum creatinine values checked annually and their blood pressure and urine checked every 3 mo until the hematuria resolves. Diagnoses to be considered in this situation include resolving postinfectious glomerulonephritis, thin basement membrane disease, IgA nephropathy, or heavy exercise/trauma. Referral to a pediatric nephrologist should be considered for patients with persistent asymptomatic hematuria greater than 1 yr duration.

Feld LG, Waz WR, Perez LM, et al: Hematuria. An integrated medical and surgical approach. *Pediatr Clin North Am* 1997; 44:1191–1210.
Feld LG, Meyers K, Kaplan BS, et al: Limited evaluation of microscopic hematuria in pediatrics. *Pediatrics* 1998; 102:e42.

Chapter 502

Isolated Glomerular Diseases with Recurrent Gross Hematuria

Approximately 10% of children with gross hematuria have either an acute or chronic form of glomerulonephritis that may be associated with a systemic illness. The gross hematuria, which is usually characterized by brown or cola-colored urine, may be painless or associated with vague flank or abdominal pain. Presentation with gross hematuria is common within 1–2 days after the onset of an apparent viral upper respiratory tract infection in many forms of glomerulonephritis, such as IgA nephropathy, and typically resolves within 5 days. This relatively short period contrasts to a latency period of 7–21 days occurring between the onset of a streptococcal pharyngitis or impetigo skin infection and the development of acute glomerulonephritis. Gross hematuria in these circumstances may last as long as 4–6 wk. Gross hematuria may also be seen in children with glomerular basement membrane (GBM) disorders such as hereditary nephritis (i.e., Alport syndrome) and thin GBM disease. However, these glomerular diseases may also present as microscopic hematuria and/or proteinuria without gross hematuria.

502.1 IgA Nephropathy (Berger Nephropathy)

IgA nephropathy is the most common chronic glomerular disease worldwide. It is characterized by a predominance of IgA within mesangial deposits of the glomerulus in the absence of systemic diseases such as systemic lupus erythematosus or Henoch-Schönlein purpura. Other diseases with prominent IgA mesangial deposition include rheumatoid arthritis, ankylosing spondylitis, Reiter syndrome, and hepatic cirrhosis.

Pathology and Pathologic Diagnosis. On light microscopy, focal and segmental mesangial proliferation and increased mesangial matrix are seen in the glomerulus (Fig. 502–1). Some children display generalized mesangial proliferation which may be associated with crescent formation and scarring. IgA is the predominant immunoglobulin deposited in the mesangium (Fig. 502–2), but lesser amounts of IgG, IgM, C3, and properdin are common. Electron microscopic studies demonstrate electron-dense mesangial deposits in most patients. Electron-dense deposits may also be seen in the subendothelial and subepithelial regions of the GBM.

Although the pathogenesis remains to be elucidated, IgA nephropathy is an immune complex disease that appears to be caused by abnormalities in the IgA immune system. Furthermore, familial clustering of IgA nephropathy cases suggests the importance of genetic factors. Genetic studies using genome-wide linkage analysis suggest linkage of IgA nephropathy to 6q22-23 in multiplex IgA nephropathy kindreds.

Clinical and Laboratory Manifestations. A majority of children with IgA nephropathy in the United States and Europe present with gross hematuria whereas microscopic hematuria and/or proteinuria is a more common presentation in Japan. Other types of presentation include acute nephritic syndrome, nephrotic syndrome, or a combined nephritic-nephrotic syndrome. Also, IgA nephropathy is seen more often in males than in females. Gross hematuria often occurs in association with an upper respiratory or gastrointestinal infection and may be associated with loin pain. Proteinuria is frequently less than 1,000 mg/24 hr in patients with asymptomatic microscopic hematuria. Mild to moderate hypertension is most often seen in patients with nephritic or nephrotic syndrome but is rarely severe enough to result in hypertensive emergencies. Normal serum levels of C3 in IgA nephropathy help to distinguish this disorder from post-streptococcal glomerulonephritis. Serum IgA levels have no diagnostic value because they are elevated in only 15% of patients.

Prognosis and Treatment. Although IgA nephropathy does not lead to significant kidney damage in most children, progressive disease develops in 20–30% of children at 15–20 yr after disease onset. Therefore, most children with IgA nephropathy will not display progressive renal dysfunction until adulthood, prompting the need for careful long-term follow-up. Poor prognostic indicators include persistent hypertension, diminished renal function, and heavy or prolonged proteinuria. A worse prognosis is suggested by histologic evidence of diffuse mesangial proliferation, extensive glomerular crescents, glomeruloscle-

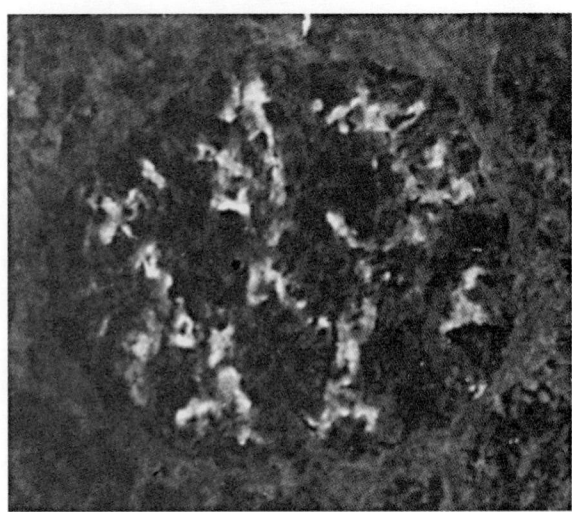

FIGURE 502–2. Immunofluorescence microscopy of the biopsy from a child having recurrent episodes of gross hematuria demonstrating mesangial deposition of IgA. (×250.)

rosis, and tubulointerstitial changes, including inflammation and fibrosis.

The primary treatment of IgA nephropathy is proper blood pressure control. A controlled study in adults with IgA nephropathy suggests that fish oil, which contains anti-inflammatory omega-3 fatty acids, may decrease the rate of renal progression. Immunosuppressive therapy with corticosteroids or more intensive, multidrug regimens may be beneficial in some patients. The benefits of angiotensin-converting enzyme inhibitors and angiotensin II receptor antagonists in reducing proteinuria and retarding the rate of renal progression remain to be determined. Prophylactic antibiotics and tonsillectomy may reduce the frequency of gross hematuria but have no proven benefit on reducing the rate of renal disease progression. Patients with IgA nephropathy may undergo successful renal transplantation. Although recurrent disease is frequent, allograft loss caused by IgA nephropathy occurs in only 15–30% of patients.

Bartosik LP, Lajoie, Sugar L, Cattran DC: Predicting progression in IgA nephropathy. *Am J Kidney Dis* 2001; 38:728–35.
Donadio JV Jr, Larson TS, Bergstralh EJ, et al: A randomized trial of high-dose compared with low-dose omega-3 fatty acids in severe IgA nephropathy. *J Am Soc Nephrol* 2001; 12:791–99.
Gharavi AG, Yan Y, Scolari F, et al: IgA nephropathy, the most common cause of glomerulonephritis is linked to 6q22–23. *Nat Genet* 2000; 26:354–57.
Wang AY, Lai FM, Yu AW, et al: Recurrent IgA nephropathy in renal transplant allografts. *Am J Kidney Dis* 2001; 38:588–96.
Wyatt RJ, Hogg RJ: Evidence-based assessment of treatment options for children with IgA nephropathies. *Pediatr Nephrol* 2001; 16:156–67.
Yoshikawa N, Tanaka R, Iijima K: Pathophysiology and treatment of IgA nephropathy in children. *Pediatr Nephrol* 2001; 16:446–57.

502.2 Alport Syndrome

Alport syndrome (AS), hereditary nephritis, is a genetically heterogeneous disease caused by mutations in the genes coding for type IV collagen, a major component of basement membranes. These genetic alterations are associated with marked variability in clinical presentation, natural history, and histologic abnormalities.

Genetics. Approximately 85% of patients have X-linked disease caused by a mutation in the *COL4A5* gene encoding the α5 chain of type IV collagen. Patients with a subtype of X-linked AS and diffuse leiomyomatosis demonstrate a contiguous mutation within the *COL4A5* and *COL4A6* genes that encodes the α5 and

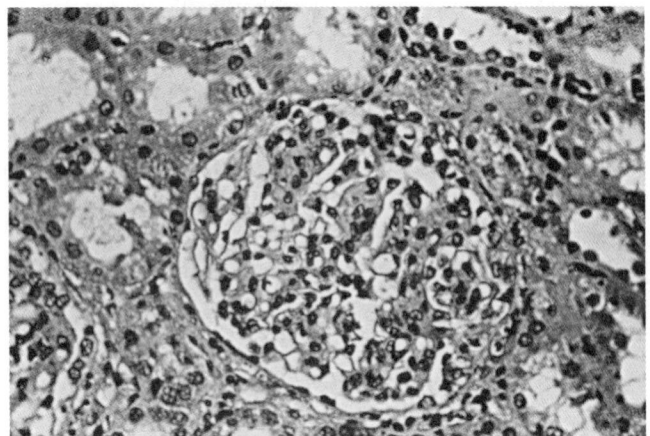

FIGURE 502–1. Light microscopy of IgA nephropathy demonstrating segmental mesangial proliferation and increased matrix. (×180.)

α6 chains, respectively, of type IV collagen. Autosomal recessive forms of AS are caused by mutations in the *COL4A3* and *COL4A4* genes on chromosome 2 encoding the α3 and α4 chains, respectively, of type IV collagen. An autosomal dominant form of AS linked to the *COL4A3-COL4A4* gene locus occurs in 5% of cases.

Pathology. Kidney biopsy specimens during the first decade of life may show few changes on light microscopy. Later, the glomeruli may develop mesangial proliferation and capillary wall thickening, leading to progressive glomerular sclerosis. Tubular atrophy, interstitial inflammation and fibrosis, and presence of lipid containing tubular or interstitial cells, referred to as foam cells, develop as the disease progresses. Immunopathologic studies are usually nondiagnostic.

In most patients, electron microscopic studies reveal diffuse thickening, thinning, splitting, and layering of the basement membranes of the glomeruli (Fig. 502–3) and tubules. However, ultrastructural analysis of the GBM may be completely normal, display nonspecific alterations, or demonstrate only uniform thinning in families that have the typical clinical manifestations of AS.

Clinical Manifestations. All patients with Alport syndrome have asymptomatic microscopic hematuria, which may be intermittent in girls and younger boys. Single or recurrent episodes of gross hematuria commonly occurring 1–2 days after an upper respiratory infection are seen in approximately 50% of patients. Proteinuria is frequently seen in males but may be absent, mild, or intermittent in females. Progressive proteinuria, often exceeding 1 g/24 hr, is common by the second decade of life and can be severe enough to cause nephrotic syndrome.

Extrarenal manifestations of AS include hearing deficits and ocular abnormalities. Bilateral sensorineural hearing loss, which is never congenital in onset, occurs in 90% of hemizygous males with X-linked AS, 10% of heterozygous females with X-linked AS, and 67% of individuals with autosomal recessive AS. This deficit begins in the high-frequency range but progresses to involve conversational speech, prompting the need for hearing aids. Ocular abnormalities, which occur in 30–40% of patients with X-linked AS, include anterior lenticonus (extrusion of the central portion of the lens into the anterior chamber), macular flecks, and corneal erosions. Leiomyomatosis of the esophagus, tracheobronchial tree, and female genitals and platelet abnormalities are rarely seen.

Diagnosis. A careful family history, a screening urinalysis of first-degree relatives, an audiogram, and an ophthalmologic examination are critical in making the diagnosis of AS. Presence of anterior lenticonus is pathognomonic. AS is highly likely in the patient with hematuria and at least two of the following characteristic clinical features: macular flecks, recurrent corneal erosions, GBM thickening and thinning, and sensorineural deafness. Absence of epidermal basement membrane staining for the α5 chain of type IV collagen in male hemizygotes and discontinuous epidermal basement membrane staining in female heterozygotes is pathognomonic for X-linked AS. Mutation screening or linkage analysis is not readily available for routine clinical use. Prenatal diagnosis is available for families with X-linked AS individuals who carry an identified mutation.

Prognosis and Treatment. The risk of progressive renal dysfunction leading to end-stage renal disease (ESRD) is highest among hemizygotes and autosomal recessive homozygotes. ESRD occurs before age 30 yr in approximately 75% of hemizygotes with X-linked AS. The risk of ESRD in X-linked heterozygotes is 12% by age 40 and 30% by age 60. Risk factors for progression are gross hematuria during childhood, nephrotic syndrome, and prominent GBM thickening. Intrafamilial variation in phenotypic expression results in significant differences in the age of ESRD among family members. No specific therapy is available to treat AS, although some studies suggest that cyclosporine and angiotensin-converting enzyme inhibitors may slow the rate of renal progression. Careful management of renal failure complications such as hypertension, anemia, and electrolyte imbalance is critical. Patients with ESRD are treated with dialysis and successful kidney transplantation. Approximately 5% of renal transplant recipients develop anti-GBM nephritis, which occurs primarily in males with X-linked AS who develop ESRD before age 30 yr.

Bernstein J: The glomerular basement membrane abnormality in Alport syndrome. *Am J Kidney Dis* 1987; 10:222.

Jais JP, Knebelman B, Giatras I, et al: X-linked Alport syndrome: Natural history in 195 families and genotype-phenotype correlations in males. *J Am Soc Nephrol* 2000; 11:649–657.

Kashtan C: Alport syndromes: Phenotypic heterogeneity of progressive hereditary nephritis. *Pediatr Nephrol* 2000, 14:502–512.

Kashtan C: Alport syndrome and thin glomerular basement membrane disease. *J Am Soc Nephrol* 1998; 9:1736–1750.

Pirson Y: Making the diagnosis of Alport syndrome. *Kidney Int* 1999; 56:760–775.

502.3 Thin Glomerular Basement Membrane Disease

Thin glomerular basement membrane disease (TGBMD) is defined by the presence of persistent microscopic hematuria and isolated thinning of the GBM on electron microscopy. Isolated hematuria in multiple family members without renal dysfunction is referred to as *benign familial hematuria*.

TGBMD may be sporadic or transmitted as an autosomal dominant trait. Mutations in the *COL4A3* and *COL4A4* genes among heterozygotes with benign familial hematuria have been reported. However, family kindreds with isolated GBM thinning and no identified mutations within the type IV collagen genes have also been reported.

Microscopic hematuria is usually persistent and often initially observed during childhood. However, hematuria may initially present in adulthood and may be intermittent. Episodic gross hematuria may also be present, particularly after a respiratory illness. There is no treatment. Progressive renal insufficiency, hypertension, proteinuria, and extrarenal manifestations of TGBMD are rare and suggest the presence of AS. GBM thinning may also be seen in IgA nephropathy.

Buzza M, Wang YY, Dagher H, et al: COL4A4 mutation in thin basement membrane disease previously described in Alport syndrome. *Kidney Int* 2001; 60:480–483.

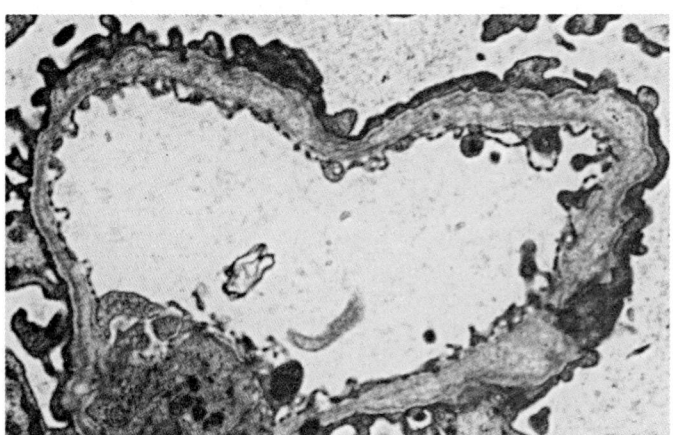

FIGURE 502–3. Electron micrograph of the biopsy specimen from a child with Alport syndrome depicting thickening, thinning, splitting, and layering of the glomerular basement membrane. (×16,250.) (From Yum M, Bergstein JM: Basement membrane nephropathy. *Hum Pathol* 14:996, 1983.)

Chapter 503
Glomerulonephritis Associated with Infections

503.1 Acute Poststreptococcal Glomerulonephritis

This disease is a classic example of the acute nephritic syndrome characterized by the sudden onset of gross hematuria, edema, hypertension, and renal insufficiency. Acute poststreptococcal glomerulonephritis is one of the most common glomerular causes of gross hematuria in children, surpassed only by IgA nephropathy.

Etiology and Epidemiology. Acute poststreptococcal glomerulonephritis follows infection of the throat or skin by certain "nephritogenic" strains of group A β-hemolytic streptococci. The factors that allow only certain strains of streptococci to be nephritogenic remain unclear. Poststreptococcal glomerulonephritis commonly follows streptococcal pharyngitis during cold weather months and streptococcal skin infections or pyoderma during warm weather months. Although epidemics of nephritis have been described in association with both throat (serotype 12) and skin (serotype 49) infections, this disease is most commonly sporadic.

Pathology. As in most forms of acute glomerulonephritis, the kidneys appear symmetrically enlarged. On light microscopy, all glomeruli appear enlarged and relatively bloodless and show diffuse mesangial cell proliferation with an increase in mesangial matrix (Fig. 503–1). Polymorphonuclear leukocytes are common in glomeruli during the early stage of the disease. Crescents and interstitial inflammation may be seen in severe cases. These changes are not specific for poststreptococcal glomerulonephritis. Immunofluorescence microscopy reveals lumpy-bumpy deposits of immunoglobulin and complement on the glomerular basement membrane (GBM) and in the mesangium. On electron microscopy, electron-dense deposits, or "humps," are observed on the epithelial side of the GBM (Fig. 503–2).

Pathogenesis. Although morphologic studies and a depression in the serum complement (C3) level strongly suggest that post-

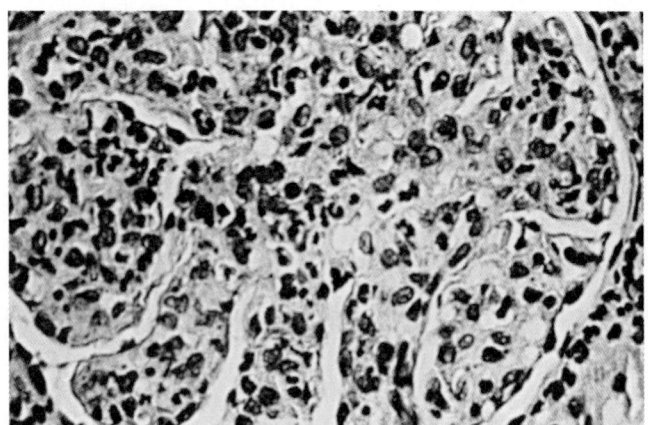

FIGURE 503–1. Glomerulus from a patient having poststreptococcal glomerulonephritis appearing enlarged and relatively bloodless and showing mesangial proliferation and exudation of neutrophils. (×400.)

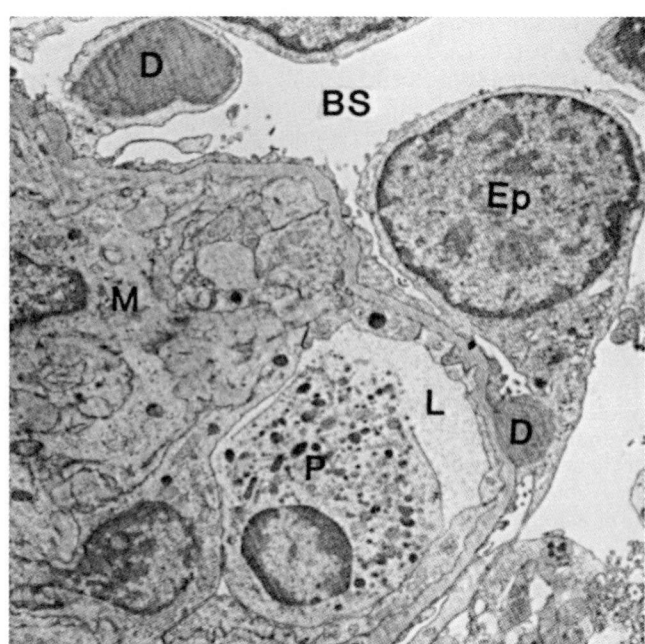

FIGURE 503–2. Electron micrograph in poststreptococcal glomerulonephritis demonstrating electron-dense deposits (D) on the epithelial cell (Ep) side of the glomerular basement membrane. A polymorphonuclear leukocyte (P) is present within the lumen (L) of the capillary. BS = Bowman space; M = mesangium.

streptococcal glomerulonephritis is mediated by immune complexes, the precise mechanisms by which nephritogenic streptococci induce complex formation remain to be determined. Despite clinical and histologic similarities to acute serum sickness in rabbits, the finding of circulating immune complexes in poststreptococcal glomerulonephritis is not uniform and complement activation is primarily through the alternative rather than the classic (immune complex activated) pathway.

Clinical Manifestations. Poststreptococcal glomerulonephritis is most common in children aged 5–12 yr and uncommon before the age of 3 yr. The typical patient develops an acute nephritic syndrome 1–2 wk after an antecedent streptococcal pharyngitis or 3–6 wk after a streptococcal pyoderma. The severity of renal involvement varies from asymptomatic microscopic hematuria with normal renal function to acute renal failure. Depending on the severity of renal involvement, patients may develop various degrees of edema, hypertension, and oliguria. Patients may develop encephalopathy and/or heart failure owing to hypertension or hypervolemia. Encephalopathy may also result directly from the toxic effects of the streptococcal bacteria on the central nervous system. Edema typically results from salt and water retention and nephrotic syndrome may develop in 10–20% of cases. Specific symptoms such as malaise, lethargy, abdominal or flank pain, and fever are common. Acute subglottic edema and airway compromise has also been reported. The acute phase generally resolves within 6–8 wk. Although urinary protein excretion and hypertension usually normalize by 4–6 wk after onset, persistent microscopic hematuria may persist for 1–2 yr after the initial presentation.

Diagnosis. Urinalysis demonstrates red blood cells (RBCs), frequently in association with RBC casts, proteinuria, and polymorphonuclear leukocytes. A mild normochromic anemia may be present from hemodilution and low-grade hemolysis. The serum C3 level is usually reduced in the acute phase and returns to normal 6–8 wk after onset.

Confirmation of the diagnosis requires clear evidence of invasive streptococcal infection. A positive throat culture report may support the diagnosis or may simply represent the carrier state. On the other hand, a rising antibody titer to streptococcal antigen(s) confirms a recent streptococcal infection. Importantly, the antistreptolysin O titer is commonly elevated after a pharyngeal infection but rarely increases after streptococcal skin infections. The best single antibody titer to document cutaneous streptococcal infection is the deoxyribonuclease (DNase) B antigen. The Streptozyme test (Wampole Laboratories, Stamford, CT) is an alternative study that detects antibodies to streptolysin O, DNase B, hyaluronidase, streptokinase, and nicotinamide-adenine dinucleotidase using a slide agglutination test.

The clinical diagnosis of poststreptococcal glomerulonephritis is quite likely in a child presenting with acute nephritic syndrome, evidence of recent streptococcal infection, and a low C3 level. However, it is important to consider other diagnoses such as systemic lupus erythematosus and an acute exacerbation of chronic glomerulonephritis. Renal biopsy should be considered only in the presence of acute renal failure, nephrotic syndrome, absence of evidence for streptococcal infection, or normal complement levels. Also, renal biopsy is considered when hematuria and proteinuria, diminished renal function, and/or a low C3 level persist more than 2 mo after onset.

The differential diagnosis of poststreptococcal glomerulonephritis includes many of the causes of hematuria listed in Box 501–2. Acute glomerulonephritis may also follow infection with coagulase-positive and coagulase-negative staphylococci, *Streptococcus pneumoniae*, and gram-negative bacteria. Also, bacterial endocarditis may produce a hypocomplementemic glomerulonephritis with renal failure. Finally, acute glomerulonephritis may occur after certain fungal, rickettsial, and viral diseases, particularly, influenza.

Complications. Acute complications of this disease result primarily from hypertension and acute renal dysfunction. Hypertension is seen in 60% of patients and may be associated with hypertensive encephalopathy in 10% of cases. Other potential complications include heart failure, hyperkalemia, hyperphosphatemia, hypocalcemia, acidosis, seizures, and uremia.

Prevention. Early systemic antibiotic therapy for streptococcal throat and skin infections does not eliminate the risk of glomerulonephritis. Family members of patients with acute glomerulonephritis should be cultured for group A β-hemolytic streptococci and treated if culture positive.

Treatment. Management is directed at treating the acute effects of renal insufficiency and hypertension (see Chapter 527.1). Although a 10-day course of systemic antibiotic therapy with penicillin is recommended to limit the spread of the nephritogenic organisms, antibiotic therapy does not affect the natural history of glomerulonephritis. Sodium restriction, diuresis, and pharmacotherapy with calcium channel antagonists, vasodilators, or angiotensin-converting enzyme inhibitors are standard therapies used to treat hypertension.

Prognosis. Complete recovery occurs in more than 95% of children with acute poststreptococcal glomerulonephritis. Mortality in the acute stage can be avoided by appropriate management of acute renal failure, cardiac failure, and hypertension. Infrequently, the acute phase may be severe and lead to glomerular hyalinization and chronic renal insufficiency. However, the diagnosis of acute poststreptococcal glomerulonephritis must be questioned in patients with chronic renal dysfunction because other diagnoses such as membranoproliferative glomerulonephritis may be present. Recurrences are extremely rare.

Clark G, White RHR, Glasgow EF, et al: Poststreptococcal glomerulonephritis in children: Clinicopathological correlations and long-term prognosis. *Pediatr Nephrol* 1988; 2:381.

Dodge WF, Spargo BH, Travis LB, et al: Poststreptococcal glomerulonephritis in children: A prospective study. *N Engl J Med* 1972; 286:273–78.

Potter EV, Lipschultz SA, Abidh S, et al: Twelve to fifteen-year follow-up of patients with poststreptococcal acute glomerulonephritis in Trinidad. N Engl J Med 1982; 307:725–29.

Vogl W, Renke M, Mayer-Eichberger D, et al: Long-term prognosis for endocapillary glomerulonephritis of poststreptococcal type in children and adults. Nephron 1986; 44:58.

503.2 Other Chronic Infections

Occurrence of glomerulonephritis has been recognized during the course of various chronic infections, including bacterial endocarditis caused by *Streptococcus viridans* and other organisms, ventriculoatrial shunts for hydrocephalus infected with *Staphylococcus epidermidis*, syphilis, hepatitis B virus, hepatitis C virus, and candidiasis. Parasitic infections associated with glomerular disease include malaria, schistosomiasis, leishmaniasis, filariasis, hydatid disease, trypanosomiasis, and toxoplasmosis. In each condition, the infecting organism has low virulence and the host is chronically infected with foreign antigen. In the presence of high levels of circulating antigen, the host's antibody response leads to formation of immune complexes that deposit in the kidneys and initiate glomerular inflammation.

The histopathologic findings may resemble poststreptococcal, membranous, or membranoproliferative glomerulonephritis. The clinical manifestations are generally those of an acute nephritic or nephrotic syndrome. The complement C3 level is frequently depressed.

Eradication of the infection before severe glomerular injury occurs usually results in resolution of the glomerulonephritis. Progression to end-stage renal failure has been described.

Chesney RW, O'Regan S, Guyda HJ, et al: *Candida* endocrinopathy syndrome with membranoproliferative glomerulonephritis: Demonstration of glomerular *Candida* antigen. *Clin Nephrol* 1976; 5:232.

Hendrickse RG, Adeniyi A: Quartan malarial nephrotic syndrome in children. *Kidney Int* 1979; 16:64.

Hunte W, Al-Ghraoui F, Cohen RJ: Secondary syphilis and the nephrotic syndrome. *J Am Soc Nephrol* 1993; 3:1351.

Johnson RJ, Couser WG: Hepatitis B infection and renal disease: Clinical, immunopathogenic and therapeutic considerations. *Kidney Int* 1990; 37:663.

Johnson RJ, Gretch DR, Yamabe H, et al: Membranoproliferative glomerulonephritis associated with hepatitis C virus infection. *N Engl J Med* 1993; 328:465.

Neugarten J, Baldwin DS: Glomerulonephritis in bacterial endocarditis. *Am J Med* 1984; 77:297.

Vella J, Carmody M, Campbell E, et al: Glomerulonephritis after ventriculo-atrial shunt. *Q J Med* 1995; 88:911.

Walters S, Levin M: Infectious diseases and the kidney. In Barratt TM, Avner ED, Harmon WE (editors): *Pediatric Nephrology*, 4th ed. Baltimore, Lippincott, Williams, and Wilkins, 1999, pp 1079–1102.

Chapter 504
Membranous Glomerulopathy (Glomerulonephritis)

Although membranous glomerulopathy is the most common cause of nephrotic syndrome in adults, it is an uncommon cause of hematuria in children. Membranous glomerulopathy typically presents as an isolated renal disease. However, it may be associated with systemic illnesses, including autoimmune diseases such as systemic lupus erythematosus or chronic immune thrombocytopenic purpura, sarcoidosis, neuroblastoma, gonadoblastoma, gold or penicillamine therapy, syphilis, and hepatitis B virus infections. These secondary causes of membranous glomerulopathy are more common in children compared to adults. Furthermore, identification of these secondary causes of membranous glomerulopathy is important because treatment of these diseases may lead to resolution of the glomerular lesions.

Pathology. By light microscopy, the glomeruli show diffuse thickening of the glomerular basement membrane (GBM), without significant proliferative changes (Fig. 504–1). The thickening presumably results from the production of membrane-like material by the visceral epithelial cells in response to immune complexes deposited on the epithelial side of the membrane. This new material may in certain areas resemble spikes on the epithelial side of the GBM. Immunofluorescent microscopy demonstrates granular deposits of IgG and C3 located on the epithelial side of the GBM when viewed under electron microscopy. Linear staining of IgG, IgA, and C3 along the tubular basement membrane may be seen on immunofluorescence.

Pathogenesis. Morphologic studies suggest that membranous glomerulopathy is an immune complex–mediated disease. However, the molecular pathogenesis of membranous nephropathy in humans remains unknown. Genetic factors may influence disease susceptibility and/or disease progression.

Clinical Manifestations. In children, membranous glomerulopathy is most common in the 2nd decade of life. The disease usually presents as nephrotic syndrome and accounts for 2–6% of childhood nephrotic syndrome cases. Most patients have microscopic hematuria and occasionally gross hematuria. Approximately 20% of children present with hypertension. C3 levels are normal except in cases of systemic lupus erythematosus in which levels may be depressed.

Diagnosis. The diagnosis of membranous nephropathy is confirmed only by kidney biopsy because no single laboratory test is diagnostic. The usual indications for biopsy include the presentation of nephrotic syndrome in a child, usually older than 10 yr, or the presence of unexplained hematuria and proteinuria. Patients with membranous glomerulopathy are at an increased risk for renal vein thrombosis.

Prognosis and Treatment. The clinical course of membranous glomerulopathy is variable, although children presenting with asymptomatic low-grade proteinuria may achieve a spontaneous remission. Follow-up studies of 1–14 yr suggest that 20% of children progress to chronic renal failure whereas 40% continue with active disease. The nephrotic state is best controlled with salt restriction and diuretic agents. Studies in adults suggest that immunosuppressive therapy with prednisone in conjunction with chlorambucil or cyclophosphamide may be beneficial in slowing the rate of progressive renal disease, particularly in patients with severe or prolonged proteinuria, renal insufficiency, or hypertension.

Cattran DC: Idiopathic membranous glomerulonephritis. *Kidney Int* 2000; 59: 1983–1994.
Makker SP: Membranous glomerulopathy. In Barratt TM, Avner ED, Harmon WE (editors): *Pediatric Nephrology,* 4th ed. Baltimore, Lippincott, Williams, and Wilkins, 1999, pp 719–30.
Muirhead N: Management of idiopathic membranous nephropathy: Evidence-based recommendations. *Kidney Int* 1999; 55(Suppl 70):S47–55.

Chapter 505

Membranoproliferative (Mesangiocapillary) Glomerulonephritis

The term *chronic glomerulonephritis* implies continuing glomerular injury that frequently leads to glomerular destruction and end-stage renal failure. Membranoproliferative glomerulonephritis (MPGN) is the most common cause of chronic glomerulonephritis in older children and young adults.

Pathology and Pathogenesis. MPGN was initially distinguished from other forms of chronic glomerulonephritis by the finding of hypocomplementemia in most patients. In some patients, hypocomplementemia results from an antibody, referred to as C3 nephritic factor, that activates the alternative complement pathway. Three histologic types of MPGN are described.

Type I MPGN is the most common form. The glomeruli reveal an accentuation of the lobular pattern, owing to a generalized increase in mesangial cells and matrix (Fig. 505–1). The glomerular capillary walls appear thickened, often containing regions of duplication or splitting from interposition of mesangial cytoplasm and matrix between the endothelial cells and

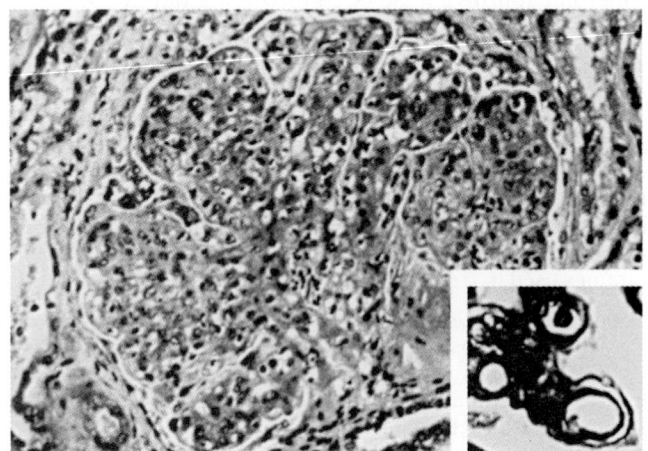

FIGURE 505–1. Glomerulus from a patient with type I membranoproliferative glomerulonephritis demonstrating an accentuated lobular pattern, a generalized increase in mesangial cells and matrix, and "splitting" of the glomerular capillary wall *(inset).* (×250.) (From Kim Y, Michael AF: Idiopathic membranoproliferative glomerulonephritis. Reproduced with permission from the *Annual Review of Medicine,* vol 31. © 1980 by Annual Reviews, Inc.)

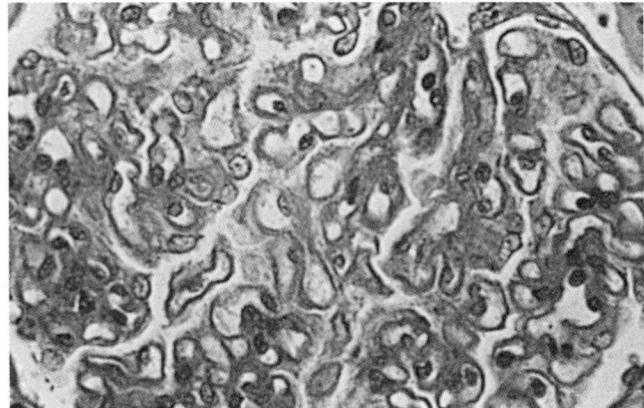

FIGURE 504–1. Glomerulus from a patient having membranous glomerulopathy, demonstrating diffuse thickening of the glomerular basement membrane in the absence of cellular proliferation. (×400.)

glomerular basement membrane (GBM). Crescents may be present and indicate a poor prognosis when detected in a high percentage of glomeruli. Immunofluorescent microscopy reveals C3 and lesser amounts of immunoglobulin in the mesangium and along the peripheral capillary walls in a lobular pattern (Fig. 505–2). Electron microscopy confirms the presence of immune complex–like deposits in the mesangial and subendothelial regions.

In *type II disease*, the mesangial changes are less prominent than in type I. The capillary walls demonstrate irregular ribbon-like thickening owing to the deposition of electron-dense deposits. Splitting of the membrane is rare, but crescents are common. On electron microscopy, the dense deposits are seen as thickenings of GBM in a region distinct from the lamina densa. The deposits are also found in Bowman capsule, mesangium, and tubular basement membranes. Immunofluorescent studies show C3 and minimal immunoglobulin along the margin of the dense deposit material.

In *type III disease*, the light and immunofluorescent microscopic findings resemble those found in type I disease. Electron microscopy reveals contiguous subepithelial and subendothelial deposits associated with disruption and layering of the lamina densa portion of the GBM.

Clinical Manifestations. MPGN is most common in the second decade of life. The majority of patients present with nephrotic syndrome, although others may present with acute nephritic syndrome characterized by gross hematuria or asymptomatic microscopic hematuria and proteinuria. Renal function may be normal or depressed. Hypertension is common. The serum C3 complement level may be decreased.

Diagnosis and Differential Diagnosis. The diagnosis of MPGN is made by renal biopsy. Indications for biopsy include nephrotic syndrome in a child older than 10 yr, significant proteinuria with microscopic hematuria, or hypocomplementemia greater than 8 wk duration in a child with acute nephritis.

Both MPGN and poststreptococcal glomerulonephritis may be associated with gross hematuria, low C3 levels, and elevated antistreptococcal antibody titers. However, patients with poststreptococcal glomerulonephritis improve dramatically within 2 mo of onset whereas nephritic syndrome, proteinuria, and hypocomplementemia persist in children with MPGN, resulting in the need for a kidney biopsy.

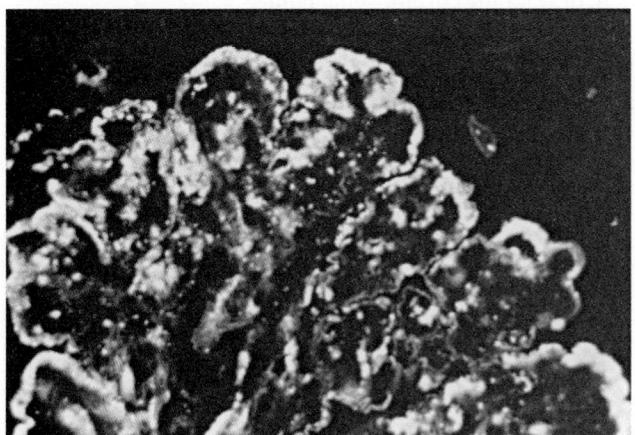

FIGURE 505–2. Immunofluorescence microscopy in type I membranoproliferative glomerulonephritis, demonstrating granular deposition of C3 along the glomerular basement membranes and in the mesangium. (×610.) (From Kim Y, Michael AF: Idiopathic membranoproliferative glomerulonephritis. Reproduced with permission from the *Annual Review of Medicine*, vol 31. © 1980 by Annual Reviews, Inc.)

Prognosis and Treatment. Although some patients recover completely, approximately 50% of patients with MPGN progress to end-stage renal disease 10 yr after their initial presentation. Prognosis appears to be affected by histologic type because patients with type II MPGN have a worse prognosis compared with those with types I and III. Recurrence of MPGN in the kidney transplant occurs in approximately 30% of patients with type I and close to 90% of patients with type II, suggesting the presence of a systemic disorder. No definitive therapy exists, although stabilization of the clinical course has been reported in many patients receiving long-term alternate-day prednisone therapy.

Bergstein JM, Andreoli SP: Response of type I membranoproliferative glomerulonephritis to pulse methylprednisolone and alternate-day prednisone therapy. *Pediatr Nephrol* 1995; 9:268.

McEnery PT: Membranoproliferative glomerulonephritis: The Cincinnati experience—cumulative renal survival from 1957 to 1989. *J Pediatr* 1990; 116:S109.

Tarshish P, Bernstein J, Tobin JN, et al: Treatment of mesangiocapillary glomerulonephritis with alternate-day prednisone—a report of The International Study of Kidney Disease in Children. *Pediatr Nephrol* 1992; 6:123.

Chapter 506
Glomerulonephritis Associated with Systemic Lupus Erythematosus

Systemic lupus erythematosus (SLE) is characterized by fever, weight loss, rash, hematologic abnormalities, arthritis, and involvement of the heart, lungs, central nervous system, and kidneys. The nonrenal manifestations are discussed in Chapter 148. Kidney disease, one of the most common manifestations of SLE in childhood, may occasionally be the only manifestation.

Pathogenesis and Pathology. Studies in a mouse strain and in humans suggest that the clinical manifestations of SLE are mediated by immune complexes. Aberrations in both B-cell and T-cell function are noted.

The classification of lupus nephritis of the World Health Organization (WHO) is based on light microscopy, immunofluorescence, and electron microscopy. In patients with WHO class I nephritis, no histologic abnormalities are detected. In WHO class II nephritis (mesangial lupus nephritis), glomeruli demonstrate mesangial deposits containing immunoglobulin and complement; light microscopy may show mild (class II-A) or moderate mesangial hypercellularity and increased matrix (class II-B).

In WHO class III nephritis (focal segmental lupus glomerulonephritis), mesangial deposits occur in almost all glomeruli and subendothelial deposits are noted between the endothelial cells and glomerular basement membrane. In addition to focal and segmental mesangial proliferation, occasional glomeruli show capillary wall necrosis, crescent formation, and sclerosis lesions.

WHO class IV nephritis (diffuse proliferative lupus nephritis) is the most common and most severe form of lupus nephritis. All glomeruli contain massive mesangial and subendothelial deposits of immunoglobulin and complement. On light microscopy, all glomeruli show mesangial proliferation. The capillary walls are frequently thickened owing to subendothelial deposits creating the wire-loop lesion and often demonstrate necrosis, crescent formation, and scarring.

WHO class V nephritis (membranous lupus nephritis) is the least common form. It resembles idiopathic membranous glomerulopathy histologically, except for mild to moderate mesangial proliferation.

Transformation of the histologic lesion from one class to another is common. This is more likely to occur among inadequately treated patients and usually results in progression to a more severe histologic lesion.

Clinical Manifestations. The majority of children with SLE are adolescent females. Clinical evidence of renal disease occurs in 30–70% of children. The clinical findings in patients having the milder forms (all class II, some class III) of lupus nephritis include hematuria, normal renal function, and proteinuria of less than 1 g/24 hr. Some patients with class III and all patients with class IV nephritis have hematuria and proteinuria, reduced renal function, nephrotic syndrome, or acute renal failure. In rare patients with proliferative glomerulonephritis, the urinalysis may be completely normal. Patients with class V nephritis commonly present with nephrotic syndrome.

Diagnosis. The diagnosis of SLE is suggested by the detection of circulating antinuclear antibodies and is confirmed by demonstrating antibodies that react with native double-stranded DNA. In most patients with active disease, C3 and C4 levels are depressed. In view of the lack of clear correlation between the clinical manifestations and the severity of the renal involvement, renal biopsy should be performed in all patients with SLE. These results are used to guide the selection of immunosuppressive therapies.

Treatment. Patients with SLE should be treated by specialists in medical centers where both medical and psychologic support can be given to both patients and their families. Immunosuppressive therapy in lupus nephritis is aimed at establishing a clinical and serologic remission as defined by normalization of anti-DNA, C3, and C4 levels. Therapy is initiated in all patients with prednisone at a dose of 1–2 mg/kg/day divided into two or three doses followed by a slow steroid taper over 4–6 mo beginning 4–6 wk after achieving a serologic remission. For patients having more severe forms of nephritis (WHO class III and class IV), six monthly intravenous infusions of cyclophosphamide at a dose of 500–1000 mg/m² followed by every-3-month dosing for 18–36 months appears to reduce the risk of progressive renal dysfunction. Azathioprine at a single daily dose of 1.5–2.0 mg/kg may be used as a steroid-sparing agent in patients with WHO class I or II lupus nephritis. Single center case reports also suggest the potential benefit of mycophenolate mofetil in patients with mild lupus nephritis.

Prognosis. Aggressive immunosuppressive therapy has dramatically improved the prognosis of SLE in childhood. Renal survival without the need for dialysis is seen in 80% of patients 10 yr after the diagnosis of SLE nephritis. Patients with diffuse proliferative WHO class IV lupus nephritis exhibit the highest risk for progression to end-stage renal disease. Concerns regarding the side effects of chronic immunosuppressive therapy and the risk of recurrent disease are lifelong. Special care must be taken to minimize the risks of osteoporosis, obesity, hypertension, and diabetes mellitus associated with chronic steroid therapy. The risk for malignancy or infertility is increased in patients receiving a cumulative dose of more than 20 g of cyclophosphamide.

Austin HA III, Boumpas DT, Vaughan EM, et al: Predicting renal outcomes in severe lupus nephritis: Contributions of clinical and histologic data. *Kidney Int* 1994; 45:544.

Baqi N, Moazami S, Singh A, et al: Lupus nephritis in children: A longitudinal study of prognostic factors and therapy. *J Am Soc Nephrol* 1996; 7:924.

Cameron JS: Lupus nephritis. *J Am Soc Nephrol* 1999; 10:413.

Illei GG, Austin HA, Crane M, et al: Combination therapy with pulse cyclophosphamide plus pulse methylprednisolone improves long-term renal outcome without adding toxicity in patients with lupus nephritis. *Ann Intern Med* 2001; 135:296–98.

Niaudet P: Treatment of lupus nephritis in children. *Pediatr Nephrol* 2000; 14:158–166.

Chapter 507
Henoch-Schönlein Purpura Nephritis

Henoch-Schönlein purpura (HSP) nephritis, also referred to as anaphylactoid purpura, is a small vessel vasculitis characterized by a purpuric rash, arthritis, abdominal pain, and glomerulonephritis (see Chapter 157.1). HSP nephritis and IgA nephropathy demonstrate identical renal findings, but systemic findings are only seen in HSP nephritis.

Pathology and Pathogenesis. Glomerular and tubulointerstitial abnormalities on light, immunofluorescence, and electron microscopy in HSP nephritis are virtually indistinguishable from the pathologic findings in IgA nephropathy. However, crescent formation is more common and more extensive in patients with HSP nephritis. Although the pathogenesis of HSP nephritis remains unknown, this disease appears to be mediated by the formation of immune complexes containing polymeric IgA1 within capillaries of the skin, intestines, and glomerulus.

Clinical and Laboratory Manifestations. The symptoms and signs of HSP nephritis typically appear 1–3 wk after an upper respiratory tract infection (see Chapter 157.1). The diagnosis of HSP is based on the constellation of clinical findings. Whereas gross hematuria is seen in 20–30% of cases, patients may also present with isolated microscopic hematuria, hematuria and proteinuria, acute nephritic syndrome, nephrotic syndrome, or renal insufficiency. Renal manifestations of HSP nephritis occur up to 12 wk after the initial presentation of HSP. An uncommon urologic manifestation of this disease is ureteritis, which is associated with loin pain and renal colic. Ureteritis is usually seen in children younger than 5 yr of age and frequently leads to ureteral stenosis and hydronephrosis requiring surgical correction.

Prognosis and Treatment. The prognosis in HSP nephritis is generally favorable, although the risk of chronic renal insufficiency is 2–5%. Presentation with isolated microscopic hematuria alone carries the best prognosis whereas presentation with acute nephritic syndrome and nephrotic syndrome carries the highest risk of developing chronic renal failure.

There are no controlled data demonstrating that steroids, cytotoxic agents, or anticoagulants alter the course of HSP nephritis. However, uncontrolled studies suggest the potential value of high doses of steroids and cytotoxic therapy with cyclophosphamide or azathioprine in patients with crescentic glomerulonephritis or significant proteinuria. Addition of dipyridamole and/or heparin/warfarin may provide additional benefit in these severe forms of nephritis. Although some studies suggest that short courses of low-dose prednisone reduce the risk of developing any clinical signs of nephritis, it is unclear whether this therapy reduces the risk for progression to severe renal disease. Tonsillectomy does not appear to alter the course of HSP nephritis.

Foster BJ, Bernard C, Drummond K, et al: Effective therapy for severe Henoch-Schönlein purpura nephritis with prednisone and azathioprine: A clinical and pathologic study. *J Pediatr* 2000; 136:370–75.

Niaudet P, Habib R: Methylprednisolone pulse therapy in the treatment of severe forms of Henoch-Schönlein purpura nephritis. *Pediatr Nephrol* 1998; 12:238–43.

Rai A, Nast C, Adler S: Henoch-Schönlein purpura nephritis. *J Am Soc Nephrol* 1999; 10:2637–44.

Chapter 508

Rapidly Progressive (Crescentic) Glomerulonephritis

"Rapidly progressive" describes the clinical course of several forms of glomerulonephritis (GN) whose unifying abnormality is the presence of crescents in the majority of glomeruli. The natural history in most forms is rapid progression to end-stage renal failure.

Classification. Crescents may be found in several well-defined types of glomerulonephritis, including (1) immune-complex–mediated forms of GN: poststreptococcal GN, lupus nephritis, membranoproliferative GN, and Henoch-Schönlein purpura/IgA nephritis; (2) anti–glomerular basement membrane–mediated GN, such as Goodpasture disease; and (3) anti–neutrophil cytoplasmic antibody (ANCA)–mediated GN: microscopic polyarteritis nodosa and Wegener granulomatosis. The typical findings on light, immunofluorescent, and electron microscopic examinations are maintained despite crescent formation. These histologic findings, in conjunction with clinical features and appropriate laboratory studies, should reveal the underlying disease. If recognized forms of glomerulonephritis are excluded, the category of idiopathic rapidly progressive disease remains.

Pathology and Pathogenesis. Crescents are found on the inside of Bowman capsule and are composed of proliferating epithelial cells of the capsule, fibrin, basement membrane–like material, and macrophages (Fig. 508–1). The stimulus for crescent formation is presumed to be the deposition of fibrin in Bowman space, probably as a result of necrosis or disruption of the glomerular capillary wall. Many patients display capillary wall immune-complex deposits or linear IgG antibody staining against glomerular basement membrane. Immunofluorescence and electron microscopy studies in patients with ANCA-mediated forms of GN typically show no evidence of immunologic injury. The complement C3 level is normal.

Clinical Manifestations. Most patients develop acute renal failure associated with acute nephritic and/or nephrotic syndrome. Progression to end-stage renal failure usually occurs within weeks to months after onset.

Diagnosis and Differential Diagnosis. Appropriate serologic studies such as antinuclear antibody, C3, and anti-deoxyribonucleotidase

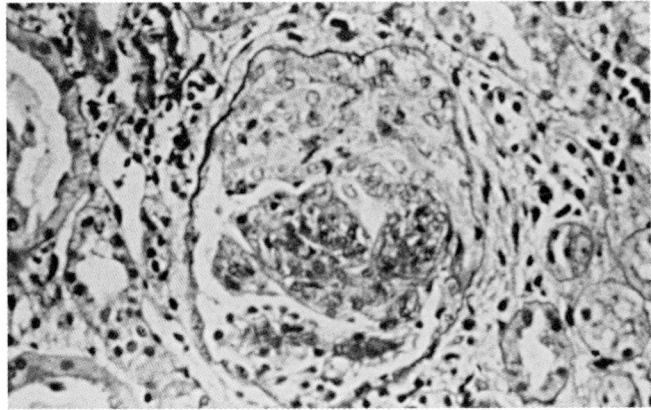

FIGURE 508–1. Light micrograph of a biopsy specimen from a child with Henoch-Schönlein purpura glomerulonephritis demonstrating a crescent overlying the glomerulus. (×180.)

B titers should be obtained to delineate specific types of glomerulonephritis. Rare forms of vasculitis, such as Wegener granulomatosis and microscopic polyarteritis nodosa, may be suggested by the detection of ANCA antibodies to either myeloperoxidase or serine proteinase-3 (PR-3) within the neutrophil cytoplasm. The diagnosis is confirmed by kidney biopsy.

Prognosis and Treatment. Children with a rapidly progressive course associated with poststreptococcal glomerulonephritis usually recover spontaneously. Excellent therapeutic response using a combination of steroids and cytotoxic therapy with cyclophosphamide often occurs in patients with systemic lupus erythematosus, IgA nephropathy, and Henoch-Schönlein purpura nephritis. Renal outcomes in other diseases causing rapidly progressive glomerulonephritis are less favorable, with end-stage renal disease occurring within 2–3 yr. However, therapy combining pulse methylprednisolone and oral cyclophosphamide may be effective, particularly in patients with Wegener granulomatosis. Plasmapheresis or lymphocytapheresis has been reported to be effective in individual cases.

Furuta T, Hotta O, Yusa N, et al: Lymphocytapheresis to treat rapidly progressive glomerulonephritis: A randomized comparison with steroid-pulse treatment. *Lancet* 1998; 352:203.

Hattori M, Kurayama H, Koitabashi Y: Antineutrophil cytoplasmic autoantibody–associated glomerulonephritis in children. *J Am Soc Nephrol* 2001; 12:1493–1500.

Savage J, Davies D, Falk RJ, et al: Antineutrophil cytoplasmic antibodies and associated diseases: A review of the clinical and laboratory features. *Kidney Int* 2000; 57:846–62.

Valentini RP, Smoyer WE, Sedman AB, et al: Outcome of antineutrophil cytoplasmic autoantibodies–positive glomerulonephritis and vasculitis in children: A single-center experience. *J Pediatr* 1998; 132:325.

von Vigier RO, Trummler SA, Laux-End R, et al: Pulmonary renal syndrome in childhood: A report of twenty-one cases and a review of the literature. *Pediatr Pulmonol* 2000; 29:382–88.

Chapter 509

Goodpasture Disease

Goodpasture disease is characterized by pulmonary hemorrhage and glomerulonephritis associated with antibodies commonly directed against specific epitopes of type IV collagen within the alveolar basement membrane of the lung and glomerular basement membrane (GBM) of the glomerulus. The etiology of these antibodies is unknown. This entity should be distinguished from Goodpasture syndrome, which is a clinical picture of pulmonary hemorrhage and glomerulonephritis that may be seen with several disorders, including systemic lupus erythematosus, Henoch-Schönlein purpura, polyarteritis nodosa, and Wegener granulomatosis. In some patients, anti-GBM nephritis occurs without pulmonary hemorrhage as one form of rapidly progressive glomerulonephritis.

Pathology. In most patients, the changes on light microscopy resemble those of rapidly progressive glomerulonephritis. Immunofluorescent microscopy demonstrates a continuous linear pattern of IgG along the GBM (Fig. 509–1).

Clinical Manifestations. Goodpasture disease is rare in childhood. Patients usually present with hemoptysis that is associated with pulmonary hemorrhage that can be life threatening. Renal manifestations include acute nephritic syndrome with hematuria, proteinuria, and hypertension. Progressive renal dysfunction occurs within days to weeks. The complement C3 level is normal.

Diagnosis. The diagnosis is suggested by kidney biopsy. Serum antibodies to the GBM confirm the diagnosis and rule out other disorders associated with Goodpasture syndrome.

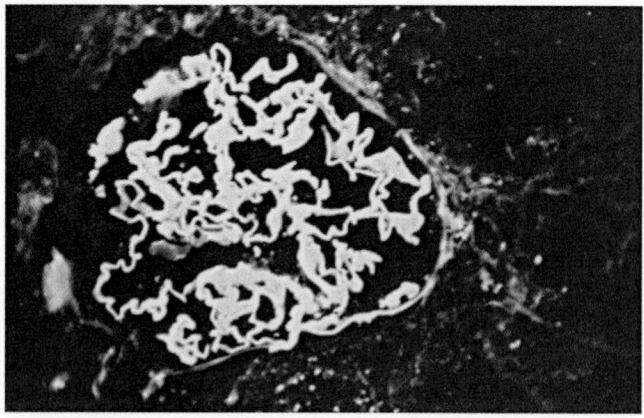

FIGURE 509–1. Immunofluorescence micrograph demonstrating the continuous linear staining of IgG along the glomerular basement membrane, as found in diseases mediated by anti–glomerular basement membrane antibody. (×250.)

Prognosis and Treatment. Patients who survive the pulmonary hemorrhage commonly progress to end-stage renal failure. Rates of survival and recovery of renal function have improved with pulse methylprednisolone, oral cyclophosphamide, and plasmapheresis therapy.

Bolton WK: Goodpasture's syndrome: *Kidney Int* 1996; 50:1753.

Gunnarsson A, Hellmark T, Wieslander J: Molecular properties of the Goodpasture epitope. *J Biol Chem* 2000; 275:30844–48.

Levy JB, Turner N, Rees AJ, et al: Long-term outcome of anti–glomerular basement membrane antibody disease treated with plasma exchange and immunosuppression. *Ann Intern Med* 2001; 134:1033–42.

McCarthy LJ, Cotton J, Danielson C, et al: Goodpasture's syndrome in childhood: Treatment with plasmapheresis and immunosuppression. *J Clin Apher* 1994; 9:116.

Chapter 510
Hemolytic-Uremic Syndrome

The hemolytic-uremic syndrome (HUS) is the most common cause of acute renal failure in young children and is characterized by microangiopathic hemolytic anemia, thrombocytopenia, and uremia. HUS has features common to thrombotic thrombocytopenic purpura, except that the latter tends to occur in young adult women as a relapsing illness with fever, serious central nervous system involvement, and thrombocytopenia.

Etiology. An acute enteritis with diarrhea caused by Shiga toxin–producing *Escherichia coli* O157:H7 precedes 80% or more of HUS cases in developed countries. The reservoir of this organism is the intestinal tract of domestic animals. It is usually transmitted by undercooked meat and unpasteurized milk. Outbreaks have followed ingestion of contaminated apple cider or bathing in a contaminated swimming pool. The organism elaborates a toxin, verotoxin, which is absorbed from the intestines and initiates endothelial cell injury. Less often, HUS is associated with other bacterial (*Shigella, Salmonella, Campylobacter, Streptococcus pneumoniae, Bartonella*) and viral (coxsackievirus, echovirus, influenza, varicella, HIV, Epstein-Barr) infections. HUS may also develop with the use of oral contraceptives, mitomycin, cyclosporine, and pyran copolymer, which is an inducer of interferon. In addition, a hemolytic-uremic type of disorder has been reported with systemic lupus erythematosus, malignant hypertension, preeclampsia, postpartum renal failure, and radiation nephritis. Several reports describe occurrence in more than one member of a family, but the role of genetic factors in predisposition to the disease is unknown.

Pathology. Initial glomerular changes include thickening of the capillary walls, narrowing of the capillary lumens, and widening of the mesangium. Electron microscopy shows these changes to be the result of subendothelial and mesangial deposition of a granular, amorphous material of unknown origin. Fibrin thrombi can be found in glomerular capillaries and arterioles and may lead to cortical necrosis.

Severely involved glomeruli progress to partial or total sclerosis. Severe vascular involvement may render other glomeruli obsolescent as a result of ischemia. In these severely involved small arteries and arterioles, concentric intimal proliferation leads to vascular occlusion.

Pathogenesis. The primary event in pathogenesis of the syndrome appears to be endothelial cell injury. Capillary and arteriolar endothelial injury in the kidney leads to localized clotting. Evidence for disseminated intravascular coagulation is unusual. The microangiopathic anemia results from mechanical damage to the red blood cells (RBCs) as they pass through the altered vasculature. Thrombocytopenia is caused by intrarenal platelet adhesion or damage. Damaged RBCs and platelets are removed from circulation by the liver and spleen. Nondiarrheal and sporadic familial cases of HUS may be caused by the absence of a plasma factor that stimulates the production of endothelial cell–derived prostacyclin, which promotes vasodilatation and inhibits thrombosis. Reduced levels of thrombomodulin, tissue plasminogen activator, and heparin-like molecules, which activate antithrombin III, result in a prothrombotic state in HUS. In addition, serum levels of prothrombotic agents, including platelet-activating factor, prothrombin fragment 1 and 2, tissue plasminogen activator antigen, tissue plasminogen activator-inhibitor (TPA-1) complex, von Willebrand factor, D-dimer, and thromboxane A_2 are increased before renal injury occurs and may be a cause of injury.

Clinical Manifestations. HUS is most common in children younger than age 4 yr. The onset is usually preceded by a gastroenteritis characterized by fever, vomiting, abdominal pain, and diarrhea that is often bloody. Less commonly, patients may present after an upper respiratory tract infection. Sudden onset of pallor, irritability, weakness, lethargy, and oliguria usually occurs 5–10 days after the initial gastrointestinal or respiratory illness. Physical examination may reveal dehydration, edema, petechiae, hepatosplenomegaly, and marked irritability.

Diagnosis and Differential Diagnosis. The diagnosis is supported by the findings of a microangiopathic hemolytic anemia, thrombocytopenia, and acute renal failure. The hemoglobin value is commonly in the range of 5–9 g/dL. The blood peripheral smear reveals helmet cells, burr cells, and fragmented RBCs (see Chapter 439). Plasma hemoglobin levels are elevated, whereas plasma haptoglobin levels are diminished. The reticulocyte count is moderately elevated, and the Coombs test result is negative. The leukocyte count may increase to 30,000/mm³. Thrombocytopenia (20,000–100,000/mm³) occurs in more than 90% of patients. Findings on urinalysis are surprisingly mild and usually consist of low-grade microscopic hematuria and proteinuria. Partial thromboplastin time and prothrombin time are usually normal. Prolongation of coagulation studies is more commonly caused by vitamin K deficiency than by disseminated intravascular coagulation. Renal manifestations vary from mild renal insufficiency to acute renal failure requiring dialysis. Barium contrast studies reveal colonic spasm and transient early filling defects. Intestinal strictures are rare sequelae.

HUS should always be considered in the child with a sudden onset of acute renal failure. The typical history, clinical picture, and laboratory findings confirm the diagnosis in most patients.

Other causes of acute renal failure, especially those that can be associated with a microangiopathic hemolytic anemia such as systemic lupus erythematosus and malignant hypertension, should be excluded. A renal biopsy is rarely indicated.

Patients with bilateral renal vein thrombosis (see Chapter 511.7) may be difficult to distinguish from those with HUS. Both disorders may be preceded by a gastrointestinal disorder associated with dehydration, pallor, and evidence of microangiopathic hemolytic anemia, thrombocytopenia, and acute renal failure. Marked renal enlargement and absence of renal vein flow by renal Doppler ultrasonography is consistent with renal vein thrombosis.

Complications. Complications include anemia, acidosis, hyperkalemia, fluid overload, heart failure, hypertension, and uremia. Extrarenal manifestations of the central nervous system, gastrointestinal tract, heart, and skeletal muscles may be life threatening. Central nervous system dysfunction includes irritability, seizures, infarcts of the basal ganglion and cerebral cortex, cortical blindness, and coma. Gastrointestinal manifestations include colitis, intestinal perforation, intussusception, and hepatitis. Focal pancreatic necrosis may result in glucose intolerance, insulin-dependent diabetes mellitus, and elevated lipase levels. Pericarditis, myocardial dysfunction, and arrhythmias may be seen in cases with cardiac involvement. Other complications such as skin necrosis, parotitis, adrenal dysfunction, and rhabdomyolysis are rarely seen.

Prognosis and Treatment. Supportive care with meticulous attention to fluid and electrolytes, control of hypertension, aggressive nutrition, and early institution of dialysis is responsible for a decrease in the mortality from this disease from 80% to less than 10% over the past 30 yr. Antibiotics should be avoided in patients with acute enteritis presumed secondary to *E. coli* 0157:H7 as they may increase the risk of developing HUS. Antithrombotic therapy has no proven therapeutic benefit in HUS. Prospective controlled studies assessing the value of plasmapheresis in HUS with a diarrheal prodrome are not available. However, plasmapheresis or administration of fresh frozen plasma may be beneficial in HUS that is not associated with a diarrheal prodrome or in children with severe central nervous system involvement. Plasmapheresis or administration of fresh frozen plasma may exacerbate HUS caused by *Streptococcus pneumoniae* and should be avoided when this infection is present. Peritoneal dialysis controls fluid and electrolyte abnormalities, maintains a normal intravascular volume, and provides the opportunity for aggressive nutritional support. Also, peritoneal dialysis may contribute to the dissolution of vascular thrombi by removing fibrinolysis inhibitors and circulating plasminogen activating inhibitor-1, thereby promoting endogenous fibrinolytic pathways. A preliminary report of a phase II clinical trial in Canada using Synsorb-PK, a silicon dioxide–derived univalent absorbent that binds Shiga toxin within the intestinal lumen, suggested a reduction in the risk of developing HUS in children when given within 3 days of the onset of a diarrheal prodrome. However, a final report of this trial has not been published. In vitro studies using more potent multivalent synthetic inhibitors of Shiga toxin or genetically engineered bacteria that neutralize large amounts of the Shiga toxin may show promise in reducing the incidence of diarrhea-associated HUS.

With aggressive management of acute renal failure, more than 90% of patients survive the acute phase of HUS with a diarrheal prodrome. End-stage renal disease occurs in approximately 9% of these patients. Patients recovering from the acute phase of HUS require long-term follow-up because complications such as hypertension, chronic renal insufficiency, and proteinuria may not be apparent for up to 20 years. Kidney transplants in patients with HUS can be successful, although disease recurrence may occur, particularly in cases without a diarrheal prodrome.

Banatvala N, Griffin PM, Greene KD, et al: The United States national prospective hemolytic-uremic syndrome study: Microbiologic, serologic, clinical, and epidemiologic findings. *J Infect Dis* 2001; 183:1063.

Brandt JR, Fouser LS, Watkins SL, et al: *Escherichia coli* 0157:H7–associated hemolytic-uremic syndrome after ingestion of contaminated hamburgers. *J Pediatr* 1994; 125:519.

Cabrera GR, Fortenberry JD, Warshaw BL, et al: Hemolytic-uremic syndrome associated with invasive *Streptococcus pneumoniae* infection. *Pediatrics* 1998; 101:699.

Chandler WL, Jelacic S, Boster DR, et al: Prothrombotic abnormalities preceding the hemolytic-uremic syndrome. *N Engl J Med* 2002; 346:23–32.

Kitov PI, Sadowski JM, Mulvey G, et al: Shiga-like toxins are neutralized by tailored multivalent carbohydrate ligands. *Nature* 2000; 403:669–72.

Paton AW, Morona R, Paton JC: A new biological agent for treatment of Shiga toxigenic *Escherichia coli* infections and dysentery in humans. *Nat Med* 2000; 6:265–72.

Safdar N, Sard A, Gagnon RE, et al: Rsik of hemolytic uremic syndrome after antibiotic treatment of *Escherichia coli* 0157:H7 enteritis. A meta-analysis. *JAMA* 2002;288:996–1001.

Siegler RL: The hemolytic-uremic syndrome. *Pediatr Clin North Am* 1995; 42:1505.

Spizzirri FD, Rahman RC, Bibiloni N, et al: Childhood hemolytic-uremic syndrome in Argentina: Long-term follow-up and prognostic features. *Pediatr Nephrol* 1997; 11:156.

Wong CS, Jelacic S, Habeeb RL, et al: The risk of the hemolytic-uremic syndrome after antibiotic treatment of *Escherichia coli* O157:H7 infections. *N Engl J Med* 2000; 342:1930–36.

Chapter 511

Upper Urinary Tract Causes of Hematuria

511.1 Interstitial Nephritis (see Chapter 524)

511.2 Toxic Nephropathy (see Chapter 525)

511.3 Cortical Necrosis (see Chapter 526)

511.4 Pyelonephritis (see Chapter 530)

511.5 Nephrocalcinosis (see Chapter 539)

511.6 Vascular Abnormalities

Hemangiomas, angiomyomas, and arteriovenous malformations of the kidneys and lower urinary tract are rare causes of hematuria. They usually present as gross hematuria and the passage of blood clots. Renal colic may develop if the upper tract is involved. The diagnosis is confirmed by angiography.

Unilateral bleeding of varicose veins of the left ureter, resulting from compression of the left renal vein between the aorta and superior mesenteric artery, is referred to as the *nutcracker syndrome*. Patients with this syndrome typically present with persistent microscopic hematuria that may be accompanied by proteinuria, lower abdominal pain, flank pain, or orthostatic hypotension. Diagnosis is confirmed by Doppler ultrasonography, computed tomography, or magnetic resonance angiography.

Takemura T, Iwasa H, Yamamoto S, et al: Clinical and radiological features in four adolescents with nutcracker syndrome. *Pediatr Nephrol* 2000; 14:1002–1005.

511.7 Renal Vein Thrombosis

Epidemiology. Renal vein thrombosis (RVT) occurs in two distinct patterns. In newborns and infants, RVT is commonly associated with asphyxia, dehydration, shock, sepsis, and infants born to mothers with diabetes mellitus. In older children, RVT is seen in patients with nephrotic syndrome, cyanotic heart disease, inherited hypercoagulable states, and following exposure to angiographic contrast agents.

Pathogenesis. RVT begins in the intrarenal venous circulation and may spread to the main renal vein and inferior vena cava. Thrombus formation is mediated by endothelial cell injury resulting from hypoxia, endotoxin, or contrast media. Other contributing factors include (1) hypercoagulability from either nephrotic syndrome or genetic mutations such as factor V Leiden; (2) hypovolemia and diminished vascular blood flow associated with septic shock, dehydration, or nephrotic syndrome; and (3) intravascular sludging due to polycythemia.

Clinical Manifestations. The development of RVT is usually heralded by the sudden onset of gross hematuria and unilateral or bilateral flank masses. Patients may also present with microscopic hematuria, flank pain, hypertension, or oliguria. RVT is usually unilateral. Bilateral RVT results in acute renal failure.

Diagnosis. The diagnosis of RVT is suggested by the development of hematuria and flank masses in a patient with predisposing clinical factors. Most patients also have a microangiopathic hemolytic anemia and thrombocytopenia. Ultrasonography shows marked enlargement, whereas radionuclide studies reveal little or no renal function in the affected kidney(s). Doppler flow studies of the inferior vena cava and renal vein confirm the diagnosis. Contrast studies should be avoided to minimize the risk of further vascular damage.

Differential Diagnosis. The differential diagnosis of RVT includes other causes of hematuria that are associated with microangiopathic hemolytic anemia or renal enlargement. These include hemolytic-uremic syndrome, hydronephrosis, polycystic kidney disease, Wilms tumor, abscess, or hematoma.

Treatment. The primary treatment of RVT consists of supportive care including correction of fluid and electrolyte imbalance and treatment of renal insufficiency. Treatment with anticoagulation or thrombolytic agents including streptokinase, urokinase, or recombinant tissue plasminogen activator remains controversial. Patients with thrombosis of the inferior vena cava may require surgical thrombectomy. Children with severe hypertension refractory to antihypertensive medications may require nephrectomy.

Prognosis. Perinatal mortality from RVT has decreased significantly over the past 20 yr. However, partial or complete renal atrophy is a common sequela of RVT in the neonate leading to renal insufficiency, renal tubular dysfunction, and systemic hypertension. These complications are also seen in older children, although recovery of renal function is common in children with RVT due to nephrotic syndrome or cyanotic heart disease.

Bokenkamp A, von Kries R, Nowak-Gottl U, et al: Neonatal renal venous thrombosis in Germany between 1992 and 1994: Epidemiology, treatment and outcome. *Eur J Pediatr* 2000; 159:44–8.
Mocan H, Beattie TJ, Murphy AV: Renal venous thrombosis in infancy: Long-term follow-up. *Pediatr Nephrol* 1991; 5:45.
Ricci MA, Lloyd DA: Renal venous thrombosis in infants and children. *Arch Surg* 1990; 125:1195.
Streif W, Andrew ME: Venous thromboembolic events in pediatric patients. Diagnosis and management. *Hematol Oncol Clin North Am* 1998; 12:1283–1312.

511.8 Idiopathic Hypercalciuria

This entity, which may be inherited as an autosomal dominant disorder, may present as recurrent gross hematuria, persistent microscopic hematuria, dysuria, or abdominal pain in the absence of stone formation. Hypercalciuria may be caused by conditions resulting in hypercalcemia, such as hyperparathyroidism, vitamin D intoxication, immobilization, and sarcoidosis. Also, hypercalciuria may be associated with Cushing syndrome, corticosteroid therapy, tubular dysfunction secondary to Fanconi syndrome (i.e., Wilson disease, oculocerebrorenal syndrome), Williams syndrome, distal renal tubular acidosis,

or Bartter syndrome. Finally, hypercalciuria may be seen in patients with Dent disease, which is an X-linked form of nephrolithiasis associated with hypophosphatemic rickets. Although microcrystal formation and irritation are believed to mediate symptoms, the precise mechanism by which the hypercalciuria causes hematuria or dysuria is unknown.

The *diagnosis* of hypercalciuria is confirmed by a 24-hour urinary calcium excretion exceeding 4 mg/kg. A screening test for hypercalciuria in patients who cannot collect a timed urine specimen may be performed on a random urine specimen by measuring the calcium and creatinine concentrations. A urine calcium to creatinine ratio (mg/mg) exceeding 0.2 suggests hypercalciuria, although normal ratios may be as high as 0.8 in infants younger than 7 mo of age.

If untreated, hypercalciuria leads to nephrolithiasis in approximately 15% of cases. Oral thiazide diuretics may normalize urinary calcium excretion by stimulating calcium reabsorption in the distal tubule. Such therapy may halt the gross hematuria or dysuria and prevent nephrolithiasis. However, the precise indications for thiazide *treatment* remain controversial. In patients with persistent gross hematuria or dysuria, therapy is initiated with hydrochlorothiazide at a dosage of 1–2 mg/kg/24 hr as a single morning dose. The dosage is titrated upward until the 24-hour urinary calcium excretion is less than 4 mg/kg and the clinical manifestations resolve. After 1 yr of treatment, hydrochlorothiazide is usually discontinued but may be resumed if gross hematuria, nephrolithiasis, or dysuria recurs. During hydrochlorothiazide therapy, the serum potassium level should be monitored periodically to avoid hypokalemia. Potassium citrate at a dose of 1 mEq/kg/24 hr may also be beneficial, particularly in patients with low urinary citrate excretion and symptomatic dysuria. Sodium restriction is important because calcium excretion parallels that of sodium excretion. Importantly, dietary calcium restriction is not recommended because of the obligate requirement for growth and lack of evidence demonstrating a reduction in urinary calcium levels.

Polito C, LaManna A, Cioce F, et al: Clinical presentation and natural course of idiopathic hypercalciuria in children. *Pediatr Nephrol* 2000; 15:211–14.
So NP, Osorio AV, Simon SD, et al: Normal urinary calcium/creatinine ratios in African-American and Caucasian children. *Pediatr Nephrol* 2001; 16:133–39.
Stapleton FB: Hematuria associated with hypercalciuria and hyperuricosuria: A practical approach. *Pediatr Nephrol* 1994; 8:756.
Stapleton FB: Making a "dent" in hereditary hypercalciuric nephrolithiasis. *J Pediatr* 1998; 132:764.
Vachvanichsanong P, Malagon M, Moore ES: Recurrent abdominal and flank pain in children with idiopathic hypercalciuria. *Acta Paediatr* 2001; 90:643–48.

Chapter 512
Hematologic Diseases Causing Hematuria

512.1 Sickle Cell Nephropathy

Gross or microscopic hematuria may be seen in children with sickle cell disease or sickle trait. Signs and symptoms resolve spontaneously in the majority of patients (see Chapter 454.1). The hematuria presumably results from microthrombosis secondary to sickling in the relatively hypoxic, acidic, hypertonic renal medulla where vascular stasis is present. Ischemia, papillary necrosis, and interstitial fibrosis may also be present in these patients. Additional clinical manifestations of sickle cell nephropathy include polyuria caused by a urinary concentrating defect, renal tubular acidosis, and proteinuria associated with a glomerular lesion resembling focal segmental glomerulosclerosis or membranoproliferative glomerulonephritis. Sickle cell nephropathy may eventually lead to hypertension and renal insufficiency that may progress to end-stage renal disease.

Pham PT, Pham PC, Wilkinson AH, at al: Renal abnormalities in sickle cell disease. *Kidney Int* 2000; 57:1–8.

Saborio P, Scheinman JI: Sickle cell nephropathy. *J Am Soc Nephrol* 1999; 10:187.

512.2 Coagulopathies and Thrombocytopenia

Gross or microscopic hematuria may be associated with inherited or acquired disorders of coagulation (hemophilia, disseminated intravascular coagulation, thrombocytopenia). In these cases, however, hematuria is not usually the presenting complaint but develops after other manifestations (see Part XX, Section 7).

Chapter 513
Anatomic Abnormalities Associated with Hematuria

513.1 Congenital Anomalies

Gross or microscopic hematuria may be associated with many types of different malformations of the urinary tract. The sudden onset of gross hematuria after minor trauma to the flank is frequently associated with ureteropelvic junction obstruction or cystic kidneys.

513.2 Autosomal Recessive Polycystic Kidney Disease

Also known as *infantile polycystic disease*, autosomal recessive polycystic kidney disease (ARPKD) is an autosomal recessive disorder occurring with an incidence of 1:10,000 to 1:40,000. Although the gene for ARPKD has not been identified, genetic linkage studies have mapped a candidate locus for this disease to the short arm of chromosome 6.

Pathology. Both kidneys are markedly enlarged and grossly show innumerable cysts throughout the cortex and medulla. Microscopic studies demonstrate microcysts radiating from the medulla to the cortex located primarily within the collecting tubules and ducts, although transient proximal tubule cysts have been reported in the fetus. Development of progressive interstitial fibrosis and tubular atrophy during advanced stages of disease eventually leads to renal failure. Liver involvement is characterized by bile duct proliferation and ectasia as well as by hepatic fibrosis that is indistinguishable from congenital hepatic fibrosis or Caroli disease.

Clinical Manifestations. The typical child presents with bilateral flank masses during the neonatal period or early infancy. ARPKD may be associated with oligohydramnios, pulmonary hypoplasia, respiratory distress, and spontaneous pneumothorax in the neonatal period. Potter facies and other components of the oligohydramnios sequence including low-set ears, micrognathia, flattened nose, limb positioning defects, and growth deficiency may be present. Hypertension is usually noted within the first few weeks of life and is often severe. Urine output is usu-

ally not diminished, although oliguria and acute renal failure may be seen. Transient hyponatremia, often in the presence of acute renal failure, is common in the neonatal period and frequently responds to diuresis. Renal function is usually impaired but may be normal in 20–30% of patients. Infrequently, ARPKD presents beyond infancy with renal insufficiency, hypertension, or hepatosplenomegaly related to hepatic fibrosis.

In the newborn, clinical evidence of liver disease by radiologic or laboratory assessment is present in about 45% of children. However, patients with ARPKD are at risk for developing (1) ascending cholangitis, varices, and hypersplenism related to portal hypertension and (2) progressive liver dysfunction, which rarely leads to overt liver failure and cirrhosis. A subset of older children with ARPKD may present with hepatosplenomegaly and display mild renal disease that is discovered incidentally during imaging studies of the abdomen.

Diagnosis. The diagnosis of ARPKD is strongly suggested by bilateral palpable flank masses in an infant with pulmonary hypoplasia, oligohydramnios, and hypertension and the absence of renal cysts in the parents. Markedly enlarged and uniformly hyperechogenic kidneys with poor corticomedullary distinction are commonly seen on ultrasonography (Fig. 513–1). Also, the diagnosis is supported by clinical/laboratory signs of hepatic fibrosis, pathologic findings of ductal plate abnormalities seen on liver biopsy, anatomic and pathologic proof of ARPKD in a sibling, or parental consanguinity. The differential diagnosis includes other causes of bilateral renal enlargement, such as multicystic dysplasia, hydronephrosis, Wilms tumor, and bilateral renal vein thrombosis. Prenatal diagnostic testing using genetic linkage analysis is available in families with at least one affected child and identified informative markers.

Treatment. The treatment of ARPKD is supportive. Aggressive ventilatory support is often necessary in the neonatal period owing to pulmonary hypoplasia and hypoventilation. Careful management of hypertension, fluid and electrolyte abnormalities, and clinical manifestations of renal insufficiency is essential. Children with severe respiratory failure or feeding intolerance from enlarged kidneys may require unilateral or bilateral nephrectomies, prompting the need for renal replacement therapy.

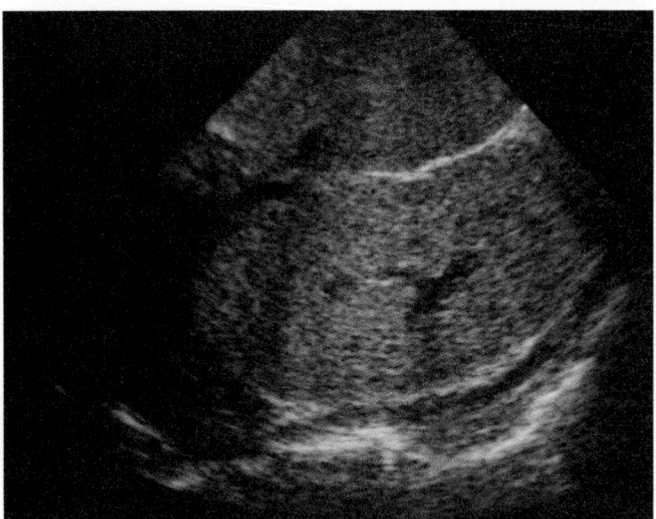

FIGURE 513–1. Ultrasound examination of a neonate with autosomal recessive polycystic kidney disease demonstrating renal enlargement (9 cm) and increased diffuse echogenicity with complete loss of corticomedullary differentiation resulting from multiple small cystic interfaces.

Prognosis. Although approximately 30% of patients die in the neonatal period of complications from pulmonary hypoplasia, modern neonatal respiratory techniques and renal replacement therapies have increased the 10-year survival of children surviving beyond the 1st year of life to over 80%. Fifteen-year survival is estimated at 70–80%. End-stage renal disease is seen in over 50% of children and usually occurs during the 1st decade of life. As a result, dialysis and renal transplantation have become standard therapies for these children. Morbidity and mortality in the older child is related to complications from chronic renal failure and liver disease.

Dell KM, Avner ED: Autosomal recessive polycystic kidney disease. In GeneClinics: Clinical Genetic Information Resource [database online]. Copyright, University of Washington, Seattle. Available at http://www.geneclinics.org.

Roy S, Dillon MJ, Trompeter RS, et al: Autosomal recessive polycystic kidney disease: Long-term outcome of neonatal survivors. *Pediatr Nephrol* 1997; 11:302.

Zerres K, Rudnik-Schoneborn S, Deget F, et al: Autosomal recessive polycystic kidney disease in 115 children: Clinical presentation, course and influence of gender. *Acta Paediatr* 1996; 85:437.

513.3 Autosomal Dominant Polycystic Kidney Disease

Autosomal dominant polycystic kidney disease (ADPKD) is the most common hereditary human kidney disease. The autosomal dominant pattern of inheritance occurs with an incidence of 1 in 500 to 1 in 1000. Approximately 85% of patients with ADPKD map to the *PKD1* gene on the short arm of chromosome 16, which encodes polycystin, a transmembrane glycoprotein. Another 10–15% of ADPKD map to the *PKD2* gene on the long arm of chromosome 4, which encodes polycystin 2, a proposed nonselective cation channel. Remaining patients may map to other loci yet to be determined.

Pathology. Both kidneys are enlarged and show cortical and medullary cysts originating from all regions of the nephron.

Clinical Presentation. Although symptomatic ADPKD commonly presents in the 4th or 5th decade of life, symptoms, including gross or microscopic hematuria, bilateral flank pain, abdominal masses, hypertension, and urinary tract infection, may be seen in children and neonates. Renal ultrasonography usually demonstrates multiple bilateral macrocysts (Fig. 513–2), although unilateral disease may be seen in the early phase of the disease.

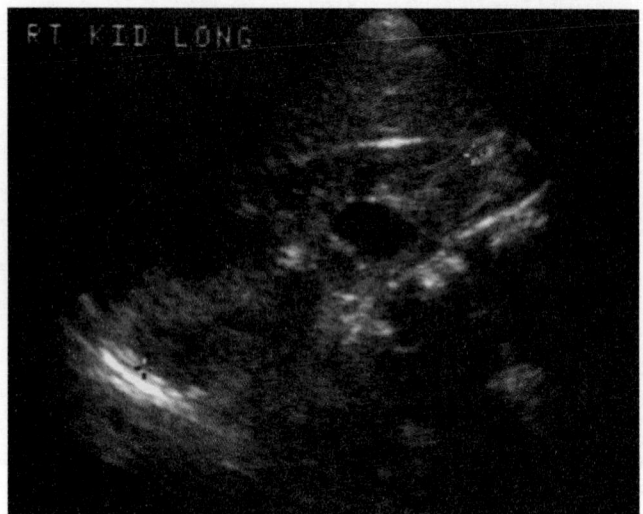

FIGURE 513–2. Ultrasound examination of an 18-mo-old boy with autosomal dominant polycystic kidney disease demonstrating renal enlargement (10 cm) and two large cysts.

ADPKD is a systemic disorder affecting many organ systems. For example, cysts may be present within the liver, pancreas, spleen, and ovaries. Intracranial aneurysms, which appear to cluster within certain families, are an important cause of mortality in adults but are rarely reported in children. Mitral valve prolapse is seen in approximately 12% of children. Hernias and intestinal diverticula may also be seen in these children.

Diagnosis. ADPKD is confirmed by the presence of enlarged kidneys with bilateral macrocysts in a patient with an affected first-degree relative. Absence of a family history of ADPKD does not preclude this diagnosis because affected family members may have silent disease or the affected child may have a new mutation that occurs in 5–10% of cases. Among patients with genetically defined ADPKD, screening renal ultrasonography results may be normal in up to 20% by 20 yr of age and less than 5% by 30 yr of age.

Prenatal diagnosis is suggested from the presence of enlarged kidneys with or without cysts on ultrasonography in families with known ADPKD. Prenatal DNA testing is available in families with affected members whose disease is linked to the *PKD1* or *PKD2* genes.

The differential diagnosis includes renal cysts associated with glomerulocystic kidney disease, tuberous sclerosis, and von Hippel-Lindau disease, which may be inherited in an autosomal dominant pattern. The neonatal manifestations of ADPKD and ARPKD may be indistinguishable.

Treatment and Prognosis. Treatment of ADPKD is primarily supportive. Control of blood pressure is critical because the rate of disease progression in ADPKD correlates with the presence of hypertension.

Although neonatal ADPKD may be lethal, long-term patient and renal survival is possible for children surviving the neonatal period. Presentation of ADPKD in older children has a favorable prognosis, with normal renal function during childhood seen in over 80% of children.

Davis ID, MacRae DK, Sweeney WS, et al: Can progression of autosomal dominant or autosomal recessive polycystic kidney disease be prevented? *Semin Nephrol* 2001; 21:430.

Fick GM, Duley IT, Johnson AM, et al: The spectrum of autosomal dominant polycystic disease in children. *J Am Soc Nephrol* 1994; 4:1654.

Fick-Brosnahan GM, Tran ZV, Johnson AM, et al: Progression of autosomal-dominant polycystic kidney disease in children. *Kidney Int* 2001; 59:1979–80.

MacDermot KD, Saggar-Malik AK, Economides DL, et al: Prenatal diagnosis of autosomal dominant polycystic kidney disease (PKD1) presenting in utero and prognosis for very early onset disease. *J Med Genet* 1998; 35:13.

Murcia NS, Sweeney WE, Avner ED: New insights into the molecular pathophysiology of polycystic kidney disease. *Kidney Int* 1999; 55:1187.

Perrone RD: Extrarenal manifestations of ADPKD. *Kidney Int* 1997; 51:2022.

Wilson PD: Polycystin: New aspects of structure, function, and regulation. *J Am Soc Nephrol* 2001; 12:834.

513.4 Trauma

Blunt or penetrating injury to the abdomen may injure a kidney. Gross or microscopic hematuria, flank pain, and abdominal rigidity may occur; associated injuries may be present. Urethral trauma may result from crushing-type injury, frequently associated with a fractured pelvis, or from direct injury. The injury is suspected when gross blood appears at the external meatus.

Dreitlein DA, Suner S, Basler J: Genitourinary trauma. *Emerg Med Clin North Am* 2001; 19:569–90.

Mirvis SE: Trauma. *Radiol Clin North Am* 1996; 34:1225.

513.5 Renal Tumors (see Chapter 491)

Chapter 514
Lower Urinary Tract Causes of Hematuria

514.1 Infectious Causes of Cystitis and Urethritis

Gross or microscopic hematuria may be associated with bacterial, mycobacterial, or viral infections of the bladder (see Chapter 530). The occurrence of hematuria may be related to the depth and severity of the inflammatory reaction within the bladder wall.

Urethritis may present as gross or microscopic hematuria, usually in conjunction with urgency and pyuria. Urine cultures occasionally reveal bacteria, *Ureaplasma*, or *Chlamydia* but are usually negative. A history of trauma should be sought. The disorder frequently resolves spontaneously. In children older than 8 yr of age, a 10-day course of doxycycline is the treatment of choice in conjunction with a urinary analgesic such as phenazopyridine for relief of pain. If conservative management fails, cystoscopy may be required to determine the nature of any underlying abnormality such as ulceration or inflammation.

514.2 Hemorrhagic Cystitis

Hemorrhagic cystitis (see also Chapter 240) is defined as acute or chronic bleeding of the bladder. Patients with hemorrhagic cystitis often present with gross hematuria and dysuria. In severe forms, bleeding may lead to a decrease in blood hemoglobin levels. Hemorrhagic cystitis may occur in response to chemical toxins (cyclophosphamide, penicillins, busulfan, thiotepa, dyes, insecticides), viruses (adenovirus types 11 and 21, polyoma BK virus, influenza A), radiation, and amyloidosis.

Hydration and the use of MESNA disulfide, which inactivates cyclophosphamide metabolites, helps to protect the bladder from the chemical irritation related to the use of intravenous cyclophosphamide. Administration of oral cyclophosphamide in the morning followed by aggressive oral hydration throughout the remainder of the day is very effective in minimizing the risk of hemorrhagic cystitis. Bladder irrigation with saline, alum, silver nitrate, or aminocaproic acid may be necessary in more severe forms of this disorder. Gross hematuria associated with viral hemorrhagic cystitis usually resolves within 1 wk.

DeVries CR, Freiha FS: Hemorrhagic cystitis: A review. *J Urol* 1990; 143:1–9.

514.3 Heavy Exercise

Gross or microscopic hematuria may follow vigorous exercise. Exercise hematuria is rare in females and can be associated with dysuria. The color of the urine may vary from red to black. Blood clots may be present in the urine. Findings on urine culture, intravenous pyelography, voiding cystourethrography, and cystoscopy are normal in most patients. This seems to be a benign condition, and the hematuria generally resolves within 48 hr after cessation of exercise. The absence of red blood cell casts or evidence of renal disease and the presence of dysuria and blood clots in some patients suggest that the source of bleeding lies in the lower urinary tract. Rhabdomyolysis with myoglobinuria or hemoglobinuria must be considered in the differential diagnosis when associated with exercise.

Abarbanel J, Benet AE, Lask D, et al: Sports hematuria. *J Urol* 1990; 143:887.
Bailey RR, Dann E, Gillies AHB, et al: What the urine contains following athletic competition. *N Z Med J* 1976; 83:309.
Gambrell RC, Blount BW: Exercise-induced hematuria. *Am Fam Physician* 1996; 53:905–11.
Siegel AJ, Hennekens CH, Solomon HS, et al: Exercise-related hematuria. *JAMA* 1979; 241:391.

514.4 Munchausen Syndrome by Proxy

(see Chapters 19 and 35.3)

SECTION 3 *Conditions Particularly Associated with Proteinuria*

Beth A. Vogt and Ellis D. Avner

Chapter 515
Introduction to the Child with Proteinuria

In a general pediatric practice the demonstration of proteinuria on a routine screening urinalysis is a common occurrence. As many as 10% of children aged 8–15 yr will test positive for proteinuria by urinary dipstick at some time. The challenge is to differentiate the child with proteinuria related to renal disease from the otherwise healthy child with transient or other benign forms of proteinuria.

Proteinuria is commonly detected by the urine dipstick test, which offers a qualitative assessment of urinary protein excretion. Dipsticks detect primarily albuminuria and are less sensitive for other forms of proteinuria (e.g., low molecular weight proteins, Bence Jones protein, gamma globulins). The depth of color of the dipstick reaction increases in a semi-quantitative manner with increasing urinary protein concentration. The dipstick is reported as negative, trace (10–20 mg/dL), 1+ (30 mg/dL), 2+ (100 mg/dL), 3+ (300 mg/dL), and 4+ (1000–2000 mg/dL).

False-negative test results may occur in patients with dilute urine (specific gravity < 1.005) or in disease states in which the predominant urinary protein is not albumin. False-positive test results may be seen in patients with gross hematuria, contamination with antiseptic agents (chlorhexidine and benzalkonium chloride), urinary pH greater than 7.0, or phenazopyridine therapy. Most importantly, the dipstick may be falsely positive in patients with highly concentrated urine. A dipstick should be considered positive for protein only if it registers greater than or equal to 1+ (30 mg/dL) in a urine sample in which the specific gravity is less than or equal to 1.015. If the specific gravity is greater than 1.015, the dipstick must read greater than or equal to 2+ to be considered clinically significant.

Because the dipstick reaction offers only a qualitative measurement of urinary protein excretion, persistent proteinuria should be quantitated using a more precise method. A timed (12–24 hr) urine collection remains the traditional method of quantitation of urinary protein excretion.

A reasonable upper limit of normal protein excretion in healthy children is 150 mg/24 hr (0.15 g/24 hr). More specifically, normal protein excretion in children is defined as less than or equal to 4 mg/m^2/hr, abnormal is defined as 4–40 mg/m^2/hr, and nephrotic range is defined as more than 40 mg/m^2/hr.

Determination of the protein/creatinine (Upr/UCr) ratio on a random urine specimen is another alternative to quantitating proteinuria and is useful when a timed urine collection is not practical. This ratio is calculated by measuring the urinary protein (mg/dL) and creatinine (mg/dL) concentrations in a random urine specimen. Ratios less than 0.5 in children younger than 2 yr of age and less than 0.2 in children 2 yr of age or older suggest normal protein excretion. A ratio greater than 3 suggests nephrotic-range proteinuria. Upr/Ucr ratios have been shown to have a high correlation with protein excretion determinations by timed urine collection.

Abitbol C, Zilleruelo G, Freundlich M, et al: Quantitation of proteinuria with urinary protein/creatinine ratios and random testing with dipsticks in nephrotic syndrome. *J Pediatr* 1990; 116:243.

Hogg R, Portman RJ, Milliner D, et al: Evaluation and management of proteinuria and nephrotic syndrome in children: Recommendations from a pediatric nephrology panel established at the National Kidney Foundation Conference of Proteinuria, Albuminuria, Risk, Assessment, Detection, and Elimination. *Pediatrics* 2000; 105:1242–49.

Vehaskari VM, Rapola J: Isolated proteinuria: Analysis of a school-age population. *J Pediatr* 1982; 101:661.

Chapter 516
Transient Proteinuria

The majority of children found to have a positive urinary dipstick for protein will subsequently have normal dipstick values. Of the 10% of children found to have proteinuria by a single dipstick measurement, only 1% had persistent proteinuria when measured on four separate occasions. This phenomenon, called transient proteinuria, may be caused by a temperature greater than 38.3°C (101°F) (see Chapter 161), exercise (see Chapter 675), dehydration, cold exposure, congestive heart failure, seizure, or stress. The proteinuria usually does not exceed 2+ on the dipstick. The mechanism of transient proteinuria is unknown. No evaluation is needed for children with transient proteinuria.

Campanacci L, Faccini L, Englaro E, et al: Exercise-induced proteinuria. *Contrib Nephrol* 1981; 26:31.

Jensen H, Henriksen K: Proteinuria in non-renal infectious disease. *Acta Med Scand* 1974; 196:75.

Marks MI, McLaine PN, Drummond KN: Proteinuria in children with febrile illnesses. *Arch Dis Child* 1970; 45:250.

Poortmans JR: Postexercise proteinuria in humans. *JAMA* 1985;253:236.

Vehaskari VM, Rapola J: Isolated proteinuria: Analysis of a school-age population. *J Pediatr* 1982;101:661.

Chapter 517
Orthostatic (Postural) Proteinuria

Orthostatic proteinuria is the most common cause of persistent proteinuria in school-aged children and adolescents, occurring

in up to 60% of children with persistent proteinuria. Children with this condition are usually asymptomatic, and the condition is discovered on routine urinalysis. Individuals with orthostatic proteinuria excrete normal or slightly increased amounts of protein in the supine position. However, in the upright position, urinary protein excretion is increased up to 10-fold, up to 1,000 mg/24 hr (1 g/24 hr). Hematuria, hypertension, and renal dysfunction are absent.

In a child with persistent asymptomatic proteinuria, orthostatic proteinuria should be ruled out before any other evaluation is undertaken. One alternative is to obtain resting (supine) and active (upright) urine samples and perform a dipstick test for protein or evaluate the protein/creatinine ratio.

The absence of proteinuria in the resting (supine) sample and the presence of proteinuria in the active (upright) sample confirms the diagnosis of orthostatic proteinuria. A less convenient, but more exact method of comparing resting and active urinary protein excretion is a split 24-hour urine collection. A finding of essentially normal protein excretion in the supine collection and increased protein excretion in the upright collection establishes the proteinuria as orthostatic.

The cause of orthostatic proteinuria is unknown, although altered renal hemodynamics, partial renal vein obstruction, and circulating immune complexes are possible causes. Long-term follow-up studies in adults suggest that orthostatic proteinuria is a benign process, but similar data are not available for children. Therefore, long-term follow-up of children is prudent to monitor patients for evidence of renal disease, including hematuria, hypertension, diminished renal function, or proteinuria exceeding 1,000 mg/24 hr.

Cho BS, Choi YM, Kang MI, et al: Diagnosis of nutcracker phenomenon using renal Doppler ultrasound in orthostatic proteinuria. *Nephrol Dial Transplant* 2001; 16:1620.

Devarajan P: Mechanisms of orthostatic proteinuria: Lessons from a transplant donor. *J Am Soc Nephrol* 1993; 4:36.

Springberg PD, Garrett LE Jr, Thompson AL, et al: Fixed and reproducible orthostatic proteinuria: Results of a 20-year follow-up study. *Ann Intern Med* 1982; 97:516.

Chapter 518
Fixed Proteinuria

Individuals found to have persistent significant proteinuria in both the resting (supine) and active (upright) positions are classified as having fixed proteinuria. Such proteinuria may be caused by either glomerular or tubular disorders.

518.1 Glomerular Proteinuria

Proteinuria may be seen in a variety of glomerular disorders as a result of increased permeability of the glomerular capillary wall (Box 518–1). Glomerular proteinuria may range from less than 1 g to more than 30 g/24 hr. Glomerular proteinuria may be termed *selective* (loss of plasma proteins of molecular weight up to and including albumin) or *nonselective* (loss of albumin and of larger molecular weight proteins such as IgG). The determination of urinary protein selectivity, however, is generally of little clinical value, because of the considerable overlap among various forms of renal disease.

Glomerular proteinuria should be suspected in any patient with protein excretion of more than 1 g/24 hr or accompanying hypertension, hematuria, or renal dysfunction. Causes include postinfectious glomerulonephritis, focal segmental glomerulosclerosis, mesangial proliferative glomerulonephritis, membranous nephropathy, membranoproliferative glomerulonephritis,

BOX 518–1. Causes of Proteinuria

TRANSIENT PROTEINURIA
Fever
Exercise
Dehydration
Cold exposure
Congestive heart failure
Seizure
Stress

ORTHOSTATIC (POSTURAL) PROTEINURIA

GLOMERULAR DISEASES
Acute postinfectious glomerulonephritis
Focal segmental glomerulosclerosis
Mesangial proliferative glomerulonephritis
Membranous nephropathy
Membranoproliferative glomerulonephritis
Lupus nephritis
IgA nephropathy
Henoch-Schönlein purpura nephritis
Amyloidosis
Diabetic nephropathy
Sickle cell nephropathy
Alport syndrome

TUBULAR DISEASES
Cystinosis
Wilson disease
Lowe syndrome
Galactosemia
Tubulointerstitial nephritis
Heavy metal poisoning
Acute tubular necrosis
Renal dysplasia
Polycystic kidney disease
Reflux nephropathy

lupus nephritis, IgA nephropathy, Henoch-Schönlein purpura nephritis, amyloidosis, diabetic nephropathy, sickle cell nephropathy, and Alport's syndrome.

Initial evaluation of a child having persistent fixed proteinuria should include measurement of serum creatinine, 24-hr urinary protein excretion, serum albumin level, and C3 level. In asymptomatic patients with low-grade proteinuria (150–1,000 mg/24 hr) in whom all other findings are normal, renal biopsy may not be indicated because the underlying process is transient/resolving (i.e., acute postinfectious glomerulonephritis) or because specific pathologic features of a chronic renal disease may not yet be apparent. Such patients should have periodic re-evaluation consisting of a physical examination and blood pressure determination, urinalysis, and measurement of serum creatinine and 24-hr urinary protein excretion. Indications for renal biopsy include increasing proteinuria in excess of 1,000 mg/24 and/or the development of hematuria, hypertension, or diminished renal function.

Dodge WF, West EF, Smith EH, et al: Proteinuria and hematuria in school-age children: Epidemiology and early natural history. *J Pediatr* 1976; 88:327.
Roy S: Proteinuria. *Pediatr Ann* 1996; 25:277–82.
Yoshikawa N, Kitagawa K, Ohta K, et al: Asymptomatic constant isolated proteinuria in children. *J Pediatr* 1991; 119:375.

518.2 Tubular Proteinuria

Fixed low-grade proteinuria (usually < 1 g/24 hr) may be a sign of a variety of renal disorders that involve the tubulointerstitial compartment of the kidney. In the healthy state, large amounts of proteins of lower molecular weight than albumin are filtered by the glomerulus and reabsorbed in the proximal tubule. Injury to the proximal tubules may result in diminished reabsorptive capacity and the loss of these low molecular weight proteins in the urine.

Tubular proteinuria (see Box 518–1) may be seen in acquired and inherited disorders and may be associated with other defects of proximal tubular function, such as glycosuria, phosphaturia, bicarbonate wasting, and aminoaciduria. Tubular proteinuria rarely presents a diagnostic dilemma because the underlying disease is usually detected before the proteinuria.

Asymptomatic patients having persistent proteinuria generally have glomerular rather than tubular proteinuria. In occult cases, glomerular and tubular proteinuria can be distinguished by electrophoresis of the urine. In tubular proteinuria, little or no albumin is detected, whereas in glomerular proteinuria the major protein is albumin.

Alt JM, Von der Heyde D, Assel E, et al: Characteristics of protein excretion in glomerular and tubular disease. *Contrib Nephrol* 1981; 24:115.
Waller KV, Ward KM, Mahan JD, et al: Current concepts in proteinuria. *Clin Chem* 1989; 35:755.

Chapter 519
Nephrotic Syndrome

Nephrotic syndrome is primarily a pediatric disorder and is 15 times more common in children than adults. The incidence is 2–3/100,000 children per year, and the vast majority of affected children will have steroid-sensitive minimal change disease. The characteristic features of nephrotic syndrome are heavy proteinuria (>3.5 g/24 hr in adults or 40 mg/m^2/hr in children), hypoalbuminemia (<2.5 g/dL), edema, and hyperlipidemia.

Etiology. Most children (90%) with nephrotic syndrome have a form of the idiopathic nephrotic syndrome. Causes of idiopathic nephrotic syndrome include minimal change disease (85%), mesangial proliferation (5%), and focal segmental glomerulosclerosis (10%). The remaining 10% of children with nephrotic syndrome have secondary nephrotic syndrome related to glomerular diseases such as membranous nephropathy or membranoproliferative glomerulonephritis (Table 519–1).

Pathophysiology. The underlying abnormality in nephrotic syndrome is an increase in permeability of the glomerular capillary wall, which leads to massive proteinuria and hypoalbuminemia. The cause of the increased permeability is not well understood. In minimal change disease, it is possible that T-cell dysfunction leads to alteration of cytokines, which causes a loss of negatively charged glycoproteins within the glomerular capillary wall.

In focal segmental glomerulosclerosis, a plasma factor, perhaps produced by lymphocytes, may be responsible for the increase in capillary wall permeability.

Although the mechanism of edema formation in nephrotic syndrome is incompletely understood, it seems likely that, in most instances, urinary protein loss leads to hypoalbuminemia, which causes a decrease in the plasma oncotic pressure and transudation of fluid from the intravascular compartment to the interstitial space. The reduction in intravascular volume decreases renal perfusion pressure, activating the renin-angiotensin-aldosterone system, which stimulates tubular reabsorption of sodium. The reduced intravascular volume also stimulates the release of antidiuretic hormone, which enhances the reabsorption of water in the collecting duct. Because of the decreased plasma oncotic pressure, fluid shifts into the interstitial space, exacerbating the edema.

This theory does not apply to all patients with nephrotic syndrome, however, because some patients actually have increased intravascular volume with diminished plasma levels of renin and aldosterone. Therefore, other factors, including a primary renal avidity for sodium and water, may be involved in

TABLE 519–1. Summary of Primary Renal Diseases That Present As Idiopathic Nephrotic Syndrome

	Minimal-Change Nephrotic Syndrome (MCNS)	Focal Segmental Sclerosis	Membranous Nephropathy	Membranoproliferative Glomerulonephritis (MPGN)	
				Type I	Type II
Frequency*					
Children	75%	10%	<5%	10%	10%
Adults	15%	15%	50%	10%	10%
Clinical Manifestations					
Age (yr)	2–6, some adults	2–10, some adults	40–50	5–15	5–15
Sex	2:1 male	1.3:1 male	2:1 male	Male-female	Male-female
Nephrotic syndrome	100%	90%	80%	60%	60%
Asymptomatic proteinuria	0	10%	20%	40%	40%
Hematuria	10–20%	60–80%	60%	80%	80%
Hypertension	10%	20% early	Infrequent	35%	35%
Rate of progression to renal failure	Does not progress	10 years	50% in 10–20 yr	10–20 yr	5–15 yr
Associated conditions	Allergy? Hodgkin disease, usually none	None	Renal vein thrombosis, cancer, SLE, hepatitis B	None	Partial lipodystrophy
Laboratory Findings	Manifestations of nephrotic syndrome ↑ BUN in 15–30%	Manifestations of nephrotic syndrome ↑ BUN in 20–40%	Manifestations of nephrotic syndrome	Low C1, C4, C3–C9	Normal C1, C4, low C3–C9
Immunogenetics	HLA-B8, B12 (3.5)†	Not established	HLA-DRw3 (12–32)†	Not established	C3 nephritic factor Not established
Renal Pathology					
Light microscopy	Normal	Focal sclerotic lesions	Thickened GBM, spikes	Thickened GBM, proliferation	Lobulation
Immunofluorescence	Negative	IgM, C3 in lesions	Fine granular IgG, C3	Granular IgG, C3	C3 only
Electron microscopy	Foot process fusion	Foot process fusion	Subepithelial deposits	Mesangial and subendothelial deposits	Dense deposits
Response to Steroids	90%	15–20%	May be slow progression	Not established	Not established

*Approximate frequency as a cause of idiopathic nephrotic syndrome. About 10% of adult nephrotic syndrome is due to various diseases that usually present as acute glomerulonephritis.
†Relative risk.
BUN = blood urea nitrogen; C = complement; GBM = glomerular basement membrane; HLA = human leukocyte antigen; Ig = immunoglobulin; SLE = systemic lupus erythematosus; hepatitis B = hepatitis B virus; ↑ = elevated.
Modified from Couser WG: Glomerular disorders. In Wyngaarden JB, Smith LH, Bennett JC (editors). Cecil Textbook of Medicine, 19th ed. Philadelphia, WB Saunders, 1992, p 560.

the formation of edema in some patients with nephrotic syndrome.

In the nephrotic state, serum lipid levels (cholesterol, triglycerides) are elevated for two reasons. Hypoalbuminemia stimulates generalized hepatic protein synthesis, including synthesis of lipoproteins. In addition, lipid catabolism is diminished, as a result of reduced plasma levels of lipoprotein lipase, related to increased urinary losses of this enzyme.

Nephrotic syndrome in children: Prediction of histopathology from clinical and laboratory characteristics at time of diagnosis. A report of the International Study of Kidney Disease in Children. *Kidney Int* 1978; 13:159.

Van de Walle JGJ, Donckerwolcke RA: Pathogenesis of edema formation in the nephrotic syndrome. *Pediatr Nephrol* 2001; 16:283.

519.1 Idiopathic Nephrotic Syndrome

Approximately 90% of children with nephrotic syndrome have idiopathic nephrotic syndrome. Idiopathic nephrotic syndrome includes three histologic types: minimal change disease, mesangial proliferation, and focal segmental glomerulosclerosis. Some experts believe that these three disorders represent three separate diseases with a similar clinical presentation, whereas others believe that these disorders represent a spectrum of a single disease.

Pathology. In *minimal change disease* (85% of total cases), the glomeruli appear normal or show a minimal increase in mesangial cells and matrix. Findings on immunofluorescence microscopy are typically negative, and electron microscopy simply reveals effacement of the epithelial cell foot processes. More than 95% of children with minimal change disease respond to corticosteroid therapy.

Mesangial proliferation (5% of total cases) is characterized by a diffuse increase in mesangial cells and matrix on light microscopy. Immunofluorescence microscopy may reveal trace to 1+ mesangial IgM and/or IgA staining. Electron microscopy reveals increased numbers of mesangial cells and matrix as well as effacement of the epithelial cell foot processes. Approximately 50% of patients with this histologic lesion respond to corticosteroid therapy.

In *focal segmental glomerulosclerosis* (10% of total cases), glomeruli show mesangial proliferation and segmental scarring on light microscopy (Fig. 519–1). Immunofluorescence microscopy shows IgM and C3 staining in the areas of segmental sclerosis. Electron microscopy shows segmental scarring of the glomerular tuft with obliteration of the glomerular capillary lumen. A similar lesion may be seen with HIV infection, vesicoureteral reflux, and intravenous heroin abuse. Approximately 20% of patients with focal segmental glomerulosclerosis respond

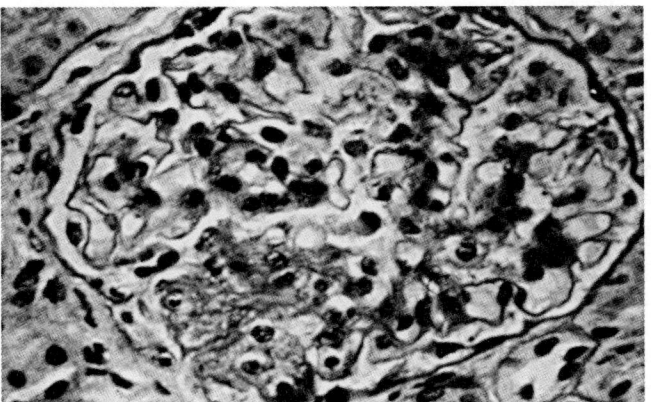

FIGURE 519–1. Glomerulus from a patient with steroid-resistant nephrotic syndrome, showing mesangial hypercellularity and an area of sclerosis in the lower portion. (×250.)

to prednisone. The disease is frequently progressive, ultimately involving all glomeruli, and leads to end-stage renal failure in most patients.

Clinical Manifestations. The idiopathic nephrotic syndrome is more common in males than in females (2:1) and most commonly appears between the ages of 2 and 6 yr. It has been reported as early as 6 mo of age and throughout adulthood. The initial episode and subsequent relapses may follow minor infections and, occasionally, reactions to insect bites, bee stings, or poison ivy. Children usually present with mild edema, which is initially noted around the eyes and in the lower extremities. Nephrotic syndrome may initially be misdiagnosed as an allergic disorder because of the periorbital swelling that decreases throughout the day. With time, the edema becomes generalized, with the development of ascites, pleural effusions, and genital edema. Anorexia, irritability, abdominal pain, and diarrhea are common; hypertension and gross hematuria are uncommon. The differential diagnosis of the child with marked edema includes protein-losing enteropathy, hepatic failure, congestive heart failure, acute or chronic glomerulonephritis, and protein malnutrition.

Diagnosis. The urinalysis reveals 3+ or 4+ proteinuria; microscopic hematuria may be present in 20% of children. Urinary protein excretion exceeds 3.5 g/24 hr in adults and 40 $mg/m^2/hr$ in children. Spot urine protein to creatinine ratio exceeds 2.0. The serum creatinine value is usually normal, but it may be increased because of diminished renal perfusion resulting from contraction of the intravascular volume. The serum albumin level is generally less than 2.5 g/dL, and the serum cholesterol and triglyceride levels are elevated. C3 and C4 levels are normal. Renal biopsy is not required for diagnosis in most children (see Treatment).

Treatment. Children with the first episode of nephrotic syndrome and mild to moderate edema may be managed as outpatients. Affected children may attend school and participate in physical activities as tolerated. The pathophysiology and treatment of nephrotic syndrome should be carefully reviewed with the family to enhance their understanding of their child's disease. Sodium intake should be reduced by the initiation of a low sodium diet and may be normalized when the child enters remission. Although there are no data to support their safety or efficacy, oral diuretics are used by many clinicians for children with nephrotic syndrome. Because of the possibility of increasing the risk of thromboembolic complications, diuretic use should be judicious and should be carefully supervised by a pediatric nephrologist.

Children with severe symptomatic edema, including large pleural effusions, ascites, or severe genital edema, should be hospitalized. In addition to sodium restriction, fluid restriction may be necessary if the child is hyponatremic. A swollen scrotum may be elevated with pillows to enhance the removal of fluid by gravity. Diuresis may be augmented by intravenous administration of chlorothiazide (10 mg/kg/dose every 12 hr) or metolazone (0.1 mg/kg/dose bid) followed by furosemide 30 min later (1–2 mg/kg/dose q 12 hr).

Intravenous administration of 25% human albumin (0.5 g/kg/12 hr) is often necessary when this potent combination is used. Such therapy mandates close monitoring of volume status, serum electrolyte balance, and renal function. Symptomatic volume overload, with hypertension and heart failure, is a potential complication of parenteral albumin therapy.

Children with onset of nephrotic syndrome between 1 and 8 yr of age are likely to have steroid-responsive minimal change disease; therefore, steroid therapy may be initiated without renal biopsy. Children with features that make minimal change disease less likely (hematuria, hypertension, renal insufficiency, hypocomplementemia, age < 1 yr or > 8 yr) should be considered for renal biopsy before treatment.

In children with presumed minimal change disease, prednisone should be administered (after confirming a negative PPD test) at a dose of 60 mg/m^2/day (maximum daily dose, 80 mg), divided into two to three doses for at least 4 consecutive weeks. There is some evidence that an initial 6 wk course of daily steroid treatment may lead to a lower relapse rate, although the frequency of steroid-induced side effects is significantly higher. Eighty to 90% of children will respond to steroid therapy (urine trace or negative for protein for 3 consecutive days), with the median time to remission of 10 days. The vast majority of children who will respond to prednisone therapy will do so within the first 4 wk of treatment.

After the initial 4–6 wk course, the prednisone dose should be tapered to 40 mg/m^2/day given every other day as a single morning dose. The alternate-day dose is then slowly tapered and discontinued over the next 2–3 mo. Children who continue to have proteinuria (2+ or greater) after 8 wk of steroid therapy are considered steroid resistant, and a diagnostic renal biopsy should be performed.

Many children with nephrotic syndrome will experience at least one relapse (3–4+ proteinuria plus edema). Although relapse rates of 60–80% have been noted in the past, the relapse rate in children treated with longer initial steroid courses may be as low as 30–40%.

Relapses should be treated with daily divided-dose prednisone at the doses noted earlier until the child enters remission (urine trace or negative for protein for 3 consecutive days). The prednisone dose is then changed to alternate-day dosing and tapered over 1–2 mo.

A subset of patients will relapse while on alternate-day steroid therapy or within 28 days of stopping prednisone therapy. Such patients are termed *steroid dependent*. Patients who respond well to prednisone therapy but relapse four or more times in a 12-mo period are termed *frequent relapsers*. Children who fail to respond to prednisone therapy within 8 wk are termed *steroid resistant*.

Steroid-dependent patients, frequent relapsers, and steroid-resistant patients may be candidates for alternative agents, particularly if the child suffers severe corticosteroid toxicity (cushingoid appearance, hypertension, cataracts, and/or growth failure). Cyclophosphamide has been shown to prolong the duration of remission and to reduce the number relapses in children with frequently relapsing and steroid-dependent nephrotic syndrome. The potential side effects of the drug (neutropenia, disseminated varicella, hemorrhagic cystitis, alopecia, sterility, and increased risk of future malignancy) should be carefully reviewed with the family before initiating treatment. The dose of cyclophosphamide is 2–3 mg/kg/24 hr given as a single dose, for a total duration of 8–12 wk. Alternate-day prednisone therapy is often continued during the course of cyclophosphamide administration. During cyclophosphamide therapy, the white blood cell count must be monitored weekly and the drug withheld if the count falls below 5,000/mm^3.

An additional option for the child with complicated nephrotic syndrome is high-dose pulse methylprednisolone. Methylprednisolone is usually given as a 30-mg/kg bolus (maximum 1,000 mg), with the first 6 doses given every other day, followed by a tapering regimen for periods up to 18 mo. Cyclophosphamide may be added to this regimen in selected patients.

Prolonged administration of cyclosporine (3–6 mg/kg/24 hr) has also been effective in maintaining a prolonged remission in children with nephrotic syndrome and is useful as a steroid-sparing agent. Children must be monitored for side effects, including hypertension, nephrotoxicity, hirsutism, and gingival hyperplasia. Unfortunately, most children who respond to cyclosporine therapy tend to relapse when the medication is discontinued.

Angiotensin-converting enzyme (ACE) inhibitors and angiotensin II blockers may be helpful as an adjunct therapy to reduce proteinuria in steroid-resistant patients.

Complications. Infection is the major complication of nephrotic syndrome. Children in relapse have increased susceptibility to bacterial infections owing to urinary losses of immunoglobulins and properdin factor B, defective cell-mediated immunity, immunosuppressive therapy, malnutrition, and edema/ascites acting as a potential "culture medium." Spontaneous bacterial peritonitis is the most frequent type of infection, although sepsis, pneumonia, cellulitis, and urinary tract infections may also be seen. Although *Streptococcus pneumoniae* is the most common organism causing peritonitis, gram-negative bacteria such as *Escherichia coli* may also be encountered. Because fever and physical findings may be minimal in the presence of corticosteroid therapy, a high index of suspicion, prompt evaluation (including cultures of blood and peritoneal fluid), and early initiation of antibiotic therapy are critical. The role of prophylactic antibiotic therapy during relapse remains controversial.

All children with nephrotic syndrome should receive polyvalent pneumococcal vaccine (if not previously immunized), ideally administered when the child is in remission and off of daily prednisone therapy. Children with a negative varicella titer should be given varicella vaccine when in remission or on a low dose of alternate-day steroids. Nonimmune nephrotic children in relapse exposed to varicella should receive varicella zoster immune globulin (VZIG) within 72 hr of exposure. Influenza vaccine should be given on a yearly basis.

Children with nephrotic syndrome are also at increased risk for thromboembolic events. The incidence of this complication in children is 2–5%, which represents a much lower risk than that of adults with nephrotic syndrome. Both arterial and venous thromboses may be seen, including renal vein thrombosis, pulmonary embolus, sagittal sinus thrombosis, and thrombosis of indwelling arterial and venous catheters. The risk of thrombosis is related to increased prothrombotic factors (fibrinogen, thrombocytosis, hemoconcentration, relative immobilization) and decreased fibrinolytic factors (urinary losses of antithrombin III, proteins C and S). Prophylactic anticoagulation is not recommended in children unless they have had a previous thromboembolic event. Overaggressive diuresis should be avoided and use of indwelling catheters limited because these factors may increase the likelihood of clotting complications.

Prognosis. The majority of children with steroid-responsive nephrotic syndrome have repeated relapses, which generally decrease in frequency as the child grows older.

Although there is no proven way to predict an individual child's course, those children who respond to steroids rapidly and those who have no relapses during the first 6 mo after diagnosis tend to follow an infrequently relapsing course. It is important to indicate to the family that the child with steroid-responsive nephrotic syndrome will not develop chronic renal failure, that the disease is generally not hereditary, and that the child (in the absence of prolonged cyclophosphamide therapy) will remain fertile. To minimize the psychological effects of the condition, the physician should emphasize that the child should be considered normal when in remission and may have unrestricted diet and activity, without the need for urine testing for protein.

Children with steroid-resistant nephrotic syndrome, most often caused by focal segmental glomerulosclerosis, generally have a much poorer prognosis (see Chapter 528). These children develop progressive renal insufficiency, ultimately leading to end-stage renal failure requiring dialysis or renal transplantation. Recurrent nephrotic syndrome develops in 30–50% of transplant recipients with focal segmental glomerulosclerosis. Plasmapheresis, plasma protein absorption onto protein A–based columns, high-dose cyclosporine or tacrolimus, and angiotensin-converting enzyme (ACE) inhibitors may reduce proteinuria in these patients.

Arbeitsgemeinschaft fur Padiatrische Nephrologie: Cyclophosphamide treatment of steroid dependent nephrotic syndrome: Comparison of eight week with 12 week course. *Arch Dis Child* 1987; 62:1102.

Cattran DC, Appel GB, Hebert LA, et al, for the North America Nephrotic Syndrome Study Group: A randomized trial of cyclosporine in patients with steroid-resistant focal segmental glomerulosclerosis. *Kidney Int* 1999; 56: 2220.

Constantinescu AR, Shah HB, Foote EF, et al: Predicting first-year relapses in children with nephrotic syndrome. *Pediatrics* 2000; 105:492–95.

Durkan AM, Hodson EM, Willis NS, et al: Immunosuppressive agents in childhood nephrotic syndrome: A meta-analysis of randomized controlled trials. *Kidney Int* 2001; 59:1919–27.

Eddy AA, Schnaper HW: The nephrotic syndrome: From the simple to the complex. *Semin Nephrol* 1998; 18:304.

Hogg R, Portman RJ, Milliner D, et al: Evaluation and management of proteinuria and nephrotic syndrome in children: Recommendations from a pediatric nephrology panel established at the National Kidney Foundation Conference of Proteinuria, Albuminuria, Risk, Assessment, Detection, and Elimination. *Pediatrics* 2000; 105:1242–49.

Kaysen G: Nonrenal complications of the nephrotic syndrome. *Annu Rev Med* 1994; 45:201.

Orth S, Ritz E: The nephrotic syndrome. *N Engl J Med* 1998; 338:1202.

Savin VI, Sharma R, Sharma M, et al: Circulating factor associated with increased glomerular permeability to albumin in recurrent focal segmental glomerulosclerosis. *N Engl J Med* 1996; 14:878.

Tarshish P, Tobin IN, Bernstein J, et al: Prognostic significance of the early course of minimal change nephrotic syndrome: Report of the International Study of Kidney Disease in Children. *J Am Soc Nephrol* 1997; 8:769–76.

Tune BM, Mendoza SA: Treatment of idiopathic nephrotic syndrome: Regimens and outcomes in children and adults. *J Am Soc Nephrol* 1997; 8:824.

519.2 Secondary Nephrotic Syndrome

Nephrotic syndrome also occurs as a secondary feature of many forms of glomerular disease. Membranous nephropathy, membranoproliferative glomerulonephritis, postinfectious glomerulonephritis, lupus nephritis, and Henoch-Schönlein purpura nephritis may all have a nephrotic component. In general, secondary nephrotic syndrome should be suspected in patients with age > 8 yr, hypertension, hematuria, renal dysfunction, extrarenal symptomatology (rash, arthralgias, etc.), or depressed serum complement levels.

In certain areas of the world, malaria and schistosomiasis are the leading causes of nephrotic syndrome. Other infectious agents associated with nephrotic syndrome include hepatitis B virus, hepatitis C virus, filaria, leprosy, and HIV.

Nephrotic syndrome has been associated with malignancy, particularly in the adult population. In patients with solid tumors, such as carcinomas of the lung and gastrointestinal tract, the renal pathology often resembles membranous glomerulopathy. Immune complexes composed of tumor antigens and tumor-specific antibodies presumably mediate the renal involvement. In patients with lymphomas, particularly Hodgkin lymphoma, the renal pathology most often resembles minimal change disease. The proposed mechanism of the nephrotic syndrome is that the lymphoma produces a lymphokine that increases glomerular capillary wall permeability. Nephrotic syndrome may develop before or after the malignancy is detected, may resolve as the tumor regresses, and may return if the tumor recurs.

Nephrotic syndrome has also developed during therapy with numerous drugs and chemicals. The histologic picture may resemble membranous glomerulopathy (penicillamine, captopril, gold, nonsteroidal anti-inflammatory drugs, mercury compounds), minimal change disease (probenecid, ethosuximide, methimazole, lithium), or proliferative glomerulonephritis (procainamide, chlorpropamide, phenytoin, trimethadione, paramethadione).

Barsoum RS: Schistosomal glomerulopathies. *Kidney Int* 1993; 44: 1–12.

Klotman FE: HIV-associated nephropathy. *Kidney Int* 1999; 56:1161–76.

Radford MG Jr, Holley KE, Grande JP, et al: Reversible membranous nephropathy associated with the use of nonsteroidal anti-inflammatory drugs. *JAMA* 1996; 276:466.

Ronco PM: Paraneoplastic glomerulopathies: New insights into an old entity. *Kidney Int* 1999; 56:355–77.

Sitprija V: Nephropathy in falciparum malaria. *Kidney Int* 1998; 34:867.

519.3 Congenital Nephrotic Syndrome

Infants who develop nephrotic syndrome within the first 3 mo of life are considered to have congenital nephrotic syndrome. The most common cause of this syndrome is Finnish type congenital nephrotic syndrome, an autosomal recessive disorder that is most common in populations of Scandinavian descent (1:8,000 incidence). This type of congenital nephrotic syndrome is caused by a mutation in the *NPHS1* gene located on chromosome 19, which encodes a protein, nephrin. Nephrin is a key component of the slit diaphragm of the glomerular epithelial cell and is thought to play an essential role in the normal function of the glomerular filtration barrier. The major pathologic features of the Finnish type of this syndrome are dilatation of the proximal tubules, mesangial hypercellularity, and glomerular sclerosis.

Infants with the Finnish type of congenital nephrotic syndrome present with massive proteinuria (detectable in utero by increased α-fetoprotein), a large placenta, and marked edema. Additional clinical features include prematurity, respiratory distress, and separation of the cranial sutures. The natural history of the disease is one of persistent edema, recurrent infections, and progressive renal failure with death by the age of 5 yr. Corticosteroids and immunosuppressive agents are of no value.

ACE inhibitors, indomethacin, and unilateral nephrectomy may diminish proteinuria and ameliorate the nephrotic state. However, the preferred treatment includes bilateral nephrectomy, chronic dialysis, aggressive nutritional support, and eventual kidney transplantation. In families at risk for the Finnish type of congenital nephrotic syndrome, antenatal diagnosis is suggested by an elevated amniotic fluid α-fetoprotein level and the diagnosis may be confirmed by DNA analysis.

Other causes of congenital nephrotic syndrome include congenital infections such as syphilis, toxoplasmosis, rubella, and cytomegalovirus. HIV and hepatitis B have also been reported to cause nephrotic syndrome in the neonatal period. The nephrotic state, which is generally less severe than the Finnish type of congenital nephrotic syndrome, may improve or resolve with treatment of the underlying infection.

Diffuse mesangial sclerosis is a rare glomerular disease seen in a minority of children with congenital nephrotic syndrome. The characteristic pathologic finding is progressive sclerosis of the glomerular mesangium, and the clinical picture is one of rapid loss of renal function, with end-stage renal disease developing within months to years. Diffuse mesangial sclerosis may occur as an isolated disease or as part of *Denys-Drash syndrome*, a condition also characterized by Wilms tumor and male pseudohermaphroditism, caused by a mutation in the Wilms tumor gene *(WT1)* on chromosome 11.

Habib R: Nephrotic syndrome in the first year of life. *Pediatr Nephrol* 1993; 7:347,

Holmberg C, Antikainen M, Ronnholm K, et al: Management of congenital nephrotic syndrome of the Finnish type. *Pediatr Nephrol* 1995; 9:87.

Lenkkeri U, Mannikko M, McCready P, et al: Structure of the gene for congenital nephrotic syndrome of the Finnish type *(NPHS 1)* and characterization of mutations. *Am J Hum Genet* 1999; 64:51–61.

Mannikko M, Kestila M, Lenkkeri U, et al: Improved prenatal diagnosis of the congenital nephrotic syndrome of the Finnish type based on DNA analysis. *Kidney Int* 1997; 51:868.

McTaggart 8J, Algar E, Chow CW, et al: Clinical spectrum of Denys-Drash and Frasier syndrome. *Pediatr Nephrol* 2001; 16:335.

SECTION 4 *Tubular Disorders*

Chapter 520

Tubular Function

Katherine MacRae Dell and Ellis D. Avner

Water and electrolytes are freely filtered at the level of the glomerulus. Thus, the electrolyte content of "ultrafiltrate" at the beginning of the proximal tubule is similar to that of plasma. Carefully regulated processes of tubular reabsorption and/or tubular secretion determine final water content and electrolyte composition of urine. As a general principle, "bulk" movement of solute tends to occur in the proximal portions of the nephron, whereas fine adjustments tend to occur distally. Modern advances in molecular biology have helped to delineate the role of specific nephron segments in regulating ion and water transport and the diseases that occur as a result of abnormalities in these processes. This chapter provides an overview of normal tubular function and tubular disorders. (See also Chapter 45.)

Sodium. Sodium is essential in maintaining extracellular fluid balance and, thus, volume status. The kidney is capable of effecting large changes in sodium excretion in a variety of normal and pathologic states. There are four main sites of sodium transport. Approximately 60% of sodium is absorbed in the proximal tubule by coupled transport with glucose or amino acids, 25% in the ascending loop of Henle (bumetanide-sensitive sodium-potassium 2 chloride transporter, NKCC2), and 15% in the distal tubule (thiazide-sensitive sodium chloride cotransporter, NCCT) and collecting tubule (epithelial sodium channel, ENaC). Under normal circumstances, the urinary excretion of sodium approximates the sodium intake (80–250 mEq/24 hr for an adult who consumes a typical American diet) minus 1–2 mEq/kg/24 hr required for normal metabolic processes. However, in states of volume depletion (e.g., dehydration, blood loss) or decreased effective circulating blood volume (e.g., septic shock, hypoalbuminemic states, or congestive heart failure), there may be a dramatic decrease in urinary sodium excretion to as low as 1 mEq/L. Changes in volume status are detected by baroreceptors in the atria, afferent arteriole, and the carotid sinus and by the macula densa, which detects changes in chloride delivery. The major hormonal mechanisms mediating sodium balance include the renin-angiotensin-aldosterone (RAA) axis, atrial natriuretic factor (ANF), and norepinephrine. Angiotensin II and aldosterone increase sodium reabsorption in the proximal tubule and distal tubules, respectively. Norepinephrine, released in response to volume depletion, does not directly act on tubular transport mechanisms but impacts on sodium balance by decreasing renal blood flow and thus decreasing the filtered load of sodium, as well as stimulating renin release. With more severe volume depletion antidiuretic hormone (ADH) is also released (see Chapter 522). Sodium excretion is promoted by atrial natriuretic factor (ANF) and suppression of renin.

Potassium. Extracellular potassium homeostasis is very tightly regulated, because small changes in plasma potassium concentrations have dramatic effects on cardiac, neural, and neuromuscular function. Essentially all filtered potassium is fully reabsorbed in the proximal tubule. Therefore, urinary excretion of potassium is completely dependent on tubular secretion by potassium channels present in the principal cells of the collect-

ing tubule. Factors that promote potassium secretion include aldosterone, increased sodium delivery to the distal nephron, and increased urine flow rate.

Calcium. A significant portion of filtered calcium (65%) is reabsorbed in the proximal tubule. Additional calcium is reabsorbed in the ascending loop of Henle by passive movement between cells (paracellular absorption) in a process driven by sodium chloride reabsorption and potassium recycling into the lumen. Calcium uptake in this nephron segment is regulated by an extracellular calcium receptor (CaR). Factors that promote calcium reabsorption include parathyroid hormone (PTH, released in response to hypocalcemia), thiazide diuretics, and volume depletion. Factors that promote calcium excretion include sodium intake (either orally or by infusion of sodium-containing intravenous fluids) and loop diuretics such as furosemide.

Phosphate. The majority of filtered phosphate is reabsorbed in the proximal tubule. Reabsorption is increased by endogenous or exogenous calcitriol (1,25-dihydroxyvitamin D) and inhibited by PTH.

Magnesium. About 25% of filtered magnesium is reabsorbed in the proximal tubule. Modulation of renal magnesium excretion occurs primarily in the ascending loop of Henle, with some contribution of the distal convoluted tubule. Although specific magnesium transporters have been identified, the precise mechanisms by which they are regulated remain unclear.

Acidification and Concentrating Mechanisms. These are addressed in the sections on renal tubular acidosis and nephrogenic diabetes insipidus (see Chapters 521 and 522).

Developmental Considerations. Tubular transport capabilities of neonates (especially premature infants) and young infants are generally less than that of adults. Although nephrogenesis (the formation of new glomerular/tubular units) is complete by about 36 wk gestation, significant tubular maturation occurs during infancy. Renal tubular immaturity, reduced glomerular filtration rate, decreased concentrating gradient, and diminished responsiveness to antidiuretic hormone are characteristic of young infants. These factors can contribute to impaired electrolyte and water regulation and acid-base homeostasis, particularly during times of acute illness.

Jones DP, Chesney RW: Tubular function: In Barratt TM, Avner ED, Harmon WE (editors): *Pediatric Nephrology*, 4th ed. Baltimore, Williams & Wilkins, 1999, pp 59–82.
Rose BD, Rennke HG: *Renal Pathophysiology—The Essentials*. Baltimore, Williams & Wilkins, 1994, pp 1–15.
Scheinman SJ, Guay-Woodford LM, Thakker RV, et al: Genetic disorders of renal electrolyte transport. *N Engl J Med* 1999;340:1177–87.
Schrier RW (editor): *Renal and Electrolyte Disorders*, 4th ed. Boston, Little, Brown & Company, 1992.
Van't Hoff WG: Molecular developments in renal tubulopathies. *Arch Dis Child* 2000;83:189–91.

Chapter 521

Renal Tubular Acidosis

Renal tubular acidosis (RTA) is a disease state characterized by a normal anion gap metabolic acidosis resulting from either impaired bicarbonate reabsorption or impaired urinary acid (hydrogen ion) excretion. Both inherited and acquired primary and secondary forms exist. There are three main forms of RTA: proximal (type II) RTA, distal (type I) RTA, and hyperkalemic (type IV) RTA. Mixed lesions (e.g., those with elements of types I and II RTA), which occur primarily in patients with inherited carbonic anhydrase deficiency, have been designated as type III RTA by some authors.

Normal Urinary Acidification. Urinary acidification involves two processes: bicarbonate reabsorption and hydrogen ion excretion. Bicarbonate reabsorption results in reclamation of the filtered bicarbonate but does not result in net acid secretion. Approximately 85% of the filtered bicarbonate is reabsorbed in the proximal tubule. In infants, bicarbonate reabsorption is less efficient, and renal bicarbonate excretion may occur at serum concentrations less than 22 mmol/L. Bicarbonate itself is not directly absorbed through a specific transporter but instead is absorbed by an indirect process. Proximal tubule reabsorption of bicarbonate begins with secretion of a hydrogen ion in exchange for a sodium ion. The hydrogen ion in the tubular lumen binds with bicarbonate and, under the influence of carbonic anhydrase, is converted to carbon dioxide and water. Carbon dioxide then diffuses into the proximal tubular cell, where a series of chemical reactions result in the creation of a bicarbonate molecule (which enters the peritubular capillary) and a hydrogen ion, which can participate in further buffering of bicarbonate in the tubular lumen. The remaining 15% of bicarbonate is reabsorbed distally. Secretion of the daily acid load (approximately 1 mEq/kg/24 hr produced during normal cellular processes) is accomplished by hydrogen ion secretion (mediated by a H^+ ATPase present in the intercalated cells of the collecting tubule), ammoniagenesis, and formation of titratable acids (formed when H^+ ions are buffered by organic acids such as phosphate).

521.1 Proximal (Type II) Renal Tubular Acidosis

Katherine MacRae Dell and Ellis D. Avner

Pathogenesis. Proximal RTA results from impaired proximal tubule bicarbonate reabsorption. Isolated forms of inherited or acquired proximal RTA occur, although they are generally rare. Isolated autosomal dominant forms, as well as an autosomal recessive form associated with ocular abnormalities, have been reported. More typically, proximal RTA occurs as a component of global proximal tubule dysfunction or Fanconi syndrome. The latter condition is characterized by low molecular weight proteinuria, glycosuria, phosphaturia, aminoaciduria, and proximal RTA. Both autosomal dominant and autosomal recessive forms of primary Fanconi syndrome occur. In addition, secondary Fanconi syndrome may occur as a component of one of several inherited renal tubular disorders or in acquired disease states. The causes of proximal RTA and Fanconi syndrome are outlined in Box 521–1. Many of these causes are inherited disorders. Two diseases, *cystinosis* and *Lowe syndrome,* are addressed in detail later. Other inherited forms of Fanconi syndrome, discussed elsewhere in the text, include *galactosemia* (see Chapter 76.2), *hereditary fructose intolerance* (see Chapter 76.3), *tyrosinemia* (see Chapter 74.2), and *Wilson disease* (see Chapters 338.2 and 590.3). *Dent disease,* or X-linked nephrolithiasis, is discussed in Chapter 523.3. In children, an important form of secondary Fanconi syndrome is exposure to ifosfamide, a component of many treatment regimens for Wilms tumor and other solid tumors.

Cystinosis is a systemic disease caused by a defect in the metabolism of cystine, which results in accumulation of cystine crystals in most of the major organs of the body, notably kidney, liver, eye, and brain. It occurs at an incidence of 1:100,000–1:200,000. In

BOX 521–1. Classification of Renal Tubular Acidosis

PROXIMAL (TYPE II)
Isolated
   Sporadic
   Hereditary
Fanconi Syndrome
   Primary
      Sporadic
      Hereditary
         Cystinosis
         Lowe syndrome
         Galactosemia
         Tyrosenemia
         Fructosemia
         Fanconi-Bickel syndrome
         Wilson disease
         Mitochondrial diseases
         Dent disease (X-linked nephrolithiasis)
   Secondary
      Heavy metals
      Outdated tetracycline
      Gentamicin
      Ifosfamide
      Cyclosporine/tacrolimus

DISTAL (TYPE I)
Primary
   Sporadic
   Hereditary
Secondary
   Interstitial nephritis
      Obstructive uropathy
      Vesicoureteral reflux
      Pyelonephritis
      Transplant rejection
      Sickle cell nephropathy
      Ehlers-Danlos syndrome
      Lupus nephritis
      Nephrocalcinosis
      Medullary sponge kidney
      Hepatic cirrhosis
   Toxins/Medications
      Amphotericin B
      Lithium
      Toluene
      Cisplatin

HYPERKALEMIC (TYPE IV)
Primary
   Sporadic
   Hereditary
Secondary
   Hypoaldosteronism
      Addison disease
      Congenital adrenal hyperplasia
      Prolonged heparinization
   Pseudohypoaldosteronism (type I or II)
   Obstructive uropathy
   Pyelonephritis
   Interstitial nephritis
   Diabetes mellitus
   Sickle cell nephropathy
   Trimethoprim/sulfamethoxazole
   Angiotensin-converting enzyme inhibitors
   Cyclosporine

certain populations, such as French Canadians, the incidence is much higher. At least three clinical patterns have been described. Young children with the most severe form of the disease *(infantile or nephropathic cystinosis)* present in the first 2 yr of life with severe tubular dysfunction and growth failure. If the disease is not treated, the children develop end-stage renal disease by the end of their first decade. A milder form of the disease presents in adolescents and is characterized by less severe tubular abnormalities and a slower progression to renal failure. A benign adult form with no renal involvement also exists. Cystinosis is caused by mutations in the *CTNS* gene, which encodes a novel protein, cystinosin. Although the precise function of cystinosin has not been fully delineated, it is thought to be an H$^+$-driven lysosomal cystine transporter. Genotype-phenotype studies in patients with severe nephropathic cystinosis demonstrate complete loss of cystinosin function, whereas patients with milder clinical disease still express partially functional protein.

Patients with nephropathic cystinosis present with *clinical manifestations* reflecting their pronounced tubular dysfunction and Fanconi syndrome, including polyuria and polydipsia, growth failure, and rickets. Fever, caused by dehydration or diminished sweat production, is common. Patients are typically fair skinned and blond, owing to diminished pigmentation. Photophobia occurs. With progressive tubulointerstitial fibrosis, renal insufficiency is invariant. Retinopathy and impaired visual acuity occur, as well as hypothyroidism, hepatosplenomegaly, and delayed sexual maturation.

The *diagnosis* of cystinosis is suggested by the detection of cystine crystals in the cornea. Confirmation is made by measurement of leukocyte cystine content. Prenatal testing is available for at-risk families.

Treatment is directed at correcting the metabolic abnormalities associated with Fanconi syndrome or chronic renal failure. In addition, specific therapy is available with cysteamine, which binds to cystine, converts it to cysteine, and facilitates transport out of the lysosome, thereby depleting cystine from tissues. Oral cysteamine does not achieve adequate levels in ocular tissues, so additional therapy with cysteamine eye drops is required. Early initiation of the drug may prevent or delay deterioration of renal function. Patients with growth failure that does not improve with cysteamine may benefit from treatment with growth hormone. Renal transplantation is a viable option in patients with renal failure; but with prolonged survival, additional complications may become evident, including central nervous system abnormalities, muscle weakness, swallowing dysfunction, and pancreatic insufficiency.

Lowe syndrome (also called *oculocerebrorenal syndrome of Lowe*) is a rare X-linked disorder characterized by congenital cataracts, mental retardation, and Fanconi syndrome. The disease is caused by mutations in the *OCRL1* gene, which encodes the phosphatidylinositol polyphosphate 5-phosphatase protein. The abnormalities seen in Lowe syndrome are thought to be due to abnormal transport of vesicles within the Golgi apparatus. Histologically, kidneys show nonspecific tubulointerstitial changes. Thickening of glomerular basement membrane and changes in the proximal tubule mitochondria are also seen.

Patients with Lowe syndrome typically present in infancy with cataracts, progressive growth failure, hypotonia, and Fanconi syndrome. Blindness and renal insufficiency often develop. Characteristic behavioral abnormalities are also seen, including tantrums, stubbornness, stereotypy (repetitive behaviors), and obsessions. There is no specific therapy for the renal disease or neurologic deficits. Cataract removal is generally required.

Clinical Manifestations of Proximal RTA and Fanconi Syndrome.
Patients with isolated, sporadic, or inherited proximal RTA commonly present with growth failure in the first year of life. Additional symptoms may include polyuria, dehydration (due to sodium losses), anorexia, vomiting, constipation, and hypotonia. Patients with primary Fanconi syndrome will have additional symptoms secondary to phosphate wasting such as rickets. Those with systemic diseases will present with additional signs and symptoms specific to their underlying disease. A non–anion gap metabolic acidosis will be present. Urinalysis in patients with isolated proximal RTA is generally unremarkable. The urine pH is acidic (<5.5), because distal acidification mechanisms are intact in these patients. In contrast, urinary indices in patients with Fanconi syndrome demonstrate varying degrees of phosphaturia, aminoaciduria, glycosuria, uricosuria, and elevated urinary sodium or potassium. Depending on the nature of the underlying disorder, laboratory evidence of chronic renal insufficiency, including elevated serum creatinine, may be present.

521.2 Distal (Type I) Renal Tubular Acidosis

Katherine MacRae Dell and Ellis D. Avner

Pathogenesis. Distal RTA occurs as the result of impaired distal urinary acidification (hydrogen ion secretion). Primary or secondary causes can result in damaged or impaired functioning of one or more transporters or proteins involved in the acidification process, including the H$^+$/ATPase, the HCO$_3^-$/Cl$^-$ anion exchangers or the components of the aldosterone pathway. Because of impaired hydrogen ion excretion, urine pH cannot be reduced below 5.5, despite the presence of severe metabolic acidosis. Loss of sodium bicarbonate results in hyperchloremia and hypokalemia. Hypercalciuria is usually present and may lead to nephrocalcinosis or nephrolithiasis. Chronic metabolic acidosis also impairs urinary citrate excretion. Hypocitraturia further increases the risk of calcium deposition in the tubules. Bone disease is common, resulting from mobilization of organic components from bone to serve as buffers to chronic acidosis. Both primary sporadic or inherited forms occur. As with proximal RTA, distal RTA can also occur as a complication of either inherited or acquired diseases of the distal tubules.

Clinical Manifestations. Patients with distal RTA share common features with those of proximal RTA, including non–anion gap metabolic acidosis and growth failure. However, distinguishing features of distal RTA include nephrocalcinosis and hypercalciuria. The phosphate and massive bicarbonate wasting characteristic of proximal RTA is generally absent.

Causes of primary and secondary distal RTA are listed in Box 521-1. Although rare, three specific inherited forms of distal RTA have been identified, including an autosomal recessive form associated with sensorineural deafness.

Medullary sponge kidney is a relatively rare sporadic disorder in children, although not uncommon in adults. It is characterized by cystic dilatation of the terminal portions of the collecting ducts as they enter the renal pyramids. Ultrasonographically, patients often have medullary nephrocalcinosis (Fig. 521–1).

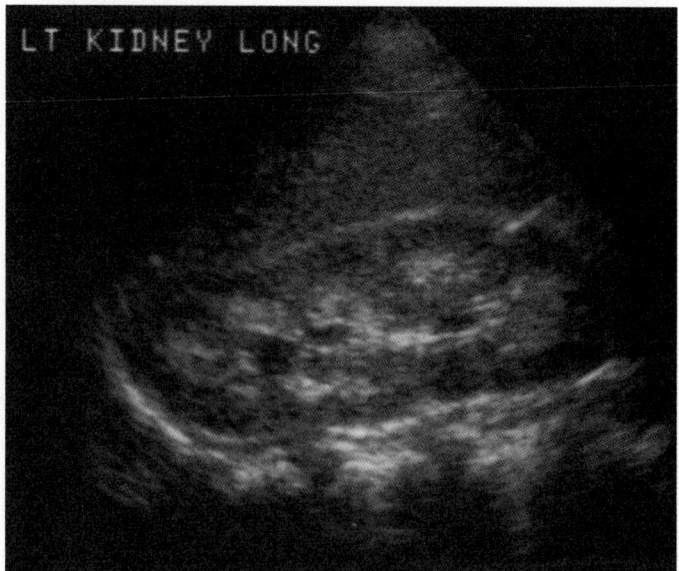

FIGURE 521–1 Ultrasound examination of a child with distal renal tubular acidosis demonstrating medullary nephrocalcinosis.

Although patients with this condition typically maintain normal renal function through adulthood, complications include nephrolithiasis, pyelonephritis, hyposthenuria (inability to concentrate urine), and distal RTA. Associations of medullary sponge kidney with Beckwith-Wiedemann syndrome or hemihypertrophy have been reported.

521.3 Hyperkalemic (Type IV) Renal Tubular Necrosis

Katherine MacRae Dell and Ellis D. Avner

Pathogenesis. Type IV RTA occurs as the result of impaired aldosterone production (hypoaldosteronism) or impaired renal responsiveness to aldosterone ("pseudo" hypoaldosteronism). Because aldosterone has a direct effect on the H$^+$ ATPase responsible for hydrogen secretion, acidosis results. In addition, aldosterone is a potent stimulant for potassium secretion in the collecting tubule. Loss of aldosterone effect results in hyperkalemia. This further affects acid-base status by inhibiting ammoniagenesis and, thus, hydrogen ion excretion. Aldosterone deficiency typically occurs as a result of adrenal gland disorders such as Addison disease or congenital adrenal hyperplasia (CAH). In children, aldosterone unresponsiveness is a more common cause of type IV RTA. This may occur transiently, during an episode of acute pyelonephritis or acute urinary obstruction, or chronically, particularly in infants and children with a history of obstructive uropathy. The latter patients may have significant hyperkalemia, even in instances when renal function is normal or only mildly impaired. Rare examples of inherited forms of type IV RTA have been identified.

Clinical Manifestations. Patients with type IV RTA, like those with types I and II RTA, may present with growth failure in the first few years of life. Polyuria and dehydration (from salt wasting) are common. Rarely, patients (especially those with pseudohypoaldosteronism type 1) will present with life-threatening hyperkalemia. Patients with obstructive uropathies may present acutely with signs and symptoms of pyelonephritis, such as fever, vomiting, and foul-smelling urine. Laboratory tests reveal a hyperkalemic non–anion gap metabolic acidosis. Urine may be alkaline or acidic. Elevated urine sodium levels with inappropriately low urine potassium levels reflect the absence of aldosterone effect.

Diagnosis. The first step in the evaluation of a patient with suspected RTA is to confirm the presence of and nature of the metabolic acidosis, identify electrolyte abnormalities, assess renal function, and rule out other causes of metabolic acidosis, such as diarrhea. Metabolic acidosis associated with diarrheal dehydration is extremely common, and acidosis will generally improve with correction of volume depletion. However, patients with protracted diarrhea may deplete their total-body bicarbonate stores and may have persistent acidosis despite apparent restoration of volume status. In those instances in which a patient has a recent history of severe diarrhea, full evaluation for RTA should be delayed for several days to permit adequate time for reconstitution of total-body bicarbonate stores. If acidosis persists beyond a few days in this setting, additional studies are indicated.

Serum electrolytes, blood urea nitrogen, calcium, phosphorus, and creatinine and pH should be obtained by venous puncture. Traumatic blood draws (such as heel stick specimens) or prolonged specimen transport time can lead to falsely low bicarbonate levels, often in association with an elevated serum potassium value. True hyperkalemic acidosis is consistent with type IV RTA, whereas the finding of normal or low potassium suggests type I or II. The anion gap should be calculated using the formula [Na$^+$] − [Cl$^-$ + HCO$_3^-$]. Values of less than 12 demonstrate the absence of an anion gap. Values more than 20 are highly suggestive of the presence of an anion gap. If such an anion gap is found, then other diagnoses (e.g., lactic acidosis, inborn errors of metabolism, or ingestions) should be investigated. If tachypnea is noted, an arterial blood gas analysis may be obtained to rule out the possibility of a primary respiratory alkalosis driving a compensatory metabolic acidosis. The finding of an acidic pH is consistent with a primary metabolic acidosis. A detailed history, with particular attention to growth and development, recent or recurrent diarrheal illnesses, and family history of mental retardation, failure to thrive, end-stage renal disease, or infant deaths or miscarriages is essential. Physical examination should determine growth parameters and volume status as well as the presence of dysmorphic features suggesting an underlying syndrome. Once the presence of a non–anion gap metabolic acidosis is confirmed, urine pH may help distinguish distal from proximal causes. A urine pH of less than 5.5 in the presence of acidosis suggests proximal RTA, whereas patients with distal RTA typically have a urine pH of more than 6.0. The urine anion gap ([Urine Na$^+$ + Urine K$^+$] − Urine Cl$^-$) is sometimes calculated to confirm the diagnosis of distal RTA. A positive gap suggests a deficiency of ammoniagenesis and, thus, the possibility of a distal RTA. A negative gap is consistent with proximal tubule bicarbonate wasting (or gastrointestinal bicarbonate wasting). A urinalysis should also be obtained to determine the presence of glycosuria, proteinuria, or hematuria suggesting the possibility of more global tubular damage or dysfunction. Random or 24-hr urine calcium and creatinine measurements will identify hypercalciuria. A renal ultrasound should be obtained to identify underlying structural abnormalities such as obstructive uropathies as well as to determine the presence of nephrocalcinosis.

Treatment and Prognosis. The mainstay of therapy in all forms of RTA is bicarbonate replacement. Patients with proximal RTA often require large quantities of bicarbonate, up to 20 mEq/kg/24 hr in the form of sodium bicarbonate or sodium citrate solution (Bicitra or Stohl's solution). The base requirement for distal RTAs is generally in the range of 2–4 mEq/kg/24 hr, although patient requirements may vary. Patients with Fanconi syndrome generally require phosphate supplementation. Patients with distal RTA should be monitored for the development of hypercalciuria. Those with symptomatic hypercalciuria (e.g., recurrent episodes of gross hematuria), nephrocalcinosis, or nephrolithiasis may require thiazide diuretics to decrease urine calcium excretion. Patients with type IV RTA may require chronic treatment for hyperkalemia with sodium-potassium exchange resin (Kayexalate®).

Prognosis is dependent to a large part on the nature of any underlying disease, if present. Patients with treated isolated proximal or distal RTA will generally demonstrate improvement in growth, provided serum bicarbonate levels can be maintained in the normal range. Patients with systemic illness and Fanconi syndrome may have ongoing difficulties with growth failure, rickets, and signs and symptoms related to their underlying disease.

Battle D, Flores G: Underlying defects in distal renal tubular acidosis: New understandings. *Am J Kidney Dis* 1996;27:896–915.

Baum M: The Fanconi syndrome of cystinosis: Insights into the pathophysiology. *Pediatr Nephrol* 1998;12:492–97.

Chan JCM, Scheinman JI, Roth KS: Renal tubular acidosis. *Pediatr Rev* 2001;22:277–86.

Charnas LR, Bernardini I, Rader I, et al: Clinical and laboratory findings in the oculocerebral syndrome of Lowe, with special reference to growth and renal function. *N Engl J Med* 1991;324:1318–25.

Kalatzis V, Cherqui S, Antignac C, et al: Cystinosin, the protein defective in cystinosis, is a H(+)-driven lysosomal cystine transporter. *EMBO J* 2001;20:5940–49.

Rodriguez-Soriano J: New insights into the pathogenesis of renal tubular acidosis—from functional to molecular studies. *Pediatr Nephrol* 2000;14:1121–36.

Suchy SF, Olivos-Glander IM, Nussbaum RL: Lowe syndrome, a deficiency of phosphatidylinositol 4,5-bisphosphate 5-phosphatase in the Golgi apparatus. *Hum Mol Genet* 1995;4:2245–50.

Wuhl E, Haffner D, Offner G, et al: Long-term treatment with growth hormone in short children with nephropathic cystinosis. *J Pediatr* 2001;138:880–887.

521.4 Rickets Associated with Renal Tubular Acidosis

Russell W. Chesney

Rickets may be present in primary renal tubular acidosis (RTA), particularly in type II or proximal RTA. See Chapters 44.10 and 697. Hypophosphatemia and phosphaturia are common in these syndromes, which are characterized by hyperchloremic metabolic acidosis, various degrees of bicarbonaturia, and, frequently, hypercalciuria and hyperkaluria. Bone demineralization without overt rickets usually is detected in type I and distal RTA. The metabolic bone disease may be characterized by bone pain, growth retardation, osteopenia, and, occasionally, pathologic fractures. Although acute metabolic acidosis in vitamin D–deficient animals may impair the conversion of 25(OH)D to 1,25(OH)$_2$D, resulting in reduced levels of this active metabolite, the circulating levels of 1,25(OH)$_2$D in patients with either type of RTA are normal. If patients with RTA have azotemia and loss of renal mass, serum 1,25(OH)$_2$D levels are often reduced.

Bone demineralization in distal RTA probably relates to dissolution of bone, because the calcium carbonate in bone may serve as a buffer against the metabolic acidosis that is due to the hydrogen ions retained by patients with RTA.

Administration of sufficient bicarbonate to reverse acidosis stops bone dissolution and the hypercalciuria that is common in distal RTA. Proximal RTA is treated with both bicarbonate and oral phosphate supplements to heal bone disease. Doses of phosphate similar to those used in familial hypophosphatemia or Fanconi syndrome should be used (see Chapter 696). Vitamin D is needed to offset the secondary hyperparathyroidism that complicates oral phosphate therapy.

Chapter 522

Nephrogenic Diabetes Insipidus *Katherine MacRae Dell and Ellis D. Avner*

Congenital nephrogenic diabetes insipidus (NDI) is a rare disorder of water metabolism characterized by an inability to concentrate urine, even in the presence of antidiuretic hormone (ADH). The most common pattern of inheritance is as an X-linked recessive disorder. Rarely, affected females are seen, presumably owing to unfavorable X chromosome inactivation. Rare autosomal recessive forms have also been described, with males and females affected equally. The clinical phenotype of autosomal recessive forms is similar to that of the X-linked form. Secondary (acquired), either partial or complete, forms of NDI may be seen in disorders affecting renal tubular function including obstructive uropathies, acute or chronic renal failure, cystic diseases, interstitial nephritis, nephrocalcinosis, or toxic nephropathy due to hypokalemia, hypercalcemia, lithium, or amphotericin B.

Pathogenesis. The ability to concentrate urine (and thus absorb water) requires the presence of an intact concentrating gradient in the renal medulla and the ability to modulate water permeability in the collecting tubule. The latter is mediated by ADH (also called arginine vasopressin [AVP]), which is synthesized in the hypothalamus and stored in the posterior pituitary. Under basal situations, the collecting tubule is impermeable to water. However, in response to increased serum osmolarity (as detected by osmoreceptors in the hypothalamus) and/or severe volume depletion, ADH is released into the systemic circulation. It then binds to its receptor, vasopressin V2 (AVPR2), on the basolateral membrane of the collecting tubule cell. Binding of the hormone to its receptor activates a cyclic adenosine monophosphate (AMP)-dependent cascade that results in movement of preformed water channels (aquaporin 2 [AQP2]) to the luminal membrane of the collecting duct, rendering it permeable to water. Defects in the *AVPR2* gene cause the more common X-linked form of NDI. Mutations in the *AQP2* gene have been identified in patients with the rarer autosomal recessive form. Prenatal testing is available for families at risk for X-linked NDI. Patients with secondary forms of NDI may have ADH resistance owing to defective aquaporin expression (e.g., lithium intoxication). More commonly, secondary ADH resistance occurs as the result of loss of the hypertonic medullary gradient due to solute diuresis or tubular damage, resulting in the inability to absorb sodium or urea.

Clinical Manifestations. Patients with congenital NDI typically present in the newborn period with massive polyuria, volume depletion, hypernatremia, and hyperthermia. Irritability and crying are common features. Constipation and poor weight gain are also seen. After multiple episodes of hypernatremic dehydration, patients may have developmental delay and mental retardation. Enuresis, caused by large urine volumes, is common. Because of the need to consume large volumes of water during the day, patients often have diminished appetite and poor food intake. However, even with adequate caloric supplementation, patients still exhibit growth abnormalities. Patients with congenital NDI also exhibit behavioral problems, including hyperactivity and short-term memory problems. Patients with the secondary form generally present later in life, primarily with hypernatremia and polyuria. Associated symptoms such as developmental delay and behavioral abnormalities are less common in this latter group.

Diagnosis. The diagnosis is suggested in a male infant with polyuria, hypernatremia, and dilute urine. Simultaneous serum and urine osmolality measurements should be obtained. If the serum osmolality value is 290 mOsm/kg or higher with a urine osmolality value of less than 290 mOsm/kg, a formal water deprivation test is not necessary. Because the differential diagnosis includes causes of central diabetes insipidus, the inability to respond to ADH (and thus the presence of NDI) should then be confirmed by the administration of vasopressin (10–20 µg intranasally or 0.1–0.2 U/kg IM) followed by serial urine and serum osmolality measurements hourly for 4 hours. In patients with possible "partial" or secondary diabetes insipidus, in whom the initial serum osmolality value may be above 290 mOsm/kg, a water deprivation test should be considered. Fluids should be withheld and urine and serum osmolalities measured periodically until the serum osmolality value is above 290 mOsm/kg; vasopressin is then given as before. Criteria for premature termination of a water deprivation test include a decrease in body weight of more than 3%. If NDI is confirmed or suspected, additional evaluation should include a detailed history to assess for toxic exposures, determination of renal function by serum creatinine and blood urea nitrogen levels, and a renal ultrasound to evaluate for obstructive uropathies or cystic disease. Because of massive urine output, patients with congenital NDI may have nonobstructive hydronephrosis of varying severity.

Treatment and Prognosis. Treatment of NDI includes (1) maintenance of adequate fluid intake and access to free water; (2) minimizing urine output by limiting solute load with a low-osmolar, low-sodium diet; and (3) administering medications directed at decreasing urine output. Human milk or a low solute formula, such as Similac PM 60/40, is preferred. Most infants with congenital NDI require gastrostomy or nasogastric feedings to ensure consistent fluid administration throughout the day and night. Sodium intake in older patients should be less than 0.7 mEq/kg/24 hr. Thiazide diuretics (2–3 mEq/kg/24 hr of hydrochlorothiazide) effectively induce sodium loss and stimulate proximal tubule reabsorption of water. Potassium-sparing diuretics, in particular, amiloride (20 mg/1.73 m²/24 hr), are often indicated. Patients who have an inadequate response to diuretics alone may benefit from the addition of indomethacin (2 mg/kg/24 hr), which has an additive effect in reducing water excretion in some patients. Renal function must be monitored closely in such patients, because indomethacin may cause deterioration in renal function over time. Patients with secondary NDI may not require medications but should have access to free water. Such patients should have serum electrolytes and volume status monitored closely, particularly during times of superimposed acute illnesses.

Prevention of recurrent dehydration and hypernatremia in patients with congenital NDI has significantly improved the neurodevelopmental outcome of these patients. However, behavioral issues remain a significant problem. In addition, chronic use of nonsteroidal anti-inflammatory drugs may predispose patients to renal insufficiency. Prognosis of patients with secondary NDI generally depends on the nature of the underlying disease.

Bichet DG, Oksche A, Rosenthal W: Congenital nephrogenic diabetes insipidus. *J Am Soc Nephrol* 1997;1951–58.
Knoers N, Monnens LAH: Amiloride-hydrochlorothiazide versus indomethacin-hydrochlorothiazide in the treatment of nephrogenic diabetes insipidus. *J Pediatr* 1990;117:499–502.
Saborio P, Tipton GA, Chan JCM: Diabetes insipidus. *Pediatr Rev* 2000;21:122–9.
Van Lieburg AF, Knoers N, Monnens LAH: Clinical presentation and follow-up of 30 patients with congenital nephrogenic diabetes insipidus. *J Am Soc Nephrol* 1999;10:1958–64.
Yamamoto T, Sasaki S: Aquaporins in the kidneys: Emerging new aspects. *Kidney Int* 1998;54:1041–51.

Chapter 523
Bartter/Gitelman Syndromes and Other Inherited Tubular Transport Abnormalities

Katherine MacRae Dell and Ellis D. Avner

Inherited tubular transport abnormalities comprise a spectrum of rare diseases, each involving distinct nephron segments. Advances in genetics and molecular biology have delineated the pathogenesis of many of these disorders and furthered the understanding of normal mechanisms of renal water and electrolyte homeostasis.

523.1 Bartter Syndrome

Bartter syndrome is a rare form of hypokalemic metabolic alkalosis with hypercalciuria, with an autosomal recessive pattern of inheritance. Two distinct clinical subtypes of Bartter syndrome are seen. Antenatal Bartter syndrome (also called hyperprostaglandin E syndrome) typically presents in infancy and has a more severe phenotype than "classic" Bartter syndrome, including polyhydramnios, salt wasting, and severe dehydration. The milder phenotype, "classic" Bartter syndrome, presents in childhood with failure to thrive and a history of recurrent episodes of dehydration. A phenotypically related disease, Gitelman syndrome, has a distinct genetic defect and is discussed in Chapter 523.2. A genetically distinct variant of antenatal Bartter syndrome associated with sensorineural deafness and chronic renal insufficiency has also been reported.

Pathogenesis. The biochemical features of Bartter syndrome, including hypokalemic metabolic alkalosis with hypercalciuria, resemble those seen with loop diuretic use and reflect a defect in sodium, chloride, and potassium transport in the ascending loop of Henle. The loss of sodium and chloride, with resultant volume contraction, stimulates the renin/angiotensin II/aldosterone (RAA) axis. Aldosterone promotes sodium uptake and potassium secretion, exacerbating the hypokalemia. It also stimulates hydrogen ion secretion distally, worsening the metabolic alkalosis. Hypokalemia stimulates prostaglandins, which further activate the RAA axis. Bartter syndrome has been associated with three distinct genetic defects in loop of Henle transporters. Each contributes, in some manner, to sodium and chloride transport. Mutations in the sodium potassium 2 chloride transporter, NKCC2 (the site of action of furosemide), or in the luminal potassium channel, ROMK, cause neonatal Bartter syndrome. Defects in the basolateral chloride channel, ClC-Kb, cause classic Bartter syndrome.

Clinical Manifestations. A history of polyhydramnios may be elicited. Dysmorphic features, including triangular facies, protruding ears, large eyes with strabismus, and drooping mouth may be present on physical examination. Consanguinity suggests the presence of an autosomal recessive disorder. Older children may have a history of recurrent episodes of dehydration, failure to thrive, and the biochemical abnormalities noted next. Hypokalemia and metabolic alkalosis are invariant features of Bartter syndrome. Urinary calcium level is typically elevated, as are urinary potassium and sodium levels. Serum renin, aldosterone, and prostaglandin E levels are often markedly elevated, particularly in the more severe antenatal form. Blood pressure is usually normal, although patients with the antenatal form may have severe salt wasting, resulting in dehydration and hypotension. Renal function is typically normal. Nephrocalcinosis, resulting from hypercalciuria, may be seen on ultrasound examination.

Diagnosis. The diagnosis is usually made on the basis of the clinical presentation and laboratory findings. The diagnosis in the neonatal infant is suggested by severe hypokalemia, usually less than 2.5 mmol/L, with metabolic alkalosis. Hypercalciuria is typical; hypomagnesemia is seen in a minority of patients but is more common in the Gitelman syndrome. Because features of Bartter syndrome resemble chronic loop diuretic use, diuretic abuse should be considered in the differential diagnosis, even in young children. Chronic vomiting may also give a similar clinical picture but can be distinguished by measurement of urinary chloride, which is elevated in Bartter syndrome and low in patients with chronic vomiting. Histologically, kidneys demonstrate hyperplasia of the juxtaglomerular apparatus. However, renal biopsy samples are rarely performed to diagnose this condition.

Treatment and Prognosis. Treatment of Bartter syndrome is directed at preventing dehydration, maintaining nutritional status, and correcting hypokalemia. Potassium supplementation, often at very high doses, is required. Even with appropriate therapy, serum potassium values may not normalize, particularly in patients with the neonatal form. Infants and young children may require sodium supplementation as well. Indomethacin, a prostaglandin inhibitor, may also be effective. With close attention to electrolyte balance, volume status, and growth, the long-term prognosis is generally good. However, in a small minority of patients, chronic hypokalemia, nephrocalcinosis, and chronic indomethacin therapy can lead to chronic interstitial nephritis and chronic renal failure.

523.2 Gitelman Syndrome

Gitelman syndrome (often called a Bartter syndrome "variant") is also a rare autosomal recessive cause of hypokalemic metabolic alkalosis, with distinct features of hypocalciuria and hypomagnesemia. Patients with Gitelman syndrome typically present later in childhood or early adulthood.

Pathogenesis. The biochemical features of Gitelman syndrome resemble those of chronic thiazide diuretic use. Thiazides act on the sodium chloride co-transporter, NCCT, present in the distal convoluted tubule. Through linkage analysis and mutational studies, defects in the gene encoding NCCT have been demonstrated in patients with Gitelman syndrome.

Clinical Manifestations. Patients with Gitelman syndrome typically present at a later age than those with Bartter syndrome. Patients often have a history of recurrent muscle cramps and spasms, presumably caused by low serum magnesium levels. They typically do not have a history of recurrent episodes of dehydration. Biochemical abnormalities include hypokalemia, metabolic alkalosis, and hypomagnesemia. The urinary calcium level is usually very low (in contrast to the elevated urinary calcium level often seen in Bartter syndrome), and the urinary magnesium level is elevated. Renin and aldosterone levels are usually normal, and prostaglandin E secretion is not elevated. Growth failure is less prominent in Gitelman syndrome than in Bartter syndrome, but it may be present.

Diagnosis. The diagnosis of Gitelman syndrome is suggested in an adolescent or adult presenting with hypokalemic metabolic alkalosis, hypomagnesemia, and hypocalciuria.

Treatment. Treatment is directed at correcting hypokalemia and hypomagnesemia with supplemental potassium and magnesium. Sodium supplementation or treatment with prostaglandin inhibitors is generally not necessary because patients typically do not have episodes of volume depletion or elevated prostaglandin E excretion.

523.3 Other Inherited Tubular Transport Abnormalities

Inherited abnormalities in distinct transporters in each segment of the nephron have now been identified and the molecular defects characterized. Renal tubular acidosis and nephrogenic diabetes insipidus are discussed in detail in Chapters 521 and 522, respectively. *Cystinuria* is an autosomal recessive disorder seen primarily in patients of Middle Eastern descent characterized by recurrent stone formation. The disease is caused by a defective high-affinity transporter for L-cystine and dibasic amino acids present in the proximal tubule.

X-linked nephrolithiasis (Dent disease) is a disease characterized by recurrent stone formation and progression to Fanconi syndrome. Consistent with the X-linked recessive inheritance, it is seen almost exclusively in males. Dent disease is caused by mutations in the voltage-gated chloride channel, CLN5, present throughout the nephron. In the loop of Henle, activating and inactivating mutations in the calcium receptor, which mediates PTH-induced calcium uptake, cause severe hypoparathyroidism or hyperparathyroidism, respectively.

In the collecting duct, gain of function mutations of the epithelial sodium channel cause an inherited form of hypertension, *Liddle syndrome*. Patients with this disorder have constitutive sodium uptake in the collecting duct, with hypokalemia and suppressed aldosterone. Conversely, loss of function mutations cause pseudohypoaldosteronism, characterized by severe sodium wasting and hyperkalemia. A variant of the latter disorder is associated with systemic abnormalities, including defects in sweat chloride, and may resemble cystic fibrosis.

Dell KM, Guay-Woodford LM: Inherited tubular transport disorders. *Semin Nephrol* 1999;19:364–73.

Jeck N, Reinalter SC, Henne T, et al: Hypokalemic salt-losing tubulopathy with chronic renal failure and sensorineural deafness. *Pediatrics* 2001;108:E5.

Kurtz I: Molecular pathogenesis of Bartter's and Gitelman's syndromes. *Kidney Int* 1998;54:1396–1410.

Langlois V, Bernard C, Scheinman SJ, et al: Clinical features of X-linked nephrolithiasis in childhood. *Pediatr Nephrol* 1998;12:625–29.

Zelkovic I: Molecular pathophysiology of tubular transport disorders. *Pediatr Nephrol* 2001;16:919–35.

Chapter 524

Tubulointerstitial Nephritis

Katherine MacRae Dell and Ellis D. Avner

Tubulointerstitial nephritis (TIN, also called interstitial nephritis) is the term applied to conditions characterized by tubulointerstitial inflammation and damage with relative sparing of glomeruli and vessels. Both acute and chronic primary forms exist. In addition, interstitial nephritis can be present with primary glomerular diseases as well as systemic diseases affecting the kidney.

ACUTE TUBULOINTERSTITIAL NEPHRITIS

Pathogenesis and Pathology. The hallmarks of acute TIN are lymphocytic infiltration of the tubulointerstitium, tubular edema, and varying degrees of tubular damage. Eosinophils may be present, especially in drug-induced TIN; occasionally, granulomas occur. The pathogenesis is not fully understood, but a T-cell–mediated immune mechanism has been postulated. A large number of medications, especially antimicrobials, anticonvulsants, and analgesics, have been implicated as etiologic agents (Box 524–1). Other causes include infections, primary glomerular diseases, and systemic diseases such as systemic lupus erythematosus (SLE).

Clinical Manifestations. The classic presentation of acute TIN is fever, rash, and arthralgia in the setting of a rising serum creatinine value. Although the full "triad" may be noted in drug-induced TIN, many patients with acute TIN do not have all of the typical features. The rash, if present, may vary from maculopapular to urticarial and is often transient. Patients often have nonspecific constitutional symptoms of nausea, vomiting, fatigue, and weight loss. Flank pain may be present from stretching of the renal capsule from kidney enlargement. If acute TIN is caused by a systemic disease such as SLE, patients may present with specific signs and symptoms of the underlying disease. Unlike the typical presentation of oliguric acute renal failure seen with glomerular diseases, 30–40% of patients with acute TIN are nonoliguric. Peripheral eosinophilia may occur, especially with drug-induced TIN. Some degree of microscopic hematuria is invariably present, but significant hematuria or proteinuria is typically absent. One exception is patients with TIN caused by nonsteroidal anti-inflammatory drugs (NSAIDs), who may present with the nephrotic syndrome. White blood cells and granular or hyaline casts may be present, but red blood cell casts, characteristic of glomerular disease, are rarely seen. Urine eosinophils are neither sensitive nor specific.

Diagnosis. The diagnosis is usually made on the basis of clinical presentation and laboratory findings. A careful history of timing of disease onset in relation to drug exposure is essential in suspected drug-induced TIN. Because of the immune-mediated nature of TIN, signs or symptoms generally appear 1–2 wk after exposure. In children, antimicrobials are a common inciting agent. Concomitant with a rise in usage, NSAIDS are being

BOX 524–1. Etiology of Interstitial Nephritis

ACUTE

Drugs
Penicillin derivatives
Cephalosporins
Sulfonamides
Trimethoprim-sulfamethoxazole
Ciprofloxacin
Tetracyclines
Erythromycin derivatives
Amphotericin B
Anticonvulsants
Diuretics
Allopurinol
Cimetidine
Cyclosporine
Nonsteroidal anti-inflammatory drugs
Protease inhibitors

Infections
Bacteria associated with acute pyelonephritis
Streptococcal species
Cytomegalovirus
Ebstein Barr virus
Hepatitis B virus
Human immunodeficiency virus
Hantavirus
Adenovirus
Toxoplasma gondii

Disease-Associated
Glomerulonephritis (e.g., systemic lupus erythematosus)
Acute allograft rejection
Tubulointerstitial nephritis and uveitis syndrome
Sarcoidosis

Idiopathic

CHRONIC

Drugs and Toxins
Analgesics
Cyclosporine
Lithium
Heavy metals

Infections (see Acute)

Disease-Associated
Metabolic/hereditary
Cystinosis
Oxalosis
Fabry disease
Wilson disease
Sickle cell nephropathy
Alport syndrome
Juvenile nephronophthisis/medullary cystic disease
Polycystic kidney disease
Immunologic
Systemic lupus erythematosus
Chronic allograft rejection
Tubulointerstitial nephritis and uveitis syndrome
Urologic
Posterior urethral valves
Eagle-Barrett syndrome
Ureteropelvic junction obstruction
Vesicoureteral reflux

Miscellaneous
Balkan nephropathy
Chinese herb nephropathy
Radiation
Sarcoidosis
Neoplasm

Idiopathic

increasingly recognized as a cause of acute TIN in children. Urinalysis and serial measurements of serum creatinine and electrolytes should be monitored. A renal ultrasound is not diag-

nostic, but it may demonstrate enlarged, echogenic kidneys. Removal of an offending agent followed by spontaneous improvement in renal function is highly suggestive of the diagnosis, and additional testing is generally not performed. In more severe cases, in which the cause is unclear or the patient's renal function deteriorates rapidly, a renal biopsy may be indicated.

Treatment and Prognosis. Treatment is generally supportive and directed at addressing complications of acute renal failure such as hyperkalemia or volume overload. Although definitive data are lacking, uncontrolled studies suggest that patients with significant renal impairment may benefit from a trial of corticosteroids. In those patients who show rapid improvement in renal function without treatment, prognosis is excellent. However, in cases with prolonged renal insufficiency, the prognosis is more guarded. Severe acute TIN from any cause that does not resolve may progress to chronic TIN.

CHRONIC TUBULOINTERSTITIAL NECROSIS

In children, chronic TIN most commonly occurs as the result of an underlying congenital renal disease, such as obstructive uropathy or vesicoureteral reflux (see Box 524–1). Chronic TIN can occur as an idiopathic disease, although this is more common in adults. *Juvenile nephronophthisis (JN)/medullary cystic disease complex (JN/MCKD)* is a group of inherited cystic diseases that share a common histologic phenotype of chronic TIN. JN is inherited as an autosomal recessive trait. Although rare in the United States, JN causes 10–20% of end-stage renal disease in Europe. Patients with JN typically present with polyuria, growth failure, "unexplained" anemia, and chronic renal failure in late childhood or adolescence. Variants of JN with extrarenal involvement include *Senior-Løken syndrome* (retinitis pigmentosa), Joubert syndrome, and oculomotor apraxia type Cogan. *MCKD* is an autosomal dominant disease that typically presents only in adulthood. *Tubulointerstitial nephritis with uveitis (TINU)* is a rare autoimmune syndrome of chronic TIN with anterior uveitis and bone marrow granulomas that occurs primarily in adolescent females. Finally, chronic TIN is seen in all forms of progressive renal disease, regardless of the underlying cause, and the severity of interstitial disease is the single most important predictor of progression to end-stage renal disease.

Pathogenesis and Pathology. As with acute TIN, the pathophysiology of chronic TIN is undefined, but data suggest that it is immune mediated. Grossly, kidneys may appear pale and small for age. Microscopically, tubular atrophy and "dropout" with interstitial fibrosis and a patchy lymphocytic interstitial inflammation are seen. Patients with juvenile nephronophthisis often have characteristic small cysts in the corticomedullary region. In primary chronic TIN, glomeruli are relatively spared until late in the disease course. Patients with chronic TIN secondary to a primary glomerular disease will have histologic evidence of the primary disease.

Clinical Manifestations. The clinical features of chronic TIN are often nonspecific and may reflect signs and symptoms of chronic renal insufficiency. Fatigue, growth failure, polyuria, polydipsia, and enuresis are often present. Anemia is common and is a particularly prominent feature of juvenile nephronophthisis. Because tubular damage often leads to renal salt wasting, significant hypertension is unusual.

Diagnosis. The diagnosis is suggested by signs or symptoms of renal tubular damage such as polyuria and an elevated serum creatinine value, coupled with a history suggestive of a chronic disease, such as long-standing enuresis or the presence of anemia resistant to iron therapy. Radiographic studies, in particular ultrasonography, may give additional evidence for chronicity, such as small, echogenic kidneys, corticomedullary cysts suggestive of juvenile nephronophthisis, or findings of obstructive uropathy. A vesicocystourethrogram (VCUG) may demonstrate the presence of vesicoureteral reflux (VUR) or bladder abnormalities. In those instances in which the cause is unclear, a renal biopsy may be performed. However, in cases of advanced disease, a renal biopsy may not be diagnostic. Many end-stage kidney diseases display a common histologic appearance of tubular fibrosis and inflammation.

Treatment and Prognosis. Treatment is directed at maintaining fluid and electrolyte balance and avoiding further exposure to nephrotoxic agents. Patients with obstructive uropathies may require salt supplementation and treatment with potassium binding resin (Kayexalate®). Prevention of infection by antibiotic prophylaxis is also important in slowing progression of renal damage in those patients. Prognosis in patients with chronic TIN is dependent, in large part, on the nature of the underlying disease. Patients with obstructive uropathy or VUR may have a variable degree of renal damage, and thus a vari-

able course. End-stage renal disease, if it occurs, may develop over months to years. Patients with juvenile nephronophthisis uniformly progress to end-stage renal disease by adolescence.

Dell KM, Kaplan BS, Meyers CM: Tubulointerstitial nephritis. In Barratt TM, Avner ED, Harmon WE (editors): *Pediatric Nephrology*, 4th ed. Baltimore, Williams & Wilkins, 1999, pp 823–34.

Ellis D, Fried WA, Yunis EJ, Blau EB: Acute interstitial nephritis in children: A report of 13 cases and review of the literature. *Pediatrics* 1981;67:862–70.

Hildebrandt F, Omram H: New insights: Nephronophthisis- medullary cystic kidney disease. *Pediatr Nephrol* 2001;16:168–76.

Rossert J: Drug-induced acute interstitial nephritis. *Kidney Int* 2001;60:804–17.

Ruffing KA, Hoppes P, Blend D, et al: Eosinophils in the urine revisited. *Clin Nephrol* 1994;41;161–66.

Schaller S, Kaplan BS: Acute nonoliguric renal failure in children associated with nonsteroidal antiinflammatory agents. *Pediatr Emerg Care* 1998;14:416–8.

Vohra S, Eddy A, Levin AV, et al: Tubulointerstitial nephritis and uveitis in children and adolescents: Four new cases and a review of the literature. *Pediatr Nephrol* 1999;13:426–32.

SECTION 5 *Toxic Nephropathies—Renal Failure*

Chapter 525

Toxic Nephropathy

Beth A. Vogt and Ellis D. Avner

Medications, diagnostic agents (iodinated radiographic contrast media), and chemicals may alter the kidneys directly (through reduction of renal blood flow, acute tubular necrosis, intratubular obstruction) or indirectly (through induction of an allergic or hypersensitivity reaction in the vessels or interstitium). Common nephrotoxic agents and their clinical manifestations are listed in Box 525–1. Nephrotoxicity is frequently reversible if the noxious agent is removed.

Useful agents should not be withheld because of potential nephrotoxicity, but the following preventive measures may reduce the risks of nephrotoxicity: (1) substitution of ultrasound, magnetic resonance imaging, or radionuclide scans for studies using contrast media in patients with pre-existing renal disease; (2) substitution of non-nephrotoxic agents for nephrotoxic agents; (3) use of the lowest effective dose of the agent in conjunction with monitoring of the blood level; (4) appropriate reduction of all drug dosing in patients with renal insufficiency, guided by well-developed nomograms; (5) avoidance of simultaneous use of several nephrotoxic agents.

Aronoff GR, Berns JS, Brier ME, et al (editors): *Drug Prescribing in Renal Failure*, 4th ed. Philadelphia, American College of Physicians, 1999.

Cayco AV, Perazella MA, Hayslett JP: Renal insufficiency after intravenous immune globulin therapy: A report of two cases and an analysis of the literature. *J Am Soc Nephrol* 1997;8:1788.

De Vriese AS, Robbrecht DL, Vanholder RC, et al: Rifampicin-associated acute renal failure: Pathophysiologic, immunologic, and clinical features. *Am J Kidney Dis* 1998;31:108.

Meyer KB, Madias NE: Cisplatin nephrotoxicity. *Miner Electrolyte Metab* 1994; 20:201.

O'Brien KL, Selanikio JD, Hecdivert C, et al: Epidemic of pediatric deaths from acute renal failure caused by diethylene glycol poisoning. *JAMA* 1998;279:1175.

Perazella MA: Crystal-induced acute renal failure. *Am J Med* 1999;106:459.

Schwartz A, Perez-Canto A: Nephrotoxicity of antiinfective drugs. *Int J Clin Pharmacol Ther* 1998;35:164–167.

Soloman R: Contrast-medium–induced acute renal failure. *Kidney Int* 1998;53: 230.

Sturmer T, Elseviers MM, De Broe ME: Nonsteroidal anti-inflammatory drugs and the kidney. *Curr Opin Nephrol Hypertens* 2001;10:161–63.

Timmer RH, Sands JM: Lithium intoxication. *J Am Soc Nephrol* 1999;10:666–74.

BOX 525–1. Renal Syndromes Produced by Nephrotoxins

NEPHROTIC SYNDROME
Angiotensin-converting enzyme (ACE) inhibitors
Gold salts
Interferon
Mercury compounds
Nonsteroidal anti-inflammatory drugs
Penicillamine

NEPHROGENIC DIABETES INSIPIDUS
Amphotericin B
Colchicine
Demeclocycline
Lithium
Methoxyflurane
Propoxyphene
Vinblastine

RENAL VASCULITIS
Hydralazine
Isoniazid
Propylthiouracil
Sulfonamides
Numerous other drugs that may cause a hypersensitivity reaction

NEPHROCALCINOSIS OR NEPHROLITHIASIS
Allopurinol
Bumetanide
Ethylene glycol
Furosemide
Methoxyflurane
Topiramate
Vitamin D

ACUTE RENAL FAILURE
Acetaminophen
Acyclovir
Aminoglycosides
Amphotericin B
Angiotensin-converting enzyme inhibitors
Cisplatin
Cyclosporine
Ethylene glycol
Halothane

Continued

BOX 525–1. Renal Syndromes Produced by Nephrotoxins *Continued*

Heavy metals
Ifosfamide
Lithium
Methoxyflurane
Nonsteroidal anti-inflammatory drugs
Radiocontrast agents
Tacrolimus
Vancomycin

FANCONI SYNDROME

Aminoglycosides
Cisplatin
Heavy metals (cadmium, lead, mercury, and uranium)
Ifosfamide
Lysol
Outdated tetracycline

RENAL TUBULAR ACIDOSIS

Amphotericin B
Lithium
Toluene

INTERSTITIAL NEPHRITIS

Amidopyrine
p-Aminosalicylate
Carbon tetrachloride
Cephalosporins
Cimetidine
Cisplatin
Colistin
Copper
Cyclosporine
Ethylene glycol
Foscarnet
Gentamicin
Gold salts
Indomethacin
Interferon-α
Iron
Kanamycin
Lithium
Mannitol
Mercury salts
Mitomycin C
Neomycin
Nonsteroidal anti-inflammatory drugs
Penicillins (especially methicillin)
Pentamidine
Phenacetin
Phenylbutazone
Poisonous mushrooms
Polymyxin B
Radiocontrast agents
Rifampin
Salicylate
Streptomycin
Sulfonamides
Tacrolimus
Tetrachloroethylene
Trimethoprim-sulfamethoxazole

placental abruption, and twin-twin or fetal- maternal transfusion. Other causes include renal vascular thrombosis and severe congenital heart disease. After the neonatal period, cortical necrosis is most commonly seen in children with septic shock or severe hemolytic-uremic syndrome as well as in adolescents with pregnancy-related acute renal failure. Less common causes of cortical necrosis include snakebites, infectious endocarditis, cefuroxime, and therapy with antifibrinolytic drugs (tranexamic acid).

Pathology. Involved portions of the cortex show infarction, with congestion of the glomeruli, thrombosis of the arterioles, and necrosis of the tubules.

Pathogenesis. Cortical necrosis develops when endothelial cell injury occurs in conjunction with diminished renal cortical blood flow. Toxins or other mediators that presumably develop during shock, hemolytic-uremic syndrome, or sepsis may injure the endothelial cells and initiate intrarenal coagulation, leading to thrombosis and cortical necrosis.

Clinical Manifestations. Cortical necrosis presents as acute renal failure developing in individuals having the previously mentioned predisposing causes. Urine output is diminished and gross and/or microscopic hematuria may be present. Hypertension is common, and thrombocytopenia may be present, as a result of renal microvascular injury.

Diagnosis. Early in the course, the diagnosis is supported by ultrasonographic detection of normal-sized or enlarged, nonobstructed kidneys. Subsequent ultrasound evaluations show a significant decrease in renal size, suggestive of renal atrophy. Radionuclide renal scans show decreased or absent renal perfusion with delayed or absent function. The differential diagnosis includes other causes of renal failure (see Box 527–1).

Treatment and Prognosis. Therapy is supportive and involves volume repletion, correction of asphyxia, and treatment of sepsis. Medical management of the complications of acute renal failure and supportive dialysis may be necessary. Children with cortical necrosis may have partial or no renal recovery, and the prognosis depends on the amount of surviving renal cortex. Those children with partial recovery are at increased risk for the subsequent development of chronic renal failure.

Agraharkar M, Fahlen M, Siddiqui M, et al: Waterhouse- Friderichsen syndrome and bilateral renal cortical necrosis in meningococcal sepsis. *Am J Kidney Dis* 2000;36:396–400.

Chevalier RL, Campbell F, Brenbridge ANAG: Prognostic factors in neonatal acute renal failure. *Pediatrics* 1984;74:265.

Lerner GR, Kurnetz R, Bernstein J, et al: Renal cortical and renal medullary necrosis in the first 3 months of life. *Pediatr Nephrol* 1992;6:516.

Manley HJ, Bailie GR, Eisele G: Bilateral renal cortical necrosis associated with cefuroxime axetil. *Clin Nephrol* 1998;49:268–70.

Palapattu GS, Barbaris Z, Raijfer J: Acute bilateral renal cortical necrosis as a cause of postoperative renal failure. *Urology* 2001;58:281.

Chapter 526
Cortical Necrosis

Beth A. Vogt and Ellis D. Avner

Renal cortical (and frequently medullary) necrosis represents a final common result of several types of renal injury. It usually affects both kidneys and may be patchy or involve the entire cortex.

Etiology. In newborns, cortical necrosis is most commonly associated with hypoxic/ischemic insults caused by perinatal asphyxia,

Chapter 527
Renal Failure

Beth A. Vogt and Ellis D. Avner

527.1 Acute Renal Failure

Acute renal failure (ARF) is a clinical syndrome in which a sudden deterioration in renal function results in the inability of the kidneys to maintain fluid and electrolyte homeostasis. ARF occurs in 2–3% of children admitted to pediatric tertiary care centers and in as many as 8% of infants in the neonatal intensive care unit.

Pathogenesis. ARF has been conventionally classified into three categories: prerenal, intrinsic renal, and postrenal (Box 527–1).

Prerenal ARF, also called prerenal azotemia, is characterized by diminished effective circulating arterial volume, which leads to inadequate renal perfusion and a decreased glomerular filtration rate (GFR). Evidence of kidney damage is absent. Common causes of prerenal ARF include dehydration, sepsis, hemorrhage, severe hypoalbuminemia, and cardiac failure. If the underlying cause of the renal hypoperfusion is reversed promptly, renal function returns to normal. If hypoperfusion is sustained, intrinsic renal parenchymal damage may develop.

Intrinsic renal ARF includes a variety of disorders characterized by renal parenchymal damage, including sustained hypoperfusion/ischemia. Many forms of glomerulonephritis, including postinfectious glomerulonephritis, lupus nephritis, Henoch-Schönlein purpura nephritis, membranoproliferative glomerulonephritis, and anti–glomerular basement membrane nephritis, may cause ARF.

Hemolytic-uremic syndrome (HUS) has been described as the most common cause of intrinsic ARF in North America (see Chapter 510). The cardinal features of HUS include ARF, microangiopathic hemolytic anemia, and thrombocytopenia. Although HUS has been linked to numerous factors, the most common predisposing factor in developed countries is hemorrhagic colitis caused by toxigenic *Escherichia coli* (OI57:H7).

Acute tubular necrosis (ATN) occurs most often in critically ill infants and children who have been exposed to nephrotoxic and/or ischemic insults. The typical pathologic process of ATN is tubular cell necrosis, although significant histologic changes are not consistently seen in patients with clinical ATN. The mechanisms of injury in ATN may include alterations in intrarenal hemodynamics, tubular obstruction, and passive backleak of the glomerular filtrate across injured tubular cells into the peritubular capillaries.

Tumor lysis syndrome is a specific form of ARF related to spontaneous or chemotherapy-induced cell lysis in patients with lymphoproliferative malignancies. This disorder is primarily caused by obstruction of the tubules by uric acid crystals (see Chapters 487 and 491).

Acute interstitial nephritis is an increasingly common cause of ARF and is usually a result of a hypersensitivity reaction to a therapeutic agent or various infectious agents (see Chapter 524).

Postrenal ARF includes a variety of disorders characterized by obstruction of the urinary tract. In neonatal infants, congenital conditions such as posterior urethral valves and bilateral ureteropelvic junction obstruction account for the majority of cases of ARF. Other conditions such as urolithiasis, tumor (intra-abdominal or within the urinary tract), hemorrhagic cystitis, and neurogenic bladder may cause ARF in older children and adolescents. In a patient with two functioning kidneys, obstruction must be bilateral to result in ARF. In general, relief of the obstruction results in recovery of renal function except in patients with associated renal dysplasia or prolonged urinary tract obstruction.

Clinical Manifestations and Diagnosis. A carefully taken history is critical in defining the cause of ARF. An infant with a 3-day history of vomiting and diarrhea most likely has prerenal ARF caused by volume depletion. A 6-yr-old child with a recent pharyngitis who presents with periorbital edema, hypertension, and gross hematuria most likely has intrinsic ARF related to acute postinfectious glomerulonephritis. A critically ill child with a history of protracted hypotension and exposure to nephrotoxic medications most likely has ATN. A neonate with a history of hydronephrosis on prenatal ultrasound and a palpable bladder most likely has congenital urinary tract obstruction, perhaps related to posterior urethral valves.

The physical examination must be thorough, with careful attention to volume status. Tachycardia, dry mucous membranes, and poor peripheral perfusion suggest inadequate circulating volume and the possibility of prerenal ARF. Peripheral edema, rales, and a cardiac gallop suggest volume overload and the possibility of intrinsic ARF from glomerulonephritis or ATN. The presence of a rash and arthritis may suggest systemic lupus erythematosus (SLE) or Henoch-Schönlein purpura nephritis. Palpable flank masses may suggest renal vein thrombosis, tumors, cystic disease, or urinary tract obstruction.

Laboratory Findings. Laboratory abnormalities may include anemia (the anemia is usually dilutional or hemolytic, as in SLE, renal vein thrombosis, and HUS); leukopenia (SLE); thrombocytopenia (SLE, renal vein thrombosis, HUS); hyponatremia (dilutional); metabolic acidosis; elevated serum concentrations of blood urea nitrogen, creatinine, uric acid, potassium, and phosphate (diminished renal function); and hypocalcemia (hyperphosphatemia).

The serum C3 level may be depressed (postinfectious, SLE, or membranoproliferative glomerulonephritis), and antibodies may be detected in the serum to streptococcal (poststreptococcal glomerulonephritis), nuclear (SLE), neutrophil cytoplasmic (antineutrophil cytoplasmic antibody; Wegener granulomatosis, microscopic polyarteritis), or glomerular basement membrane (Goodpasture disease) antigens.

The presence of hematuria, proteinuria, and red blood cell or granular urine casts suggests intrinsic ARF, in particular glomerular disease. The presence of white blood cells and white blood cell casts, with low-grade hematuria and proteinuria, suggests tubulointerstitial disease. Urinary eosinophils may be present in children with drug-induced tubulointerstitial nephritis.

Urinary indices may be useful in differentiating prerenal ARF from intrinsic ARF (Table 527–1). Patients whose urine shows an elevated specific gravity (>1.020), elevated urine osmolality (Uosm > 500 mOsm/kg), low urine sodium (UNa < 20 mEq/L), and fractional excretion of sodium (FENa) less than 1% (2.5% in neonates) most likely have prerenal ARF. Those with a specific gravity less than 1.010, low urine osmolality (Uosm < 350 mOsm/kg), high urine sodium (UNa > 40 mEq/L), and FENa

---

BOX 527–1. Common Causes of Acute Renal Failure

PRERENAL
Dehydration
Hemorrhage
Sepsis
Hypoalbuminemia
Cardiac failure

INTRINSIC RENAL
Glomerulonephritis
 Postinfectious/Poststreptococcal
 Lupus erythematosus
 Henoch-Schönlein purpura
 Membranoproliferative
 Anti–glomerular basement membrane
Hemolytic-uremic syndrome
Acute tubular necrosis
Cortical necrosis
Renal vein thrombosis
Rhabdomyolysis
Acute interstitial nephritis
Tumor infiltration
Tumor lysis syndrome

POSTRENAL
Posterior urethral valves
Ureteropelvic junction obstruction
Ureterovesicular junction obstruction
Ureterocele
Tumor
Urolithiasis
Hemorrhagic cystitis
Neurogenic bladder

TABLE 527–1. Laboratory Indices for Prerenal vs. Intrinsic Acute Renal Failure

Index	Prerenal	Intrinsic Renal
Specific gravity	>1.020	<1.010
Urine osmolality (mOsm)	>500	<350
Urine sodium (mEq/L)	<20	>40
FENa (%)	<1	>2
Blood urea nitrogen/creatinine	>20	<20

greater than 2% (> 10% in neonates) most likely have intrinsic ARF.

$$FENa\ (\%) = \frac{UNa \times PCr}{PNa \times UCr} \times 100$$

Chest roentgenography may reveal cardiomegaly and pulmonary congestion (fluid overload). Renal ultrasonography may reveal hydronephrosis and/or hydroureter, which are suggestive of urinary tract obstruction. Renal biopsy may ultimately be required to determine the precise cause of ARF in patients who do not have clearly defined prerenal or postrenal ARF.

Treatment

MEDICAL MANAGEMENT. In infants and children with urinary tract obstruction, such as in a newborn with suspected posterior urethral valves, a bladder catheter should be placed immediately to ensure adequate drainage of the urinary tract. The placement of a bladder catheter may also be considered in nonambulatory older children and adolescents to accurately monitor urine output during ARF.

Determination of the volume status is of critical importance when initially evaluating a patient with ARF. If there is no evidence of volume overload or cardiac failure, intravascular volume should be expanded by intravenous administration of isotonic saline, 20 mL/kg over 30 min. In the absence of blood loss or hypoproteinemia, colloid-containing solutions are not required for volume expansion. Severe hypovolemia may require additional fluid boluses (see Chapter 57.2). Determination of the central venous pressure may be helpful if adequacy of the blood volume is in question. After volume resuscitation, hypovolemic patients generally void within 2 hr; failure to do so points toward the presence of intrinsic or postrenal ARF.

Diuretic therapy should be considered only after the adequacy of the circulating blood volume has been established. Furosemide may be administered as a single intravenous dose of 2–4 mg/kg. Bumetanide (0.1 mg/kg) may be given as an alternative to furosemide. If urine output is not improved, then a continuous diuretic infusion may be considered. To increase renal cortical blood flow, many clinicians administer dopamine (2–3 μg/kg/min) in conjunction with diuretic therapy, although there are no controlled data to support this practice.

If there is no response to a diuretic challenge, diuretics should be discontinued and fluid restriction becomes essential. Patients with a relatively normal intravascular volume should initially be limited to 400 mL/m²/24 hr (insensible losses) plus an amount of fluid equal to the urine output for that day. Extrarenal (blood, gastrointestinal tract) fluid losses should be replaced, milliliter for milliliter, with appropriate fluids. On the other hand, markedly hypervolemic patients may require further fluid restriction, omitting the replacement of insensible fluid losses, urine output, and extrarenal losses to diminish the expanded intravascular volume. In general, glucose-containing solutions (10–30%) without electrolytes are used as maintenance fluids and the composition of the fluid modified according to the state of electrolyte balance. Fluid intake, urine and stool output, body weight, and serum chemistries should be monitored on a daily basis.

In ARF, rapid development of *hyperkalemia* (serum potassium level > 6 mEq/L) may lead to cardiac arrhythmia, cardiac arrest, and death. The earliest electrocardiographic change seen in patients with developing hyperkalemia is the appearance of peaked T waves. This may be followed by widening of the QRS intervals, ST segment depression, ventricular arrhythmias, and cardiac arrest.

Procedures to deplete body potassium should be initiated when the serum potassium value rises to 6.0 mEq/L. Exogenous sources of potassium (dietary, intravenous fluids, total parenteral nutrition) should be eliminated.

Sodium polystyrene sulfonate resin (Kayexalate®), 1 g/kg, should be given orally or by retention enema. This resin exchanges sodium for potassium and may take several hours to take effect. A single dose of 1 g/kg can be expected to lower the serum potassium level by about 1 mEq/L. Resin therapy may be repeated every 2 hr, the frequency being limited primarily by the risk of sodium overload.

More severe elevations in serum potassium (>7 mEq/L), especially if accompanied by electrocardiographic changes, require emergency measures in addition to Kayexalate®. The following agents should be administered:

1. Calcium gluconate 10% solution, 1.0 mL/kg IV, over 3–5 min
2. Sodium bicarbonate, 1–2 mEq/kg IV over 5–10 min
3. Regular insulin, 0.1 U/kg, with glucose 50% solution, 1 mL/kg, over 1 hr

Calcium gluconate counteracts the potassium-induced increase in myocardial irritability but does not lower the serum potassium level. Administration of sodium bicarbonate and insulin and glucose lowers the serum potassium level by shifting potassium from the extracellular to the intracellular compartment. Because the duration of action of these emergency measures is just a few hours, persistent hyperkalemia should be managed by dialysis.

Mild *metabolic acidosis* is common in ARF as a result of retention of hydrogen ions, phosphate, and sulfate, but it rarely requires treatment. If acidosis is severe (arterial pH < 7.15; serum bicarbonate < 8 mEq/L) or contributes to hyperkalemia, treatment is required. The acidosis should be corrected partially by the intravenous route, generally giving enough bicarbonate to raise the arterial pH to 7.20 (which approximates a serum bicarbonate level of 12 mEq/L). The remainder of the correction may be accomplished by oral administration of sodium bicarbonate after normalization of the serum calcium and phosphorus levels. Correction of metabolic acidosis with intravenous bicarbonate may precipitate tetany in patients with renal failure as rapid correction of acidosis reduces the ionized calcium concentration (see also Chapter 48.9).

Hypocalcemia is primarily treated by lowering the serum phosphorus level. Calcium should not be given intravenously, except in cases of tetany, to avoid deposition of calcium salts into tissues. Patients should be instructed to follow a low phosphorus diet, and phosphate binders should be given by mouth to bind any ingested phosphate and increase gastrointestinal phosphate excretion. Common agents include calcium carbonate (Tums tablets or Titralac suspension), calcium acetate (PhosLo), and sevelamer (Renagel). The starting dose is one to three tablets with meals. The total daily dose should be gradually increased until the serum phosphorus level falls to normal. Aluminum-based binders, which were commonly employed in the past, should be avoided because of the possibility of aluminum toxicity.

Hyponatremia is most commonly a dilutional disturbance, which must be corrected by fluid restriction rather than sodium chloride administration. Administration of hypertonic (3%) saline should be limited to those patients with symptomatic hyponatremia (seizures, lethargy) or those with serum sodium level less than 120 mEq/L. Acute correction of the serum sodium to 125 mEq/L (mmol/L) should be accomplished using the following formula:

$$\text{mEq NaCl required} = 0.6 \times \text{weight (kg)} \times (125 - \text{serum sodium [mEq/L]})$$

ARF patients are predisposed to *gastrointestinal bleeding* because of uremic platelet dysfunction, increased stress, and heparin exposure if on hemodialysis or continuous renal replacement therapy. Oral or intravenous H$_2$ blockers such as ranitidine are commonly administered to prevent this complication.

Hypertension may result from hyperreninemia associated with the primary disease process and/or expansion of the extracellular fluid volume and is most common in ARF patients with acute glomerulonephritis or HUS. Salt and water restriction is critical, and diuretic administration may be useful (see Chapter 437). Isradipine (0.05–0.15 mg/kg/dose, maximum dose 5 mg qid) or nifedipine (0.25–0.5 mg/kg PO, maximum dose 10 mg q 2–6 hr) may be administered for relatively rapid reduction in blood pressure. Longer-acting agents such as calcium channel blockers (amlodipine, 0.1–0.6 mg/kg/24 hr qd or bid), β-blockers (propranolol, 0.5–8 mg/kg/24 hr divided bid-tid; labetalol, 4–40 mg/kg/24 hr divided bid-tid) may be helpful in maintaining control of blood pressure. Children with severe symptomatic hypertension (hypertensive urgency/emergency) should be treated with continuous infusions of sodium nitroprusside (0.5–10 µg/kg/min), labetalol (0.25–3.0 mg/kg/hr), or esmolol (150–300 µg/kg/min) and converted to intermittently dosed antihypertensives when more stable.

Neurologic symptoms in ARF may include headache, seizures, lethargy, and confusion. Potential etiologic factors include hyponatremia, hypocalcemia, hypertension, cerebral hemorrhage, cerebral vasculitis, and the uremic state. Diazepam is the most effective agent in controlling seizures, and therapy should be directed toward the precipitating cause.

The *anemia* of ARF is generally mild (hemoglobin 9–10 g/dL) and primarily results from volume expansion (hemodilution). However, children with HUS, SLE, active bleeding, or prolonged ARF may require transfusion of packed red blood cells if their hemoglobin level falls below 7 g/dL. In hypervolemic patients, blood transfusion carries the risk of further volume expansion, which may precipitate hypertension, heart failure, and pulmonary edema. Slow (4–6 hr) transfusion with packed red blood cells (10 mL/kg) diminishes the risk of hypervolemia. The use of fresh, washed red blood cells minimizes the risk of hyperkalemia. In the presence of severe hypervolemia or hyperkalemia, blood transfusions are most safely administered during dialysis/ultrafiltration.

Nutrition is of critical importance in children who develop ARF. In most cases, sodium, potassium, and phosphorus should be restricted. Protein intake should be restricted moderately while maximizing caloric intake to minimize the accumulation of nitrogenous wastes. In critically ill patients with ARF, parenteral hyperalimentation with essential amino acids should be considered.

DIALYSIS. Indications for dialysis in ARF include the following:

1. Volume overload with evidence of hypertension and/or pulmonary edema refractory to diuretic therapy
2. Persistent hyperkalemia
3. Severe metabolic acidosis unresponsive to medical management
4. Neurologic symptoms (altered mental status, seizures)
5. Blood urea nitrogen greater than 100–150 mg/dL (or lower if rapidly rising)
6. Calcium/phosphorus imbalance, with hypocalcemic tetany

An additional indication for dialysis is the inability to provide adequate nutritional intake because of the need for severe fluid restriction. In patients with ARF, dialysis support may be necessary for days or for up to 12 wk. Many patients with ARF require dialysis support for 1–3 wk. The advantages and disadvantages of the three types of dialysis currently available are shown in Table 527–2.

Intermittent hemodialysis is useful in patients with relatively stable hemodynamic status. This highly efficient process accomplishes both fluid and electrolyte removal in 3–4 hr sessions using a pump-driven extracorporeal circuit and large central venous catheter. Intermittent hemodialysis may be performed three to seven times a week based on the patient's fluid and electrolyte balance.

Peritoneal dialysis is most commonly employed in neonates and infants with ARF, although this modality may be used in children and adolescents of all ages. Hyperosmolar dialysate is infused into the peritoneal cavity via a surgically or percutaneously placed peritoneal dialysis catheter. The fluid is allowed to dwell for 45–60 min and is then drained from the patient by gravity (manually or with the use of a cycler machine), accomplishing both fluid and electrolyte removal. Cycles are repeated for 8–24 hr/day based on the patient's fluid and electrolyte balance.

Anticoagulation is not necessary; peritoneal dialysis is contraindicated in patients with abdominal disorders.

Continuous renal replacement therapy (CRRT) is useful in patients with unstable hemodynamic status, concomitant sepsis, or multiorgan failure in the intensive care setting. CRRT is an extracorporeal therapy in which fluid, electrolytes, and small-and medium-sized solutes are continuously removed from the blood (24 hr/day) using a specialized pump-driven machine. Usually, a double-lumen catheter is placed into the subclavian, internal jugular, or femoral vein. The patient is then connected to the pump-driven CRRT circuit, which continuously passes the patient's blood across a highly permeable filter.

CRRT may be performed in three basic fashions. In continuous venovenous hemofiltration (CVVH), a large amount of fluid moves by pressure across the filter, bringing with it by convection other molecules such as urea, creatinine, phosphorus, and uric acid. The blood volume is reconstituted by intravenous infusion of a replacement fluid having a desirable electrolyte composition similar to the blood. Continuous venovenous dial-

TABLE 527–2. Peritoneal Dialysis (PD) vs. Intermittent Hemodialysis (IHD) vs. Continual Renal Replacement Therapy (CRRT)

	PD	IHC	CRRT
Benefits			
Fluid removal	+	++	++
Urea and creatinine clearance	+	++	+
Potassium clearance	++	++	+
Toxin clearance	+	++	+
Complications			
Abdominal pain	+	−	−
Bleeding	−	+	+
Dysequilibrium	−	+	−
Electrolyte imbalance	+	+	+
Need for heparinization	−	+	+
Hyperglycemia	+	−	-
Hypotension	+	++	+
Hypothermia	−	−	+
Central line infection	−	+	+
Inguinal/abdominal hernia	+	−	−
Peritonitis	+	−	−
Protein loss	+	−	−
Respiratory compromise	+	−	−
Vessel thrombosis	−	+	+

Adapted from Rogers MC: Textbook of Pediatric Intensive Care. Baltimore, Williams & Wilkins, 1992.

ysis (CVVH-D) utilizes the principle of diffusion by circulating dialysate in a countercurrent direction on the ultrafiltrate side of the membrane. No replacement fluid is used. Continuous hemodiafiltration (CVVH-DF) employs both replacement fluid and dialysate, offering the most effective solute removal of all forms of CRRT.

Prognosis. The mortality rate in children with ARF is variable and depends entirely on the nature of the underlying disease process rather than on the renal failure itself. In general, children with ARF caused by a renal-limited condition such as postinfectious glomerulonephritis have a very low mortality rate (<1%); those with ARF related to multiorgan failure have a very high mortality rate (>90%).

The prognosis for recovery of renal function depends on the disorder that precipitated the ARF. In general, recovery of function is likely after ARF resulting from prerenal causes, HUS, ATN, acute interstitial nephritis, or tumor lysis syndrome. On the other hand, recovery of renal function is unusual when ARF results from most types of rapidly progressive glomerulonephritis, bilateral renal vein thrombosis, or bilateral cortical necrosis.

Medical management may be necessary for a prolonged period of time to treat sequelae of ARF, including chronic renal insufficiency, hypertension, renal tubular acidosis, and urinary concentrating defect.

Aligren RL, Marbury TC, Noor Rahman S, et al: Anaritide in acute tubular necrosis. *N Engl J Med* 1997;336:828.

Bellomo R, Chapman M, Finfer S, et al: Low-dose dopamine in patients with early renal dysfunction: A placebo-controlled randomized trial. Australian and New Zealand Intensive Care Society (ANZICS) Clinical Trials Group. *Lancet* 2000;356:2139–43.

Brater DC: Diuretic therapy. *N Engl J Med* 1998;339:387.

Denton MD, Chertow GM, Brady HR: "Renal-dose" dopamine for the treatment of acute renal failure: Scientific rationale, experimental studies and clinical trials. *Kidney Int* 1996;49:4.

Gouyon JB, Guignard J-P: Management of acute renal failure in newborns. *Pediatr Nephrol* 2000;14:1037–44.

Jones DP, Mahmoud H, Chesney RW: Tumor lysis syndrome: Pathogenesis and management. *Pediatr Nephrol* 1995;9:206–12.

Manns M, Sigler MH, Teehan BP: Continuous renal replacement therapies: An update. *Am J Kidney Dis* 1998;32:185–207.

Mindell JA, Chertow GM: A practical approach to acute renal failure. *Med Clin North Am* 1997;81:731.

Niaudet P, Haj-lbrahim M, Gagnadoux M-F, et al: Outcome of children with acute renal failure. *Kidney Int* 1985;17(Suppl):148.

Thadhani R, Pascual M, Bonventre JV: Acute renal failure. *N Engl J Med* 1996;334:1448.

Toth-Heyn P, Drukker A, Guignard J-P: The stressed neonatal kidney: From pathophysiology to clinical management of neonatal vasomotor nephropathy. *Pediatr Nephrol* 2000;14:227–39.

527.2 Chronic Renal Failure

Chronic renal failure (CRF) is defined as an irreversible reduction in GFR. The prevalence of CRF in the pediatric population is approximately 18 per 1 million. The prognosis for the infant, child, or adolescent with CRF has improved dramatically over the past 4 decades because of improvements in medical management (aggressive nutritional support, recombinant erythropoietin, and recombinant growth hormone), dialysis techniques, and renal transplantation.

Etiology. In children, CRF may be the result of congenital, acquired, inherited, or metabolic renal disease, and the underlying cause correlates closely with the age of the patient at the time when the CRF is first detected. CRF in children younger than 5 yr is most commonly a result of congenital abnormalities such as renal hypoplasia, dysplasia, and/or obstructive uropathy.

After 5 yr of age, acquired diseases (various forms of glomerulonephritis) and inherited disorders (familial juvenile nephronophthisis, Alport syndrome) predominate. CRF related to metabolic disorders (cystinosis, hyperoxaluria) and certain inherited disorders (polycystic kidney disease) may present throughout the childhood years.

Pathogenesis. In addition to progressive injury with ongoing structural/metabolic genetic diseases, renal injury may progress despite removal of the original insult. Although the precise mechanisms that result in progressive deterioration of renal function are unclear, putative factors include hyperfiltration injury, persistent proteinuria, systemic or intrarenal hypertension, renal calcium-phosphorus deposition, and hyperlipidemia.

Hyperfiltration injury is proposed to be an important final common pathway of glomerular destruction, independent of the underlying cause of renal injury. As nephrons are lost, the remaining nephrons undergo structural and functional hypertrophy characterized by an increase in glomerular blood flow. The driving force for glomerular filtration is thereby increased in the surviving nephrons. Although this compensatory hyperfiltration temporarily preserves total renal function, it is theorized to cause progressive damage to the surviving glomeruli, possibly by a direct effect of the elevated hydrostatic pressure on the integrity of the capillary wall and/or the toxic effect of increased protein traffic across the capillary wall. Over time, as the population of sclerosed nephrons increases, the surviving nephrons suffer an increased excretory burden, resulting in a vicious cycle of increasing glomerular blood flow and hyperfiltration injury.

In addition to hyperfiltration injury, other factors may play a role in the progression of chronic renal insufficiency. Proteinuria itself may contribute to renal functional decline, as evidenced by studies that have shown a beneficial effect of reduction in proteinuria. Proteins that traverse the glomerular capillary wall may exert a direct toxic effect and recruit monocytes/macrophages, enhancing the process of glomerular sclerosis and tubulointerstitial fibrosis. Uncontrolled hypertension may exacerbate disease progression by causing arteriolar nephrosclerosis as well as by increasing the hyperfiltration injury described earlier.

Hyperphosphatemia may increase progression of disease by leading to calcium-phosphate deposition in the renal interstitium and blood vessels. Finally, hyperlipidemia, a common condition in CRF patients, may adversely affect glomerular function through oxidant-mediated injury.

CRF may be viewed as a continuum of disease with increasing biochemical and clinical manifestations as renal function deteriorates. The pathophysiologic manifestations of CRF are outlined in Table 527–3. Although the terminology used to describe the degrees of renal dysfunction varies, many clinicians use the following definitions:

Mild chronic renal insufficiency: GFR 50–75 mL/min/1.73 m^2
Moderate chronic renal insufficiency: GFR 25–50 mL/min/1.73 m^2
Chronic renal failure (CRF): GFR 10–25 mL/min/1.73 m^2
End stage renal disease (ESRD): GFR < 10 mL/min/1.73 m^2

Clinical Manifestations. The clinical presentation of CRF is quite varied and dependent on the underlying renal disease. Children and adolescents with CRF from glomerulonephritis, including the nephrotic syndrome, may present with edema, hypertension, hematuria, and proteinuria. Infants and children with congenital disorders such as renal dysplasia and obstructive uropathy may present in the neonatal period with failure to thrive, dehydration, urinary tract infection, or overt renal insufficiency. With the widespread use of prenatal ultrasonography, many of these infants are identified prenatally, allowing early diagnostic and therapeutic intervention. Children with familial juvenile nephronophthisis may have a very subtle presentation with nonspecific complaints such as headache, fatigue, lethargy, anorexia, vomiting, polydipsia, polyuria, and growth failure over a number of years.

The physical examination in patients with CRF may reveal pallor and a sallow appearance. Patients with long-standing

TABLE 527–3. Pathophysiology of Chronic Renal Failure

Manifestation	Mechanisms
Accumulation of nitrogenous waste products	Decrease in glomerular filtration rate
Acidosis	Decreased ammonia synthesis
	Impaired bicarbonate reabsorption
	Decreased net acid excretion
Sodium retention	Excessive renin production
	Oliguria
Sodium wasting	Solute diuresis
	Tubular damage
Urinary concentrating defect	Solute diuresis
	Tubular damage
Hyperkalemia	Decrease in glomerular filtration rate
	Metabolic acidosis
	Excessive potassium intake
	Hyporeninemic hypoaldosteronism
Renal osteodystrophy	Impaired renal production of 1,25-dihydroxycholecalciferol
	Hyperphosphatemia
	Hypocalcemia
	Secondary hyperparathyroidism
Growth retardation	Inadequate caloric intake
	Renal osteodystrophy
	Metabolic acidosis
	Anemia
	Growth hormone resistance
Anemia	Decreased erythropoietin production
	Iron deficiency
	Folate deficiency
	Vitamin B_{12} deficiency
	Decreased erythrocyte survival
Bleeding tendency	Defective platelet function
Infection	Defective granulocyte function
	Impaired cellular immune functions
	Indwelling dialysis catheters
Neurologic symptoms (fatigue, poor concentration, headache, drowsiness, memory loss, seizures, peripheral neuropathy)	Uremic factor(s)
	Aluminum toxicity
	Hypertension
Gastrointestinal symptoms (feeding intolerance, abdominal pain)	Gastroesophageal reflux
	Decreased gastrointestinal motility
Hypertension	Volume overload
	Excessive renin production
Hyperlipidemia	Decreased plasma lipoprotein lipase activity
Pericarditis/cardiomyopathy	Uremic factor(s)
	Hypertension
	Fluid overload
Glucose intolerance	Tissue insulin resistance

untreated CRF may have short stature and the bony abnormalities of renal osteodystrophy (see also Chapters 521.3 and 521.5). Children with CRF due to glomerulonephritis (or children with advanced renal failure from any cause) may have edema, hypertension, and other signs of extracellular fluid volume overload.

Laboratory findings include elevations in blood urea nitrogen and serum creatinine. The degree of renal dysfunction may be determined by applying the following formula, which provides an estimation of the patient's GFR:

$$\text{GFR (mL/min/1.73m}^2) = \frac{k \times \text{height (cm)}}{\text{serum creatinine (mg/dL)}}$$

where k is 0.33 for low-birthweight infants younger than 1 yr, 0.45 for term AGA infants younger than 1 yr, 0.55 for children and adolescent females, and 0.70 for adolescent males.

Laboratory findings may also reveal hyperkalemia, hyponatremia (if volume overloaded), acidosis, hypocalcemia, hyperphosphatemia, and an elevation in uric acid. Patients with heavy proteinuria may have hypoalbuminemia. A complete blood cell count usually shows a normochromic, normocytic anemia. Serum cholesterol and triglyceride levels are usually elevated. In children with CRF caused by glomerulonephritis, the urinalysis shows hematuria and proteinuria. In children with CRF from congenital lesions such as renal dysplasia, the urinalysis usually has a low specific gravity and minimal abnormalities.

Treatment. The treatment of CRF is aimed at (1) replacing absent/diminished renal functions, which progressively increase in parallel with the progressive loss of GFR, and (2) slowing the progression of renal dysfunction. Children with CRF should be treated at a medical center capable of supplying multidisciplinary services, including medical, nursing, social service, nutritional, and psychological support.

The management of CRF requires close monitoring of a patient's clinical and laboratory status. Blood studies to be followed routinely include the hemoglobin level and serum electrolytes, blood urea nitrogen, creatinine, calcium, phosphorus, albumin, and alkaline phosphatase. Periodic measurement of intact parathyroid hormone (PTH) levels and roentgenographic studies of bone may be of value in detecting early evidence of renal osteodystrophy. Echocardiography should be performed periodically to identify left ventricular hypertrophy and cardiac dysfunction that may occur as a consequence of the complications of CRF.

FLUID AND ELECTROLYTE MANAGEMENT. Most children with chronic renal insufficiency maintain normal sodium and water balance with the sodium intake derived from an appropriate diet. However, infants and children whose renal failure is a consequence of renal dysplasia may be polyuric with significant urinary sodium losses. These children may benefit from high volume, low caloric density feedings with sodium supplementation. On the other hand, children with high blood pressure, edema, or heart failure may require sodium restriction and diuretic therapy. Fluid restriction is rarely necessary in children with CRF until the development of end-stage renal disease (ESRD) requires the initiation of dialysis.

In most children with CRF, potassium balance is maintained until renal function deteriorates to the level at which dialysis is initiated. Hyperkalemia may develop, however, in patients with moderate renal insufficiency who have excessive dietary potassium intake, severe acidosis, or hyporeninemic hypoaldosteronism (related to destruction of the renin-secreting juxtaglomerular apparatus). Hyperkalemia may be treated by restriction of dietary potassium intake, administration of oral alkalinizing agents, and/or treatment with Kayexalate.

ACIDOSIS. Metabolic acidosis develops in almost all children with CRF owing to decreased net acid excretion by the failing kidneys. Either Bicitra (1 mEq sodium citrate/mL) or sodium bicarbonate tablets (650 mg equals 8 mEq of base) may be used to maintain the serum bicarbonate level above 22 mEq/L.

NUTRITION. Patients with CRF usually require progressive restriction of various dietary components as their renal function declines. Dietary phosphorus, potassium, and sodium should be restricted according to the individual patient's laboratory studies and fluid balance. In infants with CRF, formulas containing a reduced amount of phosphate (Similac PM 60/40) are commonly employed.

The optimal caloric intake in patients with CRF is unknown, but it is recommended to provide at least the recommended dietary allowance of caloric intake for age. Protein intake should be 2.5 g/kg/24 hr and should consist of proteins of high biologic value that are metabolized primarily to usable amino acids rather than to nitrogenous wastes. The proteins of highest biologic value are those of eggs and milk, followed by meat, fish, and fowl.

Dietary intake should be adjusted according to response, optimally through consultation with a dietitian with expertise in childhood renal failure. Caloric intake may be enhanced in infants by supplementing the formula with modular components of carbohydrates (Polycose), fat (medium chain triglycerides [MCT] oil), and protein (pro-Mod) as tolerated by the patient. In older children and adolescents, commercial enteral products (Boost) may be helpful. If oral caloric intake remains inadequate and/or weight gain and growth velocity suboptimal, enteral tube feedings should be considered. Supplemental feedings may be provided via nasogastric, gastrostomy, or gastrojejunal tube. Continuous overnight infusions with or without daytime bolus administrations are commonly employed.

Children with CRF may become deficient in water-soluble vitamins either because of inadequate dietary intake or dialysis losses. These should be routinely supplied, using preparations such as Nephrocaps (Fleming, Fenton, MO). Zinc and iron supplements should be added only if deficiencies are confirmed. Supplementation with fat-soluble vitamins A, E, and K is usually not required.

GROWTH. Short stature has emerged as one of the most significant long-term sequelae of childhood CRF. A key etiologic factor is that children with CRF have an apparent growth hormone (GH)–resistant state with elevated GH levels but decreased insulin-like growth factor-I (IGF-I) levels and major abnormalities of IGF-binding proteins.

Children with CRF who remain less than −2 SD for height despite optimal medical support (adequate caloric intake and effective treatment of renal osteodystrophy, anemia, and metabolic acidosis) may benefit from treatment with pharmacologic doses of recombinant human growth hormone (rHuGH). Treatment may be initiated with rHuGH (0.05 mg/kg/24 hr) subcutaneously, with periodic adjustment in the dose to achieve a goal of normal height velocity for age.

Treatment with rHuGH may be continued until the patient (1) reaches the 50th percentile for midparental height, (2) achieves a final adult height, or (3) undergoes renal transplantation. Long-term rHuGH treatment significantly improves final adult height and induces persistent catch-up growth, and the majority of patients achieve a normal adult height.

RENAL OSTEODYSTROPHY. The term *renal osteodystrophy* is used to indicate a spectrum of bone disorders seen in patients with CRF. The most common condition seen in children is high-turnover bone disease caused by secondary hyperparathyroidism. The skeletal pathologic finding in this condition is osteitis fibrosa cystica.

The pathophysiology of renal osteodystrophy is complex. Early in the course of CRF, when the GFR declines to approximately 50% of normal, the decrease in functional renal mass leads to a decline in renal 1α-hydroxylase activity, with decreased production of activated vitamin D (1,25- dihydroxycholecalciferol). This deficiency in activated vitamin D results in decreased intestinal calcium absorption, hypocalcemia, and increased parathyroid gland activity. Excessive PTH secretion attempts to correct the hypocalcemia by effecting an increase in bone resorption. Later in the course of CRF, when the GFR declines to 20–25% of normal, compensatory mechanisms to enhance phosphate excretion become inadequate, resulting in hyperphosphatemia, which further promotes hypocalcemia and increased PTH secretion.

Clinical manifestations of renal osteodystrophy include muscle weakness, bone pain, and fractures with minor trauma. In growing children, rachitic changes, varus and valgus deformities of the long bones, and slipped capital femoral epiphyses may be seen. Laboratory studies may demonstrate a decreased serum calcium level, increased serum phosphorus level, increased alkaline phosphatase, and a normal PTH level. Radiographs of the hands, wrists, and knees show subperiosteal resorption of bone with widening of the metaphyses.

The goals of *treatment* are to prevent bony deformity and normalize growth velocity using both dietary and pharmacologic interventions. Children and adolescents should follow a low phosphorus diet, and infants should be provided with a low-phosphorus formula such as Similac PM 60/40. Because it is impossible to fully restrict phosphorus intake, phosphate binders are used to enhance fecal phosphate excretion. Calcium carbonate (Tums) and calcium acetate (PhosLo) are the most commonly used phosphate binders, although newer, non–calcium-based binders such as sevelamer (Renagel) are increasing in use, particularly in patients prone to hypercalcemia.

Because aluminum may be absorbed from the gastrointestinal tract and can lead to aluminum toxicity, aluminum-based binders should be avoided.

The cornerstone of therapy for renal osteodystrophy is vitamin D administration. Vitamin D therapy is indicated in patients with (1) renal osteodystrophy with PTH levels greater than three times the upper limit of normal or (2) persistent hypocalcemia despite reduction of the serum phosphorus level below 6 mg/dL. Therapy may be initiated with 0.01–0.05 µg/kg/24 hr of calcitriol (Rocaltrol, 0.25-µg capsules or 1 µg/mL suspension). Rarely, dihydrotachysterol (DHT) solution (0.05–0.20 mg/24 hr) may be used. Newer noncalcemic vitamin D analogues such as paracalcitol and doxercalciferol are increasingly used, especially in patients predisposed to hypercalcemia. Phosphate binders and vitamin D should be adjusted to maintain the intact

PTH level two to three times the upper limit of normal and the serum calcium and phosphorus levels within the normal range for age. Many nephrologists also attempt to maintain the calcium/phosphorus product (Ca × PO$_4$) less than 55 to minimize the possibility of tissue deposition of calcium phosphorus salts.

ADYNAMIC BONE DISEASE. Adynamic bone disease (low-turnover bone disease) has been increasingly recognized in both children and adults with CRF. The pathologic finding in this condition is osteomalacia. This condition has been associated with oversuppression of PTH, perhaps related to the widespread use of calcium-containing phosphate binders and vitamin D analogues.

ANEMIA. Anemia in patients with CRF is primarily the result of inadequate erythropoietin production by the failing kidneys and usually becomes manifest at a GFR less than 35 mL/min/1.73 m^2.

Other possible contributory factors include iron deficiency, folic acid or vitamin B$_{12}$ deficiency, and decreased erythrocyte survival. Whereas patients with CRF often required repeated red cell transfusions in the past, the introduction of recombinant human erythropoietin (rHuEPO) therapy has dramatically decreased the need for transfusion in patients with CRF. Erythropoietin is usually initiated when the patient's hemoglobin concentration falls below 10 g/dL, at a dose of 50–150 mg/kg/dose subcutaneously one to three times weekly. The dose is adjusted to maintain the hemoglobin concentration between 11–12 g/dL. All patients receiving rHuEPO therapy should be provided with either oral or intravenous iron supplementation. Patients who appear to be resistant to rHuEPO should be evaluated for iron deficiency, occult blood loss, chronic infection/inflammatory state, vitamin B$_{12}$ or folate deficiency, and bone marrow fibrosis related to secondary hyperparathyroidism. The merits of erythropoietin therapy are summarized in Box 527–2.

HYPERTENSION. Children with CRF may have sustained hypertension related to volume overload and/or excessive renin production related to glomerular disease. Hypertensive children with suspected volume overload should follow a salt-restricted diet (2–3 g/24 hr) and may benefit from loop diuretic (furosemide) therapy. Angiotensin-converting enzyme (ACE) inhibitors (enalapril, lisinopril) are the antihypertensive medication of choice in all children with proteinuric renal disease, because of their potential ability to slow the progression to end-stage renal disease. Angiotensin-II blockers (losartan) have been shown to be effective in controlling blood pressure and in slowing disease progression in patients with diabetic nephropathy. Extreme care must be taken when using these agents, however, to monitor renal function and electrolyte balance, particularly in those children with advanced CRF. Calcium channel blockers (amlodipine, nifedipine), centrally acting agents (clonidine), and β-blockers (propranolol, atenolol) may be useful in children with CRF whose blood pressure cannot be controlled using dietary sodium restriction, diuretics, and ACE inhibitors.

IMMUNIZATIONS. Children with CRF should receive all standard immunizations according to the schedule used for healthy children. An exception must be made in withholding live vaccines from children with CRF related to glomerulonephritis during treatment with immunosuppressive medications. It is critical, however, to make every attempt to administer live virus vaccines (MMR, varicella) before renal transplantation, because these vaccines are not advised for use in immunosuppressed patients. All children with CRF should receive a yearly influenza vaccine.

Data suggest that children with CRF may respond suboptimally to immunizations.

ADJUSTMENT IN DRUG DOSAGE. Because many drugs are excreted by the kidneys, their dosing may need to be adjusted in patients with chronic renal insufficiency to maximize effectiveness and minimize the risk of toxicity (see Chapter 712). Strategies in dose adjustment include lengthening of the interval between doses, decreasing the absolute dose, or both.

PROGRESSION OF DISEASE. Although there are no definitive treatments to improve renal function in children or adults with CRF, there are several strategies that may be effective in slowing the rate of progression of renal dysfunction. Optimal control of hypertension (maintaining the blood pressure less than the 75th percentile) is critical in all patients with CRF. ACE inhibitors or angiotensin-II blockers should be the antihypertensive drug of choice in hypertensive children with chronic proteinuric renal disease. Such agents should also be strongly considered in children with CRF who have significant proteinuria, even in the absence of hypertension. Serum phosphorus should be maintained within the normal range for age and the calcium-phosphorus product less than 55 to minimize renal calcium-phosphorus deposition. Prompt treatment of infectious complications and episodes of dehydration may minimize additional loss of renal parenchyma.

Other potentially beneficial recommendations include correction of anemia with erythropoietin therapy, avoidance of cigarette smoking, minimization of regular use of nonsteroidal anti-inflammatory medications, and control of hyperlipidemia. Although dietary protein restriction has been shown to be useful in adults, this recommendation is generally not suggested for children with CRF because of the concern of adverse effects on growth and development.

527.3 End-Stage Renal Disease

End-stage renal disease (ESRD) represents the state in which a patient's renal dysfunction has progressed to the point at which homeostasis and survival can no longer be sustained with native kidney function and maximal medical management. At this point, renal replacement therapy (dialysis or renal transplantation) becomes necessary. The ultimate goal for children with ESRD is successful kidney transplantation (see Chapter 528) because it provides the most normal lifestyle and possibility for rehabilitation for the child and family. Seventy-five percent of North American children with ESRD, however, require a period of dialysis before transplantation can be performed.

The optimal time to initiate dialysis is based on a combination of the biochemical and clinical characteristics of the patient. It is the consensus opinion to arrange renal replacement therapy when the child's native kidney function falls to a GFR (measured by creatinine clearance) of 10–15 mL/min/1.73 m^2. Other specific indications include refractory fluid overload, electrolyte imbalance, acidosis, growth failure, or uremic symptoms, including fatigue, nausea, and impaired school performance. Cardiovascular death accounts for about a quarter of pediatric and young adult ESRD deaths. In general, most nephrologists

---

■ BOX 527–2. Merits of Recombinant Human Erythropoietin Therapy

BENEFITS
Avoidance/minimization of blood transfusions
   Reduced sensitization to histocompatibility antigens
   Reduced exposure to infectious diseases
   Less chance of chronic iron overload
Improved appetite
Enhanced exercise tolerance
Improved sleep
Improved well-being

POTENTIAL COMPLICATIONS
Iron deficiency
Hypertension
Seizures
Clotting of vascular access
Pure red cell aplasia (in adults due to rHuEPO anibodies)

attempt to initiate dialysis early enough to prevent the development of severe fluid and electrolyte abnormalities, malnutrition, and uremic symptoms.

The selection of dialysis modality must be individualized to fit the needs of each child. In the North America, two thirds of children with ESRD are treated with peritoneal dialysis, whereas one third are treated with hemodialysis. Age is a defining factor in dialysis modality selection: 88% of infants and children from birth to 5 yr of age are treated with peritoneal dialysis, whereas 54% of children older than 12 yr of age are treated with hemodialysis.

Peritoneal dialysis is a technique that employs the patient's peritoneal membrane as a dialyzer. Excess body water is removed by an osmotic gradient created by the high dextrose concentration in the dialysate; wastes are removed by diffusion from the peritoneal capillaries into the dialysate. Access to the peritoneal cavity is achieved by a surgically inserted, tunneled Tenckhoff catheter.

Peritoneal dialysis may be provided either as continuous ambulatory peritoneal dialysis (CAPD) or as any of several forms of automated therapies using a cycler (continuous cyclic peritoneal dialysis [CCPD], intermittent peritoneal dialysis [IPD], or nocturnal intermittent peritoneal dialysis [NIPD]). The majority of North American children treated with peritoneal dialysis use cycler-driven therapy, which allows the child and family to be free of dialysis demands during the waking hours. The exchanges are performed automatically during sleep by machine. This permits an uninterrupted day of activities, a reduction in the number of dialysis catheter connections and disconnections (which should decrease the risk of peritonitis), and a reduction in the time required by patients and parents to perform dialysis, reducing the risk of fatigue and burnout. Because peritoneal dialysis is not as efficient as hemodialysis, it must be performed on a daily basis rather than 3 times weekly as in hemodialysis. The merits of peritoneal dialysis are outlined in Box 527–3.

Hemodialysis, unlike peritoneal dialysis, is usually performed in a hospital setting. Children and adolescents typically have three 3–4 hour sessions per week during which fluid and solute wastes are removed. Access to the child's circulation is achieved by a surgically created arteriovenous fistula, graft, or indwelling subclavian or internal jugular catheter.

Aronoff GR, Berns JS, et al (editors): *Drug Prescribing in Renal Failure: Dosing Guidelines for Adults,* 4th ed. Philadelphia, American College of Physicians, 1999.

Brouhard BH, Donaldson LA, Lawry KW, et al: Cognitive functioning in children on dialysis and post-transplantation. *Pediatr Transplant* 2000;4:261–67.

Fischbach M, Terzic J, Menouer S, et al: Hemodialysis in children: Principles and practice. *Semin Nephrol* 2001;21:470–79.

Fivush BA, Neu AM: Immunization guidelines for pediatric renal disease. *Semin Nephrol* 1998;3:256–63.

Goodman WG, Goldin J, Kuizon BD, et al: Coronary artery calcification in young adults with end-stage renal disease who are undergoing dialysis. *N Engl J Med* 2000;342:1478–83.

> ### BOX 527–3. Merits of Peritoneal Dialysis in Pediatric Patients with End-Stage Renal Disease
>
> **ADVANTAGES**
> Ability to perform dialysis treatment at home
> Technically easier than hemodialysis, especially in infants
> Ability to live a greater distance from medical center
> Freedom to attend school and after-school activities
> Less restrictive diet
> Less expensive than hemodialysis
>
> **DISADVANTAGES**
> Catheter malfunction
> Catheter-related infections (peritonitis, exit-site)
> Impaired appetite (due to full peritoneal cavity)
> Negative body image
> Caregiver "burnout"

Haffner D, Schaefer F, Nissel R, et al: Effect of growth hormone treatment on the adult height of children with chronic renal failure. *N Engl J Med* 2000;343:923–30.

Hebert LA, Wilmer WA, Falkenhain ME, et al: Renoprotection: One or many therapies? *Kidney Int* 2001;59:1211–26.

Lewis EJ, Hunsicker LG, Clarke WR, et al: Renoprotective effect of the angiotensin-receptor antagonist irbesartan in patients with nephropathy due to type 2 diabetes. *N Engl J Med* 2001;345:851–60.

Lerner GR, Warady BA, Sullivan EK, et al: Chronic dialysis in children and adolescents: The 1996 Annual Report of the North American Pediatric Renal Transplant Cooperative Study. *Pediatr Nephrol* 1999;13:404–17.

Parekh RS, Carroll CE, Wolfe RA, et al: Cardiovasular mortality in children and young adults with end-stage kidney disease. *J Pediatr* 2002;141:197–207.

Parekh RS, Flynn JT, Smoyer WE, et al: Improved growth in young children with severe chronic renal insufficiency who use specified nutritional therapy. *J Am Soc Nephrol* 2001;12:2418–26.

Pastan S, Bailey J: Dialysis therapy. *N Engl J Med* 1998;338:1428.

Ruggenenti P, Perna A, Gherardi G, et al: Renoprotective properties of ACE-inhibition in non-diabetic nephropathies with non-nephrotic proteinuria. *Lancet* 1999;354:359–64.

Salusky IB, Goodman WG: Adynamic renal osteodystrophy: is there a problem? *J Am Soc Nephrol* 2001;12:1978–85.

Sanchez CP: Prevention and treatment of renal osteodystrophy in children with chronic renal insufficiency and end-stage renal disease. *Semin Nephrol* 2001;21:441–50.

Scharer K, Schmidt KG, Soergel M: Cardiac function and structure in patients with chronic renal failure. *Pediatr Nephrol* 1999; 13:951–65.

Schwartz GJ, Brion LP, Spitzer A: The use of plasma creatinine concentration for estimating glomerular filtration rate in infants, children, and adolescents. *Pediatr Clin North Am* 1987;34:571–90.

Valderrabano F, Jofre R, Lopez-Gomez JM: Quality of life in end-stage renal disease patients. *Am J Kidney Dis* 2001;38:443–64.

Warady, BA, Alexander SR, Watkins S, et al: Optimal care of the pediatric end-stage renal disease patient on dialysis. *Am J Kidney Dis* 1999;33:567–83.

Warady BA, Belden B, Kohaut E: Neurodevelopmental outcome of children initiating peritoneal dialysis in early infancy. *Pediatr Nephrol* 1999;13:759–65.

Chapter 528

RenalTransplantation

Rodrigo E. Urizar

Long-term dialysis therapy for end-stage renal disease (ESRD) is frequently associated with failure to thrive, social maladaptation, lack of sexual maturation, and chronic encephalopathy (in the very young) and explains the reluctance to dialyze children extensively unless more acceptable alternatives are unavailable. Optimal treatment for children with ESRD is early renal transplantation (RT) from a living related donor (LRD-RT). Although less successful than LRD-RT, cadaveric (CAD) grafts are also used in children.

Epidemiology. The United States Renal Data System (USRDS) documents 20 new ESRD cases per million children each year, peaking at about age 11–15 yr. Before 1 yr of age, the incidence is 0.2 patient/million per year. The North American Pediatric Renal Transplant Cooperative Study (NAPRTCS) reported the registration and sequential follow-up, through January 2001, of over 80% of American and Canadian children with chronic renal insufficiency (CRI), dialysis (D), transplantation, and post-transplant events. Of 11,973 registered children, 6,878, or 57.44%, received their first (index) transplant, whereas 667 additional cases (of 7,545 transplants, 63%) represented repeated procedures in the same patient, a cumulative effect since NAPRTCS's inception in 1987. Of the remaining patients, 3,271 had CRI (27.3%), whereas 1,340 (11.2%) of the 11,973 were on dialysis, all candidates for RT in the future. An estimated 43–45% of 2,000 pediatric RTs performed in the United States used kidneys donated by parents (37%) and by siblings or other relatives (6%). Preemptive RT (carried out without previous dialysis) constitutes 22% of LRD engraftings. Indications for RT are noted in Box 528–1.

BOX 528–1. Criteria for Performing Living Related Donor or Cadaveric Renal Transplantation in Pediatric Patients

Renal failure, chronic or end-stage renal disease of any etiology
Age, weight dependent to accommodate adult kidney
Good nutritional condition
Absence of
  Active infection
  Severe mental retardation
  Obstructed urinary tract (ileal loops, colonic diversions and bladder augmentation procedures are helpful in many instances)
  Gastrointestinal, liver, pancreas, or cardiovascular disease
  Serious psychosocial or behavioral problems, and noncompliance with medication and dietary regimen
  Sensitization in recipient
  Massive obesity

From Mauer SM, Nevins TE, Ascher N: Renal transplantation in children. In Edelman CM Jr (editor): *Pediatric Kidney Disease*. Boston, Little, Brown & Company, 1992, pp 941–81.

BOX 528–2. Most Frequent Hereditary-Metabolic Diseases of Childhood That Lead to End-Stage Renal Disease

Nephronophthisis—medullary cystic disease
Congenital nephrotic syndrome
Alport syndrome
Nephropathic and juvenile cystinosis
Primary oxalosis with oxaluria
Polycystic kidney disease (both infantile and adult varieties)
Nail-patella syndrome

A well-functioning graft (LRD or CAD) may fully rehabilitate the patient. Nonetheless, the expectant graft recipient and relatives must understand that RT is not a permanent cure for ESRD. Furthermore, a poorly functioning transplanted kidney (uncontrollable progressive rejection) is associated with serious morbidity, mortality, and prospective return to long-term dialysis or initiation of it. The transiency of renal grafts has committed transplant programs to many engraftments per patient, a goal seriously hampered by the limited availability of CAD kidneys. The latter may reflect reticence of the lay and professional community (general public, nurses, physicians) toward organ donation. Because of the large disproportion among the yearly increments in the need for RT (22%), and the number of transplants performed in the same period (8%), it is estimated that one hundred thousand kidneys will be required to be distributed among 180,000 patients on dialysis in the United States. In the present state of organ procurement, this objective cannot be met. Interim measures (i.e., optimizing living related and nonrelated, and cadaveric renal donation efforts, including kidneys obtained from children younger than 15 yr of age who have suffered brain death) and attempts at xenotransplantation (transplantation between different species) are being applied. Xenotransplants are presently only used on a purely experimental basis.

Causes of ESRD vary with the patient's age and include congenital renal diseases (53%), glomerulonephritides (20%), focal segmental glomerular sclerosis (12%), metabolic diseases (10%), and miscellaneous (5%) (Box 528–2 and Table 528–1). Although the glomerulopathies constitute a significant proportion of this population (particularly in 13–17 yr olds), congenital and obstructive processes predominate in the very young (<5 yr).

Treatment. Children weighing less than 15–20 kg have a transperitoneal graft via a midline incision; in those weighing more than 20 kg, the kidney is placed retroperitoneally in the right iliac fossa. Renal vessels are anastomosed to the recipient iliac vessels, and the ureter is reimplanted in the bladder (ureteroneocystostomy). The extraperitoneal kidney facilitates access for future percutaneous biopsies. The donor and recipient clinical laboratory evaluations before RT are summarized in Box 528–3. Very young age of the recipient may be an obstacle to RT. For both LRD and CAD recipients, age younger than 24 mo is associated with decreased graft survival. Nevertheless, some institutions accept patients 5–6 mo old weighing 5–6 kg to be engrafted with adult kidneys. In addition, pediatric patients transplanted with small kidneys do not fare as well as expected. Specifically, for CAD recipients, donor age of less than 6 yr is associated with decreased graft survival.

Kidney grafts from LRD have significantly better survival than CAD-RT. Approximately 90% of kidneys from LRD function adequately by 1 yr and 80% function by the 3rd yr; the figures for CAD-RT are 72% and 65%, respectively. Generally, CAD-RT in children is less favorable than in adults. In transplant recipients who are younger than 1 yr, the 2-yr graft survival is less than that of older children. Overall, by 39 mo after RT, 80% of LRD and 58% of CAD-RT are functional.

Approximately 50% of graft failure is due to rejection. In 26%, rejection was acute, whereas in 7% recurrence of the original renal disease induced the transplant failure. Although almost any glomerulopathy may redevelop in the graft, focal segmental glomerulosclerosis is observed most frequently (see Table 528–2). Thrombosis-related kidney failure occurs in 15% of cases. In patients with LRD-RT, thrombotic episodes developed in very young recipients, presumably because of hemodynamic and/or technical problems. Conversely, graft thrombosis in CAD-RT is unaffected by the recipient age but is proportional to the donor age. In older children, acute renal failure is frequently caused by tubular necrosis, which may contribute to graft loss. In summary, identified risks for graft loss in the pediatric population include recipient age younger than 2 yr, cadaveric donor less than 6 yr, previous renal transplantation, delayed graft function (acute tubular necrosis), and lack of antilymphocyte

---

TABLE 528–1. Individual Glomerulopathies of Childhood That May Progress to Chronic/End-Stage Renal Disease

Entity	Clinical Manifestation
Idiopathic rapidly progressive GN (crescentic GN, mediated by immune complexes)	Acute progressive renal failure
IgA nephropathies (Berger disease, anaphylactoid or Henoch-Schönlein purpura)	Chronic active GN, nephrotic syndrome, occasionally RPGN
Membranoproliferative glomerulonephritis (idiopathic; types I, II, and III)	Acute and chronic nephritic syndrome, occasionally RPGN
Focal segmental glomerulosclerosis	Nephrotic syndrome, progressive renal failure, acute/chronic active progressive GN, occasionally RPGN
Systemic lupus GN (WHO types 3 & 4)	
Microangiopathic syndromes (hemolytic, uremic, and thrombotic thrombocytopenic purpura syndromes)	Acute, chronic, and occasionally RPGN
Vasculitis (polyarteritis nodosa and Wegener granulomatosis)	Same
Anti–basement membrane antibody diseases (Goodpasture syndrome and idiopathic RPGN)	Acute, progressive renal failure, and RPGN with or without pulmonary renal syndrome

GN = Glomerulonephritis; RPGN = rapidly progressive glomerulonephritis.

therapy with antithymocyte gamma globulin (ATGAM) or OKT3.

Histocompatibility. The major histocompatibility complex (MHC) genes, present on the short arm of chromosome 6, encode the human leukocyte antigens (HLA) (Fig. 528–1). These are composed of class I proteins (tissue transplantation antigens) and cell-mediated immunotoxicity; class II proteins that control

induction of immune response; and class III proteins, which include tumor necrosis factor (TNF) and complement components (C2 and C4). Each chromosome 6 contains all three classes of proteins: HLA-A, -B, and -C for class I; HLA-DP, -DQ, and -DR for class II; and C2, C4, and TNF for class III. Multiple and co-dominant alleles (polymorphism) exist for each protein: 23(A), 47(B), 8(C), 19(D), 16(DR), 3(DQ), and 6(DP). The A, B, and DR proteins are regarded as the most important in clinical transplantation. The HLA genes concentrated within a defined area of chromosome 6 are inherited as a packet or haplotype. Each individual inherits a haplotype of HLA genes from each parent concurrently, and both contribute to the offspring's HLA profile. The parent donor and child recipient share 50% of the haplotypes; a child typically has one representative antigen from class I, II, and III loci of each parent, whereas among siblings, all, some, or no haplotypes may be shared (2 haplotype, 1 haplotype, or 0 haplotype match). By definition, in the absence of recombination, a child is a 1 haplotype match to each parent and transmission (inheritance) of haplotypes occurs in a co-dominant mendelian fashion (Fig. 528–2). In the genetically related donor/recipient pair, the probability of a good HLA match increases and graft loss decreases.

Cellular expression of class I and II antigens, restricted to B and T lymphocytic cells and macrophages, multiplies with inflammation and by the action of lymphokines (interleukins 2, 4, and 5) secreted by T cells. CD4 (T-helper) and CD8 (T-suppressor) cell surface markers have high affinity for MHC (HLA) class I (histocompatibility) antigens. When attached to cells displaying class I antigen, they transmit signals to synthesize cytokines or to lyse cells. In the acute and chronic rejection reaction, both cellular and humoral mechanisms damage the graft, whereas antibodies, preformed or induced by T-helper cells, mediate accelerated (hyperacute) forms of the rejection reaction (Fig. 528–3). In the cellular variety, the graft is infiltrated by lymphocytes—T-helper and suppressor cells, B lymphocytes, macrophages, plasma cells, and monocytes—resulting in hemorrhage, edema, accumulation of polymorphonuclear leukocytes, activated platelets, and clotting.

Clinically, rejection is manifested by swelling and tenderness of the graft, fever, oliguria, hypertension, and progressive elevation of serum creatinine level. Renal ultrasonography may reveal an enlarged graft with echogenic cortex, and a renal scan demonstrates decreased blood flow. Graft biopsy material shows signs of rejection with relatively intact glomeruli, mild ultrastructural changes, and negative glomerular immunofluorescence. Differentiation between rejection, acute tubular necrosis, cyclosporine toxicity, and de novo occurrence of the original renal disease in the graft requires a kidney biopsy. *Hyperacute* or *accelerated rejections* are seldom observed because pretransplant cross matching detects the presence of pre-existing anti-HLA

FIGURE 528–1. Organization of HLA region of chromosome 6. The loci for HLA-A, -B, and -C are found in the class I region. The loci encoding HLA-DR, -DQ, and -DP are found in the class II region, centromeric to class I. In between classes I and II are the so-called class III genes, which encode some of the complement proteins as well as some cytokines. (From Grimm PC, Laufer J, Ettenger RB: The immunobiology of renal transplantation. In Edelman CM Jr [editor]: *Pediatric Kidney Disease.* Boston, Little, Brown & Company, 1992.)

Human HLA Region on Chromosome #6

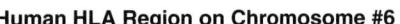
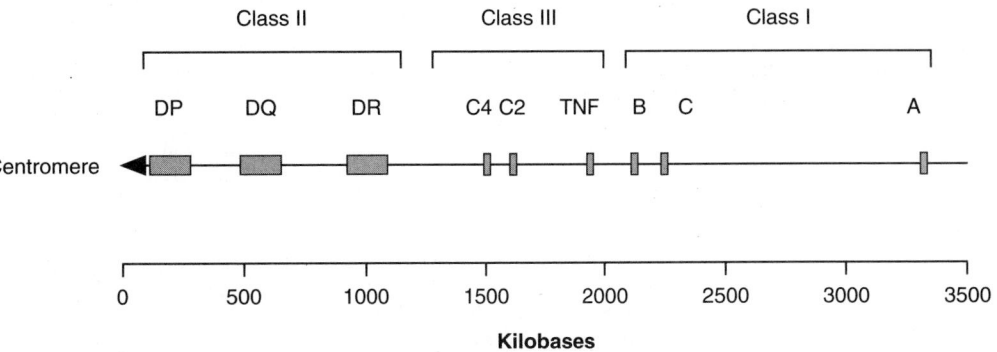

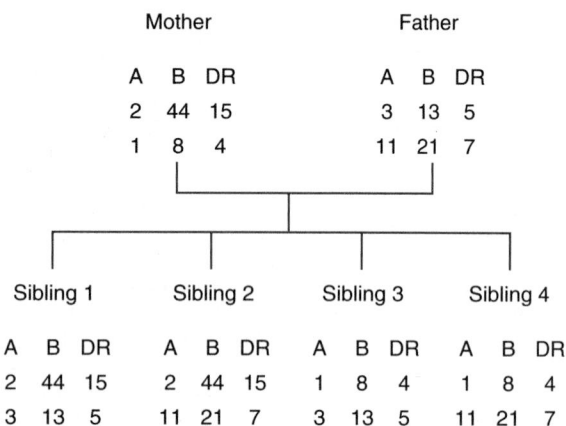

Mother

A	B	DR
2	44	15
1	8	4

Father

A	B	DR
3	13	5
11	21	7

Sibling 1

A	B	DR
2	44	15
3	13	5

Sibling 2

A	B	DR
2	44	15
11	21	7

Sibling 3

A	B	DR
1	8	4
3	13	5

Sibling 4

A	B	DR
1	8	4
11	21	7

FIGURE 528–2. Inheritance of haplotypes and HLA profile in four theoretical siblings. Sibling 1 is a 1 haplotype match to siblings 2 and 3 and a 0 haplotype match to sibling 4. (From Terasaki PI, Park MS, Danovitch GM: Histocompatibility testing, crossmatching and allocation of cadaveric kidney transplants. In Danovitch GM [editor]: *Handbook of Kidney Transplantation.* Boston, Little, Brown & Company, 1992.)

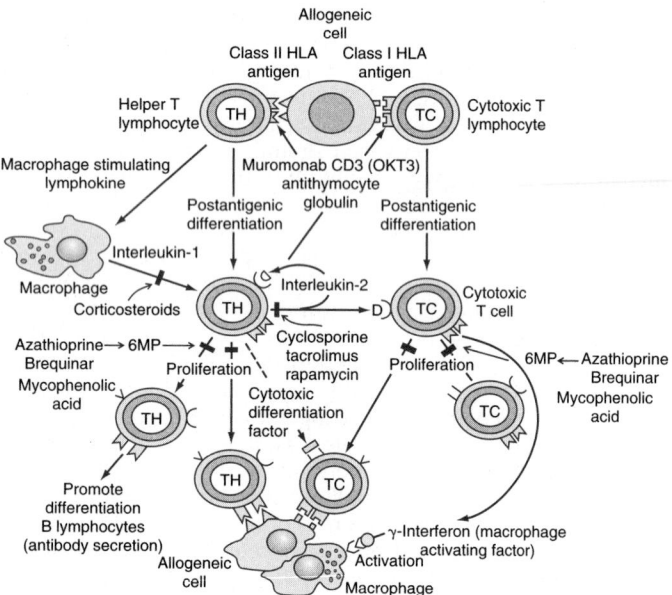

FIGURE 528–3. A representation of allograft rejection and the proposed sites of action for immunosuppressive medications. (From Shaefer MS, Collier DS: Immunosuppression for solid organ transplantation. *Dialysis Transplant* 1993;22:542.)

antibodies. In this condition, the kidney becomes dark and soft as it is revascularized. Anti-HLA antibodies bind to endothelium, and renal intravascular coagulation destroys glomeruli and peritubular capillaries. Chronic rejection damages mainly arteries and arterioles, which become thickened with obstructed lumens, while glomeruli undergo ischemic wrinkling of the basement membrane, mononuclear cells infiltrate the interstitium, and arteriolar walls may display immunoglobulin deposits.

Histocompatibility testing is considered of paramount importance in prolonging the survival of LRD and CAD-RT. Having HLA-A, -B, -C, and -D/DR identical with an MHC nonstimulatory sibling donor produces the best graft survival results. The second best is the sibling or parent donor who has 1 haplotype match.

Principles of Immunosuppression and Therapy of Rejection Reaction. Immune system stimulation by foreign protein (renal graft) results in activation of cell-mediated and humoral-mediated immune inflammation with cell destruction or rejection (see Fig. 528–3). (See also Chapter 126.) To subdue or control this process, which otherwise results in acute graft loss, the use of immunosuppressive medications is mandatory. The current drugs, doses, mechanism(s) of action, and side effects are listed in Table 528–3 and Figure 528–3.

Sequential immunosuppression with azathioprine, cyclosporine, and low-dose corticosteroids is the most frequently used protocol. However, new corticosteroid and calcineurin inhibitor–sparing protocols have been designed to avoid morbidity (prednisone-prednisolone) and nephrotoxicity (cyclosporine). Fifty percent of pediatric patients with LRD and 65% of those receiving CAD kidneys develop rejection (with one or more acute episodes in most transplants); 62% of first episodes are successfully treated, whereas only 30% can be reversed when four or more crises have occurred. Chronic rejection is relentless and unresponsive to therapy. In addition, concurrent rejection with complications, particularly infection, places patients at higher risk of graft loss or death. If complications occur as a result of immunosuppression, one should treat the complication and abandon the graft. The use of ATGAM or OKT3 prophylactically in the immediate postoperative period improves the short-term graft outcome in 50% of pediatric CAD recipients. In addition, 6 mo after LRD or CAD transplant, these children have lower mean serum creatinine levels, the interval from transplant to first rejection is lengthened, and the 1-yr graft survival is improved.

As opposed to immunosuppression, the result of medications and/or processes that block normal and fully developed T-cell immunologic response, tolerance or nonreactivity to alloantigens is generally induced during the intrauterine development of the immune system or through a variety of mechanisms (see Table 528–3). Achieving permanent immune unresponsiveness to someone else's antigens represents a more logical approach to retain a functional renal graft instead of prolonged use of dangerous medications.

Growth and Renal Transplantation. Stunted linear growth and, less often, overt malnutrition are complications of chronic renal failure and of ESRD dialysis (see Chapter 527). Although supportive care improves stamina and a sense of well-being develops, only a successful transplant adequately corrects these abnormalities. Most children awaiting RT show retarded growth of 2.8 SD when 5 yr of age or younger, whereas in those with more than one RT, stunting reaches 3.2 SD. RT-related accelerated growth, lasting 6–12 mo, is observed in younger children; in adolescents, a growth spurt has not been documented. Weight

---

BOX 528–4. Post-Transplantation Complications in Pediatric Patients

Acute tubular necrosis
Rejection reaction
Technical: vascular, urologic
Recurrence of original renal disease
Drug toxicity (immunosuppressives, antibiotics)
Infection (particularly viral, systemic); wound or urinary tract infection
Bleeding
Pancreatitis
Lymphocele
Urinoma
Bowel obstruction

From Mauer SM, Nevins TE, Ascher N: Renal transplantation in children. In Edelman CM Jr (editor): *Pediatric Kidney Disease.* Boston, Little, Brown & Company, 1992, pp 941–81.

gain, on the other hand, yields mean values similar to normal adolescents for 2–3 yr. Daily corticosteroid treatment retards growth, even at relatively small doses. Every-other-day prednisone use is unpopular in many transplant centers, allegedly because it may precipitate graft rejection. Nevertheless, the validity and success of the every-other-day corticosteroid regimen has been amply demonstrated in children. Steroids may be used daily for 6 mo in decreasing doses, then switched to every other day and tapered to 0.5–0.2 mg/kg given as a single dose every other day.

Judicious use of recombinant human growth hormone before and after RT improves linear growth significantly, although there are contradictory data indicating that graft function may decrease.

Complications. Complications that develop after RT are summarized in Box 528–4. Of these, infection is the most common cause of death during the first year after RT. Cytomegalovirus (CMV) infection is common. CMV antibody titers must be routinely screened in the donor and recipient. CMV infection may be primary, transmitted by the RT itself or by blood transfusions, or reactivated by immunosuppression in a seropositive patient (see Table 528–4). The latter disease becomes apparent 1–3 mo after RT. About 90% may be self-limited and asymptomatic, and 5–10% lead to death; direct tissue damage by CMV may also result in graft loss. In addition, CMV disease usually triggers a rejection reaction. This poses a serious therapeutic dilemma: Although immunosuppression may reactivate the disease, it is indispensable for graft retention. Low-dose immunosuppressive agents with the use of antiviral drugs (ganciclovir and anti-CMV immunoglobulin intravenously) control the infection, and kidney biopsy helps monitor the RR. Immunosuppression must be discontinued in systemic (lung, brain, liver) CMV infection. If rejection is unresponsive, the kidney should be abandoned. Concomitant infection with other viruses (varicella-zoster, Epstein-Barr [EBV], herpes simplex, hepatitis) requires thorough investigation and treatment. *Pneumocystis carinii* infection has all but disappeared, owing to prophylactic use of trimethoprim-sulfamethoxazole, which also prevents bacterial urinary tract infections. The mortality of pediatric RT recipients is 4–4.5%; in 40–45% of these, mortality is caused by infection. The 2-yr patient survivals for LRD and CAD-RT are 95% and 92%, respectively.

BOX 528–5. Consequences of EBV Growth and High-Risk Factors for the Development of PTLD in Immunosuppressed Patients

CLINICAL SYNDROMES

Mononucleosis
Meningoencephalitis
Hairy, oral leukoplakia
Smooth muscle cell tumors
T-cell lymphomas
Post-transplant lymphoproliferative disorder (PTLD, uncontrolled proliferation of EBV-infected and transformed B cells, in a polyclonal, oligoclonal, and monoclonal fashion)
Non-Hodgkin lymphoma

HIGH RISK FOR PTLD

High EBV-load
Primary EBV infection
High-dose immunosuppression (cyclosporin A, tacrolimus, antilymphocyte antibodies and steroid pulses alone or combinations)
Cardiac treatment is most commonly affected.

EBV = Epstein-Barr virus.

Immunosuppression remains an unavoidable requisite for transplantation. Unfortunately, use of such medications may result in EBV replication, leading to aggressive and potentially lethal post-transplant lymphoproliferative disorder (PTLD) in 1–2% of renal transplants. In 2001, the NAPRTCS report showed 121 cases of 7,545 transplant patients (1.7% from 1987 to 2000); the HIV-reactivity status of the affected children, however, is not stated. A single center study from France reported 16 PTLD HIV-negative cases out of 1,421 adults (1.1%, mean age 45.5 years; range 27–64 years). PTLD, a rare pre-and fully malignant condition, still is a major cause of serious morbidity and mortality when it develops in young children after the first year post transplantation. This disorder should be actively pursued and diagnosed as early as possible in the febrile transplant patient with lymphadenopathy, gastrointestinal manifestations (abdominal mass, bleeding, pain, obstruction, perforation, ascites), seizures or other central nervous system abnormalities, and asymptomatic chest or mediastinal masses. PTLD is an EBV-CMV infection-driven condition that should be sought after

TABLE 528–2. Rate of Recurrence of Glomerulopathies in Allografts and Graft Loss

Glomerulopathy	Percent Recurrence	Percent Graft Damage/Loss
FSGS (with NS)	20–40	25
IgA	50	5-10
HSP	30–80	10
MN	20	5-10
MPGN I	25	5-10
MPGN II	90	20
HUS	10–50	10-50
WG	5–20	5-20
AGBM	< 10 (rare in children)	< 1 (uncertain)
SLEGN	5–10	<5
HYPEROX	High	High losses
Cystinosis	Graft handles cystine load	Loss to rejection
IGN (de novo MPGN)	Uncertain	Uncertain

FSGS = focal segmental glomerular sclerosis; IgA = immunoglobulin A nephritis; HSP = Henoch-Schönlein purpura; MN = membranous nephropathy; MPGN I and II = membranoproliferative glomerulonephritis type I and type II; HUS = hemolytic-uremic syndrome; WG = Wegener granulomatosis; AGBM = anti–glomerular basement membrane nephritis; SLEGN = systemic lupus erythematosus glomerulonephritis; HYPEROX = hyperoxalosis/oxaluria; IGN = ideopathic glomerulonephritis.

Modified from Denton MC, Singh AK: Recurrent and de novo glomerulonephritis in the renal allograft. Semin Nephrol 2000; 20:164–75; and Mauer SM, Nevins TE, Ascher N: Renal transplantation in children. In Edelman CM Jr (editor): Pediatric Kidney Disease. Boston, Little Brown & Company, 1992, pp 941–81.

TABLE 528–3. Immunosuppressive Agents

Substance	Mechanism	Dose	Side Effects
Nonselective Antiproliferatives			
Azathioprine (Imuran)	Inhibits enzyme critical to formation of purine nucleosides, 6 thioguanine incorporated into DNA as fraudulent bases.	Alone 2–3 mg/kg/24 hr, combined 1–2 mg/kg/24 hr nonrenal excretion	Bone marrow suppression, liver cell damage, chromosomal breakage, and tumor growth
Cyclophosphamide (Cytoxan)	Radiomimetic—alkylating substance that inhibits rapidly replicating cells, by cross linking with cell DNA.	1–2 mg/kg/24 hr orally; IV pulses of 750 mg/m^2/BSA with normal GFR; decrease to 500 mg/m^2 BSA if GFR is impaired	Bone marrow suppression, infections, gastrointestinal problems, alopecia, hemorrhagic cystitis, tumors
Mycophenolate mofetil (Cell Cept)	Interferes with purine synthesis. Stops progression of activated T and B cells in S phase of cell cycle. May also alter *N*-glycosulation of cell membrane glycoproteins.	1–3 g day PO; usually combined with prednisone and cyclosporin A	Gastrointestinal: esophagitis, gastritis, diarrhea, and bleeding; increased susceptibility to CMV, infection, tumors
Selective Inhibitors			
Calcineurin inhibitors Cyclosporin A (NEORAL)	Blocks calcineurin and inhibits cytokine synthesis; T-cell selective inhibitor inhibits interleukin 2 (IL-2).	4 mg/kg/24 hr (follow trough blood levels for dose adjustments)	Hirsutism, gingival hyperplasia, arterial hypertension, renal arteriolitis, nonmyelodepressant tremors (CNS toxicity)
Tacrolimus (Prograf)	Same mechanisms.	0.15–0.20 mg/kg divided q12 hr	As above—nephrotoxic, posttransplant IDDM (higher in African American patients)
Sirolimus (Rapamycin) Rapamycin Analog (SDZ-RAD)	Blocks cytokine-driven cell proliferation and maturation.	7.5 mg/m^2 BSA × 5 days and 5 mg/m^2	Thrombocytopenia, hyperlipidemia
Polyclonal antilymphocyte antibodies (equine ATGAM and rabbit thymoglobulin)	Antibodies bind to cell surface receptors opsonizing cells for complement-induced lysis/phagocytosis	ATGAM: Infusion with in-line filter into central line only, over 4 hr, 14–21 days; thymoglobulin: peripheral IV 6 hr, 1.5 mg/kg/24 hr, 14–21 days	Profound immunosuppression <150–50 peripheral blood T-lymphocyte cell count/mm^3, chills, fever, arthralgias thrombocytopenia and leukocytopenia; CMV infection, tumors
Monoclonal antibodies (OKT3 Orthoclone)	Produced by hybridomas/murine spleen cells of mice immunized against human lymphocytes. Bind CD$_3$ receptor on T cells: modulation and immunologic inactivation of CD$_3$.	For induction therapy and reversal of steroid resistant rejection reaction, 1–5 mg/dose/24 hr	Cytokine release syndrome: tumor necrosis factor, IL-2, interferon-γ, fever, chills, tremors, chest pain, wheezing, nausea, and vomiting
Interleukin-2 receptor monoclonal antibodies Basiliximab Daclizumab	Blocks the IL-2 receptor and prevents cellular activation; does not produce cytokine release syndrome; does not induce neutralizing antibodies.	Basiliximab: 20 mg IV day of surgery and day 4 Daclizumab: 1 mg/kg/IV within 24 hr of transplant followed by same dose every 2 wk × 5	Immunosuppression
B- and T-Cell Stimulators			
Janus Kinase (JAK3) inhibitor (AG490). And C-RAF isoform specific enzyme inhibitor	Inhibits IL-2 cytokine receptors.	No clinical data yet available	
Ischemia/Reperfusion-Induced Tissue Damage Inhibitors			
Selectin-blocking agents	Interrupt and modulate effects of adhesion molecules (selectin; integrin, ICAM-1, VCAM, and VLA-4).		
KPL1 antibody (TBC-1269 and CY 1503)	Monoclonal antibody to selectin; inhibits leukocyte recruitment.	No clinical data yet available	PTT prolongation, mild complement activation
Antisense intercellular adhesion molecule-1 (ICAM-1) oligonucleotides ISIS 2302	Inhibits formation of ICAM-1 and blocks cellular adhesion.		
FTY 720 (sphyngosine-like compound)	Alters leukocyte recirculation pattern diverting them away from the graft to lymphoid tissues; inhibits lymphocyte receptors, and blocks interaction with integrins.	0.25–3.5 mg (single dose)	Lymphopenia, bradycardia
Transplantation Tolerance			
Induction of anergy by inactivation or deletion of antigen reactive cells			
Alloantigen unresponsiveness			
T-cell co-stimulation (CTLA-4Ig: competitive inhibitor of T-cell surface markers)	Insufficient clinical data		
Allochimeric molecules (derived from class I–II major histocompatibility (HLA) complex	Insufficient clinical data		
Gene therapy	Insufficient clinical data		

BSA = body surface area; CMV = cytomegalovirus; CNS = central nervous system; GFR = glomerular filtration rate; IL-2 = interleukin-2; PTT = partial thromboplastin time. Modified from Hong JC, Kahan BD: Immunosuppressive in organ transplantation: Past, present and future. Semin Nephrol 2000; 20:108–125.

TABLE 528–4. Types of Cytomegalovirus in the Pediatric Renal Transplant Recipient

Type of Infection	Type of Patient	Symptomatic	Prevention
Primary	Seronegative with seropositive kidney, transfusion of leukocytes, blood products transfusion	60%	Avoidance of CMV infection or use active immunization (live attenuated vaccine: Towne strain; not very effective)
Reactivation	Seropositive before transplantation	<20%	High titer human hyperimmune anti-CMV globulin (CytoGam)
Superinfection	Seropositive patient transplanted with CMV + kidney	40%	Human IgG concentrates (CMV nonspecific Gammagard or Polygam)

CMV-cytomegalovirus.
From Snydman DR: Prevention of cytomegalovirus-associated diseases with immunoglobulin. Transplant Proc 1991;23:131.

clinically by tissue sampling and all possible laboratory means: polymerase chain reaction (PCR)-determined EBV-CMV blood viral load, RNA or DNA positivity and clonality by Southern blot analysis, and latent membrane protein 1 (LMP 1) expression in paraffin embedded tissue samples and frozen tissue studies. The clinical consequences of EBV growth and the high risks for the development of PTLD in the immunosuppressed patient are listed earlier in Box 528–5.

PTLD that occurs less than 1 yr post transplant generally exhibits a much more benign prognosis and may respond and regress by simple reduction or by discontinuation of immunosuppressive medications. Of the 16 patients with severe disease (PTLD of late onset) in the previously mentioned French study, 11 individuals received full chemotherapy (CHOP protocol: cyclophosphamide, doxorubicin, vincristine, and prednisone) with 6 achieving complete and persistent remission. The use of the CHOP protocol by these clinicians revealed no nephrotoxicity, and most patients did not mount a renal rejection reaction when, for a variable but limited period, low or no maintenance immunosuppressive medications were given after antitumor therapy was completed.

Renal Transplant in the HIV-Infected Patient. With the development of effective antiretroviral therapy, prognosis of the HIV-infected patient has improved enough to consider renal transplant in these cases on an individual basis. The conditions to perform a renal transplant or retransplant in HIV-infected patients require that the candidate is free of opportunistic infections for 2 yr and is on a stable and well-tolerated anti-HIV/Pneumocystis regimen. Good compliance and undetectable viral load (by PCR), acceptable CD4 lymphocyte count, and no complicating illnesses are mandatory.

Recurrence of Glomerular Disease in the Graft. Potentially all glomerulopathies can recur in the transplant (see Table 528–2)

with 5–10% of all allografts lost through this mechanism. Of these, focal segmental glomerular sclerosis is perhaps the most frequent, has poorly known mechanisms, and is difficult to treat (Table 528–5).

The hemolytic-uremic syndrome (HUS) does not recur but may happen de novo in the allograft. The familial non–infection-related variety of HUS, presumably genetically transmitted, does develop de novo (1–3%) or may be associated with calcineurin-inhibitor mediation (cyclosporine and others) but is more frequent in bone marrow grafts than in renal transplants. Important predictors for the development of non–infection-related HUS occurrences in the renal graft include familial disease (autosomal dominant or recessive), transplant before 6 mo to 1 yr after primary disease remitted completely, and use of cyclosporine (low dose is recommended if recurrence developed in previous transplant). Using LRDs in cases known to have familial prostacyclin synthesis abnormalities, consumption of oral contraceptive medications, and employing ATGAM and OKT3 have been associated with post-transplant de novo HUS.

Abramowicz D, Wissing KM, Broeders N: Immunosuppressive strategies in renal transplantation at the beginning of the third millennium. Adv Nephrol Necker Hosp 2000;30:9–28.
Bartosh SM, Aronson AJ, Swanson-Prewitt EE, et al: OKT3 induction in pediatric renal transplantation. Pediatr Nephrol 1993;7:45.
Broyer M: Results and side effects of treating children with growth hormone after kidney transplantation—a preliminary report. Acta Pediatr 1996;417(Suppl):76.
Denton MD, Singh AK: Recurrent and de novo glomerulonephritis in the renal allograft. Semin Nephrol 2000;20:164–75.
Droupy S, Blanchet P, Eschwege P, et al: Functional results in kidneys procured from pediatric cadavers. Transplant Proc 2000;32:2767–68.
First MR: Long-term complications after transplantation. Am J Kidney Dis 1993; 22:477.
Fisher R, Gaynor E, Dahlberg S, et al: Comparison of a standard regimen (CHOP) with three intensive chemotherapy regimens for advanced non-Hodgkin's lymphoma. N Engl J Med 2000;328:1002–6.

TABLE 528–5. FSGS: Clinical Characteristics and Effects on the Allograft

Effects on Native Kidney	Effects on Allograft	Forms of Therapy
Severe progressive FSGS and hypercellularity. Clinically, nephrotic syndrome, chronic renal failure with progression to ESRD in 60% of cases.	Histologic recurrence of FSGS in graft 20–40% Recurrent nephrotic syndrome, renal failure, ESRD in 25%.	Avoid living related donor and high cyclosporin A dose. To treat, use plasmapheresis-exchange and immunoadsorption, cyclophosphamide, and OKT3. Pretransplant bilateral nephrectomy should not be done. All forms of treatment seem purely palliative.
Dialysis and transplantation needed.	Favor recurrence: <6 yr, rapidly progressive renal failure, glomerular hypercellularity, previous recurrence, closely matched living related donor, familial distribution of FSGS, presence of assayable high levels of permeability factor in recipient's blood.	

ESRD= end-stage renal disease; FSGS = focal segmental glomerular sclerosis.

Grinyo JM: Overcoming toxicities: New regimens. *Transplant Proc* 2001;33(Suppl 3A):45–65.

Gudmundsdotir H, Turka LA: Transplantation tolerance: Mechanisms and strategies? *Semin Nephrol* 2000;20:209–16.

Hancock WW: Xenotransplantation: Is this the future? *Semin Nephrol* 2000;20:217–29.

Harmon WE, Alexander SR, Tejani A, et al: The effect of donor age on graft survival in pediatric cadaver renal transplant recipients. A report of the North American Pediatric Renal Transplant Cooperative Study. *Transplantation* 1992;54:232.

Hong JC, Kahan BD: Immunosuppressive agents in organ transplantation: Past, present and future? *Semin Nephrol* 2000;20:108–12.

Mamzer-Brunzel M-F, Lome C, Morelon E, et al: Durable remission after aggressive chemotherapy for very late post-kidney transplant lymphoproliferation: A report of 16 cases observed in a single center. *J Clin Oncol* 2000;18:3622–32.

North American Pediatric Renal Transplant Cooperative Study (NAPRTCS) 2001 report. Renal Transplantation, Dialysis, Chronic Renal Insufficiency. Data coordination center. Stablein DM, Ho M. The Emmes Corporation: 401 North Washington Street, Suite 700, Rockville Maryland 20850.

Rieu P, Noel LH, Droz D, et al: Glomerular involvement in lymphoproliferative disorders with hyperproduction of cytokines (Castleman, POEMS). *Adv Nephrol Necker Hosp* 2000;30:305–31.

Sahota A, Gao S, Hayes J, et al: Microchimerism and rejection: A meta-analysis. *Clin Transplant* 2000;14(4 pt 1):345–50.

Sollinger H: Is tolerance a clinical reality? *Transplant Proc* 2000;32(Suppl 1A):135.

Starzl TE, Murase N: Microchimerism and tolerance. *Clin Transplant* 2000;14(4 pt 1):351–4.

Tolkoff-Rubin N, Rubin RH: Recent advances in the diagnosis and management of infection in the organ transplant recipient. *Semin Nephrol* 2000;20:148–63.

Vincenti F, Kirkman R, Light S, et al: Interleukin-2 receptor blockade with daclizumab to prevent acute rejection in renal transplantation. *N Engl J Med* 1998;338:161.

Urologic Disorders in Infants and Children *Jack S. Elder*

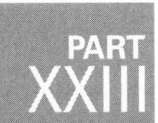

Chapter 529
Congenital Anomalies and Dysgenesis of the Kidneys

The kidney is derived from the ureteral bud and the metanephric blastema. During the 5th wk of gestation, the ureteral bud arises from the mesonephric (wolffian) duct and penetrates the metanephric blastema, which is an area of undifferentiated mesenchyme on the nephrogenic ridge. The ureteral bud undergoes a series of approximately 15 generations of divisions and by 20 wk of gestation forms the entire collecting system: the ureter, renal pelvis, calyces, papillary ducts, and collecting tubules. Under the inductive influence of the ureteral bud, nephron differentiation begins during the 7th wk of gestation. By 20 wk of gestation, when the collecting system is developed, approximately 30% of the nephrons are present. Nephrogenesis continues at a nearly exponential rate and is complete by 36 wk of gestation.

The fetal kidneys play a minor role in the maintenance of fetal salt and water homeostasis. The rate of urine production increases throughout gestation and, at term, volumes have been reported to be 51 mL/hr. The glomerular filtration rate is 25 mL/min/1.73 m^2 at term and thereafter triples by 3 mo of age. The increase in glomerular filtration rate is caused by a reduction in intrarenal vascular resistance and redistribution of intrarenal blood flow to the cortex, where more nephrons are located.

Dysgenesis of the kidney includes aplasia, dysplasia, hypoplasia, and cystic disease.

Renal Agenesis. Bilateral renal agenesis is incompatible with extrauterine life. Death occurs shortly after birth from pulmonary hypoplasia. This condition is termed *Potter syndrome*. The newborn has a characteristic facial appearance, termed *Potter facies* (Fig. 529–1). The eyes are widely separated and have epicanthic folds, the ears are low set, the nose is broad and compressed flat, the chin is receding, and there are limb anomalies. Bilateral renal agenesis should be suspected when maternal ultrasonography demonstrates oligohydramnios, nonvisualization of the bladder, and absent kidneys. The incidence is 1 in 3,000 births and represents 20% of newborns with the Potter phenotype. Other common causes of neonatal renal failure associated with the Potter phenotype include cystic renal dysplasia and obstructive uropathy. Less common causes are autosomal recessive polycystic kidney disease (infantile), renal hypoplasia, and medullary dysplasia.

Renal agenesis means that the kidney did not form because of an abnormal ureteral bud and is distinguished from aplasia, an extreme form of dysplasia in which a nubbin of nonfunctioning tissue is seen capping a normal or abnormal ureter. Clinically, this distinction may be difficult. *Hereditary renal adysplasia* is used to describe families in which renal agenesis, renal dysplasia, multicystic kidney (dysplasia), or a combination, occurs in a single family. This disorder has an autosomal dominant inheritance pattern with a penetrance of 50–90% and variable expression. Associated anorectal, cardiovascular, and skeletal abnormalities are seen in newborns with both hereditary renal adysplasia and bilateral renal agenesis.

Unilateral renal agenesis is often discovered during the course of an evaluation for other congenital anomalies or for urinary tract symptoms. Its incidence is increased in newborns with a single umbilical artery. With true agenesis, the ureter and the ipsilateral bladder hemitrigone are absent. The contralateral kidney undergoes compensatory hypertrophy, to some degree prenatally but primarily after birth. Approximately 15% have contralateral vesicoureteral reflux, and most males have an ipsilateral absent vas deferens because the wolffian duct is absent. Because the wolffian and müllerian ducts are contiguous, müllerian abnormalities in girls are also common. The *Mayer-Rokitansky-Kuster-Hauser syndrome* refers to a group of associated findings that include unilateral renal agenesis or ectopia, ipsilateral müllerian defects, and vaginal agenesis. Some individuals are diagnosed as having unilateral renal agenesis based on a finding of an absent kidney on ultrasonography or excretory urography. Some of these patients actually were born with a hypoplastic kidney or a multicystic dysplastic kidney that underwent complete cyst regression. The specific diagnosis is not critical. However, if the finding of an absent kidney is based on an ultrasonogram, a functional imaging study such as an excretory urogram or renal scan should be performed because

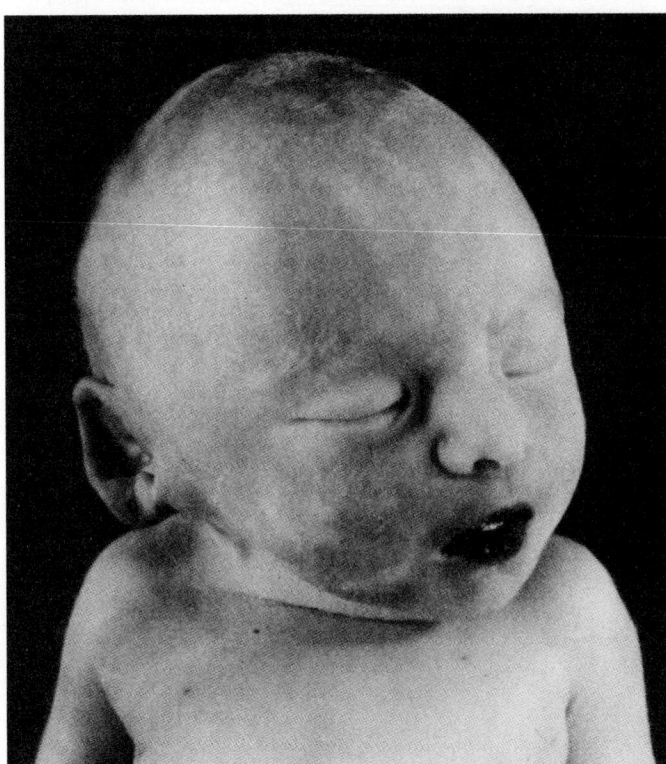

FIGURE 529–1. Stillborn with renal agenesis exhibiting the characteristic Potter facies. (Courtesy of Barbara Burke, MD, Department of Laboratory Medicine and Pathology. University of Minnesota Hospital, Minnesota.)

some of these patients may have an ectopic kidney. If there is a normal contralateral kidney, renal function should remain normal over time.

Whether individuals with a solitary kidney should avoid contact sports such as football and karate is unresolved. The arguments favoring participation are that there are other solitary organs such as the spleen, liver, and brain that do not preclude contact sport participation, and there have been few reports of individuals losing a kidney from sports injuries. The arguments against such participation are that the contralateral normal kidney is hypertrophic and not as well protected by the ribs, and a serious renal injury could have devastating life-long consequences. The American Academy of Pediatrics recommends an "individual assessment for contact, collision, and limited-contact sports."

Renal Dysplasia and Hypoplasia. The term *dysplasia* is technically a histologic diagnosis and refers to focal, diffuse, or segmentally arranged primitive structures, specifically primitive ducts, resulting from abnormal metanephric differentiation. Nonrenal elements, such as cartilage, may be present. The condition may affect all or only part of the kidney. If cysts are present, the condition is termed *cystic dysplasia*. If the entire kidney is dysplastic with a preponderance of cysts, the kidney is referred to as a *multicystic dysplastic kidney* (Fig. 529–2). The pathogenesis of dysplasia is multifactorial. The "bud" theory proposes that if the ureteral bud arises in an abnormal location, such as an ectopic ureter, there is inappropriate penetration and induction of the metanephric blastema that causes abnormal kidney differentiation-dysplasia. Renal dysplasia may also occur with severe obstructive uropathy early in gestation, as with the most severe cases of posterior urethral valves or in a multicystic dysplastic kidney, in which a portion of the ureter is absent or atretic.

A multicystic kidney is a congenital condition in which the kidney is replaced by cysts, does not function, and may result from ureteral atresia. Renal size is highly variable. The incidence is approximately 1 in 2,000. Clinicians may incorrectly assume that *multicystic kidney* and *polycystic kidney* are synonymous terms. Polycystic kidney disease is an inherited disorder that may be autosomal recessive or autosomal dominant and affects both kidneys (see Chapter 513). A multicystic kidney is usually

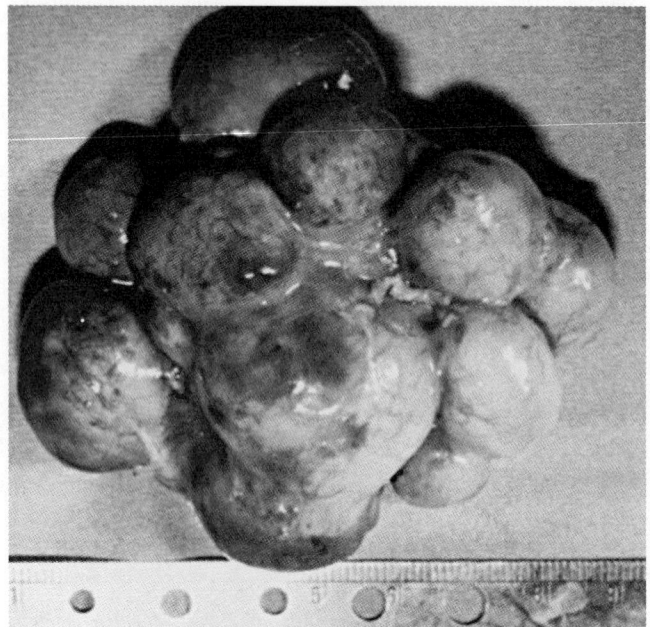

FIGURE 529–2. Surgical specimen of a multicystic dysplastic kidney associated with ureteral atresia.

unilateral and is not inherited. Bilateral multicystic kidneys are incompatible with life.

Multicystic dysplastic kidney is the most common cause of an abdominal mass in the newborn. In many cases it is discovered incidentally during antenatal sonography. In some individuals, the cysts are identified prenatally or postnatally, but no renal tissue is identified because of cyst regression in utero. Contralateral vesicoureteral reflux is identified in 15%, and contralateral hydronephrosis is present in 5–10% of patients. Sonography shows the characteristic appearance of a kidney replaced by multiple cysts of varying sizes that do not communicate, and no identifiable parenchyma is present; the diagnosis should be confirmed with a renal scan, which should demonstrate nonfunction. A voiding cystourethrogram is also advisable because of a 15% incidence of contralateral reflux. Management is controversial. There have been a few reports of renin-mediated hypertension and Wilms tumor arising in these kidneys. Neoplasms arise from the stromal, not the cystic, component. Consequently, even if the cysts regress completely, the likelihood that the kidney could develop a neoplasm is not altered. Because of the occult nature of these potential problems, annual follow-up with sonography and blood pressure measurements is recommended. If there is an abdominal mass, the cysts enlarge, the stromal core increases in size, or hypertension develops, nephrectomy is recommended. Alternatively, in lieu of follow-up screening, nephrectomy may be performed through a 2.5- to 3-cm flank incision when the child is 6–12 mo old. The Section on Urology of the American Academy of Pediatrics has an ongoing registry to determine the long-term risk of the nonoperative management of multicystic kidneys.

Renal hypoplasia refers to a small nondysplastic kidney that has less than the normal number of calyces and nephrons. The term refers to a group of conditions with an abnormally small kidney and should be distinguished from aplasia, in which the kidney is rudimentary. If the condition is unilateral, the diagnosis usually is made incidentally during evaluation for another urinary tract problem or hypertension. Bilateral hypoplasia usually presents with the manifestations of chronic renal failure and is a leading cause of end-stage renal disease during the first decade of life. A history of polyuria and polydipsia is common. Urinalysis results may be normal. A rare form of bilateral hypoplasia is called *oligomeganephronia*, in which the number of nephrons is markedly reduced but those present are markedly hypertrophied.

The *Ask-Upmark kidney*, also termed *segmental hypoplasia*, refers to small kidneys, usually weighing not more than 35 g, with one or more deep grooves on the lateral convexity, underneath which the parenchyma consists of tubules resembling those in the thyroid gland. It is unclear whether the lesion is congenital or acquired. Most patients are 10 yr or older at diagnosis and have severe hypertension. Nephrectomy usually controls the hypertension.

Anomalies in Shape and Position. During renal development the kidneys normally ascend from the pelvis into their normal position behind the ribs. The normal process of ascent and rotation of the kidney may be incomplete, resulting in renal ectopia or nonrotation. The ectopic kidney may be in a pelvic, iliac, thoracic, or contralateral position. If it is contralateral, in 90% of individuals there is fusion of the two kidneys. The incidence of renal ectopia is approximately 1 in 900.

Renal fusion anomalies are common. The lower poles of the kidneys may fuse in the midline, resulting in a *horseshoe kidney* (Fig. 529–3). Horseshoe kidneys occur in 1 in 500 births but are seen in 7% of patients with Turner syndrome. Horseshoe kidney is one of the many renal anomalies that occur in 30% of these patients. Wilms tumors are four times more frequent in children with horseshoe kidneys than in the general population. In addition, stone disease and hydronephrosis secondary to

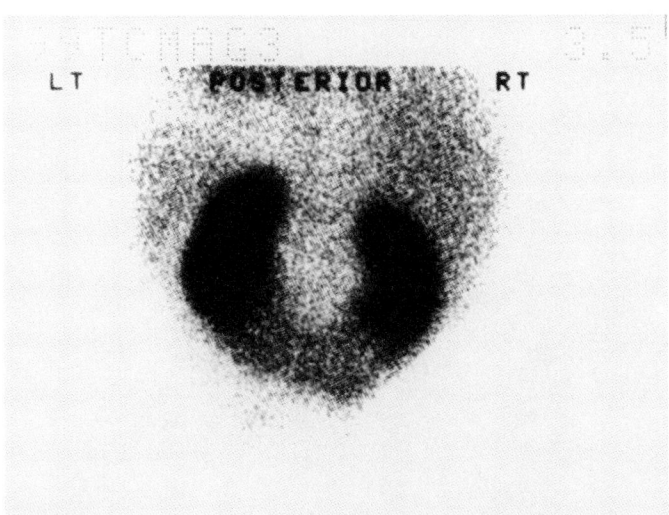

FIGURE 529–3. Isotopic renogram showing the characteristic configuration of a horseshoe kidney with an isthmus of functioning parenchyma.

ureteropelvic junction obstruction are potential late complications. There also appears to be a slightly increased incidence of multicystic dysplastic kidney affecting one of the two sides of a horseshoe kidney. With *crossed fused ectopia*, one kidney crosses over to the other side and the parenchyma of the two kidneys fuse. Renal function is generally normal. The most common finding is that the left kidney may cross over and fuse with the lower pole of the right kidney. The insertion of the ureter does not change. In addition, the adrenal glands remain in their normal positions. The clinical significance of this anomaly is that if renal surgery is necessary, the blood supply is variable and may make partial nephrectomy more difficult.

Associated Physical Findings. Upper urinary tract anomalies are more common in children with certain physical findings. For example the incidence of renal anomalies is increased if there is a single umbilical artery and an abnormality of an organ system (e.g., congenital heart disease). In addition, external ear anomalies (particularly if the child has multiple congenital anomalies), imperforate anus, and scoliosis are associated with renal anomalies. Babies with these physical findings should undergo a renal sonogram.

American Academy of Pediatrics, Committee on Sports Medicine and Fitness: Medical conditions affecting sports participation. *Pediatrics* 2001;107:1205–9.

Belk RA, Thomas DF, Mueller RF, et al: A family study and the natural history of prenatally detected unilateral multicystic dysplastic kidney. *J Urol* 2002; 167:666–69.

Feldenburg LR, Siegel NJ: Clinical course and outcome for children with multicystic dysplastic kidneys. *Pediatr Nephrol* 2000;14:1098–1101.

Glassberg KI: Normal and abnormal development of the kidney: a clinician's interpretation of current knowledge. *J Urol* 2002;167:2339–51.

Ichikawa I, Kuyayama F, Pope JC IV, et al: Paradigm shift from classic anatomic theories to contemporary cell biological views of CAKUT. *Kidney Int* 2002;61:889–98.

Li S, Qayyum A, Coakley FV, et al: Association of renal agenesis and müllerian duct anomalies. *J Comput Assist Tomogr* 2000;24:829–34.

McCallum T, Milunsky J, Munarriz R, et al: Unilateral renal agenesis associated with congenital bilateral absence of the vas deferens: Phenotypic findings and genetic considerations. *Hum Reprod* 2001;16:282–88.

Mingin GC, Gilhooly P, Sadeghi-Nejad H: Transitional cell carcinoma in a multicystic dysplastic kidney. *J Urol* 2000;162:544.

Oshima K, Miyazaki Y, Brock JW III, et al: Angiotensin type II receptor expression and ureteral budding. *J Urol* 2001;166:1848–52.

Pope JC IV, Brock JW III, Adams MC, et al: Congenital anomalies of the kidney and urinary tract—role of the loss of function mutation in the pluripotent angiotensin type 2 receptor gene. *J Urol* 2001;165:196–202.

Seeman T, John U, Blahova K, et al: Ambulatory blood pressure monitoring in children with unilateral multicystic kidney. *Eur J Pediatr* 2001;160:78–83.

Snodgrass WT: Hypertension associated with multicystic dysplastic kidney in children. *J Urol* 2000;164:472–73.

Sukthankar S, Watson AR: Unilateral multicystic dysplastic kidney disease: Defining the natural history. *Acta Paediatr* 2000;89:811–13.

Wang RY, Earl DL, Ruder RO, et al: Syndromic ear anomalies and renal ultrasounds. *Pediatrics* 2001;108(2):E32.

Chapter 530
Urinary Tract Infections

(See also Chapter 511.)

Prevalence and Etiology. Urinary tract infections (UTIs) occur in 3–5% of girls and 1% of boys. In girls, the first UTI usually occurs by the age of 5 yr, with peaks during infancy and toilet training. After the first UTI, 60–80% of girls will develop a second UTI within 18 mo. In boys, most UTIs occur during the 1st yr of life; UTIs are much more common in uncircumcised boys. The prevalence of UTIs varies with age. During the 1st yr of life, the male:female ratio is 2.8–5.4:1. Beyond 1–2 yr, there is a striking female preponderance, with a male:female ratio of 1:10.

UTIs are caused mainly by colonic bacteria. In females, 75–90% of all infections are caused by *Escherichia coli*, followed by *Klebsiella* and *Proteus*. Some series report that in males older than 1 yr of age, *Proteus* is as common as *E. coli*; others report a preponderance of gram-positive organisms in males. *Staphylococcus saprophyticus* is a pathogen in both sexes. Viral infections, particularly adenovirus, may also occur, especially as a cause of cystitis.

UTIs have been considered an important risk factor for the development of renal insufficiency or end-stage renal disease. Some have questioned the importance of UTI as a risk factor because only 2% of children with current renal insufficiency report a history of UTI. This paradox is probably secondary to better recognition of the risks of UTI and prompt diagnosis and therapy.

Clinical Manifestations and Classification. There are three basic forms of UTI: pyelonephritis, cystitis, and asymptomatic bacteriuria.

Pyelonephritis is characterized by any or all of the following: abdominal or flank pain, fever, malaise, nausea, vomiting, and occasionally diarrhea. Some newborns and infants may show nonspecific symptoms such as jaundice, poor feeding, irritability, and weight loss. These symptoms are an indication that there is bacterial involvement of the upper urinary tract. Involvement of the renal parenchyma is termed *acute pyelonephritis*, whereas if there is no parenchymal involvement, the condition may be termed *pyelitis*. Acute pyelonephritis may result in renal injury, which is termed **pyelonephritic scarring**.

Cystitis indicates that there is bladder involvement and symptoms include dysuria, urgency, frequency, suprapubic pain, incontinence, and malodorous urine. Cystitis does not cause fever and does not result in renal injury.

Asymptomatic bacteriuria refers to individuals who have a positive urine culture without any manifestations of infection and occurs almost exclusively in girls. This condition is benign and does not cause renal injury, except in pregnant women, in whom asymptomatic bacteriuria, if left untreated, can result in a symptomatic UTI. Some girls are mistakenly identified as having asymptomatic bacteriuria, whereas they actually are symptomatic, experiencing day or night incontinence or perineal discomfort.

Pathogenesis and Pathology. Nearly all UTIs are ascending infections. The bacteria arise from the fecal flora, colonize the perineum, and enter the bladder via the urethra. In uncircumcised boys, the bacterial pathogens arise from the flora beneath the prepuce. In some cases, the bacteria ascend to the kidney to cause pyelonephritis. In rare cases, renal infection may occur by hematogenous spread.

If bacteria ascend from the bladder to the kidney, acute pyelonephritis may occur. Normally the simple and compound papillae in the kidney have an antireflux mechanism that prevents urine from flowing in a retrograde manner into the collecting tubules. Some compound papillae, typically located in the upper and lower poles of the kidney, allow intrarenal reflux. Infected urine then stimulates an immunologic and inflammatory response (Fig. 530–1). The result may cause renal injury and scarring (Fig. 530–2).

Children of any age with a febrile UTI may have acute pyelonephritis with renal scarring. The exception to this observation is that if a child with UTIs has a normal 2,3-dimercaptosuccinic acid (DMSA) scan by 4 yr of age, the risk of pyelonephritogenic scarring from future UTIs is probably low.

Host risk factors for UTI are listed in Box 530–1. Vesicoureteral reflux is discussed in Chapter 531. In girls, UTIs often occur at the onset of toilet training because of voiding dysfunction that occurs at that age. The child is trying to retain urine to stay dry, yet the bladder may have uninhibited contractions forcing urine out. The result may be high-pressure, turbulent urine flow or incomplete bladder emptying, both of which increase the likelihood of bacteriuria. Voiding dysfunction may occur in the toilet-trained child who voids infrequently. Obstructive uropathy resulting in hydronephrosis increases the risk of UTI because of urinary stasis. Urethral instrumentation during a voiding cystourethrogram or nonsterile catheterization may infect the bladder with a pathogen. Constipation can increase the risk of UTI because it may cause voiding dysfunction.

The pathogenesis of UTI is based in part on the presence of bacterial pili or fimbriae on the bacterial surface. There are two types of fimbriae, type I and type II. Type I fimbriae are found on most strains of *E. coli*. Because attachment to target cells can be blocked by D-mannose, these fimbriae are referred to as "mannose-sensitive." They have no role in pyelonephritis. The attachment of type II fimbriae is not inhibited by mannose, and

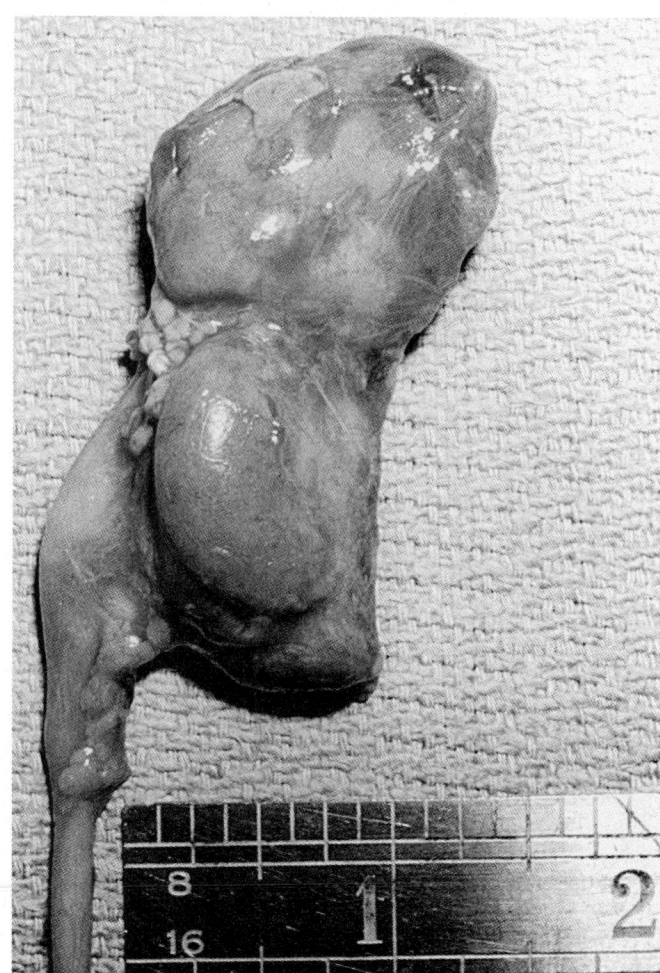

FIGURE 530–2. Scarred kidney from recurrent pyelonephritis.

these are known as "mannose-resistant." These fimbriae are expressed by only certain strains of *E. coli*. The receptor for type II fimbriae is a glycosphingolipid that is present on both the uroepithelial cell membrane and red blood cells. The Gal 1–4 Gal oligosaccharide fraction is the specific receptor. Because these fimbriae can agglutinate by P blood group erythrocytes, they are known as P fimbriae. Bacteria with P fimbriae are more likely to cause pyelonephritis. Between 76–94% of pyelonephritogenic strains of *E. coli* have P fimbriae, compared with 19–23% of cystitis strains.

Other host factors for UTI include anatomic abnormalities precluding normal micturition, such as a labial adhesion. This lesion acts as a barrier and causes vaginal voiding. A neuropathic bladder may cause UTIs if there is incomplete bladder emptying or detrusor-sphincter dyssynergia, or both. Sexual activity is associated with UTIs in girls, in part because of incomplete bladder emptying. Finally, during pregnancy 4–7% have asymptomatic bacteriuria, which can result in a symptomatic UTI. The incidence of UTI in infants who are breast fed is lower than in those fed with formula.

Xanthogranulomatous pyelonephritis is a rare type of renal infection characterized by granulomatous inflammation with giant cells and foamy histiocytes. It may present clinically as a renal mass or an acute or chronic infection. Renal calculi, obstruction, and infection with *Proteus* or *E. coli* contribute to the development of this lesion, which usually requires total or partial nephrectomy.

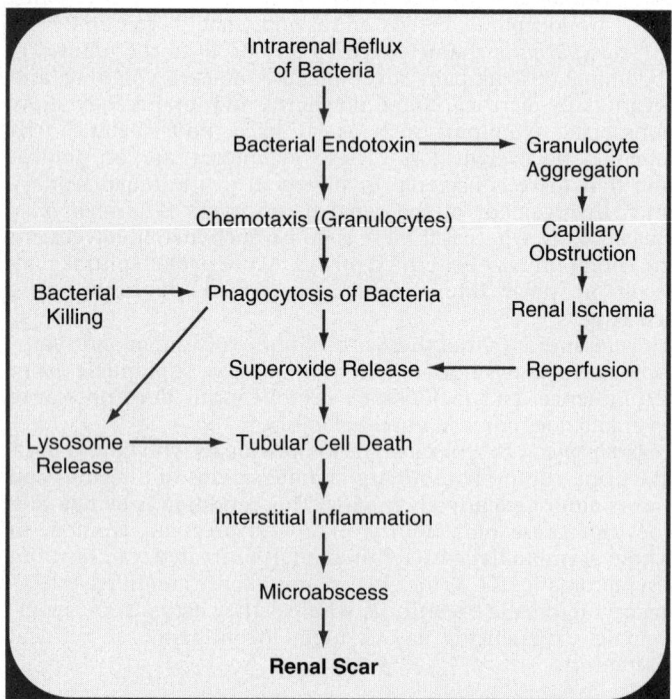

FIGURE 530–1. Pathogenesis of pyelonephritic scarring following acute pyelonephritis. (Adapted from Roberts JA: Pathogenesis of pyelonephritis. *J Urol* 1983;129:1102.)

Diagnosis. A UTI may be suspected based on the symptoms or findings on urinalysis, or both, but a urine culture is necessary

BOX 530–1. Risk Factors for Urinary Tract Infection

Female
Uncircumcised male
Vesicoureteral reflux*
Toilet training
Voiding dysfunction
Obstructive uropathy
Urethral instrumentation
Wiping from back to front
Bubble bath
Tight clothing (underwear)
Pinworm infestation
Constipation
P fimbriated bacteria*
Anatomic abnormality (e.g., labial adhesion)
Neuropathic bladder
Sexual activity
Pregnancy

*Risk increased for clinical pyelonephritis, not cystitis.

for confirmation and appropriate therapy. Thus, the diagnosis of UTI depends on having the proper sample of urine. There are several ways to obtain a urine sample; some are more accurate than others.

In toilet-trained children, a *midstream urine sample* is usually satisfactory. Most studies have failed to show any benefit to formally cleansing the introitus before obtaining the specimen. If the culture shows greater than 100,000 colonies of a single pathogen, or if there are 10,000 colonies and the child is symptomatic, it is considered a UTI. In uncircumcised males, the prepuce must be retracted; if the prepuce is not retractable, this method of urine collection is unreliable.

In infants, the application of an adhesive, sealed, *sterile collection bag* after disinfection of the skin of the genitals can be useful, particularly if the culture is negative. However, a positive culture may reflect a contaminant, particularly in girls and uncircumcised boys. In such cases, if the urinalysis result is positive, the patient is symptomatic, and there is a single organism cultured with a colony count greater than 100,000, there is a presumed UTI. However, if any of these criteria are not met, confirmation of infection with a catheterized sample is recommended (see next paragraph).

When greater assurance as to the possibility of infection is needed, a *catheterized specimen* must be obtained. Proper skin preparation and good technique of catheterization are important. The use of a No. 5 French polyethylene feeding tube in infants or a No. 8 French tube with proper lubrication in older children minimizes the chance of urethral trauma and contamination. Only a few milliliters need to be aspirated with a syringe to obtain the urine sample. Catheterization shortly after spontaneous voiding produces a measure of the residual urine in the bladder and helps assess problems related to bladder emptying.

Prompt plating of the urine sample is important because if the urine sits at room temperature for more than 60 min, overgrowth of a minor contaminant may suggest a UTI, when in fact the urine may not be infected. Placing the sample in a refrigerator is a reliable method of storing the urine until it can be cultured.

A urinalysis should be obtained from the same specimen as that cultured. Pyuria (leukocytes in the urine) suggests infection, but infection can occur in the absence of pyuria; consequently, this finding is more confirmatory than diagnostic. Conversely, pyuria can be present without UTI. Nitrites and leukocyte esterase are usually positive in infected urine. Microscopic hematuria is common in acute cystitis. White blood cell casts in the urinary sediment suggest renal involvement, but these are rarely seen. If the child is asymptomatic and the urinalysis result is normal, it is unlikely that the urine is infected. However, if the child is symptomatic, a UTI is possible, even if the urinalysis result is negative.

With acute renal infection, leukocytosis, neutrophilia, and elevated erythrocyte sedimentation rate and C-reactive protein are common. The latter two are nonspecific markers of bacterial infection, and their elevation does not mean that the child has acute pyelonephritis. With a renal abscess, the white blood cell count is markedly elevated to greater than 20,000 to 25,000/mm^3. Because sepsis is common in pyelonephritis, particularly in infants and in any child with obstructive uropathy, blood cultures should be considered.

Acute hemorrhagic cystitis is frequently caused by *E. coli*; it has been attributed also to adenovirus types 11 and 21. Adenovirus cystitis is more frequent in males; it is self-limiting, with hematuria lasting approximately 4 days.

Eosinophilic cystitis is a rare form of cystitis of obscure origin that occasionally is found in children. The usual symptoms are those of cystitis with hematuria, ureteral dilatation with occasional hydronephrosis, and filling defects in the bladder caused by masses that consist histologically of inflammatory infiltrates with eosinophils. Children with eosinophilic cystitis may have had exposure to an allergen. Frequently, bladder biopsy is necessary to exclude a neoplastic process. Treatment usually includes antihistamines and nonsteroidal anti-inflammatory agents, but in some cases intravesical dimethyl sulfoxide instillation is necessary.

Interstitial cystitis is characterized by irritative voiding symptoms such as urgency, frequency, and dysuria, and bladder and pelvic pain relieved by voiding with a negative urine culture. The disorder is most likely to affect adolescent girls and is idiopathic. Diagnosis is made by cystoscopic observation of mucosal ulcers with bladder distention. Treatments have included bladder hydrodistention and laser ablation of ulcerated areas, but no treatment yields sustained relief.

Treatment. Acute cystitis should be treated promptly to prevent its possible progression to pyelonephritis. If the symptoms are severe, a specimen of bladder urine is obtained for culture and treatment is started immediately. If the symptoms are mild or the diagnosis is doubtful, treatment can be delayed until the results of culture are known, and the culture can be repeated if the results are uncertain. For example, if a midstream culture grew between 10^4 and 10^5 colonies of a gram-negative organism, a second culture may be obtained by catheterization before treatment is initiated. If treatment is initiated before the results of a culture and sensitivities are available, a 3- to 5-day course of therapy with trimethoprim-sulfamethoxazole (see later) is effective against most strains of *E. coli*. Nitrofurantoin (5–7 mg/kg/24 hr in three to four divided doses) is also effective and has the advantage of being active against *Klebsiella-Enterobacter* organisms. Amoxicillin (50 mg/kg/24 hr) is also effective as initial treatment but has no clear advantages over the sulfonamides or nitrofurantoin.

In acute febrile infections suggestive of pyelonephritis, a 14-day course of broad-spectrum antibiotics capable of reaching significant tissue levels is preferable. Children who are dehydrated, are unable to drink fluids, or in whom sepsis is a possibility should be admitted to the hospital for intravenous rehydration and intravenous antibiotic therapy. Parenteral treatment with ceftriaxone (50–75 mg/kg/24 hr, not to exceed 2 g) or ampicillin (100 mg/kg/24 hr) with an aminoglycoside such as gentamicin (3 to 5 mg/kg/24 hr in one to three divided doses) is preferable. The potential ototoxicity and nephrotoxicity of aminoglycosides should be considered, and serum creatinine and trough gentamicin levels must be obtained before initiating treatment as well as daily thereafter as long as treatment continues. Treatment with aminoglycosides is particularly effective against *Pseudomonas*, and alkalinization of urine with sodium bicarbonate increases their effectiveness in the urinary tract. Oral third-generation cephalosporins such as cefixime are as effective as parenteral ceftriaxone against a variety of gram-negative organisms other than *Pseudomonas*, and these medications are considered by some authorities to be the treatment of choice for oral therapy.

Nitrofurantoin should not be used in children with a febrile UTI because it does not achieve significant renal tissue levels. The oral fluoroquinolone ciprofloxacin is an alternative agent for resistant microorganisms, particularly *Pseudomonas,* in patients older than 17 yr. It also has been used in younger children with cystic fibrosis and pulmonary infection secondary to *Pseudomonas* and is used on occasion for short course therapy in children with *Pseudomonas* UTI. However, the clinical use of fluoroquinolones in children should be restricted because of potential cartilage damage that occurred in research with immature animals. The safety and efficacy of oral ciprofloxacin in children is under study. In some children with a febrile UTI, intramuscular injection of a loading dose of ceftriaxone followed by oral therapy with a third-generation cephalosporin is effective.

Children with a renal or perirenal abscess or with infection in obstructed urinary tracts require surgical or percutaneous drainage in addition to antibiotic therapy and other supportive measures.

A urine culture should be performed 1 wk after the termination of treatment of any UTI to ensure that the urine is sterile. Given the tendency of urinary tract infections to recur even in the absence of predisposing anatomic factors, a follow-up urine culture should be performed periodically for 1–2 yr, even when the child is asymptomatic.

If recurrences are frequent, identifying predisposing factors to UTI is beneficial. For example, many school-aged girls have voiding dysfunction, and treatment of this condition often reduces the likelihood of recurrent UTI. Some children with urinary tract infections void infrequently, and many also have severe constipation. Counseling of parents and patients to try to establish more normal patterns of voiding and defecation may be helpful in controlling recurrences. In addition, prophylaxis against reinfection, using either the sulfamethoxazole-trimethoprim combination or nitrofurantoin at one third of the normal therapeutic dose once a day, is often effective. Prophylaxis with amoxicillin or cephalexin also may be effective, but the risk of breakthrough UTI is higher because bacterial resistance may be induced. Other indications for long-term prophylaxis (neurogenic bladder, urinary tract stasis and obstruction, reflux, and calculi) are discussed in other chapters. Cranberry juice has not proved beneficial in preventing UTI.

The main consequences of chronic renal damage caused by pyelonephritis are arterial hypertension and renal insufficiency; when they are found they should be treated appropriately (see Chapters 437 and 527).

Imaging Studies. The goal of imaging studies in children with a UTI is to identify anatomic abnormalities that predispose to infection. A renal ultrasonogram should be obtained to rule out hydronephrosis and renal or perirenal abscesses; ultrasonography also may show acute pyelonephritis (in 30–60% of cases) by demonstrating an enlarged kidney. Power Doppler ultrasonography has been slightly more sensitive but is unreliable in identifying all cases. Ultrasonography demonstrates 30% of renal scars. Normally, the difference in renal lengths between the two kidneys is less than 1 cm, and a larger disparity may be an indication of impaired renal growth. One should remember that in a child with acute pyelonephritis, a small kidney may be enlarged because of the infection, giving the erroneous impression that the kidneys are equal in size. Renal ultrasonography is also sensitive for detecting pyonephrosis, a condition that may require prompt drainage of the collecting system by percutaneous nephrostomy.

A voiding cystourethrogram (VCUG) is also indicated in all children younger than 5 yr with a UTI, any child with a febrile UTI, school-aged girls who have had two or more UTIs, and any male with a UTI. The most common finding is vesicoureteral reflux, which is identified in approximately 40% of patients (Fig. 530–3). Timing of the VCUG is controversial. In some centers the study is delayed for 2–6 wk to allow inflammation in the

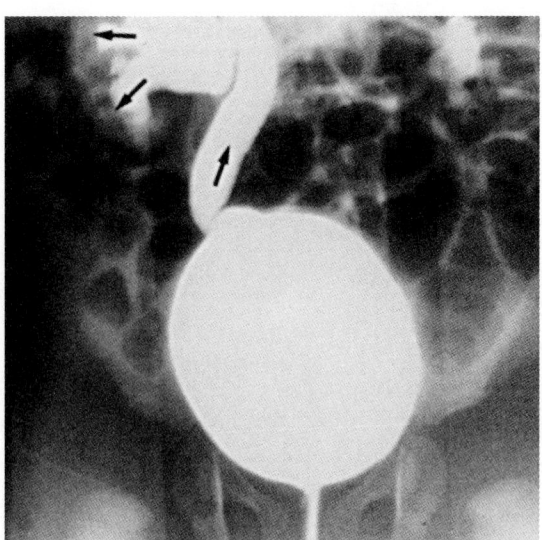

FIGURE 530–3. Intrarenal reflux. Voiding cystourethrogram in a young infant male with a past history of a urinary tract infection. Note the right vesicoureteral reflux with ureteral dilatation, with opacification of the renal parenchyma representing intrarenal reflux.

bladder to resolve. However, the incidence of reflux is identical, irrespective of whether the VCUG is obtained during treatment of the UTI or after 6 wk. Consequently, obtaining the VCUG before the child is discharged from the hospital is recommended. If available, a radionuclide VCUG instead of a contrast VCUG can be used in girls; this technique causes less radiation exposure to the gonads than does the contrast study. However, the radioisotopic VCUG does not provide anatomic definition of the bladder, allow precise grading of reflux, demonstrate a paraureteral diverticulum, or show whether reflux is occurring into a duplicated collecting system or an ectopic ureter. In boys, radiographic definition of the urethra is important; accordingly, contrast VCUG is recommended for the initial work-up.

Because of concern that the VCUG is traumatic to the child, some parents question the need for a VCUG if the ultrasonogram is normal. However, ultrasonography is insensitive in detecting reflux; only 40% of children with reflux have any abnormality on the ultrasonogram. The VCUG should not be performed using general anesthesia, because the study is incomplete without a voiding phase and it subjects the child unnecessarily to the risk and cost of anesthesia. In selected cases, oral or nasal midazolam (up to 0.5 mg/kg oral route, 0.2 mg/kg nasal route), which causes anterograde amnesia and anxiolysis, may

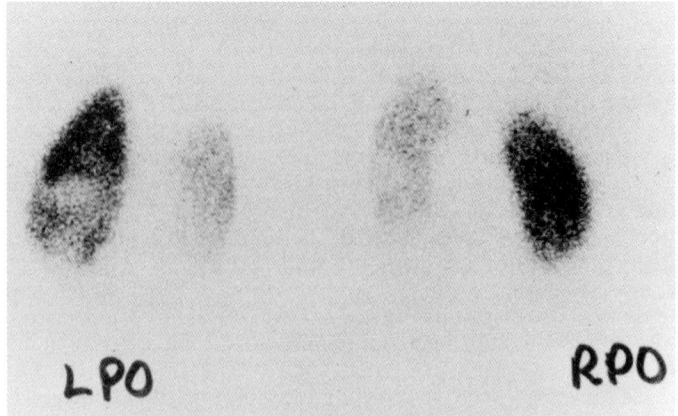

FIGURE 530–4. DMSA renal scan showing bilateral photopenic areas indicative of acute pyelonephritis and renal scarring.

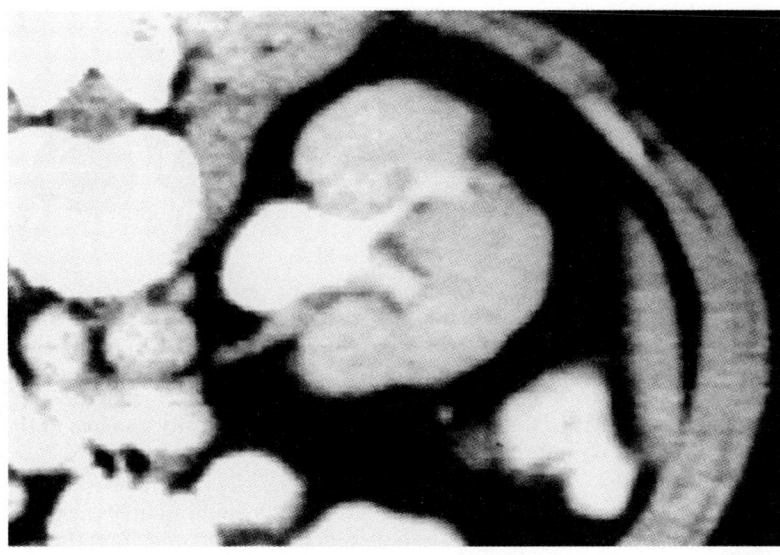

FIGURE 530–5. CT scan showing an area of parenchymal thinning corresponding to an underlying calyx, characteristic of pyelonephritic scarring or reflux nephropathy.

be used. We have found that this medication is efficacious and safe and provides an acceptable experience with VCUG. Vital signs are monitored and pulse oximetry is used; no anesthesiologist is present.

When the diagnosis of acute pyelonephritis is uncertain, renal scanning with technetium-labeled DMSA or glucoheptonate is useful. The presence of photopenia supports the diagnosis of pyelonephritis, and experienced radiologists can differentiate an acute from a chronic process. In approximately 50% of children with a febrile UTI, irrespective of age, the DMSA scan demonstrates parenchymal involvement. In children with grade III, IV, or V reflux and a febrile UTI, 80–90% show acute pyelonephritis. If the DMSA scan shows acute pyelonephritis, approximately 50% will acquire a scar in that site over the following 5 mo. However, if the DMSA scan is normal during a febrile UTI, no scarring results from that particular infection. Computed tomography is another diagnostic tool that can diagnose acute pyelonephritis, but clinical experience with DMSA is much greater.

If vesicoureteral reflux is present, a DMSA scan (Fig. 530–4) often is performed to assess whether renal scarring is present. The DMSA is the most sensitive and accurate study for demonstrating scarring. Excretory urography is not as sensitive as the DMSA scan in demonstrating renal scarring; in addition, visualization of the collecting system in infants and young children often is suboptimal, there is a slight risk of a contrast allergy, and it can take 1–2 yr for a renal scar to appear on the urogram. Computed tomography also has been used by some to evaluate the upper urinary tract because it is effective in demonstrating renal scarring (Fig. 530–5).

Frequently performed cystoscopies and measurements of urethral caliber in girls contribute nothing to the therapeutic decisions to be made in children with UTIs and are contraindicated. Narrowing of the female urethra was once postulated to be a contributing factor in the development of UTIs, but the urethras of girls with recurrent UTIs are not narrower than those of girls without infections.

Alghasham AA, Nahata MC: Clinical use of fluoroquinolones in children. *Ann Pharmacother* 2000;34:347–59.

American Academy of Pediatrics Committee on Quality Improvement. Subcommittee on Urinary Tract Infection: Practice parameter: The diagnosis, treatment, and evaluation of the initial urinary tract infection in febrile infants and young children. *Pediatrics* 1999;103:843–52.

Armengol CE, Hendley JO, Schlager TA: Should we abandon standard microscopy when screening for urinary tract infections in young children? *Pediatr Infect Dis J* 2001;20:1176–177.

Bachelard M, Verkauskas G, Bertilsson M, et al: Recognition of bladder instability on voiding cystourethrography in infants with urinary tract infection. *J Urol* 2001;166:1899–1903.

Benador D, Neuhaus TJ, Papazyan J-P, et al: Randomised controlled trial of three day versus 10 day intravenous antibiotics in acute pyelonephritis: Effect on renal scarring. *Arch Dis Child* 2001; 84:241–46.

Biggi A, Dardanelli L, Cussino P, et al: Prognostic value of the acute DMSA scan in children with first urinary tract infection. *Pediatr Nephrol* 2001;16:800–4.

Cascio S, Colhoun E, Puri P: Bacterial colonization of the prepuce in boys with vesicoureteral reflux who receive antibiotic prophylaxis. *J Pediatr* 2001;139:160–62.

Chon CH, Lai FC, Shortliffe LM: Pediatric urinary tract infections. *Pediatr Clin North Am* 2001;48:1441–59.

Christian MT, McColl JH, MacKenzie JR, et al: Risk assessment of renal cortical scarring with urinary tract infection by clinical features and ultrasonography. *Arch Dis Child* 2000;82:376–80.

Garcia FJ, Nager AL: Jaundice as an early diagnostic sign of urinary tract infection in infancy. *Pediatrics* 2002;109:846–57.

Goldman M, Bistritzer T, Horne T, et al: The etiology of renal scars in infants with pyelonephritis and vesicoureteral reflux. *Pediatr Nephrol* 2000;14:385–88.

Huicho L, Campos-Sanchez M, Alamo C: Meta-analysis of urine screening tests for determining the risk of urinary tract infection in children. *Pediatr Infect Dis* 2002;21:1–11.

Hoberman A, Wald ER, Hickey RW, et al: Oral versus initial intravenous therapy for urinary tract infections in young febrile children. *Pediatrics* 1999;105:79–86.

Jantunen ME, Saxen H, Salo E, et al: Recurrent urinary tract infections in infancy: Relapses or reinfections? *J Infect Dis* 2002;185:375–79.

Jodal U, Lindberg U: Guidelines for management of children with urinary tract infection and vesico-ureteric reflux: Recommendations from a Swedish state-of-the-art conference. *Acta Paediatr Suppl* 1999;431:87–89.

Keren R, Chan E: A meta-analysis of randomized, controlled trials comparing short- and long-course antibiotic therapy for urinary tract infections in children. *Pediatrics* 2002;109(5):e70.

Levtchenko E, Lahy C, Levy J, et al: Treatment of children with acute pyelonephritis: A prospective randomized study. *Pediatr Nephrol* 2001;16:878–84.

McDonald A, Scranton M, Gillespie R, et al: Voiding cystourethrograms and urinary tract infections: how long to wait? *Pediatrics* 2000;105(4):e50.

Mahant S, To T, Friedman J: Timing of voiding cystourethrogram in the investigation of urinary tract infections in children. *J Pediatr* 2001;139:568–71.

Markowitz JE, Bengmark S: Probiotics in health and disease in the pediatric patient. *Pediatr Clin North Am* 2002;49:127–41.

Martinell J, Hansson S, Claesson I, et al: Detection of urographic scars in girls with pyelonephritis followed for 13–38 years. *Pediatr Nephrol* 2000;14:1006–10.

Reid G, Burton J: Use of *Lactobacillus* to prevent infection by pathogenic bacteria. *Microbes Infect* 2002;4:319–24.

Schlager TA: Urinary tract infections in children younger than 5 years of age: Epidemiology, diagnosis, treatment, outcomes and prevention. *Paediatr Drugs* 2001;3:219–27.

Tran D, Muchant DG, Aronoff SC: Short-course versus conventional length antimicrobial therapy for uncomplicated lower urinary tract infections in children: A meta-analysis of 1279 patients. *J Pediatr* 2001;139:93–99.

Wennerstrom M, Hansson S, Jodal U, et al: Renal function 16 to 26 years after the first urinary tract infection in childhood. *Arch Pediatr Adolesc Med* 2000;154:339–45.

Williams G, Lee A, Craig J: Antibiotics for the prevention of urinary tract infection in children: A systematic review of randomized controlled trials. *J Pediatr* 2001;138:868–74.

Wold AE, Adlerberth I: Breast feeding and the intestinal microflora of the infant-implications for protection against infectious diseases. *Adv Exp Med Biol* 2000;478:77–93.

Chapter 531
Vesicoureteral Reflux

Vesicoureteral reflux is the retrograde flow of urine from the bladder to the ureter and renal pelvis. The ureter is normally attached to the bladder in an oblique direction, perforating the bladder muscle (detrusor) laterally and proceeding between the bladder mucosa and detrusor muscle, creating a flap-valve mechanism that prevents reflux (Fig. 531–1). Reflux occurs when the submucosal tunnel between the mucosa and detrusor muscle is short or absent. Reflux is usually congenital, occurs in families, and affects approximately 1% of children.

Reflux predisposes to renal infection (pyelonephritis) by facilitating the transport of bacteria from the bladder to the upper urinary tract. The inflammatory reaction caused by a pyelonephritic infection may result in renal injury or scarring, also termed *reflux nephropathy*. Extensive renal scarring impairs renal function and may result in renin-mediated hypertension, renal insufficiency or end-stage renal disease, impaired somatic growth, and morbidity during pregnancy. Reflux nephropathy once accounted for as much as 15–20% of end-stage renal disease in children and young adults. Currently, with greater attention to the management of urinary tract infections and a better understanding of reflux, it is much less common. Nevertheless, reflux nephropathy is one of the most common causes of hypertension in children.

Classification. Reflux severity is graded using the International Study Classification of I to V and is based on the appearance of the urinary tract on a contrast voiding cystourethrogram (VCUG) (Figs. 531–2 and 531–3). The higher the reflux grade, the greater the likelihood of renal injury. Reflux severity is an indirect indication of the degree of abnormality of the ureterovesical junction.

Reflux may be primary or secondary (Table 531–1). Primary vesicoureteral reflux results from an anatomic deformity of the ureterovesical junction (see Fig. 531–1). Conditions such as bladder instability can precipitate reflux or worsen pre-existing reflux if there is a marginally competent ureterovesical junction. In the most severe cases, there is such massive reflux into the upper tracts that the bladder becomes overdistended. This condition, termed the *megacystis-megaureter syndrome*, occurs primarily in males and may be unilateral or bilateral (Fig. 531–4). In this particular condition, reimplantation of the ureters into the bladder to correct reflux resolves the condition.

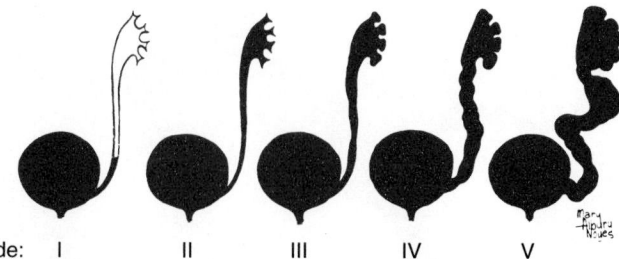

Grade: I   II   III   IV   V

FIGURE 531–2. Grading of vesicoureteral reflux. Grade I: reflux into a nondilated ureter. Grade II: reflux into the upper collecting system without dilatation. Grade III: reflux into dilated ureter and/or blunting of calyceal fornices. Grade IV: reflux into a grossly dilated ureter. Grade V: massive reflux, with significant ureteral dilatation and tortuosity and loss of the papillary impression.

Approximately 1 in 125 children has a duplication of the upper urinary tract in which two ureters rather than one drain the kidney. Duplication may be partial or complete. In partial duplication the ureters join above the bladder and there is one ureteral orifice. In complete duplication the lower pole ureter drains superolateral to the upper pole ureter in the bladder. Reflux occurs in as many as 50% of cases into the lower ureter, which typically has a less competent valve, but in some cases reflux occurs into both the lower and upper systems (Fig. 531–5). With a duplication anomaly, some patients have an ectopic ureter, in which the upper pole ureter drains outside the bladder (see Chapter 532). If the ectopic ureter drains into the bladder neck, typically it is obstructed and refluxes. Duplication anomalies also are common in children with a ureterocele, which is a cystic swelling of the intramural portion of the distal ureter. In these patients often there is reflux into the associated lower pole ureter

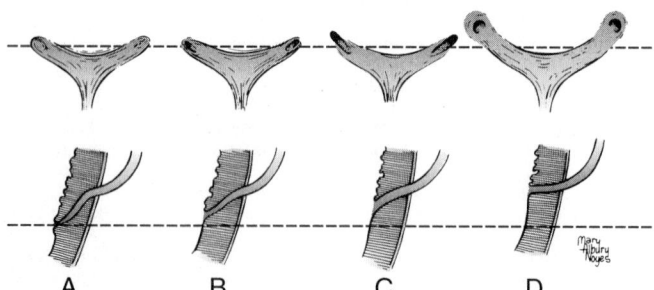

FIGURE 531–1. Normal and abnormal configuration of the ureteral orifices. Shown from *left to right,* progressive lateral displacement of the ureteral orifices and shortening of the intramural tunnels. *Top,* Endoscopic appearance. *Bottom,* Sagittal view through the intramural ureter.

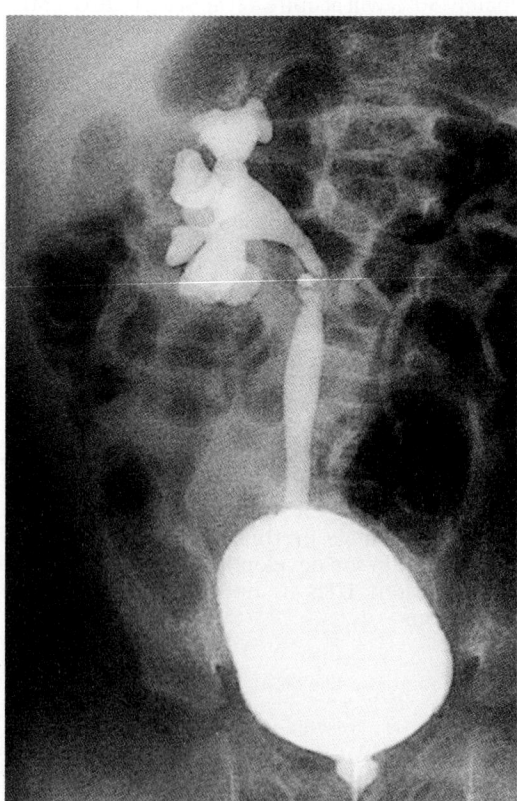

FIGURE 531–3. Voiding cystourethrogram (VCUG) showing grade IV right vesicoureteral reflux with intrarenal reflux.

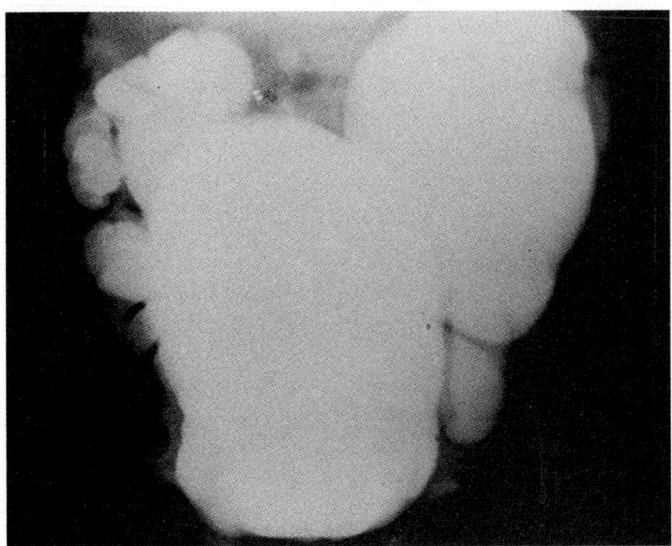

FIGURE 531–4. VCUG in male newborn with megacystic-megaureter syndrome. Note the massive ureteral dilatation due to high-grade vesicoureteral reflux. The bladder is very distended. There was no urethral obstruction or neuropathic dysfunction.

or the contralateral ureter. Reflux also typically is present when the ureter enters a diverticulum (Fig. 531–6).

In children with neuropathic bladder, as occurs in myelomeningocele, sacral agenesis, and many children with a high imperforate anus, reflux is present in 25% at birth. Reflux is seen in 50% of boys with posterior urethral valves. Clinically, reflux with increased intravesical pressure (as in detrusor-sphincter dyssynergia or bladder outlet obstruction) can result in renal injury, even in the absence of infection.

Primary reflux is found in association with several congenital urinary tract abnormalities. For example, 15% of children with a multicystic dysplastic kidney or renal agenesis have reflux into the contralateral kidney, and 10–15% of children with a ureteropelvic junction obstruction have reflux into either the hydronephrotic kidney or the contralateral kidney.

Reflux is an inherited trait. Approximately 35% of siblings of children with reflux also have reflux; the majority are asymptomatic. The likelihood of a sibling having reflux is independent of the grade of reflux or sex of the index child. Approximately 12% of asymptomatic siblings with reflux have evidence of renal scarring. In addition, in women with a history of reflux, 50% of offspring have reflux. Consequently, many believe that siblings

TABLE 531–1. Classification of Vesicoureteral Reflux

Type	Cause
1. Primary	Congenital incompetence of the valvular mechanism of the vesicoureteral junction
2. Primary associated with other malformations of the ureterovesical junction	Ureteral duplication Ureterocele with duplication Ureteral ectopia Paraureteral diverticula
3. Secondary to increased intravesical pressure	Neuropathic bladder Non-neuropathic bladder dysfunction Bladder outlet obstruction
4. Secondary to inflammatory processes	Severe bacterial cystitis Foreign bodies Vesical calculi Clinical cystitis
5. Secondary to surgical procedures involving the ureterovesical junction	

of children with reflux should be screened even if they have not had a urinary tract infection (UTI). Screening with a radionuclide cystogram of all siblings 3 yr or younger and any sibling with a UTI is appropriate. Older siblings may undergo renal ultrasonography, and if an abnormality such as hydronephrosis or disparity in renal length is found, VCUG is recommended. Primary reflux is less common in African-Americans.

Clinical Manifestations. Usually reflux is discovered during an evaluation for a urinary tract infection (see Chapter 530). In these children, 80% with reflux are female and the average age at diagnosis is 2–3 yr. In other children, VCUG is performed during evaluation of voiding dysfunction, renal insufficiency, hypertension, or other suspected pathologic process of the urinary tract. Primary reflux also may be discovered during evaluation for prenatal hydronephrosis. In this population, 80% of affected children are male and the reflux grade usually is higher than in females diagnosed with a urinary tract infection.

Diagnosis. Diagnosis of reflux generally requires catheterization of the bladder, instillation of a solution containing iodinated contrast or a radiopharmaceutical, and radiologic imaging of the lower and upper urinary tract—a contrast VCUG or radionuclide VCUG, respectively. The bladder and upper urinary tracts are imaged during bladder filling and voiding. Reflux occurring during bladder filling is termed *low-pressure* or *passive reflux*; reflux during voiding is termed *high-pressure* or *active reflux*. Children with passive reflux are less likely to show spontaneous reflux resolution than are children who exhibit only active reflux. Radiation exposure during radionuclide VCUG is significantly less compared with contrast VCUG. However, the contrast study provides more anatomic information, such as demonstration of a duplex collecting system, ectopic ureter, paraureteral (bladder) diverticulum, bladder outlet obstruction in boys, upper urinary tract stasis, and signs of voiding dysfunction, such as a spinning top urethra in girls. Furthermore, the reflux grading system is based on the appearance on VCUG. Consequently, the VCUG is used in most centers as the initial study. For follow-up evaluation, the radionuclide cystogram is often preferred because of the lower radiation exposure (Fig. 531–7).

Children undergoing cystography may be psychologically or emotionally traumatized by the catheterization, or both. Careful preparation by caregivers or administering oral or nasal midazolam (for sedation and amnesia) before the study can result in a more acceptable experience.

A technique of detecting reflux without catheterization is termed *indirect cystography* and involves injecting an intravenous radiopharmaceutical that is excreted by the kidneys, waiting for it to be excreted into the bladder, and imaging the lower urinary tract while the patient voids. This technique detects only 50% of reflux cases. Another technique, avoiding cystourethrosonography, involves the use of ultrasonographic contrast medium, which is administered through a urethral catheter. The urinary tract is imaged with ultrasonography. The advantage of this technique is the absence of radiation, but its disadvantage is that it is less accurate than contrast VCUG and reflux cannot be graded.

After reflux is diagnosed, graded, and determined to be primary or secondary, it is important to assess the upper urinary tract. The goal of upper tract imaging is to assess whether renal scarring and associated urinary tract anomalies are present. Renal imaging can be performed by ultrasonography, excretory urography (intravenous pyelogram), or renal scintigraphy. Ultrasonography is a noninvasive method of evaluating the kidney, because it can demonstrate hydronephrosis, gross renal scars, and renal duplication (possibly with an obstructed upper pole system or a thin lower pole) and allows one to monitor renal growth over time. Only 30–60% of renal scars are demonstrated with this technique. Intravenous pyelography involves

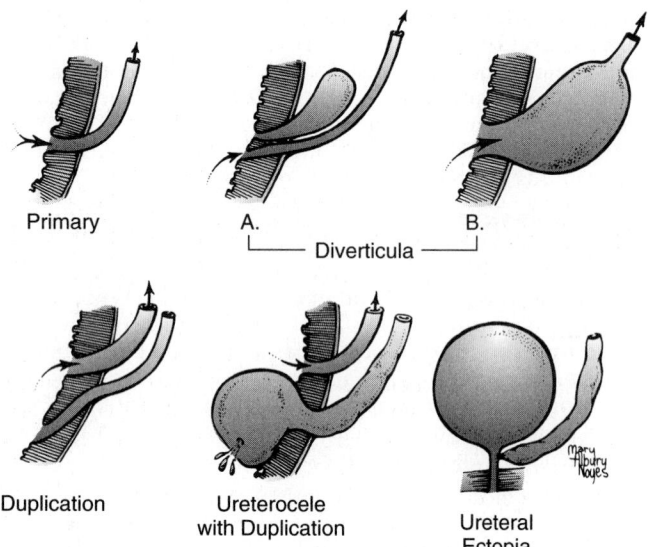

Primary

A. ──── Diverticula ──── B.

Duplication   Ureterocele with Duplication   Ureteral Ectopia

FIGURE 531–5. Various anatomic defects of the ureterovesical junction associated with vesicoureteral reflux.

injection of an iodinated contrast agent and provides good anatomic detail of the kidneys, but this study is performed infrequently in children at present. Approximately 90% of scars are demonstrated with this technique. Renal scintigraphy is usually performed with dimercaptosuccinic acid (DMSA), which demonstrates renal cortical detail well and is reliable in demonstrating nearly all renal scarring. However, it is less reliable than the other two studies in demonstrating renal anomalies such as hydronephrosis.

The child should be evaluated for voiding dysfunction, including urgency, frequency, diurnal incontinence, infrequent voiding, or a combination of these. In addition, bowel habits should be assessed. Children with bladder instability often require anticholinergic therapy and a voiding routine in addition to antibiotic prophylaxis.

After diagnosis, the child's height, weight, and blood pressure should be measured. If upper tract imaging shows renal scarring, a serum creatinine measurement should be obtained. The urine should be assessed for infection and proteinuria. Cystoscopy is of

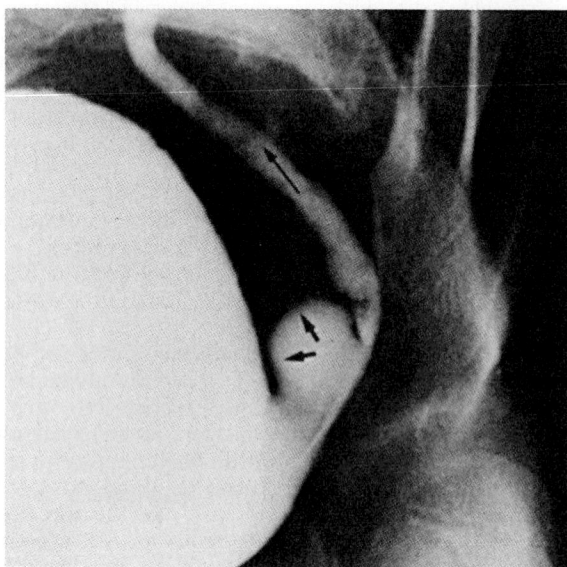

FIGURE 531–6. Reflux and bladder diverticulum. The voiding cystourethrogram demonstrates left vesicoureteral reflux and a paraureteral diverticulum.

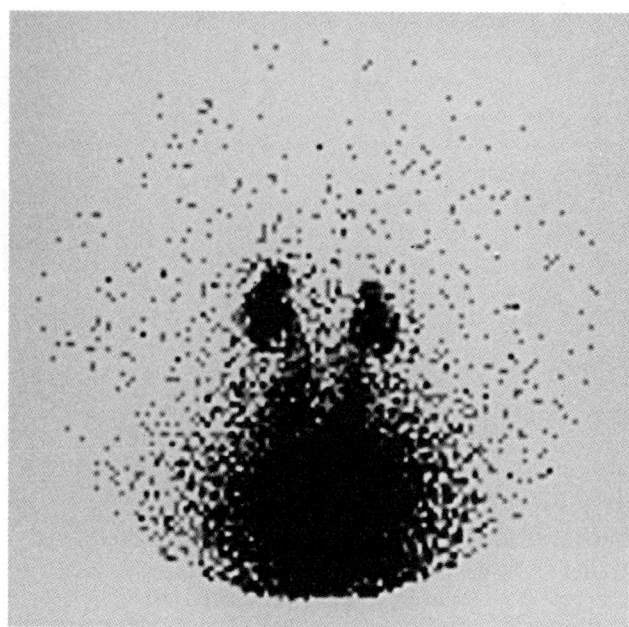

FIGURE 531–7. Radionuclide cystogram shows bilateral reflux.

no value in determining the prognosis or selecting treatment. Urethral dilatation is not beneficial.

Natural History. The incidence of renal scarring or reflux nephropathy increases with the grade of reflux. With bladder growth and maturation, there is a tendency for reflux to resolve or improve over time. Lower grades of reflux are much more likely to resolve than are higher grades. For grades I and II reflux, the likelihood of resolution is similar irrespective of age at diagnosis and whether it is unilateral or bilateral. For grade III, a younger age at diagnosis and unilateral reflux generally are associated with a higher rate of spontaneous resolution (Fig. 531–8). Bilateral grade IV reflux is much less likely to resolve than is unilateral grade IV reflux. Grade V reflux rarely resolves. The mean age at reflux resolution is 6–7 yr. Reflux is unlikely to cause renal injury in the absence of infection. However, in situations with high-pressure reflux, as in children with posterior urethral valves, neuropathic bladder, and non-neurogenic neurogenic bladder (**Hinman syndrome**), sterile reflux can cause significant renal damage. Children with high-grade reflux who acquire a UTI are at significant risk for pyelonephritis and renal scarring.

Treatment. The goals of treatment are to prevent pyelonephritis, renal injury, and other complications of reflux. Medical therapy is based on the principle that reflux often resolves over time and that the morbidity or complications of reflux may be prevented nonsurgically. The basis for surgical therapy is that in selected children, ongoing reflux has caused or has a significant potential for causing renal injury or other reflux-related complications and that elimination of reflux minimizes the likelihood of these problems.

Continuous antibiotic prophylaxis is the cornerstone in the initial management of children with reflux. Drugs commonly used for prophylaxis include sulfamethoxazole-trimethoprim, trimethoprim alone, and nitrofurantoin, generally administered once daily at a dose of one fourth to one third of the dose necessary to treat an acute infection. Prophylaxis is usually continued until reflux resolves or until the risk of reflux to the individual is considered to be low. The child's voiding and defecation habits are assessed, and voiding dysfunction and constipation should be treated (see Chapter 535). A urine culture should be performed if there are symptoms or signs of a UTI, or both. VCUG

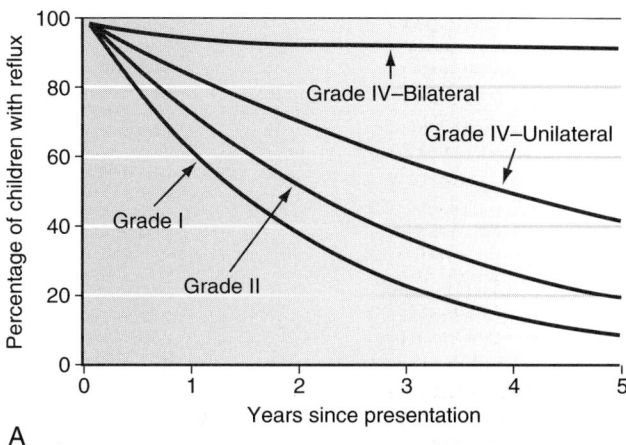
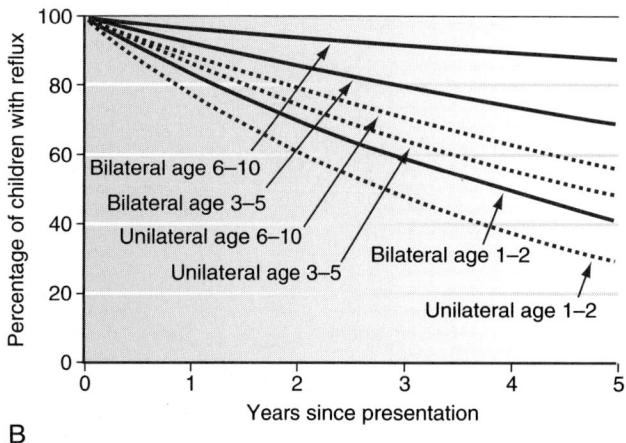

FIGURE 531–8. *A,* Percent chance of reflux persistence, grades I, II, and IV, for 1–5 yr after presentation. *B,* Percent chance of reflux persistence by age at presentation, grade III, for 1–5 yr after presentation. (From Elder JS, Peters CA, Arant BS Jr, et al: Pediatric Vesicoureteral Reflux Guidelines Panel Summary Report on the management of primary vesicoureteral reflux in children. *J Urol* 1997;157:1846.)

(contrast or radionuclide) is generally performed every 12–18 mo. Periodic upper tract imaging should be performed to monitor the status of the upper urinary tracts. Follow-up evaluation should be performed at least annually, at which time the child's height, weight, and blood pressure should be recorded.

Medical management with antibiotic prophylaxis is considered successful if the child remains free of infection and has no new renal scarring and if the reflux resolves spontaneously. Breakthrough UTI, development of new renal scars, and failure of reflux to resolve are examples of failed medical management. Noncompliance, allergic reaction, or side effects to the prescribed medication may preclude medical management or lead to its failure.

Surgical therapy can be performed either through a low abdominal incision or endoscopically. Open surgical management involves modifying the abnormal ureterovesical attachment to create a 4:1 to 5:1 ratio of intramural ureter length:ureteral diameter. Numerous techniques have been described. Some involve opening the bladder (Politano-Leadbetter, Cohen transtrigonal, Glenn-Anderson), whereas others accomplish reflux correction by an extravesical approach (Lich-Gregoir detrusorrhaphy). If there is a simple duplication anomaly, both ureters are reimplanted together, termed a *common sheath reimplant.* When reflux associated with severe ureteral dilatation, termed a **megaureter,** is corrected, the ureter must be tapered or narrowed to a more normal size to allow a normal length:width ratio for the intramural tunnel, and a corner of the bladder is attached to the psoas tendon, termed a **psoas hitch.** If the refluxing kidney is poorly functioning, nephrectomy or nephroureterectomy is indicated. Some clinicians are investigating the role of laparoscopic reflux correction via an extravesical approach.

Open surgical repair is generally performed in children who fail medical management, including those with breakthrough UTI, persistent reflux, and grade IV or V reflux. In general, blood loss is minimal and the hospital stay averages 2 days. The success rate in children with primary reflux is greater than 95–98% for grades I–IV, with 2% experiencing persistent reflux and 1% having ureteral obstruction that requires correction. The success rate is so high that many do not perform a postoperative VCUG unless the child develops clinical pyelonephritis. For grade V reflux, the success rate is approximately 80%. In lower grades of reflux, a failed reimplantation is most likely to occur in children with undiagnosed voiding dysfunction. In children with secondary reflux, the success rate is slightly lower than with primary reflux.

The technique of endoscopic repair of reflux involves injection of a bulking agent via a cystoscope under the ureteral

orifice, creating an artificial flap-valve (Fig. 531–9). This technique has been termed the *subureteral injection.* The advantage of this technique is that it is a noninvasive outpatient procedure (under general anesthesia) with no recovery time. The success rate is 70–80% and is highest for lower grades of reflux. In October 2001 the U.S. Food and Drug Administration (FDA) approved the use of dextran microspheres suspended in hyaluronic acid (Deflux) for subureteral injection. In Europe the majority of children undergoing surgical correction of reflux undergo the STING. Other bulking agents are undergoing FDA-approved clinical trials.

The International Reflux Study showed that in children with grades III–IV reflux, after 5 years of medical or surgical therapy, similar results occurred with regard to new renal scarring and renal function. However, the incidence of clinical pyelonephritis was 2.5 times higher in the children managed medically and, at the end of the study, more than half of the medically managed children still had reflux.

Evidence-based guidelines pertaining to the treatment of reflux diagnosed after a UTI were published in 1997 by the American Urological Association (Table 531–2). These guidelines were written before an endoscopic FDA-approved implant became available. A guide for parents based on the report is available to assist the physician in discussing treatment options with the parents. The decision whether to recommend medical or surgical therapy is based on the risk of reflux to the patient,

TABLE 531–2. Treatment Recommendations for Vesicoureteral Reflux Diagnosed Following a Urinary Tract Infection*

Grade	Age (yr)	Scarring	Initial Treatment	Follow-up
I–II	Any	Yes/no	Antibiotic prophylaxis	No consensus
III–IV	0–5	Yes/no	Antibiotic prophylaxis	Surgery
III–IV	6–10	Yes/no	Unilateral: antibiotic prophylaxis	Surgery
			Bilateral: surgery	
V	<1	Yes/no	Antibiotic prophylaxis	Surgery
V	1–5	No	Unilateral: antibiotic prophylaxis	Surgery
V	1–5	No	Bilateral: surgery	
V	1–5	Yes	Surgery	
V	6–10	Yes/no	Surgery	

Summary of guidelines developed by American Urological Association; age refers to age at diagnosis.

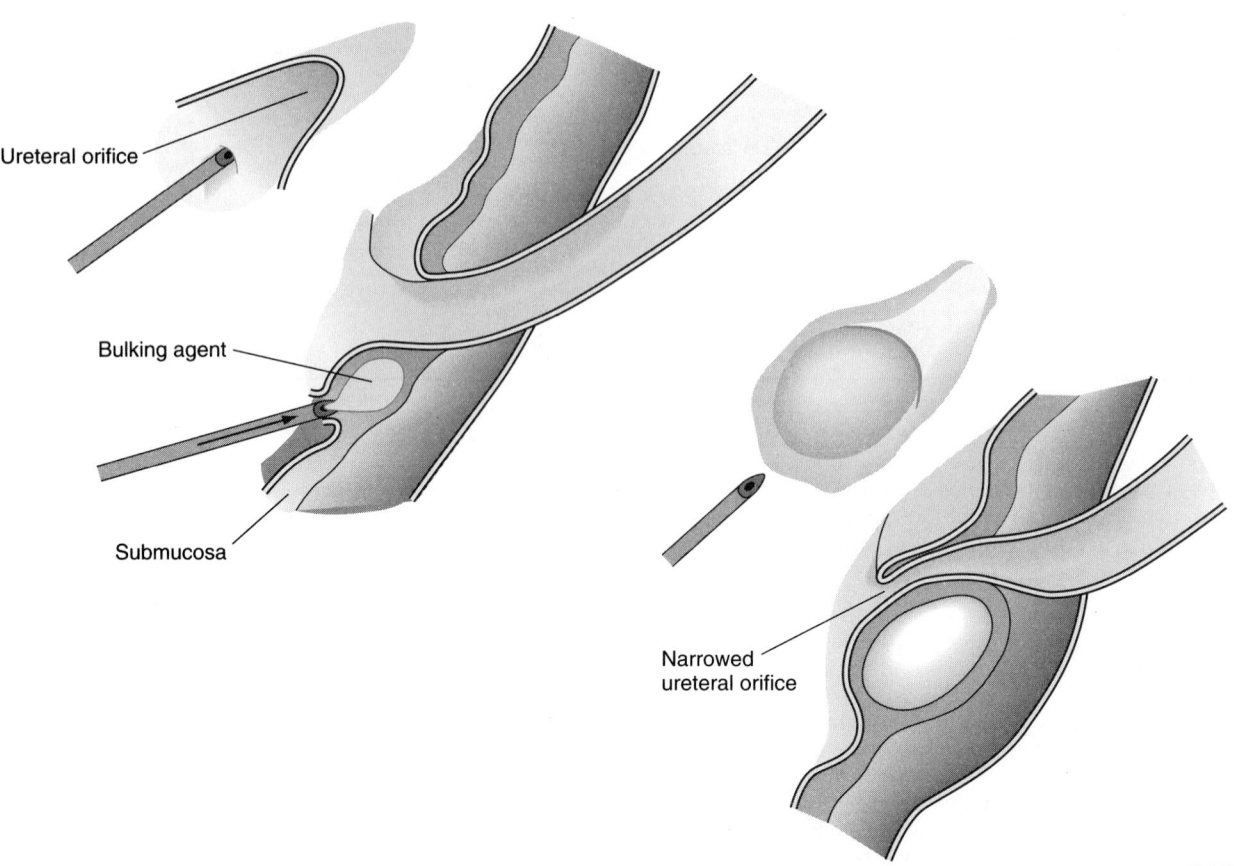

FIGURE 531–9. Endoscopic correction of reflux. Through a cystoscope, a needle is inserted into the submucosal plane deep to the ureteral orifice and bulking agent is injected, creating a flap-valve to prevent reflux. (Adapted from Ortenberg J: Endoscopic treatment of vesicoureteral reflux in children. *Urol Clin North Am* 1998;25:152).

the likelihood of spontaneous resolution, and parental-patient preferences.

Capozza N, Caione P: Dextranomer/hyaluronic acid copolymer implantation for vesicoureteral reflux: A randomized comparison with antibiotic prophylaxis. *J Pediatr* 2002;140:230–34.

Craig JC, Irwig LM, Knight JF, et al: Does treatment of vesicoureteric reflux in childhood prevent end-stage renal disease attributable to reflux nephropathy? *Pediatrics* 2000;105:1236–41.

Elder JS: Guidelines for consideration for surgical repair of vesicoureteral reflux. *Curr Opin Urol* 2000;10:579–85.

Elder JS, Peters CA, Arant BS Jr, et al: Pediatric Vesicoureteral Reflux Guidelines Panel Summary Report on the management of primary vesicoureteral reflux in children. *J Urol* 1997;157:1846–51.

Elder JS, Peters CA, Arant BS Jr, et al: *Report On the Management of Primary Vesicoureteral Reflux in Children.* Baltimore, American Urological Association, 1997.

Farhat W, McLorie G, Geary D, et al: The natural history of neonatal vesicoureteral reflux associated with antenatal hydronephrosis. *J Urol* 2000;164:1057–60.

Herz D, Hafez A, Bagli D, et al: Efficacy of endoscopic subureteral polydimethylsiloxane injection for treatment of vesicoureteral reflux in children: A North American clinical report. *J Urol* 2001;166:1880–86.

Jodal U, Hansson S, Hjalmas K: Medical or surgical management for children with vesicoureteric reflux? *Acta Paediatr Suppl* 1999;431:53–61.

Lackgren G, Wahlin N, Skoldenberg E, et al: Long-term followup of children treated with dextranomer/hyaluronic acid copolymer for vesicoureteral reflux. *J Urol* 2001;166:1887–92.

Lackgren G, Wahlin N, Stenberg A: Endoscopic treatment of children with vesicoureteric reflux. *Acta Paediatr Suppl* 1999;431:62–71.

Lama G, Russo M, De Rosa E, et al: Primary vesicoureteric reflux and renal damage in the first year of life. *Pediatr Nephrol* 2000;15:205–10.

Mathews R, Naslund M, Docimo S: Cost analysis of the treatment of vesicoureteral reflux: A computer model. *J Urol* 2000;163:561–567.

Mentzel H-J, Vogt S, John U, Kaiser WA: Voiding urosonography with ultrasonography contrast medium in children. *Pediatr Nephrol* 2002;17:272–76.

Miller OF, Bloom TL, Smith LJ, et al: Early hospital discharge for intravesical ureteroneocystostomy. *J Urol* 2002;167:2556–59.

Ogan K, Pohl HG, Carlson D, et al: Parental preferences in the management of vesicoureteral reflux. *J Urol* 2001;166:240–43.

Parekh DJ, Pope JC IV, Adams MC, Brock JC III: Outcome of sibling vesicoureteral reflux. *J Urol* 2002;167:283–84.

Smellie JM, Barratt TM, Chantler C, et al: Medical versus surgical treatment in children with severe bilateral vesicoureteric reflux and bilateral nephropathy: A randomised trial. *Lancet* 2001;357:1329–33.

Smellie JM, Sodal U, Lax H, et al: Outcome at 10 years of severe vesicoureteric reflux managed medically: Report of the International Reflux Study in Children. *J Pediatr* 2001;139:656–63.

Sweeney B, Cascio S, Velayudham M, Puri P: Reflux nephropathy in infancy: A comparison of infants presenting with and without urinary tract infection. *J Urol* 2001;166:648–50.

Chapter 532

Obstructions of the Urinary Tract

Obstructive lesions of the urinary tract occur at any level from the urethral meatus to the calyceal infundibula. Obstruction can be congenital (anatomic) or caused by trauma, neoplasia, calculi, inflammatory processes, or surgical procedures (Table 532–1). The pathophysiologic effects of obstruction depend on its level, extent of involvement, age at onset, and acute or chronic nature. In childhood, most obstructive lesions are congenital.

Etiology. Severe ureteral obstruction of early onset in fetal life results in renal dysplasia, ranging from the multicystic kidney, usually associated with ureteral or pelvic atresia (see Fig. 529–2), to various degrees of histologic renal cortical dysplasia

TABLE 532–1. Types and Causes of Urinary Tract Obstruction

Location	Cause
Infundibula	Congenital Calculi Inflammatory (tuberculosis) Traumatic Postsurgical Neoplastic
Renal pelvis	Congenital (infundibulopelvic stenosis) Inflammatory (tuberculosis) Calculi Neoplasia (Wilms tumor, neuroblastoma)
Ureteropelvic junction	Congenital stenosis Calculi Neoplasia Inflammatory Postsurgical Traumatic

Ureter	Congenital obstructive megaureter
	Midureteral structure
	Ureteral ectopia
	Ureterocele
	Retrocaval ureter
	Ureteral fibroepithelial polyps
	Ureteral valves
	Calculi
	Postsurgical
	Extrinsic compression
	  Neoplasia (neuroblastoma, lymphoma, and
	    other retroperitoneal or pelvic tumors)
	  Inflammatory (Crohn disease, chronic
	    granulomatous disease)
	  Hematoma, urinoma
	  Lymphocele
	  Retroperitoneal fibrosis

Bladder outlet and urethra	Neurogenic bladder dysfunction (functional
	  obstruction)
	Posterior urethral valves
	Anterior urethral valves
	Diverticula
	Urethral strictures (congenital, traumatic, or
	  iatrogenic)
	Urethral atresia
	Ectopic ureterocele
	Meatal stenosis (males)
	Calculi
	Foreign bodies
	Phimosis
	Extrinsic compression by tumors
	Urogenital sinus anomalies

seen with less severe obstruction. Chronic ureteral obstruction in late fetal life or after birth results in dilatation of the ureter, renal pelvis, and calyces, with alterations of renal parenchyma ranging from minimal tubular changes to dilatation of Bowman space, glomerular fibrosis, and interstitial fibrosis. After birth, infections often complicate obstruction and may increase renal damage.

Clinical Manifestations. Urinary tract obstruction generally causes hydronephrosis, which typically is asymptomatic in its early phases. An obstructed kidney secondary to a ureteropelvic junction (UPJ) or ureterovesical junction obstruction may cause upper abdominal or flank pain on the affected side; pyelonephritis may occur because of urinary stasis. Occasionally, an upper urinary tract stone occurs, which can cause abdominal and flank pain and hematuria. With bladder outlet obstruction, the urinary stream may be weak; urinary tract infection (UTI) is common. Many of these lesions are identified by antenatal ultrasonography; an abnormality involving the genitourinary tract is suspected in as many as 1 in 100 fetuses.

Obstructive renal insufficiency can manifest itself by failure to thrive, vomiting, diarrhea, or other nonspecific signs and symptoms. In older children, infravesical obstruction can be associated with overflow urinary incontinence or a poor urinary stream. Acute ureteral obstruction causes flank or abdominal

pain; there may be nausea and vomiting. Chronic ureteral obstruction can be silent or can cause vague abdominal or typical flank pain with increased fluid intake.

Diagnosis. Urinary tract obstruction is often silent. In the newborn infant, a palpable abdominal mass is most commonly a hydronephrotic or multicystic dysplastic kidney. With infravesical obstructive lesions in boys, a walnut-sized mass, representing the bladder, is palpable just above the pubic symphysis. A patent urachus should suggest urethral obstruction. Urinary ascites in the newborn usually is caused by renal or bladder urinary extravasation secondary to posterior urethral valves.

Urinary tract obstruction may be diagnosed prenatally by ultrasonography, typically showing hydronephrosis. Further ultrasonography and a more complete evaluation should be undertaken in the neonatal period. Infection and sepsis may be the first indications of an obstructive lesion of the urinary tract. The combination of infection and obstruction poses a serious threat to infants and children and usually requires parenteral administration of antibiotics and drainage of the obstructed kidney. Renal ultrasonography should be performed in all children during the acute stage of febrile urinary tract infections.

IMAGING STUDIES

Renal Ultrasonography. The common characteristic of obstruction is the presence of a dilated urinary tract. Hydronephrosis is frequently an ultrasonographic finding (Fig. 532–1). Dilatation is not always indicative of obstruction and may persist after surgical correction of an obstructive lesion. Dilatation may result from vesicoureteral reflux, or it may be a manifestation of abnormal development of the urinary tract, even when there is no obstruction. Renal length, degree of caliectasis and parenchymal thickness, and presence or absence of ureteral dilatation should be assessed. Ideally, the severity of hydronephrosis should be graded from 1 to 4 using the Society for Fetal Urology grading scale (Table 532–2). One may ascertain that the contralateral kidney is normal, and the bladder should be imaged to see whether the bladder wall is thickened, the lower ureter is dilated, and whether bladder emptying is complete. In acute or intermittent obstruction, the dilatation of the collecting system may be minimal and ultrasonography may be misleading.

Voiding Cystourethrogram (VCUG). In all cases of congenital hydronephrosis and in any child with ureteral dilatation, a VCUG should be obtained, because the dilatation is secondary to vesicoureteral reflux in 15% of cases. In males, the VCUG also is necessary to rule out urethral obstruction, particularly in cases of suspected posterior urethral valves. In infravesical obstruction in infants, the bladder may be palpable because of chronic distention and incomplete emptying. In older children, the urinary flow rate can be measured noninvasively with a

TABLE 532–2. Society for Fetal Urology Grading System for Hydronephrosis

Grade of Hydronephrosis	Renal Image	
	Central Renal Complex	*Renal Parenchymal Thickness*
0	Intact	Normal
1	Slight splitting	Normal
2	Evident splitting, complex confined within renal border	Normal
3	Wide splitting pelvis dilated outside renal border, calyces uniformly dilated	Normal
4	Further dilatation of pelvis and calyces (calyces may appear convex)	Thin

After Maizels M, Mitchell B, Kass E, et al: Outcome of nonspecific hydronephrosis in the infant: A report from the registry of the Society for Fetal Urology. J Urol 152:2324, 1994.

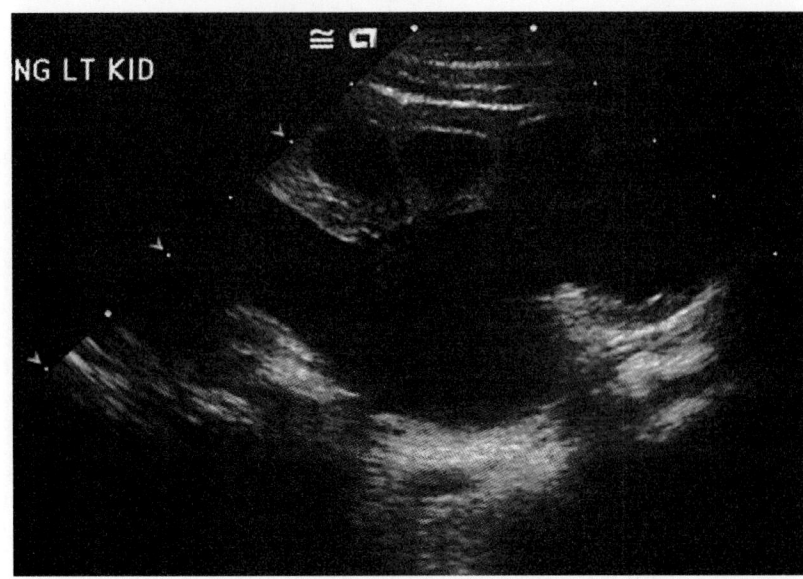

FIGURE 532–1. Ultrasonographic image of the left kidney with marked pelvic and calyceal dilatation (grade IV hydronephrosis) in a boy with ureteropelvic junction obstruction.

urinary flowmeter and decreased flow with a normal bladder contraction is suggestive of infravesical obstruction. When the urethra cannot be catheterized to obtain a VCUG, one must suspect a urethral stricture or an obstructive urethral lesion. Retrograde urethrography with contrast medium injected into the urethral meatus helps delineate the anatomy of the urethral obstruction.

Radioisotope Studies. Renal scintigraphy is used to assess renal anatomy and function. The two most common radiopharmaceuticals are mercaptoacetyl triglycine (MAG-3) and technetium-99m-labeled dimercaptosuccinic acid (DMSA). MAG-3 is excreted by renal tubular secretion; it is used to assess differential renal function and, when furosemide is administered, drainage can also be measured. An alternative to MAG-3 is diethylene tetrapentaacetic acid (DTPA), which is cleared by glomerular filtration. The background activity of DTPA is much higher than MAG-3. DMSA is a renal cortical imaging agent and is used to assess differential renal function and to demonstrate

whether renal scarring is present. It is used infrequently in children with obstructive uropathy.

In a *MAG-3 diuretic renogram*, a small dose of technetium-labeled MAG-3 is injected intravenously (Figs. 532–2 and 532–3). During the first 2 to 3 min, renal parenchymal uptake is analyzed and compared, allowing computation of differential renal function. Subsequently, excretion is evaluated. After 20 to 30 min, furosemide is injected intravenously and the rapidity and pattern of drainage from the kidneys to the bladder are analyzed. If no obstruction is present, half of the radionuclide should be cleared from the renal pelvis within 10 to 15 min, termed the half-life ($t^{1/2}$). If there is significant upper tract obstruction, the $t^{1/2}$ generally is greater than 20 min. A $t^{1/2}$ between 15 and 20 min is indeterminate. The images generated usually provide an accurate assessment of the site of obstruction. Numerous variables affect the outcome of the diuretic renogram. For example, newborn kidneys are functionally immature and, in some cases, normal kidneys may not demonstrate normal drainage after

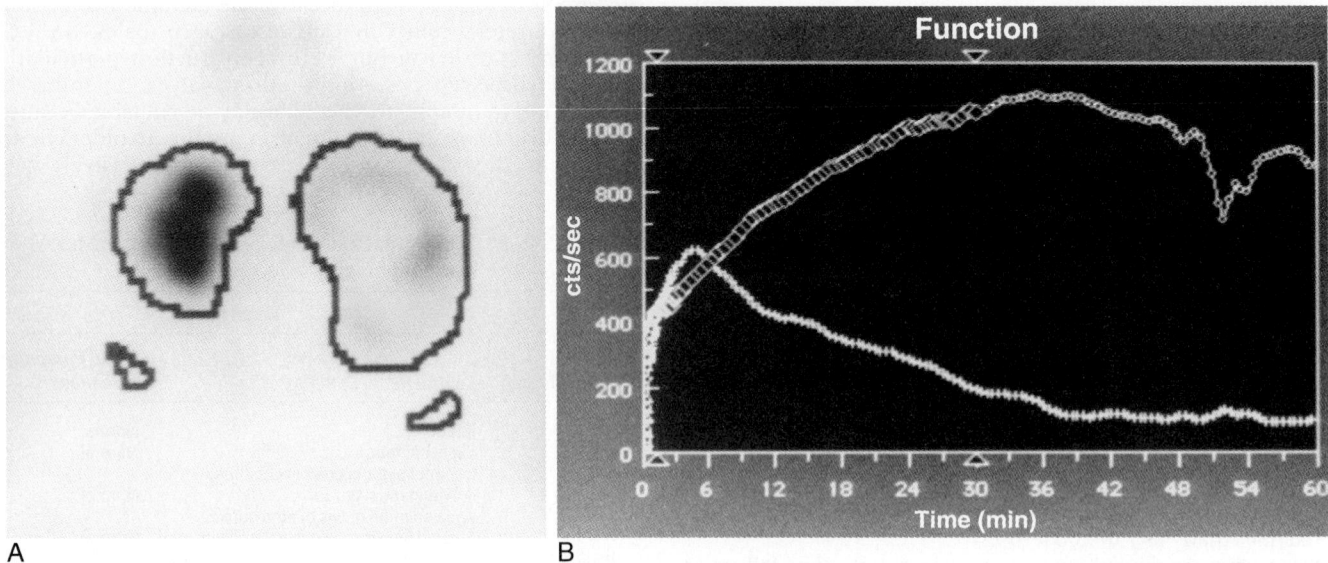

A B

FIGURE 532–2. MAG-3 diuretic renogram in a 6-wk-old infant with right hydronephrosis detected by prenatal ultrasonography. The right kidney is on the right side of the image. *A,* Differential renal function: left kidney 70%, right kidney 30%. *B,* After administration of furosemide, drainage from the left kidney was normal and drainage from the right kidney was slow, consistent with right ureteropelvic junction obstruction. Pyeloplasty was performed on the right kidney.

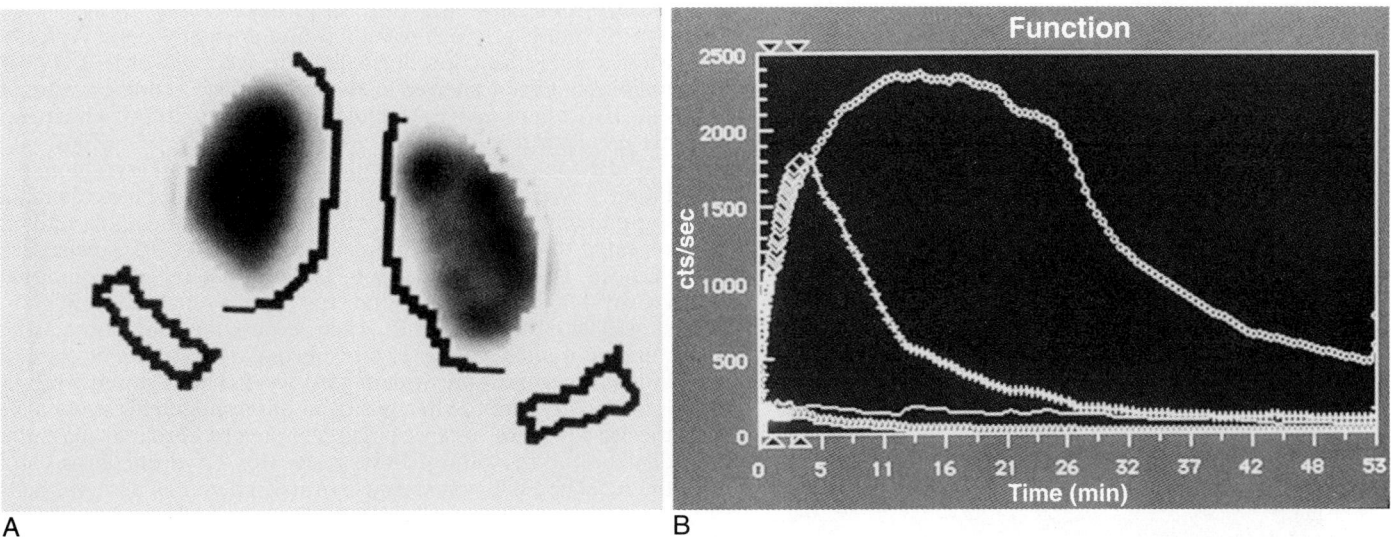

A   B

FIGURE 532–3. Same patient as in Figure 532–2. *A* and *B,* MAG-3 diuretic renogram at 14 mo of age shows equal function in the two kidneys and prompt drainage after the administration of furosemide.

diuretic administration. Dehydration prolongs parenchymal transit and can blunt the diuretic response. Giving an insufficient dose of furosemide may result in inadequate drainage. If vesicoureteral reflux is present, continuous catheter drainage is mandatory to prevent the radionuclide from refluxing from the bladder into the dilated upper tract, which would prolong the washout phase. Because of the numerous variables, the Society for Fetal Urology and the Pediatric Nuclear Medicine Club jointly developed a standardized method for performing diuretic renography in infants and children termed the *well-tempered renogram.*

The MAG-3 diuretic renogram is considered superior to the excretory urogram in infants and children with hydronephrosis because bowel gas and immaturity of renal function often cause the intravenous pyelogram (IVP) images to be suboptimal. In addition, the diuretic renogram provides an objective assessment of the relative function of each kidney.

Excretory Urogram (IVP). The IVP is used infrequently for imaging the urinary tract in children but is useful in selected cases (Fig. 532–4). The plain film of the abdomen should be inspected for calculi, spinal abnormalities, and an abnormal intestinal gas pattern or severe constipation. In infravesical obstruction, the bladder wall is irregular or trabeculated because of detrusor hypertrophy. A postvoid film may show residual bladder urine. In ureteral obstruction, there is dilatation of the collecting system above the obstruction and blunting of the calyces. Concentration of the radiopaque medium on the obstructed side is impaired, and there may be a delayed appearance of contrast medium in the collecting system with progressive increase in concentration at the point of obstruction when delayed radiographs are obtained. In high-grade obstruction, the contrast agent may remain in the collecting system after 24 hr.

Urinary extravasation can be detected in the early or delayed films of a urographic study as well as on an MAG-3 renogram. When intermittent obstruction is suspected, intravenous urography during an acute episode of pain is often the most valuable diagnostic study.

Computed Tomography. In children with a suspected ureteral calculus, noncontrast spiral computed tomography of the abdomen and pelvis provides an excellent method of demonstrating whether a calculus (or calculi) is present, its location, and whether there is significant proximal hydronephrosis. This study is the initial study of choice in these patients.

Ancillary Studies. In unusual cases, another way to assess the anatomy of the upper urinary tract is by inserting a percutaneous nephrostomy tube and injecting contrast agent, termed an ***antegrade pyelogram.*** This procedure usually requires general anesthesia. In addition, an antegrade pressure-perfusion flow study, a ***Whitaker test,*** may be performed, in

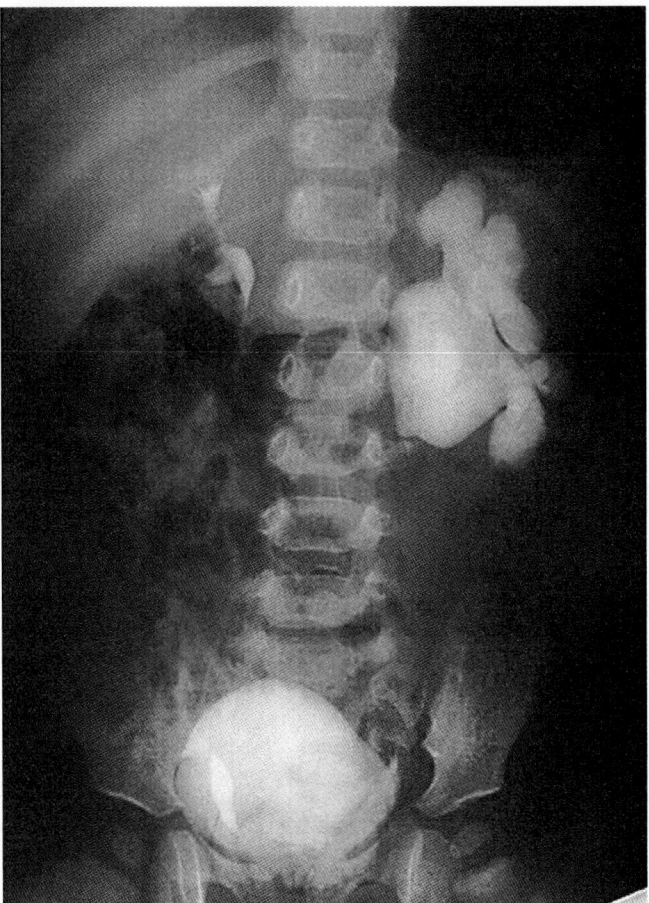

FIGURE 532–4. Ureteropelvic junction obstruction. Excretory urogram in a boy, showing dilatation of the left renal pelvis and blunting of the calyces characteristic of a ureteropelvic junction obstruction.

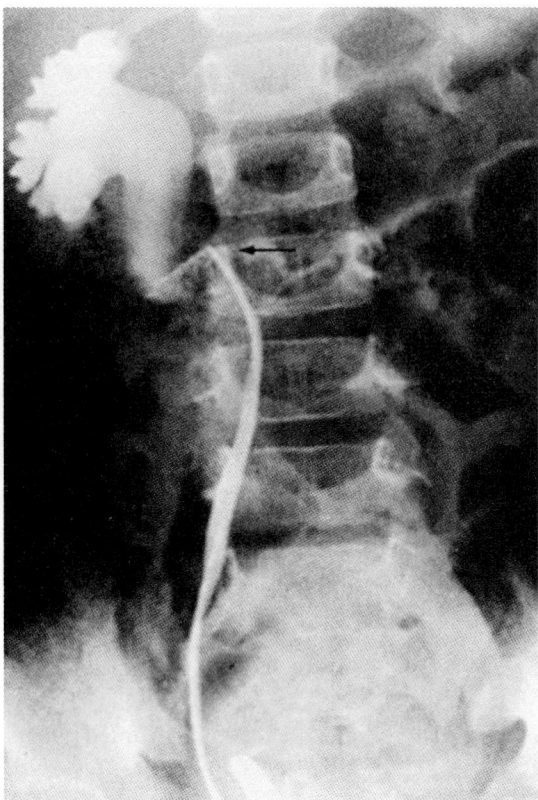

FIGURE 532–5. Retrocaval ureter. Retrograde pyelogram showing medial deviation of a dilated upper ureter to the level of the 3rd lumbar vertebra, characteristic of a retrocaval ureter.

which fluid is infused at a measured rate, usually 10 mL/min. The pressures in the renal pelvis and the bladder are monitored during this infusion, and pressure differences exceeding 20 cm H_2O are suggestive of obstruction. In other cases, cystoscopy with retrograde pyelography provides excellent images of the upper urinary tract (Fig. 532–5).

SPECIFIC TYPES OF URINARY TRACT OBSTRUCTION AND THEIR TREATMENT

Hydrocalycosis. This term refers to a localized dilatation of the calyx caused by obstruction of its infundibulum, termed *infundibular stenosis.* Such obstruction can be developmental in origin or secondary to inflammatory processes, such as UTI. When the abnormality is not discovered by antenatal ultrasonography or incidentally, it is usually discovered during evaluation for pain or UTI. The diagnosis of infundibular stenosis is usually established by IVP.

UPJ Obstruction. This is the most common obstructive lesion in childhood and is usually caused by intrinsic stenosis (see Figs. 532–1 through 532–4). At times an accessory artery to the lower pole of the kidney also causes extrinsic obstruction. The typical appearance on ultrasonography is grade 3 or 4 hydronephrosis without a dilated ureter. UPJ obstruction most commonly presents (1) on maternal ultrasonography revealing fetal hydronephrosis; (2) as a palpable renal mass in a newborn or infant; (3) as abdominal, flank, or back pain; (4) as a febrile UTI; or (5) as hematuria after minimal trauma. Approximately 60% of cases occur on the left side, and the male:female ratio is 2:1. Ten percent of UPJ obstructions are bilateral. In kidneys with UPJ obstruction, renal function may be significantly impaired from pressure atrophy. The anomaly is corrected by performing a pyeloplasty, in which the stenotic segment is excised and the normal ureter and renal pelvis are reattached. Success rates are 91–98%.

Lesser degrees of UPJ obstruction may cause mild hydronephrosis, which usually is nonobstructive, and typically these kidneys function normally. The spectrum of UPJ abnormalities has been referred to as *anomalous UPJ.* Another cause of mild hydronephrosis is fetal folds of the upper ureter, which also are nonobstructive.

The diagnosis can be difficult to establish in an asymptomatic infant in whom dilatation of the renal pelvis is found incidentally in a prenatal ultrasonogram. After birth, the sonographic study is repeated to confirm the prenatal finding. A VCUG is necessary because 10–15% of patients have ipsilateral vesicoureteral reflux. If no dilatation is found after birth, a renal ultrasonogram should be repeated at 1 mo of age because the dilatation may be minimal immediately after birth secondary to transient oliguria but may become more evident a few weeks later. Consequently, it is best to perform the first postnatal ultrasonographic study after the 3rd day of life because oliguria in the newborn may mask the dilatation. If the kidney shows grade 1 or 2 hydronephrosis and the renal parenchyma appears normal, a period of observation is usually appropriate with sequential renal ultrasonograms to monitor the severity of hydronephrosis, and disappearance of the hydronephrosis usually occurs. The child should receive antibiotic prophylaxis, usually trimethoprim-sulfamethoxazole, although amoxicillin or cephalexin is preferable before 2 mo of age. If the hydronephrosis is grade 3 or 4, spontaneous resolution is less likely and obstruction is more likely to be present. A diuretic renogram with MAG-3 is performed at 4–6 wk of age. If there is poor upper tract drainage or the differential renal function is poor, pyeloplasty is recommended. After pyeloplasty the differential renal function often improves and improved drainage with furosemide stimulation is expected.

If the differential function on renography is normal and drainage is satisfactory, the infant can be followed with serial ultrasonograms. If the hydronephrosis remains severe with no improvement, a repeat diuretic renogram after 6–12 mo may help in the decision between continued observation and surgical repair. Prompt surgical repair is indicated in infants with an abdominal mass, bilateral severe hydronephrosis, a solitary kidney, or diminished function in the involved kidney. In unusual cases the differential renal function is less than 10% but the kidney definitely has some function. In this situation, insertion of a percutaneous nephrostomy tube allows drainage of the hydronephrotic kidney for a few weeks to allow reassessment of renal function. In older children who present with symptoms, the diagnosis of UPJ obstruction usually is established by ultrasonography and diuretic renography.

In the *differential diagnosis,* the following entities should be considered: (1) megacalycosis, a congenital nonobstructive dilatation of the calyces without pelvic or ureteric dilatation; (2) vesicoureteral reflux with marked dilatation and kinking of the ureter; and (3) midureteral or distal ureteral obstruction when the ureter is not well visualized on the urogram.

Midureteral Obstruction. Congenital ureteral stenosis or a ureteral valve in the midureter is rare and is corrected by excision of the strictured segment and reanastomosing the normal upper and lower ureteral segments. A *retrocaval ureter* is an anomaly in which the upper right ureter travels posterior to the inferior vena cava. In this anomaly, the vena cava may cause extrinsic compression and obstruction. An IVP shows the right ureter to be medially deviated at the level of the 3rd lumbar vertebra. The diagnosis may be confirmed by retrograde pyelography (see Fig. 532–5). Surgical treatment consists of transection of the upper ureter, moving it anterior to the vena cava, and reanastomosing the upper and lower segments. Repair is necessary only when obstruction is present. Retroperitoneal tumors, fibrosis caused by surgical procedures, inflammatory processes (as in chronic granulomatous disease), and radiation therapy can cause acquired midureteral obstruction.

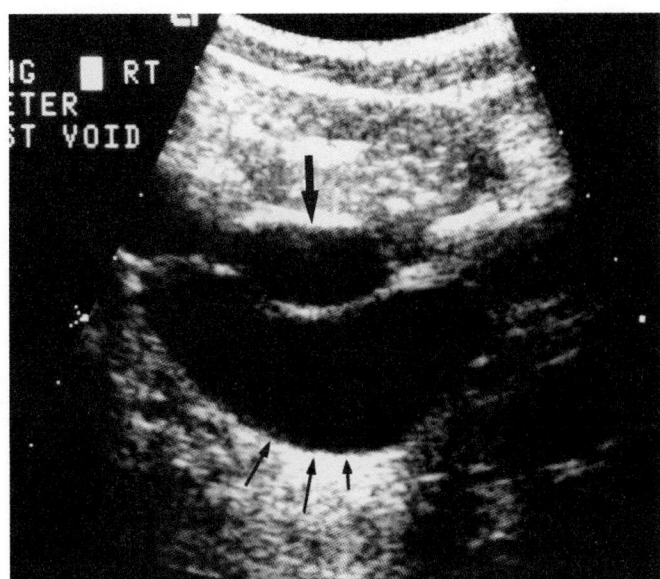

FIGURE 532–6. Ultrasonographic image of the right dilated ureter *(thin arrows)* extending behind and caudal to a nearly empty bladder *(arrow)* in a girl with urinary incontinence and ectopic ureter draining into the vagina.

Ectopic Ureter. An ectopic ureter refers to a ureter that drains outside the bladder. They are three times as common in girls as in boys. The ectopic ureter usually drains the upper pole of a duplex collecting system (i.e., two ureters). In girls, approximately 35% enter the urethra at the bladder neck, 35% enter the urethrovaginal septum, 25% enter the vagina, and a few drain into the cervix, uterus, Gartner duct, or a urethral diverticulum. With the exception of the ectopic ureter entering the bladder neck, all cause continuous urinary incontinence from the affected renal moiety. In addition, UTI is common because of urinary stasis. In boys, ectopic ureters enter the posterior urethra (above the external sphincter) in 47%, the prostatic utricle in 10%, the seminal vesicle in 33%, the ejaculatory duct in 5%, and the vas deferens in 5%. Consequently, in boys, an ectopic ureter does not cause incontinence, and most patients present with a UTI or epididymitis. Evaluation includes a renal sonogram, VCUG, and renal scan, which demonstrates whether the affected segment has significant function. The sonogram shows the affected hydronephrotic kidney or dilated upper pole and ureter down to the bladder (Fig. 532–6). If the ectopic ureter drains into the bladder neck (female), a VCUG usually shows reflux into the ureter. Otherwise, there is no reflux into the ectopic ureter, but there may be reflux into the ipsilateral lower pole ureter or contralateral collecting system.

Treatment depends on the status of the renal unit drained by the ectopic ureter. If there is satisfactory function, ureteral reimplantation into the bladder or ureteroureterostomy (anastomosing the ectopic upper pole ureter into the normally inserting lower pole ureter) is indicated. If function is poor, partial or total nephrectomy is indicated. Often this can be done laparoscopically.

Ureterocele. A ureterocele is a cystic dilatation of the terminal ureter and is obstructive because of a pinpoint ureteral orifice. Ureteroceles are much more common in females than in males. Affected children often are discovered by prenatal ultrasonography or present with a UTI. Ureteroceles may be ectopic, in which the cystic swelling extends through the bladder neck into the urethra, or orthotopic, in which the ureterocele is entirely within the bladder.

In girls, ureteroceles are nearly always associated with ureteral duplication (Fig. 532–7), whereas in boys there often is only one ureter. The ureter involved with the ureterocele drains the upper renal moiety, which frequently functions poorly or is dysplastic because of congenital obstruction. The lower pole ureter drains into the bladder superior and lateral to the upper pole ureter and frequently refluxes.

Ectopic ureteroceles extend submucosally into the urethra. Rarely, large ectopic ureteroceles may cause bladder outlet obstruction and retention of urine with bilateral hydronephrosis;

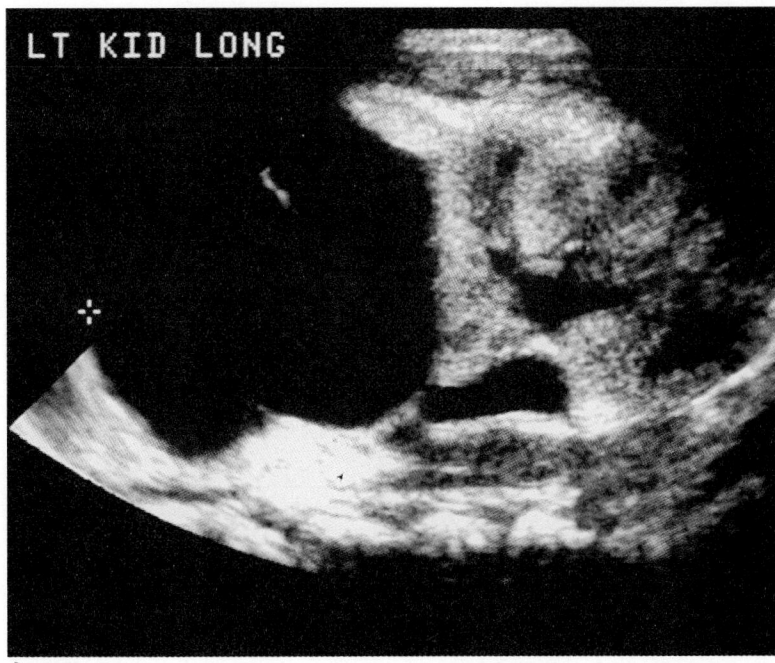

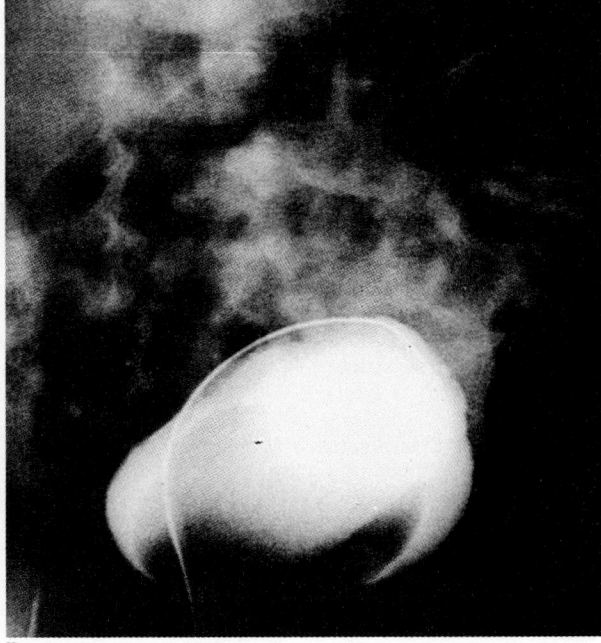

A   B

FIGURE 532–7. *A,* Infant with ectopic ureterocele. Sonogram of left kidney shows massive dilatation of the upper pole and a normal lower pole. *B,* VCUG shows large ureterocele, draining the left upper pole, in the bladder. No reflux is present.

in females, the ureterocele may prolapse from the urethral meatus (see Chapter 536). Both simple and ectopic ureteroceles can be bilateral. Ultrasonography is effective in demonstrating the ureterocele and whether the associated obstructed system is duplicated or single. VCUG usually shows a filling defect, sometimes large, in the bladder corresponding to the ureterocele, and often shows reflux into the adjacent lower pole collecting system with typical findings of a "drooping lily" appearance to the kidney. Renal scintigraphy is most accurate in demonstrating whether the affected renal moiety has significant function.

Treatment of ectopic ureteroceles is variable among different medical centers and depends on whether the upper pole functions on renal scan and whether there is reflux into the lower poleureter. If there is no function of the upper pole and there is no reflux, treatment usually involves laparoscopic or open excision of the obstructed upper pole and most of the associated ureter. If there is function in the upper pole, there is significant reflux; or if the patient is septic from infection of the hydronephrotic kidney, then transurethral incision with cautery or the holmium laser is appropriate initial therapy to decompress the ureterocele. However, reflux into the incised ureterocele is common and subsequent excision of the ureterocele and ureteral reimplantation usually is necessary.

Orthotopic ureteroceles are associated with duplicated or nonduplicated collecting systems, and the orifice is in the expected location in the bladder (Fig. 532–8). They are usually discovered during an investigation for prenatal hydronephrosis or a UTI. Ultrasonography is sensitive for detecting the ureterocele in the bladder and hydroureteronephrosis. IVP reveals varying degrees of ureteral and calyceal dilatation, and there is a round filling defect in the bladder. In delayed films, the cystic dilatation of the ureter may be clearly visible and full of contrast material. Transurethral incision of the ureterocele effectively relieves the obstruction, but it may result in vesicoureteral reflux, necessitating ureteral reimplantation later. Some prefer open excision of the ureterocele and reimplantation as the initial form of treatment. Small, simple ureteroceles incidentally discovered without upper tract dilatation may not require treatment.

Megaureter. A classification of megaureters (dilated ureter) is given in Table 532–3. There are numerous disorders that can cause ureteral dilatation, and many are nonobstructive.

Megaureters are usually discovered through screening ultrasonography of the kidneys and bladder because of a prenatal diagnosis of hydronephrosis or postnatal UTI, hematuria, or abdominal pain. A careful history, physical examination, and VCUG identify causes of secondary megaureters and refluxing megaureters as well as the prune-belly syndrome. Primary obstructed megaureters and nonobstructed megaureters probably represent varying severities of the same anomaly.

The primary obstructed nonrefluxing megaureter results from abnormal development of the distal ureter, with collagenous tissue replacing the muscle layer. There is disruption of normal ureteral peristalsis, and the proximal ureter widens. Usually there is not a true stricture. On IVP, the distal ureter is more

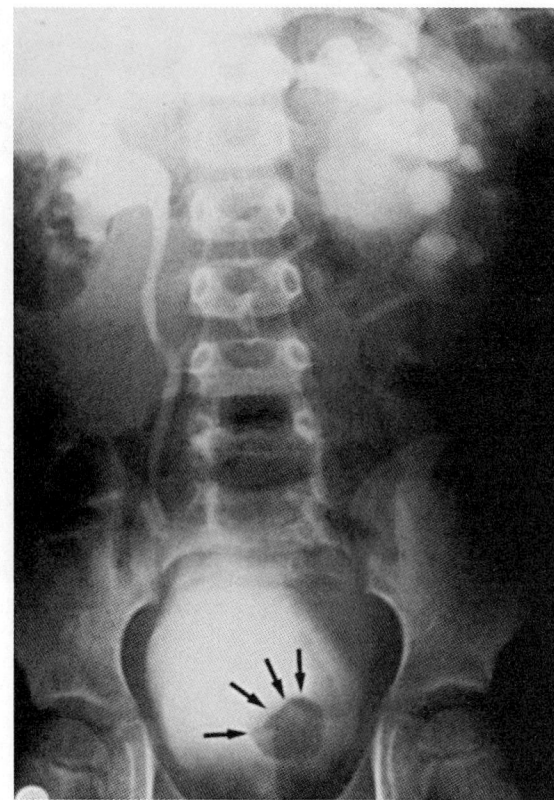

FIGURE 532–8. Simple intravesical ureterocele. Excretory urogram shows left hydronephrosis and a round filling defect on the left side of the bladder corresponding to a simple ureterocele causing left ureteral obstruction. This lesion was treated by transurethral incision and drainage of the ureterocele.

dilated in its distal segment and tapers abruptly at or above the junction of the bladder (Fig. 532–9). The lesion may be unilateral or bilateral. Dilatation of the upper collecting system and calyceal blunting are suggestive of obstruction. Megaureter predisposes to UTI, urinary stones, and flank pain because of urinary stasis. In most cases, diuretic renography and sequential sonographic studies can reliably differentiate obstructed from nonobstructed megaureters. Generally, hydronephrosis lessens and most megaureters diminish in size over time (Fig. 532–10). Truly obstructed megaureters require surgical treatment, with excision of the narrowed segment, ureteral tapering, and reimplantation of the ureter. The results of surgical reconstruction are usually good, but the prognosis depends on pre-existing renal function and whether complications develop.

If differential renal function is normal (>45%) and the child is asymptomatic, it seems safe to follow the patient with serial ultrasonography and diuretic renography to monitor renal function and drainage. These children should receive prophylactic antimicrobial therapy while there is urinary stasis in the

TABLE 532–3. Classification of Megaureter

Refluxing		Obstructed		Nonrefluxing and Nonobstructed	
Primary	*Secondary*	*Primary*	*Secondary*	*Primary*	*Secondary*
Primary reflux	Neuropathic bladder	Intrinsic (primary obstructed megaureter)	Neuropathic bladder	Nonrefluxing, nonobstructive	Diabetes insipidus
Megacystic-megaureter syndrome	Hinman syndrome		Hinman syndrome		Infection
Ectopic ureter	Posterior urethral valves	Ureteral valve	Posterior urethral valves		Persistent after relief of obstruction
Prune-belly syndrome	Bladder diverticulum	Ectopic ureter	Ureteral calculus		
	Postoperative	Ectopic uretocele	Extrinsic		
			Postoperative		

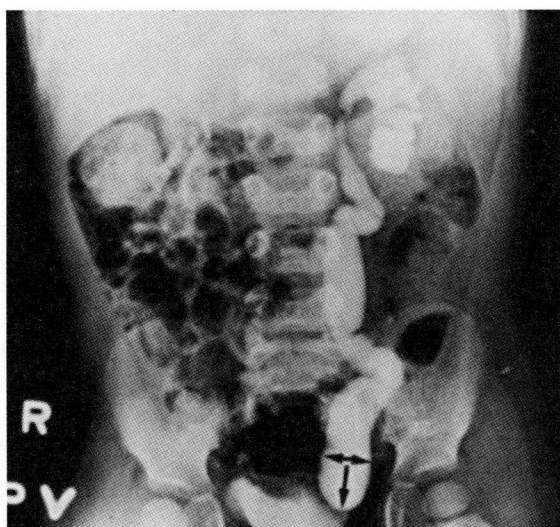

FIGURE 532–9. Obstructed nonrefluxing megaureter. Excretory urogram in a girl with a history of a febrile urinary tract infection. The right side is normal. The left side reveals hydroureteronephrosis with predominant dilatation of the distal ureter. Note the characteristic appearance of the distal ureter. There was no vesicoureteral reflux. The diagnosis of obstruction was confirmed by diuretic renography.

upper ureter and kidney. If renal function deteriorates, upper urinary tract drainage slows, or UTI occurs, ureteral reimplantation is recommended. Overall, 20–30% of children with a nonrefluxing megaureter undergo ureteral reimplantation.

Prune-Belly Syndrome. This syndrome, also called *triad syndrome* or *Eagle-Barrett syndrome*, occurs in approximately 1 in 40,000 births; 95% of affected individuals are male. The characteristic association of deficient abdominal muscles, undescended testes, and urinary tract abnormalities probably results from severe urethral obstruction in fetal life (Fig. 532–11). Oligohydramnios and pulmonary hypoplasia are frequent complications in the perinatal period. Many affected infants are stillborn. Urinary tract abnormalities include massive dilatation of the ureters and upper tracts and a very large bladder, with a patent urachus or a urachal diverticulum. Most patients have vesicoureteral reflux. The prostatic urethra is usually dilated, and the prostate is hypoplastic. The anterior urethra may be dilated, resulting in a megalourethra. Rarely, there is urethral stenosis or atresia. The kidneys usually show various degrees of dysplasia, and the testes are usually intra-abdominal. There is often malrotation of the bowel. Cardiac abnormalities occur in 10% of cases; more than 50% have abnormalities of the musculoskeletal system, including limb abnormalities and scoliosis. In females, anomalies of the urethra, uterus, and vagina are usually present.

Many neonates with prune-belly syndrome have difficulty with effective bladder emptying because the bladder musculature is poorly developed and the urethra may be narrowed. When no obstruction is present, the goal of treatment is the prevention of urinary tract infection with antibiotic prophylaxis. When obstruction of the ureters or urethra is demonstrated, temporary drainage procedures, such as a vesicostomy, may help to preserve renal function until the child is old enough for surgery. Some children with prune-belly syndrome have been found to have classic or atypical posterior urethral valves. Urinary tract infections are frequent and should be treated promptly. Correction of the undescended testes by orchidopexy can be difficult in these children because the testes are located high in the abdomen and is best accomplished in the first 6 mo of life. Reconstruction of the abdominal wall offers cosmetic and functional benefits.

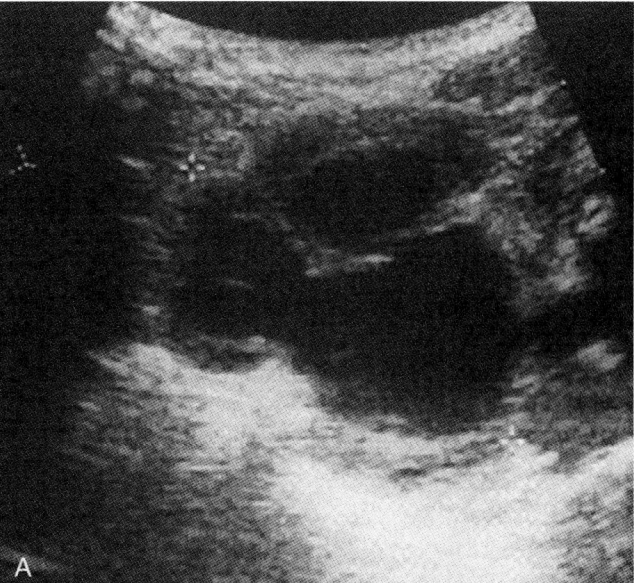

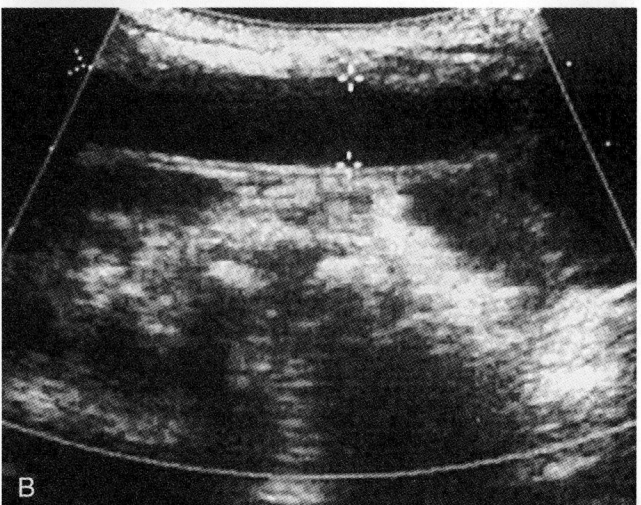

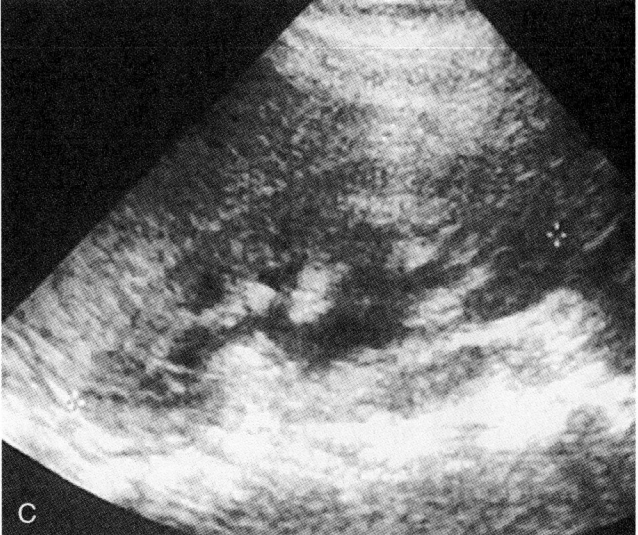

FIGURE 532–10. Neonate with primary nonrefluxing megaureter. *A,* Renal sonogram shows grade IV hydronephrosis. *B,* Dilated ureter. Renal scan showed equal function with the contralateral kidney and satisfactory drainage with diuresis stimulation. *C,* Follow-up sonogram at 10 months shows complete resolution of hydronephrosis.

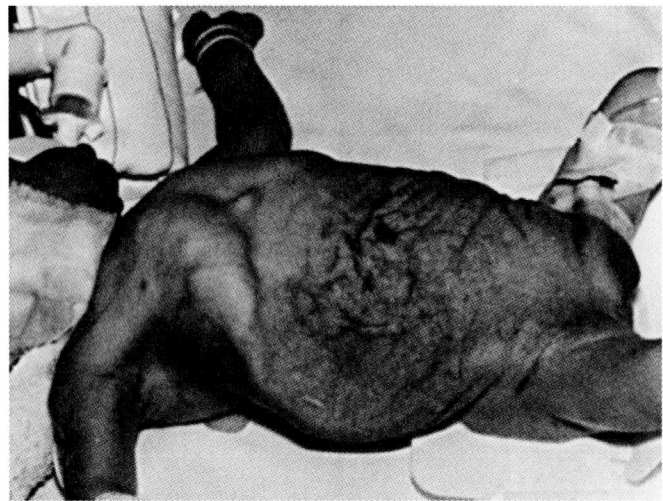

FIGURE 532–11. Prune-belly syndrome. Photograph of a 1,600-g newborn with the prune-belly syndrome. Note the lack of tonicity of the abdominal wall and the wrinkled appearance of the skin.

The prognosis ultimately depends on the degree of pulmonary hypoplasia and renal dysplasia. One third of children with prune-belly syndrome are stillborn or die in the first few months of life because of pulmonary complications. Of the long-term survivors, as many as 30% develop end-stage renal disease from dysplasia or complications of infection or reflux and eventually require renal transplantation. The results of renal transplantation in these patients are favorable.

Bladder Neck Obstruction. Bladder neck obstruction is usually secondary to ectopic ureterocele, bladder calculi, or a tumor of the prostate (rhabdomyosarcoma). The manifestations include difficulty voiding, urinary retention, urinary tract infection, and bladder distention with overflow incontinence. Apparent bladder neck obstruction is common in cases of posterior urethral valves, but it seldom has any functional significance. Primary bladder neck obstruction is extremely rare.

Posterior Urethral Valves. The most common cause of severe obstructive uropathy in children is posterior urethral valves, affecting 1 in 8,000 boys. Urethral valves refers to tissue leaflets fanning distally from the prostatic urethra to the external urinary sphincter. Typically, the leaflets are separated by a slitlike opening. Valves are of unclear embryologic origin and cause varying degrees of obstruction. Approximately 30% of patients experience end-stage renal disease or chronic renal insufficiency. The prostatic urethra dilates, and the bladder muscle undergoes hypertrophy. Vesicoureteral reflux occurs in 50% of patients, and distal ureteral obstruction may result from a chronically distended bladder or bladder muscle hypertrophy. The renal changes range from mild hydronephrosis to severe renal dysplasia; their severity probably depends on the severity of the obstruction and the time of its onset in fetal life. As in other cases of obstruction or renal dysplasia, there may be oligohydramnios and pulmonary hypoplasia.

Affected boys with posterior urethral valves are discovered prenatally when maternal ultrasonography reveals bilateral hydronephrosis, a distended bladder, and, if the obstruction is severe, oligohydramnios. Prenatal bladder decompression by percutaneous vesicoamniotic shunt or open fetal surgery has been reported. Experimental and clinical evidence of the possible benefits of fetal intervention is lacking, and few affected fetuses are candidates. Prenatally diagnosed posterior urethral valves, particularly when discovered in the second trimester, carry a poorer prognosis than those detected after birth. In the male neonate, posterior urethral valves are suspected when

there is a palpably distended bladder and the urinary stream is weak. If the obstruction is severe and goes unrecognized during the neonatal period, infants may present later in life with failure to thrive due to uremia or sepsis caused by infection in the obstructed urinary tract. With lesser degrees of obstruction, children present later in life with difficulty in achieving diurnal urinary continence or with UTI. The diagnosis is established with a VCUG (Fig. 532–12) or by perineal ultrasonography.

After the diagnosis is established, renal function and the anatomy of the upper urinary tract should be carefully evaluated. In the healthy neonate, a small polyethylene feeding tube (No. 5 or 8 French) is inserted in the bladder and left for several days. Passing the feeding tube may be difficult, because the tip of the tube may coil in the prostatic urethra. A sign of this problem is that urine drains around the catheter rather than through it. A Foley (balloon) catheter should not be used, because the balloon may cause severe bladder spasm, which may produce severe ureteral obstruction.

If the serum creatinine level remains normal or returns to normal, treatment consists of transurethral ablation of the valve leaflets, which is performed endoscopically under general anesthesia. If the urethra is too small for transurethral ablation, temporary vesicostomy is preferred, in which the dome of the bladder is exteriorized on the lower abdominal wall. When the child is older, the valves may be ablated and the vesicostomy closed.

If the serum creatinine level remains high or increases despite bladder drainage by a small catheter, secondary ureteral obstruction, irreversible renal damage, or renal dysplasia should be suspected. In such cases, a vesicostomy should be performed. Cutaneous pyelostomy rarely affords better drainage when compared with cutaneous vesicostomy, and the latter also allows continued bladder growth and gradual improvement in bladder wall compliance.

Infants presenting later in life with uremia without infection should be evaluated and treated after identical guidelines. In the septic and uremic infant, lifesaving measures must include prompt correction of the electrolyte imbalance and control of the infection by appropriate antibiotics. Drainage of the upper tracts by percutaneous nephrostomy and hemodialysis may be necessary. After the patient's condition becomes stable,

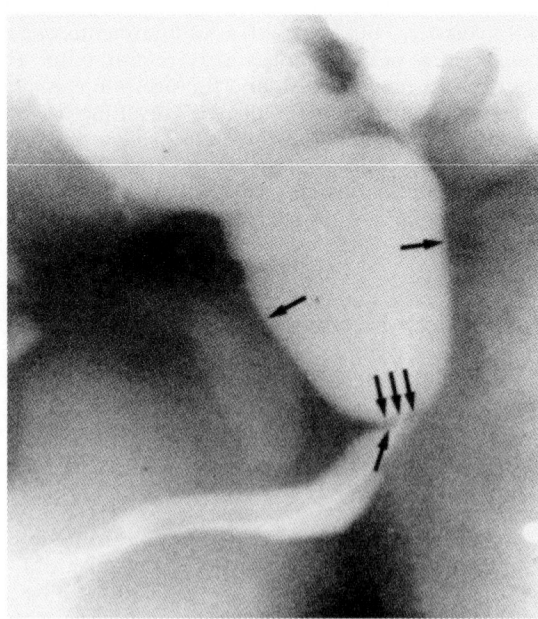

FIGURE 532–12. Posterior urethral valves. Voiding cystourethrogram in an infant with posterior urethral valves. Note the dilatation of the prostatic urethra and the transverse linear filling defect corresponding to the valves.

step-by-step evaluation and treatment can be undertaken. Most boys presenting with incontinence can be treated by primary valve ablation.

Favorable prognostic factors include having a normal prenatal ultrasonogram between 18 and 24 wk of gestation, a serum creatinine level less than 0.8 to 1.0 mg/dL after bladder decompression, and visualization of the corticomedullary junction on renal sonography. There are several situations in which a "popoff valve" may occur during urinary tract development, which preserves the integrity of one or both kidneys. For example, 15% of boys with posterior urethral valves have unilateral reflux into a nonfunctioning dysplastic kidney, termed the *VURD syndrome* (valves, unilateral reflux, dysplasia). In these boys, the high bladder pressure is dissipated into the nonfunctioning kidney, allowing normal development of the contralateral kidney. In newborn boys with urinary ascites, the urine generally leaks out from the obstructed collecting system through the renal fornices, allowing normal renal development. Unfavorable prognostic factors include the presence of oligohydramnios in utero, identification of hydronephrosis before 24 wk of gestation, a serum creatinine level greater than 1.0 mg/dL after bladder decompression, identifying cortical cysts in both kidneys, and persistence of diurnal incontinence beyond 5 yr of age.

The prognosis in the newborn is related to the degree of pulmonary hypoplasia and potential for recovery of renal function. Severely affected infants are often stillborn. Of those who survive the neonatal period, approximately 30% retain some degree of renal insufficiency and many eventually require renal transplantation. In some series, renal transplantation in children with posterior urethral valves has a lower success rate than does transplantation in children with normal bladders, presumably because of the adverse influence of altered bladder function on graft function and survival.

After valve ablation, antimicrobial prophylaxis is beneficial in preventing UTI, because hydronephrosis often persists to some degree for many years. These boys should be evaluated annually with a renal ultrasonogram, physical examination, including assessment of somatic growth and blood pressure, urinalysis, and determination of serum levels of electrolytes. Many boys have significant polyuria resulting from a concentrating defect secondary to prolonged obstructive uropathy. If these children acquire a systemic illness with vomiting or diarrhea, or both, urine output cannot be used to assess the child's hydration status. They can become dehydrated quickly, and there should be a low threshold for hospital admission for intravenous rehydration. Some of these patients have renal tubular acidosis, requiring oral bicarbonate therapy. If there is any significant degree of renal dysfunction, growth impairment, or hypertension, they should be followed closely by a pediatric nephrologist. When vesicoureteral reflux is present, expectant treatment and prophylactic doses of antibacterial drugs are advisable. If breakthrough UTI occurs, surgical correction should be undertaken.

After treatment, boys with urethral valves often do not achieve diurnal urinary continence as early as other boys. Incontinence may result from a combination of factors, including uninhibited bladder contractions, poor bladder compliance, bladder atonia, bladder neck dyssynergia, or polyuria. Often these boys need to undergo urodynamic evaluation with urodynamics or videourodynamics to plan therapy. Boys with noncompliance are at significant risk for ongoing renal damage, even in the absence of infection. Using an indwelling catheter overnight has been shown to be beneficial in boys with polyuria. Urinary incontinence usually improves with age, particularly after puberty. Meticulous attention to bladder compliance, emptying, and infection may improve results in the future.

Urethral Atresia. The most severe form of obstructive uropathy in boys is urethral atresia. In utero there is a distended bladder, bilateral hydroureteronephrosis, and oligohydramnios. In most cases, these infants are stillborn or succumb to pulmonary hypoplasia. Some boys with prune-belly syndrome also have urethral atresia. If the urachus is patent, oligohydramnios is unlikely and the infant usually survives. Urethral reconstruction is difficult, and most patients are managed with continent urinary diversion.

Urethral Hypoplasia. Urethral hypoplasia is a less severe form of obstructive uropathy than is urethral atresia in boys. In urethral hypoplasia, the urethral lumen is extremely small. This condition is rare. These neonates typically have bilateral hydronephrosis and a distended bladder. Passage of a small pediatric feeding tube through the urethra is difficult or impossible. Usually a cutaneous vesicostomy must be performed to relieve upper urinary tract obstruction, and the severity of renal insufficiency is variable. The most severely affected boys have end-stage renal disease. Treatment includes urethral reconstruction, gradual urethral dilatation, or continent urinary diversion.

Urethral Strictures. Urethral strictures *in males* usually result from urethral trauma, either iatrogenic (catheterization, endoscopic procedures, or previous urethral reconstruction) or accidental (straddle injuries or pelvic fractures). Because these lesions may develop gradually, the decrease in force of the urinary stream is seldom noticed by the child or the parents. More commonly, the obstruction causes symptoms of bladder instability, hematuria, or dysuria. Catheterization of the bladder is usually impossible. The diagnosis is made by a voiding film obtained during intravenous urography or retrograde urethrography. Ultrasonography has also been used to diagnose urethral strictures. Endoscopy is confirmatory. Endoscopic treatment of short strictures by dilatation or internal urethrotomy is usually successful. Longer strictures surrounded by periurethral fibrosis often require urethroplasty. Repeated endoscopic procedures should generally be avoided, because they may cause additional urethral damage. Noninvasive measurement of the urinary flow rate and pattern is useful for diagnosis and follow-up.

In females, true urethral strictures are exceptional because the female urethra is protected from trauma, particularly in childhood. In the past it was thought that a distal urethral ring commonly caused obstruction of the female urethra and urinary tract infection and that affected girls benefited from urethral dilatation. The diagnosis was suspected when a "spinning top" deformity of the urethra was found in the VCUG (see Fig. 535–4) and was confirmed by urethral calibration. There is no correlation between the radiologic appearance of the urethra in the VCUG and the urethral caliber and no significant difference in urethral caliber between females with recurrent cystitis and normal age-matched controls. The finding usually is secondary to detrusor-sphincter dyssynergia. Consequently, urethral dilatation in girls is rarely indicated.

Anterior Urethral Valves and Urethral Diverticula in the Male. *Anterior urethral valves* are rare. The obstruction is not obstructing valve leaflets, as occurs in the posterior urethra. Rather, it is a urethral diverticulum in the penile urethra that expands during voiding. The distal extension of the diverticulum causes extrinsic compression of the distal penile urethra, causing urethral obstruction. Typically there is a soft mass on the ventral surface of the penis at the penoscrotal junction. In addition, the urinary stream often is weak and the physical findings associated with posterior urethral valves often are present. The diverticulum may be small and minimally obstructive or in other cases may be severely obstructive and cause renal insufficiency. The diagnosis is suspected on physical examination and is confirmed by the VCUG. Treatment involves open excision of the diverticulum or transurethral excision of the distal urethral cusp. *Urethral diverticula* occasionally occur after extensive hypospadias repair.

Fusiform dilatation of the urethra or megalourethra may result from underdevelopment of the corpus spongiosum and support structures of the urethra. This condition is commonly associated with the prune-belly syndrome.

Male Urethral Meatal Stenosis. See Chapter 536.

Cromie WJ, Lee K, House K, et al: Implications of prenatal ultrasound screening in the incidence of major genitourinary malformations. *J Urol* 2001;165:1677–80.

Gonzalez RM, de Filippo R, Jednak R, et al: Urethral atresia: Long-term outcome in 6 children who survived neonatal period. *J Urol* 2001;165:2241–44.

Herndon CDA, Ferrer FA, Freedman A, et al: Consensus on prenatal management of antenatally detected urological abnormalities. *J Urol* 2000;164:1052–56.

Holmes N, Harrison MR, Baskin LS: Fetal surgery for posterior urethral valves: Long-term postnatal outcomes. *Pediatrics* 2001;107(7):e7.

Horowitz M, Shah SM, Gerzli G, et al: Laparoscopic partial upper pole nephrectomy in infants and children. *BJU Int* 2001;87:514–16.

Husmann D, Strand B, Ewalt D, et al: Management of ectopic ureterocele associated with renal duplication: A comparison of partial nephrectomy and endoscopic decompression. *J Urol* 1999;162:1406–9.

Koff SA, Mutabagani KH, Jayanthi VR: The valve bladder syndrome: Pathophysiology and treatment with nocturnal bladder emptying. *J Urol* 2002;167:291–97.

Marr L, Skoog SJ: Laser incision of ureterocele in the pediatric patient. *J Urol* 2002;167:280–82.

Misseri R, Horowitz M, Combs AJ, et al: Myogenic failure in posterior urethral valve disease: Real or imagined? *J Urol* 2002;168:1844–48.

Nichols G, Hrouda D, Kellett MJ, et al: Endopyelotomy in the symptomatic older child. *BJU Int* 2001;87:525–27.

Noh PH, Cooper CS, Winkler AC, et al: Prognostic factors for long-term renal function in boys with the prune belly syndrome. *J Urol* 1999;162:1399–1401.

Pohl HG, Rushton HG, Park J-S, et al: Early diuresis renogram findings predict success following pyeloplasty. *J Urol* 2001;165:2311–15.

Roth KS, Carter WH Jr, Chan JCM: Obstructive nephropathy in children: Long-term progression after relief of posterior urethral valve. *Pediatrics* 2001;107:1004–10.

Ulman I, Jayanthi VR, Koff SA: Long-term follow-up of newborns with severe unilateral hydronephrosis initially treated nonoperatively. *J Urol* 2000;164:1101–5.

Upadhyay J, Bolduc S, Braga L, et al: Impact of prenatal diagnosis on the morbidity associated with ureterocele management. *J Urol* 2002;167:2560–65.

Wiener JS, O'Hara SM: Optimal timing of initial postnatal ultrasonography in newborns with prenatal hydronephrosis. *J Urol* 2002;168:1826–29.

Chapter 533
Anomalies of the Bladder

BLADDER EXSTROPHY

Exstrophy of the urinary bladder occurs about once in every 35,000 to 40,000 births. The male:female ratio is 2:1. The severity ranges from a small vesicocutaneous fistula in the abdominal wall or simple epispadias to complete exstrophy of the cloaca involving exposure of the entire hindgut and the bladder.

Clinical Manifestations. These anomalies result when the mesoderm fails to invade the cephalad extension of the cloacal membrane; the extent of this failure determines the degree of the anomaly. In classic bladder exstrophy (Fig. 533–1), the bladder protrudes from the abdominal wall and its mucosa is exposed. The umbilicus is displaced downward, the pubic rami are widely separated in the midline, and the rectus muscles are separated. In males, there is complete epispadias with a wide and shallow scrotum. Undescended testes and inguinal hernias are common. Females also have epispadias, with separation of the two sides of the clitoris and wide separation of the labia. The anus is displaced anteriorly in both sexes, and there may be rectal prolapse. Individuals with exstrophy tend to be shorter than normal. The consequences of untreated bladder exstrophy are total urinary incontinence and an increased incidence of bladder cancer, usually adenocarcinoma. The genital deformities can produce sexual disability in both sexes, particularly in the male. The wide separation of the pubic rami causes a characteristic

broad-based gait but no significant disability. In classic bladder exstrophy, the upper urinary tracts usually are normal.

Treatment. Management of bladder exstrophy should start at birth. The bladder should be covered with plastic wrap to keep the bladder mucosa moist. Application of gauze or petroleum-gauze to the bladder mucosa should be avoided. The infant should then be promptly transferred to a center equipped for the treatment of such anomalies. Conventional therapy has included a series of staged reconstructive procedures, but more recently a single-stage complete reconstruction in the neonatal infant is popular.

Prompt closure of the exstrophic bladder is the preferred treatment. During this procedure the abdominal wall is mobilized and the pubic rami are brought together in the midline. If the bladder closure is performed during the first 48 hr of life, there is sufficient mobility of the pubic rami to allow approximation of the pubic symphysis. If the procedure is delayed, however, the pelvic bone must be broken (pelvic osteotomy) to allow the pubic rami to be brought together. Early bladder closure can be applied to almost all neonatal infants with classic bladder exstrophy. Treatment should be deferred in selected situations when surgery would be excessively risky or complex, such as in a premature baby.

Total reconstruction includes closure of the bladder, closure of the abdominal wall, and, in the male, correction of epispadias using the technique of penile disassembly. Postoperatively, the infant's upper urinary tract is monitored closely for the possible development of hydronephrosis and infection. The majority of such infants have vesicoureteral reflux and should receive antibiotic prophylaxis. In the male, if the epispadias is not corrected at birth, then epispadias repair is generally performed between 1–2 yr of age. At this point the child has total urinary incontinence because there is no external urinary sphincter.

The final stage of reconstruction involves creation of a sphincter muscle for bladder control and correction of the vesicoureteral reflux. In general, the child is at least 3 yr of age, the bladder capacity should be at least 80 mL, and the child must have gained rectal control.

At puberty, the pubic hair is distributed to the sides of the external genitals. A monsplasty is performed to provide a more normal escutcheon.

Prognosis. This plan of treatment has yielded more than 70% continence in some centers, with less than 15% deterioration of the upper urinary tract. This continence rate reflects not only the successful reconstruction but also the quality and size of the bladder. Children who undergo reconstructive surgery as newborns have a greater chance of obtaining a normally functioning bladder. Children who remain incontinent for more than 1 yr after bladder neck reconstruction or those who are not eligible for bladder neck reconstruction because of a small bladder capacity are candidates for an alternative reconstructive procedure to achieve dryness. Such procedures include (1) augmentation cystoplasty, in which the bladder is enlarged with a patch of small or large bowel to increase its capacity; (2) creation of a neobladder out of small and large bowel with placement of a continent abdominal stoma through which clean intermittent catheterization can be performed; (3) placement of an artificial urinary sphincter, with possible augmentation cystoplasty; and (4) ureterosigmoidostomy, in which the ureters are detached from the bladder and sutured to the sigmoid colon. Individuals with the latter procedure void from the rectum and rely on their anal sphincter for continence. This operation was popular in the past and is still employed in some centers; it is attractive because it avoids the need for external urinary diversion. However, it carries a significant risk of chronic pyelonephritis, upper urinary tract damage, metabolic acidosis resulting from absorption of hydrogen ion and chloride in the intestine, and at least a 15% long-term risk of colonic carcinoma.

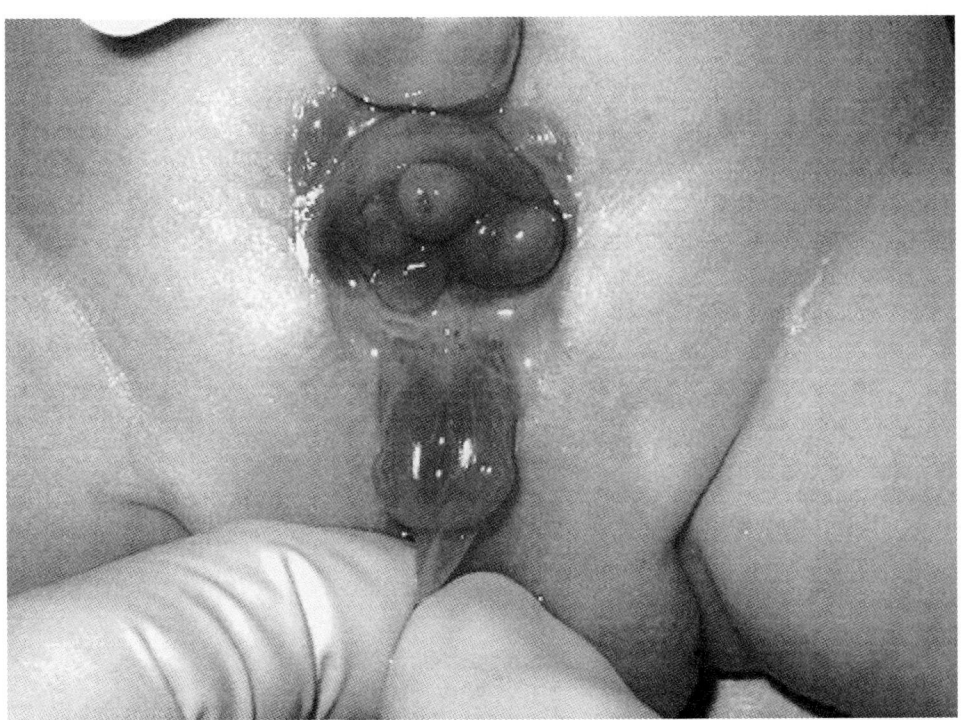

FIGURE 533–1. Classic bladder exstrophy. The bladder is exposed in the midline; the umbilical cord is displaced caudad; the penis is epispadiac; and the scrotum is broad.

Late follow-up has shown that men with exstrophy have a penis that is half normal size but experience satisfactory sexual function. Fertility has been low, possibly because of iatrogenic injury to the secondary sexual organs during reconstruction. In women, fertility is not affected but uterine prolapse during pregnancy is a problem.

OTHER EXSTROPHY ANOMALIES

Children with more complex cases of *cloacal exstrophy,* which has an incidence of 1 in 400,000, have an omphalocele and severe abnormalities of the colon and the rectum and often have short bowel syndrome. Approximately 50% of patients have an upper urinary tract anomaly, and 50% have spina bifida. Current reconstructive techniques result in a satisfactory outcome in most patients with permanent urinary diversion (either ileal conduit or continent urinary diversion) and a colostomy. Because the penis in boys with cloacal exstrophy usually is diminutive, genital reconstruction in males with cloacal exstrophy generally has been unsatisfactory. In the past most specialists recommended assigning a female gender to such infants, but currently there is debate whether these children with a 46,XY karyotype and androgen imprinting in utero can have a satisfactory female gender identity. Decisions regarding gender assignment should be made jointly by the physicians caring for the infant (surgical team, pediatric endocrinologist, child psychiatrist, and ethicist) and family.

Epispadias is in the spectrum of exstrophy anomalies, affecting approximately 1 in 117,000 boys and 1 in 480,000 girls. In boys, the diagnosis is obvious because the prepuce is distributed primarily on the ventral aspect of the penile shaft and the urethral meatus is on the dorsum of the penis. In girls, the clitoris is bifid and the urethra is split dorsally. Distal epispadias in boys usually is associated with normal urinary control and normal upper urinary tracts and should be repaired by 6–12 mo of age. In the more severe cases of epispadias, the sphincter is incompletely formed and these individuals (male and female) have total urinary incontinence and usually separation of the pubic rami. These children require surgical reconstruction procedures analogous to those of the 2nd and 3rd stages of management of patients with classic bladder exstrophy.

BLADDER DIVERTICULA

Bladder diverticula usually occur at the ureterovesical junction and are associated with vesicoureteral reflux (see Fig. 531–6), because the diverticulum interferes with the normal flap-valve attachment between the ureter and bladder. Congenital diverticula occur in other locations also. Bladder diverticula are also commonly associated with distal urethral obstruction or neurogenic bladder dysfunction. Small diverticula require no treatment other than that of the primary disease, whereas large diverticula may contribute to inefficient voiding, residual urine, urinary stasis, and urinary tract infections and should be excised.

URACHAL ANOMALIES

Urachal abnormalities are more common in males than in females. A patent urachus can occur as an isolated anomaly, or it may be associated with prune-belly syndrome. In this condition there is continuous urinary drainage from the umbilicus. The tract should be excised surgically. Another urachal anomaly is the urachal cyst, which can become infected. Typical symptoms and physical findings include suprapubic pain, fever, irritative voiding symptoms, and an infraumbilical mass, which can be erythematous. Diagnosis is made by ultrasonography or computed tomography. Treatment is intravenous antibiotic therapy and drainage and excision. Other urachal anomalies include the urachal diverticulum, which is a diverticulum of the bladder dome, and external urachal sinus, which is a blind external sinus that opens at the umbilicus. These lesions should be excised.

Capolicchio G, McLorie GA, Farhat W, et al: Population-based analysis of continence outcomes and bladder exstrophy. *J Urol* 2001;165:2418–21.

Dodson JL, Surer I, Baker LA, et al: The newborn exstrophy bladder inadequate for primary closure: Evaluation, management and outcome. *J Urol* 2001;165:1656–59.

El-Sherbiny MT, Hafez AT, Ghoneim MA: Complete repair of exstrophy: Further experience with neonates and children after failed initial bladder closure. *J Urol* 2002;168:1692–94.

Feng AH, Kaar S, Elder JS: Influence of enterocystoplasty on linear growth in children with exstrophy. *J Urol* 2002;167:2552–55.

Gearhart JP: Complete repair of bladder exstrophy in newborn: Complications and management. *J Urol* 2001;165:2431–33.

Grady RW, Mitchell ME: Complete primary repair of exstrophy. *J Urol* 1999;162:1415–20.

Gros D-A C, Dodson JL, Lopatin UA, et al: Decreased linear growth associated with intestinal bladder augmentation in children with bladder exstrophy. *J Urol* 2000;164:917–20.

Hafez AT, Elsherbiny MT, Ghoneim MA: Complete repair of bladder exstrophy: Preliminary experience with neonates and children with failed initial closure. *J Urol* 2001;165:2428–30.

Schober JM, Carmichael PA, Hines M, et al: The ultimate challenge of cloacal exstrophy. *J Urol* 2002;167:300–4.

Surer I, Baker LA, Jeffs RD, et al: Modified Young-Dees-Leadbetter bladder neck reconstruction in patients with successful primary bladder closure elsewhere: Single institution experience. *J Urol* 2001;165:2438–40.

Chapter 534
Neuropathic Bladder

Neuropathic bladder dysfunction in children is usually congenital and may result from myelomeningocele, lipomeningocele, sacral agenesis, or other spinal abnormalities. Acquired diseases and traumatic lesions of the spinal cord are less frequent. Central nervous system tumors, sacrococcygeal teratoma, and spinal abnormalities associated with imperforate anus can also result in abnormal innervation of the bladder or sphincter, or both.

Myelodysplasia. Myelodysplasia *(spina bifida)* describes various abnormal conditions of the vertebral column that affect spinal cord function, including *myelomeningocele* and *meningocele* (see Chapter 585). The incidence of myelodysplasia is 1 in 1,000 births in the United States, but with antenatal screening and abortion, the incidence is decreasing. A few medical centers have been performing selective antenatal myelomeningocele closure, but follow-up studies of the urinary tract have not shown a definite improvement in lower urinary tract function.

The most important consequences of neurogenic bladder dysfunction associated with myelodysplasia are urinary incontinence, urinary tract infections (UTIs), and upper tract deterioration. Hydronephrosis, pyelonephritis, and renal function deterioration are common causes of premature demise of affected individuals.

In the neonate, renal ultrasonography, a random check of postvoid residual urine volumes, and a voiding cystourethrogram are performed after closure of the back. Ten to 15 percent of patients have hydronephrosis and 25% have vesicoureteral reflux. A *urodynamic study* should also be performed. This study involves filling the bladder with saline and measuring the bladder volume and pressure, as well as assessing sphincter tone. During bladder filling, the bladder may show (1) uninhibited (premature) contractions at low volumes, (2) normal bladder volume with contraction at an appropriate volume, or (3) atonia (lack of bladder contraction). Bladder compliance or elasticity may also be reduced. The sphincter may show (1) normal tone with relaxation during bladder contraction, (2) reduced or absent tone, or (3) normal or increased tone that increases during bladder contraction (termed *detrusor-sphincter dyssynergia*) (Fig. 534–1).

Renal damage usually results from failure of the sphincter to relax during a bladder contraction. This dyssynergia results in functional obstruction of the bladder outlet, leading to high intravesical pressure, bladder muscle hypertrophy and trabeculation, and transmission of the high pressure into the upper urinary tract, causing hydronephrosis (Fig. 534–2). Vesicoureteral reflux and urinary tract infection (UTI) compound the problem. Treatment includes reduction of bladder pressure with anticholinergic drugs (oxybutynin, 0.2 mg/kg/24 hr in two or three divided doses) and clean intermittent catheterization every 3–4 hr. If there is vesicoureteral reflux or UTIs, antimicrobial

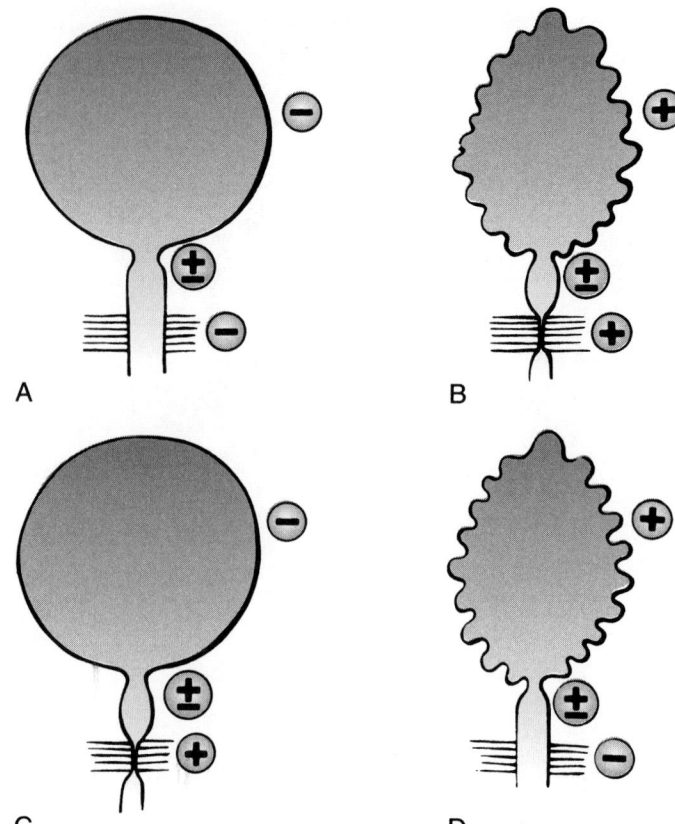

FIGURE 534–1. Grouping of neurogenic bladder dysfunction according to the innervation, tonicity, and coordination of the detrusor and sphincters described by Guzman. This grouping is based on data from imaging studies, cystometrography, and electromyography of the sphincters. Patients in group *B* are at risk of developing reflux and hydronephrosis. For guidance in the treatment of incontinence, group *A* benefits from procedures that increase outlet resistance, group *B* from anticholinergics or bladder augmentation surgery, and group *C* from intermittent catheterization and group *D* requires both increased outlet resistance and pharmacologic or surgical bladder enlargement. Most patients require intermittent catheterization to empty. (Modified from Gonzalez R: Urinary incontinence. In Kelalis PK, King LR, Belman AB [editors]: *Clinical Pediatric Urology*. Philadelphia, WB Saunders, 1992, p 387.)

prophylaxis is also prescribed. In the newborn or infant, temporary urinary diversion by cutaneous vesicostomy is a satisfactory alternative for severe reflux. Another option in the child with severe detrusor sphincter dyssynergia is botulinum toxin (Botox) injection into the sphincter. This procedure usually requires general anesthesia and results in sphincteric incompetence for 4–6 mo. Clean intermittent catheterization and anticholinergic therapy cure the reflux in up to 80% of patients without ureteral dilatation (grades I and II). Children with more severe reflux often require corrective surgery followed by intermittent catheterization and anticholinergic drugs. When intermittent catheterization is difficult or if anticholinergic agents are not well tolerated, a temporary cutaneous vesicostomy provides effective bladder decompression. Failure of these methods to relieve intravesical pressures is an indication for augmentation enterocystoplasty and intermittent catheterization.

Urinary incontinence in the child with neuropathic bladder can result from total or partial denervation of the sphincter, bladder hyperreflexia, poor bladder compliance, chronic urinary retention, or a combination of these factors. Less than

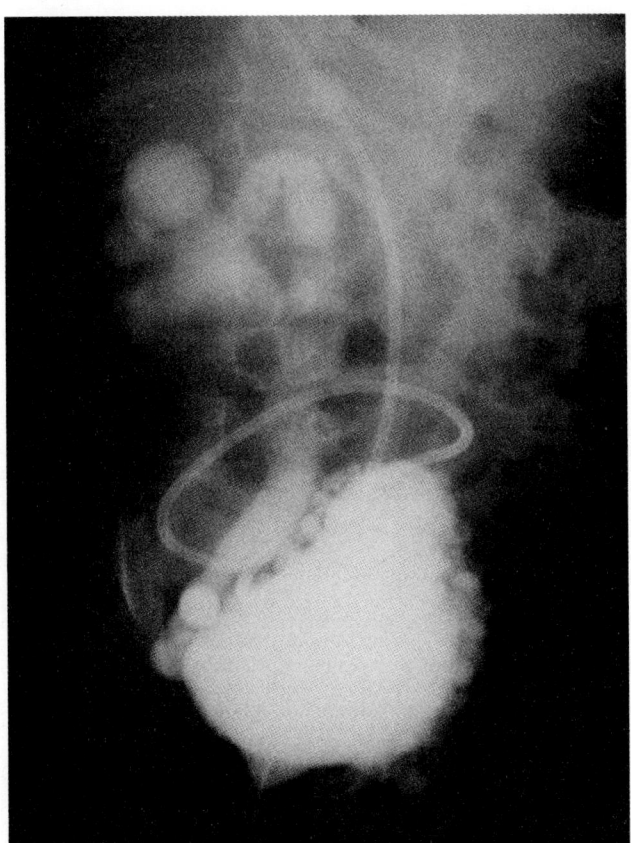

FIGURE 534–2. Voiding cystourethrogram in an infant with myelodysplasia shows a severely trabeculated bladder with multiple diverticula and grade V (out of V) right vesicoureteral reflux. Evaluation showed severe detrusor-sphincter dyssynergia.

5% of children born with myelodysplasia achieve normal continence. Supravesical diversion, commonly performed in the 1970s to prevent incontinence, has a high long-term complication rate and is now seldom employed.

Incontinence often is addressed around 4 yr of age. Nearly all children require clean intermittent catheterization to stay dry. This technique allows efficient bladder emptying with minimal risk of symptomatic UTI. The treatment of incontinence is tailored to the individual case. The urinary tract should be evaluated with renal ultrasonography, a voiding cystourethrogram, and a urodynamic study, including bladder capacity. If the sphincter tone is sufficient and the bladder has adequate compliance, intermittent catheterization every 3–4 hr is usually successful in keeping the child dry. If there are unstable bladder contractions, an anticholinergic medication such as oxybutynin chloride, hyoscyamine, or tolterodine is prescribed to increase bladder capacity. If there is sphincter incompetence, α-adrenergic medications are prescribed to enhance outlet resistance. Bacteriuria is seen in up to 50% of children using intermittent self-catheterization, but it seldom causes symptoms. In the absence of reflux, there seems to be little cause for concern. Antibacterial prophylaxis can often be effective in keeping the urine sterile while intermittent catheterization is used. With this treatment plan, 40–85% of patients are dry, depending on one's definition of continence. Some children wear a pad in their underwear or a diaper but state that they are dry.

If there is persistent incontinence despite these measures, reconstructive urinary tract surgery usually can provide complete or satisfactory continence. If urethral resistance is low, implantation of an artificial sphincter is usually successful. This sphincter consists of an inflatable cuff that is placed around the bladder neck, a pressure-regulating balloon implanted in the extraperitoneal space, and a pumping mechanism that is implanted in the scrotum of males and in the labia majora of females. Alternatively, bladder neck reconstructive procedures often are successful. If the bladder capacity or bladder compliance is low, or if there are persistent uninhibited contractions despite anticholinergic therapy, enlargement of the bladder with a patch of small or large intestine or stomach, termed **augmentation cystoplasty** or **enterocystoplasty**, is effective. These patients still need to perform clean intermittent catheterization. If urethral catheterization is difficult, a continent stoma may be incorporated into the urinary tract reconstruction. A common method is termed the **Mitrofanoff** procedure, in which the appendix is isolated from the cecum on its vascular pedicle and is interposed between the bladder and abdominal wall to allow intermittent catheterization through a dry stoma. Many of these patients also have bowel problems with constipation, and some benefit from a procedure termed the **Malone antegrade continence enema** procedure, in which the appendix is brought out to the skin to allow a catheter to be inserted into the cecum for antegrade enema.

There are important potential complications of enterocystoplasty:

1. The urine is usually colonized with gram-negative bacteria, and attempts to sterilize the urine for prolonged periods usually fail. There is no evidence that chronic bacteriuria in these patients is associated with renal damage. Therefore, only symptomatic UTIs should be treated.

2. The enteric mucosal surface in contact with the urine absorbs ammonium, chloride, and hydrogen ions and loses potassium. Hyperchloremic metabolic acidosis can result and may require medical treatment (see Chapter 45). Chronic acidosis may compromise skeletal growth. This complication is more common in patients with compromised renal function. To overcome this limitation of enterocystoplasty in patients with chronic renal insufficiency, a gastric segment can be used instead of a segment of the small or large intestine. The stomach secretes chloride and hydrogen ions; thus, pre-existing metabolic acidosis remains stable or improves. However, the possibility of intractable metabolic alkalosis and peptic ulceration of the augmentation has diminished the enthusiasm for this procedure. Composite augmentations using stomach and small or large bowel has resulted in few metabolic complications.

3. Perforation of the augmented bladder and peritonitis are serious complications that are potentially life-threatening. This complication seems to result from acute or chronic overdistention of the augmented bladder. These patients typically present with severe abdominal pain. Prompt diagnosis and treatment with exploratory laparotomy and bladder closure are necessary. Meticulous adherence to the prescribed program of intermittent catheterization to avoid bladder overdistention is important.

4. Bladder calculi have developed in as many as 70% of children followed for 10 yr after enterocystoplasty. The calculi develop because of mucus that accumulates in the bladder and acts as a nidus for stone formation.

5. The potential for malignancy secondary to enterocystoplasty is unknown, but, based on past experience with ureterosigmoidostomy and some reported cases, it is prudent to advise yearly endoscopic examinations or urine cytologic studies beginning in the 10th postoperative year.

Latex Allergy. One of the most serious problems encountered by as many as half of individuals with spina bifida and other urologic conditions that require clean intermittent catheterization and urinary tract reconstructive procedures is latex allergy. This IgE-mediated allergy is acquired and is secondary to repeated exposure to the medically associated latex allergen. Latex allergy may manifest as watery eyes, sneezing, itching, hives, or anaphylaxis when blowing up a balloon or if an examiner is using latex gloves. Intraoperatively, a sensitized individual can experience anaphylactic shock. A latex-free environment should be provided for these children in the office, during hospitalization, and during operative procedures.

Occult Spinal Dysraphism. Approximately 1 in 4,000 patients have occult spinal dysraphism, which includes lipomeningocele, intradural lipoma, diastematomyelia, tight filum terminale, dermoid cyst-sinus, aberrant nerve roots, anterior sacral meningocele, and cauda equina tumor. More than 90% of patients have a cutaneous abnormality overlying the lower spine, including a small dimple, tuft of hair, dermal vascular malformation, or a subcutaneous lipoma (Fig. 534–3). Often these children have high arched feet, discrepancy in muscle size and strength between the legs, and a gait abnormality. Newborns and young infants usually have a normal neurologic examination. Older children often have absent perineal sensation and back pain. Lower urinary tract function is abnormal in 40% of patients, including incontinence, recurrent UTI, and fecal soiling. The likelihood of a normal examination is inversely related to the age at surgical correction of the spinal lesion. In infants with abnormal urodynamics, 60% revert to normal; in older children only 27% become normal. Management of the urinary tract in other children is similar to that described for myelodysplasia.

Sacral Agenesis. Sacral agenesis is defined as the absence of part or all of two or more lower vertebral bodies. This condition is more common in the offspring of women with diabetes. These children have flattened buttocks and a low, short gluteal cleft but usually have no orthopedic deformity, although some have high arched feet. Palpation of the coccygeal area reveals the absent vertebrae. Approximately 20% of cases are undetected until the age of 3–4 yr; many are diagnosed after unsuccessful toilet training. Urodynamic studies in these children show a variety of patterns, and most need clean intermittent catheterization and pharmacotherapy to stay dry.

Imperforate Anus. Between 30% and 45% of children with a high imperforate anus have a neuropathic bladder, often because of

sacral agenesis. Newborns with imperforate anus should undergo a spinal ultrasound during their initial evaluation; and if these children have difficulty with toilet training, complete urologic evaluation with upper and lower urinary tract imaging and urodynamics should be performed. (Also see Chapter 325.)

Cerebral Palsy. Children with cerebral palsy have reasonable bladder control. However, continence is achieved at a later age than in unaffected children. Their upper urinary tracts are usually normal. Urodynamic studies have shown that most have uninhibited bladder contractions. Timed voiding and anticholinergic therapy is usually effective. Clean intermittent catheterization rarely is necessary. (Also see Chapters 37 and 591.1.)

Feng AH, Kaar S, Elder JS: Influence of enterocystoplasty on linear growth in children with exstrophy. *J Urol* 2002;167:2552–55.

Holzerbein J, Pope JC IV, Adams MC, et al: The urodynamic profile of myelodysplasia in childhood with spinal closure during gestation. *J Urol* 2000;164:1336–39.

Lopez Pereira P, Martinez Urrutia MJ, Lobato Romera R, et al: Should we treat vesicoureteral reflux in patients who simultaneously undergo bladder augmentation for neuropathic bladder? *J Urol* 2001;165:2259–61.

Lottmann HB, Margarian M, Bernuy M, et al: The effect of endoscopic injections of dextranomer based implants on continence and bladder capacity: A prospective study of 31 patients. *J Urol* 2002;168:1863–67.

Palmer JS, Kaplan WE, Firlit CF: Erectile dysfunction in patients with spina bifida is treatable condition. *J Urol* 2000;164:958–61.

Park JM, McGuire EM, Koo HP, et al: External urethral sphincter dilation for management of high risk myelomeningocele: 15-year experience. *J Urol* 2001;165:2383–88.

Smith CP, Somogyi GT, Chancellor MB: Botulinum toxin: Poisoning the spastic bladder and urethra. *Rev Urol* 2002;4:61–68.

Tackett LD, Minevich E, Benedict JF, et al: Appendiceal versus ileal segment for antegrade continence enema. *J Urol* 2002;167:683–86.

Wedderburn A, Lee RS, Denny A, et al: Synchronous bladder reconstruction and antegrade continence enema. *J Urol* 2001;165:2392–93.

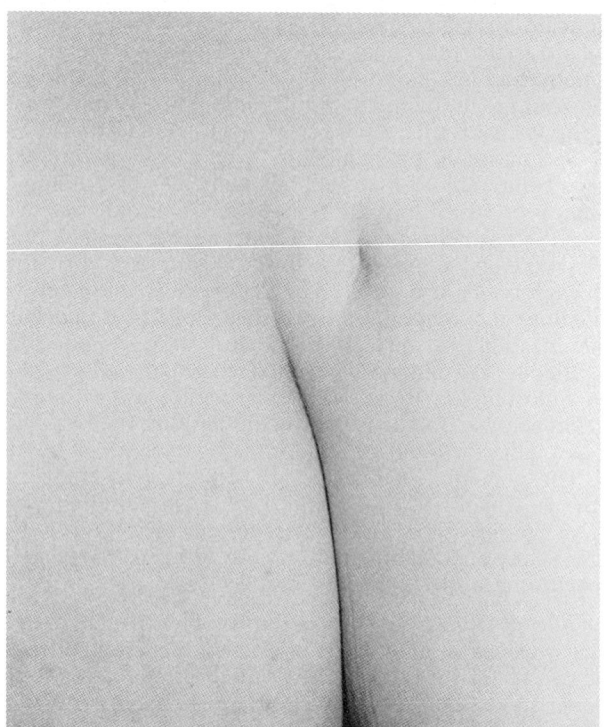

FIGURE 534–3. Buttocks of teenage boy with tethered cord secondary to lipomeningocele. Note sacral dimple and deviation of gluteal fold to the left.

Chapter 535
Voiding Dysfunction

NORMAL VOIDING AND TOILET TRAINING

In the fetus, voiding occurs by reflex bladder contraction and is "balanced," with simultaneous contraction of the bladder and relaxation of the sphincter. Urine storage consists of sympathetic and pudendal nerve–mediated inhibition of detrusor contractile activity accompanied by closure of the bladder neck and proximal urethra with increased activity of the external sphincter.

The infant has coordinated, reflex voiding as often as 15 to 20 times per day. Over time, the bladder enlarges gradually, and the average *bladder capacity* in ounces is equal to the age (in years) plus 2. This formula applies to children up to the age of 12–14 yr. At 2–4 yr, toilet training begins. To achieve normal conscious bladder control, several steps must occur: (1) awareness of bladder filling, (2) cortical inhibition (suprapontine modulation) of reflex (unstable) bladder contractions, (3) ability to consciously tighten the external sphincter to prevent incontinence, (4) normal bladder growth, and (5) motivation by the child to stay dry. The *transitional phase of voiding* refers to the period when children are acquiring bladder control. Girls typically acquire bladder control before boys, and bowel control is typically achieved before urinary control. By 5 yr of age, 90–95% are nearly completely continent during the day and 80–85% are continent at night (also see Chapter 20).

NOCTURNAL ENURESIS (See Chapter 20.3)

Nocturnal enuresis is the occurrence of involuntary voiding at night at 5 yr, the age when volitional control of micturition is expected. Enuresis may be primary (75%; nocturnal urinary control never achieved) or secondary (25%; the child was dry at night for at least a few months and then enuresis occurs). In addition, 75% of children with enuresis are wet only at night, whereas 25% are wet day and night. This distinction is important because the pathogenesis of the two patterns is different.

Epidemiology. Approximately 60% of children with nocturnal enuresis are boys. Family history is also important and is positive in 50% of cases. Although primary nocturnal enuresis may be polygenetic, candidate genes have been localized to chromosomes 12 and 13. If one parent was enuretic, each child has a 44% risk of enuresis; if both parents were enuretic, each child has a 77% likelihood of enuresis. Nocturnal enuresis without overt daytime voiding symptoms affects up to 20% of children at the age of 5 yr; it ceases spontaneously in approximately 15% of involved children every year thereafter. Its frequency among adults is less than 1%.

Pathogenesis. The pathogenesis of primary nocturnal enuresis (normal daytime voiding habits) is multifactorial and includes the following:

- Delayed maturation of the cortical mechanisms that allow voluntary control of the micturition reflex.
- Sleep disorder–enuretic children, who are classically described as being deep sleepers, although no specific sleep pattern has been described. Enuresis can occur in any stage of sleep. All children are most difficult to arouse in the first third of the night and are easiest to awaken in the last third of the night, but enuretic children are more difficult to arouse than those with normal bladder control.
- Reduced antidiuretic hormone production at night, resulting in an increased urine output, which explains why children with enuresis often are described as "soaking the bed."
- Genetic factors, with chromosomes 12 and 13q the likely sites of the gene for enuresis; family history is often positive in enuretic children, as described earlier.
- Psychologic factors, often implicated in secondary enuresis.
- Organic factors, such as urinary tract infection (UTI) or obstructive uropathy, which is an uncommon cause of enuresis.
- Sleep apnea (snoring) secondary to enlarged adenoids.

Clinical Manifestations and Diagnosis. A careful history should be obtained, especially with respect to fluid intake at night and pattern of nocturnal enuresis. Children with diabetes insipidus, diabetes mellitus, and chronic renal disease may have a high obligatory urinary output and a compensatory polydipsia. The family should be asked whether the child snores loudly at night. A complete physical examination should include palpation of the abdomen and rectal examination after voiding to assess the possibility of a chronically distended bladder. The child with nocturnal enuresis should be examined carefully for neurologic and spinal abnormalities. There is an increased incidence of bacteriuria in enuretic girls, and, if found, it should be investigated and treated (see Chapter 530), although this does not always lead to resolution of bed-wetting. Urinalysis should be obtained after an overnight fast and evaluated for specific gravity or osmolality, or both, to exclude polyuria as a cause of frequency and incontinence and to ascertain that the concentrating ability is normal. The absence of glycosuria should be confirmed. If there are no daytime symptoms and if the physical examination and urinalysis are normal, and culture is negative, further evaluation for urinary tract pathology generally is not warranted. A renal ultrasonogram is reasonable in an older child with enuresis or in children who do not respond appropriately to therapy.

Treatment. The best approach to treatment is to reassure parents that the condition is self-limited and to avoid punitive measures that may affect the child's psychologic development adversely (see Chapter 20.3). Fluid intake should be restricted to 2 oz after 6 or 7 o'clock in the evening if the child weighs less than 75 lb, 3 oz if the child weighs 75 to 100 lb, and 4 oz if the child weighs more than 100 lb. In addition, the parents should be certain that the child voids at bedtime. If the child snores and the adenoids are enlarged, referral to an otolaryngologist should be considered, because adenoidectomy may result in cure of the enuresis.

Active treatment should be avoided in children younger than age 6 yr because enuresis is extremely common in younger children. The simplest initial measure is motivational and includes a star chart for dry nights. Waking children a few hours after they go to sleep to have them void often allows them to awaken dry, although this measure is not curative. Some have recommended that children try holding their urine for longer periods during the day, but there is no evidence that this approach is beneficial. *Conditioning therapy* involves use of an auditory alarm attached to electrodes in the underwear. The alarm sounds when voiding occurs and is intended to awaken children and alert them to void. This form of therapy is considered curative and has a reported success of 30–60%. Often the alarm wakes up other family members and not the enuretic child; persistence for several months is necessary. A vibratory alarm is available also. Conditioning therapy tends to be most effective in older children. Another form of therapy to which some children respond is *self-hypnosis*. The primary role of psychological therapy is to help the child deal with enuresis psychologically and help motivate arising to void at night if the child awakens with a full bladder.

Pharmacologic therapy is intended to treat the symptom of enuresis and is not curative. One form of treatment is *desmopressin acetate*, which is a synthetic analog of antidiuretic hormone and reduces urine production overnight. It is available as a tablet, with a dosage of 0.2–0.6 mg at bedtime. In the past it was used as a nasal spray, with a dosage of 10 µg (1 spray) to 40 µg (4 sprays total) at bedtime. The lowest effective dose should be used. It is important to reduce evening fluid intake, and the drug should not be used if the child has a systemic illness with vomiting or diarrhea. Hyponatremia has been reported in a few children using the nasal spray, primarily those who were not using the medication properly. It has not been reported in children using the tablets. In children with rhinorrhea, the nasal spray is not absorbed and consequently is ineffective. Desmopressin acetate is effective in as many as 40% of children. If effective, it should be used for 3–6 mo, and then an attempt should be made to taper it. If tapering results in recurrent enuresis, the medication may be started again at the higher dosage. No adverse events have been reported with the long-term use of desmopressin acetate. Another pharmacologic agent is *imipramine*, which is a tricyclic antidepressant. This medication has mild anticholinergic and α-adrenergic effects and may alter the sleep pattern also. The dosage of imipramine is 25 mg in children age 6–8 yr, 50 mg in children age 9–12 yr, and 75 mg in teenagers. Reported success rates are 30–60%. Side effects include anxiety, insomnia, and dry mouth. In addition, the drug is one of the most common causes of poisoning by prescription medication in younger siblings. Oxybutynin chloride, a pure anticholinergic agent, has been used in some children with primary nocturnal enuresis, but the response rate is low.

DIURNAL INCONTINENCE

Daytime incontinence not secondary to neurologic abnormalities is common in children. At age 5 yr, 95% have been dry during the day at some time and 92% are dry. At 7 yr, 96% are dry, although 15% have significant urgency at times. At 12 yr, 99% are dry during the day. The most common cause of daytime incontinence is a pediatric unstable bladder (also termed *uninhibited or overactive bladder, bladder spasms*). Table 535–1 lists the causes of diurnal incontinence in children.

Important points in the history include the pattern of incontinence, including the frequency, the volume of urine lost during incontinent episodes, whether the incontinence is associated with urgency or giggling, whether it occurs after voiding, and whether the incontinence is continuous. In addition, the frequency of voiding and whether there is nocturnal enuresis, a strong, continuous urinary stream, or sensation of incomplete bladder emptying should be assessed. Other urologic problems such as UTIs, reflux, neurologic disorders, or a family history of duplication anomalies should be assessed. Bowel habits also should be evaluated, because incontinence is common in children with constipation or encopresis, or both. Diurnal incontinence may occur in girls with a history of sexual abuse. Physical examination is directed at identifying signs of organic causes of incontinence: short stature, hypertension, enlarged kidneys or bladder or both, constipation, labial adhesion, ureteral ectopy (Figs. 535–1 to 535–3), back or sacral anomalies (see Fig. 534–3), and neurologic abnormalities. A urinalysis or culture, or both, should be performed to check for infection. In some cases, assessing the postvoid residual urine volume or urinary flow rate is appropriate. Imaging is reserved for children who have significant physical findings, a family history of urinary tract anomalies, UTIs, or those who do not respond to therapy appropriately. A renal ultrasonogram with or without a voiding cystourethrogram is indicated. Urodynamics may be helpful if there is evidence of neurologic disease or if empirical therapy is ineffective.

PEDIATRIC UNSTABLE (OVERACTIVE) BLADDER

A pediatric unstable bladder is smaller than normal and exhibits strong uninhibited contractions. These children typically exhibit urinary frequency, urgency, and urge incontinence. Such symptoms are also seen in about 25% of children with nocturnal enuresis. Often girls will squat down on their foot to try to prevent incontinence ("Vincent curtsy"). Many children indicate they do not feel the need to urinate, even just before they are incontinent. In females, a history of recurrent UTI is common, but incontinence may persist long after infections are brought under control. It is not clear in these cases if the voiding dysfunction is a sequel of the infections or if the voiding dysfunction predisposes to recurrent infections. In girls, voiding cystourethrography (VCUG) often shows a dilated urethra ("spinning top deformity"; Fig. 535–4) and narrowed bladder neck with bladder wall hypertrophy. The urethral finding results from inadequate relaxation of the external urinary sphincter. In addition, constipation is common.

Initial therapy is timed voiding every 1.5–2 hr and anticholinergic therapy with oxybutynin chloride, hyoscyamine, or

TABLE 535–1. Causes of Urinary Incontinence in Childhood

Pediatric unstable bladder (uninhibited bladder)
Infrequent voiding
Detrusor-sphincter dyssynergia
Non-neurogenic neurogenic bladder (Hinman syndrome)
Vaginal voiding
Giggle incontinence
Cystitis
Bladder outlet obstruction (posterior urethral valves)
Ectopic ureter and fistula
Sphincter abnormality (epispadias, exstrophy; urogenital sinus abnormality)
Neurogenic
Overflow incontinence
Traumatic
Iatrogenic
Behavioral
Combination

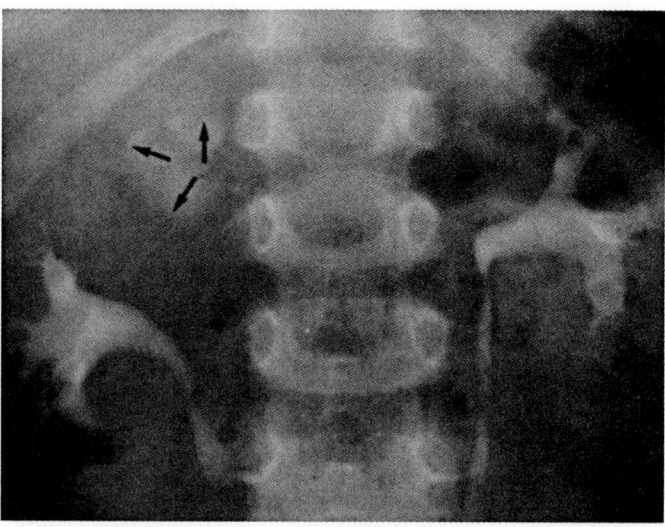

FIGURE 535–1. Duplication of the right collecting system with ectopic ureter. Excretory urogram in a female presenting with a normal voiding pattern and constant urinary dribbling. The left kidney is normal, and the right side, well visualized, is the lower collecting system of a duplicated kidney. On the upper pole opposite the first and second vertebral bodies, note the accumulation of contrast material corresponding with a poorly functioning upper pole drained by a ureter opening in the vestibule.

tolterodine. Constipation and UTIs also must be addressed. This treatment program is usually prolonged and should be interrupted periodically to determine its continued need. An alternative to pharmacologic therapy is biofeedback, in which children are taught pelvic floor exercises, because there is evidence that daily performance of these exercises may reduce or eliminate

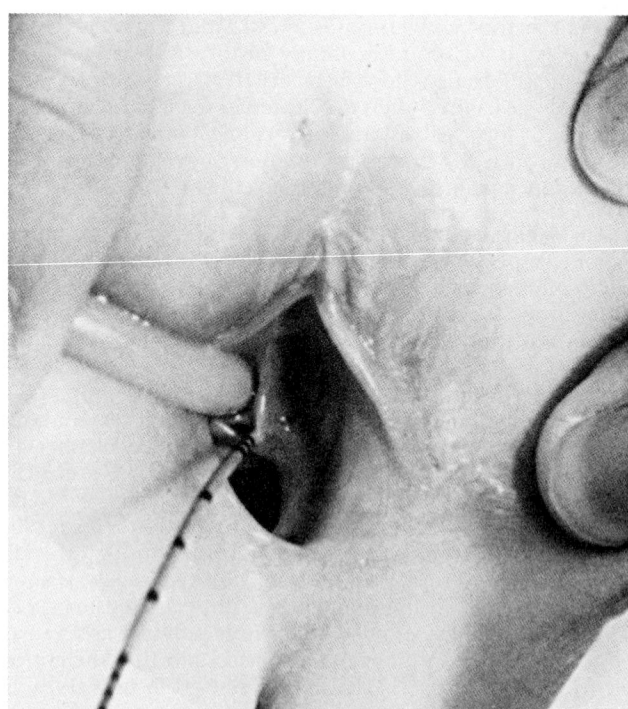

FIGURE 535–2. Ectopic ureter. The photograph shows an ectopic ureter entering the vestibule next to the urethral meatus. The thin ureteral catheter with transverse marks has been introduced into this ectopic ureter. This girl had a normal voiding pattern and constant urinary dribbling.

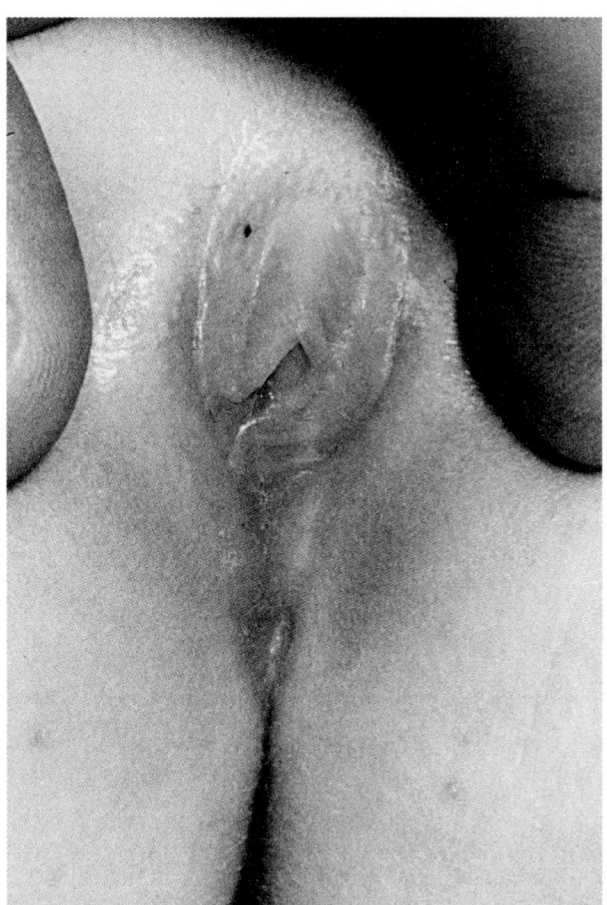

FIGURE 535–3. Labial adhesion. Note the inability to visualize the urethral meatus and vagina.

unstable bladder contractions. In some children treatment with an alpha blocker such as terazosin or doxazosin may aid in timed voiding. Children not responding to therapy should be evaluated endoscopically and urodynamically to rule out other possible forms of bladder or sphincter dysfunction.

NON-NEUROGENIC NEUROGENIC BLADDER (HINMAN SYNDROME)

Hinman syndrome is a more serious but less common disorder involving failure of the external sphincter to relax during voiding in children without neurologic abnormalities. Children with this syndrome, also called *detrusor-sphincter dyssynergia*, typically exhibit a staccato stream, day and night wetting, recurrent UTIs, constipation, and encopresis. Evaluation of affected children often reveals vesicoureteral reflux, a trabeculated bladder, and a decreased urinary flow rate with an intermittent pattern. In severe cases, hydronephrosis, renal insufficiency, and even end-stage renal disease can occur. The pathogenesis of this syndrome is thought to involve learning abnormal voiding habits during toilet training; the syndrome is rarely seen in infants. Urodynamic studies and magnetic resonance imaging of the spine are indicated to rule out a neurologic cause for the bladder dysfunction. The treatment is usually complex and may include anticholinergic and alpha blocker therapy, timed voiding, treatment of constipation, behavioral modification, and encouragement of relaxation during voiding. Biofeedback has been used successfully in older children to teach relaxation of the external sphincter. In some cases botulinum toxin (Botox) injection into the external sphincter can provide temporary sphincteric paralysis and thereby reduce outlet resistance. In severe cases, intermittent catheterization is necessary to ensure bladder emptying. In selected patients, external

urinary diversion is necessary to protect the upper urinary tract. These children require long-term treatment and careful follow-up.

INFREQUENT VOIDING

Infrequent voiding is a common disorder of micturition, usually associated with urinary tract infections. Affected children, usually girls, void only twice a day rather than the normal four to seven times. With bladder overdistention and prolonged retention of urine, growth of bacteria can lead to recurrent UTIs. Some of these children are constipated. Some also have occasional episodes of incontinence due to overflow or urgency. The disorder is behavioral. When the children have UTIs, the treatment is antibacterial prophylaxis and encouragement of frequent voiding and complete emptying of the bladder by double voiding until a normal pattern of micturition is re-established.

VAGINAL VOIDING

In girls with vaginal voiding, incontinence typically occurs after urination after the girl stands up. Usually the volume of urine is 5–10 mL. One of the most common causes is *labial adhesion* (see Fig. 535–3). This lesion is seen in young girls and can be managed either by topical application of estrogen cream to the adhesion or lysis in the office. Some girls experience vaginal voiding because they do not separate their legs widely during urination. These girls are usually overweight or do not pull their underwear down to their ankles when they urinate. Management involves encouragement of the girl to separate the legs as widely as possible during urination. The most effective way to do this is to have the child sit backward on the toilet seat during micturition.

OTHER CAUSES OF INCONTINENCE IN GIRLS

Ureteral ectopia, usually associated with a duplicated collecting system in girls, can produce urinary incontinence characterized by constant dribbling of urine during day and night, even though they void regularly. Sometimes the urine production from the renal segment drained by the ectopic ureter is small and urinary drainage is confused with watery vaginal discharge.

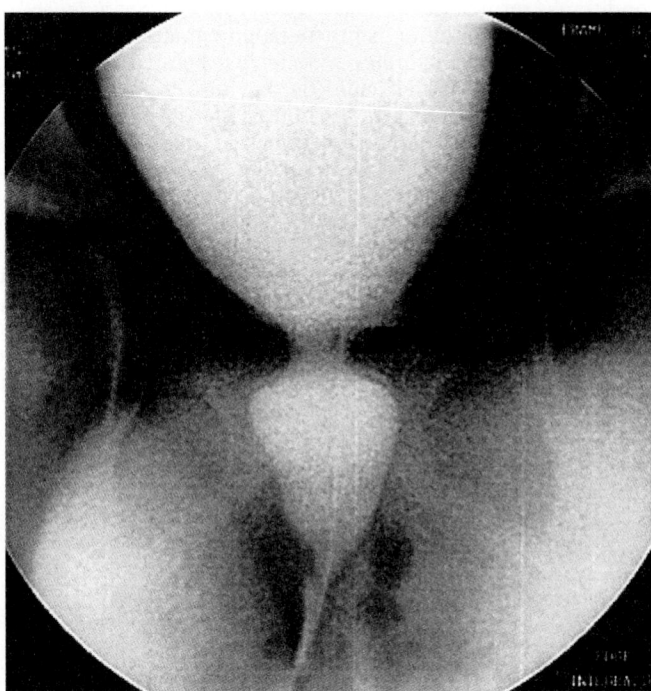

FIGURE 535–4. Spinning top deformity. VCUG demonstrating dilation of the urethra with distal urethral narrowing and contraction of the bladder neck.

Children with a history of vaginal discharge or incontinence and an abnormal voiding pattern require careful study. The ectopic orifice is usually difficult to find. On ultrasonography or intravenous urography, one may suspect duplication of the collecting system (see Fig. 535–1), but the upper collecting system drained by the ectopic ureter usually has poor or delayed function. Computed tomography of the kidneys helps rule out subtle duplication that may not be discovered on intravenous urography. Examination under anesthesia for an ectopic ureteral orifice in the vestibule or the vagina is often necessary (see Fig. 535–2). The treatment in these cases is either partial nephrectomy, with removal of the upper pole segment of the duplicated kidney and its ureter down to the pelvic brim, or ipsilateral ureteroureterostomy, in which the upper pole ectopic ureter is anastomosed to the normally positioned lower pole ureter.

Giggle incontinence is a condition that typically affects girls between 7 and 15 yr of age. The incontinence occurs suddenly during giggling, and the entire bladder volume is lost. The pathogenesis is thought to be sudden relaxation of the urinary sphincter. Anticholinergic medication and timed voiding rarely are effective. The most effective treatment is methylphenidate administration.

Total incontinence may be secondary to *epispadias*. This condition, which affects only 1 of 480,000 females, is characterized by separation of the pubic symphysis, separation of the right and left sides of the clitoris, and a patulous urethra. Treatment is bladder neck reconstruction to repair the totally incompetent urethra.

A short, incompetent urethra may be associated with certain urogenital sinus malformations. The diagnosis of these malformations requires a high index of suspicion and a careful physical examination of all incontinent girls. In these cases, urethral and vaginal reconstruction can often restore continence.

VOIDING DISORDERS WITHOUT INCONTINENCE

Some children have the abrupt onset of severe urinary frequency, voiding as often as every 10–15 min during the day, without dysuria, UTI, daytime incontinence, or nocturia. The most common age for these symptoms to occur is 4–6 yr, after the child is toilet-trained, and the vast majority are boys. This condition is termed the *daytime frequency syndrome of childhood* or *pollakiuria*. The condition is functional; no anatomic problem is detected. Often the symptoms occur just before a child starts kindergarten or if the child is having emotional family stress–related problems. These children should be checked for UTI, and the clinician should ascertain that the child is emptying the bladder satisfactorily. Occasionally, pinworms can cause these symptoms. The condition is self-limited, and symptoms generally resolve within 2–3 mo. Anticholinergic therapy rarely is effective.

Some children have the *dysuria-hematuria syndrome*, in which the child has dysuria without UTI and microscopic or gross hematuria. This condition affects children who are toilet-trained and often is secondary to hypercalciuria. A 24-hr urine sample should be obtained and calcium and creatinine excretion assessed. A 24-hr calcium excretion of more than 4 mg/kg is abnormal and deserves treatment with thiazides because some of these children may be at risk for urolithiasis.

Austin PF, Homsy YL, Masel JL, et al: Alpha-adrenergic blockade in children with neuropathic and nonneuropathic voiding dysfunction. *J Urol* 1999;162:1064–71.
Austin PF, Ritchey ML: Dysfunctional voiding. *Pediatr Rev* 2000;21:336–41.
Evans JHC: Evidence-based management of nocturnal enuresis. *BMJ* 2001;323:1167–69.
Glazener CM, Evans JH: Alarm interventions for nocturnal enuresis in children (Cochrane Review). *Cochrane Database Syst Rev* 2001;(1):CD002911.
Glazener CM, Evans JH: Tricyclic and related drugs for nocturnal enuresis in children (Cochrane Review). *Cochrane Database Syst Rev* 2000;(3):CD002117.
Hjalmas K, Hellstromj A-L, Mogren K, et al: The overactive bladder in children: A potential future indication for tolterodine. *BJU Int* 2001;87:569–74.

Herndon CDA, Decambre M, McKenna PH: Interactive computer games for treatment of pelvic floor dysfunction. *J Urol* 2001;166:1893–98.
Kodman-Jones C, Hawkins L, Schulman SL: Behavioral characteristics of children with daytime wetting. *J Urol* 2001;166:2392–95.
Leebeek-Groenewegen A, Blom J, Sukhai R, et al: Efficacy of desmopressin combined with alarm therapy for monosymptomatic nocturnal enuresis. *J Urol* 2001;166:2456–58.
Palmer LS, Franco I, Rotario P, et al: Biofeedback therapy expedites the resolution of reflux in older children. *J Urol* 2002;168:1699–1703.
Schulman SL, Colish Y, von Zuben FC, et al: Effectiveness of treatments for nocturnal enuresis in a heterogeneous population. *Clin Pediatr* 2000;39:359–64.
Schulman SL, Stokes A, Salzman PM: The efficacy and safety of oral desmopressin in children with primary nocturnal enuresis. *J Urol* 2001;166:2427–31.
Schulman SL, Von Zuben FC, Plachter N, et al: Biofeedback methodology: Does it matter how we teach children how to relax the pelvic floor during voiding? *J Urol* 2001;166:2423–26.
Schum TR, Kolb TM, McAuliffe TL, et al: Sequential acquisition of toilet-training skills: A descriptive study of gender and age differences in normal children. *Pediatrics* 2002;109(3):E48.
Smith CP, Somogyi GT, Chancellor MB: Botulinum toxin: Poisoning the spastic bladder and urethra. *Rev Urol* 2002;4:61–68.

Chapter 536
Anomalies of the Penis and Urethra

Hypospadias. Hypospadias refers to a urethral opening that is on the ventral surface of the penile shaft and affects 1 in 250 male newborns. There is incomplete development of the prepuce, termed a *dorsal hood*, in which the foreskin is on the sides and dorsal aspect of the penile shaft and absent ventrally. Some boys, particularly those with proximal hypospadias, have chordee, in which there is ventral penile curvature during erection. The incidence of hypospadias may be increasing, possibly because of in utero exposure to estrogenic or antiandrogenic endocrine-disrupting chemicals (polychlorbiphenyls, phytoestrogens).

CLINICAL MANIFESTATIONS. Hypospadias is classified according to the position of the urethral meatus after taking into account whether chordee is present (Fig. 536–1). The deformity is described as glanular (on the glans penis), coronal, subcoronal, midpenile, penoscrotal, scrotal, and perineal. Approximately 60% of cases are distal, 25% are subcoronal or midpenile, and

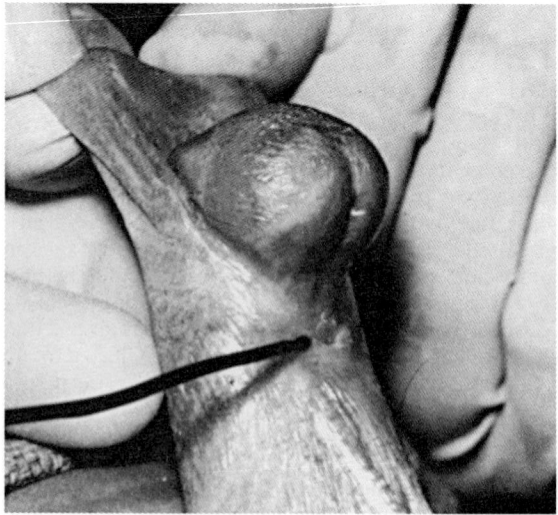

FIGURE 536–1. Subcoronal hypospadias. Note the urethral meatus in the subcoronal position and the incomplete or hooded prepuce. There was no ventral curvature of the penis in this case.

15% are proximal. In the more severe cases, the scrotum is bifid and sometimes extends to the dorsal base of the penis (scrotal engulfment) (Fig. 536–2). There is also a *megameatal variant,* in which the foreskin is normally developed, but there is either distal or subcoronal hypospadias with a "fish mouth" meatus (Fig. 536–3). These cases may not be diagnosed until after a circumcision is performed.

Hypospadias usually is an isolated anomaly. However, hypospadias is common in boys with multiple congenital anomalies. Approximately 10% of boys with hypospadias have an undescended testis, and inguinal hernias are also common. In the newborn, the differential diagnosis of proximal hypospadias with an undescended testis should include forms of ambiguous genitalia, particularly masculinization of females (congenital adrenal hyperplasia) and mixed gonadal dysgenesis. A karyotype should be obtained in patients with midpenile or proximal hypospadias and cryptorchidism (see Chapter 577). Boys with penoscrotal hypospadias should undergo a voiding cystourethrogram because 5–10% have a dilated prostatic utricle, which is a remnant of the müllerian system. The incidence of other anomalies of the genitourinary tract in boys with hypospadias is low, and with the exception of the more severe cases of perineal hypospadias, radiographic studies of the urinary tract are unnecessary.

Complications of untreated hypospadias include (1) deformity of the urinary stream, either ventral deflection or severe splaying; (2) sexual dysfunction secondary to penile curvature; (3) infertility if the urethral meatus is proximal; and (4) meatal stenosis (congenital), which is extremely rare. The goal of hypospadias surgery is to correct the functional and cosmetic deformities. Whereas hypospadias repair is recommended for boys with midpenile and proximal hypospadias, some boys with distal hypospadias will have no functional abnormality and do not need any surgical correction.

TREATMENT. Management begins in the newborn period. Circumcision should be avoided, because the foreskin is often used in the repair. The ideal age for repair in a healthy infant is 6–12 mo. This age is chosen because (1) there is no greater risk of general anesthesia at this age than at 2–3 yr, (2) penile growth over the next several years is slow, (3) the child does not remember the surgical procedure, and (4) analgesic needs are less than in older children. Nearly all cases are repaired in a single operation on an outpatient basis. In most boys with distal

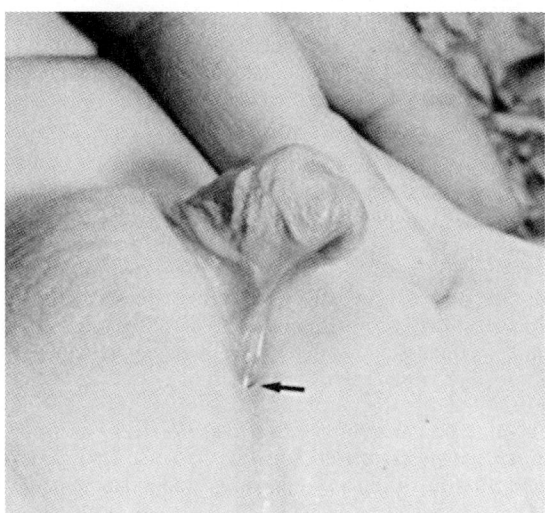

FIGURE 536–2. Severe perineoscrotal hypospadias. Note the ventral curvature and the underdeveloped ventral surface of the penis, the hooded prepuce, and the urethral meatus in the midline of the bifid scrotum. This child had palpable gonads and a normal chromosome pattern.

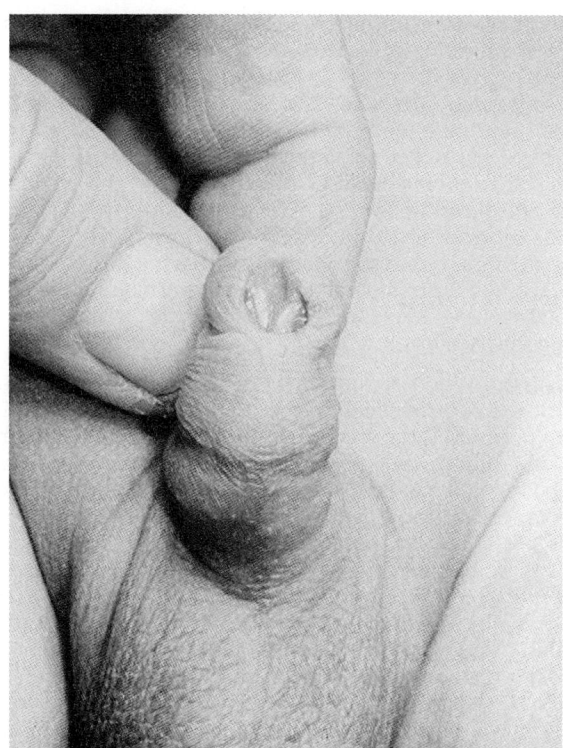

FIGURE 536–3. Megameatal variant of hypospadias. Note fishmouth meatus. This boy has been circumcised.

hypospadias the urethral plate is tubularized, whereas with more proximal cases a vascularized skin flap from the foreskin is used and the remaining foreskin covers the ventral penile surface. The complication rate is low: less than 5% for distal hypospadias, 5–10% for midpenile hypospadias, and 15% for proximal hypospadias. Complications include urethrocutaneous fistula, hematoma, wound infection, meatal stenosis, urethral diverticulum, and wound dehiscence. Repair of hypospadias is a technically demanding operation and should be performed by surgeons with special training and extensive experience.

Chordee without Hypospadias. In some boys there is ventral penile curvature (chordee) and incomplete development of the foreskin (dorsal hood), but the urethral meatus is at the tip of the glans. In most of these boys, the urethra is normal but there is insufficient ventral penile skin or prominent, inelastic ventral bands of dartos fascia that prevent a normal straight erection. In some cases, however, the urethra is short and hypoplastic, and a formal urethroplasty is necessary for repair. The only sign of this anomaly in the neonate may be the dorsal hood deformity, and delayed repair under general anesthesia at 6 mo of age is recommended.

Phimosis and Paraphimosis. *Phimosis* refers to the inability to retract the prepuce. At birth, phimosis is physiologic. Over time the adhesions between the prepuce and glans lyse and the distal phimotic ring loosens. In 90% of uncircumcised males the prepuce becomes retractable by the age of 3 yr. Accumulation of epithelial debris under the infantile prepuce is not pathologic and does not require surgical treatment. In older boys, phimosis may be physiologic, may be pathologic from inflammation and scarring at the tip of the foreskin, or may occur after circumcision (see later discussion of trapped penis). The prepuce may have been retracted forcefully on one or two occasions in the past, which can result in a cicatricial scar that prevents subsequent foreskin retraction. In boys with persistent physiologic or pathologic phimosis, application of corticosteroid cream to the foreskin three times daily for 1 mo loosens the phimotic ring in two thirds of cases. If there is ballooning of the foreskin during voiding or phimosis beyond 10 yr of age, circumcision is recommended.

Paraphimosis occurs when the foreskin is retracted behind the coronal sulcus and the prepuce cannot be pulled back over the glans (Fig. 536–4). Painful venous stasis in the retracted foreskin results, with edema leading to severe pain and inability to reduce the foreskin (pull it back over the glans). Treatment includes lubrication of the foreskin and glans and then compressing the glans and simultaneously placing distal traction on the foreskin to try to push the phimotic ring beyond the coronal sulcus. In rare cases, emergency circumcision under general anesthesia is necessary.

Circumcision. Whether the newborn male should undergo circumcision is controversial. In the United States, circumcision is usually performed for social reasons. Reasons given in support of circumcision include reducing the risk of urinary tract infection (UTI) and sexually transmitted diseases and prevention of penile cancer, phimosis, and balanitis.

UTIs are 10 to 15 times more common in uncircumcised infants than in circumcised infants, the urinary pathogens arising from bacteria that colonize the space between the prepuce and glans. The risk of febrile UTI is primarily between birth and 6 mo, but there is an increased risk of UTI at least through 5 yr of age. Many recommend circumcision in infants who are predisposed to UTI, such as those with congenital hydronephrosis and vesicoureteral reflux. Whether circumcision reduces the risk of sexually transmitted diseases, in particular acquired immunodeficiency syndrome, is unresolved, because most of the data have been acquired from countries in which the prevalence of acquired immunodeficiency syndrome is high and because it has been difficult to ascertain whether the sexual practices of the circumcised and uncircumcised subjects were similar. There have been only a handful of reports of adult men who were circumcised at birth and subsequently acquired penile carcinoma, but in Scandinavian countries, where few men are circumcised and hygiene is good, the incidence of penile cancer is low.

Complications after neonatal circumcision include bleeding, wound infection, meatal stenosis, secondary phimosis, removal of insufficient foreskin, and dense penile adhesions (skin bridge; Fig. 536–5); 0.2–3% of patients have a subsequent operative procedure. Boys with a large hydrocele or hernia are at particular risk for secondary phimosis (see later discussion of trapped penis). Potentially serious complications include sepsis,

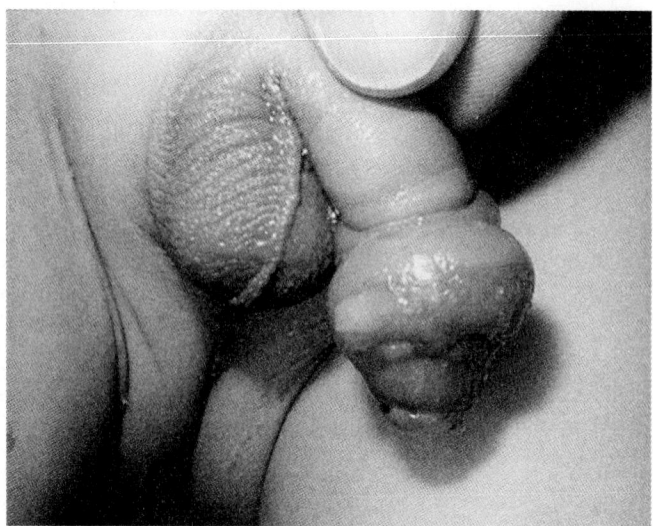

FIGURE 536–4. Paraphimosis. Foreskin has been retracted proximal to the glans penis and has become markedly swollen secondary to venous congestion.

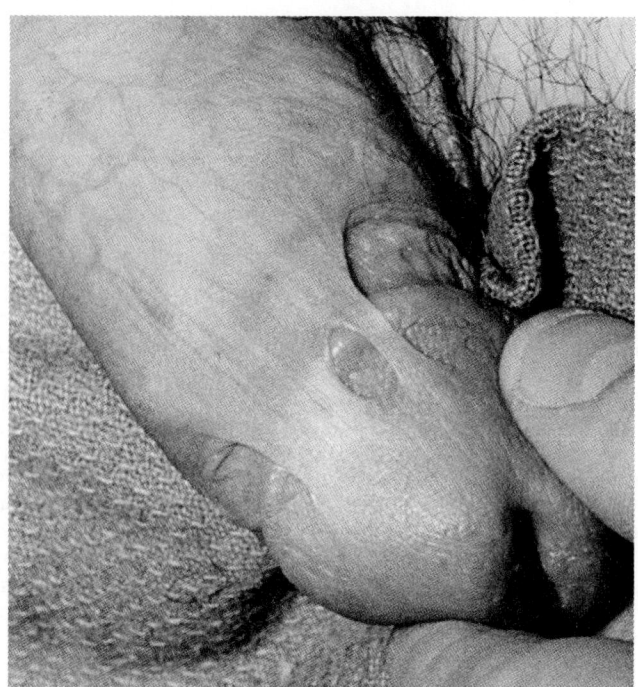

FIGURE 536–5. Skin bridges between glans and penile shaft resulting from penile adhesions forming after newborn circumcision. Skin bridges cause painful penile curvature during erection and predispose to infection under the adhesion and should be excised.

amputation of the distal part of the glans, removal of an excessive amount of foreskin, and urethrocutaneous fistula. Circumcision should not be performed in neonates with hypospadias, chordee without hypospadias, or a dorsal hood deformity (relative contraindication) or in those with a small penis.

When performing a neonatal circumcision, local analgesia, such as a dorsal nerve block or application of EMLA cream, is recommended.

Penile Torsion. Penile torsion is a rotational defect of the penile shaft. It usually occurs in a counterclockwise direction, that is, to the left side. In most cases, penile development is normal and the condition is unrecognized until circumcision is performed or the foreskin is retractable. Penile torsion also occurs in some boys with hypospadias. The defect has primarily cosmetic significance and correction is unnecessary if the rotation is less than 60 degrees from the midline.

Inconspicuous Penis. The term *inconspicuous penis* refers to a penis that appears to be small. A *webbed penis* is a condition in which the scrotal skin extends onto the ventrum of the penis. This deformity represents an abnormality of the attachment between the penis and scrotum. Although the cosmetic appearance is only mildly abnormal, if a routine circumcision is performed, the penis tends to retract into the scrotum and can result in secondary phimosis. In rare cases, the distal urethra is hypoplastic, necessitating urethral reconstruction. The *concealed (hidden or buried) penis* is a normally developed penis that is camouflaged by the suprapubic fat pad (Fig. 536–6). This anomaly may be congenital or iatrogenic after circumcision. A *trapped penis* is an acquired form of inconspicuous penis and refers to a phallus that becomes embedded in the suprapubic fat pad after circumcision (Fig. 536–7). This deformity may occur after neonatal circumcision in an infant who has significant scrotal swelling from a large hydrocele or inguinal hernia or after routine circumcision in an infant with a webbed penis. This complication can predispose to UTIs and may cause urinary retention.

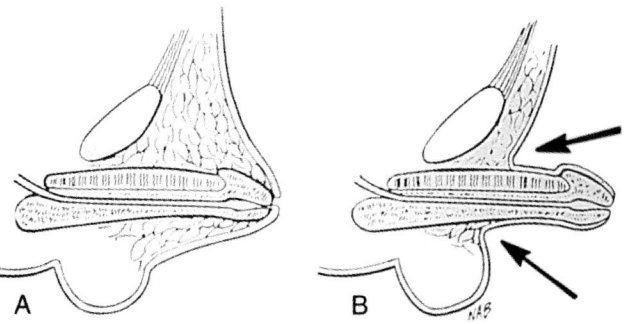

FIGURE 536–6. Concealed penis *(A)*, which may be visualized by retracting skin lateral to penile shaft *(B)*.

Micropenis. *Micropenis* is defined as a normally formed penis that is at least 2.5 standard deviations below the mean in size (Fig. 536–8). Typically, the ratio of the length of the penile shaft to its circumference is normal. The pertinent measurement is the *stretched penile length*, which is measured by gently stretching the penis and measuring the distance from the penile base under the pubic symphysis to the tip of the glans. The mean length of a newborn penis is 3.5 ± 0.7 cm and 1.1 ± 0.2 cm in diameter, and it should be at least 1.9 cm in length. Micropenis results from a hormonal abnormality that occurs after 14 wk of gestation. Common causes include (1) hypogonadotropic hypogonadism, (2) hypergonadotropic hypogonadism (primary testicular failure), and (3) idiopathic micropenis. The most common cause of micropenis is failure of the hypothalamus to produce an adequate amount of gonadotropin-releasing hormone, and typically this occurs in Kallmann syndrome, Prader-Willi syndrome, and Lawrence-Moon-Biedl syndrome. In some cases, there is

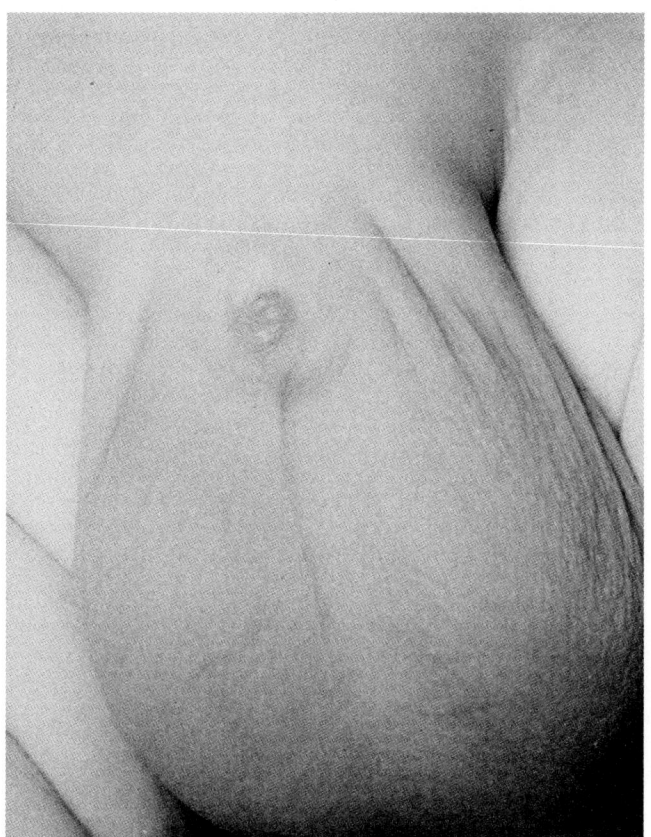

FIGURE 536–7. Concealed, trapped penis secondary to circumcision. This baby's penis is normal length; large hydroceles predisposed him to this complication.

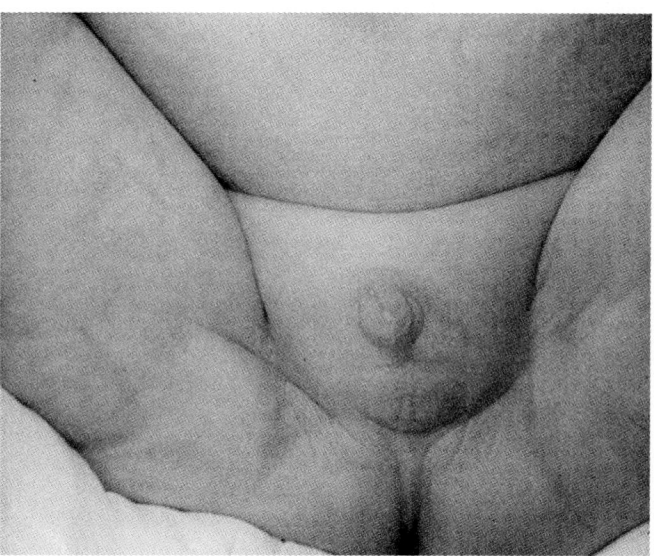

FIGURE 536–8. Infant with microphallus. Also note the small scrotum, which was empty.

growth hormone deficiency. Primary testicular failure may result from gonadal dysgenesis or rudimentary testes syndrome and also occurs in Robinow syndrome. All these children should be examined by a pediatric endocrinologist and pediatric urologist. Evaluation includes a karyotype, assessment of anterior pituitary function, testicular function, and magnetic resonance imaging to determine the anatomic integrity of the hypothalamus and the anterior pituitary gland as well as the midline structure of the brain. One of the difficult questions is whether androgen therapy is essential during childhood because stimulation of penile growth in a prepubertal boy may limit the growth potential of the penis in puberty. In addition, studies of small numbers of men with micropenis suggest that many, although not all, have satisfactory sexual function. Consequently, a decision for gender reassignment is made infrequently.

Other Penile Anomalies. Agenesis of the penis affects approximately 1 in 10 million boys. The karyotype is almost always 46,XY, and the usual appearance is that of a well-developed scrotum with descended testes and an absent penile shaft. Upper urinary tract abnormalities are common. In most cases, gender reassignment is recommended in the newborn period. *Diphallia* ranges from a small accessory penis to complete duplication. *Lateral penile curvature* usually is caused by overgrowth or hypoplasia of a corporal (erectile) body and usually is congenital. Surgical repair is recommended at age 6–12 mo.

Meatal Stenosis. Meatal stenosis is a condition that is almost always acquired and occurs after neonatal circumcision. It probably results from severe inflammation of the denuded glans. If the meatus is pinpoint, boys void with a forceful, fine stream that goes a great distance. These boys may experience dysuria, frequency, or hematuria, or a combination of these conditions, without UTI between the ages of 3 and 8 yr. Other boys have dorsal deflection of the urinary stream. Although the meatus may be small, hydronephrosis or voiding difficulty is extremely rare unless there is associated balanitis xerotica obliterans. Treatment is meatoplasty, in which the urethral meatus is opened surgically; this procedure can be performed either under anesthesia as an outpatient or in the office using local anesthesia (EMLA cream) with or without sedation. Routine cystoscopy is unnecessary.

Other Male Urethral Anomalies. Parameatal urethral cyst presents as an asymptomatic small cyst on one side of the urethral meatus. Treatment is excision under anesthesia. *Congenital*

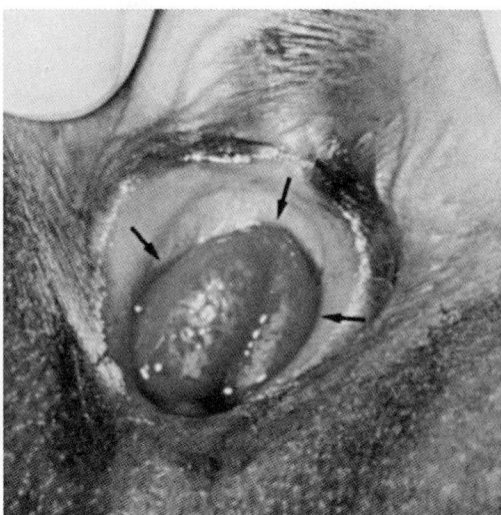

FIGURE 536–9. Urethral prolapse in a 4-yr-old black girl who had bloody spotting on her underwear.

urethral fistula is a rare deformity in which a fistula is present from the penile urethra. It is usually an isolated abnormality. Treatment is fistula closure. *Megalourethra* is a large urethra that is usually associated with abnormal development of the corpus spongiosum. This condition is most commonly associated with prune-belly syndrome. *Urethral duplication* is a rare condition in which the two urethral channels lie in the same sagittal plane, and the more normal urethra is the one positioned more ventrally. Some children have significant obstructive uropathy and require major reconstructive surgery. *Urethral hypoplasia* is a rare condition in which the urethra is extremely small but patent. In some cases, a temporary cutaneous vesicostomy is necessary for satisfactory urinary drainage. Either gradual enlargement of the urethra or major urethroplasty is necessary.

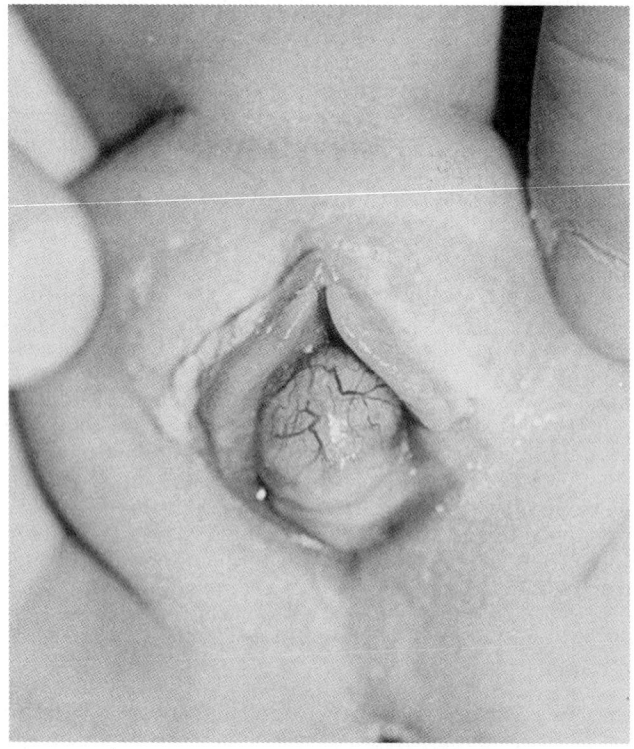

FIGURE 536–10. Paraurethral cyst in a newborn girl.

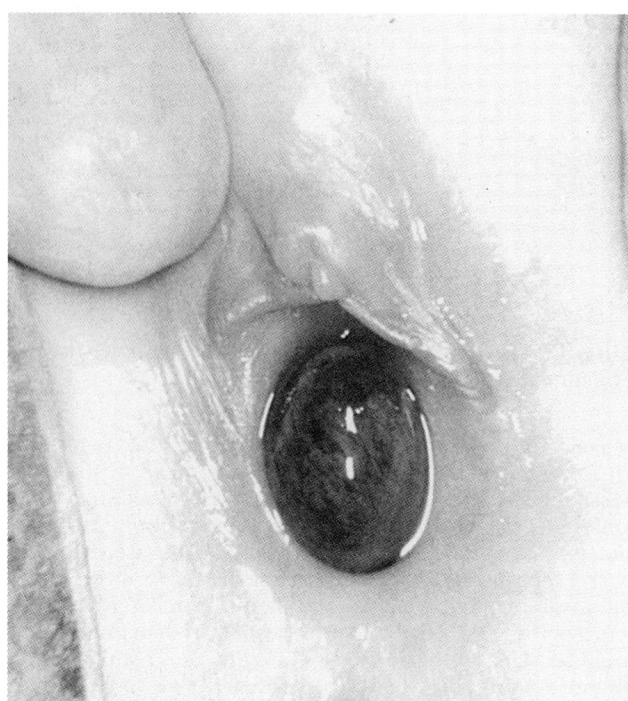

FIGURE 536–11. Prolapsed ectopic ureterocele in a female infant. She had a nonfunctioning upper pole collecting system connected to the ureterocele.

Urethral atresia refers to nondevelopment of the urethra and is nearly always fatal unless the urachus remains patent throughout gestation.

Urethral Prolapse (Female). Urethral prolapse is encountered predominantly in black females between 1 and 9 yr of age. The most common signs are bloody spotting on the underwear or diaper, although dysuria or perineal discomfort may also occur (Fig. 536–9). An inexperienced examiner may mistake the finding for sexual abuse. The usual therapy consists of application of estrogen cream two to three times daily for 3–4 wk and sitz baths. Surgical excision and reapproximation of the mucosal edges is curative.

Other Female Urethral Lesions. Paraurethral cyst results from retained secretions in the Skene glands secondary to ductal obstruction (Fig. 536–10). These lesions are present at birth and most regress in size during the first 4–8 wk, although occasionally it is necessary to incise them. A *prolapsed ectopic ureterocele* appears as a cystic mass protruding from the urethra and is a presenting symptom in 10% of girls with a ureterocele, which is a cystic swelling of the terminal ureter (Fig. 536–11). Ultrasonography should be performed to visualize the upper urinary tracts to confirm the diagnosis. Usually the ureterocele is either incised or an upper urinary tract reconstructive procedure is necessary.

American Academy of Pediatrics, Task Forced on Circumcision. Circumcision policy statement. *Pediatrics* 1999;103:686–93.

Baskin L: Hypospadias: A critical analysis of cosmetic outcomes using photography. *BJU Int* 2001:87:534–39.

Cheng EY, Vemulapalli SN, Kropp BP, et al: Snodgrass hypospadias repair with vascularized dartos flap: The perfect repair for virgin hypospadias? *J Urol* 2002;168:1723–26.

Kaefer M, Diamond D, Hendren WH, et al: Incidence of intersexuality in children with cryptorchidism and hypospadias: Stratification based on gonadal palpability and meatal position. *J Urol* 1999;162:1003–7.

McAleer IM, Kaplan GW: Is routine karyotyping necessary in the evaluation of hypospadias and cryptorchidism? *J Urol* 2001; 165:2029–31.

Palmer LS, Palmer JS, Franco I, et al: The "Long Snodgrass": Applying the tubularized incised plate urethroplasty to penoscrotal hypospadias in 1-stage or 2-stage repairs. *J Urol* 2002;168:1748–50.

Schoen EJ, Colby CJ, Ray GT: Newborn circumcision decreases incidence and costs of urinary tract infections during the first year of life. *Pediatrics* 2000;105:789–93.

Schoen EJ, Oehrli M, Colby CJ, et al: The highly protective effect of newborn circumcision against invasive penile cancer. *Pediatrics* 2000;105(3):e36.

Schoen EJ, Wiswell TE, Moses S: New policy on circumcision—cause for concern. *Pediatrics* 2000;105:620–23.

Snodgrass W, Patterson K, Plaire JC, et al: Histology of urethral plate: Implications for hypospadias repair. *J Urol* 2000;164:988–90.

Wiswell TE: The prepuce, urinary tract infections, and the consequences. *Pediatrics* 2000;106:860–61.

Chapter 537

Disorders and Anomalies of the Scrotal Contents

UNDESCENDED TESTES

Failure to find one or both testes in the scrotum may indicate that the testis is undescended, absent, or retractile.

Epidemiology. An undescended (cryptorchid) testis is the most common disorder of sexual differentiation in boys. At birth, approximately 4.5% of boys have an undescended testis. Because testicular descent occurs late in gestation, 30% of premature male infants have an undescended testis; the incidence is 3.4% at term. The majority of undescended testes descend spontaneously during the first 3 mo of life, and by 6 mo the incidence decreases to 0.8%. If the testis has not descended by 6 mo, it will remain undescended. Cryptorchidism is bilateral in 10% of cases. There is some evidence that the incidence of cryptorchidism is increasing. Some boys have secondary cryptorchidism after repair of an inguinal hernia. This complication of hernia repair is most common in neonates and young infants and affects as many as 1–2% of patients.

Pathogenesis. The process of testicular descent is regulated by an interaction between hormonal and mechanical factors, including testosterone, dihydrotestosterone, müllerian-inhibiting factor, the gubernaculum, intra-abdominal pressure, and the genitofemoral nerve. The testis develops at 7–8 wk of gestation. At 10–11 wk, the Leydig cells produce testosterone, which stimulates differentiation of the wolffian (mesonephric) duct into the epididymis, vas deferens, seminal vesicle, and ejaculatory duct. At 32–36 wk, the testis, which is anchored at the internal inguinal ring by the gubernaculum, begins its process of descent. The gubernaculum distends the inguinal canal and guides the testis into the scrotum.

Clinical Manifestations. Undescended testes are usually in the inguinal canal. Some boys have an ectopic testis, typically in the superficial inguinal pouch or perineum. Some testes are intra-abdominal; these are nonpalpable. Approximately 10% of cryptorchid boys have a nonpalpable testis; in these the testis is present and abdominal or inguinal in 50%, and it is absent secondary to perinatal testicular torsion in 50%. In a newborn with bilateral nonpalpable testes, one should suspect that the child could be a virilized female with congenital adrenal hyperplasia.

The consequences of cryptorchidism include infertility, malignancy, associated hernia, torsion of the cryptorchid testis, and the possible psychologic effects of an empty scrotum.

The undescended testis is histologically normal at birth, but pathologic changes can be demonstrated at 6–12 mo. Delayed germ cell maturation, reduction in germ cell number, hyalinization of the seminiferous tubules, and reduced Leydig cell number are typical; these changes are progressive over time if the testis remains undescended. Similar, although less severe, changes are found in the contralateral descended testis after 4–7 yr. After treatment for bilateral undescended testes, 50–65% of patients are fertile; 85% of boys treated for a unilateral undescended testis are fertile.

The risk of *malignancy* in the undescended testis is 4 to 10 times higher than that in the general population and is approximately 1 in 80 with a unilateral undescended testis and 1 in 40 to 1 in 50 for bilateral undescended testes. The peak age for this tumor is 15–45 yr. The most common tumor developing in an undescended testis is a seminoma (65%); in contrast, after orchiopexy, seminomas represent only 30% of testis tumors. Orchiopexy does not change the risk of developing cancer of the testis.

Indirect inguinal hernias usually accompany undescended testes but are rarely symptomatic. *Torsion and infarction* of the undescended testes can occur because of excessive mobility of such testes.

"Acquired" or *ascending undescended testes* are becoming recognized more frequently. These boys have a descended testis at birth, but during childhood, often between 4–10 yr of age, the testis does not remain in the scrotum. In such boys, on physical examination the testis often can be pulled into the scrotum, but there is obvious tension on the spermatic cord. This condition is thought to result from incomplete disappearance of the processus vaginalis so that the spermatic cord does not grow as rapidly as the child, resulting in the testis gradually moving out of a scrotal position.

Retractile testes often are misdiagnosed as undescended testes. Boys older than 1 yr of age frequently have a brisk cremasteric reflex; and if the child is anxious or ticklish during scrotal examination, the testis may be difficult to manipulate into the scrotum. Boys should be examined with their legs in a relaxed frog-leg position, and if the testis can be manipulated into the scrotum comfortably, it is probably retractile. It should be monitored every 6–12 mo with follow-up physical examinations, because it could be an acquired undescended testis. Boys with a retractile testis are not at increased risk for infertility or malignancy.

Treatment. The undescended testis should be treated at 9–15 mo. Most testes can be brought down to the scrotum with an operation *(orchiopexy)*. This procedure involves an inguinal incision, mobilization of the testis and spermatic cord, and correction of the indirect inguinal hernia. The procedure is typically performed on an outpatient basis with a success rate of 98%.

If the testis is *nonpalpable*, diagnostic laparoscopy is performed to determine its location. Ultrasound has been demonstrated to be ineffective in localizing the nonpalpable testis. Approximately 50% of these boys have an intra-abdominal testis or a testis that is located high in the inguinal canal; in the remaining patients, the testis is absent. When the testis is *absent*, usually an atrophic remnant is found in the scrotum or inguinal canal. The atrophy is thought to result from testicular torsion in utero. These gonads have been termed **vanishing testes**. In the majority of cases, orchiopexy of the intra-abdominal testis located immediately inside the internal inguinal ring is successful, but orchiectomy should be considered in the more difficult cases or when the testis appears to be atrophic. Two-stage orchidopexy is sometimes needed in high abdominal testes. Testicular prostheses are available for older children and adolescents when the absence of the gonad in the scrotum may have an undesirable psychologic effect.

Hormonal treatment is used infrequently. The concept is that because testicular descent is under androgen regulation human chorionic gonadotropin (which stimulates Leydig cell production of testosterone) or luteinizing hormone–releasing hormone (LHRH) may stimulate testicular descent. Although hormonal treatment has been used in Europe, randomized controlled trials have not shown either hormone to be very effective. There is some preliminary evidence that an LHRH analog, buserelin, may be helpful in increasing germ cell number and normalizing testicular histologic features.

SCROTAL SWELLING

Scrotal swelling may be acute or chronic and painful or painless. Abrupt onset of painful scrotal swelling necessitates prompt evaluation, because some conditions, such as testicular torsion and incarcerated inguinal hernia, require emergency surgical management. The differential diagnosis is shown in Tables 537–1 and 537–2.

Clinical Manifestations. A detailed history is helpful in determining the cause of the swelling and includes (1) onset of pain—with testicular torsion the pain often is sudden in onset and may be associated with exercise or minor genital trauma; (2) duration of pain; (3) radiation of pain—inguinal discomfort is common with an inguinal hernia or epididymitis and associated flank pain may occur with passage of a ureteral calculus; (4) previous episodes of similar pain, which are common in boys with intermittent testicular torsion or inguinal hernia; (5) nausea and vomiting, which are associated with testicular torsion and inguinal hernia; and (6) irritative urinary symptoms, such as dysuria, urgency, and frequency, which are indicative of a urinary tract infection that can cause epididymitis. Boys with lower urinary tract pathology may be prone to epididymitis.

Physical examination in boys with a painful scrotum may be difficult. Some have advocated performing a spermatic cord block or administering intravenous analgesia to facilitate the examination, but such measures are usually unnecessary. Scrotal wall erythema is common in testicular torsion, epididymitis, torsion of the appendix testis, and an incarcerated hernia. In boys with a normal cremasteric reflex, testicular torsion is unlikely. Absence of a cremasteric reflex, however, is nondiagnostic.

Laboratory Findings and Diagnosis. Pertinent laboratory studies include a urinalysis and culture. A positive urinalysis is suggestive of epididymitis. Serum studies generally are not helpful in establishing a diagnosis, unless a testis tumor is suspected. After initial evaluation, *imaging studies* may be helpful in establishing the diagnosis. These studies include color Doppler ultrasonography and radionuclide testicular flow scan. Imaging studies are used to assess whether testicular blood flow is normal, reduced, or increased. In addition, if a hydrocele is present and the testis is nonpalpable, or if an abnormality of the testis is found, ultrasonography may be helpful. Imaging studies are not 100% accurate; they should not be used to decide whether a boy with testicular pain should be referred for urologic care.

Color Doppler ultrasonography allows assessment of testicular blood flow and testicular morphologic features. Accuracy is 95% if the ultrasonographer is experienced. A false-negative study (i.e., demonstrates excellent testicular blood flow) may occur in a boy with testicular torsion if the degree of torsion is less than 360 degrees and the duration of torsion is short, because there may be continued testicular perfusion. In addi-

TABLE 537–1. Differential Diagnosis of Scrotal Masses in Boys and Adolescents

Painful	Painless
Testicular torsion	Hydrocele
Torsion of appendix testis	Inguinal hernia*
Epididymitis	Varicocele*
Trauma: ruptured testis, hematocele	Spermatocele*
Inguinal hernia (incarcerated)	Testicular tumor*
Mumps orchitis	Henoch-Schönlein purpura*
	Idiopathic scrotal edema

Occasionally associated with discomfort.

TABLE 537–2. Differential Diagnosis of Scrotal Swelling in Newborns

Hydrocele	Scrotal hematoma
Inguinal hernia (reducible)	Testicular tumor
Inguinal hernia (incarcerated)*	Meconium peritonitis
Testicular torsion*	Epididymitis*

Occasionally associated with discomfort.

tion, in prepubertal boys blood flow may be difficult to demonstrate in as many as 30% of normal testes.

The ^{99m}Tc-pertechnetate *testicular flow scan* can demonstrate whether there is blood flow to the testis. After intravenous injection of the radionuclide, flow and static images are obtained. Testicular torsion usually appears as a "cold spot" of absent flow to the affected testis. Inflammatory conditions usually cause hyperemia. Accuracy in demonstrating blood flow is approximately 95%. A false-negative scan may occur in a boy with testicular torsion if the degree of torsion is less than 360 degrees. The test can often be obtained on an emergent basis during the day, but at night it may take 2–3 hr to perform and interpret the study.

TESTICULAR (SPERMATIC CORD) TORSION

Testicular torsion requires prompt diagnosis and treatment to save the testis. Torsion is the most common cause of testicular pain in boys 12 yr and older and is uncommon in those younger than 10 yr. It is caused by inadequate fixation of the testis within the scrotum resulting from a redundant tunica vaginalis, allowing excessive mobility of the testis. The abnormal attachment has been termed a **bell clapper deformity** and is often bilateral. Shortly after torsion occurs, venous congestion begins; subsequently, arterial flow is interrupted. The likelihood of testis survival depends on the duration and severity of torsion. Within 4 to 6 hr of absent blood flow to the testis, spermatogenesis may be lost.

Testicular torsion produces acute pain and swelling of the scrotum. On examination, the scrotum is swollen, tender, and often difficult to examine. The cremasteric reflex is nearly always absent. The condition can be differentiated from an incarcerated hernia because swelling in the inguinal area is often absent. If the pain has lasted less than 4–6 hr, manual detorsion may be attempted. This maneuver is performed by rotating the testis outward (the left testis is rotated clockwise). Successful manual detorsion results in dramatic pain relief.

Treatment is prompt surgical exploration and detorsion. If the testis is explored within 6 hr of torsion, as many as 90% of the gonads will survive. Survival decreases rapidly with a delay of more than 6 hr. If the degree of torsion is 360 degrees or less, the testis may have sufficient arterial flow to allow the gonad to survive, even after 24–48 hr. The testis is then fixed in the scrotum with nonabsorbable sutures, termed **scrotal orchiopexy,** to prevent torsion in the future. The contralateral testis should be fixed in the scrotum because the condition may be bilateral. If the testis appears nonviable, orchiectomy is performed (Fig. 537–1).

Testicular torsion can also occur in the fetus or neonate and results from incomplete attachment of the tunica vaginalis to the scrotal wall and is "extravaginal." When torsion occurs in utero, the baby is usually born with a large, firm, nontender testis. Usually the ipsilateral hemiscrotum is ecchymotic (Fig. 537–2). In these cases, the testis is rarely viable because torsion was a remote event. However, the contralateral testis is at increased risk for torsion until 1 mo beyond term. Many pediatric urologists recommend exploration to establish the diagnosis, remove the necrotic testis, and anchor the contralateral testis. In other cases, the initial examination is normal, and

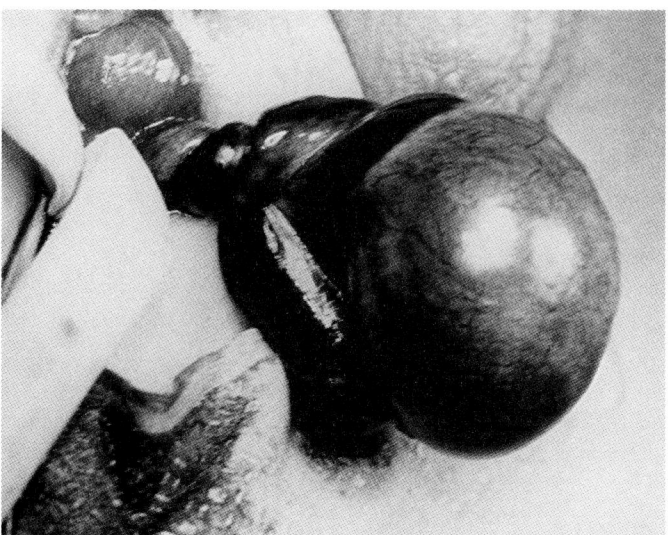

FIGURE 537–1. Left testicular torsion in an adolescent; the testis is necrotic.

acute scrotal swelling is recognized subsequently. In such cases, the testis occasionally may be saved.

TORSION OF THE APPENDIX TESTIS

Torsion of the appendix testis is the most common cause of testicular pain in boys between 2 and 11 yr but is rare in adolescents. The appendix testis is a stalklike structure that is a vestigial embryonic remnant of the müllerian (paramesonephric) ductal system that is attached to the upper pole of the testis. When it undergoes torsion, progressive inflammation and swelling of the testis and epididymis occurs, resulting in testicular pain and scrotal erythema. The onset of pain is usually gradual. Palpation of the testis usually reveals a 3–5 mm tender indurated mass on the upper pole (Fig. 537–3). In some cases, the appendage that has undergone torsion may be visible through the scrotal skin, termed the *blue dot sign*. In some boys,

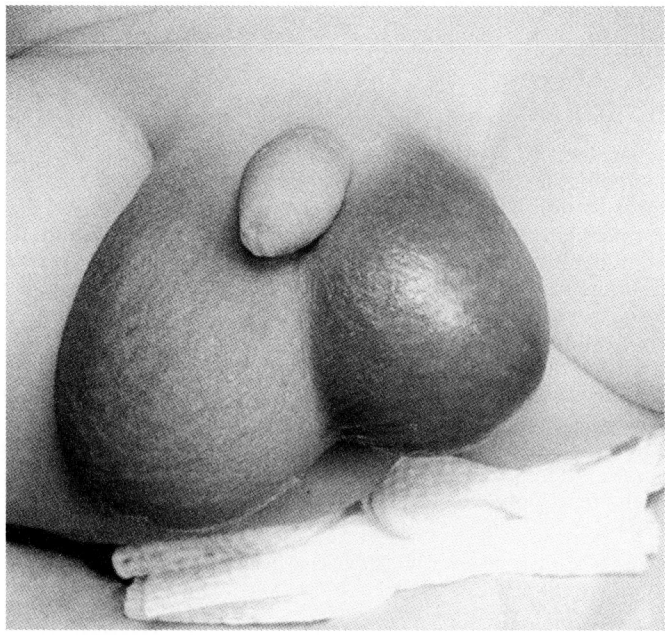

FIGURE 537–2. Left testicular torsion in a newborn. Left hemiscrotum is ecchymotic, and the testis was slightly enlarged, quite firm, and nontender.

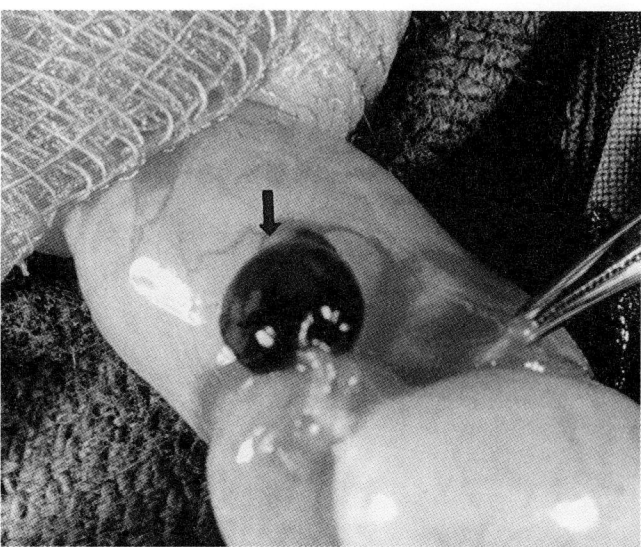

FIGURE 537–3. Torsion of the appendix testis, which is necrotic *(arrow)*.

distinguishing torsion of the appendix from testicular torsion is difficult. In such cases, a testicular flow scan or color Doppler ultrasonography may be helpful.

The natural history of torsion of the appendix testis is for the inflammation to resolve in 3–10 days. Nonoperative treatment is recommended, including bed rest and analgesia with nonsteroidal anti-inflammatory medication for 5 days. If the diagnosis is uncertain, scrotal exploration is recommended.

EPIDIDYMITIS

Acute inflammation of the epididymis is an ascending retrograde infection from the urethra, through the vas into the epididymis. This condition causes acute scrotal pain and swelling. It is rare before puberty and should raise the question of a congenital abnormality of the wolffian duct, such as an ectopic ureter entering the vas. After puberty, epididymitis becomes progressively more common and is the principal cause of acute painful scrotal swelling in young, sexually active adult men. Urinalysis usually reveals pyuria. Epididymitis can be infectious (usually gonococcus, *Chlamydia*), but often the organism remains undetermined. Treatment consists of bed rest and antibiotics. Differentiation from torsion can be difficult, and in children surgical exploration is usually required.

VARICOCELE

A varicocele is an abnormal dilatation of the pampiniform plexus in the scrotum (Fig. 537–4). Dilatation of the pampiniform venous plexus results from valvular incompetence of the spermatic vein. Approximately 15% of adult men have a varicocele; 15% are subfertile. Varicocele is the most common surgically correctable cause of subfertility in men. A varicocele is found in 5% of adolescent boys, but it is rare in boys younger than 10 yr old. Varicoceles occur predominantly on the left side, are bilateral in 10% of cases, and rarely involve the right side only. A varicocele in a boy younger than 10 yr or one on the right side may be indicative of an abdominal or retroperitoneal mass; an ultrasonographic scan should be performed.

A varicocele usually is a painless paratesticular mass, often described as a "bag of worms." Occasionally patients describe a dull ache in the affected testis. Usually the varicocele is decompressed when the patient is supine and prominent when standing. Testicular size should be documented because if the affected testis is small, spermatogenesis probably has been adversely affected.

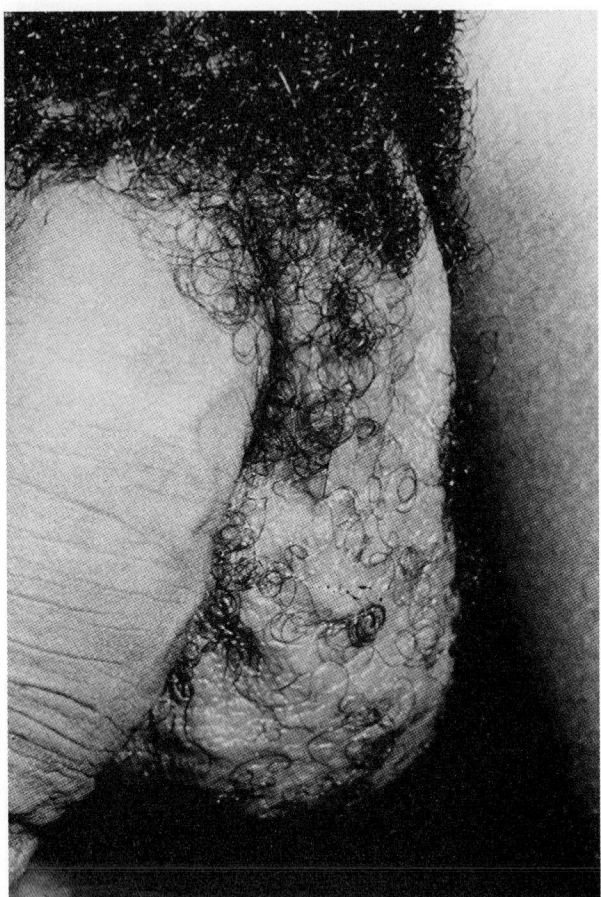

FIGURE 537–4. Left varicocele in an adolescent boy.

The goal of varicocelectomy is to maximize chances for fertility. Surgical treatment of varicoceles in children and adolescents is indicated in boys with a significant disparity in testicular size or pain in the affected testis, or if the contralateral testis is diseased or absent. Typically the involved testis enlarges and catches up with the normal testis over the following 1–2 yr. Varicocelectomy should also be considered in boys with a large varicocele, even without a disparity in testicular size. Surgical repair is performed by ligation of the veins of the pampiniform plexus through an inguinal incision or by ligating the internal spermatic vein in the retroperitoneum. The operation is carried out on an ambulatory basis.

SPERMATOCELE

A spermatocele is a cystic lesion containing sperm that is attached to the upper pole of the sexually mature testis. Spermatoceles are usually painless and are incidental findings on physical examination. Enlargement of the spermatocele or pain is an indication for removal.

HYDROCELE

A hydrocele is an accumulation of fluid in the tunica vaginalis (Fig. 537–5). One to 2% of male neonates have a hydrocele. In most cases, the hydrocele is noncommunicating (the processus vaginalis was obliterated during development). In such cases, the hydrocele fluid disappears by 1 yr of age. If there is a persistently patent processus, the hydrocele persists and becomes progressively larger during the day and is small in the morning. A rare variant of a hydrocele is the *abdominoscrotal hydrocele*, in which there is a large, tense hydrocele that extends into the lower abdominal cavity. In some older boys, a noncommunicating hydrocele may result from an inflammatory condition within the

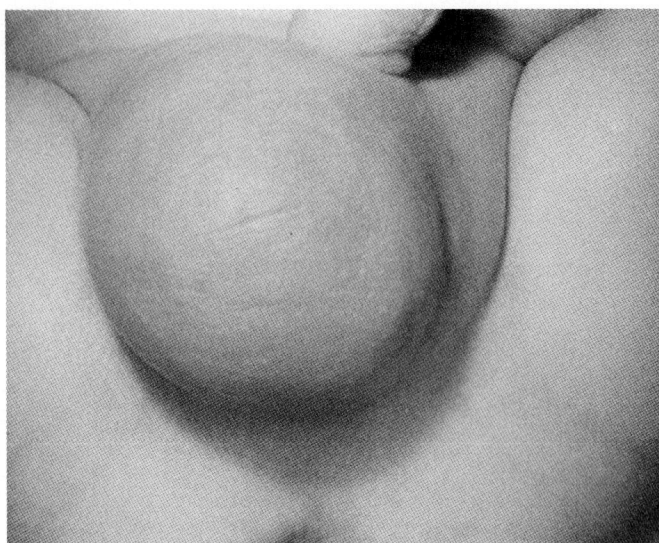

FIGURE 537–5. Newborn with large right hydrocele.

scrotum, such as testicular torsion, torsion of the appendix testis, epididymitis, or testicular tumor. The risk of a communicating hydrocele is the development of an inguinal hernia.

On examination, hydroceles are smooth and nontender. Transillumination of the scrotum confirms the fluid-filled nature of the mass. If compression of the fluid-filled mass completely reduces the size of the hydrocele, an inguinal hernia is the likely diagnosis.

Most hydroceles resolve by 12 mo of age after reabsorption of the hydrocele fluid. If the hydrocele is large and tense, however, early surgical correction is recommended because it is difficult to verify that the child does not have a hernia, and large hydroceles rarely disappear spontaneously. Hydroceles persisting beyond 12–18 mo are usually communicating and should be repaired. Surgical correction is similar to a herniorrhaphy (see Chapter 327). Through an inguinal incision, the spermatic cord is identified, the hydrocele fluid is drained, and a high ligation of the processus vaginalis is performed.

INGUINAL HERNIA

This condition is similar to hydrocele and is discussed in Chapter 327.

TESTICULAR TUMOR

Testicular and paratesticular tumors can occur at any age, including in the newborn. Approximately 65% are malignant; most commonly they are yoke sac tumors. Most present as a painless, hard testicular mass that does not transilluminate. Scrotal ultrasonography should be performed to confirm the finding of a testicular mass and may help to delineate the type of testis tumor. Serum tumor markers, α-fetoprotein and β-human chorionic gonadotropin, should be determined. Definitive therapy includes surgical exploration through an inguinal incision. In most cases a radical orchiectomy, consisting of removal of the entire testis and spermatic cord, is performed, but if the ultrasonographic study or surgical exploration suggests that the tumor is benign, such as a teratoma or epidermoid cyst, removal of the mass only may be performed.

Cortes D, Thorup J, Visfeldt J: Cryptorchidism: Aspects of fertility and neoplasms: A study including data of 1,335 consecutive boys who underwent testicular biopsy simultaneously with surgery for cryptorchidism. *Horm Res* 2001;55:21–27.

Cortes D, Thorup J, Visfeldt J: Hormonal treatment may harm the germ cells in 1- to 3-year-old boys with cryptorchidism. *J Urol* 2000;163:1290–92.

Diamond DA, Paltiel HJ, DiCanzio J, et al: Comparative assessment of pediatric testicular volume: Orchiometer versus ultrasound. *J Urol* 2000;164:1111–14.

Elder JS: Ultrasonography is unnecessary in evaluating boys with a nonpalpable testis. *Pediatrics* 2002, in press.

Gracia JS, Zalabardo JS, Garc J, et al: Clinical, physical, sperm and hormonal data in 251 adults operated on for cryptorchidism in childhood. *BJU Int* 2000;85:1100–1103.

Hadziselimovic F, Herzog B: The importance of both an early orchidopexy and germ cell maturation for fertility. *Lancet* 2001;358:1156–57.

Huff DS, Fenig DM, Canning DA, et al: Abnormal germ cell development in cryptorchidism. *Horm Res* 2001;55:11–17.

Huff DS, Snyder HM III, Rusnack SL, et al: Hormonal therapy for the subfertility of cryptorchidism. *Horm Res* 2001;55:38–40.

Kaefer M, Diamond D, Hendren WH, et al: Incidence of intersexuality in children with cryptorchidism and hypospadias: Stratification based on gonadal palpability and meatal position. *J Urol* 1999;162:1003–7.

Kass EJ, Stork BR, Steinert BW: Varicocele in adolescence induces left and right testicular volume loss. *BJU Int* 2001;87:499–501.

Lee PA, Coughlin MT: The single testis: Paternity after presentation as unilateral cryptorchidism. *J Urol* 2002;168:1680–83.

Lee PA, Coughlin MT: Fertility after bilateral cryptorchidism: Evaluation by paternity, hormone and semen data. *Horm Res* 2001;55:28–32.

Lee PA, Coughlin MT, Bellinger MF: Inhibin B: Comparison with indexes of fertility among formerly cryptorchid and control men. *J Clin Endocrinol Metab* 2001;86:2576–84.

McAleer IM, Kaplan GW: Is routine karyotyping necessary in the evaluation of hypospadias and cryptorchidism? *J Urol* 2001;165:2029–31.

Matteson JR, Stock JA, Hanna MK, et al: Medicolegal aspects of testicular torsion. *Urology* 2001;57:783–86.

Mayr JM, Lawrenz K, Berghold A: Undescended testicles: An epidemiological review. *Acta Paediatr* 1999;88:1089–93.

Nussbaum Blask AR, Bulas D, Shalaby-Rana E, et al: Color Doppler sonography and scintigraphy of the testis: A prospective, comparative analysis in children with acute scrotal pain. *Pediatr Emerg Care* 2002;18:67–71.

Sheldon CA: The pediatric genitourinary examination. Inguinal, urethral, and genital diseases. *Pediatr Clin North Am* 2001;48:1339–80.

Thomas J, Elder JS: Testicular growth arrest and adolescent varicocele: Does varicocele size make a difference? *J Urol* 2002;168:1689–91.

Chapter 538

Trauma to the Genitourinary Tract

Injuries to the genitourinary tract in children usually result from blunt trauma during falls, athletic activities, or motor vehicle accidents. In more than half of the cases there are also major injuries to the brain, spinal cord, skeleton, lungs, or abdominal organs. Children are at greater risk of blunt renal injury than are adults because of less body fat and because the kidneys are not located directly behind the ribs. Children with a pre-existing renal anomaly such as hydronephrosis secondary to a ureteropelvic junction obstruction, horseshoe kidney, or renal ectopia are also at increased risk for renal injury. Blunt abdominal or flank trauma often causes a renal injury. Falling may cause a deceleration injury that results in an injury to the renal pedicle, interrupting blood flow to the kidney. If the bladder is full, blunt lower abdominal trauma may cause a bladder rupture. Rupture of the membranous urethra occurs in 30% of cases of pelvic fractures. Straddle injuries are usually associated with trauma to the bulbous urethra. Symptoms and signs of urinary tract injury include gross or microscopic hematuria, bleeding from the urethral meatus, abdominal or flank pain, a flank mass, fractured lower ribs or lumbar transverse processes, and a perineal or scrotal hematoma.

Evaluation of the patient begins after an adequate airway has been established and the patient is hemodynamically stable (see Chapter 57). With significant abdominal injury, gross hematuria or more than 50 red blood cells per high-power field, or suspicion of renal injury (e.g., deceleration injury, flank pain or bruise), renal imaging is indicated. In addition, the bladder should be catheterized, unless blood is dripping from the urethral meatus, which is an indication of potential urethral injury. Passing the catheter in the presence of a urethral injury may

increase the extent of the damage and convert a partial membranous urethral tear into a total disruption. In these patients, a retrograde urethrogram should be performed by injecting radiopaque contrast medium into the urethral meatus. Oblique radiographs demonstrate the extent of the injury and whether urethral continuity is preserved or has been disrupted.

Spiral computed tomography is performed to evaluate the kidneys, ureters, and bladder. Delayed images are important to detect renal extravasation of blood or urine. Prompt function of both kidneys without extravasation usually excludes significant renal injury. Renal injuries are classified as minor and major. Minor renal injuries are most common and include contusion of the renal parenchyma and shallow cortical lacerations not involving the collecting system. Major renal injuries include deep lacerations involving the collecting system, the shattered kidney, and renal pedicle injuries (Fig. 538–1). Complete absence of function of one kidney without contralateral compensatory hypertrophy (indicative of congenital absence) should be regarded as an indication of major injury to the renal pedicle. Renal angiography, once used to evaluate renal injuries further, particularly if a renal pedicle injury is suspected, is now rarely used because such patients are often hemodynamically unstable, and management is not significantly affected by the findings. In some cases, a pre-existing renal anomaly may be demonstrated on the study. A ruptured ureteropelvic junction obstruction may be apparent if the kidney is intact but the distal ureter is not visualized.

Minor renal injuries such as contusions are managed by bed rest and monitoring of vital signs until abdominal or flank discomfort and gross hematuria has resolved. Children with a *major renal injury* are usually admitted to an intensive care unit for continuous monitoring of vital signs and urine output. Intravenous antibiotics are also administered. These injuries are also managed nonoperatively, because Gerota fascia often causes tamponade of bleeding from the kidney and dramatic healing of the injured parenchyma can occur even with significant urinary extravasation. Approximately 10% of children with a major renal injury undergo surgical exploration because of hemodynamic instability, persistent extravasation, or persistent hematuria or to correct a congenital renal deformity. It can be difficult to identify normal and devitalized parenchyma, and the likelihood of having to perform a nephrectomy is significant. If the child is undergoing exploration for other abdominal injuries, the injured kidney is examined. If there is persistent extravasation because of intermittent ureteral obstruction from a blood clot, passage of a temporary double-J stent endoscopically between the bladder and kidney may allow resolution. If there is a renal pedicle injury, nephrectomy is necessary. The kidney can be salvaged by emergency renal revascularization only if the kidney is explored within 2–3 hr of the injury. All penetrating injuries of the kidneys should be explored. In addition to loss of renal function, the main long-term complication of renal injury is renin-mediated hypertension. Children who sustain renal injuries must have periodic measurement of blood pressure.

Ureteral injuries are usually iatrogenic. Injuries of the ureter by blunt or penetrating trauma require immediate surgical attention.

When the bladder can be catheterized, a static cystogram is obtained, infusing a contrast solution through the catheter by gravity, ideally using fluoroscopy. Flat and oblique views are often obtained; a postvoid film also should be obtained because, in some cases, extravasation may be hidden by the full bladder.

Bladder ruptures can be intraperitoneal or extraperitoneal. All intraperitoneal ruptures require surgical repair. Minor extraperitoneal near-ruptures might be treated by catheter drainage but generally require surgical treatment.

Treatment of a **membranous urethral injury** is controversial. Erectile dysfunction, urethral stricture, and urinary

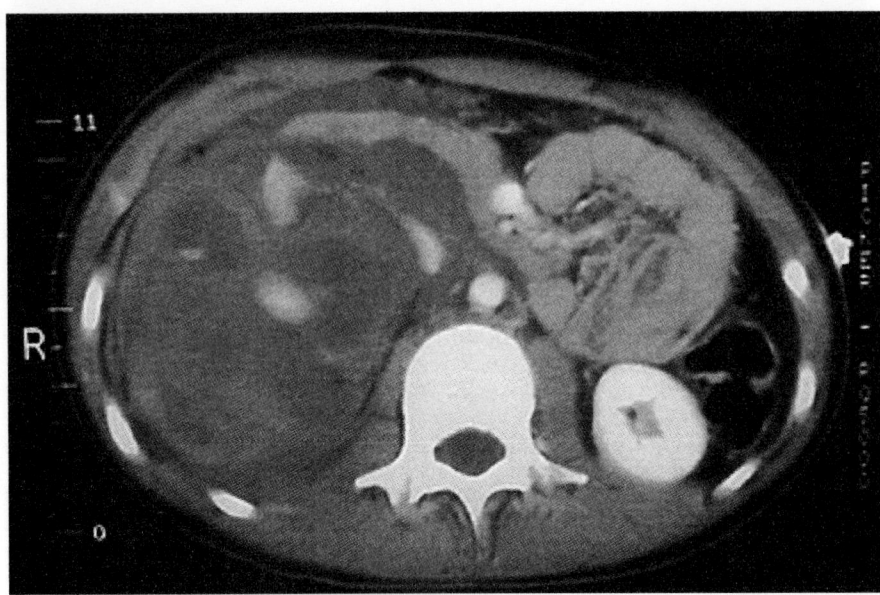

FIGURE 538–1. CT scan of girl who sustained major renal injury from falling off a bicycle demonstrates ruptured right kidney with urinary extravasation.

incontinence are the major late complications of rupture of the membranous urethra, and therapy is directed at minimizing the risk of these problems. There is often a large pelvic hematoma with tamponade, and attempting to repair the injury immediately can be technically difficult and result in significant hemorrhage. Many such injuries are initially managed by temporary suprapubic cystostomy, with continuous bladder drainage for 3–6 mo. Subsequently, open or endoscopic urethroplasty can be performed. Alternatively, some try to achieve urethral continuity under anesthesia and leave a urethral catheter for several months. These patients typically require subsequent open or endoscopic urethroplasty.

Penile injury is uncommon. Some boys who are in the process of toilet training sustain an injury to the glans penis if the lid of the toilet falls while they are urinating. These boys often have a hematoma covering the distal half of the glans. Typically, they have no difficulty urinating and do not need extensive evaluation. Adolescent boys who indulge in extremely vigorous sexual intercourse may sustain rupture of one of the corporal bodies. These boys have severe swelling of the penile shaft and require emergency exploration and repair. Boys with penetrating injuries of the penis also require emergency débridement and repair.

Testicular injuries are relatively uncommon in children because of the small size of the testes and their mobility within the scrotum. Such injuries usually result from blunt trauma during athletic activity. Typically, these boys have significant scrotal swelling, testicular pain, and tenderness. Ultrasonography demonstrates rupture of the tunica albuginea, which is the capsule of the testis, and surrounding hemorrhage. Prompt surgical treatment of testicular injuries increases the salvage rate.

American Academy of Pediatrics, Committee on Sports Medicine and Fitness: Medical conditions affecting sports participation. *Pediatrics* 2001;107: 1205–09.

Brown SL, Haas C, Dinchman KH, et al: Radiologic evaluation of pediatric blunt trauma in patients with microscopic hematuria. *World J Surg* 2001;25:1557–60.

Gerstenbluth RL, Spirnak JP, Elder JS: Sports participation and high-grade renal injuries in children. *J Urol* 2002, in press.

McAleer IM, Kaplan GW, LoSasso BE: Congenital urinary tract anomalies in pediatric renal trauma patients. *J Urol* 2002;168:1808–10.

McAleer IM, Kaplan GW, LoSasso BE: Renal and testis injuries in team sports. *J Urol* 2002;168:1805–07.

Perez-Brayfield MR, Gatti JM, Smith EA, et al: Blunt traumatic hematuria in children: Is a simplified algorithm justified? *J Urol* 2002;167:2543–47.

Podesta ML, Jordan GH: Pelvic fracture urethral injuries in girls. *J Urol* 2001;165:1660–65.

Chapter 539
Urinary Lithiasis

Urinary lithiasis in children is less common in the United States than in other parts of the world. The wide geographic variation in the incidence of lithiasis in childhood is related to climatic, dietary, and socioeconomic factors. Approximately 7% of urinary calculi occur in children younger than 16 yr of age. In the United States, most children with stone disease have a metabolic abnormality. The exceptions are patients with a neuropathic bladder, who are prone to infection-initiated renal stones, and those who have urinary tract reconstruction with intestine, which predisposes to bladder calculi. Metabolic stones are twice as common in boys as in girls and are rare in African-Americans. In Southeast Asia, urinary calculi are endemic and are related to dietary factors.

Stone Formation. The composition and site of urinary calculi vary, depending on the pathogenesis. Most stones are composed of calcium, oxalate, uric acid, cystine, ammonium, or phosphate crystals, or a combination of these substances (Box 539–1). The risk of stone formation is increased with increasing concentrations of these crystals and reduced with increasing concentrations of inhibitors. Renal calculi develop from crystals that form on the calyx and aggregate to form a calculus. Bladder calculi may be stones that formed in the kidney and traveled down the ureter, or they may form primarily in the bladder.

Stone formation depends on four factors. *Matrix* is a mixture of protein, non-amino sugars, glucosamine, water, and organic ash. Matrix makes up 2–9% of the dry weight of urinary stones and is arranged within the stones in organized concentric laminations. *Precipitation-crystallization* refers to supersaturation of the urine with specific ions comprising the crystal. Once a nucleus of crystal forms, the crystals aggregate by chemical and electrical forces. Increasing the saturation of urine with respect to the ions increases the rate of nucleation, crystal growth, and aggregation and increases the likelihood of stone formation and growth. *Epitaxy* refers to the aggregation of crystals of different composition but similar lattice structure, thus forming stones of a heterogeneous nature. The lattice structures of calcium oxalate and monosodium urate have similar structures, and calcium oxalate crystals can aggregate on a nucleus of monosodium urate crystals. Urine also contains *inhibitors* of

BOX 539–1. Classification of Urolithiasis

CALCIUM STONES (CALCIUM OXALATE AND CALCIUM PHOSPHATE)

Hypercalciuria
   Absorptive
   Renal leak
   Resorptive
   Distal renal tubular acidosis (type 1) (calcium phosphate)
   Hyperparathyroidism
   Sarcoidosis
   Furosemide administration
   Vitamin D excess
   Immobilization
   Corticosteroid administration
   Cushing disease
Hyperuricosuria
Heterozygous cystinuria
Hyperoxaluria (calcium oxalate)
   Primary hyperoxaluria, types 1 and 2
   Secondary hyperoxaluria
   Enteric hyperoxaluria
Hypocitruria
Renal tubular acidosis

CYSTINE STONES

Cystinuria

STRUVITE STONES (MAGNESIUM AMMONIUM PHOSPHATE)

Urinary tract infection (urea-splitting organism)
Foreign body
Urinary stasis

URIC ACID STONES

Hyperuricosuria
Lesch-Nyhan syndrome
Myeloproliferative disorders
After chemotherapy
Inflammatory bowel disease

INDINAVIR STONES

NEPHROCALCINOSIS

stone formation, including citrate, diphosphonate, and magnesium ion.

Clinical Manifestations. Children with urolithiasis usually have gross or microscopic hematuria. If the calculus is in the renal pelvis, calyx, or ureter and causes obstruction, then abdominal or flank pain (renal colic) occurs. Typically the pain radiates anteriorly to the scrotum or labia. Often the pain is intermittent, corresponding to periods of obstruction of urine flow, which increases the pressure in the collecting system. If the calculus is in the distal ureter, the child may have irritative symptoms of dysuria, urgency, and frequency. If the stone has passed into the bladder, the child is usually asymptomatic. If the stone is in the urethra, dysuria and difficulty voiding may result. Some children pass small amounts of gravel-like material.

Diagnosis. Approximately 90% of urinary calculi are calcified to some degree and consequently are radiopaque on a plain abdominal film. Some calculi are only a few millimeters in diameter and may not be obvious, particularly if they are in the ureter. Struvite (magnesium ammonium phosphate) stones are radiopaque. Cystine and uric acid calculi may be radiolucent but often are slightly opacified. Some children have **nephrocalcinosis**, which is calcification of the renal tissue itself. Nephrocalcinosis is seen most commonly in premature neonates receiving furosemide, which causes hypercalciuria, and in children with medullary sponge kidney.

In a child with suspected renal colic, a *nonenhanced spiral CT scan of the abdomen and pelvis* is performed in many centers. This study takes only a few minutes to perform, delineates the number and location of calculi, and demonstrates whether the involved kidney is hydronephrotic. In the past, an excretory urogram generally was performed. This test demonstrates a delay in visualization of the collecting system compared with the normal side; and if there is a ureteral calculus, there is columnization of contrast medium down to the stone. If the calculus is radiolucent or small, the urogram may not demonstrate the stone. Consequently, the noncontrast spiral CT scan is preferred. Another alternative is to obtain a plain radiograph of the abdomen and pelvis plus a renal ultrasonogram. If a small calculus is in the ureter, it may not be imaged by these two studies; and if the calculus is not causing impaired urinary flow at the time of the study, the renal ultrasonogram may not show hydronephrosis. In a child with a calculus that already has been diagnosed, however, serial plain films or renal ultrasonography can be used to follow the status of the calculus, such as whether it has grown or diminished in size or moved. If a child has a renal pelvic calculus, a ureteropelvic junction obstruction should be suspected. In some cases, it can be difficult to determine whether hydronephrosis in such a child is secondary to an obstructing stone or the ureteropelvic junction obstruction, or both. Finally, even though a ureteral or renal pelvic stone may be obstructive, a MAG-3 diuretic renogram has no role in assessing whether the stone itself is causing significant obstruction.

Any material that resembles a calculus should be sent for analysis by a laboratory that specializes in the identification of the components of urinary calculi.

METABOLIC EVALUATION. A metabolic evaluation for the most common predisposing factors should be undertaken in all children with urolithiasis, bearing in mind that structural, infectious, and metabolic factors often coexist. This evaluation should not be undertaken in a child who is in the process of passing a stone because the altered diet and hydration status, as well as the effect of obstruction on the kidney, may alter the results of the study. The basic laboratory studies required are listed in Box 539–2, and the normal values for 24-hr urine collections are shown in Table 539–1. In children with hypercalciuria, further studies of calcium excretion with dietary calcium restriction and calcium loading are necessary.

Pathogenesis of Specific Renal Calculi

CALCIUM OXALATE AND CALCIUM PHOSPHATE CALCULI. Most urinary calculi in children in the United States are composed of calcium oxalate or calcium phosphate, or both. The most common metabolic abnormality in these individuals is hypercalciuria. Between 30–60% of children with calcium stones have hypercalciuria without hypercalcemia. Other metabolic aberrations that predispose to stone disease include hyperoxaluria, hyperuricosuria, hypocitruria, heterozygous cystinuria, hypomagnesuria, hyperparathyroidism, and renal tubular acidosis.

BOX 539–2. Laboratory Tests Suggested to Evaluate Urolithiasis

SERUM

Calcium
Phosphorus
Uric acid
Electrolytes and anion gap
Creatinine
Alkaline phosphatase

URINE

Urinalysis
Urine culture
Calcium:creatinine ratio
Spot test for cystinuria
24-hr collection for
   Creatinine clearance
   Calcium
   Phosphate
   Oxalate
   Uric acid
   Dibasic amino acids (if cystine spot test result is positive)

TABLE 539–1. Normal Values for Urine Chemistries in Children

	mg/kg/24 hr
Calcium	<4.0
Oxalate	<0.57
Uric acid	<10.7
Citrate	>2.0
Cystine	
Heterozygote	1.4–2.8
Homozygote	>5.7
Phosphate	<15.0

Hypercalciuria may be absorptive, renal, or resorptive. The primary disturbance in **absorptive hypercalciuria** is intestinal hyperabsorption of calcium. In some children, an increase in 1,25-dihydroxyvitamin D is associated with the increased calcium absorption, and in others the process is independent of vitamin D. **Renal hypercalciuria** refers to impaired renal tubular reabsorption of calcium. Renal leak of calcium causes mild hypocalcemia, which triggers an increased production of parathyroid hormone, with increased intestinal absorption of calcium and increased mobilization of calcium stores. **Resorptive hypercalciuria** is uncommon and is found in patients with primary hyperparathyroidism. Excess parathyroid hormone secretion stimulates intestinal absorption of calcium and mobilization of calcium stores. A brief summary of the metabolic evaluation of children with hypercalciuria is shown in Table 539–2.

Hyperoxaluria is another potentially important cause of calcium stones. Oxalate increases the solubility product of calcium oxalate crystallization 7 to 10 times more than calcium. Consequently, hyperoxaluria significantly increases the likelihood of calcium oxalate precipitation. Oxalate is found in high concentration in tea, coffee, spinach, and rhubarb. *Primary hyperoxaluria* is a rare autosomal recessive disorder that can be subclassified into glycolic aciduria and L-glyceric aciduria. Most patients with primary hyperoxaluria have glycolic aciduria; oxalic and glycolic acids are increased in the urine of affected individuals. Both defects cause increased endogenous production of oxalate, with hyperoxaluria, urolithiasis, nephrocalcinosis, and renal injury. Death from renal failure occurs by age 20 yr in untreated patients. Oxalosis, defined as extrarenal deposition of calcium oxalate, occurs when renal insufficiency is present with elevated plasma oxalate. Calcium oxalate deposits appear first in blood vessels and bone marrow, and with time they appear throughout the body. *Secondary hyperoxaluria* is more common and can occur in patients with increased intake of oxalate and oxalate precursors such as vitamin C, in those with pyridoxine deficiency, and in children with intestinal malabsorption.

Enteric hyperoxaluria refers to disorders such as inflammatory bowel disease, pancreatic insufficiency, and biliary disease, in which there is gastrointestinal malabsorption of fatty acids, which bind intraluminal calcium and form salts that are excreted in the feces. Normally, calcium forms a complex with oxalate to reduce oxalate absorption, but if calcium is unavailable, there is increased absorption of unbound oxalate.

Hypocitruria refers to a low excretion of citrate, which is an inhibitor of calcium stone formation. Citrate acts as an inhibitor of calcium urolithiasis by forming complexes with calcium, increasing the solubility of calcium in the urine, and inhibiting the aggregation of calcium phosphate and calcium oxalate crystals. Disorders such as chronic diarrhea, intestinal malabsorption, and renal tubular acidosis may cause hypocitruria. It may also be idiopathic.

Renal tubular acidosis (RTA) is a syndrome involving a disturbance of acid-base balance within the kidney that can be classified into three types, one of which predisposes to renal calculi that are typically calcium phosphate. In type 1, the distal nephron does not secrete hydrogen ion into the distal tubule. The urine pH is never less than 5.8, and hyperchloremic hypokalemic acidosis results. Patients acquire nephrolithiasis, nephrocalcinosis, muscle weakness, and osteomalacia. Type 1 RTA can be an autosomal dominant disorder, but more often it is acquired and associated with systemic diseases such as Sjögren syndrome, Wilson disease, primary biliary cirrhosis, and lymphocytic thyroiditis, or it results from amphotericin B, lithium, or toluene (an organic solvent associated with glue sniffing).

Five to 8% of individuals with *cystic fibrosis* have urolithiasis. Typically the stones are calcium and often become manifest in adolescence or young adulthood. Microscopic nephrocalcinosis also occurs in younger children with the disease. These patients do not have hypercalciuria, and the propensity for urolithiasis has been speculated to result from an inability to excrete a sodium chloride load or from intestinal malabsorption.

Other disorders may play a role in causing calcium stones. *Hyperuricosuria* may be related to the epitactic growth of calcium oxalate crystals around a nucleus of uric acid crystals or to the action of uric acid as a counterinhibitor of urinary mucopolysaccharides, which inhibit calcium oxalate crystallization. *Heterozygous cystinuria* is found in some patients with calcium stones. The mechanism is unknown but may be similar to that of uric acid. *Sarcoidosis* causes an increased sensitivity to vitamin D_3 and thus an increased absorption of calcium from the gastrointestinal tract. In *Lesch-Nyhan syndrome*, there is excessive uric acid synthesis. These patients are more likely to form uric acid stones, but some of these stones may be calcified. *Immobility* may cause hypercalciuria by mobilization of calcium stores. High-dose *corticosteroids* may cause hypercalciuria and calcium oxalate precipitation. *Furosemide,* which is administered in the neonatal intensive care unit, also can cause severe hypercalciuria, urolithiasis, and nephrocalcinosis.

In some children, calcium calculi are *idiopathic*. This diagnosis should not be given until a complete metabolic evaluation has been performed.

CYSTINE CALCULI. Cystinuria accounts for 1% of renal calculi in children. The condition is a rare autosomal recessive disorder of the epithelial cells of the renal tubule that prevents absorption of the four dibasic amino acids (cystine, ornithine, arginine, and lysine) and results in excessive urinary excretion of these products. The only known complication of this familial disease is the formation of calculi, because of the low solubility of cystine. The patients usually have acidic urine, which leads to a higher rate of precipitation. In the homozygous patient, the daily excretion of cystine usually exceeds 500 mg, and stone

TABLE 539–2. Metabolic Evaluation of Children with Hypercalciuria

	Serum Calcium	Restricted Calcium (Urine)	Fasting Calcium (Urine)	Calcium Load (Urine)	Parathyroid Hormone (Serum)
Absorptive	N	N or I	N	I	I
Renal	N	I	I	I	N
Resorptive	I	I	I	I	I

N = Normal; I = increased.

formation occurs at an early age. Heterozygotes excrete 100 to 300 mg/day and typically do not have clinical urolithiasis. The sulfur content of cystine gives these stones their faint radiopaque appearance.

STRUVITE CALCULI. Urinary tract infections caused by urea-splitting organisms (most often *Proteus*, and occasionally *Klebsiella, Escherichia coli, Pseudomonas,* and others) result in urinary alkalinization and excessive production of ammonia, which can lead to the precipitation of magnesium ammonium phosphate (struvite) and calcium phosphate. In the kidney, often the calculi have a staghorn configuration, filling the calyces. The stones act as foreign bodies, causing obstruction, perpetuating infection, and causing gradual renal damage. Patients with struvite stones may also have metabolic abnormalities that predispose to stone formation. These stones are often seen in children with neuropathic bladder dysfunction, particularly those who have undergone an ileal conduit procedure. In children who have undergone urinary tract reconstruction with augmentation cystoplasty or continent diversion, or both, struvite stones may form in the reconstructed bladder.

URIC ACID CALCULI. Calculi containing uric acid represent less than 5% of all cases of lithiasis in children in the United States but are more common in less developed areas of the world. Hyperuricosuria with or without hyperuricemia is the common underlying factor in most cases. The stones are radiolucent. The diagnosis should be suspected when there is a persistently acid urine and urate crystalluria.

Hyperuricosuria may result from various inborn errors of purine metabolism that lead to overproduction of uric acid, the end product of purine metabolism in humans. Children with the Lesch-Nyhan syndrome and patients with glucose-6-phosphatase deficiency form urate calculi as well. In children with short-bowel syndrome, and particularly those with ileostomies, chronic dehydration and acidosis are sometimes complicated by uric acid lithiasis.

One of the most common causes of uric acid lithiasis is the rapid turnover of purine with some tumors and myeloproliferative diseases. The risk of uric acid lithiasis is especially great when treatment of these diseases causes rapid breakdown of nucleoproteins. Uric acid calculi or "sludge" can fill the entire upper collecting system and cause renal failure and even anuria. Urates are also present within calcium-containing stones. In these cases, more than one predisposing factor for stone formation may exist. A related disorder is *2,8-dihydroxyadeninelithiasis,* which results from a deficiency in adenine phosphoribosyltransferase. The stones are radiolucent and can be differentiated from uric acid calculi by mass spectrometry but not by routine chemical analysis. In contrast to uric acid, which is soluble in alkaline urine, the solubility of 2,8-dihydroxyadenine changes little within physiologic pH ranges.

INDINAVIR CALCULI. Indinavir sulfate is a protease inhibitor approved for the treatment of human immunodeficiency virus infection. As many as 4% of patients acquire symptomatic nephrolithiasis. Most of the calculi are radiolucent and composed of indinavir-based monohydrate, although calcium oxalate or phosphate, or both, have been present in some. After each dose, 12% of the drug is excreted unchanged in the urine. The urine in these patients often contains crystals of characteristic rectangles and fan-shaped or starburst crystals. Indinavir is soluble at a pH of less than 5.5. Consequently, dissolution therapy by urinary acidification with ammonium chloride or ascorbic acid should be considered.

NEPHROCALCINOSIS. Nephrocalcinosis refers to calcium deposition within the renal tissue. Often nephrocalcinosis is associated with urolithiasis. The most common causes are furosemide (administered to premature neonates), distal RTA, hyperparathyroidism, medullary sponge kidney, hypophos-

phatemic rickets, sarcoidosis, cortical necrosis, hyperoxaluria, prolonged immobilization, Cushing syndrome, hyperuricosuria, and renal candidiasis.

Treatment. In a child with a renal or ureteral calculus, the decision whether to remove the stone is dependent on the location, size, and composition (if known) and whether obstruction or infection, or both, is present. Small ureteral calculi often pass spontaneously, although the child may experience severe renal colic. The narrow parts of the ureter include the ureteropelvic junction and the midureter, where it crosses the common iliac artery; the narrowest segment is the ureterovesical junction. In some cases, passage of a ureteral stent past the stone endoscopically allows relief of pain and dilates the ureter sufficiently to allow the calculus to pass. In cases such as children with a uric acid calculus or an infant with a furosemide-associated calculus, dissolution therapy may be effective.

If the calculus does not pass or seems unlikely to pass, or if there is associated urinary tract infection, removal is necessary. Lithotripsy of bladder, ureteral, and small renal pelvic calculi using the holmium laser through a flexible or rigid ureteroscope is most effective. Extracorporeal shock wave lithotripsy has been successfully applied to children with renal and ureteral stones at a success rate of more than 75%.

In children with urolithiasis, treatment of the underlying metabolic disorder should be addressed. Because lithiasis results from having too high a concentration of specific substances in the urine, often an effective method of preventing further stones is by maintaining a continuous high urine output by maintaining a high fluid intake. The high fluid intake should be continued at night, and usually it is necessary to get up at least once at night to urinate and drink more water.

In children with hypercalciuria, some reduction in calcium and sodium intake is necessary, but caution is urged in the growing child. Thiazide diuretics also reduce renal calcium excretion. Addition of potassium citrate, an inhibitor of calcium stones, with a dosage of 1–2 mEq/kg/24 hr is beneficial. An excellent source of citrate is lemonade, because 4 ounces of lemon juice contains 84 mEq of citric acid. A daily mixture of 4 ounces of reconstituted lemon juice in 2 L of water and sweetened to taste should significantly increase the urinary citrate level. In difficult cases, neutral orthophosphate should be given also, although it is poorly tolerated.

In patients with uric acid stones, allopurinol is effective. Allopurinol is an inhibitor of xanthine oxidase and is effective in reducing the production of both uric acid and 2,8-dihydroxyadenine and can help control recurrence of both types of stones. In addition, urinary alkalinization with sodium bicarbonate or sodium citrate is beneficial. The urine pH should be at least 6.5 and can be monitored at home by the family.

Maintaining a high urine pH can also prevent recurrence of cystine calculi. Cystine is much more soluble when the urinary pH is greater than 7.5, and alkalinization of urine with sodium bicarbonate or sodium citrate is effective. Another important medication is D-penicillamine, which is a chelating agent that binds to cysteine or homocystine, increasing the solubility of the product. Although poorly tolerated by many patients, it has been reported to be effective in dissolving cystine stones and in preventing recurrences when hydration and urinary alkalinization fail. *N*-Acetylcysteine appears to have low toxicity and may be effective in controlling cystinuria, but long-term experience with it is lacking.

Treatment of type 1 RTA involves correction of the metabolic acidosis and replacement of potassium and sodium loss. Sodium or potassium citrate therapy, or both, is necessary. When the metabolic acidosis is corrected, the urinary citrate excretion returns to normal.

Treatment of primary hyperoxaluria involves hepatic transplantation because the defective enzymes are hepatic. Ideally, this procedure should be performed before renal failure occurs. In the most severe cases renal transplantation is also necessary.

Borghi L, Schiachi T, Meschi T, et al: Comparison of two diets for the prevention of recurrent stones in idiopathic hypercalciuria. *N Engl J Med* 2002;346:77–84.

Gofrit ON, Pode D, Meretyk S, et al: Is the pediatric ureter as efficient as the adult ureter in transporting fragments following extracorporeal shock wave lithotripsy for renal calculi larger than 10 mm? *J Urol* 2001;166:1862–64.

Hulton S-A: Evaluation of urinary tract calculi in children. *Arch Dis Child* 2001;84:320–23.

Landau EH, Gofrit ON, Shapiro A, et al: Extracorporeal shock wave lithotripsy is highly effective for ureteral calculi in children. *J Urol* 2001;165:2316–19.

Lottmann HB, Traxer O, Archambaud F, et al: Monotherapy extracorporeal shock wave lithotripsy for treatment of staghorn calculi in children. *J Urol* 2001;165:2324–27.

Netto NR, Longo JA, Ikonomidis JA, et al: Extracorporeal shock wave lithotripsy in children. *J Urol* 2002;167:2164–66.

Parekh DJ, Pope JC IV, Adams MC, et al: The association of an increased urinary calcium-to-creatinine ratio, and asymptomatic gross and microscopic hematuria in children. *J Urol* 2002;167:272–74.

Pietrow PK, Pope JC IV, Adams MC, et al: Clinical outcome of pediatric stone disease. *J Urol* 2002;167:670–73.

Saarela T, Lanning P, Koivisto M, et al: Nephrocalcinosis in full-term infants receiving furosemide treatment for congestive heart failure: A study of the incidence and 2-year follow up. *Eur J Pediatr* 1999;158:668–72.

Saarela T, Vaarala A, Lanning P, et al: Incidence, ultrasonic patterns and resolution of nephrocalcinosis in very low birthweight infants. *Acta Paediatr* 1999;88:655–60.

Tekin A, Tekgul S, Atsu N, et al: Cystine calculi in children: Results of metabolic evaluation and response to medical therapy. *J Urol* 2001;165:2328–30.

Van Savage JG, Palanca LG, Andersen RD, et al: Treatment of distal ureteral stones in children: Similarities to American Urological Association Guidelines in adults. *J Urol* 2000;164:1089–93.

Villanyi KK, Szekely JG, Farkas LM, et al: Short-term changes in renal function after extracorporeal shock wave lithotripsy in children. *J Urol* 2001;166:222–24.

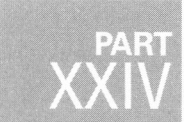
Gynecologic Problems of Childhood

Joseph S. Sanfilippo

Chapter 540

History and Physical Examination

Neonatal Infant. The initial gynecologic assessment of newborn infants should begin with the breast examination. Not uncommonly, as a result of maternal endogenous estrogen production, breast tissue is increased in neonates; nipple discharge may be noted. The abdomen is gently palpated for evidence of organomegaly, and the external genitalia are assessed for any ambiguity. The labia should be grasped gently and separated, allowing inspection of the introitus-hymenal area. Abducting the hips with the labia gently retracted frequently facilitates inspection of the introital area. A normal protuberant hymen with associated thin white mucoid discharge from the vagina is often perceptible. In the first few weeks of life, a small amount of vaginal bleeding may occur, reflecting the decline of circulating levels of maternal estrogens. On completion of the inspection segment of the examination, a rectal examination is performed. A midline structure, indicative of the uterus, is usually palpable, but the adnexa should not be palpable at this time.

Prepubertal Child. A pediatric or adolescent patient undergoing her first gynecologic examination should be treated with particular care, because the initial encounter may well set the stage for all future gynecologic examinations. If the examination is painful or uncomfortable or if there is significant lack of rapport between the patient and the examiner, the child may suffer lasting psychologic consequences. A gentle, caring attitude by the health care provider will go far in enabling the patient to relax.

The history is obtained primarily from the parent(s), who should be integrally involved in the physical examination of a child in this age group. In addition, patients should have a sense of control over the examination, be involved, and should experience no discomfort. These goals are facilitated by providing an adequate explanation before the examination.

Much information can be obtained by inspection of the vulvovaginal area. Ideally, a patient is placed in a frog-leg position. If this is not satisfactory, then a knee-chest position with a Valsalva maneuver allows adequate assessment of the introital (lower-third) vaginal area. Magnification often can be accomplished with use of a colposcope or hand-held magnifying glass; appropriate documentation is also important. Visualizing the vestibule permits assessment of any discharge. Aspiration of any fluid in the vagina and lavage should be carried out with aseptic technique: An intravenous tubing (butterfly) is passed into a soft number 12-bladder catheter, all of which is then attached to a 1-mL tuberculin syringe. Wet mounts can be obtained and evaluated as indicated. Cultures should be taken for evaluation of vulvovaginitis. Other instrumentation used for the genital examination includes an otoscope or Cameron-Myers vaginoscope. Gentle traction on the labia upward and outward further exposes the vaginal introitus for assessment. Calcium alginate (Calgi) swabs are also useful, especially for obtaining cultures from the vagina. A number of variations of the normal-appearing hymen occur, and care must be taken to determine if a patient has an imperforate, microperforate, or septate hymen. If an inadequate examination is accomplished in an office-clinic setting, then sedation or examination under anesthesia should be considered.

Adolescent. Obtaining a history in this age group may initially take place in the presence of the patient's parents. However, an adolescent should be made aware of the concept of confidentiality and be given the opportunity to provide her own history without the parents being present. This can be accomplished in the examination room before the physical examination. Concern for the presence of vaginal discharge, the potential for sexually transmitted disease, pregnancy, or menstrual aberration should be explored. Physicians should win the confidence of the adolescent, provide a relaxed atmosphere for the examination, and communicate one's availability for consultation. Also see Chapters 14, 17, and 100. Indications for the first pelvic examination in adolescents are presented in Box 540–1.

If an adolescent does not have one of the criteria listed in Box 540–1, the American College of Obstetricians and Gynecologists recommends that the first "gynecologic encounter" be between the age of 14 and 18 yr. This encounter does not necessitate a pelvic examination but is an opportunity for the physician to provide education for the adolescent.

One suggestion for the adolescent interview is the use of **HEADSS is VG.** This mnemonic is outlined below:

Home—Household, family dynamics and relationships, living arrangements.

Education—School attendance, failed a grade, grades as compared to last year's grades, attitude toward school, most difficult and best subjects, goals: college, career.

Activities—Physical activity, sports, exercise, hobbies, friends, after school, weekends.

Drugs—Cigarettes/smokeless tobacco, alcohol and/or other drugs: use at school or parties; use by friends, self; frequency, and quantity used.

Sexuality—Sexual feelings: Opposite or same sex, sexual intercourse: Age at first intercourse, number of lifetime and current partners, recent change in partners, contraception, sexually transmitted infection, prior pregnancies, abortions.

Suicide/depression—Feelings about self, history of depression or other mental health problems, prior suicidal thoughts, prior suicide attempts, sleep problems.

> **BOX 540–1. Suggested Indications for Pelvic Examination in Adolescents**
>
> Age 18
> Sexually active
> Past or current
>   Menstrual irregularities
>   Severe dysmenorrhea
>   Unexplained abdominal pain
>   Unexplained dysuria
>   Abnormal vaginal discharge
>
> ---
>
> Modified from The adolescent obstetric-gynecologic patient. *ACOG Technical Bull* 1990;145:3.

Violence—How are conflicts handled in the home (i.e., late for curfew), school, work, guns in the home, weapon carrying, nonconsensual sex, physical contact.

Gangs—Member, friends in gangs, number present in high school, gang markings on skin.

The most important factor with respect to the interview is to establish rapport. During this time the rules of confidentiality should be emphasized with the patient. Sufficient time should be allowed for the office visit. This segment of the interview process (history) should be one-on-one patient and physician.

Pelvic Examination. The teenage patient, in a manner similar to that for a pediatric patient, should be involved in the pelvic examination. The examination is best performed in the absence of the parents, but a female chaperone should be present and may serve to neutralize any adverse psychosocial aspects of the situation. Communication should occur between the physician and the patient throughout the examination. The examination should be performed in the dorsal lithotomy position with an effort made to maintain eye contact. Appropriate-sized specula should be available, including the small Pedersen's (8 cm in depth). The 4–5-cm speculum is best avoided because it usually results in inadequate visualization; however, the pediatric-sized Huffman speculum is appropriate.

Inspection of the vulva is followed by palpation of the Bartholin's–urethral Skene's glands. The clitoris, which is normally 2–4 mm wide, is then assessed. A clitoris wider than 10 mm, especially in the presence of other signs of virilization, is abnormal. The hymenal configuration should also be evaluated. A patient should be told immediately prior to the insertion of the speculum that she will experience a pressure sensation. Before touching the introitus, it is useful to touch the inner thigh with the speculum. Trauma to the urethra should be avoided, and displacement of the fourchette posteriorly further facilitates proper speculum placement. Discussion with the adolescent about techniques to relax the perineal musculature is often helpful.

Once the speculum portion of the examination is complete, a bimanual examination is undertaken. In a virginal female, a single digit examination with an appropriately lubricated, gloved finger allows proper palpation of the vaginal walls and cervix and bimanual assessment of the uterus and the adnexa. The cul-de-sac is assessed, and a rectovaginal examination performed to complete the bimanual examination.

A number of resources for education of adolescents regarding their first pelvic examination are available. These include:

- North American Society for Pediatric and Adolescent Gynecology. HTTP://www.naspag.org
- The Society for Adolescent Medicine. HTTP://www.adolescent.health.org
- Aware Foundation. HTTP://www.aware foundation.org
- Association of Reproductive Health Professionals. HTTP://www.arhp.org
- GYN101. HTTP://www.gyn101.com

A "tool kit" is available through the American College of Obstetricians and Gynecologists; it includes information on how to establish an office-friendly environment for the adolescent gynecologic evaluation, tools for adolescent assessment, suggestions about how to talk with teens, handouts for adolescents, and a number of resources for health care professionals. (Address: 409 12th Street, SW, PO Box 96920, Washington, DC 20090-6920.)

Cavanaugh R: Obtaining a personal and confidential history from adolescents. An opportunity for prevention. *J Adolesc Health Care* 1986;2:118.

Phillips S, Bohannon W, Heald F: Teenager's choices regarding the presence of family members during the examination of genitalia. *J Adolesc Health Care* 1986;7:245.

Pokorny SF: Pediatric vulvovaginitis. In Kaufman R, Friedrich E, Gardner H (editors): *Benign Diseases of the Vulva and Vagina.* Chicago, Year Book Medical Publishers, 1989, p 55.

Pokorny SF, Stormer J: Atraumatic removal of secretions from the prepubertal vagina. *Am J Obstet Gynecol* 1987;156:5.

Ricciardi R: First pelvic examination in the adolescent. *Nurse Practitioner Forum* 2000;113:161.

Saipik R: Adolescent contraception. In Sanfilippo JS, Muran D, Dewrurst J, Lee P (editors): *Pediatric Adolescent Gynecology,* 2nd edition. Philadelphia, WB Saunders, 2001, pp 305–17.

Sanders JM Jr, Durant RH, Chastain DO: Pediatricians' use of chaperones when performing gynecologic examinations on adolescent females. *J Adolesc Health Care* 1989;10:110.

Talbot CW: The gynecologic examination of the pediatric patient. *Pediatr Ann* 1986;15:501.

Chapter 541
Vulvovaginitis

Vulvovaginitis is the most common childhood or adolescent gynecologic problem. The main clinical manifestations, in order of frequency, include vaginal discharge, erythema, and pruritus. Vulvovaginal irritation results from the lack of labial fat pads and pubic hair for protection of the external genitalia. The labia minora tend to open when a child squats; this, in turn, causes exposure of the sensitive tissues within the hymenal ring. In addition, the close proximity of the anal orifice to the vagina allows transfer of fecal bacteria to the vulvovaginal area. Masturbation may also be a contributing factor.

In the relatively low estrogenic prepubertal environment, the thin atrophic vaginal epithelium is susceptible to bacterial invasion. Recurrent vulvovaginitis usually ceases once a girl reaches puberty, estrogen increases, and the pH of the vagina becomes more acidic. In part, this change results from increased production of acetic and lactic acids, a phenomenon accompanied by an increase in superficial cell proliferation and glycogen as well as by enhancement of normal bacterial flora (Table 541–1).

Vaginal culture, cytology, and vaginoscopy may be indicated for evaluation of pediatric patients with vulvovaginitis. Leukocyte esterase dipsticks are a rapid screening test for vaginitis and cervicitis. The technique has been used to identify trichomonads, *Candida*, and bacterial vaginosis and to evaluate cervical secretions for identification of gonococcal and chlamydial infections.

Physiologic Leukorrhea. This discharge reflects circulating estrogen levels. Treatment consists of reassurance that this normal process is self-limited.

Pathologic Vaginal Discharge. In pediatric patients, vaginal discharge is a common presenting complaint. It is often the primary symptom of vulvitis, vaginitis, or vulvovaginitis. Pruritus, frequent urination, dysuria, or enuresis may be associated signs and symptoms. Vulvitis is manifested primarily by dysuria and pruritus and is associated with erythema of the vulva. It commonly has a more protracted course than vaginitis; the latter is characterized by discharge without associated dysuria, pruritus, or erythema. Vulvovaginitis involves a combination of these manifestations. The color, odor, and duration of the discharge should be noted. Although there are a number of causes of vulvovaginitis in pediatric patients, the more common ones include poor perineal hygiene, *Candida* infection, and a foreign body.

Nonspecific Vulvovaginitis. Patients with poor perineal hygiene often develop a condition known as nonspecific vulvovaginitis. This condition accounts for 70% of all pediatric vulvovaginitis cases. The discharge is characteristically brown or green, has a fetid odor, and is associated with vaginal pH of 4.7–6. In 68% of reported cases, this vaginitis is associated with coliform bacteria

TABLE 541–1. Specific Vulvovaginitis

Organism	Presentation	Diagnosis	Treatment
Enterobiasis (pinworms)	Perineal pruritus (nocturnal); gastrointestinal symptoms; variable vulvovaginal contamination from feces	Adult worms in stool or eggs on perianal skin	Mebendazole; repeat in 3 wk if necessary
Giardiasis	Asymptomatic fecal contaminant, vaginal discharge, diarrhea, malabsorption syndrome	Protozoal flagellate (cyst or trophozoites) in feces	Metronidazole or quinacrine
Molluscum contagiosum	Vulvar lesions, nodules with umbilicated area; white core of curdlike material	Isolation of poxvirus	Dermal curettage of papule
Phthirus pubis (pediculosis pubis)	Pruritus, excoriation, sky-blue macules; inner thigh or lower abdomen	Nits on hair shafts, lice—skin or clothing	Lindane lotion (Kwell); also see Chapter 658
Sarcoptes scabiei (scabies)	Nocturnal pruritus, pruritic vesicles, pustules in runs	Mites; ova black, dots of feces (microscopic)	1% lindane
Shigella species (shigellosis)	Fever, malaise, fecal contamination, diarrhea; blood and mucus, cramps, pus in stool	Stools; white blood cells and red blood cells, positive for *Shigella*	Trimethoprim and sulfamethoxazole; chloramphenicol, ampicillin, or tetracycline
Staphylococcus and *Streptococcus*	Vaginal discharge to vulvovaginal area; spread from primary lesion	Positive culture results of appropriate organism	Penicillin or cephalosporin

From Sanfilippo J: Adolescent girls with vaginal discharge. Pediatr Ann *1986;15:509.*

secondary to fecal contamination. The next most common bacterial organisms associated with nonspecific vulvovaginitis are hemolytic *Streptococcus* and coagulase-positive *Staphylococcus.* These organisms are often transmitted manually from the nasopharynx. Clothing, chemicals, cosmetics, and soap products or detergents used for bathing or laundry may also cause irritation that leads to nonspecific vulvovaginitis. Tight-fitting clothing, such as jeans, leotards, and tights, as well as rubber pants or plastic-coated paper diapers, have also been implicated. Nonspecific vulvovaginitis occasionally can result in chronic infection, which may cause significant psychologic consequences for a child and her parents alike. Physical examination should emphasize the importance of avoiding "vaginal fixation," while encouraging proper perineal hygiene.

Successful treatment of nonspecific vulvovaginitis should include instruction in perineal hygiene, switching from tight-fitting underwear, the use of sitz baths with mild soap, and air-drying the vulva. Patients should be instructed in appropriate bowel and bladder habits, emphasizing the need to wipe fecal material away from the vulvovaginal area. Recurrent vulvovaginitis should be treated with systemic antibiotics such as amoxicillin or cephalosporins. Topical estrogen cream or polysporin ointment is often helpful.

Specific Vulvovaginitis. *Gardnerella vaginalis* is the most common organism cultured in pediatric or adolescent patients with vulvovaginitis, followed by *Candida.* Other identified organisms include enterococci and anaerobic bacteria such as *Peptococcus, Peptostreptococcus, Veillonella parvula, Eubacterium, Propionibacterium,* and *Bacteroides* species. Protozoa, helminths, and viruses should also be considered as etiologic agents. Treatment depends on the offending organism (see Table 541–1).

Vaginal Cysts. These cysts are uncommon and frequently incidental findings. They represent rests of the wolffian or müllerian ducts or an epithelial inclusion cyst. Management depends on their location and appearance. They are usually observed, but resection is recommended if they become symptomatic.

Gartner Duct Cyst. These represent a rudimentary portion of wolffian duct. In girls, the duct usually regresses completely. However, it may have remnants along the anterolateral walls of the vagina. The cysts have been associated with dyspareunia in sexually active adolescents. This symptomatology warrants surgical resection.

Clitoral Synechiae. These are often associated with pruritus involving the clitoral area and may result from rubbing of the anterior genital area during ambulation. Erythema is variable. The examination should attempt to gently slide the clitoral skin fold back from the glans clitoris. The clitoral hood appears to be agglutinated to the glans clitoris and may be painful when evaluated. Treatment consists of applying estrogen cream to the peri-clitoral area daily over a 1–2-wk period. This usually suffices; however, surgical intervention may be warranted.

Labial Adhesions. In this disorder, the labia minora have a central line of adherence from an area immediately inferior to the clitoris to the fourchette (Fig. 541–1). Labial adhesions are commonly seen in patients younger than 6 yr of age, and the condition is often asymptomatic. The lesions usually are associated with local inflammation and the hypoestrogenic state of preadolescents. Pooling of urine in the vagina and recurrent vulvovaginitis provide a continuous nidus for recurrent urinary tract infections. These urinary symptoms occur in 20–40% of patients and should be treated.

Topical estrogen cream applied each evening for 1 wk is the treatment of choice and is effective in over 90% of reported cases. Cleansing followed by periodic application of a bland ointment such as petrolatum or zinc oxide should continue for 1–2 mo after the adhesions separate to prevent recurrence.

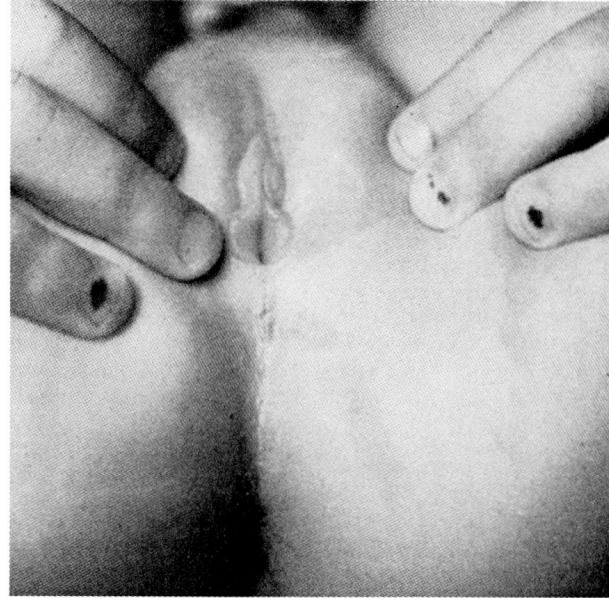

FIGURE 541–1. Labial adhesions. See also color plates.

Mechanical separation of the adhesions is advisable only if the adhesions appear to separate easily and if it does not cause significant trauma. Once the adhesions are separated, the patient should be re-examined for any predisposing cause, such as the presence of a vaginal septum.

Candidiasis. *Candida* infection is often associated with a diaper rash. *Candida* vulvovaginitis, though rare in children, must be considered, especially for girls with chronic mucocutaneous candidiasis. The presence of *Candida*-infected tissue may be indicative of significant immunosuppression. Underlying factors such as diabetes mellitus should be considered. Treatment with an imidazole cream (e.g., clotrimazole) is frequently effective, except in cases of chronic mucocutaneous candidiasis. Also see Chapter 215.

Molluscum Contagiosum. This common infection of the skin is caused by molluscum contagiosum virus, or poxvirus. Molluscum contagiosum presents as an umbilicated, dome-shaped papule. The central umbilication is usually associated with a pulpy core. Vulvar lesions appear to result from autoinoculation or from close contact (sexual or nonsexual) with an infected individual. The incubation period is 2–7 wk. Diagnosis is confirmed by light microscopic visualization of viral inclusions (molluscum bodies) in the central core. Treatment requires elimination of the lesions, usually by gentle curettage; other methods of therapy include cryosurgery or electrocautery.

Intertrigo. Intertrigo can occur in the genitocrural areas in association with friction, obesity, and moisture in the area. Miliaria and secondary infection can also occur in association with intertrigo. The affected areas are red and macerated. Careful hygiene, combined with bland emollients and sometimes a mild corticosteroid, is an effective treatment.

Impetigo. This entity is commonly identified during the first several weeks of life. It is usually caused by *Staphylococcus aureus*, often phage group II, type 71, which may be acquired from the mother, other relatives, or staff. Impetigo tends to affect the vulva and periumbilical areas, causing lesions or blisters that later become crusted. Extensive spread and complications may ensue if treatment with antibiotics is not promptly instituted. Also see Chapter 166.

Malassezia Furfur. This condition is caused by *Pityrosporum orbiculare* and is manifested by scaly macules on the trunk in postpubertal patients, but lesions have been reported on the face and genital area. The diagnosis is established by visualization of hyphae and spores on wet preparation with 10% potassium hydroxide. Treatment requires application of topical imidazoles (e.g., clotrimazole). Also see Chapter 217.

Herpes Simplex Virus. Herpes simplex virus (HSV) types 1 and 2 involve the vulvar area. The types are not exclusively site specific, but type 2 is commonly responsible for genital lesions and type 1, in general, for facial-oral lesions. The infection is characterized by papules that become vesicles, with the virus affecting the dorsal root ganglia. Differential diagnoses include any eroded or blistering lesions as well as herpes zoster. A definitive diagnosis is established by culturing the virus or visualizing it via electron microscopy. Treatment with topical acyclovir reduces viral shedding and accelerates healing. See Chapter 231.

Human Papillomavirus (HPV). HPV is associated with a number of serotypes, including 6, 11, 16, and 18, which usually are noted in the anogenital region. Types 16 and 18 are particularly associated with malignant and premalignant lesions of the vulva. Differential diagnoses include molluscum contagiosum, condyloma acuminatum, and vulvar intraepithelial neoplasia. The possibility of child sexual abuse must be strongly considered

when these lesions are identified. Treatment is based upon presenting signs and symptoms. See Chapter 243.

Lichen Sclerosus

CLINICAL MANIFESTATIONS. This is a chronic atrophic skin disease characterized by small, pink to ivory, flat-topped papules that are several millimeters in diameter. The papules appear to coalesce into plaques that become wrinkled and atrophic. The anogenital lesions frequently resemble an hourglass or a figure 8 (Fig. 541–2). Vesicles and bullae may spread over the vulva with associated hemorrhage. Lichen sclerosus commonly presents in the prepubertal patient; 10–15% of all cases of lichen sclerosus occur in children. Also see Chapter 645.

The onset of lichen sclerosus in most children usually occurs before 7 yr of age. The youngest reported patient was an infant several weeks old. The onset of menarche often results in spontaneous improvement of the lesions, but the process usually continues. Patients are often intermittently symptomatic, and there is no relationship between menarche and symptomatic improvement or resolution of the disease. Atrophy of the labia minora and clitoral phimosis, as well as contracture of the introitus, may occur.

ETIOLOGY. The cause of lichen sclerosus is unknown, but it is believed to be related to an autoimmune disorder. There is an association with certain HLA types. Family clusters have now been documented. There may be a relationship between lichen sclerosus and morphea (localized scleroderma or the spirochete *Borrelia*). Decreased 5-alpha reductase activity has also been proposed as a possible cause for lichen sclerosus. Positive immunofluorescence for fibrin, serum complement (C3), or immunoglobulin M (IgM) in the involved area has been demonstrated in 75% of patients.

TREATMENT. This is symptomatic; emollients and topical corticosteroids usually provide relief. Corticosteroids are the treatment of choice for lichen sclerosus in adults and have been efficacious in children as well. Initially, 1–2% hydrocortisone cream is used. If there is failure to respond, a short course of betamethasone dipropionate 0.05% or clotrimazole is recommended. Minimal side effects are associated with this treatment. After the initial response, a milder topical corticosteroid may be used to prevent recurrence. Topical estrogens and androgens also have been advocated, but these agents may produce a vagi-

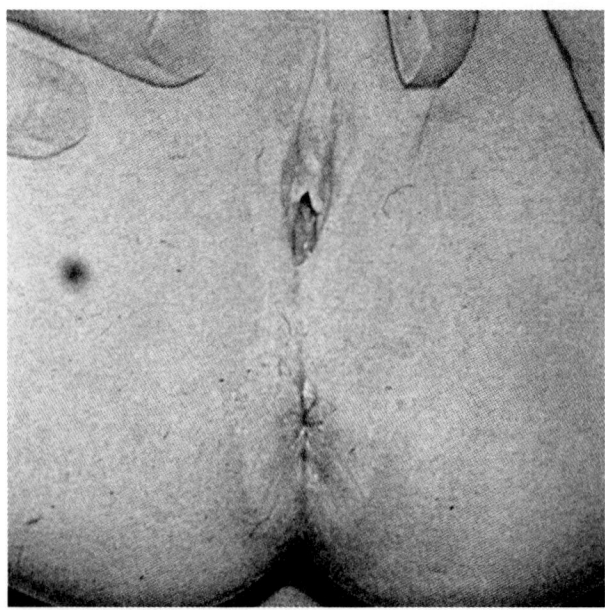

FIGURE 541–2. Lichen sclerosus.

nal discharge as well as other secondary problems, such as breast development and clitoral enlargement. Secondary infections should be treated with antibiotics. Some affected individuals demonstrate Koebner phenomenon; these individuals should avoid tight-fitting clothing and genital trauma. Laser vaporization has also been advocated.

Lichen Planus. Vulvar lichen planus is often associated with oral mucosal and subcutaneous lesions. The vulvar lesions are characterized by angular violaceous, flat-topped papules and may simulate leukoplakia. In addition, the oral lesions consist of minute white papules that form a lacy pattern and usually are located on the buccal mucosa. The lesions are intensely pruritic and may become excoriated and macerated; erosions and ulcerations may occur in severe cases. Diagnosis requires biopsy. Exacerbation or recurrence of the lesions is common.

Treatment consists of topical intralesional corticosteroids and antihistamines to control the pruritus. Squamous cell carcinoma may occur with long-standing, hypertrophic, vulvar lichen planus; therefore, long-term follow-up and histologic examination of any changes or otherwise suspicious areas is advisable.

Lichen Simplex Chronicus (Neurodermatitis). This is a chronic, lichenified plaque that causes pruritus. It results from persistent rubbing and scratching of the vulvar skin; excoriations and fissuring occur. The labia have the appearance of white, hypertrophic, edematous lesions. The changes can occur on the mons pubis as well as the labia majora. Scratching and inflammation may result, causing a vicious cycle. The condition is rare in children. Treatment with antihistamines and topical or intralesional corticosteroids is recommended. Triamcinolone (5–10 mg/mL) has been utilized for intralesional injection.

Seborrheic Dermatitis. This presents as erythematous, oily, circumscribed patches that can be found on the face, scalp and chest as well as on the intertriginous areas of the body. There may also be fissures and associated secondary infection around the vulva; secondary bacterial or candidal infection is quite common, causing pain, pruritus, dysuria, and vaginal bleeding. Acute episodes are best *treated* with sitz bath or topical aluminum acetate solution (Burow solution). Exacerbating factors, such as tight clothing or rubber pants, should be eliminated. Systemic antibiotics with appropriate topical antifungal medication should be administered for secondary infection.

Atopic Dermatitis. This affects 3% of all children (also see Chapter 135). Patients present with hay fever or asthma or both, and generally a family history is noted. The vulvar lesion is characterized as a chronic condition accompanied by intense pruritus, erythema, papules, and vesicles, with oozing and crusting of the involved areas. Associated circumscribed, lichenified scaly patches may be seen on the vulvar area. Pruritus often causes scratching, which results in excoriation of the lesions. Secondary bacterial or candidal infection is common.

Antihistamines are necessary for control of pruritus. Sitz baths with mild soap and lubricants are helpful. Topical corticosteroids such as 1% hydrocortisone are also effective. Secondary bacterial or candidal infections require specific treatment.

Dermatitis. In either allergic or irritant contact dermatitis, the vulva may be affected by edematous, erythematous, oozing lesions that are sometimes accompanied by vesicles or pustules. Chronic contact dermatitis is often associated with thickened and lichenified lesions. The clue to correct diagnosis of this condition is the limitation of the dermatitis to the area of contact with the etiologic agent. There may also be a secondary candidal or bacterial infection. Some common etiologic agents are soaps, powders, bubble baths, feminine hygiene sprays, topical medications, toilet paper, rubber, and certain types of clothing.

Treatment should include avoidance of the offending agents and sitz baths, or compresses with topical aluminum acetate solution (Burow solution) during acute episodes. Mild topical corticosteroids such as 0.5–1% hydrocortisone cream applied several times daily may further aid healing and alleviate vulvar irritation. Recurrence can be prevented by removal of the offending etiologic agent.

Folliculitis. This can occur either spontaneously or secondary to shaving or other depilatory methods such as waxing. It results in a papulopustular eruption secondary to inflammation of the hair follicle. It may occur in any hair-bearing skin. On physical examination pustules are identified ranging in size from 2–10 mm. The pustules may be pierced in the center by a visible hair. The pustules become replaced by red papules. *Staphylococcus aureus* is the most common agent; however, *Pseudomonas aeruginosa* can also occur. The latter is associated with "hot tub folliculitis." Treatment includes sitz baths and cleansing with povidone-iodine solution once or twice a day. When *Staphylococcus* infections do not respond, treatment is with doxycycline, cephalosporins, or erythromycin.

Vulvar Psoriasis. This is frequently associated with lesions of other parts of the body and is characterized by violaceous papules or plaques with a thick, adherent, silvery scale (Fig. 541–3). The intertriginous areas may show "inverse" psoriasis, a variation that does not occur on the extremities. Vulvar lesions are poorly demarcated and may present as scaly patches, most commonly on the mons pubis. The vulvar lesions are often resistant to therapy. A corticosteroid cream (e.g., 1% hydrocortisone) should be used in conjunction with control of secondary infection and pruritus.

Enterobiasis. Pinworms (*Enterobius vermicularis*) are helminths that may carry colonic bacteria to the perineum, causing recurrent vulvovaginitis (also see Chapter 271). Female pinworms emerge from the anus to deposit eggs. Vulvovaginitis develops in about 20% of girls infected with *E. vermicularis*. The plastic tape test should be used to search for the organism if it is suspected or in cases of undiagnosed recurrent vulvovaginitis. Victims typically have pruritus and nocturnal episodes of scratching. Treatment consists of pyrantel pamoate (see Table 541–1).

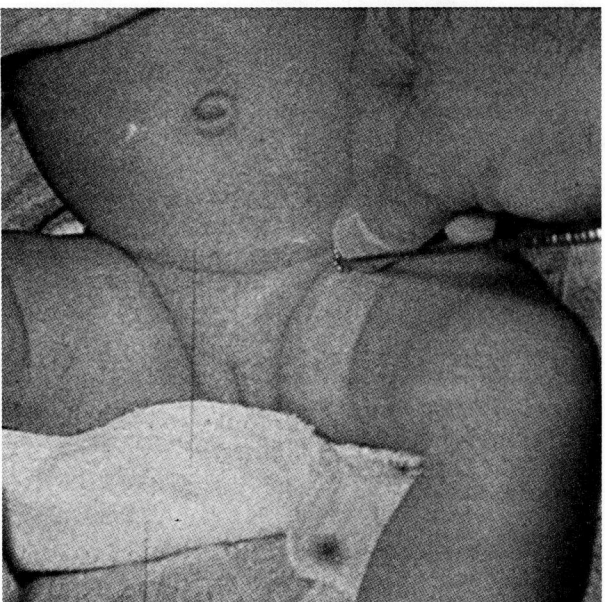

FIGURE 541–3. Vulvar psoriasis. See also color plates.

Shigellosis. *Shigella flexneri* and *S. sonnei* cause various gastrointestinal symptoms in association with vaginitis. Forty-seven per cent of patients present with a bloody vaginal discharge and 2% with diarrhea. Systemic antibiotics are the treatment of choice. Bowel colonization with *Shigella* can result in subclinical gastrointestinal symptoms in 10% of household members. See Chapter 182.

Vitiligo. This presents as sharply demarcated pink to ivory patches that tend to spread and coalesce (Fig. 541–4). The skin on the patch is smooth and shows no palpable changes. It may be differentiated from lichen sclerosus because the hyperpigmented patches are asymptomatic. No treatment is necessary unless cosmetic problems result.

Aphthous Ulcers. Aphthous ulcers of the genital region as well as oral mucosa range in size from 1–10 mm and have a grayish-yellow base. These ulcers may recur and last at least 7–10 days. The etiology remains unclear. Vulva lesions can be treated with topical corticosteroids and if necessary topical anesthetics.

Drug Reactions Associated with Vulvar Lesions. Erythema multiforme can present with genital ulcers complementing lesions on the palms, soles, and other parts of the body. The lesions usually persist for approximately 1 wk. They may represent an allergic reaction to a medication or a preceding flare-up of herpes simplex.

Stevens-Johnson Syndrome. This is a variant of erythema multiforme with more severe mucosal membrane involvement. Medications that cause Stevens-Johnson syndrome include nonsteroidal antiinflammatory agents, sulfonamides, and some anticonvulsive drugs. *Mycoplasma pneumoniae* can also cause this syndrome. In general, the prodromal period is 1–14 days and is characterized by fever, headaches, sore throat, and malaise. There may also be vomiting and diarrhea. The oral mucosa and the eyes can be affected simultaneously. Also see Chapters 138 and 139.

Toxic Epidermal Necrolysis. These lesions are secondary to a number of medications; 20–30% of patients die. The skin appears to be scalded, vulvar erosion and ulceration can be extensive. Resulting vulvar synechiae and atrophy can produce dyspareunia. See Chapter 647.

Labial Hypertrophy. Hypertrophy of the labia minora is uncommon. It may occur either unilaterally or bilaterally. Occasionally, it is symptomatic; the patient complains of irritation or discomfort with walking, riding, biking, or intercourse. In the asymptomatic patient, treatment includes reassurance. However, in the symptomatic patient the excessive tissue can be excised and the skin re-approximated with interrupted sutures or a subcuticular closure. The patient may require a Foley catheter immediately postoperatively.

Crohn Disease. This is a chronic noncaseating granulomatous disease involving the gastrointestinal tract (see Chapter 317.2). However, gynecologic problems occur in up to 24% of women with Crohn disease. These manifestations include erythema, edema, and subsequent ulcer formation. Cutaneous ulcers of the vulva are slit-like, deep, and multiple. Secondary infection may occur. The diagnosis must be distinguished from other defects such as sarcoidosis, condyloma acuminata, condyloma lata, and hidradenitis suppurativa. Biopsy confirms the diagnosis. Treatment of the gastrointestinal problem with steroids and antibiotics is the primary objective of management. Vulvar lesions are treated with local application of steroids and systemic antibiotics for secondary infections.

Behçet Disease. This is a rare chronic multisystem disease associated with occlusive vasculitis (see Chapter 151). It is a multiorgan system problem characterized by recurrent oral and genital aphthous ulcers and uveitis, cutaneous vasculitis, synovitis, and meningoencephalitis. Genital ulcers occur in 58–78% of patients. They are painful, red macular lesions. Symptomatic treatment includes topical anesthetics such as lidocaine jelly. Intralesional steroids may be necessary for symptomatic ulcers. In severe forms of the disease treatment has included colchicine or methotrexate.

Brown M, Cartwright P, Snow B: Common office problems in pediatric urology and gynecology. *Pediatr Clin North Am* 1997;44(5):1091.

Chacki MR, Rozinetz CA, Hill R, et al: Leukocyte esterase dipstick as a rapid screening test for vaginitis and cervicitis. *J Pediatr Adolesc Gynecol* 1986;9:185.

Charles V, Charles SX: A case of vulvo-vaginal diphtheria in a girl of seven years. *Indian Pediatr* 1978;15:257.

Davis AJ, Goldstein DP: Treatment of pediatric lichen sclerosus with the CO₂ laser. *Adolesc Pediatr Gynecol* 1989;2:103.

Fisher G, Rogers M: Treatment of childhood vulvar lichen sclerosus with potent topical corticosteroid. *Pediatr Dermatol* 1997;14:235.

Fivozinsky K, Laufer R: Vulvar disorders in adolescence. *Adolesc Med* 1999;10(2):305.

Gerstner G, Grunberger W, Boschitsch E, et al: Vaginal organisms in prepubertal children with and without vulvovaginitis. *Arch Gynecol* 1982;231:247.

Jones R: Childhood vulvovaginitis and vaginal discharge in general practice. *Fam Pract* 1996;13:369.

Koumantakis EE, Hassan EA, Deligeoroglou EK, et al: Vulvovaginitis during childhood and adolescence. *J Pediatr Adolesc Gynecol* 1997;10:30.

Leung AK, Robson WL, tay-Uyboco J: The incidence of labial fusion in children. *J Pediatr Child Health* 1993;29:235.

Murphy T, Nelson J: Shigella vaginitis: Report of 38 patients and review of the literature. *Pediatrics* 1979;63:511.

Paradise J, Willis E: Probability of vaginal body in girls with genital complaints. *Am J Dis Child* 1985;139:472.

Pokorny S: Pediatric and adolescent gynecology. *Compr Ther* 1997;23(5):337.

Quint E, Smith Y: Vulvar disorders in adolescent patients. *Pediatr Clin North Am* 1999;46(3):593.

Rau F, Muram D: Vulvovaginitis in children. In Sanfilippo JS, et al (editors): *Pediatric Adolescent gynecology,* 2nd editions. Philadelphia, WB Saunders, 2001, p 199.

Ridley C: Dermatologic conditions of the vulva. In Sanfilippo JS, et al (editors): *Pediatric Adolescent Gynecology,* 2nd edition. Philadelphia, WB Saunders 2001, p 216.

Schroeder B: Vulvar disorders in adolescents. *Obstet Gynecol Clin North Am* 2000;27(1):35.

Sobel JD: Vaginitis. *N Engl J Med* 1997;337:1896.

Williams T, Callen J, Owen L: Vulvar disorders in the prepubertal female. *Pediatr Ann* 1986;15:588.

Young SJ, Wells DL, Ogden EJ: Lichen sclerosus, genital trauma and child sexual abuse. *Aust Fam Physician* 1993;22:729.

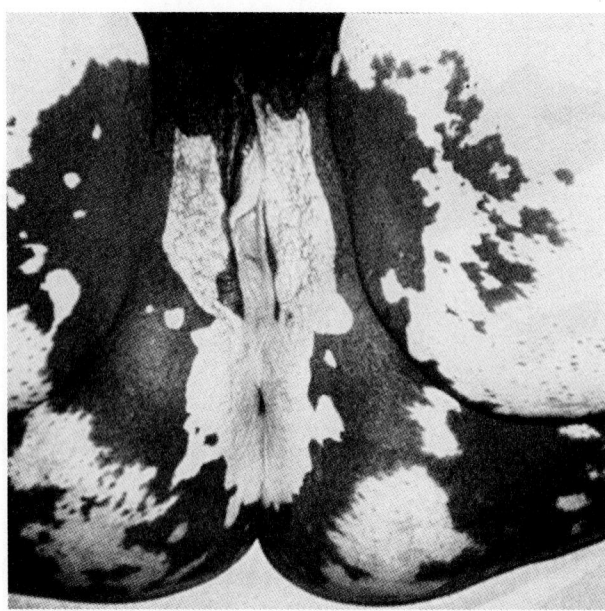

FIGURE 541–4. Vitiligo.

Chapter 542

Bleeding

The entities responsible for isolated vaginal bleeding in the pediatric patient include exposure to exogenous sex steroids; foreign body; hemorrhagic cystitis; hypothyroidism; precocious puberty; an ovarian cyst; trauma, which may or may not be associated with sexual abuse; urethral prolapse; vulvovaginitis; and neoplasms. See Chapter 107 for discussion of menstrual problems.

Foreign Body. A foreign body is commonly responsible for vaginal bleeding in pediatric patients. A foul-smelling discharge associated with vaginal bleeding suggests this possibility. Wadded toilet paper is the most common foreign body identified in the vagina. A plain roentgenogram or ultrasonography of the pelvis is often helpful. A vaginal foreign body was found in 18% of preadolescent girls with vaginal bleeding with or without discharge and in 50% of those with bleeding and no discharge.

Urethral Prolapse. Vulvar bleeding can be associated with urethral prolapse. This uncommon disorder is characterized by the urethral mucosa protruding through the meatus and forming a sensitive vulvar mass that bleeds easily. The "mass" is separate from the vagina. Patients may have difficulty with urination, depending on the size of the mass and whether or not it occludes the urethral meatus. The entity responds to topical application of estrogens because the distal urethra is estrogen sensitive. Urethral prolapse is often misdiagnosed when there is urogenital bleeding.

Genital Trauma. Although most injuries to this area are accidental, the possibility of physical or sexual abuse must be considered (see Chapter 35). Blunt injury may cause blood vessels beneath the perineal skin to rupture. Blood accumulating under the skin forms a hematoma, which may present as a round, tense, tender mass. Contusion of the vulva usually does not require treatment. A small vulvar hematoma often can be controlled by pressure with an ice pack. Analgesics may be required.

Penetrating injuries to the vaginal area warrant further careful evaluation, including serious considerations of the possibility of sexual abuse. A detailed examination is necessary, especially in the presence of active bleeding. The potential for bowel or bladder trauma must also be considered.

Genital Tumors. Benign and malignant tumors of the vulva should be considered when vaginal bleeding occurs in pediatric patients. A broad spectrum of entities, ranging from capillary hemangiomas through malignancies such as rhabdomyosarcoma, requires appropriate tissue diagnosis and treatment. The most common tumors include endodermal carcinoma, which occurs most often in young children; mesonephric carcinoma, which arises in a remnant of a mesonephric duct and occurs more often in girls 3 yr of age or older; and clear cell adenocarcinoma, which is often associated with a history of antenatal exposure to diethylstilbestrol (see Chapters 495 and 545).

Capillary Venous Malformation of the Labia Majora. Capillary venous malformation has been reported as a cause of vaginal bleeding in pediatric patients with expansion in vaginal volume on response to hormonal changes at puberty. The differential diagnosis includes hemangioma and other vascular malformation(s). Diagnosis is based on an evaluation that includes ultrasonography, magnetic resonance imaging, and abdominal arteriography. The malformation can be locally excised.

American College of Obstetricians and Gynecologists: *Dysfunctional Uterine Bleeding.* ACOG Technical Bulletin 134, Washington, DC, 1989.

Anveden-Hertzberg L, Gauderer MW, Elder JS: Urethral prolapse: An often misdiagnosed cause of urogenital bleeding in girls. *Pediatr Emerg Care* 1995;11:212.

Grant DB: Vaginal bleeding in childhood. *Pediatr Adolesc Gynecol* 1983;1:173.

Kempinaire A, De Raeve L, Roseeuw D, et al: Capillary-venous malformation in the labia majora of a 12-year-old girl. *Dermatology* 1997;194:405.

Kerns DL, Terman DL, Larson CS: The role of physicians in reporting and evaluating child sexual abuse cases. *The Future of Children* 1994;4:119.

Minjarez D, Bradshaw KD: Abnormal uterine bleeding in adolescents. *Obstet Gynecol Clin North Am* 2000;27:1.

Templeman C, Hertweck SP, Muram D, Sanfilippo JS: Vaginal bleeding in childhood and menstrual disorders in adolescence. In Sanfilippo JS, et al (editors): *Pediatric and Adolescent Gynecology.* 2nd edition. Philadelphia, WB Saunders, 2001, pp 237–47.

Chapter 543

Breast Disorders

The mammary glands are derived from the epidermal layer. Beginning at approximately 6 wk of gestation, epidermal cells migrate to the mesenchyme and form the mammary ridges. Breast buds, lactiferous ducts, and fully developed mammary glands eventually form. Breast development normally occurs in girls between the ages of $8^{1}/_{2}$ and 13 yr. The rate of breast growth varies, and development is often asymmetric. Complete development may not occur until a woman is in her early 20s.

Breast Self-Examination. Early diagnosis is central to improving health care for breast abnormalities, including carcinoma. Instruction in breast self-examination should be given to adolescents (Box 543–1).

Congenital Anomalies. Complete absence of breast, *amastia*, is rare; it is usually unilateral and often associated with other abnormalities, such as Poland syndrome (aplasia of the pectoralis muscles, rib deformities, webbed fingers, and radial nerve aplasia). Amastia can be iatrogenic, as a result of inadvertent excision of a breast bud. *Athelia* is defined as absence of one or both nipples. This condition is also rare and may not be associated with absent breast tissue. Both abnormalities require surgical correction.

Supernumerary breasts (polymastia) and *supernumerary nipples* (polythelia) are relatively common (Fig. 543–1); they occur

---

BOX 543–1. How to Do Breast Self-Examination

1. Lie down. Flatten your right breast by placing a pillow under your right shoulder. If your breasts are large, use your right hand to hold your right breast while you do the exam with your left hand.
2. Use the sensitive pads of the middle three fingers on your left hand. Feel for lumps using a rubbing motion.
3. Press firmly enough to feel different breast tissues.
4. Completely feel all of the breast and chest area to cover breast tissue that extends toward the shoulder. Allow enough time for a complete exam. Women with small breasts need at least 2 minutes to examine each breast. Larger breasts take longer.
5. Use the same pattern to feel every part of the breast tissue. Choose the method easiest for you. The three patterns preferred by women and their doctors are the circular, clock, or oval pattern; the vertical strip; and the wedge.
6. After you have completely examined your right breast, then examine your left breast using the same method. Compare what you have felt in one breast with the other.
7. You may also want to examine your breasts while bathing, when your skin is wet and lumps may be easier to feel.
8. You can check your breasts in a mirror; look for any change in size or contour, dimpling of the skin, or spontaneous nipple discharge.

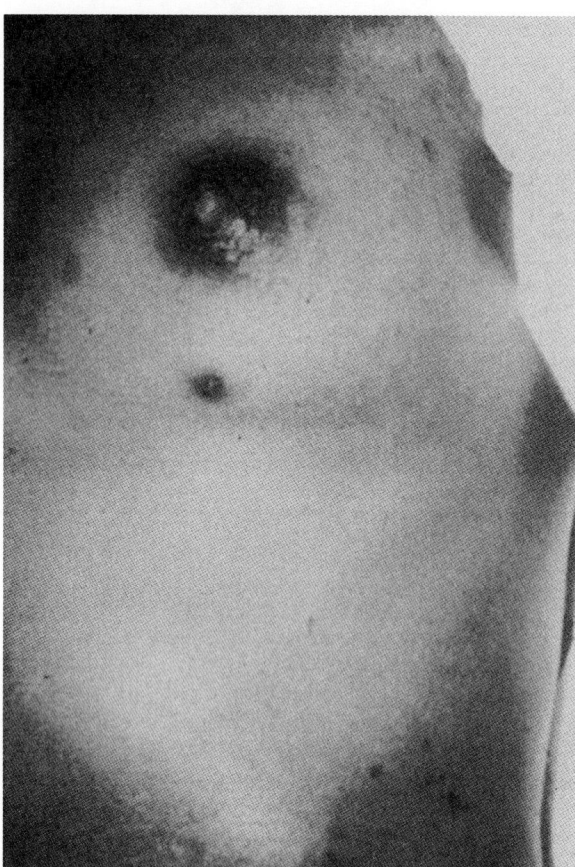

FIGURE 543–1. Polythelia.

along the milk lines and are usually asymptomatic. There is an association between polythelia and anomalies of the urinary and cardiovascular systems. In general, surgical excision of the accessory breasts or nipples is not necessary. However, if the aberrant breasts or nipples become symptomatic, excision may be indicated.

Hypoplasia of the breasts varies in degree from a nearly total absence of breast tissue to well-formed breasts that are considered by the patient to be too small. There are three general causes for poor or absent breast development: (1) The onset of breast development may be delayed, and the breasts develop slowly but are normal in all other respects; (2) a patient's family history may include late breast development; (3) ovarian function may have failed or been suppressed (see Chapter 580). Treatment depends on the underlying cause.

Breast atrophy is seen occasionally in adolescents and is almost uniformly secondary to dietary changes such as occur with anorexia nervosa. Correction of the underlying problem results in re-establishment of breast tissue.

Neonatal Breast Abnormalities. Bilateral breast hypertrophy may occur as a result of elevated circulating maternal endogenous steroid hormones in late gestation. It may be associated with discharge from the nipples known as "witch's milk." Repeated manipulation of the breast can exacerbate the condition. On occasion, the hypertrophy is associated with mastitis caused by a staphylococcal infection; antibiotics should be administered.

Mastodynia. Painful breast engorgement (mastodynia) usually is associated with ovulatory cycles; this is uncommon in adolescents until approximately 18 mo after menarche, the time that may be necessary to establish ovulatory cycles. There is frequently a cyclic pattern of the breast discomfort. Analgesics such

as nonsteroidal anti-inflammatory drugs, including ibuprofen, as well as the use of a good support bra, are often helpful in alleviating discomfort.

Breast Masses. A retrospective review of breast disease in adolescent females revealed that about 54% have fibroadenomas and 13% have virginal hypertrophy. Fibrocystic or proliferative breast disease occurs in about 24%. Primary rhabdomyosarcoma, metastatic rhabdomyosarcoma, metastatic neuroblastoma, and non-Hodgkin lymphoma occur in 2–3% of all breast masses in this age group. Other diagnoses include polythelia, accessory breast tissue, mastitis, hemangioma, fat necrosis, and intramammary lymph nodes. Breast masses during adolescence may stem from several causes:

- Fibroadenoma
- Fibrocystic disease
- Breast cyst
- Abscess/mastitis
- Intraductal papilloma
- Fat necrosis/lipoma
- Cystosarcoma phyllodes
- Adenomatous hyperplasia
- Rare lesions (hemangiomas, lymphangiomas, lymphoma)
- Normal breast tissue
- Cancer

A thorough history and physical examination are mandatory for any pediatric or adolescent patient who has a breast mass. The clinical problem should be reviewed with a radiologist before initiating any radiologic assessment. Needle aspiration and biopsy are often essential for evaluation of palpable breast abnormalities. Large breast tumors also occur in adolescents. Although malignancy is often suspected because of rapid growth of the mass and skin ulceration, the incidence is very low. Breast tumors can have varied presentations. Giant fibroadenomas in adolescence may be treated by simple enucleation.

Malignant Tumors. Although rare, *breast cancer* does occur in adolescents. Early menarche in association with anovulatory cycles is a risk factor. The estrogen-to-androgen ratio appears to be critical, with androgens having a protective effect.

Cystosarcoma phylloides, an uncommon breast tumor in adults, may occur in adolescents. It is characterized by asymmetric breast enlargement in association with a firm, mobile, circumscribed mass. The tumor often increases rapidly in size and can become quite large. Fixation of the tumor to the skin or chest wall is rare. The majority of these tumors are benign, but malignant cystosarcoma phylloides with metastases has been reported. Excision is the preferred initial therapy in adolescent patients, regardless of the histologic classification of the lesion. Malignant cystosarcoma is more likely to recur than is a benign lesion. Fatal metastatic cystosarcoma phylloides in an adolescent has occurred.

Breast tumors also may be the first manifestation of relapse (extramedullary) in *acute lymphoblastic leukemia*. Reports in the literature include a case of radiation-induced sarcoma of the breast in a female adolescent and a case of liposarcoma in a 17-yr-old black female who previously had a total mastectomy.

Macromastia (Virginal Hypertrophy). The cause of massive breast enlargement during puberty and early adolescence is unknown, but the condition probably represents an end-organ increased sensitivity to circulating estrogens. It is bilateral, often occurs over a brief period, and most commonly affects girls 13–17 yr old. Physical and psychologic problems may occur in adolescents with macromastia. Posture problems and discomfort often result. Reduction mammoplasty is the treatment of choice but should be delayed until late adolescence to allow for complete breast development. Surgical intervention often necessitates relocation of the nipple, which may result in decreased sensation and altered lactation. In addition, strong emotional support should be provided.

Tuberous Breasts. This deformity results in breasts that are reminiscent of a tuberous root plant. It may be the result of an exogenous steroid use, especially with induction of pubertal development. Surgical intervention is required for correction.

Mastitis and Abscess. Mastitis and breast abscess may require antibiotic therapy as well as incision and drainage. See Chapter 106.

Trauma and Inflammation. Breast trauma in adolescent females has become more common because of the increased number of young women participating in contact sports. The trauma usually takes the form of contusion or hematoma and often resolves with either late cystic changes in the breast or fibrosis with retraction of skin or the nipple over the injured area. These late changes may mimic those associated with malignancy; biopsy may be the only means of differentiating the two.

Mammary Dysplasia. This common lesion is characterized by changes associated with the menstrual cycle. Hormonal imbalance may cause exaggerated responses in the breast tissue, especially in the upper and outer quadrants during the premenstrual phase of the cycle. The extent of treatment depends on the degree of symptoms; ibuprofen is often helpful. In addition, methylxanthines and caffeine (e.g., coffee, tea, carbonated drinks) should be eliminated from the diet.

Nipple Discharge. This must be carefully evaluated and a distinction made between the presence of galactorrhea (spontaneous flow of milk), bloody, and other discharge (Table 543–1). Evaluation of galactorrhea in children is the same as for adults. Serum prolactin levels are obtained to rule out the presence of a pituitary prolactinoma (see Chapter 554.2). If a pituitary tumor or adenoma is suspected on the basis of markedly elevated serum hemianopsia, appropriate radiologic (computed tomography, magnetic resonance imaging) assessment is necessary. Another cause of galactorrhea is hypothyroidism in association with elevated levels of thyroid-releasing hormone, which also stimulates prolactin release. Medications may also cause galactorrhea (Table 543–2). Treatment of galactorrhea (non-thyroid related) consists primarily of dopamine agonists such as bromocriptine or cabergoline (Dostinex). Surgical intervention, usually transsphenoidal hypophysectomy, is rarely required. Galactorrhea secondary to chest wall surgery in an adolescent has also been reported. The galactorrhea occurred for 2 mo and was associated with transient amenorrhea.

Bloody nipple discharge can be indicative of duct ectasia. Cytologic assessment and surgical consultation are indicated. Nipple discharge in association with Montgomery tubercles also has been reported. These secretions can be episodic and vary in color from clear to brown, but they are usually not milky. This discharge evolves over a period of 3–5 wk, may be associated

TABLE 543–1. Differential Diagnosis of Nipple Discharge

Type	Differential Diagnosis (in Order of Frequency)
Milky	Galactorrhea
Multicolored/sticky	Duct ectasia
Purulent	Mastitis
Watery	Papilloma
	Cancer
Serous/serosanguineous	Intraductal papilloma
	Fibrocystic changes
	Cancer
	Duct ectasia

From Neinstein LS: Breast masses in adolescents. Adolesc Pediatr Gynecol 1994;7:119.

TABLE 543–2. Medications that Cause Galactorrhea

Amitriptyline	Estrogens	Narcotics
Amphetamines	Fluphenazine	Opiates
Androgens	Haloperidol	Prostaglandins
Anesthetics	Meprobamate	Reserpine
Chlorpromazine	Methyldopa	Sulpiride
Cimetidine	Metoclopramide	Trifluoperazine
Domperidone	Monoamine oxidase inhibitors	

Adapted from Yazigi RA, Quintero CH, Salameh WA: Prolactin disorders. Fertil Steril 1997;67:215, reprinted by permission of the American Society for Reproductive Medicine.

with breast lumps, and is a benign, self-limited problem. Intraductal breast papillomas have occurred in adolescents.

Breast Asymmetry. Beginning in the neonate there may be unilateral breast development. In adolescents, it is not uncommon for approximately 25% of patients to have an element of breast asymmetry that persists after the age of 18. Asymmetry is common especially between Tanner stage 2 and 4 (see Fig. 14–2).

Apter D, Vinko R: Early menarche, a risk factor for breast cancer, indicates early onset of ovulatory cycles. *J Clin Endocrinol Metab* 1983;57:82.

Briggs R, Walters M, Rosenthal D: Cystosarcoma phylloides in adolescent female patients. *Am J Surg* 1983;146:712.

Cromer B, Frankel M, Kader L: Compliance with breast self-examination and instruction in healthy adolescents. *J Adolesc Health Care* 1989;10:105.

Diehl G, Kaplan D: Breast masses in adolescent females. *J Adolesc Health Care* 1985;6:353.

Ellegaard J, Bendix-Hanson K, Boesen A, et al: Breast tumor as a first manifestation of extramedullary relapse in acute lymphoblastic leukemia. *Scand J Haematol* 1984;33:288.

Heyman R, Rauh J: Areolar gland discharge in adolescent females appears to be benign. *J Adolesc Health Care* 1983;4:285.

Letson G, Moore D: Galactorrhea secondary to chest wall surgery in an adolescent. *J Adolesc Health Care* 1984;5:277.

Neinstein L: Breast disease in adolescents and young women. *Pediatr Clin North Am* 1999;46(3):607.

Ngala J: Fatal metastatic cystosarcoma phylloides in a young woman: Report of a case. *Arch Surg* 1983;118:871.

Raganoonan C, Fairbairn J, Williams S, et al: Giant breast tumors of adolescence. *Aust N Z J Surg* 1987;57:243.

Simmons P, Wold L: Surgically treated breast disease in adolescent females: A retrospective review of 185 cases. *Adolesc Pediatr Gynecol* 1989;2:95.

Templeman C, Hertweck SP: Breast disorders in the pediatric and adolescent patient. *Obstet Gynecol Clin North Am* 2000;27(1):19.

Watkind F, Giacomantonio M, Salisbury S: Nipple discharge and breast lump related to Montgomery's tubercles in adolescent females. *J Pediatr Surg* 1988;23:718.

Chapter 544

Hirsutism and Polycystic Ovarian Syndrome

Hirsutism (excessive hair growth) must be distinguished from virilization. The latter involves increased body hair, acne, deepening of the voice, change in body habitus due to increased muscle mass, and clitoromegaly (see Chapter 570). Premature pubarche is defined as the appearance of genital hair or axillary hair or both before age 8 yr (Chapter 556). Adrenarche, the output of increased androgen from the adrenal glands, usually occurs between ages 12 and 18 yr and is discussed in Chapter 14.

Polycystic ovarian syndrome (PCOS) is believed to have its origin at puberty. Teenagers usually present with menstrual disturbances or hirsutism (Box 544–1). Ultrasonographic

BOX 544–1. Causes of Hirsutism

PERIPHERAL
Idiopathic
Partial androgen insensitivity (5-α-reductase deficiency)
HAIR-AN syndrome (hirsutism, androgenization, insulin resistance, and acanthosis nigricans)
Hyperprolactinemia

GONADAL
Polycystic ovary syndrome (polycystic ovaries, chronic anovulation)
Ovarian neoplasm (Sertoli-Leydig cell, granulosa cell, thecoma, gynandroblastoma, lipoid cell, luteoma, hypernephroma, Brenner's tumor)
Gonadal dysgenesis (Turner's mosaic with XY, or H-Y antigen positive)

ADRENAL
Cushing syndrome
Adrenal hyper-responsiveness
Congenital adrenal hyperplasia (classic, cryptic, adult onset)
21-hydroxylase deficiency
11-hydroxylase deficiency
3β-hydroxysteroid deficiency
17α-hydroxylase deficiency
Adrenal neoplasm (adenoma, cortical carcinoma)

EXOGENOUS
Minoxidil
Dilantin
Cyclosporine
Anabolic steroids
Acetazolamide (Diamox)
Penicillamine
Oral contraceptives with androgenic progestins
Danazol
Androgenic steroids
Psoralens
Hydrochlorothiazide
Phenothiazines

CONGENITAL ANOMALIES
Trisomy 18 (Edwards syndrome)
Cornelia de Lange syndrome
Hurler syndrome
Juvenile hypothyroidism

Adapted from Bailey-Pridham DD, Sanfilippo JS: Hirsutism in the adolescent female. *Pediatr Clin North Am* 1989;36:581.

cause of hirsutism, and controversy exists about whether the basic defect is central (hypothalamic or pituitary regulation of gonadotropins) or ovarian (defect in a peptide hormone, perhaps inhibin, with resultant abnormal feedback to the pituitary gland). The usual hormonal pattern of PCOS begins with altered luteinizing hormone release (a ratio of luteinizing hormone [LH] to follicle-stimulating hormone of 2:1 or 3:1, shortened pulse frequency, and slightly increased pulse amplitude of LH). Adolescents with hyperandrogenism display an exaggerated LH pulsatility similar to that found in adults with PCOS syndrome.

PCOS is associated with peripheral insulin resistance in addition to excessive levels of LH, resulting in increased ovarian androgen production. Hyperinsulinemia is associated with increased bioavailable insulin-like growth factor-1 (IGF-1) and depressed production of IGF-1 carrier protein (IGFBP-1). Activation of IGF-1 receptor may also be involved in increased ovarian androgen production. Peripheral conversion of ovarian androstenedione to testosterone contributes to the commonly identified increase in total serum testosterone levels that are an integral part of the PCOS hormonal pattern. In addition to their hyperinsulinemic state, these patients have long-term cardiovascular risks for hypertension and coronary artery disease. This patient population often also has increases in total triglyceride levels.

The insulin resistance is an integral part of the *HAIR-AN syndrome*, which consists of hyperandrogenism, hirsutism, insulin resistance, and acanthosis nigricans. Insulin receptor mutation as well as circulating antibodies to the insulin receptor and postreceptor defects occur in this syndrome. Defects in glucose transport as well as high levels of insulin stimulate the activity of cytochrome P450c 17α, an enzyme actively involved in the production of androgens by the ovary. With PCOS there is also dysregulation of the cytochrome P450c 17α enzyme system.

Hirsutism in adolescents can also be due to a heterozygous form of *21-hydroxylase deficiency* (see Chapter 570). This has been called adult-onset congenital adrenal hyperplasia (AOCAH). Various other forms of congenital adrenal hyperplasia and congenital anomalies are also associated with hirsutism. Clinically, it may be difficult to distinguish between PCOS and AOCAH.

Ovarian hyperthecosis, which can be familial, is a variant of PCOS. Hyperthecosis is defined as isolated islands of luteinized cells within the ovary, contributing to increased androgen production. Ovarian androgen production and its peripheral effects are similar to those associated with PCOS.

Medications, radiation, and chronic irritation (e.g., the placement of a cast) can also initiate localized, nonendocrinologic hair growth.

assessment often identifies multicystic ovaries, a characteristic "pearl necklace." The prevalence of polycystic ovaries increases throughout puberty and may reach as high as 26% by 15 yr of age.

PCOS (polycystic ovaries, chronic anovulation, and Stein-Leventhal syndrome) is the most commonly diagnosed ovarian

TABLE 544–1. Treatment of Hirsutism: Idiopathic and Polycystic Ovary Syndrome

Medication	Dose*	Comments
Oral contraceptives (estrogen dominant)	35 µg	Decrease in plasma testosterone, androstenedione, and DHEA-S
Spironolactone	100 mg bid	Decreased androgen production and androgen receptor competition
Medroxyprogesterone acetate depot (Depo-Provera)	150–250 mg q 2–4 wk	Decreased testosterone production and 17-ketosteroid levels
Cyproterone acetate	Diane, 2 mg Androcur, 100 mg	Decreased plasma testosterone, androstenedione, SHBG, induces "insulinemia"
Dexamethasone	0.25–0.5 mg	Dose adequate if plasma-free testosterone <15 pg/mL
Cimetidine	200–300 mg tid–qid	Decreased serum testosterone, increased serum estradiol
GnRH agonist (Flutamide)	250 mg tid	5α-reductase inhibitor; decreased testosterone and androstenedione

*Dosages given are for a 70-kg female. Daily dosages are indicated unless otherwise specified.
DHEA-S = dehydroepiandrosterone sulfate; SHBG = sex hormone–binding globulin.
From Bailey-Pridham DD, Sanfilippo JS: Hirsutism in the adolescent female. Pediatr Clin North Am *1989;36:581*, with permission.

Treatment of Hirsute Patients. Treatment alternatives for idiopathic hirsutism and PCOS are outlined in Table 544–1. Hirsutism secondary to hyperprolactinemia is best treated with bromocriptine. In patients with multicystic (polycystic) ovaries and primary hypothyroidism, the polycystic ovaries resolve rapidly with adequate doses of thyroid replacement therapy. If an exogenous cause such as a medication is producing hirsutism, the exogenous agent should be eliminated. Even when the increased tissue androgen effect is reversed by appropriate treatment, hair follicles converted to terminal hair may still produce that type of hair. Electrolysis may provide an improved cosmetic appearance, with the assurance that if the underlying abnormality is controlled, no new hair growth should ensue. Cushing syndrome or disease, androgen-producing tumors, and congenital adrenal hyperplasia are discussed in Chapters 570 and 571.

Metformin, an insulin-sensitizing agent, has been recommended for hyperinsulinemic PCOS patients. The objective is to reduce circulating insulin levels, which is associated with decreases in serum LH and testosterone with PCOS. This result occurs within 4 to 8 wk. It is imperative that treated patients have pre-therapy, as well as periodic, evaluation of liver function.

Apter D, Siegberg R, Laatikainen T: Pulsatile secretion of luteinizing hormone in adolescents with hyperandrogenism. *Adolesc Pediatr Gynecol* 1988;1:104.

Belgorosky A, Rivarola M: Progressive increase in non-sex hormone binding globulin-bound testosterone and estradiol from infancy to late prepuberty in girls. *J Clin Endocrinol Metab* 1988;67:234.

Boor JT, Herwig J, Schrezenmeir J, et al: Familial insulin resistant diabetes associated with acanthosis nigricans, polycystic ovaries, hypogonadism, pigmentary retinopathy, labyrinthine deafness, and mental retardation. *Am J Med Genet* 1993;45:649.

Franks S: Polycystic ovary syndrome. *Arch Dis Child* 1997;77:89.

Gordon C: Menstrual disorders in adolescents—excessive androgens and polycystic ovarian syndrome. *Pediatr Clin North Am* 1999;46(3);519.

Judd H, Scully R, Herbst A, et al: Familial hyperthecosis: Comparison of endocrinologic and histologic findings with polycystic ovarian disease. *Am J Obstet Gynecol* 1973;117:976.

Kamilaris T, DeBold C, Manolus K, et al: Testosterone secreting adrenal adenoma in a peripubertal patient. *JAMA* 1987;258:2558.

Lindsay A, Voorhess M, MacGillivray M: Multicystic ovaries in primary hypothyroidism. *Obstet Gynecol* 1983;61:433.

Parker L, Sack J, Fisher D, et al: The adrenarche: Prolactin, gonadotropins, adrenal androgens and cortisol. *J Clin Endocrinol Metab* 1985;60:409.

Ploufee L Jr: Disorders of excessive hair growth in the adolescent. *Obstet Gynecol Clin North Am* 2000;27(1):79.

Rosen G, Kaplan B, Lobo R: Menstrual function and hirsutism in patients with gonadal dysgenesis. *Obstet Gynecol* 1988;71:677.

Speroff L, Glass RH, Kase NG: Hirsutism. In Speroff L, Glass RH, Kase NG (editors): *Clinical Gynecologic Endocrinology and Infertility*, 4th ed. Baltimore, Williams & Wilkins, 1999, pp 523–556.

Zumogg B, Freeman R, Coupa S, et al: A chronobiologic abnormality of luteinizing hormone secretion in teenage girls with the polycystic ovary syndrome. *N Engl J Med* 1983;309:1206.

Chapter 545
Neoplasms

The most common gynecologic neoplasm found in children is of ovarian origin and usually presents as an abdominal mass. Ovarian neoplasms constitute 1% of all childhood malignancies, and 8% of all malignant and abdominal tumors in children are of ovarian origin. Furthermore, 10–30% of the ovarian neoplasms operated on during childhood or adolescence are malignant. Paraovarian tumors are next in frequency, followed by uterine neoplasms. The vagina or vulva may also be the site of a benign or malignant lesion in children. Cervical dysplasia may occur in adolescents. Breast masses are discussed in Chapter 543.

Chemotherapy, especially with alkylating agents (cyclophosphamide, busulphan, chlorambucil, and nitrogen mustard), is associated with germ cell damage in the postpubertal ovary. The prepubertal ovary, on the other hand, is markedly resistant to chemotherapeutic damage of germ cells. The effect of combined oral contraceptive therapy during chemotherapy in adolescents remains controversial.

Survivors of childhood cancer who previously underwent abdominal or gonadal irradiation have an increased rate of spontaneous abortions. However, the incidence of congenital malformations is not increased in comparison with the general population. Patients who have evidence of premature ovarian failure may be candidates for assisted reproductive technology with the use of donor ova.

OVARIES

Neonatal and Pediatric Ovarian Cysts. Most often the clinical manifestations of ovarian tumors are abdominal pain, mass, or both. Functional ovarian cysts rarely persist beyond the neonatal period. In adolescents, the most common neoplasm is the teratoma. The teratomas are usually benign, but malignant teratomas may occur. Calcification on abdominal roentgenogram is often a hallmark of a benign teratoma. During surgery, the opposite ovary should be evaluated, and if there is any question about the possibility of a neoplasm, a biopsy specimen should be obtained. Ovarian adenomas are the second most common benign tumor.

Although ovarian cancers are extremely uncommon in children, they are responsible for 1:500 ovarian malignancies. Ovarian cancers affect only 4% of women. With respect to germ cell tumors, the most common is the dysgerminoma, followed in incidence by malignant teratomas, endodermal sinus tumors, embryonal carcinomas, mixed cell neoplasms, and gonadoblastomas (see Chapter 495). Immature teratomas and endodermal sinus tumors are more aggressive malignancies than dysgerminomas and occur in a significantly higher proportion of younger girls (<10 yr of age). In this age group, 10-year survival rates were 73% for epithelial carcinomas, 44% for sex cord stromal tumors, 73% for dysgerminomas, 33% for malignant teratomas, 39% for endodermal sinus tumors, 25% for embryonal carcinomas, 30% for other germ cell neoplasms, and 100% for gonadoblastomas. Dysgerminomas usually are associated with XY gonadal dysgenesis; Y-DNA probes are important in their diagnosis. Tumor markers such as α-fetoprotein, carcinoembryonic antigen, and the antigen CA-125 are also used to assess ovarian malignancy (Table 545–1). The germ cell tumors are associated with positive alpha-fetoprotein, human chorionic gonadotropin (HCG), and chorioembryonic antigen.

Treatment consists of surgical excision followed by postoperative chemotherapy; radiotherapy is often necessary. Staging at the beginning of therapy is of the utmost importance. In many cases, a second-look procedure is indicated in order to decide about subsequent treatment of these neoplasms.

Embryonal Carcinoma. This cancer accounts for 6% of pediatric ovarian neoplasms and 8% of all germ cell tumors. The patient presents with progressive increase in abdominal pain and distention. The embryonal cell carcinoma is highly malignant with an average age of detection between 13–15 yr. Overall, 60% of patients have endocrinologic signs and symptoms, which may include precocious pseudopuberty,

TABLE 545–1. Serum Tumor Markers

Marker	Associated Tumor
CA 125	Epithelial tumors (especially serous)
	Immature teratoma (rare)
Alpha-fetoprotein	Endodermal sinus tumors
	Embryonal carcinomas
	Mixed germ cell tumors
	Immature teratoma (rare)
	Polyembryoma (rare)
Human chorionic gonadotropins	Choriocarcinoma
	Embryonal carcinomas
	Mixed germ cell tumors
	Polyembryoma
	Dysgerminoma (rare)
Lactate dehydrogenase	Dysgerminoma
	Mixed germ cell tumors
Estradiol	Thecomas
	Adult granulosa cell tumors
Testosterone	Sertoli cell tumors
	Leydig (hilus) cell tumors
F9 embryoglycan	Embryonal carcinoma
	Yolk sac tumor
	Choriocarcinoma
	Immature teratoma
Inhibin	Granulosa–theca cell tumor
Müllerian inhibiting substance	Granulosa–theca cell tumor

abnormal vaginal bleeding, and hirsutism. Both HXG and alpha-fetoprotein are produced by embryonal cell carcinoma. *Treatment* involves unilateral salpingo-oophorectomy for stage I disease.

Endodermal Sinus Tumor. These tumors are the most lethal of all ovarian cancers. The median age of presentation is 19 yr. The endodermal sinus tumor produces alpha-fetoprotein as a useful tumor marker. These tumors are radiosensitive. They may be treated surgically if they are stage I, for which a unilateral salpingo-oophorectomy is performed. Chemotherapy may be necessary independent of the stage of the disease.

Choriocarcinoma. Primary choriocarcinoma of the ovary is extremely rare and often fatal; 0.6% of germ cell tumors are choriocarcinomas.

Mixed Germ Cell Tumor. The frequency of mixed germ cell tumors is 4% of all ovarian neoplasms in children.

Sex Cord Stromal Tumor. Sex cord stromal tumors comprise 5% of ovarian neoplasms, of which the granulosa cell tumor is the most common. Isosexual precocity and occasionally virilization may be observed in the juvenile variety. The characteristic histologic features include modular architecture, follicle formation, microcysts, cell necrosis, and increased mitotic activity.

Sertoli–Leydig Cell Tumor. This tumor is also a sex cord stromal tumor and accounts for 2% of pediatric ovarian tumors. Sertoli–Leydig cell tumors are rare in prepubertal girls. The patient presents with evidence of virilization. *Treatment* includes unilateral salpingo-oophorectomy for stage I disease.

Ovarian Follicular Cysts. These cysts occur from birth to puberty and usually disappear spontaneously. On ultrasound examination, the cyst usually presents as a nonechogenic area, frequently larger than 20 mm at its greatest diameter; diffuse swelling of the ovarian parenchyma and follicular enlargement of the cortical zone are also noted.

Polycystic Ovarian Syndrome (PCOS). This syndrome presents with menstrual dysfunction and signs and symptoms of androgen excess often at the time of puberty. The menstrual irregularity can range from amenorrhea to oligomenorrhea. See Chapter 544.

Functional and Hemorrhagic Ovarian Cysts. These cysts are an integral part of follicular development during the menstrual cycle. On occasion a cyst may persist and increase in diameter. Following ovulation, it is termed a *corpus hemorrhagicum.* These are often symptomatic and best evaluated by ultrasonography. Expectant management for a presumed functional cyst is appropriate, with follow-up ultrasound imaging. Monophasic oral contraceptives can facilitate suppression of functional cysts.

Ovarian Torsion. Torsion of an adnexum is a complication that should always be considered in the differential diagnosis of ovarian tumors or abdominal pain in a female patient; prompt surgical intervention is necessary. Torsion often presents with intermittent sharp abdominal pain that, in many cases, radiates down the ipsilateral extremity. Bilateral ovarian torsion also may occur in infancy. When unilateral torsion is diagnosed, oophoropexy (plication) of the contralateral adnexa may be indicated.

The incidence of ovarian torsion in one series was 25% (16 of 63 benign ovarian masses). Color Doppler flow studies can facilitate the diagnosis. Adnexal torsion can often be evaluated and managed with the use of Doppler flow studies and laparoscopy. The underlying cause is usually an associated ovarian cyst or neoplasm. Recovery of ovarian function after laparoscopic detorsion has been reported with identification of normal follicle development on ultrasonography. Therefore, it is recommended that adnexal torsion be managed conservatively.

Autoamputation of the Ovary. This entity presents as a small, calcified, free-floating mass associated with absent adnexa. The child may be asymptomatic, and ultrasonography is often helpful in establishing the diagnosis. It has been hypothesized that antenatal or subclinical ovarian torsion leads to necrosis, calcification, and separation of the adnexa from its blood supply.

Juvenile Granulosa Cell Tumors of the Ovary (JGCT). JGCT account for 1–2% of all ovarian tumors. The median age of presentation is 7.6 yr, with a range of 6 mo–17.5 yr. The majority of patients have abdominal distention and sexual precocity. Patients appear to have increasingly better prognosis with the advent of multidrug chemotherapy, including cisplatin-based regimens. However, neurotoxicity, especially ototoxicity, and bone marrow depression are serious complications.

CERVIX

The prevalence of dysplasia and carcinoma in situ is 18.8/1,000 for those 15–19 yr of age, and biopsy-proven cases of all grades of cervical intraepithelial neoplasia (CIN) in the teenage population have a prevalence of 13.3/1,000. The Bethesda Classification System with the Papanicolaou (Pap) smear is widely used for diagnosis. The overall frequency of abnormal Pap smear results in the adolescent population is 3.8%, and 1% of all abnormal Pap smears are associated with CIN. Papillomavirus infection (Chapter 243) and altered vaginal flora are consistent findings in patients with CIN. Abnormal Pap smear results in adolescents also correlate with significant CIN and should be followed up with a biopsy. Colposcopic examination is essential when CIN is diagnosed in an adolescent. Other pathologic abnormalities of the cervix include cervical polyps and mixed mesodermal tumors. The latter may represent a mixed, heterologous, or homologous sarcoma of the uterine cervix.

UTERUS (BENIGN AND MALIGNANT TUMORS OF THE UTERINE CORPUS)

Adenocarcinoma of the corpus is rare in children and adolescents. Vaginal bleeding not associated with sexual precocity is a frequent presenting sign. Treatment consists of hysterectomy, with removal of the ovaries, followed by adjunctive radiotherapy or chemotherapy or both, depending on the operative findings. Mixed mesodermal tumors and leiomyomas of the uterus should be included in the differential diagnosis of a pelvic mass in an adolescent. Leiomyosarcoma, although extremely rare, has also been noted in an adolescent; the presentation is variable, but abnormal vaginal bleeding usually is present.

VAGINA

Gartner duct (mesonephric) cyst is a common vaginal wall abnormality. It usually is an incidental finding and requires no specific therapy. In sexually active patients, excision may be necessary if there is associated dyspareunia. Paramesonephric (müllerian) duct cysts often become symptomatic at menarche when the cavity fills with menstrual blood. Women who were exposed to diethylstilbestrol (DES) in utero have a high incidence of adenosis of the vagina and cervix. These patients also have potential reproductive abnormalities, including infertility, habitual abortion, and tubal and uterine cavity abnormalities. Clear cell adenocarcinoma of the vagina and cervix is a rare sequela of DES exposure in utero.

Sarcoma botryoides, a vaginal carcinoma that occurs primarily in pediatric patients, is best treated by surgical excision. Chemotherapy is usually administered postoperatively. Any questionable vulvar lesion should be submitted for histologic examination. Liposarcoma of the vulva has been reported in a 15 yr old girl. Malignant melanoma of the vulva has also been described in a 14 yr old patient.

Ablin A, Issacs H Jr: Germ cell tumors. In Pizzo PA, Poplack DG (editors): *Pediatric Oncology.* Philadelphia, JB Lippincott, 1989, pp 713–731.
Berenson A, Pokorny S, Dutton R: The autoamputated ovary: A rare cause of abdominal calcification. *Adolesc Pediatr Gynecol* 1989;2:99.
Brooks J, Livolsi V: Liposarcoma presenting on the vulva. *Am J Obstet Gynecol* 1987;156:73.
Calaminus G, Wessalowski R, Harms D, et al: Juvenile granulosa cell-tumors of the ovary in children and adolescents: Results from 33 patients registered in a prospective cooperative study. *Gynecol Oncol* 1997;64:447.
Cohen Z, Shinhar D, Kopernik G, et al: The laparoscopic approach to uterine adnexal torsion in childhood. *J Pediatr Surg* 1996;31:1557.
Copeland LJ, Gershenson DM, Saul PB, et al: Sarcoma botryoides of the female genital tract. *Obstet Gynecol* 1985;66:262.
Fields KR, Neinestein LS: Uterine myomas in adolescents: Case reports and a review of the literature. *J Pediatr Adolesc Gynecol* 1996;9:195.
Freedman R, Kopf A, Jones W: Malignant melanoma in association with lichen sclerosus on the vulva of a 14-year old. *Am J Dermatopathol* 1984;6:253.
Graif M, Itzchak Y: Sonographic evaluation of ovarian torsion in childhood and adolescence. *AJR Am J Roentgenol* 1988;150:647.
Gribbon M, Ein SH, Mancer K: Pediatric malignant ovarian tumors: A three year review. *J Pediatr Surg* 1992;27:480.
Guijon F, Paraskevas M, Brunham R: The association of sexually transmitted disease with cervical intraepithelial neoplasia: A case-controlled study. *Am J Obstet Gynecol* 1985;151:185.
Hassan E, Relakis C, Maralliotakis I, et al: Cervical cytology in adolescence. *Clin Exp Obstet Gynecol* 1997;24:28.
Hicks ML, Piver S: Conservative surgery plus adjuvant therapy for vulvovaginal rhabdomyosarcoma, diethylstilbestrol, clear cell adenocarcinoma of the vagina and unilateral germ cell tumors of the ovary. *Obstet Gynecol Clin North Am* 1992;19:219.
Kozlowski K: Ovarian masses. *Adolesc Med: State of the Art Reviews* 1999;10:2.
Liapi C, Evain-Biron D: Diagnosis of ovarian follicular cyst from birth to puberty: A report of 20 cases. *Acta Paediatr Scand* 1987;76:91.
Major T, Borsos A, Lampe L, et al: Ovarian malignancies in childhood and adolescence. *Eur J Obstet Gynecol Reprod Biol* 1995;63:65.
Mangan SA, Legano LA, Rosen CM, et al: Increased prevalence of abnormal Papanicolaou smears in early adolescence. *Arch Pediatr Adolesc Med* 1997;151:481.
Nicholson HS, Byrne J: Fertility and pregnancy after treatment for cancer during childhood or adolescence. *Cancer* 1993;71 (Suppl):3392.
Owens K, Honebrink A: Gynecologic care of medically complicated adolescents. *Pediatr Clin North Am* 1999;46:631.
Parker-Jones K: Gynecologic issues in pediatric oncology. *Clin Obstet Gynecol* 1997;40:200.
Pfeifer S, Gosman G: Evaluation of adnexal masses in adolescents. *Pediatr Clin North Am* 1999;46:573.
Piippo S, Mustaniemi L, Lenko H, et al: Surgery for ovarian masses during childhood and adolescence: A report of 79 cases. *J Pediatr Adolesc Gynecol* 1999;12:223.
Powell JL, Otis CN: Management of advanced juvenile granulosa cell tumor of the ovary. *Gynecol Oncol* 1997;64:282.
Rosenfeld WD, Kleinhaus S, Jutcher R, et al: Leiomyoma in a 15-year-old girl. *Adolesc Pediatr Gynecol* 1988;1:109.
Roye CF: Abnormal cervical cytology in adolescents: A literature review. *J Adolesc Health* 1993;13:643.
Sadeghi S, Hsieh E, Gonn S: Prevalence of cervical intraepithelial neoplasia in sexually active teenagers and young adults: Results of data analysis of mass Papanicolaou screening of 796,337 women in the United States in 1981. *Am J Obstet Gynecol* 1984;148:726.
Sagot P, Lopes P, Mensier A, et al: Carbon dioxide laser treatment of cervical dysplasia in teenagers. *Eur J Obstet Gynecol Reprod Biol* 1992;46:143.
Shalev E, Bustan M, Yarom I, et al: Recovery of ovarian function after laparoscopic detorsion. *Hum Reprod* 1995;10:2965.
Starceski P, Lee P, Siever W: Bilateral ovarian pathology and torsion in infancy: Assessment of pubertal and gonadal function. *Adolesc Pediatr Gynecol* 1988;1:199.
Young RH, Kozakewich WP, Scully RE: Metastatic ovarian tumors in children: A report of 14 cases and review of the literature. *Int J Gynecol Pathol* 1993;12:8.

Chapter 546
Vulvovaginal and Müllerian Anomalies

Embryology. The uterus is formed by fusion of the caudal elements of the müllerian ducts, a process that occurs at 8 wk of gestation. The fusion begins from the caudal end (Müller tubercle) and is completed at the upper level of the fundus. A median septum is present until the end of the 1st trimester of gestation.

The vagina is formed from the terminal portion of the uterovaginal canal (Müller tubercle). The tissue is of combined urogenital and müllerian duct origin and is known as the vaginal epithelial plate. Bilateral evaginations of the vaginal epithelial plate encircle the caudal aspect and form the uterine canal. Canalization of the vaginal plate occurs and proceeds in a caudal direction to form the vagina. The process elongates the vaginal structure, leaving the cranial two thirds of müllerian origin and the caudal one third of urogenital origin.

The paramesonephric system is responsible for müllerian tract development. Failure of lateral fusion or lack of resorption of the vertical midline septum results in a müllerian anomaly. Because of the intimate anatomic and embryologic development of the urinary and genital systems, the urinary tract is often also affected; skeletal defects, including spina bifida occulta, occur as well. Common müllerian duct anomalies and associated heritable disorders are presented in Tables 546–1 and 546–2.

Imperforate Hymen. The patient presents with primary amenorrhea; secondary sex characteristics are normal. The imperforate hymen requires surgical intervention. The outflow tract obstruction when relieved should include evaluation of the vaginal canal for any other defects.

Congenital Absence of the Vagina (Mayer-Rokitansky-Küster-Hauser Syndrome). The incidence is reported as 1/4,000 to 1/5,000 births. The etiology is unknown. Vaginal agenesis is characterized by primary amenorrhea, normal vulva, duplication anomaly of the uterus, attenuated fallopian tubes, normal ovaries, normal female karyotype and phenotype, and associated anomalies (most frequently renal and skeletal). The anomaly is often discovered in adolescents. Absence of the vagina has significant anatomic, physiologic, and psychologic implications for the patient and family.

TABLE 546–1. Common Müllerian Anomalies

Hydrocolpos	Accumulation of mucus or nonsanguineous fluid in the vagina
Hemihematometra	Atretic segment of vagina with menstrual fluid accumulation
Hydrosalpinx	Accumulation of serous fluid in the fallopian tube, often an end result of pyosalpinx
Didelphic uterus	Two cervices, each associated with one uterine horn
Bicornuate uterus	One cervix associated with two uterine horns
Unicornuate uterus	Result of failure of one müllerian duct to descend

Treatment is usually delayed until the patient is ready to be sexually active. The nonsurgical approach includes use of frank dilators to create a functional vagina. There is also a combined laparoscopic vulvar procedure in which an olive-tip with suture attached is placed at the introital area and sutures are brought up through the space of Retzius. Progressive increase in tension results in development of a functional vagina. Alternatively, surgical intervention with a McIndoe procedure involving a split-thickness skin graft placed in the vagina area has proved to be a successful approach.

Lesions involving other organ systems occur in association with the Mayer-Rokitansky-Küster-Hauser syndrome. The most common are urinary tract anomalies primarily involving unilateral absence of a kidney or a ureter (27%) and skeletal anomalies (12%), which primarily involve vertebral development.

Incomplete Vertical Fusion of the Vagina. Transverse and longitudinal vaginal septa represent failure of complete canalization of the vagina. Not uncommonly, the patient presents with amenorrhea and cyclical pain, which is a result of cryptomenorrhea. Müllerian agenesis must be differentiated from androgen insensitivity (testicular feminization); serum testosterone levels are usually in the male range with the latter. Müllerian agenesis, with a reported incidence of 1/50,000 to 1/20,000, is more common than androgen insensitivity and is second in frequency to gonadal dysgenesis as a cause of primary amenorrhea.

Renal anomalies are noted in 34% and skeletal anomalies in 12% of patients. Unilateral renal agenesis occurs in 15% of patients. The most frequent skeletal anomalies are vertebral. Klippel-Feil syndrome has been associated with müllerian agenesis. Patients usually have a normal female karyotype (46 XX), but autosomal translocation of chromosomes 12q and 14q also occurs. Affected siblings have been reported, as well as families with variable expression of defects in müllerian, renal, and skeletal systems.

A pelvic ultrasound examination is helpful in defining the anomaly; computed tomographic scanning and magnetic reso-

nance imaging provide increased detail. Laparoscopy is usually reserved for evaluating a pelvic mass and associated abnormalities. Radiologic or sonographic evaluation is indicated to identify associated anomalies. A karyotype should be obtained.

Vaginoplasty is best deferred until a patient has matured and should be supported by counseling for both patient and family. The McIndoe procedure involves the use of a skin graft, usually from the buttocks, to create a vagina after appropriate dissection of the vulvovaginal area. The artificial vaginal epithelium changes cytologically to an almost normal appearing vaginal mucosa. Other reconstructive procedures have included fasciocutaneous flaps. Various dilatation procedures may also result in an increased vaginal size, which ultimately permits intercourse. Squamous cell carcinoma of the reconstructed vagina has been reported and appears to be related to the type of tissue transplanted. Radiotherapy is usually the primary method of treatment for this squamous cell carcinoma.

Transverse Vaginal Septa. The incidence of this lesion is approximately 1/80,000 females. The patient usually presents with amenorrhea, which may be associated with cyclic pelvic pain, a pelvic mass, and cryptomenorrhea. Although usually asymptomatic until puberty, hydrometrocolpos may occur in children. Transverse vaginal septa may be associated with other congenital anomalies, although this occurs less often than with müllerian agenesis. The most common site of the septum is between the middle and upper thirds of the vagina. These patients have a functional uterus, although their fertility is often compromised; 47% of affected females in one retrospective series had spontaneous abortions. The prognosis is worse for higher obstructions. There is also an increased incidence of endometriosis secondary to retrograde menstruation.

Evaluation of transverse vaginal septa includes careful pelvic examination and often pelvic imaging to delineate the anatomic abnormalities. Treatment is surgical resection of the obstruction from below. Anastomosis of the upper and lower segments should be attempted, if at all possible, to prevent stenosis. A skin graft may be necessary. A Lucite stent is often placed in the vagina to maintain patency.

Disorders of Lateral Fusion. These include a number of anatomic variations of nonobstructive longitudinal septum as well as the obstructed hemivagina. The latter may be associated with a didelphic uterus and often with a pelvic mass, which represents retrograde menstruation associated with the occluded hemivagina. Menses, often cyclic, indicates an unobstructed outflow tract from one of the uterine horns.

Uterine Abnormalities. The incidence of uterine anomalies ranges from 1/100 to 1/1,000. Anomalous development of the uterine

TABLE 546–2. Heritable Disorders Associated with Müllerian Anomalies

Mode of Inheritance	Disorder	Associated Müllerian Defect
Autosomal dominant	Camptobrachydactyly	Longitudinal vaginal septa
	Hand-foot-genital	Incomplete müllerian fusion
Autosomal recessive	Kaufman-McCusick	Transverse vaginal septa
	Johanson-Blizzard	Longitudinal vaginal septa
	Renal-genital–middle ear anomalies	Vaginal atresia
	Fraser's syndrome	Incomplete müllerian fusion
	Uterine hernia syndrome	Persistent müllerian duct derivatives
Polygenic/multifactorial	Mayer-Rokitansky-Küster-Hauser syndrome	Müllerian aplasia
X linked	Uterine hernia syndrome	Persistent müllerian duct derivatives

From Shulman L, Elias S: Developmental abnormalities of the female reproductive tract: Pathogenesis and nosology. Adolesc Pediatr Gynecol 1988;1:232.

cavity may have varied clinical manifestations. Patients may present with primary amenorrhea or with irregular or even regular menses. There may be an asymptomatic pelvic mass or dysmenorrhea. In adolescents and adults, pregnancy wastage and infertility may cause the first suspicion of a uterine anomaly.

Diagnosis should include a pelvic ultrasound examination, renal tract assessment, and skeletal inspection for anomalies. Karyotyping and diagnostic laparoscopy may be necessary, depending on the presentation and laboratory assessment.

Treatment depends on the specific anomaly, and surgical repair to date has included Strassman metroplasty, Jones "wedge" metroplasty, and Tompkins metroplasty or hysteroscopic resection. The obstructions to the outflow tract must also be relieved; this may necessitate creation of a vaginal window or excision of a hemivagina. Retrograde menstruation in a uterine horn must also be evaluated and, if present, appropriate surgical correction provided.

Congenital Atresia of the Uterine Cervix. This extremely rare anomaly often presents at puberty with cryptomenorrhea, amenorrhea, and pelvic pain. It is associated with significant renal anomalies in 5–10% of patients. On examination, complete absence of a cervix but a palpable uterus is found. Pelvic imaging is helpful in defining the abnormality. Treatment may include laparotomy to create a uterovaginal fistula. If this is impossible, a hysterectomy may be necessary. Other associated anomalies include mesonephric cysts, which are remnants of the wolffian duct, incomplete reduplication of internal genitalia (e.g., didelphic uterus), and unilateral renal aplasia. In addition, gastrointestinal (42.9%), respiratory (47.6%), central nervous system (28.6%), cardiovascular (38.1%), and musculoskeletal abnormalities (33.3%) have been reported with this abnormality.

Complete Vulvar Duplication. This rare congenital anomaly presents in infancy and consists of two vulvas, vaginas, and bladders, a didelphic uterus, a single rectum and anus, and two renal systems.

Labial Hypertrophy. Elongation of the labia minora may be present at birth. This usually is of no consequence, but surgical revision may be indicated if there are symptoms of discomfort or bulging is noted when wearing tight fitting garments.

Clitoral Abnormalities. Agenesis of the clitoris is rare. Clitoral duplication occurs, often associated with pelvic organ abnormalities, including agenesis of other genital tract structures and bladder exstrophy.

Hymenal Abnormalities. An imperforate hymen may be present in pediatric patients and is often associated with mucocolpos; hydrometrocolpos may also be noted. Other hymenal abnormalities include cribriform or stenotic hymen.

Cloacal Anomalies. These lesions represent a common urogenital sinus into which both urethral and anal orifices exit. The single opening (cloaca) requires surgical correction.

MANAGEMENT OF EMERGENCIES ASSOCIATED WITH CONGENITAL MALFORMATIONS OF THE FEMALE GENITAL TRACT

The clinical manifestations of müllerian anomalies are varied. There may be a pelvic mass, which may or may not be associated with symptoms. A vaginal bulging mass or hemivagina is indicative of complete or partial outflow tract obstruction. An adolescent may present with pelvic pain, either in association with primary amenorrhea or several months after the onset of menarche. Patients also may be asymptomatic until there is evidence of repeat pregnancy wastage. When a presentation is acutely symptomatic, emergency management may be required.

Outflow Tract Obstruction

Obstruction may result from a number of distinct anomalies including the imperforate hymen, transverse vaginal septum, and noncommunicating rudimentary horn. As menstrual fluid accumulates proximal to the obstruction, the resulting hematocolpos, hematometra, or hematocolpometra causes cyclic pain or a pelvic mass. These obstructions are best considered according to the location of the obstruction.

Distal Vagina/Imperforate Hymen. This is the most common obstructive anomaly, and familial occurrences are reported. In the newborn period and early infancy, it may be diagnosed by a bulging membrane due to a mucocolpos from maternal estrogen stimulation. If not noted at this time, it is often not diagnosed until puberty, when menstrual fluid accumulates. The clinical manifestations often are a bulging blue-black membrane, pain, primary amenorrhea, and normal secondary sex characteristics. Depending on the circumstance, patients may have cyclic abdominal pain or a pelvic mass.

Treatment requires incision/resection of the membrane, thus relieving the outflow tract obstruction. Repair should be done at time of diagnosis, if a patient is symptomatic. Although the lesion may be repaired anytime during infancy, childhood, or adolescence, surgery is facilitated by estrogen stimulation and thus ideally performed in adolescence.

Proximal or Midvaginal Transverse Septum. Vertical fusion defects can result in a transverse septum, which may be imperforate and associated with hematocolpos or hematometra in adolescents, or mucocolpos in children. If there is a small, pinpoint aperture, fluid accumulates in the vagina. As with an imperforate hymen, a mass may be present. The vagina appears short or blind ended. The approach to resection of the septum depends on the presence or absence of an opening. In the presence of an opening, cannulation should be attempted with resection of the septum. Postoperatively, a vaginal stent may be necessary.

Rudimentary Horns. This emergency results from the presence of a horn with a functional endometrium and outflow tract obstruction. As with other types of outflow tract obstruction, severe lower abdominal pain with a pelvic mass is the primary clinical manifestation. In contrast to other forms of outflow tract obstruction, however, primary amenorrhea is usually not present because the opposite horn is unlikely to be obstructed. Asymptomatic rupture of a rudimentary horn in an adult has occurred.

Ultrasonography is indicated for visualizing the rudimentary horn. An intravenous pyelogram (IVP) or renal ultrasonography also should be obtained because of associated anomalies. If there is evidence of a functional endometrium, surgical extirpation is recommended.

Rudimentary Horn Pregnancy

This occurs in 1/40,000 pregnancies and 1/5,000–15,000 ectopic pregnancies. It may be a result of a fibromuscular or fibrous band connecting the unicornuate uterus and the rudimentary horn, but 80–85% of cases are noncommunicating. The latter is probably the result of transperitoneal migration of either sperm or the fertilized ovum. In contrast to tubal pregnancies, rudimentary horn pregnancies are often not detected until the second trimester. Because of the greater muscle wall thickness of most horns, rupture typically occurs later than in tubal gestation.

Most cases are diagnosed only after rupture occurs, when patients have acute abdominal pain and peritoneal signs and are often in shock. When rupture occurs, intraperitoneal hemorrhage may be massive and life threatening and requires immediate surgical intervention. Maternal mortality is about 5%, with 90% of this occurring within 10–15 min after rupture. Fetal demise occurs in 98%.

Before rupture, diagnosis of a rudimentary horn pregnancy may be difficult. It should be suspected in any gravida with a known rudimentary horn, and these patients should be closely monitored until an intrauterine pregnancy has been documented. In those who have not been previously identified as having a rudimentary horn, findings on early pelvic examination are similar to findings of tubal ectopic pregnancy and include deviation of the cervix to one side with an adnexal mass on the opposite side. Ultrasound findings before rupture include an extrauterine gestational sac and placenta within the horn next to a slightly enlarged uterus.

Treatment consists of surgical resection of the rudimentary horn.

Acute Urinary Retention

Outflow tract obstruction resulting in accumulation of fluid in the vagina or uterus may cause urinary retention as a result of mucocolpos in the first years of life or hematocolpos, hematometra, or hematocolpometra during the pubertal years. The retained fluid in the vagina compresses the urethra, and this is aggravated when the fluid-filled uterus applies pressure on the posterior wall of the bladder and changes the angle of the urethra. Pressure on the sacral plexus from the distended vagina may also be contributory.

The usual clinical manifestations in adolescents are lower abdominal pain and the inability to void. There also may be hesitancy and incomplete voiding for several days before presentation. Adolescents generally have primary amenorrhea, a history of cyclic lower abdominal pain, and a pelvic mass. However, if the obstruction is unilateral, as with a noncommunicating rudimentary horn or an obstructed hemivagina, the patient may have normal menses.

Temporary but immediate relief can be provided by urethral catheterization. If resistance occurs within an appropriately sized rubber catheter, a pediatric feeding tube may be used, or if necessary, a spinal needle may be passed suprapubically to empty the bladder. Urine should be sent for urinalysis and culture because urinary stasis promotes infection. Once the acute condition has been treated, the underlying problems and the obstructing mass should be appropriately evaluated. Urinary tract infections also have been associated with müllerian anomalies. This may result from renal anomalies with vesicourethral reflux, or it may precede retention as a result of vaginal outflow obstruction. Antibiotic treatment is indicated.

Acute Genital Trauma in the Premenarchal Girl

Acute genital trauma in children can present as superficial genital lacerations and abrasions that do not have active bleeding and may be merely observed. Active bleeding following trauma in the genital area merits appropriate evaluation, which usually includes examination under anesthesia with surgical repair. Forensic studies may be indicated, if there is any suspicion of sexual abuse. Application of topical estrogen cream appears to facilitate the healing process in the vulvovaginal area and clinicians should consider this following surgical intervention.

Achiron R, Tadmor O, Kamar R: Prerupture ultrasound diagnosis of interstitial and rudimentary horn pregnancy in the second trimester. *Int J Reprod Med* 1992;37:89.

American Fertility Society: The American Fertility Society classifications of adnexal adhesions, distal tubal occlusion, tubal occlusion secondary to tubal lig-

ation, tubal pregnancies, müllerian anomalies, and intrauterine adhesions. *Fertil Steril* 1988;49:944.

Bejanga I: Hematocolpos with imperforate hymen. *Int Surg* 1978;63:97.

Bergh P, Breen J, Gregori C: Congenital absence of the vagina—the Mayer-Rokitansky-Küster-Hauser syndrome. *Adolesc Pediatr Gynecol* 1989;2:73.

Brevetti L, Brevetti G, Lawrence J, et al: Pyocolpos: Diagnosis and treatment. *J Pediatr Surg* 1997;32:110.

Craighill M: Pediatric and adolescent gynecology for the primary care pediatrician. *Pediatr Clin North Am* 1998;45(6):659.

Fedele L, Bianchi S, Agnoli B, et al: Urinary tract anomalies associated with unicornuate uterus. *J Urol* 1996;155:847.

Folch M, Pigem I, Konge J: Müllerian agenesis: Etiology, diagnosis and management. *Obstet Gynecol Survey* 2000;55(10):644.

Freedman M: Uterine anomalies. *Semin Reprod Endocrinol* 1986;4:39.

Horejsi JA: Incomplete reduplication of internal genitalia and unilateral renal aplasia syndrome. *Adolesc Pediatr Gynecol* 1988;1:42.

Joshi N, Sotrel G: Diagnostic laparoscopy in apparent uterine agenesis. *J Adolesc Health Care* 1988;9:403.

Lewis V, Money J: Gender-identity/role. Par A:XY (androgen insensitivity) syndrome and XX (Rokitansky) syndrome, vaginal atresia compared. In Dennerstein L, Burroughs G (editors): *Handbook of Psychosomatic Obstetrics and Gynecology.* New York, Elsevier Biomedical Press, 1983, p 61.

Loong E, Yuen P: Acute urinary retention caused by a unilateral hematometra. *Arch Gynecol Obstet* 1990;247:211.

Merit D: Evaluating and managing acute genital trauma pre-menarche girls. *J Pediatr Adolesc Gynecol* 1999;12:237.

Nagele F, Langle R, Stolzlechner J, et al: Noncommunicating rudimentary horn—obstetric and gynecologic implications. *Acta Obstet Gynecol Scand* 1995;74:566.

Nisanian A: Hematocolpometra presenting as urinary retention: A case report. *J Reprod Med* 1993;38:57.

Peter J, Steinhardt G: Acute urinary retention in children. *Pediatr Emerg Care* 1993;9:205.

Robischon K, Baram D, Phipps WR: Presentation of a müllerian anomaly with outflow obstruction after tubal ligation. *Fertil Steril* 1996;65:866.

Rock J, Azziz R: Genital anomalies in childhood. *Clin Obstet Gynecol* 1987;30:682.

Rock JA, Horowitz IR: Surgical conditions of the vagina and urethra. In Rock JA, Thompson JD (editors): *TeLinde's Operative Gynecology.* Philadelphia, Lippincott-Raven, 1997, p 913.

Shulman LP, Elias S: Developmental abnormalities of the female reproductive tract: Pathogenesis and nosology. *Adolesc Pediatr Gynecol* 1987;1:230.

Stallion A: Vaginal obstruction. *Semin Pediatr Surg* 2000;9(3):128.

Yu T, Lin M: Acute urinary retention in two patients with imperforate hymen. *Scand J Urol Nephrol* 1993;27:543.

Chapter 547
Athletic Gynecologic Problems

The most common gynecologic problem in female athletes is menstrual aberration, usually manifested as amenorrhea or oligomenorrhea. Female adolescents who participate in strenuous training have low serum estradiol levels and are predisposed to bone demineralization. Puberty and menarche may be delayed.

Endogenous opiates within the hypothalamus may inhibit gonadotropin-releasing hormone neurons and thus affect luteinizing hormone secretion and reproductive function. There is also an increase in corticotropin secretion. In addition, a change in body composition and weight loss is involved in the menstrual abnormality. Amenorrheic runners tend to have less body fat than eumenorrheic runners, and menarche is delayed approximately 3 yr in ballet dancers (in comparison with nonathletic adolescents) preparing for a professional career. Delayed puberty in association with endurance training does not result in significant alteration of follicle-stimulating hormone and luteinizing hormone levels. It is important to assess nutritional status and other potential causes before delayed puberty is attributed to athletic activities.

The triad of disordered eating, amenorrhea, and osteoporosis is a common clinical entity among female athletes. Educational efforts, especially among adolescents, should focus on these potential problems and how to avoid them. Appropriate weight maintenance, dietary habits, and psychological factors should be addressed.

Baer JT, Taper LJ, Gwazdauskas FG, et al: Diet, hormonal, and metabolic factors affecting bone mineral density in adolescent amenorrheic and eumenorrheic female runners. *J Sports Med Phys Fitness* 1992;32:51.

Ding JH, Sheckter CB, Drinkwater BL, et al: High serum cortisol levels in exercise-associated amenorrhea. *Ann Intern Med* 1988;108:530.

Gidwani G: Amenorrhea in the athlete. *Adolesc Med* 1999;10(2):275.

Warren MD, Brooks-Gunn J, Hamilton LH, et al: Scoliosis and fractures in young ballet dancers. Relation to delayed menarche and secondary amenorrhea. *N Engl J Med* 1986;314:1348.

Warren M, Stiehl A: Exercise and female adolescents: Effects on the reproductive and skeletal systems. *J Am Med Womens Assoc* 1999;54(3):115.

West RV: The female athlete triad of disordered eating, amenorrhea and osteoporosis. *Sports Med* 1998;26(2):63.

Chapter 548
Special Gynecologic Needs

Mentally Handicapped Children. Perineal hygiene is a major problem for severely mentally handicapped pediatric or adolescent patients. Initially, an adequate gynecologic examination and Papanicolaou smear should be provided. A number of medical approaches should then be considered to suppress menses. Depo-medroxyprogesterone acetate, usually prescribed at a dose of 150 mg, may be injected intramuscularly every 3 mo. Alternatively, oral contraceptives do not produce amenorrhea but result in a marked decrease in the quantity of menstrual flow. Before hysterectomy, there should be a thorough discussion with parents or custodians after a trial of medical treatment has not been successful. An ethics advisory committee should be consulted to aid in decisions about sterilizing mentally handicapped patients (see also Chapters 2 and 37).

The problem of sexual abuse of the mentally handicapped child continues to be a challenge for both clinicians and those providing care for these children. Every effort should be made to prevent sexual abuse of mentally or physically handicapped girls. Contraception may be prescribed for patients at increased risk for pregnancy. This does not always require an initial pelvic examination. Sonography has been utilized in special circumstances to evaluate the pelvic organs prior to initiating contraceptive therapy.

Premature Ovarian Failure in Association with Chemotherapy and/or Radiation Therapy. The incidence of premature ovarian failure has increased with the increased survival of children and adolescent patients having neoplasms. Hormone replacement therapy in an approach similar to that of menopause, i.e., physiologic estrogen replacement therapy with the addition of progestins, provides the patient with secondary sex characteristics as well as regular menses.

Elkins T, Hoyle D, Darnton T, et al: The use of a societally based ethics class advisory committee to aid in decisions to sterilize mentally handicapped patients. *Adolesc Pediatr Gynecol* 1988;1:190.

Elkins T, McNeeley S, Rosen D, et al: A clinical observation of a program to accomplish pelvic exams in difficult-to-manage patients with mental retardation. *Adolesc Pediatr Gynecol* 1988;1:195.

Furman L: Institutionalized disabled adolescents: Gynecological care. *Clin Pediatr* 1989;28(4):163.

Owens K, Honebrink A: Gynecologic care of medically complicated adolescents. *Pediatr Clin North Am* 1999;46(3):631.

Piippo SH, Lenko HL, Laippala PJ: Experiences of special gynaecological services for children and adolescents: A descriptive study. *Acta Paediatr* 1998;87:805.

Chapter 549
Gynecologic Imaging

A transabdominal ultrasonic approach with a distended bladder serving as an imaging window facilitates identification of the uterus and the ovaries; bladder distention with urine displaces gas-filled bowel loops out of the pelvis and enhances imaging. A 7.5- or 5-MHz transducer is usually used, especially with larger children and teenagers. Ultrasonography is a key screening tool, enabling appropriate diagnosis in patients presenting with ambiguous genitalia, ovarian or uterine masses, primary amenorrhea, and abdominal or pelvic pain. Normal values are listed in Table 549–1.

Pelvic masses can be identified at any age. Ovarian cysts and hydrocolpos or hydrometrocolpos are the most common abnormalities noted in neonates. Hydrocolpos is defined as dilatation of the vagina, which usually is associated with accumulation of serous fluid or urine (if there is a urogenital sinus). Hydrometrocolpos causes dilatation of both the uterus and the vagina. It may also be associated with vaginal or cervical atresia, stenosis, or an imperforate hymen. Most large ovarian cysts (simple cystic) in children may be safely observed with serial pelvic ultrasonography and tend to decrease in size or completely resolve. A solid mass requires a tissue diagnosis.

Magnetic resonance imaging is useful in evaluating müllerian duct anomalies. It should be used in conjunction with

TABLE 549–1. Normal Ovarian and Uterine Dimensions

Ovary

Birth
15 mm long, 3 mm wide, 2.5 mm thick
Ovarian volume 0.7 cm³*

Post Puberty
22.5–50.0 mm in length
1.5–3 cm in width; 0.6–1.5 cm in thickness
Ovarian volume 1.8–5.7 cm³*

Uterus

Neonate
Length 2.3–4.6 cm
Anteroposterior diameter 0.8–2.2 cm

Infant to 7 yr of age
Length 2.5–3.3 cm
Anteroposterior diameter 0.4–1.0 cm

Post Puberty
Length 6 cm

*Ovarian volume can be determined by using the formula: length × height × width × 0.523.
From Sanfilippo JS, Lavery JP: The spectrum of ultrasound: Antenatal to adolescent years. Semin Reprod Endocrinol 1988; 6:47.

ultrasound assessment and, if necessary, such techniques as genitography. Three-dimensional ultrasonographic and Doppler assessment have been utilized with ovarian abnormalities. The three-dimensional Doppler studies more clearly differentiate benign from malignant ovarian lesions and reduce the false-positive findings with ultrasonography.

Kurjak A, Jupesic S, Sparac V, et al: Three-dimensional ultrasonographic and power Doppler characterization of ovarian lesions. *Ultrasound Obstet Gynecol* 2000;16:365.

Lang IM, Babyn P, Oliver GD: MR imaging of pediatric uterovaginal anomalies. *Pediatr Radiol* 1999;29:163.

Siegel MJ, Surratt JT: Pediatric gynecologic imaging. *Obstet Gynecol Clin North Am* 1992;19:103.

Warner BW, Kuhn JC, Barr LL: Conservative management of large ovarian cysts in children: The value of serial pelvic ultrasonography. *Surgery* 1992;112:749.

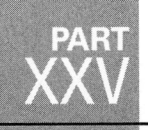
The Endocrine System

SECTION 1 *Disorders of the Hypothalamus and Pituitary Gland*

Chapter 550

Hormones of the Hypothalamus and Pituitary

John S. Parks

The anterior pituitary gland originates from the Rathke pouch as an invagination of the oral ectoderm. It then detaches from the oral epithelium and becomes an individual structure of rapidly proliferating cells. Persistent remnants of the original connection between the Rathke pouch and the oral cavity can develop into craniopharyngiomas, which are the most common type of tumor in this area. Five cell types in the anterior pituitary produce six peptide hormones. Somatotropes produce growth hormone (GH), lactotropes produce prolactin (PRL), thyrotropes make thyroid-stimulating hormone (TSH), corticotropes express pro-opiomelanocortin (POMC), the precursor of corticotropin (adrenocorticotropic hormone [ACTH]), and gonadotropes express both luteinizing hormone (LH) and follicle-stimulating hormone (FSH).

A series of sequentially expressed transcriptional activation factors directs the differentiation and proliferation of anterior pituitary cell types. These proteins are members of a large family of DNA-binding proteins resembling homeobox genes. The consequences of mutations in several of these genes are evident in human forms of multiple pituitary hormone deficiency.

The HESX1 gene is expressed in precursors of all five cell types early in development, at embryonic day 8.5 (e8.5) in the mouse. It is not expressed after day e13.5. Pituitary OTX or Ptx-1 is also expressed early. This protein is capable of activating transcription from the POMC, GH, and PRL promoters as well as from the promoter of the α-glycoprotein subunit (α-GSU) that is common to LH, FSH, and TSH. In vitro, it can also activate the β-LH and β-FSH subunits. It acts cooperatively with the transcription factor POU1F1 (formerly termed PIT1) in activation of transcription from the GH and PRL promoters. Ptx-1 appears to be necessary for expression of the next transcription factor in the cascade, termed LHX3. The protein encoded by LHX3 appears by day e9.5. It activates the α-GSU promoter and acts synergistically with POU1F1 to increase transcription from the PRL, β-TSH, and POU1F1 promoters. Targeted disruption of this gene in the mouse produces a phenotype of hypopituitarism in which the Rathke pouch develops normally, but the anterior and intermediate lobes of the pituitary fail to develop. The Ptx-2 gene, also known as the Riegl gene, is expressed from day e11 into adult life. Its DNA-binding domain differs from that of Ptx-1 by only 2 of 60 amino acids. The Ptx-2 protein is also found in developing eye, tongue, kidney, testis, and umbilicus. Expression of the "Prophet of Pit-1" or PROP1 gene begins at day e10.5 and is downregulated by day e14.5. This protein is

found in the nuclei of somatotropes, lactotropes, and thyrotropes. Its role includes turning off HESX3 and turning on POU1F1. The POU1F1 (POU-homeodomain factor 1) appears at day e14.5 and is necessary for emergence of somatotropes, lactotropes, and a definitive population of thyrotropes. This protein persists in the mature pituitary and is involved in activation of GH, PRL, and β-TSH expression.

Anterior Lobe Hormones. The protein hormones produced by the anterior pituitary act on other endocrine glands and on certain body cells to affect almost every organ. Anterior pituitary cells are themselves controlled by neuropeptide-releasing and release-inhibiting hormones that are produced by hypothalamic neurons, secreted into the capillaries of the median eminence, and carried by portal veins to the anterior pituitary. Many conditions formerly classified as pituitary in origin are caused by hypothalamic defects.

Human GH is a protein with 191 amino acids. Its gene (GH1) is the first in a cluster of five closely related genes on the long arm of chromosome 17 (q22-24). The four other genes have greater than 90% sequence identity with the GH1 gene. They consist of the CS1 and CS2 genes, which encode the same human chorionic somatomammotropin (hCS) protein, a placental growth hormone gene (GH2), and a pseudogene (CSP). Syncytiotrophoblastic cells of the fetal placenta produce large quantities of hCS, and placental GH replaces pituitary GH in the maternal circulation after 20 wk of gestation. When the fetal genome lacks the CS1, CS2, GH2, and CSP genes, hCS and placental GH are absent, but fetal growth and postpartum lactation are normal.

The GH1 gene is expressed in pituitary somatotropes under the control of three hypothalamic hormones. Growth hormone-releasing hormone (GHRH) stimulates and somatostatin inhibits GH release. Alternating secretion of GHRH and somatostatin accounts for the rhythmic secretion of GH. Peaks of GH occur when peaks of GHRH coincide with troughs of somatostatin. The secretion of GH is pulsatile, with the highest peaks occurring with sleep. A second stimulatory system, parallel to that involving the GHRH receptor, is activated by ghrelin. Ghrelin is produced in the arcuate nucleus of the hypothalamus and in much greater quantities by the stomach. GH secretion may be influenced by ghrelin levels in the hypothalamic-pituitary portal circulation and the systemic circulation. Fasting stimulates and feeding inhibits ghrelin release into the systemic circulation. Intraventricular injection of ghrelin increases feeding and weight gain in rats.

The three molecular species of GHRH contain 37, 40, or 44 amino acids. A fully active 29-amino acid synthetic GHRH is available as a diagnostic agent and for treatment of GH deficiency secondary to GHRH deficiency. Somatostatin exists in 14- and 28-amino acid forms. Somatostatin production is not limited to the hypothalamus. It also acts through autocrine and paracrine mechanisms in the islets of Langerhans and in the gastrointestinal tract. Somatostatin inhibits secretion of insulin, glucagon, secretin, gastrin, vasoactive intestinal peptide (VIP), GH, and thyrotropin. In the pancreatic islets, it is localized to the D cells. Somatostatin-secreting pancreatic tumors (somatostatinomas) occur in adults. A potent, long-acting somatostatin analog, octreotide, which inhibits GH preferentially over insulin, is available to treat patients with GH-secreting tumors. It is also useful in managing patients with gastrinomas, insulinomas, glucagonomas, VIPomas, and carcinoid tumors (see Chapters 81 and 326). ^{123}I-labeled octreotide appears to be useful in localizing somatostatin receptor-positive tumors and their metastases. Ghrelin has an unusual structure. It consists of 28 amino acids and the third amino acid, a serine, is octanoylated. This octanoyl group is essential for physiologic activity.

GH acts through binding to receptor molecules on the surface of target cells. The GH receptor is a single-chain molecule of 620 amino acids. It has an extracellular domain, a single membrane-spanning domain, and a cytoplasmic domain. Proteolytically cleaved fragments of the extracellular domain circulate in plasma and act as a GH-binding protein. As in other members of the cytokine receptor family, the cytoplasmic domain of the GH receptor lacks intrinsic kinase activity; instead, GH binding induces receptor dimerization and activation of a receptor-associated Janus kinase (Jak2). Phosphorylation of the kinase and other protein substrates initiates a series of events that leads to alterations in nuclear gene transcription.

The mitogenic actions of GH are mediated through increases in the synthesis of insulin-like growth factor-I (IGF-I), formerly named somatomedin C, a single-chain peptide with 70 amino acids coded for by a gene on the long arm of chromosome 12. IGF-I has considerable homology to insulin. Circulating IGF-I is synthesized primarily in the liver and formed locally in mesodermal and ectodermal cells, particularly in the growth plate of children, where its effect is exerted by paracrine or autocrine mechanisms. Circulating levels of IGF-I are related to blood levels of GH to a large extent, except in the fetus and during the neonatal period. IGF-I circulates bound to several different binding proteins; the major one is a 150-kd complex (IGF-BP3), which is decreased in GH-deficient children but is in the normal range in children who are short for other reasons. Human recombinant IGF-I may have therapeutic potential in conditions characterized by end organ resistance to GH. Examples include Laron syndrome, a state of resistance to GH caused by mutations in the GH receptor, and resistance caused by the development of antibodies to administered GH. IGF-II is a single-chain protein with 67 amino acids that is coded for by a gene on the short arm of chromosome 11. It has homology to IGF-I, but much less is known about its physiologic roles, although it appears to be an important mitogen in bone cells, where it occurs in a concentration many times higher than that of IGF-I.

Several disorders of growth are caused by abnormalities of the genes that code for the GHRH receptor, HESX1, POU1F1, PROP1, LHX3, GH1, the GH receptor, and IGF-I.

Prolactin is composed of 199 amino acids, and its gene is located on chromosome 6. The major prolactin-inhibiting factor is dopamine; medications that disrupt hypothalamic dopaminergic pathways result in increased serum levels of prolactin. Serum levels of prolactin are increased after administration of thyrotropin-releasing hormone (TRH), in states of primary hypothyroidism, and after disruption of the pituitary stalk, as may occur in children with craniopharyngioma. Levels are decreased by destruction of the pituitary and by mutations in PROP1 and POU1F1, which interfere with the embryonic development of lactotropes.

The main established role for prolactin is the initiation and maintenance of lactation. Concentrations in amniotic fluid are 10–100 times the levels in maternal or fetal serum. The major source of amniotic prolactin appears to be the decidua. Mean serum levels in children and in fasting adults of both sexes are about 5–20 µg/L, but levels in the fetus and in neonates during the 1st wk of life are usually higher than 200 µg/L.

TSH consists of two glycoprotein chains linked by hydrogen bonding. The α-chain is identical to that found in FSH, LH, and chorionic gonadotropin (hCG). The β-chain is unique in each of these hormones and confers specificity. The gene for the α-chain has been mapped on chromosome 6, that for the α-chain of TSH on chromosome 1, and those for the β-chains for LH and hCG on chromosome 19. TSH increases iodine uptake, iodide clearance from the plasma, iodotyrosine and iodothyronine formation, thyroglobulin proteolysis, and release of thyroxine (T_4) and triiodothyronine (T_3) from the thyroid. Most of the effects of TSH are mediated by cyclic adenosine monophosphate. Deficiency of TSH results in inactivity and atrophy of the thyroid, and excess results in hypertrophy and hyperplasia.

TRH is a tripeptide ([pyro] Glu-His-Pro-NH2). Thyroxine and triiodothyronine inhibit TSH secretion by blocking the action of TRH on the pituitary cell. TRH also stimulates the release of prolactin in both sexes. Synthetic TRH is useful for testing pituitary reserves of TSH and prolactin.

ACTH is derived by proteolytic cleavage from a large precursor glycoprotein product of the pituitary gland called POMC. Cleavage of POMC yields ACTH, a single chain of 39 amino acids, and β-lipotropin (β-LPH), a 91-amino acid glycoprotein. Further cleavage of ACTH and β-LPH in the pituitary yields yet other hormonal products. The α-melanocyte-stimulating hormone is identical to the first 13 amino acids of ACTH but has no corticotropin activity. Cleavage of β-LPH results in neurotropic peptides with morphinomimetic activity (fragment 61–91 is β-endorphin), and β-melanocyte-stimulating hormone consists of a 17-amino acid fragment of β-LPH.

ACTH acts primarily on the adrenal cortex. It produces changes in structure, chemical composition, enzymatic activity, and release of corticosteroid hormones. ACTH release has a diurnal rhythm. The level is lowest between 10 PM and 2 AM, with peak levels reached about 8 AM. Levels of β-LPH and β-endorphin are elevated in patients with increased levels of ACTH. It appears that ACTH rather than MSH is the principal pigmentary hormone in humans.

POMC peptides are also produced in nonpituitary tissues. In the testis, some peptides act as autocrine regulators of androgen-secreting Leydig cells, and others may potentiate or oppose the action of FSH on Sertoli cells.

Secretion of ACTH, β-endorphin, and other POMC-related peptides is regulated by corticotropin-releasing hormone (CRH). CRH is a 41-amino acid peptide found predominantly in the median eminence but also in other areas of the brain and in tissues outside the brain, particularly the placenta. During pregnancy, levels of CRH increase several hundred-fold, increase further during labor and delivery, and then decrease to non-pregnant levels within 24 hr. Its source is probably the placenta, which contains the peptide and its mRNA. Synthetic CRH is available for diagnostic use and it is particularly useful in differentiating the different forms of Cushing syndrome.

Gonadotropic hormones include two glycoproteins, LH and FSH. They contain the same α subunit as TSH and distinct β subunits. Receptors for FSH on the ovarian granulosa cells and on testicular Sertoli cells mediate FSH stimulation of follicular development in the ovary and of gametogenesis in the testis. On binding to specific receptors on ovarian theca cells and testicular Leydig cells, LH promotes luteinization of the ovary and Leydig cell function of the testis. The receptors for LH and FSH belong to a class of receptors with seven membrane-spanning protein domains. Receptor occupancy activates adenylyl cyclase through mediation of G proteins.

Luteinizing hormone-releasing hormone, a decapeptide, has been isolated, synthesized, and widely used in clinical studies. Because it leads to the release of LH and FSH from the same gonadotropic cells, it appears that there is only one gonadotropin-releasing hormone.

Secretion of LH is inhibited by androgens and estrogens, and secretion of FSH is suppressed by gonadal production of inhibin, a 31-kd glycoprotein produced by the Sertoli cells. Inhibin consists of α and β subunits joined by disulfide bonds. The β-β dimer (activin) also occurs, but its biologic effect is to stimulate FSH secretion. The biologic features of these newer hormones are being delineated. In addition to its endocrine effect, activin has paracrine effects in the testis. It facilitates LH-induced testosterone production, indicating a direct effect of Sertoli cells on Leydig cells analogous to the interaction of these cells through the paracrine effects of POMC.

The posterior lobe of the pituitary is part of a functional unit, the neurohypophysis, that consists of the neurons of the supraoptic and paraventricular nuclei of the hypothalamus; neuronal axons, which form the pituitary stalk; and neuronal terminals in the median eminence or in the posterior lobe.

Hormones of the Neurohypophysis. The neurohypophysis is the source of arginine vasopressin (AVP; antidiuretic hormone) and of oxytocin. Both are octapeptides, differing in only two amino acids. These hormones are produced by neurosecretion in the hypothalamic nuclei. Vasopressin derives its name from early observations of its pressor and antidiuretic activities but the latter is its physiologically important function. At levels 50–1,000 times those found in blood, it affects blood pressure, intestinal contractility, hepatic glycogenolysis, platelet aggregation, and release of factor VIII.

Vasopressin and its accompanying protein, called neurophysin II, are encoded by the same gene. A single preprohormone is cleaved and the two are transported to neurosecretory vesicles in the posterior pituitary. The two are released in equimolar amounts. Oxytocin and neurophysin I have a similar relationship.

AVP has a short half-life and responds quickly to changes in hydration. The stimuli for AVP release are increased plasma osmolality, perceived by osmoreceptors in the hypothalamus, and decreased blood volume, perceived by baroreceptors in the carotid sinus of the aortic arch. AVP changes the permeability of the renal tubular cell membrane through cyclic adenosine monophosphate. A synthetic analog, desmopressin combines high potency, selectivity for antidiuretic hormone receptors, and resistance to degradation by proteases. Desmopressin may be given by injection, by intranasal spray, or by mouth. The amount that is required for management of diabetes insipidus depends on the mode of administration. A typical dose is on the order of 1 µg for the injected, 10 µg for the intranasal, and 100 µg for the oral form.

BOX 551–1. Etiologic Classification of Hypopituitarism

ISOLATED GROWTH HORMONE DEFICIENCY
Genetic Forms of GH Deficiency and GH Resistance

GHRH Receptor	Missense and frameshifts
GH1	
Recessive	Deletions, frameshifts, missense, intron 4 splice errors
Dominant	Intron 3 splice errors
X-Linked	
Xq21.3-q22	May be associated with hypogammaglobulinemia
Xq24-q27.1	May be associated with mental retardation
GH Insensitivity	
GH Receptor	Laron syndrome
IGF-I Gene	Intrauterine and postnatal growth retardation
GH-1 Gene	Arg77Cys, intrauterine and postnatal growth retardation

Acquired GH Deficiency

Postradiation	Dependent on dose of radiation
Idiopathic	May be transient

MULTIPLE PITUITARY HORMONE DEFICIENCY
Genetic Forms

POU1F1	GH, Prl, and TSH deficiencies; normal or small pituitary
PROP1	GH, Prl, TSH, LH, FSH +/- ACTH deficiencies; normal or enlarged pituitary
LHX3	GH, Prl, TSH, LH, FSH deficiencies; normal or enlarged pituitary
HESX1	Optic nerve hypoplasia
PTX2-RIEG1	Rieger syndrome with pituitary, eye, GI, and kidney defects

Uncertain Etiology

Septo-optic dysplasia
Hall-Pallister syndrome
Single central incisor
Holoprosencephaly
Anencephaly

Acquired Disorders

Tumors	Craniopharyngioma, optic glioma, pituitary adenoma
Trauma	Shaken infant, motor vehicle injuries
Inflammatory	Histiocytosis, hypophysitis, tuberculosis

GH = growth hormone; GHRH = growth hormone–releasing hormone; TSH = thyroid-stimulating hormone; ACTH = adrenocorticotropic hormone (corticotropin); LH = luteinizing hormone; FSH = follicle-stimulating hormone; Prl = prolactin.

Chapter 551
Hypopituitarism *John S. Parks*

Hypopituitary states are associated with a deficiency of growth hormone (GH), with or without a deficiency of other pituitary hormones (Box 551–1). Affected children have in common a phenotype of postnatal growth impairment that is specifically corrected by replacement of GH.

ISOLATED DEFICIENCY OF GROWTH HORMONE

Genetic Forms. Isolated GH deficiency (IGHD) can be transmitted as an autosomal recessive (type I), autosomal dominant (type II), or X-linked recessive (type III) trait. IGHD I is caused by mutations of the GH-releasing hormone (GHRH) receptor or the GH1 gene, IGHD II by mutations in the GH1 gene, and IGHD III by mutations in two regions of the X chromosome.

Mutations in the GHRH receptor gene occur in several large kindreds from Pakistan, India, and Brazil. Homozygosity for inactivating mutations impairs the proliferation and function of somatotropes. The phenotype consists of modest compromise of fetal growth followed by severe postnatal growth failure. Puberty is delayed, and affected individuals continue to grow into their 20s and 30s. Early recognition and consistent replacement with recombinant GH enables these individuals and others with IGHD to attain normal adult heights.

Mutations and deletions in the GH1 gene produce a similar phenotype. Missense, nonsense, and frameshift mutations are described, but most cases demonstrate mutations in the fourth and final intron of the gene. These mutations eliminate the normal splice donor site used in splicing exon 4 to exon 5. An alternative donor splice site in exon 4 results in a frameshift with production of a messenger RNA encoding a protein that is longer than normal and has no biologic activity.

GH deficiency type I can also be the result of large deletions in the GH gene cluster on chromosome 17q22-24. Deletions of 6.7, 7.0, or 7.6 kb remove only the GH1 gene, whereas deletions of up to 45 kb remove one or more of the adjacent genes termed CSL, CS1, GH2, and CS2 (Chapter 550). The growth phenotype is identical with deletion of GH1 or deletion of GH1 and the other genes. Loss of the other genes without loss of GH1 causes deficiency of chorionic somatomammotropin and placental GH in the maternal circulation, but does not result in fetal or postnatal growth retardation. Homozygosity for GH1 deletion responds initially to GH treatment, but later may develop high titers of GH-binding antibodies and become resistant to GH. The term IGHD IA is applied to these cases; "A" refers to "antibodies" and is used to distinguish it from IGHD IB, which is generally less severe and is not complicated by production of blocking antibodies. This distinction persists in the OMIM classification of GH deficiency even though antibody formation is now the exception rather than the rule in persons with GH1 deletions. The reduction in risk of antibody formation is because preparations of recombinant human GH (hGH) are much less antigenic than the extracted pituitary hGH preparations used previously.

Many cases of autosomal dominant IGHD II have been associated with GH1 mutations. The most common form involves mutation in the splice donor site for intron 3. When this site is altered, exon 3 is omitted from the processed messenger RNA and amino acids 32 to 71 are omitted from the mature protein. Small amounts of the mRNA for this 17,000 molecular weight protein are made in the normal pituitary. When the protein is produced in larger quantities because of an intron 3 mutation, it interferes with production of the normal 22,000 molecular weight protein encoded by the normal allele. This interference probably occurs at the level of transport from microsomes to secretory vesicles. The severity of GH deficiency and growth impairment increases with age. It is not clear whether this progression is associated with reduction in the number of functioning somatotropes.

X-linked recessive IGHD III occurs in the sons of a normal mother and different fathers. In many cases, it is associated with hypogammaglobulinemia. The clinical expression of GH deficiency often follows the expression of immunodeficiency. The hypogammaglobulinemia mapping to Xq21.3-q22 is caused by mutations in the BTK (Bruton thymidine kinase) gene. This gene is expressed in somatotropes as well as in plasma cells. Many persons with mutations in this gene do not experience growth retardation. This may be because only limited spectrums of BTK mutations influence somatotrope function, or persons with the combined defects have disruptions of contiguous genes. In some other pedigrees, X-linked IGHD III maps to a more distal locus, at Xq24-q27.1. In these pedigrees, there is an association of IGHD with mental retardation. It is unclear whether the two features are due to mutations in a single gene or to disruption of contiguous genes.

Not all cases of heritable IGHD have been linked to the genes mentioned earlier. Although the GHRH gene is a logical candidate, extensive studies have failed to disclose any examples of mutations at this locus in either IGHD I or IGHD II pedigrees.

Acquired Forms. The GH axis is more susceptible to disruption by acquired conditions than are the other hypothalamic-pituitary axes.

Improved survival of children who receive radiotherapy for malignancies of the central nervous system or other cranial structures has resulted in a group of patients with GH deficiency. Children with acute lymphocytic leukemia who have received prophylactic cranial irradiation belong in this group. Growth typically slows during radiation therapy or chemotherapy, improves for 1–2 yr, then declines with the development of GH deficiency. Spinal irradiation contributes to disproportionately poor growth of the trunk. The dose of radiation and the fraction-

ation schedule used are important determinants of the incidence of hypopituitarism. GH deficiency is almost universal 5 yr after therapy with a total dose of 35–45 Gy. More subtle defects are seen with doses around 20 Gy. Deficiency of GH is the most common defect, but deficiencies of thyroid-stimulating hormone (TSH) and adrenocorticotropic hormone (ACTH) may also occur. In contrast to other forms of hypopituitarism, puberty is not delayed. A pubertal growth spurt at a normal to early age may lessen clinical suspicion of GH deficiency.

Diagnostic strategies for distinguishing between permanent GH deficiency and other causes of impaired growth are imperfect. Children with a combination of genetic short stature and constitutional delay of growth and pubertal development have short stature, below average growth rates, and delayed bone ages. Many of these children exhibit minimal GH secretory responses to provocative stimuli. When children who have been diagnosed with idiopathic or acquired GH deficiency are treated with hGH and are retested as adults, the majority have peak GH levels within the normal range.

PERIPHERAL RESISTANCE TO GROWTH HORMONE

Genetic Forms of Resistance to GH. There are three recognized mechanisms for end-organ insensitivity to GH. The first, described by Laron, involves abnormalities in the gene on chromosome 5p13-p12 that encodes the receptor for GH. This disease has been recognized in many individuals from many different ethnic backgrounds. Most examples show recessive inheritance, but there are also dominant forms. The second mechanism involves abnormality of the insulin-like growth factor-I (IGF-I) gene and the third involves production of an abnormal GH that serves as a competitive antagonist to the normal hormone.

Children with *Laron syndrome* have all the clinical findings of those with IGHD, but they have elevated levels of circulating GH. Levels of IGF-I are low and fail to respond to exogenous hGH. A variety of gene defects has been discovered in different families, ranging from the deletion of several exons of the gene, through nonsense mutations, to missense mutations, and to mutations that alter splicing of messenger RNA. Most of the mutations produce a loss of GH-binding activity. However, some are associated with normal or increased levels of binding. The mutant protein in at least one family retains normal affinity for GH binding but lacks the ability to form dimers of GH receptor around a single bound GH molecule. In other families, there is increased serum GH binding activity resulting from overproduction of a receptor that lacks the transmembrane domain and has no capacity for signal transduction.

Although mutations in pituitary transcription factor, GHRH receptor, GH, and GH receptor genes have minimal effects on prenatal growth, disruption of the IGF-I gene produces profound intrauterine growth retardation. The single patient described to date was 5.4 SD below the mean for length at birth and 6.9 SD below the mean for height at age 15 yr. He was homozygous for deletion of exons 3 and 4 of the IGF-I gene. There was an absence of circulating IGF-I, but elevated levels of GH and IGF-BP3.

The existence of short stature due to biologically inactive GH was proposed in the 1970s. Some patients with normal to high levels of circulating GH by immunoassay appeared to have lower levels of GH when assessed by receptor binding and cell proliferation assays. The first instance of an antagonistic GH was provided in 1996 in a child who was heterozygous for a mutation changing arginine to cysteine at position 77. The mutant protein binds to GHBP and to the GH receptor, but it does not result in activation of Jak2 kinase. Its dominant negative mechanism of action reflects a higher than normal binding affinity for the receptor. Interestingly, the patient demonstrated severe intrauterine growth retardation similar to that of the child with abnormalities of the GH1 gene. This suggests that a competitive antagonist for receptor binding has a more severe effect on fetal growth than does complete inactivation of the receptor for GH. One can speculate that inactivation of the prolactin (PRL) receptor as well as the GH receptor is necessary to eliminate endocrine stimuli to fetal production of IGF-I.

MULTIPLE PITUITARY HORMONE DEFICIENCY

Genetic Forms of Multiple Pituitary Hormone Deficiency. Quite a few genes involved in embryonic development are candidates to explain multiple pituitary hormone deficiency (MPHD) (Chapter 550). There are several distinctive heritable forms of MPHD. Mutations of transcription factor genes that are only expressed in the anterior pituitary lead to simple phenotypes with varying combinations of anterior pituitary hormone deficiencies. Mutations of transcription factor genes that are also expressed in other embryonic tissues give rise to more complex phenotypes that include multiple congenital anomalies.

POU1F1 (PIT1) was originally identified as a nuclear protein that bound to the GH and PRL promoters. Mutations in POU1F1 are responsible for combined hormone deficiencies in humans. Many different types of recessive loss of function mutations have been identified in humans. Most of the dominant cases have involved a mutation causing substitution of tryptophan for arginine at position 271. The mutant protein has normal to increased promoter-binding activity but is incapable of activating transcription. Persons with POU1F1 mutations exhibit nearly normal fetal growth but experience severe growth failure in the 1st yr of life. There are complete deficiencies of GH and PRL. The severity of TSH deficiency and resultant central hypothyroidism is variable. There is no impairment of ACTH, luteinizing hormone (LH), or follicle-stimulating hormone (FSH) production. Puberty develops spontaneously, though, at a later than normal age.

PROP1 (Prophet of PIT-1) mutations are a very common explanation for the distinctly uncommon phenotype of MPHD. Studies from Switzerland, Poland, and Russia indicate that loss of function mutations are responsible in the majority of cases with a recessive inheritance and about half of the cases with sporadic MPHD. The proportion of sporadic cases that can be explained by PROP1 mutations is even higher when a selection is made for those who have subnormal TSH responses to thyrotropin-releasing hormone (TRH) stimulation. The most common types of mutation involve one or two base pair deletions in the second of three exons. These deletions cause frame shifts and early transcriptional termination, rendering the mutant proteins incapable of binding to promoter sites or activating transcription of target genes. Missense, nonsense, and splice site mutations have also been described. The hormonal phenotypes associated with PROP1 mutations differ in several respects from those associated with POU1F1 mutations. Although the gene defects are present from conception, the hormone deficiencies show the characteristics of an acquired disease. Growth in the 1st yr of life is considerably better than with POU1F1 defects and the median age at diagnosis of GH deficiency is around 6 yr. Recognition of TSH deficiency is delayed relative to recognition of GH deficiency. Basal and TRH-stimulated PRL levels tend to be higher than in POU1F1 mutations. PROP1 mutations cause gonadotropin deficiency and POU1F1 mutations do not. Some patients with PROP1 mutations enter puberty spontaneously and then retreat from it. Girls experience secondary amenorrhea and boys show regression of testicular size and secondary sexual characteristics. There is a loss of LH and FSH responses to luteinizing hormone-releasing hormone (LHRH) stimulation. Partial deficiency of ACTH develops over time in about one third of patients with PROP1 defects. Anterior pituitary size is small in most patients, but in others there is progressive enlargement of the pituitary. A central mass clearly originates within the sella turcica but may extend above it. The cellular content of the mass during the active phase of enlargement is not known. With time, the contents of the mass appear to degenerate, with multiple cystic areas. The mass may persist as a nonenhancing structure or it may disappear completely, leaving an empty sella turcica. At different stages, the findings on MRI can suggest a macroadenoma, a microadenoma, a craniopharyngioma, or a Rathke pouch cyst.

The hormonal phenotype produced by recessive loss of function mutations in the *LHX3 gene* located on chromosome 9q34.3 resembles that produced by PROP1 mutations. There are deficiencies of GH, PRL, TSH, LH, and FSH but not of ACTH. It is not clear whether the deficiencies are present from birth or whether they appear later in childhood. There is another similarity in that some affected individuals show enlargement of the anterior pituitary. The most important distinguishing feature is that each of the cases has had a rigid cervical spine. Imaging does not show any anatomic abnormality, but the patients are only able to rotate their necks about 90 degrees compared with a normal value of 150 to 180 degrees.

Mutations in the *HESX1 gene* also result in a complex phenotype with defects in development of the optic nerve. *Septo-optic dysplasia* or *de Morsier syndrome* is a fairly common condition that combines incomplete development of the septum pellucidum with optic nerve dysplasia. Clinical observation of nystagmus and visual impairment in infancy leads to imaging studies, which, in turn, disclose the optic nerve and brain abnormalities. It is associated with anterior and/or posterior pituitary hormone deficiencies. About 25% of cases have hypopituitarism. These patients tend to show the triad of a small anterior pituitary gland, an attenuated pituitary stalk, and an ectopic posterior pituitary bright spot. The overwhelming majority of cases are sporadic. There seems to be an association with young maternal age but no specific teratogenic agents have been identified. Studies of the HESX1 gene have disclosed abnormalities in three families. Two siblings with hypopituitarism, optic nerve dysplasia, agenesis of the corpus callosum, and a history of parental consanguinity were found to be homozygotes for an inactivating mutation. More mildly affected individuals in two other families were heterozygotes for other inactivating mutations. Homozygotes (in mice) show severe optic nerve and brain abnormalities, whereas some heterozygotes show a milder phenotype.

Rieger syndrome is a complex phenotype caused by mutations in the gene for a transcription factor that is expressed in multiple tissues, including the anterior pituitary gland. In addition to variable degrees of anterior pituitary hormone deficiency, the abnormalities include colobomas of the iris, a high risk of glaucoma, and abnormal development of the kidneys, gastrointestinal tract, and umbilicus. Some cases were found to have deletions or rearrangements of a region on chromosome 4q25. Further studies identified inactivating mutations of the PTX2 (pituitary homeobox 2) gene. Because of its association with Rieger syndrome, it is also known as the *RIEG1* gene. The single normal gene copy in heterozygotes is inadequate to support normal development of a variety of organ systems.

Other Congenital Forms. Pituitary hypoplasia can occur as an isolated phenomenon or in association with more extensive developmental abnormalities, such as anencephaly or holoprosencephaly (cyclopia, cebocephaly, orbital hypotelorism). Hypoplasia of the pituitary occurs with anencephaly but may have a large residuum of normal pituitary function, suggesting that hypoplasia may be secondary to a hypothalamic defect. Midfacial anomalies (cleft lip, palate) or the finding of a solitary maxillary central incisor indicate a high likelihood of GH or other anterior or posterior hormone deficiency.

In the *Hall-Pallister syndrome*, absence of the pituitary gland is associated with hypothalamic hamartoblastoma, postaxial polydactyly, nail dysplasia, bifid epiglottis, imperforate anus, and anomalies of the heart, lungs, and kidneys.

Acquired Forms. Any lesion that damages the hypothalamus, pituitary stalk, or anterior pituitary may cause pituitary hormone deficiency. Because such lesions are not selective, multiple hormonal deficiencies are usually observed. The most common lesion is the craniopharyngioma (Chapter 489). Central nervous system germinoma, eosinophilic granuloma, tuberculosis, sarcoidosis, toxoplasmosis, and aneurysms may also cause hypothalamic-hypophyseal destruction. These lesions are frequently associated with roentgenographic changes in the skull. Besides diabetes insipidus, a deficiency of GH and other pituitary hormones may occur in children with histiocytosis. Enlargement of the sella or deformation or destruction of the clinoid processes usually indicates a tumor. Intrasellar or suprasellar calcifications usually indicate a craniopharyngioma. Trauma, including child abuse, traction at delivery, anoxia, and hemorrhagic infarction, may also damage the pituitary, its stalk, or the hypothalamus. The triad of a small anterior pituitary gland, an attenuated pituitary stalk, and an ectopic posterior pituitary bright spot on MRI has been associated with acquired as well as congenital multiple pituitary hormone deficiency.

CLINICAL MANIFESTATIONS

Congenital Hypopituitarism. The child with hypopituitarism is usually of normal size and weight at birth. Children with multiple pituitary hormone deficiencies and those with genetic defects of the GH1 or GHR gene have birth length that average 1 SD below the mean. Children with severe defects in GH production or action are more than 4 SD below the mean by 1 yr of age. Others with less severe deficiencies may have regular but slow growth in height, with the increments always less than the normal percentiles; periods of lack of growth may alternate with short spurts of growth. Delayed closure of the epiphyses permits growth beyond the age when normal persons cease to grow. Without treatment, adult heights are 4 to 12 SD below the mean.

Infants with congenital defects of the pituitary or hypothalamus usually present with neonatal emergencies such as apnea, cyanosis, or severe hypoglycemia with or without seizures. Microphallus in boys provides an additional diagnostic clue. Deficiency of GH may be accompanied by hypoadrenalism and hypothyroidism, and clinical manifestations of hypopituitarism evolve more rapidly than in the usual child with hypopituitarism. Prolonged neonatal jaundice is common. It involves elevation of conjugated and unconjugated bilirubin and may be mistaken for neonatal hepatitis.

The head is round, and the face is short and broad. The frontal bone is prominent, and the bridge of the nose is depressed and saddle-shaped. The nose is small, and the nasolabial folds are well developed. The eyes are somewhat bulging. The mandible and the chin are underdeveloped and infantile, and the teeth, which erupt late, are frequently crowded. The neck is short and the larynx is small. The voice is high-pitched and remains high after puberty. The extremities are well proportioned, with small hands and feet. The genitals are usually underdeveloped for the child's age, and sexual maturation may be delayed or absent. Facial, axillary, and pubic hair usually is lacking, and the scalp hair is fine. Length is mainly affected, giving toddlers a pudgy appearance. Symptomatic hypoglycemia, usually after fasting, occurs in 10–15% of children with panhypopituitarism and those with IGHD. Intelligence is usually normal. Affected children may become shy and retiring.

Acquired Hypopituitarism. The child is normal initially, and manifestations similar to those seen in idiopathic pituitary growth failure gradually appear and progress. When complete or almost

complete destruction of the pituitary gland occurs, signs of pituitary insufficiency are present. Atrophy of the adrenal cortex, thyroid, and gonads results in loss of weight, asthenia, sensitivity to cold, mental torpor, and absence of sweating. Sexual maturation fails to take place or regresses if already present. There may be atrophy of the gonads and genital tract with amenorrhea and loss of pubic and axillary hair. There is a tendency to hypoglycemia. Growth slows dramatically. Diabetes insipidus may be present early but tends to improve spontaneously as the anterior pituitary is progressively destroyed.

If the lesion is an expanding tumor, symptoms such as headache, vomiting, visual disturbances, pathologic sleep patterns, decreased school performance, seizures, polyuria, and growth failure may occur. Slowing of growth may antedate neurologic signs and symptoms, especially with craniopharyngiomas, but symptoms of hormonal deficit account for only 10% of presenting complaints. In other patients, the neurologic manifestations may precede the endocrinologic, or evidence of pituitary insufficiency may first appear after surgical intervention. In children with craniopharyngiomas, visual field defects, optic atrophy, papilledema, and cranial nerve palsy are common.

Laboratory Findings. The diagnosis of classic GH deficiency is suspected in cases of profound postnatal growth failure, with heights more than 3 SD below the mean for age and gender. Acquired GH deficiency can occur at any age. When the disorder is of short duration, height may still be within the normal range. A strong clinical suspicion is important in establishing the diagnosis because laboratory measures of GH sufficiency lack specificity. Observation of low serum levels of IGF-I and the GH-dependent IGF-BP3 can be helpful. Values that are in the upper part of the normal range for age effectively exclude GH deficiency. Values for normally growing and children with hypopituitarism overlap during infancy and childhood.

Definitive diagnosis rests on demonstration of absent or low levels of GH in response to stimulation. A variety of provocative tests have been devised that rapidly increase the level of GH in normal children. These include administration of L-dopa, insulin, arginine, clonidine, or glucagon. Peak levels of GH less than 10 µg/L in each of two provocative tests are compatible with GH deficiency. Stimulation with GHRH or synthetic ghrelin agonists generally produces greater responses in children with GH deficiency secondary to hypothalamic disorders and fails to elicit a response in those with GHRH receptor, GH1, POU1F1, PROP1, and LHX3 mutations. The frequency of false-negative responses to a single standard test in normally growing children is approximately 20%. One study suggests that a majority of normal prepubertal children fail to achieve GH values greater than 10 µg/L with two pharmacologic tests. The researchers suggest that 3 days of estrogen priming should be used before GH testing to achieve greater diagnostic specificity.

During the 3 decades in which hGH was obtained by extraction from human pituitary glands culled at autopsy, its supply was sharply limited and only patients with classic GH deficiency were treated. With the advent of an unlimited supply of recombinant GH, there has been a marked interest in redefining the criteria for GH deficiency to include children with lesser degrees of deficiency. It has become popular to evaluate the spontaneous secretion of GH by measuring its level every 20 min during a 24- or 12-hr (8 PM–8 AM) period. Some short children with normal levels of GH when studied by provocative tests show little spontaneous GH secretion. Such children are considered to have GH neurosecretory dysfunction. With the collection of more normative data, it is clear that frequent GH sampling also lacks diagnostic specificity. There is a wide range of spontaneous GH secretion in normally growing prepubertal children and considerable overlap with the values observed in children with classic GH deficiency. Although the clinical and laboratory criteria for GH deficiency in patients with severe (classic) hypopituitarism are well established, the diagnostic criteria are unsettled for short children with lesser degrees of GH deficiency.

In addition to establishing the diagnosis of GH deficiency, it is necessary to examine other pituitary functions. Levels of TSH, thyroxine (T_4), ACTH, cortisol, dehydroepiandrosterone sulfate, gonadotropins, and gonadal steroids may provide evidence of other pituitary hormonal deficiencies. The defect can be localized to the hypothalamus if there is a normal response to the administration of hypothalamic-releasing hormones for TSH, ACTH, or gonadotropins. When there is a deficiency of TSH, serum levels of T_4 and TSH are low. A normal increase in TSH and PRL after stimulation with TRH places the defect in the hypothalamus, and absence of such a response localizes the defect to the pituitary. An elevated level of plasma PRL taken at random in the patient with hypopituitarism is also strong evidence that the defect is in the hypothalamus rather than in the pituitary. Some children with craniopharyngioma have elevated PRL levels before surgery, but after surgery, PRL deficiency occurs because of pituitary damage. Antidiuretic hormone deficiency may be established by appropriate studies.

Roentgenographic Examination. Roentgenograms of the skull are most helpful when there is a destructive or space-occupying lesion causing hypopituitarism. Evidence of increased intracranial pressure may be found in patients with nausea, vomiting, loss of vision, headache, or an increase in circumference of the head. Enlargement of the sella, especially ballooning with erosion and calcifications within or above the sella, may be detected. MRI is indicated in all patients with hypopituitarism. In addition to providing detail about space-occupying lesions, it can define the size of the anterior and posterior pituitary lobes and the pituitary stalk. It is superior to CT in differentiating a full from an empty sella turcica. The posterior pituitary is readily recognized as a bright spot. In many cases of idiopathic MPHD with prenatal or perinatal onset, the posterior pituitary bright spot is ectopic. It appears at the base of the hypothalamus rather than in the pituitary fossa. MRI can provide timely confirmation of suspected hypopituitarism in a newborn with hypoglycemia and micropenis. MRI may also reveal pituitary gland hypoplasia or aplasia, septo-optic dysplasia, holoprosencephaly, or absence of the septum pellucidum.

Skeletal maturation is markedly delayed in patients with long-standing GH deficiency. The bone age tends to be approximately 75% of chronologic age. It may be even more delayed for patients with TSH and GH deficiency. The fontanels may remain open beyond the 2nd yr, and intersutural wormian bones may be found. Long bones are slender and osteopenic. Dual photon x-ray absorptiometry shows deficient bone mineralization, deficiencies in lean body mass, and a corresponding increase in adiposity.

Differential Diagnosis. The causes of growth disorders are legion. Systemic conditions such as inflammatory bowel disease, celiac disease, occult renal disease, and anemia must be considered. Patients with systemic conditions often have greater loss of weight than length. A few otherwise normal children are short (i.e., >3 SD below the mean for age) and grow 5 cm/yr or less but have normal levels of GH in response to provocative tests and normal spontaneous episodic secretion. Most of these children show increased rates of growth when treated with GH in doses comparable to those used to treat children with hypopituitarism. Plasma levels of IGF-I in these patients may be normal or low. Several groups of treated children have achieved final or near final adult heights. Different studies have found changes in adult height that range from −2.5 to +7.5 cm compared with pretreatment predictions. There are no methods that can reliably predict which of these children will become taller as adults as a result of GH treatment and which will have compromised adult height. Such treatment of short children without proven hypopituitarism is still undergoing experimental trials.

Constitutional growth delay is one of the variants of normal growth commonly encountered by the pediatrician. Length and weight measurements of affected children are normal at birth, and growth is normal for the first 4–12 mo of life. Growth then decelerates to near or below the 3rd percentile for height and weight. By 2–3 yr of age, growth resumes at a normal rate of 5 cm/yr or more. Studies of GH secretion and other studies are within normal limits. Bone age is closer to height age than to chronologic age. Detailed questioning often reveals other family members (frequently one or both parents) with histories of short stature in childhood, delayed puberty, and eventual normal stature. The prognosis for these children to achieve normal adult height is good. Boys with unusual degrees of delayed puberty may benefit from a short course of testosterone therapy to hasten puberty after 14 yr of age. The cause of this variant of normal growth is thought to be persistence of the relatively hypogonadotropic state of childhood (Chapter 14). Constitutional growth delay can be differentiated from genetic short stature by the level of skeletal maturation, which is consistent with chronologic age in the latter condition. Genetic short stature is usually found in other family members. Results of studies of hormones related to growth, however, are normal.

Primary hypothyroidism is usually easily diagnosed on clinical grounds. Responses to GH provocative tests may be subnormal, and enlargement of the sella may be present. Low T_4 and elevated TSH levels clearly establish the diagnosis. Pituitary hyperplasia recedes during treatment with thyroid hormone. Because thyroid hormone is a necessary prerequisite for normal GH synthesis, its levels must always be assessed before GH studies.

Emotional deprivation is an important cause of retardation of growth and mimics hypopituitarism. The condition is known as psychosocial dwarfism, maternal deprivation dwarfism, or hyperphagic short stature. The mechanisms by which sensory and emotional deprivation interfere with growth are not fully understood. Functional hypopituitarism is indicated by low levels of IGF-I and by inadequate responses of GH to provocative stimuli. Puberty may be normal or even premature in its appearance. Appropriate history and careful observations reveal disturbed mother-child or family relations and provide clues to the diagnosis (Chapter 35.2). Proof may be difficult to establish because the adults responsible often hide the true family situation from professionals, and the children rarely divulge their plight. Emotionally deprived children frequently have perverted or voracious appetites, enuresis, encopresis, insomnia, crying spasms, and sudden tantrums. The subgroup of children with hyperphagia and a normal body mass index tends to show catch-up growth when placed in a less stressful environment.

The *Silver-Russell syndrome* is characterized by short stature, frontal bossing, small triangular facies, sparse subcutaneous tissue, shortened and incurved 5th fingers, and in many cases, asymmetry (i.e., hemihypertrophy). Affected children have low birthweight for gestational age. There is some degree of GH secretory deficiency in very short children with intrauterine growth retardation, whether or not they have Silver-Russell syndrome. Short-term treatment with GH often results in increased rates of growth, particularly when higher than usual doses are used. The impact on adult height of different dosage regimens is still unknown.

Treatment. The Lawson Wilkins Pediatric Endocrine Society, Academy of Pediatrics, and the GH Research Society have published guidelines for hGH treatment. In children with classic GH deficiency, treatment should be started as soon as possible to narrow the gap in height between patients and their classmates during childhood and to have the greatest effect on mature height. The recommended dose of hGH is 0.18–0.3 mg/kg/wk. It is administered subcutaneously in six or seven divided doses. If the effect of therapy wanes, compliance should be evaluated before the dose is increased. Concurrent treatment with GH and an LHRH agonist has been used in the hope that interruption of puberty will delay epiphyseal fusion and prolong growth. This strategy may augment final height, but it can also increase the discrepancy in physical maturity between GH-deficient children and their age peers and may impair bone mineralization. Therapy should be continuous until near final height is achieved. Criteria for stopping treatment include a growth rate less than 1 inch per yr and a bone age of greater than 14 yr in girls and greater that 16 yr in boys.

Some patients treated with GH have subsequently acquired leukemia. The risk of leukemia in treated patients may be double that in the general population. There is conflicting evidence about whether GH treatment confers an increase in risk or whether the increased incidence reflects the consequences of therapeutic radiation for craniopharyngiomas and brain tumors. Other reported side effects include pseudotumor cerebri, slipped capital femoral epiphysis, gynecomastia, and worsening of scoliosis. There is an increase in total body water during the first 1–2 wk of treatment. Fasting and postprandial insulin levels are characteristically low before treatment, and they normalize during GH replacement. Development of diabetes mellitus is rare. Older GH-deficient patients treated with cadaver pituitary extracts are at risk for Creutzfeldt-Jakob disease for at least 10–15 yr after therapy. Use of recombinant GH has eliminated this risk.

Maximal response to GH occurs in the 1st yr of treatment. With each successive year of treatment, the response tends to decrease. Some patients receiving GH acquire reversible hypothyroidism. Periodic evaluation of thyroid function is indicated for all patients treated with GH. GHRH is nearly as effective as GH in the treatment of children with hypothalamic causes of hypopituitarism with a deficiency of GHRH, but daily subcutaneous injections are required. Recombinant IGF-I may prove useful in the treatment of children with Laron syndrome and possibly those with GH1 gene deletions and high titers of antibodies.

The doses of GH used to treat children with classic GH deficiency usually enhance the growth of many non–GH-deficient children as well. Intensive investigation is in progress to determine the full spectrum of short children who may benefit from treatment with GH. GH is currently approved in the United States for treatment of children with growth failure as a result of Turner syndrome, end-stage renal failure before kidney transplantation, Prader-Willi syndrome, or intrauterine growth retardation. In children with all other causes of short stature, it is unknown whether GH treatment increases their final height, and treatment of such patients should be confined to prospective clinical trials until further data establish the validity of this expensive, long-term form of therapy.

Replacement should also be directed at other hormonal deficiencies. In TSH-deficient subjects, thyroid hormone is given in full replacement doses. In ACTH-deficient patients, the optimal dose of hydrocortisone should not exceed 10 mg/m^2/24 hr. Increases are made during illness or in anticipation of surgical procedures. Therapy can often be deferred until growth has been completed if the deficiency is partial. In patients with a deficiency of gonadotropins, gonadal steroids are given when bone age reaches the age at which puberty usually takes place. For infants with microphallus, one or two 3-mo courses of monthly intramuscular injections of 25 mg of testosterone cypionate or testosterone enanthate may bring the penis to normal size without an inordinate effect on osseous maturation.

Abdul-Latif H, Leiberman E, Brown MR, et al: Growth hormone deficiency type IB caused by cryptic splicing of the GH-1 gene. *J Pediatr Endocrinol Metab* 2000; 13:21.

Berg MA, Guevara-Aguirre J, Rosenbloom AL, et al: Mutation creating a new splice site in the growth hormone receptor genes of 37 Ecuadorian patients with Laron syndrome. *Hum Mutat* 1992;1:24.

Cara JF, Kreiter ML, Rosenfield RL: Height prognosis of children with true precocious puberty and growth hormone deficiency: Effect of combination therapy with gonadotropin releasing hormone agonist and growth hormone. *J Pediatr* 1992;120:709.

Carel JC, Ecosse E, Nicolino M, et al: Adult height after long term treatment with recombinant growth hormone for idiopathic isolated growth hormone deficiency: Observational follow up of the French population based registry. *Br Med J* 2002;325:70–3.

Committee on Drugs and Committee on Bioethics: Considerations related to the use of recombinant human growth hormone in children. *Pediatrics* 1997;99:122.

Dean HJ, Bishop A, Winter JSD: Growth hormone deficiency in patients with histiocytosis. *J Pediatr* 1986;109:615.

de Zegher F, Albertsson-Wikland, Wilton P, et al: Growth hormone treatment of short children born short for gestational age: Metanalysis of four independent, randomized, controlled, multicentre studies. *Acta Paediatr Suppl* 1006;417:27.

Donaldson DL, Hallowell JG, Pan E, et al: Growth hormone secretory profiles: Variation on consecutive nights. *J Pediatr* 1989;115:51.

Duquesnoy P, Sobrier ML, Duriez B, et al: A single amino acid substitution in the exoplasmic domain of the human growth hormone (GH) receptor confers familial GH resistance (Laron syndrome) with positive GH-binding activity by abolishing receptor homodimerization. *EMBO J* 1994;13:1386.

Finkelstein BS, Imperiale TF, Speroff T, et al: Effect of growth hormone therapy on height in children with idiopathic short stature. *Arch Pediatr Adolesc Med* 2002;156:230–40.

Fluck C, Deladoey J, Rutishauser K, et al: Phenotypic variability in familial combined pituitary hormone deficiency caused by a PROP1 gene mutation resulting in the substitution of arg to cys at codon 120 (R120C). *J Clin Endocrinol Metab* 1998;84:50.

Growth Hormone Research Society: Consensus guidelines for the diagnosis and treatment of growth hormone (GH) deficiency in childhood and adolescence: Summary statement of the GH Research Society. *J Clin Endocrinol Metab* 2000;85:3998.

Guevara-Aguirre J, Rosenbloom AL, Fielder PJ, et al: Growth hormone receptor deficiency in Ecuador: Clinical and biochemical phenotype in two populations. *J Clin Endocrinol Metab* 1993;76:417.

Guidelines for the use of growth hormone in children with short stature. A report by the Drug and Therapeutics Committee of the Lawson Wilkins Pediatric Endocrine Society. *J Pediatr* 1995;127:857.

Guyda H: Four decades of growth hormone treatment for short children: What have we achieved? *J Clin Endocrinol Metab* 1990;84:4307.

Guyda HJ: Growth hormone testing and the short child. *Pediatr Res* 2000;48: 579–80.

Haverkamp F, Eiholzer U, Ranke MB, et al: Symptomatic versus substitution growth hormone therapy in short children: From auxology towards a comprehensive multidimensional assessment of short stature and related interventions. *J Pediatr Endorcrinol Metab* 2000;13:403.

Herman SP, Baggenstoss AM, Clothier MD: Liver dysfunction and histologic abnormalities in neonatal hypopituitarism. *J Pediatr* 1975;87:892.

Hintz RL, Attie KM, Baptista J, et al: Effect of growth hormone treatment on adult height of children with idiopathic short stature. Genentech Collaborative Group. *N Engl J Med* 1999;340:557.

Job JC, Chaussain JL, Job B, et al: Follow-up of three years of treatment with growth hormone and of one post-treatment year, in children with severe growth retardation of intrauterine onset. *Pediatr Res* 1996;39:354.

Kojima M, Hosoda H, Date Y, et al: Grhelin is a growth-hormone releasing acylated peptide from stomach. *Nature* 1999;409:194.

Littley MD, Shalet SM, Beardwell CG, et al: Radiation-induced hypopituitarism is dose-dependent. *Clin Endocrinol* 1989;31:363.

Lovinger RD, Kaplan SL, Grumbach MM: Congenital hypopituitarism associated with neonatal hypoglycemia and microphallus: Four cases secondary to hypothalamic hormone deficiencies. *J Pediatr* 1975;87:1171.

MacGillivary MH, Blethen SL, Buchlis JG, et al: Current dosing of growth hormone in children with growth hormone deficiency: How physiologic? *Pediatrics* 1998;102:527.

Netchine I, Sobrier ML, Krude H, et al: Mutations in LHX3 result in a new syndrome revealed by combined pituitary hormone deficiency. *Nature Genet* 2000;25:182.

Parks JS, Brown MR, Hurley DL, et al: Heritable disorders of pituitary development. *J Clin Endocrinol Metab* 1999;84:4362.

Pena-Almazan S, Buchlis J, Miller S, et al: Linear growth characteristics of congenitally GH-deficient infants from birth to one year of age. *J Clin Endocrinol Metab* 2001;86:5691–4.

Pfaffle RW, DiMattia GE, Parks JS, et al: Mutation of the POU-specific domain of Pit-1 and hypopituitarism without pituitary hypoplasia. *Science* 1992;257:1118.

Pinto G, Netchine I, Sobrier ML, et al: Pituitary stalk interruption syndrome: A clinical-biological-genetic assessment of its pathogenesis. *J Clin Endocrinol Metab* 1997;82:3450.

Radovick S, Nations M, Du Y, et al: A mutation in the POU-homeodomain of Pit-1 responsible for combined pituitary hormone deficiency. *Science* 1992;257:1115.

Ranke MB, Lindberg A: Growth hormone treatment of short children born small for gestational age or with Silver-Russell syndrome: Results from KIGS (Kabi International Growth Study), including the first report on final height. *Acta Paediatr Suppl* 1996;417:18.

Rosenbloom AR, Almonte AS, Brown MR, et al: Clinical and biochemical phenotype of familial anterior hypopituitarism from mutation of the PROP1 gene. *J Clin Endocrinol Metab* 1999;84:50.

Rosenfeld RG, Rosenbloom AL, Guevara-Aguirre J: Growth hormone (GH) insensitivity due to primary GH receptor deficiency. *Endocr Rev* 1994;15:369.

Saenger P: Growth hormone in growth hormone deficiency. *Br Med J* 2002;325:58–9.

Semina EV, Reiter R, Leysens NJ, et al: Cloning and characterization of a novel bicoid-related homeobox transcription factor gene, RIEG, involved in Rieger syndrome. *Nat Genet* 1996;14:392.

Skuse D, Albanese A, Stanhope R, et al: A new stress-related syndrome of growth failure and hyperphagia in children, associated with reversibility of growth hormone insufficiency. *Lancet* 1996;348:353.

Sorkin JA, Davis PC, Meacham LR, et al: Optic nerve hypoplasia: absence of posterior pituitary bright signal on magnetic resonance imaging correlates with diabetes insipidus. *Am J Opthalmol* 1996;122:717.

Szeto DP, Rodriguez-Estaban C, Ryan AK, et al: Role of the Bicoid-related homeodomain factor Pitx1 in specifying hindlimb morphogenesis and pituitary development. *Genes Dev* 1999;13:484.

Takahashi Y, Kaji H, Okimura Y, et al: Short stature caused by a mutant growth hormone. *N Engl J Med* 1996;334:432.

Tanaka T, Satoh M, Yasunaga T, et al: GH and GnRH analog treatment in children who enter puberty at short stature. *J Pediatr Endocrinol Metab* 1997;10:623.

Traggiai C, Stanhope R: Endocrinopathies associated with midline cerebral and cranial malformations. *J Pediatr* 2002;140:252–5.

Walker JM, Bond SA, Voss LD, et al: Treatment of short normal children with growth hormone: A cautionary tale? *Lancet* 1990;336:1331.

Wilson DM, Dotson RJ, Neely EK, et al: Effects of estrogen on growth hormone following clonidine stimulation. *Am J Dis Child* 1993;147:63.

Woods KA, Camacho-Hubner C, Savage MO, et al: Intrauterine growth retardation and postnatal growth failure associated with deletion of the insulin-like growth factor gene. *N Engl J Med* 1996;35:1363.

Wu W, Cogan JD, Pfaffle RW, et al: Mutations in PROP1 cause familial combined pituitary hormone deficiency. *Nat Genet* 1998;18:147.

Chapter 552

Diabetes Insipidus

David T. Breault and Joseph A. Majzoub

Diabetes insipidus (DI) presents clinically with polyuria and polydipsia and may result from either vasopressin deficiency (central DI) or vasopressin insensitivity at the level of the kidney (nephrogenic DI). Both central DI and nephrogenic DI can arise from inherited defects with congenital or neonatal onset, or be secondary to a variety of causes.

THE PHYSIOLOGY OF WATER BALANCE

The control of extracellular tonicity (osmolality) and volume within a narrow range is critical for normal cellular structure and function. Extracellular fluid tonicity is regulated almost exclusively by water intake and excretion, whereas extracellular volume is regulated by sodium intake and excretion. The control of plasma tonicity and intravascular volume involves a complex integration of endocrine, neural, behavioral, and paracrine systems (Fig. 552–1). Vasopressin, secreted from the posterior pituitary, is the principal regulator of tonicity, with its release largely stimulated by increases in plasma tonicity. Volume homeostasis is largely regulated by the renin-angiotensin-aldosterone system, with contributions from both vasopressin and the natriuretic peptide family.

Vasopressin, a 9-amino acid peptide, has both antidiuretic and vascular pressor activity and is synthesized in the paraventricular and supraoptic nuclei of the hypothalamus. It is transported to the posterior pituitary via axonal projections, where it is stored awaiting release into the systemic circulation. The half-life of vasopressin in the circulation is 5 min. In addition to responding to osmotic stimuli, vasopressin is secreted in response to significant decreases in intravascular volume and pressure (minimum of 8% decrement) via afferent baroreceptor pathways arising from the aortic arch (carotid sinus) and volume receptor pathways in the cardiac

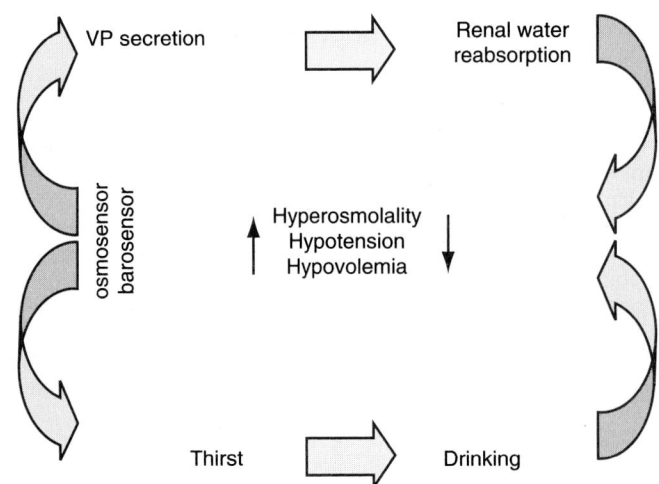

FIGURE 552–1. Regulation of vasopressin secretion and serum osmolality. Hyperosmolality, hypovolemia, and hypotension are sensed by osmosensors, volume sensors, and barosensors, respectively. These stimulate both vasopressin (VP) secretion and thirst. Vasopressin, acting on the kidney, causes increased reabsorption of water (antidiuresis). Thirst causes increased water ingestion. The results of these dual negative feedback loops cause a reduction in hyperosmolality or hypotension/hypovolemia. Additional stimuli for vasopressin secretion include nausea, hypoglycemia, and pain. (From Muglia LJ, Majzoub JA: Disorders of the posterior pituitary. In Sperling MA (editor): *Pediatric Endocrinology*, 2nd ed. Philadelphia, WB Saunders, 2002.)

atria and pulmonary veins. Osmotic and hemodynamic stimuli interact synergistically.

The sensation of thirst is regulated by cortical as well as hypothalamic neurons. The thirst threshold is approximately 10 mOsm/kg higher (~293 mOsm/kg) than the osmotic threshold for vasopressin release. Therefore, under conditions of hyperosmolality, vasopressin is released prior to the initiation of thirst, allowing for retention of ingested water. Chemoreceptors present in the oropharynx rapidly downregulate vasopressin release following water ingestion.

Vasopressin exerts its principal effect on the kidney via V2 receptors located primarily in the collecting tubule, the thick ascending limb of the loop of Henle, and the peri-glomerular tubules. The human V2 receptor gene is located on the long arm of the X chromosome (Xq28) at the locus associated with congenital, X-linked, vasopressin-resistant diabetes insipidus. Activation of the V2 receptor results in increases in intracellular cyclic adenosine monophosphate, which leads to the insertion of the aquaporin-2 water channel into the apical (luminal) membrane. This allows water movement along its osmotic gradient into the hypertonic inner medullary interstitium from the tubule lumen and excretion of concentrated urine. In contrast to aquaporin-2, aquaporins-3 and -4 are expressed on the basolateral membrane of the collecting duct cells and aquaporin-1 is expressed in the proximal tubule. These channels may also contribute to urinary concentrating ability.

Atrial natriuretic peptide (ANP), initially isolated from cardiac atrial muscle, has a number of important effects on salt and water balance, including stimulation of natriuresis, inhibition of sodium resorption, and inhibition of vasopressin secretion. ANP is expressed in endothelial cells and vascular smooth muscle where it appears to regulate relaxation of arterial smooth muscle. ANP is also expressed in brain, along with other natriuretic family members; the physiologic role of these factors has yet to be defined.

APPROACH TO THE PATIENT WITH POLYURIA, POLYDIPSIA, AND HYPERNATREMIA

The cause of pathologic polyuria or polydipsia (exceeding 2 L/m^2/24 hr) may be difficult to establish in children. Infants may present with irritability, failure to thrive, and intermittent fever. Patients with suspected DI should have a careful history, which should quantify the child's daily fluid intake and output and establish the voiding pattern, e.g., nocturia, or primary or secondary enuresis. A complete physical examination should establish the patient's hydration status and search for any evidence of visual and central nervous system dysfunction as well as other pituitary hormone deficiencies.

If pathologic polyuria or polydipsia is present, the following should be obtained: serum for osmolality, sodium, potassium, blood urea nitrogen, creatinine, glucose, and calcium; urine for osmolality, specific gravity, and glucose determination. The diagnosis of DI is established if the serum osmolality is greater than 300 mOsm/kg and the urine osmolality is less than 300 mOsm/kg. DI is unlikely if the serum osmolality is less than 270 mOsm/kg or the urine osmolality is greater than 600 mOsm/kg. If the patient's serum osmolality is less than 300 mOsm/kg (but greater than 270 mOsm/kg) and pathologic polyuria and polydipsia are present, a water deprivation test is indicated to establish the diagnosis of DI and to differentiate central from nephrogenic causes.

In the inpatient, postneurosurgical setting, central DI is likely if hyperosmolality (serum osmolality > 300 mOsm/kg) is associated with urine osmolality less than serum osmolality. It is important to distinguish between the polyuria resulting from postsurgical central DI and the polyuria resulting from the normal diuresis of fluids received intraoperatively. Both cases may be associated with a large volume (>200 mL/m^2/h) of dilute urine, although in patients with DI, the serum osmolality is high in comparison to patients undergoing a postoperative diuresis.

552.1 Causes of Hypernatremia (See Chapter 45.2)

CENTRAL DIABETES INSIPIDUS

Central diabetes insipidus can result from multiple etiologies, including genetic mutations in the vasopressin gene; trauma (accidental or surgical) to vasopressin neurons; congenital malformations of the hypothalamus or pituitary; neoplasms; infiltrative, autoimmune, and infectious diseases affecting vasopressin neurons or fiber tracts; and increased metabolism of vasopressin. In approximately 10% of children with central DI, the etiology is idiopathic. Other pituitary hormone deficiencies may be present (Chapter 551).

■ **BOX 552–1. Differential Diagnosis of Polyuria and Polydipsia**

DIABETES INSIPIDUS (DI)
  Central DI
    Genetic (autosomal dominant)
    Acquired
      Trauma (surgical or accidental)
      Congenital malformations
      Neoplasms
      Infiltrative, autoimmune, and infectious diseases
      Drugs
  Nephrogenic DI
    Genetic (X-linked, autosomal recessive, autosomal dominant)
    Acquired
      Hypercalcemia, hypokalemia
      Drugs
      Kidney disease

PRIMARY POLYDIPSIA
DIABETES MELLITUS

Autosomal dominant central DI usually presents within the first 5 yr of life and results from mutations in the vasopressin gene. A number of mutations can cause gene processing defects in a subset of vasopressin expressing neurons. *Wolfram syndrome*, which includes DI, diabetes mellitus, optic atrophy, and deafness, also results in vasopressin deficiency. The gene for this disorder is identified but its function is unknown. Congenital brain abnormalities such as septo-optic dysplasia with agenesis of the corpus callosum, the Kabuki syndrome, holoprosencephaly, and familial pituitary hypoplasia with absent stalk may be associated with central DI and defects in thirst perception. Empty sella syndrome, possibly due to unrecognized pituitary infarction, can be associated with DI in children.

Trauma (to the base of the brain) and neurosurgical intervention (in the region of the hypothalamus or pituitary) are common causes of central DI. The triphasic response following surgery refers to an initial phase of transient DI, lasting 12–48 hr, followed by a second phase of syndrome of inappropriate antidiuretic hormone secretion, lasting up to 10 days, which may be followed by permanent DI. The initial phase may be the result of local edema interfering with normal vasopressin secretion, the second phase results from unregulated vasopressin release from dying neurons, whereas in the third phase, permanent DI results if more than 90% of the neurons have been destroyed.

Given the anatomic distribution of vasopressin neurons over a large area within the hypothalamus, tumors that cause DI must either be very large and infiltrative or be strategically located near the base of the hypothalamus where vasopressin axons converge before their entry into the posterior pituitary. Germinomas and pinealomas typically arise in this region and are among the most common primary brain tumors associated with DI. Germinomas can be very small and undetectable by MRI for several years following the onset of polyuria. For this reason, quantitative measurement of the β subunit of human chorionic gonadotropin, often secreted by germinomas and pinealomas, should be performed in children with idiopathic or unexplained DI in addition to serial MRI scans. Craniopharyngiomas and optic gliomas can also cause central DI when very large, although this is more often a postoperative complication of the treatment for these tumors. Hematologic malignancies, as with acute myelocytic leukemia, can cause DI via infiltration of the pituitary stalk and sella.

Langerhans cell histiocytosis and lymphocytic hypophysitis are common types of infiltrative disorders causing central DI, with hypophysitis as the cause in 50% of "idiopathic" central DI. Infections involving the base of the brain, including meningitis (meningococcal, cryptococcal, listerial, and toxoplasma), congenital cytomegalovirus infection, and nonspecific inflammatory disease of the brain may give rise to central DI that is often transient. Drugs associated with the inhibition of vasopressin release include ethanol, phenytoin, opiate antagonists, halothane, and α-adrenergic agents.

NEPHROGENIC DIABETES INSIPIDUS

Nephrogenic (vasopressin-insensitive) DI (NDI) can result from genetic or acquired causes. Genetic causes are less common but more severe than acquired forms of NDI. The polyuria and polydipsia associated with genetic NDI usually presents within the first several weeks of life, but may only become apparent after weaning or with longer periods of nighttime sleep. Many infants initially present with fever, vomiting, and dehydration. Failure to thrive may be secondary to the ingestion of large amounts of water resulting in calorie malnutrition. Long-standing ingestion and excretion of large volumes of water may lead to nonobstructive hydronephrosis, hydroureter, and megabladder.

Congenital X-linked NDI results from inactivating mutations of the vasopressin V2 receptor. Congenital autosomal recessive NDI results from defects in the aquaporin-2 gene. An autosomal dominant form of nephrogenic DI is associated with processing mutations of the aquaporin-2 gene.

Acquired nephrogenic DI may result from hypercalcemia or hypokalemia and is associated with the following drugs: lithium, demeclocycline, foscarnet, clozapine, amphotericin, methicillin, and rifampin. Impaired renal concentrating ability can also be seen with ureteral obstruction, chronic renal failure, polycystic kidney disease, medullary cystic disease, Sjögren syndrome, and sickle cell disease. Decreased protein or sodium intake or excessive water intake, as in primary polydipsia, can lead to diminished tonicity of the renal medullary interstitium and nephrogenic DI.

TREATMENT OF CENTRAL DIABETES INSIPIDUS

Fluid Therapy

With an intact thirst mechanism and free access to oral fluids, a person with complete DI can maintain plasma osmolality and sodium in the high normal range, although at great inconvenience. Neonates and young infants are often best treated solely with fluid therapy, given their requirement for large volumes (3 L/m^2/24 hr) of nutritive fluid. The use of vasopressin analogs in patients with obligate high fluid intake is contraindicated given the risk of life-threatening hyponatremia.

Vasopressin Analogs

Treatment of central DI in older children is best accomplished with the use of the long-acting vasopressin analog dDAVP (desmopressin). dDAVP is available in an intranasal preparation (onset 5–10 min) and as tablets (onset 15–30 min). The intranasal preparation of dDAVP (10 μg/0.1 mL) can be administered by rhinal tube (allowing dose titration) or by nasal spray. The appropriate dose is determined empirically based on the desired length of antidiuresis. The nasal spray delivers 10 μg (0.1 mL) per spray and is the standard preparation used for treatment of primary enuresis in older children. Use of dDAVP in the treatment of enuresis is a temporizing measure, because it does not affect the underlying condition and should be used with caution. To prevent water intoxication, patients should have at least 1 hr of urinary breakthrough between doses each day. dDAVP tablets are available, but require at least a 10-fold increase in the dose compared with the intranasal preparation. Oral doses of 25–300 μg every 8–12 hr are safe and effective in children.

Aqueous Vasopressin

Central DI of acute onset following neurosurgery is best managed with continuous administration of synthetic aqueous vasopressin (pitressin). Under most circumstances, total fluid intake must be limited to 1 L/m^2/24 hr during antidiuresis. A typical dose for intravenous vasopressin therapy is 1.5 mU/kg/h, which results in a blood vasopressin concentration of approximately 10 pg/mL. On occasion, following hypothalamic (but not transsphenoidal) surgery, higher initial concentrations of vasopressin may be required to treat acute DI, which has been attributed to the release of a vasopressin inhibitory substance. Vasopressin concentrations greater than 1,000 pg/mL should be avoided because they may cause cutaneous necrosis, rhabdomyolysis, and cardiac rhythm disturbances. Postneurosurgical patients treated with vasopressin infusion should be switched from intravenous to oral fluids as soon as possible to allow thirst sensation, if intact, to help regulate osmolality.

TREATMENT OF NEPHROGENIC DIABETES INSIPIDUS

The treatment of acquired NDI focuses on elimination, if possible, of the underlying disorder, such as offending drugs, hypercalcemia, hypokalemia, or ureteral obstruction. Congenital nephrogenic diabetes insipidus is often difficult to treat. The main goals are to ensure the intake of adequate calories for growth and to avoid severe dehydration. Foods with the highest

ratio of caloric content to osmotic load (Na < 1 mmol/kg/24 hr) should be ingested to maximize growth and to minimize the urine volume required to excrete the solute load. Even with the early institution of therapy, however, growth failure and mental retardation are common.

Pharmacologic approaches to the treatment of NDI include the use of thiazide diuretics and are intended to decrease the overall urine output. Thiazides appear to induce a state of mild volume depletion by enhancing sodium excretion at the expense of water and by causing a decrease in the glomerular filtration rate, which results in proximal tubular sodium and water reabsorption. Indomethacin and amiloride may be used in combination with thiazides to further reduce polyuria. High-dose dDAVP therapy, in combination with indomethacin, has been used in some subjects with NDI. This treatment may prove useful in patients with genetic defects in the V2 receptor associated with a reduced binding affinity for vasopressin.

Knoers N, Monnens LH: Nephrogenic diabetes insipidus: Clinical symptoms, pathogenesis, genetics and treatment. *Pediatr Nephrol* 1992;6:476–82.
Maghnie M, Cosi G, Genovese E, et al: Central diabetes insipidus in children and young adults. *N Engl J Med* 2000;343:988–1007.
Muglia LJ, Majzoub JA: Disorders of the posterior pituitary. In Sperling MA (editor): *Pediatric Endocrinology*, 2nd ed. Philadelphia, WB Saunders, 2002.

Chapter 553

Other Abnormalities of Arginine Vasopressin Metabolism and Action

David T. Breault and Joseph A. Majzoub

Hyponatremia (serum sodium < 130 mEq/L) in children is usually associated with severe systemic disorders and is most often due to (1) intravascular volume depletion, (2) excessive salt loss, or (3) hypotonic fluid overload, especially in infants. The syndrome of inappropriate antidiuretic hormone (SIADH) is an uncommon cause of hyponatremia in children, except following vasopressin administration.

The initial approach to the patient with hyponatremia begins with the determination of the volume status. A careful review of the patient's history, physical examination, including changes in weight, and vital signs helps determine whether the patient is hypovolemic or hypervolemic. Supportive evidence includes laboratory data such as serum electrolytes, blood urea nitrogen, creatinine, uric acid, urine sodium, specific gravity, and osmolality (Chapter 45.2) (Tables 553–1 and 553–2).

CAUSES OF HYPONATREMIA

Syndrome of Inappropriate Antidiuretic Hormone Secretion

SIADH is characterized by hyponatremia, an inappropriately concentrated urine (>100 mOsm/kg), normal or slightly elevated plasma volume, a normal-to-high urine sodium, and low serum uric acid. SIADH is uncommon in children, with most cases resulting from excessive administration of vasopressin in the treatment of central diabetes insipidus. It can also occur with encephalitis, brain tumors, head trauma, psychiatric disease, in the postictal period after generalized seizures, after prolonged nausea, pneumonia, tuberculous meningitis, or AIDS. SIADH is the cause of the hyponatremic second phase of the triphasic response seen after hypothalamic-pituitary surgery

TABLE 553–1. Differential Diagnosis of Hyponatremia

TABLE 553–1. Differential Diagnosis of Hyponatremia

Disorder	Intravascular Volume Status	Urine Sodium
Systemic dehydration	Low	Low
Decreased effective plasma volume	Low	Low
Primary salt loss	Low	Low
Cerebral salt wasting	Low	Very high
SIADH	High	High
Decreased free water clearance	Normal or high	Normal or high
Primary polydipsia	Normal or high	Normal
Pseudohyponatremia	Normal	Normal
Factitious hyponatremia	Normal	Normal

SIADH = syndrome of inappropriate antidiuretic hormone secretion.

(Chapter 552). It is found in up to 35% of patients 1 wk after surgery and may result from retrograde neuronal degeneration with cell death and vasopressin release. Common drugs that have been shown to increase vasopressin secretion or mimic vasopressin action, resulting in hyponatremia, include carbamazepine, chlorpropamide, vinblastine, vincristine, and tricyclic antidepressants.

Systemic Dehydration

The initial manifestation of systemic dehydration is often hypernatremia and hyperosmolality, which subsequently lead to the activation of vasopressin secretion and a decrease in water excretion. As dehydration progresses, hypovolemia and/or hypotension become major stimuli for vasopressin release, further decreasing free water clearance. Urinary sodium excretion is low (usually <10 mEq/L) due to a low glomerular filtration rate and concomitant activation of the renin-angiotensin-aldosterone system, unless primary renal disease or diuretic therapy is present.

Primary Salt Loss

Hyponatremia can result from the primary loss of sodium chloride as seen in specific disorders of the kidney (congenital polycystic kidney disease acute interstitial nephritis, chronic renal failure), gastrointestinal tract, (gastroenteritis), or sweat glands (cystic fibrosis). The hyponatremia is not solely due to the salt loss, because the latter also causes hypovolemia, leading to an increase in vasopressin. Mineralocorticoid deficiency, pseudohypoaldosteronism (sometimes seen in children with urinary tract obstruction or infection), and diuretics can also result in loss of sodium chloride.

Decreased Effective Plasma Volume

Hyponatremia can result from decreased effective plasma volume, as found in congestive heart failure, cirrhosis, nephrotic

TABLE 553–2. Clinical Parameters to Distinguish Between SIADH, Cerebral Salt Wasting and Central Diabetes Insipidus

Clinical Parameter	SIADH	Cerebral Salt Wasting	Central DI
Serum sodium	Low	Low	High
Urine output	Normal or low	High	High
Urine sodium	High	Very high	Low
Intravascular volume status	Normal or high	Low	Low
Serum Uric acid	Low	Normal or high	High
Vasopressin level	High	Low	Low

syndrome, positive pressure mechanical ventilation, severe burns, bronchopulmonary dysplasia in neonates, cystic fibrosis with obstruction, and severe asthma. The resulting decrease in cardiac output leads to reduced water and salt excretion, as with systemic dehydration, and an increase in vasopressin secretion. In patients with impaired cardiac output and elevated atrial volume (e.g., congestive heart failure or lung disease), atrial natriuretic peptide concentrations are elevated further, leading to hyponatremia by promoting natriuresis. These patients usually have a very low urinary excretion of sodium. Unlike dehydrated patients, these patients may have excess total body sodium, from activation of the renin-angiotensin-aldosterone system, and demonstrate peripheral edema as well.

Primary Polydipsia (Increased Water Ingestion)

In patients with normal renal function, the kidney can excrete a dilute urine with an osmolality as low as 50 mOsm/kg. To excrete a daily solute load of 500 $mOsm/m^2$, the kidney must produce 10 L/m^2 of urine per day. Therefore, to avoid hyponatremia, the maximum amount of water an individual with normal renal function can consume is 10 L/m^2. Neonates, however, cannot dilute their urine to this degree, putting them at risk for water intoxication if water intake exceeds 4 $L/m^2/day$ (approximately 60 mL/h in a newborn). Many infants develop hyponatremic seizures after being fed pure water without electrolytes rather than breast milk or formula.

Decreased Free Water Clearance

Hyponatremia due to decreased renal free water clearance, even in the absence of an increase in vasopressin secretion, can result from adrenal insufficiency or thyroid deficiency, or be related to a direct effect of drugs on the kidney. Both mineralocorticoids and glucocorticoids are required for normal free water clearance in a vasopressin-independent manner. In patients with unexplained hyponatremia, adrenal and thyroid insufficiency should be considered. Also, patients with coexisting adrenal failure and diabetes insipidus may have no symptoms of the latter until glucocorticoid therapy unmasks the need for vasopressin replacement. Certain drugs may inhibit renal water excretion through direct effects on the nephron, thus causing hyponatremia; these drugs include high-dose cyclophosphamide, vinblastine, cisplatinum, and carbamazepine.

Cerebral Salt Wasting

Cerebral salt wasting appears to be the result of hypersecretion of atrial natriuretic peptide and is seen primarily with central nervous system disorders including brain tumors, head trauma, hydrocephalus, neurosurgery, cerebral vascular accidents, and brain death. Hyponatremia is accompanied by elevated urinary sodium excretion (often more than 150 mEq/L), excessive urine output, hypovolemia, normal or high uric acid, suppressed vasopressin, and elevated atrial natriuretic peptide concentrations (>20 pmol/L). Thus, it is distinguished from SIADH, in which normal or decreased urine output, euvolemia, low uric acid, only modestly elevated urine sodium concentration, and an elevated vasopressin level occur. The distinction between cerebral salt wasting and SIADH is important because the treatment of the two disorders differs markedly.

Pseudohyponatremia and Other Causes of Hyponatremia

Pseudohyponatremia may result from hypertriglyceridemia. In this condition, elevated lipid levels result in a relative decrease in serum water content. As electrolytes are dissolved in the aqueous phase of the serum, they appear low when expressed as a fraction of the total serum volume. As a fraction of serum water, however, electrolyte content is normal. Factitious hyponatremia can result from obtaining a blood sample proximal to the site of intravenous hypotonic fluid infusion.

Hyponatremia is also associated with hyperglycemia, which causes the influx of water into the intravascular space. Serum sodium decreases by 1.6 mEq/L for every 100 mg/dL increment in blood glucose greater than 100 mg/dL. Glucose is not ordinarily an osmotically active agent and does not stimulate vasopressin release, probably because it is able to equilibrate freely across plasma membranes. In the presence of insulin deficiency and hyperglycemia, however, glucose acts as an osmotic agent, presumably because its normal intracellular access to osmosensor sites is prevented. Under these circumstances, an osmotic gradient exists, stimulating vasopressin release.

TREATMENT OF HYPONATREMIA

Patients with systemic dehydration and hypovolemia should be rehydrated with salt-containing fluids such as normal saline or lactated Ringer solution. Because of activation of the renin-angiotensin-aldosterone system, the administered sodium is avidly conserved and a water diuresis quickly ensues as volume is restored and vasopressin concentrations decrease. Under these conditions, caution must be taken to prevent too rapid a correction of hyponatremia, which may result in central pontine myelinolysis characterized by discrete regions of axonal demyelination and the potential for irreversible brain damage.

Hyponatremia due to a decrease in effective plasma volume caused by cardiac, hepatic, renal, or pulmonary dysfunction is more difficult to reverse. The most effective therapy is the least easily achieved: treatment of the underlying systemic disorder. For example, patients weaned from positive pressure ventilation undergo a prompt water diuresis and resolution of hyponatremia as cardiac output is restored and vasopressin concentrations decrease.

Patients with hyponatremia due to primary salt loss require supplementation with sodium chloride and fluids. Initially, intravenous replacement of urine volume with fluid containing sodium chloride, 150 to 450 mEq/L depending on the degree of salt loss, may be necessary; oral salt supplementation may be required subsequently. This treatment contrasts with that of SIADH, in which water restriction without sodium supplementation is the mainstay.

Emergency Treatment of Hyponatremia

The development of acute hyponatremia (onset < 12 hr) or a serum sodium concentration less than 120 mEq/L may be associated with lethargy, psychosis, coma, or generalized seizures, especially in younger children. Acute hyponatremia can cause cell swelling and lead to neuronal dysfunction or to cerebral herniation. The emergency treatment of cerebral dysfunction resulting from acute hyponatremia includes water restriction and may require rapid correction with hypertonic 3% sodium chloride. If hypertonic saline treatment is undertaken, the serum sodium should be raised only high enough to cause an improvement in mental status, and in no case faster than 0.5 mEq/L/hr or 12 mEq/L/24 hr.

Treatment of SIADH

Chronic SIADH is best treated by oral fluid restriction. With full antidiuresis (urine osmolality of 1,000 mOsm/kg), a normal daily obligate renal solute load of 500 mOsmoles/m² would be excreted in 500 mL/m² water. This, plus a daily nonrenal water loss of 500 mL/m², would require that oral fluid intake be limited to 1,000 mL/m²/24 hr to avoid hyponatremia. In young children, this degree of fluid restriction may not provide adequate calories for growth (as discussed). In this situation, the

creation of nephrogenic diabetes insipidus using demeclocycline therapy may be indicated to allow sufficient fluid intake for normal growth.

Treatment of Cerebral Salt Wasting

Treatment of patients with cerebral salt wasting consists of restoring intravascular volume with sodium chloride and water, as with the treatment of other causes of systemic dehydration. The underlying cause of the disorder, which is usually due to acute brain injury, should also be treated if possible. Treatment involves the ongoing replacement of urine sodium losses (volume for volume).

Albanese A, Hindmarsh P, Stanhope R: Management of hyponatremia in patients with acute cerebral insults. *Arch Dis Child* 2001;85:246–51.

Muglia LJ, Majzoub JA: Disorders of the posterior pituitary. In Sperling MA (editor): *Pediatric Endocrinology,* 2nd ed. Philadelphia, WB Saunders, 2002.

Chapter 554

Hyperpituitarism, Tall Stature, and Overgrowth Syndromes *Pinchas Cohen*

HYPERPITUITARISM

Primary hyperpituitarism is a rare event in children, but secondary hypersecretion of pituitary hormones is an expected finding in conditions in which deficiency of a target organ gives decreased hormonal feedback, as in primary hypogonadism or hypoadrenalism. In primary hypothyroidism, pituitary hyperfunction and hyperplasia can enlarge and erode the sella and, on rare occasions, increase intracranial pressure. Such changes should not be confused with primary pituitary tumors; they disappear when the underlying thyroid condition is treated. Pituitary hyperplasia also occurs in response to stimulation by ectopic production of releasing hormones such as that seen occasionally in patients with Cushing syndrome, secondary to corticotropin-releasing hormone excess, or in children with acromegaly secondary to growth hormone-releasing hormone (GHRH) produced by a variety of systemic tumors.

Primary hypersecretion of pituitary hormones by a suspected or proven adenoma is uncommon in childhood. The most commonly encountered pituitary tumors are those that secrete corticotropin, prolactin, or growth hormone (GH). With rare exceptions, pituitary adenomas that secrete gonadotropins or thyrotropin occur in adults. Hypothalamic hamartomas that secrete gonadotropin-releasing hormone are known to cause precocious puberty. It is suspected that some pituitary tumors may result from stimulation with hypothalamic-releasing hormones and in other instances, as in McCune-Albright syndrome (MAS), the tumor is caused by constitutive activating mutation of the G-protein Gs_α gene.

TALL STATURE

The normal distribution of height predicts that 2.5% of the population will be taller than 2 SD (97.5%) above the mean. However, the social acceptability and even desirability of tallness (heightism) make tall stature an uncommon complaint. Nevertheless, it is critical to be able to identify situations in which tall stature or an accelerated growth rate provides a clue to an underlying disorder. In North America, it is extremely unusual for male patients to seek help regarding excessive height, although in Europe it is somewhat more common. Even in female patients, tall stature has become more socially acceptable, although tall girls may still approach their physician with a desire to curb their growth rate.

Differential Diagnosis of Tall Stature

Box 554–1 lists the causes of tall stature in childhood and adolescence. Of these, the normal variant familial or constitutional tall stature is by far the most common cause. Almost invariably, a family history of tallness can be elicited and no organic pathology is present. The child is often tall throughout childhood and enjoys excellent health. The parent of the constitutionally tall adolescent may reflect unhappily upon his or her own adolescence as a tall teenager. There are no abnormalities in the physical examination and the laboratory studies, if obtained, are negative.

Klinefelter syndrome (XXY syndrome) is a relatively common (1:500–1,000 live male births) abnormality associated with tall stature, mild mental retardation, gynecomastia, and decreased upper to lower body segment ratio. The testes are invariably small, although androgen production by Leydig cells is often at the low normal range. Spermatogenesis and Sertoli cell function are defective and infertility results. Similarly, excess X chromosome material containing an additional dose of the SHOX gene, whose deficiency causes short stature in Turner syndrome, can also cause tall stature. XYY syndrome is associated with tall stature and possible behavioral and mental problems. It is thought that a gene on the Y chromosome (yet to be identified) is responsible for the excess height. Marfan syndrome is an autosomal dominant connective tissue disorder consisting of tall stature, increased arm span, and decreased upper to lower body segment ratio. Additional abnormalities include arachnodactyly,

ocular abnormalities, and cardiac anomalies. Homocystinuria is an autosomal recessive inborn error of amino acid metabolism causing mental retardation when untreated, and has many features resembling Marfan syndrome, particularly ocular manifestations. Hyperthyroidism in adolescents is associated with rapid growth but normal adult height. It is almost always caused by Graves disease and is much more common in girls. Children with precocious puberty are often unusually tall but do not develop into giants, because their epiphyses close early and growth ceases prematurely. Rare cases of adrenocorticotropic hormone deficiency or resistance have been associated with tall stature. Exogenous obesity is a common condition in adolescence and may be associated with rapid linear growth and early maturation; adult height is typically normal.

The purpose of the diagnostic evaluation of tall stature is to distinguish the commonly occurring normal variant constitutional variety from the rare pathologic conditions. Often, when the history is suggestive of familial tall stature and the physical examination is entirely normal, no laboratory tests are indicated. It is valuable to obtain a bone age radiograph to predict adult height, which serves as a basis for discussions with the family and for management decisions. If, however, the history is suggestive for any of the aforementioned disorders or the physical examination reveals abnormalities, additional laboratory tests should be obtained. Insulin-like growth factor-I (IGF-I) and IGF binding protein-3 (IGFBP-3) are excellent screening tests for GH excess and can be verified with a glucose suppression test. Laboratory evidence of GH excess mandates MRI evaluation of the pituitary. Chromosome analysis is useful in boys, especially when the upper to lower body segment ratio is decreased or when mental retardation is present. If Marfan syndrome or homocystinuria is suspected from the physical examination, referral to a cardiologist and an ophthalmologist should be made. Thyroid function tests are useful to diagnose or rule out hyperthyroidism when this disorder is suspected.

PRECOCIOUS AND DELAYED PUBERTY (see Chapter 556)

Precocious puberty, whether mediated centrally (increased gonadotropin secretion) or peripherally (increased secretion of androgens, estrogens, or both), results in accelerated linear growth in childhood, mimicking the pubertal growth spurt. Because skeletal maturation is also accelerated, adult height is frequently compromised. The diagnostic evaluation and management of precocious puberty are discussed elsewhere in this book.

Although delayed puberty may be associated with short stature in childhood, as with constitutional delay, failure to eventually enter puberty and complete sexual maturation may result in sustained growth during adult life, with ultimate tall stature. The report of tall stature with open epiphyses resulting from a mutation of the estrogen receptor in a man with normal male sexual maturation underscores the fundamental role of estrogen in promoting epiphyseal fusion and termination of normal skeletal growth. Aromatase deficiency leads to tall stature through similar pathways. Furthermore, androgen insensitivity is associated with tall stature in girls, demonstrating a role for androgens in this process.

MANAGEMENT OF CONSTITUTIONAL AND SYNDROMIC TALL STATURE

Reassurance of the family and the patients is the key to the management of normal variant tall stature. The use of the bone age and a careful assessment of pubertal status to predict adult height may provide some comfort for them, as will general supportive discussions on the social acceptability of this condition. Even though treatment is available for girls and boys with excessive growth, its use should be restricted to patients with (1) predicted adult height > 3 SD above the mean (78 inches or 198 cm

---

BOX 554–1. Differential Diagnosis of Tall Stature and Overgrowth Syndromes

FETAL OVERGROWTH
Maternal diabetes mellitus
Cerebral gigantism (Sotos syndrome)
Weaver syndrome
Beckwith-Wiedemann syndrome
Other IGF-II excess syndromes

POSTNATAL OVERGROWTH LEADING TO CHILDHOOD TALL STATURE
Familial (constitutional) tall stature
Cerebral gigantism
Beckwith-Wiedemann syndrome
Exogenous obesity
Excess GH secretion (pituitary gigantism)
McCune-Albright syndrome or MEN associated with excess GH secretion
Precocious puberty
Marfan syndrome
Klinefelter syndrome (XXY)
SHOX excess syndromes
Weaver syndrome
Fragile X syndrome
Homocystinuria
XYY
Hyperthyroidism

POSTNATAL OVERGROWTH LEADING TO ADULT TALL STATURE
Familial (constitutional) tall stature
Androgen or estrogen deficiency / estrogen resistance (in males)
Testicular feminization
ACTH/cortisol deficiency/resistance
Excess GH secretion (pituitary gigantism)
Marfan syndrome
Klinefelter syndrome (XXY)
XYY

IGF = insulin-like growth factor; ACTH = adrenocorticotropic hormone; GH = growth hormone.

in male patients, 71 inches or 180 cm in female patients) and (2) evidence of significant psychosocial impairment.

For the family of a child with extreme familial tall stature or another condition such as Marfan syndrome who feel strongly about treatment, a trial of sex steroids is possible. Such therapy is designed to accelerate puberty and epiphyseal fusion, and is therefore of little benefit when given in late puberty; therapy is initiated ideally prepubertally or in early puberty. Oral estrogens in various doses have successfully reduced the predicted height of female patients by an average of 5–10 cm. This is a direct result of the known effects of sex steroids on promoting epiphyseal fusion, and therapy must begin before the bone age has reached 12 yr. Oral ethinyl estradiol at a dose of 0.15–0.5 mg/24 hr until cessation of growth occurs has been used successfully in girls. If necessary, a progestational agent can be added after 1 year of unopposed estrogen. In boys, treatment should begin before the bone age reaches 14 yr; testosterone enanthate is used at a dose of 500 mg IM every 2 wk for 6 mo. Whereas no long-term complications of sex steroid therapy have been clearly documented, short-term side effects are common. These include lipid abnormalities, thromboembolism, cholelithiasis, hypertension, nausea, menstrual irregularities, and acne fulminans. The lack of extensive experience with this form of therapy and the risks involved should be carefully weighed and discussed with the family before embarking on therapy.

The mechanism of estrogen action involves effects on both GH and IGF production. Perhaps more important, however, is the action of estrogen on the epiphysis. Recent studies have demonstrated that it is estrogen that mediates epiphyseal fusion in both girls and boys. In prepubertal girls, adult height is reportedly decreased by as much as 5–6 cm relative to pretreatment predictions. When therapy is initiated after the onset of puberty, the decrement in adult height is not likely to be as large. Therapy in boys with tall stature is even more problematic. For the reasons discussed, estrogen is likely to be most efficacious in accelerating epiphyseal fusion but is obviously undesirable in boys. Androgens also accelerate skeletal maturation, presumably via aromatization to estrogen, but at the price of rapid virilization.

PROLACTINOMA

Prolactin-secreting pituitary adenomas are the most common tumors of the pituitary in adolescents. With the advent of MRI, more of these tumors, particularly microadenomas (<1 cm), are being detected. The most common presenting manifestations are headache, amenorrhea, and galactorrhea. The disorder affects more than twice as many girls as boys; most have undergone normal puberty before becoming symptomatic. Only a few patients have delayed puberty. In some kindreds with type I multiple endocrine neoplasia, prolactinomas are the presenting features during adolescence.

Prolactin levels may be moderately (40–50 ng/mL) or markedly (10,000–15,000 ng/mL) elevated. Most prolactinomas in children have been large (macroadenomas), have caused the sella to enlarge, and, in some cases, have caused visual field defects. Approximately one third of patients with macroadenomas develop hypopituitarism, particularly GH deficiency.

Prolactinomas should not be confused with the hyperprolactinemia and pituitary hyperplasia that may occur in patients with primary hypothyroidism, which is readily treated with thyroid hormone. Moderate elevations (<200 ng/mL) of prolactin are also associated with a variety of medications (mainly psychiatric), with pituitary stalk dysfunction such as may occur with craniopharyngioma, and with other benign conditions. Treatment for most children has been surgical resection by transfrontal or transsphenoidal approach. However, the management of prolactinoma is becoming increasingly conservative. Most patients can be effectively managed by treatment with bromocriptine or long-acting cabergoline. About 80% of adult patients respond with shrinkage of the tumor and marked decreases in serum prolactin levels.

EXCESS GROWTH HORMONE SECRETION AND PITUITARY GIGANTISM

In young persons with open epiphyses, overproduction of GH results in gigantism; in persons with closed epiphyses, the result is acromegaly. Often, some acromegalic features are seen with gigantism, even in children and adolescents. After closure of the epiphyses, the acromegalic features become more prominent.

Pituitary gigantism is rare and its cause is most often a pituitary adenoma, but gigantism has been observed in a 2.5-yr-old boy with a hypothalamic tumor that presumably secreted GHRH. Other tumors, particularly in the pancreas, have produced acromegaly by secretion of large amounts of GHRH with resultant hyperplasia of the somatotrophs. The cardinal clinical feature of gigantism is longitudinal growth acceleration secondary to the GH excess. The usual manifestations consist of coarse facial features, and enlarging hands and feet. In young children, rapid growth of the head may precede linear growth. Some patients have behavioral and visual problems. In most of the recorded cases, the abnormal growth became evident at puberty, but the condition has been established as early as the newborn period in one child and at 21 mo of age in another. Giants may grow to a height of 8 ft or more. Acromegalic features consist chiefly of enlargement of the distal parts of the body, but manifestations of abnormal growth involve all portions. The circumference of the skull increases, the nose becomes broad, and the tongue is often enlarged, with coarsening of the facial features. The mandible grows excessively, and the teeth become separated. Visual field defects and neurologic abnormalities are common; signs of increased intracranial pressure appear later. The fingers and toes grow chiefly in thickness. There may be dorsal kyphosis. Fatigue and lassitude are early symptoms. GH levels are elevated and may occasionally exceed 100 ng/mL. There is typically no suppression of GH levels by the hyperglycemia of a glucose tolerance test. IGF-I and IGFBP-3 levels are consistently elevated in gigantism, whereas other growth factors are not. Gigantism is rare, with only several hundred reported cases to date. The presentation of gigantism is usually dramatic, unlike the insidious onset of acromegaly in adults. The tumor mass itself may cause headaches, visual changes due to optic nerve compression, and hypopituitarism. About half of the patients also have marked hyperprolactinemia as a result of plurihormonal adenomas that secrete GH and prolactin. This is due to the fact that mammosomatotrophs are the most common type of GH-secreting cells involved in childhood gigantism. GH-secreting tumors of the pituitary are typically eosinophilic or chromophobe adenomas. Adenomas may compromise other anterior pituitary function through growth or cystic degeneration. Secretion of gonadotropins, thyrotropin, or corticotropin may be impaired. Delayed sexual maturation or hypogonadism may occur. When GH hypersecretion is accompanied by gonadotropin deficiency, accelerated linear growth may persist for decades. In some cases, the tumor spreads outside the sella, invading the sphenoid bone, optic nerves, and brain. GH-secreting tumors in pediatric patients are more likely to be locally invasive or aggressive than are those in adult patients.

The etiology is uncertain although studies in acromegalics have suggested that many cases result from mutations that generate constitutively activated G proteins with reduced GTPase activity. The resultant increase in intracellular cyclic adenosine monophosphate in the pituitary leads to increased GH secretion. MAS, which can also be caused by mutations resulting in constitutively activated G proteins, may also include the presence of somatotrophic tumors and excess GH secretion. Approximately 20% of patients with gigantism are those with MAS (commonly consisting of a triad of precocious puberty, café au lait spots, and fibrous dyplasia). GH-secreting tumors have also been reported in multiple endocrine adenomatosis and in association with neurofibromatosis, tuberous sclerosis, and Carney complex.

Activating mutations of the stimulatory Gs_α proteins have been found in the pituitary lesions in MAS and are believed to be responsible for the other glandular adenomas observed in this condition as well. Somatic point mutations of the Gs_α protein have also been identified in somatotrophs of up to 40% of sporadic GH secreting pituitary adenomas.

Diagnosis of Growth Hormone Excess

The gold standard for making the diagnosis of GH excess is a failure to suppress serum GH levels to less than 5 ng/dL after a 1.75 g/kg oral glucose challenge (maximum, 75 g). This test measures the ability of IGF-I to suppress GH secretion because the glucose load results in insulin secretion, leading to suppression of IGFBP-1, which results in an acute increase in free IGF-I levels. The increased free IGF-I suppresses GH secretion within 30–90 min. This test can be abnormal in diabetic patients. Note that a single measurement of GH is inadequate because GH is secreted in a pulsatile manner. Therefore, the use of a random GH measurement can lead to both false-positive and false-negative results. Measurement of serum IGF-I concentration is a sensitive screening test for GH excess. An excellent linear dose-response correlation between serum IGF-I levels and 24-hr mean GH secretion has been demonstrated. An elevated IGF-I level in a patient with appropriate clinical suspicion is almost always indicative of GH excess. Potential confusion may arise when evaluating normal adolescents because significantly higher IGF-I levels occur during puberty than in adulthood. For accurate control comparison, the IGF-I level must be age- and gender-matched. Serum IGFBP-3 levels may also be useful in the diagnosis of GH excess. In patients with confirmed somatotroph adenomas, increased IGFBP-3 levels have been reported to be a sensitive marker of GH elevations and may be elevated despite normal IGF-I levels. If laboratory findings suggest GH excess, the presence of a pituitary adenoma should be confirmed using MRI. In rare cases, a pituitary mass may not be identified. This may be due to an occult pituitary microadenoma or an ectopic tumor. CT is acceptable when MRI is unavailable.

Treatment of Growth Hormone Oversecretion

The goals of therapy are to remove or shrink the pituitary mass, to restore GH and secretory patterns to normal, to restore IGF-I and IGFBP-3 levels to normal, to retain the normal pituitary secretion of other hormones, and to prevent recurrence of disease.

For well-circumscribed pituitary adenomas, transsphenoidal surgery is the treatment of choice and may be curative. The tumor should be removed completely. The likelihood of surgical cure depends greatly on the surgeon's expertise as well as on the size and extension of the mass. Intraoperative GH measurements can improve the results of tumor resection. Transsphenoidal surgery to resect the tumors has been shown to be as safe in children as in adults. At times, a transcranial approach may be necessary. The primary goal of treatment is to normalize GH levels. GH levels (<1 ng/mL within 2 hr after a glucose load) and serum IGF-I levels (age adjusted normal range) are the best tests to define a biochemical cure.

If GH secretion is not normalized by surgery, the options include pituitary radiation and medical therapy. In general, radiotherapy is recommended if GH hypersecretion is not normalized by surgery. Further growth of the tumor is prevented by radiation in more that 99% of the patients. The main disadvantage is the delayed efficacy in decreasing GH levels. GH is reduced approximately 50% from the initial concentration by 2 yr, 75% by 5 yr, and approaches 90% by 15 yr. Hypopituitarism is a predictable outcome, occurring in 40–50% of patients 10 yr after irradiation.

Surgery fails to cure a significant number of patients and therefore medical therapy has taken on a more important role in the management of patients with GH excess. Treatment has been improved by the availability of effective and well-tolerated long-acting somatostatin analogs and dopamine agonists as well as by novel GH antagonists.

The somatostatin analogs have been found to be highly effective in the treatment of patients with GH excess. Octreotide suppresses GH to less than 2.5 ng/mL in 65% of patients with acromegaly and normalizes IGF-I levels in 70%. Studies of patients for more than 14 yr have shown that the effects of octreotide are well sustained over time. Tumor shrinkage also occurs with octreotide, but it is generally modest. Consistent GH suppression was obtained with a continuous SC pump infusion of octreotide in a pubertal boy with pituitary gigantism. Long-acting formulations, including long-acting octreotide and lanreotide, produce consistent GH and IGF-I suppression in acromegalic patients with once monthly or biweekly IM depot injections. The sustained release preparations have not been formally tested in children. Sandostatin injection in the pediatric population has been used at doses of 1–40 μg/kg/24 hr.

For cases that have both GH and prolactin oversecretion, one should consider dopamine agonists, such as bromocriptine, which bind to pituitary dopamine type 2 (D_2) receptors and suppress GH secretion, although the precise mechanism of action remains unclear. Prolactin levels are often adequately suppressed; however, GH levels and IGF-I levels are rarely normalized with this treatment modality. Less that 20% of patients achieve GH levels less that 5 ng/mL and less than 10% achieve normalization of IGF-I levels. Tumor shrinkage occurs in a minority of patients. It is generally used as adjuvant medical treatment for GH excess. Its effectiveness may be additive to that of octreotide. Long-acting formulations are available; however, data on long-term control of GH and IGF-I with these agents is not yet available. The dose of bromocriptine ranges from 10–60 mg/24 hr PO divided qid. However, only a minority of patients benefit from doses greater than 20 mg/24 hr. It has been found to be safe when used in children for an extended period of time, but side effects may include nausea, vomiting, abdominal pain, arrhythmias, nasal stuffiness, orthostatic hypotension, sleep disturbances, and fatigue.

A novel GH receptor antagonist is approved for use in acromegaly (pegvisomant). It is an analog of human growth hormone that functions as a growth hormone-receptor antagonist. It effectively suppressed GH and IGF-I levels in patients with acromegaly from pituitary tumors as well as ectopic GHRH hypersecretion. Normalization of IGF-I levels occurs in up to 90% of patients treated daily with this drug for 3 mo or longer. Long-term studies need to be performed. It has not been tested in children. The adult dose is 10–30 mg via subcutaneous injection once daily.

SOTOS SYNDROME (CEREBRAL GIGANTISM)

Children with cerebral gigantism (also known as Sotos syndrome) are typically above the 90th percentile for both length and weight at birth and macrocrania may also be noted at that time. Although it is characterized by rapid growth, there is no evidence that Sotos syndrome is an endocrine disorder. A hypothalamic defect has been suggested as a cause, but none has been demonstrated functionally or at necropsy. Growth is rapid, and by 1 yr of age, affected infants are greater than the 97th percentile in height. Accelerated growth continues for the first 4–5 yr and then returns to a normal rate. Puberty usually occurs at the normal time but may occur slightly early. Adult height is usually in the upper normal range. The hands and feet are large, with thickened subcutaneous tissue. The head is large and dolichocephalic, the jaw is prominent, there is hypertelorism, and the eyes have an antimongoloid slant. Clumsiness and awkward gait are characteristic, and affected children have great difficulty in sports, in learning to ride a bicycle, and in other tasks requiring coordination. Some degree of mental retardation affects most patients; in some children, perceptual deficiencies may predominate. Osseous maturation is compatible with the patient's height. GH and IGF-I levels and results of other endocrine studies are usually normal; there are no distinctive laboratory or radiologic markers for the syndrome. Abnormal electroencephalograms are common; imaging studies frequently reveal a dilated ventricular system. Most cases are sporadic. Familial cases are usually consistent with autosomal dominant inheritance and occasionally with autosomal recessive inheritance. Affected patients may be at increased risk for neoplasia, particularly hepatic carcinoma, but Wilms, ovarian, and parotid tumors have been reported. A genetic basis for Sotos syndrome has recently been proposed to involve NSD1, a transcription factor whose function is being unraveled. A typical case is shown in Figure 554–1.

OVERGROWTH IN THE FETUS

Maternal diabetes constitutes the most common cause of infants who are large for gestational age (LGA). Even in the absence of clinical symptoms or a family history, the birth of an excessively large infant should lead to evaluation for maternal (or gestational) diabetes.

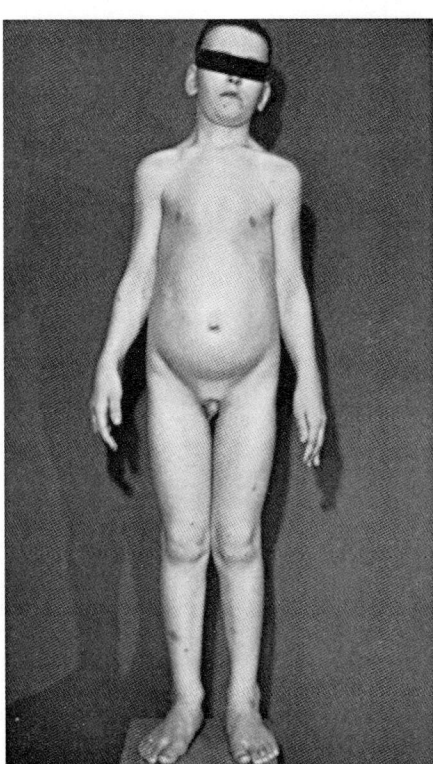

FIGURE 554–1. Cerebral gigantism in an 8-yr-old boy. The height age was 12 yr; the bone age was 12 yr. IQ was 60. The electroencephalogram had abnormal findings. Notice the prominence of the forehead and the jaw and the large hands and feet. Sexual development was consistent with chronological age. Hormone study results were normal. The adult height was 208 cm (6 ft 10 in); his sexual development was normal. He wears size 18 shoes.

A group of disorders associated with excessive somatic growth and growth of specific organs, has been described and are collectively referred to as overgrowth syndromes. These disorders appear to be caused by excess availability of IGF-II encoded by the gene Igf2. The best described of these syndromes is the *Beckwith-Wiedemann syndrome (BWS)*, which is an overgrowth malformation syndrome that occurs with an incidence of 1:13,700 births. It is manifest as a fetal overgrowth syndrome in which hypertrophy dominates the clinical picture. Typically macroglossia, omphalocele, hepatosplenomegaly, nephromegaly, and hypoglycemia secondary to pancreatic β cell hyperplasia in an LGA baby comprise the clinical picture at birth. An additional complication is that these children are predisposed to a specific subset of childhood neoplasms, among which are Wilms tumor and adrenocortical carcinoma. Overexpression of IGF-II in BWS may be caused by a number of genetic disruptions including gene duplication, loss of heterozygosity, and relaxation or loss of imprinting of the Igf2 gene. Various lines of investigation have localized "imprinted" genes involved in BWS and associated childhood tumors to chromosome 11p. These include, in addition to Igf2, the gene H19, which is involved in Igf2 suppression as well as the gene WT-1 (the Wilms tumor gene). Mutations in GPC3, a glycan gene (which code for an IGF-II neutralizing membrane receptor), cause the related *Simpson-Golabi-Behmel overgrowth syndrome*.

Abe T, Tara LA, Ludecke DK: Growth hormone-secreting pituitary adenoma in childhood and adolescence: Features and results of transnasal surgery. *Neurosurgery* 1999;45:1–10.

Barnard ND, Scialli AR, Bobela S: The current use of estrogens for growth-suppressant therapy in adolescent girls. *J Pediatr Adolesc Gynecol* 2002;15:23–6.

Drop SL, Greggio N, Cappa M, et al: Current concepts in tall stature and overgrowth syndromes. *J Pediatr Endocrinol Metab* 2001;14:975–84.

Elias LL, Huebner A, Metherell LA, et al: Tall stature in familial glucocorticoid deficiency. *Clin Endocrinol* 2000;53:423–30.

Fuqua JS, Berkovitz GD: Growth hormone excess in a child with neurofibromatosis type I and optic pathway tumor: A patient report. *Clin Pediatr* 1998;37:749–52.

Grumbach MM, Auchus RJ: Estrogen: Consequences and implications of human mutations in synthesis and action. *J Clin Endocrinol Metab* 1999;84:4677–94.

Herman-Bonert VS, Zib K, Scarlett JA, et al: Growth hormone receptor antagonist therapy in acromegalic patient resistant to somatostatin analogs. *J Clin Endocrinol Metab* 2000;85:2958–61.

Ho KK: Place of pegvisomant in acromegaly. *Lancet* 2001;358:1743.

Holl RW, Bucher P, Sorgo W, et al: Suppression of growth hormone by oral glucose in the evaluation of tall stature. *Hormone Res* 1999;51:20–5.

Kunwar S, Wilson CB:Pediatric pituitary adenomas. *J Clin Endocrinol Metab* 1999;84:4385–9.

Kurotaki N, Imaizumi K, Harada N, et al: Haploinsufficiency of NSD1 causes Sotos syndrome. *Nat Genet* 2002;30:365–6.

Lafferty AR, Chrousos GP: Pituitary tumors in children and adolescents. *J Clin Endocrinol Metab* 1999;84:4317–23.

Marcus R, Leary D, Schneider DL, et al: The contribution of testosterone to skeletal development and maintenance: Lessons for the androgen insensitivity syndrome. *J Clin Endocrinol Metab* 2000;85:1032–7.

Moran A, Pescovitz OH: Long-term treatment of gigantism with combination octreotide and bromocriptine in a child with McCune-Albright syndrome. *Endocr J* 1994;2:111–3.

Morishima A, Grumbach MM, Simpson ER, et al: Aromatase deficiency in male and female siblings caused by a novel mutation and the physiologic role of estrogens. *J Clin Endocrinol Metab* 1995;80:3689–98.

Morison IM, Becroft DM, Taniguchi T, et al: Somatic overgrowth associated with overexpression of insulin-like growth factor II. *Nat Med* 1996;2:311–6.

Nanto-Salonen K, Koskinen P, Sonninen P, et al: Suppression of GH secretion in pituitary gigantism by continuous subcutaneous octreotide infusion in a pubertal boy. *Acta Pediatr* 1999;88:29–33.

Rooman RP, Van Driessche K, Du Caju M: Growth and ovarian function in girls with 48,XXXX karyotype—Patient report and review of the literature. *J Pediatr Endocrinol Metab* 2002;15:1051–5.

Sotos JF: Overgrowth. Genetic syndromes and other disorders associated with overgrowth. *Clin Pediatr* 1997;36:157–70.

Statakis CA, Carney JA, Lin JP, et al: Carney complex, a familial multiple neoplasia and lentiginosis syndrome. *J Clin Invest* 1996;97:699–705.

Thapar K, Kovacs K, Stefanneanu L, et al: Overexpression of the growth hormone-releasing hormone gene in acromegaly-associated pituitary tumors. *Am J Pathol* 1997;151:769–84.

Trainer PJ, Drake WM, Katznelson L, et al: Treatment of acromegaly with the growth hormone-receptor antagonist pegvisomant. *N Engl J Med* 2000;342:1171–7.

Chapter 555
Physiology of Puberty

Luigi Garibaldi

Between early childhood and approximately 8–9 yr of age (i.e., *prepubertal* stage), the hypothalamic-pituitary-gonadal axis is dormant, as reflected by undetectable serum concentrations of luteinizing hormone (LH) and sex hormones (i.e., estradiol in girls, testosterone in boys). In this phase, the activity of the hypothalamus and pituitary is thought to be suppressed by poorly characterized neuronal restraint pathways.

One to 3 yr before the onset of puberty becomes clinically evident, low serum levels of LH during sleep become demonstrable (i.e., *peripubertal* period). This sleep-entrained LH secretion occurs in a pulsatile fashion and probably reflects endogenous episodic discharge of hypothalamic gonadotropin-releasing hormone (GnRH). Nocturnal pulses of LH continue to increase in amplitude and, to a lesser extent, in frequency as clinical puberty approaches. This pulsatile secretion of gonadotropins is responsible for enlargement and maturation of the gonads and the secretion of sex hormones. The appearance of the secondary sex characteristics in *early puberty* is the visible culmination of the sustained, active interaction occurring among hypothalamus, pituitary, and gonads in the peripubertal period. By *midpuberty*, LH pulses become evident even during the daytime and occur at about 90–120 min intervals.

A second critical event occurs in middle or late adolescence in girls, in whom cyclicity and ovulation occur. A positive feedback mechanism develops whereby increasing levels of estrogen in midcycle cause a distinct increase of LH.

The factors that normally activate or restrain the hypothalamic neurons responsible for GnRH secretion (i.e., neurosecretory unit known as the *GnRH pulse generator*) are unknown. In nonhuman primates, a decline in the γ aminobutyric acid (GABA)-ergic tone in hypothalamic neurons and the resultant increase in the glutamate-ergic tone have been shown to activate the GnRH pulse generator. Several other neurotransmitters are probably involved in humans and other primates.

It is clear that GnRH is the major, if not the only, hormone responsible for the onset and progression of puberty, because pubertal development can be reproduced in sexually immature or gonadotropin-deficient animals and humans by pulsed administration of GnRH.

The interpretation of the hormonal changes of puberty is complex because of several factors. First, pituitary gonadotropins are heterogeneous and circulate in multiple isoforms: more-bioactive isoforms of LH may be preponderant during puberty. Second, LH immunoreactivity is variable in different immunoassays, and the results of LH measurements vary widely among laboratories. Third, the pulsatile secretion of gonadotropins and the synergism of follicle-stimulating hormone and LH in promoting gonadal maturation make interpretation of single serum gonadotropin concentrations difficult. Measurement of gonadotropins in serially obtained (every 10–20 min for 12–24 hr) serum samples or timed urine collections is more meaningful. Fourth, important sex differences exist in the maturation of the hypothalamus and pituitary gland, and serum LH concentrations increase earlier in the course of the pubertal process in boys than in girls.

The effects of gonadal steroids (i.e., testosterone in boys, estradiol in girls) on bone growth and osseous maturation have become increasingly clear in the last decade, with the characterization of estrogen deficiency states in male patients. Both aromatase deficiency and estrogen receptor defects result in delayed epiphyseal fusion and tall stature in affected boys. These observations suggest that estrogens, rather than androgens, are responsible for the process of bone maturation that ultimately leads to epiphyseal fusion and cessation of growth. Estrogens also mediate the increased production of growth hormone, which along with a direct effect of sex steroids on bone growth, is responsible for the pubertal growth spurt.

The age of onset of puberty varies and is more closely correlated with osseous maturation than with chronological age (Chapter 14). In girls, the breast bud is usually the first sign of puberty (10–11 yr), followed by the appearance of pubic hair 6–12 mo later. The interval to menarche is usually 2–2.5 yr but may be as long as 6 yr. In the United States, at least one sign of puberty is present in approximately 95% of girls by 12 yr of age and in 99% of girls by 13 yr of age. Peak height velocity occurs early (at breast stage II–III, typically between 11 and 12 yr of age) in girls and always precedes menarche. The mean age of menarche is about 12.75 yr. There are, however, wide variations in the sequence of changes involving growth spurt, breast bud, pubic hair, and maturation of the internal and external genitalia.

In boys, growth of the testes (>3 mL in volume or 2.5 cm in longest diameter) and thinning of the scrotum are the first signs of puberty. These are followed by pigmentation of the scrotum and growth of the penis (Chapter 14). Pubic hair then appears. Appearance of axillary hair usually occurs in midpuberty. In boys, unlike girls, acceleration of growth begins after puberty is well under way and is maximal at genital stage IV–V (typically between 13 and 14 yr of age). In boys, the growth spurt occurs approximately 2 yr later than in girls, and growth may continue beyond 18 yr of age.

Genetic and environmental factors affect the onset of puberty. Following a decrease in menarcheal age in the past century, probably reflecting better nutrition and improved general health, the age of menarche has been stable for the last 30–40 yr. American black girls may be more advanced in development of secondary sex characteristics than white girls. Ballet dancers, gymnasts, runners, and other female athletes in whom leanness and strenuous physical activity have coexisted from early childhood frequently exhibit a marked delay in puberty or menarche, and frequently have oligomenorrhea or amenorrhea as adults. This observation supports the thesis that the energy balance is closely related to the activity of the GnRH pulse generator and the mechanisms initiating and sustaining puberty, perhaps via hormonal signals originating from the adipocytes (leptin and others peptides).

Adrenal cortical androgens also play a role in sexual maturation. Serum levels of dehydroepiandrosterone (DHEA) and its sulfate (DHEAS) begin to increase at approximately 6–8 yr of age, before any increase in LH or sex hormones and before the earliest physical changes of puberty are apparent; this process has been called adrenarche. DHEAS is the most abundant adrenal C-19 steroid in the blood, and its serum concentration remains fairly stable over 24 hr. A single measurement of this hormone is commonly used as a marker of adrenal androgen secretion. Although adrenarche typically antedates the onset of gonadal activity (i.e., gonadarche) by a few years, the two processes do not seem to be causally related, because adrenarche and gonadarche are dissociated in conditions such as central precocious puberty and adrenocortical failure.

Chapter 556

Disorders of Pubertal Development *Luigi Garibaldi*

Precocious puberty is generally defined as the onset of secondary sexual characteristics before 8 yr of age in girls and 9 yr in boys. This definition is somewhat arbitrary, however, because of the marked variation in the age at which puberty begins in normal children, particularly in different ethnic groups.

Precocious pubertal development may be classified as gonadotropin dependent, also called *true* or *central* precocious

puberty, or gonadotropin independent, also called *peripheral precocious puberty* or precocious *pseudopuberty* (Box 556–1). True precocious puberty is always isosexual and stems from hypothalamic-pituitary-gonadal activation. The gonadotropin-mediated increase in the size and activity of the gonads leads to increasing sex hormone secretion and progressive sexual maturation. In precocious pseudopuberty, some of the secondary sex characteristics appear, but there is no activation of the normal hypothalamic-pituitary-gonadal interplay. In this latter group, the sex characteristics may be isosexual or heterosexual ("contrasexual") (see Chapters 576 to 582).

Precocious pseudopuberty may induce maturation of the hypothalamic-pituitary-gonadal axis and eventually trigger the onset of true sexual precocity. This mixed type of precocious puberty occurs commonly in conditions such as congenital adrenal hyperplasia, McCune-Albright syndrome, and familial male-limited precocious puberty, when the bone age reaches the pubertal range (10.5–12.5 yr).

556.1　Gonadotropin-Dependent Precocious Puberty

The condition occurs at least 10-fold more frequently in girls than in boys and is usually sporadic, although some cases are familial. Despite the widespread use of CT scans and MRI, more than 90% of sexual precocity in girls is idiopathic. A structural central nervous system (CNS) abnormality can, however, be demonstrated in 25–75% of boys and in some girls with central precocious puberty. A high prevalence of idiopathic sexual precocity has been reported in girls adopted from developing countries, with the limitations that the exact date of birth may be uncertain in some cases.

Clinical Manifestations. Sexual development may begin at any age and generally follows the sequence observed in normal puberty. In girls, the first sign is development of the breast; pubic hair may appear simultaneously but more often appears later. Maturation of the external genitalia, the appearance of axillary hair, and the onset of menstruation follow. The early menstrual cycles may be more irregular than they are with normal puberty. The initial cycles are usually anovulatory, but pregnancy has been reported as early as 5.5 yr of age (Fig. 556–1).

In boys, enlargement of the testes is followed by enlargement of the penis, appearance of pubic hair, and acne. Erections are common, and nocturnal emissions may occur. The voice deepens, and linear growth is accelerated. Testicular biopsies have shown stimulation of all elements of the testes, and spermatogenesis has been observed as early as 5–6 yr of age.

In affected girls and boys, height, weight, and osseous maturation are advanced. The increased rate of bone maturation results in early closure of the epiphyses, and the ultimate stature is less than it would have been otherwise. Without treatment, approximately one third of girls and an even larger percentage of boys achieve a height less than the 5th percentile as adults. Mental development is usually compatible with chronological age. Emotional behavior and mood swings are common, but serious psychological problems are rare.

Although the clinical course is variable, three main patterns of pubertal progression can be identified. Most girls (particularly those younger than 6 yr of age at the onset) and most boys have *rapidly progressive* sexual precocity, characterized by rapid physical and osseous maturation, leading to a loss of height potential. Several girls (generally older than 6 yr of age at the onset) have a *slowly progressive variant*, characterized by parallel advancement of osseous maturation and linear growth, with preserved height potential. A slowly progressive variant of central sexual precoc-

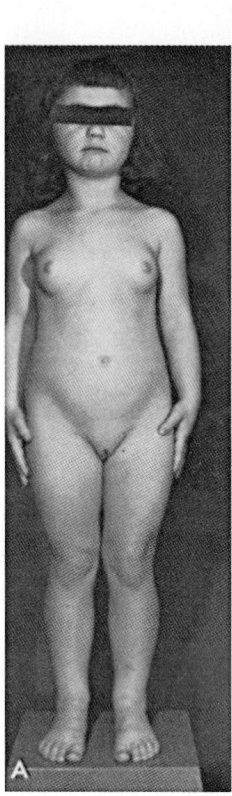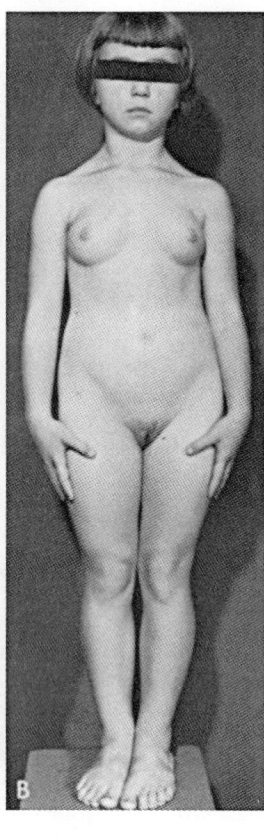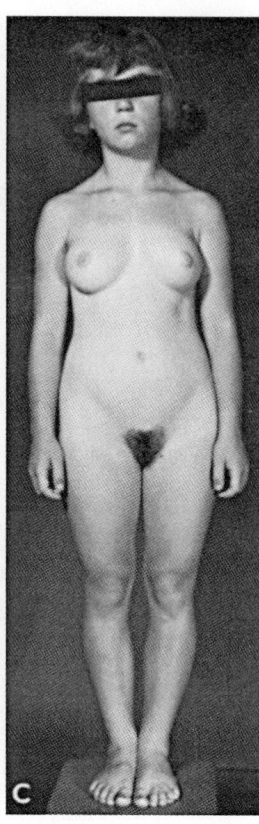

FIGURE 556–1. Idiopathic precocious puberty. Patient (*A*) at $3^{11}/_{12}$, (*B*) at $5^{8}/_{12}$, and (*C*) at $8^{1}/_{2}$ yr of age. Breast development and vaginal bleeding began at $2^{1}/_{2}$ yr of age. Osseous age was $7^{1}/_{2}$ yr at $3^{11}/_{12}$ and 14 yr at 8 yr of age. Repeated estrogen assays varied between normal prepubertal and adult female levels. Urinary gonadotropins were not demonstrable until the child was 5 yr of age. Intelligence and dental age were normal for chronological age. Growth was completed at 10 yr; ultimate height was 142 cm (56 in).

ity has recently been reported in boys, too, but it appears to be much less common than in girls. A small percentage of girls have spontaneously regressive or *unsustained* central precocious puberty. This variability in the natural course of sexual precocity underscores the need for longitudinal observation at the onset of sexual development, before treatment is considered.

Laboratory Findings. Sex hormone concentrations are usually appropriate for the stage of puberty in both sexes. Thus, serum estradiol concentrations in girls are low or undetectable in the early phase of sexual precocity, as they are in normal puberty. In boys, serum testosterone levels are detectable or clearly elevated by the time the parents seek medical attention, particularly if an early morning blood sample is obtained.

Sensitive immunometric (including immunoradiometric, immunofluorometric, and chemiluminescent) assays for luteinizing hormone (LH) have largely replaced the traditional LH radioimmunoassays and offer greater diagnostic sensitivity using random blood samples. With these new assays, serum LH concentrations are undetectable in prepubertal children, but they become detectable in 50–70% of girls and a higher percentage of boys with central sexual precocity. Measurement of LH in serial blood samples obtained during sleep has greater diagnostic power than measurement in a single random sample, and it typically reveals a well-defined pulsatile secretion of LH. Intravenous administration of gonadotropin-releasing hormone *(GnRH stimulation test)* or a GnRH agonist (leuprolide stimulation test) is a helpful diagnostic tool, particularly for boys, in whom a brisk LH response (LH peak >5–10 IU/L) with predominance of LH over follicle-stimulating hormone (FSH) occurs in the early phase of precocious puberty. In girls with sexual precocity, however, the nocturnal LH secretion and the LH response to GnRH may be quite low at breast stage II–early stage III (immunometric-LH peak, often <5 IU/L), and the LH:FSH ratio may remain low until midpuberty. In such girls with "low" LH response, the central nature of sexual precocity can be proven by detecting pubertal levels of estradiol (>50 pg/mL), 20–24 hr after stimulation with leuprolide.

Osseous maturation is variably advanced, often more than 2–3 SD. Pelvic ultrasonography in girls reveals progressive enlargement of the ovaries, followed by enlargement of the uterus to pubertal size. A CT or MRI scan usually demonstrates physiologic enlargement of the pituitary gland, as seen in normal puberty, and sometimes reveals CNS pathology (see later text).

Differential Diagnosis. Organic CNS causes of central sexual precocity should be ruled out by MRI scans, particularly in girls without pubic hair, in girls with estradiol greater than 30 pmol/L, in girls younger than 6 yr of age, and in all boys. However, in children presenting without neurologic signs or symptoms, the CNS lesions causing precocious puberty are rarely malignant and seldom require neurosurgical intervention.

Gonadotropin-independent causes of isosexual precocious puberty must be considered in the differential diagnosis (see Box 556–1). For girls, these include tumors of the ovaries, autonomously functioning ovarian cysts, feminizing adrenal tumors, McCune-Albright syndrome, and exogenous sources of estrogens. For boys, congenital adrenal hyperplasia, adrenal tumors, Leydig cell tumors, chorionic gonadotropin-producing tumors, and familial male precocious puberty should be considered.

Treatment. The observation that the pituitary gonadotropic cells require pulsatile, rather than continuous, stimulation by GnRH to maintain the ongoing release of gonadotropins provides the rationale for using GnRH agonists for treatment of central precocious puberty. By virtue of being more potent and having a longer duration of action than native GnRH, these GnRH analogs (after a brief period of stimulation) "desensitize" the gonadotropic cells of the pituitary to the stimulatory effect of endogenous GnRH and effectively halt the progression of central sexual precocity. Virtually all boys and the large subgroup of girls with rapidly progressive precocious puberty are candidates for treatment. However, girls with slowly progressive puberty do not seem to benefit in terms of height prognosis from GnRH-agonist therapy. Rare patients require treatment for psychological or social reasons alone.

Depot formulations of long-acting GnRH analogs, which maintain fairly constant serum concentration of the drug for weeks, constitute the preparations of choice for treatment of central precocious puberty. Leuprolide acetate (Lupron Depot Ped), the only depot preparation approved for this use in the United States, is given in a dose of 0.25–0.3 mg/kg (minimum, 7.5 mg) intramuscularly once every 4 wk. Other long-acting preparations (D-Trp6-GnRH [Decapeptyl]; goserelin acetate [Zoladex]) are approved for treatment of precocious puberty in other countries. Recurrent sterile fluid collections at the sites of injections is the most troublesome local side effect and occurs in less than 5% of treated patients. In children with such local reactions, treatment should be changed to subcutaneous injections of aqueous leuprolide, given once or twice daily (total dose 60 μg/kg/24 hr), or intranasal administration of the GnRH agonist nafarelin [Synarel], 800 μg bid. However, the potential for irregular compliance with daily administration, as well as the variable absorption of the intranasal route for nafarelin, may limit the long-term benefit of the latter preparations on adult height. GnRH antagonists have only recently become commercially available and are currently under study for treatment of sexual precocity.

Treatment results in decrease of the growth rate, generally to age-appropriate values, and an even greater decrease of the rate of osseous maturation. Some children, particularly those with greatly advanced (pubertal) bone age, may show marked deceleration of their growth rate and a complete arrest in the rate of osseous maturation. Treatment results in enhancement of the predicted height, although the actual adult height of patients followed to epiphyseal closure is approximately 1 SD less than their midparental height. In girls, breast development may regress in those with Tanner stage II–III development. Most commonly, the size of the breasts remains unchanged in girls with stage III–V development or may even increase slightly because of progressive adipose tissue deposition. The amount of glandular tissue decreases. Pubic hair usually remains stable in girls, or may even progress slowly during treatment, reflecting the gradual increase in adrenal androgens. Menses, if present, cease. Pelvic sonography demonstrates a decrease of the ovarian and uterine size. In boys, there is decrease of testicular size, variable regression of pubic hair, and decrease in the frequency of erections. Except for a reversible decrease in bone density (of uncertain clinical significance), no serious adverse effects of GnRH analogs have been reported in children treated for sexual precocity.

If treatment is effective, the serum sex hormone concentrations decrease to prepubertal levels (testosterone, <20 ng/dL in boys; estradiol, <10 pg/mL in girls). The serum LH and FSH concentrations, as measured by sensitive immunometric assays, decrease to less than 1 IU/L, although rarely does the LH return to truly prepubertal levels (<0.1 IU/L). Moreover, the incremental FSH and LH responses to GnRH stimulation decrease to less than 1–2 IU/L. Serum LH and sex hormone levels remain suppressed for as long as therapy is continued, but puberty resumes promptly when therapy is discontinued. In girls, menarche and ovulatory cycles generally appear within 6–18 mo of cessation of therapy. The addition of human growth hormone (hGH) to GnRH agonists has been used in children with precocious puberty, markedly advanced bone age, and poor height prediction. Preliminary data suggest that combined therapy may improve the adult height.

556.2 Precocious Puberty Resulting from Organic Brain Lesions

Etiology. With the advent of CT and especially MRI scans, *hypothalamic hamartoma* has been recognized as one of the most common brain lesions causing true precocious puberty (Fig. 556–2). This congenital malformation consists of ectopically located

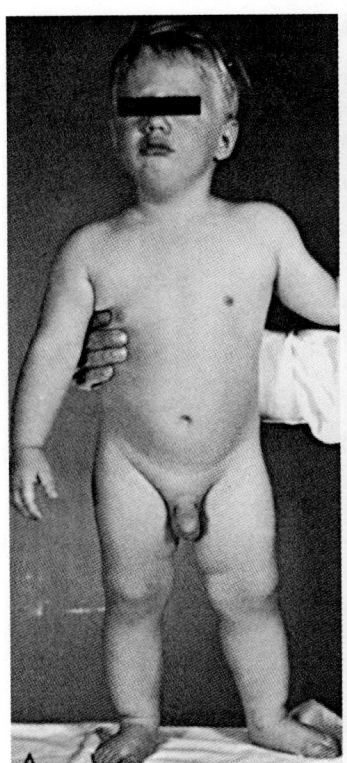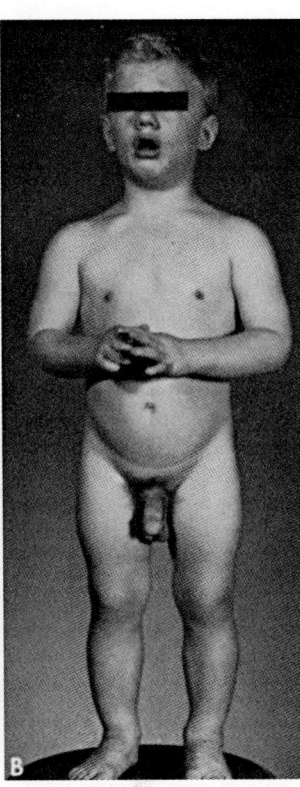

FIGURE 556–2. Precocious puberty with central nervous system lesion. Photographs at 1.5 (*A*) and 2.5 (*B*) yr of age. Accelerated growth, muscular development, osseous maturation, and testicular development were consistent with the degree of secondary sexual maturation. In early infancy, the patient began having frequent spells of rapid, purposeless motion; later in life, he had episodes of uncontrollable laughing with ocular movements. At 7 yr, he exhibited emotional lability, aggressive behavior, and destructive tendencies. Although a hypothalamic hamartoma had been suspected, it was not established until CT scanning became available, when the patient was 23 yr of age. Epiphyses fused at 9 yr of age; final height was 142 cm (56 in). At 24 yr of age, he developed an embryonal cell carcinoma of the retroperitoneum.

neural tissue containing GnRH-secretory neurons and may function as an accessory GnRH pulse generator. On MRI, it appears as a small pedunculated mass attached to the tuber cinereum or the floor of the third ventricle or, less often, as a sessile mass (Fig. 556–3), which remains static in size over years. This lesion is infrequently associated with gelastic or psychomotor seizures.

A wide variety of lesions of the CNS, usually involving the hypothalamus by scarring, invasion, or pressure, have been associated with gonadotropin-dependent sexual precocity. These lesions probably induce sexual maturation by interrupting poorly characterized pubertal restraint pathways. They include postencephalitic scars, tuberculous meningoencephalitis, tuberous sclerosis, severe head trauma, and hydrocephalus, either isolated or associated with myelomeningocele. Neoplasms causing precocious puberty include astrocytomas, ependymomas, and optic tract tumors. Tumors of the latter type (typically slowly progressive or indolent optic gliomas) are highly prevalent (15–20%) in children with neurofibromatosis type 1 (NF-1) and constitute the main etiologic factor for the central sexual precocity encountered in a small subset (approximately 3%) of children with NF-1.

About half of the tumors in the pineal region are germinomas or astrocytomas; the remainder consists of a wide variety of

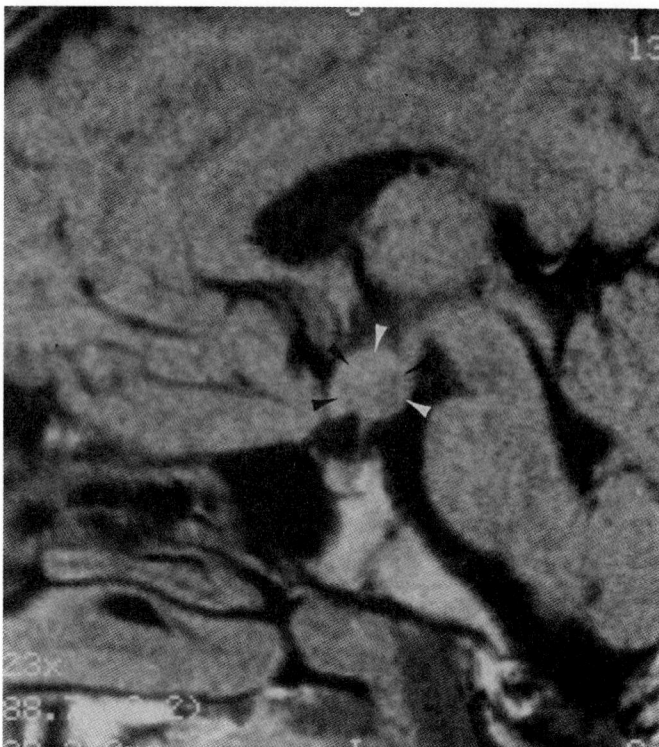

FIGURE 556–3. MRI of a central nervous system lesion in a child with central precocious puberty. A 6-yr-old girl was referred for stage IV breast development and growth acceleration. Serum luteinizing hormone and estradiol concentrations were in the adult range. The midsagittal T1-weighted image shows an isointense hypothalamic mass (*arrowheads*), typical of a hamartoma. (From Sharafuddin M, Luisiri A, Garibaldi LR, et al: MR imaging diagnosis of cerebral precocious puberty: Importance of changes in the shape and size of the pituitary gland. *Am J Roentgenol* 1994;162:1167.)

histologically distinct tumor types. These tumors, too, cause precocious puberty by interrupting CNS inhibitory pathways to the hypothalamus or, in boys only, by secreting human chorionic gonadotropin (hCG), which stimulates the Leydig cells of the testes. Intracranial hCG-secreting germinomas usually do not produce precocious puberty in girls, presumably because complete ovarian function cannot occur without FSH priming.

Clinical Manifestations. Some of these tumors or malformations (e.g., hypothalamic hamartomas) remain static in size or grow slowly, producing no signs other than precocious puberty. For lesions causing neurologic symptoms, the neuroendocrine manifestations may be present for 1–2 yr before the tumor can be detected radiologically. Hypothalamic signs or symptoms such as diabetes insipidus, adipsia, hyperthermia, unnatural crying or laughing (gelastic seizures), obesity, and cachexia should suggest the possibility of an intracranial lesion. Visual signs (e.g., proptosis) may be the first manifestation of an optic glioma.

The sexual precocity is always isosexual, and the endocrine patterns are generally those found in children without demonstrable organic lesions. Rapidly progressive sexual precocity in very young children suggests the likelihood of a hypothalamic hamartoma. In conditions other than hypothalamic hamartoma, growth hormone deficiency may occur and may be masked by the growth-promoting effect of the increased sex hormone levels.

Treatment. Neurosurgical intervention is not indicated for hypothalamic hamartomas, except in rare patients with intractable seizures. For other neurologic lesions, therapy depends on the nature and location of the pathologic process. Regardless of the cause, therapy with GnRH analogs is as effective in children with organic brain lesions causing central precocious puberty as it is in children with idiopathic sexual precocity, and the analogs are the therapy of choice to halt premature sexual development. Combined growth hormone therapy should be considered for patients with associated growth hormone deficiency.

556.3 Precocious Puberty Following Irradiation of the Brain

Radiation therapy, generally for leukemia or intracranial tumors, increases the risk of precocious puberty considerably, whether the irradiation is directed to the hypothalamic area or to areas of the brain anatomically distant from the hypothalamus. Low-dose radiation (18–24 Gy) hastens the onset of puberty almost exclusively in girls. High-dose radiation (25–47 Gy), conversely, appears to trigger precocious sexual development in both sexes, and the risk of sexual precocity is inversely proportional to the age of the child at the time radiation was given.

This type of sexual precocity often occurs in the face of growth hormone deficiency, and may be associated with other conditions (e.g., spinal radiation, hypothyroidism) adversely affecting the prognosis for a reasonable adult height. Unless careful attention is paid to early signs of pubertal development in these children, the combination of growth hormone deficiency and the growth promoting effect of sex steroids often results in a "normal" growth rate at the expense of a rapidly advancing bone age and impaired adult height potential.

Treatment. As in other types of central precocious puberty, GnRH analogs are very effective in arresting pubertal progression in this patient population. However, concomitant growth hormone deficiency (and/or thyroid hormone deficiency) need to be diagnosed and treated promptly in order for the adult height prognosis to improve.

Paradoxically, hypopituitarism with gonadotropin deficiency may subsequently develop as a late effect of high-dose CNS radiation in patients with or without a history of precocious puberty, and may require substitution therapy with sex steroids.

556.4 Syndrome of Precocious Puberty and Hypothyroidism

In children with untreated hypothyroidism, the onset of puberty is usually delayed until epiphyseal maturation has reached 12–13 yr of age. Precocious puberty in a child with untreated hypothyroidism and a prepubertal bone age presents a strikingly unphysiologic association, yet is not uncommon and may occur in as many as 50% of children with severe hypothyroidism of long duration. These children have the usual manifestations of hypothyroidism, including retardation of growth and of osseous maturation. The cause of the hypothyroidism is often undiagnosed lymphocytic thyroiditis and rarely thyroidectomy or overtreatment with antithyroid drugs.

Sexual development in girls consists primarily of breast enlargement and menstrual bleeding; the latter may occur even in girls with minimal breast enlargement. Pelvic sonography may reveal large, multicystic ovaries. Boys have testicular enlargement associated with modest or no penile enlargement and no pubic hair development. Enlargement of the sella, which is typical of long-standing primary hypothyroidism, may be demonstrated by skull film or MRI. Plasma levels of thyroid-stimulating hormone (TSH) are markedly elevated, often greater than 500 µU/mL, and those of prolactin are mildly elevated. Although serum FSH is low and LH is undetectable, when measured by specific assays, the massively elevated concentrations of TSH appear to interact with the FSH receptor ("specificity spillover"), thus inducing FSH-like effects in the absence of LH effects on the gonads. As a consequence, unlike in true precocious puberty, testicular enlargement occurs without substantial Leydig cell stimulation and testosterone secretion in affected boys. In affected girls, ovarian estrogen production occurs without a concomitant increase in androgens. Thus, the precocious puberty associated with hypothyroidism behaves as an incomplete form of gonadotropin-dependent puberty. Treatment of the hypothyroidism results in rapid return to normal of the biochemical and clinical manifestations. Macroorchidism (testicular volume > 30 mL) may persist in adult life despite adequate thyroxine therapy.

556.5 Gonadotropin-Secreting Tumors

Hepatic Tumors. Isosexual precocious puberty may be uncommonly associated with hepatoblastoma. All reported cases have been male, with the age of onset varying from 4 mo–8 yr (average, 2 yr). An enlarged liver or mass in the upper quadrant should suggest the diagnosis. The tumor cells produce hCG, which stimulates the LH receptors in the Leydig cells of the testes. The testicular histology reveals interstitial cell hyperplasia and absence of spermatogenesis. Plasma levels of hCG and α-fetoprotein are usually markedly elevated; they serve as useful markers for following the effects of therapy. Plasma levels of testosterone are elevated, and the FSH and LH levels, as measured by specific, immunometric assays, are low; in the past, LH levels were falsely elevated because of cross-reaction with hCG on radioimmunoassay.

Treatment for these tumors is the same as that for other carcinomas of the liver; prognosis for survival beyond 1–2 yr from the time of diagnosis is poor.

Other Tumors. Chorionic gonadotropin-secreting choriocarcinomas, teratocarcinomas, or teratomas (also called ectopic pinealomas or atypical teratomas), located in the CNS, mediastinum, gonads, or even adrenal glands, may cause precocious puberty, more commonly (10- to 20-fold) in boys than in girls. Affected patients often have marked elevations of hCG and α-fetoprotein. Mediastinal tumors, but not gonadal tumors, have been reported to cause precocious puberty in boys with Klinefelter syndrome.

Precocious Pseudopuberty. The adrenal causes of pseudopuberty are discussed in Chapter 570, and the gonadal causes are discussed in Chapters 578 and 581.

556.6 McCune-Albright Syndrome (Precocious Puberty with Polyostotic Fibrous Dysplasia and Abnormal Pigmentation)

This is a syndrome of endocrine dysfunction associated with patchy cutaneous pigmentation and fibrous dysplasia of the skeletal system. Although sexual precocity in girls was the major recognized endocrinopathy in the past, associated pituitary, thyroid, and adrenal aberrations are also recognized. The disorder is characterized by autonomous hyperfunction of many glands and is caused by a missense mutation in the gene encoding the α-subunit of G_s, the G protein that stimulates cyclic adenosine monophosphate (cAMP) formation, resulting in the formation of the putative *gsp* oncoprotein. Activation of receptors (e.g., corticotropin [ACTH], TSH, FSH, LH receptors) that operate with a cAMP-dependent mechanism, as well as cell prolifera-

tion, ensue. Because the mutation is somatic, rather than genomic, it is expressed differently in different glands or tissues; hence, the variability of clinical expression in different patients.

Precocious puberty has been described predominantly in girls (Fig. 556–4). The average age at onset in affected girls is about 3 yr, but vaginal bleeding has occurred as early as 4 mo of age and secondary sex characteristics have occurred as early as 6 mo. Young girls have suppressed levels of LH and FSH, and there is no response to GnRH stimulation. Estradiol levels vary from normal to markedly elevated (>900 pg/mL), are often cyclic, and may correlate with the size of the cysts. In boys, precocious puberty is less common but has been reported in several instances. Unlike ovarian enlargement in girls, testicular enlargement in boys is fairly symmetric. It is followed by the appearance of phallic enlargement and pubic hair, as in normal puberty. Testicular histology has demonstrated large seminiferous tubules and no or minimal Leydig cell hyperplasia; these findings may simply reflect the fact that biopsy specimens were obtained at an early stage of pubertal development. In girls and boys, when the bone age reaches the usual pubertal age range, gonadotropin secretion begins, and the response to GnRH becomes pubertal. True (gonadotropin-dependent) precocious puberty overrides the antecedent (gonadotropin-independent) precocious pseudopuberty. In girls, menses become more regular, but often not completely, and fertility has been documented.

Pubertal progression is variable in these patients. Functioning ovarian cysts often disappear spontaneously; aspiration or surgical excision of cysts is rarely indicated. For girls with persistent estradiol secretion, agents that interfere with the final step of estrogen biosynthesis, that is, aromatase inhibitors such as testolactone, letrozole or anastrozole, or antiestrogens (such as tamoxifen) may limit, to a variable extent, the estrogen effects on pubertal and osseous maturation. These compounds, however, have not been approved by the Food and Drug Administration for this indication; tamoxifen may be hepatotoxic. Associated therapy with long-acting analogs of GnRH is indicated only for patients whose puberty has shifted from a gonadotropin-independent to a predominantly gonadotropin-dependent mechanism.

Extragonadal Manifestations. The hyperthyroidism that occurs in this condition differs from that characteristic of Graves disease. There is an equal distribution among male and female patients; the goiters are multinodular. Clinical hyperthyroidism is uncommon in children, but goiters, mildly elevated triiodothyronine levels, suppressed TSH levels, and abnormalities on ultrasound have been reported. Only rarely is thyroidectomy necessary.

In patients with associated Cushing syndrome, bilateral nodular adrenocortical hyperplasia has occurred in early infancy, antedating the sexual precocity. ACTH levels are low, and adrenal function is not suppressed by large doses of dexamethasone. Treatment is bilateral adrenalectomy.

Increased secretion of growth hormone occurs uncommonly and is manifested clinically by gigantism or acromegaly or by increased rates of growth even in the absence of precocious puberty. Girls and boys are equally affected. Serum levels of growth hormone are elevated and increase during sleep; they are augmented by thyrotropin (TRH) and poorly inhibited by oral glucose. Serum levels of prolactin are increased in most patients, but fewer than half of the patients have a demonstrable pituitary tumor. Octreotide, a long-acting somatostatin analog, has been used to treat the hypersomatotropism. The prognosis is favorable for longevity, but deformities, repeated fractures, pain, and occasional cranial nerve compression may result from the bony lesions.

Of the extraglandular manifestations, phosphaturia, leading to rickets or osteomalacia, is the most common. Cardiovascular

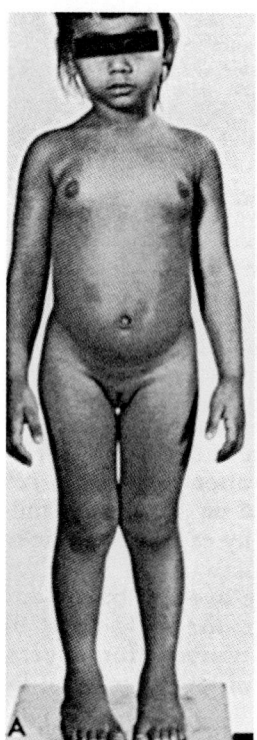 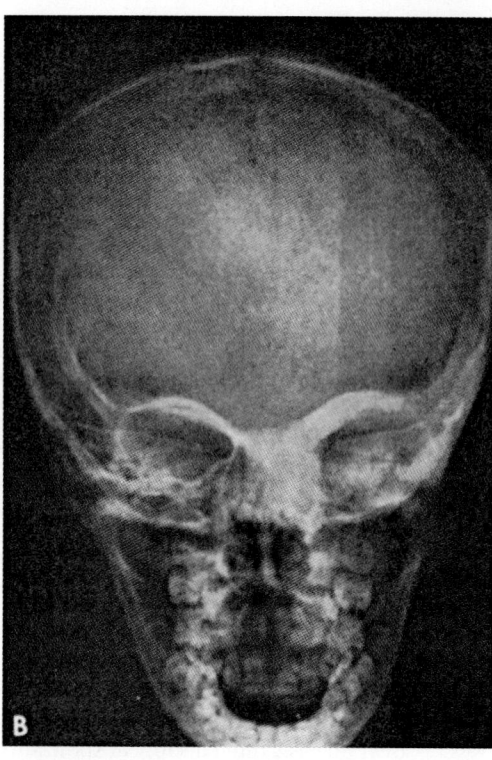

FIGURE 556–4. Precocious puberty associated with polyostotic fibrous dysplasia (McCune-Albright syndrome) in a girl 4.5 yr of age; at this time, her height age and osseous age were normal. Menarche occurred at 4 yr of age. *A*, Notice the bilateral breast development, the hyperpigmented spots on the abdomen, and the prominence of the left side of the face. *B*, Roentgenograms revealed fibrous dysplasia in the distal end of the left ulna and thickening of the bones about the left orbit and the maxillary portion of the frontal bones shown here.

and hepatic involvement is rare but may be life-threatening (e.g., severe neonatal cholestasis).

556.7 Familial Male Gonadotropin-Independent Precocious Puberty

This is a rare, autosomal dominant form of sexual precocity that is transmitted from affected males and unaffected female carriers of the gene to their male offspring. Signs of puberty appear by 2–3 yr of age. The testes are only slightly enlarged. Testicular biopsies show Leydig cell maturation and, in some instances, marked hyperplasia. Maturation of seminiferous tubules may be present. Testosterone levels are markedly elevated to the same range seen in boys with true precocious puberty; however, baseline levels of LH are prepubertal, pulsatile secretion of LH is absent, and LH does not respond to stimulation with GnRH. The cause for activation of Leydig cells independent of gonadotropin stimulation is a missense mutation of the LH receptor leading to constitutive activation of cAMP production.

Osseous maturation may be markedly advanced; when it reaches the pubertal age range, hypothalamic maturation shifts the mechanism of pubertal development to a gonadotropin-dependent one. This sequence of events is similar to that occurring in children with McCune-Albright syndrome (see earlier discussion) or in those with congenital adrenal hyperplasia (see Chapter 570.1).

Gonadotropin-independent precocious puberty has been diagnosed in a few unrelated boys with type IA pseudohypoparathyroidism who had a single mutation of the $G_s\alpha$ protein. This mutation is inactivating at normal body temperature and causes pseudohypoparathyroidism, but in the cooler temperature of the testes, it is constitutionally activating, resulting in adenyl cyclase stimulation and production of testosterone. Although this mutation differs from the constitutive LH receptor (mutation), which usually causes familial male gonadotropin-independent precocious puberty, the end result is the same.

Treatment. Young boys have been successfully treated with ketoconazole (600 mg/24 hr in 8-hr divided doses), an antifungal drug that inhibits C-17,20-lyase and testosterone synthesis. Other investigators have used a combination of spironolactone (to block androgen action) and aromatase inhibitors (such as testolactone, letrozole, or anastrozole), because estrogens derived from androgens stimulate bone maturation. These medications are unable to revert the serum testosterone to the normal (prepubertal) concentrations or completely offset the unfavorable effects of the elevated sex hormones. They slow down, but do not halt, the progression of puberty and may not improve the height prognosis. Boys whose GnRH pulse generator has matured require combined therapy with GnRH agonists.

556.8 Incomplete (Partial) Precocious Development

Isolated manifestations of precocity without development of other signs of puberty are not unusual; development of the breasts in girls and growth of sexual hair in both sexes are the two most common forms.

Premature Thelarche. This term applies to a transient condition of isolated breast development that most often appears in the first 2 yr of life; in some girls breast development is present at birth and persists. Breast development may be unilateral or asymmetric and often fluctuates in degree. Growth and osseous maturation are normal or slightly advanced. The genitalia show no evidence of estrogenic stimulation. The condition is usually sporadic and is rarely familial. Breast development may regress after 2 yr, often persists for 3–5 yr, and is rarely progressive. Menarche occurs at the expected age, and reproduction is normal. Basal serum levels of FSH and the FSH response to GnRH stimulation may be greater than that seen in normal controls. Plasma levels of LH and estradiol are consistently less than the limits of detection. Ultrasound examination of the ovaries reveals normal size, but a few small (<9 mm) cysts are not uncommon.

In some girls of the same age group, breast development may be associated with definite evidence of systemic estrogen effects, such as growth acceleration or bone age advancement. Pelvic sonography may reveal enlarged ovaries or uterus. This condition has been referred to as *exaggerated* or *atypical thelarche*. It differs from central sexual precocity because it has spontaneous regression. GnRH stimulation elicits a robust FSH response and a minimal LH response. The pathogeneses of typical and exaggerated forms of thelarche are unclear, although a delay in the transition from the activated (neonatal-infantile) to the inactive (prepubertal) pituitary-ovarian axis may underlie both conditions.

Premature thelarche is a benign condition but may be the first sign of true or pseudoprecocious puberty, or it may be caused by exogenous exposure to estrogens. In addition to a detailed history, a bone age should be obtained. The serum concentrations of FSH, LH, and estradiol are generally low and not diagnostic. Pelvic ultrasound examination is rarely indicated. Continued observation is important because the condition cannot be readily distinguished from true precocious puberty. Regression and recurrence suggest functioning follicular cysts. Occurrence of thelarche in children older than 3 yr of age most often is caused by a condition other than benign precocious thelarche.

Premature Pubarche (Adrenarche). This term applies to the appearance of sexual hair before the age of 8 yr in girls or 9 yr in boys without other evidence of maturation. It is much more frequent in girls than in boys and may occur more frequently in American black girls than in others. Hair appears on the mons and labia majora in girls, perineal and scrotal area in boys; axillary hair generally appears later. Adult-type axillary odor is common. Affected children are slightly advanced in height and osseous maturation.

Premature adrenarche is an early maturational event of adrenal androgen production. This event coincides with precocious maturation of the zona reticularis, an associated decrease in 3β-hydroxysteroid-dehydrogenase activity, and an increase in C-17,20-lyase activity. These enzymatic changes result in increased basal and ACTH-stimulated serum concentrations of the Δ^5-steroids (17-hydroxypregnenolone and DHEA) and, to a lesser extent, of the Δ^4-steroids (particularly androstenedione) compared with age-matched control subjects. The levels of these steroids and those of DHEAS are usually comparable to those of children in the early stages of normal puberty.

Premature adrenarche is a benign condition that requires no therapy. However, a subset of patients with precocious pubarche has one or more features of systemic androgen effect, such as marked growth acceleration, clitoral (girls) or phallic (boys) enlargement, cystic acne, or advanced bone age (>2 SD above the mean for age). In these patients with *atypical premature adrenarche*, an ACTH stimulation test with measurement of steroid intermediates (mainly serum 17-hydroxyprogesterone concentrations) is indicated to rule out nonclassic congenital adrenal hyperplasia due to 21-hydroxylase deficiency. Epidemiologic and molecular-genetic studies have shown that the prevalence of nonclassical 21-hydroxylase deficiency is approximately 3–6% of unselected children presenting with precocious pubarche; the prevalence of other enzyme defects (i.e., 3β-hydroxysteroid-dehydrogenase or 11β-hydroxylase deficiencies) is extremely low.

Although idiopathic premature adrenarche has been considered a benign condition, longitudinal observations suggest that approximately 50% of girls with premature adrenarche are at high risk for hyperandrogenism and polycystic ovarian syndrome, alone or, more often, in combination with other components of the so-called metabolic syndrome (insulin resistance possibly progressing to type 2 diabetes mellitus; dyslipidemia; hypertension; increased abdominal fat) as adults. An increased risk of premature adrenarche and the metabolic syndrome has been documented in children born small for their gestational age. This appears to be associated with insulin resistance and decreased beta-cell reserve, perhaps as a consequence of fetal undernutrition.

Premature Menarche. This is a very rare entity, much less frequent than premature thelarche or premature adrenarche, and is a diagnosis of exclusion. In girls presenting with isolated vaginal bleeding in the absence of other secondary sexual characteristics, more common causes such as vulvovaginitis, foreign body, or sexual abuse, and uncommon causes such as urethral prolapse and sarcoma botryoides must be carefully excluded. The majority of girls with idiopathic premature menarche have only 1–3 episodes of bleeding; puberty occurs at the usual time and menstrual cycles are normal. Plasma levels of gonadotropins are normal, but estradiol levels may be elevated, probably owing to bursts of ovarian activity. Occasional patients are found to have ovarian follicular cysts on ultrasound.

556.9 Medicational Precocity

A variety of medicaments can induce the appearance of secondary sexual characteristics that may be confused with precocious puberty. A careful history focused on exploring the possibility of accidental exposure to or ingestion of sex hormones is important. Precocious pseudopuberty has occurred in both boys and girls from the accidental ingestion of estrogens (including contraceptive pills) and from the administration of anabolic steroids. Estrogens in cosmetics, hair creams, and breast augmentation creams have caused breast development in girls and gynecomastia in boys; estrogens are readily absorbed through the skin. The high prevalence of premature thelarche and precocious pseudopuberty in Puerto Rico for the last 2 decades has been attributed to contamination of meats, particularly chicken, with estrogens used in animal husbandry but has not been proved. Exogenous estrogens may produce an intense, dark brown color in the areola of the breasts that is not usually seen in endogenous types of precocity. The precocious changes disappear after cessation of exposure to the hormones. Recently, the widespread use of testosterone gel, which is applied to the skin for treatment of male hypogonadism, has resulted in virilization of children and women following skin contact at, and systemic absorption from, the area where the gel was applied.

Anasti JN, Flack MR, Froehlich J, et al: A potential novel mechanism for precocious puberty in juvenile hypothyroidism. *J Clin Endocrinol Metab* 1995;80: 276–80.

Brann DW, Wade MF, Dhandapani KM, et al: Leptin and reproduction. *Steroids* 2002;67:95–104.

Chalumeau M, Chemaitilly W, Trivin C, et al: Central precocious puberty in girls: An evidence-based diagnosis tree to predict central nervous system abnormalities. *Pediatrics* 2002;109:61–7.

Chemaitilly W, Trivin C, Adan L, et al: Central precocious puberty: Clinical and laboratory features. *Clin Endocrinol* 2001;54:289–94.

Farel Z, Bourne HR, Taroh I: The expanding spectrum of G protein diseases. *N Engl J Med* 1999;340:1012–20.

Garibaldi LR, Aceto T Jr, Weber C: The pattern of gonadotropin and estradiol secretion in exaggerated thelarche. *Acta Endocrinol* 1993;128:345–9.

Huirne JA, Lambalk CB: Gonadotropin-releasing-hormone-receptor antagonists. *Lancet* 2001;358:1793–803.

Ibanez L, Dimartino-Nardi J, Potau N, et al: Premature adrenarche—Normal variant or forerunner of adult disease? *Endocr Rev* 2000;21:671–96.

Ibanez L, Potau N, Marcos MV, et al: Adrenal hyperandrogenism in adolescent girls with a history of low birthweight and precocious pubarche. *Clin Endocrinol* 2000;53:523–7.

Ibanez L, Potau N, Zampolli M, et al: Use of leuprolide acetate response patterns in the early diagnosis of pubertal disorders: Comparison with the gonadotropin-releasing hormone test. *J Clin Endocrinol Metab* 1994;78:30–5.

Klein K, Barnes KM, Jones JV, et al: Increase in final height in precocious puberty after long-term treatment with LHRH agonists: The National Institutes of Health experience. *J Clin Endocrinol Metab* 2001;86:4711–6.

Lahlou N, Carel JC, Chaussain JL, et al: Pharmacokinetics and pharmacodynamics of GnRH antagonists: Clinical implications for pediatrics. *J Pediatr Endocrinol Metab* 2000;13:723–37.

Latronico AC, Lins TS, Brito VN, et al: The effect of distinct activating mutations of the luteinizing hormone receptor gene on the pituitary-gonadal axis in both sexes. *Clin Endocrinol* 2000;53:609–13.

Lebrethon MC, Bourguignon JP: Management of central isosexual precocity: Diagnosis, treatment, outcome. *Curr Opin Pediatr* 2000;12:394–9.

Leger J, Reynaud R, Czernichow P: Do all girls with apparent idiopathic precocious puberty require gonadotropin-releasing hormone agonist treatment? *J Pediatr* 2000;137:819–25.

Partsch CJ, Sippell WG: Pathogenesis and epidemiology of precocious puberty. Effects of exogenous estrogens. *Hum Reprod Update* 2001;7:292–302.

Pathomvanich A, Merke DP, Chrousos GP, et al: Early puberty: A cautionary tale. *Pediatrics* 2000;105:115–6.

Pucarelli I, Segni M, Ortore M, et al: Combined therapy with GnRH analog plus growth hormone in central precocious puberty. *J Pediatr Endocrinol Metab* 2000;13:811–20.

Stanhope R: Premature thelarche: Clinical follow-up and indication for treatment. *J Pediatr Endocrinol Metab* 2000;13:827–30.

Terasawa E, Fernandez DL: Neurobiological mechanisms of the onset of puberty in primates. *Endocr Rev* 2001;22:111–51.

Trollmann R, Strehl E, Dorr HG: Precocious puberty in children with myelomeningocele: Treatment with gonadotropin-releasing hormone analogues. *Dev Med Child Neurol* 1998;40:38–43.

Van Beek JT, Sharafuddin MJ, Kao SC, et al: Prospective evaluation of pituitary size and shape on MR imaging after suppressive hormonal therapy in central precocious puberty. *Pediatr Radiol* 2000;30(7):444–6.

Virdis R, Sigorini M, Laiolo A, et al: Neurofibromatosis type 1 and precocious puberty. *J Pediatr Endocrinol Metab* 2000;13:841–4.

Virdis R, Street ME, Zampolli M, et al: Precocious puberty in girls adopted from developing countries. *Arch Dis Child* 1998;78:152–4.

Walvoord EC, Pescovitz OH: Combined use of growth hormone and gonadotropin-releasing hormone analogues in precocious puberty: Theoretic and practical considerations. *Pediatrics* 1999;104:1010–4.

Weinstein LS: The stimulatory G protein alpha-subunit gene-mutations and imprinting lead to complex phenotypes. *J Clin Endocrinol Metab* 2001;86:4622–6.

SECTION 2 *Disorders of the Thyroid Gland*
Stephen LaFranchi

Chapter 557
Thyroid Development and Physiology

FETAL DEVELOPMENT

The fetal thyroid bilobed shape is recognized by 7 wk of gestation, and characteristic thyroid follicle cell and colloid formation is seen by 10 wk. Thyroglobulin synthesis occurs from 4 wk, iodine trapping by 8–10 wk, and thyroxine (T_4) and, to a lesser extent, triiodothyronine (T_3) synthesis and secretion occur from 12 wk of gestation. There is evidence that three transcription factors, TTF-1, TTF-2, and PAX8, are important in thyroid gland morphogenesis and differentiation. These factors also bind to the promotors of thyroglobulin and thyroid peroxidase genes and so influence thyroid hormone production. Hypothalamic neurons synthesize thyrotropin-releasing hormone (TRH) by 6–8 wk, the pituitary portal vessel system begins development by 8–10 wk, and thyroid-stimulating hormone (TSH) secretion is seen by 12 wk of gestation. Maturation of the hypothalamic-pituitary-thyroid axis occurs over the second half of gestation, but normal feedback relationships are not mature until approximately 3 mo of postnatal life. Another transcription factor, Pit-1, is important for differentiation and growth of thyrotrophs, along with somatotrophs and lactotrophs.

THYROID PHYSIOLOGY

The main function of the thyroid gland is to synthesize T_4 and T_3. The only known physiologic role of iodine is in the synthesis of these hormones; the recommended dietary allowance of iodine is greater than 30 µg/kg/24 hr for infants, 70–120 µg/24 hr for children, and 150 µg/24 hr for adolescents and adults. The daily intake in North America varies from 240 to more than 700 µg. The median iodine intake in the United States has decreased by approximately 50% between the 1970s and the 1990s. Whatever the chemical form ingested, iodine eventually reaches the thyroid gland as iodide. Thyroid tissue has an avidity for iodine and is able to trap (with a gradient of 100:1), transport, and concentrate it in the follicular lumen for synthesis of

thyroid hormone. Iodine transport is carried out by the sodium-iodide symporter, the gene for which has been cloned.

Before trapped iodide can react with tyrosine, it must be oxidized; this reaction is catalyzed by thyroidal peroxidase. The thyroid cells also elaborate a specific thyroprotein, a globulin with approximately 120 tyrosine units (thyroglobulin). Iodination of tyrosine forms monoiodotyrosine and diiodotyrosine; two molecules of diiodotyrosine then couple to form one molecule of T_4 or one molecule of diiodotyrosine and one of monoiodotyrosine to form T_3. Once formed, hormones are stored as thyroglobulin in the lumen of the follicle (colloid) until ready to be delivered to the body cells. Thyroglobulin is a large globular glycoprotein with a molecular weight of about 660,000 and under normal conditions is detectable in the blood of most individuals at nanogram levels. T_4 and T_3 are liberated from thyroglobulin by activation of proteases and peptidases.

The metabolic potency of T_3 is three to four times that of T_4. In adults, the thyroid produces approximately 100 µg of T_4 and 20 µg of T_3 daily. Only 20% of circulating T_3 is secreted by the thyroid; the remainder is produced by deiodination of T_4 in the liver, kidney, and other peripheral tissues by type I 5'-deiodinase. Selenocysteine is the active center of the iodothyronine deiodinases. Thus, selenium indirectly plays a role in normal growth and development. In the pituitary and brain, approximately 80% of required T_3 is produced locally from T_4 by a different enzyme, type II 5'-deiodinase. In the fetal rat, although plasma levels of T_3 are very low, cerebral concentrations increase to almost adult levels. The level of T_3 in blood is 1/50th that of T_4, but T_3 is the physiologically active thyroid hormone.

The thyroid hormones increase oxygen consumption, stimulate protein synthesis, influence growth and differentiation, and affect carbohydrate, lipid, and vitamin metabolism. The free hormones enter cells, where T_4 may be converted to T_3 by deiodination. Intracellular T_3 then enters the nucleus, where it binds to thyroid hormone receptors. Thyroid hormone receptors are members of the steroid hormone receptor superfamily that includes glucocorticoids, estrogen, progesterone, vitamin D, and retinoids. Four different isoforms of the thyroid hormone receptor (α_1, α_2, β_1, and β_2) are expressed in different tissues; the protein product of the formerly designated *c-erb A* proto-oncogene (now called *THRA2*) has been identified as the α_2 thyroid hormone receptor in the brain and hypothalamus. Thyroid hormone receptors consist of a ligand-binding domain (binds T_3), hinge region, and DNA-binding domain (zinc finger). Binding of

T_3 activates the thyroid hormone receptor response element, resulting in production of an encoded mRNA and protein synthesis and of secretion specific for the target cell. In this manner, a single hormone, T_4, acting through tissue-specific thyroid hormone receptor isoforms and gene-specific thyroid response elements, can produce multiple effects in various tissues.

About 70% of the circulating T_4 is firmly bound to *thyroxine-binding globulin* (TBG). Less important carriers are thyroxine-binding prealbumin, called *transthyretin*, and albumin. Only 0.03% of T_4 in serum is not bound and comprises free T_4. Approximately 50% of circulating T_3 is bound to TBG, and 50% is bound to albumin; 0.30% of T_3 is unbound or free T_3. Because the concentration of TBG is altered in many clinical circumstances, its status must be considered when interpreting T_4 or T_3 levels.

THYROID REGULATION

The thyroid is regulated by TSH, a glycoprotein produced and secreted by the anterior pituitary. This hormone activates adenylate cyclase in the thyroid gland to effect release of thyroid hormones. TSH is composed of two noncovalently bound subunits (chains): α and β. The α subunit is common to luteinizing hormone, follicle-stimulating hormone, and chorionic gonadotropin; the specificity of each hormone is conferred by the β subunit. TSH synthesis and release are stimulated by TSH-releasing hormone (TRH), which is synthesized in the hypothalamus and secreted into the pituitary. TRH is found in other parts of the brain besides the hypothalamus and in many other organs; aside from its endocrine function, it may be a neurotransmitter. TRH is a simple tripeptide. In states of decreased production of thyroid hormone, TSH and TRH are increased. Exogenous thyroid hormone or increased thyroid hormone synthesis inhibits TSH and TRH production. Except in the neonate, levels of TRH in serum are very low.

Further control of the level of circulating thyroid hormones occurs in the periphery. In many nonthyroidal illnesses, extrathyroidal production of T_3 decreases; factors that inhibit thyroxine-5'-deiodinase include fasting, chronic malnutrition, acute illness, and certain drugs. Levels of T_3 may be significantly decreased, whereas levels of free T_4 and TSH remain normal. Presumably, the decreased levels of T_3 result in decreased rates of oxygen production, of substrate use, and of other catabolic processes.

Burrow GH, Fisher DA, Larsen PR: Maternal and fetal thyroid function. *N Engl J Med* 1994;331:1072.

Cavalieri RD: Iodine metabolism and thyroid physiology: Current concepts. [Review.] *Thyroid* 1997;7:177.

Fisher DA, Brown RS: Thyroid physiology in the perinatal period and during childhood. In Braverman LE, Utiger RD (editors): *Werner & Ingbar's the Thyroid: A Fundamental and Clinical Text*, 8th ed. Philadelphia, Lippincott Williams & Wilkins, 2000, p 959.

Hollowell JG, Staehling NW, Hannon WH, et al. Iodine nutrition in the United States. Trends and public health implications: Iodine excretion data from National Health and Nutrition Examination Surveys I and III (1971–1974 and 1988–1994). *J Clin Endocrinol Metab* 1998;83:3398.

557.1 Thyroid Hormone Studies

Serum Thyroid Hormones. Methods are available to measure all of the thyroid hormones in sera: T_4, free T_4, T_3, free T_3, and the diiodothyronines. A metabolically inert T_3 (3,5', 3'-triiodothyronine), called reverse T_3, is also present in sera. Age must be considered in interpreting results, particularly in the neonate.

Thyroglobulin is a glycoprotein dimer that is secreted through the apical surface of the thyrocyte into the colloid. Small amounts escape into the circulation and are measurable in serum. Levels increase with TSH (also called thyrotropin) stimulation and decrease with TSH suppression. Levels are increased in the neonate, in patients with Graves disease and other forms of autoimmune thyroid disease, and in those with endemic goiter. The most marked elevations of thyroglobulin occur in patients with differentiated carcinoma of the thyroid. Athyreotic infants may have markedly reduced levels of thyroglobulin in serum.

TSH levels in serum are an extremely sensitive indicator of primary hypothyroidism. A 3rd generation of assays (chemiluminescent assays) that can measure complete suppression of TSH below the normal range is standard. After the neonatal period, normal levels of TSH are less than 6 μU/mL. These sensitive TSH assays obviate the need for TRH stimulation in the diagnosis of most patients with thyroid disorders.

Fetal and Newborn Thyroid. Fetal serum T_4 increases progressively from midgestation to approximately 11.5 μg/dL at term. Fetal levels of T_3 are low before 20 wk and then gradually increase to about 45 ng/dL at term. Reverse T_3 levels, however, are very high in the fetus (250 ng/dL at 30 wk) and decrease to 150 ng/dL at term. Serum levels of TSH gradually increase to 10 mU/L at term. Approximately one third of maternal T_4 crosses the placenta to the fetus. Maternal T_4 may play a role in fetal development, especially that of the brain, before the synthesis of fetal thyroid hormones begins. The fetus of a hypothyroid mother may be at risk for neurologic damage, and a hypothyroid fetus may be partially protected by maternal T_4 until delivery.

At birth, there is an acute release of TSH; peak serum concentrations reach 60 mU/L in 30 min in full-term infants. A rapid decline occurs in the ensuing 24 hr and a more gradual decline within the next 5 days to less than 10 μU/mL. The acute increase in TSH produces a dramatic increase in levels of T_4 to approximately 16 μg/dL and of T_3 to approximately 300 ng/dL in about 4 hr. This T_3 seems largely derived from increased peripheral conversion of T_4 to T_3. T_4 levels gradually decrease during the first 2 wk of life to 12 μg/dL. T_3 levels then decline during the 1st wk of life to levels under 200 ng/mL. Serum free T3 concentrations are approximately 540 pg/dL in infancy and decline to 210–440 pg/dL in childhood. Reverse T_3 levels are maintained for 2 wk (200 ng/dL) and decrease by 4 wk to around 50 ng/dL. The amount of T_4 that crosses the placenta is not sufficient to interfere with a diagnosis of congenital hypothyroidism in the neonate.

Serum Thyroxine-Binding Globulin. The thyroid hormones are transported in plasma bound to TBG, a glycoprotein synthesized in the liver. Estimation of TBG levels is occasionally necessary because TBG is increased or decreased in a variety of clinical situations, with effects on the level of total thyroxine. TBG binds about 70% of T_4 and 50% of T_3. TBG levels increase in pregnancy and in the newborn period, and with administration of estrogens (oral contraceptives), perphenazine, and heroin, and decrease with androgens, anabolic steroids, glucocorticoids, and L-asparaginase. These effects are the results of modulation of hepatic synthesis of TBG. Phenytoin (diphenylhydantoin) is another cause of drug-induced abnormality of thyroid function tests. Phenytoin, an inducer of hepatic enzymes, stimulates hepatic degradation of T_4 and accelerates transport of T_4 into tissues. Phenobarbital and carbamazepine have a similar effect. Some drugs, particularly phenytoin, also inhibit binding of T_4 and T_3 to TBG. Decreased or increased levels of TBG also occur as genetic traits (see Chapter 558). TBG levels may be markedly decreased owing to decreased production with liver disease or loss in the urine, as in the congenital nephrotic syndrome.

In Vivo Radionuclide Studies. Markedly improved direct tests of thyroid function have made radioiodine uptake studies less useful. The iodine-trapping or concentrating mechanism of the thyroid can be evaluated by measuring the uptake of radioactive isotope ^{123}I (half-life of 13 hr). The technology allows doses of radioiodine (0.1–0.5 mCi) that are only a fraction of those formerly used with [131]I. Technetium (^{99m}Tc) is a particularly useful radioisotope for children, because in contrast to iodine, it is trapped but not organified by the thyroid and has a half-life of only 6 hr. Thyroid scanning may be indicated to assess the presence of thyroid tissue in questions of thyroid agenesis, to detect ectopic thyroid tissue, or to evaluate possible "hot" thyroid nodules. These studies should be performed with ^{99m}Tc as pertechnetate because it has the advantages of lower radiation exposure and high-quality scintigrams. Use of ^{131}I in children should be limited to those known to have thyroid cancer.

Thyroid Ultrasonographic Studies. Thyroid ultrasound examinations can determine the location, size, and shape of the thyroid gland, and they can assess the solid or cystic nature of nodules. Ultrasound is not as reliable as radionuclide studies in evaluating infants with suspected thyroid dysgenesis, particularly ectopic glands. Ultrasound examinations are very useful in identifying normal thyroid gland position in children with suspected thyroglossal duct cysts. In children with autoimmune thyroiditis, ultrasound reveals scattered hypoechogenicity. Ultrasound examinations are more accurate than physical examination in estimating goiter size and assessing thyroid nodules.

Fisher DA: Physiological variations in thyroid hormones: Physiological and pathophysiological considerations. *Clin Chem* 1996;42:135.

Haddow JE, Palomaki GE, Allan WC, et al: Maternal thyroid deficiency during pregnancy and subsequent neuropsychological development of the child. *N Engl J Med* 1999;341:549.

O'Reilly DS: Thyroid function tests—Time for a reassessment. *Br Med J* 2000;320:1332–4.

Pop VJ, Kuijpens JL, van Baar AL, et al. Low maternal free thyroxine concentrations during early pregnancy are associated with impaired psychomotor development in infancy. *Clin Endocrinol* 1999;50:149.

Chapter 558
Defects of Thyroxine-Binding Globulin

Abnormalities in levels of thyroxine-binding globulin (TBG) are not associated with clinical disease and do not require treatment. They are usually uncovered by a chance finding of abnormally low or high levels of thyroxine (T_4) and may be a source of confusion in the diagnosis of hypothyroidism or hyperthyroidism.

TBG deficiency occurs as an X-linked dominant disorder. Congenital TBG deficiency is most often discovered through screening programs for neonatal hypothyroidism that use levels of T_4 as the primary screen. Affected patients have low levels of T_4 and elevated resin triiodothyronine uptake (RT_3U), but levels of free T_4 and thyroid-stimulating hormone (TSH) are normal. The diagnosis is confirmed by the finding of absent or low levels of TBG. The disorder is more readily recognized in male patients because it is caused by a gene on the short arm of the X chromosome. TBG deficiency occurs in 1 in 2,400 male newborns, 36% of whom have TBG levels less than 1 mg/dL. Milder forms of TBG deficiency occur in approximately 1/42,000 heterozygous female newborns. Complete TBG deficiency (<5 µg/dL) occurs much less frequently. Three of eight families with complete TBG deficiency have been found to have a codon mutation (leucine to proline); other patients with reduced affinity of TBG for T_4 have had other point mutations that affect the tertiary structure of the protein. Acquired TBG deficiency occurs with androgen and glucocorticoid treatment, hepatic insufficiency (not hepatitis), and renal disease and proteinuria.

TBG excess is also a harmless X-linked dominant anomaly, occurring in about 1/25,000 persons. It has been recognized primarily in adults, but neonatal screening programs uncover the condition in the neonate. The level of T_4 is elevated, T_3 is variably elevated, TSH and free T_4 are normal, and RT_3U is decreased. The elevated levels of TBG confirm the diagnosis. In neonates, levels of T_4 as high as 95 µg/dL have been found, which decrease to 20–30 µg/dL after 2–3 wk. Such high levels of T_4 are thought to be related in part to the normally elevated levels of TBG in neonates during the 1st mo of life, presumably as an effect of maternal estrogens. Affected patients are euthyroid. Family studies may be indicated to alert other affected individuals. Acquired elevations of TBG occur with pregnancy, estrogen treatment, and hepatitis.

Familial dysalbuminemic hyperthyroxinemia is an autosomal dominant disorder that may be confused with hyperthyroidism. Markedly increased binding of T_4 to an abnormal albumin variant leads to increased serum concentrations of T_4. However, the levels of free T_4, free T_3, and TSH are normal. Levels of T_3 are normal or only slightly elevated. Affected patients are euthyroid.

Mandel SH, Hanna CE, Boston BA, et al: Thyroxine binding globulin deficiency detected by newborn screening. *J Pediatr* 1993;122:227–30.

Refetoff S: Inherited thyroxine-binding globulin abnormalities in man. *Endocr Rev* 1989;10:275.

Chapter 559
Hypothyroidism

Hypothyroidism results from deficient production of thyroid hormone or a defect in thyroid hormonal receptor activity (Box 559–1). The disorder may be manifested from birth. When symptoms appear after a period of apparently normal thyroid function, the disorder may be truly "acquired" or may only appear so as a result of one of a variety of congenital defects in which the manifestation of the deficiency is delayed. The term *cretinism* is often used synonymously with congenital hypothyroidism but should be avoided.

CONGENITAL HYPOTHYROIDISM

Congenital causes of hypothyroidism may be sporadic or familial, goitrous or nongoitrous. In many cases, the deficiency of thyroid hormone is severe, and symptoms develop in the early weeks of life. In others, lesser degrees of deficiency occur, and manifestations may be delayed for months.

Epidemiology. The prevalence of congenital hypothyroidism based on nationwide programs for neonatal screening is 1/4,000 infants worldwide; prevalence is lower in black Americans (1/32,000) and higher in Hispanics and Native Americans (1/2,000). Twice as many girls as boys are affected.

Etiology
THYROID DYSGENESIS. Some form of thyroid dysgenesis (aplasia, hypoplasia, or an ectopic gland) is the most common cause of congenital hypothyroidism, accounting for 85% of cases; 10% are caused by an inborn error of thyroxine synthesis, and 5% are the result of transplacental maternal thyrotropin-receptor blocking antibody. In about one third of cases of dysgenesis, even sensitive radionuclide scans can find no remnants of thyroid tissue (*aplasia*). In the other two thirds of infants, rudiments of thyroid tissue are found in an ectopic location, anywhere from the base of the tongue (*lingual thyroid*) to the normal position in the neck (*hypoplasia*).

Thyroid dysgenesis occurs sporadically, but familial cases have occasionally been reported. In neonates with congenital hypothyroidism due to thyroid dysgenesis, 2% of cases are familial; thus, 98% are sporadic.

CENTRAL (HYPOPITUITARY) HYPOTHYROIDISM

Pit-1 (homeobox protein) mutations
    Deficiency of thyrotropin, growth hormone, and prolactin
Prop-1 mutations
    Deficiency of thyrotropin, growth hormone, prolactin, LH, FSH,
    ±ACTH
Thyrotropin-releasing hormone (TRH) deficiency
    Isolated?
    Multiple hypothalamic deficiencies (e.g., craniopharyngioma)
TRH unresponsiveness
    Mutations in TRH receptor
Thyrotropin (TSH) deficiency
    Mutations in β-chain
    Multiple pituitary deficiencies
Thyrotropin unresponsiveness
    $G_s\alpha$ mutation (e.g., type IA pseudohypoparathyroidism)
    Mutation in TSH receptor

PRIMARY HYPOTHYROIDISM

Defect of fetal thyroid development
    Aplasia, ectopia (dysgenesis)
Defect in thyroid hormone synthesis (e.g., goitrous hypothyroidism)
    Thyroid oxidase mutations: homozygotic—permanent;
        heterozygotic—transient
    Iodide transport defect
    Thyroid peroxidase defect
    Thyroglobulin synthesis defect
    Deiodination defect
Iodine deficiency (endemic goiter)
    Neurologic type
    Myxedematous type
Maternal antibodies
    Thyrotropin receptor–blocking antibody (TRBAb) (also termed
        thyrotropin binding inhibitor immunoglobulin)
Maternal medications
    Radioiodine, iodides
    Propylthiouracil, methimazole
    Amiodarone

LH = luteinizing hormone; FSH = follicle-stimulating hormone; ACTH = adrenocorticotropic hormone

---

The exact cause of thyroid dysgenesis is unknown in most cases. Three transcription factors, TTF-1, TTF-2, and PAX-8, are important for thyroid morphogenesis and differentiation; of 98 neonates with congenital hypothyroidism, two had mutations in the PAX-8 gene. One infant had thyroid ectopy, whereas the other had thyroid hypoplasia. Two siblings have been reported with thyroid agenesis and mutations in the gene for TTF-2; they also had a cleft lip and choanal atresia.

The frequent finding of thyroid dysgenesis confined to only one of a pair of monozygotic twins suggests the operation of a deleterious factor during intrauterine life. Maternal antithyroid antibodies might be that factor, especially because antibodies in patients with autoimmune thyroid disease belong predominantly to the IgG class and can cross the placenta. Although thyroid peroxidase (TPO) antibodies have been detected in some mother-infant pairs, there is little evidence of their pathogenicity. The demonstration of thyroid growth-blocking and cytotoxic antibodies in some infants with thyroid dysgenesis, as well as in their mothers, suggests a more likely pathogenetic mechanism.

Ectopic thyroid tissue (lingual, sublingual, subhyoid) may provide adequate amounts of thyroid hormone for many years or may fail in early childhood. Affected children come to clinical attention because of a growing mass at the base of the tongue or in the midline of the neck, usually at the level of the hyoid. Occasionally, ectopia is associated with thyroglossal duct cysts. It may occur in siblings. Surgical removal of ectopic thyroid tissue from a euthyroid individual usually results in hypothyroidism, because most such patients have no other thyroid tissue. Newborn screening programs may detect these patients and avoid delayed diagnosis.

DEFECTIVE SYNTHESIS OF THYROXINE. A variety of defects in the biosynthesis of thyroid hormone may result in congenital hypothyroidism; when the defect is incomplete, compensation occurs, and onset of hypothyroidism may be delayed for years. A goiter is almost always present, and the defect is detected in 1/30,000–50,000 live births in neonatal screening programs. These defects are transmitted in an autosomal recessive manner.

DEFECT OF IODIDE TRANSPORT. This rare defect has been reported in nine related infants of the Hutterite sect, and about half the cases are from Japan. Consanguinity has occurred in about one third of the families. It almost certainly involves mutations in the gene coding for the sodium-iodine symporter. In the past, clinical hypothyroidism, with or without a goiter, often developed in the first few months of life; the condition has been detected in neonatal screening programs. In Japan, however, untreated patients acquire goiter and hypothyroidism after 10 yr of age, perhaps because of the very high iodine content (often 19 mg/24 hr) of the Japanese diet.

The energy-dependent mechanisms for concentrating iodide are defective in the thyroid and salivary glands. In contrast to other defects of thyroid hormone synthesis, uptake of radioiodine and pertechnetate is low; a saliva:serum ratio of ^{123}I may be required to establish the diagnosis. This condition responds to treatment with large doses of potassium iodide, but treatment with thyroxine (T_4) is preferable.

THYROID PEROXIDASE DEFECTS OF ORGANIFICATION AND COUPLING. This is the most common of the T_4 synthetic defects. After iodide is trapped by the thyroid, it is rapidly oxidized to reactive iodine, which is then incorporated into tyrosine units. This process requires generation of H_2O_2, thyroid peroxidase, and hematin (an enzyme cofactor); defects can involve each of these components, and there is considerable clinical and biochemical heterogeneity. In the Dutch neonatal screening program, 23 infants were found with a complete organification defect (1/60,000), but its prevalence in other areas is unknown. A characteristic finding in all patients with this defect is a marked decrease in thyroid radioactivity when perchlorate or thiocyanate is administered 2 hr after administration of a test dose of radioiodine. In these patients, perchlorate discharges 40–90% of radioiodine compared with less than 10% in normal individuals. Several mutations in the TPO gene have been reported in children with congenital hypothyroidism. Patients with Pendred syndrome, a disorder comprising sensorineural deafness and goiter, also have a positive perchlorate discharge. **Pendred syndrome** appears to be due to a defect in a sulfate transport protein common to the thyroid gland and the cochlea.

Thyroid oxidase 2 helps generate H_2O_2. Bi-allelic inactivating mutations produce permanent congenital hypothyroidism, whereas single gene lesions produce transient hypothyroidism.

DEFECTS OF THYROGLOBULIN SYNTHESIS. This heterogeneous group of disorders, characterized by goiter, elevated thyroid-stimulating hormone (TSH), low T_4 levels, and absent or low levels of thyroglobulin (TG), has been reported in approximately 100 patients. Studies in animal models with congenital goiter have disclosed point mutations of the gene for TG in Afrikaner cattle and in Dutch goitrous goats. Analogous molecular defects have been described in a few patients.

DEFECTS IN DEIODINATION. Monoiodotyrosine and diiodotyrosine released from thyroglobulin are normally deiodinated within the thyroid or in peripheral tissues by a deiodinase. The liberated iodine is recycled in the synthesis of TG. Patients with a deficiency of this enzyme experience severe iodine loss from the constant urinary excretion of nondeiodinated tyrosines, leading to hormonal deficiency and goiter. The deiodination defect may be limited to thyroid tissue only or to peripheral tissue only, or it may be universal.

THYROTROPIN RECEPTOR-BLOCKING ANTIBODY. Thyrotropin receptor-blocking antibody (TRBAb) is called *thyroid-binding inhibitor immunoglobulin.* An unusual cause of transitory congenital hypothyroidism is the transplacental passage of maternal antibodies that inhibit binding of TSH to its receptor in the neonate. The frequency is approximately 1/50,000–100,000 infants. It should be suspected whenever there is a history of maternal autoimmune thyroid disease, including Hashimoto thyroiditis, Graves disease, hypothyroidism while the patient is receiving replacement therapy, or recurrent congenital hypothyroidism of a transient nature in subsequent siblings. In these situations, maternal levels of TRBAb should be measured during pregnancy. Affected infants and their mothers often also have thyrotropin receptor-stimulating antibodies and TPO antibodies. Technetium pertechnetate and ^{125}I scans may fail to detect any thyroid tissue, mimicking thyroid agenesis, but after the condition remits, a normal thyroid gland is demonstrable following discontinuation of replacement treatment. The half-life of the antibody is 21 days, and remission of the hypothyroidism occurs in about 3 mo. Correct diagnosis of this cause of congenital hypothyroidism prevents protracted unnecessary treatment, alerts the clinician to possible recurrences in future pregnancies, and allows a favorable prognosis.

RADIOIODINE ADMINISTRATION. Hypothyroidism has been reported as a result of inadvertent administration of radioiodine during pregnancy for treatment of Graves disease or cancer of the thyroid. Although only a few affected infants have been reported, a 1976 mail survey of endocrinologists uncovered 237 cases of women who had inadvertently received therapeutic doses of ^{131}I during the 1st trimester of pregnancy. The fetal thyroid is capable of trapping iodide by 70–75 days. Whenever radioiodine is administered to a woman of childbearing age, a pregnancy test must be performed before a therapeutic dose of ^{131}I is given, regardless of the menstrual history or putative history of contraception. Administration of radioactive iodine to lactating women is also contraindicated because it is readily excreted in milk.

THYROTROPIN DEFICIENCY. Deficiency of TSH and hypothyroidism may occur in any of the conditions associated with developmental defects of the pituitary or hypothalamus (see Chapter 551). More often in these conditions, the deficiency of TSH is secondary to a deficiency of thyrotropin-releasing hormone (TRH). TSH-deficient hypothyroidism is found in 1/30,000–50,000 infants, but only 30–40% of these cases are detected by neonatal thyroid screening. The majority of affected infants have multiple pituitary deficiencies and present with hypoglycemia, persistent jaundice, and micropenis in association with septo-optic dysplasia, midline cleft lip, midface hypoplasia, and other midline facial anomalies.

Pit-1 mutations are a recessive cause of hypothyroidism secondary to TSH deficiency. Affected children also have deficiency of growth hormone and prolactin. Pit-1, a gene transcription factor, is essential to differentiation, maintenance, and proliferation of somatotrophs, lactotrophs, and thyrotrophs. Examination of prolactin and TSH responses to TRH stimulation can detect these patients. Failure of the prolactin response to TRH should prompt examination of the Pit-1 gene.

Isolated deficiency of TSH is a rare autosomal recessive disorder that has been reported in five sibships. DNA studies in two Japanese children and in three children in two related Greek families have revealed different point mutations in the TSH β subunit gene; studies in two German siblings revealed a mutation causing a stop codon due to a frame shift.

A mutation in the TSH-receptor gene has been reported in three siblings with elevated levels of TSH and normal levels of T$_4$; two of them had been detected during neonatal screening. Despite persistent resistance to TSH through childhood, they remained euthyroid without treatment. Patients in three other reports of presumed TSH-receptor gene mutations had severe hypothyroidism that required treatment. The disorder is inherited in an autosomal recessive fashion. Both homozygous and compound heterozygous mutations in the TSH receptor gene have been reported.

THYROTROPIN HORMONE UNRESPONSIVENESS. Mild congenital hypothyroidism has been detected in newborn infants who subsequently proved to have type Ia pseudohypoparathyroidism. The molecular cause of resistance to TSH in these patients is the generalized impairment of cyclic adenosine monophosphate activation caused by genetic deficiency of the α subunit of the guanine nucleotide regulatory protein, G$_s$ (see Chapter 566).

Several instances of isolated TSH unresponsiveness have been detected. Serum levels of T$_4$ were low, those of TSH by radioimmunoassay and bioassay were elevated, and there was no response to exogenous TSH administration.

THYROTROPIN-RELEASING HORMONE ABNORMALITY. A patient with a TRH receptor abnormality resulting in isolated TSH deficiency and hypothyroidism has been reported. This condition was suspected because of failure of both TSH and prolactin to respond to TRH stimulation. Investigations disclosed a compound heterozygote mutation in the gene coding for the TRH receptor, resulting in inability of the receptor to bind TRH.

THYROID HORMONE UNRESPONSIVENESS. An increasing number of patients are being found with resistance to the actions of endogenous and exogenous T$_4$ and triiodothyronine (T$_3$). Most patients have goiter, and levels of T$_4$, T$_3$, free T$_4$, and free T$_3$ are elevated. These findings have often led to the erroneous diagnosis of Graves disease, although most affected patients are clinically euthyroid. The unresponsiveness may vary among tissues. There may be subtle clinical features of hypothyroidism, including mild mental retardation, growth retardation, and delayed skeletal maturation. One neurologic manifestation is an increased association of attention-deficit hyperactivity disorder; the converse is not true, however, because individuals with attention-deficit hyperactivity disorder do not have an increased risk of thyroid hormone resistance. It is presumed that these patients have varying tissue resistance to thyroid hormone. TSH levels are diagnostic in that they are not suppressed as in Graves disease but instead are moderately elevated or normal but inappropriate for the levels of T$_4$ and T$_3$ when measured by a sensitive TSH assay. A TSH response to TRH occurs in these patients, unlike the situation in Graves disease. The failure of TSH suppression indicates that the resistance is generalized and affects the pituitary gland as well as peripheral tissues. The disorder is most often inherited in an autosomal dominant fashion. More than 40 distinct point mutations in the hormone-binding domain of the β-thyroid receptor have been identified. Different phenotypes do not correlate with genotypes. The same mutation has been observed in individuals with generalized or isolated pituitary resistance, even in different individuals of the same family. A child homozygous for the receptor mutation showed unusually severe resistance. These cases support the dominant negative effect of mutant receptors, in which the mutant receptor protein inhibits normal receptor action in heterozygotes. Elevated levels of T$_4$ on neonatal thyroid screening should suggest the possibility of this diagnosis. No treatment is usually required unless growth and skeletal retardation are present.

Two infants of consanguineous matings are known to have an autosomal recessive form of thyroid resistance. These infants had manifestations of hypothyroidism early in life, and DNA studies revealed a major deletion of the β-thyroid receptor in one individual. The resistance appears to be more severe in this form of the entity.

On rare occasions, resistance to thyroid hormone may selectively affect the pituitary gland. Because the peripheral tissues are not resistant to thyroid hormones, the patient presents with a goiter and manifestations of hyperthyroidism. The laboratory findings are the same as those seen with generalized thyroid hormone resistance. This condition must be differentiated from a pituitary TSH-secreting tumor. At least one young child has been successfully treated with D-thyroxine therapy. Bromocriptine administration, which interferes with TSH secretion, was reported to be successful in another patient.

IODINE EXPOSURE. Congenital hypothyroidism may result from fetal exposure to excessive iodides or antithyroid drugs. Perinatal exposure may occur with the use of iodine antiseptic to prepare the skin for cesarian section or painting of the cervix prior to delivery. These conditions are transitory and must not be mistaken for the other forms of hypothyroidism described. In the neonate, topical iodine-containing antiseptics used in nurseries and by surgeons can also cause transient congenital hypothyroidism, especially in low birthweight infants, and can lead to abnormal results on neonatal screening tests. In older children, the usual sources of iodides are proprietary preparations used to treat asthma. In a few instances, the cause of hypothyroidism was amiodarone, an antiarrhythmic drug with high iodine content. In most of these instances goiter is present (see Chapter 561.3).

IODINE DEFICIENCY-ENDEMIC GOITER. Essentially unseen in the United States, iodine deficiency or endemic goiter is the most common cause of congenital hypothyroidism worldwide. Borderline iodine deficiency is more likely to cause problems in preterm infants who depend on a maternal source of iodine.

THYROID FUNCTION IN PRETERM BABIES. Postnatal thyroid function in preterm babies is qualitatively similar but quantitatively reduced compared with that of term infants. The cord serum T_4 is decreased in proportion to gestational age and birthweight. The postnatal TSH surge is reduced, and infants with complications of prematurity, such as respiratory distress syndrome, actually experience a decrease in serum T_4 in the 1st week of life. As these complications resolve, the serum T_4 gradually increases so that generally by 6 wk of life it enters the T_4 range seen in term infants. Serum free T_4 concentrations seem less affected, and when measured by equilibrium dialysis, these levels are often normal. Preterm babies also have a higher frequency of transient TSH elevations and apparent transient primary hypothyroidism. Premature infants less than 28 wk of gestation may have problems resulting from a combination of immaturity of the hypothalamic-pituitary-thyroid axis and loss of the maternal contribution of thyroid hormone and so may be candidates for temporary thyroid hormone replacement; further studies on this issue are needed.

Clinical Manifestations. Most infants with congenital hypothyroidism are asymptomatic at birth, even if there is complete agenesis of the thyroid gland. This situation is attributed to the transplacental passage of moderate amounts of maternal T_4, which provides fetal levels that are 33% of normal at birth. These low serum levels of T_4 and concomitantly elevated levels of TSH make it possible to screen and detect most hypothyroid neonates.

The clinician is dependent on neonatal screening tests for diagnosis of congenital hypothyroidism. Laboratory errors occur, however, and awareness of early symptoms and signs must be maintained. Congenital hypothyroidism is twice as common in girls as in boys. Before neonatal screening programs, congenital hypothyroidism was rarely recognized in the newborn because the signs and symptoms are usually not sufficiently developed. It can be suspected and the diagnosis established during the early weeks of life if the initial but less characteristic manifestations are recognized. Birthweight and length are normal, but head size may be slightly increased because of myxedema of the brain. Prolongation of physiologic

icterus, caused by delayed maturation of glucuronide conjugation, may be the earliest sign. Feeding difficulties, especially sluggishness, lack of interest, somnolence, and choking spells during nursing, are often present during the 1st mo of life. Respiratory difficulties, due in part to the large tongue, include apneic episodes, noisy respirations, and nasal obstruction. Typical respiratory distress syndrome may also occur. Affected infants cry little, sleep much, have poor appetites, and are generally sluggish. There may be constipation that does not usually respond to treatment. The abdomen is large, and an umbilical hernia is usually present. The temperature is subnormal, often less than 35°C (95°F), and the skin, particularly that of the extremities, may be cold and mottled. Edema of the genitals and extremities may be present. The pulse is slow, and heart murmurs, cardiomegaly, and asymptomatic pericardial effusion are common. Anemia (macrocytic) is often present and is refractory to treatment with hematinics. Because symptoms appear gradually, the diagnosis is often delayed.

These manifestations progress; retardation of physical and mental development becomes greater during the following months, and by 3–6 mo of age, the clinical picture is fully developed (Fig. 559–1). When there is only a partial deficiency of thyroid hormone, the symptoms may be milder, the syndrome incomplete, and the onset delayed. Although breast milk contains significant amounts of thyroid hormones, particularly T_3, it is inadequate to protect the breast-fed infant with congenital hypothyroidism, and it has no effect on neonatal thyroid screening tests.

The child's growth is stunted, the extremities are short, and the head size is normal or even increased. The anterior and posterior fontanels are open widely; observation of this sign at birth may serve as an initial clue to the early recognition of congenital hypothyroidism. Only 3% of normal newborn infants have a posterior fontanel larger than 0.5 cm. The eyes appear far apart, and the bridge of the broad nose is depressed. The palpebral fissures are narrow and the eyelids swollen. The mouth is kept open, and the thick and broad tongue protrudes from it. Dentition is delayed. The neck is short and thick, and there may be deposits of fat above the clavicles and between the neck and shoulders. The hands are broad and the fingers short. The skin is dry and scaly, and there is little perspiration. Myxedema is manifested, particularly in the skin of the eyelids, the back of the hands, and the external genitals. Carotenemia may cause a yellow discoloration of the skin, but the scleras remain white. The scalp is thickened, and the hair is coarse, brittle, and scanty. The hairline reaches far down on the forehead, which usually appears wrinkled, especially when the infant cries.

Development is usually retarded. Hypothyroid infants appear lethargic and are late in learning to sit and stand. The voice is hoarse, and they do not learn to talk. The degree of physical and mental retardation increases with age. Sexual maturation may be delayed or may not take place at all.

The muscles are usually hypotonic, but in rare instances generalized muscular pseudohypertrophy occurs (*Kocher-Debré-Sémélaigne syndrome*). Affected children may have an athletic appearance because of pseudohypertrophy, particularly in the calf muscles. Its pathogenesis is unknown; nonspecific histochemical and ultrastructural changes seen on muscle biopsy return to normal with treatment. Boys are more prone to development of the syndrome, which has been observed in siblings born to a consanguineous mating. Affected patients have hypothyroidism of longer duration and severity.

Laboratory Findings. Most newborn screening programs in North America measure levels of T_4, supplemented by measurement of TSH when T_4 is low. This approach identifies infants with primary hypothyroidism, those with low levels of thyroxine-binding globulin, some with hypothalamic or pituitary hypothyroidism, and infants with a delayed increase in TSH levels.

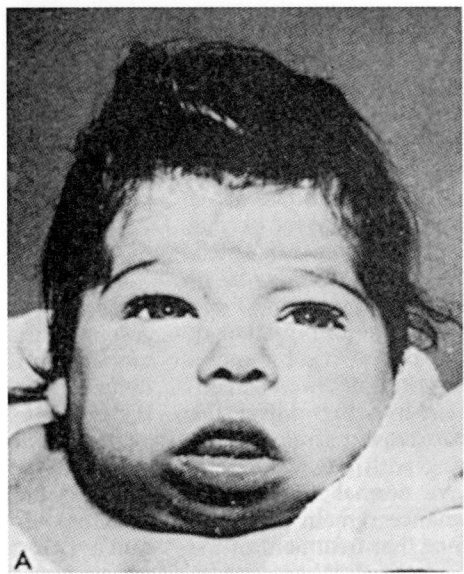
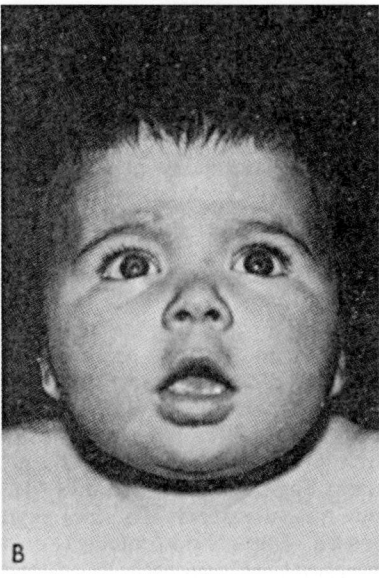

FIGURE 559-1. Congenital hypothyroidism in an infant 6 mo of age. The infant ate poorly in the neonatal period and was constipated. She had a persistent nasal discharge and a large tongue; she was very lethargic; she had no social smile and no head control. *A,* Notice the puffy face, dull expression, and hirsute forehead. Tests revealed a negligible uptake of radioiodine. Osseous development was that of a newborn. *B,* Four mo after treatment, notice the decreased puffiness of the face, the decreased hirsutism of the forehead, and the alert appearance.

European and Japanese neonatal screening programs are based on a primary measurement of TSH; some North American programs are switching to primary TSH screening. This approach detects infants with primary hypothyroidism and may detect infants with subclinical hypothyroidism (normal T_4, elevated TSH), but it misses infants with delayed TSH elevation, low thyroxine-binding globulin levels, and hypothalamic or pituitary hypothyroidism. With any of these assays, special care should be given to the normal range of values for age of the patient, particularly in the first weeks of life. Regardless of the approach used for screening, some infants escape detection because of technical or human errors; clinicians must maintain their vigilance for clinical manifestations of hypothyroidism.

Serum levels of T_4 or free T_4 are low; serum levels of T_3 may be normal and are not helpful in the diagnosis. If the defect is primarily in the thyroid, levels of TSH are elevated, often to greater than 100 mU/L. Serum levels of prolactin are elevated, correlating with those of TSH. Serum levels of TG are usually low in infants with thyroid agenesis or defects of TG synthesis or secretion, but they may be elevated with ectopic glands and other inborn errors of thyroxine synthesis.

Special attention should be paid to identical twins, because in at least four cases neonatal screening failed to detect the discordant twin with hypothyroidism, and the diagnosis was not made until the infants were 4–5 mo of age. Apparently, transfusion of euthyroid blood from the unaffected twin normalized the serum level of T_4 and TSH in the affected twin at the initial screening.

Retardation of osseous development can be shown roentgenographically at birth in about 60% of congenitally hypothyroid infants and indicates some deprivation of thyroid hormone during intrauterine life. For example, the distal femoral epiphysis, normally present at birth, is often absent (Fig. 559–2A). In untreated patients, the discrepancy between chronological age and osseous development increases. The epiphyses often have multiple foci of ossification (epiphyseal dysgenesis, Fig. 559–2B); deformity ("breaking") of the 12th thoracic or 1st or 2nd lumbar vertebra is common. Roentgenograms of the skull show large fontanels and wide sutures; intersutural (wormian) bones are common. The sella turcica is often enlarged and round; in rare instances there may be erosion and thinning. Delays in formation and eruption of teeth may occur. Cardiac enlargement or pericardial effusion may be present.

Scintigraphy can help to pinpoint the underlying cause in infants with congenital hypothyroidism, but treatment should not be unduly delayed for this study. ^{123}I-sodium iodide is superior to ^{99m}Tc-sodium pertechnetate for this purpose. Ultrasonographic examination of the thyroid is helpful, but studies show it may miss some ectopic glands shown by scintigraphy. Serum levels of TG are low with agenesis and elevated with ectopic glands and goiters, but there is a wide overlap of ranges. Demonstration of ectopic thyroid tissue is diagnostic of thyroid dysgenesis and establishes the need for lifelong treatment with T_4. Failure to demonstrate any thyroid tissue suggests thyroid aplasia, but this also occurs in neonates with TRBAb and in infants with the iodide-trapping defect. A normally situated thyroid gland with a normal or avid uptake of radionuclide indicates a defect in thyroid hormone biosynthesis. Patients with goitrous hypothyroidism may require extensive evaluation, including radioiodine studies, perchlorate discharge tests, kinetic studies, chromatography, and studies of thyroid tissue, if the biochemical nature of the defect is to be determined.

The electrocardiogram may show low-voltage P and T waves with diminished amplitude of QRS complexes and suggest poor left ventricular function and pericardial effusion. The electroencephalogram frequently shows low voltage. In children older than 2 yr of age, the serum cholesterol level is usually elevated. Brain MRI before treatment is reportedly normal, although proton magnetic resonance spectroscopy shows high levels of choline-containing compounds, which may reflect blocks in myelin maturation.

Treatment. Sodium-L-thyroxine given orally is the treatment of choice. Because 80% of circulating T_3 is formed by monodeiodination of T_4, serum levels of T_4 and T_3 in treated infants return to normal. This is also true in the brain, where 80% of required T_3 is produced locally from T_4. In neonates, the initial starting dose is 10–15 µg/kg (37.5 to 50 µg/24 hr). Thyroxine tablets should not be mixed with soy protein formulas or iron, because these can bind T_4 and inhibit its absorption. Levels of T_4 and TSH should be monitored at recommended intervals and maintained in the normal range for age. Children with hypothyroidism require about 4 µg/kg/24 hr, and adults require only 2 µg/kg/24 hr.

Later, confirmation of the diagnosis may be necessary for some infants to rule out the possibility of transient hypothyroidism. This is unnecessary in infants with proven thyroid ectopia or in those who manifest elevated levels of TSH after 6–12 mo of therapy because of poor compliance or an inade-

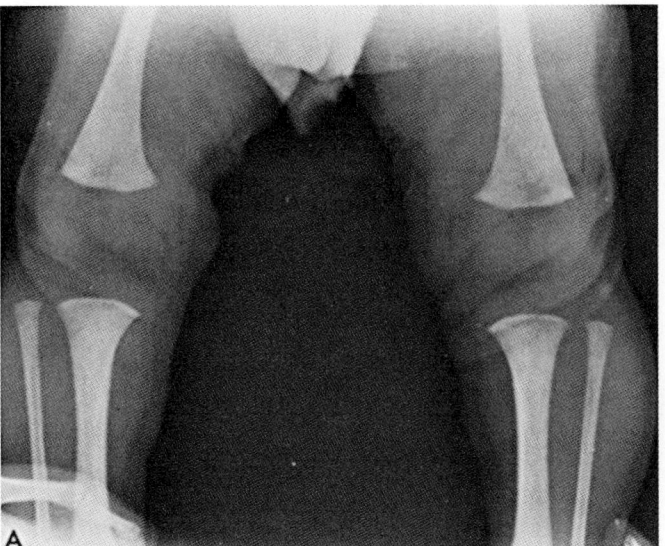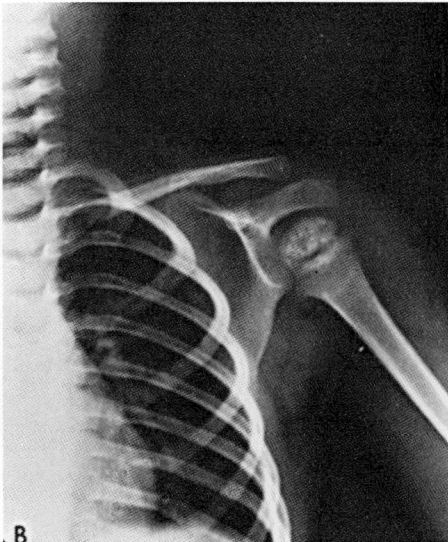

FIGURE 559–2. Congenital hypothyroidism. *A*, Absence of distal femoral epiphysis in a 3-mo-old infant who was born at term. This is evidence for the onset of the hypothyroid state during fetal life. *B*, Epiphyseal dysgenesis in the head of the humerus in a 9-yr-old girl who had been inadequately treated with thyroid hormone.

quate dose of T_4. Discontinuation of therapy at about 3 yr of age for 3–4 wk results in a marked increase in TSH levels in children with permanent hypothyroidism.

The only untoward effects of sodium-L-thyroxine are related to its dose. Overtreatment may risk craniosynostosis and temperament problems. An occasional older child (8–13 yr) with acquired hypothyroidism may experience pseudotumor cerebri within the first 4 mo of treatment. In older children, after catch-up growth is complete, the growth rate provides an excellent index of the adequacy of therapy. Parents should be forewarned about changes in behavior and activity expected with therapy, and special attention must be given to any developmental or neurologic deficits.

Prognosis. With the advent of neonatal screening programs for detection of congenital hypothyroidism, the prognosis for affected infants has improved dramatically. Early diagnosis and adequate treatment from the first weeks of life result in normal linear growth and intelligence comparable with that of unaffected siblings. Some screening programs report that the most severely affected infants, as judged by the lowest T_4 levels and retarded skeletal maturation, have slightly reduced (5–10 points) IQs and other neuropsychologic sequelae, such as incoordination, hypotonia or hypertonia, short attention span, and speech problems. Approximately 20% of children have a neurosensory hearing deficit. Without treatment, affected infants become profoundly mentally deficient dwarfs. Thyroid hormone is critical for normal cerebral development in the early postnatal months; biochemical diagnosis must be made soon after birth, and effective treatment must be initiated promptly to prevent irreversible brain damage. Delay in diagnosis, failure to correct initial hypothyroxinemia rapidly, inadequate treatment, and poor compliance in the first 2–3 yr of life result in variable degrees of brain damage. When onset of hypothyroidism occurs after 2 yr of age, the outlook for normal development is much better even if diagnosis and treatment have been delayed, indicating how much more important thyroid hormone is to the rapidly growing brain of the infant.

ACQUIRED HYPOTHYROIDISM

Epidemiology. Studies of school-aged children report that hypothyroidism occurs in approximately 0.08% (1:1,250). Acquired hypothyroidism is most commonly a result of chronic lymphocytic thyroiditis; 1.3% of children have evidence of autoimmune

thyroid disease, which occurs with a 2:1 female to male preponderance.

Etiology. The most common cause of acquired hypothyroidism (Box 559–2) is lymphocytic thyroiditis. Autoimmune thyroid disease may be part of polyglandular syndromes; children with Down, Turner, and Klinefelter syndromes and celiac disease or diabetes are at higher risk for associated autoimmune thyroid disease (see Chapter 560). Although typically seen in adolescence, it occurs as early as in the 1st yr of life. Some patients with congenital thyroid dysgenesis or with incomplete genetic defects in thyroid hormone synthesis may not display clinical manifestations until childhood and appear to have acquired hypothyroidism; these conditions are usually now detected by newborn screening programs. Subtotal thyroidectomy for thyrotoxicosis or cancer may result in hypothyroidism, as may removal of ectopic thyroid tissue. For example, *lingual thyroid, subhyoid median thyroid*, or thyroid tissue in a *thyroglossal duct cyst* usually constitutes the only source of thyroid hormone, and excision results in hypothyroidism. Because subhyoid glands usually mimic thyroglossal duct cysts, ultrasonographic examination or a radionuclide scan before surgery is indicated in these patients.

BOX 559–2. Etiologic Classification of Acquired Hypothyroidism

AUTOIMMUNE (ACQUIRED HYPOTHYROIDISM)
Hashimoto thyroiditis
Polyglandular autoimmune syndrome, types I, II, and III

IATROGENIC
Propylthiouracil, methimazole, iodides, lithium, amiodarone
Irradiation
Radioiodine
Radiographs (neck or whole body)
Thyroidectomy

SYSTEMIC DISEASE
Cystinosis
Histiocytic infiltration

HEMANGIOMAS (LARGE) OF THE LIVER (TYPE 3 IODOTHYRONINE DEIODINASE)

RESISTANCE TO THYROID HORMONE (ONLY OCCASIONAL CLINICAL MANIFESTATIONS OF HYPOTHYROIDISM)

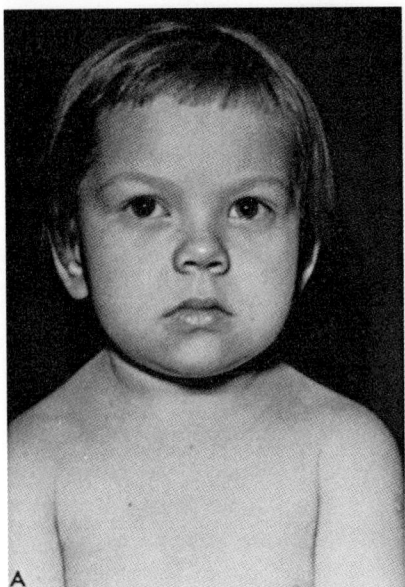
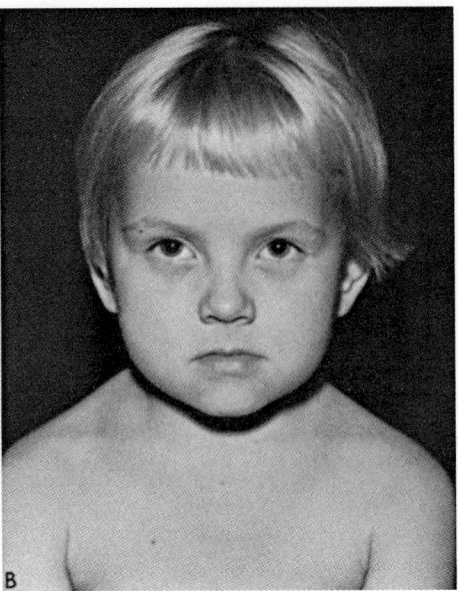

FIGURE 559–3. *A*, Acquired hypothyroidism in a girl 6 yr of age. She was treated with a wide variety of hematinics for refractory anemia for 3 yr. She had almost complete cessation of growth, constipation, and sluggishness for 3 yr. The height age was 3 yr; the bone age was 4 yr. She had a sallow complexion and immature facies with a poorly developed nasal bridge. Serum cholesterol, 501 mg/dL; radioiodine uptake, 7% at 24 hr; PBI, 2.8 mg/dL. *B*, After therapy for 18 mo, notice the nasal development, the increased luster and decreased pigmentation of hair, and the maturation of face. The height age was 5.5 yr; the bone age was 7 yr. There was a decided improvement in her general condition. Menarche occurred at 14 yr. The ultimate height was 155 cm (61 in). She graduated from high school. The disorder was well controlled with sodium-L-thyroxine daily.

Children with *nephropathic cystinosis*, a disorder characterized by intralysosomal storage of cystine in body tissues, acquire impaired thyroid function. Hypothyroidism may be overt, but subclinical forms are more common, and periodic assessment of TSH levels is indicated. By 13 yr of age, two thirds of these patients require T_4 replacement.

Histiocytic infiltration of the thyroid in children with Langerhans cell histiocytoses may result in hypothyroidism.

Irradiation of the area of thyroid that is incidental to the treatment of Hodgkin disease or other head and neck malignancies or that is administered before bone marrow transplantation often results in thyroid damage. About one third of such children acquire elevated TSH levels within a year after therapy and 15–20% progress to hypothyroidism within 5–7 yr. Some clinicians recommend periodic TSH measurements, but others recommend treatment of all exposed patients with doses of T_4 to suppress TSH.

Protracted ingestion of medications containing iodides can cause hypothyroidism, usually accompanied by goiter (see Chapter 561). Amiodarone, a drug used for cardiac arrhythmias and consisting of 37% iodine by weight, causes hypothyroidism in about 20% of treated children. It affects thyroid function directly by its high iodine content as well as by inhibition of 5'-deiodinase, which converts T_4 to T_3. Children treated with this drug should have serial measurements of T_4, T_3, and TSH.

Hypothyroidism can occur in children with large *hemangiomas* of the liver, due to increased type 3 deiodinase activity, which catalyzes conversion of T_4 to rT_3 and T_3 to T_2. Thyroid secretion is increased but is not enough to compensate for the large increase in T_4 to rT_3 degradation.

Clinical Manifestations. Deceleration of growth is usually the first clinical manifestation, but this sign often goes unrecognized (Fig. 559–3). Myxedematous changes of the skin, constipation, cold intolerance, decreased energy, and an increased need for sleep develop insidiously. Surprisingly, schoolwork and grades usually do not suffer, even in severely hypothyroid children. Osseous maturation is delayed, often strikingly, which is an indication of the duration of the hypothyroidism. Adolescents typically have delayed puberty, whereas younger children may present with galactorrhea or pseudoprecocious puberty. Galactorrhea is a result of increased TRH-stimulating prolactin secretion. The precocious puberty, characterized by

breast development in girls and macro-orchidism in boys, is thought to be the result of abnormally high TSH concentrations binding to the follicle-stimulating hormone receptor with subsequent stimulation.

Some children present with headaches and visual problems; they usually have hyperplastic enlargement of the pituitary gland, often with suprasellar extension, after long-standing hypothyroidism; this condition, believed to be the result of thyrotroph hyperplasia, may be mistaken for a pituitary tumor (see Chapter 551).

All these changes return to normal with adequate replacement of T_4, but in children with long-standing hypothyroidism, catch-up growth may be incomplete. During the first 18 mo of treatment, skeletal maturation often exceeds expected linear growth, resulting in a loss of about 7 cm of predicted adult height. The cause for this is unknown.

Diagnostic Studies and Treatment. Treatment and diagnostic studies are the same as those described for congenital hypothyroidism. Measurement of antithyroglobulin and antiperoxidase (formerly antimicrosomal) antibodies may pinpoint autoimmune thyroiditis as the cause. During the 1st yr of treatment, deterioration of schoolwork, poor sleeping habits, restlessness, short attention span, and behavioral problems may ensue, but these are transient; forewarning families about these manifestations enhances appropriate management. These may be partially ameliorated by starting at subreplacement T_4 doses and advancing slowly.

Adams A, Matthews C, Collingwood TH, et al: Genetic analysis of 29 kindreds with generalized and pituitary resistance to thyroid hormone. *J Clin Invest* 1994;94:506.

American Academy of Pediatrics: Newborn screening for congenital hypothyroidism: Recommended guidelines. *Pediatrics* 1993;91:1203.

Bakker B, Bikker H, Vulsma T, et al: Two decades of screening for congenital hypothyroidism in The Netherlands: TPO gene mutations in total iodide organification defects (an update). *J Clin Endocrinol Metab* 2000;85:3708.

Bartelena L, Bogazzi F, Braverman LE, et al: Effects of amiodarone administration during pregnancy on neonatal thyroid function and subsequent neurodevelopment. *J Endocrinol Invest* 2001;24:116.

Biebermann H, Schoneberg T, Krude H, et al: Mutations in the human thyrotropin receptor gene causing thyroid hyperplasia and persistent congenital hypothyroidism. *J Clin Endocrinol Metab* 1997;82:3471.

Biebermann H, Liesenkotter K-P, Emeis M, et al: Severe congenital hypothyroidism due to a homozygous mutation of the βTSH gene. *Pediatr Res* 1999;46:170.

Bongers-Schhokking JJ, Koot HM, Wiersma D, et al: Influence of timing and dose of thyroid hormone replacement on development in infants with congenital hypothyroidism. *J Pediatr* 2000;136:292.

Brown RS, Bellisario RL, Mitchell E, et al: Detection of thyrotropin binding inhibitory activity in neonatal blood spots. *J Clin Endocrinol Metab* 1993;77:1005.

Castanet M, Lyonnet S, Bonaiti-Pellie C, et al: Familial forms of thyroid dysgenesis among infants with congenital hypothyroidism. *N Engl J Med* 2000;343:441.

Clifton-Bligh, RJ, Wentworth, JM, Heinz, P, et al: Mutation of the gene encoding TTF-2 associated with thyroid agenesis, cleft palate and choanal atresia. *Nat Genet* 1998;19:399.

Collu R, Tang J, Castagne J, et al: A novel mechanism for isolated central hypothyroidism: Inactivating mutations in the thyroropin-releasing hormone receptor gene. *J Clin Endocrinol Metab* 1997;82:1361.

Congdon T, Nguyen LQ, Nogueira CR, et al: A novel mutation (Q40P) in PAX8 associated with congenital hypothyroidism and thyroid hypoplasia: evidence for phenotypic variability in mother and child. *J Clin Endocrinol Metab* 2001;86:3962.

Daliva AL, Lindner B, DiMartino-Nardi J, et al: Three-year follow-up of borderline congenital hypothyroidism. *J Pediatr* 2000;136:53.

Delange F: Neonatal screening for congenital hypothyroidism: Results and perspectives. [Review.] *Horm Res* 1997;48:51.

Devos, H, Rodd C, Gagne N, et al: A search for the possible molecular mechanisms of thyroid dysgenesis: Sex ratios and associated malformations. *J Clin Endocrinol Metab* 1999;84:2502.

Everett LA, Morsli H, Wu DK, Green ED: Expression pattern of the mouse ortholog of the Pendred's syndrome gene (pds) suggests a key role for pendrin in the inner ear. *Proc Natl Acad Sci U S A* 1999;96:9727.

Fisher DA, Schoen DA, LaFranchi S, et al: The hypothalamic-pituitary-thyroid negative feedback control axis in children with treated congenital hypothyroidism. *J Clin Endocrinol Metab* 2000;85:2722–7.

Frank JE, Faix JE, Hermos RJ, et al: Thyroid function in very low birth weight infants: Effects on neonatal hypothyroid screening. *J Pediatr* 1996;128:548.

Hauser P, Zametkin AJ, Martinez P, et al: Attention deficit-hyperactivity disorder in people with generalized resistance to thyroid hormone. *N Engl J Med* 1993;328:997.

Hrytsiuk I, Gilbert R, Logan S, et al: Starting dose of levothyroxine for the treatment of congenital hypothyroidism. *Arch Pediatr Adolesc Med* 2002;156:483–91.

Huang SA, Tu HM, Harney JW, et al: Severe hypothyroidism caused by type 3 iodothyronine deiodinase in infantile hemangiomas. *N Engl J Med* 2000;343:185–9.

Hunter MK, Mandel SH, Sesser DE, et al: Follow-up of newborns with low thyroxine and nonelevated thyroid-stimulating hormone-secreting concentrations: Results of the 20-year experience in the Northwest Regional Newborn Screening Program. *J Pediatr* 1998;132:70.

Karlson B, Gustafsson J, Hedov G, et al: Thyroid dysfunction in Down's syndrome: Relation to age and thyroid autoimmunity. *Arch Dis Child* 1998;79:242.

Macchia PE, Lapi P, Krude H, et al: PAX8 mutations associated with congenital hypothyroidism caused by thyroid dysgenesis. *Nat Genet* 1998;19:83.

Mandel SJ, Hermos RJ, Larson CA, et al: Atypical hypothyroidism and the very low birthweight infant. *Thyroid* 2000;10:693.

Moreno JC, Bikker H, Kempers MJE, et al: Inactivating mutations in the gene for thyroid oxidase 2 (THOX2) and congenital hypothyroidism. *N Engl J Med* 2002;347:95–102.

New England Congenital Hypothyroidism Collaborative: Correlation of cognitive test scores and adequacy of treatment in adolescents with congenital hypothyroidism. *J Pediatr* 1994;124:383.

Oakley GA, Muir T, Ray M, et al: Increased incidence of congenital malformations in children with transient thyroid-stimulating hormone elevation on neonatal screening. *J Pediatr* 1998;132:726.

Parks JS, Kinoshita EI, Pfaffle RW: Pit-1 and hypopituitarism. *Trends Endocrinol Metab* 1993;4:81.

Pohlenz J, Rosenthal IM, Weiss RE, et al: Congenital hypothyroidism due to mutations in the sodium/iodide symporter. Identification of a nonsense mutation producing a downstream cryptic 3' splice site. *J Clin Invest* 1998;101:1028.

Reuss ML, Paneth N, Pinto-Martin JA, et al: The relation of transient hypothyroxinemia in preterm infants to neurologic development at two years of age. *N Engl J Med* 1996;334:821.

Rivkees SA, Bode HH, Crawford JD: Long-term growth in juvenile acquired hypothyroidism: The failure to achieve normal adult stature. *N Engl J Med* 1988;318:519.

Rovet JF, Ehrlich R: Psychological outcome in children with early-treated congenital hypothyroidism. *Pediatrics* 2000;105:515.

Scott DA, Wang R, Kreman VC, et al: The Pendred syndrome is caused by mutations in a putative sulphate transporter gene (PDS). *Nat Genet* 1999;17:411.

Siragusa V, Boffelli S, Weber G, et al: Brain magnetic resonance imaging in congenital hypothyroid infants at diagnosis. *Thyroid* 1997;7:761.

VanDop C, Conte FA, Koch TK, et al: Pseudotumor cerebri associated with initiation of levothyroxine therapy for juvenile hypothyroidism. *N Engl J Med* 1983;308:1076.

Van Vliet G: Treatment of congenital hypothyroidism. *Lancet* 2001;358:86–7.

Van Wassenaer AG, Kok JH, de Vijlder JJ, et al: Effects of thyroxine supplementation on neurologic development in infants born at less than 30 weeks' gestation. *N Engl J Med* 1997;336:21.

Vilain C, Rydlewski, Duprez, L, et al: Autosomal dominant transmission of congenital thyroid hypoplasia due to loss-of-function mutation of PAX-8. *J Clin Endocrinol Metab* 2001;86:234.

Chapter 560
Thyroiditis

LYMPHOCYTIC THYROIDITIS (HASHIMOTO THYROIDITIS; AUTOIMMUNE THYROIDITIS)

Lymphocytic thyroiditis is the most common cause of thyroid disease in children and adolescents and accounts for many of the enlarged thyroids formerly designated "adolescent" or "simple" goiter. It is also the most common cause of acquired hypothyroidism, with or without goiter. There are 1.3% of school-aged children who have evidence for autoimmune thyroid disease.

Etiology. This typical organ-specific autoimmune disease is characterized histologically by lymphocytic infiltration of the thyroid. Early in the course of the disease, there may be hyperplasia only; this is followed by infiltration of lymphocytes and plasma cells between the follicles and by atrophy of the follicles. Lymphoid follicle formation with germinal centers is almost always present; the degree of atrophy and fibrosis of the follicles varies from mild to moderate.

Intrathyroidal lymphocyte subsets differ from those in blood. About 60% of infiltrating lymphoid cells are T cells, and about 30% express B-cell markers; the T-cell population is represented by helper (CD4+) and cytotoxic (CD8+) cells. The participation of cellular events in the pathogenesis is clear. Certain HLA haplotypes (HLA-DR4, HLA-DR5) are associated with an increased risk of goiter and thyroiditis, and others (HLA-DR3) are associated with the atrophic variant of thyroiditis.

A variety of different thyroid antigen autoantibodies are also involved. Thyroid antiperoxidase antibodies (TPOAbs), formerly called "antimicrosomal antibodies," are demonstrable in the sera of 90% of children with lymphocytic thyroiditis and in many patients with Graves disease. TPOAbs inhibit enzyme activity and stimulate natural killer cell cytotoxicity. Antithyroglobulin antibodies occur in a smaller percentage of affected children but are much more common in adults. Thyrotropin receptor-blocking antibodies are frequently present, especially in patients with hypothyroidism, and it is now believed that they are related to the development of hypothyroidism and thyroid atrophy in patients with autoimmune thyroiditis.

Clinical Manifestations. The disorder is four to seven times more frequent in girls than in boys. It may occur during the first 3 yr of life but becomes sharply more common after 6 yr of age and reaches a peak incidence during adolescence. The most common clinical manifestations are goiter and growth retardation. The goiter may appear insidiously and may be small or large. In most patients, the thyroid is diffusely enlarged, firm, and nontender. In about one third of patients, the gland is lobular and may seem to be nodular. Most of the affected children are clinically euthyroid and asymptomatic; some may have symptoms of pressure in the neck. Some children have clinical signs of hypothyroidism, but others who appear clinically euthyroid have laboratory evidence of hypothyroidism. A few children have manifestations suggestive of hyperthyroidism, such as nervousness, irritability, increased sweating, or hyperactivity, but results of laboratory studies are not necessarily those of hyperthyroidism. Occasionally, the disorder may coexist with Graves disease. Ophthalmopathy may occur in lymphocytic thyroiditis in the absence of Graves disease.

The clinical course is variable. The goiter may become smaller or may disappear spontaneously, or it may persist unchanged for years while the patient remains euthyroid. Most children who are euthyroid at presentation remain euthyroid, although a percentage of patients acquire hypothyroidism gradually within months or years. Over several years, about half of children with subclinical hypothyroidism revert to euthyroidism, while the other half develop overt hypothyroidism. Thyroiditis is the cause of most cases of nongoitrous (atrophic) hypothyroidism.

Familial clusters of lymphocytic thyroiditis are common; the incidence in siblings or parents of affected children may be as high as 25%. Autoantibodies to thyroglobulin and human thyroid peroxidase in these families appear to be inherited in an autosomal dominant fashion, with reduced penetrance in males. The concurrence within families of patients with lymphocytic thyroiditis, "idiopathic" hypothyroidism, and Graves disease provides cogent evidence for a basic relationship among these three conditions. The disorder has been associated with many of the other autoimmune disorders. Autoimmune thyroiditis occurs in 10% of patients with *type I polyglandular autoimmune syndrome*, which consists of hypoparathyroidism, Addison disease, and mucocutaneous candidiasis ("HAM" syndrome). The association of Addison disease with insulin-dependent diabetes mellitus or autoimmune thyroid disease, or both, is known as *Schmidt syndrome* or *type II polyglandular autoimmune disease*. Autoimmune thyroid disease also tends to be associated with pernicious anemia, vitiligo, or alopecia. TPOAbs are found in approximately 20% of white and 4% of black children with diabetes mellitus. Autoimmune thyroid disease has an increased incidence in children with congenital rubella. Lymphocytic thyroiditis is also associated with certain chromosomal disorders, particularly Turner syndrome and Down syndrome. In children with Down syndrome, one study reported that 28% had antithyroid antibodies (predominantly anti-TPOs), 7% had subclinical hypothyroidism, 7% had overt hypothyroidism, and 5% had hyperthyroidism. In a study of girls with Turner syndrome, 41% had antithyroid antibodies (again, predominantly anti-TPOs), 18% had goiter, and 8% had subclinical or overt hypothyroidism. Another study of 75 girls with Turner syndrome found that autoimmune thyroid disease increased from the first (15%) to the third (30%) decade of life. Boys with Klinefelter syndrome are also at risk for autoimmune thyroid disease.

Laboratory Findings. The definitive diagnosis can be established by biopsy of the thyroid, but this procedure is rarely indicated for clinical purposes alone. Thyroid function tests are often normal, although the level of thyroid-stimulating hormone (TSH) may be slightly or even moderately elevated in some individuals, termed *subclinical hypothyroidism*. The fact that many children with lymphocytic thyroiditis do not have elevated levels of TSH indicates that the goiter may be caused by the lymphocytic infiltrations or by thyroid growth-stimulating immunoglobulins. In 50% of children, thyroid scans reveal irregular and patchy distribution of the radioisotope, and in about 60% or more, the administration of perchlorate results in a greater than 10% discharge of iodide from the thyroid gland. Thyroid ultrasonography shows scattered hypoechogenicity in most patients. Most patients with lymphocytic thyroiditis have serum antibody titers to TPO, but the antithyroglobulin test for thyroid antibodies is positive in fewer than 50%. When both tests are used, approximately 95% of patients with thyroid autoimmunity are detected. In general, levels in children and adolescents are lower than those in adults with lymphocytic thyroiditis, and repeated measurements are indicated in questionable instances because titers may increase later in the course of the disease.

Antithyroid antibodies may also be found in almost half the siblings of affected patients and in a significant percentage of the mothers of children with Down syndrome or Turner syndrome without demonstrable thyroid disease. They are also found in 20% of children with diabetes mellitus and in 23% of children with the congenital rubella syndrome.

Treatment. If there is evidence of hypothyroidism, replacement treatment with sodium-L-thyroxine (50–150 µg daily) is indicated. The goiter usually shows some decrease in size but may persist for years. Antibody levels fluctuate in both treated and untreated patients and persist for years. Because the disease may be self-limited in some instances, the need for continued therapy requires periodic re-evaluation. Untreated patients should also be checked periodically. Prominent nodules that persist despite suppressive therapy should be examined histologically because thyroid cancer has occurred in patients with lymphocytic thyroiditis.

OTHER CAUSES OF THYROIDITIS

Specific conditions such as tuberculosis, sarcoidosis, mumps, and cat-scratch disease are rare causes of thyroiditis.

Acute suppurative thyroiditis is uncommon; it is usually preceded by a respiratory infection. The left lower lobe is affected predominantly. Abscess formation may occur. Anaerobic organisms, with or without aerobes, are the most common organisms; *Eikenella corrodens* has been reported. Recurrent episodes or the detection of a mixed bacterial flora suggests that the infection arises from a thyroglossal duct remnant or, more often, from a piriform sinus fistula. Exquisite tenderness of the gland, swelling, erythema, dysphagia, and limitation of head motion are characteristic findings. Systemic manifestations are often absent, and leukocytosis is present. Scintigrams of the thyroid often reveal decreased uptake in the affected areas, and ultrasonography may show a complex echogenic mass. Thyroid function is usually normal, but thyrotoxicosis due to escape of thyroid hormone has been encountered in a child with suppurative thyroiditis resulting from *Aspergillus*. When suppuration occurs, incision and drainage and administration of antibiotics are indicated. After the infection subsides, a barium esophagram is indicated to search for a fistulous tract; if one is found, exteriorization is indicated.

Subacute nonsuppurative thyroiditis (de Quervain disease) is rare in children. It is thought to have a viral cause and remits spontaneously. The disorder becomes manifested by a vague tenderness over the thyroid and low-grade fever or by severe pain in the region of the thyroid and systemic manifestations with chills and high fever. Inflammation results in leakage of preformed thyroid hormone from the gland into the circulation. Serum levels of T_4 and T_3 are elevated, and mild symptoms of hyperthyroidism may be present, but radioiodine uptake is depressed. The erythrocyte sedimentation rate is increased. The course is variable, usually passing through a euthyroid to a hypothyroid phase; remission usually occurs in several months. Occasionally, this condition is superimposed on lymphocytic thyroiditis.

Boyages SC, Halpern JP, Maberly GF, et al: Possible role for thyroid autoimmunity. *Lancet* 1989;2:529.

Chiovato L, Vitti P, Santini F, et al: Incidence of antibodies blocking thyrotropin effect in vitro in patients with euthyroid or hypothyroid autoimmune thyroiditis. *J Clin Endocrinol Metab* 1990;71:40.

Foley TP Jr, Abbassi V, Copeland KC, et al: Brief report: Hypothyroidism caused by chronic autoimmune thyroiditis in very young infants. *N Engl J Med* 1993;330:466.

Gruneiro de Papendieck L, Iorcansky S, Coco R: High incidence of thyroid disturbances in 49 children with Turner syndrome. *J Pediatr* 1987;111:258.

Gutekunst R, Hafermann W, Mansky T, et al: Ultrasonography related to clinical and laboratory findings in lymphocytic thyroiditis. *Acta Endocrinol* 1989;121:129.

Hayashi Y, Tamai H, Fukata S, et al: A long-term clinical, immunological, and histological follow-up study of patients with goitrous chronic lymphocytic thyroiditis. *J Clin Endocrinol Metab* 1985;61:1172.

Jaruratanasirikul S, Leethanaporn K, Khuntigij P, et al: The clinical course of Hashimoto's thyroiditis in children and adolescents: 6 years longitudinal follow-up. *J Pediatr Endocrinol Metab* 2001;14:177.

Mangklabruks A, Cox N, DeGroot IJ: Genetic factors in autoimmune thyroid disease analyzed by restriction fragment length polymorphisms of candidate genes. *J Clin Endocrinol Metab* 1991;73:236.

Matsuura N, Konishi J, Yuri K, et al: Comparison of atrophic and goitrous autoimmune thyroiditis in children: Clinical, laboratory and TSH-receptor antibody studies. *Eur J Pediatr* 1990;149:529.

Perheentupa J: Autoimmune polyendocrinopathy-candidiasis- ectodermal dystrophy (APECED). [Review.] *Horm Metab Res* 1996;28:353.

Phillips D, McLachlan S, Stephenson A, et al: Autosomal dominant transmission of autoantibodies to thyroglobulin and thyroid peroxidase. *J Clin Endocrinol Metab* 1990;70:742.

Pueschel SM, Pezzallo JC: Thyroid dysfunction in Down syndrome. *Am J Dis Child* 1985;139:636.

Queen JS, Clegg HW, Council JC, et al: Acute suppurative thyroiditis caused by *Eikenella corrodens*. *J Pediatr Surg* 1988;23:359.

Rallison ML, Dobyns BM, Keating FR, et al: Occurrence and natural history of chronic lymphocytic thyroiditis in childhood. *J Pediatr* 1975;86:675.

Rallison ML, Dobyns BM, Meikle AW, et al: Natural history of thyroid abnormalities: Prevalence, incidence, and regression of thyroid diseases in adolescents and young adults. *Am J Med* 1991;91:363.

Rich EJ, Mendelman PM: Acute suppurative thyroiditis in pediatric patients. *Pediatr Infect Dis J* 1987;6:936.

Weetman AP: Autoimmune thyroiditis: Predisposition and pathogenesis. *Clin Endocrinol* 1992;36:307.

Chapter 561
Goiter

A goiter is an enlargement of the thyroid gland. Persons with enlarged thyroids may have normal function of the gland *(euthyroidism)*, thyroid deficiency *(hypothyroidism)*, or overproduction of the hormones *(hyperthyroidism)*. Goiter may be congenital or acquired, endemic or sporadic.

The goiter often results from increased pituitary secretion of thyrotropic hormone in response to decreased circulating levels of thyroid hormones. Thyroid enlargement may also result from infiltrative processes that may be inflammatory or neoplastic. Goiter in patients with thyrotoxicosis is caused by thyrotropin receptor-stimulating antibodies.

561.1 Congenital Goiter

Congenital goiter is usually sporadic and may result from a fetal *thyroxine (T₄) synthetic defect* or the administration of *antithyroid drugs* or *iodides* during pregnancy for the treatment of thyrotoxicosis. Goitrogenic drugs and iodides cross the placenta and at high doses may interfere with synthesis of thyroid hormone, resulting in goiter and hypothyroidism in the fetus. The concomitant administration of thyroid hormone with the goitrogen does not prevent this effect, because insufficient amounts of T_4 cross the placenta. Iodides are included in many proprietary preparations used to treat asthma; these preparations must be avoided during pregnancy because they have often been a cause of unexpected congenital goiter. Amiodarone, an antiarrhythmic drug with a 37% iodine content, has also caused congenital goiter with hypothyroidism. Even when the infant is clinically euthyroid, there may be retardation of osseous maturation, low levels of T_4, and elevated levels of thyroid-stimulating hormone (TSH). In women with Graves disease on antithyroid drugs, these effects can occur when the mother takes only 100–200 mg of propylthiouracil/24 hr; all such infants should undergo thyroid studies at birth. Administration of thyroid hormone to affected infants may be indicated to treat clinical hypothyroidism, to hasten the disappearance of the goiter, and to prevent brain damage. Because the condition is rarely permanent, thyroid hormone may be safely discontinued after the antithyroid drug has been excreted by the neonate, usually after a week.

Enlargement of the thyroid at birth may occasionally be sufficient to cause respiratory distress that interferes with nursing and may even cause death. The head may be maintained in extreme hyperextension. When respiratory obstruction is severe, partial thyroidectomy rather than tracheostomy is indicated (Fig. 561–1).

Goiter is almost always present in the *congenitally hyperthyroid* infant. These goiters usually are not large; the infant manifests

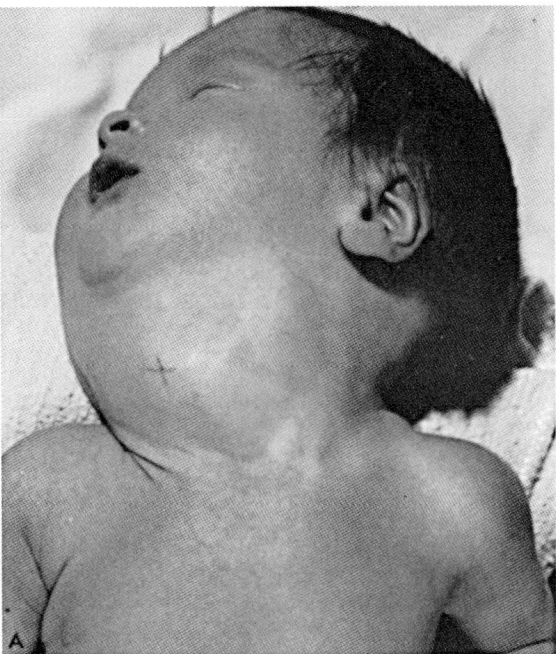
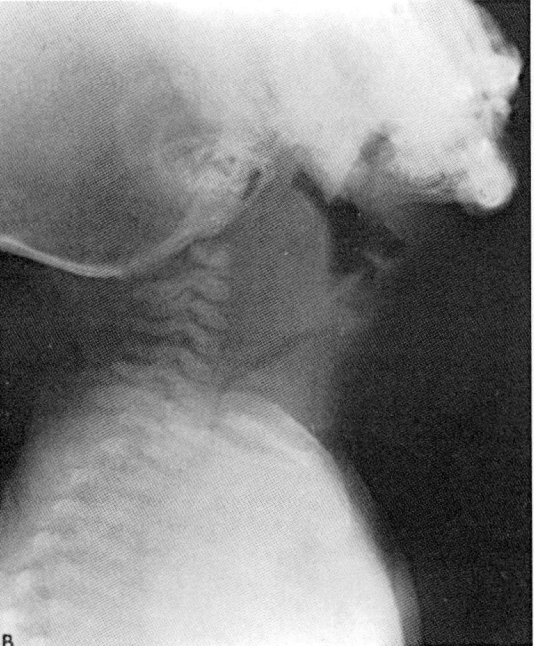

FIGURE 561–1. Congenital goiter in infancy. *A,* Large congenital goiter in an infant born to a mother with thyrotoxicosis who had been treated with iodides and methimazole during pregnancy. *B,* A 6-wk-old infant with increasing respiratory distress and cervical mass since birth. The operation revealed a large goiter that almost completely encircled the trachea. Notice the anterior deviation and posterior compression of the trachea. Partial thyroidectomy completely relieved the symptoms. It is apparent why a tracheostomy is not adequate treatment for these infants. The cause for the goiter was not found.

clinical symptoms of hyperthyroidism, and the mother often has a history of Graves disease (see Chapter 562.1). TSH receptor-activating mutations are also a recognized cause of congenital goiter.

When no causative factor is identifiable, a *defect in synthesis of thyroid hormone* should be suspected. Neonatal screening programs find congenital hypothyroidism caused by such a defect in 1/30,000–50,000 live births. If the infant is hypothyroid, it is advisable to treat immediately with thyroid hormone and to postpone more detailed studies for later in life. Because these defects are transmitted by recessive genes, a precise diagnosis is helpful for genetic counseling. Monitoring subsequent pregnancies with ultrasonography can be useful in detecting fetal goiters (see Chapters 85.2).

Iodine deficiency as a cause of congenital goiters is rare in developed countries, but persists in isolated endemic areas (see below). More important is the recent recognition that severe iodine deficiency early in pregnancy may cause neurologic damage during fetal development, even in the absence of goiter. The iodine deficiency may result in maternal and fetal hypothyroidism, preventing the partially protective transfer of maternal thyroid hormones.

When the "goiter" is lobulated, asymmetric, firm, or large to an unusual degree, a *teratoma* within or in the vicinity of the thyroid must be considered in the differential diagnosis (see Chapter 563).

561.2 Endemic Goiter and Cretinism

Etiology

IODINE DEFICIENCY. The association between dietary deficiency of iodine and the prevalence of goiter or cretinism has been recognized for more than half a century. A moderate deficiency of iodine can be overcome by increased efficiency in the synthesis of thyroid hormone. Iodine liberated in the tissues is returned rapidly to the gland, which resynthesizes triiodothyronine (T_3) preferentially at a higher rate than normal. This increased activity is achieved by compensatory hypertrophy and hyperplasia, which satisfy the demands of the tissues for thyroid hormone. In geographic areas where deficiency of iodine is severe, decompensation and hypothyroidism may result. It is estimated that 2 billion individuals in developing countries live in areas of iodine deficiency.

Seawater is rich in iodine, and the iodine content of fish and shellfish is also high. Endemic goiter is rare therefore in populations living along the sea. Iodine is deficient in the water and native foods in the Pacific West and the Great Lakes areas of the United States. Deficiency of dietary iodine is even greater in certain Alpine valleys, the Himalayas, the Andes, the Congo, and the highlands of Papua New Guinea. In areas such as the United States, where iodine is provided in foods from other areas and in iodized salt, endemic goiter has disappeared. Iodized salt in the United States contains potassium iodide ($100 \mu g/g$) and provides excellent prophylaxis. Further iodine intake in the United States is contributed by iodates used in baking, iodine-containing coloring agents, and iodine-containing disinfectants used in the dairy industry. The recommended daily allowance of iodine for infants is greater than $30 \mu g/kg/24$ hr; this amount is exceeded fourfold in breast-fed infants and 10-fold in infants fed cow's milk in the United States.

Clinical Manifestations. If the deficiency of iodine is mild, thyroid enlargement does not become noticeable except when there is increased demand for the hormone during periods of rapid growth, as in adolescence and during pregnancy. In regions of moderate iodine deficiency, goiter observed in schoolchildren may disappear with maturity and reappear during pregnancy or lactation. Iodine-deficient goiters are more common in girls than in boys. In areas where iodine deficiency is severe, as in the hyperendemic highlands of Papua New Guinea, nearly half the population has large goiters, and endemic cretinism is common.

Serum T_4 levels are often low in individuals with endemic goiter, although clinical hypothyroidism is rare. This is true in New Guinea, the Congo, the Himalayas, and South America. Despite low serum levels of thyroid hormone, serum TSH concentrations are often only moderately increased. In such patients, circulating levels of T_3 are elevated. Moreover, T_3 levels are also elevated in patients with normal T_4 levels, indicating a preferential secretion of T_3 by the thyroid in this disease.

Endemic cretinism is the most serious consequence of iodine deficiency; it occurs only in geographic association with endemic goiter. The term *endemic cretinism* includes two different but overlapping syndromes—a neurologic type and a myxedematous type. The frequency of the two types varies among different populations. In Papua New Guinea, the neurologic type occurs almost exclusively, but in Zaire, the myxedematous type predominates. Both types are found in all endemic areas, and some individuals have intermediate or mixed features.

The neurologic syndrome is characterized by mental retardation, deaf-mutism, disturbances in standing and gait, and pyramidal signs such as clonus of the foot, the Babinski sign, and patellar hyperreflexia. Affected individuals are goitrous but euthyroid, have normal pubertal development and adult stature, and have little or no impaired thyroid function. Individuals with the myxedematous syndrome also are mentally retarded and deaf and have neurologic symptoms, delayed sexual development and growth, myxedema, and absence of goiter; serum T_4 levels are low, and TSH levels are markedly elevated. Delayed skeletal maturation may extend into the 3rd decade or later. Ultrasonographic examination shows thyroid atrophy.

Pathogenesis. The pathogenesis of the neurologic syndrome has been attributed to iodine deficiency and hypothyroxinemia during pregnancy, leading to fetal and postnatal hypothyroidism. Although some investigators have attributed brain damage to a direct effect of elemental iodine deficiency in the fetus, most believe the neurologic symptoms are caused by fetal and maternal hypothyroxinemia. There is evidence that the human fetal brain has receptors for thyroid hormone before development of the fetal thyroid, and there is also evidence of transplacental passage of maternal thyroid hormone into the fetus, which normally might ameliorate the effects of fetal hypothyroidism on the developing nervous system. The pathogenesis of the myxedematous syndrome leading to thyroid atrophy is more bewildering. Searches for additional environmental factors that may provoke continuing postnatal hypothyroidism have led to incrimination of selenium deficiency, goitrogenic foods, thiocyanates, and *Yersinia*. Studies from Western China suggest that thyroid autoimmunity may play a role. Myxedematous cretins with thyroid atrophy, but not euthyroid cretins, were found to have thyroid growth-blocking immunoglobulins of the kind found in infants with sporadic congenital hypothyroidism. Others are skeptical about any role of thyroid growth-blocking immunoglobulins to explain these findings.

Treatment. In many developing countries, administration of a single intramuscular injection of iodinated poppy seed oil to women prevents iodine deficiency during future pregnancies for about 5 yr. This form of therapy given to children younger than 4 yr of age with myxedematous cretinism results in a euthyroid state in 5 mo. However, older children respond poorly and adults not at all to iodized oil injections, indicating an inability of the thyroid gland to synthesize hormone; these patients require treatment with T_4. In the Xinjiang province of China, where the usual methods of iodine supplementation had failed, iodination of irrigation water has increased iodine levels in soil, animals, and human beings.

561.3 Sporadic Goiter

The term *sporadic goiter* encompasses goiters developing from a variety of causes; patients are usually euthyroid but may be hypothyroid. The most common cause of sporadic goiter is **lymphocytic thyroiditis** (see Chapter 560). Intrinsic biochemical defects in the synthesis of thyroid hormone are almost always associated with goiter. The occurrence of the disorder in siblings, onset in early life, and possible association with hypothyroidism (goitrous hypothyroidism) are important clues to the diagnosis.

Iodide Goiter. A small percentage of patients treated with iodide preparations for prolonged periods acquire goiters. Iodides are commonly included for their expectorant effect in cough medicines and in proprietary mixtures for asthma. Goiters resulting from iodine administration are firm and diffusely enlarged, and in some instances hypothyroidism may develop. In normal individuals, acute administration of large doses of iodine inhibits the organification of iodine and the synthesis of thyroid hormone (Wolff-Chaikoff effect). This effect is short-lived and does not lead to hypothyroidism. When iodide administration continues, an autoregulatory mechanism in normal persons limits iodine trapping and permits the level of iodide in the thyroid to decrease and organification to proceed normally. In patients with iodide-induced goiter, this escape does not occur because of an underlying abnormality of biosynthesis of thyroid hormone. The persons most susceptible to the development of iodide goiter are those with lymphocytic thyroiditis or with a subclinical inborn error in thyroid hormone synthesis and those who have had a partial thyroidectomy.

Lithium carbonate also causes goiters; it is currently widely used as a psychotropic drug. Lithium competes with iodide; the mechanism producing the goiter or hypothyroidism is similar to that described earlier for iodide goiter. Lithium and iodide also act synergistically to produce goiter; their combined use should be avoided.

Amiodarone, a drug used to treat cardiac arrhythmias, can cause thyroid dysfunction with goiter because it is rich in iodine. It is also a potent inhibitor of 5′-deiodinase, preventing conversion of T_4 to T_3. It can cause hypothyroidism, particularly in patients with underlying autoimmune disease; in other patients, it may cause hyperthyroidism.

Simple Goiter (Colloid Goiter). A few children with euthyroid nontoxic goiters have simple goiters, a condition of unknown cause not associated with hypothyroidism or hyperthyroidism and not caused by inflammation or neoplasia. The condition predominates in girls and has a peak incidence before and during the pubertal years. Histologic examination of the thyroid either is normal or reveals variable follicular size, dense colloid, and flattened epithelium. The goiter may be small or large. It is firm in half the patients and is occasionally asymmetric or nodular. Levels of TSH are normal or low, scintiscans are normal, and thyroid antibodies are absent. Differentiation from lymphocytic thyroiditis may not be possible without a biopsy, but biopsy ordinarily is not indicated. Therapy with thyroid hormone may help avoid progression to a large multinodular goiter, although it is difficult to separate any treatment effects from the natural history, which is for the goiter to decrease in size. Untreated patients should be re-evaluated periodically. This condition must be differentiated from lymphocytic thyroiditis (see Chapter 560).

Multinodular Goiter. Rarely, a firm goiter with a lobulated surface and single or multiple palpable nodules is encountered. Areas of cystic change, hemorrhage, and fibrosis may be present. The incidence of this condition has decreased markedly with the use of iodine-enriched salt. A mild goitrogenic stimulus, acting over a long time, is thought to be the cause. Ultrasonographic examination may reveal multiple echo-free and echogenic lesions that are nonfunctioning on scintiscans. Thyroid studies are usually normal, but TSH may be elevated and thyroid antibodies may be present. The condition occurs in children with McCune-Albright syndrome (usually resulting in hyperthyroidism) and has been described in three children (including two siblings) with digital anomalies and cystic renal disease. Dominant nodules within a multinodular goiter, particularly those not suppressed by replacement therapy with T_4, may be an indication for evaluation by fine-needle aspiration because malignancy cannot readily be ruled out.

Toxic Goiter (Hyperthyroidism). See Chapter 562.

561.4 Intratracheal Goiter

One of the many ectopic locations of thyroid tissue is within the trachea. The intraluminal thyroid lies beneath the tracheal mucosa and is frequently continuous with the normally situated extratracheal thyroid. The thyroid tissue is susceptible to goitrous enlargement, which involves the normally situated and the ectopic thyroid. When there is obstruction of the airway associated with a goiter, it must be ascertained whether the obstruction is extratracheal or endotracheal. If obstructive manifestations are mild, administration of sodium-L-thyroxine usually causes the goiter to decrease in size. When symptoms are severe, surgical removal of the endotracheal goiter is indicated (also see Chapter 561.1).

Goiter

Brix TH, Kyvik KO, Hegedus L: Major role of genes in the etiology of simple goiter in females: A population-based twin study. *J Clin Endocrinol Metab* 1999;84:3071.

Daneman D, Davy T, Mancer K, et al: Association of multinodular goiter, cystic renal disease, and digital anomalies. *J Pediatr* 1985;107:270.

Feuillan PP, Shawker T, Rose SR, et al: Thyroid abnormalities in the McCune-Albright syndrome. Ultrasonography and hormonal studies. *J Clin Endocrinol Metab* 1990;71:1596.

Jaruratanasirkul S, Leethanaporn K, Suchat K: The natural clinical course of children with an initial diagnosis of simple goiter: A 5-year longitudinal follow-up. *J Pediatr Endocrinol Metab* 2000;13:1109.

Lisboa HR, Gross JL, Orsolin A, et al: Clinical examination is not an accurate method of defining the presence of goiter in schoolchildren. *Clin Endocrinol* 1996;45:471.

Pharoah POD, Buttfield IH, Hetzel BS: Neurological damage to the foetus resulting from severe iodine deficiency during pregnancy. *Lancet* 1971;1:308.

Vade A, Gottschalk ME, Yetter EM, et al: Sonographic measurements of the neonatal thyroid gland. *J Ultrasound Med* 1997;16:395.

Vicens-Calvet E, Potau N, Carreras E, et al: Diagnosis and treatment in utero of goiter with hypothyroidism caused by iodine overload. *J Pediatr* 1998;133:147.

Goitrous Cretinism

Abramowicz MJ, Targovnik HM, Cochaux P, et al: Identification of a mutation in the coding sequence of the human thyroid peroxidase gene causing congenital goiter. *J Clin Invest* 1992;90:1200.

Aghini-Lombardi, F, Antonangeli L, Pinchera, A, et al: Effect of iodized salt on thyroid volume of children living in an area previously characterized by moderate iodine deficiency. *J Clin Endocrinol Metab* 1997;82:1136.

Benmiloud M, Chaouki ML, Gutekunst R, et al: Oral iodized oil for correcting iodine deficiency: Optimal dosing and outcome indicator selection. *J Clin Endocrinol Metab* 1994;79:20.

Bikker H, den Hartog MT, Baas F, et al: A 20-base pair duplication in the human thyroid peroxidase gene results in a total iodide organification defect and congenital hypothyroidism. *J Clin Endocrinol Metab* 1994;79:248.

Boyages SC, Halpern JP, Maberly GF, et al: A comparative study of neurological and myxedematous endemic cretinism in western China. *J Clin Endocrinol Metab* 1988;67:1262.

Boyages SC, Halpern JP, Maberly GF, et al: Endemic cretinism: Possible role for thyroid autoimmunity. *Lancet* 1989;2:529.

Boyages SC, Halpern JP, Maberly GF, et al: Supplementary iodine fails to reverse hypothyroidism in adolescents and adults with endemic cretinism. *J Clin Endocrinol Metab* 1990;70:336.

Couch RM, Dean HJ, Winter JS: Congenital hypothyroidism caused by defective iodide transport. *J Pediatr* 1985;106:950.

Gattereau A, Bernard B, Bellabarba D, et al: Congenital goiter in four euthyroid siblings with glandular and circulating iodoproteins and defective iodothyronine synthesis. *J Clin Endocrinol Metab* 1973;37:118.

Illum P, Kiaer HW, Hvidberg-Hansen J, et al: Fifteen cases of Pendred's syndrome. Congenital deafness and sporadic goiter. *Arch Otolaryngol* 1972;96:297.

Medeiros-Neto G, Targovnik HM, Vassart G: Defective thyroglobulin synthesis and secretion causing goiter and hypothyroidism. *Endocr Rev* 1993;14:165.

Weetman AP: Is endemic goiter an autoimmune disease? [Editorial.] *J Clin Endocrinol Metab* 1994;78:1017.

Chapter 562
Hyperthyroidism

Hyperthyroidism results from excessive secretion of thyroid hormone and, with few exceptions, is due to diffuse toxic goiter (Graves disease) during childhood. Germ line mutations of the thyroid-stimulating hormone (TSH) receptor resulting in constitutively activating (i.e., gain of function) mutations have been reported in both familial (autosomal dominant) and sporadic cases of non-autoimmune hyperthyroidism. These patients, who may present in the neonatal period or in later childhood, have thyroid hyperplasia with goiters and suppressed levels of TSH. Different activating mutations have been identified in some cases of thyroid adenomas. Hyperthyroidism occurs in some patients with McCune-Albright syndrome, which is the result of an activating mutation of the α subunit of the G protein; these patients tend to have a multinodular goiter. Other rare causes of hyperthyroidism that have been observed in children include toxic uninodular goiter (Plummer disease), hyperfunctioning thyroid carcinoma, thyrotoxicosis factitia, subacute thyroiditis, and acute suppurative thyroiditis. Suppression of plasma TSH indicates that the hyperthyroidism is not pituitary in origin. Hyperthyroidism due to excess thyrotropin secretion is rare and, in most cases, is caused by pituitary unresponsiveness to thyroid hormone. TSH-secreting pituitary tumors have been reported only in adults. In infants born to mothers with Graves disease, hyperthyroidism is almost always a transitory phenomenon; classic Graves disease during the neonatal period is rare. Choriocarcinoma, hydatidiform mole, and struma ovarii have caused hyperthyroidism in adults but have not been recognized as causes in children.

562.1 Graves Disease

Epidemiology. Graves disease occurs in approximately 0.02% of children (1:5,000). It has a peak incidence in the 11–15 year old; there is a 5:1 female to male ratio. Most children with Graves disease have a positive family history of some form of autoimmune thyroid disease.

Etiology. Enlargement of the thymus, splenomegaly, lymphadenopathy, infiltration of the thyroid gland and retro-orbital tissues with lymphocytes and plasma cells, and peripheral lymphocytosis are well-established findings in Graves disease. In the thyroid gland, T helper cells ($CD4^+$) tend to predominate in dense lymphoid aggregates; in areas of lower cell density, cytotoxic T cells ($CD8^+$) predominate. The percentage of activated B lymphocytes infiltrating the thyroid is higher than in peripheral blood. A postulated failure of T suppressor cells allows expression of T helper cells, sensitized to the TSH antigen, which interact with B cells. These cells differentiate into plasma cells, which produce thyrotropin receptor-stimulating antibody (TRSAb). TRSAb binds to the receptor for TSH and stimulates cyclic adenosine monophosphate, analogous to TSH itself. In addition to TRSAb, thyrotropin receptor-blocking antibody (TRBAb) may also be produced, and the clinical course of the disease usually correlates with the ratio between the two antibodies.

The ophthalmopathy occurring in Graves disease appears to be caused by antibodies against antigens shared by the thyroid and eye muscle. TSH receptors have been identified in retro-orbital adipocytes and may represent a target for antibodies. The antibodies that bind to the extraocular muscles and orbital fibroblasts stimulate the synthesis of glycosaminoglycans by orbital fibroblasts and produce cytotoxic effects on muscle cells.

In whites, Graves disease is associated with HLA-B8 and HLA-DR3; the latter carries a sevenfold relative risk for Graves disease. Therefore, it is not surprising that Graves disease is also associated with other HLA-D3–related disorders such as Addison disease, insulin-dependent diabetes mellitus, myasthenia gravis, and celiac disease. Systemic lupus erythematosus, rheumatoid arthritis, vitiligo, idiopathic thrombocytopenic purpura, and pernicious anemia have been described in children with Graves disease. In family clusters, the conditions associated most frequently with Graves disease are lymphocytic thyroiditis, autoimmune hypothyroidism, and neonatal hyperthyroidism.

Clinical Manifestations. About 5% of all patients with hyperthyroidism are younger than 15 yr of age; the peak incidence in these children occurs during adolescence. Graves disease has begun between 6 wk and 2 yr of age in children born to mothers without a history of hyperthyroidism. The incidence is about five times higher in girls than in boys.

The clinical course in children is highly variable but usually is not as fulminant as it is in many adults (Box 562–1). Symptoms develop gradually; the usual interval between onset and diagnosis is 6–12 mo and may be longer in prepubertal children compared with adolescents. The earliest signs in children may be emotional disturbances accompanied by motor hyperactivity. The children become irritable, excitable, and cry easily because of emotional lability. Their schoolwork suffers as a result of a short attention span. Tremor of the fingers can be noticed if the arm is extended. There may be a voracious appetite combined with loss of or no increase in weight. The size of the thyroid is variable. It may be enlarged so little that it escapes detection initially, but with careful examination, a goiter is found in almost all patients. Exophthalmos is noticeable in most patients but is usually mild. Lagging of the upper eyelid as the eye looks downward, impairment of convergence, and retraction of the upper eyelid and infrequent blinking may be present (Fig. 562–1). The skin is smooth and flushed, with excessive sweating. Muscular weakness is uncommon but may be severe enough to result in falling spells. Tachycardia, palpitations, dyspnea, and cardiac enlargement and insufficiency cause discomfort but rarely endanger the patient's life. Atrial fibrillation is a rare complication. Mitral regurgitation, probably resulting from papillary muscle dysfunction, is the cause of the apical systolic murmur present in some patients. The systolic blood pressure and the pulse pressure are increased. Many of the findings in Graves disease result from hyperactivity of the sympathetic nervous system.

Thyroid "crisis," or "storm," is a form of hyperthyroidism manifested by an acute onset, hyperthermia, and severe tachycardia and restlessness. There may be rapid progression to delirium, coma, and death. "Apathetic," or "masked," hyperthyroidism is another variety of hyperthyroidism characterized by extreme listlessness, apathy, and cachexia. A combination of both forms may also occur. These symptom complexes are rare in children.

Laboratory Findings. Serum levels of thyroxine (T_4), triiodothyronine (T_3), free T_4, and free T_3 are elevated. In some patients, levels of T_3 may be more elevated than those of T_4. Levels of TSH are suppressed to less than normal levels. Thyroid peroxidase antibodies are often present. Most patients with newly diagnosed Graves disease have measurable TRSAb, and its disappearance predicts remission of the disease. Assays of TSH receptor antibodies are generally not necessary for diagnosis or management of Graves disease, but can be helpful in equivocal cases. Radioiodine is rapidly and diffusely concentrated in the thyroid, but this study is rarely necessary. Very young children

BOX 562–1. Major Symptoms and Signs of Hyperthyroidism and of Graves Disease and Conditions Associated with Graves Disease

MANIFESTATIONS OF HYPERTHYROIDISM

Symptoms
 Hyperactivity, irritability, altered mood, insomnia
 Heat intolerance, increased sweating
 Palpitations
 Fatigue, weakness
 Dyspnea
 Weight loss with increased appetite (weight gain in 10% of patients)
 Pruritus
 Increased stool frequency
 Thirst and polyuria
 Oligomenorrhea or amenorrhea, loss of libido
Signs
 Sinus tachycardia, atrial fibrillation
 Fine tremor, hyperkinesis, hyperreflexia
 Warm, moist skin
 Palmar erythema, onycholysis
 Hair loss
 Muscle weakness and wasting
 High-output heart failure, chorea, periodic paralysis
  (primarily in Asian men), psychosis*

MANIFESTATIONS OF GRAVES DISEASE

Diffuse goiter
Ophthalmopathy
 A feeling of grittiness and discomfort in the eye
 Retrobulbar pressure or pain
 Eyelid lag or retraction
 Periorbital edema, chemosis, scleral injection
 Exophthalmos (proptosis)
 Extraocular muscle dysfunction
 Exposure keratitis
 Optic neuropathy
Localized dermopathy
Lymphoid hyperplasia
Thyroid acropachy

CONDITIONS ASSOCIATED WITH GRAVES DISEASE

Type 1 diabetes mellitus
Addison disease
Vitiligo
Pernicious anemia
Alopecia areata
Myasthenia gravis
Celiac disease
Other autoimmune disorders associated with the HLA-DR3 haplotype

---

*These signs are rare.
Adapted from Weetman AP: Graves disease, *N Engl J Med* 2000;343: 1236–48.

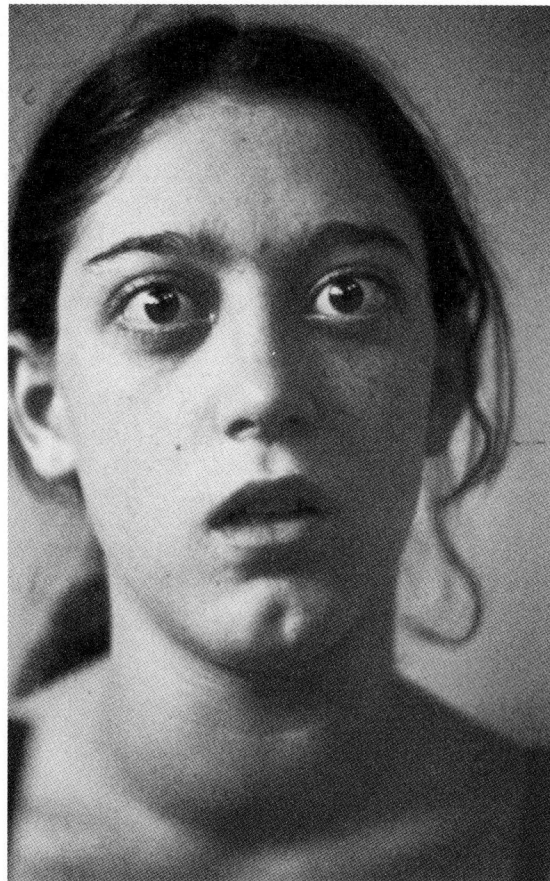

FIGURE 562–1. A 15-yr-old girl with classic Graves disease. Clinical features include a goiter and exophthalmos. She was treated with antithyroid drugs, to which she had a good response.

with Graves disease often have advanced skeletal maturation and craniostenosis. Bone density may be reduced at diagnosis but returns to normal with treatment.

Differential Diagnosis. Diagnosis is rarely difficult once hyperthyroidism is considered. Elevated levels of T_4 and free T_4 in association with suppressed levels of TSH are usually diagnostic. The presence of TRSAb establishes the cause as Graves disease.

Most other causes of hyperthyroxinemia are rare but may result in erroneous diagnosis. Patients with elevated thyroxine-binding globulin (TBG) levels or familial dysalbuminemic hyperthyroxinemia have normal levels of free T_4 and TSH. If a thyroid nodule is palpable, or if T_3 is preferentially elevated, a functional thyroid nodule must be considered; radionuclide study is diagnostic. If precocious puberty, polyostotic fibrous dysplasia, or café-au-lait pigmentation is present, the autonomous thyroid disorder of McCune-Albright syndrome is likely. Patients with generalized thyroid hormone unresponsiveness have elevated levels of free T_4, but levels of TSH are inappropriately elevated or normal. Patients with pituitary unresponsiveness to thyroid hormone also have clinical hyperthyroidism, but their levels of TSH are elevated or normal, and they must be differentiated from patients with TSH-secreting pituitary tumors who have elevated serum levels of the TSH α chain.

When hyperthyroxinemia is caused by exogenous thyroid hormone, levels of free T_4 and TSH are the same as those seen in Graves disease, but the level of thyroglobulin is very low, whereas in patients with Graves disease, it is elevated.

Treatment. Most pediatric endocrinologists recommend medical therapy using *antithyroid drugs* rather than radioiodine or subtotal thyroidectomy. The two antithyroid drugs in widest use are propylthiouracil (PTU) and methimazole (Tapazole). Both compounds inhibit incorporation of trapped inorganic iodide into organic compounds, and they may also suppress levels of TRSAb by directly affecting intrathyroidal autoimmunity. However, there are important differences between the two drugs. Methimazole is at least 10 times more potent than PTU on a weight basis and has a much longer serum half-life (6–8 hr vs 0.5 hr); PTU generally is administered three times daily, but methimazole can be given once daily. Unlike methimazole, PTU is heavily protein-bound and has a lesser ability to cross the placenta and to pass into breast milk; theoretically, PTU is the preferred drug during pregnancy and for nursing mothers. PTU, more than methimazole, inhibits extrathyroidal conversion of T_4 to T_3; this may be advantageous in the treatment of neonatal thyrotoxicosis.

Toxic reactions occur with both drugs; most are mild, but some are life-threatening. They are unpredictable and can occur after therapy of any duration. There is increasing evidence that these reactions may be fewer in patients treated with methimazole. Transient leukopenia ($<4,000/\text{mm}^3$) is common; it is asymptomatic and is not a harbinger of agranulocytosis, and it usually is not a reason to discontinue treatment. Transient urticarial rashes are common. They can be managed by a short period off therapy, restarting with the alternate antithyroid drug. The most severe reactions are hypersensitive and include agranulocytosis, hepatitis, hepatic failure, a lupus-like syndrome, glomerulonephritis, and a vasculitis involving the skin and other organs. Although uncommon, these reactions have been reported with both drugs, and it is probably best to treat unusually hypersensitive patients with radioiodine or thyroidectomy. Cases of congenital skin defects (aplasia cutis) have been seen in infants exposed in fetal life to methimazole, but this association does not appear to be a strong one.

The initial dosage of PTU is 5–10 mg/kg/24 hr given three times daily, and that of methimazole is 0.25–1.0 mg/kg/24 hr given once or twice daily. Smaller initial dosages should be used in early childhood. Careful surveillance is required after treatment is initiated. Rising serum levels of TSH to greater than normal indicates overtreatment and leads to increased size of the goiter. Clinical response becomes apparent in 2–3 wk, and adequate control is evident in 1–3 mo. The dose is decreased to the minimal level required to maintain a euthyroid state.

Drug therapy may be necessary for 5 yr or longer because there appears to be a remission rate of about 25% every 2 yr. If a relapse occurs, it usually appears within 3 mo and almost always within 6 mo after therapy has been discontinued. Therapy may be resumed in case of a relapse. Patients older than 13 yr of age, boys, those with a higher body mass index, and those with small goiters and modestly elevated T_3 levels appear to have earlier remissions.

A β-adrenergic blocking agent such as propranolol (0.5–2.0 mg/kg/24 hr po, given three times daily) is a useful supplement in the management of severely toxic patients. Thyroid hormones potentiate the actions of catecholamines, which include tachycardia, tremor, excessive sweating, lid lag, and stare. These symptoms abate with the use of propranolol, which does not, however, alter thyroid function or exophthalmos.

Surgery or radioiodine treatment is indicated when adequate cooperation for medical management is not possible or when adequate trial of medical management has failed to result in permanent remission or severe side effects preclude further use of antithyroid drugs. Subtotal thyroidectomy, a rather safe procedure if performed by an experienced team, is performed only after the patient has been brought to a euthyroid state. This may be accomplished with PTU or methimazole over 2–3 mo. After a euthyroid state has been attained, 5 drops of a saturated solution of potassium iodide/24 hr are added to the regimen for 2 wk before surgery to decrease the vascularity of the gland. Complications of surgical treatment are rare and include hypoparathyroidism (transient or permanent) and paralysis of the vocal cords. The incidence of residual or recurrent hyperthyroidism or hypothyroidism depends on the extent of the surgery. Most recommend near-total thyroidectomy. The incidence of recurrence is low, but that of hypothyroidism may exceed 50%.

Radioiodine is an effective, relatively safe first or alternate therapy for Graves disease in children over 10yr old. Pretreatment with antithyroid drugs is unnecessary; if a patient is taking them, they should be stopped a week before radioiodine administration. Most children become euthyroid after one dose (88% in one study), but a few may require a second or third dose. Because the full effects of treatment may not be complete for 2–3 mo, adjunctive therapy with a β-adrenergic antagonist and lower doses of antithyroid drugs are recommended. Although there have been concerns about radiation oncogenesis and genetic damage, follow-up of treated children for as long as 50 yr has not shown this. The risk of benign adenoma may be increased (0.6–1.9% in one study). The major consequence of radioiodine is hypothyroidism, which occurs in 10–20% of patients after the first year and in about 3% per year thereafter.

The ophthalmopathy remits gradually and usually independently of the hyperthyroidism. Severe ophthalmopathy may require treatment with prednisone or radiotherapy.

562.2 Congenital Hyperthyroidism

Etiology and Pathogenesis. Onset of neonatal hyperthyroidism usually begins prenatally and is present at birth, although it may not be noticed until a few days after birth; occasionally, onset may be delayed for several weeks or more. The mothers of these infants have active Graves disease, Graves disease in remission or, rarely, hypothyroidism, and a history of lymphocytic thyroiditis. The condition is caused by transplacental passage of TRSAb, but the clinical onset, severity, and course may be modified by the concurrent presence of TRBAb and by the transplacental passage of antithyroid drugs taken by the mother. Very high levels of TRSAb usually result in classic neonatal hyperthyroidism, but if the infant has been exposed to the antithyroid drugs, onset of symptoms is delayed 3–4 days to allow degradation of the maternally derived antithyroid drug. If TRBAb is also present, onset of hyperthyroid symptoms may be delayed for several weeks.

Neonatal hyperthyroidism occurs in only about 2% of infants born to mothers with a history of Graves disease. The finding of very high levels of TRSAb in these mothers usually predicts the occurrence of an affected infant. Fetal tachycardia and goiter may allow prenatal diagnosis. Unlike Graves disease at all other ages, neonatal hyperthyroidism affects boys as often as girls. The disorder usually remits spontaneously within 6–12 wk but may persist longer, depending on the levels of TRSAb. Mild asymptomatic hyperthyroxinemia also occurs. Rarely, classic neonatal Graves' disease does not remit but persists for several years or longer. These children have impressive family histories of Graves' disease. In these infants, TRSAb transfer from the mother apparently blends with the infantile onset of autonomous Graves disease.

Clinical Manifestations. Many of the infants are premature and appear to have intrauterine growth retardation. Most have goiters. The infant is extremely restless, irritable, and hyperactive, and appears anxious and unusually alert. Microcephaly and ventricular enlargement may be present. The eyes are opened widely and appear exophthalmic (Fig. 562–2). There may be extreme tachycardia and tachypnea, and the temperature is elevated. In severely affected infants, there is a progression of symptoms; weight loss occurs despite a ravenous appetite, hepatosplenomegaly increases, and jaundice may become manifested. Cardiac decompensation is common, and severe hypertension may occur. The infant may die if therapy is not instituted promptly. The serum level of T_4 is markedly elevated and TSH is suppressed. Advanced bone age, frontal bossing with triangular facies, and cranial synostosis are common, especially in infants with persistent clinical manifestations of hyperthyroidism.

Treatment. Treatment consists of oral administration of propranolol (1–2 mg/kg/24 hr, orally in three divided doses) and PTU (5–10 mg/kg/24 hr given every 8 hr); Lugol solution (1 drop every 8 hr) may be added. When propranolol is used during pregnancy to treat thyrotoxicosis, it crosses the placenta and may cause respiratory depression in the newborn infant. If the thyrotoxic state is severe, parenteral fluid therapy and corticosteroids may be indicated. If heart failure occurs, digitalization is indicated. After a euthyroid state is reached, only PTU treatment is necessary. The dose should be gradually tapered to keep the infant euthyroid. Most cases remit by 3–4 mo of age.

Occasionally, neonatal hyperthyroidism does not remit but persists into childhood. These patients may have an impressive family history of hyperthyroidism. Several cases of neonatal

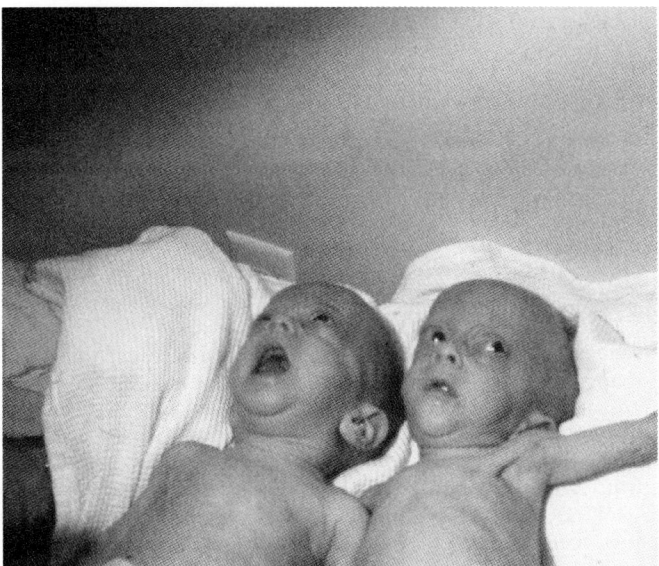

FIGURE 562–2. Twin boys with neonatal hyperthyroidism confirmed by abnormal thyroid function tests. Clinical features include lack of subcutaneous tissue due to a hypermetabolic state and a wide-eyed, anxious stare. They were given the diagnosis of neonatal Graves disease, but, in fact, their mother did not have Graves disease; they had persistent, not transient, hyperthyroidism. At age 8 yr, they were treated with radioiodine. They are now believed to have had some other form of neonatal hyperthyroidism, such as a constitutive activation of the TSH receptor.

hyperthyroidism, without evidence for autoimmune disease in infant or mother, have now been reported due to a mutation in the TSHR gene, which produced constitutive activation of the receptor. Hyperthyroidism recurs when antithyroid drugs are discontinued; these children must be treated with radioiodine or surgery.

Prognosis. Advanced osseous maturation, microcephaly, and mental retardation occur when treatment is delayed. Prognosis for intellectual development is guarded in infants with neonatal Graves disease.

Bahn RS, Heufelder AE: Pathogenesis of Graves' ophthalmopathy. *N Engl J Med* 1993;329:1468.

Botero D, Brown RS. Bioassay of the thyrotropin receptor antibodies with Chinese hamster ovary cells transfected with recombinant human thyrotropin receptor: Clinical utility in children and adolescents with Graves' disease. *J Pediatr* 1998;132:612.

Bowman ML, Bergmann M, Smith JF: Intrapartum labetalol for the treatment of maternal and fetal thyrotoxicosis. *Thyroid* 1998;8:795.

Cheron RG, Kaplan MM, Larsen PR, et al: Neonatal thyroid function after propylthiouracil therapy for maternal Graves' disease. *N Engl J Med* 1981;304:525.

Clark JD, Gelfand MJ, Elgazzar AH: Iodine-131 therapy of hyperthyroidism in pediatric patients. *J Nucl Med* 1995;36:442.

Daneman D, Howard NJ: Neonatal thyrotoxicosis: Intellectual impairment and craniosynostosis in later years. *J Pediatr* 1980;97:257.

DeLuca G, Chaussain JL, Job JC: Hyperfunctioning thyroid nodules in children and adolescents. *Acta Paediatr Scand* 1986;75:118.

Duprez L, Parma J, Van Sande J, et al: Germline mutations in the thyrotropin receptor gene cause non-autoimmune autosomal dominant hyperthyroidism. *Nat Genet* 1994;7:396.

Glaser NS, Styne DM: Predictors of early remission of hyperthyroidism in children. *J Clin Endocrinol Metab* 1997;82:1719.

Hashizume K, Ichikawa K, Sakurai A, et al: Administration of thyroxine in treated Graves' disease. Effects on the level of antibodies to thyroid-stimulating hormone receptors and on the risk of recurrence of hyperthyroidism. *N Engl J Med* 1991;324:947.

Kopp P, van Sande J, Parma J, et al: Brief report: Congenital hyperthyroidism caused by a mutation in the thyrotropin-receptor gene. *N Engl J Med* 1995;332:150.

Levy WJ, Schumacher P, Gupta M: Treatment of childhood Graves' disease: A review with emphasis on radioiodine treatment. *Cleve Clin J Med* 1988;55:373.

Mastorakos G, Mitsiades NS, Doufas AG, et al: Hyperthyroidism in McCune-Albright syndrome with a review of thyroid abnormalities sixty years after the first report. *Thyroid* 1997;7:433.

Milham S Jr: Scalp defects in infants of mothers treated for hyperthyroidism with methimazole or carbimazole during pregnancy. *Teratology* 1985;32:321.

Mouritis MP, van Kempen-Hartveld ML, Garcia MB, et al: Radiotherapy for Graves orbitopathy: Randomized placebo-controlled study. *Lancet* 2000;355:1505–10.

Polak M, Leger J, Luton D, Oury JF, et al: Fetal cord blood sampling in the diagnosis and the treatment of fetal hyperthyroidism in the offspring of the euthyroid mother producing thyroid-stimulating immunoglobulins. *Ann Endocrinol* 1997;58:338.

Polak M: Hyperthyroidism in early infancy: Pathogenesis, clinical features and diagnosis with a focus on neonatal hyperthyroidism. *Thyroid* 1998;8:1171.

Rivkees SA, Sklar C, Freemark M: The management of Graves' disease in children, with special emphasis on radioiodine treatment. *J Clin Endocrinol Metab* 1998;83:3767.

Segni M, Leonardi E, Mazzoncini B, et al. Special features of Graves' disease in early childhood. *Thyroid* 1999;9:871.

Shulman DI, Muhar I, Jorgensen EV, et al: Autoimmune hyperthyroidism in prepubertal children and adolescents: Comparison of clinical and biochemical features at diagnosis and responses to medical therapy. *Thyroid* 1997;7:755.

Sills IN: Hyperthyroidism. *Pediatr Rev* 1994;15:417.

Skuza KA, Sills IN, Stene M, et al: Prediction of neonatal hyperthyroidism in infants born to mothers with Graves' disease. *J Pediatr* 1996;128:264.

Soreide JA, van Heerden JA, Lo CY, et al: Surgical treatment of Graves' disease in patients younger than 18 years. *World J Surg* 1996;20:794.

Stenszky V, Kozma L, Balazs C, et al: The genetics of Graves disease: HLA and disease susceptibility. *J Clin Endocrinol Metab* 1985;61:835.

Volpe R, Ehrlich R, Steiner G, et al: Graves' disease in pregnancy years after hypothyroidism with recurrent passive-transfer neonatal Graves disease in offspring. Therapeutic considerations. *Am J Med* 1984;77:572.

Weetman AP: Graves Disease. *N Engl J Med* 2000;343:1236–48.

Zimmerman D, Lteif AN. Thyrotoxicosis in children. *Endocrinol Metab Clin North Am* 1998;27:109.

Chapter 563

Carcinoma of the Thyroid

Epidemiology. Carcinoma of the thyroid is rare in childhood; the annual incidence in children younger than 15 yr of age is approximately 0.5 cases/million, compared with an annual incidence at all ages around the world ranging from 0.5 to 10 cases/million. Unlike other malignancies in childhood, thyroid cancer usually has an indolent course, even after pulmonary metastases have developed.

Pathogenesis. Genetic factors and radiation exposure are important factors in the pathogenesis of thyroid cancer. Rearrangements of the RET proto-oncogene are found in 3–33% of papillary carcinomas and 60–80% of those occurring after irradiation, as in children in Belarus exposed to radiation after the nuclear accident at Chernobyl or in those who were exposed to external radiation in childhood. Inactivating point mutations of the p53 tumor-suppressor gene are rare in patients with differentiated thyroid carcinoma but are common in those with anaplastic thyroid cancer. Overall, 5–10% of cases of papillary thyroid carcinoma are familial and are usually inherited in an autosomal dominant manner. The thyroid gland of children is unusually sensitive to exposure to external radiation. There probably is no threshold dose; 1 Gy results in a 7.7 relative risk of thyroid cancer. In the past, about 80% of children with cancer of the thyroid had received irradiation of the neck and adjacent areas during infancy for benign conditions such as "enlarged" thymus, hypertrophied tonsils and adenoids, hemangiomas, nevi, eczema, tinea capitis, and "cervical adenitis." With the discontinuation of irradiation for benign conditions, this cause of thyroid cancer has vanished. However, the long-term survival of children who have received therapeutic irradiation of areas of the neck for neoplastic disease has now made this cause of thyroid cancer and nodules increasingly prevalent; increased dose, younger age at time of treatment, and female sex are factors that increase the risk of thyroid cancer developing. Long-term risk data for cancer are sparse, but 15–50% of children who have received irradiation and chemotherapy for Hodgkin disease, leukemia, and other malignancies of the head and neck have elevated levels of thyroid-stimulating hormone (TSH) within the 1st yr of therapy, and 5–20% progress to hypothyroidism during the next 5–7 yr. Most large groups of treated children have a 10–30% incidence of benign thyroid nodules and an increased incidence of thyroid cancer. The latter begins to appear within 3–5 yr after radiation treatment and reaches a peak in 15–25 yr. It is unknown whether there is a period after which no more tumors develop. Administration of iodine-131 for diagnostic or therapeutic purposes does not appear to increase the risk of thyroid cancer.

Histologically, the carcinomas are papillary (80%), follicular (17%), medullary (2%), or mixed differentiated tumors. These are usually slow-growing tumors and may remain dormant for years. The type of tumor and the natural course of disease in irradiated and nonirradiated patients are the same, except that multicentricity is more frequent in irradiation-induced cancer. Undifferentiated (anaplastic) thyroid neoplasms are rare in children and usually have a rapidly fatal course.

Clinical Manifestations. Girls are affected twice as often as boys. The average age at diagnosis is 9 yr, but the onset may be as early as the 1st yr of life. A painless nodule in the thyroid or in the neck is the usual first evidence of disease. Cervical lymph node involvement is often present at the time of initial diagnosis. Any unexplained cervical lymph node enlargement requires examination of the thyroid, which occasionally has a primary tumor too small to be felt; the diagnosis is based on biopsy results of the lymph node. The lungs are the most common site of metastases beyond the neck. There may be no clinical manifestations referable to them; roentgenographically, they appear as diffuse miliary or nodular infiltrations, principally in the basal portions. They may be mistaken for tuberculosis, histoplasmosis, or sarcoidosis. Other sites of metastases include the mediastinum, long bones, skull, and axilla. Almost all children are euthyroid, but rarely, the carcinoma may be functional and produce symptoms of hyperthyroidism.

Diagnosis. The most helpful diagnostic test in the case of a solitary nodule is fine needle aspiration (FNA). An ultrasonographic examination of the thyroid can provide information on the consistency of the nodule (solid vs cystic) and whether other nonpalpable nodules are present. A thyroid scan, preferably using ^{123}I or ^{99m}Tc-pertechnetate, can provide information on trapping function, and whether the nodule is "cold," "warm," or "hot." The majority of cold nodules are benign. Neither ultrasound nor a thyroid scan can differentiate between a benign or malignant lesion. FNAs may be interpreted as benign tumor, malignant tumor, indeterminate, or inadequate specimen. Experience in children using FNA generally shows a 5–10% false-negative rate and a 1–2% false-positive rate, with an overall diagnostic accuracy of 90–95%. Generally tests of thyroid function are normal, but Hashimoto's thyroiditis has been associated with thyroid cancer.

Treatment. Because differentiated thyroid carcinoma is a chronic disease with a long survival, optimal therapy is still evolving. There is increasing evidence that small (<1 cm) papillary carcinoma, the least aggressive type, is effectively treated by subtotal thyroidectomy and suppressive doses of thyroid hormone. Papillary carcinomas tend to be multicentric, and several studies show that half these children have regional lymph node involvement at presentation. For larger papillary carcinomas, follicular carcinoma, or with regional lymph node involvement, near-total thyroidectomy with excision of regional lymph nodes appears to be the treatment of choice. There is no role for radical

neck dissection. Thyroidectomy is usually followed by an ablative dose (30–100 mCi) of ^{131}I.

After surgery, all patients should be treated with sodium-L-thyroxine in doses sufficient to suppress TSH to the lower range of normal. Serum thyroglobulin (Tg) is an excellent marker for tumor recurrence, and periodic determinations of Tg levels should be performed. If the patient has undergone a total thyroidectomy or ^{131}I ablation, the serum Tg level should be less than 5 ng/mL when thyroxine (T$_4$) suppressive therapy is being received. Patients with an elevated serum Tg should undergo radioactive iodine uptake and scan to locate the source of Tg and plan appropriate management.

Prognosis. For any form of therapy, survival or recurrence does not appear to be different for patients with or without involvement of the cervical nodes. Even patients with cervical or pulmonary metastases have survived many years. More than 95% of patients are alive 25 yr after initial treatment if the tumor was intrathyroid, less than 2 cm in diameter, and classified as grade 1. Greater tumor size, distant spread, and greater atypia are associated with increased cumulative mortality.

563.1   Solitary Thyroid Nodule

Solitary nodules of the thyroid are uncommon in children. Most are the result of benign tumors, such as follicular adenoma. In the past, it was estimated that as many as half were carcinomas, but later studies indicated that there is an approximately 15% incidence of malignancy, perhaps because of decreasing exposure of children to radiation (Box 563–1). Children exposed to radiation have a high incidence of benign adenoma and carcinoma of the thyroid.

Benign disorders that may present as solitary thyroid nodules include benign adenomas (e.g., follicular, embryonal, Hürthle cell), colloid (adenomatous) nodule, lymphocytic thyroiditis, thyroglossal duct cyst, ectopically located normal thyroid tissue, a single median thyroid, agenesis of one of the lateral thyroid lobes with hypertrophy of the contralateral lobe, thyroid cysts, and abscess. A suddenly appearing or rapidly enlarging thyroid mass may indicate hemorrhage into a benign adenoma. In most cases, the child is euthyroid, and thyroid function studies are normal. When lymphocytic thyroiditis is the cause of the nodule, T$_4$ may be low, TSH may be elevated, and thyroid antibodies are usually present. Radionuclide imaging, if performed, may reveal a moth-eaten appearance. Rarely, lymphocytic thyroiditis may be associated with carcinoma of

---

BOX 563–1. Etiologic Classification of Solitary Thyroid Nodules

Lymphoid follicle, as part of chronic lymphocytic thyroiditis
Thyroid developmental anomalies
  Hemiagenesis
  Intrathyroidal thyroglossal duct cyst
Thyroid abscess (acute suppurative thyroiditis)
Simple cyst
Neoplasms
  Benign
    Colloid (adenomatous) nodule
    Follicular adenoma
    Toxic adenoma
    Nonthyroidal (e.g., lymphohemangioma)
  Malignant
    Papillary carcinoma
    Follicular carcinoma
    Mixed papillary-follicular carcinoma
    Undifferentiated (anaplastic)
    Medullary carcinoma
    Nonthyroidal
      Lymphoma
      Teratoma

the thyroid. Ultrasonography is particularly useful in detecting cystic lesions.

The *diagnostic studies* to delineate the underlying cause include serum thyroid function tests, antithyroid antibody determinations, ultrasonographic examination of the thyroid, radionuclide uptake and scan, and FNA. Response to a trial of suppressive T_4 treatment to look for shrinkage of nodule size is not reliable. Although *thyroid carcinomas* generally present as a solid, cold nodule, most cold nodules are benign lesions. FNA is useful in avoiding surgery for benign nodules. However, surgery without delay is indicated when the nodule is hard or has grown rapidly, when there is evidence of tracheal or vocal cord involvement, or when there is enlargement of adjacent lymph nodes. All persons with a history of head or neck irradiation should have careful examinations of the thyroid at least every 2 yr indefinitely.

Rarely, thyroid nodules may be functional, producing hyperthyroidism *(Plummer disease)*. The uptake of radionuclide is concentrated in the nodule ("hot" or "warm" nodule), and thyroid function studies indicate that the nodule is functioning autonomously. Such nodules are usually benign, but a few instances of carcinoma in such cases have been reported. T_4 levels are usually normal, but triiodothyronine (T_3) levels are elevated (T_3 toxicosis), and TSH levels are suppressed. Treatment consists of surgical removal of the nodule.

563.2 Medullary Carcinoma

Medullary carcinoma of the thyroid arises from the parafollicular cells (C cells) of the thyroid and accounts for about 2% of thyroid malignancies. The most common symptom is goiter or a palpable thyroid nodule. Roentgenograms may reveal dense, conglomerate, homogeneous calcification in the thyroid. Metastases to the regional lymph nodes and to the liver are common, and these also may calcify. Death may result, but long survivals are common.

The tumors occur sporadically, as a familial autosomal dominant disorder, and as components of two distinct autosomal dominant syndromes. The susceptibility for all these disorders has been associated with germ line mutations of the RET proto-oncogene, which maps to chromosome 10q11.2. When the tumor occurs sporadically, it is usually unicentric, but in the familial form, it is usually multicentric, and it begins as hyperplasia of parafollicular cells. The tumors are often too small to be found by palpation, scintigraphy, or ultrasonographic examination in at-risk patients in these families. Diagnosis of medullary carcinoma should lead to a careful search for associated tumors, particularly pheochromocytoma. No clinically recognizable manifestations result from the elevated serum levels of calcitonin or from the calcitonin gene-related peptide.

Multiple Endocrine Neoplasia, Type IIA. When hyperplasia or carcinoma of C cells is associated with adrenal medullary hyperplasia or pheochromocytoma and parathyroid hyperplasia, it is known as multiple endocrine neoplasia (MEN) IIA. The inheritance pattern for MEN IIA is autosomal dominant, with a high degree of penetrance and variable expressivity. At least 19 different specific missense mutations of exon 10 or 11 of the extracellular domain of the RET gene have been described for MEN IIA and for cases of familial medullary thyroid carcinoma. DNA analysis permits unambiguous identification of carriers of the RET proto-oncogene gene. C-cell hyperplasia or tumors usually appear earlier than pheochromocytoma. Pheochromocytomas are frequently bilateral and may be multiple. Adrenal medullary hyperplasia is known to precede pheochromocytoma, but the detectable latent period is short. Hypercalcemia is a late manifestation and indicates hyperparathyroidism. The parathyroid glands may reveal chief-cell hyperplasia or only hypercellularity.

Multiple Endocrine Neoplasia, Type IIB. The distinguishing feature of MEN IIB, also called the *mucosal neuroma syndrome,* is the occurrence of multiple neuromas and a characteristic phenotype associated with medullary carcinoma and pheochromocytoma. This condition is also autosomal dominant, and 93% of families have a missense mutation of the RET proto-oncogene. However, the mutation is in exon 16, the tyrosine catalytic domain of RET; all patients have had the same point mutation.

The neuromas most often occur on the tongue, buccal mucosa, lips, and conjunctivae. Peripheral neurofibromas and café-au-lait patches may be present, and intestinal ganglioneuromatosis is common. Diffuse proliferation of nerves and ganglion cells is found in mucosal, submucosal, myenteric, and subserosal plexus involving the small and large bowel as well as the esophagus. The patients may be tall, with arachnodactyly and a Marfan-like appearance. Scoliosis, pectus excavatum, pes cavus, and muscular hypotonia are common. The eyelids may be thickened and everted, the lips patulous and blubbery, the jaw prognathic. Feeding difficulties, poor sucking, diarrhea, constipation, and failure to thrive may begin in infancy or early childhood, many years before the appearance of neuromas or endocrine symptoms.

Treatment. Total thyroidectomy is indicated for all children who are shown by DNA studies to carry the gene. Recognition of familial forms of this tumor is critical to the early diagnosis in children at risk. Evidence suggests that thyroidectomy must be performed early because medullary carcinoma has been seen in a 6-mo-old child with MEN IIB and in a 3-yr-old child with MEN IIA. Monitoring the levels of calcitonin is useful in following the course of the disease after operation and detecting metastatic lesions. Periodic screening for the development of pheochromocytoma is indicated.

Corrias A, Einaudi E, Chiorboli G, et al. Accuracy of fine needle aspiration biopsy of thyroid nodules in detecting malignancy in childhood: Comparison with conventional clinical, laboratory, and imaging approaches. *J Clin Endocrinol Metab* 2001;86:4644.

Crom DB, Kaste SC, Tubergen DG, et al: Ultrasonography for thyroid screening after head and neck irradiation in childhood cancer survivors. *Med Pediatr Oncol* 1997;28:15.

Degnan BM, McClellan DR, Francis GL: An analysis of fine-needle aspiration biopsy of the thyroid in children and adolescents. *J Pediatr Surg* 1996;31:903.

Eng C, Smith DP, Mulligan LH, et al: Point mutation within the tyrosine kinase domain of the *RET* proto-oncogene in multiple endocrine neoplasia type 2B and related sporadic tumors. *Hum Mol Genet* 1994;3:237.

Feinmesser R, Lubin E, Segal K, et al: Carcinoma of the thyroid in children—a review. *J Pediatr Endocrinol Metab* 1997;10:561.

Flannery TK, Kirkland JL, Copeland KC, et al: Papillary thyroid cancer: A pediatric perspective. *Pediatrics* 1996;98:464.

Fleming ID, Black TL, Thompson EI, et al: Thyroid dysfunction and neoplasia in children receiving neck irradiation for cancer. *Cancer* 1985;55:1190.

Heshmati HM, Gharib H, Khosla S, et al: Genetic testing in medullary thyroid carcinoma syndromes: Mutation types and clinical significance. *Mayo Clin Proc* 1997; 72:430.

Hopwood NJ, Kelch RP: Thyroid masses: Approach to diagnosis and management in childhood and adolescence. *Pediatr Rev* 1993;14:481.

Hung W, Anderson KD, Chandra RS, et al: Solitary thyroid nodules in 71 children and adolescents. *J Pediatr Surg* 1992;27:1407.

Keiser HR, Beaven MA, Doppham J, et al: Sipple's syndrome: Medullary thyroid carcinoma, pheochromocytoma and parathyroid disease. *Ann Intern Med* 1973; 78:561.

Kendall-Taylor P: Managing differential thyroid cancer. *Br Med J* 2002;324:988–9.

Kirk JM, Mort C, Grand DB, et al: The usefulness of serum thyroglobulin in the follow-up of differentiated thyroid carcinoma in children. *Med Pediatr Oncol* 1992;20:201.

Lafferty AR, Batch JA: Thyroid nodules in childhood and adolescence—Thirty years of experience. *J Pediatr Endocrinol Metab* 1997;10:479.

Lips CJ, Landsvater RM, Hoppener JW, et al: Clinical screening as compared with DNA analysis in families with multiple endocrine neoplasia type 2A. *N Engl J Med* 1994;331:828.

Mazzaferri EL: Management of a solitary thyroid nodule. *N Engl J Med* 1993;328: 553.

Nikiforov YE, Rowland JM, Bove KE, et al: Distinct pattern of ret oncogene rearrangements in morphological variants of radiation-induced and sporadic thyroid papillary carcinomas in children. *Cancer Res* 1997;57:1690.

Raab SS, Silverman JF, Elsheikh TM, et al: Pediatric thyroid nodules: Disease demographics and clinical management as determined by fine needle aspiration biopsy. *Pediatrics* 1995;95:46.

Schlumberger MJ: Papillary and follicular thyroid carcinoma. *N Engl J Med* 1998; 338:297.

Scott MD, Crawford JD: Solitary thyroid nodules in childhood: Is the incidence of thyroid carcinoma declining? *Pediatrics* 1976;58:521.

Stjernholm MR, Freudenborg JC, Mooney HS, et al: Medullary carcinoma of the thyroid before age 2 years. *J Clin Endocrinol Metab* 1980;51:252.

Vane D, King DR, Boles ET Jr: Secondary thyroid neoplasm in pediatric cancer patients: Increased risk with improved survival. *J Pediatr Surg* 1984;19: 855.

Zimmerman D: Thyroid neoplasia in children. *Curr Opin Pediatr* 1997;9:407.

SECTION 3 *Disorders of the Parathyroid*

Daniel A. Doyle and Angelo M. DiGeorge

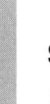

Chapter 564

Hormones and Peptides of Calcium Homeostasis and Bone Metabolism

Parathyroid hormone (PTH) and vitamin D are the principal regulators of calcium homeostasis (see Chapters 44, 48, and 691). Calcitonin and PTH-related peptide (PTHrP) appear to be important primarily in the fetus.

Parathyroid Hormone. PTH is an 84-amino acid chain (9,500 d), but its biologic activity resides in the first 34 residues. In the parathyroid gland, a pre-pro-PTH (115-amino acid chain) and a proparathyroid hormone (90 amino acids) are synthesized. Pre-pro-PTH is converted to pro-PTH and pro-PTH to PTH. PTH (1–84) is the major secretory product of the gland, but it is rapidly cleaved in the liver and kidney into smaller COOH-terminal, mid-region, and NH$_2$-terminal fragments.

The occurrence of these fragments in serum has led to the development of a variety of assays. The 1–34 amino-terminal (N-terminus) fragments possess biologic activity but are present in low amounts in the circulation; assay of these fragments is most useful for detecting acute secretory changes. The carboxy-terminal (C-terminus) and mid-region fragments, although biologically inert, are cleared more slowly from the circulation and represent 80% of plasma immunoreactive PTH; values of the C-terminal fragment are 50–500 times the level of the active hormone. The C-terminal assays are effective in detecting patients with hyperparathyroidism, but because C-terminal fragments are removed from the circulation by glomerular filtration, these assays are less useful for evaluating the secondary hyperparathyroidism characteristic of renal disease. Only certain sensitive radioimmunoassays for PTH can differentiate the subnormal concentrations that occur in hypoparathyroidism from normal levels. A sensitive 15-min immunochemiluminometric assay, developed for intraoperative use, can provide the surgeon with useful information.

When serum levels of calcium fall, the signal is transduced through the calcium-sensing receptor and secretion of PTH increases (Fig. 564–1). PTH stimulates activity of 1α-hydroxylase in the kidney, enhancing production of 1,25-dihydroxycholecalciferol (1,25[OH]$_2$D$_3$). The increased level of 1,25[OH]$_2$D$_3$ induces synthesis of a calcium-binding protein *(calbindin-D)* in the intestinal mucosa with resultant absorption of calcium. PTH also mobilizes calcium by directly enhancing bone resorption, an effect that requires 1,25[OH]$_2$D$_3$. The effects of PTH on bone and kidney are mediated through binding to specific receptors on the membranes of target cells and through activation of a transduction pathway involving a G protein coupled to the adenylate cyclase system (also see Chapter 566).

The *calcium-sensing receptor* regulates the secretion of PTH and the reabsorption of calcium by the renal tubules in response to alterations in serum calcium concentrations. The gene for the receptor is located on chromosome 3q13.3-q21 and encodes a cell surface protein of 1,078 amino acids that is expressed in parathyroid glands and kidneys and belongs to the family of G protein–coupled receptors. In the normally functioning calcium-sensing receptor, hypocalcemia induces increased secretion of PTH and hypercalcemia depresses PTH secretion. Loss of function mutations result in an increased set point with respect to serum calcium, resulting in hypercalcemia and in the conditions of familial hypocalciuric hypercalcemia and neonatal severe hyperparathyroidism. Gain of function mutations result in depressed secretion of PTH in response to hypocalcemia, leading to the syndrome of familial hypocalcemia with hypercalciuria (see Fig. 564–1).

Parathyroid Hormone-Related Peptide. PTHrP is homologous to PTH only in the first 13 amino acids of its amino terminus, 8 of which are identical to PTH. Its gene is on the short arm of chromosome 12, and that of PTH is on the short arm of chromosome 11.

PTHrP, like PTH, activates PTH receptors in kidney and bone cells and increases urinary cyclic adenosine monophosphate and renal production of 1,25[OH]$_2$D$_3$. It is produced in almost every type of cell of the body, including every tissue of the embryo at some stage of development. PTHrP is critical for normal fetal development. Inactivating mutations of the receptor for PTH/PTHrP result in a lethal bone disorder characterized by short limbs and markedly advanced bone maturation known as *Blomstrand chondrodysplasia* (see Fig. 564–1). It appears to have a paracrine or autocrine role because serum levels are low except in a few clinical situations. Cord blood contains levels of PTHrP that are threefold higher than in serum from adults; it is produced by the fetal parathyroid glands and appears to be the main agent stimulating maternal-fetal calcium transfer. PTHrP appears to be essential for normal skeletal maturation of the fetus, which requires 30 g of calcium. During pregnancy, maternal absorption of calcium increases from about 150 mg daily to 400 mg during the second trimester.

As in cord blood, PTHrP levels are increased during lactation and in patients with benign breast hypertrophy. Breast milk and pasteurized bovine milk have levels of PTHrP that are 10,000 times higher than those of normal plasma. Most instances of the hormonal hypercalcemia syndrome of malignancy are caused by elevated concentrations of PTHrP.

Vitamin D. See Chapters 44 and 48.

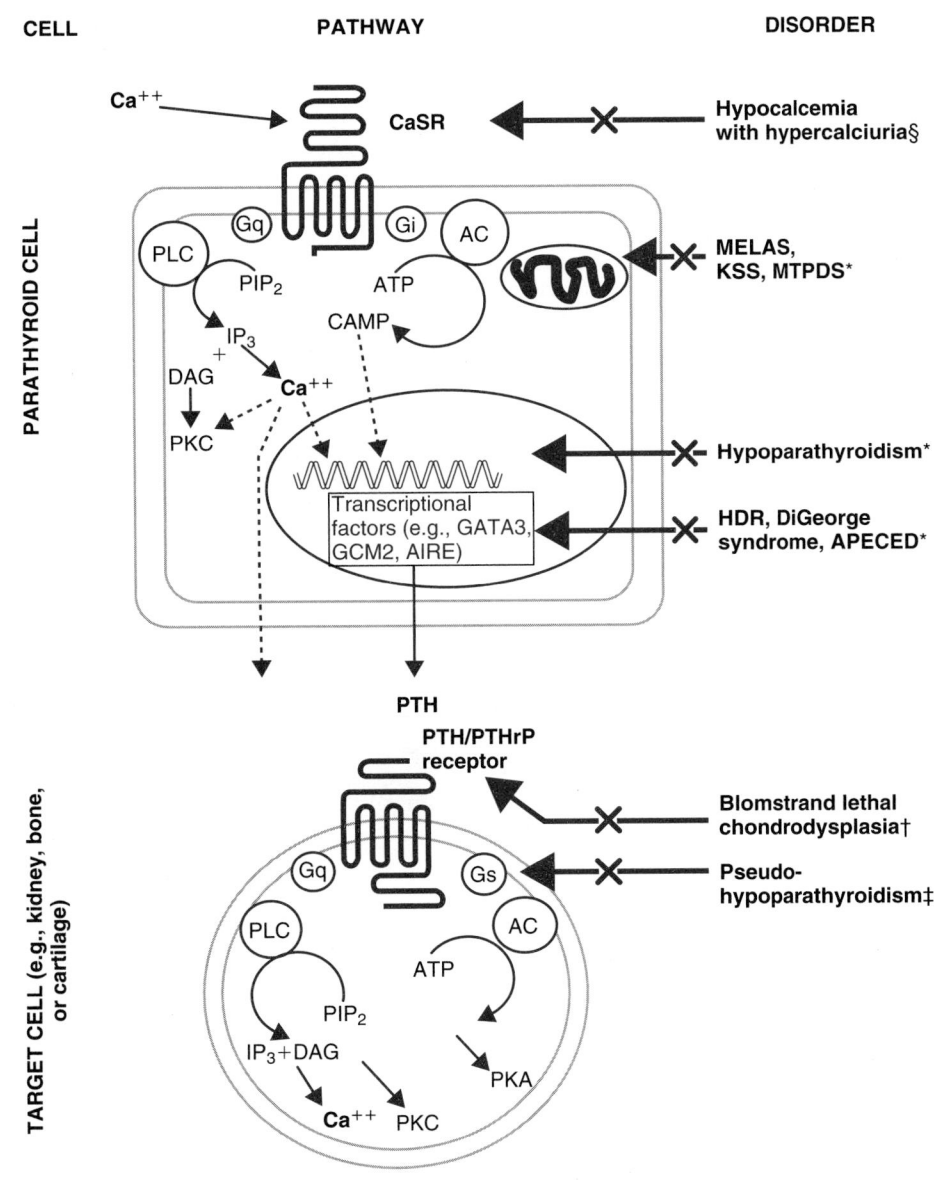

CaSR and PTH/PTHrP-receptor mediate their effects through G protein-coupled signaling pathways, which in turn activate the adenyl cyclase (AC) and phospholipase C (PLC) systems. Gq = G-pertussis-toxin-insensitive protein; Gi = G inhibitory protein; PIP_2 = phosphatidyl inositol 4,5-bisphosphate; IP_3 = inositol 1,4,5-triphosphate; DAG = diacylglycerol; PKC = protein kinase C.
*Disorders due to PTH deficiency.
†Defect due to defect in the PTH/PTHrP receptor.
‡Defect due to insensitivity to PTH caused by defects downstream of the PTH/PTHrP receptor.
§Defect due to altered set-point in the Ca^{++}/PTH axis, associated with a gain-of-function mutation of the CaSR.
MELAS = mitochondrial encephalopathy, stroke-like episodes, and lactic acidosis.
KSS = Kearns Sayre syndrome (progressive external opthalmoplegia, pigmentary retinopathy, heart block, and cardiomyopathy).
MTPDS = mitochondrial trifunctional protein-deficiency syndrome.
HDR = hypoparathyroidism, deafness, and renal anomalies.
APECED = autoimmune polyendocrinopathy-candidosis-ectodermal dystrophy.

FIGURE 564–1. Some components involved in calcium homeostasis. (From Thakker RV: Genetic development in hypoparathyroidism. *Lancet* 2001;357:974–76, with permission.)

Calcitonin. Calcitonin (CT) is a 32-amino acid polypeptide. Its gene is on chromosome 11p and is tightly linked to that of PTH. The gene for CT encodes three peptides: CT, a 21-amino acid carboxy-terminal flanking peptide (katacalcin), and a CT gene-related peptide. Katacalcin and CT are co-secreted in equimolar amounts by the parafollicular cells (C cells) of the thyroid gland. CT appears to be of little consequence in children and adults because very high levels in patients with medullary carcinoma of the thyroid (a tumor arising from the C cells) does not cause hypercalcemia. In the fetus, however, circulating levels are high and appear to augment bone metabolism and skeletal growth; these high levels are probably stimulated by the normally high fetal calcium levels. Unlike the high levels in cord blood and circulating concentrations in young children, levels in older children and adults are low. Infants and children with congenital hypothyroidism (and presumed deficiency of C cells) have lower levels of CT than do normal children.

Its action appears to be independent of PTH and vitamin D. Its main biologic effect appears to be the inhibition of bone resorption by decreasing the number and activity of bone-resorbing osteoclasts. This action of CT is the rationale behind its use in treatment of Paget disease. CT is synthesized in other organs, such as the gastrointestinal tract, pancreas, brain, and pituitary. In these organs, CT is thought to behave as a neurotransmitter to impose a local inhibitory effect on cell function.

Chapter 565
Hypoparathyroidism

Etiology (Box 565–1). Hypocalcemia is common between 12–72 hr of life, especially in premature infants, in infants with asphyxia at birth, and in infants of diabetic mothers (*early neonatal hypocalcemia*) (see Chapter 95). After the 2nd–3rd day and during the 1st wk of life, the type of feeding is also a determinant of the level of serum calcium (*late neonatal hypocalcemia*). The role played by the parathyroid glands in these hypocalcemic infants remains to be clarified, although functional immaturity of the parathyroid glands has often been invoked as one pathogenetic factor. In a group of infants with *transient idiopathic hypocalcemia* (1–8 wk of age), serum levels of parathyroid hormone (PTH) are significantly lower than those in normal infants. It is possible that the functional immaturity is a manifestation of a delay in development of the enzymes that convert glandular PTH to secreted PTH; other mechanisms are also possible.

APLASIA OR HYPOPLASIA OF THE PARATHYROID GLANDS. This is often associated with the *DiGeorge/velocardiofacial syndrome* (see Fig. 564–1). This syndrome occurs in 1/4,000 newborns. In 90% of patients the condition is caused by a deletion of chromosome 22q11.2. Approximately 25% of these patients inherit the chromosomal abnormality from one of their parents. Neonatal hypocalcemia occurs in 60% of affected patients, but it is transitory in the majority; hypocalcemia may recur later or may have its onset later in life. Associated abnormalities of the 3rd and 4th pharyngeal pouches are common; these include conotruncal defects of the heart in 25%, velopharyngeal insufficiency in 32%, cleft palate in 9%, renal anomalies in 35%, and aplasia of the thymus with severe immunodeficiency in 1%. This syndrome has also been reported in a small number of patients with a deletion of chromosome 10p13, in infants of diabetic mothers, and in infants born to mothers treated with retinoic acid for acne early in pregnancy.

X-LINKED RECESSIVE HYPOPARATHYROIDISM. Familial clusters of hypoparathyroidism with various patterns of transmission have been described. In two large North American pedigrees, this disorder appears to be transmitted by an *X-linked recessive gene* located on Xq26-q27. In these families, the onset of afebrile seizures characteristically occurs in infants from 2 wk–6 mo of age. The absence of parathyroid tissue after detailed examination of a boy with this condition suggests it is a defect in embryogenesis.

AUTOSOMAL RECESSIVE HYPOPARATHYROIDISM WITH DYSMORPHIC FEATURES. This syndrome has been described in Middle Eastern children. Parental consanguinity

occurred for almost all of several dozen affected patients. Profound hypocalcemia occurs early in life, and dysmorphic features include microcephaly, deep-set eyes, beaked nose, micrognathia, and large floppy ears. Intrauterine and postnatal growth retardation are severe, and mental retardation is common. The putative gene is on chromosome 1q42-43. The autosomal recessive form of hypoparathyroidism that occurs with type I polyglandular autoimmune disease is described subsequently. In a few patients with autosomal recessive inheritance of isolated hypoparathyroidism, mutations of the *PTH* gene have been found.

HDR SYNDROME. Hypoparathyroidism, sensorineural *deafness* and *renal* anomaly occurs due to mutations of the *GATA3* gene. The protein encoded by this gene is essential in the development of the parathyroids, auditory system, and kidneys. The *GATA3* gene is located at chromosome 10p14 and is nonoverlapping with the DiGeorge critical region at 10p13 (see Fig. 564–1).

SUPPRESSION OF NEONATAL PTH SECRETION DUE TO MATERNAL HYPERPARATHYROIDISM. This may result in transient hypocalcemia of the newborn infant. It appears that neonatal hypocalcemia results from suppression of the fetal

---

BOX 565–1. Etiologic Classification of Hypocalcemia

Parathyroid hormone (PTH) deficiency
  Aplasia or hypoplasia of parathyroids
    With 22q11 deletion
      DiGeorge syndrome
      Velocardiofacial syndrome
      Conotruncal-face syndrome
    With 10p13 deletion
    With maternal diabetes mellitus or retinoic acid embryopathy
    With X-linked isolated hypoparathyroidism
    With mutation of *GCMB* (Glial Cell Missing B) autosomal recessive
    With retardation and dysmorphism (Sanjad-Sakati syndrome) autosomal recessive
    With deafness and renal dysplasia (*GATA3* mutation)
    With osteosclerosis (Kenny-Caffey syndrome), TBCE mutation
  Suppression of neonatal PTH secretion due to maternal hyperparathyroidism
  Preproparathyroid hormone gene mutation
    Autosomal dominant
  Ca^{2+}-sensing receptor activating mutation
    Sporadic
    Autosomal dominant
  Autoimmune parathyroiditis
    Isolated
    With type 1 autoimmune polyendocrinopathy, APECED
      Mutation of *AIRE* gene
  Infiltrative lesions
    Hemosiderosis (treatment of thalassemia)
    Copper deposition (Wilson disease)
PTH receptor defects (pseudohypoparathyroidism)
  Type 1a (inactivating mutation of Gs_a)
    With gonadotropin-independent precocious puberty
  Type 1b (paternal imprinting of *GNAS1*)
  Type 2 (normal cAMP response)
Mitochondrial DNA mutations
  Kearns-Sayre syndrome
  Pearson marrow pancreas syndrome
  Mutation of long-chain 3-hydroxyacylcoenzyme A dehydrogenase
Magnesium deficiency
  Renal magnesium loss (autosomal dominant)
  Magnesium malabsorption (autosomal recessive)
  Aminoglycoside therapy
Exogenous inorganic phosphate excess
  Laxatives
  Soft drinks with phosphoric acid
Vitamin D deficiency
  Nutritional
  Vitamin D dependency (rickets)
    Mutation of 1-α (OH)ase (P450)

parathyroid glands by exposure to elevated levels of calcium in maternal serum. Tetany usually develops within 3 wk but may be delayed 1 mo or more if the infant is breast-fed. Hypocalcemia may persist for weeks or months. When the cause of hypocalcemia in infants is unknown, measurements of calcium, phosphorus, and PTH should be obtained from the mothers. Most affected mothers are asymptomatic, and the cause of their hyperparathyroidism is usually a parathyroid adenoma.

AUTOSOMAL DOMINANT HYPOPARATHYROIDISM. These patients have an activating (gain of function) mutation of the Ca^{2+}-sensing receptor, forcing the receptor to an "on" state with subsequent depression of PTH secretion even during hypocalcemia. The patients have hypercalciuria. The hypocalcemia is usually mild and may not require treatment beyond childhood (see Fig. 564–1).

HYPOPARATHYROIDISM ASSOCIATED WITH MITOCHONDRIAL DISORDERS. Mitochondrial DNA mutations in Kearns-Sayre syndrome and in mitochondrial trifunctional protein have been associated with hypoparathyroidism. A diagnosis of mitochondrial cytopathy should be considered in patients with unexplained symptoms such as ophthalmoplegia, sensorineural hearing loss, cardiac conduction disturbances, and tetany (see Fig. 564–1).

SURGICAL HYPOPARATHYROIDISM. Removal or damage of the parathyroid glands may complicate thyroidectomy. Hypoparathyroidism has developed even when the parathyroid glands have been identified and left undisturbed at the time of operation. This presumably is the result of interference with the blood supply or of postoperative edema and fibrosis. Symptoms of tetany may occur abruptly postoperatively and may be temporary or permanent. In some instances, symptoms may develop insidiously and go undetected until months after thyroidectomy. Occasionally, the first evidence of surgical hypoparathyroidism may be the development of cataracts. The status of parathyroid function should be carefully monitored in all patients undergoing thyroidectomy.

Deposition of iron pigment or of copper in the parathyroid glands (e.g., thalassemia, Wilson disease) may produce hypoparathyroidism.

AUTOIMMUNE HYPOPARATHYROIDISM. An autoimmune mechanism for hypoparathyroidism is strongly suggested by the finding of parathyroid antibodies and by its frequent association with other autoimmune disorders or organ-specific antibodies. Autoimmune hypoparathyroidism is often associated with Addison disease and chronic mucocutaneous candidiasis. The association of at least two of these three conditions has been tentatively classified as *autoimmune polyglandular disease type I*. It is also known as *autoimmune polyendocrinopathy/candidiasis/ectodermal dystrophy*. This syndrome is inherited in an autosomal recessive fashion and is not related to any single HLA-associated haplotype. One third of patients with this syndrome have all three components; two thirds have only two of three conditions. The candidiasis almost always precedes the other disorders (70% of cases occur in children younger than 5 yr of age); the hypoparathyroidism (90% after 3 yr of age) usually occurs before Addison disease (90% after 6 yr of age). A variety of other disorders occur at various times and include alopecia areata or totalis, malabsorption disorder, pernicious anemia, gonadal failure, chronic active hepatitis, vitiligo, and insulin-dependent diabetes. Some of these associations may not appear until adult life. Autoimmune thyroid disease is a rare concomitant finding.

Affected siblings may have the same or different constellations of disorders (e.g., hypoparathyroidism and Addison disease). The disorder is exceptionally prevalent among Finns and Iranian Jews. The gene for this disorder is designated *AIRE* (autoimmune regulator); it is located on chromosome 21q22. It appears to be a transcription factor that plays an essential role in

the development of immunologic tolerance. Patients with Addison disease as part of polyendocrinopathy syndrome type I have demonstrated adrenal-specific autoantibody reactivity directed against the side-chain cleavage enzyme.

IDIOPATHIC HYPOPARATHYROIDISM. This term should be reserved for the small residuum of children with hypoparathyroidism for whom no causative mechanism can be defined. Most children in whom onset of hypoparathyroidism occurs after the first few years of life have an autoimmune condition. Autoantibodies to the extracellular domain of the calcium-sensing receptor have been identified in some patients with acquired hypoparathyroidism. One should always consider incomplete forms of DiGeorge syndrome or an activating calcium-sensing receptor mutation in the differential diagnosis.

Clinical Manifestations. There is a spectrum of parathyroid deficiencies with clinical manifestations varying from no symptoms to those of complete and long-standing deficiency. Mild deficiency may be revealed only by appropriate laboratory studies. Muscular pain and cramps are early manifestations; they progress to numbness, stiffness, and tingling of the hands and feet. There may be only a positive Chvostek or Trousseau sign or laryngeal and carpopedal spasms. Convulsions with or without loss of consciousness may occur at intervals of days, weeks, or months. These episodes may begin with abdominal pain, followed by tonic rigidity, retraction of the head, and cyanosis. Hypoparathyroidism is frequently mistaken for epilepsy. Headache, vomiting, increased intracranial pressure, and papilledema may be associated with convulsions and may suggest a brain tumor.

In patients with long-standing hypocalcemia, the teeth erupt late and irregularly. Enamel formation is irregular, and the teeth may be unusually soft. The skin may be dry and scaly, and the nails of the fingers and toes may have horizontal lines. Mucocutaneous candidiasis, when present, antedates the development of hypoparathyroidism; the candidal infection most often involves the nails, the oral mucosa, the angles of the mouth, and, less often, the skin.

Cataracts in patients with long-standing untreated disease are a direct consequence of hypoparathyroidism; other autoimmune ocular disorders such as keratoconjunctivitis may also occur. Manifestations of Addison disease, lymphocytic thyroiditis, pernicious anemia, alopecia areata or totalis, hepatitis, and primary gonadal insufficiency may also be associated with those of hypoparathyroidism.

Permanent physical and mental deterioration occur if initiation of treatment is long delayed.

Laboratory Findings. The serum calcium level is low (5–7 mg/dL), and the phosphorus level is elevated (7–12 mg/dL). Blood levels of ionized calcium (usually approximately 45% of the total) more nearly reflect physiologic adequacy but are also low. The serum level of alkaline phosphatase is normal or low, and the level of $1,25[OH]_2D_3$ is usually low, but high levels have been found in some children with severe hypocalcemia. The level of magnesium is normal but should always be checked in hypocalcemic patients. Levels of PTH are low when measured by immunometric assay. Administration of the synthetic 1–34 fragment of human PTH (teriparatide acetate) results in increased urinary levels of cyclic adenosine monophosphate and phosphate. This response differentiates hypoparathyroidism from pseudohypoparathyroidism. With the advent of very sensitive PTH assays, this test is usually not necessary. Radiographs of the bones occasionally reveal an increased density limited to the metaphyses, suggestive of heavy metal poisoning, or an increased density of the lamina dura. Radiographs or CT of the skull may reveal calcifications in the basal ganglia. There is a prolongation of the QT interval on the electrocardiogram, which disappears when the hypocalcemia is corrected. The electroencephalogram usually reveals widespread slow activity; the tracing returns to normal after the serum calcium concentration has been within the normal range for a few weeks, unless irreversible brain damage has occurred or unless the parathyroid insufficiency is associated with epilepsy. When hypoparathyroidism occurs concurrently with Addison disease, the serum level of calcium may be normal, but hypocalcemia appears after effective treatment of the adrenal insufficiency.

Treatment. Emergency treatment of neonatal tetany consists of intravenous injections of 5–10 mL of a 10% solution of calcium gluconate at the rate of 0.5–1 mL/min while the heart rate is monitored. Additionally, 1,25-dihydroxycholecalciferol (calcitriol) should be given. The initial dosage is 0.25 μg/24 hr; the maintenance dosage ranges from 0.01–0.10 μg/kg/24 hr, to a maximum of 1–2 μg/24 hr. Calcitriol has a short half-life and should be given in two equal divided doses; it has the advantages of rapid onset of effect (1–4 days) and rapid reversal of hypercalcemia after discontinuation in the event of overdosage (i.e., calcium levels begin to fall in 3–4 days). Calcitriol is now supplied as an oral solution (1 μg/mL, Roche Pharmaceuticals).

After normocalcemia has been achieved, one may wish to continue therapy with vitamin D_2 because it is considerably less expensive than calcitriol. The usual dosage is 0.1–0.5 mg/24 hr in infants and young children. One milligram of vitamin D_2 has a biologic activity of 40,000 IU. Older children require 1.25–2.50 mg (50,000–100,000 IU) once daily. Vitamin D_2 has a slow onset of effect, and reversal of hypercalcemia after discontinuation of treatment is markedly delayed; its main advantage is its low cost.

An adequate intake of calcium should be ensured. Supplemental calcium can be given in the form of calcium gluconate or calcium glubionate (Neo-Calglucon) to provide 800 mg of elemental calcium daily, but it is rarely essential. Foods with a high phosphorus content such as milk, eggs, and cheese should be reduced in the diet.

Clinical evaluation of the patient and frequent determinations of the serum calcium levels are indicated in the early stages of treatment to determine the requirement for calcitriol or vitamin D_2. If hypercalcemia occurs, therapy should be discontinued and resumed at a lower dose after the serum calcium level has returned to normal. In long-standing cases, repair of cerebral and dental changes is not likely. Pigmentation, lowering of the blood pressure, or weight loss may indicate adrenal insufficiency, which requires specific treatment. Patients with autosomal dominant hypocalcemic hypercalciuria may develop nephrocalcinosis and renal impairment if treated with vitamin D.

Differential Diagnosis. Magnesium deficiency must be considered in patients with unexplained hypocalcemia. Concentrations of serum magnesium less than 1.5 mg/dL (1.2 mEq/L) are usually abnormal. *Familial hypomagnesemia* with secondary hypocalcemia has been reported in about 50 patients, most of whom developed tetany and seizures at 2–6 wk of age. Administration of calcium is ineffective, but administration of magnesium promptly corrects both calcium and magnesium levels. Oral supplements of magnesium are necessary to maintain levels of magnesium in the normal range. Two genetic forms have been described. One is caused by an autosomal recessive gene on chromosome 9, resulting in a specific defect in absorption of magnesium. The other is caused by an autosomal dominant gene on chromosome 11q23, resulting in renal loss of magnesium.

Hypomagnesemia also occurs in malabsorption syndromes such as granulomatous colitis and cystic fibrosis. Patients with autoimmune polyglandular disease type I and hypoparathyroidism may also have concurrent steatorrhea and low magnesium levels. Therapy with aminoglycosides causes hypomagnesemia by increasing urinary losses.

It is not clear how low levels of magnesium lead to hypocalcemia. Evidence suggests that hypomagnesemia impairs release of PTH and induces resistance to the effects of the hormone, but other mechanisms also may be operative.

Poisoning with inorganic phosphate leads to hypocalcemia and tetany. Infants administered large doses of inorganic phosphates, either as laxatives or as sodium phosphate enemas, have had sudden onset of tetany, with serum calcium levels less than 5 mg/dL and markedly elevated levels of phosphate. Symptoms are quickly relieved by intravenous administration of calcium. The mechanism of the hypocalcemia is not clear (see Chapter 48.9).

Hypocalcemia may occur early in the course of treatment of *acute lymphoblastic leukemia.* Hypocalcemia is usually associated with hyperphosphatemia resulting from destruction of lymphoblasts.

Episodic symptomatic hypocalcemia occurs in the *Kenny-Caffey syndrome,* which is characterized by medullary stenosis of the long bones, short stature, delayed closure of the fontanel, delayed bone age, and eye abnormalities. Idiopathic hypoparathyroidism and abnormal PTH levels have been found. Autosomal dominant and autosomal recessive modes of inheritance have been reported. Mutations of the TBCE gene (1q 43-44) perturb microtubule organization in diseased cells.

Chapter 566
Pseudohypoparathyroidism (Albright Hereditary Osteodystrophy)

In contrast to the situation in hypoparathyroidism, in pseudohypoparathyroidism (PHP), the parathyroid glands are normal or hyperplastic and they can synthesize and secrete parathyroid hormone (PTH). Serum levels of immunoreactive PTH are elevated even when the patient is hypocalcemic and may be elevated when the patient is normocalcemic. Neither endogenous nor administered PTH raises the serum levels of calcium or lowers the levels of phosphorus. The genetic defects in the hormone receptor adenylate cyclase system are classified into various types depending on the phenotypic and biochemical findings.

Type IA. This type accounts for the majority of patients with PHP. Affected patients have a genetic defect of the α subunit of the stimulatory guanine nucleotide-binding protein ($G_{s\alpha}$). This coupling factor is required for PTH bound to cell surface receptors to activate cyclic adenosine monophosphate (AMP). Heterogeneous mutations of the $G_{s\alpha}$ gene have been documented; the gene is located on chromosome 20q13.2. Deficiency of the $G_{s\alpha}$ subunit is a generalized cellular defect and accounts for the association of other endocrine disorders with type IA PHP. The defect is inherited as an autosomal dominant trait, and the paucity of father-to-son transmissions is thought to be due to decreased fertility in males.

Tetany is often the presenting sign. Affected children have a short, stocky build and a round face. Brachydactyly with dimpling of the dorsum of the hand is usually present. The 2nd metacarpal is involved least often. As a result, the index finger may occasionally be longer than the middle finger. Likewise, the 2nd metatarsal is only rarely affected. There may be other skeletal abnormalities such as short and wide phalanges, bowing, exostoses, and thickening of the calvaria. These patients frequently have calcium deposits and metaplastic bone formation subcutaneously. Moderate degrees of mental retardation, calcification of the basal ganglia, and lenticular cataracts are common in patients who are diagnosed late.

Some members of affected kindreds may have the usual anatomic stigmata of PHP, but serum levels of calcium and phosphorus are normal despite reduced $G_{s\alpha}$ activity; however, PTH levels may be slightly elevated. Such patients have been labeled as having *pseudopseudohypoparathyroidism*. Transition from normocalcemia to hypocalcemia often occurs with increasing age of the patient. These phenotypically similar but metabolically dissimilar patients may occur in the same family and have the same mutations of $G_{s\alpha}$ protein. It is not known what other factors cause clinically overt hypocalcemia in some affected patients and not in others. There is some evidence to suggest that the $G_{s\alpha}$ mutation is paternally transmitted in pseudopseudohypoparathyroidism and maternally transmitted in patients with type Ia disease. The gene may be imprinted in a tissue-specific manner.

In addition to resistance to PTH, resistance to other G protein–coupled receptors for thyroid-stimulating hormone (TSH), gonadotropins, and glucagon may result in various metabolic effects. Clinical hypothyroidism is uncommon, but basal levels of TSH are elevated and thyrotropin-releasing hormone–stimulated TSH responses are exaggerated. Moderately decreased levels of thyroxine and increased levels of TSH have been detected by newborn thyroid screening programs, leading to the detection of type IA PHP in infancy. In adults, gonadal dysfunction is common, as manifested by sexual immaturity, amenorrhea, oligomenorrhea, and infertility. Each of these abnormalities can be related to deficient synthesis of cyclic AMP secondary to a deficiency of $G_{s\alpha}$, but it is not clear why resistance to other G protein–dependent hormones (e.g., corticotropin, vasopressin) is much less affected.

Serum levels of calcium are low, and those of phosphorus and alkaline phosphatase are elevated. Clinical diagnosis can be confirmed by demonstration of a markedly attenuated response in urinary phosphate and cyclic AMP after intravenous infusion of the synthetic 1–34 fragment of human PTH (teriparatide acetate), but this compound is no longer commercially available in the United States. Definitive diagnosis is established by demonstration of the mutated G protein.

TYPE IA WITH PRECOCIOUS PUBERTY. Two boys have been reported with both type IA PHP and gonadotropin-independent precocious puberty (see Chapter 556.6). They were found to have a temperature-sensitive mutation of the G_s protein. Thus, at normal body temperature (37°C), the G_s is degraded, resulting in PHP, but in the cooler temperature of the testes (33°C) the G_s mutation results in constitutive activation of the luteinizing hormone receptor and precocious puberty.

Type IB. Affected patients have normal levels of G protein activity and a normal phenotypic appearance. These patients have tissue-specific resistance to PTH but not to other hormones. Serum levels of calcium, phosphorus, and immunoreactive PTH are the same as those in patients with type IA PHP. These patients also show no rise in cyclic AMP in response to exogenous administration of PTH. Bioactive PTH is not increased. The pathophysiology of the disorder in this group of patients is caused by paternal uniparental isodisomy of chromosome 20q and resulting GNAS1 methylation. This, along with the loss of the maternal *GNAS1* gene, leads to PTH resistance in the proximal renal tubules, which leads to impaired mineral ion homeostasis.

Type II. This type of pseudohypoparathyroidism has been detected in only a few patients and differs from type I in that the urinary excretion of cyclic AMP is elevated both in the basal state and after stimulation with PTH, but phosphaturia does not increase. Phenotypically, patients are normal and hypocalcemia is present. The defect appears to be distal to cyclic AMP because it is normally activated, but the cell is unable to respond to the signal.

Chapter 567
Hyperparathyroidism

Excessive production of parathyroid hormone (PTH) may result from a primary defect of the parathyroid glands such as an adenoma or hyperplasia *(primary hyperparathyroidism)*.

More often, the increased production of PTH is compensatory, usually aimed at correcting hypocalcemic states of diverse origins *(secondary hyperparathyroidism)*. In vitamin D–deficient rickets and the malabsorption syndromes, intestinal absorption of calcium is deficient but hypocalcemia and tetany may be averted by increased activity of the parathyroid glands. In pseudohypoparathyroidism, PTH levels are elevated because a mutation in the $G_{s\alpha}$ protein interferes with response to PTH. Early in chronic renal disease, hyperphosphatemia results in a reciprocal fall in the calcium concentration with a consequent increase in PTH, but in advanced stages of renal failure, production of $1,25[OH]_2D_3$ is also decreased, leading to worsening hypocalcemia and further stimulation of PTH. In some instances, if stimulation of the parathyroid glands has been sufficiently intense and protracted, the glands may continue to secrete increased levels of PTH for months or years after renal transplantation, with resulting hypercalcemia.

Etiology. Childhood hyperparathyroidism is rare. Onset during childhood is usually the result of a single benign adenoma. It usually becomes manifested after 10 yr of age. There have been a number of kindreds in which multiple members have hyperparathyroidism transmitted in an autosomal dominant fashion. Most of the affected family members are adults, but children have been involved in about a third of the pedigrees. Some affected patients in these families are asymptomatic and are detected only by careful study. In other kindreds, hyperparathyroidism occurs as part of the constellation known as the *multiple endocrine neoplasia (MEN) syndromes* or of the *hyperparathyroidism/ jaw tumor syndrome*.

Neonatal severe hyperparathyroidism has been reported in approximately 50 infants. Symptoms develop shortly after birth and consist of anorexia, irritability, lethargy, constipation, and failure to thrive. Radiographs reveal subperiosteal bone resorption, osteoporosis, and pathologic fractures. Symptoms may be mild, resolving without treatment, or may have a rapidly fatal course if diagnosis and treatment are delayed. Histologically, the parathyroid glands show diffuse hyperplasia. Affected siblings have been observed in some kindreds, and parental consanguinity has been reported in several kindreds. Most cases have occurred in kindreds with the clinical and biochemical features of *familial hypocalciuric hypercalcemia*. Infants with neonatal severe hyperparathyroidism may be homozygous or heterozygous for the mutation in the Ca^{2+}-sensing receptor gene, whereas most individuals with one copy of this mutation exhibit autosomally dominant familial hypocalciuric hypercalcemia.

MEN type I is an autosomal dominant disorder characterized by hyperplasia or neoplasia of the endocrine pancreas (which secretes gastrin, insulin, pancreatic polypeptide, or occasionally glucagon), the anterior pituitary (which usually secretes prolactin), and the parathyroid glands. In most kindreds, hyperparathyroidism is usually the presenting manifestation, with a prevalence approaching 100% by 50 yr of age but occurring only rarely in children younger than 18 yr of age. In the past, after an affected family was identified, it was necessary to perform repeated metabolic screening for many years to detect other affected family members. With appropriate DNA probes, it is now possible to detect carriers of the gene with 99% accuracy at birth, avoiding unnecessary biochemical screening programs.

The gene for MEN type I is on chromosome 11q13; it appears to function as a tumor suppressor gene and follows the two-hit hypothesis of tumor development. The first mutation (germinal) is inherited and is recessive to the dominant allele; this does not result in tumor formation. A second mutation (somatic) is required to eliminate the normal allele, which then leads to tumor formation.

Hyperparathyroidism/jaw tumor syndrome is an autosomal dominant disorder characterized by parathyroid adenomas and fibro-osseous jaw tumors. Affected patients may also have polycystic kidney disease, renal hamartomas, and Wilms tumor. Although the condition affects adults primarily, it has been diagnosed as early as age 10 yr.

MEN type II may also be associated with hyperparathyroidism (see Chapter 563.2).

Transient neonatal hyperparathyroidism has occurred in a few infants born to mothers with hypoparathyroidism (idiopathic or surgical) or with pseudohypoparathyroidism. In each case, the maternal disorder had been undiagnosed or inadequately treated during pregnancy. The cause of the condition is chronic intrauterine exposure to hypocalcemia with resultant hyperplasia of the fetal parathyroid glands. In the newborn, manifestations involve the bones primarily and healing occurs between 4 and 7 mo of age.

Clinical Manifestations. At all ages, the clinical manifestations of hypercalcemia of any cause include muscular weakness, anorexia, nausea, vomiting, constipation, polydipsia, polyuria, loss of weight, and fever. When hypercalcemia is of long duration, calcium may be deposited in the renal parenchyma (nephrocalcinosis), with progressively diminished renal function. Renal calculi may occur and may produce renal colic and hematuria. Osseous changes may produce pain in the back or extremities, disturbances of gait, genu valgum, fractures, and tumors. Height may decrease from compression of vertebrae; the patient may become bedridden. Detection of completely asymptomatic patients is increasing with the advent of automated panel assays that include serum calcium determinations.

Abdominal pain is occasionally prominent and may be associated with acute pancreatitis. Parathyroid crisis may occur, manifested by serum calcium levels greater than 15 mg/dL and progressive oliguria, azotemia, stupor, and coma. In infants, failure to thrive, poor feeding, and hypotonia are common. Mental retardation, convulsions, and blindness may occur as sequelae of long-standing hypercalcemia.

Laboratory Findings. The serum calcium level is elevated; 39 of 45 children with adenomas had levels greater than 12 mg/dL. The hypercalcemia is more severe in infants with parathyroid hyperplasia; concentrations ranging from 15–20 mg/dL are common, and values as high as 30 mg/dL have been reported. Even when the total serum calcium level is borderline or only slightly elevated, ionized calcium levels are often increased. The serum phosphorus level is reduced to about 3 mg/dL or less, and the level of serum magnesium is low. The urine may have a low and fixed specific gravity, and serum levels of nonprotein nitrogen and uric acid may be elevated. In patients with adenomas who have skeletal involvement, serum phosphatase levels are elevated, but in infants with hyperplasia the levels of alkaline phosphatase may be normal even when there is extensive involvement of bone.

Serum levels of PTH measured by carboxy-terminal antisera are elevated, especially in relation to the level of calcium. Results may vary markedly from one laboratory to another, depending on the antibody used. Calcitonin levels are normal. Acute hypercalcemia can stimulate calcitonin release; but with prolonged hypercalcemia, hypercalcitoninemia does not occur.

The most consistent and characteristic radiographic finding is resorption of subperiosteal bone, best seen along the margins of the phalanges of the hands. In the skull, there may be gross trabeculation or a granular appearance resulting from focal rarefaction; the lamina dura may be absent. In more advanced disease, there may be generalized rarefaction, cysts, tumors, fractures, and deformities. About 10% of patients have radiographic signs of rickets. Radiographs of the abdomen may reveal renal calculi or nephrocalcinosis.

Differential Diagnosis. Other causes of hypercalcemia may result in a similar clinical pattern and must be differentiated from hyperparathyroidism (Box 567–1). A low serum phosphorus level with hypercalcemia is characteristic of primary hyperparathyroidism; elevated levels of PTH are also diagnostic. With hypercalcemia of any cause except hyperparathyroidism and familial hypocalciuric hypercalcemia, PTH levels are suppressed. Pharmacologic doses of corticosteroids lower the serum calcium level to normal in patients with hypercalcemia from other causes but generally do not affect the calcium level in patients with hyperparathyroidism.

Treatment. Surgical exploration is indicated in all instances. All glands should be carefully inspected; if an adenoma is discovered, it should be removed; very few instances of carcinoma are known in children. Most neonates with severe hypercalcemia require total parathyroidectomy; less severe hypercalcemia may remit spontaneously in others. A portion of a parathyroid gland may be autografted into the forearm; four infants treated in this fashion were able to maintain normocalcemia without supplementary treatment, but no long-term outcome has yet been reported. The patient should be carefully observed postoperatively for the development of hypocalcemia and tetany; intravenous administration of calcium gluconate may be required for a few days. The serum calcium level then gradually returns to normal, and, under

---

BOX 567–1. Etiologic Classification of Hypercalcemia

Parathyroid hormone (PTH) excess
  Primary hyperparathyroidism
    Adenoma
      Sporadic
      Autosomal dominant
      Hyperparathyroidism-jaw tumor syndrome
    Hyperplasia or adenoma
      Multiple endocrine neoplasia type1
        Mutation in *MEN1* gene (11q13)
      Parathyroid hyperplasia of infancy
        Inactivating mutation of Ca^{2+}-sensing receptor
        Secondary to maternal hypoparathyroidism
  Ectopic PTH production
    Nonendocrine malignancies
Parathyroid hormone–related peptide (PTHrP) excess
  Nonendocrine malignancies
  Benign hypertrophy of breasts
Ca^{2+}-sensing receptor inactivating mutation
  Heterozygous-familial hypocalciuric hypercalcemia
  Neonatal severe hyperparathyroidism
Activating mutation of PTH/PTHrP receptor
  Autosomal dominant
    Jasen-type metaphyseal chondrodysplasia
Inactivating mutation of PTH/PTHrP receptor
  Autosomal recessive
    Blomstrand chondrodysplasia
Vitamin D excess
  Iatrogenic
  Ectopic production
    Sarcoidosis, tuberculosis, granulomatous lesions, subcutaneous
      fat necrosis
  Excessively fortified milk
Unknown cause
  Williams syndrome (7q11.23 deletion)
Other
  Hypophosphatasia
    Mutation of tissue nonspecific alkaline phosphatase gene
  Prolonged immobilization
  Thyrotoxicosis
  Hypervitaminosis A
  Leukemia

ordinary circumstances, a diet high in calcium and phosphorus must be maintained for only several months after operation.

Arteriography and selective venous sampling with radioimmunoassay of PTH for preoperative localization and differentiation of a single adenoma from hyperplasia have been replaced by imaging methods. CT, real-time ultrasonography, and subtraction scintigraphy using sestamibi/Tc-pertechnetate alone and in combination have proved effective in 50–90% of adults. These procedures are rarely required by the expert parathyroid surgeon but may be advisable before re-exploration in cases of persistent or recurrent hyperparathyroidism.

Prognosis. The prognosis is good if the disease is recognized early and there is appropriate surgical treatment. When extensive osseous lesions are present, deformities may be permanent. A search for other affected family members is indicated.

Other Causes of Hypercalcemia

FAMILIAL HYPOCALCIURIC HYPERCALCEMIA (FAMILIAL BENIGN HYPERCALCEMIA). Patients with this disorder are usually asymptomatic, and the hypercalcemia comes to light by chance during routine investigation for other conditions. The parathyroid glands are normal, PTH levels are inappropriately normal, and subtotal parathyroidectomy does not correct the hypercalcemia. Serum levels of magnesium are high normal or mildly elevated. The rate of calcium to creatinine clearance is usually decreased despite hypercalcemia. The disorder is inherited in an autosomal dominant manner and is caused by a mutant gene on chromosome 3q2. Penetrance is near 100%, and affected individuals can be diagnosed early in childhood by serum and urinary calcium concentrations. Detection of other affected family members is important to avoid inappropriate parathyroid surgery. The basic defect in this condition results from inactivating mutations in the Ca^{2+}-sensing receptor gene. This G protein–coupled receptor senses the level of free Ca^{2+} in the blood and triggers the pathway to increase extracellular Ca^{2+} in the face of hypocalcemia. This receptor functions in the parathyroid and kidney to regulate calcium homeostasis; inactivating mutations lead to an increased set point with respect to serum Ca^{2+}, resulting in mild to moderate hypercalcemia in heterozygotes.

GRANULOMATOUS DISEASES. Hypercalcemia occurs in 30–50% of children with sarcoidosis and less often in patients with other granulomatous diseases such as tuberculosis. Levels of PTH are suppressed, and levels of 1,25[OH]$_2$D$_3$ are elevated. The source of ectopic 1,25[OH]$_2$D$_3$ is the activated macrophage, through stimulation by interferon-α from T lymphocytes, which are present in abundance in granulomatous lesions. Unlike renal tubular cells, the 1α-hydroxylase in macrophages is unresponsive to homeostatic regulation. Oral administration of prednisone (2 mg/kg/24 hr) lowers serum levels of 1,25[OH]$_2$D$_3$ to normal and corrects the hypercalcemia.

HYPERCALCEMIA OF MALIGNANCY. Hypercalcemia frequently occurs in adults with a wide variety of solid tumors but is identified much less often in children. It has been reported in infants with malignant rhabdoid tumors of the kidney or congenital mesoblastic nephroma and in children with neuroblastoma, medulloblastoma, leukemia, Burkitt lymphoma, dysgerminoma, and rhabdomyosarcoma. Serum levels of PTH are rarely elevated. In most patients, the hypercalcemia associated with malignancy is caused by elevated levels of parathyroid hormone–related peptide (PTHrP) and not PTH. Rarely, tumors produce 1,25[OH]$_2$D$_3$ or PTH ectopically.

MISCELLANEOUS CAUSES OF HYPERCALCEMIA. Hypercalcemia may occur in infants with subcutaneous *fat necrosis*. Levels of PTH are normal. In one infant, the level of 1,25[OH]$_2$D$_3$ was elevated and biopsy of the skin lesion revealed granulomatous infiltration, suggesting that the mechanism of the hypercalcemia was akin to that seen in patients with other granulomatous disease. In another infant, although the level of 1,25[OH]$_2$D$_3$ was normal, PTH was suppressed, suggesting the

hypercalcemia was not PTH related. Treatment with prednisone is effective.

Hypophosphatasia, especially the severe infantile form, is usually associated with mild to moderate hypercalcemia (see Chapter 694). Serum levels of phosphorus are normal, and those of alkaline phosphatase are subnormal. The bones exhibit rachitic-like lesions on radiographs. Urinary levels of phosphoethanolamine, inorganic pyrophosphate, and pyridoxal 5′-phosphate are elevated; each is a natural substrate to a *tissue-nonspecific* (liver, bone, kidney) *alkaline phosphatase enzyme.* Missense mutations of the tissue-nonspecific alkaline phosphatase enzyme gene result in an inactive enzyme in this autosomal recessive disorder.

Idiopathic hypercalcemia of infancy is manifested by failure to thrive and hypercalcemia during the 1st yr of life, followed by spontaneous remission. Serum levels of phosphorus and PTH are normal. The hypercalcemia results from increased absorption of calcium. Vitamin D may be involved in the pathogenesis. Both normal and elevated levels of 1,25[OH]$_2$D$_3$ have been reported. An excessive rise in the level of 1,25[OH]$_2$D$_3$ in response to PTH administration years after the hypercalcemic phase suggests that vitamin D has a role in the pathogenesis. A blunted calcitonin response to intravenous calcium has also been reported.

Ten per cent of patients with *Williams syndrome* also exhibit associated infantile hypercalcemia. The phenotype consists of feeding difficulties, slow growth, elfin facies, renovascular disorders, and a gregarious personality. The IQ score of 50 to 70 is curiously accompanied by enhanced quantity and quality of vocabulary, auditory memory, and social use of language. A submicroscopic deletion at chromosome 7q11.23, which includes deletion of one elastin allele, occurs in 90% of patients and seems to account for the vascular problems. Definitive diagnosis can be established by specific fluorescent in situ hybridization. The hypercalcemia and central nervous system symptoms may be caused by deletion of adjacent genes. Hypercalcemia has been successfully controlled with either prednisone or calcitonin.

Hypervitaminosis D resulting in hypercalcemia from drinking milk that has been incorrectly fortified with vitamin D has been reported. Serum levels of 25[OH]D are a better indicator of hypervitaminosis D than 1,25[OH]$_2$D$_3$ because 25[OH]D has a longer half-life.

Prolonged immobilization may lead to hypercalcemia and occasionally to decreased renal function, hypertension, and encephalopathy. Children having hypophosphatemic rickets and undergoing surgery with subsequent long-term immobilization are at risk for hypercalcemia and should therefore have their vitamin D supplementation decreased or discontinued.

Jansen-type metaphyseal chondrodysplasia is a rare genetic disorder characterized by short-limbed dwarfism and severe but asymptomatic hypercalcemia (see Chapter 692). Circulating levels of PTH and PTHrP are undetectable. These patients have an activating PTH-PTHrP receptor mutation that results in aberrant calcium homeostasis and abnormalities of the growth plate.

Aaltonen J, Bjorses P, Su Lee Y, et al: An autoimmune disease, APECED, caused by mutations in a novel gene featuring two PHD-type zinc-finger domains. *Nat Genet* 1997;17:399.

Ahonen P, Myllarniemi S, Sipla I, et al: Clinical variation of autoimmune polyendocrinopathy-candidiasis-ectodermal dystrophy (APECED) in a series of 68 patients. *N Engl J Med* 1990;322:1829.

Bassett JH, Forbes SA, Thakker RV, et al: Characterization of mutations in patients with multiple endocrine neoplasia type I. *Am J Hum Genet* 1998;62:232.

Brown EM, Pollak M, Hebert SC, et al: Calcium-ion-sensing cell-surface receptors (review). *N Engl J Med* 1995;333:234.

Burgess JR, Shepherd JJ, Greenaway TM, et al: Spectrum of pituitary disease in multiple endocrine neoplasia type I (MEN 1): Clinical, biochemical, and radiological features of pituitary disease in a large MEN 1 kindred. *J Clin Endocrinol Metab* 1996;81:2642.

Clapman DS: Why testicles are cool. *Nature* 1994;371:109.

Cook JS, Stone MS, Hansen JR: Hypercalcemia in association with subcutaneous fat necrosis of the newborn: Studies of calcium-regulating hormones. *Pediatrics* 1992;90:93.

Cooper L, Wertheimer J, Levey R, et al: Severe primary hyperparathyroidism in a neonate with two hypercalcemic parents: Management with parathyroidectomy and heterotopic autotransplantation. *Pediatrics* 1986;78:263.

Damiani D, Agwar CH, Bueno VS, et al: Primary hyperparathyroidism in children: Patient report and review of literature. *J Pediatr Endocrinol Metab* 1998;11:83.

Ewart AK, Morris CA, Atkinson D, et al: Hemizygosity at the elastin locus in a developmental disorder, Williams syndrome. *Nat Genet* 1993;5:11.

Fedde KN, Michell MP, Whyte MP, et al: Aberrant properties of alkaline phosphatase in patients with clinical expressivity in severe forms of hypophosphatasia. *J Clin Endocrinol Metab* 1996;81:2587.

Gillis D, Hirsch HJ, Peylan-Ramu N, et al: Parathyroid adenoma after radiation in an 8-year old boy. *J Pediatr* 1998;132:892.

Hobbs MR, Pole AR, Pidisirng GN, et al: Hyperparathyroidism-jaw tumor syndrome: The HRPT2 locus is within a 0.7-cM region on chromosome 1q. *Am J Hum Genet* 1999;64:518.

Iiri T, Herzmark P, Nakimoto JM, et al: Rapid GDP release from Gsα in patients with gain and loss of endocrine function. *Nature* 1994;371:164.

Irvin GL, Carneiro DM: Management changes in primary hyperparathyroidism. *JAMA* 2000;284:934–36.

Jacabus CH, Holick MF, Shao G, et al: Hypervitaminosis D associated with drinking milk. *N Engl J Med* 1992;326:1173.

Jobert AS, Zhang P, Courineau A, et al: Absence of functional receptors for parathyroid hormone and parathyroid hormone–related peptide in Blomstrand chondrodysplasia. *J Clin Invest* 1998;102:34.

Kahn KT, Uma R, Farag TI, et al: Kenny-Caffey syndrome in six Bedouin sibships: Autosomal recessive inheritance is confirmed. *Am J Med Genet* 1997;69:126.

Key LL, Thorne M, Pitzer B, et al: Management of neonatal hyperparathyroidism with parathyroidectomy and autotransplantation. *J Pediatr* 1990;116:923.

Kovacs CS, Kronenberg HM: Maternal-fetal calcium and bone metabolism during pregnancy, puerperium and lactation. *Endocr Rev* 1997;18:832.

Learoyd DL, Twigg SM, Robinson BG, et al: The practical management of multiple endocrine neoplasia. *Trends Endocrinol Metab* 1995;6:273.

Levitt M, Gessert C, Finberg L: Inorganic phosphate (laxative) poisoning resulting in tetany in an infant. *J Pediatr* 1973;82:479.

Li Y, Song Y-H, Muir A, et al: Autoantibodies to the extracellular domain of the calcium-sensing receptor in patients with acquired hypoparathyroidism. *J Clin Invest* 1996;97:910.

Liu J, Litman D, Weinstein LS, et al: A GNAS1 imprinting defect in pseudohypoparathyroidism type 1B. *J Clin Invest* 2000;107:793.

Marx SJ: Hyperparathyroid and hypoparathyroid disorders. *N Engl J Med* 2000;343:1863.

McKay C, Furman WL: Hypercalcemia complicating childhood malignancies. *Cancer* 1993;72:256.

Meij IC, Saar K, vanden Heuvel LPS, et al: Hereditary isolated renal magnesium loss maps to chromosome 11q23. *Am J Hum Genet* 1999;64:180.

Miric A, Vechio JD, Levine MA: Heterogeneous mutations in the gene encoding the α-subunit of the stimulatory G protein of adenylyl cyclase in Albright hereditary osteodystrophy. *J Clin Endocrinol Metab* 1993;76:1560.

Nagamine K, Peterson P, Shimizu N, et al: Positional cloning of the APECED gene. *Nat Genet* 1997;17:393.

Nakamoto JM, Sandstrom AT, Van Dop C, et al: Pseudohypoparathyroidism type Ia from maternal but not paternal transmission of a Gsα gene mutation. *Am J Med Genet* 1998;77:261.

Parvari R, Hershkovitz F, Grossman N, et al: Mutation of TBCE causes hypoparathyroidism-retardation-dysmorphism and autosomal recessive Kenny-Caffey syndrome. *Nat Genet* 2002;32:448.

Pearce SH: Multiple endocrine neoplasia type I (MEN 1): Recent advances (commentary). *Clin Endocrinol* 1997;47:513.

Pearce SH, Williamson C, Thaker RV, et al: A familial syndrome of hypocalcemia with hypercalciuria due to mutations in the calcium-sensing receptor. *N Engl J Med* 1996;335:1115.

Pollak MR, Brown EM, Wu Chou YH, et al: Mutations in the human Ca²⁺-sensing receptor gene cause familial hypocalciuric hypercalcemia and neonatal severe hyperthyroidism. *Cell* 1992;75:1297.

Pollak MR, WuChou YH, Marx SJ, et al: Familial hypocalciuric hypercalcemia and neonatal severe hyperparathyroidism: Effects of mutant gene dosage on phenotype. *J Clin Invest* 1994;93:1108.

Ryan AK, Goodship JA, Wilson DI, et al: Spectrum of clinical features associated with interstitial chromosome 22q11 deletions: a European collaborative study. *J Med Genet* 1997;34:708.

Sanjad SA, Sakati NA, Abu-Osba YK, et al: A new syndrome of congenital hypoparathyroidism, severe growth failure and dysmorphic features. *Arch Dis Child* 1992;66:193.

Schipani E, Langman CB, Juppner H, et al: Constitutively activated receptors for parathyroid hormone and parathyroid hormone–related peptide in Jansen's metaphyseal chondrodysplasia. *N Engl J Med* 1996;335:708.

Shalev H, Phillip M, Landau D, et al: Clinical presentation and outcome in primary familial hypomagnesaemia. *Arch Dis Child* 1998;78:127.

Tean BT, Farnebo F, Larson C, et al: Familial isolated hyperparathyroidism maps to the hyperparathyroidism-jaw tumor locus in 1q21-q32 in a subset of families. *J Clin Endocrinol Metab* 1998;83:2114.

Tengan CH, Kiyomoto BH, Moraes CT, et al: Mitochondrial encephalomyopathy and hypoparathyroidism associated with a duplication and a deletion of mitochondrial deoxyribonucleic acid. *J Clin Endocrinol Metab* 1998;83:125.

Thakker RV: Genetic developments in hypoparathyroidism. *Lancet* 2001;357:974–76.

Thomas BR, Bennett JD: Symptomatic hypocalcemia and hypoparathyroidism in two infants of mothers with hyperparathyroidism and familial benign hypercalcemia. *J Perinatol* 1995;15:23.

Toft AD: Surgery for primary hyperparathyroidism—sooner rather than later. *Lancet* 2000;355:1478–79.

Trump D, Dixon PH, Mumm S, et al: Localization of X-linked idiopathic hypoparathyroidism to a 1.5 Mb region on Xq26-q27. *J Med Genet* 1998;35:905.

Tyni T, Rapola J, Pihko H: Hypoparathyroidism in a patient with long-chain 3-hydroxyacyl-coenzyme A dehydrogenase deficiency caused by the G1528C mutation. *J Pediatr* 1997;131:766.

Van Esch H, Groenen P, Devriendt K, et al: GATA3 haplo-insufficiency causes human HDR syndrome. *Nature* 2000;406:419.

Walder RY, Shalev H, Sheffield VC, et al: Familial hypomagnesemia maps to chromosome 9q not to the X chromosome: Genetic linkage mapping and analysis of a balanced translocation breakpoint. *Hum Mol Genet* 1997;6:1491.

Watanabe T, Bai M, Yasuda T, et al: Familial hypoparathyroidism: Identification of a novel gain of function mutation in transmembrane domain 5 of the calcium-sensing receptor. *J Clin Endocrinol Metab* 1998;83:2497.

Weinstein LS, Yu S: The role of genomic imprinting of G_{sα} in the pathogenesis of Albright hereditary osteodystrophy. *Trends Endocrinol Metab* 1999;10:81.

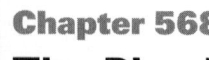

SECTION 4 *Disorders of the Adrenal Glands*

Lenore S. Levine and Perrin C. White

Chapter 568

The Physiology of the Adrenal Gland

568.1 Histology and Embryology

The adrenal gland is composed of two endocrine tissues, the medulla and the cortex. The chromaffin cells of the adrenal medulla are derived from neuroectoderm, whereas the cells of the adrenal cortex are derived from mesoderm. Mesodermal cells also contribute to the development of the gonads. The adrenal glands and gonads have certain common enzymes involved in steroid synthesis; an inborn error in steroidogenesis in one tissue may also be present in the other.

The adrenal cortex consists of three zones: the zona glomerulosa, the outermost zone located immediately beneath the capsule; the zona fasciculata, the middle zone; and the zona reticularis, the innermost zone, lying next to the adrenal medulla. The zona fasciculata is the largest of the zones, constituting about three fourths of the cortex; the zona glomerulosa comprises about 15% and the zona reticularis about 10%. Glomerulosa cells are small with a lower cytoplasmic:nuclear ratio, intermediate number of lipid inclusions, and smaller nuclei containing more condensed chromatin than the cells of the other two zones. The cells of the zona fasciculata are large with a high cytoplasmic:nuclear ratio and many lipid inclusions that give the cytoplasm a foamy, vacuolated appearance. The cells are arranged in radial cords. The cells of the zona reticularis are arranged in irregular anastomosing cords. The cytoplasmic:nuclear ratio is intermediate, and the compact cytoplasm has relatively little lipid content.

The zona glomerulosa synthesizes aldosterone, the most potent natural mineralocorticoid in humans. The zona fasciculata produces cortisol, the most potent natural glucocorticoid in humans, and the zona fasciculata and zona reticularis synthesize the adrenal androgens.

The adrenal medulla consists mainly of neuroendocrine (chromaffin) cells and glial (sustentacular) cells with some connective tissue and vascular cells. Neuroendocrine cells are polyhedral with abundant cytoplasm and small, pale-staining nuclei. Under the electron microscope, the cytoplasm contains many large secretory granules that contain catecholamines. Glial cells have less cytoplasm and more basophilic nuclei.

The primordium of the fetal adrenal gland can be recognized at 3–4 wk of gestation just cephalad to the developing mesonephros. At 5–6 wk, the gonadal ridge develops into the steroidogenic cells of the gonads and adrenal cortex; the adrenal and gonadal cells separate, the adrenal cells migrate retroperitoneally, and the gonadal cells migrate caudad. At 6–8 wk of gestation, the gland rapidly enlarges, the cells of the inner cortex differentiate to form the fetal zone, and the outer subcapsular rim remains as the definitive zone. The primordium of the adrenal cortex is invaded at this time by sympathetic neural elements that differentiate into the chromaffin cells capable of synthesizing and storing catecholamines. Catechol-O-methyltransferase, which converts norepinephrine to epinephrine, is expressed later in gestation. By the end of the 8th wk of gestation, the encapsulated adrenal gland is associated with the upper pole of the kidney. By 9–12 wk of gestation, the cells of the fetal zone are capable of active steroidogenesis. In the fetus of 2 mo, the adrenals are larger than the kidneys, but from the 4th mo, the kidneys grow rapidly, becoming twice as large as the adrenals by the end of the 6th mo. In the full-term infant, the adrenal gland is one third the size of the kidney and the combined weight of both glands is 7–9 g. At birth, the inner fetal cortex makes up about 80% of the gland and the outer "true" cortex, 20%. Within a few days the fetal cortex begins to involute, undergoing a 50% reduction by 1 mo of age. Conversely, the adrenal medulla is relatively small at birth and undergoes a proportionate increase in size over the first 6 postnatal months. By 1 yr, the adrenal glands each weigh less than 1 g. Adrenal growth thereafter results in adult adrenal glands reaching a combined weight of 8 g. The zonae fasciculata and glomerulosa are fully differentiated by about 3 yr of age. The zona reticularis may not be fully differentiated until puberty.

Early fetal adrenal growth appears to be independent of adrenocorticotropic hormone (ACTH), but, at least from midterm until term, ACTH is essential for adrenal growth and maturation. At which stage of fetal development feedback regulation of ACTH by cortisol is established has not been fully defined, but clinical experience suggests that normal pituitary-adrenal feedback relationships are operative in the first trimester. Additional factors important in fetal growth and steroidogenesis include placental chorionic gonadotropins and a number of peptide growth factors produced by the placenta and fetus.

Two transcription factors are critical for the development of the adrenal glands: steroidogenic factor-1 (SF-1) and DAX-1 (*d*osage-sensitive sex reversal, *a*drenal hypoplasia congenita, *X*-chromosome). SF-1 is also important in the transcriptional regulation of several genes coding for enzymes of steroidogenesis. Disruption of SF-1, encoded on chromosome 9q33, results in adrenal and gonadal agenesis, absence of pituitary gonadotropes, and an underdeveloped ventral medial hypothalamus. Mutations in the *DAX1* gene, encoded on Xp21, result in congenital adrenal hypoplasia and hypogonadotropic hypogonadism. DAX-1 also plays an important role in regulating steroidogenesis.

568.2 Adrenal Steroid Biosynthesis

Cholesterol is the starting substrate for all steroid biosynthesis (Fig. 568–1). Although adrenal steroid cells can synthesize cholesterol de novo from acetate, 80% of the cholesterol precursor for adrenal cortex hormone formation is provided by the circulating plasma lipoproteins. Specific cell surface receptors for low-density lipoprotein (LDL) bind the circulating LDL and internalize it by receptor-mediated endocytosis. Cholesterol is stored as cholesteryl esters in vesicles and subsequently hydrolyzed by cholesteryl ester hydrolase to liberate free cholesterol to be used for steroid hormone synthesis.

The rate-limiting step of adrenal steroidogenesis is importation of cholesterol across the mitochondrial outer and inner membrane. This requires several proteins, including the peripheral benzodiazepine receptor and the steroidogenic acute regulatory (StAR) protein. StAR protein has a very short half-life, and its synthesis is rapidly induced by trophic factors (e.g., corticotropin); thus, it is the main short-term (min to hr) regulator of steroid hormone biosynthesis.

At the mitochondrial inner membrane, the side-chain of cholesterol is cleaved to yield pregnenolone. This is catalyzed by cholesterol side-chain cleavage enzyme (cholesterol desmolase, P450scc, CYP11A1), a cytochrome P450 (CYP) enzyme. Like other P450s, this is a membrane-bound hemoprotein with a molecular mass of about 50 kd. It accepts electrons from an NADPH-dependent mitochondrial electron transport system consisting of two accessory proteins, adrenodoxin reductase (a flavoprotein) and adrenodoxin (a small protein containing nonheme iron). P450 enzymes utilize electrons and O_2 to hydroxylate the substrate and form H_2O. In the case of the cholesterol side-chain cleavage reaction, three successive oxidative reactions are performed to cleave the C20,22 carbon bond. Pregnenolone then diffuses out of mitochondria and enters the endoplasmic reticulum. The subsequent reactions that occur depend on the zone of the adrenal cortex.

Zona Glomerulosa. In the zona glomerulosa, pregnenolone is converted to progesterone by 3β-hydroxysteroid dehydrogenase (HSD3B2), an NAD+-dependent enzyme of the "short chain dehydrogenase" type. Progesterone is converted to 11-deoxycorticosterone by steroid 21-hydroxylase (P450c21, CYP21), which is another cytochrome P450. Like other P450s in the endoplasmic reticulum, it utilizes an electron transport system with only one accessory protein, cytochrome P450 reductase.

Deoxycorticosterone then re-enters mitochondria and is converted to aldosterone by aldosterone synthase (P450aldo, CYP11B2), another P450 enzyme structurally related to cholesterol desmolase. Aldosterone synthase also carries out three successive oxidations: 11β-hydroxylation, 18-hydroxylation, and further oxidation of the 18-methyl carbon to an aldehyde.

Zona Fasciculata. In the endoplasmic reticulum of the zona fasciculata, pregnenolone and progesterone are converted by 17α-hydroxylase (P450c17, CYP17) to 17-hydroxypregnenolone and 17-hydroxyprogesterone, respectively. This enzyme is not expressed in the zona glomerulosa, which consequently cannot synthesize 17-hydroxylated steroids. 17-Hydroxypregnenolone is converted to 17-hydroxyprogesterone and 11-deoxycortisol by the same 3β-hydroxysteroid and 21-hydroxylase enzymes, respectively, as are active in the zona glomerulosa. Thus, inherited disorders in these enzymes affect both aldosterone and cortisol synthesis (see Chapter 570). Finally, 11-deoxycortisol re-enters mitochondria and is converted to cortisol by steroid 11β-hydroxylase (P450c11, CYP11B1). This enzyme is closely related to aldosterone synthase but has low 18-hydroxylase and nonexistent 18-oxidase

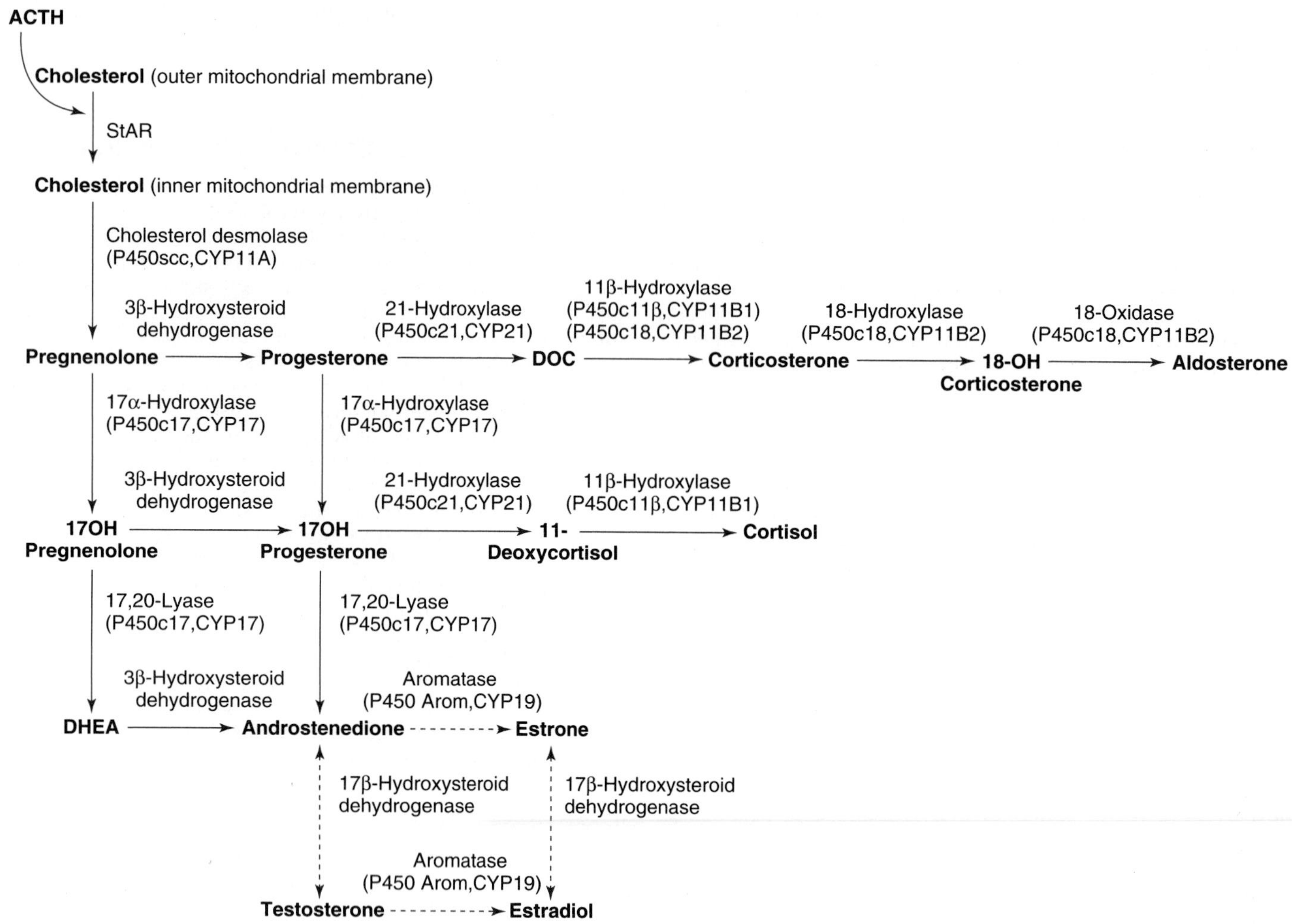

ACTH

FIGURE 568–1. Pathways of steroid biosynthesis. The pathways for adrenal synthesis of mineralocorticoids (aldosterone), glucocorticoids (cortisol) and androgens (DHEA, androstenedione) are arranged vertically. The enzymatic activity for each bioconversion is indicated. The systematic name for the activities mediated by specific cytochromes P450 is indicated in parentheses. The reactions shown with dotted arrows occur primarily in gonads, not in adrenals. P450c11β mediates 11β-hydroxylase activity in the zona fasciculata to convert DOC to corticosterone and 11-deoxycortisol to cortisol. P450c18 mediates 11β-hydroxylase, 18-hydroxylase and 18-oxidase activities in the zona glomerulosa for the conversion of DOC to aldosterone.

activity. Thus, under normal circumstances the zona fasciculata cannot synthesize aldosterone.

Zona Reticularis. In the zona reticularis and to some extent in the zona fasciculata, the 17-hydroxylase (CYP17) enzyme has an additional activity, cleavage of the 17,20 carbon-carbon bond. This converts 17-hydroxypregnenolone to dehydroepiandrosterone (DHEA). Dehydroepiandrosterone is converted by 3β-hydroxysteroid dehydrogenase to androstenedione. This may be further converted in other tissues to testosterone and estrogens.

Fetoplacental Unit. Steroid synthesis in the fetal adrenal differs from that in the postnatal gland. LDL cholesterol synthesized by the fetal liver is the major cholesterol source for steroid synthesis in the fetal adrenal gland. The fetal adrenal gland has low 3β-hydroxysteroid dehydrogenase activity and high steroid sulfokinase activity. Thus, the major steroid products of the fetal adrenal gland are DHEA and DHEA sulfate (DHEAS) and, by 16α-hydroxylation in the liver, 16α-hydroxy DHEAS. The placenta, which has high steroid sulfatase activity, uses DHEA and DHEAS as substrates for estrone and estradiol and 16α-OH DHEAS as a substrate for estriol. Placental estrone and estradiol are derived equally from fetal and maternal precursors; estriol is

almost exclusively produced from substrates of fetal origin. In addition to providing substrate for the placental synthesis of estrogens, the fetal adrenal gland also produces significant amounts of cortisol, much of which is converted to cortisone by the enzyme 11β-hydroxysteroid dehydrogenase. As term approaches, fetal cortisol concentration increases as a result of increased cortisol secretion and decreased conversion of cortisol to cortisone. Low levels of aldosterone are produced in mid gestation, but aldosterone secretory capacity increases near term.

568.3 Regulation of the Adrenal Cortex

Regulation of Cortisol Secretion. Glucocorticoid secretion is regulated mainly by adrenocorticotropic hormone (corticotropin, ACTH), a 39-amino acid peptide that is produced in the anterior pituitary. It is synthesized as part of a larger molecular weight precursor peptide known as pro-opiomelanocortin (POMC). This precursor peptide is also the source of β-lipotropin (β-LPH). In addition, ACTH and β-LPH are cleaved further to yield α- and β-melanocyte-stimulating hormone, corticotropin-like intermediate lobe peptide (CLIP), γ-LPH, β- and γ-endorphin, and enkephalin (see Chapter 550).

ACTH is released in secretory bursts of varying amplitude throughout the day and night. The normal diurnal rhythm of cortisol secretion is caused by the varying amplitudes of ACTH pulses. Pulses of ACTH and cortisol occur every 30–120 min, are highest at about the time of waking, are low in late afternoon and evening, and reach their lowest point 1 or 2 hr after sleep begins.

Corticotropin-releasing hormone (CRH), synthesized by neurons of the parvicellular division of the hypothalamic paraventricular nucleus, is the most important stimulator of ACTH secretion. Arginine vasopressin (AVP) augments CRH action. Neural stimuli from the brain cause the release of CRH and AVP (see Chapter 550). AVP and CRH are secreted in the hypophyseal-portal circulation in a pulsatile manner. This pulsatile secretion appears to be responsible for the pulsatile (ultradian) release of ACTH. The circadian rhythm of corticotropin release is probably induced by a corresponding circadian rhythm of hypothalamic CRH secretion, regulated by the suprachiasmatic nucleus with input from other areas of the brain. Cortisol exerts a negative feedback effect on the synthesis and secretion of ACTH, CRH, and AVP. ACTH inhibits its own secretion, a feedback effect mediated at the level of the hypothalamus. Thus the secretion of cortisol is a result of the interaction of the hypothalamus, pituitary, and adrenal glands and other neural stimuli.

ACTH acts through a specific G protein–coupled receptor to activate adenylate cyclase and increase levels of cyclic adenosine monophosphate (AMP). Cyclic AMP has short-term (minutes to hours) effects on cholesterol transport into mitochondria by increasing expression of steroidogenesis acute regulatory (StAR) protein. The long-term effects (hours to days) of ACTH stimulation are to increase the uptake of LDL cholesterol and the expression of genes encoding the enzymes required to synthesize cortisol. These transcriptional effects occur at least in part through increased activity of protein kinase A, which phosphorylates several transcriptional regulatory factors.

Regulation of Aldosterone Secretion. The rate of aldosterone synthesis, which is normally 100- to 1000-fold less than that of cortisol synthesis, is regulated mainly by the renin-angiotensin system and by potassium levels, with ACTH having only a short-term effect. In response to decreased intravascular volume, renin is secreted by the juxtaglomerular apparatus of the kidney. Renin is a proteolytic enzyme that cleaves angiotensinogen (renin substrate), an α_2-globulin produced by the liver, to yield the inactive decapeptide angiotensin I. Angiotensin-converting enzyme in the lungs and other tissues rapidly cleaves angiotensin I to the biologically active octapeptide angiotensin II. Cleavage of angiotensin II produces the heptapeptide angiotensin III. Angiotensin II and III are potent stimulators of aldosterone secretion; angiotensin II is a more potent vasopressor agent. Angiotensin II and III occupy a G protein–coupled receptor activating phospholipase C. The latter protein hydrolyzes phosphatidylinositol bisphosphate to produce inositol triphosphate and diacylglycerol, which raise intracellular calcium levels and activate protein kinase C and calmodulin-activated (CaM) kinases. Similarly, increased levels of extracellular potassium depolarize the cell membrane and increase calcium influx through voltage-gated L-type calcium channels. Phosphorylation of as yet unidentified factors by CaM kinases increases transcription of the aldosterone synthase (CYP11B2) enzyme required for aldosterone synthesis.

Regulation of Adrenal Androgen Secretion. The mechanisms by which the adrenal androgens dehydroepiandrosterone and androstenedione are regulated are not completely understood. *Adrenarche* is a maturational process in the adrenal gland that results in increased adrenal androgen secretion between the ages of 5 and 20 years. The process begins before the earliest signs of puberty and continues throughout the years when puberty is occurring. Histologically, it is associated with the appearance of the zona reticularis. Whereas ACTH stimulates adrenal androgen production acutely and clearly is the primary stimulus for cortisol release (see later), additional factors have been implicated in the stimulation of the adrenal androgens. These include a relative decrease in expression of 3β- hydroxysteroid dehydrogenase in the zona reticularis and possibly increases in 17,20-lyase activity owing to phosphorylation or increased cytochrome b5 expression.

568.4 Adrenal Steroid Hormone Actions

Steroid hormones act through several distinct receptors corresponding to the known biologic activities of the steroid hormones: glucocorticoid, mineralocorticoid, progestin, estrogen, and androgen. These receptors belong to a larger superfamily of nuclear transcriptional factors that include, among others, thyroid hormone and retinoic acid receptors. They have a common structure that includes a carboxy-terminal ligand-binding domain and a mid-region DNA-binding domain. The latter domain contains two "zinc fingers," each of which consists of a loop of amino acids stabilized by four cysteine residues chelating a zinc ion.

Unliganded glucocorticoid and mineralocorticoid receptors are found mainly in the cytosol. Hormone molecules diffuse through the cell membrane and bind receptors, changing their conformation and causing them to be translocated to the nucleus where they bind DNA at specific hormone response elements. Bound receptors may recruit other transcriptional co-regulatory factors to DNA.

Whereas different steroids may share bioactivities because of their ability to bind to the same receptor, a given steroid may exert diverse biologic effects in different tissues. The diversity of hormonal responses is determined by the different genes that are regulated by the hormone in different tissues. Additionally, different combinations of co-regulators are expressed in different tissues, allowing each steroid hormone to have many different effects. Moreover, enzymes may increase or decrease the affinity of steroids for their receptors and thus modulate their activity.

Actions of Glucocorticoids. Glucocorticoids are essential for survival. The term *glucocorticoid* refers to the glucose-regulating properties of these hormones. However, the glucocorticoids have multiple effects on carbohydrate, lipid, and protein metabolism. They also regulate immune, circulatory, and renal function. They influence growth, development, bone metabolism, and central nervous system activity.

In stress situations, glucocorticoid secretion can increase up to 10-fold. This increase is believed to enhance survival through increased cardiac contractility, cardiac output, sensitivity to the pressor effects of the catecholamines and other pressor hormones, work capacity of the skeletal muscles, and capacity to mobilize energy stores.

METABOLIC EFFECTS. The primary action of the glucocorticoids on carbohydrate metabolism is to increase glucose production by increasing hepatic gluconeogenesis. In addition to inducing gluconeogenic enzymes, glucocorticoids stimulate glycolysis, proteolysis, and lipolysis, which provides more substrate for gluconeogenesis. Glucocorticoids also increase cellular resistance to insulin, thereby decreasing entry of glucose into the cell. This inhibition of glucose uptake occurs in adipocytes, muscle cells, and fibroblasts. In addition to opposing insulin action, glucocorticoids may work in parallel with insulin to protect against long-term starvation by stimulating glycogen deposition and production in liver. Both hormones stimulate glycogen synthetase activity and decrease glycogen breakdown.

Thus, glucocorticoid excess may cause hyperglycemia, whereas glucocorticoid deficiency may cause hypoglycemia.

Glucocorticoids increase free fatty acid levels by enhancing lipolysis, decreasing cellular glucose uptake and decreasing glycerol production, which is necessary for re-esterification of fatty acids. This increase in lipolysis is also stimulated through the permissive enhancement of lipolytic action of other factors such as epinephrine. This action affects adipocytes differently according to their anatomic locations. In the patient with glucocorticoid excess, fat is lost in the extremities, but it is increased in the trunk (centripetal obesity), neck, and face (moon facies). This may involve effects on adipocyte differentiation.

Glucocorticoids generally exert a catabolic/antianabolic effect on protein metabolism. Proteolysis in fat, skeletal muscle, bone, lymphoid, and connective tissue increases amino acid substrates that can be used in gluconeogenesis. Cardiac muscle and the diaphragm are almost entirely spared from this catabolic effect.

CIRCULATORY AND RENAL EFFECTS. Glucocorticoids have a positive inotropic influence on the heart, increasing the left ventricular work index. Moreover, they have a permissive effect on the actions of epinephrine and norepinephrine on both the heart and the blood vessels. In the absence of glucocorticoids, decreased cardiac output and shock may develop; in states of glucocorticoid excess, hypertension is frequently observed. This may be due to activation of the mineralocorticoid receptor (see later), which occurs when renal 11β-hydroxysteroid dehydrogenase is saturated by excessive levels of glucocorticoids.

GROWTH. In excess, glucocorticoids inhibit linear growth and skeletal maturation in children. This results primarily from the direct inhibitory effect of glucocorticoids on the epiphyses. This may in part be mediated by decreasing levels of growth hormone and insulin-like growth factor-1 (IGF-1) and by increasing IGF binding protein-1 (IGFBP-1), which inhibits somatic growth by decreasing circulating levels of free IGF-1.

Although excess glucocorticoids clearly impair growth, they are also necessary for normal growth and development. In the fetus and neonate, they accelerate the differentiation and development of various tissues. These actions include the development of the hepatic and gastrointestinal systems, as well as the production of surfactant in the fetal lung. Glucocorticoids are routinely given to pregnant women at risk for delivery of premature infants in an effort to accelerate these maturational processes.

IMMUNOLOGIC EFFECTS. Glucocorticoids play a major role in immune regulation. They inhibit synthesis of glycolipids and prostaglandin precursors and the actions of bradykinin. They also block histamine and proinflammatory cytokine (tumor necrosis factor-α, interleukin-1, and interleukin-6) secretion and effects. These actions diminish the inflammatory process. High doses of glucocorticoids deplete monocytes, eosinophils, and lymphocytes, especially T cells. They do so at least in part by inducing cell cycle arrest in the G1 phase and by activating apoptosis through glucocorticoid receptor–mediated effects. The effects on lymphocytes are primarily exerted on T helper 1 cells and hence on cellular immunity, whereas the T helper 2 cells are spared, leading to a predominantly humoral immune response. Pharmacologic doses of glucocorticoids may also decrease the size of immunologic tissues (i.e., the spleen, thymus, and lymph nodes).

Glucocorticoids increase circulating polymorphonuclear cell counts, mostly by preventing their egress from the circulation. Glucocorticoids decrease diapedesis, chemotaxis, and phagocytosis of polymorphonuclear cells. Thus, the mobility of these cells is altered such that they do not arrive at the site of inflammation to mount an appropriate immune response. High levels of glucocorticoids decrease inflammatory and cellular immune responses and increase susceptibility to certain bacterial, viral, fungal, and parasitic infections.

EFFECTS ON SKIN, BONE, AND CALCIUM. Glucocorticoids inhibit fibroblasts, leading to increased bruising and poor wound healing through cutaneous atrophy. This effect explains the thinning of the skin and striae that are seen in patients with Cushing syndrome.

Glucocorticoids have the overall effect of decreasing serum calcium and have been used in emergency therapy for certain types of hypercalcemia. This hypocalcemic effect probably results from a decrease in the intestinal absorption of calcium and a decrease in the renal reabsorption of calcium and phosphorus. The serum calcium level, however, generally does not fall below normal because of the secondary increase in parathyroid hormone secretion.

The most significant effect of long-term glucocorticoid excess on calcium and bone metabolism is osteoporosis. Glucocorticoids inhibit osteoblastic activity by decreasing the number and activity of osteoblasts. Glucocorticoids also decrease osteoclastic activity, but to a lesser extent, leading to low bone turnover with an overall negative balance. The tendency of glucocorticoids to lower serum calcium and phosphate levels causes secondary hyperparathyroidism. These actions decrease bone accretion and cause a net loss of bone mineral.

CENTRAL NERVOUS SYSTEM EFFECTS. Glucocorticoids readily penetrate the blood-brain barrier and have direct effects on brain metabolism. They decrease certain types of CNS edema and are frequently used to treat increased intracranial pressure. They stimulate appetite and cause insomnia with a reduction in rapid eye movement sleep. There is an increase in irritability and emotional lability, with an impairment of memory and ability to concentrate. Mild to moderate glucocorticoid excess for a limited period of time often causes a feeling of euphoria or well-being, but glucocorticoid excess and deficiency may both be associated with clinical depression. Furthermore, glucocorticoid excess may produce psychosis in some patients.

Glucocorticoid effects in brain are mediated largely through interactions with both the mineralocorticoid and glucocorticoid receptors (sometimes referred to in this context as type I and type II corticosteroid receptors, respectively). Activation of type II receptors increases sensitivity of hippocampal neurons to the neurotransmitter serotonin, which may help explain the euphoria associated with high doses of glucocorticoids. Glucocorticoids suppress release of corticotropin-releasing hormone (CRH) in the anterior hypothalamus, but stimulate it in the central nucleus of the amygdala and lateral bed nucleus of the stria terminalis, where it may mediate fear and anxiety states. In addition, glucocorticoids and other steroids may have nongenomic effects by modulating activities of both γ-aminobutyric acid (GABA) and N-methyl-D-aspartate (NMDA) receptors.

Actions of Mineralocorticoids. The most important mineralocorticoids are aldosterone and, to a lesser degree, 11-deoxycorticosterone; corticosterone and cortisol are normally not important as mineralocorticoids unless secreted in excess. As a class of hormones, mineralocorticoids have more limited actions than glucocorticoids. Their major function is to maintain intravascular volume by conserving sodium and eliminating potassium and hydrogen ions. They exert these actions in kidney, gut, and salivary and sweat glands. In addition, aldosterone may have distinct effects in other tissues. Mineralocorticoid receptors are found in the heart and vascular endothelium, and aldosterone increases myocardial fibrosis in heart failure.

The distal convoluted tubules and cortical collecting ducts of the kidney are the major sites of action of the mineralocorticoids where they induce reabsorption of sodium and secretion of potassium. In the medullary collecting duct, they act in a permissive fashion to allow vasopressin to increase osmotic water flux. Thus, patients with mineralocorticoid deficiency may develop weight loss, hypotension, hyponatremia, and hyperkalemia, whereas patients with mineralocorticoid excess may develop hypertension, hypokalemia, and metabolic alkalosis (see Chapters 569–572).

The mechanisms by which aldosterone affects sodium excretion are incompletely understood. Most effects of aldosterone are presumably due to changes in gene expression mediated by the mineralocorticoid receptor, and indeed levels of subunits of both the Na+/K+ ATPase and the epithelial sodium channel (ENaC) increase in response to aldosterone.

The mineralocorticoid receptor has similar affinities in vitro for cortisol and aldosterone, yet cortisol is a weak mineralocorticoid in vivo. This discrepancy results from the action of 11β-hydroxysteroid dehydrogenase, which converts cortisol to cortisone. Cortisone is not a ligand for the receptor, whereas aldosterone is not a substrate for the enzyme. Pharmacologic or genetic inhibition of this enzyme allows cortisol to occupy renal mineralocorticoid receptors and produce sodium retention and hypertension.

Actions of the Adrenal Androgens. Many actions of adrenal androgens are exerted through their conversion to active androgens or estrogens such as testosterone, dihydrotestosterone, estrone, and estradiol. In adult men, less than 2% of the biologically important androgens are derived from adrenal production, whereas in women about 50% of androgens are of adrenal origin. The adrenal contribution to circulating estrogen levels is mainly important in pathologic conditions, such as feminizing adrenal tumors. Adrenal androgens contribute to the physiologic

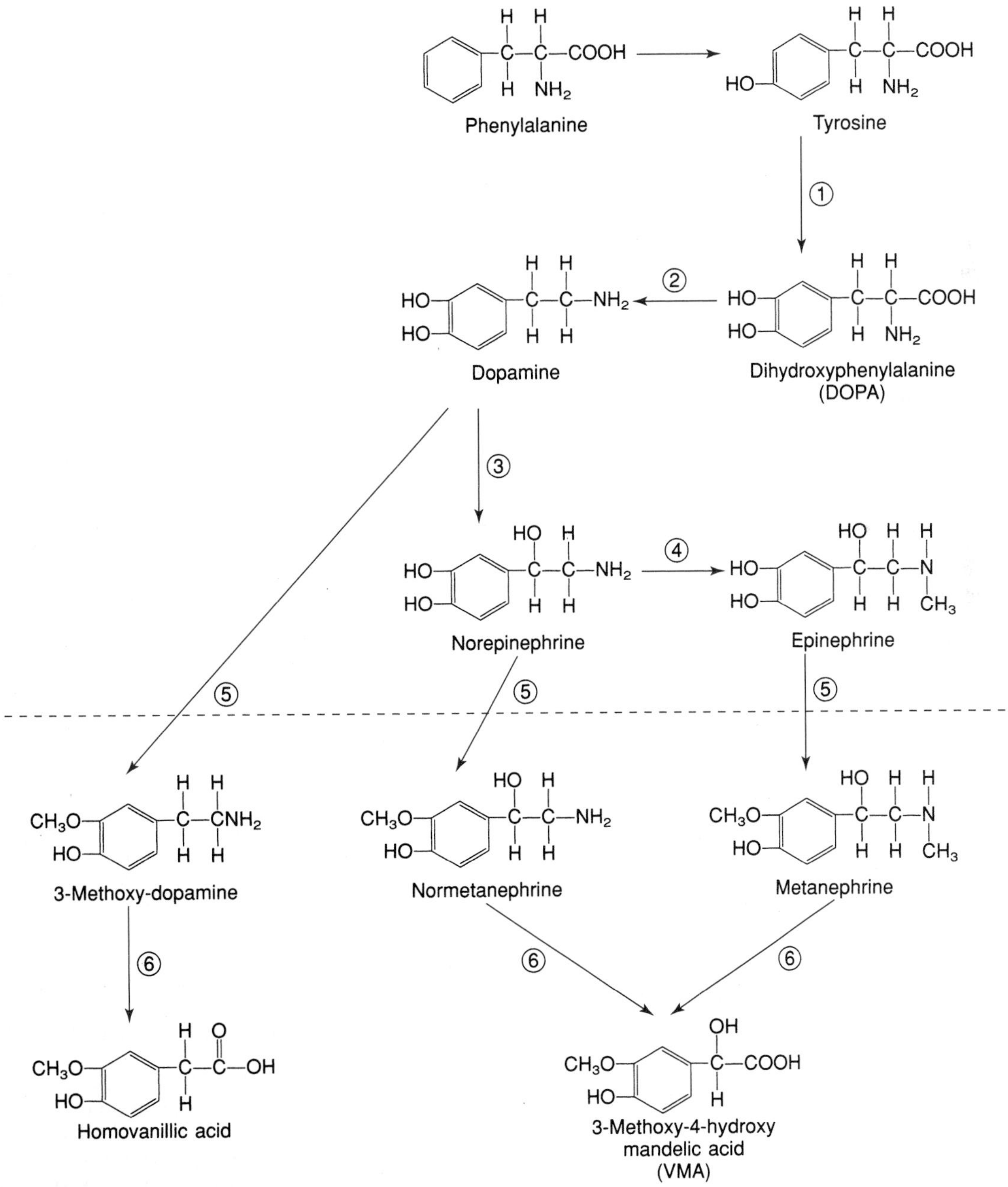

FIGURE 568–2. Biosynthesis *(above dashed line)* and metabolism *(below dashed line)* of the catecholamines norepinephrine and epinephrine. Enzymes: 1, tyrosine hydroxylase; 2, dopa decarboxylase; 3, dopamine β-oxidase; 4, phenylethanolamine-*N*-methyltransferase; 5, catechol-O-methyltransferase; 6, monoamine oxidase.

development of pubic and axillary hair during normal puberty. They also play an important role in the pathophysiology of congenital adrenal hyperplasia, premature adrenarche, adrenal tumors, and Cushing syndrome (see Chapters 570, 571, 573).

In humans, circulating levels of DHEA and DHEAS, the chief adrenal androgens, reach a peak in early adulthood and then decline. This has led to speculation that age-related physiologic changes might be reversed by DHEA administration, and beneficial effects have been proposed on insulin sensitivity, bone mineral density, muscle mass, cardiovascular risk, obesity, cancer risk, autoimmunity, and the central nervous system.

SYNTHETIC CORTICOSTEROIDS. Many synthetic analogues of cortisone and hydrocortisone are available. Prednisone and prednisolone are derivatives with an additional double bond in ring A. They are 4–5 times as potent in anti-inflammatory and carbohydrate activity but have slightly less effect on retention of water and sodium. Halogenated derivatives have different effects. Betamethasone and dexamethasone have 25–40 times the glucocorticoid potency of cortisol but have little mineralocorticoid effect. These analogues are usually used in pharmacologic doses for their anti-inflammatory or immunosuppressive properties. In contrast, fludrocortisone has about 15 times greater anti-inflammatory activity than does hydrocortisone but is more than 125 times as active a mineralocorticoid; it is used to treat aldosterone deficiency.

568.5   Adrenal Medulla

The principal hormones of the adrenal medulla are the physiologically active catecholamines: dopamine, norepinephrine, and epinephrine (Fig. 568–2). Catecholamine synthesis also occurs in the brain, in sympathetic nerve endings, and in chromaffin tissue outside the adrenal medulla. Metabolites of catecholamines are excreted in the urine. The principal ones are 3-methoxy-4-hydroxymandelic acid (VMA), metanephrine, and normetanephrine. Measurement of metanephrine and catecholamines is used to detect functioning tumors of the adrenal medulla.

The proportions of epinephrine and norepinephrine in the adrenal gland vary with age. In early fetal stages, there is practically no epinephrine; and at birth, norepinephrine is predominant. In adults, norepinephrine makes up only 10–30% of the pressor amines in the medulla.

The effects of catecholamines are mediated through a series of G protein–coupled adrenergic receptors. Both epinephrine and norepinephrine raise the mean arterial blood pressure, but only epinephrine increases cardiac output. By increasing peripheral vascular resistance, norepinephrine increases systolic and diastolic blood pressures with only a slight reduction in the pulse rate. Epinephrine increases the pulse rate and, by decreasing the peripheral vascular resistance, decreases the diastolic pressure. The hyperglycemic and calorigenic effects of norepinephrine are much less pronounced than are those of epinephrine.

Aguilera G, Rabadan-Diehl C: Vasopressinergic regulation of the hypothalamic-pituitary-adrenal axis: Implications for stress adaptation. *Regul Pept* 2000;96: 23–29.

Allen DB: Growth suppression by glucocorticoid therapy. *Endocrinol Metab Clin North Am* 1996;25:699–717.

Ashwell JD, Lu FW, Vacchio MS: Glucocorticoids in T cell development and function. *Annu Rev Immunol* 2000;18:309–45.

Bamberger CM, Schulte HM, Chrousos GP: Molecular determinants of glucocorticoid receptor function and tissue sensitivity to glucocorticoids. *Endocr Rev* 1996;17:245.

de Kloet ER, Vreugdenhil E, Oitzl MS, et al: Brain corticosteroid receptor balance in health and disease. *Endocr Rev* 1998;19:269–301.

Itoi K, Seasholtz AF, Watson SJ: Cellular and extracellular regulatory mechanisms of hypothalamic corticotropin-releasing hormone neurons. *Endocr J* 1998;45: 13–33.

Jenkins BD, Pullen CB, Darimont BD: Novel glucocorticoid receptor coactivator effector mechanisms. *Trends Endocrinol Metab* 2001;12:122–26.

Lamberts SW, Bruining HA, de Jong FH: Corticosteroid therapy in severe illness. *N Engl J Med* 1997;337:1285–92.

Lane NE, Lukert B: The science and therapy of glucocorticoid-induced bone loss. *Endocrinol Metab Clin North Am* 1998;27:465–83.

Lupien SJ, McEwen BS: The acute effects of corticosteroids on cognition: Integration of animal and human model studies. *Brain Res Brain Res Rev* 1997;24: 1–27.

Manelli F, Giustina A: Glucocorticoid-induced osteoporosis. *Trends Endocrinol Metab* 2000;11:79–85.

Matsusaka T, Ichikawa I: Biological functions of angiotensin and its receptors. *Annu Rev Physiol* 1997;59:395–412.

Miller WL: Early steps in androgen biosynthesis: From cholesterol to DHEA. *Baillieres Clin Endocrinol Metab* 1998;12:67–81.

Peter M, Dubuis JM: Transcription factors as regulators of steroidogenic P-450 enzymes. *Eur J Clin Invest* 2000;30:Suppl-20.

Rainey WE, White PC: Functional adrenal zonation and regulation of aldosterone biosynthesis. *Curr Opin Endocrinol Diab* 1998;5:175–82.

Stocco DM: StAR protein and the regulation of steroid hormone biosynthesis. *Annu Rev Physiol* 2001;63:193–213.

Wallberg AE, Wright A, Gustafsson JA: Chromatin-remodeling complexes involved in gene activation by the glucocorticoid receptor. *Vitam Horm* 2000;60:75–122.

White PC: Genetic diseases of steroid metabolism. *Vitam Horm* 1994;49:131–95.

White PC: Abnormalities of aldosterone synthesis and action in children. *Curr Opin Pediatr* 1997;9:424–30.

White PC, Mune T, Agarwal AK: 11β-Hydroxysteroid dehydrogenase and the syndrome of apparent mineralocorticoid excess. *Endocr Rev* 1997;18:135–56.

Yanovski JA, Cutler GBJ: Glucocorticoid action and the clinical features of Cushing's syndrome. *Endocrinol Metab Clin North Am* 1994;23:487–509.

■ **Chapter 569**
Adrenocortical Insufficiency

In primary adrenal insufficiency, congenital or acquired lesions of the adrenal cortex prevent production of cortisol and often aldosterone (Box 569–1). Acquired primary adrenal insufficiency is termed *Addison disease*. Dysfunction of the hypothalamus or anterior pituitary gland may cause a deficiency of corticotropin (ACTH) and lead to hypofunction of the adrenal cortex; this is termed *secondary adrenal insufficiency*.

569.1   Primary Adrenal Insufficiency

Primary adrenal insufficiency may be caused by genetic conditions that are not always manifested in infancy and by acquired problems such as autoimmune conditions. However, susceptibility to autoimmune conditions often has a genetic basis, and so these distinctions are not absolute.

Inherited Etiologies

INBORN DEFECTS OF STEROIDOGENESIS. The most common causes of adrenocortical insufficiency in infancy are the salt-losing forms of congenital adrenal hyperplasia (see Chapter 570). Approximately 75% of infants with 21-hydroxylase deficiency, almost all infants with lipoid adrenal hyperplasia, and most infants with a deficiency of 3β-hydroxysteroid dehydrogenase manifest salt-losing symptoms in the newborn period because they are unable to synthesize either cortisol or aldosterone.

ADRENAL HYPOPLASIA CONGENITA. Hypoadrenalism usually presents acutely in the neonatal period but may be delayed until later childhood or even adulthood with a more insidious onset. Histologic examination of the hypoplastic adrenal cortex reveals disorganization and cytomegaly. The disorder affects primarily boys and is caused by mutation of the *DAX1* gene, a member of the nuclear hormone receptor family, located on Xp21. Boys with adrenal hypoplasia congenita (AHC) do not undergo puberty, owing to hypogonadotropic hypogonadism; both AHC and hypogonadotropic hypogonadism are caused by

BOX 569–1. Etiologic Classification of Adrenocortical Hypofunction

Corticotropin-releasing hormone deficiency
  Isolated deficiency
  Multiple deficiencies
    Congenital defects (e.g., anencephaly, septo-optic dysplasia)
    Destructive lesions (e.g., tumor)
    Idiopathic (e.g., idiopathic hypopituitarism)
Corticotropin deficiency
  Isolated
  Autosomal recessive
  Multiple deficiencies
    Pituitary hypoplasia or aplasia
    Destructive lesions (e.g., craniopharyngioma)
    Autoimmune hypophysitis
Primary adrenal hypoplasia or aplasia
  X-linked
    With Duchenne muscular dystrophy and glycerol kinase
      deficiency (Xp21 deletion)
    With hypogonadotropic hypogonadism (*DAX1* mutation)
Familial glucocorticoid deficiency
  Corticotropin-receptor mutations (ACTH unresponsiveness)
    With alacrima, achalasia, and neurologic disorders (triple A
      syndrome)
Defects of steroid biosynthesis
  Lipoid adrenal hyperplasia (StAR mutation)
  3β-Hydroxysteroid dehydrogenase deficiency
    Classic
      Salt loser
      Non–salt loser
    Mild or nonclassic
  21-Hydroxylase (P450C21) deficiency
    Classic
      Salt loser
      Non–salt loser
    Nonclassic or mild
  Isolated aldosterone (P450C18) deficiency
Pseudohypoaldosteronism (aldosterone unresponsiveness)
Adrenoleukodystrophy (peroxisomal membrane protein defect)
  Isolated adrenal involvement
  With neurologic involvement
Acid lipase deficiency
  Wolman disease, fatal neonatal form
Destructive lesions of adrenal cortex
  Granulomatous lesions (e.g., tuberculosis)
Autoimmune adrenalitis (idiopathic Addison disease)
  Isolated
  Associated with hypoparathyroidism or mucocutaneous
    candidiasis (type I autoimmune polyglandular syndrome), or both
  Associated with autoimmune thyroid disease and insulin-
    dependent diabetes (type II autoimmune polyglandular syndrome)
Neonatal hemorrhage
Severe prematurity
Acute infection (Waterhouse-Friderichsen syndrome)
Mitochondrial disorders
Acquired immunodeficiency syndrome
Iatrogenic
  Abrupt cessation of exogenous corticosteroids or corticotropin
  Removal of functioning adrenal tumor
  Adrenalectomy for Cushing disease
  Drugs
    Aminoglutethimide
    Mitotane (o, p'-DDD)
    Metyrapone
    Ketoconazole
Fetal adrenal suppression–maternal hypercortisolism
  Endogenous
  Therapeutic

the same mutated *DAX1* gene. Cryptorchidism, often noted in these boys, is probably an early manifestation of hypogonadotropic hypogonadism.

AHC also occurs as part of a contiguous gene deletion syndrome together with Duchenne muscular dystrophy, glycerol kinase deficiency, mental retardation, or a combination of these conditions.

ADRENOLEUKODYSTROPHY. In this disorder, adrenocortical deficiency is associated with demyelination in the central nervous system (see Chapters 75.2 and 592.3). High levels of very long-chain fatty acids are found in tissues and body fluids, resulting from their impaired β-oxidation in the peroxisomes.

The most frequent form of ALD is an X-linked disorder with various presentations. The most common clinical picture is of a degenerative neurologic disorder appearing in childhood or adolescence and progressing to severe dementia and deterioration of vision, hearing, speech, and gait, with death occurring within a few years. A milder form of X-linked ALD is adrenomyeloneuropathy (ALM), which begins in later adolescence or early adulthood. Many patients have evidence of adrenal insufficiency at the time of neurologic presentation, but Addison disease may precede neurologic symptoms by many years. X-linked ALD may present as isolated Addison disease. X-linked adrenal leukodystrophy (X-ALD) is caused by mutations in the *ABCD1* gene located on Xq28. The gene encodes a transmembrane transporter involved in the importation of very long-chain fatty acids into peroxisomes. More than 400 mutations have been described in patients with X-ALD; the majority of X-ALD families have a unique mutation. Clinical phenotypes can vary even within families, perhaps owing to modifier genes or other unknown factors. There is no correlation between the degree of neurologic impairment and severity of adrenal insufficiency. Prenatal diagnosis by DNA analysis and family screening by very long-chain fatty acids assays and mutation analysis are available. Women who are heterozygous carriers of the *X-ALD* gene may develop symptoms in midlife or later. Adrenal insufficiency is rare. Therapeutic approaches of uncertain efficacy include administration of glycerol trioleate and glycerol trierucate (Lorenzo's oil), bone marrow transplantation, lovastatin, fenofibrate, and gene therapy.

Neonatal ALD is a rare autosomal recessive disorder. Infants present with neurologic deterioration and have or acquire evidence of adrenocortical dysfunction. Most patients have severe mental retardation and die before 5 yr of age. This disorder is a subset of Zellweger (cerebro-hepato-renal) syndrome, in which peroxisomes do not develop at all owing to mutations in any of several genes controlling the development of this organelle.

FAMILIAL GLUCOCORTICOID DEFICIENCY. This form of chronic adrenal insufficiency is characterized by isolated deficiency of glucocorticoids, elevated levels of ACTH, and normal aldosterone production. The salt-losing manifestations present in most other forms of adrenal insufficiency do not occur; instead, patients present primarily with hypoglycemia, seizures, and increased pigmentation during the 1st decade of life. The disorder affects both sexes equally and is inherited in an autosomal recessive manner. There is marked adrenocortical atrophy with relative sparing of the zona glomerulosa. A number of mutations in the gene for the ACTH receptor have been described in some (approximately 40%) but not all of these patients.

Another syndrome of ACTH resistance occurs in association with achalasia of the gastric cardia and alacrima (triple A or Allgrove syndrome). These patients often have a progressive neurologic disorder that includes autonomic dysfunction, mental retardation, deafness, and motor neuropathy. This syndrome is also inherited in an autosomal recessive fashion, and the gene has been mapped to chromosome 12q13.

DISORDERS OF CHOLESTEROL SYNTHESIS/METABOLISM. Patients with disorders of cholesterol synthesis or metabolism, including abetalipoproteinemia with deficient lipoprotein B–containing lipoproteins, and familial hypercholesterolemia, with decreased or impaired LDL receptors, have been demonstrated to have limited adrenal cortical function. Adrenal insufficiency has been reported in patients with Smith-Lemli-Opitz syndrome (SLOS), an autosomal recessive disorder presenting with facial anomalies, microcephaly, limb anomalies, and developmental delay. Mutations in the gene coding for sterol Δ7-reductase, mapped to 11q12-q13, resulting in impairment of the final step in cholesterol synthesis with marked elevation of 7-dehydrocholesterol, abnormally low cholesterol, and adrenal insufficiency have been identified in SLOS. Wolman disease is a rare autosomal recessive disorder caused by mutations in the gene encoding human lysosomal acid lipase. There is marked intralysosomal accumulation of cholesterol esters throughout most organ systems and ultimately organ failure. Infants present during the first or second month of life with hepatosplenomegaly, steatorrhea, abdominal distention, and failure to thrive. Adrenal insufficiency and bilateral adrenal calcification are present and death usually occurs in the first year of life. The gene for lysosomal acid lipase has been mapped to chromosome 10q23.2-23.3; the genetic defects in patients with Wolman disease have been elucidated.

CORTICOSTEROID BINDING GLOBULIN (CBG) DEFICIENCY AND DECREASED CORTISOL-BINDING AFFINITY. These disorders result in low levels of plasma cortisol but normal urinary free cortisol and normal plasma ACTH levels. A high prevalence of hypotension and fatigue has been reported in some adults with abnormalities of CBG.

Acquired Etiologies

AUTOIMMUNE ADDISON DISEASE. The most common cause of Addison disease is autoimmune destruction of the glands. The glands may be so small that they are not visible at autopsy, and only remnants of tissue are found in microscopic sections. Usually the medulla is not destroyed, and there is marked lymphocytic infiltration in the area of the former cortex. In advanced disease, all adrenal cortical function is lost, but early in the clinical course, isolated cortisol deficiency may occur. Most patients have antiadrenal cytoplasmic antibodies in their plasma; 21-hydroxylase (CYP21) is the most frequently occurring autoantigen.

Addison disease often occurs as a component of two syndromes, each consisting of a constellation of autoimmune disorders. *Type I autoimmune polyendocrinopathy* (APS-1) is also known as the *autoimmune polyendocrinopathy/candidiasis/ectodermal dystrophy* (APECED) syndrome. Chronic mucocutaneous candidiasis is most often the first manifestation, followed by hypoparathyroidism and then by Addison disease, which typically develops in early adolescence. Other closely associated autoimmune disorders include gonadal failure, alopecia, vitiligo, keratopathy, enamel hypoplasia, nail dystrophy, intestinal malabsorption, and chronic active hepatitis. Hypothyroidism and type I diabetes mellitus occur in fewer than 10% of affected patients. Some components of the syndrome continue to develop as late as the 5th decade. The presence of antiadrenal antibodies and steroidal cell antibodies in these patients usually indicates a high likelihood of the development of Addison disease or, in females, ovarian failure. Adrenal failure may evolve rapidly in APS-1; death in patients previously diagnosed and unexplained deaths in siblings of patients with APS-1 have been reported, indicating the need to closely monitor patients with APS-1 and to thoroughly evaluate apparently unaffected siblings of patients with this disorder.

Autoantibodies to the CYP21, CYP17, and CYP11A1 enzymes have been reported in patients with APS-1. The disorder is inherited as an autosomal recessive disorder, and the gene, designated autoimmune regulator-1 (AIRE1), has been mapped to chromosome 21q22.3. The *AIRE1* gene encodes a protein, which appears to be a transcription factor having an important role in immune response. Approximately 40 different mutations in the *AIRE1* gene have been described in patients with APS-1, with two mutations (R257X and a 3-bp deletion) being most frequent. There has been autosomal dominant transmission in one kindred owing to a specific missense mutation (G228W).

Type II autoimmune polyendocrinopathy (APS-2) consists of Addison disease associated with autoimmune thyroid disease (Schmidt syndrome) or type-1 diabetes (Carpenter syndrome). Gonadal failure, vitiligo, alopecia, and chronic atrophic gastritis, with or without pernicious anemia, may occur. HLA-D3 and HLA-D4 are increased in these patients and appear to confer an increased risk of developing this disease; alleles at the major histocompatibility complex class I chain-related genes A and B (MICA and MICB) have also been associated with this disorder. The disorder is most common in middle-aged females and may occur in many generations of the same family. Antiadrenal antibodies, specifically antibodies to the CYP21, CYP17, and CYP11A1 enzymes, are also found in these patients.

INFECTION. Tuberculosis was a common cause of adrenal destruction in the past but is much less prevalent now. The most frequent infectious etiology for adrenal insufficiency is meningococcemia (see Chapter 176); adrenal crisis from this cause is referred to as the Waterhouse-Friderichsen syndrome. Patients with AIDS may have a variety of subclinical abnormalities in the hypothalamic-pituitary-adrenal axis, but frank adrenal insufficiency is rare. However, drugs used in the treatment of AIDS may affect adrenal hormone homeostasis.

DRUGS. Ketoconazole, an antifungal drug, can cause adrenal insufficiency by inhibiting adrenal enzymes. Rifampicin and anticonvulsive drugs such as phenytoin and phenobarbital reduce the effectiveness and bioavailability of corticosteroid replacement therapy by inducing steroid-metabolizing enzymes in the liver. Mitotane (o,p'-DDD), used in the treatment of adrenal carcinoma and refractory Cushing syndrome (see Chapters 571, 573), is cytotoxic to the adrenal cortex and may also alter extra-adrenal cortisol metabolism. Signs of adrenal insufficiency occur in a substantial percentage of patients treated with mitotane.

HEMORRHAGE INTO ADRENAL GLANDS. This may occur in the neonatal period as a consequence of difficult labor (especially breech presentation), or its etiology may not be apparent. An incidence rate of 3 per 100,000 live births has been suggested. The hemorrhage may be sufficiently extensive to result in death from exsanguination or hypoadrenalism. An abdominal mass, anemia, unexplained jaundice, or scrotal hematoma may be the presenting sign. Often, the hemorrhage is asymptomatic initially and is identified later by calcification of the adrenal gland. Fetal adrenal hemorrhage has also been reported. Postnatally, adrenal hemorrhage most often occurs in patients being treated with anticoagulants. It may also occur as a result of child abuse.

Clinical Manifestations. Primary adrenal insufficiency leads to cortisol and often aldosterone deficiency. The signs and symptoms of adrenal insufficiency are most easily understood in the context of the normal actions of these hormones, which were discussed in Chapter 568.

Hypoglycemia is a prominent feature of adrenal insufficiency. It is often accompanied by ketosis as the body attempts to utilize fatty acids as an alternative energy source. It is aggravated by anorexia, nausea, and vomiting, all of which occur frequently.

Cortisol deficiency decreases cardiac output and vascular tone; moreover, catecholamines such as epinephrine have decreased inotropic and pressor effects in the absence of cortisol. These problems are initially manifested as orthostatic hypotension in older children and may progress to frank shock in patients of any age. They are exacerbated by aldosterone deficiency, which results in hypovolemia due to decreased resorption of sodium in the distal nephron.

Hypotension and decreased cardiac output decrease glomerular filtration and thus decrease the ability of the kidney to excrete free water. Vasopressin (AVP) is secreted by the posterior pituitary in response to hypotension and also as a direct consequence of lack of inhibition by cortisol. These factors decrease plasma osmolality and lead in particular to hyponatremia. Hyponatremia is also caused by aldosterone deficiency and may be much worse when both cortisol and aldosterone are deficient.

In addition to hypovolemia and hyponatremia, aldosterone deficiency causes hyperkalemia by decreasing potassium excretion in the distal nephron. However, cortisol deficiency alone does not cause hyperkalemia.

Finally, cortisol deficiency decreases negative feedback on the hypothalamus and pituitary, leading to increased secretion of ACTH. Hyperpigmentation is caused by ACTH and other peptide hormones (e.g., γ-melanocyte stimulating hormone) arising from the ACTH precursor pro-opiomelanocortin. In patients with a fair complexion, the skin may have a bronze cast. Pigmentation may be more prominent in skin creases, mucosa, and scars. In dark-skinned patients, it may be most readily appreciated in the gingival and buccal mucosa.

The clinical presentation of adrenal insufficiency depends on the age of the patient, whether both cortisol and aldosterone secretion are affected, and to some extent on the underlying etiology. The most common causes in early infancy are inborn errors of steroid biosynthesis, sepsis, adrenal hypoplasia congenita, and adrenal hemorrhage. Infants have a relatively greater requirement for aldosterone than older children, possibly owing to immaturity of the kidney and also to the low sodium content of human breast milk and infant formula. Hyperkalemia, hyponatremia, and hypoglycemia are prominent presenting signs of adrenal insufficiency in infants. Ketosis is not consistently present because infants generate ketones less well than older children. Hyperpigmentation is not usually seen because this takes weeks or months to develop, and orthostatic hypotension is obviously difficult to demonstrate in infants.

Infants can become ill very quickly. There may be only a few days of decreased activity, anorexia, and vomiting before critical electrolyte abnormalities develop.

In older children with Addison disease, the onset is usually more gradual and is characterized by muscle weakness, malaise, anorexia, vomiting, weight loss, and orthostatic hypotension. Hyperpigmentation is often but not necessarily present. Hypoglycemia and ketosis are common, as is hyponatremia. Hyperkalemia tends to occur later in the course of the disease in older children than in infants. Thus, the clinical presentation can be easily confused with gastroenteritis or other acute infections. Chronicity of symptoms may alert the clinician to the possibility of Addison disease, but this diagnosis should be considered in any child with orthostatic hypotension, hyponatremia, hypoglycemia, and ketosis.

Laboratory Findings. Hypoglycemia, ketosis, hyponatremia, and hyperkalemia have been discussed. An electrocardiogram is useful for quickly detecting hyperkalemia in a critically ill child. Acidosis is frequently present, and the blood urea nitrogen level is elevated if the patient is dehydrated.

Cortisol levels may sometimes be at the low end of the normal range but are invariably low when the patient's degree of illness is considered. ACTH levels are high in primary adrenal insufficiency but may take time to be reported by the laboratory. Similarly, aldosterone levels may be within the normal range but inappropriately low considering the patient's hyponatremia, hyperkalemia, and hypovolemia. Plasma renin activity is elevated. Blood eosinophils may be increased in number, but this is rarely useful diagnostically.

Urinary excretion of sodium and chloride are increased and urinary potassium is decreased, but these are difficult to assess on random urine samples. Accurate interpretation of urinary electrolytes requires more prolonged (24 hr) urine collections and knowledge of the patient's sodium and potassium intake.

The most definitive test for adrenal insufficiency is measurement of serum levels of cortisol before and after administration of ACTH; resting levels are low and do not increase normally after administration of ACTH. Occasionally, normal resting levels that do not increase after administration of ACTH may indicate an absence of adrenocortical reserve. A low initial level

followed by a significant response to ACTH may indicate secondary adrenal insufficiency. Traditionally, this test has been performed by measuring cortisol levels before and 30 or 60 minutes after giving 0.250 mg of cosyntropin (ACTH 1-24) by rapid intravenous infusion. Aldosterone will transiently increase in response to this dose of ACTH and may also be measured. A low-dose test (0.5–1 μg ACTH 1–24/1.73 m^2) is a more sensitive test of pituitary-adrenal reserve but has somewhat lower specificity (i.e., more false-positive tests).

Additional testing is directed at identifying the specific cause for adrenal insufficiency. When congenital adrenal hyperplasia is suspected, serum levels of cortisol precursors (e.g., 17-hydroxyprogesterone) should be measured along with cortisol in an ACTH stimulation test. This is discussed further in Chapter 570. Elevated levels of very long-chain fatty acids are diagnostic of adrenoleukodystrophy. The presence of antiadrenal antibodies suggests an autoimmune pathogenesis. Patients with autoimmune Addison disease must be closely observed for the development of other autoimmune disorders. In children, hypoparathyroidism is the most frequently associated disorder, and is suspected if hypocalcemia and elevated phosphate levels are noted.

Ultrasonography, CT, or MRI may help define the size of the adrenal glands.

Treatment. Treatment of acute adrenal insufficiency must be immediate and vigorous. If the diagnosis of adrenal insufficiency has not been established, a blood sample should be obtained before therapy for determination of electrolytes, glucose, ACTH, cortisol, aldosterone, and plasma renin activity. If the patient's condition permits, an ACTH stimulation test can be performed while initial fluid resuscitation is underway. Intravenous administration of 5% glucose in 0.9% saline solution should be given to correct hypoglycemia, hypovolemia, and hyponatremia. If hyperkalemia is severe, it may require treatment with intravenous calcium and/or bicarbonate, intrarectal potassium-binding resin (Kayexalate), or intravenous infusion of glucose and insulin. A water-soluble form of hydrocortisone, such as hydrocortisone sodium succinate, should be given intravenously. As much as 10 mg for infants, 25 mg for toddlers, 50 mg for older children, and 100 mg for adolescents should be administered at 6-hr intervals for the first 24 hr. These doses may be reduced during the next 24 hr if progress is satisfactory. Adequate fluid and sodium repletion is achieved by intravenous saline administration, aided by the mineralocorticoid effect of high doses of hydrocortisone.

After the acute manifestations are under control, most patients require chronic replacement therapy for their cortisol and aldosterone deficiencies. Hydrocortisone (i.e., cortisol) may be given orally in daily doses of 10 mg/M^2/24 hr in three divided doses. Equivalent doses (20–25% of the hydrocortisone dose) of prednisone or prednisolone may be used, divided twice daily. ACTH levels may be used to monitor adequacy of glucocorticoid replacement in primary adrenal insufficiency; in congenital adrenal hyperplasia, levels of precursor hormones are used instead (see Chapter 570). During situations of stress, such as periods of infection or minor operative procedures, the dose of hydrocortisone should be increased 2–3 fold. Major surgery under general anesthesia requires high intravenous doses of hydrocortisone similar to those used for acute adrenal insufficiency. If aldosterone deficiency is present, fludrocortisone (Florinef), a mineralocorticoid, is given orally in doses of 0.05–0.3 mg daily. Measurements of plasma renin activity are useful in monitoring the adequacy of mineralocorticoid replacement. Chronic overdosage with glucocorticoids leads to obesity, short stature, and osteoporosis, whereas overdosage with fludrocortisone results in tachycardia, hypertension, and occasionally hypokalemia.

569.2 Secondary Adrenal Insufficiency

Etiology

ABRUPT CESSATION OF ADMINISTRATION OF CORTICOSTEROIDS. Secondary adrenal insufficiency most commonly occurs when the hypothalamic-pituitary-adrenal axis is suppressed by prolonged administration of high doses of a potent glucocorticoid and that agent is suddenly withdrawn or the dose is tapered too quickly. Patients at risk for this problem include those with leukemia, asthma (particularly when patients are transitioned from oral to inhaled corticosteroids), and collagen vascular disease or other autoimmune conditions and those who have undergone tissue transplants or neurosurgical procedures. The maximum duration and dose of glucocorticoid that can be administered before encountering this problem is not known, but it is assumed that high dose glucocorticoids (the equivalent of >10 times physiologic cortisol secretion) can be administered for at least a week without requiring a subsequent taper of dose. On the other hand, when high doses of dexamethasone are given to children with leukemia, it can take up to 2 mo or longer after therapy is stopped before tests of adrenal function return to normal. Signs and symptoms of adrenal insufficiency are most likely in patients who are subsequently subjected to stresses such as severe infections or additional surgical procedures.

CORTICOTROPIN (ACTH) DEFICIENCY. Pituitary or hypothalamic dysfunction can cause corticotropin deficiency (see Chapter 557), usually associated with deficiencies of other pituitary hormones such as growth hormone and thyrotropin. Destructive lesions in the area of the pituitary, such as craniopharyngioma and germinoma, are the most common causes of corticotropin deficiency. In many cases the pituitary or hypothalamus are further damaged during surgical removal or radiotherapy of tumors in the midline of the brain. In very rare instances, autoimmune hypophysitis has been the cause of corticotropin deficiency.

Congenital lesions of the pituitary also occur. The pituitary alone may be affected, or additional midline structures may be involved, such as the optic nerves or septum pellucidum. The latter type of abnormality is termed *septo-optic dysplasia* or *de Morsier syndrome*. More severe developmental anomalies of the brain, such as anencephaly and holoprosencephaly, can also affect the pituitary. These disorders are usually sporadic, although a few cases of autosomal recessive inheritance have occurred. Isolated deficiency of corticotropin has been reported, including in several sets of siblings. Patients with multiple pituitary hormone deficiencies due to mutations in the *PROP1* gene have been described with progressive ACTH/cortisol deficiency. Isolated deficiency of corticotropin-releasing hormone has been documented in an Arabic kindred as an autosomal recessive trait.

Clinical Presentation. Because the adrenal gland is, by definition, intact in secondary adrenal insufficiency, and the renin-angiotensin system is not involved, aldosterone secretion is unaffected. Thus, signs and symptoms are those of cortisol deficiency. Newborns often present with hypoglycemia. Older children may have orthostatic hypotension or weakness. Electrolytes are usually normal.

When secondary adrenal insufficiency is due to an inborn or acquired anatomic defect involving the pituitary, there may be signs of associated deficiencies of other pituitary hormones. The penis may be small in male infants if gonadotropins are also deficient. Infants with secondary hypothyroidism are often jaundiced. Children with associated growth hormone deficiency grow poorly after the 1st yr of life.

Some children with pituitary abnormalities have hypoplasia of the midface. Children with optic nerve hypoplasia may have obvious visual impairment. They usually have a characteristic wandering nystagmus, but this is often not apparent until several months of age.

Treatment. Iatrogenic secondary adrenal insufficiency (i.e., caused by chronic glucocorticoid administration) is best avoided by using the smallest effective doses of systemic glucocorticoids for the shortest period of time. When a patient is thought to be at risk, tapering the dose rapidly to a level equivalent to or slightly less than physiologic replacement ($\sim$10 mg/M^2/24h) and further tapering over several weeks may allow the adrenal cortex to recover without signs of adrenal insufficiency developing. Patients with anatomic lesions of the pituitary should be treated indefinitely with glucocorticoids. Mineralocorticoid replacement is not required.

Abdu TAM, Clayton RN: The low-dose synacthen test for the assessment of secondary adrenal insufficiency. *Curr Opin Endocrinol* 2000;7:116–21.

Anderson RA, Bryson GM, Parks JS: Lysosomal acid lipase mutations that determine phenotype in Wolman and cholesterol ester storage disease. *Mol Genet Metab* 1999;68:333–45.

Berberogly M, Aycan Z, Oeal G, et al: Syndrome of congenital adrenocortical unresponsiveness to ACTH: Report of six patients. *J Pediatr Endocrinol Metabol* 2001;14:1113–18.

Betterle C, Volpato M, Smith BR, et al: II. Adrenal cortex and steroid 21-hydroxylase autoantibodies in children with organ-specific autoimmune diseases: Markers of high progression to clinical Addison's disease. *J Clin Endocrinol Metab* 1997;82:939–42.

Boles RG, Roe T, Senadheera D, et al: Mitochondrial DNA deletion with Kearns-Sayre syndrome in a child with Addison disease. *Eur J Pediatr* 1998;157:643–7.

Burris TP, Weiwen G, McCabe ERB: The gene responsible for adrenal hypoplasia congenita, DAX-1, encodes a nuclear hormone receptor that defines a new class within the superfamily. *Recent Prog Horm Res* 1996;51:241–59.

Clark AJL, Metherell L, Swords FM, Elias LLK: The molecular pathogenesis of ACTH insensitivity syndromes. *Ann Endocrinol* 2001;62:207–11.

Coursin DB, Wood KE: Corticosteroid supplementation for adrenal insufficiency. *JAMA* 2002;287:236–40.

Dickstein G: Hypothalamo-pituitary-adrenal axis testing: Nothing is sacred and caution in interpretation is needed. *Clin Endocrinol* 2001;54:15–6.

Drake AJ, Howells RJ, Shield PH, et al: Symptomatic adrenal insufficiency presenting with hypoglycaemia in asthmatic children with asthma receiving high dose inhaled fluticasone propionate. *BMJ* 2002;324:1081–82.

Eledrisi MS, Verghese AC: Adrenal insufficiency in HIV infection: A review and recommendations. *Am J Med Sci* 2001;321:137–44.

Heino M, Peterson P, Kudoh J, et al: APECED mutations in the autoimmune regulator (AIRE) gene. *Hum Mutat* 2001;18:205–11.

Huysman MWA, Hokken-Koelega ACS, De Ridder MAJ, et al: Adrenal function in sick very preterm infants. *Pediatr Res* 2000;48:629–33.

Kemp S, Pujol A, Waterham HR, et al: ABCD1 mutations and the X-linked adrenoleukodystrophy mutation database: Role in diagnosis and clinical correlations. *Hum Mutat* 2001;18:499–515.

Krivit W, Peters C, Dusenbery K, et al: Case report: Wolman disease successfully treated by bone marrow transplantation. *Bone Marrow Trans* 2000;26:567–70.

Myhre AG, Undlien DE, Lovas K, et al: Autoimmune adrenocortical failure in Norway autoantibodies and human leukocyte antigen class II associations related to clinical features. *J Clin Endocrinol Metab* 2002;87:618–23.

Pai GS, Khan M, Barbosa E, et al: Lovastatin therapy for X-linked adrenoleukodystrophy: Clinical and biochemical observations on 12 patients. *Mol Genet Metab* 2000;69:312–22.

Pearce SHS, Cheetham TD: Autoimmune polyendocrinopathy syndrome type 1: Treat with kids gloves. *Clin Endocrinol* 2001;54:433–35.

Peter M, Partsch C-J, Sippell WG: Multisteroid analysis in children with terminal aldosterone biosynthesis defects. *J Clin Endocrinol Metab* 1995;80:1622–27.

Peter M, Viemann M, Partsch CJ, et al: Congenital adrenal hypoplasia: Clinical spectrum, experience with hormonal diagnosis, and report on new point mutations of the DAX-1 gene. *J Clin Endocrinol Metab* 1998;83:2666–74.

Sandrini F, Farmakidis C, Kirschner LS, et al: Spectrum of mutations of the *AAAS* gene in Allgrove syndrome: Lack of mutations in six kindreds with isolated resistance to corticotropin. *J Clin Endocrinol Metab* 2001;86:5433–37.

Ten S, New M, Maclaren N: Clinical review: Addison's disease 2001. *J Clin Endocrinol Metab* 2001;86:2909–22.

Torpy DJ, Bachmann AW, Grice JE, et al: Familial corticosteroid-binding globulin deficiency due to a novel null mutation: Association with fatigue and relative hypotension. *J Clin Endocrinol Metab* 2001;86:3692–3700.

Vaidya B, Pearce S, Kendall-Taylor P: Recent advances in the molecular genetics of congenital and acquired primary adrenocortical failure. *Clin Endocrinol* 2000;53:403–18.

Vallette-Kasic S, Barlier A, Teinturier B, et al: *PROP1* gene screening in patients with multiple pituitary hormone deficiency reveals two sites of hypermutability and a high incidence of corticotropin deficiency. *J Clin Endocrinol Metab* 2001;86:4529–35.

Velaphi SC, Perlman JM: Neonatal adrenal hemorrhage: Clinical and abdominal sonographic findings. *Clin Pediatr* 2001;40:545–48.

Congenital Adrenal Hyperplasia and Related Disorders

Congenital adrenal hyperplasia (CAH) is a family of autosomal recessive disorders of cortisol biosynthesis (normal adrenal steroidogenesis is discussed in Chapter 568). Cortisol deficiency increases secretion of corticotropin (ACTH), which in turn leads to adrenocortical hyperplasia and overproduction of intermediate metabolites. Depending on the enzymatic step that is deficient, there may be signs, symptoms, and laboratory findings of mineralocorticoid deficiency or excess; incomplete virilization or premature puberty in affected males; and virilization or sexual infantilism in affected females (Figs. 570–1 and 570–2; Table 570–1).

570.1 Congenital Adrenal Hyperplasia due to 21-Hydroxylase Deficiency

More than 90% of CAH cases are caused by 21-hydroxylase deficiency. This P450 enzyme (CYP21, P450c21) hydroxylates progesterone and 17-hydroxyprogesterone (17-OHP) to yield 11-deoxycorticosterone (DOC) and 11-deoxycortisol, respectively (see Fig. 568–1). These conversions are required for synthesis of aldosterone and cortisol, respectively. Both hormones are deficient in the most severe, "salt wasting" form of the disease. Slightly less severely affected patients are able to synthesize adequate amounts of aldosterone but have elevated levels of androgens of adrenal origin; this is termed *simple virilizing* disease. These two forms are collectively termed *classic* 21-hydroxylase deficiency. Patients with *nonclassic* disease have relatively mildly elevated levels of androgens and may have signs of androgen excess postnatally.

Classic 21-hydroxylase deficiency occurs in about 1 in 15,000–20,000 births in most populations. Approximately 75% of affected infants have the salt-losing form, whereas 25% have the simple virilizing form of the disorder. Nonclassic disease has a prevalence of about 1/1,000 in the general population but occurs more frequently in specific ethnic groups such as Ashkenazi Jews.

Genetics. There are two steroid 21-hydroxylase genes, *CYP21P (CYP21A1P, CYP21A)* and *CYP21 (CYP21A2, CYP21B)*, which alternate in tandem with two genes for the fourth component of complement *(C4A* and *C4B)* in the human leukocyte antigen major histocompatibility complex on chromosome 6p21.3 between the HLA-B and HLA-DR loci. Many other genes are located in this cluster. *CYP21* is the active gene; *CYP21P* is 98% identical in DNA sequence to *CYP21* but is a pseudogene due to nine different mutations. More than 90% of mutations causing 21-hydroxylase deficiency are recombinations between *CYP21* and *CYP21P.* Approximately 20% are deletions generated by unequal meiotic crossing-over between *CYP21* and *CYP21P,* whereas the remainder are nonreciprocal transfers of deleterious mutations from *CYP21P* to *CYP21,* a phenomenon termed *gene conversion.*

The deleterious mutations in *CYP21P* have varying effects on enzymatic activity when transferred to *CYP21.* Several mutations completely prevent synthesis of a functional protein, whereas others are missense mutations (i.e., they result in amino acid substitutions) that yield enzymes with 1–50% of normal activity. Disease severity correlates well with the muta-

tions carried by an affected individual; for example, patients with salt-wasting disease usually carry mutations on both alleles that completely destroy enzymatic activity. When patients are compound heterozygotes for different types of mutations, the severity of disease expression is largely determined by the activity of the less severely affected of the two alleles.

Clinical Manifestations

ALDOSTERONE AND CORTISOL DEFICIENCY. Because both cortisol and aldosterone require 21-hydroxylation for their synthesis, both hormones are deficient in the most severe, "salt wasting" form of the disease. This form constitutes about 75% of cases of classic 21-hydroxylase deficiency. The signs and symptoms of cortisol and aldosterone deficiency, and the pathophysiology underlying them, are essentially those described in Chapter 569. These include progressive weight loss, anorexia, vomiting, dehydration, weakness, hypotension, hypoglycemia, hyponatremia and hyperkalemia. These problems typically first develop in affected infants at approximately 2 wk of age. Without treatment, shock, cardiac arrhythmias, and death may occur within days or weeks.

CAH differs from other causes of primary adrenal insufficiency in that precursor steroids accumulate proximal to the blocked enzymatic conversion. Because cortisol is not synthesized efficiently, ACTH levels are high, leading to hyperplasia of the adrenal cortex and levels of precursor steroids that may be hundreds of times normal. In the case of 21-hydroxylase deficiency, these precursors include 17-hydroxyprogesterone and progesterone. Progesterone and perhaps other metabolites act as antagonists of the mineralocorticoid receptor and thus may exacerbate the effects of aldosterone deficiency in untreated patients.

PRENATAL ANDROGEN EXCESS. The most important problem caused by accumulation of steroid precursors is that 17-hydroxyprogesterone is shunted into the pathway for androgen biosynthesis, leading to high levels of androstenedione that are converted outside the adrenal gland to testosterone. This problem begins in affected fetuses by 8–10 wk of gestation and leads to abnormal genital development in females (see Figs. 570–1 and 570–2).

The external genitalia of males and females normally appear identical early in gestation (see Chapter 576). In normal females, the genital tubercle becomes the clitoris; the urethral folds develop into the labia minora, and the labioscrotal swellings become the labia majora. In males, development of the external genitalia is normally controlled by testosterone secreted by the fetal testes. The genital tubercle enlarges to become the glans of the penis; the urethral folds fuse to form the shaft of the penis and penile urethra, and the labioscrotal swellings fuse to form the scrotum. Testosterone also controls the development of the wolffian ducts into male internal genital structures such as the prostate, spermatic ducts, and epididymis, but higher levels of testosterone are required than for development of the male external genitalia. In contrast, testosterone has no effect on development of female internal reproductive structures (cervix, uterus, and fallopian tubes) from müllerian ducts. In male fetuses, these structures involute under the influence of anti-müllerian hormone (müllerian inhibitory factor) secreted by the testes.

Thus, affected females, who are exposed in utero to high levels of androgens of adrenal origin, have masculinized external genitalia. This is manifested by enlargement of the clitoris and by partial or complete labial fusion. The vagina usually has a common opening with the urethra (urogenital sinus). The clitoris may be so enlarged that it resembles a penis and, because the urethra opens below this organ, some affected females may be mistakenly presumed to be males with hypospadias and cryptorchidism. The severity of virilization is greatest in females with the salt-losing form of 21-hydroxylase deficiency. The internal genital organs are normal, because affected females

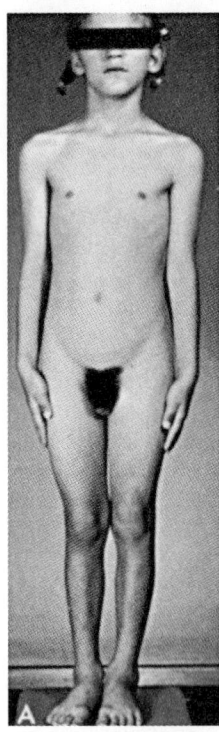 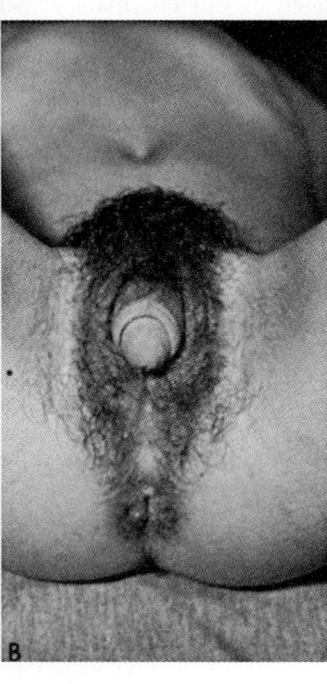 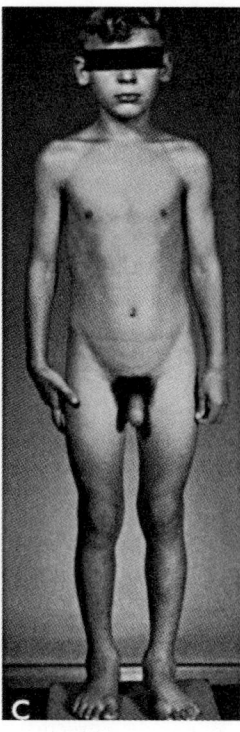

FIGURE 570–1. *A,* A 6-yr-old girl with congenital virilizing adrenal hyperplasia. The height age was 8.5 yr; the bone age was 13 yr; and urinary 17-ketosteroids were 50 mg/24 hr. *B,* Notice the clitoral enlargement and labial fusion. *C,* Five-yr-old brother of girl in *A* was not considered to be abnormal by the parents. The height age was 8 yr; the bone age was 12.5 yr; and the urinary 17-ketosteroids were 36 mg/24 hr.

have normal ovaries and not testes and thus do not secrete anti-müllerian hormone.

Prenatal exposure of the brain to high levels of androgens may influence subsequent sexually dimorphic behaviors in affected females. Girls tend to be interested in masculine toys such as cars and trucks and often show decreased interest in playing with dolls. Women may have decreased interest in maternal roles. There is an increased frequency of homosexuality in affected females, but most function heterosexually. It is unusual for affected females to assign themselves a male role.

Male infants appear normal at birth. Thus, the diagnosis may not be made in boys until signs of adrenal insufficiency develop. Because patients with this condition can deteriorate quickly,

infant boys are much more likely to die than girls. For this reason, many states and countries have instituted newborn screening for this condition (see later).

POSTNATAL ANDROGEN EXCESS. Untreated or inadequately treated children of both sexes develop additional signs of androgen excess after birth. Boys with the simple virilizing form of 21-hydroxylase deficiency often have delayed diagnosis because they appear normal and rarely develop adrenal insufficiency.

Signs of androgen excess include rapid somatic growth and accelerated skeletal maturation. Thus, affected patients are tall in childhood but premature closure of the epiphyses causes growth to stop relatively early, and adult stature is stunted (see Fig. 570–1). Muscular development may be excessive. Pubic and

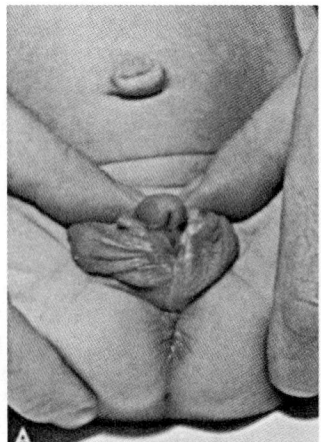 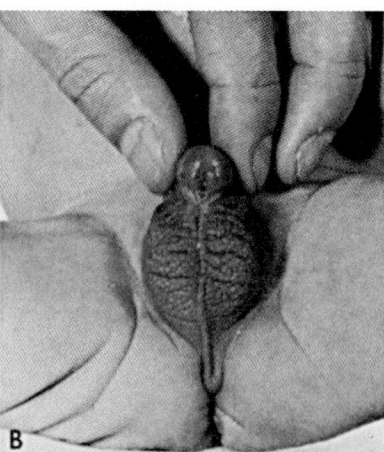 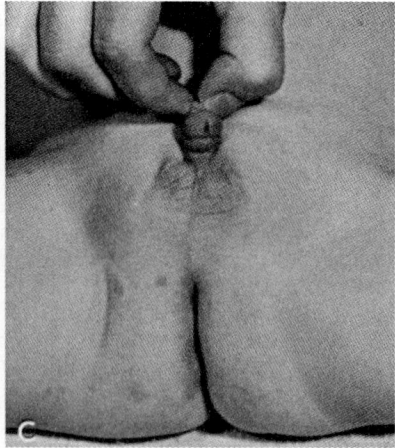

FIGURE 570–2. Three female pseudohermaphrodites with untreated congenital adrenal hyperplasia. All were erroneously assigned male sex at birth, and each had normal female sex-chromosome complement. Infants *A* and *B* were salt losers and were diagnosed in early infancy. Infant *C* was referred at 1 yr of age because of bilateral cryptorchidism. Notice the completely penile urethra; such complete degrees of masculinization in females with adrenal hyperplasia are rare; most of these infants are salt losers.

TABLE 570–1. Diagnosis and Treatment of Congenital Adrenal Hyperplasia

Disorder	Signs and Symptoms	Laboratory Findings	Therapeutic Measures
Lipoid congenital adrenal hyperplasia	Salt-wasting crisis Male pseudohermaphoditism	Low levels of all steroid hormones, with decreased or absent response to ACTH Decreased or absent response to hCG in male pseudohermaphroditism ↑ ACTH ↑ PRA	Glucocorticoid and mineralocorticoid administration Sodium chloride supplementation Gonadectomy of male pseudohermaphrodite Sex hormone replacement consonant with sex of rearing
3β-HSD deficiency	Classic form: Salt-wasting crisis Male and female pseudohermaphroditism Precocious pubarche Disordered puberty	↑↑ Baseline and ACTH-stimulated Δ5 steroids (pregnenolone, 17-OH pregnenolone, DHEA, and their urinary metabolites) ↑ ACTH ↑ PRA Suppression of elevated adrenal steroids after glucocorticoid administration	Glucocorticoid and mineralocorticoid administration Sodium chloride supplementation Surgical correction of genitals and sex hormone replacement as necessary consonant with sex of rearing
3β-HSD deficiency	Nonclassic form: Precocious pubarche, disordered puberty, menstrual irregularity, hirsutism, acne, infertility	↑ Baseline and ACTH-stimulated Δ5 steroids (pregnenolone, 17-OH pregnenolone, DHEA, and their urinary metabolites) ↑ Δ5/Δ4 serum and urinary steroids Suppression of elevated adrenal steroids after glucocorticoid administration	Glucocorticoid administration
21-OH deficiency	Classic form: Salt-wasting crisis Female pseudohermaphroditism Postnatal virilization	↑↑ Baseline and ACTH-stimulated 17-OH progesterone and pregnanetriol ↑↑ Serum androgens and urinary metabolites ↑ ACTH ↑ PRA Suppression of elevated adrenal steroids after glucocorticoid administration	Glucocorticoid and mineralocorticoid replacement Sodium chloride supplementation Vaginoplasty and clitoral recession in female pseudohermaphroditism
21-OH deficiency	Nonclassic form: Precocious pubarche, disordered puberty, menstrual irregularity, hirsutism, acne, infertility	↑ Baseline and ACTH-stimulated 17-OH progesterone and pregnanetriol ↑ Serum androgens and urinary metabolities Suppression of elevated adrenal steroids after glucocorticoid administration	Glucocorticoid administration
11β-Hydroxylase deficiency	Classic form: Female pseudohermaphroditism Postnatal virilization in males and females Hypertension	↑↑ Baseline and ACTH-stimulated compound S and DOC and their urinary metabolites ↑↑ Serum androgens and their urinary metabolites ↑ ACTH ↓ PRA Hypokalemia Suppression of elevated steroids after glucocorticoid administration	Glucocorticoid administration Vaginoplasty and clitoral recession in female pseudohermaphroditism
11β-Hydroxylase deficiency	Nonclassic form: Precocious pubarche, disordered puberty, menstrual irregularity, hirsutism, acne, infertility	↑ Baseline and ACTH-stimulated compound S and DOC and their urinary metabolites ↑ Serum androgens and their urinary metabolites Suppression of elevated steroids after glucocorticoid administration	Glucocorticoid administration
17α-OH/17,20-lyase deficiency	Male pseudohermaphroditism Sexual infantilism Hypertension	↑↑ DOC, 18-OH DOC, corticosterone, 18-hydroxycorticosterone Low 17-α-hydroxylated steroids and poor response to ACTH Poor response to hCG in male pseudohermaphroditism ↓ PRA ↑ ACTH Hypokalemia Suppression of elevated adrenal steroids after glucocorticoid administration	Glucocorticoid administration Surgical correction of genitals and sex hormone replacement in male pseudohermaphroditism consonant with sex of rearing Sex hormone replacement in female

ACTH = adrenocorticotropic hormone (corticotropin); hCG = human chorionic gonadotropin; PRA = plasma renin activity; DOC = deoxycorticosterone.
Adapted from Miller WL, Levine LS: Molecular and clinical advances in congenital adrenal hyperplasia. J Pediatr 1987;111:1.

axillary hair may appear; and acne and a deep voice may develop. The penis, scrotum, and prostate may become enlarged in affected boys; however, the testes are usually prepubertal in size so that they appear relatively small in contrast to the enlarged penis. Occasionally, ectopic adrenocortical cells in the testes of patients become hyperplastic similar to the adrenal glands, producing testicular adrenal rest tumors (see Chapter 578). The clitoris may become further enlarged in affected females (see Fig. 570–1). Although the internal genital structures are female, breast development and menstruation do not occur unless the excessive production of androgens is suppressed by adequate treatment.

Similar but milder signs of androgen excess may occur in nonclassic 21-hydroxylase deficiency. In this attenuated form, cortisol and aldosterone levels are normal and affected females have normal genitalia at birth. Males and females may present with precocious pubarche and early development of pubic and axillary hair. Hirsutism, acne, menstrual disorders, and infertility may develop later in life. However, many females and males are completely asymptomatic.

Laboratory Findings (see Table 570–1). Patients with salt-losing disease have typical laboratory findings associated with cortisol and aldosterone deficiency, including hyponatremia, hyperkalemia, acidosis, and often hypoglycemia, but these abnormalities can take 1–2 wk or longer to develop after birth. Blood levels of 17-hydroxyprogesterone are markedly elevated. However, levels of this hormone are high during the first 2–3 days of life, even in unaffected infants and especially if they are sick or premature. After infancy, once the circadian rhythm of cortisol is established, 17-hydroxyprogesterone levels vary in the same circadian pattern, being highest in the morning and lowest at night. Blood levels of cortisol are usually low in patients with the salt-losing type of disease. They are often normal in those with the simple virilizing type but inappropriately low in relation to the ACTH and 17-hydroxyprogesterone levels. In addition to 17-hydroxyprogesterone, levels of androstenedione and testosterone are elevated in affected females; testosterone is not elevated in affected males because normal infant males have high testosterone levels compared with those seen later in childhood. Levels of urinary 17-ketosteroids and pregnanetriol are elevated but are now rarely used clinically because blood samples are easier to obtain than 24-hr urine collections. Corticotropin (ACTH) levels are elevated but have no diagnostic utility over 17-hydroxyprogesterone levels. Plasma levels of renin are elevated, and serum aldosterone is inappropriately low for the renin level. However, renin levels are normally high in the first few days of life.

Diagnosis of 21-hydroxylase deficiency is most reliably established by measuring 17-hydroxyprogesterone before and 30 or 60 min after an intravenous bolus of 0.125–0.25 mg of cosyntropin (ACTH 1–24). Nomograms exist that readily distinguish normals and patients with nonclassic and classic 21-hydroxylase deficiency. Heterozygous carriers of this autosomal recessive disorder tend to have higher ACTH-stimulated 17-hydroxyprogesterone levels than genetically unaffected individuals, but there is significant overlap between subjects in these two categories.

ADDITIONAL STUDIES. Intersex conditions are discussed more generally in Chapter 582. The initial step in evaluating an infant with ambiguous genitalia is a thorough physical examination to define the anatomy of the genitalia, locate the urethral meatus, palpate the scrotum or labia and the inguinal regions for testes (palpable gonads almost always indicate the presence of testicular tissue and thus that the infant is a genetic male), and look for any other anatomic abnormalities. Ultrasonography is helpful in demonstrating the presence or absence of a uterus and can often locate the gonads. A rapid karyotype (such as fluorescent in situ hybridization of interphase nuclei for X and Y chromosomes) can quickly determine the genetic sex of the infant. These results are all likely to be available before the results of hormonal testing and together allow the clinical team to advise the parents as to the genetic sex of the infant and the anatomy of internal reproductive structures. Injection of contrast medium into the urogenital sinus of female pseudohermaphrodites demonstrates a vagina and uterus and is essential for the surgeon to formulate a plan for surgical management.

Prenatal Diagnosis and Treatment. Prenatal diagnosis of 21-hydroxylase is possible late in the first trimester by analysis of DNA obtained by chorionic villus sampling or during the second trimester by amniocentesis. This is usually done because the parents already have an affected child. Most often, the *CYP21* gene is analyzed for frequently occurring mutations, but closely linked, highly polymorphic microsatellite markers may be used instead if an affected child (i.e., the proband) is available for genetic comparison.

Besides genetic counseling, the main goal of prenatal diagnosis is to facilitate appropriate prenatal treatment of affected females. Recommendations for pregnancies at risk consist of administration of dexamethasone, a steroid that readily crosses the placenta, in an amount of 20 μg/kg prepregnancy maternal weight daily in two or three divided doses. This suppresses secretion of steroids by the fetal adrenal, including secretion of adrenal androgens. If started by 6 wk of gestation, this ameliorates the virilization of the external genitalia in affected females. Chorionic villus biopsy is then performed to determine the sex and genotype of the fetus; therapy is continued only if the fetus is an affected female. DNA analysis of fetal cells isolated from maternal plasma for sex determination and *CYP21* gene analysis may permit earlier identification of the affected female fetus, but this is not yet widely used. No specific deleterious effects have been observed in children exposed to this therapy, but at present there is insufficient information to determine whether there are any long-term risks, particularly in the males and unaffected females who derive no benefit from the treatment. Maternal side effects of prenatal treatment have included edema, excessive weight gain, hypertension, glucose intolerance, cushingoid facial features, and severe striae.

Newborn Screening. Because 21-hydroxylase deficiency is often undiagnosed in affected males until they have severe adrenal insufficiency, many American states and other countries have instituted newborn screening programs. These programs analyze 17-hydroxyprogesterone levels in dried blood obtained by heel-stick and absorbed on filter paper cards; the same cards are screened in parallel for other congenital conditions such as hypothyroidism and phenylketonuria. Potentially affected infants are typically recalled for additional testing (e.g., electrolytes and repeat 17-hydroxyprogesterone determination) at approximately 2 wk of age. Infants with salt-wasting disease often have abnormal electrolytes by this age but are usually not severely ill. Thus, screening programs seem to be effective in preventing many cases of adrenal crisis in affected males. The nonclassic form of the disease is not reliably detected by newborn screening, but this is of little clinical significance because adrenal insufficiency does not occur in this type of 21-hydroxylase deficiency.

The main problem with current newborn screening programs is that to reliably detect all affected infants, the cut-off 17-hydroxyprogesterone levels for recalls are set so low that there is a very high frequency of false-positive results (i.e., the test has high sensitivity and low specificity). This problem is worst in premature infants. Genotyping for *CYP21* might improve specificity but is not routinely available.

Treatment

GLUCOCORTICOID REPLACEMENT. Cortisol deficiency is treated with glucocorticoids. Treatment also suppresses excessive production of androgens by the adrenal cortex and thus minimizes problems such as excessive growth and skeletal maturation and virilization. This often requires larger glucocorticoid doses than are needed in other forms of adrenal insufficiency, typically 10–20 mg/m^2/24 hr of hydrocortisone daily administered orally in three divided doses. Double or triple doses are indicated during periods of stress, such as infection or surgery.

Glucocorticoid treatment must be continued indefinitely in all patients with classic 21-hydroxylase deficiency but may not be necessary in patients with nonclassic disease unless signs of androgen excess are present. Therapy must be individualized. It is desirable to maintain linear growth along percentile lines; crossing to higher height percentiles may suggest undertreatment, whereas loss of height percentiles often indicates overtreatment with glucocorticoids. Overtreatment is also suggested by excessive weight gain. Pubertal development should be monitored by periodic examination, and skeletal maturation is evaluated by serial radiographs of the hand and wrist for bone age. Hormone levels, particularly 17-hydroxyprogesterone and androstenedione, should be measured early in the morning, before taking the morning medications, or at a consistent time in relation to medication dosing. In general, desirable 17-hydroxyprogesterone levels are in the high normal range or several times normal; low-normal levels can usually be achieved only with excessive glucocorticoid doses.

Menarche occurs at the appropriate age in most girls in whom good control has been achieved. However, it may be delayed in girls with suboptimal control.

Children with simple virilizing disease, particularly males, are frequently not diagnosed until 3–7 yr of age, at which time skeletal maturation may be 5 yr or more in advance of chronologic age. In some children, especially if the bone age is 12 yr or more, spontaneous gonadotropin-dependent puberty may occur when treatment is instituted, because therapy with hydrocortisone has suppressed production of adrenal androgens and stimulated release of pituitary gonadotropins if the appropriate level of hypothalamic maturation is present. This form of superimposed true precocious puberty may be treated with a gonadotropin hormone–releasing hormone analogue such as leuprolide.

Males with 21-hydroxylase deficiency who have had inadequate corticosteroid therapy may develop adrenal rest testicular tumors, which usually regress with increased steroid dosage. Testicular MRI, ultrasonography, and color flow Doppler examination help define the character and extent of disease. Testis-sparing surgery for steroid-unresponsive tumors has been reported.

MINERALOCORTICOID REPLACEMENT. Patients with salt-wasting disease (i.e., aldosterone deficiency) require mineralocorticoid replacement with fludrocortisone. Infants may have very high mineralocorticoid requirements in the first few months of life, usually 0.1–0.3 mg daily in two divided doses but occasionally up to 0.4 mg daily, and often require sodium supplementation (sodium chloride, 1–3 g) in addition to the mineralocorticoid. Older infants and children are usually maintained with 0.05–0.1 mg daily of fludrocortisone. In some patients, simple virilizing disease may be easier to control with a low dose of fludrocortisone in addition to hydrocortisone even when these patients have normal aldosterone levels in the absence of mineralocorticoid replacement. Therapy is evaluated by monitoring of vital signs; tachycardia and hypertension are signs of overtreatment with mineralocorticoids. Serum electrolytes should be measured frequently in early infancy as therapy is adjusted. Plasma renin activity is a useful way to determine adequacy of therapy; it should be maintained in or near the normal range but not suppressed.

Additional approaches to improve outcome include an antiandrogen with an aromatase inhibitor (blocks conversion of androgens to estrogen); growth hormone with or without LHRH agonists; and adrenalectomy for poor controlled patients.

SURGICAL MANAGEMENT OF AMBIGUOUS GENITALIA. Significantly virilized females usually undergo surgery between 4–12 mo of age. If there is marked clitoromegaly, the clitoris is reduced in size, with partial excision of the corporal bodies and preservation of the neurovascular bundle. Vaginoplasty and correction of the urogenital sinus usually are performed at the time of clitoral surgery; revision in adolescence is often necessary.

Risks and benefits of surgery should be fully discussed with parents of affected females. There is limited long-term follow-up of functional outcomes in patients who have undergone modern surgical procedures. Sex assignment of infants with intersex conditions is usually based on expected sexual functioning and fertility in adulthood with early surgical correction of the external genitals to conform with the sex assignment. However, lay and medical opponents of this practice state that it ignores any prenatally biased gender role predisposition and precludes the patient from having any decision as to his or her own preferred sexual identity and what surgical correction of the genitals should be performed. These individuals and groups say treatment should be aimed primarily at educating patient, family, and others about the medical condition, its treatment, and how to deal with the intersex condition. They propose that surgery should be delayed until the patient decides on what, if any, correction should be performed. Whether this would be a successful practice in our society requires long-term follow-up studies.

570.2 Congenital Adrenal Hyperplasia due to 11β-Hydroxylase Deficiency

Etiology. Deficiency of 11β-hydroxylase is due to a mutation in the *CYP11B1* gene located on chromosome 8q24. *CYP11B1* mediates 11-hydroxylation of 11-deoxycortisol to cortisol. Because 11-deoxycortisol is not converted to cortisol, levels of corticotropin are high. In consequence, precursors—particularly 11-deoxycortisol and deoxycorticosterone—accumulate and are shunted into androgen biosynthesis in the same manner as occurs in 21-hydroxylase deficiency. However, the adjacent *CYP11B2* gene encoding aldosterone synthase is unaffected in this disorder, and so patients are able to synthesize aldosterone normally.

11β-Hydroxylase deficiency accounts for 5–8% of cases of adrenal hyperplasia; its incidence has been estimated as 1/250,000 to 1/100,000. More than 30 different mutations in *CYP11B1* have been identified. The disorder occurs relatively frequently in Israeli Jews of North African origin (1 in 15,000–17,000 live births); in this ethnic group almost all alleles carry a Arg448 to His (R448H) mutation. This disorder presents in a classic, severe form and rarely in a nonclassic, milder form.

Clinical Manifestations. Although cortisol is not synthesized efficiently, aldosterone synthetic capacity is normal, and some corticosterone is synthesized from progesterone by the intact aldosterone synthase enzyme. Thus, it is unusual for patients to manifest signs of adrenal insufficiency, such as hypotension, hypoglycemia, hyponatremia, and hyperkalemia. Approximately two thirds of patients become hypertensive, although this can take several years without treatment to develop. Hypertension is probably a consequence of elevated levels of deoxycorticosterone, which has mineralocorticoid activity, or metabolites thereof. Infants may transiently develop signs of mineralocorticoid deficiency after treatment with hydrocortisone is instituted. This is presumably due to sudden suppression of deoxycorticosterone secretion in a patient with atrophy of the zona glomerulosa caused by chronic suppression of renin activity.

All signs and symptoms of androgen excess that are found in 21-hydroxylase deficiency may also occur in 11-hydroxylase deficiency.

Laboratory Findings. Plasma levels of 11-deoxycortisol and deoxycorticosterone are elevated. Because deoxycorticosterone and metabolites have mineralocorticoid activity, plasma renin activity is suppressed. Consequently, aldosterone levels are low even though the ability to synthesize aldosterone is intact. Hypokalemic alkalosis occasionally occurs.

Treatment. Patients are treated with hydrocortisone in doses similar to those used for 21-hydroxylase deficiency. Mineralocorticoid replacement is sometimes transiently required in infancy but is rarely necessary otherwise. Hypertension often resolves with glucocorticoid treatment but may require additional therapy if it is of long standing. Calcium channel blockers may be beneficial under these circumstances.

570.3 Congenital Adrenal Hyperplasia due to 3β-Hydroxysteroid Dehydrogenase Deficiency

Etiology. Deficiency of 3β-hydroxysteroid dehydrogenase (3β-HSD) occurs in fewer than 2% of patients with adrenal hyperplasia. This enzyme is required for conversion of Δ5 steroids (pregnenolone, 17-hydroxypregnenolone, dehydroepiandrosterone [DHEA]) to Δ4 steroids (progesterone, 17-hydroxyprogesterone, and androstenedione). Thus, deficiency of the enzyme results in decreased synthesis of cortisol, aldosterone, and androstenedione but increased secretion of DHEA (see Fig. 568–1). The 3β-HSD enzyme expressed in the adrenal cortex and gonad is encoded by the *HSD3B2* gene located on chromosome 1. Over 30 mutations in the *HSD3B2* gene have been described in patients with 3β-HSD deficiency.

Clinical Manifestations. Because cortisol and aldosterone are not synthesized in patients with the classic form of the disease, infants are prone to salt-wasting crises. Because androstenedione and testosterone are not synthesized, boys are incompletely virilized. Varying degrees of hypospadias may occur, with or without bifid scrotum or cryptorchidism. Because DHEA levels are elevated and this hormone is a weak androgen, girls are mildly virilized, with slight to moderate clitoral enlargement. Postnatally, continued excessive DHEA secretion can cause precocious adrenarche. During adolescence and adulthood, hirsutism, irregular menses, and polycystic ovarian disease occur in females. Males manifest variable degrees of hypogonadism, although appropriate male secondary sexual development may occur. A persistent defect of testicular 3β-HSD is demonstrated, however, by the high Δ5:Δ4 steroid ratio in testicular effluent.

Laboratory Findings. The hallmark of this disorder is the marked elevation of the Δ5 steroids (such as 17-hydroxypregnenolone and DHEA) preceding the enzymatic block. Patients may also have elevated levels of 17-hydroxyprogesterone because of the extra-adrenal 3β-HSD activity that occurs in peripheral tissues; these patients may be mistaken for patients with 21-hydroxylase deficiency. However, the ratio of 17-hydroxypregnenolone:17-hydroxyprogesterone is markedly elevated in 3β-HSD deficiency, in contrast to the decreased ratio in 21-hydroxylase deficiency. Plasma renin activity is elevated in the salt-wasting form.

It is not unusual for children with premature adrenarche, or women with signs of androgen excess, to have mild to moderate elevations in DHEA levels. It has been suggested that such individuals have "nonclassic 3β-HSD deficiency." However, mutations in the *HSD3B2* gene are not found in most such individuals and the nonclassic form of this deficiency must be quite rare.

Treatment. Patients require glucocorticoid and mineralocorticoid replacement with hydrocortisone and fludrocortisone, respectively, as in 21-hydroxylase deficiency. Incompletely virilized genetic males in whom a male sex of rearing is contemplated may benefit from several injections of a depot form of testosterone early in infancy to increase the size of the phallus. They may also require testosterone replacement at puberty.

570.4 Congenital Adrenal Hyperplasia due to 17-Hydroxylase Deficiency

Etiology. Fewer than 1% of CAH cases are caused by 17-hydroxylase deficiency. A single polypeptide, CYP17, catalyzes two distinct reactions: 17-hydroxylation of pregnenolone and progesterone to 17-hydroxypregnenolone and 17-hydroxyprogesterone, respectively, and the 17,20-lyase reaction mediating conversion of 17-hydroxypregnenolone to DHEA and, to a lesser extent, 17-hydroxyprogesterone to Δ4-androstenedione. DHEA and androstenedione are steroid precursors of testosterone and estrogen (see Fig. 568–1). The enzyme is expressed in both the adrenal cortex and the gonads and is encoded by a gene on chromosome 10. Most mutations affect both the hydroxylase and lyase activities, but rare mutations can affect either activity alone.

Clinical Manifestations and Laboratory Findings. Patients with 17-hydroxylase deficiency cannot synthesize cortisol, but their ability to synthesize corticosterone is intact. Because corticosterone is an active glucocorticoid, patients do not develop adrenal insufficiency. However, deoxycorticosterone, the immediate precursor of corticosterone, is synthesized in excess. This can cause hypertension, hypokalemia, and suppression of renin and aldosterone secretion, as occurs in 11-hydroxylase deficiency. However, in contrast to 11-hydroxylase deficiency, patients with 17-hydroxylase deficiency are unable to synthesize sex hormones. Affected males are incompletely virilized and present as phenotypic females (but gonads are usually palpable in the inguinal region or the labia) or with sexual ambiguity (male pseudohermaphroditism). Affected females usually present with failure of sexual development at the expected time of puberty. 17-Hydroxylase deficiency in females must be considered in the differential diagnosis of primary hypogonadism (see Chapter 580). In addition to the increased DOC, suppressed renin and aldosterone, and decreased 17-hydroxylated steroids, cortisol and sex steroids are unresponsive to stimulation with ACTH and human chorionic gonadotropin, respectively.

Treatment. Patients with 17-hydroxylase deficiency require cortisol replacement to suppress secretion of deoxycorticosterone and thus control hypertension. Additional antihypertensive medication may be required. Females require estrogen replacement at puberty. Genetic males may require either estrogen or androgen supplementation depending on the sex of rearing. As with androgen insensitivity syndrome (see Chapter 582), genetic males with severe 17-hydroxylase deficiency being reared as females require gonadectomy at or before adolescence because of the chance of malignant transformation of abdominal testes.

570.5 Lipoid Adrenal Hyperplasia

Etiology. Lipoid adrenal hyperplasia is a rare disorder, reported in fewer than 100 patients, the majority of whom are Japanese. In this disorder there is marked accumulation of cholesterol and lipids in the adrenal cortex and gonads, associated with severe impairment of all steroidogenesis. Lipoid adrenal hyperplasia is usually caused by mutations in the gene for steroidogenic acute regulatory protein (StAR), a mitochondrial protein that promotes the movement of cholesterol from the outer to the inner mitochondrial membrane. Mutations in the P450scc gene have been reported in two patients with lipoid adrenal hyperplasia.

Some cholesterol is able to enter mitochondria even in the absence of StAR, so it might be supposed that this disorder would not completely impair steroid biosynthesis. However, the accumulation of cholesterol in the cytoplasm is cytotoxic, eventually leading to death of all steroidogenic cells in which StAR is normally expressed. This occurs prenatally in the adrenals and testes. However, the ovaries do not normally synthesize steroids until puberty, so cholesterol does not accumulate and the ovaries can retain the capacity to synthesize estrogens until adolescence.

Although estrogens synthesized by the placenta are required to maintain pregnancy, the placenta does not require StAR for steroid biosynthesis. Thus, mutations of StAR are not prenatally lethal.

Clinical Manifestations. Patients with lipoid adrenal hyperplasia are usually unable to synthesize any adrenal steroids. Thus, affected infants are likely to be confused with those with adrenal hypoplasia. Salt-losing manifestations are usual, and many infants die in early infancy. Genetic males are unable to synthesize androgens and thus are phenotypically female but with gonads. Genetic females appear normal at birth and may undergo feminization at puberty with menstrual bleeding. They too, however, progress to hypergonadotropic hypogonadism when accumulated cholesterol kills granulosa (i.e., steroid synthesizing) cells in the ovary.

Laboratory Findings. Adrenal and gonadal steroid hormone levels are low in lipoid adrenal hyperplasia, with a decreased or absent response to stimulation (ACTH, human chorionic gonadotropin). Plasma renin levels are increased.

Imaging studies of the adrenal gland demonstrating massive adrenal enlargement in the newborn help establish the diagnosis of lipoid adrenal hyperplasia.

Treatment. Patients require glucocorticoid and mineralocorticoid replacement. Genetic males are usually assigned a female sex of rearing; thus both genetic males and females require estrogen replacement at the expected age of puberty.

570.6 Aldosterone Synthase Deficiency

Etiology. This is a rare autosomal recessive disorder in which conversion of corticosterone to aldosterone is impaired; a group of Iranian Jewish patients has been most thoroughly studied. Most cases result from mutations in the *CYP11B2* gene coding for aldosterone synthase; however, linkage to *CYP11B2* has been excluded in other kindreds. Aldosterone synthase mediates the three final steps in the synthesis of aldosterone from deoxycorticosterone (11-hydroxylation, 18-hydroxylation, 18-oxidation). Although 11-hydroxylation is required to convert deoxycorticosterone to corticosterone, this conversion can also be catalyzed by the related enzyme, CYP11B1, located in the fasciculata, which is unaffected in this disorder. For the same reason, these patients have normal cortisol biosynthesis.

The disease has previously been divided into two types termed *corticosterone methyloxidase deficiency types I and II.* They differ only in levels of the immediate precursor of aldosterone, 18-hydroxycorticosterone; levels are low in type I deficiency and elevated in type II deficiency. These differences do not correspond in a simple way to particular mutations and are of limited clinical importance.

Clinical Manifestations. Infants with aldosterone synthase deficiency may have severe electrolyte abnormalities with hyponatremia, hyperkalemia, and acidosis. However, because cortisol synthesis is unaffected, infants rarely become as ill as untreated infants with salt-losing forms of congenital adrenal hyperplasia such as 21-hydroxylase deficiency. Thus, some infants escape diagnosis. They may present later in infancy or in early childhood with failure to thrive and poor growth. Adults often are asymptomatic, although they may develop electrolyte abnormalities when depleted of sodium through procedures such as bowel preparation for a barium enema.

Laboratory Findings. Infants have elevated plasma renin activity. Aldosterone levels are decreased; they may be at the lower end of the normal range but are always inappropriately low for the degree of hyperkalemia or hyperreninemia. Corticosterone levels are often elevated. As mentioned, some but not all patients have marked elevation of 18-hydroxycorticosterone but low levels of this steroid do not exclude the diagnosis. In kindreds in which 18-hydroxycorticosterone levels are elevated in affected individuals, this biochemical abnormality persists in adults even when they have no electrolyte abnormalities.

Treatment. Treatment consists of giving enough fludrocortisone (0.05–0.3 mg daily), sodium chloride, or both to return plasma renin levels to normal. With increasing age, salt-losing signs usually improve and drug therapy can often be discontinued.

570.7 Glucocorticoid-Suppressible Hyperaldosteronism

Etiology. Glucocorticoid-suppressible aldosteronism (glucocorticoid-remediable aldosteronism, familial hyperaldosteronism type I) is an autosomal dominant form of low-renin hypertension in which hyperaldosteronism is rapidly suppressed by glucocorticoid administration. This unusual effect of glucocorticoids suggests that in this disorder is regulated by ACTH aldosterone secretion instead of by the renin-angiotensin system. In addition to abnormally regulated secretion of aldosterone, there is marked overproduction of 18-hydroxycortisol and 18-oxocortisol. The synthesis of these steroids requires both 17-hydroxylase *(CYP17)* activity, which is expressed only in the zona fasciculata, and aldosterone synthase *(CYP11B2)* activity, which is normally expressed only in the zona glomerulosa. Together, these features imply that aldosterone synthase is being expressed in a manner similar to the closely related enzyme steroid 11-hydroxylase *(CYP11B1)*. The disorder is caused by unequal meiotic crossing over events between the *CYP11B1* and *CYP11B2* genes, which are closely linked on chromosome 8q24. An additional "hybrid" gene is produced, having regulatory sequences of *CYP11B1* juxtaposed with coding sequences of *CYP11B2*. This results in the inappropriate expression of a *CYP11B2*-like enzyme with aldosterone synthase activity in the adrenal fasciculata.

Clinical Manifestations. Some affected children have no symptoms, the diagnosis being established after incidental discovery of moderate hypertension, typically about 30 mm Hg higher than unaffected family members of the same age. Others have more symptomatic hypertension with headache, dizziness, and visual disturbances. A strong family history of early-onset hypertension or early strokes may alert the clinician to the diagnosis. Some patients have chronic hypokalemia, but this is not a consistent finding and is usually mild.

Administration of dexamethasone, 25 μg/kg/day in divided doses, suppresses aldosterone secretion. Hypertension resolves in patients in whom the hypertension is not severe or of long standing.

Laboratory Findings. Patients have elevated plasma and urine levels of aldosterone and suppressed plasma renin activity. As mentioned, hypokalemia is not consistently present. Urinary and plasma levels of 18-oxocortisol and 18-hydroxycortisol are markedly increased. The hybrid *CYP11B1/CYP11B2* gene can be readily detected by molecular genetic methods. However, these assays are not routinely available.

Treatment. Glucocorticoid-suppressible hyperaldosteronism is managed by daily administration of a glucocorticoid, usually prednisone or dexamethasone. If necessary, effects of aldosterone can be blocked with a potassium-sparing diuretic such as spironolactone, eplerenone, or amiloride. If hypertension is of long standing, additional antihypertensive medication may be required, such as a calcium channel blocker.

Because of the autosomal dominant mode of inheritance, at-risk family members should be investigated for this easily treated cause of hypertension.

Auchus RJ: The genetics, pathophysiology, and management of human deficiencies of P450c17. *Endocrinol Metab Clin North Am* 2001;30:101–19.

Berenbaum SA: Cognitive function in congenital adrenal hyperplasia. *Endocrinol Metab Clin North Am* 2001;30:173–92.

Bose HS, Sato S, Aisenberg J, et al: Mutations in the steroidogenic acute regulatory protein (StAR) in six patients with congenital lipoid adrenal hyperplasia. *J Clin Endocrinol Metab* 2000;85:3636–39.

Collett-Solberg PF: Congenital adrenal hyperplasia: From genetics and biochemistry to clinical practice: I. *Clin Pediatr* 2001;40:1–16.

Collett-Solberg PF: Congenital adrenal hyperplasia: From genetics and biochemistry to clinical practice: II. *Clin Pediatr* 2001;40:125–32.

Dluhy RG: Glucocorticoid-remediable aldosteronism. *Endocrinologist* 2001;11:263–68.

Forest MG: Prenatal diagnosis, treatment, and outcome in infants with congenital adrenal hyperplasia. *Curr Opin Endocrinol Diabetes* 1997;4:209–17.

Giacaglia LR, Mendonca BB, Madureira G, et al: Adrenal nodules in patients with congenital adrenal hyperplasia due to 21-hydroxylase deficiency: Regression after adequate hormonal control. *J Pediatr Endocrinol Metab* 2001;14:415–19.

Gmyrek GA, New MI, Sosa RE, Poppas DP: Bilateral laparoscopic adrenalectomy as a treatment for classic congenital adrenal hyperplasia attributable to 21-hydroxylase deficiency. *Pediatrics* 2002;109:E28.

Katsumata N, Ohtake M, Hojo T, et al: Compound heterozygous mutations in the cholesterol side chain cleaving enzyme (CYP11A) causing congenital adrenal insufficiency in humans. *J Clin Endocrinol Metab* 2002;87:3808–13.

Krege S, Walz KH, Hauffa BP, et al: Long-term follow-up of female patients with congenital adrenal hyperplasia from 21-hydroxylase deficiency, with special emphasis on the results of vaginoplasty. *BJU Int* 2000;86:253–59.

Levine LS: Congenital adrenal hyperplasia. *Pediatr Rev* 2000;21:159–70.

Merke DP, Chrousos GP, Eisenhofer G, et al: Adrenomedullary dysplasia and hypofunction in patients with classic 21–hydroxylase deficiency. *N Engl J Med* 2000;343:1362–68.

Merke DP, Cutler GBJ: New ideas for medical treatment of congenital adrenal hyperplasia. *Endocrinol Metab Clin North Am* 2001;30:121–35.

Meyer-Bahlburg HF: Gender and sexuality in classic congenital adrenal hyperplasia. *Endocrinol Metab Clin North Am* 2001;30:155–71.

Migeon CJ, Wisniewski AB: Congenital adrenal hyperplasia owing to 21-hydroxylase deficiency: Growth, development, and therapeutic considerations. *Endocrinol Metab Clin North Am* 2001;30:193–206.

New MI: Prenatal treatment of congenital adrenal hyperplasia: The United States experience. *Endocrinol Metab Clin North Am* 2001;30:1–13.

Nordenstrom A, Wedell A, Hagenfeldt L, et al: Neonatal screening for congenital adrenal hyperplasia: 17-Hydroxyprogesterone levels and CYP21 genotypes in preterm infants. *Pediatrics* 2001;108:E68.

Pang S: Congenital adrenal hyperplasia owing to 3 beta-hydroxysteroid dehydrogenase deficiency. *Endocrinol Metab Clin North Am* 2001;30:81–99.

Premawardhana LD, Hughes IA, Read GF, et al: Longer term outcome in females with congenital adrenal hyperplasia (CAH): The Cardiff experience. *Clin Endocrinol* 1997;46:327–32.

Quintos JBQ, Vogiatzi MG, Harbison MD, et al: Growth hormone therapy alone or in combination with gonadotropin-releasing hormone analog therapy to improve the height deficit in children with congenital adrenal hyperplasia. *J Clin Endocrinol Metab* 2001;86:1511–17.

Schnitzer JJ, Donahoe PK: Surgical treatment of congenital adrenal hyperplasia. *Endocrinol Metab Clin North Am* 2001;30:137–54.

Simard J, Ricketts ML, Moisan AM, et al: A new insight into the molecular basis of 3β-hydroxysteroid dehydrogenase deficiency. *Endocr Res* 2000;26:761–70.

Tajima T, Fujieda K, Kouda N, et al: Heterozygous mutation in the cholesterol side chain cleavage enzyme (P450scc) gene in a patient with 46,XY sex reversal and adrenal insufficiency. *J Clin Endocrinol Metab* 2001;86:3820–25.

Therrell BL: Newborn screening for congenital adrenal hyperplasia. *Endocrinol Metab Clin North Am* 2001;30:15–30.

Van Wyk JJ, Gunther DF, Ritzen EM, et al: The use of adrenalectomy as a treatment for congenital adrenal hyperplasia. *J Clin Endocrinol Metab* 1996;81:3180–90.

White PC: Steroid 11-beta-hydroxylase deficiency and related disorders. *Endocrinol Metab Clin North Am* 2001;30:61–79.

White PC, Speiser PW: Congenital adrenal hyperplasia due to 21-hydroxylase deficiency. *Endocr Rev* 2000;21:245–91.

Chapter 571
Cushing Syndrome

Cushing syndrome is the result of abnormally high blood levels of cortisol or other glucocorticoids. This can be iatrogenic or the result of endogenous cortisol secretion, either due to an adrenal tumor or to hypersecretion of corticotropin (adrenocorticotropic hormone [ACTH]) by the pituitary (Cushing disease) or by a tumor (Box 571–1).

Etiology. By far the most common cause of Cushing syndrome is prolonged exogenous administration of glucocorticoid hormones, especially in the high doses used to treat lymphoproliferative disorders. This rarely represents a diagnostic challenge, but management of hyperglycemia, hypertension, weight gain, linear growth retardation, and osteoporosis often complicates therapy with corticosteroids.

Endogenous Cushing syndrome is most often caused in infants by a *functioning adrenocortical tumor*, usually a malignant carcinoma but occasionally a benign adenoma (see Chapter

---

BOX 571–1. Etiologic Classification of Adrenocortical Hyperfunction

Excess androgen
  Congenital adrenal hyperplasia
    21-Hydroxylase (P450c21) deficiency
    11 β-Hydroxylase (p450c11) deficiency
    3β-Hydroxysteroid dehydrogenase defect
  Tumor
    Carcinoma
    Adenoma
Excess cortisol (Cushing syndrome)
  Bilateral adrenal hyperplasia
    Hypersecretion of corticotropin (Cushing disease)
    Ectopic secretion of corticotropin
    Exogenous corticotropin
  Adrenocortical nodular dysplasia
  Pigmented nodular adrenocortical disease (Carney complex)
  Tumor
    Carcinoma
    Adenoma
Excess mineralocorticoid (hypertensive hypokalemic syndrome)
  Primary hyperaldosteronism
    Aldosterone-secreting adenoma
    Bilateral micronodular adrenocortical hyperplasia
    Glucocorticoid-suppressible aldosteronism
  Tumor
    Adenoma
    Carcinoma
  Desoxycorticosterone excess
    Congenital adrenal hyperplasia
      11β-Hydroxylase (P450c11)
      17α-Hydroxylase (P450c17)
    Tumor (carcinoma)
  Apparent mineralocorticoid excess
    11β-Hydroxysteroid dehydrogenase deficiency
Excess estrogen (adrenal feminization syndrome)
  Carcinoma
  Adenoma
Mixed hypercorticism-tumor

---

573). Patients with these tumors often exhibit signs of hypercortisolism mixed with signs of hypersecretion of other steroids such as androgens, estrogens, and aldosterone.

Although extremely rare in infants, the most common etiology of endogenous Cushing syndrome in children older than 7 yr of age is Cushing disease, in which excessive ACTH secreted by a pituitary adenoma causes bilateral adrenal hyperplasia. Such adenomas are often too small to detect by imaging techniques and are termed *microadenomas*. They consist principally of chromophobe cells and frequently have positive immunostaining for ACTH and its precursor, pro-opiomelanocortin (POMC).

ACTH-dependent Cushing syndrome may also result from *ectopic production of ACTH*, although this is uncommon in children. Ectopic ACTH secretion in children has been associated with islet cell carcinoma of the pancreas, neuroblastoma or ganglioneuroblastoma, hemangiopericytoma, Wilms tumor, and thymic carcinoid.

Primary pigmented nodular adrenocortical disease (PPNAD) is a distinctive form of ACTH-independent Cushing syndrome, usually presenting before 20 yr of age. It may occur as an isolated event or, more commonly, as a familial disorder with other manifestations. The adrenal glands are small and have characteristic multiple, small (<4 mm in diameter), pigmented (black) nodules containing large cells with cytoplasm and lipofuscin; between the nodules, there is cortical atrophy. This adrenal disorder occurs as a component of **Carney complex,** an autosomal dominant disorder also consisting of centrofacial lentigines and blue nevi, cardiac and cutaneous myxomas, pituitary, thyroid, and testicular tumors, and pigmented melanotic schwannomas. Carney complex is inherited in an autosomal dominant manner, although sporadic cases occur. Genetic loci for Carney complex have been mapped to chromosome 2p16 and to the gene for the type 1α regulatory subunit of protein kinase A on chromosome 17q22-24.

ACTH-independent Cushing syndrome with nodular hyperplasia and adenoma formation occurs rarely in cases of *McCune-Albright syndrome,* with symptoms beginning in infancy or childhood. McCune-Albright syndrome is caused by a somatic mutation of a G protein, $G_{s\alpha}$, resulting in inhibition of guanosine triphosphatase activity and constitutive activation of adenylate cyclase. When the mutation is present in adrenal tissue, cortisol and cell division are stimulated independently of ACTH. Other tissues in which activating mutations may occur are bone (producing fibrous dysplasia), gonads, thyroid, and pituitary. Clinical manifestations depend on which tissues are affected.

Adrenocortical lesions including diffuse hyperplasia, nodular hyperplasia, adenoma, or, rarely, carcinoma, may occur as part of the multiple endocrine neoplasia type 1 syndrome, an autosomal dominant disorder, in which there is homozygous inactivation of a putative tumor suppressor gene on chromosome 11q13.

Clinical Manifestations. Symptoms have been recognized in infants younger than 1 yr of age. The disorder appears to be more severe and the clinical findings more flagrant in infants than when the onset occurs in older children. The face is rounded, with prominent cheeks and a flushed appearance (moon facies). Generalized obesity is common in younger children. In children with adrenal tumors, signs of abnormal masculinization occur frequently; accordingly, there may be hypertrichosis on the face and trunk, pubic hair, acne, deepening of the voice, and enlargement of the clitoris in girls. Growth is impaired, with length falling below the 3rd percentile, except when significant virilization produces normal or even accelerated growth. Hypertension is common and may occasionally lead to heart failure. An increased susceptibility to infection may also lead to fatal sepsis.

In older children, in addition to obesity, short stature is a common presenting feature. Gradual onset of obesity and deceleration or cessation of growth may be the only early manifestations. Older children most often have more severe obesity of the face and trunk compared with the extremities. Purplish striae on the hips, abdomen, and thighs are common. Pubertal development may be delayed, or amenorrhea may occur in girls past menarche. Weakness, headache, and emotional lability may be prominent. Hypertension and hyperglycemia usually occur; hyperglycemia may progress to frank diabetes. Osteoporosis is common and may cause pathologic fractures.

Laboratory Findings. Cortisol levels in blood are normally elevated at 8 AM and decrease to less than 50% by midnight except in infants and young children in whom a diurnal rhythm is not always established. In patients with Cushing syndrome this circadian rhythm is lost, and cortisol levels at midnight and 8 AM are usually comparable. Obtaining diurnal blood samples presents logistical difficulties as part of an outpatient evaluation, but cortisol can be measured in saliva samples, which can be obtained at home at the appropriate times of day. Nighttime salivary cortisol levels are elevated and may be a screening test in obese children.

Urinary excretion of free cortisol is increased. This is best measured in a 24-hr urine sample and is expressed as a ratio of micrograms of cortisol excreted per gram of creatinine. This ratio is independent of body size and completeness of the urine collection.

A single-dose dexamethasone suppression test is often helpful; a dose of 25–30 µg/kg (maximum of 2 mg) given at 11 PM results in a plasma cortisol level of less than 5 µg/dL at 8 AM the next morning in normal individuals but not in patients with Cushing syndrome.

A glucose tolerance test is often abnormal despite elevated levels of insulin. Levels of serum electrolytes are usually normal, but potassium may be decreased, especially in tumors with ectopic ACTH secretion.

After the diagnosis of Cushing syndrome has been established, it is necessary to determine whether it is caused by a pituitary adenoma, an ectopic ACTH-secreting tumor, or a cortisol-secreting tumor. ACTH concentrations are usually suppressed in patients with cortisol-secreting tumors, are very high in patients with ectopic ACTH-secreting tumors, but may be normal in patients with ACTH-secreting pituitary adenomas. After an intravenous bolus of corticotropin-releasing hormone (CRH), patients with ACTH-dependent Cushing syndrome have an exaggerated ACTH and cortisol response but those with adrenal tumors show no increase in ACTH and cortisol. The two-step dexamethasone suppression test consists of administration of dexamethasone, 30 and 120 µg/kg/24 hr in four divided doses, on consecutive days. In children with pituitary Cushing syndrome, the larger dose, but not the smaller dose, suppresses serum levels of cortisol. Typically, patients with ACTH-independent Cushing syndrome do not show suppressed cortisol levels with dexamethasone.

CT detects virtually all adrenal tumors larger than 1.5 cm in diameter. MRI may detect ACTH-secreting pituitary adenomas, but many are too small to be seen; the addition of gadolinium contrast increases the sensitivity of detection. Bilateral inferior petrosal blood sampling to measure concentrations of ACTH before and after CRH administration may be required to localize the tumor when a pituitary adenoma is not visualized.

Differential Diagnosis. Cushing syndrome is frequently suspected in children with obesity, particularly when striae and hypertension are present. Children with simple obesity are usually tall, whereas those with Cushing syndrome are short or have a decelerating growth rate. Although urinary excretion of cortisol is often elevated in simple obesity, salivary nighttime levels of cortisol are normal and cortisol secretion is suppressed by oral administration of low doses of dexamethasone.

Elevated levels of cortisol and ACTH without clinical evidence of Cushing syndrome occur in patients with generalized glucocorticoid resistance. Affected patients may be asymptomatic or exhibit hypertension, hypokalemia, and precocious pseudopuberty; these manifestations are caused by increased mineralocorticoid and adrenal androgens in response to elevated ACTH levels. Mutations in the glucocorticoid receptor have been identified. Absence of cushingoid phenotype in a patient with a pituitary adenoma and biochemically proven Cushing disease has been reported. In this patient, defective cortisone to cortisol conversion resulted in increased cortisol clearance, protecting the patient from cortisol excess.

Treatment. Transsphenoidal pituitary microsurgery is the treatment of choice in pituitary Cushing disease in children. The overall success rate with follow-up of less than 10 yr is 60–80%. Low postoperative serum or urinary cortisol concentrations appear to be predictive of long-term remission in the majority of cases. Reoperation or pituitary irradiation is performed when relapse occurs.

Cyproheptadine, a centrally acting serotonin antagonist that blocks ACTH release, has been used to treat Cushing disease in adults; remissions are usually not sustained after discontinuation of therapy. This agent is rarely used in children. Inhibitors of adrenal steroidogenesis (metyrapone, ketoconazole, aminoglutethimide) have been used preoperatively to normalize circulating cortisol levels and reduce perioperative morbidity and mortality.

If a pituitary adenoma does not respond to treatment or if ACTH is secreted by an ectopic metastatic tumor, the adrenal glands may need to be removed. This can often be accomplished laparoscopically. Adrenalectomy may lead to increased ACTH secretion by an unresected pituitary adenoma, evidenced mainly by marked hyperpigmentation; this is termed *Nelson syndrome.*

If the lesion is a benign cortical adenoma, unilateral adrenalectomy is indicated. Such adenomas are occasionally bilateral;

then the treatment of choice is subtotal adrenalectomy. In either instance, an excellent therapeutic result is achieved by removing the tumor. Adrenocortical carcinomas frequently metastasize, especially to the liver and lungs, and the prognosis may be unfavorable despite removal of the primary lesion. Rarely, the tumors are bilateral and require total adrenalectomy. It is often impossible to differentiate benign from malignant tumors by histologic appearance alone.

Management of patients undergoing adrenalectomy requires adequate preoperative and postoperative replacement therapy with a corticosteroid. Tumors that produce corticosteroids usually lead to atrophy of the normal adrenal tissue, and replacement with cortisol is required until there is recovery of the hypothalamic-pituitary-adrenal axis. Postoperative complications have included sepsis, pancreatitis, thrombosis, poor wound healing, and sudden collapse, particularly in infants with Cushing syndrome. Substantial catch-up growth, pubertal progress, and increased bone density occur, but bone density remains abnormal and adult height is often compromised.

Bourdeau I, D'amour P, Hamet P, et al: Aberrant membrane hormone receptors in incidentally discovered bilateral macronodular adrenal hyperplasia with subclinical Cushing's syndrome. *J Clin Endocrinol Metab* 2001;86:5534–40.

Castro M, Elias PC, Quidute ARP, et al: Outpatient screening for Cushing's syndrome: The sensitivity of the combination of circadian rhythm and overnight dexamethasone suppression salivary cortisol tests. *J Clin Endocrinol Metab* 1999;84:878–82.

Devoe DJ, Miller WL, Conte FA, et al: Long-term outcome in children and adolescents after transsphenoidal surgery for Cushing's disease. *J Clin Endocrinol Metab* 1997;82:3196–202.

Gafni RI, Papanicolaou DA, Nieman LK: Nighttime salivary cortisol measurement as a simple, noninvasive, outpatient screening test for Cushing's syndrome in children and adolescents. *J Pediatr* 2000;137:30–35.

Hiroi N, Chrousos GP, Kohn B, et al: Clinical Case Seminar: Adrenocortical-pituitary hybrid tumor causing Cushing's syndrome. *J Clin Endocrinol Metab* 2001;86:2631–37.

Kirk JMW, Brain CE, Carson DJ, et al: Cushing's syndrome caused by nodular adrenal hyperplasia in children with McCune-Albright syndrome. *J Pediatr* 1999;134:789–92.

Lacroix A, N'Diaye N, Tremblay J, et al: Ectopic and abnormal hormone receptors in adrenal Cushing's syndrome. *Endocr Rev* 2001;22:75–110.

Lienhardt A, Grossman AB, Dacie JE, et al: Relative contributions of inferior petrosal sinus sampling and pituitary imaging in the investigation of children and adolescents with ACTH-dependent Cushing's syndrome. *J Clin Endocrinol Metab* 2001;86:5711–14.

Raffin-Sanson ML, de Keyzer Y, Bertagna X: Syndromes of ectopic ACTH secretion: Recent pathophysiological progresses and their clinical implications. *Endocrinologist* 2000;10:97–106.

Stratakis CA, Kirschner LS, Carney JA: Clinical and molecular features of the Carney complex: Diagnostic criteria and recommendations for patient evaluation. *J Clin Endocrinol Metab* 2001;86:4041–46.

Chapter 572
Primary Aldosteronism

Primary aldosteronism encompasses disorders caused by excessive aldosterone secretion independent of the renin-angiotensin system. These disorders are characterized by hypertension, hypokalemia, and suppression of the renin-angiotensin system.

Aldosterone-secreting adenomas are unilateral and have been reported in children as young as 3.5 yr of age; they mainly affect girls. *Bilateral micronodular adrenocortical hyperplasia* tends to occur in older children and is more frequent in males. Primary aldosteronism due to *unilateral adrenal hyperplasia* may also occur. All are very rare in children. Glucocorticoid-suppressible hyperaldosteronism is discussed in Chapter 570.

Clinical Manifestations. Some affected children have no symptoms, the diagnosis being established after incidental discovery of moderate hypertension. Others have severe hypertension (up

to 240/150 mm Hg), with headache, dizziness, and visual disturbances. Chronic hypokalemia, if present, may lead to polyuria, nocturia, enuresis, and polydipsia. Muscle weakness and discomfort, tetany, intermittent paralysis, fatigue, and growth failure affect children with severe hypokalemia.

Laboratory Findings. Hypokalemia occurs frequently. Serum pH and the carbon dioxide and sodium concentrations may be elevated and the serum chloride and magnesium levels decreased. Serum levels of calcium are normal, even in children who manifest tetany. The urine is neutral or alkaline, and kaliuresis is present. Plasma levels of aldosterone may be normal or elevated. Aldosterone concentrations in 24 hr urine collections are always increased. Plasma levels of renin are persistently low, and the ratio of plasma aldosterone concentration to renin activity is always high. Aldosterone does not decrease with sodium chloride administration, and renin does not respond to salt and fluid restriction. Urinary and plasma levels of 18-oxocortisol and 18-hydroxycortisol may be increased but not to the extent seen in glucocorticoid-suppressible hyperaldosteronism.

Treatment. The treatment of an aldosterone-producing adenoma is surgical removal. This has been performed primarily by laparotomy and adrenalectomy. However, successful enucleation of aldosterone-producing adenomas as well as laparoscopic adrenalectomy are reported. Pharmacologic treatment of hyperaldosteronism due to bilateral adrenal hyperplasia with spironolactone often results in normalization of blood pressure and serum potassium levels.

If the side effects of spironolactone are unacceptable, amiloride may be used and other antihypertensive agents added as necessary. In patients whose condition cannot be controlled medically, unilateral adrenalectomy may be considered.

Chapter 573
Adrenal Tumors

Adrenocortical tumors are rare in childhood. They occur in all age groups but most commonly in children younger than 10 yr of age. In 2–10% of cases, the tumors are bilateral. Symptoms of endocrine hyperfunction are present in more than 90% of children with adrenal tumors (see Table 571–1). Tumors may be associated with hemihypertrophy, usually occurring during the first few years of life. They are also associated with the Beckwith-Wiedemann syndrome and other congenital defects, particularly genitourinary tract and central nervous system abnormalities and hamartomatous defects.

Germ line mutations in p53 (on chromosome 17p13.1) have been found in patients with isolated adrenal carcinoma as well as in patients with familial clustering of unusual malignancies. Loss of heterozygosity involving chromosomes 2, 4, 11, and 18 and *IGF2* gene overexpression (chromosome 11p15.5) have also been reported in sporadic adrenocortical carcinomas.

573.1 Virilizing Adrenocortical Tumors

Virilization is the most common presenting symptom. In males, this produces a clinical picture similar to that of simple virilizing congenital adrenal hyperplasia: accelerated growth velocity and muscle development, acne, penile enlargement, and the precocious development of pubic and axillary hair. In females, virilizing tumors of the adrenal gland cause masculinization of a previously normal female with clitoral enlargement, growth acceleration, acne, deepening of the voice, and premature pubic and axillary hair development.

In addition to virilization, 20–40% of children with adrenal cortical tumors also have Cushing syndrome (see Chapter 571). Although virilization may occur alone (50–80%), it is unusual to have Cushing syndrome alone in children with adrenal tumors.

Serum levels of dehydroepiandrosterone (DHEA), DHEA sulfate, and androstenedione are usually elevated, often markedly. Serum levels of testosterone are often increased, usually as a result of peripheral conversion of androstenedione, but infants with predominantly testosterone-secreting adenomas have been reported. Urinary 17-ketosteroids (sex steroid metabolites) are also increased. Many adrenocortical tumors have a relative deficiency of 11β-hydroxylase activity and secrete increased amounts of deoxycorticosterone; these patients are hypertensive, and their tumors are often malignant.

Tumors can usually be detected by ultrasonography, CT, or MRI. Preoperatively the presence of metastatic disease should be determined by MRI or CT of the chest, abdomen, and pelvis. Differentiation between benign and malignant tumors by histologic criteria often is not possible.

The treatment is surgical. A transperitoneal approach has usually been recommended, but laparoscopic removal is possible. Some of these neoplasms are highly malignant and metastasize widely, but cure with regression of the masculinizing features may follow removal of less malignant encapsulated tumors. Incomplete resection, tumors weighing more than 100 g, tumors larger than 200 cm^3, age greater than 3.5 yr at diagnosis, symptoms for more than 6 mo, and a marked increase in urinary 17-ketosteroids and 17-hydroxysteroids have been associated with poor prognosis. Postoperatively, patients should be closely monitored biochemically, with frequent determinations of adrenal androgen levels and imaging studies. Recurrent symptoms or biochemical abnormalities should prompt a careful search for metastatic disease. Metastases primarily involve liver, lung, and regional lymph nodes. The majority of metastatic recurrences appear within 1 yr of tumor resection. Repeat surgical resection of metastatic lesions should be performed if possible and adjuvant therapy instituted. Radiation therapy has not been generally helpful. Antineoplastic agents, such as cisplatin and etoposide, ifosfamide and carboplatin, and 5-fluorouracil and leucovorin have had limited use in children, and their success is not established. Therapy with o,p'-DDD (mitotane), an adrenolytic agent, may relieve the symptoms of hypercortisolism or virilization in recurrent disease but does not appear to improve survival. Other agents that interfere with adrenal steroid synthesis, such as ketoconazole, aminoglutethimide, and metyrapone, may also relieve symptoms of steroid excess but do not improve survival.

A neoplasm of one adrenal gland may produce atrophy of the other, because excessive production of cortisol by the tumor suppresses adrenocorticotropic hormone stimulation of the normal gland. Consequently, adrenal insufficiency may follow surgical removal of the tumor. This situation can be avoided by giving 10–25 mg of hydrocortisone every 6 hr, starting on the day of operation and continuing for 3–4 days postoperatively. Adequate quantities of water, sodium chloride, and glucose must also be provided.

573.2 Feminizing Adrenal Tumors

Feminizing adrenocortical tumors may be either carcinomas or benign adenomas. They may produce only estrogens or, in addition, androgens, cortisol, or mineralocorticoids (see Fig. 568–1). High levels of aromatase activity and expression of the CYP19 (P450arom) gene, absent in normal adrenal tissue, are found in these tumors.

Such tumors may become symptomatic at any age after 6 mo. Gynecomastia in males or premature thelarche in girls is often the initial manifestation. Growth and development may be otherwise normal, or concomitant virilization may occur, evidenced by acne, deep voice, penile or clitoral enlargement, and advanced osseous maturation. Hypertension is common in affected adults but has not been observed in children.

In addition to elevated plasma and urinary levels of estrogens, there are often elevated levels of adrenal androgens (i.e., dehydroepiandrosterone and its sulfate) in plasma and 17-ketosteroids in urine. Plasma gonadotropin levels are suppressed, and gonadotropin-releasing hormone stimulation does not elicit a response. Tumors may appear calcified on radiographs but are usually localized by CT.

If the tumor can be resected, gynecomastia regresses and hormone values return to normal.

Chapter 574
Pheochromocytoma

Pheochromocytoma, a catecholamine-secreting tumor, arises from chromaffin cells. The most common site of origin (approximately 90%) is the adrenal medulla; however, tumors may develop anywhere along the abdominal sympathetic chain and are likely to be located near the aorta at the level of the inferior mesenteric artery or at its bifurcation. They also appear in the periadrenal area, the urinary bladder or ureteral walls, the thoracic cavity, and the cervical region. Ten per cent occur in children, in whom they present most frequently between 6 and 14 yr of age. Tumors vary from 1–10 cm in diameter; they are found more often on the right side than on the left. In more than 20% of affected children, the adrenal tumors are bilateral; and in 30–40% of children, tumors are found in both the adrenal and extra-adrenal areas or only in an extra-adrenal area.

Pheochromocytoma may be inherited as an autosomal dominant trait. In affected families, the ages of patients at the time of diagnosis have varied from the 1st to 5th decades of life; more than half the patients have had multiple tumors.

Pheochromocytomas may also be associated with other syndromes such as neurofibromatosis and von Hippel-Lindau disease and as a component of multiple endocrine neoplasia (MEN) syndromes MEN-2A and MEN-2B. The NF1 neurofibromatosis gene is a tumor suppressor gene mapping to chromosome 17q11.2. Germ line mutations of the RET proto-oncogene on chromosome 10 (10q11.2) have been found in families with MEN-2A and MEN-2B, and germ line mutations in a tumor suppressor gene on chromosome 3p25-26 have been identified in von Hippel-Lindau syndrome. Pheochromocytoma is also associated with tuberous sclerosis, Sturge-Weber syndrome, and ataxia-telangiectasia. Somatic mutations of genes associated with familial cancer syndromes have been found in nonfamilial forms of pheochromocytoma.

Clinical Manifestations. The clinical features of pheochromocytoma result from excessive secretion of epinephrine and norepinephrine. All patients have hypertension at some time. Paroxysmal hypertension should particularly suggest pheochromocytoma as a diagnostic possibility. However, the hypertension in children is more often sustained rather than paroxysmal, in contrast to adults. When there are paroxysms of hypertension, the attacks are usually infrequent at first but become more frequent and eventually give way to a continuous hypertensive state. Between attacks of hypertension, the patient may be free of symptoms. During attacks, the patient complains of headache, palpitations, abdominal pain, and dizziness; pallor, vomiting, and sweating also occur. Convulsions and other manifestations of hypertensive encephalopathy may occur. In severe cases, precordial pains radiate into the arms and pulmonary edema and cardiac and hepatic enlargement may develop. The child has a good appetite but because of hypermetabolism does not gain weight, and severe cachexia may develop. Polyuria and polydipsia can be sufficiently severe to suggest diabetes insipidus. Growth failure may be striking. The blood pressure may range from 180–260 mm Hg systolic and 120–210 mm Hg diastolic, and the heart may be enlarged. Ophthalmoscopic examination may reveal papilledema, hemorrhages, exudate, and arterial constriction.

Laboratory Findings. The urine may contain protein, a few casts, and occasionally glucose. Gross hematuria suggests that the tumor is in the bladder wall. Polycythemia is occasionally observed. The diagnosis is established by demonstration of elevated blood or urinary levels of catecholamines and their metabolites.

Pheochromocytomas produce norepinephrine and epinephrine. Normally, norepinephrine in plasma is derived from both the adrenal gland and adrenergic nerve endings whereas epinephrine is derived primarily from the adrenal gland. In contrast to adults with pheochromocytoma in whom both norepinephrine and epinephrine are elevated, children with pheochromocytoma predominantly excrete norepinephrine. Total urinary catecholamine excretion usually exceeds 300 μg/24 hr. Urinary excretion of vanillylmandelic acid (VMA, 3-methoxy-4-hydroxymandelic acid), the major metabolite of epinephrine and norepinephrine, is increased, as is excretion of metanephrine (see Fig. 568–2). Catecholamine levels can be measured by radioimmunoassay and high-performance liquid chromatography methods. Excretion of catecholamine metabolites may be similar in children with neuroblastoma and pheochromocytoma, but neuroblastoma does not usually produce hypertension. Urinary levels of most catecholamines are higher in those with pheochromocytoma, although levels of dopamine and homovanillic acid are usually higher in neuroblastoma. Daily urinary excretion of these compounds by unaffected children increases with age; and vanilla-containing foods and fruits can produce falsely elevated levels of VMA. Certain drugs interfere with fluorometric determinations of catecholamines.

Most tumors in the area of the adrenal gland are readily localized by ultrasonography or by CT or MRI; their frequent bilateral occurrence must not be forgotten. Extra-adrenal tumors may be difficult to detect. ^{131}I-Metaiodobenzylguanidine (MBIG) is taken up by chromaffin tissue anywhere in the body and is useful for localizing small tumors. Venous catheterization with sampling of blood at different levels for catecholamine determinations is now only rarely necessary for localizing the tumor.

Differential Diagnosis. Various causes of hypertension in children must be considered, such as renal or renovascular disease, coarctation of the aorta, hyperthyroidism, Cushing syndrome, deficiencies of 11β-hydroxylase, 17β-hydroxylase, or 11β-hydroxysteroid dehydrogenase, primary aldosteronism, adrenal cortical tumors, and essential hypertension (see Chapter 437). A nonfunctioning kidney may result from compression of a ureter or of a renal artery by a pheochromocytoma. Paroxysmal hypertension may be associated with porphyria or familial dysautonomia. Urinary excretion of VMA is low in familial dysautonomia because of a defect in release rather than in synthesis of catecholamines. Cerebral disorders, diabetes insipidus, diabetes mellitus, and hyperthyroidism must also be considered in the differential diagnosis. Hypertension in patients with neurofibromatosis may be caused by renal vascular involvement and by concurrent pheochromocytoma.

Neuroblastoma, ganglioneuroblastoma, and ganglioneuroma frequently produce catecholamines. Secreting neurogenic tumors commonly produce hypertension, excessive sweating, flushing, pallor, rash, polyuria, and polydipsia. Chronic diarrhea may be associated with these tumors, particularly with ganglioneuroma, and at times may be sufficiently persistent to suggest the celiac syndrome.

Treatment. Removal of these tumors results in cure, but the operation is very high risk. Careful preoperative, intraoperative, and postoperative management is essential. Preoperative α- and β-adrenergic blockade and fluid administration are required. Because these tumors are often multiple in children, a thorough transabdominal exploration of all the usual sites offers the best chance of finding all of them. Appropriate choice of anesthesia and expansion of blood volume with appropriate fluids during surgery are critical to avoid a precipitous drop in blood pressure during operation or within 48 hr postoperatively. Manipulation and excision of these tumors result in marked increases in catecholamine secretion that cause rises in blood pressure and heart rate. Surveillance must continue postoperatively.

Although these tumors often appear malignant histologically, the only accurate indicators of malignancy are the presence of metastatic disease, local invasiveness that precludes complete resection, or both. Approximately 10% of all adrenal pheochromocytomas are malignant. Such tumors are very rare in childhood; pediatric malignant pheochromocytomas occur more frequently in extra-adrenal sites. Prolonged follow-up is indicated because functioning tumors at other sites may be manifested many years after the initial operation. Examination of relatives of affected patients may reveal other persons harboring unsuspected tumors; such individuals may be asymptomatic.

Chapter 575
Adrenal Masses

575.1 Adrenal Incidentaloma

As a result of the widespread use of CT and MRI, adrenal masses are discovered with increasing frequency in patients undergoing abdominal imaging for reasons unrelated to the adrenal gland. The rate of detection of single adrenal masses has ranged from less than 1% to more than 4% of abdominal CT examinations in adults. The unexpected discovery of such a mass presents the clinician with a dilemma in terms of diagnostic steps to undertake and treatment interventions to recommend. The differential diagnosis of adrenal incidentaloma includes benign lesions such as cysts, hemorrhagic cysts, hematomas, and myelolipomas. These lesions can usually be identified on CT or MRI. If the nature of the lesion is not readily apparent, additional evaluation is required. Included in the differential diagnosis of lesions requiring additional evaluation are benign adenomas, pheochromocytomas, adrenocortical carcinoma, and metastasis from an extra-adrenal primary carcinoma. Benign hormonally inactive adrenocortical adenomas comprise the majority of incidentalomas. Careful history, physical examination, and endocrine evaluation must be performed to seek evidence of autonomous cortisol, androgen, mineralocorticoid, or catecholamine secretion. Functional tumors require removal. If the adrenal mass is nonfunctional and larger than 6 cm, recommendations are to proceed with surgical resection of the mass. A recent recommendation has been made of 4 cm diameter as the threshold for removal. Lesions of 3 cm or less should be followed clinically with periodic re-imaging. Treatment, however, must be individualized; nonsecreting adrenal incidentalomas may enlarge and become hyperfunctioning. Nuclear scan, and occasionally fine-needle aspiration, may be helpful in defining the mass.

575.2 Adrenal Calcification

Calcification within the adrenal glands may occur in a wide variety of situations, some serious and others of no obvious consequence. Adrenal calcifications are often detected as incidental findings in radiographic studies of the abdomen in infants and children. The physician may elicit a history of anoxia or trauma at birth. Hemorrhage into the adrenal gland at or immediately after birth is probably the most common factor that leads to subsequent calcification. Although it is advisable to assess the adrenocortical reserve of such patients, there is rarely any functional disorder.

Neuroblastomas, ganglioneuromas, cortical carcinomas, pheochromocytomas, and cysts of the adrenal gland may be responsible for calcifications, particularly if hemorrhage has occurred within the tumor. Calcification in such lesions is almost always unilateral.

In the past, tuberculosis was a common cause both of calcification within the adrenals and of Addison disease. Calcifications may also develop in the adrenal glands of children who recover from the Waterhouse-Friderichsen syndrome; such patients are usually asymptomatic. Infants with *Wolman disease*, a rare lipid disorder due to deficiency of lysosomal acid lipase, have extensive bilateral calcifications of the adrenal glands (see Chapter 75.2).

Agrons GA, Lonergan GJ, Dickey GE, et al: Adrenocortical neoplasms in children: Radiologic-pathologic correlation. *Radiographics* 1999;19:989–1008.

Barzon L, Boscaro M: Diagnosis and management of adrenal incidentalomas. *J Urol* 2000;163:398–407.

Bilal MM, Brown JJ: MR imaging of renal and adrenal masses in children. *Magn Reson Imaging Clin North Am* 1997;5:179–97.

Bornstein SR, Stratakis CA, Chrousos GP: Adrenocortical tumors: Recent advances in basic concepts and clinical management. *Ann Intern Med* 1999;130:759–71.

Bravo EL: Evolving concepts in the pathophysiology, diagnosis and treatment of pheochromocytoma. *Endocr Rev* 1994;15:356–68.

Brunt LM, Moley JF: Adrenal incidentaloma. *World J Surg* 2001;25:905–913.

Ciftci AO, Senocak ME, Tanyel FC, et al: Adrenocortical tumors in children. *J Pediatr Surg* 2001;36:549–54.

Ein SH, Weitzman S, Thorner P, et al: Pediatric malignant pheochromocytoma. *J Pediatr Surg* 1994;29:1197–201.

Eisenhoffer G, Lenders JWM, Linehan WM, et al: Plasma normetanephrine and metanephrine for detecting pheochromocytoma in von Hippel-Lindau

disease and multiple endocrine neoplasia type 2. *N Engl J Med* 1999;340: 1872–79.

Ghazi AAM, Mofid D, Rahimi F, et al: Oestrogen and cortisol producing adrenal tumour. *Arch Dis Child* 1994;71:358–59.

Kjellman M, Roshani L, Teh BT, et al: Genotyping of adrenocortical tumors: Very frequent deletions of the MEN1 locus in 11q13 and of a 1-centimorgan region in 2p16. *J Clin Endocrinol Metab* 1999;84:730–35.

Koch CA, Vortmeyer AO, Huang SC, et al: Genetic aspects of pheochromocytoma. *Endocr Regul* 2001;35:43–52.

LaFranchi SH, Hanna CE, Mandel SH: Feminizing adrenal adenoma secreting estrone presenting as prepubertal gynecomastia. *J Pediatr Endocrinol* 1989;3: 261–65.

Latronico AC, Pinto EM, Domenice S, et al: An inherited mutation outside the highly conserved DNA-binding domain of the p53 tumor suppressor protein in children and adults with sporadic adrenocortical tumors. *J Clin Endocrinol Metab* 2001;86:4970–73.

Magill SB, Raff H, Shaker JL, et al: Comparison of adrenal vein sampling and computed tomography in the differentiation of primary aldosteronism. *J Clin Endocrinol Metab* 2001;86:1066–71.

Mayer SK, Oligny LL, Deal C, et al: Childhood adrenocortical tumors: Case series and reevaluation of prognosis—a 24-year experience. *J Pediatr Surg* 1997;32: 911–15.

Mendonca BB, Lucon AM, Menezes CAV, et al: Clinical, hormonal and pathological findings in a comparative study of adrenocortical neoplasms in childhood and adulthood. *J Urol* 1995;154:2004–9.

Moneva MH, Gomez-Sanchez CE: Establishing a diagnosis of primary hyperaldosteronism. *Curr Opin Endocrinol Diabet* 2001;8:124–29.

Phornphutkul C, Okubo T, Wu K, et al: Aromatase P450 expression in a feminizing adrenal adenoma presenting as isosexual precocious puberty. *J Clin Endocrinol Metab* 2001;86:649–52.

Prys-Roberts C: Phaeochromocytoma—recent progress in its management. *Br J Anaesth* 2000;85:44–57.

Reincke M, Beuschlein F, Slawik M, et al: Molecular adrenocortical tumourigenesis. *Eur J Clin Invest* 2000;30:63–68.

Ross JH: Pheochromocytoma: Special considerations in children. *Urol Clin North Am* 2000;27:393–402.

Sandrini R, Ribeiro RC, DeLacerda L: Childhood adrenocortical tumors. *J Clin Endocrinol Metab* 1997;82:2027–31.

Siren J, Tervahartiala P, Sivula A, et al: Natural course of adrenal incidentalomas: Seven-year follow-up study. *World J Surg* 2000;24:579–82.

Wajchenberg BL, Albergaria Pereira MA, Medonca BB, et al: Adrenocortical carcinoma: Clinical and laboratory observations. *Cancer* 2000;88:711–36.

Wilkin F, Gagne N, Paquette J, et al: Pediatric adrenocortical tumors: Molecular events leading to insulin-like growth factor II gene overexpression. *J Clin Endocrinol Metab* 2000;85:2048–56.

Young J, Bulun SE, Agarwal V, et al: Aromatase expression in a feminizing adrenocortical tumor. *J Clin Endocrinol Metab* 1996;81:3173–76.

Young WFJ: Pheochromocytoma and primary aldosteronism: Diagnostic approaches. *Endocrinol Metab Clin North Am* 1997;26:801–27.

SECTION 5 *Disorders of the Gonads*

Robert Rapaport

Chapter 576

Development and Function of the Gonads

Embryonic Gonadal Differentiation. The undifferentiated, bipotential fetal gonad arises from a thickening of the urogenital ridge, close to the region that forms the kidney and adrenal cortex. At 6 wk of gestation, the gonad contains germ cells, stromal cells that will become Leydig cells in testes, or theca, interstitial or hilar cells in the ovary, and supporting cells that will develop into Sertoli cells in testes or granulosa cells in ovaries. In the absence of a testis-determining factor, thought to be the SRY (sex-determining region on the Y chromosome), the gonad develops into an ovary.

A 46,XX complement of chromosomes is necessary for the development of normal ovaries. Both the long and the short arms of X chromosomes bear genes for normal ovarian development. The *DSS* (dosage sensitive/sex reversal) locus associated with the *DAX1* gene responsible for X-linked congenital adrenal hypoplasia and hypogonadotropic hypogonadism, a member of the nuclear receptor superfamily, acts as a repressor of male gene expression. *DAX1* acts by binding to a related nuclear receptor SF-1 (steroidogenic factor-1). The signaling gene *WNT4* in vitro upregulates *DAX1*, resulting in enhanced interference with Leydig cell formation. WNTs are secreted ligands that activate receptor-mediated signal transduction pathways and are involved in modulating gene expression as well as cell behavior, adhesion, and polarity. Alternative splicing of the Wilms tumor 1 *(WT1)* gene may also be involved in sex differentiation. *WT1* mutations are associated with the Dennis-Drash syndrome (early-onset renal failure with abnormal external genitalia and Wilms tumor). Haploinsufficiency of a 3-amino acid (KTS) form of *WT1* has been implicated in the gonadal dysgenesis of patients with Fraser syndrome (late-onset progressive glomerulopathy and 46,XY gonadal dysgenesis). Autosomal genes also play a role in normal ovarian organogenesis and testicular development. Several conditions of gonadal dysgenesis are associated with chromosomal abnormalities. A deletion affecting the short arm of the X chromosome produces the typical somatic anomalies of Turner syndrome.

Development of the testis requires a Y chromosome, but the short arm of the Y chromosome is critical for sex determination; a testis-determining factor at this site has been identified, and the gene for it has been cloned and designated *SRY*. During male meiosis, the Y chromosome must segregate from the X chromosome so that both X and Y chromosomes do not occur in the same spermatozoa. The major portion of the Y chromosome is composed of Y-specific sequences that do not pair with the X chromosome. However, a minor portion of the Y chromosome shares sequences with the X chromosome and pairing does occur in this region. The genes and sequences in this area recombine between the sex chromosomes, behaving like autosomal genes. Therefore, the term *pseudoautosomal* is used to describe the genetic behavior of these genes. The *SRY* gene is localized to the 35-kb portion proximal to this pairing and exchange (pseudoautosomal) region of the Y chromosome. It contains a high-mobility group nonhistone protein (HMG box), suggesting that *SRY* may be a transcriptional regulator of other, some as yet unidentified, genes involved in sex differentiation. These include *SOX9*, an *SRY*-related gene, containing a shared motif homologous with the high-mobility group box 9 (HMG box 9) of *SRY*, located on chromosome 17, that results in sex reversal and campomelic dysplasia, steroidogenic factor 1 (SF-1) on chromosome 9q33, and the Wilms tumor genes *(WTI)* especially the -KSTiso form on chromosome 11p13 needed for early gonadal, adrenal, and renal development, fibroblast growth factor-9 (FGF-9), GATA-4, and XH-2. When recombination events extend beyond the pseudoautosomal region, X- and Y-specific DNA may be transferred between the chromosomes. Such aberrant recombinations result in X chromosomes carrying SRY, resulting in XX males, or Y chromosomes that have lost SRY, resulting in XY females. SRY acts as a transcriptional regulator to increase cellular proliferation, attract interstitial cells from adjacent mesonephros into the genital ridge and stimulates Sertoli cell differentiation. Sertoli cells act as organizer of steroidogenic and germ cell lines and produce anti-müllerian hormone (AMH) that causes the female duct system to regress.

Function of the Testes. In the 1st trimester of pregnancy, levels of placental chorionic gonadotropin peak (8–12 wk) and stimulate the fetal Leydig cells to secrete testosterone, the main hormonal product of the testis. This period is critical for normal virilization of the XY fetus. Defects in this process lead to different forms of male pseudohermaphroditism (see Chapter 582.2). After virilization occurs, fetal levels of testosterone decrease but are maintained at low levels in the latter half of pregnancy by luteinizing hormone (LH) secreted by the fetal pituitary; this is required for continued penile growth.

As part of the normal transition from intrauterine to extrauterine life, likely as a result of the abrupt withdrawal of maternal and placental hormones, the newborn experiences a transient postnatal surge of gonadotropins and sex steroids. In males, LH and testosterone peak at 1–2 mo of age and reach prepubertal levels by 4–6 months of age. Follicle-stimulating hormone (FSH), along with inhibin B peak at 3 mo and decline to prepubertal levels by 9 and 15 mo, respectively. The LH rise is, however, dominant. In females, the FSH surge predominates. FSH peaks around 3–6 mo of age, declines by 12 mo, but remains detectable for 24 mo. Under LH influence, estradiol peaks at 2–6 mo of age. The inhibin B response is variable, peaking between 2–12 mo and remaining at above prepubertal levels

until 24 mo. The neonatal surge may be important for postnatal maturation of the gonads, stabilization of male external genitalia, and perhaps also for gender identity and sexual behaviors. The postnatal surge in LH and testosterone is absent or blunted in infants with hypopituitarism, cryptorchidism, and complete androgen insensitivity syndrome (CAIS). The development of nocturnal pulsatile secretion of LH marks the advent of puberty (see Chapter 555).

Within specific target cells, 6–8% of testosterone is converted by 5-reductase to dihydrotestosterone, another potent androgen (see Fig. 582–1) and about 0.3% is acted on by aromatase to produce estradiol (see Fig. 568–1). Approximately half of circulating testosterone is bound to *sex hormone-binding globulin* (SHBG) and half to albumin; only 2% circulates in the free form. Plasma levels of SHBG are low at birth, rise rapidly during the 1st 10 days of life, and then remain stable until the onset of puberty. Thyroid hormone may play a role in this physiologic increase because neonates with athyreosis have very low levels of SHBG.

Anti-müllerian hormone (AMH, previously referred to as müllerian inhibitory substance [MIS]), inhibin, and activin are members of the transforming growth factor-β (TGF-β) superfamily of growth factors, which has over 45 members, including bone morphogenic proteins (BMPs). Members of the TGF-β superfamily are involved in the regulation of developmental processes and multiple human disease states, including chondrodysplasias and cancer.

AMH, a 140-kd homodimeric glycoprotein hormone, is the earliest secreted product of the Sertoli cells of the fetal testis. Produced as a prohormone, its carboxyl-terminal fragment needs to be removed before it is active by way of a plasma membrane receptor. The gene for AMH is on chromosome 19. Its transcription is initiated by SOX-9 acting through the HMG box while its expression is upregulated by SF-1 binding to its promoter and further interacting with SOX-9, WT-I, and GATA-4. Two distinct serine/threonine receptors with a single transmembrane domain have been identified. The activated type 1 receptor signals to the SMAD family of intracellular mediators.

The gene for the AMH receptor (on chromosome 12) is expressed in Sertoli cells and also in fetal müllerian duct and fetal and postnatal granulosa cells. During sexual differentiation, AMH causes involution of the embryologic precursors of the cervix, uterus, and fallopian tubes (müllerian ducts).

AMH is secreted in males by Sertoli cells during both fetal and postnatal life. In females, it is secreted by granulosa cells from 36 wk of gestation to menopause but at lower levels. The serum concentration of AMH in males is highest at birth, whereas in females it is highest at puberty. After puberty, both sexes have similar serum concentrations of AMH.

Inhibin is another glycoprotein hormone secreted by the Sertoli cells of the testes and granulosa and theca cells of the ovary. Inhibin A consists of an α-subunit disulfide linked to the β A subunit, whereas inhibin B consists of the same α subunit linked to the β B subunit.

Activins are dimers of the B subunits, either homodimers (BA/BA, BB/BB) or heterodimers (BA/BB). Inhibins selectively inhibit whereas activins stimulate pituitary FSH secretion. By means of immunoassays specific for inhibin A or B, it has been shown that inhibin A is absent in males and is present mostly in the luteal phase in women. Inhibin B is the principal form of inhibin in males and females during the follicular phase. Inhibin B may be used as a marker of Sertoli cell function in males. FSH stimulates inhibin B secretion in females and males, but only in males is there also evidence for a gonadotropin-independent way of its regulation.

Like inhibin and activin, follistatin (a single-chain glycosylated protein) is produced by gonads and other tissues such as the hypothalamus, kidney, adrenal gland, and placenta. Follistatin inhibits FSH secretion principally by binding activins, thus blocking the effects of activins at the level of both ovary and pituitary.

An additional plethora of peptides are known to be involved as mediators of the development and function of the testis. They include neurohormones such as growth hormone–releasing hormone, gonadotropin-releasing hormone (GnRH), corticotropin-releasing hormone, oxytocin, arginine vasopressin, somatostatin, substance P, and neuropeptide Y; growth factors such as insulin-like growth factors (IGFs) and IGF-binding proteins, TGF-β, and fibroblast, platelet-derived, and nerve growth factors; vasoactive peptides; and immune-derived cytokines such as tumor necrosis factor and interleukins IL-1, IL-2, IL-4, and IL-6.

Considerable attention will continue to be focused on the complex endocrine and, especially, paracrine, autocrine, and intracrine effects of these regulatory peptides.

Clinical patterns of pubertal changes vary widely (see Chapters 14 and 555). In 95% of boys, enlargement of the genitals begins between 9.5 and 13.5 yr, reaching maturity from 13–17 yr. In a minority of normal boys, puberty begins after 15 yr of age. In some boys, pubertal development is completed in less than 2 yr, but in others, it may take longer than 4.5 yr. The adolescent growth spurt occurs later in boys than in girls at corresponding levels of sexual maturation; for example, the peak velocity of change in height is not attained in boys until the genitals are well developed, but in girls the growth rate is usually at its maximum when the nipple and areola have developed but before there is any other significant breast development.

The median age of sperm production *(spermarche)* is 14 yr. This event occurs in mid puberty as judged by pubic hair, testis size, evidence of growth spurt, and testosterone levels. Nighttime levels of FSH are in the adult male range at the time of spermarche; the first conscious ejaculation occurs at about the same time.

Function of the Ovaries. Without the presence of the *SRY* gene, the undifferentiated gonad can be identified histologically as an ovary by 10–11 wk of gestation. Oocytes are present from the 4th mo of gestation and reach a peak of 7 million by 5 mo of gestation. For normal maintenance, oocytes need granulosa cells to form primordial follicles. Functional FSH (but not LH) receptors are present in oocytes of primary follicles during follicular development. Normal X chromosomes are needed for the maintenance of the oocytes. In contrast to somatic cells, in which only one X chromosome is active, both are active in germ cells. At birth, the ovaries contain about 1 million active follicles, which decrease to 0.5 million by menarche. Thereafter, they decrease at a rate of 1000/mo, and at an even higher rate after the age of 35 yr.

The hormones of the fetal ovary are provided in most part by the fetoplacental unit. As in males, peak gonadotropin secretion occurs in fetal life and then again at 2–3 mo of life, with the lowest levels at about 6 yr of age. In both infancy and childhood, gonadotropin levels are higher in females than in males.

The most important estrogens produced by the ovary are estradiol-17 (E_2) and estrone (E_1); estriol is a metabolic product of these two, and all three estrogens may be found in the urine of mature females. Estrogens also arise from androgens in the adrenal gland and in the testis; the pathway for this conversion is shown in Figure 568–1. This conversion explains why in certain types of male pseudohermaphroditism, feminization occurs at puberty; in 17-ketosteroid reductase deficiency, for example, the enzymatic block results in markedly increased secretion of androstenedione, which is converted in the peripheral tissues to estradiol and estrone; these estrogens, in addition to those directly secreted by the testis, result in gynecomastia. Estrogen regulates a host of functionally different activities in multiple tissues. There are two distinct estrogen receptors with different expression patterns. The ovary also synthesizes progesterone, a progestational steroid; the adrenal cortex and testis synthesize progesterone as a precursor for other adrenal and testicular hormones.

As in the testis, a host of other hormones with autocrine, paracrine, and intracrine effects have been identified in the ovary. They include inhibins, activins, relaxin, and growth factors IGF-1, TGF-α and TGF-β, and cytokines.

Plasma levels of estradiol increase slowly but steadily with advancing sexual maturation and correlate well with clinical evaluation of pubertal development, skeletal age, and rising levels of FSH. Levels of LH do not rise until secondary sexual characteristics are well developed. Estrogens, like androgens, inhibit secretion of both LH and FSH (negative feedback). In females, estrogens also provoke the surge of LH secretion that occurs in the mid-menstrual cycle. The capacity for this positive feedback is another maturational milestone of puberty.

The average age at menarche in American girls is 12.5–13 yr, but the range of "normal" is wide, and 1–2% of "normal" girls have not menstruated by 16 yr of age. The age at onset of pubertal signs varies, with recent studies suggesting earlier ages then previously thought, especially in the United States African American population (see Chapter 14). Menarche generally correlates closely with skeletal age (see Chapters 14 and 555). Maturation and closure of the epiphyses is at least partially estrogen dependent, as demonstrated by a 28-yr-old, normally masculinized male with incomplete closure of the epiphyses who proved to have complete estrogen insensitivity because of an estrogen-receptor defect.

Diagnostic Aids. Improved, sensitive, and specific assays for pituitary and gonadal hormones that can be measured in small amounts of blood have contributed to rapid advances in the understanding of normal and aberrant hypothalamic-pituitary-gonadal interactions. For example, in male infants, measurements of LH, FSH, and testosterone can detect pituitary-testicular defects. Leydig cell integrity in childhood can be determined by the testosterone response following human chronic gonadotropic administration (e.g., 5,000 IU daily for 3 days). The integrity as well as the maturity of the hypothalamic-pituitary-gonadal axis in males and females can be assessed by the administration of gonadotropin-releasing hormone (GnRH) or a GnRH analog. An ultrasensitive LH assay has been shown to differentiate between boys with delayed puberty and those with complete but not partial hypogonadotropic hypogonadism.

Normal inhibin B levels have been documented in infant boys; inhibin B may be a marker of spermatogenesis and also of tumors such as granulosa cell tumors. Inhibin may be involved in tumor suppression. Estrogen-receptor assays may be clinically useful in the management of various ovarian cancers. AMH measurements are useful in the evaluation of children with nonpalpable gonads and intersex problems.

Therapeutic Aids. Phytoestrogens, a family of plant compounds such as soy and flax products, have been shown to have both estrogenic and antiestrogenic properties. Their potential health consequences, so far based largely on population studies, are being investigated. Polyhalogenated aromatic hydrocarbons (PHAHs) are environmental pollutants acting as endocrine disruptors by interfering with reproductive and endocrine function in birds, fish, reptiles, and mammals. The estrogenic effects of PHAHs may in part be due to inhibition of estradiol sulfation by estrogen sulfotransferase (SULTIE), an important pathway of estradiol inactivation. Naturally occurring estrogens administered orally are rapidly destroyed by gastrointestinal and liver enzymes; accordingly, they are usually given as conjugates or esters. The most widely used oral preparations are equine conjugated estrogens (e.g., Premarin) and ethinyl estradiol. Estrogen-containing skin patches for transdermal absorption are also used. With improvements in the understanding of estrogen and estrogen receptor interactions, a new class of compounds called selective estrogen-receptor modulators have been synthesized. For example, raloxifene, a nonsteroidal benzothiophene derivative acts as an estrogen agonist in bone and liver and as an estrogen antagonist in breast and uterus. Androgens such as testosterone are generally injected intramuscularly as long-acting esters (enanthate or cypionate, most commonly) because of their potency and steady response. Transdermal testosterone patches applied to the scrotal or nonscrotal areas and a cutaneously applied gel have to date been used mostly in adults with hypogonadism because of the difficulty in titrating the doses needed during childhood and adolescence. Oral preparations, such as methyltestosterone or fluoxymesterone, do not produce as potent an androgenic response and may be hepatotoxic. Testosterone undecenoate, another oral preparation, is used in Europe but not in the United States. Sublingual (microspheres or pellets) and buccal (absorption via the buccal mucosa) preparations of testosterone are in development.

Attisano L, Wrana JL: Signal transduction by the TGF-β superfamily. *Science* 2002;296:1646–47.

Bergada I, Bergada C, Campo S: Role of inhibins in childhood and puberty. *J Pediatr Endcrinol Metab* 2001;14:343–53.

Bouvattier C, Carel JC, Lecointre C, et al: Postnatal changes of T, LH, and FSH in 46,XY infants with mutations in the *AR* gene. *J Pediatr Endocrinol Metab* 2002; 87:29–32.

Habert R, Lejeune H, Saez J: Origin, differentiation and regulation of fetal and adult leydig cells. *Mol Cell Endocrinol* 2001;179:47–74.

Hastie ND: Lief, Sex and WT1 Isoforms—Three amino acids can make all the difference. *Cell* 2001;106:391–94.

Josso N, diClemente N, Gouedard L: Anti-müllerian hormone and its receptors. *Mol Cell Endocrinol* 2001;179:25–32.

Kester MH, Bulduk S, van Toor H, et al: Potent inhibition of estrogen sulfotransferase by hydroxylated metabolites of polyhalogenated aromatic hydrocarbons reveals alternative mechanism for estrogenic activity of endocrine disrupters. *J Clin Endocrinol Metab* 2002;87:1142–50.

Ketola I, Pentikäinen V, Vaskivuo T, et al: Expression of transcription factor GATA-4 during human testicular development and disease. *J Clin Endocrinol Metab* 2000;85:3925–31.

Koopman P: The genetics and biology of vertebrate sex determination. *Cell* 2001; 105:843–47.

McDonnell DP, Norris JD: Connections and regulation of the human estrogen receptor. *Science* 2002;296:1642–44.

Moon RT, Bowerman B, Boutros M, et al: The promise and perils of Wnt signaling through β-catenin. *Science* 2002;296:1644–46.

Ostrer H: Sex determination: Lessons from families and embryos. *Clin Genet* 2001; 59:207–15.

Pierik FH, Vreeburg JTM, Stijnen T, et al: Serum inhibin B as a marker of spermatogenesis. *J Clin Endocrinol Metab* 1998;83:3110–14.

Quigley CA: Editorial: The postnatal gonadotropin and sex steroid surge: Insights from the androgen insensitivity syndrome. *J Clin Endocrinol Metab* 2002; 87: 24–28.

Rajpert-De Meyts E: Expression of anti-müllerian hormone during normal and pathological gonadal development: Association with differentiation of Sertoli and granulosa cells. *J Clin Endocrinol Metab* 1999;84:3836–44.

Rey RA, Belville C, Nihoul-Fékété C, et al: Evaluation of gonadal function in 107 intersex patients by means of serum anti-müllerian hormone measurements. *J Clin Endocrinol Metab* 1999;84:627–31.

Risbridger GP, Schmitt JF, Robertson DM: Activins and inhibins in endocrine and other tumors. *Endocr Rev* 2001;22:836–58.

Sequera AM, Fideleff HL, Boquete HR, et al: Basal ultra sensitive LH assay: A useful tool in the early diagnosis of male pubertal delay? *J Pediatr Endocrinol Metab* 2002;15:589–96.

Stark A, Madar Z: Phytoestrogens: A review of recent findings. *J Pediatr Endocrinol Metab* 2002;15:561–72.

Swain A, Narvaez V, Burgoyne P, et al: *Dax1* antagonizes *Sry* action in mammalian sex determination. *Nature* 1998;391:761–67.

Swerdloff RS, Wang C, Cunningham G, et al: Long-term pharmacokinetics of transdermal testosterone gel in hypogonadal men. *J Clin Endocrinol Metab* 2000;85:4500–10.

Teixeira J, Maheswaran S, Donahue PK: Müllerian inhibiting substance: An instructive development hormone with diagnostic and possible therapeutic applications. *Endocr Rev* 2001;22:657–74.

Veitia RA, Salas-Cortés L, Ottolenghi C, et al: Testis determination in mammals: More questions than answers. *Mol Cell Endocrinol* 2001;179:3–16.

Chapter 577

Hypofunction of the Testes

Testicular hypofunction may be primary in the testis (primary hypogonadism) or secondary to deficiency of pituitary gonadotropic hormones (secondary hypogonadism). Patients with primary hypogonadism have elevated levels of gonadotropin (hypergonadotropic); those with secondary hypogonadism have low or absent levels (hypogonadotropic).

577.1 Hypergonadotropic Hypogonadism in the Male (Primary Hypogonadism)

Defects of androgen production involving the fetal testis and resulting in male pseudohermaphroditism are discussed in Chapter 582.1.

Etiology. Congenital anorchia occurs in 0.6% of boys with non-palpable testes (1/20,000 males). These boys have normal external genitals, indicating that a noxious factor damaged the fetal testes of the genetic male fetus at some time after sexual differentiation had taken place (14th wk of fetal life). Hence, some refer to this condition as *vanishing testes syndrome*. The condition has been reported in monozygotic twins. Familial occurrence of this condition suggests a genetic etiology. Low levels of testosterone (<10 ng/dL) and markedly elevated levels of luteinizing hormone (LH) and follicle-stimulating hormone (FSH) are found in the early postnatal months; thereafter, levels of gonadotropins tend to decrease even in agonadal children, rising to very high levels as the pubertal years approach. Stimulation with human chorionic gonadotropin (hCG) fails to evoke an increase in the levels of testosterone. Serum levels of anti-müllerian hormone (AMH) are undetectable or low.

A syndrome of *rudimentary testes* has been described in which the testes are exceedingly small; this appears to be inherited as an autosomal or X-linked recessive trait. The cause is unknown. Atrophy of the testes may follow damage to the vascular supply as a result of unskillful manipulation of the testes during surgical procedures for correction of cryptorchidism or as a result of bilateral torsion of the testes. Acute orchitis in pubertal or adult males with mumps may also damage the testes; usually, only the reproductive function of the testes is impaired. The routine immunization of all prepubertal males with mumps vaccine should prevent this complication.

Testicular damage is a frequent consequence of chemotherapy and radiotherapy for cancer. The frequency and extent of damage depend on the agent used, total dosage, duration of therapy, and post-therapy interval of observation. Another important variable is age at therapy; germ cells are less vulnerable in prepubertal than in pubertal and postpubertal boys. Chemotherapy is most damaging if more then one agent is used. The use of alkylating agents such as cyclophosphamide in prepubertal children does not impair pubertal development, even though there may be biopsy evidence of germ cell damage. Most chemotherapeutic agents produce azoospermia and infertility more commonly then Leydig cell damage. Interleukin-2 can depress Leydig cell function, whereas interferon-α does not seem to affect gonadal function.

Radiation damage is dose dependent (see Chapter 700). Temporary azoospermia can be seen with doses greater then 0.3 Gy, with permanent azoospermia seen with doses greater then 8 Gy. Leydig cells are more resistant to radiation. Mild damage as determined by elevated LH levels can be seen with up to 6 Gy;

doses greater then 30 Gy cause hypogonadism in most. Whenever possible, testes should be shielded from radiation. Testicular function should be carefully evaluated in adolescents after multimodal treatment for cancer in childhood. Replacement therapy with testosterone and counseling concerning fertility may be indicated.

The term *hypogonadism* has been widely used to describe aspects in children with a variety of multiple malformation syndromes. The term often refers simply to cryptorchidism, a small phallus, or a scrotal anomaly. In many of these syndromes little is known about the function of the testes; hypergonadotropic or hypogonadotropic hypogonadism has been proved in some instances.

In patients with *Prader-Willi syndrome*, both hypogonadotropic hypogonadism and hypergonadotropic hypogonadism, perhaps secondary to cryptorchidism and its treatment, have been reported. Growth hormone treatment has resulted in improved body composition, physical and psychomotor function, as well as growth in patients with Prader-Willi syndrome. Small testes and azoospermia are seen in patients with *Sertoli cell-only syndrome* (germ cell aplasia or Del Castillo syndrome).

Various degrees of hypogonadism also occur in a significant percentage of patients with chromosomal aberrations such as Klinefelter syndrome or XX males.

Clinical Manifestations. Primary hypogonadism may be suspected at birth if the testes and penis are abnormally small. The condition often is not noticed until puberty when secondary sex characteristics fail to develop. Facial, pubic, and axillary hair is scant or absent; there is neither acne nor regression of scalp hair; and the voice remains high pitched. The penis and scrotum remain infantile and may be almost obscured by pubic fat; the testes are small or absent. Fat accumulates in the region of the hips and buttocks and sometimes in the breasts and on the abdomen. The epiphyses close late in life; therefore, extremities are long. The span is several inches longer than the height, and the distance from the symphysis pubis to the soles of the feet is much greater than that from the symphysis to the vertex. The proportions of the body are described as *eunuchoid*. (The upper to lower segment ratio is considerably less than 0.9.) Many individuals with milder degrees of hypogonadism may be detected only by appropriate studies of the pituitary-gonadal axis. Examination of the testes should be performed routinely by pediatricians; testicular volumes as determined by comparison with standard orchidometers should be recorded.

Diagnosis. Levels of serum FSH and, to a lesser extent, of LH are elevated to greater than age-specific normal values. These elevated levels indicate that even in the prepubertal child there is an active hypothalamic-gonadal feedback relationship. After the age of 11 yr, FSH and LH levels rise significantly, reaching the castrate range. Measurements of random plasma testosterone levels in prepubertal boys are not helpful because they are ordinarily low in normal prepubertal children, rising during puberty to attain adult levels. During puberty, these levels correlate better with testicular size, stage of sexual maturity, and bone age than with chronologic age. In patients with primary hypogonadism, testosterone levels remain low at all ages. There is an attenuated rise or no rise after administration of hCG, in contrast to normal males in whom hCG produces a significant rise in plasma testosterone at any stage of development. Measurements of serum AMH and inhibin levels may give an indication of gonadal presence and function.

NOONAN SYNDROME

Etiology. The term *Noonan syndrome* has been applied to males and females who have certain phenotypic features that occur also in females with Turner syndrome. These boys and girls have normal karyotypes. Noonan syndrome occurs in 1:1000–2500 live births. The disorder is autosomal dominant with variable expression. Sporadic and autosomal recessive occurrence has been reported. Missense mutations in *PTPN11*—a gene on chromosome 12q24.1 encoding the nonreceptor protein tyrosine phosphatase SHP-2—are seen in the majority of studied cases.

Clinical Manifestations. The most common abnormalities are short stature, webbing of the neck, pectus carinatum or pectus excavatum, cubitus valgus, right-sided congenital heart disease, and characteristic facies. Hypertelorism, epicanthus, downward slanted palpebral fissures, ptosis, micrognathia, and ear abnormalities are common. Other abnormalities such as clinodactyly, hernias, and vertebral anomalies occur less frequently. The mean IQ of school-aged children with the condition is 86, with a range of 53 to 127. Verbal IQ tends to be better than performance IQ. High-frequency sensorineural hearing loss is common. The cardiac defect is most often pulmonary valvular stenosis, hypertrophic cardiomyopathy, or atrial septal defect. Hepatosplenomegaly and several hematologic diseases, including low clotting factors XI and XII, acute lymphoblastic leukemia, and chronic myelomonocytic leukemia, are noted. Features of both Noonan syndrome and type 1 neurofibromatosis have been reported, but linkage has been excluded. Noonan-like features can be part of the phenotypic variation of the *NF1* gene mutation, suggesting the possible existence of a Noonan syndrome locus also on chromosome 17q. A few patients with *NF1* and features of Noonan syndrome were subsequently reported as having Turner syndrome. Males frequently have cryptorchidism and small testes; they may be hypogonadal or normal. Puberty is delayed 2 yr; adult height is achieved by the end of the 2nd decade and usually reaches the lowest limit of the normal population. Prenatal diagnosis should be suspected in fetuses with normal karyotype, edema, or hydrops and short femur length.

Treatment. Human growth hormone has resulted in improvement in growth velocity comparable to that seen in patients with Turner syndrome without adverse effects on cardiac ventricular wall thickness. Adult height after growth hormone treatment, resulting in improved height, has only been reported in fewer than 12 patients.

KLINEFELTER SYNDROME

Also see Chapters 70 and 554.

Etiology. Approximately 1/500 newborn males has a 47,XXY chromosome complement, representing the most common sex chromosomal aneuploidy in males. The incidence approximates 1% among the mentally retarded, clustering among patients with IQs greater than 50 and among children admitted to psychiatric hospitals or referred to psychiatric clinics. In infertile males, the incidence is 3%. The chromosomal aberration most often results from meiotic nondisjunction of an X chromosome during parental gametogenesis; the extra X chromosome is maternal in origin in 54% and paternal in origin in 46% of patients. Increased maternal age predisposes to meiotic nondisjunction and to this syndrome, but in most instances maternal age is not advanced.

The 47,XXY complement is the most common chromosomal pattern in persons with Klinefelter syndrome (80%); some have mosaic patterns: 46,XY/47,XXY, 46,XY/48,XXYY, 45,X/46,XY/47,XXY, or 46,XX/47,XXY. Rarely, occurrence of more than two X chromosomes may result in Klinefelter variants: 48,XXXY, 49,XXXYY, 49,XXXXY, 50,XXXXYY, 47,XXY/48,XXXY, 47,XXY/49,XXXXY, or 48,XXYY karyotype. Even with as many as four X chromosomes, the Y chromosome determines a male phenotype. In most patients with four or five X chromosomes, all the additional chromosomes come from the same parent and are not associated with increased parental age.

Clinical Manifestations. The diagnosis is rarely made before puberty because of the paucity or subtleness of clinical manifestations in childhood. Because behavioral or psychiatric disorders may often be apparent long before defects in sexual development, the condition should be considered in all boys with mental retardation and in children with psychosocial, learning, or school adjustment problems. Affected children may be anxious, immature, excessively shy, or aggressive, and they may engage in antisocial acts. Fire-setting behavior has been observed in some of these children. In a prospective study, a group of children with 47,XXY karyotypes identified at birth exhibited relatively mild deviations from normal during the first 5 yr of life. None had major physical, intellectual, or emotional disabilities; some were inactive, with poorly organized motor function and mild delay in language acquisition. Problems often first become apparent after the child begins school. Full-scale IQ scores may be normal, with verbal IQ being somewhat decreased. Verbal cognitive defects and underachievement in reading, spelling, and mathematics are common. By late adolescence, most boys with Klinefelter syndrome have generalized learning disabilities, most of which are language based, and are four to five grade levels behind. Despite these difficulties, most complete high school. High-resolution MRI has shown reduction in left temporal lobe gray matter volumes (less so in testosterone-treated subjects).

The patients tend to be tall, slim, and underweight and to have relatively long legs, but body habitus can vary markedly. The testes tend to be small for age, but this sign may become apparent only after puberty, when normal testicular growth fails to occur. The phallus tends to be smaller than average, and cryptorchidism or hypospadias may occur in a few patients.

Pubertal development may be delayed. Some degree of androgen deficiency is usually detected, although some children may undergo almost normal virilization. About 80% of adults have gynecomastia; they have sparser facial hair, most shaving less often than daily. The most common testicular lesions are spermatogenic arrest and Sertoli cell predominance. The sperm have a high incidence of sex chromosomal aneuploidy. Azoospermia and infertility are usual, although rare instances of fertility are known. Testicular sperm extraction followed by intracytoplasmic sperm injection can result in the birth of healthy infants. Antisperm antibodies have been detected in one quarter of tested specimens. In nonmosaic Klinefelter patients, most testicular sperm (94%) have a normal pattern of sex chromosome segregation.

The height of patients with Klinefelter syndrome tends to be increased. There is an increased incidence of pulmonary disease, varicose veins, and cancer of the breast. Among 93 unselected male breast cancer patients, 7.5% were found to have Klinefelter syndrome. Mediastinal germ cell tumors have been reported; some of these tumors produce hCG and cause precocious puberty in young boys. They may also be associated with leukemia, lymphoma, and other hematologic neoplasia. The highest cancer risk (relative risk 2.7) occurs in the 15–30 yr age group.

In adults with XY/XXY mosaicism, the features of Klinefelter syndrome are decreased in severity and frequency. Children with mosaicism have a better prognosis for virilization, fertility, and psychosocial adjustment.

KLINEFELTER VARIANTS. When the number of X chromosomes exceeds two, the clinical manifestations, including mental retardation and impairment of virilization, are more severe. The XXYY variant is the most common variant (1/50,000 male births). In most, mental retardation occurs with IQ scores between 60 and 80, but 10% have IQs greater then 110. The XXYY male phenotype is not distinctively different from that of the XXY patient, except that XXYY adults tend to be taller than the average XXY patient. The 49,XXXXY variant is sufficiently distinctive to be detected in childhood. Its incidence is estimated to be 1/80,000 to 1/100,000 male births. The disorder arises from sequential nondisjunction in meiosis. Affected patients are severely retarded and have short necks and typical coarse facies with wide-set eyes with a mild upward slant of the fissures, epicanthus, strabismus, a wide and flat upturned nose, a large open mouth, and large malformed ears. The testes are small and may be undescended, the scrotum is hypoplastic, and the penis is very small. Defects suggestive of Down syndrome (e.g., short incurved terminal 5th phalanges, single palmar creases, and hypotonia) and other skeletal abnormalities (including defects in the carrying angle of the elbows and restricted supination) are common. The most frequent radiographic abnormalities are radioulnar synostosis or dislocation, elongated radius, pseudoepiphyses, scoliosis or kyphosis, coxa valga, and retarded osseous age. Most patients with such extensive changes have a 49,XXXXY chromosome karyotype; several mosaic patterns have also been observed: 48,XXXY/49,XXXXY (Fig. 577–1); 48,XXXY/49,XXXXY/50,XXXXXY; and 48,XXXY/49,XXXXY/50, XXXXYY. Prenatal diagnosis of a 49,XXXXY infant has been reported. The fetus had intrauterine growth retardation, edema, and cystic hygroma colli.

The 48,XXXY variant is relatively rare. The characteristic features are generally less severe then in those patients with 49,XXXXY and more severe than in 47,XXY patients. Mild mental retardation, delayed speech and motor development, and immature but passive and pleasant behavior are associated with this condition.

Very few patients have been described with 49,XYYY and 49,XXYYY karyotypes. Dysmorphic features and mental retardation are common to both.

Laboratory Findings. Most males with this condition go through life undiagnosed. The chromosomes should be examined in all patients suspected of having Klinefelter syndrome, particularly

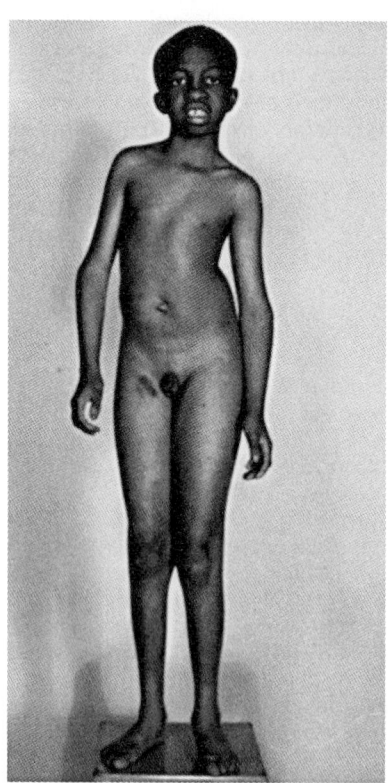

FIGURE 577–1. A 12-yr-old boy with 48,XXXY/49,XXXXY mosaicism who has prognathism, epicanthal folds, scoliosis, very small testes, severe mental retardation, clinodactyly, and radioulnar synostoses.

those attending child guidance, psychiatric, and mental retardation clinics. Before 10 yr of age, boys with 47,XXY Klinefelter syndrome have normal basal plasma levels of FSH and LH. Responses to gonadotropin-stimulating hormone and to hCG are also normal. The testes show normal growth early in puberty, but by mid puberty the testicular growth stops, gonadotropins become elevated, and testosterone levels are slightly low. Inhibin B levels are low in men with the syndrome. Elevated levels of estradiol, resulting in a high estradiol:testosterone ratio, account for the development of gynecomastia during puberty. Despite hypogonadism, most have normal bone mass.

Testicular biopsy before puberty may reveal only a deficiency or absence of germinal cells. After puberty, the seminiferous tubular membranes are hyalinized, and there is adenomatous clumping of Leydig cells. Sertoli cells predominate. Azoospermia is characteristic, and infertility is the rule.

Treatment. Replacement therapy with a long-acting testosterone preparation depends on the age of the patient. It should begin at 11–12 yr of age. The enanthate ester may be used in a starting dose of 25–50 mg injected intramuscularly every 3–4 wk, with 50-mg increments every 6–9 mo until a maintenance dose for adults (200–250 mg every 3–4 wk) is achieved. At that time, testosterone patches or testosterone gel may be substituted for the injections. For older boys, larger initial doses and increments can achieve more rapid virilization. Testosterone treatment leads to an increase in prostate volume and prostate-specific antigen levels. Fertility can be accomplished by an intracytoplasmic sperm injection technique.

XX MALES

This disorder is thought to occur in 1 of 20,000 newborn males. Affected individuals have a male phenotype, small testes, a small phallus, and no evidence of ovarian or müllerian duct tissue; they appear, therefore, to be distinct from the XX true hermaphrodite (see Chapter 582.3). This disorder resembles Klinefelter syndrome, but stature is greater in the latter. Undescended testes and hypospadias occur in a minority of patients. The histologic features of the testes are essentially the same as in Klinefelter syndrome. Patients with the condition usually come to medical attention in adult life because of hypogonadism, gynecomastia, or infertility. Hypergonadotropic hypogonadism occurs secondary to testicular failure. A few cases have been diagnosed perinatally as a result of discrepancies between prenatal ultrasonography and karyotype findings.

In 80% of XX males with normal male external genitals, one of the X chromosomes carries the *SRY* gene. The exchange from the Y to the X chromosome occurs during paternal meiosis, when the short arms of the Y and X chromosomes pair. XX males inherit one maternal X chromosome and one paternal X chromosome containing the translocated male-determining gene. Such exchanges occur because of the proximity of the *SRY* gene to the pseudoautosomal region where recombination between X and Y chromosomes normally occurs in meiosis. Most XX males who are identified before puberty have hypospadias or micropenis; this group of patients usually lacks Y-specific sequences, suggesting other mechanisms for virilization (see Chapter 576). Fluorescent in situ hybridization and primed in situ labeling (PRINS) have been used to identify small *SRY* DNA segments. Yp fragment abnormalities may result in sexually ambiguous phenotypes.

45,X MALES

Also see Chapter 576.

Of the few male patients recognized with a 45,X karyotype, Yp sequences have been translocated to an autosomal chromo-

some. In one instance, the terminal short arm of the Y chromosome was translocated onto an X chromosome. In another, *SRY*/autosomal translocation was postulated. A male with 45,X karyotype and Leri-Weill dyschondrosteosis, *SHOX* gene loss, and *SRY* to Xp translocation was also described.

47,XXX MALES

A Japanese male with poor pubic hair development, hypoplastic scrotal testes (4 mL), normal penis and normal height, gynecomastia, and severe mental retardation had 47,XXX karyotype due to abnormal X-Y interchange during paternal meiosis and X-X nondisfunction during maternal meiosis.

XYY MALES

The 47,XYY male does not have hypogonadism; this condition is discussed here for easy comparison with the XXY and the XX male syndromes.

Approximately 1/1,000 male newborns has an XYY chromosome pattern. In most, the extra Y is generated by nondisjunction at meiosis II after a normal chiasmate meiosis I. When this disorder was first discovered in adults, studies of XYY individuals in mental or penal institutions created a stereotype of affected individuals as having deviant behavior marked by physical aggressiveness and violence. The rate at which XYY males are found in mental or penal settings may be 20 times higher than the rate of the condition of birth. Adults with this karyotype may be relatively impulsive, antisocial, and likely to break the law, but they are not especially aggressive. Unselected 47,XYY boys detected in screening programs tend to exhibit attention deficits, impulsive behavior, inadequate interactions, and poor self-image. Patients with 48,XXYY and 48,XYYY karyotypes tend to have similar deviant behavior.

The XYY adult has few phenotypic manifestations. He tends to be tall and to have severe nodulocystic acne. In affected persons, genital abnormalities have been observed, but cryptic mosaicism, such as X/XYY, is a possibility in these instances. Prolonged PR intervals on electrocardiography and radioulnar synostosis occur more often than in the general population. Renal agenesis and cystic dysplasia of the kidney, as well as hematologic malignancies, have been reported. No clear-cut endocrine abnormalities have been found. This condition poses a serious dilemma for counseling of parents of infants or children discovered to have this sex chromosome complement. The risks for some developmental disability may not be trivial, but neither do they appear to be as dire as earlier thought. Still, the most common reason for a 47,XYY male to be karyotyped is developmental delay or behavioral problems, or both. Children with sex chromosome abnormalities are at an increased risk of learning disabilities, cognitive skill impairments, and difficulties in psychosocial adaptation. Stable, supportive, and compassionate family environments promote improved adaptation of these children and adolescents.

577.2 Hypogonadotropic Hypogonadism in the Male (Secondary Hypogonadism)

In hypogonadotropic hypogonadism, there is deficiency of FSH or LH, or both. The primary defect may lie in the anterior pituitary or in the hypothalamus as a deficiency of gonadotropin-releasing hormone (GnRH). The testes are normal but remain in the prepubertal state because stimulation by gonadotropins is lacking. The disorder may be recognized in infancy, around the time of puberty, or, rarely, in adulthood. Several different gene defects have been described in patients with hypogonadotropic hypogonadism.

Etiology

HYPOPITUITARISM. Most causes of hypopituitarism may be associated with deficiency of gonadotropins and hypogonadotropic hypogonadism (see Chapter 551). In patients with organic lesions in or near the pituitary, whether congenital or acquired, the gonadotropin deficiency is pituitary in origin. In most patients with "idiopathic" hypopituitarism, the defect is in the hypothalamus, caused by a deficiency of GnRH. In patients with multiple pituitary hormone deficiencies, defects in pituitary transcription factors such as PROP-1, HESX-1, and LHX-3 have been described. Microphallus (<2.5 cm) in the newborn male with growth hormone deficiency suggests the likelihood of gonadotropin deficiency, and diagnostic confirmation is feasible; after 6 mo of age, gonadotropin deficiency can rarely be established with certainty until the teenage years.

ISOLATED DEFICIENCY OF GONADOTROPIN. Usually, this disorder involves the hypothalamus rather than the pituitary. It affects about 1/10,000 males and 1/50,000 females and encompasses a heterogeneous group of entities. GnRH deficiency may be complete or partial; it may occur sporadically or in families. *Kallmann syndrome*, one of the most frequent genetic forms of hypogonadotropic hypogonadism, is characterized by its association with anosmia or hyposmia. The X-linked disorder is caused by several mutations of the *KAL* gene at Xp22.3. The association reflects the failure of olfactory axons and GnRH-expressing neurons to migrate from their common origin in the olfactory placode to the brain. The *KAL* gene product anosmin-1, an extracellular matrix glycoprotein, facilitates neuronal growth and migration. The *KAL* gene is also expressed in various parts of the brain, facial mesenchyme, and mesonephros and metanephros, thus explaining some of the associated findings in patients with Kallman syndrome, and as synkinesia, midfacial defects, and renal agenesis.

Some kindreds contain anosmic individuals with or without hypogonadism; others contain hypogonadal individuals who are anosmic. Cleft lip and palate, hypotelorism, median facial clefts, sensorineural hearing loss, unilateral renal aplasia, neurologic deficits, and other findings occur in some affected patients. When Kallmann syndrome is caused by terminal or interstitial deletions of the Xp22.3 region, it may be associated with other contiguous gene syndromes, such as steroid sulfatase deficiency, chondrodysplasia punctata, X-linked ichthyosis, or ocular albinism. Autosomal recessive and autosomal dominant forms of Kallmann syndrome have been reported.

As in patients with Kallmann syndrome, children with *X-linked congenital adrenal hypoplasia* have associated hypogonadotropic hypogonadism (HHG) owing to impaired gonadotropin-releasing hormone (GnRH) secretion. In these patients, there is a mutation of the *DAX1* gene at Xp21.2-21.3. Conditions occasionally associated with these patients because of the contiguous gene syndrome include glycerol kinase deficiency, Duchenne muscular dystrophy, and ornithine transcarbamyl transferase deficiency. Most boys with *DAX1* mutations develop HHG in adolescence, although a patient with adult-onset adrenal insufficiency and partial HHG and two females with HHG and delayed puberty have also been described, the latter as part of extended families with males with classic HHG. The *DAX1* gene defect is, however, rare in patients with delayed puberty or HHG without at least a family history of adrenal failure.

Several genetic defects involving the hypothalamic-pituitary-gonadal axis have been identified. They involve the function of either hormones or their receptors. Depending on both the level and nature of the mutation, hypogonadism, precocious puberty, or sexual ambiguity may develop. To date, eight different GnRH-receptor gene mutations, most compound heterozygotes, have been identified as the cause of HHG. The phenotype, however, varies from partial to complete hypogonadism. A mutation in the gene for the β-subunit of LH at the level of the pituitary causes HHG. At the level of the gonads, LH-receptor defects have led to Leydig cell hypoplasia and undervirilization in genetic males. A boy was reported with micropenis and normal testes that did not produce testosterone even after repeated courses of hCG. Vanishing Leydig cell syndrome was thought to be a possibility (by analogy with the vanishing testes syndrome). Normally functioning Leydig cells must have been present in the first trimester of pregnancy, but because of LH receptor defect, inadequate testosterone production in the 2nd and 3rd trimesters led to an underdeveloped penis at birth. A novel mutation of the β-subunit of FSH also has been described as the cause of hypogonadism in an 18-yr-old man evaluated for delayed puberty and three women with delayed puberty and primary amenorrhea (Table 577–1). Mutations in leptin, in the leptin receptor as well as in the endopeptidase prohormone convertase-1 (PC-1), have been associated with HHG.

OTHER DISORDERS. HHG has been observed in a few patients with polyglandular autoimmune syndrome, in some with elevated melatonin levels, and in a variety of other syndromes, such as Bardet-Biedl, Prader-Willi, multiple lentigines, and several syndromes of ataxia.

Diagnosis. Levels of gonadotropins and gonadal steroids remain in the prepubertal range, and nocturnal pulsatile secretion of LH does not occur. The gonadotropin response to stimulation with GnRH or a more potent analogue of GnRH is markedly blunted. These findings are also consistent with those observed in normal adolescents with the variant known as constitutional delayed puberty; it is difficult to distinguish between the two conditions. Many different tests, including stimulation tests with GnRH, thyrotropin-releasing hormone, metoclopramide, and domperidone, have yielded inconclusive results. The measurement of a single, 8 AM testosterone level may be a good indicator of impending puberty. A value of more then 0.7 nmol/L (20 mg/dL) was noted in boys, all of whom had an increase in testicular volume to greater than 4 mL by 15 mo and 77% by 12 mo. In contrast, of boys with testosterone levels lower then 0.7 nmol/L, only 25% entered puberty by 15 yr of age. The use of a GnRH analogue or the GnRH test after 36 hr of "priming" of the hypothalamic-pituitary-gonadal axis with pulsatile GnRH administration may distinguish adolescents with hypogonadism from those with delayed puberty.

Gonadotropin deficiency is likely if the patient has evidence of another pituitary deficiency, such as a deficiency of growth hormone, particularly if it is associated with corticotropin (adrenocorticotropic hormone [ACTH]) deficiency. The presence of

TABLE 577–1. Known Gene Defects Causing Hypogonadism

Defect	Clinical Condition	Affected Gender
Gonadotropin-Releasing Hormone		
KAL-1	Kallmann syndrome	Both
DAX-1	X-linked adrenal hypoplasia and hypogonadotropic hypogonadism	Male
Receptor	Familial hypogonadotropic hypogonadism	Both
Luteinizing Hormone		
β Subunit	Pubertal delay, Leydig cell hypoplasia, infertility	Male
Receptor	Male pseudohermaphroditism, Leydig cell hypoplasia, micropenis Amenorrhea	Both
Follicle-Stimulating Hormone		
β Subunit	Pubertal delay Amenorrhea	Both
Receptor	Ovarian failure Ovarian germ cell tumors	Female

anosmia usually indicates permanent gonadotropin deficiency, but occasional instances of markedly delayed puberty (18–20 yr of age) have been observed in anosmic individuals. Although anosmia may be present in the family or in the patient from early childhood, its existence is rarely volunteered, and direct questioning is necessary in all patients with delayed puberty. MRI may detect anomalous olfactory lobes and sulci in some patients. Prolactinomas are increasingly recognized as a cause of delayed puberty and should be excluded by determination of serum levels of prolactin.

Probes are available to establish the diagnosis in heterozygotes and newborn infants with the X-linked form of Kallmann syndrome. During the first 3–4 mo of life, unaffected infants demonstrate the usual physiologic rise in gonadotropins and gonadal steroids, and the response to GnRH exceeds that seen in prepubertal children.

Treatment. Constitutional delayed puberty should be ruled out before a diagnosis of isolated deficiency of GnRH is established and treatment is initiated. Testicular volume of less than 4 mL by 14 yr of age occurs in about 3% of boys, but true hypogonadotropic hypogonadism is a rare condition. Even relatively moderate delays in sexual development and growth may result in significant psychologic distress and require attention. Initially, an explanation of the variations characteristic of puberty and reassurance suffice for the majority of boys. If by 15 yr of age there is no clinical evidence of puberty beginning, and the testosterone level is less than 50 ng/dL, a brief course of testosterone is indicated. Testosterone enanthate, 100 mg intramuscularly once monthly for 4–6 mo, usually results in an increase in the signs of secondary sexual characteristics and an increase in growth velocity; it may initiate puberty and may differentiate constitutional delay in puberty from isolated gonadotropin deficiency. The age of initiation of this treatment must be individualized.

Patients with established deficiency of gonadotropins should be treated with the same program of repository testosterone as that used for those with primary testicular deficiency (see Chapter 577.1). With this therapy, the testes will remain small. Treatment with hCG, given subcutaneously or intramuscularly in doses of 500–1,000 IU, three times weekly, stimulates growth of the testes and spermatogenesis. If, after 6–12 mo of therapy, sufficient growth of the testes has not occurred, human menopausal gonadotropin may be added in doses of 37.5–150 IU, three times weekly. It may require up to 2 yr of treatment to achieve adequate spermatogenesis in adults. Recombinantly produced gonadotropins are able to stimulate gonadal growth and function.

A more physiologic, but cumbersome, form of treatment consists of episodic administration (subcutaneously or intravenously) of GnRH. Long-term therapy has been provided with a programmable peristaltic infusion pump. Most patients require about 2 yr of treatment to maximize testicular growth and achieve spermatogenesis.

Achermann JC, Jameson JL: Advances in the molecular genetics of hypogonadotropic hypogonadism. *J Pediatr Endocrinol Metab* 2001;14:3–15.

Bader-Meunier B, Tchernia G, Mielot F, et al: Occurrence of myeloproliferative disorder in patients with Noonan syndrome. *J Pediatr* 1997;130:885.

Bahuau M, Houdayer C, Assouline B, et al: Novel recurrent nonsense mutation causing neurofibromatosis type 1 (NF1) in a family segregating both NF1 and Noonan syndrome. *Am J Med Genet* 1998;75:254.

Carrel AL, Myers SE, Whitman BY, et al: Growth hormone improves body composition, fat utilization, physical strength and agility, and growth in Prader-Willi syndrome: A controlled study. *J Pediatr* 1000;134:215–21.

Chen CP, Chern SR, Chang CL, et al: Prenatal diagnosis and genetic analysis of X chromosome polysomy 49, XXXXY. *Prenat Diagn* 2000;20:754–7.

Cotterill AM, McKenna WJ, Brady AF, et al: The short-term effects of growth hormone therapy on height velocity and cardiac ventricular wall thickness in children with Noonan syndrome. *J Clin Endocrinol Metab* 1996;81:2291.

DeRoux N, Young J, Misrahi M, et al: A family with hypogonadotropic hypogonadism and mutations in the gonadotropin-releasing hormone receptor. *N Engl J Med* 1997;337:1597.

Dobs AS, Hoover DR, Chen MC, et al: Pharmacokinetic characteristics, efficacy, and safety of buccal testosterone in hypogonadal males: A pilot study. *J Clin Endocrinol Metab* 1998;83:33.

Domenice S, Nishi MY, Billerbeck AE, et al: Molecular analysis of *SRY* gene in Brailizan 46,XXX sex reversed patients: Absence of SRY sequence in gonadal tissue. *Med Sci Monit* 2001;7:238–41.

Foresta C, Galeazzi C, Bettella A, et al: High incidence of sperm sex chromosomes aneuploidies in two patients with Klinefelter's syndrome. *J Clin Endocrinol Metab* 1998;83:203.

Fuleihan GEH: Tissue-specific estrogens—the promise for the future. *N Engl J Med* 1997;337:1686.

Geschwind DH, Boone KB, Miller BL, et al: Neurobehavioral phenotype of Klinefelter syndrome. *Ment Retard Dev Disabil Res Rev* 2000;6:107–16.

Gnessi J, Fabbri A, Spera G: Gonadal peptides as mediators of development and functional control of the testis: An integrated system with hormones and local environment. *Endocr Rev* 1997;18:541.

Goodfellow PN, Camerino G: DAX-1, an "antitestis" gene. *EXS* 2001;91:57–69.

Hardelin J: Kallmann syndrome: Towards molecular pathogenesis. *Mol Cell Endocrinol* 2001;179:75–81.

Hayes FJ, Hall JE, Boepple PA, et al: Differential control of gonadotropin secretion in the human: Endocrine role of inhibin. *J Clin Endocrinol Metab* 1998;826:1835.

Hultborn R, Hanson C, Kopf I, et al: Prevalence of Klinefelter's syndrome in male breast cancer patients. *Anticancer Res* 1997;17:4293.

Kadandale JS, Wachtel SS, Tunca Y, et al: Localization of SRY by primed in situ labeling in XX and XY sex reversal. *Am J Med Genet* 2000;95:71–74.

Khorram O, Patrizio P, Wang C, et al: Reproductive Technologies for Male infertility. *J Clin Endocrinol Metab* 2001;86:2373–79.

Kotlar TJ, Young RH, Albanese C, et al: A mutation in the follicle-stimulating hormone receptor occurs frequently in human ovarian sex cord tumors. *J Clin Endocrinol Metab* 1997;82:1020.

Latronico AC, Anasti J, Arnhold IJ, et al: Brief report: Testicular and ovarian resistance to luteinizing hormone caused by inactivating mutations of the luteinizing hormone-receptor gene. *N Engl J Med* 1996;334:507.

Layman LC, Lee EJ, Peak DB, et al: Delayed puberty and hypogonadism caused by mutations in the follicle stimulating hormone β-subunit gene. *N Engl J Med* 1997;337:607.

Lee MM, Donahoe PK, Silverman BL, et al: Measurements of serum mullerian inhibiting substance in the evaluation of children with nonpalpable gonads. *N Engl J Med* 1997;336:1480.

MacLean HE, Warne GL, Zajac JD: Intersex disorders: Shedding light on male sexual differentiation beyond SRY. *Clin Endocrinol* 1997;46:101.

Matthews CH, Borgato S, Beck-Peccoz, et al: Primary amenorrhea and infertility due to a mutation in the β-subunit of follicle-stimulating hormone. *Nat Genet* 1993;5:83.

Maya-Nunez G, Janovick JA, Ulloa-Aguirre A, et al: Molecular basis of hypogonadotropic hypogonadism: Restoration of mutant ($E^{90}K$) GnRH receptor function by a deletion at a distant site. *J Clin Endocrinol Metab* 2002;87:2144–49.

McCabe ERB: Vulnerability within a robust complex system—DAX1 mutations and steroidogenic axis development. *J Clin Endocrinol Metab* 2002;87:41–43.

Merke DP, Tajima T, Baron J, et al: Hypogonadotropic hypogonadism in a female caused by an X-linked recessive mutation in the DAX1 gene. *N Engl J Med* 1999;340:1248–52.

Meyer J, Sudbeck P, Held M, et al: Mutational analysis of the *SOX9* gene in campomelic dysplasia and autosomal sex reversal: Lack of genotype/phenotype correlations. *Hum Mol Genet* 1997;6:9108.

Miller SP, Riley P, Shevell MI: The neonatal presentation of Prader-Willi syndrome revisited. *J Pediatr* 1999;134:226–28.

Misrahi M, Meduri G, Pissard S, et al: Comparison of immunocytochemical and molecular features with the phenotype in a case of incomplete male pseudohermaphroditism associated with a mutation of the luteinizing hormone receptor. *J Clin Endocrinol Metab* 1997;82:2159.

Muller J: Hypogonadism and endocrine metabolic disorders in Prader-Willi syndrome. *Acta Paediatr Suppl* 1997;423:58.

Nisbet DL, Griffin DR, Chitty LS: Prenatal features of Noonan syndrome. *Prenat Diagn* 1999;19:642–47.

Noonan JA: Noonan syndrome revisited. *J Pediatr* 1999;135:667–68.

Ogata T, Matsuo M, Muroya K, et al: 47,XXX male: A clinical and molecular study. *Am J Med Genet* 2001;98:353–56.

Palermo GD, Schlegel PN, Sills ES: Births after intracytoplasmic injection of sperm obtained by testicular extraction from men with nonmosaic Klinefelter's syndrome. *N Engl J Med* 1998;338:588.

Patwardhan AJ, Eliez S, Bender B, et al: Brain morphology in Klinefelter syndrome: Extra X chromosome and testosterone supplementation. *Neurology* 2000;54:2218–23.

Phillip M, Arbelle JE, Segev Y, Parvari R: Male hypogonadism due to a mutation in the gene for the β-subunit of follicle-stimulating hormone. *N Engl J Med* 1998;338:1729.

Robinson DO, Jacobs PA: The origin of the extra Y chromosome in males with a 47,XYY karyotype. *Hum Mol Genet* 1999;8:2205–9.

Romano AA, Blethen SL, Dana K, et al: Growth hormone treatment in Noonan syndrome: The National Cooperative Growth Study experience. *J Pediatr* 1996;128:S18.

Rovet J, Netley C, Keenan M, et al: The psychoeducational profile of boys with Klinefelter syndrome. *J Learn Disabil* 1996;29:180.

Smals AGH, Hermus ARM, Boers GHJ, et al: Predictive value of luteinizing hormone releasing hormone (LHRH) bolus testing before and after 36-hour pulsatile LHRH administration in the differential diagnosis of constitutional delay of puberty and male hypogonadotropic hypogonadism. *J Clin Endocrinol Metab* 1994;78:602.

Stavrou SS, Zhu YS, Cai LQ, et al: A novel mutation of the human luteinizing hormone receptor in 46XY and 46XX sisters. *J Clin Endocrinol Metab* 1998;83:2091.

Stuppia L, Calabrese G, Borrelli P, et al: Loss of the *SHOX* gene associated with Leri-Weill dyschondrosteosis in a 45,X male. *J Med Genet* 1999;36:711–13.

Toledo SPA, Brunner HG, Kraaij R, et al: An inactivating mutation of the luteinizing hormone receptor causes amenorrhea in a 46,XX female. *J Clin Endocrinol Metab* 1996;81:3850.

VanDop C, Burstein S, Conte FA, et al: Isolated gonadotropin deficiency in boys: Clinical characteristics and growth. *J Pediatr* 1987;111:684.

Wu FC, Brown DC, Butler GE, et al: Early morning plasma testosterone is an accurate predictor of imminent pubertal development in prepubertal boys. *J Clin Endocrinol Metab* 1993;76:26.

Chapter 578

Pseudoprecocity Resulting from Tumors of the Testes

Leydig cell tumors of the testes are rare causes of precocious pseudopuberty and cause asymmetric enlargement of the testes. They account for 3% of all testicular tumors. Leydig cells are sparse before puberty; tumors derived from them are more common in the adult. The reported cases in children include one member in each of two pairs of identical twins. These tumors are usually unilateral and benign; 10% may become malignant. Reinke crystalloids are a characteristic microscopic feature but occur in fewer than 50% of Leydig cell tumors. A gsp mutation was described in one testicular Leydig cell tumor. In adult testes, testicular germ cell tumors, but not Sertoli cell tumors or Leydig cell tumors, exhibit biallelic expression of the human *H19* gene.

The *clinical manifestations* are those of puberty in the male; onset occurs usually from 5–9 yr of age. Gynecomastia has been described. The tumor of the testis can usually be readily felt; the contralateral unaffected testis is normal in size for the age of the patient.

Plasma levels of testosterone are markedly elevated. Follicle-stimulating hormone and luteinizing hormone levels are suppressed, and there is no response to gonadotropin-releasing hormone. Ultrasonography may aid in the detection of small nonpalpable tumors. Fine-needle aspiration biopsy may help define the diagnosis.

Treatment consists of surgical removal of the affected testis. Progression of virilization ceases, and partial reversal of the signs of precocity may occur.

Testicular adrenal rests may develop into tumors that mimic Leydig cell tumors; in the absence of Reinke crystals, these two tumors cannot be differentiated histologically. Adrenal rest tumors are usually bilateral and occur in children with congenital adrenal hyperplasia, usually salt-losing patients, during adolescence or young adult life. The stimulus for the growth of the adrenal rests is inadequate corticosteroid suppressive therapy, and treatment with adequate doses almost always results in their regression. Definite evidence of the origin of these tumors has been achieved by demonstrating their 21-hydroxylase activity. The misdiagnosis of these tumors in patients with congenital adrenal hyperplasia has led to unnecessary orchidectomy.

Fragile X syndrome is the most frequent cause of hereditary mental retardation, with an incidence of 1/2,000 births. It is caused by the amplification of a polymorphic CGG repeat in the 5′ untranslated region of the *FMRI* gene at Xp17.3. Amplified beyond 200 units, the repeat CGG sequence leads to methylation of the promoter region of FMRI and to a lack of gene product (FMRP). A cardinal characteristic of the condition is testicular enlargement (macro-orchidism), reaching 40–50 mL after puberty. Although the condition has been recognized in a child as young as 5 mo of age, affected boys younger than 6 yr of age rarely have testicular enlargement; by 8–10 yr of age, most have testicular volumes greater than 3 mL. The testes are enlarged bilaterally, are not nodular, and are histologically normal. Results of hormonal studies are normal. Direct DNA analysis searching for CGG repeat sequences permits definitive diagnosis (see Chapter 70).

Sex cord tumors with annular tubules of the testes can cause breast development in young boys. These tumors usually are associated with Peutz-Jeghers syndrome; they occur bilaterally, are multifocal, and are detectible by ultrasonography. Excessive production of aromatase (P450$_{arom}$) causes feminization of these boys.

In boys with *unilateral cryptorchidism*, the contralateral testis is about 25% larger than normal for age. Testicular enlargement has also been noted in boys with Henoch-Schönlein purpura and lymphangiectasia. Epidermoid and dermoid cysts of the testes have been reported rarely.

Assi A, Sironi M, Bacchioni AM, et al: Leydig cell tumor of the testis: A cytohistological, immunohistochemical, and ultrastructural case study. *Diagn Cytopathol* 1997;16:2626.

Clark RV, Albertson BD, Monabi A, et al: Steroidogenic enzyme activities, morphology and receptor studies of a testicular rest in a patient with congenital adrenal hyperplasia. *J Clin Endocrinol Metab* 1990;70:1408.

Coen P, Kulin H, Ballantine T, et al: An aromatase-producing sex-cord tumor resulting in prepubertal gynecomastia. *N Engl J Med* 1991;324:317.

Combes-Moukousky ME, Kottler ML, Valensi P, et al: Gonadal and adrenal catheterization during adrenal suppression and gonadal stimulation in a patient with bilateral testicular tumors and congenital adrenal hyperplasia. *J Clin Endocrinol Metab* 1994;79:1390.

Fragoso MCBV, Latronico AC, Carvalho FM, et al: Activating mutation of the stimulatory G protein (gsp) as a putative cause of ovarian and testicular human stromal Leydig cell tumors. *J Clin Endocrinol Metab* 1998;83:2074.

Hoogeveen AT, Oostra BA: The fragile X syndrome. *J Inherit Metab Dis* 1997;20:139.

Nisula BC, Loriaux DL, Sherins RJ, et al: Benign bilateral testicular enlargement. *J Clin Endocrinol Metab* 1974;38:440.

Rosenberg T, Gilboa Y, Golik A, et al: Pseudoprecocious puberty in a young boy due to interstitial cell adenomas of the testis. *Helv Paediatr Acta* 1984;39:79.

Chapter 579

Gynecomastia

Gynecomastia, the occurrence of mammary tissue in the male, is a common condition. True gynecomastia (the presence of granular breast tissue) needs to be distinguished from pseudogynecomastia (consisting of only adipose tissue) seen in overweight boys. Gynecomastia is usually a sign of estrogen-androgen imbalance; its cause is often obscure. It occurs in most newborn males as a result of stimulation by maternal hormones; the effect disappears in a few weeks.

During early to mid puberty, approximately two thirds of boys develop various degrees of subareolar hyperplasia of the breasts. *Physiologic pubertal gynecomastia* may involve only one breast, and it is not unusual for both breasts to enlarge at disproportionate rates or at different times. Tenderness of the breast is common but transitory. Spontaneous regression may occur within a few months; it rarely persists longer than 2 yr. Mean concentrations of follicle-stimulating hormone, luteinizing hormone, prolactin, testosterone, estrone, and estradiol are the same as in boys without gynecomastia. When levels are correlated with stage of puberty, a decreased ratio of testosterone to estradiol is found in boys with gynecomastia. Cultured pubic skin fibroblasts from boys with gynecomastia show excessive aromatase activity. *Treatment* usually consists of reassuring the boy and his family of the physiologic and transient nature of the phenomenon. When the enlargement is striking and persistent and causes serious emotional disturbance to the patient, treatment may be justified. Medical treatment is generally aimed at decreasing the estrogen/androgen ratio. Danazol has anti-estrogenic effects but also numerous untoward side effects. Aromatase inhibitors such as testolactone and anastrozole are being evaluated for use in patients with gynecomastia. Surgical removal of the enlarged breast tissue is rarely indicated. One technique involves endoscopically assisted transaxillary removal of glandular tissue.

Benign, self-limited, and usually transient gynecomastia has been reported in prepubertal children during the initiation of therapy with human growth hormone.

Occasionally, breast development may mimic female breast development (to Tanner stages 3–5) and fails to regress. *Familial gynecomastia* has occurred in several kindreds as an X-linked or autosomal dominant sex-limited trait. Levels of gonadotropins, testosterone, prolactin, and steroid-binding globulins are normal. Increased peripheral conversion of C19-steroids to estrogens (increased aromatization) has been found in familial and sporadic cases of gynecomastia and may explain some instances of this condition.

A report of the *syndrome of aromatase excess* in a father and his son and daughter suggests autosomal dominant inheritance. There was gynecomastia in the 9-yr-old boy and macromastia and isosexual precocity in his 7.5-yr-old sister. Excess aromatase activity was shown in skin fibroblasts and transformed lymphocytes in vitro. This was associated with $P450_{arom}$ polymorphism that suggested a sequence change in the $P450_{arom}$ promoter region. In mice, disruption of the *dax1* gene causes increased aromatase expression.

In prepubertal children with gynecomastia, an *exogenous source of estrogens* must be sought. Accidental or therapeutic exposure to small amounts of exogenous estrogens by inhalation, percutaneous absorption, or ingestion may cause gynecomastia. Three boys developed gynecomastia after indirect exposure to their mothers' custom-compounded topical estrogen-containing creams. Increased pigmentation of the nipple and areola should suggest this cause. Exposure to medications that decrease levels of androgens, especially free androgens, increase estradiol, or displace androgens from breast androgen receptors may result in gynecomastia.

Several other pathologic conditions may cause gynecomastia. It has been observed in children with congenital virilizing adrenal hyperplasia (e.g., 11β-hydroxylase deficiency). It may be associated with Leydig cell tumors of the testis or with feminizing tumors of the adrenal gland. Several boys with the *Peutz-Jeghers syndrome* and gynecomastia had *sex-cord tumors with annular tubules* of the testes. The testes may not be enlarged; the tumor is usually multifocal and bilateral. Excessive aromatase production accounts for the gynecomastia. This condition occurs in patients with Klinefelter syndrome and with other types of testicular failure (hypergonadotropic states). It is a common finding in boys with certain types of male pseudohermaphroditism (particularly Reifenstein syndrome), with the androgen insensitivity syndromes, and with the 17-ketosteroid reductase defect. When gynecomastia is associated with galactorrhea, a prolactinoma should be considered. In a pubertal boy with fibrolamellar carcinoma of the liver, the associated gynecomastia and elevated estrogen level were attributed to increased aromatization of circulating androgens by the tumor. In an 8-yr-old boy with a calcifying Sertoli cell tumor, the gynecomastia was postulated to be the result of peripheral aromatization of androgens derived from Leydig cells newly differentiated from interstitial cells stimulated by the tumor. Hyperthyroidism alters the androgen:estrogen ratio by increasing bound androgen and decreasing the free testosterone and may result in gynecomastia.

In adults, gynecomastia occurs with liver cirrhosis, with digitalis therapy for congestive heart failure, bronchogenic carcinoma, administration of various nonsteroidal therapeutic agents, and heavy marijuana smoking. Ketoconazole, an antifungal drug, causes gynecomastia by directly inhibiting testosterone synthesis. Spironolactone, methyldopa, phenothiazines, antidepressants, coumadin, digitalis, and heroin have all been associated with gynecomastia.

Braunstein GD: Gynecomastia. *N Engl J Med* 1993;328:490.

Bulard J, Mowszowicz I, Schaison G: Increased aromatase in pubic skin fibroblasts from patients with isolated gynecomastia. *J Clin Endocrinol Metab* 1987;64:618.

Felner EI, White PC: Prepubertal gynecomastia: Indirect exposure to estrogen cream. *Pediatrics* 2000;105:1–3.

Hochberg Z, Even L, Zadik Z: Mineralocorticoids in the mechanism of gynecomastia in adrenal hyperplasia caused by 11β-hydroxylase deficiency. *J Pediatr* 1991; 118:258.

Lazala C, Saenger P: Pubertal gynecomastia. *J Pediatr Endocrinol Metab* 2002; 15:553–60.

Maclaren NK, Migeon CJ, Raiti S: Gynecomastia with congenital virilizing adrenal hyperplasia (11β-hydroxylase deficiency). *J Pediatr* 1975;86:579.

Malozowski S, Stadel BV: Prepubertal gynecomastia during growth hormone therapy. *J Pediatr* 1995;126:659.

Ohyama T, Takada A, Fujikawa M, et al: Endoscope-assisted transaxillary removal of glandular tissue in gynecomastia. *Ann Plast Surg* 1998;40:62.

Stratakis CA, Vottero A, Brodies A, et al: The aromatase excess syndrome is associated with feminization of both sexes and autosomal dominant transmission of aberrant P450 aromatase gene transcription. *J Clin Endocrinol Metab* 1998;83:1348–57.

Chapter 580

Hypofunction of the Ovaries

Hypofunction of the ovaries may be caused by congenital failure of development, postnatal destruction (primary or hypergonadotropic hypogonadism), or lack of stimulation by the pituitary and or hypothalamus (secondary or tertiary hypogonadotropic hypogonadism). Many chronic diseases may result in hypogonadotropic hypogonadism.

580.1 Hypergonadotropic Hypogonadism in the Female (Primary Hypogonadism)

Diagnosis of hypergonadotropic hypogonadism before puberty is difficult. Except in the case of Turner syndrome, most affected patients have no prepubertal clinical manifestations.

TURNER SYNDROME

Turner described a syndrome consisting of sexual infantilism, webbed neck, and cubitus valgus in adult females (also see Chapter 70). Ullrich described an 8-yr-old girl with short stature and many of the same phenotypic features. The term *Ullrich-Turner syndrome* is frequently used in Europe but rarely used in the United States. The condition is defined as the combination of the characteristic phenotypic features accompanied by complete or partial absence of the second X chromosome with or without mosaicism.

Pathogenesis. Half the patients with Turner syndrome have a 45,X chromosomal complement. About 15% of patients are mosaics for 45,X and a normal cell line (45,X/46,XX). Other mosaics with isochromosomes, 45,X/46,X,i(Xq); with rings, 45,X/46,X,r(X); or with fragments, 45,X/46fra, occur less often. The single X is of maternal origin in 50–70% of 45,X patients. The mechanism of chromosome loss is unknown, and the risk for the syndrome does not increase with maternal age. The genes involved in the Turner phenotype are X-linked genes that escape inactivation. A major locus involved in the control of linear growth has been mapped within the pseudoautosomal region of the X chromosome (PAR 1). *SHOX*, a homeobox-containing gene of 170 kb of DNA within the PAR 1, is thought to be important for controlling growth in children with Turner syndrome, in patients having idiopathic short stature, and in the Leri-Weill syndrome. Genes for the control of normal ovarian function are postulated to be on Xp and perhaps two "supergenes" on Xq.

Turner syndrome occurs in about 1/1,500–2,500 liveborn females. The frequency of the 45,X karyotype at conception is about 3.0%, but 99% of these are spontaneously aborted, accounting for 5–10% of all abortuses. Mosaicism (45,X/46,XX) occurs in a proportion higher than that seen with any other aneuploid state, but the mosaic Turner constitution is rare among the abortuses; these findings indicate preferential survival for mosaic forms.

The normal fetal ovary contains about 7 million oocytes, but these begin to disappear rapidly after the 5th mo of gestation. At birth, there are only 2 million (1 million active follicles); by menarche, there are 400,000–500,000; and at menopause, 10,000 remain. In the absence of one X chromosome, this process is accelerated, and nearly all oocytes are gone by 2 yr of age. In aborted 45,X fetuses, the number of primordial germ cells in the gonadal ridge appears to be normal, suggesting that the normal process is accelerated in patients with Turner syndrome. Eventually, the ovaries are described as "streaks" and consist only of connective tissue, but a few germ cells may persist.

Clinical Manifestations. Many patients with Turner syndrome are recognizable at birth because of a characteristic edema of the dorsa of the hands and feet and loose skinfolds at the nape of the neck. Low birthweight and decreased length are common. Clinical manifestations in childhood include webbing of the neck, a low posterior hairline, small mandible, prominent ears, epicanthal folds, high arched palate, a broad chest presenting the illusion of widely spaced nipples, cubitus valgus, and hyperconvex fingernails. The diagnosis is often first suspected at puberty when sexual maturation fails to occur.

Short stature, the cardinal finding in all girls with Turner syndrome, may be present with minimal other clinical manifestations. The growth deceleration begins in infancy and young childhood, gets progressively more pronounced in later childhood and adolescence, and results in significant adult short stature. Sexual maturation fails to occur at the expected age. The mean adult height is 143–144 cm in the United States and most of northern Europe, but 140 cm in Argentina and 147 cm in Scandinavia (Fig. 580–1). The height is well correlated with the midparental height (average of the parents' heights). Specific growth curves have been developed for girls with Turner syndrome.

Associated defects are common. Complete cardiologic evaluation, including echocardiography, reveals isolated nonstenotic bicuspid aortic valves in one third to one half of patients. In later life, bicuspid aortic valve disease can progress to dilatation of the aortic root. Less frequent defects include aortic coarctation (20%), aortic stenosis, mitral valve prolapse, and anomalous pulmonary venous drainage. In a study of 170/393 females with Turner syndrome in Denmark, 38% of patients with 45,X chromosomes had cardiovascular malformations compared with 11% of those with mosaic monosomy X; the most common were aortic valve abnormalities and aortic coarctation. Webbed neck in patients with or without recognized syndromes is associated with both flow- and non–flow-related heart defects. Among patients with Turner syndrome, those with webbed neck have a much greater chance of having coarctation of the aorta than do those without webbed necks. Repeat cardiac evaluation should be considered even in those without prior findings of cardiac abnormalities during adolescence, and certainly before pregnancy is contemplated. Blood pressure should be routinely monitored even in the absence of cardiac or renal lesions and especially in those with suggestions of aortic root dilatation.

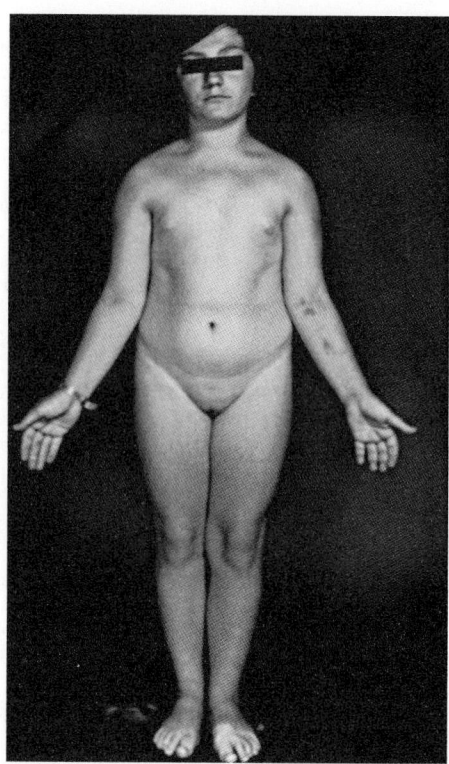

FIGURE 580–1. Turner syndrome in a 15-yr-old girl exhibiting failure of sexual maturation, short stature, cubitus valgus, and a goiter. There is no webbing of the neck. Karyotyping revealed 45,X/46,XX chromosome complement, and the urinary gonadotropin level was over 96 mouse units/24 hr; T_4 was 2.2 µg/dL.

One fourth to one third of patients have renal malformations on ultrasonographic examination (50% of those with 45,X karyotypes). The more serious defects include pelvic kidney, horseshoe kidney, double collecting system, complete absence of one kidney, and ureteropelvic junction obstruction. Idiopathic hypertension is also common. When the ovaries were examined by ultrasonography, older studies found a significant decrease in percentage of detectable ovaries from infancy to later childhood. A subsequent report found no such age-related differences in a cross sectional (N = 142) and longitudinal study (N = 38) conducted in Italy; 27–46% of patients had detectable ovaries at various ages; 76% of those with X mosaicism and 26% of those with 45,X karyotypes had detectable ovaries.

Sexual maturation usually fails to occur, but 10–20% of girls have spontaneous breast development, and a small percentage may have menstrual periods. Pregnancies have been reported for spontaneously menstruating patients with Turner syndrome. Premature menopause, increased risk of miscarriage, and offspring with increased risk of trisomy 21 have been reported in some of these women. A woman with a 45, X/46, X, r(X) karyotype treated with hormone replacement therapy had three pregnancies, resulting in a normal 46,XY male infant, a spontaneous abortion, and a healthy term female with Turner syndrome 45X/46Xr(X).

Antithyroid antibodies, thyroid peroxidase, or thyroglobulin antibodies occur in 30–50% of patients. The prevalence increases with advancing age. Ten to 30% have autoimmune thyroid disease, with or without the presence of a goiter. Age-dependent abnormalities in carbohydrate metabolism characterized by abnormal glucose tolerance and insulin resistance and, only rarely, frank type 2 diabetes occur in patients with

Turner syndrome. Cholesterol levels are elevated in adolescence, regardless of body mass index or karyotype.

Inflammatory bowel disease, both Crohn disease and ulcerative colitis; gastrointestinal bleeding due to abnormal mesenteric vasculature; and delayed gastric emptying time have all been reported.

Sternal malformations can be detected by lateral chest radiography. An increased carrying angle at the elbow is usually not clinically significant. Scoliosis occurs in about 10% of adolescent girls. Reported eye findings include anterior segment dysgenesis and keratoconus. Pigmented nevi become more prominent with age; melanocytic nevi are common. Essential hyperhidrosis, torus mandibularis, and alopecia areata occur rarely.

Recurrent bilateral otitis media develops in about 75% of patients. Sensorineural hearing deficits are common, and the frequency increases with age. Problems with gross and fine motor-sensory integration, failure to walk before 15 mo of age, and early language dysfunction often raise questions about developmental delay, but intelligence is normal in most patients. However, mental retardation does occur in patients with 45,X/46,X,r(X); the ring chromosome is unable to undergo inactivation and leads to two functional X chromosomes. In adults, deficits in perceptual spatial skills are more common than they are in the general population. Evidence suggests the existence of an imprinted X-linked locus that affects cognitive function. Patients with Turner syndrome with a 45,X karyotype whose X chromosome was of paternal origin were significantly better adjusted and had superior verbal and higher-order executive function skills then did those whose X chromosome was of maternal origin.

The prevalence of mosaicism depends in large part on the techniques used for studying chromosomal patterns. The use of fluorescent in situ hybridization and reverse transcription-polymerase chain reaction (PCR) has increased the reported prevalence of mosaic patterns to as high as 60–74%.

Mosaicism involving the Y chromosome occurs in 5%. A population study of 114 Danish women (mean age 27 ± 13 yr) using PCR with five different primer sets found Y chromosome material in 12.2%. Gonadoblastoma among Y-positive patients occurred in 7–10%. Therefore, the current recommendation that prophylactic gonadectomy should be performed even in the absence of MRI or CT evidence of tumors may need to be re-evaluated in the future. The gonadoblastoma locus on the Y chromosome (GBY) maps close to the Y centromere. The presence of only the *SRY* (sex determining region on Y) locus is not sufficient to confer increased susceptibility for the development of gonadoblastoma. A careful study of 53 patients with Turner syndrome by nested PCR excluded low-level Y mosaicism in almost all cases. A second round of PCR detected *SRY* on the distal short arm of the Y chromosome in only two subjects. Therefore, routine PCR for Y chromosome detection for the purpose of assigning gonadoblastoma risk does not seem indicated.

In patients with 45,X/46,XX mosaicism, the abnormalities are attenuated and fewer; short stature is as frequent as it is in the 45,X patient and may be the only manifestation of the condition other than ovarian failure (see Fig. 580–1).

Laboratory Findings. Chromosomal analysis must be considered in all short girls. In a systematic search, using Southern blot analysis of leukocyte DNA, Turner syndrome was detected in 4.8% of girls referred to an endocrinology service because of short stature. Girls referred with already recognized Turner phenotypes were excluded from analysis. Patients with a marker chromosome in some or all cells should be tested for DNA sequences at or near the centromere of the Y chromosome.

Ultrasonography of the heart, kidneys, and ovaries is indicated after the diagnosis is established. The most common skeletal abnormalities are shortening of the 4th metatarsal and metacarpal bones, epiphyseal dysgenesis in the joints of the knees and elbows, Madelung deformity, scoliosis, and, in older patients, inadequate osseous mineralization.

Plasma levels of gonadotropins, particularly follicle-stimulating hormone (FSH), are markedly elevated to greater than those of age-matched controls during infancy; at 2–3 yr of age, a progressive decrease in levels occurs until they reach a nadir at 6–8 yr of age, and by 10–11 yr, they rise to adult castrate levels.

Thyroid antiperoxidase antibodies should be checked periodically and, if positive, levels of thyroxine and thyroid-stimulating hormone should be obtained. Extensive studies have failed to establish that growth hormone deficiency plays a primary role in the pathogenesis of the growth disorder. Defects in normal secretory patterns of growth hormone are seen in adolescents but not younger girls with Turner syndrome. In vitro, monocytes and lymphocytes show decreased sensitivity to insulin-like growth factor-1 (IGF-1).

The American Academy of Pediatrics has published a comprehensive guide to the health supervision of children with Turner syndrome.

Treatment. Treatment with recombinant human growth hormone increases height velocity and ultimate stature in most but not all children. Many girls achieve heights of greater than 150 cm with early initiation of treatment. By adjusting growth hormone doses according to growth velocity measures, 80% of 14 patients achieved final adult height better than 2 SD less than the mean for the general population (mean height 155 cm). In a large multicenter placebo-controlled U.S. clinical trial, 99 patients with Turner syndrome who started receiving growth hormone at a mean age of 10.9 yr at doses between 0.27 and 0.36 mg/kg/wk achieved a mean height of 149 cm, with nearly one third reaching heights greater than 152.4 cm (60 in). In the Netherlands, higher doses of growth hormone (up to 0.63 mg/kg/wk in the 3rd yr of treatment) resulted in 85% of the subjects reaching adult heights in the normal range for the Dutch reference population. Growth hormone treatment should be initiated in early childhood and/or when there is evidence of growth velocity attenuation on specific Turner syndrome growth curves. The starting dose of growth hormone is 0.375 mg/kg/wk. Growth hormone therapy does not significantly aggravate carbohydrate tolerance and does not result in marked adverse events in patients with Turner syndrome. Serum levels of IGF-1 should be routinely monitored during growth hormone treatment.

Replacement therapy with estrogens is indicated, but there is little consensus about the optimal age at which to initiate treatment. The psychologic preparedness of the patient to accept therapy must be taken into account. The improved growth achieved by girls treated with growth hormone in childhood permits initiation of estrogen replacement at 12–13 yr. For greater gains in height, especially for those in whom growth hormone treatment is not initiated until later in childhood or adolescence, estrogen treatment may need to be delayed until 14–15 yr of age. Careful consideration should be given to the sometimes conflicting psychologic consequences of delaying estrogen therapy for the purpose of achieving better ultimate height. The effects on bone accretion should also be considered. The availability of very low dose estrogen replacement therapy in the future may obviate the need to choose between appropriate pubertal replacement and optimizing height potential. Estrogen therapy improves verbal and nonverbal memory in girls with Turner syndrome.

Premarin, a conjugated estrogen, 0.3–0.625 mg, or Estrace, 0.5 mg (micronized estradiol), given daily for 3–6 mo is usually effective in inducing puberty. The estrogen then is cycled (taken on days 1–23), and Provera, a progestin, is added (taken on days 10–23) in a dose of 5–10 mg daily. In the remainder of the calendar month, during which no treatment is given, withdrawal bleeding usually occurs.

Prenatal chromosome analysis for advanced maternal age has revealed a frequency of 45,X/46,XX that is 10 times higher than when diagnosed postnatally. Most of these patients have no clinical manifestations of Turner syndrome, and levels of gonadotropins are normal. Awareness of this mild phenotype is important in counseling patients.

Psychosocial support for these girls is an integral component of treatment. The Turner Syndrome Society, which has local chapters in the United States, and similar groups in Canada and other countries provide a valuable support system for these patients and their families in addition to that given by the health care team.

Successful pregnancies have been carried to term using ovum donation and in vitro fertilization.

In adult women with Turner syndrome, there seems to be a high prevalence of undiagnosed bone mineral density, lipid, and thyroid abnormalities. Glucose intolerance, diminished first-phase insulin response, elevated blood pressure, and lowered fat free mass are common. Glucose tolerance worsens, but fat free mass and blood pressure and general physical fitness improve with sex hormone replacement.

In an analysis of a cohort of 597 women with cytogenetically proven Turner syndrome in Denmark (Danish Cytogenetic Register), neoplasms were identified in 20 women. Only one case, a Wilms tumor, was diagnosed in childhood. Colon cancer was observed in five patients for a relative risk of 6.9. No case of dysgerminoma or gonadoblastoma was found even in the 20 women with Y chromosomes.

Careful and appropriate health maintenance should be continued for patients with Turner syndrome throughout their lives.

XX GONADAL DYSGENESIS

Some phenotypically and genetically normal females have gonadal lesions identical to those in 45,X patients but without somatic features of Turner syndrome; their condition is termed *pure gonadal dysgenesis* or *pure ovarian dysgenesis*. Here we discuss only those with the XX chromosome constitution. XY gonadal dysgenesis, also termed *Swyer syndrome*, is discussed later in the section on male pseudohermaphroditism. These two conditions are distinct entities; XX and XY gonadal dysgenesis have not been reported in the same family.

The disorder is rarely recognized in children because the external genitals are normal, no other abnormalities are visible, and growth is normal. At pubertal age, sexual maturation fails to take place. Plasma gonadotropin levels are elevated. Delay of epiphyseal fusion results in a eunuchoid habitus. Pelvic ultrasonography reveals streak ovaries.

Affected siblings, parental consanguinity, and failure to uncover mosaicism all point to female-limited autosomal recessive inheritance. The disorder appears to be especially frequent in Finland (1/8,300 liveborn girls). In this population, several mutations in the FSH receptor gene (on chromosome 2p) were demonstrated as the cause of the condition. FSH receptor gene mutations were not detected in Mexican women with 46,XX gonadal dysgenesis. In some patients, XX gonadal dysgenesis has been associated with sensorineural deafness *(Perrault syndrome)*. A patient with this condition and concomitant growth hormone deficiency and virilization has also been reported. There may be distinct genetic forms of this disorder. Müllerian agenesis, or the Mayer-Rokitansky-Küster-Hauser syndrome, second to gonadal dysgenesis as the most common cause of primary amenorrhea occurring in 1:4,000–1:5,000 females, has been reported in association with 46,XX gonadal dysgenesis in a 17-yr-old adolescent with primary amenorrhea and lack of breast development. One case of dysgerminoma with syncytiotrophoblastic giant cells was reported. Treatment consists of estrogen replacement therapy.

45,X/46,XY GONADAL DYSGENESIS

45,X/46,XY gonadal dysgenesis, also called *mixed gonadal dysgenesis*, has extreme phenotypic variability postnatally that may extend from a Turner-like syndrome to a male phenotype with a penile urethra; it is possible to delineate three major clinical phenotypes. Short stature is a major finding in all affected children. Ninety per cent of prenatally diagnosed cases have a normal male phenotype.

Some patients have no evidence of virilization; they have a female phenotype and often have the somatic signs of Turner syndrome. The condition is discovered prepubertally when chromosomal studies are made in short girls, or later when chromosomal studies are made because of failure of sexual maturation. Fallopian tubes and the uterus are present. The gonads consist of intra-abdominal undifferentiated streaks; chromosome study of the streak often reveals an XY cell line. The streak gonad differs somewhat from that in girls with Turner syndrome; in addition to wavy connective tissue, there are often tubular or cordlike structures, occasional clumps of granulosa cells, and, frequently, mesonephric or hilar cells.

Some children have mild virilization manifested only by prepubertal clitorimegaly. Normal müllerian structures are present, but at puberty virilization occurs. These patients usually have an intra-abdominal testis, a contralateral streak gonad, and bilateral fallopian tubes.

Most children present with frank ambiguity of the genitals in infancy. A testis and vas deferens are found on one side in the labioscrotal fold, and a streak gonad is identified on the contralateral side. Despite the presence of a testis, fallopian tubes are often present bilaterally. An infantile or rudimentary uterus is almost always present.

Other genotypes and phenotypes have been described. About 25% of 200 analyzed patients have a dicentric Y chromosome (45,X/46,X,dic Y). In some patients, the Y chromosome may be represented by only a fragment (45,X/45,X +fra); application of Y-specific probes can establish the origin of the fragment. It is not clear why the same genotype (45,X/46,XY) can result in such diverse phenotypes.

Children with a female phenotype present no problem in gender of rearing. Patients who are only slightly virilized are usually assigned a female gender of rearing before a diagnosis is established. Patients with ambiguity of the genitals are readily confused with various types of male pseudohermaphrodism. In most but not all instances, these children are best reared as females; the short stature, the ease of genital reconstruction, and the predisposition of the gonad to the development of malignancy favor this choice. In some patients followed to adulthood, the putative normal testis proves to be dysgenetic with eventual loss of Leydig and Sertoli cell function (see also Chapter 577). In an analysis of 22 Australian patients with mixed gonadal dysgenesis, no significant associations or correlations were found between internal and external phenotypes or endocrine function and gonadal morphologic features. The sex of rearing was determined by the appearance of the external genitals. In 11 patients, basal and human chorionic gonadotropin–stimulated testosterone levels were lower than in control subjects.

Gonadal tumors, usually gonadoblastomas, occur in about 25% of these children. A gonadoblastoma locus has been localized to a region near the centromere of the Y chromosome (GBY). These germ cell tumors are preceded by the changes of carcinoma in situ. Accordingly, both gonads should be removed in all patients reared as girls, and the undifferentiated gonad should be removed in the patients reared as boys.

There is no correlation between the proportion of 45,X/46,XY cell lives in either blood or fibroblasts and phenotype. In the past, all patients came to clinical attention because of their abnormal phenotypes. However, 45,X/46,XY mosaicism is found in about 7% of fetuses with true chromosome mosaicism encountered prenatally. Of 76 infants with 45,X/46,XY mosaicism diagnosed prenatally, 72 had a normal male phenotype, 1 had a female phenotype, and only 3 males had hypospadias. Of 12 males whose gonads were examined, only 3 were abnormal. These data must be taken into account when counseling a family in which a 45,X/46,XY infant is discovered prenatally.

XXX, XXXX, AND XXXXX FEMALES

XXX Females. Trisomy (autosome or sex chromosome) is the most common chromosomal abnormality in humans occurring in 4% of recognized pregnancies. The 47,XXX chromosomal constitution is the most frequent X chromosome abnormality in females, occurring in almost 1/1,000 liveborn females. In 68%, this condition is caused by maternal meiotic nondisjunction, but most 45,X and half of 47,XXY constitutions are caused by paternal sex chromosome errors. The phenotype is that of a normal female; affected infants and children are not recognized.

Sexual development and menarche are normal. Most pregnancies have resulted in normal infants. By 2 yr of age, delays in speech and language become evident and lack of coordination, poor academic performance, and immature behavior are seen. These girls tend to be tall and gangly, manifest behavior disorders, and are placed in special education classes. Using high-resolution MRI, 10 47,XXX subjects had lower amygdala volumes than 20 euploid controls; ten 47,XXY subjects had even lower amygdala volumes. There is marked variability within the syndrome, and a small proportion of affected girls are well coordinated, socially outgoing, and academically superior.

XXXX and XXXXX Females. The great majority of females with these rare karyotypes have been mentally retarded. Commonly associated defects are epicanthal folds, hypertelorism, clinodactyly, transverse palmar creases, radioulnar synostosis, and congenital heart disease. Sexual maturation is often incomplete and may not occur at all. Nevertheless, three women with the tetra-X syndrome gave birth, but no pregnancies were reported in 49,XXXXX women. Most 48,XXXX women tend to be tall, with an average height of 169 cm, whereas short stature is a common feature of the 49,XXXXX phenotype.

NOONAN SYNDROME

Girls with Noonan syndrome show certain anomalies that also occur in girls with 45,X Turner syndrome, but they have normal 46,XX chromosomes. The most common abnormalities are the same as those described for males with Noonan syndrome (see Chapter 577.1). The phenotype differs from Turner syndrome in several respects. Mental retardation is often present, the cardiac defect is most often pulmonary valvular stenosis or an atrial septal defect rather than an aortic defect, normal sexual maturation usually occurs but is delayed 2 yr on average, and premature ovarian failure has been reported.

OTHER OVARIAN DEFECTS

Some young women with no chromosomal abnormality are found to have streak gonads that may contain only occasional or no germ cells. Gonadotropins are increased. *Cytotoxic drugs*, especially alkylating agents such as cyclophosphamide and busulfan, procarbazine, etoposide, and exposure of the ovaries to radiation for the treatment of malignancy are increasingly frequent causes of ovarian failure. Young women with Hodgkin disease demonstrate that combination chemotherapy and pelvic irradiation may be more deleterious than either therapy alone. Teenagers are more likely than older women to retain or recover ovarian function after irradiation or combined chemotherapy; normal pregnancies have occurred after such treatment. Current treatment regimens may result in some ovarian damage in most

girls treated for cancer. The LD_{50} for the human oocyte has been estimated to be about 4 Gy; doses as low as 6 Gy have produced primary amenorrhea. Ovarian transposition before abdominal and pelvic irradiation in childhood can preserve ovarian function by decreasing the ovarian exposure to less then 4–7 Gy.

Autoimmune ovarian failure occurs in 60% of children older than 13 yr of age with *type I autoimmune polyendocrinopathy* (Addison disease, hypoparathyroidism, candidiasis). This condition, also known as polyglandular autoimmune disease (PGAD) type 1 is rare worldwide but not in Finland, where, as a result of a founder gene effect, it occurs in 1:25,000 people. The gene for this disorder is located on chromosome 21 and is associated with HLA-DR5. In patients with PGAD-1 and ovarian failure an association with HLA-A3 has been described. Affected girls may not develop sexually, or secondary amenorrhea may occur in young women. The ovaries may have lymphocytic infiltration or appear simply as streaks. Most affected patients have circulating steroid cell antibodies and autoantibodies to 21-hydroxylase.

The condition also occurs in young women as an isolated event or in association with other autoimmune disorders, leading to secondary amenorrhea *(premature ovarian failure [POF])*. It occurs in 0.2–0.9% of women younger than 40 years of age. Premature ovarian failure is a heterogeneous disorder with many causes: chromosomal, genetic, enzymatic, infectious, or iatrogenic. When associated with autoimmune adrenal disease, steroid cell autoantibodies are always present. These antibodies react with P450scc, 17α-OH, or 21-OH enzymes. When associated with an entire host of endocrine and nonendocrine autoimmune diseases and not adrenal autoimmunity, steroid cell autoantibodies are rarely found. A second autoimmune disorder, often subclinical, is found in 10–39% of adult patients with POF. One 17 yr old with idiopathic thrombocytopenic purpura and 47,XXX chromosomes had autoimmune POF.

Galactosemia, particularly the classic form of the disease, usually results in ovarian damage, beginning during intrauterine life. Levels of FSH and luteinizing hormone (LH) are elevated early in life. Ovarian damage may be due to deficient uridine diphosphate-galactose (see Chapter 76.2). The Denys-Drash syndrome, caused by a *WT1* mutation, can result in ovarian dysgenesis.

Ataxia-telangiectasia may be associated with ovarian hypoplasia and elevated gonadotropins; the cause is unknown. Gonadoblastomas and dysgerminomas have occurred in a few girls.

Hypergonadotrophic hypogonadism has been postulated to also occur because of the resistance of the ovary to both endogenous and exogenous gonadotropins (Savage syndrome). This condition occurs also in women with POF. Antiovarian antibodies or FSH receptor abnormalities may cause this condition. Mutation of the FSH receptor gene has been reported as an autosomal recessive condition (see under XX Gonadal Dysgenesis). A few females with 46,XX chromosomes presenting in primary amenorrhea with elevated gonadotropin levels were found to have inactivating mutations of the LH receptor gene. This suggests that LH action is needed for normal follicular development and ovulation.

580.2 Hypogonadotropic Hypogonadism in the Female (Secondary Hypogonadism)

Hypofunction of the ovaries can result from failure to secrete normal levels of gonadotropins. The defect may lie in the anterior pituitary or, more commonly, in the hypothalamus.

Etiology

HYPOPITUITARISM (also see Chapter 551). Congenital or acquired lesions in or near the pituitary almost always result in impaired secretion of gonadotropins and other pituitary hormones. In children with multiple pituitary hormone defects including gonadotropin deficiency, pituitary transcription factor defects such as in PROP-1 have been described. In children with idiopathic hypopituitarism, the defect is usually found in the hypothalamus. In these patients, administration of gonadotropin-releasing hormone (GnRH) results in increased plasma levels of FSH and LH, establishing the integrity of the pituitary gland.

ISOLATED DEFICIENCY OF GONADOTROPINS. This heterogeneous group of disorders is sorted out with the help of the GnRH test. In most children, the pituitary is normal, with the defect residing in the hypothalamus.

Several sporadic instances of anosmia with hypogonadotropic hypogonadism have been reported. Anosmic hypogonadal females have also been reported in kindreds with Kallmann syndrome, but hypogonadism more frequently affects the males in these families. Mutations in the gene for the β-subunit of FSH and LH have been reported.

Some autosomal recessive disorders such as the Laurence-Moon-Biedl, multiple lentigines, and Carpenter syndromes appear in some instances to include gonadotropic hormone deficiency. Girls with Prader-Willi syndrome may have hypogonadotropic hypogonadism. Girls with severe thalassemia may have gonadotropin deficiency from pituitary damage caused by chronic iron overload secondary to multiple transfusions. Anorexia nervosa frequently results in hypogonadotropic hypogonadism (see Chapter 104).

Diagnosis. The diagnosis may be apparent in patients with other deficiencies of pituitary tropic hormones, but, as in males, it is difficult to differentiate isolated hypogonadotropic hypogonadism from physiologic delay of puberty. Repeated measurements of FSH and LH, particularly during sleep, may reveal the rising levels that herald the onset of puberty. Stimulation testing with GnRH or one of its analogues may help establish the diagnosis.

POLYCYSTIC OVARIES (STEIN-LEVENTHAL SYNDROME)

The classic polycystic ovaries syndrome (PCOS) is characterized by obesity, hirsutism, and secondary amenorrhea, with bilaterally enlarged polycystic ovaries, but these manifestations may not all be present (also see Chapter 544). Onset usually occurs at puberty or shortly thereafter; menstrual irregularities and hirsutism are the most frequent complaints. In the reproductive years, the condition is the most common cause of anovulatory infertility. Several terms have gained acceptance in describing these patients: *functional ovarian hyperandrogenism* and, especially in adults, *chronic hyperandrogenic anovulation.* There seems to be a strong relationship between premature adrenarche and the subsequent development of PCOS. The enlarged ovaries can often be felt on combined rectal and abdominal palpation and are always demonstrable by ultrasonography (see Chapter 544).

The cause of the disorder in most patients is unsettled despite intensive investigation. PCOS is a heterogeneous condition that may be associated with several distinct entities, such as 21-hydroxylase deficiency, deficiency of 3-hydroxysteroid dehydrogenase, and deficiency of ovarian 17-ketoreductase, the enzyme that converts androstenedione to testosterone and estrone to estradiol. Conversion of cholesterol to pregnenolone by the cholesterol side-chain cleavage enzyme P450scc, encoded by the gene *CYP11A*, occurs after cholesterol enters the mitochondria aided by the steroidogenic acute regulatory protein (StAR). DAX-1 can repress StAR gene expression, and SF-1 regulates SF-1. *CYP11A* or DAX-1 were found in hyperandrogenic hirsute women with and without menstrual disturbances. In most patients with PCOS, the elevated plasma level of free testosterone or androstenedione is not suppressed by dexamethasone, ruling out an adrenal cause of the disorder. In some

patients, serum levels of total testosterone may not be elevated but serum levels of free testosterone are, and sex hormone-binding globulins are markedly diminished. About 75% of patients have an increased ratio of LH to FSH levels, an increased amplitude and frequency of plasma LH levels, and an exaggerated response to GnRH. Inhibin B levels are high at baseline and lack normal pulsatile changes. Premenarcheal girls may have an early morning rise in LH rather than the characteristic nocturnal one. The perturbances of LH secretion are believed to bring about hyperplasia of theca cells, arrested follicular development, and impaired estradiol production. Aberrant follicular development, one of the hallmarks of PCOS, may be related to dysregulation of oocyte growth differentiation factor-9 (GDF-9) but not bone morphogenic factor-15 (BMP-15), both known oocyte growth factors. These effects lead to hyperandrogenemia and irregular cycles or amenorrhea. In children having congenital virilizing syndromes, the hypothalamic-pituitary axis appears to be programmed for hypersecretion of LH at puberty, leading to hyperandrogenism even when adrenal androgens are thought to be adequately suppressed. Several common polymorphisms in the interlukin-6 gene promoter are associated with hyperandrogenism.

There is an association between hyperandrogenism and insulin resistance. Especially in obese patients, PCOS may be associated with hyperinsulinism, insulin resistance, and acanthosis nigricans. Because of the high prevalence of PCOS, it needs to be counted among the most common conditions associated with glucose intolerance and type II diabetes. Adolescents with PCOS tend to have a higher incidence (7/27 in one study) of impaired glucose tolerance. The insulin resistance seems to be related to excessive serine phosphorylation of the insulin receptor. The same process, serine phosphorylation, is important in regulating the activity of P450c17, a major enzyme involved in androgen biosynthesis. Therefore, some have postulated this defect as the single abnormality that may be responsible for both the insulin resistance and hyperandrogenism seen in PCOS. Variations in the gene encoding the cysteine protease calpain-10 may be associated with increased susceptibility to type 2 diabetes. The 112/121 haplotype is associated with both insulin levels and a 2-fold risk of PCOS in white and African American women.

For *diagnosis* of PCOS, measurements of serum LH, FSH, prolactin, free testosterone, and sex hormone–binding globulin as well as dehydroepiandrosterone sulfate (DHEAS) are helpful. Brothers of women with PCOS have elevated DHEAS levels, whereas in sisters of women with PCOS markers of insulin resistance (elevated fasting insulin levels and decreased fasting glucose/insulin ratios) are associated with hyperandrogenemia but not menstrual irregularities. Measures of insulin resistance however, may have significant intraindividual variations in women with PCOS. Complex stimulation and inhibitory pharmacologic manipulation have been used to distinguish between adrenal and ovarian causes of hyperandrogenism. Basal and adrenocorticotropic hormone stimulated adrenal steroid levels may reveal subtle adrenal steroidogenic defects.

A deficiency of 17-ketoreductase is suggested when there are affected brothers or when the estrone:estradiol and androstenedione:testosterone ratios are increased. Women treated with valproate for epilepsy before 20 yr of age often have PCOS and elevated serum testosterone levels, but their levels of LH are normal.

The optimal method of *treatment* is still evolving. The mainstay of therapy is ovarian suppression with oral contraceptives containing nonandrogenic progestins such as desogestrel (Desogen). Spironolactone, in addition to oral contraceptives, has been the main pharmacologic agent available in the United States to diminish hirsutism. Further suppression can be achieved with testolactone, a compound with antiandrogen and weak progestin properties. Electrolysis and laser therapy are the main nonpharmacologic treatment modalities for hirsutism. Attention to the obesity is important because its correction often leads to correction of the insulin resistance. Oral agents to treat type II diabetes are beginning to be used to improve insulin resistance in patients with PCOS. Insulin-sensitizing agents such as metformin and troglitazone decrease hyperinsulinemia and ovarian hyperandrogenism in women. Three months of metformin treatment improves insulin resistance and the exaggerated adrenal androgen responses to ACTH. D-*Chiro*-inositol treatment of women with PCOS improves insulin action, thus enhancing ovarian function while decreasing serum androgen levels. This approach stimulates postreceptor insulin action. Naltrexone, an opioid antagonist, decreases insulin secretion in hyperinsulinemic patients with PCOS.

Aittomaki K, Lucena JLD, Pakarinen P, et al: Mutation in the follicle-stimulating hormone receptor gene causes hereditary hypergonadotropic ovarian failure. *Cell* 1995;82:959.

Arslanian SA, Lewy V, Danadian K, et al: Metformin therapy in obese adolescents with polycystic ovary syndrome and impaired glucose tolerance: Amelioration of exaggerated adrenal response to adrenocorticotropin with reduction of insulinemia/insulin resistance. *J Clin Endocrinol Metab* 2002;87:1555–59.

Berdahl LD, Wenstrom KD, Hanson JW: Web neck anomaly and its association with congenital heart disease. *Am J Med Genet* 1995;56:304.

Betterle C, Volpato M: Adrenal and ovarian autoimmunity. *Eur J Endocrinol* 1998;138:16–25.

Binder G, Kock A, Wajs E, et al: Nested polymerase chain reaction study of 53 cases with Turner syndrome: Is cytogenetically undetected Y mosaicism common? *J Clin Endocrinol Metab* 1995;80:3532.

Calvo RM, Asuncion M, Telleria D, et al: Screening for mutations in the steroidogenic acute regulatory protein and steroidogenic factor-1 genes, and in *CYP11A* and dosage-sensitive sex reversal-adrenal hypoplasia gene on the X chromosome, gene-1 *(DAX-1)*, in hyperandrogenic hirsute women. *J Clin Endocrinol Metab* 2001;86:1746–49.

Carel JC, Mathivon L, Gendrel C, et al: Near normalization of final height with adapted doses of growth hormone in Turner syndrome. *J Clin Endocrinol Metab* 83:1462, 1998.

Chang HJ, Clark RD, Bachman H: The phenotype of 45,X/46,XY mosaicism: An analysis of 92 prenatally diagnosed cases. *Am J Hum Genet* 1990;46:156.

De la Chesnayae E, Canto P, Ulloa-Aguirre A, et al: No evidence of mutations in the follicle-stimulating hormone receptor gene in Mexican women with 46,XX pure gonadal dysgenesis. *Am J Med Genet* 2001;98:125–28.

Doherty E, Pakarinen P, Tiitinen A, et al: A novel mutation in the FSH receptor inhibiting signal transduction and causing primary ovarian failure. *J Clin Endocrinol Metab* 2002;87:1151–55.

Dunaif A: Insulin resistance and the polycystic ovary syndrome: Mechanism and implications for pathogenesis. *Endocr Rev* 1997;18:774.

Ehrmann DA, Schwarz PEH, Hara M, et al: Relationship of calpain-10 genotype to phenotype features of polycystic ovary syndrome. *J Clin Endocrinol Metab* 2002;87:1669–73.

Gicquel C, Gaston V, Cabrol S, et al: Assessment of Turner syndrome by molecular analysis of the X chromosome in growth-retarded girls. *J Clin Endocrinol Metab* 1998;83:1472.

Gorgojo JJ, Almodovar F, Lopez E, et al: Gonadal agenesis 46, associated with the atypical form of Rokitansky syndrome. *Fertil Steril* 2002;77:185–87.

Gravholt CH, Juul S, Naeraa RW, et al: Prenatal and postnatal prevalence of Turner syndrome: A registry study. *BMJ* 1996;312:16.

Gravholt CH, Fedder J, Naeraa RW, et al: Occurrence of gonadoblastoma in females with Turner syndrome and Y chromosome material: A population study. *J Clin Endocrinol Metab* 2000;85:3199–3202.

Gravholt CH, Naeraa RW, Nyhold B, et al: Glucose metabolism, lipid metabolism and cardiovascular risk factors in adult Turner syndrome. *Diabetes Care* 1998;21:1062.

Guido M, Pavone V, Ciampelli M, et al: Involvement of ovarian steroids in the opioid-mediated reduction of insulin secretion in hyperinsulinemic patients with polycystic ovary syndrome. *J Clin Endocrinol Metab* 1998;83:1742.

Hochberg Z, Aviram M, Rubin D, et al: Decreased sensitivity to insulin-like growth factor I in Turner syndrome: A study of monocytes and T lymphocytes. *Eur J Clin Invest* 1997;27:543.

Hoek A, Schoemaker J, Dreshage HA: Premature ovarian failure and ovarian autoimmunity. *Endocr Rev* 1997;18:107.

Holland CM: 47,XXX in an adolescent with premature ovarian failure and autoimmune disease. *J Pediatr Adolesc Gynecol* 2001;14:77–80.

Iezzoni JC, Kap-Herr CV, Golden W, et al: Gonadoblastomas in 45,X/46,XY mosaicism. *Am J Clin Pathol* 1997;108:197–203.

Jayagopal V, Kilpatrick ES, Holding S, et al: The biological variation of insulin resistance in polycystic ovarian syndrome. *J Clin Endocrinol Metab* 2002;87:1560–62.

Legro RS, Kunselman AR, Demers L, et al: Elevated dehydroepiandrosterone sulfate levels as the reproductive phenotype in the brothers of women with polycystic ovary syndrome. *J Clin Endocrinol Metab* 2002;87:2134–38.

Lin AE, Lippe B, Rosenfeld RD: Further delineation of aortic dilation, dissection, and rupture in patients with Turner syndrome. *Pediatrics* 1998;102:e12.

Linssen WHJP, Bent MJV, Brunner HG, et al: Deafness, sensory neuropathy, and ovarian dysgenesis: A new syndrome or a broader spectrum of Perrault syndrome. *Am J Med Genet* 1994;51:81.

Lopes F, Filho T, Baracat EC, et al: Aberrant expression of growth differentiation factor-9 in oocytes of women with polycystic ovary syndrome. *J Clin Endocrinol Metab* 2002;87:1337–44.

Matthews CH, Borgato S, Beck-Peccoz P, et al: Primary amenorrhea and infertility due to a mutation in the β-subunit of follicle-stimulating hormone. *Nat Genet* 1993;5:83.

Mazzanti L, Cacciari E, Bergamaschi R, et al: Pelvic ultrasonography in patients with Turner syndrome: Age-related findings in different karyotypes. *J Pediatr* 1997;131:135.

Melner MH, Feltus FA: Autoimmune premature ovarian failure—endocrine aspects of a T-cell disease: Review. *Endocrinology* 1999;140:3401–3.

Merke DP, Tajima T, Baron J, et al: Hypogonadotropic hypogonadism in a female caused by an X-linked recessive mutation in the *Dax1* gene. *N Engl J Med* 1999;340:1248–52.

Migeon BR, Luo S, Jani M, et al: The severe phenotype of females with tiny ring X chromosomes are associated with inability of these chromosomes to undergo X inactivation. *Am J Med Genet* 1994;55:497.

Muller J, Shakkeback NE, Ritzen M, et al: Carcinoma in situ of the testis in children with 45,X/46,XY gonadal dysgenesis. *J Pediatr* 1985;106:431.

Nester J, Jakubowicz D, Reamer P, et al: Ovulatory and metabolic effects of D-*chiro*-inositol in polycystic ovary syndrome. *N Engl J Med* 1999;340:1314.

Palmert MR, Gordon CM, Kartashov AI, et al: Screening for abnormal glucose tolerance in adolescent with polycystic ovary syndrome. *J Clin Endocrinol Metab* 2002;87:1017–23.

Pasquino AM, Passeri F, Pucarelli I, et al: Spontaneous pubertal development in Turner syndrome. *J Clin Endocrinol Metab* 1997;82:1810.

Patwardham AJ, Brown WE, Bender BG, et al: Reduced size of the amygdala in individuals with 47,XXY and 47,XXX karyotypes. *Am J Med Genet* 2002;114:93–98.

Quigley CA, Crowe BJ, Anglin DG, et al: Growth hormone and low dose estrogen in Turner syndrome: Results of a United States multi-center trial to near-final height. *J Clin Endocrinol Metab* 2002;87:2033–41.

Rongen-Westerlaken C, Corel K, van den Broeck J, et al: Reference values for height, height velocity and weight in Turner syndrome. *Acta Paediatr* 1997;86:937.

Rosenfeld RL, Pesovic N, Deveine N, et al: Optimizing estrogen replacement treatment on Turner syndrome. *Pediatrics* 1998;102:486.

Ross JL, Roeltgen D, Feuillan P, et al: Use of estrogen in young girls with Turner syndrome. *Neurology* 2000;54:164–70.

Schorry EK, Lovell AM, Milatovich A, et al: Ullrich-Turner syndrome and neurofibromatosis-1. *Am J Med Genet* 1996;66:423.

Seashore MR, Cho S, Desposito F, et al: Health supervision for children with Turner syndrome. *Pediatrics* 1995;96:1166.

Sempe M, Hansson Bodallaz C, Limoni C: Growth curves in untreated Ullrich-Turner syndrome: French reference standards 1–22 years. *Eur J Pediatr* 1996;155:862.

Skuse DH, James RS, Bishop DVM, et al: Evidence from Turner syndrome of an imprinted X-linked locus affecting cognitive function. *Nature* 1997;387:705.

Sills I, Rapaport R, Skuza K, et al: 46,XX pure gonadal dysgenesis with growth hormone deficiency and impaired 3β-hydroxysteroid dehydrogenase activity. *Am J Med Genet* 1992;42:100.

Sybert VP: Cardiovascular malformations and complications in Turner syndrome. *Pediatrics* 1998;101:E11.

Tanaka Y, Sasaki Y, Nishihira H, et al: Ovarian juvenile granulosa cell tumor associated with Maffucci's syndrome. *Am J Clin Pathol* 1992;97:523.

Telvi L, Lebar A, DelPino O, et al: 45,X/46,XY mosaicism: Report of 27 cases. *Pediatrics* 1999;104:304–8.

Thibaud E, Ramirez M, Brauner R, et al: Preservation of ovarian function by ovarian transposition performed before pelvic irradiation during childhood. *J Pediatr* 1992;121:880.

Villuendas G, San Millan JL, Sancho J, et al: The -597 G→A and -174 G→C polymorphisms in the promoter of the IL-6 gene are associated with hyperandrogenism. *J Clin Endocrinol Metab* 2002;87:1134–41.

Zinn AR, Page DC, Fisher EMC: Turner syndrome: The case of the missing X chromosome. *Trends Genet* 1993;9:90.

Chapter 581

Pseudoprecocity Due to Lesions of the Ovary

Ovarian tumors are rare in pediatrics, thought to occur at a rate of 2.6/100,000. Ovarian malignancies, the most common genital neoplasms in adolescence, account for 1% of childhood cancers. More then 60% are germ cell tumors, most of which are dysgerminomas that can secrete tumor markers and hormones (see Chapter 495). Next most common are epithelial cell tumors (~20%), and nearly 10% are sex cord/stromal tumors (granulosa, Sertoli cell, and mesenchymal tumors). Multiple tumor markers can be seen in ovarian tumors, including α-fetoprotein, human chorionic gonadotropin (hCG), carcinoembryonic antigen, oncoproteins, p105, p53, *KRAS* mutations, cyclin D1, epidermal growth factor–related proteins and receptors, cathepsin B, and others. Various levels of inhibin-activin subunit gene expression were detected in ovarian tumors.

Functioning lesions of the ovary consist of benign cysts or malignant tumors. The majority synthesize estrogens; a few synthesize androgens.

Estrogenic Lesions of the Ovary. These lesions cause isosexual precocious sexual development but account for only a small percentage of all cases of precocity. Benign ovarian follicular cysts are the most common tumors associated with isosexual precocious puberty in girls; they may rarely be gonadotropin dependent.

JUVENILE GRANULOSA CELL TUMOR. In childhood, the most common neoplasm of the ovary with estrogenic manifestations is the granulosa cell tumor, although it composes 1–10% of all ovarian tumors. These tumors have distinctive histologic features that differ from those encountered in older women (adult granulosa cell tumor). The cells have high mitotic activity, follicles are often irregular, Call-Exner bodies are rare, and luteinization is frequent. The tumor may be solid or cystic, or both. They are usually benign. In a few instances, this tumor has been associated with multiple enchondromas *(Ollier disease)* and, in fewer still, with multiple subcutaneous hemangiomas *(Maffucci syndrome)*.

CLINICAL MANIFESTATIONS AND DIAGNOSIS. The tumor has been observed in newborns and may manifest with sexual precocity at 2 yr of age or younger; about half of these tumors have occurred before 10 yr of age. The mean age at diagnosis is 7.5 yr. The tumors are almost always unilateral. The breasts become enlarged, rounded, and firm and the nipples prominent. The external genitals resemble those of a normal girl at puberty, and the uterus is enlarged. A white vaginal discharge is followed by irregular or cyclic menstruation. Ovulation, however, does not occur. The presenting manifestation may be abdominal pain or swelling. Pubic hair is usually absent unless there is mild virilization.

A mass is readily palpable in the lower portion of the abdomen in most children by the time sexual precocity is evident. The tumor may be small, however, and escape detection even on careful rectal and abdominal examination; the tumors may be detected by ultrasonography, but multidetector CT scans are most sensitive. Most such tumors (90%) are diagnosed at very early stages of malignancy (FIGO, International Federation of Gynecology and Obstetrics, stage I).

Plasma estradiol levels are markedly elevated. Plasma levels of gonadotropins are suppressed and do not respond to gonadotropin-releasing hormone stimulation. Levels of müllerian-inhibiting substance (anti-müllerian hormone), inhibin, and α-fetoprotein may be elevated. Osseous development is moderately advanced.

TREATMENT AND PROGNOSIS. The tumor should be removed as soon as the diagnosis is established. Prognosis is excellent because fewer than 5% of these tumors in children are malignant. Advanced stage tumors, however, behave very aggressively and require difficult decisions regarding surgical approaches as well the use of radiation and chemotherapy. In adults with granulosa cell tumors, *p53* expression is associated with unfavorable prognosis. Vaginal bleeding immediately after removal of the tumor is common. Signs of precocious puberty abate and may disappear within a few months after the operation. The secretion of estrogens returns to normal.

Sex cord tumor with annular tubules is a distinctive tumor, thought to arise from granulosa cells, that occurs primarily in patients with Peutz-Jeghers syndrome. These tumors are multifocal, bilateral, and usually benign. The presence of calcifications aids ultrasonographic detection. Increased aromatase production by these tumors results in gonadotropin-independent precocious puberty. Inhibin A and B levels are elevated and decrease after tumor removal. In one study, 9 of 13 sex cord/stromal tumors exhibited follicle-stimulating hormone receptor mutations, suggesting a role for such mutation in the development of these tumors.

Chorioepithelioma has been reported only rarely. This very malignant tumor is thought to arise from a pre-existing teratoma. The usually unilateral tumor produces large amounts of hCG, which stimulates the contralateral ovary to secrete estrogens and progesterone. Elevated levels of hCG are diagnostic.

FOLLICULAR CYST. Small ovarian cysts (<0.7 cm in diameter) are common in prepubertal children. At puberty and in girls with true isosexual precocious puberty, larger cysts (1–6 cm) are often seen; these are secondary to stimulation by gonadotropins. However, similar larger cysts occur occasionally in young girls with precocious puberty in the absence of luteinizing hormone and follicle-stimulating hormone. Because surgical removal or spontaneous involution of these cysts results in regression of pubertal changes, there is little doubt that they are its cause. The mechanism of production of these autonomously functioning cysts is unknown. Such cysts may form only once, or they may disappear and recur, resulting in waxing and waning of the signs of precocious puberty. They may be unilateral or bilateral. The sexual precocity that occurs in young girls with McCune-Albright syndrome is usually associated with autonomous follicular cysts caused by a somatic-activating mutation of the G protein occurring early in development (see Chapter 556.6). Gonadotropins are suppressed, and estradiol levels are often markedly elevated, but they may fluctuate widely and even return to normal. Gonadotropin-releasing hormone stimulation fails to evoke an increase in gonadotropins. Because gonadotropins are suppressed in these children, the mechanism of ovarian stimulation is unknown. Ultrasonography is the method of choice for the detection and monitoring of such cysts. A short period of observation to ascertain a lack of spontaneous resolution is advisable before cyst aspiration or cystectomy is considered. Cystic neoplasms must be considered in the differential diagnosis.

Androgenic Lesions of the Ovary. Virilizing ovarian tumors are rare at all ages but particularly so in prepubertal girls. The *arrhenoblastoma* has been reported as early as 14 days of age, but few cases have been reported in girls younger than 16 yr of age.

The *gonadoblastoma* occurs exclusively in dysgenetic gonads, particularly in phenotypic females who have a Y chromosome in their genotype (46,XY; 45,X/46,XY; 45,X/46,X fra). The tumor may be bilateral. Virilization occurs with some but not all tumors. The clinical features are the same as those seen in patients with virilizing adrenal tumors and include accelerated growth, acne, clitoral enlargement, and growth of sexual hair. A palpable, abdominal mass is found in only about 50% of patients. Plasma levels of testosterone and androstenedione are elevated, and those of gonadotropins are suppressed. Ultrasonography, CT, and MRI usually localize the lesion. The dysgenetic gonad of phenotypic females with a Y chromosome should be removed prophylactically. When a unilateral tumor is removed, the contralateral dysgenetic gonad should also be removed. In an immunohistochemical study of two gonadoblastomas, expression of *WT1*, *p53*, and *MIS* as well as inhibin were all demonstrated.

Virilizing manifestations occur occasionally in girls with *juvenile granulosa cell tumors*. Adrenal rests and hilus cell tumors rarely lead to virilization. Activating mutations of G protein genes have been described in ovarian (and testicular) tumors. *GSP* mutations, usually seen in gonadal tumors associated with

McCune-Albright syndrome, were also noted in four of six Leydig cell tumors (three ovarian, one testicular). Two granulosa cell tumors and one thecoma of 10 ovarian tumors studied were found to have *GIP-2* mutations.

Sertoli-Leydig cell tumors, rare sex cord/stromal neoplasms, comprise less than 1% of ovarian tumors. In one 12 mo old with Sertoli-Leydig cell tumor presenting with isosexual precocity the only detectable tumor marker was the serum inhibin level, with elevations in both A and B subunits. Of 102 consecutive patients who underwent surgery because of ovarian masses over a 15-yr period the presenting symptoms were acute abnormal peak in 56% and abdominal or pelvic mass in 22%. Of 9 children whose cause for surgery was presumed malignancy, 3 had dysgerminomas, 2 had teratomas, 2 had juvenile granulose cell tumors, 1 had a Sertoli-Leydig cell tumor, and 1 had a yolk sac tumor.

Calaminus G, Wessalowski R, Harms D, et al: Juvenile granulosa cell tumors of the ovary in children and adolescents: Results from 33 patients registered in a prospective cooperative study. *Gynecol Oncol* 1997;65:447.

Cass DL, Hawkins E, Brandt ML, et al: Surgery for ovarian masses in infants, children, and adolescents: 102 consecutive patients treated in a 15-year period. *J Pediatr Surg* 2001;36:693–99.

Choong CS, Fuller PJ, Chu S, et al: Sertoli-Leydig cell tumor of the ovary, a rare cause of precocious puberty in a 12 month-old infant. *J Clin Endocrinol Metab* 2002;87:49–56.

Fink D, Kubik-Huch RA, Wildetmuth S: Juvenile granulose cell tumor. *Abdom Imaging* 2001;26:550–52.

Fotiou SK: Ovarian malignancies in adolescence. *Ann NY Acad Sci* 1997;816:338.

Fuller PJ, Zumpe ET, Chu S, et al: Inhibin-activ receptor subunit gene expression in ovarian tumors. *J Clin Endocrinol Metab* 2002;87:1395–1401.

Hussong J, Crussi FG, Chou PM: Gonadoblastoma: Immunohistochemical localization of müllerian-inhibiting substance, inhibin, WT-1, and p53. *Mod Pathol* 1997; 10:1101.

Kotlar TJ, Young RH, Albanese C, et al: A mutation in the follicle-stimulating hormone receptor occurs frequently in human ovarian sex cord tumors. *J Clin Endocrinol Metab* 1997;82:1020.

Lazar EL, Stolar CJ: Evaluation and management of pediatric solid ovarian tumors. *Semin Pediatr Surg* 1998;7:29.

Powell JL, Connor GP, Henderson GS: Management of recurrent juvenile granulose cell tumor of the ovary. *Gynecol Oncol* 2001;81:113–16.

Silverman LA, Gitelman SE: Immunoreactive inhibin, müllerian inhibitory substance, and activin as biochemical markers for juvenile granulosa cell tumors. *J Pediatr* 1996;129:918.

Zalel Y, Piura B, Elchalal U, et al: Diagnosis and management of malignant germ cell ovarian tumors in young females. *Int J Gynecol Obstet* 1996;55:1.

Chapter 582
Intersex

Intersex, formerly known as hermaphroditism, implies a discrepancy between the morphology of the gonads and that of the external genitals. Many chromosomal aberrations resulting in ambiguity of the external genitals are discussed earlier in this section. In this chapter, conditions of aberrant sexual differentiation that are imposed on the XX or XY genotype—46,XX intersex and 46,XY intersex—are discussed (Box 582–1). An increasing number of such conditions are understood through advances in the knowledge about molecular biology of normal sexual differentiation. The category of true gonadal intersex, previously known as true hermaphroditism, with few exceptions, is still a poorly understood heterogeneous group of disorders.

Sexual Differentiation (see also Chapter 576). In normal differentiation, the final form of all sexual structures is consistent with normal sex chromosomes (either XX or XY). A 46,XX complement of chromosomes as well as genetic factors such as DAX-1 and the signaling molecule WNT-4 are necessary for the development of normal ovaries. Development of the male phenotype is even more complex. It requires a Y chromosome and, specifi-

cally, an intact *SRY* gene, which, in association with other genes such as *SOX9, SF1,* and *WT1,* and more (see Chapter 576), directs the undifferentiated gonad to become a testis. Aberrant recombinations may result in X chromosomes carrying *SRY,* resulting in XX males, or Y chromosomes that have lost *SRY,* resulting in XY females.

Anti-müllerian hormone (AMH) also known as müllerian-inhibiting substance, the first testicular hormone produced at 6–7 wk of gestation, causes the müllerian ducts to regress; in its absence, they persist. AMH activation in the testes may require the *SF1* gene for activation. By about 8 wk of gestation, the Leydig cells of the testis begin to produce testosterone. During this critical period of male differentiation, testosterone secretion is stimulated by placental human chorionic gonadotropin (hCG), which peaks at 8–12 wk. In the latter half of pregnancy, lower levels of testosterone are maintained by luteinizing hormone secreted by the fetal pituitary. Testosterone initiates virilization of the wolffian duct into the epididymis, vas deferens, and seminal vesicle. Development of the external genitals also requires dihydrotestosterone (DHT), an active metabolite of testosterone. DHT is necessary to fuse the genital folds to form

---

BOX 582–1. Etiologic Classification of Intersex Conditions

46,XX -INTERSEX (46,XX —VIRILIZED)
Androgen Exposure
Fetal Source
21-Hydroxylase (P450 c21) deficiency
11β-Hydroxylase (P450 c11) deficiency
3β-Hydroxysteroid dehydrogenase II (3β-HSD II) deficiency
Aromatase (P450$_{arom}$) deficiency
Glucocorticoid receptor gene mutation
Maternal Source
Virilizing ovarian tumor
Virilizing adrenal tumor
Androgenic drugs
Undetermined Origin
Associated with genitourinary and gastrointestinal tract defects

46,XY-INTERSEX (46,XY — UNDERVIRILIZED)
Defects in Testicular Differentiation
Denys-Drash syndrome (mutation in *WT1* gene)
WAGR syndrome (*W*ilms tumor, *a*niridia, *g*enitourinary malformation, *r*etardation)
Deletion of 11p13
Camptomelic syndrome (autosomal gene at 17q24.3–q25.1) and *SOX9* mutation
XY pure gonadal dysgenesis (Swyer syndrome)
Mutation in *SRY* gene
Unknown cause
XY gonadal agenesis

Deficiency of Testicular Hormones
Leydig cell aplasia
Mutation in LH receptor
Lipoid adrenal hyperplasia (P450 scc) deficiency; mutation in StAR (steroidogenic acute regulatory protein)
3β-HSDII deficiency
17-Hydroxylase/17,20-lyase (P450 c17) deficiency
Persistent müllerian duct syndrome
Gene mutations, anti-müllerian hormone
Receptor defects for anti-müllerian hormone

Defect in Androgen Action
5α-Reductase II mutations
Androgen receptor defects
Complete androgen insensitivity syndrome
Partial androgen insensitivity syndrome (Reifenstein and other syndromes)
Smith-Lemli-Opitz syndrome
Defect in conversion of 7-dehydrocholesterol to cholesterol

TRUE GONADAL INTERSEX
XX
XY
XX/XY chimeras

the penis and scrotum. A functional androgen receptor, controlled by an X-linked gene, is required for testosterone and DHT to produce these virilizing changes.

In the XX fetus with normal long and short arms of the X chromosome, the bipotential gonad develops into an ovary by about the 10th–11th wk. This occurs only in the absence of *SRY*, testosterone, and AMH and requires a normal gene in the *DSS* locus DAX-1, and the WNT-4 molecule. The female phenotype develops independently of the fetal gonads, but maleness is imposed on a basically female potential by the hormones of the fetal testis. Estrogen is unnecessary for normal prenatal sexual differentiation, as demonstrated by 46,XX patients with aromatase deficiency and by mice without estradiol receptors.

582.1 46,XX Intersex (46,XX with Virilization)

In this condition, formerly referred to as female pseudohermaphroditism, the genotype is XX and the gonads are ovaries, but the external genitals are virilized. Because there is no AMH (the gonads are ovaries not testes), the uterus, tubes, and ovaries develop. The varieties and causes of this condition are relatively few. Most instances result from exposure of the female fetus to excessive exogenous or endogenous androgens during intrauterine life. The changes consist principally of virilization of the external genitals (clitoral hypertrophy and labioscrotal fusion).

Congenital Adrenal Hyperplasia (see Chapter 570.1). This is the most common cause of genital ambiguity and 46,XX intersex. Females with the 21-hydroxylase and 11-hydroxylase defects are the most highly virilized, although minimal virilization also occurs with the type II 3β-hydroxysteroid dehydrogenase defect. Salt losers tend to have greater degrees of virilization than do non–salt-losing patients. Masculinization may be so intense that a complete penile urethra results, and the condition may mimic a male with cryptorchidism (see Chapter 570.1).

Aromatase Deficiency. In genotypic females, aromatase deficiency during fetal life leads to 46,XX intersex and results in hypergonadotropic hypogonadism at puberty because of ovarian failure to synthesize estrogen (see Section 4 and Fig. 568–1).

Two 46,XX infants had enlargement of the clitoris and posterior labial fusion at birth. In one instance, maternal serum and urinary levels of estrogen were very low and serum levels of androgens were high. Cord serum levels of estrogen were also extremely low, but those of androgen were elevated. The second patient also had virilization of unknown cause since birth, but the aromatase deficiency was not diagnosed until 14 yr of age, when she had further virilization and failed to go into puberty. At that time, she had elevated levels of gonadotropins and androgens but low estrogen levels, and ultrasonography revealed large ovarian cysts bilaterally. These two patients demonstrate the important role of aromatase in the conversion of androgens to estrogens. Additional female and male patients with aromatase deficiency due to mutations in the P450$_{arom}$ *(CYP19)* gene are known. Two siblings were described. The 28-yr-old XY proband was 177.6 cm tall (+2.5 SD) after having received hormonal replacement therapy; her 24-yr-old brother was 204 cm tall (+3.7 SD), and had a bone age of 14 yr. Low-dose estradiol replacement, carefully adjusted to maintain normal age-appropriate levels, may be indicated for affected females even prepubertally.

Glucocorticoid Receptor Gene Mutation. A 9-yr-old girl with 46,XX intersex, thought to be due to 21-OHase deficiency (congenital adrenal hyperplasia) since the age of 5 yr, had elevated cortisol levels at baseline and after dexamethasone, hypertension, and hypokalemia suggestive of the diagnosis of generalized glucocorticoid resistance. A novel homozygous mutation in exon 5 of the glucocorticoid receptor was demonstrated. In this Brazilian family the condition was autosomal recessive.

Virilizing Maternal Tumors. Rarely, the female fetus has been virilized during fetal life by a maternal androgen-producing tumor. In a few cases, the lesion was a benign adrenal adenoma, but all others were ovarian tumors, particularly androblastomas, luteomas, and Krukenberg tumors. Maternal virilization may be manifested by enlargement of the clitoris, acne, deepening of the voice, decreased lactation, hirsutism, and elevated levels of androgens. In the infant, there is enlargement of the clitoris of varying degrees, often with labial fusion. Mothers of children with unexplained 46,XX intersex should undergo measurements of their own levels of plasma testosterone, dehydroepiandrosterone sulfate, and androstenedione.

Administration of Androgenic Drugs to Women During Pregnancy. Testosterone and 17-methyltestosterone have been reported to cause 46,XX intersex in some instances. The greatest number of cases has resulted from the use of certain progestational compounds for the treatment of threatened abortion. These progestins have been replaced by nonvirilizing ones.

Infants with virilization and 46,XX chromosomes and caudal anomalies have been reported for whom no virilizing agent could be identified. In such instances, the disorder is usually associated with other congenital defects, particularly of the urinary and gastrointestinal tracts. Y-specific DNA sequences, including SRY, are absent. In one case, a scrotal raphe and elevated testosterone levels were found, but the cause remains unknown.

582.2 46,XY Intersex (46,XY with Undervirilization)

In this condition, formerly referred to as male pseudohermaphroditism, the genotype is XY, but the external genitals are incompletely virilized, ambiguous, or completely female. When gonads can be found, they are invariably testes; their development may range from rudimentary to normal. Because the process of normal virilization in the fetus is so complex, it is not surprising that there are many varieties of undervirilized 46,XY individuals.

DEFECTS IN TESTICULAR DIFFERENTIATION

The first step in male differentiation is conversion of the indifferent gonad to a testis. In the XY fetus, if there is a deletion of the *short arm of the Y chromosome* or of the *SRY* gene, male differentiation does not occur. The phenotype is female; müllerian ducts are well developed because of the absence of AMH, but gonads consist of undifferentiated streaks. By contrast, even extreme deletions of the *long arm of the Y chromosome* (Yq-) have been found in normally developed males, most of whom are azoospermic and have short stature, indicating that the long arm of the Y chromosome normally has genes that prevent these manifestations. In other syndromes in which the testes fail to differentiate, Y chromosomes are morphologically normal.

Denys-Drash Syndrome. The constellation of nephropathy with ambiguous genitals and bilateral Wilms tumor are the major characteristics of this syndrome. Most reported cases have been 46,XY. Müllerian ducts are often present, indicating a global deficiency of fetal testicular function. Patients with 46,XX karyotype have normal external genitals. The onset of proteinuria in infancy progresses to nephrotic syndrome and end-stage renal failure by 3 yr of age, with focal or diffuse mesangial sclerosis being the most consistent histopathologic finding. Wilms tumor usually develops in children younger than 2 yr of age and is frequently bilateral. Gonadoblastomas have been reported.

Several mutations of the Wilms tumor gene *(WT1)*, located on chromosome 11p13, have been found. *WT1* functions as a tumor-suppressor gene and transcriptional factor and is expressed in the genital ridge and fetal gonads. Nearly all reported mutations have been near or within the zinc finger coding region. One report found a zinc finger domain mutation in the *WT1* alleles of a patient without any genitourinary abnormalities, suggesting that some cases of sporadic Wilms tumor may carry the *WT1* mutation. Different mutations of the *WT1* gene have been described in Fraser syndrome, a condition of nonspecific focal and segmental glomerulosclerosis, 46,XY gonadal dysgenesis, and frequent gonadoblastoma, without Wilms tumor.

WAGR Syndrome. This acronymic contiguous gene syndrome consists of *W*ilms tumor, *a*niridia, *g*enitourinary malformations, and *r*etardation. These children have a deletion of one copy of chromosome 11p13, which may be visible on karyotype analysis. The deleted region encompasses the aniridia gene *(PAX6)* and the Wilms tumor suppressor gene *(WT1)*. Only 46,XY males have genital abnormalities, ranging from cryptorchidism to severe deficiency of virilization. Gonadoblastomas have developed in the dysgenetic gonads. Wilms tumor usually occurs by 2 yr of age. Three cases also had unexplained obesity, raising the question of an obesity-associated gene in this region of chromosome 11.

Camptomelic Syndrome (see Chapter 692). This form of short-limbed dysplasia is characterized by anterior bowing of the femur and tibia and by malformations of other organs. It is usually lethal in early infancy. About 75% of reported 46,XY patients exhibit sex reversal with a completely female phenotype; the external and internal genitals are female. Some 46,XY patients have ambiguous genitals. The gonads appear to be ovaries but histologically may contain elements of ovaries and testes.

The gene responsible for the condition is *SOX9* (*SRY*-related HMG-box gene) and is on 17q24-q25. This gene is structurally related to *SRY* and also directly regulates the type II collagen gene *(COL2A1)* development. The same mutations may result in different gonadal phenotypes. Gonadoblastoma was reported in a patient with this condition. The inheritance is autosomal dominant. Adrenal insufficiency and 46,XY gonadal dysgenesis was described in a patient with mutation of the *SF1* gene.

46,XY sex reversal has been described in patients with deletions of parts of autosomal loci on chromosomes 2q, 9p, and 10q.

XY Pure Gonadal Dysgenesis (Swyer Syndrome). The designation "pure" distinguishes this condition from forms of gonadal dysgenesis that are of chromosomal origin and associated with somatic anomalies. Affected patients have normal stature and a female phenotype, including vagina, uterus, and fallopian tubes, but at pubertal age, breast development and menarche fail to occur. None of the defects associated with 45,X children is present. Patients present at puberty with hypergonadotropic primary amenorrhea. Familial cases suggest an X-linked or a sex-limited dominant autosomal transmission. Most of the patients examined have had mutations of the *SRY* gene. None had a *SOX9* gene mutation. The gonads consist of almost totally undifferentiated streaks despite the presence of a cytogenetically normal Y chromosome. The primitive gonad cannot accomplish any testicular function, including suppression of müllerian ducts. There may be hilar cells in the gonad capable of producing some androgens; accordingly, some virilization, such as clitoral enlargement, may occur at the age of puberty. The streak gonads may undergo neoplastic changes, such as gonadoblastomas and dysgerminomas and should be removed shortly after diagnosis, regardless of age.

Pure gonadal dysgenesis also occurs in XX individuals (see Chapter 580.).

XY Gonadal Agenesis Syndrome (Embryonic Testicular Regression Syndrome). In this rare syndrome, the external genitals are slightly ambiguous but more nearly female. Hypoplasia of the labia, some degree of labioscrotal fusion, a small clitoris-like phallus, and a perineal urethral opening are present. No uterus, no gonadal tissue, and usually no vagina can be found. At the age of puberty, no sexual development occurs and gonadotropin levels are elevated. Most children have been reared as females. In several patients with XY gonadal agenesis in whom no gonads could be found on exploration, significant rises in testosterone followed stimulation with hCG, indicating Leydig cell function somewhere. Siblings with the disorder are known.

It is presumed that testicular tissue was active long enough during fetal life for AMH to inhibit development of müllerian ducts but not long enough for testosterone production to result in virilization. In one patient, no deletion of the Y chromosome was found using Y-specific DNA probes. Testicular degeneration seems to occur between the 8th and the 12th fetal wk. Regression of the testis before the 8th wk of gestation results in Swyer syndrome; between the 14th and the 20th wk of gestation, it results in the rudimentary testis syndrome; and after the 20th wk, it results in anorchia.

In *bilateral anorchia*, testes are absent, but the male phenotype is complete; it is presumed that tissue with fetal testicular function was active during the critical period of genital differentiation but that sometime later it was damaged. Bilateral anorchia in identical twins and unilateral anorchia in identical twins and in siblings suggest a genetic predisposition. Coexistence of anorchia and the gonadal agenesis syndrome in a sibship is evidence for a relationship between the disorders. *SRY* defects have not yet been reported for patients with anorchia.

A retrospective review of urologic explorations revealed absent testes in 21% of 691 testes. Of those, 73% had blind-ending cord structures with the suggested site of the vanishing testes being the inguinal canal (59%), the abdomen (21%), superficial inguinal ring (18%), and scrotum (2%). It was suggested that the presence of cord structures on laparoscopy should prompt inguinal exploration because viable testicular tissue was found in four of these children. No hormonal data (hCG stimulation tests, AMH levels) were reported.

DEFECTS IN TESTICULAR HORMONES

Five genetic defects have been delineated in the enzymatic synthesis of testosterone by fetal testis, and a defect in Leydig cell differentiation has been described. These defects produce 46,XY males with inadequate masculinization (Fig. 582–1). Because levels of testosterone are normally low before puberty, an hCG stimulation test must be used in children to assess the ability of the testes to synthesize testosterone.

Leydig Cell Aplasia. Patients with aplasia or hypoplasia of the Leydig cells usually have female phenotypes, but there may be mild virilization. Testes, epididymis, and vas are present; the uterus and fallopian tubes are absent. There are no secondary sexual changes at puberty; pubic hair may be normal. Plasma levels of testosterone are low and do not respond to hCG; luteinizing hormone (LH) levels are elevated. The Leydig cells of the testes are absent or markedly deficient. The defect may involve a lack of receptors for LH. In children, hCG stimulation is necessary to differentiate the condition from the androgen insensitivity syndromes (AIS). There is male-limited autosomal recessive inheritance. The human LH receptor is a member of the G protein–coupled superfamily of receptors that contains seven transmembrane domains. Several inactivating mutations of the LH receptor have been described in males with hypogonadism suspected of having Leydig cell hypoplasia or aplasia.

High serum LH and low follicle-stimulating hormone (FSH) were noted in one male with hypogonadism owing to a mutation in the gene for the β-subunit of FSH (see Table 577–1]).

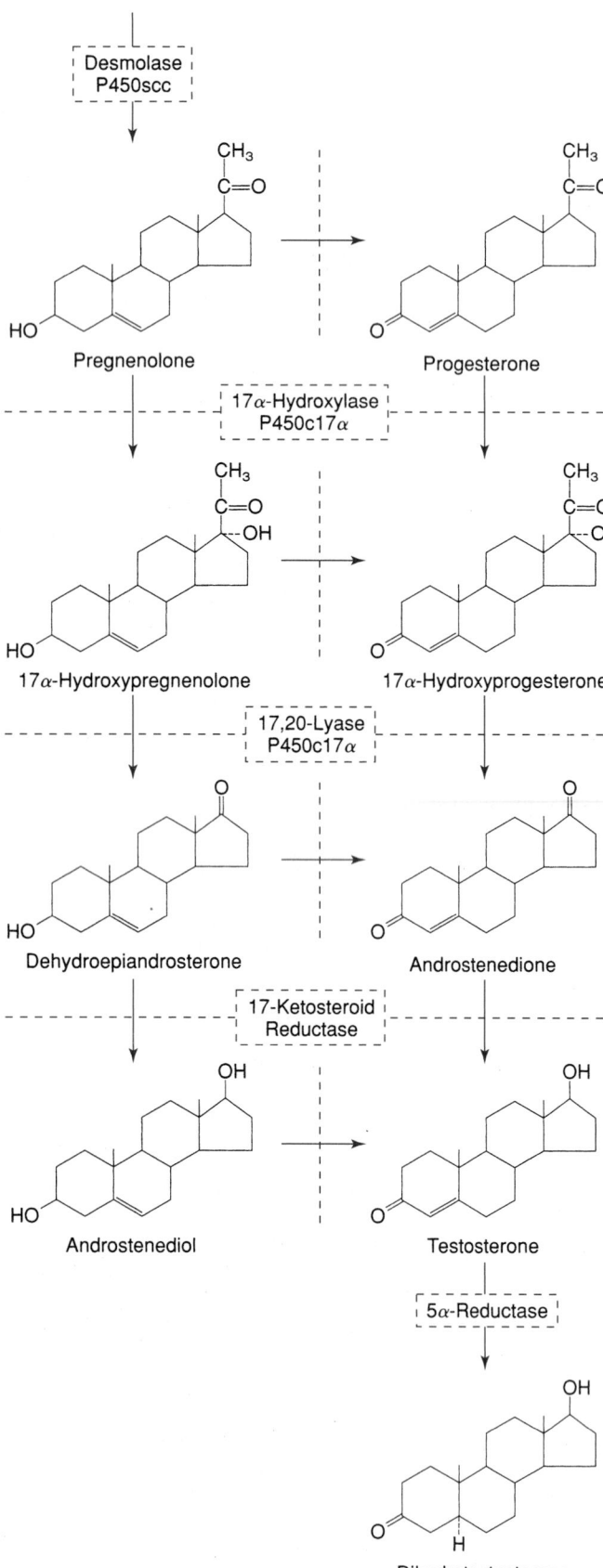

FIGURE 582–1. Biosynthesis of androgens. The *dotted lines* indicate enzymatic defects associated with male pseudohermaphroditism. The *vertical dotted line* indicates a defect in 3β-hydroxysteroid dehydrogenase. A single polypeptide, P450c17, catalyzes both 17α-hydroxylase and 17,20-lyase activities.

Lipoid Adrenal Hyperplasia (also see Chapter 570). The most severe form of congenital adrenal hyperplasia derives its name from the appearance of the enlarged adrenal glands resulting from accumulation of cholesterol and cholesterol esters. It was previously thought to be due to defective P450scc activity, the enzyme responsible for side-chain cleavage of a carbon unit from cholesterol to form pregnenolone. It has now been proved that it is due to diminished delivery of the substrate cholesterol to the inner mitochondrial membrane and to the P450scc system. That process is regulated by steroidogenic acute regulatory protein (StAR), mutations of which were documented in children with lipoid adrenal hyperplasia.

All serum steroid levels are low or undetectable, whereas corticotropin and plasma renin levels are elevated. The phenotype is female in genetic females and males; genetic males have no müllerian structures because the testes can produce normal AMH but no steroid. These children present with acute adrenal crisis and salt wasting in infancy. Most patients are 46,XY. In a few patients, ovarian steroidogenesis is present at puberty.

The regulatory role of StAR-independent steroidogenesis is illustrated by 46,XX 4-mo-old twins with lipoid adrenal hyperplasia. One died at 15 mo because of cardiac complications related to coarctation of the aorta. The adrenal glands had characteristic lipid deposits. The surviving twin had spontaneous puberty with feminization at 11.5 yr with menarche at 13.8 yr. When restudied at the age of 15 yr, a homozygous frameshift-inactivating mutation in her StAR gene was discovered. This and the fact that she survived as an infant until 4 mo of age without replacement therapy with detectable serum aldosterone levels supports the hypothesis that StAR-independent steroidogenesis was able to proceed until enough intracellular lipid accumulated to destroy steroidogenic activity. Partial defects in only partially virilized males and delayed onset of salt wasting have been described. Complete P450scc defects may be incompatible with life because only this enzyme can convert cholesterol to pregnenolone, which then becomes progesterone, a hormone essential for the maintenance of normal mammalian pregnancy. Heterozygous mutation in P450scc was described in a 4 yr old with 46,XY sex reversal and late-onset form of lipoid adrenal hyperplasia. At 6–7 wk of gestation, when maternal corpus luteum progesterone synthesis stops, the placenta, which does not express StAR, produces progesterone by StAR-independent steroidogenesis using the P450scc enzyme system.

3β-Hydroxysteroid Dehydrogenase Deficiency. Males with this form of congenital adrenal hyperplasia (see Chapter 570) have various degrees of hypospadias, with or without bifid scrotum and cryptorchidism and, rarely, a complete female phenotype. Affected infants usually acquire salt-losing manifestations shortly after birth. Incomplete defects, occasionally seen in boys with premature pubarche, as well as late-onset nonclassic forms have been reported. These children have point mutations of the gene for type II 3β-hydroxysteroid enzyme, resulting in impairment of steroidogenesis in the adrenals and gonads; the impairment may be unequal between adrenals and gonads. Normal pubertal changes in some boys could be explained by the normally present type I 3β-hydroxysteroid dehydrogenase present in many peripheral tissues. Infertility is not infrequent. More than 31 different mutations are reported. There is no correlation between degree of salt wasting and degree of phenotypic abnormality.

Deficiency of 17-Hydroxylase/17,20 Lyase. A single enzyme (P450c17) encoded by a single gene on chromosome 10q24.3 has both 17-hydroxylase and 17,20 lyase activities in adrenal and gonadal tissues (see Chapter 570). Many different genetic lesions have been reported. Genetic males usually present with a complete female phenotype or, less often, with various degrees of undervirilization from labioscrotal fusion to perineal hypospadias and cryptorchidism. Pubertal development fails to occur in both genetic sexes.

In the classic disorder, there is decreased synthesis of cortisol by the adrenals and of sex steroids by the adrenals and gonads (see Fig. 582–1 and Fig. 568–1). Levels of deoxycorticosterone (DOC) and corticosterone are markedly increased and lead to the hypertension and hypokalemia characteristic of this form of male pseudohermaphroditism. Although levels of cortisol are low, the elevated corticotropin and corticosterone levels maintain a eucorticoid state. The renin-aldosterone axis is suppressed because of the strong mineralocorticoid effect of elevated DOC. Virilization does not occur at puberty; levels of testosterone are low, and those of gonadotropins are increased. Because fetal production of AMH is normal, no müllerian duct remnants are present. In phenotypic XY females, gonadectomy and replacement therapy with hydrocortisone and sex steroids are indicated.

The defect follows autosomal recessive inheritance. Affected XX females are usually not detected until young adult life, when they fail to experience normal pubertal changes and are found to have hypertension and hypokalemia. This condition should be suspected in patients presenting with primary amenorrhea and hypertension whose chromosomal complement is either 46,XX or 46,XY.

Deficiency of 17-Ketosteroid Reductase.

This enzyme, also called 17β-hydroxysteroid dehydrogenase (17β-HSD), is the last in the testosterone biosynthetic pathway; it is necessary to convert androstenedione to testosterone and also dehydroepiandrosterone to androstenediol and estrone to estradiol. Enzymatic defects in fetal testicular tissue give rise to males with complete or near-complete female phenotype in 46,XY males. Müllerian ducts are absent, and a shallow vagina is present. The diagnosis is based on the ratio of testosterone to androstenedione; in prepubertal children, prior stimulation with hCG is necessary.

The defect is inherited in an autosomal recessive fashion. At least four different types of 17β-HSD are recognized, each coded by a different gene or different chromosomes. Type III is the enzyme defect that is especially common in a highly inbred Arab population in Gaza. The gene for the disorder is at 9q22 and is expressed only in the testes, where it converts androstenedione to testosterone. Most patients are diagnosed at puberty because of the failure to menstruate and virilization. Testosterone levels at puberty may approach normal, presumably as a result of peripheral conversion of androstenedione to testosterone; at this time, some patients spontaneously adopt a male gender role.

Type I 17β-HSD, encoded by a gene on chromosome 17q21, converts estrone to estradiol and is found in placenta, ovary, testis, liver, prostate, adipose tissue, and endometrium. Type II, whose gene is on chromosome 16q24, has activities that are opposite to those of types I and III (convert testosterone to androstenedione and estrone to estradiol). Type IV is similar in action to type II. A late-onset form of 17-ketosteroid reductase deficiency presents as gynecomastia in young adult males.

Persistent Müllerian Duct Syndrome.

In this disorder, there is persistence of müllerian duct derivatives in otherwise completely virilized males. Cases have been reported in siblings and identical twins. Cryptorchidism is present in 80% of affected males; and during surgery for this or inguinal hernia, the condition is uncovered when a fallopian tube and uterus are found. The degree of müllerian development is variable and may be asymmetric. Testicular function is normal in most, but testicular degeneration has been reported. Some affected males acquire testicular tumors after puberty. In a study of 38 families, 16 families had defects in the AMH gene, located on the short arm of chromosome 19. They had low AMH levels. In 16 families with high AMH levels, the defect was in the AMH type II receptor gene, with 10/16 having identical 27-bp deletions on exon 10 in at least one allele.

Treatment consists of removal of as many of the müllerian structures as possible without causing damage to the testis, epididymis, or vas deferens.

DEFECTS IN ANDROGEN ACTION

In the following group of disorders, fetal synthesis of testosterone is normal and defective virilization results from inherited abnormalities in androgen action.

5α-Reductase Deficiency.

Decreased production of dihydrotestosterone (DHT) in utero results in severe ambiguity of the external genitals of the affected male fetus. Biosynthesis and peripheral action of testosterone are normal.

The phenotype most commonly associated with this condition results in boys who have a small phallus, bifid scrotum, urogenital sinus with perineal hypospadias, and a blind vaginal pouch. Testes are in the inguinal canals or labioscrotal folds and are normal histologically. There are no müllerian structures. Wolffian structures—the vas deferens, epididymis, and seminal vesicles—are present. Most affected patients have been identified as females. At puberty, virilization occurs; the phallus enlarges, the testes descend and grow normally, and spermatogenesis occurs. There is no gynecomastia. Beard growth is scanty, acne is absent, the prostate is small, and recession of the temporal hairline fails to occur. Virilization of the wolffian duct is caused by the action of testosterone itself, although masculinization of the urogenital sinus and external genitals depends on the action of DHT during the critical period of fetal masculinization. Growth of facial hair and of the prostate also appears to be DHT dependent.

The adult height reached is close to that of the father and other male siblings. There is, however, significant phenotypic heterogeneity. This has led to a classification of such patients into five types of steroid 5α-reductase deficiency (SRD) ranging from complete female (type 5), to partial female (type 4), ambiguous (type 3), predominantly male with micropenis (type 2), and completely male phenotype without apparent undervirilization (type 1).

Several different gene defects leading to steroid 5α-reductase deficiency have been identified in the 5α-reductase type 2 gene, located on the short arm of chromosome 2, in patients from throughout the world. Familial clusters have been reported from the Dominican Republic, Turkey, Papua New Guinea, Brazil, Mexico, and the Middle East. There is no correlation between severity of the genetic defect and phenotype.

The disorder is inherited as an autosomal recessive trait but is limited to males; normal homozygous females with normal fertility indicate that in females DHT has no role in sexual differentiation or in ovarian function later in life. The clinical diagnosis should be made as early as possible in infancy; it should be distinguished from androgen insensitivity syndrome. The biochemical diagnosis is based on finding normal serum testosterone levels, normal or low DHT levels with markedly increased basal and, especially, hCG-stimulated testosterone:DHT ratios (>17), and high ratios of urinary etiocholanolone to androsterone and 5β to 5α metabolites. Children with androgen insensitivity have normal hepatic 5α reduction and, thus, a normal ratio of tetrahydrocortisol to 5α-tetrahydrocortisol as opposed to those with SRD.

Most but, importantly, not all children reared as females in childhood have changed to male around the time of puberty. It appears that exposures to testosterone in utero, neonatally, and at puberty contribute to the formation of male gender identity. Much more needs to be learned about the influences of hormones such as androgens as well as the influences of cultural, social, psychologic, genetic, and other biologic factors in gender identity and behavior. Infants with this condition should be reared as boys whenever practical. Treatment of male infants with DHT results in phallic enlargement.

Androgen Insensitivity Syndromes.

The AIS compose the most common forms of male pseudohermaphroditism, occurring with a presumed frequency of 1/20,000 genetic males. This group of heterogeneous X-linked disorders is due to more than 150 different mutations in the androgen receptor gene, located on Xq11-12: single point mutations resulting in amino acid substitutions or premature stop codons, frameshift and premature terminations, gene deletions, and splice site mutations.

CLINICAL MANIFESTATIONS. The clinical spectrum of patients with AIS, all of whom have a 46,XY chromosomal complement, range from phenotypic females (in complete AIS) to males with various forms of ambiguous genitals and undervirilization (partial AIS, or clinical syndromes such as Reifenstein syndrome) to phenotypically normal-appearing males with infertility. In addition to normal 46,XY chromosomes, the presence of testes and normal or elevated testosterone levels are common to all such children.

In complete AIS, an extreme form of failure of virilization, genetic males appear female at birth and are invariably reared accordingly. The external genitals are female. The vagina ends blindly in a pouch, and the uterus is absent. In about one third of patients, unilateral or bilateral fallopian tube remnants are found. The testes are usually intra-abdominal but may descend into the inguinal canal; they consist largely of seminiferous tubules. Twin girls with inguinal hernias containing testes were described. At puberty, there is normal development of breasts, and the habitus is female, but menstruation does not occur and sexual hair is absent. Adult heights of these women are commensurate with those of normal males despite profound congenital deficiency of androgenic effects.

The testes of affected adult patients produce normal male levels of testosterone and DHT. Failure of normal male differentiation during fetal life reflects defective response to androgens at that time, but the absence of müllerian ducts indicates normal fetal testicular production of AMH. The absence of androgenic effects is caused by a striking resistance to the action of endogenous or exogenous testosterone at the cellular level.

Prepubertal children with this disorder are often detected when inguinal masses prove to be testes or when a testis is unexpectedly found during herniorrhaphy in a phenotypic female. About 1–2% of girls with an inguinal hernia prove to have this disorder. In infants, elevated gonadotropin levels should suggest the diagnosis. In adults, amenorrhea is the usual presenting symptom. In prepubertal children, the condition must be differentiated from other types of XY undervirilized males in which there is complete feminization. These include XY gonadal dysgenesis (Swyer syndrome), true agonadism, Leydig cell aplasia including LH receptor defects, and 17-ketosteroid reductase deficiency; all of these conditions, unlike complete AIS, are characterized by low levels of testosterone as neonates and during adult life and by failure to respond to hCG during the prepubertal years. Although patients with complete AIS present with unambiguously female external genitals at birth, those with partial AIS have a wide variety of phenotypic presentations ranging from perineoscrotal hypospadias, bifid scrotum, and cryptorchidism to extreme undervirilization appearing as clitoromegaly and labial fusion. Some forms of partial AIS have been known as specific syndromes. Patients with *Reifenstein syndrome* have incomplete virilization characterized by hypogonadism, severe hypospadias, and gynecomastia. *Gilbert-Dreyfuss* and *Lubs* are additional syndromes classified as partial AIS. In all cases, abnormalities in the androgen receptor gene have been identified.

DIAGNOSIS. The diagnosis of patients with partial AIS may be particularly difficult in infancy. In some, especially those sufficiently virilized in infancy, the diagnosis is not suspected until puberty when there is inadequate virilization with lack of facial hair or voice change and the appearance of gynecomastia. Azoospermia and infertility are common. Increasingly, androgen receptor defects are being recognized in adults who have a small phallus and testes and infertility. A single amino acid substitution in the androgen receptor was reported in a large Chinese family in whom some affected members were fertile while others had gynecomastia and/or hypospadias.

TREATMENT AND PROGNOSIS. In patients with complete AIS whose sexual orientation is unambiguously female, the testes should be removed as soon as they are discovered. Laparoscopic removal of Y-chromosome bearing gonads has been performed in patients with AIS and in those with gonadal dysgenesis. In one third of patients, malignant tumors, usually seminomas, develop by 50 yr of age. Several teenaged girls have acquired seminomas. Replacement therapy with estrogens is indicated at the age of puberty.

Normal breasts develop in affected girls who have not had their testes removed by the age of puberty. In these individuals, production of estradiol results from aromatase activity. The absence of androgenic activity also contributes to the feminization of these women.

The psychosexual and surgical management of patients with partial AIS is extremely complex and depends in large part on the presenting phenotype. Osteopenia is now recognized as a feature of AIS.

Molecular analyses have suggested that phenotype may depend in part on somatic mosaicism of the androgen receptor gene. This was based on the case of a 46,XY patient who had a premature stop codon in exon 1 of the *AR* gene but who also had evidence of virilization (pubic hair and clitoral enlargement) explained by the discovery of the wild-type alleles on careful examination of the sequencing gel. The presence of mosaicism shifts the phenotype to a higher degree of virilization than expected from the genotype of the mutant allele alone.

Genetic counseling is difficult in families with androgen receptor gene mutation. In addition to lack of genotype-phenotype correlations, there is a high rate (27%) of de novo mutations in families.

Sex hormone–binding globulin reduction after exogenous androgen administration (stanozolol) has been shown to correlate with the severity of the receptor defect and may become a useful clinical tool. Successful therapy with supplemental androgens has been reported in patients with partial AIS and various mutations of the androgen receptor in the DNA-binding domain and the ligand-binding domain.

Mutated androgen receptors are also reported in patients with spinal and bulbar muscular atrophy in whom clinical manifestations including testicular atrophy, infertility, gynecomastia, and elevated LH, FSH, and estradiol levels usually manifest between the 3rd–5th decades of life. Androgen receptor mutations have also been described in patients with prostate cancer.

UNDETERMINED CAUSES

Other XY undervirilized males display great variability of the external and internal genitals and various degrees of phallic and müllerian development. Testes may be histologically normal or rudimentary, or there may only be one. Even the newer techniques may find no recognized cause of intersex in a substantial number of children. Some ambiguity of genitals is associated with a wide variety of chromosomal aberrations, which must always be considered in the differential diagnosis, the most common being the 45,X/46,XY syndrome (see Chapter 580.1). It may be necessary to examine several tissues to establish mosaicism. Other complex genetic syndromes, many resulting from single gene mutations, are associated with varying degrees of ambiguity of the genitals, particularly in the male. These entities must be identified on the basis of the associated extragenital malformations.

Smith-Lemli-Opitz syndrome is an autosomal recessive disorder characterized by prenatal and postnatal growth retardation, microcephaly, ptosis, anteverted nares, broad alveolar ridges, syndactyly of the 2nd–3rd toes, and severe mental retardation (see Chapter 75.3). Genotypic males usually have genital ambiguity and, occasionally, complete sex reversal with female genital ambiguity or complete sex reversal with female external genitals. Müllerian duct derivatives are usually absent. Affected 46,XX patients have normal genitals. Two types of Smith-Lemli-Opitz syndrome have been recognized: the classic form (type I) described earlier and the acrodysgenital syndrome, which is usually lethal within 1 yr and is associated with severe malformations, postaxial polydactyly, and extremely abnormal external genitals (type II). Pyloric stenosis is associated with Smith-Lemli-Opitz syndrome type I and Hirschsprung disease with type II. Cleft palate, skeletal abnormalities, and one case of a lipoma of the pituitary gland have been seen in type II cases.

Low plasma cholesterol with elevated 7-dehydrocholesterol, its precursor, are found in both types (see Chapter 75.3 for treatment).

46,XY Intersex subjects also have been described in siblings with the α-thalassemia/mental retardation syndrome.

582.3 True Gonadal Intersex

In true gonadal intersex, formerly known as true hermaphroditism, both ovarian and testicular tissues are present, either in the same or in opposite gonads. Affected patients have ambiguous genitals, varying from normal female with only slight enlargement of the clitoris to almost normal male external genitals.

About 70% of all patients have a 46,XX karyotype; 97% of affected African blacks are 46,XX. Fewer than 10% of persons with true intersex are 46,XY. About 20% have 46,XX/46,XY mosaicism. Half of these are derived from more than one zygote and are chimeras (chi 46,XX/46,XY). The presence of paternal and both maternal alleles for some blood groups is demonstrated. A true gonadal intersex chimera, 46,XX/46,XY, was reported as resulting from embryo amalgamation after in vitro fertilization. Each embryo was derived from an independent, separately fertilized ovum.

Examination of 46,XX true gonadal intersex patients with Y-specific probes has detected fewer than 10% with a portion of the Y chromosome including the SRY gene. True gonadal intersex is usually sporadic, but a number of siblings have been reported. The cause of most cases of true gonadal intersex is unknown.

The most frequently encountered gonad in true gonadal intersex is an ovotestis, which may be bilateral; if unilateral, the contralateral gonad is usually an ovary but may be a testis. The ovarian tissue is normal, but the testicular tissue is dysgenetic. The presence and function of testicular tissue can be determined by measuring basal and hCG-stimulated testosterone levels and AMH levels. Patients who are highly virilized, have good testicular function, and have no uterus are usually reared as males. If a uterus exists, virilization is mild, and testicular function minimal, assignment of female sex may be indicated. Selective removal of gonadal tissue inconsistent with sex of rearing is indicated. In a few families, 46,XY true gonadal intersex subjects and 44,XX males have been in the same sibship.

Pregnancies with living offspring have been reported in 46,XX true intersex individuals reared as females, but only very few intersex males with true gonadal intersex have fathered children. About 5% of patients acquire gonadoblastomas, dysgerminomas, or seminomas.

Diagnosis and Management. In the neonate, ambiguity of the genitals requires immediate attention to decide on the sex of rearing as early in life as possible. The family of the infant needs to be informed of the child's condition as early, completely, compassionately, and honestly as possible. Caution must be used to avoid feelings of guilt, shame, and discomfort. Guidance needs to be provided to alleviate both short-term and long-term concerns and allow the child to grow up in a completely supportive environment. The initial care is best provided by a team of professionals that include neonatologists and pediatric specialists, endocrinologists, radiologists, urologists, psychologists, and geneticists, all of whom remain focused foremost on the needs of the child. Management of the potential psychologic upheaval that these disorders can generate in the child or the family is of paramount importance and requires physicians and other health care professionals with sensitivity, training, and experience in this field.

While awaiting the results of chromosomal analysis, pelvic ultrasonography or MRI is indicated to determine the presence of a uterus and ovaries. Presence of a uterus and absence of palpable gonads usually suggests a virilized XX female. A search for the source of virilization should be undertaken; this includes studies of adrenal hormones to rule out varieties of congenital adrenal hyperplasia, and studies of androgens and estrogens occasionally may be necessary to rule out aromatase deficiency. Virilized XX females are generally reared as females even when highly virilized.

The absence of a uterus, with or without palpable gonads, almost always indicates an undervirilized male and an XY karyotype. Measurements of levels of gonadotropins, testosterone, AMH, and DHT are necessary to determine whether testicular production of androgen is normal. Undervirilized males who are totally feminized may be reared as females. However, certain significantly feminized infants, such as those with 5α-reductase deficiency, should be reared as males because these children virilize normally at puberty. An infant with a comparable degree of feminization resulting from an androgen receptor defect is best reared as a female. Infants with 45,XX/46,XY karyotype whose phenotype varies from almost completely male to completely female are usually reared as females because they are generally short in stature and have a uterus; they require gonadectomy.

When receptor disorders are suspected in the XY male with a small phallus (micropenis), a course of three monthly intramuscular injections of testosterone enanthate (25–50 mg) may assist in the differential diagnosis as well as in treatment.

In some mammals, the female exposed to androgens prenatally or in early postnatal life exhibits nontraditional sexual behavior in adult life. Most, but not all, girls who have undergone fetal masculinization from congenital adrenal hyperplasia or from maternal progestin therapy have no such problems in sexual identity, although during childhood they may appear to prefer male playmates and activities over female playmates and feminine play with dolls in mothering roles.

Advances in visualization procedures, hormonal assays, molecular methodology, as well as surgical techniques should make for more rapid, accurate, and appropriate diagnosis and management of the infant and child with intersex. It has been thought that it is more feasible to reconstruct the external genitals to create a functional female, particularly when a vagina is present, than to create a functional male phallus. Hence, in the absence of reasonable prospects for a well-functioning male phallus, the intersex infants have in the past always been assigned a female gender. Considerable controversy currently exists regarding these decisions. A poorly functioning female external genital system may be no better then a poorly functioning male phallus. In addition, sexual functioning is to a large extent more dependent on other neurohormonal and behavioral factors then the physical appearance and functional ability of the genitals. This concept is given added support by a case report of a 46,XY subject whose penis was accidentally ablated and was subsequently reared as a female. At puberty this individual switched to male and continues to successfully live as such.

Similarly, controversy exists regarding the timing of the performance of invasive and definitive procedures, such as surgery. Whenever possible without endangering the physical or psychological health of the child, an expert multidisciplinary team should consider deferring elective surgical repairs and gonadectomies until the child can participate in the informed consent for the procedure. Long-term prospective as well as retrospective science- and evidence-based studies in sufficient numbers of individuals born with intersex are necessary to evaluate their anatomic, psychosexual, social, as well as functional status.

The pediatrician and pediatric endocrinologist, along with the appropriate additional specialists, should provide ongoing compassionate, supportive care to the patient and the patient's family throughout childhood, adolescence, and even young adulthood. Support groups are available for patients and families with many of the conditions discussed.

Affara NA, Chalmers IJ, Ferguson-Smith MA: Analysis of the *SRY* gene in 22 sex-reversed XY females identifies four new point mutations in the conserved DNA binding domain. *Hum Mol Genet* 1993;2:785.

Alo N, Moisan AM, Ward L, et al: A novel A10E homozygous mutation in the *HSD3B2* gene causing severe salt-wasting 3β-hydroxysteroid dehydrogenase deficiency in 46,XX and 46,XY French-Canadians: Evaluation of gonadal function after puberty. *J Clin Endocrinol Metab* 2000;85:1968–74.

Battiloro E, Angeletti B, Tozzi MC, et al: A novel double nucleotide substitution in the HMG box of the *SRY* gene associated with Swyer syndrome. *Hum Genet* 1997; 100:585–7.

Bell DM, Leung KK, Wheatley SC, et al: SOX9 directly regulates the type-II collagen gene. *Nat Genet* 1997;16:174.

Bose HS, Pescovitz OH, Miller WL: Spontaneous feminization in a 46,XX female patient with congenital lipoid adrenal hyperplasia due to a homozygous frameshift mutation in the steroidogenic acute regulatory protein. *J Clin Endocrinol Metab* 1997;82:1511.

Brinkmann AO: Molecular basis of androgen insensitivity. *Mol Cell Endocrinol* 2001;179:105–9.

Cameron FJ, Montalto J, Byrt E, et al: Gonadal dysgenesis: Associations between clinical features and sex of rearing. *Endocr J* 1997;44:95.

Canto P, Vilchis F, Chavez B, et al: Mutations of the 5α-reductase type 2 gene in eight Mexican patients from six different pedigrees with 5α-reductase-2 deficiency. *Clin Endocrinol* 1997;46:155.

Castro-Magana M, Angulo M, Uy J: Male hypogonadism with gynecomastia caused by late-onset deficiency of testicular 17-ketosteroid reductase. *N Engl J Med* 1993;328:1297.

Chu J, Zhang R, Zhao Z, et al: Male fertility is compatible with an Arg840 Cys substitution in the AR in a large Chinese family affected with divergent phenotypes of AR insensitivity syndrome. *J Clin Endocrinol Metab* 2002;87:347–51.

Conte FA, Grumbach MM, Ito Y, et al: A syndrome of female pseudohermaphroditism, hypergonadotropic hypogonadism, and multicystic ovaries associated with missense mutations in the gene encoding aromatase (P450$_{arom}$). *J Clin Endocrinol Metab* 1994;78:1287.

Creighton S, Minto C: Managing intersex. *BMJ* 2001;323:1264–65.

Daaboul J, Frader J: Ethics and the management of the patient with intersex: A middle way. *J Pediatr Endocrinol Metab* 2001;14:1575–83.

Damiani D, Fellous M, McElreavey K, et al: True hermaphroditism: Clinical aspects and molecular studies in 16 cases. *Eur J Endocr* 1997;136:201.

Diamond M, Sigmundson K: Sex reassignment at birth. *Arch Pediatr Adolesc Med* 1997;151:298.

Frade Costa EM, Bilharinho Mendonca B, Inacio M, et al: Management of ambiguous genitalia in pseudohermaphrodites: New perspectives on vaginal dilation. *Fertil Steril* 1997;67:229.

Geissler WM, Davis DL, Wu L, et al: Male pseudohermaphroditism caused by mutation of testicular 17β-hydroxysteroid dehydrogenase 3. *Nat Genet* 1994;7:34.

Ghahremani M, Chan CB, Bistritzer T, et al: A novel mutation H373Y in the Wilms tumor suppressor gene, *WT1*, associated with Denys-Drash syndrome. *Hum Hered* 1996;46:336.

Gul D: Third case of WAGR syndrome with severe obesity and constitutional deletion of chromosome (11)(p12p14). *Am J Med Genet* 2002;107:70–1.

Hiort O, Sinnecker GHG, Holterbus PM, et al: Inherited and de novo androgen receptor gene mutations: Investigation of single-case families. *J Pediatr* 1998; 132:939.

Hochberg Z, Chayen R, Reiss N, et al: Clinical, biochemical and genetic findings in a large pedigree of male and female patients with 5α-reductase 2 deficiency. *J Clin Endocrinol Metab* 1996;81:2821.

Holterhus PM, Bruggenwirth HT, Hiort O, et al: Mosaicism due to a somatic mutation of the androgen receptor gene determines phenotype in androgen insensitivity syndrome. *J Clin Endocrinol Metab* 1997;82:3584.

Imbeaud S, Belville C, Messika-Zeitoun L, et al: A 27 base-pair deletion of the anti-müllerian type II receptor gene is the most common cause of the persistent müllerian duct syndrome. *Hum Mol Genet* 1996;5:1269.

Kremer H, Karaaij R, Toledo SPA, et al: Male pseudohermaphroditism due to a homozygous missense mutation of the luteinizing hormone receptor gene. *Nat Genet* 1995;9:160.

Krob G, Braun A, Kuhnle U: True hermaphroditism: Geographical distribution, clinical findings, chromosomes and gonadal histology. *Eur J Pediatr* 1994;153:2.

McPherson EW, Clemens MM, Gibbons RJ, et al: X-linked α-thalassemia/mental retardation (ATR-X) syndrome: A new kindred with severe genital anomalies and mild hematologic expression. *Am J Med Genet* 1995;55:302.

Mebarki F, Sanchez R, Rheaumes E, et al: Non–salt-losing male pseudohermaphroditism due to the novel homozygous N100S mutation in the type II 3β-hydroxysteroid dehydrogenase gene. *J Clin Endocrinol Metab* 1995;80: 2127.

Mendonca BB, Inacio M, Costa EMF, et al: Male pseudohermaphroditism due to steroid 5α-reductase 2 deficiency. *Medicine* 1996;75:64.

Mendonca BB, Leite MV, DeCastro M, et al: Female pseudohermaphroditism caused by a novel homozygous mutation of the *GR* gene. *J Clin Endocrinol Metab* 2002;87:1805–9.

Moisan AM, Ricketts ML, Tardy V, et al: New insight into the molecular basis of 3β-hydroxysteroid dehydrogenase deficiency: Identification of eight mutations in the *HSD3* gene in eleven patients from seven new families and comparison of the functional properties of twenty-five mutant enzymes. *J Clin Endocrinol Metab* 1999;84:4410–25.

Mongan NP, Jaaskelainen J, Green K, et al: Two de novo mutations in the *AR* gene cause the complete androgen insensitivity syndrome in a pair of monozygotic twins. *J Clin Endocrinol Metab* 2002;87:1057–61.

Monno S, Mizushima Y, Toyoda N, et al: A new variant of the cytochrome P450c17 *(CYP17)* gene mutation in three patients with 17 α-hydroxylase deficiency. *Ann Hum Genet* 1997;61:275.

Morishima A, Grumbach MM, Simpson ER, et al: Aromatase deficiency in male and female siblings caused by a novel mutation and the physiological role of estrogens. *J Clin Endocrinol Metab* 1995;80:3689.

Mueller RF: The Denys-Drash syndrome. *J Med Genet* 1994;31:471.

Mullis PE, Yoshimura N, Kuhlmann B, et al: Aromatase deficiency in a female who is compound heterozygote for two new point mutations in the P450$_{arom}$ gene: Impact of estrogens on hypergonadotropic hypogonadism, multicystic ovaries, and bone densitometry in childhood. *J Clin Endocrinol Metab* 1997;82:1739.

Quigley CA, French FS: Androgen insensitivity syndromes. *Curr Ther Endocrinol Metab* 1994;5:342.

Reardon W, Gibbons RJ, Winter RM, et al: Male pseudohermaphroditism in sibs with the α-thalassemia/mental retardation (ATR-X) syndrome. *Am J Med Genet* 1995;55:285.

Saenger P: New developments in congenital lipoid adrenal hyperplasia and steroidogenic acute regulatory protein. *Pediatr Clin North Am* 1997;44:397.

Sarafoglou K, Ostrer H: Clinical Review 111—Familial sex reversal: A review. *J Clin Endocrinol Metab* 2000;85:483–93.

Sinnecker GHG, Hirot O, Nitsche EM: Functional assessment and clinical classification of androgen sensitivity in patients with mutations of the androgen receptor gene. *Eur J Pediatr* 1997;156:7.

Smith EP, Boyd J, Frank GR, et al: Estrogen resistance caused by a mutation in the estrogen-receptor gene in a man. *N Engl J Med* 1994;331:1056.

Tajima T, Fujieda K, Kouda N, et al: Heterozygous mutation in the cholesterol side chain cleavage enzyme (P450scc) gene in a patient with 46,XY sex reversal and adrenal insufficiency. *J Clin Endocrinol Metab* 2001;86:3820–5.

Warne GL, Zajac JD, MacLean HE: Androgen insensitivity syndrome in the era of molecular genetics and the Internet: A point of view. *J Pediatr Endocrinol Metab* 1998;11:3.

Weidemann W, Peters B, Romalo G, et al: Response to androgen treatment in a patient with partial androgen insensitivity and a mutation in the deoxyribonucleic acid-binding domain of the androgen receptor. *J Clin Endocrinol Metab* 1998;83:1173.

White PC, Speiser PW: Congenital adrenal hyperplasia due to 21-hydroxylase deficiency. *Endocr Rev* 2000;21:245–91.

SECTION 6 *Diabetes Mellitus in Children*

Ramin Alemzadeh and David T. Wyatt

Chapter 583

Diabetes Mellitus

583.1 Introduction and Classification

Diabetes mellitus (DM) is a common, chronic, metabolic syndrome characterized by hyperglycemia as a cardinal biochemical feature. The major forms of diabetes are divided into those caused by deficiency of insulin secretion due to pancreatic β-cell damage (type 1 DM), and those that are a consequence of insulin resistance occurring at the level of skeletal muscle, liver, and adipose tissue, with various degrees of β-cell impairment (type 2 DM). Type 1 DM is the most common endocrine-metabolic disorder of childhood and adolescence, with important consequences for physical and emotional development. Individuals with type 1 DM confront serious lifestyle alterations that include an absolute daily requirement for exogenous insulin, the need to monitor their own glucose control, and the need to pay attention to dietary intake. Morbidity and mortality stem from acute metabolic derangements and from long-term complications (usually in adulthood) that affect small and large vessels resulting in retinopathy, nephropathy, neuropathy, ischemic heart disease, and arterial obstruction with gangrene of the extremities. The acute clinical manifestations are due to hypoinsulinemic hyperglycemic ketoacidosis. Autoimmune mechanisms are factors in the genesis of type 1 DM; the long-term complications are related to metabolic disturbances (hyperglycemia).

DM is not a single entity but rather a heterogeneous group of disorders in which there are distinct genetic patterns as well as other etiologic and pathophysiologic mechanisms that lead to impairment of glucose tolerance. A classification of diabetes and other categories of glucose intolerance is presented in Table 583–1. Three major forms of diabetes and several forms of carbohydrate intolerance are identified.

Type 1 Diabetes Mellitus. Formerly called insulin-dependent diabetes mellitus (IDDM) or juvenile diabetes, type 1 DM is characterized by low or absent levels of endogenously produced insulin and dependence on exogenous insulin to prevent development of ketoacidosis, an acute life-threatening complication of type 1 DM. The natural history includes preketotic, non–insulin-dependent phases both before and after the initial diagnosis. The onset occurs predominantly in childhood, with median age of 7 to 15 yr, but it may present at any age. Type 1 DM is characterized by autoimmune destruction of pancreatic islet β cells. Both genetic susceptibility and environmental factors contribute to the pathogenesis of type. Susceptibility to type 1 DM is genetically controlled by alleles of the major histocompatability complex (MHC) class II genes expressing human leukocyte antigens (HLAs). It is also associated with autoantibodies to islet cell cytoplasm (ICA), insulin (IAA), antibodies to glutamic acid decarboxylase (GADA or GAD65), and ICA512 (IA2). Type 1 DM is associated with other autoimmune diseases such as thyroiditis, celiac disease, multiple sclerosis, and Addison disease. In some children and adolescents with apparent type 1 DM, the β-cell destruction is not immune-mediated. This subtype of diabetes occurs in patients of African or Asian origin and is distinct from known causes of β-cell destruction,

TABLE 583–1. Etiologic Classifications of Diabetes Mellitus

Type I diabetes* (β-cell destruction, usually leading to absolute insulin deficiency)	*Drug- or chemical-induced*
Immune mediated	Vacor
Idiopathic	Pentamidine
Type II diabetes* (may range from predominantly insulin resistance with relative insulin deficiency to a predominantly secretory defect with insulin resistance)	Nicotinic acid
	Glucocorticoids
	Thyroid hormone
	Diazoxide
	β-Adrenergic agonists
Other specific types	Thiazides
Genetic defects of β-cell function	Dilantin
Chromosome 12, HNF-1α (formerly MODY-3)	β-Interferon
	Others—cyclosporine, tacrolimus
Chromosome 7, glucokinase (formerly MODY-2)	*Infections*
	Congenital rubella
Chromosome 20, HNF-4α (formerly MODY-1)	Cytomegalovirus
	Others—hemolytic uremic syndrome
Mitochondrial DNA	*Uncommon forms of immune-mediated diabetes*
Others	"Stiff-man" syndrome
Genetic defects in insulin action	Cytomegalovirus
Type A insulin resistance	Others
Leprechaunism	*Other genetic syndromes sometimes associated with diabetes*
Rabson-Mendenhall syndrome	Down syndrome
Lipoatrophic diabetes	Klinefelter syndrome
Others	Turner syndrome
Diseases of the exocrine pancreas	Wolfram syndrome
Pancreatitis	Friedreich ataxia
Trauma, pancreatectomy	Huntington chorea
Neoplasia	Laurence-Moon-Biedl syndrome
Cystic fibrosis	Myotonic dystrophy
Hemochromatosis	Porphyria
Fibrocalculous pancreatopathy	Prader-Willi syndrome
Pancreatic resection	Others
Others	**Gestational diabetes mellitus**
Endocrinopathies	**Neonatal diabetes mellitus**
Acromegaly	Transient—without recurrence
Cushing disease	Transient—recurrence 7–20 yr later
Glucagonoma	Permanent from onset
Pheochromocytoma	
Hyperthyroidism	
Somatostatinoma	
Aldosteronoma	
Others	

*Patients with any form of diabetes may require insulin treatment at some stage of the disease. Such use of insulin does not, of itself, classify the patient.

which include drugs or chemicals, viruses, mitochondrial gene defects, pancreatectomy, and ionizing radiation. These individuals may present with ketoacidosis but have extensive periods of remission with variable insulin deficiency, similar to patients with type 2 DM.

Type 2 Diabetes Mellitus. The children and adolescents with this type of diabetes are usually obese but are not insulin-dependent and infrequently develop ketosis. Some may develop ketosis during severe infections or other stresses and may then need insulin for correction of symptomatic hyperglycemia. This category includes the most prevalent form of diabetes in adults, which is characterized by insulin resistance and often a progressive defect in insulin secretion. This type of diabetes was formerly known as adult-onset diabetes mellitus, non–insulin-dependent diabetes mellitus (NIDDM), or maturity-onset diabetes of the young (MODY).

The presentation of type 2 DM is typically more insidious than that with type 1 DM. In contrast to patients with type 1 DM who are usually ill at the time of diagnosis, children with type 2 DM often seek medical care because of excessive weight gain and fatigue as a result of insulin resistance and/or incidental finding of glycosuria during routine physical examination. A history of polyuria and polydipsia is relatively uncommon in these patients. The incidence of type 2 DM in children has increased by more than 10-fold in many diabetes centers, in part as a result of the epidemic of childhood obesity. Pediatric type 2 DM may account for as many as 30% of the new cases of diabetes, especially in obese African and Mexican American adolescents. *Acanthosis nigricans* (dark pigmentation of skin creases/flexural areas), a sign of insulin resistance, is present in the majority of patients with type 2 DM and is accompanied by a relative hyperinsulinemia at the time of the diagnosis (see Chapter 642). However, the serum insulin elevation is usually disproportionately lower than that of age-, weight-, and sex-matched nondiabetic children and adolescents, suggesting a state of insulin insufficiency. In some individuals, it may represent slowly evolving type 1 DM.

In some children with strong family history of type 2 DM, impaired glucose tolerance may occur in a pattern implying dominant inheritance. This pattern of diabetes has been termed *maturity-onset diabetes of the young* (MODY) and may require insulin treatment. In MODY, there is no apparent autoimmune destruction of β cells and no association with HLAs. This subclass of type 2 DM consists of specific genetic disorders involving mutations in the gene encoding pancreatic β-cell and liver glucokinase (GK) or in the nuclear transcription factors hepatocyte nuclear factor (HNF)-4α or hepatic nuclear factor (HNF)-1α. A defect in the gene regulating glucose transport into the pancreatic β cell, GLUT-2 transporter, may be responsible for other forms of type 2 DM. The genetic basis of type 2 DM also includes defects in glycogen synthase, insulin receptors, Rad (Ras associated with diabetes), and possibly apolipoprotein C-III.

Other Specific Types of Secondary Diabetes. Examples include diabetes secondary to exocrine pancreatic diseases (e.g., cystic fibrosis), endocrine diseases other than pancreatic diseases (e.g., Cushing syndrome), and ingestion of certain drugs or poisons (e.g., the rodenticide Vacor). Certain genetic syndromes, including those with abnormalities of the insulin receptor, also are included in this category. There are no associations with HLAs, autoimmunity, or islet cell antibodies among the entities in this subdivision.

Table 583–2 details the current criteria for the diagnosis of DM. It should be noted that a fasting blood glucose that exceeds 126 mg/dL (7.0 mM) is the accepted criterion for diagnosing diabetes.

TABLE 583–2. Diagnostic Criteria for Impaired Glucose Tolerance and Diabetes Mellitus

Impaired Glucose Tolerance (IGT)	Diabetes Mellitus (DM)
Fasting glucose 110–125 mg/dL (6.1–7.0 mmol/L)	Symptoms* of DM plus random plasma glucose ≥ 200 mg/dL (11.1 mmol/L) *or*
2-hr plasma glucose during the OGTT <200 mg/dL (11.1 mmol/L) but ≤140 mg/dL	Fasting plasma glucose ≥ 126 mg/dL (7.0 mmol/L) *or* 2-hr plasma glucose during the OGTT ≥ 200 mg/dL

*Symptoms include polyuria, polydipsia, and unexplained weight loss with glucosuria and ketonuria.
OGTT, oral glucose tolerance test.
From Report of the Expert Committee on the Diagnosis and Classification of Diabetes Mellitus. Diabetes Care 1999; 20(Suppl 1):S5.

Impaired Glucose Tolerance. The term *impaired glucose tolerance* (IGT) refers to a metabolic stage that is intermediate between normal glucose homeostasis and diabetes. A fasting glucose concentration of 109 mg/dL (6.1 mmol/L) is the upper limit of "normal." This choice is near the level above which acute-phase insulin secretion is lost in response to intravenous administration of glucose and is associated with a progressively greater risk of the development of microvascular and macrovascular complications.

Many individuals with IGT are euglycemic in their daily lives and may have normal or nearly normal glycated hemoglobin levels. Individuals with IGT often manifest hyperglycemia only when challenged with the oral glucose load used in the standardized oral glucose tolerance test.

In the absence of pregnancy, IGT is not a clinical entity but rather a risk factor for future diabetes and cardiovascular disease. This may be observed as an intermediate stage in any of the disease processes listed in Table 583–1. IGT is associated with the *insulin resistance syndrome* (also known as syndrome X or the metabolic syndrome), which consists of insulin resistance, compensatory hyperinsulinemia to maintain glucose homeostasis, obesity (especially abdominal or visceral obesity), dyslipidemia of the high-triglyceride or low-high-density lipoprotein type, or both, and hypertension. Insulin resistance is directly involved in the pathogenesis of type 2 DM. IGT appears as a risk factor for this type of diabetes at least in part because of its correlation with insulin resistance. The diagnostic criteria for IGT are presented in Table 583–2.

583.2 Type 1 Diabetes Mellitus (Immune Mediated)

Epidemiology: Genetics and Environment. The incidence of type 1 DM is rapidly increasing in specific regions and shows a trend toward earlier age of onset. The incidence of type 1 DM is highly variable among different ethnic groups. The overall age-adjusted incidence of type 1 DM varies from 0.7/100,000 per year in Karachi (Pakistan) to about 40/100,000 per year in Finland (Fig. 583–1). This represents more than a 400-fold variation in the incidence among about 100 populations analyzed. The increased incidence is seen in nations with a previous low incidence of autoimmune diabetes. For instance, the incidence of type 1 DM in Thailand increased markedly from 0.2/100,000 in 1984–1985 to 1.65/100,000 10 yr later. It is predicted that the overall incidence of type 1 DM will be about 40% higher in 2010 than in 1997.

Data from Western European diabetes centers suggest that the annual rate increase in type 1 DM incidence is 3–4%, whereas some central and eastern European countries demonstrate a significantly more rapid increase. The rates of increase in type 1 DM incidence as a function of age at onset are 6.3%, 3.1%, and 2.4% in age groups of children 0–4 yr, 5–9 yr, and 10–14 yr, respectively. In the United States, the prevalence of diabetes among school-aged children is about 1.9/1,000. The frequency, however, is highly correlated with increasing age; the range is 1 case/1,430 children at 5 yr of age to 1 in 360 children at 16 yr. Among African Americans, the occurrence of type 1 DM is between one third and two thirds of that seen in American whites. The annual incidence in the United States is about 14.9 new cases/100,000 of the child population. Girls and boys are almost equally affected; there is no apparent correlation with socioeconomic status. Peaks of presentation occur in two age groups: at 5–7 yr of age and at the time of puberty. Nonetheless, a growing number of patients are presenting between 1 and 2 yr of age. The first peak may correspond to the time of increased exposure to infectious agents coincident with the beginning of school; the latter may correspond to the pubertal growth spurt induced by gonadal steroids and the increased pubertal growth

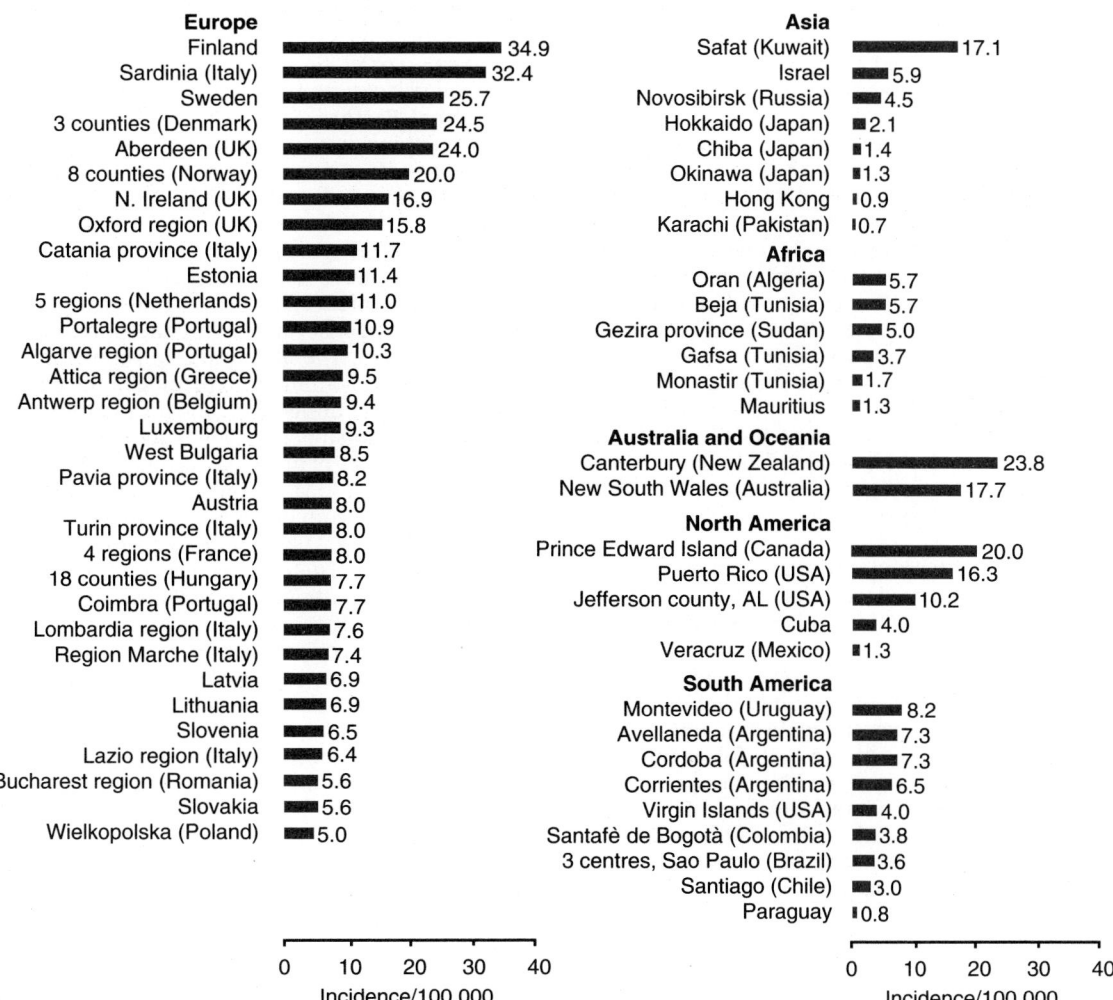

FIGURE 583–1. Incidence rates of type 1 diabetes mellitus by region and country. (From LaPorte RA, et al: The DiaMond Project. *Pract Diabetes Int* 1995;12:93.)

hormone secretion (which antagonizes insulin). These possible cause-and-effect relationships remain to be proved.

GENES. Genes for type 1 DM may provide both susceptibility to, and protection from, the disease. Although many chromosomal loci associated with such activities have been located, few true genes have been identified. The genetics of type 1 DM cannot be classified according to a specific model of inheritances. The most important genes are located within the MHC HLA class II region on chromosome 6p21, formally termed (IDDM1), accounting for about 60% genetic susceptibility for the disease; their specific contribution to the pathogenesis of type 1 DM remains unclear. The importance of the class II haplotypes not only depends on the well-known risk for disease associated with HLA-DR3 and HLA-DR4 but also on additional susceptibility associated with DQ α-chains and DQ β-chains. Inheritance of HLA-DR3 or -DR4 antigens appears to confer a twofold to threefold increased risk for the development of type 1 DM. When both DR3 and DR4 are inherited, the relative risk for the development of diabetes is increased 7–10-fold. Analysis of DNA polymorphisms after digestion by specific restriction endonucleases has revealed further heterogeneity in the HLA-DR region among individuals with and without diabetes despite the possession of both DR3 or DR4 markers, suggesting a yet to be defined "susceptibility" locus within these markers.

In whites, at least one major susceptibility locus may reside in the $DQ\beta_1$ gene. The homozygous absence of aspartic acid at position 57 of the HLA DQ β-chain (nonAsp/nonAsp) confers an approximately 100-fold relative risk for the development of type 1 diabetes. Those who are heterozygous with a single aspartic acid at position 57 (nonAsp/Asp) are far less likely to acquire diabetes and only marginally more susceptible than individuals who have aspartic acid on both DQ β-chains, that is, homozygous Asp/Asp. Thus, the presence of aspartic acid at one or both alleles of DQ β protects against the development of autoimmune diabetes. Indeed, the incidence of type 1 DM in any given population appears to be proportional to the gene frequency of nonAsp alleles in that population. In addition, arginine at position 52 of the DQ β-chain confers marked susceptibility to type 1 DM. Position 57 of the DQ β and position 52 of DQ β are at critical locations of the HLA molecule that permit or prevent antigen presentation to T-cell receptors and activate the autoimmune cascade. However, type 1 DM seems unique among autoimmune diseases, in that, in addition to forming susceptibility, certain MHC haplotypes provide significant protection. The HLA-DRB1*0301, HLA-DRB1*0401, HLA-DQB1*0302, and HLA-DQA1*0301 alleles of MHC (IDDM1) confer high-risk susceptibility in humans, whereas other alleles such as HLA-DRB1*0403, HLA-DQB1*0602, and HLA-DQA1*0102 are negatively associated with type 1 DM and may confer resistance.

The observation that 20% of individuals from Europe or the United States carry protective HLA-DR2 haplotype, yet fewer than 1% of children with type 1 DM are DR2 (DQB1*0602) positive, signifies the importance of genetics in disease development.

Type 1 DM represents a heterogeneous and polygenic disorder. About 20 non-HLA loci contributing to disease susceptibility have been identified. The function of only two non-HLA loci is known. IDDM2 on chromosome 11p5.5 is a polymorphic region that maps to a variable number of tandem minisatellite repeats (VNTR), with short class I VNTR alleles predisposing to type 1 DM and the longer class III alleles providing dominant protective effect. This locus contributes about 10% toward disease susceptibility. Another locus associated with type 1 DM in some populations is IDDM12 on chromosome 2q33, which maps close to two T-cell markers involved in the T-cell activation: cytotoxic T lymphocyte–associated protein4 (CTLA-4) and CD28. Studies in Italian and Spanish families have shown that a polymorphism at CTL4 gene (A-G transition at position 49 of exon 1) called G allele, is preferentially transmitted to the affected siblings.

Factors other than pure inheritance of HLA markers or other genes must also be involved in producing diabetes. For example, HLA-DR3 or -DR4 is found in approximately 50% of the general population, and (nonAsp/nonAsp) is found in approximately 20% of nondiabetic whites in the United States, yet the risk for type 1 DM in these subjects is only one tenth of that in an HLA identical sibling of an index case possessing these markers. Even siblings sharing only one haplotype have a 6–10-fold greater risk of development of type 1 DM compared with the normal population. In addition, about 10% of patients with type 1 DM do not possess either HLA-DR3 or -DR4, although most white diabetic patients lack at least one aspartic acid at position 57 of the DQ β chain. The concordance rate among identical twins of whom one has type 1 DM is only 30–50%, suggesting the participation of environmental triggering factors or other genetic factors such as the postnatal selection of certain autoreactive T-cell clones that bear receptors recognizing "self." This postnatal process occurs within the thymus and implies that identical twins are not identical with respect to the T-cell receptor repertoire they possess.

Type 1 DM among African Americans is associated with the same HLA genes as it is in whites. If a sibling shares both HLA-D haplotypes with an index case, the risk for type 1 DM in that individual is 12–20%; for a sibling sharing one haplotype, the risk is 5–7%; with no haplotypes in common, the risk is only 1–2%. It can be assumed that in whites, the overall risks to siblings is approximately 6% if the proband is younger than 10 yr of age and 3% if the proband is older at the time of diagnosis. The risk to offspring of a diabetic parent is 2–5%, with the higher risk occurring in the offspring of a diabetic father. In African Americans, these risks are only one half to two thirds of those in whites.

ENVIRONMENT. Factors such as infections, chemicals, seasonality, and geographic locations have been suspected of contributing to differences in the incidence and prevalence of type 1 DM in various ethnic populations. No dominant environmental agent or agents responsible for triggering type 1 DM have been uncovered. Environmental risk determinants that have been vigorously investigated can be classified into viral infections, early infant diet, and chemicals.

Viral Infections and Vaccinations. Although the etiologic role of viral infections in human type 1 DM is controversial, coxsackie B3, coxsackie B4, cytomegalovirus, rubella, and mumps can infect human β cells. Only congenital rubella infection is associated with diabetes in later life. It is estimated that 10–12% of patients infected with congenital rubella develop type 1 DM and that up to 40% develop impaired glucose tolerance. The diabetes induced by rubella resembles type 1 DM because it is associated to HLA-DR3 and/or HLA-DR4 and is mediated by immune responses against β-cell antigens. There has been no convincing correlation between timing of childhood vaccinations and risk of type 1 DM.

Seasonal Factors. Seasonal and long-term cyclic variations occur in the incidence of IDDM. Newly recognized cases appear with greater frequency in the autumn and winter months in the northern and southern hemispheres. Seasonal variations are most apparent in the adolescent years. Attempts to link a pattern of long-term cyclicity with the incidence of mumps or other viral infections have not been successful.

Dietary Factors. Feeding cow's milk to animal models of type 1 DM has been associated with the development of diabetes in these animals. The likely mechanism is the molecular mimicry between a 17-amino acid peptide of the bovine serum albumin and the islet antigen 69. Even though there appears to be a strong relationship between cow's milk consumption and national incidence of diabetes in children, the role of cow's milk in human type 1 DM is controversial. N-nitroso compounds, derived from the conversion of nitrates from dietary vegetables and meat in the gut, have also been involved in the development of diabetes. The role of these compounds as a significant risk factor in the pathogenesis of diabetes remains controversial.

Chemicals. Drugs such as alloxan, streptozotocin (STZ), pentamidine, and Vacor are directly cytotoxic to β cells and cause diabetes in experimental animals and humans. In susceptible animals, multiple subdiabetogenic doses of STZ induce primary β-cell damage and subsequently immune responses against β cells, providing mechanistic evidence that a β-cell insult can elicit specific autoimmunity. Autoimmunity against β cells has also been reported in humans after intoxication with the human rodenticide Vacor.

Figure 583–2 summarizes current concepts of the etiology of type 1 DM as an autoimmune disease, with a genetic component inherited through the HLA system, in which autoimmune destruction of β cells is triggered by an as yet unidentified agent. The slope of decline in insulin varies, and the point at which clinical features appear corresponds to an approximately 80% destruction of the insulin secretory reserve. This process may take months to years, usually in adolescent and older patients, and weeks in the very young patient. Higher titers of spontaneous autoinsulin antibodies and islet cell antibodies are characteristic of the more active islet cell destruction typically seen in the younger patient and may prove useful in predicting evolving diabetes.

Environmental agents may serve as modifiers of disease pathogenesis rather than triggers. These include infectious agents, dietary factors, environmental toxins as well as other influencing variables such as sanitation, health care access, and vaccinations. Multiple infections during the 1st yr of life are associated with a decreased risk of type 1 DM. Increased risk has been associated with perinatal infections coupled with a protective effect of preschool daycare with a possible link to the age-dependent modifying effect of infections on the developing immune system. Environmental exposures could act to promote and attenuate disease during different stages of development, with effect dependent on both timing and quantity of encounters.

Pathogenesis

AUTOIMMUNE INJURY. Genetic predisposition and environmental factors lead to initiation of an autoimmune process against the pancreatic islets. It is also assumed that the autoimmune response needs to be sustained and diversified against multiple target proteins (epitope spreading) for prolonged periods of time to overcome protective mechanisms. The autoimmune attack on the pancreatic islets leads to a gradual and progressive destruction of β cells with loss of insulin secretion. It is estimated that, at the onset of clinical diabetes, 80–90% of the pancreatic islets are destroyed. Regeneration of new islets has

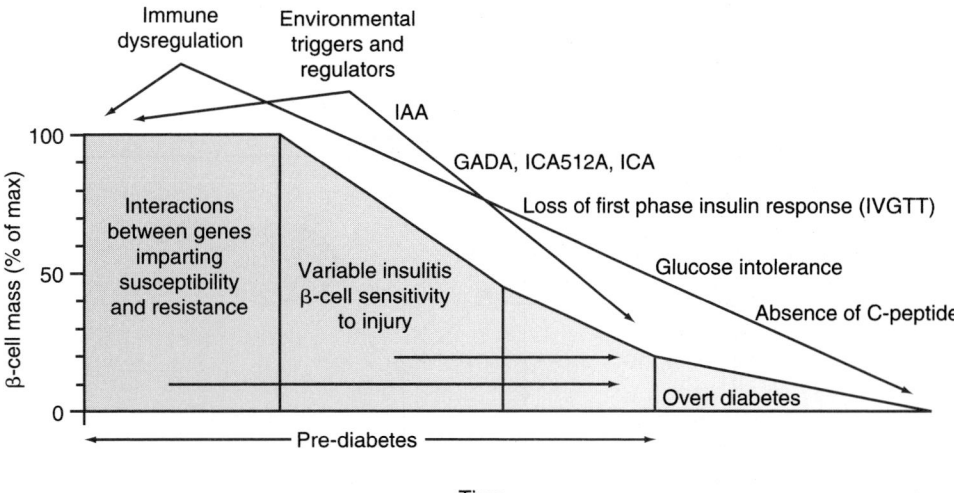

FIGURE 583–2. Proposed model of the pathogenesis and natural history of type 1 DM. IVGTT = intravenous glucose tolerance test; GADA = glutamic acid decarboxylase antibody; IAA = insulin autoantibodies; ICA = islet cell antibody. (Adapted from Atkinson MA, Eisenbarth GS: Type 1 diabetes: New perspectives on disease pathogenesis and treatment. *Lancet* 2001; 358:221–9.)

been detected at onset of type 1 DM, and it is thought to be responsible for the honeymoon phase (a transient decrease in insulin requirement associated with improved β-cell function). In young diabetic children, especially those of DR3/DR4 haplotypes, the destruction of β cells is almost complete during the first 3 yr after the onset of hyperglycemia, whereas in older patients the β-cell destruction may take up to 10 yr. These observations indicate that the impairment of β-cell function at the onset of hyperglycemia is the consequence of both β-cell destruction and cytokine-mediated inhibition of insulin secretion. The distinction between β-cell destruction and inhibition of insulin secretion is important, since a fraction of β-cells may be recovered providing that effective therapeutic interventions can be implemented at the onset of the disease. Once islet cell autoimmunity has begun, progression to islet cell destruction is quite variable, with some patients rapidly progressing to clinical diabetes while others remain in a nonprogressive state. Antigenic/epitope spreading of the autoantibody responses is an important marker of impending progression; those with but a single autoantibody progress slowly, whereas those with autoantibodies to multiple antigens most often progress rapidly. Most individuals progressing to overt diabetes express multiple anti-islet antibodies (GAD65, ICA512/IA-2, and IAA) by the time of diabetes onset. The autoimmune response against the pancreatic β cells is believed to consist of four phases: (1) environmental insult, (2) priming of T cells, (3) T-cell differentiation, and (4) β-cell destruction (Fig. 583–3).

Environment. Pathogens can initiate or precipitate the self-reactive process by three possible mechanisms. First, molecular mimicry between viral proteins and self-proteins expressed by β cells (i.e., PC2 protein of coxsackie virus and GAD65, rubella virus capsid protein and 52-kd islet protein, cytomegalovirus and 38-kd islet protein). Second, after acute β-cell infection or β-cell damage induced by cytokines during inflammatory responses against pathogens, the released proteins can be taken up by antigen presenting cells (APCs), which present the self-peptides to T cells. Third, cytokines secreted during a viral infection can upregulate the expression of co-stimulatory and MHC molecules on the surface of the facultative or nonfacultative APCs, enabling them to present self-peptides in immunogenic form to T cells. Exposure to microbial and viral pathogens early in life may also be protective against the development of type 1 DM.

Priming of T Cells. The presentation of β cell–specific autoantigens by APC macrophages or dendritic cells [DCs]) to CD4 T helper (Th) cells in association with MHC class II molecules is considered the first step in the initiation of disease process (see Fig. 583–3). Macrophages secrete interleukin (IL)-12, stimulating CD4 T cells to secret interferon-γ and IL-2. Interferon-γ stimulates other resting macrophages to release, in turn, other cytokines such as IL-1β, tumor necrosis factor (TNF)-α, and free radicals (NO, O^-_2), which are toxic to pancreatic β cells. During this process, cytokines induce the migration of β-cell autoantigen-specific CD8 cytotoxic cells. On recognizing specific autoantigens on β cells in association with class 1 molecule, these CD8 cytotoxic T cells cause β-cell damage by releasing perforin and granzyme and by Fas-mediated apoptosis of the β cells.

Differentiation of T Cells. Immune-mediated diabetes is associated with polyclonal populations of T cells reactive against multiple β-cell antigens. Thus T cells reactive against specific glutamic acid decarboxylase 65 (GAD65), proinsulin, tyrosine phosphatase (ICA512/IA-2), heat shock protein 60 (hsp60), and islet antigen 69 (ICA69) have been detected in type 1 DM patients. Among these antigens, GAD65 appears to be the early target of T cells. Because GAD65 is an intracellular protein, β-cell injury may be required to initiate the autoimmune process. The association between MHC class II and type 1 DM strongly suggests a pathogenic role of CD4 T cells, because MHC class II molecules are required for thymic education of precursors and for the restriction of CD4 T-cell responses. There is a correlation between the binding affinity of the peptide to MHC class II and antigenicity. Whereas the type 1 DM protective class II molecules bind self-peptides with high affinity and delete thymic precursors, type 1 DM–susceptible class II molecules bind self-peptides with low affinity, leading to a failure of central tolerance and escape of self-reactive T cells to periphery. T cells are differentiated into Th1 and Th2 effector cells. Th1 cells protect against intracellular microbes and parasites, and mediate delayed-type hypersensitivity and acute allograft rejection, whereas Th2 cells regulate humoral immune responses (IgE and IgG1), mediate allergic reactions, and protect against organ-specific autoimmune diseases such as type 1 DM, multiple sclerosis, thyroiditis, and Crohn disease. CD4 Th1 cells secrete IL-2 and interferon-γ and are associated with cell-mediated immunity. Th2 cells secrete IL-4 and IL-10, and are associated with humoral and anti-inflammatory responses. A subset of regulatory T cells known as natural killer T (NKT) cells prevents diabetes by secretion of IL-4 and/or IL-10. The regulatory Th3 (CD4) cells also tend to exert antidiabetogenic effect by the secretion of the suppressive cytokine tumor growth factor-β. Functional abnormalities in these regulatory cells may also play a role in the pathogenesis of type 1 DM.

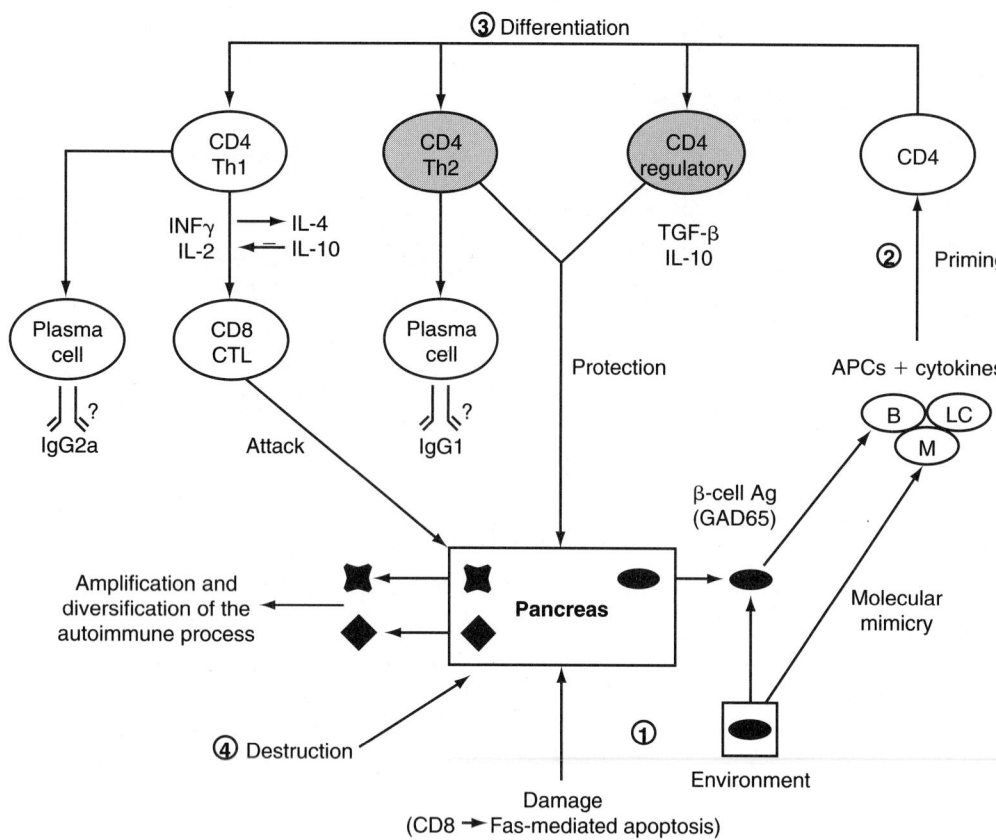

FIGURE 583–3. Schematic representation of the autoimmune response against the pancreatic β cells. An insult on the pancreas leads to the release of β-cell antigens (GAD65), which are taken up by antigen-presenting cells (APCs) and the epitopes presented to the CD4 T cells. Type and stages of activation of APCs as well as the cytokine environment, in which the CD4 T cell priming takes place, dictate the differentiation of autoreactive T cells toward diabetogenic T helper-1 (Th1) cells, Th2 cells, or antigen-specific regulatory T cells. A predominant Th1 autoimmune response results in the recruitment and differentiation of cytotoxic CD8 cells, which attack the pancreatic β cells, leading to a massive release of β-cell antigens, epitope spreading, and destruction of the pancreatic islets. B, B cell; DC, dendritic cell; M, macrophage; CTL, cytotoxic cell; TGF-β, tumor growth factor-β; INFγ, interferon-γ; IL, interleukin. (Adapted from Casares S, Brumeanu TD: Insights into the pathogenesis of type 1 diabetes: A hint for novel immunospecific therapies. *Curr Molec Med* 2001;1:357–78.)

β-Cell Destruction. Mononuclear cell infiltration into the pancreatic islets (insulitis) and a reduction of insulin-producing β cells are recognized as key pathologic features of type 1 DM. Pancreatic biopsy samples obtained from prediabetic patients and from those with recent-onset type 1 DM have shown various degrees of reduction in β-cell volume in all patients, yet insulitis could not be identified in about 50%. When insulitis is detected, the infiltrate is composed of CD8 and CD4 T cells, B cells, and macrophages, with a predominance of CD8 T cells. Inflamed islet cells show hyperexpression of MHC class I molecules. The degree of insulitis and hyperexpression of MHC class I molecules correlates with deteriorating glycemic control and GAD65 antibody levels. Fas is detected on β cells within inflamed cells, whereas islet-infiltrating mononuclear cells express Fas ligand. An interaction between Fas on β cells and Fas ligand on infiltrating cells might trigger selective apoptotic β-cell death in inflamed cells, leading to type 1 DM.

Prediction and Prevention. Autoimmunity precedes clinical type 1 DM, and indicators of maturing autoimmune responses may be useful markers for disease prediction. Individuals at risk for type 1 DM can be identified using a combination of genetic, immunologic, and metabolic markers. The most informative genetic locus, HLA class II, confers about half of the total genetic risk but has a low positive predictive value (PPV) when used in the general population. Autoantibodies provide a practical readout of β-cell autoimmunity, are easily sampled in venous blood, and have become the mainstay of type 1 DM prediction efforts. Initially described in terms of the islet cell antibody (ICA) immunofluorescence assay on pancreatic sections, autoantibod-

ies are described in terms of defined ICA target antigens, such as insulin (IAA), glutamic acid dehydrogenase (GAD65), and the tyrosine phosphatase homologue ICA512/IA-2.

Autoantibodies are useful for detecting developing type 1 DM in close relatives of diabetic patients whose risk for diabetes is about 3.5–5.0%. However, most cases are sporadic rather than familial, necessitating general population screening. This has been difficult, in part, because the observed autoantibody prevalence greatly exceeds the low disease prevalence in nonrelatives, leading to high false-positive rates. Single defined autoantibody (d-aab) positivity may result from persistent memory B cells in lymph nodes or bone marrow after brief transient insulitis not resulting in clinical diabetes. It has been suggested that because different d-aab appear sequentially over time during prediabetes, the presence of multiple d-aab may mark more persistent insulitis and greater diabetes risk. In the first-degree relatives of patients with type 1 DM, the number of positive d-aab can help estimate the risk of developing type 1 DM: low risk (single d-aab: PPV of 2–6%), moderate risk (2 d-aab: PPV of 21–40%), and high risk (>2 d-aab: PPV of 59%–80%) over a 5-yr period. In children carrying the type 1 DM highest-risk genotype (HLA-DQB1*0201-DQA1*05/DQB1*0302-DQA1*03), insulitis is almost 10 times more frequent (PPV 21%) than in children with other genotypes (PPV 2.2%). On the other hand, in general populations of children, some studies have suggested a very low overall PPV for single d-aab (0–0.5%), whereas overall PPV for multiple (≥2) d-aab has been reported to be as high as 19–50% (high risk) over a 2–8 yr period.

There is no known agent capable of preventing type 1 DM. There are several obstacles to finding a plausible prevention strategy. These include (1) ethical issues surrounding prediction, (2) treatment dilemma, (3) selection of populations at risk and treatment strategies, and (4) finding new preventive agents. The ability to predict future cases of type 1 DM, although a major benefit to knowledge about the natural history of this disease, in the absence of a preventing agent raises ethical considerations related to induction of stress, lifestyle changes, and potential effects on insurability.

A second challenge facing the diabetes prevention efforts is treatment dilemma. It is well recognized that the most effective interventions are those that are started early in the autoimmune process. However, the process of disease prediction, using immunologic, genetic, and metabolic markers, is most accurate in the period close to the onset of overt diabetes. Consequently, many health care providers and researchers are faced with ethical and clinical conflicts wherein the most effective forms of therapy might involve treatment of individuals in a period in which disease prediction is less accurate. Also, it has been very difficult to find safe and benign forms of therapy that can be used in individuals who may never develop type 1 DM.

Another obstacle is the selection of type of populations and appropriate therapeutic approaches. Attempts to prevent type 1 DM need to address therapy of high-risk population (relatives of type 1 DM patients with positive immune markers) versus the general population with low risk of developing diabetes. Whereas clinical trials in high-risk populations may be more efficient and cost-effective, the general population approach may be more important because about 85% of new cases of type 1 DM have no family history of the disease. In the general population, a safe and benign therapy capable of interrupting adverse immune events and environmental agents or alterations in lifestyle providing avoidance of disease risk factors would ideally be implemented. There is a considerable cost associated with screening general populations. Vitamin D supplementation of infants and maternal intake of cod liver oil during pregnancy have been shown to be associated with the reduced risk of type 1 DM in children. This protective effect of vitamin D is believed to be due to its immunosuppressive action, reducing lymphocyte proliferation and cytokine production. Therefore, age-appropriate vitamin D supplementation of all infants can be a relatively inexpensive strategy in the general population.

Another issue is the lack of an obvious therapeutic agent for diabetes prevention. For instance, the United States Diabetes Prevention Trial I (DPT-I) was started in 1994 to determine whether antigen-based therapies with insulin (i.e., low-dose parenteral insulin therapy to high-risk relatives or oral insulin vs placebo to intermediate-risk relatives) would prevent or delay the onset of diabetes. Therapy did not provide evidence for disease prevention, and the 2-yr results of oral insulin and low-dose parenteral insulin will be released soon.

IMMUNOTHERAPY IN NEW-ONSET TYPE 1 DM. Type 1 DM is a T-cell–mediated autoimmune disease that begins, in many cases, 3–5 yr before the onset of clinical symptoms, continues after diagnosis, and can recur after islet transplantation. The effector mechanisms responsible for the destruction of β-cells involve cytotoxic T cells as well as soluble T-cell products, such as interferon-γ and TNF-α. Such observations have led to clinical trials with immunomodulatory drugs such as cyclosporine, azathioprine, prednisone, and antithymocyte globulin, which were shown to cause transient improvement in clinical measures and to increase the rate of non–insulin-requiring remissions when initiated soon after diagnosis. Unfortunately, the toxic effects of such drugs, concern about the risk associated with immune suppression, and the need for continuous treatment in an otherwise healthy, young population limit the use of these agents.

Immunotherapy using modified monoclonal antibody against CD3 hOKT3γ1 has efficacy in patients with renal-allograft rejection. Treatment with hOKT3γ1 infusions mitigates the deterio-

ration in insulin production and improves metabolic control during the 1st yr of type 1 DM in a majority of patients. The side effects include transient fever, gastrointestinal symptoms, and pruritic rash, without any long-term toxic effects up to 2 yr. The mechanisms of action of the anti-CD3 monoclonal antibody may involve direct effects on pathogenic T cells and/or the induction of populations of regulatory cells.

Pathophysiology. Insulin performs a critical role in the storage and retrieval of cellular fuel. Its secretion in response to feeding is exquisitely modulated by the interplay of neural, hormonal, and substrate-related mechanisms to permit controlled disposition of ingested foodstuff as energy for immediate or future use. Insulin levels must be lowered to then mobilize stored energy during the fasted state. Thus, in normal metabolism, there are regular swings between the postprandial, high-insulin anabolic state and the fasted, low-insulin catabolic state that affect liver, muscle, and adipose tissue (Table 583–3). Type 1 DM is a progressive low-insulin catabolic state in which feeding does not reverse but rather exaggerates these catabolic processes. With moderate insulinopenia, glucose utilization by muscle and fat decreases and postprandial hyperglycemia appears. At even lower insulin levels, the liver produces excessive glucose via glycogenolysis and gluconeogenesis, and fasting hyperglycemia begins. Hyperglycemia produces an osmotic diuresis (glucosuria) when the renal threshold is exceeded (180 mg/dL; 10 mmol/L). The resulting loss of calories and electrolytes, as well as the persistent dehydration, produce a physiologic stress with hypersecretion of stress hormones (epinephrine, cortisol, growth hormone, and glucagon). These hormones, in turn, contribute to the metabolic decompensation by further impairing insulin secretion (epinephrine), by antagonizing its action (epinephrine, cortisol, growth hormone), and by promoting glycogenolysis, gluconeogenesis, lipolysis, and ketogenesis (glucagon, epinephrine, growth hormone, and cortisol) while decreasing glucose utilization and glucose clearance (epinephrine, growth hormone, cortisol).

The combination of insulin deficiency and elevated plasma values of the counter-regulatory hormones is also responsible for accelerated lipolysis and impaired lipid synthesis, with resulting increased plasma concentrations of total lipids, cholesterol, triglycerides, and free fatty acids. The hormonal interplay of insulin deficiency and glucagon excess shunts the free fatty acids into ketone body formation; the rate of formation of these ketone bodies, principally β-hydroxybutyrate and acetoacetate, exceeds the capacity for peripheral utilization and renal excretion. Accumulation of these ketoacids results in

TABLE 583–3.	**Influence of Feeding (High Insulin) or of Fasting (Low Insulin) on Some Metabolic Processes in Liver, Muscle, and Adipose Tissue***	
	High Plasma Insulin (Postprandial State)	**Low Plasma Insulin (Fasted State)**
Liver	Glucose uptake	Glucose production
	Glycogen synthesis	Glycogenolysis
	Absence of gluconeogenesis	Gluconeogenesis
	Lipogenesis	Absence of lipogenesis
	Absence of ketogenesis	Ketogenesis
Muscle	Glucose uptake	Absence of glucose uptake
	Glucose oxidation	Fatty acid and ketone oxidation
	Glycogen synthesis	Glycogenolysis
	Protein synthesis	Proteolysis and amino acid release
Adipose tissue	Glucose uptake	Absence of glucose uptake
	Lipid synthesis	Lipolysis and fatty acid release
	Triglyceride uptake	Absence of triglyceride uptake

*Insulin is considered to be the major factor governing these metabolic processes. Diabetes mellitus may be viewed as a permanent low-insulin state that, untreated, results in exaggerated fasting.

metabolic acidosis (diabetic ketoacidosis, DKA) and compensatory rapid deep breathing in an attempt to excrete excess CO_2 (Kussmaul respiration). Acetone, formed by nonenzymatic conversion of acetoacetate, is responsible for the characteristic fruity odor of the breath. Ketones are excreted in the urine in association with cations and thus further increase losses of water and electrolyte. With progressive dehydration, acidosis, hyperosmolality, and diminished cerebral oxygen utilization, consciousness becomes impaired, and the patient ultimately becomes comatose.

Clinical Manifestations. As diabetes develops, symptoms steadily increase, reflecting the decreasing β-cell mass, worsening insulinopenia, progressive hyperglycemia, and eventual ketoacidosis. Initially, when only insulin reserve is limited, occasional hyperglycemia occurs. When the serum glucose increases above the renal threshold, intermittent polyuria or nocturia begins. With further β-cell loss, chronic hyperglycemia causes a more persistent diuresis, often with nocturnal enuresis; polydipsia becomes more apparent. Female patients may develop monilial vaginitis due to the chronic glucosuria. Calories are lost in the urine (glucosuria), triggering a compensatory hyperphagia. If this hyperphagia does not keep pace with the glucosuria, loss of body fat ensues, with clinical weight loss and diminished subcutaneous fat stores. An average healthy 10-yr-old child consumes about 50% of 2,000 daily calories as carbohydrate. As that child becomes diabetic, daily losses of water and glucose may be 5 L and 250 g, respectively, representing 1,000 calories, or 50%, of the average daily caloric intake. Despite the child's compensatory increased intake of food, the body starves, because unused calories are lost in the urine.

When extremely low insulin levels are reached, ketoacids accumulate. At this point, the child quickly deteriorates. Ketoacids produce abdominal discomfort, nausea, and emesis, preventing oral replacement of urinary water losses. Dehydration accelerates, causing weakness or orthostasis—but polyuria persists. As in any hyperosmotic state, the degree of dehydration may be clinically underestimated because intravascular volume is conserved at the expense of intracellular volume. Ketoacidosis exacerbates prior symptoms and leads to Kussmaul respirations (deep heavy rapid breathing), fruity breath odor (acetone), diminished neurocognitive function, and possible coma. About 20–40% of children with new-onset diabetes progress to DKA before diagnosis.

This entire progression happens much more quickly (over a few weeks) in younger children, probably due to a more aggressive autoimmune destruction of β cells. In infants, most of the weight loss is acute water loss, because they will not have had a prolonged caloriuria when diagnosed, and there will be an increased incidence of DKA at diagnosis. In adolescents, the course is usually more prolonged (over months), and most of the weight loss represents fat loss due to prolonged starvation. Additional weight loss due to acute dehydration may occur just before diagnosis. In any child, the progression of symptoms may be accelerated by the stress of an intercurrent illness or trauma, when counter-regulatory (stress) hormones overwhelm the limited insulin secretory capacity.

Diagnosis. The diagnosis of type 1 diabetes is usually straightforward *if considered in the differential diagnosis*. Although most symptoms are nonspecific, the most important clue is an inappropriate polyuria in any child with dehydration, poor weight gain, or "the flu." Hyperglycemia, glucosuria, and ketonuria can be determined quickly. Nonfasting blood glucose greater than 200 mg/dL (11.1 mmol/L) with typical symptoms is diagnostic with or without ketonuria. In the obese child, type 2 diabetes must be considered (see later text). Once hyperglycemia is confirmed, it is prudent to determine whether DKA is present (especially if ketonuria is found) and to evaluate electrolyte abnormalities—even if signs of dehydration are minimal.

A baseline glycohemoglobin (HbA_{1c}) allows an estimate of the duration of hyperglycemia and provides an initial value by which to compare the effectiveness of subsequent therapy.

In the nonobese child, testing for autoimmunity to β cells is not necessary. Other autoimmunities associated with type 1 diabetes should be screened, including celiac disease (tissue transglutaminase IgA and total IgA) and thyroiditis (antithyroid peroxidase and antithyroglobulin antibodies). Because significant physiologic distress can disrupt the pituitary-thyroid axis, a free thyroxine (T_4) and TSH should be checked after the child is stable for a few weeks.

Rarely, a child has transient hyperglycemia with glucosuria while under substantial physical stress. This usually resolves permanently during recovery from the stressors. However, such stress hyperglycemia could reflect a limited insulin reserve temporarily revealed by counter-regulatory hormones. A child with temporary hyperglycemia should therefore be monitored for the development of symptoms of persistent hyperglycemia and tested if such symptoms occur. Formal testing in a child who remains clinically asymptomatic is not necessary.

Routine screening procedures, such as postprandial determinations of blood glucose or screening oral glucose tolerance tests, have yielded low detection rates in healthy, asymptomatic children, even among those considered at risk, such as siblings of diabetic children. Accordingly, such screening procedures are not recommended in children.

DIABETIC KETOACIDOSIS. DKA is the end result of the metabolic abnormalities resulting from a severe deficiency of insulin or insulin effectiveness. The latter occurs during stress as counter-regulatory hormones block insulin action. DKA occurs in 20–40% of children with new-onset diabetes, and in children with known diabetes who omit insulin doses or who do not successfully manage an intercurrent illness. DKA may be arbitrarily classified as mild, moderate, or severe (Table 583–4), and the range of symptoms depends on the depth of ketoacidosis. There is a large ketonuria, an increased ion gap, a decreased serum bicarbonate (or total CO_2) and pH, and an elevated effective serum osmolality indicating hypertonic dehydration.

Treatment. Therapy is tailored to the degree of insulinopenia at presentation. Most children with new diabetes (60–80%) have mild to moderate symptoms, minimal dehydration with no history of emesis, and have not progressed to ketoacidosis. Once DKA has resolved in the newly diagnosed child, therapy is transitioned to that described for children with nonketotic onset. Children with previously diagnosed diabetes who develop DKA are usually transitioned to their previous insulin regimen.

NEW ONSET DIABETES WITHOUT KETOACIDOSIS. Excellent diabetes control involves many goals: to maintain a balance between tight glucose control and avoiding hypoglycemia, to eliminate polyuria and nocturia, to prevent ketoacidosis, and to

TABLE 583–4. **Classification of Diabetic Ketoacidosis**

	Normal	Mild	Moderate	Severe[†]
CO_2 (mEq/L, venous)*	20–28	16–20	10–15	<10
pH (venous)*	7.35–7.45	7.25–7.35	7.15–7.25	< 7.15
Clinical	No change	Oriented, alert but fatigued	Kussmaul respirations; oriented but sleepy; arousable	Kussmaul or depressed respirations; sleepy to depressed sensorium to coma

*CO_2 and pH measurement are method dependent; normal ranges may vary.
[†]Severe hypernatremia (corrected Na > 150 mEq/L) would also be classified as severe DKA.

permit normal growth and development with minimal effect on lifestyle. Therapy encompasses initiation and adjustment of insulin, extensive teaching of the child and caretakers, and reestablishing the routine of life. Each aspect should be addressed early in the overall care for the family. Ideally, therapy can begin in the outpatient setting, with complete team staffing by a pediatric endocrinologist, experienced nursing staff, dietitians with training as diabetes educators, and a social worker. Close contact between the diabetes team and family must be assured. Otherwise, initial therapy should be done in the hospital setting.

INSULIN. Several factors influence the initial daily insulin dose per kilogram of body weight. The dose is usually higher in pubertal children. It is higher in those who have to restore greater deficits of body glycogen, protein, and fat stores and who, therefore, have higher initial caloric capacity. On the other hand, most children with new-onset diabetes have some residual β-cell function (the "honeymoon" period), which reduces exogenous insulin needs. Children with longstanding diabetes and no insulin reserve require about 0.7 units/kg/d if prepubertal, 1.0 unit/kg/d at midpuberty, and 1.2 units/kg/d by the end of puberty. A reasonable dose in the newly diagnosed child, then, is about 60–70% of the full replacement dose based on pubertal status. The optimal insulin dose can only be determined empirically, with frequent self-monitored blood glucose levels and insulin adjustment by the diabetes team. Residual β-cell function usually fades within a few months and is reflected as a steady increase in insulin requirements and wider glucose excursions.

The initial insulin *schedule* should be directed toward the optimal degree of glucose control in an attempt to duplicate the activity of the β cell. There are inherent limits to our ability to mimic the β cell. Exogenous insulin does not have a first pass to the liver, whereas 50% of pancreatic portal insulin is taken up by the liver, a key organ for the disposal of glucose; absorption of an exogenous dose continues despite hypoglycemia, whereas endogenous insulin release ceases and serum levels quickly lower with a normally rapid clearance; and absorption rate from an injection varies by injection site and patient activity level, whereas endogenous insulin is secreted directly into the portal circulation. Despite these fundamental physiologic differences, quite acceptable glucose control can be obtained with new insulin analogs used in a basal-bolus regimen, that is, with slow onset, long duration background insulin for between meal glucose control, and rapid-onset insulin at each meal.

All preanalog insulins form hexamers, which must dissociate into monomers subcutaneously before being absorbed into the circulation. Thus, a detectable effect for regular (R) insulin is delayed by 30–60 min after injection. This, in turn, requires delaying the meal 30–60 min after the injection for optimal effect—a delay rarely attained in a busy child's life. R has a wide peak and a long tail for bolus insulin (Figs. 583–4 and 583–5). This profile limits postprandial glucose control, produces prolonged peaks with excessive hypoglycemic effects between meals, and increases the risk of nighttime hypoglycemia. These unwanted between-meal effects often necessitate "feeding the insulin" with snacks and limiting the overall degree of blood glucose control. NPH and Lente insulins also have inherent limits because they do not create a peakless background insulin level (see Fig. 583–4C–E). This produces significant hypoglycemic effect during the midrange of their duration. Thus, it is often difficult to predict their interaction with fast-acting insulins. When R is combined with NPH or lente (see Fig. 583–4E), the composite insulin profile poorly mimics normal endogenous insulin secretion. There are broad areas of excessive insulin effect alternating with insufficient effect throughout the day and night.

Lispro (L) and aspart (A), insulin analogs, are absorbed much quicker because they do not form hexamers. They provide discrete pulses with little if any overlap and short tail effect. This allows better control of postmeal glucose increase and reduces between meal or nighttime hypoglycemia (Fig. 583–4A). The long-acting analog glargine (G) creates a much flatter 24-hr profile, making it easier to predict the combined effect of a rapid bolus (L or A) on top of the basal insulin, producing a more physiologic pattern of insulin effect (see Fig. 583–4A). Postprandial glucose elevations are better controlled, and between meal and nighttime hypoglycemia are reduced.

Ultralente (UL) given twice a day can provide a reasonable basal profile (see Fig. 583–5C) and is quite effective when used with lispro or aspart (see Fig. 583–4B). This combination may be used in children for whom glargine does not produce a complete 24-hr basal coverage.

The basal insulin glargine should be 25–30% of the total dose in toddlers and 40–50% in older children. The remaining portion of the total daily dose is divided evenly as bolus injections for the three meals. A simple three- or four-step dosing schedule is begun based on the blood glucose level (Table 583–5). As soon as the family is taught to calculate the carbohydrate content of meals, bolus insulin can be more accurately dosed by both the carbohydrate content of the meal as well as ambient glucose (see Table 583–5).

Frequent blood glucose monitoring and insulin adjustment are necessary in the first weeks as the child returns to routine activities and adapts to a new nutritional schedule, and as the total daily insulin requirements are determined. The major physiologic limit to tight control is hypoglycemia. Intensive control dramatically reduces the risk of long-term vascular complications; it is associated with a three-fold increase in severe hypoglycemia. Use of insulin analogs moderates but does not eliminate this problem.

Some families may be unable to administer four daily injections. In these cases, a compromise may be needed. A three-injection regimen combining the basal insulin ultralente (at breakfast and supper) with a rapid analog bolus at each meal may provide good glucose control. Further compromise to a two-injection regimen may occasionally be needed. This would require NPH or lente combined with a rapid analog bolus at breakfast and supper. However, such a schedule would provide poor coverage for lunch and early morning, and would increase the risk of hypoglycemia at midmorning and early night.

INSULIN PUMP THERAPY. Continuous subcutaneous insulin infusion (CSII) via battery-powered pumps provides a closer approximation of normal plasma insulin profiles and increased flexibility regarding timing of meals and snacks compared to conventional insulin injection regimens. Insulin pump therapy in adolescents with type 1 DM is associated with improved metabolic control and reduced risk of severe hypoglycemia without affecting psychosocial outcomes. The use of overnight CSII improves the metabolic control in children ages 7–10 yr. CSII has also been useful in toddlers. Others have demonstrated that CSII was associated with improved metabolic control in only 39% of patients and that the remainder of the patients either did not show reduction in HbA$_{1c}$ (41%) or showed deterioration in metabolic control (20%). These investigators reported a mean HbA$_{1c}$ of 8.3%, which is similar to that reported by the Diabetes Control and Complications Trial (DCCT) adolescents of 8.1%. The degree of glycemic control is mainly dependent on how closely patients adhere to the principles of diabetes self-care, regardless of the type of intensive insulin regimen. A greater proportion of patients on insulin pump therapy experience decreased seizure and hypoglycemic frequency as well as severe hypoglycemic episodes. CSII therapy is not associated with an abnormal increase in body weight.

INHALED AND ORAL INSULIN THERAPIES. Preprandial inhaled insulin is being evaluated in adults with type 1 and type 2 DM. The preliminary metabolic data is promising. Patients on premeal inhaled insulin in combination with once daily bedtime long-acting insulin (ultralente) injection achieved similar

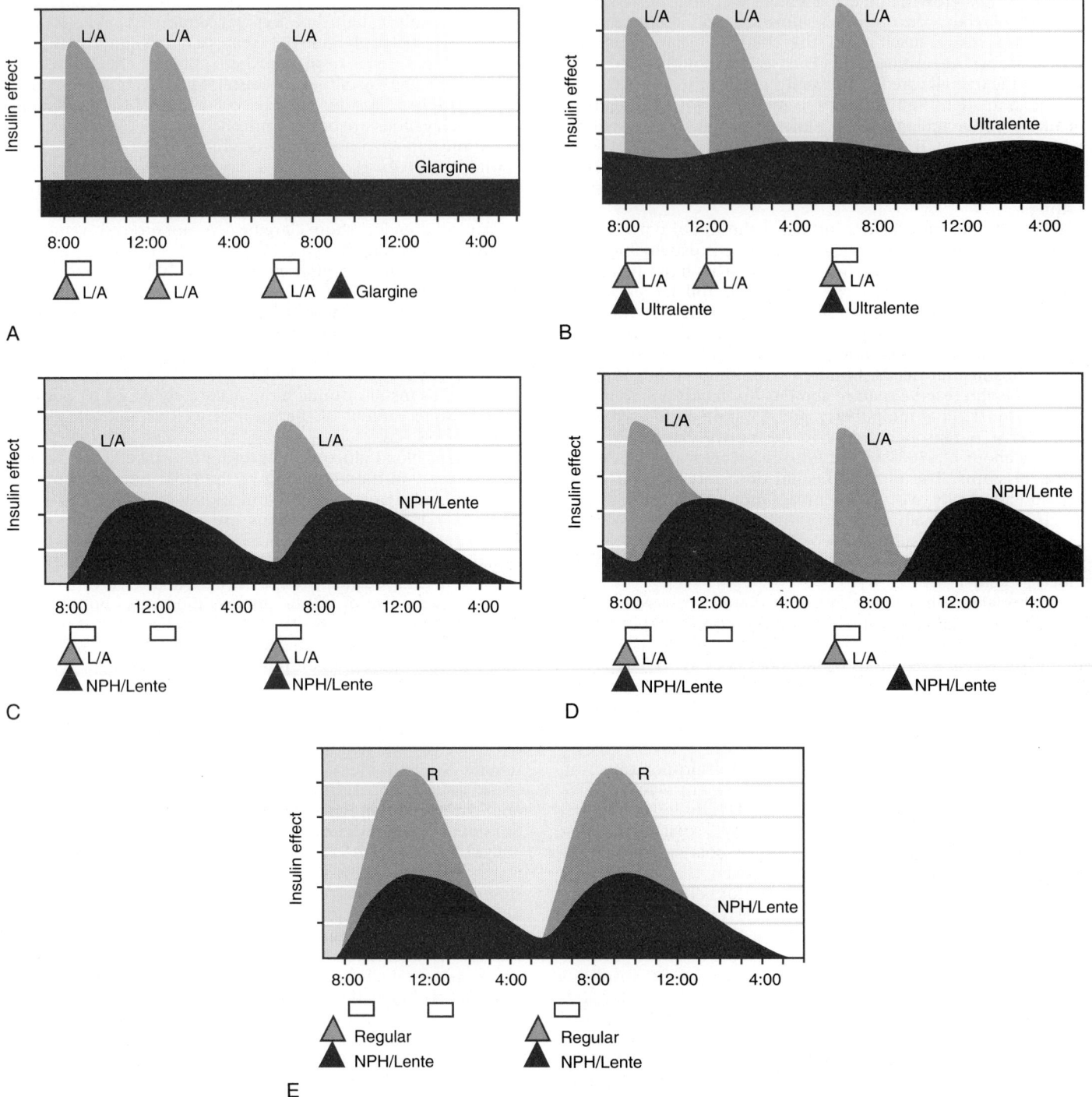

FIGURE 583–4. Approximate composite insulin effect profiles. Meals are shown as rectangles below time axis. Injections are shown as labeled triangles. L/A = lispro or aspart. Even though the fast and long-acting insulins are shaded differently to show the addition of one insulin effect to another, the profile is changed to show the combined effect. For example, in the breakfast injection in C, the quick decline of L/A effect is blunted by the rising NPH/lente effect, producing a broad tail, which slowly declines to baseline at supper. All profiles are idealized using average absorption and clearance rates. In typical clinical situations, these profiles vary among patients. A given patient has varying rates of absorption depending on the injection site, physical activity, and other variables. *A,* L or A pre-meal; glargine at bedtime. The rapid onset and short duration of L or A reduce overlap between pre-meal injections, and there is no extended nighttime action. This reduces the risk of hypoglycemia. Glargine provides a steady basal profile that simplifies prediction of bolus insulin effect. *B,* L or A pre-meal; ultralente at breakfast and supper. Ultralente produces a basal profile similar to that seen with glargine. Some excessive insulin effect, however, is seen before supper and at nighttime. *C,* L or A pre-meal; NPH or lente at breakfast and supper. The broad peak of NPH or lente produces substantial risk of hypoglycemia before lunch and during the early hours of the night. The waning insulin effect before supper and breakfast may also allow breakthrough hyperglycemia. *D,* L or A pre-meal; NPH or lente at breakfast and bedtime. Moving the evening long-acting insulin helps to cover the pre-breakfast hours, but the risk of nighttime lows persists. *E,* Regular and NPH or lente at breakfast and supper. This produces the least physiologic profile, with large excesses before lunch and during the early night, combined with poor coverage before supper and breakfast.

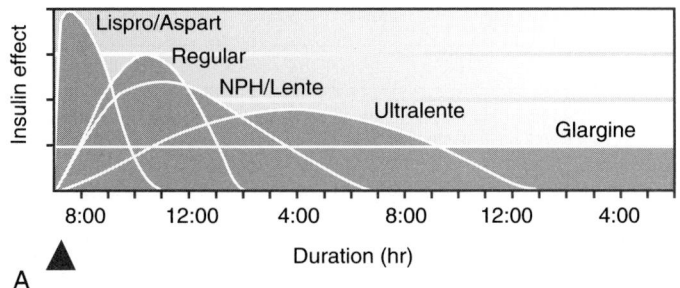

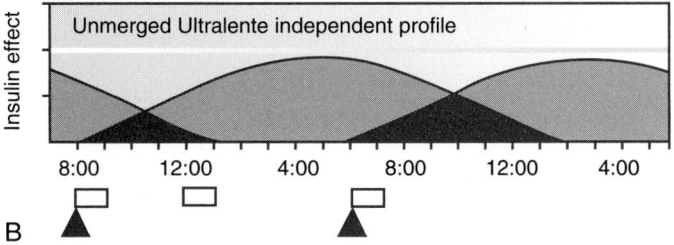

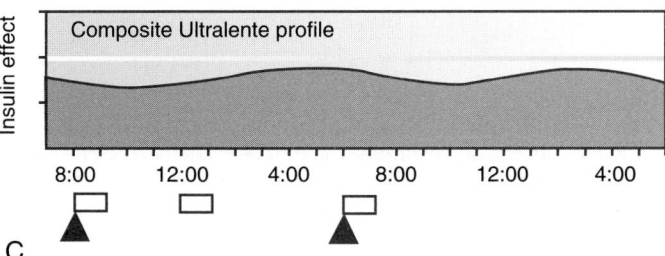

FIGURE 583–5. Approximate insulin effect profiles. *A,* The following relative peak effect and duration units are used: lispro/aspart, peak 20 for 4 hours; regular, peak 15 for 7 hours; NPH/lente, peak 12 for 12 hours; ultralente, peak 9 for 18 hours; glargine, peak 5 for 24 hours. ▲,Injection time. *B,* Two ultralente injections given at breakfast and supper. Note overlap of profiles. *C,* Composite curve showing approximate cumulative insulin effect for the two ultralente injections. This composite view is much more useful to the patient, parents, and medical personnel because it shows important combined effects of multiple insulin injections with variable absorption characteristics and overlapping durations.

metabolic control compared to patients on two to three daily injections of insulin. There was no significant difference in the frequency of hypoglycemic episodes between the two groups. There have been reports of pulmonary fibrosis in a small number of patients, necessitating further monitoring and evaluation of patients on inhaled insulin before this route of insulin administration is deemed safe.

Premeal oral insulin (Oralin) has been evaluated in comparison with oral hypoglycemic agents, mostly in patients with type 2 DM. The clinical data appears promising, but further evaluation of its efficacy in type 1 DM is needed.

BASIC EDUCATION. Therapy consists not only of initiation and adjustment of insulin dose but also of education of the patient and family. Teaching is most efficiently provided by experienced diabetes educators and nutritionists. In the acute phase, the family must learn the "basics," which includes monitoring the child's blood glucose and urine ketones, preparing and injecting the correct insulin dose subcutaneously at the proper time, recognizing and treating low blood glucose reactions, and having a basic meal plan. Most families trying to

adjust psychologically to the new diagnosis of diabetes in their child consequently have a limited ability to retain new information. Written materials covering these basic topics help the family during the first few days.

KETOACIDOSIS. Severe insulinopenia (or lack of effective insulin action) results in a physiologic cascade of events in three general pathways.

1. Excessive glucose production coupled with reduced glucose utilization raises serum glucose. This produces an osmotic diuresis, with loss of fluid and electrolytes, dehydration, and activation of the renin-angiotensin-aldosterone axis with accelerated potassium loss. If glucose elevation and dehydration are severe and persist for several hours, the risk of cerebral edema increases.

2. Increased catabolic processes result in cellular losses of sodium, potassium, and phosphate.

3. Increased release of free fatty acids from peripheral fat stores supplies substrate for hepatic ketoacid production. When ketoacids accumulate, buffer systems are depleted and a metabolic acidosis ensues. Therapy must address both the initiating event in this cascade (insulinopenia) and the subsequent physiologic disruptions.

Reversal of DKA is associated with inherent risks that include hypoglycemia, hypokalemia, and cerebral edema. Any protocol must be used with caution and close monitoring of the patient. Adjustments based on sound medical judgment may be necessary for any given level of DKA (Table 583–6).

HYPERGLYCEMIA AND DEHYDRATION. Insulin must be given at the beginning of therapy to accelerate movement of glucose into cells, to subdue hepatic glucose production, and to halt the movement of fatty acids from the periphery to the liver. However, an initial insulin bolus does not speed recovery and may increase the risk of hypokalemia and hypoglycemia. Therefore, insulin infusion is begun without a bolus at a rate of 0.1 unit/kg/h. This approximates maximal insulin output in normal subjects during an oral glucose tolerance test. Rehydration also lowers glucose levels by improving renal perfusion and enhancing renal excretion. The combination of these therapies usually causes a rapid initial decline in serum glucose levels. Once glucose goes below 180 mg/dL (10 mmol/L), the osmotic diuresis stops and rehydration accelerates without further increase in the infusion rate.

Repair of hyperglycemia occurs well before correction of acidosis. Therefore, insulin is still needed to control fatty acid release after normal glucose levels are reached. To continue the

TABLE 583–5. **Subcutaneous Insulin Dosing**

Age (years)	Target Glucose (mg/dL)	Total Daily Insulin (units/kg/d)*	Basal Insulin, % of Total Daily Dose	Bolus† Insulin Units Added per 100 mg/dL above Target	Units Added Per 15 g at Meal
0–5	100–200	0.6–0.7	25–30	0.50	0.50
5–12	80–150	0.7–1.0	40–50	0.75	0.75
12–18	80–150	1.0–1.2	40–50	1.0–2.0‡	1.0–2.0

*Newly diagnosed children in the "honeymoon" may only need 60–70% of a full replacement dose. Total daily dose per kg increases with puberty.

†Newly diagnosed children who do not use carbohydrate dosing should divide the nonbasal portion of the daily insulin dose into equal doses for each meal. A dosing scale is then added for each dose. **For example:** a 6-yr-old child who weighs 20 kg needs about (0.7 units/kg/24 hr × 20 kg) = 14 units/24 hr with 7 units (50%) as basal and 7 units as total daily bolus. Give basal as glargine at hs. Give 2 units lispro or aspart before each meal if the blood glucose is within target; subtract 1 unit if below target; add 0.75 unit for each 100 mg/dL above target (round the dose to the nearest 0.5 unit).

‡For more finessed control, extra insulin may be dadded for 50-mg/dL increments.

TABLE 583–6. Diabetic Ketoacidosis Treatment Protocol

Time	Therapy	Comments
1st hour	10–20 mL/kg IV bolus 0.9% NaCl or LR Insulin drip at 0.05 to 0.10 u/kg/hr	Quick volume expansion; may be repeated. NPO. Monitor I/O, neurologic status. Use flow sheet. Have mannitol at bedside; 1 g/kg IV push for cerebral edema.
2nd hour until DKA resolution	0.45 % NaCl: plus continue insulin drip 20 mEq/L KPhos and 20 mEq/L KAc 5% glucose if blood sugar <250 mg/dL (14 mmol/L)	IV rate $= \dfrac{85\ mL/kg + maintenance - bolus}{23\ hr}$ If K <3 mEq/L, give 0.5 to 1.0 mEq/kg as oral K solution *OR* increase IV K to 80 mEq/L
Variable	Oral intake with subcutaneous insulin	No emesis; $CO_2 \geq 16$ mEq/L; normal electrolytes

Note that the initial IV bolus is considered part of the total fluid allowed in the first 24 hr and is subtracted before calculating the IV rate.
Maintenance (24 hr) = 100 mL/kg (for the 1st 10 kg) + 50 mL/kg (for the 2nd 10 kg) + 25 mL/kg (for all remaining kg)
Sample calculation for a 30-kg child:
1st hour = 300 mL IV bolus 0.9% NaCl or LR

2nd and subsequent hours $= \dfrac{(85\ mL \times 30) + 1750\ mL - 300\ mL}{23\ hr} = \dfrac{175\ mL}{hr}$ (0.45% NaCl with 20 mEq/L KPhos and 20 mEq/L Kac)

NaCl, sodium chloride; LR, lactated Ringer solution; KPhos, potassium phosphate; KAc, potassium acetate; I/O, input and output (urine, emesis).

insulin infusion without causing hypoglycemia, glucose must be added to the infusion, usually as 5% solution. Glucose should be added when the serum glucose has decreased to about 250 mg/dL (14 mmol/L) so that there is sufficient time to adjust the infusion before the serum glucose falls further. The insulin infusion can also be lowered from the initial maximal rate once hyperglycemia has resolved.

Repair of fluid deficits must be tempered by the potential risk of cerebral edema. It is prudent to approach any child in any hyperosmotic state with cautious rehydration. The effective serum osmolality ($E_{osm} = 2 \times [Na_{uncorrected}] + [glucose]$) is an accurate index of tonicity of the body fluids, reflecting intracellular and extracellular hydration better than measured plasma osmolality. It is calculated with sodium and glucose in mmol/L. This value is usually elevated at the beginning of therapy and should steadily normalize. A rapid decline, or a slow decline to a subnormal range, may indicate an excess of free water entering the vascular space and an increasing risk of cerebral edema. Therefore, patients should not be allowed oral fluids until rehydration is well progressed and significant electrolyte shifts are no longer likely. Limited ice chips may be given as a minimal oral intake. All fluid intake and output should be closely monitored.

Calculation of fluid deficits using clinical signs is difficult in children with DKA because intravascular volume is better maintained in the hypertonic state. For any degree of tachycardia, delayed capillary refill, decreased skin temperature, or orthostatic blood pressure change, the child with DKA will be more dehydrated than the child with a normotonic fluid deficit. The protocol in Table 583–6 corrects a deficit of 85 mL/kg (8.5% dehydration) for all patients in the first 24 hr. Children with mild DKA rehydrate earlier and can be switched to oral intake, whereas those with severe DKA and a greater volume deficit require 30–36 hr with this protocol. This more gradual rehydration of the child with severe DKA is an inherent safety feature. The initial intravenous bolus (20 mL/kg of glucose-free isotonic sodium salt solution such as Ringer lactate or 0.9% sodium chloride) for all patients ensures a quick volume expansion and may be repeated if clinical improvement is not quickly seen. This bolus is given as isotonic saline because the patient is inevitably hypertonic, keeping most of the initial infusion in the intravascular space. Subsequent fluid is hypotonic to repair the free water deficit, to allow intracellular rehydration, and to allow a more appropriate replacement of ongoing hypotonic urine losses.

The initial serum sodium is usually normal or low because of the osmolar dilution of hyperglycemia and the effect of an elevated sodium-free lipid fraction. An estimate of the reconstituted, or "true," serum sodium for any given glucose level above 100 mg/dL (5.6 mmol/L) is calculated as follows:

$$[Na^+] + \left[\frac{Glucose - 100}{100}\right] \times 1.6$$

where glucose is in mg/dL, or

$$[Na^+] + \left[\frac{Glucose - 5.6}{5.6}\right] \times 1.6$$

where glucose is in mmol/L.

One should expect the sodium to increase about 1.6 mmol/L for each 100 mg/dL decline in the glucose. The corrected sodium is usually normal or slightly elevated and indicates a moderate hypernatremic dehydration. If the corrected value is greater than 150 mmol/L, severe hypernatremic dehydration may be present and may require slower fluid replacement. The sodium should steadily increase with therapy. Declining sodium may indicate excessive free water accumulation and a risk of cerebral edema.

CATABOLIC LOSSES. Both the metabolic shift to a catabolic predominance and the acidosis move potassium and phosphate from the cell to the serum. The osmotic diuresis, the kaliuretic effect of the hyperaldosteronism, and the ketonuria then accelerate renal losses of potassium and phosphate. Sodium is also lost with the diuresis, but free water losses are greater than isotonic losses. With prolonged illness and severe DKA, total body losses can approach 10–13 mEq/kg of sodium, 5–6 mEq/kg of potassium, and 4–5 mEq/kg of phosphate. These losses continue for several hours during therapy until the catabolic state is reversed and the diuresis is controlled. For example, 50% of infused sodium may be lost in the urine during IV therapy. Even though the sodium deficit may be repaired within 24 hr, intracellular potassium and phosphate may not be completely restored for several days.

Although patients with DKA have a total body potassium deficit, the initial serum level is often normal or slightly elevated. This is due to the movement of potassium from the intracellular space to the serum, both as part of the ketoacid buffering process and as part of the catabolic shift. These effects are reversed with therapy and potassium returns to the cell. (Note that therapy for hyperkalemia uses insulin and glucose in the same manner, i.e., to promote the anabolic movement of potassium into the cell.) Improved hydration increases renal blood flow, allowing for increased excretion of potassium in the elevated aldosterone state. The net effect is often a dramatic decline in serum potassium levels, especially in severe DKA, and can precipitate changes in cardiac conductivity, flattening of T waves, prolongation of the QRS complex, and cause skeletal muscle weakness or an ileus. The risk of myocardial dysfunction is increased with shock and acidosis. Potassium levels must be closely followed and electrocardiographic monitoring continued until DKA is substantially resolved. If needed, the parenteral potassium can be increased to 80 mEq/L or an oral supplement can be given if there is no emesis. Rarely, the IV insulin must be temporarily stopped.

It is unclear whether phosphate deficits contribute to symptoms of DKA such as generalized muscle weakness. In pediatric patients, a deficit has not been shown to compromise oxygen delivery via a deficiency of 2,3-diphosphoglycerate (2,3-DPG). Because the patient will receive an excess of chloride, which may aggravate acidosis, it is prudent to use potassium phosphate rather than potassium chloride as a potassium source. Potassium acetate is also used, because it provides an additional source of metabolic buffer.

Pancreatitis is occasionally seen with DKA, especially if prolonged abdominal distress is present; serum amylase may be elevated. If, however, the serum lipase is not elevated, the amylase is likely nonspecific or salivary in origin. Serum creatinine adjusted for age may be falsely elevated due to interference by ketones in the autoanalyzer methodology. An initial elevated value rarely indicates renal failure and should be rechecked when the child is less ketonemic. Blood urea nitrogen (BUN) may be elevated with prerenal azotemia and should be rechecked as the child is rehydrated. Mildly elevated creatine or BUN is not reason to withhold potassium therapy if good urinary output is present.

KETOACID ACCUMULATION. Low insulin infusion rates (0.02–0.05 units/kg/h) are sufficient to stop peripheral release of fatty acids, thus eliminating the flow of substrate for ketogenesis. Therefore, the initial infusion rate may be decreased if blood glucose levels go below 150 mg/dL (8 mmol/L) despite the addition of glucose to the infusion. Ketogenesis continues until fatty acid substrates already in the liver are depleted, but this production declines much more quickly without new substrate inflow. Bicarbonate buffers, regenerated by the distal renal tubule and by metabolism of ketone bodies, steadily repair the acidosis once ketoacid production is controlled. Bicarbonate therapy is rarely necessary and may even increase the risk of hypokalemia and cerebral edema.

There should be a steady increase in pH and serum bicarbonate as therapy progresses. Kussmaul respirations should abate and abdominal pain resolve. Persistent acidosis may indicate inadequate insulin or fluid therapy, infection, or, rarely, lactic acidosis. Urine ketones may be positive long after ketoacidosis has resolved because the nitroprusside reaction routinely used to measure urine ketones by dipstick only measures acetoacetate. During DKA, most excess ketones are β-hydroxybutyrate, which increases the normal ratio to acetoacetate from 3:1 to as high as 8:1. With resolution of the acidosis, β-hydroxybutyrate converts to acetoacetate, which is excreted into the urine and detected by the dipstick test. Therefore, persistent ketonuria may not accurately reflect the degree of clinical improvement and should not be relied upon as an indicator of therapeutic failure.

All patients with DKA should be checked for initiating events that triggered the metabolic decompensation, for example, an infection.

DKA PROTOCOL. (See Table 583–6.) Even though DKA can be of variable severity, a common approach to all cases simplifies the therapeutic regimen and can be safely used for most children. Fluids are best calculated based on weight, not body surface area (M^2), because heights are rarely available for the calculation. The Milwaukee protocol has been used for more than 20 yr in a large clinic setting with no deaths and no neurologic sequelae in any child treated with this protocol. It can be used for children of all ages and with all degrees of DKA. It is designed to restore most electrolyte deficits, to reverse the acidosis, and to rehydrate the moderately ill child in about 24 hr. A standard water deficit (85 mL/kg) is assumed. This amount, when added to maintenance, yields about 4 L/M^2 for children of all sizes. Children with milder DKA recover in 10 to 20 hr (and

need less total IV fluid before switching to oral intake), whereas those with more severe DKA require 30 to 36 hr with this protocol. Any child can be easily transitioned to oral intake and subcutaneous insulin when DKA has essentially resolved (total CO_2 > 15 mEq/L; pH > 7.30; sodium stable between 135–145 mEq/L; no emesis). The IV is capped, and the first dose of subcutaneous insulin is given with a meal. Children with mild DKA can often be discharged after a few hours of therapy in the emergency department if adequate follow-up is provided.

A flow sheet is mandatory for accurate monitoring of changes in acidosis, electrolytes, fluid balance, and clinical status, especially if the patient is transferred from the emergency department to an inpatient setting with new caretakers. This flow sheet is best implemented by a central computer system, which allows for rapid update and wide availability of results, as well as rule-driven highlighting of critical values. A paper flow sheet suffices if it stays with the patient, is kept current, and is reviewed frequently by the physician. Any flow sheet should include columns for serial electrolytes, pH, glucose, and fluid balance. Blood testing should occur hourly for children with severe DKA and every 3–4 hr for those with mild to moderate DKA.

Even though this protocol has a long safety record, one must continue to *closely monitor each patient*. For all but the mildest cases, this should include frequent neurologic checks for any signs of increasing intracranial pressure, such as a change of consciousness, depressed respiration, worsening headache, bradycardia, apnea, pupillary changes, papilledema, posturing, or seizures. Mannitol must be readily available for use at the earliest sign of cerebral edema. One must also keep informed of the laboratory changes; hypokalemia or hypoglycemia can occur rapidly. Children with moderate to severe DKA have a higher overall risk and should be treated in an intensive care environment. Finally, this protocol may not be appropriate for some patients such as the severely hypernatremic child (corrected sodium greater than 150 mEq/L) who may need slower rehydration with a longer duration of isotonic fluids.

Some residual β-cell function is seen even in children presenting with DKA. This function may improve as the child recovers from the effects of hyperglycemia and elevated counter-regulatory hormones. This residual secretion may necessitate a reduction in the initial total subcutaneous insulin dose used in the first few days of therapy.

NONKETOTIC HYPEROSMOLAR COMA. This syndrome is characterized by severe hyperglycemia (blood glucose greater than 800 mg/dL), absence of or only slight ketosis, nonketotic acidosis, severe dehydration, depressed sensorium or frank coma, and various neurologic signs that may include grand mal seizures, hyperthermia, hemiparesis, and positive Babinski signs. Respirations are usually shallow, but coexistent metabolic (lactic) acidosis may be manifested by Kussmaul breathing. Serum osmolarity is commonly 350 mOsm/kg or greater. This condition is uncommon in children; among adults, mortality rates have been as high as 40–70%, possibly in part because of delays in recognition and institution of appropriate therapy. In children, there has been a high incidence of pre-existing neurologic damage. Profound hyperglycemia may develop over a period of days and, initially, the obligatory osmotic polyuria and dehydration may be partially compensated for by increasing fluid intake. With progression of disease, thirst becomes impaired, possibly because of alteration of the hypothalamic thirst center by hyperosmolarity and, in some instances, because of a pre-existing defect in the hypothalamic osmoregulating mechanism.

The low production of ketones is attributed mainly to the hyperosmolarity, which in vitro blunts the lipolytic effect of epinephrine and the antilipolytic effect of residual insulin; blunting of lipolysis by the therapeutic use of β-adrenergic blockers may contribute to the syndrome. Depression of consciousness is closely correlated with the degree of hyperosmolarity in this condition as well as in DKA; hemoconcentration may also predispose to cerebral arterial and venous thromboses.

Treatment of nonketotic hyperosmolar coma is directed at rapid repletion of the vascular volume deficit and very slow correction of the hyperosmolar state. One-half isotonic saline (0.45% NaCl; some use normal saline) is administered at a rate estimated to replace 50% of the volume deficit in the first 12 hr, and the remainder is administered during the ensuing 24 hr. The rate of infusion and the saline concentration are titrated to result in a slow decline of serum osmolality. When the blood glucose concentration approaches 300 mg/dL, the hydrating fluid should be changed to 5% dextrose in 0.2 normal (N) saline. Approximately 20 mEq/L of potassium chloride should be added to each of these fluids to prevent hypokalemia. Serum potassium and plasma glucose concentrations should be monitored at 2-hr intervals for the first 12 hr and at 4-hr intervals for the next 24 hr to permit appropriate adjustments of administered potassium and insulin.

Insulin can be given by continuous IV infusion beginning with the 2nd hr of fluid therapy. Blood glucose may decrease dramatically with fluid therapy alone. IV insulin dose should be 0.05 U/kg/h of regular (fast-acting) rather than 0.1 U/kg/h as advocated for patients with DKA.

NUTRITIONAL MANAGEMENT. Nutrition plays an essential role in the management of patients with type 1 DM. This is of critical importance during childhood and adolescence, when appropriate energy intake is required to meet the needs for energy expenditure, growth, and pubertal development. Nutritional treatment alone or in combination with appropriate insulin therapy averts or relieves symptoms of hyperglycemia in diabetic patients. Moreover, nutritional practices may influence the development of long-term complications of diabetes (i.e., diabetic nephropathy). There are no special nutritional requirements for the diabetic child other than those for optimal growth and development. In outlining nutritional requirements for the child on the basis of age, sex, weight, and activity, food preferences, including any based on cultural and ethnic backgrounds, must be considered.

Total recommended *caloric intake* is based on size or surface area and can be obtained from standard tables (Tables 583–7 and 583–8). The caloric mixture should comprise approximately 55% carbohydrate, 30% fat, and 15% protein. Approximately 70% of the carbohydrate content should be derived from complex carbohydrates such as starch; intake of sucrose and highly refined sugars should be limited. Complex carbohydrates require prolonged digestion and absorption so that plasma glucose levels increase slowly, whereas glucose from refined sugars,

TABLE 583–7. Calorie Needs for Children and Young Adults

Age	Kcal Required/Kg Body Weight*
Children	
0–12 mo	120
1–10 yr	100–75
Young women	
11–15 yr	35
≥16 yr	30
Young men	
11–15 yr	80–50 (65)
16–20 yr	
Average activity	40
Very physically active	50
Sedentary	30

Numbers in parentheses are means.
Gradual decline in calories per unit weight as age increases.
From Nutrition Guide for Professionals: Diabetes Education and Meal Planning. *Alexandria, VA, and Chicago, IL, The American Diabetes Association and The American Dietetic Association, 1988.*

TABLE 583–8. Summary of Nutrition Guidelines for Children and/or Adolescents with Type 1 Diabetes Mellitus

Nutrition Care Plan
Promotes optimal compliance.
Incorporates goals of management: normal growth and development, control of blood glucose, maintenance of optimal nutritional status, and prevention of complications. Uses staged approach.

Nutrient Recommendations and Distribution

Nutrient	(%) of Calories	Recommended Daily Intake
Carbohydrate	Will vary	High fiber, especially soluble fiber; optimal amount unknown
Fiber	>20 g per day	
Protein	12–20	
Fat	<30	
Saturated	<10	
Polyunsaturated	6–8	
Monounsaturated	Remainder of fat allowance	
Cholesterol		300 mg
Sodium		Avoid excessive; limit to 3,000–4,000 mg if hypertensive

Additional Recommendations

Energy: If using measured diet, re-evaluate prescribed energy level at least every 3 mo.
Protein: High-protein intakes may contribute to diabetic nephropathy. Low intakes may reverse preclinical nephropathy. Therefore, 12–20% of energy is recommended; lower end of range is preferred. In guiding toward the end of the range, a staged approach is useful.
Alcohol: Safe use of moderate alcohol consumption should be taught as routine anticipatory guidance as early as junior high.
Snacks: Snacks vary according to individual needs (generally three snacks per day for children; midafternoon and bedtime snacks for junior high children or teens).
Alternative sweeteners: Use of a variety of sweeteners is suggested.
Educational techniques: No single technique is superior. Choice of educational method used should be based on patient needs. Knowledge of variety of techniques is important. Follow-up education and support are required.
Eating disorders: Best treatment is prevention. Unexplained poor control or severe hypoglycemia may indicate a potential eating disorder.
Exercise: Education is vital to prevent delayed or immediate hypoglycemia and to prevent worsened hyperglycemia and ketosis.

From Connell JE, Thomas-Doberson D: *Nutritional management of children and adolescents with insulin-dependent diabetes mellitus: A review by the Diabetes Care and Education Dietetic Practice Group.* J Am Diet Assoc 1991; 91:1556.

including carbonated beverages, is rapidly absorbed and may cause wide swings in the metabolic pattern; carbonated beverages should be sugar-free. Priority should be given to total calories and total carbohydrate consumed rather than its source. *Carbohydrate counting* has become a mainstay in the nutrition education and management of patients with DM. Each carbohydrate exchange unit is 15 g. Patients and their families are provided with information regarding the carbohydrate contents of different foods and food label reading. This allows patients to adjust their insulin dosage to their mealtime carbohydrate intake. The use of carbohydrate counting and insulin to carbohydrate ratios and the use of fast-acting insulin analogs and long-acting basal insulins (ultralente and glargine) provide many children with less rigid meal planning. Flexibility in the use of insulin in relation to carbohydrate content of food improves the quality of life.

Although in children there is concern about the potential cumulative effect of saccharin, available data do not support an association of moderate amounts with bladder cancer. Other non-nutritive sweeteners such as aspartame are used in a variety of products. Sorbitol and xylitol should not be used as artificial sweeteners; they are products of the polyol pathway and are implicated in some of the complications of diabetes.

Diets with *high fiber content* are useful in improving control of blood glucose. Moderate amounts of sucrose consumed with fiber-rich foods such as whole meal bread may have no more glycemic effect than their low-fiber, sugar-free equivalents. The concept of biologic equivalence or of a "glycemic index" of foods is under investigation.

The *intake of fat* is adjusted so that the polyunsaturated:saturated ratio is increased to about 1.2:1.0, in contrast to the estimated American average of 0.3:1.0. Dietary fats derived from animal sources are, therefore, reduced and replaced by polyunsaturated fats from vegetable sources. Substituting margarine for butter, vegetable oil for animal oils in cooking, and lean cuts of meat, poultry, and fish for fatty meats, such as bacon, is advisable. The intake of cholesterol is also reduced by these measures and by limiting the number of egg yolks consumed. These simple measures reduce serum low-density lipoprotein cholesterol, a predisposing factor to atherosclerotic disease. Less than 10% of calories should be derived from saturated fats, up to 10% from polyunsaturated fats, and the remaining fat-derived calories from monounsaturated fats. Table 583–8 summarizes current nutritional guidelines.

The total daily caloric intake is divided to provide 20% at breakfast, 20% at lunch, and 30% at dinner, leaving 10% for each of the midmorning, midafternoon, and evening snacks, if they are desired. In older children, the midmorning snack may be omitted and its caloric equivalent added to lunch. Special brochures and pamphlets describing sample meal plans for children are usually available from regional diabetes associations; their use should be encouraged as part of the educational process. Meal plans are often based on groups of food exchanges; within each of the exchange lists of the foods that are principal sources of carbohydrates, proteins, and fats, there is a wide variety of foods that can be substituted or exchanged. There are few restrictions so that each child can select a diet based on personal taste or preferences with the help of the physician or dietitian, or both. Emphasis should be placed on regularity of food intake and on constancy of carbohydrate intake. Occasional excesses for birthdays and other parties are permissible and tolerated to not foster rebellion and stealth in obtaining desired food. Cakes and even candies are permissible on special occasions as long as the food exchange value and carbohydrate content are adjusted in the meal plan. Adjustments in meal planning must constantly be made to meet the needs as well as the desires of each child, although a consistent eating pattern with appropriate supplements for exercise, the pubertal growth spurt, and pregnancy in a diabetic adolescent are important for metabolic control. There is also an increased frequency of eating disorders among young women with diabetes. Thus, expectations and educational advice regarding nutrition must be dealt with in a sensitive careful manner, especially in adolescents.

MONITORING. Success in the daily management of the diabetic child can be measured by the competence acquired by the family, and subsequently by the child, in assuming responsibility for daily "diabetic care." Their initial and ongoing instruction in conjunction with their supervised experience can lead to a sense of confidence in making intermittent adjustments in insulin dosage for dietary deviations, unusual physical activity, and even for some minor intercurrent illnesses, as well as for otherwise unexplained repeated hypoglycemic reactions and excessive glucosuria. Such acceptance of responsibility should make them relatively independent of the physician for their ordinary care. The physician must maintain ongoing interested supervision and shared responsibility with the family and the child.

Self-monitoring of blood glucose (SMBG) is an essential component of managing diabetes and necessitates a regimen that includes measurements of blood glucose and, at times, urinary ketones, as well as the keeping of a standardized record of these results and the corresponding data of dietary deviations, unusual physical activity, hypoglycemic reactions, intercurrent illness, the daily dose of insulin, and other items of possible relevance. When the physician mistrusts the patient's record, physicians may make their own evaluations. If these data are counter to those in the parent or child's report, the physician can then attempt to clarify the situation in a manner that does not undermine their mutual confidence.

Daily blood glucose monitoring has been markedly enhanced by the availability of strips impregnated with glucose oxidase that permit blood glucose measurement from a drop of blood. A portable calibrated reflectance meter can approximate the blood glucose concentration accurately. Many meters contain a memory "chip" enabling recall of each measurement, its average over a given interval, and the ability to display the pattern on a computer screen. Such information is a useful educational tool for verifying degree of control and modifying recommended regimens. A small spring-loaded device that automates capillary blood letting (lancing device) in a relatively painless fashion is commercially available. Parents and patients should be taught to use these devices and measure blood glucose three to four times daily—before breakfast, lunch, and supper, and at bedtime. Initially, at diagnosis, the blood glucose measurement should also be performed at 12 AM and 3 AM to exclude inappropriate nocturnal hypoglycemia and avoid the Somogyi phenomenon. Ideally, the blood glucose concentration should range from approximately 80 mg/dL in the fasting state to 140 mg/dL after meals. In practice, however, a range of 60–220 mg/dL is acceptable, based on age of the patient. Blood glucose measurements that are consistently at or outside these limits, in the absence of an identifiable cause such as exercise or dietary indiscretion, are an indication for a change in the insulin dose. If the fasting blood glucose is high, the evening dose of long-acting insulin is increased by 10–15% and/or the insulin (lispro or aspart) coverage for bedtime snack may be considered; if the noon glucose level exceeds set limits, the morning fast-acting insulin (lispro or aspart) is increased by 10–15%; if the presupper glucose is high, the noon dose fast-acting insulin is increased by 10–15%; and if the prebedtime glucose measurement is high, the presupper dose of fast-acting insulin is increased by 10–15%. Similarly, reductions in the insulin type and dose should be made if the corresponding blood glucose measurements are consistently below desirable limits.

A minimum of four daily blood glucose measurements should be performed. However, some children and adolescents may need to have more frequent blood glucose monitoring based on their level of physical activity and history of frequent hypoglycemic reactions. Families should be encouraged to become sufficiently knowledgeable about managing their diabetes. They can maintain near-normal glycemia for prolonged periods of time by self-monitoring of blood glucose levels before and 2 hr after meals, and in conjunction with multiple daily injections of insulin, adjusted as necessary, can maintain near-normal glycemia for prolonged periods.

The *continuous glucose monitoring system (CGMS)* records data obtained from a subcutaneous sensor every 5 min for up to 72 hr and provides the clinician with a continuous profile of tissue glucose levels. The interstitial glucose levels lag 13 min behind the blood glucose values independent of level in ambient blood glucose. The CGMS values tend to have high correlation coefficient for blood glucose values ranging between 40 and 400 mg/dL. CGMS is minimally invasive and entails the placement of a small, subcutaneous catheter that can be easily worn by adults and children. The system provides information that allows the patient and healthcare team to adjust the insulin regimen and the nutrition plan to improve glycemic control. CGMS can be helpful in detecting asymptomatic nocturnal hypoglycemia as well as in lowering HbA_{1c} values without increasing the risk for severe hypoglycemia. While there are potential pitfalls in CGMS use including suboptimal compliance, human error, incorrect technique and sensor failure, the implementation of CGMS in ambulatory diabetes practice allows the clinician to diagnose abnormal glycemic patterns in a more precise manner.

Glucowatch Biographer uses reverse iontophoresis to analyze the glucose content of interstitial fluid, which is extracted through a membrane patch on the patient's wrist beneath the Glucowatch device. Glucowatch provides realtime interstitial fluid glucose values, in the range of 40–400 mg/dL, that are the average of blood glucose values for the preceding 20 min. Glucose values in the range of 70–280 mg/dL have the highest correlation coefficient with blood glucose values. Additionally, Glucowatch alarm can be set for monitoring nocturnal hypoglycemia as needed.

A reliable index of long-term glycemic control is provided by measurement of *glycosylated hemoglobin*. HbA_{1c} represents the fraction of hemoglobin to which glucose has been nonenzymatically attached in the bloodstream. The formation of HbA_{1c} is a slow reaction that is dependent on the prevailing concentration of blood glucose; it continues irreversibly throughout the red blood cell's life span of approximately 120 days. The higher the blood glucose concentration and the longer the red blood cell's exposure to it, the higher is the fraction of HbA_{1c}, which is expressed as a percentage of total hemoglobin. Because a blood sample at any given time contains a mixture of red blood cells of varying ages, exposed for varying times to varying blood glucose concentrations, an HbA_{1c} measurement reflects the average blood glucose concentration of the preceding 2–3 mo. When measured by standardized methods to remove labile forms, the fraction of HbA_{1c} is not influenced by an isolated episode of hyperglycemia. Consequently, as an index of long-term glycemic control, a measurement of HbA_{1c} is superior to measurements of glycosuria or a single blood glucose determination. It is recommended that HbA_{1c} measurements be obtained three to four times per year to obtain a profile of long-term glycemic control. The more consistently lower the HbA_{1c} level, and hence the better the metabolic control, the more likely it is that microvascular complications such as retinopathy and nephropathy will be less severe, delayed in appearance, or avoided. Depending on the method used for determination, HbA_{1c} values may be spuriously elevated in thalassemia (or other conditions with elevated hemoglobin F) and spuriously lower in sickle cell disease. Although values of HbA_{1c} may vary according to the method used for measurement, in nondiabetic individuals, the HbA_{1c} fraction is usually less than 6%; in diabetics, values of 6–8.5% represent good metabolic control, values of 9–10%, fair control, and values of 11% or higher, poor control (Table 583–9).

EXERCISE. No form of exercise, including competitive sports, should be forbidden to the diabetic child. A major complication of exercise in diabetic patients is the presence of a hypoglycemic reaction during or within hours after exercise. If hypoglycemia does not occur with exercise, adjustments in diet or insulin are not necessary, and glucoregulation is likely to be improved through the increased utilization of glucose by muscles. The major contributing factor to hypoglycemia with exercise is an increased rate of absorption of insulin from its injection site.

Higher insulin levels dampen hepatic glucose production so that it is inadequate to meet the increased glucose utilization of exercising muscle. Regular exercise also improves glucoregulation by increasing insulin receptors. In patients who are in poor metabolic control, vigorous exercise may precipitate ketoacidosis because of the exercise-induced increase in the counterregulatory hormones.

In anticipation of vigorous exercise, one additional carbohydrate exchange may be taken before exercise, and glucose from orange juice, carbonated nondietetic beverage, or candy should be available during and after exercise. With experience and trial and error, each patient, guided by the physician, should develop an appropriate regimen for regularly planned exercise that is frequently associated with hypoglycemia; in such instances, the total dose of insulin may be reduced by about 10–15% on the day of the scheduled exercise. Prolonged exercise, such as long-distance running may require reduction of as much as 50% or more of the usual insulin dose.

BENEFITS OF IMPROVED GLYCEMIC CONTROL. The DCCT established conclusively the association between higher glucose levels and long-term microvascular complications. Intensive management produced dramatic reductions of retinopathy, nephropathy, and neuropathy by 47–76%. The data from the adolescent cohort demonstrated the same degree of improvement and the same relationship between the outcome measures of microvascular complications. Adolescents gained more weight and experienced significantly more frequent episodes of severe hypoglycemia and ketoacidosis than did adults. Other studies of children and adolescents have not documented increased frequency or severity of hypoglycemia.

The beneficial effect of intensified treatment was determined by the degree of blood glucose normalization, independent of the type of intensified treatment used. Frequent blood glucose monitoring was considered an important factor in achieving better glycemic control for the intensively treated adolescents and adults. Patients who were intensively treated had individualized glucose targets, frequent adjustments based on ongoing capillary blood glucose monitoring, and a team approach that focused on the person with diabetes as the prime initiator of ambulatory care. Care was constantly adjusted toward reaching normal or near normal glycemic goals, while avoiding or minimizing severe episodes of hypoglycemia. Teaching emphasized a proactive (preventive) approach to blood glucose fluctuations with constant readjustment (reactive approach) to counterbalance any high or low blood glucose readings. Target blood glucose goals were adjusted upward if hypoglycemia could not be prevented.

Total duration of diabetes contributes to development and severity of complications. Nonetheless, many professionals have concerns about applying the results of the DCCT to preschool-aged children, who often have hypoglycemia unawareness with unique safety issues and to prepubertal school-aged children, who were not included in the DCCT.

CURRENT INTENSIVE INSULIN REPLACEMENT REGIMENS. The goal of physiologic insulin replacement for type 1 DM is accomplished with short-acting insulins that more closely mimic the sharp increase and short duration of pancreatic insulin secreted with nutrient intake. The rapid-acting insulin analog lispro has superior pharmacokinetic properties for the control of postprandial glucose. Improved postprandial glucose responses occur when treated with twice-daily injections (conventional insulin, CI), multiple daily injections (MDI), or CSII. The use of lispro or aspart insulin reduces the frequency of between-meal hypoglycemic events, especially when it is carefully balanced with the carbohydrate content of meal. This has improved how insulin is given to toddlers as well as when a flexible meal plan is desired.

The carbohydrate content of food does not influence glycemic control if premeal rapid-acting insulin (bolus) is adjusted to the

TABLE 583–9. Target Premeal and 30-Day Average Blood Glucose Ranges and the Corresponding Hemoglobin A_{1c} for each Age Group

Age Group (yr)	Target Premeal BG Range (mg/dL)	30-Day Average BG Range (mg/dL)	Target HbA$_{1c}$ (%)
<5	100–200	180–250	7.5–9.0
5 to 11	80–150	150–200	6.5–8.0
12 to 15	80–130	120–180	6.0–7.5
16 to 18	70–120	100–150	5.5–7.0

In our laboratory the nondiabetic reference range for HbA$_{1c}$ is 4.5–5.7% (95% confidence interval).

BG, blood glucose; HBA$_{1c}$, hemoglobin A$_{1c}$.

carbohydrate content of meal. Wide variations in carbohydrate intake do not modify long-acting (ultralente/glargine) or basal insulin requirement. Insulin replacement strategies stress the importance of administering smaller doses of insulin throughout the day. This approach allows insulin doses to be changed as needed to correct hyperglycemia, supplement for additional anticipated carbohydrate intake, or subtract for exercise. Indeed, bolus-basal treatment with multiple injections is better adapted to the physiologic profiles of insulin and glucose and can therefore provide better glycemic control than the conventional two- to three-dose regimen. Age-adjusted and individualized insulin to carbohydrate ratios and insulin dosage adjustment algorithms have been developed to normalize elevated blood glucose levels and to compensate for alterations in carbohydrate intake. The use of flexible multiple daily injections (FMDIs) and CSII in children with type 1 DM improves glycemic control without an increase in the incidence of severe hypoglycemia.

HYPOGLYCEMIC REACTIONS. Hypoglycemia is the major limitation to tight control of glucose levels. Once injected, insulin absorption and action are independent of the glucose level, thus creating a unique risk of hypoglycemia from an unbalanced insulin effect. Insulin analogs may help reduce but cannot eliminate this risk. Most children with type 1 diabetes can expect mild hypoglycemia each week, moderate hypoglycemia a few times each year, and severe hypoglycemia every few years. These episodes are usually not predictable, although exercise, delayed meals or snacks, and wide swings in glucose levels increase the risk. Infants and toddlers are at higher risk because they have more variable meals and activity levels, are unable to recognize early signs of hypoglycemia, and are limited in their ability to seek a source of oral glucose to reverse the hypoglycemia. The very young have an increased risk of permanently reduced cognitive function as a long-term sequela of severe hypoglycemia. For this reason, a more relaxed degree of glucose control is necessary until the child matures (see Table 583–9).

Hypoglycemia can occur at any time of day or night. Early symptoms and signs (mild hypoglycemia) may occur with a sudden decrease in blood glucose to levels that do not meet standard criteria for hypoglycemia in nondiabetic children (see Chapter 81). The child may show pallor, sweating, apprehension or fussiness, hunger, tremor, and tachycardia, all due to the surge in catecholamines as the body attempts to counter the excessive insulin effect. Behavioral changes such as tearfulness, irritability, aggression, and naughtiness are more prevalent in children. As glucose levels decline further, cerebral glucopenia occurs with drowsiness, personality changes, mental confusion, impaired judgment (moderate hypoglycemia), progressing to an inability to seek help, and seizures or coma (severe hypoglycemia). Prolonged severe hypoglycemia can result in a depressed sensorium or strokelike focal motor deficits that persist after the hypoglycemia has resolved. Although permanent sequelae are rare, severe hypoglycemia is frightening for the child and family, and can result in a significant reluctance to attempt even moderate glycemic control afterward.

Important counter-regulatory hormones in children include growth hormone, cortisol, epinephrine, and glucagon. The latter two seem more critical in the older child. Many older patients with long-standing type 1 diabetes lose their ability to secrete glucagon in response to hypoglycemia. In the young adult, epinephrine deficiency may also develop as part of a general autonomic neuropathy. This substantially increases the risk of hypoglycemia because the early warning signals of a declining glucose level are due to catecholamine release. Recurrent hypoglycemic episodes associated with tight metabolic control may aggravate partial counter-regulatory deficiencies, producing a syndrome of *hypoglycemia unawareness* and reduced ability to restore euglycemia (hypoglycemia-associated autonomic fail-

ure). Avoidance of hypoglycemia allows some recovery from this unawareness syndrome.

The most important factors in the management of hypoglycemia are an understanding by the patient and family of the symptoms and signs of the reaction and an anticipation of known precipitating factors such as gym or sports activities. Tighter glucose control increases the risk. Families should be taught to look for typical hypoglycemic scenarios or patterns in the home blood glucose log, so that they may adjust the insulin dose and avert predictable episodes. A source of emergency glucose should be available at all times and places, including at school and during visits to friends. If possible, it is initially important to document the hypoglycemia before treating, because some symptoms may not always be due to hypoglycemia. Most families and children develop a good sense for true hypoglycemic episodes and can institute treatment before testing. Any child suspected of having a moderate to severe hypoglycemic episode should also be treated before testing. It is important not to give too much glucose; 5–10 g should be given as juice or a sugar-containing carbonated beverage or candy and the blood glucose checked 15–20 minutes later. Patients, parents, and teachers should also be instructed in the administration of *glucagon* when the child cannot take glucose orally. An injection kit should be kept at home and school. The intramuscular dose is 0.5 mg if the child weighs less than 20 kg and 1.0 mg if more than 20 kg. This produces a brief release of glucose from the liver. Glucagon often causes emesis, which precludes giving oral supplementation if the blood glucose declines after the glucagon effect has waned. Caretakers must then be prepared to take the child to the hospital for IV glucose administration, if necessary.

THE SOMOGYI PHENOMENON, THE DAWN PHENOMENON, AND BRITTLE DIABETES. There are several reasons that blood glucose levels increase in the early morning hours before breakfast. The most common is a simple decline in insulin levels and is seen in many children using NPH or lente as the basal insulin at supper or bedtime. This usually results in routinely elevated morning glucose. The *dawn phenomenon* is thought to be due mainly to overnight growth hormone secretion and increased insulin clearance. It is a normal physiologic process seen in most nondiabetic adolescents, who compensate with more insulin output. A child with type 1 diabetes cannot compensate and may actually have declining insulin levels if using evening NPH or lente. The dawn phenomenon is usually recurrent and modestly elevates most morning glucose levels.

Rarely, high morning glucose is due to the Somogyi phenomenon, a theoretical rebound from late night or early morning hypoglycemia, thought to be due to an exaggerated counter-regulatory response. It is unlikely to be a common cause, in that most children remain hypoglycemic once nighttime glucose levels decline. Continuous glucose monitoring systems should allow clarification of ambiguously elevated morning glucose levels.

The term *brittle diabetes* has been used to describe the child, usually an adolescent female, with unexplained wide fluctuations in blood glucose, often with recurrent DKA, who is on large doses of insulin. An inherent physiologic abnormality is rarely present because these children usually show normal insulin responsiveness when in the hospital environment. Psychosocial or psychiatric problems, including eating disorders, and dysfunctional family dynamics are usually present, which preclude effective diabetes therapy. Hospitalization is usually needed to confirm the environmental effect, and aggressive psychosocial or psychiatric evaluation is essential.

BEHAVIORAL/PSYCHOLOGICAL ASPECTS AND EATING DISORDERS. Diabetes in a child affects the lifestyle and interpersonal relationships of the entire family. Feelings of anxiety and guilt are common in parents. Similar feelings, coupled with denial and rejection, are equally common in children, particularly during the rebellious teenage years. Family conflict has been associated with poor treatment adherence and poor metabolic control among youths with type 1 DM. No specific personality disorder or psychopathology is characteristic of diabetes; similar feelings are observed in families with other chronic disorders.

Nonadherence. Family conflict, denial, and feelings of anxiety find expression in nonadherence to instructions regarding nutritional and insulin therapy and in noncompliance with self-monitoring. Deliberate overdosage with insulin, resulting in hypoglycemia, or omission of insulin, often in association with excesses in nutritional intake and resulting in ketoacidosis, may be pleas for psychological help or manipulative attempts to escape an environment perceived as undesirable or intolerable; occasionally, they may be manifestations of suicidal intent. Frequent admissions to the hospital for ketoacidosis or hypoglycemia should arouse suspicion of an underlying emotional conflict. Overprotection on the part of parents is common and often is not in the best interest of the patient. Feelings of being different or of being alone, or both, are common and may be justified in view of the restrictive schedules imposed by testing of urine and blood, administration of insulin, and nutritional limitations. Furthermore, concern about the likelihood of complications developing and the decreased life span of patients with diabetes fosters anxiety. Unfortunately, misinformation abounds about the risks of the development of diabetes in siblings or off-spring and of pregnancy in young diabetic women. Even appropriate information often causes further anxiety.

Many of these problems can be averted through continued empathic counseling based on correct information and attempts to build attitudes of normality in the patient and a feeling of being a productive member of society. Recognizing the potential impact of these problems, peer discussion groups have been organized in many locales; feelings of isolation and frustration tend to be lessened by the sharing of common problems. Summer camps for diabetic children afford an excellent opportunity for learning and sharing under expert supervision. Education about the pathophysiology of diabetes, insulin dose, technique of administration, nutrition, exercise, and hypoglycemic reactions can be reinforced by medical and paramedical personnel. The presence of numerous peers with similar problems offers new insights to the diabetic child. Residential treatment for children and adolescents with difficult to manage type 1 DM is an option available only in some centers.

Anxiety and Depression. It has been shown that there are significant correlations between a poor metabolic control and depressive symptoms, a high level of anxiety, or a previous psychiatric diagnosis. In a similar way, poor metabolic control is related to higher levels of personal, social, school maladjustment, or family environment dissatisfaction. It is estimated that between 20–26% of adolescent patients may develop major depressive disorder (MDD), which is similar to the occurrence rate of MDD in nondiabetic adolescents. The course characteristics of MDD in young diabetic subjects and psychiatric control subjects appear to be similar; however, eventual propensity of diabetic youths for more protracted depressions is greater and there is higher risk of recurrence among young diabetic females. Therefore, the health care providers managing a child or adolescent with diabetes should be aware of their pivotal role as counselor and advisor and should closely monitor the mental health of patients with diabetes.

Fear of Self-injecting and Self-testing. Extreme fear of self-injecting (FSI) insulin (injection phobia) is likely to compromise glycemic control as well as emotional well-being. Likewise, fear of finger pricks can be a source of distress and may seriously hamper self-management. Children and adolescents with FSI either omit insulin dosing and/or refuse to rotate their injection sites because repeated injections in the same site is associated with less pain sensation. Failure to rotate injection sites results in subcutaneous scar formation (lipohypertrophy). Insulin injection into the lipohypertrophic skin is usually associated with poor insulin absorption and/or insulin leakage with resultant suboptimal glycemic control.

Eating Disorders. Treatment of type 1 DM involves constant monitoring of food intake. In addition, improved glycemic control is commonly associated with increased weight gain. In adolescent females, these two factors, along with individual, familial, and socioeconomic factors, can lead to an increased incidence of both nonspecific and specific eating disorders, which can disrupt glycemic control and increase the risk of long-term complications. Eating disorders and subthreshold eating disorders are almost twice as common in adolescent females with type 1 DM as in their nondiabetic peers. The reports of the frequencies of specific (anorexia or bulimia nervosa) eating disorders vary between 1–6.9% among female patients with type 1 DM. The prevalence of nonspecific and subthreshold eating disorders is 9% and 14%, respectively. About 11% of type 1 DM adolescent females take less insulin than prescribed to lose weight. Among adolescent females with an eating disorder, about 42% of patients misuse insulin, whereas the estimates of insulin misuse prevalence in subthreshold and nondisordered eating groups are 18% and 6%, respectively. While there is little information regarding the prevalence of eating disorders among male adolescents with type 1 DM, available data suggest normal eating attitudes in this group of patients. Among healthy adolescent males who participate in wrestling, however, the drive to lose weight has led to the seasonal, transient development of abnormal eating attitudes and behaviors, which may lead to insulin dose omission in order to lose weight.

When behavioral/psychological problems and/or eating disorders are assumed to be responsible for poor compliance with the medical regimen, referral for psychological evaluation and management is indicated. Children and adolescents with injection phobia and fear of self-testing can be counseled by a trained behavioral therapist and benefit from such techniques as desensitization and biofeedback to attenuate pain sensation and psychological distress associated these procedures. Behavioral therapists and psychologists usually form part of the pediatric diabetes team in most centers, and can help assess and manage emotional and behavioral disorders in diabetic children.

MANAGEMENT DURING INFECTIONS. While infections are no more common in diabetic children than in nondiabetic ones, they can often disrupt glucose control and may precipitate DKA. In addition, the diabetic child is at increased risk of dehydration if hyperglycemia causes an osmotic diuresis or if ketosis causes emesis. Counter-regulatory hormones associated with stress blunt insulin action and elevate glucose levels. If anorexia occurs, however, lack of caloric intake increases the risk of hypoglycemia. Although children younger than 3 yr tend to become hypoglycemic and older children tend toward hyperglycemia, the overall effect is unpredictable. Therefore, frequent blood glucose monitoring and adjustment of insulin doses are essential elements of sick day guidelines (Table 583–10).

The overall goals are to maintain hydration, control glucose levels, and avoid ketoacidosis. This can usually be done at home if proper sick day guidelines are followed and with telephone contact with health care providers. The family should seek advice if home treatment does not control ketonuria, hyperglycemia, or hypoglycemia, or if the child shows signs of dehydration. A child with large ketonuria and emesis should be seen in the emergency department for a general examination, to evaluate hydration, and to determine whether ketoacidosis is present by checking serum electrolytes, glucose, pH, and total CO_2. A child whose blood glucose declines to less than 50–60 mg/dL (2.8–3.3 mmol/L) and who cannot maintain oral intake may need IV glucose, especially if further insulin is needed to control ketonemia.

TABLE 583–10. Guidelines for Sick Day Management

Urine Ketone Status	Glucose Testing and Extra Insulin	Rapid-Acting Insulin Correction Doses*	Comments
Neg or small†	q2 hr	q2 hr for glucose > 250 mg/dL	Check ketones every other void.
Moderate to large‡	q1 hr	q1 hr for glucose > 250 mg/dL	Check ketones each void. Go to hospital if emesis occurs.

Basal insulin: glargine or ultralente basal insulin should be given at the usual dose and time. NPH and lente should be reduced by one half if blood glucose <150 mg/dL and the oral intake is limited.

Oral fluids: sugar free if blood glucose > 250 mg/dL (14 mmol/L); sugar-containing if blood glucose <250 mg/dL.

Call physician or nurse if blood glucose remains elevated after three extra doses; if blood glucose remains less than 70 mg/dL and child cannot take oral supplement; if dehydration occurs.

*Give insulin based on individualized dosing schedule. Also give usual dose for carbohydrate intake if glucose > 150 mg/dL.

†For home serum ketones <1.5 mmol/L per commercial kit.

‡For home serum ketones > 1.5 mmol/L.

TABLE 583–11. Guidelines for Intravenous Insulin Coverage During Surgery

Blood Glucose Level (mg/dL)	Insulin Infusion (units/kg/hr)	Blood Glucose Monitoring
<120	0.00	1 hr
121–200	0.03	2 hr
200–300	0.06	2 hr
300–400	0.08	1 hr*
400	0.10	1 hr*

An infusion of 5% glucose and 0.45% saline solution with 20 mEq/L of potassium acetate is given at 1.5 times maintenance rate.

*Check urine ketones.

MANAGEMENT DURING SURGERY. Surgery can disrupt glucose control in the same way as can intercurrent infections. Stress hormones associated with the underlying condition as well as with surgery itself decrease insulin sensitivity. This increases glucose levels, exacerbates fluid losses, and may initiate DKA. On the other hand, caloric intake is usually restricted, which decreases glucose levels. The net effect is as difficult to predict as during an infection. Vigilant monitoring and frequent insulin adjustments are required to maintain euglycemia and avoid ketosis.

Maintaining glucose control and avoiding DKA are best accomplished with IV insulin and fluids. A simple insulin adjustment scale based on the patient's weight and blood glucose level can be used in most situations (Table 583–11). The IV insulin is continued after surgery as the child begins to take oral fluids; the IV fluids can be steadily decreased as oral intake increases. When full oral intake is achieved, the IV may be capped and subcutaneous insulin begun. When surgery is elective, it is best performed early in the day, allowing the patient maximal recovery time to restart oral intake and subcutaneous insulin therapy. When elective surgery is brief (less than 1 hr) and full oral intake is expected shortly afterward, one may simply monitor the blood glucose hourly and give a rapid analog according to the child's home glucose correction scale. If glargine is used as the basal insulin, a full dose is given the evening before planned surgery. If NPH, lente, or ultralente are used, one half of the morning dose is given before surgery. The child should not be discharged until blood glucose levels are stable and oral intake is tolerated.

Long-Term Complications: Relation to Glycemic Control. The increasingly prolonged survival of the diabetic child is associated with an increasing prevalence of complications. Complications of DM can be divided into three major categories—(1) microvascular complications, specifically retinopathy and nephropathy; (2) macrovascular complications, particularly accelerated coronary artery disease, cerebrovascular disease, and peripheral vascular disease; and (3) neuropathies, both peripheral and autonomic, affecting a variety of organs and systems. Cataracts affect the lens.

Diabetic retinopathy is the leading cause of blindness in the United States in adults aged 20–65 yr. The risk of diabetic retinopathy after 15 yr duration of diabetes is 98% for individuals with type 1 DM and 78% for those with type 2 DM. Lens opacities (due to glycation of tissue proteins and activation of polyol pathway) are present in at least 5% of those younger than 19 yr of age. Although the metabolic control has an impact on the development of this complication, genetic factors also have a role, because only 50% of patients develop proliferative retinopathy. The earliest clinically apparent manifestations of diabetic retinopathy are classified as nonproliferative or background diabetic retinopathy—microaneurysms, dot and blot hemorrhages, hard and soft exudates, venous dilation and beading, and intraretinal microvascular abnormalities. These changes do not impair vision. The more severe form is proliferative diabetic retinopathy—manifested by neovascularization, fibrous proliferation, and preretinal and vitreous hemorrhages. Proliferative retinopathy, if not treated, is relentlessly progressive and impairs vision, leading to blindness. The mainstay of treatment is panretinal laser photocoagulation. In advanced diabetic eye disease—manifested by severe vitreous hemorrhage or fibrosis, often with retinal detachment—vitrectomy is an important therapeutic modality. Eventually, the eye disease becomes quiescent, a stage termed *involutional retinopathy*. A separate subtype of retinopathy is diabetic maculopathy, which is manifested by severe macular edema impairing central vision, for which focal laser photocoagulation may be effective.

Guidelines suggest that diabetic patients have an initial dilated and comprehensive examination by an ophthalmologist shortly after the diagnosis of diabetes is made in patients with type 2 DM, and within 3–5 yr after the onset of type 1 DM (but not before age 10 yr). Any patients with visual symptoms or abnormalities should be referred for ophthalmologic evaluation. Subsequent evaluations for both type 1 and type 2 DM patients should be repeated annually by an ophthalmologist who is experienced in diagnosing the presence of diabetic retinopathy and is knowledgeable about its management.

Diabetic nephropathy is the leading known cause of end-stage renal disease (ESRD) in the United States. Most ESRD from diabetic nephropathy is preventable. Diabetic nephropathy affects 20–30% of patients with type 1 DM and 15–20% of type 2 DM patients 20 yr after onset. The mean 5-yr life expectancy for patients with diabetes-related ESRD is less than 20%. The increased mortality risk in long-term type 1 DM may be due to nephropathy, which may account for about 50% of deaths. The risk of nephropathy increases with duration of diabetes, up until 25–30 yr duration (after which this complication rarely begins), degree of metabolic control, and genetic predisposition to essential hypertension. Only 30–40% of patients affected by type 1 DM eventually experience ESRD. The glycation of tissue proteins results in glomerular basement membrane thickening. The course of diabetic nephropathy is slow. An increased urinary albumin excretion rate (AER) of 30–300 mg/24 hr (20–200 µg/min)—so-called microalbuminuria—can be detected and constitutes an early stage of nephropathy from intermittent to persistent (incipient), which is commonly associated with glomerular hyperfiltration and blood pressure elevation. As nephropathy evolves to early overt stage with proteinuria (AER > 300 mg/24 hr or > 200 µg/min), it is accompanied by hypertension. Advanced stage nephropathy is defined by a progressive decline in renal function (declining glomerular filtration rate and elevation of serum blood urea and creatinine), progressive proteinuria, and hypertension. Progression to ESRD is recognized by the appearance of uremia, the nephritic syndrome, and the need for renal replacement (transplantation or dialysis).

Screening for diabetic nephropathy is a routine aspect of diabetes care. The American Diabetes Association (ADA) recommends yearly screening for individuals with type 2 DM and yearly screening for those with type 1 DM after 5 yr duration of disease (but not before puberty). Twenty-four hour AER (urinary albumin and creatinine) or timed (overnight) urinary AER are acceptable techniques. Positive results should be confirmed by a second measurement of AER because of the high variability of albumin excretion in patients with diabetes. Short-term hyperglycemia, exercise, urinary tract infections, marked hypertension, heart failure, and acute febrile illness can cause transient elevation urinary albumin excretion. There is marked day-to-day variability in albumin excretion, so at least two of three collections done in a 3–6 mo period should show elevated levels before a patient is diagnosed with microalbuminuria and treatment is started. Once albuminuria is diagnosed, a number of factors attenuate the effect of hyperfiltration on kidneys: (1) meticulous control of hyperglycemia, (2) aggressive control of systemic blood pressure, (3) selective control of arteriolar dilation by use of angiotensin-converting enzyme (ACE) inhibitors (thus decreasing transglomerular capillary pressure), and (4) dietary protein restriction (because high protein intake increases renal perfusion rate).

Diabetic Neuropathy. Both the peripheral and autonomic nervous systems can be involved, and adolescents with diabetes can show early evidence of neuropathy. This complication can be traced to the metabolic effects of hyperglycemia and/or other effects of insulin deficiency on the various constituents of the peripheral nerve. The polyol pathway, nonenzymatic glycation, and/or disturbances of myoinositol metabolism affecting one or more cell types in the multicellular constituents of the peripheral nerve appear likely to have an inciting role. The role of other factors, such as possible direct neurotrophic effects of insulin, insulin-related growth factors, nitric oxide, and stress proteins, seems to be relevant. Peripheral neuropathy may first present in some adolescents with long-standing history of diabetes. Using quantitative sensory testing (QST), abnormal cutaneous thermal perception is a common finding in both upper and lower limbs in neurologically asymptomatic young diabetic patients. Heat-induced pain threshold in the hand is correlated with the duration of the diabetes. There is no correlation between QST scores and metabolic control. Subclinical motor nerve impairment as manifested by reduced sensory nerve conduction velocity and sensory nerve action potential amplitude can be detected during late puberty and after puberty in about 10% of adolescents. Poor metabolic control during puberty appears to induce deteriorating peripheral neural function in young patients. An early sign of autonomic neuropathy such as decreased heart rate variability may present in adolescents with a history of long-standing disease and poor metabolic control. A number of therapeutic strategies have been attempted with variable results. These treatment modalities include (1) improvement in metabolic control, (2) use of aldose reductase inhibitors to reduce by-products of polyol pathway, (3) use of α-lipoic acid (an antioxidant) that enhances tissue nitric oxide and its metabolites, and use of anticonvulsants (e.g., lorazepam, valproate, carbamazepine, tiagabine, and topiramate) for treatment of neuropathic pain.

Other complications in diabetic children include dwarfism associated with a glycogen-laden enlarged liver (Mauriac syndrome), osteopenia, and a *syndrome of limited joint mobility* associated with tight, waxy skin, growth impairment, and maturational delay. The Mauriac syndrome is related to under-insulinization; it is rare because of the availability of the longer-acting insulins. Clinical features of Mauriac syndrome include moon face, protuberant abdomen, proximal muscle wasting, and enlarged liver due to fat and glycogen infiltration. The syndrome of limited joint mobility is frequently associated with the early development of diabetic microvascular complications, such as retinopathy and nephropathy, which may appear before 18 yr of age.

Prognosis. Type 1 DM is not a benign disease. It has been estimated that average life span of individuals with diabetes is about 10 yr shorter than nondiabetic population. Visual, renal, neuropathic, and other complications were relatively frequent. Furthermore, although diabetic children eventually attain a height within the normal adult range, puberty may be delayed, and the final height may be less than the genetic potential. From studies in identical twins, it is apparent that despite seemingly satisfactory control, the diabetic twin manifests delayed puberty and a substantial reduction in height when onset of disease occurs before puberty. These observations indicate that, in the past, conventional criteria for judging control were inadequate and that adequate control of type 1 DM was almost never achieved by routine means.

The introduction of portable devices (insulin pumps) that can be programmed to provide CSII with meal-related pulses is one approach to the resolution of these long-term problems. In selected individuals, nearly normal patterns of blood glucose and other indices of metabolic control, including HbA_{1c}, have been maintained for several years. This approach, however, should be reserved for highly motivated persons committed to rigorous self-monitoring of blood glucose, who are alert to the potential complications such as mechanical failure of the infusion device causing hyperglycemia or hypoglycemia and to infections at the site of catheter insertion.

The changing pattern of metabolic control is having a profound influence on reducing the incidence and the severity of certain complications. For example, after 20 yr of diabetes, there is a decline in the incidence of nephropathy in type 1 DM in Sweden among children diagnosed in 1971–1975 compared with those diagnosed in the preceding decade. Also, in most patients with microalbuminuria in whom it was possible to obtain good glycemic control, microalbuminuria disappeared. Thus, prognosis is related to metabolic control.

Pancreas and Islet Transplantation and Regeneration. In an attempt to cure type 1 DM, transplantation of a segment of the pancreas or of isolated islets has been performed. These procedures are both technically demanding and associated with the risks of disease recurrence and complications of rejection and its treatment by immunosuppression. Hence, segmental pancreas transplantation is generally performed in association with transplantation of a kidney for a patient with ESRD due to diabetic nephropathy in which the immunosuppressive regimen is indicated for the renal transplantation. Several thousand such transplants have been performed in adults. With experience and newer immunosuppressive agents, functional survival of the pancreatic graft may be achieved for up to several years, during which time patients may be in metabolic control with no or minimal exogenous insulin and reversal of some of the microvascular complications. However, because children and adolescents with DM are not likely to have ESRD from their diabetes, pancreas transplantation as a primary treatment in children cannot be recommended or its risk justified. Complications of immunosuppression include the development of malignancy. Some antirejection drugs, notably cyclosporine and tacrolimus, are themselves toxic to the islets of Langerhans, impairing insulin secretion and even causing diabetes. Attempts to transplant isolated islets have been equally challenging because of rejection. Research continues to improve techniques for the yield, viability, and reduction of immunogenicity of the islets of Langerhans for transplantation.

An islet transplantation strategy (Edmonton-protocol) infuses isolated pancreatic islets into the portal vein of a group of adults with type 1 DM. This therapeutic strategy also involved the use of a new generation of immunosuppressive medications that apparently have lower side-effect profiles than other drugs. Out of 15 consecutive patients with at least 1 yr of follow-up after the initial transplant, 12 (80%) were insulin independent at 1 yr. Although patients experienced minimal side effects from immunosuppressive medications, some complications associated with islet transplantation procedures were observed that included portal vein thrombosis, bleeding related to the percutaneous portal vein access, an expanding intrahepatic and subscapular hemorrhage on anticoagulation (requiring transfusion and surgery). Elevated liver function test results were found in 46% of subjects but resolved in all.

Regeneration of islets is an approach that could potentially cure type 1 DM. It is classified into three categories:

1. In vitro therapy using transplanted cultured cells, including embryonic stem cells, pancreatic stem cells, and β cell lines, in conjunction with immunosuppressive therapy or immunoisolation.
2. Ex vivo regeneration therapy, patients' own cells, such as bone marrow stem cells, which are transiently removed and induced to differentiate into β cells in vitro. At present, however, insulin-producing cells cannot be generated from bone marrow stem cells.
3. In vivo regeneration therapy, in which impaired tissues regenerate from patients' own cells in vivo. β-cell neogenesis from non–β cells and β-cell proliferation in vivo has been considered, particularly as regeneration therapies for type 2 DM.

Regeneration therapy of pancreatic β cells can be combined with various other therapeutic strategies, including islet transplantation, cell-based therapy, gene therapy, and drug therapy to promote β-cell proliferation and neogenesis, and it is hoped that these strategies will, in the future, provide a cure for diabetes.

583.3 Type 2 Diabetes Mellitus

Type 2 DM is considered a polygenic disease aggravated by environmental factors, such as low physical activity or hypercaloric lipid-rich diet. Obese type 2 diabetic patients show insulin resistance of skeletal muscle, enhanced hepatic glucose production, and decreased glucose-induced insulin secretion. Over time, hyperglycemia worsens, a phenomenon that has been attributed to deleterious effect of chronic hyperglycemia (glucotoxicity) or chronic hyperlipidemia (lipotoxicity) on β-cell function and is often accompanied by increased triglyceride content and decreased insulin gene expression. This category of diabetes has been considered a disease of obese and sedentary adults after age 40 yr. Numerous studies describe type 2 DM in Native American youth, as well as their African American, Hispanic, and white peers. Pediatric type 2 DM in adolescents represents one of the most rapidly growing forms of diabetes. The incidence of type 2 DM among children diagnosed with diabetes at one medical center increased from 4% before 1992 to 16% in 1994. In that report, among those aged 10–19 yr, type 2 DM accounted for one third of all newly diagnosed children with diabetes in 1994. Overall, the incidence of adolescent type 2 DM increased 10-fold from 0.7 to 7.2/100,000 per year in the reported Midwest metropolitan area. The mean age of presentation was 13.8 yr; most children were markedly obese. We have observed a more than 10-fold increase in incidence of type 2 DM (from less than 2% to about 22% of new cases of DM) in children aged 10–18 yr in the past decade. African American, Hispanic, and white adolescents are usually affected. African Americans constitute almost 70% of the type 2 DM cases.

The epidemic of type 2 DM in children and adolescents parallels the emergence of the obesity epidemic. Although obesity itself is associated with insulin resistance, diabetes does not develop until there is some degree of failure of insulin secretion. Thus, when measured, insulin secretion in response to glucose or other stimuli is always lower in persons with type 2 DM than in control subjects matched for age, sex, weight, and equivalent glucose concentration. Although it is generally believed that autoimmune destruction of pancreatic β cells does not occur in type 2 DM diabetes, autoimmune markers of type 1 DM, namely GAD65, ICA512, and IAA may be positive in up to one third of the cases of adolescent type 2 DM. These findings reflect a broad spectrum of pancreatic and peripheral abnormalities that could lead to type 2 DM and the presence of these autoimmune markers does not rule out type 2 DM in children and adolescents.

In type 2 DM, insulin deficiency is rarely absolute, so patients usually do not need insulin to survive, although glycemic control may be improved by exogenous insulin. DKA, when it occurs, is associated with the stress of another illness such as severe infection and may resolve when the stressful illness resolves. DKA tends to be more common in African American patients than in other ethnic groups. Most patients with type 2 DM remain asymptomatic for months to years because hyperglycemia is so moderate that symptoms are not as dramatic as the polyuria and weight loss accompanying type 1 DM; weight gain may continue. The prolonged hyperglycemia may be accompanied, in time, by the development of microvascular and macrovascular complications. Type 2 DM occurs more frequently in certain ethnic or racial groups, such as Pacific Islanders, Pima Indians, and African Americans. It also occurs in individuals with hypertension and dyslipidemia. Type 2 DM has a stronger genetic component than in type 1 DM. Concordance rates among identical twins are virtually 100% for type 2 and only 30–50% for type 1 DM. The genetic basis for type 2 DM is complex and incompletely defined; no single identified defect predominates as does the HLA association with type 1 DM. *Acanthosis nigricans* may be a marker for insulin resistance, hyperinsulinemia, and eventually type 2 DM. Hirsutism, associated with the *polycystic ovary syndrome*, premature adrenarche, or mild mutations in steroidogenic enzymes, is frequently associated with insulin resistance in children and adolescents and may be a forerunner of the future development of type 2 DM (see Chapter 580).

Type A insulin resistance with acanthosis nigricans is characterized by severe insulin resistance and acanthosis nigricans in the absence of obesity or lipoatrophy; affected females also have hyperandrogenism, possibly as a secondary manifestation of the hyperinsulinemia with stimulation of androgen synthesis by ovarian theca cells (see Chapter 580). Glucose intolerance is variable and includes symptomatic diabetes. The hyperandrogenism presents with clinical and biochemical findings suggestive of polycystic ovary syndrome. Some patients, predominantly African American females with obesity, acanthosis nigricans, and accelerated growth suggestive of gigantism, may represent insulin resistance due to obesity with downregulation of the insulin receptor. The gigantism may represent a "spillover" effect of insulin acting via the insulin growth factor 1 receptor rather than as the insulin receptor.

Treatment. Nutritional education is a cornerstone of therapy for children and adolescents with type 2 DM. These children often come from a household environment with a poor understanding of healthy eating habits. Commonly observed behaviors include skipping meals, heavy snacking, and excessive daily television viewing, video game playing, and computer use. Adolescents engage in non-appetite–based eating (i.e., emotional eating, television-cued eating, boredom) and cyclic dieting ("yo-yo"). Treatment for type 2 DM should target weight loss and increasing physical activity as an initial approach. These approaches, however, are frequently unsuccessful.

The only universally accepted pharmacologic agent available for type 2 DM in children is insulin. Although optimal glycemic control can be obtained with insulin therapy, it often results in significant weight gain. At the time of diagnosis and depending on presentation, insulin therapy may be necessary, but with close medical follow-up, it can often be reduced, substituted, or even discontinued within a few weeks after glucose control is achieved. Once a patient is nonacidotic and well hydrated, an effective therapy is to initiate insulin management in combination with metformin (a biguanide), which decreases hepatic glucose production. The starting dose of metformin is usually 500 mg, twice daily with meals. Metformin is contraindicated if there is significant renal or liver impairment. Therefore, proper assessment of liver and renal function is essential before initiating therapy. A class of pharmaceutical agents, the thiozolidinediones, enhances insulin action by decreasing hepatic glucose production and facilitating glucose disposal in muscle and fat. Because they act as insulin enhancers, they are used in conjunction with exogenous insulin and metformin. These agents, the "glitazones," are not approved for use in children in the United States; undue liver toxicity has been reported.

Prevention. The difficulties in achieving good glucose control and preventing diabetes complications make prevention a compelling strategy. This is particularly true for type 2 DM, which is clearly linked to modifiable risk factors, i.e., obesity, and a sedentary lifestyle. The Diabetes Prevention Program (DPP) was designed to prevent or delay the development of type 2 DM in adult individuals at high risk for its development by virtue of their having impaired glucose tolerance (IGT). The DPP results demonstrated that intensified lifestyle or drug intervention in individuals with IGT prevented or delayed the onset of type 2 DM. The results were striking. Lifestyle intervention reduced diabetes incidence by 58%; metformin reduced the incidence by 31% compared with placebo. The effects were similar for men and women and for all racial and ethnic groups. Lifestyle interventions are believed to have similar beneficial effects in obese adolescents with IGT.

Impaired Glucose Tolerance. The term *impaired glucose tolerance* (IGT) is suggested as a replacement for terms such as asymptomatic diabetes, chemical diabetes, subclinical diabetes, borderline diabetes, or latent diabetes in order to avoid the stigma associated with the term *diabetes mellitus*, which may influence the choice of vocation, eligibility for health or life insurance, and self-image. Although IGT represents a biochemical intermediate between normal glucose metabolism and that of diabetes, experience has shown that few children with IGT go on to acquire diabetes; estimates range from 0–10%. There is disagreement about whether the degree of glucose intolerance is useful as a prognostic index of the likelihood of progression, but there is evidence that among the few instances of progression, the insulin response during glucose tolerance testing is severely impaired. Islet cell or insulin autoantibodies as well as the HLA-DR3 or -DR4 haplotype are commonly found in those who go on to develop clinical diabetes. In most obese children with IGT, insulin responses during oral glucose tolerance tests are higher than the mean for age-adjusted but not weight-adjusted control subjects; these individuals have some resistance to the effects of insulin rather than a total inability to secrete it.

In healthy nondiabetic children, the glucose response during an oral glucose tolerance test is similar at all ages. In contrast, plasma insulin responses during the test increase progressively within the age span of about 3–15 yr and are significantly higher during puberty so that interpretation of these responses requires comparison with age- and puberty-adjusted responses.

The performance of the glucose tolerance test should be standardized according to currently accepted criteria. These include

at least 3 days of a well-balanced diet containing approximately 50% of calories from carbohydrates, fasting from midnight until the time of the test in the morning, and a dose of glucose for the test of 1.75 g/kg but not more than 75 g. Plasma samples are obtained before ingestion of the glucose and at 1, 2, and 3 hr thereafter. The arbitrarily designated response to the test that identifies IGT is a fasting plasma glucose value of less than 126 mg/dL and a value at 2 hr of more than 140 mg/dL but less than 200 mg/dL (see Table 583–2). Determination of serum insulin responses during the glucose tolerance test is not a prerequisite for reaching a diagnosis; the magnitude of the response, however, may have prognostic value.

In children with IGT but without fasting hyperglycemia, repeated oral glucose tolerance tests are not recommended. Investigations in such children indicate that the degree of impaired glucose tolerance tends to remain stable or may actually improve over a period of years, except in patients with markedly subnormal insulin responses. Consequently, apart from reduction in weight for the obese child, no therapy is indicated. In particular, the use of oral hypoglycemic agents should be restricted to investigational studies. If fasting hyperglycemia or characteristic symptoms of diabetes develop, the affected children have the characteristics of type 2 DM, previously known as NIDDM (see Table 583–1).

583.4 Other Specific Types of Diabetes

Genetic Defects of β-Cell Function

MATURITY-ONSET DIABETES OF YOUTH. This subtype of DM contains a group of heterogeneous genetic and clinical entities, which are characterized by early onset between the ages of 9 and 25 yr of age, autosomal dominant inheritance (AD), and a primary defect in insulin secretion. Three types of maturity-onset diabetes of youth (MODY) genes have been identified. MODY 1 results from a mutation in the hepatocyte nuclear factor (HNF)-4α gene located on the long arm of chromosome 20. MODY 2 is caused by a mutation in the gene for glucokinase located on the short arm of chromosome 7. MODY 3 is due to a gene mutation for HNF-1α located on the long arm of chromosome 12. Strict criteria for the diagnosis of MODY include diabetes in at least three generations with AD transmission and diagnosis before age 25 yr in at least one affected subject.

Mutations in the glucokinase gene responsible for MODY 2 result in mild, chronic hyperglycemia due to mild reductions in pancreatic β-cell response to glucose. As a result, this is usually a relatively mild form of diabetes with mild fasting hyperglycemia and IGT in the majority of patients, which can be treated with small doses of exogenously administered insulin. Patients affected with mutations in HNF-4α or -1α show more severe abnormalities of carbohydrate metabolism, varying from impaired glucose tolerance to severe diabetes and often progressing from a mild to a severe form over time. About one third of these patients will require insulin and are prone to the development of vascular complications. Patients with MODY 2 and defects in the glucokinase gene may demonstrate normal insulin responses to intravenous glucose when blood glucose concentrations are maintained at greater than 7 mM. Defective glucokinase activity has been likened to a defective glucose sensor in the pancreatic β cell. By contrast, patients with MODY 1 and MODY 3 have more severe impairment of insulin secretion, and this defect cannot be overcome by priming with glucose infusion.

By definition, the absence of a family history suggestive of AD inheritance makes a diagnosis of MODY virtually untenable. In such circumstances, the appearance of diabetes in a relatively young person would most likely represent evolving type 1 DM, and therefore evaluation for markers of autoimmunity are warranted. Milder, slowly evolving type 1 DM could be confused with type 2 DM.

Distinction among the present forms of MODY has clinical relevance in counseling because of the lesser likelihood of vascular complications in MODY 2 and, therefore, the need to treat appropriately with insulin, if necessary, in patients with MODY 1 and MODY 3. Molecular analysis for the currently known gene mutations on chromosomes 20, 7, and 12 are likely to become available for routine clinical use in the future to facilitate diagnosis and management. An additional form of MODY due to heterozygous mutation in a homeodomain transcription factor called insulin promoter factor-1 has also been described.

Primary or secondary defects in *GLUT-2 type of glucose transporter,* an insulin-independent form, may also be associated with diabetes. GLUT-2 rapidly transports glucose into β cells for subsequent phosphorylation by glucokinase, which eventually leads to insulin secretion. The phenomenon of glucose toxicity, in which there is a loss or reduction in the first-phase insulin response to a pulse of glucose, may be the result of secondary downregulation of GLUT-2 transporters.

MODY also may be a manifestation of a *polymorphism in the glycogen synthase gene.* This enzyme is crucially important for storage of glucose as glycogen in muscle. Patients with this defect are notable for marked resistance to insulin and hypertension as well as a strong family history of diabetes.

MITOCHONDRIAL GENE DEFECTS. Point mutations in mitochondrial DNA are sometimes associated with DM and deafness. One mutation is identical to the mutation in MELAS (myopathy, encephalopathy, lactic acidosis, and stroke–like syndrome), but this syndrome is not associated with diabetes so that the phenotypic expression of the same defect varies. Another form of IDDM, sometimes associated with mitochondrial mutations, is the Wolfram syndrome.

Wolfram syndrome is characterized by diabetes insipidus, DM, optic atrophy, and deafness—thus the acronym DIDMOAD. Wolfram syndrome is caused by mitochondrial dysfunction, possibly by a nuclear gene mapped to the short arm of chromosome 4. Some patients with diabetes appear to have severe insulinopenia, whereas others have significant insulin secretion as judged by C-peptide. In two patients who were tested, islet cell antibodies were not detected, whereas HLA typing revealed DR2, which is generally considered "protective" for diabetes. In some patients with diabetes and deafness, a mutation in mitochondrial tRNA has been detected; in others, this mutation is absent. The overall prevalence is 1/770,000. The sequence of appearance of the stigmata was as follows: nonautoimmune IDDM in the 1st decade; central diabetes insipidus and sensorineural deafness in two thirds to three fourths of the patients in the 2nd decade; renal tract anomalies in about one half of the patients in the 3rd decade; and neurologic complications such as cerebellar ataxia and myoclonus in one half to two thirds of the patients in the 4th decade. Other features included primary gonadal atrophy in the majority of males and a progressive neurodegenerative course with neurorespiratory death at a median age of 30 yr. Absence of maternal diabetes or deafness and absence of the previously reported mitochondrial gene defect suggests autosomal recessive inheritance.

DIABETES MELLITUS OF THE NEWBORN

Transient. Onset of persistent type 1 DM before the age of 6 mo is most unusual. The syndrome of transient DM in the newborn infant has its onset in the 1st wk of life and persists only several weeks to months before spontaneous resolution. It occurs most often in infants who are small for gestational age and is characterized by hyperglycemia and pronounced glycosuria, resulting in severe dehydration and, at times, metabolic acidosis but with only minimal or no ketonemia or ketonuria. Insulin responses to glucose or tolbutamide are low to absent; basal plasma insulin concentrations are normal. After sponta-

neous recovery, the insulin responses to these same stimuli are brisk and normal, implying a functional delay in β-cell maturation with spontaneous resolution. Occurrence of the syndrome in consecutive siblings has been reported. Abnormalities of chromosome 6 are common in transient neonatal DM. There are also reports of patients with classic type 1 DM who formerly had transient diabetes of the newborn. It remains to be determined whether this association of transient diabetes in the newborn followed much later in life by classic type 1 DM is a chance occurrence or causally related. This syndrome should be distinguished from severe hyperglycemia that may occur in hypertonic dehydration; this condition usually occurs in infants beyond the newborn period who respond promptly to rehydration with a minimal requirement for insulin.

Administration of insulin is mandatory during the active phase of DM in the newborn. One to 2 U/kg/24 hr of an intermediate-acting insulin in two divided doses usually results in dramatic improvement and accelerated growth and gain in weight. Attempts at gradually reducing the dose of insulin may be made as soon as recurrent hypoglycemia becomes manifested or after 2 mo of age.

Permanent. DM in the newborn period may be permanent if associated with the rare syndrome of pancreatic agenesis. Long-term follow-up of a cohort of patients with neonatal diabetes revealed that almost one half had permanent diabetes, one third had transient diabetes, and about one fourth had transient diabetes that recurred when they were 7–20 yr old. The majority of all these infants were small at birth. Instances of affected twins and families with more than one affected infant have been reported. Some cases of permanent neonatal DM are initially euglycemic and present within the first month of life.

ABNORMALITIES OF THE INSULIN GENE. Diabetes of variable degrees may also result from *defects in the insulin gene* from faulty processing of proinsulin to insulin, an autosomal dominant defect, to various amino acid substitutions that impair the effectiveness of insulin at the receptor level. However, these defects are notable for the high concentration of insulin as measured by radioimmunoassay, whereas defects in glucokinase, MODY-1, MODY-3, and GLUT-2 are characterized by relative or absolute deficiency of insulin secretion for the prevailing glucose concentrations.

Genetic Defects of Insulin Action. Two mutations in the insulin receptor gene with relevance for children are leprechaunism and Rabson-Mendenhall syndrome.

LEPRECHAUNISM. This is a syndrome characterized by intrauterine growth retardation, fasting hypoglycemia, and postprandial hyperglycemia in association with profound resistance to insulin, whose serum concentrations may be 100-fold that of comparable age-matched infants during an oral glucose tolerance test. Various defects of the insulin receptor have been described, thereby attesting to the important role of insulin and its receptor in fetal growth and possibly in morphogenesis. However, even probable complete absence of functional insulin receptors due to homozygous inheritance of a missense mutation in the insulin-receptor gene resulted in normal organogenesis and a liveborn infant who had a severe form of leprechaunism. Most of these patients die in the 1st yr of life.

RABSON-MENDENHALL SYNDROME. This entity is defined by clinical manifestations that appear to be intermediate between those of acanthosis nigricans with insulin resistance type A and leprechaunism. The features include extreme insulin resistance, acanthosis nigricans, abnormalities of the teeth and nails, and pineal hyperplasia. It is not clear whether this syndrome is entirely distinct from leprechaunism; however, patients with Rabson-Mendenhall tend to live beyond the 1st yr of life. Defects in the insulin-receptor gene have been described in this syndrome.

Cystic Fibrosis-Related Diabetes. Because of improvements in the medical care of children with cystic fibrosis (CF), many survive to the late teenage and early adult years. On the other hand, as the annual screening of patients for diabetes among CF centers has become routine, the number of CF-related diabetes (CFRD) cases has almost more than doubled. It is estimated that up to 25% of adolescents with CF have diabetes. The care of these patients is very different from that of patients with type 1 or type 2 DM, because CFRD patients have distinct pathophysiology and complicated nutritional and medical problems.

Patients with CFRD are slender and have insulin deficiency. The clinical presentation is similar to that of type 2 DM in that the onset of the disease is insidious and the occurrence of ketoacidosis is rare. Islet antibody titers are negative. The prevalence of microvascular complications in CFRD in relationship to duration of diabetes, glycemic control, and pulmonary diseases are not well characterized. Macrovascular complications do not appear to be of concern in CFRD. Several factors unique to CF influence both the onset and the course of diabetes: (1) frequent acute or chronic infections are associated with waxing and waning of insulin resistance; (2) energy needs are increased because of infection and pulmonary disease; (3) malnutrition is associated with poor survival; (4) malabsorption is caused by pancreatic exocrine insufficiency, despite enzyme supplementation; (5) altered nutrient absorption is caused by abnormal intestinal transit time; (6) liver disease is present; (7) anorexia and nausea are common as a result of illness, gastroesophageal reflux, delayed gastric emptying, intestinal obstruction, increased work of breathing, and psychosocial factors; (8) there is a wide variation in daily food intake based on the patient's acute health status; and (9) insulin and glucagon secretion are impaired.

In the pancreas, exocrine tissue is replaced by fibrosis and fat; many of the pancreatic islets are destroyed. The remaining islets demonstrate diminished numbers of β-, α-, and pancreatic polypeptide-secreting cells. Secretion of the islet hormones insulin, glucagon, and pancreatic polypeptide is impaired in patients with CF in response to a variety of secretagogues. It has been suggested that insulin resistance may also play a role in the development of CFRD, especially in the setting of acute infection.

In Denmark, oral glucose tolerance screening of the entire CF population demonstrated no diabetes in patients younger than 10 yr, 12% diabetes in patients aged 10–19 yr, and 48% diabetes in adults aged 20 yr and older. At a Midwestern center where routine annual oral glucose tolerance screening is performed, only about one half of children and one fourth of adults have normal glucose tolerance. Diabetes is seen in 9% of CF children, 26% of adolescents, and 35% of adults aged 20–29 yr. About one third of patients with CFRD have fasting hyperglycemia and two thirds have CFRD without fasting hyperglycemia. The fasting hyperglycemia is exacerbated chronically, or intermittently with infection or glucocorticoid therapy in 3% of children, 11% of adolescents, and 15% of adults.

When hyperglycemia develops, the accompanying metabolic derangements are usually mild and, if insulin therapy becomes necessary, relatively low doses usually suffice for adequate management. Ketoacidosis is uncommon but may occur with progressive deterioration of islet cell function. Treatment with insulin is as outlined for type 1 DM, but dietary management may be limited by the constraints of the primary disturbance.

Autoimmune Diseases. *Chronic lymphocytic thyroiditis (Hashimoto thyroiditis)* is frequently associated with type 1 DM in children (Chapter 559). As many as one in five insulin-dependent diabetic patients may have thyroid antibodies in their serum; the prevalence is 2–20 times greater than that observed in control populations. Only a small proportion of these patients, however, acquire clinical hypothyroidism; the interval between diagnosis of diabetes and thyroid disease averages about 5 yr. Periodic palpation of the thyroid gland is indicated in all diabetic children; if the gland feels firm or enlarged, or both, serum measurements of thyroid antibodies and thyroid-stimulating hormone (TSH) should be obtained. A TSH level of greater than 10 μU/mL indicates existing or incipient thyroid dysfunction that warrants replacement with thyroid hormone. Deceleration in the rate of growth may also be due to thyroid failure and is, in itself, a reason for securing serum measurements of thyroxine and TSH concentrations.

When diabetes and thyroid disease coexist, the possibility of *adrenal insufficiency* should also be considered. It may be heralded by decreasing insulin requirements, increasing pigmentation of the skin and buccal mucosa, salt craving, weakness, asthenia and postural hypotension, or even frank addisonian crisis as evidence of primary adrenal failure. This syndrome is most unusual in the 1st decade of life, but it may become apparent in the 2nd decade or later.

Celiac disease, formerly known as nontropical sprue, another autoimmune disorder, is due to hypersensitivity to dietary gluten that occurs with significant frequency in children with type 1 DM (Chapter 320.8). It is estimated that about 7.0% of children with type 1 DM develop celiac disease within the first 6 yr from the diagnosis. Young children with type 1 DM and celiac disease usually present with gastrointestinal symptoms (abdominal cramping, diarrhea, and gastroesophageal reflux), growth failure due to suboptimal weight gain, and unexplained hypoglycemic reactions due to nutrient malabsorption, whereas adolescents may remain asymptomatic for the most part. The diagnosis of celiac disease is considered if serum antiendomysial and/or tissue transglutaminase antibody titers are positive in the presence of normal serum total IgA level. However, the diagnosis is confirmed on endoscopic evaluation and biopsy of small bowel revealing characteristic histopathologic (atrophic) changes of intestinal villi.

Circulating antibodies to gastric parietal cells and to intrinsic factor are two to three times more common in patients with type 1 DM than in control subjects. There are good correlations of antibodies to gastric parietal cells with atrophic gastritis and of antibodies to intrinsic factor with *malabsorption of vitamin B_{12}.* Although the possibility of megaloblastic anemia should be considered in children with type 1 diabetes, its occurrence is rare.

A *variant of the multiple endocrine deficiency syndrome* is characterized by type 1 diabetes-idiopathic intestinal mucosal atrophy with associated inflammation and severe malabsorption, IgA deficiency, and circulating antibodies to multiple endocrine organs including the thyroid, adrenal, pancreas, parathyroid, and gonads. In addition, nondiabetic family members have an increased frequency of vitiligo, Graves disease, and multiple sclerosis as well as low complement levels and antibodies to endocrine tissues.

Endocrinopathies. The endocrinopathies listed in Table 583–1 are only rarely encountered as a cause of diabetes in childhood. They may accelerate the manifestations of diabetes in those with inherited or acquired defects in insulin secretion or action.

Drugs. The immunosuppressive agents cyclosporin and tacrolimus are toxic to β cells, causing IDDM in a significant proportion of patients treated with these agents. Their toxicity to pancreatic β cells was a contributing factor in limiting their usefulness to arrest ongoing autoimmune destruction of β cells. Streptozotocin and the rodenticide Vacor also are toxic to β cells, causing diabetes.

Genetic Syndromes Associated with Diabetes Mellitus. A number of rare genetic syndromes associated with IDDM or carbohydrate intolerance have been described (see Table 583–1). These syndromes represent a broad spectrum of diseases ranging from premature cellular aging, as in the Werner and Cockayne syndromes (see Chapter 79), to excessive obesity associated with hyperinsulinism, resistance to insulin action, and carbohydrate intolerance as in the Prader-Willi syndrome (see Chapter 69). Some of these syndromes are characterized by primary disturbances in the insulin receptor or in antibodies to the insulin receptor without any impairment in insulin secretion. Although rare, these syndromes provide unique models to understand the multiple causes of disturbed carbohydrate metabolism from defective insulin secretion or from defective insulin action at the cell receptor or postreceptor level.

Epidemiology, Etiology, Pathology, Classification, and Prevention

Atkinson MA, Eisenbarth GS: Type 1 diabetes: New perspectives on disease pathogenesis and treatment. *Lancet* 2001;358:221–9.

Atkinson MA, Ellis TM: Infants diets and insulin-dependent diabetes: Evaluating the "cows' milk hypothesis" and a role for anti-bovine serum albumin immunity. *J Am Coll Nutr* 1997;16:334.

Atkinson MA, Maclaren NK: The pathogenesis of insulin-dependent diabetes mellitus. *N Engl J Med* 1994;331:1.

Bach JF: Insulin-dependent diabetes mellitus as an autoimmune disease. *Endocr Rev* 1994;15:516.

Casares S, Brumeanu TD: Insights into the pathogenesis of type 1 diabetes: A hint for novel immunospecific therapies. *Curr Molec Med* 2001;1:357–78.

Ferner RE: Drug-induced diabetes. *Baillieres Clin Endocrinol Metab* 1992;6:849.

Froguel P, Zouali H, Vionnet N, et al: Familial hyperglycemia due to mutations in glucokinase. *N Engl J Med* 1993;328:697.

Gottlieb PA, Eisenbarth GS: Diagnosis and treatment of pre-insulin dependent diabetes. *Annu Rev Med* 1998;49:391.

Kahn BB: Type 2 diabetes: When insulin secretion fails to compensate for insulin resistance. *Cell* 1998;92:593.

Karvonen M, Tuomilehto J, Libman I, et al: A review of the recent epidemiological data on the worldwide incidence of type 1 (insulin-dependent) diabetes mellitus. World Health Organization DIAMOND Project Group. *Diabetologia* 1993;36:883.

Mandrup-Poulsen T: Diabetes. *Br Med J* 1998;316:1221.

Report of the Expert Committee on the Diagnosis and Classification of Diabetes Mellitus. *Diabetes Care* 1999;22:55.

Schatz DA, Maclaren NK: Cow's milk and insulin-dependent diabetes mellitus. *JAMA* 1996;276:647.

Solimena M, DeCamilli P: Coxsackieviruses and diabetes. *Nat Med* 1995;1:25.

Weir GC: A defective β-cell glucose sensor as a cause of diabetes. *N Engl J Med* 1993;328:729.

Yoon JW: The role of viruses and environmental factors in the induction of diabetes. *Curr Top Microbiol Immunol* 1990;164:95.

Genetics

Cordell HJ, Todd JA: Multifactorial inheritance in type 1 diabetes. *Trends Genet* 1995;11:499.

Faas S, Trucco M: The genes influencing the susceptibility to IDDM in humans. *J Endocrinol Invest* 1994;17:477.

Ghosh S, Schork NJ: Genetic analysis of NIDDM. The study of quantitative traits. *Diabetes* 1996;45:1.

Johns DR: Mitochondrial DNA and disease. *N Engl J Med* 1995;333:638.

Owerbach D, Gabbay KH: The search for IDDM susceptibility genes: The next generation. *Diabetes* 1996;45:544.

Pratley RE, Thompson DB, Prochazka M, et al: An autosomal genomic scan for loci linked to prediabetic phenotypes in Pima Indians. *J Clin Invest* 1998;101:1757.

Velho G, Froguel P: Genetic, metabolic and clinical characteristics of maturity onset diabetes of the young. *Eur J Endocrinol* 1998;138:233.

Zamani M, Cassiman JJ: Reevaluation of the importance of polymorphic HLA class II alleles and amino acids in the susceptibility of individuals of different populations to type 1 diabetes. *Am J Med Genet* 1998;76:183.

Diabetic Ketoacidosis

Duck SC, Wyatt DT: Factors associated with brain herniation in the treatment of diabetic ketoacidosis. *J Pediatr* 1988;113:10–4.

Durr JA, Hoffman, WH, Sklar AH, et al: Correlates of brain edema in uncontrolled IDDM. *Diabetes* 1992;41:627.

Felner EI, White PC: Improving management of diabetic ketoacidosis in children. *Pediatrics* 2001;108:735–40.

Finberg L: Fluid management of diabetic ketoacidosis. *Pediatr Rev* 1996;17:46.

Genuth SM: Diabetic ketoacidosis and hyperglycemic hyperosmolar coma. *Curr Ther Endocrinol Metab* 1997;6:438.

Glaser N, Barnett P, McCaslin I, et al: Risk factors for cerebral edema in children with diabetic ketoacidosis. *N Engl J Med* 2001;344:264–9.

Glaser N, Kuppermann N, Yee C, et al: Variation in the management of pediatric diabetic ketoacidosis by specialty training. *Arch Pediatr Adolesc Med* 1997;151:1125–32.

Green SM, Rothrock SG, Ho JD, et al: Failure of adjunctive bicarbonate to improve outcome in severe pediatric diabetic ketoacidosis. *Ann Emerg Med* 1998;31:41–8.

Hale PM, Rezvani I, Braunstein AW, et al: Factors predicting cerebral edema in young children with diabetic ketoacidosis and new onset type 1 diabetes. *Acta Paediatr* 1997;86:626.

Harris GD, Fiordalisi I: Physiologic management of diabetic ketoacidemia. A 5-year prospective pediatric experience in 231 episodes. *Arch Pediatr Adolesc Med* 1994;148:1046–52.

Linares M, Schunk JE, Lindsay R: Laboratory presentation in diabetic ketoacidosis and duration of therapy. *Pediatr Emerg Care* 1996;12:347–51.

Okuda Y, Adrogue J, Field JB, et al: Counterproductive effects of sodium bicarbonate in diabetic ketoacidosis. *J Clin Endocrinol Metab* 1996;81:314–20.

Rosenbloom AL, Hanas R: Diabetic ketoacidosis treatment guidelines. *Clin Pediatr* 1996;261–6.

Rosenbloom AL: Intracerebral crisis during treatment of diabetic ketoacidosis. *Diabetes Care* 1990;13:22.

Tattersall RB: Brittle diabetes revisited: The Third Arnold Bloom Memorial Lecture. *Diabet Med* 1997;14:99.

Management of Type 1 Diabetes in Children

Arslanian S, Ohki Y, Becker DJ, Drash AL. The dawn phenomenon: comparison between normal and insulin-dependent diabetic adolescents. *Pediatr Res* 1992;31:203–6.

Bolli GB, Gerich JE: The "dawn phenomenon"—A common occurrence in both non-insulin and insulin-dependent diabetes mellitus. *N Engl J Med* 1984;310:746.

Bolli GB, Gottesman IS, Campbell PJ, et al: Glucose counter regulation and waning of insulin in the Somogyi phenomenon (posthypoglycemic hyperglycemia). *N Engl J Med* 1984;311:1214.

Goldstein DE: Understanding GHb assays: A guided tour for clinicians. *Clin Diabetes* 1986;4:7.

Kaufman FR, Devgan S, Roe TF, et al: Perioperative management with prolonged intravenous insulin infusion versus subcutaneous insulin in children with type 1 diabetes mellitus. *J Diab Comp* 1996;10:6–11.

Litton J, Rice A, Friedman N, et al: Insulin pump therapy in toddlers and preschool children with type 1 diabetes mellitus. *J Pediatr* 2002;141:490–5.

Rami B, Schober E: Postprandial glycaemia after regular and lispro insulin in children and adolescents with diabetes. *Eur J Pediatr* 1997;156:838.

Rutledge KS, Chase HP, Klingensmith GJ, et al: Effectiveness of postprandial Humalog in toddlers with diabetes. *Pediatrics* 1997;100:968.

Zinman B: The physiologic replacement of insulin. *N Engl J Med* 1989;321:363.

Long-Term Outcome of Childhood Diabetes: Relation of Control to Development of Complications

Bojestig M, Arnqvist HJ, Hermansson G, et al: Declining incidence of nephropathy in insulin-dependent diabetes mellitus. *N Engl J Med* 1994;330:15.

Bojestig M, Arnqvist HJ, Karlberg BE: Glycemic control and prognosis in type 1 diabetic patients with microalbuminuria. *Diabetes Care* 1996;19:313.

Diabetes Control and Complications Trial: Are continuing studies of metabolic control and microvascular complications in insulin-dependent diabetes mellitus justified? *N Engl J Med* 1988;318:246–50.

Leslie ND, Sperling MA: Relation of metabolic control to complications in diabetes mellitus. *J Pediatr* 1986;108:491.

Lewis EJ, Hunsicker LG, Bain RP, et al: The effect of angiotensin-converting enzyme inhibition on diabetic nephropathy. *N Engl J Med* 1993;329:1456.

Makita Z, Radoff S, Rayfield EJ, et al: Advanced-glycosylation end products in patients with diabetic nephropathy. *N Engl J Med* 1991;325:936.

Nathan DM: Long-term complications of diabetes mellitus. *N Engl J Med* 1993;328:1676.

Reichard P, Nilsson BY, Rosenqvist U: The effect of long-term intensified insulin treatment on the development of microvascular complications of diabetes mellitus. *N Engl J Med* 1993;329:304.

Rosenbloom AL: Skeletal and joint manifestations of childhood diabetes. *Pediatr Clin North Am* 1984;31:569.

Sandman DD, Shore AC, Tooke JE: Relation of skin capillary pressure in patients with insulin-dependent diabetes mellitus to complications and metabolic control. *N Engl J Med* 1992;327:760.

The absence of a glycemic threshold for the development of long-term complications: The perspective of the Diabetes Control and Complications Trial. *Diabetes* 1996;45:1289.

Wang PH: Tight glucose control and diabetic complications. *Lancet* 1993;342:129.

Diseases and Syndromes Associated with Diabetes

Barrett TG, Bundey SE: Wolfram (DIAMOAD) syndrome. *J Med Genet* 1997;34:838.

DeFronzo RA: Classification and diagnosis of diabetes mellitus. In DeFronzo RA (editor): *Current Management of Diabetes Mellitus.* St. Louis, CV Mosby, 1998, pp 8–13.

Jones KL: Non-insulin dependent diabetes in children and adolescents: The therapeutic challenge. *Clin Pediatr* 1998;37:103.

Krook A, Brueton L, O'Rahilly S: Homozygous nonsense mutation in the insulin receptor gene in an infant with leprechaunism. *Lancet* 1993;342:277.

Low L, Chernausek SD, Sperling MA: Acromegaloid patients with type-A insulin resistance: Parallel defects in insulin and insulin-like growth factor-I receptors and biological responses in cultured fibroblasts. *J Clin Endocrinol Metab* 1989;69:329.

Morrison EY, McKenzie K: The Mauriac syndrome. *West Indian Med J* 1989;38:180.

Pinhas-Hamiel O, Dolan LM, Daniels SR: Increased incidence of non-insulin-dependent diabetes mellitus among adolescents. *J Pediatr* 1996;128:608.

Pinhas-Hamiel O, Dolan LM, Zeitler PS: Diabetic ketoacidosis among obese African American adolescents with NIDDM. *Diabetes Care* 1997;20:484.

Rotig A, Cormier V, Chatelain P, et al: Deletion of mitochondrial DNA in a case of early-onset diabetes mellitus, optic atrophy, and deafness. *J Clin Invest* 1993;91:1095.

Sullivan MM, Denning CR: Diabetic microangiopathy in patients with cystic fibrosis. *Pediatrics* 1989;84:642.

Taylor SI, Cama A, Accili D, et al: Mutations in the insulin receptor gene. *Endocr Rev* 1992;13:566.

Watkins PB, Whitcomb RW: Hepatic dysfunction associated with troglitazone. *N Engl J Med* 1998;338:916.

Winter WE, Maclaren NK, Riley WJ, et al: Congenital pancreatic hypoplasia: A syndrome of exocrine and endocrine pancreatic insufficiency. *J Pediatr* 1986; 109:465.

Winter WE, Maclaren NK, Riley WJ, et al: Maturity-onset diabetes of youth in black Americans. *N Engl J Med* 1987;316:285.

Diabetes of the Newborn

Alcolado JC, Thomas AW: Maternally inherited diabetes mellitus: The role of mitochondrial DNA defects. *Diabetic Med* 1995;12:102.

Blethen SL, White NH, Santiago JV, et al: Plasma somatomedins, endogenous insulin secretion, and growth in transient neonatal diabetes mellitus. *J Clin Endocrinol Metab* 1981;52:144.

Geffner ME, Clare-Salzler M, Kaufman DL, et al: Permanent diabetes developing after transient neonatal diabetes. *Lancet* 1993;341:1095.

Metz C, Cavé H, Bertrand AM, et al: Neonatal diabetes mellitus: Chromosomal analysis in transient and permanent cases. *J Pediatr* 2002;141:483–9.

Pagliara AS, Karl IE, Kipnis DB: Transient neonatal diabetes: Delayed maturation of the pancreatic beta cell. *J Pediatr* 1973;82:97.

Schiff D, Colle E, Stern L: Metabolic and growth patterns in transient neonatal diabetes. *N Engl J Med* 1972;287:119.

Shield JPH, Baum JD: Is transient neonatal diabetes a risk factor for diabetes in later life? *Lancet* 1993;341:693.

von Muhlendahl KR, Herkenhoff H: Long-term course of neonatal diabetes. *N Engl J Med* 1995;333:704.

Hypoglycemia and Diabetes

Amiel SA, Tamborlane WV, Simonson DC, et al: Defective glucose counter regulation after strict glycemic control of insulin-dependent diabetes mellitus. *N Engl J Med* 1987;316:1376.

Bergada I, Suissa S, Dufresne J, et al: Severe hypoglycemia in IDDM children. *Diabetes Care* 1989;12:239.

Bolli GB, Fanelli CG: Unawareness of hypoglycemia. *N Engl J Med* 1995;333:1771.

Cryer PE, Fisher JN, Shamoon H: Hypoglycemia. *Diabetes Care* 1994;17:734–55.

Diabetes Control and Complications Trial Research Group: Hypoglycemia in the diabetes control and complications trial. *Diabetes* 1997;46:271–86.

Gerich JE: Lilly Lecture, 1988. Glucose counterregulation and its impact on diabetes mellitus. *Diabetes* 1988;37:1608.

Gschwend S, Ryan C, Atchinson J, et al: Effects of acute hyperglycemia on mental efficiency and counterregulatory hormones in adolescents with insulin-dependent diabetes mellitus. *J Pediatr* 1995;126:178–84.

McCrimmon RJ, Gold AE, Deary IJ, et al: Symptoms of hypoglycemia in children with IDDM. *Diabetes Care* 1995;18:858–61.

Porter PA, Keating B, Byrne G, et al: Incidence and predictive criteria of nocturnal hypoglycemia in young children with insulin-dependent diabetes mellitus. *J Pediatr* 1997;130:366–72.

Ryan C, Vega A, Drash A. Cognitive deficits in adolescents who developed diabetes early in life. *Pediatrics* 1985;75:921–7.

Shalwitz RA, Farkas-Hirsch R, White NH, et al: Prevalence and consequences of nocturnal hypoglycemia among conventionally treated children with diabetes mellitus. *J Pediatr* 1990;116:685–9.

Silverstein JH, Gordon G, Pollock BH, et al: Long-term glycemic control influences the onset of limited joint mobility in type I diabetes. *J Pediatr* 1998;132:944.

Wayne EA, Dean HJ, Booth F, et al: Focal neurologic deficits associated with hypoglycemia in children with diabetes. *J Pediatr* 1990;117:575–7.

Pancreas and Islet Transplantation

Alejandro R, Lehmann R, Ricordi C, et al: Long-term function (6 years) of islet allografts in type 1 diabetes. *Diabetes* 1997;46:1983.

Brouhard BH, Rogers DG: Pancreatic and islet replacement therapy for insulin-dependent diabetes mellitus. *Clin Pediatr* 1993;32:258.

Humar A, Gruessner RW, Sutherland DE: Living related donor pancreas and pancreas-kidney transplantation. *Br Med Bull* 1997;53:879.

Larsen JL, Stratta RJ: Consequences of pancreas transplantation. *J Invest Med* 1994;42:62.

Mitanchez D, Doiron B, Chen R, et al: Glucose-stimulated genes and prospects of gene therapy for type 1 diabetes. *Endocr Rev* 1997;18:520.

Robertson RP, Kendall D, Teuscher A, et al: Long-term metabolic control with pancreatic transplantation. *Transplant Proc* 1994;26:386.

Ryan EA, Lakey JR, Paty BW, et al: Successful islet transplantation: continued insulin reserve provides long-term glycemic control. *Diabetes* 2002; 51:2148.

Soon-Shiong P, Heintz RE, Merideth N, et al: Insulin independence in a type 1 diabetic patient after encapsulated islet transplantation. *Lancet* 1994;343:950.

Sutherland DE: Present status of pancreas transplantation alone in non-uremic diabetic patients. *Transplant Proc* 1994;26:379.

Chapter 584

Neurologic Evaluation

Robert H. A. Haslam

The neurologic evaluation seeks to assess the integrity of the central nervous system (CNS) by means of a thorough history and physical examination and thus to determine the location (and causes) of abnormal function.

HISTORY

The history is the most important component of the evaluation of a child with a neurologic problem. The history should carefully document in chronological order the onset of symptoms and a thorough description of their frequency, duration, and associated characteristics. Most children beyond the age of 3–4 yr are capable of contributing to their history, particularly about facts relating to the present illness. It is essential to obtain a comprehensive review of the function and interaction of all organ systems, because abnormalities of the CNS may initially present with clinical manifestations (e.g., vomiting, pain, constipation, or urinary tract disorders) implicating other systems. A detailed history might suggest that the child's vomiting is due to increased intracranial pressure (ICP), that the pain behind the eye may be caused by migraine headaches or multiple sclerosis, and that the constipation and urinary dribbling may be due to a spinal cord tumor.

It is important to start with a concise description of the chief complaint within its developmental context. For example, parents may be concerned that their child cannot talk. The seriousness of this problem depends on many factors, including the age of the patient, the normal range of language development for age, the parent-child interaction, function of the auditory system, and the intellectual level of the child. A comprehensive understanding of developmental milestones is essential in order to ascertain the relative importance of the parents' observations (see Chapters 9–16).

After the chief complaint and history of present illness are elicited, a review of the pregnancy, labor, and delivery is indicated, particularly if a congenital disorder is suspected (see Chapters 82–98). Was the mother exposed to a viral illness during the pregnancy, and what is the mother's rubella, HIV, and syphilis immune status? The history should also include information about the quantity of cigarette and alcohol consumption, toxin exposure, and drug use (legal and illicit) that are known to have adverse effects on fetal development. Decreased or absent fetal activity may be associated with the congenital myopathies and other neuromuscular disorders. Seizures in utero occasionally occur and suggest placental insufficiency or rare inborn errors of metabolism, such as pyridoxine dependence. Seizure activity in utero is difficult to evaluate, particularly in a primigravida. The fact that fetal seizures occurred during pregnancy is often realized retrospectively after the mother has had an opportunity to observe her infant's seizures. The mother's postpartum health may provide a clue to the cause of her infant's neurologic problem, e.g., maternal fever, drug dependence, cervical or vaginal vesicles (e.g., herpes simplex), hemorrhage, petechiae, or the presence of an abnormal placenta.

The history of the birthweight, length, and head circumference is particularly important. It may be necessary to obtain the infant's hospital records to determine the head circumference, particularly if congenital microcephaly is a consideration, and the Apgar score, for suspected asphyxia. Several indicators of neurologic dysfunction during the newborn period can reliably be obtained from the history. The fact that a full-term infant was unable to breathe spontaneously and required ventilatory assistance may suggest a CNS abnormality. Poor, uncoordinated sucking or a full-term infant who requires an inordinate amount of time to feed suggests a neurologic disorder requiring careful evaluation. If such an infant requires gavage feeding, there is almost certainly a significant problem. All of the aforementioned abnormalities may be common to a premature infant, particularly a very low birthweight infant, and do not necessarily signify a poor neurologic outcome. Additional important information in the newborn period includes the presence of jaundice, its degree, and management. The physician should also attempt to assess the activity, sleep patterns, the nature of the cry, and the general well-being of the newborn infant from the history.

The most important component of a neurologic history is a child's developmental assessment (see Chapters 7 and 16). Careful evaluation of a child's developmental milestones usually determines the presence of a global delay in language and gross and fine motor or social skills or a delay in a particular subset of development. An abnormality in development from birth suggests an intrauterine or perinatal cause. Slowing of the rate of acquisition of skills later in infancy or childhood may imply an acquired abnormality of the nervous system. A loss of skills (regression) over time strongly suggests an underlying degenerative disease of the CNS. The ability of parents to precisely recall the timing of their children's developmental milestones is extremely variable. Some are very reliable and others are uncertain, particularly if the patient in question has a significant neurodevelopmental problem. Table 584–1 provides some guidelines with regard to the upper range of normal skills that are usually recalled by the parents and that, if not present, should alert the physician. It is often helpful to request photographs taken at an earlier age or to review the family's baby book, because milestones for a child may have been dutifully recorded. Parents (particularly mothers) are usually aware when their children have a developmental problem, and the physician should show appropriate concern.

Family history is extremely important in the neurologic evaluation of a child. Parents are sometimes unwilling to discuss family members with debilitating neurologic disorders or may be unaware of them, particularly if they are institutionalized. However, most parents are extremely cooperative in securing medical information about family members, particularly if it may have relevance for their child. The history should document the ages and well-being of all close relatives and the presence of neurologic disease, including epilepsy, migraine, cerebrovascular accidents, developmental delay, and heredofamilial disorders. The sex and age at death of miscarriages or live-born siblings, including the results of postmortem examinations, should be obtained because this information may have a direct bearing on the patient's condition. It should also be determined whether the parents are related, because the incidence of metabolic and degenerative disorders affecting the CNS is increased significantly in children of consanguineous marriages.

1973

TABLE 584–1. Screening Scheme for Developmental Delay: Upper Range

Age (mo)	Gross Motor	Fine Motor	Social Skills	Language
3	Supports weight on forearms	Opens hands spontaneously	Smiles appropriately	Coos, laughs
6	Sits momentarily	Transfers objects	Shows likes and dislikes	Babbles
9	Pulls to stand	Pincer grasp	Plays pat-a-cake, peek-a-boo	Imitates sounds
12	Walks with one hand held	Releases an object on command	Comes when called	1–2 meaningful words
18	Walks upstairs with assistance	Feeds from a spoon	Mimics actions of others	At least 6 words
24	Runs	Builds a tower of six blocks	Plays with others	2–3 word sentences

Finally, an attempt should be made to learn about the patient as a person. The child's performance in school, both academically and socially, may shed light on the diagnosis, particularly if there has been an abrupt change. A description of the child's personality before and after the onset of symptoms may provide a clue to the cause of the disorder. Discussions with the daycare worker or kindergarten or school teacher may provide useful information that is not available from the parent.

NEUROLOGIC EXAMINATION

Neurologic examination of a child begins at the outset of the interview. Observation during interaction with the parents, while playing, or during the time when little attention is directed to the child can provide useful information (see Chapters 6 and 17). It may be obvious that the child has characteristic facies, an unusual posture, or an abnormality of motor function manifested by a gait disturbance or hemiparesis. Furthermore, much can be learned from observing the child's behavior during the interview. A normally inquisitive child or toddler may play independently but soon wishes to become involved with the interview process. A child with an attention disorder may display inappropriate behaviors in the examining room, whereas a neurologically abnormal child may appear lethargic or disinterested or may show complete lack of awareness of the environment. The degree of interaction between the parent and the child should be noted. Because the neurologic examination of a newborn or premature infant requires a somewhat modified approach from that of an older child, the differences in the examination are highlighted for both age groups (see also Chapters 6 and 83).

The examination should be conducted in a setting that is nonthreatening and enjoyable for a child. The more it seems like a game, the greater will be the degree of cooperation. Children may be most comfortable on a parent's lap or interacting on the floor of the examination room. It is unwise to force a child to sit on the examining table or to demand that all clothes be removed at the beginning of the procedure. Cooperation is essential for a comprehensive neurologic examination; as a child's confidence increases, so too does the level of participation. Several methods may be used to assess *mental status, cognitive function*, and the level of *alertness*, depending on the age of the child. Simple puzzles may be useful. A child's ability to tell a story or to draw a picture is often a powerful method for assessing cognitive function or for determining developmental level. The manner in which a child plays with toys or explores the function of a new object or game is an excellent indicator of intellectual curiosity. The level of alertness of a newborn infant depends on many factors, including the time of the last feeding, the room temperature, and the gestational age. Sequential assessment of the infant is valuable in determining changes in neurologic function. Premature infants of less than 28 wk of gestation do not consistently demonstrate periods of alertness, whereas gentle physical stimulation applied to a slightly older infant arouses the child from sleep and results in a brief period of alertness. Sleep and waking patterns are well developed at term.

The examiner must take advantage of the opportunities provided by the patient; if the circumstances permit, evaluation of muscle power and tone or cerebellar function might precede the cranial nerve examination. However, if a hearing assessment is considered to be important from the historical information, attention should be directed initially to that portion of the examination so that full cooperation can be achieved before the interest and curiosity of the child are lost.

The Head. The *size* and *shape* of the head should be documented carefully. A tower-head, or oxycephalic skull, suggests premature closure of sutures and is associated with various forms of inherited craniosynostosis (see Chapter 585.12). A broad forehead may indicate hydrocephalus and a small head microcephaly. The observation of a square or a box-shaped skull should suggest chronic subdural hematomas because the long-standing presence of fluid in the subdural space causes enlargement of the middle fossa. Inspection of the scalp should include observation of the venous pattern, because increased ICP and thrombosis of the superior sagittal sinus can produce marked venous distention.

An infant has two *fontanels* at birth: a diamond-shaped open anterior fontanel that is situated in the midline at the junction of the coronal and sagittal sutures and a posterior fontanel between the intersection of the occipital and parietal bones that may be closed at birth or, at the most, admit the tip of a finger. The posterior fontanel is usually closed and nonpalpable after the first 6–8 wk of life; its persistence suggests underlying hydrocephalus or the possibility of congenital hypothyroidism. The anterior fontanel varies greatly in size, but the usual measurement approximates 2 by 2 cm. The average time of closure is 18 mo, but the fontanel may normally close as early as 9 mo. A very small or absent anterior fontanel at birth may indicate premature fusion of the sutures or microcephaly, whereas a very large fontanel could signify a variety of problems. *The fontanel is normally slightly depressed and pulsatile and is best evaluated when an infant is held upright while asleep or feeding.* A bulging fontanel is a reliable indicator of increased ICP, but vigorous crying can cause a protuberant fontanel in a normal infant.

Palpation of a newborn's skull characteristically shows overriding of the cranial sutures for the first several days of life as a result of the pressures exerted on the skull during its descent through the pelvis. Marked overriding of the sutures beyond a few days is cause for alarm and suggests the possibility of an underlying abnormality of the brain. Palpation may uncover cranial defects or *craniotabes,* a peculiar softening of the parietal bone so that gentle pressure produces a sensation similar to indenting a ping-pong ball. Craniotabes is often associated with prematurity.

Auscultation of the skull is an important adjunct to a neurologic examination. *Cranial bruits* are most prominent over the anterior fontanel, temporal region, or the orbits and are best heard through the diaphragm of the stethoscope. Soft symmetric bruits may be discovered in normal children younger than 4 yr or in association with a febrile illness. Arteriovenous malformations of the middle cerebral artery or vein of Galen may produce a loud bruit. Murmurs arising from the heart or great vessels frequently are transmitted to the cranium. A child with severe anemia is often found to have a skull bruit that disappears when the anemia is corrected. Increased ICP resulting from hydrocephalus, tumor, subdural effusions, or purulent meningitis frequently produces significant intracranial bruits. *Demonstration of a loud or localized bruit is usually significant and warrants further investigation.*

Correct *measurement of the head circumference* is important. It should be performed on every patient, at every visit, and should be recorded on a suitable head growth chart. A nondistensible plastic measuring tape should be used. The tape is placed over the midforehead and is extended circumferentially to include the most prominent portion of the occiput so that the greatest volume of the cranium is measured. The head circumferences of the parents and siblings should also be recorded if the patient is found to have an abnormal skull. Errors in the accurate measurement of a newborn skull are frequent and result from scalp edema, overriding of the sutures, intravenous fluid infiltration, and the presence of a cephalohematoma. The average rate of head growth in a healthy premature infant is 0.5 cm in the first 2 wk, 0.75 cm during the 3rd wk, and 1.0 cm in the 4th wk and thereafter until the 40th wk of development. The head circumference of a term infant at birth measures 34–35 cm, 44 cm by 6 mo, and 47 cm by 1 yr of age (see Chapters 9 and 10).

Cranial Nerves

OLFACTORY NERVE (1). Anosmia, loss of smell, is most commonly found in association with an upper respiratory tract infection in children and therefore is a transient abnormality. A fracture of the base of the skull and cribriform plate as well as a frontal lobe tumor also may produce anosmia. Occasionally, a child who recovers from purulent meningitis or in whom hydrocephalus develops has a diminished sense of smell. Rarely, anosmia is congenital. Although not a routine component of the examination, smell can be tested reliably as early as the 32nd wk of gestation. Care should be taken to use appropriate stimuli, such as coffee, peppermint, and other substances that are familiar to the child; strongly aromatic substances should be avoided.

OPTIC NERVE (2). Examination of the optic disc and retina is an important component of the neurologic examination. To visualize a good portion of the retina, dilation of the pupil is necessary. One drop of a combination of 1% cyclopentolate hydrochloride, 2.5% phenylephrine hydrochloride, and 1% tropicamide repeated every 15 min three times effectively produces mydriasis. Mydriatics should not be used if a patient's pupil reaction is necessary to follow the level of consciousness or if a cataract is present. Examination of an infant's retina is enhanced by providing a nipple or soother and by placing the head on one side. The physician gently strokes the patient to maintain arousal, while examining the closest eye. An older child should be placed in the parent's lap and should be distracted by bright objects or toys that are presented during the ophthalmologic examination. The optic nerve is salmon-pink in a child but is gray-white in the newborn, particularly in a blond infant. This normal finding may cause confusion and may lead to the improper diagnosis of optic atrophy.

Papilledema rarely occurs in infancy because the skull sutures are capable of separating to accommodate the expanding brain. Papilledema in an older child may be recognized by the following progressive changes in the optic nerve and surrounding retina (Fig. 584–1):

1. The optic nerve becomes hyperemic.
2. The small capillaries that normally cross the optic nerve are no longer visualized as they become constricted.
3. The larger veins become dilated, and the accompanying arterioles become constricted.
4. The border of the optic nerve becomes indistinct from the surrounding retina, particularly along the temporal edge.
5. Subhyaloid, flame-shaped hemorrhages appear in the retina surrounding the optic nerve.
6. In some cases, a macular star develops owing to retinal edema in the region of the macula. Visual acuity and color vision

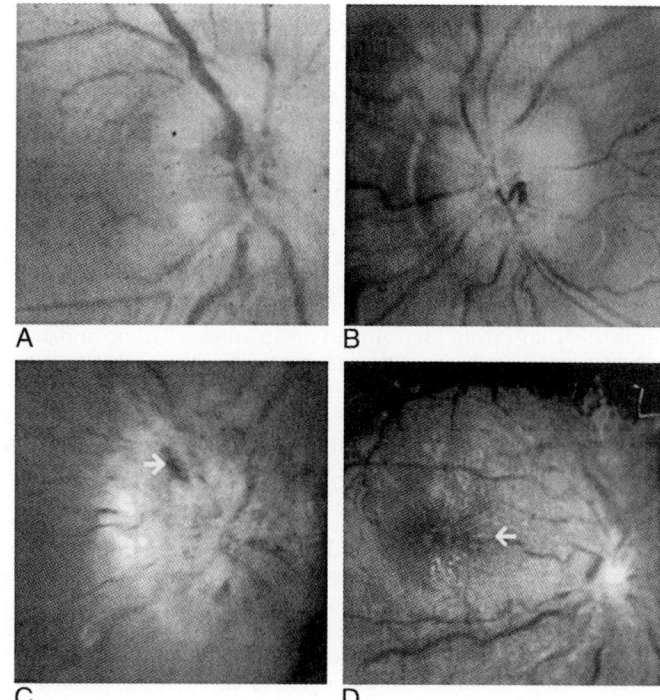

FIGURE 584–1. *A,* Mild papilledema. Blurred disc margins and venous congestion. *B,* Moderate papilledema. Disc edematous and raised. Vessels buried within substance of nerve tissue. *C,* Severe papilledema. Hemorrhages are evident within disc (*arrow*), and there are microinfarcts (soft exudates) in the nerve fiber layer. *D,* Macular star (*arrow*) with edema residues distributed within the Henle layer of the macula. See also color plates.

remain intact in acute papilledema as contrasted with optic neuritis, but the blind spot is increased in both.

Retinal hemorrhages occur in 30–40% of all full-term newborn infants. The hemorrhages are more common after vaginal delivery than after cesarean section and are not associated with birth injury or with neurologic complications. They disappear spontaneously by 1–2 wk of age.

Vision (see also Part XXVIII). Normal 28-wk-old premature infants blink when a bright light is directed to the eyes, and by 32 wk, infants maintain eye closure until the light source is removed. At 37 wk, normal premature infants turn the head and the eyes to a soft light, and by term, visual fixation and the ability to follow a brilliant target are present. During a period of alertness, optokinetic nystagmus can be demonstrated in a newborn. Visual acuity in term infants approximates 20/150 and reaches the adult level of 20/20 by about 6 mo of age. Children who are too young to read the standard letters on the Snellen Eye Chart may learn the "E game" by pointing a finger in the direction that the "E" is oriented. Children as young as 2½ or 3 yr of age with normal vision identify the objects on the Allen Chart at a distance of 15–20 ft. Peripheral vision may be tested in an infant by bringing an object from behind the patient into the peripheral field of vision that normally produces a visual recognition response. The examiner should be sure that the object rather than a sound produces the visual response.

The *pupil* is difficult to examine in premature infants owing to the poorly pigmented iris and the resistance to lid opening. The pupil reacts to light by the 29th–32nd wk of gestation. The equality of the pupils, their size, and their reaction to light may be affected by drugs, a space-occupying brain lesion, metabolic disorders, and abnormalities of the midbrain and optic nerves.

Horner syndrome is characterized by miosis, ptosis, enophthalmos, and ipsilateral anhidrosis of the face. It may be congenital or may result from a lesion involving the sympathetic nervous system in the brainstem, cervical spinal cord, or the sympathetic plexus in juxtaposition to the carotid artery. Localization of the lesion within the sympathetic nervous system is aided by the pupillary response to a series of topical drugs, including cocaine, epinephrine, hydroxyamphetamine, and phenylephrine. Visual fields are tested in an infant by advancing a brightly colored (red) object from behind the child's head through the peripheral field of vision and noting when the child first looks at the object. Suspension of the object by a string prevents the infant from focusing on the examiner's hand and arm.

OCULOMOTOR (3), TROCHLEAR (4), AND ABDUCENS NERVES (6). The eye is moved by the extraocular muscles that are innervated by the oculomotor, trochlear, and abducens nerves. The oculomotor nerve innervates the superior, inferior, and medial rectus as well as the inferior oblique and the levator palpebrae superioris muscles. Complete paralysis of the oculomotor nerve causes ptosis, dilation of the pupil, displacement of the eye outward and downward, and impairment of adduction and elevation. The trochlear nerve supplies the superior oblique muscle, and isolated paralysis causes the eye to deviate upward and outward, often with an associated head tilt. The abducens nerve innervates the lateral rectus muscle so that its paralysis causes medial deviation of the eye and the inability to abduct beyond the midline. In an older child, the **red glass test** is used to assess extraocular palsies. A red glass is placed over one eye, and the patient is requested to follow a white light in all fields of direction. The child sees only one red/white light in the direction of normal muscle function but notes a separation of the red and white images that is greatest in the plane of action of the affected muscle. *Internuclear ophthalmoplegia* results from a lesion in the brainstem and consists of paralysis of medial rectus function of the adducting eye and nystagmus confined to the abducting eye. *Internal ophthalmoplegia* refers to a dilated pupil that is unreactive to light and accommodation but has normal extraocular function, and *external ophthalmoplegia* is associated with ptosis and paralysis of all eye muscles with preservation of the pupillary response. *Nystagmus* is an involuntary rapid movement of the eye that may be horizontal, vertical, rotatory, pendular, or mixed. Jerk nystagmus is used to describe a fast and slow phase. As a general rule, horizontal nystagmus occurs with an abnormality of the peripheral labyrinth or with a lesion of the vestibular system in the brainstem or cerebellum and as a consequence of drugs, particularly phenytoin. Vertical nystagmus is indicative of brainstem dysfunction.

Complete ocular movement may be demonstrated as early as 25 wk of gestation using the **doll's eye maneuver**. This technique is used to examine horizontal and vertical eye movements in an infant or an uncooperative or comatose patient. If the head is suddenly turned to the right, the eyes look to the left in a symmetric fashion. Horizontal eye movements in the opposite direction may then be evaluated if the head is turned to the left. Vertical movements may be assessed in a similar fashion by rapid flexion and extension of the head. Normal infants and children follow a toy or interesting object in all directions. The rapid on-off occlusion ("blinking light") of a light source is a reliable test for visual following in uncooperative children. The examiner observes the completeness and flow of the eye movements and determines the presence or absence and the direction of nystagmus, diplopia, opsoclonus (chaotic, jerky oscillations of the eyes, often associated with neuroblastoma or viral infections), ocular bobbing, or other abnormal eye positions. Premature infants tend to have slightly disconjugate eyes at rest, with one eye horizontally displaced from the other by 1 or 2 mm. Skew deviation of the eyes (vertical displacement) is always abnormal and requires investigation. Strabismus is discussed in Chapter 614.

TRIGEMINAL NERVE (5). The sensory distribution of the face is divided into three areas: the ophthalmic area, the maxillary area, and the mandibular area. Each region may be tested by light touch and by pinprick, and may be compared with the opposite side. The corneal response is elicited by touching the cornea with a small pledget of cotton and by observing the eye closure response. Trigeminal nerve function in premature infants is best documented by facial grimacing from a pinprick (away from the eye) or by stimulating the nostril with a cotton tip. Motor function may be tested by examination of the masseters, pterygoid, and temporalis muscles during mastication as well as by evaluation of the jaw jerk.

FACIAL NERVE (7). Decreased voluntary movement of the lower face with flattening of the nasolabial angle on the ipsilateral side indicates an upper motor neuron or supranuclear corticospinal lesion. A lower motor neuron lesion tends to involve upper and lower facial muscles equally. Facial nerve paralysis may be congenital or secondary to trauma, infection, intracranial tumor, hypertension, toxins, or myasthenia gravis. Taste for the anterior two thirds of the tongue may be tested in a cooperative child by placing a solution of saline or glucose on one side of the extended tongue. Normal children can identify the substance with little difficulty.

AUDITORY NERVE (8). Screening for hearing loss is an important component of the neurologic examination, because a hearing deficit is not readily recognized by parents (see Chapter 627). Normal newborns pause briefly during sucking when a bell is presented, but after several stimuli the pauses cease as habituation occurs. Neurologically abnormal infants do not habituate. Normal hearing infants turn their head toward a bell, rattle, or crumpled paper and by 3 mo of age look in the direction of the sound source. Normally intelligent, hearing-impaired toddlers are visually alert and respond appropriately to physical stimuli. Temper tantrums and abnormal speech are common symptoms in a hearing-impaired child. Audiometry or brainstem–evoked potential testing is mandatory for any child suspected of having a hearing loss (see Chapter 627). The risk factors that indicate a need for testing during the first few months of life include a family history of deafness, prematurity, severe asphyxia, use of ototoxic drugs in the newborn period, hyperbilirubinemia, congenital anomalies of the head or neck, bacterial meningitis, and congenital infections due to rubella, toxoplasmosis, herpes, and cytomegalovirus. Parental concern is often a reliable indicator of hearing impairment and warrants a formal hearing assessment.

Vestibular function may be evaluated by the *caloric test*. Approximately 5 mL of ice water is delivered by syringe into the external auditory canal with the patient's head elevated 30 degrees from the horizontal position. In obtunded or comatose patients with an intact brainstem, there is prompt deviation of the eyes to the side of the stimulus. A much smaller quantity of ice water (0.5 mL) is used in alert, awake subjects. In normal subjects, introduction of ice water produces nystagmus with the quick component in the opposite direction to the stimulated labyrinth. No response implies severe dysfunction of the brainstem and medial longitudinal fasciculus. If the otoscopic examination reveals a ruptured tympanic membrane, the test should not be performed in that ear.

GLOSSOPHARYNGEAL NERVE (9). This nerve supplies innervation to the stylopharyngeus muscle. An isolated lesion of the 9th cranial nerve is rare. The nerve is tested by observing the gag response to tactile stimulation of the posterior pharyngeal wall. Taste for the posterior one third of the tongue is provided by the sensory portion of the glossopharyngeal nerve.

VAGUS NERVE (10). A unilateral injury of the vagus nerve produces weakness and asymmetry of the ipsilateral soft palate and a hoarse voice due to paralysis of a vocal cord. Bilateral lesions may produce respiratory distress as a result of vocal cord paralysis as well as nasal regurgitation of fluids, pooling of secretions, and an immobile, low-lying soft palate. Isolated lesions of the vagus nerve may occur postoperatively after a thoracotomy due to separation of the recurrent laryngeal nerve, and these lesions are not uncommon during the neonatal period in children with the type II Chiari malformation. If a lesion involving the vagus nerve is suspected, visualization of the vocal cords is necessary. To test for a cough in a neonate/infant, the examiner applies gentle pressure to the trachea at the suprasternal notch.

ACCESSORY NERVE (11). Paralysis and atrophy of the sternomastoid and trapezius muscles result from lesions of the accessory nerve. The sternomastoid muscle has two origins, sternal and clavicular, and is tested by forceful rotation of the head and neck against the examiner's hand. Motor neuron disease, myotonic dystrophy, and myasthenia gravis are the most common conditions producing weakness and atrophy of these muscles.

HYPOGLOSSAL NERVE (12). The hypoglossal nerve innervates the tongue. Examination of the tongue includes an assessment of its motility, size, and shape and the presence of atrophy or fasciculations. Malfunction of the hypoglossal nucleus or nerve produces wasting, weakness, and fasciculations of the tongue. If the injury is bilateral, tongue protrusion is not possible and dysphagia may be present. Werdnig-Hoffmann disease (infantile spinal muscular atrophy, or SMA type 1) and congenital anomalies in the region of the foramen magnum are the principal causes of hypoglossal nerve involvement.

Motor Examination. The motor examination includes an assessment of the integrity of the musculoskeletal system and a search for abnormal movements that may indicate a disorder of the peripheral nervous system or the CNS. The components of the motor examination include testing of strength (power), muscle bulk, tone, posture, locomotion and motility, deep tendon reflexes, and the presence of primitive reflexes, when applicable.

STRENGTH. Testing of muscle strength is relatively straightforward in cooperative children. It may begin by requesting that the child squeeze the examiner's fingers, flex and extend the wrist and elbow, and adduct and abduct the shoulder against resistance. Shoulder girdle muscle strength may be evaluated in a newborn or infant by supporting the child by the axillae. Patients with weakness are unable to support body weight and slip through the examiner's hands. Distal power can be tested in an infant by evaluating the palmar grasp; a child with weakness does not adequately grasp or shows abnormalities in the manipulation of objects. A normal 3- to 4-yr-old child cooperates in testing extension or flexion of the muscles of the foot, knee, and hip. Examination of the pelvic girdle and proximal lower extremity muscles is also performed by observing the child climb steps or stand up from a prone position. Weakness in these muscles causes the child to use the hands to "climb up" the legs in order to assume an upright position, a maneuver called *Gowers sign* (Fig. 584–2). Infants with diminished power in the lower extremities tend to have decreased spontaneous activity in the legs and refuse to support body weight when suspended by the axillae. It is important not only to assess individual muscle groups but also to carefully compare muscle power between the upper and lower extremities as well as the opposite extremities. Muscle power in a cooperative child is graded on a scale of 0–5 as follows: 0 = no contraction; 1 = flicker or trace of contraction; 2 = active movement, with gravity eliminated; 3 = active movement against gravity; 4 = active movement against gravity and resistance; 5 = normal power. Examination of muscle power should include the muscles of respiration. Observation of the action of the intercostal muscles, diaphragmatic movement, and the use of accessory muscles of respiration should be

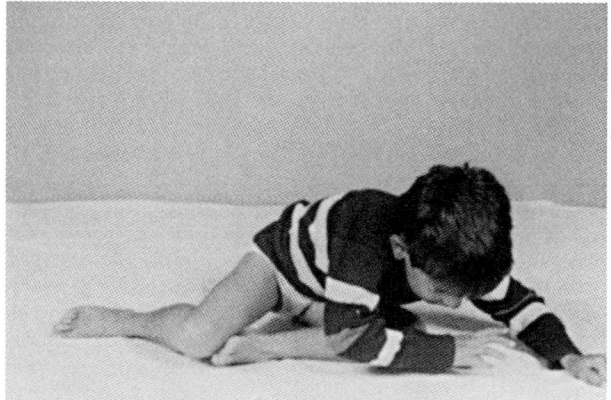
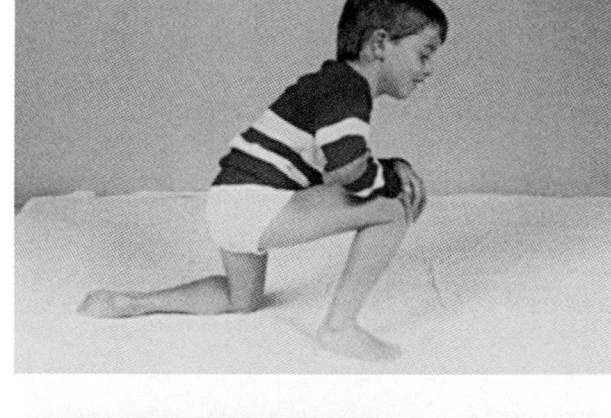
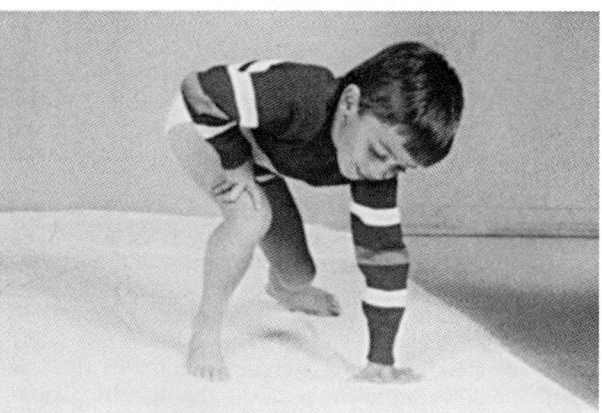
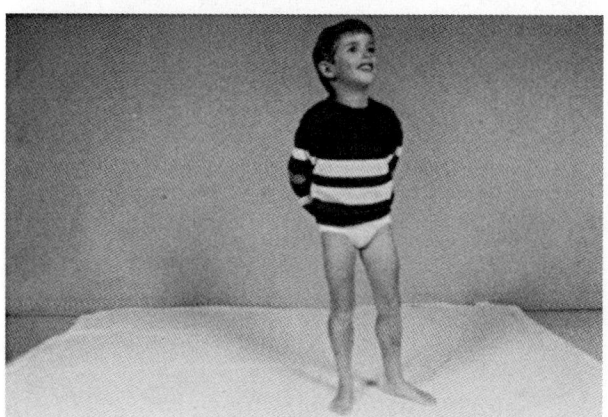

FIGURE 584–2. Gowers sign. A boy with hip girdle weakness due to Duchenne muscular dystrophy.

documented. Finally, evaluation of power should include an assessment of muscle bulk and nutrition. Weakness may be associated with muscle atrophy and fasciculations. Because most infants have excess body fat, muscle fasciculations and atrophy are most commonly demonstrated in the denervated tongue in this age group.

TONE. Muscle tone is tested by assessing the degree of resistance when an individual joint is moved passively. Tone undergoes considerable change and assumes different forms depending on age. A premature or newborn infant is relatively hypotonic compared with a child. Tone in this age group is tested by various maneuvers (see Chapter 86). When the upper extremity of a normal term infant is pulled gently across the chest, the elbow normally does not quite reach the midsternum (*scarf sign*). The elbow of a hypotonic infant extends beyond the midline with ease. Measurement of the popliteal angle is a useful method to document tone in the legs of a newborn. The examiner flexes the child's lower extremity on the abdomen and extends the knee. Normal term infants allow extension of the knee to approximately 80 degrees. Abnormalities of tone consist of spasticity, rigidity, and hypotonia.

Spasticity is characterized by an initial resistance to passive movement, followed by a sudden release called the **clasp-knife** phenomenon. Spasticity is most apparent in the upper extremity flexors and lower extremity extensor muscles. It is associated with brisk tendon reflexes and an extensor plantar reflex, clonus, diminished active movements, and disuse atrophy. *Clonus* may be demonstrated in the lower extremity by sudden dorsiflexion of the foot with the knee partially flexed. Whereas sustained clonus is always abnormal, 5–10 beats in a newborn is a normal finding unless the clonus is asymmetric. Spasticity results from a lesion that involves upper motor neuron tracts and may be unilateral or bilateral. *Rigidity*, the result of a basal ganglia lesion, is characterized by constant resistance to passive movement of both extensor and flexor muscles. As the extremity is undergoing passive movement, a typical **cogwheel** (caused by superimposition of an extrapyramidal tremor on rigidity) sensation may be evident. The rigidity persists with repetitive passive extension and flexion of a joint and does not give way or release, such as with spasticity. Children with spastic lower extremities drag the legs while crawling (commando style) or walk on tiptoes. Patients with marked spasticity or rigidity develop a posture of *opisthotonos*, in which the head and the heels are bent backward and the body bowed forward (Fig. 584–3). *Decerebrate* rigidity is characterized by marked extension of the extremities resulting from dysfunction or injury to the brainstem at the level of the superior colliculi. *Hypotonia* refers to abnormally diminished tone and is the most common abnor-

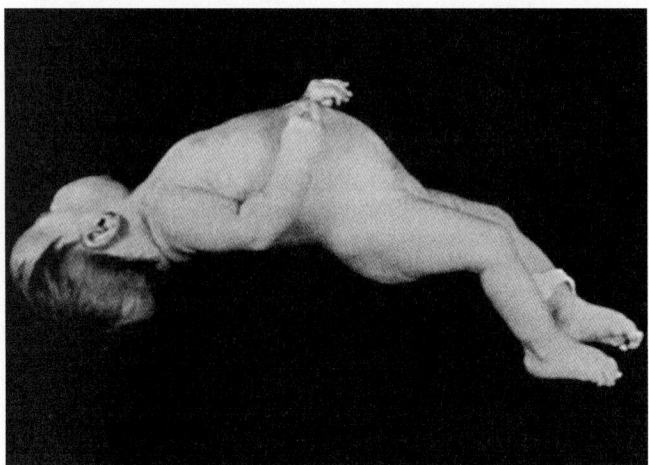

FIGURE 584–3. Opisthotonus in a brain-injured infant.

mality of tone in neurologically compromised premature or full-term neonates. Demonstration of hypotonia may reflect pathology of the cerebral hemispheres, cerebellum, spinal cord, anterior horn cell, peripheral nerve, myoneural junction, or muscle. An unusual position or posture in an infant is a reflection of abnormal tone. A hypotonic infant is *floppy* and may have difficulty in maintaining head support or a straight back while sitting. Such infants may assume a **frog-leg posture** in the supine position. Premature infants of 28 wk of gestation tend to extend all extremities at rest, but by 32 wk there is evidence of flexion, particularly in the lower extremities. A normal full-term infant's posture is characterized by flexion of all extremities.

MOTILITY AND LOCOMOTION. Premature infants of less than 32 wk of gestation display random, slow, writhing movements interspersed with rapid, myoclonic-like activity of the extremities. Beyond 32 wk, the motor activity is primarily flexor. Observation of crawling, walking, or running may uncover movement disorders, most of which are likely to be apparent during motion and to disappear with rest or sleep. *Ataxia* refers to incoordination of movement or a disturbance of balance. It may be primarily truncal or may be limited to the extremities. Truncal ataxia is characterized by unsteadiness during sitting or standing and results primarily from involvement of the cerebellar vermis. Abnormalities of the cerebellar hemispheres characteristically cause intention tremor unaffected by visual attention. Ataxia may be demonstrated by the finger-to-nose and heel-to-shin tests, heel-to-toe or tandem walking, and, in infants by observation of reaching for or playing with toys. Additional abnormalities associated with cerebellar lesions include dysmetria (errors in measuring distances), rebound (inability to inhibit a muscular action, such as when the examiner suddenly releases the flexed arm and the patient inadvertently strikes the face), and disdiadochokinesia (diminished performance of rapid alternating movements). Hypotonia, dysarthria, nystagmus, and decreased deep tendon reflexes are common features of cerebellar abnormalities. Sensory ataxia is found with diseases of the spinal cord and peripheral nerves. In these disorders, the **Romberg sign** is positive (patient is unsteady with eyes closed but not open), and there are often related sensory findings including abnormalities in joint position and vibration sense.

Chorea is characterized by involuntary movements of the major joints, trunk, and the face that are rapid and jerky. Affected children are incapable of extending their arms without producing abnormal movements. They have a tendency to pronate the arms when held above the head. The hand grip contracts and relaxes (**milkmaid sign**), the speech is explosive and inarticulate, the deep tendon reflexes of the knee are "hung up," and patients may have difficulty in maintaining protrusion of the tongue. *Athetosis* is a slow, writhing movement that is often associated with abnormalities of muscle tone. It is most prominent in the distal extremities and is enhanced by voluntary activity or emotional upset. Speech and swallowing may be affected. Chorea and athetosis are the result of basal ganglia lesions and are difficult to separate clinically. Both may be prominent in the same patient. *Dystonia* is an involuntary, slow, twisting movement that primarily involves the proximal muscles of the extremities, trunk, and neck.

DEEP TENDON REFLEXES AND THE PLANTAR RESPONSE. The deep tendon reflexes are readily elicited in most infants and children. In premature and term infants, the biceps, knee, and ankle jerks are the most reliable deep tendon reflexes. They are graded from 0 (absent) to 4 (markedly hyperactive), with 2 being normal. The ankle reflex is difficult to obtain by percussing the Achilles tendon in this age group. Gentle dorsiflexion of the foot and tapping the plantar surface with the reflex hammer usually elicits a response. The knee jerk in an infant may produce a crossed adductor response (tapping the patellar tendon in one leg causes contraction in the opposite extremity), which, if present, does not become abnormal until 6–7 mo of age. The deep tendon reflexes are absent or decreased in primary disorders of the muscle (myopathy), nerve (neuropathy), and myoneural junction and in abnormalities of the cerebellum. They are characteristically increased in upper motor neuron lesions. Asymmetry of deep tendon reflexes suggests a lateralizing lesion. The plantar response is obtained by stimulation of the external portion of the sole of the foot, beginning at the heel and extending to the base of the toes. Firm pressure from the examiner's thumb is a useful method for eliciting the response. The *Babinski reflex* is characterized by extension of the great toe and by fanning of the remaining toes. Too vigorous stimulation may produce withdrawal, which may be misinterpreted as a Babinski response. Most newborn infants show an initial flexion of the great toe on plantar stimulation. As with adults, asymmetry of the plantar response between extremities is a useful lateralizing sign in infants and children.

PRIMITIVE REFLEXES. Primitive reflexes appear and disappear in sequence during specific periods of development (Table 584–2). Their absence or persistence beyond a given time frame signifies dysfunction of the CNS. Some primitive reflexes, such as the snout or *rooting reflex*, reappear during old age or with specific degenerative diseases involving the cerebral cortex. Although many primitive reflexes have been described, the Moro, grasp, tonic neck, and parachute reflexes are the most important. The *Moro reflex* is obtained by placing the infant in a semi-upright position. The head is momentarily allowed to fall backward, with immediate resupport by the examiner's hand. The child symmetrically abducts and extends the arms and flexes the thumbs, followed by flexion and adduction of the upper extremities. An asymmetric response may signify a fractured clavicle, brachial plexus injury, or a hemiparesis. Absence of the Moro reflex in a term newborn is ominous, suggesting significant dysfunction of the CNS. The *grasp* response is elicited by placing a finger or object in the open palm of each hand. Normal infants grasp the object, and with attempted removal, the grip is reinforced. The *tonic neck* reflex is produced by manually turning the head to one side while supine. Extension of the arm occurs on that side of the body corresponding to the direction of the face, while flexion develops in the contralateral extremities. An obligatory tonic neck response, by which the infant remains "locked" in the fencer's position, is always abnormal and implies a CNS disorder. The *parachute reflex* is demonstrated by suspending the child by the trunk and by suddenly producing forward flexion as if the child were to fall. The child spontaneously extends the upper extremities as a protective mechanism. The parachute reflex appears before the onset of walking.

Sensory Examination. Sensory examination is difficult to perform in an infant or uncooperative child. Furthermore, the understanding child soon tires of the examination because it requires considerable attention to repetitious and uninteresting tasks. The more this part of the neurologic examination can be made to simulate a game, the greater is the likelihood that a child will cooperate. Fortunately, disorders involving the sensory system are less common in the pediatric population than among adults; thus, this component of the neurologic assessment is less important for infants and children than for adolescents and adults.

While the infant is distracted by a parent or an interesting toy, the examiner touches the patient with a piece of cotton or a fragment of a tongue depressor. Normal children indicate an awareness of the stimulus by pausing during play, withdrawing the extremity, crying, or looking at and touching the stimulated area. Unfortunately, a child quickly loses patience and soon begins to disregard the examiner. It is critical, therefore, that the area in question is tested efficiently and, if necessary, re-examined at an appropriate time.

Identification of a sensory level in association with a *spinal cord lesion* can be very difficult in an infant. Observation may suggest a difference in color, temperature, or perspiration, with the skin cooler and dry below the spinal cord level. Touching the skin lightly above the level evokes a response that is usually in the form of a squirming movement or physical withdrawal. The superficial abdominal reflexes may be absent. A child with a spinal cord lesion may have evidence of rectal sphincter incontinence that is manifested by a patulous anus, by the absence of contraction of the sphincter when the skin in the anal region is stimulated with a sharp object (anal wink), and by a lack of contraction of the anal sphincter during the rectal examination. In boys, the presence of the cremasteric reflex is also a valuable finding. Children 4–5 yr of age are capable of detailed sensory testing, including joint position, vibration, temperature, stereognosis, two-point discrimination, double simultaneous extinction, light touch, and pain. The success of the sensory examination depends on the ingenuity and the patience of the examiner.

Gait and Station. Observation of a child's gait is an important aspect of a neurologic examination. The *spastic gait* is characterized by stiffness and by stepping like a tin soldier. Spastic children may walk on tiptoes because of tightness or contractures of the Achilles tendons. *Hemiparesis* is associated with a decreased arm swing on the affected side and a lateral circular motion of the leg (*circumduction gait*). Extrapyramidal movements, such as dystonia or chorea, may become apparent while the child is walking or running. Cerebellar ataxia produces a broad-based unsteady gait, and if severe, the child requires support to prevent falling. Heel-to-toe or tandem walking is performed poorly in patients with abnormalities of the cerebellum. A *waddling gait* results from weakness of the proximal hip girdle. Affected children often develop a compensatory lordosis and have difficulty in climbing stairs. Weakness or hypotonia of the lower extremities may result in genu recurvatum and flat feet, which causes a clumsy, tentative gait. *Scoliosis* may cause an abnormal gait and can result from disorders of muscle and spinal cord.

GENERAL EXAMINATION

Physical examination of other organ systems is an essential component of a neurologic examination. For example, cutaneous lesions suggest a neurocutaneous syndrome (see Chapter 589); hepatosplenomegaly suggests inborn errors of metabolism, storage diseases, HIV, or malignancy; and dysmorphic features suggest various syndromes (see Chapter 97). Heart murmurs raise the possibility of rheumatic fever (chorea), tuberous sclerosis (cardiac rhabdomyoma), cerebral abscess or thrombosis (cyanotic heart disease), or cerebral vascular occlusion (endocarditis).

Soft Neurologic Signs. These signs should be interpreted cautiously because they are present in normal children during various stages of neurodevelopment. A soft neurologic sign may be defined as a particular form of deviant performance on a motor or sensory test in the neurologic examination that is abnormal for a particular age. Testing for the presence of soft neurologic signs involves the observation of a series of timed motor tasks and a comparison of the quality and the precision of the patient's movement with normal controls of similar age and sex.

TABLE 584–2. **Timing of Selected Primitive Reflexes**

Reflex	Onset	Fully Developed	Duration
Palmar grasp	28 wk	32 wk	2–3 mo
Rooting	32 wk	36 wk	Less prominent after 1 mo
Moro	28–32 wk	37 wk	5–6 mo
Tonic neck	35 wk	1 mo	6–7 mo
Parachute	7–8 mo	10–11 mo	Remains throughout life

The tests include repetitive and successive finger movements, hand pats, arm pronation-supination movements, foot taps, hopping, and tandem walking. There is considerable variation in the expression of these signs, depending on age, sex, and maturation of the nervous system. For example, minimal choreoathetoid movements in the fingers of the extended arms are normal at 4 yr of age but disappear by 7 or 8 yr of age. Neurodevelopment of girls is more accelerated than that of boys for many motor tasks, including hopping, skipping, and fine balance maneuvers. Although intellectually normal children may demonstrate a soft neurologic sign, the finding of two or more persistent soft signs correlates significantly with neurologic dysfunction, including attention deficit disorder, learning disorders, and cerebral palsy. Because specific soft signs lack association with a particular disability and can occur in a normal child, it is unwise to label a child who shows several soft neurologic signs. It is more appropriate to monitor such a patient closely and to ensure that a developmental disability has been precluded.

SPECIAL DIAGNOSTIC PROCEDURES

Lumbar Puncture and Cerebrospinal Fluid Examination. Examination of the cerebrospinal fluid (CSF) is essential in confirming the diagnosis of meningitis, encephalitis, and subarachnoid hemorrhage and is often helpful in evaluating demyelinating, degenerative, and collagen vascular diseases and the presence of tumor cells within the subarachnoid space. Preparation of a patient is important in order to successfully complete the procedure. An experienced assistant has a vital role in positioning, restraining, and comforting the patient. The skin is thoroughly prepared with a cleansing agent, and the patient is placed in the lateral recumbent position. The physician should be gowned and gloved; the patient should be draped. The neck and legs of the patient are flexed by an assistant to enlarge the intervertebral spaces. The ideal interspace for lumbar puncture (LP) is L3-L4 or L4-L5, which is determined by drawing an imaginary horizontal line from one anterior superior spine of the ilium to the other. The skin and underlying tissue are anesthetized with a local anesthetic or by placing on the skin 30 min before the procedure a patch that contains a eutectic mixture of local anesthetics including lidocaine and prilocaine (EMLA). A 22-gauge, 1- to 2-in, sharp, beveled spinal needle with a properly fitting stylet is introduced into the midsagittal plane directed slightly in the cephalic direction. The stylet is removed frequently as the needle is slowly advanced to determine whether CSF is present. A pop is felt as the needle penetrates the dura and enters the subarachnoid space. A manometer and a three-way stopcock may be attached to obtain an opening pressure. The opening pressure in the recumbent and relaxed position averages 100 mm of fluid; the range in the flexed lateral decubitus position is 60–180 mm of fluid. The most common cause of an elevated opening pressure is a crying, uncooperative, and struggling patient. The pressure is recorded most reliably with a child positioned comfortably with the head and the legs extended. Sick neonates may be placed in the upright position for a spinal tap, because decreased ventilation and perfusion abnormalities leading to respiratory arrest are more common in the recumbent position in this age group.

Contraindications for performing an LP include: (1) elevated ICP owing to a suspected mass lesion of the brain or spinal cord, (2) symptoms and signs of pending cerebral herniation in a child with probable meningitis, (3) critical illness (on rare occasions), (4) skin infection at the site of the LP, and (5) thrombocytopenia.

In the first instance, transtentorial herniation or herniation of the cerebellar tonsils may develop after the procedure. Inspection of the eyegrounds for the presence of papilledema is mandatory before proceeding with an LP.

In the second instance, symptoms and signs include decerebrate or decorticate posture, a generalized tonic seizure, abnormalities of pupil size and reaction, with absence of the oculocephalic response and fixed oculomotor deviation of the eyes. Pending herniation is also associated with respiratory abnormalities, including hyperventilation, Cheyne-Stokes respiration, ataxic breathing, apnea, and respiratory arrest. These children must be treated immediately with appropriate intravenous antibiotics and transported to a critical care unit for stabilization and imaging studies before an LP is contemplated. LP is the primary diagnostic procedure in children with suspected bacterial meningitis in the absence of overwhelming sepsis or shock, or symptoms and signs of brain herniation. Because the clinical status of children with untreated bacterial meningitis may rapidly deteriorate, deferral of the LP and initiation of appropriate antibiotic therapy while awaiting the results of a CT scan could be the determining factor between recovery or severe complications and death.

In the third case, *on rare occasions*, an LP is temporarily withheld from a critically ill, moribund patient because the procedure may produce cardiorespiratory arrest. In this situation, blood cultures are drawn, antibiotics and supportive care are administered, and when the patient is stabilized, an LP may be accomplished safely under more controlled circumstances.

In the fourth instance, if examination of the CSF is urgent in a patient with skin infection at the site of the LP, a ventricular or cisterna magna tap performed by a skilled physician is indicated.

In the fifth instance, thrombocytopenia, with a platelet count less than 20×10^9/L, may cause uncontrolled bleeding in the subarachnoid or subdural space.

Normal CSF is the color of water. Cloudy CSF results from an elevated white blood cell (WBC) or red blood cell (RBC) count. Normal CSF contains up to 5/mm^3 WBCs, and a newborn may have as many as 15/mm^3. Polymorphonuclear (PMN) cells are always abnormal in a child, but 1–2/mm^3 may be present in a normal neonate. The presence of PMN cells raises suspicion of a pathologic process. An elevated PMN count suggests bacterial meningitis or the early phase of an aseptic meningitis (see Chapter 594). CSF lymphocytosis indicates aseptic, tuberculous, or fungal meningitis; demyelinating diseases; brain or spinal cord tumor; immunologic disorders including collagen vascular diseases; and chemical irritation (e.g., postmyelogram, intrathecal methotrexate).

A Gram stain of the CSF is essential in the investigation of suspected bacterial meningitis; an acid-fast stain or India ink preparation is used if tuberculous or fungal meningitis is a possibility. The fluid is placed on appropriate culture media based on the clinical findings and on the CSF analysis.

Normal CSF contains no RBCs. The presence of RBCs indicates a traumatic tap or a subarachnoid hemorrhage. Bloody CSF should be centrifuged immediately. The supernatant of a bloody tap is clear, but it is xanthochromic in the presence of a subarachnoid hemorrhage. Progressive clearing of bloody CSF is noted during collection of the fluid in the case of a traumatic tap. The presence of crenated RBCs does not differentiate a traumatic tap from a subarachnoid hemorrhage. In addition to a subarachnoid hemorrhage, xanthochromia may result from hyperbilirubinemia, carotenemia, and a markedly elevated CSF protein.

The normal *CSF protein* ranges from 10–40 mg/dL in a child to as high as 120 mg/dL in a neonate. The CSF protein falls to the normal childhood range by 3 mo of age. The CSF protein may be elevated in many processes, including infectious, immunologic, vascular, and degenerative diseases as well as tumors of the brain and spinal cord. The CSF protein is increased after a bloody tap by approximately 1 mg/dL for every 1,000 mm^3. Elevation of CSF immunoglobulin G (IgG), which normally represents approximately 10% of the total protein, is observed in subacute sclerosing panencephalitis, postinfectious encephalomyelitis, and in some cases of multiple sclerosis. If the diagnosis of multiple sclerosis is suspected, the CSF should be tested for the presence of oligoclonal bands.

The *CSF glucose* content is about 60% of the blood glucose in a healthy child. To prevent a spuriously elevated blood/CSF glucose ratio in a case of suspected meningitis, it is advisable to collect the blood glucose before the LP when the child is relatively calm. Hypoglycorrhachia is found in association with diffuse meningeal disease, particularly bacterial and tuberculous meningitis. In addition, widespread neoplastic involvement of the meninges, subarachnoid hemorrhage, fungal meningitis, and, on occasion, aseptic meningitis can produce a low CSF glucose level.

The CSF may also be examined for specific *antigens* (e.g., latex agglutination for suspected meningitis) and in investigation of a series of metabolic diseases (e.g., lactate, amino acids, endolase determination).

Subdural Tap. This procedure may be indicated to establish the diagnosis of a subdural effusion or hematoma. A blunt, short-beveled 20-gauge needle and stylet are used for the procedure. The subdural space is approached at the lateral border of the anterior fontanel or along the upper margin of the coronal suture at least 2–3 cm from the midline to prevent injury to the underlying sagittal sinus. After adequate cleansing and preparation of the skull, including shaving of the hair from the operative site, the patient is placed in the supine position and is firmly held by an attendant. After a local anesthetic, the needle and stylet are slowly advanced through the skin and underlying tissue with a z-like movement until the dura is entered with a sudden popping sensation. Considerable care is taken to prevent advancement of the needle into the cerebral cortex, which in an infant is approximately 1.5 cm from the skin surface. A hemostat attached approximately 5–7 mm from the beveled end of the needle should provide an adequate safeguard. The subdural fluid, which may squirt out under pressure, is collected and sent for protein analysis, cell count, and culture. The color of the fluid may be xanthochromic, bright red, or oily brown (depending on the age of the subdural collections). Bilateral subdural taps may be indicated, because subdural collections are bilateral in most cases. The amount of fluid removed with each tap should be limited to a total of 15–20 mL from each side in order to prevent rebleeding from a sudden shift of the intracranial contents. At the termination of the procedure, a sterile dressing is applied, and the child is placed in a sitting position that tends to prevent leakage of fluid from the puncture site. (See Chapter 594 for a discussion of subdural fluid associated with meningitis.)

Ventricular Tap. A ventricular tap is used for the removal of CSF in the management of life-threatening increased ICP associated with hydrocephalus, when conservative measures have failed. The procedure should not be undertaken by a pediatrician except when the patient's life is in jeopardy and a neurosurgeon is not available. For an infant, the procedure is similar to a subdural tap. A 20-gauge ventricular needle with a stylet is placed in the lateral border of the anterior fontanel and is directed toward the inner canthus of the ipsilateral eye. The needle is advanced slowly, and the stylet is removed frequently to determine the presence of CSF. The ventricle is usually encountered about 4 cm from the skin surface.

Neuroradiologic Procedures. A *skull roentgenogram* is occasionally a useful diagnostic procedure. It may demonstrate fractures, intracranial calcification, craniosynostosis, congenital anomalies, or bony defects and evidence of increased ICP. Acute increased ICP is characterized by separation of the sutures, whereas erosion of the posterior clinoid processes, enlargement of the sella turcica, and an increase in convolutional markings indicate long-standing intracranial hypertension.

CT scanning is an important diagnostic procedure for emergencies and for less emergent disorders. CT scanning is a noninvasive procedure that uses conventional x-ray techniques. Sedation is usually required for infants and young children, because a lack of head movement is essential during the study. Pentobarbital, 4 mg/kg IM 30 min before the CT scan, with a supplementary dose of 2 mg/kg IM 1–1½ hr later if necessary, is usually effective. Chloral hydrate, 50–75 mg/kg PO 45 min before the procedure, is an alternative method of sedation. CT scanning is useful in demonstrating congenital malformations of the brain, including hydrocephalus and porencephalic cysts, subdural collections, cerebral atrophy, intracranial calcification, intracerebral hematoma, brain tumors and areas of cerebral edema, infarction, and demyelination (Table 584–3). Intravenous injection of radiographic contrast medium enhances areas of increased vascular permeability due to abnormalities of the blood-brain barrier and highlights abnormal collections of blood vessels in an arteriovenous malformation.

MRI is a noninvasive procedure and is especially well suited for the study of neoplasms, cerebral edema, demyelination, degenerative diseases, and congenital anomalies, particularly of the posterior fossa and spinal cord (see Table 584–3). MRI is capable of detecting small plaques in patients with multiple sclerosis and areas of localized gliosis in children with uncontrolled

---

TABLE 584–3. Preferred Imaging Procedures in Neurologic Diseases

Neurologic Disease	Imaging Procedure
Cerebral or cerebellar ischemic infarction	CT in the first 12–24 hr; MRI after 12–24 hr (diffusion-weighted and perfusion-weighted MRI augments the findings, especially in the first 24 hr, and even before 8 hr)
Cerebral or cerebellar hemorrhage	CT in the first 24 hr; MRI after 24 hr; MRI and endovascular angiography for suspected arteriovenous malformation
Transient ischemic attack	MRI to identify lacunar or other small lesions; ultrasound studies of the carotid arteries; magnetic resonance angiography
Arteriovenous malformation	CT for acute hemorrhage; MRI and endovascular angiography as early as possible
Cerebral aneurysm	CT for acute subarachnoid hemorrhage; CT angiography or endovascular angiography to identify the aneurysm; TCD to detect vasospasm
Brain tumor	MRI without and with injection of contrast material
Craniocerebral trauma	CT initially; MRI after initial assessment and treatment
Multiple sclerosis	MRI without and with injection of contrast material
Meningitis or encephalitis	CT without and with injection of contrast material initially; MRI after initial assessment and treatment
Cerebral or cerebellar abscess	CT without and with injection of contrast material for initial diagnosis or, if stable, MRI instead of CT; MRI without and with injection of contrast material subsequently
Granuloma	MRI without and with injection of contrast material
Dementia	MRI; PET; SPECT
Movement disorders	MRI; PET
Neonatal and development disorders	Ultrasonography in unstable premature neonates; otherwise MRI
Epilepsy	MRI; PET; SPECT
Headache	CT in patients suspected of having structural disorders

PET = positron-emission tomography; SPECT = single-photon-emission computed tomography; TCD = transcranial Doppler ultrasonography. From Gilman S: Imaging the brain. N Engl J Med 1998; 338:812.

seizures. MRI is routinely used in the evaluation of children who are potential candidates for epilepsy surgery. Intracerebral calcifications are not detected by MRI. The contrast agent, gadolinium-DTPA, is useful during MRI, especially to highlight lesions associated with a disrupted blood-brain barrier. Functional MRI (fMRI) is a noninvasive technique for detecting and mapping with high resolution the hemodynamic changes produced by localized brain activity during specific cognitive and/or sensorimotor function. It is useful for presurgical localization of critical brain functions (and is very promising as a tool for investigating the development and plasticity of these functions).

Radionuclide brain scan uses a radioactive material such as ^{99}Tc, which concentrates in regions where the blood-brain barrier has been disrupted. It is useful in the investigation of herpes encephalitis and cerebral abscess. *Positron-emission tomography* (PET) provides unique information on brain metabolism and perfusion by measuring blood flow, oxygen uptake, and glucose consumption. PET is an expensive technique that has been used primarily in adults, but it is increasingly used in many pediatric centers, particularly those with active epilepsy surgery programs. *Single-photon-emission computerized tomography* (SPECT), using ^{99m}Tc hexamethyl propylenamine oxime (Tc 99m-HMPAO) is a sensitive and inexpensive technique to study regional cerebral blood flow. SPECT is particularly useful in investigating cerebral vascular disease in children (systemic lupus erythematosus), as well as herpes encephalitis, and for localization of focal epileptiform discharges and recurrent brain tumors. *Cerebral angiography* is reserved for the study of vascular disorders. The procedure requires a general anesthetic in most children. Cerebral angiography, using subtraction techniques, is particularly useful for the delineation of arteriovenous malformations, aneurysms, arterial occlusions, and venous thrombosis. In most cases, a four-vessel study (internal carotids and vertebral arteries) is accomplished. *MRA* (angiography) may reduce the need for contrast invasive angiography. *Cranial ultrasonography* for the detection of periventricular leukomalacia, intracranial hemorrhage, hydrocephalus, and intracranial tumors, is limited to infants with a patent fontanel. The procedure is used intraoperatively in older children for placing shunts, locating small tumors, and directing needle biopsies. *Myelography* was used in the past for demonstrating congenital anomalies, tumors, and vascular malformations of the spinal cord. MRI is superior in most cases to contrast myelography and is not associated with arachnoiditis, which occasionally complicates injection of contrast material into the subarachnoid space.

Electroencephalography. An *electroencephalogram* (EEG) provides a continuous recording of electrical activity between reference electrodes placed on the scalp. Although the genesis of the electrical activity is not certain, it likely originates from postsynaptic potentials in the dendrites of cortical neurons. Even with amplification of the electrical activity, not all potentials are recorded because there is a buffering effect of the scalp, muscles, bone, vessels, and subarachnoid fluid. The EEG waves are classified according to their frequency as delta (1–3/sec), theta (4–7/sec), alpha (8–12/sec), and beta (13–20/sec). These waves are altered by many factors, including age, state of alertness, eye closure, drugs, and disease states. High-voltage slow and sharp waves (K complexes) and sleep spindles (regular 12–14/sec waves) confined to the central regions occur during sleep in a normal EEG. Abnormalities of waveform include spikes and slow waves. Spikes are characteristically paroxysmal, sharp, and of high voltage followed by a slow wave. Spikes and slow waves are associated with epilepsy, but some normal patients may have this EEG finding. Focal spikes are often associated with irritative lesions, including cysts, slow-growing tumors, and glial scar tissue. Epileptiform activity may be enhanced by activation procedures, including hyperventilation, photic stimulation, and

sleep deprivation. Slow waves may be focal, in which case a circumscribed lesion such as a hematoma, tumor, infarction, or a localized infectious process may be considered; generalized slow waves suggest a metabolic, inflammatory, or more widespread process.

EEG/polygraphic/video monitoring provides precise characterization of seizure types, which allows for specific medical or surgical management. In addition, the physician is more accurately able to differentiate epileptic seizures from paroxysmal events that mimic epilepsy, including pseudoseizures. EEG/polygraphic/video monitoring provides for measurement of seizure discharges and for study of the efficacy of various therapeutic regimens. Finally, polygraphic/EEG with video monitoring simultaneously records physiologic and EEG changes; it is particularly useful in neonates in whom the characterization of seizures is difficult.

Magnetoencephalography (MEG) detects magnetic fields associated with the intracellular current flow within neurons. *Magnetic source imaging (MSI)* is an advanced neurophysiologic technique that combines MEG and MRI to measure the magnetic field generated by a series of neurons. MSI is particularly useful for the investigation of patients who may be candidates for epilepsy surgery.

Evoked Potentials. An evoked potential is an electrical response that follows stimulation of the CNS by a specific stimulus of the visual, auditory, or sensory system. Clinical application of evoked potentials in infants and children has increased dramatically during the past decade. Stimulation of the visual system by a flash or patterned stimulus, such as a black-and-white checkerboard, produces *visual-evoked potentials* (VEPs), which are recorded over the occiput and averaged in a computer. Abnormal VEPs result from lesions involving the visual system from the retina to the visual cortex. Neurodegenerative diseases, such as Tay-Sachs, Krabbe, Pelizaeus-Merzbacher disease, and neuronal ceroid lipofuscinoses, show characteristic VEP abnormalities. Lesions of the optic nerve and chiasm also produce abnormalities in the VEP response. The VEP, using patterned stimuli, is useful particularly in assessing visual function in at-risk neonates. Flash VEPs are also very useful in predicting outcome in term infants after asphyxia. *Brainstem auditory-evoked potentials* (BAEPs) may be used to objectively measure hearing acuity, particularly in a neonate or uncooperative child when routine hearing assessment techniques have failed. BAEPs are abnormal in many neurodegenerative diseases in children and are an important tool in evaluating patients with suspected tumors of the cerebellopontine angle. BAEPs are helpful in the assessment of brainstem function in comatose patients, because the waveforms are unaffected by drugs or by the level of consciousness. They are not accurate in predicting neurologic recovery and outcome. *Somatosensory-evoked potentials* (SSEPs) are obtained by stimulating a peripheral nerve (peroneal, median) and by recording the electrical response over the cervical region and contralateral parietal somatosensory cortex. The SSEP determines the functional integrity of the dorsal column-medial-lemniscal system and is useful in monitoring spinal cord function during operative procedures, such as scoliosis, the repair of coarctation of the aorta, and myelomeningocele. SSEPs are abnormal in many neurodegenerative disorders in children and are the most accurate evoked potential in the assessment of neurologic outcome following a severe CNS insult.

Ellis R: Lumbar cerebrospinal fluid opening pressure measured in a flexed lateral decubitus position in children. *Pediatrics* 1994;93:622.

Gilman S: Imaging the brain. Parts I and II. *N Engl J Med* 1998;338:812.

Haslam RH: Role of computed tomography in the early management of bacterial meningitis. *J Pediatr* 1991;119:157.

Mizrahi EM: Electroencephalographic/polygraphic/video monitoring in childhood epilepsy. *J Pediatr* 1984;105:1.

Otsubo H, Snead C: Magnetoencephalography and magnetic source imaging in children. *J Child Neurol* 2001;16:227–35.

Packer RJ, Zimmerman RA, Sutton LN, et al: Magnetic resonance imaging of spinal cord disease of childhood. *Pediatrics* 1986;78:251.

Portnoy JM, Olson LC: Normal cerebrospinal fluid values in children: Another look. *Pediatrics* 1985;75:484.

Taylor MJ: Evoked potentials in paediatrics. In Halliday AM (editor): *Evoked Potentials in Clinical Testing*, 2nd ed. Edinburgh, Churchill Livingstone, 1993, p 489.

Chapter 585

Congenital Anomalies of the Central Nervous System

Michael V. Johnston and Stephen Kinsman

585.1 Neural Tube Defects (Dysraphism)

Neural tube defects account for most congenital anomalies of the central nervous system (CNS) and result from failure of the neural tube to close spontaneously between the 3rd and 4th wk of in utero development. Although the precise cause of neural tube defects remains unknown, evidence suggests that many factors, including radiation, drugs, malnutrition, chemicals, and genetic determinants (mutations in folate-responsive or folate-dependent pathways), may adversely affect normal development of the CNS from the time of conception. In some cases, an abnormal maternal nutritional state or exposure to radiation before conception may increase the likelihood of a CNS congenital malformation. The major neural tube defects include spina bifida occulta, meningocele, myelomeningocele, encephalocele, anencephaly, dermal sinus, tethered cord, syringomyelia, diastematomyelia, and lipoma involving the conus medullaris.

The human nervous system originates from the primitive ectoderm that also develops into the epidermis. The ectoderm, endoderm, and mesoderm form the three primary germ layers that are developed by the 3rd wk. The endoderm, particularly the notochordal plate and the intraembryonic mesoderm, induces the overlying ectoderm to develop the neural plate during the 3rd wk of development (Fig. 585–1A). Failure of normal induction is responsible for most of the neural tube defects. Rapid growth of cells within the neural plate causes further invagination of the neural groove and differentiation of a conglomerate of cells, the neural crest, which migrate laterally on the surface of the neural tube (see Fig. 585–1B). The notochordal plate becomes the centrally placed notochord, which acts as a foundation around which the vertebral column ultimately develops. With formation of the vertebral column, the notochord undergoes involution and becomes the nucleus pulposus of the intervertebral disks. The neural crest cells differentiate to form the peripheral nervous system, including the spinal and autonomic ganglia as well as the ganglia of cranial nerves V, VII, VIII, IX, and X. In addition, the neural crest forms the leptomeninges, as well as Schwann cells, which are responsible for myelinization of the peripheral nervous system. The dura is believed to arise from the paraxial mesoderm.

During the 3rd wk of embryonic development, invagination of the neural groove is completed and the neural tube is formed by separation from the overlying surface ectoderm (see Fig. 585–1C). Initial closure of the neural tube is accomplished in the area corresponding to the future junction of the spinal cord and medulla and moves rapidly both caudally and rostrally. For a brief period, the neural tube is open at both ends, and the neural canal communicates freely with the amniotic cavity (see Fig. 585–1D). Failure of closure of the neural tube allows excretion of fetal substances (e.g., α-fetoprotein [AFP], acetylcholinesterase) into the amniotic fluid, serving as biochemical markers for a neural tube defect. Prenatal screening of maternal serum for AFP during 16–18 wk of gestation is an effective method for identifying pregnancies at risk for fetuses with neural tube defects in utero. Normally, the rostral end of the neural tube closes on the 23rd day and the caudal neuropore closes by a process of secondary neurulation by the 27th day of development, before the time that many women realize they are pregnant.

585.2 Spina Bifida Occulta

This common anomaly consists of a midline defect of the vertebral bodies without protrusion of the spinal cord or meninges. Most individuals are asymptomatic and lack neurologic signs, and the condition is usually of no consequence. In some cases, patches of hair, a lipoma, discoloration of the skin, or a dermal sinus in the midline of the low back signifies an underlying malformation of the spinal cord. A spine roentgenogram shows a defect in closure of the posterior vertebral arches and laminae, typically involving L5 and S1. There is no abnormality of the meninges, spinal cord, or nerve roots. Spina bifida occulta is occasionally associated with more significant developmental abnormalities of the spinal cord, including syringomyelia, diastematomyelia, and a tethered cord. A *dermoid sinus* usually forms a small skin opening, which leads into a narrow duct, sometimes indicated by protruding hairs, a hairy patch, or a vascular nevus. Dermoid sinuses occur in the midline at the site of occurrence of meningoceles or encephaloceles, that is, the lumbosacral region or occiput. Dermoid sinus tracts may pass through the dura, acting as a conduit for the spread of infection. Recurrent meningitis of occult origin should prompt careful examination for a small sinus tract in the posterior midline region, including the back of the head.

585.3 Meningocele

A meningocele is formed when the meninges herniate through a defect in the posterior vertebral arches. The spinal cord is usually normal and assumes a normal position in the spinal canal, although there may be tethering, syringomyelia, or diastematomyelia. A fluctuant midline mass that may transilluminate occurs along the vertebral column, usually in the low back. Most meningoceles are well covered with skin and pose no threat to the patient. Careful neurologic examination is mandatory. Asymptomatic children with normal neurologic findings and full-thickness skin covering the meningocele may have surgery delayed. Before surgical correction of the defect, the patient must be thoroughly examined with the use of plain roentgenograms, ultrasonography, and MRI to determine the extent of neural tissue involvement, if any, and associated anomalies, including diastematomyelia, tethered spinal cord, and lipoma. Those patients with leaking cerebrospinal fluid (CSF) or a thin skin covering should undergo immediate surgical treatment to prevent meningitis. A CT scan of the head is recommended for children with a meningocele because of the association with hydrocephalus in some cases. An anterior meningocele projects into the pelvis through a defect in the sacrum. Symptoms of constipation and bladder dysfunction develop due to the increasing size of the lesion. Female patients may have associated anomalies of the genital tract, including a rectovaginal fistula and vaginal septa. Plain roentgenograms demonstrate a defect in the sacrum, and CT scanning or MRI outlines the extent of the meningocele.

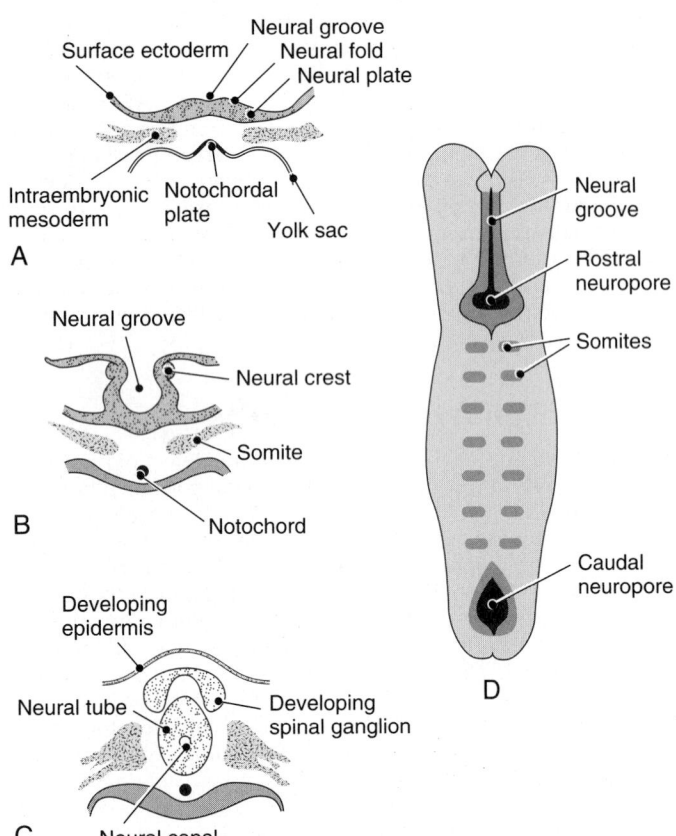

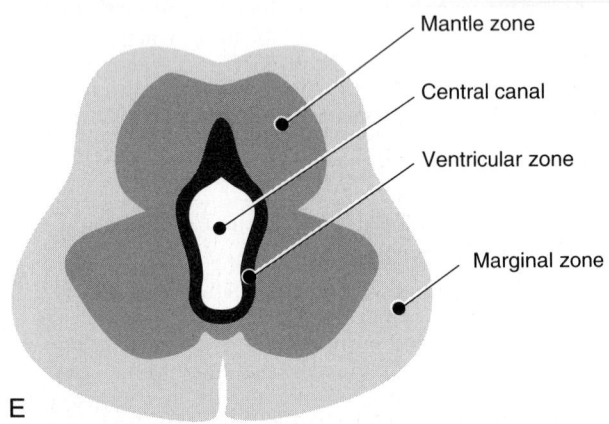

FIGURE 585–1. Diagrammatic illustration of the developing nervous system. *A,* Transverse sections of the neural plate during the 3rd wk. *B,* Formation of the neural groove and the neural crest. *C,* The neural tube is developed. *D,* Longitudinal drawing showing the initial closure of the neural tube in the central region. *E,* Cross-sectional drawing of the embryonic neural tube (primitive spinal cord).

585.4 Myelomeningocele

Myelomeningocele represents the most severe form of dysraphism involving the vertebral column and occurs with an incidence of approximately 1/4,000 live births.

Etiology. The cause of myelomeningocele is unknown, but as with all neural tube closure defects, a genetic predisposition exists; the risk of recurrence after one affected child increases to 3–4% and increases to approximately 10% with two previous abnormal pregnancies. Nutritional and environmental factors undoubtedly have a role in the etiology of myelomeningocele. There is strong evidence that maternal periconceptional use of folic acid supplementation reduces the incidence of neural tube defects in pregnancies at risk by at least 50%. To be effective, folic acid supplementation should be initiated before conception and continued until at least the 12th wk of gestation when neurulation is complete. The U.S. Public Health Service has recommended that all women of childbearing age and who are capable of becoming pregnant take 0.4 mg of folic acid daily and that women who have previously had a pregnancy resulting in a neural tube defect be treated with 4 mg of folic acid daily, beginning 1 mo before the time the pregnancy is planned. The modern diet provides about half the daily requirement of folic acid. In order to increase folic acid intake, fortification of flour, pasta, rice, and cornmeal with 0.15 mg folic acid per 100 g was mandated in the United States and Canada in 1998. Unfortunately, the added folic acid will be insufficient to meet the minimal requirements to prevent neural tube defects. Therefore, informative educational programs remain essential for women planning a pregnancy. Certain drugs—including drugs that antagonize folic acid such as trimethoprim and the anticonvulsants carbamazepine, phenytoin, phenobarbital, and primidone—increase the risk of myelomeningocele. The anticonvulsant valproic acid causes neural tube defects in approximately 1–2% of pregnancies if the drug is administered during pregnancy. Some epilepsy clinicians recommend that all female patients of childbearing potential who take anticonvulsant medications should also receive folic acid supplements.

Clinical Manifestations. The condition produces dysfunction of many organs and structures, including the skeleton, skin, and genitourinary tract, in addition to the peripheral nervous system and the CNS. A myelomeningocele may be located anywhere along the neuraxis, but the lumbosacral region accounts for at least 75% of the cases. The extent and degree of the neurologic deficit depend on the location of the myelomeningocele. A lesion in the low sacral region causes bowel and bladder incontinence associated with anesthesia in the perineal area but with no impairment of motor function. Newborns with a defect in the midlumbar region typically have a saclike cystic structure covered by a thin layer of partially epithelialized tissue (Fig. 585–2). Remnants of neural tissue are visible beneath the membrane, which may occasionally rupture and leak CSF. Examination of the infant shows a flaccid paralysis of the lower extremities, an absence of deep tendon reflexes, a lack of response to touch and pain, and a high incidence of postural abnormalities of the lower extremities (including clubfeet and subluxation of the hips). Constant urinary dribbling and a relaxed anal sphincter may be evident. Thus, a myelomeningocele in the midlumbar region tends to produce lower motor neuron signs due to abnormalities and disruption of the conus medullaris. Infants with myelomeningocele typically have an increasing neurologic deficit as the myelomeningocele extends higher into the thoracic region. However, patients with a myelomeningocele in the upper thoracic or the cervical region usually have a very minimal neurologic deficit and in most cases do not have hydrocephalus.

Hydrocephalus in association with a type II Chiari defect develops in at least 80% of patients with myelomeningocele. Generally, the lower the deformity in the neuraxis (e.g., sacrum), the less likely is the risk of hydrocephalus. Ventricular enlargement may be indolent and slow growing or may be rapid, causing a bulging anterior fontanel, dilated scalp veins, setting-sun appearance of the eyes, irritability, and vomiting associated with an increased head circumference. Not infrequently, infants with hydrocephalus and Chiari II malformation develop symptoms of hindbrain dysfunction, including difficulty feeding, choking, stridor, apnea, vocal cord paralysis, pooling of secretions, and spasticity of the upper extremities, which, if untreated, can lead to death. This *Chiari crisis* is due to downward herniation of the medulla and cerebellar tonsils through the foramen magnum.

Treatment. Management and supervision of a child and family with a myelomeningocele require a *multidisciplinary team approach*, including surgeons, physicians, and therapists, with one individual (often a pediatrician) acting as the advocate and coordinator of the treatment program. The news that a newborn child has a devastating condition such as myelomeningocele causes parents to feel considerable grief and anger. They need time to learn about the handicap and the associated complications and to reflect on the various procedures and treatment plans. The parents must be given the facts by a knowledgeable individual in an unhurried and nonthreatening setting. If possible, discussions with other parents of children with neural tube defects are helpful in resolving important questions and issues.

Surgery can be delayed for several days (except when there is a CSF leak) to allow the parents time to begin to adjust to the shock and to prepare for the multiple procedures and inevitable problems that lie ahead. Evaluation of other congenital anomalies and renal function can also be initiated before surgery. Most pediatric centers aggressively treat the majority of infants with myelomeningocele. After repair of a myelomeningocele, most infants require a shunting procedure for hydrocephalus. If symptoms or signs of hindbrain dysfunction appear, early surgical decompression of the medulla and cervical cord is indicated. Clubfeet may require casting, and dislocated hips may require operative procedures.

Careful evaluation and reassessment of the *genitourinary system* are some of the most important components of the management. Teaching the parents, and ultimately the patient, to regularly catheterize a neurogenic bladder is a crucial step in maintaining a low residual volume that prevents urinary tract infections and reflux leading to pyelonephritis and hydronephrosis. Periodic urine cultures and assessment of renal function, including serum electrolytes and creatinine as well as renal scans, intravenous pyelograms, and ultrasonography, are obtained according to the progress of the patient and the results of the physical examination. This approach to urinary tract management has greatly reduced the need for surgical diversionary procedures and has significantly decreased the morbidity and mortality associated with progressive renal disease in these patients. Some children can become continent with surgical implantation of an artificial urinary sphincter or bladder augmentation at a later age. Although *incontinence of fecal matter* is common and is socially unacceptable during the school years, it does not pose the same risks as urinary incontinence. Many children can be bowel-trained with a regimen of timed enemas or suppositories that allows evacuation at a predetermined time once or twice a day. Appendicostomy for antegrade enemas may also be helpful. Also see Chapter 20.4.

Functional *ambulation* is the wish of each child and parent and may be possible, depending on the level of the lesion and on intact function of the iliopsoas muscles. Almost every child with a sacral or lumbosacral lesion obtains functional ambulation; approximately half the children with higher defects ambulate with the use of braces and canes.

Prognosis. For a child who is born with a myelomeningocele and who is treated aggressively, the mortality rate is approximately 10–15%, and most deaths occur before age 4 yr. At least 70% of survivors have normal intelligence, but learning problems and seizure disorders are more common than in the general population. Previous episodes of meningitis or ventriculitis adversely affect the ultimate intelligence quotient. Because myelomeningocele is a chronic handicapping condition, periodic multidisciplinary follow-up is required for life.

585.5 Encephalocele

Two major forms of dysraphism affect the skull, resulting in protrusion of tissue through a bony midline defect, called *cranium bifidum*. A *cranial meningocele* consists of a CSF-filled meningeal sac only, and a *cranial encephalocele* contains the sac plus cerebral cortex, cerebellum, or portions of the brainstem. Microscopic examination of the neural tissue within an encephalocele often reveals abnormalities. The cranial defect occurs most commonly

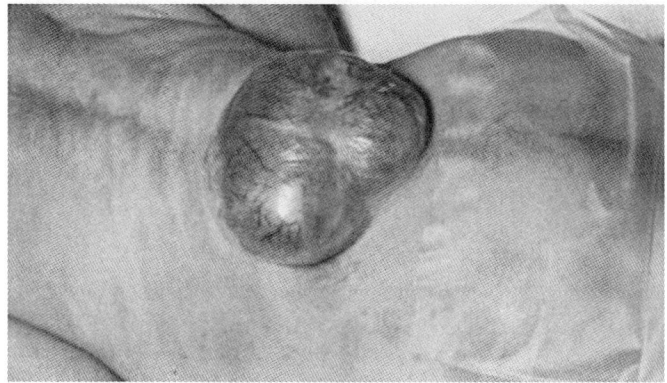

FIGURE 585–2. A lumbar myelomeningocele is covered by a thin layer of skin.

in the occipital region at or below the inion, but in certain parts of the world frontal or nasofrontal encephaloceles are more prominent. These abnormalities are one tenth as common as neural tube closure defects involving the spine. The etiology is presumed to be similar to that for anencephaly and myelomeningocele, because examples of each have been reported in the same family.

Infants with a cranial encephalocele are at increased risk for developing hydrocephalus due to aqueduct stenosis, Chiari malformation, or the Dandy-Walker syndrome. Examination may show a small sac with a pedunculated stalk or a large cystlike structure that may exceed the size of the cranium. The lesion may be completely covered with skin, but areas of denuded skin can occur and require urgent surgical management. Transillumination of the sac may indicate the presence of neural tissue. A plain roentgenogram of the skull and cervical spine is indicated to define the anatomy of the vertebra. Ultrasonography is most helpful in determining the contents of the sac, obviating the need for a CT scan in most cases. Children with a cranial meningocele generally have a good prognosis, whereas patients with an encephalocele are at risk for visual problems, microcephaly, mental retardation, and seizures. Generally, children with neural tissue within the sac and associated hydrocephalus have the poorest prognosis. *Meckel-Gruber syndrome* is a rare autosomal recessive condition that is characterized by an occipital encephalocele, cleft lip or palate, microcephaly, microphthalmia, abnormal genitalia, polycystic kidneys, and polydactyly. Encephaloceles may be diagnosed in utero by determination of AFP levels and ultrasound measurement of the biparietal diameter.

585.6 Anencephaly

An anencephalic infant presents a distinctive appearance with a large defect of the calvarium, meninges, and scalp associated with a rudimentary brain, which results from failure of closure of the rostral neuropore. The primitive brain consists of portions of connective tissue, vessels, and neuroglia. The cerebral hemispheres and cerebellum are usually absent, and only a residue of the brainstem can be identified. The pituitary gland is hypoplastic, and the spinal cord pyramidal tracts are missing owing to the absence of the cerebral cortex. Additional anomalies include folding of the ears, cleft palate, and congenital heart defects in 10–20% of cases. Most anencephalic infants die within several days of birth. The incidence of anencephaly approximates 1/1,000 live births, and the greatest frequency is in Ireland and Wales. The recurrence risk is approximately 4% and increases to 10% if a couple has had two previously affected pregnancies. Many factors have been implicated as the cause of anencephaly (in addition to a genetic basis), including low socioeconomic status, nutritional and vitamin deficiencies, and a large number of environmental and toxic factors. It is very likely that several noxious stimuli interact on a genetically susceptible host to produce anencephaly. Fortunately, the frequency of anencephaly has been decreasing during the past 2 decades. Approximately 50% of cases of anencephaly are associated with polyhydramnios. Couples who have had an anencephalic infant should have successive pregnancies monitored, including amniocentesis, determination of AFP levels, and ultrasound examination between the 14th and 16th wk of gestation.

Aksnes G, Diseth TH, Helseth A, et al: Appendicostomy for antegrade enema: Effects on somatic and psychosocial functioning in children with myelomeningocele. *Pediatrics* 2002;109:484-9.

Charney EB, Weller SC, Sutton LN, et al: Management of the newborn with myelomeningocele: Time for a decision-making process. *Pediatrics* 1985;75:58.

Fernandes ET, Reinberg Y, Vernier R, et al: Neurogenic bladder dysfunction in children: Review of pathophysiology and current management. *J Pediatr* 1994;124:1.

Haddow JE, Palomaki GE, Knight GJ, et al: Reducing the need for amniocentesis in women 35 years of age or older with serum markers for screening. *N Engl J Med* 1994;330:1114.

Hannigan KF: Teaching intermittent self-catheterization to young children with myelodysplasia. *Dev Med Child Neurol* 1979;21:365.

Hernandez-Diaz S, Werler MM, Walker AM, et al: Folic acid antagonists during pregnancy and the risk of birth defects. *N Engl J Med* 2000;343:1608.

Lemire RJ, Beckwith JB, Warkany J: *Anencephaly.* New York, Raven Press, 1978.

Lorber J, Salfiedl S: Results of selective treatment of spina bifida cystica. *Arch Dis Child* 1981;56:822.

McLone DG: Results of treatment of children born with a myelomeningocele. *Clin Neurosurg* 1983;30:407.

McLone DG, Czyzewski D, Raimondi AJ, et al: Central nervous system infections as a limiting factor in the intelligence of children with myelomeningocele. *Pediatrics* 1982;70:338.

MRC Vitamin Study Research Group: Prevention of neural tube defects: Results of the Medical Research Council Vitamin Study. *Lancet* 1991;338:131.

Norman D, Brant-Zawadski M, Yeates A, et al: Magnetic resonance imaging of the spinal cord and canal: Potentials and limitations. *AJNR* 1985;5:9.

Opitz JM, Howe JJ: The Meckel syndrome. *Birth Defects* 1969;5:167.

Robert E, Guibaud P: Maternal valproic acid and congenital neural tube defects. *Lancet* 1982;2:937.

585.7 Disorders of Neuronal Migration

Disorders of neuronal migration may result in minor abnormalities with little or no clinical consequence (e.g., small heterotopia of neurons) or devastating abnormalities of the CNS (e.g., mental retardation, lissencephaly, schizencephaly) (Fig. 585–3). One of the most important mechanisms in the control of neuronal migration is the radial glial fiber system that guides neurons to their proper site. Migrating neurons attach to the radial glial fiber and then disembark at predetermined sites to ultimately form the precisely designed six-layered cerebral cortex. The product of a mouse gene called *reelin* directs the new neuron to reach its final destination in the brain. Another mouse gene (*mdab1*) may act as a signaling pathway triggered by *reelin*. Mutations of these genes in mice produce major neuronal migration abnormalities. The severity and the extent of the dis-

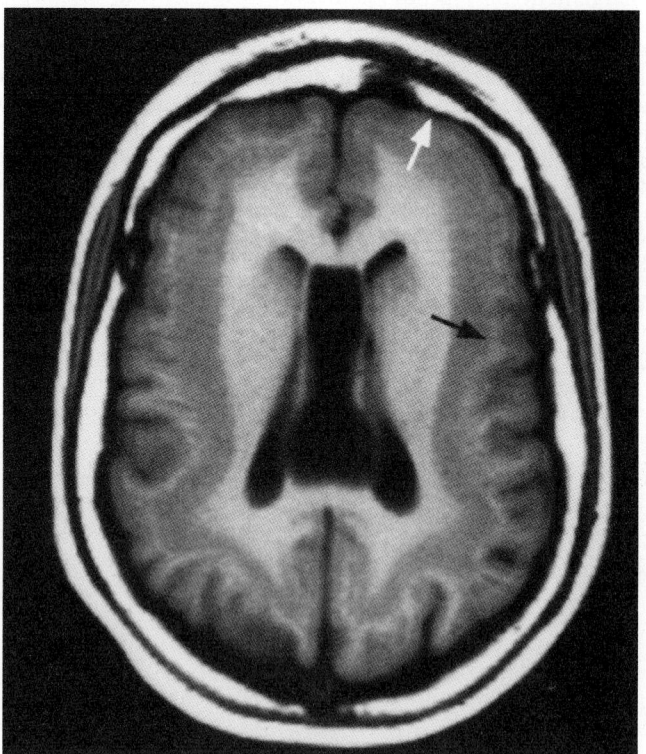

FIGURE 585–3. T1 weighted MRI scan demonstrating band heterotopia. A thin layer of white matter (*black arrow*) lies between the band of heterotopic gray matter and the cortical surface. Failure of cortical organization with lissencephaly is present in both frontal lobes (*white arrow*).

order are related to numerous factors, including the timing of a particular insult and a host of environmental and genetic factors.

The embryonic neural tube consists of three zones: ventricular, mantle, and marginal (see Fig. 585–1E). The ependymal layer consists of a pluripotential, pseudostratified, columnar neuroepithelium. Specific neuroepithelial cells differentiate into primitive neurons or neuroblasts that form the mantle layer. The marginal zone is formed from cells in the outer layer of the neuroepithelium, which ultimately becomes the white matter. Glioblasts, which act as the primitive supportive cells of the CNS, also arise from the neuroepithelial cells in the ependymal zone. They migrate to the mantle and marginal zones and become future astrocytes and oligodendrocytes. It is likely that microglia originate from mesenchymal cells at a later stage of fetal development when blood vessels begin to penetrate the developing nervous system. Continued advancement of an understanding of the molecular bases of cortical development is leading to new classifications of malformations of cortical development.

Lissencephaly. Lissencephaly, or agyria, is a rare disorder that is characterized by the absence of cerebral convolutions and a poorly formed sylvian fissure, giving the appearance of a 3–4 mo fetal brain. The condition is probably a result of faulty neuroblast migration during early embryonic life and is usually associated with enlarged lateral ventricles and heterotopias in the white matter. There is a four-layered cortex, rather than the usual six-layered one, with a thin rim of periventricular white matter and numerous gray heterotopia visible by microscopic examination. Clinically, these infants present with failure to thrive, microcephaly, marked developmental delay, and a severe seizure disorder. Ocular abnormalities are common, including hypoplasia of the optic nerve and microphthalmia. Lissencephaly can occur as an isolated finding, but it is associated with *Miller-Dieker syndrome* (MDS) in about 15% of cases. These children have characteristic facies, including a prominent forehead, bitemporal hollowing, anteverted nostrils, a prominent upper lip, and micrognathia. About 90% of children with MDS have visible or submicroscopic chromosomal deletions of 17p13.3. The gene *LIS-1* (lissencephaly 1) in 17p13.3 is deleted in patients with MDS. CT and MRI scans typically show a smooth brain with an absence of sulci (Fig. 585–4).

Schizencephaly. Schizencephaly is the presence of unilateral or bilateral clefts within the cerebral hemispheres due to an abnormality of morphogenesis. The cleft may be fused or unfused and, if unilateral and large, may be confused with a porencephalic cyst. Not infrequently, the borders of the cleft are surrounded by abnormal brain, particularly microgyria. CT scan is diagnostic and clearly demonstrates the size and extent of the cleft. Many patients are severely mentally retarded, with seizures that are difficult to control, and microcephalic, with spastic quadriparesis when the clefts are bilateral.

Porencephaly. This is the presence of cysts or cavities within the brain that result from developmental defects or acquired lesions, including infarction of tissue. *True porencephalic* cysts are most frequently located in the region of the sylvian fissure and typically communicate with the subarachnoid space, the ventricular system, or both. They represent developmental abnormalities of cell migration and are often associated with other malformations of the brain, including microcephaly, abnormal patterns of adjacent gyri, and encephalocele. Affected infants tend to have many problems, including mental retardation, spastic quadriparesis, optic atrophy, and seizures. *Pseudoporencephalic cysts* characteristically develop during the perinatal or postnatal period and result from abnormalities (infarction, hemorrhage) of arterial or venous circulation. These cysts tend to be unilateral, they do not communicate with a fluid-filled cavity, and

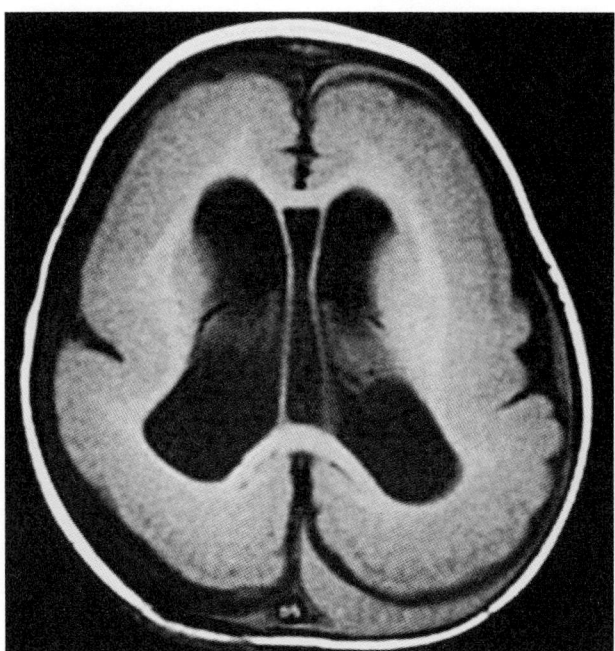

FIGURE 585–4. MRI of an infant with lissencephaly. Note the absence of cerebral sulci and the maldeveloped sylvian fissures associated with enlarged ventricles.

they are not associated with abnormalities of cell migration or CNS malformations. Infants with pseudoporencephalic cysts present with hemiparesis and focal seizures during the 1st year of life.

Holoprosencephaly. This developmental disorder of the brain results from defective cleavage of the prosencephalon. The abnormality, which represents a spectrum of severity, is classified into three groups: alobar, semilobar, and lobar, depending on the degree of the cleavage abnormality (Fig. 585–5). A fourth type, the middle interhemispheric fusion (MIHF variant) or syntelencephaly, involves a segmental area of noncleavage of the posterior frontal and parietal lobes. Facial abnormalities including cyclopia, cebocephaly, and premaxillary agenesis are common in severe cases, in that the prechordal mesoderm that induces the prosencephalon is also responsible for induction of the median facial structures. The most severe form, alobar holoprosencephaly, is typically associated with neuronal migration disorders. Alobar holoprosencephaly is characterized by a single ventricle, an absent falx, and fused basal ganglia. Affected infants have high mortality rates, but some children live for years. Mortality and morbidity with milder types are more variable and less severe. Care must be taken not to prognosticate in these cases. The incidence of holoprosencephaly ranges from 1/5,000 to 1/16,000. A prenatal diagnosis can be confirmed by ultrasonography after the 10th wk of gestation for more severe types. The cause for holoprosencephaly is usually not identified, although there appears to be an association with maternal diabetes in many cases. Chromosomal abnormalities, including deletions of chromosomes 7q and 3p, 21q, 2p, 18p, and 13q, as well as trisomy 13 and 18, account for the minority of cases. Mutations in the "sonic hedgehog" gene at 7q have been shown to cause holoprosencephaly.

585.8 Agenesis of the Corpus Callosum

Agenesis of the corpus callosum consists of a heterogeneous group of disorders that vary in expression from severe intellectual and neurologic abnormalities to the asymptomatic and normally intelligent individual. The corpus callosum develops from

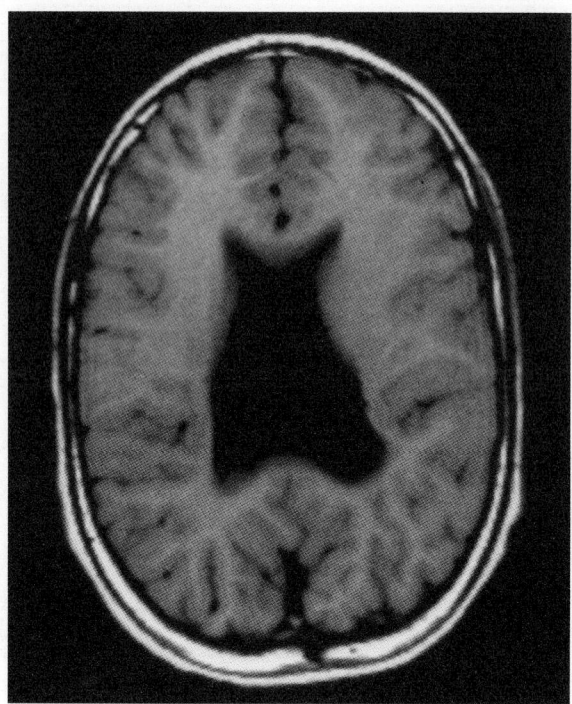

FIGURE 585–5. Lobar holoprosencephaly. T1 weighted MRI scan demonstrates failure of separation of the hemispheres and a persistent fused ventricle.

the commissural plate that lies in proximity to the anterior neuropore. An insult to the commissural plate during early embryogenesis causes agenesis of the corpus callosum. When agenesis of the corpus callosum is an isolated phenomenon, the patient may be normal, whereas individuals with neurologic symptoms, including mental retardation, microcephaly, hemiparesis, diplegia, and seizures, have associated brain anomalies due to cell migration defects, such as heterotopias, microgyria, and pachygyria (broad, wide gyri) in addition to the absence of the corpus callosum. The anatomic features are best depicted on a CT scan or by MRI and show widely separated frontal horns with an abnormally high position of the third ventricle between the lateral ventricles. MRI precisely outlines the extent of the corpus callosum defect. Absence of the corpus callosum may be inherited as an X-linked recessive trait or as an autosomal dominant trait. The condition may be associated with specific chromosomal disorders, particularly 8-trisomy and 18-trisomy.

Aicardi syndrome represents a complex disorder that affects many systems and is typically associated with agenesis of the corpus callosum. Patients are almost all female, suggesting a genetic abnormality of the X chromosome (it may be lethal in males during fetal life). Seizures become evident during the first few months and are typically resistant to anticonvulsants. An electroencephalogram (EEG) shows independent activity recorded from both hemispheres as a result of the absent corpus callosum. All patients are severely mentally retarded and may have abnormal vertebrae that may be fused or only partially developed (e.g., hemivertebra). Abnormalities of the retina, including circumscribed pits or lacunae and coloboma of the optic disc, are the most characteristic findings of Aicardi syndrome.

585.9 Agenesis of the Cranial Nerves

Absence of the cranial nerves or the corresponding central nuclei has been described in several conditions and includes the optic nerve, congenital ptosis, Marcus Gunn phenomenon

(sucking jaw movements causing simultaneous eyelid blinking; this congenital synkinesis results from abnormal innervation of the trigeminal and oculomotor nerves), the trigeminal and auditory nerves, and cranial nerves IX, X, XI, and XII. *Möbius syndrome* is characterized by bilateral facial weakness, which is often associated with abducens nerve paralysis. Hypoplasia or agenesis of brainstem nuclei as well as absent or decreased numbers of muscle fibers has been reported. Affected infants present in the newborn period with facial weakness, causing feeding difficulties due to a poor suck. The immobile, dull facies may give the incorrect impression of mental retardation; the prognosis for normal development is excellent in most cases.

585.10 Microcephaly

Microcephaly is defined as a head circumference that measures more than three standard deviations below the mean for age and sex. This condition is relatively common, particularly among the mentally retarded population. Although there are many causes of microcephaly, abnormalities in neuronal migration during fetal development, including heterotopias of neuronal cells and cytoarchitectural derangements, are found in many brains. Microcephaly may be subdivided into two main groups: primary (genetic) microcephaly and secondary (nongenetic) microcephaly. A precise diagnosis is important for genetic counseling and for prediction for future pregnancies.

Etiology. Primary microcephaly refers to a group of conditions that usually have no other malformations and follow a mendelian pattern of inheritance or are associated with a specific genetic syndrome. Affected infants are usually identified at birth because of a small head circumference. The more common types include familial and autosomal dominant microcephaly and a series of chromosomal syndromes that are summarized in Table 585–1. Secondary microcephaly results from a large number of noxious agents that may affect a fetus in utero or an infant during periods of rapid brain growth, particularly the first 2 yr of life.

Clinical Manifestations and Diagnosis. A thorough family history should be taken, seeking additional cases of microcephaly or disorders affecting the nervous system. It is important to measure a patient's head circumference at birth. A very small head circumference implies a process that began early in embryonic or fetal development. An insult to the brain that occurs later in life, particularly beyond the age of 2 yr, is less likely to produce severe microcephaly. Serial head circumference measurements are more meaningful than a single determination, particularly when the abnormality is minimal. In addition, the head circumference of each parent and sibling should be recorded.

Laboratory investigation of a microcephalic child is determined by the history and physical examination. If the cause of the microcephaly is unknown, the mother's serum phenylalanine level should be determined. High phenylalanine serum levels in an asymptomatic mother can produce marked brain damage in an otherwise normal nonphenylketonuric infant. A karyotype is obtained if a chromosomal syndrome is suspected or if the child has abnormal facies, short stature, and additional congenital anomalies. CT scanning or MRI may be useful in identifying structural abnormalities of the brain or intracerebral calcification. Additional studies include a fasting plasma and urine amino acid analysis; serum ammonium determination; *t*oxoplasmosis, *r*ubella, *c*ytomegalovirus, and *h*erpes simplex (TORCH) titers of the mother and child; and a urine sample for the culture of cytomegalovirus.

Treatment. Once the cause of microcephaly has been established, the physician must provide accurate and supportive genetic and family counseling. Because many children with microcephaly are also mentally retarded, the physician must assist with place-

TABLE 585–1. Causes of Microcephaly

Causes	Characteristic Findings
Primary (Genetic)	
1. Familial (autosomal recessive)	• Incidence 1/40,000 births
	• Typical appearance with slanted forehead, prominent nose and ears; severely mentally retarded and prominent seizures; surface convolutional markings of the brain poorly differentiated and disorganized cytoarchitecture
2. Autosomal dominant	• Nondistinctive facies, up-slanting palpebral fissures, mild forehead slanting, and prominent ears
	• Normal linear growth, seizures readily controlled, and mild or borderline mental retardation
3. Syndromes	
Down (21-trisomy)	• Incidence 1/800
	• Abnormal rounding of occipital and frontal lobes and a small cerebellum; narrow superior temporal gyrus, propensity for Alzheimer's neurofibrillary alterations, and ultrastructure abnormalities of cerebral cortex
Edward (18-trisomy)	• Incidence 1/6,500
	• Low birthweight, microstomia, micrognathia, low-set malformed ears, prominent occiput, rocker-bottom feet, flexion deformities of fingers, congenital heart disease, increased gyri, heterotopias of neurons
Cri-du-chat (5 p-)	• Incidence 1/50,000
	• Round facies, prominent epicanthic folds, low-set ears, hypertelorism, and characteristic cry
	• No specific neuropathology
Cornelia de Lange	• Prenatal and postnatal growth delay, synophrys, thin down-turning upper lip
	• Proximally placed thumb
Rubinstein-Taybi	• Beaked nose, downward slanting of palpebral fissures, epicanthic folds, short stature with broad thumbs and toes
Smith-Lemli-Opitz	• Ptosis, scaphocephaly, inner epicanthic folds, anteverted nostrils
	• Low birthweight, marked feeding problems
Secondary (Nongenetic)	
1. Radiation	• Microcephaly and mental retardation most severe if exposure before 15th wk of gestation
2. Congenital infections	
Cytomegalovirus	• Small for dates, petechial rash, hepatosplenomegaly, chorioretinitis, deafness, mental retardation, and seizures
	• Central nervous system calcification and microgyria
Rubella	• Growth retardation, purpura, thrombocytopenia, hepatosplenomegaly, congenital heart disease, chorioretinitis, cataracts, and deafness
	• Perivascular necrotic areas, polymicrogyria, heterotopias, subependymal cavitations
Toxoplasmosis	• Purpura, hepatosplenomegaly, jaundice, convulsions, hydrocephalus, chorioretinitis, and cerebral calcification
3. Drugs	
Fetal alcohol	• Growth retardation, ptosis, absent philtrum and hypoplastic upper lip, congenital heart disease, feeding problems, neuroglial heterotopia, and disorganization of neurons
Fetal hydantoin	• Growth delay, hypoplasia of distal phalanges, inner epicanthic folds, broad nasal ridge, and anteverted nostrils
4. Meningitis/encephalitis	• Cerebral infarcts, cystic cavitation, diffuse loss of neurons
5. Malnutrition	• Controversial cause of microcephaly
6. Metabolic	• Maternal diabetes mellitus and maternal hyperphenylalaninemia
7. Hyperthermia	• Significant fever during 1st 4–6 wk has been reported to cause microcephaly, seizures, and facial anomalies
	• Pathologic studies show neuronal heterotopias
	• Further studies showed no abnormalities with maternal fever
8. Hypoxic-ischemic encephalopathy	• Initially diffuse cerebral edema; late stages characterized by cerebral atrophy

ment in an appropriate program that will provide for maximum development of the child (see Chapter 37.2).

Barkovich AJ, Quint DJ: Middle hemispheric fusion: An unusual variant of holoprosencephaly. *AJNR* 1993;14:431.

Barkovich AJ, Kuzniecky RI, Jackson MD, et al: Classification system for malformations of cortical development. *Neurology* 2001;57:2168.

Barr M, Cohen MM: Holoprosencephaly survival and performance. *Am J Med Genet* 1999;89:116.

Barth PG: Disorders of neuronal migration. *Can J Neurol Sci* 1987;14:1.

Dobyns WB, Reiner O, Carrozzo R, et al: A human brain malformation associated with deletion of LIS1 gene located at chromosome 17p13. *JAMA* 1993;270:2838.

Harwood-Nash DC: Congenital craniocerebral abnormalities and computed tomography. *Semin Roentgenol* 1977;12:39.

Haslam RH: Microcephaly. In Vinken PJ, Bruyn G, Klawans HL (editors): *Handbook of Clinical Neurology*. Amsterdam, Elsevier Science Publishers, 1987, pp 267–84.

Kinsman SL, Plawner LL, Hahn JS: Holoprosencephaly: Recent advances and insights. *Curr Opin Neurol* 2000;13:127.

Miller GM, Stears JC, Guggenheim MA, et al: Schizencephaly: A clinical and CT study. *Neurology* 1984;34:997.

Molina JA, Mateos F, Merino M, et al: Aicardi syndrome in two sisters. *J Pediatr* 1989;115:282.

Nerdich JA, Nussbaum RL, Packer TC, et al: Heterogeneity of clinical severity and molecular lesions in Aicardi syndrome. *J Paediatr* 1990;116:911.

Parrish ML, Roessmann U, Levinsohn MW: Agenesis of the corpus callosum: A study of the frequency of associated malformations. *Ann Neurol* 1979;6:349.

Reiner D, Carrozzo R, Shen Y, et al: Isolation of a Miller-Dieker lissencephaly gene containing G protein β-subunit-like repeats. *Nature* 1993;364:717.

Sheldon M, Rice DS, D'Arcangelo G, et al: Scrambler and yotari disrupt the disabled gene and produce a reeler-like phenotype in mice. *Nature* 1997;389:730.

Sudarshan A, Goldie WD: The spectrum of congenital facial diplegia (Moebius syndrome). *Pediatr Neurol* 1985;1:180.

585.11 Hydrocephalus

Hydrocephalus is not a specific disease; rather, it represents a diverse group of conditions that result from impaired circulation and absorption of CSF or, in the rare circumstance, from increased production by a choroid plexus papilloma.

Physiology. The CSF is formed primarily in the ventricular system by the choroid plexus, which is situated in the lateral, third, and fourth ventricles. Although most CSF is produced in the lateral ventricles, approximately 25% originates from extrachoroidal sources, including the capillary endothelium within the brain parenchyma. There is active neurogenic control of CSF formation as the choroid plexus is innervated by adrenergic and cholinergic nerves. Stimulation of the adrenergic system diminishes CSF production, whereas excitation of the cholinergic nerves may double the normal CSF production rate. In a normal child, approximately 20 mL/hr of CSF is produced. The total volume of CSF approximates 50 mL in an infant and 150 mL in an adult. Most of the CSF is extraventricular. CSF is formed by the choroid plexus in several stages; through a series of intricate steps, a plasma ultrafiltrate is ultimately processed into a secretion, the CSF.

CSF flow results from the pressure gradient that exists between the ventricular system and venous channels. Intraventricular pressure may be as high as 180 mm H_2O in the normal state, whereas the pressure in the superior sagittal sinus is in the range of 90 mm H_2O. Normally, CSF flows from the lateral ventricles through the foramina of Monro into the third ventricle. It then traverses the narrow aqueduct of Sylvius, which is approximately 3 mm long and 2 mm in diameter in a child, to enter the fourth ventricle. The CSF exits the fourth ventricle through the paired lateral foramina of Luschka and the midline foramen of Magendie into the cisterns at the base of the brain. Hydrocephalus resulting from obstruction within the ventricular system is called *obstructive* or *noncommunicating hydrocephalus*. The CSF circulates from the basal cisterns posteriorly through the cistern system and over the convexities of the cerebral hemispheres. CSF is absorbed primarily by the arachnoid villi through tight junctions of their endothelium by the pressure forces that were noted earlier. CSF is absorbed to a much lesser extent by the lymphatic channels directed to the paranasal sinuses, along nerve root sleeves, and by the choroid plexus itself. Hydrocephalus resulting from obliteration of the subarachnoid cisterns or malfunction of the arachnoid villi is called *nonobstructive* or *communicating hydrocephalus*.

Pathophysiology and Etiology. Obstructive or noncommunicating hydrocephalus develops most commonly in children because of an abnormality of the aqueduct or a lesion in the fourth ventricle. *Aqueductal stenosis* results from an abnormally narrow aqueduct of Sylvius that is often associated with branching or forking. In a small percentage of cases, aqueductal stenosis is inherited as a sex-linked recessive trait. These patients occasionally have minor neural tube closure defects, including spina bifida occulta. Rarely, aqueductal stenosis is associated with neurofibromatosis. *Aqueductal gliosis* may also give rise to hydrocephalus. As a result of neonatal meningitis or a subarachnoid hemorrhage in a premature infant, the ependymal lining of the aqueduct is interrupted and a brisk glial response results in complete obstruction. Intrauterine viral infections may also produce aqueductal stenosis followed by hydrocephalus, and mumps meningoencephalitis has been reported as a cause in a child. A vein of Galen malformation can expand to become large and, because of its midline position, obstruct the flow of CSF. Lesions or malformations of the posterior fossa are prominent causes of hydrocephalus, including posterior fossa brain tumors, Chiari malformation, and the Dandy-Walker syndrome.

Nonobstructive or communicating hydrocephalus most commonly follows a subarachnoid hemorrhage, which is usually a result of intraventricular hemorrhage in a premature infant. Blood in the subarachnoid spaces may cause obliteration of the cisterns or arachnoid villi and obstruction of CSF flow. Pneumococcal and tuberculous meningitis have a propensity to produce a thick, tenacious exudate that obstructs the basal cisterns, and intrauterine infections may also destroy the CSF pathways. Finally, leukemic infiltrates may seed the subarachnoid space and produce communicating hydrocephalus.

Clinical Manifestations. The clinical presentation of hydrocephalus is variable and depends on many factors, including the age at onset, the nature of the lesion causing obstruction, and the duration and rate of increase of the intracranial pressure (ICP). In an infant, an accelerated rate of enlargement of the head is the most prominent sign. In addition, the anterior fontanel is wide open and bulging, and the scalp veins are dilated. The forehead is broad, and the eyes may deviate downward because of impingement of the dilated suprapineal recess on the tectum, producing the setting-sun eye sign. Long-tract signs including brisk tendon reflexes, spasticity, clonus (particularly in the lower extremities), and Babinski sign are common owing to stretching and disruption of the corticospinal fibers originating from the leg region of the motor cortex. In an older child, the cranial sutures are partially closed so that the signs of hydrocephalus may be more subtle. Irritability, lethargy, poor appetite, and vomiting are common to both age groups, and headache is a prominent symptom in older patients. A gradual change in personality and deterioration in academic productivity suggest a slowly progressive form of hydrocephalus. Serial

measurements of the head circumference indicate an increased velocity of growth. Percussion of the skull may produce a "cracked-pot" or **Macewen Sign,** indicating separation of the sutures. A foreshortened occiput suggests Chiari malformation, and a prominent occiput suggests the Dandy-Walker malformation. Papilledema, abducens nerve palsy, and pyramidal tract signs, which are most evident in the lower extremities, are apparent in most cases.

Chiari malformation consists of two major subgroups; type I typically produces symptoms during adolescence or adult life and is usually not associated with hydrocephalus. Patients complain of recurrent headache, neck pain, urinary frequency, and progressive lower extremity spasticity. The deformity consists of displacement of the cerebellar tonsils into the cervical canal. Although the pathogenesis is unknown, the prevailing theory suggests that obstruction of the caudal portion of the fourth ventricle during fetal development is responsible. The type II Chiari malformation is characterized by progressive hydrocephalus and a myelomeningocele. This lesion represents an anomaly of the hindbrain, probably due to a failure of pontine flexure during embryogenesis, and results in elongation of the fourth ventricle and kinking of the brainstem, with displacement of the inferior vermis, pons, and medulla into the cervical canal (Fig. 585–6). Approximately 10% of type II malformations produce symptoms during infancy consisting of stridor, weak cry, and apnea, which may be relieved by shunting or by posterior fossa decompression. A more indolent form consists of abnormalities of gait, spasticity, and increasing incoordination during childhood. Plain skull radiographs show a small posterior fossa and a widened cervical canal. CT scanning with contrast and MRI display the cerebellar tonsils protruding downward into the cervical canal and the hindbrain abnormalities. The anomaly is treated by surgical decompression.

The *Dandy-Walker malformation* consists of a cystic expansion of the fourth ventricle in the posterior fossa, which results from a developmental failure of the roof of the 4th ventricle during embryogenesis (Fig. 585–7). Approximately 90% of patients

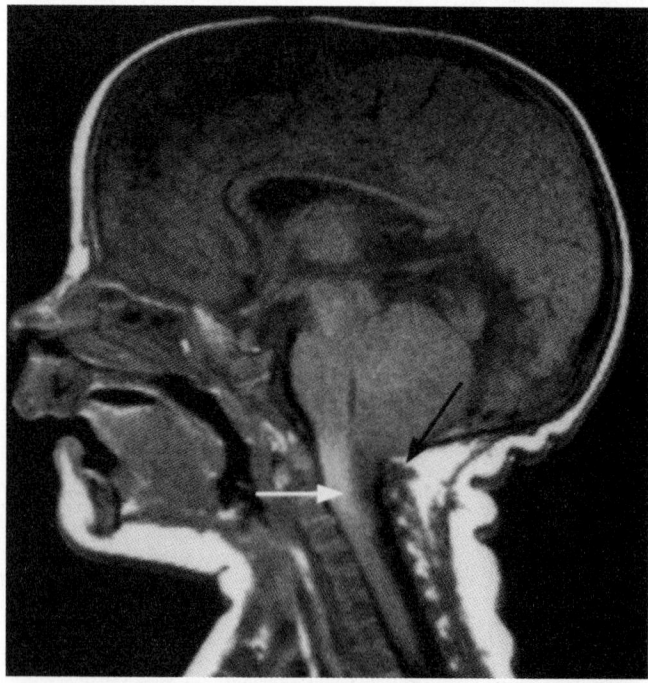

FIGURE 585–6. A midsagittal T1 weighted MRI of a patient with type II Chiari malformation. The cerebellar tonsils (*white arrow*) have descended below the foramen magnum (*black arrow*). Note the small slitlike 4th ventricle, which has been pulled into a vertical position.

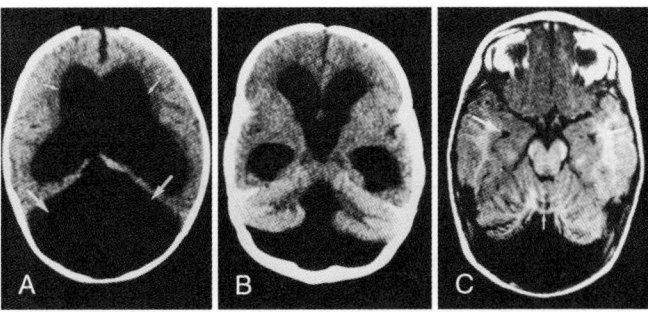

FIGURE 585–7. Dandy-Walker cyst. *A,* Axial CT scan (preoperative) showing large posterior fossa cyst (Dandy-Walker cyst; *large arrows*) and dilated lateral ventricles (*small arrows*), a complication secondary to CSF pathway obstruction at the 4th ventricular outlet. *B,* Same patient, with a lower axial CT scan showing splaying of the cerebellar hemispheres by the dilated 4th ventricle (Dandy-Walker cyst). The dilated ventricles proximal to the 4th ventricle again show CSF obstruction due to the Dandy-Walker cyst. *C,* MRI of the same patient showing decreased size of the Dandy-Walker cyst and temporal horns (*arrows*) following shunting. The incomplete vermis (*small arrow*) now becomes recognizable.

have hydrocephalus, and a significant number of children have associated anomalies, including agenesis of the posterior cerebellar vermis and corpus callosum. Infants present with a rapid increase in head size and a prominent occiput. Transillumination of the skull may be positive. Most children have evidence of long-tract signs, cerebellar ataxia, and delayed motor and cognitive milestones, probably due to the associated structural anomalies. The Dandy-Walker malformation is managed by shunting the cystic cavity (and on occasion the ventricles as well) in the presence of hydrocephalus.

Diagnosis and Differential Diagnosis. Investigation of a child with hydrocephalus begins with the history. Familial cases suggest X-linked hydrocephalus secondary to aqueductal stenosis. A past history of prematurity with intracranial hemorrhage, meningitis, or mumps encephalitis is important to ascertain. Multiple café-au-lait spots and other clinical features of neurofibromatosis point to aqueductal stenosis as the cause of hydrocephalus. Examination includes careful inspection, palpation, and auscultation of the skull and spine. The occipitofrontal head circumference is recorded and compared with previous measurements. The size and configuration of the anterior fontanel are noted, and the back is inspected for abnormal midline skin lesions, including tufts of hair, lipoma, or angioma that might suggest spinal dysraphism. The presence of a prominent forehead or abnormalities in the shape of the occiput may suggest the pathogenesis of the hydrocephalus. A cranial bruit is audible in association with many cases of vein of Galen arteriovenous malformation. Transillumination of the skull is positive with massive dilatation of the ventricular system or in the Dandy-Walker syndrome. Inspection of the eyegrounds is mandatory because the finding of chorioretinitis suggests an intrauterine infection such as toxoplasmosis as a cause of the hydrocephalus. Papilledema is observed in older children but is rarely present in infants because the cranial sutures separate as a result of the increased pressure. Plain skull films typically show separation of the sutures, erosion of the posterior clinoids in an older child, and an increase in convolutional markings (beaten-silver appearance) with long-standing increased ICP. The CT scan and/or MRI along with ultrasonography in an infant are the most important studies to identify the specific cause of hydrocephalus.

The head may appear enlarged and be confused with hydrocephalus secondary to a thickened cranium resulting from chronic anemia, rickets, osteogenesis imperfecta, and epiphyseal dysplasia. Chronic subdural collections can produce bilateral parietal bone prominence. Various metabolic and degenerative disorders of the CNS produce megalencephaly due to abnormal storage of substances within the brain parenchyma. These disorders include lysosomal diseases (e.g., Tay-Sachs, gangliosidosis, and the mucopolysaccharidoses), the aminoacidurias (e.g., maple syrup urine disease), and the leukodystrophies (e.g., metachromatic, Alexander disease, and Canavan disease). In addition, cerebral gigantism and neurofibromatosis are characterized by increased brain mass. Familial megalencephaly is inherited as an autosomal dominant trait and is characterized by delayed motor milestones and hypotonia but normal or near-normal intelligence. Measurement of the parent's head circumference is necessary to establish the diagnosis.

Hydranencephaly may be confused with hydrocephalus. The cerebral hemispheres are absent or represented by membranous sacs with remnants of frontal, temporal, or occipital cortex dispersed over the membrane. The midbrain and brainstem are relatively intact (Fig. 585–8). The cause of hydranencephaly is unknown, but bilateral occlusion of the internal carotid arteries during early fetal development would explain most of the pathologic abnormalities. Affected infants may have a normal or enlarged head circumference at birth that grows at an excessive rate postnatally. Transillumination shows an absence of the cerebral hemispheres. The child is irritable, feeds poorly, develops seizures and spastic quadriparesis, and has little or no cognitive development. A ventriculoperitoneal shunt prevents massive enlargement of the cranium.

Treatment. Therapy for hydrocephalus depends on the cause. Medical management, including the use of acetazolamide and furosemide, may provide temporary relief by reducing the rate of CSF production, but long-term results have been disappointing. Most cases of hydrocephalus require extracranial shunts, particularly a ventriculoperitoneal shunt (occasionally a ventriculostomy suffices). The major complication of shunts is bacterial infection, usually due to *Staphylococcus epidermidis* (see Chapter 166). With meticulous preparation, the shunt infection rate can be reduced to less than 5%. The results of intrauterine surgical management of fetal hydrocephalus have been poor, possibly because of the high rate of associated cerebral malformations in addition to the hydrocephalus.

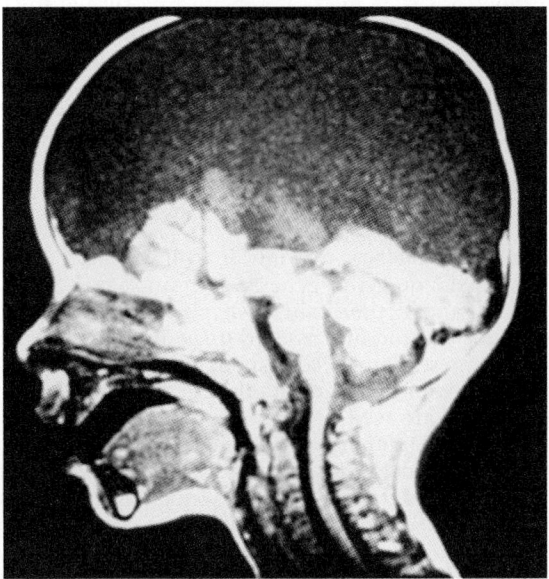

FIGURE 585–8. Hydranencephaly. MRI scan showing the brainstem and spinal cord with remnants of the cerebellum and the cerebral cortex. The remainder of the cranium is filled with CSF.

Prognosis. This depends on the cause of the dilated ventricles and not on the size of the cortical mantle at the time of operative intervention. Hydrocephalic children are at increased risk for various developmental disabilities. The mean intelligence quotient is reduced compared with the general population, particularly for performance tasks as compared with verbal abilities. Most children have abnormalities in memory function. Visual problems are common, including strabismus, visuospatial abnormalities, visual field defects, and optic atrophy with decreased acuity secondary to increased ICP. The visual-evoked potential latencies are delayed and take some time to recover after correction of the hydrocephalus. Although most hydrocephalic children are pleasant and mild mannered, some children show aggressive and delinquent behavior. Accelerated pubertal development in patients with shunted hydrocephalus or meningomyelocele is relatively common, possibly because of increased gonadotropin secretion in response to increased ICP. It is imperative that hydrocephalic children receive long-term follow-up in a multidisciplinary setting.

Chumas P, Tyagi A, Livingston J: Hydrocephalus–What's new? *Arch Dis Child Fetal Neonatal Ed* 2001;85:F149–54.

Cochrane DD, Myles ST, Nimrod C, et al: Intrauterine hydrocephalus and ventriculomegaly: Associated abnormalities and fetal outcome. *Can J Neurol Sci* 1985;12:51.

Cull C, Wyke MA: Memory function of children with spina bifida and shunted hydrocephalus. *Dev Med Child Neurol* 1984;26:177.

De Myer W: Megalencephaly in children. *Neurology* 1972;22:634.

Dennis M, Fitz CR, Netley CT, et al: The intelligence of hydrocephalic children. *Arch Neurol* 1981;38:607.

Fernell E, Hagberg G, Hagberg B: Infantile hydrocephalus epidemiology: An indicator of enhanced survival. *Arch Dis Child* 1994;70:123.

Fitzsimmons JS: Laryngeal stridor and respiratory obstruction in association with myelomeningocele. *Dev Med Child Neurol* 1973;15:553.

Greene M, Benacerraf B, Crawford J: Hydranencephaly: US appearance during in utero evolution. *Radiology* 1985;156:779.

Hirsch JF, Pierre-Kahn A, Renier D, et al: The Dandy-Walker malformation. *J Neurosurg* 1984;61:515.

Hoffman HJ, Hendrick EB, Humphreys RP: Manifestations and management of Arnold-Chiari malformations in patients with myelomeningocele. *Childs Brain* 1975;1:255.

Jackson JC, Blumhagen JD: Congenital hydrocephalus due to prenatal intracranial hemorrhage. *Pediatrics* 1983;72:344.

Löppönen T, Saukkonen A-L, Serlo W, et al: Accelerated pubertal development in patients with shunted hydrocephalus. *Arch Dis Child* 1996;74:490.

585.12 Craniosynostosis

Craniosynostosis is defined as premature closure of the cranial sutures and is classified as primary or secondary. *Primary craniosynostosis* refers to closure of one or more sutures due to abnormalities of skull development, whereas *secondary craniosynostosis* results from failure of brain growth and expansion and is not discussed here. The incidence of primary craniosynostosis approximates 1/2,000 births. The cause is unknown in the majority of children; however, genetic syndromes account for 10–20% of cases.

Development and Etiology. A review of skull development is helpful in understanding the genesis of craniosynostosis. During early development, the brain is enveloped by a film of mesenchyme. By the 2nd mo, osseous tissue is evident in that portion of the mesenchyme corresponding to the cranium, and cartilaginous tissue is formed at the base of the skull. The bones of the cranium are well developed by the 5th mo of gestation (frontal, parietal, temporal, and occipital) and are separated by sutures and fontanels. The brain grows rapidly during the first several years of life and is normally not impeded because of equivalent growth along the suture lines. The cause of craniosynostosis is unknown, but the prevailing hypothesis suggests that abnormal development of the base of the skull creates exaggerated forces on the dura that act to disrupt normal cranial suture development. Dysfunctional osteoblasts or osteoclasts are not responsible for craniosynostosis.

Clinical Manifestations and Treatment. Most cases of craniosynostosis are evident at birth and are characterized by a skull deformity that is a direct result of premature suture fusion. Palpation of the suture reveals a prominent bony ridge, and fusion of the suture may be confirmed by plain skull roentgenograms or bone scan in ambiguous cases.

Premature closure of the sagittal suture produces a long and narrow skull, or *scaphocephaly*, the most common form of craniosynostosis. Scaphocephaly is associated with a prominent occiput, a broad forehead, and a small or absent anterior fontanel. The condition is sporadic and more common in males and often causes difficulties during labor because of cephalopelvic disproportion. Scaphocephaly does not produce increased ICP or hydrocephalus, and results of neurologic examination of affected patients are normal.

Frontal plagiocephaly is the next most common form of craniosynostosis and is characterized by unilateral flattening of the forehead, elevation of the ipsilateral orbit and eyebrow, and a prominent ear on the corresponding side. The condition is more common in females and is the result of premature fusion of a coronal and sphenofrontal suture. Surgical intervention produces a cosmetically pleasing result.

Occipital plagiocephaly is most often a result of positioning during infancy and is more common in an immobile or handicapped child, but fusion or sclerosis of the lambdoid suture can cause unilateral occipital flattening and bulging of the ipsilateral frontal bone. *Trigonocephaly* is a rare form of craniosynostosis due to premature fusion of the metopic suture. These children have a keel-shaped forehead and hypotelorism and are at risk for associated developmental abnormalities of the forebrain. *Turricephaly* refers to a cone-shaped head due to premature fusion of the coronal and often sphenofrontal and frontoethmoidal sutures. The *kleeblattschädel deformity* is a peculiarly shaped skull that resembles a cloverleaf. Affected children have very prominent temporal bones, and the remainder of the cranium is constricted. Hydrocephalus is a common complication.

Premature fusion of only one suture rarely causes a neurologic deficit. In this situation, the sole indication for surgery is to enhance the child's cosmetic appearance, and the prognosis depends on the suture involved and on the degree of disfigurement. Neurologic complications, including hydrocephalus and increased ICP, are more likely to occur when two or more sutures are prematurely fused, in which case operative intervention is essential.

The most prevalent genetic disorders associated with craniosynostosis include Crouzon, Apert, Carpenter, Chotzen, and Pfeiffer syndromes. *Crouzon syndrome* is characterized by premature craniosynostosis and is inherited as an autosomal dominant trait. The shape of the head depends on the timing and order of suture fusion but most often is a compressed back-to-front diameter or brachycephaly due to bilateral closure of the coronal sutures. The orbits are underdeveloped, and ocular proptosis is prominent. Hypoplasia of the maxilla and orbital hypertelorism are typical facial features.

Apert syndrome has many features in common with Crouzon syndrome. However, Apert syndrome is usually a sporadic condition, although autosomal dominant inheritance may occur. It is associated with premature fusion of multiple sutures, including the coronal, sagittal, squamosal, and lambdoid sutures. The facies tend to be asymmetric, and the eyes are less proptotic than in Crouzon syndrome. Apert syndrome is characterized by syndactyly of the 2nd, 3rd, and 4th fingers, which may be joined to the thumb and the 5th finger. Similar abnormalities often occur in the feet. All patients have progressive calcification and fusion of the bones of the hands, feet, and cervical spine.

Carpenter syndrome is inherited as an autosomal recessive condition, and the many fusions of sutures tend to produce the kleeblattschädel skull deformity. Soft-tissue syndactyly of the hands and feet is always present, and mental retardation is common. Additional but less common abnormalities include congenital heart disease, corneal opacities, coxa valga, and genu valgum.

Chotzen syndrome is characterized by asymmetric craniosynostosis and plagiocephaly. The condition is the most prevalent of the genetic syndromes and is inherited as an autosomal dominant trait. It is associated with facial asymmetry, ptosis of the eyelids, shortened fingers, and soft tissue syndactyly of the 2nd and 3rd fingers.

Pfeiffer syndrome is most often associated with turricephaly. The eyes are prominent and widely spaced, and the thumbs and great toes are short and broad. Partial soft tissue syndactyly may be evident. Most cases appear to be sporadic, but autosomal dominant inheritance has been reported.

Mutations of the fibroblast growth factor receptor (FGFR) gene family have been shown to be associated with phenotypically specific types of craniosynostosis. Mutations of the $FGFR_1$ gene located on chromosome 8 result in Pfeiffer syndrome; a similar mutation of the $FGFR_2$ gene causes Apert syndrome. Identical mutations of the $FGFR_2$ gene may result in both Pfeiffer and Crouzon phenotypes.

Each of the genetic syndromes poses a risk of additional anomalies, including hydrocephalus, increased ICP, papilledema, optic atrophy due to abnormalities of the optic foramina, respiratory problems secondary to a deviated nasal septum or choanal atresia, and disorders of speech and deafness. Craniectomy is mandatory for management of increased ICP, and a multidisciplinary craniofacial team is essential for the long-term follow-up of affected children. Craniosynostosis may be surgically corrected with good outcomes and relatively low morbidity and mortality, especially for nonsyndromic infants.

Cohen MM: Craniosynostosis update. *Am J Med Genet* 1987;4(suppl):99.
Rutland P, Pulleyn LJ, Reardon W, et al: Identical mutations in the FGFR$_2$ gene cause both Pfeiffer and Crouzon syndrome phenotypes. *Nature Genet* 1995;56:334.
Sloan GM, Wells KC, Raffel C, et al: Surgical treatment of craniosynostosis: Outcome analysis of 250 consecutive patients. *Pediatrics* 1997;100:1.

Chapter 586
Seizures in Childhood

Michael V. Johnston

A seizure or convulsion is a paroxysmal, time-limited change in motor activity and/or behavior that results from abnormal electrical activity in the brain. Seizures are common in the pediatric age group and occur in approximately 10% of children. Most seizures in children are provoked by somatic disorders originating outside the brain, such as high fever, infection, syncope, head trauma, hypoxia, toxins, or cardiac arrhythmias. Other events, such as breath-holding spells and gastroesophageal reflux, can cause events that simulate seizures (see Chapter 587). A few children also exhibit psychogenic seizures of psychiatric origin. Less than one third of seizures in children are caused by epilepsy, a condition in which seizures are triggered recurrently from within the brain. For epidemiologic classification purposes, epilepsy is considered to be present when two or more unprovoked seizures occur at an interval greater than 24 hr apart. The cumulative lifetime incidence of epilepsy is 3% and more than half of cases begin in childhood. However, the annual prevalence of epilepsy is lower (0.5–0.8%) because many children outgrow epilepsy. Although the outlook for most children with symptomatic seizures or those associated with epilepsy is generally good, the seizures may signal a potentially serious underlying systemic or central nervous system (CNS) disorder that requires thorough investigation and management. For children with epilepsy, the prognosis is generally good, but 10–20% have persistent seizures refractory to drugs, and those cases pose a diagnostic and management challenge.

Evaluation of the First Seizure. Initial evaluation of an infant or child during or shortly after a suspected seizure should include an assessment of the adequacy of the airway, ventilation, and cardiac function as well as measurement of temperature, blood pressure, and glucose concentration. For acute evaluation of the first seizure, the physician should search for potentially life-threatening causes of seizures such as meningitis, systemic sepsis, accidental and nonaccidental head trauma, and ingestion of drugs of abuse and other toxins. The *history* should attempt to define factors that may have promoted the convulsion and to provide a detailed description of the seizure and the child's postictal state. Most parents vividly recall their child's initial convulsion and can describe it in detail.

The first step in an evaluation is to determine whether the seizure has a focal onset or is generalized. *Focal seizures* may be characterized by motor or sensory symptoms and include forceful turning of the head and eyes to one side, unilateral clonic movements beginning in the face or extremities, or a sensory disturbance such as paresthesias or pain localized to a specific area. Focal seizures in an adult usually indicate a localized lesion, but investigation of focal seizures during childhood may be nondiagnostic. Motor seizures may be focal or generalized and tonic-clonic, tonic, clonic, myoclonic, or atonic. *Tonic seizures* are characterized by increased tone or rigidity, and *atonic seizures* are characterized by flaccidity or lack of movement during a convulsion. *Clonic seizures* consist of rhythmic muscle contraction and relaxation, and *myoclonus* is most accurately described as shocklike contraction of a muscle. The duration of the seizure and state of consciousness (retained or impaired) should be documented. The history should determine whether an aura preceded the convulsion and the behavior of the child immediately preceding the seizure. The most common aura experienced by children consists of epigastric discomfort or pain and a feeling of fear. The posture of the patient, presence and distribution of cyanosis, vocalizations, loss of sphincter control (particularly of the urinary bladder), and postictal state (including sleep and headache) should be noted.

In addition to the assessment of cardiorespiratory and metabolic status described above, *examination* of a child with a seizure disorder should be geared toward the search for an organic cause. The child's head circumference, length, and weight are plotted on a growth chart and compared with previous measurements. A careful general and neurologic examination should be performed. The eyegrounds must be examined for the presence of papilledema, retinal hemorrhages, chorioretinitis, coloboma, and macular changes, as well as retinal phakoma. The finding of unusual facial features or associated physical findings such as hepatosplenomegaly point to an underlying metabolic or storage disease as the cause of the neurologic disorder. A search for vitiliginous lesions of tuberous sclerosis using an ultraviolet light source, examination for adenoma sebaceum, shagreen patch, multiple café-au-lait spots, or a nevus flammeus, and the presence of retinal phakoma would indicate a neurocutaneous disorder as the cause of the seizure.

Localizing neurologic signs such as a subtle hemiparesis with hyperreflexia, an equivocal Babinski sign, and a downward-drifting extended arm with eyes closed might suggest a contralateral hemispheric structural lesion, such as a slow-growing temporal lobe glioma, as the cause of the seizure disorder. Unilateral growth arrest of the thumbnail, hand, or extremity in a child with a focal seizure disorder suggests a chronic condition such as a porencephalic cyst, arteriovenous malformation, or cortical atrophy in the opposite hemisphere.

586.1 Febrile Seizures

Febrile convulsions, the most common seizure disorder during childhood, generally have an excellent prognosis but may also signify a serious underlying acute infectious disease such as sepsis or bacterial meningitis. Therefore, each child with a seizure associated with fever must be carefully examined and appropriately investigated for the cause of the fever (see Chapter 162), especially when it is the first seizure. Febrile seizures are age dependent and are rare before 9 mo and after 5 yr of age. The peak age of onset is approximately 14–18 mo of age, and the incidence approaches 3–4% of young children. A strong family history of febrile convulsions in siblings and parents suggests a genetic predisposition. Linkage studies in several large families have mapped the febrile seizure gene to chromosomes 19p and 8q13-21. An autosomal dominant inheritance pattern is demonstrated in some families.

Clinical Manifestations. A simple febrile convulsion is usually associated with a core temperature that increases rapidly to 39°C or greater. The seizure is usually generalized, is tonic-clonic and lasts a few seconds to 10-min, and is followed by a brief postictal period of drowsiness. A febrile seizure is described as atypical or complicated when the duration is longer than 15 min, when repeated convulsions occur within the same day, or when focal seizure activity or focal findings are present during the postictal period.

Approximately 30–50% of children have recurrent seizures with later episodes of fever and a small minority have numerous recurrent seizures. Although children with simple febrile seizures are at no greater risk of later epilepsy than the general population, some factors are associated with increased risk. These include the presence of atypical features of the seizure or postictal period, a positive family history of epilepsy, an initial febrile seizure before 9 mo of age, delayed developmental milestones, or a pre-existing neurologic disorder. The incidence of epilepsy is approximately 9% when several risk factors are present, compared with an incidence of 1% in children who have febrile convulsions and no risk factors.

During the acute evaluation, a physician's most important responsibility is to determine the cause of the fever and to rule out meningitis. *If any doubt exists about the possibility of meningitis, a lumbar puncture with examination of the cerebrospinal fluid (CSF) is indicated.* Seizure-induced CSF abnormalities are rare in children and all patients with abnormal CSF after a seizure should be thoroughly evaluated for other causes. The possibility of viral meningoencephalitis should also be kept in mind, especially that caused by herpes simplex. Viral infections of the upper respiratory tract, roseola, and acute otitis media are most frequently the causes of febrile convulsions.

Aside from glucose determination, laboratory testing such as serum electrolytes and toxicology screening should be ordered based on individual clinical circumstances such as evidence of dehydration. An electroencephalogram (EEG) is not warranted after a simple febrile seizure but may be useful for evaluating patients with an atypical feature or with other risk factors for later epilepsy. Similarly, neuroimaging is also not useful for children with simple febrile convulsions, but may be considered for children with atypical features, including focal neurologic signs or pre-existing neurologic deficits.

Treatment. Routine treatment of a normal infant with simple febrile convulsions includes a careful search for the cause of the fever, active measures to control the fever, including the use of antipyretics, and reassurance of the parents. Prolonged anticonvulsant prophylaxis for preventing recurrent febrile convulsions is controversial and no longer recommended. Antiepileptics such as phenytoin and carbamazepine have no effect on febrile seizures. Phenobarbital can be effective in preventing recurrent febrile seizures but may also decrease cognitive function in treated children compared with untreated children. Sodium valproate is also effective in the management of febrile seizures, but the potential risks of the drug do not justify its use in a disorder with an excellent prognosis regardless of treatment. The incidence of fatal valproate-induced hepatotoxicity is highest in children younger than 2 yr of age. Oral diazepam is an effective and safe method of reducing the risk of recurrence of febrile seizures. At the onset of each febrile illness, oral diazepam, 0.3 mg/kg q8h (1 mg/kg/24 hr), is administered for the duration of the illness (usually 2–3 days). The side effects are usually minor, but symptoms of lethargy, irritability, and ataxia may be reduced by adjusting the dose. This strategy may be useful when parental anxiety associated with febrile seizures is severe.

586.2 Unprovoked Seizures

First Seizure. Although the occurrence of a seizure in a child without a provocative stimulus such as high fever is often considered a harbinger of a chronic seizure disorder or epilepsy, less than half of these children go on to develop a second seizure. A careful history is warranted to ascertain a potential family history of epilepsy, a prior neurologic disorder, or history of seizure with fever, which may increase the likelihood of recurrence. As for febrile seizures, laboratory testing of serum electrolytes, toxicology screening, or urine and serum metabolic testing should be chosen based on individual clinical circumstances rather than on a routine basis. In the child with a first nonfebrile seizure, a lumbar puncture is of limited value and should be used primarily when there is concern about possible meningitis, encephalitis, sepsis, subarachnoid hemorrhage, or a demyelinating disorder. An EEG, however, is recommended as part of the neurodiagnostic evaluation of the child with an apparent first unprovoked seizure because it is useful for diagnosis of the event, prediction of recurrence risk, and identification of specific focal abnormalities and/or epileptic syndromes. Neuroimaging is generally not recommended after a first unprovoked seizure unless there is an indication for it on neurologic examination. If it is obtained, however, MRI of the brain is recommended over CT scanning. Anticonvulsant medication is generally not recommended after a single seizure.

Recurrent Seizures. Two unprovoked seizures greater than 24 hours apart suggest the presence of an epileptic disorder within the brain that will lead to future recurrences. It is important to perform a careful evaluation to look for the cause of the seizures as well as to assess the need for treatment with antiepileptic drugs and estimate the potential for response to treatment and remission of seizures in the future.

The *history* can provide important information about the type of seizures. Some parents can precisely act out or re-create a seizure. Children who have a propensity to develop epilepsy may experience the first convulsion in association with a viral illness or a low-grade fever. Seizures that occur during the early morning hours or with drowsiness, particularly during the initial phase of sleep, are common in childhood epilepsy. In retrospect, irritability, mood swings, headache, and subtle personality changes may precede a seizure by several days. Some parents can accurately predict the timing of the next seizure on the basis of changes in the child's disposition. The physical portrayal of the convulsion by the parent or caregiver is often surprisingly similar to the actual convulsion and is much more accurate than the verbal description. Aside from the description of the seizure pattern, the frequency, time of day, precipitating factors, and alternation in the type of convulsive disorder are important. Although generalized tonic-clonic seizures are readily documented, the frequency of absence seizures is often underestimated by parents. A prolonged personality change or intellectual deterioration may suggest a degenerative disease of the CNS, whereas constitutional symptoms, including vomiting and failure to thrive, might indicate a primary metabolic disorder or a structural lesion. It is essential to obtain details of prior anticonvulsant medication and the child's response to the regimen and to determine whether drugs that may potentiate seizures, including chlorpromazine or methylphenidate, were prescribed. The description of the seizure along with the family history can provide clues to the presence of possible genetic epileptic syndromes. These include autosomal dominant nocturnal frontal lobe epilepsy, familial benign neonatal convulsions, familial benign infantile convulsions, autosomal dominant febrile seizures, partial epilepsy with auditory symptoms, autosomal dominant frontal lobe progressive epilepsy with mental retardation, absence epilepsy, and febrile seizures with later partial complex seizures.

The physical, ophthalmologic, and neurologic *examination* can provide information about the presence of increased intracranial pressure, neurocutaneous syndromes, and structural brain abnormalities including malformations, injuries, infections, or tumors.

The EEG is useful for determining the type of epilepsy and the future prognosis. Measurement of serum electrolytes including calcium and magnesium is not recommended as a routine practice. Metabolic testing, including administration of pyridoxine for suspected pyridoxine-responsive seizures, serum lactate and pyruvate, and urine organic acids, is also not recommended routinely but should be dictated by clinical circumstances. Lumbar puncture should be considered for children with repeated seizures and other evidence of neurodevelopmental disability. It may be useful for detecting low CSF glucose in the glucose transporter disorder, alterations in amino acids, neurotransmitters, or cofactors in metabolic disorders, or evidence of chronic infection. Neuroimaging with MRI should be considered during the evaluation of children with newly diagnosed epilepsy, especially for those with neurologic deficits or partial seizures or focal EEG abnormalities that are not part of an idiopathic localization-related epilepsy syndrome.

Classification of Seizures. It is important to classify the type of seizure for several reasons. First, the seizure type may provide a clue to the cause of the seizure disorder. In addition, precise delineation of the seizure may allow a firm basis for making a prognosis and choosing the most appropriate treatment. Anticonvulsants may readily control generalized tonic-clonic epilepsy in a child, but a patient with multiple seizure types or partial seizures may fare less well with the same type of therapy.

BOX 586–1. International Classification of Epileptic Seizures

PARTIAL SEIZURES
Simple partial (consciousness retained)
  Motor
  Sensory
  Autonomic
  Psychic
Complex partial (consciousness impaired)
  Simple partial, followed by impaired consciousness
  Consciousness impaired at onset
Partial seizures with secondary generalization

GENERALIZED SEIZURES
Absences
  Typical
  Atypical
Generalized tonic-clonic
Tonic
Clonic
Myoclonic
Atonic
Infantile spasms

UNCLASSIFIED SEIZURES

Infants with benign myoclonic epilepsy have a more favorable outlook than patients with infantile spasms. Similarly, a school-aged child who has benign partial epilepsy with centrotemporal spikes (rolandic epilepsy) has an excellent prognosis and is unlikely to require a prolonged course of anticonvulsants. Clinical classification of seizures may be difficult because the manifestations of different seizure types may be similar. For example, the clinical features of a child with absence seizures may be almost identical to those of another patient with complex partial epilepsy. An EEG is a useful adjunct to the classification of epilepsy because of the variability of seizure expressivity in this age group. A classification combining the clinical description of the seizure with the EEG findings has improved the delineation of childhood epilepsy (Box 586–1).

Epilepsy in children has also been classified by syndrome. Using the age at onset of seizures, cognitive development and neurologic examination, description of seizure type, and EEG findings, including the background rhythm, it has been possible to classify approximately 50% of childhood seizures into specific syndromes. The *syndromic* classification of seizures provides a distinct advantage over previous classifications by improving management with appropriate anticonvulsant medication, identifying potential candidates for epilepsy surgery, and providing patients and families with a reliable and accurate prognosis. Examples of epilepsy syndromes include infantile spasms (West syndrome), benign myoclonic epilepsy of infancy, the Lennox-Gastaut syndrome, febrile convulsions, Landau-Kleffner syndrome, benign childhood epilepsy with centrotemporal spikes (rolandic epilepsy), Rasmussen encephalitis, juvenile myoclonic epilepsy (Janz syndrome), and Lafora disease (progressive myoclonic epilepsy).

586.3 Partial Seizures

Partial seizures account for a large proportion of childhood seizures, up to 40% in some series. Partial seizures may be classified as *simple* or *complex*; consciousness is maintained with simple seizures and is impaired in patients with complex seizures.

Simple Partial Seizures (SPS). Motor activity is the most common symptom of SPS. The movements are characterized by asynchronous clonic or tonic movements, and they tend to involve the face, neck, and extremities. *Versive seizures* consisting of head turning and conjugate eye movements are particularly common in SPS. Automatisms do not occur with SPS, but some patients complain of aura (e.g., chest discomfort and headache), which may be the only manifestation of a seizure. Children have difficulty in describing aura and often refer to it as "feeling funny" or "something crawling inside me." The average seizure persists for 10–20 sec. *The distinguishing characteristic of SPS is that the patients remain conscious and may verbalize during the seizure. Furthermore, no postictal phenomenon follows the event.* SPS may be confused with tics; however, *tics* are characterized by shoulder shrugging, eye blinking, and facial grimacing and primarily involve the face and shoulders (see Chapter 21). Tics can be briefly suppressed, but partial seizures cannot be controlled. The EEG may show spikes or sharp waves unilaterally or bilaterally or a multifocal spike pattern in patients with SPS.

Complex Partial Seizures (CPS). A CPS may begin with a simple partial seizure with or without an aura, followed by impaired consciousness; conversely, the onset of the CPS may coincide with an altered state of consciousness. An *aura* consisting of vague, unpleasant feelings, epigastric discomfort, or fear is present in approximately one third of children with SPS and CPS. *The presence of an aura always indicates a focal onset of the seizure.* Because partial seizures are difficult to document in infants and children, the frequency of their association with CPS may be underestimated. Impaired consciousness in infants and children is difficult to appreciate. There may be a brief blank stare or a sudden cessation or pause in activity that is frequently overlooked by the parent. Furthermore, the child is unable to communicate or to describe the periods of impaired consciousness in most cases. Finally, the periods of altered consciousness may be brief and infrequent, and only an experienced observer or an EEG may be able to identify the abnormal event.

Automatisms are a common feature of CPS in infants and children, occurring in approximately 50–75% of cases; the older the child, the greater is the frequency of automatisms. Automatisms develop after the loss of consciousness and may persist into the postictal phase, but they are not recalled by the child. The automatic behavior observed in infants is characterized by alimentary automatisms, including lip smacking, chewing, swallowing, and excessive salivation. These movements can represent normal infant behavior and are difficult to distinguish from the automatisms of CPS. Prolonged and repetitive alimentary automatisms associated with a blank stare or with a lack of responsiveness almost always indicate CPS in an infant. Automatic behavior in older children consists of semi-purposeful, incoordinated, and unplanned gestural automatisms, including picking and pulling at clothing or bed sheets, rubbing or caressing objects, and walking or running in a nondirective, repetitive, and often fearful fashion.

Spreading of the epileptiform discharge during CPS can result in secondary generalization with a tonic-clonic convulsion. During the spread of the ictal discharge throughout the hemisphere, contralateral versive turning of the head, dystonic posturing, and tonic or clonic movements of the extremities and face including eye blinking may be noted. The average duration of a CPS is 1–2 min, which is considerably longer than an SPS or an absence seizure.

CPSs are associated with interictal EEG anterior temporal lobe sharp waves or focal spikes, and multifocal spikes are a frequent finding. Approximately 20% of infants and children with CPS have a normal routine interictal EEG. In these patients, a sleep-deprived EEG study, zygomatic leads during EEG, prolonged EEG recording, or video EEG study of the hospitalized patient weaned from anticonvulsants are techniques that can be used to increase the identification of spikes and sharp waves (Fig. 586–1A). In addition, some children with CPS have interictal sharp waves or spikes originating from the frontal, parietal, or occipital lobes. Radiographic studies including CT scanning and especially MRI are most likely to identify an abnormality in the temporal lobe of a child with CPS. These lesions include mesial temporal sclerosis, hamartoma, postencephalitic gliosis, subarachnoid cysts, infarction, arteriovenous malformations, and slow-growing glioma.

Benign Partial Epilepsy with Centrotemporal Spikes (BPEC). BPEC is a common type of partial epilepsy in childhood and has an excellent prognosis. The clinical features, EEG findings (rolandic foci), and lack of a neuropathologic lesion are characteristic and readily separate BPEC from CPS. BPEC occurs between the ages of 2 and 14 yr and has a peak age of onset of 9–10 yr. The disorder occurs in normal children with an unremarkable history and

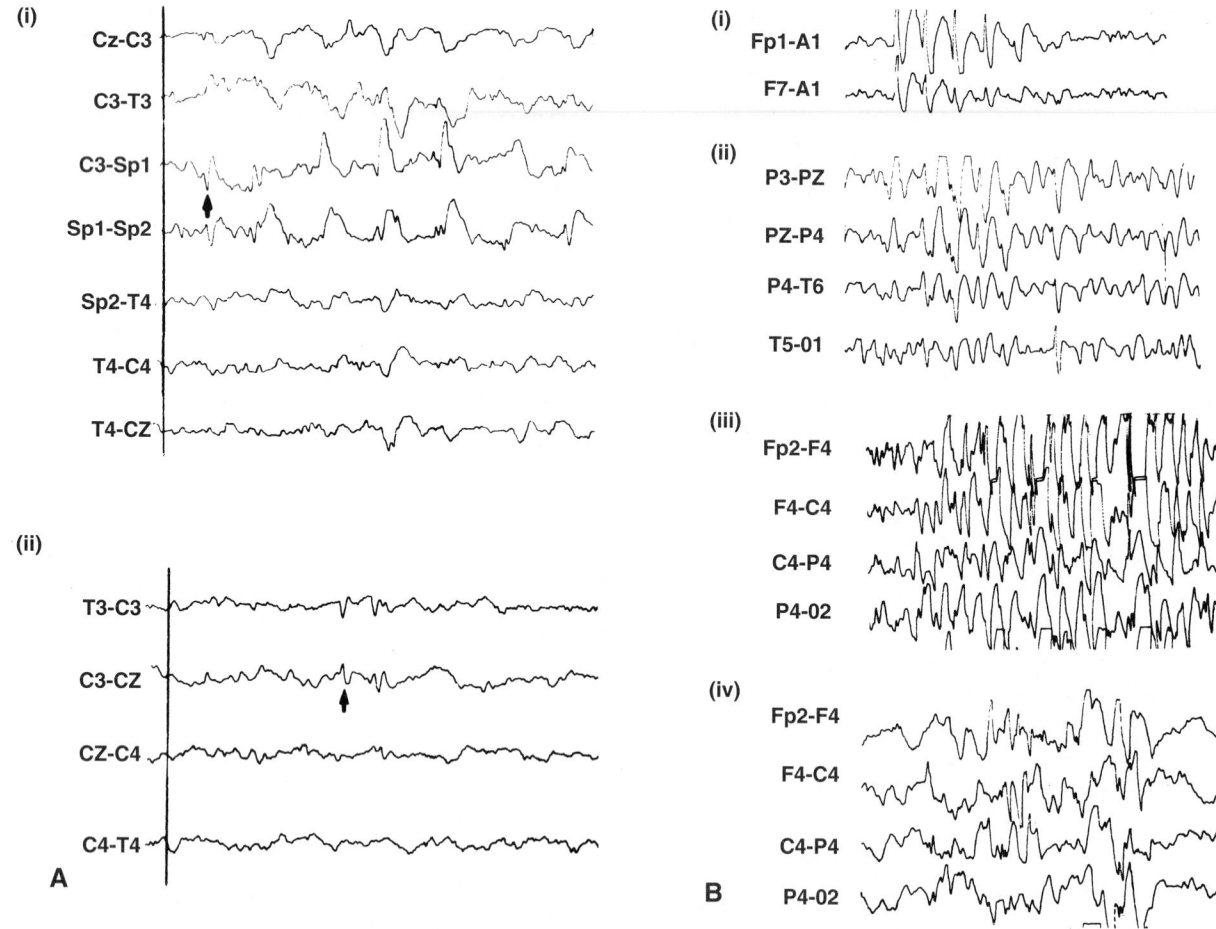

FIGURE 586–1. *A,* An EEG of partial seizures: (i) spike discharges from the left temporal lobe (*arrow*) in a patient with CPS, (ii) left parietal central spikes (*arrow*) characteristic of BPEC. *B,* Representative EEGs of generalized seizures: (i) 3/sec spike and wave discharge of absence seizures with normal background activity, (ii) complex myoclonic epilepsy (Lennox-Gastaut syndrome) with interictal slow spike waves, (iii) juvenile myoclonic epilepsy showing 6/sec spike and waves enhanced by photic stimulation, and (iv) hypsarrhythmia with an irregular high-voltage spike and wave activity.

normal neurologic examination. There is often a positive family history of epilepsy. The seizures are usually partial, and motor signs and somatosensory symptoms are often confined to the face. Oropharyngeal symptoms include tonic contractions and paresthesias of the tongue, unilateral numbness of the cheek (particularly along the gum), guttural noises, dysphagia, and excessive salivation. Unilateral tonic-clonic contractures of the lower face frequently accompany the oropharyngeal symptoms, as do clonic movements or paresthesias of the ipsilateral extremities. Consciousness may be intact or impaired, and the partial seizure may proceed to secondary generalization.

Approximately 20% of children experience only one seizure, the majority have infrequent seizure, and about one fourth have repeated clusters of seizures. BPEC occurs during sleep in 75% of patients, whereas CPS tends to be observed during waking hours. The EEG pattern is diagnostic for BPEC and is characterized by a repetitive spike focus localized in the centrotemporal or rolandic area with normal background activity (see Fig. 586–1*A*). Anticonvulsants are necessary for patients who have frequent seizures but should not be prescribed automatically after the initial convulsion. Carbamazepine is the preferred drug, which is continued for at least 2 yr or until 14–16 yr of age, when spontaneous remission of BPEC usually occurs.

Rasmussen Encephalitis. This subacute inflammatory encephalitis is one cause of *epilepsia partialis continua*. A nonspecific febrile illness may have preceded the onset of focal seizures, which may be frequent or continuous. The onset is usually before age 10 yr. Sequelae include hemiplegia, hemianopia, and aphasia. The EEG reveals diffuse paroxysmal activity with a slow background. The disease is progressive and potentially lethal but more often becomes self-limited with significant neurologic deficits. The disease may be due to autoantibodies that bind to and stimulate the glutamate receptors. Studies have identified cytomegalovirus in several surgical specimens of patients with Rasmussen encephalitis.

586.4 ■ Generalized Seizures

Absence Seizures. Simple (typical) absence (petit mal) seizures are characterized by a sudden cessation of motor activity or speech with a blank facial expression and flickering of the eyelids. These seizures, which are uncommon before age 5 yr, are more prevalent in girls, they are never associated with an aura, they rarely persist longer than 30 sec, and they are not associated with a postictal state. These features tend to differentiate absence seizures from complex partial seizures. Children with absence seizures may experience countless seizures daily, whereas complex partial seizures are usually less frequent. Patients do not lose body tone, but their head may fall forward slightly. Immediately after the seizure, patients resume preseizure activity with no indication of postictal impairment. Automatic behavior frequently accompanies simple absence seizures. Hyperventilation for 3–4 min routinely produces an absence seizure. The EEG shows a typical 3/sec spike and generalized wave discharge (see Fig. 586–1*B*). Complex (atypical) absence seizures have associated motor components consisting of myoclonic movement of the face, fingers, or extremities and, on occasion, loss of body tone. These seizures produce atypical EEG spike and wave discharges at 2–2.5/sec.

Generalized Tonic-Clonic Seizures. These seizures are extremely common and may follow a partial seizure with a focal onset (second generalization) or occur de novo. They may be associated with an aura, suggesting a focal origin of the epileptiform discharge. It is important to inquire about the presence of an aura, because its presence and site of origin may indicate the area of pathology. Patients suddenly lose consciousness and in some cases emit a shrill, piercing cry. Their eyes roll back, their

entire body musculature undergoes tonic contractions, and they rapidly become cyanotic in association with apnea. The clonic phase of the seizure is heralded by rhythmic clonic contractions alternating with relaxation of all muscle groups. The clonic phase slows toward the end of the seizure, which usually persists for a few minutes, and patients often sigh as the seizure comes to an abrupt stop. During the seizure, children may bite their tongue but rarely vomit. Loss of sphincter control, particularly the bladder, is common during a generalized tonic-clonic seizure.

Tight clothing and jewelry around the neck should be loosened, the patient should be placed on one side, and the neck and jaw should be gently hyperextended to enhance breathing. The mouth should not be opened forcibly by an object or by a finger because the patient's teeth may be dislodged and aspirated, or significant injury to the oropharyngeal cavity may result. Postictally, children initially are semicomatose and typically remain in a deep sleep from 30 min to 2 hr. If patients are examined during the seizure or immediately postictally, they may demonstrate truncal ataxia, hyperactive deep tendon reflexes, clonus, and a Babinski reflex. The postictal phase is often associated with vomiting and an intense bifrontal headache.

Idiopathic seizure is a term applied when the cause of a generalized seizure cannot be ascertained. Many factors are known to precipitate generalized tonic-clonic seizures in children, including low-grade fever associated with infections, excessive fatigue or emotional stress, and various drugs including psychotropic medications, theophylline, and methylphenidate, particularly if the seizures are poorly controlled by anticonvulsant drugs.

Myoclonic Epilepsies of Childhood. This disorder is characterized by repetitive seizures consisting of brief, often symmetric muscular contractions with loss of body tone and falling or slumping forward, which has a tendency to cause injuries to the face and mouth. Myoclonic epilepsies include a heterogeneous group of conditions with multiple causes and variable outcomes. However, at least five distinct subgroupings can be identified; these represent the broad spectrum of myoclonic epilepsies in the pediatric population.

BENIGN MYOCLONUS OF INFANCY. Benign myoclonus begins during infancy and consists of clusters of myoclonic movements confined to the neck, trunk, and extremities. The myoclonic activity may be confused with infantile spasms; however, the EEG is normal in patients with benign myoclonus. The prognosis is good, with normal development and the cessation of myoclonus by 2 yr of age. An anticonvulsant is not indicated.

TYPICAL MYOCLONIC EPILEPSY OF EARLY CHILDHOOD. Children who develop typical myoclonic epilepsy are near normal before the onset of seizures, with an unremarkable pregnancy, labor, and delivery and intact developmental milestones. The mean age of onset is approximately 2 yr, but the range spreads from 6 mo to 4 yr. The frequency of myoclonic seizures varies; they may occur several times daily, or children may be seizure-free for weeks. A few patients have febrile convulsions or generalized tonic-clonic afebrile seizures that precede the onset of myoclonic epilepsy. Approximately half of patients occasionally have tonic-clonic seizures in addition to the myoclonic epilepsy. The EEG shows fast spike wave complexes of 2.5 Hz or greater and a normal background rhythm in most cases. At least one third of the children have a positive family history of epilepsy, which suggests a genetic etiology in some cases. The long-term outcome is relatively favorable. Mental retardation develops in the minority, and more than 50% are seizure-free several years later. However, learning and language problems and emotional and behavioral disorders occur in a significant number of these children and require prolonged follow-up by a multidisciplinary team.

COMPLEX MYOCLONIC EPILEPSIES. These consist of a heterogeneous group of disorders with a uniformly poor prognosis. Focal or generalized tonic-clonic seizures beginning during the 1st year of life typically antedate the onset of myoclonic epilepsy. The generalized seizure is often associated with an upper respiratory tract infection and a low-grade fever and frequently develops into status epilepticus. Approximately one third of these patients have evidence of delayed developmental milestones. A history of hypoxic-ischemic encephalopathy in the perinatal period and the finding of generalized upper motor neuron and extrapyramidal signs with microcephaly constitute a common pattern among these children. A family history of epilepsy is much less prominent in this group compared with typical myoclonic epilepsy.

Some children display a combination of frequent myoclonic and tonic seizures, and when interictal slow spike waves are evident in the EEG, the seizure disorder is classified as the *Lennox-Gastaut syndrome*. This syndrome is characterized by the triad of intractable seizures of various types, a slow spike wave EEG during the awake state, and mental retardation. Patients with complex myoclonic epilepsy routinely have interictal slow spike waves and are refractory to anticonvulsants (see Fig. 586–1B). The seizures are persistent, and the frequency of mental retardation and behavioral problems is approximately 75% of all patients. Treatment with valproic acid or benzodiazepines may decrease the frequency or intensity of the seizures. The ketogenic diet should be considered for patients whose seizures are refractory to anticonvulsants.

JUVENILE MYOCLONIC EPILEPSY (JANZ SYNDROME). Juvenile myoclonic epilepsy usually begins between the ages of 12 and 16 yr and accounts for approximately 5% of the epilepsies. A gene locus has been identified on chromosome 6p21. Patients note frequent myoclonic jerks on awakening, making hair combing and tooth brushing difficult. As the myoclonus tends to abate later in the morning, most patients do not seek medical advice at this stage and some deny the episodes. A few years later, early morning generalized tonic-clonic seizures develop in association with the myoclonus. The EEG shows a 4–6/sec irregular spike and wave pattern, which is enhanced by photic stimulation (see Fig. 586–1B). The neurologic examination is normal, and the majority respond dramatically to valproate, which is required lifelong. Discontinuance of the drug causes a high rate of recurrence of seizures.

PROGRESSIVE MYOCLONIC EPILEPSIES. This heterogeneous group of rare genetic disorders uniformly has a grave prognosis. These conditions include Lafora disease, myoclonic epilepsy with ragged-red fibers (MERRF) (see Chapter 591.2), sialidosis type 1 (see Chapter 592.4), ceroid lipofuscinosis (see Chapter 592.2), juvenile neuropathic Gaucher disease, and juvenile neuroaxonal dystrophy.

Lafora disease presents in children between 10 and 18 yr with generalized tonic-clonic seizures. Ultimately, myoclonic jerks appear; these become more apparent and constant with progression of the disease. Mental deterioration is a characteristic feature and becomes evident within 1 yr of the onset of seizures. Neurologic abnormalities, particularly cerebellar and extrapyramidal signs, are prominent findings. The EEG shows polyspike-wave discharges, particularly in the occipital region, with progressive slowing and a disorganized background. The myoclonic jerks are difficult to control, but a combination of valproic acid and a benzodiazepine (e.g., clonazepam) is effective in controlling the generalized seizures. Lafora disease is an autosomal recessive disorder, and the diagnosis may be established by examination of a skin biopsy specimen for characteristic periodic acid-Schiff positive inclusions, which are most prominent in the eccrine sweat gland duct cells. The gene for Lafora disease is located on 6p24 and it encodes a protein, tyrosine phosphatase.

Infantile Spasms. Infantile spasms usually begin between the ages of 4 and 8 mo and are characterized by brief symmetric contrac-

tions of the neck, trunk, and extremities. There are at least three types of infantile spasms: flexor, extensor, and mixed. *Flexor spasms* occur in clusters or volleys and consist of sudden flexion of the neck, arms, and legs onto the trunk, whereas *extensor spasms* produce extension of the trunk and extremities and are the least common form of infantile spasm. *Mixed infantile spasms*, consisting of flexion in some volleys and extension in others, is the most common type of infantile spasm. Clusters or volleys of seizures may persist for minutes, with brief intervals between each spasm. A cry may precede or follow an infantile spasm, accounting for the confusion with colic in a few cases. The spasms occur during sleep or arousal but have a tendency to develop while patients are drowsy or immediately on awakening. The EEG that is most commonly associated with infantile spasms is referred to as *hypsarrhythmia*, which consists of a chaotic pattern of high-voltage, bilaterally asynchronous, slow-wave activity (see Fig. 586–1B), or a modified hypsarrhythmia pattern.

Infantile spasms are typically classified into two groups: *cryptogenic* and *symptomatic*. A child with cryptogenic infantile spasms has an uneventful pregnancy and birth history as well as normal developmental milestones before the onset of seizures. The neurologic examination and the CT and MRI scans of the head are normal, and there are no associated risk factors. Approximately 10–20% of infantile spasms are classified as cryptogenic, and the remainder are classified as symptomatic. Symptomatic infantile spasms are related directly to several prenatal, perinatal, and postnatal factors. Prenatal and perinatal factors include hypoxic-ischemic encephalopathy with periventricular leukomalacia, congenital infections, inborn errors of metabolism, neurocutaneous syndromes such as tuberous sclerosis, cytoarchitectural abnormalities including lissencephaly and schizencephaly, and prematurity. Postnatal conditions include CNS infections, head trauma (especially subdural hematoma and intraventricular hemorrhage), and hypoxic-ischemic encephalopathy. The fact that infantile spasms and immunizations often occur simultaneously around 6 mo of age is a coincidence of timing rather than a cause and effect of any immunization antigen.

Infants with cryptogenic infantile spasms have a good prognosis, whereas those with the symptomatic type have an 80–90% risk of mental retardation. The underlying CNS disorder has a major role in the neurologic outcome. Several theories have been advanced with regard to the pathogenesis of infantile spasms, including dysfunction of the monoaminergic neurotransmitter system in the brainstem, derangement of neuronal structures in the brainstem, and an abnormality of the immune system. One hypothesis implicates corticotropin-releasing hormone (CRH), a putative neurotransmitter, metabolized in the inferior olive. CRH acts on the pituitary to enhance the release of adrenocorticotropic hormone (ACTH); ACTH and glucocorticoids suppress the metabolism and secretion of CRH by a feedback mechanism. It is proposed that specified stresses or injury to an infant during a critical period of neurodevelopment causes CRH overproduction, resulting in neuronal hyperexcitability and seizures. The number of CRH receptors reaches a maximum in an infant's brain followed by spontaneous reduction with age, perhaps accounting for the eventual resolution of infantile spasms, even without therapy. Exogenous ACTH and glucocorticoids suppress CRH synthesis, which may account for their effectiveness in treating infantile spasms. Therapy for infantile spasms is discussed in the section on treatment

Landau-Kleffner Syndrome (LKS). This is a rare condition of unknown cause. It is more common in boys and has a mean onset of 51/2 yr. LKS is often confused with autism, in that both conditions are associated with a loss of language function. LKS is characterized by loss of language skills in a previously normal child. At least 70% have an associated seizure disorder. Language regression may be sudden or the speech loss protracted. The aphasia may be primarily receptive or expressive, and auditory agnosia may be so severe that the child is oblivious to everyday sounds. Hearing is normal, but behavioral problems, including irritability and poor attention span, are particularly common. Formal testing often shows normal performance and visual-spatial skills despite poor language. The seizures are of several types, including focal or generalized tonic-clonic, atypical absence, partial complex, and occasionally myoclonic. High-amplitude spike and wave discharges predominate and tend to be bitemporal, but they can be multifocal or generalized. In the evolutionary stages of the condition, the EEG findings may be normal. The spike discharges are always more apparent during non–rapid eye movement (REM) sleep; thus, a child suspected of LKS should have an EEG during sleep, particularly if the awake record is normal. If the sleep EEG is normal but a high index of suspicion for the diagnosis of LKS continues, the child should be referred to a tertiary pediatric epilepsy center for prolonged EEG recording and specific neuroimaging studies. CT and MRI studies typically yield normal results, and positron-emission tomography (PET) scans have demonstrated either unilateral or bilateral hypometabolism or hypermetabolism. Microscopic examination of surgical specimens has shown minimal gliosis but no evidence of encephalitis.

Valproic acid is the anticonvulsant of choice; however, some children require a combination of valproic acid and clobazam to control their seizures. If the seizures and aphasia persist, a trial of steroids should be considered. One recommended schedule consists of oral prednisone, 2 mg/kg/24 hr for 1 mo, tapered to 1 mg/kg/24 hr for an additional month. With clinical improvement, the prednisone is reduced further to 0.5 mg/kg/24 hr for up to 6–12 mo. It is imperative to initiate speech therapy and maintain treatment for several years, because improvement in language function occurs over a prolonged period. Some centers advocate an operative procedure—subpial transection—when medical management fails. Methylphenidate should be considered for patients with severe hyperactivity and inattention. Seizures, if poorly controlled, may be potentiated by methylphenidate; however, anticonvulsants are usually protective. Intravenous immunoglobulin may be helpful in LKS. Some children experience a recurrence of aphasia and seizures after apparent recovery. Most children with LKS have a significant abnormality of speech function during adulthood. The onset of LKS at an early age (<2 yr) uniformly tends to be associated with a poor prognosis for recovery of speech.

586.5 Mechanisms of Seizures

Although the precise mechanisms of seizures are unknown, several physiologic factors are responsible for the development of a seizure. To initiate a seizure, there must be a group of neurons that are capable of generating a significant burst discharge and a GABAergic inhibitory system. Seizure discharge transmission ultimately depends on excitatory glutamatergic synapses. Evidence suggests that excitatory amino acid neurotransmitters (glutamate, aspartate) may have a role in producing neuronal excitation by acting on specific cell receptors. Seizures may arise from areas of neuronal death, and these regions of the brain may promote development of novel hyperexcitable synapses that can cause seizures. For example, lesions in the temporal lobe (including slow-growing gliomas, hamartomas, gliosis, and arteriovenous malformations) cause seizures, and when the abnormal tissue is removed surgically, the seizures are likely to cease. Further, convulsions may be produced in experimental animals by the phenomenon of *kindling*. In this model, repeated subconvulsive stimulation of the brain (e.g., amygdala) ultimately leads to a generalized convulsion. Kindling may be responsible for the development of epilepsy in humans after an injury to the brain. In humans, it has been proposed that recur-

rent seizure activity from an abnormal temporal lobe may produce seizures in the contralateral normal temporal lobe by transmission of the stimulus via the corpus callosum.

Seizures are more common in infants and in immature experimental animals. Certain seizures in the pediatric population are age specific (e.g., infantile spasms); this observation suggests that the underdeveloped brain is more susceptible to specific seizures than is the brain of an older child or adult. Genetic factors account for at least 20% of all cases of epilepsy. Using linkage analyses, the chromosomal location of several familial epilepsies has been identified, including benign neonatal convulsions (20q and 8q), juvenile myoclonic epilepsy (6p), and progressive myoclonic epilepsy (21q22.3). The genetic defect of benign familial neonatal convulsions has been characterized by the identification of submicroscopic deletion of chromosome 20q13.3. Study of the cDNAs spanning the deleted region identified one encoding a novel voltage-gated potassium channel, $KCNQ_2$. Furthermore, the substantia nigra has an integral role in the development of generalized seizures. Electrographic seizure activity spreads within the substantia nigra, causing an increase in uptake of 2-deoxyglucose in adult animals, but there is little or no metabolic activity within the substantia nigra when immature animals have a convulsion. It has been proposed that the functional immaturity of the substantia nigra may have a role in the increased seizure susceptibility of the immature brain. Additionally, the γ-aminobutyric acid (GABA)-sensitive substantia nigra pars reticulata neurons play a part in preventing seizures. It is likely that substantia nigra outflow tracts modulate and regulate seizure dissemination but are not responsible for the onset of seizures.

Use of the EEG to Diagnose Epilepsy. The investigation of a seizure depends on many factors, including the age of the patient, the type and frequency of the seizure, and the presence or absence of neurologic findings and constitutional symptoms. Demonstration of paroxysmal discharges on the EEG during a clinical seizure is diagnostic of epilepsy, but seizures rarely occur in the EEG laboratory. A normal EEG does not preclude the diagnosis of epilepsy, because the interictal recording is normal in approximately 40% of patients. Activation procedures, including hyperventilation, eye closure, photic stimulation, and, when indicated, sleep deprivation and special electrode placement (e.g., zygomatic leads) substantially increase the positive yield. Seizure discharges are more likely to be recorded in infants and children than in adolescents or adults. Patients who are taking an anticonvulsant and who are scheduled for a routine EEG should not have the medication decreased or discontinued before the study, because status epilepticus could result.

Prolonged EEG monitoring with simultaneous closed-circuit video recording is reserved for complicated cases of protracted and unresponsive seizures. It provides an invaluable method for recording ictal seizure events that are rarely obtained during routine EEG studies. This technique is extremely helpful in the classification of seizures because it can accurately determine the location and frequency of seizure discharges while recording alterations in the level of consciousness and the presence of clinical signs. Patients with pseudoseizures can be readily distinguished from those with true epilepsy, and seizure type (e.g., complex partial vs generalized) can be more precisely identified. Determination of seizure type is critical in the investigation of a child who may be a candidate for epilepsy surgery.

586.6 Treatment of Epilepsy

The first step in the management of epilepsy is to ensure that the patient has a seizure disorder and not a condition that mimics epilepsy (see Chapter 587). It is sometimes difficult to be certain about the cause of a paroxysmal event in a normal child. A negative result on a neurologic examination and EEG usually supports the approach of watchful waiting rather than administration of an anticonvulsant. The true cause of the paroxysmal disorder eventually becomes apparent. Although there is not uniform agreement, most would concur that antiepileptics should be withheld from a previously healthy child with the first afebrile convulsion if there is a negative family history, normal results of an examination and EEG, and a cooperative and compliant family. Approximately 70% of these children will not experience another convulsion. Approximately 75% of those patients with two or three unprovoked seizures have additional seizures. A recurrent seizure, particularly if it occurs in close proximity to the first seizure, is an indication to begin an anticonvulsant. Figure 586–2 suggests an approach to a child with a suspected seizure disorder.

The second step involves choosing an anticonvulsant. The drug of choice depends on the classification of the seizure, determined by the history and EEG findings. The goal for every patient should be the use of only one drug with the fewest possible side effects for the control of seizures. The drug is increased slowly until seizure control is accomplished or until undesirable side effects develop. The child's serum anticonvulsant level should be monitored during this stage, and the dose should be altered accordingly. Table 586–1 summarizes the common antiepileptic drugs used in childhood epilepsy and highlights the recommended daily dose, therapeutic serum levels, and common side effects. A suggested loading dose is indicated for drugs that are useful for the treatment of status epilepticus. Physicians should be familiar with the pharmacokinetics of the anticonvulsant and its toxic actions and should monitor the child on a regular basis to gauge the seizure control while watching for unwanted side effects.

Routine serum monitoring of anticonvulsant levels is not recommended because the practice is not cost effective. There are several important indications for anticonvulsant drug monitoring: (1) at the onset of anticonvulsant therapy to confirm that the drug level is within the therapeutic range; (2) for noncompliant patients and families; (3) at the time of status epilepticus; (4) during accelerated growth spurts; (5) for patients on polytherapy, especially valproic acid, phenobarbital, and lamotrigine

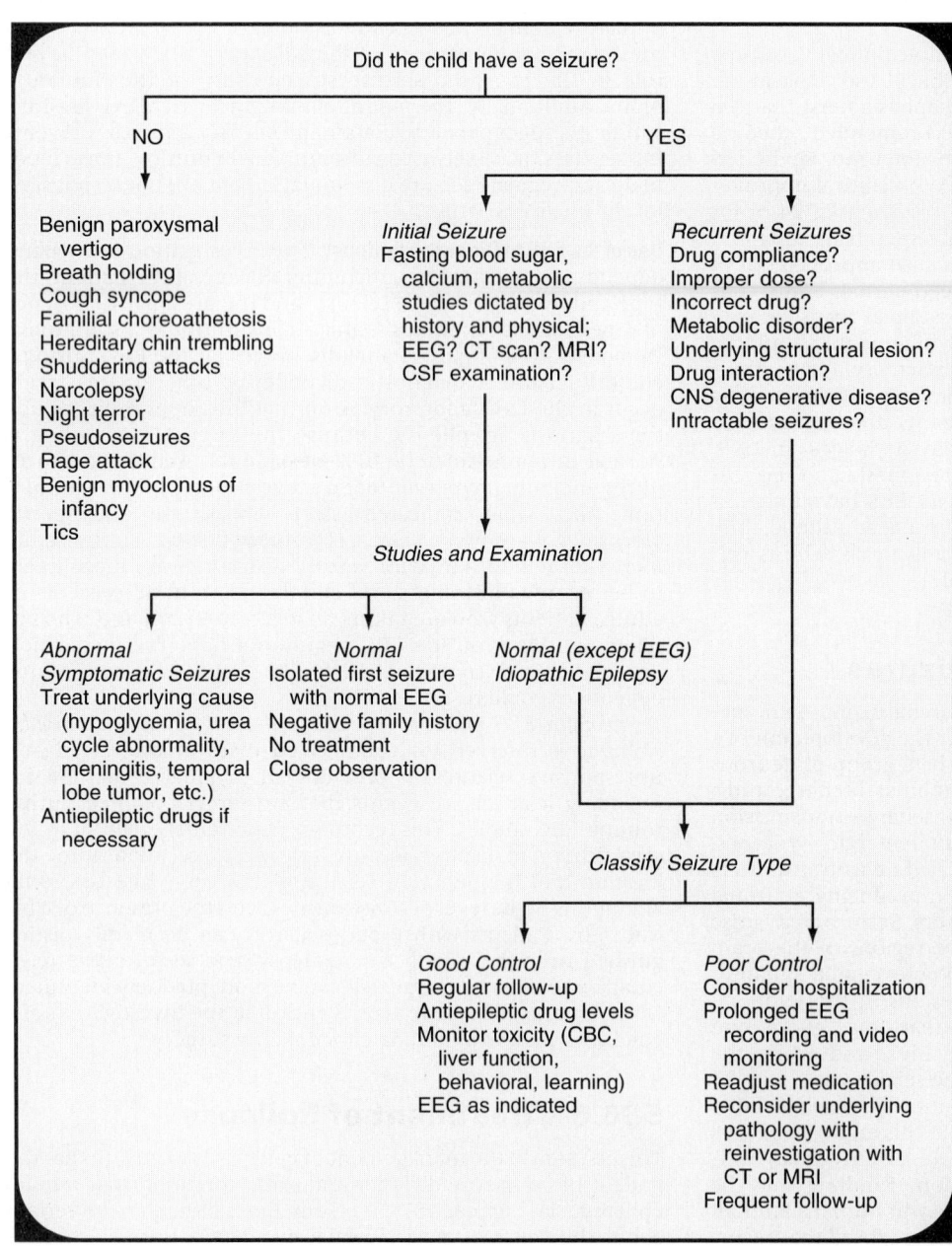

FIGURE 586–2. An approach to the child with a suspected convulsive disorder.

TABLE 586–1. Common Anticonvulsant Drugs

Drug	Seizure Type	Oral Dose	Loading Dose (IV)	Therapeutic Serum Level (μg/mL)	Side Effects and Toxicity
Carbamazepine (Tegretol)	Generalized tonic-clonic Partial	Begin 10 mg/kg/24 hr Increase to 20–30 mg/kg/24 hr tid	—	8–12	Dizziness, drowsiness, diplopia, liver dysfunction, anemia, neutropenia, SIADH, blood dyscrasias rare, hepatotoxic effects
*Clobazam (Frisium)	Adjunctive therapy when seizures poorly controlled	0.25–1 mg/kg/24 hr bid or tid	—	—	Dizziness, fatigue, weight gain, ataxia and behavior problems
Clonazepam (Rivotril)	Absence Myoclonic Infantile spasms Partial Lennox-Gastaut Akinetic	Children <30 kg: Begin 0.05 mg/kg/24 hr Increase by 0.05 mg/kg/wk Maximum 0.2 mg/kg/24 hr bid or tid Children >30 kg: 1.5 mg/kg/24 hr tid, not to exceed 20 mg/24 hr	—	>0.013	Drowsiness, irritability, agitation, behavioral abnormalities, depression, excessive salivation
Ethosuximide (Zarontin)	Absence May increase tonic-clonic seizures	Begin 20 mg/kg/24 hr Increase to maximum of 40 mg/kg/24 hr or 1.5 g/24 hr, whichever is less	—	40–100	Abdominal discomfort, skin rash, liver dysfunction, leukopenia
Gabapentin (Neurontin)	Adjunctive therapy when seizures poorly controlled	Children: 20–50 mg/kg/24 hr tid Adolescence: 900–3,600 mg/24 hr tid	—	Not necessary to monitor	Somnolence, dizziness, ataxia, headache, tremor, vomiting, nystagmus, fatigue and weight gain
Lamotrigine (Lamictal)	Adjunctive therapy when seizures poorly controlled Broad-spectrum anticonvulsant activity in various seizure types including: complex partial, absence, myoclonic, clonic, tonic-clonic, and Lennox-Gastaut	Individualized based on age and additional anticonvulsants (see Chapter 586.6)	—	—	Rash, dizziness, ataxia, somnolence, diplopia, headache, nausea, vomiting
*Nitrazepam (Mogadon)	Absence Myoclonic Infantile spasms	Begin 0.2 mg/kg/24 hr Increase slowly to 1 mg/kg/24 hr tid	—	—	Similar to clonazepam, hallucinations
Paraldehyde	Generalized status epilepticus	Make a 5% solution by adding 1.75 mL of paraldehyde to D5W with total volume of 35 mL	150–200 mg/kg Maintenance, 20 mg/kg/hr	—	
Phenobarbital	Generalized tonic-clonic Partial Status epilepticus	3–5 mg/kg/24 hr bid	20 mg/kg 20–30 mg/kg in the neonate	15–40	Hyperactivity, irritability, short attention span, temper tantrums, altered sleep pattern, Stevens-Johnson syndrome, depression of cognitive function
Phenytoin (Dilantin)	Generalized tonic-clonic Partial Status epilepticus	3–9 mg/kg/24 hr bid	20 mg/kg	10–20	Hirsutism, gum hypertrophy, ataxia, skin rash, Stevens-Johnson syndrome, nystagmus, nausea, vomiting, drowsiness, coarsening facial features, blood dyscrasias
Primidone (Mysoline)	Generalized tonic-clonic Partial	Children <8 yr: 10–25 mg/kg/24 hr tid or qid Children >8 yr: usual maintenance dose, 750–1,500 mg/24 hr tid or qid 1–9 mg/kg/24 hr bid	—	5–12	Aggressive behavior, personality changes, similar to phenobarbital
Topiramate (Topimax)	Adjunctive therapy for poorly controlled seizures		—	—	Fatigue, cognitive depression
Tiagabine (Gabitril)	Refractory complex partial seizures Adjunctive therapy for complex partial seizures	Average dose, 6 mg tid	—	—	Asthenia, dizziness, poor attention span, nervousness, tremor
Valproic acid (Depakene, Epival)	Generalized tonic-clonic Absence Myoclonic Partial Akinetic	Begin 10 mg/kg/24 hr Increase by 5–10 mg/kg/wk Usual dose, 30–60 mg/kg/24 hr tid or qid	Intravenous preparation now available Studies in children under way	50–100	Nausea, vomiting, anorexia, amenorrhea, sedation, tremor, weight gain, alopecia, hepatotoxicity
*Vigabatrin (Sabril)	Infantile spasms Adjunctive therapy for poorly controlled seizures	Begin 30 mg/kg/24 hr once daily or bid Maintenance dose, 30–100 mg/kg/24 hr once daily or bid	—	—	Hyperactivity, agitation, excitement, somnolence, weight gain Note: Reports of visual field constriction, optic pallor or atrophy, and optic neuritis

*Not available in the United States.
SIADH = syndrome of inappropriate secretion of antidiuretic hormone.

because of drug interactions; (6) for uncontrolled seizures or seizures that have changed in type; (7) for symptoms and signs of drug toxicity (e.g., toxicity due to a metabolite of carbamazepine, carbamazepine-10,11 epoxide); (8) for patients with hepatic or renal disease; and (9) for children with cognitive and physical disabilities, especially those taking phenytoin, in whom toxicity may be difficult to evaluate. Good clinical judgment is more reliable in achieving seizure control than over-reliance on therapeutic drug monitoring.

There is controversy about whether routine blood tests (complete blood count [CBC], liver function studies) are indicated during anticonvulsant therapy. Because most serious adverse anticonvulsant drug reactions develop during the initial 2–3 mo of therapy, monthly blood screening for the first 3 mo is recommended. Subsequently, routine blood tests are ordered only when clinically indicated.

Anticonvulsants that are introduced during childhood may be required during adolescence and the childbearing years. Unfortunately, some anticonvulsants, including phenytoin, valproic acid, carbamazepine, and primidone, are associated with the occurrence of specific birth defects, including facial and limb anomalies and spinal dysraphism. Whether the teratogenic effect is secondary to the mother's epilepsy or the anticonvulsant medication is still debated. Meanwhile, the pediatrician should counsel the family about the possible relationship and should avoid prescribing an anticonvulsant to a pregnant patient unless it is absolutely necessary.

If complete seizure control is accomplished by an anticonvulsant, a minimum of 2 seizure-free years is an adequate and safe period of treatment for a patient with no risk factors. Prominent risk factors include age greater than 12 yr at onset, neurologic dysfunction (motor handicap or mental retardation), a history of prior neonatal seizures, and numerous seizures before control is achieved. In a child with complete seizure control for a minimum of 2 yr and low risk factors, the chance of recurrence is approximately 20–25%, particularly during the first 6 mo after discontinuation of the anticonvulsant. Those children with the best prognosis following anticonvulsant withdrawal are those with benign epilepsy with rolandic spikes and those with idiopathic generalized seizures. CPS and juvenile myoclonic seizures are more likely to recur. When the decision is made to discontinue the drug, the weaning process should occur for 3–6 mo, because abrupt withdrawal may cause status epilepticus.

Possible sites of action, dose, and side effects of anticonvulsants are noted in Figure 586–3 and Table 586–1.

Benzodiazepines. The benzodiazepines exert anticonvulsant activity by binding to a specific GABA site that enhances the opening frequency of the chloride channel without affecting open or burst duration (see Fig. 586–3). The drugs *diazepam* and *lorazepam* IV are used for initial management of status epilepticus. Rectal *diazepam* gel has been demonstrated to be an effective and safe treatment to abort episodes of acute repetitive seizures in children and is available as Diastat gel in 2.5, 5, and

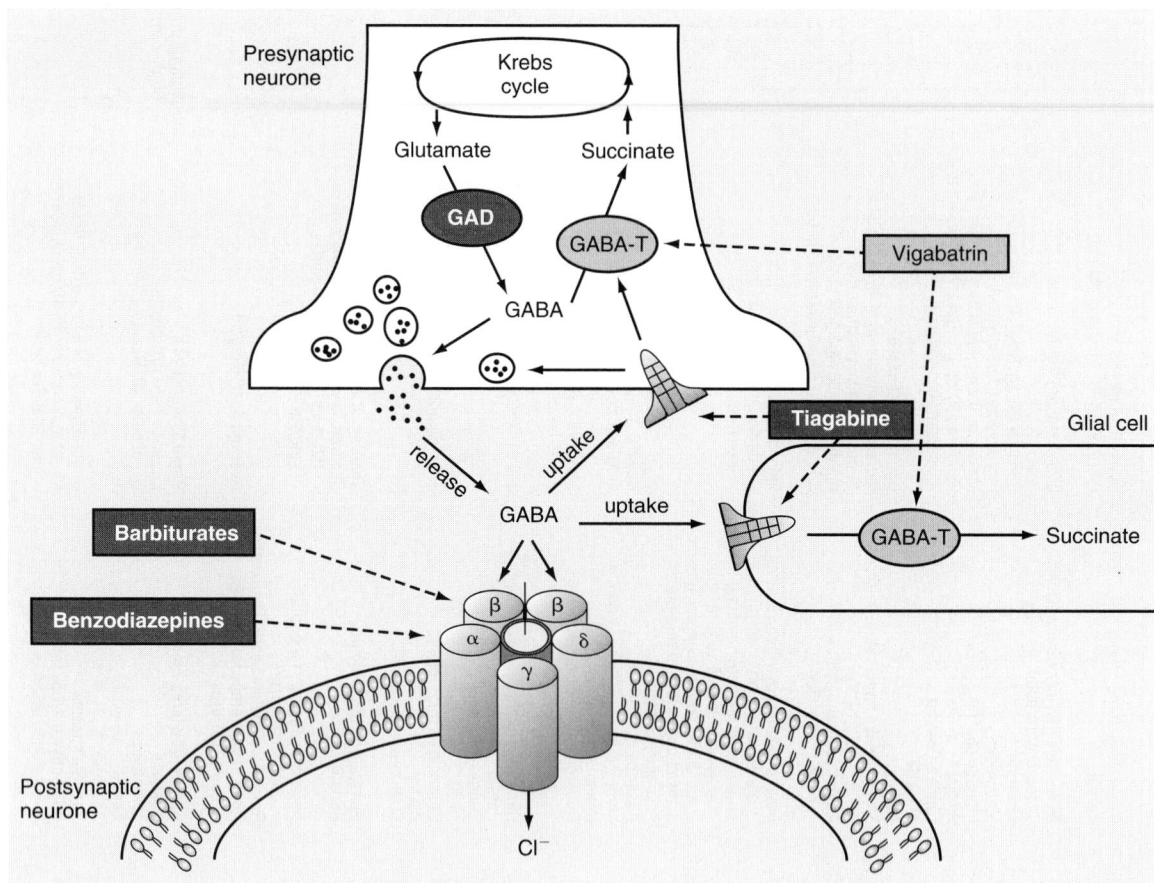

FIGURE 586–3. Pharmacologic effects of antiepileptic drugs at GABA$_A$ receptor. GABA = γ-aminobutyric acid; GAD = glutamic acid decarboxylase; GABA-T = GABA transaminase. Barbiturates bind to β-subunit of GABA$_A$ receptor to potentiate action of endogenous agonist GABA and prolong opening time of chloride ion channel. Benzodiazepines bind to an α-subunit of GABA$_A$ to potentiate action of GABA and increase frequency of opening of chloride ion channel. Vigabatrin irreversibly binds to GABA-transaminase to inhibit degradation of inhibitory neurotransmitter GABA. Tiagabine blocks uptake of synaptically released GABA into both presynaptic neurons and glial cells, allowing GABA to remain at site of action for longer periods. (From Leach JP, Brodie MJ: Tiagabine. *Lancet* 1998;351:203.)

10 mg doses for children. *Clonazepam* is useful for the management of the Lennox-Gastaut syndrome, myoclonic, akinetic, and absence seizures. The elimination half-life is 18–50 hr. Clonazepam may increase serum phenytoin concentrations when used together, and additional CNS depression may occur when combined with other CNS depressant drugs. Clonazepam is supplied in 0.5 and 2 mg tablets. *Nitrazepam* is useful for the management of myoclonic seizures. The elimination half-life is 18–57 hr. The drug may increase CNS depression when used with additional depressants. Nitrazepam is supplied in 5 and 10 mg tablets. *Clobazam* is indicated as adjunctive therapy for complex partial seizures. The half-life is 10–30 hr. Clobazam may increase the serum drug levels of carbamazepine, phenytoin, phenobarbital, and valproic acid when used concomitantly. Clobazam is supplied in 10 mg tablets.

Carbamazepine. This drug is effective for the management of generalized tonic-clonic and partial seizures. Carbamazepine acts similarly to phenytoin by decreasing the sustained repetitive firing of neurons by blocking sodium-dependent channels and by decreasing depolarization-dependent calcium uptake. Significant leukopenia (<1,000 neutrophils/mL^3) and hepatotoxicity may rarely develop, particularly during the initial 3–4 mo of therapy. Therefore, a CBC with differential and AST and ALT levels should be obtained on a monthly basis during this period, although serious idiosyncratic drug reactions may develop despite normal liver function tests results and routine blood work. Subsequent laboratory testing is determined by the presence of adverse symptoms or signs. The parents should be informed of untoward drug effects and instructed to report them immediately to the physician. Erythromycin should be used cautiously with carbamazepine because the two drugs compete for metabolism by the liver. The plasma concentration of carbamazepine is lowered by phenytoin, phenobarbital, and valproic acid. Carbamazepine-10,11-epoxide, which is an active metabolite of carbamazepine, may produce toxicity despite therapeutic carbamazepine levels, particularly when valproic acid is added to the drug regimen. Hyponatremia has also been reported as a side effect of this drug. Carbamazepine is supplied in suspension, 20 mg/mL; chew tabs, 100 and 200 mg tablets; and controlled release (CR) form, 200 and 400 mg tablets. The half-life is 8–20 hr, and the drug should be given two or three times daily.

Ethosuximide. Ethosuximide provides its anticonvulsant action by blocking calcium channels associated with thalamocortical circuitry. Ethosuximide is an effective drug for the management of typical absence epilepsy and has a half-life of 60 hr. When used with phenobarbital or primidone, ethosuximide may reduce the serum levels of those anticonvulsants. Ethosuximide is supplied in syrup, 50 mg/mL, and in 250 mg capsules.

Gabapentin. This anticonvulsant is used as an add-on drug for patients with refractory complex partial and secondarily generalized tonic-clonic seizures. The mechanism of action results from binding of the drug to neuronal membranes (glutamate synapses) and increased brain GABA turnover. The plasma half-life of gabapentin is 5–7 hr. The drug is rapidly absorbed from the gastrointestinal tract, does not bind to plasma proteins, and is not metabolized. Gabapentin has no significant drug interactions and is relatively free of dose-related CNS adverse effects. Gabapentin is recommended for children 12 yr and older. Gabapentin is supplied in 100, 300, and 400 mg capsules.

Lamotrigine. Lamotrigine is a phenyltriazine compound used as an add-on drug for the management of complex partial and generalized tonic-clonic seizures. Lamotrigine is effective as monotherapy for some children with the Lennox-Gastaut syndrome and generalized absence seizures. Pharmacologic studies suggest the drug acts at voltage-sensitive sodium channels to stabilize neuronal membranes and inhibit neuronal release, particularly glutamate. The plasma elimination half-life is 22–37 hr.

In children, the recommended starting dose is 2 mg/kg/24 hr for 2 wk divided into two doses, followed by 5 mg/kg/24 hr for an additional 2 wk. The maintenance dose is 5–15 mg/kg/24 hr. If lamotrigine is added to valproate therapy, the starting dose of lamotrigine should be reduced to 0.5 mg/kg/24 hr because valproate inhibits the metabolism of lamotrigine. In this case, the maintenance dose of lamotrigine is 1–5 mg/kg/24 hr. The therapeutic serum level is 1–4 mg/L or 3.9–15.6 μmol/L. Common side effects include nausea, headache, dizziness, blurred vision, diplopia, and ataxia. A maculopapular skin rash develops in about 3% of patients. The Stevens-Johnson syndrome, angioedema, or toxic epidermal necrolysis occasionally results, usually during the first month of therapy, especially in association with valproate. Because these skin disorders may be fatal, the anticonvulsants must be immediately discontinued. Lamotrigine is supplied in 25, 50, 100, and 200 mg tablets.

Phenobarbital and Primidone. These are relatively safe anticonvulsants that are particularly useful for generalized tonic-clonic seizures. However, approximately 25% of children undergo severe behavioral changes on these drugs. Neurologically abnormal children are at greater risk. Furthermore, there is evidence that phenobarbital may adversely affect the cognitive performance of children treated on a long-term basis. Valproic acid interferes with the metabolism of phenobarbital, causing elevated phenobarbital plasma levels and toxicity despite the usual daily doses. Phenobarbital acts on the GABA receptor to increase the chloride channel open duration (see Fig. 586–3). The plasma half-life is 48–150 hr. Phenobarbital is supplied in an elixir, 4 mg/mL; tablets, 15, 30, 60, and 100 mg; and injectable, 30 and 120 mg/mL. Primidone is prepared in a suspension, 50 mg/mL, and in 125 and 250 mg tablets. The plasma half-life of primidone is 10–21 hr. Phenobarbital is prescribed twice daily, and primidone is prescribed three times a day. Routine blood tests are not indicated for these anticonvulsants.

Phenytoin. Phenytoin acts by decreasing the sustained repetitive firing of single neurons by blocking sodium-dependent channels and decreasing depolarization-dependent calcium uptake. Phenytoin is used for primary and secondary generalized tonic-clonic seizures, partial seizures, and status epilepticus. The plasma half-life is 7–42 hr. Phenytoin has many drug interactions that may increase or decrease other concomitantly used anticonvulsants (see Table 586–1). Phenytoin is supplied in a suspension, 6 and 25 mg/mL; chewable tablets, 50 mg; capsules, 100 mg; and injectable, 100 mg/2 mL and 250 mg/5 mL. Fosphenytoin, a water-soluble prodrug of phenytoin for intramuscular or intravenous use, is available in a concentration of 75 mg/mL, equivalent to 50 mg/mL of phenytoin.

Tiagabine. Tiagabine inhibits seizure activity by blocking reuptake of the neuroinhibitory transmitter GABA into neuronal and glial cells (see Fig. 586–3). The drug is effective in the management of complex partial seizures as an add-on drug. Tiagabine is supplied in 4, 12, 16, and 20 mg tablets.

Topiramate. Topiramate produces anticonvulsant action by blocking voltage-dependent sodium channels. The drug is used as adjunctive therapy for refractory complex seizures with or without secondary generalization. The elimination half-life is 21 hr. Phenytoin, carbamazepine, and valproic acid may decrease the concentration of topiramate. Topiramate is dispensed in 25, 100, and 200 mg tablets.

Valproic Acid. Valproic acid is a broad-spectrum anticonvulsant. It acts by blocking voltage-dependent sodium channels and increases calcium-dependent potassium conductance. The elimination half-life is 6–16 hr. This drug is useful for the management of many seizure types, including generalized tonic-clonic, absence, atypical absence, and myoclonic seizures. It rarely induces behavioral changes but is associated with mild gastrointestinal disturbances, alopecia, tremor, and hyperphagia. Two rare but serious side effects of valproate are a Reye-like syndrome and irreversible hepatotoxicity. A small number of children develop progressive lethargy and coma with elevated serum ammonia and decreased levels of serum carnitine. Valproic acid may block the metabolism of carnitine, producing the altered state of consciousness in these patients. Discontinuation of valproic acid leads to recovery over several days.

Another small group of patients, particularly children younger than 2 yr and having specific neurologic syndromes, who are treated with several anticonvulsants simultaneously, are at significant risk (1:800) for developing an idiosyncratic potentially fatal hepatotoxic syndrome, characterized by abdominal pain, anorexia, weight loss, and retching within a few weeks to months of beginning valproate therapy. These patients have normal results of liver function studies during the initial stages; thus, significant and persistent gastrointestinal symptoms are cause for alarm during the initial few months of valproate therapy. If reduction in the valproate dose does not provide immediate relief, the physician should discontinue the drug. To decrease the risk of fatal hepatotoxicity, a series of screening tests for an underlying metabolic disorder is indicated for a child younger than 2 yr and having a seizure disorder of unknown cause, before initiation of valproic acid therapy. The tests include determinations of serum ammonium, amino acids, blood gases, a lactate-pyruvate ratio, urinary organic acids, and free and total serum carnitine. The incidence of fatal valproic acid–induced hepatotoxicity has decreased dramatically in recent years due to less use of the drug in epileptic children younger than 2 yr and the knowledge that monotherapy is much less likely to result in fatal liver disease.

Valproic acid also may cause a decrease in serum-free carnitine levels by inhibition of plasmalemmal carnitine uptake. Some studies suggest that carnitine deficiency is a major cause of valproate hepatotoxicity and that supplementation with L-carnitine, 50–100 mg/kg/24 hr, may prevent this fatal complication. Until further data are available, it is recommended that L-carnitine supplementation be provided to those children at greatest risk for hepatotoxicity (see earlier). In older children on valproic acid therapy, L-carnitine supplementation should be administered if there are clinical symptoms suggestive of carnitine deficiency (weakness, lethargy, hypotonia) or if a significant decrease in the serum-free carnitine levels is measured on a periodic basis. Valproic acid is available in a syrup, 50 mg/mL; capsules, 250 and 500 mg; and tablets, 125, 250, and 500 mg.

Depakote sprinkle capsules (divalproex sodium, a stable coordination compound composed of sodium valproate and valproic acid) are useful for children who are unable to tolerate valproate suspension, tablets, or capsules. The contents of the Depakote capsule are sprinkled onto soft food that does not require chewing. Depakote sprinkle capsules are supplied in 125 mg capsules.

Vigabatrin. Vigabatrin acts by binding to the degradative enzyme GABA transaminase receptor, causing an increase in GABA levels and inhibition of neurotransmission (see Fig. 586–3). The drug is effective in the management of infantile spasms, particularly in children with tuberous sclerosis. Vigabatrin is also useful as adjunctive therapy for poorly controlled seizures. The plasma half-life is 5–8 hr. Vigabatrin may cause a reduction in plasma phenobarbital and phenytoin levels. Visual field constrictions have also been reported. The drug is supplied in 500 mg tablets and 500 mg sachets.

Leviractam. Leviracetam acts by an unknown mechanism and is indicated for use as an adjunctive treatment for partial seizures. Plasma half-life is approximately 8 hr. It is supplied in 250, 500, and 750 mg tablets as Keppra.

Oxcarbazepine. Oxcarbazepine has some similarity to carbamazepine in its action and is useful as an adjunctive treatment for partial seizures in adults and children. The half-life of the drug is 2 hr, whereas that of its major metabolite, 10-monohydroxy oxcarbazepine (MHD), is 9 hr. A total of 30% of patients with allergic reactions to carbamazepine also react to oxcarbazepine; hyponatremia occurs in 2.5% of patients. Oxcarbazepine is supplied as Trileptal in tablets, 150, 300, and 600 mg, and in suspension, 300 mg/5 mL.

Zonisamide. Zonisamide is useful as an adjunctive treatment for partial seizures and may also be useful for myoclonic syndromes, but its mechanism of action is unclear. As a single drug, its half-life is 60 hr; half-life is shortened to 30 hr when used with drugs metabolized by the liver. Zonisamide has been associated with development of renal calculi. It is supplied as Zonegran in 100 mg tablets.

ACTH. This is the preferred drug for the management of infantile spasms, although the dose and duration of therapy are not uniform. Prednisone is equally effective. A common schedule includes ACTH, 20 U/day IM for 2 wk, and if no response occurs, the dosage is increased to 30 and then 40 U/day IM for an additional 4 wk. Unless seizure control is complete, ACTH is replaced with oral prednisone, 2 mg/kg/24 hr for 2 wk. If the seizures persist, prednisone is given for an additional 4 wk. The side effects of ACTH include hyperglycemia, hypertension, electrolyte abnormalities, gastrointestinal disturbances, infection, and transient brain shrinkage observed by CT scanning. ACTH and prednisone are equally effective for the treatment of cryptogenic and symptomatic seizures, and control can be expected in approximately 70% of patients. There is no relationship between the ease or degree of seizure control and ultimate neurologic and cognitive outcome. The response to medication is usually apparent within a few weeks of therapy, but one third of patients who respond suffer relapse when the ACTH or prednisone is discontinued.

Ketogenic Diet. This treatment should be considered for the management of recalcitrant seizures, particularly for children with complex myoclonic epilepsy with associated tonic-clonic convulsions. The diet is also the primary therapy for infants with pyruvate dehydrogenase deficiency and glucose transporter protein deficiency and appears safe and effective for infants with epilepsy who are younger than 2 yr of age. The diet restricts the quantity of carbohydrate and protein, and most calories are provided as fat. Some children older than 2–3 yr will not tolerate this fatty, unpalatable diet. Because the diet demands precise weighing of foodstuffs and is time consuming to prepare, it is not accepted by all families. Some children respond to a liberalized ketogenic diet that substitutes medium-chain triglycerides for the high-fat content of the former diet. Although the mechanism of action of the ketogenic diet is unknown, some evidence shows that it exerts an anticonvulsant effect secondary to elevated levels of β-hydroxybutyrate and acetoacetate resulting from the ketosis. The use of valproic acid is contraindicated in association with the ketogenic diet, because the risk of hepatotoxicity is enhanced.

Surgery for Epilepsy. Surgery should be considered for children with intractable seizures unresponsive to anticonvulsants. Certain children, particularly those with focal seizures, are candidates for surgery. Although the history and neurologic examination may suggest a focal onset of seizure activity, an EEG is critical in documenting the localization and extent of the epileptogenic discharges. Prolonged EEG recording with video monitoring, which may be frequently necessary, is essential for precise localization of the epileptogenic area. It is often helpful to decrease or discontinue the anticonvulsant in hospitalized patients to increase the probability of recording ictal and interictal epileptogenic activity. When the EEG used with sphenoidal electrodes does not adequately localize the focus, placement of subdural electrodes may provide invaluable information. Subdural electrodes are particularly useful in the investigation of epileptogenic foci in sites other than the temporal lobe. EEG studies are complemented by neuropsychologic testing, the Wada (intracarotid injection of amobarbital to establish the dominant hemisphere) test, single-photon-emission CT (SPECT) or PET scanning, and neuroimaging procedures, including CT scanning, MRI, and functional MRI (fMRI). Some centers use magnetic source imaging/magnetoelectroencephalograms (MSI/MEG), which localize seizure discharges more precisely than other techniques. The results of surgery in children with a well-defined focus of epileptogenic activity supported by an identical structural lesion on CT scanning or MRI scan are extremely favorable and are comparable to those in adults with similar pathology.

Vagal Nerve Stimulation. Animal experiments have suggested that electrical stimulation of the left vagal nerve will interrupt or prevent seizures. In a double-blind trial in 60 children, 16 of whom were younger than 12 yr of age, left vagal nerve stimulation produced by an implanted device reduced seizures by 31–42% over 18 mo, suggesting that it may be a safe adjunctive therapy for patients refractory to other therapies.

Counseling the Parents. Most parents are initially frightened by the diagnosis of epilepsy and require support and accurate information. Physicians should anticipate questions, including inquiries about the duration of the seizure disorder, side effects of medication and convulsions, etiology, social and academic repercussions, and parental guilt. Parents usually wish to know if restrictions should be placed on the child and whether the teacher should be informed. Others inquire about the genetic implications, including the risks for future children. Parents should be encouraged to treat their child as normally as possible. For most children with epilepsy, restriction of physical activity is unnecessary except that they must be attended by a responsible adult while bathing and swimming. The mechanism of the seizure and what epilepsy means should be explained, and the purpose and side effects of the specific anticonvulsant should be reviewed. Parents who understand the fundamental action and purpose of anticonvulsants and the need for a specific drug regimen are generally compliant. Counseling should include first-aid measures to be used if the seizure recurs. Fortunately, most parents and children readily adapt to the seizure disorder and to the requirement for long-term anticonvulsants. Most cases of epilepsy in children are well controlled with medication; the children have normal intelligence and can be expected to lead normal lives. These children require careful monitoring of their academic performance because learning disabilities are more common in children with epilepsy than in the general population. Cooperation and understanding among the parents, physician, teacher, and child enhance the outlook for patients with epilepsy.

Baram TZ, Mitchell WG, Tournay A, et al: High-dose corticotropin (ACTH) versus prednisone for infantile spasms: A prospective, randomized, blinded study. *Pediatrics* 1996;97:375.

Baumann RJ, Duffner PK: Treatment of children with simple febrile seizures: the AAP practice parameter. *Pediatr Neurol* 2000;23:11.

Berg AT, Testa FM, Levy SR, et al: Neuroimaging in children with newly diagnosed epilepsy: A community-based study. *Pediatrics* 2000;196:527.

Berkovic SF, Andermann F, Carpenter S, et al: Progressive myoclonus epilepsies: Specific causes and diagnosis. *N Engl J Med* 1986;315:296.

Camfield PR, Camfield CS, Dooley JM, et al: Epilepsy after a first unprovoked seizure in childhood. *Neurology* 1985;35:1657.

Duchowny M, Harvey AS: Pediatric epilepsy syndromes: An update and critical review. *Epilepsia* 1996;37(Suppl 1):S26.

Hirtz D, Ashwal MD, Berg A, BettisD, et al: Practice parameter: Evaluating a first nonfebrile seizure in children. *Neurology* 2000;55:616.

Kriel RL, Cloyd JC, Pellock JM, et al: Rectal diazepam gel for treatment of acute repetitive seizures. *Pediatr Neurol* 1999;20:282.

Minassian BA: Lafora's disease: Towards a clinical, pathologic,and molecular sythensis. *Pediatr Neurol* 2001;25:21–9.

Minassian BA, Lee JR, Henbrick JA, et al: Mutations in a gene encoding a novel protein tyrosine phosphate cause progressive myoclonus epilepsy. *Nat Genet* 1998;20:171.

Murphy JV, et al: Left vagal nerve stimulation in children with medically refractory epilepsy. *J Pediatr* 1994;134:563.

Nordli DR, Kuroda MM, Carroll J, et al: Experience with the ketogenic diet in infants. *Pediatrics* 2001;198:129.

Robinson R, Gardiner M: Genetics of childhood epilepsy. *Arch Dis Child* 2000;82:121.

Shinnar S, Berg AT, Moshe SL, et al: The risk of seizure recurrence following a first unprovoked seizure in childhood: An extended followup. *Pediatrics* 1996;98:216.

Shinnar S, Pellock JM: Update on the epidemiology and prognosis of pediatric epilepsy. *J Child Neurol* 2002;17:S54-17.

Singh NA, Charlier C, Stauffer D, et al: A novel potassium channel gene, KCNQ$_2$, is mutated in an inherited epilepsy of newborns. *Nat Genet* 1998;18:25.

Vining EP, Freeman JM, Pillas DJ, et al: Why would you remove half a brain? The outcome of 58 children after hemispherectomy—The Johns Hopkins experience: 1968 to 1996. *Pediatrics* 1997;100:163.

Wallace SJ: First tonic-clonic seizures in childhood. *Lancet* 1997;349:1009.

Wiebe S, Blume WT, Girvin JP, et al: A randomized, controlled trial of surgery for temporal-lobe epilepsy. *N Engl J Med* 2110;345:311.

Wong M, Schlaggar BL, Landt M: Postictal cerebrospinal fluid abnormalities in children. *J Pediatr* 2001;138:373.

586.7 Neonatal Seizures (see Chapters 86–89)

Neonates are at particular risk for the development of seizures because metabolic, toxic, structural, and infectious diseases are more likely to be manifested during this time than at any other period of life. Neonatal seizures are dissimilar from those in a child or adult because generalized tonic-clonic convulsions tend not to occur during the 1st mo of life. The arborization of axons and dendritic processes as well as myelination is incomplete in the neonatal brain. A seizure discharge, therefore, cannot readily be propagated throughout the neonatal brain to produce a generalized seizure. At least five seizure types are recognizable in newborn infants.

Clinical Manifestations and Classification. *Focal seizures* consist of rhythmic twitching of muscle groups, particularly those of the extremities and face. These seizures are often associated with localized structural lesions as well as with infections and subarachnoid hemorrhage. *Multifocal clonic* convulsions are similar to focal clonic seizures but differ in that many muscle groups are involved, frequently several simultaneously. *Tonic seizures* are characterized by rigid posturing of the extremities and trunk and are sometimes associated with fixed deviation of the eyes. *Myoclonic seizures* are brief focal or generalized jerks of the extremities or body that tend to involve distal muscle groups. *Subtle seizures* consist of chewing motions, excessive salivation, and alterations in the respiratory rate including apnea, blinking, nystagmus, bicycling or pedaling movements, and changes in color.

Neonatal seizures may be difficult to recognize clinically, and some neonatal behaviors that were considered previously to be convulsions are not substantiated by the EEG recording. Nonetheless, several clinical features distinguish seizures from nonepileptic activity in neonates. Autonomic changes such as tachycardia and elevation of the blood pressure are common with seizures but do not occur with nonepileptic events. Nonepileptic movements are suppressed by gentle restraint, but true seizures are not. Nonepileptic phenomena are enhanced by sensory stimuli that have no influence on seizures. Correct classification of neonatal seizures is important for appropriate selection of anticonvulsant therapy. Studies using polygraphic EEG recording with video monitoring have greatly enhanced the characterization of neonatal seizures and their medical management.

EEG Classification of Neonatal Seizures
    CLINICAL SEIZURE WITH A CONSISTENT EEG EVENT. In this category, a clinical seizure occurs in relationship to seizure activity recorded on the EEG and includes focal clonic, focal tonic, and some myoclonic seizures. These seizures are clearly epileptic and are likely to respond to an anticonvulsant.

CLINICAL SEIZURES WITH INCONSISTENT EEG EVENTS. Neonates may have a clinical seizure without a corresponding seizure discharge. This is observed with all generalized tonic seizures and subtle seizures and with some myoclonic seizures. These infants tend to be neurologically depressed or comatose as a result of hypoxic-ischemic encephalopathy. Seizures in this category are likely to be of nonepileptic origin and may not require or respond to antiepileptics.

ELECTRICAL SEIZURES WITH ABSENT CLINICAL SEIZURES. Electrical seizures associated with a markedly abnormal background EEG may develop in comatose infants who are not on anticonvulsants. Conversely, electrical seizures may persist in patients with focal tonic or clonic seizures without clinical signs after the introduction of an anticonvulsant.

Etiologic Diagnosis. The most common cause of neonatal seizures, hypoxic-ischemic encephalopathy, is discussed in Chapter 88.7. Many additional disorders are likely to cause seizures, including metabolic, infectious, traumatic, structural, hemorrhagic, embolic, and maternal disturbances. Because seizures in neonates may indicate a serious, life-threatening, and potentially reversible disease, it is imperative that a timely and organized approach to the investigation of neonatal seizures be carried out.

Careful neurologic examination of the infant may uncover the cause of the seizure disorder. Examination of the retina may show the presence of chorioretinitis, suggesting a congenital infection in which case TORCH titers of mother and infant are indicated. The **Aicardi syndrome,** which occurs exclusively in infant girls, is associated with coloboma of the iris and retinal lacunae, refractory seizures, and absence of the corpus callosum. Inspection of the skin may show hypopigmented lesions characteristic of tuberous sclerosis or the typical crusted vesicular lesions of incontinentia pigmenti; both neurocutaneous syndromes are associated with generalized myoclonic seizures beginning early in life. An unusual body odor suggests an inborn error of metabolism.

Blood should be obtained for determinations of glucose, calcium, magnesium, electrolytes, and blood urea nitrogen. If hypoglycemia is a possibility, a serum Dextrostix testing is indicated so that treatment can be initiated immediately. See Chapter 96.2 for a discussion of the diagnosis and treatment of hypoglycemia. Hypocalcemia may occur in isolation or in association with hypomagnesemia. A lowered serum calcium level is often associated with birth trauma or a CNS insult in the perinatal period. Additional causes include maternal diabetes, prematurity, DiGeorge syndrome, and high-phosphate feedings. See Chapters 48.9 and 95 for a full discussion. Hypomagnesemia (<1.5 mg/dL) is often associated with hypocalcemia and occurs particularly in infants of malnourished mothers. In this situation, the seizures are resistant to calcium therapy but respond to intramuscular magnesium, 0.2 mL/kg of a 50% solution of $MgSO_4$. See Chapter 95 for diagnosis and treatment of hypomagnesemia. Serum electrolyte measurement may indicate significant hyponatremia (serum sodium <135 mEq/L) or hypernatremia (serum sodium >150 mEq/L) as a cause of the seizure disorder.

A *lumbar puncture* is indicated in virtually all neonates with seizures, unless the cause is obviously related to a metabolic disorder such as hypoglycemia or hypocalcemia secondary to feeding of high concentrations of phosphate. These latter infants are normally alert interictally and usually respond promptly to appropriate therapy. The CSF findings may indicate a bacterial meningitis or aseptic encephalitis (see Chapters 98 and 594). Prompt diagnosis and appropriate therapy improve the outcome for these infants. Bloody CSF indicates a traumatic tap or a subarachnoid/intraventricular bleed. Immediate centrifugation of the specimen may assist in differentiation of the two disorders. A clear supernatant suggests a traumatic tap, and a xanthochromic color suggests a subarachnoid bleed. However, mildly jaundiced normal infants may have a yellowish discoloration of the CSF that makes inspection of the supernatant less reliable in the newborn period.

Many *inborn errors of metabolism* cause generalized convulsions in the newborn period. Because these conditions are often inherited in an autosomal recessive or X-linked recessive fashion, it is imperative that a careful family history be obtained to determine whether siblings or close relatives developed seizures or died at an early age. Serum ammonia determination is useful for screening for suspected urea cycle abnormalities, such as ornithine transcarbamylase, arginosuccinic lysate, and carbamoylphosphate synthetase deficiencies. In addition to having generalized clonic seizures, these infants present during the first few days of life with increasing lethargy progressing to coma, anorexia and vomiting, and a bulging fontanel. If the blood gases show an anion gap and a metabolic acidosis with hyperammonemia, urine organic acids should be immediately determined to investigate the possibility of methylmalonic or propionic acidemia. Maple syrup urine disease (MSUD) should be suspected when a metabolic acidosis occurs in association with generalized clonic seizures, vomiting, and muscle rigidity during the 1st wk of life. The result of a rapid screening test using 2,4-dinitrophenylhydrazine that identifies ketoderivatives in the urine is positive in MSUD. Additional metabolic causes of neonatal seizures include nonketotic hyperglycemia, a lethal condition characterized by markedly elevated plasma and CSF glycine levels, persistent generalized seizures, and lethargy rapidly leading to coma; ketotic hyperglycinemia in which seizures are associated with vomiting, fluid and electrolyte disturbances, and a metabolic acidosis; and Leigh disease suggested by elevated levels of serum and CSF lactate or an increased lactate/pyruvate ratio. Biotinidase deficiency should also be considered. A comprehensive description of the diagnosis and management of these metabolic diseases is discussed in Part X.

Unintentional *injection of a local anesthetic* into a fetus during labor can produce intense tonic seizures. These infants are often thought to have had a traumatic delivery because they are flaccid at birth, they have abnormal brainstem reflexes, and they show signs of respiratory depression that sometimes requires ventilation. Examination may show a needle puncture of the skin or a perforation or laceration of the scalp. An elevated serum anesthetic level confirms the diagnosis. The treatment consists of supportive measures and promotion of urine output by administering intravenous fluids with appropriate monitoring to prevent fluid overload.

Benign familial neonatal seizures, an autosomal dominant condition, begins on the 2nd–3rd day of life, with a seizure frequency of 10–20/day. Patients are normal between seizures, which stop in 1–6 mo. *Fifth-day fits* occur on day 5 of life (4–6 days) in normal-appearing neonates. The seizures are multifocal and are present for less than 24 hr. The prognosis is good.

Pyridoxine dependency, a rare disorder, must be considered when generalized clonic seizures begin shortly after birth with signs of fetal distress in utero. These seizures are particularly resistant to conventional anticonvulsants, such as phenobarbital or phenytoin. The history may suggest that similar seizures occurred in utero. Some cases of pyridoxine dependency are reported to begin later in infancy or in early childhood. This condition is inherited as an autosomal recessive. Although the precise biochemical defect is unknown, pyridoxine is essential for the synthesis of glutamic acid decarboxylase, which, in turn, is required for the synthesis of GABA. In affected infants, large amounts of pyridoxine are required to maintain adequate production of GABA. When pyridoxine-dependent seizures are suspected, pyridoxine, 100–200 mg IV, should be administered intravenously during the EEG, which should be promptly completed once the diagnosis is considered. The seizures abruptly cease, and the EEG normalizes during the next few hours.

However, not all cases of pyridoxine dependency respond dramatically to the initial bolus of IV pyridoxine. Therefore, A 6-wk trial of oral pyridoxine (10–20 mg/day) is recommended for infants in whom a high index of suspicion continues after a negative response to IV pyridoxine. In the future, measurement of CSF and plasma pyridoxal-5-phosphate may prove to be the more precise method of confirming the diagnosis of pyridoxine dependency. These children require lifelong supplementation of oral pyridoxine, 10 mg/day. Generally, the earlier the diagnosis and therapy with pyridoxine, the more favorable is the outcome. Untreated children have persistent seizures and are uniformly severely mentally retarded (see also Chapter 44.6).

Drug withdrawal seizures can present in the newborn nursery but may take several weeks to develop because of prolonged excretion of the drug by the neonate. The incriminated drugs include barbiturates, benzodiazepines, heroin, and methadone. The infant may be jittery, irritable, and lethargic and may show myoclonus or frank clonic seizures. The mother may deny the use of drugs; a serum or urine analysis may identify the responsible agent (see Chapter 95).

Infants with focal seizures, suspected stroke or intracranial hemorrhage, and severe *cytoarchitectural abnormalities* of the brain—including lissencephaly and schizencephaly—who clinically may appear normal or microcephalic should undergo MRI or CT scan. Indeed, many recommend imaging of all neonates with seizures unexplained by serum glucose, calcium, or electrolyte disorders. Infants with chromosome abnormalities and adrenoleukodystrophy are also at risk for seizures and should be evaluated with investigation of a karyotype and serum long-chain fatty acids, respectively.

Treatment. Anticonvulsants should be used in the treatment of infants with seizures secondary to hypoxic-ischemic encephalopathy or an acute intracranial bleed (see Chapters 88.2 and 88.7). The dose and administration of phenobarbital, diazepam, and other medications for the treatment of neonatal seizures are discussed in Chapter 88.7. Phenytoin and phenobarbital are equally but incompletely effective as anticonvulsants in neonates, controlling seizures in less than half of cases. The greater use of EEG recording in infants with subtle seizures has identified a number of patients with abnormal movements unrelated to seizure discharges.

Prognosis. This depends mainly on the primary cause of the disorder or the severity of the insult. In the case of hypoglycemic infants of a diabetic mother or hypocalcemia associated with excessive phosphate feedings, the prognosis is excellent. Conversely, a child with intractable seizures due to severe hypoxic-ischemic encephalopathy or a cytoarchitectural abnormality of the brain usually does not respond to anticonvulsants and is susceptible to status epilepticus and early death. The challenge for the physician is to identify patients who will recover with prompt treatment and to avoid delays in diagnosis that could lead to severe, irreversible neurologic damage.

Donn S, Grasela T, Goldstein G: Safety of a higher loading dose of phenobarbital in the term newborn. *Pediatrics* 1985;74:1061.

Gilman JT, Gal P, Duchowny MS, et al: Rapid sequential phenobarbital treatment of neonatal seizures. *Pediatrics* 1989;83:674.

Gospe SM, Olin KL, Keen CL: Reduced GABA synthesis in pyridoxine-dependent seizures. *Lancet* 1994;343:1133.

Herzlinger RA, Krandall SR, Vaughan HG: Neonatal seizures associated with narcotic withdrawal. *J Pediatr* 1977;91:683.

Hillman L, Hillman R, Dodson WE: Diagnosis, treatment and follow-up of neonatal mepivacaine intoxication secondary to paracervical and pudendal blocks during labor. *J Pediatr* 1979;95:472.

Hunt AD, Stokes J, McCrory WW, et al: Pyridoxine dependency: Report of a case of intractable convulsions in an infant controlled by pyridoxine. *Pediatrics* 1964;13:140.

Legido A, Clancy RR, Berman P: Neurologic outcome after electroencephalographically proven neonatal seizures. *Pediatrics* 1991;88:583.

Mizrahi E, Kellaway P: Characterizations and classification of neonatal seizures. *Neurology* 1987;37:1837.

Painter MJ, Scher MS, Stein AD, et al: Phenobarbital compared with phenytoin for treatment of neonatal seizures. *N Engl J Med* 1999;341:485.

Sillanpää M, Jalava M, Kaleva O, et al: Long-term prognosis of seizures with onset in childhood. *N Engl J Med* 1998;338:1715.

Torres OA, Miller VS, Buist NM, et al: Folinic acid-responsive neonatal seizures. *J Child Neurol* 1999;14:529.

Volpe JJ: Neonatal seizures: Current concepts and revised classification. *Pediatrics* 1989;84:422.

586.8 Status Epilepticus

Status epilepticus is defined as a continuous convulsion lasting longer than 30 min or the occurrence of serial convulsions between which there is no return of consciousness. Status epilepticus may be classified as generalized (tonic-clonic, absence) or partial (simple, complex, or with secondary generalization). Generalized tonic-clonic seizures predominate in cases of status epilepticus. Status epilepticus is a medical emergency that requires an organized and skillful approach to minimize the associated mortality and morbidity.

Etiology. There are three major subtypes of status epilepticus in children: prolonged *febrile seizures; idiopathic status epilepticus,* in which a seizure develops in the absence of an underlying CNS lesion or insult; and *symptomatic status epilepticus,* when the seizure occurs as a result of an underlying neurologic disorder or a metabolic abnormality. A febrile seizure lasting for more than 30 min, particularly in a child younger than 3 yr of age, is the most common cause of status epilepticus. The idiopathic group includes epileptic patients who have had sudden withdrawal of anticonvulsants (especially benzodiazepines and barbiturates) followed by status epilepticus. Epileptic children who are given anticonvulsants on an irregular basis or who are noncompliant are more likely to develop status epilepticus. Status epilepticus may also be the initial presentation of epilepsy. Sleep deprivation and an intercurrent infection tend to render epileptic patients more susceptible to status epilepticus. The mortality and morbidity among patients with prolonged febrile seizures and idiopathic status epilepticus are low.

Status epilepticus owing to other causes has a much higher mortality rate, and the cause of death usually is directly attributable to the underlying abnormality. Unlike those with idiopathic status epilepticus, many of these children have not previously had a convulsion. Severe anoxic encephalopathy presents with seizures during the first few days of life, and the ultimate prognosis relates partly to the ease in controlling the seizures. A prolonged convulsion may be the initial manifestation of encephalitis, and epilepsy may be a long-term complication of meningitis. Infants with congenital malformations of the brain (e.g., lissencephaly or schizencephaly) may have recurrent episodes of status epilepticus that are frequently refractory to anticonvulsants. Inborn errors of metabolism may present with status epilepticus in newborns. Affected infants often have a progressive loss of consciousness associated with failure to thrive and excessive vomiting. Electrolyte abnormalities, hypocalcemia, hypoglycemia, drug intoxication, Reye syndrome, lead intoxication, extreme hyperpyrexia, and brain tumors, particularly in the frontal lobe, are additional causes of status epilepticus.

Pathophysiology. The relationship between the neurologic outcome and the duration of status epilepticus is unknown in children and adults. Some evidence shows that the period of status epilepticus that produces neuronal injury in a child is less than that for an adult. In primates, pathologic changes can occur in the brain of ventilated animals after 60 min of constant seizure activity when metabolic homeostasis is maintained. Cell death may result from excessive release of the excitatory neurotransmitter glutamate and excessive stimulation of glutamate receptors, a process known as "excitotoxicity." The most vulnerable areas of the brain include the hippocampus, amygdala, cerebellum, middle cortical area, and thalamus. Characteristic acute pathologic changes consist of venous congestion, small petechial hemorrhages, and edema. Ischemic cellular changes are the earliest histologic finding, followed by neuronophagia, microglial proliferation, cell loss, and increased numbers of reactive astrocytes. Neuronal concentrations of calcium, arachidonic acid, and prostaglandins increase and may promote cell death. Prolonged generalized seizure activity may lead to dysfunction of the autonomic nervous system with hypotension and shock as well as to lactic acidosis, myoglobinuria, elevated lactic acid levels, and acute tubular necrosis.

Several investigations have shown that seizures become more difficult to stop and the chances of neuronal injury increase when seizures persist beyond a *transitional period* that varies between 20 and 60 min in animals during constant seizure activity. Treatment of children should be directed to supporting vital functions and to controlling the convulsions as expeditiously as possible, because the precise transitional period in humans is unknown.

Treatment. *Initial treatment* of patients begins with an assessment of the respiratory and cardiovascular systems. Children should be transferred to an intensive care unit if possible. The oral airway is secured and inspected for patency, and the pulse, temperature, respirations, and blood pressure are recorded. Excessive oral secretions are removed by gentle suction, and a properly fitting face mask attached to oxygen is applied. If patients do not respond to oxygen by mask or are difficult to ventilate by an Ambu bag, consideration should be given to intubation and assisted ventilation. A nasogastric tube is placed in position, and an IV catheter is immediately inserted. If hypoglycemia is confirmed by Dextrostix, a rapid infusion of 5 mL/kg of 10% dextrose is provided. Blood is obtained for a CBC and for determination of electrolytes (including calcium, phosphorus, and magnesium), glucose, creatinine, lactate, and anticonvulsant levels, if indicated. Blood and urine may be obtained for metabolic studies and toxicology, keeping in mind that some drugs potentiate or precipitate status epilepticus (e.g., amphetamines, cocaine, phenothiazines, theophylline in toxic levels, and tricyclic antidepressants). Arterial blood gases should be determined, and it is wise to monitor oxygen saturation (SaO_2) with an oximeter. Examination of the CSF is imperative if meningitis or encephalitis is considered, unless there is a contraindication to the procedure. In this case, appropriate antibiotics should be administered, followed by imaging studies, before a lumbar puncture is attempted. If the seizures are refractory to the front-line anticonvulsants or if the patient is paralyzed and is on a respirator, continuous EEG monitoring is important to assess the frequency of seizure discharges, their location, and the response to anticonvulsant therapy.

A physical and neurologic examination should be carried out concurrently to assess the following: evidence of trauma; papilledema, a bulging anterior fontanel, or lateralizing neurologic signs suggesting increased ICP; manifestations of sepsis or meningitis; retinal hemorrhages that may indicate a subdural hematoma; Kussmaul breathing and dehydration suggestive of metabolic acidosis or irregular respirations signifying brainstem dysfunction; evidence of failure to thrive, a peculiar body odor, or abnormal hair pigmentation that suggests an inborn error of metabolism; and constriction or dilatation of pupils suggesting a toxin or drugs as the cause of the status epilepticus. A comprehensive examination should be undertaken once the seizures are under control. Further investigation of the patient including neuroradiologic studies depends on the physical and neurologic findings and on a precise history of the seizure type and frequency.

Drugs should always be administered IV in the management of status epilepticus; the IM route is unreliable because some drugs are sequestered by muscle. One of the major problems in the management of status epilepticus is the inappropriate use of anticonvulsants. An unsuitably low drug dose is too often given, and with lack of response, another antiepileptic is introduced immediately. Care should be given with regard to how the anticonvulsant is administered. Phenytoin forms a precipitate in glucose solutions and is rendered ineffective. Other drugs interact with plastic containers or are altered by sunlight (e.g., paraldehyde). It is essential to have resuscitation equipment at the bedside and the ability to intubate and ventilate the patient immediately if respiratory depression occurs.

A *benzodiazepine* (diazepam, lorazepam, or midazolam) may be used initially, because these are effective for immediate control of prolonged tonic-clonic seizures in most children. Diazepam should be given IV directly into the vein (not the tubing) in a dose of 0.1–0.3 mg/kg at a rate no greater than 2 mg/min for a maximum of three doses. Respiratory depression and hypotension can occur, especially if administered with a barbiturate. Benzodiazepines may be as effective as pentobarbital with fewer side effects. Diazepam is effective in the management of tonic-clonic status, but the drug has a short half-life and seizures thus recur unless a longer acting anticonvulsant is administered simultaneously. Lorazepam is an equally effective short-term anticonvulsant, with a greater duration of action and decreased likelihood of producing hypotension and respiratory arrest. The recommended dose is 0.05–0.1 mg/kg IV administered slowly. The dose of midazolam is 0.15–0.3 mg/kg IV. If an IV line cannot be established or the child is some distance from a medical center, rectal diazepam or lorazepam can be used safely. Diazepam diluted in 3 mL 0.9% NaCl is placed into the rectum by a syringe and a flexible tube at a dose of 0.3–0.5 mg/kg. The effective dose of rectal lorazepam is 0.05–0.1 mg/kg. Therapeutic serum levels occur within 5–10 min. Sublingual lorazepam may be used to treat children with serial seizures that tend to develop into status epilepticus while the children are at home. The dose of sublingual lorazepam is 0.05–0.1 mg/kg. The tablet is placed under the patient's tongue and dissolves in a few seconds. Rectal diazepam gel (Diastat, pediatric doses of 2.5, 5, or 10 mg) may also be useful.

After administration of diazepam or lorazepam, several options are available for further management. If the convulsive activity ceases after diazepam or lorazepam therapy or if the seizures persist, *phenytoin* is given immediately. The loading dose of phenytoin is 15 up to 30 mg/kg IV (given in 10 mg/kg increments) at the rate of 1 mg/kg/min. The phenytoin prodrug fosphenytoin has advantages over the older formulation because it is water soluble, less irritating after IV injection, and well absorbed after intramuscular injection. Parenteral fosphenytoin (Cerebyx) is formulated in phenytoin equivalent (PE) units to allow the administration of the same amount of phenytoin despite its higher molecular weight (150 mg of fosphenytoin equals 100 mg of phenytoin). The dosage in PE units is the same as for the older phenytoin preparation. The older preparation of phenytoin may be safely added to half-normal or normal saline but not to glucose solutions; the undiluted drug can cause pain, irritation, and phlebitis of the vein. Electrocardiography is recommended during the loading phase to identify arrhythmias and bradycardia, a rare complication in children. Systemic hypotension may also complicate IV phenytoin. If the seizures do not recur, a maintenance dose of 3–9 mg/kg divided into two equal doses daily is begun 12–24 hr later. Serum phenytoin levels should be monitored because the maintenance dose varies considerably with age. Phenytoin is not always effective in controlling tonic-clonic status epilepticus, in which case an alternative drug is necessary. In some centers, *phenobarbital* is initiated before phenytoin. It is given in a loading dose of 15–20 mg/kg or in neonates 20–30 mg/kg IV during 10–30 min. With control of the seizures, the maintenance dose is 3–5 mg/kg/24 hr divided into two equal doses.

If the status epilepticus is not controlled by the preceding strategy, the physician must make some important therapeutic decisions, because it is likely the *transitional period* has passed. The choices for further drug management include paraldehyde, a diazepam infusion, barbiturate coma, or general anesthesia. By this stage, the patient is usually sedated and may show signs of respiratory depression, necessitating elective intubation and assisted ventilation.

Constant IV infusion of either midazolam (0.20 mg/kg bolus, 20–400 μg/kg/hr infusion) or propofol (1–2 mg/kg, 2–10 mg/kg/hr infusion) has been effective in managing seizures during status epilepticus unresponsive to other anticonvulsants. If seizures continue, serious consideration is given to induction of barbiturate coma. In an intensive care unit, the patient is placed on a ventilator and a continuous EEG monitor. The initial IV loading dose of thiopental is 2–4 mg/kg and is then titrated to achieve a burst suppression EEG pattern. Barbiturate coma is continued for at least 48 hr, followed by cessation of thiopental until the serum phenobarbital level falls to the therapeutic range. Barbiturate coma requires careful monitoring because hypotension due to myocardial depression often requires pressor therapy.

Paraldehyde is relatively safe for administration to children. A 5% solution of paraldehyde is prepared by adding 1.75 mL of paraldehyde (1 g/mL) to D5W to a total volume of 35 mL. The loading dose is 150–200 mg/kg IV slowly for 15–20 min, and then seizure control is maintained with an infusion of 20 mg/kg/hr in a 5% concentration in a glass bottle, because the drug is incompatible with plastic. The IV drip rate may be lowered as the seizures and EEG improve. The drug should be freshly opened, because outdated paraldehyde can deteriorate to acetylaldehyde and acetic acid.

General anesthesia is an alternative adjunct to the management of status epilepticus if conventional drug therapy is not effective or if barbiturate coma is not an option. Several agents have been used successfully, including halothane and isoflurane. General anesthesia probably acts by reversing cerebral anoxia and the concomitant metabolic abnormalities, allowing the previously administered anticonvulsants to exert their effect. The major disadvantage of general anesthesia is that it must be administered by well-trained personnel with anesthetic gas scavenging equipment for prolonged periods.

Valproic acid has been an effective anticonvulsant in the management of several types of seizures. Valproic acid is available as an injectable and may be given IV. Preliminary studies recommend a loading dose of IV valproic acid, 10–15 mg/kg. IV valproic acid may become a useful drug for status epilepticus.

The use of anticonvulsant therapy after status epilepticus is controversial. There is little question that a long-term antiepileptic should be maintained in children with a progressive neurologic disorder or with a history of recurrent seizures before the onset of status epilepticus. However, it is unlikely that a lengthy period of anticonvulsant treatment is necessary after an initial attack of idiopathic status epilepticus, particularly when a prolonged febrile seizure was the cause. Anticonvulsant therapy is maintained arbitrarily for 3 mo in this case and is discontinued if the child remains asymptomatic.

Prognosis. Status epilepticus produces potentially life-threatening disturbances in physiologic function and the mortality rate of status epilepticus is approximately 5%. The greatest number of deaths occur in the symptomatic group, most of whom have a serious and life-threatening CNS disorder known before the onset of status epilepticus. In the absence of a progressive neurologic insult (e.g., herpes encephalitis) or metabolic disorder, the morbidity from status epilepticus is low. The fact that long-term sequelae such as hemiplegia, extrapyramidal syndromes, mental retardation, and epilepsy are more common in children younger than 1 yr following status epilepticus is related to the fact that this group is more likely to have a premorbid underlying CNS disorder than are older children. Nevertheless, there remains considerable debate over whether prolonged status epilepticus can damage the brain as has been shown in animal experiments. It is noteworthy that febrile status epilepticus in a neurologically impaired child is a risk factor for subsequent febrile as well as nonfebrile seizures, but febrile status in an otherwise normal child does not increase the risk of seizures. MRI brain scan performed in several infants demonstrated that complex febrile convulsions can occasionally be associated with acute hippocampal injury progressing to atrophy. In some of these infants, pathology and brain imaging also demonstrated evidence of pre-existing cerebral dysgenesis. These cases suggest that hippocampal sclerosis associated with status epilepticus may reflect interaction between pre-existing and acquired processes.

Aicardi J, Chevrie JJ: Consequences of status epilepticus in infants and children. *Adv Neurol* 1983;34:115.

Claassen J, Hirsch LJ, Emerson RG, et al: Treatment of refractory status epilepticus with pentobarbitol, propofol, or midazolam: A systemic review. *Epilepsia* 2002;43:146.

Hanhan UA, Fiallos MR, Orlowski JP: Status epilepticus. *Pediatr Clin North Am* 2001;48:683.

Holmes GL, Riviello JJ: Midazolam and pentobarbital for refractory status epilepticus. *Pediatr Neurol* 1999;20:259.

Lowenstein DH, Alldredge BK: Status epilepticus. *N Engl J Med* 1998;338:970.

Maytal J, Shinnar S: Febrile status epilepticus. *Pediatrics* 1990;86:611.

Maytal J, Shinnar S, Moshe SL, et al: Low morbidity and mortality of status epilepticus in children. *Pediatrics* 1989;83:323.

Perez ER, Maeder P, Villemure KM, et al: Acquired hippocampal damage after temporal lobe seizures in 2 infants. *Ann Neurol* 2000;48:384.

Sabin M, Menache CC. Holmes GL, et al: Outcome of severe refractory status epilepticus in children. *Epilepsia* 2001;42:1161.

Shinnar S, Pellock JM, Berg AT, et al: Short-term outcomes of children with febrile status epilepticus. *Epilepsia* 2001;42:47.

VanLandingham KE, Heinz ER, Cavazos JE, et al: Magnetic resonance imaging evidence of hippocampal injury after prolonged focal febrile convulsions. *Ann Neurol* 1998;43:413.

Working Group on Status Epilepticus: Treatment of convulsive status epilepticus. *JAMA* 1993;270:854.

Chapter 587
Conditions that Mimic Seizures

Michael V. Johnston

Several conditions share common features with epilepsy. Because these disorders may be associated with altered levels of consciousness, tonic or clonic movements, or cyanosis, they are often confused with epilepsy. Affected children may be inappropriately placed on many anticonvulsants with no response and some risk; conditions that mimic epilepsy are refractory to antiepileptic drugs. The treatment of these children differs significantly from those with epilepsy.

Benign Paroxysmal Vertigo. Benign paroxysmal vertigo (BPV) typically develops in toddlers and is relatively rare beyond 3 yr of age. The attacks develop suddenly and are associated with ataxia, causing the child to fall or refuse to walk or sit. Horizontal nystagmus may be evident during the duration of the attack. The child appears frightened and pale. Nausea and vomiting may be prominent. Consciousness and the ability to verbalize are not disturbed; lethargy or drowsiness do not follow completion of the episode. The attacks vary in duration (seconds to minutes), frequency (daily to monthly), and intensity. A rotational sensation (vertigo) is verbalized by older children with BPV. These children are susceptible to motion sickness and may develop migraine headaches several years later, suggesting a relationship between BPV and migraine. Neurologic evaluation characteristically yields negative results, except for the finding of abnormal vestibular function detected by ice water caloric testing. Patients with clusters of attacks usually respond to diphenhydramine, 5 mg/kg/24 hr with a maximum of 300 mg/24 hr PO, IM, IV, or per rectum.

Night Terrors. Night terrors are common, particularly in boys between 5 and 7 yr of age (see Chapter 22). They occur in 1–3% of children and are usually short-lived. A night terror has a sudden onset, usually between midnight and 2:00 AM during stage 3 or 4 of slow-wave sleep. The child screams and appears frightened, with dilated pupils, tachycardia, and hyperventilation. There is little or no verbalization; the child may thrash violently, cannot be consoled, and is unaware of parents or surroundings. Sleep follows in a few minutes, and there is total amnesia the following morning. Approximately one third of children with night terrors experience somnambulism. An underlying emotional disorder should be explored in children with persistent and prolonged night terrors. A short course of diazepam or imipramine may be considered for treatment of protracted night terrors while the family dynamics are under investigation.

Breath-Holding Spells. A breath-holding spell can be a frightening experience for parents because the infant becomes lifeless and unresponsive owing to cerebral anoxia at the height of the attack. There are two major types of breath-holding spells: the more common cyanotic form and the pallid form. Also see Chapter 25.

CYANOTIC SPELLS. A cyanotic breath-holding spell is usually predictable and is always provoked by upsetting or scolding an infant. The episode is heralded by a brief, shrill cry followed by forced expiration and apnea. There is rapid onset of generalized cyanosis and a loss of consciousness that may be associated with repeated generalized clonic jerks, opisthotonos, and bradycardia. Results of an interictal electroencephalogram (EEG) are normal. A breath-holding spell can occur repeatedly within a few hours or it can recur sporadically, but it is always stereotyped. Breath-holding spells are rare before 6 mo of age, they peak at about 2 yr of age, and they abate by 5 yr of age. The management of breath-holding spells concentrates on the support and reassurance of the parents. Some parents feel that whatever the physician recommends, they must splash cold water on the face, turn the child upside down, or initiate mouth-to-mouth resuscitation and even cardiopulmonary resuscitation. A thorough examination followed by an explanation of the mechanism of breath-holding spells is reassuring for most parents. The counseling session should emphasize the need for both parents to be consistent and not reinforce the child's behavior after the child recovers from the spell. This may be accomplished by placing the child safely in bed and by refusing to cuddle, play, or hold the child for a given period of time until recovery is complete.

PALLID SPELLS. These spells are much less common than cyanotic breath-holding spells, but they share several characteristics. Pallid spells are typically initiated by a painful experience, such as falling and striking the head or a sudden startle. The child stops breathing, rapidly loses consciousness, becomes pale and hypotonic, and may have a tonic seizure. Bradycardia with periods of asystole of longer than 2 sec may be recorded. The interictal EEG is normal. Pallid spells can in some cases be induced spontaneously in the laboratory by ocular compression that produces the oculocardiac reflex, afferent stimulation of the trigeminal nerve, and efferent inhibition of the heart by way of the vagus nerve. This procedure should not be attempted by an inexperienced physician, and appropriate resuscitation equipment should be readily available. Most children respond to conservative measures as outlined for cyanotic spells, but a trial of an anticholinergic, oral atropine sulfate 0.01 mg/kg/24 hr in divided doses with a maximum daily dose of 0.4 mg, which increases the heart rate by blocking the vagus nerve, may be considered in refractory cases. Atropine should not be pre-scribed during very hot weather because an episode of hyperpyrexia may be initiated.

Syncope

SIMPLE SYNCOPE. Syncope follows an alteration in brain metabolism, the consequence of decreased cerebral blood flow, usually secondary to systemic hypotension. Decreased blood flow causes loss of consciousness, and the concomitant ischemia influences the higher cortical centers to release their inhibiting influence on the reticular formation within the brainstem. Neuronal discharges from the reticular formation then produce brief tonic contractions of the muscles of the face, trunk, and extremities in approximately 50% of patients with syncope. During a syncopal episode, a child may have fixed upward deviation of the eyes that can be confused with epilepsy. Simple syncope results from vasovagal stimulation and is precipitated by pain, fear, excitement, and extended periods of standing still, particularly in a warm environment. The EEG shows transient slowing during the attack but no seizure discharges. Simple syncope is uncommon before age 10–12 yr but is quite prevalent in adolescent girls. Tilt-table testing is an effective method of producing symptoms, including hypotension, in the majority of children with unexplained syncope. Most patients with positive tilt-table test results have vasovagal syncope, which if recurrent responds favorably to oral β-adrenergic blocking agents. Syncope can usually be differentiated from a seizure because of its short duration, associated symptoms of nausea and perspiration, and complete orientation after the event.

COUGH SYNCOPE. This is most common in asthmatic children. It often occurs shortly after the onset of sleep, and the coughing paroxysm abruptly awakens the child. The patient's face becomes plethoric, and the child perspires, becomes agitated, and is frightened. Loss of consciousness is associated with generalized muscle flaccidity, vertical upward gaze, and clonic muscle contractions lasting for several seconds. Urinary incontinence is frequent. Recovery begins within seconds, and consciousness is usually restored a few minutes later. The child has no recollection of the attack except for the events surrounding the paroxysm of coughing. Coughing produces a marked increase in intrapleural pressure followed by a lowered venous return to the right side of the heart and an associated decrease in right ventricular output. Reduction of left ventricular filling follows, and a rapidly diminished cardiac output results in altered cerebral blood flow, cerebral hypoxia, and a loss of consciousness. The cornerstone of management for asthmatic children with cough syncope is an aggressive approach to the prevention of bronchoconstriction.

PROLONGED QT SYNDROME. The incidence of the prolonged QT syndrome is 1/10,000 to 1/15,000. The prolonged QT syndrome is characterized by sudden loss of consciousness during exercise or an emotional and stressful experience (see Chapter 428.4). Loss of consciousness in association with exercise or stress is rarely due to epilepsy, and in every case a cardiac cause must be considered. The onset of the condition is typically in late childhood or adolescence, although onset in infancy may mimic sudden infant death syndrome. During the period of syncope, various cardiac arrhythmias are evident, particularly ventricular fibrillation. The child may recover within minutes or die during the event. Electrocardiography may show prolongation of the QT interval due to abnormal lengthening of the QT interval, especially during carefully monitored exercise. QT intervals corrected for heart rate of 0.46 msec or greater support the diagnosis. There are at least two varieties of the syndrome: those due to acquired heart disease (myocarditis, mitral valve prolapse, electrolyte abnormalities, drug induced) and two congenital forms. The QT syndrome may be inherited as an autosomal recessive trait (Jervell and Lange-Nielsen syndrome) that is associated with deafness or as autosomal dominant (Romano-Ward syndrome). Mutations in a cardiac potassium channel gene [KvLQT1], linked to chromosome 11p15.5, account for about 50% of the long QT syndrome inherited as an autosomal dominant (type 1 or LQT1). LQT2 results from a mutation in a second potassium channel gene (HERG), which is linked to chromosome 7q35-36. Type 3 long QT syndrome is the result of a mutation to a cardiac sodium channel gene (SCN5A) linked to chromosome 3p21-24, and a fourth type of long QT syndrome has been linked to chromosome 4q25-27. The gene for type 4 LQT has not been determined. All family members of an affected patient should have a 12-lead electrocardiogram. Further testing may include carefully supervised exercise tests or Holter monitoring. β-Adrenergic-antagonist drugs are usually effective and may be lifesaving. Permanent implantable cardiac pacing or left cervicothoracic sympathectomy may also be considered if drug therapy is not effective. Parents should be taught cardiopulmonary resuscitation, because exercise restriction and drug therapy may be ineffective for some children.

Paroxysmal Kinesigenic Choreoathetosis. This disorder is characterized by a sudden onset of unilateral or occasionally bilateral choreoathetosis or dystonic posturing of a leg or an arm and associated facial grimacing and dysarthria. The condition is precipitated by sudden movement, particularly on arising from a sitting position, or by excitement and stress. The attacks rarely persist for longer than a minute and are never associated with loss of consciousness. The age of onset is typically between 8 and 14 yr, but the condition may begin as early as 2 yr. The child may have several attacks daily, or they may be intermittent, occurring once or twice a month. Results of neurologic examination, EEG, and neuroimaging studies are normal, and neuropathologic studies in a few cases showed no abnormalities. Most reported cases are familial, suggestive of autosomal recessive inheritance. The attacks can be prevented by the use of anticonvulsants, particularly phenytoin. The attacks of paroxysmal kinesigenic choreoathetosis tend to diminish in frequency during adulthood, and the anticonvulsant can be successfully weaned at that time.

Shuddering Attacks. Shuddering attacks have their onset at 4–6 mo of age and may persist to 6–7 yr of age. They produce an interesting posture, with sudden flexion of the head and trunk and shuddering or shivering movements similar to what must occur if ice-cold water is poured down the back of an unsuspecting individual. These children may have 100 attacks/day followed by several symptom-free weeks. Shuddering attacks may be the childhood precursor of benign essential tremor, because examination of parents and relatives reveals a high incidence of that common condition.

Benign Paroxysmal Torticollis of Infancy. Infants with benign paroxysmal torticollis have recurrent attacks of head tilt associated with pallor, agitation, and vomiting with an onset between 2 and 8 mo of age. During the attack, the child resists passive head movement. There is no loss of consciousness, and spontaneous remission occurs by 2–3 yr of age. As with benign paroxysmal vertigo, abnormalities in vestibular function have been documented in these patients. Children with persistent torticollis should be investigated for abnormalities of the cervical vertebrae including dislocation or fracture, or a tumor located in the posterior fossa. Some infants with benign paroxysmal torticollis develop migraine headaches later in childhood.

Hereditary Chin Trembling. Hereditary chin trembling may be confused with epilepsy due to repeated episodes of rapid 3/sec chin trembling movements. These brief attacks are precipitated by stress, anger, and frustration and are inherited as an autosomal dominant trait. Findings on the neurologic examination and EEG are normal.

Narcolepsy and Cataplexy. See also Chapters 20.5 and 369. Narcolepsy is a disorder that rarely begins before adolescence and is characterized by paroxysmal attacks of irrepressible day-time sleep, which is sometimes associated with transient loss of muscle tone (cataplexy). The incidence of narcolepsy is 1/2,000. An EEG shows that the recurrent sleep attacks consist of rapid eye movement (REM) sleep. Patients with narcolepsy are easily aroused and become spontaneously alert, whereas a convulsion is followed by a deep sleep, postictal drowsiness, lethargy, and often a headache. Modafinil acetamide, 200 mg/day PO, is superior to the stimulant drugs in the management of narcolepsy and has fewer adverse side effects. Cataplexy is also occasionally confused with epilepsy. Patients with cataplexy experience sudden loss of muscle tone and fall to the floor because of laughter, stress, or frightening experiences. Cataplectic patients do not lose consciousness but lie without moving for a few minutes until normal body tone returns. Treatment consists of scheduled naps, amphetamines, methylphenidate, tricyclic antidepressants, and counseling with respect to occupational safety and driving. The stimulant and antidepressant drugs commonly produce side effects including anxiety, euphoria, hypersomnolence, and the development of tolerance.

Rage Attacks or Episodic Dyscontrol Syndrome. The *episodic dyscontrol syndrome*, a nonepileptic condition, can be confused with complex partial seizures. Patients develop sudden and recurrent attacks of violent physical behavior with minimal provocation. The attacks consist of kicking, scratching, biting, and shouting (including abusive and profane language). An affected child or adolescent cannot seem to control the behavior and may seem momentarily psychotic throughout the attack. The episode is followed by fatigue, amnesia, and sincere remorse. A routine EEG may show nonspecific abnormalities in patients with the rage syndrome. The EEG in such patients during the attack remains normal; this condition is thus distinguished from complex partial seizures, which always show an abnormal EEG during an attack.

Masturbation. Masturbation or self-stimulation behavior may occur in girls between the ages of 2 mo and 3 yr. These children have repetitive stereotyped episodes of tonic posturing associated with copulatory movements, but without manual stimulation of the genitalia. The child suddenly becomes flushed and perspires, may grunt and breathe irregularly, but has no loss of consciousness. The masturbatory activity has a sudden onset, usually persists for a few minutes (rarely hours), and tends to occur during periods of stress or boredom. The examination should include a search for evidence of sexual abuse or abnormalities of the perineum, but in most cases a cause is not found. Treatment consists of reassurance that the self-stimulatory activity will subside by 3 yr of age and that no specific therapy is required.

Pseudoseizures. The diagnosis of a pseudoseizure should be made only after a thorough history and physical examination and exclusion of "true" seizures by prolonged EEG recording when indicated. Pseudoseizures occur typically between 10 and 18 yr of age and are more frequent among girls. Pseudoseizures occur in many patients with a past history of epilepsy and in some with ongoing true seizures. A pseudoseizure may be quite realistic but frequently is bizarre, with unusual postures, verbalizations, and uncharacteristic tonic or clonic movements. There are several distinguishing features of a pseudoseizure, including lack of cyanosis, normal reaction of the pupil to light, no loss of sphincter control, normal plantar responses, and the absence of tongue biting or injury during the attack. Many patients moan or cry during a pseudoseizure, and some patients can be persuaded to have an attack on request by the physician. Patients with pseudoseizures are likely to have a neurotic personality documented by formal psychologic testing. It is not unusual to find a patient taking three or four anticonvulsants, which, of course, have no effect. The most reliable method of differentiating epilepsy from suspected pseudoseizures is to record an attack. The EEG shows an excess of muscle artifact during the pseudoseizure but a normal background rhythm devoid of seizure discharges. After a true epileptic seizure, there is a significant increase in serum prolactin, whereas there is no change from the baseline at the termination of a pseudoseizure.

Ackerman MJ, Clapham DE: Ion channels-basic science and clinical disease. *N Engl J Med* 1997;336:1575.

Broughton RJ, Fleming JA, George CF, et al: Randomized double-blind placebo-controlled crossover trial of modafinil in the treatment of excessive daytime sleepiness in narcolepsy. *Neurology* 1997;49:444.

Fleisher DR, Morrison A: Masturbation mimicking abdominal pain or seizures in young girls. *J Pediatr* 1990;116:810.

Grossman BJ: Trembling of the chin—an inheritable dominant character. *Pediatrics* 1957;19:453.

Haslam RH, Freigang B: Cough syncope mimicking epilepsy in asthmatic children. *Can J Neurol Sci* 1985;12:45.

Kertesz A: Paroxysmal kinesigenic choreoathetosis. An entity within the paroxysmal choreoathetosis syndrome. Description of 10 cases, including 1 autopsied. *Neurology* 1967;17:680.

Koenigsberger MR, Chutorian AM, Gold AP, et al: Benign paroxysmal vertigo of childhood. *Neurology* 1970;20:1108.

Lombroso CT, Lerman P: Breath-holding spells (cyanotic and pallid infantile syncope). *Pediatrics* 1967;39:563.

Mount LA, Reback S: Familial paroxysmal choreoathetosis. *Arch Neurol Psychiatry* 1940;44:841.

O'Marcaigh AS, MacLellan-Tobert SG, Porter CJ: Tilt-table testing and oral metoprolol therapy in young patients with unexplained syncope. *Pediatrics* 1994;93:278.

Pritchard PB, Wannamaker BB, Sagel J, et al: Serum prolactin and cortisol levels in evaluation of pseudoepileptic seizures. *Ann Neurol* 1985;18:87.

Ruckman RN: Cardiac causes of syncope. *Pediatr Rev* 1987;9:101.

Schneider S, Rice DR: Neurologic manifestations of childhood hysteria. *J Pediatr* 1979;94:153.

Snyder CH: Paroxysmal torticollis in infancy. *Am J Dis Child* 1969;117:458.

Vanasse M, Bedard P, Andermann F: Shuddering attacks in children: An early clinical manifestation of essential tremor. *Neurology* 1976;26:1027.

Zarcone V: Narcolepsy. *N Engl J Med* 1973;288:1156.

Chapter 588

Headaches *Robert H. A. Haslam*

Headache is a common problem in pediatrics. The effect of headaches on a child's academic performance, memory, personality, and interpersonal relationships, as well as school attendance, depends on their etiology, frequency, and intensity. A headache may occasionally indicate a severe underlying disorder (e.g., a brain tumor), and thus careful evaluation of children with recurrent, severe, or unconventional headaches is mandatory. Infants and children respond to a headache in an unpredictable fashion. Most toddlers cannot communicate the characteristics of a headache; rather they may become irritable and cranky, vomit, prefer a darkened room because of photophobia, or repeatedly rub their eyes and head. Children are poor historians when describing a headache and its associated symptoms. The most important causes of headache in children include migraine, increased intracranial pressure (ICP), and psychogenic factors or stress. Refractive errors, strabismus, sinusitis, and malocclusion of the teeth are much less common causes of significant headaches in children.

588.1 Migraine

Migraine is defined as a recurrent headache with symptom-free intervals and at least three of the following symptoms or associated findings: abdominal pain, nausea or vomiting, throbbing headache, unilateral location, associated aura (visual, sensory, motor), relief following sleep, and a positive family history. It is the most important and frequent type of headache in the pediatric population. School children with migraine report neck-shoulder pain, abdominal pain, back pain, and otalgia more

frequently than those with nonmigrainous headache. Most migraine headaches are not severe and are readily managed by conservative measures without requiring medical attention. The youngest child reported to have developed migraine was 1 yr of age. The incidence of migraine among school-aged children between 7 and 15 yr of age was 4% in a comprehensive Swedish study. Girls are more likely to develop a migraine as adolescents, whereas boys are in the slight majority among children younger than 10 yr with migraine headaches. More than half undergo spontaneous prolonged remission after the 10th birthday. As adults, 5–10% of men and 15–20% of women have migraines. The cause of migraine headaches is unknown, but an inherited predisposition to vasomotor instability appears to be an important underlying factor. Hormonal changes, food allergies, personality traits characterized by high achievement, stress, bright flashing lights, and excessive sound all have been implicated. Increased levels of circulating serotonin and substance P, a vasodilating polypeptide, may act directly on the extracranial and intracranial vessels.

Clinical Manifestations and Classification. Migraine may be classified into subgroups, including common and classic migraine, migraine variants, cluster headaches, and complicated migraine. Cluster headaches rarely occur in children.

COMMON MIGRAINE (MIGRAINE WITHOUT AURA). This migraine is not associated with an aura and is the most prevalent type of migraine in children. The headache is throbbing or pounding and tends to be unilateral at onset or throughout its duration and is located in the bifrontal or temporal regions. It may not be hemicranial in children and is less intense compared with the migraine in adults. The headache usually persists for 1–3 hr, although the pain may last for as long as 24 hr. The pain may inhibit daily activity, because physical activity aggravates the pain. A characteristic feature of childhood migraine is intense nausea and vomiting, which may be more bothersome than the headache. The vomiting may be associated with abdominal pain and fever; thus, conditions such as appendicitis and a systemic infection may be erroneously confused with the primary diagnosis. Additional symptoms include extreme paleness, photophobia, lightheadedness, phonophobia, osmophobia (aversion to odors), and paresthesias of the hands and feet. A family history, particularly on the maternal side, is present in approximately 90% of children with common migraine. Thus, considerable caution should be exercised when making the diagnosis of a common migraine in the absence of a positive family history.

Additional features of all migraines may include near synchrony with perimenstrual or periovulation timing, gradual appearance after sustained exercise, relief with sleep, stereotypical prodromes (hypersomnia, food craving, irritability, moodiness), precipitation by food or odors, and onset after a letdown or high period of stress. Manifestations suggestive of a more serious condition include rapid onset of the first or worst headache of the patient's life, a change in the characteristics of the headaches, a progressive headache lasting for days, headache associated with Valsalva maneuver, chronic systemic signs (weight loss, fever), persistent focal neurologic manifestations, seizures, loss of consciousness, nuchal rigidity, cranial bruits, abnormal visual fields, or papilledema (Box 588–1).

CLASSIC MIGRAINE (MIGRAINE WITH AN AURA). In this disorder, an aura precedes the onset of the headache. Visual auras are rarely present in young children with migraine, but when they occur they may take the form of blurred vision, scotoma (an area of depressed vision within the visual field), photopsia (flashes of light), fortification spectra (brilliant white zigzag lines), or irregular distortion of objects. Some patients also have vertigo and lightheadedness during this stage of the headache. Sensory symptoms include perioral paresthesias and numbness of the hands and feet. Distortions of body image may predominate as a prelude to a classic migraine headache. After the aura, a patient with classic migraine develops typical symptoms of a common migraine as described earlier.

MIGRAINE VARIANTS. These variants include cyclic vomiting, acute confusional states, and benign paroxysmal vertigo. The last condition is discussed in Chapter 587. *Cyclic vomiting* is characterized by recurrent, sometimes monthly bouts of severe vomiting that may be so intense that dehydration and electrolyte abnormalities occur, particularly in infants. Systemic manifestations such as fever, abdominal pain, and diarrhea are initially absent, but they may become prominent in association with excessive fluid losses secondary to vomiting. The vomiting may be protracted and persist for several days. The child may appear pale and frightened but does not lose consciousness. After a period of deep sleep, the child awakens and resumes normal play and eating habits as if the vomiting had not occurred. Many children with cyclic vomiting have a positive family history of migraine, and as they grow older and become verbal, they describe a typical migraine headache that leaves little doubt about the diagnosis and the association of the cyclic vomiting with the condition. Cyclic vomiting is treated with rectally administered antiemetics such as dimenhydrinate or ondansetron and careful attention to fluid replacement if the vomiting is excessive. Additional causes of cyclic vomiting include intestinal obstruction (e.g., malrotation, intermittent volvulus, duodenal web, duplication cysts, superior mesenteric artery compression, and internal hernias), peptic ulcer, gastritis, giardiasis, chronic pancreatitis, and Crohn disease. Abnormal gastrointestinal motility and pelvi-ureteric junction obstruction also can cause cyclic vomiting. Metabolic causes include disorders of amino acid metabolism (i.e., heterozygote ornithine transcarbamylase deficiency), organic acidurias (e.g., propionic acidemia, methylmalonic acidemia), fatty acid oxidation defects (e.g., medium-chain acyl-CoA dehydrogenase deficiency), disorders of carbohydrate metabolism (e.g., hereditary fructose intolerance), acute intermittent porphyria, and structural central nervous system (CNS) lesions (e.g., posterior fossa brain tumors, subdural hematoma or effusions).

Acute confusional states may also be a manifestation of migraine. Migraine may present in a bizarre fashion, particularly in children, characterized by confusion, hyperactivity, disorientation, unresponsiveness, memory disturbances, vomiting, and lethargy. The neurologic examination shows defects of the sensorium, delayed responses to stimuli including touch and pain, and occasionally plantar extensor responses. The differential diagnosis

includes toxic (drugs of abuse, ingestions) encephalopathy (particularly in an adolescent), encephalitis, acute psychosis, postictal state, petit mal (absence) status epilepticus, head trauma, and sepsis. The episode of acute confusion may persist for several hours and characteristically clears spontaneously after sleep; patients have no recall of the confusional state. The diagnosis is usually made in retrospect as a patient or family recalls the onset of a severe headache or visual symptoms preceding the acute attack of confusion, and a family history of migraine is established. Acute confusional states as a component of migraine probably result from localized cerebral edema due to increased vascular permeability during the headache. The electroencephalogram (EEG) shows regional areas of slowing (2–4 cps) during and shortly after the attack but routinely returns to normal within a few days.

COMPLICATED MIGRAINE. Complicated migraine refers to the development of neurologic signs during a headache that persist after termination of the headache. The presence of neurologic signs in association with a headache suggests the possibility of an underlying structural lesion and requires a thorough investigation. There are three subsets of complicated migraine.

Brainstem signs predominate in patients with *basilar migraine* because of vasoconstriction of the basilar and posterior cerebral arteries. The major symptoms include vertigo, tinnitus, diplopia, blurred vision, scotoma, ataxia, and an occipital headache. The pupils may be dilated, and ptosis may be evident. Alterations in consciousness followed by a generalized seizure may result. After the attack there is a complete resolution of the neurologic symptoms and signs. Most affected children have a strongly positive family history of migraine. Many develop classic migraine as adolescents or adults. Relatively minor head trauma may precipitate an episode of basilar migraine. The condition has been described in children of both sexes, with girls younger than 4 yr being at particular risk.

Ophthalmoplegic migraine is relatively rare in children. These patients develop a third-nerve palsy ipsilateral to the headache during the attack, which is caused by altered blood supply to the oculomotor nerve. The major differential diagnosis is a congenital aneurysm compressing the oculomotor nerve. *Amaurosis fugax* (acute, reversible, monocular blindness) may also be a variant of complicated migraine.

Hemiplegic migraine is characterized by the onset of unilateral sensory or motor signs during an episode of migraine. Hemisyndromes are more common in children than in adults and may be characterized by numbness of the face, arm, and leg; unilateral weakness; and aphasia. More than one attack is uncommon in the pediatric age group. The neurologic signs may be transient or may persist for days. It is unusual for a child to develop a completed stroke after a single episode. Hemiplegic migraine in an older child or adolescent has a relatively good prognosis, and a positive family history of similar hemiplegic events is often elicited. Familial hemiplegic migraine (FHM) is an autosomal dominant disorder. FHM is characterized by hemiplegia during the headache and, in some kindreds, progressive cerebellar atrophy. Mutations of the CACNL1A4 gene located on chromosome 19p13.1 are found in the majority of patients with FHM. Additional mutations may be identified in the calcium channel gene CACNL1A4, which would establish the genetic basis of the more common types of migraine.

Some children with migraine develop the syndrome of *alternating hemiplegia*, which has its onset during infancy. Acute hemiplegia may be the initial manifestation of migraine and may recur, affecting one side and then the other. Frequent episodes of vasoconstriction associated with ischemia may result in irreversible cerebral injury leading to mental retardation and epilepsy in this subgroup of children.

Diagnosis and Differential Diagnosis. A thorough history and physical examination suffice to establish the diagnosis in most cases. Basilar migraine may be confused with several conditions, including congenital malformations of the skull and cervical vertebrae, posterior fossa tumors, toxins and drugs, and metabolic abnormalities including Leigh disease and pyruvate decarboxylase deficiency. In children with hemiplegic migraine, an arteriovenous malformation, MELAS (mitochondrial myopathy, encephalopathy, lactic acidosis, and stroke), cerebral tumor, Todd paralysis, clotting disorders, hemoglobinopathies such as sickle cell disease, and metabolic conditions including homocystinuria should be considered. A lipid profile should be obtained in children with migraine and a positive family history of premature myocardial infarction or cerebrovascular accident. Migraines may occur in patients with systemic lupus erythematosus and patients abusing cocaine. The organization of laboratory tests and radiologic studies depends on the constellation of symptoms and findings during the neurologic examination. A CT or MRI study is indicated if the headache is associated with an unusual constellation of symptoms or signs (see earlier) or when increased ICP is suspected (see Box 588–1).

Treatment. Migraine may be prevented or ameliorated by *avoiding certain initiating stimuli*. A few children can identify specific factors that uniformly result in a headache. The most common precipitators of migraine headaches are stress, fatigue, and anxiety. An affected child may be under undue stress because of difficulties at home or school, particularly when unrealistic pressures or demands are placed on the patient. Children who experience recurrent migraine headaches during the school year may have a learning disability or may have been placed in a too highly competitive classroom. Reassessment of the child's school placement and academic abilities may be the most important step in the management of the headache disorder. Some studies implicate certain foods as a cause of migraine, particularly nuts, chocolate, cola drinks, hot dogs, spicy meats, kippers, and Chinese food (monosodium glutamate). Elimination of the incriminating foodstuff is indicated if the history suggests a relationship between the ingestion of a particular food and the onset of headache. Avoidance of bright flashing lights, sun exposure, excessive physical exertion, mild head trauma, loud noises, hunger, fatigue, motion sickness, and drugs (including alcohol and oral contraceptives) is indicated when the history suggests a direct relationship. The frequency and severity of migraine headaches are reduced significantly in at least 50% of pediatric patients who undergo a careful history and neurologic examination followed by reassurance from the physician.

Management of an acute attack of migraine should include the use of *analgesics* and *antiemetics*. Most migraine headaches in children can be treated by the judicious use of *acetaminophen* or *ibuprofen*, particularly if the headaches are mild, infrequent, and of short duration. Additional agents for more severe migraine include naproxen, ketorolac, codeine, butorphanol, and meperidine. The *ergotamine preparations* (ergotamine tartrate or dihydroergotamine) should be considered for older children and adolescents with severe, classic migraine headaches and are most efficacious during the early stages of the migraine attack. The usual dose is 1 mg, which may be administered orally, subcutaneously, or per rectum in the form of a suppository. A repeat dose may be given 30 min later. Ergotamine should not be prescribed for patients with hemiplegic episodes. The ergotamines are frequently ineffective in children because they must be used early in the evolution of the headache. Most children either are unaware of an aura or fail to communicate the onset of the headache to their parents. An antiemetic such as *dimenhydrinate*, 5 mg/kg/24 hr in four divided doses, is the mainstay of treatment when vomiting is the major symptom. The child usually prefers to rest in a quiet, darkened room and typically awakens, refreshed and headache free, several hours later after a deep sleep. *Sumatriptan*, a specific and selective 5-hydroxytryptamine receptor agonist, is effective in treating the acute phase of both classic and common migraine headaches in adults. The drug may be administered subcutaneously, nasally, or orally, and the adverse effects, including hot flushes, nausea and vomiting, fatigue, and drowsiness, are usually minor and transient. In one well-controlled study, a 20 mg dose of sumatriptan administered by nasal spray was effective and well tolerated in treating acute migraine in adolescents. Hypertension and coronary vasospasm have been reported in adults. The drug is not licensed at present for patients younger than 18 yr. Studies in young children have shown that sumatriptan is much less effective than in adolescents and adults and that there is no difference between the drug and placebo.

Children may develop severe intractable migraine attacks or status migrainosus, which are unresponsive to conventional drug regimens. *Chlorpromazine* is a useful drug in the short term (5–6 days) to "break-up" the migraine. The dose is 2 mg/kg/24 hr PO divided every 4–6 hr or 4 mg/kg/24 hr per rectum divided every 6–8 hr. Intravenous chlorpromazine, 0.5–1.0 mg/kg/dose every 6–8 hr, is often effective in the management of acute migraine in an ambulatory setting. In one study, intravenous *prochlorperazine*, 0.13–0.15 mg/kg, was highly effective in aborting intractable migraine in children with no significant side effects.

The decision to use *continuous daily medication* is based on the severity and frequency of the headaches and on the impact of the migraine on the child's daily activities, including school attendance and performance as well as participation in recreation. The use of prophylactic drugs should be considered if a child experiences more than two to four severe episodes monthly or is unable to attend school regularly. Although few drugs have been subjected to well-designed clinical trials in children, propranolol, a β-adrenergic blocker, is the drug of choice in most centers. The dose of propranolol is 10–20 mg tid (beginning with 10 mg/24 hr and gradually increasing the drug to the maximum dose or until the desired therapeutic effect is achieved) in children 7–8 yr and older. A common mistake is to discontinue the drug prematurely, because it often takes several weeks to a month until the drug is effective. Additional β-blockers include atenolol, metoprolol, and nadolol. Other drugs used for migraine prophylaxis include calcium channel blockers (flunarizine, verapamil), tricyclic antidepressants (amitriptyline, nortriptyline), nonsteroidal anti-inflammatory agents, and serotonin receptor antagonists (methysergide [not used in children younger than age 10 yr and not for more than 3 mo because retroperitoneal or pulmonary fibrosis has been reported following 6 mo of continuous use] or pizotyline). If a drug is effective, it is usually maintained for 1 yr, particularly during the school term.

Behavior management is an effective method for the treatment of migraine in some children and adolescents. Biofeedback and self-hypnosis are replacing pharmacologic treatment in some centers because of the undesirable side effects of drugs and the concern that some may produce chemical dependency. Biofeedback can be mastered by most children older than 8 yr and has been effective in many clinical trials. Several studies of migrainous children show a significant decrease in frequency and no change in intensity of headaches in those treated by self-hypnosis compared with those taking the placebo or propranolol. Many pediatric headache clinics employ social workers skilled in pain management. Children respond favorably to being taught imagery and may often learn to control the pain associated with migraine without the use of medication.

588.2 Organic Headaches

A headache may be the earliest symptom of increased ICP. The headache results from tension or traction of the cerebral blood vessels and dura and occurs initially in a sporadic fashion, primarily in the early hours in the morning or shortly after the patient arises. The headache is diffuse and generalized and is more prominent over the frontal and occipital regions. Its onset may be insidious, and the pain is enhanced by any activity that elevates the ICP (e.g., coughing, sneezing, or straining during a bowel movement). As the ICP increases, the child becomes lethargic and irritable, and the headache becomes constant. Early morning vomiting is often associated with increased ICP. Causes of organic headaches in children include brain tumors, particularly those located in the posterior fossa, hydrocephalus, meningitis and encephalitis, cerebral abscess, subdural hematoma, chronic lead poisoning, and pseudotumor cerebri. Additional causes of organic headaches in children that may not be associated with increased ICP include arteriovenous malformations, berry aneurysm, collagen vascular diseases affecting the CNS, hypertensive encephalopathy, acute subarachnoid hemorrhage, and stroke. The management of organic headaches depends on the cause. The initial step includes a thorough history and physical examination, including recording of the blood pressure and inspection of the eyegrounds. Ordering of laboratory tests and neuroradiologic procedures depends on the clues provided by the history and physical examination.

588.3 Tension or Stress Headaches

Stress or tension headaches are relatively uncommon in the pediatric age group, particularly before puberty, and are often difficult to differentiate from migraine headaches. The two are often associated in the same patient. Tension headaches infrequently appear in the morning hours but are most apparent during the school day, particularly coinciding with a test or similarly anxiety-provoking circumstance. Although these headaches can be continuous and persist for weeks, they tend to wax and wane and build in intensity during the day. The headache is described as hurting or aching but is rarely perceived as throbbing. Most tension headaches in children are distributed in the frontal region, but they may localize over the vertex or the occipital area. Unlike migraine or headaches associated with increased ICP, tension headaches are not, as a rule, associated with nausea and vomiting.

The *diagnosis* of tension headache is made by exclusion at the completion of the history and physical examination. Studies such as an EEG or a CT scan are rarely necessary. Management consists of a search for possible underlying emotional or stressful factors. Most children have considerable insight into the origin of tension headaches and, when given the opportunity, will share concerns and conflicts. A poor self-image, fear of school failure, and lack of self-confidence are common factors. A depressed child occasionally presents with severe headaches. These patients may also complain of sudden mood changes, weight loss, anorexia, disturbed sleep, fatigue, and withdrawal from social activities.

Treatment of tension headaches begins with reassurance and an explanation about how stress may cause a headache. Anxiety and stress may unconsciously produce constant isometric contraction of the temporalis, masseter, or trapezius muscles, which leads to the characteristic dull, aching headache. Steps should be introduced to remove obvious anxiety-provoking situations. Acetaminophen and other mild analgesics are often all that are required to treat a tension headache. Sedatives and antidepressants are rarely necessary. Children with severe tension headaches may benefit from a brief hospitalization, particularly if an underlying depressive illness is under consideration. In the hospital setting, the child's interaction with other patients, nursing and medical staff, and family is observed while a plan is formulated for counseling or psychiatric intervention. In most cases, the child's headaches are considerably relieved during the period of observation. As with migraine headaches, biofeedback

and self-hypnosis exercises are effective in the treatment of some patients with tension headaches.

Anttila P, Metabonkalu L, Mikkelsson M, et al: Comorbidity of other pains in school children with migraine or nonmigrainous headache. *J Pediatr* 2001;138:176.

Borge AIH, Nordhagen R, Moe B, et al: Prevalence and persistence of stomach ache and headache among children. Follow-up of a cohort of Norwegian children from 4 to 10 years of age. *Acta Paediatr* 1994;83:433.

Forsythe WI, Gillies D, Sills MA: Propranolol in the treatment of childhood migraine. *Dev Med Child Neurol* 1984;26:737.

Gardner K, Barmada MM, Ptacek LJ, et al: A new locus for hemiplegic migraine maps to chromosome 1q31. *Neurology* 1997;49:1231.

Gascon G, Barlow C: Juvenile migraine, presenting as an acute confusional state. *Pediatrics* 1970;45:628.

Goodsby PJ, Lipton RB, Ferrari MD: Migraine—Current understanding and treatment. *N Engl J Med* 2002;346(4):257–70.

Hämäläinen ML, Hoppu K, Santavuori P: Sumatriptan for migraine attacks in children: A randomized placebo-controlled study. *Neurology* 1997;48:1100.

Hämäläinen ML, Hoppu K, Valkeila E, et al: Ibuprofen and acetaminophen for the acute treatment of migraine in children: A double-blind, randomized, placebo controlled, crossover study. *Neurology* 1997;48:103.

Igarashi M, May WN, Golden GS: Pharmacologic treatment of childhood migraine. *J Pediatr* 1992;120:653.

Kabbouche MA, Vockell A-LB, LeCates SL, et al: Tolerability and effectiveness of prochlorperazine for intractable migraine in children. *Pediatrics* 2001;107:e62.

Olness H, MacDonald JT, Uden DL: Comparison of self-hypnosis and propranolol in the treatment of juvenile classic migraine. *Pediatrics* 1987;79:593.

Pryse-Phillips WE, Dodick DW, Edmeads JG, et al: Guidelines for the diagnosis and management of migraine in clinical practice. *Can Med Assoc J* 1997;156:1273.

Schwartz BS, Stewart WF, Simon D, et al: Epidemiology of tension-type headache. *JAMA* 1998;279:381.

Verret S, Steel JC: Alternating hemiplegia of childhood: A report of eight patients with complicated migraine beginning in infancy. *Pediatrics* 1971;47:675.

Wasiewski WW: Preventive therapy in pediatric migraine. *J Child Neurol* 2001;16:71–8.

Winner P, Rothner AD, Saper J, et al: A randomized double-blind placebo-controlled study of sumatriptan nasal spray in the treatment of acute migraine in adolescents. *Pediatrics* 2000;106:989.

Chapter 589
Neurocutaneous Syndromes *Robert H. A. Haslam*

The neurocutaneous syndromes include a heterogeneous group of disorders characterized by abnormalities of both the integument and central nervous system (CNS). Most disorders are familial and believed to arise from a defect in differentiation of the primitive ectoderm. Disorders classified as neurocutaneous syndromes include neurofibromatosis, tuberous sclerosis, Sturge-Weber disease, von Hippel-Lindau disease, ataxia telangiectasia, linear nevus syndrome, hypomelanosis of Ito (see Chapter 643), and incontinentia pigmenti (see Chapter 642).

589.1 Neurofibromatosis

Neurofibromatosis (NF), von Recklinghausen disease, is a common autosomal dominant disorder. The condition is protean, because virtually every system and organ may be affected, and progressive in that distinctive features may be present at birth but the development of complications is delayed for decades. NF is the consequence of an abnormality of neural crest differentiation and migration during the early stages of embryogenesis (see also Chapter 642).

Clinical Manifestations and Diagnosis. There are two distinct forms of NF. NF-1 is the most prevalent type, with an incidence of 1/4,000, and is diagnosed when any two of the following signs are present. (1) *Six or more café-au-lait macules over 5 mm in greatest diameter in prepubertal individuals and over 15 mm in greatest diameter in postpubertal individuals.* Café-au-lait spots are the hallmark of neurofibromatosis and are present in almost 100% of patients. They are present at birth but increase in size, number, and pigmentation, especially during the first few years of life. The spots are scattered over the body surface, with predilection for the trunk and extremities, with sparing of the face. (2) *Axillary or inguinal freckling* consists of multiple hyperpigmented areas 2–3 mm in diameter. (3) *Two or more iris Lisch nodules*. Lisch nodules are hamartomas located within the iris and are best identified with a slit-lamp examination. They are present in more than 74% of patients with NF-1 but are not a component of NF-2. The prevalence of Lisch nodules increases with age, from only 5% of children younger than 3 yr of age, to 42% among children 3–4 yr of age, to 100% of adults 21 yr of age or older. (4) *Two or more neurofibromas or one plexiform neurofibroma*. Neurofibromas typically involve the skin, but they may be situated along peripheral nerves and blood vessels and within viscera including the gastrointestinal tract. These cutaneous lesions appear characteristically during adolescence or pregnancy, suggesting a hormonal influence. They are usually small, rubbery lesions with a slight purplish discoloration of the overlying skin. Plexiform neurofibromas are usually evident at birth and result from diffuse thickening of nerve trunks that are frequently located in the orbital or temporal region of the face. The skin overlying a plexiform neurofibroma may be hyperpigmented to a greater degree than a café-au-lait spot. Plexiform neurofibromas may produce overgrowth of an extremity and a deformity of the corresponding bone. (5) *A distinctive osseous lesion* such as sphenoid dysplasia (which may cause pulsating exophthalmos) or cortical thinning of long bones with or without pseudoarthrosis. Scoliosis is the most common orthopedic manifestation of NF-1, although it is not specific enough to be included as a diagnostic criterion. (6) *Optic gliomas* are present in approximately 15% of patients with NF-1. These relatively benign tumors consist of glial cells and a mucinous material. Most patients with optic gliomas are asymptomatic and have normal or near-normal vision, but approximately 20% have visual disturbances or evidence of precocious sexual development secondary to tumor invasion of the hypothalamus. Children rarely are aware of unilateral visual loss; thus, diagnosis may be delayed. Patients with a unilateral optic glioma typically display an afferent pupillary defect. To test for this, each eye is alternately stimulated by a bright light source (swinging flashlight test). The affected pupil dilates rather than constricts, whereas light in the unaffected eye causes both pupils to constrict equally. Patients with NF-1 and a plexiform neuroma of the eyelid have a high association with an ipsilateral optic glioma. The MRI findings of an optic glioma include diffuse thickening, localized enlargement, or a distinct focal mass originating from the optic nerve or chiasm. (7) *A first-degree relative with NF-1 whose diagnosis was based on the aforementioned criteria*. The majority of mutations in NF-1 occur in the paternal germline. The NF-1 gene on chromosome region 17q11.2 encodes all mRNA of 11–13 kb containing at least 59 exons that produces a protein neurofibromin.

Children with NF-1 are susceptible to *neurologic complications*. MRI studies of selected children have shown abnormal signals in the globus pallidus, thalamus, and internal capsule. These probably represent low-grade glioma or hamartoma that is not detected by CT scanning (Fig. 589–1). These findings may account for the high incidence of learning disabilities, attention deficit disorders, and abnormalities of speech among affected children. Complex partial and generalized tonic-clonic seizures are a frequent complication. Hydrocephalus is a rare manifestation secondary to aqueductal stenosis, whereas macrocephaly with normal-sized ventricles is a common finding. The cerebral vessels may develop stenosis, aneurysms, or stenosis resulting in moyamoya disease (see Fig. 593–1). Neurologic sequelae include transient cerebrovascular ischemic attacks, hemiparesis, and cognitive defects. Not surprisingly, *psychologic disturbances*

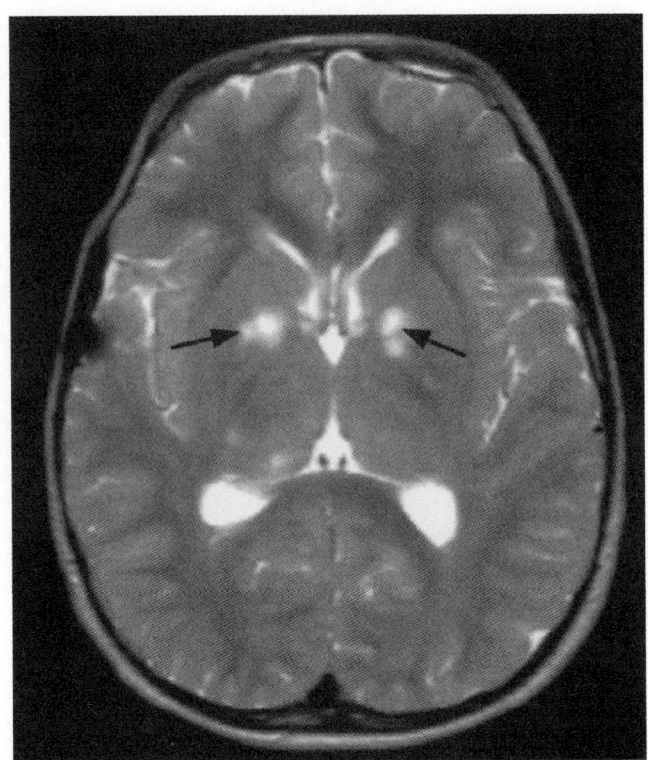

FIGURE 589–1. T2 weighted MRI scan of a patient with neurofibromatosis. Note the high-signal areas in the basal ganglia (*black arrows*), which represent hamartomas.

are prevalent owing to the seriousness and uncertainty of the disease. Precocious puberty may become evident in the presence or absence of lesions of the optic chiasm and hypothalamus. *Malignant neoplasms* are also a significant problem in patients with NF-1. A neurofibroma occasionally differentiates into a neurofibrosarcoma or malignant schwannoma. Patients with NF-1 are at risk for hypertension, which may result from renal vascular stenosis or a pheochromocytoma. The incidence of pheochromocytoma, rhabdomyosarcoma, leukemia, and Wilms' tumor is higher than in the general population. There is an unusual association involving myeloid leukemia, juvenile xanthogranuloma, and NF-1. However, tumors of the CNS (including optic gliomas, meningiomas of the brain and spinal cord, neurofibromas, astrocytomas, and neurilemmomas) account for significant morbidity and mortality because of their increased frequency in patients with NF-1.

NF-2 accounts for 10% of all cases of NF, with an incidence of 1/50,000, and may be diagnosed when one of the following is present: (1) *Bilateral eighth nerve masses* consistent with acoustic neuromas as demonstrated by CT scanning or MRI. (2) *A parent, sibling, or child with NF-2* and either unilateral eighth nerve masses or any two of the following: neurofibroma, meningioma, glioma, schwannoma, or juvenile posterior subcapsular lenticular opacities. **Bilateral acoustic neuromas** are the most distinctive feature of NF-2. Symptoms of hearing loss, facial weakness, headache, or unsteadiness may appear during childhood, although signs of a cerebellopontine angle mass are more commonly present in the 2nd and 3rd decades of life. Although café-au-lait spots and skin neurofibromas are classic findings in NF-1, they are much less common in NF-2. Posterior subcapsular lens opacities are identified in approximately 50% of patients with NF-2. As with NF-1, CNS tumors, including Schwann cell and glial tumors, and meningiomas are common in patients with NF-2. Linkage analysis has shown that the gene for NF-2 is located near the center of the long arm of chromosome 22q1.11.

Treatment. Because there is no specific treatment for NF, management includes genetic counseling and early detection of treatable conditions or complications. The National Institutes of Health (NIH) consensus statement suggests that tests should be dictated by findings on clinical evaluation. Laboratory tests in asymptomatic patients are unlikely to be of value, particularly evoked potentials, an electroencephalogram (EEG), CT, or MRI. There is a lack of consensus concerning the indications for neuroimaging studies in NF-1, although there is unanimous agreement that all symptomatic cases (i.e., visual loss or disturbance, proptosis, symptoms and signs of increased intracranial pressure) must be studied without delay. The NIH Consensus Development Conference advised against routine imaging studies, because treatment in these asymptomatic NF-1 children is rarely required. It is recommended that the child have a detailed history and physical examination by a pediatrician and a thorough annual ophthalmologic examination by a pediatric ophthalmologist. A parent with NF has a 50% chance of transmitting the disease with each pregnancy. The type of NF (NF-1 and NF-2) "breeds true" for successive generations. Because approximately half of all cases of NF result from fresh mutations, each parent should be carefully examined (including a search for Lisch nodules) before counseling for the risk of affected future pregnancies. Standard DNA diagnostic analysis is not practical for the prenatal diagnosis of the NF-1 gene because of the large size of the gene and the significant number of mutations. However, prenatal diagnosis is feasible if the mutation causing the condition is known in the affected parent. The majority of NF-2 cases are the result of a mutation. Examination of fetal DNA for the characteristic single-strand conformational polymorphism of an altered DNA sequence provides accurate prenatal testing. In familial cases, when affected and unaffected family members are available, linkage can be established, making prenatal diagnosis available with a certain degree of accuracy.

589.2 Tuberous Sclerosis

Tuberous sclerosis (TS) is inherited as an autosomal dominant trait with an estimated frequency of 1/6,000. Molecular genetic studies have identified two foci for the TS complex. In TSC 1, the abnormality is located on chromosome 9q34, and in TSC 2, the genetic abnormality is on chromosome 16p13. At least half of the cases are sporadic owing to new mutations. The 8.6-kb TSC_1 transcript encodes a protein of 130 kd called *hamartin*. The TSC_2 gene encodes the protein *tuberin*. TS is an extremely heterogeneous disease with a wide clinical spectrum varying from severe mental retardation and incapacitating seizures to normal intelligence and a lack of seizures, often within the same family. As a rule, the younger the patient presents with symptoms and signs of TS, the greater is the likelihood of mental retardation. The disease affects many organ systems other than the skin and brain, including the heart, kidney, eyes, lungs, and bone.

Pathology. The characteristic brain lesions consist of tubers. Tubers are located in the convolutions of the cerebral hemispheres and are typically present in the subependymal region, where they undergo calcification and project into the ventricular cavity, producing a candle-dripping appearance. Tubers in the region of the foramen of Monro may cause obstruction of cerebrospinal fluid (CSF) flow and hydrocephalus. The microscopic appearance of the tuber consists of decreased numbers of neurons, a proliferation of astrocytes, and the presence of oddly shaped multinucleated giant neurons. MRI is useful for identification of the lesions. Generally, the greater the number of tubers, the more neurologically impaired is the patient.

Clinical Manifestations. TS may present during infancy with infantile spasms and a hypsarrhythmic EEG pattern. Careful examination of the skin on the trunk and extremities shows the typical hypopigmented skin lesions that have been likened to an ash leaf in more than 90% of cases in this age group. Visualization of the hypopigmented lesions is enhanced by the use of a Wood ultraviolet lamp (see Chapter 545). The CT scan typically shows calcified tubers in the periventricular area, but these may not be apparent until 3–4 yr of age (Fig. 589–2). The seizures may be difficult to control, and at a later age they may develop into myoclonic epilepsy. In Europe and Canada, infantile spasms associated with TS are often treated with vigabatrin (rather than adrenocorticotropic hormone), with good results. Vigabatrin is not available in the United States. There is a high incidence of mental retardation in young patients with TS and infantile spasms.

During childhood, TS presents most often with a generalized seizure disorder and pathognomonic skin lesions. Sebaceous adenomas develop between 4 and 6 yr of age; they appear as tiny red nodules over the nose and cheeks and are sometimes confused with acne. Later, they enlarge, coalesce, and assume a fleshy appearance. A *shagreen patch* is also characteristic of TS and consists of a roughened, raised lesion with an orange-peel consistency located primarily in the lumbosacral region. Subungual or periungual fibromas arise from the stratum lucidum of the finger and toe in many patients with TS during adolescence. Retinal lesions consist of two types: mulberry tumors that arise from the nerve head or round, flat gray lesions (phakoma) in the region of the disc (Fig. 589–3). Brain tumors are much less common in TS compared with NF, but a tuber occasionally differentiates into a malignant astrocytoma. Approximately 50% of children with TS have rhabdomyomas of the heart, which may be detected in a fetus at risk by an echocardiogram. The rhabdomyomas may be numerous or located at the apex of the left ventricle, and although they can cause congestive heart failure and arrhythmias, they tend to slowly resolve spontaneously. The kidneys in most patients are involved by hamartomas or polycystic disease, resulting in hematuria, pain, and, in some cases, renal failure. Angiomyolipomas may produce generalized cystic or fibrous pulmonary changes in the lung and lead to spontaneous pneumothorax.

Diagnosis. Diagnosis of TS relies on a high index of suspicion when assessing a child with infantile spasms. A careful search for the typical skin and retinal lesions should be completed in all patients with a seizure disorder. Head CT scan or MRI confirms the diagnosis in most cases.

Treatment. Management consists of seizure control and baseline studies, including renal ultrasonography, an echocardiogram, and a chest roentgenogram with follow-up as indicated. Symptoms and signs of increased intracranial pressure suggest obstruction of the foramen of Monro by a tuber or malignant transformation of a tuber, and warrant immediate investigation and surgical intervention.

589.3 Sturge-Weber Disease

Sturge-Weber disease consists of a constellation of symptoms and signs including a facial nevus (port-wine stain), seizures, hemiparesis, intracranial calcifications, and, in many cases, mental retardation. It occurs sporadically, with a frequency of approximately 1/50,000.

Etiology. The condition is thought to result from anomalous development of the primordial vascular bed during the early stages of cerebral vascularization. At this stage, the blood supply to the brain, meninges, and face is undergoing reorganization, while the primitive ectoderm in the region differentiates into the skin of the upper face and the occipital lobe of the cerebrum. The overlying leptomeninges are richly vascularized, and the brain beneath becomes atrophic and calcified, particularly in the molecular layer of the cortex, in patients with Sturge-Weber disease.

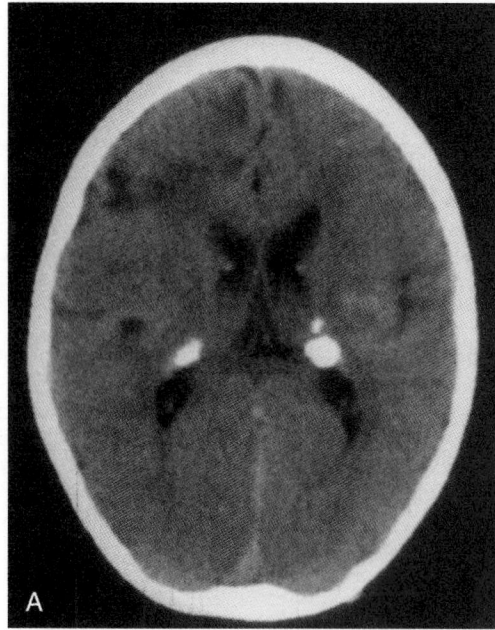
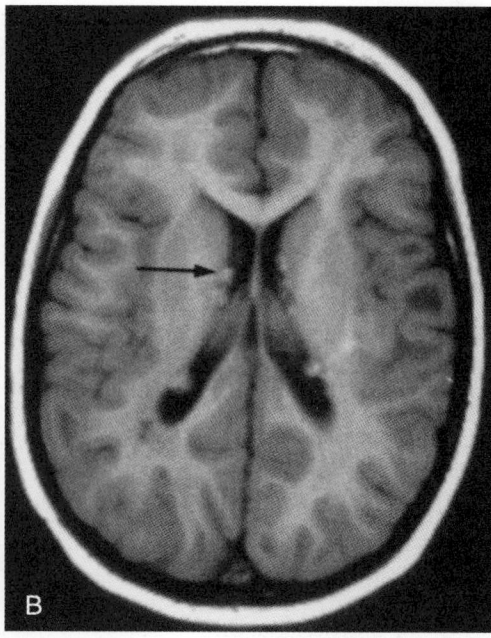

FIGURE 589–2. Tuberous sclerosis. *A,* CT scan with subependymal calcifications characteristic of tuberous sclerosis. *B,* The MRI demonstrates multiple subependymal nodules in the same patient (*black arrow*). Parenchymal tubers are also visible on both the CT and the MRI scan as low-density areas in the brain parenchyma.

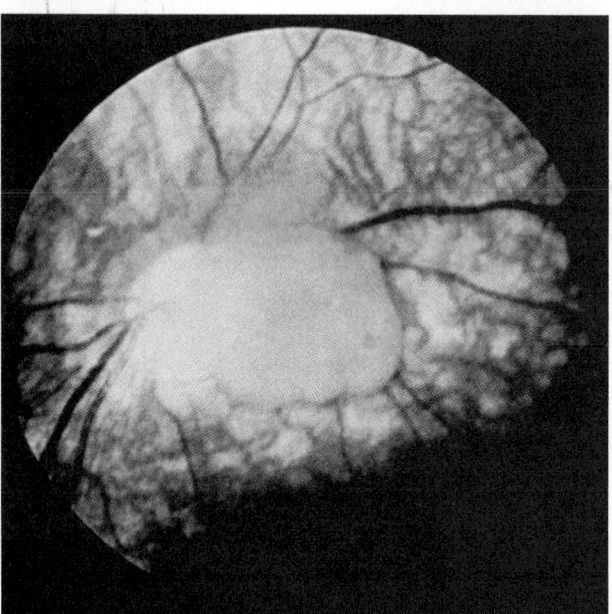

FIGURE 589–3. An astrocytoma of the retina (mulberry tumor) in a patient with tuberous sclerosis.

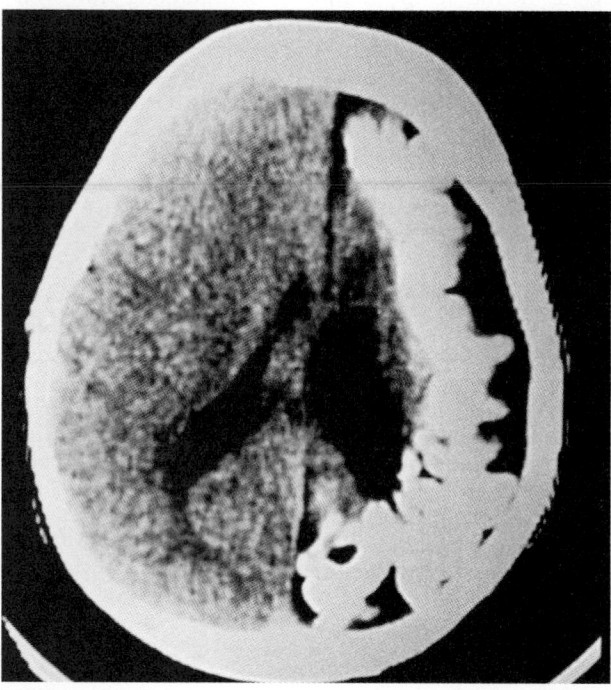

FIGURE 589–4. A CT scan of a patient with Sturge-Weber syndrome showing unilateral calcification and atrophy of a cerebral hemisphere.

Clinical Manifestations. The facial nevus is present at birth and tends to be unilateral and always involves the upper face and eyelid. The nevus may also be evident over the lower face, trunk, and in the mucosa of the mouth and pharynx. Not all children with facial nevi have Sturge-Weber disease (see Chapter 640). Buphthalmos and glaucoma of the ipsilateral eye are a common complication. Seizures develop in most patients during the 1st year of life. They are typically focal tonic-clonic and contralateral to the side of the facial nevus. The seizures tend to become refractory to anticonvulsants and are associated with a slowly progressive hemiparesis in many cases. Although neurodevelopment appears to be normal during the 1st year of life, mental retardation or severe learning disabilities are present in at least 50% during later childhood, probably the result of prolonged generalized seizures and increasing cerebral atrophy secondary to local hypoxia and use of numerous anticonvulsants.

Diagnosis. The skull radiograph shows intracranial calcification in the occipitoparietal region in most patients. This characteristically assumes a serpentine or railroad-track appearance. The CT scan highlights the extent of the calcification that is usually associated with unilateral cortical atrophy and ipsilateral dilatation of the lateral ventricle (Fig. 589–4).

Treatment. Management of Sturge-Weber disease is multifaceted and somewhat controversial. Seizure frequency and the significant risk for mental retardation influence the treatment plan. For patients with well-controlled seizures and normal or near-normal development, management is straightforward and conservative. However, increasing evidence shows that a hemispherectomy or lobectomy may prevent the development of mental retardation, in patients with recalcitrant seizures, particularly if the surgery is accomplished during the 1st year of life. Because of the risk of glaucoma, regular measurements of intraocular pressure with a tenonometer is indicated. The facial nevus is often a target for ridicule by classmates, leading to psychologic trauma. Flashlamp-pulsed laser therapy holds considerable promise for clearing of the port-wine stain. Finally, because of the high frequency of developmental disabilities, special educational facilities are frequently required.

589.4   von Hippel-Lindau Disease

As with most of the neurocutaneous syndromes, von Hippel-Lindau disease affects many organs, including the cerebellum, spinal cord, medulla, retina, kidney, pancreas, and epididymis. von Hippel-Lindau disease is inherited as an autosomal dominant trait with variable penetrance and delayed expression. The gene for von Hippel-Lindau disease has been mapped to chromosome 3p25. The major neurologic features of the condition include cerebellar hemangioblastomas and retinal angiomata. Patients with cerebellar hemangioblastoma present in early adult life or beyond with symptoms and signs of increased intracranial pressure. A smaller number of patients have hemangioblastoma of the spinal cord, producing abnormalities of proprioception and disturbances of gait and bladder dysfunction. The CT scan typically shows a cystic cerebellar lesion with a vascular mural nodule. Total surgical removal of the tumor is curative. Approximately 25% of patients with cerebellar hemangioblastoma have retinal angiomas.

Retinal angiomas are characterized by small masses of thin-walled capillaries that are fed by large and tortuous arterioles and venules. They are usually located in the peripheral retina so that vision is unaffected. However, exudation in the region of the angiomas may lead to retinal detachment and visual loss. Retinal angiomas are treated with photocoagulation and cryocoagulation, with good results. Cystic lesions of the kidneys, pancreas, liver, and epididymis as well as pheochromocytoma are frequently associated with von Hippel-Lindau disease. Renal carcinoma is the most common cause of death. Regular follow-up and appropriate imaging studies are necessary to identify lesions that may be treated at an early stage.

589.5   Linear Nevus Syndrome

This sporadic condition is characterized by a facial nevus and neurodevelopmental abnormalities. The nevus is located on the forehead and nose and tends to be midline in its distribution. It may be quite faint during infancy but later becomes hyperkeratotic, with a yellow-brown appearance. More than half of the patients have a seizure disorder and are mentally retarded. The seizures may be generalized, myoclonic, or focal motor. Most patients have normal CT studies, although hemimeganencephaly with hamartomatous changes has been reported. Focal neurologic signs including hemiparesis and homonymous hemianopia are more common in this group.

589.6   PHACE Syndrome

Large facial hemangiomas may be associated with a Dandy-Walker malformation, vascular anomalies (coarctation of aorta, aplasia or hypoplastic carotid arteries, aneurysmal carotid dilation, aberrant left subclavian artery), glaucoma, cataracts, microphthalmia, optic nerve hypoplasia, and ventral defects (sternal clefts). There is a female predominance. Airway hemangiomas may produce obstruction. The syndrome denotes *p*osterior fossa malformations, *h*emangiomas, *a*rterial anomalies, *c*oarctation of

the aorta and other cardiac defects, and *e*ye abnormalities. Interferon-α is of value in the management of the hemangiomas.

American Academy of Pediatrics Committee on Genetics: Health supervision for children with neurofibromatosis. *Pediatrics* 1995;96:368.
Cnossen MH, de Goede-Bolder A, van den Broek KM, et al: A prospective 10 year follow up study of patients with neurofibromatosis type 1. *Arch Dis Child* 1998;78:408.
Frieden IJ, Reese V, Cohen D: The association of posterior fossa brain malformations, hemangiomas, arterial anomalies, coarctation of the aorta and cardiac defects, and eye abnormalities. *Arch Dermatol* 1996;132:307.
Gutmann DH, Aylsworth A, Carey JC, et al: The diagnostic evaluation and multidisciplinary management of neurofibromatosis 1 and neurofibromatosis 2. *JAMA* 1997;278:51.
Hoffman KJ, Harris EL, Bryan RN, et al: Neurofibromatosis type 1: The cognitive phenotype. *J Pediatr* 1994;124:51.
Hurst RW, Newman SA, Cail WS: Multifocal intracranial MR abnormalities in neurofibromatosis. *AJNR* 1988;9:293.
Jozwiak S, Pedich M, Rajszys P, et al: Incidence of hepatic hamartomas in tuberous sclerosis. *Arch Dis Child* 1992;67:1363.
Jozwiak S, Kawalec W, Dluzewska J, et al: Cardiac tumors in tuberous sclerosis: Their incidence and course. *Eur J Pediatr* 1994;153:155.
Latif F, Tory K, Gmarra J, et al: Identification of the von Hippel-Landau disease tumor suppressor gene. *Science* 1993;260:1317.
Lazaro C, Gaona A, Ravella A, et al: Prenatal diagnosis of neurofibromatosis 1: From flanking RFLPS to intragene microsatellite markers. *Prenat Diagn* 1995;15:129.
Lovejoy FH, Boyle LE: Linear nevus sebaceous syndrome: Report of two cases and a review of the literature. *Pediatrics* 1973;52:382.
Maher ER, Kaelin WG Jr: von Hippel-Lindau disease. *Medicine* 1997;76:381.
O'Callaghan FJK, Shiell AW, Osborne JP, et al: Prevalence of tuberous sclerosis estimated by capture-recapture analysis. *Lancet* 1998;351:1490.
Parain D, Penniello MJ, Berquen P, et al: Vagal nerve stimulation in tuberous sclerosis complex patients. *Pediatr Neurol* 2001;25(3):213–6.
Rizzo JF, Lessell S: Cerebrovascular abnormalities in neurofibromatosis type 1. *Neurology* 1994;44:1000.
Roach ES, Williams MD, Laster MD: Magnetic resonance imaging in tuberous sclerosis. *Arch Neurol* 1987;44:301.
Seizinger BR, Martuza RL, Gusella JF: Loss of genes on chromosome 22 in tumorigenesis of human acoustic neuroma. *Nature* 1986;322:644.
Stumpf DA, Alksne JF, Annegers JF, et al: NIH Development Conference. Neurofibromatosis: Conference statement. *Arch Neurol* 1988;45:575.
Tan OT, Sherwood K, Gilchrest BA: Treatment of children with port-wine stains using the flashlamp-pulsed tunable dye laser. *N Engl J Med* 1989;320:416.
Webb DW, Clarke A, Fryer A, et al: The cutaneous features of tuberous sclerosis: A population study. *Br J Dermatol* 1996;135:1.

Chapter 590
Movement Disorders
Michael V. Johnston

Movement disorders cause involuntary movements and/or abnormalities in posture, tone, balance, or fine motor control. The type of movement disorder assists in localizing the pathologic process, whereas the onset, age, and degree of abnormal motor activity and associated neurologic findings help classify the disorder and organize the investigation.

590.1   Ataxias

Ataxia is the inability to make smooth, accurate and coordinated movements, usually due to a disorder of the cerebellum and/or sensory pathways in the posterior columns of the spinal cord. Ataxias may be generalized or primarily affect gait or the hands and arms. *Congenital anomalies* of the posterior fossa, including the Dandy-Walker syndrome, Chiari malformation, and encephalocele, are prominently associated with ataxia because of their destruction or replacement of the cerebellum (see Chapter 585). **Agenesis of the cerebellar vermis** presents in infancy with generalized hypotonia and decreased deep tendon reflexes. Delayed motor milestones and truncal ataxia are typical. A familial variety (Joubert disease) is inherited as an autosomal recessive trait. Affected children typically have abnormalities of respiration during infancy, characterized by alternating periods of hyperpnea and apnea. In addition to ataxia, mental retardation and abnormal eye movements have been described. MRI is the method of choice for investigating congenital abnormalities of the cerebellum, vermis, and related structures.

The major *infectious causes of ataxia* include cerebellar abscess, acute labyrinthitis, and acute cerebellar ataxia. **Acute cerebellar ataxia** occurs primarily in children 1–3 yr of age and is a diagnosis by exclusion. The condition often follows a viral illness, such as varicella, coxsackievirus, or echovirus infection, by 2–3 wk and is thought to represent an autoimmune response to the viral agent affecting the cerebellum (see Chapters 229, 232, and 594). The onset is sudden, and the truncal ataxia can be so severe that the child is unable to stand or sit. Vomiting may occur initially, but fever and nuchal rigidity are absent. Horizontal nystagmus is evident in approximately 50% of cases, and if the child is able to speak, dysarthria may be impressive. Examination of the cerebrospinal fluid (CSF) is typically normal at the onset of ataxia; however, a slight pleocytosis of lymphocytes (10–30/mm^3) is not unusual. Later in the course, the CSF protein undergoes a moderate elevation. The ataxia begins to improve in a few weeks but may persist for as long as 2 mo. The prognosis for complete recovery is excellent; however, a small number have long-term sequelae, including behavioral and speech disorders as well as ataxia and incoordination. **Acute labyrinthitis** may be difficult to differentiate from acute cerebellar ataxia in a toddler. The condition is associated with middle-ear infections and intense vertigo, vomiting, and abnormalities in labyrinthine function, particularly ice water caloric testing.

Toxic causes of ataxia include alcohol, thallium (which is used occasionally in homes as a pesticide), and the anticonvulsants, particularly phenytoin when serum levels reach or exceed 30 µg/mL (120 µmol/L).

Brain tumors, including tumors of the cerebellum and frontal lobe, as well as neuroblastoma, may present with ataxia. Frontal lobe tumors may cause ataxia owing to destruction of the association fibers connecting the frontal lobe with the cerebellum. Neuroblastoma may be associated with an encephalopathy characterized by progressive ataxia, myoclonic jerks, and opsoclonus (nonrhythmic horizontal and vertical oscillations of the eyes).

Several *metabolic disorders* are characterized by ataxia, including abetalipoproteinemia, arginosuccinic aciduria, and Hartnup disease. **Abetalipoproteinemia** (Bassen-Kornzweig disease) begins in childhood with steatorrhea and failure to thrive (see Chapter 75.3). A blood smear shows acanthocytosis and decreased serum levels of cholesterol and triglycerides, and the serum β-lipoproteins are absent. Neurologic signs become evident by late childhood and consist of ataxia, retinitis pigmentosa, peripheral neuritis, abnormalities in position and vibration sense, muscle weakness, and mental retardation. Vitamin E is undetectable in the serum of patients with neurologic symptoms.

Degenerative diseases of the central nervous system (CNS) represent an important group of ataxic disorders of childhood because of the genetic consequences and poor prognosis. **Ataxia-telangiectasia,** an autosomal recessive condition, is the most common of the degenerative ataxias and is heralded by ataxia beginning at about age 2 yr and progressing to loss of ambulation by adolescence (see Chapter 116.12). Ataxia-telangiectasia is caused by mutations in the ATM gene located at 11q22-q23. Oculomotor apraxia, defined as having difficulty fixating smoothly on an object and therefore overshooting the target with lateral movement of the head, followed by refixating the eyes, is a frequent finding, as is horizontal nystagmus. The telangiectasia becomes evident by midchildhood and is found on the bulbar conjunctiva, over the bridge of the nose, and on the ears and exposed surfaces of the extremities. Examination of the skin shows a loss of elasticity. Abnormalities of immunologic function that lead to frequent sinopulmonary infections include decreased serum and secretory IgA as well as diminished IgG$_2$, IgG$_4$, and IgE levels in more than 50% of patients. Children with ataxia-telangiectasia have a 50- to 100-fold greater chance over the normal population of developing lymphoreticular tumors (lymphoma, leukemia, and Hodgkin disease) as well as brain tumors. Additional laboratory abnormalities include an increased incidence of chromosome breaks, particularly of chromosome 14, and elevated levels of α-fetoprotein. Death results from infection or tumor dissemination.

Friedreich ataxia is inherited as an autosomal recessive trait. The majority of patients are homozygous for a GAA repeat expansion in the noncoding region of the X25 gene, which is located on chromosome 9q13. The gene encodes a 210 amino acid, frataxin. The onset of ataxia is somewhat later than in ataxia-telangiectasia but usually occurs before age 10 yr. The ataxia is slowly progressive and involves the lower extremities to a greater degree than the upper extremities. The Romberg test result is positive; the deep tendon reflexes are absent (particularly the Achilles), and the plantar response is extensor. Patients develop a characteristic explosive, dysarthric speech, and nystagmus is present in most children. Although patients may appear apathetic, their intelligence is preserved. They may have significant weakness of the distal musculature of the hands and feet. Typically noted is a marked loss of vibration and position sense caused by degeneration of the posterior columns and indistinct sensory changes in the distal extremities. Friedreich ataxia is also characterized by skeletal abnormalities, including high-arched feet (pes cavus) and hammer toes, as well as progressive kyphoscoliosis. Results of electrophysiologic studies including visual, auditory brainstem, and somatosensory-evoked potentials are often abnormal. Hypertrophic cardiomyopathy with progression to intractable congestive heart failure is the cause of death for most patients. Several forms of *spinocerebellar ataxia* are similar to Friedreich ataxia. **Roussy-Levy disease** has, in addition, atrophy of the muscles of the lower extremity with a similar pattern of wasting observed in Charcot-Marie-Tooth disease; **Ramsay Hunt syndrome** has an associated myoclonic epilepsy.

The **olivopontocerebellar** atrophies (OPCA) include at least five familial subtypes with dominant inheritance that usually have the onset of ataxia, cranial nerve palsies, and abnormal sensory findings in the 2nd or 3rd decade. However, some cases have been described in children, particularly of Finnish ancestry, with rapidly progressive ataxia, nystagmus, dysarthria, and seizures. Classifications of the hereditary ataxias are based on biochemical analysis; aspartic acid and glutamic acid content in the inferior olive and the Purkinje cell layer of the cerebellum are significantly decreased.

Additional degenerative ataxias include **Pelizaeus-Merzbacher disease,** neuronal ceroid lipofuscinoses, and late onset GM$_2$ gangliosidosis (see Chapter 592). Rare forms of progressive cerebellar ataxia have been described in association with **vitamin E deficiency.** A number of new inherited forms of progressive ataxia have been defined at the molecular level, including those caused by unstable trinucleotide repeat expansions.

590.2 Chorea, Athetosis, Tremor

Chorea, which means *dance* in Greek, refers to irregular, rapid, uncontrolled, involuntary movements. Choreic movements are often incorporated into semipurposeful acts in an attempt to mask the abnormality or may result in bizarre movements of the hands and arms as well abnormal gait. *Sydenham chorea* is the most common acquired chorea of childhood and is the sole neurologic manifestation of rheumatic fever (see Chapter 168.1).

The pathogenesis is probably an autoimmune response of the CNS to group A streptococcal organisms. The majority of children with Sydenham chorea have antineuronal antibodies, which develop in response to group A β-hemolytic streptococcal infections. Antineuronal antibodies cross react with the cytoplasm of subthalamic and caudate nuclei neurons. Some pediatric patients with tics and obsessive-compulsive disorder (features also associated with Sydenham chorea) have antineuronal antibodies suggesting that Tourette syndrome and other childhood neuropsychiatric disorders in some cases may be secondary to an autoimmune process. The disorder in these patients has been given the acronym PANDAS (pediatric autoimmune neuropsychiatric disorders associated with streptococcal infections). The primary pathologic findings, possibly the result of the cellular response to antineuronal antibodies, consist of vasculitis of the cortical arterioles with round cell infiltration of the gray and white matter in the surrounding area. The cerebral cortex, caudate nucleus, and subthalamic nuclei are most prominently involved. Chorea is likely a result of functional overactivity of the dopaminergic system.

The three major clinical manifestations of Sydenham chorea include chorea, hypotonia, and emotional lability. The chorea is usually symmetric, although children may have the choreic movements limited to one side of the body. The movements, which are rapid and jerky, are prominent in the face, trunk, and distal extremities and dart from one muscle group to another; they are increased by stress and disappear during sleep. The onset may be abrupt, but the chorea typically has a slowly progressive course. Hypotonia may be a prominent sign, and when combined with severe chorea, the child may be incapable of feeding, dressing, or walking. The speech is often involved and is sometimes unintelligible. Periods of uncontrollable crying and extreme mood swings are characteristic, perhaps in part as a result of the motor handicap and feelings of helplessness. Several typical signs are associated with Sydenham chorea, including the "milkmaid's grip" (relaxing and tightening hand shake), the "choreic hand" (spooning of the extended hand by flexion at the wrist and extension of the fingers), the "darting tongue" (the tongue cannot be protruded for longer than a few seconds), and the "pronator sign" (the arms and palms turn outward when held above the head). Sydenham chorea may persist for several months and as long as 1–2 yr. About 20% of children experience a recurrence of chorea within 2 yr of the initial episode. Cases with minimal signs are treated conservatively with avoidance of stress as much as possible. Incapacitating chorea is managed with a trial of diazepam followed by valproic acid, phenothiazines, or haloperidol, if the diazepam therapy is unsuccessful.

Although the phenothiazines and haloperidol are effective drugs in the treatment of Sydenham chorea, long-term use may be complicated by the development of another movement disorder, **tardive dyskinesia**. Tardive dyskinesia is characterized by stereotypical facial movements, particularly by lip smacking and protrusion and retraction of the tongue. The movement disorder may gradually disappear but in some patients persists after discontinuing the drug. Because patients with Sydenham chorea are at risk for the development of rheumatic carditis, particularly mitral stenosis, a regimen of daily penicillin prophylaxis should be instituted and maintained until adulthood. A much rarer cause of chorea during childhood, *paroxysmal kinesigenic choreoathetosis*, is discussed in Chapter 587.

Systemic lupus erythematosus (SLE) may present or be associated with neurologic symptoms and signs including seizures, organic brain syndromes (psychoses), aseptic meningitis, and various isolated neurologic signs including chorea. Chorea may be the presenting sign of SLE, particularly in children. Antiphospholipid antibodies are present in the serum in the majority of these patients. The presence of circulating antiphospholipid antibodies is associated with a high incidence of venous and arterial occlusions. Any child with chorea of unknown cause should be investigated for the possibility of antiphospholipid antibodies.

Huntington disease is a dominantly inherited degenerative disorder of the CNS cause by an expanded sequence of CAG repeats in a gene on chromosome 4p16.3, resulting in mutations in the huntingtin protein. Huntingtin forms abnormal inclusions within the nuclei of neurons and this interaction may sequester and reduce levels of proteins such as CREB binding protein (CBP) needed to activate the transcription of other genes. The onset of symptoms of progressive chorea and presenile dementia occurs most typically between 35 and 55 yr of age. Fewer than 1% of cases begin in children younger than 10 years of age with rigidity, dystonia, and seizures. Mental deterioration and behavioral problems are prominent in children. Generalized tonic-clonic seizures are common and are typically resistant to anticonvulsants. Cerebellar signs are present in 50% and oculomotor apraxia occurs in approximately 20% of cases. The course of the disease is more rapid in children, with an average duration of 8 yr until death compared with 14 yr in adults. CT scanning, although nondiagnostic, shows the mean bifrontal to bicaudate ratio to be decreased, indicating atrophy of the caudate nucleus and putamen. MRI shows hyperdensity of the putamen in adults with the akinetic-rigid form. There is no specific therapy for Huntington disease, but once the diagnosis is confirmed, the pediatrician should provide genetic counseling to the family so that risks for additional cases in future generations are understood. Molecular biologic testing (CAG trinucleotide repeat) is available but is inappropriate for children under the age of consent. Presymptomatic adult patients who test positive respond similarly to patients with cancer when the diagnosis is confirmed.

Other causes of chorea include atypical seizures, drug intoxication (e.g., phenytoin, amitriptyline, and fluphenazine), hormonally induced seizures (e.g., oral contraceptives, pregnancy/chorea gravidarum), Lyme disease, hypoparathyroidism, hyperthyroidism, and Wilson disease (see Chapter 338.2)

Athetosis or distal writhing movements of the extremities, sometimes combined with chorea (choreoathetosis), is often seen as part of extrapyramidal cerebral palsy caused by asphyxia, kernicterus, or genetic metabolic disorders such as glutaric aciduria. Athetosis is also seen with cerebral palsy associated with prematurity. Chorea and choreoathetosis may also occur after circulatory arrest is used as a support technique for complex cardiac surgery or as a complication of dopamine-blocking neuroleptic drugs such as phenothiazines. Patients with athetosis also often have *rigidity* characterized by muscle stiffness throughout the range of motion in both flexors and extensors in contrast to spasticity in which the increased tone is velocity dependent. Like athetosis and chorea, rigidity results from dysfunction of the basal ganglia, in contrast to spasticity, which reflects upper motor neuron dysfunction.

Tremor is an involuntary movement characterized by rhythmic oscillations of a part of the body, which may be more prominent during rest or with movement. *Jitteriness,* defined as rhythmic tremors of equal amplitude around a fixed axis, is the most common involuntary movement of healthy full-term infants. Jitteriness is most apparent when an infant is crying or being examined (e.g., Moro response) and is abnormal when an infant is awake and alert and when the tremor persists beyond the second week of life. Organic causes of jitteriness include sepsis, intracranial hemorrhage, hypoxic encephalopathy, hypoglycemia, hypocalcemia, hypomagnesemia, prenatal exposure to maternal marijuana, and the narcotic abstinence syndrome. *Essential tremor* is a familial condition, inherited as an autosomal dominant trait. It may begin during childhood and usually is slowly progressive. The tremor has a frequency of 4–9 Hz, primarily affects the distal upper extremities, is typically postural, and commonly disappears with rest. If the tremor causes difficulty in writing or activities of daily living, a trial of propranolol hydrochloride or primidone usually provides a favorable response. *Primary writing tremor* occurs only during the action of writing and is characterized by a jerky tremor, often responsive to β–blockers or anticholinergics. Drugs that can cause tremor include amphetamines, valproic acid, neuroleptics, tricyclic antidepressants, caffeine, and theophylline. Tremor may be the initial manifestation of a metabolic disorder, including hypoglycemia, thyrotoxicosis, neuroblastoma, and pheochromocytoma. Children recovering from a severe head injury may develop a proximal tremor that is enhanced by movement and responds to propranolol. Wilson disease often presents with a postural tremor associated with kinetic movement. These patients may also develop a wing-beating tremor of the shoulders when the upper arms are abducted and the elbows flexed. Hereditary dystonia-parkinsonism syndrome often displays a proximal tremor in addition to the characteristic dystonic movements. *Myoclonus*, sudden, brief, jerky, shocklike, involuntary movements, may be superimposed on tremor to cause a myoclonic tremor as is seen after hypoxic injury to the cerebellum or in certain neurodegenerative diseases.

590.3 Dystonia

Dystonia is a syndrome of sustained muscle contractions, frequently causing twisting and repetitive movements or abnormal postures. Major causes of dystonia include perinatal asphyxia (see Chapters 88.2 and 88.7), kernicterus, generalized primary dystonia, drugs, Wilson disease (hepatolenticular degeneration), and Hallervorden-Spatz disease and numerous other genetic mutations. Dystonia may be a prominent feature of children with extrapyramidal cerebral palsy who have had basal ganglia injury from asphyxia, kernicterus, or insults from metabolic disorders such as glutaric aciduria. Dystonia may develop gradually over many years in older children and teenagers after basal ganglia injury.

Generalized primary dystonia, also referred to as torsion dystonia or *dystonia musculorum deformans* (DMD), is caused by a group of genetic disorders that begin to progress in childhood. One form, which occurs in the Ashkenazi Jewish population, is caused by a dominantly acting mutation in the DYT_1 gene coding for the ATP binding protein Torsin A. The initial manifestation of the disease during childhood is often unilateral posturing of the lower extremity, particularly the foot, which assumes an extended and rotated position, causing tiptoe walking. Because the dystonic movement is initially intermittent and is aggravated by stress, patients are often labeled as hysterical. Ultimately, all four extremities and the axial musculature are affected as well as the muscles of the face and tongue, and thus speech and swallowing become impaired. Other forms of torsion dystonia are caused by mutations in the genes for tyrosine hydroxylase and for epsilon-sarcoglycan, causing the myoclonus dystonia syndrome.

More than a dozen loci for genes for torsion dystonia have been identified. One of these is *dopa-responsive dystonia* (DRD), also called **hereditary progressive dystonia with marked diurnal variation**, or **Segawa disease**. It is inherited as a dominant disorder more common in females. The gene for dopa-sensitive dystonia codes for GTP cyclohydrolase 1, the synthetic enzyme for the cofactor tetrahydrobiopterin that is required for synthesis of the neurotransmitters dopamine and serotonin. The dystonia is usually diurnal, improving with sleep but becoming apparent and sometimes incapacitating during the daytime. However early onset cases can easily be confused with extrapyramidal cerebral palsy. DRD responds remarkably to small daily doses (50–250 mg) of levodopa given with an inhibitor of peripheral catabolism. DRD and dystonia due to mutations in TH can be diagnosed by assaying CSF neurotransmitter metabolites for serotonin and dopamine and biopterin cofactor levels.

Segmental dystonia, including writer's cramp, blepharospasm, and buccomandibular dystonia, is more common in adults and tends to be limited to a specific group of muscles. Segmental dystonia may be seen in patients with genetic forms of torsion dystonia or may be idiopathic or acquired from overuse of muscles such as in the hands of musicians.

Certain *drugs* are capable of producing an acute dystonic reaction in children. Therapeutic doses of phenytoin or carbamazepine may rarely cause progressive dystonia in children with epilepsy, particularly in those who have an underlying structural abnormality of the brain. Children may have an idiosyncratic reaction to the phenothiazines, characterized by acute dystonic posturing that is sometimes confused with encephalitis. Intravenous diphenhydramine, 1–2 mg/kg/dose, may rapidly reverse the drug-related dystonia. Severe rigidity combined with high fever and delirium may also occur as part of the **neuroleptic malignant syndrome** a few days after starting neuroleptic drugs.

Wilson disease is a rare (incidence of 1/40,000 to 1/100,000 live births) autosomal recessive inborn error of copper transport characterized by cirrhosis of the liver and degenerative changes in the CNS, particularly the basal ganglia (see Chapter 338.2). The gene (WND) for Wilson disease has been mapped to chromosome 13q14-21. It has been determined that there are multiple mutations in the Wilson disease gene, accounting for the variability in presentation of the condition. The precise cause is unknown, but the basic mechanism relates to decreased excretion of biliary copper, owing partly to a lysosomal defect of the liver cells. The initial symptoms and signs in children younger than 10 yr relate to acute or subacute hepatic failure, which is frequently misinterpreted as infectious hepatitis. The neurologic manifestations of Wilson disease rarely appear before age 10 yr, and the initial sign is often progressive dystonia. Tremors of the extremities develop, unilaterally at first, but they eventually become coarse, generalized, and incapacitating (the so-called wing-beating tremor). Signs of progressive basal ganglia destruction include drooling, a fixed smile caused by retraction of the upper lip, dysarthria, dysphonia, rigidity, contractures, dystonia, and choreoathetosis. The Kayser-Fleischer ring, which is best seen with the slit lamp, is pathognomonic and results from deposition of copper in the Descemet membrane. In the untreated state, patients typically become bedridden and demented and die in coma within a few years from the onset of the disease. The MRI or CT scan shows ventricular dilatation in advanced cases with atrophy of the cerebrum and lesions in the thalamus and basal ganglia. The treatment of Wilson disease is discussed in Chapter 338.2.

Hallervorden-Spatz disease is a rare degenerative disorder inherited as an autosomal recessive trait. Linkage analysis indicates that the gene is located on chromosome 20p13. The condition usually begins during childhood and is characterized by progressive dystonia, rigidity, and choreoathetosis. Spasticity, extensor plantar responses, dysarthria, and intellectual deterioration become evident during adolescence, and death usually occurs by early adulthood. MRI shows lesions of the globus pallidus, including low signal intensity in T2 weighted images (corresponds to iron pigments) and an anteromedial area of high signal intensity, or "eye-of-the-tiger" sign (corresponding to areas of vacuolation). Neuropathologic examination indicates excessive accumulation of iron-containing pigments in the globus pallidus and substantia nigra.

Therapy for dystonia has progressed over the last decade. Children with generalized dystonia, including those with involvement of the muscles of swallowing, may respond to large doses of trihexyphenidyl (Artane). The initial dose is 2 mg/24 hr, slowly increasing to 60–80 mg/24 hr or until untoward side effects (urinary retention, mental confusion, or blurred vision) occur. Additional drugs that have been effective include carbamazepine, levodopa, bromocriptine, and diazepam. Segmental dystonia such as torticollis often responds well to botulinum toxin injections. Intrathecal baclofen delivered through implantable constant infusion pump may be helpful in some patients. Stereotaxic surgery or electrical deep brain stimulation in the thalamus or globus pallidus also appears to be helpful for some children with severe dystonia.

590.4 ■ Tics

Tics are spasmodic, involuntary, repetitive, stereotyped movements that are nonrhythmic, often exacerbated by stress, and may affect any muscle group. Tics can be classified into three subgroups: transient tics of childhood, chronic tics, and Gilles de la Tourette syndrome (TS). **Transient tic disorder** is the most common movement abnormality of childhood (see Chapter 21). The tics are more prevalent in boys, and the family history is often positive. They consist of eye blinking or facial movements and occasional throat-clearing noises. The disorder persists from weeks to less than a year and does not require drug therapy. **Chronic motor tic disorder** occurs in children and persists throughout adult life. The tics characteristically involve up to three muscle groups simultaneously and may occur throughout life. Evidence shows that the gene for TS may be expressed as simple transient tic of childhood and chronic motor tics, suggesting considerable overlap of these conditions.

Gilles de la Tourette syndrome is a lifelong condition, with a prevalence of approximately 1/2,000, that has an onset between 2 and 21 yr of age (see Chapter 21). TS is probably inherited in most cases as autosomal dominant, and the gene has been tentatively mapped to chromosome 18q22.1. TS is diagnosed in children who have multiple motor tics in different parts of the body with at least one vocal tic beginning before age 21 yr and waxing and waning over a period of more than a year. Obsessive-compulsive behavior and attention deficit hyperactivity disorder (ADHD) are also frequently present. Motor tics are associated with numerous fluctuating movements of the face, eyelids, neck, and shoulders. Ultimately, the tics are accompanied by vocalizations (vocal tics), including throat clearing, sniffling, barking, coprolalia (obscene words), echolalia (repetition of words addressed to the patient), palilalia (repetition of one's own words), and echokinesis (imitation of movement of others). The vocalizations are uncontrollable and frequently jeopardize patients' social interaction with other children. TS is a lifelong condition, and the ultimate prognosis can often be determined by the severity of the symptoms during adolescence.

Medication should be considered when the motor tics or vocalizations interfere significantly with a child's social and academic interactions, although behavior management and biofeedback programs have been successful for some patients. Several reports implicate stimulant medications (methylphenidate) as the cause of TS. Methylphenidate may unmask TS but not cause it. All children who have ADHD and who are treated with stimulant medication should be monitored closely for the onset of tics. The decision to continue the stimulant medication should be determined by the severity of the ADHD and tic disorder. Haloperidol, a dopamine-blocking agent, is effective in the treatment of approximately 50% of children with TS. The initial dose is 0.25 mg/24 hr, and the drug is increased weekly by 0.25 mg to the usual dose range of 2–6 mg/24 hr, although some children can tolerate larger doses. Side effects include cognitive impairment, lethargy, fatigue, depression, restlessness, acute dystonic reactions, drug-induced parkinsonism, akathisia, and tardive dyskinesia syndromes, including tardive dystonia in children. Additional drugs that may prove useful include penfluridol, pimozide, and clonidine. Clonidine, an α_2-presynaptic noradrenergic agonist, is begun at a dose of 0.05 mg/24 hr and gradually increased to a maximum of 0.125–0.2 mg/24 hr. Several weeks of clonidine therapy may be needed to control the vocal and motor tics. The major side effects

are lethargy, fatigue, and drowsiness. Approximately 50% of patients with TS experience obsessive-compulsive symptoms. The tricyclic antidepressant clomipramine is effective in approximately 60% of patients. Other useful antidepressant drugs include sertraline, fluoxetine, and fluvoxamine. Because TS is a chronic disorder associated with many social, behavioral, and learning problems, pediatricians can have an important role in the multidisciplinary management as an advocate for children.

Aron AM, Freeman JM, Carter S: The natural history of Sydenham's chorea. *Am J Med* 1965;38:83.

Bebin EM, Bebin J, Currier RD, et al: Morphometric studies in dominant olivopontocerebellar atrophy: Comparison of cell losses with amino acid decreases. *Arch Neurol* 1990;47:188.

Bray PF: Coincidence of neuroblastoma and acute cerebellar encephalopathy. *J Pediatr* 1969;75:983.

Burd L, Kerbeshian J, Berth A, et al: Long-term follow-up of an epidemiologically defined cohort of patients with Tourette syndrome. *J Child Neurol* 2001;16: 431–7.

Campuzano V, Montermini L, Malto MD, et al: Friedreich's ataxia: Autosomal recessive disease caused by an intronic GAA triplet repeat expansion. *Science* 1996;271:1423.

Cervera R, Asherson RA, Font J, et al: Chorea in the antiphospholipid syndrome. *Medicine* 76:203, 1997.

Eldridge R: The torsion dystonia: Literature review and genetic and clinical studies. *Neurology* 1970;20:1.

Fahn S: High dose anticholinergic therapy in dystonia. *Neurology* 1983;33:1255.

Golden GS: Tics and Tourette's: A continuum of symptoms? *Ann Neurol* 1978;4:145.

Hansotia P, Cleeland CS, Chun RWM: Juvenile Huntington's chorea. *Neurology* 18:217, 1968.

Harris MC, Bernbaum JC, Polin JR: Developmental follow-up of breastfed term infants with marked hyperbilirubinemia. *Pediatrics* 2001;107:1075.

Holinski-Feder E, Baldwin K, Hörtnagel K: Large intergenerational variation in age of onset in two young patients with Huntington's disease presenting as dyskinesia. *Pediatrics* 1997;100:896.

Hyland, K, Arnold, LA: Value of lumbar puncture in the diagnosis of genetic metabolic encephalopathies. *J Child Neurol* 1999;14:S9.

Ichinose H, Ohye T, Takahashi E: Hereditary progressive dystonia with marked diurnal fluctuation caused by mutations in the GTP cyclohydrolase I gene. *Nat Genet* 1994;8:236.

Joubert M, Eisenring JJ, Robb JP, et al: Familial agenesis of the cerebellar vermis. *Neurology* 1969;19:824.

Kids Move: *www.wemove.org/kidsmove/* [A good description of movement disorders in children and their treatment.]

Konigsmark BW, Weiner LP: The olivopontocerebellar atrophies: A review. *Medicine* 1970;49:227.

Misbahuddin A, Warner TT: Dystonia: An update on genetics and treatment. *Curr Opin Neurol* 2001;14:471.

Parker S, Zuckerman B, Bauchner H, et al: Jitteriness in full-term neonates: Prevalence and correlates. *Pediatrics* 1990;85:17.

Paulson H, Ammache Z: Ataxia and hereditary disorders. *Neurol Clin* 2001;19:759.

Swedo SE, Leonard HL, Milttleman BB, et al: Identification of children with pediatric autoimmune neuropsychiatric disorders associated with streptococcal infections by a marker associated with rheumatic fever. *Am J Psychiatry* 1997;154:110 and 1998;155:264.

Thomas GR, Forbes JR, Roberts EA, et al: The Wilson disease gene: Spectrum of mutations and their consequences. *Nat Genet* 1995;9:210.

Vakili S: Hallervorden-Spatz syndrome *Arch Neurol* 1977;34:729.

Weiss S, Carter S: Course and prognosis of acute cerebellar ataxia in children. *Neurology* 1959;9:711.

Wong PC, Barlow CF, Hickey PR, et al: Factors associated with choreoathetosis after cardiopulmonary bypass in children with congenital heart disease. *Circulation* 1992;86(Suppl II):118.

Zimprich A, Grabowski M, Asmus F, et al: Mutations in the gene encoding epsilon-sarcoglycan cause myoclonus-dystonia syndrome. *Nat Genet* 2001;29:66.

Chapter 591
Encephalopathies
Michael V. Johnston

Encephalopathy is a generalized disorder of cerebral function that may be acute or chronic, progressive or static. The etiology of the encephalopathies in children includes infectious, toxic (e.g., carbon monoxide, drugs, lead), metabolic, and ischemic causes. Hypoxic-ischemic encephalopathy is discussed in Chapter 88.7.

591.1 Cerebral Palsy

See also Chapters 37 and 86.2.

Cerebral palsy (CP) is a diagnostic term used to describe a group of motor syndromes resulting from disorders of early brain development. CP is caused by a broad group of developmental, genetic, metabolic, ischemic, infectious, and other acquired etiologies that produce a common group of neurologic phenotypes. Although it has historically been considered a *static encephalopathy*, this term is now inaccurate because of the recognition that the neurologic features of CP often change or progress over time. In addition, although CP is often associated with epilepsy and abnormalities of speech, vision, and intellect, it is the selective vulnerability of the brain's motor systems that defines the disorder. Many children and adults with CP function at a high educational and vocational level, without any sign of the type of cognitive dysfunction that is generally implied by the term *encephalopathy*.

Epidemiology and Etiology. CP is the most common and costly form of chronic motor disability that begins in childhood with a prevalence of 2/1000. The Collaborative Perinatal Project, in which approximately 45,000 children were regularly monitored from pregnancy to the age of 7 yr, found that most children with CP had been born at term with uncomplicated labors and deliveries. In 80% of cases, features were identified pointing to antenatal factors causing abnormal brain development. A substantial number of children with CP had congenital anomalies external to the central nervous system (CNS). Fewer than 10% of children with CP had evidence of intrapartum asphyxia. Intrauterine exposure to maternal infection (e.g., chorioamnionitis, inflammation of placental membranes, umbilical cord inflammation, foul-smelling amniotic fluid, maternal sepsis, temperature greater than 38°C during labor, and urinary tract infection) is associated with a significant increase in the risk of CP in normal birthweight infants. Another study found elevated levels of inflammatory cytokines in heelstick blood collected at birth from children who later were identified with CP. The prevalence of CP is increased among low birthweight infants, particularly those weighing less than 1,000 g at birth, primarily because of intracerebral hemorrhage and periventricular leukomalacia (PVL). Cramped synchronized general movements may be an early clinical finding in these infants. Although the incidence of intracerebral hemorrhage has declined significantly, PVL remains a major problem. PVL appears to reflect the enhanced vulnerability of immature oligodendroglia in premature infants to oxidative stress caused by ischemia or infectious/inflammatory insults. This information suggests that attempts to reduce the incidence of CP in term born infants should be directed toward increasing understanding of fetal developmental biology and that for premature infants strategies need to be developed to protect the vulnerable developing white matter.

Clinical Manifestations. CP is generally divided into several major motor syndromes that differ according to the pattern of neurologic involvement, neuropathology, and etiology (Table 591–1). The physiologic classification identifies the major motor abnormality, whereas the topographic taxonomy indicates the involved extremities. CP is also commonly associated with a spectrum of developmental disabilities, including mental retardation, epilepsy, and visual, hearing, speech, cognitive, and behavioral abnormalities. The motor handicap may be the least of the child's problems.

Infants with *spastic hemiplegia* have decreased spontaneous movements on the affected side and show hand preference at a very early age. The arm is often more involved than the leg and difficulty in hand manipulation is obvious by 1 yr of age. Walking is usually delayed until 18–24 mo, and a circumductive gait is apparent. Examination of the extremities may show growth arrest, particularly in the hand and thumbnail, especially if the contralateral parietal lobe is abnormal, because extremity growth is influenced by this area of the brain. Spasticity is apparent in the affected extremities, particularly the ankle, causing an equinovarus deformity of the foot. An affected child often walks on tiptoes because of the increased tone, and the affected upper extremity assumes a dystonic posture when the child runs. Ankle clonus and a Babinski sign may be present, the deep tendon reflexes are increased, and weakness of the hand and foot dorsiflexors is evident. About one third of patients with spastic hemiplegia have a seizure disorder that usually develops during the first year or two, and approximately 25% have cognitive abnormalities including mental retardation. A CT scan or MRI study may show an atrophic cerebral hemisphere with a dilated lateral ventricle contralateral to the side of the affected extremities. An MRI is far more sensitive than CT for most lesions seen with CP, although a CT scan may be useful for detecting calcifications associated with congenital infections. Focal cerebral infarction secondary to intrauterine or perinatal thromboembolism related to thrombophilic disorders, especially anticardiolipin antibodies, is an important cause of hemiplegic CP. Family histories suggestive of thrombosis and inherited clotting disorders may be present and evaluation of the mother may provide information valuable for future pregnancies and other family members.

Spastic diplegia is bilateral spasticity of the legs greater than in the arms. The first indication of spastic diplegia is often noted when an affected infant begins to crawl. The child uses the arms in a normal reciprocal fashion but tends to drag the legs behind more as a rudder (commando crawl) rather than using the normal four-limbed crawling movement. If the spasticity is severe, application of a diaper is difficult because of the excessive

TABLE 591–1. Classification of Cerebral Palsy and Major Causes

Motor Syndrome	Neuropathology	Major Causes
Spastic Diplegia	Periventricular Leukomalacia (periventricular leukomalacic [PVL])	Prematurity Ischemia Infection Endocrine/metabolic (e.g., thyroid)
Spastic quadriplegia	PVL Multicystic encephalomalacia Malformations	Ischemia Infection Endocrine/metabolic Genetic/developmental
Hemiplegia	Stoke: in utero or neonatal	Thrombophilic disorders Infection Genetic/developmental Periventricular hemorrhagic infarction
Extrapyramidal (athetoid, dyskinetic)	Basal ganglia Pathology: putamen, globus pallidus, thalamus	Asphyxia Kernicterus Mitochondrial Genetic/metabolic

adduction of the hips. Examination of the child reveals spasticity in the legs with brisk reflexes, ankle clonus, and a bilateral Babinski sign. When the child is suspended by the axillae, a scissoring posture of the lower extremities is maintained. Walking is significantly delayed, the feet are held in a position of equinovarus, and the child walks on tiptoes. Severe spastic diplegia is characterized by disuse atrophy and impaired growth of the lower extremities and by disproportionate growth with normal development of the upper torso. The prognosis for normal intellectual development is excellent for these patients, and the likelihood of seizures is minimal. The most common neuropathologic finding is periventricular leukomalacia, particularly in the area where fibers innervating the legs course through the internal capsule. MRI is very useful for evaluating the severity of white matter injury and for excluding other brain lesions.

Spastic quadriplegia is the most severe form of CP because of marked motor impairment of all extremities and the high association with mental retardation and seizures. Swallowing difficulties are common as a result of supranuclear bulbar palsies, often leading to aspiration pneumonia. The most common lesions seen on pathologic examination or on MRI scanning are severe PVL and multicystic cortical encephalomalacia. Neurologic examination shows increased tone and spasticity in all extremities, decreased spontaneous movements, brisk reflexes, and plantar extensor responses. Flexion contractures of the knees and elbows are often present by late childhood. Associated developmental disabilities, including speech and visual abnormalities, are particularly prevalent in this group of children. Children with spastic quadriparesis often have evidence of athetosis and may be classified as having mixed CP.

Athetoid CP, also called *choreoathetoid* or *extrapyramidal* CP, is less common than spastic cerebral palsy. Affected infants are characteristically hypotonic with poor head control and marked head lag and develop increased variable tone with rigidity and dystonia over several years. Feeding may be difficult, and tongue thrust and drooling may be prominent. Speech is typically affected because the oropharyngeal muscles are involved. Speech may be absent or sentences are slurred, and voice modulation is impaired. Generally, upper motor neuron signs are not present, seizures are uncommon, and intellect is preserved in many patients. This form of CP is also referred to as dyskinetic CP in Europe and is the type most likely to be associated with birth asphyxia. Extrapyramidal CP secondary to acute intrapartum near-total asphyxia is associated with bilaterally symmetric lesions in the posterior putamen and ventrolateral thalamus. These lesions appear to be the correlate of the neuropathologic lesion called *status marmoratus* in the basal ganglia. Athetoid CP can also be caused by kernicterus secondary to high levels of bilirubin, and in this case the MRI scan shows lesions in the globus pallidus bilaterally. Extrapyramidal CP can also be associated with lesions in the basal ganglia and thalamus caused by metabolic genetic disorders such as mitochondrial disorders and glutaric aciduria. MRI scanning and possibly metabolic testing are important in the evaluation of children with extrapyramidal CP to make a correct diagnosis of etiology.

Diagnosis. A thorough history and physical examination should preclude a progressive disorder of the CNS, including degenerative diseases, metabolic disorders, spinal cord tumor, or muscular dystrophy. The possibility of anomalies at the base of the skull or other disorders affecting the cervical spinal cord needs to be considered in patients with little involvement of the arms or cranial nerves. An MRI scan of the brain is generally indicated to determine the location and extent of structural lesions or associated congenital malformations, and an MRI scan of the spinal cord is worthwhile if there is any question about spinal cord pathology. Additional studies may include tests of hearing and visual function. Genetic evaluation should be considered in patients with congenital malformations or evidence of metabolic disorders. Because CP is usually associated with a wide spectrum of developmental disorders, a multidisciplinary approach is most helpful in the assessment and treatment of such children.

Treatment. A team of physicians from various specialties, as well as occupational and physical therapists, speech pathologists, social workers, educators, and developmental psychologists provide important contributions to the treatment of these children. Parents should be taught how to handle their child in daily activities such as feeding, carrying, dressing, bathing, and playing in ways that limit the effects of abnormal muscle tone. They also need to be instructed in the supervision of a series of exercises designed to prevent the development of contractures, especially a tight Achilles tendon. There is no proof that physical or occupational therapy prevents development of CP in infants at risk or that it corrects the neurologic deficit, but ample evidence shows that therapy optimizes the development of an abnormal child.

Children with spastic diplegia are treated initially with the assistance of adaptive equipment, such as walkers, poles, and standing frames. If a patient has marked spasticity of the lower extremities or evidence of hip dislocation, consideration should be given to performing surgical soft tissue procedures that reduce muscle spasm around the hip girdle, including an adductor tenotomy or psoas transfer and release. A rhizotomy procedure in which the roots of the spinal nerves are divided has produced considerable improvement in selected patients with severe spastic diplegia. A tight heel cord in a child with spastic hemiplegia may be treated surgically by tenotomy of the Achilles tendon. Quadriplegia is managed with motorized wheelchairs, special feeding devices, modified typewriters, and customized seating arrangements.

Communication skills may be enhanced by the use of Bliss symbols, talking typewriters, and specially adapted computers including artificial intelligence computers to augment motor and language function. Significant behavior problems may substantially interfere with the development of a child with CP; their early identification and management are important, and the assistance of a psychologist or psychiatrist may be necessary. Learning and attention deficit disorders and mental retardation are assessed and managed by a psychologist and educator. Strabismus, nystagmus, and optic atrophy are common in children with CP; thus, an ophthalmologist should be included in the initial assessment. Lower urinary tract dysfunction should receive prompt assessment and treatment.

Several drugs have been used to treat spasticity, including dantrolene sodium, the benzodiazepines, and baclofen. These medications are generally ineffective but should be considered if severe spasticity is not controlled by other measures. Intrathecal baclofen has been used successfully in selected children with severe spasticity. This experimental therapy requires a team approach and constant follow-up for complications of the infusion pumping mechanism and infection. Botulinum toxin is undergoing study for the management of spasticity in specific muscle groups, and the preliminary findings show a positive response in those patients studied. Patients with rigidity, dystonia, and spastic quadriparesis sometimes respond to levodopa, and children with dystonia may benefit from carbamazepine or trihexyphenidyl. Hyperbaric oxygen does not improve the condition of children with CP.

591.2 Mitochondrial Encephalomyopathies*

Mitochondrial diseases are a complex family of disorders with many clinical manifestations that can be caused by mutations of nuclear DNA (nDNA) or mitochondrial DNA (mtDNA). They can affect various developmental stages, tissues, or systems,

---

*Written with the collaboration of Dr. Ingrid Tein.

resulting in a diversity of clinical phenotypes that span all age groups. Biochemically, they can present with a tissue-specific or generalized monoenzymopathy, tissue-specific multienzymopathy, or generalized multienzymopathy. In the respiratory chain, oxidative phosphorylation is mediated by five intramitochondrial enzyme complexes (complexes I–V) that are responsible for producing the adenosine triphosphate (ATP) required for normal cellular function. The maintenance and assembly of oxidative phosphorylation require coordinated regulation of nuclear DNA and mitochondrial DNA genes. Human mtDNA is a small (16.5 kb), circular, double-stranded molecule that has been completely sequenced and encodes 13 structural proteins, all of which are subunits of the respiratory chain complexes, as well as two ribosomal RNAs and 22 tRNAs needed for translation. The nuclear DNA is responsible for synthesizing approximately 70 subunits, transporting them to the mitochondria via chaperone proteins, ensuring their passage across the inner mitochondrial membrane, and coordinating their correct processing and assembly.

mtDNA is unique from nDNA for the following reasons: (1) Its genetic code differs from nDNA, (2) it is tightly packed with information because it contains no introns, (3) it is subject to spontaneous mutations at a higher rate than nDNA, (4) it has less efficient repair mechanisms, and (5) it is present in hundreds or thousands of copies per cell and is transmitted by maternal inheritance. mtDNA is contributed only by the oocyte in the formation of the zygote. If a mutation in mtDNA occurs in the ovum or zygote, it may be passed on randomly to subsequent generations of cells. Some receive few or no mutant genomes (normal or wild-type homoplasmy), others receive a mixed population of mutant and wild-type mtDNAs (heteroplasmy), and others receive primarily or exclusively mutant genomes (mutant homoplasmy). The important implications of maternal inheritance and heteroplasmy are as follows: (1) Inheritance of the disease is maternal, but both sexes are equally affected; (2) phenotypic expression of an mtDNA mutation depends on the relative proportions of mutant and wild-type genomes, with a minimum critical number of mutant genomes being necessary for expression (threshold effect); (3) at cell division, the proportion may shift in daughter cells (mitotic segregation), leading to a corresponding phenotypic change; and (4) subsequent generations are affected at a higher rate than in autosomal dominant diseases. The critical number of mutant mtDNAs required for the threshold effect may vary, depending on the vulnerability of the tissue to impairments of oxidative metabolism as well as on the vulnerability of the same tissue over time that may increase with aging. Diseases of mitochondrial oxidative phosphorylation can be divided into three groups: (1) defects of nDNA, (2) defects of mtDNA, and (3) defects of communication between the nuclear and mitochondrial genome.

Using a broader classification system, mitochondrial diseases caused by defects of nDNA include defects of substrate transport (plasmalemmal carnitine transporter, carnitine palmitoyltransferase I and II, carnitine acylcarnitine translocase defects), defects of substrate oxidation (pyruvate dehydrogenase complex, pyruvate carboxylase, intramitochondrial fatty acid oxidation defects), defects of the Krebs cycle (α-ketoglutarate dehydrogenase, fumarase, aconitase defects), and defects of the respiratory chain (complexes I to V) including defects of oxidation/phosphorylation coupling (Luft syndrome) and defects of mitochondrial protein transport. These diseases follow mendelian inheritance. Diseases caused by defects of mtDNA can be divided into those due to point mutations that are maternally inherited (Leber hereditary optic neuropathy and MELAS, MERRF, and NARP syndromes—see later text) and those due to deletions or duplications that tend to be sporadic (Kearns-Sayre and Pearson marrow/pancreas syndromes). Finally, diseases caused by defects of communication between the nuclear and mitochondrial genome follow mendelian inheritance and include multiple mtDNA deletions, which are autosomal dominant, and mtDNA depletion syndromes, which are generally autosomal recessive.

Mitochondrial Encephalomyopathy, Encephalomyopathy, Lactic Acidosis, and Strokelike Episodes (MELAS). Children with MELAS may be normal for the first several years, but they gradually display delayed motor and cognitive development and short stature. The clinical syndrome is characterized by (1) strokelike episodes most commonly in the posterior temporal, parietal, and occipital lobes (with CT or MRI evidence of focal brain abnormalities); (2) lactic acidosis, ragged red fibers (RRF), or both; and (3) at least two of the following: focal or generalized seizures, dementia, recurrent migraine headaches, and vomiting. In one series, onset was before age 15 yr in 62% of patients and hemianopia or cortical blindness was the most common manifestation. Cerebrospinal fluid protein is often increased. The MELAS 3243 mutation can also be associated with different combinations of exercise intolerance, myopathy, ophthalmoplegia, pigmentary retinopathy, hypertrophic or dilated cardiomyopathy, cardiac conduction defects, deafness, endocrinopathy (diabetes mellitus), and proximal renal tubular dysfunction. MELAS is a progressive disorder that has been reported in siblings. It is punctuated with episodes of stroke leading to dementia. Also see Chapter 602.4.

Regional hypoperfusion can be detected by single-photon-emission CT (SPECT) studies. Neuropathology may show cortical atrophy with infarct-like lesions in both cortical and subcortical structures, basal ganglia calcifications, and ventricular dilatation. Muscle biopsy specimens usually show RRF. Mitochondrial accumulations and abnormalities have been shown in smooth muscle cells of intramuscular vessels and of brain arterioles and in the epithelial cells and blood vessels of the choroid plexus, producing a mitochondrial angiopathy. Muscle biochemistry has shown complex I deficiency in many cases; however, multiple defects have also been documented involving complexes I, III, and IV. Inheritance is maternal, and there is a highly specific, although not exclusive, point mutation at nt 3243 in the tRNA$^{Leu (UUR)}$ gene of mtDNA in approximately 80% of patients. An additional 7.5% have a point mutation at nt 3271 in the tRNA$^{Leu (UUR)}$ gene. A third mutation has been identified at nt 3252 in the tRNA$^{leu (UUR)}$ gene. Because the number of mutant genomes is lower in blood than in muscle, muscle is the preferable tissue for examination.

The prognosis in patients with the full syndrome is poor. Therapeutic trials have included corticosteroids and coenzyme Q10. Lowering the serum lactate concentration with dichloroacetate has led to marked clinical improvement in some cases.

Myoclonus Epilepsy and Ragged-Red Fibers (MERRF). This syndrome is characterized by progressive myoclonic epilepsy, mitochondrial myopathy, and cerebellar ataxia with dysarthria and nystagmus. Onset may be in childhood or in adult life, and the course may be slowly progressive or rapidly downhill. Other features include dementia, sensorineural hearing loss, optic atrophy, peripheral neuropathy, and spasticity. Because some patients have abnormalities of deep sensation and pes cavus, the condition may be confused with Friedreich ataxia. As with MELAS syndrome, a significant number of patients have a positive family history and short stature. This condition is maternally inherited.

Pathologic findings include elevated serum lactate concentrations, RRF on muscle biopsy, and marked neuronal loss and gliosis affecting in particular the dentate nucleus and inferior olivary complex with some dropout of Purkinje cells and neurons of the red nucleus. Pallor of the posterior columns of the spinal cord and degeneration of the gracile and cuneate nuclei are noted. Muscle biochemistry has shown variable defects of complex III, complexes II and IV, complexes I and IV, or complex IV alone. More than 80% of cases are caused by a heteroplasmic

G to A point mutation at nt 8344 of the tRNA^{Lys} gene of mtDNA. Additional patients have been reported with a T to C mutation at nt 8356 in the tRNA^{Lys} gene.

There is no specific therapy, although coenzyme Q10 appeared to be beneficial in a mother and daughter with the MERRF mutation.

Leber Hereditary Optic Neuropathy (LHON). LHON is characterized by onset usually between the ages of 18 and 30 yr of acute or subacute visual loss caused by severe bilateral optic atrophy, although children as young as 5 yr have been reported to have LHON. At least 85% of patients are young men. This suggests an X-linked factor that modulates the expression of the mitochondrial DNA point mutation. The classic ophthalmologic features include circumpapillary telangiectatic microangiopathy and pseudoedema of the optic disc. Variable features may include cerebellar ataxia, hyperreflexia, Babinski sign, psychiatric symptoms, peripheral neuropathy, or cardiac conduction abnormalities (pre-excitation syndrome). Some cases have been associated with widespread white matter lesions as seen with multiple sclerosis. Lactic acidosis and RRF tend to be conspicuously absent in LHON. More than 11 mtDNA point mutations have been described, including a usually homoplasmic G to A transition at nt 11,778 of the ND4 subunit gene of complex I. The latter leads to replacement of a highly conserved arginine residue by histidine at the 340th amino acid and accounts for approximately 50–70% of cases in Europe and more than 90% of cases in Japan. Certain LHON pedigrees with other point mutations are associated with complex neurologic disorders and may have features in common with MELAS syndrome and with infantile bilateral striatal necrosis.

ATPase Subunit 6 Mutation (NARP). This maternally inherited disorder presents with either Leigh syndrome or with developmental delay, retinitis pigmentosa, dementia, seizures, ataxia, proximal weakness, and sensory neuropathy (NARP syndrome). It is due to a point mutation at nt 8993 within the ATPase subunit 6 gene. The severity of the disease presentation appears to have close correlation with the percentage of mutant mtDNA in leukocytes.

Kearns-Sayre Syndrome (KSS). The criteria for KSS include a triad of (1) onset before age 20 yr, (2) progressive external ophthalmoplegia (PEO) with ptosis, and (3) pigmentary retinopathy. In addition, there must be at least one of the following: heart block, cerebellar syndrome, or cerebrospinal fluid protein greater than 100 mg/dL. Other nonspecific but common features include dementia, sensorineural hearing loss, and multiple endocrine abnormalities, including short stature, diabetes mellitus, and hypoparathyroidism. The prognosis is poor, despite placement of a pacemaker, and progressively downhill, with death resulting by the 3rd or 4th decade. Unusual clinical presentations can include renal tubular acidosis and Lowe syndrome. There are also a few overlap cases of children with KSS and strokelike episodes. Muscle biopsy shows RRF and variable cytochrome oxidase (COX)-negative fibers. Most patients have mtDNA deletions, and some have duplications. These may be new mutations accounting for the generally sporadic nature of KSS. A few pedigrees have shown autosomal dominant transmission.

Sporadic PEO with RRF is a clinically benign condition characterized by adolescent or young adult–onset ophthalmoplegia, ptosis, and proximal limb girdle weakness. It is slowly progressive and compatible with a relatively normal life. The muscle biopsy material demonstrates RRF and COX-negative fibers. Approximately 50% of patients with PEO have mtDNA deletions, and there is no family history.

Leigh Disease (Subacute Necrotizing Encephalomyopathy). There are at least four known genetically determined causes of Leigh disease: pyruvate dehydrogenase complex deficiency, complex I deficiency, complex IV (COX) deficiency, and complex V (ATPase) deficiency. These defects may occur sporadically or be inherited by autosomal recessive transmission, as in the case of COX deficiency; by X-linked transmission, as in the case of PDH E$_1\alpha$ deficiency; or by maternal transmission, as in complex V (ATPase 6 nt 8993 mutation) deficiency. Most cases become apparent during infancy with feeding and swallowing problems, vomiting, and failure to thrive. Delayed motor and language milestones may be evident, and generalized seizures, weakness, hypotonia, ataxia, tremor, pyramidal signs, and nystagmus are prominent findings. Intermittent respirations with associated sighing or sobbing are characteristic and suggest brainstem dysfunction. Some patients have external ophthalmoplegia, ptosis, optic atrophy, and decreased visual acuity. Abnormal results on CT or MRI scan consist of bilaterally symmetric areas of low attenuation in the basal ganglia. Pathologic changes consist of focal symmetric areas of necrosis in the thalamus, basal ganglia, tegmental gray matter, periventricular and periaqueductal regions of the brainstem, and posterior columns of the spinal cord. Microscopically, these *spongiform* lesions show cystic cavitation with neuronal loss, demyelination, and vascular proliferation. Elevations in serum lactate levels are characteristic. The overall outlook is poor, but a few patients experience prolonged periods of remission.

Reye Syndrome. This encephalopathy, which has become quite uncommon, is associated with pathologic features characterized by fatty degeneration of the viscera (microvesicular steatosis) and mitochondrial abnormalities and biochemical features consistent with a disturbance of mitochondrial metabolism (see Chapter 342). Sporadic Reye syndrome can occur in the context of influenza B virus and salicylate ingestion, in the idiosyncratic valproic acid hepatotoxicity reaction in individuals who may have an underlying genetic predisposition, and in Jamaican vomiting sickness (caused by the hypoglycin toxin).

Recurrent Reye-like syndrome is encountered in children with genetic defects of fatty acid oxidation, such as deficiencies of the plasmalemmal carnitine transporter, carnitine palmitoyltransferase I and II, carnitine acylcarnitine translocase, medium- and long-chain acyl-CoA dehydrogenase, multiple acyl CoA dehydrogenase, and long-chain L-3 hydroxyacyl-CoA dehydrogenase or trifunctional protein. These disorders are manifested by recurrent hypoglycemic and hypoketotic encephalopathy, and they are inherited in an autosomal recessive pattern. Other potential inborn errors of metabolism presenting with Reye syndrome include urea cycle defects (e.g., ornithine transcarbamylase, carbamyl phosphate synthetase) and certain of the organic acidurias (e.g., glutaric aciduria type I), respiratory chain defects, and defects of carbohydrate metabolism (e.g., fructose intolerance).

591.3 Other Encephalopathies

AIDS Encephalopathy. Encephalopathy is an unfortunate and common manifestation in infants and children with HIV infection (see Chapter 254). Neurologic signs in congenitally infected patients may appear during early infancy or may be delayed to as late as 5 yr of age. The primary features of AIDS encephalopathy include an arrest in brain growth, evidence of developmental delay, and the evolution of neurologic signs including weakness with pyramidal tract signs, ataxia, myoclonus, pseudobulbar palsy, and seizures.

Acute Disseminated Encephalomyelitis (ADEM). ADEM is a monophasic, immune-mediated illness that follows immunizations or infections including rubeola, rubella, varicella, herpes zoster, mumps, mycoplasma pneumoniae, or other upper respiratory tract infections. Clinical features include lethargy, delirium, coma, seizures, bilateral optic neuritis, myelopathy, and other focal neurologic signs. MRI typically shows disseminated multifocal lesions in white matter, basal ganglia, and brainstem consistent with edema, inflammation, and demyelination, which may enhance with gadolinium. Hemorrhagic white matter lesions are sometimes seen. Some cases may respond to corticosteroids or immunoglobulin therapy.

Lead Encephalopathy. See Chapter 703.

Burn Encephalopathy. An encephalopathy develops in approximately 5% of children with significant burns during the first several weeks of hospitalization (see also Chapter 62). There is no single cause of burn encephalopathy but rather a combination of factors that include anoxia (smoke inhalation, carbon monoxide poisoning, laryngospasm), electrolyte abnormalities, bacteremia and sepsis, cortical vein thrombosis, a concomitant head injury, cerebral edema, drug reactions, and emotional distress. Seizures are the most common clinical manifestation of burn encephalopathy, but altered states of consciousness, hallucinations, and coma may also occur. Management of burn encephalopathy is directed to a search for the underlying cause and treatment of hypoxemia, seizures, specific electrolyte abnormalities, or cerebral edema. The prognosis for complete neurologic recovery is generally excellent, particularly if seizures are the primary abnormality.

Hypertensive Encephalopathy. Hypertensive encephalopathy is most commonly associated with renal disease in children, including acute glomerulonephritis, chronic pyelonephritis, and end-stage renal disease (see Chapters 437 and 527). In some cases, hypertensive encephalopathy is the initial manifestation of underlying renal disease. Marked systemic hypertension produces vasoconstriction of the cerebral vessels, which leads to vascular permeability, causing areas of focal cerebral edema and hemorrhage. The onset may be acute, with seizures and coma, or more indolent, with headache, drowsiness and lethargy, nausea and vomiting, blurred vision, transient cortical blindness, and hemiparesis. Examination of the eyegrounds may be nondiagnostic in children, but papilledema and retinal hemorrhages may occur. Treatment is directed at restoration of a normotensive state and control of seizures with appropriate anticonvulsants.

Radiation Encephalopathy. Although techniques for administering radiation therapy to the brain have improved considerably and the incidence of serious side effects has decreased significantly, radiation encephalopathy remains an important complication. *Acute radiation encephalopathy* is most likely to develop in young patients who have received large daily doses. Excessive radiation injures vessel endothelium, resulting in enhanced vascular permeability, cerebral edema, and numerous hemorrhages. The child may suddenly become irritable and lethargic, complain of headache, or present with focal neurologic signs and seizures. Patients occasionally develop hemiparesis due to an infarct secondary to vascular occlusion of the cerebral vessels. Steroids are often beneficial in reducing the cerebral edema and reversing the neurologic signs. *Late radiation encephalopathy* is characterized by headaches and slowly progressive focal neurologic signs, including hemiparesis and seizures. Some children with acute lymphatic leukemia treated with a combination of intrathecal methotrexate and cranial irradiation develop neurologic signs months or years later; signs consist of increasing lethargy, loss of cognitive abilities, dementia, and focal neurologic signs and seizures (see Chapter 486). The CT scan shows calcifications in the white matter, and the postmortem examination demonstrates a necrotizing encephalopathy. This devastating complication of the treatment of leukemia has prompted re-evaluation of the use of cranial radiation in the treatment of these children.

Zellweger Syndrome (Cerebrohepatorenal Syndrome [CHRS]). This rare, lethal disorder is inherited as an autosomal recessive trait.

It represents the prototype of a group of peroxisomal disorders that have overlapping symptoms, signs, and biochemical abnormalities (see Chapter 75.2). Infants with Zellweger syndrome have dysmorphic facies consisting of frontal bossing and a large anterior fontanel. The occiput is flattened, and the external ears are abnormal. A high-arched palate, excessive skinfolds of the neck, severe hypotonia, and areflexia are usually evident. Examination of the eyes reveals searching nystagmoid movements, bilateral cataracts, and optic atrophy. Generalized seizures become evident early in life, associated with severe global developmental delay and a significant bilateral hearing loss. The cause of the severe neurologic abnormalities is related to an arrest of migrating neuroblasts during early development, resulting in cerebral pachygyria with neuronal heterotopia (see Chapter 585.7). Hepatomegaly is a prominent finding shortly after birth, often associated with a history of prolonged neonatal jaundice. Patients with Zellweger syndrome rarely survive beyond 1 yr of age.

Bottos M, Feliciangeli A, Sciuto LS, et al: Functional status of adults with cerebral palsy and implications for treating children. *Dev Med Child Neurol* 2001;431:516–28.

Brunstrom JE, Bastion AJ, Wong M, et al: Motor benefit from levodopa in spastic quadriplegic cerebral palsy. *Ann Neurol* 2000;47:662.

Brunstrom JE: Clinical considerations on cerebral palsy and spasticity. *J Child Neurol* 2001;16:10–5.

Butler C, Darrah J: Effects of neurodevelopmental treatment (NDT) for cerebral palsy: An AACPDM evidence report. *Dev Med Child Neurol* 2001;43:778–90.

Chong SK: Gastrointestinal problems in the handicapped child. *Eur Opin Pediatr* 2001;13:441–6.

Ciafaloni E, Ricci E, Shanske S, et al: MELAS: Clinical features, biochemistry and molecular genetics. *Ann Neurol* 1992;31:391.

Collet J, Vanasse M, Marois P, et al: Hyperbaric oxygen for children with cerebral palsy: A randomized multicenter trial. *Lancet* 2001;357:582–6.

Croen LA, Grether JK, Curry CJ: Congenital abnormalities among children with cerebral palsy: More evidence for prenatal antecedents. *J Pediatr* 2001;138:804.

Dammann O, Leviton A: Maternal intrauterine infection, cytokines, and brain damage in the preterm newborn. *Pediatr Res* 1997;42:1.

Edgar TS: Clinical utility of botulinum toxin in the treatment of cerebral palsy: Comprehensive review. *J Child Neurol* 2001;16:37–46.

Fehlings D, Rang M, Glazier J, et al: An evaluation of botulinum-A toxin injections to improve upper extremity function in children with hemiplegic cerebral palsy. *J Pediatr* 2000;137:331.

Ferrari F, Cioni G, Einspieler C, et al: Cramped synchronized general movements in preterm infants as early markers for cerebral palsy. *Arch Pediatr Adolesc Med* 2002;156:460–7.

Gilmartin R, Bruce D, Storrs BB, et al: Intrathecal baclofen for management of spastic cerebral palsy: Multicenter trial. *J Child Neurol* 2000;15:71.

Golomb MR, MacGregor DL, Domi T, et al: Presumed pre- or perinatal arterial ischemic stroke: Risk factors and outcomes. *Ann Neurol* 2001;50:163.

Goto Y, Nonaka I, Horai S: A mutation in the tRNA$^{Leu(UUR)}$ gene associated with the MELAS subgroup of mitochondrial encephalomyopathies. *Nature* 1990; 348:651.

Grether JK, Nelson KB: Maternal infection and cerebral palsy in infants of normal birth weight. *JAMA* 1997;278:207.

Harum KH, Hoon AH, Kato GJ, et al: Homozygous factor-V mutation as a genetic cause of perinatal thrombosis and cerebral palsy. *Dev Med Child Neuro* 1999; 41:777.

Hoon AH, Reinhardt EM, Kelley RI, et al: Brain MR imaging in suspected extrapyramidal cerebral palsy: Observations in distinguishing genetic-metabolic from acquired etiologies. *J Pediatr* 1997;131:159.

Hoon AH, Freese PO, Reinhardt EM, et al: Age-dependent effects of trihexyphenidyl in extrapyramidal cerebral palsy. *Pediatr Neurol* 2001;25:55.

Hyland K, Arnold LA: Value of lumbar puncture in the diagnosis of genetic metabolic encephalopathies. *J Child Neurol* 1999;14:S9.

Karpati G, Carpenter S, Larbrisseau A, et al: The Kearns-Sayre syndrome: A multisystem disease with mitochondrial abnormality demonstrated in skeletal muscle and skin. *J Neurol Sci* 1973;19:133.

Kobayashi M, Morishita H, Sugiyama N, et al: Two cases of NADH-coenzyme Q reductase deficiency: Relationship to MELAS syndrome. *J Pediatr* 1987;110:223.

Koman LA, Brashear A, Rosenfeld S, et al: Botulinum toxin type A neuromuscular blockade in the treatment of equinus foot deformity in cerebral palsy: A multicenter, open-label clinical trial. *Pediatrics* 2001;108(5):1062–70.

Krach LE: Pharmacotherapy of spasticity: Oral medications and intrathecal baclofen. *J Child Neurol* 2001;16(1):31–6.

McLaughlin J, Bjornson KI, Temkin N, et al: Selective dorsal rhizotomy: Meta-analysis of three randomized controlled trials. *Dev Med Child Neurol* 2002;44: 17–25.

Mohnot D, Snead OC, Benton JW: Burn encephalopathy in children. *Ann Neurol* 12:42, 1982.

Moraes CT, DiMauro S, Zeviani M, et al: Mitochondrial DNA deletions in progressive external ophthalmoplegia and Kearns-Sayre syndrome. *N Engl J Med* 1989;320:1293.

Nasr JT, Andriola MR, Coyle PK: ADEM: Literature review and case report of acute psychosis presentation. *Pediatr Neurol* 2000;22:8.

Nelson KB, Dambrosia JM, Grether JK, et al: Neonatal cytokines and coagulation factors in children with cerebral palsy. *Ann Neurol* 1998;44:665.

Pavlakis SG, Phillips PC, Di Mauro S, et al: Mitochondrial myopathy, encephalopathy, lactic acidosis, and strokelike episodes: A distinctive clinical syndrome. *Ann Neurol* 1984;16:481.

Robinson BH, Taylor J, Sherwood WG: The genetic heterogeneity of lactic acidosis: Occurrence of recognizable inborn errors of metabolism in a pediatric population with lactic acidosis. *Pediatr Res* 1980;14:956.

Shoffner JM, Lott M, Lezza AM, et al: Myoclonic epilepsy and ragged-red fiber disease (MERRF) is associated with a mitochondrial DNA tRNA^{Lys} mutation. *Cell* 1990;61:931.

Ubhi T, Bhakta BB, Allgar V, et al: Randomised double blind placebo controlled trail of the effect of botulinum toxin on walking in cerebral palsy. *Arch Dis Child* 2000;83:481.

Wallace DC, Singh G, Lott MT, et al: Mitochondrial DNA mutation associated with Leber's hereditary optic neuropathy. *Science* 1988;242:1427.

Chapter 592

Neurodegenerative Disorders of Childhood

Michael V. Johnston

Neurodegenerative disorders of childhood encompass a large number of heterogeneous diseases that result from specific genetic and biochemical defects, chronic viral infections, and a significant group of conditions of unknown cause. In the past, children with suspected neurodegenerative disorders were subjected to brain and rectal biopsies, but with the advent of modern neuroimaging techniques and specific biochemical molecular diagnostic tests, these invasive procedures are rarely necessary. Nevertheless, the most important component of the investigation continues to be a thorough history and physical examination. The hallmark of a neurodegenerative disease is progressive deterioration of neurologic function with loss of speech, vision, hearing, or locomotion, often associated with seizures, feeding difficulties, and impairment of intellect. The age of onset, rate of progression, and principal neurologic findings determine whether the disease is primarily affecting the white or gray matter. Upper motor neuron signs are prominent early in the former, and convulsions, intellectual, and visual impairment in the latter. A precise history confirms regression of developmental milestones, and the neurologic examination localizes the process within the nervous system. Although the outcome is usually fatal and current therapeutic attempts have been unsuccessful, it is important to make the correct diagnosis

so that genetic counseling may be offered and prevention strategies can be implemented. Bone marrow transplantation and other forms of cell and gene therapies are also becoming useful for preventing the progression of disease in presymptomatic individuals. For all conditions in which the specific enzyme defect is known, prevention by prenatal diagnosis (chorionic villus sampling or amniocentesis) is possible. Carrier detection is also often possible by enzyme assay. Table 592–1 summarizes the heredity, biochemical defects, and specific diagnostic abnormality in the inherited neurodegenerative disorders. Additional age of onset-related categorization is noted in Table 592–2.

The inherited neurodegenerative disorders include the sphingolipidoses, neuronal ceroid lipofuscinoses, adrenoleukodystrophy, and sialidosis. The sphingolipidoses are characterized by intracellular storage of a normal lipid component of the cell membrane that results from a defect in catabolism of the compound. The sphingolipidoses are subclassified into six categories: Niemann-Pick disease, Gaucher disease, GM$_1$ gangliosidosis, GM$_2$ gangliosidosis, Krabbe disease, and metachromatic leukodystrophy. Niemann-Pick disease and Gaucher disease are discussed in Chapter 75.4. The spinocerebellar degenerative diseases (Friedreich ataxia, ataxia-telangiectasia, olivopontocerebellar atrophy, and abetalipoproteinemia) and degenerative disorders of the basal ganglia (Huntington disease, dystonia musculorum deformans, Wilson disease, and Hallervorden-Spatz disease) are discussed in Chapter 590. Finally, a miscellaneous group of degenerative diseases is discussed in this section, including multiple sclerosis, Pelizaeus-Merzbacher disease, Alexander disease, Canavan spongy degeneration, kinky hair disease, Rett syndrome, and subacute sclerosing panencephalitis.

592.1 Sphingolipidoses

GANGLIOSIDOSES

See also Chapter 75.4.

Gangliosides are glycosphingolipids, normal constituents of the neuronal and synaptic membranes. The basic structure of GM$_1$ ganglioside consists of an oligosaccharide chain attached to a hydroxyl group of ceramide and sialic acid bound to galactose. The gangliosides are catabolized by sequential cleavage of the sugar molecules by specific exoglycosidases. Abnormalities in catabolism result in an accumulation of the ganglioside within the cell. Defects in ganglioside degradation can be classified into two groups: the GM$_1$ gangliosidoses and the GM$_2$ gangliosidoses.

GM$_1$ Gangliosidoses. The three subtypes of GM$_1$ gangliosidoses are classified according to age at presentation: infantile (type 1), juvenile (type 2), and adult (type 3). The condition is inherited as an autosomal recessive trait and results from a marked

TABLE 592–1. Heredity and Biochemical Defects in the Neurodegenerative Disorders

Neurodegenerative Disorder	Mode of Inheritance	Biochemical Defect	Specimen for Analysis
Sphingolipidosis			
GM$_1$ gangliosidosis	AR	β-Galactosidase	Serum, leukocytes, skin fibroblasts
GM$_2$ gangliosidosis			
Tay-Sachs disease	AR	Hexosaminidase A	Serum, leukocytes, skin fibroblasts
Sandhoff disease	AR	Hexosaminidase A and B	Serum, leukocytes, skin fibroblasts
Krabbe disease	AR	Galactocerebrosidase	Leukocytes and skin fibroblasts
Metachromatic leukodystrophy	AR	Arylsulfatase A	Leukocytes and skin fibroblasts
Neuronal Ceroid Lipofuscinoses	AR	Pamitoyl-protein thioesterase (PPT) Tripeptidyl peptidasel (TPP1)	EM of skin biopsy
Adrenoleukodystrophy	XLR	VLCFA oxidation	Plasma, skin fibroblasts
Sialidosis	AR	Neuraminidase	Skin fibroblasts

AR = autosomal recessive; EM = electron microscopy; XLR = X-linked recessive; VLCFA = very long chain fatty acid.

TABLE 592–2. Select "Intrinsic" Conditions Associated with Developmental Regression

Age at Onset (yr)	Condition	Comments
<2—with hepatomegaly (see Chapter 76.3)	Fructose intolerance	Vomiting, hypoglycemia, poor feeding, failure to thrive (when given fructose)
	Galactosemia	Lethargy, hypotonia, icterus, cataract, hypoglycemia (when given lactose)
	Glycogenosis (glycogen storage disease) types I–IV	Hypoglycemia, cardiomegaly (II)
	Mucopolysaccharidosis types I and II	Coarse facies, stiff joints
	Niemann-Pick disease, infantile type	Gray matter disease, failure to thrive
	Tay-Sachs disease	Seizures, cherry red macula, edema, coarse facies
	Zellweger (cerebrohepatorenal) syndrome	Hypotonia, high forehead, flat facies
	Gaucher disease type II	Extensor posturing, irritability
<2—without hepatomegaly	Krabbe disease	Irritability, extensor posturing, optic atrophy and blindness
	Rett syndrome	Girls with deceleration of head growth, loss of hand skills, hand wringing, impaired language skills, gait apraxia
	Maple syrup urine disease	Poor feeding, tremors, myoclonus, opisthotonos
	Phenylketonuria	Light pigmentation, eczema, seizures
	Menkes kinky hair disease	Hypertonia, irritability, seizures, abnormal hair
	Subacute necrotizing encephalopathy of Leigh	White matter disease
	Cerebro-oculofacioskeletal syndrome (of Pena and Shokeir)	Reduced white matter, failure to thrive
	Canavan disease	White matter disease
	Pelizaeus-Merzbacher disease	White matter disease
2–5	Niemann-Pick disease types III and IV	Hepatosplenomegaly, gait difficulty
	Wilson disease	Liver disease, Kayser-Fleischer ring, deterioration of cognition is late
	Gangliosidosis type II	Gray matter disease
	Ceroid lipofuscinosis	Gray matter disease
	Mitochondrial encephalopathies (e.g., myoclonic epilepsy, ragged-red fibers [MERRF])	Gray matter diseases
	Ataxia-telangiectasia	Basal ganglia disease
	Huntington's disease (chorea)	Basal ganglia disease
	Hallervorden-Spatz syndrome	Basal ganglia disease
	Metachromatic leukodystrophy	White matter disease
	Adrenoleukodystrophy	White matter disease, behavior problems, falling school performance, quadriparesis
5–15	Subacute sclerosing panencephalitis	Diffuse encephalopathy, myoclonus, may occur years after measles
	Adrenoleukodystrophy	See above for adrenoleukodystrophy
	Multiple sclerosis	White matter disease
	Neuronal ceroid lipofuscinosis, juvenile and adult (Spielmeyer-Vogt and Kuf disease)	Gray matter disease
	Schilder disease	White matter disease, focal neurologic symptoms
	Refsum disease	Peripheral neuropathy, ataxia, retinitis pigmentosa
	Sialidosis II, juvenile form	Cherry red macula, myoclonus, ataxia, coarse facies

From Liptak G: In Kliegman R (editor): Practical Strategies in Pediatric Diagnosis and Therapy. *Philadelphia, WB Saunders, 1996, p 503.*

deficiency of acid β-galactosidase. This enzyme may be assayed in leukocytes and cultured fibroblasts. The acid β-galactosidase gene has been mapped to chromosome 3p14.2. Prenatal diagnosis is possible by measurement of acid β-galactosidase in cultured amniotic cells.

Infantile GM₁ gangliosidosis presents at birth or during the neonatal period with anorexia, poor sucking, and inadequate weight gain. Development is globally retarded, and generalized seizures are prominent. The phenotype is striking and shares many characteristics with Hurler syndrome. The facial features are coarse, the forehead is prominent, the nasal bridge is depressed, the tongue is large (macroglossia), and the gums are hypertrophied. Hepatosplenomegaly is present early in the course as a result of accumulation of foamy histiocytes, and kyphoscoliosis is evident because of anterior beaking of the vertebral bodies. The neurologic examination is dominated by apathy, progressive blindness, deafness, spastic quadriplegia, and decerebrate rigidity. A cherry red spot in the macular region is visualized in approximately 50% of cases. The **cherry red spot** is characterized by an opaque ring (sphingolipid-laden retinal ganglion cells) encircling the normal red fovea (Fig. 592–1). Children rarely survive beyond age 2–3 yr, and death is due to aspiration pneumonia.

Juvenile GM₁ gangliosidosis has a delayed onset beginning about 1 yr of age. The initial symptoms consist of incoordination, weakness, ataxia, and regression of language. Thereafter, convulsions, spasticity, decerebrate rigidity, and blindness are the major findings. Unlike the infantile type, this type is not usually marked by

coarse facial features and hepatosplenomegaly. Radiographic examination of the lumbar vertebrae may show minor beaking. Children rarely survive beyond 10 yr of age. *Adult GM₁ gangliosidosis* is a slowly progressive disease consisting of spasticity, ataxia, dysarthria, and a gradual loss of cognitive function.

GM₂ Gangliosidoses. The GM₂ gangliosidoses are a heterogeneous group of autosomal recessive inherited disorders that consist of several subtypes, including Tay-Sachs disease (TSD), Sandhoff disease, juvenile GM₂ gangliosidosis, and adult GM₂ gangliosidosis. *Tay-Sachs disease* is most prevalent in the Ashkenazi Jewish population and has a carrier rate of approximately 1/30. TSD is due to mutations in the HEXA gene located on chromosome 15q23-q24. Affected infants appear normal until approximately 6 mo of age, except for a marked startle reaction to noise that is evident soon after birth. Affected children then begin to lag in developmental milestones, and by 1 yr of age they lose the ability to stand, sit, and vocalize. Early hypotonia develops into progressive spasticity, and relentless deterioration follows, with convulsions, blindness, deafness, and cherry red spots in almost all patients (see Fig. 592–1). Macrocephaly becomes apparent by 1 yr of age and results from the 200- to 300-fold normal content of GM₂ ganglioside deposited within the brain. Few children live beyond 3–4 yr of age, and death is usually associated with aspiration or bronchopneumonia. A deficiency of the isoenzyme hexosaminidase A is found in tissues of patients with TSD. Mass screening for prenatal diagnosis of TSD is a reliable and cost-effective method of prevention because the

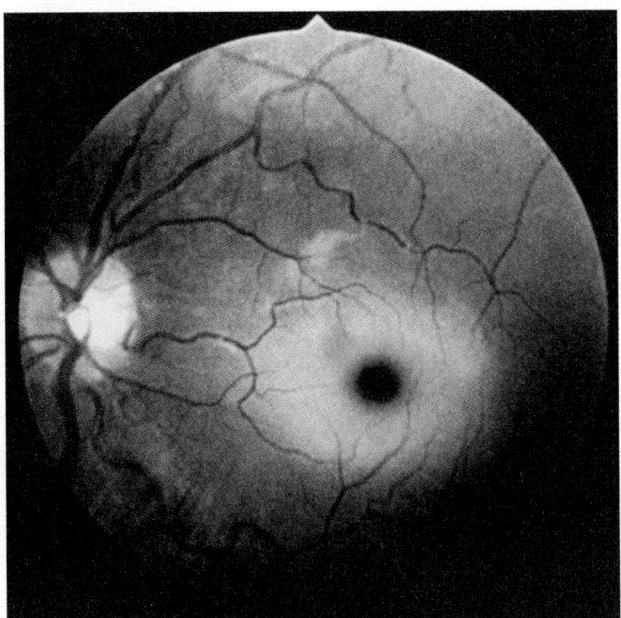

FIGURE 592–1. A cherry red spot in a patient with GM₁ gangliosidosis. Note the whitish ring of sphingolipid-laden ganglion cells surrounding the fovea.

condition occurs in a defined population (Ashkenazi Jews). An accurate and inexpensive carrier detection test is available (serum or leukocyte hexosaminidase A), and the disease can be reliably diagnosed by chorionic villus sampling during the 1st trimester of pregnancy in couples at risk (heterozygote parents).

Sandhoff disease is very similar to TSD in the mode of presentation, including progressive loss of motor and language milestones beginning at 6 mo of age. Seizures, cherry red spots, macrocephaly, and doll-like facies are present in most patients; however, children with Sandhoff disease may also have splenomegaly. The visual-evoked potentials (VEPs) are normal early in the course of Sandhoff disease and TSD but become abnormal or absent as the disease progresses. The auditory brainstem responses (ABRs) show prolonged latencies. The diagnosis of Sandhoff disease is established by finding deficient levels of hexosaminidase A and B in serum and leukocytes. Children usually die by 3 yr of age. Sandhoff disease is due to mutations in the HEXB gene located on chromosome 5q13.

Juvenile GM₂ gangliosidosis develops in midchildhood, initially with clumsiness followed by ataxia. Signs of spasticity, athetosis, loss of language, and seizures gradually develop. Progressive visual loss is associated with optic atrophy, but cherry red spots rarely occur in juvenile GM₂ gangliosidosis. A deficiency of hexosaminidase is variable (total deficiency to near normal) in these patients. Death occurs around 15 yr of age.

Adult GM₂ gangliosidosis is characterized by a myriad of neurologic signs, including slowly progressive gait ataxia, spasticity, dystonia, proximal muscle atrophy, and dysarthria. Generally, visual acuity and intellectual function are unimpaired. Hexosaminidase A or A and B activity is reduced significantly in the serum and leukocytes.

Krabbe Disease (Globoid Cell Leukodystrophy). Krabbe disease (KD) is a rare autosomal recessive neurodegenerative disorder characterized by severe myelin loss and the presence of globoid bodies in the white matter. The gene for KD (GALC) is located on chromosome 14q24.3-q32.1. The disease results from a marked deficiency of the lysosomal enzyme galactocerebroside β-galactosidase, which cleaves a galactose moiety from the ceramide portion of galactocerebroside. KD is a disorder of myelin destruction rather than abnormal myelin formation.

Normally, myelination begins during the 3rd trimester, corresponding with a rapid increase of galactocerebroside β-galactosidase activity in the brain. In patients with KD, galactocerebroside cannot be metabolized during the normal turnover of myelin because of deficiency of galactocerebroside β-galactosidase. When galactocerebroside is injected into the brains of experimental animals, a globoid cell reaction ensues. It has been postulated that a similar phenomenon occurs in humans; nonmetabolized galactocerebroside stimulates the formation of globoid cells that reflect the destruction of oligodendroglial cells. Because oligodendroglial cells are responsible for the elaboration of myelin, their loss results in myelin breakdown, thus producing additional galactocerebroside and causing a vicious circle of myelin destruction.

The symptoms of KD become evident during the first few months of life and include excessive irritability and crying, unexplained episodes of hyperpyrexia, feeding problems, vomiting, and failure to thrive. During the initial stage of KD. children are often treated for colic or "milk allergy" with frequent formula changes. Generalized seizures may appear early in the course of the disease. Alterations in body tone with rigidity and opisthotonos and visual inattentiveness due to optic atrophy become apparent as the disease progresses. During the later stages of the illness, blindness, deafness, absent deep tendon reflexes, and decerebrate rigidity constitute the major physical findings. A nonenhanced CT scan of the head may show symmetric increased densities in the caudate nuclei and thalami. Most patients die by 2 yr of age.

Late-onset KD has been described beginning in childhood or during adolescence. Patients present with optic atrophy and cortical blindness, and their condition is often confused with the adrenoleukodystrophies. Slowly progressive gait disturbances, including spasticity and ataxia, are prominent. As with classic KD, globoid cells are abundant in the white matter, and leukocytes are deficient in galactocerebroside β-galactosidase. An examination of the cerebrospinal fluid (CSF) shows an elevated protein content, and the nerve conduction velocities are markedly delayed due to segmental demyelination of the peripheral nerves. The VEPs decrease gradually in amplitude with no response in the late stages of the disease, and the ABRs are characterized by the presence of only waves I and II. CT scans and MRI studies highlight the marked decrease in white matter, especially of the cerebellum and centrum semiovale, with sparing of the subcortical u fibers. Prenatal diagnosis is possible by the assay of galactocerebroside β-galactosidase activity in chorionic villi or in cultured amniotic fluid cells.

Metachromatic Leukodystrophy (MLD). This disorder of myelin metabolism is inherited as an autosomal recessive trait and is characterized by a deficiency of arylsulfatase A activity. Several mutations in the gene encoding for arylsulfatase A have been identified. The gene is located on chromosome 22q13-13qter, and DNA diagnosis is possible. The absence or deficiency of arylsulfatase A leads to accumulation of cerebroside sulfate within the myelin sheath of the central nervous system (CNS) and peripheral nervous system due to the inability to cleave sulfate from galactosyl-3-sulfate ceramide. The excessive cerebroside sulfate is thought to cause myelin breakdown and destruction of oligodendroglia. Prenatal diagnosis of MLD is made by assay of arylsulfatase A in chorionic villi or cultured amniotic fluid cells. Cresyl violet applied to tissue specimens produces metachromatic staining of the sulfatide granules, giving the disease its name. Six disorders are included in the MLD group of diseases, classified by the age at onset and enzyme deficiency. Three conditions are briefly discussed: the classic or late infantile, juvenile, and adult leukodystrophies.

Late infantile MLD begins with insidious onset of gait disturbances between 1 and 2 yr of age. The child initially appears awkward and frequently falls, but locomotion is gradually impaired significantly and support is required in order to walk. The extremities are hypotonic, and the deep tendon reflexes are absent or diminished. Within the next several months, the child can no longer stand, and deterioration in intellectual function becomes apparent. The speech is slurred and dysarthric, and the child appears dull and apathetic. Visual fixation is diminished, nystagmus is present, and examination of the retina shows optic atrophy. Within 1 yr from the onset of the disease, the child is unable to sit unsupported, and progressive decorticate postures develop. Feeding and swallowing are impaired due to pseudobulbar palsies, and a feeding gastrostomy is required. Patients ultimately become stuporous and die of aspiration or bronchopneumonia by age 5–6 yr. Neurophysiologic evaluation shows progressive changes in the VEPs, ABRs, and somatosensory-evoked potentials (SSEPs), and the nerve conduction velocities (NCVs) of the peripheral nerves are significantly reduced. CT and MRI images of the brain indicate diffuse symmetric attenuation of the cerebellar and cerebral white matter, and examination of the CSF shows an elevated protein content. Bone marrow transplantation is a promising experimental therapy for the management of late infantile MLD. Favorable outcomes have been reported only in patients treated very early in the course of the disease. The total number of patients treated is relatively small and the follow-up too short to draw conclusions about the efficacy of bone marrow transplantation.

Juvenile MLD has many features in common with late infantile MLD, but the onset of symptoms is delayed to 5–10 yr of age. Deterioration in school performance and alterations in personality may herald the onset of the disease. This is followed by incoordination of gait, urinary incontinence, and dysarthria. Muscle tone becomes increased, and ataxia, dystonia, or tremor may be present. During the terminal stages, generalized tonic-clonic convulsions are prominent and are difficult to control. Patients rarely live beyond midadolescence.

Adult MLD occurs from the 2nd to 6th decade. Abnormalities in memory, psychiatric disturbances, and personality changes are prominent features. Slowly progressive neurologic signs, including spasticity, dystonia, optic atrophy, and generalized convulsions, lead eventually to a bedridden state characterized by decorticate postures and unresponsiveness.

592.2 Neuronal Ceroid Lipofuscinoses

Neuronal ceroid lipofuscinoses constitutes the most common class of neurodegenerative diseases in children and consist of three disorders inherited as autosomal recessive traits. They are autosomal recessive disorders characterized by the storage of an autofluorescent substance within lysosomes of neurons and other tissues. Eight genes have been identified. In the infantile forms and some early childhood forms, mutations have been identified in the lysosomal enzyme palmitoyl-protein thioesterase-1 (PPT).

Infantile type (Haltia-Santavuori) begins near the end of the 1st year of life with myoclonic seizures, intellectual deterioration, and blindness. Optic atrophy and brownish discoloration of the macula are evident on examination of the retina, and cerebellar ataxia is prominent. The electroretinogram (ERG) typically shows small-amplitude or absent waveforms. Death occurs at approximately 10 yr of age. The gene defect causing the infantile form has been assigned to chromosome 1p32. *Late infantile type (Jansky-Bielschowsky)* is the most common type of neuronal ceroid lipofuscinosis. The presenting manifestation is myoclonic seizures beginning between 2 and 4 yr of age in a previously normal child. Dementia and ataxia are combined with a progressive loss of visual acuity and microcephaly. Examination of the retina shows marked attenuation of vessels, peripheral black "bone spicule" pigmentary abnormalities, optic atrophy, and a subtle brown pigment in the macular region. The ERG is abnormal early in the course as a result of deposition of the abnormal

storage substance within the rod and cone area of the retina. VEPs are characteristic and consist of markedly enlarged responses followed by absent waveforms with progression of the disease. The autofluorescent material is deposited in neurons, fibroblasts, and secretory cells. Electron microscopic examination of the storage material in skin or conjunctival biopsy material typically shows curvilinear bodies or "fingerprint profiles."

Juvenile type (Spielmeyer-Vogt) is characterized by progressive visual loss and intellectual impairment beginning between 5 and 10 yr of age. The funduscopic changes are similar to those for the late infantile type. The ERG is also abnormal early in the course of the disease, but in the juvenile type the VEPs typically are characterized by small-amplitude waves and, later, absence of waveforms as the disease progresses. Myoclonic seizures are not as prominent as in the late infantile type of neuronal ceroid lipofuscinosis, but dystonic posturing is marked during the late stages of the disease. Elevated urine dolichol levels are a nonspecific finding. Ultrastructural abnormalities of skin biopsy samples are present in most cases. CLN2, which encodes the lysosomal enzyme tripeptidyl peptidase 1, and several others have been identified in juvenile forms.

592.3 Adrenoleukodystrophy

See Chapter 75.2.

The adrenoleukodystrophies consist of a group of CNS degenerative disorders that are often associated with adrenal cortical insufficiency and are inherited by X-linked recessive transmission. *Classic adrenoleukodystrophy* (ALD) becomes symptomatic between 5 and 15 yr of age with evidence of academic deterioration, behavioral disturbances, and gait abnormalities. ALD is caused by mutations in the ABCD 1 gene located on Xq28, which encodes peroxisomal transporter involved in the import of very long chain fatty acids into the peroxisome. The incidence of ALD approximates 1/20,000 boys. Generalized seizures are common in the early stages. Upper motor neuron signs include spastic quadriparesis and contractures, ataxia, and marked swallowing disturbances secondary to pseudobulbar palsy. These dominate the terminal stages of the illness. Hypoadrenalism is present in approximately 50% of cases, and adrenal insufficiency characterized by abnormal skin pigmentation (tanning without exposure to sun) may precede the onset of neurologic symptoms. CT scans and MRI studies of patients indicate periventricular demyelination beginning posteriorly; this advances progressively to the anterior regions of the cerebral white matter. ABRs, VEPs, and SSEPs may be normal initially but ultimately show prolonged latencies and abnormal waveforms. Death supervenes within 10 yr of the onset of the neurologic signs; however, long-term follow-up has shown that bone marrow transplant can prevent the progress of the disease when done at an early stage.

Adrenomyeloneuropathy begins with a slowly progressive spastic paraparesis, urinary incontinence, and onset of impotence during the 3rd or 4th decade, even though adrenal insufficiency may have been present since childhood. Cases of typical ALD have occurred in families in whom the propositus presented with adrenomyeloneuropathy. One of the most difficult problems in the management of X-linked ALD is the common observation that affected individuals in the same family may have quite different clinical courses. For example, in one family, one affected boy had severe classic ALD culminating in death by age 10 yr; another affected male (a brother) had late-onset adrenomyeloneuropathy, and a third had no symptoms at all. Counseling families with presymptomatic males is extraordinarily difficult because there is no reliable method for predicting the clinical course.

Neonatal ALD is characterized by marked hypotonia, severe psychomotor retardation, and early onset of seizures. It is inherited as an autosomal recessive condition. Visual inattention is secondary to optic atrophy. Results of adrenal function tests are normal, but adrenal atrophy is evident postmortem. Correction of adrenal insufficiency is ineffective in halting neurologic deterioration.

592.4 Sialidosis

Sialidosis is inherited as an autosomal recessive trait and results from accumulation of a sialic acid-oligosaccharide complex secondary to a deficiency in the lysosomal enzyme neuraminidase. The lysosomal sialidase gene has been mapped to chromosome 6p21.3. Urinary excretion of sialic acid–containing oligosaccharides is increased significantly in affected patients.

Sialidosis type I, the cherry red spot–myoclonus syndrome (CRSM), usually presents during the 2nd decade of life, when a patient complains of visual deterioration. Inspection of the retina shows a cherry red spot, but, unlike patients with TSD, visual acuity declines slowly in individuals with CRSM. Myoclonus of the extremities is gradually progressive and often debilitating and eventually renders patients nonambulatory. The myoclonus is triggered by voluntary movement, touch, and sound and is not controlled with anticonvulsants. Generalized convulsions responsive to antiepileptic drugs occur in most patients.

Sialidosis type II may be subdivided into infantile and juvenile forms, depending on the age at presentation. In addition to cherry red spots and myoclonus, these patients have somatic involvement, including coarse facial features, corneal clouding (rarely), and dysostosis multiplex, producing anterior beaking of the lumbar vertebrae. Examination of lymphocytes shows vacuoles in the cytoplasm, biopsy of the liver demonstrates cytoplasmic vacuoles in Kupffer cells, and membrane-bound vacuoles are found in Schwann cell cytoplasm, all attesting to the multiorgan nature of sialidosis type II. No distinctive neuroimaging findings or abnormalities in electrophysiologic studies are noted in this group of disorders. Patients with sialidosis have been reported to live beyond the 5th decade.

Some cases of what appears to be sialidosis type II are the result of combined deficiencies of β-galactosidase and α-neuraminidase due to deficiency of a "protective protein" that prevents premature intracellular degradation of the two enzymes. Clinically, affected patients are indistinguishable from those with sialidosis type II, either the infantile or juvenile form, caused by isolated α-neuraminidase deficiency. The diagnosis may be missed if β-galactosidase testing is done and testing of α-neuraminidase activity in fibroblasts is not completed.

592.5 Miscellaneous Disorders

Multiple Sclerosis. Multiple sclerosis (MS) is a chronic, remitting disorder characterized by multiple white lesions in the CNS separated by time and location. The condition is rare in the pediatric population; onset before age 10 yr occurs in 0.2–2% of all cases. There is a greater incidence of MS in females in the pediatric age group compared with adults. The cause of MS is unknown, but interactive genetic, immunologic, and infectious factors are probably responsible. The most frequent presenting symptom is unilateral weakness or ataxia. Headache is an important early component of the disease and is often severe, prolonged, and generalized. Ill-defined paresthesias involving the lower extremities, distal portions of the hands and feet, and the face are common. Visual symptoms including diplopia, blurred vision, or sudden visual loss secondary to optic neuritis are also important early manifestations of MS. Vertigo, dysarthria, and sphincter disturbances are relatively uncommon. *Neuromyelitis optica* (*Devic disease*) is a variant of classic MS and consists of optic neuritis and transverse myelitis, which occur conjointly.

The *pathology* of MS consists of demyelination with the formation of plaques. No reliable laboratory test unequivocally confirms the diagnosis of MS, except for an autopsy. MRI is the neuroimaging technique of choice; small plaques of 3–4 mm can be identified, particularly those located in the brainstem and spinal cord (Fig. 592–2).

The *treatment* of MS is supportive, and particular attention is given to the management of a neurogenic bladder. No evidence shows that corticosteroids alter the long-term course of the disease, but they may expedite recovery after an acute attack. Studies indicate that interferon β-1b given subcutaneously every other day or interferon β-1a given intramuscularly every day on a weekly basis are effective in the treatment of MS by decreasing disease activity and disease burden, as shown by serial gadolinium-enhanced lesions in brain MRI scan in adults.

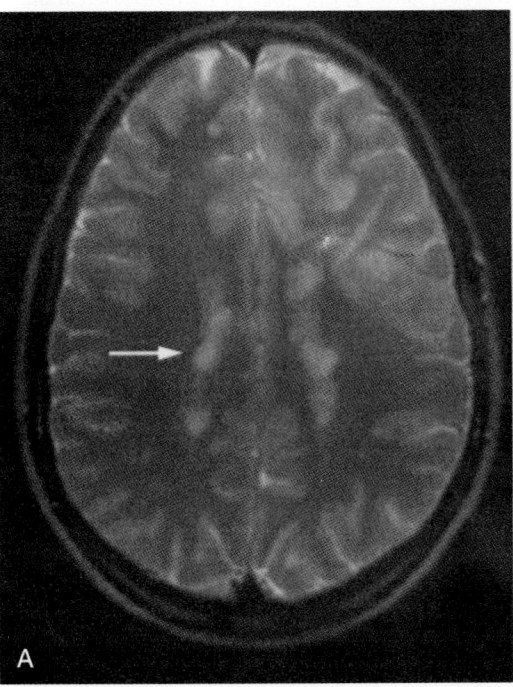
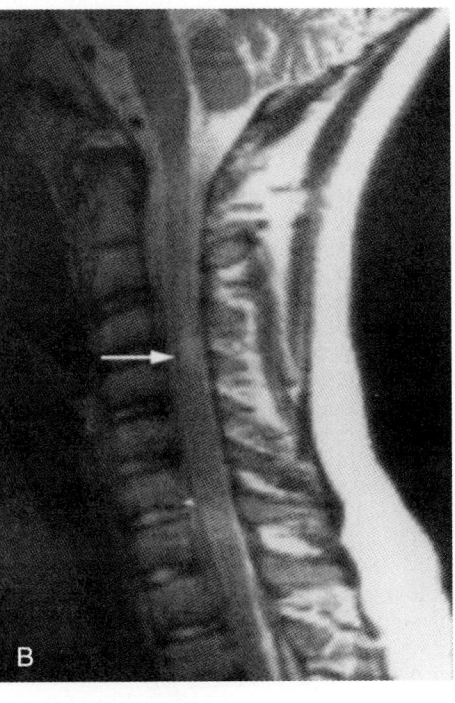

FIGURE 592–2. Multiple sclerosis. *A*, T2 weighted MRI scan of brain demonstrates multiple lesions located in the white matter characteristic of multiple sclerosis (*white arrow*). *B*, T1 weighted MRI scan of spine indicates a demyelinating plaque of multiple sclerosis in the midcervical region (*white arrow*).

The *prognosis* for childhood MS is similar to that in adults; recovery is often complete, and progression of the disease tends to be slow, with long periods of remission in most cases. Promising immunologic therapy, including the use of intravenous immunoglobulins, is currently being investigated.

Pelizaeus-Merzbacher Disease. This disease consists of a group of disorders that are characterized by nystagmus and abnormalities of myelin. The classic form is inherited as an X-linked recessive trait caused by abnormalities in the proteolipid protein (PLP) gene, which is essential for CNS myelin formation and oligodendrocyte differentiation. Mutations in the same gene can cause *familial spastic paraparesis*. It is recognized by nystagmus and roving eye movements with head nodding during infancy. The gene is located on chromosome Xq22. Molecular diagnosis of Pelizaeus-Merzbacher disease is possible using mutation analysis. However, as with most X-linked diseases, the molecular diagnosis of Pelizaeus-Merzbacher disease is complex because exonic mutations are present in only 10–25% of patients with the disease. A child's developmental milestones are delayed, and ataxia, choreoathetosis, and spasticity ultimately develop. Optic atrophy and dysarthria are associated findings, and death occurs in the 2nd or 3rd decade. The major pathologic finding is a loss of myelin with intact axons, suggesting a defect in the function of oligodendroglia. Studies point to a genetic defect in the biosynthesis of proteolipid apoprotein, a protein that is concerned with the differentiation and maintenance of oligodendrocytes. An MRI scan shows a symmetric pattern of delayed myelination. Multimodal-evoked potential studies demonstrate early in the course a pattern consisting of loss of waves III–V on the ABR. This finding is useful in the investigation of nystagmus in infant boys. VEPs show prolonged latencies, and SSEPs show absent cortical responses or delayed latencies.

Alexander Disease. This is a rare disorder that occurs sporadically and causes progressive macrocephaly during the 1st year of life. It is caused by mutations in the glial fibrillary acidic protein (GFAP) gene. Pathologic examination of the brain discloses deposition of eosinophilic hyaline bodies in a perivascular distribution throughout the brain and beneath the pia mater. Degeneration of white matter is most prominent in the frontal lobes, and a CT scan during this stage shows corresponding attenuation of the cerebral white matter. Affected children develop progressive loss of intellect, spasticity, and unresponsive seizures causing death by 5 yr of age.

Canavan Spongy Degeneration. See Chapter 74.14.

Menkes Disease. Menkes disease (kinky hair disease) is a progressive neurodegenerative condition inherited as a sex-linked recessive trait. The Menkes gene codes for a copper transporting P-type ATPase, and mutations in the protein are associated with low serum copper and ceruloplasmin levels as well as a defect in copper absorption and transport across the intestines. Symptoms begin during the first few months of life and include hypothermia, hypotonia, and generalized myoclonic seizures. The facies are distinctive, with chubby, rosy cheeks and kinky, colorless, friable hair. Microscopic examination of the hair shows several abnormalities, including trichorrhexis nodosa (fractures along the hair shaft) and pili torti (twisted hair). Feeding difficulties are prominent and lead to failure to thrive. Severe mental retardation and optic atrophy are constant features of the disease. Neuropathologic changes include tortuous degeneration of the gray matter and marked changes in the cerebellum with loss of the internal granule cell layer and necrosis of the Purkinje cells. Death occurs by 3 yr of age in untreated patients.

Copper-histidine therapy has been shown to be effective in preventing neurologic deterioration in some patients with Menkes' disease, particularly when treatment is begun during the neonatal period or, preferably, with the fetus. Copper is essential during the early stages of CNS development, and its absence probably accounts for the neuropathologic changes. Copper-histidine is given subcutaneously in a dose of 50–150 µg elemental copper/kg/24 hr for the duration of the child's life. The serum copper and ceruloplasmin levels return to the normal range within 2–3 wk of commencing therapy.

The *occipital horn syndrome*, a skeletal dysplasia caused by different mutations in the same gene as that involved in Menkes disease, is a relatively mild disease. The two diseases are often confused, because the biochemical abnormalities are identical. Resolution of the uncertainty about treatment of patients with Menkes disease will require careful genotype-phenotype correlation, along with further clinical trials of copper therapy.

Rett Syndrome. Rett syndrome (RS) is a disorder of developmental regression and deceleration of brain growth over the first year of life after a relatively normal neonatal course occurring predominantly in girls. The frequency is approximately 1/15,000 to 1/22,000. RS is caused by mutations in MeCP2, a transcription factor that binds to methylated CpG islands and silences transcription. Development proceeds normally until 1 yr of age, when regression of language and motor milestones and acquired microcephaly become apparent. An ataxic gait or fine tremor of hand movements is an early neurologic finding. Most children develop peculiar sighing respirations with intermittent periods of apnea that may be associated with cyanosis. The hallmark of Rett syndrome is repetitive hand-wringing movements and a loss of purposeful and spontaneous use of the hands; these may not appear until 2–3 yr of age. Autistic behavior is a typical finding in all patients. Generalized tonic-clonic convulsions occur in the majority and are usually well controlled by anticonvulsants. Feeding disorders and poor weight gain are common. After the initial period of neurologic regression, the disease process appears to plateau, with persistence of the autistic behavior. Death occurs during adolescence or during the 3rd decade. Cardiac arrhythmias may result in sudden, unexpected death.

Postmortem studies show significantly reduced brain weight (60–80% of normal) with a decrease in the number of synapses, associated with a decrease in dendritic length and branching. The phenotype may be related to failure to suppress expression of genes that normally are silent during the early phases of postnatal development. Although very few males survive with the classic RS phenotype, genotyping of boys without the classic RS phenotype but with mental retardation and other atypical neurologic features has detected a significant number with mutations in MeCP2. Some data indicate that mutations in MeCP2 may be as common in mentally retarded populations as fragile X syndrome. This suggests that mutations in the Rett gene may cause a far broader spectrum of neurodevelopmental disability than once thought.

Subacute Sclerosing Panencephalitis. This is a rare, progressive, slow-virus infection of the CNS caused by a measles-like virus (Chapter 225.1). The number of reported cases has decreased dramatically to 0.06 cases/million population, paralleling the decline in reported measles cases. The initial clinical manifestations include personality changes, aggressive behavior, and impaired cognitive function. Myoclonic seizures soon dominate the clinical picture. Later, generalized tonic-clonic convulsions, hypertonia, and choreoathetosis become evident, followed by progressive bulbar palsy, hyperthermia, and decerebrate postures. Funduscopic examination early in the course of the disease reveals papilledema in approximately 20% of the cases. Optic atrophy, chorioretinitis, and macular pigmentation are observed in most patients. The *diagnosis* is established by the typical clinical course and one of the following: (1) measles antibody detected in the CSF, (2) a characteristic electroencephalogram consisting of bursts of high-voltage slow waves interspersed with a normal background in the early stages, and (3) typical histologic findings in the brain biopsy or postmortem specimen. *Treatment* with a series of antiviral agents has been attempted without success. Death occurs usually within 1–2 yr from the onset of symptoms.

Amir RE, Van den Veyver IB, Wan M, et al: Rett syndrome is caused by mutations in X-linked MeCP2, encoding methyl-CpG-binding protein 2. *Nat Genet* 1999;23:185.

Aoki Y, Haginoya K, Munakata M, et al: A novel mutation in glial fibrillary acidic protein gene in a patient with Alexander disease. *Neurosci Lett* 2001;312:71.

Baram TZ, Goldman AM, Percy AK: Krabbe disease: Specific MRI and CT findings. *Neurology* 1986;36:111.

Berger J, Moser HW, Forss-Petter S: Leukodystrophies: Recent developments in genetics, molecular biology, pathogenesis and treatment. *Curr Opin Neurol* 2001;14:305.

Boustany RM, Alroy J, Kolodny EH: Clinical classification of neuronal ceroid lipofuscinosis subtypes. *Am J Med Genet* 1988;5(Suppl):47.

Chelly J, Tümer Z, Tonnesen T, et al: Isolation of a candidate gene for Menkes disease that encodes a potential heavy binding protein. *Nat Genet* 1993;3:14.

Couvert P, Bienvenu T, Aquaviva C: MeCP2 is highly mutated in X-linked mental retardation. *Hum Mol Genet* 2001;10:941.

Duquette P, Murray TJ, Pleines J, et al: Multiple sclerosis in childhood: Clinical profile in 125 patients. *J Pediatr* 1987;111:359.

Dyken PR, Cunningham SC, Ward LC: Changing character of subacute sclerosing panencephalitis in the United States. *Pediatr Neurol* 1989;5:339.

Inoue K, Osaka H, Sugiyama N, et al: A duplicated PLP gene causing Pelizaeus-Merzbacher disease detected by comparative multiplex PCR. *Am J Hum Genet* 1996;59:32.

Johnson WG: The clinical spectrum of hexosaminidase deficiency disease. *Neurology* 1981;31:1453.

Johnston MV, Jeon OH, Pevsner J, et al: Neurobiology of Rett syndrome: A genetic disorder of synapse development. *Brain Dev* 2001;23:S206.

Julu PO, Kerr AM, Apartopoulos F, et al: Characterisation of breathing and associated central autonomic dysfunction in Rett disorder. *Arch Dis Child* 2001;85:29.

Kaye EM: Update on genetic disorders affecting white matter. *Pediatr Neurol* 2001;24:11.

Kelley RI, Datta NS, Dobyns WB, et al: Neonatal adrenoleukodystrophy: New cases, biochemical studies and differentiation from Zellweger and related peroxisomal polydystrophy syndromes. *Am J Med Genet* 1986;23:869.

Krivit W, Shapiro EG, Peters C, et al: Hematopoietic stem-cell transplantation in globoid-cell leukodystrophy. *N Engl J Med* 1998;338:1119.

Lonnqvist T, Vanhanen SL, Vettenranta K: Hematopoietic stem cell transplantation in infantile neuronal ceroid lipofuscinosis. *Neurology* 2001;57:1411.

Mobley WC, White CL, Tennekoon G, et al: Neonatal adrenoleukodystrosphy. *Ann Neurol* 1982;12:204.

Mole SE: Batten's disease: Eight genes and still counting. *Lancet* 1999;354:443.

Moser HW, Loes DJ, Melhem ER, et al: X-linked adrenoleukodystrophy: Overview and prognosis as a function of age and brain MRI abnormality. A study involving 372 patients. *Neuropediatrics* 2000;31:227.

Moser J, Douar A-M, Sarde C-D, et al: Putative X-linked adrenoleukodystrophy gene shares unexpected homology with ABC transporters. *Nature* 1993;361:726.

Neufeld EF: Lysosomal storage diseases. *Annu Rev Biochem* 1991;60:259.

Percy AK: The inherited neurodegenerative disorders of childhood: Clinical assessment. *J Child Neurol* 1987;2:82.

Pshezhetsky AV, Richard C, Michaud L, et al: Cloning, expression and chromosomal mapping of human lysosomal sialidase and characterization of mutations in sialidoses. *Nat Genet* 1997;15:316.

Sarkar B, Lingertat-Walsh K, Clarke JT: Copper-histidine therapy for Menkes disease. *J Pediatr* 1993;123:828.

Shapiro E, Krivit W, Lockman L, et al: Long-term effect of bone-marrow transplantation for childhood-onset cerebral X-linked adrenoleukodystrophy. *Lancet* 2000;356:713.

Wisniewski KE, Kida E, Golabek AA, et al: Neuronal lipofuscinosis: Classification and diagnosis. *Adv Genet* 2001;45:1.

Wood AJ: Management of multiple sclerosis. *N Engl J Med* 1997;337:1604.

Chapter 593
Acute Stroke Syndromes
Michael V. Johnston

Hemiplegia secondary to vascular disorders occurs in children with an incidence of 1–3/100,000 per year. The pediatric causes of stroke are distinctive compared with adult causes. Types of stroke include arterial and venous thrombosis, intracranial hemorrhage, arterial embolism, and various miscellaneous conditions. The cause of stroke in children is established in approximately 75% of cases (Box 593–1). Because the mode of presentation of acute stroke syndromes is not uniform, a brief description of the most prevalent forms of pediatric stroke follows.

593.1 Arterial Thrombosis/Embolism

Arterial thrombosis and embolism may involve major cerebral arteries (internal carotid or anterior, middle, and posterior cerebral artery occlusion) or smaller cerebral arteries. Certain thrombotic processes affect large vessels and others more commonly involve small arteries. *Thrombosis of the internal carotid artery* may result from blunt trauma to the posterior pharynx caused by a fall on a pencil or popsicle stick in the child's mouth. The injury produces a tear in the intima of the vessel wall, which may lead to formation of a dissecting aneurysm. Cerebral symptoms result from shedding of emboli from the thrombus. The onset of symptoms may be delayed for up to 24 hr after the accident, with a stuttering but progressive flaccid hemiplegia, lethargy, and aphasia if the dominant hemisphere is involved. Focal motor seizures are a common complication. Dissection of vessels in the vertebral basilar circulation can lead to acute signs of brainstem dysfunction.

A *retropharyngeal abscess* may produce an identical clinical picture, but in this case the arterial thrombosis results from inflammation of the intima. A cerebral angiogram or MRI/magnetic resonance angiography (MRA) typically demonstrates occlusion of the internal carotid artery, and a CT/MRI scan shows a hypodense lesion outlining the area of infarction.

Embolization of cerebral vessels may also produce acute hemiparesis. Cardiac abnormalities are the most common overall cause of thromboembolic stroke in children. Cardiac causes include arrhythmias (particularly atrial fibrillation), myxoma, paradoxical emboli through a patent foramen ovale, and bacterial endocarditis that results in a mycotic aneurysm. Air emboli may complicate surgery, and fat emboli occur with fracture of long bones. Septic emboli may seed the cerebral vessels and evolve into an area of cerebritis leading to a cerebral abscess.

Cyanotic congenital heart disease in children younger than 2 yr may cause thrombosis, particularly of the middle cerebral artery. These patients are particularly vulnerable when the oxygen saturation is significantly decreased together with a viral illness or dehydration. Cardiac procedures, including catheterization and complex cardiac surgery operations (e.g., Fontan), can result in arterial thrombosis from embolization of a clot. If a cardiac cause of arterial thrombosis is suspected, the child must have an echocardiogram as part of the investigation.

Occlusive vascular disorders are also important causes of acute hemiplegia in the pediatric population. *Basal arterial occlusion with telangiectasia* or *moyamoya ("puff of smoke") disease* has a characteristic angiogram (Fig. 593–1). The condition is more common in girls and often presents with headache and bilateral upper motor neuron signs. It may also present with chorea. Intermittent episodes of transient ischemic attacks can produce progressive neurologic signs and severe disability. Surgical procedures designed to enhance cerebral flow (superficial temporal artery to middle cerebral artery shunt and laying the superficial temporal artery on the arachnoid membrane) have variable results.

Sickle cell disease is the most common cause of stroke in black children and is associated with large vessel stenosis of the proximal middle cerebral or distal internal carotid arteries.

Coagulation disorders are an important risk factor for stroke in children and neonates. Mutations in factor V Leiden and prothrombin, deficiencies in protein C, protein S, and antithrombin III, as well as antiphospholipid antibodies, have been identified in up to 50% of infants and children with cerebral thromboembolism (see Chapters 470 and 471). *Occlusion of small arteries* is also associated with diabetes mellitus,

BOX 593–1. Causes of Stroke in Children

I. Cardiac Disease
  A. Congenital
    1. Aortic stenosis
    2. Mitral stenosis; mitral prolapse
    3. Ventricular septal defects
    4. Patent ductus arteriosus
    5. Cyanotic congenital heart disease involving right-to-left shunt
  B. Acquired
    1. Endocarditis (bacterial, systemic lupus erythematosus)
    2. Kawasaki disease
    3. Cardiomyopathy
    4. Atrial myxoma
    5. Arrhythmia
    6. Paradoxical emboli through patent foramen ovale
    7. Rheumatic fever
    8. Prosthetic heart valve
II. Hematologic Abnormalities
  A. Hemoglobinopathies
    1. Sickle cell (SS) disease
    2. Sickle (SC) disease
  B. Polycythemia
  C. Leukemia/lymphoma
  D. Thrombocytopenia
  E. Thrombocytosis
  F. Disorders of coagulation
    1. Protein C deficiency
    2. Protein S deficiency
    3. Factor V Leiden
    4. Antithrombin III deficiency
    5. Lupus anticoagulant
    6. Oral contraceptive pill use
    7. Pregnancy and the postpartum state
    8. Disseminated intravascular coagulation
    9. Paroxysmal nocturnal hemoglobinuria
    10. Inflammatory bowel disease (thrombosis)
III. Inflammatory Disorders
  A. Meningitis
    1. Viral
    2. Bacterial
    3. Tuberculosis
  B. Systemic infection
    1. Viremia
    2. Bacteremia
    3. Local head and neck infections

C. Drug-induced inflammation
    1. Amphetamine
    2. Cocaine
  D. Autoimmune disease
    1. Systemic lupus erythematosus
    2. Juvenile rheumatoid arthritis
    3. Takayasu arteritis
    4. Mixed connective tissue disease
    5. Polyarteritis nodosum
    6. Primary central nervous system vasculitis
    7. Sarcoidosis
    8. Behçet's syndrome
    9. Wegener granulomatosis
IV. Metabolic Disease Associated with Stroke
  A. Homocystinuria
  B. Pseudoxanthoma elasticum
  C. Fabry disease
  D. Sulfite oxidase deficiency
  E. Mitochondrial disorders
    1. MELAS
    2. Leigh syndrome
  F. Ornithine transcarbamylase deficiency
V. Intracerebral Vascular Processes
  A. Ruptured aneurysm
  B. Arteriovenous malformation
  C. Fibromuscular dysplasia
  D. Moyamoya disease
  E. Migraine headache
  F. Postsubarachnoid hemorrhage vasospasm
  G. Hereditary hemorrhagic telangiectasia
  H. Sturge-Weber syndrome
  I. Carotid artery dissection
  J. Post varicella
VI. Trauma and Other External Causes
  A. Child abuse
  B. Head trauma/neck trauma
  C. Oral trauma
  D. Placental embolism
  E. ECMO therapy

ECMO = extracorporeal membrane oxygenation; MELAS = mitochondrial encephalomyopathy, lactic acidosis, and stroke.
From Riukin M: In Kliegman R (editor): *Practical Strategies in Pediatric Diagnosis and Therapy.* Philadelphia, WB Saunders, 1996.

neurofibromatosis, postvaricella angiopathy, head and neck radiation, oral contraceptives, and illicit drug use (amphetamines, cocaine). Patients present with unilateral neurologic signs, and recovery is often complete because of the small area of infarction. Patients with *thrombosis of small arteries*, including the perforating striate vessels, which result from polyarteritis nodosa and homocystinuria, generally have a progressive debilitating course characterized by bilateral signs and high mortality rate.

593.2 Venous Thrombosis

Venous sinus thrombosis may be subdivided into septic and nonseptic causes. The symptoms and signs may evolve over days and in neonates are characterized by diffuse neurologic signs and seizures, whereas focal neurologic signs are more prominent in children. Dilated scalp veins, a bulging anterior fontanel, and symptoms and signs of increased intracranial pressure may be present.

Septic causes of venous sinus thrombosis include encephalitis and bacterial meningitis. Hemiplegia is a relatively common complication of **bacterial meningitis** caused by thrombosis of the superficial cortical and deep penetrating veins. Additional infectious causes of septic sinus thrombosis in children include **otitis media** and **mastoiditis** with involvement of the dural

vessels, as well as retrograde orbital infections producing **cavernous sinus thrombosis**.

Aseptic causes include **severe dehydration** in infancy, which may cause thrombosis of the superior sagittal sinus and the superficial cortical veins that result from hyperviscosity and sludging of blood. Conditions resulting in hypercoagulopathy, cyanotic congenital heart diseases, and leukemic infiltrates of cerebral veins are additional causes of nonseptic acute hemiplegia of childhood. Prothrombotic disorders including deficiencies of inhibitors of coagulation such as protein C, protein S, antithrombin III, mutations in Leiden factor V, and anticardiolipin antibodies are found in 12–50% of cases (see Chapters 470 and 471).

593.3 Intracranial Hemorrhage

Intracranial hemorrhage may occur in the subarachnoid space, or the bleeding may be primarily located in the parenchyma of the brain. Subarachnoid bleeding is characterized by severe headache, nuchal rigidity, and progressive loss of consciousness, and intracerebral bleeding is characterized by focal neurologic signs and seizures. Intracranial hemorrhage is a common event in premature infants and is discussed in Chapter 88.2.

Arteriovenous malformations result from failure of normal capillary bed development between arteries and veins during

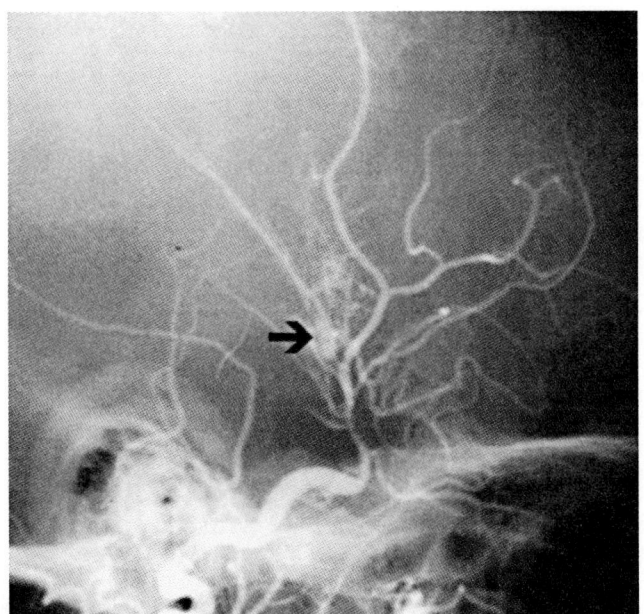

FIGURE 593–1. Cerebral angiogram showing idiopathic supraclinoid-internal carotid arteriopathy with classic moyamoya collaterals (*arrow*).

embryogenesis. Arteriovenous malformations produce abnormal shunting of blood, causing an expansion of vessels and a space-occupying effect or rupture of a vein and intracerebral bleeding. Arteriovenous malformations are typically located in the cerebral hemisphere, but they may be situated in the cerebellum, brainstem, or spinal cord. Although the malformation may remain asymptomatic throughout life, rupture and bleeding can occur at any age. Children with arteriovenous malformations frequently have a history of seizures and migraine-like headaches. Typical migraine alternates from one side of the head to the other, whereas headaches associated with an arteriovenous malformation classically remain on the same side. Auscultation of the skull is positive for a high-pitched bruit in approximately 50% of cases. Rupture of an arteriovenous malformation causes a severe headache, vomiting, nuchal rigidity caused by subarachnoid bleeding, progressive hemiparesis, and a focal or generalized seizure. Cavernous angiomas may be familial and are of lower risk for spontaneous hemorrhage. An **arteriovenous malformation of the vein of Galen** during infancy can cause high-output congestive heart failure secondary to shunting of large volumes of blood or progressive hydrocephalus and increased intracranial pressure secondary to obstruction of the cerebrospinal fluid (CSF) pathways. Vein of Galen malformations are difficult to treat and are associated with a poor prognosis.

Cerebral aneurysms producing symptoms in children are relatively rare. In contrast to those in adults, aneurysms in children tend to be large and are located at the carotid bifurcation or on the anterior and posterior cerebral arteries rather than the circle of Willis. The aneurysmal dilatation results from a congenital weakness of the vessel, and in some cases a deficiency of type III collagen has been demonstrated. In children, there is an association between cerebral aneurysms and coarctation of the aorta and bilateral polycystic kidney disease. Although most ruptured aneurysms bleed into the subarachnoid space, causing an intense headache, nuchal rigidity, and coma, intracerebral hemorrhage and progressive hemiparesis also occur. Additional causes of intracerebral hematoma include hematologic disorders, particularly thrombocytopenic purpura and hemophilia. Finally, trauma can produce hemiparesis due to intracerebral bleeding or a subdural or epidural hematoma. A contrast CT scan or MRI with gadolinium and MRA is useful for identifying large arteriovenous malformations; however, four-vessel cerebral angiography is the study of choice for investigating arteriovenous malformations and cerebral aneurysm.

593.4 Differential Diagnosis of Strokelike Events

Etiology and Clinical Manifestations. *Alternating hemiplegia of childhood* is occasionally associated with migraine, but in most cases the cause is unknown. It develops in infants between 2 and 18 mo of age and is characterized by intermittent episodes of hemiplegia alternating from one side of the body to the other. Rarely, both sides are involved during an attack. Choreoathetosis and dystonic movements are commonly observed in the hemiparetic extremity. Signs spontaneously regress with sleep but recur with awakening. The hemiplegia persists for minutes to weeks and then resolves spontaneously. The condition has a poor prognosis with progressive mental retardation and developmental disabilities. Results of neuroimaging and metabolic studies are negative.

Several **metabolic diseases** are associated with strokelike episodes in children, including mitochondrial encephalomyelopathy (MELAS; see Chapter 591.2), ornithine transcarbamylase deficiency, pyruvate dehydrogenase deficiency, and homocystinuria.

Todd paralysis may be confused initially with a stroke. The hemiparesis follows a focal seizure, but the weakness and neurologic signs disappear completely within 24 hr of the convulsion. Although the cause of Todd paralysis remains unknown, the hemiparesis probably results from an inhibitory phenomenon, possibly related to neurotransmitter dysfunction.

Additional causes of hemiparesis include *cerebral tumor*, *encephalitis* (particularly herpes), *focal postviral encephalitis*, and *status epilepticus*. In some pediatric series of unexplained stroke, *lipid abnormalities*, including elevated triglycerides and low levels of high-density lipoprotein cholesterol, have been found in approximately 20% of the cases. The family histories of these children reveal an increased incidence of premature coronary heart disease and early ischemic cerebrovascular diseases. Screening of at-risk families identifies children who may benefit from long-term dietary management.

Diagnosis. The most critical component of the investigation is a thorough history and physical examination, searching for an underlying disease process; evidence of trauma; an infectious, metabolic, or hematologic disorder; neurocutaneous syndrome; increased intracranial pressure; or hydrocephalus. Appropriate tests for infectious diseases, metabolic disorders, and hematologic disorders are based on the results of the history and physical examination. An electroencephalogram (EEG) may be helpful in localizing the disease process but rarely establishes the diagnosis. A brain scan is extremely useful in cases of focal encephalitis, cerebritis, cerebral abscess, and infarction. A CT scan can detect recent bleeding or a large area of infarction, but diffusion weighted MRI and MRA are superior for early detection of cerebral ischemia and assessment of cerebral vessels. A cerebral angiogram may be useful in some cases in which MRI studies are nondiagnostic, such as to detect vasculitis or sites of intracranial hemorrhage. In these cases, a four-vessel cerebral angiogram is indicated. Electrocardiography and echocardiography may help to exclude intrinsic cardiac diseases or an arrhythmia as a cause of the stroke. Finally, the basic investigations for a child with an unexplained stroke syndrome should be organized to eliminate the following conditions: (1) vasculitis and connective tissue diseases (ESR, C3, C4, RF, ANA), (2) lipid disorders, (3) coagulation disorders, (4) hematologic disorders (sickle cell disease, thrombocytopenia), (5) metabolic disorders (homocystinuria, Fabry disease, MELAS), and (6) an infectious etiology (meningitis and encephalitis).

Treatment. Specific therapies include low molecular weight heparin for venous sinus thrombosis and prevention of recurrent cardiac emboli. Thrombolytic therapies (e.g., tissue plasminogen activator) are useful within 3 hr after stokes in adults but have not been studied in children. The contraindications for the use of an antithrombotic agent include significant intracerebral hemorrhage and hypertension. Regular blood transfusions reduce the incidence of stroke in sickle cell disease. Immunosuppressant therapy for vasculitis and surgical evacuation of a large blood clot are other examples of specific therapies. Rehabilitation requirements after a stroke can include speech therapy, occupational and physical therapy, psychologic services, and special education. These treatment regimens are most effectively provided in a multidisciplinary setting.

Bourgeois M, Aicardi J, Goutières F: Alternating hemiplegia of childhood. *J Pediatr* 1993;122:673.

Christodoulou J, Qureshi IA, McInnes RR, et al: Ornithine transcarbamylase deficiency presenting with strokelike episodes. *J Pediatr* 1993;122:423.

David M, Andrew M: Venous thromboembolic complications in children. *J Pediatr* 1993;123:337.

DeVeber G, Andrew M, Adams C, et al: Cerebral sinovenous thrombosis in children. *N Engl J Med* 2001;345:417.

Fisher M, Bogousslavsky J: Further evolution toward effective therapy for acute ischemic stroke. *JAMA* 1998;279:1298.

Ganesan V, Kirkham FJ: Mechanisms of ischaemic stroke after chickenpox. *Arch Dis Child* 1997;76:522.

Kelly JJ, Mellinger JF, Sundt TM: Intracranial arteriovenous malformations in childhood. *Ann Neurol* 1978;3:338.

Lynch JK, Hirtz DG, DeVeber G, et al: Report on the National Institute of Neurological Diseases and Stroke Workshop on perinatal and childhood stroke. *Pediatrics* 2002;109:116.

Lynch JK, Nelson KB, Curry CJ, et al: Cerebrovascular disorders in children with the Leiden factor V mutation. *J Child Neurol* 2001;16:735.

Martin PJ, Enevoldson TP, Humphrey PR: Causes of ischaemic stroke in the young. *Postgrad Med J* 1997;73:855.

Rivkin MJ, Volpe JJ: Strokes in children. *Pediatr Rev* 1996;17:265.

Seeler RA, Royal JE, Powe L, et al: Moya-moya in children with sickle cell anemia and cerebrovascular occlusion. *J Pediatr* 1978;93:808.

Tomsick TA, Lukin RR, Chambers AA, et al: Neurofibromatosis and intracranial arterial occlusive disease. *Neuroradiology* 1976;11:229.

Watanabe K, Negoro T, Maehara M, et al: Moyamoya disease presenting with chorea. *Pediatr Neurol* 1990;6:40.

Chapter 594
Central Nervous System
Infections *Charles G. Prober*

Acute infection of the central nervous system (CNS) is the most common cause of fever associated with signs and symptoms of CNS disease in children. Infection may be caused by virtually any microbe, the specific pathogen being influenced by the age and immune status of the host and the epidemiology of the pathogen. In general, viral infections of the CNS are much more common than bacterial infections, which, in turn, are more common than fungal and parasitic infections. Infections caused by rickettsiae (e.g., Rocky Mountain spotted fever and *Ehrlichia*) are relatively uncommon but assume important roles under certain epidemiologic circumstances. *Mycoplasma* spp also can cause infections of the CNS, although their precise contribution often is difficult to determine.

Regardless of etiology, most patients with acute CNS infection have similar clinical syndromes. Common symptoms include headache, nausea, vomiting, anorexia, restlessness, and irritability; however, most of these symptoms are nonspecific. Common signs of CNS infection, in addition to fever, include

photophobia, neck pain and rigidity, obtundation, stupor, coma, seizures, and focal neurologic deficits. The severity and constellation of signs are determined by the specific pathogen, the host, and the area of the CNS affected. Infection of the CNS may be diffuse or focal. Meningitis and encephalitis are examples of diffuse infection. Meningitis implies primary involvement of the meninges, whereas encephalitis indicates brain parenchymal involvement. Because these anatomic boundaries are often not distinct, many patients have evidence of both meningeal and parenchymal involvement and should be considered to have meningoencephalitis. Brain abscess is the best example of a focal infection of the CNS. The neurologic expression of this infection is determined by the site and extent of the abscess(es).

The diagnosis of diffuse CNS infections depends on careful examination of cerebrospinal fluid (CSF) obtained by lumbar puncture (LP). Table 594–1 provides an overview of the expected CSF abnormalities with various CNS disorders.

594.1 Acute Bacterial Meningitis Beyond the Neonatal Period

Bacterial meningitis is one of the most potentially serious infections occurring in infants and older children. This infection is associated with a high rate of acute complications and risk of long-term morbidity. The etiology of bacterial meningitis and its treatment during the neonatal period (0–28 days) are generally distinct from those in older infants and children (Chapter 98). Nonetheless, the etiology of meningitis in the neonatal and postneonatal periods may overlap, especially in 1–2 mo old patients, in whom group B *Streptococcus*, *Streptococcus pneumoniae* (pneumococcus), *Neisseria meningitidis* (meningococcus), and *Haemophilus influenzae* type b all may cause meningitis.

The incidence of bacterial meningitis is sufficiently high in febrile infants that it should be included in the differential diagnosis of altered mental status or other neurologic dysfunction.

Etiology. During the first 2 mo of life, the bacteria that cause meningitis in normal infants reflect the maternal flora and the environment to which the infant is exposed. The most common pathogens include groups B and D streptococci, gram-negative enteric bacilli, and *Listeria monocytogenes*. In addition, meningitis in this age group may occasionally be due to *H. influenzae* (both type b and nonencapsulated strains) and the other pathogens more typically found in older patients.

Bacterial meningitis in children 2 mo–12 yr of age is usually caused by *S. pneumoniae*, *N. meningitidis*, or *H. influenzae* type b. Before the widespread use of *H. influenzae* type b vaccines, approximately 70% of cases of bacterial meningitis among children younger than 5 yr were due to *H. influenzae* type b. Subsequent to the implementation of universal immunization against this bacterium, beginning at about 2 mo of age, the incidence of *H. influenzae* type b meningitis dropped precipitously. The median age of bacterial meningitis in the United States increased from age 15 mo in 1986 to 25 yr in 1995. Meningitis now is most commonly caused by *S. pneumoniae* and *N. meningitidis*. However, subsequent to the licensure of conjugated pneumococcal vaccine in 2000 and the recommendation for its universal use beginning at 2 mo of age, the incidence of meningitis caused by this pathogen is decreasing.

Alterations of host defense due to anatomic defects or immune deficits increase the risk of meningitis from less common pathogens such as *Pseudomonas aeruginosa*, *Staphylococcus aureus*, coagulase-negative staphylococci, *Salmonella* spp, and *L. monocytogenes*.

Epidemiology. A major risk factor for meningitis is the lack of immunity to specific pathogens associated with young age. Additional risks include recent colonization with pathogenic bacteria, close contact (e.g., household, daycare centers, mili-

TABLE 594–1. Cerebrospinal Fluid Findings in Central Nervous System Disorders

Condition	Pressure (mm H$_2$O)	Leukocytes (mm³)	Protein (mg/dL)	Glucose (mg/dL)	Comments
Normal	50–80	<5, ≥75% lymphocytes	20–45	>50 (or 75% serum glucose)	
Common Forms of Meningitis					
Acute bacterial meningitis	Usually elevated (100–300)	100–10,000 or more; usually 300–2,000; PMNs predominate	Usually 100–500	Decreased, usually <40 (or <50% serum glucose)	Organisms usually seen on Gram stain and recovered by culture.
Partially treated bacterial meningitis	Normal or elevated	5–10,000; PMNs usual but mononuclear cells may predominate for extended period of time	Usually 100–500	Normal or decreased	Organisms may be seen on Gram stain. Pretreatment may render CSF sterile. Antigen may be detected by agglutination test
Viral meningitis or meningoencephalitis	Normal or slightly elevated (80–150)	Rarely >1,000 cells. Eastern equine encephalitis and lymphocytic choriomeningitis (LCM) may have cell counts of several thousand. PMNs early but mononuclear cells predominate through most of the course	Usually 50–200	Generally normal; may be decreased to <40 in some viral diseases, particularly mumps (15–20% of cases)	HSV encephalitis is suggested by focal seizures or by focal findings on CT or MRI scans or EEG. Enteroviruses and HSV infrequently recovered from CSF. HSV and enteroviruses may be detected by PCR of CSF
Uncommon Forms of Meningitis					
Tuberculous meningitis	Usually elevated	10–500; PMNs early, but lymphocytes predominate through most of the course	100–3,000; may be higher in presence of block	<50 in most cases; decreases with time if treatment is not provided	Acid-fast organisms almost never seen on smear. Organisms may be recovered in culture of large volumes of CSF. *Mycobacterium tuberculosis* may be detected by PCR of CSF
Fungal meningitis	Usually elevated	5–500; PMNs early but mononuclear cells predominate through most of the course. Cryptococcal meningitis may have no cellular inflammatory response	25–500	<50; decreases with time if treatment is not provided	Budding yeast may be seen. Organisms may be recovered in culture. Cryptococcal antigen (CSF and serum) may be positive in cryptococcal infection
Syphilis (acute) and leptospirosis	Usually elevated	50–500; lymphocytes predominate	50–200	Usually normal	Positive CSF serology. Spirochetes not demonstrable by usual techniques of smear or culture; darkfield examination may be positive
Amebic (*Naegleria*) meningoencephalitis	Elevated	1,000–10,000 or more; PMNs predominate	50–500	Normal or slightly decreased	Mobile amebae may be seen by hanging-drop examination of CSF at room temperature
Brain and Parameningeal Abscesses					
Brain abscess	Usually elevated (100–300)	5–200; CSF rarely acellular; lymphocytes predominate; if abscess ruptures into ventricle, PMNs predominate and cell count may reach >100,000	75–500	Normal unless abscess ruptures into ventricular system	No organisms on smear or culture unless abscess ruptures into ventricular system
Subdural empyema	Usually elevated (100–300)	100–5,000; PMNs predominate	100–500	Normal	No organisms on smear or culture of CSF unless meningitis also present; organisms found on tap of subdural fluid
Cerebral epidural abscess	Normal to slightly elevated	10–500; lymphocytes predominate	50–200	Normal	No organisms on smear or culture of CSF
Spinal epidural abscess	Usually low, with spinal block	10–100; lymphocytes predominate	50–400	Normal	No organisms on smear or culture of CSF
Chemical (drugs, dermoid cysts, myelography dye)	Usually elevated	100–1,000 or more; PMNs predominate	50–100	Normal or slightly decreased	Epithelial cells may be seen within CSF by use of polarized light in some children with dermoids
Noninfectious Causes					
Sarcoidosis	Normal or elevated slightly	0–100; mononuclear	40–100	Normal	No specific findings
Systemic lupus erythematosus with CNS involvement	Slightly elevated	0–500; PMNs usually predominate; lymphocytes may be present	100	Normal or slightly decreased	No organisms on smear or culture. LE preparation may be positive. Positive neuronal and ribosomal P protein antibodies in CSF
Tumor, leukemia	Slightly elevated to very high	0–100 or more; mononuclear or blast cells	50–1,000	Normal to decreased (20–40)	Cytology may be positive

PMN = polymorphonuclear neutrophils; CSF = cerebrospinal fluid; EEG = electroencephalogram; HSV = herpes simplex virus; PCR = polymerase chain reaction.

tary barracks) with individuals having invasive disease caused by *H. influenzae* type b and *N. meningitidis*, crowding, poverty, black race, and male gender. The mode of transmission is probably person to person contact through respiratory tract secretions or droplets. The risk of meningitis is increased among infants and young children with occult bacteremia (see Chapter 162); the odds ratio is greater for meningococcus (85 times) and *H. influenzae* type b (12 times) relative to that for pneumococcus.

Specific host defense defects due to altered immunoglobulin production in response to encapsulated pathogens may be responsible for the increased risk of bacterial meningitis in Native Americans and Eskimos, whereas defects of the complement system (C5-C8) have been associated with recurrent meningococcal infection, and defects of the properdin system have been associated with a significant risk of lethal meningococcal disease. Splenic dysfunction (sickle cell anemia) or asplenia (due to trauma, congenital defect, staging of Hodgkin disease) is associated with an increased risk of pneumococcal, *H. influenzae* type b (to some extent), and, rarely, meningococcal sepsis and meningitis. T-lymphocyte defects (congenital or acquired by chemotherapy, AIDS, or malignancy) are associated with an increased risk of *L. monocytogenes* infections of the CNS.

Congenital or acquired CSF leak across a mucocutaneous barrier, such as cranial or midline facial defects (cribriform plate) and middle ear (stapedial foot plate) or inner ear fistulas (oval window, internal auditory canal, cochlear aqueduct), or CSF leakage through a rupture of the meninges due to a basal skull fracture into the cribriform plate or paranasal sinus, is associated with an increased risk of pneumococcal meningitis. Lumbosacral dermal sinus and meningomyelocele are associated with staphylococcal and gram-negative enteric bacterial meningitis. CSF shunt infections increase the risk of meningitis due to staphylococci (especially coagulase-negative species) and other cutaneous bacteria.

STREPTOCOCCUS PNEUMONIAE. The epidemiology of infections caused by *S. pneumoniae* is being dramatically altered by the widespread use of conjugated pneumococcal vaccine, licensed in the United States in February 2000. This vaccine is recommended for routine administration to all children 23 mo of age and younger at 2, 4, 6, and 12 to 15 mo of age. Immunization targets this population because the incidence of invasive pneumococcal infections peaks during the first 2 yr of life, reaching rates of 228/100,000 in children 6 to 12 mo of age. Children with anatomic asplenia or functional asplenia secondary to sickle cell disease and those infected with HIV have infection rates that are 20- to 100-fold higher than in those of healthy children during the first 5 years of life. Additional risk factors for contracting pneumococcal meningitis include otitis media, sinusitis, pneumonia, CSF otorrhea or rhinorrhea, and chronic graft versus host disease following bone marrow transplantation.

NEISSERIA MENINGITIDIS. Meningococcal meningitis may be sporadic or may occur in epidemics. In the United States, serogroups B, C, and Y each account for approximately 30% of cases, although serogroup distribution may vary by location and time. Epidemic disease, especially in developing countries, usually is caused by serogroup A. Cases occur throughout the year but may be more common in the winter and spring. Nasopharyngeal carriage of *N. meningitidis* occurs in 1–15% of adults. Colonization may last weeks to months; recent colonization places nonimmune younger children at greatest risk for meningitis. The incidence of disease occurring in association with an index case in the family is 1%, a rate that is 1,000-fold the risk in the general population. The risk of secondary cases occurring in contacts at daycare centers is about 1/1,000. Most infections of children are acquired from a contact in a daycare facility, a colonized adult family member, or an ill patient with meningococcal disease. College freshmen living in dormitories have an increased incidence of infection compared to noncollege-attending, age-matched controls.

HAEMOPHILUS INFLUENZAE **TYPE B.** Before universal *H. influenzae* type b vaccination in the United States, invasive infections occurred primarily in infants 2 mo–2 yr of age; peak incidence was at 6–9 mo of age, and 50% of cases occurred in the 1st yr of life. The risk to children was markedly increased among family or daycare center contacts of patients with *H. influenzae* type b disease. Unvaccinated individuals and those with blunted immunologic responses to vaccine (e.g., children with HIV infection) remain at risk for *H. influenzae* type b meningitis.

Pathology and Pathophysiology. A meningeal exudate of varying thickness may be distributed around the cerebral veins, venous sinuses, convexity of the brain, and cerebellum and in the sulci, sylvian fissures, basal cisterns, and spinal cord. Ventriculitis with bacteria and inflammatory cells in ventricular fluid may be present, as may subdural effusions and, rarely, empyema. Perivascular inflammatory infiltrates also may be present, and the ependymal membrane may be disrupted. Vascular and parenchymal cerebral changes characterized by polymorphonuclear infiltrates extending to the subintimal region of the small arteries and veins, vasculitis, thrombosis of small cortical veins, occlusion of major venous sinuses, necrotizing arteritis producing subarachnoid hemorrhage, and, rarely, cerebral cortical necrosis in the absence of identifiable thrombosis have been described at autopsy. Cerebral infarction, resulting from vascular occlusion due to inflammation, vasospasm, and thrombosis, is a frequent sequela. Infarct size ranges from microscopic to involvement of an entire hemisphere.

Inflammation of spinal nerves and roots produces meningeal signs, and inflammation of the cranial nerves produces cranial neuropathies of optic, oculomotor, facial, and auditory nerves. Increased intracranial pressure (ICP) also produces oculomotor nerve palsy due to the presence of temporal lobe compression of the nerve during tentorial herniation. Abducens nerve palsy may be a nonlocalizing sign of elevated ICP.

Increased ICP is due to cell death (cytotoxic cerebral edema), cytokine-induced increased capillary vascular permeability (vasogenic cerebral edema), and, possibly, increased hydrostatic pressure (interstitial cerebral edema) after obstructed reabsorption of CSF in the arachnoid villus or obstruction of the flow of fluid from the ventricles. ICP often exceeds 300 mm H_2O; cerebral perfusion may be further compromised if the cerebral perfusion pressure (mean arterial pressure minus ICP) is less than 50 cm H_2O owing to reduced cerebral blood flow. The syndrome of inappropriate antidiuretic hormone secretion (SIADH) may produce excessive water retention, increasing the risk of elevated ICP. (See Chapter 553.1.) Hypotonicity of brain extracellular spaces may cause cytotoxic edema after cell swelling and lysis. Tentorial, falx, or cerebellar herniation does not usually occur because the increased ICP is transmitted to the entire subarachnoid space and there is little structural displacement. Furthermore, if the fontanels are still patent, increased ICP is readily dissipated.

Hydrocephalus can occur as an acute complication of bacterial meningitis. It most often takes the form of a communicating hydrocephalus due to adhesive thickening of the arachnoid villi around the cisterns at the base of the brain. Thus, there is interference with the normal resorption of CSF. Less often, obstructive hydrocephalus develops after fibrosis and gliosis of the aqueduct of Sylvius or the foramina of Magendie and Luschka.

Raised CSF protein levels are due in part to increased vascular permeability of the blood-brain barrier and the loss of albumin-rich fluid from the capillaries and veins traversing the subdural space. Continued transudation may result in subdural effusions, usually found in the later phase of acute bacterial meningitis. Hypoglycorrhachia (reduced CSF glucose levels) is due to decreased glucose transport by the cerebral tissue.

Damage to the cerebral cortex may be due to the focal or diffuse effects of vascular occlusion (infarction, necrosis, lactic acidosis), hypoxia, bacterial invasion (cerebritis), toxic encephalopathy (bacterial toxins), elevated ICP, ventriculitis, and transudation (subdural effusions). These pathologic factors result in the clinical manifestations of impaired consciousness, seizures, cranial nerve deficits, motor and sensory deficits, and later psychomotor retardation.

Pathogenesis. Bacterial meningitis most commonly results from hematogenous dissemination of microorganisms from a distant site of infection; bacteremia usually precedes meningitis or occurs concomitantly. Bacterial colonization of the nasopharynx with a potentially pathogenic microorganism is the usual source of the bacteremia. There may be prolonged carriage of the colonizing organisms without disease or, more likely, rapid invasion after recent colonization. Prior or concurrent viral upper respiratory tract infection may enhance the pathogenicity of bacteria producing meningitis.

N. meningitidis and *H. influenzae* type b attach to mucosal epithelial cell receptors by pili. After attachment to epithelial cells, bacteria breach the mucosa and enter the circulation. *N. meningitidis* may be transported across the mucosal surface within a phagocytic vacuole after ingestion by the epithelial cell. Bacterial survival in the bloodstream is enhanced by large bacterial capsules that interfere with opsonic phagocytosis and are associated with increased virulence. Host-related developmental defects in bacterial opsonic phagocytosis also contribute to the bacteremia. In young, nonimmune hosts, the defect may be due to an absence of preformed IgM or IgG anticapsular antibodies, whereas in immunodeficient patients, various deficiencies of components of the complement or properdin system may interfere with effective opsonic phagocytosis. Splenic dysfunction also may reduce opsonic phagocytosis by the reticuloendothelial system.

Bacteria gain entry to the CSF through the choroid plexus of the lateral ventricles and the meninges and then circulate to the extracerebral CSF and subarachnoid space. Bacteria rapidly multiply because the CSF concentrations of complement and antibody are inadequate to contain bacterial proliferation. Chemotactic factors then incite a local inflammatory response characterized by polymorphonuclear cell infiltration. The presence of bacterial cell wall lipopolysaccharide (endotoxin) of gram-negative bacteria (*H. influenzae* type b, *N. meningitidis*) and of pneumococcal cell wall components (teichoic acid, peptidoglycan) stimulates a marked inflammatory response, with local production of tumor necrosis factor, interleukin-1, prostaglandin E, and other cytokine inflammatory mediators. The subsequent inflammatory response is characterized by neutrophilic infiltration, increased vascular permeability, alterations of the blood-brain barrier, and vascular thrombosis. Excessive cytokine-induced inflammation continues after the CSF has been sterilized and is thought to be partly responsible for the chronic inflammatory sequelae of pyogenic meningitis.

Meningitis rarely may follow bacterial invasion from a contiguous focus of infection such as paranasal sinusitis, otitis media, mastoiditis, orbital cellulitis, or cranial or vertebral osteomyelitis or may occur after introduction of bacteria via penetrating cranial trauma, dermal sinus tracts, or meningomyeloceles. Meningitis may occur during endocarditis, pneumonia, or thrombophlebitis. It also may be associated with severe burns, indwelling catheters, or contaminated infusion equipment.

Clinical Manifestations. The onset of acute meningitis has two predominant patterns. The more dramatic and, fortunately, less common presentation is sudden onset with rapidly progressive manifestations of shock, purpura, disseminated intravascular coagulation (DIC), and reduced levels of consciousness frequently resulting in death within 24 hr. More often, meningitis is preceded by several days of fever accompanied by upper respiratory tract or gastrointestinal symptoms, followed by nonspecific signs of CNS infection such as increasing lethargy and irritability.

The signs and symptoms of meningitis are related to the nonspecific findings associated with a systemic infection and to manifestations of meningeal irritation. Nonspecific findings include fever, anorexia and poor feeding, symptoms of upper respiratory tract infection, myalgias, arthralgias, tachycardia, hypotension, and various cutaneous signs, such as petechiae, purpura, or an erythematous macular rash. Meningeal irritation is manifested as nuchal rigidity, back pain, Kernig sign (flexion of the hip 90 degrees with subsequent pain with extension of the leg), and Brudzinski sign (involuntary flexion of the knees and hips after passive flexion of the neck while supine). In some children, particularly in those younger than 12–18 mo, Kernig and Brudzinski signs are not consistently present. Increased ICP is suggested by headache, emesis, bulging fontanel or diastasis (widening) of the sutures, oculomotor or abducens nerve paralysis, hypertension with bradycardia, apnea or hyperventilation, decorticate or decerebrate posturing, stupor, coma, or signs of herniation. Papilledema is uncommon in uncomplicated meningitis and should suggest a more chronic process, such as the presence of an intracranial abscess, subdural empyema, or occlusion of a dural venous sinus. Focal neurologic signs usually are due to vascular occlusion. Cranial neuropathies of the ocular, oculomotor, abducens, facial, and auditory nerves also may be due to focal inflammation. Overall, about 10–20% of children with bacterial meningitis have focal neurologic signs.

Seizures (focal or generalized) due to cerebritis, infarction, or electrolyte disturbances occur in 20–30% of patients with meningitis. Seizures that occur on presentation or within the first 4 days of onset are usually of no prognostic significance. Seizures that persist after the 4th day of illness and those that are difficult to treat may be associated with a poor prognosis.

Alterations of mental status are common among patients with meningitis and may be due to increased ICP, cerebritis, or hypotension; manifestations include irritability, lethargy, stupor, obtundation, and coma. Comatose patients have a poor prognosis. Additional manifestations of meningitis include photophobia and tache cérébrale, which is elicited by stroking the skin with a blunt object and observing a raised red streak within 30–60 sec.

Diagnosis. The diagnosis of acute pyogenic meningitis is confirmed by analysis of the CSF, which typically reveals microorganisms on Gram stain and culture, a neutrophilic pleocytosis, elevated protein, and reduced glucose concentrations (see Table 594–1). LP should be performed when bacterial meningitis is suspected. Contraindications for an immediate LP include (1) evidence of increased ICP (other than a bulging fontanel), such as 3rd or 6th cranial nerve palsy with a depressed level of consciousness, or hypertension and bradycardia with respiratory abnormalities; (2) severe cardiopulmonary compromise requiring prompt resuscitative measures for shock or in patients in whom positioning for the LP would further compromise cardiopulmonary function; and (3) infection of the skin overlying the site of the LP. Thrombocytopenia is a relative contraindication for LP. If an LP is delayed, empirical antibiotic therapy should be initiated. CT scanning for evidence of a brain abscess or increased ICP also should not delay therapy. LP may be performed after increased ICP has been treated or a brain abscess has been excluded.

Blood cultures should be performed in all patients with suspected meningitis. Blood cultures reveal the responsible bacteria in 80–90% of cases of meningitis.

LUMBAR PUNCTURE. LP usually is performed with a patient in the flexed lateral decubitus position; the styletted needle is passed into the L3-L4 or L4-L5 intervertebral space. After entry into the subarachnoid space, the patient's position is changed to a more extended one to measure the opening CSF pressure, although an accurate reading may not be determined in a crying child. When the pressure is high, only a small volume of CSF should be removed to avoid a precipitous decline in ICP. Also see Chapter 584.

The CSF leukocyte count in bacterial meningitis is usually elevated to greater than 1,000/mm^3 and typically there is a neutrophilic predominance (75–95%). Turbid CSF is present when the CSF leukocyte count exceeds 200–400/mm^3. Normal healthy neonates may have as many as 30 leukocytes/mm^3, but older children without viral or bacterial meningitis have <5 leukocytes/mm^3 in the CSF; in both age groups there is a predominance of lymphocytes or monocytes.

A CSF leukocyte count less than 250/mm^3 may be present in as many as 20% of patients with acute bacterial meningitis; pleocytosis may be absent in patients with severe overwhelming sepsis and meningitis and is a poor prognostic sign. Pleocytosis with a lymphocyte predominance may be present during the early stage of acute bacterial meningitis; conversely, neutrophilic pleocytosis may be present in patients during the early stages of acute viral meningitis. The shift to lymphocytic-monocytic predominance in viral meningitis invariably occurs within 8 to 24 hr of the initial LP. The Gram stain is positive in most (70–90%) patients with bacterial meningitis.

Traumatic LP complicates the diagnosis of meningitis. Repeat LP at a higher interspace may produce less hemorrhagic fluid, but this fluid usually also contains red blood cells. Interpretation of CSF leukocytes and protein concentration are affected by LPs that are traumatic, although the Gram stain, culture, and glucose level may not be influenced. Although methods for correcting for the presence of red blood cells have been proposed, it is prudent to rely on the bacteriologic results rather than to attempt to interpret the CSF leukocyte and protein results of a traumatic LP.

Differential Diagnosis. In addition to *S. pneumoniae, N. meningitidis,* and *H. influenzae* type b, many other microorganisms can cause generalized infection of the CNS with similar clinical manifestations. These organisms include less typical bacteria, such as *Mycobacterium tuberculosis, Nocardia, Treponema pallidum* (syphilis), and *Borrelia burgdorferi* (Lyme disease); fungi, such as those endemic to specific geographic areas (*Coccidioides, Histoplasma,* and *Blastomyces*) and those responsible for infections in compromised hosts (*Candida, Cryptococcus,* and *Aspergillus*); parasites, such as *Toxoplasma gondii* and those that cause cysticercosis and, most frequently, viruses. Focal infections of the CNS including brain abscess and parameningeal abscess (subdural empyema, cranial and spinal epidural abscess) also may be confused with meningitis. Noninfectious illnesses also can cause generalized inflammation of the CNS. Relative to infections, these disorders are uncommon and include malignancy, collagen vascular syndromes, and exposure to toxins.

Determining the specific cause is facilitated by careful examination of the CSF with specific stains (e.g., Kinyoun carbol fuchsin for mycobacteria, India ink for fungi), cytology, antigen detection (bacteria, *Cryptococcus*), serology (syphilis), and viral culture (enterovirus). Other potentially valuable diagnostic tests include CT or MRI of the brain, blood cultures, serologic tests, and possibly brain biopsy. Acute viral meningoencephalitis is the most likely infection to be confused with bacterial meningitis. Although, in general, children with viral meningoencephalitis appear less ill than those with bacterial meningitis, both types of infection have a spectrum of severity. Some children with bacterial meningitis may have relatively mild signs and symptoms, whereas some with viral meningoencephalitis may be critically ill. Although classic CSF profiles associated with bacterial versus viral infection tend to be distinct (see Table 594–1), specific test results may have considerable overlap.

Another diagnostic conundrum in the evaluation of children with suspected bacterial meningitis is the analysis of CSF obtained from children already receiving antibiotic therapy. This is an important issue, because 25–50% of children being evalu-ated for bacterial meningitis are receiving oral antibiotics when their CSF is obtained. Such partial treatment of a patient with acute bacterial meningitis usually does not substantially alter the typical bacterial CSF profile. Although the frequency of positive CSF Gram stain results and ability to grow the bacteria may be reduced, the concentration of CSF glucose and protein and the neutrophil profile are not substantially altered by pretreatment.

Treatment. The therapeutic approach to patients with presumed bacterial meningitis depends on the nature of the initial manifestations of the illness. A child with rapidly progressing disease of less than 24-hr duration, in the absence of increased ICP, should receive antibiotics immediately after an LP is performed. If there are signs of increased ICP or focal neurologic findings, antibiotics should be given without performing an LP and before obtaining a CT scan. Increased ICP should be treated simultaneously. Immediate treatment of associated multiple organ system failure, such as shock and adult respiratory distress syndrome, also is indicated.

Patients who have a more protracted subacute course and become ill over a 1–7 day period should also be evaluated for signs of increased ICP and focal neurologic deficits. Unilateral headache, papilledema, and other signs of increased ICP suggest a focal lesion such as a brain or epidural abscess, or subdural empyema. Under these circumstances, antibiotic therapy should be initiated before LP and CT scanning. If no signs of increased ICP are evident, an LP should be performed.

INITIAL ANTIBIOTIC THERAPY. The initial (empirical) choice of therapy for meningitis in immunocompetent infants and children is primarily determined by the antibiotic susceptibilities of *S. pneumoniae.* Selected antibiotics should achieve bactericidal levels in the CSF. Although there are substantial geographic differences in the frequency of resistance of *S. pneumoniae* to antibiotics, rates are increasing throughout the world. In the United States, 25–50% of strains of *S. pneumoniae* are currently resistant to penicillin; relative resistance (MIC, 0.1–1.0 ug/mL) is more common than high-level resistance (MIC ≥ 2.0 ug/mL). Resistance to cefotaxime and ceftriaxone also is evident in up to 25% of isolates. In contrast, most strains of *N. meningitidis* are sensitive to penicillin and cephalosporins, although rare resistant isolates have been reported. Approximately 30–40% of isolates of *H. influenzae* type b produce β-lactamases and therefore are resistant to ampicillin. These β-lactamase-producing strains remain sensitive to the extended-spectrum cephalosporins.

Based on the substantial rate of resistance of *S. pneumoniae* to β-lactam drugs recommended empirical therapy is vancomycin (60 mg/kg/24 hr, given every 6 hr) in combination with either of the third-generation cephalosporins, cefotaxime (200 mg/kg/24 hr, given every 6 hr) or ceftriaxone (100 mg/kg/24 hr administered once per day or 50 mg/kg/dose, given every 12 hr). Patients allergic to β-lactam antibiotics can be treated with chloramphenicol, 100 mg/kg/24 hr, given every 6 hr.

If *L. monocytogenes* infection is suspected, as in infants 1–2 mo old or patients with a T-lymphocyte deficiency, ampicillin (200 mg/kg/24 hr, given every 6 hr) should be given with ceftriaxone or cefotaxime because cephalosporins are inactive against *L. monocytogenes.* Intravenous trimethoprim-sulfamethoxazole is an alternative treatment for *L. monocytogenes.*

If a patient is immunocompromised and gram-negative bacterial meningitis is suspected, initial therapy might include ceftazidime and an aminoglycoside.

DURATION OF ANTIBIOTIC THERAPY. Therapy for uncomplicated penicillin-sensitive *S. pneumoniae* meningitis should be completed with a third-generation cephalosporin or intravenous penicillin (400,000 U/kg/24 hr, given every 4–6 hr) for 10–14 days. If the isolate is resistant to penicillin and the third-generation cephalosporin, therapy should be completed with vancomycin. Intravenous penicillin (400,000 U/kg/24 hr) for

5–7 days is the treatment of choice for uncomplicated *N. meningitidis* meningitis. Uncomplicated *H. influenzae* type b meningitis should be treated for a total of 7–10 days. Ampicillin should be used to complete the course of therapy if the isolate is found to be sensitive.

Patients who receive intravenous or oral antibiotics before LP and who do not have an identifiable pathogen but do have evidence of an acute bacterial infection on the basis of their CSF profile should continue to receive therapy with ceftriaxone or cefotaxime for 7–10 days. If focal signs are present or the child does not respond to treatment, a parameningeal focus may be present and a CT or MRI scan should be performed.

A routine repeat LP is not indicated in patients with uncomplicated meningitis due to antibiotic-sensitive *S. pneumoniae*, *N. meningitidis*, or *H. influenzae* type b. Repeat examination of CSF is indicated in some neonates, in patients with gram-negative bacillary meningitis, or in infection caused by a β-lactam-resistant *S. pneumoniae*. The CSF should be sterile within 24–48 hr of initiation of appropriate antibiotic therapy.

Meningitis due to *Escherichia coli* or *P. aeruginosa* requires therapy with a third-generation cephalosporin active against the isolate in vitro. Most isolates of *E. coli* are sensitive to cefotaxime or ceftriaxone, and most isolates of *P. aeruginosa* are sensitive to ceftazidime. Gram-negative bacillary meningitis should be treated for 3 wk or for at least 2 wk after CSF sterilization, which may occur after 2–10 days of treatment.

Side effects of antibiotic therapy of meningitis include phlebitis, drug fever, rash, emesis, oral candidiasis, and diarrhea. Ceftriaxone may cause reversible gallbladder pseudolithiasis, detectable by abdominal ultrasonography. This is usually asymptomatic but may be associated with emesis and right upper quadrant pain.

CORTICOSTEROIDS. Rapid killing of bacteria in the CSF effectively sterilizes the meningeal infection but releases toxic cell products after cell lysis (cell wall endotoxin) that precipitates the cytokine-mediated inflammatory response. The resultant edema formation and neutrophilic infiltration may produce additional neurologic injury with worsening of CNS signs and symptoms. Therefore, agents that limit production of inflammatory mediators may be of benefit to patients with bacterial meningitis.

Data support the use of intravenous dexamethasone, 0.15 mg/kg/dose given every 6 hr for 2 days, in the treatment of children older than 6 wk with acute bacterial meningitis caused by *H. influenzae* type b. However, data are inconclusive regarding the benefit, if any, of corticosteroids in the treatment of meningitis caused by other bacteria. Therefore, their use is controversial. Among children with meningitis due *H. influenzae* type b, corticosteroid recipients had less fever, lower CSF protein and lactate levels, and a reduction in permanent auditory nerve damage, as manifested by sensorineural hearing loss, than did placebo recipients, enrolled in randomized, controlled trials. Corticosteroids appear to have maximum benefit if given 1–2 hr before antibiotics were initiated. Corticosteroids are not harmless; complications of their use may include gastrointestinal bleeding, hypertension, hyperglycemia, leukocytosis, and rebound fever, after the last dose.

SUPPORTIVE CARE. Repeated medical and neurologic assessments of patients with bacterial meningitis are essential to identify early signs of cardiovascular, CNS, and metabolic complications. Pulse rate, blood pressure, and respiratory rate should be monitored frequently. Neurologic assessment, including pupillary reflexes, level of consciousness, motor strength, cranial nerve signs, and evaluation for seizures, should be made frequently during the first 72 hr, when the risk of neurologic complications is greatest. Important laboratory studies include an assessment of blood urea nitrogen; serum sodium, chloride, potassium, and bicarbonate levels; urine output and specific gravity; complete blood and platelet counts; and, in the presence of petechiae, purpura, or abnormal bleeding, measure of coagulation function (fibrinogen, prothrombin, and partial thromboplastin times).

Patients should initially receive nothing by mouth. If a patient is judged to be normovolemic, with normal blood pressure, intravenous fluid administration should be restricted to one half to two thirds of maintenance, or 800–1,000 mL/m²/24 hr, until it can be established that increased ICP or SIADH is not present. Fluid administration may be returned to normal (1,500–1,700 mL/m²/24 hr) when serum sodium levels are normal. Fluid restriction is not appropriate in the presence of systemic hypotension because reduced blood pressure may result in reduced cerebral perfusion pressure and CNS ischemia. Therefore, shock must be treated aggressively to prevent brain and other organ dysfunction (acute tubular necrosis, adult respiratory distress syndrome). Patients with shock, a markedly elevated ICP, coma, and refractory seizures require intensive monitoring with central arterial and venous access and frequent vital signs, necessitating admission to a pediatric intensive care unit. Patients with septic shock require fluid resuscitation and therapy with vasoactive agents such as dopamine, epinephrine, and sodium nitroprusside (Chapter 163). The goal of such therapy in patients with meningitis is to avoid excessive increases in ICP without compromising blood flow and oxygen delivery to vital organs.

Neurologic complications include increased ICP with subsequent herniation, seizures, and an enlarging head circumference due to a subdural effusion or hydrocephalus. Signs of increased ICP should be treated emergently with endotracheal intubation and hyperventilation (to maintain the PCO_2 at approximately 25 mm Hg). In addition, intravenous furosemide (Lasix, 1 mg/kg) and mannitol (0.5–1 g/kg) osmotherapy may reduce ICP (Chapter 57.7). Furosemide may reduce brain swelling by venodilation and diuresis without increasing intracranial blood volume, whereas mannitol produces an osmolar gradient between the brain and plasma, thus shifting fluid from the CNS to the plasma, with subsequent excretion during an osmotic diuresis.

Seizures are common during the course of bacterial meningitis. Immediate therapy for seizures includes intravenous diazepam (0.1–0.2 mg/kg/dose) or lorazepam (0.05 mg/kg/dose), paying careful attention to the risk of respiratory suppression. Serum glucose, calcium, and sodium levels should be monitored to rule out a metabolic etiology. After immediate management of seizures, patients should receive phenytoin (15–20 mg/kg loading dose, 5 mg/kg/24 hr maintenance) to reduce the likelihood of recurrence. Phenytoin is preferred to phenobarbital because it produces less CNS depression and permits assessment of a patient's level of consciousness. Serum phenytoin levels should be monitored to maintain them in the therapeutic range (10–20 μg/mL).

Complications. During the treatment of meningitis, acute CNS complications can include seizures, increased ICP, cranial nerve palsies, stroke, cerebral or cerebellar herniation, and thrombosis of the dural venous sinuses.

Collections of fluid in the subdural space develop in 10–30% of patients with meningitis and are asymptomatic in 85–90% of patients. Subdural effusions are especially common in infants. Symptomatic subdural effusions may result in a bulging fontanel, diastasis of sutures, enlarging head circumference, emesis, seizures, fever, and abnormal results of cranial transillumination. CT or MRI scanning confirms the presence of a subdural effusion. In the presence of increased ICP or a depressed level of consciousness, symptomatic subdural effusion should be treated by aspiration through the open fontanel. Fever alone is not an indication for aspiration.

SIADH occurs in the majority of patients with meningitis, resulting in hyponatremia and reduced serum osmolality in

30–50% of infected children. This may exacerbate cerebral edema or independently produce hyponatremic seizures.

Fever associated with bacterial meningitis usually resolves within 5–7 days of the onset of therapy. Prolonged fever (>10 days) is noted in about 10% of patients. Prolonged fever usually is due to intercurrent viral infection, nosocomial or secondary bacterial infection, thrombophlebitis, or drug reaction. Secondary fever refers to the recrudescence of elevated temperature after an afebrile interval. Nosocomial infections are especially important to consider in the evaluation of these patients. Pericarditis or arthritis may occur in patients being treated for meningitis. Involvement of these sites may result either from bacterial dissemination or from immune complex deposition. In general, infectious pericarditis or arthritis occurs earlier in the course of treatment than does immune-mediated disease.

Thrombocytosis, eosinophilia, and anemia may develop during therapy for meningitis. Anemia may be due to hemolysis or bone marrow suppression. DIC is most often associated with the rapidly progressive pattern of presentation and is noted most commonly in patients with shock and purpura. The combination of endotoxemia and severe hypotension initiates the coagulation cascade; the coexistence of ongoing thrombosis may produce symmetric peripheral gangrene.

Prognosis. Appropriate recognition, prompt antibiotic therapy, and supportive care have reduced the mortality of bacterial meningitis after the neonatal period to less than 10%. The highest mortality rates are observed with pneumococcal meningitis. Severe neurodevelopmental sequelae may occur in 10–20% of patients recovering from bacterial meningitis, and as many as 50% have some, albeit subtle, neurobehavioral morbidity. The prognosis is poorest among infants younger than 6 mo and in those with more than 10^6 colony-forming units of bacteria/mL in their CSF. Those with seizures occurring more than 4 days into therapy or with coma or focal neurologic signs on presentation have an increased risk of long-term sequelae. There does not appear to be a correlation between duration of symptoms before diagnosis of meningitis and outcome.

The most common neurologic sequelae include hearing loss, mental retardation, seizures, delay in acquisition of language, visual impairment, and behavioral problems. Sensorineural hearing loss is the most common sequela of bacterial meningitis. It is due to labyrinthitis following cochlear infection and occurs in as many as 30% of patients with pneumococcal meningitis, 10% with meningococcal, and 5–20% of those with *H. influenzae* type b meningitis. Hearing loss also may be due to direct inflammation of the auditory nerve. All patients with bacterial meningitis should undergo careful audiologic assessment before or soon after discharge from the hospital. Frequent reassessment on an outpatient basis is indicated for patients who have a hearing deficit.

Prevention. Vaccination and antibiotic prophylaxis of susceptible at-risk contacts represent the two available means of reducing the likelihood of bacterial meningitis. The availability and application of each of these approaches depend upon the specific infecting bacteria.

NEISSERIA MENINGITIDIS. Chemoprophylaxis is recommended for all close contacts of patients with meningococcal meningitis regardless of age or immunization status. Close contacts should be treated with rifampin 10 mg/kg/dose every 12 hr (maximum dose of 600 mg) for 2 days as soon as possible after identification of a case of suspected meningococcal meningitis or sepsis. Close contacts include household, daycare center, and nursery school contacts and health care workers who have direct exposure to oral secretions (e.g., mouth-to-mouth resuscitation, suctioning, intubation). Exposed contacts should be treated immediately on suspicion of infection in the index patient; bacteriologic confirmation of infection should not be awaited. In addition, all contacts should be educated about the early signs of meningococcal disease and the need to seek prompt medical attention if these signs develop.

Meningococcal quadrivalent vaccine against serogroups A, C, Y, and W135 is recommended for high-risk children older than 2 yr. High-risk patients include those with anatomic or functional asplenia or deficiencies of terminal complement proteins. Use of meningococcal vaccine should be considered for college freshmen, especially those who live in dormitories, because of an observed increased risk of invasive meningococcal infections compared to the risk in noncollege-attending, age-matched controls. The vaccine also may be used as an adjunct with chemoprophylaxis for exposed contacts and during epidemics of meningococcal disease.

HAEMOPHILUS INFLUENZAE **TYPE B.** Rifampin prophylaxis should be given to all household contacts, including adults, if any close family member younger than 48 mo has not been fully immunized or if an immunocompromised child resides in the household. A household contact is one who lives in the residence of the index case or who has spent a minimum of 4 hr with the index case for at least 5 of 7 days preceding the patient's hospitalization. Family members should receive rifampin prophylaxis immediately after the diagnosis is suspected in the index case because more than 50% of secondary family cases occur in the 1st wk after the index patient has been hospitalized.

The dose of rifampin is 20 mg/kg/24 hr (maximum dose of 600 mg) given once each day for 4 days. Rifampin discolors the urine and sweat red-orange, stains contact lenses, and reduces the serum concentrations of some drugs, including oral contraceptives. Rifampin is contraindicated during pregnancy.

The most striking advance in the prevention of childhood bacterial meningitis followed the development and licensure of vaccines against *H. influenzae* type b. Four conjugate vaccines are licensed in the United States. Although each vaccine elicits different profiles of antibody response in infants immunized at 2–6 mo of age, all result in protective levels of antibody with efficacy rates, against invasive infections, that range from 70–100%. Efficacy is not as consistent in Native American populations, a group recognized as having an extremely high incidence of disease. All children should be immunized with *H. influenzae* type b conjugate vaccine beginning at 2 mo of age. See Chapter 282.

STREPTOCOCCUS PNEUMONIAE. A heptavalent conjugate vaccine against *S. pneumoniae* was licensed for use in the United States in 2000. Routine administration of this vaccine is recommended for all children younger than 2 yr of age. The initial dose is given at approximately 2 mo of age. Children who are at high risk of invasive pneumococcal infections should also receive the vaccine, including those with functional or anatomic asplenia and those with underlying immunodeficiency, such as infection with HIV, primary immunodeficiency, and those receiving immunosuppressive therapy.

594.2 Viral Meningoencephalitis

Viral meningoencephalitis is an acute inflammatory process involving the meninges and, to a variable degree, brain tissue. These infections are relatively common and may be caused by a number of different agents. The CSF is characterized by pleocytosis and the absence of microorganisms on Gram stain and routine bacterial culture. In most instances, the infections are self-limited. However, in some cases, substantial morbidity and mortality occur.

Etiology. Enteroviruses cause more than 80% of all cases of meningoencephalitis. Enteroviruses are small RNA-containing viruses; more than 80 serotypes have been identified. The severity of disease ranges from mild, self-limited illness with primarily meningeal involvement to severe encephalitis with death or significant sequelae.

Arboviruses are arthropod-borne agents, responsible for some cases of meningoencephalitis during summer months. Mosquitoes and ticks are the most common vectors, spreading disease to humans and other vertebrates, such as horses, after biting infected birds or small animals. Encephalitis in horses ("blind staggers") may be the first indication of an incipient epidemic. Although rural exposure is most common, urban and suburban outbreaks are also frequent. The most common arboviruses responsible for CNS infection in the United States are St. Louis and California encephalitis viruses (Chapter 244). West Nile virus recently made its appearance in the Western hemisphere, causing two successive outbreaks of encephalitis in 1999 and 2000 in the northeastern United States. Although most of the 78 cases during these two epidemics were in adults, two children were hospitalized. The incidence of West Nile virus infections continues to increase across the United States.

Several members of the herpes family of viruses can cause meningoencephalitis. Herpes simplex virus type 1 (HSV-1) is an important cause of severe, sporadic encephalitis in children and adults. Brain involvement usually is focal; progression to coma and death occurs in 70% of cases without antiviral therapy. Severe encephalitis with diffuse brain involvement is caused by herpes simplex virus type 2 (HSV-2) in neonates who usually contract the virus from their mothers at delivery. A mild transient form of meningoencephalitis may accompany genital herpes infection in sexually active adolescents; most of these infections are caused by HSV-2. Varicella-zoster virus (VZV) may cause CNS infection in close temporal relationship with chickenpox. The most common manifestation of CNS involvement is cerebellar ataxia, and the most severe is an acute encephalitis. After primary infection, VZV becomes latent in spinal and cranial nerve roots and ganglia, expressing itself later as herpes zoster, often with accompanying mild meningoencephalitis. Cytomegalovirus (CMV) infection of the CNS may be part of congenital infection or disseminated disease in immunocompromised hosts, but it does not cause meningoencephalitis in normal infants and children. Epstein-Barr virus (EBV) has been associated with myriad CNS syndromes (Chapter 233).

Mumps is a common pathogen in regions where mumps vaccine is not widely used. Mumps meningoencephalitis is mild, but deafness due to damage of the 8th cranial nerve may be a sequela. Meningoencephalitis is caused occasionally by respiratory viruses, rubeola, rubella, or rabies.

Epidemiology. The epidemiologic pattern of viral meningoencephalitis is primarily determined by the prevalence of enteroviruses, the most common etiology. Infection with enteroviruses is spread directly from person to person, with a usual incubation period of 4–6 days. Most cases in temperate climates occur in the summer and fall. Epidemiologic considerations in aseptic meningitis due to agents other than enteroviruses also include season, geography, climatic conditions, animal exposures, and factors related to the specific pathogen.

Pathogenesis. Neurologic damage is caused by direct invasion and destruction of neural tissues by actively multiplying viruses or by a host reaction to viral antigens. Most neuronal destruction is probably due directly to viral invasion, whereas the host's vigorous tissue response induces demyelination and vascular and perivascular destruction.

Tissue sections of the brain generally are characterized by meningeal congestion and mononuclear infiltration, perivascular cuffs of lymphocytes and plasma cells, some perivascular tissue necrosis with myelin breakdown, and neuronal disruption in various stages, including ultimately neuronophagia and endothelial proliferation or necrosis. A marked degree of demyelination with preservation of neurons and their axons is considered predominantly to represent "postinfectious" or "allergic" encephalitis. The cerebral cortex, especially the temporal lobe, is often severely affected by HSV; the arboviruses tend to affect the entire brain; rabies has a predilection for the basal structures. Involvement of the spinal cord, nerve roots, and peripheral nerves is variable.

Clinical Manifestations. The progression and severity of disease are determined by the relative degree of meningeal and parenchymal involvement, which in part is determined by the specific etiology. However, the clinical course resulting from infection with the same pathogen varies widely. Some children may appear to be mildly affected initially, only to lapse into coma and die suddenly. In others, the illness may be ushered in by high fever, violent convulsions interspersed with bizarre movements, and hallucinations alternating with brief periods of clarity, followed by complete recovery.

The onset of illness is generally acute, although CNS signs and symptoms often are preceded by a nonspecific febrile illness of a few days' duration. The presenting manifestations in older children are headache and hyperesthesia, and in infants, irritability and lethargy. Headache is most often frontal or generalized; adolescents frequently complain of retrobulbar pain. Fever, nausea and vomiting, photophobia, and pain in the neck, back, and legs are common. As body temperature increases, there may be mental dullness, progressing to stupor in combination with bizarre movements and convulsions. Focal neurologic signs may be stationary, progressive, or fluctuating. Loss of bowel and bladder control and unprovoked emotional bursts may occur.

Exanthems often precede or accompany the CNS signs, especially with echoviruses, coxsackieviruses, VZV, measles, and rubella. Examination often reveals nuchal rigidity without significant localizing neurologic changes, at least at the onset.

Specific forms or complicating manifestations of CNS viral infection include Guillain-Barré syndrome, transverse myelitis, hemiplegia, and cerebellar ataxia.

Diagnosis. The diagnosis of viral encephalitis is usually made on the basis of the clinical presentation of nonspecific prodrome followed by progressive CNS symptoms. The diagnosis is supported by examination of the CSF, which usually shows a mild mononuclear predominance (see Table 594–1). Other tests of potential value in the evaluation of patients with suspected viral meningoencephalitis include an electroencephalogram (EEG) and neuroimaging studies. The EEG typically shows diffuse slow-wave activity, usually without focal changes. Neuroimaging studies (CT or MRI) may show swelling of the brain parenchyma. Focal seizures or focal findings on EEG or CT or MRI, especially involving the temporal lobes, suggest HSV encephalitis.

Differential Diagnosis. A number of clinical conditions that cause CNS inflammation mimic viral meningoencephalitis. The most important group of alternative infectious agents to consider is bacteria. Most children with acute bacterial meningitis appear more critically ill than those with CNS viral infection. Parameningeal bacterial infections, such as brain abscess or subdural or epidural empyema, may have features similar to viral CNS infections. Infections caused by *M. tuberculosis*, *T. pallidum* (syphilis), *Borrelia burgdorferi* (Lyme disease), and *Bartonella henselae*, the bacillus associated with cat-scratch disease, tend to result in indolent courses. Analysis of CSF and appropriate serologic tests are necessary to differentiate these various pathogens.

Infections due to fungi, rickettsiae, *Mycoplasma*, protozoa, and other parasites also need to be included in the differential diagnosis. Consideration of these agents usually arises as a result of accompanying symptoms, geographic locality of infection, or host immune factors.

Various noninfectious disorders may be associated with CNS inflammation and have manifestations overlapping with those associated with viral meningoencephalitis. Some of these disorders include malignancy, collagen vascular diseases, intracranial hemorrhage, and exposure to certain drugs or toxins. Attention to history and other organ involvement usually allows elimination of these diagnostic possibilities.

Laboratory Findings. The CSF contains from a few to several thousand cells per cubic millimeter. Early in the disease, the cells are often polymorphonuclear; later, mononuclear cells predominate. This change in cellular type is often demonstrated in CSF samples obtained as little as 8–12 hr apart. The protein concentration in CSF tends to be normal or slightly elevated, but concentrations may be very high if brain destruction is extensive, such as that caused by HSV encephalitis. The glucose level is usually normal, although with certain viruses, for example, mumps, a substantial depression of CSF glucose concentrations may be observed.

The CSF should be cultured for viruses, bacteria, fungi, and mycobacteria; in some instances, special examinations are indicated for protozoa, *Mycoplasma,* and other pathogens. The success of isolating viruses from the CSF of children with viral meningoencephalitis is determined by the time in the clinical course that the specimen is obtained, the specific etiologic agent, whether the infection is a meningitic as opposed to a localized encephalitic process, and the skill of the diagnostic laboratory. Isolating a virus is most likely early in the illness, and the enteroviruses tend to be the easiest to isolate, although recovery of these agents from the CSF rarely exceeds 70%. To increase the likelihood of identifying the putative viral pathogen, specimens for culture also should be obtained from nasopharyngeal swabs, feces, and urine. Although isolating a virus from one or more of these sites does not prove causality, it is highly suggestive.

A serum specimen should be obtained early in the course of illness and, if viral cultures are not diagnostic, again 2–3 wk later for serologic studies. Serologic methods are not practical for diagnosing CNS infections caused by the enteroviruses because there are too many serotypes. However, this approach may be useful to confirm that a case is caused by a known circulating viral type. Serologic tests also may be of value in determining the etiology of nonenteroviral CNS infection. Detection of viral DNA or RNA by polymerase chain reaction may be useful in the diagnosis of CNS infection caused by HSV and enteroviruses, respectively.

Treatment. With the exception of the use of acyclovir for HSV encephalitis, treatment of viral meningoencephalitis is supportive. Treatment of mild disease may require only symptomatic relief. Headache and hyperesthesia are treated with rest, non-aspirin–containing analgesics, and a reduction in room light, noise, and visitors. Acetaminophen is recommended for fever. Codeine, morphine, and the phenothiazine derivatives may be necessary for pain and vomiting, but if possible, their use in children should be minimized because they may induce misleading signs and symptoms. Intravenous fluids are occasionally necessary because of poor oral intake. More severe disease may require hospitalization and intensive care.

It is important to anticipate and be prepared to manage convulsions, cerebral edema, hyperpyrexia, inadequate respiratory exchange, disturbed fluid and electrolyte balance, aspiration and asphyxia, and cardiac or respiratory arrest of central origin. Therefore, all patients with severe encephalitis should be monitored closely. In patients with evidence of increased ICP, placement of a pressure transducer in the epidural space may be indicated. The risks of cardiac and respiratory failure or arrest are high with severe disease. All fluids, electrolytes, and medications are initially given parenterally. In prolonged states of coma, parenteral alimentation is indicated. SIADH is common in acute CNS disorders; frequent monitoring of serum sodium concentrations is required for early detection (see Chapter 553.1). Normal blood levels of glucose, magnesium, and calcium must

be maintained to minimize the likelihood of convulsions. If cerebral edema or seizures become evident, vigorous treatment should be instituted.

Prognosis. Supportive and rehabilitative efforts are very important after patients recover. Motor incoordination, convulsive disorders, total or partial deafness, and behavioral disturbances may follow viral CNS infections. Visual disturbances due to chorioretinopathy and perceptual amblyopia also may occur. Special facilities and, at times, institutional placement may become necessary. Some sequelae of infection may be very subtle. Therefore, neurodevelopmental and audiologic evaluations should be part of the routine follow-up of children who have recovered from viral meningoencephalitis.

Most children completely recover from viral infections of the CNS, although the prognosis depends on the severity of the clinical illness, the specific cause, and the age of the child. If the clinical illness is severe and substantial parenchymal involvement is evident, the prognosis is poor, with potential deficits being intellectual, motor, psychiatric, epileptic, visual, or auditory in nature. Severe sequelae also should be anticipated in those with infection caused by HSV. Although some literature suggests that infants who contract viral meningoencephalitis have a poorer long-term outcome than older children, other data refute this observation. Approximately 10% of children younger than 2 yr with enteroviral CNS infections suffer an acute complication such as seizures, increased ICP, or coma. However, almost all have favorable long-term neurologic outcomes.

Prevention. Widespread use of effective viral vaccines for polio, measles, mumps, rubella, and varicella has almost eliminated CNS complications from these diseases in the United States. The availability of domestic animal vaccine programs against rabies has reduced the frequency of rabies encephalitis. Control of encephalitis due to arboviruses has been less successful because specific vaccines for the arboviral diseases that occur in North America are not available. However, control of insect vectors by suitable spraying methods and eradication of insect breeding sites reduces the incidence of these infections.

594.3 Eosinophilic Meningitis

Eosinophilic meningitis is defined as 10 or more eosinophils/mm^3 of CSF. The most common cause worldwide of eosinophilic pleocytosis is CNS infection with helminthic parasites. However, in countries such as the United States, where helminthic infestation is uncommon, the differential diagnosis of CSF eosinophilic pleocytosis is broad.

Etiology. Although any tissue-migrating helminth may cause eosinophilic meningitis, the most common cause is human infection with the rat lungworm *Angiostrongylus cantonensis* (Chapter 274). Other parasites that can cause eosinophilic meningitis include *Gnathostoma spinigerum* (dog and cat roundworm) (Chapter 274), *Baylisascaris procyonis* (raccoon roundworm), *Ascaris lumbricoides* (human roundworm), *Trichinella spiralis, Toxocara canis, Toxoplasma gondii, Paragonimus westermani, Echinococcus granulosus, Schistosoma japonicum, Onchocerca volvulus,* and *T. solium.* Eosinophilic meningitis also may occur as an unusual manifestation of more common viral, bacterial, or fungal infections of the CNS. Noninfectious causes of eosinophilic meningitis include multiple sclerosis, malignancy, hypereosinophilic syndrome, or a reaction to medications or a ventriculoperitoneal shunt.

Epidemiology. *A. cantonensis* is found in Southeast Asia, the South Pacific, Japan, Taiwan, Egypt, Ivory Coast, and Cuba. Infection is acquired by eating raw or undercooked freshwater snails, slugs, prawns, or crabs containing infectious third-stage larvae. *Gnathostoma* infections are found in Japan, China, India,

Bangladesh, and Southeast Asia. Gnathostomiasis is acquired by eating undercooked or raw fish, frog, bird, or snake meat.

Clinical Manifestations. When eosinophilic meningitis results from helminthic infestation, patients become ill 1–3 wk after exposure, because the parasites migrate from the gastrointestinal tract to the CNS. Common concomitant findings include fever, peripheral eosinophilia, vomiting, abdominal pain, creeping skin eruptions, or pleurisy. Neurologic symptoms may include headache, meningismus, ataxia, cranial nerve palsies, and paresthesias. Paraparesis or incontinence can result from radiculitis or myelitis.

Diagnosis. The presumptive diagnosis of helminth-induced eosinophilic meningitis is made by travel and exposure history in the presence of typical clinical and laboratory findings.

Treatment. Treatment is supportive, because infection is self-limited and anthelmintic drugs do not appear to influence the outcome of infection. Analgesics should be given for headache and radiculitis, and CSF removal or shunting should be performed to relieve hydrocephalus, if present. Steroids may decrease the duration of headaches in adults with eosinophilic meningitis.

Prognosis. The prognosis is good; 70% of patients improve sufficiently to leave the hospital in 1–2 wk. Mortality associated with eosinophilic meningitis is less than 1%.

Acute Bacterial Meningitis
Arditi M, Mason EO, Bradley JS, et al: Three-year multicenter surveillance of pneumococcal meningitis in children: Clinical characteristics and outcome related to penicillin susceptibility and dexamethasone use. *Pediatrics* 1998;102;1087–97.
Baraff LJ, Lee SI, Schriger DL: Outcomes of bacterial meningitis in children: A meta-analysis. *Pediatr Infect Dis J* 1993;12:389–94.
Blazer S, Berant M, Alon U: Bacterial meningitis: Effect of antibiotic treatment on cerebrospinal fluid. *J Clin Pathol* 1983;80:386–7.
Bonsu BK, Harper MB: Fever interval before diagnosis, prior antibiotic treatment, clinical outcome for young children with bacterial meningitis. *Clin Infect Dis* 2001;32:566–72.
Committee on Infectious Diseases: Policy Statement: Recommendations for the prevention of pneumococcal infections, including the use of pneumococcal conjugate vaccine (Prevnar), pneumococcal polysaccharide vaccine, and antibiotic prophylaxis. *Pediatrics* 2000;106:362–6.
Dawson KG, Emerson JC, Burns JL: Fifteen years of experience with bacterial meningitis. *Pediatr Infect Dis J* 1999;18:816–22.
Dodge PR, Davis H, Feigin RD, et al: Prospective evaluation of hearing impairment as a sequela of acute bacterial meningitis. *N Engl J Med* 1984;311:869–74.
Feigin RD, McCracken GH, Klein JO: Diagnosis and management of meningitis. *Pediatr Infect Dis J* 1992;11:785–814.
Grimwood K, Anderson P, Anderson V, et al: Twelve year outcome following bacterial meningitis: Further evidence for persisting effects. *Arch Dis Child* 2000;83:111–6.
Kilpi T, Anttila M, Kallio MJ, et al: Severity of childhood bacterial meningitis and duration of illness before diagnosis. *Lancet* 1991;338:406–9.
Kilpi T, Anttila M, Kallio MJ, et al: Length of prediagnostic history related to the course and sequelae of childhood bacterial meningitis. *Pediatr Infect Dis J* 1993;12:184–8.
McIntyre PB, Berkey CS, King SM, et al: Dexamethasone as adjunctive therapy in bacterial meningitis. A meta-analysis of randomized clinical trials since 1988. *JAMA* 1997;278:925–31.
Pomeroy SL, Holmes SJ, Dodge PR, et al: Seizures and other neurologic sequelae of bacterial meningitis in children. *N Engl J Med* 1990;323:1651–57.
Quagliarello V, Sheld WM: Treatment of bacterial meningitis. *N Engl J Med* 1997;336:708–16.
Radetsky M: Duration of symptoms and outcome in bacterial meningitis: An analysis of causation and the implications of a delay in diagnosis. *Pediatr Infect Dis J* 1992;11:694–8.
Syrogiannopoulos GA, Nelson JD, McCracken GH: Subdural collections of fluid in acute bacterial meningitis: A review of 136 cases. *Pediatr Infect Dis* 1986;5:343–52.
Talan DA, Guterman JJ, Overturf GD, et al: Analysis of emergency department management of suspected bacterial meningitis. *Ann Emerg Med* 1989;18:856–62.

Viral Meningoencephalitis
Gutierrez KM, Prober CG: Encephalitis: Identifying the specific cause is key to effective management. *Postgrad Med* 1998;103:123–43.
Rautonen J, Koskiniemi M, Vaheri A: Prognostic factors in childhood encephalitis. *Pediatr Infect Dis J* 1991;10:441–6.
Rorabaugh ML, Berlin LE, Heldrich F, et al: Aseptic meningitis in infants younger than 2 years of age: Acute illness and neurologic complications. *Pediatrics* 1993;92:206–11.
Tyler KL: West Nile virus encephalitis in America. *N Engl J Med* 2001;344:1858–59.
Whitley RJ: Viral encephalitis. *N Engl J Med* 1990;323:242–50.
Wilfert CM, Lehrman SN, Katz SL: Enteroviruses and meningitis. *Pediatr Infect Dis* 1983;2:333–41.

Eosinophilic Meningitis
Chotmongkol V, Sawanyawisuth K, Thavornpitak Y: Corticosteroids treatment of eosinophilic meningitis. *Clin Infect Dis* 2000;31:660–2.
Hsu W, Chen J, Chien C, et al: Eosinophilic meningitis caused by *Angiostrongylus cantonensis*. *Pediatr Infect Dis J* 1990;9:443–5.
Weller PF: Eosinophilic meningitis. *Am J Med* 1993;95:250–3.

Chapter 595
Brain Abscess *Robert H. A. Haslam*

Brain abscesses can occur in children of any age but are most common in children between 4 and 8 yr. The causes of brain abscess include embolization due to congenital heart disease with right-to-left shunts (especially tetralogy of Fallot), meningitis, chronic otitis media and mastoiditis, sinusitis, soft tissue infection of the face or scalp, orbital cellulitis, dental infections, penetrating head injuries, immunodeficiency states, and infection of ventriculoperitoneal shunts. The pathogenesis is undetermined in 10–15% of cases. Cerebral abscesses are evenly distributed between the two hemispheres, and approximately 80% of cases are divided equally between the frontal, parietal, and temporal lobes. Brain abscesses in the occipital lobe, cerebellum, and brainstem account for about 20% of the cases. Most brain abscesses are single, but 30% are multiple and may involve more than one lobe. An abscess in the frontal lobe is often caused by extension from sinusitis or orbital cellulitis, whereas abscesses located in the temporal lobe or cerebellum are frequently associated with chronic otitis media and mastoiditis. Abscesses resulting from penetrating injuries tend to be singular and caused by *Staphylococcus aureus*, whereas those resulting from septic emboli, congenital heart disease, or meningitis often have several causal organisms.

Etiology. The responsible bacteria include *S. aureus*, streptococci (*viridans*, pneumococci, microaerophilic), anaerobic organisms (gram-positive cocci, *Bacteroides* spp, *Fusobacterium* spp, *Prevotella* spp, *Actinomyces* spp, and *Clostridium* spp), and gram-negative aerobic bacilli (enteric rods, *Proteus* spp, *Pseudomonas aeruginosa*, *Citrobacter diversus*, and *Haemophilus* spp). One organism is cultured in the majority of abscesses (70%), two in 20%, and three or more in 10% of cases. Abscesses associated with mucosal infections (sinusitis) frequently have anaerobic bacteria.

Clinical Manifestations. The early stages of cerebritis and abscess formation are associated with nonspecific symptoms, including low-grade fever, headache, and lethargy. The significance of these symptoms is generally not recognized, and an oral antibiotic is often prescribed with resultant transient relief. As the inflammatory process proceeds, vomiting, severe headache, seizures, papilledema, focal neurologic signs (hemiparesis), and coma may develop. A cerebellar abscess is characterized by nystagmus, ipsilateral ataxia and dysmetria, vomiting, and headache. If the abscess ruptures into the ventricular cavity, overwhelming shock and death usually ensue.

Diagnosis. The peripheral white blood cell count can be normal or elevated, and the blood culture is positive in approximately 10% of cases. Examination of the cerebrospinal fluid (CSF) shows variable results; the white blood cells and protein may be minimally elevated or normal. The glucose level may be slightly low, and CSF cultures are rarely positive. Aspiration of the abscess is much more likely to establish a bacteriologic diagnosis. Because examination of the CSF is seldom useful and a lumbar puncture may cause herniation of the cerebellar tonsils, the procedure should not be undertaken in a child suspected of having a brain abscess. The electroencephalogram (EEG) shows corresponding focal slowing, and the radionuclide brain scan indicates an area of enhancement due to disruption of the blood-brain barrier in greater than 80% of cases. CT and MRI are the most reliable methods of demonstrating cerebritis and abscess formation (Fig. 595–1). The CT findings of cerebritis are characterized by a parenchymal low-density lesion, and MRI T2 weighted images indicate increased signal intensity. An abscess cavity shows a ring-enhancing lesion by contrast CT, and the MRI also demonstrates an abscess capsule with gadolinium administration.

Treatment. The initial management of a brain abscess includes prompt diagnosis and institution of an antibiotic regimen that is based on the probable pathogenesis and most likely organism. When the cause is unknown, the dual combination of a third-generation cephalosporin and metronidazole is commonly used. If there is a history of head trauma or neurosurgery, a combination of nafcillin or vancomycin with a third-generation cephalosporin and metronidazole is given. The choice of antibiotics should be altered when the culture and sensitivity results become available. An abscess resulting from a penetrating injury, head trauma, or sinusitis should be treated with a combination of nafcillin or vancomycin, cefotaxime or ceftriaxone, and metronidazole. Monotherapy with meropenem, which has good activity against gram-negative bacilli, anaerobes, staphylococci, and streptococci, including virtually all antibiotic-resistant pneumococci, is a reasonable alternative. In contrast, the initial treatment of a lesion resulting from cyanotic heart disease is penicillin and metronidazole. Abscesses secondary to an infected ventriculoperitoneal shunt may be initially treated with vancomycin and ceftazidime. When otitis media, sinusitis, or mastoiditis is the likely cause, vancomycin, because of the increasing incidence of penicillin resistance among *S. pneumoniae*, in combination with a third-generation cephalosporin and metronidazole is initially indicated until the culture results become available. When *Citrobacter* meningitis (often in neonates) leads to abscess formation, a third-generation cephalosporin is used, typically in combination with an aminoglycoside. In immunocompromised patients, broad-spectrum antibiotic coverage is used, and amphotericin B therapy should be considered.

Surgical management of brain abscesses has changed since the advent of CT. In the early stages of cerebritis or with multiple abscesses, antibiotics may be used alone. An encapsulated abscess, particularly if the lesion is causing a mass effect or increased intracranial pressure, should be treated by a combination of antibiotics and aspiration. Surgical excision of an abscess is rarely required, because the procedure may be associated with greater morbidity compared with aspiration of a cavity. Surgery is indicated when the abscess is larger than 2.5 cm in diameter, gas is present in the abscess, the lesion is multiloculated, the lesion is located in the posterior fossa, or a fungus is identified. Associated infectious processes, such as mastoiditis, sinusitis, or a periorbital abscess, may require surgical drainage. The duration of antibiotic therapy depends on the organism and response to treatment, but it is usually is 4–6 wk.

Prognosis. Mortality rate associated with brain abscess has decreased significantly, to approximately 5–10% with the use of CT or MRI and prompt antibiotic and surgical management. Factors associated with high mortality rate at the time of admission include multiple abscesses, coma, and lack of CT facilities. Long-term sequelae occur in at least 50% of survivors and include hemiparesis, seizures, hydrocephalus, cranial nerve abnormalities, and behavior and learning problems.

Brook I: Aerobic and anaerobic bacteriology of intracranial abscesses. *Pediatr Neurol* 1992;8:210.

Saez-Lloreus XJ, Umana NA, Odio CN, et al: Brain abscesses in infants and children. *Pediatr Infect Dis J* 1989;8:449.

Sjolin J, Lilja A, Erikson N, et al: Treatment of brain abscess with cefotaxime and metronidazole: Prospective study on 15 consecutive patients. *Clin Infect Dis* 1993;17:857.

Smith RR: Neuroradiology of intracranial infection. *Pediatr Neurosurg* 1992;18:92.

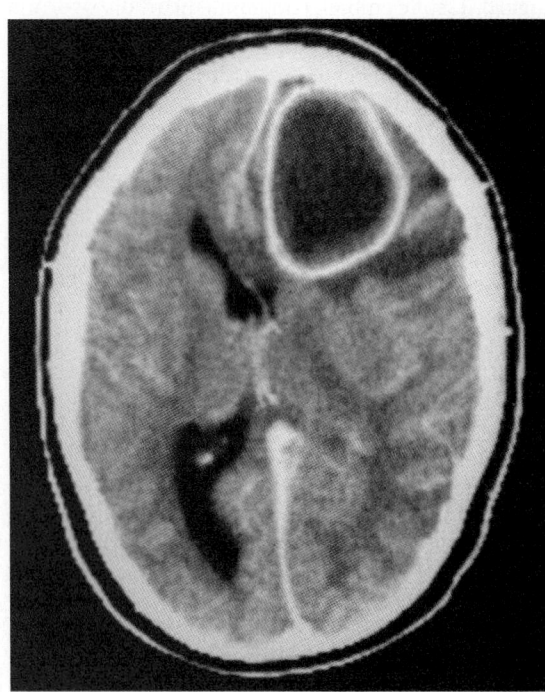

FIGURE 595–1. CT with contrast. Note the large wall-enhancing abscess in the left frontal lobe. The lesion is causing a shift of the brain to the right. The patient had no neurologic signs until just before the CT scan because the abscess is located in the frontal lobe, a "silent" area of the brain.

Chapter 596

Pseudotumor Cerebri

Robert H. A. Haslam

Pseudotumor cerebri is a clinical syndrome that mimics brain tumors and is characterized by increased intracranial pressure (ICP) with a normal cerebrospinal fluid (CSF) cell count and protein content and normal ventricular size, anatomy, and position.

Etiology. There are many explanations for the development of pseudotumor cerebri, including alterations in CSF absorption and production, cerebral edema, abnormalities in vasomotor control and cerebral blood flow, and venous obstruction. The causes of pseudotumor are numerous and include *metabolic disorders* (galactosemia, hypoparathyroidism, pseudohypoparathyroidism, hypophosphatasia, prolonged corticosteroid therapy or too rapid corticosteroid withdrawal, possibly growth hormone treatment, refeeding of a significantly malnourished child, hypervitaminosis A, vitamin A deficiency, Addison disease, obesity, menarche, oral contraceptives, and pregnancy), *infections* (roseola infantum, chronic otitis media and mastoiditis, Guillain-Barré syndrome), *drugs* (nalidixic acid, tetracycline, nitrofurantoin, isotretinoin), *hematologic disorders* (polycythemia, hemolytic and iron-deficiency anemia, Wiskott-Aldrich syndrome), *obstruction of intracranial drainage by venous thrombosis* (lateral sinus or posterior sagittal sinus thrombosis), head injury, and obstruction of the superior vena cava.

Clinical Manifestations. The most frequent symptom is headache, and although vomiting also occurs, it is rarely as persistent and pernicious as that associated with a posterior fossa tumor. Diplopia secondary to paralysis of the abducens nerve is a frequent complaint. Most patients are alert and lack constitutional symptoms. Examination of the infant characteristically reveals a bulging fontanel and a "cracked-pot sound" or Macewen sign (percussion of the skull produces a resonant sound) due to separation of the cranial sutures. Papilledema with an enlarged blind spot is the most consistent sign in a child beyond infancy. Early optic nerve edema may be noted with ultrasonography. An inferior nasal defect may be detected on formal tangent screen testing. The presence of focal neurologic signs indicates a process other than pseudotumor cerebri.

Treatment. The prime goal in management should be discovery and treatment of the underlying cause. Pseudotumor cerebri is mainly a self-limited condition, but optic atrophy and blindness are the most significant complications. Consideration should be given to treating sinus thrombosis with anticoagulation. For many patients, repeated follow-up and monitoring of the visual acuity are all that is required. Serial visual-evoked potentials are useful if the visual acuity cannot be reliably documented. For others, the initial lumbar tap that follows a CT or MRI scan is diagnostic and therapeutic. The spinal needle produces a small rent in the dura that allows CSF to escape the subarachnoid space, thus reducing the ICP. Several additional lumbar taps and the removal of sufficient CSF to reduce the opening pressure by 50% occasionally lead to resolution of the process. Acetazolamide, 10–30 mg/kg/24 hr, and corticosteroids have been effective for some patients. Rarely, a lumboperitoneal shunt or subtemporal decompression is necessary if the aforementioned approaches are unsuccessful and optic nerve atrophy supervenes. Some centers perform optic nerve sheath fenestration. Finally, any patient whose increased ICP proves to be refractory to treatment warrants consideration for repeat neuroradiologic studies. A slow-growing tumor or obstruction of a venous sinus may become evident at the time of reinvestigation.

Baker R, Baumann R, Buncic J: Idiopathic intracranial hypertension (pseudotumor cerebri) in pediatric patients. *Pediatr Neurol* 1989;5:5.

Shuper A, Snir M, Barash D: Ultrasonography of the optic nerves: Clinical application in children with pseudotumor cerebri. *J Pediatrics* 1997;131:734.

Soler D, Cox T, Bullock P, et al: Diagnosis and management of benign intracranial hypertension. *Arch Dis Child* 1998;78:89.

Chapter 597
Spinal Cord Disorders
Robert H. A. Haslam

597.1 Spinal Cord Tumors

In children, spinal cord tumors account for approximately 20% of neuraxial tumors and are classified according to anatomic position (Fig. 597–1). *Intramedullary tumors* arise within the substance of the cord and grow slowly by infiltration, usually in the cervical region. The most common intramedullary tumor is a low-grade astrocytoma, followed by an ependymoma. *Extramedullary intradural tumors* tend to be benign and arise from neural crest tissue. Tumors in this area include neurofibroma, ganglioneuroma, and meningioma. *Extramedullary extradural tumors* characteristi-

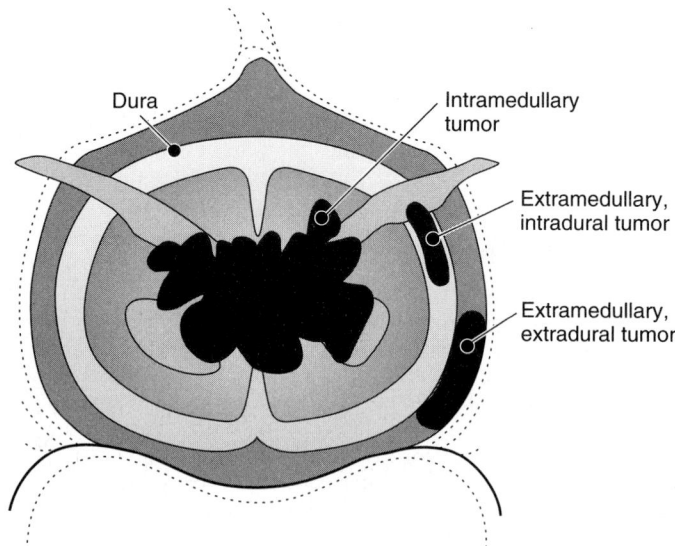

FIGURE 597–1. Diagram of the location of spinal cord tumors in children.

cally are metastatic lesions, particularly neuroblastoma, sarcoma, and lymphoma.

Clinical Manifestations. Most children with spinal cord tumors present with a combination of gait disturbance, scoliosis, and back pain, depending on tumor location. Intramedullary gliomas are slow growing. Progressive difficulties in locomotion and sphincter disturbances are the earliest symptoms. Glial tumors in the cervical cord produce lower motor neuron signs in the upper extremities and upper motor neuron signs in the legs. Denervation of the intercostal muscles decreases chest wall movement and results in a weak cough. Loss of pain, temperature, and light touch sensation is evident in the lower extremities, and a cord level on occasion may be documented by light touch and pain sensation or by somatosensory-evoked potentials. With extramedullary tumors, the presenting symptom is often back pain. The child has difficulty sleeping because of pain and maintains a tripod posture while attempting to assume the supine position. If the tumor is attached to a nerve root, segmental pain, paresthesia, and weakness are evident. Extramedullary extradural tumors have a propensity to cause an acute block of the cerebrospinal fluid (CSF) pathways owing to rapid growth within a confined space. Such children present with a flaccid paraplegia, urinary retention, and a patulous anus. Some extramedullary tumors produce the Brown-Séquard syndrome, which consists of ipsilateral weakness, spasticity, and ataxia, with contralateral loss of pain and temperature sensation. Papilledema is observed in a few patients, usually in association with markedly elevated CSF protein levels that presumably interfere with normal CSF flow dynamics.

Diagnosis. It is important to establish the diagnosis of a spinal cord tumor as early as possible, because surgical management is facilitated and irreversible damage to the cord may be prevented. In approximately 40% of the cases, routine roentgenograms show abnormalities including widening of the interpediculate distance, destruction or sclerosis of the adjacent vertebral bodies or pedicles, and widening of the vertebral the foramen on an oblique view in the case of a neurofibroma or ganglioneuroma. MRI is the most important diagnostic test to establish the diagnosis. Intramedullary tumors produce a fusiform swelling of the cord, often with a complete block of the CSF (Fig. 597–2). Neurofibromas tend to create a circular indentation of the cord, and extramedullary tumors show various degrees of blockage.

Treatment. With modern surgical techniques, many tumors can be totally and safely resected. Surgical removal of benign extramedullary tumors is associated with a good prognosis. For children with a primary neuroblastoma presenting with a sudden onset of paraplegia secondary to metastases in the extradural space, immediate radiation therapy may circumvent the need for a laminectomy.

597.2 Spinal Cord Trauma

(See also Chapters 51 and 88.3.)

Acute spinal cord injuries in children may result from indirect trauma caused by hyperflexion, hyperextension, or vertical compression accidents; however, fracture dislocation of the vertebral column or epidural bleeding may also compromise spinal cord integrity secondary to a mass effect. As with the brain, the degree of injury to the spinal cord is variable and includes concussion, contusion, laceration, and transection. Recovery depends on the extent of the trauma as well as on the immediate and long-term management. Common causes of spinal cord injury include traumatic breech deliveries, physical abuse (as in the shaken baby syndrome), automobile and diving accidents, falls from playground equipment, and congenital defects such as the underlying vertebral abnormality in Down syndrome (DS).

Individuals with DS are susceptible to atlantoaxial instability resulting from laxity of the transverse ligaments. Atlantoaxial instability has been defined as a distance greater than 4.5 mm between the odontoid process of the axis and the anterior arch of the atlas. Spinal cord compression (myelopathy) may be a consequence of atlantoaxial instability. There is no consensus about the usefulness of radiograph screening in predicting spinal cord injury in children with DS. It is recommended that (1) lateral roentgenograms of the neck in the flexion position be obtained at 5–8 yr, 10–12 yr, and 18 yr in individuals with DS, because atlantoaxial instability can develop during periods of growth; (2) children with atlantoaxial instability be advised not to participate in risky sports, such as tumbling, diving, and football; (3) radiographs of the neck be obtained before operative procedures or therapeutic programs that involve active neck movement or manipulation; (4) parents and physicians be made aware of the symptoms and signs of cord compression (neck pain, urinary and fecal incontinence, head tilt, gait abnormalities, ataxia, hyperreflexia, weakness, spasticity, and quadriplegia); and (5) there be prompt investigation (neck radiographs, CT scan, MRI study) followed by consideration for operative intervention in patients with signs of myelopathy.

A patient with *severe cord injury* presents with **spinal shock**, consisting of flaccidity, areflexia, and loss of sensation. This may persist for up to 4 wk and results from dysfunction of synaptic activity in the pathways caudal to the injury. Ultimately, reflex flexor movements develop, followed by extensor reflex activity associated with hyperactive deep tendon reflexes, spasticity, and an automatic bladder. *Fracture dislocations at the C5-C6 level* are the most common acute cause of spinal cord injuries and are characterized by a flaccid quadriparesis, loss of sphincter function, and a sensory level corresponding to the upper sternum. A transverse injury in the high cervical cord level (C1-C2) causes respiratory arrest and death in the absence of ventilatory support. Fractures in the low thoracic (T12-L1) region may produce the **conus medullaris syndrome,** which includes a loss of urinary and rectal sphincter control, flaccid weakness, and sensory disturbances of the legs. Spinal cord injury may occur in the absence of a vertebral fracture. A **central cord lesion** may result from contusion and hemorrhage and typically involves the upper extremities to a greater degree than the legs. There are lower motor neuron signs in the upper extremities and upper motor neuron signs in the legs, bladder dysfunction, and loss of sensation caudal to the lesion. Recovery may be considerable, particularly in the lower extremities.

Spinal cord injuries should be managed by stabilization and immobilization of the spine at the accident site using a cervical collar or sandbags. An adequate airway should be maintained, respiratory support should be provided, and shock should be treated with appropriate volume expanders. High-dose intravenous methylprednisolone (30 mg/kg bolus followed by 5.4 mg/kg/hr for 24 hr) should be started immediately, even before transport. If steroids are started within 3–8 hr of the injury, they should be continued for 48 hr. After transportation, roentgenograms of the spine, including oblique views, should be obtained. Approximately 50% of children with severe cord injuries show no abnormality on the spine roentgenogram. Fracture dislocations are treated with traction, immobilization, and, if the injury is unstable, vertebral fusion. Laminectomy and inspection of the cord are reserved for patients with progression of neurologic signs and appearance on CT or MRI scan that suggests an epidural or intraspinal hemorrhage. Additional therapeutic measures include management of bladder and gastrointestinal disturbances, nutritional and skin care, and a rigorous multidisciplinary rehabilitation program. The prognosis following spinal cord trauma is directly related to the extent of the injury. Recovery may occur over an extended period of months to years. Central cord injuries have a better prognosis than those injuries producing transverse lesions.

597.3 Tethered Cord

During fetal development, the spinal cord occupies the entire length of the vertebral column, but due to differential growth, the conus medullaris in a child ultimately assumes a position at the level of L1. Normal regression of the distal embryonic spinal cord produces a slender, threadlike filum terminale that is attached to the coccyx. A tethered cord results when a thickened ropelike filum terminale persists and anchors the conus at or below the L2 level. Neurologic signs may develop as a result of abnormal tension on the spinal cord, compromising blood

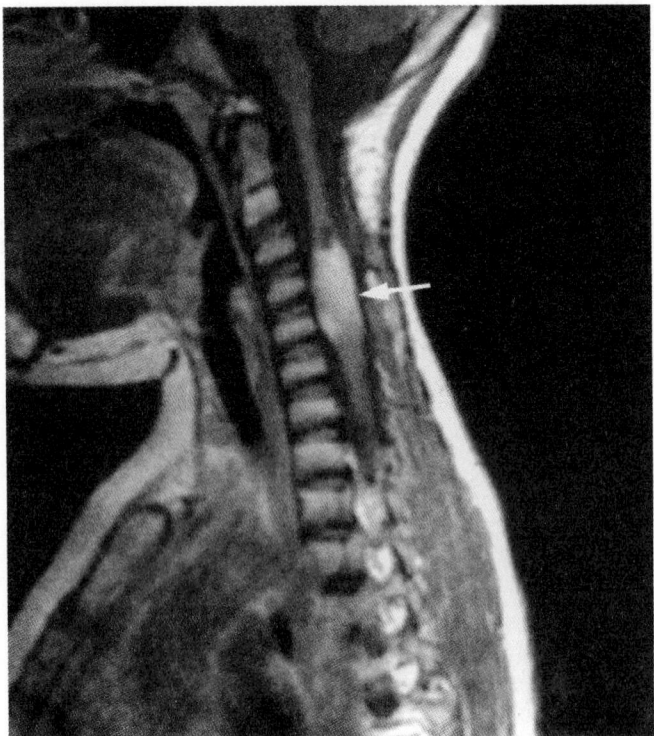

FIGURE 597–2. T1 weighted MRI scan of a spinal cord tumor (*white arrow*). The fusiform expansion of the cervical cord enhances following intravenous gadolinium injection.

supply, particularly during flexion and extension movements. Diastematomyelia may coexist with a tethered cord. Inspection of the back shows a midline skin lesion in approximately 70% of cases, such as a lipoma, cutaneous hemangioma, tuft of hair, hyperpigmentation, or dermal pit. The clinical presentation varies, and signs may be evident at birth or may be delayed until adulthood. Infants may have asymmetric growth in a foot or leg associated with talipes cavus deformities and muscle wasting due to prolonged denervation. Abnormalities in bladder function with overflow incontinence, progressive scoliosis, and diffuse pain in the lower extremities are more common findings in a child. Plain roentgenograms of the lumbosacral spine demonstrate spina bifida in most cases. MRI precisely outlines the level of the conus medullaris and the filum terminale. Surgical transection of the thickened filum terminale tends to halt progression of neurologic signs and prevents the development of dysfunction in asymptomatic patients.

597.4 Diastematomyelia

Diastematomyelia is division of the spinal cord into two halves by projection of a fibrocartilaginous or bony septum originating from the posterior vertebral body and extending posteriorly. It represents a disorder of neural tube fusion with the persistence of mesodermal tissue from the primitive neurenteric canal acting as the septum. The defect involves the lumbar vertebrae (L1-L3) in approximately 50% of cases and tends to be associated with abnormalities of the vertebral bodies, including fusion defects, hemivertebra, hypoplasia, kyphoscoliosis, spina bifida, and myelomeningocele. A midline abnormality of the skin, such as a cutaneous hemangioma, provides a clue to the possibility of an underlying abnormality. The neurologic signs are thought to result from flexion and extension movements of the cord, which produce traction and additional trauma by the impaling septum. The clinical presentation of diastematomyelia varies, and in some cases patients may remain asymptomatic. Most often, unilateral foot abnormalities, including talipes equinovarus, claw toes, atrophy of the gastrocnemius, and loss of pain and temperature sensation, are apparent in a preschool child. A more progressive course may ensue, characterized by bilateral weakness and muscle atrophy in the lower extremities, absent ankle jerks, urinary incontinence, and low back pain. Plain roentgenograms of the vertebrae may not detect the septum due to lack of calcification; thus, CT scanning or MRI is the study of choice. The treatment of symptomatic patients is excision of the bony spur or septum and lysis of the adjacent adhesions.

597.5 Syringomyelia

Syringomyelia is a cystic cavity within the spinal cord that may communicate with the CSF pathways or remain localized and noncommunicating. *Syringobulbia* exists when the cystic cavity extends into the medulla. Although the pathogenesis of communicating syringomyelia is unknown, the prevailing hypothesis suggests a constriction of the central canal at the level of the foramen magnum during embryogenesis. CSF may pass caudad through the narrowed canal, especially during periods of increased intracranial pressure (e.g., sneezing, coughing), and produce dilatation of the central canal. Because of the constriction, CSF is prevented from flowing in a cephalic direction. Communicating syringomyelia is frequently associated with the Chiari type I malformation, whereas the noncommunicating syrinx is associated with cord tumors, vascular accidents, trauma, and arachnoiditis. Because of its slow evolution, syringomyelia rarely produces symptoms during childhood.

Interruption of the anterior white commissure at the level of the cervical cord disrupts the lateral spinothalamic tracts, causing an asymmetric loss of pain and temperature sensation in the

upper extremities, with preservation of light touch (dissociation of sensation). Progressive enlargement of the cavity impinges on the anterior horn cells and corticospinal tracts, resulting in muscle wasting of the hands, absent deep tendon reflexes in the upper extremities, and upper motor neuron signs in the lower extremities. A rapidly progressive scoliosis may be the initial manifestation of syringomyelia. Trophic ulcers associated with vasomotor disturbances of the hands and arms indicate the loss of appreciation of pain. CT scanning with intrathecal injection of metrizamide outlines an enlarged spinal cord in the region of the syrinx, and a delayed scan displays the contrast medium within the cavity. MRI is the study of choice (Fig. 597–3). The management is surgical and depends on the site and cause of the syringomyelia. Decompression of the foramen magnum and the upper cervical vertebrae is recommended when the syrinx is associated with a Chiari type I or II anomaly. Additional procedures include insertion of a tissue plug in the open end of the central canal, draining the cystic cavity into the subarachnoid space, and percutaneous aspiration of the syrinx, which may result in marked improvement in neurologic function for prolonged periods.

597.6 Transverse Myelitis

Transverse myelitis is characterized by abrupt onset of progressive weakness and sensory disturbances in the lower extremities. A history of a preceding viral infection accompanied by fever and malaise is documented in most cases. Several viruses have been implicated, including Epstein-Barr virus and herpes, influenza, rubella, mumps, and varicella viruses. Additional infectious agents include Lyme disease and *Mycoplasma pneumoniae*. At least three hypotheses have been proposed to explain the pathogenesis of transverse myelitis: cell-mediated autoimmune response, direct viral invasion of the spinal cord, and autoimmune vasculitis. Pathologic examination of the cord

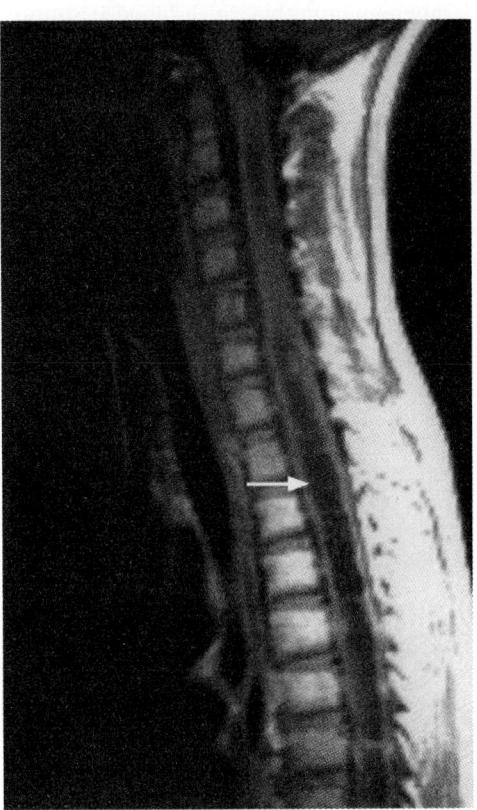

FIGURE 597–3. T1 weighted MRI scan of upper spinal cord showing an extensive syringomyelia (*white arrow*).

shows marked softening and perivascular cuffing by lymphocytes, supporting an immunologic basis for the disorder.

Low back or abdominal pain and paresthesias of the legs are prominent symptoms in the early stages. The leg muscles are weak and flaccid, and a sensory level is present, usually in the midthoracic region. Pain, temperature, and light touch sensation are affected, but joint position and vibration sense may be preserved. Sphincter disturbances are common, in which case catheterization of the bladder is necessary. Fever and nuchal rigidity are present early in most cases. The neurologic deficit evolves for 2–3 days and then plateaus, with flaccidity gradually changing to spasticity and with the concomitant development of upper motor neuron signs in the lower extremities. Examination of the CSF shows moderate lymphocyte pleocytosis and a normal or slightly elevated protein level. MRI is always indicated in a suspected case of transverse myelitis to rule out a compressive lesion compromising the cord. CT scanning or MRI reveals mild fusiform swelling in the affected region. Spontaneous recovery occurs over a period of weeks or months and is complete in approximately 60% of cases. Residual deficits include bowel and bladder dysfunction and weakness in the lower extremities. Management is directed to bladder care and physiotherapy. There is no evidence that steroids influence the course or the outcome of transverse myelitis. The differential diagnosis includes meningitis, infectious polyneuropathy (Guillain-Barré syndrome), poliomyelitis, neuromyelitis optica (Devic disease), spinal cord neoplasm, epidural abscess, and a vascular malformation.

597.7 Arteriovenous Malformation

An arteriovenous malformation of the spinal cord consists of a collection of tortuous dilated veins that are usually located on the dorsal aspect of the thoracic cord. The malformation may cause neurologic symptoms by its mass effect on the cord or by the "steal" phenomenon, by which blood is shunted through the abnormal veins, bypassing the spinal cord, which produces transient and in some cases progressive loss of neurologic function. Patients occasionally present with acute paraparesis and a sensory deficit due to a subarachnoid bleed from the malformation. More commonly, gradual onset of gait abnormalities, low back pain, and bowel and bladder dysfunction are noted. The deep tendon reflexes are absent or reduced in the lower extremities, and the Babinski reflex is present. In approximately one third of cases, a midline cutaneous angioma overlies the arteriovenous malformation, and a spinal bruit may occasionally be auscultated. Roentgenograms of the spine may show erosion of the pedicles; however, contrast myelography and selective spinal angiography are required to delineate the blood supply and the extent of the malformation. The malformation is removed by surgical excision with the use of an operating microscope or is obliterated by embolization.

Bracken MB, Shepard MJ, Holford TR, et al: Administration of methylprednisolone for 24 or 48 hours or tirilazad mesylate for 48 hours in the treatment of acute spinal cord injury. *JAMA* 1997;277:1597.

Cahan LD, Bentson JR: Considerations in the diagnosis and treatment of syringomyelia and Chiari malformation. *J Neurosurg* 1982;57:24.

Committee on Sports Medicine and Fitness 1994–1995, American Academy of Pediatrics: Atlantoaxial instability in Down syndrome: Subject review. *Pediatrics* 1995;96:151.

Cremers MJ, Bol E, deRoos F, et al: Risk of sports activities in children with Down's syndrome and atlantoaxial instability. *Lancet* 1993;342:511.

DiJunno JF, Formal CS: Chronic spinal cord injury. *N Engl J Med* 1994;330:550.

Haft H, Ransohoff J, Carter S: Spinal cord tumors in children. *Pediatrics* 1959;23:1152.

Hendrick EB, Hoffman HJ, Humphreys RP: The tethered spinal cord. *Clin Neurosurg* 1982;30:457.

Hilal S, Marton D, Pollack E: Diastematomyelia in children. *Radiology* 1974;112:609.

McAtee-Smith J, Hebert AA, Rapini R, et al: Skin lesions of the spinal axis and spinal dysraphism. *Arch Pediatr Adolesc Med* 1994;148:740.

Pueschel SM, Findley TW, Furia J, et al: Atlantoaxial instability in Down syndrome: Roentgenographic, neurologic and somatosensory evoked potential studies. *J Pediatr* 1987;110:515.

Riche MC, Modenesi-Freitas J, Djindjian M, et al: Arteriovenous malformations (AVM) of the spinal cord in children: Review of 38 cases. *Neuroradiology* 1982;22:171.

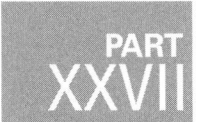
The term *neuromuscular disease* defines disorders of the motor unit and excludes influences on muscle function from the brain, such as in spasticity. The motor unit has four components: (1) a motor neuron in the brainstem or ventral horn of the spinal cord; (2) its axon that, together with other axons, forms the peripheral nerve; (3) the neuromuscular junction; and (4) all muscle fibers innervated by a single motor neuron. The size of the motor unit varies among different muscles and with the precision of muscular function required. In large muscles, such as the glutei and quadriceps femoris, hundreds of muscle fibers are innervated by a single motor neuron; in small finely tuned muscles, such as the stapedius or the extraocular muscles, a 1:1 ratio may prevail. The motor unit is influenced by suprasegmental or upper motor neuron control that alters properties of muscle tone, precision of movement, reciprocal inhibition of antagonistic muscles during movement, and sequencing of muscle contractions to achieve smooth, coordinated movements. Suprasegmental impulses also augment or inhibit the monosynaptic stretch reflex; the corticospinal tract is inhibitory upon this reflex.

Diseases of the motor unit are common in children. These neuromuscular diseases may or may not be genetically determined, congenital or acquired, acute or chronic, and progressive or static. Because specific therapy is available for many diseases and because of genetic and prognostic implications, precise diagnosis is important; laboratory confirmation is required for most diseases because of overlapping clinical manifestations.

Many chromosomal loci have been identified with specific neuromuscular diseases as a result of genetic linkage studies and the isolation and cloning of a few specific genes. In some cases, such as Duchenne muscular dystrophy, the genetic defect has been shown to be a deletion of nucleotide sequences and is associated with a defective protein product, dystrophin; in other cases, such as myotonic muscular dystrophy, the genetic defect is an expansion or repetition, rather than a deletion, in a codon (a set of three consecutive nucleotide repeats that encodes for a single amino acid), with many copies of a particular codon, in this example also associated with abnormal mRNA. Some diseases present as autosomal dominant and autosomal recessive traits in different pedigrees; these distinct mendelian genotypes may result from different genetic mutations on different chromosomes (e.g., nemaline rod myopathy) or may be small differences in the same gene at the same chromosomal locus (e.g., myotonia congenita), despite many common phenotypic features and shared histopathologic findings in a muscle biopsy specimen. Among the several clinically defined mitochondrial myopathies, specific mtDNA deletions and tRNA point mutations are recognized. The inheritance patterns and chromosomal and mitochondrial loci of common neuromuscular diseases affecting infants and children are summarized in Table 599–1.

Chapter 598
Evaluation and Investigation

Clinical Manifestations. Examination of the neuromuscular system includes an assessment of muscle bulk, tone, and strength. Tone and strength should not be confused: Passive tone is range of motion around a joint; active tone is physiologic resistance to movement. Head lag when an infant is pulled to a sitting position from supine is a sign of weakness, not of low tone. Hypotonia may be associated with normal strength or with weakness; enlarged muscles may be weak or strong; thin, wasted muscles may be weak or have unexpectedly normal strength. The distribution of these components is of diagnostic importance. In general, myopathies follow a proximal distribution of weakness and muscle wasting (with the notable exception of myotonic muscular dystrophy); neuropathies are generally distal in distribution (with the notable exception of juvenile spinal muscular atrophy). Involvement of the face, tongue, palate, and extraocular muscles provides an important distinction in the differential diagnosis. Tendon stretch reflexes are generally lost in neuropathies and in motor neuron diseases and are diminished but preserved in myopathies. A few specific clinical features are important in the diagnosis of some neuromuscular diseases. Fasciculations of muscle, which are often best seen in the tongue, are a sign of denervation. Sensory abnormalities indicate neuropathy. Fatigable weakness is characteristic of neuromuscular junctional disorders. Myotonia is specific for a few myopathies.

Some features do not distinguish myopathy from neuropathy. Muscle pain or myalgias are associated with acute disease of either myopathic or neurogenic origin. Both acute dermatomyositis and acute polyneuropathy (Guillain-Barré syndrome) are characterized by myalgias. Muscular dystrophies and spinal muscular atrophies are not associated with muscle pain. Myalgias also occur in several metabolic diseases of muscle and in ischemic myopathy. Contractures of muscles, whether present at birth or developing later in the course of an illness, occur in both myopathic and neurogenic diseases.

Infant boys who are weak in late fetal life and in the neonatal period often have undescended testes. The testes are actively pulled into the scrotum from the anterior abdominal wall by a pair of cords that consist of smooth and striated muscle called the gubernaculum (Fig. 598–1). The gubernaculum is weakened in many congenital neuromuscular diseases, including spinal muscular atrophy, myotonic muscular dystrophy, and many congenital myopathies.

The thorax of infants with congenital neuromuscular disease often has a funnel shape, and the ribs are thin and radiolucent, owing to intercostal muscle weakness during intrauterine growth. This phenomenon is characteristically found in infantile spinal muscular atrophy but also occurs in myotubular myopathy, neonatal myotonic dystrophy, and other disorders. Because of the small muscle mass, birth weight may be low for gestational age.

Generalized hypotonia and motor developmental delay are the most common presenting manifestations of neuromuscular disease in infants and young children. These features may also be expressions of neurologic disease, endocrine and systemic metabolic diseases, and Down syndrome, or they may be nonspecific neuromuscular expressions of malnutrition or chronic systemic illness. A prenatal history of decreased fetal movements and intrauterine growth retardation is often found in patients who are symptomatic at birth.

Laboratory Findings
SERUM ENZYMES. Several lysosomal enzymes are released by damaged or degenerating muscle fibers and may be measured in serum. The most useful of these enzymes is the *creatine kinase* (CK), which is found in only three organs and may be separated into corresponding isozymes: MM for skeletal muscle, MB for cardiac muscle, and BB for brain. Serum CK determination is by no means a universal screening test for neuromuscular disease because many diseases of the motor unit may not be associated with elevated enzymes. However, the CK level is characteristically elevated in certain diseases, such as Duchenne

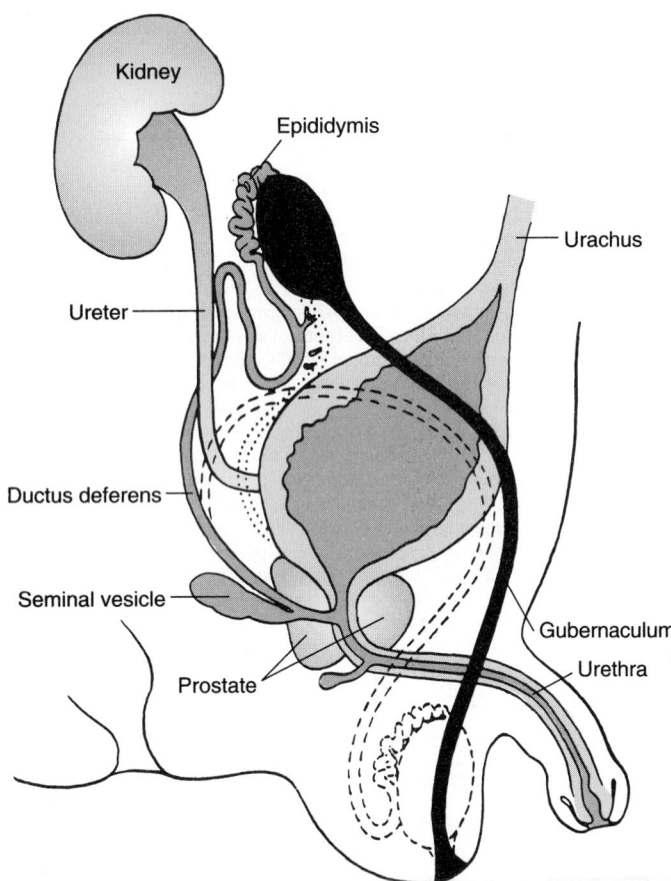

FIGURE 598–1. Undescended testes are common in male neonates with neuromuscular disease already symptomatic at birth, regardless of the cause. The gubernaculum is a cylinder of striated muscle surrounding a core of smooth muscle that actively pulls the testis into the scrotum in late gestation. Weakness of the gubernaculum in a generalized myopathy of fetal life prevents or delays the descent of the testis. (Reproduced with permission from Sarnat HB, Sarnat MS: Disorders of muscle in the newborn. In Moss AJ, Stern L [editors]: *Pediatrics Update,* 4th ed. New York, Elsevier-North Holland, 1983.)

muscular dystrophy, and the magnitude of increase is characteristic for particular diseases.

MOLECULAR GENETIC MARKERS. Many DNA markers of hereditary myopathies and neuropathies are now available from blood samples. If the clinical manifestations cause suspicion of a particular disease, these tests may provide a definitive diagnosis and not subject the child to more invasive procedures, such as muscle biopsy. Other molecular markers are available only in muscle biopsy tissue. Genetic blood tests, whether ordered individually or in "panels," are expensive and often are excluded in health insurance plans.

NERVE CONDUCTION VELOCITY (NCV). Motor and sensory nerve conduction may be measured electrophysiologically by using surface electrodes. Neuropathies of various types are detected by decreased conduction. The site of a traumatic nerve injury may also be localized. The nerve conduction at birth is about half of the mature value achieved by age 2 yr. Tables are available for normal values at various ages in infancy, including for preterm infants. Because the NCV study measures only the fastest conducting fibers in a nerve, 80% of the total nerve fibers must be involved before slowing in conduction is detected.

ELECTROMYOGRAPHY (EMG). EMG requires insertion of a needle into the belly of a muscle and recording the electric potentials in various states of contraction. It is less useful in pediatrics than in adult medicine, in part because of technical difficulties in recording these potentials in young children and in part because the best results require the patient's cooperation for full relaxation and maximal voluntary contraction of a muscle. Most children are too frightened to provide such cooperation. Characteristic EMG patterns distinguish denervation from myopathic involvement. The specific type of myopathy is not usually definitively diagnosed, but certain specialized myopathic conditions, such as myotonia, may be demonstrated. An EMG may transiently raise the serum CK level.

EMG combined with repetitive electrical stimulation of a motor nerve supplying a muscle to produce tetany is useful in demonstrating myasthenic decremental responses. Small muscles, such as the abductor digiti quinti of the hypothenar eminence, are used for such studies.

MUSCLE BIOPSY. The muscle biopsy is the most important and specific diagnostic study of most neuromuscular disorders, if the definitive diagnosis of a hereditary disease is not provided by molecular genetic testing in blood. Not only are neurogenic and myopathic processes distinguished, but also the type of myopathy and specific enzymatic deficiencies may be determined. The vastus lateralis (quadriceps femoris) is the muscle that is most commonly sampled. The deltoid muscle should be avoided in most cases because it normally has a 60–80% predominance of type I fibers so that the distribution patterns of fiber types are difficult to recognize. Muscle biopsy is a simple outpatient procedure that may be performed under local anesthesia with or without femoral nerve block. Needle biopsies are not recommended because they require an incision in the skin similar to open biopsy, numerous samples must be taken to conduct an adequate examination of the tissue, and they provide inferior specimens.

Histochemical studies of frozen sections of the muscle are obligatory in all pediatric muscle biopsies because many congenital and metabolic myopathies cannot be diagnosed from paraffin sections using conventional histologic stains. Immunohistochemistry is a useful supplement in some cases, such as for demonstrating dystrophin in suspected Duchenne muscular dystrophy or merosin in congenital muscular dystrophy. A portion of the biopsy specimen should be fixed for potential electron microscopy, but ultrastructure has additional diagnostic value only in selected cases. Muscle biopsy sample interpretation is complex and should be performed by an experienced pathologist. A portion of frozen muscle tissue should also be routinely saved for possible biochemical analysis (e.g., mitochondrial cytopathies, carnitine palmityltransferase, acid maltase).

NERVE BIOPSY. The most commonly sampled nerve is the sural nerve, which is a pure sensory nerve that supplies a small area of skin on the lateral surface of the foot. Whole or fascicular biopsy specimens of this nerve may be taken. When the sural nerve is severed behind the lateral malleolus of the ankle, regeneration of the nerve occurs in more than 90% of cases so that permanent sensory loss is not experienced. The sural nerve is often involved in many neuropathies whose clinical manifestations are predominantly motor.

Electron microscopy is performed on most nerve biopsy specimens because many morphologic alterations cannot be appreciated at the resolution of a light microscope. Teased fiber preparations are sometimes useful in demonstrating segmental demyelination, axonal swellings, and other specific abnormalities, but this time-consuming procedure is not done routinely. Special stains may be applied to ordinary frozen or paraffin sections of nerve biopsy material to demonstrate myelin, axoplasm, and metabolic products.

ELECTROCARDIOGRAPHY (ECG). Cardiac evaluation is important if myopathy is suspected because of involvement of the heart in muscular dystrophies and in inflammatory and metabolic myopathies. ECG often detects early cardiomyopathy or conduction defects that are clinically asymptomatic. At times, a more complete cardiac work-up, such as echocardiography and consultation with a pediatric cardiologist, may be indicated. Serial pulmonary function tests also should be performed in muscular dystrophies and in other chronic or progressive diseases of the motor unit.

Chapter 599
Developmental Disorders of Muscle

A heterogeneous group of congenital neuromuscular disorders is sometimes known as the *congenital myopathies*, but in some of these disorders the assumption that the pathogenesis is primarily myopathic is unjustified. Most congenital myopathies are nonprogressive conditions, but some patients show slow clinical deterioration accompanied by additional changes in their muscle biopsy specimen. Most of the diseases in the category of congenital myopathies are hereditary; others are sporadic. Although clinical features, including phenotype, may raise a strong suspicion of a congenital myopathy, the definitive diagnosis is determined by the histopathologic findings in the muscle biopsy specimen. In conditions for which the defective gene has been identified, the diagnosis may be established by the specific molecular genetic probe on lymphocytes. The morphologic and histo-chemical abnormalities differ considerably from those of the muscular dystrophies, spinal muscular atrophies, and neuropathies. Many are reminiscent of the embryologic development of muscle, thus suggesting possible defects in the genetic regulation of muscle development.

Myogenic Regulatory Genes and Genetic Loci of Inherited Diseases of Muscle (Table 599–1) A family of four myogenic regulatory genes shares encoding transcription factors of "basic helix-loop-helix" (bHLH) proteins associated with common DNA nucleotide sequences. These proto-oncogenes direct the differentiation of striated muscle from any undifferentiated mesodermal cell; some are so strongly expressed that they convert partially differentiated mesenchymal cells, such as fibroblasts or chondroblasts, into myoblasts. The earliest bHLH gene to program the differentiation of myoblasts is myogenic factor 5 *(Myf5)*. The second gene, *myogenin*, promotes fusion of myoblasts to form myotubes. *Herculin* (also known as *MYF6*) and *MYOD1* are the other two myogenic genes. *Myf5 cannot support myogenic differentiation without myogenin, MyoD, and MYF6.* Each of these four genes can activate the expression of at least one other and, under certain circumstances, can autoactivate as well. The expression of *MYF5* and of *herculin* is transient in early ontogenesis but returns later in fetal life and persists into adult life. The human locus of the *MYOD1* gene is on chromosome 11, very near to the domain associated with embryonal rhabdomyosarcoma. The genes encoding *Myf5* and *herculin* are on chromosome 12 and that for *myogenin* is on chromosome 1. The myogenic genes are activated during muscle regeneration, recapitulating the developmental process; *MyoD* in particular is required for myogenic stem cell (i.e., satellite cell) activation in

TABLE 599–1. Inheritance Patterns and Chromosomal or Mitochondrial Loci of Neuromuscular Diseases Affecting the Pediatric Age Group

Disease	Transmission	Locus
Duchenne/Becker muscular dystrophy	XR	Xp21.2
Emery-Dreifuss muscular dystrophy	XR	Xq28
Myotonic muscular dystrophy (Steinert)	AD	19q13
Facio-scapulo-humeral muscular dystrophy	AD	4q35
Limb-girdle muscular dystrophy	AD	5q
Limb-girdle muscular dystrophy	AR	15q
Congenital muscular dystrophy with merosin deficiency	AR	6q2
Congenital muscular dystrophy (Fukuyama)	AR	8q31–33
Myotubular myopathy	XR	Xq28
Myotubular myopathy	AR	Unknown
Nemaline rod myopathy	AD	1q21–q23
Nemaline rod myopathy	AR	2q21.2–q22
Congenital muscle fiber–type disproportion	AR	Unknown
Central core disease	AD	19q13.1
Myotonia congenita (Thomsen)	AD	7q35
Myotonia congenita (Becker)	AR	7q35
Paramyotonia congenita	AD	17q13.1–13.3
Hyperkalemic periodic paralysis	AD	17q13.1–13.3
Hypokalemic periodic paralysis	AD	1q31–q32
Glycogenosis II (Pompe; acid maltase deficiency)	AR	17q23
Glycogenosis V (McArdle; myophosphorylase deficiency)	AR	11q13
Glycogenosis VII (Tarui; phosphofructokinase deficiency)	AR	1cenq32
Glycogenosis IX (phosphoglycerate kinase deficiency)	XR	Xq13
Glycogenosis X (phosphoglycerate mutase deficiency)	AR	7p12–p13
Glycogenosis XI (lactate dehydrogenase deficiency)	AR	11p15.4
Muscle carnitine deficiency	AR	Unknown
Muscle carnitine palmityltransferase deficiency 2	AR	1p32
Spinal muscular atrophy (Werdnig-Hoffmann; Kugelberg-Welander)	AR	5q11–q13
Familial dysautonomia (Riley-Day)	AR	9q31–33
Hereditary motor-sensory neuropathy (Charcot-Marie-Tooth; Dejerine-Sottas)	AD	17p11.2
Hereditary motor-sensory neuropathy (axonal type)	AD	1p35–p36
Hereditary motor-sensory neuropathy (Charcot-Marie-Tooth-X)	XR	Xq13.1
Mitochondrial myopathy (Kearns-Sayre)	Maternal; sporadic	Single large mtDNA deletion
Mitochondrial myopathy (MERRF)	Maternal	tRNA point mutation at position 8344
Mitochondrial myopathy (MELAS)	Maternal	tRNA point mutation at positions 3243 and 3271

AD = autosomal dominant; AR = autosomal recessive; XR = X-linked recessive; MERRF = mitochondrial encephalomyopathy with ragged-red fibers; MELAS = mitochondrial encephalomyopathy with lactic acidosis and strokelike episodes; mtDNA = mitochondrial deoxyribonucleic acid; tRNA = transfer ribonucleic acid.

adult muscle. The *PAX3* gene also plays an important role in myogenesis and interacts with each of the four basic genes mentioned above. Another gene, *myostatin*, is a negative regulator of muscle development by preventing myocytes from differentiating. The precise role of the myogenic genes in developmental myopathies is not yet defined.

599.1 Myotubular Myopathy

The term *myotubular myopathy* implies a maturational arrest of fetal muscle during the myotubular stage of development at 8–15 wk of gestation. It is based on the morphologic appearance of myofibers: A row of central nuclei lie within a core of cytoplasm; contractile myofibrils form a cylinder around this core (Fig. 599–1). Many challenge this interpretation and use the more neutral term *centronuclear myopathy* when referring to this myopathy. But this term is too nonspecific because internal nuclei occur in many unrelated myopathies.

Pathogenesis. Although the pathogenesis has sometimes been suggested to be neurogenic, spinal motor neurons are normal in number and morphology. Peripheral nerves also usually have normal ultrastructure and conduction velocity. Persistently high fetal concentrations of vimentin and desmin are demonstrated in myofibers of infants with myotubular myopathy, although not reproduced in cultured myocytes of patients. These intermediate filament proteins serve as cytoskeletal elements in fetal myotubes, attaching nuclei and mitochondria to the sarcolemmal membranes to preserve their central positions. As intracellular organization changes with maturation, the nuclei move to the periphery and mitochondria are redistributed between myofibrils. At the same time, vimentin and desmin diminish. Vimentin disappears altogether by term, and desmin remains

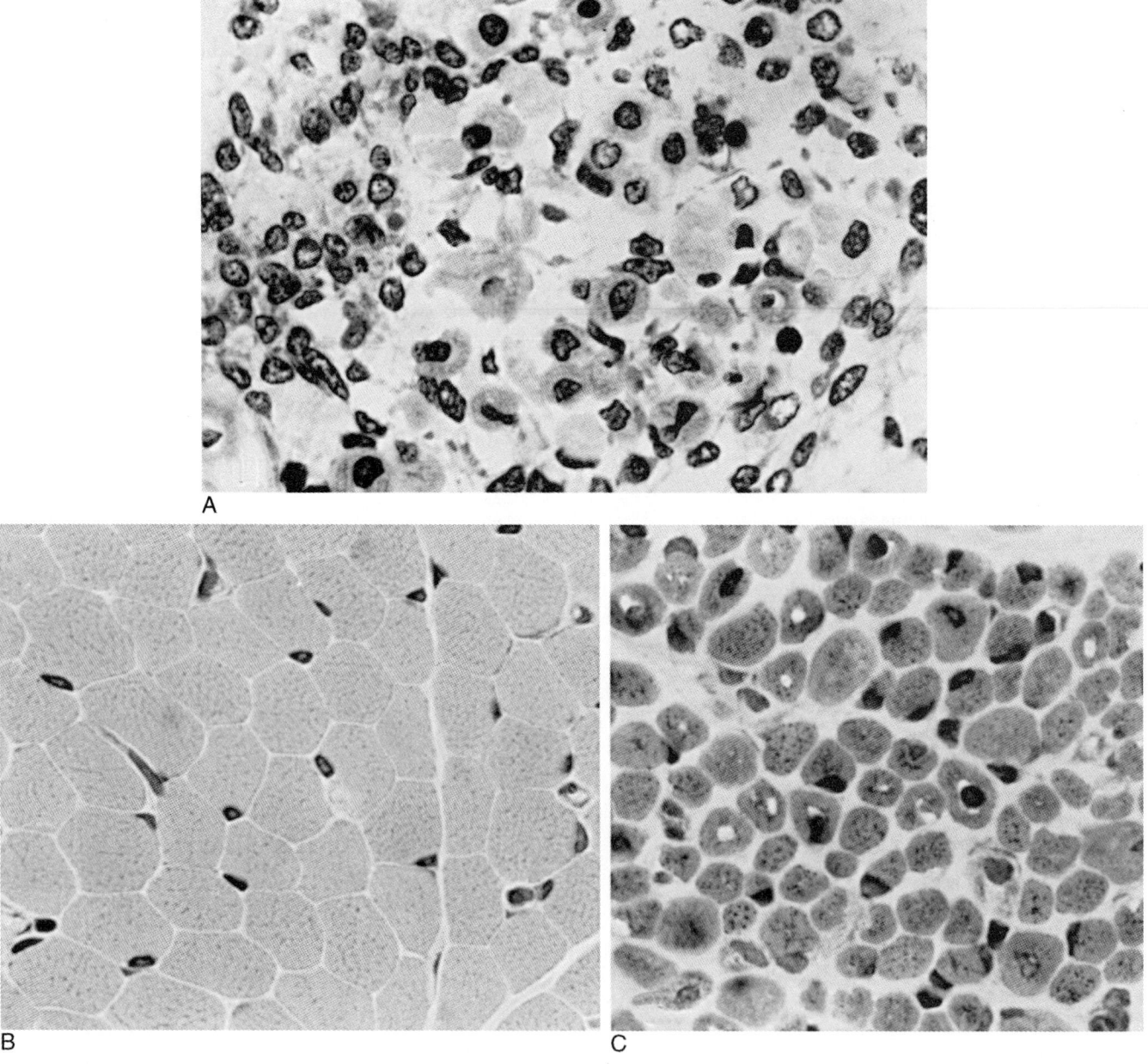

FIGURE 599–1. *A*, Cross-section of muscle from a 14-wk-old human fetus; *B*, normal full-term neonate; and *C*, term neonate with X-linked recessive myotubular myopathy. Myofibers have large central nuclei in the fetus and in myotubular myopathy, and nuclei are at the periphery of the muscle fiber in the term neonate as in the adult. (Hematoxylin & eosin, ×500.)

only in trace amounts. Persistent fetal vimentin and desmin in muscle fibers may be one mechanism of "maturational arrest." A secondary myasthenia-like defect in neuromuscular transmission also occurs in some infants with myotubular myopathy. Myocytes of patients co-cultured with nerve in vitro develop normal innervation and mature normally, not reproducing the in vivo pathologic changes.

Clinical Manifestations. Decreased fetal movements may occur in late gestation. Polyhydramnios is a common complication because of pharyngeal weakness of the fetus and inability to swallow amniotic fluid. At birth, affected infants have a thin muscle mass involving axial, limb girdle, and distal muscles; severe generalized hypotonia; and diffuse weakness. Respiratory efforts may be ineffective, requiring ventilatory support. Gavage feeding may be required because of weakness of the muscles of sucking and deglutition. The testes are often undescended. Facial muscles may be weak, but infants do not have the characteristic facies of myotonic dystrophy. Ophthalmoplegia is observed in a few cases. The palate may be high. The tongue is thin, but fasciculations are not seen. Tendon stretch reflexes are weak or absent. Myotubular myopathy is not associated with cardiomyopathy; mature cardiac muscle fibers normally have central nuclei. Congenital anomalies of the central nervous system or of other systems are not associated.

Older children and adults may develop centronuclear myopathy with variable weakness. The relation of this disorder to the severe neonatal disease is uncertain.

Laboratory Findings. Serum levels of creatine phosphokinase (CK) are normal. The electromyogram (EMG) does not show evidence of denervation; results are usually normal or show minimal nonspecific myopathic features in early infancy. Nerve conduction velocity may be slow but is usually normal. The electrocardiogram (ECG) appears normal. Roentgenograms of the chest show no cardiomegaly; the ribs may be thin.

Diagnosis. The muscle biopsy findings are diagnostic at birth, even in premature infants. More than 90% of muscle fibers are small and have centrally placed, large vesicular nuclei in a single row. Spaces between nuclei are filled with sarcoplasm containing mitochondria. Histochemical stains for oxidative enzymatic activity and glycogen reveal a central distribution as in fetal myotubes. The cylinder of myofibrils shows mature histochemical differentiation with adenosine triphosphatase (ATPase) stains. The connective tissue of muscle, spindles, blood vessels, intramuscular nerves, and motor end plates are mature. Ultrastructural features in neonatal myotubular myopathy, other than those that define the disease, are also mature. Vimentin and desmin show strong immunoreactivity in muscle fibers in myotubular myopathy and no demonstrable activity in normal term neonatal muscle. The molecular genetic marker in blood is available and is useful not only for confirming the diagnosis but also for early prenatal diagnosis.

Genetics. X-linked recessive inheritance is the most common trait; most patients are boys. The mothers of affected infants are clinically asymptomatic, but their muscle biopsy specimen shows minor alterations. Autosomal dominant and autosomal recessive forms are also reported but are rarer.

Genetic linkage on the X chromosome has been localized to the Xq28 site, a locus different from the Xp21 gene of Duchenne and Becker muscular dystrophies. A deletion in the responsible *MTM1* gene has been identified. It encodes a protein, myotubularin, with a putative tyrosine phosphatase domain. Although only a single gene is involved, five distinct point mutations of the *MTM1* gene out of 242 known mutations account for only 27% of cases; many different alleles may produce the same clinical disease.

Treatment. Only supportive and palliative treatment is available.

Prognosis. About 75% of severely affected neonates die within the first few weeks or months of life. Survivors do not experience a progressive course but have major physical handicaps, rarely walk, and remain severely hypotonic.

599.2 Congenital Muscle Fiber-Type Disproportion (CMFTD)

This condition occurs as an isolated "congenital myopathy" but also develops in association with various unrelated disorders that include nemaline rod disease, Krabbe disease (globoid cell leukodystrophy) early in the course before expression of the neuropathy, cerebellar hypoplasia and certain other brain malformations (see later), fetal alcohol syndrome, some glycogenoses, multiple sulfatase deficiency, Lowe's syndrome, rigid spine myopathy, and some infantile cases of myotonic muscular dystrophy.

Pathogenesis. The association of CMFTD with cerebellar hypoplasia (see later) suggests that the pathogenesis may be an abnormal suprasegmental influence on the developing motor unit during the stage of histochemical differentiation of muscle between 20 and 28 wk of gestation. Muscle fiber types and growth are determined by innervation and are mutable even in adults. Although CMFTD does not actually correspond with any normal stage of development, it appears to be an embryologic disturbance of fiber type differentiation and growth.

Clinical Manifestations. As an isolated condition not associated with other diseases, CMFTD is a nonprogressive disorder present at birth. Patients have generalized hypotonia and weakness, but the weakness is usually not severe and respiratory distress and dysphagia are rare. Mild congenital contractures are often present. Poor head control and developmental delay for gross motor skills are common in infancy. Walking is usually delayed until 18–24 mo but is eventually achieved. Because of the hypotonia, subluxation of the hips may occur. Muscle bulk is reduced. The muscle wasting and hypotonia are proportionately greater than the weakness, and the child may be stronger than expected during examination. Cardiomyopathy is a rare complication.

The facies of children with CMFTD often raise suspicion, especially if the child is referred for assessment of developmental delay and hypotonia. The head is dolichocephalic, and facial weakness is present. The palate is usually high arched. Thin muscles of the trunk and extremities give a thin, wasted appearance. Patients do not complain of myalgias. The clinical course is benign and nonprogressive. The facies and body habitus of many children with CMFTD may be indistinguishable from those of nemaline rod myopathy (see later), which also includes CMFTD as a component.

Laboratory Findings. Serum CK, ECG, EMG, and nerve conduction velocity results are normal in simple CMFTD. If other diseases are associated, laboratory investigation of those conditions discloses the specific features.

Diagnosis. CMFTD is diagnosed by a muscle biopsy that shows a disproportion in both size and relative ratios of histochemical fiber types: Type I fibers are uniformly small, and type II fibers are hypertrophic; type I fibers are more numerous than those of type II. Degeneration of myofibers and other primary myopathic features are absent. The biopsy is diagnostic at birth.

Genetics. Many cases of simple CMFTD are sporadic, although autosomal recessive inheritance is well documented in some families and an autosomal dominant trait is suspected in others. CMFTD also may be associated with cerebellar hypoplasia.

Treatment. No drug therapy is available. Physiotherapy may be helpful for some patients in strengthening muscles that do not receive sufficient exercise in daily activities. Mild congenital contractures often respond well to gentle range of motion exercises and rarely require plaster casting or surgery.

599.3 ■ Nemaline Rod Myopathy

Nemaline rods (derived from the Greek *nema*, meaning "thread") are rod-shaped inclusion-like abnormal structures within muscle fibers. They are difficult to demonstrate histologically with conventional hematoxylin-eosin stain but are easily seen with special stains. They are not foreign inclusion bodies but rather consist of excessive Z-band material with a similar ultrastructure (Fig. 599–2). Chemically, the rods are composed of actin, α-actinin, tropomyosin-3, and the protein nebulin. Nemaline rod formation may be an unusual reaction of muscle fibers to injury because these rod structures have rarely been found in other diseases. They are most abundant in the congenital myopathy known as nemaline rod disease. Most rods are within the myofibrils (cytoplasmic), but intranuclear rods are occasionally demonstrated by electron microscopy; how they form in the nucleus is unknown.

Clinical Manifestations. Severe infantile and juvenile forms of the disease are known. Patients resemble those with CMFTD, except that they are more severely affected. Generalized hypotonia, weakness including bulbar-innervated and respiratory muscles, and a very thin muscle mass are characteristic (Fig. 599–3). The head is dolichocephalic, and the palate high arched or even cleft. Muscles of the jaw may be too weak to hold it closed (Fig. 599–4). Infants may be severely weak at birth; some die in the neonatal period. Decreased fetal movements are reported by the mother, and neonates suffer from hypoxia and dysphagia and sometimes have arthrogryposis.

Laboratory Findings. Serum CK level is normal. The muscle biopsy sample shows CMFTD or at least fiber type I predominance in addition to the nemaline rods. In some patients, uniform type I fibers are seen with few or no type II fibers. Focal myofibrillar degeneration and an increase in lysosomal enzymes have been found in a few severe cases associated with progressive symptoms. Intranuclear nemaline rods correlate with the most severe clinical manifestations.

Genetic Aspects. Autosomal dominant and autosomal recessive forms of nemaline rod disease occur, and an X-linked dominant form in girls also may occur. Autosomal dominant nemaline rod

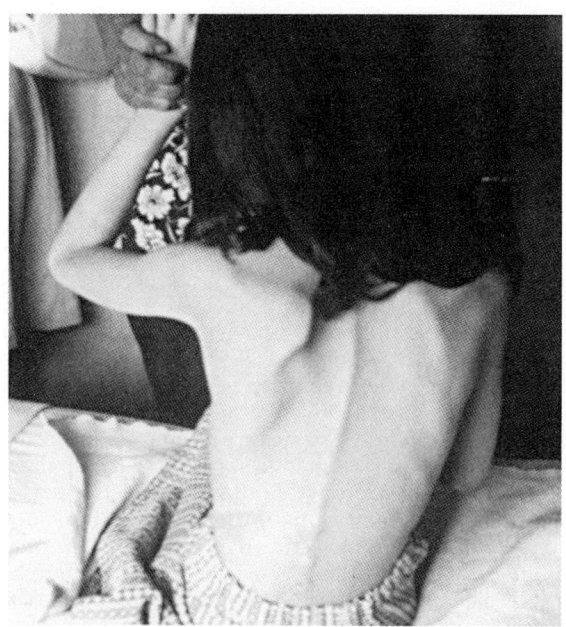

FIGURE 599–3. Back of a 13-yr-old girl with juvenile form of nemaline rod disease. The paraspinal muscles are very thin, and winging of the scapulae is evident. The muscle mass of the extremities is also greatly reduced both proximally and distally.

myopathy has been mapped to the 1q21-23 locus; the responsible gene, *TPM3*, programs tropomyosin-3, an important component of the Z band. The more common autosomal recessive form results from a defective gene at the 2q21.2-q22 locus that produces *nebulin*, a large molecule also needed for Z-band integrity.

Treatment and Prognosis. Therapy is supportive. Survivors are confined to an electric wheelchair and are usually unable to overcome gravity. Both proximal and distal muscles are involved.

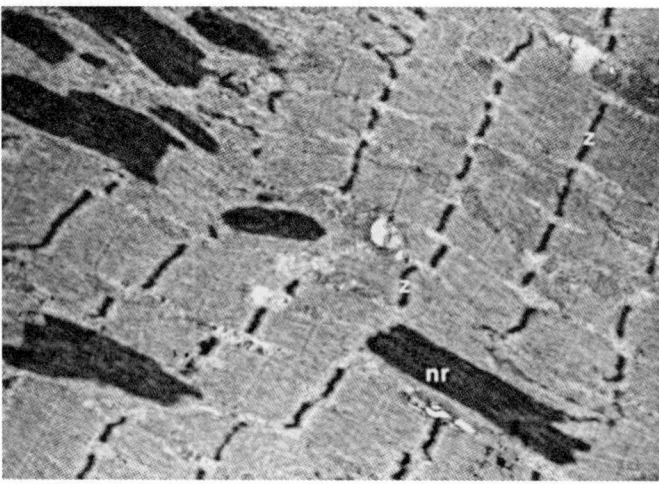

FIGURE 599–2. Electron micrograph of the muscle from a patient shown in Figure 599–4. Nemaline rods (nr) are seen within many myofibrils. They are identical in composition to the normal Z bands (z). (×6000.)

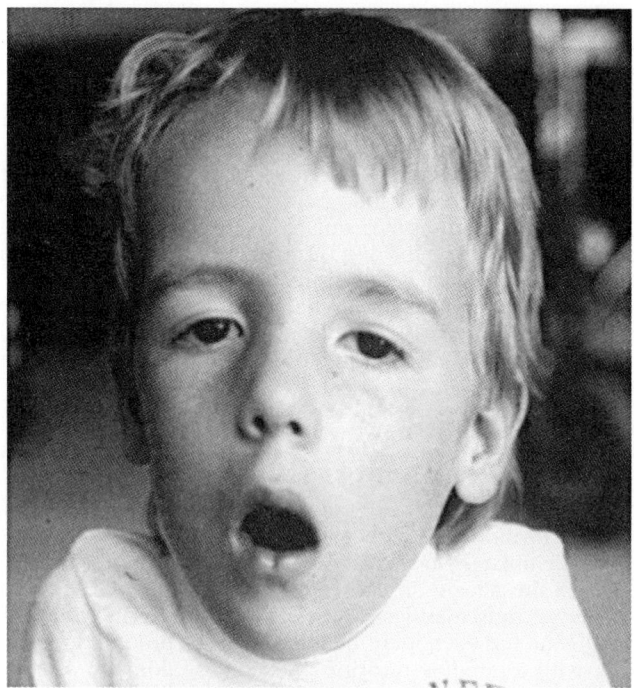

FIGURE 599–4. Infantile form of nemaline rod disease in a 6-yr-old boy. Facial weakness and generalized muscle wasting are severe. The head is dolichocephalic. The mouth is usually open because the masseters are too weak to lift the mandible against gravity for more than a few seconds.

Gastrostomy may be needed for chronic dysphagia. In the juvenile form, patients are ambulatory and are able to perform most tasks of daily living. Weakness is not usually progressive, but some patients have more difficulty over time or enter a phase of progressive weakness. Cardiomyopathy is an uncommon complication. Pneumonia occurs frequently.

599.4 Central Core Disease

This autosomal dominant disease, caused by an abnormal gene at the 19q13.1 locus, is characterized pathologically by central cores within muscle fibers in which only amorphous, granular cytoplasm is found with an absence of myofibrils and organelles. Histochemical stains show a lack of enzymatic activities of all types within these cores. Infantile hypotonia, proximal weakness, muscle wasting, and involvement of facial muscles and neck flexors are the typical features. The course is nonprogressive, and the weakness is not usually severely disabling. Congenital dislocated hips and skeletal deformities are common. Scoliosis occurs even without much axial weakness.

Central core disease is consistently associated with malignant hyperthermia, and all patients should have special precautions with pretreatment by dantrolene before an anesthetic agent is administered. The serum CK value is normal in central core disease except during crises of malignant hyperthermia. See Chapter 602.2.

Variants of central cores, called *minicores* and *multicores*, are described in some families, but minicore myopathy is probably a different genetic disease. Children with this disorder are hypotonic in early infancy and have a benign course but often develop progressive kyphoscoliosis or a rigid spine in adolescence. Some children with Prader-Willi syndrome have focal loss of myofilaments resembling early central cores.

599.5 Brain Malformations and Muscle Development

Infants with *cerebellar hypoplasia* are hypotonic and developmentally delayed. Muscle biopsy is sometimes performed to exclude a congenital myopathy. A biopsy specimen may show delayed maturation of muscle, fiber-type predominance, or CMFTD. Other malformations of the brain may also be associated with abnormal histochemical patterns, but supratentorial lesions are less likely than brain stem or cerebellar lesions to alter muscle development. Abnormal descending impulses along bulbospinal pathways probably alter discharge patterns of lower motor neurons that determine the histochemical differentiation of muscle. The corticospinal tract does not participate because it is not yet functional during this period of fetal life.

599.6 Amyoplasia

Congenital absence of individual muscles is common and is often asymmetric. A common aplasia is the *palmaris longus muscle* of the ventral forearm, which is absent in 30% of normal subjects and is fully compensated by other flexors of the wrist. Unilateral absence of a *sternocleidomastoid muscle* is one cause of congenital torticollis. Absence of one *pectoralis major muscle* is part of the Poland anomalad.

When innervation does not develop, such as in the lower limbs in severe cases of *myelomeningocele*, muscles may fail to develop. In *sacral agenesis*, the abnormal somites that fail to form bony vertebrae may also fail to form muscles from the same defective mesodermal plate, a disorder of induction resulting in segmental amyoplasia. Skeletal muscles of the extremities fail to differentiate from embryonic myomeres if the long bones do not

form. Absence of one long bone, such as the radius, is associated with variable aplasia or hypoplasia of associated muscles, such as the *carpi flexor radialis*. End-stage neurogenic atrophy of muscle is sometimes called *amyoplasia*, but this use is semantically incorrect.

Generalized amyoplasia usually results in fetal death, and liveborn neonates rarely survive. A mutation in one of the myogenic genes is the suspected etiology because of genetic knockout studies in mice, but it has not been proven in humans.

599.7 Muscular Dysgenesis (Proteus Syndrome Myopathy)

The *Proteus syndrome* is a disturbance of cellular growth involving ectodermal and mesodermal tissues. The cause is unknown, but it is not a mendelian trait. It presents as asymmetric overgrowth of the extremities, verrucous cutaneous lesions, angiomas of various types, thickening of bones, hemimegalencephaly, and excessive growth of muscles without weakness. Histologically, the muscle is a unique *muscular dysgenesis*. Abnormal zones are adjacent to zones of normal muscle formation and do not follow anatomic boundaries. The disorder may be due to abnormal paracrine growth factors. Historically the "elephant man," who was exploited for his grotesque features in late 19th century London and became a popular sensation, was long misdiagnosed as having neurofibromatosis but is now recognized to have had Proteus syndrome.

599.8 Benign Congenital Hypotonia

Benign congenital hypotonia is not a disease but is a descriptive term for infants or children with nonprogressive hypotonia of unknown origin. The hypotonia is not usually associated with weakness or developmental delay, although some children acquire gross motor skills more slowly than normal. Tendon stretch reflexes are normal or hypoactive. There are no cranial nerve abnormalities, and intelligence is normal.

The *diagnosis* is one of exclusion after results of laboratory studies, including muscle biopsy and imaging of the brain with special attention to the cerebellum, are normal. No known molecular genetic basis for this syndrome has been identified.

The *prognosis* is generally good; no specific therapy is required. Contractures do not develop. Hypotonia persists into adult life. The disorder is not always as "benign" as its name implies, because a common complication is recurrent dislocation of joints, especially the shoulders. Excessive motility of the spine may result in stretch injury, compression, or vascular compromise of nerve roots or of the spinal cord. These are particular hazards for patients who perform gymnastics or who become circus performers because of agility of joints without weakness or pain.

599.9 Arthrogryposis

Arthrogryposis multiplex congenita is not a disease but is a descriptive term that signifies numerous congenital contractures. The causes encompass both neurogenic and primary myopathic diseases, but most cases, and indeed the most severe cases, are not due to neuromuscular disease. Myopathies that have a high incidence of either minor congenital contractures or extensive arthrogryposis include myotonic muscular dystrophy, many congenital myopathies, and intrauterine viral myositis. Neurogenic diseases causing arthrogryposis include infantile spinal muscular atrophy and the Pena-Shokeir and Marden-Walker syndromes (see Chapter 672).

Barth PG, Dubowitz V: X-linked myotubular myopathy: A long-term follow-up study. *Eur J Paediatr Neurol* 1998;1:49.

De Gouyon BM, Zhao W, Laporte J, et al: Characterization of mutations in the myotubularin gene in twenty-six patients with X-linked myotubular myopathy. *Hum Mol Genet* 1997;6:1499.

Iannaccone ST: Myogenes and myotubes. *J Child Neurol* 1992;7:180.

Martinez BA, Lake BD: Childhood nemaline myopathy: A review of clinical presentation in relation to prognosis. *Dev Med Child Neurol* 1987;29:815.

Miller JB: Myoblasts, myosins, MyoDs, and the diversification of muscle fibers. *Neuromuscul Disord* 1991;1:7.

Sarnat HB: Cerebral dysgeneses and their influence on fetal muscle development. *Brain Dev* 1986;8:495.

Sarnat HB: New insights into the pathogenesis of congenital myopathies. *J Child Neurol* 1994;9:193.

Sarnat HB: Ontogenesis of striated muscle. In Polin RA, Fox WW (editors): *Neonatal and Fetal Medicine: Physiology and Pathophysiology*, 3rd ed. Philadelphia, WB Saunders, 2003 (in press).

Shimomura C, Nonaka I: Nemaline myopathy: Comparative muscle histochemistry in the severe neonatal, moderate congenital, and adult-onset forms. *Pediatr Neurol* 1989;5:25.

Valdez MR, Richardson JA, Klein WH, et al: Failure of Myf5 to support myogenic differentiation without myogenin, MyoD and MRF4. *Dev Biol* 2000;219:287.

Wallgren-Pattersson C, Clarke A, Samson F, et al: The myotubular myopathies: Differential diagnosis of the X-linked recessive, autosomal dominant and autosomal recessive forms and present state of DNA studies. *J Med Genet* 1995;32:673.

Chapter 600
Muscular Dystrophies

The term *dystrophy* means abnormal growth, derived from the Greek *trophe*, meaning "nourishment." *Muscular dystrophy* implies much more than simply aberrant growth or nutrition of muscle fibers. A muscular dystrophy is distinguished from all other neuromuscular diseases by four obligatory criteria: (1) It is a primary myopathy; (2) it has a genetic basis; (3) the course is progressive; (4) degeneration and death of muscle fibers occur at some stage in the disease. This definition excludes neurogenic diseases such as spinal muscular atrophy, nonhereditary myopathies such as dermatomyositis, nonprogressive and non-necrotizing congenital myopathies such as congenital muscle fiber–type disproportion (CMFTD), and nonprogressive inherited metabolic myopathies. Some metabolic myopathies may fulfill the definition of a progressive muscular dystrophy but are not traditionally classified as dystrophies. An example is muscle carnitine deficiency. Conversely, all muscular dystrophies might eventually be reclassified as metabolic myopathies once the biochemical defects are better defined.

Muscular dystrophies are a group of unrelated diseases, each transmitted by a different genetic trait and each differing in its clinical course and expression. Some are severe diseases at birth or lead to early death; others follow very slow progressive courses over many decades, may be compatible with normal longevity, or may not even become symptomatic until late adult life. Some categories of dystrophies, such as limb-girdle muscular dystrophy, are not homogeneous diseases but rather syndromes encompassing several distinct myopathies. Relationships between the various muscular dystrophies are resolved by molecular genetics rather than by similarities or differences in clinical and histopathologic features.

600.1 ■ Duchenne and Becker Muscular Dystrophies

Duchenne muscular dystrophy is the most common hereditary neuromuscular disease affecting all races and ethnic groups. Its incidence is 1:3,600 liveborn infant boys. This disease is inherited as an X-linked recessive trait. The abnormal gene is on the X chromosome at the Xp21 locus and is one of the largest genes identified. Becker muscular dystrophy is the same fundamental disease as Duchenne dystrophy, with a genetic defect at the same locus, but clinically it follows a milder and more protracted course.

Duchenne recognized most of the characteristic clinical features in 1861: hypertrophy of the calves, progressive weakness, intellectual impairment, and proliferation of connective tissue in muscle.

Clinical Manifestations. Infant boys are only rarely symptomatic at birth or in early infancy, although some are already mildly hypotonic. Early gross motor skills, such as rolling over, sitting, and standing, are usually achieved at the appropriate ages or may be mildly delayed. Poor head control in infancy may be the first sign of weakness. Distinctive facies are not a feature because facial muscle weakness is a late event. Walking is often accomplished at the normal age of about 12 mo, but hip girdle weakness may be seen in subtle form as early as the 2nd year. Toddlers may assume a lordotic posture when standing to compensate for gluteal weakness. An early Gowers sign is often evident by age 3 yr and is fully expressed by age 5 or 6 yr (see Fig. 584–2). A Trendelenburg gait, or hip waddle, appears at this time.

The length of time that a patient remains ambulatory varies greatly. Some patients are confined to a wheelchair by 7 yr of age; most patients continue to walk with increasing difficulty until age 10 yr without orthopedic intervention. With orthotic bracing, physiotherapy, and sometimes minor surgery (e.g., Achilles tendon lengthening), most are able to walk until age 12 yr. Ambulation is important not only for postponing the psychologic depression that accompanies the loss of an aspect of personal independence but also because scoliosis usually does not become a major complication as long as a patient remains ambulatory, even for as little as 1 hr/day; scoliosis often becomes rapidly progressive after confinement to a wheelchair.

The relentless progression of *weakness* continues into the 2nd decade. The function of distal muscles is usually relatively well enough preserved, allowing the child to continue to use eating utensils, a pencil, and a computer keyboard. Respiratory muscle involvement is expressed as a weak and ineffective cough, frequent pulmonary infections, and decreasing respiratory reserve. Pharyngeal weakness may lead to episodes of aspiration, nasal regurgitation of liquids, and an airy or nasal voice quality. The function of the extraocular muscles remains well preserved. Incontinence due to anal and urethral sphincter weakness is an uncommon and very late event.

Contractures most often involve the ankles, knees, hips, and elbows. Scoliosis is common. The thoracic deformity further compromises pulmonary capacity and compresses the heart. Scoliosis may be uncomfortable or painful. Enlargement of the calves (pseudohypertrophy) and wasting of thigh muscles is a classic feature. The enlargement is caused by hypertrophy of some muscle fibers, infiltration of muscle by fat, and proliferation of collagen. After the calves, the next most common site of muscular hypertrophy is the tongue, followed by muscles of the forearm. Fasciculations of the tongue do not occur.

Unless ankle contractures are severe, ankle jerks remain well preserved until terminal stages. The knee jerks may be present until about 6 yr of age but are less brisk than the ankle jerks and are eventually lost. In the upper extremities, the brachioradialis reflex is usually stronger than the biceps or triceps brachii reflexes.

Cardiomyopathy is a constant feature of this disease. The severity of cardiac involvement does not necessarily correlate with the degree of skeletal muscle weakness. Some patients die early of severe cardiomyopathy while still ambulatory; others in terminal stages of the disease have well-compensated cardiac function.

Intellectual impairment occurs in all patients, although only 20–30% have an IQ less than 70. The majority have learning disabilities that still allow them to function in a regular classroom, particularly if remedial help is available. A few patients are profoundly mentally retarded, but there is no correlation with the severity of the myopathy. Epilepsy is slightly more common than in the general pediatric population.

The degenerative changes and fibrosis of muscle constitute a painless process. Myalgias and muscle spasms do not occur. Calcinosis of muscle is rare.

Death occurs usually at about 18 yr of age. The causes of death are respiratory failure in sleep, intractable heart failure, pneumonia, or occasionally aspiration and airway obstruction.

In *Becker muscular dystrophy*, boys remain ambulatory until late adolescence or early adult life. Calf pseudohypertrophy, cardiomyopathy, and elevated serum levels of creatine phosphokinase (CK) are similar to those of patients with Duchenne dystrophy. Learning disabilities are less frequent. The onset of weakness is later in Becker than in Duchenne dystrophy. Death often occurs in the mid to late 20s; fewer than half of patients are still alive by age 40 yr; these survivors are severely disabled.

Laboratory Findings. The serum CK level is consistently greatly elevated in Duchenne muscular dystrophy, even in presymptomatic stages, including at birth. The usual serum concentration is 15,000–35,000 IU/L (normal <160 IU/L). A normal serum CK level is incompatible with the diagnosis of Duchenne dystrophy, although in terminal stages of the disease the serum CK value may be considerably lower than it was a few years earlier because there is less muscle to degenerate. Other lysosomal enzymes present in muscle, such as aldolase and aspartate aminotransferase, are also increased but are less specific.

Cardiac assessment by echocardiography, electrocardiogram (ECG), and chest roentgenogram is essential and should be repeated periodically. After the diagnosis is established, patients should be referred to a pediatric cardiologist for long-term cardiac care.

Electromyography (EMG) shows characteristic myopathic features but is not specific for Duchenne muscular dystrophy. No evidence of denervation is found. Motor and sensory nerve conduction velocities are normal.

Diagnosis. A specific *molecular genetic diagnosis* is possible by demonstrating deficient or defective dystrophin by immunohistochemical staining of sections of muscle biopsy tissue or by DNA analysis from peripheral blood. Confirmation of the diagnosis by one of these methods should be done in every case. If the blood PCR is diagnostic, muscle biopsy may be deferred, but if it is normal and clinical suspicion is high, the more specific dystrophin immunocytochemistry test performed on muscle biopsy sections detects the one third of cases that do not show a PCR abnormality. Dystroglycans and other sarcolemmal regional proteins, such as merosin and sarcoglycans, also can be tested, because they may be secondarily decreased.

The *muscle biopsy* is diagnostic and shows characteristic changes (Figs. 600–1 and 600–2). Myopathic changes include endomysial connective tissue proliferation, scattered degenerating and regenerating myofibers, foci of mononuclear inflammatory cell infiltrates as a reaction to muscle fiber necrosis, mild architectural changes in still functional muscle fibers, and many dense fibers. These hypercontracted fibers probably result from segmental necrosis at another level, allowing calcium to enter the site of breakdown of the sarcolemmal membrane and trigger a contraction of the whole length of the muscle fiber. Calcifications within myofibers are correlated with secondary β-dystroglycan deficiency.

The decision about whether muscle biopsy should be performed to establish the diagnosis sometimes presents problems. If there is a family history of the disease, particularly in the case of an involved brother whose diagnosis has been confirmed, a patient with typical clinical features of Duchenne muscular dystrophy and high concentrations of serum CK probably does not need to undergo biopsy. The result of the polymerase chain

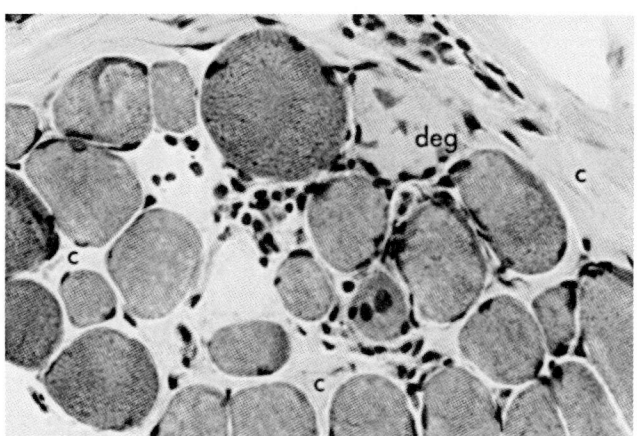

FIGURE 600–1. Muscle biopsy of a 4-yr-old boy with Duchenne muscular dystrophy. Both atrophic and hypertrophic muscle fibers are seen, and some fibers are degenerating (deg). Connective tissue (c) between muscle fibers is increased. (Hematoxylin & eosin, ×400.)

reaction (PCR) may also influence whether to perform a muscle biopsy. A first case in a family, even if the clinical features are typical, should have the diagnosis confirmed to ensure that another myopathy is not masquerading as Duchenne dystrophy. The most common muscles sampled are the vastus lateralis (quadriceps femoris) and the gastrocnemius.

Genetic Etiology and Pathogenesis. Despite the X-linked recessive inheritance in Duchenne muscular dystrophy, about 30% of patients are new mutations, and the mother is not a carrier. The female carrier state usually shows no muscle weakness or any clinical expression of the disease, but affected girls are occasionally encountered, usually having much milder weakness than boys. These symptomatic girls are explained by the Lyon hypothesis in which the normal X chromosome becomes inactivated and the one with the gene deletion is active (see Chapter 69). The full clinical picture of Duchenne dystrophy has occurred in several girls with Turner syndrome in whom the single X chromosome must have had the Xp21 gene deletion.

The asymptomatic carrier state of Duchenne dystrophy is associated with elevated serum CK values in 80% of cases. The level of increase is usually in the magnitude of hundreds or a few thousand but does not have the extreme values noted in affected males. Prepubertal girls who are carriers of the dystrophy also have increased serum CK values, with highest levels at 8–12 yr of age. Approximately 20% of carriers have normal serum CK values. If the mother of an affected boy has normal CK levels, it is unlikely that her daughter can be identified as a carrier by measuring CK. Muscle biopsy of suspected female carriers may detect an additional 10% in whom serum CK is not elevated; a specific genetic diagnosis using PCR on peripheral blood is definitive.

Detection of the carrier state by serum CK or muscle biopsy will become obsolete because of discoveries in the molecular genetics of Duchenne muscular dystrophy. The Xp21 site of the Duchenne gene has more than 2,000 kb, but Duchenne DNA encompasses only 14 kb; the entire gene sequence has been mapped.

A 427-kd cytoskeletal protein known as *dystrophin* is encoded by the gene at the Xp21.2 locus. This subsarcolemmal protein attaches to the sarcolemmal membrane overlying the A band and M band of the myofibrils and consists of four distinct regions or domains: the amino terminus contains 250 amino acids and is related to the *N*-actin binding site of α-actinin; the second domain is the largest, with 2,800 amino acids, and contains many repeats, giving it a characteristic rod shape; a third

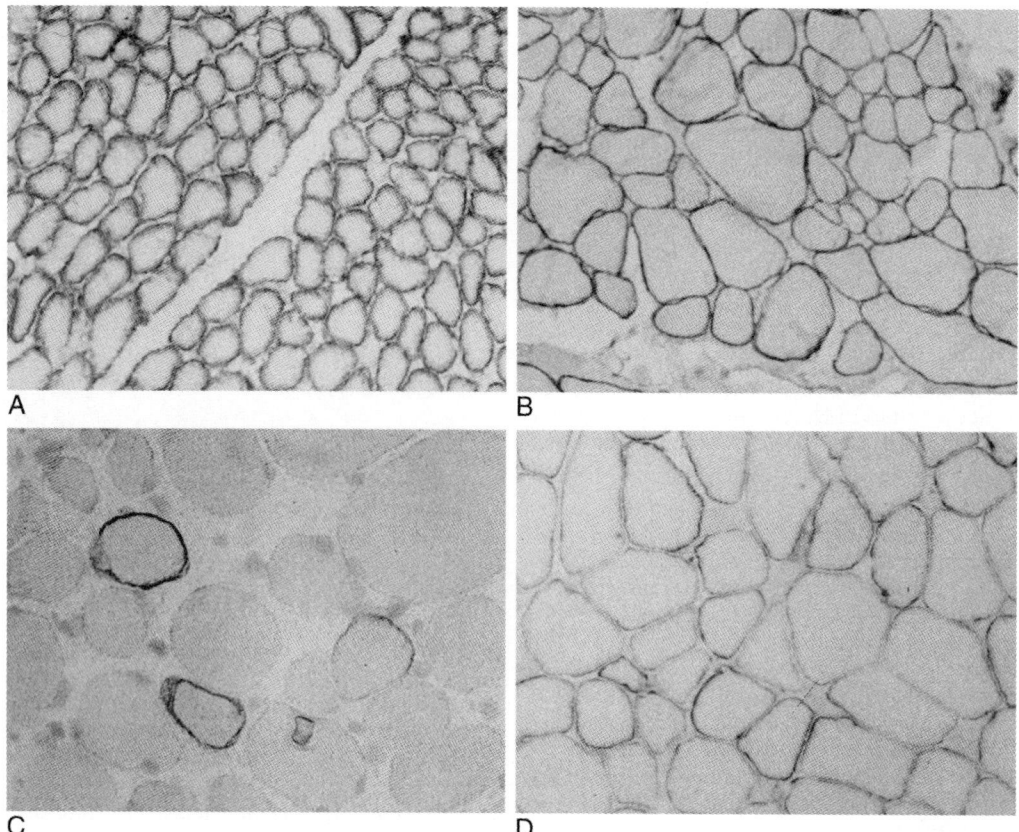

FIGURE 600–2. Dystrophin is demonstrated by immunohistochemical reactivity in the muscle biopsies of a normal term male neonate *(A)*; a 10-yr-old boy with limb-girdle muscular dystrophy *(B)*; a 6-yr-old boy with Duchenne muscular dystrophy *(C)*; and a 10-yr-old boy with Becker muscular dystrophy *(D)*. In the normal condition and also in non–X-linked muscular dystrophies in which dystrophin is not affected, the sacrolemmal membrane of every fiber is strongly stained, including atrophic and hypertrophic fibers. In Duchenne dystrophy, most myofibers express no detectable dystrophin, but a few scattered fibers known as "revertant fibers" show near-normal immunoreactivity. In Becker muscular dystrophy, the abnormal dystrophin molecule is expressed as thin, pale-staining of the sarcolemma in which reactivity varies not only between myofibers but also along the circumference of individual fibers (×250).

cysteine-rich domain is related to the carboxyl terminus of α-actinin; and the final carboxyl-terminal domain of 400 amino acids is unique to dystrophin and to a dystrophin-related protein encoded by chromosome 6. Dystrophin is first detected in developing human fetal muscle at the 11th wk of gestation. Dystrophin mRNA normally is detected in cardiac and smooth muscle as well as in skeletal muscle and brain. All of these tissues show various degrees of clinical involvement.

The molecular defects in the dystrophinopathies are of various types: intragenic deletions, duplications, or point mutations of nucleotides. About 65% of patients have deletions, and only 7% exhibit duplications. The site or size of the intragenic abnormality does not always correlate well with the phenotypic severity; in both Duchenne and Becker forms the mutations are mainly near the middle of the gene, involving deletions of exons 46–51. Phenotypic or clinical variations are explained by the alteration of the translational reading frame of mRNA, which results in unstable, truncated dystrophin molecules and severe, classic Duchenne dystrophy; mutations that preserve the reading frame still permit translation of coding sequences further downstream on the gene and produce a semifunctional dystrophin, expressed clinically as Becker muscular dystrophy. An even milder form of adult onset, formerly known as *quadriceps myopathy*, is also caused by an abnormal dystrophin molecule. The clinical spectrum of the dystrophinopathies not only includes the classic Duchenne and Becker forms but ranges from a severe neonatal muscular dystrophy to asymptomatic children with persistent elevation of serum CK levels greater than 1,000 IU/L.

The absence of dystrophin leads to a secondary reduction in several dystrophin-associated glycoproteins in the sarcolemma, which results in loss of linkage to the extracellular matrix and renders the sarcolemma even more susceptible to necrosis. Dystroglycan, often secondarily reduced in Duchenne muscular dystrophy, also is essential for normal brain development, for anchoring radial glia, and for intercellular adhesion in particular.

Analysis of the dystrophin protein requires a muscle biopsy and is demonstrated by Western blot analysis or in tissue sections by immunohistochemical methods using either fluorescence or light microscopy of antidystrophin antisera (see Fig. 600–2). In classic Duchenne dystrophy, levels of less than 3% of normal are found; in Becker muscular dystrophy, the molecular weight of dystrophin is reduced to 20–90% of normal in 80% of patients, but in 15% the dystrophin is of normal size but reduced in quantity, and 5% have an abnormally large protein caused by excessive duplications or repeats of codons. Selective immunoreactivity of different parts of the dystrophin molecule in sections of muscle biopsy material distinguishes the Duchenne and Becker forms (Fig. 600–3). The demonstration of deletions and duplications also can be made from blood samples by the more rapid PCR, which identifies as many as 98% of deletions by amplifying 18 exons but cannot detect duplications. The diagnosis can thus be confirmed at the molecular genetic level from either the muscle biopsy material or from peripheral blood, although as many as one third of boys with Duchenne or Becker dystrophy have a false-normal blood PCR; all cases of dystrophinopathy are detected by muscle biopsy.

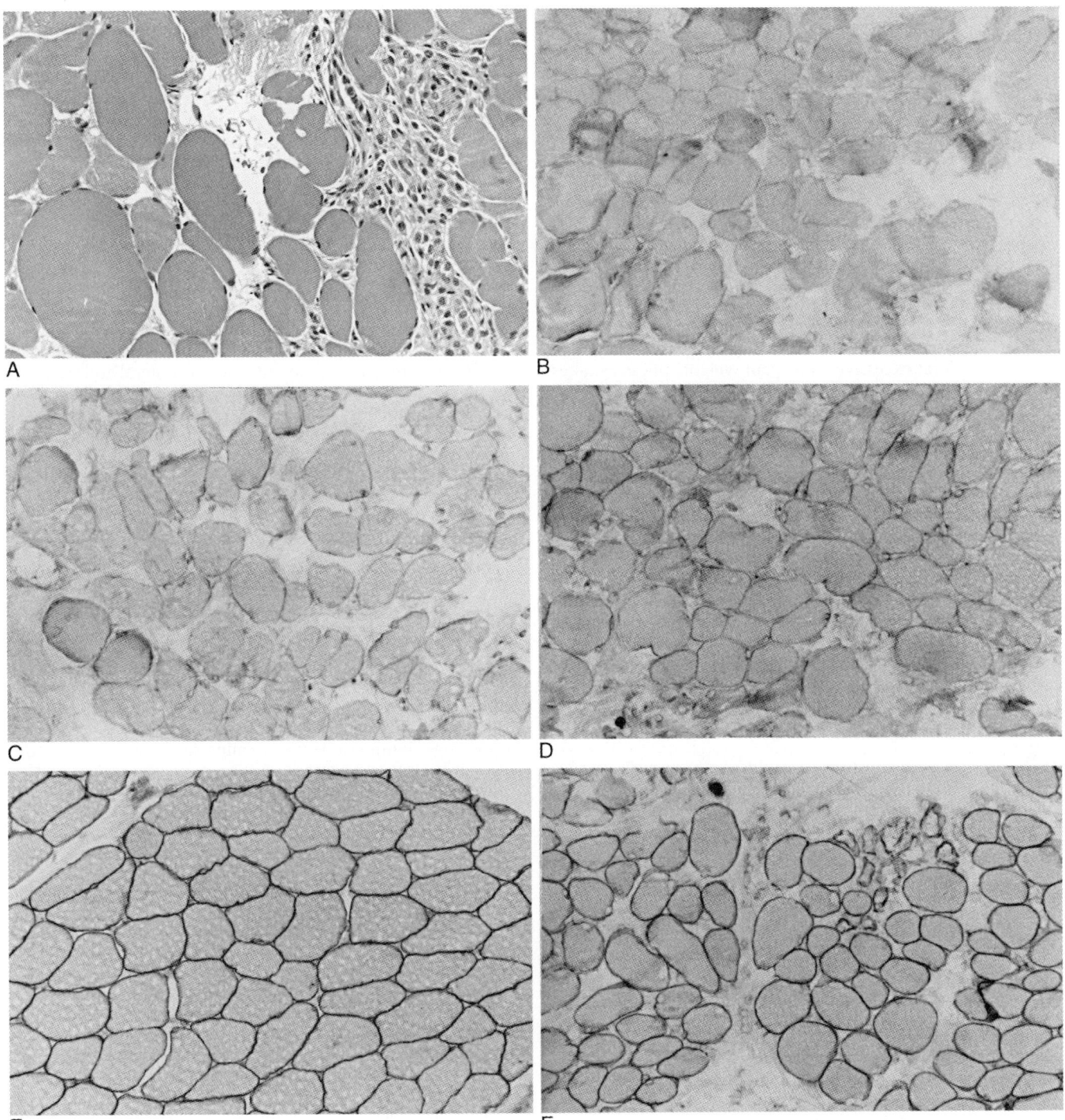

FIGURE 600–3. Quadriceps femoris muscle biopsy specimens from a 4-yr-old boy with Becker muscular dystrophy. *A,* Myofibers vary greatly in size, with both atrophic and hypertrophic forms; at the right is a zone of degeneration and necrosis infiltrated by macrophages, similar to Duchenne muscular dystrophy. (Hematoxylin-eosin, ×250.) Immunoreactivity using antibodies against the dystrophin molecule in the rod domain *(B),* carboxyl-terminus *(C),* and amino terminus *(D)* all show deficient but not totally absent dystrophin expression; most fibers of all sizes retain some dystrophin in parts of the sarcolemma but not around the entire circumference in cross section. Alternatively, the prominence of dystrophin is less, appearing weak, when compared with the simultaneously incubated normal control from another child of similar age *(E).* F, Merosin expression is normal in this patient with Becker dystrophy, in both large and small myofibers, and is lacking only in frankly necrotic fibers. Compare with classic Duchenne muscular dystrophy illustrated in Figure 600–2C and with Figure 600–5.

The same methods of DNA analysis from blood samples may be applied for carrier detection in female relatives at risk, such as sisters and cousins, and to determine whether the mother is a carrier or whether a new mutation occurred in the embryo.

Prenatal diagnosis is possible as early as the 12th wk of gestation by sampling chorionic villi for DNA analysis by Southern blot or PCR and is confirmed in aborted fetuses with Duchenne dystrophy by immunohistochemistry for dystrophin in muscle.

Treatment. There is neither a medical cure for this disease nor a method of slowing its progression. Much can be done to treat complications and to improve the quality of life of affected children. *Cardiac decompensation* often responds well to digoxin, at least in early stages. *Pulmonary infections* should be promptly treated. Patients should avoid contact with children who have obvious respiratory or other contagious illnesses. Immunizations for influenza virus and routine vaccinations are indicated.

Preservation of a good *nutritional state* is important. Duchenne muscular dystrophy is not a vitamin deficiency disease, and excessive doses of vitamins should be avoided. Adequate calcium intake is important to minimize osteoporosis in boys confined to a wheelchair, and fluoride supplements may also be given, particularly if the local drinking water is not fluoridated. Because sedentary children burn fewer calories than active children and because of depression as an additional factor, these children tend to eat excessively and gain weight. Obesity makes a patient with myopathy even less functional because part of the limited reserve muscle strength is dissipated in lifting the weight of excess subcutaneous adipose tissue. Dietary restrictions with supervision may be needed.

Physiotherapy delays but does not always prevent contractures. At times, contractures may actually be useful in functional rehabilitation. For example, if contractures prevent extension of the elbow beyond 90 degrees and the muscles of the upper limb no longer are strong enough to overcome gravity, the elbow contractures are functionally beneficial in fixing an otherwise flail arm and in allowing the patient to eat and write. Surgical correction of the elbow contracture may be technically feasible, but the result may be deleterious. Physiotherapy contributes little to muscle strengthening because patients usually are already using their entire reserve for daily function, and exercise cannot further strengthen involved muscles. Excessive exercise may actually accelerate the process of muscle fiber degeneration.

The discovery of the dystrophin molecule, its encoding gene, and the specific mutations in Duchenne and Becker muscular dystrophies raises the theoretical potential of a cure by molecular genetic engineering. One experimental approach is *myoblast transfer therapy*, in which normal myoblasts from the muscle of a genetically close relative, usually the father, are cultured in vitro and then injected into dystrophic muscles with the expectation that they will form healthy myofibers with normal dystrophin to replace degenerating fibers. A major drawback is the requirement for immunosuppression to prevent rejection of the foreign cells. The results in cases without rejection phenomena have not been encouraging. Another potential but unproven approach is the introduction by intramuscular injection or a viral vector of a recombinant dystrophin gene.

Other treatment of human patients with Duchenne dystrophy involves the use of prednisone, prednisolone, deflazacort, or other steroids. Glucocorticoids decrease the rate of apoptosis or programmed cell death of myotubes during ontogenesis and theoretically may decelerate the myofiber necrosis in muscular dystrophy. Strength usually improves initially, but the long-term complications of chronic steroid therapy, including considerable weight gain and osteoporosis, may offset this advantage or even result in greater weakness than might have occurred in the natural course of the disease. Also, fluorinated steroids, such as dexamethasone, induce myopathy by altering the myotube abundance of ceramide.

600.2 Emery-Dreifuss Muscular Dystrophy

Emery-Dreifuss muscular dystrophy, also known as *scapuloperoneal* or *scapulohumeral muscular dystrophy*, is a rare X-linked recessive dystrophy. The locus is on the long arm within the large Xq28 region that includes other mutations that cause myotubular myopathy, neonatal adrenoleukodystrophy, and the Bloch-Sulzberger type of incontinentia pigmenti; it is far from the gene for Duchenne muscular dystrophy on the short arm of the X chromosome. Another, rarer, form of Emery-Dreifuss dystrophy is transmitted as an autosomal dominant trait and is localized at 1q. This form may present quite late, in adolescence or early adult life, although the muscular and cardiac symptoms and signs are similar, and sudden death from ventricular fibrillation is a risk.

Clinical manifestations begin in middle childhood, but many patients survive to late adult life because of the slow progression of its course. Hypertrophy of muscles does not occur. Contractures of elbows and ankles develop early, and muscle becomes wasted in a scapulohumeroperoneal distribution. Facial weakness does not occur; this disease is thus distinguished clinically from autosomal dominant scapulohumeral and scapuloperoneal syndromes of neurogenic origin. Myotonia is absent. Intellectual function is normal. Cardiomyopathy is severe and is often the cause of death, more frequently from conduction defects and sudden ventricular fibrillation than from intractable myocardial failure. The serum CK value is only mildly elevated, further distinguishing this disease from other X-linked recessive muscular dystrophies.

Nonspecific myofiber necrosis and endomysial fibrosis are seen in the muscle biopsy. Many centronuclear fibers and selective histochemical type I muscle fiber atrophy may cause confusion with myotonic dystrophy. The defective gene in the X-linked form is called emerin and, unlike other dystrophies in which the defective gene is expressed at the sarcolemmal membrane, emerin is expressed at the nuclear membrane; the emerin protein may be demonstrated immunocytochemically in the muscle biopsy for definitive diagnosis. Emerin also may be tested as a genetic marker in blood. The defective protein in the autosomal dominant form is called lamin-A-C and also is a nuclear membrane protein with several subtypes and different mutations demonstrated. Treatment should be supportive, with special attention to cardiac conduction defects, and may require medications or a pacemaker.

600.3 Myotonic Muscular Dystrophy

Myotonic dystrophy (Steinert disease) is the second most common muscular dystrophy in North America, Europe, and Australia, having an incidence of 1:30,000 general population. It is inherited as an autosomal dominant trait.

Myotonic dystrophy is an example of a genetic defect causing dysfunction in multiple organ systems. Not only is striated muscle severely affected, but smooth muscle of the alimentary tract and uterus is also involved; cardiac function is altered; and patients have multiple and variable endocrinopathies, immunologic deficiencies, cataracts, dysmorphic facies, intellectual impairment, and other neurologic abnormalities.

Clinical Manifestations. In the usual clinical course, excluding the severe neonatal form, infants may appear almost normal at birth, or facial wasting and hypotonia may already be early expressions of the disease. The facial appearance is characteristic, consisting of an inverted V-shaped upper lip, thin cheeks, and scalloped, concave temporalis muscles (Fig. 600–4). The head may be narrow, and the palate is high and arched because the weak temporal and pterygoid muscles in late fetal life do not exert sufficient lateral forces on the developing head and face.

Weakness is mild in the first few years. Progressive wasting of distal muscles becomes increasingly evident, particularly involving intrinsic muscles of the hands. The thenar and hypothenar eminences are flattened, and the atrophic dorsal interossei leave deep grooves between the fingers. The dorsal forearm muscles

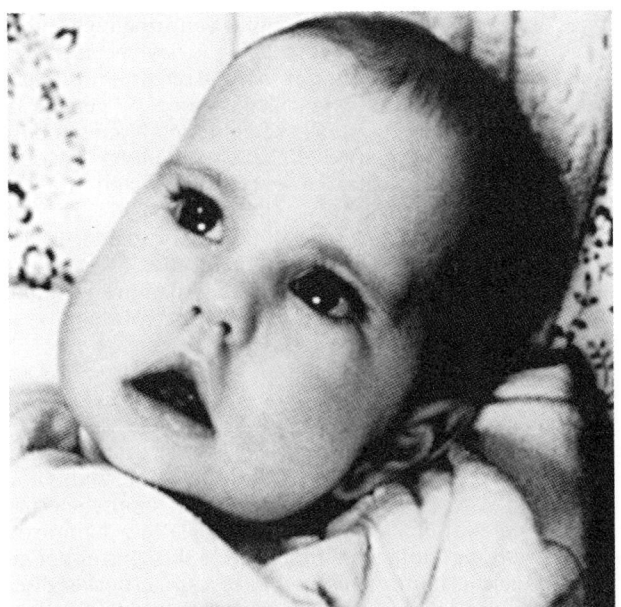

FIGURE 600–4. Facial weakness, inverted V-shaped upper lip, and loss of muscle mass in the temporal fossae are characteristic of myotonic muscular dystrophy, even in infancy, as seen in this 8-mo-old girl.

and anterior compartment muscles of the lower legs also become wasted. The tongue is thin and atrophic. Wasting of the sternocleidomastoids gives the neck a long, thin, cylindric contour. Proximal muscles also eventually undergo atrophy, and scapular winging appears. Difficulty with climbing stairs and Gowers sign are progressive. Tendon stretch reflexes are usually preserved.

The distal distribution of muscle wasting in myotonic dystrophy is an exception to the general rule of myopathies having proximal and neuropathies having distal distribution patterns. The muscular atrophy and weakness in myotonic dystrophy are slowly progressive throughout childhood and adolescence and continue into adulthood. It is rare for patients with myotonic dystrophy to lose the ability to walk even in late adult life, although splints or bracing may be required to stabilize the ankles.

Myotonia, a characteristic feature shared by few other myopathies, does not occur in infancy and is usually not clinically or even electromyographically evident until about age 5 yr. Exceptional patients develop it as early as age 3 yr. Myotonia is a very slow relaxation of muscle after contraction, regardless of whether that contraction was voluntary or was induced by a stretch reflex or electrical stimulation. During physical examination, myotonia may be demonstrated by asking the patient to make tight fists and then to quickly open the hands. It may be induced by striking the thenar eminence with a rubber percussion hammer, and it may be detected by watching the involuntary drawing of the thumb across the palm. Myotonia may also be demonstrated in the tongue by pressing the edge of a wooden tongue blade against its dorsal surface and by observing a deep furrow that disappears slowly. The severity of myotonia does not necessarily parallel the degree of weakness, and the weakest muscles often have only minimal myotonia. Myotonia is not a painful muscle spasm. Myalgias do not occur in myotonic dystrophy.

The *speech* of patients with myotonic dystrophy is often articulated poorly and is slurred because of the involvement of the muscles of the face, tongue, and pharynx. Difficulties with swallowing sometimes occur. Aspiration pneumonia is a risk in severely involved children. Incomplete external ophthalmoplegia may sometimes result from extraocular muscle weakness.

Smooth muscle involvement of the *gastrointestinal tract* results in slow gastric emptying, poor peristalsis, and constipation. Some patients have encopresis associated with anal sphincter weakness. Women with myotonic dystrophy may have ineffective or abnormal uterine contractions during labor and delivery.

Cardiac involvement is usually manifested as heart block in the Purkinje conduction system and arrhythmias rather than as cardiomyopathy, unlike most other muscular dystrophies.

Endocrine abnormalities involve many glands and appear at any time during the course of the disease so that re-evaluation of endocrine status must be done annually. Hypothyroidism is common; hyperthyroidism may occur rarely. Adrenocortical insufficiency may lead to an addisonian crisis even in infancy. Diabetes mellitus is common in patients with myotonic dystrophy; some children have a disorder of insulin release rather than defective insulin production. Onset of puberty may be precocious or, more often, delayed. Testicular atrophy and testosterone deficiency are common in adults and are responsible for a high incidence of male infertility. Ovarian atrophy is rare. Frontal baldness is also characteristic in males and often begins in adolescence.

Immunologic deficiencies are common in myotonic dystrophy. The plasma IgG level is often low.

Cataracts occur frequently in myotonic dystrophy. They may be congenital, or they may begin at any time during childhood or adult life. Early cataracts are detected only by slit lamp examination; periodic examination by an ophthalmologist is recommended. Visual evoked potentials are often abnormal in children with myotonic dystrophy and are unrelated to cataracts. They are not usually accompanied by visual impairment.

About half of the patients with myotonic dystrophy are intellectually impaired, but severe mental retardation is unusual. The remainder are of average or occasionally above average intelligence. Epilepsy is not common.

A severe neonatal form of myotonic dystrophy appears in a minority of involved infants born to mothers with myotonic dystrophy. Clubfoot deformities alone or more extensive congenital contractures of many joints may involve all extremities and even the cervical spine. Generalized hypotonia and weakness are present at birth. Facial wasting is prominent. Some infants require gavage feeding or even ventilator support for respiratory muscle weakness or apnea. One or both leaves of the diaphragm may be nonfunctional. The abdomen becomes distended with gas in the stomach and intestine because of poor peristalsis from smooth muscle weakness. The distention further compromises respiration. Inability to empty the rectum may compound the problem. About 75% of severely affected neonates die within the first year.

Laboratory Findings. The classic myotonic EMG is not found in infancy but may appear in toddlers or during the early school years. The levels of serum CK and other serum enzymes from muscle may be normal or only mildly elevated in the hundreds (never the thousands).

An ECG should be performed annually in early childhood. Ultrasonic imaging of the abdomen may be indicated in affected infants to determine diaphragmatic function. Roentgenograms of the chest and abdomen and contrast studies of gastrointestinal motility may be needed.

Endocrine assessment should be undertaken to determine thyroid and adrenal cortical function and to verify carbohydrate metabolism (glucose tolerance test). Immunoglobulins should be examined, and, if needed, more extensive immunologic studies should be performed.

Diagnosis. The primary diagnostic test is a DNA analysis of blood to demonstrate the abnormal expansion of the CTG repeat. Prenatal diagnosis also is feasible. The muscle biopsy in older children shows many muscle fibers with central nuclei and selective atrophy of histochemical type I fibers, but degenerating fibers are usually few and widely scattered, and there is little or no fibrosis of muscle. Intrafusal fibers of muscle spindles are also abnormal. In young children with the common form of the disease, the biopsy specimen may even appear normal or may at least not show myofiber necroses, which is a striking contrast with Duchenne muscular dystrophy. In the severe neonatal form of myotonic dystrophy, the muscle biopsy reveals maturational arrest in various stages of development in some and congenital muscle fiber–type disproportion in others. It is likely that the sarcolemmal membrane of muscle fibers not only has abnormal properties of electrical polarization but is also incapable of responding to trophic influences of the motor neuron. Muscle biopsy is not usually required for diagnosis, which in typical cases can be based on the clinical manifestations.

Genetics. The genetic defect in myotonic muscular dystrophy is on chromosome 19 at the 19q13 locus. It consists of an expansion of the *DM* gene that encodes a serine-threonine kinase *(DMPK)*, with numerous repeats of the cytosine-thymine-guanine (CTG) codon. Expansions range from 50 to over 2,000, with the normal alleles of this gene ranging in size from 5 to 37; the larger the expansion, the more severe the clinical expression, with the largest expansions seen in the severe neonatal form. Rarely, the disease is associated with no detectable repeats, perhaps a spontaneous correction of a previous expansion but a phenomenon still incompletely understood. A second type of myotonic dystrophy (PROMM) is a clinical entity linked to at least two different chromosomal loci than classic myotonic dystrophy but one that shares a common unique pathogenesis in being mediated by a mutant mRNA. Defects in RNA splicing explain the insulin resistance in myotonic dystrophies as well as the myotonia.

Both clinical and genetic expression may vary between siblings or between an affected parent and child. In the severe neonatal form of the disease, the mother is the transmitting parent in 94% of cases, a fact not explained by increased male infertility alone. Genetic analysis reveals that such infants usually have many more repeats of the CTG codon than do patients with the more classic form of the disease. Myotonic dystrophy often exhibits a pattern of *anticipation* in which each successive generation has a tendency to be more severely involved than the previous generation.

Treatment. There is no specific medical treatment, but the cardiac, endocrine, gastrointestinal, and ocular complications can often be treated. Physiotherapy and orthopedic treatment of contractures in the neonatal form of the disease may be beneficial.

Myotonia may be diminished, and function may be restored by drugs that raise the depolarization threshold of muscle membranes, such as mexiletine, phenytoin, carbamazepine, procainamide, and quinidine sulfate. These drugs also have cardiotropic effects; thus, cardiac evaluation is important before prescribing them. Phenytoin and carbamazepine are used in doses similar to their use as anticonvulsants (see Chapter 586.4); serum concentrations of 40–80 µmol/L for phenytoin and 35–50 µmol/L for carbamazepine should be maintained. If a patient's disability is caused mainly by weakness rather than by myotonia, these drugs will be of no value.

OTHER MYOTONIC SYNDROMES

Most patients with myotonia have myotonic dystrophy. Myotonia is not specific for this disease and occurs in several rarer conditions.

Myotonic chondrodystrophy (Schwartz-Jampel disease) is a rare congenital disease characterized by generalized muscle hypertrophy and weakness. Dysmorphic phenotypical features and the roentgenographic appearance of long bones are reminiscent of Morquio disease (see Chapter 77), but abnormal mucopolysac-

charides are not found. Dwarfism, joint abnormalities, and blepharophimosis are present. Several patients have been the products of consanguinity, suggesting autosomal recessive inheritance. The muscle protein perlecan, encoded by the *SJS1* gene, a large heparan sulfate proteoglycan of basement membranes and cartilage, is defective in some cases of Schwartz-Jampel disease and explains both the muscular hyperexcitability and the chondrodysplasia.

EMG reveals continuous electrical activity in muscle fibers closely resembling or identical to myotonia. Muscle biopsy reveals nonspecific myopathic features, which are minimal in some cases and pronounced in others. The sarcotubular system is dilated.

Myotonia congenita (Thomsen disease) is a channelopathy and is characterized by weakness and generalized muscular hypertrophy so that affected children resemble bodybuilders. Myotonia is prominent and may develop at age 2–3 yr, earlier than in myotonic dystrophy. The disease is clinically stable and is apparently not progressive for many years. Muscle biopsy specimens show minimal pathologic changes, and the EMG demonstrates myotonia. Various families are described as showing either autosomal dominant (Thomsen disease) or recessive (Becker disease, not to be confused with Becker/Duchenne muscular dystrophy) inheritance. Rarely, myotonic dystrophy and myotonia congenita coexist in the same family. Both the autosomal dominant and autosomal recessive forms of myotonia congenita have been mapped to the same 7q35 locus. This gene is important for the integrity of chloride channels of the sarcolemmal and T-tubular membranes.

Paramyotonia is a temperature-related myotonia that is aggravated by cold and alleviated by warm external temperatures. Patients have difficulty when swimming in cold water or if they are dressed inadequately in cold weather. Paramyotonia congenita is a defect in a gene at the 17q13.1-13.3 locus, the identical locus identified in hyperkalemic periodic paralysis. By contrast with myotonia congenita, paramyotonia is a disorder of the sodium channel. Myotonic dystrophy also is a sodium channelopathy.

In sodium channelopathies, exercise produces increasing myotonia, whereas in chloride channelopathies, exercise reduces the myotonia. This is easily tested during examination by asking patients to close the eyes forcefully and open them repeatedly; it becomes progressively more difficult in sodium channel disorders and progressively easier in chloride channel disorders.

600.4 Limb-Girdle Muscular Dystrophy

This term encompasses a group of progressive hereditary myopathies that mainly affect muscles of the hip and shoulder girdles. Distal muscles also eventually become atrophic and weak. Hypertrophy of the calves and ankle contractures develop in some forms, causing potential confusion with Becker muscular dystrophy.

The initial *clinical manifestations* rarely appear before middle or late childhood or may be delayed until early adult life. Low back pain may be a presenting complaint because of the lordotic posture resulting from gluteal muscle weakness. Confinement to a wheelchair usually becomes obligatory at about 30 yr of age. The rate of progression varies from one pedigree to another but is uniform within a kindred. Although weakness of neck flexors and extensors is universal, facial, lingual, and other bulbar-innervated muscles are rarely involved. As weakness and muscle wasting progress, tendon stretch reflexes become diminished. Cardiac involvement is unusual. Intellectual function is generally normal. The clinical differential diagnosis of limb-girdle muscular dystrophy includes juvenile spinal muscular atrophy

(Kugelberg-Welander disease), myasthenia gravis, and metabolic myopathies.

Most cases of limb-girdle muscular dystrophy are of autosomal recessive inheritance, but some families express an autosomal dominant trait. The latter often follows a benign course with little functional impairment.

The EMG and muscle biopsy show confirmatory evidence of muscular dystrophy, but none of the findings is specific enough to make the definitive *diagnosis* without additional clinical criteria. In some cases, adhalen, a dystrophin-related glycoprotein of the sarcolemma, is deficient; this specific defect may be demonstrated in the muscle biopsy by immunocytochemistry. Increased serum CK level is usual, but the magnitude of elevation varies among families. The ECG is usually unaltered.

In one autosomal dominant form of limb-girdle muscular dystrophy, a *genetic defect* has been localized to the long arm of chromosome 5. In the autosomal recessive disease, it is on the long arm of chromosome 15. A mutated dystrophin-associated protein in the sarcoglycan complex (sarcoglycanopathy) is responsible for some cases of autosomal recessive limb-girdle muscular dystrophy. Adhalen is α-sarcoglycan; other limb-girdle dystrophies due to deficiencies in β-, γ-, and δ-sarcoglycan also occur. In normal smooth muscle, α- is replaced by ε-sarcoglycan and the others are the same.

Another group of limb-girdle dystrophies are caused by allelic mutations of the dysferlin *(DYSF)* gene, another gene expressing a protein essential to structural integrity of the sarcolemma, though not associated with the dystrophin-glycoprotein complex. *DYSF* interacts with caveolin-3 or calpain-3, and *DYSF* deficiency may be secondary to defects in these other gene products. Autosomal recessive (Miyoshi myopathy) and autosomal dominant traits are documented. Both are slowly progressive myopathies with onset in adolescence or young adult life and may affect distal as well as proximal muscles. Cardiomyopathy is rare. Chronically elevated serum CK in the thousands is found in dysferlinopathies. Ultrastructure shows a thickened basal lamina over defects in the sarcolemma and replacement of the sarcolemma by multiple layers of small vesicles. Regenerating myofibers outnumber degenerating myofibers.

600.5 Facioscapulohumeral Muscular Dystrophy

Facioscapulohumeral muscular dystrophy, also known as **Landouzy-Dejerine disease,** is probably not a single disease entity but a group of diseases with similar clinical manifestations. Autosomal dominance is the rule; *genetic anticipation* is often found within several generations of a family, the succeeding more severely involved at an earlier age than the preceding. The genetic mechanism in autosomal dominant facioscapulohumeral dystrophy involves integral deletions of a 3.3-kb tandem repeat (D4Z4) in the subtelomeric region at the 4q35 locus. A closely homologous 3.3-kb repeat array at the subtelomeric locus 10q26, with chromosomal translocation or sequence conversion between these two regions, possibly predisposes to the DNA rearrangement causing facioscapulohumeral dystrophy.

Clinical Manifestations. Facioscapulohumeral dystrophy shows the earliest and most severe weakness in facial and shoulder girdle muscles. The facial weakness differs from that of myotonic dystrophy; rather than an inverted V-shaped upper lip, the mouth in facioscapulohumeral dystrophy is rounded and appears puckered because the upper and lower lips protrude. Inability to close the eyes completely in sleep is a common expression of upper facial weakness; some patients have extraocular muscle weakness, although ophthalmoplegia is rarely complete. Facioscapulohumeral dystrophy has been asso-

ciated with Möbius syndrome on rare occasions. Pharyngeal and tongue weakness may be absent and is never as severe as the facial involvement. Hearing loss, which may be subclinical, and retinal vasculopathy (indistinguishable from Coat syndrome) are associated features, particularly in *severe* cases of facioscapulohumeral dystrophy with early childhood onset.

Scapular winging is prominent, often even in infants. Flattening or even concavity of the deltoid contour is seen, and the biceps and triceps brachii muscles are wasted and weak. Muscles of the hip girdles and thighs also eventually lose strength and undergo atrophy, and Gowers sign and a Trendelenburg gait appear. Contractures are rare. Finger and wrist weakness occasionally is the first symptom. Weakness of the anterior tibial and peroneal muscles may lead to footdrop; this complication usually occurs only in advanced cases with severe weakness. Lumbar lordosis and kyphoscoliosis are common complications of axial muscle involvement. Calf hypertrophy is not a feature.

Facioscapulohumeral muscular dystrophy may also be a mild disease causing minimal disability. Clinical manifestations may not be expressed in childhood and are delayed into middle adult life. Unlike most other muscular dystrophies, asymmetry of weakness is common.

Laboratory Findings. Serum levels of CK and other enzymes vary greatly, ranging from normal or near normal to elevations of several thousand. ECG should be performed, although the anticipated findings are usually normal. EMG reveals nonspecific myopathic muscle potentials. Diagnostic molecular testing in both individual cases and within families is indicated for prediction.

Diagnosis and Differential Diagnosis. Muscle biopsy distinguishes more than one form of facioscapulohumeral dystrophy, consistent with clinical evidence that several distinct diseases are embraced by the term *FSH dystrophy*. Muscle biopsy and EMG also distinguish the primary myopathy from a neurogenic disease with a similar distribution of muscular involvement. The general histopathologic findings in the muscle biopsy material are extensive proliferation of connective tissue between muscle fibers, extreme variation in fiber size with many hypertrophic as well as atrophic myofibers, and scattered degenerating and regenerating fibers. An "inflammatory" type of facioscapulohumeral muscular dystrophy is also distinguished, characterized by extensive lymphocytic infiltrates within muscle fascicles. Despite the resemblance of this form to inflammatory myopathies, such as polymyositis, there is no evidence of autoimmune disease, and steroids and immunosuppressive drugs do not alter the clinical course. A precise histopathologic diagnosis has important therapeutic implications. Mononuclear cell "inflammation" in a muscle biopsy sample of infants younger than 2 yr is usually facioscapulohumeral dystrophy.

Treatment. Physiotherapy is of no value in regaining strength or in retarding progressive weakness or muscle wasting. Footdrop and scoliosis may be treated by orthopedic measures. Cosmetic improvement of the facial muscles of expression may be achieved by reconstructive surgery, which grafts a fascia lata to the zygomatic muscle and to the zygomatic head of the quadratus labiae superioris muscle.

600.6 Congenital Muscular Dystrophy

The term *congenital muscular dystrophy* is misleading because all muscular dystrophies are genetically determined. It is used to encompass several distinct diseases with a common characteristic of severe involvement at birth but that ironically usually follow a benign clinical course. Autosomal recessive inheritance is the rule.

Clinical Manifestations. Infants often have contractures or arthrogryposis at birth and are diffusely hypotonic. The muscle mass is thin in the trunk and extremities. Head control is poor. Facial muscles may be mildly involved, but ophthalmoplegia, pharyngeal weakness, and weak sucking are not common. A minority have severe dysphagia and require gavage or gastrostomy. Tendon stretch reflexes may be hypoactive or absent. Arthrogryposis is common in all forms of congenital muscular dystrophy (see Chapter 599.9).

One form of congenital muscular dystrophy, the Fukuyama type, is the 2nd most common muscular dystrophy in Japan (after Duchenne dystrophy); it has also been reported in children of Dutch, German, Scandinavian, and Turkish ethnic backgrounds. In the Fukuyama variety, severe cardiomyopathy and malformations of the brain usually accompany the skeletal muscle involvement. Signs and symptoms related to these organs are prominent: cardiomegaly and heart failure, mental retardation, seizures, microcephaly, and failure to thrive. The genetic defect in Fukuyama congenital muscular dystrophy has been identified at the 8q31-33 locus in Japanese patients.

Neurologic disease may accompany forms of congenital muscular dystrophy other than Fukuyama disease. Mental and neurologic status are the most variable features; an apparently normal brain and normal intelligence do not preclude the diagnosis if other manifestations indicate this myopathy. The cerebral malformations that occur are not consistently of one type and vary from severe dysplasias (holoprosencephaly, lissencephaly) to milder conditions (agenesis of the corpus callosum, focal heterotopia of the cerebral cortex and subcortical white matter, cerebellar hypoplasia). Congenital muscular dystrophy is a consistent association with cerebral dysgenesis in the *Walker-Warburg syndrome* and in *muscle-eye-brain disease of Santavuori*. The neuropathologic findings are those of neuroblast migratory abnormalities in the cerebral cortex, cerebellum, and brain stem. Another separate form of congenital muscular dystrophy is characterized by microcephaly and mental retardation.

Laboratory Findings. Serum CK level is usually moderately elevated from several hundred to many thousand IU/L; only marginal increases are sometimes found. EMG shows nonspecific myopathic features. Investigation of all forms of congenital muscular dystrophy should include cardiac assessment and an imaging study of the brain. Muscle biopsy is essential for the diagnosis.

Diagnosis. Muscle biopsy is diagnostic in the neonatal period or thereafter. An extensive proliferation of endomysial collagen envelops individual muscle fibers even at birth, also causing them to be rounded in cross-sectional contour by acting as a rigid sleeve, especially during contraction. The perimysial con-

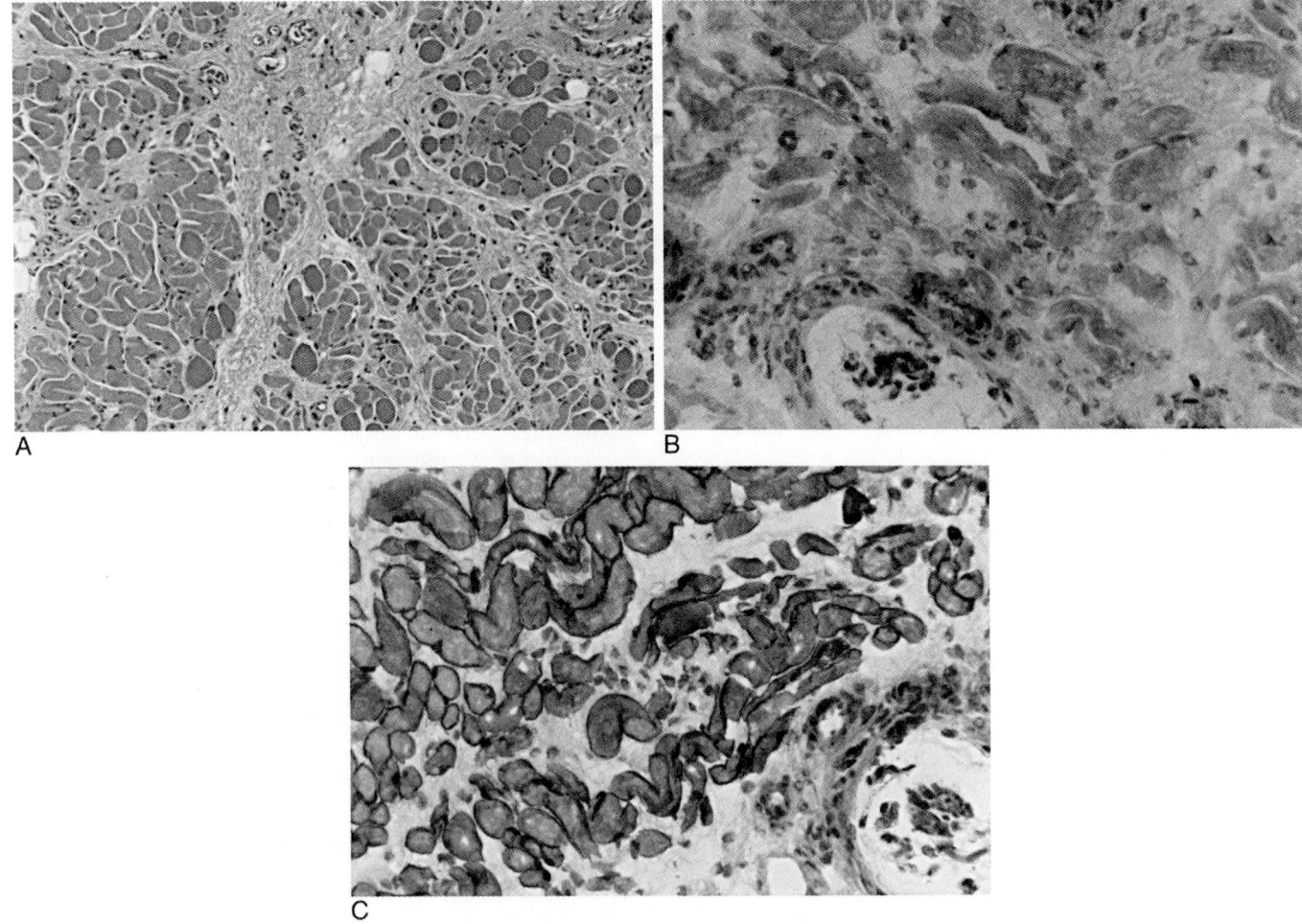

FIGURE 600–5. Quadriceps femoris muscle biopsy of a 6-mo-old girl with congenital muscular dystrophy associated with merosin (α_2-laminin) deficiency. *A,* Histologically, the muscle is infiltrated by a great proliferation of collagenous connective tissue; myofibers vary in diameter, but necrotic fibers are rare. *B,* Immunocytochemical reactivity for merosin (α_2-laminin) is absent in all fibers, including the intrafusal myofibers of a muscle spindle seen at bottom. *C,* Dystrophin expression (rod domain) is normal. Compare with Figures 600–2, 600–3, and 600–6.

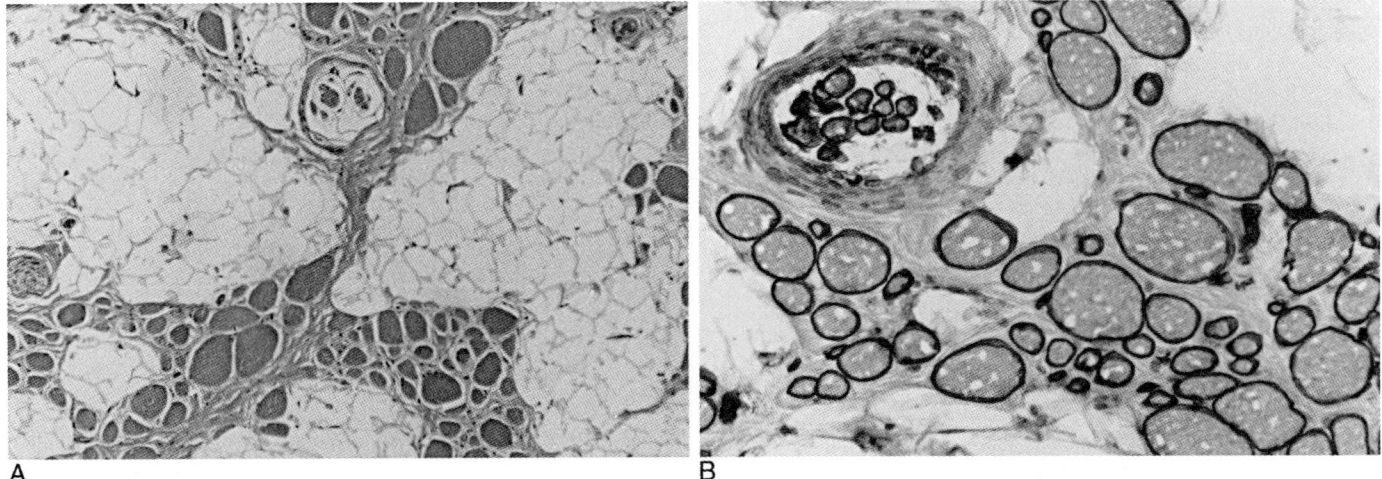

FIGURE 600–6. Quadriceps femoris muscle biopsy of a 2-yr-old girl with congenital muscular dystrophy. *A*, The fascicular architecture of the muscle is severely disrupted, and muscle is replaced by fat and connective tissue; remaining small groups of myofibers of variable size are seen, including a muscle spindle at top. *B*, Merosin expression is normal in both extrafusal fibers of all sizes and in intrafusal spindle fibers. The severity of the myopathy does not relate to the presence or absence of merosin in congenital muscular dystrophy. Compare with Figure 600–5.

nective tissue and fat are also increased, and the fascicular organization of the muscle may be disrupted by the fibrosis. Tissue cultures of intramuscular fibroblasts exhibit increased collagen synthesis, but the structure of the collagen is normal. Muscle fibers vary in diameter, and many show central nuclei, myofibrillar splitting, and other cytoarchitectural alterations. Scattered degenerating and regenerating fibers are seen. No inflammation or abnormal inclusions are found.

Immunocytochemical reactivity for merosin (α_2 chain of laminin) at the sarcolemmal region is absent in about half the cases and normally expressed in the others (Figs. 600–5 and 600–6). Merosin is a protein that binds the sarcolemmal membrane of the myofiber to the basal lamina or basement membrane. Its defect is a mutation of the *LAMA2* gene at the 6q22-q23 locus. The presence or absence of merosin does not always correlate with the severity of the myopathy or predict its course, but cases with merosin deficiency tend to have more severe cerebral involvement and myopathy. Adhalen (α-dystroglycan) may be secondarily reduced in some cases.

Treatment. Only supportive therapy is available.

Angelini C, Fanin N, Freda MP, et al: The clinical spectrum of sarcoglycanopathies. *Neurology* 1999;52:176.

Bonne G, Muchin A, Helbling-Lecleerc A, et al: Clinical and genetical heterogeneity of laminopathies. *Acta Myologica* 2001;20:138.

Brook JD, McCurrach ME, Harley HG, et al: Molecular basis of myotonic dystrophy: Expansion of a trinucleotide (CTG) repeat at the 3N end of a transcript encoding a protein kinase family member. *Cell* 1992;68:799.

Brouwer OF, Padberg GW, Wijmenga C, et al: Facioscapulohumeral muscular dystrophy in early childhood. *Arch Neurol* 1994;51:387.

Colomer J, Iturriaga C, Bonne G, et al: Autosomal dominant Emery-Dreifuss muscular dystrophy; a new family with late diagnosis. *Neuromusc Disord* 2002;12:19.

Duggan DJ, Gorospe JR, Fanin N, et al: Mutations in the sarcoglycan genes in patients with myopathy. *N Engl J Med* 1997;336:618.

Miller G, Wessel HB: Diagnosis of dystrophinopathies: Review for the clinician. *Pediatr Neurol* 1993;9:3.

Monsieurs KG, Van Broeckhoven C, Martin JJ, et al: Gly241Arg mutation indicating malignant hyperthermia susceptibility: Specific cause of chronically elevated serum creatine kinase activity. *J Neurol Sci* 1998;154:62.

Moxley RT, Meola G: Myotonic dystrophy. In Deymeer F (editor): Neuromuscular Disorders: From Basic Mechanisms to Clinical Management. *Monogr Clin Neurosci* 2000;18:61–78.

Nicole S, Vicart S, Davoine CS, et al: Mutations of perlecan, the major proteoglycan of basement membranes, cause Schwartz-Jampel syndrome: a new mechanism for myotonia? *Acta Myologica* 2001;20:130.

Rose MR: Neurological channelopathies. *BMJ* 1998;316:1104.

Ruggieri V, Lubieniecki F, Meli F, et al: Merosin-positive congenital muscular dystrophy with mental retardation, microcephaly and central nervous system

abnormalities unlinked to the Fukuyama muscular dystrophy and muscular-eye-brain loci: Report of three siblings. *Neuromusc Disord* 2001;11:570.

Santavuori P, Valanne L, Autti T, et al: Muscle-eye-brain disease: Clinical features, visual evoked potentials and brain imaging in 20 patients. *Eur J Paediatr Neurol* 1998;1:41.

Sewry CA, Brown BC, Mercuri E, et al: Skeletal muscle pathology in autosomal dominant Emery-Dreifuss muscular dystrophy with lamin A/C mutations. *Neuropathol Appl Neurobiol* 2001;27:241.

Tokgozoglu LS, Ashizawa T, Pacifico A, et al: Cardiac involvement in a large kindred with myotonic dystrophy. *JAMA* 1995;274:813.

Tsilfidis C, MacKenzie AE, Mettler G, et al: Correlation between CTG trinucleotide repeat length and frequency of severe congenital myotonic dystrophy. *Nat Genet* 1992;1:192.

van Deutekom JC, Baaker E, Lemmers RJ, et al: Evidence for subtelomeric exchange of 3.3 kb tandemly repeated units between chromosomes 4q35 and 10q26: Implications for genetic counselling and etiology of *FSHD1*. *Hum Mol Genet* 1996;5:1997–2003.

Voit T: Congenital muscular dystrophies: 1997 update. *Brain Dev* 1998;20:65.

Chapter 601
Endocrine Myopathies

Thyroid Myopathies. (See also Part XXV, Section 2.) Thyrotoxicosis causes proximal weakness and wasting accompanied by myopathic electromyographic changes. Thyroxine binds to myofibrils and, if in excess, impairs contractile function. Hyperthyroidism may also induce myasthenia gravis and hypokalemic periodic paralysis.

Hypothyroidism, whether congenital or acquired, consistently produces hypotonia and a proximal distribution of weakness. Although muscle wasting is most characteristic, one form of cretinism, the Kocher-Debré-Sémélaigne syndrome, is characterized by generalized pseudohypertrophy of weak muscles. Infants may have a herculean appearance reminiscent of myotonia congenita. The serum creatine phosphokinase (CK) level is elevated in hypothyroid myopathy and returns to normal after thyroid replacement therapy. Muscle biopsy material reveals myopathic changes, including myofiber necrosis and sometimes central cores.

Both the clinical and pathologic features of hyperthyroid myopathy and hypothyroid myopathy resolve after appropriate treatment of the thyroid disorder.

Hyperparathyroidism (see Chapter 567). Most patients with primary hyperparathyroidism develop weakness, fatigability, and muscle wasting that are reversible after removal of the parathyroid adenoma.

Steroid-Induced Myopathy. Both natural Cushing disease and iatrogenic Cushing syndrome due to exogenous corticosteroid administration may cause progressive proximal weakness, increased serum CK levels, and a myopathic electromyogram and muscle biopsy specimen (see Chapter 571). Myosin filaments may be selectively lost. Fluorinated steroids, such as dexamethasone, are the most likely to produce *steroid myopathy*. Dexamethasone alters the abundance of ceramides in myotubes in developing muscle. In patients with dermatomyositis or other myopathies treated with steroids, it is sometimes difficult to distinguish refractoriness of the disease from steroid-induced weakness, especially after long-term steroid administration. All patients who have been taking steroids for long periods develop a reversible type II myofiber atrophy; this is a *steroid effect* but is not steroid myopathy unless it progresses to become a necrotizing myopathy.

Hyperaldosteronism (Conn syndrome) is accompanied by episodic and reversible weakness similar to that of periodic paralysis. The proximal myopathy may become irreversible in chronic cases. Elevated CK levels and even myoglobinuria sometimes occur during acute attacks.

Gellerra C, Verderio E, Floridia G, et al: Assignment of the human carnitine palmitoyltransferase (CPT1) to chromosome 1p32. *Genomics* 1994;24:195.

Hilton-Jones D, Squier M, Taylor D, et al: *Metabolic Myopathies.* Philadelphia, WB Saunders, 1995.

Lestienne P, Ponsot G: Kearns-Sayre syndrome with muscle mitochondrial DNA deletion. *Lancet* 1988;1:885.

Mastaglia FL, Ojeda VJ, Sarnat HB, et al: Myopathies associated with hypothyroidism. *Aust N Z J Med* 1988;18:799.

Tsujino S, Shanske S, DiMauro S, et al: Molecular genetic heterogeneity of myophosphorylase deficiency (McArdle's disease). *N Engl J Med* 1993;329:241.

Chapter 602
Metabolic Myopathies

602.1 Periodic Paralyses (Potassium-Related)

Episodic, reversible weakness or paralysis known as *periodic paralysis* is associated with transient alterations in serum potassium levels, usually hypokalemia but occasionally hyperkalemia. All familial forms of periodic paralysis are caused by mutations in genes encoding voltage-gated ion channels in muscle: sodium, calcium, and potassium. During attacks, myofibers are electrically inexcitable, although the contractile apparatus can respond normally to calcium. The disorder is inherited as an autosomal dominant trait. It is precipitated in some patients by a heavy carbohydrate meal, insulin, adrenaline including that induced by emotional stress, hyperaldosteronism or hyperthyroidism, administration of amphotericin B, or ingestion of licorice. The defective genes are at the 17q13.1-13.3 locus in *hyperkalemic periodic paralysis*, the same as in paramyotonia congenita, and at the 1q31-32 locus in *hypokalemic periodic paralysis*.

In childhood, periodic paralysis is often an episodic event; patients are unable to move after awakening and gradually recover muscle strength during the next few minutes or hours. Muscles that remain active in sleep, such as the diaphragm and cardiac muscle, are not affected. Patients are normal between attacks, but in adult life the attacks become more frequent, and the disorder causes progressive myopathy with permanent weakness even between attacks.

Alterations in serum potassium level occur only during acute episodes and are accompanied by T-wave changes in the electrocardiogram (ECG). Hypokalemia may be due to alterations in calcium gradients. The creatine kinase (CK) level may be mildly elevated at those times. Muscle biopsy findings are often normal between attacks, but during an attack a vacuolar myopathy is demonstrated. Pathologic changes in the periodic paralyses are similar whether the disease is due to a sodium or potassium channel defect, suggesting that they may result from the recurrent paralytic state rather than the specific channelopathy. The vacuoles are dilated sarcoplasmic reticulum and invaginations of the extracellular space into the cytoplasm, and they may be filled with glycogen. Hypoglycemia does not occur.

602.2 Malignant Hyperthermia

(See also Chapters 65 and 599.4.)

This syndrome is usually inherited as an autosomal dominant trait. It occurs in all patients with central core disease but is not limited to that particular myopathy. The gene is at the 19q13.1 locus in both central core disease and malignant hyperthermia without this specific myopathy. At least 15 separate mutations in this gene are associated with malignant hyperthermia. The gene programs the ryanodine receptor, a tetrameric calcium release channel in the sarcoplasmic reticulum, apposed to the voltage-gated calcium channel of the transverse tubule. It occurs rarely in Duchenne and other muscular dystrophies, in various other myopathies, and in an isolated syndrome not associated with other muscle disease. Affected children sometimes have peculiar facies. All ages are affected, including premature infants whose mothers underwent general anesthesia for cesarean section.

Acute episodes are precipitated by exposure to general anesthetics and occasionally to local anesthetic drugs. Patients suddenly develop extreme fever, rigidity of muscles, and metabolic and respiratory acidosis; the serum CK level rises to as high as 35,000 IU/L. Myoglobinuria may result in tubular necrosis and acute renal failure.

The muscle biopsy during an episode of malignant hyperthermia or shortly afterward shows widely scattered necrosis of muscle fibers known as rhabdomyolysis. Between attacks, the muscle biopsy is normal unless there is an underlying chronic myopathy.

It is important to recognize patients at risk for malignant hyperthermia because the attacks may be prevented by administering dantrolene sodium before an anesthetic is given. Identification of patients at risk, such as siblings of those who have experienced an episode, is done by the caffeine contracture test: A portion of fresh muscle biopsy tissue in a saline bath is attached to a strain gauge and exposed to caffeine and other drugs; an abnormal spasm is diagnostic. The syndrome receptor also may be demonstrated by immunochemistry in frozen sections of the muscle biopsy. The gene defect of the ryanodine receptor is present in 50% of patients; gene testing is available only for this genetic group. Another candidate gene is at the 1q31 locus.

Apart from the genetic disorder of malignant hyperthermia, some drugs may induce acute rhabdomyolysis with myoglobinuria and potential renal failure, but this usually occurs in patients who are predisposed by some other metabolic disease. Valproic acid, for example, may induce this process in children with mitochondrial cytopathies or with carnitine palmitoyltransferase deficiency.

602.3 Glycogenoses

(See also Chapter 76.)

Glycogenosis I (von Gierke disease) is not a true myopathy because the deficient liver enzyme, glucose-6-phosphatase, is not normally present in muscle. Nevertheless, children with this disease are hypotonic and mildly weak for unknown reasons.

Glycogenosis II (Pompe disease) is an autosomal recessively inherited deficiency of the glycolytic lysosomal enzyme acid maltase. Of the 12 known glycogenoses, type II is the only one with a defective lysosomal enzyme. The defective gene is at locus 17q23. Two forms are described. The infantile form is a severe generalized myopathy and cardiomyopathy. Patients have cardiomegaly and hepatomegaly and are diffusely hypotonic and weak. The serum CK level is greatly elevated. Muscle biopsy reveals a vacuolar myopathy with abnormal lysosomal enzymatic activities such as acid and alkaline phosphatases. Death in infancy or early childhood is usual.

The late childhood or adult form is a much milder myopathy without cardiac or hepatic enlargement. It may not become clinically expressed until later childhood or early adult life but may be symptomatic as myopathic weakness and hypotonia even in early infancy. The serum CK level is greatly elevated, and the muscle biopsy findings are diagnostic even in the presymptomatic stage.

The diagnosis of glycogenosis II is confirmed by quantitative assay of acid maltase activity in muscle or liver biopsy specimens. A rare KM variant of the milder form of acid maltase deficiency may show muscle acid maltase activity in the low normal range with only intermittent decreases to subnormal values, but the muscle biopsy findings are similar although milder. In another form, *Danon disease,* transmitted as an X-linked recessive trait at the Xq24 locus, the primary deficiency is *lysosomal membrane protein-2 (LAMP2)* and results in hypertrophic cardiomyopathy, proximal myopathy, and mental retardation.

Glycogenosis III (Cori-Forbes disease), deficiency of debrancher enzyme (amylo-1,6-glucosidase), is the most common of the glycogenoses but also the least severe. Hypotonia, weakness, hepatomegaly, and fasting hypoglycemia in infancy are common, but these features often resolve spontaneously, and patients become asymptomatic in childhood and adult life. Others experience slowly progressive distal muscle wasting, hepatic cirrhosis, and heart failure. Minor myopathic findings including vacuolation of muscle fibers are found in the muscle biopsy specimen.

Glycogenosis IV (Andersen disease) is a deficiency of brancher enzyme, resulting in the formation of an abnormal glycogen molecule, amylopectin, in the liver, reticuloendothelial cells, and skeletal and cardiac muscle. Hypotonia, generalized weakness, muscle wasting, and contractures are the usual signs of myopathic involvement. Most patients die before age 4 yr because of hepatic or cardiac failure. A few children without neuromuscular manifestations have been described.

Glycogenosis V (McArdle disease) is due to muscle phosphorylase deficiency inherited as an autosomal recessive trait at locus 11q13. Exercise intolerance is the cardinal clinical feature. Physical exertion results in cramps, weakness, and myoglobinuria, but strength is normal between attacks. The serum CK level is elevated only during exercise. A characteristic clinical feature is lack of the normal rise in serum lactate level during ischemic exercise because of inability to convert pyruvate to lactate under anaerobic conditions in vivo. Myophosphorylase deficiency may be demonstrated histochemically and biochemically in the muscle biopsy tissue.

A rare *neonatal form of myophosphorylase deficiency* causes feeding difficulties in early infancy, may be severe enough to result in neonatal death, or may follow a course of slowly progressive weakness resembling a muscular dystrophy.

The long-term prognosis is good. Patients must learn to moderate their physical activities, but they do not develop severe chronic myopathic handicaps or cardiac involvement.

Glycogenosis VII (Tarui disease) is muscle phosphofructokinase deficiency. Although this disease is rarer than glycogenosis V, the symptoms of exercise intolerance, clinical course, and inability to convert pyruvate to lactate are identical. The distinction is made by biochemical study of the muscle biopsy specimen. It is transmitted as an autosomal recessive trait at the 1cenq32 locus.

602.4 Mitochondrial Myopathies

(See also Chapter 591.2.)

Several diseases involving muscle, brain, and other organs are associated with structural and functional abnormalities of mitochondria, producing defects in aerobic cellular metabolism, the electron transport chain, and the Krebs cycle. The structural aberrations are best demonstrated by electron microscopy of the muscle biopsy sample, revealing abnormally shaped cristae and fusion of cristae to form paracrystalline structures. Histochemical study of the muscle biopsy reveals abnormal clumping of oxidative enzymatic activity, sometimes increased neutral lipids because of impaired lipid metabolism, and ragged-red muscle fibers with accumulations of membranous material beneath the muscle fiber membrane, best demonstrated by special stains. These characteristic histochemical and ultrastructural changes are most consistently seen only with point mutation in mitochondrial tRNA. The large mtDNA deletions of 5 or 7.4 kb (the single mitochondrial chromosome has 16.5 kb) are associated with defects in mitochondrial respiratory oxidative enzyme complexes, if as few as 2% of the mitochondria are affected, but minimal or no morphologic or histochemical changes may be noted in the muscle biopsy specimen, even by electron microscopy; hence, the quantitative biochemical studies of the muscle tissue are needed to confirm the diagnosis.

Several distinct mitochondrial diseases that primarily affect striated muscle or muscle and brain are identified. The *Kearns-Sayre syndrome* is characterized by the triad of progressive external ophthalmoplegia, pigmentary degeneration of the retina, and onset before age 20 yr. Heart block, cerebellar deficits, and high cerebrospinal fluid protein content are often associated. Visual evoked potentials are abnormal. Patients usually do not experience weakness of the trunk or extremities or dysphagia. Most cases are sporadic.

Chronic progressive external ophthalmoplegia may be isolated or accompanied by limb muscle weakness, dysphagia, and dysarthria. A few patients described as having *ophthalmoplegia plus* have additional central nervous system (CNS) involvement. Autosomal dominant inheritance is found in some pedigrees, but most cases are sporadic.

Myoclonic epilepsy and ragged-red fibers (MERRF) and the *MELAS syndrome,* an acronym for mitochondrial myopathy, encephalopathy, lactic acidosis, and strokelike episodes, are other mitochondrial disorders affecting children. The latter is characterized by stunted growth, episodic vomiting, seizures, and recurrent cerebral insults causing hemiparesis, hemianopia or even cortical blindness, and dementia. The disease behaves as a degenerative disorder, and children die within a few years. Ragged-red fibers are characteristic of combined defects in oxidative respiratory complexes I and IV, although a few cases with complex V deficiency exhibit ragged-red fibers.

Other "degenerative" diseases of the CNS that also involve myopathy with mitochondrial abnormalities include *Leigh subacute necrotizing encephalopathy* (see Chapter 76.4) and *cerebrohepatorenal (Zellweger) disease* (see Chapter 75.2). Another recognized mitochondrial myopathy is *cytochrome-c-oxidase deficiency. Oculopharyngeal muscular dystrophy* is also fundamentally a mitochondrial myopathy. Many other rare diseases with only a few case reports are suspected of being mitochondrial disorders.

Mitochondrial DNA is distinct from the DNA of the cell nucleus and is inherited exclusively from the mother; mitochondria are present in the cytoplasm of the ovum but not in the head of the sperm, the only part that enters the ovum at fertilization. The rate of mutation of mitochondrial DNA is 10 times higher than that of nuclear DNA. The mitochondrial respiratory enzyme complexes each have subunits encoded either in mtDNA or in nuclear DNA. For example, complex II (succinate dehydrogenase, a Krebs cycle enzyme) has 4 subunits, all encoded in nuclear DNA; complex III (ubiquinol or cytochrome-b-oxidase) has 9 subunits, only one of which is encoded by mtDNA and 8 of which are programmed by nuclear DNA; complex IV (cytochrome-c-oxidase) has 13 subunits, only 3 of which are encoded by mtDNA. For this reason, mitochondrial diseases of muscle may be transmitted as autosomal recessive traits rather than by strict maternal transmission even though all mitochondria are inherited from the mother.

In the Kearns-Sayre syndrome, a single large mtDNA deletion has been identified, but other genetic variants are known; in the MERRF and MELAS syndromes of mitochondrial myopathy, point mutations occur in tRNA (see Table 599–1).

There is no effective treatment of mitochondrial cytopathies, but various "cocktails" are often used empirically to try to overcome the metabolic deficits. These include oral carnitine supplements, riboflavin, coenzyme Q_{10}, ascorbic acid (vitamin C), vitamin E, and other antioxidants. Although some anecdotal reports are encouraging, no controlled studies that prove efficacy are published.

602.5   Lipid Myopathies

(See Chapter 75.4.)

Considered as metabolic organs, skeletal muscles are the most important sites in the body for long-chain fatty acid metabolism because of their large mass and their rich density of mitochondria where fatty acids are metabolized. Hereditary disorders of lipid metabolism that cause progressive myopathy are an important, relatively common, and often treatable group of muscle diseases.

Muscle carnitine deficiency is an autosomal recessive disease involving deficient transport of dietary carnitine across the intestinal mucosa. Carnitine is acquired from dietary sources but is also synthesized in the liver and kidneys from lysine and methionine; it is the obligatory carrier of long- and medium-chain fatty acids into muscle mitochondria.

The clinical course may be one of sudden exacerbations of weakness or may resemble a progressive muscular dystrophy with generalized proximal myopathy and sometimes facial, pharyngeal, and cardiac involvement. Symptoms usually begin in late childhood or adolescence or may be delayed until adult life. Progression is slow but may end in death.

Serum CK level is mildly elevated. Muscle biopsy material shows vacuoles filled with lipid within muscle fibers in addition to nonspecific changes suggestive of a muscular dystrophy. Mitochondria may appear normal or abnormal. Carnitine measured in muscle biopsy tissue is reduced, but serum carnitine level is normal.

Treatment stops the progression of the disease and may even restore lost strength if the disease is not too advanced. It consists of special diets low in long-chain fatty acids. Steroids may enhance fatty acid transport. Specific therapy with L-carnitine taken orally in large doses overcomes the intestinal barrier in some patients. Some patients also improve when given supplementary riboflavin, and other patients seem to improve with propranolol.

Systemic carnitine deficiency is a disease of impaired renal and hepatic synthesis of carnitine rather than a primary myopathy. Patients with this autosomal recessive disease experience progressive proximal myopathy and show muscle biopsy changes similar to those of muscle carnitine deficiency; however, the onset of weakness is earlier and may be evident at birth. Endocardial fibroelastosis also may occur. Episodes of acute hepatic encephalopathy resembling Reye syndrome may occur. Hypoglycemia and metabolic acidosis complicate acute episodes.

The concentration of carnitine is reduced in serum as well as in muscle and liver. A similar clinical syndrome may be a complication of renal Fanconi syndrome, because of excessive urinary loss of carnitine or loss during chronic hemodialysis.

Treatment with L-carnitine improves the maintenance of blood glucose and serum carnitine levels but does not reverse the ketosis or acidosis or improve exercise capacity.

Muscle carnitine palmitoyltransferase (CPT) deficiency presents as episodes of rhabdomyolysis, coma, and elevated serum CK level that may be indistinguishable from Reye syndrome. CPT transfers long-chain fatty acid acyl-CoA residues to carnitine on the outer mitochondrial membrane for transport into the mitochondria. Exercise intolerance and myoglobinuria resemble glycogenoses V and VII. Fasting hypoglycemia may also occur. Genetic transmission is autosomal recessive, owing to a defect on chromosome 1 at the 1p32 locus. Administration of valproic acid may precipitate acute rhabdomyolysis with myoglobinuria in patients with CPT deficiency; it should be avoided in the treatment of seizures or migraine if they occur.

602.6   Vitamin E Deficiency Myopathy

Deficiency of vitamin E (α-tocopherol; an antioxidant also important in mitochondrial superoxide generation) in experimental animals produces a progressive myopathy closely resembling a muscular dystrophy. Myopathy and neuropathy are recognized in humans who lack adequate intake of this antioxidant. Patients with chronic malabsorption, those undergoing long-term dialysis, and premature infants who do not receive vitamin E supplements are particularly vulnerable. Treatment with high doses of vitamin E may reverse the deficiency. Myopathy due to chronic hypervitaminosis E also occurs.

Cannon SC: An expanding view for the molecular basis of familial periodic paralysis. *Neuromusc Disord* 2000;12:533.

Chow CK: Vitamin E regulation of mitochondrial superoxide generation. *Biol Signals Recept* 2001;10:112.

Kottlors M, Jaksch M, Ketelsen U-P, et al: Valproic acid triggers acute rhabdomyolysis in a patient with carnitine palmitoyltransferase type II deficiency. *Neuromusc Disord* 2001;11:757.

Nishino I, Yamamoto A, Sugie K, et al: Danon disease and related disorders. *Acta Myologica* 2001;20:120.

Chapter 603

Disorders of Neuromuscular Transmission and of Motor Neurons

603.1   Myasthenia Gravis

Myasthenia gravis is a disease caused by an immune-mediated neuromuscular blockade. The release of acetylcholine (ACh) into the synaptic cleft by the axonal terminal is normal, but the postsynaptic muscle membrane or *motor end plate* is less responsive than normal. A decreased number of available ACh receptors is due to circulating receptor-binding antibodies in most cases of acquired myasthenia. The disease is generally nonhereditary and is an autoimmune disorder. A rare familial myasthenia gravis is probably an autosomal recessive trait and is not associated with plasma anti-ACh antibodies. One familial form is a deficiency of motor end plate ACh, designated AChE. Infants born to myasthenic mothers may have a transient neonatal myasthenic syndrome secondary to placentally transferred anti-ACh receptor antibodies, distinct from congenital myasthenia gravis.

Clinical Manifestations. Ptosis and some degree of extraocular muscle weakness are the earliest and most constant signs in myasthenia gravis. Older children may complain of diplopia, and young children may hold open their eyes with their fingers or thumbs if the ptosis is severe enough to obstruct vision. The pupillary responses to light are preserved. Dysphagia and facial weakness are also common, and in early infancy feeding difficulties are often the cardinal sign of myasthenia. Poor head control because of weakness of the neck flexors is also prominent. Involvement may be limited to bulbar-innervated muscles, but the disease is systemic and weakness involves limb-girdle muscles and distal muscles of the hands in most cases. Fasciculations of muscle, myalgias, and sensory symptoms do not occur. Tendon stretch reflexes may be diminished but are rarely lost.

Rapid fatigue of muscles is a characteristic feature of myasthenia gravis that distinguishes it from most other neuromuscular diseases. Ptosis increases progressively as patients are asked to sustain an upward gaze for 30–90 sec. Holding the head up from the surface of the examining table while lying supine is very difficult, and gravity cannot be overcome for more than a few seconds. Repetitive opening and closing of the fists produces rapid fatigue of hand muscles, and patients cannot elevate their arms for more than 1–2 min because of fatigue of the deltoids. Patients are more symptomatic late in the day or when tired. Dysphagia may interfere with eating, and the muscles of the jaw soon tire when an affected child chews.

If untreated, myasthenia gravis is usually progressive and may become life threatening because of respiratory muscle involvement and the risk of aspiration, particularly at times when the child is otherwise unwell with an upper respiratory tract infection. Familial myasthenia gravis usually is not progressive.

Infants born to myasthenic mothers may have respiratory insufficiency, inability to suck or swallow, and generalized hypotonia and weakness. They may show little spontaneous motor activity for several days to weeks. Some require ventilatory support and feeding by gavage during this period. After the abnormal antibodies disappear, the infants have normal strength and are not at increased risk for developing myasthenia gravis in later childhood. The syndrome of *transient neonatal myasthenia gravis* is to be distinguished from a rare and often hereditary *congenital myasthenia gravis* not related to maternal myasthenia that is nearly always a permanent disorder without spontaneous remission. Three presynaptic congenital myasthenic syndromes are recognized, all as autosomal recessive traits, but their molecular genetic basis remains unknown. Another synaptic form is caused by absence or marked deficiency of AChE in the synaptic basal lamina, and postsynaptic forms of congenital myasthenia are caused by mutations in AChR (acetylcholine receptor) subunit genes that alter the synaptic response to ACh. An abnormality of the ACh receptor channels appearing as high conductance and excessively fast closure may be the result of a point mutation in a subunit of the receptor affecting a single amino acid residue. Children with congenital myasthenia gravis do not experience myasthenic crises and rarely exhibit elevations of anti-ACh antibodies in plasma.

Myasthenia gravis is occasionally secondary to hypothyroidism, usually due to *Hashimoto thyroiditis*. Other collagen vascular diseases may also be associated. Thymomas, noted in some adults, rarely coexist with myasthenia gravis in children; nor do carcinomas of the lung occur, which produce a unique form of myasthenia in adults, the *Eaton-Lambert syndrome*.

Laboratory Findings and Diagnosis. Myasthenia gravis is one of the few neuromuscular diseases in which an *electromyogram* (EMG) is more specifically diagnostic than a muscle biopsy. A decremental response is seen in response to repetitive nerve stimulation; the muscle potentials diminish rapidly in amplitude until the muscle becomes refractory to further stimulation. Motor nerve conduction velocity remains normal. This unique EMG pattern is the electrophysiologic correlate of the fatigable weak-

ness observed clinically and is reversed after a cholinesterase inhibitor is administered. A myasthenic decrement may be absent or difficult to demonstrate in muscles that are not involved clinically. This feature may be confusing in early cases or in patients showing only weakness of extraocular muscles. Microelectrode studies of end plate potentials and currents reveal whether the transmission defect is presynaptic or postsynaptic. Special electrophysiologic studies are required in the classification of congenital myasthenic syndromes and involve the estimation of the number of AChR per end-plate and in vitro study of end plate function. These special studies and patch-clamp recordings of kinetic properties of channels are performed on special biopsies of intercostal muscle strips that include both origin and insertion of the muscle but are only performed in specialized centers.

Anti-ACh antibodies should be assayed in the plasma but are inconsistently demonstrated. About one third of adolescents show elevations, but anti-ACh receptor antibodies are only occasionally demonstrated in the plasma of prepubertal children. Other serologic tests of autoimmune disease, such as antinuclear antibodies and abnormal immune complexes, should also be sought. If these are positive, more extensive autoimmune disease involving vasculitis or tissues other than muscle is likely. A thyroid profile should always be examined. The serum creatine kinase (CK) level is normal in myasthenia gravis.

The heart is not involved, and the electrocardiogram (ECG) findings remain normal. Roentgenograms of the chest often reveal an enlarged thymus, but the hypertrophy is not a *thymoma*. It may be further defined by tomography or by CT scanning of the anterior mediastinum.

The role of conventional *muscle biopsy* in myasthenia gravis is limited. It is not required in most cases, but about 17% of patients show inflammatory changes sometimes called *lymphorrhages* that are interpreted by some physicians as a mixed myasthenia-polymyositis immune disorder. Muscle biopsy tissue in myasthenia gravis shows nonspecific type II muscle fiber atrophy, similar to that seen with disuse atrophy, steroid effects on muscle, polymyalgia rheumatica, and many other conditions. The ultrastructure of motor end plates shows simplification of the membrane folds.

A *clinical test for myasthenia gravis* is administration of a short-acting cholinesterase inhibitor, usually edrophonium chloride. Ptosis and ophthalmoplegia improve within a few seconds, and fatigability of other muscles decreases.

RECOMMENDATIONS ON THE USE OF CHOLINESTERASE INHIBITORS AS A DIAGNOSTIC TEST FOR MYASTHENIA GRAVIS IN INFANTS AND CHILDREN
For Children 2 Yr of Age or Older

1. Child should have a specific fatigable weakness that can be measured, such as ptosis of the eyelids, dysphagia, inability of cervical muscles to support head; nonspecific generalized weakness without cranial nerve motor deficits is not a criterion.

2. An intravenous infusion should be started to enable the administration of medications in the event of an adverse reaction.

3. ECG monitoring during test is recommended.

4. A dose of atropine sulfate (0.01 mg/kg) should be available in a syringe, ready for intravenous administration at the bedside during the edrophonium test, to block acute muscarinic effects of the cholinesterase inhibitor (mainly abdominal cramps and/or sudden diarrhea from increased peristalsis, profuse bronchotracheal secretions that may obstruct the airway, or, rarely, cardiac arrhythmias, if needed. Some physicians pretreat all patients with atropine before administering edrophonium, but this is not recommended unless there is a history of reaction from previous tests. Remember that atropine may cause the pupils to be dilated and fixed for as long as 14 days after a single dose, and the pupillary effects of homatropine may last 4–7 days.

5. Edrophonium chloride (Tensilon) is administered intravenously. Initially, a test dose of 0.04 mg/kg is given to ensure that the patient does not have an allergic reaction or is otherwise very sensitive to muscarinic side effects. If this test dose is well tolerated, the diagnostic dose administered is 0.1 to 0.2 mg/kg (maximum single dose 10 mg, regardless of weight; in children weighing less than 30 kg, 2 mg is the maximum dose; a typical dose for a 3–5-yr-old child is 5 mg). These same doses may be given intramuscularly or subcutaneously, but these routes are not recommended because the results are much more variable because of unpredictable absorption, and the test may be ambiguous or falsely negative.

6. Effects should be seen within 10 seconds and disappear within 120 seconds; weakness is measured (e.g., distance between upper and lower eyelids before and after administration; degree of external ophthalmoplegia; ability to swallow a sip of water).

7. Long-acting cholinesterase inhibitors, such as pyridostigmine (Mestinon) are generally not as useful for the acute assessment of myasthenic weakness. The prostigmine test may be used (as outlined later) but may not be as definitively diagnostic as the edrophonium test.

For Infants Younger than 2 Yr of Age

1. Infant ideally should have a specific fatigable weakness that can be measured, such as ptosis of the eyelids, dysphagia, inability of cervical muscles to support head; nonspecific generalized weakness without cranial nerve motor deficits is less easy to assess results but may be a criterion at times.

2. An intravenous infusion should be started as a rapid route for medications in the event of an adverse effect of the test medication.

3. ECG monitoring is recommended during test.

4. Pretreatment with atropine sulfate to block the muscarinic effects of the test medication is not recommended but should be available at the bedside in a prepared syringe. If needed, it should be administered intravenously in a dose of 0.1 mg/kg.

5. Edrophonium is not recommended for use in infants; its effect is too brief for objective assessment and an increased incidence of acute cardiac arrhythmias is reported in infants, especially neonates, with this drug.

6. Prostigmine methylsulfate (Neostigmine) is administered intramuscularly at a dose of 0.04 mg/kg; if the result is negative or equivocal, another dose of 0.04 mg/kg may be administered 4 hours after the first dose (a typical dose is 0.5–1.5 mg). The peak effect is seen in 20–40 minutes. Intravenous prostigmine is not recommended because of risk of cardiac arrhythmias.

7. Long-acting cholinesterase inhibitors administered orally, such as pyridostigmine (Mestinon), are generally not as useful for the acute assessment of myasthenic weakness because onset and duration are less predictable.

WHERE SHOULD TEST BE PERFORMED? The setting may be the emergency department, hospital ward, or, at times, a physician's office; the important issue is preparation for potential complications such as cardiac arrhythmia or cholinergic crisis, as previously outlined.

Treatment. Some patients with mild myasthenia gravis require no treatment. *Cholinesterase-inhibiting drugs* are the primary therapeutic agents. Neostigmine methylsulfate (0.04 mg/kg) may be given intramuscularly every 4–6 hr, but most patients tolerate oral neostigmine bromide, 0.4 mg/kg every 4–6 hr. If dysphagia is a major problem, the drug should be given about 30 min before meals to improve swallowing. Pyridostigmine is an alternative; the dose required is about four times greater than that of neostigmine, but it may be slightly longer acting. Overdoses of cholinesterase inhibitors produce cholinergic crises; atropine blocks the muscarinic effects but does not block the nicotinic effects that produce additional skeletal muscle weakness. In the

rare familial myasthenia gravis caused by absence of end-plate AChE, cholinesterase inhibitors are not helpful and often cause increased weakness; these patients can be treated with ephedrine or with an experimental drug, diaminopyridine (DAP), both of which increase ACh release from terminal axons.

Because of the autoimmune basis of the disease, long-term *steroid treatment* with prednisone may be effective. *Thymectomy* should be considered and may provide a cure. Thymectomy is most effective in patients with high titers of anti-ACh-receptor antibodies in the plasma and who are symptomatic for less than 2 yr. Thymectomy is ineffective in congenital and familial forms of myasthenia gravis. Treatment of hypothyroidism usually abolishes an associated myasthenia without the use of cholinesterase inhibitors or steroids.

Plasmapheresis is effective treatment in some children, particularly those who do not respond to steroids, but plasma exchange therapy may provide only temporary remission. *Intravenous immunoglobulin* (IVIG) is sometimes beneficial and might be tried before plasmapheresis because it is less invasive. Both plasmapheresis and IVIG appear to be most effective in patients with high circulating levels of anti-ACh receptor antibodies.

Neonates with transient maternally transmitted myasthenia gravis require cholinesterase inhibitors for only a few days or occasionally for a few weeks, especially to allow feeding. No other treatment is usually necessary.

Complications. Children with myasthenia gravis do not tolerate neuromuscular blocking drugs, such as succinylcholine and pancuronium, and may be paralyzed for weeks after a single dose. An anesthesiologist should carefully review myasthenic patients who require a surgical anesthetic. Also, certain antibiotics may potentiate myasthenia and should be avoided; these include the aminoglycosides (gentamicin and others).

Prognosis. This is difficult to predict. Some patients undergo spontaneous remission after a period of months or years; others have a permanent disease extending into adult life. Immunosuppression, thymectomy, and treatment of associated hypothyroidism may provide a cure.

OTHER CAUSES OF NEUROMUSCULAR BLOCKADE

Organophosphate chemicals, commonly used as insecticides, may cause a myasthenia-like syndrome in children exposed to these toxins (see Chapter 704).

Botulism results from ingestion of food containing the toxin of *Clostridium botulinum*, a gram-positive, spore-bearing, anaerobic bacillus (see Chapter 193). Honey is a frequent source of contamination. The incubation period is short, only a few hours, and symptoms begin with nausea, vomiting, and diarrhea. Cranial nerve involvement soon follows, with diplopia, dysphagia, weak suck, facial weakness, and absent gag reflex. Generalized hypotonia and weakness then develop and may progress to respiratory failure. Neuromuscular blockade is documented by EMG with repetitive nerve stimulation. Respiratory support may be required for days or weeks until the toxin is cleared from the body. No specific antitoxin is available. Guanidine, 35 mg/kg/24 hr, may be effective for extraocular and limb muscle weakness but not for respiratory muscle involvement.

Tick paralysis is a disorder of ACh release from axonal terminals due to a neurotoxin that blocks depolarization. It also affects large myelinated motor and sensory nerve fibers. This toxin is produced by the wood tick or dog tick, insects common in the Appalachian and Rocky Mountains of North America. The tick embeds its head into the skin, usually the scalp, and neurotoxin production is maximal about 5–6 days later. Motor symptoms include weakness, loss of coordination, and sometimes an ascending paralysis resembling Guillain-Barré syndrome. Tendon reflexes are lost. Sensory symptoms of tingling paresthesias may occur in the face and extremities. The diagnosis is confirmed by EMG and nerve conduction studies and by identifying the tick. The tick must be removed completely, and the buried head not left beneath the skin. Patients then recover completely within hours or days.

603.2 ■ Spinal Muscular Atrophies

Spinal muscular atrophies (SMA) are degenerative diseases of motor neurons that begin in fetal life and continue to be progressive in infancy and childhood. The progressive denervation of muscle is compensated in part by re-innervation from an adjacent motor unit, but giant motor units are thus created with subsequent atrophy of muscle fibers when the re-innervating motor neuron eventually becomes involved. Upper motor neurons remain normal.

SMA is classified into a severe infantile form, also known as *Werdnig-Hoffmann disease* or SMA type 1; a late infantile and more slowly progressive form, SMA type 2; and a more chronic or juvenile form, also called *Kugelberg-Welander disease*, or SMA type 3. These distinctions are clinical and are based on age at onset, severity of weakness, and clinical course; muscle biopsy does not distinguish types 1 and 2, although type 3 shows a more adult than perinatal pattern of denervation/re-innervation. Some patients are transitional between types 1 and 2 or between types 2 and 3 in terms of clinical function. A variant of SMA, *Fazio-Londe disease*, is a progressive bulbar palsy resulting from motor neuron degeneration more in the brain stem than the spinal cord.

Etiology. The cause of SMA is a pathologic continuation of a process of programmed cell death that is normal in embryonic life. A surplus of motor neuroblasts and other neurons is generated from primitive neuroectoderm, but only about half survive and mature to become neurons; the excess cells have a limited life cycle and degenerate. If the process that arrests physiologic cell death fails to intervene by a certain stage, neuronal death may continue in late fetal life and postnatally. The survivor motor neuron *(SMN)* gene arrests apoptosis (programmed cell death) of motor neuroblasts. Unlike most genes that are highly conserved in evolution, *SMN* is a unique mammalian gene.

Clinical Manifestations. The cardinal features of SMA type 1 are severe hypotonia; generalized weakness; thin muscle mass; absent tendon stretch reflexes; involvement of the tongue, face, and jaw muscles; and sparing of extraocular muscles and sphincters. Infants who are symptomatic at birth may have respiratory distress and are unable to feed. Congenital contractures, ranging from simple clubfoot to generalized arthrogryposis, occur in about 10% of severely involved neonates. Infants lie flaccid with little movement, unable to overcome gravity. They lack head control. More than two thirds die by 2 yr of age, and many die early in infancy.

In type 2 SMA, affected infants are usually able to suck and swallow and respiration is adequate in early infancy. These infants show progressive weakness, but many survive into the school years or beyond, although confined to an electric wheelchair and severely handicapped. Nasal speech and problems with deglutition develop later. Scoliosis becomes a major complication in many patients with long survival.

Kugelberg-Welander disease is the mildest SMA (type 3), and patients may appear normal in infancy. The progressive weakness is proximal in distribution, particularly involving shoulder girdle muscles. Patients are ambulatory. Symptoms of bulbar muscle weakness are rare. About 25% of patients with this form of SMA have muscular hypertrophy rather than atrophy, and it may easily be confused with a muscular dystrophy. Longevity may extend well into middle adult life. Fasciculations are a specific clinical sign of denervation of muscle. In thin children, they

may be seen in the deltoid, biceps brachii, and occasionally the quadriceps femoris, but the continuous involuntary wormlike movements may be masked by a thick pad of subcutaneous fat. Fasciculations are best observed in the tongue, where almost no subcutaneous connective tissue separates the muscular layer from the epithelium. If the intrinsic lingual muscles are contracted, such as in crying or when the tongue protrudes, fasciculations are more difficult to see than when the tongue is relaxed.

The outstretched fingers of children with SMA often show a characteristic tremor owing to fasciculations and weakness. It should not be confused with a cerebellar tremor. Myalgias are not a feature of SMA.

The heart is not involved in SMA. Intelligence is normal, and children often appear brighter than their normal peers because the effort they cannot put into physical activities is redirected to intellectual development, and they are often exposed to adult speech more than to juvenile language because of the social repercussions of the disease.

Laboratory Findings. The serum CK level may be normal but more commonly is mildly elevated in the hundreds. A CK level of several thousand is rare. Results of motor nerve conduction studies are normal, except for mild slowing in terminal stages of the disease, an important feature distinguishing SMA from peripheral neuropathy. The EMG shows fibrillation potentials and other signs of denervation of muscle.

Diagnosis. The simplest, most definitive diagnostic test is a molecular genetic marker in blood for the *SMN* gene. Muscle biopsy reveals a characteristic pattern of perinatal denervation that is unlike that of mature muscle. Groups of giant type I fibers are mixed with fascicles of severely atrophic fibers of both histochemical types (Fig. 603–1). Scattered immature myofibers resembling myotubes also are demonstrated. In juvenile SMA, the pattern may be more similar to adult muscle that has undergone many cycles of denervation and re-innervation. Neurogenic changes in muscle also may be demonstrated by EMG, but the results are less definitive than by muscle biopsy in infancy. Sural nerve biopsy sometimes shows mild sensory neuropathic changes, and sensory nerve conduction

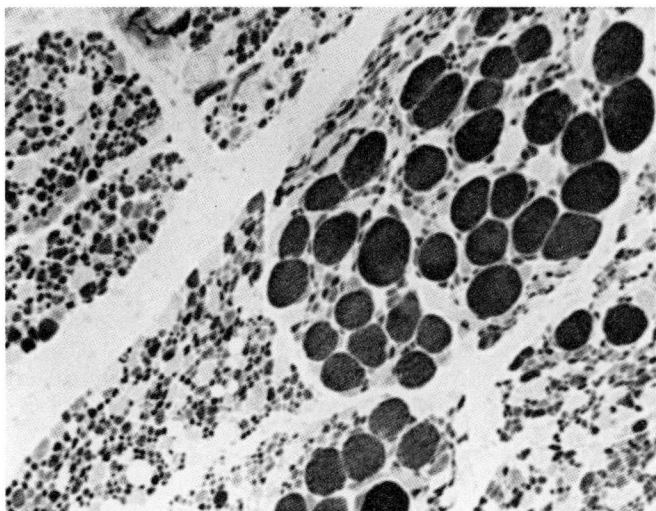

FIGURE 603–1. Muscle biopsy of neonate with infantile spinal muscular atrophy. Groups of giant type I (darkly stained) fibers are seen within muscle fascicles of severely atrophic fibers of both histochemical types. This is the characteristic pattern of perinatal denervation of muscle. Myofibrillar ATPase, preincubated at pH 4.6. (×400.)

velocity may be slowed. At autopsy, mild degenerative changes are seen in sensory neurons of dorsal root ganglia and in somatosensory nuclei of the thalamus, but these alterations are not perceived clinically as sensory loss or paresthesias. The most pronounced neuropathologic lesions are the extensive neuronal degeneration and gliosis in the ventral horns of the spinal cord and brain stem motor nuclei, especially the hypoglossal nucleus.

Genetics. Molecular genetic diagnosis by DNA probes in blood samples or in muscle biopsy or chorionic villi tissues is available not only for diagnosis of suspected cases but also for prenatal diagnosis. Most cases are inherited as an autosomal recessive trait. The incidence of SMA is 10–15 per 100,000 live births, affecting all ethnic groups; it is the second most common neuromuscular disease, following Duchenne muscular dystrophy. The incidence of heterozygosity for autosomal recessive SMA is 1:50. The genetic locus for all three of the common forms of SMA is on chromosome 5, a deletion at the 5q11-q13 locus, indicating that they are variants of the same disease rather than different diseases. The affected *SMN* gene contains 8 exons that span 20 kb, with telomeric and centromeric exons that differ only by 5 bp and produce a transcript encoding 294 amino acids. Another gene, the *neuronal apoptosis inhibitory gene (NAIP)* is located next to the *SMN* gene and in many cases there is an inverted duplication with two copies, telomeric and centromeric, of both genes; isolated mutations or deletions of *NAIP* do not produce clinical SMA.

Infrequent families with autosomal dominant inheritance are described, and a rare X-linked recessive form is reported. Carrier testing by dosage analysis is available.

Treatment. No medical treatment is able to delay the progression. Supportive therapy includes orthopedic care with particular attention to scoliosis and joint contractures, mild physiotherapy, and mechanical aids for assisting the child to eat and to be as functionally independent as possible. Most children learn to use a computer keyboard with great skill but cannot use a pencil easily.

603.3 Other Motor Neuron Diseases

Motor neuron diseases other than SMA are rare in children. *Poliomyelitis* used to be a major cause of chronic disability, but since the routine use of polio vaccine, this viral infection is now rare (see Chapter 228). *Other enteroviruses*, such as Coxsackieviruses and Echoviruses, or the live polio vaccine virus, may also cause an acute infection of motor neurons with symptoms and signs similar to poliomyelitis, although usually milder. Specific polymerase chain reaction tests and viral cultures of cerebrospinal fluid are diagnostic.

A *juvenile form of amyotrophic lateral sclerosis* is rare. Upper motor neuron loss as well as lower motor neuron loss is evident clinically, unlike SMA. The course is progressive and is ultimately fatal.

The *Pena-Shokeir* and *Marden-Walker syndromes* are progressive motor neuron degenerations associated with severe arthrogryposis and congenital anomalies of many organ systems. *Pontocerebellar hypoplasias* are progressive degenerative diseases of the central nervous system that begin in fetal life; one form also involves motor neuron degeneration resembling a spinal muscular atrophy, but the *SMN* gene or chromosome 5 is normal.

Motor neurons become involved in several metabolic diseases of the nervous system, such as gangliosidosis (Tay-Sachs disease), ceroid lipofuscinosis (Batten disease), and glycogenosis II (Pompe disease), but the signs of denervation may be minor or obscured by the more prominent involvement of other parts of the central nervous system or of muscle.

Disorders of Neuromuscular Transmission

Afifi AK, Bell WE: Tests for juvenile myasthenia gravis: Comparative diagnostic yield and prediction of outcome. *J Child Neurol* 1993;8:403.

Anlar B, Özdirim E, Renda Y, et al: Myasthenia gravis in childhood. *Acta Paediatr* 1996;85:838.

Engel AG, Olino K, Stans AA: Congenital myasthenic syndromes. In Deymeer F (editor): Neuromuscular Disorders: From Basic Mechanisms to Clinical Management. *Monogr Clin Neurosci* 2000;18:96–112.

Milstein JM, Sarnat HB: Myasthenia gravis. In Burg FD, Ingelfinger JR, Wald ER, Polin RA (editors): *Current Pediatric Therapy,* 16th ed. Philadelphia, WB Saunders, 1999, pp 949–51.

Spinal Muscular Atrophies

Hageman G, Willemse J, van Ketel BA, et al: The heterogeneity of the Pena-Shokeir syndrome. *Neuropediatrics* 1987;18:45.

Hausmanowa-Petrusewicz I, Zaremba J: Proximal spinal muscular atrophy of childhood. In Deymeer F (editor): Neuromuscular Disorders: From Basic Mechanisms to Clinical Management. *Monogr Clin Neurosci* 2000;18:163–76.

Roy N, Mahedevan N, McLean M, et al: The gene for neuronal apoptosis inhibitory protein is partially deleted in individuals with spinal muscular atrophy. *Cell* 1995;80:167.

Sees JN Jr, Towfighi J, Robins DB, et al: Marden-Walker syndrome: Neuropathologic findings in two siblings. *Pediatr Pathol* 1990;10:807.

Souchon F, Simard LR, Lebrun S, et al: Clinical and genetic study of chronic (types II and III) childhood onset spinal muscular atrophy. *Neuromuscul Disord* 1996;6:419.

Talbot K: What's new in the molecular genetics of spinal muscular atrophy? *Eur J Paediatr Neurol* 1997;5/6:149.

Chapter 604
Hereditary Motor-Sensory Neuropathies

The hereditary motor-sensory neuropathies (HMSN) are a group of progressive diseases of peripheral nerves. Motor components generally dominate the clinical picture, but sensory and autonomic involvement are expressed later.

604.1 Peroneal Muscular Atrophy (Charcot-Marie-Tooth Disease; HMSN Type I)

This disease is the most common genetically determined neuropathy and has an overall prevalence of 3.8/100,000. It is transmitted as an autosomal dominant trait with 83% expressivity; the 17p11.2 locus is the site of the abnormal gene. The gene product is *peripheral myelin protein P22* (PMP22). A much rarer X-linked HMSN type I results from a defect at the Xq13.1 locus, causing mutations in the gap junction protein *connexin-32.*

Clinical Manifestations. Most patients are asymptomatic until late childhood or early adolescence, but young children sometimes show signs of gait disturbance as early as the 2nd yr. The peroneal and tibial nerves are the earliest and most severely affected. Children with the disorder are often described as being clumsy, falling easily, or tripping over their own feet. The onset of symptoms may be delayed until after the 5th decade.

Muscles of the anterior compartment of the lower legs become wasted, and the legs have a characteristic storklike contour. The muscular atrophy is accompanied by progressive weakness of dorsiflexion of the ankle and eventual footdrop. The process is bilateral but may be slightly asymmetric. Pes cavus deformities may develop because of denervation of intrinsic foot muscles, further destabilizing the gait. Atrophy of muscles of the forearms and hands is usually not as severe as that of the lower extremities, but in advanced cases contractures of the wrists and fingers produce a claw hand. Proximal muscle weakness is a late manifestation and is usually mild. Axial muscles are not involved.

The disease is slowly progressive throughout life, but patients occasionally show accelerated deterioration of function over a few years. Most patients remain ambulatory and have normal longevity, although orthotic appliances are required to stabilize the ankles.

Sensory involvement mainly affects large myelinated nerve fibers that convey proprioceptive information and vibratory sense, but the threshold for pain and temperature may also increase. Some children complain of tingling or burning sensations of the feet, but pain is rare. Because the muscle mass is reduced, the nerves are more vulnerable to trauma or compression. Autonomic manifestations may be expressed as poor vasomotor control with blotching or pallor of the skin of the feet and inappropriately cold feet.

Nerves often become palpably enlarged. Tendon stretch reflexes are lost distally. Cranial nerves are not affected. Sphincter control remains well preserved. Autonomic neuropathy does not affect the heart, gastrointestinal tract, or bladder. Intelligence is normal.

Davidenkow syndrome is a variant of HMSN type I with a scapuloperoneal distribution.

Laboratory Findings and Diagnosis. Motor and sensory nerve conduction velocities are greatly reduced, sometimes as slow as 20% of normal conduction time. In new cases without a family history, both parents should be examined, and nerve conduction studies should be performed.

Electromyography (EMG) and muscle biopsy are not usually required for diagnosis, but they show evidence of many cycles of denervation and reinnervation. Serum creatine kinase (CK) level is normal. Cerebrospinal fluid (CSF) protein may be elevated, but no cells appear in the CSF.

Sural nerve biopsy is diagnostic. Large- and medium-sized myelinated fibers are reduced in number, collagen is increased, and characteristic *onion bulb formations* of proliferated Schwann cell cytoplasm surround axons. This pathologic finding is called *interstitial hypertrophic neuropathy*. Extensive segmental demyelination and remyelination also occur.

The definitive molecular genetic diagnosis may be made in blood.

Treatment. Stabilization of the ankles is a primary concern. In early stages, stiff boots that extend to the mid-calf often suffice, particularly when patients walk on uneven surfaces such as ice and snow or stones. As the dorsiflexors of the ankles weaken further, lightweight plastic splints may be custom made to extend beneath the foot and around the back of the ankle. They are worn inside the socks and are not visible, reducing self-consciousness. External short-leg braces may be required when footdrop becomes complete. Surgical fusion of the ankle may be considered in some cases.

The leg should be protected from traumatic injury. In advanced cases, compression neuropathy during sleep may be prevented by placing soft pillows beneath or between the lower legs. Burning paresthesias of the feet are not common but are often abolished by phenytoin or carbamazepine. No medical treatment is available to arrest or slow the progression.

604.2 Peroneal Muscular Atrophy (Axonal Type)

This disease is clinically similar to HMSN type I, but the rate of progression is slower and the disability is less. EMG shows denervation of muscle. Sural nerve biopsy reveals axonal degeneration rather than the demyelination and whorls of Schwann cell processes typical in type I. The locus is on chromosome 1 at 1p35-p36; this is a different disease than HMSN type I, although both are transmitted as autosomal dominant traits.

604.3 Dejerine-Sottas Disease (HMSN Type III)

This interstitial hypertrophic neuropathy of autosomal dominant transmission is similar to HMSN type I but is more severe. Symptoms develop in early infancy and are rapidly progressive. Pupillary abnormalities, such as lack of reaction to light or *Argyll Robertson pupil*, are common. Kyphoscoliosis and pes cavus deformities complicate about 35% of cases. Nerves become palpably enlarged at an early age.

The onion-bulb formations seen in the sural nerve biopsy specimen are more pronounced. Hypomyelination also occurs.

The genetic locus of 17p11.2 is identical to that of HMSN type I or Charcot-Marie-Tooth disease. The clinical and pathologic differences may be phenotypic variants of the same disease, analogous to the situation in Duchenne and Becker muscular dystrophies. An autosomal recessive form of Dejerine-Sottas disease is also described but is incompletely documented.

604.4 Roussy-Lévy Syndrome

This syndrome is defined as a combination of HMSN type I and cerebellar deficit resembling Friedreich ataxia, but it does not have cardiomyopathy.

604.5 Refsum Disease

(See Chapter 75.2.)

This rare disease is due to an enzymatic block in β-oxidation of phytanic acid to pristanic acid. Phytanic acid is a branched-chain fatty acid that is derived mainly from dietary sources: spinach, nuts, and coffee. Levels of phytanic acid are greatly elevated in plasma, CSF, and brain tissue. The CSF shows an albuminocytologic dissociation with a protein concentration of 100–600 mg/dL.

Clinical onset is usually between 4 and 7 yr of age, with intermittent motor and sensory neuropathy. Ataxia, progressive neurosensory hearing loss, retinitis pigmentosa and loss of night vision, ichthyosis, and liver dysfunction also develop in various degrees. Motor and sensory nerve conduction velocities are delayed. Treatment is by dietary management and periodic plasma exchange.

604.6 Fabry Disease

(See Chapter 75.4.)

This rare X-linked recessive trait results in storage of *ceramide trihexose* because of deficiency of the enzyme *ceramide trihexosidase*, which cleaves the terminal galactose from ceramide trihexose (ceramide-glucose-galactose-galactose), resulting in tissue accumulation of this trihexose lipid in central nervous system (CNS) neurons, Schwann cells and perineurial cells, ganglion cells of the myenteric plexus, skin, kidneys, blood vessel endothelial and smooth muscle cells, heart, sweat glands, cornea, and bone marrow.

Clinical Manifestations. The presentation is in late childhood or adolescence, with recurrent episodes of burning pain and paresthesias of the feet and lower legs so severe that patients are unable to walk. These episodes are often precipitated by fever or by physical activity. Objective sensory and motor deficits are not demonstrated on neurologic examination, and reflexes are preserved. Characteristic skin lesions are seen in the perineal region, scrotum, buttocks, and periumbilical zone as flat or raised red-black telangiectases known as *angiokeratoma corporis diffusum*. Hypohidrosis may be present. Corneal opacities, cataracts, and necrosis of the femoral heads are inconstant features. The disease is progressive. Hypertension and renal failure are usually delayed until early adult life. Recurrent strokes result from vascular wall involvement. Death occurs in the 5th decade owing to cerebral infarction or renal failure.

Laboratory Findings. Motor and sensory nerve conduction velocities are normal to only mildly slow, showing preservation of large myelinated nerve fibers. CSF protein is normal. Proteinuria is present early in the course.

Pathologic features are usually first detected in skin or sural nerve biopsy specimens. Crystalline glycosphingolipids appear as *zebra bodies* in lysosomes of endothelial cells, in smooth myocytes of arterioles, and in Schwann cells, best demonstrated by electron microscopy. Nerves show a selective loss of small myelinated fibers and relative preservation of large and medium-sized axons, contrasting to most axonal neuropathies in which large myelinated fibers are most involved.

Assay for the deficient enzyme may be performed from skin fibroblasts, leukocytes, and other tissues. This test permits detection of the asymptomatic female carrier state and provides a reliable means of prenatal diagnosis.

Treatment. See Chapter 75.4.

604.7 Giant Axonal Neuropathy

This rare autosomal recessive disease with onset in early childhood is a progressive mixed peripheral neuropathy and degeneration of central white matter, similar to the leukodystrophies. Ataxia and nystagmus are accompanied by signs of progressive peripheral neuropathy. Some affected children have frizzy hair, which microscopically shows variation in diameter of the shaft or may appear normal. Focal axonal enlargements are seen in both the peripheral nervous system and the CNS, but the myelin sheath is intact. The disease is a general proliferation of intermediate filaments, including neurofilaments in axons, glial filaments (i.e., Rosenthal fibers) in brain, cytokeratin in hair, and vimentin in Schwann cells and fibroblasts. A homozygous mutation in the *GAN* gene at 16q24 is responsible for defective synthesis of the protein gygaxonin.

604.8 Congenital Hypomyelinating Neuropathy

This disorder is a lack of normal myelination of motor and sensory peripheral nerves but not of CNS white matter. It is not a degeneration or loss of previously formed myelin, thus differentiating it from a leukodystrophy. Schwann cells are preserved, and axons are normal. Cases in siblings suggest autosomal recessive inheritance.

The condition is present from birth; hypotonia and developmental delay are the hallmark clinical findings. Many patients present clinically as having congenital insensitivity to pain. Cranial nerves are inconsistently involved, and respiratory distress and dysphagia are rare complications. Tendon reflexes are absent. Arthrogryposis is present at birth in at least half the cases. It is uncertain whether the condition is progressive; myelination of nerves proceeds at a slow rate and remains incomplete. Motor and sensory nerve conduction velocities are slow. The diagnosis is confirmed by sural nerve biopsy, which shows lack of myelination of large and small fibers and sometimes interstitial hypertrophic reactive changes. Muscle biopsy may show mild neurogenic atrophy but not the characteristic alterations of spinal muscular atrophy. No inflammation is demonstrated in muscle or nerve. Treatment is supportive.

604.9 Tomaculous Neuropathy

This hereditary neuropathy is characterized by redundant overproduction of myelin around each axon in an irregular segmental fashion so that tomaculous (i.e., sausage-shaped) bulges occur in the individual myelinated nerve fibers. The nerves are particularly prone to pressure palsies, and patients present with recurrent mononeuropathies secondary to minor trauma. It is transmitted as an autosomal dominant trait, and the locus has been identified at 17p11.2. Sural nerve biopsy is diagnostic, but special "teased fiber" preparations should be made to demonstrate the myelin abnormalities most clearly. The genetic defect is a deletion of exons in the *PMP22* gene. Treatment is supportive.

604.10 Leukodystrophies

Several hereditary degenerative diseases of white matter of the CNS also cause peripheral neuropathy. The most important are Krabbe disease (globoid cell leukodystrophy), metachromatic leukodystrophy, and adrenoleukodystrophy (see Chapter 75).

Balestrini MR, Cavaletti G, D'Angelo A, et al: Infantile hereditary neuropathy with hypomyelination. *Neuropediatrics* 1991;22:65.
Boylan KB, Ferriero DM, Greco CM, et al: Congenital hypomyelination neuropathy with arthrogryposis multiplex congenita. *Ann Neurol* 1992;31:337.
Chance PF, Alderson MK, Leppig KA, et al: DNA deletion associated with hereditary neuropathy with liability to pressure palsies. *Cell* 1993;72:143.
Flanigan KM, Crawford TO, Griffin JW, et al: Localization of the giant axonal neuropathy gene to chromosome 16q24. *Ann Neurol* 1998;43:143.
Ouvrier RA: Giant axonal neuropathy: A review. *Brain Dev* 1989;11:207.
Roa BB, Garcia CA, Pentao L, et al: Evidence for a recessive PMP22 point mutation in Charcot-Marie-Tooth disease type 1A. *Nat Genet* 1993;5:189.
Ronen GM, Lowry N, Wedge JH, et al: Hereditary motor-sensory neuropathy type I presenting as scapuloperoneal atrophy (Davidenkow syndrome): Electrophysiological and pathological studies. *Can J Neurol Sci* 1986;13:264.

Chapter 605
Toxic Neuropathies

Many *chemicals* (organophosphates), *toxins*, and *drugs* are capable of causing peripheral neuropathy. *Heavy metals* are well-known neurotoxins. Lead poisoning, especially if chronic, causes mainly a motor neuropathy selectively involving large nerves, such as the common peroneal, radial, or median nerves, a condition known as *mononeuritis multiplex* (see Chapter 703). Arsenic produces painful burning paresthesias and motor polyneuropathy. Exposure to industrial and agricultural chemicals is a less common cause of toxic neuropathy in children than in adults.

Antimetabolic and immunosuppressive drugs, such as vincristine, cisplatin, and taxol, produce polyneuropathies as complications of chemotherapy for neoplasms. This "iatrogenic" cause is the most frequent etiology of toxic neuropathies in children. It is usually an axonal degeneration rather than primary demyelination, unlike autoimmune neuropathies such as Guillain-Barré syndrome.

Chronic uremia is associated with toxic neuropathy and myopathy. The neuropathy is caused by excessive levels of circulating parathyroid hormone. Reduction in serum parathyroid hormone levels is accompanied by clinical improvement and a return to normal of nerve conduction velocity.

Chapter 606
Autonomic Neuropathies

606.1 Familial Dysautonomia

Familial dysautonomia (Riley-Day syndrome) is an autosomal recessive disorder that is common in Eastern European Jews, among whom the incidence is 1/10,000–20,000, and the carrier state is estimated to be 1%. It is rare in other ethnic groups. The defective gene is at the 9q31-q33 locus.

Pathology. This disease of the peripheral nervous system is characterized pathologically by a reduced number of small unmyelinated nerve fibers that carry pain, temperature, and taste sensations and that mediate autonomic functions. Large myelinated afferent nerve fibers that relay impulses from muscle spindles and Golgi tendon organs are also deficient. The degree of demonstrable anatomic change in peripheral and especially autonomic nerves is variable. Fungiform papillae of the tongue (taste buds) are absent or reduced in number.

Clinical Manifestations. The disease is expressed in infancy by poor sucking and swallowing. Aspiration pneumonia may occur. Feeding difficulties remain a major symptom throughout childhood. Vomiting crises may occur. Excessive sweating and blotchy erythema of the skin are common, especially at mealtime or when the child is excited. Breath-holding spells followed by syncope are common in the first 5 yr. As affected children become older, insensitivity to pain becomes evident and traumatic injuries are frequent. Corneal ulcerations are common. Newly erupting teeth cause tongue ulcerations. Walking is delayed or clumsy or appears ataxic because of poor sensory feedback from muscle spindles. The ataxia is probably related more to deficient muscle spindle feedback and to vestibular nerve dysfunction than to cerebellar involvement. Tendon stretch reflexes are absent. Scoliosis is a serious complication in the majority of patients and usually is progressive. Normal overflow tearing with crying does not normally develop until 2–3 mo of age but fails to develop after that time or is severely reduced in children with familial dysautonomia.

About 40% of patients have generalized major motor seizures, some of which are associated with acute hypoxia during breath-holding, some with extreme fevers, but most without an apparent precipitating event. Body temperature is poorly controlled; both hypothermia and extreme fevers occur. Intellectual function is usually impaired but is unrelated to epilepsy. Puberty is often delayed, especially in girls. Speech is often slurred or nasal.

After 3 yr of age, autonomic crises begin, usually with attacks of cyclic vomiting lasting 24–72 hr or even several days. Retching and vomiting occur every 15–20 min and are associated with hypertension, profuse sweating, blotching of the skin, apprehension, and irritability. Prominent gastric distention may occur, causing abdominal pain and even respiratory distress. Hematemesis may complicate pernicious vomiting.

Allgrove syndrome is a clinical variant, involving alacrima, achalasia, autonomic dysfunction with orthostatic hypotension and altered heart rate variability, and sensorimotor polyneuropathy, usually presenting in adolescence. Cholinergic dysfunction may be demonstrated.

Laboratory Findings. Electrocardiography discloses prolonged correcting QT intervals with lack of appropriate shortening with exercise, a reflection of the aberration in autonomic regulation of cardiac conduction. Chest roentgenograms show atelectasis and pulmonary changes resembling cystic fibrosis. Urinary vanillylmandelic acid level is decreased, and homovanillic acid level is increased. Plasma level of dopamine β-hydroxylase (the enzyme that converts dopamine to epinephrine) is diminished. Sural nerve biopsy shows a decreased number of unmyelinated fibers. An electroencephalogram is useful for evaluating seizures.

Diagnosis. Slow intravenous infusion of norepinephrine produces an exaggerated pressor response. The hypotensive response to infusion of methacholine is increased. Intradermal injection of 1:1,000 histamine phosphate fails to produce a normal axon flare, and local pain is absent or diminished. Because the skin of a normal infant reacts more intensely to histamine, a 1:10,000 dilution should be used. Instillation of 2.5% methacholine into the conjunctival sac produces miosis in patients with familial dysautonomia and no detectable effect on a normal pupil; this is a nonspecific sign of parasympathetic denervation due to any cause. Methacholine is applied to only one eye in this test, with the other eye serving as a control; the pupils are compared at 5-min intervals for 20 min.

Treatment. Symptomatic treatment includes special attention to the respiratory and gastrointestinal systems, methylcellulose eye drops or topical ocular lubricants to replace tears and prevent corneal ulceration, orthopedic management of scoliosis and joint problems, and appropriate anticonvulsants for epilepsy. Chlorpromazine is an effective antiemetic and may be given as rectal suppositories during autonomic crises. It also reduces apprehension and lowers the blood pressure. Dehydration and electrolyte disturbances should be anticipated. Bethanechol may be an alternative drug for cyclic vomiting. It is also useful for enuresis, another common complication, and augments tear production. Protection from injuries is important because of the lack of pain as a protective mechanism. Scoliosis often requires surgical treatment.

Intravenous gamma globulin results in dramatic improvement in the hypotension and pupillary areflexia in some cases and may deserve a clinical trial in severely disabled children, but most patients would be expected to have little benefit.

Prognosis. Most patients die in childhood, usually of chronic pulmonary failure or aspiration.

606.2 Other Autonomic Neuropathies

Myenteric Plexus Neuropathies. *Aganglionic megacolon (Hirschsprung disease)* is a failure of embryonic development of parasympathetic neurons in the submucosal and myenteric plexuses of segments of the colon and rectum. Nerves between the longitudinal and circular layers of smooth muscle of the gut wall are hypertrophic; ganglion cells are absent (see Chapter 313.3).

Congenital Insensitivity to Pain and Anhidrosis. This hereditary disorder of uncertain genetic transmission affects boys much more frequently than girls and presents in early infancy. Patients have episodes of high fever related to warm environmental temperatures because they do not perspire. Frequent burns and traumatic injuries result from apparent lack of pain perception. Intelligence is normal. Nerve biopsy reveals an almost total absence of unmyelinated nerve fibers that convey impulses of pain, temperature, and autonomic functions. Some cases of hypomyelinating neuropathy present clinically as congenital insensitivity to pain (see Chapter 604.8). The sympathetic skin response as an electrophysiologic study is a reliable diagnostic test in cases associated with a mutation at the TrKA receptor for nerve growth factor (NGF).

Reflex Sympathetic Dystrophy. This disorder is a form of local causalgia, usually involving a hand or foot but not corresponding to the anatomic distribution of a peripheral nerve. A continuous burning pain and hyperesthesia are associated with vasomotor instability in the affected zone, resulting in increased skin temperature, erythema, and edema due to vasodilatation and hyperhidrosis. In the chronic state, atrophy of skin appendages, cool and clammy skin, and disuse atrophy of underlying muscle and bone occur. More than one extremity is occasionally involved. The pain is disabling and is exacerbated by the movement of an associated joint, although no objective signs of arthritis are seen; immobilization provides some relief. The most common preceding event is local trauma in the form of a contusion, laceration, sprain, or fracture that occurred days or weeks earlier.

Several theories of pathogenesis have been proposed to explain this phenomenon. The most widely accepted is reflexive overactivity of autonomic nerves in response to injury, and regional sympathetic blockade often affords temporary relief. Physiotherapy also is helpful. Some cases resolve spontaneously after weeks or months, but others continue to be symptomatic and require sympathectomy. A psychogenic component is suspected in some cases but is difficult to prove.

Axelrod FB, Gouge TH, Ginsburg HB, et al: Fundoplication and gastrostomy in familial dysautonomia. *J Pediatr* 1991;118:388.

Axelrod FB, Nachtigal P, Dancis J: Familial dysautonomia: Diagnosis, pathogenesis and management. *Adv Pediatr* 21:75, 1974.

Blumenfeld A, Slaugenhaupt SA, Axelrod FB, et al: Localization of the gene for familial dysautonomia on chromosome 9 and definition of DNA markers for genetic diagnosis. *Nat Genet* 1993;4:160.

Bonica JJ: Causalgia and other reflex sympathetic dystrophies. In Bonica JJ (editor): *The Management of Pain*, 2nd ed. Philadelphia, Lea & Febiger, 1990, pp 220–43.

Chu ML, Berlin D, Axelrod FB: Allgrove syndrome: Documenting cholinergic dysfunction by autonomic testing. *J Pediatr* 1996;129:156.

Heafield MTE, Gammage MD, Nightingale S, et al: Idiopathic dysautonomia treated with intravenous gamma globulin. *Lancet* 1996;347:28.

Shorer Z, Moses SW, Hershkovitz E, et al: Neurophysiologic studies in congenital insensitivity to pain with anhidrosis. *Pediatr Neurol* 2001;25:397.

Chapter 607
Guillain-Barré Syndrome

Guillain-Barré syndrome is a postinfectious polyneuropathy involving mainly motor but sometimes also sensory and autonomic nerves. This syndrome affects people of all ages and is not hereditary. The disorder closely resembles experimental allergic polyneuritis in animals. Most patients have a demyelinating neuropathy, but primarily axonal degeneration is documented in some cases.

Clinical Manifestations. The paralysis usually follows a nonspecific viral infection by about 10 days. The original infection may have caused only gastrointestinal (especially *Campylobacter jejuni*) or respiratory tract (especially *Mycoplasma pneumoniae*) symptoms. Weakness begins usually in the lower extremities and progressively involves the trunk, the upper limbs, and finally the bulbar muscles, a pattern known as **Landry ascending paralysis**. Proximal and distal muscles are involved relatively symmetrically, but asymmetry is found in 9% of patients. The onset is gradual and progresses over days or weeks. Particularly in cases with an abrupt onset, tenderness on palpation and pain in muscles is common in the initial stages. Affected children are irritable. Weakness may progress to inability or refusal to walk and later to flaccid tetraplegia. Paresthesias occur in some cases.

Bulbar involvement occurs in about half of cases. Respiratory insufficiency may result. Dysphagia and facial weakness are often impending signs of respiratory failure. They interfere with eating and increase the risk of aspiration. The facial nerves may be involved. Some young patients may exhibit symptoms of viral meningitis or meningoencephalitis. Extraocular muscle involvement is rare, but in an uncommon variant, oculomotor and other cranial neuropathies are severe early in the course. **The Miller-Fisher syndrome** consists of acute external ophthalmoplegia, ataxia, and areflexia. Papilledema is found in some cases, although visual impairment is not clinically evident. Urinary incontinence or retention of urine is a complication in about 20% of cases but is usually transient. The Miller-Fisher syndrome overlaps with Bickerstaff brainstem encephalitis, which also shares many features with Guillain-Barré syndrome with lower motor neuron involvement and may indeed be the same basic disease.

Tendon reflexes are lost, usually early in the course, but are sometimes preserved until later. This variability may cause confusion when attempting early diagnosis. The autonomic nervous system may also be involved in some cases. Lability of blood pressure and cardiac rate, postural hypotension, episodes of profound bradycardia, and occasional asystole occur. Cardiovascular monitoring is important. A few patients require insertion of a temporary venous cardiac pacemaker.

Prognosis. The clinical course is usually benign, and spontaneous recovery begins within 2–3 wk. Most patients regain full muscular strength, although some are left with residual weakness. The tendon reflexes are usually the last function to recover. Improvement usually follows a gradient inverse to the direction of involvement, with recovery of bulbar function first and lower extremity weakness resolving last. Bulbar and respiratory muscle involvement may lead to death if the syndrome is not recognized and treated. Although prognosis is generally good with the majority of children recovering completely, three clinical features are predictive of poor outcome with sequelae: cranial nerve involvement, intubation, and maximum disability at the time of presentation. An electrophysiologic feature of conduction block, by contrast, is predictive of good outcome.

Chronic relapsing polyradiculoneuropathy (sometimes called chronic inflammatory demyelinating polyradiculoneuropathy) or *chronic unremitting polyradiculoneuropathy* are chronic varieties of Guillain-Barré syndrome that recur intermittently or do not improve for a period of months or years. About 7% of children with Guillain-Barré syndrome suffer relapse. Patients are usually severely weak and may have a flaccid tetraplegia with or without bulbar and respiratory muscle involvement.

Congenital Guillain-Barré syndrome is described rarely, presenting as generalized hypotonia, weakness, and areflexia in an affected neonate, fulfilling all electrophysiologic and cerebrospinal fluid (CSF) criteria, and in the absence of maternal neuromuscular disease. Treatment may not be required, and there is gradual improvement over the first few months and no evidence of residual disease by a year of age. In one case, the mother had ulcerative colitis treated with prednisone and mesalamine from the 7th month until delivery at term.

Laboratory Findings and Diagnosis. CSF studies are essential for diagnosis. The CSF protein is elevated to more than twice the upper limit of normal, glucose level is normal, and there is no pleocytosis. Fewer than 10 white blood cells/mm^3 are found. The results of bacterial cultures are negative, and viral cultures rarely isolate specific viruses. The dissociation between high CSF protein and a lack of cellular response in a patient with an acute or subacute polyneuropathy is diagnostic of Guillain-Barré syndrome.

Motor nerve conduction velocities are greatly reduced, and sensory nerve conduction time is often slow. An electromyogram shows evidence of acute denervation of muscle. Serum creatine phosphokinase (CK) level may be mildly elevated or normal. Antiganglioside antibodies, mainly against GM1 and GD1, are sometimes elevated in the serum in Guillain-Barré syndrome, particularly in cases with primarily axonal rather than demyelinating neuropathy, and suggest that they may play a role in disease propagation and/or recovery in some cases. Muscle biopsy is not usually required for diagnosis; specimens appear normal in early stages and show evidence of denervation atrophy in chronic stages. Sural nerve biopsy tissue shows segmental demyelination, focal inflammation, and wallerian degeneration but also is usually not required for diagnosis.

Serologic testing for *Campylobacter* infection helps establish the cause if results are positive but does not alter the course of treatment. Results of stool cultures are rarely positive because the infection is self-limited and only occurs for about 3 days, and the neuropathy follows the acute gastroenteritis.

Treatment. Patients in early stages of this *acute* disease should be admitted to the hospital for observation because the ascending paralysis may rapidly involve respiratory muscles during the next 24 hr. Patients with slow progression may simply be observed for stabilization and spontaneous remission without treatment. Rapidly progressive ascending paralysis is treated with intravenous immunoglobulin (IVIG), administered for 2, 3, or 5 days. Plasmapheresis, steroids, and/or immunosuppressive drugs are alternatives, if IVIG is ineffective. Combined administration of immunoglobulin and interferon is effective in some patients. Supportive care, such as respiratory support, prevention of decubiti in children with flaccid tetraplegia, and treatment of secondary bacterial infections, is important.

Chronic relapsing polyradiculoneuropathy or unremitting chronic neuropathy is also treated with IVIG. Plasma exchange, sometimes requiring as many as 10 exchanges daily, is an alternative. Remission in these cases may be sustained, but relapses may occur within days, weeks, or even after many months; relapses usually respond to another course of plasmapheresis. Steroid and immunosuppressive drugs are another alternative, but their effectiveness is less predictable. High-dose pulsed methylprednisolone given intravenously is successful in some cases. The prognosis in chronic forms of the Guillain-Barré syndrome is more guarded than in the acute form, and many patients are left with major residual handicaps.

Even if *Campylobacter jejuni* infection is documented by stool culture or serologic tests, treatment of the infection is not necessary because it is self-limited, and the use of antibiotics does not alter the course of the polyneuropathy.

Abd-Allah SA, Jansen PW, Ashwan S, et al: Intravenous immunoglobulin as therapy for pediatric Guillain-Barré syndrome. *J Child Neurol* 1997;12:376.

Ammache Z, Afini AK, Brown CK, et al: Childhood Guillain-Barré syndrome: Clinical and electrophysiologic features predictive of outcome. *J Child Neurol* 2001;16:477.
Bradshaw DY, Jones HR: Pseudomeningoencephalitic presentation of pediatric Guillain-Barré syndrome. *J Child Neurol* 2001;16:505.
Diener HC, Haupt WF, Kloss TM, et al: A preliminary, randomized, multicenter study comparing intravenous immunoglobulin, plasma exchange and immune adsorption in Guillain-Barré syndrome. *Eur Neurol* 2001;46:107.
Hartung HP, Kieseier BC, Kiefer R: Progress in Guillain-Barré syndrome. *Curr Opin Neurol* 2001;14:597.
Jackson AH, Barquis GD, Shah BL: Congenital Guillain-Barré syndrome. *J Child Neurol* 1996;11:407.
Press R, Mata S, Lolli F, et al: Temporal profile of anti-ganglioside antibodies and their relation to clinical parameters and treatment in Guillain-Barré syndrome. *J Neurol Sci* 2001;190:41.
Schaller B, Radziwill AJ, Steck AJ: Successful treatment of Guillain-Barré syndrome with combined administration of interferon-β-1a and intravenous immunoglobulin. *Eur Neurol* 2001;46:167.
Winer JB: Bickerstaff's encephalitis and the Miller-Fisher syndrome. *J Neurol Neurosurg Psychiatry* 2001;71:433.

Chapter 608
Bell Palsy

Bell palsy is an acute unilateral facial nerve palsy that is not associated with other cranial neuropathies or brainstem dysfunction. It is a common disorder at all ages from infancy through adolescence and usually develops abruptly about 2 wk after a systemic viral infection. The preceding infection is due to the Epstein-Barr virus in about 20% of cases; Lyme disease, herpes simplex virus, and mumps virus are identified in many others. The disease is believed to be a postinfectious allergic or immune demyelinating facial neuritis rather than an active viral invasion of the nerve or of its motor neurons of origin. At times, it is associated with hypertension.

Clinical Manifestations. The upper and lower portions of the face are paretic, and the corner of the mouth droops. Patients are unable to close the eye on the involved side and may develop an exposure keratitis at night. Taste on the anterior two thirds of the tongue is lost on the involved side in about half of cases; this finding helps to establish the anatomic limits of the lesion as being proximal or distal to the chorda tympani branch of the facial nerve. Numbness and paresthesias do not occur.

Treatment. Protection of the cornea with methylcellulose eye drops or an ocular lubricant is especially important at night. Studies do not support the efficacy of steroids to induce remission, and they are not recommended. Surgical decompression of the facial canal, theoretically to provide more space for the swollen facial nerve, is not of value.

Prognosis. The prognosis is excellent. More than 85% of cases recover spontaneously with no residual facial weakness; another 10% have mild facial weakness as a sequela; only 5% are left with permanent severe facial weakness. In patients with chronic cases who do not recover within a few weeks, electrophysiologic examination of the facial nerve helps to determine the degree of neuropathy and regeneration. In chronic cases, other causes of facial neuropathy should be considered, including facial nerve tumors such as schwannomas and neurofibromas, infiltration of the facial nerve by leukemic cells or by a rhabdomyosarcoma of the middle ear, brainstem infarcts or tumors, and traumatic injury of the facial nerve.

Facial Palsy at Birth. This is usually a compression neuropathy from forceps application during delivery and recovers spontaneously in a few days or weeks in most cases. Congenital Bell palsy should not be diagnosed. *Congenital absence of the depressor angularis oris muscle* causes facial asymmetry, especially when an affected infant cries. It is not a facial nerve lesion but is a cosmetic defect that does not interfere with feeding. Infants with *Möbius syndrome* may have bilateral or, less commonly, unilateral facial palsy; this syndrome is usually caused by symmetric calcified infarcts in the tegmentum of the pons and medulla oblongata during midgestation or late fetal life, although it rarely may be a developmental anomaly of the brainstem.

Eidlitz-Markus T, Gilai A, Mimouri M, et al: Recurrent facial nerve palsy in pediatric patients. *Eur J Pediatr* 2001;160:659–63.

Salman MS, MacGregor DL: Should children with Bell's palsy be treated with corticosteroids? A systematic review. *J Child Neurol* 2001;26:565.

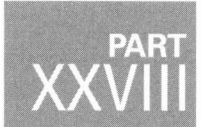

PART XXVIII

Disorders of the Eye

Scott E. Olitsky and Leonard B. Nelson

Chapter 609

Growth and Development

At birth, the eye of a normal full-term infant is approximately 65% of adult size. Postnatal growth is maximal during the 1st yr, proceeds at a rapid but decelerating rate until the 3rd yr, and continues at a slower rate thereafter until puberty, after which little change occurs. In general, the anterior structures of the eye are relatively large at birth but thereafter grow proportionately less than the posterior structures. This results in a progressive change in the shape of the globe; it becomes more spherical.

In an infant, the *sclera* is thin and translucent, with a bluish tinge. The *cornea* is relatively large in newborns (averaging 10 mm) and attains adult size (nearly 12 mm) by the age of 2 yr or earlier. Its curvature tends to flatten with age, with progressive change in the refractive properties of the eye. A normal cornea is perfectly clear. In infants born prematurely, the cornea may have a transient opalescent haze. The anterior chamber in a newborn appears shallow, and the angle structures, important in the maintenance of normal intraocular pressure, must undergo further differentiation after birth. The *iris*, typically light blue or gray at birth in white individuals, undergoes progressive change of color as the pigmentation of the stroma increases in the first 6 mo of life. The pupils of a newborn infant tend to be small and are often difficult to dilate. Remnants of the pupillary membrane (anterior vascular capsule) are often evident on ophthalmoscopic examination, appearing as cobweb-like lines crossing the pupillary aperture, especially in preterm infants.

The *lens* of a newborn infant is more spherical than that of an adult; its greater refractive power helps to compensate for the relative shortness of the young eye. The lens continues to grow throughout life; new fibers added to the periphery continually push older fibers toward the center of the lens. With age, the lens becomes progressively more dense and more resistant to change of shape during accommodation.

The *fundus* of a newborn's eye is less pigmented than that of an adult; the choroidal vascular pattern is highly visible, and the retinal pigmentary pattern often has a fine peppery or mottled appearance. In some darkly pigmented infants, the fundus has a gray or opalescent sheen. In a newborn, the macular landmarks, particularly the foveal light reflex, are less well defined and may not be readily apparent. The peripheral retina appears pale or grayish, and the peripheral retinal vasculature is immature, especially in premature infants. The optic nerve head color varies from pink to slightly pale, sometimes grayish. Within 4–6 mo, the appearance of the fundus approximates that of the mature eye.

Superficial retinal hemorrhages may be observed in many newborn infants. These are usually absorbed promptly and rarely leave any permanent effect. Conjunctival hemorrhages also may occur at birth and are resorbed spontaneously without consequence.

Remnants of the primitive hyaloid vascular system may also be seen as small tufts or wormlike structures projecting from the disc (Bergmeister papilla) or as a fine strand traversing the vitreous; in some cases, only a small dot (Mittendorf dot) remains on the posterior aspect of the lens capsule.

An infant's eye is somewhat hyperopic (farsighted). The general trend is for hyperopia to increase from birth until 7 yr. Thereafter, the level of hyperopia tends to decrease rapidly until age 14. Elimination of the hyperopic state may occur during this time. If the process continues, myopia (nearsightedness) develops. A slower continuation of the decrease in hyperopia, or increase in myopia, continues into the 3rd decade of life. The refractive state at any time in life depends on the net effect of many factors: the size of the eye, the state of the lens, and the curvature of the cornea.

Newborn infants tend to keep their eyes closed much of the time, but normal newborns can see, respond to changes in illumination, and fixate points of contrast. The *visual acuity* in newborns is estimated to be in the range of 20/400. One of the earliest responses to a formed visual stimulus is an infant's regard for the mother's face, evident especially during feeding. By 2 wk of age, an infant shows more sustained interest in large objects, and by 8–10 wk of age a normal infant can follow an object through an arc of 180 degrees. The acuity improves rapidly and may reach 20/30–20/20 by the age of 2–3 yr.

Many normal infants may have imperfect coordination of the *eye movements* and *alignment* during the early days and weeks, but proper coordination should be achieved by 3–6 mo, usually sooner. Persistent deviation of an eye in an infant requires evaluation.

Tears often are not present with crying until after 1–3 mo. Preterm infants have reduced reflex and basal tear secretion, which may allow topically applied medications to become concentrated and lead to rapid drying of their corneas.

Archer SM, Sondhi N, Helveston EM: Strabismus in infancy. *Ophthalmology* 1989;96:133.

Friendly DS: Development of vision in infants and young children. *Pediatr Clin North Am* 1993;40:693.

Gordon RA, Donzis PB: Refractive development of the human eye. *Arch Ophthalmol* 1985;103:785.

Isenberg SJ, Apt L, McCarty J: Development of tearing in preterm and term infants. *Arch Ophthalmol* 1998;116:773.

Khodadoust AA, Ziai M, Biggs SL: Optic disc in normal newborns. *Am J Ophthalmol* 1968;66:502.

Krishnamohan VK, Wheeler MB, Testa MA, et al: Correlation of postnatal regression of the anterior vascular capsule of the lens to gestational age. *J Pediatr Ophthalmol Strabismus* 1982;19:28.

Roarty JD, Keltner JL: Normal pupil size and anisocoria in newborn infants. *Arch Ophthalmol* 1990;108:94.

Spieres A, Isenberg SJ, Inkelis SH: Characteristics of the iris in 100 neonates. *J Pediatr Ophthalmol Strabismus* 1989;26:28.

Chapter 610
Examination of the Eye

Examination of the eyes is a routine part of the periodic pediatric assessment beginning in the newborn period. The primary care physician is very important in detecting both obvious and insidious, asymptomatic eye diseases. Screening in schools and community programs can also be effective in detecting problems early. The American Academy of Ophthalmology recommends preschool vision screening as a means of reducing preventable visual loss (Table 610–1). This testing should be done by pediatricians during well child visits. Children should be examined by an ophthalmologist whenever a significant ocular abnormality or vision defect is noted or suspected. Children who are at high risk for ophthalmologic problems, such as genetically inherited ocular conditions and various systemic disorders, should also be examined by an ophthalmologist.

Basic examination, whether done by a pediatrician or an ophthalmologist, must include evaluation of visual acuity and the visual fields, assessment of the pupils, ocular motility and alignment, a general external examination, and an ophthalmoscopic examination of the media and fundi. When indicated, biomicroscopy (slit-lamp examination), cycloplegic refraction, and tonometry are performed by an ophthalmologist. Special diagnostic procedures, such as ultrasonic examination, fluorescein angiography, electroretinography, or visual evoked response (VER) testing, are also indicated for specific conditions.

Visual Acuity. There are many tests of visual acuity. Which test is used depends on a child's age and ability to cooperate, as well as a clinician's preference and experience with each test. The most common visual acuity test in infants is an assessment of their ability to fixate and follow a target. If appropriate targets are used, this reflex can be demonstrated by about 6 wk of age. The test is performed by seating the child comfortably in the caretaker's lap. The object of visual interest, usually a bright-colored toy, is slowly moved to the right and to the left. The examiner observes whether the infant's eyes turn toward the object and follow its movements. The examiner can use a thumb to occlude one of the infant's eyes in order to test each eye separately. Although a sound-producing object might compromise the purity of the visual stimulus, in practice, toys that squeak or rattle heighten an infant's awareness and interest in the test.

The human face is a better target than test objects. The examiner can exploit this by moving his or her face slowly in front of the infant's face. If the appropriate following movements are not elicited, the test should be repeated with the caretaker's face as the test stimulus. It should be remembered that even children with poor vision may follow a large object without apparent difficulty, especially if only one eye is affected.

An objective measurement of visual acuity is usually possible when children reach $2\frac{1}{2}$–3 yr of age. Children this age are tested using a schematic picture or other illiterate eye chart. Each eye should be tested separately. It is essential to prevent peeking. The examiner should hold the occluder in place and observe the child throughout the test. The child should be reassured and encouraged throughout the test, because many children are intimidated by the procedure and fear a "bad grade" or punishment for errors.

The **E test,** in which a child points in the direction of the letter, is the most widely used visual acuity test for preschool children. Right-left presentations are more confusing than up-down presentations. With pretest practice, this test can be performed by most children 3–4 yr of age.

An adult-type **Snellen acuity chart** can be used at about 5 or 6 yr of age if the child knows letters. An acuity of 20/40 is generally accepted as normal for 3-yr-old children. At 4 yr of age, 20/30 is typical. By 5 or 6 yr of age, most children attain 20/20 vision.

Optokinetic nystagmus (the response to a sequence of moving targets; "railroad" nystagmus) can also be used to assess vision; this can be calibrated by targets of various sizes (stripes or dots) or by a rotating drum at specified distances. The visual evoked response (VER), an electrophysiologic method of evaluating the response to light and special visual stimuli, such as calibrated stripes or a checkerboard pattern, can also be used to study visual function in selected cases. Preferential looking tests are also used for evaluating vision in infants and children who cannot respond to standard acuity tests. This is a behavioral technique based on the observation that, given a choice, an infant prefers to look at patterned rather than unpatterned stimuli. Preferential looking tests cannot be directly correlated to standard visual acuity data. Because these tests require the presence of a skilled examiner, their use is often limited to research protocols involving preverbal children.

Visual Field Assessment. Like visual acuity testing, visual field assessment must be geared to a child's age and abilities. Formal visual field examination (perimetry and scotometry) can often be accomplished in school-aged children. The examiner must often rely on confrontation techniques and finger counting in quadrants of the visual field. In many children, only testing by attraction can be accomplished; the examiner observes a child's response to familiar objects brought into each of the four quadrants of the visual field of each eye in turn. The child's bottle, a favorite toy, and lollipops are particularly effective attention-getting items. These gross methods can often detect diagnostically significant field changes such as the bitemporal hemianopia of a chiasmal lesion or the homonymous hemianopia of a cerebral lesion.

Color Vision Testing. This can be accomplished whenever a child is able to name or trace the test symbols; these may be either numbers or X's, O's, triangles, or other symbols. Color vision testing is not frequently necessary in young children, but parents sometimes request it, particularly if their child seems to be slow in learning colors. Parents are often reassured to know that color "deficient" children do not misname colors and that true "color blindness" is very rare and not compatible with normal vision. Defective color vision is common in male patients but is rare in female patients. Achromatopsia, a total color vision defect with subnormal visual acuity, nystagmus, and photophobia, is encountered occasionally. A change in color discrimination can be a sign of optic nerve or retinal disease.

TABLE 610–1. Vision Screening Schedule for Infants and Children

Age	Screening Test	Findings Requiring Referral
Newborn–3 mo	Red reflex test	Opacity of the cornea, cataract, retinal detachment or disorder
	Corneal light reflex test	Ocular misalignment (strabismus)
	External examination	Structural defect
6–12 mo	Red reflex test	As above
	Corneal light reflex test	As above
	Occlusion of each eye separately	Amblyopia if child resists occlusion unequally
	Fixation and following	Amblyopia if unable to do
3 yr	Red reflex test	As above
	Corneal light reflex test	As above
	Visual acuity test	Refractive error, amblyopia
	Stereoacuity	Refractive error, amblyopia
5 yr	Same as 3 yr	As above

From Catalano RA, Nelson LB: Pediatric Ophthalmology. A Text Atlas. Norwalk, CT, Appleton & Lange, 1994.

Pupillary Examination. This includes evaluation of both the direct and consensual reactions to light, the reaction on near gaze, and the response to reduced illumination, noting the size and symmetry of the pupils under all conditions. Special care must be taken to differentiate the reaction to light from the reaction to near gaze. A child's natural tendency is to look directly at the approaching light, inducing the near gaze reflex when one is attempting to test only the reaction to light; accordingly, every effort must be made to control fixation. The swinging flashlight test is especially useful for detecting unilateral or asymmetric prechiasmatic afferent defects in children (see Marcus Gunn Pupil, Chapter 613).

Ocular Motility. This is tested by having a child follow an object into the various positions of gaze. Movements of each eye individually (ductions) and of the two eyes together (versions, conjugate movements, and convergence) are assessed. Alignment is judged by the symmetry of the corneal light reflexes and by the response to alternate occlusion of each eye (see discussion on cover tests for strabismus in Chapter 614).

Binocular Vision. A determination of the degree of binocular vision is commonly performed by an ophthalmologist. The **Titmus test** is probably the most frequently used test; a series of three-dimensional images are shown to the child while he or she wears a set of Polaroid glasses. The level of difficulty with which these images can be detected correlates with the degree of binocular vision that is present. Other tests may also be used to detect the presence of abnormal binocular adaptations secondary to poor vision or strabismus.

External Examination. This begins with general inspection in good illumination, noting size, shape, and symmetry of the orbits, position and movement of the lids, and position and symmetry of the globes. Viewing the eyes and lids from above aids in detecting orbital asymmetry, lid masses, proptosis (exophthalmos), and abnormal pulsations. Palpation is also important in detecting orbital and lid masses.

The lacrimal apparatus is assessed by looking for evidence of tear deficiency, overflow of tears (epiphora), erythema, and swelling in the region of the tear sac or gland. The sac is massaged to check for reflux when obstruction is suspected. The presence and position of the puncta are also checked.

The lids and conjunctiva are specifically examined for focal lesions, foreign bodies, and inflammatory signs; loss and maldirection of lashes should also be noted. When necessary, the lids can be everted in the following manner: (1) instruct the patient to look down; (2) grasp the lashes of the patient's upper lid between the thumb and index finger of one hand; (3) place a probe, a cotton-tipped applicator, or the thumb of the other hand at the upper margin of the tarsal plate; and (4) pulling the lid down and outward, evert it over the probe, using the instrument as a fulcrum. Foreign bodies commonly lodge in the concavity just above the lid margin and are exposed only by fully everting the lid.

The anterior segment of the eye is then evaluated with oblique focal illumination, noting luster and clarity of the cornea, depth and clarity of the anterior chamber, and features of the iris. Transillumination of the anterior segment aids in detecting opacities and in demonstrating atrophy or hypopigmentation of the iris; these latter signs are important when ocular albinism is suspected. When necessary, fluorescein dye can be used to aid in diagnosing abrasions, ulcerations, and foreign bodies.

Biomicroscopy (Slit-Lamp Examination). This provides a highly magnified view of the various structures of the eye and an optical section through the media of the eye—the cornea, aqueous humor, lens, and vitreous. Lesions can be identified and localized according to their depth within the eye; the resolution is sufficient to detect individual inflammatory cells in the aqueous and vitreous. With the addition of special lenses and prisms, the angle of the anterior chamber and regions of the fundus also can be examined with a slit lamp. Biomicroscopy is often crucial in trauma and in examining for iritis. It is also helpful in diagnosing many metabolic diseases of childhood.

Fundus Examination (Ophthalmoscopy). This is best done with the pupil dilated unless there are neurologic or other contraindications. Tropicamide (Mydriacyl), 0.5–1%, and phenylephrine (Neo-Synephrine), 2.5%, are recommended as mydriatics of short duration. These are safe for most children, but the possibility of adverse systemic effects must be recognized. For very small infants, more dilute preparations may be advisable. Beginning with posterior landmarks, the disc and the macula, the four quadrants are systematically examined by following each of the major vessel groups to the periphery. More of the fundus can be seen if a child is directed to look up, down, right, and left. Even with care, only a limited amount of the fundus can be seen with a direct or handheld ophthalmoscope. For examination of the far periphery, an indirect ophthalmoscope is used, and full dilation of the pupil is essential.

Refraction. This determines the refractive state of the eye—the degree of nearsightedness, farsightedness, or astigmatism. Retinoscopy provides an objective determination of the amount of correction needed and can be performed at any age. In young children, it is best done with cycloplegia. Subjective refinement of refraction involves asking patients for preferences in the strength and axis of corrective lenses; it can be accomplished in many school-aged children. Refraction and determination of visual acuity with appropriate corrective lenses in place are essential steps in deciding whether or not a patient has a visual defect or amblyopia. Photoscreening cameras aid ancillary medical personnel in screening for abnormal refractive errors in preverbal children. The accuracy and practical usefulness of these devices are still being investigated.

Tonometry. This measures intraocular pressure; it may be performed with a portable, stand-alone instrument or by the applanation method with the slit lamp. Alternative methods are pneumatic and electronic tonometry. When accurate measurement of the pressure is necessary in a child who cannot cooperate, it may be performed with sedation or general anesthesia. A gross estimate of pressure can be made by palpating the globe with the index fingers placed side by side on the upper lid above the tarsal plate.

American Academy of Ophthalmology Preferred Practice Patterns Committee, Pediatrics Ophthalmology Panel: Pediatric eye evaluations: Preferred practice pattern. Abstracts of Clinical Care Guidelines, April 7, 1998.

American Academy of Ophthalmology: *Preferred Practice Pattern: Comprehensive Pediatric Eye Evaluation.* San Francisco, American Academy of Ophthalmology, 1992.

American Academy of Pediatrics, Committee on Practice and Ambulatory Medicine, Section on Ophthalmology: Eye examination and vision screening in infants, children and young adults. *Pediatrics* 1996;98:153.

Fulton A: Screening preschool children to detect visual and ocular disorders. *Arch Ophthalmol* 1992;110:1553.

Isenberg SJ: Clinical application of the pupil examination in neonates. *J Pediatr* 1991;118:650.

Reinecke RD: Screening 3-year olds for visual problems: Are we gaining or falling behind? *Arch Ophthalmol* 1987;105:1497.

Simons K: Preschool vision screening: Rationale, methodology and outcome. *Surv Ophthalmol* 1996;41:3.

Teller DY, McDonald MA, Preston KI, et al: Assessment of visual acuity in infants and children: The acuity card procedure. *Dev Med Child Neurol* 1986;28:779.

Tong PY, Enke-Miyazaki E, Bassin RE, et al: Screening for amblyopia in preverbal children with photoscreening photographs. *Ophthalmology* 1998;105:856–63.

Chapter 611
Abnormalities of Refraction and Accommodation

Emmetropia is the state in which parallel rays of light come to focus on the retina with the eye at rest (nonaccommodating). Such an ideal optical state is common, but the opposite condition, ametropia, often exists. Three principal types occur: hyperopia (farsightedness), myopia (nearsightedness), and astigmatism. The majority of children are physiologically hyperopic at birth, but a significant number, especially those born prematurely, are myopic, and they often have some degree of astigmatism. With growth, the refractive state tends to change and should be evaluated periodically.

Measurement of the refractive state of the eye (refraction) can be accomplished objectively and subjectively. The objective method involves focusing a beam of light from a retinoscope onto a patient's retina through lenses of various powers placed in front of the eye. This method is precise and can be carried out at any age because it requires no response from a patient. In infants and children, it is best done after instillation of eye drops that produce *mydriasis* (dilatation of the pupil) and *cycloplegia* (relaxation of accommodation); those used most commonly are tropicamide (Mydriacyl), cyclopentolate (Cyclogyl), homatropine hydrobromide, and atropine sulfate. The subjective method involves placing various lenses in front of the eye and having the patient report which lenses provide the clearest image of the letters on the chart. This method depends on a patient's ability to discriminate and communicate, but it can be used for some children and can be helpful in determining the best refractive correction for children who are developmentally capable.

Hyperopia. If parallel rays of light come to focus posterior to the retina with the eye in a state of rest (nonaccommodating), hyperopia or farsightedness exists. This may result because the anteroposterior diameter of the eye is too short, because the refractive power of the cornea or lens is less than normal, or because the lens is dislocated posteriorly.

In hyperopia, accommodation is used to bring objects into focus for both far and near gaze. If the accommodative effort required is not too great, the child has clear vision and is comfortable with both distant and close work. In high degrees of hyperopia requiring greater accommodative effort, vision may be blurred, and the child may complain of eyestrain, headaches, or fatigue. Squinting, eye rubbing, and lack of interest in reading are frequent manifestations. If the induced discomfort is great enough, a child does not make an effort to see well and may develop bilateral amblyopia (ametropic amblyopia). Esotropia may also be associated (see discussion on convergent strabismus, accommodative esotropia, in Chapter 614). Convex lenses (spectacles or contact lenses) of sufficient strength to provide clear vision and comfort are prescribed when indicated. Even children who have high degrees of hyperopia but who have good vision will happily wear glasses because they provide comfort by eliminating the excessive accommodation required to see well. Preverbal children should also be given glasses for high levels of hyperopia to prevent the development of esotropia or amblyopia. Children with normal levels of hyperopia do not require correction in the majority of cases.

Myopia. In myopia, parallel rays of light come to focus anterior to the retina. This may result because the anteroposterior diameter of the eye is too long, because the refractive power of the cornea or lens is greater than normal, or because the lens is dislocated forward. The principal symptom is blurred vision for distant objects. The far point of clear vision varies inversely with the degree of myopia; as the myopia increases, the far point of clear vision comes closer. With myopia of 1 diopter, for example, the far point of clear focus is 1 m from the eye; with myopia of 3 diopters, the far point of clear vision is only $1/3$ m from the eye. Thus, myopic children tend to hold objects and reading matter close, prefer to be close to the blackboard, and may be uninterested in distant activities. Frowning and squinting are common, because the visual acuity is improved when the lid aperture is reduced; the effect is similar to that achieved by closing or "stopping down" the aperture of the diaphragm of a camera.

Myopia is infrequent in infants and preschool children. It is more common in preterm infants and in infants with a history of retinopathy of prematurity. A hereditary tendency to myopia is also observed, and children of myopic parents should be examined at an early age. The incidence of myopia increases during the school years, especially during the preteen and teen years. The degree of myopia also increases with age during the growing years.

Concave lenses (spectacles or contact lenses) of appropriate strength to provide clear vision and comfort are prescribed. Changes are usually needed periodically, sometimes in 1–2 yr, sometimes every few months. Excessive accommodation during near work has been considered by some to lead to progression of myopia. Based on this philosophy, some practitioners advocate the use of cycloplegic agents, bifocals, intentional undercorrection of myopic refractive errors, or mandatory removal of myopic glasses for near work in an effort to retard the progression of myopia. The value of such treatment has not been scientifically proved.

In most cases, myopia is not a result of pathologic alteration of the eye and is referred to as simple or physiologic myopia. Some children may have pathologic myopia, a rare condition caused by a pathologically abnormal axial length of the eye; this is usually associated with thinning of the sclera, choroid, and retina and often with some degree of uncorrectable visual impairment. Tears or breaks in the retina may occur as it becomes increasingly thin, leading to the development of retinal detachments. Myopia may also occur as a result of other ocular abnormalities, such as keratoconus, ectopia lentis, congenital stationary night blindness, and glaucoma and is also a major feature of the *Stickler syndrome*.

Astigmatism. In astigmatism, the refractive power of the various meridians of the eye differs. Most cases are caused by irregularity in the curvature of the cornea; some astigmatism results from changes in the lens. Mild degrees of astigmatism are common and may produce no symptoms. With greater degrees, there may be distortion of vision. To achieve a clearer image, a person with astigmatism uses accommodation or frowns or squints to obtain a pinhole effect. Symptoms include eyestrain, headache, and fatigue. Eye rubbing, indifference to schoolwork, and holding reading matter close are common manifestations in childhood. Cylindric or spherocylindric lenses are used to provide optical correction when indicated. Glasses may be needed constantly or only part time, depending on the degree of astigmatism and the severity of the attendant symptoms. In some cases, contact lenses are used.

Infants and children with corneal irregularity resulting from injury, periorbital and eyelid hemangiomas, and ptosis are at increased risk for astigmatism and attendant amblyopia.

Anisometropia. When the refractive state of one eye is significantly different from the refractive state of the other eye, anisometropia exists. If uncorrected, one eye may always be out of focus, leading to the development of amblyopia, or lazy eye. Early detection and correction are essential if normal visual development in both eyes is to be achieved.

Accommodation. During accommodation, the ciliary muscle contracts, the suspensory fibers of the lens relax, and the lens assumes a more rounded shape to bring rays of light into focus on the retina. The amplitude of accommodation is greatest during childhood and gradually diminishes with age. The physiologic decrease in accommodative ability that occurs with age is called *presbyopia.*

Disorders of accommodation in children are relatively rare. Premature presbyopia is occasionally encountered in youngsters. The most common cause of paralysis of accommodation in children is intentional or inadvertent use of cycloplegic substances, topically or systemically; included are all the anticholinergic drugs and poisons, as well as plants and plant substances having these effects. Neurogenic causes of accommodative paralysis include lesions affecting the oculomotor nerve (3rd cranial nerve) in any part of its course. Differential diagnosis includes tumors, degenerative diseases, vascular lesions, trauma, and infectious diseases. Systemic disorders that may cause impairment of accommodation include botulism, diphtheria, Wilson disease, diabetes mellitus, and syphilis. Adie tonic pupil may also lead to a deficiency of accommodation after some viral illnesses (see Chapter 613). Rarely, inability to accommodate is caused by a congenital defect of the ciliary muscle. An apparent defect in accommodation may be psychogenic in origin; it is common for a child to feign inability to read when it can be demonstrated that visual acuity and ability to focus are normal.

Brodstein RS, Brodstein DE, Olson RJ, et al: The treatment of myopia with atropine and bifocals: A long-term prospective study. *Ophthalmology* 1984;91:1373.

Curtin BJ: The etiology of myopia. In Curtin BJ (editor): *The Myopias: Basic Science and Clinical Management.* Philadelphia, Harper & Row, 1985, pp 113–24.

Fulton AB, Dobson V, Salem D, et al: Cycloplegic refractions in infants and young children. *Am J Ophthalmol* 1980;90:239.

Gordon RA, Donzis PB: Refractive development of the human eye. *Arch Ophthalmol* 1985;103:785.

Gordon RA, Donzis PB: Myopia associated with retinopathy of prematurity. *Ophthalmology* 1986;93:1593.

Mantyjarvi MI: Changes in refraction in schoolchildren. *Arch Ophthalmol* 1985;103:790.

Schoenleber DB, Crouch ER: Bilateral hypermetropic amblyopia. *J Pediatr Ophthalmol Strabismus* 1987;24:75.

Slataper FJ: Age norms of refraction and vision. *Arch Ophthalmol* 1950;43:466.

Spencer JB, Mets MB: Refractive abnormalities in childhood. *Ophthalmol Clin North Am* 1990;2:265.

Chapter 612
Disorders of Vision

Amblyopia. Amblyopia is the decrease in visual acuity, unilateral or bilateral, that occurs in visually immature children as a result of a lack of a clear image falling on the retina. The unformed retinal image may occur secondary to a deviated eye (strabismic amblyopia), an unequal need for vision correction between the eyes (anisometropic amblyopia), a high refractive error in both eyes (ametropic amblyopia), or a media opacity within the visual axis (deprivation amblyopia).

Under normal conditions, the development of visual acuity proceeds rapidly in infancy and early childhood. Anything that interferes with the formation of a clear retinal image during this early developmental period can produce amblyopia. Amblyopia may occur only during the critical period of development, before the cortex has become visually mature, within the first decade of life. The younger a child, the more susceptible he or she is to the development of amblyopia.

The *diagnosis* of amblyopia is confirmed when a complete ophthalmologic examination reveals reduced acuity that is unexplained by an organic abnormality. If the history and ophthalmologic examination do not support the diagnosis of amblyopia in a child with poor vision, consideration must be given to other causes (i.e., neurologic, psychologic). Amblyopia is usually asymptomatic and detected only by screening programs. Screening is easier in older children. However, just as amblyopia is less likely to occur in an older child, it is also more resistant to treatment at that age. Amblyopia is reversed more rapidly in younger children whose visual system is less mature, although screening is more difficult. The key to the successful treatment of amblyopia is early detection and prompt intervention.

Treatment generally first consists of removing any media opacity or prescribing appropriate glasses, if needed, so that a well-formed retinal image can be produced in each eye. The sound eye is then covered (occlusion therapy) or blurred with glasses or drops (penalization therapy) to stimulate proper visual development of the more severely affected eye. In many cases, best results are achieved with complete and constant occlusion throughout the waking hours by the use of adhesive eye patches; in some cases, part-time occlusion is sufficient or preferred. Occluders placed on spectacles allow peeking, and the adjustable headband type of cloth or plastic occluder is too easily removed by a child. In selected cases, an opaque contact lens or a contact lens of sufficiently high power to blur the vision in the better eye is used. Most children and their families tolerate occlusion therapy well. In some cases, a child resists therapy because of the severity of the vision defect, the cosmetic blemish of the patching, or related psychologic disturbances. The goals of treatment must be thoroughly understood and the treatment carefully supervised. Close monitoring of amblyopia therapy is essential, especially in the very young, to avoid deprivation amblyopia in the good eye. Many families need reassurance and support throughout the trying course of treatment.

Diplopia. Diplopia, or double vision, is most frequently a result of malalignment of the visual axes, for example, displacement or deviation of the eye. It is common in heterophoria, in heterotropia of recent onset (particularly when caused by acquired nerve palsy), and in proptosis. Occluding one eye relieves the diplopia; affected children commonly squint, cover one eye with a hand, or assume abnormal head postures (a face turn or head tilt) to alleviate the bothersome sensation. These mannerisms, especially in preverbal children, are important clues to diplopia. The onset of diplopia in any child warrants prompt evaluation; it may signal the onset of a serious problem such as increased intracranial pressure, a brain tumor, an orbital mass, or myasthenia gravis.

Monocular diplopia results from dislocation of the lens, cataract, or some defect in the media or macula.

Suppression. In the presence of strabismus, diplopia occurs secondary to the same image falling on two different regions of the retina. In a visually immature child, a process that may occur in the cortex eliminates the disability of seeing double. This active process is termed *suppression,* and it occurs only in children. Although suppression eliminates the annoying symptom of diplopia, it is the potential awareness of a second image that tends to keep eyes properly aligned. Once suppression develops, it may allow an intermittent strabismus to become constant or strabismus to redevelop later in life even after successful treatment during childhood.

Amaurosis. Amaurosis is partial or total loss of vision; the term is usually reserved for profound impairment, blindness, or near blindness. When amaurosis exists from birth, primary consideration in differential diagnosis must be given to developmental malformations, damage consequent to gestational or perinatal infection, anoxia or hypoxia, perinatal trauma, and the genetically determined diseases that can affect the eye itself or the visual pathways (Table 612–1). In certain cases, the reason for amaurosis can be readily determined by objective ophthalmic examination; examples are severe microphthalmia, corneal opacification, dense cataracts, chorioretinal scars, macular defects, retinal dysplasia, and severe optic nerve hypoplasia. In some cases, an intrinsic retinal disease may not be apparent on initial ophthalmoscopic examination; an example is **Leber congenital retinal amaurosis**. In this retinal dystrophy, the fundus may appear normal or near normal for some time before ophthalmoscopically appreciable signs of retinal degeneration (e.g., pigmentary deposits, arteriolar attenuation, optic disc pallor) develop. In such cases, electroretinography is important in diagnosis, because the electroretinographic response in this condition is markedly reduced or absent. In many cases of amaurosis, the defect lies not in the eye or optic nerve but in the brain, requiring neurologic and neuroradiologic evaluation, including CT or MRI.

Amaurosis that develops in a child who once had useful vision has different implications (see Table 612–1). In the absence of obvious ocular disease (e.g., cataract, chorioretinitis, retinoblastoma, retinitis pigmentosa), consideration must be given to many neurologic and systemic disorders that can affect the visual pathways. Amaurosis of rather rapid onset may indicate an encephalopathy (hypertension), infectious or parainfectious processes, vasculitis, migraine, leukemia, toxins, or trauma. It may be caused by acute demyelinating disease affecting the optic nerves, chiasm, or cerebrum. In some cases, precipitous loss of vision is a result of increased intracranial pressure, rapidly progressive hydrocephalus, or dysfunction of a shunt. More slowly progressive visual loss suggests tumor or neurodegenerative disease. Gliomas of the optic nerve and chiasm and craniopharyngiomas are primary diagnostic considerations in children who show progressive loss of vision.

Clinical manifestations of impairment of vision vary with the age and abilities of a child, the mode of onset, and the laterality and severity of the deficit. The first clue to amaurosis in an infant may be nystagmus or strabismus, the vision defect itself passing undetected for some time. Timidity, clumsiness, or behavioral change may be the initial clues in the very young. Deterioration in school progress and indifference to school activities are common signs in an older child. School-aged children often try to hide their disability and, in the case of very slowly progressive disorders, may not themselves realize the severity of the problem; some detect and promptly report small changes in their vision.

Any evidence of loss of vision requires prompt and thorough ophthalmic evaluation. Complete delineation of childhood amaurosis and its cause usually requires extensive investigation involving neurologic evaluation, electrophysiologic tests, neuroradiologic procedures, and sometimes metabolic and genetic studies. Furthermore, attendant special educational, social, and emotional needs must be met.

TABLE 612–1. Etiologies of Childhood Amaurosis (Blindness)

Congenital

Optic nerve hypoplasia or aplasia
Optic coloboma
Congenital hydrocephalus
Hydranencephaly
Porencephaly
Micrencephaly
Encephalocele, particularly occipital type
Morning glory disc
Aniridia
Anterior microphthalmia
Peter anomaly
Persistent pupillary membrane
Glaucoma
Cataracts
Persistent hyperplastic primary vitreous

Phakomatoses

Tuberous sclerosis
Neurofibromatosis (special association with optic glioma)
Sturge-Weber syndrome
von Hippel–Lindau disease

Tumors

Retinoblastoma
Optic glioma
Perioptic meningioma
Craniopharyngioma
Cerebral glioma
Posterior and intraventricular tumors when complicated by hydrocephalus
Pseudotumor cerebri

Neurodegenerative Diseases

Cerebral storage disease
Gangliosidoses, particularly Tay-Sachs disease (infantile amaurotic familial idiocy), Sandhoff variant, generalized gangliosidosis
Other lipidoses and ceroid lipofuscinoses, particularly the late-onset amaurotic familial idiocies such as those of Jansky-Bielschowsky and of Batten-Mayou-Spielmeyer-Vogt
Mucopolysaccharidoses, particularly Hurler syndrome and Hunter syndrome
Leukodystrophies (dysmyelination disorders), particularly metachromatic leukodystrophy and Canavan disease
Demyelinating sclerosis (myelinoclastic diseases), especially Schilder disease and Devic neuromyelitis optica

Special types: Dawson disease, Leigh disease, the Bassen-Kornzweig syndrome, Refsum disease
Retinal degenerations: retinitis pigmentosa and its variants, and Leber congenital type
Optic atrophies: congenital autosomal recessive type, infantile and congenital autosomal dominant types, Leber disease, and atrophies associated with hereditary ataxias—the types of Behr, of Marie, and of Sanger-Brown

Infectious Processes

Encephalitis, especially in the prenatal infection syndromes due to *Toxoplasma gondii*, cytomegalovirus, rubella virus, *Treponema pallidum*, herpes simplex
Meningitis; arachnoiditis
Chorioretinitis
Endophthalmitis
Keratitis

Hematologic Disorders

Leukemia with central nervous system involvement

Vascular and Circulatory Disorders

Collagen vascular diseases
Arteriovenous malformations—intracerebral hemorrhage, subarachnoid hemorrhage
Central retinal occlusion

Trauma

Contusion or avulsion of optic nerves, chiasm, globe, cornea
Cerebral contusion or laceration
Intracerebral, subarachnoid, or subdural hemorrhage

Drugs and Toxins

Quinine
Ethambutol
Methanol
Many others

Other

Retinopathy of prematurity
Sclerocornea
Conversion reaction
Optic neuritis
Osteopetrosis

Modified from Kliegman R: Practical Strategies in Pediatric Diagnosis and Therapy. *Philadelphia, WB Saunders, 1996.*

Nyctalopia. Nyctalopia, or night blindness, is vision that is defective in reduced illumination. It generally implies impairment in function of the rods, particularly in dark adaptation time and perceptual threshold. *Stationary congenital night blindness* may occur as an autosomal dominant, autosomal recessive, or X-linked recessive condition. It may be associated with myopia, nystagmus, and disc anomaly. *Progressive night blindness* usually indicates primary or secondary retinal, choroidal, or vitreoretinal degeneration (see Chapter 621); it occurs also in vitamin A deficiency or as a result of retinotoxic drugs such as quinine.

Psychogenic Disturbances. Vision problems of psychogenic origin are common in school-aged children. Both conversion reactions and willful feigning are encountered. The usual manifestation is a report of reduced visual acuity in one or both eyes. Another common manifestation is constriction of the visual field. In some cases, the symptom is diplopia or polyopia. See Chapters 19 and 22.

Important clues to the diagnosis are inappropriate affect, excessive grimacing, inconsistency in performance, and suggestibility. Thorough ophthalmologic examination is essential to differentiate organic from functional visual disorders.

Affected children usually fare well with reassurance and positive suggestion. In some cases, psychiatric care is indicated. In all cases, the approach must be supportive and nonpunitive.

Dyslexia. Dyslexia is the inability to develop the capability to read at an expected level despite an otherwise normal intellect. The terms *reading disability* and *dyslexia* are often used interchangeably. Most dyslexic individuals also display poor writing ability. Dyslexia is a primary reading disorder and should be differentiated from secondary reading difficulties due to mental retardation, environmental or educational deprivation, and physical or organic diseases. Because there is no one standard test for dyslexia, the diagnosis is usually made by comparing reading ability with intelligence and standard reading expectations. Dyslexia is a language-based disorder and is not caused by any defect in the eye or visual acuity per se, nor is it attributable to a defect in ocular motility or binocular alignment. Although ophthalmologic evaluation of children with a reading problem is recommended to diagnose and correct any concurrent ocular problems such as a refractive error, amblyopia, or strabismus, treatment directed to the eyes themselves cannot be expected to correct developmental dyslexia (Chapter 29.3).

American Academy of Ophthalmology: *Policy Statement: Learning Disabilities, Dyslexia, and Vision.* San Francisco, American Academy of Ophthalmology, 1992.
Barnet AB, Manson JI, Wilmer E: Acute cerebral blindness in childhood. Six cases studied clinically and electrophysiologically. *Neurology* 1970;30:1147.
Brooks SE: Amblyopia. Ophthalmol Clin North Am 1996;2:171.
Catalano RA, Simon JW, Krohel GB, et al: Functional visual loss in children. *Ophthalmology* 1986;93:385.
Flynn JT: Amblyopia revisited. *J Pediatr Ophthalmol Strabismus* 1991;28:171.
Francois J: Diagnosis of blindness in the infant. *Ann Ophthalmol* 1970;2:533.
Hittner HM, Borda RP, Justice J Jr: X-linked recessive congenital stationary night blindness, myopia, and tilted discs. *J Pediatr Ophthalmol* 1981;18:15.
Jastrzebski GR, Hoyt CS, Marg E: Stimulus deprivation amblyopia in children: Sensitivity, plasticity, and elasticity (SPE). *Arch Ophthalmol* 1984;102:1030.
Kushner BJ: Functional amblyopia associated with organic ocular lesions. *Am J Ophthalmol* 1981;91:39.
Mellor DH, Fields AR: Dissociated visual development: Electrodiagnostic studies in infants who are "slow to see." *Dev Med Child Neurol* 1980;22:327.
Olitsky SE, Nelson LB: Reading disorders in children. *Ophthalmol Clin North Am* 1996;2:309.
Stager DR: Amblyopia and the pediatrician. *Pediatr Ann* 1977;8:91.
Tong PY, Enke-Miyazaki E, Bassin RE, et al: Screening for amblyopia in preverbal children with photoscreening photographs. *Ophthalmology* 1998;105:856.
Tongue AC: Low vision examination in children with visual impairment. *J Pediatr Ophthalmol Strabismus* 1980;17:175.
Vellutino F: Dyslexia. *Sci Am* 1987;25:20.
Von Noorden GK: Amblyopia: A multidisciplinary approach. *Invest Ophthalmol Vis Sci* 1985;26:1704.
Wiesel TN, Hubel DH: Effects of visual deprivation on morphlogy and physiology of cells in the cat's lateral geniculate body. *J Neurophysiol* 1963;26:978.

Chapter 613
Abnormalities of Pupil and Iris

Aniridia. The term aniridia is a misnomer because iris tissue is usually present, although it is hypoplastic (Fig. 613–1). Two thirds of the cases are dominantly transmitted with a high degree of penetrance. The other one third of cases are sporadic and are considered to be new mutations. The condition is bilateral in 98% of all patients regardless of the means of transmission and is found in approximately 1/50,000 persons.

Aniridia is a panocular disorder and should not be thought of as an isolated iris defect. Macular and optic nerve hypoplasia are commonly present and lead to decreased vision and sensory nystagmus. The visual acuity is measured as 20/200 in most patients, although the vision may occasionally be better. Other ocular deformities are common and may involve the lens and cornea. The cornea may be small, and a cellular infiltrate (pannus) occasionally develops in the superficial layers of the peripheral cornea. Clinically this appears as a gray opacification. Lens abnormalities include cataract formation and partial or total lens dislocation. Glaucoma develops in as many as 75% of individuals with aniridia.

One fifth of sporadic aniridic patients may develop **Wilms tumor** (Chapter 491.1). Of particular interest is the association of aniridia, genitourinary anomalies, mental retardation, and a partial deletion of the short arm of chromosome 11. Among individuals thus affected, the appearance of Wilms tumor is more common. It is thought that only patients with sporadic aniridia are at risk for developing Wilms tumor, although Wilms tumor has occurred in a patient with familial aniridia. Wilms tumor usually presents before the 3rd yr. Therefore, these children should be screened using renal ultrasonography every 3–6 mo, until approximately age 5 yr of age.

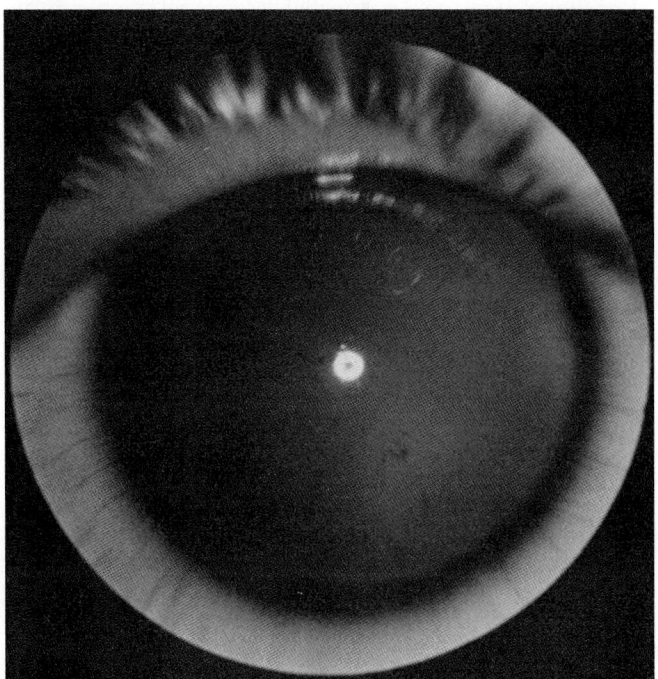

FIGURE 613–1. Aniridia. Minimal iris tissue. (From Nelson LB, Spaeth GL, Nowinski TS, et al: Aniridia: A review. *Surv Ophthalmol* 1984;28:621.)

The gene for aniridia had been localized to the 11p13 region. This gene may be involved in properly directing the interactions between the optic cup, surface ectoderm, and neural crest cells during early formation of the iris and other ocular structures.

Coloboma of the Iris. This developmental defect may present as a defect in a sector of the iris, a hole in the substance of the iris, or a notch in the pupillary margin. Simple colobomas are frequently transmitted as an autosomal dominant trait and may occur alone or in association with other anomalies. A coloboma is formed when the embryonic fissure fails to close completely. Because of the anatomic location of the embryonic fissure, an iris coloboma is always located inferiorly, giving the iris a keyhole appearance. An iris coloboma may be the only externally visible part of an extensive malclosure of the embryonic fissure that also involves the fundus and optic nerve. When this occurs, vision is likely to be severely affected. Therefore, all children with an iris coloboma should undergo a full ophthalmologic examination.

Microcoria. Microcoria (congenital miosis) appears as a small pupil that does not react to light or accommodation and that dilates poorly, if at all, with medication. The condition may be unilateral or bilateral. In bilateral cases, the degree of miosis may be different in each eye. The eye may be otherwise normal or may demonstrate other abnormalities of the anterior segment. Congenital microcoria is usually transmitted as an autosomal dominant trait, although it may occur sporadically.

Congenital Mydriasis. In this disorder, the pupils appear dilated, do not constrict significantly to light or near gaze, and respond minimally to miotic agents. The iris is otherwise normal, and affected children are usually healthy. Trauma, pharmacologic mydriasis, and neurologic disorders should be considered. Many apparent cases of congenital mydriasis show abnormalities of the central iris structures and may be considered a form of aniridia.

Dyscoria and Corectopia. Dyscoria is abnormal shape of the pupil, and corectopia is abnormal pupillary position. They may occur together or independently as congenital or acquired anomalies.

Congenital corectopia is usually bilateral and symmetric and rarely occurs as an isolated anomaly; it is usually accompanied by dislocation of the lens (ectopia lentis et pupillae), and the lens and pupil are commonly dislocated in opposite directions. Ectopia lentis et pupillae is transmitted as an autosomal recessive disorder; consanguinity is common.

When acquired, distortion and displacement of the pupil are frequently a result of trauma or intraocular inflammation. Prolapse of the iris after perforating injuries of the eye leads to peaking of the pupil in the direction of the perforation. Posterior synechiae (adhesions of the iris to the lens) are commonly seen when inflammation due to any cause occurs in the anterior segment.

Anisocoria. This is inequality of the pupils. The difference in size may be due to local or neurologic disorders. As a rule, if the inequality is more pronounced in the presence of bright focal illumination or on near gaze, there is a defect in pupillary constriction and the larger pupil is abnormal. If the anisocoria is worse in reduced illumination, a defect in dilation exists and the smaller pupil is abnormal. Neurologic causes of anisocoria (parasympathetic or sympathetic lesions) must be differentiated from local causes such as synechiae (adhesions), congenital iris defects (colobomas, aniridia), and pharmacologic effects. Simple central anisocoria may occur in otherwise healthy individuals.

Dilated Fixed Pupil. Differential diagnosis of a dilated unreactive pupil includes internal ophthalmoplegia caused by a central or peripheral lesion, Hutchinson pupil of transtentorial herniation, tonic pupil, pharmacologic blockade, and iridoplegia secondary to ocular trauma.

The most common cause of a dilated unreactive pupil is purposeful or accidental instillation of a cycloplegic agent, particularly atropine and related substances. Central lesions, such as a pinealoma, may cause internal ophthalmoplegia in children. Because the external surface of the oculomotor nerve carries the fibers responsible for pupillary constriction, compression of the nerve along its intracranial course may be associated with internal ophthalmoplegia, even before the development of ptosis or an ocular motility deficit. Although ophthalmoplegic migraine is a common cause of a 3rd nerve palsy with pupillary involvement in children, an intracranial aneurysm must also be considered in the differential diagnosis. The "blown pupil" of transtentorial herniation, occurring with increasing intracranial pressure, is generally unilateral, and patients usually are obviously ill. The pilocarpine test can help differentiate neurologic iridoplegia from pharmacologic blockade. In the case of neurologic iridoplegia, the dilated pupil constricts within minutes after instillation of 1 or 2 drops of 0.5–1% pilocarpine; if the pupil has been dilated with atropine, pilocarpine has no effect. Because pilocarpine is a long-acting drug, this test is not to be used in acute situations in which pupillary signs must be carefully monitored. Because of the consensual pupil response to light, even complete uniocular blindness does not cause a unilaterally dilated pupil.

Tonic Pupil. This is typically a large pupil that reacts poorly to light (the reaction may be very slow or essentially nil), reacts poorly and slowly to accommodation, and redilates in a slow, tonic manner. The features of tonic pupil are explained by cholinergic supersensitivity of the sphincter after peripheral (postganglionic) denervation and imperfect reinnervation. A distinctive feature of a tonic pupil is its sensitivity to dilute cholinergic agents. Instillation of 0.125% pilocarpine causes significant constriction of the involved pupil and has little or no effect on the unaffected side. The condition is usually unilateral.

Tonic pupil may develop after the acute stage of a partial or complete iridoplegia. It can be seen after trauma to the eye or orbit and may occur in association with toxic or infectious conditions. In those in the pediatric age group, tonic pupil is uncommon. Infectious processes (primarily viral syndromes) and trauma are the primary causes. Features of tonic pupil may also be seen in infants and children with familial dysautonomia (Riley-Day syndrome), although the significance of these findings has been questioned. Tonic pupil has also been reported in young children with Charcot-Marie-Tooth disease. The occurrence of tonic pupil in association with decreased deep tendon reflexes in young women is referred to as **Adie syndrome**.

Marcus Gunn Pupil. This relative afferent pupillary defect indicates an asymmetric, prechiasmatic, afferent conduction defect. It is best demonstrated by the swinging flashlight test; this allows comparison of the direct and consensual pupillary responses in both eyes. With patients fixing on a distant target (to control accommodation), a bright focal light is directed alternately into each eye in turn. In the presence of an afferent lesion, both the direct response to light in the affected eye and the consensual response in the fellow eye are subnormal. Swinging the light to the better or normal eye causes both pupils to react (constrict) normally. Swinging the light back to the affected eye causes both pupils to redilate to some degree, reflecting the defective conduction. This is a very sensitive and useful test for detecting and confirming optic nerve and retinal disease. This test is only abnormal if there is a "relative" difference in the conduction properties of the optic nerves. Therefore, patients with bilateral and symmetrical optic nerve disease will not demonstrate an afferent pupillary defect. A subtle relative afferent defect may be found in some children with amblyopia.

Horner Syndrome. The principal signs of oculosympathetic paresis (Horner syndrome) are homolateral miosis, mild ptosis, and apparent enophthalmos with slight elevation of the lower lid. Patients may also have decreased facial sweating, increased amplitude of accommodation, and transient decrease in intraocular pressure. If paralysis of the ocular sympathetic fibers occurs before the age of 2 yr, heterochromia iridis with hypopigmentation of the iris may occur on the affected side.

Oculosympathetic paralysis may be caused by a lesion in the midbrain, brainstem, upper spinal cord, neck, middle fossa, or orbit. Congenital oculosympathetic paresis, often as part of Klumpke brachial palsy, is common, although the ocular signs, particularly the anisocoria, may pass undetected for years. Horner syndrome is also seen in some children after thoracic surgery, such as for congenital heart disease. Congenital Horner syndrome may occur in association with vertebral anomalies and with enterogenous cysts. In some infants and children, Horner syndrome is the presenting sign of tumor in the mediastinal or cervical region, particularly neuroblastoma. Rare causes of Horner syndrome, such as vascular lesions, also occur in the pediatric age group. In some cases, no cause of Horner syndrome can be identified. Occasionally, the condition is familial.

When the cause of Horner syndrome is in question, investigative procedures should be implemented, including chest radiography, CT, MRI of the head and neck, and 24-hr urinary catecholamine assay. Examining old photographs and old records can sometimes be helpful in establishing the age of onset of Horner syndrome.

The *cocaine test* is useful in diagnosing oculosympathetic paralysis; a normal pupil dilates within 20–45 min after instillation of 1 or 2 drops of 4% cocaine, whereas the miotic pupil of an oculosympathetic paresis dilates poorly, if at all, with cocaine. In some cases there is denervation supersensitivity to dilute phenylephrine; 1 or 2 drops of a 1% solution dilates the affected but not the normal pupil. Furthermore, instillation of 1% hydroxyamphetamine hydrobromide dilates the pupil only if the postganglionic sympathetic neuron is intact.

Paradoxical Pupil Reaction. Some children exhibit paradoxical constriction of the pupils to darkness. An initial brisk constriction of the pupils occurs when the light is turned off, followed by slow redilation of the pupils. The response to direct light stimulation and the near response are normal. The mechanism is not clear, but paradoxical constriction of the pupils in reduced light can be a sign of retinal or optic nerve abnormalities. The phenomenon has been observed in children with congenital stationary night blindness, albinism, retinitis pigmentosa, Leber congenital retinal amaurosis, and Best disease. It has also been observed in those with optic nerve anomalies, optic neuritis, optic atrophy, and possibly amblyopia.

Persistent Pupillary Membrane. Involution of the pupillary membrane and anterior vascular capsule of the lens is usually completed during the 5th–6th mo of fetal development. It is common to see some remnants of the pupillary membrane in newborns, particularly in premature infants. These membranes are nonpigmented strands of obliterated vessels that cross the pupil and may secondarily attach to the lens or cornea. The remnants tend to atrophy in time and usually present no problem. In some cases, however, significant remnants that remain obscure the pupil and interfere with vision. Rarely, there is patency of the vascular elements; hyphema may result from rupture of persistent vessels.

Intervention must be considered to minimize amblyopia in infants with extensive persistent pupillary membrane of sufficient degree to interfere with vision in the early months of life. In some cases, mydriatics and occlusion therapy may be effective, but in others surgery may be needed to provide an adequate pupillary aperture.

Heterochromia. In heterochromia, the two irides are of different color (heterochromia iridium), or a portion of an iris differs in color from the remainder (heterochromia iridis). Simple heterochromia may occur as an autosomal dominant characteristic. Congenital heterochromia is also a feature of **Waardenburg syndrome,** an autosomal dominant condition characterized principally by lateral displacement of the inner canthi and puncta, pigmentary disturbances (usually a median white forelock and patches of hypopigmentation of the skin), and defective hearing. Change in the color of the iris may occur as a result of trauma, hemorrhage, intraocular inflammation (iridocyclitis, uveitis), intraocular tumor (especially retinoblastoma), intraocular foreign body, glaucoma, iris atrophy, oculosympathetic palsy (Horner syndrome), melanosis oculi, previous intraocular surgery, and some glaucoma medications.

Other Iris Lesions. Discrete nodules of the iris, referred to as **Lisch nodules**, are commonly seen in patients with neurofibromatosis. Lisch nodules represent melanocytic hamartomas of the iris and vary from slightly elevated pigmented areas to distinct balllike excrescences. Lisch nodules are found in 92–100% of individuals older than 5 yr of age and having neurofibromatosis. Slit-lamp identification of these nodules may help to fulfill the criteria required to confirm the diagnosis of neurofibromatosis.

In leukemia there may be infiltration of the iris, sometimes with hypopyon, an accumulation of white blood cells in the anterior chamber, which may herald relapse or involvement of the central nervous system.

The lesion of juvenile xanthogranuloma (nevoxanthoendothelioma) may occur in the eye as a yellowish fleshy mass or plaque of the iris. Spontaneous hyphema (blood in the anterior chamber), glaucoma, or a red eye with signs of uveitis may be associated. A search for the skin lesions of xanthogranuloma (see also Chapter 75.3) should be made in any infant or young child with spontaneous hyphema. In many cases, the ocular lesion responds to topical corticosteroid therapy.

Leukokoria. This includes any white pupillary reflex, or so-called *cat's-eye reflex.* Primary diagnostic considerations in any child with leukokoria are cataract, persistent hyperplastic primary vitreous, cicatricial retinopathy of prematurity, retinal detachment and retinoschisis, larval granulomatosis, and retinoblastoma (Fig. 613–2). Also to be considered are endophthalmitis, organized vitreous hemorrhage, leukemic ophthalmopathy, exudative retinopathy (as in *Coats disease*), and less common conditions such as medulloepithelioma, massive retinal gliosis, the retinal pseudotumor of Norrie disease, the so-called pseudoglioma of the *Bloch-Sulzberger syndrome,* retinal dysplasia, and the retinal lesions of the phakomatoses. A white reflex may also be seen with fundus coloboma, large atrophic chorioretinal scars, and ectopic medullation of retinal nerve fibers. Leukokoria is an indication for prompt and thorough evaluation.

The diagnosis can often be made by direct examination of the eye by ophthalmoscopy and biomicroscopy. Ultrasonographic and radiologic examinations are often helpful. In some cases, the final diagnosis rests with a pathologist.

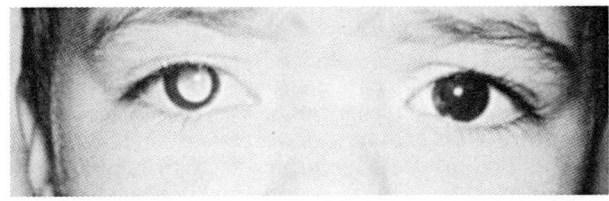

FIGURE 613–2. Leukocoria. White pupillary reflex in a child with retinoblastoma.

Cross HE: Ectopia lentis et pupillae. *Am J Ophthalmol* 1979;88:381.

Francois J: Differential diagnosis of leukokoria in children. *Ann Ophthalmol* 1978;10:1375.

Frank JW, Kushner BJ, France TD: Paradoxic pupillary phenomenon: A review of patients with pupillary constriction to darkness. *Arch Ophthalmol* 1988;106:1564.

Greenwald MJ, Folk ER: Afferent pupillary defects in amblyopia. *J Pediatr Ophthalmol Strabismus* 1983;20:63.

Hersh JH, Douglas C, Houston J, et al: Familial iridoplegia. *J Pediatr Ophthalmol Strabismus* 1982;24:49.

Ivanov I, Shuper A, Shohat M, et al: Aniridia: Recent achievements in paediatric practice. *Eur J Pediatr* 1995;154:795.

Jaffe N, Cassady JR, Filler RM, et al: Heterochromia and Horner syndrome associated with cervical and mediastinal neuroblastoma. *J Pediatr* 1975;87:75.

Jeffery AR, Ellis FJ, Repka MX, et al: Pediatric Horner syndrome. *J Amer Assoc Pediatr Ophthalmol Strabismus* 1998;2:129.

Krishnamohan VK, Wheeler MD, Testa MA, et al: Correlation of postnatal regression of the anterior vesicular capsule of the lens to gestational age. *J Pediatr Ophthalmol Strabismus* 1982;19:28.

Lewis RA, Riccardi VM: Von Recklinghausen neurofibromatosis: Incidence of iris hamartomata. *Ophthalmology* 1981;88:348.

Lowenfeld IE: "Simple, central" anisocoria: A common condition seldom recognized. *Trans Am Acad Ophthalmol Otolaryngol* 1977;83:832.

Maloney WF, Younge BR, Moyer NJ: Evaluation of the causes and accuracy of pharmacologic localization in Horner syndrome. *Am J Ophthalmol* 1980;90:394.

Schachat AP, Jabs DA, Graham ML, et al: Leukemic iris infiltration. *J Pediatr Ophthalmol Strabismus* 1988;25:135.

Thompson HS: Segmental palsy of the iris sphincter in Adie's syndrome. *Arch Ophthalmol* 1978;96:1615.

Thompson HS, Newsome DA, Loewenfeld IE: The fixed dilated pupil: Sudden iridoplegia or mydriatic drops? A simple diagnostic test. *Arch Ophthalmol* 1971;86:21.

Woodruff G, Buncic JR, Morin JD: Horner syndrome in children. *J Pediatr Ophthalmol Strabismus* 1988;25:40.

Chapter 614

Disorders of Eye Movement and Alignment

STRABISMUS

Strabismus, or misalignment of the eyes, is one of the most common eye problems encountered in children, affecting approximately 4% of children younger than 6 yr of age. This important ocular disorder can result in vision loss (amblyopia) in one eye and can have significant psychologic effects. Early detection and treatment of strabismus is essential to prevent permanent visual impairment. Of children with strabismus, 30–50% develop secondary visual loss (amblyopia). Restoration of proper alignment of the visual axis must occur at an early stage of visual development to allow these children a chance to develop normal binocular vision.

Definitions. The word *strabismus* means "to squint or to look obliquely." Many terms are used in discussing strabismus.

Orthophoria is the ideal condition of exact ocular balance. It implies that the oculomotor apparatus is in perfect equilibrium so that the eyes remain coordinated and aligned in all positions of gaze and at all distances. Even when fusion is interrupted, as by occlusion of one eye, truly orthophoric individuals maintain perfect alignment. Orthophoria is seldom encountered, because the majority of individuals have a small latent deviation (heterophoria).

Heterophoria is a latent tendency for the eyes to deviate. This latent deviation is normally controlled by fusional mechanisms that provide binocular vision or avoid diplopia (double vision). The eye deviates only under certain conditions, such as fatigue, illness, or stress, or during tests that interfere with maintenance of these normal fusional abilities (such as covering one eye). If the amount of heterophoria is large, it may give rise to bothersome symptoms, such as transient diplopia (double

vision), headaches, or asthenopia (eyestrain). Some degree of heterophoria is found in normal individuals; it is usually asymptomatic.

Heterotropia is a misalignment of the eyes that is constant. It occurs because of an inability of the fusional mechanism to control the deviation. Tropias can be alternating, involving both eyes, or unilateral. In an alternating tropia, there is no preference for fixation of either eye, and both eyes drift at an equal rate. Vision usually develops normally in both eyes because each eye is used in turn. A unilateral tropia is a more serious situation because only one eye is constantly malaligned. The undeviated eye becomes the preferred eye, resulting in loss of vision or amblyopia of the deviated eye.

It is common in ocular misalignments to describe the type of deviation present because this indicates different causes and treatments of the strabismus. The prefixes *eso-*, *exo-*, *hyper-*, and *hypo-* are added to the terms *phoria* and *tropia* to delineate further the type of deviation. *Esophorias* and *esotropias* are inward or convergent deviations of the eyes, commonly known as *crossed eyes*. *Exophorias* and *exotropias* are divergent or outward-facing eye deviations, *walleyed* being the lay term. Hyperdeviations and hypodeviations designate upward or downward deviations of an eye. In cases of unilateral strabismus, the deviating eye is often part of the description of the misalignment (left esotropia).

Diagnosis. Many techniques are used to assess ocular alignment and movement of the eyes to aid in diagnosing strabismic disorders. In a child with strabismus or any other ocular disorder, assessment of visual acuity is mandatory. Decreased vision in one eye requires evaluation for ocular deviation or other ocular abnormalities, which may be difficult to discern on a brief screening evaluation. Even strabismic deviations of only a few degrees in magnitude, too small to be evident by gross inspection, may lead to amblyopia and devastating vision loss.

Corneal light reflex tests are perhaps the most rapid and easily performed diagnostic tests for strabismus. They are particularly useful in children who are uncooperative and in those who have poor ocular fixation. To perform the Hirschberg corneal reflex test, the examiner projects a light source onto the cornea of both eyes simultaneously as a child looks directly at the light. Comparison should then be made of the placement of the corneal light reflex in each eye. In straight eyes, the light reflection appears symmetric and, because of the relationship between the cornea and the macula, slightly nasal to the center of each pupil. If strabismus is present, the reflected light is asymmetric and appears off center in one eye. Krimsky's method of the corneal reflex test uses prisms placed over one or both eyes to align the light reflections. The amount of prism needed to align the reflections is used to measure the degree of deviation of the eye. Although it is a useful screening test, corneal light reflex testing may not detect a small angle or an intermittent strabismus.

Cover tests for strabismus require a child's attention and cooperation, good eye movement capability, and reasonably good vision in each eye. If any of these are lacking, the results of these tests may not be valid. These tests consist of the cover-uncover test and the alternate cover test. In the cover-uncover test, a child looks at an object in the distance, preferably 6 m away. An eye chart is commonly used for fixation in children older than 3 yr of age. For younger children, a brightly colored or noise-making toy helps hold their attention for the test. As the child looks at the distant object, the examiner covers one eye and watches for movement of the uncovered eye. If no movement occurs, there is no apparent misalignment of that eye. After one eye is tested, the same procedure is repeated on the other eye. When performing the alternate cover test, the examiner rapidly covers and uncovers each eye, shifting back and forth from one eye to another like a windshield wiper. If the child has any ocular deviation, the eye rapidly moves as the cover is shifted to the other eye. Both the cover-uncover test and the alternate cover test should be performed at both distance and near fixation, with and without glasses. The cover-uncover test differentiates tropias, or manifest deviations, from latent deviations, called *phorias*.

Clinical Manifestations and Treatment. The etiologic classification of strabismus is complex, and the causative types must be distinguished; these are nonparalytic and paralytic types.

NONPARALYTIC STRABISMUS. Nonparalytic strabismus is the most common type. The individual extraocular muscles usually have no defect. The amount of deviation is constant, or relatively constant, in the various directions of gaze.

Esodeviations. Esodeviations are the most common type of ocular misalignment in children and represent well over 50% of all ocular deviations.

Pseudostrabismus (pseudoesotropia) is one of the most common reasons a pediatric ophthalmologist is asked to evaluate an infant. This condition is characterized by the false appearance of strabismus when the visual axes are aligned accurately. This appearance may be caused by a flat, broad nasal bridge, prominent epicanthal folds, or a narrow interpupillary distance. The observer may see less white sclera nasally than would be expected, and the impression is that the eye is turned in toward the nose, especially when the child gazes to either side. Parents frequently comment that when their child looks to the side, the eye almost disappears from view. Pseudoesotropia can be differentiated from a true misalignment of the eyes when the corneal light reflex is centered in both eyes and when the cover-uncover test shows no refixation movement. Once pseudoesotropia has been confirmed, parents can be reassured that the child will outgrow the appearance of esotropia. As the child grows, the bridge of the nose becomes more prominent and displaces the epicanthal folds, and the medial sclera becomes proportional to the amount visible on the lateral aspect. It is the appearance of crossing that the child will outgrow. Many parents of children with pseudoesotropia erroneously believe that their child has an actual esotropia that will resolve on its own. Because true esotropia can develop later in children with pseudoesotropia, parents and pediatricians should be cautioned that reassessment is required if the apparent deviation does not improve.

Congenital esotropia is a confusing term. Few children who are diagnosed with this disorder are actually born with an esotropia. Most reports in the literature have therefore considered infants with confirmed onset earlier than 6 mo as having the same condition, which some observers have redesignated infantile esotropia.

The characteristic angle of congenital esodeviations is large and constant. Because of the large deviation, cross-fixation is frequently encountered. This is a condition in which the child looks to the right with the left eye and to the left with the right eye. With cross-fixation, each eye is reluctant to turn away from the nose (abduction); this condition simulates a 6th nerve palsy. Abduction can be demonstrated by the doll's head maneuver or by patching one eye for a short time. Children with congenital esotropia tend to have refractive errors similar to those of normal children of the same age. This contrasts with the characteristic high level of farsightedness associated with accommodative esotropia (see later text). Amblyopia is common in children with congenital esotropia.

The primary goal of treatment in congenital esotropia is to eliminate or reduce the deviation as much as possible. Ideally, this results in normal sight in each eye, in straight-looking eyes, and in the development of binocular vision. Early treatment is more likely to lead to the development of binocular vision, which helps to maintain long-term ocular alignment. Once any associated amblyopia is treated, surgery is performed to align the eyes. Even with successful surgical alignment, it is common for vertical deviations to develop in children with a history of congenital esotropia. One form of vertical deviation results from overaction of the inferior oblique muscles. When this occurs, side gaze produces an upshoot of the eye closest to the nose. Dissociated vertical deviation also develops in children with infantile esotropia. In this type of deviation, one eye drifts up slowly with no movement of the other eye. Surgery may be necessary to treat either or both of these conditions.

It is important that parents realize that early successful surgical alignment is only the beginning of the treatment processes. Because many children may redevelop strabismus or amblyopia, they need to be monitored closely during the visually immature period of life.

Accommodative esotropia is defined as a "convergent deviation of the eyes associated with activation of the accommodative (focusing) reflex." It usually occurs in a child who is between 2 and 3 yr of age and who has a history of acquired intermittent or constant crossing. Amblyopia occurs in the majority of cases.

The mechanism of accommodative esotropia involves uncorrected hyperopia, accommodation, and accommodative convergence. The image entering a hyperopic (farsighted) eye is blurred. If the amount of hyperopia is not significant, the blurred image can be sharpened by accommodating (focusing of the lens of the eye). Accommodation is closely linked with convergence (eyes turning inward). If a child's hyperopic refractive error is large or if the amount of convergence that occurs in response to each unit of accommodative effort is great, esotropia may develop.

To treat accommodative esotropia, the full hyperopic (farsighted) correction is initially prescribed. These glasses eliminate a child's need to accommodate and therefore eliminate the esotropia (Fig. 614–1). Although many parents are initially concerned that their child will not want to wear glasses, the benefits of binocular vision and decreasing the focusing effort required to see clearly provide a strong stimulus to wear glasses, and they are generally accepted well. The full hyperopic correction sometimes straightens the eye position at distance fixation but leaves a residual deviation at near fixation; this may be observed or treated with bifocal lenses, antiaccommodative drops, or surgery.

It is important to warn parents of children with accommodative esotropia that the esodeviation may appear to increase without glasses after the initial correction is worn. Parents frequently state that before wearing glasses, their child had a small esodeviation, whereas after removal of the glasses the esodeviation becomes quite large. Parents often blame the increased esodeviation on the glasses. This apparent increase is due to a child's using the appropriate amount of accommodative effort after the glasses have been worn. When these children remove their glasses, they continue to use an accommodative effort to bring objects into proper focus and increase the esodeviation.

Most children maintain straight eyes once initially treated. Because hyperopia generally decreases with age, many patients outgrow the need to wear glasses to maintain alignment. In some patients, a residual esodeviation persists even when wearing their glasses. This condition commonly occurs when there is a delay between the onset of accommodative esotropia and treatment. In others, the esotropia may initially be eliminated with glasses but crossing redevelops and is not correctable with glasses. The crossing that is no longer correctable with glasses is the deteriorated or nonaccommodative portion. Surgery for this portion of the crossing is indicated to regain binocular vision.

Exodeviations. Exodeviations are the second most common type of misalignment. The divergent deviation may be intermittent or constant. **Intermittent exotropia** is the most common exodeviation in childhood. It is characterized by outward drifting of one eye, which usually occurs when a child is fixating at distance. The deviation is generally more frequent with fatigue or illness. Exposure to bright light may cause reflex closure of the exotropic eye. Because the eyes initially can be kept straight

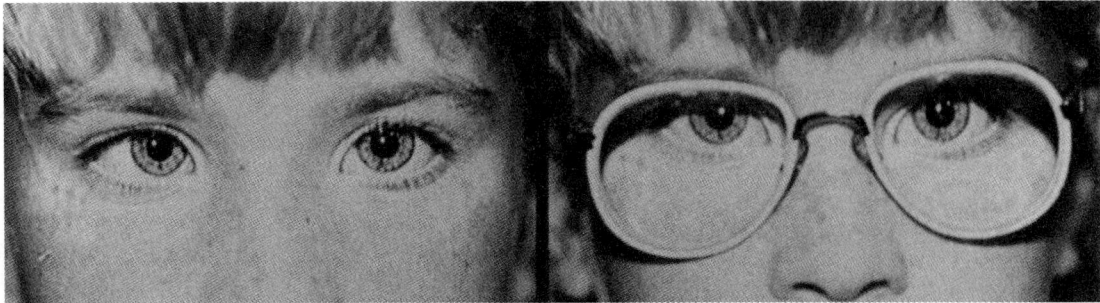

FIGURE 614–1. Accommodative esotropia; control of deviation with corrective lenses.

most of the time, visual acuity tends to be good in both eyes and binocular vision is initially normal.

The age of onset of intermittent exotropia varies but is often between age 6 mo and 4 yr. The decision to perform eye muscle surgery is based on the amount and frequency of the deviation. If the deviation is small and infrequent, it is reasonable just to observe the child. If the exotropia is large or increasing in frequency, surgery is indicated to maintain normal binocular vision.

Constant exotropia may rarely be congenital. Exotropia also may be associated with neurologic disease or abnormalities of the bony orbit, as in Crouzon syndrome. Exotropia that occurs later in life may represent a deterioration of an intermittent exotropia that was present in childhood. Surgery can restore binocular vision even in long-standing cases.

PARALYTIC STRABISMUS. When an eye muscle is paretic or palsied, a characteristic muscle imbalance occurs in which the deviation of the eye varies according to the direction of gaze. Recent onset of a paretic muscle can be suggested by the symptom of double vision that increases in one direction, the findings of an ocular deviation that increases in the field of action of the paretic muscle, and an increase in the deviation when the child fixates with the paretic eye. It is important to differentiate an extraocular muscle paresis or palsy from a comitant deviation because noncomitant forms of strabismus are often associated with trauma, systemic disorders, or neurologic abnormalities.

3rd Nerve Palsy. In the pediatric population, 3rd nerve palsies are usually congenital. The congenital form is often associated with a developmental anomaly or birth trauma. Acquired 3rd nerve palsies in children can be an ominous sign and may indicate a neurologic abnormality such as an intracranial neoplasm or an aneurysm. Other less serious causes include an inflammatory or infectious lesion, head trauma, postviral syndromes, and migraines.

A 3rd nerve palsy, whether congenital or acquired, usually results in an exotropia. In this situation, the exotropia is associated with a hypotropia, or downward deviation of the affected eye, as well as complete or partial ptosis of the upper lid. This characteristic deviation results from the action of the remaining unopposed muscles, the lateral rectus muscle and the superior oblique muscle. If the internal branch of the 3rd nerve is involved, pupillary dilation may be noted as well. Eye movements are usually limited nasally, in elevation and in depression. In addition, clinical findings and treatment may be complicated in congenital and traumatic cases of 3rd nerve palsy owing to misdirection of regenerating nerve fibers, referred to as **aberrant regeneration**. This results in anomalous and paradoxical eyelid, eye, and pupil movement such as elevation of the eyelid, constriction of the pupil, or depression of the globe on attempted medial gaze.

4th Nerve Palsy. These palsies can be congenital or acquired. Because the 4th nerve has a long intracranial course, it is susceptible to damage resulting from head trauma. In children, however, 4th nerve palsies are more frequently congenital than

traumatic. A palsied 4th nerve results in weakness in the superior oblique muscle, which causes an upward deviation of the eye, a hypertropia. Because the antagonist muscle, the inferior oblique, is relatively unopposed, the affected eye demonstrates an upshoot when looking toward the nose. Children typically present with a head tilt to the shoulder opposite the affected eye, their chin down and their face turned away from the affected side. This position is assumed to minimize the deviation and the associated double vision. Because the abnormal head posture maintains the child's ocular alignment, amblyopia is uncommon. Because no abnormality exists in the neck muscles, attempts to correct the head tilt by exercises and neck muscle surgery are ineffective. Recognition of a superior oblique paresis can be difficult because deviation of the head and the eye may be minimal. Eye muscle surgery can be performed to improve the ocular alignment and eliminate the abnormal head posture.

6th Nerve Palsy. These palsies produce markedly crossed eyes with limited ability to move the afflicted eye laterally. Children frequently present with their head turned toward the palsied muscle, a position that helps preserve binocular vision. The esotropia is largest when the eye is moved toward the affected muscle.

Congenital 6th nerve palsies are rare. Decreased lateral gaze in infants is often associated with other disorders, such as congenital esotropia or Duane retraction syndrome. In neonates, a transient 6th nerve paresis can occur; it usually clears spontaneously by 6 wk. It is believed that increased intracranial pressure associated with labor and delivery is the contributing factor.

Acquired 6th nerve palsies in childhood are often an ominous sign because the 6th nerve is susceptible to increased intracranial pressure associated with hydrocephalous and intracranial tumors. Other causes of 6th nerve defects in children include trauma, vascular malformations, meningitis, and **Gradenigo syndrome.** In this latter syndrome, otitis media precipitates a mastoiditis with associated petrositis and edema of the dura. These events result in pinching the 6th nerve against the petrosphenoidal ligament as the nerve passes between the ligament and the dura on its intracranial course. The 6th nerve palsy resolves with antibiotic treatment. A benign 6th nerve palsy, which is painless and acquired, can be noted in infants and older children. This is frequently preceded by a febrile illness or upper respiratory tract infection and may be recurrent. Complete resolution of the palsy is usual. Although not uncommon, other causes of an acute 6th nerve palsy should be eliminated before this diagnosis is made.

STRABISMUS SYNDROMES. Special types of strabismus have unusual clinical features. Most of these disorders are caused by structural anomalies of the extraocular muscles or adjacent tissues.

Double Elevator Palsy. A monocular elevation deficit in both abduction and adduction is referred to as double elevator palsy. It may represent a paresis of both elevators, the superior rectus and inferior oblique muscles, or a possible restriction to elevation from a fibrotic inferior rectus muscle. When an affected child fixates with the nonparetic eye, the paretic eye is hypotropic and the ipsilateral upper eyelid may appear ptotic. Fixation with the paretic eye causes a hypertropia of the nonparetic eye and a disappearance of the ptosis.

Duane Syndrome. This congenital disorder of ocular motility is characterized by retraction of the globe on adduction. This is attributed to anomalous innervation, which results in cocontraction of the medial and lateral rectus muscles on attempted adduction of the affected eye. Within the spectrum of Duane syndrome, patients may exhibit impairment of abduction, impairment of adduction, or upshoot or downshoot of the involved eye on adduction. They may have esotropia, exotropia, or relatively straight eyes. Many exhibit compensatory posturing for the defect in horizontal eye movement. Some develop amblyopia. Surgery to improve ocular motility and alignment or to reduce a noticeable face turn can be helpful in selected cases.

Duane syndrome usually occurs sporadically. It is sometimes inherited as an autosomal dominant trait. It usually occurs as an isolated condition but may occur in association with various other ocular and systemic anomalies.

Möbius Syndrome. The distinctive features of Möbius syndrome are congenital facial paresis and abduction weakness. The facial palsy is commonly bilateral, frequently asymmetric, and often incomplete, tending to spare the lower face and platysma. Ectropion, epiphora, and exposure keratopathy may develop. The abduction defect may be unilateral or bilateral. Esotropia is common. The cause is unknown. Whether the primary defect is maldevelopment of cranial nerve nuclei, hypoplasia of the muscles, or a combination of central and peripheral factors is unclear. Gestational factors such as trauma, illness, and intake of various drugs, particularly thalidomide, have been implicated. Some familial cases have been reported. Associated developmental defects may include ptosis, palatal and lingual palsy, hearing loss, pectoral and lingual muscle defects, micrognathia, syndactyly, supernumerary digits, or the absence of hands, feet, fingers, or toes. Surgical correction of the esotropia is indicated in selected cases, and any attendant amblyopia should be treated.

Brown Syndrome. In this syndrome, elevation of the eye in the adducted position is restricted or absent. An associated downward deviation of the affected eye in adduction is common. A compensatory tilt of the head may occur. Various causes have been described. Some cases have been attributed to structural abnormalities such as a tight superior oblique tendon, congenital shortening or thickening of the superior oblique tendon sheath, or connective tissue trabeculae between the superior oblique tendon and the trochlea. Sometimes, no anatomic abnormality is found.

Acquired Brown syndrome may follow trauma to the orbit involving the region of the trochlea or sinus surgery. It may also occur with inflammatory processes, particularly sinusitis and juvenile rheumatoid arthritis.

Acquired inflammatory Brown syndrome may respond to treatment with steroids. Surgery may be helpful for children with true congenital Brown syndrome.

Parinaud Syndrome. This eponym designates a palsy of vertical gaze, isolated or associated with pupillary or nuclear oculomotor (cranial nerve III) paresis. It indicates a lesion affecting the mesencephalic tegmentum. The ophthalmic signs of midbrain disease include vertical gaze palsy, dissociation of the pupillary responses to light and to near focus, general pupillomotor paralysis, corectopia, dyscoria, accommodative disturbances, pathologic lid retraction, ptosis, extraocular muscle paresis, and convergence paralysis. Some cases have associated spasms of convergence, convergent retraction nystagmus, and vertical nystagmus, particularly on attempted vertical gaze. Combinations of these signs are referred to as the Koerber-Salus-Elschnig or sylvian aqueduct syndrome.

A principal cause of vertical gaze palsy and associated mesencephalic signs in children is tumor of the pineal gland or 3rd ventricle. Differential diagnosis includes trauma and demyelinating disease. In children with hydrocephalus, impairment of vertical gaze and pathologic lid retraction are referred to as the *setting-sun sign.* A transient supranuclear disorder of gaze is sometimes seen in healthy neonates.

CONGENITAL OCULAR MOTOR APRAXIA

This congenital disorder of conjugate gaze is characterized by a defect in voluntary horizontal gaze, compensatory jerking movement of the head, and retention of slow pursuit and reflexive eye movements. Additional features are absence of the fast (refixation) phase of optokinetic nystagmus and obligate contraversive deviation of the eyes on rotation of the body. Affected children typically are unable to look quickly to either side voluntarily in response to a command or in response to an eccentrically presented object but may be able to follow a slowly moving target to either side. To compensate for the defect in purposive lateral eye movements, children jerk their head to bring the eyes into the desired position and may also blink repetitively in an attempt to change fixation. The signs tend to become less conspicuous with age.

The pathogenesis of congenital ocular motor apraxia is unknown. It may be a result of delayed myelination of the ocular motor pathways. Structural abnormalities of the central nervous system have been found in a few patients, including agenesis of the corpus callosum and cerebellar vermis, porencephaly, hamartoma of the foramen of Monro, and macrocephaly. Many children with congenital ocular motor apraxia show delayed motor and cognitive development.

A disorder of eye movement resembling congenital ocular motor apraxia may occur in patients with certain metabolic neurodegenerative diseases (particularly Gaucher disease) or with ataxia-telangiectasia, or as a sign of brain tumor.

NYSTAGMUS

Nystagmus (rhythmic oscillations of one or both eyes) may be caused by an abnormality in any one of the three basic mechanisms that regulate position and movement of the eyes: the fixation, conjugate gaze, or vestibular mechanisms. In addition, physiologic nystagmus may be elicited by appropriate stimuli (Table 614–1).

Congenital pendular nystagmus is generally associated with ocular abnormalities that lead to decreased visual acuity; common disorders that lead to early onset nystagmus include albinism, aniridia, achromatopsia, congenital cataracts, congenital macular lesions, congenital optic atrophy, and high refractive errors. In some instances, pendular nystagmus occurs as a dominant or X-linked characteristic without obvious ocular abnormalities. Rhythmic movements of the head may be associated.

Congenital idiopathic motor nystagmus is characterized by horizontal jerky oscillations with gaze preponderance; the nystagmus is coarser in one direction of gaze than in the other, with the jerk toward the direction of gaze. There are no ocular anatomic defects that cause the nystagmus and the visual acuity is generally near normal. There may be a point of reversal or a null point in which the nystagmus lessens and the vision improves; compensatory posturing, turning the head to bring the eyes into the position of least nystagmus, is characteristic. The cause of congenital jerky nystagmus is unknown; in some instances it is familial. Eye muscle surgery may be performed to eliminate abnormal head postures by bringing the point of best vision into straight-ahead gaze.

Acquired nystagmus requires prompt and thorough evaluation. Worrisome pathologic types are the gaze-paretic or gaze-evoked oscillations of cerebellar, brainstem, or cerebral disease.

TABLE 614–1. Specific Patterns of Nystagmus

Pattern	Description	Associated Conditions
Latent nystagmus	Conjugate jerk nystagmus toward viewing eye	Congenital vision defects, occurs with occlusion of eye
Manifest latent nystagmus	Fast jerk to viewing eye	Strabismus, congenital idiopathic nystagmus
Periodic alternating	Cycles of horizontal or horizontal-rotary that change direction	Caused by both visual and neurologic conditions
Seesaw nystagmus	One eye rises and intorts as other eye falls and extorts	Usually associated with optic chiasm defects
Nystagmus retractorius	Eyes jerk back into orbit or toward each other	Caused by pressure on mesencephalic tegmentum (Parinaud syndrome)
Gaze-evoked nystagmus	Jerk nystagmus in direction of gaze	Caused by medications, brainstem lesion, or labyrinthine dysfunction
Gaze-paretic nystagmus	Eyes jerk back to maintain eccentric gaze	Cerebellar disease
Downbeat nystagmus	Fast phase beating downward	Posterior fossa disease, drugs
Upbeat nystagmus	Fast phase beating upward	Brainstem and cerebellar disease; some visual conditions
Vestibular nystagmus	Horizontal-torsional or horizontal jerks	Vestibular system dysfunction
Asymmetric or monocular nystagmus	Pendular vertical nystagmus	Disease of retina and visual pathways
Spasmus nutans	Fine, rapid, pendular nystagmus	Torticollis, head nodding; idiopathic or gliomas of visual pathways

From Kliegman R: Practical Strategies in Pediatric Diagnosis and Therapy. *Philadelphia, WB Saunders, 1996.*

TABLE 614–2. Specific Patterns of Non-Nystagmus Eye Movements

Pattern	Description	Associated Conditions
Opsoclonus	Multidirectional conjugate movements of varying rate and amplitude	Hydrocephalus, diseases of brainstem and cerebellum, neuroblastoma
Ocular dysmetria	Overshoot of eyes on rapid fixation	Cerebellar dysfunction
Ocular flutter	Horizontal oscillations with forward gaze and sometimes with blinking	Cerebellar disease, hydrocephalus, or central nervous system neoplasm
Ocular bobbing	Downward jerk from primary gaze, remain for a few seconds, then drift back	Pontine disease
Ocular myoclonus	Rhythmic to-and-fro pendular oscillations of the eyes, with synchronous nonocular muscle movement	Damage to red nucleus, inferior olivary nucleus, and ipsilateral dentate nucleus

From Kliegman R: Practical Strategies in Pediatric Diagnosis and Therapy. *Philadelphia, WB Saunders, 1996.*

Nystagmus retractorius or *convergent nystagmus* is repetitive jerking of the eyes into the orbit or toward each other. It is usually seen with vertical gaze palsy as a feature of **Parinaud** or **Koerber-Salus-Elschnig** (sylvian aqueduct) **syndrome**. The causal condition may be neoplastic, vascular, or inflammatory. In children, nystagmus retractorius suggests particularly the presence of pinealoma or hydrocephalus.

Spasmus nutans is a special type of acquired nystagmus in childhood (see also Chapter 590). In its complete form, it is characterized by the triad of pendular nystagmus, head nodding, and torticollis. The nystagmus is characteristically very fine, very rapid, horizontal, and pendular; it is often asymmetric, sometimes unilateral. Signs usually develop within the 1st year or 2 of life. Components of the triad may develop at various times. In many cases, the condition is benign and self-limited, usually lasting a few months, sometimes years. The cause of this classic type of spasmus nutans, which usually resolves spontaneously, is unknown. Many children exhibiting signs resembling those of spasmus nutans have underlying brain tumors, particularly hypothalamic and chiasmal optic gliomas. Appropriate neurologic and neuroradiologic evaluation and careful monitoring of infants and children with nystagmus are therefore recommended.

OTHER ABNORMAL EYE MOVEMENTS

To be differentiated from true nystagmus are certain special types of abnormal eye movements, particularly opsoclonus, ocular dysmetria, and flutter (Table 614–2).

Opsoclonus. Opsoclonus and ataxic conjugate movements are spontaneous, nonrhythmic, multidirectional, chaotic movements of the eyes. The eyes appear to be in agitation, with bursts of conjugate movement of varying amplitude in varying directions. Opsoclonus is most often associated with encephalitis. It may be the first sign of neuroblastoma.

Ocular Motor Dysmetria. This is analogous to dysmetria of the limbs. Affected individuals show a lack of precision in performing movements of refixation, characterized by an overshoot (or undershoot) of the eyes with several corrective to-and-fro oscillations on looking from one point to another. Ocular motor dysmetria is a sign of cerebellar or cerebellar pathway disease.

Flutter-Like Oscillations. These intermittent to-and-fro horizontal oscillations of the eyes may occur spontaneously or on change of fixation. They are characteristic of cerebellar disease.

Anthony JH, Ouvrier RA, Wise G: Spasmus nutans: A mistaken identity. *Arch Neurol* 1980;37:373.

Awner S, Catalano RA: Nystagmus. In Nelson LB (editor): *Harley's Pediatric Ophthalmology,* 4th ed. Philadelphia, WB Saunders, 1998.

Birch EE, Stager DR, Everett ME: Random dot stereoacuity following surgical correction of infantile esotropia. *J Pediatr Ophthalmol Strabismus* 1995;32:231.

Bixenman WW, von Noorden GK: Benign recurrent VI nerve palsy in childhood. *J Pediatr Ophthalmol Strabismus* 1981;18:29.

Cogan DG: Heredity of congenital ocular motor apraxia. *Trans Am Acad Ophthalmol Otolaryngol* 1972;76:60.

DeRespinis PA, Caputo AR, Wagner RS, et al: Duane's retraction syndrome. *Surv Ophthalmol* 1993;38:257.

Harley RD: Paralytic strabismus in children: Etiologic incidence and management of the third, fourth and sixth nerve palsies. *Ophthalmology* 1980;87:24.

Hoyt CS, Mousel DK, Weber AA: Transient supranuclear disturbance of gaze in healthy neonates. *Am J Ophthalmol* 1980;89:708.

Ing M: Early surgical alignment for congenital esotropia. *Ophthalmology* 1983;90:132.

Kushner BJ: Ocular causes of abnormal head postures. *Ophthalmology* 1979;86:2115.

Kushner BJ: Atropine vs patching for treatment of amblyopia in children. *JAMA* 2002;287:2145–6.

Lavery MA, O'Neill JF, Chau FC, et al: Acquired nystagmus in early childhood: A presenting sign of intracranial tumor. *Ophthalmology* 1984;91:425.

Lee MS, Galetta SL, Volpe NJ, et al: Sixth nerve palsies in children. *Pediatr Neurol* 1999;20:49.

Metz HS: Double elevator palsy. *Arch Ophthalmol* 1979;97:901.

Miller MT, Ray V, Owens P, et al: Möbius and Möbius-like syndromes (TTV-OFM, OMLH). *J Pediatr Ophthalmol Strabismus* 1989;26:176.

Miller NR: Solitary oculomotor nerve palsy in children. *Am J Ophthalmol* 1977;83:106.

Mohindra I, Zwann J, Held R, et al: Development of acuity and stereopsis in infants with esotropia. *Ophthalmology* 1985;92:691.

Morre RT, Morin JD: Bilateral acquired inflammatory Brown's syndrome. *J Pediatr Ophthalmol Strabismus* 1985;22:26.

Morris RJ, Scott WE, Dickey CF: Fusion after surgical alignment of longstanding strabismus in adults. *Ophthalmology* 1993;100:135.

Nelson LB, Wagner RS, Simon JW, et al: Congenital esotropia. *Surv Ophthalmol* 1987;31:363.

Norton EW, Cogan DG: Spasmus nutans: A clinical study of twenty cases followed two years or more since onset. *Arch Ophthalmol* 1954;52:442.

Olitsky SE, Nelson LB: Strabismus disorders. In Nelson LB (editor): *Harley's Pediatric Ophthalmology*, 4th ed. Philadelphia, WB Saunders, 1998.

Pediatric Eye Disease Investigator Group: A randomized trial of atropine vs patching for treatment of moderate amblyopia in children. *Arch Ophthalmol* 2002;120:268–78.

Raab EL: Etiologic factors in accommodative esodeviation. *Trans Am Ophthalmol Soc* 1982;80:657.

Rappaport L, Urlon D, Strand K, et al: Concurrence of congenital oculomotor apraxia and other motor problems: An expanded syndrome. *Dev Med Child Neurol* 1987;29:85.

Richard JM, Parks M: Intermittent exotropia: Surgical results in different age groups. *Ophthalmology* 1983;90:1172.

Richards BW, Jones FR, Younge BR: Causes and prognosis in 4,278 cases of paralysis of the oculomotor, trochlear and abducens cranial nerves. *Am J Ophthalmol* 1992;113:489.

Shetty T, Rosman NP: Opsoclonus in hydrocephalus. *Arch Ophthalmol* 1972;88:585.

von Noorden GK, Murray E, Wong SY: Superior oblique paralysis: A review of 270 cases. *Arch Ophthalmol* 1986;104:1771.

Wang FM, Wertenbaker C, Behrens MM, et al: Acquired Brown's syndrome in children with juvenile rheumatoid arthritis. *Ophthalmology* 1984;91:23.

Wilson ME, Eustis HS, Parks MM: Brown's syndrome. *Surv Ophthalmol* 1989;34:153.

Chapter 615
Abnormalities of the Lids

Ptosis. In *blepharoptosis,* the upper eyelid droops below its normal level. Congenital ptosis is usually a result of a localized dystrophy of the levator muscle in which the striated muscle fibers are replaced with fibrous tissue. The condition may be unilateral or bilateral and can be familial, transmitted as a dominant trait.

Parents often comment that the eye looks smaller because of the drooping eyelid. The lid crease is decreased or absent where the levator muscle would normally insert below the skin surface. Because the levator is replaced by fibrous tissue, the lid does not move downward fully in downgaze (lid lag). If the ptosis is severe, affected children often attempt to raise the lid by lifting their brow or adapting a chin-up head posture to maintain binocular vision. **Marcus Gunn jaw-winking ptosis** accounts for 5% of ptosis in children. In this syndrome, an abnormal synkinesis exists between the 5th and 3rd cranial nerves; this causes the eyelid to elevate with movement of the jaw. The wink is produced by chewing or sucking and may be more noticeable than the ptosis itself.

Although ptosis in children is often an isolated finding, it may occur in association with other ocular or systemic disorders. Systemic disorders include myasthenia gravis, muscular dystrophy, and botulism. Ocular disorders include mechanical ptosis secondary to lid tumors, blepharophimosis syndrome, congenital fibrosis syndrome, combined levator/superior rectus maldevelopment, and congenital or acquired 3rd nerve palsy. A complete ophthalmic and systemic examination is therefore important in the evaluation of a child with ptosis.

Amblyopia may occur in children with ptosis. The amblyopia may be secondary to the lid's covering the visual axis (deprivation) or induced astigmatism due to the weight of the lid on the globe (anisometropia). When amblyopia occurs, it should generally be treated before treating the ptosis.

Treatment of ptosis in a child is indicated for elimination of an abnormal head posture, improvement in the visual field, prevention of amblyopia, and restoration of a normal eyelid appearance. The timing of surgery depends on the degree of ptosis, its cosmetic and functional severity, the presence or absence of compensatory posturing, the wishes of the parents, and the discretion of the surgeon. Surgical treatment is determined by the amount of levator function that is present. A levator resection may be used in children with moderate to good function. In patients with poor or absent function, a frontalis suspension procedure may be necessary. This technique requires that a suspension material be placed between the frontalis muscle and the tarsus of the eyelid. It allows patients to use their brow and frontalis muscle more effectively to raise their eyelid. Amblyopia remains a concern even after surgical correction and should be monitored closely.

Epicanthal Folds. These vertical or oblique folds of skin extend on either side of the bridge of the nose from the brow or lid area, covering the inner canthal region. They are present to some degree in most young children and become less apparent with age. The folds may be sufficiently broad to cover the medial aspect of the eye, making the eyes appear crossed (pseudo-esotropia). Epicanthal folds are a common feature of many syndromes, including chromosomal aberrations (trisomies) and disorders of single genes.

Lagophthalmos. This is a condition in which complete closure of the lids over the globe is difficult or impossible. It may be paralytic, because of a facial palsy involving the orbicularis muscle, or spastic, as in thyrotoxicosis. It may be structural when retraction or shortening of the lids results from scarring or atrophy consequent to injury (burns) or disease. Infants with collodion membrane may have temporary lagophthalmos caused by the restrictive effect of the membrane on the lids. Lagophthalmos may accompany proptosis or buphthalmos when the lids, although normal, cannot effectively cover the enlarged or protuberant eye. A degree of physiologic lagophthalmos may occur normally during sleep, but functional lagophthalmos in an unconscious or debilitated patient can be a problem.

In patients with lagophthalmos, exposure of the eye may lead to drying, infection, corneal ulceration, or perforation of the cornea; the result may be loss of vision, even loss of the eye. In lagophthalmos, protection of the eye by artificial tear preparations, ophthalmic ointment, or moisture chambers is essential. Gauze pads are to be avoided, because the gauze may abrade the cornea. In some cases, surgical closure of the lids (tarsorrhaphy) may be necessary for long-term protection of the eye.

Lid Retractions. Pathologic retraction of the lid may be myogenic or neurogenic. Myogenic retraction of the upper lid occurs in thyrotoxicosis, in which it is associated with three classic signs: a staring appearance **(Dalrymple sign),** infrequent blinking **(Stellwag sign),** and lag of the upper lid on downward gaze **(von Graefe sign).**

Neurogenic retraction of the lids may occur in conditions affecting the anterior mesencephalon. Lid retraction is a feature of the **syndrome of the sylvian aqueduct.** In children, it is commonly a sign of hydrocephalus. It may occur with meningitis. Paradoxical retraction of the lid is seen in the Marcus Gunn jaw-winking syndrome. It may also be seen with attempted eye movement after recovery from a 3rd nerve palsy, if aberrant regeneration of the oculomotor nerve fibers has occurred.

Simple staring and the physiologic or reflexive lid retraction ("eye popping"), in contrast to pathologic lid retractions, occur in infants in response to a sudden reduction in illumination or as a startle reaction.

Ectropion, Entropion, and Epiblepharon. *Ectropion* is eversion of the lid margin; it may lead to overflow of tears (epiphora) and subsequent maceration of the skin of the lid, to inflammation of exposed conjunctiva, or to superficial exposure keratopathy. Common causes are scarring consequent to inflammation, burns, or trauma, or weakness of the orbicularis muscle as a result of facial palsy; these forms may be corrected surgically. Protection of the cornea is essential. Ectropion is also seen in certain children who have faulty development of the lateral canthal ligament; this may occur in Down syndrome.

Entropion is inversion of the lid margin, which may cause discomfort and corneal damage because of the inward turning of the lashes (trichiasis). A principal cause is scarring secondary to inflammation such as occurs in trachoma or as a sequela of Stevens-Johnson syndrome. There is also a rare congenital form. Surgical correction is effective in many cases.

Epiblepharon is commonly seen in childhood and may be confused with entropion. In epiblepharon, a roll of skin beneath the lower eyelid lashes causes the lashes to be directed vertically and to touch the cornea. Unlike entropion, the eyelid margin itself is not rotated toward the cornea. Epiblepharon usually resolves spontaneously. If corneal scarring begins to occur, surgical correction may be necessary.

Blepharospasm. This spastic or repetitive closure of the lids may be caused by irritative disease of the cornea, conjunctiva, or facial nerve; fatigue or uncorrected refractive error; or common tic. Thorough ophthalmic examination for pathologic causes, such as trichiasis, keratitis, conjunctivitis, or foreign body, is indicated. Local injection of botulinum toxin may give relief but frequently must be repeated.

Blepharitis. This inflammation of the lid margins is characterized by erythema and crusting or scaling; the usual symptoms are irritation, burning, and itching. The condition is commonly bilateral and chronic or recurrent. The two main types are staphylococcal and seborrheic. In *staphylococcal blepharitis*, ulceration of the lid margin is common, the lashes tend to fall out, and conjunctivitis and superficial keratitis are often associated. In *seborrheic blepharitis*, the scales tend to be greasy, the lid margins are less red, and ulceration usually does not occur. The blepharitis is often of mixed type.

Thorough daily cleansing of the lid margins with a cloth or moistened cotton applicator to remove scales and crusts is important in the treatment of both forms. Staphylococcal blepharitis is treated with an antistaphylococcal antibiotic applied directly to the lid margins. When a child also has seborrhea, concurrent treatment of the scalp is important.

Pediculosis of the eyelashes may produce a clinical picture of blepharitis. The lice can be smothered with ophthalmic-grade petrolatum ointment applied to the lid margin and lashes. Nits should be mechanically removed from the lashes.

Hordeolum. Infection of the glands of the lid may be acute or subacute; tender focal swelling and redness are noted. The usual agent is *Staphylococcus aureus*. When the meibomian glands are involved, the lesion is referred to as an *internal hordeolum;* the abscess tends to be large and may point through either the skin or the conjunctival surface. When the infection involves the glands of Zeis or Moll, the abscess tends to be smaller and more superficial and points at the lid margin; it is then referred to as an *external hordeolum* or *stye.*

Treatment is frequent warm compresses and, if necessary, surgical incision and drainage. In addition, topical antibiotic preparations are often used. Untreated, the infection may progress to cellulitis of the lid or orbit, requiring the use of systemic antibiotics.

Chalazion. A chalazion is a granulomatous inflammation of a meibomian gland characterized by a firm, nontender nodule in the upper or lower lid. This lesion tends to be chronic and differs from internal hordeolum in the absence of acute inflammatory signs. Although many chalazia subside spontaneously, excision may be necessary if they become large enough to distort vision (by inducing astigmatism by exerting pressure on the globe) or to be a cosmetic blemish.

Coloboma of the Eyelid. This cleftlike deformity may vary from a small indentation or notch of the free margin of the lid to a large defect involving almost the entire lid. If the gap is extensive, xerosis, ulceration, and corneal opacities may result from exposure. Early surgical correction of the lid defect is recommended. Other deformities frequently associated with lid colobomas include dermoid cysts or dermolipomas on the globe; they often occur in a position corresponding to the site of the lid defect. Lid colobomas may also be associated with extensive facial malformation, as in mandibulofacial dysostosis (Franceschetti or Treacher Collins syndrome).

Tumors of the Lid. A number of lid tumors arise from surface structures (the epithelium and sebaceous glands). *Nevi* may appear in early childhood; most are junctional. Compound nevi tend to develop in the prepubertal years and dermal nevi at puberty. *Malignant epithelial tumors* (basal cell carcinoma, squamous cell carcinoma) are rare in children, but the basal cell nevus syndrome and the malignant lesions of xeroderma pigmentosum and of Rothmund-Thomson syndrome may develop in childhood.

Other lid tumors arise from deeper structures (the neural, vascular, and connective tissues). *Capillary hemangiomas* are especially common in children. Many tend to regress spontaneously, although they may show alarmingly rapid growth in infancy. In many cases, the best management of such hemangiomas is patient observation, allowing spontaneous regression to occur (see Chapter 640). In the case of a rapidly expanding lesion, which may cause amblyopia by obstructing the visual axis or inducing astigmatism, corticosteroid, interferon, or surgical treatment should be considered. *Nevus flammeus* (portwine stain), a noninvoluting hemangioma, occurs as an isolated lesion or in association with other signs of Sturge-Weber syndrome. Affected patients should be monitored for the development of glaucoma. *Lymphangiomas* of the lid appear as firm masses at or soon after birth and tend to enlarge slowly during the growing years. Associated conjunctival involvement, appearing as a clear, cystic, sinuous conjunctival mass, may provide a clue to the diagnosis. In some cases there is also orbital involvement. The treatment is surgical excision. *Plexiform neuromas* of the lids occur in children with neurofibromatosis, often with ptosis as the first sign. The lid may take on an S-shaped configuration. The lids may also be involved by other tumors, such as retinoblastoma, neuroblastoma, and rhabdomyosarcoma of the orbit; these conditions are discussed elsewhere.

Anderson RL, Baumgarten SA: Amblyopia in ptosis. *Arch Ophthalmol* 1980;98:1068.

Crawford JS: Congenital eyelid anomalies in children. *J Pediatr Ophthalmol Strabismus* 1984;21:140.

Crawford JS, Iliff CE, Stasier OG: Symposium on congenital ptosis. *J Pediatr Ophthalmol Strabismus* 1982;19:245.

Johnson CC: Epicanthus and epiblepharon. *Arch Ophthalmol* 1978;96:1030.

Masaki S: Congenital bilateral facial paralysis. *Arch Otolaryngol* 1971;94:260.

McCully JP, Dougherty JM, Deneau DG: Classification of chronic blepharitis. *Ophthalmology* 1982;89:1173.

Moainie R, Kopelowitz N, Rosenfeld W, et al: Congenital eversion of the eyelids: A report of two cases treated with conservative management. *J Pediatr Ophthalmol Strabismus* 1982;19:326.

Pico G: Congenital ectropion and distichiasis. Etiologic and hereditary factors. A report of cases and review of the literature. *Am J Ophthalmol* 1959;47:363.

Pratt SG, Beyer CK, Johnson CC: The Marcus Gunn phenomenon: A review of 71 cases. *Ophthalmology* 1984;91:27.

Schaefer DP, Schaefer AJ: Blepharoptosis: Classification, evaluation and treatment in the pediatric age group. *Ophthalmol Clin North Am* 1996;2:277.

Stigmar G, Crawford JS, Ward CM, et al: Ophthalmic sequelae of infantile hemangiomas of the eyelid and orbit. *Am J Ophthalmol* 1978;85:806.

Chapter 616
Disorders of the Lacrimal System

The Tear Film. The tear film, which bathes the eye, is actually a complex structure composed of three layers. The innermost mucin layer is secreted by the goblet and epithelial cells of the conjunctiva and the acinar cells of the lacrimal gland. It adds stability and provides an attachment for the tear film to the conjunctiva and cornea. The middle aqueous layer constitutes 98% of the tear film and is produced by the main lacrimal gland and accessory lacrimal glands. It contains various electrolytes and proteins as well as antibodies. The outermost lipid layer is produced largely from the sebaceous meibomian glands of the eyelid and retards evaporation of the tear film. Tears drain medially into the punctal openings of the lid margin and flow through the canaliculi into the lacrimal sac and then through the nasolacrimal duct into the nose.

Dacryostenosis and Dacryocystitis. *Congenital nasolacrimal duct obstruction* (CNLDO), or dacryostenosis, is the most common disorder of the lacrimal system, occurring in up to 6% of newborn infants. It is usually caused by a failure of canalization of the epithelial cells that form the nasolacrimal duct as it enters the nose (valve of Hasner). Signs of CNLDO may be present at the time of birth, although the condition may not become evident until normal tear production develops. Signs of CNLDO include an excessive tear lake, overflow of tears onto the lid and cheek, and reflux of mucoid material that is produced in the lacrimal sac. Erythema or maceration of the skin may result from irritation and rubbing produced by dripping of tears and discharge. If the blockage is complete, these signs may be severe and continuous. If obstruction is only partial, the nasolacrimal duct may be capable of draining the basal tear film that is produced. However, under periods of increased tear production (exposure to cold, wind, sunlight) or increased closure of the distal end of the nasolacrimal duct (nasal mucosal edema), tear overflow may become evident or may increase.

Infants with CNLDO may develop acute infection and inflammation of the nasolacrimal sac (dacryocystitis), inflammation of the surrounding tissues (pericystitis), or rarely periorbital cellulitis. With dacryocystitis, the sac area is swollen, red, and tender, and patients may have systemic signs of infection such as fever and irritability.

The primary treatment of uncomplicated nasolacrimal obstruction is a regimen of nasolacrimal massage, usually 2–3 times a day, accompanied by cleansing of the lids with warm water. Topical antibiotics are used for significant mucopurulent drainage. Most cases of CNLDO resolve spontaneously, 96% before 1 yr of age. For cases that do not resolve by 1 yr, the nasolacrimal duct may be probed, with a cure rate of approximately 90%.

Acute dacryocystitis or *cellulitis* requires prompt treatment with antibiotics. In such cases, some form of definitive surgical intervention is usually indicated.

A *mucocele* is an unusual presentation of a nonpatent nasolacrimal sac that is obstructed both proximally and distally. Mucoceles can be seen at birth or shortly after birth as a bluish subcutaneous mass just below the medial canthal tendon. Initial treatment should include warm compresses and gentle massage of the lacrimal sac. If an infection develops, systemic administration of antibiotics is required. A probing of the nasolacrimal system may then be necessary to prevent further infection or treat abscess formation.

Not all tearing in infants and children is caused by nasolacrimal obstruction. Tearing may also be a sign of glaucoma, intraocular inflammation, or external irritation, such as that from a corneal abrasion or foreign body.

Dacryoadenitis. Dacryoadenitis, or inflammation of the lacrimal gland, is uncommon in childhood. It may occur with mumps (in which case it is usually acute and bilateral, subsiding in a few days or weeks) or with infectious mononucleosis. *Staphylococcus aureus* may produce a suppurative dacryoadenitis. Chronic dacryoadenitis is associated with certain systemic diseases, particularly sarcoidosis, tuberculosis, and syphilis. Some systemic diseases may produce enlargement of the lacrimal and salivary glands (**Mikulicz syndrome**).

Alacrima and "Dry Eye." Marked deficiency of tears may occur as an isolated unilateral or bilateral congenital defect or in association with other nervous system anomalies, such as aplasia of cranial nerve nuclei. It occurs congenitally in familial dysautonomia (Riley-Day syndrome) and in the anhidrotic type of ectodermal dysplasia; it may occur with glucocorticoid deficiency, sometimes in association with swallowing dysfunction. An acquired abnormality of any layer of the tear film may produce a dry eye. Commonly acquired disorders that may lead to a decreased or unstable tear film include Sjögren syndrome, Stevens-Johnson syndrome, vitamin A deficiency, ocular pemphigoid, trachoma, chemical burns, irradiation, and meibomian gland dysfunction. Any tear deficiency can lead to corneal ulceration, scarring, or infection. Treatment includes correction of the underlying disorder when possible and frequent instillation of an artificial tear preparation. In some cases, occlusion of the lacrimal puncta is helpful. In severe cases, tarsorrhaphy may be necessary to protect the cornea.

Caccamise WC, Townes PL: Congenital absence of the lacrimal puncta associated with alacrima and aptyalism. *Am J Ophthalmol* 1980;89:62.
El-Mansoury J, Calhoun JH, Nelson LB, et al: Results of late probing for congenital nasolacrimal duct obstruction. *Ophthalmology* 1986;93:1052.
Geffner ME, Lippe BM, Kaplan SA, et al: Selective ACTH insensitivity, achalasia, and alacrima: A multisystem disorder presenting in childhood. *Pediatr Res* 1983;17:532.
MacEwen CJ, Young JD: Epiphora during the first year of life. *Eye* 1991;5:596.
Manson AM, Cheng KP, Mumma JV, et al: Congenital dacryocele. *Ophthalmology* 1991;98:1744.
Mondino BJ, Brown SI: Hereditary congenital alacrima. *Arch Ophthalmol* 1976;94:1478.
Paul TO: Medical management of congenital nasolacrimal duct obstruction. *J Pediatr Ophthalmol Strabismus* 1985;22:68.
Robb RM: Success rates of nasolacrimal duct probing at time intervals after 1 year of age. *Ophthalmology* 1998;105:1307.
Schnall BM, Christian CJ: Conservative treatment of congenital dacryocele. *J Pediatr Ophthalmol Strabismus* 1996;33:219.
Wagner RS: Lacrimal disorders. *Ophthalmol Clin North Am* 1996;2:229.
Young JD, MacEwen CJ: Managing congenital lacrimal obstruction in general practice. *Br Med J* 1997;315:293.

Chapter 617
Disorders of the Conjunctiva

Conjunctivitis. The conjunctiva reacts to a wide range of bacterial and viral agents, allergens, irritants, toxins, and systemic diseases. Conjunctivitis is common in childhood and may be infectious or noninfectious (Table 617–1).

Ophthalmia Neonatorum. Ophthalmia neonatorum, a form of conjunctivitis occurring in infants younger than 4 wk of age, is the most common eye disease of newborns. Its many different etiologic agents vary greatly in their virulence and outcome. For instance, silver nitrate instillation may result in a mild self-limited conjunctivitis, whereas *Neisseria gonorrhoeae* and

TABLE 617–1. The Red Eye

Condition	Etiology	Signs and Symptoms	Treatment
Bacterial conjunctivitis	*Haemophilus influenzae, Haemophilus aegyptius, Streptococcus pneumoniae, Neisseria gonorrhoeae*	Mucopurulent unilateral or bilateral discharge, normal vision, photophobia Conjunctival injection and edema (chemosis); gritty sensation	Topical antibiotics, parenteral ceftriaxone for gonococcus, *H. influenzae*
Viral conjunctivitis Neonatal conjunctivitis	Adenovirus, ECHO virus, coxsackievirus *Chlamydia trachomatis*, gonococcus, chemical (silver nitrate), *Staphylococcus aureus*	As above; may be hemorrhagic, unilateral Palpebral conjunctival follicle or papillae; as above	Self- limited Ceftriaxone for gonococcus and erythromycin for *C. trachomatis*
Allergic conjunctivitis	Seasonal pollens or allergen exposure	Itching, incidence of bilateral chemosis (edema) greater than that of erythema, tarsal papillae	Antihistamines, steroids, cromolyn
Keratitis	Herpes simplex, adenovirus, *Streptococcus pneumoniae, Staphylococcus aureus, Pseudomonas, Acanthamoeba,* chemicals	Severe pain, corneal swelling, clouding, limbus erythema, hypopyon, cataracts; contact lens history with amebic infection	Specific antibiotics for bacterial/fungal infections; keratoplasty, acyclovir for herpes
Endophthalmitis	*S. aureus, S. pneumoniae, Candida albicans,* associated surgery or trauma	Acute onset, pain, loss of vision, swelling, chemosis, redness; hypopyon and vitreous haze	Antibiotics
Anterior uveitis (iridocyclitis)	JRA, Reiter syndrome, sarcoidosis, Behçet disease, Kawasaki's disease, inflammatory bowel disease	Unilateral/bilateral; erythema, ciliary flush, irregular pupil, iris adhesions; pain, photophobia, small pupil, poor vision	Topical steroids, plus therapy for primary disease
Posterior uveitis (choroiditis) Episcleritis/scleritis	Toxoplasmosis, histoplasmosis, *Toxocara canis* Idiopathic autoimmune disease (e.g., SLE, Henoch-Schönlein purpura)	No signs of erythema, decreased vision Localized pain, intense erythema, unilateral; blood vessels bigger than in conjunctivitis; scleritis may cause globe perforation	Specific therapy for pathogen Episcleritis is self-limiting; topical steroids for fast relief
Foreign body Blepharitis	Occupational exposure *S. aureus, Staphylococcus epidermidis,* seborrheic, blocked lacrimal duct; rarely molluscum contagiosum, *Phthirus pubis, Pediculus capitis*	Unilateral, red, gritty feeling; visible or microscopic size Bilateral, irritation, itching, hyperemia, crusting, affecting lid margins	Irrigation, removal; check for ulceration Topical antibiotics, warm compresses
Dacryocystitis	Obstructed lacrimal sac: *S. aureus, H. influenzae,* pneumococcus	Pain, tenderness, erythema and exudate in area of lacrimal sac (inferomedial to inner canthus); tearing (epiphora); possible orbital cellulitis	Systemic, topical antibiotics; surgical drainage
Dacryoadenitis	*S. aureus, Streptococcus,* CMV, measles, EBV, enteroviruses; trauma, sarcoidosis, leukemia	Pain, tenderness, edema, erythema over gland area (upper temporal lid); fever, leukocytosis	Systemic antibiotics; drainage of orbital abscesses
Orbital cellulitis (postseptal cellulitis)	Paranasal sinusitis: *H. influenzae, S. aureus, S. pneumoniae,* streptococci Trauma: *S. aureus* Fungi: *Aspergillus, Mucor* spp. if immunodeficient	Rhinorrhea, chemosis, vision loss, painful extraocular motion, proptosis, ophthalmoplegia, fever, lid edema, leukocytosis	Systemic antibiotics, drainage of orbital abscesses
Periorbital cellulitis (preseptal cellulitis)	Trauma: *S. aureus,* streptococci Bacteremia: pneumococcus, streptococci, *H. influenzae*	Cutaneous erythema, warmth, normal vision, minimal involvement of orbit; fever, leukocytosis, toxic appearance	Systemic antibiotics

CMV = cytomegalovirus; EBV = Epstein-Barr virus; JRA = juvenile rheumatoid arthritis; SLE = systemic lupus erythematosus.
From Behrman R, Kliegman R: Nelson's Essentials of Pediatrics, 3rd ed. Philadelphia, WB Saunders, 1998.

Pseudomonas are capable of causing corneal perforation, blindness, and death. The risk of conjunctivitis in newborns depends on frequencies of maternal infections, prophylactic measures, circumstances during labor and delivery, and postdelivery exposures to microorganisms.

EPIDEMIOLOGY. Conjunctivitis during the neonatal period is usually acquired during vaginal delivery and reflects the sexually transmitted diseases prevalent in the community. In 1880, 10% of European children developed gonococcal conjunctivitis at birth. Ophthalmia neonatorum was the leading cause of blindness during that period. The epidemiology of this condition changed dramatically in 1881, when Crede reported that 2% silver nitrate solution instilled in the eyes of newborns reduced the incidence of gonococcal ophthalmia from 10% to 0.3%.

During the 20th century, the incidence of gonococcal ophthalmia neonatorum decreased in industrialized countries secondary to widespread use of silver nitrate prophylaxis and prenatal screening and treatment of maternal gonorrhea. Gonococcal ophthalmia neonatorum has an incidence of 0.3/1,000 live births in the United States. In comparison, *Chlamydia trachomatis* is the most common organism causing ophthalmia neonatorum in the United States, with an incidence of 8.2/1,000 births.

CLINICAL MANIFESTATIONS. The clinical manifestations of the various forms of ophthalmia neonatorum are not specific enough to allow an accurate diagnosis. Although the timing and character of the signs are somewhat typical for each cause of this condition, there is considerable overlap and physicians should not rely solely on clinical findings. Regardless of its cause, ophthalmia neonatorum is characterized by redness and chemosis (swelling) of the conjunctiva, edema of the eyelids, and discharge, which may be purulent.

Ophthalmia neonatorum is a potentially blinding condition. The infection may also have associated systemic manifestations that require treatment. Therefore, any newborn infant who develops signs of conjunctivitis needs a prompt and comprehensive evaluation to determine the agent causing the infection and the appropriate treatment.

The onset of inflammation caused by silver nitrate drops usually occurs within 6–12 hr after birth, with clearing by 24–48 hr. The usual incubation period for conjunctivitis due to *N. gonorrhoeae* is 2–5 days and for that due to *C. trachomatis* is 5–14 days. Gonococcal infection may be present at birth or delayed beyond 5 days of life owing to partial suppression by ocular prophylaxis. Gonococcal conjunctivitis may also begin in infancy after inoculation by the contaminated fingers of adults. The time of onset of disease with other bacteria is highly variable.

Gonococcal conjunctivitis begins with mild inflammation and a serosanguineous discharge. Within 24 hr, the discharge becomes thick and purulent, and tense edema of the eyelids with marked chemosis occurs. If proper treatment is delayed, the infection may spread to involve the deeper layers of the conjunctivae and the cornea. Complications include corneal ulceration and perforation, iridocyclitis, anterior synechiae, and rarely panophthalmitis. Conjunctivitis caused by *C. trachomatis* (inclusion blennorrhea) may vary from mild inflammation to severe swelling of the eyelids with copious purulent discharge. The process involves mainly the tarsal conjunctivae; the corneas are rarely affected. Conjunctivitis due to *Staphylococcus aureus* or other organisms is similar to that produced by *C. trachomatis*. Conjunctivitis due to *Pseudomonas aeruginosa* is uncommon, is acquired in the nursery, and is a potentially serious process. It is characterized by the appearance on day 5–18 of edema, erythema of the lids, purulent discharge, pannus formation, endophthalmitis, sepsis, shock, and death.

DIAGNOSIS. Conjunctivitis appearing after 48 hr should be evaluated for a possibly infectious cause. Gram stain of the purulent discharge should be performed and the material cultured. If a viral etiology is suspected, a swab should be submitted in tissue culture media for virus isolation. In chlamydial conjunctivitis, the diagnosis is made by examining Giemsa-stained epithelial cells scraped from the tarsal conjunctivae for the characteristic intracytoplasmic inclusions, by isolating the organisms from a conjunctival swab using special tissue culture techniques, by immunofluorescent staining of conjunctival scrapings for chlamydial inclusions, or by tests for chlamydial antigen. The differential diagnosis includes dacryocystitis caused by congenital lacrimal duct obstruction with lacrimal sac distention (dacryocystocele).

TREATMENT. Treatment of infants in whom gonococcal ophthalmia is suspected and the Gram stain shows the characteristic intracellular gram-negative diplococci should be initiated immediately with ceftriaxone, 50 mg/kg/24 hr for one dose not to exceed 125 mg. In addition, the eye should be irrigated initially with saline every 10–30 min, gradually increasing to 2-hr intervals until the purulent discharge has cleared. An alternative regimen includes cefotaxime (100 mg/kg/24 hr given IV or IM every 12 hr for 7 days or 100 mg/kg as a single dose). Treatment is extended if sepsis or other extraocular sites are involved (meningitis, arthritis). Inclusion blennorrhea is treated with oral erythromycin (50 mg/kg/24 hr in four divided doses) for 2 wk. This cures conjunctivitis and may prevent subsequent chlamydial pneumonia. *Pseudomonas* neonatal conjunctivitis is treated with systemic antibiotics, including an aminoglycoside, plus local saline irrigation and gentamicin ophthalmic ointment. Staphylococcal conjunctivitis is treated with parenteral methicillin and local saline irrigation.

PROGNOSIS AND PREVENTION. Before the institution of topical ophthalmic prophylaxis at birth, gonococcal ophthalmia was a common cause of blindness or permanent eye damage. If properly applied, this form of prophylaxis is highly effective unless infection is present at birth. Drops of 0.5% erythromycin or 1% silver nitrate are instilled directly into the open eyes at birth using wax or plastic single-dose containers. Saline irrigation after silver nitrate application is unnecessary. Silver nitrate is ineffective against active infection. Povidone-iodine (2% solution) is also an effective prophylactic agent.

Identification of maternal gonococcal infection and appropriate treatment has become a standard element of routine prenatal care. An infant born to a woman who has untreated gonococcal infection should receive a single dose of ceftriaxone, 50 mg/kg (maximum 125 mg) IV or IM, in addition to topical prophylaxis. The dose should be reduced for premature infants. Penicillin (50,000 units) should be used if the mother's gonococcal isolate is known to be penicillin sensitive.

Neither topical prophylaxis nor topical treatment prevents the afebrile pneumonia that occurs in 10–20% of infants exposed to *C. trachomatis*. Although chlamydial conjunctivitis is often a self-limiting disease, chlamydial pneumonia may have serious consequences. It is important that infants with chlamydial disease receive systemic treatment. Treatment of colonized pregnant women with erythromycin may prevent neonatal disease.

Acute Purulent Conjunctivitis. This is characterized by more or less generalized conjunctival hyperemia, edema, mucopurulent exudate, and various degrees of ocular discomfort. It is usually a result of bacterial infection. The most frequent causes are nontypable *Haemophilus influenzae* (associated with ipsilateral otitis media), pneumococci, staphylococci, and streptococci. Conjunctival smear and culture are helpful in differentiating specific types. These common forms of acute purulent conjunctivitis usually respond well to warm compresses and frequent topical instillation of antibiotic drops. **Brazilian purpuric fever** due to *Haemophilus aegyptius* manifests as conjunctivitis and sepsis. *N. gonorrhoeae* and *Chlamydia* are relatively common causes of acute purulent conjunctivitis in children beyond the newborn period, especially in adolescents. These infections require specific testing and treatment.

Viral Conjunctivitis. This is generally characterized by a watery discharge. Follicular changes (small aggregates of lymphocytes) are often found in the palpebral conjunctiva. Conjunctivitis resulting from adenovirus infection is relatively common, sometimes with corneal involvement (see later text). Outbreaks of conjunctivitis caused by enterovirus are also encountered; this type may be hemorrhagic. Conjunctivitis is commonly associated with such systemic viral infections as the childhood exanthems, particularly measles. These types are self-limited.

Epidemic Keratoconjunctivitis. This is caused by adenovirus type 8 and is transmitted by direct contact. It initially presents as a sensation of a foreign body beneath the lids, with itching and burning. Edema and photophobia develop rapidly, and large oval follicles appear within the conjunctiva. Preauricular adenopathy and a pseudomembrane on the conjunctival surface occur frequently. Subepithelial corneal infiltrates may develop and may cause blurring of vision; these usually disappear but may permanently reduce visual acuity. Corneal complications are less common in children than in adults. Children may have associated upper respiratory tract infection and pharyngitis. Although antibacterial drops are often prescribed, these are generally not indicated. No specific medical therapy is available to decrease the symptoms or shorten the course of the disease. Emphasis must be placed on prevention of spread of the disease. Replicating virus is present in 95% of patients 10 days after the appearance of symptoms.

Membranous and Pseudomembranous Conjunctivitis. These types can be encountered in a number of diseases. The classic membranous conjunctivitis is that of diphtheria, accompanied by a fibrin-rich exudate that forms on the conjunctival surface and permeates the epithelium; the membrane is removed with difficulty and leaves raw bleeding areas. In pseudomembranous conjunctivitis, the layer of fibrin-rich exudate is superficial and can often be stripped easily, leaving the surface smooth. This type occurs with many bacterial and viral infections, including staphylococcal, pneumococcal, streptococcal, or chlamydial conjunctivitis, and in epidemic keratoconjunctivitis. It is also found in vernal conjunctivitis and in Stevens-Johnson disease.

Allergic Conjunctivitis. This is usually accompanied by intense itching, tearing, and conjunctival edema. It is commonly seasonal. Cold compresses and decongestant drops give symptomatic relief. Topical mast cell stabilizers or prostaglandin inhibitors may also help. In selected cases, topical corticosteroids are used under an ophthalmologist's supervision.

Vernal Conjunctivitis. This usually begins in the prepubertal years and may recur for many years. Atopy appears to have a role in its origin, but the pathogenesis is uncertain. Extreme itching and tearing are the usual complaints. Large, flattened, cobblestone-like papillary lesions of the palpebral conjunctivae are characteristic. A stringy exudate and a milky conjunctival pseudomembrane are frequently present. Small elevated lesions of the bulbar conjunctiva adjacent to the limbus (limbal form) may be found. Smear of the conjunctival exudate reveals many eosinophils. Topical corticosteroid therapy and cold compresses afford some relief. Topical mast cell stabilizers or prostaglandin inhibitors are useful when long-term control is needed. The long-term use of corticosteroids should be avoided.

Chemical Conjunctivitis. This can result when an irritating substance enters the conjunctival sac (as in the acute but benign conjunctivitis caused by silver nitrate in newborns). Other common offenders are household cleaning substances, sprays, smoke, smog, and industrial pollutants. Alkalis tend to linger in the conjunctival tissues and continue to inflict damage for hours or days. Acids precipitate the proteins in tissues and so produce

their effect immediately. In either case, prompt, thorough, and copious irrigation is crucial. Extensive tissue damage, even loss of the eye, can result, especially if the offending agent is an alkali.

Other Conjunctival Disorders. *Subconjunctival hemorrhage* is manifested by bright or dark red patches in the bulbar conjunctiva and may result from injury or inflammation. It commonly occurs spontaneously. It may occasionally result from severe sneezing or coughing. Rarely it may be a manifestation of a blood dyscrasia.

Pinguecula is a yellowish-white, slightly elevated mass on the bulbar conjunctiva, usually in the interpalpebral region. It represents elastic and hyaline degenerative changes of the conjunctiva. No treatment is required except for cosmetic reasons, in which case simple excision suffices.

Pterygium is a fleshy triangular conjunctival lesion that may encroach on the cornea. It typically occurs in the nasal interpalpebral region. The pathologic findings are similar to those of a pinguecula. The development of pterygia is related to exposure to ultraviolet light, and it therefore is more commonly found among people who live near the equator. Removal is suggested when the lesion encroaches far onto the cornea. Recurrence after removal is common.

Dermoid cyst and *dermolipoma* are benign lesions, clinically similar in appearance. They are smooth, elevated, round to oval lesions of various sizes. The color varies from yellowish white to fleshy pink. The most frequent site is the upper outer quadrant of the globe; they also commonly occur near or straddling the limbus. Dermolipoma is composed of adipose and connective tissue. Dermoid cysts may also contain glandular tissue, hair follicles, and hair shafts. Excision for cosmetic reasons is feasible. Dermolipomas are often connected to the extraocular muscles, making their complete removal impossible without sacrificing ocular motility.

Conjunctival nevus is a small, slightly elevated lesion that may vary in pigmentation from pale salmon to dark brown. It is usually benign, but careful observation for progressive growth or changes suggestive of malignancy is advised.

Symblepharon is a cicatricial adhesion between the conjunctiva of the lid and the globe; the lower lid is usually affected. It follows operation or injuries, especially burns from lye, acids, or molten metals. It is a serious complication of Stevens-Johnson syndrome. It may interfere with motion of the eyeball and may cause diplopia. The adhesions should be separated and the raw surfaces kept from uniting during healing. Grafts of oral mucous membrane may be necessary.

Abelson MB, Schaefer K: Conjunctivitis of allergic origin: Immunologic mechanisms and current approaches to therapy. *Surv Ophthalmol* 1993;38:115.

Arstikaitis MJ: Ocular aftermath of Stevens-Johnson syndrome. *Arch Ophthalmol* 1973;90:376.

Brook I: Anaerobic and aerobic bacterial flora of acute conjunctivitis in children. *Arch Ophthalmol* 1980;98:833.

Catalano RA, Nelson LB: Conjunctivitis. In Dershervitz RA (editor): *Ambulatory Pediatric Care*, 2nd ed. Philadelphia, JB Lippincott, 1992.

Fischer MC: Conjunctivitis in children. *Pediatr Clin North Am* 1987;34:1447.

Hammerschlag MR, Cummings C, Roblin PM, et al: Efficacy of neonatal ocular prophylaxis for the prevention of chlamydial and gonococcal conjunctivitis. *N Engl J Med* 1989;320:769.

Isenberg SJ, Apt L, Wood M: A controlled trial of povidone-iodine as prophylaxis against ophthalmia neonatorum. *N Engl J Med* 1995;332:562.

Isenberg SJ, Apt L, Yoshimura R, et al: Bacterial flora of the conjunctiva at birth. *J Pediatr Ophthalmol Strabismus* 1986;23:284.

Knopf HL, Hierholzer JC: Clinical and immunologic responses in patients with viral keratoconjunctivitis. *Am J Ophthalmol* 1975;80:661.

Matobu A: Ocular viral infections. *Pediatr Infect Dis* 1984;3:358.

O'Hara MA: Ophthalmia neonatorum. *Pediatr Clin North Am* 1993;40:715.

Roba LA, Kowalski RP, Romanowski E, at al: How long are patients with epidemic keratoconjunctivitis infectious? *Invest Ophthalmol Vis Sci* 1993;34:848.

Schnall BM, Nelson LB: Ophthalmia neonatorum. *Semin Ophthalmol* 1990;5:107.

Shiuey Y, Ambati BK, Adamis AP, and the Viral Conjunctivitis Study Group: A randomized, double-masked trial of topical ketorolac versus artificial tears for treatment of viral conjunctivitis. *Ophthalmology* 2000;107:1512.

Chapter 618
Abnormalities of the Cornea

Megalocornea. This is a nonprogressive symmetric condition characterized by an enlarged cornea (>12 mm in diameter) and an anterior segment in which there is no evidence of previous or concurrent ocular hypertension. High myopia is frequently present and may lead to reduced vision. A frequent complication is the development of lens opacities in adult life. All modes of inheritance have been described, although X-linked recessive is most common; therefore, this disorder most commonly afflicts males. Systemic abnormalities that may be associated with megalocornea include Marfan syndrome, craniosynostosis, and Alport syndrome. The cause of the enlargement of the cornea and the anterior segment is unknown, but possible explanations include a defect in the growth of the optic cup and an arrest of congenital glaucoma. The region on the X chromosome responsible for this disorder has been identified.

Pathologic corneal enlargement caused by glaucoma is to be differentiated from this anomaly. Any progressive increase in the size of the cornea, especially when accompanied by photophobia, lacrimation, or haziness of the cornea, requires prompt ophthalmologic evaluation.

Microcornea. Microcornea, or *anterior microphthalmia,* is an abnormally small cornea in an otherwise relatively normal eye. It may be familial, with transmission being dominant more often than recessive. More commonly, a small cornea is just one feature of an otherwise developmentally abnormal or microphthalmic eye; associated defects include colobomas, microphakia, congenital cataract, glaucoma, and aniridia.

Keratoconus. This is a disease of unclear pathogenesis characterized by progressive thinning and bulging of the central cornea, which becomes cone shaped. Although familial cases are known, most cases are sporadic. Eye rubbing and contact lens wear have been implicated as pathogenic, but the evidence to support this is equivocal. The incidence is increased in individuals with atopy, Down syndrome, Marfan syndrome, and retinitis pigmentosa.

Most cases are bilateral, but involvement may be asymmetric. The disorder usually presents and progresses rapidly during adolescence; progression slows and stabilizes when patients reach full growth. Descemet membrane may occasionally be stretched beyond its elastic breaking point, causing an acute rupture in the membrane with resultant sudden and marked corneal edema (acute hydrops) and decrease in vision. The corneal edema resolves as endothelial cells cover the defective area. Some degree of corneal scarring occurs, but the visual acuity is often better than before the initial incident. Signs of keratoconus include Munson sign (bulging of the lower eyelid on looking downward) and the presence of a Fleischer ring (a deposit of iron in the epithelium at the base of the cone). Corneal transplantation is indicated if satisfactory visual acuity cannot be attained with the use of contact lenses.

Neonatal Corneal Opacities. Loss of the normal transparency of the cornea in neonates may occur secondary to either intrinsic hereditary or extrinsic environmental causes (Table 618–1).

Sclerocornea. In sclerocornea, the normal translucent cornea is replaced by sclera-like tissue. Instead of a clearly demarcated cornea, white, feathery, often ill-defined and vascularized tissue develops in the peripheral cornea, appearing to blend with and extend from the sclera. The central cornea is usually clearer, but total replacement of the cornea with sclera may occur. The curvature of the cornea is often flatter, similar to the sclera. Potentially coexisting abnormalities include a shallow anterior chamber, iris abnormalities, and microphthalmos. This condition is usually bilateral. In approximately 50% of cases, a dominant or recessive inheritance has been described. Sclerocornea has been reported in association with numerous systemic abnormalities including limb deformities, craniofacial defects, and genitourinary disorders. In generalized sclerocornea, early keratoplasty should be considered in an effort to provide vision.

Peters Anomaly. Peters anomaly is a central corneal opacity (leukoma) that is present at birth. It is often associated with iridocorneal adhesions that extend from the iris collarette to the border of the corneal opacity. Approximately one half of patients have other ocular abnormalities, which may include cataracts, glaucoma, and microcornea. As many as 80% of cases may be bilateral, and 60% are associated with systemic malformations that may affect any major organ system. Some investigators have divided Peter anomaly into two types: a mesodermal or neuroectodermal form (type I), which shows no associated lens changes, and a surface ectodermal form (type II), which does. Histologic findings include a focal absence of Descemet membrane and corneal endothelium in the region of the opacity. Peters anomaly may be caused by incomplete migration and differentiation of the precursor cells of the central corneal endothelium and Descemet membrane or a defective separation between the primitive lens and cornea during embryogenesis.

Dermoids. Epibulbar dermoids are choristomas. They are often present at birth and may increase in size with age. They occur most frequently in the lower temporal quadrant. They most commonly straddle the limbus and extend into the peripheral cornea. Rarely, they may be confined entirely to the cornea or conjunctiva. Epibulbar dermoids may cause visual disturbance by encroaching on the visual axis or by contributing to the development of astigmatism.

A dermoid usually appears as a well-circumscribed rounded or oval, gray or pinkish-yellow mass with a dry surface from which short hairs may protrude. It may affect only the superficial layers of the cornea, although full-thickness involvement is common. Associated ocular anomalies include eyelid and iris colobomas, microphthalmos, and retinal and choroidal defects. A total of 30% of dermoids are associated with systemic abnormalities. Many of the associated anomalies involve developmental defects of the first branchial arch (vertebral anomalies, dystosis of the facial bones and dental anomalies, and Goldenhar syndrome). Epibulbar dermoids are found in 75% of cases of Goldenhar syndrome.

Dendritic Keratitis. Infection of the cornea with the virus of herpes simplex produces a characteristic lesion of the corneal epithelium, referred to as a *dendrite*; it has a branching treelike pattern that can be demonstrated by fluorescein staining. The acute episode is accompanied by pain, photophobia, tearing, blepharospasm, and conjunctival infection. Specific treatment may include mechanical debridement of the involved corneal epithelium to remove the source of infection and eliminate an antigenic stimulus to inflammation in the adjacent stroma. Medical treatment involves the use of 5-iodo-2'-deoxyuridine (IDU), topical vidarabine, or, most commonly, trifluridine. In addition, a cycloplegic agent is useful to relieve pain from spasm of the ciliary muscle. Overly aggressive topical antiviral treatment itself can be toxic to the cornea and should be avoided. Recurrent infection and deep stromal involvement can lead to corneal scarring and loss of vision.

Topical use of corticosteroids causes exacerbation of superficial herpetic disease of the eye and may lead to corneal perforation; eye drops combining steroids and antibiotics are therefore to be avoided in treatment of red eye unless there are clear-cut indications for their use and close supervision during therapy.

Infants born to mothers infected with herpes simplex virus should be examined carefully for signs of ocular involvement.

TABLE 618–1. STUMPED: Differential Diagnosis of Neonatal Corneal Opacities

Diagnosis	Laterality	Opacity	Ocular Pressure	Other Ocular Abnormalities	Natural History	Inheritance
S–Sclerocornea	Unilateral or bilateral	Vascularized, blends with sclera, clearer centrally	Normal (or elevated)	Cornea plana	Nonprogressive	Sporadic
T–Tears in endothelium and Descemet's membrane						
Birth trauma	Unilateral	Diffuse edema	Normal	Possible hyphema, periorbital ecchymoses	Spontaneous improvement in 1 mo	Sporadic
Infantile glaucoma	Bilateral	Diffuse edema	Elevated	Megalocornea, photophobia and tearing, abnormal angle	Progressive unless treated	Autosomal recessive
U–Ulcers						
Herpes simplex keratitis	Unilateral	Diffuse with geographic epithelial defect	Normal	None	Progressive	Sporadic
Congenital rubella	Bilateral	Disciform or diffuse edema, no frank ulceration	Normal or elevated	Microphthalmos, cataract, pigment epithelial mottling	Stable, may clear	Sporadic
Neurotrophic—exposure	Unilateral or bilateral	Central ulcer	Normal	Lid anomalies, congenital sensory neuropathy	Progressive	Sporadic
M–Metabolic (rarely present at birth) (mucopolysaccharidoses IH, IS; mucolipidoses type IV)*	Bilateral	Diffuse haze, denser peripherally	Normal	Few	Progressive	Autosomal dominant
P–Posterior corneal defect	Unilateral or bilateral	Central, diffuse haze or vascularized leukoma	Normal or elevated	Anterior chamber cleavage syndrome	Stable, sometimes early clearing or vascularization	Sporadic, autosomal recessive
E–Endothelial dystrophy						
Congenital hereditary endothelial dystrophy	Bilateral	Diffuse corneal edema, marked corneal thickening	Normal	None	Stable	Autosomal dominant or recessive
Posterior polymorphous dystrophy	Bilateral	Diffuse haze, normal corneal thickness	Normal	Occasional peripheral anterior synechiae	Slowly progressive	Autosomal dominant
Congenital hereditary stromal dystrophy	Bilateral	Flaky, feathery stromal opacities; normal corneal thickness	Normal	None	Stable	Autosomal dominant
D–Dermoid	Unilateral or bilateral	White vascularized mass, hair, lipid arc	Normal	None	Stable	Sporadic

Mucopolysaccharidosis IH (Hurler's syndrome); mucopolysaccharidosis IS (Scheie's syndrome).
From Nelson LB, Calhoun JH, Harley RD: Pediatric Ophthalmology, 3rd ed. Philadelphia, WB Saunders, 1991, p 210.

Intravenous acyclovir is required for treatment of ocular herpes in newborns.

Corneal Ulcers. The usual signs and symptoms are focal or diffuse corneal haze, hyperemia, lid edema, pain, photophobia, tearing, and blepharospasm. *Hypopyon* (pus in the anterior chamber) is common. Corneal ulcers require prompt treatment. They result most frequently from traumatic lesions that become secondarily infected. Many organisms are capable of infecting the cornea. One of the most troublesome is *Pseudomonas aeruginosa*; it can rapidly destroy stromal tissue and lead to corneal perforation. *Neisseria gonorrhoeae* also is particularly damaging to the cornea. Indolent ulcers may be caused by fungi, often in association with the use of contact lenses. In each case, scrapings of the cornea must be studied in an effort to identify the infectious agent and to determine the best therapy. Although aggressive local treatment is generally needed to save the eye, systemic treatment may be necessary in some cases as well. Perforation or scarring resulting from corneal ulceration is an important cause of blindness throughout the world and is estimated to be responsible for 10% of blindness in the United States.

Unexplained corneal ulcers in infants and young children should raise the question of a sensory defect, as in Riley-Day or Goldenhar-Gorlin syndrome, or of a metabolic disorder such as tyrosinemia.

Phlyctenules. These are small, yellowish, slightly elevated lesions usually located at the corneal limbus; they may encroach on the cornea and extend centrally. A small corneal ulcer is often found at the head of the advancing lesion, with a fascicle of blood vessels behind the head of the lesion. Although once thought to represent a sign of systemic tuberculin infection, phlyctenular keratoconjunctivitis is now accepted as a morphologic expression of delayed hypersensitivity to diverse antigens. In children, it commonly occurs as a result of a hypersensitivity reaction of the conjunctiva or cornea to bacterial products. Treatment usually consists of eliminating the underlying disorder, usually staphylococcal blepharitis or meibomianitis, and suppressing the immune response with the use of topical corticosteroid therapy. A superficial stromal pannus and scarring sometimes remain after treatment.

Interstitial Keratitis. This denotes inflammation of the corneal stroma. The most common cause is syphilis, interstitial keratitis being one of the characteristic late manifestations of congenital syphilis. The corneal changes in congenital syphilis occur in two phases. The acute phase presents between the ages of 5 and 10 yr, with an intense keratitis that may last for several months and causes a severe reduction in vision. The acute effects of syphilis are due in most part to the host immune response, such as mononuclear cell infiltrates, proliferative vascular changes, and occasionally granuloma formation. The deep inflammation produces pain, photophobia, tearing, circumcorneal injection, and corneal haze. The acute episode is followed by a chronic stage with significant regression in the corneal findings along with a parallel improvement in visual acuity. Although the corneal findings may regress with time, "ghost vessels," which represent the previous vascular changes, and patchy corneal scarring remain and serve as permanent stigmata of the disease.

Cogan syndrome is a nonluetic interstitial keratitis associated with hearing loss and vestibular symptoms. Although its cause is unknown, a systemic vasculitis is suspected. Prompt treatment is required to avoid permanent hearing loss. Both the corneal changes and the auditory involvement may respond to the use of immunosuppressive agents.

Less frequently, interstitial keratitis is caused by other infectious diseases, such as tuberculosis or leprosy.

Corneal Manifestations of Systemic Disease. Several metabolic diseases produce distinctive corneal changes in childhood. Refractile polychromatic crystals are deposited throughout the cornea in cystinosis. Corneal deposits producing various degrees of corneal haze also occur in certain of the mucopolysaccharidoses, particularly MPS IH (Hurler), MPS IS (Scheie), MPS I H/S (Hurler-Scheie compound), MPS IV (Morquio), MPS VI (Maroteaux-Lamy), and sometimes MPS VII (Sly). Corneal deposits may develop in patients with GM_1 (generalized) gangliosidosis. In Fabry disease, fine opacities radiating in a whorl or fanlike pattern occur, and corneal changes can be important in identifying the carrier state. A spraylike pattern of corneal opacities may also be seen in the Bloch-Sulzberger syndrome. In Wilson disease, the distinctive corneal sign is the Kayser-Fleischer ring, a golden brown ring in the peripheral cornea resulting from changes in Descemet membrane. Pigmented corneal rings may develop in neonates with cholestatic liver disease. Corneal changes may occur in autoimmune hypoparathyroidism and band keratopathy in patients with hypercalcemia. Transient keratitis may occur with rubeola and sometimes with rubella.

Allen NB, Cox CC, Cobo M, et al: Use of immunosuppressive agents in the treatment of severe ocular and vascular manifestations of Cogan's syndrome. *Am J Med* 1990;88:296.

Beauchamp GR, Gillette TE, Friendly DS: Phlyctenular keratoconjunctivitis. *J Pediatr Ophthalmol Strabismus* 1981;18:22.

Dunn LL, Annable WL, Kliegman RM: Pigmented corneal rings in neonates with liver disease. *J Pediatr* 1987;110:771.

Elliott JH, Feman SS, O'Day DM, et al: Hereditary sclerocornea. *Arch Ophthalmol* 1985;103:676.

Goldberg MF, Payne JW, Brunt PW: Ophthalmologic studies of familial dysautonomia. *Arch Ophthalmol* 1966;80:732.

Kraft SP, Judisch GF, Grayson DM: Megalocornea: A clinical and echographic study of an autosomal dominant pedigree. *J Pediatr Ophthalmol Strabismus* 1984;21: 190.

Mackey DA, Buttery RG, Wise GM, et al: Description of X-linked megalocornea with identification of the gene locus. *Arch Ophthalmol* 1991;109:829.

Mohandessan MM, Romano PE: Neuroparalytic keratitis in Goldenhar-Gorlin syndrome. *Am J Ophthalmol* 1978;85:111.

Ndiaye IC, Rassi SJ, Wiener-Vacher SR: Cochleovestibular impairment in pediatric Cogan's syndrome. *Pediatrics* 2002;109(2):e38. (Pediatrics.org/cgi/content/full/109/2/e38)

Reidy JJ: Congenital corneal opacities. *Ophthalmol Clin North Am* 1996;2:199.

Schanzlin DJ, Goldberg DB, Brown SI: Transplantation of congenitally opaque corneas. *Ophthalmology* 1980;87:1253.

Traboulsi EI, Maumenee IH: Peters' anomaly and associated congenital malformations. *Arch Ophthalmol* 1992;110:1739.

Tso MO, Fine BS, Thorpe HE: Kayser-Fleischer ring and associated cataract in Wilson's disease. *Am J Ophthalmol* 1975;79:479.

Yang LL, Lambert SR, Fernhoff PM, et al: Peters' anomaly: Associated congenital malformations and etiology. *Invest Ophthalmol Vis Sci* 1995;36:S41.

Yang LL, Lambert SR, Lynn MJ, et al: Long-term results of corneal graft survival in infants and children with peters anomaly. *Ophthalmology* 1999;106:833.

Chapter 619
Abnormalities of the Lens

Cataracts. A cataract is any opacity of the lens. Some are clinically unimportant, others significantly affect visual function, and many are associated with ocular or systemic disease.

DIFFERENTIAL DIAGNOSIS. The differential diagnosis of cataracts in infants and children includes a wide range of developmental disorders, infectious and inflammatory processes, metabolic diseases, and toxic and traumatic insults (Table 619–1). Cataracts may also develop secondary to intraocular processes, such as retinopathy of prematurity, persistent hyperplastic primary vitreous, retinal detachment, retinitis pigmentosa, and uveitis.

Developmental Variants. Early developmental processes may lead to various congenital lens opacities. Discrete dots or white plaquelike opacities of the lens capsule are common and sometimes involve the contiguous subcapsular region. Small opacities of the posterior capsule may be associated with persistent remnants of the primitive hyaloid vascular system (the common Mittendorf dot), whereas those of the anterior capsule may be associated with persistent strands of the pupillary membrane or vascular sheath of the lens. Congenital cataracts of this type are usually stationary and rarely interfere with vision; in some, progression occurs.

Prematurity. A special type of lens change seen in some preterm newborns is the so-called cataract of prematurity. The appearance is of a cluster of tiny vacuoles in the distribution of the Y sutures of the lens. They can be visualized with an ophthalmoscope and are best seen with the pupil well dilated. The pathogenesis is unclear. In most cases, the opacities disappear spontaneously, often within a few weeks.

Mendelian Inheritance. Many cataracts unassociated with other diseases are hereditary. The most common mode of inheritance is autosomal dominant. Penetrance and expressivity vary. Autosomal recessive inheritance occurs less frequently; it is sometimes found in populations with high rates of consanguinity. X-linked inheritance of cataracts unassociated with disease is relatively rare, whereas cataracts occurring in association with X-linked disease are seen in Lowe syndrome, Alport syndrome, and Fabry disease.

Congenital Infection Syndrome. Cataracts in infants and children frequently are a result of prenatal infection. Lens opacity may occur in any of the major congenital infection syndromes (e.g., toxoplasmosis, cytomegalovirus, syphilis, rubella, herpes simplex virus). Cataracts may also occur secondary to other perinatal infections, including measles, poliomyelitis, influenza, varicella-zoster, and vaccinia.

Metabolic Disorders. Cataracts are a prominent manifestation of many metabolic diseases, particularly certain disorders of carbohydrate, amino acid, calcium, and copper metabolism. A primary consideration in any infant with cataracts is the possibility of galactosemia (see Chapter 76.2). In classic infantile galactosemia, galactose-1-phosphate uridyl transferase deficiency, the cataract is typically of the zonular type, with haziness or opacification of one or more of the perinuclear layers of the lens; haziness or clouding of the nucleus also often occurs. In its early stages, the cataract generally has a distinctive oil droplet appearance and is best detected with the pupil fully dilated. Progression to complete opacification of the lens may occur within weeks. With early treatment (galactose-free diet), the lens changes may be reversible.

In galactokinase deficiency, cataracts are the sole clinical manifestation. The cataracts are usually zonular and may appear in the first months or years of life or later in childhood.

In children with juvenile-onset diabetes mellitus, lens changes are uncommon. Some develop snowflake-like white opacities and vacuoles of the lens. Others develop cataracts that may progress and mature rapidly, sometimes in a matter of days, especially during adolescence. An antecedent event may be the sudden development of myopia caused by changes in the optical density of the lens.

Congenital lens opacities may be seen in children of diabetic and prediabetic mothers. Hypoglycemia in neonates can also be associated with early development of cataracts. Ketotic hypoglycemia is also associated with cataracts.

TABLE 619–1. Differential Diagnosis of Cataracts

Developmental Variants

Prematurity (Y suture vacuoles) with or without retinopathy of prematurity

Genetic Disorders

Simple Mendelian Inheritance

Autosomal dominant (most common)
Autosomal recessive
X-linked

Major Chromosomal Defects

Trisomy disorders (13, 18, 21)
Turner syndrome (45 X)
Deletion syndromes (11p13, 18p, 18q)
Duplication syndromes (3q, 20p, 10q)

Multisystem Genetic Disorders

Alport syndrome (hearing loss, renal disease)
Alström syndrome (nerve deafness, diabetes mellitus)
Apert disease (craniosynostosis, syndactyly)
Cockayne syndrome (premature senility, skin photosensitivity)
Conradi disease (chondrodysplasia punctata)
Crouzon disease (dysostosis craniofacialis)
Hallermann-Streiff syndrome (microphthalmia, small pinched nose, skin atrophy, and hypotrichosis)
Hypohidrotic ectodermal dysplasia (anomalous dentition, hypohidrosis, hypotrichosis)
Ichthyosis (keratinizing disorder with thick, scaly skin)
Incontinentia pigmenti (dental anomalies, mental retardation, cutaneous lesions)
Lowe syndrome (oculocerebrorenal syndrome: hypotonia, renal disease)
Marfan syndrome
Meckel-Gruber syndrome (renal dysplasia, encephalocele)
Myotonic dystrophy
Nail-patella syndrome (renal dysfunction, dysplastic nails, hypoplastic patella)
Marinesco-Sjögren syndrome (cerebellar ataxia, hypotonia)
Nevoid basal cell carcinoma syndrome (autosomal dominant, basal cell carcinoma erupts in childhood)
Peters anomaly (corneal opacifications with iris-corneal dysgenesis)
Reiger syndrome (iris dysplasia, myotonic dystrophy)
Rothmund-Thomson syndrome (poikiloderma: skin atrophy)
Rubinstein-Taybi syndrome (broad great toe, mental retardation)
Smith-Lemli-Opitz syndrome (toe syndactyly, hypospadias, mental retardation)
Sotos syndrome (cerebral gigantism)
Spondyloepiphyseal dysplasia (dwarfism, short trunk)
Werner syndrome (premature aging in 2nd decade of life)

Inborn Errors of Metabolism

Abetalipoproteinemia (absent chylomicrons, retinal degeneration)
Fabry disease (α-galactosidase A deficiency)
Galactokinase deficiency
Galactosemia (galactose-1-phosphate uridyltransferase deficiency)
Homocystinemia (subluxation of lens, mental retardation)
Mannosidosis (acid α-mannosidase deficiency)
Niemann-Pick disease (sphingomyelinase deficiency)
Refsum disease (phytanic acid α-hydrolase deficiency)
Wilson disease (accumulation of copper leads to cirrhosis and neurologic symptoms)

Endocrinopathies

Hypocalcemia (hypoparathyroidism)
Hypoglycemia
Diabetes mellitus

Congenital Infections

Toxoplasmosis
Cytomegalovirus infection
Syphilis
Rubella
Perinatal herpes simplex infection
Measles (rubeola)
Poliomyelitis
Influenza
Varicella-zoster

Ocular Anomalies

Microphthalmia
Coloboma
Aniridia
Mesodermal dysgenesis
Persistent pupillary membrane
Posterior lenticonus
Persistent hyperplastic primary vitreous
Primitive hyaloid vascular system

Miscellaneous Disorders

Atopic dermatitis
Drugs (corticosteroids)
Radiation
Trauma

Idiopathic

An association between cataracts and hypocalcemia is well established. Various lens opacities may be seen in patients with hypoparathyroidism.

The oculocerebral renal syndrome of Lowe is associated with cataracts in infants. Affected male children frequently have dense bilateral cataracts at birth, often in association with glaucoma and miotic pupils. Punctate lens opacities are frequently present in heterozygous females.

The distinctive sunflower cataract of Wilson disease is not commonly seen in children. Various lens opacities may be seen in children with certain of the sphingolipidoses, mucopolysaccharidoses, and mucolipidoses, particularly Niemann-Pick disease, mucosulfatidosis, Fabry disease, and aspartylglycosaminuria.

Chromosomal Defects. Lens opacities of various types may occur in association with chromosomal defects, including 13-, 18-, and 21-trisomy; Turner syndrome; and a number of deletion (11p13, 18p, 18q) and duplication syndromes (3q, 20p, 10q).

Drugs, Toxic Agents, and Trauma. Of the various drugs and toxic agents that may produce cataracts, corticosteroids are of major importance in the pediatric age group. Steroid-related cataracts characteristically are posterior subcapsular lens opacities. The incidence and severity vary. The relative significance of dose, mode of administration, duration of treatment, and individual susceptibility is controversial, and the pathogenesis of steroid-induced cataracts is unclear. The effect on vision depends on the extent and density of the opacity. In many cases, the acuity is only minimally or moderately impaired. Reversibility of steroid-induced cataracts may occur in some cases. All children being treated with long-term steroids should have periodic eye examinations.

Trauma to the eye is a major cause of cataracts in children. Opacification of the lens may result from contusion or penetrating injury. Cataracts are an important manifestation of child abuse. Other physical agents, such as radiation, can also damage the lens and produce cataracts.

Miscellaneous Disorders. The list of multisystem syndromes and diseases associated with lens opacities and other eye anomalies is extensive. The clinical features of some of the major disorders are presented in Table 619–2.

TREATMENT. The treatment of cataracts that significantly interfere with vision includes the following: (1) surgical removal of lens material to provide an optically clear visual axis; (2) correction of the resultant aphakic refractive error with spectacles, contact lenses, or, in appropriate cases, intraocular lens implantation; and (3) correction of any associated sensory deprivation amblyopia. Because the use of spectacles may not be possible or may be contraindicated in children after cataract removal, the use of contact lenses for visual rehabilitation is a medical necessity. They should not be thought of as a cosmetic alternative to glasses. Treatment of the amblyopia may be the most demanding and difficult step in the visual rehabilitation of infants or children with cataracts.

PROGNOSIS. Prognosis depends on many factors, including the nature of the cataract, the underlying disease, age of onset,

TABLE 619–2.   Clinical Features and Ocular Changes in Developmental Pediatric Syndromes

CNS Anomalies

Anencephaly (see Chapter 585.6)
  Optic nerve aplasia or hypoplasia
Holoprosencephaly (see Chapter 585.7)
  Hypotelorism; in extreme form, cyclopia; in some cases, iris coloboma
Cyclopia
  A single eye of variable complexity, usually accompanied by a proboscis-like
    structure on the forehead; often associated with holoprosencephaly; sometimes
    fusion of both eyes with duplication of lenses, corneas, and other structures;
    rosette formation in the retina; optic nerve rudimentary or absent; orbit diamond
    shaped
Arnold-Chiari malformation (see Chapter 585.11)
  Nystagmus, usually vertical, often downbeat; ocular motor palsies with diplopia;
    sometimes skew deviation
Dandy-Walker syndrome (see Chapter 585.11)
  Ophthalmic manifestations of increased intracranial pressure
Septo-optic dysplasia (deMorsier syndrome)
  Malformation of anterior midline structures (agenesis of septum pellucidum,
    primitive optic ventricle, with hypoplasia of optic nerves, chiasm, and
    infundibulum); sometimes associated endocrine abnormalities; vision defects,
    strabismus, nystagmus; in some cases, other anomalies of eyes

Craniostenosis Syndromes (see Chapter 585.12)

Apert syndrome (acrocephalosyndactyly)
  Orbits shallow, eyes protuberant (proptosis) and widely spaced; antimongoloid
    slant of palpebral fissures; ocular motor abnormalities (strabismus, partial
    ophthalmoplegia, nystagmus); papilledema; optic atrophy; cataracts; sometimes
    dislocated lenses; occasionally iris and fundus colobomas
Carpenter syndrome (acrocephalopolysyndactyly)
  Orbits shallow; lateral displacement of medial canthi; epicanthus; antimongoloid
    slant of palpebral fissures; optic atrophy; microcornea and corneal opacities in
    some cases
Crouzon disease (dysostosis craniofacialis)
  Eyes protuberant (proptosis) and widely spaced; luxation of globe may occur;
    antimongoloid slant of palpebral fissures; strabismus; papilledema; optic
    atrophy; vision loss; cataracts in some patients
Kleeblattschädel syndrome (cloverleaf skull)
  Shallow orbits with proptosis; high risk of corneal ulceration

Miscellaneous Craniofacial Defects and Syndromes

Frontonasal dysplasia (median cleft-face syndrome)
  Hypertelorism (radiographic interorbital distance 2 SD above normal for age); in
    some cases, anophthalmia, microphthalmia, epibulbar dermoids, lid colobomas,
    congenital cataracts
Opitz syndrome
  Hypertelorism, particularly associated with hypospadias; antimongoloid slant of
    palpebral fissures; epicanthus; strabismus
Waardenburg syndrome
  Lateral displacement of medial canthi and inferior puncta; heterochromia iridis,
    total or partial; in some cases both irides completely blue (isochromia); fundus
    pigmentary changes in some cases
Oculodentodigital dysplasia (Meyer-Schwickerath syndrome)
  Hypotelorism, microphthalmos, microcornea, dental anomalies and enamel
    hypoplasia, camptodactyly, syndactyly, and other skeletal defects; persistent
    pupillary membrane; glaucoma
Hallermann-Streiff syndrome (dyscephalia oculomandibulofacialis)
  Microphthalmos, cataract, sparse eyebrows and lashes, blue sclerae,
    nystagmus
Pierre Robin syndrome
  Congenital glaucoma; retinal detachment; strabismus
Treacher Collins syndrome (mandibulofacial dysostosis; Franceschetti-Klein
    syndrome)
  Antimongoloid slant of palpebral fissures; underdevelopment of supraorbital
    ridges, colobomas of lower eyelids and in some cases of iris or choroid
Goldenhar syndrome (oculoauriculovertebral dysplasia)
  Antimongoloid slant of palpebral fissures; colobomata of eyelid, upper lid more
    commonly involved than lower; hypoplasia or coloboma of iris; hypertelorism;
    sometimes microphthalmos

Chromosomal Abnormalities

21-Trisomy (Down syndrome; see Chapter 70)
  Mongoloid slant of palpebral fissures; epicanthus; dacryostenosis; blepharitis;
    Brushfield spots of iris; peripheral thinning of iris stroma; keratoconus and
    corneal hydrops; cataracts; high refractive errors; strabismus; nystagmus;
    increased vessels at disc
18-Trisomy (Edwards syndrome; see Chapter 70)
  Ptosis; short palpebral fissures; epicanthus; hypoplastic supraorbital ridges;
    microphthalmia; corneal opacities; anisocoria; cataracts; fundus and disc
    colobomas; retinal hypopigmentation
13-Trisomy (Patau syndrome; see Chapter 70)
  Microphthalmos; anophthalmos; cyclopia in some cases; dysgenesis of anterior
    segment (iris hypoplasia, iris adhesions, chamber angle abnormalities); corneal
    opacities; congenital glaucoma; cataracts; persistent hyperplastic primary

vitreous; retinal dysplasia; colobomas of iris, ciliary body, fundus; intraocular
    cartilage, optic nerve hypoplasia
9-Trisomy
  Antimongoloid slant of palpebral fissures; deeply set eyes; corectopia; strabismus
8-Trisomy
  Dysmorphic skull; strabismus
Syndrome 45X (Turner and mosaic variants; see Chapter 70)
  Ptosis; epicanthus; blue sclerae; defective color vision; cataracts; strabismus;
    nystagmus
47, XXY; 48,XXXY; 49,XXXY (Klinefelter) syndromes (see Chapter 577)
  Hypertelorism; epicanthus; Brushfield spots of iris; myopia; strabismus
Partial deletion short arm chromosome 4 (4p −) (see Chapter 70)
  Ptosis; hypertelorism; epicanthus; colobomata
Partial deletion short arm chromosome 5 (5p −) (cri-du-chat syndrome; see Chapter 70)
  Antimongoloid slant of palpebral fissures; hypertelorism; epicanthus; strabismus
Partial deletion short arm chromosome 9 (9p −) (see Chapter 70)
  Mongoloid slant of palpebral fissures; epicanthus; arched brows
Partial deletion long arm chromosome 13 (13q −)
  Ptosis; epicanthus; hypertelorism; microphthalmos; colobomas; retinoblastoma
Partial deletion long arm chromosome 18 (18q −) (see Chapter 70)
  Horizontal palpebral fissures; epicanthus; deeply set eyes; optic disc pallor;
    tapetoretinal degeneration; nystagmus
Partial deletion long arm chromosome 21 (21q −)
  Downward slanting palpebral fissures
Partial deletion long arm chromosome 22 (22q −)
  Ptosis; epicanthus
Extrachromosomal material (cat-eye syndrome)
  Antimongoloid slant of palpebral fissures; epicanthus; hypertelorism;
    microphthalmos; colobomas of iris, fundus, optic nerve; macular defects; pale
    discs; cataracts; strabismus; nystagmus

Disorders of Amino Acid Metabolism

Albinism*
  Defect in the formation of melanin; several forms:
  (1) *Oculocutaneous albinism, tyrosinase negative;* generalized hypopigmentation;
      iris blue or gray; generalized hypopigmentation of eye; typical pink or orange
      reflex; fundus bright, with increased choroidal vascular pattern; macula/fovea
      poorly defined (hypoplastic); photophobia; nystagmus; subnormal vision; often
      high refractive error
  (2) *Oculocutaneous albinism, tyrosinase positive;* pigmentation may increase with
      age; iris blue, yellow, or brownish; color increases with age; photophobia;
      nystagmus; subnormal vision, which may improve with age
  (3) *Amish* or *yellow mutant;* generalized albinism in which a yellowish pigment is
      produced instead of melanin, providing some skin and hair color
  (4) *Hermansky-Pudlak syndrome;* tyrosine-negative albinism associated with a
      hemorrhagic diathesis; iris blue-gray to brown; photophobia; nystagmus; slight
      to moderate vision defect
  (5) *Cross syndrome;* tyrosine positive; a syndrome of hypopigmentation, gingival
      fibromatosis, spasticity, athetoid movements, and microphthalmos; iris blue-
      gray, microphthalmos; cataracts; severe vision defect; nystagmus
  (6) *Ocular albinism;* pigment deficiency limited to the eye; generalized ocular
      hypopigmentation; macular hypoplasia; nystagmus (in blacks, fundus
      tessellated)
Alkaptonuria (see Chapter 74.2)
  Black discoloration of sclera, most noticeable at insertion of extraocular muscles
Tyrosinemia (Richner-Hanhart syndrome; see Chapter 74.2)
  Corneal ulceration, "herpetiform"
Cystinosis (see Chapter 521.3)
  Accumulation of refractile crystals in cornea (best seen with slit lamp, but corneal
    haze may be detected grossly); photophobia; pigmentary retinopathy; fundi
    generally hypopigmented, with fine to coarse spotty pigmentation, most marked
    peripherally; vision usually normal to nearly normal
Homocystinemia, type I (see Chapter 74.3)
  Ectopia lentis; cataract; secondary glaucoma; peripheral cystic degeneration of
    retina
Sulfite oxidase deficiency (see Chapter 74.4)
  Subluxation of lens; spherophakia; strabismus
Hartnup disease (see Chapter 74.5)
  Photophobia; nystagmus; strabismus
Maple syrup urine disease (see Chapter 74.6)
  Strabismus, varying with condition of child

The Mucopolysaccharidoses (MPS)

Hurler syndrome (MPS IH; α-L-iduronidase deficiency; see Chapter 77)
  Hypertelorism, prominent eyes; puffy lids; heavy brows; deposition of MPS and
    attendant cellular changes throughout most regions of eye, particularly the
    conjunctiva, cornea, sclera, iris, ciliary body, retina, and optic nerve;
    characteristic corneal clouding, clinically evident early in life, and progressing
    to dense milky "ground-glass" haze, often with associated photophobia;
    progressive retinal degeneration with pigmentary dispersion and clumping,
    arteriolar attenuation and disc pallor, and reduced ERG; optic atrophy; vision
    loss, principally because of corneal, retinal, and optic nerve changes;
    hydrocephalus and cerebral changes; glaucoma in some cases

Table continued on following page

TABLE 619–2. **Clinical Features and Ocular Changes in Developmental Pediatric Syndromes** *Continued*

Scheie syndrome (MPS IS; α-ʟ-iduronidase deficiency; see Chapter 77)
Progressive corneal clouding, diffuse but sometimes more dense peripherally than centrally; progressive retinal degeneration; visual symptoms, field loss, and night blindness often commencing in 2nd or 3rd decade; glaucoma in some cases
Hurler-Scheie Compound (MPS IH/S; α-ʟ-iduronidase deficiency; see Chapter 77)
Corneal clouding, diffuse and progressive; glaucoma in some cases; vision loss because of corneal clouding or optic nerve effects of arachnoid cysts
Hunter (MPS II; iduronosulfate sulfatase deficiency)
Phenotypically similar to MPS IH; both mild and severe forms occur; progressive retinal degeneration with pigmentary changes, arteriolar attenuation, optic atrophy, vision, loss, reduced ERG; corneas macroscopically (clinically) clear, but microscopic corneal changes documented; papilledema secondary to hydrocephalus in some cases
Sanfilippo syndrome (MPS III; type A [heparin sulfate sulfatase deficiency, B [N-acetyl-α-ᴅ-glucosaminidase deficiency], and C [acetyl-Co A:α-glucosaminide N-acetyl transferase deficiency])
Retinal changes in some patients—arteriolar narrowing; reduced ERG; corneas clinically clear but some microscopic changes reported
Morquio syndrome (MPS IV; galactosamine-6-sulfate sulfatase deficiency in classic form, β-galactosidase deficiency reported in variants; see Chapter 77)
Fine corneal clouding in many patients; slowly progressive; often not clinically apparent for several years
Maroteaux-Lamy syndrome (MPS VI; arylsulfatase-B deficiency; see Chapter 77)
Diffuse corneal clouding, usually evident within 1st few yr of life; tortuosity of retinal vessels in some patients; papilledema and 6th nerve paresis in some patients with hydrocephalus
Sly syndrome (MPS VII; β-ᴅ-glucuronidase deficiency)
Some diversity of phenotype; corneas clear or cloudy; corneal haze of either fine or coarse type
Di Ferrenti syndrome (MPS VIII; N-acetylglucosamine-6-sulfate sulfatase deficiency)
Short stature; mild dysostosis multiplex; odontoid hypoplasia; hepatosplenomegaly; mental retardation; ophthalmologic abnormalities not yet described

The Sphingolipidoses

Generalized gangliosidosis (GM₁ gangliosidosis type 1; β-galactosidase deficiency; see Chapter 592.1)
Diffuse corneal clouding (MPS accumulation); macular cherry red spot of retinal ganglioside accumulation; retinal vascular tortuosity and retinal hemorrhages; optic atrophy; vision loss, nystagmus, strabismus
Juvenile GM₁ gangliosidosis (GM₁ gangliosidosis type 2; β-galactosidase deficiency; see Chapter 592.1)
Corneas clinically clear; histologic changes of retinal ganglioside storage without clinically obvious signs; optic atrophy and vision loss; nystagmus and strabismus
Tay-Sachs disease (GM₂ gangliosidosis type 1; hexosaminidase A deficiency; see Chapter 592.1)
Macular cherry red spot; optic atrophy (demyelination and degeneration of optic nerves, chiasm, and tracts); progressive loss of vision, caused by ocular and cerebral abnormalities; sequential deterioration of eye movements
Sandhoff variant (GM₂ gangliosidosis type 2; hexosaminidase A and B deficiency; see Chapter 592.1)
Macular cherry red spot; optic atrophy and progressive loss of vision; corneas clinically clear or slightly opalescent; histologic evidence of storage cytosomes in cornea
Juvenile GM₂ gangliosidosis (GM₂ gangliosidosis type 3; partial deficiency of hexosaminidase; see Chapter 592.1)
Retinal pigmentary degeneration; macular changes (cherry red spot type) in some cases; optic atrophy; blindness later in course of disease
Krabbe globoid cell leukodystrophy (galactosyl ceramide lipidosis; galactosylceramide β-galactosidase deficiency)
Cortical blindness and optic atrophy caused by degenerative changes in brain and visual pathways; nystagmus; strabismus
Gaucher's disease (glycosyl ceramide lipidosis; glucosyl ceramide β-glucosidase deficiency; see Chapter 75.4)
Paralytic strabismus caused by brainstem and cranial nerve involvement in neuronopathic forms; nystagmus; macular changes (grayness) in some cases; retinal hemorrhages secondary to anemia, thrombocytopenia; discrete white spots in or on retina reported in juvenile form; pingueculae (wedge-shaped conjunctival lesions) in chronic non-neuronopathic form; possibly corneal clouding
Niemann-Pick disease (sphingomyelin lipidoses; sphingomyelinase deficiency; see Chapter 75.4)
Grayish macular haze in classic infantile neuronopathic form (type A), and in subacute neurovisceral or juvenile form (type C); corneal clouding, lens opacities in some cases (type A); vertical gaze palsy in some patients
Fabry disease (glycosphingolipid lipidosis; α-galactosidase A deficiency; see Chapter 75.4)
Corneal dystrophy related to epithelial lipid deposits (radiating lines/whorls in affected males and in carrier females); aneurysmal dilatation and tortuosity of conjunctival and retinal vessels; renovascular signs of renal hypertension; papilledema; orbital and lid edema; cataracts (spokelike posterior cortical lens opacities—anterior lens opacities in some cases)

Farber disease (ceramide lipidosis; ceramidase deficiency; see Chapter 75.4)
Cherry red–like spot; grayish posterior pole; retinal pigmentary mottling; granulomas in and around eye

Ceroid Lipofuscinoses (see also Chapters 75.4 and 592.2)

Infantile (Finnish variant; unsaturated fatty acid lipidosis)
Microcephaly; marked atrophy of brain; loss of vision; granular inclusions; ataxia; myoclonus; profound dementia, decorticate state; onset 1–2 yr; death by 10 yr
Late infantile (Jansky-Bielschowsky)
Intellectual deterioration, seizures, ataxia; pigmentary retinal degeneration, in some cases, predominantly macular; ERG abnormal; optic atrophy; inclusions of curvilinear type; onset 2–4 yr; death by 10 yr
Juvenile (Batten-Mayou-Spielmeyer-Vogt)
Intellectual deterioration, seizures, ataxia, progressive loss of motor function; pigmentary retinal degeneration, resembling retinitis pigmentosa, with progressive loss of vision; in some cases predominantly macular degeneration; ERG abnormal; optic atrophy as a late manifestation; mixed inclusion bodies including curvilinear and fingerprint types, and lipofuscin in brain; onset 5–8 yr, sometimes later; death in teens or 20s
Late juvenile or adult (Kuf)
Behavior disturbances and intellectual impairment; ataxia, spasticity, myoclonic seizures; vision and fundi usually normal; macular degeneration in some cases; mostly lipofuscin in brain; onset in childhood, adolescence, or early adult life
Cherry red spot myoclonus syndrome
Macular cherry red spot; vision loss; intention myoclonus; variable inclusions in brain; light inclusions in hepatocytes and Kupffer cells; onset in childhood; survival to adulthood

Leukodystrophies (see also Chapter 592.1)

Metachromatic leukodystrophy (arylsulfatase A deficiency)
Retinal degeneration resembling retinitis pigmentosa; in some cases, early macular involvement (macular grayness with accentuation of central red spot); optic atrophy; vision loss; strabismus and nystagmus
Pelizaeus-Merzbacher disease
"Eye rolling" (rhythmic eye movements) noted soon after birth, sometimes with rotary movements of the head; optic atrophy as a late manifestation
Canavan disease
Vacuolation of ganglion cell layer of retina reportedly detectable with slit lamp; retinal pigmentary changes; optic atrophy; blindness early in course; ERG normal; VER reduced; strabismus, roving eye movements, and nystagmus

Demyelinating Scleroses (see Chapter 592.5)

Schilder disease (encephalitis periaxialis diffusa)
Involvement of visual pathways, producing retrobulbar neuritis, optic atrophy, central scotomas, chiasmal syndromes, homonymous field defects; disorders of cortical gaze functions; nystagmus
Multiple sclerosis
Optic neuritis (episodic loss of vision, typically a central scotoma, unilateral more often than bilateral, often with retrobulbar pain); other visual pathway lesions (various field defects); internuclear ophthalmoplegia; supranuclear gaze palsies; nystagmus; sheathing of peripheral retinal vessels in some cases
Neuromyelitis optica (Devick disease)
Optic neuritis (usually papillitis with visible disc edema), with resultant optic atrophy; other visual pathway lesions (various visual field defects); in some cases extraocular muscle palsies, conjugate gaze palsies, nystagmus, pupil abnormalities

Hamartomatoses and Phakomatoses

Tuberous sclerosis (Bourneville disease; see Chapter 589.2)
Retinal phakomas (glial hamartomas, ranging from small flat or slightly elevated white or yellowish lesions to large elevated refractile yellowish multinodular or cystic masses often likened to an unripe mulberry); fibroangioma of the lids; in some, papilledema or optic atrophy, vision defects, pupil or ocular motor signs related to CNS changes (tumors, hydrocephalus); occasionally iris or pigmentary changes
Neurofibromatosis (von Recklinghausen syndrome; see Chapter 589.1)
Plexiform neuromas of eyelids, often producing ptosis; episcleral and conjunctival neurofibromas; prominent corneal nerves; Lisch iris nodules; uveal hypercellularity; glaucoma (related to angle anomalies, uveal hypercellularity, neovascularization, or synechiae); hamartomas (phakomas) of disc and retina; fundus pigmentary changes likened to café-au-lait spots; optic gliomas and vision loss (presenting with proptosis, strabismus, nystagmus if intraorbital—with signs of increased intracranial pressure, hydrocephalus, or diencephalic syndrome when intracranial); orbital asymmetry; orbital wall defects; pulsatile exophthalmos, intraorbital neurofibromas, with proptosis
Angiomatosis of the retina and cerebellum (von Hippel–Lindau disease; see Chapter 589.4)
Retinal hemangioblastoma (reddish or yellowish globular mass with paired vessels coursing to and from the lesion, sometimes likened to a toy balloon in the fundus); may lead to hemorrhage, exudates, retinal detachment
Encephalofacial angiomatosis (Sturge-Weber syndrome; see Chapter 589.3)
Lid and conjunctival involvement of facial nevus flammeus; choroidal hemangioma; dilated and tortuous retinal vessels; glaucoma, congenital or later in infancy or

TABLE 619–2. Clinical Features and Ocular Changes in Developmental Pediatric Syndromes *Continued*

childhood (related to possible angle anomalies, vascular lesion, or hypersecretion); visual field defects associated with CNS lesions; hemianopia in some cases)
Angiomatosis of mid-brain and retina (Wyburn-Mason syndrome)
   Extensive vascular malformations involving principally the midbrain and eye; angiomatosis of the retina; vessels dilated and tortuous; angiomatosis affecting optic nerve and orbit

Neurocutaneous Syndromes

Ataxia-telangiectasia (Louis-Barr syndrome; see Chapter 590.1)
   Telangiectasias of bulbar conjunctivae, usually by the age of 4–6 yr; apraxic disorder of conjugate eye movements; horizontal and vertical gaze performed in halting dyssynergic fashion; difficulty in maintaining eccentric gaze; sometimes convergence defect; nystagmus
Sjögren-Larsson syndrome
   Chorioretinal lesions; discrete defects in retinal pigment epithelium of unknown cause; circumscribed symmetric lesions of varying size in and about the macula in approximately 25% of cases
Incontinentia pigmenti (Bloch-Sulzberger syndrome; see Chapter 642)
   Intraocular retrolental masses ("pseudogliomas") and membranes, apparently secondary to an underlying retinal vascular disorder characterized by aneurysmal dilatation, abnormal arteriovenous connections, and vasoproliferative changes; sometimes intraocular hemorrhage and inflammation; microphthalmos; corneal opacities; cataracts; optic atrophy
Linear nevus sebaceus of Jadassohn (see Chapter 642)
   Coloboma of the eyelids, iris, and fundus; corectopia; epibulbar lipodermoids; orbital teratomas; proptosis; aberrant lacrimal gland; corneal vascularization; ocular motor palsies; nystagmus; defective vision
Xerodermic idiocy of de Sanctis and Cacchione (see Chapter 642)
   Atrophy of eyelids; loss of cilia, ectropion, entropion, symblepharon, ankyloblepharon; drying and infection of conjunctiva; ulceration of cornea; iritis; photophobia
Klippel-Trénaunay-Weber syndrome (see Chapter 640)
   Conjunctival telangiectasia; choroidal hemangioma; iris coloboma; heterochromia; glaucoma; strabismus

Special Neurobiothrophies

Subacute sclerosing panencephalitis (Dawson excephalitis; Van Bogaert encephalitis; see Chapter 225)
Focal retinitis (edema, hemorrhage, pigmentary changes), with chorioretinal scarring (usually macular or paramacular, usually bilateral)—may precede other neurologic manifestations; papilledema; optic atrophy; visual symptoms of retinal and optic nerve involvement; field defects of cerebral involvement; nystagmus; extraocular muscle palsies; ptosis
Subacute necrotizing encephalomyopathy (Leigh disease; see Chapter 591)
   Abnormal eye movements (bizarre rolling eye movements, disconjugate eye movements, horizontal and vertical nystagmus, saccadic ocular movements); extraocular muscle palsies (sometimes complete external ophthalmoplegia); blepharoptosis; progressive optic atrophy and vision loss; sometimes retinal changes (diminished macular reflex); afferent and efferent pupil defects
Hepatolenticular degeneration (Wilson disease; see Chapter 338.2)
   Kayser-Fleischer ring of cornea (copper deposition in periphery of Descemet's membrane, particularly in deepest zone adjacent to endothelium, seen as granules of golden, greenish, grayish, or brown hue); Sonnenblumenkatarakt ("sunflower" cataract); occasionally ocular motor abnormalities (jerky oscillations of eyes, involuntary upward deviation of eyes, or paresis of upward gaze); accommodation sometimes affected; in some cases, optic neuritis secondary to penicillamine therapy
Trichopoliodystrophy (Menkes syndrome; kinky hair disease)
   Decrease in retinal ganglion cells, thinning of retinal nerve fiber layer, and partial atrophy of optic nerve; progressive vision loss; abnormal ERG; microcysts of pigment epithelium of iris
Abetalipoproteinemia (acanthocytosis; Bassen-Kornzweig syndrome; see Chapter 75.3)
   Pigmentary retinal degeneration with progressive impairment of visual function (pigment dispersion, arteriolar attenuation, disc pallor, impaired dark adaptation); cataracts, ptosis, and ocular motor abnormalities; in some cases, progressive exotropia, paresis of medial recti, and dissociated nystagmus on lateral gaze
Heredopathia atactica polyneuritiformis (Refsum disease; phytanic acid α-hydrolase deficiency; see Chapter 75.2)
   Pigmentary retinal degeneration (pigmentary clumping, arteriolar attenuation, optic atrophy, progressive impairment of night vision and visual field); ERG abnormal; sometimes vitreous opacities, cataracts, cornea guttata, miosis; ophthalmoparesis; nystagmus
Familial dysautonomia (Riley-Day syndrome; see Chapter 606.1)
   Depressed or absent corneal sensation, with corneal ulceration and scarring common; defective lacrimation; tortuosity of retinal vessels; tonic pupil in some cases; myopia and exotropia common
Congenital familial sensory neuropathy with anhidrosis (Pinsky-DiGeorge syndrome; see Chapter 606.2)
   Defective corneal sensation, with defective lacrimation; corneal ulceration and scarring may result

Disorders of Connective Tissues, Bones, and Joints

Arachnodactyly (Marfan syndrome; see Chapter 690)

Ectopia lentis (lens dislocation, usually upward) and iridodonesis (tremulous iris); microphakia, spherophakia; cataract; myopia; glaucoma; retinal changes, degeneration, detachment
Cutis hyperelastica (Ehlers-Danlos syndrome; see Chapter 649)
   Epicanthus; blue sclera; keratoconus; subluxation of lens; retinal detachment
Pseudoxanthoma elasticum (see Chapter 649
   Angioid streaks (breaks in Bruch's membrane appearing as dark lines in the fundus radiating from the disc); tendency to retinal hemorrhage
Osteogenesis imperfecta (see Chapter 689)
   Blue sclera; prominent eyes; in some cases, megalocornea, keratoconus, corneal opacities
Polyostotic fibrous dysplasia (McCune-Albright syndrome; see Chapter 556.6)
   Thickening of bones of orbit
Osteopetrosis (Albers-Schönberg disease; "marble bones"; see Chapter 687)
   Vision loss and extraocular muscle palsies, caused by bony overgrowth of cranial foramina; in some cases, retinal degeneration, optic atrophy
Chondrodystrophia calcificans congenita (Conradi syndrome; see Chapter 648)
   Cataract, optic atropy; hypertelorism
Spondyloepiphyseal dysplasia congenita (see Chapter 683)
   Myopia; retinal detachment; cataract; buphthalmos
Spondyloepiphyseal dysplasia variants (see Chapter 683)
   Punctate corneal dystrophy without impairment of vision
Hereditary onycho-osteodysplasia (nail-patella syndrome; see Chapter 683)
   Dark "cloverleaf" pigmentation of iris; cataract; microphakia; microcornea; keratoconus; ptosis
Progressive arthro-ophthalmopathy (Stickler's syndrome)
   Pain and stiffness of joints with bony enlargement; kyphosis, cleft palate; Pierre Robin anomaly; deafness; progressive myopia; retinal detachment; glaucoma

Dermatologic Disorders

Focal dermal hypoplasia (Goltz syndrome; see Chapter 638)
   Nystagmus; strabismus; microphthalmos; coloboma
Hypohidrotic (anhidrotic) ectodermal dysplasia (see Chapter 638)
   Deficiency of tears, leading to keratopathy, photophobia; stenosis of the lacrimal puncta; cataracts; lashes and brows sparse
Dyskeratosis congenita (see Chapter 638)
   Bullous conjunctivitis, with minimal scarring of cornea; chronic blepharitis; loss of lashes and ectropion; keratinization of lacrimal puncta
Ichthyosis (see Chapter 648)
   Conjunctivitis, ectropion, and corneal erosions in lamellar and sex-linked forms; cataracts in congenital and vulgaris forms
Basal cell nevus syndrome (see Chapter 660)
   Prominent supraorbital ridges; hypertelorism or dystopia canthorum; cataracts; coloboma; vision defects; strabismus
Juvenile xanthogranuloma (nevoxanthoendothelioma; see Chapter 660)
   Xanthogranuloma in ocular tissues, as infiltrates in orbit, iris, episclera, ciliary body; presenting signs may be proptosis, heterochromia, spontaneous hyphema, uveitis, glaucoma
Poikiloderma congenitale (Rothmund-Thomson syndrome; see Chapter 646)
   Sparse eyebrows and eyelashes; cataracts (onset 2–7 yr); corneal dystrophy
Bloom syndrome (see Chapter 646)
   Conjunctivitis; conjunctival telangiectasias; drusen at posterior pole of fundus

Syndromes of Multiple Developmental Abnormalities

Cornelia de Lange syndrome
   Microbrachycephaly, short neck, low hairline, anteverted nares, micrognathism, and low-set ears; physical and mental retardation; limb defects including micromelia-phocomelia, oligodactyly, polydactyly; cardiac and urogenital anomalies; synophrys (confluent eyebrows) and long, curly eyelashes; ptosis; epicanthus; microphthalmos with eccentric pupils; corneal opacities; optic atrophy; strabismus
Fraser syndrome
   Facial, genitourinary, skeletal anomalies (including lateral cleft of nostril, ear deformity, renal agenesis, hydronephrosis, hypospadias, cryptorchidism, syndactyly); cerebral defects, meningoencephalocele; cryptophthalmos (eye hidden, fused lids—absence of palpebral fissure), sometimes with symblepharon (adhesion of lid to globe); microphthalmos in some cases; flat supraorbital ridge
Rieger syndrome
   Various dental and limb anomalies; occasionally intellectual retardation, muscular dystrophy, and myotonic dystrophy; dysplasia of anterior segment of the eye; posterior embryotoxon (prominence and anterior displacement of Schwalbe's line), often with bands of iris tissue attached (Axenfeld syndrome); iris hypoplasia; glaucoma; cataracts; ectopia lentis; colobomas; micro-or megalocornea; strabismus; ptosis; optic atrophy
Peters syndrome
   Skeletal anomalies; developmental defects of the gastrointestinal tract and CNS; hydrocephalus and mental retardation; central defect of Descemet membrane, with central corneal leukoma, shallow anterior chamber, peripheral anterior synechia; cataracts
Lenz syndrome
   Microcephaly, mental retardation; short stature, digital anomalies, and dental defects; colobomatous microphthalmos; blepharoptosis; nystagmus; strabismus
Meckel syndrome (Meckel-Gruber syndrome)
   Microcephaly, occipital encephalocele, or anencephaly; polycystic kidneys; polydactyly; congenital heart disease; genital abnormalities; microphthalmos,

Table continued on following page

TABLE 619–2. **Clinical Features and Ocular Changes in Developmental Pediatric Syndromes** *Continued*

anophthalmos, cryptophthalmos; sclerocornea; partial aniridia; cataract; retinal dysplasia; optic nerve hypoplasia

Otopalatodigital syndrome (Rubinstein-Taybi syndrome)
Intellectual and growth retardation; abnormally broad thumbs and broad great toes; characteristic facies with hypoplasia of maxilla and mandible, beaked nose, posterior rotation of ears; hypertrichosis; cryptorchidism; cardiac and renal anomalies; hypertelorism, with epicanthus, ptosis, and antimongoloid slant of palpebral fissures; cataract, colobomas, strabismus

Seckel syndrome
Growth retardation with small head circumference and characteristic face, narrow with beaklike nose ("bird head"); micrognathia and apparent prominence of maxilla; sometimes musculoskeletal and genitourinary anomalies; hypertelorism, with antimongoloid slant of palpebral fissures, prominent eyes; strabismus

Freeman-Sheldon syndrome
Syndrome characterized by masklike face with small pursed mouth, "whistling face"; ulnar deviation of the hand and fingers; talipes equinovarus; deep-set eyes; epicanthus, blepharophimosis, ptosis; strabismus

Aicardi's syndrome
Agenesis of the corpus callosum, with cortical heterotopia; seizures; mental retardation; costovertebral anomalies; multiple discrete chorioretinal defects of varying size; sometimes microphthalmos

Wildervanck syndrome
Association of the Klippel-Feil malformation with congenital deafness and Duane syndrome; unilateral or bilateral (congenital defect in abduction with retraction of the globe or attempted adduction of the affected eye); epibulbar dermoid cysts

Falls-Kertesz syndrome
Pterygium coli; later onset of lymphedema of lower extremities; distichiasis of all four lids; partial ectropion of lower lids

Kartagener syndrome (see Chapter 403)
Pigmentary retinal disorder; cataracts

Miscellaneous Multisystem Disorders

Oculocerebrorenal syndrome (Lowe syndrome; see Chapter 521.4)
Congenital cataracts in affected males; fine lens opacities in carrier females; glaucoma; rarely, microphthalmos

Cerebrohepatorenal syndrome (Zellweger syndrome) (congenital adrenoleukodystrophy)
Profound hypotonia, growth retardation, and failure to thrive; hepatomegaly, jaundice, hypoprothrombinemia; renal cortical cysts; characteristic facies, flat profile; accumulation of iron in various organs; mild hypertelorism, flat supraorbital ridges, and epicanthal folds, cataracts; glaucoma (also, nonglaucomatous corneal haze); vitreous opacities; optic nerve hypoplasia; retinal pigmentary disorder (fundi generally hypopigmented with fine to coarse spotty pigmentation, most marked peripherally)

Laurence-Moon-Biedl syndrome (see Chapter 43)
Pleomorphic pigmentary retinal degeneration (retinitis pigmentosa type, with prominent macular involvement in some cases), with progressive vision impairment

Prader-Willi syndrome
Hypotonia, hypomentia, hypogonadism, and obesity, with tendency to diabetes mellitus; strabismus

Cockayne syndrome (see Chapter 646)
Pigmentary retinal degeneration; optic atrophy, cataracts; photophobia

Werner syndrome
Syndrome of premature aging, in the 2nd decade, with cessation of growth, graying of the hair, alopecia, scleroderma-like changes of the skin,

atherosclerosis, and diabetes mellitus; hypogonadism, increased risk of neoplasia; cataracts, juvenile onset; pigmentary retinal degeneration ("retinitis pigmentosa"); macular degeneration; glaucoma

Asphyxiating thoracic dysplasia (Jeune syndrome; see Chapter 409)
Pigmentary retinal degeneration, with progressive vision impairment in some cases

Alström syndrome
Nerve deafness, diabetes mellitus, and obesity in childhood; pigmentary retinal degeneration; cataracts

Renal-retinal dystrophy
Interstitial nephritis; progressive pigmentary retinal degeneration, with attenuation of arterioles, reduced ERG, optic atrophy, and loss of vision

Usher syndrome
Nerve deafness; pigmentary retinal degeneration ("retinitis pigmentosa"); cataracts

Norrie disease
A syndrome of retinal malformation, mental retardation, and deafness; congenital retinal pseudoglioma; persistent hyperplastic primary vitreous, with vision loss; degenerative changes with phthisis bulbi; corneal opacities; cataracts

Congenital Infection Syndromes

Congenital rubella (see Chapter 226)
Ophthalmic sequelae, both teratogenic and inflammatory; bilateral or unilateral effects; persistence of virus in the eye for months or years; microphthalmia; cataract (usually a dense, pearly, nuclear opacity with relatively clearer cortical rim); iris hypoplasia, atrophy synechiae (pupils often difficult to dilate); congenital glaucoma; transient nonglaucomatous corneal clouding in a newborn; retinopathy (pigmentary "salt and pepper" mottling, focal or generalized, without loss of function); acute maculopathy (submacular neovascularization) as a delayed complication later in childhood in some cases, with attendant vision impairment; optic atrophy; vision defects and ocular motor abnormalities (nystagmus, strabismus) related not only to ocular involvement but also to effects of encephalomyelitis

Congenital cytomegalovirus infection (see Chapter 234)
Chorioretinitis (single or multifocal atrophic and pigmented fundus lesions, more often peripheral than macular—sometimes perivascular retinal exudates and hemorrhages); anterior uveitis, conjunctivitis, and corneal clouding; optic atrophy; optic nerve hypoplasia; coloboma; microphthalmos; vision defects with strabismus, nystagmus

Congenital toxoplasmosis (see Chapter 266)
Retinochoroditis (retinitis, with secondary choroiditis; often with exudate into vitreous in early stages, resulting in single or multifocal atrophic and pigmented scars); often large macular lesions; satellite lesions and recurrent inflammation common in later years caused by persistence of organism in eye; vision loss, optic atrophy, retinal detachment, cataract, and glaucoma common; attendant oculomotor abnormalities (strabismus, nystagmus) attributed to ocular and/or CNS involvement; congenital anomalies of eye (e.g., microphthalmos)

Congenital syphilis (see Chapter 200)
Perivascular infiltration by *T. pallidum*, with inflammation in the cornea, uvea, retina, and optic nerve; persistence of the organism in the eye for years; interstitial keratitis, usually appearing after age 5 or 6 yr (iridocyclitis and intense photophobia in acute phase, vascularization and corneal opacification later, with decreased vision); retinopathy ("salt and pepper" pigmentary changes, frequently with arteriolar attenuation and disc pallor); retinal periphlebitis, sometimes with vascular occlusion; exudative uveitis in some cases; phthisis may result; disc edema; optic atrophy

---

To be differentiated from these forms of albinism is the Chédiak-Higashi syndrome in which the defect is in the morphology of the melanosomes, not in the formation of melanin. Ocular signs include hypopigmentation of iris and fundus, photophobia, nystagmus, and papilledema with lymphocytic infiltration of the optic nerve.

ERG = electroretinogram; VER = visual evoked response; CNS = central nervous system.

---

age of intervention, duration and severity of any attendant amblyopia, and presence of any associated ocular abnormalities (e.g., microphthalmia, retinal lesions, optic atrophy, glaucoma, nystagmus, strabismus). Persistent amblyopia is the most common cause of poor visual recovery after cataract surgery in children. Secondary conditions and complications may develop in children who have had cataract surgery, including inflammatory sequelae, secondary membranes, glaucoma, retinal detachment, and changes in the axial length of the eye. All these should be considered in planning treatment.

Ectopia Lentis. Normally, the lens is suspended in place behind the iris diaphragm by the zonular fibers of the ciliary body. Abnormalities of the suspensory system resulting from a devel-

opmental defect, disease, or trauma may result in instability or displacement of the lens. Displacement of the lens is classified as luxation (dislocation—complete displacement of the lens) or as subluxation (partial displacement—shifting or tilting of the lens). Symptoms include blurring of vision, which is often the result of refractive changes such as myopia, astigmatism, or aphakic hyperopia. Some patients experience diplopia. An important sign of displacement is iridodonesis, a tremulousness of the iris caused by the loss of its usual support. Also, the anterior chamber may appear deeper than normal. Sometimes the equatorial region ("edge") of the displaced lens may be visible in the pupillary aperture. On ophthalmoscopy, this may appear as a black crescent. Also, the difference between the phakic and aphakic portions can be appreciated when focusing on the fundus.

DIFFERENTIAL DIAGNOSIS. A major cause of lens displacement is trauma. Displacement may occur as a result of ocular disease, such as uveitis, intraocular tumor, congenital glaucoma, high myopia, megalocornea, or aniridia, or in association with cataract. There are also heritable forms of ectopia lentis and those associated with systemic disease.

Displacement of the lens occurring as a heritable ocular condition unassociated with systemic abnormalities is referred to as *simple ectopia lentis*. Simple ectopia lentis is usually transmitted as an autosomal dominant condition. The lens is generally displaced upward and temporally. The ectopia may be present at birth or may appear later in life. Another form of heritable dislocation is *ectopia lentis et pupillae*. In this condition, both the lens and pupil are displaced, usually in opposite directions. This condition is generally bilateral, with one eye being almost a mirror image of the other. Ectopia lentis et pupillae is a recessive condition, although variable expression with some intermingling with simple ectopia lentis has been reported.

Systemic disorders associated with displacement of the lens include Marfan syndrome, homocystinuria, Weill-Marchesani syndrome, and sulfite oxidase deficiency. Ectopia lentis occurs in approximately 80% of patients with Marfan syndrome, and in about 50% of patients, the ectopia is evident by the age of 5 yr. In most cases, the lens is displaced superiorly and temporally; it is almost always bilateral and relatively symmetric. In homocystinuria, the lens is usually displaced inferiorly and somewhat nasally. It occurs early in life and is often evident by 5 yr of age. In Weill-Marchesani syndrome, the displacement of the lens is often downward and forward, and the lens tends to be small and round.

Ectopia lentis is also associated occasionally with other conditions, including Ehlers-Danlos, Sturge-Weber, Crouzon, and Klippel-Feil syndrome; oxycephaly; and mandibulofacial dysostosis. A syndrome of dominantly inherited blepharoptosis, high myopia, and ectopia lentis has also been described.

TREATMENT AND PROGNOSIS. Displacement of the lens often results only in optical problems; in other cases, however, more serious complications may develop, such as glaucoma, uveitis, retinal detachment, or cataract. Management must be individualized according to the type of displacement, its etiology, and the presence of any complicating ocular or systemic conditions. For many patients, optical correction by spectacles or contact lenses can be provided. Manipulation of the iris diaphragm with mydriatic or miotic drops may sometimes help improve vision. In selected cases, the best treatment is surgical removal of the lens. In many children, treatment of any associated amblyopia must be instituted early. In addition, for children with ectopia lentis, safety precautions should be taken to prevent injury to the eye.

Microspherophakia. The term *microspherophakia* refers to a small, round lens that may occur as an isolated anomaly (probably autosomal recessive) or in association with other ocular abnormalities, such as ectopia lentis, myopia, or retinal detachment (possibly autosomal dominant). Microspherophakia may also occur in association with various systemic disorders, including Marfan syndrome, Marchesani syndrome, Alport syndrome, mandibulofacial dysostosis, and Klinefelter syndrome.

Anterior Lenticonus. Anterior lenticonus is a rare bilateral condition in which the anterior surface of the lens bulges centrally. It may be accompanied by lens opacities or other eye anomalies and is a prominent feature of Alport syndrome. The increased curvature of the central area may cause high myopia.

Posterior Lenticonus. Posterior lenticonus, which occurs more commonly than anterior lenticonus, is characterized by a circumscribed round or oval bulge of the posterior lens capsule and cortex, restricted to the 2–7 mm central (axial) region. In the early stages, by the red reflex test, this may look like an oil droplet. It occurs in infants and young children, and it tends to increase with age. Usually the lens material within and surrounding the capsular bulge eventually becomes opacified. Posterior lenticonus usually occurs as an isolated ocular anomaly. It is generally unilateral but may be bilateral. It is believed to be sporadic, although autosomal dominant heredity has been suggested in some cases. Infants or children with posterior lenticonus may require lens surgery for progressive cataract, optical correction, amblyopia treatment, and care of secondary conditions, such as strabismus.

Bateman JB, Spence MA, Marazita ML, et al: Genetic linkage analysis of autosomal dominant congenital cataracts. *Am J Ophthalmol* 1986;101:218.

Buckley EG: Pediatric cataracts and lens anomalies. In Nelson LB (editor): *Harley's Pediatric Ophthalmology*, 4th ed. Philadelphia, WB Saunders, 1998.

Casper DS, Simon JW, Nelson LB, et al: Familial simple ectopia lentis. A case study. *J Pediatr Ophthalmol Strabismus* 1985;22:227.

Cheng KP, Hiles DA, Biglan AW, et al: Visual results after early surgical treatment of unilateral congenital cataracts. *Ophthalmology* 1991;98:903.

Chugh KS, Sakhuja V, Agarwal A, et al: Hereditary nephritis (Alport's syndrome)–Clinical profile and inheritance in 28 kindreds. *Nephrol Dial Transplant* 1993;8:690.

Cross HE, Jensen AD: Ocular manifestations in the Marfan syndrome and homocystinuria. *Am J Ophthalmol* 1973;75:405.

Cumming RG, Mitchell P, Leeder SR: Use of inhaled corticosteroids and the risk of cataracts. *N Engl J Med* 1997;337:8.

Forman AR, Loreto JA, Tina LU: Reversibility of corticosteroid-associated cataracts in children with the nephrotic syndrome. *Am J Ophthalmol* 1977;84:75.

Gelbart SS, Hoyt CS, Jastrebski G, et al: Long-term visual results in bilateral congenital cataracts. *Am J Ophthalmol* 1982;93:615.

Goldberg MF: Clinical manifestations of ectopia lentis et pupillae in 16 patients. *Ophthalmology* 1988;95:1080.

Hiles DA: Intraocular lens implantation in children with monocular cataracts, 1974–1983. *Ophthalmology* 1984;91:1231.

Jaafar MS, Robb RM: Congenital anterior polar cataract: A review of 63 cases. *Ophthalmology* 1984;91:249.

Khalil M, Saheb N: Posterior lenticonus. *Ophthalmology* 1984;91:1429.

Levin AV, Edmonds SA, Nelson LB, et al: Extended-wear contact lenses for the treatment of pediatric aphakia. *Ophthalmology* 1988;95:1107.

Nelson LB: Diagnosis and management of congenital and developmental cataracts. *Semin Ophthalmol* 1990;5:154.

Nelson LB, Calhoun JH, Simon JW, et al: Progression of congenital anterior polar cataracts in childhood. *Arch Ophthalmol* 1985;103:1842.

Nelson LB, Maumenee IH: Ectopia lentis. *Surv Ophthalmol* 1982;27:143.

Olitsky SE, Nelson LB: Intraocular lens implantation in children. In Wilson RP (editor): *Year Book of Ophthalmology*, St. Louis, CV Mosby, 1997, p 227.

Parks MM: Visual results in aphakic children. *Am J Ophthalmol* 1982;94:441.

Rasoby R, Ben Ezra D: Congenital and traumatic cataracts: The effect on ocular axial length. *Arch Ophthalmol* 1988;106:1066.

Simon JW, Mehta N, Simmons ST, et al: Glaucoma after pediatric lensectomy/vitrectomy. *Ophthalmology* 1991;98:670.

Wets B, Milot JA, Polomeno RC, et al: Cataracts and ketotic hypoglycemia. *Ophthalmology* 1982;89:999.

Chapter 620
Disorders of the Uveal Tract

Uveitis (Iritis, Cyclitis, Chorioretinitis). The uveal tract (the inner vascular coat of the eye, consisting of the iris, ciliary body, and choroid) is subject to inflammatory involvement in a number of systemic diseases, both infectious and noninfectious, and in response to exogenous factors, including trauma and toxic agents (Box 620–1). Inflammation may affect any one portion of the uveal tract preferentially or all parts together.

Iritis may occur alone or in conjunction with inflammation of the ciliary body as iridocyclitis or in association with pars planitis. Pain, photophobia, and lacrimation are the characteristic symptoms of acute anterior uveitis, but the inflammation may develop insidiously without disturbing symptoms. Signs of anterior uveitis include conjunctival hyperemia, particularly in the perilimbal region (ciliary flush), and cells and protein ("flare") in the aqueous humor (Fig. 620–1). Inflammatory deposits on

BOX 620–1. UVEITIS IN CHILDHOOD

ANTERIOR UVEITIS

Juvenile rheumatoid arthritis (pauciarticular)
Sarcoidosis
Trauma
Tuberculosis
Kawasaki disease
Ulcerative colitis
Reiter syndrome
Spirochetal (syphilis, leptospiral)
Heterochromic iridocyclitis (Fuchs)
Viral (herpes simplex, herpes zoster)
Ankylosing spondylitis
Stevens-Johnson syndrome
Idiopathic
Drugs

POSTERIOR UVEITIS (Choroiditis—may involve retina)

Toxoplasmosis
Parasites (toxocariasis)
Sarcoidosis
Tuberculosis
Viral (rubella, herpes simplex, HIV, cytomegalovirus)
Subacute sclerosing panencephalitis
Idiopathic

ANTERIOR AND/OR POSTERIOR UVEITIS

Sympathetic ophthalmia (trauma to other eye)
Vogt-Koyanagi-Harada syndrome (uveo-otocutaneous syndrome: poliosis, vitiligo, deafness, tinnitus, uveitis, aseptic meningitis, retinitis)
Behçet syndrome
Lyme disease

the posterior surface of the cornea (keratic precipitates [KPs]) and congestion of the iris may also be seen. More chronic cases may show degenerative changes of the cornea (band keratopathy), lenticular opacities (cataract), development of glaucoma, and impairment of vision. The cause of anterior uveitis is often obscure; primary considerations in children are rheumatoid disease, particularly pauciarticular rheumatoid arthritis, Kawasaki disease, Reiter syndrome, and sarcoidosis. Iritis may be secondary to corneal disease, such as herpetic keratitis or a bacterial or fungal corneal ulcer, or to a corneal abrasion or foreign body. Traumatic iritis and iridocyclitis are especially common in children.

Iridocyclitis that occurs in children with arthritis deserves special mention. Unlike most forms of anterior uveitis, it rarely creates pain, photophobia, or conjunctival hyperemia. Loss of vision may not be noticed until severe and irreversible damage

has occurred. Because of the lack of symptoms and the high incidence of uveitis in these children, routine periodic screening is necessary.

Choroiditis, inflammation of the posterior portion of the uveal tract, invariably also involves the retina; when both are obviously affected, the condition is termed *chorioretinitis*. The causes of posterior uveitis are numerous; the more common are toxoplasmosis, histoplasmosis, cytomegalic inclusion disease, sarcoidosis, syphilis, tuberculosis, and toxocariasis (Fig. 620–2). Depending on the etiology, the inflammatory signs may be diffuse or focal. Vitreous reaction often occurs as well. With many types, the result is atrophic chorioretinal scarring demarcated by pigmentation, often with visual impairment. Secondary complications include retinal detachment, glaucoma, and phthisis.

Panophthalmitis is inflammation involving all parts of the eye. It is frequently suppurative, most often as a result of a perforating injury or of septicemia. It produces severe pain, marked congestion of the eye, inflammation of the adjacent orbital tissues and eyelids, and loss of vision. In many cases, the eye is lost despite intensive treatment of the infection and inflammation. Enucleation of the eye or evisceration of the orbit may be necessary.

Sympathetic ophthalmia is a rare type of inflammatory response that affects the uninjured eye after a perforating injury. It may occur weeks, months, or even years after the injury. A hypersensitivity phenomenon is the most probable cause. Loss of vision in the uninjured (sympathizing) eye may result. Removal of the injured eye prevents the development of sympathetic ophthalmia but does not stop the progression of the disease once it has occurred. Therefore, early enucleation should be considered if there is no hope of visual recovery after a severe injury.

TREATMENT. The various forms of intraocular inflammation are treated according to their etiologic factors. When infection is proved or suspected, appropriate systemic antimicrobial therapy is used. In some cases, subconjunctival or intravitreal injection of antibiotics is indicated. Prevention or reduction of inflammatory sequelae is also important; in selected cases, topical or systemic corticosteroids are used. Systemic immunosuppressive agents may also be required. Cycloplegic agents, particularly atropine, are also used to reduce inflammation and to prevent adhesion of the iris to the lens, especially in anterior uveitis.

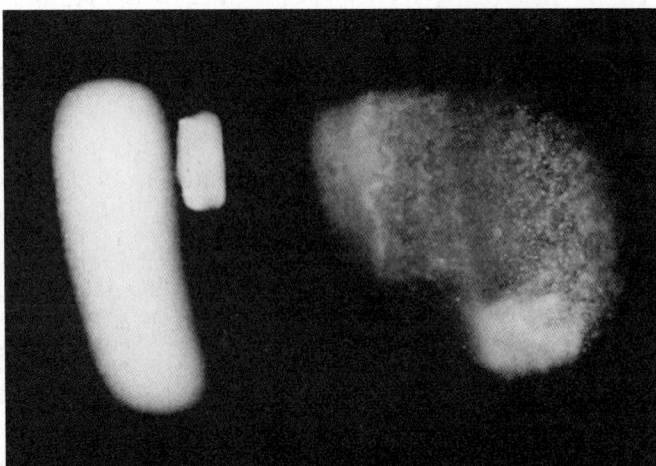

FIGURE 620–1. Cell and flare in the anterior chamber. The flare represents protein leakage. (Courtesy of Peter Buch, C.R.A.)

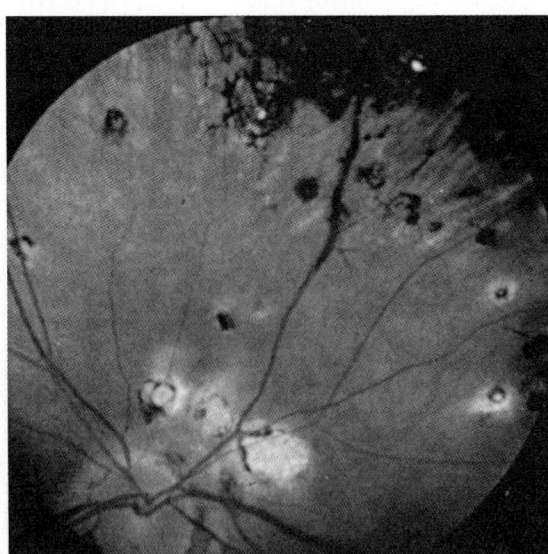

FIGURE 620–2. Focal atrophic and pigmented scars of chorioretinitis.

Albert DM, Diaz-Rohena R: A historical review of sympathetic ophthalmia and its epidemiology. *Surv Ophthalmol* 1989;34:1.

Cochereau-Massin I, LeHoang P, Lautier-Frau M, et al: Efficacy and tolerance of intravitreal ganciclovir in cytomegalovirus retinitis in acquired immune deficiency syndrome. *Ophthalmology* 1991;98:1348.

Contreras F, Pereda J: Congenital syphilis of the eye with lens involvement. *Arch Ophthalmol* 1978;96:1052.

Giannini EH, Brewer EJ, Kuzmina N, et al: Methotrexate in resistant juvenile rheumatoid arthritis: Results of the U.S.A.-U.S.S.R. double-blind, placebo-controlled trial. *N Engl J Med* 1992;326:1043.

Giles CL: Uveitis in children. In Nelson LB (editor): *Harley's Pediatric Ophthalmology*, 4th ed. Philadelphia, WB Saunders, 1998.

Guidelines for ophthalmic examinations in children with juvenile rheumatoid arthritis: Section on rheumatology and section on ophthalmology. *Pediatrics* 1993;92:295.

Hoover DL, Khan JA, Giangiacomo J: Pediatric ocular sarcoidosis. *Surv Ophthalmol* 1986;30:215.

Kanski JJ: Juvenile arthritis and uveitis. *Surv Ophthalmol* 1990;34:253.

Kimura SJ: Uveitis in children: Analysis of 274 cases. *Trans Am Ophthalmol Soc* 1964;62:171.

Oren B, Sehgal A, Simon JW, et al: The prevalence of uveitis in juvenile rheumatoid arthritis. *J Amer Assoc Pediatr Ophthalmol Strabismus* 2001;5:2.

Regillo CD, Shields CL, Shields JA, et al: Ocular tuberculosis. *JAMA* 1991;266:1490.

Shields JA: Ocular toxocariasis: A review. *Surv Ophthalmol* 1984;28:361.

Stern GA, Romano PE: Congenital ocular toxoplasmosis: Possible occurrence in siblings. *Arch Ophthalmol* 1978;96:615.

Winterkorn JM: Lyme disease: Neurologic and ophthalmologic manifestations. *Surv Ophthalmol* 1990;35:191.

Chapter 621
Disorders of the Retina and Vitreous

Retinopathy of Prematurity (ROP). This retinal vasculopathy occurs almost exclusively in preterm infants (see Chapter 86.2). It may be acute (early stages) or chronic (late stages). Clinical manifestations range from mild, usually transient changes of the peripheral retina to severe progressive vasoproliferation, scarring, and potentially blinding retinal detachment. ROP includes all stages of the disease and its sequelae. Retrolental fibroplasia (RLF), the previous name for this disease, described only the cicatricial stages.

PATHOGENESIS. Beginning at 16 wk of gestation, retinal angiogenesis normally proceeds from the optic disc to the periphery, reaching the outer rim of the retina (ora serrata) nasally at about 36 wk and extending temporally by approximately 40 wk. Injury to the process results in various pathologic and clinical changes. The first observation in the acute phase is cessation of vasculogenesis. Rather than a gradual transition from vascularized to avascular retina, there is an abrupt termination of the vessels, marked by a line in the retina. The line may then grow into a ridge composed of mesenchymal and endothelial cells. Cell division and differentiation may later resume, and vascularization of the retina may proceed. Alternatively, there may be progression to an abnormal proliferation of vessels out of the plane of the retina, into the vitreous, and over the surface of the retina. Cicatrization and traction on the retina may follow, leading to detachment.

The risk factors associated with ROP are not fully known, but prematurity and the associated retinal immaturity at birth represent the major factors. Hyperoxia is also a major factor, but other problems, such as respiratory distress, apnea, bradycardia, heart disease, infection, hypoxia, hypercarbia, acidosis, anemia, and the need for transfusion are thought by some to be contributory factors. Generally, the lower the birthweight and the sicker the infant, the greater the risk for ROP.

The basic pathogenesis of ROP is still unknown. Exposure to the extrauterine environment including the necessarily high inspired oxygen concentrations produces cellular damage, perhaps mediated by free radicals. Later in the course of the disease, peripheral hypoxia develops and vascular endothelial growth factors are produced in the nonvascularized retina. These growth factors stimulate abnormal vasculogenesis, and neovascularization may occur. This may then lead to scarring and vision loss.

CLASSIFICATION. The currently used international classification of ROP describes the location, extent, and severity of the disease. To delineate location, the retina is divided into three concentric zones, centered on the optic disc. Zone I, the posterior or inner zone, extends twice the disc-macular distance, or 30 degrees in all directions from the optic disc. Zone II, the middle zone, extends from the outer edge of zone I to the ora serrata nasally and to the anatomic equator temporally. Zone III, the outer zone, is the residual crescent that extends from the outer border of zone II to the ora serrata temporally, this area of the retina being vascularized. The extent of involvement is described by the number of circumferential clock hours involved.

The phases and severity of the disease process are classified into five stages. Stage 1 is characterized by a demarcation line that separates vascularized from avascular retina. This line lies within the plane of the retina and appears relatively flat and white. Often noted is abnormal branching or arcading of the retinal vessels that lead into the line. Stage 2 is characterized by a ridge; the demarcation line has grown, acquiring height, width, and volume and extending up and out of the plane of the retina. It may change from white to pink. Vessels may leave the plane of the retina to enter the ridge. Stage 3 is characterized by the presence of a ridge and by the development of extraretinal fibrovascular tissue (Fig. 621–1A). Stage 4 is characterized by subtotal retinal detachment caused by traction from the proliferating tissue in the vitreous or on the retina. Stage 4 is subdivided into two phases: (1) subtotal retinal detachment not involving the macula and (2) subtotal retinal detachment involving the macula. Stage 5 is total retinal detachment.

When signs of posterior retinal vascular changes accompany the active stages of ROP, the term *plus disease* is used (see Fig. 621-1B). Patients reaching the point of dilatation and tortuosity of the retinal vessels also frequently demonstrate the associated findings of engorgement of the iris, pupillary rigidity, and vitreous haze.

CLINICAL MANIFESTATIONS AND PROGNOSIS. In more than 90% of at-risk infants, the course is one of spontaneous arrest and regression of the usually asymmetric disease process, with little or no residual effects or visual disability. Fewer than 10% of infants have progression toward severe disease, with significant extraretinal vasoproliferation, cicatrization, detachment of the retina, and impairment of vision.

Some children with arrested or regressed ROP are left with demarcation lines, undervascularization of the peripheral retina, or abnormal branching, tortuosity, or straightening of the retinal vessels. Some are left with retinal pigmentary changes, dragging of the retina (so-called dragged disc), ectopia of the macula, retinal folds, or retinal breaks. Others proceed to total retinal detachment, which commonly assumes a funnel-like configuration. The clinical picture is often that of a retrolental membrane, producing leukokoria (a white reflex in the pupil). Some patients develop cataract, glaucoma, and signs of inflammation. The end stage is often a painful blind eye or a degenerated phthisical eye. The spectrum of ROP also includes myopia, which is often progressive and of significant degree in infancy. The incidence of anisometropia, strabismus, amblyopia, and nystagmus may also be increased.

DIAGNOSIS. Systematic ophthalmologic examination of infants at risk is recommended. Guidelines vary but generally include infants weighing less than 1,500 g at birth and those born before 28 wk of gestational age. Infants born weighing

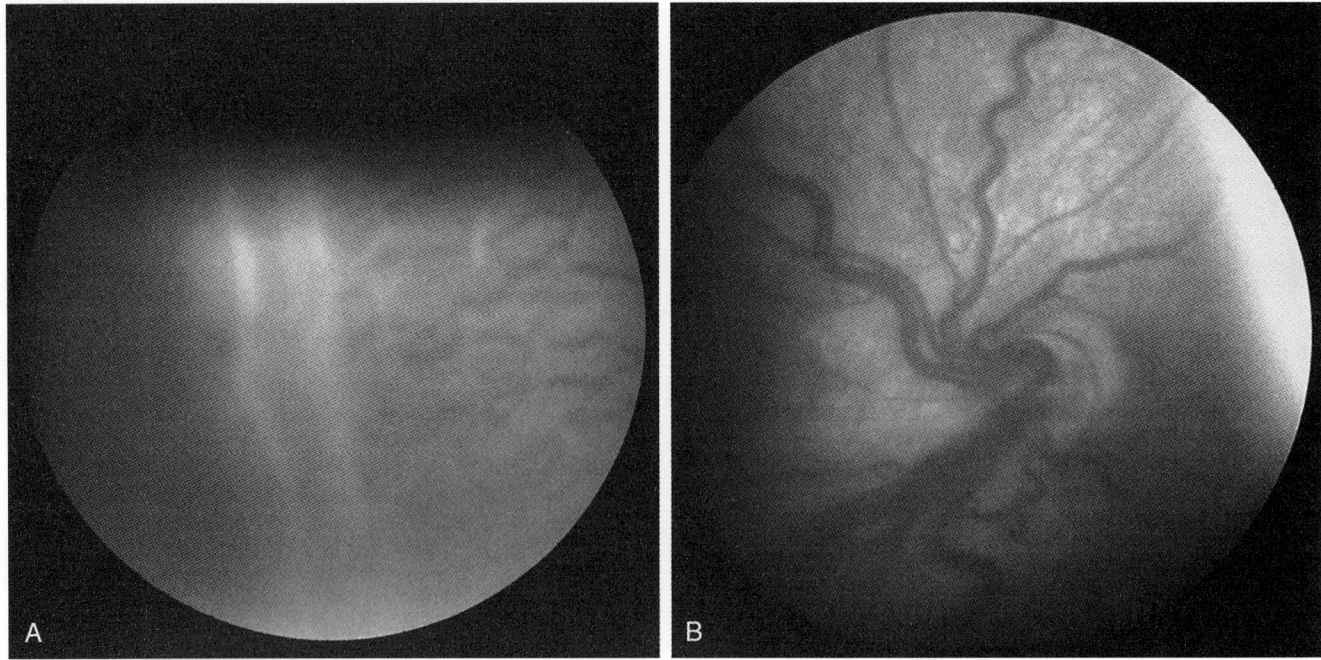

FIGURE 621–1. Retinopathy of prematurity (ROP). *A,* In stage 3, there is a ridge and extraretinal vascular tissue. *B,* Retinal vessels are dilated and tortuous in active ROP plus disease.

more than 1,500 g, who have an unstable clinical course and who are thought to be at high risk, should also be examined for ROP. The initial examination should be performed at 4–6 wk of chronological age or at 31–33 wk postconceptional age. ROP is diagnosed most often at 32–44 wk after conception. The examination can be stressful to fragile preterm infants, and the dilating drops can have untoward side effects; thus, discretion must be used in timing the eye examination, and infants must be carefully monitored during and after the examination. Follow-up is based on the initial findings and risk factors but is usually 2 wk or less.

TREATMENT. In selected cases, cryotherapy or laser photocoagulation of the avascular retina reduces the more severe complications of progressive ROP. Advances in vitreoretinal surgical techniques have led to limited success in reattaching the retina in infants with total retinal detachment (stage 5 ROP), but the visual results are often disappointing. The efficacy of laser photocoagulation in infants with earlier stages of ROP is being evaluated.

PREVENTION. Prevention of ROP ultimately depends on prevention of premature birth and its attendant problems. Despite advances in technology and the meticulous care given to high-risk infants in modern nurseries, ROP continues to occur. Oxygen alone is neither sufficient nor necessary to produce ROP, and no safe level of oxygen has yet been determined. Each infant must be treated with whatever is necessary to sustain life and neurologic function. Some investigators have suggested the use of supplemental vitamin E for its antioxidant properties in infants at risk for ROP. Its efficacy has not been proven; at certain dosage levels, it may produce untoward side effects (see Chapter 86.2).

Persistent Hyperplastic Primary Vitreous (PHPV). PHPV includes a spectrum of manifestations caused by the persistence of various portions of the fetal hyaloid vascular system and associated fibrovascular tissue.

During development of the eye, the hyaloid artery extends from the optic disc to the posterior aspect of the lens; it sends branches into the vitreous and ramifies to form the posterior portion of the vascular capsule of the lens. The posterior portion of the hyaloid system normally regresses by the 7th fetal mo and the anterior portion by the 8th fetal mo. Small remnants of the system, such as a tuft of tissue at the disc (Bergmeister papilla) or a tag of tissue on the posterior capsule of the lens (Mittendorf dot), are common findings in healthy persons. More extensive remnants and associated complications constitute PHPV. Two major forms are described, anterior PHPV and posterior PHPV. Variability is great, and mixed or intermediate forms occur.

The usual *clinical manifestation* of anterior PHPV is the presence of a vascularized plaque of tissue on the back surface of the lens in an eye that is microphthalmic or slightly smaller than normal. The condition is usually unilateral and may occur in infants with no other abnormalities and no history of prematurity. The fibrovascular tissue tends to undergo gradual contracture. The ciliary processes become elongated, and the anterior chamber may become shallow. The lens usually is smaller than normal and may be clear but often becomes cataractous and may swell or absorb fluid. Large or anomalous vessels of the iris may be present. The anterior chamber angle may have abnormalities. In time, the cornea may become cloudy.

Anterior PHPV is usually noted in the 1st wk or mo of life. The most frequent presenting signs are leukokoria (white pupillary reflex), strabismus, and nystagmus. The course is usually progressive and the outcome poor. Major complications are spontaneous intraocular hemorrhage, swelling of the lens caused by rupture of the posterior capsule, and glaucoma. The eye may eventually deteriorate.

Surgery is performed in an effort to prevent complications, to preserve the eye and a reasonably good cosmetic appearance, and, in some cases, to salvage vision. Surgical *treatment* usually involves aspirating the lens and excising the abnormal tissue. If useful vision is to be attained, refractive correction and aggressive amblyopia therapy are required. In some cases, the affected eye is enucleated, because distinguishing between this white mass and retinoblastoma can be difficult. Ultrasonography and CT are valuable diagnostic aids.

The spectrum of posterior PHPV includes fibroglial veils around the disc and macula, vitreous membranes and stalks containing hyaloid artery remnants projecting from the disc, and meridional retinal folds. Traction detachment of the retina may occur. Vision may be impaired, but the eye is usually retained.

Retinoblastoma (also see Chapter 494). Retinoblastoma (Fig. 621–2) is the most common primary malignant intraocular tumor of childhood. It occurs in approximately 1/18,000 infants; 250–300 new cases are diagnosed in the United States annually. Hereditary and nonhereditary patterns of transmission occur; there is no sex or race predilection. The hereditary form is usually bilateral and multifocal, whereas the nonhereditary form is generally unilateral and unifocal. Fifteen percent of unilateral cases are hereditary. Bilateral cases often present earlier than unilateral cases. Unilateral tumors are often large by the time they are discovered. The average age at diagnosis is 15 mo for bilateral cases, compared with 25 mo for unilateral cases. It is unusual for a child to present with a retinoblastoma after 2 yr of age. Rarely, the tumor is discovered at birth, during adolescence, or even in adulthood.

The *clinical manifestations* of retinoblastoma vary, depending on the stage at which the tumor is detected. The initial sign in the majority of patients is a white pupillary reflex (leukokoria). Leukokoria results because of the reflection of light off the white tumor. The second most frequent initial sign of retinoblastoma is strabismus. Less frequent presenting signs include pseudohypopyon (tumor cells layered inferiorly in front of the iris), caused by tumor seeding in the anterior chamber of the eye; hyphema (blood layered in front of the iris), secondary to iris neovascularization; vitreous hemorrhage; or signs of orbital cellulitis. On examination, the tumor appears as a white mass, sometimes small and relatively flat, sometimes large and protuberant. It may appear nodular. Vitreous haze or tumor seeding may be evident.

The retinoblastoma gene is a recessive suppressor gene located on chromosome 13 at the 13q14 region. Because of the hereditary nature of retinoblastoma, family members of affected children should undergo a complete ophthalmologic examination and genetic counseling. Newborn siblings and children of affected patients should be referred to an ophthalmologist shortly after birth, when the peripheral retina can be evaluated without the need for an examination under anesthesia.

The *diagnosis* of a retinoblastoma is made by direct observation by an experienced ophthalmologist. Ancillary testing such as CT scanning or ultrasonography may help to confirm the diagnosis and demonstrate calcification within the mass. A definitive diagnosis occasionally cannot be made, and removal of the eye must be considered to avoid the possibility of lethal metastasis of the tumor. Because a biopsy can lead to spread of the tumor, histologic confirmation before enucleation is not possible in most cases. Therefore, removal of a blind eye in which the diagnosis of retinoblastoma is likely may be appropriate.

Treatment varies, depending on the size and location of the tumor as well as whether it is unilateral or bilateral. Advanced tumors may be treated by enucleation. Other treatment modalities include the use of external beam irradiation, radiation plaque therapy, laser or cryotherapy, and chemotherapy.

The *prognosis* for children with retinoblastoma depends on the size and extension of the tumor. When confined to the eye, most tumors can be cured. The prognosis for long-term survival is poor when the tumor has extended into the orbit or along the optic nerve.

Retinitis Pigmentosa. This progressive retinal degeneration is characterized by pigmentary changes, arteriolar attenuation, usually some degree of optic atrophy, and progressive impairment of visual function. Dispersion and aggregation of the retinal pigment produce various ophthalmoscopically visible changes, ranging from granularity or mottling of the retinal pigment pattern to distinctive focal pigment aggregates with the configuration of bone spicules (Fig. 621–3). Other ocular findings include subcapsular cataract, glaucoma, and keratoconus.

Impairment of night vision or dark adaptation is often the first *clinical manifestation*. Progressive loss of peripheral vision, often in the form of an expanding ring scotoma or concentric contraction of the field, is usual. There may be loss of central vision. Retinal function, as measured by electroretinography (ERG), is characteristically reduced. Manifestations commonly begin in childhood. The disorder may be autosomal recessive, autosomal dominant, or sex linked.

A special form of retinitis pigmentosa is **Leber congenital retinal amaurosis**, in which the retinal changes tend to be pleomorphic, with various degrees of pigment disorder, arteriolar attenuation, and optic atrophy. The retina may appear normal during infancy. Vision impairment is usually evident soon after birth, and the ERG findings are abnormal early.

Clinically similar, secondary pigmentary retinal degenerations to be differentiated from retinitis pigmentosa occur in a wide variety of metabolic diseases, neurodegenerative processes, and multifaceted syndromes. Examples include the

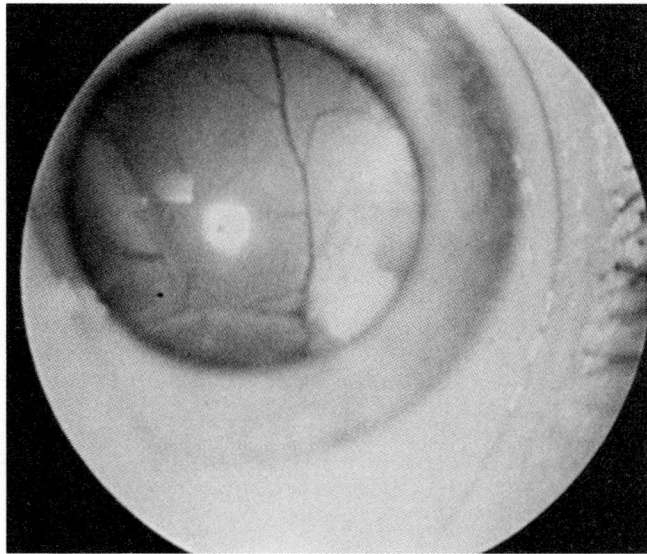
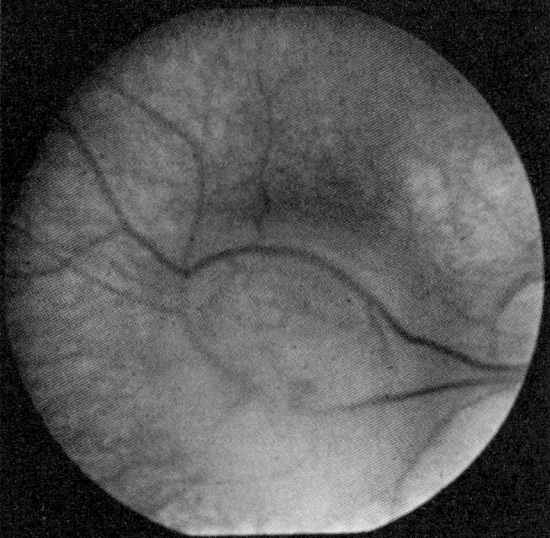

FIGURE 621–2. Retinoblastoma.

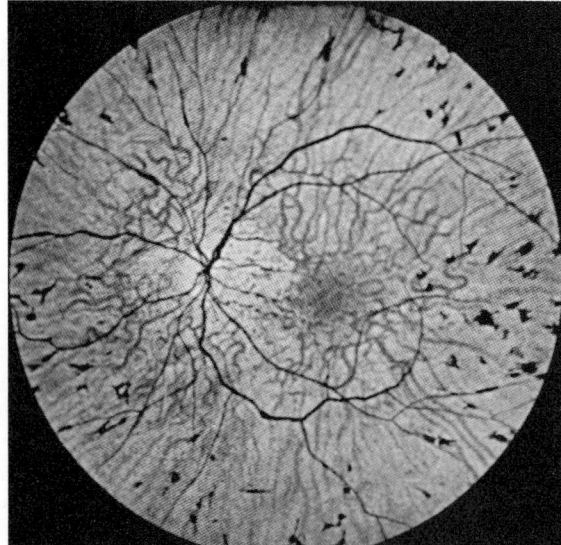

FIGURE 621–3. Retinitis pigmentosa.

progressive retinal changes of the mucopolysaccharidoses (particularly Hurler, Hunter, Scheie, and Sanfilippo syndromes) and certain of the late-onset gangliosidoses (Batten-Mayou, Spielmeyer-Vogt, and Jansky-Bielschowsky diseases), the progressive retinal degeneration that is associated with progressive external ophthalmoplegia (Kearns-Sayre syndrome), and the retinitis pigmentosa-like changes in the Laurence-Moon and Bardet-Biedl syndromes. The retinal manifestations of abeta-lipoproteinemia (Bassen-Kornzweig syndrome) and Refsum disease are similar to those found in retinitis pigmentosa. The diagnosis of these latter two disorders in a patient with presumed retinitis pigmentosa is important because treatment is possible. There is also an association of retinitis pigmentosa and congenital hearing loss, as in Usher syndrome.

Stargardt Disease (Fundus Flavimaculatus). This autosomal recessive retinal disorder is characterized by slowly progressive bilateral macular degeneration and vision impairment. It usually appears at 8–14 yr of age, and affected children are often initially misdiagnosed as having functional visual loss. The foveal reflex becomes obtunded or appears grayish, pigment spots develop in the macular area, and macular depigmentation and chorioretinal atrophy eventually occur. Macular hemorrhages also may develop. Some patients also have white or yellow spots beyond the macula or pigmentary changes in the periphery; the term *fundus flavimaculatus* is commonly used for this condition. It is now recognized that Stargardt disease and fundus flavimaculatus represent different parts on the spectrum of the same disease. Central visual acuity is reduced, often to 20/200, but total loss of vision does not occur. ERG findings vary. The condition is not associated with central nervous system abnormalities and is to be differentiated from the macular changes of many progressive metabolic neurodegenerative diseases. The genetic mutation responsible for Stargardt macular dystrophy has been identified.

Best Vitelliform Degeneration. This macular dystrophy is characterized by a distinctive yellow or orange discoid subretinal lesion in the macula, resembling the intact yolk of a fried egg. Diagnosis is usually made at 3–15 yr of age, with a mean age of presentation of 6 yr. Vision is usually normal at this stage. The condition may be progressive; the yolklike lesion may eventually degenerate ("scramble") and result in pigmentation, chorioretinal atrophy, and vision impairment. The condition is usually bilateral. There is no association with systemic abnormalities. Inheritance is usually autosomal dominant. In vitelli-form macular degeneration, the ERG response is normal. The electrooculogram findings are abnormal in affected patients and carriers, and this test is useful in diagnosis and in genetic counseling.

Cherry Red Spot. Because of the special histologic features of the macula, certain pathologic processes affecting the retina produce an ophthalmoscopically visible sign referred to as a cherry red spot, a bright to dull red spot at the center of the macula surrounded and accentuated by a grayish-white or yellowish halo. The halo is a result of a loss of transparency of the retinal ganglion cell layer secondary to edema, lipid accumulation, or both. Because ganglion cells are not present in the fovea, the retina surrounding the fovea is opacified but the fovea transmits the normal underlying choroidal color (red), accounting for the presence of the cherry red spot. A cherry red spot typically occurs in certain sphingolipidoses, principally in Tay-Sachs disease (GM_2 type 1), in the Sandhoff variant (GM_2 type 2), and in generalized gangliosidosis (GM_1 type 1). Similar but less distinctive macular changes occur in some cases of metachromatic leukodystrophy (sulfatide lipidosis), in some forms of neuronopathic Niemann-Pick disease, and in certain mucolipidoses. The cherry red spot that characteristically occurs as a result of retinal ischemia secondary to vasospasm, ocular contusion, or occlusion of the central retinal artery must be differentiated from the cherry red spot of neurodegenerative disease.

Phakomas. These are the herald lesions of the hamartomatous disorders. In Bourneville disease (**tuberous sclerosis**), the distinctive ocular lesion is a refractile, yellowish, multinodular cystic lesion arising from the disc or retina; the appearance of this typical lesion is often compared with that of an unripe mulberry (Fig. 621–4). Equally characteristic and more common in tuberous sclerosis are flatter, yellow to whitish retinal lesions, varying in size from minute dots to large lesions approaching the size of the disc. These lesions are benign astrocytic proliferations. Rarely, similar retinal phakomas occur in von **Recklinghausen disease (neurofibromatosis)**. In von Hippel-Lindau disease (angiomatosis of the retina and cerebellum), the distinctive fundus lesion is a hemangioblastoma; this vascular lesion usually appears as a reddish globular mass with large paired arteries and veins passing to and from the lesion. In **Sturge-Weber syndrome** (encephalofacial angiomatosis), the fundus abnormality is a choroidal hemangioma; the hemangioma may impart a dark color to the affected area of the fundus, but the lesion is best seen with fluorescein angiography.

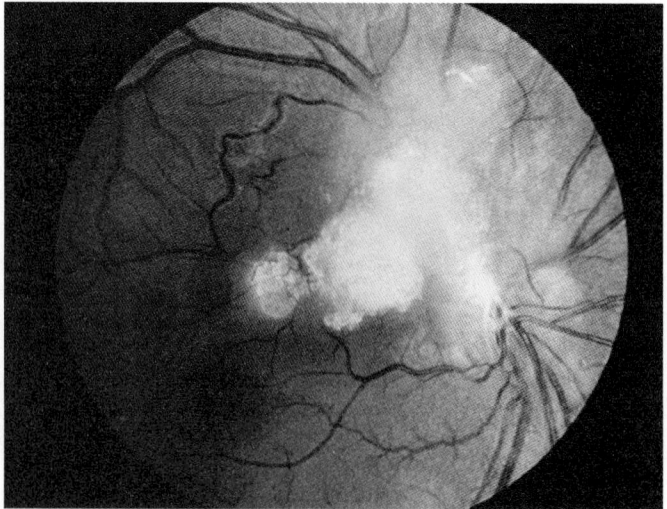

FIGURE 621–4. Retinal phakoma of tuberous sclerosis.

Retinoschisis. *Congenital hereditary retinoschisis*, also referred to as *juvenile X-linked retinoschisis*, is a bilateral vitreoretinal dystrophy that appears early in life, often in infancy. It is characterized by splitting of the retina into inner and outer layers. The usual ophthalmoscopic finding in affected males is an elevation of the inner layer of the retina, most commonly in the inferotemporal quadrant of the fundus, often with round or oval holes visible in the inner layer. Schisis of the fovea is virtually pathognomonic and is found in almost 100% of patients. Ophthalmoscopically, this appears in early stages as small, fine striae in the internal limiting membrane. These striae radiate outward in a petaloid or spoke wheel configuration. In some cases, frank retinal detachment or vitreous hemorrhage occurs.

Vision impairment varies from mild to severe; visual acuity may worsen with age, but good vision is often retained. Carrier females are asymptomatic, but linkage studies may be useful to help detect carriers.

Retinal Detachment. A retinal detachment is a separation of the outer layers of the retina from the underlying retinal pigment epithelium (RPE). During embryogenesis, the retina and RPE are initially separated. During ocular development, they join together and are held in apposition to each other by various physiologic mechanisms. Pathologic events leading to a retinal detachment return the retina-RPE to its former separated state. The detachment can occur as a congenital anomaly but more commonly arises secondary to other ocular abnormalities or trauma. Three types of detachment are described; each may occur in children. *Rhegmatogenous detachments* result from a break in the retina that allows fluid to enter the subretinal space. In children, these are usually a result of trauma (such as child abuse) but may occur secondary to myopia or ROP or after congenital cataract surgery. *Tractional retinal detachments* result when vitreoretinal membranes pull on the retina. They can occur in diabetes, sickle cell disease, and ROP. *Exudative retinal detachments* result when exudation exceeds absorption. This can be seen in Coats disease, retinoblastoma, and ocular inflammation.

The presenting sign of retinal detachment in an infant or child may be loss of vision, secondary strabismus or nystagmus, or leukokoria (white pupillary reflex). In addition to direct examination of the eye, special diagnostic studies such as ultrasonography and neuroimaging (CT, MRI) may be necessary to establish the cause of the detachment and the appropriate treatment. Prompt care is essential if vision is to be salvaged.

Coats Disease. This exudative retinopathy of unknown cause is characterized by telangiectasis of retinal vessels with leakage of plasma to form intraretinal and subretinal exudates and by retinal hemorrhages and detachment. The condition is usually unilateral. It predominantly affects boys, usually appearing in the first decade. The condition is nonfamilial and for the most part occurs in otherwise healthy children. The most frequent presenting signs are blurring of vision, leukokoria, and strabismus. Rubeosis of the iris, glaucoma, and cataract may develop. Treatment with photocoagulation or cryotherapy may be helpful.

Familial Exudative Vitreoretinopathy (FEV). This progressive retinal vascular disorder is of unknown cause, but clinical and angiographic findings suggest an aberration of vascular development. Avascularity of the peripheral temporal retina is a significant finding in most cases, with abrupt cessation of the retinal capillary network in the region of the equator. The avascular zone often has a wedge- or V-shaped pattern in the temporal meridian. Glial proliferation or well-marked retinochoroidal atrophy may be found in the avascular zone. Excessive branching of retinal arteries and veins, dilatation of the capillaries, arteriovenous shunt formation, neovascularization, and leakage from retinal vessels of the farthest vascularized retina occur. Vitreoretinal

adhesions are usually present at the peripheral margin of the vascularized retina. Traction, retinal dragging and temporal displacement of the macula, falciform retinal folds, and retinal detachment are common. Intraretinal or subretinal exudation, retinal hemorrhage, and recurrent vitreous hemorrhages may develop. Patients may also develop cataracts and glaucoma. Vision impairment of varying severity occurs. The condition is usually bilateral. FEV is usually an autosomal dominant condition with incomplete penetrance. Asymptomatic family members often display a zone of avascular peripheral retina.

The findings in FEV may resemble those of ROP in the cicatricial stages, but unlike ROP, the neovascularization of FEV seems to develop years after birth and most patients with FEV have no history of prematurity, oxygen therapy, prenatal or postnatal injury or infection, or developmental abnormalities. FEV is also to be differentiated from Coats disease, angiomatosis of the retina, peripheral uveitis, and other disorders of the posterior segment.

Hypertensive Retinopathy. In the early stages of hypertension, no retinal changes may be observable. Generalized constriction and irregular narrowing of the arterioles are usually the first signs in the fundus. Other alterations include retinal edema, flame-shaped hemorrhages, cotton-wool spots (retinal nerve fiber layer infarcts), and papilledema (Fig. 621–5). These changes are reversible if the disease can be controlled in the early stages, but in long-standing hypertension, irreversible changes may occur. Thickening of the vessel wall may produce a silver- or copper-wire appearance. Hypertensive retinal changes in a child should alert the physician to renal disease, pheochromocytoma, collagen disease, and cardiovascular disorders, particularly coarctation of the aorta.

Diabetic Retinopathy. The retinal changes of diabetes mellitus are classified as nonproliferative or proliferative. *Nonproliferative diabetic retinopathy* is characterized by retinal microaneurysms, venous dilatation, retinal hemorrhages, and exudates. The microaneurysms appear as tiny red dots. The hemorrhages may be of both the dot and blot type, representing deep intraretinal bleeding, and the splinter or flame-shaped type, involving the superficial nerve fiber layer. The exudates tend to be deep and to appear waxy. There may also be superficial nerve fiber infarcts called *cytoid bodies* or cotton-wool spots, as well as retinal edema. These signs may wax and wane. They are seen primarily in the posterior pole, around the disc and macula, well within the range of direct ophthalmoscopy. Involvement of the macula may lead to decreased vision.

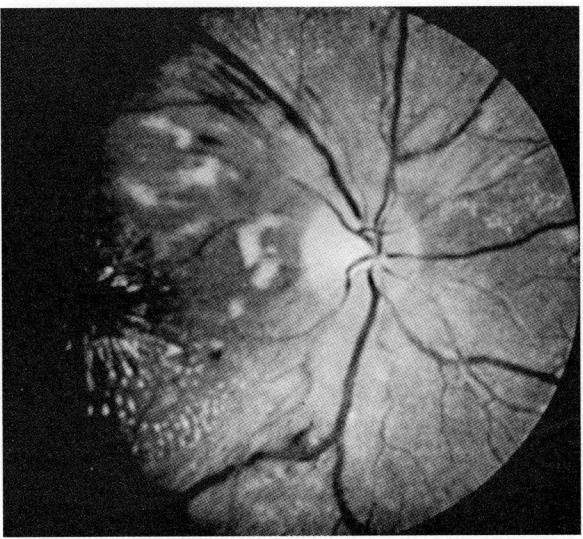

FIGURE 621–5. Hypertensive retinopathy.

Proliferative retinopathy, the more serious form, is characterized by neovascularization and proliferation of fibrovascular tissue on the retina, extending into the vitreous. Neovascularization may occur on the optic disc (NVD), elsewhere on the retina (NVE), or on the iris and in the anterior chamber angle (NVI, or rubeosis irides) (Fig. 621–6). Traction on these new vessels leads to hemorrhage and eventually scarring. The vision-threatening complications of proliferative diabetic retinopathy are retinal and vitreous hemorrhages, cicatrization, traction, and retinal detachment. Neovascularization of the iris may lead to secondary glaucoma if not treated promptly.

Diabetic retinopathy involves the alteration and nonperfusion of retinal capillaries, retinal ischemia, and neovascularization, but its pathogenesis is not yet completely understood, either in terms of location of the primary pathogenetic mechanism (retinal vessels vs surrounding neuronal or glial tissue) or the specific biochemical factors involved. The better the degree of long-term metabolic control, the lower the risk of diabetic retinopathy.

Clinically, the prevalence and course of retinopathy relate to a patient's age and to duration of disease. Detectable microvascular changes are rare in prepubertal children, with the prevalence of retinopathy increasing significantly after puberty, especially after the age of 15 yr. The incidence of retinopathy is low during the first 5 yr of disease and increases progressively thereafter, with the incidence of proliferative retinopathy becoming substantial after 10 yr and with increased risk of visual impairment after 15 yr or more. Periodic ophthalmologic evaluation is recommended for all patients with diabetes mellitus.

In addition to retinopathy, patients with juvenile-onset diabetes may develop optic neuropathy, characterized by swelling of the disc and blurring of vision. Patients with diabetes may also develop cataracts, even at an early age, sometimes with rapid progression.

Macular edema is the leading cause of visual loss in diabetic persons. Photocoagulation may be used to decrease the risk of continued vision loss in patients with macular edema. Proliferative retinopathy causes the most severe vision loss and can lead to total loss of vision and even loss of the eye.

Patients who have proliferative disease and who display certain high-risk characteristics should undergo panretinal photocoagulation (PRP) to preserve their central vision. Neovascularization of the iris is also treated with PRP to stop the development of neovascular glaucoma. Vitrectomy and other intraocular surgery may be necessary in patients with nonresolving vitreous hemorrhage or traction retinal detachment.

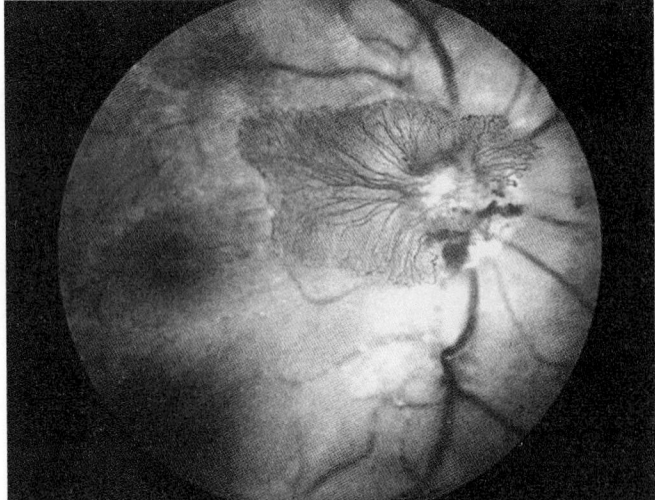

FIGURE 621–6. Proliferative diabetic retinopathy with neovascularization of the disc (NVD).

The value of technologic advances, such as insulin infusion pumps and pancreatic transplants, in preventing ocular complications is under investigation (see Chapter 583).

Subacute Bacterial Endocarditis. At some time during the course of the disease, retinopathy is present in approximately 40% of cases of subacute bacterial endocarditis. The lesions include hemorrhages, hemorrhages with white centers *(Roth spots)*, papilledema, and, rarely, embolic occlusion of the central retinal artery.

Blood Disorders. In primary and secondary anemias, retinopathy in the form of hemorrhages and cotton-wool patches may occur. Vision can be affected if hemorrhage occurs in the macular area. The hemorrhages may be light and feathery or dense and preretinal. In polycythemia vera, the retinal veins are dark, dilated, and tortuous. Retinal hemorrhages, retinal edema, and papilledema may be observed. In leukemia, the veins are characteristically dilated, with sausage-shaped constrictions; hemorrhages, particularly white-centered hemorrhages and exudates, are common during the acute stage. In the sickling disorders, fundus changes include vascular tortuosity, arterial and venous occlusions, "salmon patches," refractile deposits, pigmented lesions, arteriolar-venous anastomoses, and neovascularization (with "sea-fan" formations), sometimes leading to vitreous hemorrhage and retinal detachment. Individuals with Hb SC and Hb S-β-thalassemia hemoglobinopathies are at a higher risk for the development of retinopathy than are those with HbSS disease. It is thought that the more anemic state of those patients with SS disease offers protection from vascular occlusions in the retina.

Trauma-Related Retinopathy. Retinal changes may occur in patients who suffer trauma to other parts of the body. The occurrence of retinal hemorrhages in infants who have been physically abused is well documented (see Chapter 35). Retinal, subretinal, subhyaloid, and vitreous hemorrhages have been described. Often there are no signs of direct trauma to the eye, periocular region, or head. Such cases may result from violent shaking of an infant, and permanent retinal damage may result. Retinal, subhyaloid, and vitreous hemorrhages are common in patients with traumatic and nontraumatic subarachnoid hemorrhage, an association referred to as **Terson syndrome**.

In patients with head or chest trauma, a traumatic retinal angiopathy known as **Purtscher retinopathy** may occur. This is characterized by retinal hemorrhage, cotton-wool spots, possible disc swelling, and decreased vision. The pathogenesis is unclear, but there is evidence for arteriolar obstruction in this condition. A Purtscher-like fundus picture may also occur in several nontraumatic settings, such as acute pancreatitis, lupus erythematosus, and childbirth.

Medullated Nerve Fibers. Myelination of the optic nerve fibers normally terminates at the level of the disc, but in some individuals, ectopic medullation extends to nerve fibers of the retina. The condition is most commonly seen adjacent to the disc, although more peripheral areas of the retina may be involved. The characteristic ophthalmoscopic picture is a focal white patch with a feathered edge or brush-stroke appearance. Because the macula is generally unaffected, the visual prognosis is good. A relative or absolute visual field defect corresponding to areas of ectopic medullation is usually the only associated ocular abnormality. Extensive unilateral involvement, however, has been associated with ipsilateral myopia, amblyopia, and strabismus. If unilateral high myopia and amblyopia are present, appropriate optical correction and occlusion therapy should be instituted. For unknown reasons, the disorder is more commonly encountered in patients with craniofacial dysostosis, oxycephaly, neurofibromatosis, and Down syndrome.

Coloboma of The Fundus. The term *coloboma* describes a defect such as a gap, notch, fissure, or hole. The typical fundus coloboma is a result of malclosure of the embryonic fissure, which leaves a gap in the retina, RPE, and choroid, thus baring the underlying sclera. The defect may be extensive, involving the ciliary body, iris, and even lens, or it may be localized to one or more portions of the fissure. The usual appearance is of a well-circumscribed, wedge-shaped white area extending inferonasally below the disc, sometimes involving or engulfing the disc. In some cases there is ectasia or cyst formation in the area of the defect. Less extensive colobomatous defects may appear as only single or multiple focal punched-out chorioretinal defects or anomalous pigmentation of the fundus in the line of the embryonic fissure. Colobomas may occur in one or both eyes. A visual field defect usually corresponds to the chorioretinal defect. Visual acuity may be impaired, particularly if the defect involves the disc or macula.

Fundus colobomas may occur in isolation as sporadic defects or as an inherited condition. Isolated colobomatous anomalies are commonly inherited in an autosomal dominant manner with highly variable penetrance and expressivity. Family members of affected patients should receive appropriate genetic counseling. Colobomas may also be associated with such abnormalities as microphthalmia, glioneuroma of the eye, cyclopia, or encephale. They occur in children with various chromosomal disorders, including 13-trisomy, 18-trisomy, triploidy, cat's eye syndrome, and 4p-. Ocular colobomata also occur in many multisystem disorders, including the CHARGE* association; Joubert, Aicardi, Meckel, Warburg, and Rubinstein-Taybi syndromes; linear sebaceous nevus; Goldenhar and Lenz microphthalmia syndromes; and Goltz focal dermal hypoplasia.

Aaby AA, Kushner BJ: Acquired and progressive myelinated nerve fibers. *Arch Ophthalmol* 1985;103:542.

Abramson DH, Frank CM, Susman M, et al: Presenting signs of retinoblastoma. *J Pediatr* 1998;132:505.

Barr CC, Glaser JS, Blankenship G: Acute disc swelling in juvenile diabetes: Clinical profile and natural history of 12 cases. *Arch Ophthalmol* 1980;98:2185.

Bateman JB, Riedner E, Levin LS, et al: Heterogeneity of retinal degeneration and hearing impairment syndromes. *Am J Ophthalmol* 1980;90:755.

Berson EL, Rosner B, Siminoff E: Risk factors for genetic typing and detection in retinitis pigmentosa. *Am J Ophthalmol* 1980;89:763.

Burns RP, Lourien EW, Cibis AB: Juvenile sex-linked retinoschisis: Clinical and genetic studies. *Trans Am Acad Ophthalmol Otolaryngol* 1971;75:1011.

Chang M, McLean IW, Merritt JC: Coats' disease: A study of 62 histologically confirmed cases. *J Pediatr Ophthalmol Strabismus* 1984;21:163.

Cryotherapy for Retinopathy of Prematurity Cooperative Group: Multicenter trial of cryotherapy for retinopathy of prematurity outcomes at 10 years. *Arch Ophthalmol* 2001;119:1110.

Dass AB, Trese MT: Surgical results of persistent hyperplastic primary vitreous. *Ophthalmology* 1999;106:280.

Drack AV: Preventing blindness in premature infants. *N Engl J Med* 1998;338:1620.

Duane TD, Osher RH, Green WR: White-centered hemorrhages: Their significance. *Ophthalmology* 1980;87:66.

Eagle RC, Lucier AC, Bernardino VB Jr, et al: Retinal pigment epithelial abnormalities in fundus flavimaculatus. *Ophthalmology* 1980;87:1189.

Early Treatment Diabetic Retinopathy Research Study Group: Photocoagulation for diabetic macular edema. Early treatment diabetic retinopathy study report 1. *Arch Ophthalmol* 1985;103:1796.

Goldberg MF, Mafee M: Computed tomography for diagnosis of persistent hyperplastic primary vitreous (PHPV). *Ophthalmology* 1983;90:442.

Hardwig P, Robertson DM: Von Hippel-Lindau disease: A familial, often lethal, multi-system phakomatosis. *Ophthalmology* 1984;91:263.

Jackson RL, Ide CH, Guthrie RA, et al: Retinopathy in adolescents and young adults with onset of insulin-dependent diabetes in childhood. *Ophthalmology* 1982;89:7.

Juan Verdaguer T: Juvenile retinal detachment. *Am J Ophthalmol* 1982;93:145.

Knobloch WH, Layer JM: Clefting syndromes associated with retinal detachment. *Am J Ophthalmol* 1972;73:517.

---

*C = coloboma; H = heart disease; A = atresia choanae; R = retarded growth and development and/or central nervous system anomalies; G = genetic anomalies and/or hypogonadism; E = ear anomalies and/or deafness.

Kushner BJ, Sondheimer S: Medical treatment of glaucoma associated with cicatricial retinopathy of prematurity. *Am J Ophthalmol* 1982;94:313.

Mann E, Kut LJ, Lee CB: Rheumatogenous retinal detachment in infancy. *Arch Ophthalmol* 1971;95:1774.

Matthews JD, Weiter JJ, Kolodny EH: Macular halos associated with Niemann-Pick type B disease. *Ophthalmology* 1986;93:933.

Miyakulo H, Hashimoto K, Miyakulo S: Retinal vascular pattern in familial exudative vitreoretinopathy. *Ophthalmology* 1984;91:1524.

Mohler CW, Fine SL: Long-term evaluation of patients with Best's vitelliform dystrophy. *Ophthalmology* 1981;88:688.

Noble KG, Carr RE: Leber's congenital amaurosis: A retrospective study of 33 cases and a histopathological study of one case. *Arch Ophthalmol* 1978;96:818.

Noble KG, Carr RE: Stargardt's disease and fundus flavimaculatus. *Arch Ophthalmol* 1979;97:1281.

Nyboer JH, Robertson DM, Gomez MR: Retinal lesions in tuberous sclerosis. *Arch Ophthalmol* 1976;94:1277.

Pagon RA: Ocular coloboma. *Surv Ophthalmol* 1981;25:223.

Pierce EA, Foley ED, Smith LE: Regulation of vascular endothelial growth factor by oxygen in a model of retinopathy of prematurity. *Arch Ophthalmol* 1996;114:1219.

Quinn GE, Dobson V, Repka MX, et al: Development of myopia in infants with birthweights less than 1251 grams. *Ophthalmology* 1992;99:329.

Reynolds JD: Retinopathy of prematurity. *Ophthalmol Clin North Am* 1996;2:149.

Reynolds JD, Hardy RJ, Kennedy KA, et al: Lack of efficacy of light reduction in preventing retinopathy of prematurity. *N Engl J Med* 1998;338:1572.

Ridgeway EW, Jaffe N, Walton DS: Leukemic ophthalmopathy in children. *Cancer* 1976;38:1744.

Riley FC, Campbell RJ: Double phakomatosis. *Arch Ophthalmol* 1979;97:518.

Rosenthal AR: Ocular manifestations of leukemia. *Ophthalmology* 1983;90:899.

Salazar FG, Lamiell JM: Early identification of retinal angiomas in a large kindred with von Hippel-Lindau disease. *Am J Ophthalmol* 1980;89:540.

Screening examination of premature infants for retinopathy of prematurity. A joint statement of the American Academy of Pediatrics, the American Association for Pediatric Ophthalmology and Strabismus and the American Academy of Ophthalmology. *Pediatrics* 1997;100:273.

Shalev B, Farr A, Repka MX: Randomized comparison of diode laser photocoagulation versus cryotherapy for threshold retinopathy of prematurity: Seven year outcome. *Am J Ophthalmol* 2001;132:76.

Shields CL, De Potter P, Himelstein BP, et al: Chemoreduction in the initial management of intraocular retinoblastoma. *Arch Ophthalmol* 1996;114:1330.

Shields CL, Shields JA: Genetics of retinoblastoma. In Tasman WS, Jaeger EA (editors): *Duane's Foundation of Clinical Ophthalmology*. Philadelphia, JB Lippincott, 1997.

The STOP-ROP Multicenter Study Group: Supplemental Therapeutic Oxygen for Pre-Threshold Retinopathy of Prematurity (STOP-ROP), a randomized, controlled trial. I: Primary outcomes. *Pediatrics* 2000;105:295.

Straatsma BR, Foos RY, Heckenlively JR, et al: Myelinated retinal nerve fibers. *Am J Ophthalmol* 1981;91:25.

Walsh JB: Hypertensive retinopathy: Description, classification and prognosis. *Ophthalmology* 1982;89:1127.

Wright K, Anderson ME, Walker E, et al: Should fewer premature infants be screened for retinopathy of prematurity in the managed care era? *Pediatrics* 1998;102:31.

Chapter 622
Abnormalities of the Optic Nerve

Optic Nerve Aplasia. This rare congenital anomaly is typically unilateral. The optic nerve, retinal ganglion cells, and retinal blood vessels are absent. A vestigial dural sheath usually connects with the sclera in a normal position, but no neural tissue is present within this sheath. Optic nerve aplasia typically occurs sporadically in an otherwise healthy person. A wide variety of ocular abnormalities may occur, but colobomas are the most frequent associated finding.

Optic Nerve Hypoplasia. Hypoplasia of the optic nerve is a nonprogressive condition characterized by a subnormal number of optic nerve axons with normal mesodermal elements and glial supporting tissue. In typical cases, the nerve head is small and pale, with a pale or pigmented peripapillary halo or double ring sign.

This anomaly is associated with defects of vision and of visual fields of varying severity, ranging from blindness to normal or near-normal vision. It may be associated with systemic anomalies that most commonly involve the central nervous system (CNS). Protean CNS defects such as hydranencephaly or anencephaly or more focal lesions compatible with continued development of a patient may accompany optic nerve hypoplasia, but unilateral or bilateral optic nerve hypoplasia may be found without any concomitant defects.

Optic nerve hypoplasia is a principal feature of **septo-optic dysplasia of de Morsier,** a developmental disorder characterized by the association of anomalies of the midline structures of the brain with hypoplasia of the optic nerves, optic chiasm, and optic tracts; typically noted are agenesis of the septum pellucidum, partial or complete agenesis of the corpus callosum, and malformation of the fornix, with a large chiasmatic cistern. Patients may have hypothalamic abnormalities and endocrine defects, ranging from panhypopituitarism to isolated deficiency of growth hormone, hypothyroidism, or diabetes insipidus. Neonatal hypoglycemia and seizures are important presenting signs in affected infants.

Bilateral subtle hypoplasia may be difficult to diagnose from the appearance of the disc alone because no comparison with a contralateral uninvolved eye is possible. However, it is important to establish the diagnosis because this eliminates confusion with optic atrophy or glaucoma and may explain the cause of decreased vision in a patient unresponsive to amblyopia therapy. Endocrine function should be watched closely in patients with optic nerve hypoplasia.

The etiology of optic nerve hypoplasia remains unclear. Early gestational injuries to midline CNS structures with secondary axonal injury or a disruption of normal neuronal guidance mechanisms that affect both optic nerve and cerebral neurons may account for these commonly associated disorders. Optic nerve hypoplasia may occur with somewhat increased frequency in infants of diabetic mothers and has been associated with maternal use of dilantin, quinine, LSD (lysergic acid diethylamide), and alcohol during pregnancy.

Morning Glory Disc Anomaly. This term describes a congenital malformation of the optic nerve characterized by an enlarged, excavated, funnel-shaped disc with an elevated rim, resembling a morning glory flower. White glial tissue is present in the central part of the disc. The retinal vessels are abnormal and appear at the peripheral disc and course over the elevated pink rim in a radial fashion. Pigmentary mottling of the peripapillary region is usually seen. Most cases are unilateral. Females are affected twice as often as males. Visual acuity is usually severely reduced, and retinal detachment occurs in approximately one third of involved eyes. The association between basal encephaloceles and the morning glory disc anomaly has been well established.

Tilted Disc. In this congenital anomaly, the vertical axis of the optic disc is directed obliquely, so that the upper temporal portion of the nerve head is more prominent and anterior to the lower nasal portion of the disc. The retinal vessels emerge from the upper temporal portion of the disc rather than from the nasal side. Often noted is a peripapillary crescent or conus. Associated visual field defects and myopic astigmatism may be found. Clinical recognition of the tilted disc syndrome is important to avoid confusion of its disc and visual field signs with those of papilledema and intracranial tumor.

Drusen of the Optic Nerve. These globular, acellular bodies are thought to arise from axoplasmic derivatives of disintegrating nerve fibers. Drusen may be buried within the optic nerve, producing elevation of the optic nerve head (which can be confused with papilledema), or they may be partially or completely exposed, appearing as refractile bodies at the surface of the disc. Visual field defects and spontaneous peripapillary nerve fiber layer hemorrhages may occur in association with drusen. Drusen may occur as an autosomal dominant condition. They have also been observed in children with various neurologic disorders, including primary megalencephaly, seizures, learning disorders, mental retardation, schizophrenia, tuberous sclerosis, Down syndrome, and intracranial tumors.

Papilledema. The term *papilledema* ("choked disc") is reserved to describe swelling of the nerve head secondary to increased intracranial pressure (ICP). *Clinical manifestations* of papilledema include edematous blurring of the disc margins, fullness or elevation of the nerve head, partial or complete obliteration of the disc cup, capillary congestion and hyperemia of the nerve head, generalized engorgement of the veins, loss of spontaneous venous pulsation, nerve fiber layer hemorrhages around the disc, and peripapillary exudates (see Fig. 584–1). In some cases, edema extending into the macula may produce a fan- or star-shaped figure. In addition, concentric peripapillary retinal wrinkling (Paton lines) may be noted. Transient obscuration of vision may occur, lasting seconds and associated with postural changes. Vision, however, is usually normal in acute papilledema. Normally, when the ICP is relieved, the papilledema resolves and the disc returns to a normal or nearly normal appearance within 6–8 wk. Sustained chronic papilledema or long-standing unrelieved increased ICP may, however, lead to permanent nerve fiber damage, atrophic changes of the disc, macular scarring, and impairment of vision. In cases of impending or progressive vision loss caused by papilledema in patients with benign intracranial hypertension, decompression of the optic nerve by slitting the sheath may preserve vision.

The *pathophysiology* of papilledema is probably as follows: elevation of intracranial subarachnoid cerebrospinal fluid (CSF) pressure, elevation of CSF pressure in the sheath of the optic nerve, elevation of tissue pressure in the optic nerve, stasis of axoplasmic flow and swelling of the nerve fibers in the optic nerve head, and secondary vascular changes and the characteristic ophthalmoscopic signs of venous stasis. Associated neuroophthalmic signs of increased ICP in infants and children include abducent palsy and attendant esotropia, lid retraction, paresis of upward gaze, tonic downward deviation of the eyes, and convergent nystagmus.

The common *etiologies* of papilledema in childhood are intracranial tumors and obstructive hydrocephalus, intracranial hemorrhage, the cerebral edema of trauma, meningoencephalitis and toxic encephalopathy, and certain metabolic diseases. Whatever the cause, the optic disc signs of increased ICP in early childhood may occasionally be modified by the distensibility of the young skull. In the absence of conditions associated with early closure of sutures and early obliteration of the fontanel (craniosynostosis, Crouzon disease, and Apert syndromes), infants with increased ICP may not develop papilledema.

The *differential diagnosis* of papilledema includes structural changes of the disc ("pseudopapilledema," "pseudoneuritis," drusen, and medullated fibers), with which it may be confused, and the disc swelling of hypertension and diabetes mellitus. Unless retinal hemorrhage or edema involves the macular area, the preservation of good central vision and the absence of an afferent pupillary defect (Marcus Gunn pupil) help to differentiate acute papilledema from the edema of the optic nerve head found in acute optic neuritis.

Papilledema is a neurologic emergency. It can be accompanied by other signs of increased ICP, including headaches, nausea, and vomiting. Neuroimaging should be performed; if no intracranial masses are detected, a lumbar puncture and determination of CSF pressure should follow.

Optic Neuritis. This is any inflammation, demyelinization, or degeneration of the optic nerve with attendant impairment of function. The process is usually acute, with rapidly progressive loss of vision. It may be unilateral or bilateral. Pain on movement of the globe or pain on palpation of the globe may precede or accompany the onset of visual symptoms.

When the retrobulbar portion of the nerve is affected without ophthalmoscopically visible signs of inflammation at the disc, the term *retrobulbar neuritis* is applied. When there is ophthalmoscopically visible evidence of inflammation of the nerve head, the term *papillitis* or *intraocular optic neuritis* is used. When there is involvement of both the retina and papilla, the term *optic neuroretinitis* is used.

In childhood, optic neuritis may occur as an isolated condition or as a manifestation of a neurologic or systemic disease. It may occur with bacterial meningitis or with viral infection (often accompanying encephalomyelitis following an exanthem). It may signify one of the many demyelinating diseases of childhood. Although a significant percentage of adults who experience an episode of optic neuritis eventually develop other symptoms associated with multiple sclerosis, children with optic neuritis are seemingly at less risk. Bilateral optic neuritis in children may be associated with neuromyelitis optica (Devic disease). This syndrome is characterized by rapid and severe bilateral visual loss accompanied by transverse myelitis and paraplegia. Optic neuritis may also be secondary to an exogenous toxin or drug, such as with lead poisoning or as a complication of long-term high-dose treatment with chloramphenicol or vincristine therapy. Extensive pediatric neurologic and ophthalmic investigation, including neuroradiologic and electrophysiologic studies, is usually required.

In most cases of acute optic neuritis, some improvement in vision begins within 1–4 wk after onset, and vision may improve to normal or near normal within weeks or months. The course varies with etiology. Although central vision may fully recover, it is common to find permanent defects in other areas of visual function (contrast sensitivity, color, brightness sense, and motion perception).

A *treatment* trial demonstrated that intravenous corticosteroids may help to speed the visual recovery in young adults but do not alter the long-term visual outcome. Therefore, their use has been reserved by some physicians for cases with severe vision loss or significant discomfort. Orally administered corticosteroids should not be used because they are associated with a significant increase in the recurrence rate of optic neuritis. It is unknown to what degree the results of the aforementioned trial may be extrapolated to optic neuritis in childhood.

Leber Optic Neuropathy. This entity is characterized by sudden loss of central vision occurring in the 2nd and 3rd decades of life, primarily affecting young males. A characteristic peripapillary telangiectatic microangiopathy occurs not only in the presymptomatic phase of involved eyes but also in a high number of asymptomatic offspring in the female line. Disc hyperemia and edema mark the acute phase of visual loss. One eye is usually affected before the other. In time, progressive optic atrophy and vision loss usually ensue. The tortuous angiopathy becomes less obvious. Although visual function after the initial loss generally remains stable, a significant and sometimes complete recovery may occur in as many as one third of affected individuals. This recovery may take place years or decades after the initial episode of acute vision loss. The peripapillary angiopathy, the lack of short-term remission, and the degree of symmetry serve to distinguish most cases of Leber disease from the optic neuritis of multiple sclerosis.

Leber optic neuropathy is maternally inherited and is caused by defective cytoplasmic mitochondrial DNA. Multiple point mutations in the mitochondrial DNA that lead to the development of the disorder have been found. Because of the mitochondrial nature of the disorder, skeletal and cardiac muscle disorders, including electrocardiographic abnormalities, may also be encountered in affected individuals.

Optic Atrophy. This denotes degeneration of optic nerve axons, with attendant loss of function. The ophthalmoscopic signs of optic atrophy are pallor of the disc and loss of substance of the nerve head, sometimes with enlargement of the disc cup. The associated vision defect varies with the nature and site of the primary disease or lesion.

Optic atrophy is the common expression of a wide variety of congenital or acquired pathologic processes. The cause may be traumatic, inflammatory, degenerative, neoplastic, or vascular; intracranial tumors and hydrocephalus are principal causes of optic atrophy in children. In some cases, progressive optic atrophy is hereditary. Dominantly inherited infantile optic atrophy is a relatively mild heredodegenerative type that tends to progress through childhood and adolescence. Autosomal recessively inherited congenital optic atrophy is a rare condition that is evident at birth or develops at a very early age; the visual defect is usually profound. Behr optic atrophy is a hereditary type associated with hypertonia of the extremities, increased deep tendon reflexes, mild cerebellar ataxia, some degree of mental deficiency, and possibly external ophthalmoplegia. This disorder afflicts principally boys age 3–11 yr. Some forms of heredodegenerative optic atrophy are associated with sensorineural hearing loss, as may occur in some children with juvenile-onset (insulin-dependent) diabetes mellitus. In the absence of an obvious cause, optic atrophy in an infant or child warrants extensive etiologic investigation.

Optic Nerve Glioma. Optic nerve glioma, more properly referred to as juvenile pilocytic astrocytoma, is the most frequent tumor of the optic nerve in childhood. This neuroglial tumor may develop in the intraorbital, intracanalicular, or intracranial portion of the nerve; the chiasm is often involved.

The tumor is a cytologic benign hamartoma that is generally stationary or only slowly progressive. The principal manifestations when the tumor occurs in the intraorbital portion of the nerve are unilateral loss of vision, proptosis, and deviation of the eye; optic atrophy or congestion of the optic nerve head may occur. Chiasmal involvement may be attended by defects of vision and visual fields (often bitemporal hemianopia), increased ICP, papilledema or optic atrophy, hypothalamic dysfunction, pituitary dysfunction, and sometimes nystagmus or strabismus. Juvenile pilocytic astrocytomas occur with increased frequency in patients with neurofibromatosis.

Treatment of optic pathway gliomas is controversial. The best management is usually periodic observation. Surgical removal may be appropriate when the tumor is confined to the intraorbital, intracanalicular, or prechiasmal portion of the nerve if a patient has unsightly proptosis with complete or nearly complete loss of vision of the affected eye. When the chiasm is involved, resection is not usually indicated and radiation and chemotherapy may be necessary.

Traumatic Optic Neuropathies. Injury to the optic nerve may result from both direct and indirect trauma. Direct trauma to the optic nerve is a result of a penetrating injury to the orbit with transection or contusion of the nerve. Blunt trauma to the orbit may also lead to severe visual loss if the traumatic force is transmitted to the optic canal and causes disruption of the blood supply to the intracanalicular portion of the nerve. Treatment may include high-dose corticosteroids or optic canal decompression.

Anderson RL, Panje WR, Gross CE: Optic nerve blindness following blunt forehead trauma. *Ophthalmology* 1982;89:445.
Barr CC, Glaser JS, Blankenship G: Acute disc swelling in juvenile diabetes: Clinical profile and natural history of 12 cases. *Arch Ophthalmol* 1980;98:2185.

Brown MD, Voljavec AS, Lott MT, et al: Leber's hereditary optic neuropathy: A model for mitochondrial neurodegenerative diseases. *FASEB J* 1992;6:2791.

Costin G, Murgpree AL: Hypothalamic-pituitary function in children with optic nerve hypoplasia. *Am J Dis Child* 1985;139:249.

Haik BG, Greenstein SH, Smith ME, et al: Retinal detachment in the morning glory anomaly. *Ophthalmology* 1984;91:1638.

Hayreh SS: Optic disc edema in raised intracranial pressure: VI. Associated visual disturbances and their pathogenesis. *Arch Ophthalmol* 1977;95:1566.

Hoover DL, Robb RM, Petersen RA: Optic disc drusen and primary megalencephaly in children. *J Pediatr Ophthalmol Strabismus* 1989;26:81.

Hotchkiss ML, Green WR: Optic nerve aplasia and hypoplasia. *J Pediatr Ophthalmol Strabismus* 1979;16:225.

Hoyt CS: Autosomal dominant optic atrophy: A spectrum of disability. *Ophthalmology* 1980;87:245.

Kazarian EL, Gager WE: Optic neuritis complicating measles, mumps and rubella vaccination. *Am J Ophthalmol* 1978;86:544.

Leys D, Petit H, Block AM, et al: Neuromyelitis optica (Devic's disease). Four cases. *Rev Neurol (Paris)* 1987;143:722.

Listernick R, Louis DN, Packer RJ, et al: Optic pathway gliomas in children with neurofibromatosis 1: Consensus statement from the NF1 optic pathway glioma task force. *Ann Neurol* 1997;41:143.

Margalith D, Jan JE, McCormick AQ, et al: Clinical spectrum of congenital optic nerve hypoplasia: Review of 51 patients. *Dev Med Child Neurol* 1984;26:311.

Nikoskelainen E, Hoyt WF, Nummelin K: Ophthalmoscopic findings in patients with Leber's hereditary optic neuropathy. I. Fundus findings in asymptomatic family members. *Arch Ophathalmol* 1982;100:1597.

Optic Neuritis Study Group: Visual function 5 years after optic neuritis. Experience of the optic neuritis treatment trial. *Arch Ophthalmol* 1997;115:1545.

Repka MX, Miller NR: Optic atrophy in children. *Am J Ophthalmol* 1988;106:191.

Rosenberg MA, Savino PJ, Glaser JS: A clinical analysis of pseudopapilledema. I: Population, laterality, acuity, refractive error, ophthalmoscopic characteristics, and coincident disease. *Arch Ophthalmol* 1979;97:65.

Sergott RC, Savino PJ, Bosley TM: Modified optic nerve sheath decompression provides long-term visual improvement for pseudotumor cerebri. *Arch Ophthalmol* 1988;106:1384.

Singh G, Lott MT, Wallace DC: A mitochondrial DNA mutation as a cause of Leber's hereditary optic neuropathy. *N Engl J Med* 1989;320:1300.

Skarf B, Hoyt CS: Optic nerve hypoplasia in children: Association with anomalies of the endocrine and CNS. *Arch Ophthalmol* 1984;102:62.

Traboulsi EI, O'Neill JE: The spectrum in the morphology of the so-called "morning glory disc anomaly." *J Pediatr Ophthalmol Strabismus* 1988;25:93.

Weiss AH, Beck RW: Neuroretinitis in childhood. *J Pediatr Ophthalmol Strabismus* 1989;26:198.

Chapter 623
Childhood Glaucoma

Glaucoma is a general term used to indicate damage to the optic nerve with visual field loss that is caused by or related to elevated pressure within the eye. It is classified according to the age of the affected individual at presentation and the association of other ocular or systemic conditions. Glaucoma that begins within the first 3 yr of life is called *infantile* (congenital); that which begins between the ages of 3 and 30 yr is called *juvenile.*

Primary glaucoma indicates that the cause is an isolated anomaly of the drainage apparatus of the eye (trabecular meshwork). More than 50% of infantile glaucoma is primary. In secondary glaucoma, other ocular or systemic abnormalities are associated, even if a similar developmental defect of the trabecular meshwork is also present. Primary infantile glaucoma occurs with an incidence of only 0.03%.

Clinical Manifestations. The symptoms of infantile glaucoma include the classic triad of epiphora (tearing), photophobia (sensitivity to light), and blepharospasm (eyelid squeezing). Each can be attributed to corneal irritation. Only about 30% of affected infants demonstrate the classic symptom complex. Other signs include corneal edema, corneal and ocular enlargement, conjunctival injection, and visual impairment.

The sclera and cornea are more elastic in early childhood than later in life. An increase in intraocular pressure (IOP), therefore, leads to an expansion of the globe, including the cornea, and the development of buphthalmos ("ox eye"). If the cornea continues to enlarge, breaks occur in the endothelial basement membrane (Descemet membrane) and may lead to permanent corneal scarring. These breaks in Descemet membrane (Haab striae) are visible as horizontal edematous lines that cross or curve around the central cornea. They rarely occur beyond 3 yr of age or in corneas less than 12.0 mm in diameter. The cornea also becomes edematous and cloudy, with increased IOP. The corneal edema leads to tearing and photophobia. Glaucoma should be considered in a child suspected of having a nasolacrimal duct obstruction if any of these other signs or symptoms are present.

Children with unilateral glaucoma generally present early because the difference in the corneal size between the eyes can be noticed. When the disease is bilateral, parents may not recognize the increased corneal size. Many parents view the large eyes as attractive and do not seek help until other symptoms develop.

Cupping of the optic nerve head is detected by ocular examination. The optic nerve of an infant is easily distended by excessive pressure. Deep, central cupping readily occurs and may regress with normalization of pressure.

Some infants and children with early onset glaucoma have more extensive maldevelopment of the anterior segment of the eye. The **neurocristopathies**, once known as mesodermal dysgenesis, comprise a spectrum of conditions relating to abnormal embryologic development of the anterior segment. They are usually bilateral and may include abnormalities of the iris, cornea, and lens. Other ocular anomalies that may be associated with glaucoma in infants and children are aniridia, cataract, spherophakia, and ectopia lentis. Glaucoma may also develop secondary to persistent hyperplastic primary vitreous or retinopathy of prematurity.

Trauma, intraocular hemorrhage, ocular inflammatory disease, and intraocular tumor are also important causes of glaucoma in the pediatric population. Systemic disorders associated with glaucoma in infants and children are Sturge-Weber syndrome, von Recklinghausen disease, Lowe syndrome, Marfan syndrome, congenital rubella, a number of chromosomal syndromes, and juvenile xanthogranuloma.

Diagnosis and Treatment. The diagnosis of infantile glaucoma is made on recognition of the signs and symptoms. Although measurement of IOP may be helpful in monitoring treatment response, it is not a vital part of the diagnostic process. Once the diagnosis is established, treatment is started promptly. Unlike adult glaucoma, in which medication is often the first line of therapy, for infantile glaucoma the treatment is primarily surgical. Procedures used to treat glaucoma in children include surgery to establish a more normal anterior chamber angle (goniotomy and trabeculotomy), to create a site for aqueous fluid to exit the eye (trabeculectomy and seton surgery), or to reduce aqueous fluid production (cyclocryotherapy and photocyclocoagulation). Many children frequently require several operations to lower and maintain their IOP adequately, and long-term medical therapy may be necessary as well. Although vision may be reduced secondary to glaucomatous optic nerve damage or corneal scarring, amblyopia is the most common cause of loss of vision in these children.

Bardelli AM, Hadjistilianou T: Congenital glaucoma associated with other abnormalities in 150 cases. *Glaucoma* 1987;9:10.

Barsoum-Homsy M, Chevrette L: Incidence and prognosis of childhood glaucoma: A study of 63 cases. *Ophthalmology* 1986;93:1323.

Cibis GW, Tripathi RC, Tripathi BJ: Glaucoma in Sturge-Weber syndrome. *Ophthalmology* 1984;91:1061.

Ginsberg J, Bove KE, Fogelson MH: Pathological features of the eye in the oculo-cerebrorenal (Lowe) syndrome. *J Pediatr Ophthalmol Strabismus* 1981;18:16.

Kushner BJ, Sondheiner S: Medical treatment of glaucoma associated with cicatricial retinopathy of prematurity. *Am J Ophthalmol* 1982;94:313.

McPherson SD Jr, Berry DP: Goniotomy vs external trabeculotomy for developmental glaucoma. *Am J Ophthalmol* 1983;95:427.

Mullaney PB, Selleck C, Al-Awad A, et al: Combined trabeculotomy and trabeculectomy as an initial procedure in uncomplicated congenital glaucoma. *Arch Ophthalmol* 1999;117:457.

Netland P, Walton D: Glaucoma drainage implants in pediatric patients. *Ophthalmic Surg Lasers* 1993;24:723.

Neely DE, Plager DA: Endocyclophotocoagulation for management of difficult pediatric glaucomas. *J Am Assoc Pediatr Ophthalmol Strabismus* 2001;5:221.

Quigley HA: Childhood glaucoma: Results with trabeculotomy and study of reversible cupping. *Ophthalmology* 1982;89:219.

Rubin SE, Marcus CH: Glaucoma in childhood. *Ophthalmol Clin North Am* 1996;2:215.

Seidman DJ, Nelson LB, Calhoun JH, et al: Signs and symptoms in the presentation of primary infantile glaucoma. *Pediatrics* 1986;77:399.

Stern JH, Catalono RA: Current status of diagnostic and therapeutic measures in infantile glaucoma. *Semin Ophthalmol* 1990;5:166.

Chapter 624
Orbital Abnormalities

Hypertelorism and Hypotelorism. *Hypertelorism* is wide separation of the eyes or an increased interorbital distance, which may occur as a morphogenetic variant, a primary deformity, or a secondary phenomenon in association with developmental abnormalities, such as frontal meningocele or encephalocele or the persistence of a facial cleft. Often associated are strabismus, generally exotropia, and sometimes optic atrophy.

Hypotelorism refers to narrowness of the interorbital distance, which may occur as a morphogenetic variant alone or in association with other anomalies, such as epicanthus or holoprosencephaly or secondary to a cranial dystrophy, such as scaphocephaly.

Exophthalmos and Enophthalmos. Protrusion of the eye is referred to as *exophthalmos* or *proptosis*. It may be caused by shallowness of the orbits, as in many craniofacial malformations, or by increased tissue mass within the orbit, as with neoplastic, vascular, and inflammatory disorders. Ocular complications include exposure keratopathy, ocular motor disturbances, and optic atrophy with loss of vision.

Posterior displacement or sinking of the eye back into the orbit is referred to as *enophthalmos*. This may occur with orbital fracture or with atrophy of orbital tissue.

Orbital Cellulitis. This is a condition involving inflammation of the tissues of the orbit, with proptosis, limitation of movement of the eye, edema of the conjunctiva (chemosis), and inflammation and swelling of the eyelids. Patients often feel some discomfort, usually with general symptoms of toxicity, fever, and leukocytosis. Also see Chapter 178.

Orbital cellulitis may follow direct infection of the orbit from a wound, metastatic deposition of organisms during bacteremia, or more often direct extension or venous spread of infection from contiguous sites such as the lids, conjunctiva, globe, lacrimal gland, nasolacrimal sac, or commonly the paranasal sinuses. In some cases, primary or metastatic tumor in the orbit can produce the clinical picture of orbital cellulitis. The most common cause of orbital cellulitis in children is paranasal sinusitis. Frequent pathogenic organisms include nontypable *Haemophilus influenzae*, *Staphylococcus aureus*, group A β-hemolytic streptococci, *Streptococcus pneumoniae*, and anaerobic bacteria.

The orbital inflammatory *clinical manifestations* of paranasal sinusitis vary with the location and extent of involvement. Stage 1 is swelling of the lids—the edema of impaired venous drainage or the reactive inflammation of underlying periostitis; in this stage, the infection is still confined to the sinus. The 2nd stage is subperiosteal abscess, a collection of pus between the periosteum and the wall of the orbit, often with localized tenderness, displacement of the globe, and some limitation of eye movement. The 3rd stage is true orbital cellulitis, diffuse inflammation of the tissues within the orbit, with proptosis and impairment of ocular motility. The 4th stage is orbital abscess, resulting from localization of infection in the orbit or from extension of a subperiosteal abscess through the periosteum.

The potential for complications is great. Involvement of the optic nerve may result in loss of vision. Extension of infection from the orbit into the cranial cavity may lead to cavernous sinus thrombosis or meningitis or to epidural, subdural, or brain abscesses.

Orbital cellulitis must be recognized promptly and treated aggressively (see Chapter 178). Hospitalization and systemic antibiotic therapy are usually indicated. In some cases, surgical intervention is necessary to drain infected sinuses or a subperiosteal or orbital abscess.

Periorbital Cellulitis. Inflammation of the lids and periorbital tissues without signs of true orbital involvement (such as proptosis or limitation of eye movement) is generally referred to as periorbital or preseptal cellulitis. This is common in young children and may be caused by trauma, by an infected wound, or by abscess of the lid or periorbital region (e.g., pyoderma, hordeolum, conjunctivitis, dacryocystitis, or insect bite). It may be associated with respiratory infection or more often bacteremia, often with *H. influenzae* type b, streptococci, or pneumococci. What initially appears to be periorbital or preseptal cellulitis may be the first sign of sinusitis that may occasionally progress to true orbital cellulitis. Prompt antibiotic therapy and careful monitoring for signs of sepsis and local progression are essential. See Chapter 365.

Orbital Inflammation. Inflammatory disease involving the orbit may be primary or secondary to systemic disease. Idiopathic orbital inflammation (orbital pseudotumor) represents a wide spectrum of clinical entities. Symptoms at the time of presentation may include pain, eyelid swelling, proptosis, and fever. The inflammation may involve a single extraocular muscle (myositis) or the entire orbit. Confusion with orbital cellulitis is common but can be differentiated by the lack of associated sinus disease, its appearance on CT scan, and lack of improvement with systemic antibiotics. Treatment includes the use of high-dose systemic corticosteroids. Immunotherapy or radiation treatment may be necessary for resistant or recurrent cases.

Thyroid-related ophthalmopathy (TRO) is believed to be secondary to an immune mechanism, leading to inflammation and deposition of mucopolysaccharides and collagen in the extraocular muscles and orbital fat. Involvement of the extraocular muscles may lead to a restrictive strabismus. Lid retraction and exophthalmos may cause corneal exposure and infection or perforation. Involvement of the posterior orbit can compress the optic nerve. Treatment of TRO may include the use of systemic corticosteroids, radiation of the orbit, eyelid surgery, strabismus surgery, or orbital decompression to eliminate symptoms and protect vision. The degree of orbital involvement is often independent of the status of the systemic disease. Also see Chapter 562.

Other systemic disorders that may cause inflammatory disease within the orbit include lymphoma, sarcoidosis, amyloidosis, polyarteritis nodosa, systemic lupus erythematosus, dermatomyositis, Wegener granulomatosis, and juvenile xanthogranuloma.

Tumors of the Orbit. Various tumors occur in and about the orbit in childhood. Among benign tumors, the most common are vascular lesions (principally hemangiomas) and dermoids. Among malignant neoplasms, rhabdomyosarcoma, lymphosarcoma, and metastatic neuroblastoma are the most frequent. Optic gliomas and retinoblastomas that extend into the orbit also occur.

The effects of orbital tumors vary with their locations and growth patterns. The principal signs are proptosis, resistance to retroplacement of the eye, and impairment of eye movement. A palpable mass may be found. Other significant signs are ptosis, optic nerve head congestion, optic atrophy, and loss of vision. Bruit and visible pulsation of the globe are important clues to vascular lesions.

Evaluation of orbital tumors includes ultrasonography, MRI, and CT. Pseudotumor of the orbit also must be considered in children with signs of a mass lesion.

Barone SR, Aiuto LT: Periorbital and orbital cellulitis in the *Haemophilus influenzae* vaccine era. *J Pediatr Ophthalmol Strabismus* 1997;34:293.

Haik BG, Jakobiec FA, Ellsworth RM, et al: Capillary hemangioma of the lids and orbit: An analysis of the clinical features and therapeutic results in 101 cases. *Ophthalmology* 1979;86:760.

Hawkins DB, Clark RW: Orbital involvement in acute sinusitis: Lessons from 24 childhood patients. *Clin Pediatr* 1977;16:464.

Mottow LS, Jakobiec FA: Idiopathic inflammatory orbital pseudotumor in childhood. *Arch Ophthalmol* 1978;96:1410.

Shields JA, Bakewell B, Augsberger JJ, et al: Space-occupying orbital masses in children: A review of 250 consecutive biopsies. *Ophthalmology* 1988;93:379.

Utresky SH, Kennerdell JS, Gupta JP: Graves' ophthalmopathy in childhood and adolescence. *Arch Ophthalmol* 1980;98:1963.

Weiss A, Friendly D, Eglin K, et al: Bacterial periorbital cellulitis in childhood. *Ophthalmology* 1983;90:195.

Chapter 625
Injuries to the Eye

About one third of all blindness in children results from trauma. Children and adolescents account for a disproportionate number of episodes of ocular trauma. Boys ages 11–15 yr are the most vulnerable; their injuries outnumber those in girls by a ratio of about 4:1. The majority of injuries are related to sports, toy darts, other projectiles, sticks, stones, fireworks, and air-powered BB guns. The last causes particularly devastating ocular and orbital injuries. Much of the trauma is avoidable. See Chapter 50.

Ecchymoses and Swelling of the Eyelids. These are common after blunt trauma. Hemorrhage into the lids and periorbital region ("black eye" or "shiner") is usually of no consequence and absorbs spontaneously, but it should prompt careful examination of the eye for deeper, more serious injury, such as a blowout fracture of the orbit, an intraocular hemorrhage, or rupture of the globe.

Lacerations of the Eyelids. These require careful management. Horizontal laceration of the upper lid may involve the levator, the tarsal plate, or the orbital septum. Faulty repair can result in ptosis, distortion of the lid, or herniation of orbital fat. Lacerations involving the lid margins require meticulous surgical apposition to prevent notching, eversion, or inversion of the margin or misdirection of the lashes that might lead to epiphora (tear overflow), wetting defects of the cornea, and chronic irritation. Lacerations situated near the medial canthus may involve the punctum, canaliculi, or nasolacrimal duct and require microsurgical repair by an experienced ophthalmic surgeon. In all cases of lid laceration, examination of the globe for perforating injury is mandatory.

Superficial Abrasions of the Cornea. When the corneal epithelium is scratched, abraded, or denuded, it exposes the underlying epithelial basement layer and superficial corneal nerves. This is accompanied by pain, tearing, photophobia, and decreased vision. Corneal abrasions are detected by instilling fluorescein dye and inspecting the cornea using a blue-filtered light. A slit lamp is ideal for this examination, but a hand-held Wood's lamp is adequate for young children.

Treatment of a corneal abrasion is directed at promoting healing and relieving pain. Abrasions are treated with frequent applications of a topical antibiotic ointment until the epithelium is completely healed. The use of a semi-pressure patch does not improve healing time or decrease pain. Furthermore, an improperly applied patch may itself abrade the cornea. A topical cycloplegic agent (cyclopentolate hydrochloride 1%) can relieve the pain from ciliary spasm in patients with large abrasions. Topical anesthetics should not be given at home because they retard epithelial healing and inhibit the natural blinking reflex.

Foreign Body on or in the Cornea or Conjunctiva. This usually produces acute discomfort, lacrimation, and inflammation. Most foreign bodies can be detected by examination in good light with the aid of magnification; a direct ophthalmoscope set on a high plus lens (+10 or +12) is helpful. In many cases, slit-lamp examination is necessary, especially if the particle is deep or metallic. Some conjunctival foreign bodies tend to lodge under the upper eyelid, causing the sensation of corneal foreign body as they come into contact with the globe on eyelid movement; they may also produce vertically oriented linear corneal abrasions. Finding these abrasions should lead to a suspicion of such a foreign body, and eversion of the lid may be necessary (Chapter 610). If a foreign body is suspected but not found, further examination is indicated. If the history suggests injury with a high-velocity particle, roentgenographic examination of the eye may be needed to explore the possibility of intraocular foreign body.

Removal of a foreign body can be facilitated by instillation of a drop of topical anesthetic. Many foreign bodies can be removed by irrigating or by gently wiping them away with a moistened cotton-tipped applicator. Embedded foreign bodies should be treated by an ophthalmologist. Removal of corneal foreign bodies may leave epithelial defects, which are treated as corneal abrasions. Metallic foreign bodies may cause rust to form in the corneal tissues; examination by an ophthalmologist a day or two after removal of a foreign body is recommended, because a rust ring would require further treatment (curettage).

Lacerations and Perforating Wounds of the Cornea or Sclera. These require immediate referral to an ophthalmologist and prompt surgical repair if the eye and vision are to be saved. Important clues to perforating injury of the eye are collapse of the anterior chamber, distortion and displacement of the pupil, and protrusion of dark tissue (uvea) into the wound. Emergency treatment consists of protecting the injured eye from further damage by applying a sterile bandage and a rigid eye shield. If these medical supplies are not on hand, an adequate eye shield can be fashioned from a plastic or Styrofoam cup or from a piece of cardboard bent into a box or cone shape. Manipulation should be kept to a minimum, and no medication should be instilled except under the direction of an ophthalmologist.

Hyphema. This is the presence of blood in the anterior chamber of the eye. It may occur with either a blunt or perforating injury. Hyphema appears as a bright or dark red fluid level between the cornea and iris or as a diffuse murkiness of the aqueous humor. Children with hyphema have pain and may be somnolent. The treatment of hyphema usually includes bed rest, with the head elevated 30–45 degrees to promote settling and resorption of the blood. Hospitalization and sedation may be necessary to ensure compliance in some children. In most cases, topical mydriatics, topical or oral corticosteroids, or oral aminocaproic acid are used to prevent rebleeding. Secondary bleeding typically occurs 3–5 days after the initial hemorrhage, increasing the risk of sequelae. The blood in the anterior chamber may produce elevation of intraocular pressure and blood staining of the cornea. These complications may affect vision. In such cases, surgical evacuation of the clot and irrigation of the anterior chamber may be necessary. Patients with sickle cell disease or trait are at higher risk for acute loss of vision and rebleeding and may require more aggressive intervention. Individuals with a history of traumatic hyphema have an increased incidence of glaucoma later in life.

Chemical Injuries. Chemical burns of the cornea and adnexal tissue are among the most urgent of ocular emergencies. Alkali burns are usually more destructive than acid burns because they react with fats to form soaps, which damage cell membranes, allowing further penetration of the alkali into the eye. Acids generally cause less severe, more localized tissue damage. The corneal epithelium offers moderate protection against weak acids, and little damage occurs unless the pH is 2.5 or less. Most stronger acids precipitate tissue proteins, creating a physical barrier against their further penetration.

Mild acid or alkali burns are characterized by conjunctival injection and swelling and mild corneal epithelial erosions. The corneal stroma may be mildly edematous, and the anterior chamber may have mild to moderate cell and flare reactions. With strong acids, the cornea and conjunctiva rapidly become white and opaque. The corneal epithelium may slough, leaving a relatively clear stroma; this appearance may initially mask the severity of the burn. Severe alkali burns are characterized by corneal opacification.

Emergency treatment of a chemical burn begins with copious immediate irrigation with water or saline. Local debridement and removal of foreign particles should be performed while still irrigating. If the nature of the chemical injury is unknown, the use of pH test paper is helpful in determining whether the agent was basic or acidic. Irrigation should continue for at least 30 min or until 2 L of irrigant has been instilled in mild cases and for 2–4 hr or until 10 L of irrigant has been instilled in severe cases. At the end of irrigation, the pH should be within a normal range (7.3–7.7). The pH should be checked again approximately 30 min after irrigation to ensure that it has not changed.

Fractures. A *direct orbital floor fracture* is a floor fracture associated with an orbital rim fracture. An *indirect orbital floor fracture* is an isolated floor fracture and is more commonly known as a blowout fracture. Floor fractures are common when objects larger than the orbital opening, such as a ball, fist, or the dashboard of an automobile, strike the orbit, particularly the inferior lateral orbit.

The most obvious clinical sign of an orbital floor fracture is limitation of upward gaze. Additional signs include lower eyelid ecchymosis, nosebleed, orbital emphysema, and hypesthesia of the ipsilateral cheek and upper lip. The last results from disruption of the infraorbital nerve as it traverses the orbital floor.

The best imaging techniques to visualize orbital fractures are plain-film radiography and CT. The Waters' view best demonstrates the orbital floor and maxillary sinus.

Treatment for children with acute orbital fractures includes antibiotic prophylaxis, nasal decongestants, and ice packs. If entrapment of the extraocular muscles (resulting in restriction of movement of the eye and diplopia) and herniation of orbital fat or of the eye itself (resulting in enophthalmos) occur, then surgical repair may be necessary.

Penetrating Wounds of the Orbit. These demand careful evaluation for possible damage to the eye, the optic nerve, or the brain. Examination should include investigation for retained foreign body. Orbital hemorrhage and infection are common with penetrating wounds of the orbit; such injuries must be treated as emergencies.

Child Abuse. This is a major cause of injuries to the eye and orbital region. The manifestations are numerous and may have a prominent role in recognition of this syndrome. The possibility of nonaccidental trauma must be considered in any child with ecchymosis or laceration of the lids, hemorrhage in or about the eye, cataract or dislocated lens, retinal detachment, or fracture of the orbit (Fig. 625–1). Also see Chapter 35.

Fireworks-Related Injuries. Injuries related to the use of fireworks can be the most devastating of all ocular trauma that occurs in children. At least one fifth of emergency room visits for fireworks-related injuries are for ocular trauma. In the United States, a majority of these injuries take place around Independence Day, and most occur despite adult supervision.

Sports-Related Ocular Injuries and Their Prevention. Although sports injuries occur in all age groups, far more children and adolescents participate in high-risk sports than do adults. The greater number of participating children, their athletic immaturity, and the increased likelihood of their using inadequate or improper eye protection account for their disproportionate share of sports-related eye injuries. See Chapters 677 and 681.

The sports with the highest risk of eye injury are those in which no eye protection can be worn, including boxing, wrestling, and martial arts. High-risk sports include those that use a rapidly moving ball or puck, bat, stick, racquet, or arrow (baseball, hockey, lacrosse, racquet sports, and archery) or involve aggressive body contact (football and basketball). Related to both risk and frequency of participation, the highest percentage of eye injuries are in basketball and baseball.

Protective eyewear, designed for a specific activity, is available for most sports. For basketball, racquet sports, and other recreational activities that do not require a helmet or face mask, molded polycarbonate sports goggles that are secured to the head by an elastic strap are suggested. For hockey, football, lacrosse, and baseball (batter), specific helmets with polycarbonate face shields and guards are available. Children should also wear sports goggles under the helmets. For baseball, goggles and helmets should be worn for batting, catching, and base running; goggles alone are usually sufficient for other positions.

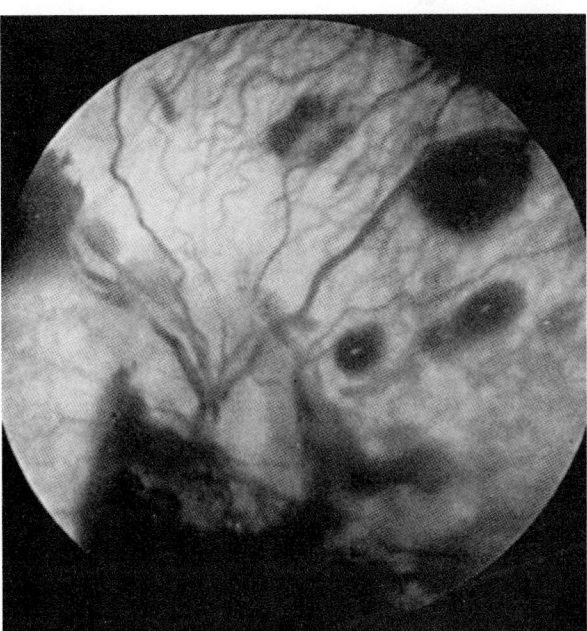

FIGURE 625–1. Retinal hemorrhages in an abused child with subdural hematoma.

American Academy of Pediatrics Committee on Sports Medicine and Fitness, American Academy of Ophthalmology Committee on Eye Safety and Sports Ophthalmology: Protective eyewear for young athletes. *Pediatrics* 1996;98 :311.

Catalono RA: Eye injuries and prevention. *Pediatr Clin North Am* 1993;40: 827.

Deutsch TA, Weinreb RN, Goldberg MF: Indications for surgical management of hyphema in patients with sickle cell trait. *Arch Ophthalmol* 1984;102:566.

Hofman RF, Paul TO, Pentelei-Molner J: The management of corneal birth trauma. *J Pediatr Ophthalmol Strabismus* 1981;18:45.

Kaiser PK: A comparison of pressure patching versus no patching for corneal abrasions due to trauma or foreign body removal. Corneal Abrasion Patching Study Group. *Ophthalmology* 1995;102:1936.

Lavrich JB, Goldberg DS, Nelson LB, et al: Visual outcome of severe eye injuries during the amblyopiagenic years. *Binocular Vision* 1994;9:39.

Levin AV: Ocular manifestations of child abuse. *Ophthalmol Clin North Am* 1990;3:249.

Nelson LB, Wilson TW, Jeffers JB: Eye injuries in childhood: Demography, etiology and prevention. *Pediatrics* 1989;84:438.

Pfister RR: Chemical injuries of the eye. *Ophthalmology* 1983;90:1246.

Serious eye injuries associated with fireworks—United States, 1990–1994. *MMWR Morbid Mortal Wkly Rep* 1995;44:449.

Smith GA, Knapp JF, Barnett TM, et al: The rocket's red glare, the bombs bursting in air: Fireworks-related injuries to children. *Pediatrics* 1996;98:1.

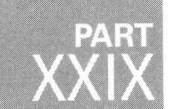

Chapter 626
Clinical Manifestations

Joseph Haddad Jr.

Eight prominent signs and symptoms are associated primarily with diseases of the ear and temporal bone. They are as follows:

Otalgia. This is usually associated with inflammation of the external or middle ear, but it may represent pain referred from involvement of the teeth, temporomandibular joint, or pharynx. In young infants, pulling or rubbing the ear with general irritability or poor sleep, especially when associated with fever, may be the only sign of ear pain. Ear pulling alone is not diagnostic of ear pathology.

Purulent Otorrhea. This is a sign of otitis externa, otitis media with perforation of the tympanic membrane (TM), and/or drainage from the middle ear through a patent tympanostomy tube. Bloody discharge may be associated with acute or chronic inflammation (often with granulation tissue), trauma, neoplasm, foreign body, or blood dyscrasia. Clear drainage suggests a perforation of the TM with a serous middle-ear effusion or, rarely, a cerebrospinal fluid leak draining through defects (congenital or traumatic) in the external auditory canal or from the middle ear.

Hearing Loss. This results from disease of either the external or middle ear (conductive hearing loss) or from pathology in the inner ear, retrocochlear structures, or central auditory pathways (sensorineural hearing loss). The most common cause of hearing loss in children is otitis media (OM).

Swelling. Swelling around the ear is most commonly a result of inflammation (external otitis, perichondritis, mastoiditis), trauma (hematoma), benign cystic masses, or neoplasm.

Vertigo. This is an uncommon complaint in children; the child or parent may not volunteer information about balance unless asked directly. *Vertigo*, a specific type of dizziness, is defined as any hallucination, illusion, or sensation of motion; *dizziness* refers to an altered orientation in space and is less specific than vertigo. The most frequent cause of dizziness in young children is eustachian tube–middle-ear disease, but true vertigo may also be caused by labyrinthitis, perilymphatic fistula between the inner and middle ear due to trauma or a congenital inner ear defect, cholesteatoma in the mastoid or middle ear, vestibular neuronitis, benign paroxysmal vertigo, Meniere disease, or disease of the central nervous system. Older children may describe a feeling of room-spinning or turning; younger children may express the dysequilibrium only by falling, stumbling, or clumsiness.

Nystagmus. Unidirectional, horizontal, or jerk nystagmus, usually associated with vertigo, is vestibular in origin.

Tinnitus. Although infrequently described spontaneously by children, tinnitus is common, especially in patients with eustachian tube–middle-ear disease or with sensorineural hearing loss (SNHL). Children may describe tinnitus if asked directly about it, including laterality and the quality of the sound.

Facial Paralysis. The facial nerve may be dehiscent in its course through the middle ear in up to 50% of patients; infection with local inflammation (most commonly in acute OM) may lead to a temporary paralysis of the facial nerve. It may also be due to cholesteatoma, Bell palsy, the Ramsay Hunt syndrome (herpes zoster oticus), Lyme disease, fracture, neoplasm, or infection of the temporal bone. Congenital facial paralysis may be due to birth trauma or congenital abnormality of the 7th nerve or may be associated with other cranial nerve abnormalities and craniofacial anomalies.

Physical Examination. Complete examination with special attention to the head and neck may reveal a condition that may predispose to or be associated with ear disease in children. The facial appearance and the character of speech may give clues to an abnormality of the ear or hearing. Many craniofacial anomalies, such as cleft palate, mandibulofacial dysostosis (Treacher Collins syndrome), and trisomy 21 (Down syndrome), are associated with disorders of the ear and eustachian tube. Mouth breathing and hyponasality may indicate intranasal or postnasal obstruction; hypernasality is a sign of velopharyngeal insufficiency. Examining the oropharyngeal cavity may uncover an overt cleft palate or a submucous cleft (usually associated with a bifid uvula), both of which predispose to OM with effusion. A nasopharyngeal tumor with nasal and eustachian tube blockage may be associated with OM.

The *position* of the patient for examination of the ear, nose, and throat depends on the patient's age, ability to cooperate, clinical setting, and examiner preference. The child can be examined on an examination table or in the parent's lap. The presence of a parent or assistant is usually necessary to minimize movement and improve the examination (Fig. 626–1) An examining table may be desirable for uncooperative older infants or when a procedure, such as microscopic evaluation or tympanocentesis, is performed. Lap examination is adequate and preferable in most infants and young children; the parent

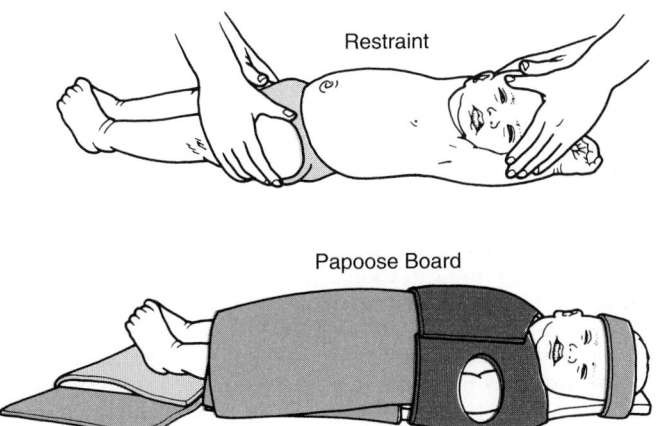

FIGURE 626–1. Methods of restraining an infant for examination and for procedures such as tympanocentesis or myringotomy. (From Bluestone CD, Klein JO: *Otitis Media in Infants and Children*, 2nd ed. Philadelphia, WB Saunders, 1995, p 91.)

may assist in restraining the child by folding the child's wrists and arms over the child's own abdomen with one hand and holding the child's head against the parent's chest with the other hand. If necessary, the child's legs can be held between the parent's knees. To avoid ear trauma with movement, the examiner should hold the otoscope with the hand placed firmly against the child's head or face, so that the otoscope moves with the head. Pulling up and out on the pinna straightens the ear canal and allows better exposure of the TM.

When *examining the ear,* inspection of the auricle and external auditory meatus for infection may aid in the evaluation of complications of OM. For instance, external otitis may result from acute OM with discharge, or inflammation of the posterior auricular area may indicate a periosteitis or subperiosteal abscess extending from the mastoid air cells. The presence of preauricular pits or skin tags should also be noted, because affected children have a slightly higher incidence of SNHL.

The presence of wax in the ear canal may interfere with examination. **Removal of cerumen** is usually done with the surgical head of the otoscope, which allows passage of a wire loop or a blunt curette under direct visualization. Other methods include gentle irrigation of the ear canal with warm water (irrigate only when the TM is intact) or instillation of a solution such as diluted hydrogen peroxide in the ear canal for a few minutes to soften the wax for suction removal or irrigation. Some commercial preparations (trolamine polypeptide oleate-condensate [Cerumenex]) may cause dermatitis of the external canal with chronic use and should be used only under a physician's supervision.

Inflammation of the ear canal with associated pain often indicates external otitis. Abnormalities of the external auditory canal include stenosis (common in children with trisomy 21), bony exostoses, otorrhea, and the presence of foreign bodies. Cholesteatoma of the middle ear may manifest in the canal as intermittent foul-smelling drainage, sometimes associated with white debris; cholesteatoma of the external canal may appear as a white pearl-like mass in the canal skin. White or gray debris of the canal suggests fungal external otitis. Newborn ear canals are filled with vernix caseosa, which is soft and pale yellow and should disappear shortly after birth.

The TM and its mobility are best assessed with a pneumatic otoscope. The normal TM is in a neutral position; a bulging TM may be caused by increased middle-ear air pressure, with or without pus or effusion in the middle ear; visualization of the malleus and annulus may be obscured by a bulging drum. Retraction of the TM usually indicates negative middle-ear pressure, but it may also result from previous middle-ear disease with fixation of the ossicles, ossicular ligaments, or TM. When retraction is present, the bony malleus appears more prominent and the incus may be more visible posterior to the malleus.

The normal TM has a silvery-gray waxed paper appearance; a white or yellow TM may indicate a middle-ear effusion. A red TM alone may not indicate pathology, because the blood vessels of the membrane may be engorged as a result of crying, sneezing, or nose-blowing. A normal TM is translucent, allowing the observer to visualize the middle-ear landmarks—incus, promontory, round window niche, and frequently the chorda tympani nerve. If a middle-ear effusion is present, an air-fluid level or bubbles may be visible. Inability to visualize the middle-ear structures indicates opacification of the drum, usually caused by thickening of the TM, a middle-ear effusion, or both. Assessment of the light reflex is generally not helpful, as a middle ear with effusion reflects light as well as a normal ear.

TM mobility is helpful in assessing middle ear pressures and the presence or absence of fluid. To best perform pneumatic otoscopy, a speculum of adequate size is used to obtain a good seal and allow air movement in the canal. A rubber ring around the tip of the speculum may help to obtain a better canal seal. Normal middle-ear pressure is characterized by a neutral TM position and brisk TM movement to both positive and negative pressures.

Eardrum retraction is most common when negative middle-ear pressure is present; with even moderate negative middle-ear pressure there is no visible inward movement with applied positive pressure in the ear canal. However, negative canal pressure, which is produced by releasing the rubber bulb of the pneumatic otoscope, may cause the TM to bounce out toward the neutral position. A retracted TM may occur in both the presence and absence of middle-ear fluid, and if the middle-ear fluid is mixed with air, the TM may still have some mobility. Outward eardrum movement is less likely in the presence of severe negative middle-ear pressure or middle-ear effusion.

The TM that exhibits fullness (bulging) moves to applied positive pressure but not to applied negative pressure if the pressure within the middle ear is positive and some air is present. A full TM and positive middle-ear pressure without an effusion may be seen in young infants who are crying during the otoscopic examination, in older infants and children with nasal obstruction, and in the early stage of acute OM. When the middle-ear–mastoid air cell system is filled with an effusion and little or no air is present, the mobility of the TM is severely decreased or absent in response to both applied positive and negative pressures.

Aspiration of the middle ear is the definitive method of verifying the presence and type of a middle-ear effusion. Diagnostic tympanocentesis is performed by inserting, through the inferior portion of the TM, an 18-gauge spinal needle attached to a syringe or a collection trap (Fig. 626–2). Culturing of the ear canal and alcohol cleansing should precede tympanocentesis and culture of the middle-ear aspirate; a canal culture is taken to help determine whether organisms cultured from the middle ear are contaminants from the external canal or true pathogens.

Further diagnostic studies of the ear and hearing include audiometric evaluation, impedance audiometry (tympanometry), acoustic reflectometry, and specialized eustachian tube function studies. Diagnostic imaging studies, including computed tomography and magnetic resonance imaging, often provide further information about anatomic abnormalities and the extent of inflammatory processes or neoplasms. Specialized assessment of labyrinthine function should be considered in the evaluation of a child with a suspected vestibular disorder (Chapter 631).

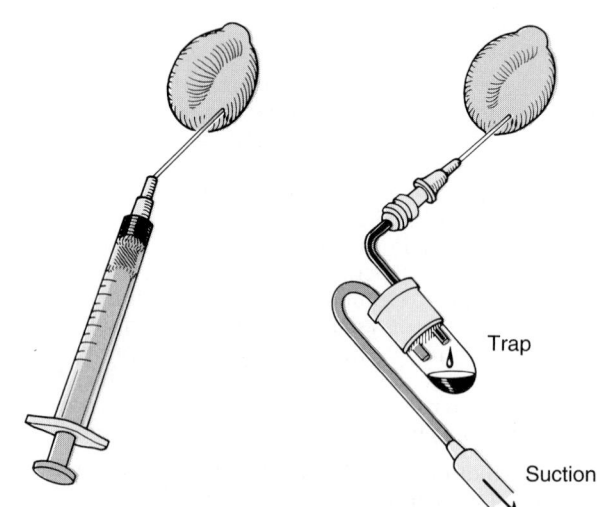

FIGURE 626–2. Tympanocentesis can be performed with a needle attached to a tuberculin syringe *(left)* or by using an Alden-Senturia collection trap (Storz Instrument Co, St. Louis). (From Bluestone CD, Klein JO: *Otitis Media in Infants and Children,* 2nd ed. Philadelphia, WB Saunders, 1995, p 127.)

Chapter 627
Hearing Loss *Joseph Haddad Jr.*

Incidence and Prevalence. Although estimates vary because of differences in criteria for defining hearing impairment, the age group surveyed, and the testing methods used, from 1–2 newborns/1,000 live births have moderate (30–50 dB), severe (50–70 dB), or profound (70 dB or greater) bilateral sensorineural hearing loss (SNHL), including 0.5–1/1,000 with bilateral SNHL exceeding 75 dB. An additional 1–2/1,000 may have milder or unilateral impairments; by age 19 yr, the prevalence doubles. Unilateral SNHL of 45 dB or greater occurs in 3/1,000 U.S. school children; hearing loss of 26 dB or greater occurs in 13/1,000. Onset of hearing loss can occur at any time in childhood. When considering less severe hearing loss, or the transient conductive hearing loss (CHL) that commonly accompanies middle-ear disease in young children, the number of affected children increases substantially.

Types of Hearing Loss. Hearing loss can be peripheral or central in origin. Peripheral hearing loss is commonly caused by dysfunction in the transmission of sound through the external or middle ear or by abnormal transduction of sound energy into neural activity in the inner ear and the 8th nerve. Peripheral hearing loss can be conductive, sensorineural, or mixed. *CHL* is the most common type in children and occurs when sound transmission is physically impeded in the external and/or middle ear. Common causes of CHL in the ear canal include atresia or stenosis, impacted cerumen, or foreign bodies; in the middle ear, perforation of the tympanic membrane (TM), discontinuity or fixation of the ossicular chain, otitis media (OM) with effusion, otosclerosis, and cholesteatoma can cause CHL. Damage to or maldevelopment of structures in the inner ear can cause *SNHL*; these include hair cell destruction from noise, disease, or ototoxic agents; cochlear malformation; perilymphatic fistula of the round or oval window membrane; and lesions of the acoustic division of the 8th nerve. A combined CHL and SNHL is considered a *mixed hearing loss.*

Auditory deficits originating along the central auditory nervous system pathways from the proximal 8th nerve to the cerebral cortex are generally considered central (or retrocochlear) hearing losses. Tumors or demyelinating disease of the 8th nerve and cerebellopontine angle can cause hearing deficits but spare the outer, middle, and inner ear. These causes of hearing loss are rare in children. Other forms of central auditory deficits, known as *central auditory processing disorders*, include those that make it difficult even for children with normal hearing to listen selectively in the presence of noise, to combine information from the two ears properly, to process speech when it is slightly degraded, and to integrate auditory information that is delivered faster than at a slow rate. These deficits may manifest as poor attention, or academic or behavior problems in school. Strategies for coping with such disorders are available in older children, and identification and documentation of the central auditory processing disorder is often valuable because parents and teachers are made aware of a valid reason for the child's poor attention or behavior and adjustments can be made.

Etiology. The etiology of a hearing impairment depends on whether the hearing loss is conductive or sensorineural. Most CHL is acquired, with middle ear fluid the most common cause. Congenital causes include anomalies of the pinna, external ear canal, TM, and ossicles. Rarely, congenital cholesteatoma or other masses in the middle ear may present as CHL. TM perforation (trauma, OM), ossicular discontinuity (infection, cholesteatoma, trauma), tympanosclerosis, acquired cholesteatoma, or masses in the ear canal or middle ear (Langerhans' cell histiocytosis, salivary gland tumors, glomus tumors, rhabdomyosarcoma) may also present as CHL. Uncommon diseases affecting the middle ear and temporal bone that may present with CHL include otosclerosis, osteopetrosis, fibrous dysplasia, and osteogenesis imperfecta.

SNHL may be congenital or acquired. Causes of SNHL include genetic, infectious, autoimmune, anatomic, traumatic, ototoxic, and idiopathic factors. The most common *infectious* cause of congenital SNHL is cytomegalovirus (CMV), which infects 1/100 newborns in the United States. Of these, 6,000–8,000 infants per year will have clinical manifestations, including approximately 75% with SNHL. Congenital CMV warrants special attention because it is associated with hearing loss in its symptomatic and asymptomatic forms; the hearing loss may be progressive. Some children with congenital CMV have suddenly lost residual hearing at age 4–5 yr. Other less common congenital infectious causes of SNHL include toxoplasmosis and syphilis. Congenital CMV, toxoplasmosis, and syphilis may also present with delayed onset of SNHL, months to years after birth. Rubella, once the most common viral cause of congenital SNHL, is now very uncommon because of effective vaccination programs. Prenatal infection with herpes is rare, and hearing loss as the only manifestation is very unusual.

Other postnatal infectious causes of SNHL include Group B streptococcal sepsis in newborns and bacterial meningitis. *Streptococcus pneumoniae* is the most common cause of bacterial meningitis that results in SNHL after the neonatal period; this cause may become less frequent with the routine administration of pneumococcal conjugate vaccine. *Haemophilus influenzae*, once the most common cause of meningitis resulting in SNHL, is now rare owing to the Hib vaccine. Uncommon infectious causes of SNHL include Lyme disease, parvovirus B19, and varicella. Mumps, rubella, and rubeola, all once common causes of SNHL in children, are rare owing to vaccination programs.

Genetic causes of SNHL are probably responsible for as many as 50% of SNHL cases. These disorders may be associated with other abnormalities, may be part of a named syndrome, or may exist in isolation. SNHL often occurs with abnormalities of the ear and eye and with disorders of the metabolic, musculoskeletal, integumentary, renal, and nervous systems. Autosomal dominant hearing losses account for about 10% of all cases of childhood SNHL. Waardenburg (types I and II) and branchiootorenal syndromes represent two of the most common autosomal dominant syndromic types of SNHL. Autosomal recessive genetic SNHL, both syndromic and nonsyndromic, accounts for about 80% of all childhood cases of SNHL. Usher syndrome (types I, II, and III), Pendred syndrome, and the Jervell and Lange-Nielsen syndromes (a form of the long Q-T syndrome) are three of the most common syndromic recessive types of SNHL. Whereas children with an easily identified syndrome or with anomalies of the outer ear may be identified as being at risk for hearing loss and monitored adequately, nonsyndromic children present greater difficulty. Mutations of the connexin-26 and -30 genes have been identified in autosomal recessive and autosomal dominant and in sporadic nonsyndromic patients with SNHL. Sex-linked disorders associated with SNHL, thought to account for 1–2% of SNHL, include Norrie disease, the otopalatal digital syndrome, and Alport syndrome. Chromosomal abnormalities such as 13–15-trisomy, 18-trisomy, and 21-trisomy can also be accompanied by hearing impairment. Patients with Turner syndrome have monosomy for all or part of one X chromosome and may have CHL, SNHL, or mixed hearing loss. The hearing loss may be progressive. Mitochondrial genetic abnormalities may also result in SNHL.

Agenesis or malformation of cochlear structures, including the Scheibe, Mondini, Alexander, and Michel anomalies, and enlarged vestibular aqueducts and semicircular canal anomalies may be genetic. These anomalies probably occur before the 8th wk of gestation and result from arrest in normal development, aberrant development, or both. Many of these anomalies have also been described in association with other congenital conditions such as intrauterine infections (CMV, rubella). These abnormalities are quite common; in as many as 20% of children with SNHL, obvious or subtle temporal bone abnormalities are seen on high-resolution computed tomography scanning or magnetic resonance imaging.

CHL can also be genetic. Conditions, diseases, or syndromes that include craniofacial abnormalities are often associated with conductive hearing loss and possibly with SNHL. Pierre Robin, Treacher Collins, Klippel-Feil, Crouzon, and branchio-otorenal syndromes and osteogenesis imperfecta are often associated with hearing loss. Congenital anomalies causing CHL include malformations of the ossicles and middle-ear structures and atresia of the external auditory canal.

Many genetically determined causes of hearing impairment, including both syndromic and nonsyndromic, do not express themselves until some time after birth. Alport, Alström, and Down syndromes, von Recklinghausen disease, and Hunter-Hurler syndrome are genetic diseases that may have SNHL as a late manifestation.

SNHL may also occur secondary to exposure to *toxins, chemicals, and antimicrobials.* Early in pregnancy, the embryo is particularly vulnerable to the effects of toxic substances. Ototoxic drugs, including aminoglycosides, loop diuretics, and chemotherapeutic agents (cisplatin) may also cause SNHL. Congenital SNHL may occur secondary to exposure to these drugs as well as to thalidomide and retinoids. Certain chemicals, such as quinine, lead, and arsenic, may cause hearing loss both prenatally and postnatally.

Trauma, including temporal bone fractures, inner ear concussion, head trauma, iatrogenic trauma (surgery, extracorporeal membrane oxygenation [ECMO]), radiation, and noise may also cause SNHL. Other uncommon causes of SNHL in children include immune disease (systemic or limited to the inner ear), metabolic abnormalities, and neoplasms of the temporal bone.

Box 627–1 lists some factors that place a newborn at risk for hearing impairment. These factors account for about 50% of cases of moderate to profound SNHL in neonates.

Effects of Hearing Impairment. These depend on the nature and degree of the hearing loss and on the individual characteristics of the child. Hearing loss may be unilateral or bilateral, conductive, sensorineural, or mixed; mild, moderate, severe, or profound; of sudden or gradual onset; stable, progressive, or fluctuating; and affecting a part, or all, of the audible spectrum. Other factors such as intelligence, medical or physical condition (including accompanying syndromes), family support, age at onset, age at time of identification, and promptness of intervention also affect the impact of hearing loss on a child.

Most hearing-impaired children have some usable hearing. Only 6% of those in the hearing-impaired population have bilateral profound hearing loss. Hearing loss very early in life can affect the development of speech and language, social and emotional development, behavior, attention, and academic achievement. Some cases of hearing impairment are misdiagnosed because affected children have sufficient hearing to respond to environmental sounds and can learn some speech and language but when challenged in the classroom cannot perform to full potential.

Even mild or unilateral hearing loss may have a detrimental effect on the development of a young child and on school performance. Children with such hearing impairments have greater difficulty when listening conditions are unfavorable (background noise and poor acoustics), as may occur in a classroom. The fact that schools are auditory-verbal environments is unappreciated by those who minimize the impact of hearing impairment on learning. Hearing loss should be considered in any child with speech and language difficulties or below-par performance, poor behavior, or inattention in school (Table 627–1).

BOX 627–1. Indicators Associated With Sensorineural and/or Conductive Hearing Loss

For use with neonates (birth through age 28 days) when universal screening is not available
Family history of hereditary childhood sensorineural hearing loss
In utero infection, such as cytomegalovirus, rubella, syphilis, herpes simplex, or toxoplasmosis
Craniofacial anomalies, including those with morphologic abnormalities of the pinna and ear canal
Birth weight less than 1500 g (3.3 lb)
Hyperbilirubinemia at a serum level requiring exchange transfusion
Ototoxic medications, including but not limited to the aminoglycosides, used in multiple courses or in combination with loop diuretics
Bacterial meningitis
Apgar scores of 0 to 4 at 1 min or 0 to 6 at 5 min
Mechanical ventilation lasting 5 days or longer
Stigmata or other findings associated with a syndrome known to include a sensorineural and/or conductive hearing loss
For use with infants (age 29 days through 2 yr) when certain health conditions develop that require rescreening
Parent/caregiver concern regarding hearing, speech, language, and/or developmental delay
Bacterial meningitis and other infections associated with sensorineural hearing loss
Head trauma associated with loss of consciousness or skull fracture
Stigmata or other findings associated with a syndrome known to include a sensorineural and/or conductive hearing loss
Ototoxic medications, including but not limited to chemotherapeutic agents or aminoglycosides used in multiple courses or in combination with loop diuretics
Recurrent or persistent otitis media with effusion for at least 3 mo
For use with infants (age 29 days through 3 yr) who require periodic monitoring of hearing
(Some newborns and infants may pass initial hearing screening but require periodic monitoring of hearing to detect delayed-onset sensorineural and/or conductive hearing loss. Infants with these indicators require hearing evaluation at least every 6 mo until age 3 yr, and at appropriate intervals thereafter.)
Indicators associated with delayed-onset sensorineural hearing loss include:
Family history of hereditary childhood hearing loss
In utero infection, such as cytomegalovirus, rubella, syphilis, herpes simplex, or toxoplasmosis
Neurofibromatosis type II and neurodegenerative disorders
Indicators associated with conductive hearing loss include:
Recurrent or persistent otitis media with effusion
Anatomic deformities and other disorders that affect eustachian tube function
Neurodegenerative disorders

Adapted from American Academy of Pediatrics, Joint Committee on Infant Hearing: Joint Committee on Infant Hearing 1994 Position Statement. *Pediatrics* 1995;95:152.

Children with moderate, severe, or profound hearing impairment and those with other handicapping conditions are often educated in classes or schools for children with special needs. The auditory management and choices about modes of communication and education for children with hearing handicaps must be individualized because these children are not a homogeneous group. A team approach to individual case management is essential because each child and family unit represents unique needs and abilities.

Hearing Screening. Hearing impairment can have a major impact on the development of a child and because early identification improves prognosis, screening programs have been widely and strongly advocated. Data from the Colorado newborn screening program suggest that if hearing-impaired infants are identified and treated by age 6 mo, these children (with the exception of those with bilateral profound impairment) should develop the same level of language as their age-matched peers who are not hearing impaired. This is compelling support for the establishment of mandated newborn hearing screening programs for all children. The American Academy of Pediatrics endorses the goal of universal

TABLE 627–1. Hearing Handicap as a Function of Average Hearing Threshold Level of the Better Ear

Average Threshold Level (dB) at 500–2,000 Hz (ANSI)	Description	Common Causes	What Can Be Heard Without Amplification	Degree of Handicap (if Not Treated in 1st yr of Life)	Probable Needs
0–15	Normal range	Conductive hearing loss	All speech sounds	None	None
16–25	Slight hearing loss	Otitis media, TM perforation, tympanosclerosis; eustachian tube dysfunction; some SNHL	Vowel sounds heard clearly, may miss unvoiced consonant sounds	Mild auditory dysfunction in language learning. Difficulty in perceiving some speech sounds	Consideration of need for hearing aid; speech reading; auditory training Speech therapy Preferential seating Appropriate surgery
25–30	Mild	Otitis media, TM perforation, tympanosclerosis, severe eustachian dysfunction, SNHL	Hears only some of speech sounds, the louder voiced sounds	Auditory learning dysfunction Mild language retardation Mild speech problems Inattention	Hearing aid Lip reading Auditory training Speech therapy Appropriate surgery
30–50	Moderate hearing loss	Chronic otitis, ear canal/middle ear anomaly, SNHL	Misses most speech sounds at normal conversational level	Speech problems Language retardation Learning dysfunction Inattention	All of the above, plus consideration of special classroom situation
50–70	Severe hearing loss	SNHL or mixed loss due to a combination of middle-ear disease and sensorineural involvement	Hears no speech sound of normal conversations	Severe speech problems Language retardation Learning dysfunction Inattention	All of the above; probable assignment to special classes
70+	Profound hearing loss	SNHL or mixed	Hears no speech or other sounds	Severe speech problems Language retardation Learning dysfunction Inattention	All of the above; probable assignment to special classes or schools

ANSI = American National Standards Institute; TM = tympanic membrane; SNHL = sensorineural hearing loss.
Modified from Northern JL, Downs MP: Hearing in Children, 4th ed. Baltimore, Williams & Wilkins, 1991.

detection of hearing loss in infants before 3 mo of age, with appropriate intervention no later than 6 mo of age. At present, hearing screening has been mandated in 32 states in the United States.

Until mandated screening programs are universally established, many hospitals will continue to use other criteria to screen for hearing loss. Some use the high-risk criteria (see Box 627–1) to decide which infants to screen, some screen all infants who require intensive care, and some both. The problem with using high-risk criteria to screen is that 50% of the cases of hearing impairment will be missed because the infants are hearing impaired but do not meet any of the high-risk criteria, or they develop hearing loss after the neonatal period.

The recommended hearing screening techniques are either otoacoustic emissions (OAE) testing or auditory brainstem evoked responses (ABR). The ABR test, an auditory evoked electrophysiologic response that correlates highly with hearing, has been used successfully and cost-effectively to screen newborns and to identify further the degree and type of hearing loss. OAE tests, used successfully in many newborn screening programs, are quick, easy to administer and inexpensive, and provide a sensitive indication of the presence of hearing loss. Results are relatively easy to interpret. OAEs are absent if hearing is worse than 30–40 dB, no matter what the cause; those children who fail OAEs undergo an ABR for a more definitive evaluation. Screening methods such as observing behavioral responses to uncalibrated noisemakers or using automated systems such as the Crib-o-gram or the auditory response cradle (in which movement of the infant in response to sound is recorded by motion sensors) are not recommended.

Many children become hearing impaired after the neonatal period and, therefore, are not identified by newborn screening programs. It is often not until children are in preschool or kindergarten that further hearing screening takes place. Consequently, primary care physicians and pediatricians should be alert to the signs and symptoms of childhood hearing impairment, so that those with hearing impairment who are not screened formally can be identified as early as possible.

IDENTIFICATION OF HEARING IMPAIRMENT. The impact of hearing impairment is greatest on an infant who has yet to develop language; therefore, identification, diagnosis, description, and treatment should begin as soon as possible. In general, infants with a prenatal or perinatal history that puts them at risk (see Box 627–1) or those who have failed a formal hearing screening should be closely monitored by an experienced clinical audiologist until a reliable assessment of auditory function has been obtained. Pediatricians should encourage families to cooperate with the follow-up plan. Infants who are born at risk but who have not been screened as neonates (often because of transfer from one hospital to another) should have a hearing screening by age 3 mo.

Hearing-impaired infants who are born at risk or screened for hearing loss in a neonatal hearing screening program account for only a portion of those in the pediatric hearing-impaired population. Those who are congenitally deaf because of autosomal recessive inheritance or subclinical congenital infection are often not identified until the 2nd or 3rd yr of life. Usually, the more severe the hearing loss, the earlier is the age at identification, but identification often occurs later than the age necessary for an optimal outcome. Children with normal hearing have developed an extensive language by age 3 yr. Parental concern about hearing and any delayed development of speech and language should alert the pediatrician; parental concern usually precedes formal identification and diagnosis of hearing impairment by 6 mo–1 yr. Table 627–2 presents guidelines for screening language development in young children, and Table 627–3 provides guidelines for identifying children with abnormal auditory behavior. Failure to fulfill these criteria should be reason for an audiologic evaluation.

Clinical Audiologic Evaluation. Even the youngest infants can be evaluated for auditory function. When hearing impairment is suspected in a young child, reliable and valid estimates of auditory function can be obtained. Successful treatment strategies for hearing-impaired children rely on prompt identification and

TABLE 627–2. Criteria for Referral for Audiologic Assessment

Age (mo)	Referral Guidelines for Children with "Speech" Delay
12	No differentiated babbling or vocal imitation
18	No use of single words
24	Single-word vocabulary of ≤ 10 words
30	Fewer than 100 words; no evidence of two-word combinations; unintelligible
36	Fewer than 200 words; no use of telegraphic sentences, clarity < 50%
48	Fewer than 600 words; no use of simple sentences; clarity ≤ 80%

From Matkin ND: Early recognition and referral of hearing-impaired children. Pediatr Rev *1984;6:151. Reproduced by permission of* Pediatrics.

ongoing assessment to define the dimensions of auditory function. Cooperation among the pediatrician and those specializing in such areas as audiology, speech and language pathology, education, and child development is necessary to optimize auditory-verbal development. Therapy for hearing-impaired children includes considering (and often fitting) an amplification device; monitoring hearing and auditory skills, counseling parents and families, advising teachers, and dealing with public agencies.

AUDIOMETRY. The technique of the audiologic evaluation varies as a function of the age or developmental level of the child, the reason for the evaluation, and the child's otologic condition or history. An audiogram provides the fundamental description of hearing sensitivity (Fig. 627–1). Hearing thresholds are assessed as a function of frequency using pure tones (sine waves) at octave intervals from 250–8,000 Hz. Earphones are typically used, and hearing is assessed independently for each ear. *Air-conducted* signals are presented through earphones (or loudspeakers) and are used to provide information about the sensitivity of the auditory system. These same test sounds can be delivered to the ear through an oscillator that is placed on the head, usually on the mastoid. Such signals are considered *bone-conducted* because the bones of the skull transmit vibrations as sound energy directly to the inner ear, essentially bypassing the outer and middle ears. In a normal ear, the air and bone conduction thresholds are the same; they are also the same in those with SNHL. In those with CHL, the air and bone conduction thresholds differ. This is called the *air-bone gap*; it indicates the amount of hearing loss attributable to dysfunction in the outer and/or middle ear. With mixed hearing loss, both the bone and air conduction thresholds are abnormal, and there is an air-bone gap.

SPEECH RECOGNITION THRESHOLD. Another measure useful in describing auditory function is the speech recognition threshold (SRT), which is the lowest intensity level at which a score of approximately 50% correct is obtained on a task of recognizing spondee words. Spondee words are two-syllable words

TABLE 627–3. Guidelines for Referral of Children Suspected of Having Hearing Loss

Age (mo)	Normal Development
0–4	Should startle to loud sounds, quiet to mother's voice, momentarily cease activity when sound is presented at a conversational level
5–6	Should correctly localize to sound presented in a horizontal plane, begin to imitate sounds in own speech repertoire or at least reciprocally vocalize with an adult
7–12	Should correctly localize to sound presented in any plane Should respond to name, even when spoken quietly
13–15	Should point toward an unexpected sound or to familiar objects or persons when asked
16–18	Should follow simple directions without gestural or other visual cues; can be trained to reach toward an interesting toy at midline when a sound is presented
19–24	Should point to body parts when asked; by 21–24 mo, can be trained to perform play audiometry

From Matkin ND: Early recognition and referral of hearing-impaired children. Pediatr Rev *1984;6:151. Reproduced by permission of* Pediatrics.

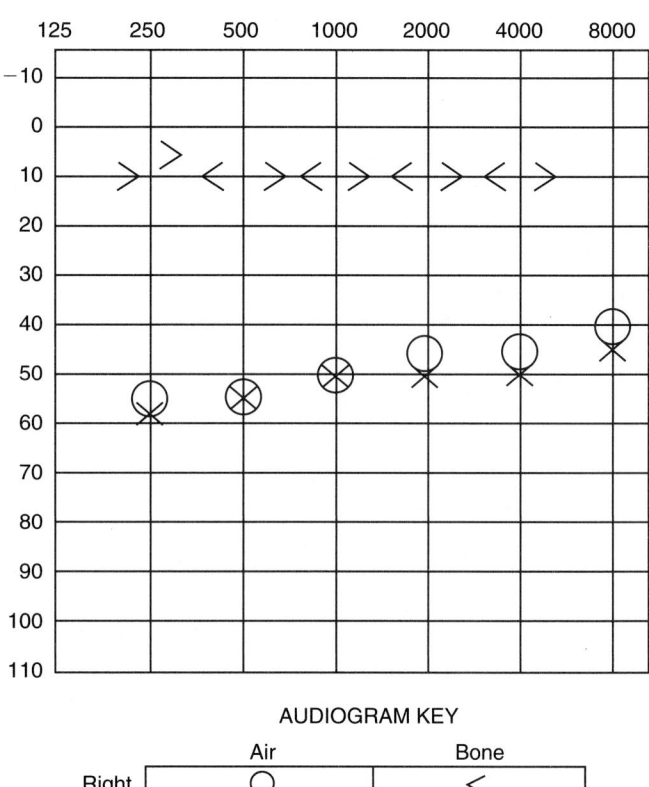

PURE-TONE AUDIOGRAM
Frequency (cycles/sec)

	Air	Bone
Right	○	<
Left	×	>

AUDIOGRAM KEY

FIGURE 627–1. Audiogram showing bilateral conductive hearing loss.

or phrases that have equal stress on each syllable (baseball, hotdog, pancake). Listeners must be familiar with all the words for a valid test result to be obtained. The SRT should correspond to the average of pure-tone thresholds at 500, 1,000, and 2,000 Hz, the pure-tone average (PTA). The SRT is relevant as an indicator of a child's potential for development and use of speech and language; it also serves as a check of the validity of a test because children with nonorganic hearing loss (malingerers) may show a discrepancy between the PTA and SRT.

The basic battery of hearing tests concludes with an assessment of a child's ability to understand monosyllabic words when presented at a comfortable listening level. Performance on such word intelligibility tests assists in the differential diagnosis of hearing impairment and provides a measure of how well a child performs when speech is presented at loudness levels similar to those encountered in the environment.

PLAY AUDIOMETRY. Hearing testing is age-dependent. For children at or above the developmental level of a 5 or 6 yr old, conventional test methods can be used. For children 2 1/2–5 yr old, play audiometry can be used. Responses in play audiometry are usually conditioned motor activities associated with a game, such as dropping blocks in a bucket, placing rings on a peg, or completing a puzzle. The technique can be used to obtain a reliable audiogram for a preschool child. For those who will not or cannot repeat words clearly for the SRT and word intelligibility tasks, pictures can be used with a pointing response.

VISUAL REINFORCEMENT AUDIOMETRY. For those between the ages of about 6 mo and 2 1/2 yr, visual reinforcement audiometry (VRA) is commonly used. In this technique, the child is observed for a head-turning response upon activation of an animated (mechanical) toy reinforcer. If infants are properly conditioned, by giving sounds associated with the visual toy cue, VRA can provide reliable estimates of hearing sensitivity for tones and speech sounds. In most applications of VRA, sounds are presented by loudspeakers in a sound field, so no ear-specific information is obtained. Assessment of an infant is often designed to rule out hearing loss that would affect the development of speech and language. Normal sound field response levels of infants indicate sufficient hearing for this purpose despite the possibility of different hearing levels in the two ears.

BEHAVIORAL OBSERVATION AUDIOMETRY. Used as a screening device for infants younger than 5 mo, behavioral observation audiometry (BOA) is limited to unconditioned, reflexive responses to complex (not frequency-specific) test sounds, such as noise, speech, or music presented using calibrated signals from a loudspeaker or uncalibrated noisemakers. Response levels can vary widely within and among infants and usually do not represent a reliable estimate of sensitivity.

Assessment of a child with suspected hearing loss is not complete until pure-tone hearing thresholds and SRTs (a reliable audiogram) have been obtained in each ear. BOA and VRA in sound-field testing give estimates of hearing responsivity in the better hearing ear.

ACOUSTIC IMMITANCE TESTING. This is a standard part of the clinical audiologic test battery and includes tympanometry. Acoustic immitance testing is a useful objective assessment technique that provides information about the status of the middle ear. Tympanometry can be performed in a physician's office and is helpful in the diagnosis and management of OM with effusion, a common cause of mild to moderate hearing loss in young children.

Tympanometry. This technique provides a graph of the ability of the middle ear to transmit sound energy (admittance, or compliance) or impede sound energy (impedance) as a function of air pressure in the external ear canal. Because most immitance test instruments measure acoustic admittance, the term *admittance* is used here. The principles apply to whatever units of measurement are used.

A probe is inserted into the entrance of the external ear canal so that an airtight seal is obtained. The probe varies air pressure, presents a tone, and measures sound pressure level in the ear canal through the probe assembly. The sound pressure measured in the ear canal relative to the known intensity of the probe signal is used to estimate the acoustic admittance of the ear canal and middle-ear system. Admittance can be expressed in a unit called a millimho (mmho) or as a volume of air (mL) with equivalent acoustic admittance. The test is performed so that an estimate of the volume of air enclosed between the probe tip and TM can be made. The acoustic admittance of this volume of air is deducted from the overall admittance measure to obtain a measure of the admittance of the middle-ear system alone. Estimating ear canal volume also has a diagnostic benefit because an abnormally large value is consistent with the presence of an opening in the TM (perforation or tube).

With elimination of the admittance of the air mass in the external auditory canal, it is assumed that the remaining admittance measure accurately reflects the admittance of the entire middle-ear system. Its value is largely controlled by the dynamics of the TM. Abnormalities of the TM can dictate the shape of tympanograms and thus obscure abnormalities medial to the TM. In addition, the frequency of the probe tone, the speed and direction of the air pressure change, and the air pressure at which the tympanogram is initiated can all influence the outcome.

When air pressure in the ear canal is equal to that in the middle ear, the middle-ear system is functioning optimally. Therefore, the ear canal pressure at which there is the greatest flow of energy (admittance) should be a reasonable estimate of the air pressure in the middle-ear space. This pressure is determined by finding the admittance maximum (peak) on the tympanogram and obtaining its value on the x-axis. The value on the y-axis at the tympanogram peak is an estimate of peak admittance. This peak measure is sometimes referred to as static acoustic admittance, even though it is estimated from a dynamic measure (Fig. 630–6A). Table 627–4 presents the norms for peak admittance based on admittance tympanometry for normal adults and children.

Tympanometry in Otitis Media with Effusion. Children with OME often have reduced peak admittance or high negative tympanometric peak pressures (Fig. 630–6C); however, in the diagnosis of effusion, the tympanometric measure with the greatest sensitivity and specificity is the tympanogram shape rather than its peak pressure or admittance. This shape is sometimes referred to as the tympanometric gradient or width; it measures the degree of roundness or "peakedness" of the tympanogram. The more rounded the peak (or "flat" in an absent peak), the higher is the probability that an effusion is present (Fig. 630–6B). It is important to know which instrument is used, as some compute gradient automatically but others do not.

Acoustic Reflex Test (ART). This is also part of the immitance test battery. With a properly functioning middle-ear system, admittance at the TM changes on activation of the stapedius and tensor tympani muscles. In healthy ears, the stapedial reflex occurs after exposure to loud sounds. Admittance instruments are designed to present reflex activating signals (pure tones of various frequencies or noise), either to the same or the contralateral ear, while monitoring admittance. Very small admittance changes that are time locked to presentations of the signal are considered to be a result of middle-ear muscle reflexes. Absence of admittance changes can occur when the hearing loss is sufficient to prevent the signal from reaching the loudness level necessary to elicit the reflex or when a middle-ear condition affects the ability to monitor a small admittance change. Reflexes are usually absent in those with CHL due to the presence of an abnormal transfer system; thus, the ART is useful in the differential diagnosis of hearing impairment. ART also is used in the assessment of SNHL and the integrity of the neurologic components of the reflex arc, including cranial nerves VII and VIII.

AUDITORY BRAINSTEM RESPONSE. The ABR test is used for newborn hearing screening, to confirm hearing loss in young children, to obtain ear-specific information in young children, and to test children who cannot, for whatever reason, cooperate with behavioral test methods. It is also important in the diagnosis of auditory dysfunction and of disorders of the auditory nervous system. The ABR test is a far-field recording of minute electrical discharges from numerous neurons.

TABLE 627–4. Norms for Peak (Static) Admittance (in mL) Using a 226-Hz Probe Tone for Children and Adults

		Speed of Air Pressure Sweep	
		≤50 daPa/sec*	200 daPa/sec†
Children (3–5 yr)	Lower limit	0.30	0.36
	Median	0.55	0.61
	Upper limit	0.90	1.06
Adults	Lower limit	0.56	0.27
	Median	0.85	0.72
	Upper limit	1.36	1.38

*Ear canal volume measurement based on admittance at lowest tail of tympanogram.
†Ear canal measurement based on admittance at lowest tail of tympanogram for children and at +200 daPa for adults.
daPa = decaPascals.
Adapted from Margolis RH, Shanks JE: Tympanometry: Basic principles of clinical application. In Rintelman WS (editor): Hearing Assessment, 2nd ed. Austin, TX, PRODED, 1991, pp 179–245.

The stimulus, therefore, must be able to cause simultaneous discharge of the large numbers of neurons involved. Stimuli with very rapid onset, such as clicks or tone bursts, must be used. Unfortunately, the rapid onset required to create a measurable ABR also causes energy to be spread in the frequency domain, reducing the frequency-specificity of the response.

The ABR result is not affected by sedation or general anesthesia. Infants and children from about 4 mo-4 yr of age are routinely sedated to minimize electrical interference caused by muscle activity during testing. The ABR also can be performed in the operating room when a child is anesthetized for another procedure.

The ABR is recorded as 5–7 waves. Waves I, III, and V can be obtained consistently in all age groups; Waves II and IV appear less consistently. The latency of each wave (time of occurrence of the wave peak after stimulus onset) increases, and the amplitude decreases with reductions in stimulus intensity or loudness; latency also decreases with increasing age, with the earliest waves reaching mature latency values earlier in life than the later waves.

The ABR test has two major uses in a pediatric setting. As an audiometric test, it provides information on the ability of the peripheral auditory system to transmit information to the auditory nerve and beyond. It is used also in the differential diagnosis or monitoring of central nervous system pathology. For audiometry, the goal is to find the minimum stimulus intensity that yields an observable ABR. Plotting latency versus intensity for various waves also aids in the differential diagnosis of hearing impairment. A major advantage of auditory assessment using the ABR test is that ear-specific threshold estimates can be obtained on infants or difficult-to-test patients. ABR thresholds using click stimuli correlate best with behavioral hearing thresholds in the higher frequencies (1,000–4,000 Hz); responsivity in the low frequencies requires different stimuli (tone bursts or filtered clicks) or the use of masking, neither of which isolates the low-frequency region of the cochlea in all cases, and this may affect interpretation.

The ABR test does not assess "hearing." It reflects auditory neuronal electric responses that can be correlated to behavioral hearing thresholds, but a normal ABR result only suggests that the auditory system, up to the level of the midbrain, is responsive to the stimulus used. Conversely, a failure to elicit an ABR indicates an impairment of the system's synchronous response but does not necessarily mean that there is no "hearing." The behavioral response to sound is sometimes normal when no ABR can be elicited, such as in neurologic demyelinating disease. The ABR test may be used to infer whether and at what level of the auditory system an impairment exists.

Hearing losses that are sudden, progressive, or unilateral are indications for ABR testing. Although it is believed that the different waves of the ABR reflect activity in increasingly rostral levels of the auditory system, the neural generators of the response have not been precisely determined. Each ABR wave beyond the earliest waves is probably the result of neural firing at many levels of the system, and each level of the system probably contributes to several ABR waves. High-intensity click stimuli are used for the neurologic application. The morphology of the response and wave and interwave latencies are examined in respect to age-appropriate forms. Delayed or missing waves in the ABR result often have diagnostic significance.

The ABR and other electrical responses are extremely complex and difficult to interpret. A number of factors, including instrumentation design and settings, environment, degree and configuration of hearing loss, and patient characteristics, may influence the quality of the recording. Therefore, testing and interpretation of electrophysiologic activity as it possibly relates to hearing should be carried out by trained audiologists to avoid the risk that unreliable or erroneous conclusions will affect a patient's care.

OTOACOUSTIC EMISSIONS. During normal hearing, OAEs originate from the hair cells in the cochlea and are detected by sensitive amplifying processes. They travel from the cochlea through the middle ear to the external auditory canal, where they can be detected using miniature microphones. Transient evoked OAEs (TEOAEs) may be used to check the integrity of the cochlea. In the neonatal period, detection of OAEs can be accomplished during natural sleep, and TEOAEs can be used as screening tests in infants and children for hearing at the 30 dB level of hearing loss. They are less time consuming and elaborate than ABR and are more sensitive than behavioral tests in young children. TEOAEs are reduced or absent owing to various dysfunctions in the middle and inner ears. They are absent in patients with more than 30 dB of hearing loss and are not used to determine hearing threshold; rather, they provide a screen for whether hearing is present at greater than 30–40 dB. Diseases such as OM or congenitally abnormal middle ear structures reduce the transfer of TEOAEs and may incorrectly indicate a cochlear hearing disorder. If a hearing loss is suspected by the absence of OAE, the ears should be examined for evidence of pathology, and then ABR testing should be used for confirmation and identification of the type, degree, and laterality of hearing loss.

ACOUSTIC REFLECTOMETRY. In this test, a hand-held instrument is placed next to the opening of a child's ear canal and 80-dB sound is delivered that varies in frequency from 2,000–4,500 Hz in a 100-msec period. The instrument measures the total level of reflected and transmitted sound. Some physicians have found this device useful to help gauge the presence or absence of middle-ear fluid, and a commercial version is being marketed to parents as a way to monitor ear fluid. The instrument does not provide any information about hearing; if the presence of chronic fluid is suggested, audiometric evaluation should be obtained.

Treatment. Once a hearing loss is identified, a full developmental and speech and language evaluation is needed. Parental counseling and involvement is required in all stages of the evaluation and treatment or rehabilitation. A conductive hearing loss can often be corrected through treatment of a middle-ear effusion (ear tube placement) or surgical correction of the abnormal sound-conducting mechanism. Children with SNHL should be evaluated for possible hearing aid use by a pediatric audiologist. Hearing aids may be fitted for children as young as 2 mo. Compelling evidence from the hearing screening program in Colorado shows that identification and amplification before age 6 mo makes a very significant difference in the speech and language abilities of affected children, compared with those cases identified and amplified after the age of 6 mo. In these children, repeat audiologic testing is needed to reliably identify the degree of hearing loss and to fine-tune the use of hearing aids.

The best educational approach to children with significant hearing loss is a subject of ongoing controversy. Because we live in a predominantly speaking world, some have advocated a pure auditory and oral approach to hearing therapy. However, because affected children often are slow to develop communication skills, many advocate a total communication approach; depending on the individual child's needs, this technique uses a mixture of sign language, lip-reading, hearing aids, and speech. The appropriate program for each child depends on the patient, family, and available resources.

The use of a surgically placed cochlear implant in children with severe to profound hearing loss and little or no help from conventional hearing aids improves the development of communication skills. The device is currently approved for use in the United States in children age 2 yr and older. However, because of a possible increased risk of pneumococcal meningitis, children with implants should receive age-appropriate vaccination against pneumococcal disease. Some members of the hearing-impaired community have objected to its use in children who have no decision in the matter; they argue that the child may develop excellent communication abilities using more conventional therapeutic strategies.

Chapter 628
Congenital Malformations

Joseph Haddad Jr.

The external and middle ears, derived from the 1st and 2nd branchial arches and grooves, grow throughout puberty, but the inner ear, which develops from the otocyst, reaches adult size and shape by mid-fetal development. The ossicles are derived from the 1st and 2nd arches (malleus and incus), and the stapes arises from the 2nd arch and the otic capsule. The ossicles achieve adult size and shape by the 15th wk of gestation for the malleus and incus and 18th wk for the stapes. Although the pinna, ear canal, and tympanic membrane (TM) continue to grow after birth, congenital abnormalities of these structures develop during the 1st half of gestation. Malformed external and middle ears may be associated with serious renal anomalies, mandibulofacial dysostosis, hemifacial microsomia, and other craniofacial malformations. Facial nerve abnormalities may be associated with any of the congenital abnormalities of the ear and temporal bone. Malformations of the external and middle ears may also be associated with abnormalities of the inner ear and both conductive (CHL) and sensorineural hearing loss (SNHL). Any child born with an abnormality of the pinna, external auditory canal, or TM should have a complete audiologic evaluation in the neonatal period.

Pinna Malformations. Severe malformations of the external ear are rare, but minor deformities are common. Isolated abnormalities of the external ear occur in approximately 1% of children. A *pit*-like depression just in front of the helix and above the tragus may represent a cyst or an epidermis-lined fistulous tract; these are common, with an incidence of approximately 8/1,000 children, and may be unilateral or bilateral and familial. The pits only require surgical removal if there is recurrent infection. Accessory *skin tags*, with an incidence of 1–2/1,000, can be removed for cosmetic reasons by simple ligation if they are attached by a narrow pedicle; if the pedicle is broad-based or contains cartilage, the defect should be corrected surgically. An unusually prominent or *"lop" ear* results from lack of bending of the cartilage that creates the antihelix. It may be improved cosmetically in the neonatal period by applying a firm framework (sometimes soldering wire is used) attached by Steri-Strips to the pinna and worn continuously for weeks to months. Otoplasty for cosmetic correction can be considered in children age 5 yr or older; by this time, the pinna has reached about 80% of its adult size.

The term *microtia* may indicate subtle abnormalities of the size, shape, and location of the pinna and ear canal, or major abnormalities with only small nubbins of skin and cartilage and absence of the ear canal opening; *anotia* indicates complete absence of the pinna and ear canal. Microtic ears are often more anterior and inferior in placement than normal auricles; the facial nerve location and function may be abnormal. Surgery to correct microtia is considered for both cosmetic and functional reasons; children who have some pinna can wear regular glasses, a hearing aid, and earrings and feel more normal in appearance. If the microtia is severe, some patients may opt for creation and attachment of a prosthetic ear, which cosmetically closely resembles a real ear. Surgery to correct severe microtia may involve a multistage procedure including carving and

transplantation of autogenous cartilage rib grafts, and local soft tissue flaps. Cosmetic reconstruction of the auricle is customarily done between ages 5 and 7 and is performed before canal atresia repair in the child deemed appropriate for this surgery (see later discussion).

Congenital External Auditory Canal Stenosis/Atresia. Stenosis or atresia of the ear canal often occurs in association with malformation of the auricle and middle ear; minor stenoses may occur in isolation. In some genetic syndromes, such as trisomy 21, ear canals are narrow. Audiometric evaluation of these children should be undertaken as early in life as possible. Most children with significant CHL secondary to bilateral atresia wear bone conduction hearing aids for the first several years of life. Diagnosis, evaluation, and surgical planning are often aided by computed tomography (CT), and sometimes magnetic resonance imaging (MRI), of the temporal bone. Mild cases of ear canal stenosis do not require surgical enlargement unless the patient develops chronic external otitis or severe cerumen impaction that affects hearing.

Reconstructive ear canal and middle-ear surgery for atresia is generally considered for patients older than 5 yr with bilateral deformities resulting in a significant CHL. The aim of reconstructive surgery is to improve hearing to a point where the child may not need a hearing aid or to provide an ear canal and pinna so that the child can derive improved benefit from an air conduction hearing aid. CT evidence of an adequate middle-ear cleft and mastoid is required to perform the surgery; the position of the facial nerve, which is frequently in an abnormal location in these children, also needs to be considered. The use of bone-anchored hearing aids may provide an option for some of these children when they are older.

Congenital Middle-Ear Malformations. Children may have congenital abnormalities of the middle ear as an isolated defect or in association with other abnormalities of the temporal bone, especially the ear canal and pinna, or as part of a syndrome. Affected children usually have CHL but may have mixed CHL and SNHL. Most malformations involve the ossicles, with the incus being the most commonly affected. Other less common abnormalities of the middle ear include persistent stapedial artery, high-riding jugular bulb, and abnormalities of the shape and volume of the aerated portion of the middle ear and mastoid; all present problems for a surgeon. Depending on the type of abnormality and the presence of other anomalies, surgery may be considered to improve hearing.

Congenital Inner Ear Malformations. Congenital inner ear malformations have been identified and classified as a result of improvements in imaging modalities, especially CT and MRI. As many as 20% of children with SNHL may have anatomic abnormalities identified on CT or MRI. Congenital malformations of the inner ear are usually associated with SNHL of various degrees from mild to profound. These malformations may occur as isolated anomalies or in association with other syndromes, genetic abnormalities, or structural abnormalities of the head and neck. Enlarged vestibular aqueducts have been identified on imaging studies in association with SNHL; although no therapy exists for this condition, it may be associated with progressive SNHL in some children, and, therefore, diagnosis may have some prognostic value.

Congenital perilymphatic fistula (PLF) of the oval or round window membrane may present as a rapid-onset, fluctuating, or progressive SNHL with or without vertigo and is often associated with congenital inner ear abnormalities. Middle ear exploration may need to be performed to confirm this diagnosis, inasmuch as no reliable nonoperative diagnostic test exists. PLFs may need to be repaired to prevent possible spread of infection from the middle ear to the labyrinth, to stabilize hearing loss, and to improve vertigo when present.

Congenital Cholesteatoma. A congenital cholesteatoma usually appears as a white, round, cystlike structure medial to an intact TM; cysts are most commonly seen in the anterior-superior portion of the middle ear, although they can present in other locations and within the TM or in the skin of the ear canal. Affected children frequently have no prior history of otitis media (OM). A common theory for pathogenesis is that the cyst derives from a congenital rest of epithelial tissue that persists beyond 33 wk of gestation, when it would ordinarily disappear. Other theories include squamous metaplasia of the middle ear, entrance of squamous epithelium through a nonintact eardrum into the middle ear, ectodermal implants between the 1st and 2nd branchial arch remnants, and residual amniotic fluid squamous debris. Congenital or acquired cholesteatoma should be suspected when deep retraction pockets, keratin debris, chronic drainage, aural granulation tissue, or a mass behind or involving the TM is present. Besides acting as a benign tumor causing local bone destruction, the keratinaceous debris of a cholesteatoma is a good culture medium and may become a focus of infection for chronic OM. Complications include ossicular erosion with hearing loss, bone erosion into the inner ear with dizziness, or exposure of the dura with consequent meningitis or a brain abscess. Cholesteatoma should be removed surgically after CT scan and hearing evaluation, and appropriate antibiotic therapy.

Chapter 629
Diseases of the External Ear
Joseph Haddad Jr.

EXTERNAL OTITIS (OTITIS EXTERNA)

In an infant, the outer two thirds of the ear canal is cartilaginous and the inner third is bony, whereas in an older child and adult only the outer third is cartilaginous. In the bony portion the epithelium is thinner than in the cartilaginous portion, there is no subcutaneous tissue, and epithelium is tightly applied to the underlying periosteum; hair follicles, sebaceous glands, and apocrine glands are scarce or absent. The skin in the cartilaginous area has well-developed dermis and subcutaneous tissue and contains hair follicles, sebaceous glands, and apocrine glands. The highly viscid secretions of the sebaceous glands and the watery, pigmented secretions of the apocrine glands in the outer portion of the canal combine with exfoliated surface cells of the skin to form a protective, waxy, water-repellent coating (cerumen).

The normal flora of the external canal consists mainly of aerobic bacteria and includes coagulase-negative staphylococci, *Corynebacterium* (diphtheroids), *Micrococcus* species, and occasionally *Staphylococcus aureus*, viridans streptococci, and *Pseudomonas aeruginosa*. Excessive wetness (swimming, bathing, or increased environmental humidity), dryness (dry canal skin and lack of cerumen), and the presence of other skin pathology (previous infection, eczema or other forms of dermatitis) and trauma (digital or foreign body) make the skin of the canal vulnerable to infection by the normal flora or exogenous bacteria.

Etiology. External otitis (also called "swimmer's ear," although it can occur without swimming) is most commonly caused by *P. aeruginosa*, but *S. aureus, Enterobacter aerogenes, Proteus mirabilis, Klebsiella pneumoniae*, streptococci, coagulase-negative staphylococci, diphtheroids, and fungi such as *Candida* and *Aspergillus* may also be isolated. External otitis results from chronic irritation and maceration from excessive moisture in the canal; loss of protective cerumen may play a role, but cerumen impaction with trapping of water can also cause infection. Inflammation of the ear canal due to herpesvirus, varicella-zoster, other skin exanthems, and eczema may also predispose to external otitis.

Clinical Manifestations. The predominant symptom is ear pain, often severe, accentuated by manipulation of the pinna or by pressure on the tragus. The severity of the pain and tenderness may be disproportionate to the degree of inflammation, because the skin of the external ear canal is closely adherent to the underlying perichondrium and periosteum. Itching is a frequent precursor of pain and is usually characteristic of chronic inflammation of the canal or resolving acute otitis externa. Conductive hearing loss may result from edema of the skin and tympanic membrane (TM), serous or purulent secretions, or the canal skin thickening associated with chronic external otitis.

Edema of the ear canal, erythema, and thick, clumpy otorrhea are prominent signs of the acute disease. The cerumen is usually white and soft in consistency, as opposed to its usual yellow color and firmer consistency. The canal frequently is so tender and swollen that the entire ear canal and TM cannot be adequately visualized, and complete otoscopic examination may be delayed until the acute swelling subsides. If the TM can be visualized, it may appear either normal or opaque; TM mobility may be normal or, if thickened, reduced in response to positive and negative pressure.

Other physical findings may include palpable and tender lymph nodes in the periauricular region, and erythema and swelling of the pinna and periauricular skin. Rarely, facial paralysis, other cranial nerve abnormalities, vertigo, and/or sensorineural hearing loss are present. If these occur, *necrotizing (malignant) external otitis* is probable. This invasive infection of the temporal bone and skull base requires immediate culture, intravenous antibiotics, and imaging studies to evaluate the extent of the disease. Surgical intervention to obtain cultures or debride devitalized tissue may be necessary. *P. aeruginosa* is the most common causative organism of necrotizing otitis externa; fortunately, this disease is rare in children and is seen only in association with immunocompromise or severe malnourishment.

Diagnosis. Diffuse external otitis may be confused with furunculosis, otitis media (OM), and mastoiditis. Furuncles occur in the lateral hair-bearing part of the ear canal; furunculosis usually causes a localized swelling of the canal limited to one quadrant, whereas external otitis is associated with concentric swelling and involves the entire ear canal. In OM, the TM may be perforated, severely retracted, or bulging and immobile; hearing is usually impaired. If the middle ear is draining through a perforated TM or tympanostomy tube, secondary external otitis may occur; if the TM is not visible owing to drainage or ear canal swelling, it may be difficult to distinguish acute OM with drainage from an acute external otitis. Pain on manipulation of the auricle and significant lymphadenitis are not common features of OM, and these findings assist in the differential diagnosis. In some patients with external otitis, the periauricular edema is so extensive that the auricle is pushed forward, creating a condition that may be confused with acute mastoiditis and a subperiosteal abscess; in mastoiditis, the postauricular fold is obliterated, whereas in external otitis the fold is usually better preserved. In acute mastoiditis, a history of OM and hearing loss is usual; tenderness is noted over the mastoid and not on movement of the auricle; and otoscopic examination may show sagging of the posterior canal wall.

Treatment. Topical otic preparations containing neomycin (active against gram-positive organisms and some gram-negative organisms, notably *Proteus* species) with either colistin or polymyxin (active against gram-negative bacilli, notably *Pseudomonas* species) and corticosteroids are effective in treating most forms of acute external otitis. Newer preparations of ear drops are available that do not contain potentially ototoxic antibiotics. If canal edema is marked, a wick should be inserted into the ear canal and the topical drops applied to the wick 3 times a day for 24–48 hr; the wick can be removed after this time and topical antibiotic is continued. After 2 or 3 days of this treatment, the edema of the ear canal is usually markedly improved and the ear canal and TM are better seen. When the pain is severe, oral analgesics (ibuprofen, codeine) may be necessary.

As the inflammatory process subsides, cleaning the canal with a suction or cotton-tipped applicator to remove the debris enhances the effectiveness of the topical medications. In subacute and chronic infections, periodic cleansing of the canal is essential. In severe, acute external otitis associated with fever and lymphadenitis, oral or parenteral antibiotics may be indicated; an ear canal culture should be done, and empiric antibiotic treatment can then be modified if necessary, based on susceptibility of the organism cultured. A fungal infection (otomycosis) of the external auditory canal is characterized by fluffy white debris, sometimes with black spores seen; treatment includes cleaning and application of antifungal solutions such as clotrimazole or nystatin; other antifungal agents include *m*-cresyl acetate 25%, gentian violet 2%, and thimerosal 1:1,000.

Prevention. Preventing external otitis may be necessary for individuals susceptible to recurrences, especially children who swim. The most effective prophylaxis is instillation of dilute alcohol or acetic acid (2%) immediately after swimming or bathing. During an acute episode of otitis externa, patients should not swim and the ears should be protected from water during bathing.

OTHER DISEASES OF THE EXTERNAL EAR

Furunculosis. This is caused by *S. aureus* and affects only the hair-containing outer third of the ear canal. Mild forms are treated with oral antibiotics active against *S. aureus*; if an abscess develops, incision and drainage may be necessary.

Acute Cellulitis. Acute cellulitis of the auricle and external auditory canal is usually caused by group A *Streptococcus* and occasionally by *S. aureus*. The skin is red, hot, and indurated, without a sharply defined border. Fever may be present with little or no exudate in the canal. Parenteral administration of penicillin G or a penicillinase-resistant penicillin is the therapy of choice.

Perichondritis/Chondritis. Perichondritis is an infection involving the skin and perichondrium of the auricular cartilage; extension of infection to the cartilage is termed *chondritis*. The ear canal, especially the lateral aspect, may also be involved. Early perichondritis may be difficult to differentiate from cellulitis because both are characterized by skin that is red, edematous, and tender. The main cause of perichondritis/chondritis and cellulitis is trauma (accidental or iatrogenic, laceration or contusion), including ear piercing (especially through the cartilage). The most commonly isolated organism in perichondritis/chondritis is *P. aeruginosa*, although other gram-negative and occasionally gram-positive organisms may be found. Treatment involves systemic, often parenteral, antibiotics; surgery to drain an abscess or remove nonviable skin or cartilage may also be needed. Removal of all ear jewelry is mandatory in the presence of infection.

Dermatoses. Various dermatoses (seborrheic, contact, infectious eczematoid, or neurodermatoid) are common causes of inflammation of the external canal; acute external otitis in these conditions is caused by scratching and the introduction of infecting organisms.

Seborrheic dermatitis is characterized by greasy scales that flake and crumble as they are detached from the epidermis; associated changes in the scalp, forehead, cheeks, brow, postauricular areas, and concha are usual.

Contact dermatitis of the auricle or canal may be caused by earrings, or by topical otic medications such as neomycin, which may produce erythema, vesiculation, edema, and weeping. Poison ivy, oak, and sumac may also produce contact dermatitis. Hair care products have been implicated in sensitive individuals.

Infectious eczematoid dermatitis is caused by a purulent infection of the external canal, middle ear, or mastoid; the purulent drainage infects the skin of the canal, auricle, or both. The lesion is weeping, erythematous, or crusted.

Atopic dermatitis occurs in children with a familial or personal history of allergy; the auricle, particularly the postauricular fold, becomes thickened, scaly, and excoriated.

Neurodermatitis is recognized by the intense itching and erythematous, thickened epidermis localized to the concha and orifice of the meatus.

Treatment of these dermatoses depends on the type but should include application of an appropriate topical medication, elimination of the source of infection or contact when identified, and management of any underlying dermatologic problem. In addition to topical antibiotics (or antifungals), topical steroids are helpful if contact dermatitis, atopic dermatitis, or eczematoid dermatitis is suspected.

Herpes Simplex. This may appear as vesicles on the auricle and lips. The lesions eventually become encrusted and dry and may be confused with impetigo. Topical application of a 10% solution of carbamide peroxide in anhydrous glycerol is symptomatically helpful. The **Ramsay Hunt syndrome** (herpes zoster oticus) may present with herpes vesicles in the ear canal and on the pinna and with facial paralysis and pain. Other cranial nerves may be affected as well, especially the 8th nerve. The current recommended treatment of herpes zoster oticus includes systemic antiviral agents, such as acyclovir, and corticosteroids. As many as 50% of patients with Ramsay Hunt syndrome do not have complete recovery of their facial nerve function.

Bullous Myringitis. Commonly associated with an acute upper respiratory tract infection, this condition presents as an ear infection with more severe pain than usual. On examination, hemorrhagic or serous blisters (bullas) may be seen on the TM. The disease is sometimes difficult to differentiate from acute OM, because a large bulla may be confused with a bulging TM. The organisms involved are the same as those causing acute OM, including both bacteria and viruses. Treatment consists of empiric antibiotic therapy and pain medications; in addition to ibuprofen or codeine for severe pain, a topical anesthetic eardrop may also provide some relief. Incision of the bullae, although not necessary, promptly relieves the pain.

Exostoses and Osteomas. Exostoses represent benign hyperplasia of the perichondrium and underlying bone of the external ear canal and are frequently found in people who swim often in cold water. Exostoses are broad based, often multiple and bilateral. Osteomas are benign bony growths in the ear canal; their cause is uncertain. They are usually solitary and attached by a narrow pedicle to the tympanosquamous or tympanomastoid suture line. Both are more common in males; exostoses are more common than osteomas. Surgical treatment is recommended when large masses cause cerumen impaction, ear canal obstruction, or hearing loss.

Chapter 630

Otitis Media *Jack L. Paradise*

General Considerations. Next to the common cold, otitis media is the most commonly diagnosed and probably the most prevalent illness of children in the United States, with peak incidence and prevalence from 6–20 mo of age. Otitis media figures importantly in the differential diagnosis of fever, is the most common reason for prescribing antimicrobial drugs to children, and often serves as the sole or the main basis for undertaking the most frequently performed operations in infants and young children, namely, myringotomy with insertion of tympanostomy tubes, adenoidectomy, and adenotonsillectomy. An important characteristic of otitis media is its propensity to become chronic and recur. Generally, the earlier in life a child experiences a first episode, the greater the degree of subsequent difficulty as measured by frequency of recurrence, severity, and persistence of middle-ear effusion.

Otitis media challenges the clinician in a number of ways. Accurate diagnosis in infants and young children is often difficult. Symptoms may be absent or inapparent, especially in early infancy and in chronic stages of the disease. The eardrum may be obscured by cerumen, removal of which may be arduous and time-consuming. Abnormalities of the eardrum may be subtle and difficult to appreciate. In the face of these difficulties, both underdiagnosis and overdiagnosis occur commonly. Once a diagnosis of otitis media has been established—whatever the type of the disease—its significance to the child's health and well-being and its optimal method of management remain open to question and the subjects of continuing controversy. Underlying the uncertainties are incomplete knowledge and lack of consensus among authorities concerning benefit-risk ratios of available medical and surgical treatments and the likelihood of long-term consequences of otitis media. These include possible direct effects in the form of middle-ear damage, inner-ear damage, and hearing impairment, and possible indirect effects in the form of lasting impairments of speech, language, cognitive, and psychosocial development. Whether developmental effects actually occur remains the subject of ongoing investigation.

The spectrum of middle-ear disease subsumed under the term otitis media has two main components: infection, which is termed **suppurative or acute otitis media (AOM)**; and usually noninfective inflammation accompanied by effusion, termed **nonsuppurative or secretory otitis media, or otitis media with effusion (OME)**. These two main types of otitis media are interrelated: Infection usually is succeeded by residual, noninfective inflammation and effusion that, in turn, predispose children to recurrent infection. In one study, infants monitored closely during the first year of life commonly developed OME de novo, often followed by the development of AOM. These findings suggest that, most commonly, OME may be the form of otitis media that young infants first develop. Middle-ear effusion (MEE) is a feature both of AOM and of OME, and, in both conditions, is an expression of the underlying middle-ear mucosal inflammation. In children with otitis media, mucosal inflammation is generally also present in the mastoid air cells, which are in continuity with the middle-ear cavity.

Otitis media is accompanied by a variable degree of conductive hearing loss ranging from none to as much as 50 decibels hearing level (dB HL). Losses of 21–30 dB HL are usual. Although most individual episodes of otitis media subside within several weeks, middle-ear effusion persists for 3 mo or longer in approximately 10–25% of cases.

Epidemiology. Many studies of the epidemiology of otitis media have been conducted, varying widely in design, methodology,

outcome measures, scope, and generalizability. Their findings also have varied. The differences in findings may have been attributable to population or secular differences, or to differences in the intensity of surveillance, in the accuracy of disease detection, or to combinations of these factors. Factors known or believed to affect the occurrence of otitis media include age, sex, race, genetic background, socioeconomic status, type of milk used in infant feeding, degree of exposure to tobacco smoke, degree of exposure to other children, presence or absence of respiratory allergy, and season of the year. Children with certain types of congenital craniofacial anomalies are particularly prone to otitis media.

AGE. Most prospective studies of the prevalence of otitis media in infants have involved those from families of low socioeconomic status largely or exclusively. In these studies, one or more episodes of otitis media reportedly developed in 61–73% of infants by the age of 6 mo, in 77–85% by 1 yr, and in 77–99% by 2 yr; the median cumulative proportions of days with MEE ranged from 12–27% during the first year of life and from 15–18% during the second year of life. Reported rates in infants from middle-class families have been somewhat lower: one or more episodes of otitis media in 36–46% by the age of 6 mo, 63–77% by 1 yr, and 66–90% by 2 yr. The median cumulative proportions of days with MEE in these infants ranged from 5% to 15% during the first year of life and from 6% to 11% during the second year of life. Across groups, rates were highest during 6–20 mo of age. After the age of 2 yr, the incidence and prevalence of otitis media decline progressively, although the disease remains relatively common into the early school-age years. Possible reasons for the higher rates in infants and younger children include less well-developed immunologic defenses, more abundant nasopharyngeal lymphoid tissue, less favorable eustachian tubal factors involving both the structure and function of the tube, and greater proportions of time spent in the horizontal position.

SEX. Although some studies have found no sex-related differences in the occurrence of otitis media, other, more convincing studies have found the incidence greater in boys than in girls. In a large Pittsburgh child development/otitis media study involving close monitoring in a sociodemographically diverse population, male infants consistently had higher mean cumulative proportions of days with MEE than female infants, even after controlling for confounding variables, but the differences were not large. Supporting a greater predilection for the disease in boys, and also suggesting greater severity in boys, are the facts that boys have predominated in most reported studies of the treatment of otitis media, and, compared with girls, consistently had higher rates of operations aimed at relieving the effects or reducing the occurrence of otitis media, namely, tympanostomy tube insertion, tympanoplasty, and adenoidectomy.

RACE. Otitis media is especially prevalent and severe among Native American, Inuit, and Indigenous Australian children. Studies comparing the occurrence of otitis media in white children and black children have given conflicting results: Most of the studies have reported higher rates in white children. However, in the Pittsburgh study, at the practice sites that included substantial numbers of both black infants and white infants, the cumulative proportion of days with MEE during the first year of life was higher in black infants; during the second year of life the values in black and in white infants were identical. Overall, findings suggesting race-based differences in occurrence rates seem most likely attributable to differences in socioeconomic status and related factors, in access to or utilization of care, in intensity of surveillance or accuracy of diagnosis, or to combinations of these factors.

GENETIC BACKGROUND. That middle-ear disease tends to "run in families" is a commonplace observation, and a number of studies have suggested that otitis media has a heritable component. The strongest supporting evidence to date is provided by the finding that the degree of concordance for the occurrence of otitis media is much greater among monozygotic than among dizygotic twins.

SOCIOECONOMIC STATUS. Poverty has long been considered an important contributing factor to both the development and the severity of otitis media. Although study results in the past have been divided on whether associations exist, recent evidence suggests strongly that low socioeconomic status is one of the most important, if not the most important, identifiable risk factor for the disease. Various component elements contributing to this relationship can be surmised to include crowding, limited hygienic facilities, suboptimal nutritional status, limited access to medical care, and limited resources for complying with prescribed medical regimens.

BREAST MILK VS FORMULA FEEDING. Most studies examining this question have found a protective effect of breast milk feeding against otitis media. The effect is probably limited at best, but may be greater in socioeconomically disadvantaged than in more advantaged children. That the protective effect is attributable to the milk itself rather than to the mechanics of breastfeeding was shown in a study of infants with cleft palate to whom all feeding—whether of breast milk or formula—was delivered via an artificial, compressible nurser.

EXPOSURE TO TOBACCO SMOKE. A positive relation between the occurrence of otitis media and household exposure to tobacco smoke has been found in some studies but not others. In these studies generally, measures used to estimate the degree of exposure have been problematic. Additionally, because household smoking correlates inversely with socioeconomic status, possible confounding by socioeconomic factors further complicates valid assessment of risk. Despite the uncertainty, it seems prudent at present to include exposure to tobacco smoke on the list of accepted risk factors.

EXPOSURE TO OTHER CHILDREN. Many studies have established that a strong, positive relationship exists between the occurrence of otitis media and the extent of repeated exposure to other children—measured mainly by the number of other children involved—whether at home or in out-of-home group daycare. Together, but independently, family socioeconomic status and the extent of exposure to other children appear to constitute the two most important identifiable risk factors for developing otitis media.

SEASON. In temperate climates, in keeping with the pattern of occurrence of upper respiratory tract infections in general, highest rates of occurrence of otitis media are observed during cold weather months and lowest rates during the heat of summer.

CONGENITAL ANOMALIES. Otitis media is virtually universal among infants with unrepaired palatal clefts, and is also highly prevalent among children with submucous cleft palate, other craniofacial anomalies, and Down syndrome. The presence of submucous cleft palate should be suspected in children with hypernasal speech, a bifid uvula, or a history of nasal regurgitation during feeding.

OTHER FACTORS. A reported study suggesting that restricting pacifier use results in a reduction in the occurrence of otitis media cannot be considered conclusive. Neither maternal age nor birthweight nor season of birth appears to influence the occurrence of otitis media once other demographic factors are taken into account.

Etiology

ACUTE OTITIS MEDIA. Pathogenic bacteria can be isolated from middle-ear exudate in approximately 65–75% of cases of well-documented AOM; in the remaining cases bacterial culture shows either no growth or the presence of organisms generally considered nonpathogenic. Three pathogens predominate: *Streptococcus pneumoniae* is found in approximately 40% of cases, nontypable *Haemophilus influenzae* in approximately 25–30%, and *Moraxella catarrhalis* in approximately 10–15%.

Other pathogens that, together, account for approximately 5% of cases include group A *Streptococcus, Staphylococcus aureus,* and Gram-negative organisms such as *Pseudomonas aeruginosa. S. aureus* and Gram-negative organisms are found most commonly in neonates and very young infants who are hospitalized; in outpatient settings, the distribution of pathogens in these young infants is similar to that in older infants. Evidence suggests that *H. influenzae* more commonly causes recurrent episodes than initial episodes of AOM.

Respiratory viruses (or virus-derived RNA) may also be found in middle-ear exudates of children with AOM, either alone or, more commonly, in association with pathogenic bacteria. Of these viruses, rhinovirus and respiratory syncytial virus (RSV) are found most often. AOM is a usual complication in children who develop bronchiolitis; however, middle-ear aspirates in such children regularly contain bacterial pathogens, suggesting that RSV is rarely, if ever, the sole cause of their AOM. It remains uncertain whether viruses alone can cause AOM under any circumstances, or whether, as discussed earlier, their role is limited to setting the stage for bacterial invasion, and perhaps also to amplifying the inflammatory process and interfering with resolution of the bacterial infection. Finally, it is possible that, in cases of AOM from which bacterial pathogens cannot be recovered, pathogens had nonetheless been present initially but were rendered nonviable as a result of host reaction, or were lost because of problems in collection, handling, or laboratory methods.

OTITIS MEDIA WITH EFFUSION. Middle-ear fluid cultures from children with OME are usually sterile, but the pathogens typically found in AOM are recoverable also in approximately 30% of children with OME. In addition, in various studies of children with OME involving polymerase chain reaction (PCR) assay, middle-ear fluids have been found to contain bacterial DNA and/or viral RNA in much larger proportions of the children. In studies using special techniques, *Chlamydia pneumoniae* and *Alloiococcus otitidis* have also been identified in the effusions of children with OME. The significance of these various positive identifications is debatable; it is not clear that the organisms or materials found are indicative of actual current or past infection.

Pathogenesis. AOM is usually caused by bacterial pathogens and may also be caused by viruses. However, central to an understanding of how otitis media develops is consideration of the eustachian tube. Under usual circumstances the tube is passively closed and is opened by contraction of the tensor veli palatini muscle. In relation to the middle ear, the tube appears to have three main functions: ventilation, protection, and clearance. The most important appears to be ventilation. The middle-ear mucosa depends on a continuing supply of air from the nasopharynx delivered by way of the eustachian tube. Interruption of this ventilatory process by tubal obstruction initiates a complex inflammatory response that includes secretory metaplasia, compromise of the mucociliary transport system, and effusion of liquid into the tympanic cavity. Impaired middle-ear ventilation probably underlies all cases of OME and at least contributes to the development of most cases of AOM. Whether middle-ear infection, as distinct from sterile inflammation, can develop in the absence of pre-existing eustachian tube obstruction is uncertain; if so, the infection would undoubtedly lead quickly to tubal obstruction as a consequence of both inflammatory edema and the accumulation of middle-ear secretions.

It seems likely that tubal obstruction might result in a number of ways: extraluminally, from hypertrophied nasopharyngeal lymphoid tissue, or tumor; or intraluminally, from inflammatory edema of the tubal mucosa, most commonly as a consequence of upper respiratory tract infection; or intramurally, from impairment of the opening mechanism of the tube, attributable in turn to abnormal tubal muscular function, or excessive tubal wall compliance, or both. Progressive reduction in tubal wall compliance with increasing age may help explain the progressive decline in the occurrence of otitis media as children grow older. The protection and clearance functions of the eustachian tube may also be involved in the pathogenesis of otitis media. Thus, if the tubes are patulous or excessively compliant, they may fail to protect the middle ear from reflux of infective nasopharyngeal secretions, whereas impairment of the mucociliary clearance function of the tube might contribute to both the establishment and persistence of infection. The shorter and more horizontal orientation of the tube in infants and young children may increase the likelihood of reflux from the nasopharynx, but on the other hand may facilitate the ventilatory function of the tube.

Although otitis media may develop and certainly may persist in the absence of apparent respiratory tract infection, many if not most episodes are initiated by viral or bacterial upper respiratory tract infection. In a study of children in group daycare, AOM was observed in approximately 30–40% of children with respiratory illness caused by RSV, influenza viruses, or adenoviruses, and in approximately 10–15% of children with respiratory illness caused by parainfluenza viruses, rhinoviruses, or enteroviruses. Viral infection of the upper respiratory tract results in release of cytokines and inflammatory mediators, some of which may cause eustachian tubal dysfunction. Respiratory viruses also may enhance nasopharyngeal bacterial colonization and adherence and impair host immune defenses against bacterial infection. In children with bacterial infection of the middle ear, evidence is mixed as to whether viruses, if present, may amplify the inflammatory process or interfere with resolution of the infection.

IgA deficiency is found in some children with recurrent AOM but the significance is questionable, inasmuch as IgA deficiency is also found not infrequently in children without recurrent AOM. Selective IgG subclass deficiencies (despite normal total serum IgG) may be found in children with recurrent AOM in association with recurrent sinopulmonary infection, which probably underlie the susceptibility to infection. Children with recurrent otitis media that is not associated with recurrent infection at other sites rarely have a readily identifiable immunologic deficiency. Nonetheless, evidence that subtle immune deficits play a role in the pathogenesis of recurrent AOM is provided by studies involving antibody responses to various types of infection and immunization; by the observation that breast milk feeding, as opposed to formula feeding, confers limited protection against the occurrence of otitis media in infants with cleft palate; and by studies in which young children with recurrent AOM achieved a measure of protection from intramuscularly administered bacterial polysaccharide immune globulin or intravenously administered polyclonal immunoglobulin.

In children with cleft palate, the main factor underlying the chronic middle-ear inflammation appears to be impairment of the opening mechanism of the eustachian tube, due perhaps to greater-than-normal compliance of the tubal wall. Another possible factor is defective velopharyngeal valving, which may result in disturbed aerodynamic and hydrodynamic relationships in the nasopharynx and proximal portions of the eustachian tubes. Finally, as noted earlier, infection and related immunologic factors appear to play a role. In children with other craniofacial anomalies and with Down syndrome, the high prevalence of otitis media is presumably attributable to structural and/or functional eustachian tubal abnormalities. No convincing evidence exists that respiratory allergy plays a role in the pathogenesis of otitis media; however, in children with both conditions it seems possible that the otitis is aggravated by the allergy.

Clinical Manifestations. Symptoms and signs of AOM are highly variable, especially in infants and young children. There may be rupture of the tympanic membrane with purulent otorrhea, or

evidence of ear pain, often manifested by holding or tugging at the ear, or fever, irritability, or other systemic symptoms, or there may be no symptoms, the disease having been discovered at a routine health examination. OME is usually not accompanied by apparent symptoms, and the associated conductive hearing loss usually goes undetected, especially in younger children. Older children may complain of mild discomfort or a sense of fullness in the ear. Also see Chapter 626.

EXAMINATION OF THE EARDRUM

Otoscopy. For clinicians other than otolaryngologists, who may use an operating microscope, the eardrum is ordinarily viewed by means of an otoscope. Two types of otoscope heads are available: **surgical or operating**, and **diagnostic or pneumatic** (Fig. 630–1). The surgical head embodies a lens that can swivel over a wide arc and an unenclosed light source, thus providing ready access of the examiner's instruments to the external auditory canal and tympanic membrane. A suitable instrument is the Welch Allyn (Skaneateles Falls, NY) model 21700. Use of the surgical head is optimal for removing cerumen or debris from the canal under direct observation, and is necessary for satisfactorily performing tympanocentesis or myringotomy. The diagnostic head incorporates a larger lens, an enclosed light source, and a nipple for the attachment of a rubber bulb and tubing. When an attached speculum is fitted snugly into the external auditory canal, an airtight chamber is created comprising the vault of the otoscope head, the bulb and tubing, the speculum, and the proximal portion of the external canal. A suitable instrument is the Welch Allyn model 20200. Reusable specula such as those supplied with the otoscope afford less discomfort to the patient than thinner, sharper-edged disposable specula, and using a rubber-tipped speculum or adding a small sleeve of rubber tubing to the tip of the plastic speculum may serve to minimize patient discomfort and enhance the ability to achieve a proper fit and an airtight seal. By observing as the bulb is alternately squeezed gently and released, the degree of tympanic membrane mobility in response to both positive and negative pressure can be estimated. With both types of otoscope heads, bright illumination is critical to adequate visualization of the tympanic membrane.

Clearing the External Auditory Canal. If the tympanic membrane is obscured by cerumen, the cerumen may be removed under direct observation through the surgical head of

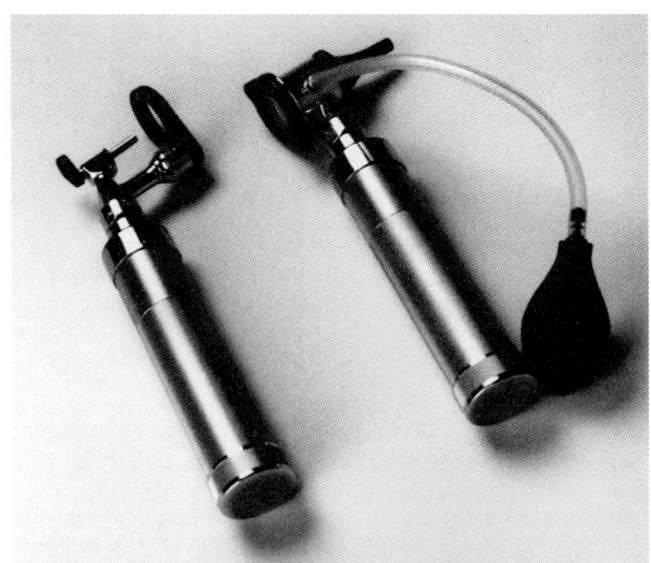

FIGURE 630–1. Otoscope types. *Left:* Otoscope embodying surgical or operating head. *Right:* Otoscope embodying diagnostic head, with rubber bulb attachment for pneumatic otoscopy.

the otoscope, using a Buck curette (N-400-0, Storz Instrument Co) (Fig. 630–2). Remaining bits can then be wiped away using a Farrell applicator (N-2001A, Storz Instrument Co) (Fig. 630–2), with its tip (triangular in cross section) wrapped with a bit of dry or alcohol-moistened cotton to create a dry or wet "mop." Alternatively, gentle suction may be applied, using a No. 7 French ear suction tube. During this procedure it may be most advantageous to restrain the infant or young child in the prone position, turning the child's head to the left or right as each ear is cleared. One adult, usually a parent, can place one hand on each of the child's buttocks and brace the child's hips against the examining table, using his or her own weight for additional bracing if necessary. Another adult can restrain the child's head with one hand and the child's free arm with the other, changing hands for the opposite ear. In children old enough to cooperate, usually beginning at about 5 yr of age, clearing of the external canal can often be achieved more easily and safely and less traumatically by lavage than by mechanical removal, provided one can be certain that a tympanic membrane perforation is not present. A convenient device for accomplishing lavage is the Welch-Allyn Ear Wash System (Model 29300).

Tympanic Membrane Findings. Important characteristics of the tympanic membrane consist of contour, color, translucence, structural changes if any, and mobility. Normally the contour of the membrane is **slightly concave**; abnormalities consist of fullness or bulging, or conversely, extreme retraction. The normal color of the tympanic membrane is **pearly gray**. Erythema may be a sign of inflammation, but unless intense, erythema alone may result from crying or vascular flushing. Abnormal whiteness of the membrane may result from either scarring or the presence of liquid in the middle-ear cavity; liquid also may impart an amber, pale yellow, or (rarely) bluish color. Normally, the membrane is translucent, although some degree of opacity may be normal in the first few months of life; later, opacification denotes either scarring, or more commonly, underlying effusion. Structural changes include scars, perforations, and retraction pockets. Of all the visible characteristics of the tympanic

membrane, mobility is the most sensitive and specific in determining the presence or absence of MEE. Importantly, mobility is not an all-or-none phenomenon; although total absence of mobility (in the absence of a tympanic membrane perforation) is virtually always indicative of MEE, substantial impairment of mobility is the more common finding.

Diagnosis. Distinguishing between AOM and OME on clinical grounds is straightforward in most cases, but because each condition may evolve into the other without any clearly differentiating physical findings, any schema for distinguishing between them is to some extent arbitrary. Nonetheless, in an era of increasing bacterial resistance, distinguishing between AOM and OME has become increasingly important in determining treatment. Obviously, purulent otorrhea of recent onset is indicative of AOM; thus, difficulty in distinguishing clinically between AOM and OME is limited to circumstances in which purulent otorrhea is not present. Both AOM without otorrhea and OME are accompanied by physical signs of MEE, namely, the presence of at least two of three tympanic membrane abnormalities: white, yellow, amber, or (rarely) blue discoloration; opacification other than that due to scarring; and decreased or absent mobility. Alternatively in OME, either air-fluid levels or air bubbles outlined by small amounts of fluid may be visible behind the tympanic membrane, a condition often indicative of impending resolution.

To support a diagnosis of AOM in a child with MEE, distinct fullness or bulging of the tympanic membrane should also be present, with or without accompanying erythema, or, at minimum, MEE should be accompanied by ear pain that appears clinically important. Unless intense, erythema alone is insufficient; erythema without other abnormalities may result from crying or vascular flushing. The malleus may be obscured, and the tympanic membrane may resemble a bagel without a hole but with a central depression (Fig. 630–3), or may be obscured by surface bullae, or may have a cobblestone appearance. **Bullous myringitis** is a physical manifestation of AOM and not an etiologically discrete entity. Within days after onset, fullness

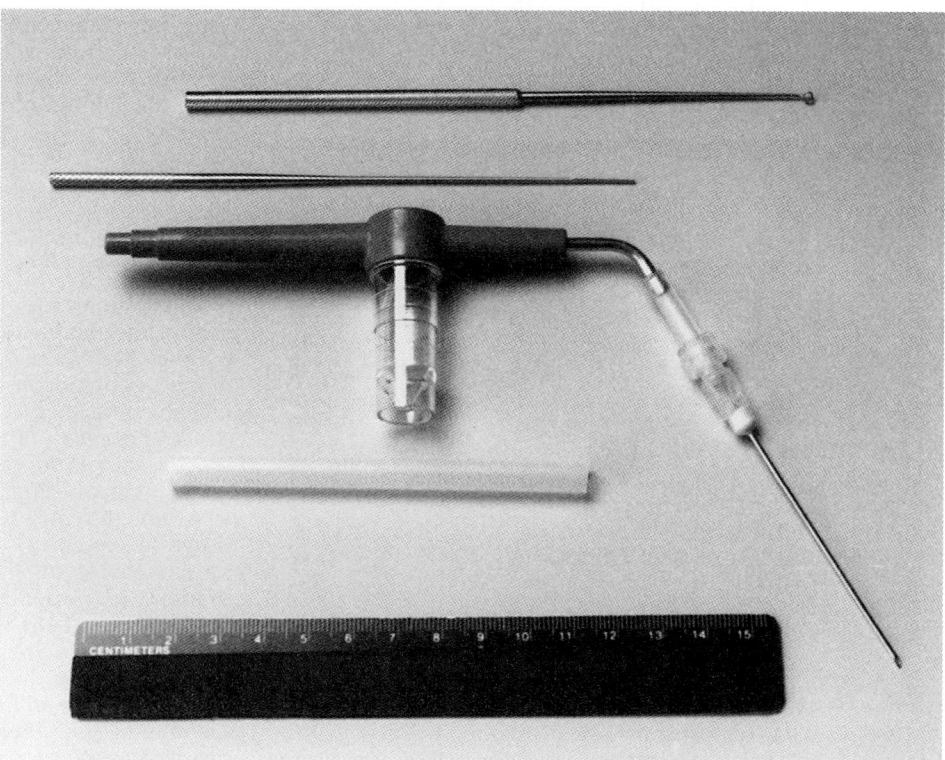

FIGURE 630–2. *Top:* Buck curette. Note the narrow caliber of the metal forming the end loop. *Center:* Farrell applicator. Its tip is triangular in cross-section. *Bottom:* Tympanocentesis aspirator.

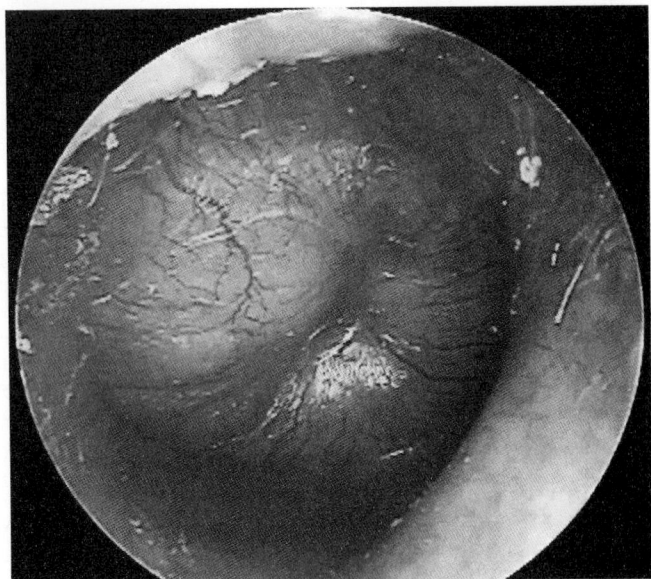

FIGURE 630–3. Tympanic membrane in acute otitis media (AOM). See also color plates.

of the membrane may diminish, even though infection may still be present. Exceptionally, early in the course of AOM, effusion may not yet have become evident, in which case ear pain and intense erythema of the tympanic membrane are the only localizing clinical manifestations.

In OME, fullness of the tympanic membrane is absent or slight or the membrane may be retracted (Fig. 630–4); erythema also is absent or slight, but may increase with crying or with superficial trauma to the external auditory canal incurred in clearing the canal of cerumen or during otoscopic examination. In children with MEE but without tympanic membrane fullness or bulging, the presence of unequivocal ear pain is usually indicative of AOM, but a diagnosis of AOM is not justified by the associated presence of only nonspecific symptoms such as fever, irritability, anorexia, vomiting, and diarrhea. A simplified differentiating schema calls for a diagnosis of AOM when, in addition to having MEE, a child gives evidence of recent, clinically important ear pain or the tympanic membrane shows marked redness or distinct fullness or bulging (Fig. 630–5).

Commonly, both before and after episodes of otitis media and also in the absence of otitis media, the tympanic membrane may be retracted as a consequence of negative middle-ear air pressure. Presumably, the cause is more rapid diffusion of air from the middle-ear cavity than its replacement via the eustachian tube. Mild retraction cannot be considered pathologic, although in some children it is accompanied by mild conductive hearing loss. More extreme retraction, however, is of concern, as discussed later in the section on sequelae of otitis media.

TYMPANOMETRY. Tympanometry, also termed **acoustic immittance testing**, is a simple, rapid, atraumatic test that offers objective evidence of the presence or absence of MEE. The tympanogram provides information about tympanic membrane compliance in electroacoustic terms that can be thought of as roughly equivalent to tympanic membrane mobility as perceived visually during pneumatic otoscopy. The test depends on the facts that the absorption of sound by the tympanic membrane varies inversely with its stiffness and that the stiffness of the membrane is least, and accordingly its compliance is greatest, when the air pressures impinging on each of its surfaces—middle-ear air pressure and external canal air pressure—are equal. Anything tending to stiffen the tympanic membrane—for example, stretching (if the pressures on the two surfaces become unequal), scarring (of either the membrane or its attachments), or an accumulation of middle-ear liquid—increases its acoustic impedance, or stated reciprocally, reduces its acoustic **admittance**, which was formerly termed **compliance**.

Tympanograms may be grouped into one of three categories:

1. Tracings characterized by high admittance (measured by the height of the peak), relatively steep gradient (i.e., sharp-angled peak), and middle-ear air pressure (location of the peak in terms of air pressure) that approximates atmospheric pressure (Fig. 630–6A). Such tracings are generally assumed to indicate normal middle-ear status.

2. Tracings characterized by low admittance and by negative or indeterminate middle-ear air pressure, and often termed *flat* (Fig. 630–6B). Such tracings are generally assumed to indicate the presence of a middle-ear abnormality that is causing heightened impedance. By far the most common such abnormality in infants and children is MEE.

3. Tracings characterized by intermediate findings—somewhat low admittance, often in association with a gradual gradient (obtuse-angled peak) or negative middle-ear air pressure, or combinations of these features (Fig. 630–6C). Such tracings may or may not be associated with MEE, and must be considered nondiagnostic or equivocal. In general, the lower the admittance, the more gradual the gradient, and the more negative the middle-ear air pressure, the greater the likelihood of MEE.

In addition to providing information concerning middle-ear status, the tympanometer also measures and records the volume of the external auditory canal, and if a tympanic membrane perforation or a patent tympanostomy tube is present, the volume of the middle ear and mastoid air cells as well. A volume reading in excess of 1.0 mL, particularly if associated with a flat tracing, should suggest the presence of either a perforation or a patent tympanostomy tube.

Although tympanometry is quite sensitive in detecting MEE, its positive predictive value is limited. Accordingly, abnormal or questionable tympanograms are not infrequently found in association with normal middle-ear status, especially in infants. On the other hand, the tympanogram is sometimes normal early in the course of AOM. Use of tympanometry may be helpful in office screening, by obviating the need for routine otoscopic examination in difficult-to-examine patients whose tympanic membranes have been visualized previously, who are asymptomatic, and whose tympanograms are classified as normal, and

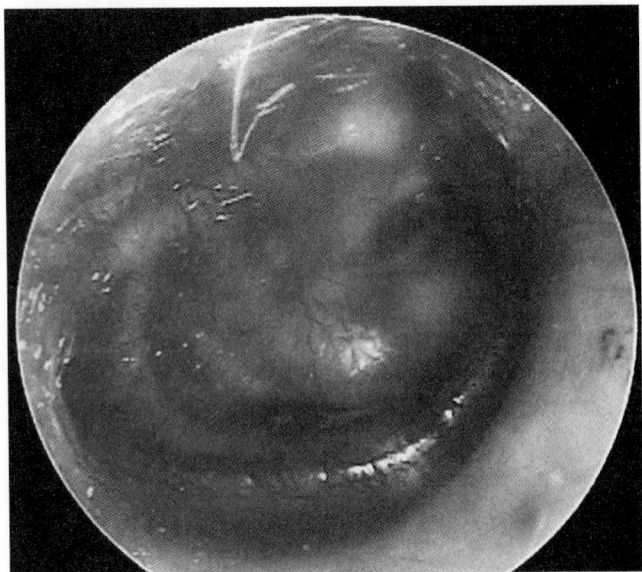

FIGURE 630–4. Tympanic membrane in otitis media with effusion (OME). See also color plates.

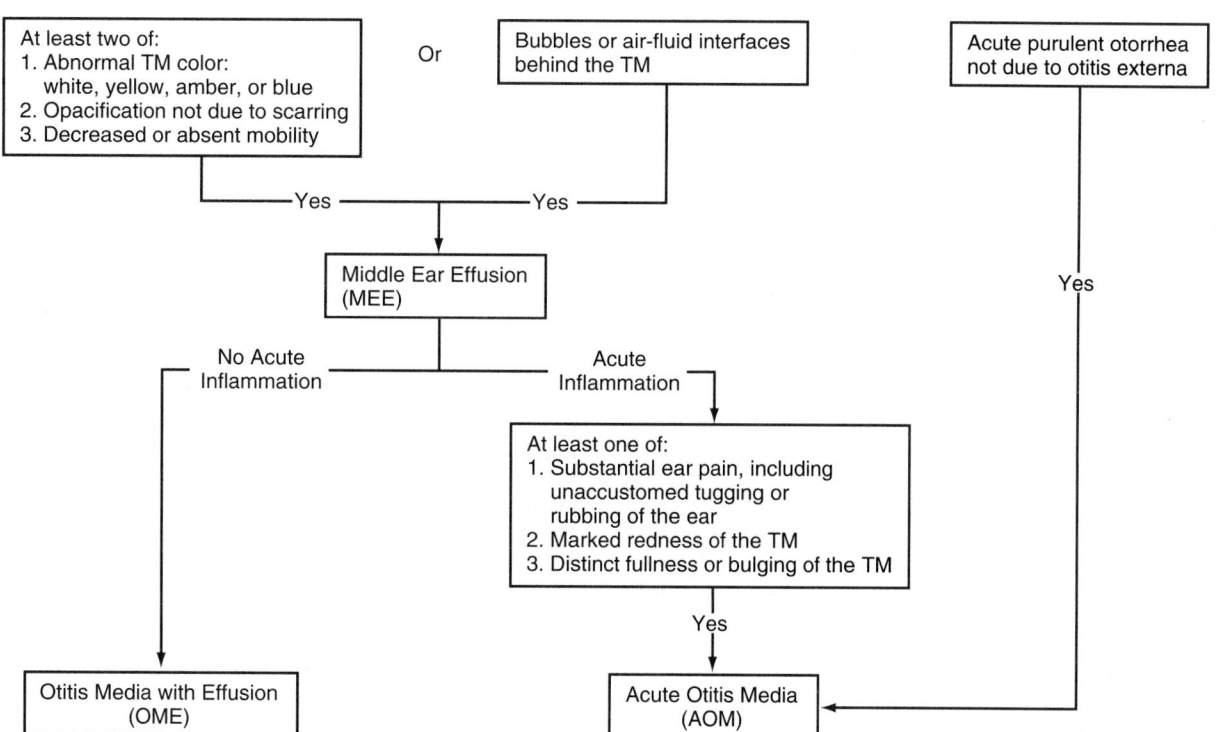

FIGURE 630–5. Algorithm for distinguishing between acute otitis media (AOM) and otitis media with effusion (OME). (TM = tympanic membrane.)

by identifying patients who require further attention because their tympanograms are abnormal. Tympanometry also may be used to help confirm, refine, or clarify questionable otoscopic findings; to objectify the follow-up evaluation of patients with known middle-ear disease; and to serve as validators (or invalidators) of otoscopic diagnoses of MEE. Importantly, even though tympanometry can predict the probability of MEE, it cannot distinguish the effusion of OME from that of AOM.

SPECTRAL GRADIENT ACOUSTIC REFLECTOMETRY (SGAR). Reflectometry is a more newly developed acoustic test that estimates the condition of the middle ear by assessing the response of the tympanic membrane to a sound stimulus (also see Chapter 627). The instrument analyzes the reflectance of sound waves with respect to frequency and presents results as spectral gradient angles that correlate with the likelihood that MEE is present. An angle of greater than 95 degrees indicates a low risk of

MEE, and an angle of less than 49 degrees indicates a high risk of MEE. The instrument is small and portable, and gives readings rapidly. However, the information provided concerning middle-ear status is more limited than that provided by tympanometry. Results regarding the accuracy of reflectometry as compared with that of tympanometry in predicting the presence or absence of MEE have been mixed. As in the case of tympanometry, SGAR cannot distinguish the effusion of OME from that of AOM.

Treatment. The management of otitis media is based on the diagnosis of the illness as either AOM or OME.

MANAGEMENT OF ACUTE OTITIS MEDIA. Individual episodes of AOM have customarily been treated with antimicrobial drugs. However, concern about increases in bacterial resistance has prompted some authors to recommend withholding antimicrobial treatment in some or most cases unless

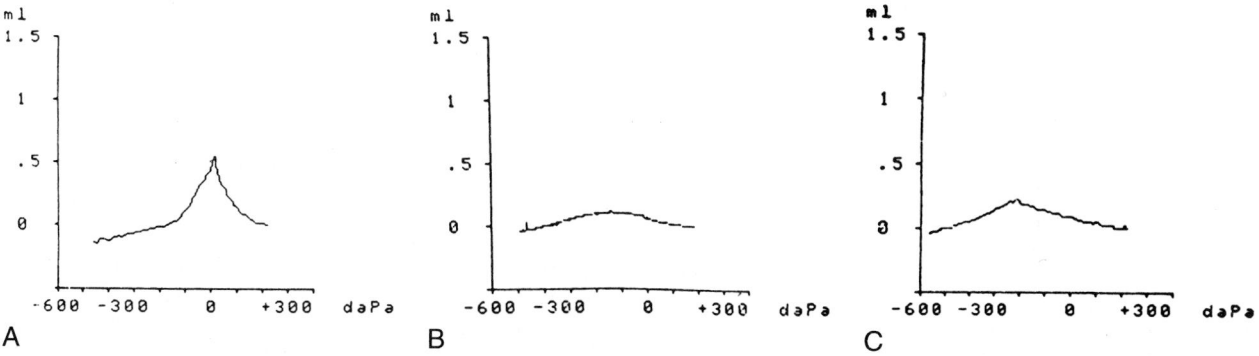

FIGURE 630–6. Tympanograms obtained with a Grason-Stadler GSI 33 Middle Ear Analyzer, exhibiting *(A)* high admittance, steep gradient (i.e., sharp-angled peak), and middle ear air pressure approximating atmospheric pressure (zero decaPascals [daPa]); *(B)* low admittance and indeterminate middle-ear air pressure; and *(C)* somewhat low admittance, gradual gradient, and markedly negative middle-ear air pressure.

symptoms persist for 2 or 3 days, or worsen. This recommendation must be viewed in light of the fact that much of the use of antimicrobials for otitis media has been directed not at treating individual episodes of AOM but, instead, at treating OME or at attempting to prevent recurrent episodes of AOM. Avoidance of inappropriate antimicrobial use for these latter purposes should go far toward reducing antimicrobial use for otitis media generally.

Three factors argue in favor of routinely treating children who have bona fide AOM with an antimicrobial drug. First, pathogenic bacteria cause a large majority of cases. Second, symptomatic improvement and resolution of infection occur more promptly and more consistently with antimicrobial treatment than without (even though most untreated cases eventually also resolve). Third, prompt and adequate antimicrobial treatment may prevent the development of suppurative complications. The sharp decline in such complications during the last half-century seems likely attributable, at least in part, to the widespread routine use of antimicrobials for AOM. In the Netherlands, where initial antibiotic treatment is routinely withheld from most children older than 6 mo of age, and where only approximately 30% of children with AOM currently receive antibiotics at all, the incidence of acute mastoiditis, although low (in children < 14 yr, 3.8 per 100,000 person years), is substantially higher than rates in the United States and in many other countries with higher antibiotic prescription rates. It is also the case that follow-up of children in the Netherlands is generally more assiduous than is customary in the United States, where failure to improve or worsening might not be detected as promptly. Accordingly, it seems advisable to continue the present policy of routine antimicrobial treatment for AOM. In particular, antimicrobials should not be withheld initially from children with AOM who are younger than 2 yr of age, or who are ill systemically or appear to have severe infections, or who have recent histories of recurrent AOM, or in whom satisfactory follow-up cannot be assured. Admittedly, the policy of withholding treatment initially in milder cases in children at lower risk will deserve further consideration if the prevalence of bacterial resistance continues to escalate.

Bacterial Resistance. Bacteria have a remarkable ability to develop resistance to antimicrobial drugs. Adaptive mechanisms include mutations in their β-lactamases that enable these enzymes to inactivate new β-lactam drugs, development of an intracellular pump that removes antibiotics before they can act upon the bacteria, changes in their cell wall proteins that serve to keep antibiotics out, and development of substitute proteins that are not targeted by antibiotics. Bacterial resistance in general has been an increasing problem in the past decade. Children at greatest risk of harboring resistant bacteria are those who are younger than 2 yr of age, in regular contact with large groups of other children, or have recently received antimicrobial treatment. Bacterial resistance is a problem in relation particularly to otitis media on two counts. First, both the development of resistant bacterial strains and their rapid spread have been fostered and facilitated by selective pressure resulting from extensive use of antimicrobial drugs, the most common target of which, in children, is otitis media. Second, many strains of each of the pathogenic bacteria that commonly cause AOM are resistant to certain commonly used antimicrobial drugs.

Currently, approximately 40% of strains of nontypable *H. influenzae* and almost all strains of *M. catarrhalis* are resistant to aminopenicillins (ampicillin and amoxicillin). In most cases the resistance is attributable to production of β-lactamase, and can be overcome by combining amoxicillin with a β-lactamase inhibitor, namely, clavulanate, or by using a β-lactamase-stable antibiotic such as cefixime. However, occasional strains of nontypable *H. influenzae* that do not produce β-lactamase are resistant to aminopenicillins and other β-lactam antibiotics by virtue of alterations in their penicillin-binding proteins.

Currently also, approximately 50% of strains of *S. pneumoniae* are penicillin-nonsusceptible, divided approximately equally between penicillin-intermediate and penicillin-resistant strains. Resistance by *S. pneumoniae* to the penicillins and other β-lactam antibiotics is mediated not by β-lactamase production, but by alterations in penicillin-binding proteins. There are at least six known penicillin-binding proteins, and the greater the number of alterations in these proteins the greater the degree of resistance. This mechanism of resistance can be overcome, however, if higher concentrations of β-lactam antibiotics at the site of infection can be achieved for a sufficient time interval. Many penicillin-resistant strains of *S. pneumoniae* are also resistant to other antimicrobial drugs, including sulfonamides, macrolides, and the newer cephalosporins. In general, as penicillin resistance increases, so also does resistance to other antimicrobial classes. Resistance to macrolides by *S. pneumoniae* has been increasing rapidly; approximately 30% of strains are currently macrolide-resistant. Two mechanisms of macrolide resistance have been identified: one, mediated by the mef(A) gene, involves an efflux pump that decreases intracellular accumulation of macrolides and results in low-level resistance; the other mechanism, mediated by the erm(B) gene, involves production of ribosomal methylases that modify ribosomal RNA and result in high-level resistance. The latter mechanism also results in resistance to clindamycin, which otherwise is generally effective against resistant strains of *S. pneumoniae*. Unlike resistance to β-lactam antibiotics, macrolide resistance cannot be overcome by increasing the dose. Currently, the only antimicrobial to which resistance by *S. pneumoniae* has not been reported is vancomycin.

First-Line Antimicrobial Treatment. Currently, amoxicillin remains the drug of first choice for uncomplicated AOM under most circumstances because of its excellent record of safety, relative efficacy, palatability, and low cost. In particular, amoxicillin is the most efficacious of available oral antimicrobial drugs against both penicillin-susceptible and penicillin-nonsusceptible strains of *S. pneumoniae*. Increasing the dose from the traditional 40 mg/kg/24 hr to 80–100 mg/kg/24 hr will generally provide efficacy against penicillin-intermediate and some penicillin-resistant strains. This higher dose should be used particularly in children younger than 2 yr old, in children who have recently received treatment with β-lactam drugs, and in children who are exposed to large numbers of other children, because, as noted earlier, it is in these children that the prevalence of nonsusceptible strains of *S. pneumoniae* is highest. A limitation of amoxicillin is that it may be inactivated by the β-lactamases produced by many strains of nontypable *H. influenzae* and most strains of *M. catarrhalis*. Fortunately, episodes of AOM caused by these pathogens often, although by no means always, resolve spontaneously. For children who are allergic to β-lactams, or in whom palatability or convenience of administration are of overriding importance, azithromycin, which also has an excellent safety record, is an appropriate alternative first-line drug. Resistance to trimethoprim-sulfamethoxazole (TMP-SMZ) by many strains of both *H. influenzae* and *S. pneumoniae* and a reported high clinical failure rate in children with AOM treated initially with TMP-SMZ argue against its use as first-line treatment.

Duration of Treatment. The duration of treatment of AOM has often been set at 10 days, in an apparent extrapolation from the optimal duration of treatment of streptococcal pharyngitis with penicillin. However, 10 days may be unduly long for some children while not long enough for others. Studies comparing shorter with longer durations of treatment suggest that short-course treatment will often prove inadequate in children younger than 6 yr of age, and particularly in children younger than 2 yr. Thus, for most episodes in most children, treatment that provides tissue concentrations of an antimicrobial for at least 10 days would seem advisable. Treatment for shorter periods, of 3–5 days, may be appropriate for older children with mild episodes who improve quickly, whereas treatment for longer than 10 days will often be required for children who are very young or are having severe episodes or whose previous experience with otitis media has been problematic.

Follow-Up. The principal goals of follow-up are to assess the outcome of treatment and to differentiate between inadequate response to treatment and early recurrence. Accordingly, the appropriate interval for follow-up should be individualized. Follow-up within days is advisable in the young infant with a severe episode or in a child of any age with continuing pain. Follow-up within 2 wk is appropriate for the infant or young child who has apparently been having frequent recurrences. At that point, the tympanic membrane is not likely to have returned to normal, but substantial improvement in its appearance should be evident. In the child with only a sporadic episode of AOM and prompt symptomatic improvement, follow-up 1 mo after initial examination is early enough, or in older children, no follow-up may be necessary. Importantly, the continuing presence of MEE alone following an episode of AOM is not an indication for additional or second-line antimicrobial treatment.

Unsatisfactory Response to First-Line Treatment. AOM is essentially a closed-space infection and its resolution depends both on eradication of the offending organism and restoration of middle-ear ventilation. Factors contributing to unsatisfactory response to first-line treatment, in addition to inadequate antimicrobial efficacy, include poor compliance with treatment regimens, concurrent or intercurrent viral infection, persistent eustachian tube dysfunction and middle-ear under-aeration, reinfection from other sites or from outside sources, and immature or impaired host defenses. Despite these many potential factors, switching to an alternative or second-line drug would seem reasonable when there has been inadequate improvement in symptoms or in middle-ear status as reflected in the appearance of the tympanic membrane, or when the persistence of purulent nasal discharge suggests that the antimicrobial drug being used has less than optimal efficacy. Second-line drugs may also appropriately be used when AOM develops in a child already receiving antimicrobial prophylaxis, or in an immunocompromised child, or in a child with severe symptoms whose previous experience with otitis media has been problematic.

Second-Line Treatment. When treatment of AOM with a first-line antimicrobial drug has proven inadequate, a number of second-line alternatives are available. As recently emphasized by the Drug-resistant *Streptococcus pneumoniae* Therapeutic Working Group of the U.S. Centers for Disease Control and Prevention (CDC), drugs chosen for second-line treatment should be effective against β-lactamase-producing strains of *H. influenzae* and *M. catarrhalis* and against susceptible and most nonsusceptible strains of *S. pneumoniae*. Based on available evidence, the CDC Working Group concluded that only three drugs had been clearly shown to meet that requirement: amoxicillin-clavulanate, cefuroxime axetil, and intramuscular ceftriaxone. Because high-dose amoxicillin is effective against most strains of *S. pneumoniae* and because the addition of clavulanate extends the effective antibacterial spectrum of amoxicillin to include β-lactamase-producing bacteria, high-dose amoxicillin-clavulanate is particularly well-suited as a second-line drug for treating AOM. The 14:1 amoxicillin-clavulanate formulation contains twice as much amoxicillin as the previously available 7:1 formulation. Diarrhea, especially in infants and young children, is a common adverse effect, but may perhaps be ameliorated in some cases by feeding yogurt, and usually is not severe enough to require cessation of treatment. Unfortunately, amoxicillin-clavulanate is quite expensive. The two other drugs identified by the CDC Working Group have important limitations for use in young children. The currently available suspension of cefuroxime axetil is not palatable and its acceptance is low. Ceftriaxone treatment entails both the pain of intramuscular injection and substantial cost, and the injection may need to be repeated once or twice at 2- or 3-day intervals to achieve the desired degree of effectiveness. Nonetheless, use of ceftriaxone is appropriate in severe cases of

AOM when oral treatment is not feasible, or in highly selected cases after treatment failure using orally administered second-line antimicrobials (i.e., amoxicillin-clavulanate or cefuroxime axetil), or when highly resistant *S. pneumoniae* is found in aspirates obtained from diagnostic tympanocentesis.

In cases of treatment failure specifically, the clinical effectiveness of the various available drugs has not been tested in appropriately designed studies. The newer macrolides, clarithromycin and azithromycin, have only limited activity against nonsusceptible strains of *S. pneumoniae* and against β-lactamase-producing strains of *H. influenzae*. Macrolide use also appears to be a major factor in causing increases in rates of resistance to macrolides by group A *Streptococcus* and *S. pneumoniae*. Of the cephalosporins other than cefuroxime axetil, cefpodoxime and cefdinir seem most promising, with antibacterial spectrums similar to those of cefuroxime axetil. The liquid preparation of cefdinir is quite palatable, but that of cefpodoxime is not. Cefprozil possesses somewhat less β-lactamase stability than either cefuroxime or cefpodoxime. Cefaclor and loracarbef have limited activity against β-lactamase-producing bacteria and nonsusceptible pneumococci, and cefaclor may occasionally cause serum sickness. Cefixime has excellent activity against β-lactamase-producing bacteria but limited activity against even penicillin-susceptible pneumococci. All of the cephalosporins are expensive. TMP-SMZ is relatively inexpensive, but its efficacy is limited and its use for treating AOM is not recommended. Additionally, this drug rarely may cause severe reactions such as bone-marrow suppression or Stevens-Johnson syndrome. Erythromycin-sulfisoxazole also may cause such reactions and is not active against penicillin-nonsusceptible pneumococci. Clindamycin is active against most strains of *S. pneumoniae*, including resistant strains, but is not active against *H. influenzae* or *M. catarrhalis*. It should therefore be reserved for patients known to have infection caused by penicillin-nonsusceptible pneumococci.

Because comparative studies of antibiotics in children who have experienced treatment failure are lacking, the choice of drugs to use in such cases should be guided by the limited clinical evidence available concerning the efficacy of individual drugs; by available in vitro, pharmacokinetic, and pharmacodynamic data; and, because bacterial resistance patterns vary geographically, by personal clinical experience.

Myringotomy and Tympanocentesis. Myringotomy is a time-honored treatment for AOM but is rarely necessary in children receiving antimicrobials initially. In a clinical trial limited to children with severe AOM, those who received amoxicillin plus myringotomy fared no better overall than those who received amoxicillin only, but the study population was not large enough to have excluded the possibility that myringotomy had been marginally beneficial. Indications for myringotomy in children with AOM include severe, refractory pain; hyperpyrexia; complications of AOM such as facial paralysis, mastoiditis, labyrinthitis, or central nervous system infection; and immunologic compromise from any source. In children with AOM in whom clinical response to vigorous, second-line treatment has been unsatisfactory, either diagnostic tympanocentesis or myringotomy is indicated to enable identification of the offending organism and its sensitivity profile. Either procedure, but more reliably, myringotomy, may be additionally helpful in effecting relief of pain. Tympanocentesis with culture of the middle-ear aspirate is also indicated as part of the sepsis work-up in very young infants with AOM who show systemic signs of illness such as fever, vomiting, or lethargy, and whose illness accordingly cannot be presumed to be limited to infection of the middle ear. "In an era of increasing antimicrobial resistance," the CDC Working Group wrote, "clinicians treating children with AOM should consider developing the capacity to perform tympanocentesis themselves or establish ready referral mechanisms to a clinician with this capacity." Performing tympanocentesis is much facilitated by use of a specially designed tympanocentesis aspirator (No. 91-19010, Xomed Surgical Products, Jacksonville, FL) (see Fig. 630–2).

Early Recurrence After Treatment. Recurrence of AOM after apparent resolution may be due either to incomplete eradication of infection in the middle ear or upper respiratory tract or to reinfection by the same or a different bacterium or bacterial strain. Recurrence within several days is usually caused by the same organism, and thus treatment may be best guided by the response to treatment of the antecedent episode: if it had seemed to respond to a first-line antimicrobial, that drug would again be appropriate; if it had failed to respond to a first-line drug but seemed to respond to a second-line drug, use of a second-line drug from the outset might be advisable. Recurrence developing 2 wk or more after a treated episode of AOM is usually caused by a different organism; accordingly, use of a first-line antimicrobial irrespective of previous responses to treatment is usually appropriate.

Tube Otorrhea. Otorrhea through a previously inserted tympanostomy tube must be considered evidence of middle-ear infection, although in some cases it may result from reflux of secretions from the nasopharynx via the eustachian tube. When accompanied by pain or fever, tube otorrhea should be treated as described earlier for AOM because the causative organisms tend to be the same as those that cause AOM. However, in many cases, especially those that become persistent, *Pseudomonas aeruginosa* is the main offending pathogen; in such cases the drugs commonly used for AOM are not effective. When tube otorrhea develops without associated pain or fever, ototopical treatment may suffice. Currently, ofloxacin otic solution is the only preparation approved for use in the middle ear because of its lack of ototoxicity. Polymixin B-neomycin-hydrocortisone otic suspension is also relatively effective, but carries a theoretical risk in humans of ototoxicity. Prompt adjunctive treatment of tube otorrhea with a short course of oral prednisolone has recently been reported to result in more rapid resolution. In all cases, attention to aural toilet, that is, cleansing the external auditory canal of secretions, is important. When children with tube otorrhea fail to improve satisfactorily with conventional outpatient management, they may require tube removal, or hospitalization to receive parenteral antibiotic treatment, or both.

MANAGEMENT OF OTITIS MEDIA WITH EFFUSION. To determine the course of an episode of OME, and to distinguish between persistence and recurrence, examination should be conducted monthly until resolution, and hearing should be assessed if effusion has been present for 3 mo or more. Rational management of OME depends in considerable degree on an understanding of its natural history and its possible complications and sequelae. Unfortunately, information in each of these areas is limited. Most cases of OME resolve with or without treatment within 3 mo; however, virtually no data are available concerning the subsequent long-term course of children in whom resolution does not occur within that time frame and who do not receive surgical intervention.

Except in the few children who are troubled by the variable accompanying conductive hearing loss, the occasional mild discomfort, or the unusual tinnitus or disturbance of balance, the main rationale for treating OME is to prevent possible complications and sequelae. These have been thought to include, variously, a heightened risk of developing AOM; pathologic middle-ear changes, namely, atelectasis of the tympanic membrane and retraction pocket, adhesive otitis media, ossicular discontinuity, and cholesteatoma; conductive and sensorineural hearing loss; and long-term adverse effects on speech, language, cognitive, and psychosocial development.

Many uncertainties remain about the extent to which these constitute risks of OME under most circumstances. Physical damage, when it occurs, is more often a consequence of

repeated or chronic infection than of OME. Whether persistent early-life MEE during the first few years of life results in later developmental impairment has been addressed in many studies over more than 3 decades. Specifically at issue has been whether the mild-to-moderate hearing impairment commonly associated with MEE, occurring during supposedly "critical" or "sensitive" developmental periods, leaves in its wake what might be thought of as developmental scars, persisting into later childhood long after both otitis media and hearing loss have been resolved. Impairments of development associated with persistent early-life otitis media have been reported in four domains: speech, language, cognition, and psychosocial development.

Most of the reported studies of developmental outcomes of early-life otitis media have had important limitations, and as a group, their results have been inconclusive and contradictory. Moreover, because of the studies' uniformly associational designs, they have been unsuited to address the question of causality. Results from a more recent study incorporating a randomized clinical trial suggest that in otherwise healthy children, effusion developing at common levels of frequency and duration (e.g., up to 9 mo continuously in both ears) during the first 3 yr of life poses no developmental risks measurable at 3 and 4 yr of age. At present writing, all results in the study children at age 6 yr are not yet available, and few of the children have reached 9 yr of age, when another battery of tests will be administered. Whether adverse developmental consequences will emerge or become apparent at later ages, or whether there are adverse consequences of more prolonged periods of effusion, remains uncertain.

Variables Influencing OME Management Decisions. In deciding whether to intervene in individual cases of OME, and if so, how vigorously, it may be useful to take into account a number of variables. Patient-related variables include the child's age; the frequency and severity of previous episodes of AOM and the interval since the last episode; the child's language development; the presence or absence of a history of adverse drug reactions, concurrent medical problems, or risk factors such as daycare attendance or other exposure to infectious disease; and the parents' wishes. Disease-related variables include whether the effusion is unilateral or bilateral; the apparent quantity of effusion; the duration, if known; the degree of hearing impairment; the presence or absence of other possibly related symptoms, such as tinnitus, vertigo, or disturbance of balance; and the presence or absence of mucopurulent or purulent rhinorrhea, which, if sustained for 2 wk or more, would suggest that concurrent nasopharyngeal or paranasal sinus infection is contributing to continuing compromise of middle-ear ventilation.

Medical Treatment. Antimicrobials have definite but limited efficacy in resolving OME, presumably because they help eradicate nasopharyngeal infection or inapparent middle-ear infection or both. However, mainly because of the short-term nature of their benefit and because of the contribution of antimicrobial usage to the development of bacterial resistance, routine antimicrobial treatment of OME, previously recommended by some authorities, no longer seems reasonable. Instead, treatment should be limited to cases in which there is evidence of associated bacterial upper respiratory tract infection, or in which chronicity and/or troubling hearing loss are prompting consideration of tympanostomy tube insertion. In the latter circumstance, a 2–4-wk course of antimicrobial treatment may bring about resolution of OME and thereby avert surgery. For this purpose, the most broadly effective drug available should be used as recommended for AOM.

The efficacy of corticosteroids in the treatment of OME remains debatable and is probably short-term at best. Antihistamine-decongestant combinations are not effective in treating children in general with OME, but their efficacy has not been tested in allergic children specifically. Antihistamines alone, decongestants alone, and mucolytic agents are unlikely to be effective. Allergic management might prove helpful in children with problematic OME who also have evidence of upper respiratory allergy, but supporting data are lacking. In children without such evidence, allergy testing is not indicated. Inflation of the eustachian tubes by the Valsalva maneuver or other means has no proven long-term efficacy.

Myringotomy and Insertion of Tympanostomy Tubes. When OME persists despite both adequate antimicrobial treatment and an ample period of watchful waiting, the question arises as to surgical intervention. Myringotomy alone, without tympanostomy tube insertion, permits evacuation of middle-ear effusion and may sometimes be effective, but often, because the incision heals before eustachian tube ventilatory function has been restored, effusion soon reaccumulates. Adding tube insertion offers the likelihood that middle-ear ventilation will be sustained for at least as long as the tube remains in place and functional, about 12 mo on average. However, tube placement is not consistently innocuous. Common complications include obstruction of the tube lumen, premature extrusion, and tube otorrhea. Sequelae following tubal extrusion include residual perforation of the eardrum, tympanosclerosis, localized or diffuse atrophic scarring of the eardrum that may predispose to the development of atelectasis or a retraction pocket or both, residual conductive hearing loss, and cholesteatoma. Fortunately, the more serious of these sequelae are the exception rather than the rule. Recurrence of middle-ear effusion following the extrusion of tubes develops not infrequently, especially in younger children.

Given the uncertainties concerning possible consequences of long-standing OME, and given the risks and cost of tube insertion, the point at which tube insertion should be considered remains debatable. A reasonable approach is to consider myringotomy with tube insertion after 6–12 mo of continuous bilateral OME or after 9–18 mo of continuous unilateral OME. Importantly, because even previously persistent OME usually clears spontaneously during the summer months, watchful waiting through at least one summer season is advisable in all children with OME who are otherwise well.

Complications. Most complications of AOM consist of the spread of infection to adjoining or nearby structures or the development of chronicity, or both. Suppurative complications are relatively uncommon in children in developed countries, but occur not infrequently in disadvantaged children whose medical care is limited or nonexistent. The complications of AOM may be classified as either intratemporal or intracranial.

INTRATEMPORAL COMPLICATIONS. Direct but limited extension of otitis media leads to complications within the temporal bone.

Infectious Eczematoid Dermatitis. This is an infection of the skin of the external auditory canal resulting from contamination by purulent discharge from the middle ear. The skin is often erythematous, edematous, and tender. Management consists of proper hygiene combined with systemic antimicrobials and ototopical drops as appropriate for treating AOM and tube otorrhea. Also see Chapter 629.

Chronic Suppurative Otitis Media. This consists of persistent middle-ear infection with discharge through a tympanic membrane perforation. The disease is initiated by an episode of AOM with rupture of the membrane. The mastoid air cells are invariably involved. The most common etiologic organisms are *P. aeruginosa* and *S. aureus*. Treatment is guided by the results of microbiologic investigation. If an associated cholesteatoma is not present, parenteral antimicrobial treatment combined with assiduous aural cleansing is likely to be successful in clearing the infection, but in refractory cases, tympanomastoidectomy is required.

Acute Mastoiditis. All cases of AOM are technically accompanied by mastoiditis by virtue of the associated inflammation of the mastoid air cells. However, early in the course of the disease, no signs or symptoms of mastoid infection are present, and the inflammatory process usually is readily reversible, along with the AOM, in response to antimicrobial treatment. Spread of the infection to the overlying periosteum, but without involvement of bone, constitutes **acute mastoiditis with periosteitis**. In such cases, signs of mastoiditis are usually present, namely, inflammation in the postauricular area, often with displacement of the pinna inferiorly and anteriorly. If instituted promptly, treatment with myringotomy and parenteral antibiotics usually results in satisfactory resolution. In **acute mastoid osteitis**, infection has progressed further to cause destruction of the bony trabeculae of the mastoid. Frank signs and symptoms of mastoiditis are usually, but not always, present. If, as is often the case, an associated subperiosteal abscess has also developed, fluctuation at the site or a fistula from the mastoid to the postauricular area may be present. In **acute petrositis**, infection has extended further to involve the petrous portion of the temporal bone. Eye pain is a prominent symptom, due to irritation of the ophthalmic branch of the fifth cranial nerve, and later, sixth nerve palsy develops. **Gradenigo syndrome** is the triad of suppurative otitis media, paralysis of the external rectus muscle, and pain in the ipsilateral orbit. Rarely, mastoid infection spreads to the neck muscles that attach to the mastoid tip, resulting in an abscess in the neck, termed a **Bezold abscess**.

When mastoiditis is suspected or diagnosed clinically, computed tomography (CT) scan of the temporal bone should be carried out to further clarify the nature and extent of the disease. Bony destruction of the mastoid must be differentiated from the simple clouding of mastoid air cells that is found often in uncomplicated cases of otitis media. The most common causative organisms in all variants of acute mastoiditis are *S. pneumoniae*, nontypable *H. influenzae*, and *P. aeruginosa*. Children with acute mastoid osteitis require intravenous antimicrobial treatment and mastoidectomy, with the extent of the surgery dependent on the extent of the disease process. Insofar as possible, choice of the antimicrobial regimen should be guided by the findings of microbiologic examination.

Each of the variants of mastoiditis may also occur in subacute or chronic form. Symptoms are correspondingly less prominent. **Chronic mastoiditis** is always accompanied by chronic suppurative otitis media, and occasionally will respond to the conservative regimen recommended for that condition. In most cases, however, mastoidectomy also will be required.

Facial Paralysis. The facial nerve, as it traverses the middle ear and mastoid bone, may be affected by adjacent infection. Facial paralysis occurring as a complication of AOM is uncommon, and usually resolves rapidly after myringotomy and parenteral antibiotic treatment. However, if facial paralysis develops in a child with mastoid osteitis or with chronic suppurative otitis media, mastoidectomy should be undertaken urgently.

Acquired Cholesteatoma. Cholesteatoma is a cyst-like growth within the middle ear or other pneumatized portions of the temporal bone, lined by keratinized, stratified squamous epithelium and containing desquamated epithelium and/or keratin. Acquired, as distinct from congenital (Chapter 628), cholesteatoma develops most often as a complication of long-standing chronic otitis media. However, the condition also may develop from a deep retraction pocket of the tympanic membrane or as a consequence of epithelial implantation in the middle-ear cavity from traumatic perforation of the tympanic membrane or insertion of a tympanostomy tube. Cholesteatomas tend to expand progressively, causing bony resorption, and may extend intracranially with potentially life-threatening consequences. Cholesteatoma should be suspected if otoscopy shows a discrete, whitish opacity of the eardrum or a polyp protruding through a defect in the eardrum; or a white, caseous debris persistently overlies the eardrum, especially its superior portion; or persistent malodorous aural discharge is present. When cholesteatoma is suspected, CT scan of the temporal bone should be carried out to define the presence and extent of the disease. The required treatment for cholesteatoma is tympanomastoid surgery.

Labyrinthitis. This occurs uncommonly as a result of the spread of infection from the middle ear and/or mastoid to the inner ear. Cholesteatoma or chronic suppurative otitis media is the usual source. Symptoms and signs include vertigo, tinnitus, nausea, vomiting, hearing loss, nystagmus, and clumsiness. Treatment is directed at the underlying condition and must be undertaken promptly to preserve inner ear function and prevent the spread of infection. Also see Chapter 631.

INTRACRANIAL COMPLICATIONS. Meningitis, epidural abscess, subdural abscess, focal encephalitis, brain abscess, and lateral sinus thrombosis each may develop as a complication of acute or chronic middle-ear or mastoid infection, through direct extension, hematogenous spread, or thrombophlebitis. Bony destruction adjacent to the dura is often involved, and a cholesteatoma may be present. In a child with middle-ear or mastoid infection, the presence of any systemic symptom, such as fever, headache, or lethargy, of extreme degree, or a finding of meningismus or of any central nervous system sign on physical examination, should prompt suspicion of an intracranial complication.

When an intracranial complication is suspected, lumbar puncture should be performed only after imaging studies establish that there is no evidence of mass effect or hydrocephalus. In addition to examination of the cerebrospinal fluid, culture of middle ear exudate obtained via tympanocentesis may identify the causative organism, thereby helping guide the choice of antimicrobial drugs, and myringotomy should be performed to permit middle-ear drainage. Lateral sinus thrombosis, diagnosis of which is facilitated through imaging studies, may be complicated by dissemination of infected thrombi with resultant development of septic infarcts in various organs. Intravenous antibiotic treatment of all intracranial complications, and surgical drainage of any abscess, are urgently required. If mastoiditis is present, mastoidectomy should be undertaken as soon as feasible. When meningitis develops as a complication of AOM, investigation should be directed at the possible presence of a perilymphatic fistula.

Otitic Hydrocephalus. This condition, also termed **benign intracranial hypertension**, consists of increased intracranial pressure without dilatation of the cerebral ventricles, occurring in association with acute or chronic otitis media or mastoiditis. The pathogenesis is uncertain, but the condition is commonly also associated with lateral sinus thrombosis, and the pathophysiology may involve obstruction by thrombus of intracranial venous drainage into the neck, producing a rise in cerebral venous pressure and a consequent increase in cerebrospinal fluid pressure. Symptoms are those of increased intracranial pressure. Signs may include, in addition to evidence of otitis media, paralysis of one or both lateral rectus muscles and papilledema. The diagnosis is confirmed by magnetic resonance imaging (MRI) scan. Treatment measures include the use of antimicrobials and drugs such as acetazolamide or furosemide to reduce intracranial pressure, mastoidectomy, repeated lumbar puncture, lumboperitoneal shunt, and ventriculoperitoneal shunt. If left untreated, otitic hydrocephalus may result in loss of vision secondary to optic atrophy.

PHYSICAL SEQUELAE. Physical sequelae of otitis media consist of structural middle-ear abnormalities resulting from long-standing middle-ear inflammation. In most instances, these sequelae are consequences of severe and/or chronic infection, but some may also result from the presumably noninfective inflammation of long-standing OME. The various sequelae may occur singly, or interrelatedly in various combinations.

Tympanosclerosis consists of whitish plaques in the tympanic membrane and nodular deposits in the submucosal layers of the middle ear. The changes involve hyalinization with deposition of calcium and phosphate crystals. Uncommonly, there may be associated conductive hearing loss. In developed countries, probably the most common cause of tympanosclerosis is tympanostomy tube insertion.

Atelectasis of the tympanic membrane is a descriptive term applied to either severe retraction of the tympanic membrane caused by high negative middle-ear pressure or loss of stiffness and medial prolapse of the membrane, presumably as a consequence of long-standing retraction or severe or chronic inflammation. A **retraction pocket** is a localized area of atelectasis. Atelectasis is often transient and usually unaccompanied by symptoms, but a deep retraction pocket may lead to erosion of the ossicles and adhesive otitis, and may serve as the nidus of a cholesteatoma. For a deep retraction pocket, and for the unusual instance in which atelectasis is accompanied by symptoms such as otalgia, tinnitus, or conductive hearing loss, the required treatment is tympanostomy tube insertion.

Adhesive otitis media consists of proliferation of fibrous tissue in the middle-ear mucosa, which may in turn result in impaired movement of the ossicles, rarefying osteitis and **ossicular discontinuity**, conductive hearing loss, and cholesteatoma. The hearing loss may be amenable to surgical correction.

Cholesterol granuloma is an uncommon condition in which the tympanic membrane appears to be dark blue, reflecting the presence of thick, granulomatous material in the middle-ear cavity. The condition appears to result more often from long-standing OME than from frank middle-ear infection. Tympanostomy tube insertion alone does not provide satisfactory relief, and the required treatment is middle-ear and mastoid surgery.

Chronic perforation may develop after spontaneous rupture of the tympanic membrane during an episode of AOM or as a sequela of chronic suppurative otitis media. In developed countries, however, probably the most common cause is tympanostomy tube insertion (see earlier). A chronic perforation may be amenable to surgical repair, usually after the child has been free of otitis media for an extended period.

Permanent **conductive hearing loss** may result from any of the conditions just described. Rarely, permanent **sensorineural hearing loss** may occur in association with acute or chronic otitis media, presumably from the spread of infection or products of inflammation through the round window membrane, or as a consequence of suppurative labyrinthitis.

POSSIBLE DEVELOPMENTAL SEQUELAE. Continuous, bilateral MEE for up to 9 mo during the first 3 yr of life poses no measurable developmental risk by 4 yr of age. However, it remains possible that effects not measurable by then will become apparent at older ages. In addition, it seems reasonable to assume that substantially longer periods of effusion or a sustained degree of hearing loss greater than the usual mild-to-moderate level might indeed have adverse effects. Fortunately, such circumstances are not common.

Prevention. General measures to prevent otitis media consist of breast milk feeding; avoidance, insofar as possible, of exposure to individuals with respiratory infection; and, probably, avoidance of environmental tobacco smoke. The administration of xylitol, a natural sugar, in chewing gum or syrup has been reported to provide a measure of protection against AOM by inhibiting the growth of *S. pneumoniae*, but the studies have had important limitations. Moreover, the current unavailablility of xylitol-containing products in the United States, the required frequency and duration of administration, and the absence of adequate safety data concerning the high doses of xylitol required preclude its general use.

IMMUNOPROPHYLAXIS. Pneumococcal polysaccharide vaccine is relatively ineffective in protecting against otitis media in children younger than 2 yr of age, and provides only limited protection in older children. The newer heptavalent pneumococcal conjugate vaccine was found in one study to effect a 7% overall reduction in the number of episodes of AOM, but reductions of 9–23% in children with histories of frequent episodes and a 20% reduction in the number of children undergoing tympanostomy tube insertion. In another study, the same vaccine effected a 57% reduction in serotype-specific episodes, but a reduction of only 6% in the number of overall episodes of AOM. The further development of vaccines against the pathogens that cause AOM offers promise of improved overall protection. Influenza vaccine may also provide a measure of protection against otitis media, but further studies are necessary to clarify its degree of efficacy. Passive immunization by exogenously administered immunoglobulin is not practicable because of the discomfort, risks, cost, and inconvenience entailed.

ANTIMICROBIAL PROPHYLAXIS. In children who have developed frequent episodes of AOM, antimicrobial prophylaxis with subtherapeutic doses of an aminopenicillin or a sulfonamide offers variable protection against recurrences of AOM (although not of OME). However, because of the contribution of antimicrobial usage to bacterial resistance, the risks of sustained antimicrobial prophylaxis now appear, in general, to outweigh the likely benefits, particularly for children in daycare who in any case are at increased risk of colonization with multiply resistant *S. pneumoniae*. Prophylaxis may, nonetheless, be an appropriate option for the child with recurrent AOM who is cared for at home and usually away from other young children.

MYRINGOTOMY AND INSERTION OF TYMPANOSTOMY TUBES. In children with persistent OME, several studies have shown tympanostomy tube insertion to be effective in reducing the children's subsequent proportion of time with MEE and also their recurrence rate of AOM. In the one study in children who had recurrent AOM but not persistent MEE, tube insertion was effective in reducing time with MEE, but a reduction in the recurrence rate of symptomatic episodes of AOM was offset by the occurrence of episodes of tube otorrhea. However, anecdotal evidence and personal clinical experience suggest that in children more severely affected than those enrolled in the study, tube insertion offers a greater degree of benefit than that reported.

How best to manage the individual child who is severely affected with recurrent AOM must remain a matter of individual judgment, with the alternatives to prophylaxis being either continued reliance on episodic treatment alone, which seems preferable where feasible, or referral for tympanostomy tube insertion with its attendant risks.

ADENOIDECTOMY. In children who have undergone tube insertion and in whom, after extrusion of tubes, otitis media continues to be a problem, adenoidectomy is efficacious to some extent in reducing the risk of subsequent recurrences both of AOM and of OME. Efficacy appears to be independent of adenoid size, and probably derives from removal of a focus of infection. On the other hand, in children with recurrent AOM who have not previously undergone tube insertion, the benefit of adenoidectomy is quite limited. In such children, if the burden of illness becomes intolerable, tube insertion alone is the preferred first surgical recourse.

Bluestone CD, Klein JO: *Otitis Media in Infants and Children*, 3rd ed. Philadelphia, WB Saunders, 2001.

Casselbrant ML, Kaleida PH, Rockette HE, et al: Efficacy of antimicrobial prophylaxis and of tympanostomy tube insertion for prevention of recurrent acute otitis media: Results of a randomized clinical trial. *Pediatr Infect Dis J* 1992;11:278–86.

Dowell SF, Butler JC, Giebink GS, et al: Acute otitis media: Management and surveillance in an era of pneumococcal resistance—A report from the Drug-resistant *Streptococcus pneumoniae* Therapeutic Working Group. *Pediatr Infect Dis J* 1999;18:1–9.

Heikkinen T, Thint M, Chonmaitree T: Prevalence of various respiratory viruses in the middle ear during acute otitis media. *N Engl J Med* 1999;340:260–4.

Hoberman A, Paradise JL: Acute otitis media: Diagnosis and management in the year 2000. *Pediatr Ann* 2000;29:609–20.

Paradise JL: Short-course antimicrobial treatment for acute otitis media: Not best for babies and young children. *JAMA* 1997;278:1640–2.

Paradise JL, Bluestone CD, Colborn DK, et al: Adenoidectomy and adenotonsillectomy for recurrent acute otitis media: Parallel randomized clinical trials in children not previously treated with tympanostomy-tube placement. *JAMA* 1999;282:945–53.

Paradise JL, Elster BA, Tan L: Evidence in infants with cleft palate that breast milk protects against otitis media. *Pediatrics* 1994;94:853–60.

Paradise JL, Feldman HM, Campbell TF, et al: Effect of early or delayed insertion of tympanostomy tubes for persistent otitis media on developmental outcomes at the age of three years. *N Engl J Med* 2001;344:1179–87.

Paradise JL, Rockette HE, Colborn DK, et al: Otitis media in 2253 Pittsburgh-area infants: Prevalence and risk factors during the first two years of life. *Pediatrics* 1997;99:318–33.

Chapter 631

The Inner Ear and Diseases of the Bony Labyrinth

Joseph Haddad Jr.

The function and anatomy of the inner ear may be affected by infectious organisms, including viruses, bacteria, and protozoa. Genetic abnormalities may also be responsible for abnormal anatomy and function. Other acquired diseases of the labyrinthine capsule include otosclerosis, osteopetrosis, Langerhans cell histiocytosis, fibrous dysplasia, and other types of bony dysplasia. All of these can cause hearing loss, both conductive and sensorineural, as well as vestibular dysfunction.

Viruses. Viral causes of sensorineural hearing loss (SNHL) include congenital rubella and congenital cytomegalovirus (CMV), as well as mumps, postnatal rubella, and rubeola (measles). Fifth disease, caused by parvovirus B19, is an infrequent cause of SNHL. Many other viruses are occasionally associated with SNHL. The most common cause of congenital viral sensorineural hearing loss is CMV (Chapter 627). In as many as 50%, hearing loss, which is usually bilateral though often asymmetric, progresses and worsens over weeks to years. Stabilization or improvement in the hearing loss may be possible by using ganciclovir in very young infants with congenital CMV (Chapter 234).

Before the introduction of an effective vaccine, rubella was responsible for as many as 60% of the newly identified cases of childhood SNHL. Vaccination in most developed countries has reduced the rate of rubella by more than 97%. Similarly, measles and mumps are now uncommon causes of SNHL in the United States because of successful vaccination programs.

Herpes simplex encephalitis may also be associated with SNHL; the hearing loss is more common in those children with congenital herpesvirus infection. Acyclovir and other antiviral agents may help the hearing loss and other central nervous system manifestations (Chapter 231).

Toxoplasmosis. *Toxoplasma gondii* is a protozoan that may cause congenital SNHL. About 3,000 children are born in the United States yearly with congenital toxoplasmosis; approximately 25% of untreated patients have SNHL. If infection is documented during the fetal period, medical therapy may be able to prevent some of the clinical manifestations, including SNHL (Chapter 266).

Bacterial Meningitis. Since the introduction of the Hib vaccine, *Streptococcus pneumoniae* and *Neisseria meningitidis* have become the leading causes of bacterial meningitis in children in the United States. Hearing loss occurs more commonly with *S. pneumoniae*, with an estimated incidence of 15–20%. Approximately 60% of those hearing losses are bilateral, though often asymmetric. If the hearing loss is present at the time of presentation with meningitis, and especially if it is severe to profound, the likelihood of significant improvement is small. However, if the hearing loss develops after admission for treatment and is not severe, stabilization or improvement is possible. Late progression of SNHL has also been noted in some children years after meningitis. In the United States and many other developed countries, bacterial meningitis is one of the major causes of profound deafness leading to cochlear implantation in children. The introduction of pneumococcal conjugate vaccine is expected to lead to a reduction in SNHL due to pneumococcal meningitis.

Studies have shown favorable trends in the course and outcome after administration of dexamethasone for hearing loss and other neurologic deficits associated with bacterial meningitis (Chapter 594.1), although the effectiveness, especially for *S. pneumoniae* and *N. meningitidis* meningitis, generally has not reached statistical significance because of the small number of cases in the trials. A meta-analysis of 11 studies conducted from 1988 to 1996 showed dexamethasone reduced severe hearing loss associated with *H. influenzae* type b meningitis regardless of the timing of administration of dexamethasone (before or with antibiotics vs. later) or of the antibiotic used. For pneumococcal meningitis, the meta-analysis showed a benefit of dexamethasone only when given early and only for protection against severe hearing loss. Too few cases of meningococcal meningitis were included to assess the effect of dexamethasone on this entity.

Syphilis. Congenital syphilis may cause SNHL in 3–38% of children; the exact incidence is difficult to ascertain, because the hearing loss may not occur until adolescence or even adulthood. When the condition is identified, treatment with antibiotics and steroids may improve the hearing loss.

Other Diseases of the Inner Ear. *Labyrinthitis* may be a complication of direct spread of infection from acute or chronic otitis media (OM) or mastoiditis but may also complicate bacterial meningitis as a result of organisms entering the labyrinth through the internal auditory meatus, endolymphatic duct, perilymphatic duct, vascular channels, or hematogenous spread. Clinical manifestations of labyrinthitis may include vertigo, disequilibrium, deep-seated ear pain, nausea, vomiting, nystagmus, and SNHL. Acute suppurative labyrinthitis, characterized by abrupt, severe onset of these symptoms, requires intensive antimicrobial therapy. If it is secondary to OM, it may require otologic surgery to remove underlying cholesteatoma or drain the middle ear and mastoid, in addition to antibiotics. Acute serous labyrinthitis, with milder symptoms of vertigo and hearing loss, may occur secondary to middle-ear infection as well. It usually responds well to antibiotics and steroids, with improvement in both the vertigo and hearing. Chronic labyrinthitis, most commonly associated with cholesteatoma, presents with SNHL and vestibular dysfunction that develops over time; surgery is required to remove the cholesteatoma. Chronic labyrinthitis may also uncommonly occur secondary to long-standing OM, with the slow development of SNHL, usually starting in the higher frequencies, and possibly with vestibular dysfunction. Additionally, and more commonly, children with chronic middle-ear fluid are often unsteady or off balance, a situation that immediately improves when the fluid resolves.

Otosclerosis, an autosomal dominant disease that affects only the temporal bones, causes abnormal bone growth that can result in fixation of the stapes in the oval window, leading to progressive hearing loss. The hearing loss is usually conductive at first, but SNHL may develop. White females are affected most commonly, with onset of otosclerosis in teenagers or young adults, often associated with pregnancy. Corrective surgery to replace the stapes with a mobile prosthesis is often successful.

Osteogenesis imperfecta (OI) is a systemic disease that may involve both the middle and inner ears (Chapter 689). Hearing loss occurs in about 20% of young children and as many as 90% of adults with this disease. The hearing loss is most commonly conductive because of abnormalities of the ossicles, but SNHL may occur if other areas of the otic capsule become affected. If the hearing loss is severe enough, a hearing aid may be a preferable alternative to surgical correction of the fixed stapes, because stapedectomy in children with OI can be technically very difficult, and the disease and the hearing loss may be progressive.

Osteopetrosis, a very uncommon skeletal dysplasia, may involve the temporal bone, including the middle ear and ossicles, resulting in a moderate to severe, usually conductive hearing loss. Recurrent facial nerve paralysis may also occur as a result of excess bone deposition; each time it occurs, less facial function may return (Chapter 687).

Chapter 632

Traumatic Injuries of the Ear and Temporal Bone

Joseph Haddad Jr.

Auricle and External Auditory Canal. *Hematoma*, an accumulation of blood between the perichondrium and the cartilage, may follow trauma to the pinna; this is a common sports injury in teenagers related to wrestling or boxing. Immediate needle aspiration or, when the hematoma is extensive or recurrent, incision and drainage and a pressure dressing are necessary to prevent perichondritis, which can result in a cauliflower ear deformity.

Frostbite of the auricle should be managed by rapidly rewarming the exposed pinna with warm irrigation or warm compresses.

Foreign bodies in the external canal are common in childhood. These can often be removed without general anesthesia if the child is informed about the procedure (if old enough to understand it) and is properly restrained; if an adequate headlight, surgical head otoscope, or otomicroscope is used for visualizing the object; and if appropriate instruments, such as alligator forceps, wire loops or a blunt cerumen curette, or suction are used, depending on the shape of the object. Gentle irrigation of the ear canal with body temperature water or saline may be used to remove very small objects, but only if the tympanic membrane (TM) is intact. Attempted removal of an object from a struggling child, or with poor visualization and inadequate tools, results in a terrified child with a swollen and bleeding ear canal and may then mandate general anesthesia for removal of the object. More difficult foreign bodies, especially those that are large, deeply embedded or associated with canal swelling, are best removed under general anesthesia. Disk batteries are removed emergently because they leach a basic fluid that can cause severe tissue destruction. Insects in the canal are first killed with mineral oil or lidocaine, and are then removed under otomicroscopic examination.

After a foreign body is removed from the external canal, the TM should be carefully inspected for possible traumatic perforation or for a pre-existing middle-ear effusion. If a foreign body has resulted in acute inflammation of the canal, treatment as described for acute external otitis should be instituted.

Tympanic Membrane and Middle Ear. Traumatic perforation of the TM usually occurs as a result of a sudden external compression (a slap) or penetration by a foreign object (a stick or cotton-tipped applicator). The perforation may be linear or stellate and is most frequently in the anterior portion of the pars tensa when it is caused by compression; it may be in any quadrant of the TM when caused by a foreign object. Systemic antibiotics and topical otic medications are not required unless suppurative otorrhea is present. Close follow-up examination is necessary to ensure that spontaneous healing occurs. If the TM does not heal within several months, surgical graft repair should be considered. As long as the perforation is present, otorrhea may occur from water entering the middle ear from the ear canal, which can occur during swimming or bathing; appropriate precautions should be taken. Perforations resulting from penetrating foreign bodies are less likely to heal than those caused by compression. Audiometric examination reveals a conductive hearing loss (CHL), with larger air-bone gaps seen in larger perforations. Immediate surgical exploration is indicated if the injury is accompanied by one or more of the following: vertigo, nystagmus, severe tinnitus, moderate to severe hearing loss, or cerebrospinal fluid (CSF) otorrhea. At the time of exploration, it is necessary to inspect the ossicles, especially the stapes, because they may have been dislocated or fractured; examination also is made for sharp objects that may have penetrated the oval or round windows. If the stapes has been subluxed or dislocated into the oval window or if either the oval or round window has been penetrated, sensorineural hearing loss (SNHL) results.

Perilymphatic fistula (PLF) may occur after sudden barotrauma or an increase in CSF pressure. This condition is suspected in a child who develops a sudden SNHL or vertigo after physical exertion, deep water diving, air travel, playing a wind instrument, or significant head trauma. The leak characteristically is at the oval or the round window and may be associated with congenital abnormalities of these structures or an anatomic abnormality of the cochlea or semicircular canals. PLFs occasionally close spontaneously, but immediate surgical repair of the fistula is recommended to control vertigo and to stop any progression of the SNHL; even timely surgery does not usually restore the SNHL. No reliable test is known for PLF, so middle-ear exploration is required for diagnosis and treatment.

Temporal Bone Fractures. Children are particularly prone to basilar skull fractures, which usually involve the temporal bone. From 70% to 80% of temporal bone fractures are longitudinal and are commonly manifested by bleeding from a laceration of the external canal or tympanic membrane; postauricular ecchymosis (**Battle sign**); hemotympanum (blood behind an intact TM); CHL resulting from TM perforation, hemotympanum, or ossicular injury; delayed onset of facial paralysis (which usually improves spontaneously); and temporary CSF otorrhea or rhinorrhea (from CSF running down the eustachian tube). Transverse fractures of the temporal bone have a graver prognosis than longitudinal fractures and are often associated with immediate facial paralysis. Facial paralysis may improve if caused by edema, but surgical decompression of the nerve is often recommended, if there is no evidence of clinical recovery and facial nerve studies are unfavorable. If the facial nerve has been transected, surgical decompression and anastomosis offer the possibility of some functional recovery. Transverse fractures are also associated with severe SNHL, vertigo, nystagmus, tinnitus, nausea, and vomiting associated with loss of cochlear and vestibular function; hemotympanum; rarely, external canal bleeding; and CSF otorrhea, either in the external auditory canal or behind the TM, which may exit the nose via the eustachian tube.

If temporal bone fracture is suspected or seen on radiographs, gentle examination of the pinna and ear canal is indicated; lacerations or avulsion of soft tissue is common with temporal bone fractures. Vigorous removal of external auditory canal blood clots or tympanocentesis is not indicated, because clot removal may further dislodge the ossicles or reopen CSF leaks. Some have advocated prophylactic parenteral administration of antibiotics when CSF otorrhea or rhinorrhea is present, but this is controversial. If a patient is afebrile and the drainage is not cloudy, watchful waiting without antibiotics is indicated. Surgical intervention is reserved for children who require repair of a nonhealing TM perforation, who have suffered dislocation of the ossicular chain, or who need decompression of the facial nerve. SNHL can also follow a blow to the head without an obvious fracture of the temporal bone (labyrinthine concussion).

Acoustic Trauma. This results from exposure to high-intensity sound (fireworks, gunfire, rock music, heavy machinery) and is initially manifested by a temporary decrease in hearing threshold, most commonly at 4,000 Hz on an audiometric examination, and tinnitus. If the sound exceeds 85 dB but is less than 140 dB, the loss is usually temporary (after a rock concert), but both the hearing loss and the tinnitus may become permanent with chronic noise exposure; the frequencies from 3,000 to 6,000 Hz are most often involved. Sudden, extremely loud (>140 dB), short-duration noises with loud peak components (gunfire, bombs) may cause permanent hearing loss after a single exposure. Ear protection and avoidance of chronic exposure to loud noise are preventive measures. Hearing loss due to chronic noise exposure should be entirely preventable.

Chapter 633
Tumors of the Ear and Temporal Bone
Joseph Haddad Jr.

Benign tumors of the external canal include *osteomas* and *monostotic* and *polyostotic fibrous dysplasia*. Osteomas present as bony masses in the canal and require removal only if hearing is impaired or external otitis results; osteomas may be confused clinically with exostoses.

Eosinophilic granuloma, which may occur in isolation or as part of the systemic Langerhans cell histiocytosis, should be suspected in patients with otalgia, otorrhea (sometimes bloody), hearing loss, abnormal tissue within the middle ear or ear canal, and roentgenographic findings of a sharply delineated destructive lesion of the temporal bone. Definitive diagnosis is made by biopsy. Treatment depends on the site of the lesion and whether it is "eosinophilic granuloma," a unifocal or multifocal lesion of the bone that has a more benign course. Depending on the site, it may be treated by surgical excision, curettage, or local radiation (Chapter 499). If the lesion is part of a systemic presentation of Langerhans cell histiocytosis, chemotherapy in addition to local therapy (surgery with or without radiation) is indicated. Long-term follow-up is necessary whether the temporal bone lesion is a single isolated one or part of a multisystem disease.

Symptoms and signs of *rhabdomyosarcoma* originating in the middle ear or ear canal include a mass or polyp in the middle ear or ear canal, bleeding from the ear, otorrhea, otalgia, facial paralysis, and hearing loss. Other cranial nerves also may be involved. Diagnosis is based on biopsy, but the extent of disease is determined by both CT and MRI of the temporal bone, skull base, and brain. Classification is generally according to the stage as outlined in the current International Rhabdomyosarcoma Study group system. Management usually involves a combination of chemotherapy, radiation, and surgery (Chapter 492.1).

Non-Hodgkin lymphoma and *leukemia* may also present in the temporal bone, although it is rare as the initial presentation in these diseases. Although primary neoplasms of the middle ear are very uncommon in children, they include adenoid cystic carcinoma, adenocarcinoma, and squamous cell carcinoma. Benign tumors of the temporal bone include glomus tumors. The initial signs and symptoms of the more common nasopharyngeal neoplasms (angiofibroma, rhabdomyosarcoma, epidermoid carcinoma) may be associated with insidious onset of chronic otitis media with effusion (often unilateral); a high index of suspicion is needed for diagnosing these tumors accurately.

Adair-Bischoff CE, Sauve RS: Environmental tobacco smoke and middle ear disease in preschool-age children. *Arch Pediatr Adolesc Med* 1998;152:127.

American Academy of Otolaryngology—Head and Neck Surgery Subcommittee on Cochlear Implants. Status of cochlear implantation in children. *J Pediatr* 1991;118:1.

American Academy of Pediatrics; Joint Committee on Infant Hearing: 1994 Position Statement. *Pediatrics* 1995;95:152.

American Academy of Pediatrics, Task Force on Newborn and Infant Hearing: Newborn and infant hearing loss: Detection and intervention. *Pediatrics* 103:527, 1999.

Barnett ED, Klein JO, Hawkins KA, et al: Comparison of spectral gradient acoustic reflectometry and other diagnostic techniques for detection of middle ear effusion in children with middle ear disease. *Pediatr Infect Dis J* 1998;17:556.

Barsky-Firkser L, Sun S: Universal newborn hearing screenings: A three-year experience. *Pediatrics* 1997;99:1.

Bluestone CD, Klein JO: *Otitis Media in Infants and Children*, 3rd ed. Philadelphia, WB Saunders, 2001.

Bluestone CD, Klein JO: Intracranial suppurative complications of otitis media and mastoiditis. In Bluestone CD, Stool SE, Kenna MA (editors): *Pediatric Otolaryngology*, 3rd ed. Philadelphia, WB Saunders, 1996, pp 636–648.

Bluestone CD, Klein JO: Intratemporal complications and sequelae of otitis media. In Bluestone CD, Stool SE, Kenna MA (editors): *Pediatric Otolaryngology*, 3rd ed. Philadelphia, WB Saunders, 1996, pp 583–635.

Bluestone CD, Klein JO: Otitis media, atelectasis, and eustachian tube dysfunction. In Bluestone CD, Stool SE, Kenna MA (editors): *Pediatric Otolaryngology*, 3rd ed. Philadelphia, WB Saunders, 1996, pp 388–582.

Bluestone CD: Otitis media and congenital perilymphatic fistula as a cause of sensorineural hearing loss in children. *Pediatr Infect Dis J* 1988;7:S141.

Cox LC: Otoacoustic emissions as a screening tool for sensorineural hearing loss. *J Pediatr* 1997;130:685.

Del Castillo I, Villamar M, Moreno-Pelayo MA, et al: A deletion involving the connexin 30 gene in nonsyndromic hearing impairments. *N Engl J Med* 2002;346:243–9.

Eilers RE, Oller DK: Infant vocalizations and early diagnosis of severe hearing impairment. *J Pediatr* 1994;124:199.

Fugazzola L, Cerutti N, Mannavola D, et al: Differential diagnoses between Pendred and pseudo-Pendred syndromes: Clinical, radiologic, and molecular studies. *Pediatr Res* 2002;51:479–84.

Grote JJ: Neonatal screening for hearing impairment. *Lancet* 2000;355:513.

Haddad J Jr.: Care of the draining ear in children. *Emerg Peds* 1995;8:75.

Haddad J Jr.: Office procedures in pediatric otolaryngology. In Blitzer A, Pillsbury HC, Jahn AF, Binder WJ (editors): *Operative Techniques in Office-Based Otolaryngology*. New York, Thieme Medical Publishers, 1998.

Haddad J Jr.: Treatment of acute otitis media and its complications. *Otolaryngol Clin North Am* 1994;27:431.

Herbert RL, King GE, Bent JP: Tympanostomy tubes and water exposure. *Arch Otolaryngol Head Neck Surg* 1998;124:1118.

Hough JVD, Stuart WD: Middle ear injuries in skull trauma. *Laryngoscope* 1968;78:899.

Isaacson G, Rosenfeld RM: Care of the child with tympanostomy tubes: A visual guide for the pediatrician. *Pediatrics* 1994;93:924.

Kemper AR, Downs SM: A cost-effectiveness analysis of newborn hearing screening strategies. *Arch Pediatr Adolesc Med* 2000;154:484.

Konigsmark BW, Gorlin RJ: *Genetic and Metabolic Deafness*. Philadelphia, WB Saunders, 1976.

Lench N, Houseman M, Newton V, et al: Connexin-26 mutations in sporadic nonsyndromal sensorineural deafness. *Lancet* 1998;351:415.

Mandel EM, Rockette HE, Bluestone CD, et al: Myringotomy with and without tympanostomy tubes for chronic otitis media with effusion. *Arch Otolaryngol Head Neck Surg* 1989;115:1217.

Maniglia AJ, Goodwin WJ, Arnold JE, et al: Intracranial abscesses secondary to nasal, sinus and orbital infections in adults and children. *Arch Otolaryngol Head Neck Surg* 1989;115:1424.

Mason JA, Herrmann KR: Universal infant hearing screening by automated auditory brainstem response measurement. *Pediatrics* 1998;101:221.

Moeller MP: Early intervention and language development in children who are deaf and hard of hearing. *Pediatrics* 2000;106:594.

Morell RJ, Kim HJ, Hood LJ, et al: Mutations in the connexin 26 gene (GJB2) among Ashkenazi Jews with nonsyndromic recessive deafness. *N Engl J Med* 1998;339:1500.

Niskar AS, Kieszak SM, Holmes A, et al: Prevalence of hearing loss among children 6 to 19 years of age. *JAMA* 1998;279:1071.

Nozza RJ: The assessment of hearing and middle ear function in children. In Bluestone CD, Stool SE, Kenna MA (editors): *Pediatric Otolaryngology*, 3rd ed. Philadelphia, WB Saunders, 1996, pp 165–206.

Samuel J, Fernandes CMC, Steinberg JL: Intracranial otogenic complications: A persisting problem. *Laryngoscope* 1986;96:272.

Teele DW, Klein JO, Rosner BA: Otitis media with effusion during the first three years of life and development of speech and language. *Pediatrics* 1984;74:282.

Thompson DC, McPhillips H, Davis RL, et al: Universal newborn hearing screening: Summary of evidence. *JAMA* 2001;286:2000.

Willems PJ: Genetic causes of hearing loss. *N Engl J Med* 2000;342:1101.

Wolf B, Spencer R, Gleason T: Hearing loss is a common feature of symptomatic children with profound biotinidase deficiency. *Pediatrics* 2002;140:242–6.

Yoshinaga-Itano C, Sedey AL, Coulter DK, et al: Language of early- and later-identified children with hearing loss. *Pediatrics* 1998;102:1161.

Zorowka PG: Otoacoustic emissions: A new method to diagnose hearing impairment in children. *Eur J Pediatr* 1993;152:626.

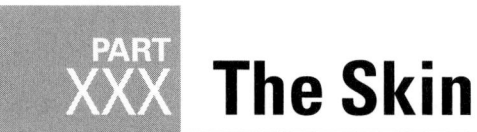

PART XXX The Skin

Gary L. Darmstadt and Robert Sidbury

Chapter 634
Morphology of the Skin

Epidermis. The mature epidermis is a stratified epithelial tissue composed predominantly of *keratinocytes*. The lowest keratinocyte layer, the basal cell layer, is constantly renewing the epidermis by mitotic division of the basal cells. Keratinocyte stem cells originate from hair follicles. Individual keratinocytes mature through a process of epidermal differentiation that results in the barrier portion of the epidermis, the stratum corneum. When composed of mature, differentiated keratinocytes, the stratum corneum is 10–50 µm thick. Damage to the stratum corneum increases skin permeability and may increase the potential for skin or systemic infection or systemic toxicity to topically applied medications or chemicals.

The continuous renewal of the surface keratinocytes of the epidermis normally proceeds in an orderly fashion as the cells of the basal cell layer move upward to the stratum corneum. The total life span from mitotic division of the basal cell until loss from the stratum corneum is approximately 28 days. In hyperproliferative diseases such as psoriasis, the movement of the cells is more rapid. The newly arrived keratinocytes in the stratum corneum are not fully differentiated and form a defective barrier. Keratinocytes are joined together by attachment plaques, the desmosomes. Cytoplasmic tonofibrils project to the desmosome and aid in cell attachment. Autoantibodies to various desmosomal adhesion molecules cause acantholysis (detachment of joined keratinocytes with bullae formation).

In addition to keratinocytes, the epidermis contains three additional cell types. The *melanocytes* are pigment-forming cells, which are responsible for skin color. Melanocytes produce melanosomes containing melanin. Epidermal melanocytes are derived from the neural crest and migrate to the skin during embryonic life. They reside in the interfollicular epidermis and in the hair follicles and increase in number in the epidermis by mitosis or migration of additional cells into the epidermis. *Merkel cells* are nerve-associated epidermal cells that may be important in the sensation of touch and in skin development. *Langerhans cells* are dendritic cells of the mononuclear phagocyte system. They contain a specific organelle, the Birbeck granule. These cells are derived from bone marrow and participate in immune reactions in the skin, playing an active part in antigen presentation and processing.

Dermis. The dermis forms a tough, pliable, fibrous supporting structure between the epidermis and the subcutaneous fat. It consists of collagen and elastic and reticulin fibers embedded in an amorphous ground substance; it contains blood vessels, lymphatics, neural structures, eccrine and apocrine sweat glands, hair follicles, sebaceous glands, and smooth muscle. Morphologically, the dermis can be divided into two layers: the superficial papillary layer that interdigitates with the rete ridges of the epidermis and the deeper reticular layer that lies beneath the papillary dermis. The papillary layer is less dense and more cellular, whereas the reticular layer appears more compact because of the coarse network of interlaced collagen and elastic fibers.

The junction of the epidermis and dermis is the *basement membrane zone*. This complex structure is a result of contributions from both epidermal and mesenchymal cells. The dermoepidermal junction extends from the basal cell plasma membrane to the uppermost region of the dermis. Ultrastructurally, the basement membrane appears as a trilaminar structure, consisting of a *lamina lucida* immediately adjacent to the basal cell plasma membrane, a central *lamina densa*, and the *subbasal lamina* on the dermal side of the lamina densa. Several structures within this zone act to anchor the epidermis to the dermis. The plasma membrane of basal cells contains electron-dense plates known as hemidesmosomes; tonofilaments course within basal cells to insert at these sites. Anchoring filaments originate in the plasma membrane, primarily near the hemidesmosomes, and insert into the lamina densa. Anchoring fibrils, composed predominantly of type VII collagen, extend from the lamina densa into the uppermost dermis where they insert into anchoring plaques. The composition of the basement membrane as well as its role in skin disease, particularly the vesiculobullous disorders, is the subject of intensive investigation. Molecular defects in basement membrane components have been shown to underlie several of the blistering diseases (see Chapter 644).

The predominant dermal cell is a spindle-shaped *fibroblast* that is responsible for the synthesis of collagen, elastic fibers, and mucopolysaccharides. Phagocytic histiocytes, mast cells, and motile leukocytes are also present. The gelatinous ground substance serves as a supporting medium for the fibrillar and cellular components and as a storage place for a substantial portion of body water. Nutrients are supplied to both epidermis and dermis by the dermal blood vessels.

Subcutaneous Tissue. Panniculus, or subcutaneous tissue, consists of fat cells and fibrous septa that divide it into lobules and anchor it to the underlying fascia and periosteum. Blood vessels and nerves are also present in this layer, which serves as a storage depot for lipid, an insulator to conserve body heat, and a protective cushion against trauma.

Appendageal Structures. These structures are derived from aggregates of epidermal cells that become specialized during early embryonic development. Small buds (primary epithelial germs) appear during the 3rd fetal mo and give rise to hair follicles, sebaceous and apocrine glands, and the attachment bulges for the arrector pili muscles. Eccrine sweat glands are derived from separate epidermal downgrowths that arise during the 2nd fetal mo and are completely formed by the 5th mo. Formation of nails is initiated during the 3rd intrauterine mo.

Hair Follicles. The hair follicle is the most prominent structure in the pilary complex, which includes the sebaceous gland, the arrector pili muscle, and, in areas such as the axillae, an apocrine gland. Hair follicles are distributed throughout the skin, except in the palms, soles, lips, and glans penis; if destroyed, they cannot regenerate. Individual follicles extend from the surface of the epidermis to the deep dermis, where the matrix cells with the dermal papilla form a bulbous hair root. The growing hair consists of a bulb and a matrix from which the keratinized hair shaft is generated; the shaft consists of an inner medulla, a cortex, and an outer cuticular layer.

Human hair growth is cyclic, with alternate periods of growth (anagen) and rest (telogen). The length of the anagen phase varies from months to years. At birth, all hairs are in the anagen phase. Subsequent generative activity lacks synchrony, so that an overall random pattern of growth and shedding prevails. Scalp hair usually grows about 1 cm/mo.

The types of hair are fetal lanugo, terminal, and vellus. *Lanugo* hair is thin and short; this hair is shed before term and is replaced by vellus hair by 36–40 wk of gestation. *Terminal hair* is long and coarse and is found on the scalp, beard, eyebrows, eyelashes, and axillary and pubic areas. *Vellus hair* is short, soft, and frequently unpigmented and is distributed over the rest of the body. During puberty, androgenic hormone stimulation causes pubic, axillary, and beard hair to change from vellus hair to terminal hair.

Sebaceous Glands. These glands occur in all areas except the palms of the hands and soles and dorsa of the feet, but they are most numerous on the face, upper chest, and back. Their ducts open into the hair follicles except on the lips, prepuce, and labia minora, where they emerge directly onto the mucosal surface. These holocrine glands are saccular structures that are often branched and lobulated and consist of a proliferative basal layer of small flat cells peripheral to the central mass of lipidized cells. The latter cells disintegrate as they move toward the duct and form the lipid secretion known as sebum, which consists of cellular debris, triglycerides, phospholipids, and cholesterol esters. Sebaceous glands depend on hormonal stimulation and are activated by androgens at puberty. Fetal sebaceous glands are stimulated by maternal androgens, and their lipid secretion, together with desquamated stratum corneum cells, constitutes the vernix caseosa.

Apocrine Glands. The apocrine glands are located in the axillae, areolae, perianal and genital areas, and the periumbilical region. These large, coiled, tubular structures continuously secrete an odorless milky fluid that is discharged in response to adrenergic stimuli, usually a result of emotional stress. Bacterial decomposition of apocrine sweat accounts for the unpleasant odor associated with perspiration. Apocrine glands remain dormant until puberty, when they enlarge and secretion begins in response to androgenic activity. The secretory coil of the gland consists of a single layer of cells enclosed by a layer of contractile myoepithelial cells. The duct is lined with a double layer of cuboidal cells and opens into the pilosebaceous complex. Although apocrine glands do not function in thermoregulation, they are involved in certain disease processes.

Eccrine Sweat Glands. These glands are distributed over the entire body surface, including the palms and soles, where they are most abundant. Those on the hairy skin respond to thermal stimuli and serve to regulate body temperature by delivering water to the skin surface for evaporation; in contrast, sweat glands on the palms and soles respond mainly to psychophysiologic stimuli.

Each eccrine gland consists of a secretory coil located in the reticular dermis or subcutaneous fat and a secretory duct that opens onto the skin surface. Sweat pores can be identified on the epidermal ridges of the palm and fingers with a magnifying lens but are not readily visualized elsewhere. Two types of cells compose the single-layered secretory coil: small dark cells and large clear cells; these rest on a layer of contractile myoepithelial cells and a basement membrane. The glands are supplied by sympathetic nerve fibers, but the pharmacologic mediator of sweating is acetylcholine rather than epinephrine. Sweat consists of water, sodium, potassium, calcium, chloride, phospho-

rus, lactate, and small quantities of iron, glucose, and protein. The composition varies with the rate of sweating but is always hypotonic in normal children.

Nails. Nails are specialized protective epidermal structures that form convex, translucent, tight-fitting plates on the distal dorsal surfaces of the fingers and toes. The nail plate, which is derived from a metabolically active matrix of multiplying cells situated beneath the posterior nail fold, grows forward at a rate of approximately 1 cm every 3 mo. The nail plate is bounded by the lateral and posterior nail folds; a thin eponychium (the cuticle) protrudes from the posterior fold over a crescent-shaped white area called the lunula. The pink color reflects the underlying vascular bed.

Holbrook KA, Sybert VP: Basic science. In Schachner LA, Hansen RC (editors): *Pediatric Dermatology*, 2nd ed. New York, Churchill Livingstone, 1995, p 1.

Loomis CA, Birge MB: Fetal skin development. In Eichenfield LF, Frieden IJ, Esterly NB (editors): *Textbook of Neonatal Dermatology*. Philadelphia, WB Saunders, 2001, p 1.

Mancini AJ: Structure and function of newborn skin. In Eichenfield LF, Frieden IJ, Esterly NB (editors): *Textbook of Neonatal Dermatology*. Philadelphia, WB Saunders, 2001, p 18.

Chapter 635
Evaluation of the Patient

History and Physical Examination. Although many skin disorders are easily recognized by simple inspection, the history and physical examination are often necessary for accurate assessment. The entire body surface, mucous membranes, conjunctiva, hair, and nails should always be examined thoroughly under adequate illumination. The color, turgor, texture, temperature, and moisture of the skin and the growth, texture, caliber, and luster of the hair and nails should be noted. Skin lesions should be palpated, inspected, and classified on the bases of morphology, size, color, texture, firmness, configuration, location, and distribution. One must also decide whether the changes are those of the primary lesion itself or whether the clinical pattern has been altered by a secondary factor such as infection, trauma, or therapy.

Primary lesions are classified as macules, papules, patches, plaques, nodules, tumors, vesicles, bullae, pustules, wheals, and cysts. A *macule* represents an alteration in skin color but cannot be felt. When the lesion is larger than 1 cm, the term *patch* is used. *Papules* are palpable solid lesions smaller than 0.5–1 cm, whereas *nodules* are larger in diameter. *Tumors* are usually larger than nodules and vary considerably in mobility and consistency. *Vesicles* are raised, fluid-filled lesions less than 0.5 cm in diameter; when larger, they are called *bullae*. *Pustules* contain purulent material. *Wheals* are flat-topped, palpable lesions of variable size, duration, and configuration that represent dermal collections of edema fluid. *Cysts* are circumscribed, thick-walled lesions that are located deep in the skin; they are covered by a normal epidermis and contain fluid or semisolid material. Aggregations of papules and pustules are referred to as *plaques*.

Primary lesions may change into secondary lesions, or secondary lesions may develop over time where no primary lesion existed. Primary lesions are usually more helpful for diagnostic purposes than secondary lesions. Secondary lesions include scales, ulcers, erosions, excoriations, fissures, crusts, and scars. *Scales* consist of compressed layers of stratum corneum cells that are retained on the skin surface. *Erosions* involve focal loss of the epidermis, and they heal without scarring. *Ulcers* extend into the dermis and tend to heal with scarring. Ulcerated lesions inflicted by scratching are often linear or angular in configuration and are called *excoriations*. *Fissures* are caused by splitting or cracking;

they usually occur in diseased skin. *Crusts* consist of matted, retained accumulations of blood, serum, pus, and epithelial debris on the surface of a weeping lesion. *Scars* are end-stage lesions that can be thin, depressed and atrophic, raised and hypertrophic, or flat and pliable; they are composed of fibrous connective tissue. *Lichenification* is a thickening of skin with accentuation of normal skin lines that is caused by chronic irritation (rubbing, scratching) or inflammation.

If the diagnosis is not clear after a thorough examination, one or more diagnostic procedures may be indicated. Besides those discussed here, others are identified in appropriate subsections (e.g., biopsies or scrapings of scabies lesions and smears, cultures of vesicles and pustules for detection of virus or bacteria).

Biopsy of Skin. Biopsy of skin is required for diagnosis in children only occasionally. *Punch biopsy* is a simple, relatively painless procedure and usually provides adequate tissue for examination if the appropriate lesion is sampled. The selection of a fresh, well-developed primary lesion is extremely important to obtain an accurate diagnosis. The site of the biopsy should have relatively low risk for damage to underlying dermal structures. The skin is anesthetized by application of EMLA cream and/or intradermal injection of 1–2% lidocaine (Xylocaine), with or without epinephrine, with a 27- or 30-gauge needle after cleansing of the site. A punch, 3 or 4 mm in diameter, is pressed firmly against the skin and rotated until it sinks to the proper depth. All three layers (epidermis, dermis, subcutis) should be contained in the plug. The plug should be lifted gently with forceps or extracted with a needle and separated from the underlying tissue with an iris scissors. Bleeding abates with firm pressure and with suturing. The biopsy specimen should be placed in 10% formaldehyde solution (Formalin) for appropriate processing.

Wood Lamp. The Wood lamp transmits ultraviolet light mainly in a wavelength of 365 nm. The examination, which is performed in a darkened room, is useful in detecting hypopigmented macules and certain superficial fungal infections of the scalp. Blue-green fluorescence is detectable at the base of each infected hair shaft in ectothrix and in some endothrix infections. Scales and crusts may appear pale yellow, but this is not evidence of a fungal infection. Dermatophyte lesions of the skin (tinea corporis) do not fluoresce; macules of tinea versicolor, however, have a golden fluorescence under a Wood lamp. *Erythrasma*, an intertriginous infection caused by *Corynebacterium minutissimum*, may fluoresce pink-orange, whereas *Pseudomonas aeruginosa* is yellow-green under a Wood lamp. Discrete areas of altered pigment can often be visualized more clearly by using a Wood lamp, particularly if the pigmentary change is epidermal. Hyperpigmented lesions appear darker, and hypopigmented lesions (as in tuberous sclerosis) lighter than the surrounding skin.

Potassium Hydroxide (KOH) Preparation. This provides a rapid and reliable method for detecting fungal elements of both yeasts and dermatophytes. Scaly lesions should be scraped at the active border for optimal recovery of mycelia and spores. Vesicles should be unroofed, and the blister top should be clipped and placed on a slide for examination. In tinea capitis, infected hairs must be plucked from the follicle; scales from the scalp do not usually contain mycelia. A few drops of 20% KOH are added to the specimen, which is then gently heated over an alcohol lamp until it begins to bubble; alternatively, ample time (approximately 10–20 min) can be allowed for dissolution of the keratin. Alternatively, dimethyl sulfoxide (DMSO) can be included in the KOH solution. The preparation is examined under low-intensity light for fungal elements.

Tzanck Smear. This is useful in the diagnosis of some viral infections (herpes simplex, varicella, herpes zoster, eczema herpeticum) and for the detection of acantholytic cells in pemphigus. An intact, fresh blister should be ruptured and drained of fluid. The base of the blister is then scraped with a dull-edged instrument, taking care to avoid drawing a significant amount of blood; the material is smeared on a clear glass slide and air dried. Staining with Giemsa stain is preferable, but Wright stain is acceptable. Balloon cells and multinucleated giant cells are diagnostic of herpesvirus infection; acantholytic epidermal cells are characteristic of pemphigus.

The *direct fluorescent assay* is more sensitive and specific. The keratinocytes are scraped from the base of the blister as described earlier. The laboratory stains the slide with labeled antibodies specific for varicella-zoster virus or herpes simplex virus. Observation of the slide with a fluorescence microscope documents the presence of the specific virus within the cells.

Immunofluorescence Studies. Immunofluorescence studies of skin can be used to detect tissue-fixed antibodies to skin components and complement; characteristic staining patterns are specific for certain skin disorders. Serum can be used for identifying circulating antibodies. Skin biopsy specimens for direct immunofluorescence preparations should be obtained from involved sites except in those diseases for which perilesional skin or uninvolved skin is required (Table 635–1). A punch biopsy sample is obtained, and the tissue is placed in a special transport medium or immediately frozen in liquid nitrogen for transport or storage. Thin cryostat sections of the specimen are incubated with fluorescein-conjugated antibodies to the specific antigens.

Serum of patients can be examined by indirect immunofluorescence techniques using sections of normal human skin, guinea pig lip, or monkey esophagus as substrate. The substrate is incubated with fresh or thawed frozen serum and then with fluorescein-conjugated antihuman globulin. If the serum contains antibody to epithelial components, its specific staining pattern can be seen on fluorescence microscopy. By serial dilution, the titer of circulating antibody can be estimated.

Gately LE, Nesbitt LT: Update on immunofluorescent testing in bullous diseases and lupus erythematosus. *Dermatol Clin* 1994;12:133.
Morrison LH: Direct immunofluorescent microscopy in the diagnosis of autoimmune bullous dermatoses. *Clin Dermatol* 2001;19:607.

635.1 Cutaneous Manifestations of Systemic Diseases

Selected diseases have signature skin findings, often as the presenting sign of illness, which can facilitate the assessment of complex medical patients (Table 635–2).

CONNECTIVE TISSUE DISEASES

Lupus Erythematosus. Lupus erythematosus (LE) (see Chapter 148) is an idiopathic autoimmune inflammatory disease that may be multisystemic or confined to the skin.

SYSTEMIC LUPUS ERYTHEMATOSUS. Systemic LE (SLE) is a multisystem disease but may present with erythematous patches in a photo distribution. The classic malar or "butterfly" rash of SLE may be the initial presentation and must be distinguished from other causes of a "red face," most notably seborrheic dermatitis, atopic dermatitis, and rosacea. Other cutaneous findings may help confirm the diagnosis of SLE including purpuric lesions, livedo reticularis, mucosal ulcerations, Raynaud phenomena, and nonscarring alopecia. The degree of cutaneous involvement often reflects the activity of underlying disease.

Histologically, cutaneous LE demonstrates varying degrees of epidermal atrophy, plugging of hair follicles, and a vacuolar alteration at an inflamed dermoepidermal junction. Immunoglobulin (IgM, IgG) and complement deposition in lesional skin may help confirm the diagnosis (see Table 635–1). Immune deposits in nonlesional sun-exposed skin are found in the majority of patients with SLE (lupus band test). Treatment of skin lesions includes sun protection and low-potency topical corticosteroids.

TABLE 635–1. Immunofluorescent Findings in Immune-Mediated Cutaneous Diseases

Disease	Involved Skin	Uninvolved Skin	Direct IF	Indirect IF	Circulating Antibodies
Dermatitis herpetiformis	Negative	Positive	Granular IgA ± C in papillary dermis	None	IgA antireticulum in 20–70%. Antiendomysial (IgA, IgG) and transglutaminase antibodies with celiac disease
Bullous pemphigoid	Positive	Positive	Linear IgG and C band in BMZ, occasionally IgM, IgA, IgE	IgG to BMZ in 70%	None
Pemphigus (all variants)	Positive	Positive	IgG in intercellular spaces of epidermis between keratinocytes	IgG to intercellular space	None
Pemphigus foliaceus	Positive	Positive	IgG to desmosomal glycoprotein, desmoglein$_1$	Same as direct IF	None
Herpes gestationis	Positive	Positive	C3 at BMZ, occasionally IgG	IgG anti-BMZ	None
Linear IgA bullous dermatosis (chronic bullous dermatosis of childhood)	Positive	Positive	Linear IgA at BMZ, occasionally C	Low titer, rare IgA, anti-BMZ	None
Discoid lupus erythematosus	Positive	Negative	Linear IgG, IgM, IgA, and C3 at BMZ (lupus band)	None	ANA negative
Systemic lupus erythematosus	Positive	Variable; exposed to sun, 30–50%; nonexposed, 10–30%	Linear IgG, IgM, C3 at BMZ (lupus band)	None	ANA Anti-Ro (SSA) Anti-RNP Anti-DNA Anti-Sm
Henoch-Schönlein purpura	Positive	Negative	IgA around vessel walls	None	IgA rheumatoid factor, occasionally

C = complement; IF = immunofluorescent findings; Ig = immunoglobulin; ANA = antinuclear antibody; BMZ = basement membrane zone at the dermoepidermal junction.

NEONATAL LUPUS ERYTHEMATOSUS. Neonatal LE (NLE) (see Chapter 148) presents during the first weeks to months of life as annular, erythematous, scaly plaques typically on the head, neck, and upper trunk. Ultraviolet light, including phototherapy for hyperbilirubinemia, may exacerbate or initiate cutaneous lesions. NLE is often misdiagnosed as infantile eczema, seborrheic dermatitis, or tinea corporis. Passive transfer of maternal IgG (e.g., anti-Ro) antibodies cause the transient skin lesions; antibody levels wane by 6 mo, generally resulting in clearance of the rash. Congenital heart block occurs in 50% of affected infants, but only 10% of affected infants have both skin and cardiac abnormalities. Noncardiac extracutaneous manifestations such as anemia, thrombocytopenia, and cholestatic liver disease are uncommon; later progression to SLE is rare. Maternal antibody (ANA) testing is indicated.

DISCOID LUPUS ERYTHEMATOSUS. Discoid LE (DLE) is uncommon in early childhood and presents in late adolescence. The signature skin findings in DLE are chronic, erythematous, scaly, atrophic, telangiectatic plaques on sun-exposed skin that frequently heal with scarring and dyspigmentation. Extracutaneous features may include involvement of the nasal and oral mucosa, eyes, and nails. The differential diagnosis includes other photo dermatoses such as polymorphous light eruption, juvenile springtime eruption, and juvenile dermatomyositis. There is a distinct overlap between SLE and DLE with common histopathologic features and photo exacerbation; most patients with DLE have normal laboratory studies and do not progress to systemic disease. Topical sunscreens and steroids may be helpful; intralesional steroids and oral antimalarials (e.g., hydroxychloroquine) are used with severe disease.

Juvenile Dermatomyositis. Characteristic skin findings are often the presenting sign of juvenile dermatomyositis (JDMS) (see Chapter 149). An ill-defined, erythematous to violaceous scaly, minimally pruritic eruption occurs in photo-distributed areas such as the face, upper trunk, and extensor extremities. Circumscribed periocular involvement of this "heliotrope" rash may take the appearance of "raccoon eyes," particularly in young children. Distinctive papules overlying the knuckles (Gottron papules) are helpful in suggesting the diagnosis in the absence of associated muscle weakness. Other cutaneous features include nail fold and gingival margin telangiectasia, palmar hyperkeratosis (or "mechanic's hands"), and a poikilodermatous (dyspigmentation and telangiectasia) eruption over the shoulder girdle ("shawl sign"). Cutaneous features may precede the systemic illness, reflecting disease activity. The differential diagnosis includes atopic dermatitis, other connective tissue diseases, lichen planus, medication reactions, and infectious exanthems. The paucity of itch in JDMS may help eliminate some considerations. Histologically, lesional skin demonstrates epidermal atrophy and vacuolar degeneration at the dermoepidermal junction. JDMS is distinct from adult dermatomyositis in both presentation and prognosis. Pediatric patients have more difficulty with gastrointestinal vasculopathy and cutaneous calcifications, but are not at increased risk of malignancy.

Treatment includes both steroidal and nonsteroidal immunosuppressants, and photoprotection is vital to prevent skin flares.

Scleroderma. Scleroderma (see Chapter 150) is an inflammatory disorder of unknown etiology that, like LE, can be either localized to the skin or affect multiple organ systems. Localized scleroderma, or *morphea*, has several distinctive presentations. The most common is a solitary circumscribed patch of erythema that evolves into an indurated, sclerotic, atrophic plaque, later healing, or "burning out" with pigment change. Morphea can affect any area of skin, but when confined to the frontal scalp, forehead, and midface in a linear band, is referred to as linear scleroderma or "en coup de sabre." This form of morphea carries a poorer prognosis because of the associated underlying musculoskeletal atrophy that can be cosmetically disfiguring. The differential diagnosis includes granuloma annulare, necrobiosis lipoidica, lichen sclerosis et atrophicus, and late stage Lyme disease (acrodermatitis chronica atrophicans). Histology is characterized by thickening or sclerosis of the dermis with collagen degeneration. Morphea tends to persist with gradual outward expansion on the skin until spontaneous or induced cessation of the inflammatory phase after months to years. Topical steroids

TABLE 635–2. **Characteristics of Cutaneous Signs of Systemic Diseases**

Disease	Age of Onset	Skin Lesions	Distribution	Diagnostic Evaluations	Associated Symptoms/Signs	Differential Diagnosis
Systemic lupus erythematosus	Any	Erythematous patches; palpable purpura; livedo reticularis; Raynaud phenomenon; thrombocytopenic and non-thrombocytopenic purpura	Photodistribution; "malar" face	ANA panel Anti-Double stranded DNA Leukopenia/ lymphopenia Thrombocytopenia Complement levels Urinalysis	Arthritis Nephritis Cerebritis Serositis	Seborrheic dermatitis Rosacea Atopic dermatitis Juvenile dermatomyositis Vasculitis
Discoid lupus	Adolescents	Annular, scaly plaques; atrophy; dyspigmentation	Photodistribution	ANA	Scarring	Subacute cutaneous lupus Polymorphous light eruption Juvenile dermatomyositis
Neonatal lupus	Newborn to 6 mo	Annular, erythematous, scaly plaques	Photodistribution; head/neck	ANA Anti-ro	Heart block Thrombocytopenia	Tinea capitis Atopic dermatitis Seborrheic dermatitis
Juvenile dermatomyositis	Any	Erythematous to violaceous scaly, macules; discrete papules overlying knuckles	Periocular face; shoulder girdle; extensor extremities; knuckles; palms	ANA Jo-1 Ab Aldolase CK LDH	Proximal muscle weakness Calcifications Vasculopathy	Atopic dermatitis Allergic contact dermatitis Lupus erythematosus Viral exanthem Drug eruption
Henoch-Schönlein purpura	Children and adolescents	Purpuric papules and plaques	Buttocks; lower extremities	Urinalysis Bun/Cr Skin biopsy	Abdominal pain Arthritis	Vasculitis Drug eruption Infantile hemorrhagic edema Viral exanthem
Kawasaki disease	Infants, children	Erythematous maculopapular to urticarial plaques; acral and groin erythema, edema, desquamation	Diffuse	Leukocytosis ESR CRP Thrombocytosis	Strawberry tongue Conjunctivitis Lymphadenopathy Cardiovascular complications	Viral syndrome Drug eruption Staphylococcal/streptococcal illness
Inflammatory bowel disease	Children and adolescents	Aphthae; erythema nodosum; pyoderma gangrenosum; thrombophlebitis	Oral ulcers; perianal fissures	ESR Thrombocytosis Radiographic abnormalities	Abdominal pain Diarrhea Cramping Arthritis Conjunctivitis	Behçet syndrome Vasculitis *Yersinia colitis*
Sweet syndrome	Any	Infiltrated erythematous, edematous plaques	Diffuse	Skin biopsy Leukocytosis ESR	Fever Flulike illness Conjunctivitis	Infection Urticaria Erythema multiforme Urticarial vasculitis
Graft versus host disease	Any	Acute: erythema, papules, vesicles, bulla	Head and neck; palms/soles; diffuse	Skin biopsy Liver function	Fever Mucositis Hepatitis	Drug eruption Infectious exanthem
Hypersensitivity reaction	Any	Erythema; urticarial macules and plaques	Diffuse	Liver function Eosinophilia Atypical lymphocytosis	Perioral edema Lymphadenopathy Fever Hepatitis	Stevens-Johnson syndrome Infectious exanthem
Serum sickness-like reaction	Any	Edematous, purpuric plaques	Acral; diffuse	ESR	Fever Lymphadenopathy Arthritis, nephritis	Kawasaki disease Connective tissue disease

ESR = erythrocyte sedimentation rate; ANA = antinuclear antibodies; LDH = lactate dehydrogenase; CK = creatine kinase; CRP = C-reactive protein.

may help shorten the disease course; however, significant postinflammatory pigment alteration often persists.

Systemic scleroderma frequently presents with acral (e.g., sclerodactyly, ulceration, nail fold telangiectasia, or Raynaud phenomena) and other cutaneous changes (e.g., pinched nose, furrowed perioral skin, or "scleroderma facies") (see Chapter 150). Overlap syndromes such as CREST and mixed connective tissue disease may include some physical and laboratory features of scleroderma.

VASCULITIDES

The vasculitides (see Chapter 157) encompass a broad group of disorders having considerable overlap with connective tissue diseases. Immune-mediated inflammation of blood vessels of varying size may be caused by an underlying inflammatory state, infection, medication, or malignancy. Common clinical features include palpable nonthrombocytopenic purpuric skin lesions, arthritis, fever, myalgia, fatigue, and weight loss, as well as an elevated erythrocyte sedimentation rate. Extracutaneous organ involvement includes the joints, lungs, kidneys, and central nervous system.

Henoch-Schönlein Purpura. Henoch-Schönlein purpura (HSP) is a vasculitis that presents with purpuric lesions prominently on the buttocks and lower extremities of school-aged children. Infantile hemorrhagic edema (IHE) shares some clinical features with HSP but appears in infants and toddlers. IHE is characterized by circumscribed purpuric papules and plaques on the trunk and extremities, but unlike HSP, commonly affects the face and lacks systemic signs or symptoms. HSP must also be differentiated from infectious causes of purpuric skin lesions such as meningococcemia, Rocky Mountain spotted fever, and purpuric viral exanthems such as those caused by enteroviruses, as well as from juvenile rheumatoid arthritis and other vasculitides.

Kawasaki Disease. Kawasaki disease (KD), (see Chapter 156), is a clinical diagnosis based on both cutaneous and extracutaneous features. The skin eruption of KD may be polymorphic, presenting variously with urticarial, maculopapular, or morbilliform patches and plaques on the trunk and extremities, but early involvement in the groin region may be an initial clue to the diagnosis. Acral edema and desquamation also are prominent features, but typically occur later. Conjunctivitis, often with sparing of the limbus, and lingual plaques ("white strawberry tongue") that shed to produce denuded, erythematous patches with prominent papilla ("strawberry tongue") are classic mucocutaneous features. Histopathologic findings in the skin are nonspecific and generally do not assist in distinguishing other differential considerations such as a viral or bacterial exanthem or medication reaction.

Behçet Disease. Behçet disease (see Chapter 151) is multisystemic disease that includes oral and genital ulceration and ocular disease (uveitis, relapsing iridocyclitis). Recurrent aphthous stomatitis is present in up to 98% of patients, and is commonly the presenting symptom. Genital ulcerations may resemble aphthae and can occur on the penis or scrotum, and may be particularly painful in females. Additional skin findings may include folliculitis, purpuric lesions, erythema nodosum, and pustule formation after venipuncture or skin trauma ("pathergy"). Differential diagnosis of oral lesions includes recurrent aphthous stomatitis, herpes simplex, and less common oculocutaneous syndromes (e.g., MAGIC syndrome: mouth and genital ulcers with inflamed cartilage). Skin biopsy demonstrates either leukocytoclastic or lymphocytic vasculitis. Oral lesions may respond to swish and spit/swallow preparations variably including corticosteroids, antihistamines, antibiotics, and analgesics.

GASTOINTESTINAL DISEASES

Inflammatory Bowel Disease. *Ulcerative colitis* (see Chapter 317) presents with cutaneous manifestations in up to 30% of patients. Aphthous ulcers are common and seem to worsen with gastrointestinal symptoms. Erythema nodosum, occurring in up to 10%, presents as warm, erythematous plaques often on the distal, lower extremities. Pyoderma gangrenosum is a focal, ulcerative process that has distinctive, inflamed, "undermined" borders and a purulent, boggy center. Thrombophlebitis also occurs at an increased rate in patients with ulcerative colitis. In most cases, treatment of the underlying disease state improves the cutaneous sequelae.

Crohn disease, or regional enteritis (see Chapter 317), classically presents with perianal fissures, abscesses, sinuses, and fistulas, and these features may be presenting signs of illness. Like ulcerative colitis, aphthae, erythema nodosum, and pyoderma gangrenosum occur at increased frequency and may improve with treatment of underlying disease. Noncaseating granulomatous inflammation is seen on routine histopathology, and when found in skin not contiguous with the intestinal tract, is labeled "metastatic Crohn disease." Metastatic lesions may present as solitary or multiple, localized, plaques or nodules and may be on perianal, perioral, or other cutaneous surfaces, including scars or ileostomy sites. Standard therapy includes immunosuppressive medications, nutritional support, and surgery for complications.

CUTANEOUS MANIFESTATIONS OF MALIGNANCY

Internal malignancies may find cutaneous expression by several mechanisms. Cutaneous metastases may present as firm nodules at any cutaneous site, including the scalp. Distinctive paraneoplastic reaction patterns may result in sometimes striking rashes. Some genetic syndromes have increased malignancy risk that may be suggested initially by cutaneous signs.

Sweet Syndrome. Also known as acute febrile neutrophilic dermatosis, Sweet syndrome (see Chapter 157) presents abruptly with tender, erythematous, edematous plaques or nodules on any area of the skin, often accompanied by fever, anemia, and leukocytosis. Diagnosis is confirmed by the presence of a dense neutrophilic infiltrate without evidence of vasculitis. The differential diagnosis includes pyoderma gangrenosum, cellulites, erythema multiforme, Behçet syndrome, and erythema nodosum. The etiology of Sweet syndrome is unknown but may

be due to a hypersensitivity reaction to a bacterial, viral, or tumor antigen, and may occur in association with Behçet disease. Even though Sweet syndrome may occur without an identifiable etiology, investigation for infection or malignancy is warranted. In children, Sweet syndrome has been associated with otitis media, osteomyelitis, aseptic meningitis, HIV, and leukemia. In adults, 15% of patients have an associated malignancy, most commonly hematologic. Sweet syndrome is sensitive to oral corticosteroids.

Necrolytic Migratory Erythema. Necrolytic migratory erythema (NME), or glucagonoma syndrome, is a distinctive migratory erythema that may signal an underlying neoplasm, such as an alpha-cell pancreatic tumor underlying the eruption of NME. Polycyclic erythematous patches and plaques on the trunk, extremities, and groin occur in association with glossitis, and cheilitis. Elevated glucagon levels, glucose intolerance, and hypoaminoacidemia confirm the diagnosis, and tumor resection leads to resolution of the rash.

Other cutaneous findings that may signal an underlying malignancy include pruritus, ichthyosis, acanthosis nigricans, urticaria, pemphigus, and erythroderma.

CUTANEOUS REACTIONS IN THE SETTING OF IMMUNOSUPPRESSION

Rashes in immunosuppressed patients are a diagnostic challenge. Medication reactions, infectious etiologies, and graft vs host disease (GVHD) are included in the differential diagnosis; cutaneous and histologic similarities can be confounding. The majority of medication reactions are mild morbilliform or exanthematous eruptions of little clinical consequence. Identifying the suspect medication may be difficult owing to the typically lengthy medication lists in this population. Features that may help identify suspect medications include rash onset relative to exposure, character of distribution and spread, associated symptoms, and laboratory data. Medication eruptions begin on the trunk 7–10 days after exposure, spread peripherally, and are associated with pruritus, and less commonly fever, arthralgia, and lymphadenopathy. Eosinophilia may support a diagnosis of drug eruption, but may be absent in the setting of bone marrow suppression. Antibiotics including penicillins, sulfa drugs, cephalosporins, nonsteroidal anti-inflammatory agents, anticonvulsants and, on occasion, aminoglycoside, are common offenders. Medication eruptions may resolve despite continued use of the offending agent, or they may progress to more severe involvement. A careful drug history, elimination of all nonessential suspect medications or change to medications of dissimilar class, and treatment of pruritus with emollients, topical steroids, antihistamines, and antipruritics are indicated. Skin biopsies are rarely useful in distinguishing medication eruptions from infectious exanthems, although GVHD, if sufficiently advanced, may have signature histopathologic findings.

Graft vs Host Disease. GVHD (see Chapter 127) may have florid cutaneous expression in addition to characteristic extracutaneous features such as fever, mucositis, diarrhea, and hepatitis. Acute GVHD may be mistaken for a medication reaction or infectious exanthem based on the nonspecific erythematous maculopapular eruption that often starts focally and generalizes. Features that may suggest GVHD include timing of eruption (typically 1–3 wk post-transplant at the time of hematopoietic reconstitution), initial involvement of the head and neck including the ears, and subsequent spread to the trunk, extremities, and palms and soles. Chronic GVHD, which occurs in approximately 20% of long-term transplant survivors, is seen most often in patients who have previously experienced acute disease. Cutaneous manifestations of chronic GVHD are distinctive, with sclerotic, dyspigmented scaly plaques and lichenoid papules predominating. Treatment includes systemic immunosuppression supplemented by topical steroids, antihistamines, antipruritics, and emollients. Chronic disease may also respond to photochemotherapy (e.g., PUVA), plasmapheresis, and thalidomide. Topical immunomodulators such as tacrolimus may offer new avenues of therapy for this difficult condition. The pediatrician should also be mindful of GVHD in susceptible nontransplant settings, such as in the severely immunosuppressed neonate or infant in response to therapeutic transfusion of blood products, the fetus with congenital immunodeficiency secondary to transplacental passage of maternal lymphocytes, and the older child with malignancy who has received nonirradiated blood products.

MULTISYSTEMIC MEDICATION REACTIONS (see Chapter 139)

Most cutaneous reactions that result from the use of systemic medications are confined to the skin and resolve without sequelae after discontinuation of the offending agent. More severe drug eruptions may be life threatening, making rapid recognition vital. (See *Stevens-Johnson syndrome* and *toxic epidermal necrolysis*.)

Hypersensitivity Syndrome. This syndrome is classically seen 1–4 wk after initial exposure to an aromatic anticonvulsant and often presents with the triad of fever, rash, and hepatitis. The skin rash is characterized by a pruritic, diffuse, erythematous to urticarial eruption of coalescing plaques. Prominent periocular edema, cervical lymphadenopathy, pharyngitis, and malaise accompany this dramatic cutaneous eruption. Eosinophilia occurs in up to 30% of patients; atypical lymphocytosis is common. Hepatitis ranging from mild transaminitis to frank hepatic failure may be accompanied by interstitial nephritis, pneumonitis, and encephalitis. Late-onset (several months) thyroiditis and hypothyroidism may occur as a result of antimicrosomal antibodies directed against thyroid peroxidases involved in drug metabolism. A heritable defect in the epoxide hydrolase pathway, in the case of anticonvulsants, leads to accumulation of toxic metabolites, which react with lymphocytes. Anticonvulsants having the distinctive aromatic structure (carbamazepine, phenobarbital, Dilantin) have a high risk of triggering hypersensitivity syndrome in susceptible individuals and their first-degree relatives. The differential diagnosis includes Stevens-Johnson syndrome, into which some of these cases can evolve, viral exanthem, or GVHD in the appropriate clinical setting. In addition to anticonvulsants, sulfonamides may cause a similar constellation of symptoms on first exposure due to abnormalities in glutathione transferase pathways.

Withdrawal of the medication is the primary therapeutic intervention, with symptomatic treatment of itch and/or pain being universal. The use of corticosteroids is controversial in Stevens-Johnson syndrome, but it is useful in the setting of rapidly evolving hepatic or renal involvement in hypersensitivity syndrome. The role of intravenous immunoglobulin in hypersensitivity syndrome is unclear. Counseling regarding increased risk with like medications and sibling risk is important. Hypersensitivity reaction can flare, both in the skin and other organ systems, well after the medication has been withdrawn and initial improvement achieved, necessitating close follow-up for several months.

Serum Sickness–Like Reaction. Serum sickness–like reaction (SSLR) presents with urticarial to purpuric, sharply marginated coalescing plaques and acral erythema/edema, often in association with arthritis, lymphadenopathy, and fever. Unlike true serum sickness, laboratory evidence of circulating immune complexes and multisystem involvement of vasculitis are typically absent. The differential diagnosis includes Kawasaki disease, connective tissue diseases, and hypersensitivity syndrome. SSLR is most commonly seen following exposure to cefaclor. The cause is unknown but a toxic metabolite is suspected. In contrast to hypersensitivity reaction, SSLR typically occurs after

repeated drug exposures. Symptomatic treatment and medication withdrawal are recommended.

Choy EH, Isenberg DA: Treatment of dermatomyositis and polymyositis. *Rheumatology* 2002;41:7.

Goker H, Haznadaroglu K, Chao NJ: Acute graft versus host disease: Pathobiology and management. *Exp Hematol* 2001;29:259.

Roujeau JC, Stern RS: Severe adverse cutaneous reactions to drugs. *N Engl J Med* 1994;331:1272.

Vogelsang GB: How I treat chronic graft vs host disease. *Blood* 2001;97:1196.

Weston WL, Morelli JG, Lee LA: The clinical spectrum of anti-Ro positive cutaneous neonatal lupus erythematosus. *J Am Acad Dermatol* 1999;40:675.

Yalcindag A, Sundel R: Vasculitis in childhood. *Curr Opin Rheum* 2001;13:422.

Chapter 636
Principles of Therapy

Competent skin care requires a specific diagnosis, knowledge of the natural course of the disease, and appreciation of primary versus secondary lesions. If the diagnosis is uncertain, it is better to err on the side of less rather than more aggressive treatment. Even when the diagnosis is clear, an acute dermatitis may require gentle and bland therapy initially.

In the use of topical medication, consideration of vehicle is as important as the specific therapeutic agent. Acute weeping lesions respond best to wet compresses, followed by lotions or creams. For dry, thickened, scaly skin or when treating a contact-allergic reaction possibly due to a component of a topical medication, an ointment base is preferable. Gels and solutions are most useful for the scalp and other hairy areas. The site of involvement is of considerable importance because the most desirable vehicle may not be cosmetically or functionally appropriate, such as an ointment on the face or hands. A patient's preference should also play a part in the choice of vehicle because compliance is poor if a medication is not acceptable to a patient.

Most *lotions* are mixtures of water and oil that can be poured. After the water evaporates, the small amount of remaining oil covers the skin. Some *shake lotions* are a suspension of water and insoluble powder; as the water evaporates, cooling the skin, a thin film of powder covers the skin. *Creams* are emulsions of oil and water that are viscous and do not pour (more oil than in lotions). *Ointments* have oils and a small amount of water or no water at all; they feel greasy, lubricate dry skin, trap water, and may be occlusive. Ointments without water usually require no preservatives because microorganisms require water to survive.

Therapy should be kept as simple as possible, and specific written instructions about the frequency and duration of application should be provided. Physicians should become familiar with one or two preparations in each category and should learn to use them appropriately. Prescribing nonspecific proprietary medications that may contain sensitizing agents should be avoided. Certain preparations such as topical antihistamines and sensitizing anesthetics are never indicated.

Wet Dressings. These dressings decrease pruritus, burning, and stinging sensations; they are indicated for acutely inflamed moist or oozing dermatitis. Although various astringent and antiseptic substances may be added to the solution, tap water compresses are just as effective.

OPEN WET DRESSINGS. These dressings cool and dry the skin by evaporation and cleanse by removing crusts and exudate that cause further irritation if permitted to remain. The solution should be cool or tepid and consist of tap water, isotonic saline, or aluminum acetate (Burow solution) in a 1:20 or 1:40 dilution. Potassium permanganate is messy and offers no advantage. Boric acid can be toxic if absorbed and should ***never*** be used for compresses. Dressings of multiple layers of Kerlix, gauze or soft cotton material should be saturated with the solution and remoistened as often as necessary. Compresses should be applied for 10–20 min at least every 4 hr and should be continued usually for 24–48 hr.

CLOSED WET DRESSINGS. These dressings are indicated for abscesses. The solution should be warm, and the dressings should be covered with plastic to prevent evaporation. Closed wet dressings, if prolonged, cause maceration because they prevent evaporation and heat loss.

Bath Oils, Colloids, Soaps. *Bath oil* has little benefit in the treatment of children. It offers little moisturizing effect while increasing the risk of injury during a bath. Bath oil may lubricate the surface of the bathtub, causing an adult or child to fall when stepping into the tub. Tar bath solutions (Balnetar, Zetar) can be prescribed and may be helpful for psoriasis and atopic dermatitis. *Colloids* such as starch powder or colloidal oatmeal (Aveeno) are soothing and antipruritic for some patients when added to the bath water. Oilated Aveeno contains mineral oil and lanolin derivatives for lubrication if the skin is dry. These can also lubricate the bathtub surface. Ordinary toilet *soaps* may be irritating and drying if patients have dry skin or dermatitis. Examples of soaps that are usually not harmful to skin are Dove, Lowila, Aveeno, Neutrogena, Basis, Alpha Keri, and Oilatum. When skin is acutely inflamed, avoidance of soap is advised. Some patients find that lipid-free cleansers containing cetyl alcohol (Cetaphil) are soothing.

Lubricants. Lubricants, such as lotions, creams, and ointments, can be used as emollients for dry skin and as vehicles for topical agents such as corticosteroids and keratolytics. In general, ointments are the most effective emollients. Numerous commercial preparations are available in addition to standard products such as petrolatum, cold cream, stearin-lanolin cream, and hydrophilic ointment. Some patients do not tolerate ointments, and some may be sensitized to a component of the lubricant; some preservatives of creams (most commonly parabens) are sensitizers. Useful lubricating lotions include Lubriderm, Nutraderm, and Nivea. Creams include Eucerin, Neutrogena, Nutraderm, Purpose, Vanicream, and Complex 15. Aquaphor is a cosmetically acceptable alternative to petrolatum. These preparations can be applied several times a day if necessary. Maximal effect is achieved when they are applied *immediately* to damp skin after a bath or shower. Sarna lotion contains menthol and camphor in an emollient vehicle for control of pruritus and dryness.

Shampoos. Special shampoos containing sulfur, salicylic acid, antiseptics, and selenium sulfide (Selsun, Exsel) are useful for conditions in which there is scaling of the scalp. Most shampoos also contain surfactants and detergents. Shampoos with sulfur or salicylic acid include Ionil, Sebulex, Fostex, and Vanseb. Those with only antiseptic agents include DHS-Zinc, Danex, and Head and Shoulders. Tar-containing shampoos such as T-Gel, Ionil-T, Sebutone, and Polytar are useful for psoriasis and severe seborrheic dermatitis. They can be used as frequently as necessary to control scaling, but use should be limited to avoid irritation. Patients should be instructed to leave the lathered shampoo in contact with the scalp for 5–10 min.

Shake Lotions. These lotions are useful antipruritic agents; they consist of a suspension of powder in a liquid vehicle. A water-dispersible oil may be added for lubrication. Calamine lotion is acceptable but tends to cake on the skin. A prototype lotion is zinc oxide 20 g, talc 20 g, glycerin 20 g, Alpha Keri 5 g, and water to make 120 g. These preparations can be used effectively in combination with wet dressings for exudative dermatitis. Cooling occurs as the lotion evaporates and moisture is absorbed by the powder deposited on the skin.

Powders. Powders are hygroscopic and serve as absorptive agents in areas of excessive moisture. When dry, powders decrease friction between two surfaces. They are most useful in the intertriginous areas and between the toes, where maceration and abrasion may result from friction on movement. Coarse powders may cake; therefore, they should be of fine particle size and inert unless medication has been incorporated in the formulation. Zeasorb is a bland, finely milled, general purpose powder that can be applied to any area of the body.

Pastes. These contain a fine powder in an ointment vehicle and are not often prescribed in current dermatologic therapy; in certain situations, however, they can be used effectively to protect vulnerable or damaged skin. A stiff zinc oxide paste is bland and inert and can be applied to the diaper area to prevent further irritation due to diaper dermatitis. Zinc paste should be applied in a thick layer completely obscuring the skin and is removed more easily with mineral oil than with soap and water.

Keratolytic Agents. *Urea-containing agents* are hydrophilic; they hydrate the stratum corneum and make the skin more pliable. In addition, because urea dissolves hydrogen bonds and epidermal keratin, it is effective in treating scaling disorders. Concentrations of 10–25% are available in several commercial lotions and creams (Carmol 20, Carmol 10, Nutraplus, Aquacare HP), which can be applied once or twice daily as tolerated. *Salicylic acid* is an effective keratolytic agent and can be incorporated into various vehicles in concentrations up to 6% to be applied two to three times daily. Salicylic acid preparations should not be used in treating small infants or on large surface areas or denuded skin; percutaneous absorption may result in salicylism. The α-*hydroxy acids*, particularly *lactic acid* and *glycolic acid*, are available in commercial preparations (LactiCare, LacHydrin, Aqua Glycolic) or can be incorporated in an ointment vehicle such as petrolatum or Aquaphor in concentrations up to 5%. Eucerin Plus Creme contains both urea and lactic acid. The α-hydroxy acid preparations are useful for the treatment of keratinizing disorders and may be applied once or twice daily. Some patients complain of burning; in this case, the frequency of application should be decreased.

Tar Compounds. Tars are obtained from bituminous coal, shale, petrolatum (coal tars), and wood. They are antipruritic and astringent and appear to promote normal keratinization. They may be useful for chronic eczema and psoriasis, and their efficacy may be increased if the affected area is exposed to ultraviolet (UV) light after the tar has been removed. *Tars should not be used in acute inflammatory lesions.* Tars are often messy and unacceptable because they may stain and they have an odor. Tars may be incorporated into shampoos, bath oils, lotions, and ointments. A useful preparation for pediatric patients is liquor carbonis detergens 2–5% in a cream or ointment vehicle. Tar gels (PsoriGel, Estargel, AquaTar) and tar in a light body oil (T-Derm) are relatively pleasant cosmetic preparations that cause minimal staining of skin and fabrics. Tars can also be incorporated into a vehicle with a topical corticosteroid. The frequency of application varies from one to three times daily, according to tolerance. Many children refuse to use tar preparations because of their odor and staining characteristics.

Antifungal Agents. These agents are available as powders, lotions, creams, and ointments for the treatment of dermatophyte and yeast infections. Nystatin, naftifine (Naftin), and amphotericin B are specific for *Candida* and are ineffective in other fungal disorders. Tolnaftate is effective against dermatophytes but not effective for yeast. The spectrum for ciclopirox olamine includes the dermatophytes, *Malassezia furfur,* and *Candida albicans.* The azoles—miconazole, clotrimazole, econazole, oxiconazole, and ketoconazole (Nizoral)—have a similar broad spectrum. Terbinafine has greater activity against dermatophytes but poorer activity against yeasts than the azoles. The topical antifungal agents should be applied one to two times a day for most fungal infections. All have low sensitizing potential; however, additives such as preservatives and stabilizers in the vehicles may cause allergic contact dermatitis. Whitfield's ointment (6% benzoic acid and 3% salicylic acid) is a potent keratolytic agent that has also been used for the treatment of dermatophyte infections. Irritant reactions are common.

Topical Antibiotics. Topical antibiotics have been used to treat local cutaneous infections for many years, although their efficacy, with the exception of mupirocin (Bactroban), has been questioned. Ointments are the preferred vehicles, and combinations with other topical agents, such as corticosteroids, are in general inadvisable. Whenever possible, the etiologic agent should be identified and treated specifically. Antibiotics in wide use as systemic preparations should be avoided because of the risk of sensitization. The sensitizing potential of certain other antibiotics, such as neomycin and nitrofurazone (Furacin), should be kept in mind. Mupirocin is the most effective topical agent currently available and is as effective as oral erythromycin in treatment of mild to moderate impetigo. Polysporin and bacitracin are not as effective as mupirocin or oral antibiotics.

Topical Corticosteroids. Topical corticosteroids are potent antiinflammatory agents and effective antipruritic agents. Successful therapeutic results are achieved in a wide variety of skin conditions. Corticosteroids fall into two classes: nonfluorinated preparations, such as hydrocortisone (Hytone), desonide (Tridesilon, Des Owen), hydrocortisone butyrate (Locoid), and mometasone furoate (Elocon), and fluorinated compounds, including triamcinolone (Kenalog, Aristocort), flurandrenolide (Cordran), fluocinolone (Synalar), betamethasone (Valisone, Benisone, Flurobate), and amcinonide (Cyclocort). The nonfluorinated steroids are usually of lesser potency and may cause fewer local and systemic side effects, whereas fluorinated steroids are potentially more harmful, particularly with long-term use. Other fluorinated compounds, for example, fluorocinonide (Lidex), halcinonide (Halog), betamethasone dipropionate (Diprolene), and clobetasol propionate (Temovate), are extremely potent and should be prescribed with care. Some of these compounds are formulated in several strengths based on their clinical efficacy and degree of vasoconstriction. Physicians using topical steroids should become familiar with several preparations and with the potency of the preparations used.

All corticosteroids can be obtained in various vehicles, including creams, ointments, solutions, gels, and aerosols. Absorption is enhanced by an ointment or gel vehicle, but the vehicle should be selected on the basis of the type of disorder and the site of involvement. Frequency of application should be determined by the potency of the preparation and the severity of the eruption. Applying a *thin film* two times daily usually suffices. Adverse local effects include cutaneous atrophy, striae, telangiectasia, hypopigmentation, and increased hair growth.

In selected circumstances, corticosteroids may be administered by intralesional injection (acne cysts, keloids, psoriatic plaques, alopecia areata, persistent insect bite reactions). This method of administration should be used only by experienced physicians.

Sunscreens. Sunscreens are of two general types: (1) those that reflect all wavelengths of UV and visible spectrums, such as zinc oxide and titanium dioxide, and (2) a heterogeneous group of chemicals that selectively absorb energy of various wavelengths within the UV spectrum. Some sunscreens permit tanning without burning; others prevent both. In addition to the spectrum of light that is blocked, other factors to be considered include cosmetic acceptance, sensitizing potential, retention on skin while swimming or sweating, required frequency of application, and cost. Effective opaque total barrier agents are zinc oxide ointment, Covermark, Dermablend, and RVPaque. Para-aminoben-

zoic acid (PABA)-ethanol (Pabanol, PreSun) and cinnamate-benzophenone combinations (Maxafil, Solbar, Uval) effectively prevent transmission of solar UVB and at least some UVA wavelengths. PABA esters (Eclipse, Pabafilm, Sundown) afford partial protection. Lip protectants that absorb in the UVB range (Sunstick, Blistik, PreSun) are also available for patients with photo-induced lip disorders such as recurrent herpesvirus infections. Sunscreens are designated by sun protection factor (SPF). The SPF is defined as the amount of time to develop a mild sunburn with the sunscreen compared with the amount of time without the sunscreen. A minimum SPF factor of 15 is required for most fair-skinned individuals to prevent sunburn. The higher the SPF, the better the protection is against UVB rays. Examples of sunscreens offering maximal protection are Supershade, Photoplex, and Total Eclipse. The efficacy of these agents depends on careful attention to instructions for use. PABA-containing sunscreens should be applied at least 30 min before sun exposure to permit penetration of the epidermis. Most patients with photosensitivity eruptions require protection by agents that absorb UVB wavelengths; patients with porphyria, phototoxic eruptions, and some types of solar urticaria require agents with a broader spectrum of prevention (see Chapters 136 and 646).

Although sunscreens do confer photoprotection and may decrease the development of nevi, protection is incomplete against all harmful UV light. Sun avoidance is also important during the times when the sun is most intense, such as during midday. Clothing and hats offer additional sun protection.

Darmstadt GL: Oral antibiotics for uncomplicated bacterial skin infections in children. *Pediatr Infect Dis J* 1997;16:227.

Darmstadt GL, Dinulos JG: Neonatal skin care. *Pediatr Clin North Am* 2000;47(4):757.

Gallagher RP, Rivers JK, Lee TK, et al: Broad spectrum sunscreen use may decrease the development of new nevi in white children. *JAMA* 2000;283:2955.

McGregor J, Young A: Sunscreens, suntans and skin cancer. *Br Med J* 1996;312:1621.

Morelli JG, Weston WL: Soaps and shampoos in pediatric practice. *Pediatrics* 1987;80:634.

Nilsson EJ, Henning CG, Magnusson J: Topical corticosteroids and *Staphylococcus aureus* in atopic dermatitis. *J Am Acad Dermatol* 1992;27:29.

Scherschum L, Lim HW: Photoprotection by sunscreens. Am J Clin Dermatol 2001;2:131.

Siegfried EC: Neonatal skin care and toxicology. In Eichenfield LF, Frieden IJ, Esterly NB (editors): *Textbook of Neonatal Dermatology*. Philadelphia, WB Saunders, 2001, p. 62.

Weinstein JM, Yarnold PR, Hornung RL: Parental knowledge and practice of primary skin cancer prevention: gaps and solutions. *Pediatr Dermatol* 2001;18:473.

Yohn JJ, Weston WL: Topical glucocorticoids. *Curr Probl Dermatol* 1990;2:33.

Chapter 637
Diseases of the Neonate

Minor evanescent lesions of newborn infants, particularly when florid, may cause undue concern. Most neonatal rashes of the entities described in this chapter are relatively common, benign, and transient; they do not require therapy.

Sebaceous Hyperplasia. Minute, profuse, yellow-white papules are frequently found on the forehead, nose, upper lip, and cheeks of a term infant; they represent hyperplastic sebaceous glands. These tiny papules diminish gradually in size and disappear entirely within the first few weeks of life.

Milia. Milia are superficial epidermal inclusion cysts that contain laminated keratinized material. The lesion is a firm papule, 1–2 mm in diameter, and pearly, opalescent white. Milia may occur at any age but in neonates are most frequently scattered over the face and gingivae and on the midline of the palate, where they are called *Epstein pearls*. Milia exfoliate spontaneously in most infants and may be ignored; those that appear in scars or sites of trauma in older children may be gently unroofed and the contents extracted with a fine-gauge needle.

Sucking Blisters. Solitary or scattered superficial bullae on the upper limbs of infants at birth are presumed to be induced by vigorous sucking on the affected part in utero. Common sites are the radial aspect of the forearm, thumb, and index finger. These bullae resolve rapidly without sequelae and should be distinguished from sucking pads (calluses), which are found on the lips in the first few months and are due to combined intracellular edema and hyperkeratosis. The diagnosis can be confirmed by observing the neonate suck the affected area.

Cutis Marmorata. When a newborn infant is exposed to low environmental temperatures, an evanescent, lacy, reticulated red and/or blue cutaneous vascular pattern appears over most of the body surface. This vascular change represents an accentuated physiologic vasomotor response that disappears with increasing age, although it is sometimes discernible even in older children. Persistent and pronounced cutis marmorata occurs in Menkes disease, familial dysautonomia, and Cornelia de Lange, Down, and trisomy 18 syndromes. *Cutis marmorata telangiectatica congenita* is clinically similar, but the lesions are more intense, may be segmental, are persistent, and may be associated with loss of dermal tissue, epidermal atrophy, and ulceration. The condition improves in the 1st yr year of life, however, with half showing decreased vascular markings. The congenital form is associated with microcephaly, micrognathia, cleft palate, dystrophic teeth, glaucoma, short stature, and skull asymmetry.

Harlequin Color Change. This rare but dramatic vascular event occurs in the immediate newborn period and is most common in low birthweight infants. It probably reflects an imbalance in the autonomic vascular regulatory mechanism. When the infant is placed on the side, the body is bisected longitudinally into a pale upper half and a deep red dependent half. The color change lasts only for a few minutes and occasionally affects only a portion of the trunk or face. Changing the infant's position may reverse the pattern. Muscular activity causes generalized flushing and obliterates the color differential. Repeated episodes may occur but do not indicate permanent autonomic imbalance.

Salmon Patch (Nevus Simplex). Salmon patches are small, pale pink, ill-defined, vascular macules that occur most commonly on the glabella, eyelids, upper lip, and nuchal area of 30–40% of normal newborn infants. These lesions, which represent localized vascular ectasia, persist for several months and may become more visible during crying or changes in environmental temperature. Most lesions on the face eventually fade and disappear completely, but those on the posterior neck and occipital areas often persist. The facial lesions should not be confused with a port-wine stain, which is a permanent lesion. The salmon patch is usually symmetric, with lesions on both eyelids or both sides of midline. Port-wine stains are often larger and unilateral, and they usually end along the midline (see Chapter 640).

Mongolian Spots. These blue or slate-gray macular lesions have variably defined margins; they occur most commonly in the presacral area but may be found over the posterior thighs, legs, back, and shoulders. They may be solitary or numerous and often involve large areas. More than 80% of black, Asian, and East Indian infants have these lesions, whereas the incidence in white infants is less than 10%. The peculiar hue of these macules is due to the dermal location of melanin-containing melanocytes that are presumably arrested in their migration from neural crest to epidermis. Mongolian spots usually fade during the first few years of life but occasionally persist. Malignant degeneration does not occur. Widespread numerous lesions, particularly those in unusual sites, are unlikely to disap-

pear. The characteristic appearance and congenital onset distinguish these spots from the bruises of child abuse.

Erythema Toxicum. This benign, self-limited, evanescent eruption occurs in approximately 50% of full-term infants; preterm infants are affected less commonly. The lesions are firm, yellow-white, 1–2 mm papules or pustules with a surrounding erythematous flare (Fig. 637–1). At times, splotchy erythema is the only manifestation. Lesions may be sparse or numerous and clustered in several sites or widely dispersed over much of the body surface. Palms and soles are usually spared. Peak incidence occurs on the 2nd day of life, but new lesions may erupt during the first few days as the rash waxes and wanes. Onset may occasionally be delayed for a few days to weeks in premature infants. The pustules form below the stratum corneum or deeper in the epidermis and represent collections of eosinophils that also accumulate around the upper portion of the pilosebaceous follicle. The eosinophils can be demonstrated in Wright-stained smears of the intralesional contents. Cultures are sterile.

The cause of erythema toxicum is unknown. The lesions can mimic pyoderma, candidosis, herpes simplex, transient neonatal pustular melanosis, and miliaria but can be differentiated by the characteristic infiltrate of eosinophils and the absence of organisms on a stained smear. The course is brief, and no therapy is required. Incontinentia pigmenti and eosinophilic pustular folliculitis also have eosinophilic infiltration but can be distinguished by their distribution, histologic type, and chronicity.

Transient Neonatal Pustular Melanosis. Pustular melanosis, which is more common in black than in white infants, is a transient, benign, self-limited dermatosis of unknown cause that is characterized by three types of lesions: (1) evanescent superficial pustules, (2) ruptured pustules with a collarette of fine scale, at times with a central hyperpigmented macule, and (3) hyperpigmented macules (Fig. 637–2). Lesions are present at birth, and one or all types of lesions may be found in a profuse or sparse distribution. Pustules represent the early phase of the disorder, and macules, the late phase. The pustular phase rarely lasts more than 2–3 days; hyperpigmented macules may persist for as long as 3 mo. Sites of predilection are the anterior neck, forehead, and lower back, although the scalp, trunk, limbs, palms, and soles may be affected.

The active phase shows an intracorneal or subcorneal pustule filled with polymorphonuclear leukocytes, debris, and an occasional eosinophil. The macules are characterized only by increased melanization of epidermal cells. Cultures and smears can be used to distinguish these pustules from those of erythema toxicum and pyoderma because they do not contain bacteria or dense aggregates of eosinophils. No therapy is required.

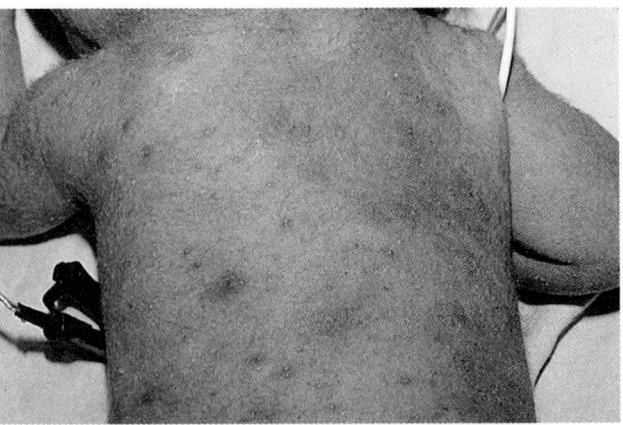

FIGURE 637–1. Erythema toxicum on the trunk of a newborn infant. See also color plates.

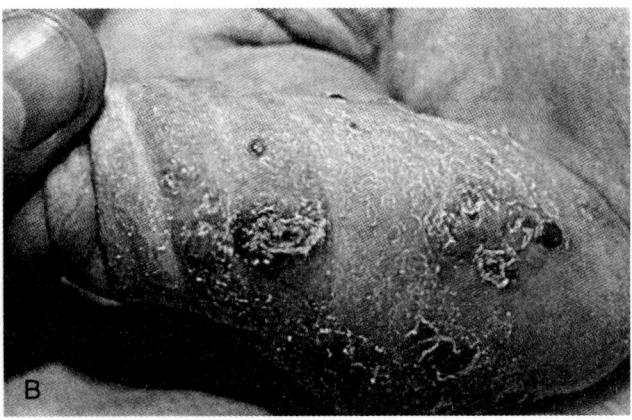

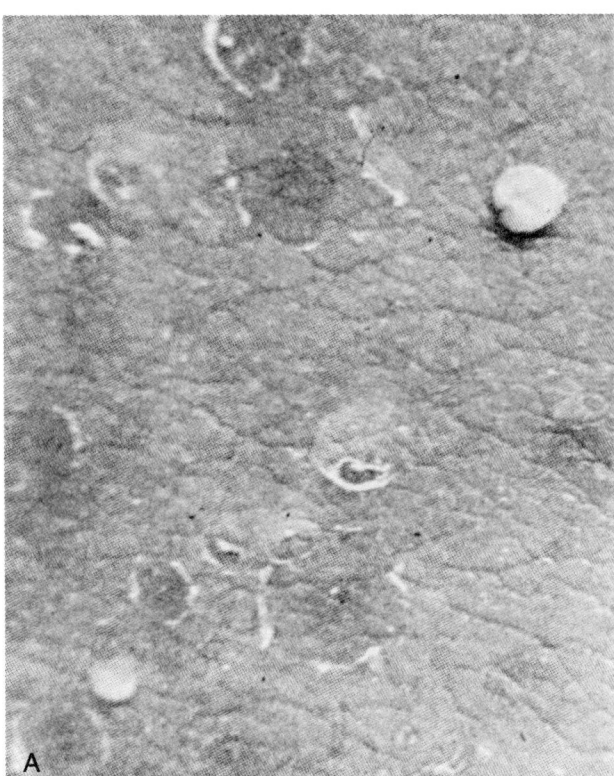

FIGURE 637–2. *A* and *B,* Transient neonatal pustular melanosis showing pustules, rings of scales, and hyperpigmented macules.

Infantile Acropustulosis. Infantile acropustulosis generally has its onset at 2–10 mo of age; lesions are occasionally noted at birth. Black males have a predisposition for this eruption, but infants of both sexes and all races may be affected. The cause is unknown.

The lesions are initially discrete erythematous papules that become vesiculopustular within 24 hr and subsequently crust before healing. They are intensely pruritic, and a fresh outbreak is usually accompanied by fretfulness and irritability. Preferred sites are the palms of the hands and soles and sides of the feet, where the lesions may develop in profusion. A less dense eruption may be found on the dorsum of the hands and feet, ankles, and wrists. Pustules occasionally may occur elsewhere on the body. Each episode lasts 7–14 days, during which time pustules continue to appear in crops. After a 2–4 wk remission, a new outbreak follows. This cyclic pattern continues for about 2 yr; permanent resolution is often preceded by longer intervals of remission between periods of activity. Infants with acropustulosis are otherwise well.

Wright-stained smears of intralesional contents show abundant neutrophils or, occasionally, a predominance of eosinophils. Histologically, well-circumscribed, subcorneal, neutrophilic pustules, with or without eosinophils, are noted.

The *differential diagnosis* in neonates includes transient neonatal pustular melanosis, erythema toxicum, milia, cutaneous candidosis, and staphylococcal pustulosis. In older infants and toddlers, additional diagnostic considerations include scabies, and a history of previous scabies infection is common; dyshidrotic eczema; pustular psoriasis; subcorneal pustular dermatosis; and hand-foot-and-mouth disease. A therapeutic trial of a scabicide is warranted in equivocal cases.

Therapy is directed at minimizing discomfort for infants. Topical corticosteroid preparations or oral antihistamines decrease the severity of the pruritus and an infant's irritability. Dapsone 2 mg/kg/24 hr PO bid has been effective but has poten-

tially serious side effects—notably, hemolytic anemia and methemoglobinemia—and should be used with caution.

Eosinophilic Pustular Folliculitis. This is described as recurrent crops of pruritic, coalescing, follicular papulopustules on the face, trunk, and extremities. Fifty per cent of patients have peripheral eosinophilia exceeding 5%, and about one third (32%) have leukocytosis (>10,000/mm³).

Infants make up less than 10% of all cases. The clinical and histologic appearance of this disorder in infants closely resembles that in immunocompetent adults, with minor exceptions. In infants, the lesions are most prominent on the scalp, although they also occur on the trunk and extremities and occasionally are found on the palms and soles. The classic annular and polycyclic appearance with centrifugal enlargement is not seen in infants. Adults have an eosinophilic infiltrate that invades sebaceous glands and the outer root sheath of hair follicles, often leading to spongiosis in the outer root sheath. The eosinophilic infiltrate in most infants, however, is perifollicular, without spongiosis in the outer root sheath. Because of the slightly different clinical findings and course in immunocompetent adults compared with infants or patients with acquired immunodeficiency syndrome, it has been proposed that eosinophilic pustular folliculitis (EPF) be subclassified into classic, human immunodeficiency virus–related, and infantile forms. The differential diagnosis includes erythema toxicum neonatorum, infantile acropustulosis, localized pustular psoriasis, pustular folliculitis, and transient neonatal pustular melanosis.

The pathogenesis of EPF is linked epidemiologically to sebaceous gland activity because lesions appear most commonly in association with hair follicles in areas of the body with a high density of sebaceous glands. Most theories on the pathogenesis of EPF invoke immunologic mechanisms in the initiation of lesions. Proposed etiologic factors in EPF include a cyclo-oxygenase–generated metabolite with chemotactic properties; an exaggerated response to skin saprophytes or dermatophytes, leading to eosinophilic infiltration and destruction of the follicle; or autoantibodies directed against the intercellular substance of the lower epidermis or the cytoplasm of basal cells of the epidermis and the outer sheath of hair follicles.

Response of EPF to therapy is variable; no one specific treatment is the therapy of choice. Antimicrobials and medicated shampoos have been ineffective; mid-potency topical corticosteroids are modestly effective in the treatment of scalp lesions in infants.

Alper JC, Holmes LB: The incidence and significance of birthmarks in a cohort of 4,641 newborns. *Pediatr Dermatol* 1983;1:58.

Jacobs AH, Walton RG: The incidence of birthmarks in the neonate. *Pediatrics* 1976;58:281.

Jennings JL, Burrows WM: Infantile acropustulosis. *J Am Acad Dermatol* 1983;9:733.

Karlsson J, Telang G, Tunnessen W: Cutis marmorata telangiectatica congenita. *Arch Pediatr Adolesc Med* 1997;151:950.

Mancini AJ, Frieden IJ, Paller AS: Infantile acropustulosis revisited: History of scabies and response to topical corticosteroids. *Pediatr Dermatol* 1998;15:337.

Chapter 638
Cutaneous Defects

Skin Dimples. Cutaneous depressions over bony prominences and in the sacral area, at times associated with pits and creases, may occur in normal children and in association with dysmorphologic syndromes. Skin dimples may develop in utero as a result of interposition of tissue between a sharp bony point and the uterine wall, which leads to decreased subcutaneous tissue formation. A rare benign autosomal dominant anomaly presents with dimples near the acromion bilaterally in association with deletion of the long arm of chromosome 18. Dimples tend to occur over the patella in congenital rubella, over the lateral aspects of the knees and elbows in prune-belly syndrome, on the pretibial surface in camptomelic dwarfs, and in the shape of an H on the chin in whistling-face syndrome.

Sacral dimples are common, and may occur as an isolated finding or occur as part of multiple syndromes, including Bloom syndrome, Smith-Lemli-Opitz syndrome, 4p deletion syndrome, spina bifida occulta, and diastomyelia. Large size (>5 mm), increased distance from the anus (>2.5 cm), or association with a mass or other cutaneous stigmata (e.g., hair, nevus flammeus, hemangioma) should increase concern for underlying spinal dysraphism. Ultrasonography during the first 3 mo of life, before ossification of the posterior elements of the lower spine, may provide a cost-effective, noninvasive method for assessment of any associated lumbosacral abnormalities.

Redundant Skin. Loose folds of skin must be differentiated from a congenital defect of elastic tissue or collagen such as cutis laxa, Ehlers-Danlos syndrome, or pseudoxanthoma elasticum. Redundant skin over the posterior part of the neck is common in the Turner, Noonan, Down, and Klippel-Feil syndromes; more generalized folds of skin occur in infants with trisomy 18 and short-limbed dwarfism.

Amniotic Constriction Bands. Partial or complete constriction bands that produce defects in extremities and digits are found in 1/10,000–1/45,000 otherwise normal infants. Constrictive tissue bands are caused by primary amniotic rupture, with subsequent entanglement of fetal parts, particularly limbs, in shriveled fibrotic amniotic strands. This event is probably sporadic, with negligible risk of recurrence. Formation of constrictive tissue bands is associated with abdominal trauma, amniocentesis, and hereditary defects of collagen such as Ehlers-Danlos syndrome or osteogenesis imperfecta.

Constriction bands on the limbs may be removed by plastic surgical procedures (Chapter 97).

Adhesive bands involve the craniofacial area and are associated with severe defects such as encephalocele and facial clefts. Adhesive bands result from broad fusion between disrupted fetal parts and an intact amniotic membrane. The craniofacial defects do not appear to be caused by constrictive amniotic bands but result from a vascular disruption sequence with or without cephaloamniotic adhesion.

The *limb-body wall complex* (LBWC) involves vascular disruption early in development, affecting several embryonic structures; it includes at least two of the following three characteristics: exencephaly or encephalocele with facial clefts, thoracoschisis and/or abdominoschisis, and limb defects. Amniotic rupture may be the cause of embryonic vascular disruption, leading to the LBWC; however, LBWC has been reported in the absence of amniotic rupture.

Preauricular Sinuses and Pits. Pits and sinus tracts anterior to the pinna may be a result of imperfect fusion of the tubercles of the first and second branchial arches. These anomalies may be unilateral or bilateral, may be familial, are more common in females and blacks, and at times are associated with other anomalies of the ears and face. Preauricular pits are present in branchio-otorenal dysplasia, an autosomal dominant disorder that consists of external ear malformations, branchial fistulas, hearing loss, and renal anomalies. When the tracts become chronically infected, retention cysts may form and drain intermittently; such lesions may require excision.

Accessory Tragi. An accessory tragus typically appears as a single pedunculated, flesh-colored papule in the preauricular region anterior to the tragus. Less commonly, accessory tragi are multiple, are unilateral or bilateral, and may be located in the preauricular area, on the cheek along the line of the mandible, or on the lateral aspect of the neck anterior to the sternocleidomastoid muscle. In contrast to the rest of the pinna, which develops from the second branchial arch, the tragus and accessory tragi derive from the first branchial arch. Accessory tragi may occur as isolated defects or in chromosomal first branchial arch syndromes that include anomalies of the ears and face such as cleft lip, cleft palate, and mandibular hypoplasia. Accessory tragus is consistently found in *oculoauriculovertebral syndrome (Goldenhar syndrome)*. Surgical excision is appropriate.

Branchial Cleft and Thyroglossal Cysts and Sinuses. Cysts and sinuses in the neck may be formed along the course of the first, second, third, or fourth branchial clefts as a result of improper closure during embryonic life. Second branchial cleft cysts are the most common. The lesions may be unilateral or bilateral (2–3%) and may open onto the cutaneous surface or drain into the pharynx. Secondary infection is an indication for systemic antibiotic therapy. These anomalies may be inherited as autosomal dominant traits.

Thyroglossal cysts and fistulas are similar defects located in or near the midline of the neck; they may extend to the base of the tongue. A pathognomonic sign is vertical motion of the mass with swallowing and tongue protrusion. Cysts in the tongue base may be differentiated from an undescended lingual thyroid by radionuclide scanning. Unlike branchial cysts, a thyroglossal duct cyst often appears after an upper respiratory infection.

Supernumerary Nipples. Solitary or multiple accessory nipples may occur in a unilateral or bilateral distribution along a line from the anterior axillary fold to the inguinal area. They are more common in black (3.5%) than white (0.6%) children. Accessory nipples may or may not have an areola and may be mistaken for congenital nevi. They may be excised for cosmetic reasons. Rarely, they undergo malignant change. Renal or urinary tract anomalies may occur in children with this finding.

Aplasia Cutis Congenita (Congenital Absence of Skin). Developmental absence of skin is usually noted on the scalp as multiple or solitary (70%), noninflammatory, well-demarcated, oval or circular 1–2 cm ulcers. The appearance of lesions varies, depending on when they occurred during intrauterine development. Those that form early in gestation may heal before delivery and appear as an atrophic, fibrotic scar with associated alopecia, whereas more recent defects may present as an ulceration. Most occur at the vertex just lateral to the midline, but similar defects may also occur on the face, trunk, and limbs, where they are often symmetric. The depth of the ulcer varies. Only the epidermis and upper dermis may be involved, resulting in minimal scarring or hair loss, or the defect may extend to the deep dermis, subcutaneous tissue, and, rarely, to the periosteum, skull, and dura.

No unifying theory can account for all lesions of aplasia cutis congenita. *Diagnosis* is made on the basis of physical findings indicative of in utero disruption of skin development. Lesions are sometimes mistakenly attributed to scalp electrodes or obstetric trauma. Rather, they appear to be due to various factors, including genetic factors, teratogens, compromised vasculature to the skin, and trauma.

Although most individuals with aplasia cutis congenita have no other abnormalities, these lesions may be associated with isolated physical anomalies or with a number of malformation syndromes. Scalp lesions may be seen in association with distal limb reduction anomalies, generally with autosomal dominant inheritance, or sporadically in association with epidermal and organoid nevi. Aplasia cutis congenita may also be found in association with an overt or underlying embryologic malformation, such as meningomyelocele, gastroschisis, omphalocele, or spinal dysraphism. Aplasia cutis congenita in association with fetus papyraceus is apparently due to ischemic or thrombotic events in the placenta and fetus. Blistering or skin fragility and/or absence or deformity of nails in association with aplasia cutis congenita is a well-recognized presentation of epidermolysis bullosa. Maternal ingestion of the teratogen methimazole or intrauterine herpes simplex virus or varicella-zoster virus infection may also be associated with lesions of aplasia cutis congenita. Finally, aplasia cutis congenita may also occur in the setting of a malformation syndrome such as several of the ectodermal dysplasias, trisomy 13 or 14, deletion of the short arm of chromosome 4, Johanson-Blizzard syndrome, focal facial dermal dysplasia, or focal dermal hypoplasia. Cutis aplasia may be confused with traumatic skin injury from monitoring devices and spontaneous atrophic patches (anetoderma) of prematurity.

Major *complications* are hemorrhage, secondary local infection, and meningitis. If the defect is small, recovery is uneventful, with gradual epithelialization and formation of a hairless atrophic scar over a period of several weeks (Fig. 638–1). Small bony defects usually close spontaneously during the 1st yr of life. Large or numerous scalp defects may require excision and primary closure if feasible, rotation of a flap to fill the defect, or the use of tissue expanders. Truncal and limb defects, despite large size, usually epithelialize and form atrophic scars, which can later be revised.

Focal Facial Ectodermal Dysplasia (Bitemporal Aplasia Cutis Congenita, Ectodermal Dysplasia of the Face). This rare disorder is characterized by congenital atrophic scarlike lesions on the temples. Sweating is absent over the defects, the lateral one third of the eyebrows is sparse, and linear vertical wrinkles are present on the forehead. Autosomal dominant and autosomal recessive inheritance have been documented; both subgroups of patients lack associated facial anomalies. A subgroup, identified as *Setler syndrome*, is marked by full lips, coarse facies, and rugae around the lips and chin. Growth and development are generally normal.

Focal Dermal Hypoplasia (Goltz Syndrome). This rare congenital mesoectodermal and ectodermal disorder is characterized by dys-

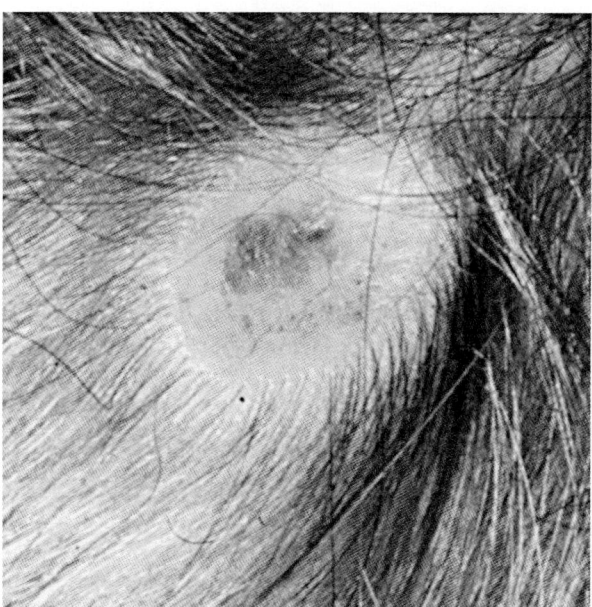

FIGURE 638–1. Healing solitary lesion of aplasia cutis congenita.

plasia of connective tissue in the skin and skeleton. It presents with numerous soft tan papillomas. Other cutaneous findings include linear atrophic lesions; reticulated hypopigmentation and hyperpigmentation; telangiectasias; congenital absence of skin; angiofibromas presenting as verrucous excrescences; and papillomas of the lips, tongue, circumoral region, vulva, anus, and the inguinal, axillary, and periumbilical areas. Partial alopecia, sweating disorders, and dystrophic nails are additional less common ectodermal anomalies. The most frequent skeletal defects include syndactyly, clinodactyly, polydactyly, and scoliosis. Osteopathia striata are fine parallel vertical stripes noted on radiographs in the metaphyses of long bones; these are highly characteristic of focal dermal hypoplasia but are not pathognomonic. Many ocular abnormalities, the most common of which are colobomas, strabismus, nystagmus, and microphthalmia, are also characteristic. Small stature, dental defects, soft tissue anomalies, and peculiar dermatoglyphic patterns are also common. Mental deficiency occurs occasionally.

This familial disorder occurs principally in girls. It has been postulated that an X-linked dominant gene, lethal in hemizygous males, may account for the sex distribution. The linear pattern of skin and bone lesions may be due to random X-inactivation in females. Cases of father-daughter transmission, evidence for an autosomal locus on chromosome 9q32-qter, and the unexpectedly high (10%) proportion of males with the disorder, however, argue against X-linked dominance with lethality in males. Affected males may have an early half chromatid mutation or autosomal dominant inheritance affecting the germ line.

The primary defect may be due to a deficiency of collagen caused by a fibroblastic defect. Others suggest that the cutaneous defects represent heterotopic proliferations of fatty nevi within the dermis, resulting from dysplasia, not hypoplasia, followed by herniation of subcutaneous fat.

This disorder is often confused with incontinentia pigmenti because of the sex predilection for females, the linear distribution of skin lesions, and the initial inflammatory phase, which are features of both disorders. The cutaneous lesions may also superficially resemble epidermal nevi. *Treatment* should be directed at amelioration of specific anomalies; genetic counseling is advisable.

Dyskeratosis Congenita (Zinsser-Engman-Cole Syndrome). This rare familial syndrome consists classically of the triad of reticulated hyperpigmentation of the skin, dystrophic nails, and mucous membrane leukoplakia. It usually affects males and is inherited most often in an X-linked recessive fashion, although autosomal recessive or dominant inheritance has been reported. The gene for the X-linked form of dyskeratosis congenita, DKC1, is on Xq28. Onset occurs during childhood, most commonly as nail dystrophy, at age 5–13 yr. The nails become atrophic and ridged longitudinally, and there is considerable loss of the nail plate. Skin changes usually appear 2–3 yr after onset of nail changes and consist of reticulated gray-brown pigmentation, atrophy, and telangiectasia, especially on the neck, face, and chest. Hyperhidrosis and hyperkeratosis of the palms and soles, acrocyanosis, and occasional bullae on the hands and feet are also characteristic. Blepharitis, ectropion, and excessive tearing as a result of atresia of the lacrimal ducts are occasional manifestations. Vesiculobullous lesions may occur on the oral mucous membranes and result in ulceration, formation of epithelial tags, atrophic changes of the tongue, and oral leukokeratosis. Oral leukokeratosis generally presents after the 3rd decade of life and may give rise to squamous cell carcinoma. Similar changes have been noted in the urethral and anal mucosae. The scalp hair, eyebrows, and lashes may become sparse. Hypoplastic anemia, at times of the Fanconi variety, may present at age 10 yr or older in up to 50% of patients. Impaired cell-mediated immunity has been noted. The primary causes of death are infections, including *Pneumocystis carinii*, and carcinoma. In one large series, approximately 12% of patients had tumors, most commonly oral and anal squamous cell carcinoma, pancreatic adenocarcinoma, or Hodgkin disease. The *differential diagnosis* includes the ectodermal dysplasias, pachyonychia congenita, poikilodermas, epidermolysis bullosa, keratoderma of the palms and soles, and lichen sclerosus et atrophicus. The abnormalities noted in skin biopsy specimens are those of poikiloderma.

Treatment includes biopsy of leukoplakic sites to identify malignancies. Etretinate may cause regression of leukoplakia, and orally administered β-carotene has some utility for treatment of leukoplakia and as a preventive agent for oral cancer. Aplastic anemia may be treated by administration of androgens or granulocyte-macrophage colony-stimulating factor or bone marrow transplantation.

Cutis Verticis Gyrata. This unusual alteration of the scalp, which is more common in males, may be present from birth or may develop during adolescence. The scalp is characterized by convoluted elevated folds, 1–2 cm in thickness, usually in the fronto-occipital axis. Unlike the lax skin of other disorders, the convolutions cannot generally be flattened by traction. Primary cutis gyrata is often associated with mental retardation, ocular defects, abnormal size and shape of the head, seizures, and spasticity. Secondary cutis gyrata may be due to chronic inflammatory diseases, tumors, nevi, acromegaly, and pachydermoperiostosis, a syndrome characterized by hypertrophy of the skin and bones.

Drachtman RA, Alter BP: Dyskeratosis congenita: Clinical and genetic heterogeneity. *Am J Pediatr Hematol Oncol* 1992;14:297.

Drolet BA: Developmental abnormalities. In Eichenfield LF, Frieden IJ, Esterly NB (editors): *Textbook of Neonatal Dermatology*. Philadelphia, WB Saunders, 2001, p. 117.

Frieden IJ: Aplasia cutis congenita: A clinical review and proposal for classification. *J Am Acad Dermatol* 1986;14:646.

Heiss NS, Knight SW, Vulliamy TJ, et al: X-linked dyskeratosis congenital is caused by mutations in highly conserved gene with putative nucleolar functions. *Nat Genet* 1998;19:32.

Kriss VM, Desai NS: Occult spinal dysraphism in neonates: Assessment of high-risk cutaneous stigmata by sonography. *AJR* 1998;171:1687.

Kowalski DC, Fenske NA: The focal facial dermal dysplasias: Report of a kindred and proposed new classification. *J Am Acad Dermatol* 1992;27:575.

Moerman P, Fryns JP, Vandenberghe K, et al: Constrictive amniotic bands, amniotic adhesions, and limb-body wall complex: Discrete disruption sequences with pathogenetic overlap. *Am J Med Genet* 1992;42:470.

Prizant T, Lucky A, Frieden I, et al: Spontaneous atrophic patches in extremely premature infants. *Arch Dermatol* 1996;132:671.

Sebben JE: The accessory tragus—No ordinary skin tag. *J Dermatol Surg Oncol* 1989;15:304.

Chapter 639
Ectodermal Dysplasias

Ectodermal dysplasia is a heterogeneous group of disorders characterized by a constellation of findings involving defects of two or more of the following: the teeth, skin, and appendageal structures, including hair, nails, and eccrine and sebaceous glands. Disturbances in tissue derived from embryologic layers other than ectoderm are common.

Hypohidrotic (Anhidrotic) Ectodermal Dysplasia. This syndrome is manifested as a triad of defects: partial or complete absence of sweat glands, anomalous dentition, and hypotrichosis. It is usually inherited as an X-linked recessive trait, with full expression only in males; however, an autosomal recessive mode of inheritance may be operative in some families. Mutations in ectodysplasin, the protein product of the EDA or ED1 gene, cause the X-linked form of hypohidrotic ectodermal dysplasia.

Heterozygotic females may have no or variable *clinical manifestations*, including dental defects, sparse hair, and reduced sweating; because of random X-inactivation, they are mosaics of functionally normal and abnormal cells. Affected children, unable to sweat, may experience episodes of high fever in warm environments and may be mistakenly considered to have fever of unknown origin. This is particularly the case in infancy, when the facial changes are not easily appreciated. The typical facies is characterized by frontal bossing; malar hypoplasia; a flattened nasal bridge; recessed columella; thick, everted lips; wrinkled, hyperpigmented periorbital skin; and prominent, low-set ears (Fig. 639–1). The skin over the entire body is dry, finely wrinkled, and hypopigmented, often with a prominent venous pattern. Extensive peeling of the skin is a clinical clue to diagnosis in the newborn period. The paucity of sebaceous glands may account for the dry skin. The hair is sparse, unruly, and lightly pigmented, and eyebrows and lashes are sparse or absent. Anodontia or hypodontia with widely spaced, conical teeth is a consistent feature (see Fig. 639–1). Less commonly, stenotic lacrimal puncta, corneal opacity, cataracts, hypoplastic or absent mammary glands, and conductive hearing loss have been observed. The incidence of atopic diseases in these children is relatively high. Poor development of mucous glands in the respiratory and gastrointestinal tract may result in increased susceptibility to respiratory infection, purulent rhinitis, dysphonia, dysphagia, and diarrhea. Sexual development is usually normal. Approximately 30% of affected boys die during the first 2 yr of life of hyperpyrexia or respiratory infection.

The sweating deficit is a reflection of hypoplasia or absence of eccrine glands; this may be *diagnosed* by skin biopsy. The palmar skin is an appropriate site for biopsy. Reduction or absence of sweating can be documented by pilocarpine iontophoresis or by topical application of *o*-phthalaldehyde to the palmar skin. Sweat pores are not visible in the palmar ridges of affected children and are decreased in number in carrier females. Applying a 2% solution of iodine in alcohol to the back, followed by applying a suspension of cornstarch in castor oil, also allows highlighting of sweat glands by the appearance of a black dot; this test may be useful for detecting female carriers. Linkage analysis has been used for prenatal and early neonatal diagnosis.

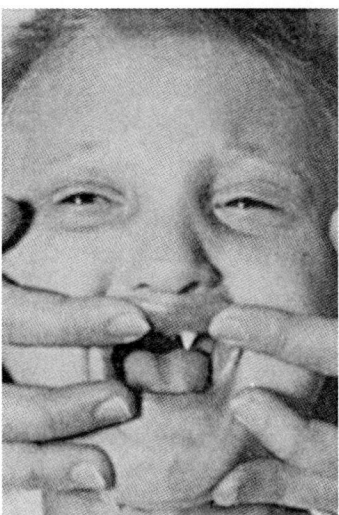

FIGURE 639–1. Hypohidrotic ectodermal dysplasia is characterized by pointed ears, wispy hair, periorbital hyperpigmentation, midfacial hypoplasia, and pegged teeth.

Treatment of these children includes protecting them from exposure to high ambient temperatures. Early dental evaluation is necessary so that prostheses can be provided for cosmetic reasons and for adequate nutrition. The use of artificial tears prevents damage to the cornea in patients with defective lacrimation. Alopecia may necessitate the wearing of a wig to improve appearance.

Hidrotic Ectodermal Dysplasia (Clouston Syndrome). Dystrophic, hypoplastic, or absent nails; sparse hair; and hyperkeratosis of the palms and soles are the salient features of this autosomal dominant disorder. The dentition is usually normal, although small teeth and numerous caries are occasionally found. Conjunctivitis and blepharitis are common. Sweating is always normal. Absence of eyebrows and lashes and hyperpigmentation over the knees, elbows, and knuckles have been noted in some affected individuals. Mutations in the GJB6 gene encoding the gap junction protein connexin 30, are responsible for this disorder.

EEC Syndrome. Ectrodactyly (split hand and foot), ectodermal dysplasia, cleft lip and palate, and tear duct abnormalities constitute the EEC syndrome, which is probably inherited as an autosomal dominant trait of low penetrance and variable expressivity. The ectodermal dysplasia consists of dry, poorly pigmented skin; light-colored, wispy, sparse scalp hair and eyebrows; and absence of lashes. Decreased numbers of hair follicles and sebaceous glands have been demonstrated by biopsy. Nails may be dystrophic. Clinical expression of the EEC syndrome is variable; any one of these signs may be absent, except the ectodermal signs. Associated defects include anomalies of the hands and feet, nail hypoplasia, granulomatous perlèche frequently complicated by candidosis, defective dentition, deafness, ocular abnormalities (blepharophimosis, strabismus), and abnormalities of the urinary tract. Sweating usually is normal.

Clarke A, Burn J: Sweat testing to identify female carriers of X linked hypohidrotic ectodermal dysplasia. *J Med Genet* 1991;28:330.

Clarke A, Phillips DI, Brown R, et al: Clinical aspects of X-linked hypohidrotic ectodermal dysplasia. *Arch Dis Child* 1987;62:989.

Freire-Maia N, Pinheiro M: Ectodermal dysplasias. Some recollections and a classification. In Salinas CF, Opitz JM, Paul NW (editors): *Recent Advances in Ectodermal Dysplasias*, vol 24. New York, Alan R. Liss, 1988, p. 3.

Kere J, Srivastava AK, Montonen O, et al: X-linked anhidrotic (hypohidrotic) ectodermal dysplasia is caused by a mutation in a novel transmembrane protein. *Nat Genet* 1996;13:409.

Lamartine J, Munhoz Essenfelder G, Kibar Z, et al: Mutations in GJB6 cause hidrotic ectodermal dysplasia. *Nat Genet* 2000;26:142.

Rodini ES, Richieri-Costa A: EEC syndrome: Report on 20 new patients, clinical and genetic considerations. *Am J Med Genet* 1990;37:42.

Zonana J: Hypohidrotic (anhidrotic) ectodermal dysplasia: Molecular genetic research and its clinical application. *Semin Dermatol* 1993;12:241.

Chapter 640
Vascular Disorders

Developmental vascular anomalies may occur as isolated defects or as part of a syndrome. They can be separated into two major categories: hemangiomas and vascular malformations. Hemangiomas are proliferative hamartomas of vascular endothelium that are present at birth or, more commonly, become apparent in the first few (e.g., 3–5) weeks of life, predictably enlarge, and then spontaneously involute. Hemangiomas are the most common tumor of infancy, occurring in 1–2% of newborns and 10% of white infants in the 1st yr of life. Vascular anomalies occur sporadically and occasionally have a genetic basis (Table 640–1). Malformations are present at birth and are derived from capillaries, veins, arteries, or lymphatics or any combination thereof. Malformations do not regress but usually enlarge over time.

Port-Wine Stain (Nevus Flammeus, Port-Wine Nevus). Port-wine stains are present at birth. These vascular malformations consist of mature dilated dermal capillaries and represent a permanent developmental defect. The lesions are macular, sharply circumscribed, pink to purple, and tremendously varied in size (Fig. 640–1). The head and neck region is the most common site of predilection, and most lesions are unilateral. The mucous membranes can be involved. As a child matures into adulthood, the port-wine stain may become darker in color and pebbly in consistency, and it may occasionally develop elevated areas that bleed spontaneously.

True port-wine stains should be distinguished from the most common vascular malformation, the salmon patch of neonates, which is, in contrast, a relatively transient lesion (see Chapter 637). Stretching the skin horizontally or placing firm pressure on a glass slide over the involved skin decreases the red color of both lesions and is not diagnostic. When a port-wine stain is localized to the trigeminal area of the face, specifically around the eyelids, the diagnosis of *Sturge-Weber syndrome* (glaucoma, leptomeningeal venous angioma, seizures, hemiparesis contralateral to the facial lesion, intracranial calcification) must be considered (see Chapter 589.3). Early screening for glaucoma is important to prevent additional damage to the eye. Port-wine stains also occur as a component of *Klippel-Trenaunay-Weber syndrome* and with moderate frequency in other syndromes, including the *Cobb* (spinal arteriovenous malformation, port-wine stain), *Proteus*, *Beckwith-Wiedemann*, and *Bonnet-Dechaume-Blanc* syndromes. In the absence of associated anomalies, morbidity from these lesions may include a poor self-image, hypertrophy of underlying structures, and traumatic bleeding.

The most effective treatment for port-wine stains is the flash-lamp-pumped-pulsed dye laser. This therapy is targeted at the lesion and avoids thermal injury to the surrounding normal tissue. After such treatment, the texture and pigmentation of the skin are generally normal without scarring. Therapy can begin in infancy when the surface area of involvement is smaller, although the response appears to be similar regardless of age when treated. Other therapies include masking with cosmetics (Covermark, Dermablend), cryosurgery, excision, grafting, and tattooing.

Hemangioma. Superficial hemangiomas are bright red, protuberant, compressible, sharply demarcated lesions that may occur on any area of the body. Although sometimes present at birth, they

TABLE 640–1. Familial Vascular Anomalies with Identified Genetic Mutations

Disorder	Chromosome	Gene	Function
Hereditary hemorrhagic telangiectasia	9q3	Endoglin	TGF β binding proteins
	12q	activin receptor-like kinase 1 (ALK-1)	
Cerebral cavernous malformations	7q (Hispanic)	KRIT 1	RAPIA GTPase signal transduction pathway
	7p		
	3q		
Familial glomus tumors			
Paragangliomas	11q23		
Disseminated cutaneous glomangioma	1p21–22		
Familial lymphedema	5q34–q35	VEGFR3 (FLT4)	Lymphatic development
Familial venous malformation	9p	Tie-2	Endothelial cell/smooth muscle cell interaction
Familial hemangioma	5q33–34	VEGFR	

From Blei F: Vascular Anomalies: From Bedside to Bench and Back Again. Curr Prob Pediatr Adoles Health *2002;32:67–102.*

more often appear within the first 2 mo and are heralded by an erythematous or blue mark or an area of pallor, which subsequently develops a fine telangiectatic pattern before the phase of expansion. The presenting sign may occasionally be an ulceration of the perineum or lip. Girls are affected more often than boys. Favored sites are the face, scalp, back, and anterior chest; lesions may be solitary or multiple. Most superficial hemangiomas undergo a phase of rapid expansion, followed by a stationary period, and finally by spontaneous involution. Regression may be anticipated when the lesion develops blanched or pale gray areas that indicate fibrosis. The course of a particular lesion is unpredictable, but approximately 60% of

these lesions involute completely by the age 5 yr, with 90–95% by age 9 yr. Spontaneous involution cannot be correlated with size or site of involvement, but lip lesions seem to persist most often. Complications include ulceration, secondary infection, and, rarely, hemorrhage. The location of a lesion may interfere with a vital function (e.g., eyelid with vision, urethra with urination). Hemangiomas in a "beard" distribution may be associated with upper airway or subglottic involvement. Respiratory symptoms should suggest a tracheobronchial lesion. Large hemangiomas may be complicated by coexistent hypothyroidism due to type-3 iodothyronine deiodinase, and symptoms may be difficult to detect in this age group (Table 640–2).

In the usual patient who has no serious complications or extensive overgrowth that results in tissue destruction and severe disfigurement, *treatment* consists of expectant observation. Because almost all lesions resolve spontaneously, therapy is rarely indicated and may cause further harm. Parents require repeated reassurance and support. After spontaneous resolution, approximately 10% of patients are left with small cosmetic defects, such as puckering or discoloration of skin. These defects can be eliminated or minimized by judicious plastic repair if desired. In the rare case in which intervention is required, early therapy by the flashlamp-pumped-pulsed dye laser may be beneficial in decreasing growth of the hemangioma and in inducing more rapid resolution of an ulcerated hemangioma. Excision may be advisable in lesions that have remained large for several years; the extent of scarring anticipated should influence the final decision. Radiation can be hazardous and should be considered only in life-threatening situations, such as the Kasabach-Merritt syndrome (see later discussion). Elastic bandages may reduce the amount of tissue distortion resulting from rapid growth, but they are appropriate only in selected patients with large hemangiomas. Systemic or intralesional administration of corticosteroids and interferon-α (IFN-α) may be indicated for infants at risk for serious sequelae from exceptionally large or rapidly growing hemangiomas in vital areas (see later text) (Table 640–3).

Hemangiomas that are more deeply situated appear more diffuse and ill defined than superficial hemangiomas. The lesions are cystic, firm, or compressible, and the overlying skin may appear normal in color or have a bluish hue. Mixed hemangiomas have both superficial and deep components. Deep hemangiomas progress from a growth phase to a stationary phase to a period of involution. These lesions are as likely to regress as superficial hemangiomas, and the outcome cannot be predicted from size or site of involvement. A course of expectant observation should be followed in most cases. If involvement of underlying structures is

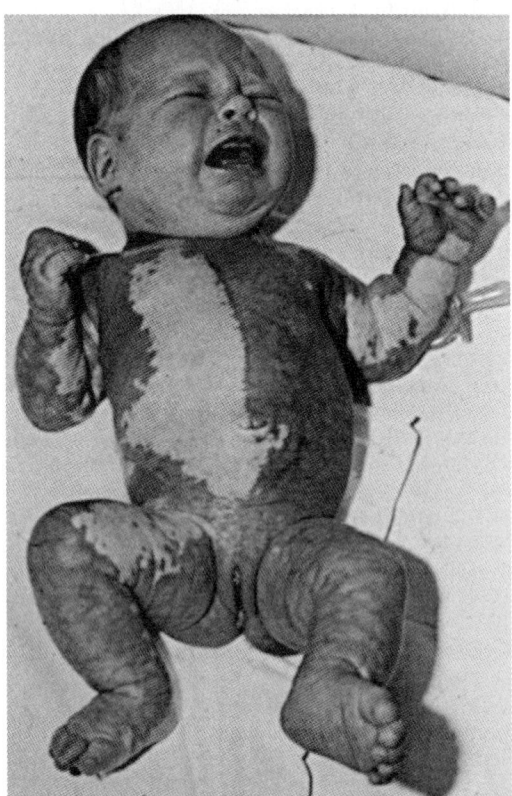

FIGURE 640–1. Widespread nevus flammeus in an infant with Klippel-Trenaunay-Weber syndrome.

TABLE 640-2. **Clinical Red Flags Associated with Hemangiomas**

Clinical Finding	Recommended Evaluation
Facial hemangioma involving significant area of face	Evaluate for PHACES—MRI for orbital hemangioma ± posterior fossa malformation Cardiac, ophthalmologic evaluation Evaluate for midline abnormality—supraumbilical raphe, sternal atresia, cleft palate, thyroid abnormality
Cutaneous hemangiomas in *beard* distribution	Evaluate for airway hemangioma, especially if presenting with stridor
Periocular hemangioma	MRI of orbit Ophthalmologic evaluation
Paraspinal midline vascular lesion	Ultrasound or MRI to evaluate for occult spinal dysraphism
Hemangiomatosis—multiple small cutaneous hemangiomas	Evaluate for parenchymal hemangiomas, especially hepatic/CNS Guaiac stool
Large hemangioma, especially hepatic	U/S with doppler flow MRI Thyroid function studies
Thrill and/or bruit associated with hemangioma	Consider cardiac evaluation and echo to r/o diastolic reversal of flow in aorta MRI to evaluate extent and flow characteristics
Head tilting	Evaluate appropriately for specific site of lesion, plus consider physical therapy evaluation
Delayed milestones	Consider side effect of corticosteroids (myopathy, weight-related) Consider side effect of interferon (especially spastic diplegia)

MRI, magnetic resonance imaging; U/S, ultrasound
From Blei F: Vascular anomalies: From bedside to bench and back again. Curr Prob Pediatr Adolesc Health *2002;32:67–102.*

suspected, appropriate radiologic studies should be performed for elucidation. Rarely, these lesions impinge on vital structures, interfere with functions such as vision or feeding (Fig. 640–2), cause grotesque disfigurement because of rapid growth, or are associated with life-threatening complications such as thrombocytopenia and hemorrhage (see Kasabach-Merritt syndrome).

If *treatment* becomes necessary, a course of prednisone (2–5 mg/kg/24 hr) is effective in some infants. Termination of growth and sometimes regression may be evident after approximately 4 wk of therapy. When a response is obtained, the dose should be decreased gradually. Alternate-day corticosteroid therapy has also been administered with success. Intralesional corticosteroid injection with the patient anesthetized can also induce rapid involution of a localized hemangioma. Pulsed dye laser therapy is also beneficial in managing complicated (cervicofacial, periorbital, parotid, lumbosacral) hemangiomas. IFN-α therapy may also be effective and may be the next therapeutic action. Spastic diplegia is a rare complication of interferon therapy.

Syndromes associated with hemangiomas include PHACES (*p*osterior fossa defects such as Dandy-Walker malformation or cerebellar hypoplasia, large plaque-like facial *h*emangioma, *a*rterial abnormalities such as aneurysms and stroke, *c*oarctation of the aorta, *e*ye abnormalities, and *s*ternal raphe defects such as pits or scars), disseminated hemangiomatosis, Klippel-Trenaunay-

Weber, Gorham (cutaneous hemangiomas with massive osteolysis), and Bannayan-Riley-Ruvalcaba (macrocephaly lipomas, hemangiomas–autosomal dominant inheritance).

Disseminated Hemangiomatosis. This is a serious condition in which numerous hemangiomas are widely distributed. The skin usually has many small red or purple papular hemangiomas, but infrequently they may be sparse or absent. The internal hemangiomas may involve any of the viscera; the liver, gastrointestinal tract, central nervous system, and lungs are the most common sites. Although involvement falls along a continuum, three entities have been described: (1) benign neonatal hemangiomatosis, with widespread cutaneous hemangiomas in the absence of apparent visceral involvement; (2) disseminated neonatal hemangiomatosis, with myriad small (2 mm–2 cm) papular hemangiomas of the skin and internal organs; and (3) hemangiomatosis of the liver. In cases of benign neonatal hemangiomatosis, spontaneous regression of the lesions without complications is probable. Multiple hemangiomas may also occur in several rare syndromes, such as macrocephaly combined with pseudopapilledema or with lipomas. Ultrasound and CT scanning are indicated to determine the extent of visceral or

TABLE 640-3. **Hemangioma Complications and Their Treatment**

Clinical Finding	Recommended Treatment
Severe ulceration/maceration	Encourage twice daily cleansing regimen Dilute sodium bicarbonate soaks ± Flashlamp pulsed dye laser ± Oral corticosteroids ± Metronidazole cream
Bleeding (not KMP)	Gelfoam or Surgifoam Compression therapy ± embolization
Hemangioma with ophthalmologic sequelae	Patching therapy as directed by ophthalmologist Topical vs intralesional vs oral corticosteroids
Subglottic hemangioma	Oral corticosteroids ± KtP laser Tracheotomy if required
KMP	Corticosteroids, aminocaproic acid, vincristine, interferon alpha ± embolization
High flow hepatic hemangioma	Corticosteroids or interferon ± embolization

KMP, Kasabach-Merritt phenomenon.
From Blei F: Vascular anomalies: From bedside to bench and back again. Curr Prob Pediatr Adolesc Health *2002;32:67–102.*

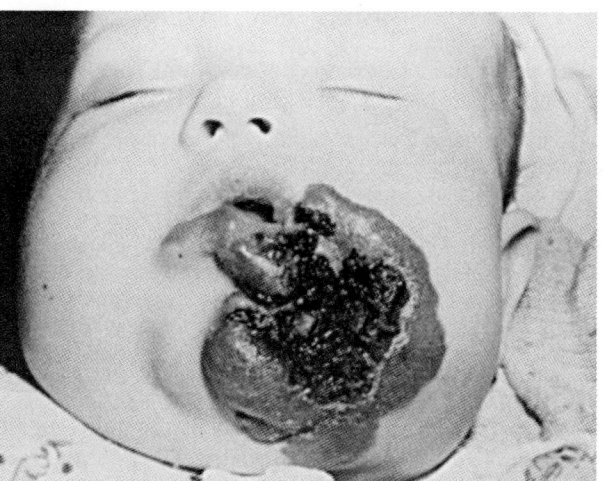

FIGURE 640–2. Large hemangioma with central crusted ulcer.

neural involvement. The disorder is often fatal because of high-output cardiac failure, visceral hemorrhage, obstruction of the respiratory tract, or compression of central neural tissue. In some cases, systemic corticosteroid therapy alone or in combination with IFN-α, surgery, or irradiation has been lifesaving.

Kasabach-Merritt Syndrome. This syndrome is a combination of a rapidly enlarging vascular anomaly, thrombocytopenia, microangiopathic hemolytic anemia, and an acute or chronic consumption coagulopathy. The vascular lesion is most likely either a tufted angioma or a kaposiform hemangioendothelioma with lymphatic-like vessels. The lesions may not spontaneously regress; both lesions are uncommon compared to hemangiomas. The *clinical manifestations* are usually evident during early infancy, but the onset occasionally is later. The vascular lesion is usually cutaneous and is only rarely located in viscera. The associated platelet defect may lead to precipitous hemorrhage accompanied by ecchymoses, petechiae, and a rapid increase in size of the vascular lesion. Severe anemia as a result of hemorrhage or microangiopathic hemolysis may ensue. The platelet count is depressed, but the bone marrow contains increased numbers of normal or immature megakaryocytes. The thrombocytopenia has been attributed to sequestration or increased destruction of platelets within the lesion hemangioma. Hypofibrinogenemia and decreased levels of consumable clotting factors are relatively common (see Chapter 474).

Treatment includes management of thrombocytopenia, anemia, and consumptive coagulopathy by administering platelets and by transfusion of red blood cells and fresh frozen plasma. Heparinization is controversial but has benefited some patients when combined with transfusions. Arteriovenous shunts in large lesions may produce high-output heart failure requiring digitalization (see Chapter 436). Treatment of these lesions includes systemic steroids, embolization, radiation therapy, vincristine, aminocaproic acid (inhibits fibrinolysis), cyclophosphamide, pentoxifylline, or recombinant IFN-α, which may inhibit proliferation of endothelial and smooth muscle cells. The mortality rate is 20–30%.

Blue Rubber Bleb Nevus. This syndrome consists of numerous vascular malformations of the skin, mucous membranes, and gastrointestinal tract. Typical lesions are blue-purple and rubbery in consistency; they vary in size from a few millimeters to a few centimeters in diameter. They are sometimes painful or tender. The nodules occasionally are present at birth but usually appear in childhood. New lesions may continue to develop throughout life. Large disfiguring and irregular blue marks may also occur. The lesions, which can rarely be located in the liver, spleen, and central nervous system in addition to the skin and gastrointestinal tract, do not involute spontaneously. Recurrent gastrointestinal hemorrhage may lead to severe anemia. Palliation can be achieved by excision of involved bowel. Cutaneous angiomas have been successfully removed by laser therapy.

Pyogenic Granuloma (Lobular Capillary Hemangioma, Telangiectatic Granuloma). A pyogenic granuloma is a small red, glistening, sessile, or pedunculated papule that often has a discernible epithelial collarette (Fig. 640–3). The surface may be weeping and crusted or completely epithelialized. Pyogenic granulomas initially grow rapidly, may ulcerate, and bleed easily when traumatized because they consist of exuberant granulation tissue. They are relatively common in children, particularly on the face, arms, and hands. Those located on a finger or hand may appear as a subcutaneous nodule. Lesions that develop on the oral mucosa during pregnancy are called *granuloma gravidarum.* Pyogenic granulomas generally arise at sites of injury, but a history of trauma often cannot be elicited. Clinically, they resemble and are often indistinguishable from small hemangiomas. Microscopically, an early lesion resembles an early capillary

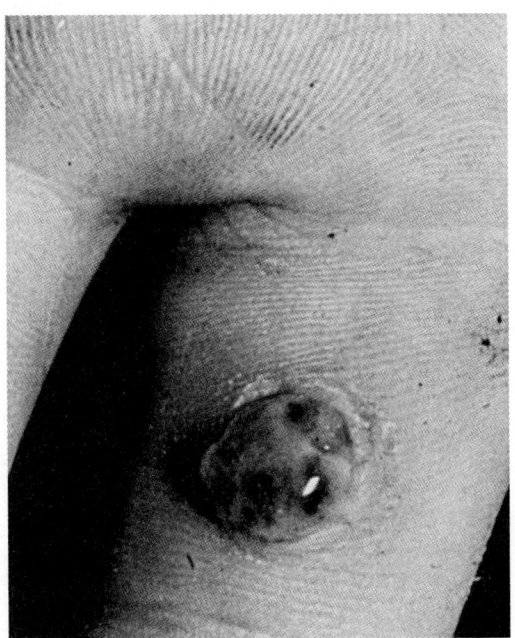

FIGURE 640–3. Pyogenic granuloma with a moist surface and epithelial collarette at the base.

hemangioma. Collarette formation at the base of the tumor and edema of the stroma may allow differentiation from a capillary hemangioma.

Pyogenic granulomas are benign but a nuisance because they bleed easily with trauma and may recur if incompletely removed. Numerous satellite papules have developed after incomplete removal of pyogenic granulomas from the back, particularly in the interscapular region. Small lesions may regress after cauterization with silver nitrate; larger lesions require excision and electrodesiccation of the base of the granuloma. They also have been treated successfully with the flashlamp-pumped-pulsed dye laser.

Maffucci Syndrome. The association of numerous vascular and, occasionally, lymphatic malformations with nodular enchondromas in the metaphyseal or diaphyseal portion of long bones is known as Maffucci syndrome. Vascular lesions typically are soft, compressible, asymptomatic blue-to-purple subcutaneous masses that grow in proportion to a child's growth and stabilize by adult life. Mucous membranes or viscera also may be involved. Onset occurs during childhood. Bone lesions may produce limb deformities and pathologic fractures. Malignant transformation of enchondromas (chondrosarcoma, angiosarcoma) or primary malignancies (ovarian, fibrosarcoma, glioma, pancreatic) may be a complication (Chapters 492 and 493).

Klippel-Trenaunay-Weber Syndrome. A cutaneous vascular malformation in combination with bony and soft tissue hypertrophy and venous varicosities constitutes the triad of defects of this nonheritable disorder. The anomaly is present at birth and usually involves a lower limb but may involve more than one and portions of the trunk or face (see Fig. 640–1). Enlargement of the soft tissues may be gradual and may involve the entire extremity, a portion of it, or selected digits. The vascular lesion most often is a nevus flammeus, generally localized to the hypertrophied area. Venous blebs and/or vesicular lymphatic lesions may be present on their surface. Thick-walled venous varicosities typically become apparent ipsilateral to the vascular malformation after the child begins to ambulate. The deep venous system may be absent, hypoplastic, or obstructed, resulting in lymphedema. Arteriovenous fistulas can develop, and bruits may be audible in the affected part. This disorder can be confused with Maffucci syndrome or, if the surface vascular lesion is minimal, with Milroy disease. Pain, limb swelling, and cellulitis may occur. Thrombophlebitis, dislocations of joints, gangrene of the affected extremity, congestive heart failure, hematuria secondary to angiomatous involvement of the urinary tract, rectal bleeding from lesions of the gastrointestinal tract, pulmonary lesions, and malformations of the lymphatic vessels are infrequent complications. Arteriograms, venograms, and CT or MRI scans may delineate the extent of the anomaly, but surgical correction or palliation is often difficult. The indications for radiologic studies of viscera and bones are best determined by clinical evaluation. Supportive care includes compression bandages for varicosities; surgical treatment may help carefully selected patients. Leg-length differences should be treated with orthotic devices to prevent the development of spinal deformities. Corrective bone surgery may eventually be needed to treat significant leg-length discrepancy.

Phakomatosis Pigmentovascularis. This rare disorder is characterized by the association of a nevus flammeus and melanocytic lesions. Typically, the nevus flammeus is extensive, and associated pigmentary lesions may include dermal melanocytosis (i.e., Mongolian spots), café-au-lait macules, or a nevus spilus (speckled nevus). Nonpigmented skin lesions that may occur in this setting include nevus anemicus and epidermal nevi. Systemic anomalies include ocular abnormalities, colonic polyposis, renal angiomas, granular cell tumors, moyamoya disease, and selective IgA deficiency.

Hereditary Hemorrhagic Telangiectasia (Osler-Weber-Rendu Disease). This disorder is inherited as an autosomal dominant trait. One involved gene encodes endoglin, a membrane glycoprotein on endothelial cells that binds transforming growth factor-β. Affected children may experience recurrent epistaxis before detection of the characteristic skin and mucous membrane lesions. The mucocutaneous lesions, which usually develop at puberty, are 1–4 mm, sharply demarcated red to purple macules, papules, or spider-like projections, each composed of a tightly woven mat of tortuous telangiectatic vessels. The nasal mucosa, lips, and tongue are usually involved; less commonly, cutaneous lesions occur on the face, ears, palms, and nail beds. Vascular ectasias may also arise in the conjunctivae, larynx, pharynx, gastrointestinal tract, bladder, vagina, bronchi, brain, and liver.

Massive hemorrhage is the most serious complication and may result in severe anemia. Bleeding may occur from the nose, mouth, gastrointestinal tract, genitourinary tract, and lungs; epistaxis often is the only complaint, however, occurring in 80% of patients. Approximately 15–20% of patients with arteriovenous malformations in the lungs present with stroke due to embolic abscesses. Persons with hereditary hemorrhagic telangiectasia have normal levels of clotting factors and an intact clotting mechanism. In the absence of serious complications, life span is normal. Local lesions may be ablated temporarily with chemical cautery or electrocoagulation. More drastic surgical measures may be required for lesions in critical sites such as the lung or gastrointestinal tract. Anemia should be treated with iron.

Spider Angiomas. A vascular spider (nevus araneus) consists of a central feeder artery with many dilated radiating vessels and a surrounding erythematous flush, varying from a few millimeters to several centimeters in diameter. Pressure over the central vessel causes blanching; pulsations visible in larger nevi are evidence for the arterial source of the lesion. Spider angiomas are associated with conditions in which there are increased levels of circulating estrogens, such as cirrhosis and pregnancy, but they also occur in up to 15% of normal preschool-aged children and 45% of school-aged children. Sites of predilection in children

are the dorsum of the hand, forearm, face, and ears. Angiomas can be obliterated by application of liquid nitrogen, electrocoagulation, or pulsed dye laser; they may also regress spontaneously.

Generalized Essential Telangiectasia. A rare and presumably nevoid anomaly of unknown cause, essential telangiectasia may have its onset in childhood or adulthood. Mild expression consists of patchy retiform telangiectases, particularly on the limbs, with occasional progression to involve large areas of the body surface. The condition must be distinguished from the secondary telangiectasias of connective tissue diseases, xeroderma pigmentosum, poikiloderma, and ataxia-telangiectasia. There is no treatment; however, patients can be reassured that their health will not be affected by the cutaneous disorder.

Unilateral Nevoid Telangiectasia. This unusual entity is characterized by the appearance of telangiectasia in a unilateral distribution, primarily on the face, neck, chest, and arms. The acquired form occurs particularly in females at onset of menses or during pregnancy. The congenital form predominantly affects males who lack endocrine abnormalities. The appearance of these lesions usually coincides with elevated levels of circulating estrogens, whatever the cause. When initiated by pregnancy, the telangiectasia may fade or disappear postpartum.

Hereditary Benign Telangiectasia. This rare disorder is inherited as an autosomal dominant trait and develops during childhood. The face, upper trunk, and arms are the areas of predilection. The condition is progressive but remains limited to the skin.

Cutis Marmorata Telangiectatica Congenita (Congenital Generalized Phlebectasia). This benign vascular anomaly represents dilatation of superficial capillaries and veins and is apparent at birth. Involved areas of skin have a reticulated red or purple hue that resembles physiologic cutis marmorata but is more pronounced and relatively unvarying (Fig. 640–4). The lesions may be restricted to a single limb and a portion of the trunk or may be more widespread. Port-wine stain may also be associated. The lesions become more pronounced during changes in environmental temperature, physical activity, or crying. In some cases, the underlying subcutaneous tissue is underdeveloped, and ulceration may occur within the reticulated bands. Rarely, defective growth of bone and other congenital abnormalities may be present. No specific therapy is indicated; the expected

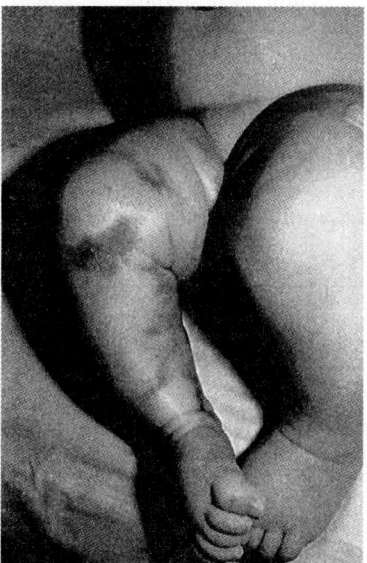

FIGURE 640–4. Marbled pattern of cutis marmorata telangiectatica congenita on the right leg. See also color plates.

course is one of gradual improvement, with partial or complete resolution by adolescence.

Ataxia-Telangiectasia (see Chapter 116.12). This disorder *(Louis-Bar syndrome)* is transmitted as an autosomal recessive trait due to a mutation in the ATM gene. The characteristic telangiectasias develop at about 3 yr of age, first on the bulbar conjunctivae and later on the nasal bridge, malar areas, external ears, hard palate, upper anterior chest, and antecubital and popliteal fossae. Additional cutaneous stigmata include café-au-lait spots, premature graying of the hair, and sclerodermatous changes.

Angiokeratomas. Several forms of angiokeratomas have been described, but some do not occur during childhood or adolescence. Angiokeratomas, characterized by ectasia of superficial dermal vessels and hyperkeratosis of the overlying epidermis, look like flat hemangiomas with a verrucous, irregular surface. *Angiokeratoma of Mibelli,* probably transmitted in an autosomal dominant pattern, is characterized by 1–8 mm red, purple, or black scaly, verrucous, occasionally crusted papules and nodules that appear on the dorsum of the fingers and toes and on the knees and the elbows. Less commonly, palms, soles, and ears may be affected. In many patients, onset has followed frostbite or chilblains. These nodules bleed freely after injury and may involute in response to trauma. *Angiokeratoma circumscriptum* is a rare solitary lesion that presents as a plaque of blue-red papules or nodules with a verrucous surface. These usually develop during infancy and early childhood, and they increase in size at adolescence. The lower limb is the site of predilection. They may be effectively eradicated by cryotherapy, fulguration, excision, or laser ablation.

Angiokeratoma Corporis Diffusum (Fabry Disease) (see Chapter 75). This inborn error of glycolipid metabolism is an X-linked recessive disorder that is fully penetrant in males and is of variable penetrance in carrier females. Angiokeratomas have their onset before puberty and occur in profusion over the genitalia, hips, buttocks, and thighs and in the umbilical and inguinal regions. They consist of 0.1–3 mm red to blue-black papules that may have a hyperkeratotic surface. Telangiectasias are seen in the mucosa and conjunctiva. On light microscopy, these angiokeratomas appear as blood-filled, dilated, endothelium-lined vascular spaces. Granular lipid deposits are demonstrable in dermal macrophages, fibrocytes, and endothelial cells.

Additional *clinical manifestations* include recurrent episodes of fever and agonizing pain, cyanosis and flushing of the acral limb areas, paresthesias of the hands and feet, corneal opacities detectable by slit-lamp examination, and hypohidrosis. Renal and cardiac involvement are the usual causes of death. The biochemical defect is a deficiency of the lysosomal enzyme α-galactosidase, with accumulation of ceramide trihexoside in tissues, particularly vascular endothelium, and excretion in urine. Similar cutaneous lesions have also been described in another lysosomal enzyme disorder, α-L-fucosidase deficiency, and in sialidosis, a storage disease with neuraminidase deficiency. See Chapter 75 for therapy.

Nevus Anemicus. Although present at birth, nevus anemicus may not be detectable until early childhood. The nevus consists of solitary or numerous sharply delineated pale macules that are most often on the trunk but may also occur on the neck or limbs. These nevi may simulate plaques of vitiligo, leukoderma, or nevoid pigmentary defects, but they can be readily distinguished by their response to firm stroking. Stroking evokes an erythematous line and flare in normal surrounding skin, but the skin of a nevus anemicus does not redden. Although the cutaneous vasculature appears normal histologically, the blood vessels within the nevus do not respond to injection of vasodilators. It has been postulated that the persistent pallor may represent a sustained localized adrenergic vasoconstriction.

Lymphangiomas. See Chapter 481.

Barlow CF, Priebe CJ, Mulliken JB, et al: Spastic diplegia as a complication of interferon alfa-2a treatment of hemangiomas of infancy. *J Pediatr* 1998;132:527.

Batta K, Goodyear HM, Moss C, et al: Randomised controlled study of early pulsed dye laser treatment of uncomplicated childhood haemangiomas: Results of a 1-year analysis. *Lancet* 2002;360:521–7.

Blei F: Vascular anomalies: From bedside to bench and back again. *Curr Prob Pediatr Adolesc Health Care* 2002;32:67–102.

Boon LM, Enjolras O, Mulliken JB, et al: Congenital hemangioma: Evidence of accelerated involution. *J Pediatr* 1996;128:329.

Drolet BA, Esterley NB, Frieden IJ: Hemangiomas in children. *N Engl J Med* 1999;341:173.

Drolet BA, Scott LA, Esterly NB, et al: Early surgical intervention in a patient with Kasabach-Merritt phenomenon. *J Pediatr* 2001;138:756–8.

Enjolras O, Garzon MC: Vascular stains, malformations, and tumors. In Eichenfield LF, Frieden IJ, Esterly NB (editors): *Textbook of Neonatal Dermatology.* Philadelphia, WB Saunders, 2001, p. 324.

Enjolras O, Wassef M, Mazoyer E, et al: Infants with Kasabach-Merritt syndrome do not have "true" hemangiomas. *J Pediatr* 1997;130:631.

Frieden IJ, Reese V, Cohen D: PHACE syndrome. The association of posterior fossa brain malformations, hemangioma, arterial anomalies, coarctation of the aorta, and cardiac defects, and eye abnormalities. *Arch Dermatol* 1996;132:307.

Guttmacher AE, Marchuk DA, White RI: Hereditary hemorrhagic telangiectasia. *N Engl J Med* 1995;333:918.

Hohenleutner U, Landthaler M: Laser treatment of childhood haemangioma: Progress or not? *Lancet* 2002;30:502–3.

Huang SA, Tu HM, Harney JW, et al: Severe hypothyroidism caused by type 3 iodothyronine deiodinase in infantile hemangioma. *N Engl J Med* 2000;343:185.

Klein JA, Barr RJ: Bannayan-Zonana syndrome associated with lymphangiomyomatous lesions. *Pediatr Dermatol* 1990;7:48.

Lacour M, Syed S, Linward J, et al: Role of the pulsed dye laser in the management of ulcerated capillary haemangiomas. *Arch Dis Child* 1996;74:161.

Metry DW, Dowd CF, Barkovich AJ, et al: The many faces of PHACE syndrome. *J Pediatr* 2001;139:117–23.

Metry DW, Herbert AA: Benign cutaneous vascular tumors of infancy. *Arch Dermatol* 2000;136:905–14.

Orlow SJ, Isakoff MS, Blei F: Increased risk of symptomatic hemangiomas of the airway in association with cutaneous hemangiomas in a "beard" distribution. *J Pediatr* 1997;131:643.

Picascia DD, Easterly NB: Cutis marmorata telangiectatica congenita: A report of 22 cases. *J Am Acad Dermatol* 1989;20:1098.

Sadan N, Wolach B: Treatment of hemangiomas of infants with high doses of prednisone. *J Pediatr* 1996;128:141.

Tallman B, Tan OT, Morelli JG, et al: Location of port-wine stains and the likelihood of ophthalmic and/or central nervous system complications. *Pediatrics* 1991;87:323.

Tay YK, Weston WL, Morelli JG: Treatment of pyogenic granuloma in children with the flashlamp-pumped pulsed dye laser. *Pediatrics* 1997;99:368.

Van der Horst CM, Koster PH, De Borgie CA, et al: Effect of the timing of treatment of port-wine stains with the flash-lamp-pumped pulsed dye laser. *N Engl J Med* 1998;338:1028.

Chapter 641
Cutaneous Nevi

Nevus skin lesions are characterized histopathologically by collections of well-differentiated cell types normally found in the skin. Vascular nevi are described in Chapter 640. Melanocytic nevi are subdivided into two broad categories: those that appear after birth, or acquired nevi, and those that are present at birth, the congenital nevi.

Acquired Melanocytic Nevus. Melanocytic nevi are a benign cluster of melanocytic nevus cells that arise as a result of proliferation of melanocytes at the epidermal-dermal junction. Nevus cells may have the same origin as melanocytes and are probably identical to them. An alternative, less popular theory is that nevus cells are of dual origin, with superficially located cells arising from melanocytes *(melanocytic nevus)* and cells in the deeper layers arising from Schwann cells *(neuroid nevus).*

EPIDEMIOLOGY. The number of acquired melanocytic nevi increases gradually during childhood, sharply at adolescence, and more slowly in early adulthood. It reaches a plateau in number during the 3rd or 4th decade and then slowly decreases thereafter. The mean number of melanocytic nevi in an adult is

25–35. The greater the number of nevi present, the greater is the risk for development of melanoma. Sun exposure during childhood, particularly intermittent, intense exposure of an individual with light skin, and a propensity to burn and freckle rather than tan are important determinants of the number of melanocytic nevi that develop. Increased numbers of nevi are also associated with immunosuppression and administration of chemotherapy.

CLINICAL MANIFESTATIONS. Nevocellular nevi have a well-defined life history and are classified as junctional, compound, or dermal in accordance with the location of the nevus cells in the skin. In childhood, more than 90% of nevi are junctional; melanocyte proliferation occurs at the junction of the epidermis and dermis to form nests of cells. *Junctional nevi* appear anywhere on the body in various shades of brown; they are relatively small, discrete, flat, and variable in shape. The melanized nevus cells are cuboidal or epithelioid in configuration and occur in nests on the epidermal side of the basement membrane. Although some nevi, particularly those on the palms, soles, and genitalia, remain junctional throughout life, most become compound as melanocytes migrate into the papillary dermis to form nests at both the epidermal-dermal junction and within the dermis. If the junctional melanocytes stop proliferating, nests of melanocytes remain only within the dermis, forming an intradermal nevus. With maturation, *compound* and *intradermal nevi* may become raised, dome shaped, verrucous, or pedunculated. Slightly elevated lesions are usually compound. Distinctly elevated lesions are usually intradermal. With age, the dermal melanocytic nests regress and the nevi gradually disappear.

PROGNOSIS AND TREATMENT. Acquired pigmented nevi are benign, but a very small percentage undergo malignant transformation. Suspicious changes such as rapid increase in size; development of satellite lesions; variegation of color, particularly with shades of red, brown, gray, black, and blue; pigmentary incontinence; notching or irregularity of the borders; changes in texture such as scaling, erosion, ulceration, and induration; and regional lymphadenopathy are indications for excision and histopathologic evaluation. Most of these changes are due to irritation, infection, or maturation; darkening and gradual increase in size and elevation normally occur during adolescence and should not be cause for concern. Consideration should be given to the presence of risk factors for development of melanoma and the parents' wishes about removal of the nevus. If doubt remains about the benign nature of a nevus, excision is a safe and simple outpatient procedure that may be justified to allay anxiety.

Atypical Melanocytic Nevus. Atypical nevocellular nevi occur both in an autosomal dominant familial melanoma-prone setting (familial mole-melanoma syndrome, dysplastic nevus syndrome, BK mole syndrome) and as a sporadic event. Only 2% of all pediatric melanomas occur in individuals with this familial syndrome, and 10% of those with the syndrome have a melanoma develop before age 20 yr. Malignant melanoma has been reported in children with the dysplastic nevus syndrome as early as age 10 yr. Risk for development of melanoma is essentially 100% in individuals with dysplastic nevus syndrome and two family members who have had melanomas. The term *atypical mole syndrome* has been proposed to describe lesions in those individuals without an autosomal dominant familial history of melanoma but with more than 50 nevi, some of which are atypical. The lifetime risk of melanoma associated with dysplastic nevi in this context is estimated to be 5–10%.

Atypical nevi tend to be large (5–15 mm) and round to oval. They have irregular margins, variegated color, and elevation of a portion of the lesion. These nevi are most common on the posterior trunk, suggesting that intermittent, intense sun exposure has a role in their genesis. They may also occur, however, in sun-protected areas such as the breasts, buttocks, and scalp. Atypical nevi do not usually develop until puberty, although scalp lesions may be present earlier. Atypical nevi demonstrate disordered proliferation of atypical intraepidermal melanocytes, lymphocytic infiltration, fibroplasia, and angiogenesis. It may be helpful to obtain histopathologic documentation of dysplastic change by biopsy to identify these individuals. It is prudent to excise borderline atypical nevi in immunocompromised children or in those treated with irradiation or chemotherapeutic agents. Although chemotherapy has been associated with the development of a greater number of melanocytic nevi, it has not been directly linked to increased risk for development of melanoma. The threshold for removal of clinically atypical nevi is also lower at sites that are difficult to observe, such as the scalp. Children with atypical nevi should have a complete skin examination every 6–12 mo. Parents must be counseled about the importance of sun protection and avoidance and be instructed to look for early signs of melanoma on a regular basis, approximately every 3–4 mo.

Congenital Melanocytic Nevus. Congenital melanocytic nevi are present in approximately 1% of newborn infants. These nevi have been categorized by size: giant congenital nevi are more than 20 cm in diameter (adult size), small congenital nevi are less than 2 cm in diameter, and intermediate nevi are in between in size. Congenital nevi are characterized by the presence of nevus cells in the lower reticular dermis; between collagen bundles; surrounding cutaneous appendages, nerves, and vessels in the lower dermis; and occasionally extending to the subcuticular fat. Identification is often uncertain, however, because they may have the histologic features of ordinary junctional, compound, or intradermal nevi. Some nevi that were not present at birth display histopathologic features of congenital nevi. Furthermore, congenital nevi may be difficult to distinguish clinically from other types of pigmented lesions, adding to the difficulty that parents may have in identifying nevi that were present at birth. The clinical differential diagnosis includes mongolian spots, café-au-lait spots, smooth muscle hamartoma, and dermal melanocytosis (nevi of Ota and Ito).

Sites of predilection of *small congenital nevi* are the lower trunk, upper back, shoulders, chest, and proximal limbs. The lesions may be flat, elevated, verrucous, or nodular and may be various shades of brown, blue, or black. Given the difficulty in identifying small congenital nevi with certainty, data regarding their malignant potential are controversial. Based on historical criteria, it is estimated that approximately 15% of melanomas arise within small congenital nevi. With histopathologic criteria, a congenital nevus has been found in association with approximately 3–8% of melanomas. Removal of all small congenital nevi is not warranted, particularly in view of the fact that development of melanoma in a small congenital nevus is an exceedingly rare event before puberty. A number of factors must be weighed in the decision about whether or not to remove a nevus, including its location and ability to be monitored clinically, the potential for scarring, the presence of other risk factors for melanoma, and the presence of atypical clinical features.

Giant congenital pigmented nevi (<1/20,000 births) occur most commonly on the posterior trunk but may also appear on the head or the extremities. These nevi are of special significance because of their association with leptomeningeal melanocytosis and their predisposition for development of malignant melanoma. Leptomeningeal involvement occurs most often when the nevus is located on the head or midline on the trunk, particularly when associated with "satellite" melanocytic nevi. Nevus cells within the leptomeninges and brain parenchyma may cause increased intracranial pressure, hydrocephalus, seizures, retardation, and motor deficits and may result in melanoma. Malignancy can be identified by careful cytologic examination of the cerebrospinal fluid for melanin-containing cells. Asymptomatic leptomeningeal melanosis on MRI scans is seen in approximately 30% of individuals with a giant congenital nevus. The overall incidence of malignant melanoma arising in a giant congenital nevus is estimated to be approximately 5–10%; approximately 3% of all melanomas arise within a giant congenital nevus. Half of all melanomas that arise within a giant congenital nevus do so by age 5 yr. The mortality rate is 45%. Management of giant congenital nevi remains controversial and should involve the parents, pediatrician, dermatologist, and plastic surgeon. If the nevus lies over the head or spine, an MRI scan may allow detection of neural melanosis; its presence makes gross removal of a nevus from the skin a futile effort. In the absence of neural melanosis, early excision and repair aided by tissue expanders or grafting may reduce the burden of nevus cells and thus the potential for development of melanoma, but at the cost of many potentially disfiguring surgeries. Even then, nevus cells deep within subcutaneous tissues may evade excision. Random biopsies of the nevus are not helpful, but biopsy of newly expanding nodules is indicated. Follow-up is recommended every 6 mo for 5 yr and every 12 mo thereafter. Serial photographs of the nevus may aid in detecting changes.

Melanoma. Malignant melanoma accounts for 1–3% of all pediatric malignancies and is the most common cancer in young adults age 25–29 yr. The incidence of melanoma has increased 150% since 1973. Melanoma develops primarily in white individuals, on the head and trunk in males and on the extremities in females. Risk factors for development of melanoma include the presence of the familial atypical mole-melanoma syndrome or xeroderma pigmentosum; increased number of melanocytic nevi, consisting of acquired nevi, giant congenital nevus, or atypical nevi; fair complexion; excessive sun exposure, especially intense sunlight intermittently; a personal or family (i.e., first-degree relative) history of a previous melanoma; and immuno-suppression. In previously well children, UV radiation is responsible for most melanomas. Fewer than 5% of childhood melanomas develop within giant congenital nevi or in those with the familial atypical mole-melanoma syndrome. Approximately 40–50% of the time, melanoma develops at a site where there was no apparent nevus. The mortality rate from melanoma is related primarily to tumor thickness and the level of invasion into the skin. The overall mortality rate reaches approximately 40%, regardless of whether it arises in a child or adult. Given the lack of effective therapy for melanoma, prevention and early detection are the most effective measures. Avoidance of intense midday sun exposure between 10 A.M. and 3 P.M.; use of protective clothing such as a hat, long sleeves, and pants; and use of sunscreen should be emphasized. Early detection includes frequent clinical and photographic examinations for patients at risk (dysplastic nevus syndrome) and prompt response to rapid changes in nevi (size, shape, color, inflammation, bleeding or crusting, and sensation).

Halo Nevus (Leukoderma Acquisitum Centrifugum). Halo nevi occur primarily in children and young adults, most commonly on the back (Fig. 641–1). Development of the halo may coincide with puberty or pregnancy. Several pigmented nevi frequently develop a halo simultaneously. Subsequent disappearance of the central nevus over several months is the usual outcome, and the depigmented area may or may not become repigmented. Excision and histopathologic examination of the lesion is indicated only when the nature of the central lesion is in question. An acquired melanocytic nevus occasionally develops a peripheral zone of depigmentation over a period of days to weeks. There is a dense inflammatory infiltrate of lymphocytes and histiocytes in addition to the nevus cells. The pale halo reflects disappearance of the melanocytes. This phenomenon is associated with congenital nevi, blue nevi, Spitz nevi, dysplastic nevi, neurofibromas, and primary and secondary malignant melanoma

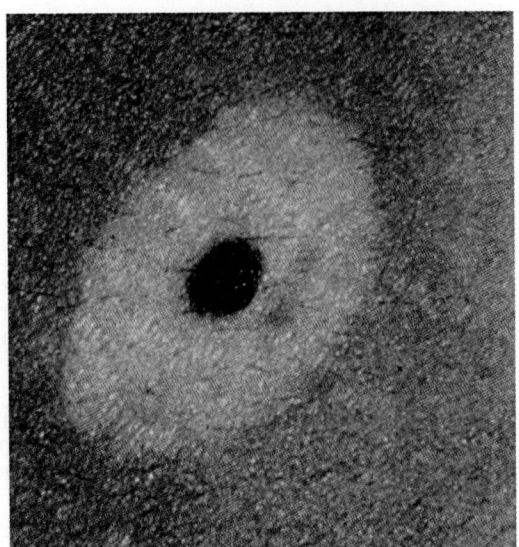

FIGURE 641–1. Well-developed halo nevus.

and occasionally with poliosis, Vogt-Koyanagi-Harada syndrome, and pernicious anemia. Patients with vitiligo have an increased incidence of halo nevi. Individuals with halo nevi have circulating antibodies against the cytoplasm of malignant melanoma cells, and their lymphocytes display enhanced killing of melanoma cells in culture.

Spitz Nevus (Spindle and Epithelioid Cell Nevus). Spitz nevus presents most commonly during the first 2 decades of life as a pink to red, smooth, dome-shaped, firm, hairless papule on the face, shoulder, or upper limb. Most are less than 1 cm in diameter, but they can achieve a size of 3 cm. Rarely, they occur as numerous grouped lesions. Visually similar lesions include pyogenic granuloma, hemangioma, nevocellular nevus, juvenile xanthogranuloma, and basal cell carcinoma, but histologically these entities are distinguishable. Spitz nevus may be difficult to distinguish histopathologically from malignant melanoma because nuclear atypia is a common feature, particularly after local recurrence of the nevus. Local recurrence after excision may occur up to 5% of the time. If a nevus arouses clinical suspicion that it may be a melanoma, an excisional biopsy of the entire lesion is recommended. If the margins of excision of a Spitz nevus are positive, re-excision of the site is prudent to avoid difficulties in histopathologic interpretation of the lesion in the future.

Zosteriform Lentiginous Nevus (Agminated Lentigines). This nevus is a unilateral, linear, bandlike collection of numerous 2–10 mm brown or black macules on the face, trunk, or limbs. The nevus may be present at birth or may develop during childhood. Seen histopathologically are increased numbers of melanocytes in elongated rete ridges of the epidermis.

Nevus Spilus (Speckled Lentiginous Nevus). This nevus is a flat brown patch within which are darker, flat or raised brown melanocytic elements. These nevi vary considerably in size and can occur anywhere on the body. Nevus spilus is rare at birth and is commonly acquired during late infancy or early childhood. Dark elements within the nevus are usually present initially and tend to increase in number gradually over time. The darker macules represent nevus cells in a junctional or dermal location; the patch has increased numbers of melanocytes in a lentiginous epidermal pattern. The malignant potential of these nevi is uncertain; nevus spilus is found more commonly in individuals with melanoma than in matched control subjects. The nevi need not be excised, unless atypical features or recent clinical changes are noted.

Nevus of Ota. Nevus of Ota is more common in females and in Asian and black patients. This nevus consists of a permanent patch composed of blue, black, and brown, partially confluent macules. The intensity of pigmentation may vary from day to day, and enlargement and darkening may occur with time. Some areas of the nevus occasionally are raised. The macular nevi resemble mongolian spots in color and occur unilaterally in the areas supplied by the 1st and 2nd divisions of the trigeminal nerve. Nevus of Ota differs from a mongolian spot, not only by its distribution but also by having a speckled rather than a uniform appearance. It also has a greater concentration of elongated, dendritic dermal melanocytes located in the upper rather than the lower portion of the dermis. Nevus of Ota is sometimes present at birth; in other cases, it may arise during the 1st or 2nd decade of life. Patchy involvement of the conjunctiva, hard palate, pharynx, nasal mucosa, buccal mucosa, or tympanic membrane occurs in some patients. Malignant change is exceedingly rare. Laser therapy may effectively decrease the pigmentation.

Nevus of Ito is localized to the supraclavicular, scapular, and deltoid regions. This nevus tends to be more diffuse in its distribution and less mottled than the nevus of Ota. The only available treatment is masking with cosmetics or laser therapy.

Blue Nevi. The *common blue nevus* is a solitary, asymptomatic, smooth, dome-shaped, blue to blue-gray papule less than 10 mm in diameter on the dorsal aspect of the hands and feet. Rarely, common blue nevi form large plaques. Blue nevus is nearly always acquired, often during childhood and more commonly in females. Microscopically, it is characterized by groups of intensely pigmented spindle-shaped melanocytes in the dermis. This nevus is benign.

The *cellular blue nevus* is typically 1–3 cm in diameter and occurs most frequently on the buttocks and in the sacrococcygeal area. In addition to collections of deeply pigmented dermal dendritic melanocytes, cellular islands composed of large spindle-shaped cells are noted in the dermis and may extend into the subcutaneous fat. The cellular blue nevus has a low but definite incidence of malignant transformation; therefore, excision is the treatment of choice. A *combined nevus* is the association of a blue nevus with an overlying melanocytic nevus.

The blue-gray that is characteristic of these nevi is an optical effect caused by dermal melanin. Longer wavelengths of visible light penetrate to the deep dermis and are absorbed there by melanin; shorter-wavelength blue light cannot penetrate deeply but instead is reflected back to the observer.

Achromic Nevus (Nevus Depigmentosus). These nevi are usually present at birth; they are localized macular hypopigmented patches or streaks, often with bizarre, irregular borders. They can resemble hypomelanosis of Ito clinically, except that they are more localized and often unilateral. Small lesions may also resemble the white leaf macules of tuberous sclerosis. They appear to represent a focal defect in transfer of melanosomes to keratinocytes.

Epidermal Nevi. These may be visible at birth or may develop within the first months or years of life. They affect both sexes equally and usually occur sporadically. Epidermal nevi are hamartomatous lesions characterized by hyperplasia of the epidermis and/or adnexal structures in a focal area of the skin. Proliferation of nevocellular nevus cells is not present in these lesions.

Epidermal nevi are classified into a number of variants, depending on the morphology and extent of the nevus and the epidermal structure that is predominant. An epidermal nevus may appear initially as a discolored, slightly scaly patch that, with maturation, becomes more linear, thickened, verrucous, and hyperpigmented. *Systematized* refers to a diffuse or extensive distribution of lesions, and *ichthyosis hystrix* indicates that the distribution is extensive and bilateral. Morphologic types include pigmented papillomas, often in a linear distribution; unilateral hyperkeratotic streaks involving a limb and perhaps a portion of the trunk; velvety hyperpigmented plaques; and whorled or marbled hyperkeratotic lesions in localized plaques (Fig. 641–2) or over extensive areas of the body along Blaschko lines. An inflammatory linear verrucous variant is markedly pruritic and tends to become erythematous, scaling, and crusted.

The histologic pattern evolves as the lesion matures, but epidermal hyperplasia of some degree is apparent in all stages of development. One or another dermal appendage may predominate in a particular lesion. These nevi must be distinguished from lichen striatus, lymphangioma circumscriptum, shagreen patch of tuberous sclerosis, congenital hairy nevi, linear porokeratosis, linear lichen planus, linear psoriasis, the verrucous stage of incontinentia pigmenti, and nevus sebaceus (Jadassohn). Keratolytic agents such as retinoic acid or salicylic acid may be moderately effective in reducing scaling and controlling pruritus, but definitive *treatment* requires full-thickness excision; recurrence is usual if more superficial removal is attempted. Alternatively, the nevus may be left intact. Rarely, basal cell carcinoma or squamous cell carcinoma has developed in a verrucous epidermal nevus that shows sudden growth, nodularity, or erosions.

Epidermal nevi are occasionally associated with other abnormalities of the skin and soft tissues, eyes, and nervous, cardiovascular, musculoskeletal, and urogenital systems. In these instances, referred to as *epidermal nevus syndrome*, a mosaic phenotype is expressed. This syndrome, however, is not a distinct clinical entity. The well established syndromes that involve a type of epidermal nevus and distinct birth defects include the sebaceous nevus, *Proteus*, and CHILD (congenital *h*emidysplasia with *i*chthyosiform erythroderma and *l*imb *d*efects) syndromes.

NEVUS SEBACEUS (JADASSOHN). This is a relatively small, sharply demarcated, oval or linear, yellow-orange, elevated plaque that is usually devoid of hair and occurs on the head and neck of infants. It may occur occasionally on the trunk. Although the lesion is characterized histopathologically by an abundance of sebaceous glands, all elements of the skin are represented. It is frequently flat and inconspicuous in early childhood. With maturity, usually during adolescence, the lesions become verrucous and studded with large rubbery nodules. The changing clinical appearance reflects the histologic pattern, which is characterized by a variable degree of hyperkeratosis, hyperplasia of the epidermis, malformed hair follicles, and often a profusion of sebaceous glands and the presence of

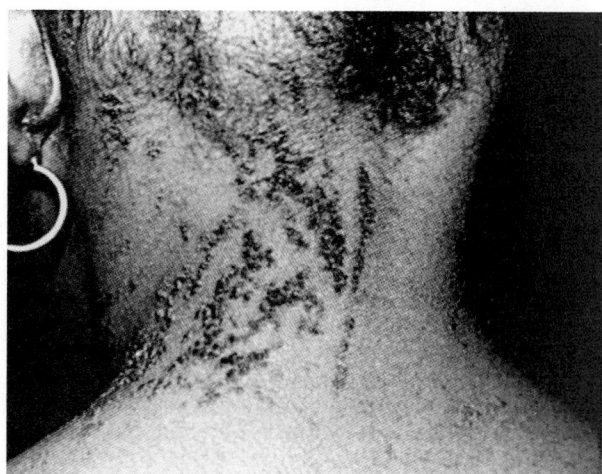

FIGURE 641–2. Verrucous streaky epidermal nevus on the neck.

ectopic apocrine glands. It is believed that these nevi form from pluripotential primary epithelial germ cells, which can dedifferentiate into various epithelial tumors. Consequently, during adulthood, these nevi are frequently complicated by secondary malignancies and benign adnexal tumors, most commonly basal cell carcinoma or syringocystadenoma papilliferum. The risk of malignancy may be smaller than previously recognized. The risk of basal cell carcinoma may be close to 1%, with a significantly greater risk of benign neoplasia. Deletions in the PTCH gene, the putative gene defect in basal cell carcinoma, have been found in sebaceous nevi. Diagnosis can be established by biopsy; the treatment of choice is total excision before adolescence. Sebaceous nevi associated with central nervous system, skeletal, and ocular defects represent a variant of the epidermal nevus syndrome.

BECKER NEVUS (BECKER MELANOSIS). This form of epidermal nevus develops predominantly in males, during childhood or adolescence, initially as a hyperpigmented patch. The lesion commonly develops hypertrichosis, limited to the area of hyperpigmentation, and evolves into a unilateral, slightly thickened, irregular, hyperpigmented plaque. The most common sites are the upper torso and upper arm. The nevus shows an increased number of basal melanocytes and variable epidermal hyperplasia. Becker melanosis is commonly associated with a smooth muscle hamartoma, which may appear as slight perifollicular papular elevations or slight induration. Stroking such a lesion may induce smooth muscle contraction and make the hairs stand up. Androgen sensitivity may have a role in the development of Becker melanosis. The nevus is benign, has no risk for malignant change, and is rarely associated with other anomalies.

Nevus Comedonicus. This is an uncommon organoid nevus of epithelial origin that consists of linear plaques of plugged follicles that simulate comedones; they may be present at birth or may appear during childhood. The horny plugs represent keratinous debris within dilated, malformed pilosebaceous follicles. The lesions are most often unilateral and may develop at any site. Rarely, they are associated with other congenital malformations, including skeletal defects, cerebral anomalies, and cataracts. Although these lesions are often asymptomatic, some individuals experience recurrent inflammation, resulting in cyst formation, fistulas, and scarring. There is no effective treatment except full-thickness excision; palliation of larger lesions may be achieved by regular applications of a retinoic acid preparation.

Connective Tissue Nevus. This is a hamartoma of collagen, elastin, and/or glycosaminoglycans of the dermal extracellular matrix. It may occur as a solitary defect or as a manifestation of an associated disorder. These nevi may occur at any site but are most common on the back, buttocks, arms, and thighs. They are skin-colored, ivory, or yellow plaques, 2–15 cm in diameter, composed of many tiny papules or grouped nodules that are frequently difficult to appreciate visually because of the subtle color changes. The plaques have a rubbery or cobblestone consistency on palpation. Biopsy findings are variable and include increased amounts and/or degeneration or fragmentation of dermal collagen, elastic tissue, or ground substance. Similar lesions occurring with tuberous sclerosis are called shagreen patches; however, shagreen patches consist only of excessive amounts of collagen. The association of many small papular connective tissue nevi with osteopoikilosis is called *dermatofibrosis lenticularis disseminata* (Buschke-Ollendorf syndrome).

Smooth Muscle Hamartoma. This hamartoma is a developmental anomaly resulting from hyperplasia of the smooth muscle (arrector pili) associated with hair follicles. It is usually evident at birth or shortly thereafter as a flesh-colored or lightly pigmented plaque with overlying hypertrichosis on the trunk or limbs. Transient elevation or a rippling movement of the lesion,

caused by contraction of the muscle bundles, can sometimes be elicited by stroking the surface. Smooth muscle hamartoma can be mistaken for congenital pigmented nevus, but the distinction is important because it has no risk for malignant melanoma and need not be removed.

Berg P, Lindelöf B: Differences in malignant melanoma between children and adolescents. *Arch Dermatol* 1997;133:295.

Bittencourt FV, Marghoob AA, Kopf AW, et al: Large congenital melanocytic nevi and the risk for development of malignant melanoma and neurocutaneous melanocytosis. *Pediatrics* 2000;106:736.

Casso EM, Grin-Jorgensen CM, Grant-Kels JM: Spitz nevi. *J Am Acad Dermatol* 1992;27:901.

Ceballos PI, Ruiz-Maldonado R, Mihm MC: Melanoma in children. *N Engl J Med* 1995;332:656.

Cribier B, Scrivener Y, Grosshans E: Tumors arising in nevus sebaceus: A study of 596 cases. *J Am Acad Dermatol* 2000;42:263.

De David M, Orlow SJ, Provost N, et al: Neurocutaneous melanosis: Clinical features of large congenital melanocytic nevi in patients with manifest central nervous system melanosis. *J Am Acad Dermatol* 1996;35:529.

Frieden IJ, Williams ML, Barkovich AJ: Giant congenital melanocytic nevi: Brain magnetic resonance findings in neurologically asymptomatic children. *J Am Acad Dermatol* 1994;31:423.

Fry A, Verne J: Preventing skin cancer. *BMJ* 2003;326:114–5.

Gallagher RP, McClean DI, Yang CP, et al: Anatomic distribution of acquired melanocytic nevi in white children. *Arch Dermatol* 1990;125:466.

Gallagher RP, McClean DI, Yang CP, et al: Suntan, sunburn, and pigmentation factors and the frequency of acquired melanocytic nevi in children. *Arch Dermatol* 1990;126:770.

Glanz K, Saraiya M, Wechsler H, et al: Guidelines for school programs to prevent skin cancer. *MMWR* 2002;51:1–19.

Green MH, Clark WH, Tucker MA, et al: Acquired precursors of cutaneous malignant melanoma. (The familial dysplastic nevus syndrome.) *N Engl J Med* 1985;312:91.

Jacobs AH, Walton RG: The incidence of birthmarks in the neonate. *Pediatrics* 1976;58:2811.

Marghoob AA, Orlow SJ, Kopf AW: Syndromes associated with melanocytic nevi. *J Am Acad Dermatol* 1993;29:373.

Ruiz-Maldonado R, Orozco-Covarrubias ML: Malignant melanoma in children. *Arch Dermatol* 1997;133:363.

Shpall S, Frieden I, Chesney M, et al: Risk of malignant transformation of congenital melanocytic nevi in blacks. *Pediatr Dermatol* 1994;11:204.

Tucker M, Halpern A, Holly E, et al: Clinically recognized dysplastic nevi. *JAMA* 1997;277:1439.

Vandeweyer E, Sales F, Deraemaecker: Cutaneous malignant melanoma in children. *Eur J Pediatr* 2000;159:582–4.

Williams ML, Pennella R: Melanoma, melanocytic nevi, and other melanoma risk factors in children. *J Pediatr* 1994;124:833.

Xin H, Matt D, Burg G, et al: Deletions in the PTCH gene in sebaceous nevi. *J Invest Dermatol* 1999;112:587.

Chapter 642
Hyperpigmented Lesions

Disorders of Pigment. Increased skin color may be generalized or localized and may result from various defects in melanocyte formation, differentiation, migration, or distribution or in the production or distribution of melanin. Some of these aberrations are a manifestation of systemic disease (hyperpigmentation of Addison disease); others represent generalized or focal developmental defects (piebaldism); still others may be nonspecific and the result of cutaneous inflammation (postinflammatory hyperpigmentation).

Ephelides (Freckles). These are light or dark brown macules usually less than 3 mm in diameter, with a poorly defined margin that occur in sun-exposed areas, such as the face, upper back, arms, and hands. They are induced by exposure to sun, particularly during the summer, and may fade or disappear during the winter. They are more common in fair-haired individuals, appear first during the preschool years, and are determined by an autosomal dominant gene. Histologically, they are marked by increased melanin pigment in epidermal basal cells, which have more numerous and larger dendritic processes than the melanocytes of the surrounding paler skin. The lack of melanocytic proliferation or elongation of epidermal rete ridges distinguishes them from lentigines. Freckles have been identified as a risk factor for melanoma independent of melanocytic nevi.

Lentigines. Lentigines, often mistaken for freckles or junctional nevi, are small (<3 cm), round, dark-brown macules that can appear anywhere on the body. They are unrelated to sun exposure and remain permanently. Histologically, they have elongated, club-shaped, epidermal rete ridges with increased numbers of melanocytes and dense epidermal deposits of melanin. No nests of melanocytes are found. The lesions are benign and, when few, may be viewed as a normal occurrence.

Lentigines may increase in number and darken excessively in Addison disease and during pregnancy. *Lentiginosis profusa* involves innumerable small, pigmented macules that are present at birth or appear during childhood. There are no associated abnormalities, and mucous membranes are spared. *LAMB syndrome* consists of *l*entigines of the face and vulva, *a*trial myxoma, *m*ucocutaneous myxomas, and *b*lue nevi. The *multiple lentigines (LEOPARD) syndrome* is an autosomal dominant entity consisting of a generalized, symmetric distribution of *l*entigines in association with *e*lectrocardiogram abnormalities, *o*cular hypertelorism, *p*ulmonary stenosis, *a*bnormal genitals (cryptorchidism, hypogonadism, hypospadias), growth *r*etardation, and sensorineural *d*eafness. Other features include hypertrophic obstructive cardiomyopathy and pectus excavatum or carinatum.

The *Peutz-Jeghers syndrome* is characterized by melanotic macules on the lips and mucous membranes and by gastrointestinal (GI) polyposis. It is inherited as an autosomal dominant trait. The causative gene encodes a nuclear serine/threonine kinase, LKB1, which functions as a tumor suppressor. Onset is noted during infancy and early childhood when pigmented macules appear on the lips and buccal mucosa. The macules are usually a few millimeters in size but may be as large as 1–2 cm. Macules also appear occasionally on the palate, gums, tongue, and vaginal mucosa. Cutaneous lesions may develop on the nose, hands, and feet; around the mouth, eyes, and umbilicus; and as longitudinal bands or diffuse hyperpigmentation of the nails. Pigmented macules often fade from the lips and skin during puberty and adulthood but generally do not disappear from mucosal surfaces. Buccal mucosal macules are the most constant feature of the disorder; in some families, however, occasional members may be affected only with the pigmentary changes. Indistinguishable pigmentary changes beginning in adult life also occur sporadically in individuals without intestinal involvement.

Polyposis usually involves the jejunum and ileum but may also occur in the stomach, duodenum, colon, and rectum (Chapter 326). Episodic abdominal pain, diarrhea, melena, and intussusception are frequent complications. Patients have a significantly increased risk of GI tract and non-GI tract tumors at a young age. GI cancer has been reported in approximately 2–3% of patients; the lifetime relative risk of GI malignancy is 13. The relative risk of non-GI tract malignancies is 9, including ovarian, cervical, and testicular tumors. Peutz-Jeghers syndrome must be differentiated from other syndromes associated with multiple lentigines *(Laugier-Hunziker syndrome)*, from ordinary freckling, from *Gardner syndrome*, and from *Cronkhite-Canada syndrome*, a disorder characterized by GI polyposis; alopecia; onychodystrophy; and diffuse pigmentation of the palms, volar aspects of the fingers, and dorsal hands. Treatment of Peutz-Jeghers melanotic macules has been successful, in some cases, with carbon dioxide, ruby, or argon lasers.

Café-au-Lait Spots. These are uniformly hyperpigmented, sharply demarcated macular lesions, the hues of which vary with the normal degree of pigmentation of the individual: They are tan or light brown in white individuals and may be dark brown in black children. Café-au-lait spots vary tremendously in size and may be large, covering a significant portion of the trunk or limb. Generally, the borders are smooth, but some have an exceedingly irregular border. The lesions are characterized by increased numbers of melanocytes and melanin in the epidermis but lack the clubbed rete ridges that typify lentigines. One to three café-au-lait spots are common in normal children; approximately 10% of normal children have café-au-lait macules. They may be present at birth or develop during childhood.

Large, often asymmetric café-au-lait spots with irregular borders are characteristic of patients with *McCune-Albright syndrome* (see Chapter 556.6). This disorder includes polyostotic fibrous dysplasia of bone, leading to pathologic fractures; precocious puberty; and numerous hyperfunctional endocrinopathies. The macular hyperpigmentation may be present at birth or develop late in childhood. Cutaneous pigmentation typically is most extensive on the side showing the most severe bone involvement. The full syndrome with precocious puberty occurs only in girls. A mutation in the gene for the α subunit of G_s, resulting in stimulation of cyclic adenosine monophosphate formation, occurs in these patients.

NEUROFIBROMATOSIS TYPE 1 (VON RECKLINGHAUSEN DISEASE). The café-au-lait spot is the most familiar cutaneous hallmark of this autosomal dominant neurocutaneous syndrome (see Chapter 589.1). These lesions also occur with certain other disorders, including other types of neurofibromatosis (Box 642–1). Included in the criteria for this diagnosis is the presence of five or more café-au-lait spots more than 5 mm in diameter in prepubertal patients or six or more café-au-lait spots more than 15 mm in diameter in postpubertal children. Multiple café-au-lait macules commonly produce a freckled appearance of non–sun-exposed areas such as the axillae (Crowe sign), the inguinal and inframammary regions, and under the chin.

Incontinentia Pigmenti (Bloch-Sulzberger Disease). This rare, heritable, multisystem ectodermal disorder features dermatologic, dental, and ocular abnormalities. The phenotype is produced by functional mosaicism caused by random X-inactivation of an X-linked dominant gene that is lethal in males. The paucity of affected males, the occurrence of female-to-female transmission, and an increased frequency of spontaneous abortions in carrier females supports this supposition. The gene, nuclear factor kappa B essential modulator (NEMO), is located at Xq28.

CLINICAL MANIFESTATIONS. This disease has four phases, not all of which may occur in a given patient. The *first phase* is evident at birth or during the first few weeks of life and consists of erythematous linear streaks and plaques of vesicles that are most pronounced on the limbs and circumferentially on the trunk. The lesions may be confused with those of herpes simplex, bullous impetigo, or mastocytosis, but the linear configuration is unique. Histopathologically, epidermal edema and eosinophil-filled intraepidermal vesicles are present. Eosinophils also infiltrate the adjacent epidermis and dermis. Blood eosinophilia up to 65% also is common. The first stage generally resolves by 4 mo of age, but mild, short-lived recurrences of

---

BOX 642–1. Disorders with Café-au-Lait Spots

Neurofibromatosis	Basal cell nevus syndrome
McCune-Albright syndrome	Gaucher disease
Russell-Silver syndrome	Chédiak-Higashi syndrome
Ataxia telangiectasia	Hunter syndrome
Fanconi anemia	Maffucci syndrome
Tuberous sclerosis	Multiple mucosal neuroma
Bloom syndrome	syndrome
	Watson syndrome

blisters may develop during febrile illnesses of childhood. In the *second phase,* as blisters on the distal limbs resolve, they become dry and hyperkeratotic, forming verrucous plaques. The verrucous plaques rarely affect the trunk or face and generally involute within 6 mo. Epidermal hyperplasia, hyperkeratosis, and papillomatosis are characteristic. The *third* or *pigmentary stage* is the hallmark of incontinentia pigmenti. It generally develops over weeks to months and may overlap the earlier phases, be evident at birth, or, more commonly, begin to appear within the first few weeks of life. Hyperpigmentation more often is apparent on the trunk than the limbs and is distributed in macular whorls, reticulated patches, flecks, and linear streaks that follow Blaschko lines. The axillae and groin are invariably affected. The sites of involvement are not necessarily those of the preceding vesicular and warty lesions. The pigmented lesions, once present, persist throughout childhood (Fig. 642–1). They generally begin to fade by early adolescence, however, and often have disappeared by age 16 yr. Occasionally, the pigmentation remains permanently, particularly in the groin. The lesion, histopathologically, shows vacuolar degeneration of the epidermal basal cells and melanin in melanophages of the upper dermis as a result of incontinence of pigment. In the *fourth stage,* hypopigmented, hairless, anhidrotic patches or streaks occur as a late manifestation of incontinentia pigmenti; they may develop, however, before the hyperpigmentation of stage three has resolved. The lesions develop mainly on the flexor aspect of the lower legs and less often on the arms and trunk.

Although skin lesions may constitute the only manifestation, approximately 80% of affected children have other defects. Alopecia, which may be scarring and patchy or diffuse, is most common on the vertex and occurs in up to 40% of patients. Hair may be lusterless, wiry, and coarse. Dental anomalies, which are present in up to 80% of patients and are persistent throughout life, consist of late dentition, hypodontia, conical teeth, and impaction. Central nervous system manifestations, including motor and cognitive developmental retardation, seizures, microcephaly, spasticity, and paralysis, are found in up to one third of affected children. Ocular anomalies, such as neovascularization, microphthalmos, strabismus, optic nerve atrophy, cataracts, and retrolenticular masses, occur in more than 30% of children. Nonetheless, more than 90% of patients have normal vision. The ocular and central nervous system lesions may be secondary to an occlusive vasculopathy. Less common abnormalities include dystrophy of nails (ridging, pitting) and skeletal defects.

Diagnosis of incontinentia pigmenti is made on clinical grounds, although major and minor criteria have been established to aid in diagnosis. Wood lamp examination may be useful in older children and adolescents to highlight pigmentary abnormalities.

TREATMENT. The choice of investigative studies and the plan of management depend on the occurrence of particular noncutaneous abnormalities because the skin lesions are benign. The high incidence of associated major anomalies warrants genetic counseling.

Postinflammatory Pigmentary Changes. Either hyperpigmentation or hypopigmentation can occur as a result of cutaneous inflammation. Alteration in pigmentation usually follows a severe inflammatory reaction but may result from mild dermatitis. Dark-skinned children are more likely to show these changes than fair-skinned ones. Although altered pigmentation may persist for weeks to months, patients can be reassured that these lesions are usually temporary. These changes must be distinguished from nevoid lesions and diseases manifested by pigmentary alterations such as vitiligo.

Bolognia JL, Orlow SJ, Glick SA: Lines of Blaschko. *J Acad Dermatol* 1994;31:157.
Eichenfield LF, Gibbs NF: Hyperpigmentation disorders. In Eichenfield LF, Frieden IJ, Esterly NB (editors): *Textbook of Neonatal Dermatology.* Philadelphia, WB Saunders, 2001, p. 370.
Gutman D, Aylsworth A, Carey J, et al: The diagnostic evaluation and multidisciplinary management of neurofibromatosis 1 and neurofibromatosis 2. *JAMA* 1997;278:51.
Hizawa K, Iida M, Matsumoto T, et al: Neoplastic transformation arising in Peutz-Jeghers polyposis. *Dis Colon Rectum* 1993;36:953.
Hyer W: Polyposis syndromes: Pediatric implications. *Gastrointest Endosc Clin North Am* 2001;11:659.
Landy SJ, Donnai D: Incontinentia pigmenti (Bloch-Sulzberger syndrome). *J Med Genet* 1993;30:53.
Lee A, Goldberg M, Gillard J, et al: Intracranial assessment of incontinentia pigmenti using magnetic resonance imaging, angiography, and spectroscopic imaging. *Arch Pediatr Adolesc Med* 1995;149:573.
Smahi A, Courtois G, Vabres P, et al: Genomic rearrangement in NEMO impairs NF-kappa B activation and is a cause of incontinentia pigmenti. The International Incontinentia Pigmenti Consortium. *Nature* 2000;405:466.

Chapter 643
Hypopigmented Lesions

Albinism. Several types of congenital oculocutaneous albinism consist of partial or complete failure of melanin production in the skin, hair, and eyes despite the presence of normal number, structure, and distribution of melanocytes. The various forms of albinism, including nine autosomal recessive and one rare autosomal dominant variants, may be distinguished by clinical manifestations, morphology of the melanosomes, and the hair bulb incubation test, in which hair bulbs are plucked and incubated with tyrosine to determine whether tyrosinase is present. Tyrosinase is the copper-containing enzyme that catalyzes at least three steps in melanin biosynthesis (see Chapter 74.2). Tyrosinase-positive variants, which are characterized by darkening of the hair bulb on incubation with tyrosine, are most common.

Ocular albinism, which involves only the eyes, presents in X-linked and autosomal dominant forms, and one autosomal recessive form. Two of these types are associated with deafness.

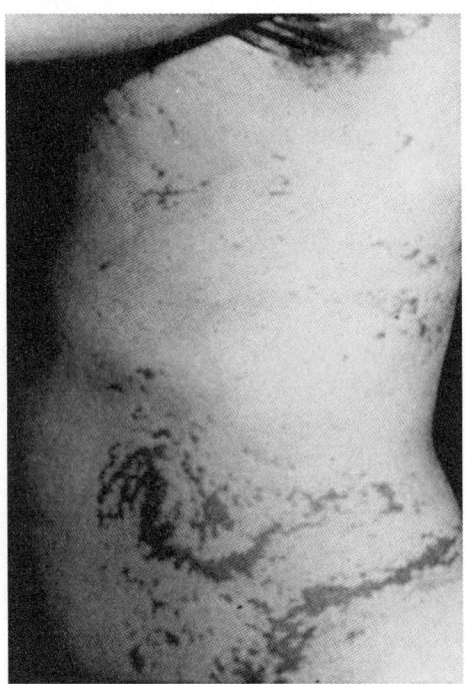

FIGURE 642–1. Whorled macular hyperpigmentation of incontinentia pigmenti.

Female carriers of the X-linked types may show irregular retinal pigmentation.

Tyrosinase-negative or type 1 oculocutaneous albinism is characterized by greatly reduced or absent tyrosinase activity. Type 1A albinism, the most severe form, is characterized by a lack of visible pigment in hair, skin, and eyes. This is manifested as photophobia, nystagmus, defective visual acuity, white hair, and white skin. The irises are blue-gray in oblique light and prominent pink in reflected light. Type 1B or yellow mutant albinism presents at birth with white hair, pink skin, and gray eyes. This type is particularly prevalent in Amish communities. Progressively, however, the hair becomes yellow-red, the skin tans lightly on exposure to the sun, and the irises may accumulate some brown pigment, with a resultant improvement in visual acuity. Photophobia and nystagmus are present but are mild. Numerous different allelic mutations in the tyrosinase gene account for types 1A and 1B albinism. In whites, no single mutant tyrosinase allele accounts for a significant fraction of the total, and this fact complicates molecular approaches to carrier detection and prenatal diagnosis.

The phenotype of *tyrosinase-positive or type 2 albinism* ranges from nearly normal to closely resembling type 1 albinism. Little or no melanin is present at birth, but pigment, particularly red-yellow pigment, may accumulate rapidly during childhood to produce straw-colored or light brown skin in whites. Progressive improvement in visual acuity and nystagmus occurs with aging. Blacks may have yellow-brown skin, dark-brown freckles in sun-exposed areas, and brown coloration of the irises. The defect in type 2 albinism has been mapped to chromosome 15 (the P gene) and may involve a tyrosine-specific transport protein. Deletions in this region also result in the Prader-Willi and Angelman syndromes, which include hypopigmentation.

The *Hermansky-Pudlak syndrome, due to mutations in the HPS gene,* is tyrosinase-positive albinism, with variable pigmentation, in association with a platelet storage pool deficiency and a hemorrhagic diathesis. Additional features include accumulation of a ceroid-like pigment in cells of the reticuloendothelial system, pulmonary fibrosis, and granulomatous colitis.

The *Cross-McKusick-Breen syndrome* consists of tyrosinase-positive albinism with ocular abnormalities, retardation, spasticity, and athetosis. Some patients have darkly pigmented hairs distributed among hair without color in the eyebrows and eyelashes.

Because of the absence of normal protection by adequate amounts of epidermal melanin, persons with albinism are predisposed to develop actinic keratoses and cutaneous carcinoma secondary to skin damage by ultraviolet light. Protective clothing and a broad-spectrum sunscreen preparation (see Chapter 646) should be worn during exposure to sunlight.

Partial Albinism (Piebaldism). This congenital autosomal dominant disorder is characterized by sharply demarcated amelanotic patches that occur most frequently on the forehead, anterior scalp (producing a white forelock), ventral trunk, elbows, and knees. Islands of normal pigmentation may be present within the amelanotic areas. The plaques are a result of a permanent localized absence of melanocytes and melanosomes or reduced numbers of abnormally large melanocytes. Piebaldism results from mutations in the *KIT* proto-oncogene, which encodes the cellular transmembrane tyrosinase kinase for mast/stem cell growth factor. The pattern of depigmentation is thought to stem from defective melanocyte proliferation or migration from the neural crest during development. Piebaldism must be differentiated from vitiligo, which may be progressive and is not usually congenital; nevus depigmentosus; and Waardenburg syndrome.

Waardenburg Syndrome. Waardenburg syndrome is an autosomal dominantly inherited disorder characterized by pigmentary abnormalities and defects in other tissues derived from the neu-

ral crest. Mutations in one of three transcription factors, PAX3, MITF, and SOX 10, lead to several distinctive presentations. Common features include lateral displacement of the medial canthi with dystopia canthorum (99%), broad nasal root (80%), heterochromic irises (25%), congenital deafness (20%), a white forelock (17%), and cutaneous hypopigmentation. A few patients have skin changes identical to piebaldism. Premature graying may develop in the 3rd decade. Waardenburg syndrome is inherited as an autosomal dominant trait with variable penetrance. It is due to defective migration and differentiation of neural crest cells.

Chédiak-Higashi Syndrome. See Chapter 120.3.

Tuberous Sclerosis. See Chapter 589.2 This disorder is a multisystemic disorder affecting primarily tissues derived from ectoderm but also involving organs of mesodermal and endodermal origin, particularly the eyes, kidneys, and heart. The classic clinical triad is skin lesions in association with epilepsy and mental retardation.

ETIOLOGY AND EPIDEMIOLOGY. This is an autosomal dominant condition with variable expression. Mutations have been mapped to chromosome 9q34.3 (TSC1) and 16p13.3 (TSC2). The TSC2 product is tubern, which has sequence homology with a GTPase-activating protein and may have a role in regulating cellular growth by acting as a growth suppressor gene. TSC1 also is postulated to act as a growth suppressor. Approximately half of cases are due to new mutations. The most reliable early cutaneous sign is the white- or ash-leaf macule, which presents at birth or in early infancy, often years before other signs of the disease. Ash-leaf macules also appear in 2–3/1,000 normal newborns. They are sharply demarcated, pale, 0.5–3 cm lesions that often assume the shape of a mountain ash leaflet.

CLINICAL MANIFESTATIONS. Single or multiple ash-leaf lesions are most often found on the trunk (Fig. 643–1A) but also occur on the face and limbs. Small, confetti-like hypopigmented macules are also present in some instances, reflecting inadequate melanization of the melanosomes in melanocytes. *Adenoma sebaceum* is the most commonly recognized cutaneous marker of tuberous sclerosis; the lesions appear on the face during middle to late childhood or adolescence in approximately 80% of patients. These red-brown or flesh-colored, smooth, glistening, telangiectatic 1–10 mm papules may extend from the nasolabial folds to the cheeks and chin (see Fig. 643–1B). The presence of telangiectasias and the lack of comedones and pustules help to distinguish this eruption from acne vulgaris. Adenoma sebaceum is a misnomer because these growths are angiofibromas rather than tumors of the sebaceous gland tumors. Similar fibromatous nodules may be scattered on the forehead, trunk, and limbs. Large, skin-colored, irregularly thickened plaques with an orange peel or cobblestone texture *(shagreen patch)* may occur in the lumbosacral area. At puberty, firm, flesh-colored *periungual fibromas* (see Fig. 643–1C) emerge on the nail folds of some children; gingival fibromas may also occur, unassociated with the administration of anticonvulsant medications. Café-au-lait spots occur with increased frequency but are not as numerous as in neurofibromatosis. Mental deficiency occurs in 60–70%; nearly all have epilepsy. Epilepsy is also present in approximately 70% of those patients without mental retardation. Epilepsy begins in infancy or early childhood and is often progressively more severe. Cardiac rhabdomyomas are present in approximately one half of infants and usually regress; mechanical obstruction is a potential complication. Rarely, the presenting sign of tuberous sclerosis is hematuria, caused by a renal angiomyolipoma, which is characteristic of this condition. Seventy-five per cent of patients with tuberous sclerosis die before the age of 25 yr, most commonly as a complication of epilepsy, of intercurrent infection, or occasionally of cardiac failure or pulmonary fibrosis.

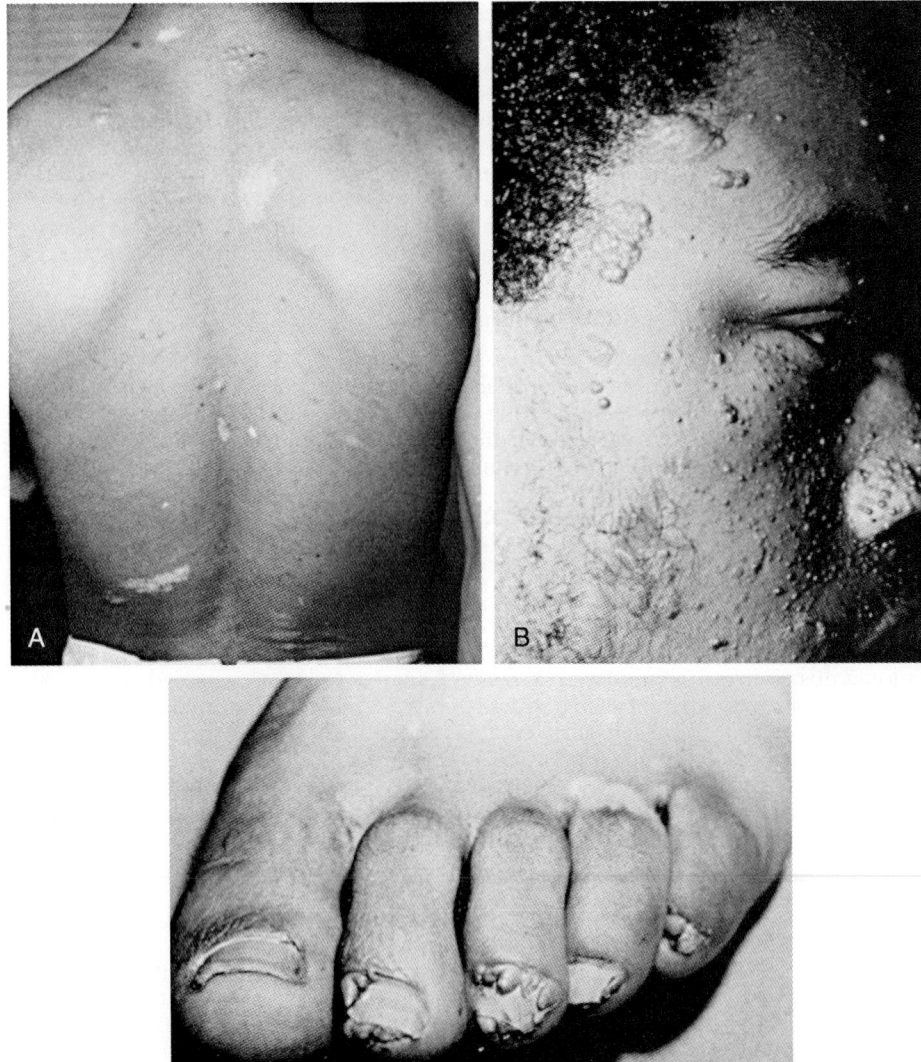

FIGURE 643–1. Tuberous sclerosis. *A*, Multiple white-leaf macules, small papular fibromas, and shagreen patch on lower back. *B*, Angiofibromas and angiofibromatous plaques on the temple. *C*, Periungual fibromas.

Hypomelanosis of Ito (Incontinentia Pigmenti Achromians). This congenital skin disorder affects children of both sexes and is frequently associated with defects in several organ systems. There is no evidence for genetic transmission; chromosomal mosaicism and chromosomal translocations have been reported. Hypomelanosis of Ito currently is a descriptive rather than definitive diagnosis.

The skin lesions of hypomelanosis of Ito are generally present at birth but may be acquired within the first 2 yr of life. The lesions are similar to a negative image of that present in incontinentia pigmenti, consisting of bizarre, patterned, hypopigmented macules arranged over the body surface in sharply demarcated whorls, streaks, and patches that follow the lines of Blaschko (Fig. 643–2). The palms, soles, and mucous membranes are spared. The hypopigmentation remains unchanged throughout childhood but fades during adulthood. The degree of depigmentation varies from hypopigmented to achromic. Neither inflammatory nor vesicular lesions precede the development of the pigmentary changes as in incontinentia pigmenti. The hypopigmented areas demonstrate fewer and smaller melanocytes and a decreased number of melanin granules in the basal cell layer than normal. Inflammatory cells and pigment incontinence are lacking.

The most commonly associated abnormalities involve the nervous system, including mental retardation (70%), seizures (40%), microcephaly (25%), and muscular hypotonia (15%). The musculoskeletal system is the second most frequently involved system, affected by scoliosis and thoracic and limb deformities. Minor ophthalmologic defects (strabismus, nystagmus) are present in 25% of patients, and 10% have cardiac defects. The differential diagnosis includes systematized nevus depigmentosus, which is a stable leukoderma not associated with systemic manifestations. Differentiation from incontinentia pigmenti, particularly the hypopigmented fourth stage, is critical for genetic counseling because incontinentia pigmenti, unlike hypomelanosis of Ito, is inherited.

Vitiligo. Approximately half of cases of this acquired pigmentary defect present before age 20 yr. The lesions are sharply circumscribed, depigmented macules that vary in size and shape.

EPIDEMIOLOGY AND ETIOLOGY. Although no clear-cut pattern of genetic transmission is established, 30–40% of patients have a positive family history. Associated abnormalities include uveitis and premature graying of hair. *Vogt-Koyanagi syndrome* presents with vitiligo, uveitis, and premature graying of hair but also involves the central nervous system. Vitiligo is

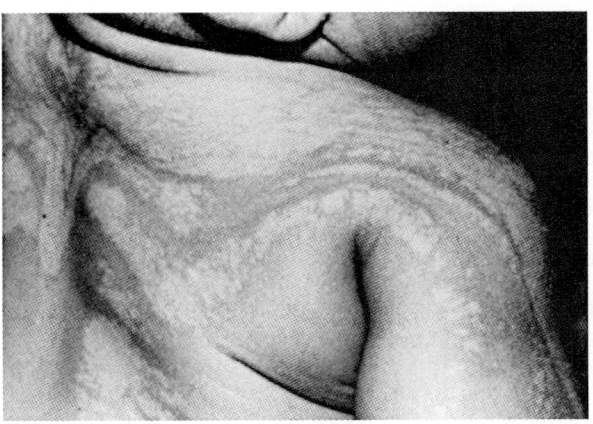

FIGURE 643–2. Marbled hypopigmented streaks of hypomelanosis of Ito (incontinentia pigmenti achromians).

more prevalent in patients with thyroid disease (hypothyroidism or hyperthyroidism), adrenal insufficiency, pernicious anemia, and diabetes mellitus. The cause of vitiligo is unknown, but trauma appears to have a role in induction of the lesions. A popular theory on the pathogenesis of vitiligo proposes an autoimmune mechanism, based on the finding that organ-specific autoantibodies to thyroid, gastroparietal, and adrenal tissue are found more frequently in the serum of patients with vitiligo than in the general population. Alternatively, a neurogenic theory purports that a compound that is released at peripheral nerve endings in the skin may inhibit melanogenesis; a self-destruct theory suggests that melanocytes destroy themselves as a result of a defective protective mechanism that normally would remove toxic melanin precursors.

CLINICAL MANIFESTATIONS. Areas of predilection are normally relatively hyperpigmented, such as the face, particularly around the eyes or mouth, the axillae, the inguinal region and genitals, and the areolas. Sites that are frequently subjected to trauma and friction are also likely to be affected, including the hands and feet, elbows, knees, and ankles (Fig. 643–3). When the scalp or brow is affected, the hair may lose pigment. The distribution of involvement is generally symmetric but occasionally is unilateral or dermatomal.

The course of vitiligo varies; some lesions may remit spontaneously while others are developing, but relentlessly progressive depigmentation may occur. Spontaneous repigmentation occurs in 10–20% of patients, most commonly in lesions that are in a sun-exposed distribution. Histopathologically, melanocytes are absent from involved sites and repopulate the epidermis from the hair follicle epithelium when repigmentation occurs. Although the diagnosis is usually made clinically, the disappearance of melanocytes can be confirmed by DOPA stains or electron microscopy of specimens obtained from depigmented skin.

TREATMENT. Treatment of vitiligo is challenging. In adults, treatment usually involves administration of oral or topical psoralen compounds in conjunction with exposure to sunlight or an ultraviolet light source. Repigmentation may be partial or complete, but many months of therapy may be required. In the pediatric population, the risk/benefit ratio of phototherapy for vitiligo is less clear. High-potency topical steroids are sometimes effective in repigmenting small areas of vitiligo or early lesions in areas not amenable to phototherapy (lips). Small lesions may be camouflaged by application of a specially prepared makeup (Covermark, Dermablend). Because of the absence of melanin, vitiliginous skin burns readily on sun exposure and should be protected at all times with an appropriate sunscreen. Therapies that have anecdotal support include vitamin supplementation, pseudocatalase cream in association with ultraviolet light, and topical immunomodulators such as tacrolimus, but controlled trials are lacking.

Bologna J, Pawelek JM: Biology of hypopigmentation. *J Am Acad Dermatol* 1988;19:217.

Bondurand N, Pingault V, Goerich DE, et al: Interaction among SOX 10, PAX 3, MITF, three genes altered in Waardenburg syndrome. *Hum Mol Genet* 2000;9:1907.

Ellis SS, Mallory SB: Hypopigmentation disorders. In Eichenfield LF, Frieden IJ, Esterly NB (editors): *Textbook of Neonatal Dermatology.* Philadelphia, WB Saunders, 2001, p. 353.

Grimes PE: Vitiligo: An overview of therapeutic approaches. *Dermatol Clin* 1993;11:325.

Kuster W, Happle R: Neurocutaneous disorders in children. *Curr Opin Pediatr* 1993;5:436.

Naughton GK, Reggiardo D, Bystryn J-C: Correlation between vitiligo antibodies and extent of depigmentation in vitiligo. J Am Acad Dermatol 15:978, 1986.

Nordlund JJ, Halder RM, Grimes P: Management of vitiligo. *Dermatol Clin* 1993;11:27.

Northrup H, Wheless JW, Bertin TK, et al: Variability of expression in tuberous sclerosis. *J Med Genet* 1993;30:411.

Selvaag E, Aas ALM, Heide S: Structural hair shaft abnormalities in hypomelanosis of Ito and other ectodermal dysplasia. *Acta Paediatr* 2000;89:610–2.

Spritz RA: Molecular genetics of oculocutaneous albinism. *Semin Dermatol* 1993;12:167.

Thibaut H, Parizel PM, Van Goethem J, et al: Tuberous sclerosis: CT and MRI characteristics. *Eur J Radiol* 1993;16:176.

Vanderhooft S, Francis J, Pagon R: Prevalence of hypopigmented macules in a healthy population. *J Pediatr* 1996;129:355.

Winship I, Young K, Martell P, et al: Piebaldism: An autonomous autosomal dominant entity. *Clin Genet* 1991;39:330.

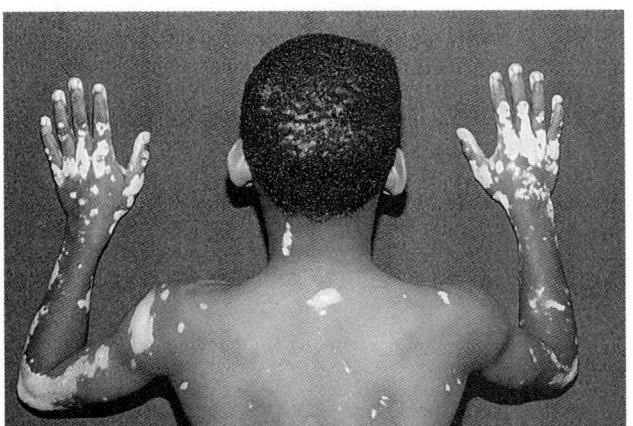

FIGURE 643–3. Multiple, sharply demarcated, symmetric, depigmented areas of vitiligo.

Chapter 644
Vesiculobullous Disorders

Many diseases are characterized by vesiculobullous lesions; they vary considerably in cause, age of onset, and pattern. Some of them (varicella) are discussed in other chapters; some are described in other chapters of this part because the vesiculobullous lesions represent only a transient stage of the disease (incontinentia pigmenti) or are seen only on occasion (mastocytosis). The morphology of the blister often provides a visual clue to the location of the lesion within the skin. Blisters localized to the epidermal layers are thin walled, relatively flaccid, and easily ruptured. Subepidermal blisters are tense, thick walled, and more durable. Biopsies of blisters can be diagnostic because the level of cleavage within the skin and associated findings such as the nature of the inflammatory infiltrate are characteristic for a particular disorder. Other diagnostic procedures such as immunofluorescence and electron microscopy can often help distinguish vesiculobullous disorders that have nearly identical histopathologic findings (Table 644–1).

Erythema Multiforme. Erythema multiforme (EM) has numerous morphologic manifestations on the skin, varying from erythematous macules, papules, vesicles, bullae, or urticaria-appearing plaques to patches of confluent erythema. The eruption appears most commonly in patients between the ages of 10 and 30 yr and usually is asymptomatic, although a burning sensation or pruritus may be present. The *diagnosis* of EM is established by finding the classic lesion: doughnut-shaped, target-like (iris, or bull's eye) papules with an erythematous outer border, an inner pale ring, and a dusky purple to necrotic center.

EM is characterized by an abrupt, symmetric cutaneous eruption, most commonly on the extensor upper extremities; lesions are relatively sparse on the face, trunk, and legs. The eruption often appears initially as red macules or urticarial plaques that expand centrifugally to form lesions up to 2 cm in diameter with a dusky to necrotic center. Lesions of a particular episode typically appear within 72 hr and remain fixed in place. Oral lesions may occur, but other mucosal surfaces are spared. Approximately 25% of cases of EM appear to be confined to the oral mucosa, with a predilection for the vermilion border of the lips and the buccal mucosa, generally sparing the gingivae. Prodromal symptoms generally are absent. Lesions typically resolve without sequelae in about 2 wk; progression to Stevens-Johnson syndrome does not occur.

Although EM may present initially with urticarial lesions, unlike urticaria, a given lesion of EM does not fade within 24 hr. Serum sickness–like reaction (SSLR) to cefaclor also may present with EM-like lesions. Although the lesions may develop a dusky to purple center, in most cases the eruption of cefaclor-induced SSLR is pruritic, transient, and migratory and is probably urticarial rather than true EM.

The *differential diagnosis* of EM also includes bullous pemphigoid, pemphigus, linear IgA dermatosis, graft vs host disease, bullous drug eruption, urticaria, viral infections such as herpes simplex, Reiter disease, Kawasaki disease, Behçet disease, allergic vasculitis, erythema annulare centrifugum, and periarteritis nodosa. EM that primarily involves the oral mucosa may be confused with a handful of other conditions, including bullous pemphigoid, pemphigus vulgaris, vesiculobullous or erosive lichen planus, Behçet syndrome, recurrent aphthous stomatitis, and primary herpetic gingivostomatitis.

Among the numerous factors implicated in the *etiology* of EM, infection with herpes simplex virus (HSV) is the most common. HSV labialis and, less commonly, HSV genitalis have been implicated in 60% of episodes of EM and are believed to trigger nearly all episodes of recurrent EM, frequently in association with sun exposure, despite the presence of robust HSV-specific immunity. HSV antigens and DNA are present in skin lesions of EM but are absent in nonlesional skin. Presence of the human leukocyte antigens B62, B35, and DR53 is associated with an increased risk of HSV-induced EM, particularly the recurrent form. Most patients experience a single self-limited episode of EM. Lesions of HSV-induced recurrent EM typically develop 10–14 days after onset of recurrent HSV eruptions, have a similar appearance from episode to episode, but may vary in frequency and duration in a given patient. Not all episodes of recurrent HSV evolve into EM in susceptible patients.

The *pathogenesis* of EM is unclear, but it may be a host-specific cell-mediated immune response to an antigenic stimulus, resulting in damage to keratinocytes. Cytokines released by activated mononuclear cells and keratinocytes may contribute to epidermal cell death and constitutional symptoms.

TABLE 644–1. Sites of Blister Formation and Diagnostic Studies for the Vesiculobullous Disorders

Disorder	Blister Cleavage Site	Cutaneous Diagnostic Studies
Acrodermatitis enteropathica	IE	–
Bullous impetigo	GL	Smear, culture
Bullous pemphigoid	SE (junctional)	Direct and indirect immunofluorescence studies
Candidosis	SC	KOH preparation, culture
Chronic bullous dermatosis of childhood	SE	Direct immunofluorescence studies
Dermatitis herpetiformis	SE	Direct immunofluorescence studies
Dermatophytosis	IE	KOH preparation, culture
Dyshidrotic eczema	IE	–
EB simplex	IE	Electron microscopy; immunofluorescence mapping
Hands and feet	IE	Electron microscopy; immunofluorescence mapping
Junctional EB (letalis)	SE (junctional)	Electron microscopy; immunofluorescence mapping
Recessive dystrophic EB	SE	Electron microscopy; immunofluorescence mapping
Dominant dystrophic EB	SE	Electron microscopy; immunofluorescence mapping
Epidermolytic hyperkeratosis	IE	–
Erythema multiforme	SE	–
Erythema toxicum	SC, IE	Smear for eosinophils
Incontinentia pigmenti	IE	Smear for eosinophils
Insect bites	IE	–
Mastocytosis	SE	Smear for mast cells
Miliaria crystallina	IC	–
Pachyonychia congenita	IC	–
Pemphigus foliaceus	GL	Direct and indirect immunofluorescence studies Tzanck smear
Pemphigus vulgaris	SB	Direct and indirect immunofluorescence studies Tzanck smear
Pseudomonas infection	IE, SE	Smear, culture
Scabies	IE	Scraping
Staphylococcal scalded skin syndrome	GL	Frozen section biopsy
Syphilis	SE	Dark-field preparation
Toxic epidermal necrolysis (Lyell)	SE	Frozen section biopsy
Transient neonatal pustular melanosis	SC, IE	Smear for cells
Viral blisters	IE	Tzanck smear for herpesvirus infections

GL = granular layer; IC = intracorneal; IE = intraepidermal; SB = suprabasal; SC = subcorneal; SE = subepidermal; EB = epidermolysis bullosa; KOH = potassium hydroxide.

Microscopic findings of EM, as with the gross appearance of the cutaneous eruption, are variable but are significant *diagnostically*. Early lesions typically show slight intercellular edema, rare dyskeratotic keratinocytes, and basal vacuolation in the epidermis and a perivascular lymphohistiocytic infiltrate with edema in the upper dermis. More mature lesions show an accentuation of these characteristics and the development of lymphocytic exocytosis and an intense, perivascular and interstitial mononuclear infiltrate, lacking in significant numbers of eosinophils or neutrophils, in the upper third of the dermis. The entire epidermis becomes necrotic in severe cases.

Treatment of EM is supportive. Topical emollients and systemic antihistamines and nonsteroidal anti-inflammatory agents do not alter the course of the disease but may provide symptomatic relief. No controlled, prospective studies support the use of corticosteroids in the management of EM. Rather, glucocorticoid therapy may be permissive of HSV replication and make EM episodes more frequent or continuous. Prophylactic oral acyclovir given for 6 mo may be effective in controlling recurrent episodes of HSV-associated EM. On discontinuation of acyclovir, both HSV and EM may recur, although episodes may be less frequent and more mild.

Stevens-Johnson Syndrome. Cutaneous lesions in Stevens-Johnson syndrome generally consist initially of erythematous macules that rapidly and variably develop central necrosis to form vesicles, bullae, and areas of denudation on the face, trunk, and extremities. The skin lesions typically are more widespread than in EM and are accompanied by involvement of two or more mucosal surfaces, namely the eyes, oral cavity, upper airway or esophagus, gastrointestinal tract, or anogenital mucosa. A burning sensation, edema, and erythema of the lips and buccal mucosa are often the presenting signs, followed by development of bullae, ulceration, and hemorrhagic crusting. Lesions may be preceded by a flulike upper respiratory illness. Pain from mucosal ulceration is often severe, but skin tenderness is minimal to absent, in contrast to toxic epidermal necrolysis. Corneal ulceration, anterior uveitis, panophthalmitis, bronchitis, pneumonitis, myocarditis, hepatitis, enterocolitis, polyarthritis, hematuria, and acute tubular necrosis leading to renal failure may occur. Disseminated cutaneous bullae and erosions may result in significant blood loss, increased insensible fluid loss, and a high risk of bacterial superinfection and sepsis. New lesions occur in crops, and complete healing may take 4–6 wk; ocular scarring and visual impairment and strictures of the esophagus, bronchi, vagina, urethra, or anus may remain. Nonspecific laboratory abnormalities in Stevens-Johnson syndrome include leukocytosis, elevated erythrocyte sedimentation rate and liver transaminase levels, and decreased serum albumin values. *Toxic epidermal necrolysis* is the most severe disorder in the clinical spectrum of the disease, involving considerable constitutional toxicity and extensive necrolysis of the mucous membranes and more than 30% of the body surface area.

Mycoplasma pneumoniae is the most convincingly demonstrated infectious cause of Stevens-Johnson syndrome; the organism also has been detected in lesional skin. Drugs, particularly sulfonamides, nonsteroidal anti-inflammatory agents (butazones, pyrazolones, ibuprofen, piroxicam, and salicylates), and anticonvulsants (phenytoin), are the agents most commonly precipitating Stevens-Johnson syndrome and toxic epidermal necrolysis (Box 644–1).

TREATMENT. Management of Stevens-Johnson syndrome is supportive and symptomatic. Potentially offending drugs must be discontinued as soon as possible. Ophthalmologic consultation is mandatory because ocular sequelae such as corneal scarring can lead to vision loss. Oral lesions should be managed with mouthwashes and glycerin swabs. Vaginal lesions should be observed closely and treated to prevent vaginal stricture or

---

BOX 644–1. Potential Causes of Erythema Multiforme, Stevens-Johnson Syndrome, and Toxic Epidermal Necrolysis

INFECTIOUS AGENTS
Herpes simplex 1, 2[*]
Mycoplasma pneumoniae
Mycobacterium tuberculosis
Group A streptococci
Hepatitis B
Epstein-Barr virus
Francisella tularensis
Yersinia
Enteroviruses
Histoplasma
Coccidioides

NEOPLASIA
Leukemia
Lymphoma

ANTIBIOTICS
Penicillin
Sulfonamides
Isoniazid
Tetracyclines
Cephalosporins
Quinolones

ANTICONVULSANTS
Phenytoin
Phenobarbital
Carbamazepine
Lamotrigine
Valproic acid

OTHER
Radiation therapy
Captopril
Etoposide
Nonsteroidal anti-inflammatory agents
Aspirin
Sunlight
Pregnancy
Allopurinol

---
[*]*Recurrent erythema multiforme.*
Drug reactions occur 1–3 wk after exposure.

---

fusion. Topical anesthetics (diphenhydramine, dyclonine, and viscous lidocaine) may provide relief from pain, particularly when applied before eating. Denuded skin lesions can be cleansed with saline or Burow solution compresses. Antibiotic therapy is appropriate for secondary bacterial infection. Treatment may require admission to an intensive care unit; intravenous fluids; nutritional support; sheepskin or air-fluid bedding; daily saline or Burow solution compresses; paraffin gauze or hydrogel dressing of denuded areas; saline compresses on the eyelids, lips, or nose; analgesics; and urinary catheterization (when needed). A daily examination for infection and ocular lesions, which constitute the major cause of long-term morbidity, is essential. Systemic antibiotics are indicated for urinary or cutaneous infections and for suspected bacteremia because infection is the leading cause of death. Prophylactic systemic antibiotics, however, are not necessary. Although corticosteroids are sometimes advocated in early, severe cases of Stevens-Johnson syndrome, no prospective double-blind studies evaluating their efficacy have been reported. Most authorities discourage their use because of reports of increased morbidity and mortality (sepsis) with their administration. Intravenous immunoglobulin has been used anecdotally.

Toxic Epidermal Necrolysis (Lyell Syndrome)
EPIDEMIOLOGY AND ETIOLOGY. The pathogenesis of toxic epidermal necrolysis is not proved but may involve a hypersensitivity phenomenon that results in damage primarily to the basal cell layer of the epidermis. Epidermal damage appears to result from Fas-mediated keratinocyte apoptosis. This condition is triggered by many of the same factors that are thought to be responsible for Stevens-Johnson syndrome, principally drugs such as the sulfonamides, amoxicillin, phenobarbital, hydantoin, butazones, and allopurinol. Toxic epidermal necrolysis is defined by (1) widespread blister formation and morbilliform or confluent erythema, associated with skin tenderness; (2) absence of target lesions; (3) sudden onset and generalization within 24–48 hr; (4) histologic findings of full-thickness epidermal necrosis and a minimal to absent dermal infiltrate. These criteria categorize toxic epidermal necrolysis as a

separate entity from EM; some authorities, however, contend that toxic epidermal necrolysis represents the most severe form of the spectrum of EM. This condition is exceedingly rare in infants younger than 6 mo; only three such cases have been documented.

CLINICAL MANIFESTATIONS. The prodrome consists of fever, malaise, localized skin tenderness, and diffuse erythema. Inflammation of the eyelids, conjunctivae, mouth, and genitals may precede skin lesions. Flaccid bullae may develop, although this is not a prominent feature. Characteristically, full-thickness epidermis is lost in large sheets. *Nikolsky sign* (denudation of the skin with gentle tangential pressure) is present but only in the areas of erythema. Conjunctivitis and oral lesions are usually not as severe as in Stevens-Johnson syndrome. Healing takes place over 14 or more days. Scarring, particularly of the eyes, may result in corneal opacity. The course may be relentlessly progressive, complicated by severe dehydration, electrolyte imbalance, shock, and secondary localized infection and septicemia. Loss of nails and hair may also occur. Long-term morbidity includes alterations in skin pigmentation, eye problems (lack of tears, conjunctival scarring, loss of lashes), and strictures of mucosal surfaces. The differential diagnosis includes staphylococcal scalded skin syndrome, in which the blister cleavage plane is intraepidermal; graft versus host disease; chemical burns; drug eruptions; and pemphigus.

Anticonvulsant hypersensitivity syndrome is a multisystem reaction that appears approximately 4 wk to 3 mo after starting phenytoin, carbamazepine, phenobarbitone, or primidone. The mucocutaneous eruption may be identical to that of EM, Stevens-Johnson syndrome, or toxic epidermal necrolysis, but the reaction typically also includes lymphadenopathy, as well as fever, hepatitis, eosinophilia, and leukocytosis.

TREATMENT. Appreciation of the specific etiologic factor is crucial; particularly when the disorder is drug induced, its administration must be discontinued as soon as possible. Management is similar to that for severe burns and may be best accomplished in a burn unit. It may include strict reverse isolation, meticulous fluid and electrolyte therapy, use of an air-fluid bed, and daily cultures. Systemic antibiotic therapy is indicated when secondary infection is evident or suspected. Skin care consists of cleansing with isotonic saline or Burow solution and applications of mupirocin ointment. Biologic or hydrogel dressings alleviate pain and reduce fluid loss. Narcotics are often required for pain relief. Mouth and eye care may be necessary, such as for EM major. Early high-dose systemic corticosteroids are not of proven benefit; pulse methylprednisolone alone or in concert with intravenous immunoglobulin have produced positive results in small uncontrolled series.

Epidermolysis Bullosa. Diseases categorized under this general term are a heterogeneous group of congenital, hereditary blistering disorders. They differ in severity and prognosis, clinical and histologic features, and inheritance patterns (Table 644–2) but are all characterized by induction of blisters by trauma and exacerbation of blistering in warm weather. The disorders can be categorized under three major headings: epidermolysis bullosa simplex, junctional epidermolysis bullosa, and dystrophic epidermolysis bullosa.

EPIDERMOLYSIS BULLOSA SIMPLEX. This is a nonscarring, autosomal dominant disorder. The defect in all types of epidermolysis bullosa simplex is in the central α-helical coil of keratin 5 or 14, which makes up intermediate filaments of the basal keratinocytes. Keratin 5 and 14 genes are located on chromosomes 17q and 12q, respectively. The intraepidermal bullae result from cytolysis of the basal cells.

Blisters are usually present at birth or during the neonatal period. Sites of predilection are the hands, feet, elbows, knees, legs, and scalp. Intraoral lesions are minimal, nails rarely become dystrophic and usually regrow even when they are shed, and dentition is normal. Bullae heal with minimal to no scar or milia formation. Secondary infection is the primary complication. The propensity to blister decreases with age, and the long-term prognosis is good. Blisters should be drained by puncturing, but the blister top should be left intact to protect the underlying skin. Erosions may be covered with mupirocin if there is evidence of infection and with a semipermeable dressing. Genetic counseling should be offered to families of affected children.

Localized *epidermolysis bullosa simplex of hands and feet* (Weber-Cockayne type) often presents when a child begins to walk; onset may be delayed, however, until puberty or early adulthood when heavy shoes are worn or the feet are subjected to increased trauma. Bullae are usually restricted to the hands and feet; rarely, they occur elsewhere such as the dorsal aspect of the arms and the shins. The disorder ranges from mildly incapacitating to crippling at times of severe exacerbations. *Generalized epidermolysis bullosa simplex* (Koebner type) is characterized at birth or during early infancy by blisters on the occiput, back, and legs and in childhood by blisters on the hands, feet, and other friction points. The *herpetiformis (Dowling-Meara) variant of epidermolysis bullosa simplex* is characterized by grouped blisters. During infancy, blistering may be severe and extensive, may involve mucous membranes, and may result in shedding of nails, formation of milia, and mild pigmentary changes, without scarring. After the first few months of life, warm temperatures do not appear to exacerbate blistering. Hyperkeratosis and hyperhidrosis of the palms and soles may develop, but generally, the condition improves with age.

TABLE 644–2. **Characteristics of Epidermolysis Bullosa**

Type	Predominant Inheritance	Level of Blister Formation	Features
Simplex (epidermolytic)	Autosomal dominant	Superficial; basal cell layer; above hemidesmosomes	Usually congenital onset; hands and feet involved; minimal mucosal lesions; no scarring; defects in keratins 5 or 14 of basal keratinocytes
Junctional (letalis)	Autosomal recessive	Lamina lucida, between bullous pemphigoid antigen and laminin; absent or rare hemidesmosomes	Congenital; localized or progressive; heals with scarring; pyloric atresia; mucosal lesions; dysplastic teeth; loss of nails; defects in basement membrane–associated proteins, e.g., laminin 5, bullous pemphigoid antigen 2, α6β4 integrin
Recessive dystrophic (dermolytic)	Autosomal recessive	Deep in dermis below the lamina densa; excessive production of abnormal dermal collagenase; absent anchoring fibrils	Congenital; mitten scarring of the hands and feet; marked deformities; mucosal lesions produce esophageal stricture or gastrointestinal perforation; varied clinical course; risk for aggressive squamous cell cancer of the skin, tongue, esophagus; defects in type VII collagen
Dominant dystrophic (dermolytic)	Autosomal dominant	Deep in dermis below the lamina densa, below type IV collagen layer; sparse anchoring fibrils	Congenital; hyperkeratotic lesions; variable severity; risk for squamous cell cancer; defects in type VII collagen

JUNCTIONAL EPIDERMOLYSIS BULLOSA. *Epidermolysis bullosa letalis* (Herlitz type) is an autosomal recessive condition that is life threatening; serious morbidity and disfigurement can be predicted from the complications. An afflicted infant is usually blistered at birth or develops lesions during the neonatal period, particularly on the perioral area, scalp, legs, diaper area, and thorax. In contrast to other variants of epidermolysis bullosa, the hands and feet tend to be relatively spared, with the exception of the distal digits and the nail plates; these are dystrophic or permanently lost. Mucous membrane involvement may be severe, and ulceration of the respiratory, gastrointestinal, and genitourinary epithelium has been documented in many affected children, although less frequently than in severe, recessive dystrophic epidermolysis bullosa. Healing is delayed, and vegetating granulomas, particularly in the generalized (Herlitz) variant, may persist for a long time. Large, moist, erosive plaques may provide a portal of entry for bacteria, and septicemia is a frequent cause of death. Mild atrophy may be seen in areas of recurrent blistering. Defective dentition with early loss of teeth as a result of rampant caries is characteristic. Growth retardation and recalcitrant anemia are almost invariable. In addition to infection, cachexia and circulatory failure are common causes of death. Most patients die within the first 3 yr of life.

A subepidermal blister is found on light microscopic examination, and electron microscopy demonstrates a cleavage plane in the lamina lucida, between the plasma membranes of the basal cells and the basal lamina. Absent or greatly reduced anchoring filaments are seen on electron micrographs, along with diminished or absent laminin 5. Junctional epidermolysis bullosa is due to mutations in proteins in the basement membrane zone involved in keratinocyte-lamina densa adherence, particularly laminin 5, a glycoprotein associated with anchoring filaments beneath the hemidesmosomes. Defects have also been described in other hemidesmosomal components, such as bullous pemphigoid antigen 2 and $\alpha 6\beta 4$ integrin, a subset of patients that may have associated pyloric stenosis. Absence of laminin in amniocytes has been shown to be a prenatal marker for the Herlitz type of junctional epidermolysis bullosa.

Generalized atrophic benign epidermolysis bullosa, a milder autosomal recessive variant, presents with blistering at birth, is also nonscarring, and is characterized by identical histologic changes as the Herlitz type. It may be impossible to distinguish from the Herlitz variety for up to 2–3 yr. Pattern baldness with significant scalp atrophy is a prominent feature. The course is compatible with normal growth and life span. Mutations in collagen XVII (bullous pemphigoid antigen 180) cause this form of epidermolysis bullosa.

Treatment for junctional epidermolysis bullosa is supportive. The diet should provide adequate calories and supplemental iron. Infections should be treated promptly. Transfusions of packed red blood cells may be required if the patient does not respond to iron and erythropoietin therapy. Tissue engineered skin grafts (artificial skin derived from human keratinocytes and fibroblasts) may be beneficial.

DYSTROPHIC EPIDERMOLYSIS BULLOSA. *Dominant dystrophic epidermolysis bullosa* occurs sporadically in some cases, although an autosomal dominant mode of transmission has been documented in many families. All forms of dystrophic epidermolysis bullosa result from mutations in collagen VII, a major component of anchoring fibrils that tether the basement membrane and overlying epidermis to its dermal foundation. The type and location of the mutation dictates the severity of the phenotype. Blisters may be present at birth and are often limited to the hands, feet, and sacrum. The lesions heal promptly, with the formation of soft, wrinkled scars, milia, and alterations in pigmentation. The general health is unimpaired; in many cases, the blistering process is mild, causing little restriction of activity and unimpaired growth and development. Mucous membrane involvement tends to be minimal, but nail loss is common.

The *Cockayne-Touraine variant* of dominant dystrophic epidermolysis bullosa presents during infancy or early childhood with blisters predominantly on the extremities, although widespread blistering may occur. The *albopapuloid Pasini form* presents during adolescence with blistering that may be widespread but occurs predominantly on the hands, feet, elbows, and knees and with flesh-colored papules called albopapuloid lesions on the trunk. Transient bullous dermolysis of the newborn affects a rare subset of patients with self-limited dystrophic disease; inheritance in most cases is autosomal dominant. Blistering at birth tends to be generalized but ceases within the first 1–2 yr. Resolution of clinical blistering and the immunohistochemically altered distribution of type VII collagen occur coincidentally. The blister is subepidermal in all variants, with separation beneath the basement membrane. On electron microscopy, anchoring fibrils, a major component of which is type VII collagen, are abnormal and decreased in number over the entire skin in the Pasini type but only in areas of blister predilection in the Cockayne-Touraine variant. The type VII collagen gene, located on the short arm of chromosome 3, is the major candidate gene for dystrophic epidermolysis bullosa.

Recessive dystrophic epidermolysis bullosa is probably the most incapacitating form of epidermolysis bullosa, although the clinical spectrum is wide. Some patients have blisters, scarring, and milia formation primarily on the hands, feet, elbows, and knees. Others at birth have extensive erosions and blister formation that seriously impede their care and feeding. Mucous membrane lesions are common and may cause severe nutritional deprivation, even in older children, whose growth may be retarded. During childhood, esophageal erosions and strictures, scarring of the buccal mucosa, flexion contractures of joints secondary to scarring of the integument, development of cutaneous carcinomas, and the development of digital fusion (Fig. 644–1) may significantly limit the quality of life. The subepidermal bullae are located beneath the basement membrane, where anchoring fibrils are absent.

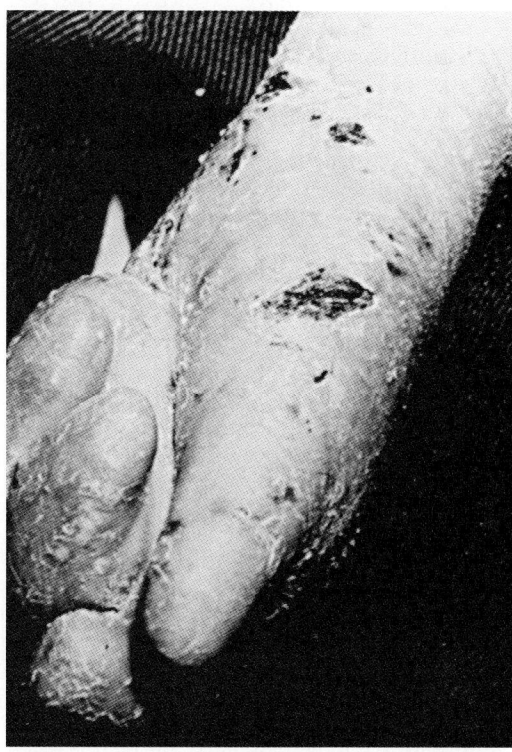

FIGURE 644–1. Mitten-hand deformity of recessive dystrophic epidermolysis bullosa.

Although the skin becomes less sensitive to trauma with aging, the progressive and permanent deformities complicate management, and the overall prognosis is poor. Foods that traumatize the buccal or esophageal mucosa should be avoided. If esophageal scarring develops, a semiliquid diet and esophageal dilatations may be required. Stricture excision or colonic interposition may be needed to relieve esophageal obstruction. In infants, severe oropharyngeal involvement may necessitate the use of special feeding devices such as a button gastrostomy tube. Continuous iron therapy for anemia; intermittent antibiotic therapy for secondary infections, which are a common cause of death; and periodic surgery for release of digits may reduce morbidity. Tissue engineered skin grafts containing keratinocytes and fibroblasts are of some benefit.

Pemphigus. Pemphigus occurs during childhood as pemphigus vulgaris or pemphigus foliaceus.

PEMPHIGUS VULGARIS. This usually first appears as painful oral ulcers, which may be the only evidence of the disease for weeks or months. Subsequently, large, flaccid bullae emerge on nonerythematous skin, most commonly on the face, trunk, pressure points, groin, and axillae. Nikolsky sign is present. The lesions rupture and enlarge peripherally, producing painful raw, denuded areas that have little tendency to heal. When healing occurs, it is without scarring, but hyperpigmentation is common. Malodorous, verrucous, and granulomatous lesions may develop at sites of ruptured bullae, particularly in the skinfolds; as this becomes more pronounced, the condition may be more properly referred to as pemphigus vegetans.

Biopsy is best performed of a fresh small blister, which reveals a suprabasal (intraepidermal) blister containing loose, acantholytic epidermal cells that have lost their intercellular bridges and thus their contact with one another. IgG antibody to epidermal intercellular substance produces a characteristic pattern on direct immunofluorescence preparations of both involved and uninvolved skin of essentially all patients (see Table 635–1). Serum IgG antibody titers to the epidermal intercellular substance correlate with the clinical course of many patients; thus, serial determinations may have predictive value. Pemphigus antibodies are pathogenic. The antigen recognized by pemphigus vulgaris antibodies is a 130-kd glycoprotein known as desmoglein III that is complexed with plakoglobin, a plaque protein of desmosomes. The desmogleins are a subfamily of the cadherin cell adhesion molecules.

Neonatal pemphigus vulgaris develops in utero as a result of placental transfer of maternal antibodies from women who have active pemphigus vulgaris, although it may occur when the mother is in remission. High antepartum maternal titers of pemphigus vulgaris antibodies and increased maternal disease activity correlate with a poor fetal outcome, including demise.

The *differential diagnosis* includes EM, bullous pemphigoid, Stevens-Johnson syndrome, and toxic epidermal necrolysis. Because the course may rapidly lead to debility, malnutrition, and death, prompt diagnosis is essential. The disease is best treated initially with high-dose systemic corticosteroid therapy. Azathioprine, cyclophosphamide, methotrexate, and gold therapy all have been useful in maintenance regimens.

PEMPHIGUS FOLIACEUS. This extremely rare disorder is characterized by intraepidermal blistering; the site of cleavage, however, is high in the epidermis rather than suprabasal as in pemphigus vulgaris. The superficial blisters rupture quickly, leaving erosions surrounded by erythema that heal with crusting and scaling. Nikolsky sign is present. Focal lesions are usually localized to the scalp, face, neck, and upper trunk. Mucous membrane lesions are minimal or absent. Pruritus, pain, and a burning sensation are frequent complaints. When generalized, the eruption may resemble exfoliative dermatitis or any of the chronic blistering disorders, but localized erythematous plaques simulate seborrheic dermatitis, psoriasis, impetigo, eczema, or lupus erythematosus. The clinical course varies but is generally more benign than that of pemphigus vulgaris. *Fogo selvagem*, which is ecdemic in certain areas of Brazil, is identical clinically, histopathologically, and immunologically to pemphigus foliaceus.

An intraepidermal acantholytic bulla high in the epidermis is diagnostic; it is imperative, however, to select an early lesion for biopsy. Tissue-bound and circulating intercellular epidermal antibodies bind to a 50-kd portion of the 160-kd desmosomal glycoprotein, desmoglein I (see Table 635–1). Long-term remission is usual after suppression of the disease by systemic corticosteroid therapy. Dapsone or a topical corticosteroid preparation is occasionally sufficient.

Bullous Pemphigoid. Bullous pemphigoid rarely occurs in children but must be considered in the differential diagnosis of any chronic blistering disorder.

CLINICAL MANIFESTATIONS. The blisters typically arise in crops on a normal, erythematous, eczematous, or urticarial base. Bullae appear predominantly on the flexural aspects of the extremities, in the axillae, and on the groin and central abdomen. Infants have involvement of the palms, soles, and face more frequently than older children. Individual lesions vary greatly in size, are tense, and are filled with serous fluid that may become hemorrhagic or turbid. Oral lesions occur less frequently (50%) and are less severe than in pemphigus vulgaris but are found more commonly in children than in adults with bullous pemphigoid. Pruritus, a burning sensation, and subcutaneous edema may accompany the eruption, but constitutional symptoms are not prominent.

DIAGNOSIS AND DIFFERENTIAL DIAGNOSES. Biopsy material should be taken from an early bulla arising on an erythematous base. A subepidermal bulla and a dermal inflammatory infiltrate, predominantly of eosinophils, can be identified histopathologically. In sections of a blister or perilesional skin, a band of immunoglobulin (usually IgG) and C3 can be demonstrated in the basement membrane zone by direct immunofluorescence (see Table 635–1). Indirect immunofluorescence studies of serum have positive results in approximately 70% of cases for IgG antibodies to the basement membrane zone; the titers, however, do not correlate well with the clinical course. The differential diagnosis includes bullous erythema multiforme, pemphigus, linear IgA dermatosis, bullous drug eruption, dermatitis herpetiformis, herpes simplex infection, and bullous impetigo, which can be differentiated by histologic examination, immunofluorescence studies, and cultures. The large, tense bullae of bullous pemphigoid can generally be distinguished from the smaller, flaccid bullae of pemphigus vulgaris. The major targets for bullous pemphigoid autoantibodies are proteins of 230 and 180 kd. The 230-kd protein is part of the hemidesmosome, whereas the 180-kd antigen localizes to both the hemidesmosome and the upper lamina lucida and is a transmembrane collagenous protein.

TREATMENT. Bullous pemphigoid can be successfully suppressed with topical or systemic corticosteroid therapy alone or in combination with azathioprine, sulfapyridine, or dapsone. Topical clobetasol improves outcome with fewer side effects. Ultimately, the condition usually remits permanently.

Dermatitis Herpetiformis. This is seen most commonly in children 2–7 yr of age. It is characterized by symmetric, grouped, small, tense, erythematous, stinging, intensely pruritic papules and vesicles. The eruption is pleomorphic, including erythematous, urticarial, papular, vesicular, and bullous lesions. Sites of predilection are the knees, elbows, shoulders, buttocks, and scalp; mucous membranes are usually spared. Hemorrhagic lesions may develop on the palms and soles. When pruritus is severe, excoriations may be the only visible sign.

ETIOLOGY. Dermatitis herpetiformis, like celiac disease, has a strong genetic association with HLA DQ on chromosome 6.

IgA antibodies directed at the endomysial antigen transglutaminase (tissue transglutaminase, epidermal transglutaminase) appear to cause both gastrointestinal and cutaneous symptoms. This is unknown; however, an association with gluten-sensitive enteropathy is found in 75–90% of patients. Aggressive gluten challenge generally unmasks the condition in the remainder of patients with dermatitis herpetiformis (see Chapter 320.8). Subepidermal blisters composed predominantly of neutrophils are found in dermal papillae on skin biopsy, and IgA and C3 can be detected in the dermal papillary tips of normal and perilesional skin in the sublamina densa region of the dermoepidermal junction by immunofluorescence studies. The frequent finding of immune complexes and autoimmune antibodies in serum and the association with histocompatibility antigen HLA-B8 in approximately 85% of patients suggest an immune mechanism. An antibody to smooth muscle endomysium is found in 70% of patients with dermatitis herpetiformis-associated gluten-sensitive enteropathy. Antibody titers correlate with the severity of intestinal disease; they decline rapidly on institution of a gluten-free diet. Enteric infection with adenovirus type 12 or 40 may increase the risk of developing gluten-sensitive enteropathy and dermatitis herpetiformis in genetically susceptible individuals.

TREATMENT. Dermatitis herpetiformis may mimic other chronic blistering diseases and may also resemble scabies, papular urticaria, insect bites, contact dermatitis, and papular eczema. The most effective treatment is oral administration of sulfapyridine or dapsone. These drugs provide immediate relief from the intense pruritus but must be used with caution because of possible serious side effects. Local antipruritic measures may also be useful. Jejunal biopsy is indicated to diagnose gluten-sensitive enteropathy because cutaneous manifestations may precede malabsorption. Enteropathy responds to a gluten-free diet more rapidly than skin lesions.

Linear IgA Dermatosis (Chronic Bullous Dermatosis of Childhood).

This rare dermatosis is most common in the 1st decade of life, with a peak incidence during the preschool years. The eruption consists of many large, tense bullae filled with clear or hemorrhagic fluid that develop on a normal or erythematous, urticarial base. Areas of predilection are the genitals and buttocks, the perioral region, and the scalp. Sausage-shaped bullae may be arranged in an annular or rosette-like fashion around a central crust (Fig. 644–2). Erythematous plaques with gyrate margins bordered by intact bullae may develop over larger areas. Pruritus may be absent or very intense, and systemic signs or symptoms are absent. Gluten-sensitive enteropathy is not present, but there is a strong association with HLA-B8.

ETIOLOGY. The cause of the eruption is unknown. The subepidermal bulla are infiltrated with a mixture of inflammatory cells. Neutrophilic abscesses may be noted in the dermal papillary tips, indistinguishable from those of dermatitis herpetiformis. The infiltrate may also be largely eosinophilic, resembling bullous pemphigoid. Therefore, direct immunofluorescence studies are required for a definitive diagnosis; lesional or perilesional skin demonstrates linear deposition of IgA and sometimes C3 at the dermoepidermal junction (see Table 635–1). Results of indirect immunofluorescence studies are sometimes positive for circulating antibodies. Immunoelectron microscopy has localized the immunoreactants to the sublamina densa, although a combined sublamina densa and lamina lucida pattern has also been seen. The linear IgA bullous dermatosis antigen has a molecular mass of 120 kd. The eruption can be distinguished by histopathologic and immunofluorescence studies from pemphigus, bullous pemphigoid, dermatitis herpetiformis, and EM. Gram stain and culture preclude the diagnosis of bullous impetigo, with which dermatitis herpetiformis is often confused on initial presentation. The lack of bullous formation in response to trauma differentiates epidermolysis bullosa.

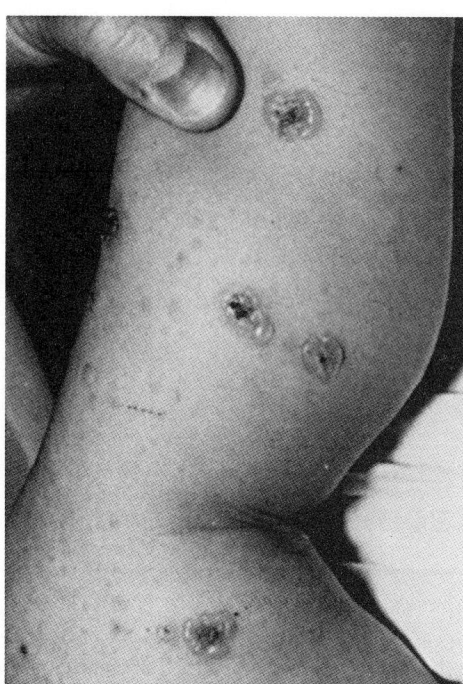

FIGURE 644–2. Rosette-like blisters around a central crust typical of linear IgA dermatosis (chronic bullous dermatosis of childhood).

TREATMENT. Many patients respond favorably to oral sulfapyridine or dapsone. During therapy with sulfapyridine, attention should be paid to maintaining urinary output and alkalization to avoid crystal formation within the renal parenchyma. Hematologic and biochemical studies must be obtained at regular intervals during treatment with either drug to avoid serious side effects. Children who do not respond to either of these drugs may benefit from oral therapy with a corticosteroid or a combination of these drugs. The usual course is 2–4 yr, although some children have persistent or recurrent disease; there are no long-term sequelae.

Assier H, Bastuji-Garin S, Revuz J, et al: Erythema multiforme with mucous membrane involvement and Stevens-Johnson syndrome are clinically different disorders with distinct causes. Arch Dermatol 1995;131:539.

Becker DS: Toxic epidermal necrolysis. Lancet 1998;351:1417.

Christiano AM, Uitto J: Molecular complexity of the cutaneous basement membrane zone. Exp Dermatol 1996;5:1.

Côté B, Wechsler J, Bastuji-Garin S, et al: Clinicopathologic correlation in erythema multiforme and Stevens-Johnson syndrome. Arch Dermatol 1995;131: 1268.

Falabella AF, Valencia IC, Eaglstein WH, et al: Tissue-engineered skin (Apligraf) in the healing of patients with epidermolysis bullosa wounds. Arch Dermatol 2000;136:1225–30.

Fine JD: Management of acquired bullous skin diseases. N Engl J Med 1995;333: 1475.

Fridge JL, Vichinsky EP: Correction of the anemia of epidermolysis bullosa with intravenous iron and erythropoietin. J Pediatr 1998;132:871.

Garcia-Doval I, LeCleach L, Bocquet H, et al: Toxic epidermal necrolysis and Stevens Johnson syndrome. Arch Dermatol 2000;136:323–7.

Jiang QI, Izakovic J, Zenker M, et al: Treatment of two patients with Herlitz junctional epidermolysis bullosa with artificial skin bioequivalents. J Pediatr 2002;141:553–9.

Joly P, Roujeau JC, Benichou J, et al: A comparison of oral and topical corticosteroids in patients with bullous pemphigoid. N Engl J Med 2002;346:321–7.

Kakourou T, Klontza D, Soteropoubu F, et al: Corticosteroid treatment of erythema multiforme major (Stevens-Johnson syndrome) in children. Eur J Pediatr 1997;156:90.

Morici MV, Galen WK, Shetty AK, et al: Intravenous immunoglobulin therapy for children with Stevens-Johnson syndrome. J Rheumatol 2000;27:2494–7.

Nakano A, Pulkkinen L, Murrell D, et al: Epidermolysis bullosa with congenital pyloric atresia: Novel mutations in the β4 integrin gene (ITGB4) and genotype/phenotype correlations. Pediatr Res 2001;49:618–26.

Nemeth AJ, Klein AD, Gould EW, et al: Childhood bullous pemphigoid: Clinical and immunologic features, treatment, and prognosis. Arch Dermatol 1991;127: 378.

Paller AS: The genetic basis of hereditary blistering disorders. *Curr Opin Pediatr* 1996;8:367.

Rabinowitz LG, Esterly NB: Inflammatory bullous diseases in children. *Dermatol Clin* 1993;11:565.

Roujeau JC, Kelly JP, Naldi L, et al: Medication use and the risk of Stevens-Johnson syndrome or toxic epidermal necrolysis. *N Engl J Med* 1995;333:1600.

Sahn EE: Vesiculopustular lesions of neonates and infants. *Curr Opin Pediatr* 1994;6:442.

Sheridan RL, Schulz JT, Ryan CM, et al: Long-term consequences of toxic epidermal necrolysis in children. *Pediatrics* 2002;109:74–8.

Spies M, Sanford AP, Low JFA, et al: Treatment of extensive toxic epidermal necrolysis in children. *Pediatrics* 2001;108:1162–8.

Tay YK, Huff C, Weston WL: *Mycoplasma pneumoniae* infection is associated with Stevens-Johnson syndrome, not erythema multiforme (von Hebra). *J Am Acad Dermatol* 1996;35:757.

Weston WL, Morelli JG: Herpes simplex virus-associated erythema multiforme in prepubertal children. *Arch Pediatr Adolesc Med* 1997;151:1014.

Chapter 645
Eczematous Disorders

Eczematous skin disorders are characterized by exudation, lichenification, and pruritus. Acute eczematous lesions demonstrate erythema, weeping, oozing, and the formation of microvesicles within the epidermis. Chronic lesions are generally thickened, dry, and scaly, with coarse skin markings (lichenification) and altered pigmentation. Many types of eczema occur in children; the most common is atopic dermatitis (see Chapter 135), although seborrheic dermatitis, allergic and irritant contact dermatitis, nummular eczema, and dyshidrosis also are relatively common in childhood. Various dermatoses that have pruritus as a common feature may become eczematized owing to scratching. Atopic skin is sensitive to many factors that increase pruritus, such as soap, wool, cool air, and food allergens.

Once the diagnosis of eczema has been established, it is important to classify the eruption more specifically for proper management. Pertinent historical data often provide the clue. In some instances, the subsequent course and character of the eruption permit classification. Histologic changes are relatively nonspecific, but all types of eczematous dermatitis are characterized by intraepidermal edema known as spongiosis.

Contact Dermatitis. This form of eczema can be subdivided into irritant dermatitis, resulting from nonspecific injury to the skin, and allergic contact dermatitis, in which the mechanism is a delayed hypersensitivity reaction. Irritant dermatitis is more frequent in children, particularly during the early years of life.

Irritant contact dermatitis can result from prolonged or repetitive contact with various substances that include saliva, citrus juices, bubble bath, detergents, abrasive materials, strong soaps, and proprietary medications. Saliva is probably one of the most common offenders; it may cause dermatitis on the face and in the neck folds of a drooling infant or a retarded child. Older children who habitually lick their lips, frequently without awareness, because of dryness may develop a striking, sharply demarcated perioral rash (Fig. 645–1A). Among the exogenous irritants, citrus juices, proprietary medications, and bubble bath preparations are relatively common; bubble bath dermatitis can be a cause of severe pruritus. Excessive accumulation of sweat and moisture as a result of wearing occlusive shoes may also cause irritant dermatitis.

Clinically, irritant contact dermatitis may be indistinguishable from atopic dermatitis or allergic contact dermatitis. A detailed history and consideration of the sites of involvement, the age of the child, and contactants usually provide clues to the etiologic agent. The propensity to develop irritant dermatitis varies considerably among children; some may respond to minimal injury, making it difficult to identify the offending agent by history. In general, irritant contact dermatitis clears after removal of the stimulus and after temporary treatment with a topical corticosteroid preparation. Education of patients and parents about the causes of contact dermatitis is crucial to successful therapy.

Diaper dermatitis can be regarded as the prototype of irritant contact dermatitis. As a reaction to overhydration of the skin, friction, maceration, and prolonged contact with urine and feces, retained diaper soaps, and topical preparations, the skin of the diaper area may become erythematous and scaly, often

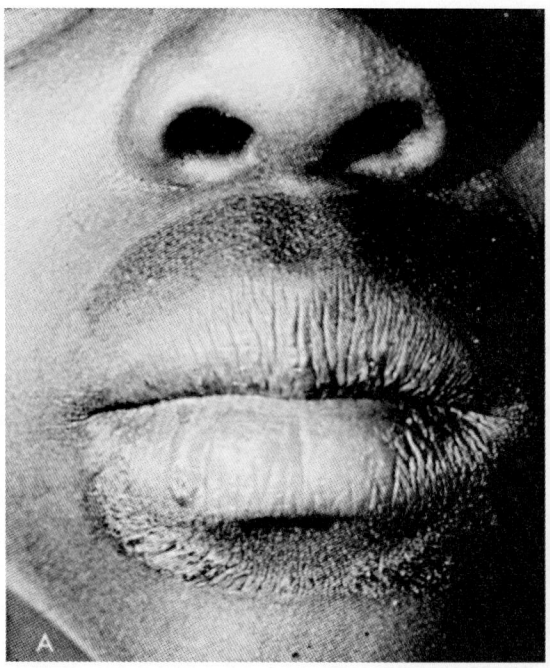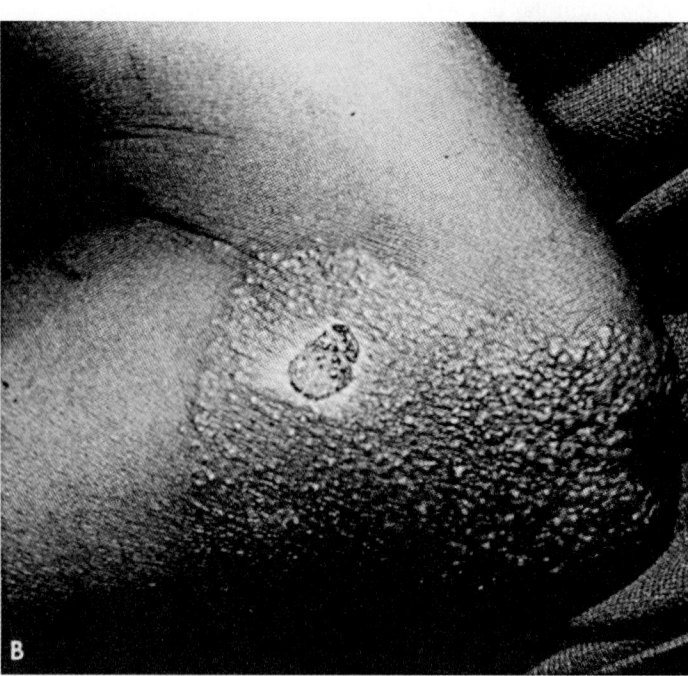

FIGURE 645–1. *A,* Perioral irritant contact dermatitis from lip licking. *B,* Allergic contact dermatitis to Merthiolate spray. Note the sharp angular border of vesicular eruption.

with papulovesicular or bullous lesions, fissures, and erosions. The eruption can be patchy or confluent, but the genitocrural folds are often spared. Chronic hypertrophic, flat-topped papules and infiltrative nodules may simulate syphilitic lesions. Secondary infection with bacteria and yeasts is common; discomfort may be marked because of intense inflammation. Such conditions as allergic contact dermatitis, seborrheic dermatitis, candidosis, atopic dermatitis, and rare disorders such as histiocytosis X (Langerhan cell histiocytosis) and acrodermatitis enteropathica should be considered when the eruption is persistent or recalcitrant to simple therapeutic measures.

Diaper dermatitis often responds to simple measures; however, some infants seem predisposed to diaper dermatitis, and management may be difficult. The damaging effects of overhydration of the skin and prolonged contact with feces and ammoniac urine can be obviated by frequent changing of diapers and meticulous washing of the genitals. Disposable diapers containing a superabsorbent material may help to maintain a relatively dry environment. Frequent topical applications of a bland protective barrier agent (petrolatum or zinc oxide paste) after thorough gentle cleansing may suffice to prevent dermatitis. When the aforementioned measures are not sufficient to promote healing, a light application of 0.5–1% topical hydrocortisone ointment after each diaper change for a limited time is often effective. Secondary complications can result from prolonged use of corticosteroids, especially fluorinated compounds. Before initiating such therapy, the possibility of candidal infection should be considered. Candidal infection can be identified by red-pink tender skin that has numerous 1–2 mm pustules and papules at the periphery of the dermatitis. Treatment with a topical anticandidal agent may be helpful.

Juvenile plantar dermatosis is a common form of irritant contact dermatitis occurring mainly in prepubertal children. The dermatitis characteristically involves the weight-bearing surfaces, is painful rather than pruritic, and causes a glazed appearance of the plantar skin. Fissuring may become extensive, producing considerable discomfort. The dermatitis results from alternating excessive hydration and rapid moisture loss, which causes chapping of the skin and cracking of the stratum corneum. Affected children often have hyperhidrosis, wear occlusive synthetic footwear, and subject their feet to rapid drying without moisturization. Immediate application of a thick emollient when socks and shoes are removed or immediately after swimming usually prevents this condition.

Allergic contact dermatitis is a T-cell–mediated hypersensitivity reaction that is provoked by application of an antigen to the skin surface. The antigen penetrates the skin, where it is conjugated with a cutaneous protein, and the hapten-protein complex is transported to the regional lymph nodes by antigen-presenting Langerhans cells. A primary immunologic response occurs locally in the nodes and becomes generalized, presumably because of dissemination of sensitized T cells. Sensitization requires several days and, when followed by a fresh antigenic challenge, is manifested as allergic contact dermatitis. Generalized distribution may also occur if enough antigen finds its way into the circulation. Once sensitization has occurred, each new antigenic challenge may provoke an inflammatory reaction within 8–12 hr; sensitization to a particular antigen usually persists for many years.

Acute allergic contact dermatitis is an erythematous, intensely pruritic, eczematous dermatitis, which, if severe, may be edematous and vesiculobullous. The chronic condition has the features of long-standing eczema: lichenification, scaling, fissuring, and pigmentary change. The distribution of the eruption often provides a clue to the diagnosis. Volatile sensitizers usually affect exposed areas, such as the face and arms. Jewelry, topical agents, shoes, clothing, and plants cause dermatitis at points of contact.

Rhus dermatitis (poison ivy, poison sumac, poison oak) is often vesiculobullous and may be distinguished by linear streaks of vesicles where the plant leaves have brushed against the skin. Contrary to popular opinion, fluid from ruptured cutaneous vesicles does not spread the eruption; however, antigen retained on the skin, under the fingernails, and on clothing initiates new plaques of dermatitis if not removed by washing with soap and water. Antigen may also be carried by animals on their fur. The saplike allergen (oleoresin) is present on live and dead leaves, and sensitization to one plant produces cross reactions with the others.

Nickel dermatitis usually develops from contact with jewelry or metal closures on clothing and is seen most frequently on the earlobes, such as when nickel-containing posts rather than nonmetallic materials or stainless steel are used to keep a pierced tract open. Some children are exquisitely sensitive to nickel, with even the trace amounts found in gold jewelry provoking eruptions.

Shoe dermatitis typically affects the dorsum of the feet and toes, sparing the interdigital spaces; it is usually symmetric. Other forms of allergic contact dermatitis, in contrast to irritant dermatitis, rarely involve the palms and soles. Common allergens are the antioxidants and accelerators in shoe rubber and the chromium salts in tanned leather or shoe dyes. These substances are often leached out by excessive sweating.

Wearing apparel contains a number of sensitizers, including dyes, mordants, fabric finishes, fibers, resins, and cleaning solutions. Dye may be poorly fixed to clothing and leached out with sweating, as are the partially cured formaldehyde resins. The elastic in garments is also a frequent cause of clothing dermatitis.

Topical medications and cosmetics may be unsuspected as allergens, particularly if the medication is being used for a pre-existing dermatitis. The most common offenders are neomycin, thimerosal (Merthiolate) (see Fig. 645–1*B*), topical antihistamines (Caladryl), anesthetics (dibucaine [Nupercainal] and cyclomethycaine [Surfacaine]), preservatives (parabens), and ethylenediamine, a stabilizer present in many medications. All types of cosmetics can cause facial dermatitis; involvement of the eyelids is characteristic for nail polish sensitivity.

Contact dermatitis can be confused with other types of eczema, dermatophytoses, and vesiculobullous diseases. Patch testing may clarify the etiology. The essential principle in *treatment* is elimination of contact with the allergen. Acute dermatitis responds to cool compresses and topical application of a corticosteroid ointment. An antihistamine may be useful when taken orally. Massive acute bullous reactions or reactions that cause swelling around the eyes or genitals such as those of poison ivy may require treatment with a 2-wk tapering course of oral corticosteroids. If secondary infection has occurred, appropriate systemic antibiotic therapy should be given. Desensitization therapy is rarely indicated.

Nummular Eczema. This disorder is unrelated to other types of eczema and is characterized by more or less coin-shaped eczematous plaques. Common sites are the extensor surfaces of the extremities (Fig. 645–2), buttocks, and shoulders. The plaques are relatively discrete, boggy, vesicular, severely pruritic, and exudative; when chronic, they often become thickened and lichenified. The cause is unknown. Most frequently, these lesions are mistaken for tinea corporis, but plaques of nummular eczema are distinguished by the lack of a raised, sharply circumscribed border, the lack of fungal organisms on a potassium hydroxide (KOH) preparation, and frequent weeping or bleeding when scraped. Secondary infection is common. Control of pruritus is usually achieved with a fluorinated corticosteroid preparation. Steroid-impregnated tapes may simultaneously treat and provide barrier protection to these circumscribed eczematous plaques. Sedation with an antihistamine may be

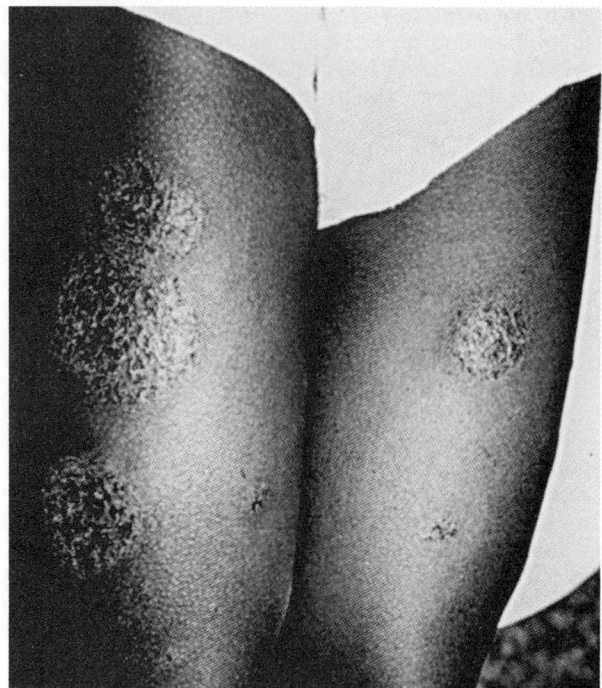

FIGURE 645–2. Multiple hyperpigmented scaly plaques of nummular eczema.

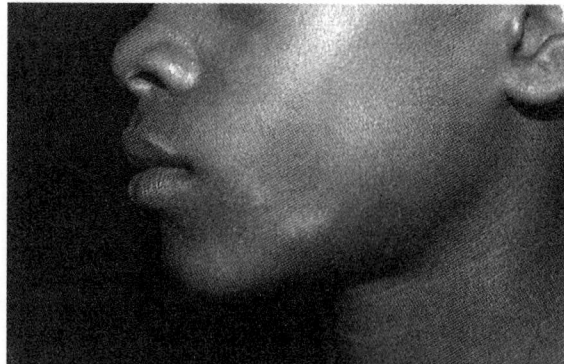

FIGURE 645–3. Patchy hypopigmented lesions with diffuse borders characteristic of pityriasis alba. See also color section.

helpful, particularly at night. Antibiotics are indicated for secondary infection.

Pityriasis Alba. This occurs mainly in children; the lesions are hypopigmented, round or oval, macular or slightly elevated patches with fine adherent scale (Fig. 645–3). They may be mildly erythematous and relatively well defined but lack a sharply marginated border. Lesions occur on the face, neck, upper trunk, and proximal portions of the arms. Itching is minimal or absent. The cause is unknown, but the eruption appears to be exacerbated by dryness and is often regarded as a mild form of eczema. Pityriasis alba is frequently misdiagnosed as tinea versicolor or corporis, each of which can be readily precluded by performing a KOH examination of surface scale. The lesions wax and wane but eventually disappear. Application of a lubricant may ameliorate the condition; if pruritus is troublesome, a topical 1% hydrocortisone preparation applied three to four times daily may be more effective. Normal pigmentation returns in weeks to months.

Lichen Simplex Chronicus. This lesion is characterized by a chronic pruritic, eczematous, circumscribed, solitary plaque that is usually lichenified and hyperpigmented. The most common sites are the posterior aspect of the neck, the dorsum of the feet, the wrists, and ankles. Trauma from rubbing and scratching accounts for persistence of the plaque, although the initiating event may be a transient lesion, such as an insect bite. Pruritus must be controlled to permit healing. A topical fluorinated corticosteroid preparation is often helpful, but constant irritation of the skin must be avoided. A covering to prevent scratching may be necessary.

Dyshidrotic Eczema (Dyshidrosis, Pompholyx). This is a recurrent, sometimes seasonal, blistering disorder of the hands and feet; it occurs in all age groups but is uncommon in infancy. The pathogenesis is unknown; no genetic factor has been identified, although an increased incidence of atopy has been recorded in patients and their relatives. The disease is characterized by recurrent crops of intensely pruritic small vesicles on the hands and feet. Sites of predilection are the palms, soles, and lateral aspects of the fingers and toes. Primary lesions are noninflammatory and filled with clear fluid, which, unlike sweat, has a physiologic pH and contains protein. Larger vesicobullae may occur, and maceration and secondary infection are frequent because of scratching (Fig. 645–4). The chronic phase is characterized by thickened, fissured plaques that may cause considerable discomfort. Hyperhidrosis is common in many patients, but the association may be fortuitous. The diagnosis is made clinically. The disorder may be confused with allergic contact dermatitis, which usually affects the dorsal rather than the volar surfaces, and with dermatophytosis, which can be distinguished by a KOH preparation of the roof of a vesicle and by appropriate cultures.

Dyshidrotic eczema responds to wet dressings, followed by a topical corticosteroid preparation during the acute phase. Control of the chronic stage is difficult; lubricants containing mild keratolytic agents in conjunction with a potent topical fluorinated corticosteroid preparation may be indicated. Secondary bacterial infection should be treated systemically with an appro-

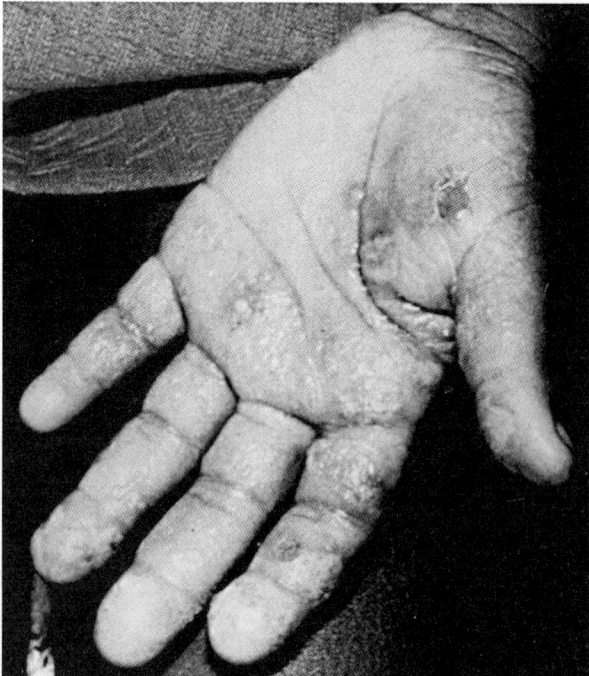

FIGURE 645–4. Vesicular palmar lesions of dyshidrotic eczema that have become secondarily infected.

priate antibiotic. Patients should be told to expect recurrence and should protect their hands and feet from the damaging effects of excessive sweating, chemicals, harsh soaps, and adverse weather.

Seborrheic Dermatitis. This chronic inflammatory disease is most common in the pediatric age group, during infancy and adolescence, paralleling the distribution, size, and activity of the sebaceous glands. The cause is unknown, as is the role of the sebaceous glands in this disease. A generalized eruption with features of seborrheic dermatitis is extremely common in HIV-infected children and adolescents.

CLINICAL MANIFESTATIONS. The disorder may begin within the 1st mo of life and may be most troublesome during the 1st yr. Diffuse or focal scaling and crusting of the scalp, sometimes called *cradle cap,* may be the initial and at times the only manifestation. A greasy, scaly, erythematous papular dermatitis, which is usually nonpruritic, may involve the face, neck, retroauricular areas, axillae, and diaper area. The dermatitis may be patchy and focal or may spread to involve almost the entire body (Fig. 645–5). Postinflammatory pigmentary changes are common, particularly in black infants. When the scaling becomes pronounced, the condition may resemble psoriasis and, at times, can be distinguished only with difficulty. The possibility of coexistent atopic dermatitis must be considered when there is an acute weeping dermatitis with pruritus. An intractable seborrhea-like dermatitis with chronic diarrhea and failure to thrive *(Leiner disease)* may reflect dysfunction of the immune system. A chronic seborrhea-like pattern, which responds poorly to treatment, may also result from cutaneous histiocytic infiltrates in infants with Langerhans cell histiocytosis X. Seborrheic dermatitis is a common cutaneous manifestation of AIDS among young adults and is characterized by thick, greasy scales on the scalp and large hyperkeratotic erythematous plaques on the face, chest, and genitals.

During adolescence, seborrheic dermatitis is more localized and may be confined to the scalp and intertriginous areas. Also noted may be marginal blepharitis and involvement of the external auditory canal. Scalp changes may vary from diffuse, brawny scaling to focal areas of thick, oily, yellow crusts with underlying erythema. Loss of hair is not uncommon, and pruritus may be absent to marked. When the dermatitis is severe, erythema and scaling may occur at the frontal hairline, at the medial aspects of the eyebrows, and in the nasolabial and retroauricular folds. Red, scaly plaques may appear in the axillae, inguinal region, gluteal cleft, and umbilicus. On the extremities, seborrheic plaques may be more eczematous and less erythematous and demarcated.

ETIOLOGY. Seborrheic dermatitis is a condition that is reactivated in some patients by stressful situations, poor hygiene, and excessive perspiration. *Malassezia furfur* has also been implicated as a causative agent, although its role in the etiology of infantile seborrheic dermatitis is unclear. The *differential diagnosis* includes psoriasis, atopic dermatitis, dermatophytosis, and candidosis. Secondary bacterial infections and superimposed candidosis are not uncommon.

TREATMENT. Scalp lesions should be controlled with an antiseborrheic shampoo (selenium sulfide, sulfur, salicylic acid, zinc pyrithion, tar), used daily if necessary. Inflamed lesions usually respond promptly to topical corticosteroid therapy given two to four times daily. Topical immunomodulatory agents (e.g. tacrolimus, pimecrolimus) approved for the treatment of atopic dermatitis in children 2 years of age and older (see Chapter 135) may have a role in the treatment of other eczematous disorders such as seborrheic dermatitis. Concerns for systemic absorption and potential immunosuppression are higher in the younger patient population typically afflicted with seborrheic dermatitis. Topical or oral antifungal agents (terbinafine) effective against *Malassezia* have also been advocated as therapy. Wet compresses should be applied to the moist or fissured lesions before application of the steroid ointment. Many patients require continued use of an antiseborrheic shampoo for control. Response to therapy is usually rapid unless there are complicating factors or the diagnosis is in error.

Faergemann J: Treatment of seborrhoeic dermatitis with oral terbinafine? *Lancet* 2001;358:170.

Fergusson DM, Horwood J, Shannon FT: Early solid feeding and recurrent childhood eczema: A 10-year longitudinal study. *Pediatrics* 1990;86:541.

Krafchik BR: Eczematous disorders. In Eichenfield LF, Frieden IJ, Esterly NB (editors): *Textbook of Neonatal Dermatology.* Philadelphia, WB Saunders, 2001, p. 241.

Paller AS: Use of non-steroidal topical immunomodulators for the treatment of atopic dermatitis in the pediatric population. *J Pediatr* 2001;138:163.

Rothe M, Grant-Kels J: Diagnostic criteria for atopic dermatitis. *Lancet* 1996;348: 769.

Tollesson A, Frithz A, Stenlund K: *Malassezia furfur* in infantile seborrheic dermatitis. *Pediatr Dermatol* 1997;14:423.

Chapter 646
Photosensitivity

Photosensitivity denotes a qualitatively or quantitatively abnormal cutaneous reaction to sunlight or artificial light.

Acute Sunburn Reaction. The most common photosensitive reaction seen in children is acute sunburn. Sunburn is caused mainly by ultraviolet (UV) B radiation (290–320 nm wavelength). Sunlight contains many times more UVA (320–400 nm) than UVB radiation, but UVA must be encountered in much larger quantities than UVB radiation to produce sunburn.

PATHOPHYSIOLOGY AND CLINICAL MANIFESTATIONS. Transmitted radiation below 300 nm is largely absorbed in the epidermis, whereas that above 300 nm is mostly transmitted to the dermis after variable epidermal melanin absorption. Children vary in susceptibility to UV radiation, depending on their skin type (amount of pigment) (Table 646–1). Immediate pigment darkening is due to UVA radiation–induced photo-oxidative darkening of existing melanin and its transfer from melanocytes to keratinocytes. This effect generally lasts for a few hours, and, like a UVA-induced tanning salon tan, is not photoprotective. UVB-induced effects appear 6–12 hr after initial exposure and reach a peak in 24 hr. Effects include redness, tenderness, edema, and blistering. The vasodilatation seen in UVB-induced erythema is mediated by prostaglandins E_2 and F_2. Delayed melanogenesis as a result of UVB radiation begins in 2–3 days and lasts several days to a few weeks. Manufacture of new melanin in melanocytes, transfer of melanin from melanocytes to keratinocytes, increase in size

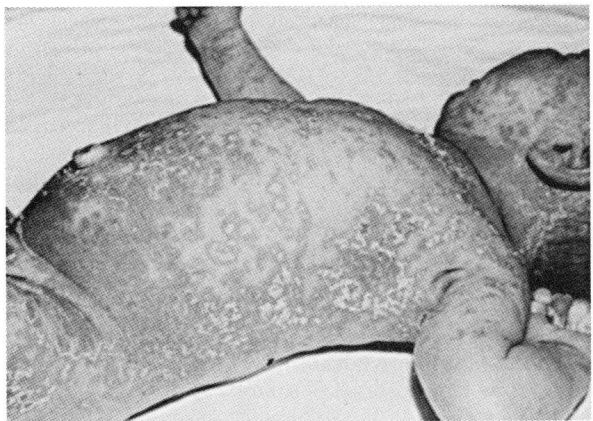

FIGURE 645–5. Widespread seborrheic dermatitis in an infant.

TABLE 646–1. Sun-Reactive Skin Types

Type	Demographics	Sunburn, Tanning History
I	Red hair, freckles, Celtic origin	Always burns easily, no tanning
II	Fair skin, fair-haired, blue-eyed, white	Usually burns, minimal tanning
III	Darker skinned white	Sometimes burns, gradual light brown tan
IV	Mediterranean background	Minimal to no burning, always tans
V	Middle eastern white, Mexican	Rarely burns, tans profusely dark brown
VI	Blacks	Never burns, pigmented black

and arborization of melanocytes, and activation of quiescent melanocytes produces delayed melanogenesis. This effect reduces skin sensitivity to development of erythema by approximately twofold to threefold. Additional effects and possible complications of sun exposure include increased thickness of the stratum corneum, recurrence or exacerbation of herpes simplex labialis, lupus erythematosus, and many other conditions (Box 646–1).

TREATMENT. Acute severe sunburn should be managed with cool compresses; topical corticosteroids may diminish inflammation and pain, and oral prostaglandin inhibitors such as ibuprofen and indomethacin may decrease erythema and pain. Proprietary preparations containing topical anesthetics are relatively ineffective and potentially hazardous because of their propensity to cause contact dermatitis. A bland emollient is effective in the desquamative phase.

PROGNOSIS AND PREVENTION OF SEQUELAE. The long-term sequelae of chronic and intense sun exposure are not often seen in children, but most individuals receive more than 50% of their lifetime UV dose by age 20 yr. Therefore, pediatricians have a pivotal role in educating patients and their parents about the harmful effects, potential malignancy risks, and irreversible skin damage that result from unduly prolonged exposure to the sun and tanning lights. Premature aging, senile elastosis, actinic keratoses, squamous and basal cell carcinomas, and melanomas all occur with greater frequency in sun-damaged skin. In particular, blistering sunburns in childhood and adolescence significantly increase the risk for development of *malignant melanoma*. Protection is enhanced by a wide variety of sunscreen agents. Physical opaque sunscreens (zinc oxide, titanium dioxide) block UV light, whereas chemical sunscreens (*p*-aminobenzoic acid [PABA], PABA esters, salicylates, benzophenones, dibenzoylmethanes, cinnamates) absorb damaging radiation. The benzophenones and dibenzoylmethanes provide protection in both the UVA and UVB ranges. Children with skin types I to III (see Table 646–1) require sunscreens with a sun protection factor (SPF) of at least 15. SPF is defined as the minimal dose of sunlight required to produce cutaneous erythema after applying a sunscreen, divided by the dose required with no use of sunscreen. Protective clothing (hats) and avoidance of sun exposure between 10:00 A.M. and 2:00 P.M. are additional prudent practices.

Photosensitive Reactions. Photosensitizers in combination with a particular wavelength of light cause dermatitis that can be classified as a phototoxic or a photoallergic reaction. Contact of the skin with the photosensitizer may occur externally, internally by enteral or parenteral administration, or by host synthesis of photosensitizers in response to an administered drug.

Photoallergic reactions occur in only a small percentage of persons exposed to photosensitizers and light and require a time interval for sensitization to take place. Thereafter, dermatitis appears within approximately 24 hr of re-exposure to the photosensitizer and light. Photoallergic dermatitis is a T-cell-mediated delayed hypersensitivity reaction in which the drug, acting as a hapten, may combine with a skin protein to form the antigenic substance. Photoallergic reactions vary in morphology

BOX 646–1. Cutaneous Reactions to Sunlight

SUNBURN
PHOTOALLERGIC DRUG ERUPTIONS
Systemic drugs include tetracyclines, psoralens, chlorthiazides, sulfonamides, barbiturates, griseofulvin, thiazides, quinidine, phenothiazines
Topical agents include coal tar derivatives, psoralens, halogenated salicylanilides (soaps), perfume oils (e.g., oil of bergamot), sunscreens (e.g., PABA, cinnamates, benzophenones)

PHOTOTOXIC DRUG ERUPTIONS
High doses of agents causing photoallergic eruptions; nalidixic acid, 5-fluorouracil, psoralens, furosemide, nonsteroidal anti-inflammatory agents (naproxen, piroxicam), sulfonamides, tetracyclines, phenothiazines, furocoumarins (e.g., lime, lemon, carrot, celery, dill, parsnip, parsley)

GENETIC DISORDER WITH PHOTOSENSITIVITY
Xeroderma pigmentosum
Bloom syndrome
Cockayne syndrome
Rothmund-Thomson syndrome

INBORN ERRORS OF METABOLISM
Porphyrias
Hartnup disease
Pellagra

INFECTIOUS DISEASES ASSOCIATED WITH PHOTOSENSITIVITY
Recurrent herpes simplex infection
Lymphogranuloma venereum
Viral exanthems (accentuated photodistribution; e.g., varicella)

SKIN DISEASE EXACERBATED OR PRECIPITATED BY LIGHT
Lichen planus
Darier disease
Lupus erythematosus
Dermatomyositis
Scleroderma
Solar urticaria
Polymorphous light eruptions (?)
Hydroa aestivale and vacciniforme (?)
Granuloma annulare
Psoriasis
Erythema multiforme
Sarcoid
Atopic dermatitis
Hailey-Hailey disease
Pemphigus
Acne rosacea
Bullous pemphigoid

DEFICIENT PROTECTION DUE TO LACK OF PIGMENT
Vitiligo
Oculocutaneous albinism
Partial albinism
Phenylketonuria
Chédiak-Higashi syndrome
Piebaldism

and may occur on partially covered and on light-exposed skin. Some of the important classes of drugs and chemicals responsible for photosensitivity reactions are listed in Box 646–1.

Phototoxic reactions occur in all individuals who accumulate adequate amounts of a photosensitizing drug or chemical within the skin. Prior sensitization is not required. Dermatitis develops within hours after exposure to radiation in the range of 285–450 nm. The eruption is confined to light-exposed areas and often resembles an exaggerated sunburn, but it may be urticarial or bullous. It results in postinflammatory hyperpigmentation. All the drugs that cause photoallergic reactions may also cause a phototoxic dermatitis if given in sufficiently high doses. Several additional drugs and contactants cause phototoxic reactions, notably the plant-derived furocoumarins (see Box 646–1). Differentiation from contact dermatitis as a result of poison ivy or oak may be difficult, but itching is prominent in contact dermatitis. In phytophotodermatitis, burning is prominent and is confined to sun-exposed areas, sparing the upper eyelids, beneath the nose and chin, and the retroauricular areas.

Although photodermatitis caused by drugs or chemicals may be diagnosed by photopatch testing, facilities for this diagnostic procedure are not widely available. A high index of suspicion combined with an appreciation of the distribution pattern of the eruption and a history of application or ingestion of a known photosensitizing agent is all that is required to make a diagnosis. Discontinuation of the offending medication or avoidance of sun exposure, oral administration of an antihistamine, and application of a topical corticosteroid to alleviate pruritus are appropriate therapeutic measures. Severe reactions may necessitate systemic corticosteroid therapy for a brief time.

Porphyrias (see Chapter 80). Porphyrias are acquired or inborn disorders due to abnormalities of specific enzyme mutations in the heme biosynthetic pathway; they are diverse in their clinical manifestations. Two in particular occur in children and have photosensitivity as a consistent feature. Signs and symptoms may be negligible during the winter, when sun exposure is minimal.

Congenital erythropoietic porphyria (Günther disease) is a rare autosomal recessive disorder caused by a deficiency of uroporphyrinogen III cosynthase, which presents within the first few months of life with exquisite sensitivity to light and which may induce repeated severe bullous eruptions that result in mutilating scars. Hyperpigmentation, hyperkeratosis, vesiculation, and fragility of skin develop in light-exposed areas. Hirsutism in areas of mild involvement, scarring alopecia in severely affected areas, pink to red urine, brown teeth, hemolytic anemia, splenomegaly, and increased amounts of uroporphyrin I in urine, plasma, and erythrocytes and of coproporphyrin I in feces are additional characteristic manifestations. Urine from affected patients fluoresces reddish pink under a Wood light.

Erythropoietic protoporphyria, an autosomal dominant trait, is due to decreased activity of ferrochelatase, which converts protoporphyrin to heme. Photosensitivity becomes apparent in early childhood and is manifested by pain, tingling, and a burning sensation within approximately 30 min of sun exposure, followed by erythema, edema, urticaria, and, rarely, vesicles on light-exposed areas. Nail changes consist of opacification of the nail plate, onycholysis, pain, and tenderness. Mild systemic symptoms of malaise, chills, and fever may accompany the acute skin reaction. Recurrent sun exposure produces a chronic eczematous dermatitis with thickened, lichenified skin, especially over the finger joints, and persistent violaceous erythema, ulcers, and pitted or linear, crusted atrophic scars on the face and rims of the ears. Pigmentation, hypertrichosis, skin fragility, and mutilation are uncommon. Liver disease is generally mild. Symptoms often improve spontaneously after age 10–11 yr.

The wavelengths of light mainly responsible for eliciting cutaneous reactions in porphyria are in the region of 400 nm. Window glass, which transmits wavelengths greater than 320 nm, is not protective, and artificial lights of a certain wavelength may be pathogenic. Patients must avoid direct sunlight, wear protective clothing, and use a sunscreen agent that effectively blocks wavelengths in the region of 400 nm. Administration of β-carotene (Solatene) quenches the fluorescence of the porphyrin molecule by yellowing the skin; its effectiveness in reducing photosensitivity in patients with protoporphyria has onset within 1–3 mo and is variable.

Colloid Milium. This is a rare, asymptomatic disorder that occurs on the face (nose, upper lip, upper cheeks) and may extend to the dorsum of the hands and the neck as a profuse eruption of ivory to yellow, firm, tiny, grouped papules. Lesions appear before puberty on otherwise normal skin, unlike the adult variant that develops on sun-damaged skin. Onset may follow an acute sunburn or chronic sun exposure. Most cases reach maximal severity within approximately 3 yr and remain unchanged thereafter, although the condition may remit spontaneously after puberty. Histopathologic changes include well-circumscribed accumulations of fissured eosinophilic material, primarily in the upper dermis in contact with the epidermis. Basal cells, which are transformed into these colloid bodies, appear to be abnormally susceptible to degeneration after actinic exposure.

Hydroa Vacciniforme. This vesicobullous disorder is more common in boys than in girls, begins in early childhood, but may remit at puberty. The peak incidence is in the spring and summer. Erythematous, pruritic macules develop symmetrically within hours of sun exposure over the ears, nose, lips, cheeks, and dorsal surfaces of the hands and forearms. Lesions progress to stinging tender papules and hemorrhagic vesicles and bullae. Severe lesions of hydroa vacciniforme resemble the vesicles of chickenpox; they become umbilicated, ulcerated, and crusted and heal with pitted scars and telangiectasias. Fever and malaise are noted occasionally during the acute phase. Histopathologically, lesions show intraepidermal multilocular vesicles, leading to focal epidermal and dermal necrosis. Noted early is a dermal perivascular mononuclear cell infiltrate that later surrounds areas of necrosis. This eruption should be distinguished from erythropoietic protoporphyria, which rarely shows vesicles. Pathogenesis of hydroa vacciniforme is unknown, but typical lesions have been reproduced with repeated doses of UVA light. A topical corticosteroid may be useful for the inflammatory phase of the eruption. Prophylactic broad-spectrum sunscreens may also be helpful, as may low-dose courses of UVB or psoralen with UVA (PUVA) therapy. β-Carotene and antimalarial agents are sometimes beneficial.

Actinic Prurigo. This is a chronic familial photodermatitis that is inherited as an autosomal dominant trait among the Native Americans of North and South America. The first episode generally occurs in early childhood several hours to 2 days after intense sun exposure. Most patients are female and are sensitive to UVA radiation. Lesions are intensely pruritic, erythematous papules on the face, lower lip, distal extremities, and, in severe cases, buttocks. Facial lesions may heal with minute pitted or linear scarring. Lesions often become chronic, without periods of total clearing, merging into eczematous plaques that lichenify and may become secondarily infected. Associated features that distinguish this disorder from other photoeruptions and atopic dermatitis include cheilitis, conjunctivitis, and traumatic alopecia of the outer half of the eyebrows. Actinic prurigo is a chronic condition that generally persists into adult life, although it may improve spontaneously in the late teenage years. Broad-spectrum sunscreens such as butyl methoxydibenzoylmethane may be helpful in preventing the eruption, but antimalarials and β-carotene afford little to no protection. Topical corticosteroids palliate the pruritus and inflammation; thalidomide also may be effective.

Solar Urticaria. This is a rare disorder induced by UV or visible irradiation. Primary solar urticaria is probably mediated by allergic type 1 hypersensitivity to a cutaneous or circulating irradiation-induced allergen, leading to mast cell degranulation and histamine release. This reaction occurs within 5–10 min of sun exposure, fades within 1–2 hr, and is characterized by widespread severe wheal formation, which may lead to faintness, headache, nausea, syncope, or bronchospasm. H_1-blocking antihistamines may be useful to prevent or abate the eruption. Secondary solar urticaria is due to photosensitization to exogenous chemicals or systemic drugs and may rarely be a presenting sign of erythropoietic protoporphyria. Treatment consists of avoidance of the photosensitizing wavelength of light and/or the drug.

Polymorphous Light Eruption. Polymorphous light eruption develops most commonly in females younger than 30 yr. The first eruption typically appears after prolonged sun exposure during the spring or summer. Onset of the eruption is delayed by hours to days after sun exposure and lasts for hours to sometimes weeks. Areas of involvement tend to be symmetric and are characteristic for a given patient, including some but not all of the exposed or lightly covered skin on the face, neck, upper chest, and distal extremities. Lesions have various morphologies but most commonly are pruritic, 2–5 mm grouped erythematous papules or papulovesicles or edematous plaques that are more than 5 cm in diameter. Most cases involve sensitivity to UVA radiation, although some are UVB induced. Therapeutic approaches include sun avoidance, broad-spectrum sunscreens, topical or systemic corticosteroids, β-carotene, nicotinamide, antimalarials, or prophylactic UVB or PUVA phototherapy.

Cockayne Syndrome. Onset of this autosomal recessive disorder is characterized by the appearance, at approximately 1 yr of age, of facial erythema in a butterfly distribution after sun exposure, followed by loss of adipose tissue and development of thin, atrophic, hyperpigmented skin, particularly over the face. Associated features include dwarfism; mental retardation; large, protuberant ears; long limbs; disproportionately large hands and feet, which are sometimes cool and cyanotic; pinched nose; carious teeth; unsteady gait with tremor; limitation of joint mobility; progressive deafness; cataracts; retinal degeneration; optic atrophy; decreased sweating and tearing; and premature graying of the hair. Diffuse extensive demyelination of the peripheral and central nervous systems ensues, and patients generally die of atheromatous vascular disease before the 3rd decade. Photosensitivity is due to deficient rates of repair of UV-induced damage, specifically within actively transcribing regions of DNA. The syndrome is distinguished from progeria (see Chapter 79) by photosensitivity and the ocular abnormalities.

Xeroderma Pigmentosum. This is a rare autosomal recessive disorder that results from a defect in nucleotide excision repair. Ten complementation groups have been recognized, based on each group's separate defect in the ability to repair damaged DNA. The wavelength of light that induces the DNA damage ranges from 280–340 nm. Skin changes are first noted during infancy or early childhood in sun-exposed areas such as the face, neck, hands, and arms; lesions may occur, however, at other sites, including the scalp. The skin lesions consist of erythema, scaling, bullae, crusting, ephelides, telangiectasia, keratoses, basal and squamous cell carcinomas, and malignant melanomas. Ocular manifestations include photophobia, lacrimation, blepharitis, symblepharon, keratitis, corneal opacities, tumors of the lids, and possible eventual blindness. Neurologic abnormalities such as mental deterioration and sensorineural deafness may develop in approximately 20% of patients. Some patients with xeroderma pigmentosum have the clinical phenotype of Cockayne syndrome, suggesting that these two disorders may represent an overlapping spectrum of excision-repair defects. The association of xeroderma pigmentosum with microcephaly, mental retardation, dwarfism, and hypogonadism is known as *De Sanctis-Cacchione syndrome*.

This disease is a serious mutilating disorder, and the life span is often brief. Affected families should have genetic counseling. The disorder is detectable in cells cultured from amniotic fluid. Affected children should be totally protected from sun exposure; protective clothing, eyeglasses, and opaque broad-spectrum sunscreens should be used even for mildly affected children. Light from unshielded fluorescent bulbs and sunlight passing through glass windows are also harmful. Early detection and removal of malignancies is mandatory. Grafting of skin from non–light-exposed areas may be helpful, as is the use of topical antimitotic agents such as 5-fluorouracil.

Rothmund-Thomson Syndrome. This syndrome is also known as *poikiloderma congenitale* because of the striking skin changes; it is inherited as an autosomal recessive trait, although a preponderance of affected females has been reported. Skin changes are noted as early as 3 mo of age. Plaques of erythema and edema appear on the cheeks, forehead, ears, neck, dorsal portions of the hands, extensor surfaces of the arms, and buttocks are replaced gradually by reticulated, atrophic, hyperpigmented, telangiectatic plaques. Light sensitivity is present in many cases, and exposure to the sun may provoke formation of bullae. Areas of involvement, however, are not strictly photodistributed. Short stature; frontal bossing; saddle nose; prognathism; small hands and feet; sparse eyebrows, eyelashes, pubic and axillary hair; sparse, fine, prematurely gray hair or alopecia; dystrophic nails; defective dentition; bony defects; and hypogenitalism are common. Cataracts commonly become apparent at 2–7 yr of age. Most patients have normal mental development and life expectancy. Keratoses and later squamous cell carcinomas may develop on exposed skin. In addition, the incidence of noncutaneous malignancies, particularly osteosarcoma, is higher than in the general population.

Hartnup Disease (see Chapter 74.5). This is a rare inborn error of metabolism with autosomal recessive inheritance. Neutral amino acids, including tryptophan, are not transported across the brush border epithelium of the intestine and kidneys, resulting in deficiency of synthesis of nicotinamide and causing a photo-induced pellagra-like syndrome. The urine contains increased amounts of monoamine monocarboxylic amino acids. Cutaneous signs, which precede neurologic manifestations, initially develop during the early months of life when an eczematous, occasionally vesicobullous eruption is noted on the face and extremities in a glove-and-stocking photodistribution. Hyperpigmentation and hyperkeratosis may supervene and are intensified by further exposure to sunlight. Episodic flares may be precipitated by febrile illness, sun exposure, emotional stress, and poor nutrition. In most cases, mental development is normal, but some patients display emotional instability and episodic cerebellar ataxia. Neurologic symptoms are fully reversible. Administration of nicotinamide and protection from sunlight result in improvement of both cutaneous and neurologic manifestations. Neomycin may also be beneficial in abating neurologic symptoms by reducing the intestinal bacterial flora and minimizing formation of indole and indican.

Bloom Syndrome. The defect in Bloom syndrome is inherited in an autosomal recessive manner on chromosome 15, perhaps owing to absence of a DNA helicase. Erythema and telangiectasia develop during infancy in a butterfly distribution on the face after exposure to sunlight. A bullous eruption on the lips and telangiectatic erythema on the hands and forearms may develop. Café-au-lait spots, ichthyosis, acanthosis nigricans, and hypertrichosis are less constant cutaneous manifestations. Prenatal and postnatal short stature and a distinctive facies consisting of a prominent nose and ears and a small, narrow face are generally found. Defective dentition, pilonidal cysts, sacral dimples, syndactyly, polydactyly, clinodactyly of the fifth fingers, shortened lower extremities, and clubfeet are additional inconstant features. Intellect is normal. Patients frequently have low levels of IgA, IgM, and IgG and are susceptible to infections. They are sensitive to UV radiation, and their rate of chromosomal breaks and sister chromatid exchanges is markedly increased. Affected children have an unusual tendency to develop lymphoreticular malignancies.

Council on Scientific Affairs: Harmful effects of ultraviolet radiation. *JAMA* 1989;262:380.

Garzon MC, DeLeo VA: Photosensitivity in the pediatric patient. *Curr Opin Pediatr* 1997;9:377.

Glanz K, Saraiya M, Wechsler H, et al: Guidelines for school programs to prevent skin cancer. *MMWR* 2002;51:1–18.

Gonzales E, Gonzales S: Drug photosensitivity, idiopathic photodermatoses, and sunscreens. *J Am Acad Dermatol* 1996;35:871.

Gould JW, Mercurio MG, Elmets CA: Cutaneous photosensitivity disease induced by exogenous agents. *J Am Acad Dermatol* 1995;33:551.

Holzle E, Plewig G, von Kries R, et al: Polymorphous light eruption. *J Invest Dermatol* 1987;88:32s.

Lane PR, Hogan DJ, Martel MJ, et al: Actinic prurigo: Clinical features and prognosis. *J Am Acad Dermatol* 1992;26:683.

Poh-Fitzpatrick MB, Ramsay CA, Frain-Bell W, et al: Photodermatoses in infants and children. *Pediatr Dermatol* 1988;5:189.

Soter NA: Acute effects of ultraviolet radiation on the skin. *Semin Dermatol* 1990;9:11.

Vennos EM, Collins M, James WD: Rothmund-Thomson syndrome: Review of the world literature. *J Am Acad Dermatol* 1992;27:750.

Chapter 647
Diseases of the Epidermis

Psoriasis. This common, chronic skin disorder is first evident in approximately one third of affected individuals within the first 2 decades of life. When the onset occurs during childhood, about 50% have a positive family history of the disease, and girls are more frequently affected. The mode of transmission is unknown; a multifactorial type of inheritance has been proposed. There is an association with histocompatibility antigens (HLA)-BW17, -B13, -B16, -BW37, and most often -CW6. The disease develops in 10% of HLA-CW6–positive patients. These HLA types are not associated with the pustular form of the disease. The pathogenesis is also unknown; epidermal turnover time, however, is distinctly accelerated compared with that of normal epidermis. In addition, infiltrating effector T lymphocytes and tumor necrosis factor may be involved, as evidenced by improvement after therapy, which block these cellular or humoral aspects of inflammation.

CLINICAL MANIFESTATIONS. The lesions consist of erythematous papules that coalesce to form plaques with sharply demarcated, irregular borders. If they are unaltered by treatment, a thick silvery or yellow-white scale (resembling mica) develops; removal of it may result in pinpoint bleeding (Auspitz sign). The *Koebner*, or isomorphic, *response*, in which new lesions appear at sites of trauma, is a valuable diagnostic feature. Lesions may occur anywhere, but preferred sites are the scalp, knees (Fig. 647–1*A*), elbows, umbilicus, superior intergluteal fold, and genitals. Scalp lesions may be confused with seborrheic dermatitis, atopic dermatitis, or tinea capitis. Small raindrop-like lesions on the face are moderately common. Nail involvement, a valuable diagnostic sign, is characterized by pitting of the nail plate (see Fig. 647–1*B*), detachment of the plate (onycholysis), yellowish-brown subungual discoloration, and accumulation of subungual debris.

Age is an important factor in determining the clinical pattern. Psoriasis is rare in neonates but may be severe and recalcitrant and pose a diagnostic problem. The initial lesions may involve the diaper area and mimic seborrheic dermatitis, eczematous diaper dermatitis, perianal streptococcal disease, or candidosis. Biopsy or prolonged observation may be required for definitive diagnosis. Other rare forms include psoriatic erythroderma, localized or generalized pustular psoriasis, and linear psoriasis. Hospitalization may be required for severe forms of the disease. *Guttate psoriasis*, a variant that occurs predominantly in children, is characterized by an explosive eruption of profuse, small, oval or round lesions that morphologically are identical to the larger plaques of psoriasis (see Fig. 647–1*C*). Sites of predilection are the trunk, face, and proximal portions of the limbs. The onset frequently follows a recent streptococcal respiratory infection; a culture of the throat and serologic titers should be obtained. Guttate psoriasis has also been observed after perianal streptococcal infection, viral infections, sunburn, and withdrawal of systemic corticosteroid therapy. Psoriatic skin lesions may be induced, in a genetically susceptible host, by CD4+ T cells that were initially activated by streptococcal pyrogenic exotoxins acting as superantigens. The source of the streptococcal antigens can be the throat or the skin. Some of the superantigen-activated T cells recognize streptococcal M protein in the skin and appear to have cross reactivity with an abnormal keratin that has homology with streptococcal M protein. The autoreactive T cells may be responsible for the formation and maintenance of psoriatic skin lesions. The lesions may be confused with viral exanthems and guttate parapsoriasis (see later).

DIAGNOSIS. This is based on the clinical manifestations. The differential diagnosis includes Reiter syndrome, which, in contrast to psoriasis, involves mucous membranes, and pityriasis rubra pilaris. When in doubt, histopathologic examination of an untreated lesion reveals characteristic changes of psoriasis.

TREATMENT. The therapeutic approach varies with the age of the child, type of psoriasis, sites of involvement, and extent of the disease. Therapy is mainly palliative and should not be overly aggressive. Physical and chemical trauma to the skin should be avoided as much as possible (see the Koebner response discussed earlier).

Tar preparations may be used in the form of an emulsion added to the daily bath, gel preparations, or ointments such as crude coal tar (1–5%) and liquor carbonis detergens (5–15%) in an emollient base alone or in conjunction with ultraviolet (UV) B light or natural sunlight. Sunlight occasionally has an adverse rather than a beneficial effect, and the use of tar preparations may have to be decreased during the summer to avoid phototoxic reactions. Salicylic acid ointment (1–3%) may provide an alternative for removal of scale, but extensive application may result in toxicity, particularly in small children. Topical corticosteroid preparations are effective during the first several weeks of therapy for an individual lesion, and then their effectiveness tends to decrease. Topical corticosteroids must be used with caution. Fluorinated compounds produce cutaneous atrophy if applied excessively or if occluded with polyethylene film for prolonged periods, and adrenal suppression may occur if systemic absorption is excessive. The preparation that is least potent but effective should be applied one to two times daily. The topical vitamin D analog calcipotriene may also be effective for limited lesions. It appears to have much less impact on calcium metabolism (e.g., 100-fold less) than calcitriol. Calcipotriene can burn and sting, which limits its usefulness in children. In addition, several weeks of therapy are necessary before benefit is seen. For scalp lesions, applications of a phenol and saline solution (Baker P & S) followed by a tar shampoo are effective in the removal of scales. A corticosteroid in a solution, lotion, or gel base may be applied when the scaling is diminished. Rarely, the more severe forms of psoriasis may require systemic therapy.

The use of psoralens and UV light (PUVA) is effective in severe psoriasis in adults, but the safety of PUVA has not been established for children. Methotrexate, oral retinoids (in combination with PUVA), and cyclosporine are used for the rare severe and generalized forms of psoriasis. The retinoid etretinate is useful in severe disorders, has a half-life of approximately 120 days, and may have serious side effects; dermatologic consultation is essential when its use is being considered. Acitretin may hold more promise for pediatric patients, because the half-life of this synthetic retinoid is 2–4 days. Psoriasis in infants and acute guttate psoriasis may flare with vigorous treatment and should be managed conservatively. Nail lesions are usually recalcitrant to therapy. Potentially beneficial therapies include 308 nm excimer laser UV-B radiation, inhibition of tumor necrosis factor with infliximab, and inhibition of CD45RO+ memory T cells with alefacept.

PROGNOSIS. This is best for children with limited disease. Psoriasis is characterized by remissions and exacerbations; if present during adolescence, it is a lifelong disease. Arthritis may be an extracutaneous complication.

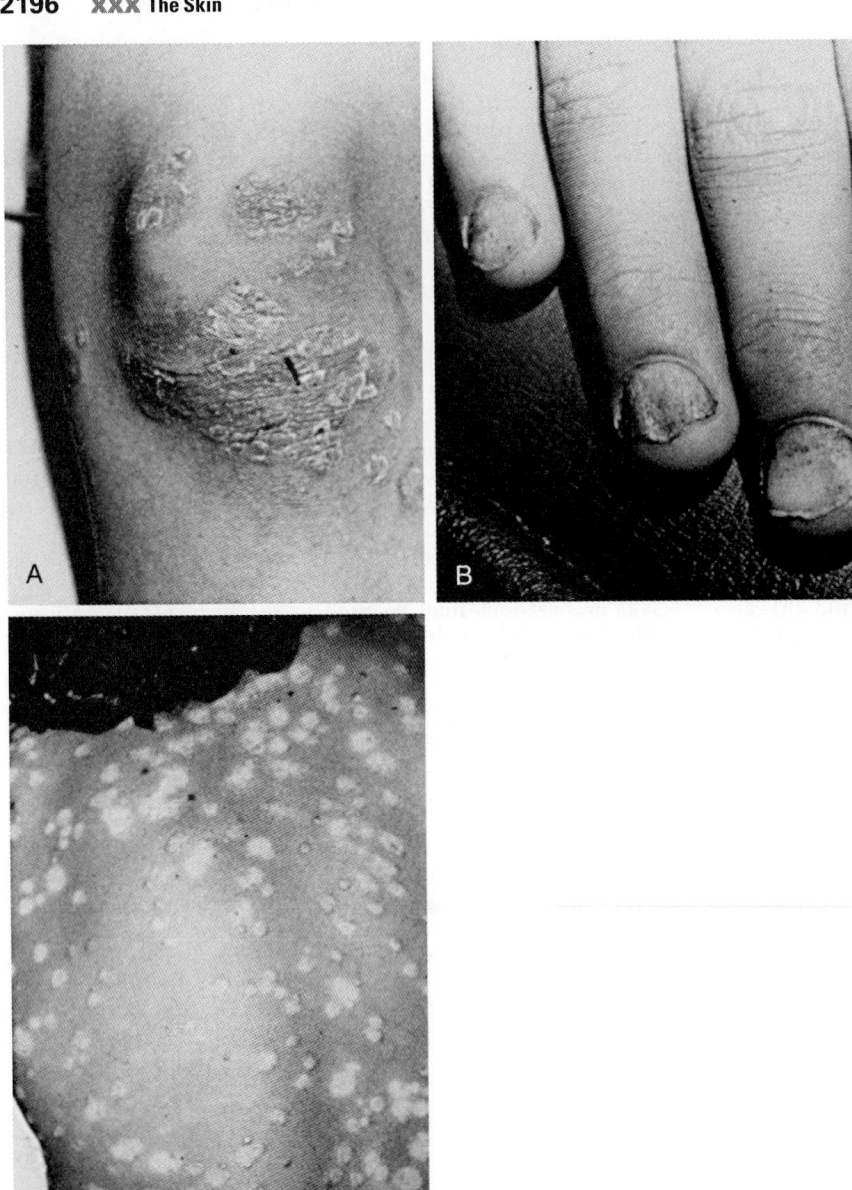

FIGURE 647–1. *A*, Chronic psoriatic plaques on the knee. *B*, Psoriatic nail changes of pitting and dystrophy. *C*, Guttate psoriasis in widespread distribution over the trunk.

Pityriasis Lichenoides. This has historically encompassed pityriasis lichenoides et varioliformis acuta (PLEVA, Mucha-Habermann disease), which tends to develop acutely, and pityriasis lichenoides chronica (PLC), which follows a chronic course. The designation of pityriasis lichenoides as acute or chronic may more properly refer to morphologic appearance of the lesions, which is often hemorrhagic or necrotic in PLEVA, than to the duration of the disease. No correlation is found between the type of lesion at the onset of the eruption and the duration of the disease. Many patients have both acute and chronic lesions simultaneously, and transition of lesions from one form into another occurs occasionally. There is a correlation between the distribution of lesions and the duration of disease: (1) disease characterized by diffusely distributed lesions may resolve relatively quickly (mean disease duration 11 mo); (2) centrally distributed lesions on the trunk, neck, and/or proximal extremities are intermediate in duration; and (3) disease located peripherally or acrally usually persists the longest (mean

31 mo). Pityriasis lichenoides most commonly presents in the 2nd and 3rd decades; approximately one third of cases present before age 20 yr.

CLINICAL MANIFESTATIONS. PLC presents with generalized, multiple, asymptomatic 3–5 mm brown-red papules that are covered by a grayish mica-like scale. A useful clinical sign is the easy detachment of the adherent scale, revealing a shining surface. Lesions may be asymptomatic or may cause minimal pruritus and occasionally become infiltrated, vesicular, hemorrhagic, and crusted. Individual papules become flat and brownish over 2–6 wk, ultimately leaving a hyperpigmented or hypopigmented macule. Scarring is unusual. Lesions are most common on the trunk and extremities and generally spare the face, palmoplantar surfaces, scalp, and mucous membranes. The eruption persists for months to years and is characterized by polymorphous lesions in various stages of evolution. PLC histologically shows a parakeratotic, thickened corneal layer; epidermal spongiosis; a superficial perivascular infiltrate of macrophages and predominantly CD8+ lymphocytes, which may extend into the epidermis; and small numbers of extravasated erythrocytes in the papillary dermis.

PLEVA presents with an abrupt eruption of numerous papules that have a vesiculopustular and then a purpuric center, are covered by a dark adherent crust, and are surrounded by an erythematous halo. Constitutional symptoms of fever, malaise, headache, and arthralgias may be present for 2–3 days after the initial outbreak. Lesions are distributed diffusely on the trunk and extremities, as in PLC. Individual lesions heal within a few weeks, sometimes leaving a varioliform scar, and successive crops of papules produce the characteristic polymorphous appearance of the eruption. The condition is generally self-limited from several weeks to months. The histopathologic changes of PLEVA reflect its more severe nature compared with PLC. Intercellular and intracellular edema in the epidermis may lead to degeneration of keratinocytes. A dense perivascular mononuclear cell infiltrate that extends upward into the epidermis and downward into the reticular dermis, endothelial cell swelling, and extravasation of erythrocytes into the epidermis and dermis are additional characteristic features. Severe changes of vasculitis are exceptional. Differential diagnosis includes guttate psoriasis, pityriasis rosea, drug eruptions, secondary syphilis, viral exanthems, and lichen planus. The chronicity of pityriasis lichenoides helps to preclude pityriasis rosea, viral exanthems, and some drug eruptions. A skin biopsy helps to preclude other differential diagnoses.

A rare form of PLEVA has been described as presenting with fever and ulceronecrotic plaques up to 1 cm in diameter; those are most common on the anterior trunk and flexors of the proximal upper extremities. Arthritis and superinfection of cutaneous lesions with *Staphylococcus aureus* may also develop. The ulceronecrotic lesions appear within papules of PLEVA and heal with hypopigmented scarring in a few weeks. Leukocytoclastic vasculitis is occasionally seen histopathologically. The eruption may resemble erythema multiforme, but it generally spares the mucous membranes.

ETIOLOGY. The cause of pityriasis lichenoides is unknown, but sporadic outbreaks have led to an unsuccessful search for an infectious agent; human-to-human transmission has not been documented. A popular hypothesis is that pityriasis lichenoides is a hypersensitivity reaction to an infectious organism. Cell-mediated mechanisms appear to be important in the pathogenesis because most infiltrating cells are cytotoxic-suppressor cells. Clonal gene rearrangement studies of the T-cell receptor and immunohistologic studies have led to the suggestion that PLEVA may be a T-cell lymphoproliferative process. The condition in two children with PLEVA was reported to evolve into cutaneous T-cell lymphoma. It has been postulated that the relatively greater proportion of cytotoxic-suppressor cells than helper-inducer T cells in lesions of PLEVA compared with those of lymphomatoid papulosis or T-cell lymphoma reflects the more effective host response in PLEVA.

TREATMENT. In general, pityriasis lichenoides should be considered a benign condition that does not alter the health of the child. A lubricant to remove excessive scaling may be all that is necessary if the patient is asymptomatic. The most appropriate treatment includes erythromycin (30–50 mg/kg/24 hr for 2 mo) in combination with natural sunlight. If this regimen is effective, erythromycin should then be tapered slowly over several months. The rare febrile ulceronecrotic form may be controlled effectively by systemic corticosteroids. Additional modalities that have been effective in some adult patients but are rarely appropriate for children include PUVA, tetracycline, dapsone, and methotrexate.

Keratosis Pilaris. This moderately common papular eruption may vary in extent from sparse lesions over the extensor aspects of the limbs to involvement of most of the body surface; typical areas of involvement include the upper extensor arms and the thighs, cheeks, and buttocks. The lesions may resemble gooseflesh; they are noninflammatory, scaly, follicular papules that do not coalesce. Irritation of the follicular plugs occasionally causes folliculitis. Because the lesions are associated with and accentuated by dry skin, they are often more prominent during the winter. They are more frequent in patients with atopic dermatitis and are most common during childhood and early adulthood, tending to subside during the 3rd decade of life. Mild or localized eruptions respond to lubrication with a bland emollient; more pronounced or widespread lesions require regular applications of a 10–25% urea cream, an α-hydroxy acid preparation such as lactic acid in an emollient or in combination with a corticosteroid, or topical retinoic acid. Therapy may improve the condition but does not cure it.

Lichen Spinulosus. This uncommon disorder occurs principally in children and more frequently in boys. The cause is unknown. The lesions consist of sharply circumscribed irregular plaques of spiny, keratinous projections that protrude from the orifices of the pilosebaceous canals (Fig. 647–2). Plaques may occur anywhere on the body and are often distributed symmetrically on the trunk, elbows, knees, and extensor surfaces of the limbs. Although sometimes erythematous, the lesions are usually skin colored. They are readily palpable and represent keratotic follicular plugs. Lichen spinulosus is easily differentiated from keratosis pilaris because the latter lesions are never grouped to form plaques. More commonly, it is confused with papular eczema.

Treatment is usually unnecessary. For patients who regard the eruption as a cosmetic defect, keratolytic agents such as salicylic acid ointment (3–7%), urea-containing lubricants (10–25%), and retinoic acid preparations are often effective in flattening the projections. The plaques usually disappear spontaneously after several months or years.

Pityriasis Rosea. This benign, common eruption occurs most frequently in children and young adults. Although a prodrome of fever, malaise, arthralgia, and pharyngitis may precede the eruption, children rarely complain of such symptoms. The cause of pityriasis rosea is unknown; a viral agent is suspected.

CLINICAL MANIFESTATIONS. A *herald patch*, a solitary, round or oval lesion that may occur anywhere on the body and is often but not always identifiable by its large size, usually precedes

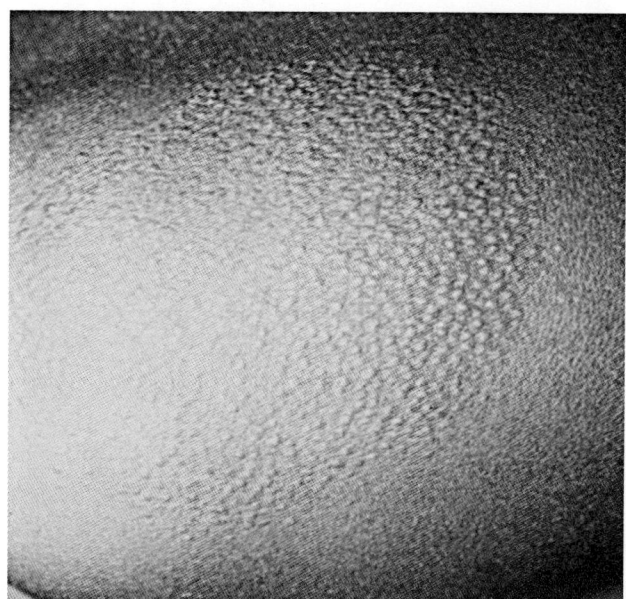

FIGURE 647–2. Sharply circumscribed plaque of follicular papules characteristic of lichen spinulosus.

the generalized eruption. Herald patches vary from 1–10 cm in diameter; they are annular in configuration and have a raised border with fine, adherent scales. Approximately 5–10 days after the appearance of the herald patch, a widespread, symmetric eruption becomes evident involving mainly the trunk and proximal limbs (Fig. 647–3). When the disease is extensive, the face, scalp, and distal limbs may be involved, or, in the inverse form of pityriasis rosea, only those sites may be affected. Lesions may appear in crops for several days. Typical lesions are oval or round, less than 1 cm in diameter, slightly raised, and pink to brown. The developed lesion is covered by a fine scale that gives the skin a crinkly appearance; some lesions clear centrally, producing a collarette of scale that is attached only at the periphery. Papular, vesicular, urticarial, hemorrhagic, and large annular lesions are unusual variants. The long axis of each lesion is usually aligned with the cutaneous cleavage lines, a feature that creates the so-called Christmas tree pattern on the back. Actually, conformation to skin lines is often more discernible in the anterior and posterior axillary folds and supraclavicular areas. Duration of the eruption varies from 2–12 wk. The lesions may be asymptomatic or mildly to severely pruritic.

DIAGNOSIS. This is clinical. The herald patch may be mistaken for tinea corporis, a pitfall that can be avoided if testing with a potassium hydroxide preparation is carried out. The generalized eruption resembles a number of other diseases; of these, secondary syphilis is the most important. Drug eruptions, viral exanthems, guttate psoriasis, PLC, and eczema can also be confused with pityriasis rosea.

TREATMENT. Therapy is unnecessary for asymptomatic patients. If scaling is prominent, a bland emollient may suffice. Pruritus may be suppressed by a lubricating lotion containing menthol and camphor or by an oral antihistamine for sedation, particularly at night, when itching may be troublesome. Occasionally, a nonfluorinated topical corticosteroid preparation may be necessary to alleviate pruritus. After the eruption has resolved, postinflammatory hypopigmentation or hyperpigmentation may be pronounced, particularly in black patients; these changes disappear during subsequent weeks to months.

Pityriasis Rubra Pilaris. This rare chronic dermatosis often has an insidious onset with diffuse scaling and erythema of the scalp, which is indistinguishable from seborrheic dermatitis, and with thick hyperkeratosis of the palms and soles. The characteristic primary lesion is a firm, dome-shaped, tiny, acuminate papule,

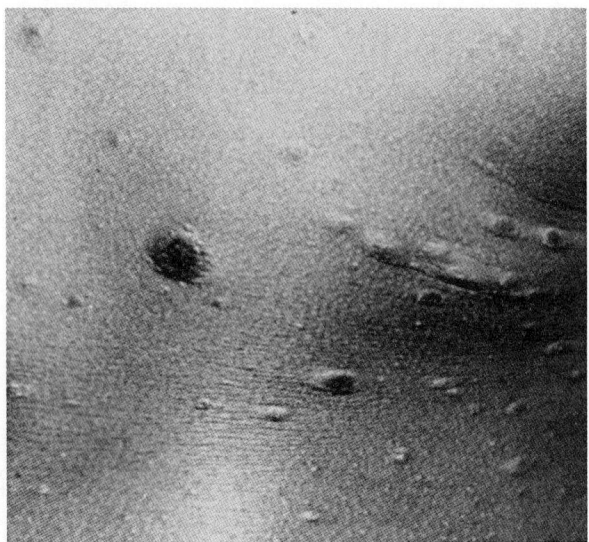

FIGURE 647–3. Ovoid, maculopapular lesions of pityriasis rosea. Note the distribution along the skin lines and the herald patch on the chest.

which is pink to red and has a central keratotic plug pierced by a vellus hair. Masses of these papules coalesce to form large, erythematous, sharply demarcated orangish plaques, within which islands of normal skin can be distinguished, creating a bizarre effect. Typical papules on the dorsum of the proximal phalanges are readily palpated. Gray plaques or papules resembling lichen planus may be found in the oral cavity. Dystrophic changes in the nails may occur and mimic those of psoriasis. In advanced stages, marked hyperkeratosis of the scalp and face may cause alopecia and ectropion. Differential diagnosis includes ichthyosis, seborrheic dermatitis, keratoderma of the palms and soles, and psoriasis.

ETIOLOGY. The cause is unknown. A genetic form with autosomal dominant transmission may account for some cases in childhood, but most appear to be sporadic. Attempts to link the disease with a defect in vitamin A metabolism have not been definitive. Skin biopsy may help to differentiate this condition from psoriasis and seborrheic dermatitis, which it resembles most closely.

TREATMENT. The numerous therapeutic regimens recommended are difficult to evaluate because the disease has a capricious course with exacerbations and remissions. Oral and topical retinoids and vitamin A have been used most frequently. When vitamin A or synthetic retinoids are administered orally, the child should be observed carefully for signs of toxicity (see earlier discussion on treatment of psoriasis). In childhood, the *prognosis* for eventual resolution is relatively good.

Darier Disease (Keratosis Follicularis). This rare genetic disorder is inherited as an autosomal dominant trait. Onset occurs usually during late childhood. Typical lesions are small, firm, skin-colored papules that are not always follicular in location. The lesions eventually acquire yellow, malodorous crusts; coalesce to form large, gray-brown, vegetative plaques; and usually involve the face, neck, shoulders, chest, back, and limb flexures in a symmetric distribution. Papules, fissures, crusts, and ulcers may appear on the mucous membranes of the lips, tongue, buccal mucosa, pharynx, larynx, and vulva. Hyperkeratosis of the palms and soles and nail dystrophy with subungual hyperkeratosis are variable features. Severe pruritus, secondary infection, offensive odor, and aggravation of the dermatosis on exposure to sunlight may occur. Darier disease is most likely to be confused with seborrheic dermatitis or juvenile flat warts. Histologic changes are diagnostic: Hyperkeratosis, intraepidermal separation with formation of suprabasal clefts, and dyskeratotic epidermal cells are characteristic features.

Treatment is nonspecific. Some patients have responded to topical vitamin A or retinoic acid, with or without occlusive dressings. Severe disease may be controlled with oral synthetic retinoids. Secondary infection may require local cleansing and systemically administered antibiotics. Affected individuals usually suffer more during the summer.

Lichen Nitidus. This chronic, benign, papular eruption is characterized by minute (1–2 mm), flat-topped, shiny, firm papules of uniform size; these are most often skin colored but may be pink or red. In black individuals, they are usually hypopigmented. Sites of predilection are the genitals, abdomen, chest, forearms, wrists, and inner aspects of the thighs. The lesions may be sparse or numerous and form large plaques; careful examination usually discloses linear papules in a line of scratch (Koebner phenomenon), a valuable clue to the diagnosis because it occurs in only a few diseases (Fig. 647–4). Lichen nitidus occurs in all age groups. The cause is unknown. Patients are usually asymptomatic and constitutionally well. The lesions may be confused with those of lichen planus and rarely coexist with them.

Widespread keratosis pilaris can also be confused with lichen nitidus, but the follicular localization of the papules and the absence of Koebner phenomenon in the former distinguish them. Verruca plana (flat warts), if small and uniform in size,

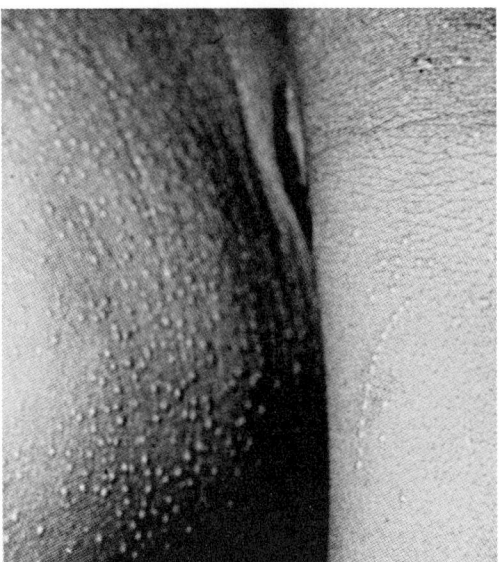

FIGURE 647–4. Tiny flat-topped papules of lichen nitidus on the arm and trunk. Note the Koebner response on the arm (papules in a line of scratch).

may occasionally resemble lichen nitidus. Although the diagnosis can be made clinically, a biopsy is occasionally indicated. Histopathologically, the lichen nitidus papule consists of sharply circumscribed nests of lymphocytes and histiocytes in the upper dermis enclosed by clawlike epidermal rete ridges. The course of lichen nitidus spans months to years, but the lesions eventually involute completely. There is no effective therapy.

Lichen Striatus. This benign, self-limited eruption consists of a continuous or discontinuous linear band of papules in a zosteriform distribution. The primary lesion is a flat-topped, red to violaceous papule covered with fine scale. Aggregates of these papules form multiple bands or plaques (Fig. 647–5). In black patients, the lesions may be hypopigmented. The cause and explanation for the linear distribution are unknown. The eruption evolves over a period of days or weeks in an otherwise

healthy child, remains stationary for weeks to months, and finally remits without sequelae. Symptoms are usually absent; some children complain of itching. Nail dystrophy may occur when the eruption involves the posterior nail fold and matrix.

Lichen striatus is occasionally confused with other disorders. The initial plaque may resemble papular eczema or lichen nitidus until the linear configuration becomes apparent. Linear lichen planus and linear psoriasis are usually associated with typical individual lesions elsewhere on the body. Linear epidermal nevi are permanent lesions that often become more hyperkeratotic and hyperpigmented than those of lichen striatus. A lubricating lotion containing menthol and camphor or a mild corticosteroid preparation provides sufficient relief when pruritus is a problem.

Lichen Planus. This is a rare disorder in young children and uncommon in older ones. The primary lesion is a violaceous, sharply demarcated, polygonal papule with fine lines or thin white scales on the surface; papules may coalesce to form large plaques. The papules are intensely pruritic, and additional ones are often induced by scratching (Koebner phenomenon) so that lines of them are often detected (Fig. 647–6). Sites of predilection are the flexor surfaces of the wrists, forearms, and inner aspects of the thighs. Characteristic lesions of mucous membranes consist of pinhead-sized white papules that coalesce to form reticulated and lacy patterns on the oral mucosa and sometimes on the lips and tongue.

Acute eruptive lichen planus is probably the most common form in children. The lesions erupt in an explosive fashion, much like a viral exanthem, and spread to involve most of the body surface. Hypertrophic, linear, bullous, atrophic, annular, follicular, erosive, and ulcerative forms of lichen planus may also occur. Nail involvement may develop in the chronic forms but is rarely evident in children (see Chapter 653). The disorder may persist for months to years, but the acute eruptive form is most likely to involute permanently. Intense hyperpigmentation frequently persists for a long time after the resolution of lesions. The histopathologic findings of lichen planus are specific, and a biopsy is indicated if the diagnosis is unclear.

Treatment is directed at alleviation of the intense pruritus and amelioration of the skin lesions. Oral antihistamines and/or

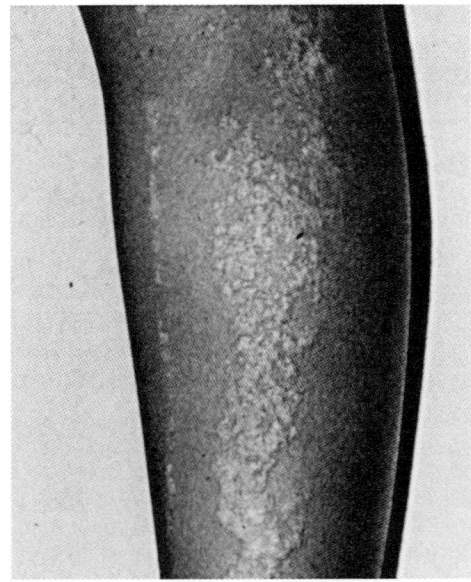

FIGURE 647–5. Multiple linear plaques and streaks of lichen striatus.

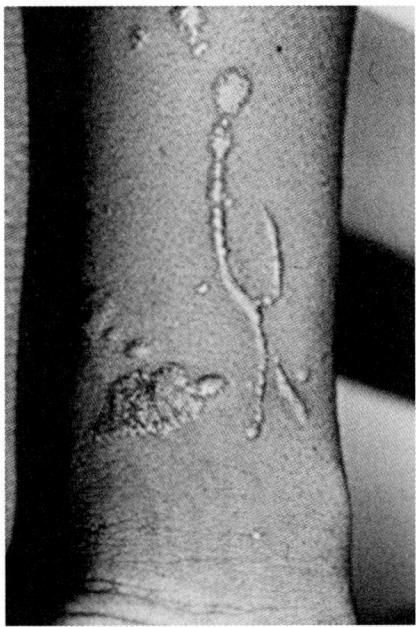

FIGURE 647–6. Violaceous polygonal papules of lichen planus. Note the striking Koebner response.

tranquilizers are often helpful. The skin lesions respond best to regular applications of a topical corticosteroid preparation. Rarely, systemic corticosteroid therapy is necessary to gain control of widespread, intractable lesions.

Porokeratosis. This rare, chronic, progressive disease is inherited as an autosomal dominant trait. Several forms have been delineated: solitary plaques, linear porokeratosis, hyperkeratotic lesions of the palms and soles, disseminated eruptive lesions, and superficial actinic porokeratosis. The last form, probably induced by excessive sun exposure, occurs more commonly in women. Other types of porokeratosis are more common in males and begin during childhood. Sites of predilection are the limbs, face, neck, and genitals. The primary lesion is a small, keratotic papule that enlarges peripherally so that the center becomes depressed, with the edge forming an elevated wall or collar. The configuration of the plaque may be round, oval, or gyrate; its elevated border is split by a thin groove from which minute cornified projections protrude. The enclosed central area is yellow, gray, or tan and sclerotic, smooth, and dry, whereas the hyperkeratotic border is a darker gray, brown, or black.

The differential diagnosis includes warts, epidermal nevi, lichen planus, granuloma annulare, and elastosis perforans serpiginosa. A skin biopsy discloses the characteristic cornoid lamella (plug of stratum corneum cells with retained nuclei), which is responsible for the invariable linear ridge of the lesion. The disease is slowly progressive but relatively asymptomatic. Lesions are sometimes responsive to applications of liquid nitrogen or occasionally may be surgically excised. Topical agents such as retinoic acid and 5-fluorouracil may be effective in some patients.

Papular Acrodermatitis of Childhood (Gianotti-Crosti Syndrome). This distinctive eruption is occasionally associated with malaise and low-grade fever but few other constitutional symptoms. The incidence peaks in early childhood. Occurrences are usually sporadic, but epidemics have been recorded. The skin lesion is a monomorphous, usually nonpruritic, dusky or coppery red, flat-topped, firm papule ranging in size from 1–5 mm. The papules appear in crops and may become profuse but remain discrete, forming a symmetric eruption on the face, buttocks, and limbs, including the palms and soles. The papules often have the appearance of vesicles; when opened, however, no fluid is obtained. The papules sometimes become hemorrhagic. Lines of papules (Koebner phenomenon) may be noted on the extremities. The trunk is relatively spared, as are the scalp and mucous membranes. Generalized lymphadenopathy and hepatomegaly (in those with hepatitis B viremia) constitute the only other abnormal physical findings. The eruption resolves spontaneously in about 15–60 days. Lymphadenopathy and hepatomegaly, if present, may persist for several months. This eruption in Italy was initially associated with primary liver infection by hepatitis B virus and surface antigenemia. Elevation of serum transaminase and alkaline phosphatase values without concomitant hyperbilirubinemia was usual. Skin biopsy was characterized by a perivascular mononuclear cell infiltrate and capillary endothelial swelling.

Generally, the disease is benign and is not associated with hepatitis in the United States. This eruption has been seen in children infected with Epstein-Barr virus, coxsackievirus A16, parainfluenza virus, and other viral infections. Papular acrodermatitis can be confused with lichen planus, erythema multiforme, histiocytosis X, and Henoch-Schönlein purpura.

Acanthosis Nigricans. This is characterized by hyperpigmented, velvety, hyperkeratotic plaques that are most often localized to the neck, axillae, inframammary areas, groin, inner thighs, and anogenital region. The histologic changes are those of papillomatosis and hyperkeratosis rather than acanthosis or excessive pigment formation. Acanthosis nigricans has classically

been associated with obesity; drugs such as nicotinic acid; endocrinopathies, including diabetes mellitus, Addison disease, Cushing syndrome, acromegaly, hypothyroidism, hyperthyroidism, Stein-Leventhal syndrome, and hyperandrogenic or hypogonadal syndromes; many different syndromes such as Bloom, Crouzon, or Rud syndromes, Wilson disease, lipoatrophic diabetes, partial lipodystrophy, and leprechaunism; and malignancies, usually in adults with an abdominal adenocarcinoma. It may occasionally be familial, with autosomal dominant inheritance. Acanthosis nigricans is found in 7% of children and is usually associated with obesity; this form is termed pseudoacanthosis nigricans.

The skin lesions appear to be a manifestation of insulin resistance. The clinical severity and histopathologic features of acanthosis nigricans correlate positively with the degree of hyperinsulinism. It has been hypothesized that insulin resistance, with compensatory hyperinsulinism, leads to insulin binding to and activation of insulin-like growth factor receptors, promoting epidermal growth. In the malignant form, tumor-secreted growth factors and hyperinsulinemia could be pathogenic.

This skin disorder is extremely difficult to treat but may be improved by palliation of the underlying disorder, weight loss in the case of pseudoacanthosis nigricans, reduction in insulin resistance, and topical or oral retinoids.

Asawananda P, Anderson RR, Chang Y, et al: 308-nm excimer laser for the treatment of psoriasis. *Arch Dermatol* 2000;136:619–24.

Caputo R, Gelmetti C, Ermacora E, et al: Gianotti-Crosti syndrome: A retrospective analysis of 308 cases. *J Am Acad Dermatol* 1992;26:207.

Chaudhari U, Romano P, Mulcahy LD, et al: Efficacy and safety of infliximab monotherapy for plaque-type psoriasis: a randomized trial. *Lancet* 2001;357:1842–7.

Elder JT, Nair RP, Henseler T, et al: The genetics of psoriasis 2001. *Arch Dermatol* 2001;137:1447–54.

Ellis CN, Krueger GG: Treatment of chronic plaque psoriasis by selective targeting of memory effector T lymphocytes. *N Engl J Med* 2001;345:248–55.

Forston JS, Schroeter AL, Esterly NB: Cutaneous T-cell lymphoma (parapsoriasis en plaque). An association with pityriasis lichenoides et varioliformis acuta in young children. *Arch Dermatol* 1990;126:1449.

Gelmetti C, Rigoni C, Alessi E, et al: Pityriasis lichenoides in children: A long term follow-up of eighty-nine cases. *J Am Acad Dermatol* 1990;23:473.

Rogers M: Pityriasis lichenoides and lymphomatoid papulosis. *Semin Dermatol* 1992;11:73.

Stern R: Psoriasis. *Lancet* 1997;350:349.

Taieb A, Youbi E, Grosshans E, et al: Lichen striatus: A Blaschko linear acquired inflammatory skin eruption. *J Am Acad Dermatol* 1991;25:637.

Chapter 648
Disorders of Keratinization

Disorders of Cornification. Disorders of cornification (ichthyoses) are a primary group of inherited conditions characterized clinically by patterns of scaling and histopathologically by hyperkeratosis. They are usually distinguishable on the basis of inheritance patterns, clinical features, associated defects, and histopathologic changes. Because some of these conditions cause disfigurement and considerable psychosocial stress, early diagnosis is helpful to predict probable course and prognosis and to provide supportive management for patients and families.

Harlequin Fetus. This rare keratinizing disorder probably represents several genotypes with similar clinical manifestations. At birth, markedly thickened, ridged, and cracked skin forms horny plates over the entire body, disfiguring the facial features and constricting the digits. Severe ectropion and chemosis obscure the orbits, the nose and ears are flattened, and the lips are everted and gaping. Nails and hair may be absent. Joint mobility is restricted, and the hands and feet appear fixed and ischemic. Affected neonates have respiratory difficulty, suck poorly, and are subject to severe cutaneous infection. Most die within the 1st days to weeks of life, but patients occasionally survive beyond infancy and have severe ichthyosis and variable neurologic impairment. Ectropion and eclabium resolve, and the cracked, horny plated skin is replaced by large, thin scales with surrounding erythema.

Inheritance is autosomal recessive. Common morphologic abnormalities include hyperkeratosis, accumulation of lipid droplets within corneocytes, and absence of normal lamellar granules. One type has an altered catalytic subunit of 2A protein phosphorylase, which is encoded on chromosome 11. The basic defect of all types is suggested to be an abnormality of lamellar granules, which have an important role in desquamation.

Initial treatment includes high fluid intake to avoid dehydration from transepidermal water loss and use of a humidified heated incubator, emulsifying ointments, careful attention to hygiene, and oral retinoids such as etretinate. Survivors after retinoid therapy have shown severe congenital ichthyosiform erythroderma. Prenatal diagnosis has been accomplished by fetoscopy, fetal skin biopsy, and microscopic examination of cells from amniotic fluid taken at the 17th and 21st wk of gestation.

Collodion Baby. These infants are covered at birth by a thick, taut membrane resembling oiled parchment or collodion, which is subsequently shed. The condition is usually a manifestation of congenital ichthyosiform erythroderma or lamellar ichthyosis; like a harlequin fetus, a collodion baby appears to be one phenotype for several genotypes. Less commonly collodion babies evolve into other forms of ichthyosis, Gaucher disease, and a small subset is otherwise healthy without chronic skin disease. Infrequently, an affected infant has normal skin after the membrane is shed. Affected neonates have ectropion, flattening of the ears and nose, and fixation of the lips in an O-shaped config-

uration (Fig. 648–1). Hair may be absent or may perforate the horny covering. The membrane cracks with initial respiratory efforts and, shortly after birth, begins to desquamate in large sheets. Complete shedding may take several weeks, and a new membrane may occasionally form in localized areas.

Neonatal morbidity and deaths may be due to cutaneous infection, aspiration pneumonia (squamous material), hypothermia, or hypernatremic dehydration from excessive transcutaneous fluid losses as a result of increased skin permeability. The outcome is uncertain, and accurate prognosis is impossible with respect to the subsequent development of ichthyosis. Treatment with a high-humidity environment and application of nonocclusive lubricants may facilitate shedding of the membrane.

Lamellar Ichthyosis and Congenital Ichthyosiform Erythroderma (Nonbullous Congenital Ichthyosiform Erythroderma). There are two major forms of autosomal recessively inherited ichthyosis. Both forms are present soon or shortly after birth and are the most common forms of ichthyosis to present as collodion babies, although most infants present with erythroderma and scaling.

After shedding of the collodion membrane, if present, *lamellar ichthyosis*, evolves into large, quadrilateral dark scales that are free at the edges and adherent at the center. Scaling is often pronounced and involves the entire body surface, including flexural surfaces (Fig. 648–2). The face is often markedly involved, including ectropion and crumpled, small ears. The palms and soles are generally hyperkeratotic. The hair may be sparse and fine, but the teeth and mucosal surfaces are normal. In contrast to congenital ichthyosiform erythroderma, there is little erythema. Neither form includes blistering. Autosomal recessive lamellar ichthyosis (ARLI) is a clinically and genetically heterogeneous disorder. In many cases, mutations in TGM1 gene encoding transglutaminase have been found.

In *congenital ichthyosiform erythroderma*, erythroderma tends to be persistent, and scales, although they are generalized, are finer and whiter than in lamellar ichthyosis. Erythema decreases in later life and may disappear in middle age, whereas scaling persists and may even worsen with age. Hyperkeratosis is particularly

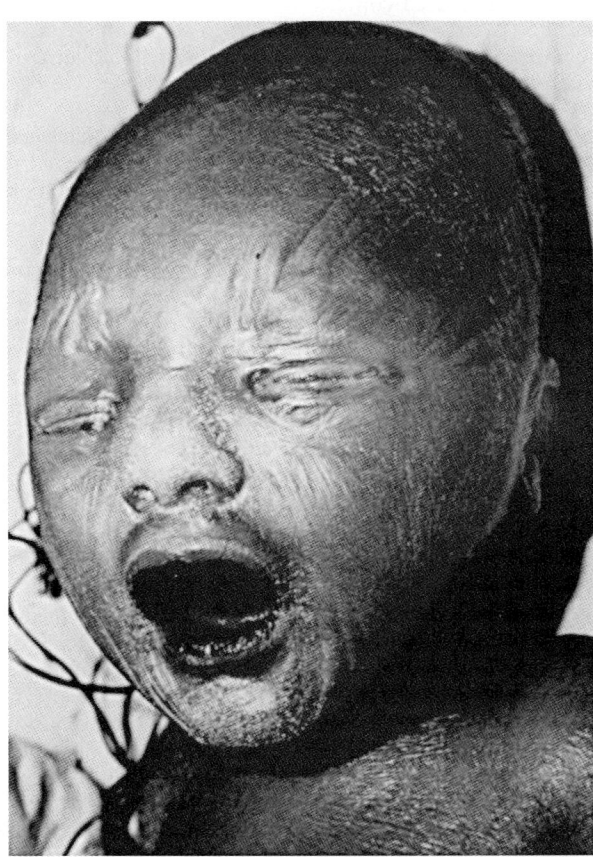

FIGURE 648–1. Typical facial appearance of a collodion baby.

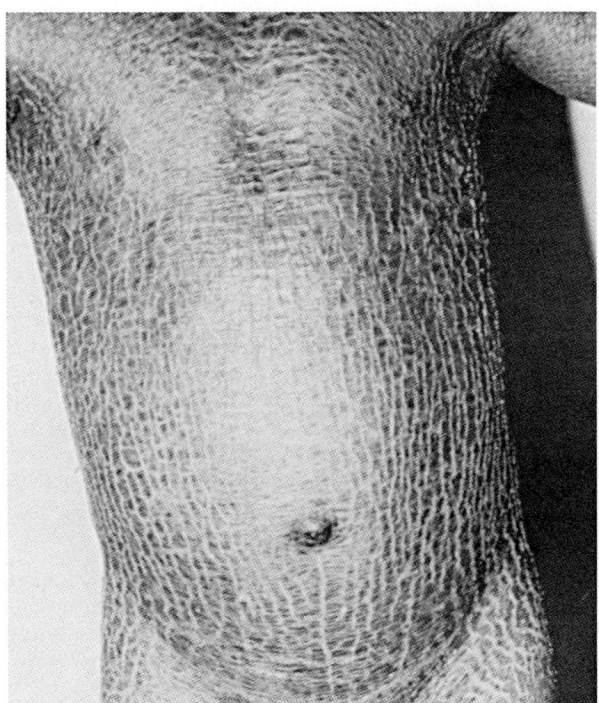

FIGURE 648–2. Generalized scaling of lamellar ichthyosis. Note the involvement of the axillary areas.

noticeable around the knees, elbows, and ankles. Palms and soles are uniformly hyperkeratotic. Some patients have sparse hair; cicatricial alopecia and nail dystrophy are found occasionally.

On histopathologic examination, lamellar ichthyosis is characterized by a markedly thickened stratum corneum and mild irregular epidermal thickening. Congenital ichthyosiform erythroderma has more epidermal thickening with parakeratosis but less hyperkeratosis and hypergranulosis than in lamellar ichthyosis. In congenital ichthyosiform erythroderma, there is a marked increase in the rate of epidermal cell production, considerably greater than the slightly increased rate observed in patients with lamellar ichthyosis.

Pruritus may be severe and responds minimally to antipruritic therapy. The unattractive appearance of the child and the malodor from bacterial colonization of macerated scales may create serious psychologic problems. Effective *treatment* includes prolonged baths with bath oil to remove excessive scales. Restriction of bathing, on the erroneous premise that accentuation of dryness will occur, only promotes malodor and accumulation of keratinous debris and contributes to pruritus and discomfort. A high-humidity environment in winter and air conditioning in summer reduce discomfort. Generous and frequent applications of emollients and keratolytic agents such as lactic or glycolic acid (5%), urea (10–25%), and retinoic acid (0.1% cream) may lessen the scaling to some extent, although these agents produce stinging if applied to fissured skin. Oral retinoids have a beneficial effect in these conditions but do not alter the underlying defect and, therefore, must be administered indefinitely. The long-term risks of these compounds (e.g., teratogenic effects and toxicity to bone) limit their usefulness. Ectropion requires ophthalmologic care and, at times, plastic procedures. Genetic counseling should be provided.

Ichthyosis Vulgaris. This autosomal dominant ichthyosis is the most common of the disorders of keratinization, with an incidence of approximately 1/300 live births. Onset generally occurs sometime after birth during the 1st yr of life and, in most cases, is trivial, consisting only of slight roughening of the skin surface. In rare cases, infants have presented as collodion babies. Scaling is most prominent on the extensor aspects of the extremities, particularly the legs and back. Flexural surfaces are spared, and the abdomen, neck, and face are relatively uninvolved. Keratosis pilaris, particularly on the upper arms and thighs, accentuated markings and hyperkeratosis on the palms and soles, and atopy are relatively common. Scaling is most pronounced during the winter months and may abate completely during warm weather. The condition may improve and even disappear with age. There is no accompanying disorder of hair, teeth, mucosal surfaces, or other organ systems.

The histopathologic changes differ from those of other types of ichthyosis in that the hyperkeratosis is associated with a decreased or absent granular layer. Abnormally small and crumbly keratohyalin granules are found in epidermal cells on electron microscopy. The rate of epidermal proliferation is normal; rather, the hyperkeratosis is due to defective desquamation. Profilaggrin, which has a role in desmosome dissolution, is deficient.

Scaling may be diminished by use of bath oil and daily applications of an emollient or a lubricant containing urea, salicylic acid, or an α-hydroxy acid, such as lactic acid.

X-Linked Ichthyosis. X-linked ichthyosis is largely limited to males, although female carriers may display some clinical manifestations of the disorder. Skin peeling may be present at birth but typically abates until 3–6 mo of life. Scaling is most pronounced on the sides of the neck, lower face, preauricular areas, anterior trunk, and the limbs, particularly the legs. The elbow and knee flexures are generally spared but may be mildly involved. The palms and soles may be slightly thickened but are

also usually spared. The condition gradually worsens in severity and extent. Keratosis pilaris is not present, and there is no increased incidence of atopy. Deep corneal opacities that do not interfere with vision develop during late childhood or adolescence and are a useful marker for the disease because they may also be present in carrier females. Cryptorchidism occurs in approximately 25% of affected males, although this may reflect an association with Kallmann syndrome, which also involves deletion on the short arm of the X chromosome. Testicular carcinoma occurs in some patients. Histologic changes include hyperkeratosis of the stratum corneum, a well-developed granular layer, and a hyperplastic epidermis.

The rate of epidermal proliferation is normal, and the hyperkeratosis is due to retention of corneocytes and delayed dissolution of the desmosomal disks. X-linked ichthyosis, however, involves a deficiency of steroid sulfatase, which hydrolyzes cholesterol sulfate and other sulfated steroids to cholesterol; cholesterol sulfate accumulates in the stratum corneum and plasma and may cause hyperkeratosis by inhibiting desmosomal proteolysis. Elevated cholesterol sulfate levels can be demonstrated in the serum, erythrocyte membranes, and epidermal cells and scales of affected males. Reduced enzyme activity can be detected in fibroblasts, keratinocytes, and leukocytes and, prenatally, in amniocytes or chorionic villus cells. In affected families, an affected male can be detected by restriction enzyme analysis of cultured chorionic villus cell DNA or amniocytes or by in situ hybridization, which identifies steroid sulfatase gene deletions prenatally in chorionic villus cells. A placental steroid sulfatase deficiency in carrier mothers results in low urinary and serum estriol values, prolonged labor, and insensitivity of the uterus to oxytocin and prostaglandins. The gene for steroid sulfatase is located on the short arm of the X chromosome (Xp22.3). Correction of steroid sulfatase deficiency is accomplished by gene transfer into tissue-cultured keratinocytes.

Hydration by bathing with bath oil and daily application of emollients and a urea-containing lubricant are usually effective *treatments*. Glycolic or lactic acid (5%) in an emollient base and propylene glycol 40–60% in water with occlusion overnight are alternative forms of therapy.

Epidermolytic Hyperkeratosis (Bullous Congenital Ichthyosiform Erythroderma). Epidermolytic hyperkeratosis is inherited as an autosomal dominant trait, although many cases are sporadic. The *clinical manifestations* are characterized by the onset at birth of generalized erythroderma and severe hyperkeratosis. The scales are small, hard, and verrucous; distinctive, parallel hyperkeratotic ridges develop over the joint flexures, including the axillary, popliteal, and antecubital fossas, and on the neck and hips. Erythema becomes less prominent after infancy; however, the hyperkeratosis persists throughout adult life. Recurrent blistering may be widespread in neonates and may cause diagnostic confusion with other blistering disorders. Blistering becomes accentuated at sites of trauma such as the knees, elbows, and lower limbs but is not problematic after age 7–8 yr. The palms and soles may be thickened, but the hair, nails, mucosa, and sweat glands are normal. Secondary bacterial infection is common and requires appropriate antibiotic therapy. Severely affected patients may have crumpled ears and ectropion.

The histopathologic pattern is *diagnostic* and consists of hyperkeratosis, a markedly thickened granular layer with an increased number of keratohyalin granules, clear spaces around nuclei, and indistinct cellular boundaries of cells in the upper epidermis. On electron microscopic examination, keratin intermediate filaments are clumped, and many desmosomes are attached to only one keratinocyte instead of connecting neighboring keratinocytes. Epidermolytic hyperkeratosis has been shown to be due to defects in either keratin 1 or 10 encoded in chromosome 12p, where the type II keratin genes are clustered. These keratins are required to form the keratin intermediate filaments in cells of the suprabasilar layers of the epidermis. Localized forms of the disease may resemble epidermal nevi (ichthyosis hystrix) or keratoderma of the palms and soles but share the distinctive histopathologic changes of epidermolytic hyperkeratosis. Prenatal diagnosis for affected families is possible by examination of DNA extracts from chorionic villus cells or amniocytes, provided that the specific mutation in the affected parent is known.

Treatment is difficult. Morbidity is increased in the neonatal period as a result of prematurity, sepsis, and fluid and electrolyte imbalance. Bacterial colonization of macerated scales produces a distinctive malodor that can be controlled somewhat by use of an antibacterial cleanser. Intermittent oral antibiotics generally are necessary. Keratolytic agents are often poorly tolerated. Oral retinoids (e.g., etretinate, acitretin, isotretinoin) may produce significant improvement, even at relatively low doses. Genetic counseling should be provided.

Ichthyosis Linearis Circumflexa. This rare autosomal recessive disorder presents at birth or in the first few months of life with generalized erythema and scaling. The trunk and limbs have diffuse erythema and superimposed migratory, polycyclic, and serpiginous hyperkeratotic lesions, some with a distinctive double-edged margin of scale. Lichenification or hyperkeratosis tends to persist in the antecubital and popliteal fossas. The face and scalp may remain erythematous and scaling. Many hair shaft deformities, most notably trichorrhexis invaginata, have been described in more than half of patients. This type of ichthyosis is characteristic of patients with Netherton syndrome (see later). Nonspecific psoriasiform changes are found on histopathologic examination.

Erythrokeratoderma Variabilis. This autosomal dominant disorder with genetic linkage to the Rh blood group usually presents in the early months of life, progresses in childhood, and stabilizes in adolescence. It is characterized by sharply demarcated hyperkeratotic plaques with geographic borders that develop in areas of normal skin or within discrete erythematous patches. Patches of erythema change shape or size within minutes to hours or days or migrate, and they may gradually became hyperkeratotic and fixed. The distribution is generalized but sparse; sites of predilection are the face, buttocks, axillae, and extensor surfaces of the limbs. The palms and soles may be thickened, but hair, teeth, and nails are normal. Histopathologic changes include hyperkeratosis, papillomatosis, and irregular hyperplasia of the epidermis.

Symmetric progressive erythrokeratoderma is an autosomal dominant disorder that presents in childhood with large, fixed, geographic and symmetric fine, scaling, hyperkeratotic, erythematous plaques primarily on the extremities, buttocks, face, ankles, and wrists. Palmoplantar keratoderma is also present. The primary feature distinguishing this from erythrokeratoderma variabilis is the lack of variable erythema, as seen in the latter condition. These two conditions may be manifestations of the same disorder.

Ichthyosiform Dermatoses. Several syndromes that include ichthyosis as a constant feature have been established as rare but distinct entities.

SJÖGREN-LARSSON SYNDROME. This autosomal recessive inborn error of metabolism consists of ichthyosis of the lamellar or congenital ichthyosiform erythroderma types, mental retardation, and spasticity. The ichthyosis is generalized but is accentuated on the flexures and the lower abdomen and consists of erythroderma, fine scaling, larger platelike scales, and dark hyperkeratosis. A degenerative defect of retinal pigment epithelium has been detected in 20–30% of affected individuals. Glistening dots in the foveal area are a cardinal ophthalmologic sign. Motor and speech developmental delays are usually noted before 1 yr of age, and spastic diplegia or tetraplegia, epilepsy,

and mental retardation generally become evident within the first 3 yr of life. Some patients may walk with the aid of braces, but most are confined to a wheelchair. The primary defect is an abnormality of fatty alcohol oxidation as a result of a deficiency of fatty aldehyde dehydrogenase, a component of the fatty alcohol-nicotinamide adenine dinucleotide oxidoreductase enzyme complex. This deficiency can be demonstrated in cultured skin fibroblasts of affected patients and carriers and, prenatally, in cultured chorionic villus cells and amniocytes from affected fetuses. Elevation of urinary leukotriene B4 (LTB4) may provide an easier approach to diagnosis.

NETHERTON SYNDROME. This autosomal recessive disorder is characterized by ichthyosis (usually ichthyosis linearis circumflexa but, occasionally, the lamellar or congenital ichthyosiform erythroderma types), trichorrhexis invaginata, and other hair shaft anomalies such as pili torti or trichorrhexis nodosa, and atopic diathesis (see Chapter 652). Mutations in the gene SPINK 5, which encodes a serine protease inhibitor, have been identified in patients with Netherton syndrome. The ichthyosis is present in the first 10 days of life and may be especially marked around the eyes, mouth, and perineal area. The erythroderma often is intensified after infection. Infants may suffer from failure to thrive, recurrent bacterial and candidal infections, elevated serum IgE levels, and marked hypernatremic dehydration. Scalp hair is sparse and short and fractures easily; eyebrows, eyelashes, and body hair are also abnormal. The most frequent allergic manifestations are urticaria, angioedema, atopic dermatitis, and asthma. Some patients are mentally retarded. The characteristic hair abnormality is seen on electron microscopy as invagination of the distal end of the hair shaft into the proximal end.

REFSUM SYNDROME (see Chapter 75.2). This multisystem disorder is inherited as an autosomal recessive trait and becomes symptomatic during the 2nd or 3rd decade of life. The ichthyosis may be generalized, is relatively mild, and resembles ichthyosis vulgaris. The ichthyosis may also be localized to the palms and soles. Chronic polyneuritis with progressive paralysis and ataxia, atypical retinitis pigmentosa, anosmia, deafness, bony abnormalities, and electrocardiographic changes are the most characteristic features. This condition is diagnosed by lipid analysis of the blood or skin, which shows elevated phytanic acid levels. Dietary avoidance of phytanic acid-containing green vegetables and dairy products produces clinical improvement.

CHONDRODYSPLASIA PUNCTATA (see Chapter 75.2). This includes several genetically heterogeneous disorders marked by ichthyosis and bone changes, principally *Conradi-Hunermann syndrome,* an X-linked dominant form affecting females only, and *rhizomelic dwarfism,* transmitted as an autosomal recessive trait. Nearly all with the X-linked dominant form and approximately 25% of patients with the recessive type have cutaneous lesions, ranging from severe, generalized erythema and scaling to mild hyperkeratosis. Rhizomelic chondrodysplasia punctata is associated with cataracts, hypertelorism, optic nerve atrophy, disproportionate shortening of the proximal extremities, psychomotor retardation, failure to thrive, and spasticity; most patients die during infancy. Numerous dysfunctional peroxisomal enzymes are found in patients with rhizomelic chondrodysplasia. Patients with the X-linked dominant form have asymmetric, variable shortening of the limbs and a distinctive ichthyosiform eruption at birth. Thick, yellow, tightly adherent keratinized plaques are distributed in a whorled pattern over the entire body, which may be intensely erythematous. The histologic changes include hyperkeratosis that penetrates to the depths of the hair follicles. The eruption typically resolves during infancy and may be superseded by a follicular atrophoderma and patchy alopecia.

Additional features in all variants include cataracts and abnormal facies with saddle nose and frontal bossing. The pathognomonic defect, termed chondrodysplasia punctata, is stippled epiphyses in the cartilaginous skeleton. This defect, which is seen in various settings and inherited disorders, often in association with peroxisomal deficiency, disappears by approximately age 3–4 yr.

Recessive X-linked chondrodysplasia punctata is due to a contiguous gene deletion affecting the recessive X-linked ichthyosis locus. These patients are deficient in steroid sulfatase activity, and their scaling resembles that in X-linked ichthyosis; peroxisomal function is normal.

RUD SYNDROME. This consists of mental retardation, epilepsy, ichthyosis (type uncertain), and sexual infantilism. Associated defects of the skeleton, eyes, dentition, and hearing have also been reported.

A number of other rare syndromes with ichthyosis as a consistent feature include the following: ichthyosis with keratitis and deafness (KID syndrome); ichthyosis with defective hair having a banded pattern under polarized light and a low sulfur content (trichothiodystrophy), hypogonadism, and mental and growth retardation (Tay syndrome); multiple sulfatase deficiency; neutral lipid storage disease with ichthyosis (Chanarin-Dorfman syndrome); and CHILD syndrome (congenital hemidysplasia with ichthyosiform erythroderma and limb defects).

Keratoderma of Palms and Soles (Keratosis Palmaris et Plantaris).

Excessive hyperkeratosis of the palms and soles may occur as a manifestation of a focal or generalized congenital hereditary skin disorder or may result from such chronic skin diseases as psoriasis, eczema, pityriasis rubra pilaris, lupus erythematosus, or Reiter disease. The names of individual disorders have been based on descriptive titles, modes of inheritance, histopathologic findings, and biochemical defects.

DIFFUSE HYPERKERATOSIS OF PALMS AND SOLES (UNNA-THOST SYNDROME, TYLOSIS). This autosomal dominant disorder presents in the first few months of life with erythema that gradually progresses to sharply demarcated hyperkeratotic scaling plaques over the palms and soles. The margins of the plaques often remain red; plaques may extend along the lateral aspects of the hands and feet and onto the volar wrists and the heels. Hyperhidrosis is usually present, but hair, teeth, and nails are usually normal. Dermatophyte infections are common and difficult to treat. Mutations in the gene for keratin 1 on chromosome 12 appear to underlie the disorder. Striate and punctate forms of palmar and plantar hyperkeratosis represent distinct entities.

EPIDERMOLYTIC HYPERKERATOSIS. This type of hyperkeratosis, which is localized to the palms and soles, is an autosomal dominant defect involving mutations in the gene for keratin 9 with clinical findings identical to those of the Unna-Thost type. There is no hyperhidrosis, however, and affected areas may blister. Histopathologic changes are characteristic.

MAL DE MELEDA (KERATODERMA PALMOPLANTARIS TRANSGREDIENS). This rare, progressive autosomal recessive condition is characterized by erythema and thick scales on the palms, fingers, soles, and flexor aspects of the wrists, knees, and elbows. Hyperhidrosis, nail thickening or koilonychia, and eczema may also occur.

MUTILATING KERATODERMA (VOHWINKEL SYNDROME). This is a progressive autosomal dominant disease with honeycombed hyperkeratosis of palms and soles, sparing the arches; starfish-like and linear keratoses on the dorsum of the hands, fingers, feet, and knees; and ainhum-like constriction of the digits that sometimes leads to autoamputation. This disorder may be associated with alopecia and hearing loss. Mutations of the gene for loricrin, a major protein of the cornified cell envelope, have been identified.

PAPILLON-LEFÈVRE SYNDROME. This autosomal recessive erythematous hyperkeratosis of the palms and soles sometimes extends to the dorsal hands and feet, elbows, and knees later in childhood. This syndrome is characterized by periodontal inflammation, leading to loss of teeth by age 4–5 yr if untreated; a tendency to frequent pyogenic skin infections; nail dystrophy, including transverse nail grooves; hyperhidrosis; and ectopic calcification of the dura.

Keratoderma of palms and soles also occurs as a feature of some forms of ichthyosis and ectodermal dysplasia. *Richner-Hanhart syndrome* is an autosomal recessive palmoplantar keratoderma with corneal ulcers, progressive mental impairment, and a deficiency of tyrosine aminotransferase, which leads to tyrosinemia. *Pachyonychia congenita* is transmitted as an autosomal dominant trait with variable expressivity. The classic type I form *(Jadassohn-Lewandowski syndrome)* is due to mutations in the gene for keratin 16. Major features of the syndrome are onychogryphosis; palmoplantar keratoderma; follicular hyperkeratosis, especially of the elbows and knees; and oral leukokeratosis. The nail dystrophy is the most striking feature and may be present at birth or develop early in life. The nails are thickened and tubular, projecting upward at the free edge to form a conical roof over a mass of subungual keratotic debris. Repeated paronychial inflammation may result in shedding of the nails. The feature seen most consistently among patients with this condition is keratoderma of the palms and soles. Additional associated features include hyperhidrosis of the palms and soles, and bullae and erosions on the palms and soles. Some patients have shown a selective cell-mediated defect in recognition and processing of candida. Surgical removal of the nails and excision of the nail matrix have been helpful in some patients.

Patients with palmoplantar hyperhidrosis may have macerated plaques that become secondarily infected and malodorous. Morbidity is lessened if the hyperkeratosis can be controlled by *treatment*; however, only mild palliation is achieved with applications of lubricants, keratolytic agents (urea, salicylic acid, lactic acid), and oral retinoids including etretinate, isotretinoin, and acitretin. Soaking in saline solution followed by debridement is a mainstay of treatment.

DiGiovanna JJ, Bale SJ: Epidermolytic hyperkeratosis: Applied molecular genetics. *J Invest Dermatol* 1994;102:390.

Huber M, Rettler I, Bernasconi K, et al: Mutations of keratinocyte transglutaminase in lamellar ichthyosis. *Science* 1995;267:525.

Paller AS: Disorders of cornification (ichthyosis). In Eichenfield LF, Frieden IJ, Esterly NB (editors): *Textbook of Neonatology.* Philadelphia, WB Saunders, 2001, p. 276.

Proksch E, Holleran WM, Menon GK, et al: Barrier function regulates epidermal lipid and DNA synthesis. *Br J Dermatol* 1993;128:473.

Rabinowitz LG, Esterly NB: Atopic dermatitis and ichthyosis vulgaris. *Pediatr Rev* 1994;15:220.

Rizzo WB: Sjögren-Larsson syndrome. *Semin Dermatol* 1993;12:210.

Russell LJ, DiGiovanna JJ, Rogers GR, et al: Mutations in the gene transglutaminase 1 in autosomal recessive lamellar ichthyosis. *Nat Genet* 1995;9:279.

Willemsen MAAP, deJong JGN, van Domburg PHMI, et al: Defective inactivation of leukotriene B4 in patients with Sjögren-Larsson syndrome. *J Pediatr* 2000;136:258.

Williams ML: Ichthyosis: Mechanisms of disease. *Pediatr Dermatol* 1992;9:365.

Williams ML, Elias PM: From basket weave to barrier. Unifying concepts for the pathogenesis of the diseases of cornification. *Arch Dermatol* 1993;129:626.

Chapter 649
Diseases of the Dermis

Keloid. A keloid is a sharply demarcated, benign, dense growth of connective tissue that forms in the dermis after trauma. The lesions are firm, raised, pink, and rubbery; they may be tender or pruritic. Sites of predilection are the face, earlobes, neck, shoulders, upper trunk, sternum, and lower legs. Keloids are usually induced by trauma and commonly follow ear piercing, burns, scalds, and surgical procedures. Certain individuals, especially blacks, seem predisposed to keloid formation. In some cases, a familial tendency (recessive or dominant inheritance) or the presence of foreign material in the wound appears to have a pathogenic role. Keloids are a rare feature of Ehlers-Danlos syndrome, Rubinstein-Taybi syndrome, and pachydermoperiostosis. In both keloids and hypertrophic scars, new collagen forms over a much longer period than in wounds that heal normally. Histopathologically, a keloid consists of whorled and interlaced hyalinized collagen fibers.

Keloids should be differentiated from hypertrophic scars, which remain confined to the site of injury and gradually involute over time. Young keloids may diminish in size if injected intralesionally at 4-wk intervals with triamcinolone suspension (10 mg/mL). At times, a more concentrated suspension is required. Large or old keloids may require surgical excision followed by intralesional injections of corticosteroid. The risk of recurrence at the same site argues against surgical excision alone. Placement of topical silicon gel sheeting over the keloid for several hours per day for several weeks may help some patients.

Striae Cutis Distensae. These thinned, depressed, erythematous bands of atrophic skin eventually become silvery, opalescent, and smooth. They occur most frequently in areas that have been subject to distention, such as the lower back, buttocks, thighs, breasts, abdomen, and shoulders. The most frequent causes are rapid growth, pregnancy, obesity, Cushing disease, or prolonged corticosteroid therapy. Adolescent striae tend to become less conspicuous with time. Histopathologically, striae distensae resemble scars.

Corticosteroid-Induced Atrophy. Both topical and systemic corticosteroid treatment can result in cutaneous atrophy. This is particularly common when a potent topical corticosteroid is applied under occlusion or to the intertriginous areas for a prolonged period. Affected skin is thin, fragile, smooth, and semitransparent, with telangiectasias and loss of normal skin markings. Histopathologically, one sees thinning of the stratum corneum and malpighii. Spaces between dermal collagen and elastic fibers are small, producing a more compact but thin dermis. The mechanism involves inhibition of synthesis of collagen type I, noncollagenous proteins, and total protein content of the skin; progressive reduction of dermal proteoglycans and glycosaminoglycans; and possibly prolonged vasoconstriction-induced ischemia. Retinoids applied topically restore these steroid-induced biochemical changes in the dermal connective tissue of the hairless mouse, without abrogating the beneficial anti-inflammatory effects.

Granuloma Annulare. This common dermatosis occurs predominantly in children and young adults. Typical lesions begin as erythematous, firm, smooth papules; they gradually enlarge to form annular plaques with a papular border and a normal, slightly atrophic or discolored central area (Fig. 649–1) up to several centimeters in size. Lesions may occur anywhere on the body, but mucous membranes are spared. Favored sites include the dorsum of the hands and feet. *Annular lesions* are often mistaken for tinea corporis because of the elevated advancing border; they differ in that they are not scaly. *Papular lesions*, another variant, may simulate rheumatoid nodules, particularly when grouped on the fingers and elbows. The disseminated papular form, which is provoked by light in some cases, is rare in children. *Subcutaneous granuloma annulare* is especially common in children; it tends to develop on the scalp and limbs, particularly in the pretibial area. These lesions are firm, usually nontender, skin-colored nodules. *Perforating granuloma annulare* is characterized by the development of a yellowish center in some of the superficial papular lesions as a result of transepidermal elimination of altered collagen.

A biopsy is occasionally required for diagnosis. The lesions consist of a granuloma with a central area of necrotic collagen;

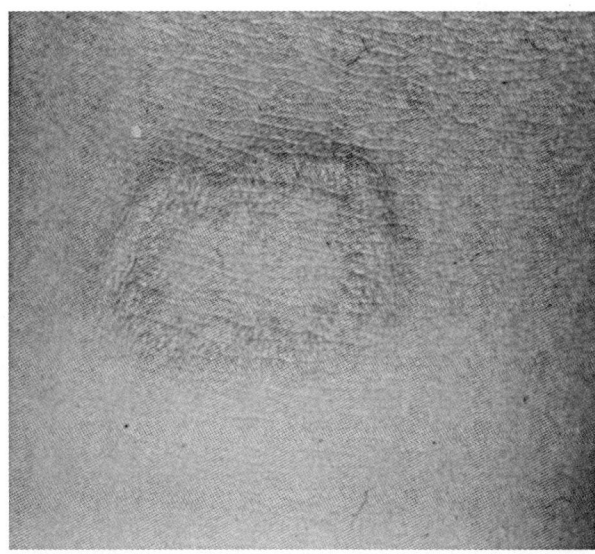

FIGURE 649–1. Annular lesion with a raised papular border and depressed center, characteristic of granuloma annulare.

mucin deposition; and a peripheral palisading infiltrate of lymphocytes, histiocytes, and foreign body giant cells. The pattern resembles that of necrobiosis lipoidica and rheumatoid nodule (see Chapter 145), but subtle histologic differences usually permit differentiation. The cause of granuloma annulare is unknown. Affected children are usually healthy. Some cases of granuloma annulare, particularly the generalized form, may be associated with diabetes mellitus. The eruption persists for months to years, but spontaneous resolution without residual change is usual; 75% of lesions clear within 2 yr. Application of a potent topical corticosteroid preparation or intralesional injections of corticosteroid may hasten involution, but nonintervention is acceptable.

Necrobiosis Lipoidica. This rare disorder presents as erythematous papules that evolve into irregularly shaped, sharply demarcated, yellow, sclerotic plaques with central telangiectasia and a violaceous border. Scaling, crusting, and ulceration are frequent. Lesions develop most commonly on the shins. Slow extension of a given lesion over the years is usual, but long periods of quiescence or complete healing with scarring may occur.

Histopathologically, poorly defined areas of necrobiotic collagen are seen throughout, but primarily low in the dermis, associated with mucin deposition. Surrounding the necrobiotic, disordered areas of collagen is a palisading lymphohistiocytic granulomatous infiltrate. Some lesions are more characteristically granulomatous, with limited necrobiosis of collagen. Necrobiosis lipoidica must be differentiated clinically from xanthomas, morphea, granuloma annulare, and pretibial myxedema. Fifty to 75% of patients have diabetes mellitus; necrobiosis lipoidica occurs in 0.3% of all diabetic patients. The lesions persist despite good control of the diabetes but may improve minimally after applications of high-potency topical steroids or local injection of a corticosteroid.

Lichen Sclerosus et Atrophicus. This presents initially with ivory-colored, shiny, indurated papules, often with a violaceous halo. The surface shows prominent dilated pilosebaceous or sweat duct orifices that often contain yellow or brown horny plugs. The papules coalesce to form irregular plaques of variable size, which may develop hemorrhagic bullae in their margins. In the latter stages, atrophy results in a depressed plaque with a wrinkled surface. This disorder occurs more commonly in girls than in boys. Sites of predilection in girls are the vulvar, perianal, and perineal skin. Extensive involvement may produce a sclerotic, atrophic plaque of hourglass configuration; shrinkage of the labia and stenosis of the introitus may result. Vaginal discharge precedes vulvar lesions in approximately 20% of patients. In boys, the prepuce and glans penis are often involved, usually in association with phimosis; most boys with the disorder were not circumcised early in life. Sites elsewhere on the body that are most commonly involved include the upper trunk, the neck, the axillae, the flexor surfaces of wrists, and the areas around the umbilicus and the eyes. Pruritus may be severe.

In children, this disorder is most frequently confused with focal scleroderma (morphea) (see Chapter 150), with which it may coexist. In the genital area, it may be mistakenly attributed to sexual abuse. Biopsy is diagnostic, revealing hyperkeratosis with follicular plugging, hydropic degeneration of basal cells, a bandlike dermal lymphocytic infiltrate, homogenized collagen, and thinned elastic fibers in the upper dermis. The lesions may involute spontaneously, usually before or at the time of menarche; involution is more likely to occur in those in whom the disorder developed at a younger age. Leukoplakia and squamous cell carcinoma may rarely develop. Potent topical corticosteroids may provide relief from pruritus and produce clearing of lesions, including those in the genital area. Topical progesterone 1% and testosterone 2% preparations have also been used for genital lesions.

Scleredema (Scleredema Adultorum, Scleredema of Buschke). Approximately 30% of cases of scleredema develop before the age of 10 yr. Onset is sudden, with brawny edema of the face and neck that spreads rapidly to involve the thorax and arms in a sweater distribution; the abdomen and legs are usually spared. The face acquires a waxy, masklike appearance; the involved areas feel indurated and woody, are nonpitting, and are not sharply demarcated from normal skin. The overlying skin is normal in color and is not atrophic. Systemic involvement, which is uncommon, is marked by thickening of the tongue; dysarthria; dysphagia; restriction of eye and joint movements; and pleural, pericardial, and peritoneal effusions. Electrocardiographic changes may also be observed.

In 65–90% of cases, the disease follows an infection such as tonsillitis, pharyngitis, influenza, scarlet fever, measles, mumps, impetigo, or cellulitis after an interval of days or weeks; most cases follow a streptococcal infection. Onset may be heralded by a prodrome of fever, arthralgia, myalgia, and malaise. Onset in diabetic patients may occur insidiously. Laboratory data are not helpful. Some cases, however, are associated with immunoglobulin (Ig)G or IgA paraproteinemia. Skin biopsy demonstrates an increase in dermal thickness as a result of swelling and homogenization of the collagen bundles, which are separated by large interfibrous spaces. Increased amounts of mucopolysaccharides in the dermis can be identified by special stains.

The active phase of the disease persists for 2–8 wk; spontaneous and complete resolution usually occurs in 6 mo–2 yr. Recurrent attacks are unusual. The disorder must be differentiated from scleroderma, morphea, myxedema, trichinosis, dermatomyositis, sclerema neonatorum, and subcutaneous fat necrosis. There is no specific therapy.

Lipoid Proteinosis (Urbach-Wiethe Disease, Hyalinosis Cutis et Mucosae). This autosomal recessive disorder consists of infiltration of hyaline material into the skin, oral cavity, larynx, and internal organs. It may be noted initially in early infancy as hoarseness. Skin lesions appear during childhood and consist of yellowish papules and nodules that may coalesce to form plaques on the face, forearms, neck, genitals, dorsum of the fingers, and scalp, where they result in patchy alopecia. Similar deposits are found on the lips, undersurface of the tongue, fauces, uvula, epiglottis, and vocal cords. The tongue becomes enlarged and feels firm on palpation; patients may be unable to protrude their tongue. Translucent nodules along the margins of the eyelids, causing thickening of the eyelids, are the most char-

acteristic clinical manifestation. Pock-like atrophic scars may develop on the face. Hypertrophic, hyperkeratotic nodules occur at sites of friction such as the elbows and knees; the palms may be diffusely thickened. The disease progresses until early adult life, but the prognosis is good. Involvement of the larynx can lead to respiratory compromise, particularly in infancy, necessitating tracheostomy. Associated anomalies include dental abnormalities, epilepsy, and recurrent parotitis as a result of infiltrates in the Stensen duct; virtually any organ can be involved. There is no specific treatment.

The distinctive histologic pattern includes dilatation of dermal blood vessels and infiltration of homogeneous eosinophilic extracellular hyaline material along capillary walls and around sweat glands. Hyaline material in homogeneous bundles, diffusely arranged in the upper dermis, produces a thickened dermis. The infiltrates appear to contain both lipid and mucopolysaccharide substances. Symmetric ossification lateral to the sella turcica in the medial temporal region, identifiable roentgenographically, is pathognomonic but is not always present. The biochemical defect is unknown but may represent a lysosomal storage disorder caused by single or numerous enzyme defects. Alterations in the distribution of collagens I, III, IV, and V have also been described.

Macular Atrophy (Anetoderma). Anetoderma is characterized by circumscribed areas of slack skin associated with loss of dermal substance. This disorder may have no associated underlying disease (primary macular atrophy) or may develop after an inflammatory skin condition (secondary macular atrophy) such as syphilis, lupus erythematosus, acne, varicella, leprosy, urticaria pigmentosa, or *Staphylococcus epidermidis* folliculitis. Lesions vary from 0.5–1 cm in diameter and, if inflammatory, may initially be erythematous. They subsequently become thin, wrinkled, and blue-white or hypopigmented. The lesions often protrude as small outpouchings that, on palpation, may be readily indented into the subcutaneous tissue because of the dermal atrophy. Sites of predilection include the trunk, thighs, upper arms, and less commonly the neck and face. Lesions remain unchanged for life; new lesions often continue to develop for years. There is no effective therapy, although some authorities have reported benefit from penicillin or pentoxifylline.

All types of macular atrophy show focal loss of elastic tissue on histopathologic examination, a change that is not recognizable unless special stains are used. The elastolysis may be due to release of elastase from inflammatory cells, such as macrophages, in contact with elastic fibers. Lesions of anetoderma occasionally resemble morphea, lichen sclerosus et atrophicus, focal dermal hypoplasia, atrophic scars, or end-stage lesions of chronic bullous dermatoses.

Cutis Laxa (Dermatomegaly, Generalized Elastolysis). Cutis laxa is a congenital autosomal recessive or autosomal dominant disorder. Affected newborn infants may appear prematurely aged. When onset appears to occur during childhood or adulthood, the disorder is termed *acquired cutis laxa*. Cutis laxa has developed after a febrile illness, inflammatory skin diseases such as lupus erythematosus or erythema multiforme, amyloidosis, urticaria, angioedema, and hypersensitivity reactions to penicillin, and in infants born to women who were taking penicillamine.

CLINICAL MANIFESTATIONS. There may be widespread folds of lax skin, or changes may be mild and limited in extent, resembling anetoderma. Patients with severe cutis laxa have characteristic facial features, including an aged appearance with sagging jowls (bloodhound appearance), a hooked nose with everted nostrils, a short columella, a long upper lip, and everted lower eyelids. The skin is also lax elsewhere on the body and may resemble an ill-fitting suit (Fig. 649–2). Hyperelasticity and hypermobility of the joints are not present as they are in the Ehlers-Danlos syndrome. Many infants have a hoarse cry, probably as a

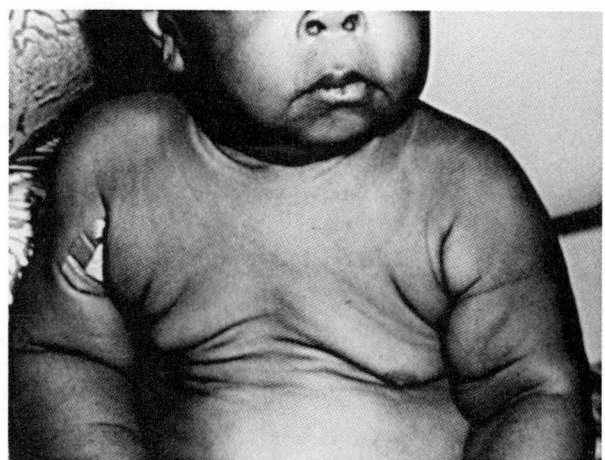

FIGURE 649–2. Pendulous folds of skin of an infant with cutis laxa. Note the long upper lip and upturned nose.

result of laxity of the vocal cords. Tensile strength of the skin is normal. Histologically, elastic tissue is reduced throughout the dermis, with fragmentation, distention, and clumping of the elastic fibers.

The dominant form of cutis laxa may develop at any age and is generally benign and mainly of cosmetic significance. When it presents in infancy, it may be associated with intrauterine growth retardation, ligamentous laxity, and delayed closure of fontanels. Affected males may be impotent and have infantile genitals and scanty body hair. Pulmonary emphysema and mild cardiovascular manifestations may also occur. In contrast, those with the more common recessive form of the disease are susceptible to severe complications, such as multiple hernias, rectal prolapse, diaphragmatic atony, diverticula of the gastrointestinal and genitourinary tracts, cor pulmonale, emphysema, pneumothoraces, peripheral pulmonary artery stenosis, and aortic dilatation. Characteristic facial features include downward slanting palpebral fissures; a broad, flat nose; and large ears. Skeletal anomalies, dental caries, growth retardation, and developmental delay also occur. Such patients often have a shortened life span.

The *pathogenesis* of cutis laxa is not well known. Abnormalities that have been described include excessive enzymatic destruction of elastin, decreased elastase inhibitor levels, and decreased elastin messenger RNA levels in fibroblasts.

Ehlers-Danlos Syndrome. This is a group of genetically (usually autosomal dominant) heterogeneous connective tissue disorders. Affected children appear normal at birth, but skin hyperelasticity, fragility of the skin and blood vessels, delayed wound healing, and joint hypermobility develop. The essential defect is a quantitative deficiency of fibrillar collagen. Many patients have haploinsufficiency of the type V collagen (*COL5A1*) gene. Others may have mutations in collagen modifying genes such as a recessive form with tenascin-X deficiency. Ehlers-Danlos syndrome has been classified into 10 clinical forms.

I. GRAVIS TYPE. This autosomal dominant disorder is characterized by premature birth caused by rupture of membranes, skin hyperelasticity and fragility, easy bruising, generalized and severe joint hypermobility, scoliosis, and mitral valve prolapse. Insignificant lacerations may form gaping wounds that leave broad, atrophic, papyraceous scars. Additional cutaneous manifestations include molluscoid pseudotumors over pressure points from accumulations of connective tissue. Life expectancy is not reduced.

II. MITIS TYPE. This autosomal dominant form is characterized by mild skin and joint manifestations, the latter limited to hands and feet. The incidence of premature birth is not increased.

III. BENIGN, HYPERMOBILE TYPE. This disorder has autosomal dominant inheritance and is manifested as generalized severe joint hypermobility and minimal skin manifestations. Osteoarthritis may develop prematurely.

IV. ECCHYMOTIC (SACK) TYPE. This form may have autosomal dominant or autosomal recessive inheritance and shows the most pronounced dermal thinning of all; consequently, the underlying venous network is prominent. The skin has minimal hyperextensibility, and the joints are not hypermobile, except perhaps during childhood. Premature birth; extensive ecchymoses from trauma; a high incidence of keloids; rupture of the bowel, especially the colon; uterine rupture during pregnancy; rupture of the great vessels; dissecting aortic aneurysm; and stroke all contribute to the increased morbidity and shortened life span. Patients should be advised to avoid becoming pregnant, avoid activities such as trumpet playing that raise intracranial pressure as a result of a Valsalva maneuver, and minimize trauma to the skin. Defects that have been identified in affected patients include multiple deletions, exon skipping, or point mutations in the *COL3A1* gene of collagen III.

V. X-LINKED TYPE. This is characterized by minimal joint hypermobility and skin hyperelasticity and moderate bruising, skin fragility, and scarring. The life span is normal. Lysyl oxidase was deficient in one family with this disorder.

VI. AUTOSOMAL RECESSIVE OCULAR TYPE. These patients have joint hyperextensibility, hypotonia, kyphoscoliosis, fragile cornea, keratoconus, skin hyperelasticity, and fragile bones. There is a mutation affecting a collagen structural protein. Patients lack lysyl hydroxylase, a crucial enzyme in collagen biosynthesis that catalyzes the formation of hydroxylysine, which cross-links collagen. Prenatal diagnosis is available by measuring lysyl hydroxylase activity in amniocytes. The diagnosis can also be confirmed by detecting decreased lysyl hydroxylase activity in cultured dermal fibroblasts. This form may respond to oral ascorbic acid.

VII. ARTHROCHALASIS MULTIPLEX CONGENITA. The A type is an autosomal recessive disorder characterized by short stature, marked joint hyperextensibility and dislocation, and moderate hyperelasticity and bruisability of skin. The defect is a failure of cleavage of the N-terminus propeptide of type I procollagen chains by procollagen N-proteinase caused by a mutation in the *COL1A1* gene that results in loss of the procollagen N-proteinase cleavage site. The B type, possibly autosomal dominant, is characterized by skin hyperelasticity and marked joint hypermobility. Mutations in the *COL1A2* gene cause loss of the N-proteinase cleavage site in the pro-α_2 (I) collagen chain. The type C disorder, known as dermatosparaxis, includes premature rupture of membranes; delayed closure of fontanels; skin fragility and laxity; easy bruisability; growth retardation; short limbs; umbilical hernia; and characteristic facies with micrognathia, jowls, and prominent, puffy eyelids. This disorder is due to a lack of N-proteinase activity.

VIII. PERIODONTITIS TYPE. This autosomal dominant disorder is characterized by mild skin hyperelasticity, small joint hypermobility, bruisability, moderate cutaneous fragility, abnormal scarring, and severe periodontitis, leading to premature loss of teeth and alveolar bone. The proportion of type III collagen is reduced.

IX. X-LINKED RECESSIVE SKELETAL TYPE. This form is characterized by occipital exostoses; widening and bowing of long bones at tendinous and ligamentous insertion sites; short, broad clavicles; mild skin hyperelasticity; bladder diverticula with spontaneous rupture; inguinal hernias; and chronic diarrhea. Defective copper transport results in low serum copper and ceruloplasm levels and diminished lysyl oxidase activity, an important copper-dependent enzyme required for collagen cross-linking. Menkes disease and X-linked cutis laxa also have altered copper metabolism and defective collagen fibril formation; these may be examples of type IX Ehlers-Danlos syndrome.

X. DYSFIBRONECTINEMIC TYPE. This autosomal recessive disorder is characterized by fibronectin-correctable failure of platelet aggregation, easy bruisability, joint hypermobility, and skin hyperextensibility.

DIFFERENTIAL DIAGNOSIS. Ehlers-Danlos syndrome has been confused with cutis laxa, but the features of the two disorders differ considerably. The skin of patients with cutis laxa hangs in redundant folds, whereas the skin in Ehlers-Danlos syndrome is hyperextensible and snaps back into place when stretched. Because of the marked skin fragility in Ehlers-Danlos syndrome, minor trauma results in ecchymoses, bleeding, and poor healing with atrophic cigarette-paper scars, which are most prominent on the forehead and lower legs, and over pressure points. Surgical procedures are fraught with risk; dehiscence of wounds is common.

Pseudoxanthoma Elasticum. This disorder of elastic tissue primarily affects the dermis, retina, and cardiovascular system.

CLINICAL MANIFESTATIONS. Onset of skin manifestations often occurs during childhood, but the changes produced by early lesions are subtle and may not be recognized. The characteristic pebbly "plucked chicken skin" cutaneous lesions are asymptomatic, 1–2-mm yellow papules that are arranged in a linear or reticulated pattern or in confluent plaques. Preferred sites are the flexural neck, axillary and inguinal folds, umbilicus, thighs, and antecubital and popliteal fossas. As the lesions become more pronounced, the skin acquires a velvety texture and droops in lax, inelastic folds. The face is usually spared. Mucous membrane lesions may involve the lips, buccal cavity, rectum, and vagina. Involvement of the connective tissue of the media and intima of blood vessels, Bruch membrane of the eye, and endocardium or pericardium may result in visual disturbances, angioid streaks in Bruch membrane, intermittent claudication, cerebral and coronary occlusion, hypertension, and hemorrhage from the gastrointestinal tract, uterus, or mucosal surfaces. Affected women have an increased risk of miscarriage in the first trimester. Arterial involvement generally presents in adulthood, but claudication and angina have occurred in early childhood. There is no effective *treatment*, although laser therapy may help to prevent retinal hemorrhage.

PATHOLOGY AND PATHOGENESIS. Histopathologic examination shows fragmented, swollen, and clumped elastic fibers in the middle and lower third of the dermis. The fibers stain positively for calcium. Collagen in the vicinity of the altered elastic fibers is reduced in amount and is split into small fibers. Aberrant calcification of the elastic fibers of the internal elastic lamina of arteries leads to narrowing of vessel lumina. It is hypothesized that an abnormal glycosaminoglycan is secreted by fibroblasts and deposited on the surface of elastic fibers, leading to fragmentation and calcification of the coated fibers. Candidate genes for pseudoxanthoma elasticum include the genes encoding elastin; the fibrillins, which form a microfibrillar coating around elastin; and lysyl oxidase, which catalyzes formation of the desmosines, the covalent interchain cross links that stabilize elastin polypeptides into their fibrillar structure. There are two autosomal dominant and two autosomal recessive forms of the disease. However, all affected patients tend to merge into a single classic phenotype involving the skin, eyes, and cardiovascular system, with considerable variability in expression of the disorder, particularly in the vascular and ophthalmologic complications.

Elastosis Perforans Serpiginosa. This is an unusual skin disorder in which 1–3 mm, skin-colored, keratotic, firm papules tend to cluster in arcuate and annular patterns on the posterolateral neck and limbs and, occasionally, on the face and trunk. Onset usually occurs during childhood or adolescence. Histopathologically, a papule consists of a circumscribed area of epidermal hyperplasia that communicates with the underlying dermis by a narrow channel. Elastotic material is extruded from the channel. There is a great increase in the amount and size of elastic fibers in the upper dermis, particularly in the dermal papillae. The primary abnormality is probably in the dermal elastin, which provokes a cellular response that ultimately leads to extrusion of the abnormal elastic tissue. Approximately one third of cases occur in association with osteogenesis imperfecta, Marfan syndrome, pseudoxanthoma elasticum, Ehlers-Danlos syndrome, Rothmund-Thomson syndrome, and Down syndrome. It has also occurred in association with penicillamine therapy. Differential diagnosis includes tinea corporis, perforating granuloma annulare, reactive perforating collagenosis, lichen planus, creeping eruption, and porokeratosis of Mibelli. Treatment is ineffective; however, the lesions are asymptomatic and disappear spontaneously.

Reactive Perforating Collagenosis. This usually presents in early childhood with small papules on the dorsal areas of the hands and forearms, elbows, knees, and sometimes face and trunk. The condition is often familial and may be inherited in an autosomal recessive pattern. Over a period of several weeks, the papules increase in size to 5–10 mm, become umbilicated, and develop a keratotic plug in the center. Individual lesions resolve spontaneously in 2–4 mo, leaving a hypopigmented macule or scar. Lesions may recur in crops; may undergo a linear Koebner reaction; and may form in response to cold temperatures or superficial trauma such as abrasions, insect bites, and acne lesions. Histopathologically, collagen in the papillary dermis is engulfed within a cup-shaped perforation in the epidermis. The central crater contains pyknotic inflammatory cells and keratinous debris. The process appears to represent transepidermal elimination of altered collagen. Topical retinoic acid may reduce the number of lesions.

Xanthomas. See Chapter 75.3.

Fabry Disease. See Chapter 75.4.

Mucopolysaccharidoses. See Chapter 77. In several of these disorders, thick, inelastic, rough skin, particularly on the extremities, and generalized hirsutism are characteristic but nonspecific features. Telangiectasias on the face, forearms, trunk, and legs have been observed in Scheie and Morquio syndromes. In some patients with Hunter syndrome, distinctive ivory-colored, firm papulonodules with a corrugated surface texture are grouped into symmetric plaques on the upper trunk, arms, and thighs. Onset of these unusual lesions occurs during the 1st decade of life, and spontaneous disappearance has been noted.

Mastocytosis. Mastocytosis encompasses a spectrum of disorders that range from solitary cutaneous nodules to diffuse infiltration of skin associated with involvement of other organs (Box 649–1). All the disorders are characterized by aggregates of mast cells in the dermis. Mast cell growth factor, which can be secreted by keratinocytes, stimulates the proliferation of mast cells and increases the production of melanin by melanocytes. Mastocytosis may be due to altered cutaneous metabolism of mast cell growth factor and, thus, may represent a hyperplastic rather than a neoplastic disorder. Mutations in c-KIT are seen in pediatric onset mastocytosis with extracutaneous involvement.

CLINICAL MANIFESTATIONS. Affected children can have intense pruritus. Systemic signs of histamine release, such as hypotension, syncope, headache, episodic flushing, tachycardia, wheezing, colic, and diarrhea, occur most frequently in the more severe types of mastocytosis. The local and systemic manifestations of the disease are due, at least partially, to release of histamine and heparin from mast cell granules; although heparin is present in significant amounts in mast cells, coagulation disturbances occur only rarely. The vasodilator prostaglandin D_2 or its

BOX 649–1. Mastocytosis Classification

CUTANEOUS MASTOCYTOSIS

1. Urticaria pigmentosa
2. Diffuse cutaneous mastocytosis
3. Mastocytoma of the skin

SYSTEMIC MASTOCYTOSIS (WITHOUT AHNMD OR LEUKEMIC MAST CELL DISEASE)

1. Systemic indolent mastocytosis
2. Systemic smoldering mastocytosis

SYSTEMIC MASTOCYTOSIS WITH AN AHNMD

1. Myeloproliferative syndrome
2. Myelodysplastic syndrome
3. Acute myeloid leukemia
4. Non–Hodgkin lymphoma

SYSTEMIC AGGRESSIVE MASTOCYTOSIS
MAST CELL LEUKEMIA
MAST CELL SARCOMA
EXTRACUTANEOUS MASTOCYTOMA

Classification adopted from World Health Organization classification. AHNMD, associated hematologic non–mast cell disorder.
Adapted from Carter MC, Metcalfe DD: Paediatric mastocytosis. *Arch Dis Child* 2002; 86:315–9.

---

metabolite appears to exacerbate the flushing response. Serum trypase levels are often elevated.

Mastocytomas are solitary lesions 1–5 cm in diameter. Lesions may be present at birth or arise during early infancy at any site; the wrist, neck, and trunk are sites of predilection. The lesions may present as recurrent, evanescent wheals or bullae; in time, however, an infiltrated, rubbery, pink, yellow, or tan plaque develops at the site of whealing or blistering (Fig. 649–3*A*). The surface acquires a pebbly, orange peel-like texture, and hyperpigmentation may become prominent. Stroking or trauma to the nodule may result in urtication (Darier sign) as a result of local histamine release; rarely, systemic signs of histamine release become apparent. The differential diagnosis includes recurrent bullous impetigo, nevi, and juvenile xanthogranuloma. Mastocytomas usually involve spontaneously during early childhood; troublesome lesions can be excised and do not recur. Only rarely do multiple cutaneous lesions develop.

Urticaria pigmentosa is the most common form of mastocytosis and occurs primarily in infants and children. Lesions may be present at birth but more often erupt in crops during the first several months to 2 yr of age. In some cases, early bullous or urticarial lesions fade, only to recur at the same site, ultimately becoming fixed and hyperpigmented; in others, the initial lesions are hyperpigmented. Vesiculation usually abates by 2 yr of age. Individual lesions range in size from a few millimeters to

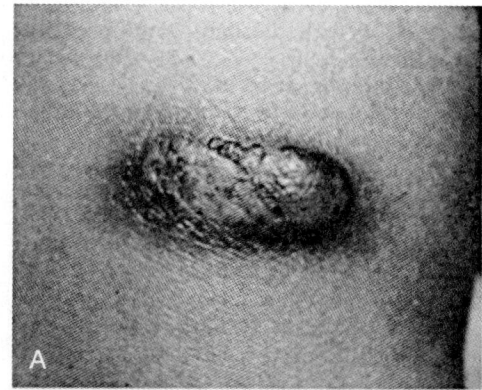

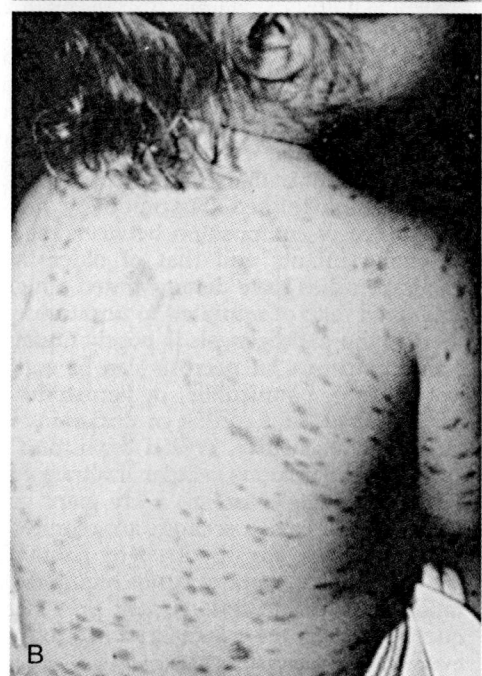

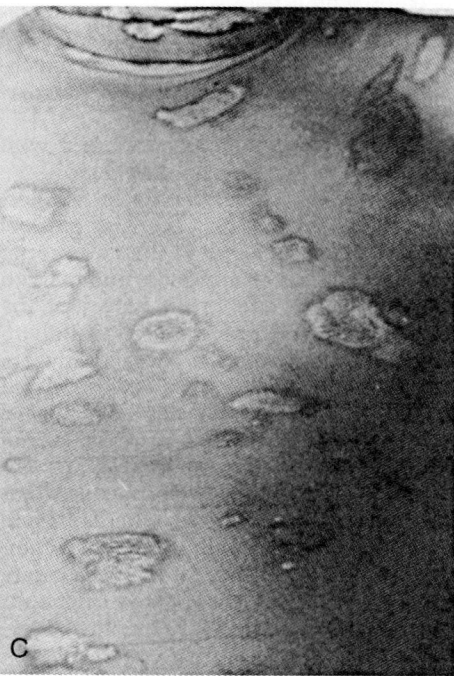

FIGURE 649–3. *A,* Solitary mastocytoma that is partially blistered. *B,* Hyperpigmented papular lesions of urticaria pigmentosa, some of which exhibit a surrounding flare. *C,* Infiltrated plaques of urticaria pigmentosa.

several centimeters and may be macular, papular, or nodular; they range in color from yellow-tan to chocolate brown and often have ill-defined borders (see Fig. 649–3B). Larger nodular lesions, like mastocytomas, may have a characteristic orange peel texture (see Fig. 649–3C). Lesions of urticaria pigmentosa may be sparse or numerous and are often symmetrically distributed. Palms, soles, and face are sometimes spared, as are the mucous membranes. The rapid appearance of erythema and whealing in response to vigorous stroking of a lesion can usually be elicited; dermographism of intervening normal skin is also common. Urticaria pigmentosa can be confused with drug eruptions, postinflammatory pigmentary change, juvenile xanthogranuloma, pigmented nevi, ephelides, xanthomas, chronic urticaria, insect bites, and bullous impetigo.

PROGNOSIS. Spontaneous involution occurs in about 50% of patients by puberty; another 25% have partial resolution by adulthood. The incidence of systemic manifestations is very low.

Diffuse Cutaneous Mastocytosis. This variant is characterized by diffuse involvement of the skin rather than discrete hyperpigmented lesions. Affected patients are usually normal at birth and develop features of the disorder after the first few months of life. Rarely, the condition may present with intense generalized pruritus in the absence of visible skin changes. The skin usually appears thickened and pink to yellow and may have a doughy feel and a texture resembling an orange peel. Surface changes are accentuated in flexural areas. Recurrent bullae, intractable pruritus, and flushing attacks are common, as is systemic involvement.

Telangiectasia macularis eruptiva perstans is another variant that consists of telangiectatic hyperpigmented macules that are usually localized to the trunk. These lesions do not urticate when stroked. This form of the disease is seen in adolescents and adults primarily.

Systemic Mastocytosis. This disorder is marked by an abnormal increase in the number of mast cells in other than cutaneous tissues. It occurs in approximately 5–10% of patients with mastocytosis and is more common in adults than in children. Bone lesions may be silent but are detectable radiologically as osteoporotic or osteosclerotic areas, principally in the axial skeleton. Gastrointestinal tract involvement may produce diarrhea and steatorrhea. Mucosal infiltrates may be detectable by barium studies or by small bowel biopsy. Peptic ulcers also occur. Hepatosplenomegaly as a result of mast cell infiltrates and fibrosis has been described, as has mast cell proliferation in lymph nodes, kidneys, periadrenal fat, and bone marrow. Abnormalities in the peripheral blood, such as anemia, leukocytosis, and eosinophilia, are noted in approximately one third of patients.

TREATMENT. Flushing can be precipitated by excessively hot baths, vigorous rubbing of the skin, and certain drugs, such as codeine, aspirin, morphine, atropine, ketorolac, alcohol, tubocurarine, iodine-containing radiographic dyes, and polymyxin B. Avoidance of these triggering factors is advisable. For patients who are symptomatic, oral antihistamines may be palliative. H_1 receptor antagonists (hydroxyzine) are the initial drugs of choice for systemic signs of histamine release. If H_1 antagonists are unsuccessful, H_2 receptor antagonists may be helpful in controlling pruritus or gastric hypersecretion. Oral mast cell-stabilizing agents, such as cromolyn sodium or ketotifen, may also be effective for diarrhea or abdominal cramping and some systemic symptoms such as headache or muscle pain.

Carter MC, Metcalfe DD: Paediatric mastocytosis. *Arch Dis Child* 2002;86:315–9.
Golkar L, Bernhard J: Mastocytosis. *Lancet* 1997;349:1379.
Hacker SM, Ramos-Caro FA, Beers BB, et al: Juvenile pseudoxanthoma elasticum: Recognition and management. *Pediatr Dermatol* 1993;10:19.
Helm KF, Gibson LE, Muller SA: Lichen sclerosus et atrophicus in children and young adults. *Pediatr Dermatol* 1991;8:97, 1991.
Lebwohl M, Neldner K, Pope M, et al: Classification of pseudoxanthoma elasticum: Report of a consensus conference. *J Am Acad Dermatol* 1994;30:103.

Lucky AW, Prose NS, Bove K, et al: Papular umbilicated granuloma annulare. A report of four pediatric cases. *Arch Dermatol* 1992;128:1375.
Mulbauer JE: Granuloma annulare. *J Am Acad Dermatol* 1980;3:217.
Murray JC: Keloids and hypertrophic scars. *Clin Dermatol* 1994;12:27.
Schalkwijk J, Zweers MC, Steijlen PM, et al: A recessive form of the Ehlers-Danlos syndrome caused by tenascin-X deficiency. *N Engl J Med* 2001;345:1167–75.
Tilstra DJ, Byers PH: Molecular basis of hereditary disorders of connective tissue. *Annu Rev Med* 1994;45:149.
Yeowell HN, Pinnell SR: The Ehlers-Danlos syndromes. *Semin Dermatol* 1993;12:229.

Chapter 650
Diseases of Subcutaneous Tissue

Diseases involving the subcutis are usually characterized by necrosis and/or inflammation; they may occur either as a primary event or as a secondary response to various stimuli or disease processes. Unfortunately, these disorders cannot all be distinguished by their histopathologic changes, which may merely reflect the stage of the lesion at the time of biopsy. The principal diagnostic criteria are the appearance and distribution of the lesions, associated symptoms, results of laboratory studies, and the natural history and exogenous provocative factors of these conditions.

Corticosteroid-Induced Atrophy. Injection of a corticosteroid intradermally can produce deep atrophy accompanied by surface pigmentary changes and telangiectasia. These changes occur approximately 2 wk after injection and may last for months. The deltoid area is most susceptible to this complication (see Chapter 649).

Panniculitis. Inflammation of fibrofatty subcutaneous tissue may primarily involve the fat lobule or, alternatively, the fibrous septum that compartmentalizes the fatty lobules. Lobular panniculitis that spares the subcutaneous vasculature includes poststeroid panniculitis, lupus erythematosus profundus, relapsing nodular nonsuppurative panniculitis *(Weber-Christian syndrome)*, pancreatic panniculitis, α_1-antitrypsin deficiency, subcutaneous fat necrosis of the newborn, sclerema neonatorum, cold panniculitis, subcutaneous sarcoidosis, and factitial panniculitis. Lobar panniculitis with vasculitis occurs in erythema induratum and occasionally as a feature of Crohn disease (see Chapter 317.2). Inflammation predominantly within the septum, sparing the vasculature, may be seen in erythema nodosum, necrobiosis lipoidica, scleroderma (see Chapter 150), and subcutaneous granuloma annulare (see Chapter 649). Septal panniculitis that includes inflammation of the vessels is found primarily in leukocytoclastic vasculitis and polyarteritis nodosa (see Chapter 157.3).

Poststeroid panniculitis has been observed in children who received high-dose corticosteroids orally for relatively short periods, usually for rheumatic fever. Within 1–2 wk after discontinuation of the drug, multiple subcutaneous nodules may appear on the cheeks, trunk, and arms. Nodules range in size from 0.5–4 cm, are erythematous or skin colored, and may be pruritic. The mechanism of the inflammatory reaction in the fat is unknown. Treatment is unnecessary because the lesions remit spontaneously over a period of months without scarring.

Lupus erythematosus profundus (lupus erythematosus panniculitis) presents with one to several firm, well-defined plaques or nodules 1 to several centimeters in diameter, most commonly on the face, buttocks, or proximal extremities. This condition may occur in patients with systemic or discoid lupus erythematosus and may precede or follow the development of other cutaneous lesions. The overlying skin is usually normal but may be erythematous, atrophic, poikilodermatous, or hyperkeratotic. Lesions may be painful and may ulcerate. On healing, a shallow depression generally remains; rarely, soft pink areas of anetoderma may result. The histopathologic changes are distinctive and may allow one to make the diagnosis in the absence of other cutaneous lesions of lupus erythematosus. The lupus band and antinuclear antibody test results are usually positive. Nodules tend to be persistent but may respond to antimalarials, oral or intralesional corticosteroids, or, in debilitating cases, immunosuppressive agents such as azathioprine or cyclophosphamide. Avoidance of sun exposure and trauma is also important.

α_1-*Antitrypsin deficiency* may present with cellulitis-like areas or red, tender nodules on the trunk or proximal extremities (see Chapter 393.4). Nodules tend to ulcerate spontaneously and discharge an oily yellow fluid. Trauma is an inciting factor in some patients. Affected individuals have severe homozygous deficiency or rarely a partial deficiency of the protease inhibitor α_1-antitrypsin, which inhibits trypsin activity and the activity of elastase, serine proteases, collagenase, factor VIII, and kallikrein. Accordingly, panniculitis may be associated with panacinar emphysema, noninfectious hepatitis, cirrhosis, persistent cutaneous vasculitis, cold-contact urticaria, or acquired angioedema. Diagnosis can be substantiated by a decreased level of serum α_1-antitrypsin activity, although, because the protein behaves as an acute-phase reactant, the level may be elevated spuriously during an acute attack of pancreatitis. Some patients respond to dapsone or infusion of random-donor–derived α_1-protease inhibitor concentrate.

Pancreatic panniculitis presents most commonly on the pretibial regions, thighs, or buttocks as tender, erythematous nodules that may be fluctuant and occasionally discharge a yellowish oily substance. It presents most often in males with alcoholism but may also occur in patients with pancreatitis as a result of cholelithiasis or abdominal trauma, with rupture of a pancreatic pseudocyst, with pancreatic ductal adenocarcinoma, or with pancreatic acinar cell carcinoma. Associated features may include arthropathy and synovitis, particularly in the ankles; eosinophilia; polyserositis; and painful osteolytic bone lesions with medullary necrosis. Microscopic changes consist of multiple foci of fat necrosis that contain ghost cells with thick, shadowy walls and no nuclei. A polymorphous inflammatory infiltrate surrounds the areas of fat necrosis. Pathogenesis of the panniculitis appears to be multifactorial, involving liberation of the lipolytic enzymes lipase, trypsin, and amylase into the circulation, causing adipocyte membrane damage and intracellular lipolysis. There is no correlation, however, between the occurrence of pancreatitis and the serum concentration of pancreatic enzymes.

Subcutaneous fat necrosis is an inflammatory disorder of adipose tissue that occurs primarily in the first 4 wk of life in full-term or post-term infants. Affected infants may have a history of perinatal asphyxia or a difficult labor and delivery. Typical lesions are asymptomatic, rubbery to firm, erythematous to violaceous plaques or nodules on the cheeks, buttocks, back, thighs, or upper arms (Fig. 650–1). Lesions may be focal or extensive and are generally asymptomatic, although they may be tender during the acute phase. Histopathologic changes are diagnostic and consist of necrosis of fat; a granulomatous cellular infiltrate composed of lymphocytes, histiocytes, multinucleated giant cells, and fibroblasts; and radially arranged clefts of crystalline triglyceride within fat cells and multinucleated giant cells. Calcium deposits are commonly found in areas of fat necrosis. Subcutaneous fat necrosis in infants may be due to ischemic injury under various circumstances such as maternal preeclampsia, birth trauma, asphyxia, and prolonged hypothermia; in many affected infants, however, no provocative factors are identified. Susceptibility has been attributed to differences in composition between the

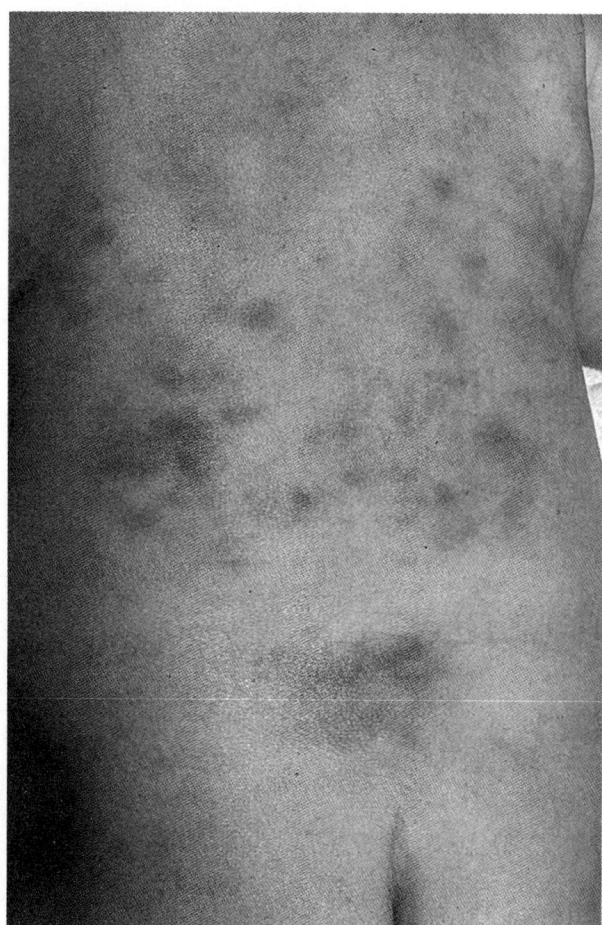

FIGURE 650–1. Red-purple nodular infiltration of skin of back caused by subcutaneous fat necrosis. See also color plates.

subcutaneous tissue of young infants and that of older infants, children, and adults. Neonatal fat solidifies at a relatively high temperature because of its relatively greater concentration of high melting point saturated fatty acids such as palmitic and stearic acids.

Uncomplicated lesions involute spontaneously within weeks to months, usually without scarring or atrophy. Calcium deposition may occasionally occur within areas of fat necrosis, and this may sometimes result in rupture and drainage of liquid material. A rare but potentially life-threatening complication is *hypercalcemia*. This presents at 1–6 mo of age with lethargy, poor feeding, vomiting, failure to thrive, irritability, seizures, shortening of the QT interval, or renal failure. The origin of the hypercalcemia is unknown but is postulated to involve excess bone resorption through elevated levels of prostaglandin E or increased intestinal calcium uptake by unregulated extrarenal production of 1,25 dihydroxyvitamin D by macrophages in the granulomatous infiltrate. Subcutaneous fat necrosis can be confused with sclerema neonatorum, panniculitis, cellulitis, or hematoma. Because the lesions are self-limited, therapy is not required for uncomplicated cases. Needle aspiration of fluctuant lesions may prevent rupture and subsequent scarring. Treatment of hypercalcemia is aimed at enhancing renal calcium excretion by hydration and furosemide administration and at limiting dietary calcium and vitamin D intake. Reduction of intestinal calcium absorption and alteration of vitamin D metabolism may be accomplished by administration of corticosteroids.

Sclerema neonatorum is an uncommon disorder of adipose tissue that presents abruptly in preterm, gravely ill infants as diffuse, yellowish-white woody induration of the skin. Affected skin becomes stony in consistency, cold, and nonpitting. The face assumes a masklike expression, and joint mobility may be compromised because of inflexibility of the skin. Histopathologic changes in sclerema neonatorum consist of an increase in the size of fat cells and an increase in the width of the fibrous connective tissue septa. In contrast to subcutaneous fat necrosis, with which it is most apt to be confused, fat necrosis, inflammation, giant cells, and calcium crystals are generally absent. Sclerema neonatorum almost always is associated with serious illness, such as sepsis, congenital heart disease, multiple congenital anomalies, or hypothermia. The appearance of sclerema in a sick infant should be regarded as an ominous prognostic sign. The outcome depends on the response of the underlying disorder to treatment.

Cold panniculitis may result in localized lesions in infants after prolonged cold exposure, especially on the cheeks, or after prolonged application of a cold object such as an ice cube, ice bag, or Popsicle to any area of the skin. Erythematous to bluish, indurated, ill-defined plaques or nodules arise within hours to a couple days of exposure, persist for 2–3 wk, and heal without residua. Recurrence of the lesions is common, however, thus emphasizing the importance of parental education in treating these patients. Histopathologic examination reveals an infiltrate of lymphoid and histiocytic cells around blood vessels at the dermal-subdermal junction; by the 3rd day, some of the fat cells in the subcutis may have ruptured and coalesced into cystic structures. Cold panniculitis may be confused with facial cellulitis caused by *Haemophilus influenzae* type b. Unlike the situation with buccal cellulitis, however, the area may be cold to the touch, and the patient is afebrile. Chilblains (pernio), a condition of acute or chronic cold injury, is characterized by localized symmetric erythematous to purplish edematous plaques and nodules in areas exposed to cold, typically acral areas (distal hands and feet, ears, face) (see Chapter 63). Lesions develop 12–24 hr after cold exposure and may be associated with itching, burning, or pain. Blister formation and ulceration are rare. Vasospasm of arterioles due to cold exposure with resultant hypoxemia and localized perivascular mononuclear inflammation appears to be responsible for the disease. Frostbite due to extreme cold exposure is painful and histopathologically involves the epidermis, dermis, and subcutaneous fat. The pathogenic mechanism of cold panniculitis may be similar to that of subcutaneous fat necrosis, involving an increased propensity of fat to solidify in infants compared with that in older children and adults as a result of the higher percentage of saturated fatty acids in the subcutaneous fat of infants.

Factitial panniculitis results from subcutaneous injection by self or proxy of a foreign substance, the most common types of which include organic materials such as milk or feces; drugs such as the opiates or pentazocine; oily materials such as mineral oil or paraffin; and the synthetic polymer povidone. Indurated plaques, ulcers, or nodules that liquefy and drain may be noted clinically. The histopathologic picture is variable, depending on the injected substance, but may include the presence of birefringent crystals, oil cysts surrounded by fibrosis and inflammation, and an acute inflammatory reaction with fat necrosis. Vessels are characteristically spared.

Lipodystrophy. Several rare conditions are associated with loss of fatty tissue in a partial or generalized distribution.

Partial lipodystrophy occurs more commonly in females than in males and generally begins during the 1st decade of life. There is gradual symmetric loss of subcutaneous tissue. Although the sites of loss are heterogeneous, loss of fat may occur primarily on the trunk and extremities, sparing the face; on the extremities, sparing both the face and trunk; or on the extremities and buttocks. The most common variant involves loss of fat from the face and the upper half of the body, resulting in a cadaverous facies and marked disproportion between the upper and lower halves of the body (*Weir-Mitchell type*). In some cases, there is a concurrent hypertrophy of the subcutaneous fat of the lower part of the body (*Laignel-Lavastine* and *Viard types*); others have hemilipodystrophy involving one half of the face or body. Loss of adipose tissue is not preceded by an inflammatory phase, and histopathologic examination reveals only absence of subcutaneous fat. Some patients have had hypocomplementemia (i.e., low C3) and associated renal disease, particularly progressive membranous mesangiocapillary glomerulonephritis, disordered glucose metabolism, or abnormal serum lipid profiles. The cause of the disorder is not understood, and there is no effective treatment, although dietary restrictions of fats and carbohydrates may be prudent. *Generalized lipodystrophy* may be congenital (*Berardinelli-Seip syndrome*) or acquired (*Seip-Lawrence syndrome*).

Congenital generalized lipodystrophy is a progressive multisystem disorder inherited as an autosomal recessive trait. The earliest manifestation is generalized loss of subcutaneous and visceral fat; it may be evident at birth or may occur during infancy. Associated cutaneous changes include prominent superficial veins, hirsutism, abundant curly scalp hair, and acanthosis nigricans. Patients have an anabolic syndrome with a voracious appetite; accelerated skeletal growth, resulting in tall stature; skeletal sclerosis; enlarged joints, especially of the hands and feet; accelerated muscle growth, resulting in a protuberant abdomen; and hypertrophic cardiomyopathy. Precocious enlargement of the genitals and mental deficiency and hemiplegia are seen commonly. Insulin resistance is present from birth. Hyperlipidemia, hyperinsulinism, and insulin-resistant nonketotic diabetes mellitus develop gradually and are reflected by increasing hepatomegaly caused by fatty infiltration and cirrhosis. Serum levels of growth hormone may be normal, but its secretion in response to stimuli may be disturbed. Hypothalamic releasing factors that are not ordinarily found in plasma have been identified in affected patients and suggest a lack of hypothalamic regulation. The underlying problem may be an insulin receptor or postreceptor defect. The acquired form is preceded by an undefined illness or an infection. Pathogenesis appears to involve autoimmune destruction of adipose tissue that results secondarily in an anabolic syndrome with insulin-resistant diabetes. When fat loss becomes generalized, the disease resembles the congenital form, although the anabolic features tend to be less striking. Pimozide, a selective dopamine blocker, or fenfluramine, a serotonergic agonist, may be helpful to some patients. Control of the diabetes with insulin is difficult to achieve, does not affect the course of the lipodystrophy, and is considered contraindicated by some authorities. Dietary fat regulation of energy consumption is the most important and efficacious intervention.

Localized lipoatrophy is an idiopathic condition that presents as annular atrophy at the ankles, a bandlike semicircular depression 2–4 cm in diameter on the thighs or, rarely, on the abdomen and upper groin as a centrifugally spreading, bluish, depressed plaque with an erythematous margin. It occurs predominantly in Japanese children.

Insulin lipoatrophy usually occurs approximately 6 mo–2 yr after initiation of relatively high doses of insulin. A dimple or well-circumscribed depression at the site of injection is typically seen, although loss of fat may extend beyond the site of injection, leading to an extensive, depressed plaque. Biopsy reveals a marked decrease or absence of subcutaneous tissue, without inflammation or fibrosis. In some patients, hypertrophy occurs clinically. In these cases, the mid-dermal collagen is replaced by hypertrophic fat cells on histopathologic sections. The mechanism of insulin lipoatrophy may be cross reaction of insulin antibodies with fat cells; the incidence of this condition has decreased since the implementation of widespread use of highly purified insulins. Lesions may also be prevented by frequent alteration of injection sites.

Aronson IK, Zeitz HJ, Variakojis D: Panniculitis in childhood. *Pediatr Dermatol* 1988;5:216.

Koransky JS, Esterly NB: Lupus panniculitis (profundus). *J Pediatr* 1981;98:241.

Seip M, Trygstad O: Generalized lipodystrophy, congenital and acquired (lipoatrophy). *Acta Paediatr* 1996;413(Suppl):26.

Senior B, Gellis SS: The syndromes of total lipodystrophy and of partial lipodystrophy. *Pediatrics* 1964;33:593.

Silverman RA, Newman AJ, LeVine MJ: Post-steroid panniculitis; a case report. *Pediatr Dermatol* 1988;5:92.

Chapter 651
Disorders of the Sweat Glands

Eccrine glands are found over nearly the entire skin surface and provide the primary means, through evaporation of the water in sweat, for cooling the body. These glands have no anatomic relationship to hair follicles and secrete a relatively large amount of odorless aqueous sweat. In contrast, apocrine glands are limited in distribution to the axillae, anogenital skin, mammary glands, ceruminous glands of the ear, Moll glands in the eyelid, and selected areas of the face and scalp. The apocrine gland duct enters the pilosebaceous follicle at the level of the infundibulum and secretes a small amount of a complex, viscous fluid that, on alteration by microorganisms, produces a distinctive body odor. Some disorders of these two sweat glands are similar pathogenetically, whereas others are unique to a given gland.

Anhidrosis. *Neuropathic anhidrosis* results from a disturbance in the neural pathway from the control center in the brain to the peripheral efferent nerve fibers that activate sweating. Disorders in this category, which are characterized by generalized anhidrosis, include tumors of the hypothalamus and damage to the floor of the third ventricle. Pontine or medullary lesions may produce anhidrosis of the ipsilateral face or neck and ipsilateral or contralateral anhidrosis of the rest of the body. Peripheral or segmental neuropathies, caused by leprosy, amyloidosis, diabetes mellitus, alcoholic neuritis, or syringomyelia, may be associated with anhidrosis of the innervated skin. Various autonomic disorders are also associated with altered eccrine sweat gland function.

At the *level of the sweat gland,* drugs such as the anticholinergics atropine and scopolamine may paralyze the sweat glands. Acute intoxication with barbiturates or diazepam has produced necrosis of sweat glands, resulting in anhidrosis with or without erythema and bullae. Eccrine glands are largely absent throughout the skin or are present in a localized area among patients with anhidrotic ectodermal dysplasia or localized congenital absence of sweat glands, respectively. Infiltrative or destructive disorders that may produce atrophy of sweat glands by pressure or scarring include scleroderma, acrodermatitis chronica atrophicans, radiodermatitis, burns, Sjögren disease, multiple myeloma, and lymphoma. Obstruction of sweat glands may occur in miliaria and in a number of inflammatory and hyperkeratotic disorders such as the ichthyoses, psoriasis, lichen planus, pemphigus, porokeratosis, atopic dermatitis, and seborrheic dermatitis. Occlusion of the sweat pore may also occur with the topical agents aluminum and zirconium salts, formaldehyde, or glutaraldehyde.

Diverse *disorders that are associated with anhidrosis by unknown mechanisms* include dehydration; toxic overdose with lead, arsenic, thallium, fluorine, or morphine; uremia; cirrhosis; endocrine disorders such as Addison disease, diabetes mellitus, diabetes insipidus, or hyperthyroidism; and inherited conditions such as Fabry disease, Franceschetti-Jadassohn syndrome, which combines features of incontinentia pigmenti and anhidrotic ectodermal dysplasia, and familial anhidrosis with neurolabyrinthitis.

Whereas anhidrosis may be complete, in many cases, what appears clinically to be anhidrosis is actually *hypohidrosis* caused by anhidrosis of many but not all eccrine glands. Compensatory, localized *hyperhidrosis* of the remaining functional sweat glands may occur, particularly in diabetes mellitus and miliaria. The primary complication of anhidrosis is hyperthermia, seen primarily in anhidrotic ectodermal dysplasia or in otherwise normal preterm or full-term *neonates* who have immature eccrine glands.

Hyperhidrosis. The numerous disorders that may be associated with increased production of eccrine sweat may also be classified into those with neural mechanisms involving an abnormality in the pathway from the neural regulatory centers to the sweat gland and those that are non-neurally mediated by direct effects on the sweat glands (Box 651–1). Excessive sweating of the palms and soles in response to emotional stimuli (volar hyperhidrosis) may respond to 10% glutaraldehyde soaks, 20% aluminum chloride in anhydrous ethanol applied under occlusion for several hours, iontophoretic therapy with anticholinergics, or in severe, refractory cases, cervicothoracic or lumbar sympathectomy. Axillary hyperhidrosis does not respond to topical glutaraldehyde or salts of aluminum, zirconium, or zinc. Aluminum chloride (Drysol) applied to the axillae at bedtime under occlusion, aided, if necessary, by oral administration of an anticholinergic agent such as glycopyrrolate, may produce a prompt and significant reduction in sweating. Local injection of botulism toxin may also be effective. Cervicothoracic sympathectomy or selective surgical removal of the most highly

---

BOX 651–1. Causes of Hyperhidrosis

CORTICAL
Emotional
Familial dysautonomia
Congenital ichthyosiform
  erythroderma
Epidermolysis bullosa
Nail-patella syndrome
Jadassohn-Lewandowsky
  syndrome
Pachyonychia congenita
Palmoplantar keratoderma

HYPOTHALAMIC

Drugs
Antipyretics
Emetics
Insulin
Meperidine

Exercise

Infection
Defervescence
Chronic illness

Metabolic
Debility
Diabetes mellitus
Hyperpituitarism
Hyperthyroidism
Hypoglycemia
Obesity
Porphyria
Pregnancy
Rickets
Infantile scurvy

Cardiovascular
Heart failure
Shock

Vasomotor
Cold injury
Raynaud phenomenon
Rheumatoid arthritis

Neurologic
Abscess
Familial dysautonomia
Postencephalitic
Tumor

Miscellaneous
Chédiak-Higashi syndrome
Compensatory
Phenylketonuria
Pheochromocytoma
Vitiligo

MEDULLARY
Physiologic gustatory
  sweating
Encephalitis
Granulosis rubra nasi
Syringomyelia
Thoracic sympathetic trunk
  injury

SPINAL
Cord transection
Syringomyelia

CHANGES IN BLOOD FLOW
Maffucci syndrome
Arteriovenous fistula
Klippel-Trenaunay
  syndrome
Glomus tumor
Blue rubber bleb nevus
  syndrome

sudoriferous eccrine glands in the axillae may be effective in refractory cases.

Miliaria. This results from retention of sweat in occluded eccrine sweat ducts as a result of a keratinous plug in the sweat duct. Retrograde pressure may result in rupture of the duct and leakage of sweat into the epidermis and/or the dermis. The eruption is most often induced by hot, humid weather, but it may also be caused by high fever. Infants who are dressed too warmly may develop this eruption indoors, even during the winter.

In *miliaria crystallina,* asymptomatic, noninflammatory, pinpoint clear vesicles may suddenly erupt in profusion over large areas of the body surface, leaving brawny desquamation on healing (Fig. 651–1). The clarity of the fluid, superficiality of the vesicles, and absence of inflammation permit differentiation from other blistering disorders. This type of miliaria occurs most frequently in newborn infants because of the relative immaturity and delayed patency of the sweat duct and the tendency for infants to be nursed in relatively warm, humid conditions. It may also occur in older patients with hyperpyrexia. Histopathologically, an intracorneal or subcorneal vesicle is seen in communication with the sweat duct.

Miliaria rubra is a less superficial eruption characterized by erythematous, minute papulovesicles that may impart a prickling sensation. The lesions are usually localized to sites of occlusion or to flexural areas, such as the neck, groin, and axillae, where friction may have a role in their pathogenesis. Involved skin may become macerated and eroded. This lesion may be confused with or superimposed on other diaper area eruptions, including candidosis and folliculitis; lesions of miliaria rubra, however, are extrafollicular. Histopathologically, one sees focal areas of spongiosis and spongiotic vesicle formation in close proximity to sweat ducts that generally contain a keratinous plug. The keratinous plug does not form, however, until the later stages of the disease and therefore does not appear to be the primary cause of sweat duct obstruction. The initial obstruction is postulated to be due to swelling of the ductal epidermal cells, perhaps from imbibition of water. Miliaria rubra is generally reversible. Supplemental vitamin C may help restore normal sweating in refractory cases. Prophylactic use of antibacterial agents may prevent development of miliaria rubra. Repeated attacks of miliaria rubra may lead to *miliaria profunda,* which is

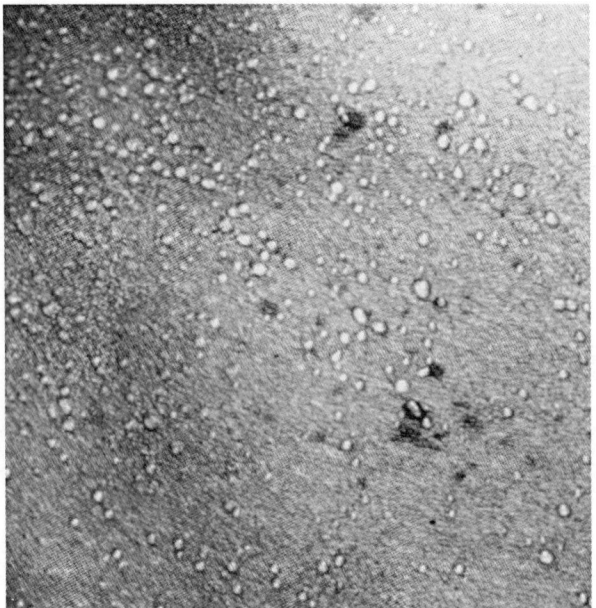

FIGURE 651–1. Superficial clear vesicles of miliaria crystallina in a patient with hyperpyrexia and lymphoma.

due to rupture of the sweat duct deeper in the skin at the level of the dermoepidermal junction. Severe, extensive miliaria rubra or miliaria profunda may result in disturbance of heat regulation. Lesions of miliaria rubra may become infected, particularly in malnourished or debilitated infants, leading to development of periporitis staphylogenes, which involves extension of the process from the sweat duct into the sweat gland.

All forms of miliaria respond dramatically to cooling the patient by regulation of environmental temperatures and by removal of excessive clothing; administration of antipyretics is also beneficial to patients with fever. Topical agents are usually ineffective and may exacerbate the eruption.

Bromhidrosis. The excessive odor that characterizes bromhidrosis may result from alteration of either apocrine or eccrine sweat. Apocrine bromhidrosis develops after puberty as a result of the formation of short-chain fatty acids and ammonia by the action of anaerobic diphtheroids on axillary apocrine sweat. Treatments that may be helpful include cleansing with germicidal soaps; topical application of aluminum, zirconium, or zinc salts or gentamicin cream, all of which have antibacterial action; and axillary shaving. Eccrine bromhidrosis is caused by microbiologic degradation of stratum corneum that has become softened by excessive eccrine sweat. The soles of the feet and the intertriginous areas are the primary affected sites. Hyperhidrosis, warm weather, obesity, intertrigo, and diabetes mellitus are predisposing factors. In addition to local measures, oral anticholinergic drugs such as propantheline (Pro-Banthine) may decrease eccrine sweating but do not alter apocrine gland secretion. Topical aluminum chloride preparations such as Drysol are particularly useful for plantar eccrine bromhidrosis.

Hidradenitis Suppurativa. This is a chronic, inflammatory, suppurative disorder of the apocrine glands in the axillae, the anogenital area, and occasionally the scalp, posterior aspect of the ears, female breasts, and periumbilical area. Onset of clinical manifestations, sometimes preceded by pruritus or discomfort, usually occurs during puberty or early adulthood. Solitary or multiple painful erythematous nodules, deep abscesses, and contracted scars are sharply confined to areas of skin containing apocrine glands. When the disease is severe and chronic, sinus tracts, ulcers, and thick, linear fibrotic bands develop. Hidradenitis suppurativa tends to persist for many years, punctuated by relapses and partial remissions. Complications include cellulitis, ulceration, and burrowing abscesses that may perforate adjacent structures, forming fistulas to the urethra, bladder, rectum, or peritoneum. Episodic inflammatory arthritis develops in some patients. A minority of patients have the follicular occlusion triad, which includes acne and perifolliculitis capitis. Early lesions are often mistaken for infected epidermal cysts, furuncles, scrofuloderma, actinomycosis, cat-scratch disease, granuloma inguinale, or lymphogranuloma venereum. Sharp localization to areas of the body that bear apocrine glands, however, should suggest hidradenitis. When involvement is limited to the anogenital region, the condition may be difficult to distinguish from Crohn disease and may coexist with it.

Histopathologically, early lesions are characterized by a keratinous plug in the apocrine duct or hair follicle orifice and by cystic distention of the follicle. The process generally but not necessarily extends into the apocrine gland. Later changes include inflammation within and around apocrine glands and the presence of groups of cocci within apocrine glands and in the adjacent dermis. Skin appendages may become obliterated by scarring. The disease is probably initiated by plugging of apocrine gland ducts with keratinous debris. Bacterial infection, particularly with *Staphylococcus aureus, Streptococcus milleri, Escherichia coli,* and possibly anaerobic streptococci, appears to be important in the progressive dilatation below the obstruction, leading to rupture of the duct, inflammation, sinus tract formation, and destructive scarring. Pathogenesis of hidradenitis suppurativa is controversial, but it appears to be an androgen-dependent condition.

Patients should be counseled to avoid tight-fitting clothes, because occlusion may exacerbate the condition. *Treatment* with topical antibiotic agents such as chlorhexidine, erythromycin, or clindamycin or with topical retinoids may be effective in early, indolent disease. Systemic antibiotics, chosen on the basis of bacterial culture (usually staphylococcal and streptococcal pathogens) and sensitivity tests, should be administered in the acute phase. Empirical therapy may be initiated with tetracycline, doxycycline, or minocycline if the patient is 8 yr or older; clindamycin and cephalosporins also are effective. Some patients require long-term treatment with tetracycline or erythromycin. Intralesional triamcinolone acetonide (5–10 mg/mL) is often helpful in early disease. The addition of prednisone, 40–60 mg/day for 7–10 days, tapering gradually as inflammation subsides, to the regimen of patients who respond poorly to antibiotics may decrease fibrosis and scarring. Oral contraceptive agents, which contain a high estrogen-to-progesterone ratio and low androgenicity of the progesterone, or oral retinoids may be helpful in some patients. Warm compresses encourage spontaneous rupture of abscesses; those that are "pointing" should be incised and drained. Ultimately, surgical measures may be required for control or cure.

Fox-Fordyce Disease. This disease is most common in females and presents during puberty or the 3rd decade of life with pruritus in the axillae and, occasionally, in the anogenital region and around the breasts. Pruritus is exacerbated by emotional stress and stimuli that induce apocrine sweating. Skin-colored to slightly hyperpigmented dome-shaped follicular papules develop in the pruritic areas. Histopathologically, one sees keratinous plugging of the distal apocrine duct, rupture of the intraepidermal portion of the apocrine duct, paraductal microvesicle formation, and paraductal acanthosis. The condition generally remits during pregnancy, particularly in the third trimester. Oral contraceptive pills and topical corticosteroids or retinoic acid may help some patients.

Barth JH, Kealey T: Androgen metabolism by isolated human axillary apocrine glands in hidradenitis suppurativa. *Br J Dermatol* 1991;125:304.
Holzle E, Kligman AM: The pathogenesis of miliaria rubra. *Br J Dermatol* 1978;99:117.
Jackman PJ: Body odor—the role of skin bacteria. *Semin Dermatol* 1982;1:143.
Sato K, Kang WH, Saga K, et al: Biology of sweat glands and their disorders. *J Am Acad Dermatol* 1989;20:537.

Chapter 652
Disorders of Hair

Disorders of hair in infants and children may be due to intrinsic disturbances of hair growth, underlying biochemical or metabolic defects, inflammatory dermatoses, or structural anomalies of the hair shaft. Excessive and abnormal hair growth is referred to as hypertrichosis or hirsutism. Hypertrichosis is excessive hair growth at inappropriate locations; hirsutism is an androgen-dependent male pattern of hair growth in women. Hypotrichosis is deficient hair growth, and hair loss, partial or complete, is called alopecia. Alopecia may be classified as non-scarring or scarring; the latter type is rare in children and, if present, is most often due to prolonged or untreated inflammatory conditions such as pyoderma or tinea capitis.

Hypertrichosis

Hypertrichosis is rare in children and may be localized or generalized and permanent or transient. Hypertrichosis has many causes, some of which are listed in Box 652–1.

BOX 652–1. Causes of and Conditions Associated with Hypertrichosis

INTRINSIC FACTORS
Racial and familial forms such as hairy ears, hairy elbows, intraphalangeal hair, or generalized hirsutism

EXTRINSIC FACTORS
Local trauma
Malnutrition
Anorexia nervosa
Long-standing inflammatory dermatoses
Drugs
    Diazoxide, phenytoin, corticosteroids, Cortisporin, cyclosporine, androgens, anabolic agents, hexachlorobenzene, minoxidil, psoralens, penicillamine, streptomycin

HAMARTOMAS OR NEVI
Congenital pigmented nevocytic nevus, nevus pilosus, Becker nevus, congenital smooth muscle hamartoma, fawn-tail nevus associated with diastematomyelia

ENDOCRINE DISORDERS
Virilizing ovarian tumors, Cushing syndrome, acromegaly, hyperthyroidism, hypothyroidism, congenital adrenal hyperplasia, adrenal tumors, gonadal dysgenesis, male pseudohermaphroditism, nonendocrine hormone-secreting tumors, polycystic ovary syndrome

CONGENITAL AND GENETIC DISORDERS
Hypertrichosis lanuginosa, mucopolysaccharidosis, leprechaunism, congenital generalized lipodystrophy, de Lange syndrome, trisomy 18, Rubinstein-Taybi syndrome, Bloom syndrome, congenital hemihypertrophy, gingival fibromatosis with hypertrichosis, Winchester syndrome, lipoatrophic diabetes (Lawrence-Seip syndrome), fetal hydantoin syndrome, fetal alcohol syndrome, congenital erythropoietic or variegate porphyria (sun-exposed areas), porphyria cutanea tarda (sun-exposed areas), Cowden syndrome, Seckel syndrome, Gorlin syndrome, partial trisomy 3 q, Ambra syndrome

---

HYPOTRICHOSIS AND ALOPECIA

Some of the disorders associated with hypotrichosis and alopecia are listed in Box 652–2. True alopecia is rarely congenital; it is more often related to an inflammatory dermatosis, mechanical factors, drug ingestion, infection, endocrinopathy, nutritional disturbance, or disturbance of the hair cycle. Any inflammatory condition of the scalp, such as atopic dermatitis or seborrheic dermatitis, if severe enough, may result in partial alopecia; hair growth returns to normal if the underlying condition is treated successfully, unless the hair follicle has been permanently damaged.

Telogen Effluvium. Telogen effluvium presents with sudden loss of large amounts of hair, often with brushing, combing, and washing of hair. Diffuse loss of scalp hair occurs from premature conversion of growing, or anagen, hairs, which normally constitute 80–90% of hairs, to resting, or telogen, hairs. Hair loss is noted 6 wk to 3 mo after the precipitating cause, which may include childbirth; a febrile episode; surgery; acute blood loss, including blood donation; sudden severe weight loss; discontinuation of high-dose corticosteroids or oral contraceptives; and psychiatric stress. Telogen effluvium also accounts for the loss of hair by infants during the first few months of life; friction from bed sheets, particularly in infants with pruritic, atopic skin, may exacerbate the problem. There is no inflammatory reaction; the hair follicles remain intact, and telogen bulbs can be demonstrated microscopically on shed hairs. Because more than 50% of the scalp hair is rarely involved, alopecia is usually not severe. Parents should be reassured that normal hair growth will return within approximately 6 mo.

Toxic Alopecia (Anagen Effluvium). Anagen effluvium is an acute, severe, diffuse inhibition of growth of anagen follicles, resulting

BOX 652–2. Disorders Associated with Alopecia and Hypotrichosis

Congenital total alopecia: isolated autosomal recessive abnormality, progeria, hidrotic ectodermal dysplasia, Moynahan syndrome, atrichia with keratin cysts, Baraitser syndrome
Congenital localized alopecia: aplasia cutis, alopecia triangularis, epidermal nevus, hair follicle hamartoma, facial hemiatrophy (Romberg syndrome), male pattern baldness
Hereditary hypotrichosis: hypotrichosis with keratosis pilaris, Marie-Unna syndrome, phenylketonuria, arginosuccinic aciduria, hyperlysinemia, homocystinuria, orotic aciduria, Cockayne syndrome, Rothmund-Thomson syndrome, dyskeratosis congenita, Seckel syndrome, cartilage-hair hypoplasia, Conradi syndrome, pachyonychia congenita, Hallermann-Streiff syndrome, Treacher Collins syndrome, oculodentodigital, orofaciodigital, incontinentia pigmenti, focal dermal hypoplasia, keratosis follicularis, epidermolysis bullosa, ectodermal dysplasias, ichthyoses, loose anagen hair
Diffuse alopecia of endocrine origin: hypopituitarism, hypothyroidism, hypoparathyroidism, hyperthyroidism, diabetes mellitus
Alopecia of nutritional origin: marasmus, kwashiorkor, iron deficiency, zinc deficiency (acrodermatitis enteropathica), gluten-sensitive enteropathy, essential fatty acid deficiency, biotinidase deficiency
Disturbances of the hair cycle: telogen effluvium
Toxic alopecia: anagen effluvium
Autoimmune alopecia: alopecia areata
Traumatic alopecia: traction alopecia, trichotillomania
Cicatricial alopecia: lupus erythematosus, lichen planus pilaris, pseudopelade, scleroderma, dermatomyositis, infection (kerion, favus, tuberculosis, syphilis, folliculitis, leishmaniasis, herpes zoster, varicella), acne keloidalis, follicular mucinosis, cicatricial pemphigoid, lichen sclerosus et atrophicus, sarcoidosis
Hair shaft abnormalities: monilethrix, pili annulati, pili torti, trichorrhexis invaginata, trichorrhexis nodosa, woolly hair syndrome, Menkes disease, trichothiodystrophy, trichodento-osseous syndrome, trichorhinophalangeal syndrome, uncombable hair syndrome (spun glass hair, pili trianguli et canaliculi)

in loss of greater than 80–90% of scalp hair. Hairs become dystrophic, and the hair shaft breaks at the narrowed segment. Loss is diffuse, rapid (1–3 wk after treatment), and temporary, as regrowth occurs after the offending agent is discontinued. Causes of anagen effluvium include radiation; cancer chemotherapeutic agents such as antimetabolites, alkylating agents, and mitotic inhibitors; thallium; thiouracil; heparin; the coumarins; boric acid; and hypervitaminosis A.

Traction Alopecia (Marginal or Traumatic Alopecia). Traction alopecia is due to trauma to hair follicles by tight braids or ponytails, headbands, rubber bands, curlers, and rollers (Fig. 652–1*A*). Broken hairs and inflammatory follicular papules in circumscribed patches at the scalp margins are characteristic and may be subtended by regional lymphadenopathy. Children and parents must be encouraged to avoid devices that cause trauma to the hair and, if necessary, to alter the hair style. Otherwise, scarring of hair follicles may occur.

Trichotillomania. Compulsive pulling, twisting, and breaking of hair produces irregular areas of incomplete hair loss, most often on the crown and in the occipital and parietal areas of the scalp (see Fig. 652–1*B*). Occasionally, eyebrows, eyelashes, and body hair are traumatized. Some plaques of alopecia may have a linear outline. The hairs remaining within the areas of loss are of various lengths and are typically blunt tipped because of breakage. The scalp appears normal, although chronic folliculitis may also occur. Trichophagy, resulting in trichobezoars, may complicate this disorder. The lifetime occurrence is 3% in girls and 1% in boys.

The *diagnosis* of trichotillomania is often difficult and may require biopsy confirmation. The *Diagnostic and Statistical Manual of Mental Disorders* diagnostic criteria include visible hair loss attributable to pulling; mounting tension preceding hair pulling;

gratification or release of tension after hair pulling; and absence of hair pulling attributable to hallucinations, delusions, or an inflammatory skin condition. Histologic changes include coexistent normal and damaged follicles, perifollicular hemorrhage, atrophy of some follicles, and catagen transformation of hair. In late stages, perifollicular fibrosis may occur. Long-term repeated trauma may result in irreversible damage and permanent alopecia. Tinea capitis and alopecia areata must be considered in the differential diagnosis.

Trichotillomania is closely related to, and may be an expression of, obsessive-compulsive disorder in some children; in others, it is a benign habit disorder. *Treatment* of concurrent thumb sucking may be effective in the latter children. When trichotillomania occurs secondary to obsessive-compulsive disorder, clomipramine, fluoxetine, or trazodone may be helpful, particularly when combined with behavioral interventions.

Alopecia Areata. Alopecia areata is characterized by rapid and complete loss of hair in round or oval patches on the scalp (see Fig. 652–1*C*) and on other body sites. In *alopecia totalis,* all the scalp hair is lost; *alopecia universalis* involves all body and scalp hair. The lifetime incidence of alopecia areata is 1% of the population; approximately 60% of patients are younger than 20 yr of age.

CLINICAL MANIFESTATIONS. Peripheral spread and confluence of plaques of alopecia areata often result in bizarre patterns. At the margin of active patches, the hairs can often be extracted with gentle traction and, on examination, demonstrate an attenuated or catagen bulb at the termination of a tapered, poorly pigmented shaft (i.e., exclamation hair). The skin within the plaques of hair loss appears normal. A perifollicular infiltrate of inflammatory round cells is found in biopsy specimens from active areas. In the chronic stages, the number of telogen hairs is increased, the diameter of hair fibers is reduced, and trichodystrophies such as trichorrhexis nodosa and trichomalacia may be found. Alopecia areata is associated with atopy; nail changes such as pits, ridges, opacification, serration of the free nail edge, dystrophy, and a red lunula; cataracts or lens opacification; and autoimmune diseases such as Hashimoto thyroiditis, Addison disease, pernicious anemia, ulcerative colitis, myasthenia gravis, collagen vascular diseases, and vitiligo. An increased incidence of alopecia areata has been reported in patients with Down syndrome (5–10%).

ETIOLOGY. The cause of alopecia areata is unknown. Emotional factors and stress have been suggested as triggering factors, but supportive evidence is tenuous. About 10–20% of patients have a family history of alopecia areata; the estimated risk for first-degree relatives is 6%. Inheritance is thought to be autosomal dominant with variable penetrance. The infrequent but striking association with autoimmune diseases has suggested an autoimmune pathogenesis. Some patients have serum antibodies to thyroglobulin, parietal cells, and adrenal gland, and autoantibodies to hair follicle antigens has been demonstrated. Interleukin 1 alpha (IL-1α) and IL-1β) are important inhibitors of hair growth in vitro, and genes of the IL-1 cluster are candidate genes for alopecia areata.

DIFFERENTIAL DIAGNOSIS AND PROGNOSIS. Tinea capitis, seborrheic dermatitis, trichotillomania, traumatic alopecia, and lupus erythematosus should be considered. The course is unpredictable, but spontaneous resolution within 6–12 mo is usual, particularly when relatively small, stable patches of alopecia are present. Recurrences, however, are common. In general, onset at a young age, extensive or prolonged hair loss, numerous episodes, and associated atrophy are poor prognostic signs. Alopecia universalis, totalis, and *ophiasis*, a type of alopecia areata in which hair loss is circumferential, are also less likely to resolve.

TREATMENT. This is difficult to evaluate because the course is erratic and unpredictable. The use of high-potency topical

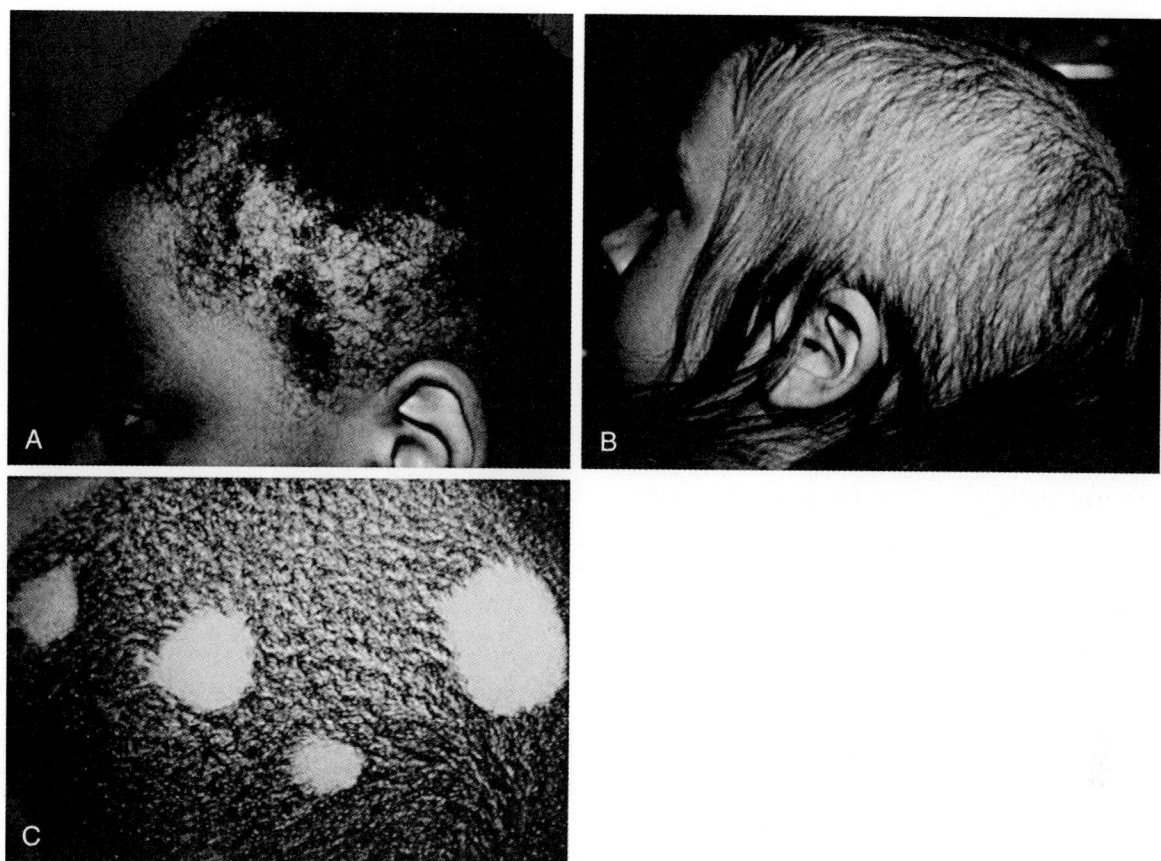

FIGURE 652–1. *A,* Marginal alopecia caused by traction. *B,* Partial alopecia with bizarre pattern typical of trichotillomania. *C,* Multiple areas of alopecia characteristic of alopecia areata. The scalp is normal.

fluorinated corticosteroids with occlusion at night is effective in some patients. Intradermal injections of steroid may also stimulate hair growth locally, but this mode of treatment is impractical in young children or in those with extensive hair loss. Systemic corticosteroid therapy has, on occasion, been associated with good results; however, the permanence of cure is questionable, and the side effects are a serious deterrent. Additional therapies that are sometimes effective include short-contact anthralin, topical minoxidil, and contact sensitization with squaric acid dibutylester or diphencyprone. Psoralen and ultraviolet A phototherapy may also be effective but has limited applicability in children. In general, parents and patients can be reassured that spontaneous remission usually occurs. New hair growth may initially be of finer caliber and lighter color, but replacement by normal terminal hair can be expected.

Structural Defects of Hair. Structural defects of the hair shaft may be congenital, reflect known biochemical aberrations, or relate to damaging grooming practices. All the defects can be demonstrated by microscopic examination of affected hairs, particularly by scanning and transmission electron microscopy.

Trichorrhexis Nodosa. This is the most common of all hair shaft abnormalities. The hair is dry, brittle, and lusterless, with irregularly spaced grayish-white nodes on the hair shaft. Microscopically, the nodes have the appearance of two interlocking brushes. The defect results from a fracture of the hair shaft at the nodal points caused by disruption of the cells in the hair cortex. Trichorrhexis nodosa has been noted as an isolated congenital defect in some families, has been observed in some infants with Menkes syndrome or argininosuccinic aciduria, and may occur in Netherton syndrome or in association with ectodermal dysplasia and other hair shaft abnormalities such as pili annulati.

ACQUIRED TRICHORRHEXIS NODOSA. This, the most common cause of hair breakage, occurs in two forms. *Proximal defects* are found most frequently in black children, whose complaint is not of alopecia but of failure of their hair to grow. The hair is short, and longitudinal splits, knots, and whitish nodules can be demonstrated in hair mounts. Easy breakage is demonstrated by gentle traction on the hair shafts. A history of other affected family members may be obtained. The problem may be caused by a combination of genetic predisposition and the cumulative mechanical trauma of rough combing and brushing, hair-straightening procedures, and "permanents." Patients must be cautioned to avoid damaging grooming techniques. A soft natural-bristle brush and a wide-toothed comb should be used. The condition is self-limited, with resolution in 2–4 yr if patients avoid damaging practices. *Distal trichorrhexis nodosa* is seen more frequently in white and Asian children. The distal portion of the hair shaft is thinned, ragged, and faded; white specks, sometimes mistaken for nits, may be noted along the shaft. Hair mounts reveal the paintbrush defect and the sites of excessive fragility and breakage. Localized areas of the moustache or beard may also be affected. Avoidance of traumatic grooming, regular trimming of affected ends, and the use of cream rinses to lessen tangling ameliorate this condition.

Pili Torti. This is the second most common hair shaft abnormality. At age 3 mo–2 yr, patients present with spangled, brittle, coarse hair of different lengths over the entire scalp or with circumscribed alopecia. There is a structural defect in which the hair shaft is grooved and flattened at irregular intervals and is twisted on its axis to various degrees. Minor twists that occur in normal hair should not be misconstrued as pili torti. Curvature of the hair follicle apparently leads to the flattening and rotation of the hair shaft. Most cases of classic, isolated pili torti of early onset have autosomal dominant inheritance. Autosomal recessive forms have been described, however, and many cases are sporadic. Keratosis pilaris, nail dystrophy, and corneal opacity develop in some patients. Syndromes in which the hair shaft abnormalities of pili torti are seen in association with other cutaneous and systemic abnormalities include Menkes kinky hair, Bazex syndrome, Björnstad syndrome (pili torti with deafness), Crandall and Rapp-Hodgkin ectodermal dysplasia syndrome, and trichothiodystrophy. It has also occurred in children treated with retinoids.

Monilethrix. This rare defect of the hair shaft is inherited as an autosomal dominant trait with variable age of onset, severity, and course. The hair appears dry, lusterless, and brittle, and it fractures spontaneously or with mild trauma. Eyebrows, lashes, body and pubic hair, and scalp hair may be affected. Monilethrix may be present at birth, but the hair is usually normal at birth and is replaced over the first few months of life by abnormal hairs; the condition sometimes is first apparent in childhood. Follicular papules may appear on the nape of the neck and the occiput and, occasionally, over the entire scalp. Short, fragile beaded hairs that emerge from the horny follicular plugs give a distinctive appearance. Keratosis pilaris and koilonychia of fingernails and toenails may also be present. Microscopically, a distinctive, regular beading pattern of the hair shaft is evident, characterized by elliptic nodes that are separated by narrower internodes. Not all hairs have nodes, and both normal and beaded hairs may break. Patients should be advised to handle the hair gently to minimize breakage. Treatment is generally ineffective, although topical minoxidil and oral etretinate have helped some patients. Spontaneous improvement may occur at puberty, during pregnancy, and with use of oral contraceptive pills.

Trichothiodystrophy. Hair in trichothiodystrophy is sparse, short, brittle, and uneven; the scalp hair, eyebrows, or eyelashes may be affected. Microscopically, the hair is flattened, folded, and variable in diameter; has longitudinal grooving; and has nodal swellings that resemble those of trichorrhexis nodosa. Under a polarizing microscope, distinctive alternating dark and light bands are seen. The abnormal hair has a cystine content that is less than 50% of normal because of a major reduction and altered composition of constituent high-sulfur matrix proteins. Trichothiodystrophy may occur as an isolated finding or in association with various syndrome complexes that include intellectual impairment, short stature, ichthyosis, nail dystrophy, dental caries, cataracts, decreased fertility, neurologic abnormalities, bony abnormalities, and immunodeficiency. Some patients are photosensitive and have impaired DNA repair mechanisms, similar to that seen in group D xeroderma pigmentosum; the incidence of skin cancers, however, is not increased. Patients with trichothiodystrophy tend to resemble one another, with a receding chin, protruding ears, raspy voice, and sociable, outgoing personality. *Trichoschisis*, a fracture perpendicular to the hair shaft, is characteristic of the many syndromes that are associated with trichothiodystrophy. Perpendicular breakage of the hair shaft has also been described in association with other hair abnormalities, particularly monilethrix.

Trichorrhexis Invaginata (Bamboo Hair). Short, sparse, fragile hair without apparent growth is characteristic of this condition, which is found primarily in association with Netherton syndrome (see Chapter 648). It has also been reported in other ichthyosiform dermatoses. The distal portion of the hair is invaginated into the cuplike proximal portion, forming a fragile nodal swelling. The abnormality is thought to result from a transient defect in keratinization of the inner root sheath and/or a

partial defect in the conversion of sulfhydryl groups to disulfide bonds in the cortex. The abnormality may be identified in body and scalp hair and seems to abate as the child matures.

Menkes Kinky Hair Syndrome (Trichopoliodystrophy). Males with this sex-linked recessive trait are born to an unaffected mother after a normal pregnancy. Neonatal problems include hypothermia, hypotonia, poor feeding, seizures, and failure to thrive. Hair is normal to sparse at birth but is replaced by short, fine, brittle, light-colored hair that may have features of trichorrhexis nodosa, pili torti, or monilethrix. The skin is hypopigmented and thin cheeks typically appear plump, and the nasal bridge is depressed. Heterozygotes may have loss of skin pigmentation. Progressive psychomotor retardation is noted in early infancy. Mutations in the ATP7A gene, encoding a copper transporting ATPase protein cause Menkes kinky hair syndrome. The disorder has been localized by linkage analysis to chromosome Xq13.3 and is due to a maldistribution of copper in the body. Copper uptake across the brush border of the small intestine is increased, but copper transport from these cells into the plasma is defective, resulting in low total body copper stores. Variable treatment success has been achieved with subcutaneous or intramuscular injection of copper salts.

Pili Annulati. Pili annulati is characterized by alternate light and dark bands of the hair shaft. When one is viewing the hair under the light microscope, the region that appeared bright in reflected light instead appears dark in the transmitted light as a result of focal aggregates of abnormal air-filled cavities within the hair shaft. The hair is not fragile. The defect may be autosomal dominant or sporadic. *Pseudopili annulati* is a variant of normal blond hair; an optical effect caused by the refraction and reflection of light from the partially twisted and flattened shaft creates the impression of banding.

Woolly Hair Disease. This disorder presents at birth with peculiarly tight, curly, abnormal hair in a nonblack person. It becomes worse in childhood and ameliorates in adulthood. An autosomal dominant form, evident at birth or in infancy, consists of excessively curly, fragile hair. An autosomal recessive type includes scalp hair that is brittle, has a bleached appearance, and is markedly reduced in diameter; body hair is short and pale. Woolly hair nevus, a sporadic form, involves only a circumscribed portion of the scalp hair. The affected hair is fine, tightly curled, and light colored, and it grows poorly. It may be associated with a pigmented or epidermal nevus in another site of the body or with ocular defects. Microscopically, affected hairs are oval and show twisting 180 degrees on their axis.

Uncombable Hair Syndrome (Spun Glass Hair). The hair of patients with this syndrome appears disorderly, is often silvery blond, and may break because of repeated, futile efforts to control it. The condition is probably autosomal dominant in inheritance, is usually first noticed in the first 3 yr of life, and may spontaneously improve in childhood. Eyebrows and eyelashes are normal. A longitudinal depression along the hair shaft is a constant feature, and most hair follicles and shafts are triangular (pili trianguli et canaliculi). The shape of the hair varies along its length, however, preventing the hairs from lying flat.

Baumeister F, Schwarz H, Stengel-Rutkowski S: Childhood hypertrichosis: Diagnosis and management. *Arch Dis Child* 1995;72:457.

Headington JT: Telogen effluvium. New concepts and review. *Arch Dermatol* 1993;129:356.

Price VH: Trichothiodystrophy: Update. *Pediatr Dermatol* 1992;9:369.

Rittmaster R: Hirsutism. *Lancet* 1997;349:191.

Rogers M: Hair disorders. In Eichenfield LF, Frieden IJ, Esterly NB (editors): *Textbook of Neonatal Dermatology.* Philadelphia, WB Saunders, 2001, p. 487.

Tazi-Ahnini R, McDonagh AJ, Cox A, et al: Association analysis of IL-1α and IL-1β variants in alopecia areata. *Heredity* 2001;87:215.

Tobin DJ, Orentreich N, Fenton DA, et al: Antibodies to hair follicles in alopecia areata. *J Invest Dermatol* 1994;102:721.

Verbov J: Hair loss in children. *Arch Dis Child* 1993;68:702, 1993.

Chapter 653
Disorders of the Nails

Nail abnormalities in children may be manifestations of generalized skin disease, skin disease localized to the periungual region, systemic disease, drugs, trauma, or localized bacterial and fungal infections. Nail anomalies are also common in certain congenital disorders (Box 653–1).

Anonychia is absence of the nail plate, usually a result of a congenital disorder or trauma. It may be an isolated finding or may be associated with malformations of the digits. *Koilonychia* is flattening and concavity of the nail plate with loss of normal contour, producing a spoon-shaped nail. Koilonychia occurs as an autosomal dominant trait or in association with hypochromic anemia, Plummer-Vinson syndrome, and hemochromatosis. The nail plate is relatively thin during the first 1–2 yr of life and consequently may be spoon-shaped in otherwise normal children.

Leukonychia is a white opacity of the nail plate that may involve the entire plate or may be punctate or striate. The nail plate itself remains smooth and undamaged. Leukonychia can be traumatic or associated with infections such as leprosy and tuberculosis, dermatoses such as lichen planus and Darier disease, malignancies such as Hodgkin disease, anemia, and arsenic poisoning (Mees lines). Leukonychia of all nail surfaces is an uncommon hereditary autosomal dominant trait that may be associated with congenital epidermal cysts, renal calculi, and deafness. Paired parallel white bands that do not change position with growth of the nail and thus reflect a change in the nail bed are associated with hypoalbuminemia and are called Muehrcke lines. When the proximal portion of the nail is white and the distal 20–50% of the nail is red, pink, or brown, the condition is called half-and-half nails or Lindsay nails; this is seen most commonly in patients with renal disease but may occur as a normal variant. White nails of cirrhosis, or Terry nails, are characterized by a white ground-glass appearance of the entire or the proximal end of the nail and a normal pink distal 1–2 mm of the nail; this is associated with hypoalbuminemia.

Onycholysis indicates separation of the nail plate from the distal nail bed. Common causes are trauma, chronic exposure to moisture, hyperhidrosis, cosmetics, psoriasis, fungal infection (distal onycholysis), atopic or contact dermatitis, porphyria, drugs (bleomycin, vincristine, retinoid agents, indomethacin, Thorazine), and drug-induced phototoxicity from tetracyclines or chloramphenicol. *Beau lines* are transverse grooves in the nail plate that represent a temporary disruption of formation of the nail plate. The lines first appear a few weeks after the event that caused the disruption in nail growth. A single transverse ridge appears at the proximal nail fold in most 4–6 wk old infants and works its way distally as the nail grows; this line may reflect metabolic changes after delivery. At other ages, Beau lines are usually indicative of periodic trauma or episodic shutdown of

the nail matrix secondary to a systemic disease such as measles, mumps, pneumonia, or zinc deficiency.

Nail changes may be particularly associated with various other diseases. Nail changes of *psoriasis* most characteristically include pitting, onycholysis, yellow-brown discoloration, and thickening. Nail changes in *lichen planus* include violaceous papules in the proximal nail fold and nail bed, leukonychia, longitudinal ridging, thinning of the entire nail plate, and *pterygium* formation, which is abnormal adherence of the cuticle to the nail plate or, if the plate is destroyed focally, to the nail bed. *Reiter disease* may include painless erythematous induration of the base of the nail fold; subungual parakeratotic scaling; and thickening, opacification, or ridging of the nail plate. *Dermatitis* that involves the nail folds may produce dystrophy, roughening, and coarse pitting of the nails. Nail changes are more common in atopic dermatitis than in other forms of dermatitis that affect the hands. *Darier disease* is characterized by red or white streaks that extend longitudinally and cross the lunula. Where the streak meets the distal end of the nail, a V-shaped notch may be present. Total leukonychia may also occur. Transverse rows of fine pits are characteristic of *alopecia areata*. In severe cases, the entire nail surface may be rough. Patients with *acrodermatitis enteropathica* may have transverse grooves (Beau lines) and nail dystrophy as a result of periungual dermatitis.

Twenty-nail dystrophy is characterized by longitudinal ridging, pitting fragility, thinning, distal notching, and opalescent discoloration of all the nails. Patients have no associated skin or systemic diseases and no other ectodermal defects. Its occasional association with alopecia areata has led some authorities to suggest that 20-nail dystrophy may reflect an abnormal immunologic response to the nail matrix, whereas histopathologic studies have suggested that it may be a manifestation of lichen planus or spongiotic (eczematous) inflammation of the nail matrix. It also can be a feature of vitiligo or psoriasis. The disorder must be differentiated from fungal infections, psoriasis, nail changes of alopecia areata, and nail dystrophy secondary to eczema. Eczema and fungal infections rarely produce changes of all the nails simultaneously. The disorder is self-limited and eventually remits by adulthood.

Congenital nail dysplasia, an autosomal dominant disorder, manifests with onset at birth and longitudinal streaks and thinning of the nail plate. There is platonychia, koilonychia, which may overgrow the lateral folds and involve all nails of the toes and fingers.

Black pigmentation of an entire nail plate or linear bands of pigmentation (melanonychia striata) are common in black (90%) and Asian (10–20%) individuals but are unusual in whites (<1%). Most often, the pigment is melanin, which is produced by melanocytes of a junctional nevus in the nail matrix and nail bed and is of no consequence. Extension or alteration in the pigment should be evaluated by biopsy because of the possibility of malignant change. Bluish-black to greenish nails may be caused by pseudomonas infection, particularly in association with onycholysis or chronic paronychia. The coloration is due to subungual debris and pyocyanin pigment from the bacterial organisms.

Splinter hemorrhages most often result from minor trauma but may also be associated with subacute bacterial endocarditis, vasculitis, severe rheumatoid arthritis, peptic ulcer disease, hypertension, chronic glomerulonephritis, cirrhosis, scurvy, trichinosis, malignant neoplasms, and psoriasis.

Clubbing of the nails (hippocratic nails) is characterized by swelling of the distal digit, an increase in the angle between the nail plate and the proximal nail fold (Lovibond angle) to greater than 180 degrees, and a spongy feeling when one pushes down and away from the interphalangeal joint because of an increase in fibrovascular tissue between the matrix and the phalanx. The pathogenesis is not known, but altered prostaglandin metabolism has been described. Nail clubbing is seen in association with

---

BOX 653–1. Congenital Disease with Nail Defects

Large nails: Pachyonychia congenita, Rubinstein-Taybi syndrome, hemihypertrophy
Small or absent nails: Ectodermal dysplasias, nail-patella, dyskeratosis congenita, focal dermal hypoplasia, cartilage-hair hypoplasia, Ellis–van Creveld, Larsen, epidermolysis bullosa, incontinentia pigmenti, Rothmund-Thomson, Turner, popliteal web, trisomy 13, trisomy 18, Apert, Gorlin-Pindborg, long arm 21 deletion, otopalatodigital, fetal alcohol, fetal hydantoin, elfin facies, anonychia, acrodermatitis enteropathica
Other: Congenital malalignment of the great toenails, familial dystrophic shedding of the nails

diseases of numerous organ systems, including pulmonary, cardiovascular, gastrointestinal, and hepatic systems, and in healthy individuals as an idiopathic finding.

Habit tic deformity consists of a depression down the center of the nail with numerous horizontal ridges extending across the nail from it. One or both thumbs are usually involved as a result of chronic rubbing and picking at the nail with an adjacent finger.

Fungal infection of the nails has been classified into four types. *White superficial onychomycosis* presents with diffuse or speckled white discoloration of the surface of the toenails. It is caused primarily by *Trichophyton mentagrophytes*, which invades the nail plate. The organism may be scraped off the nail plate with a blade, but treatment is best accomplished by the addition of a topical azole antifungal agent. *Distal subungual onychomycosis* presents with foci of onycholysis under the distal nail plate or along the lateral nail groove, followed by development of hyperkeratosis and yellow-brown discoloration. The process extends proximally, resulting in nail plate thickening, crumbling, and separation from the nail bed. *Trichophyton rubrum* and occasionally *T. mentagrophytes* are most common on toenails; fingernail disease is almost exclusively due to *T. rubrum*, which may be associated with superficial scaling of the plantar surface of the feet and often of one hand. These dermatophytes are found most readily at the most proximal area of the nail bed or adjacent ventral portion of the nail plates that are involved. Topical therapies alone are ineffective in most cases, but nail evulsion in combination with topical antifungal agents may be effective. Because of their long half-life in the nail, terbinafine or itraconazole may be effective when given as pulse therapy (1 wk of each mo for 3–4 mo). Either agent is superior to griseofulvin or ketoconazole. The risks, most concerning of which is hepatic toxicity, and costs of oral therapy must be weighed carefully against the benefits of treatment for a condition that generally causes only cosmetic problems.

Proximal white subungual onychomycosis occurs when the organism, generally *T. rubrum*, enters the nail through the proximal nail fold, producing yellow-white portions of the undersurface of the nail plate. The surface of the nail is unaffected. This occurs almost exclusively in immunocompromised patients and is a well-recognized manifestation of AIDS.

Candidal onychomycosis involves the entire nail plate in patients with chronic mucocutaneous candidiasis. It is also commonly seen in patients with AIDS. The organism, generally *Candida albicans*, enters distally or along the lateral nail folds, rapidly involves the entire thickness of the nail plate, and produces thickening, crumbling, and deformity of the plate. Topical azole antifungal agents may be sufficient for treatment of candidal onychomycosis in an immunocompetent host, but oral antifungal agents are necessary for treatment of those with immune deficiencies.

Paronychial inflammation may be acute or chronic and generally involves one or two nail folds on the fingers. Acute paronychia presents with erythema, warmth, edema, and tenderness of the proximal nail fold, most commonly as a result of pathogenic staphylococci or streptococci. Warm soaks and oral antibiotics such as clindamycin or amoxicillin plus clavulanic acid are generally effective; incision and drainage may be necessary in some cases. Development of chronic paronychia is favored by prolonged immersion in water, such as occurs in finger or thumb sucking; exposure to irritating solutions; nail fold trauma; or diseases including Raynaud phenomenon, collagen vascular diseases, or diabetes. Swelling of the proximal nail fold is followed by separation of the nail fold from the underlying nail plate and suppuration. Foreign material, embedded in the dermis of the nail fold, becomes a nidus for inflammation and infection with *Candida* species and mixed bacterial flora. A combination of attention to predisposing factors, meticulous drying of the hands, including use of 4% thymol solution, and long-term

antifungal, antibacterial, and topical anti-inflammatory agents may be required for successful treatment of chronic paronychia. The primary chancre of syphilis also may present on the finger as a relatively nontender paronychia.

Ingrown nails occur when the lateral edge of the nail, including spicules that have separated from the nail plate, penetrates the soft tissue of the lateral nail fold. Erythema, edema, and pain, most often involving the lateral great toes, are noted acutely; recurrent episodes may lead to formation of granulation tissue. Predisposing factors include (1) compression of the side of the toe from poorly fitting shoes, particularly if the great toes are abnormally long and the lateral nail folds are prominent, and (2) improper cutting of the nail in a curvilinear manner rather than straight across. Management includes proper fitting of shoes; allowing the nail to grow out beyond the free edge before cutting it straight across; warm water soaks; oral antibiotics if cellulitis affects the lateral nail fold; and, in severe, recurrent cases, application of silver nitrate to granulation tissue, nail avulsion, or excision of the lateral aspect of the nail followed by matricectomy.

Tumors in the paronychial area include pyogenic granulomas, mucous cysts, subungual exostoses, and junctional nevi. Periungual fibromas that appear during late childhood should suggest a diagnosis of tuberous sclerosis.

Nail-patella syndrome is an autosomal dominant disorder in which the nails are 30–50% their normal size and often have triangular or pyramidal lunulae. The thumbnails are always involved, although in some cases only the ulnar half of the nail may be affected or may be missing. The nails from the index finger to the little finger are progressively less damaged. The patella is also smaller than usual, and this anomaly may lead to knee instability. Bony spines arising from the posterior aspect of the iliac bones, overextension of joints, skin laxity, hyperhidrosis, and renal anomalies may also be present. Nail patella syndrome is caused by mutations in the transcription factor LMX1B gene.

Pachyonychia congenita (see Chapter 648).

Yellow nail syndrome presents with thickened, excessively curved, slow-growing yellow nails without lunulae. All nails are affected in most cases. Associated systemic disease includes bronchiectasis, recurrent bronchitis, chylothorax, and focal edema of the limbs and face. Deficient lymphatic drainage, due to hypoplastic lymphatic vessels, is believed to lead to the manifestations of this syndrome.

DeCoste SD, Imber MJ, Baden HP: Yellow nail syndrome. *J Am Acad Dermatol* 1990;22:608.

Dreyer SD, Zhou G, Baldini A, et al: Mutation in LMx1B cause abnormal skeletal patterning and renal dysplasia in nail patella syndrome. *Nat Genet* 1998;19:82.

Hamm H, Karl S, Brocker EB: Isolated congenital nail dysplasia. *Arch Dermatol* 2000;136:1239–43.

Juhlin L, Baran R. In Baran R, Dawber RP (editors): *Diseases of the Nails and Their Management*. Oxford, Blackwell Scientific, 1984, p 303.

Peluso AM, Tosti A, Piraccini BM, et al: Lichen planus limited to the nails in childhood: Case report and literature review. *Pediatr Dermatol* 1993;10:36.

Silverman RA. Nail defects. In Eichenfield LF, Frieden IJ, Esterly NB (editors): *Textbook of Neonatal Dermatology*. Philadelphia, 2001, p 504.

Chapter 654
Disorders of the Mucous Membranes

The mucous membranes may be involved in developmental disorders, infections, acute and chronic skin diseases, genodermatoses, and benign and malignant tumors. Some of the more common and distinctive diseases specific to mucous membranes are presented in this chapter.

Cheilitis. Inflammation of the lips (cheilitis) and angles of the mouth (angular cheilitis or perlèche) are most commonly due to dryness, chapping, and lip licking; excessive salivation and drooling, particularly in children with neurologic deficits, may also cause chronic irritation. Lesions of oral thrush may occasionally extend to the angles of the mouth. Protection can be provided by frequent applications of a bland ointment such as petrolatum. Candidosis should be treated with an appropriate antifungal agent, and contact dermatitis of the perioral skin should be treated with a mild topical corticosteroid preparation and an emollient.

Fordyce Spots. These are asymptomatic, minute, yellow-white papules on the vermilion border of the lips and buccal mucosa. These ectopic sebaceous glands may be found in otherwise normal individuals and require no therapy.

Mucocele. Mucus retention cysts are painless, bluish, fluctuant, tense, 2–10 mm papules on the lips, tongue, palate, or buccal mucosa. Traumatic severance of the duct of a minor salivary gland leads to submucosal retention of mucus secretion. Those on the floor of the mouth are known as *ranulas* when the submaxillary or sublingual salivary ducts are involved. Fluctuations in size are usual, and the lesions may disappear temporarily after traumatic rupture. Recurrence is prevented by excising the mucocele.

Aphthous Stomatitis (Canker Sores). Solitary or multiple painful ulcerations occur on the labial, buccal, or lingual mucosa and on the sublingual, palatal, or gingival mucosa. Lesions may present initially as erythematous, indurated papules that erode rapidly to form sharply circumscribed, necrotic ulcers with a gray fibrinous exudate and an erythematous halo. Minor aphthous ulcers are 2–10 mm in diameter and heal spontaneously in 7–10 days. Major aphthous ulcers are greater than 10 mm in diameter and take 10–30 days to heal. A third type of aphthous ulceration is herpetiform in appearance, presenting with a few to numerous grouped 1–2 mm lesions that tend to coalesce into plaques that heal over 7–10 days. Approximately one third of patients with recurrent lesions have a family history of the disorder. (See Chapter 296 for differential diagnosis.)

The *etiology* of aphthous stomatitis is probably multifactorial; the condition probably represents an oral manifestation of a number of conditions. Altered local regulation of the cell-mediated immune system, after activation and accumulation of cytotoxic T cells, may contribute to the localized mucosal breakdown. Predisposing factors include trauma, emotional stress, low serum iron or ferritin levels, deficiency of vitamin B_{12} or folate, malabsorption in association with celiac or Crohn disease, menstruation accompanied by a decrease in progestogens during the luteal phase, food hypersensitivity, and allergic or toxic drug reactions. It is a common misconception that aphthous stomatitis is a manifestation of herpes simplex virus infection. Recurrent herpes infections remain localized to the lips and rarely cross the mucocutaneous junction; involvement of the oral mucosa occurs only in primary infections.

Treatment of aphthous stomatitis is palliative. Use of 0.2% aqueous chlorhexidine gluconate mouthwash helps to maintain oral hygiene. Relief of pain, particularly before eating, may be achieved by use of a topical anesthetic such as viscous lidocaine (Xylocaine) or an oral rinse with a solution of elixir of diphenhydramine, viscous lidocaine, and 0.5% dyclonine hydrochloride. A topical corticosteroid in a mucosal adhering agent (0.1% triamcinolone in Orabase) may help to reduce inflammation, and topical tetracycline mouthwash may also hasten healing. In severe, debilitating cases, systemic therapy with corticosteroids, colchicine, or dapsone may be helpful.

Cowden Syndrome (Multiple Hamartoma Syndrome). This is an autosomal dominant condition that usually presents during the 2nd or 3rd decade with smooth, pink or whitish papules on the palatal, gingival, buccal, and labial mucosae. Mutations in the tumor suppressor gene PTEN cause Cowden syndrome. These benign fibromas may coalesce into a cobblestone appearance. Numerous flesh-colored papules also develop on the face, particularly around the mouth, nose, and ears; these papules most commonly are trichilemmomas, a benign neoplasm of the hair follicle. Associated findings may include acral keratotic papules, thyroid goiter, gastrointestinal polyps, fibrocystic breast nodules, and carcinoma of the breast or thyroid.

Epstein Pearls (Gingival Cysts of the Newborn). These are white keratin-containing cysts on the palatal or alveolar mucosa of approximately 80% of neonates. They cause no symptoms and are generally shed within a few weeks.

Geographic Tongue (Benign Migratory Glossitis). This consists of single or multiple sharply demarcated, irregular, smooth red plaques on the dorsum of the tongue caused by transient atrophy of the filiform papillae and the surface epithelium, often with elevated gray margins composed of intervening filiform papillae that are increased in thickness. Symptoms of mild burning or irritation may occasionally be bothersome. Onset is rapid, and the pattern may change over hours to days. Geographic tongue is associated with scrotal tongue in nearly 50% of patients. Some patients have atopy; some feel that the condition is exacerbated by stress or by hot or spicy foods; and some have anemia, diabetes mellitus, Reiter disease, seborrheic dermatitis, or pustular psoriasis. Geographic tongue may be an oral manifestation of pustular psoriasis, with which it shares histologic features. No therapy other than reassurance is necessary.

Scrotal (Fissured) Tongue. Approximately 1% of infants and 2.5% of children have many folds with deep grooves on the dorsal tongue surface. These impart a pebbled or wrinkled appearance. Some cases are congenital, caused by incomplete fusion of the two halves of the tongue; others develop in association with infection, trauma, malnutrition, or low vitamin A levels. Many patients with fissured tongue also have geographic tongue. Food particles and debris may become trapped in the fissures, resulting in irritation, inflammation, and halitosis. Careful cleansing with a mouth rinse and soft-bristled toothbrush is recommended.

Black Hairy Tongue. This is a dark coating on the dorsum of the tongue caused by hyperplasia and elongation of the filiform papillae; overgrowth of chromogenic bacteria and fungi and entrapped pigmented residues that adsorb to microbial plaque and desquamating keratin may contribute to the dark coloration. Changes often begin posteriorly and extend anteriorly on the dorsum of the tongue. The condition is most common in adults but may also present during adolescence. Poor oral hygiene and bacterial overgrowth, treatment with systemic antibiotics such as tetracycline (which promotes the growth of *Candida* species), and smoking are predisposing factors. Improved oral hygiene and brushing with a soft-bristled toothbrush may be all that are necessary for treatment. The filiform hyperplasia may also be decreased with topical keratolytic agents such as trichloroacetic acid, urea, or podophyllin.

Oral Hairy Leukoplakia. This occurs in approximately 25% of patients with AIDS but is rare in the pediatric population. It presents as a mostly asymptomatic white thickening and accentuation of the normal vertical folds of the lateral margins of the tongue. The mucosa is white and irregularly thickened but remains soft. Spread may occur occasionally to the ventral tongue surface, the floor of the mouth, the tonsillar pillars, and the pharynx. The condition appears to be due to Epstein-Barr virus, which is present in the upper layer of the affected epithelium. The plaques have no malignant potential. The disorder occurs predominantly in HIV-infected patients but may also be found in individuals who are immunosuppressed for other reasons, such as organ transplantation or leukemia and chemotherapy. The condition is generally asymptomatic and does not require therapy. Resolution of the plaques may be hastened, however, by use of antiviral agents such as acyclovir or local application of 0.1% vitamin A acid twice daily.

Vincent Gingivitis (Acute Necrotizing Ulcerative Gingivitis, Fusospirochetal Gingivitis, Trench Mouth). This disorder presents with punched-out ulceration, necrosis, and bleeding of interdental papillae. A grayish-white pseudomembrane may cover the ulcerations. Lesions may spread to involve the buccal mucosa, lips, tongue, tonsils, and pharynx and may be associated with dental pain, a bad taste, low-grade fever, and lymphadenopathy. It presents most commonly during the 2nd or 3rd decade, particularly in the context of poor dental hygiene, scurvy, or pellagra. A synergistic association between fusospirochetal organisms *(Fusobacterium nucleatum)* and *Borrelia vincenti* has been proposed to contribute to the pathogenesis.

Noma is a severe form of fusospirillary gangrenous stomatitis that presents primarily in malnourished children 2–5 yr of age who have had a preceding illness such as measles, scarlet fever, tuberculosis, malignancy, or immunodeficiency. It presents as a painful red, indurated papule on the alveolar margin, followed by ulceration and mutilating gangrenous destruction of tissue in the oronasal region. The process may also involve the scalp, neck, shoulders, perineum, and vulva. *Noma neonatorum* presents in the 1st mo of life with gangrenous lesions of the lips, nose, mouth, and anal regions. Affected infants are usually small for gestational age, malnourished, premature, and frequently ill, particularly with *Pseudomonas aeruginosa* sepsis. Care consists of nutritional support, conservative debridement of necrotic soft tissues, empirical broad-spectrum antibiotics such as penicillin and metronidazole, and in the case of noma neonatorum, antipseudomonal antibiotics.

Herbert AA, Berg JH: Oral mucous membrane diseases of childhood: I. Mucositis and xerostomia. II. Recurrent aphthous stomatitis. III. Herpetic stomatitis. *Semin Dermatol* 1992;11:80.

Itin PH, Bircher AJ, Litzisdorf Y, et al: Oral hairy leukoplakia in a child: Confirmation of the clinical diagnosis by ultrastructural examination of exfoliative cytologic specimens. *Dermatology* 1994;189:167.

Liaw D, Marsh DJ, Li J, et al: Germline mutations of the PTEN gene in Cowden disease, an inherited breast and thyroid cancer syndrome. *Nat Genet* 1997;16:64.

Metry DW, Hebert AA. Neonatal mucous membrane disorders. In Eichenfield LF, Frieden IJ, Esterly NB (editors): *Text book of Neonatal Dermatology*. Philadelphia, WB Saunders, 2001, p. 473.

Prose NS: Mucocutaneous disease in pediatric human immunodeficiency virus infection. *Pediatr Clin North Am* 1991;38:977.

Chapter 655
Cutaneous Bacterial Infections

Skin complaints or findings are noted in 20–30% of children who attend general pediatric clinics. Bacterial skin infection is the single most common diagnosis among children with skin problems, accounting for 17% of all clinic visits. The most common bacterial skin infection of children is impetigo, which makes up approximately 10% of all skin problems.

IMPETIGO

See Chapters 166 and 168.

Clinical Manifestations

NONBULLOUS IMPETIGO. There are two classic forms of impetigo: nonbullous and bullous. Nonbullous impetigo accounts for more than 70% of cases. Lesions typically begin on the skin of the face or on extremities that have been traumatized. The most common lesions that precede nonbullous impetigo include insect bites, abrasions, lacerations, chickenpox, scabies pediculosis, and burns. A tiny vesicle or pustule forms initially (Fig. 655–1*A*) and rapidly develops into a honey-colored crusted plaque that is generally less than 2 cm in diameter (see Fig. 655–1*B*). The infection may be spread to other parts of the body by the fingers, clothing, and towels. Lesions are associated with little to no pain or surrounding erythema, and constitutional symptoms are generally absent. Pruritus occurs occasionally, regional adenopathy is found in up to 90% of cases, and leukocytosis is present in approximately 50% of patients. Without treatment, most cases resolve spontaneously without scarring within approximately 2 wk. The differential diagnosis of nonbullous impetigo includes viral (herpes simplex, varicella-zoster), fungal (tinea corporis, kerion), and parasitic infections (scabies, pediculosis capitis), all of which may become impetiginized.

Staphylococcus aureus is the predominant organism of nonbullous impetigo in the United States; group A β-hemolytic streptococci (GABHS) are implicated in the development of some lesions. Staphylococci generally spread from the nose to normal skin and then infect the skin. In contrast, the skin becomes colonized with GABHS an average of 10 days before development of impetigo. GABHS then colonize the nasopharynx an average of 2–3 wk after the appearance of lesions of impetigo. The skin serves as the source for acquisition of GABHS in the respiratory tract and the probable primary source for spread of impetigo. Lesions of nonbullous impetigo that grow staphylococci in culture cannot be distinguished clinically from those that grow pure cultures of GABHS. Whereas *S. aureus* can be cultured from lesions of impetigo in children of all ages, GABHS is most commonly cultured from children of preschool age and is unusual before 2 yr of age, except in highly endemic areas. The staphylococcal types that cause nonbullous impetigo are variable but are not generally from phage group 2, the group that is associated with scalded skin and toxic shock syndromes. Several serotypes of GABHS, termed "impetigo strains," are found most frequently in lesions of nonbullous impetigo and are different from those that cause pharyngitis.

BULLOUS IMPETIGO. This is mainly an infection of infants and young children. Bullous impetigo is always caused by coagulase-positive *S. aureus*; approximately 80% are from phage group 2, among which 60% are type 71, and most of the remainder are types 3A, 3B, 3C, and 55. Flaccid, transparent bullae develop most commonly on skin of the face, buttocks, trunk, perineum, and extremities; neonatal bullous impetigo can begin in the diaper area. Rupture of bullae occurs easily, leaving a narrow rim of scale at the edge of a shallow, moist erosion. Surrounding erythema and regional adenopathy are generally absent. Unlike those of nonbullous impetigo, lesions of bullous impetigo are a manifestation of localized staphylococcal scalded skin syndrome and develop on intact skin.

Diagnosis. Cultures of fluid from an intact blister or moist plaque should yield the causative agent; if the patient appears ill, blood cultures should also be obtained. On histopathologic examination, lesions of bullous impetigo show vesicle formation in the subcorneal or granular region, neutrophils and occasionally acantholytic cells within the blister, spongiosis, edema of the papillary dermis, and a mixed infiltrate of lymphocytes and neutrophils around blood vessels of the superficial plexus. Unless staphylococci can be cultured from the bullae or, less commonly, can be seen on Gram stain, it may be impossible to differentiate bullous impetigo from pemphigus foliaceous or subcorneal pustular dermatosis histopathologically. Nonbullous impetigo has histopathologic findings similar to those of the bullous variant, except that blister formation is slight.

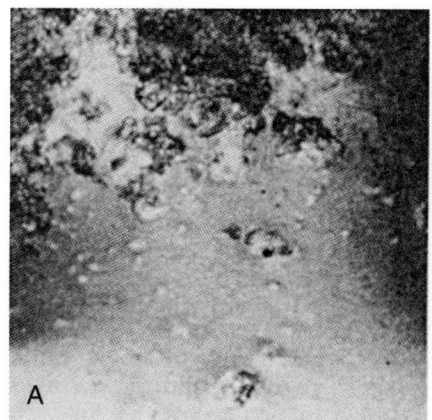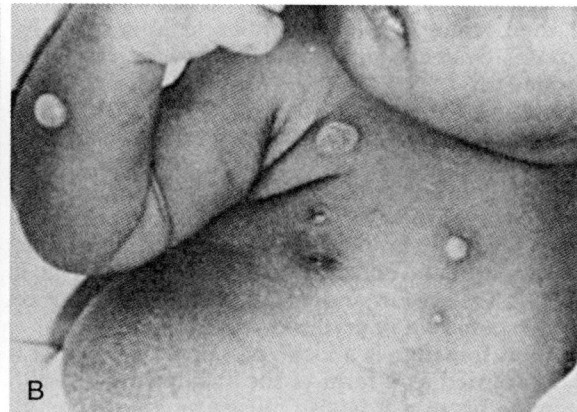

FIGURE 655–1. *A,* Multiple crusted and oozing lesions of streptococcal impetigo. *B,* Multiple tense and flaccid blisters of bullous impetigo on the trunk and arm of an infant.

The *differential diagnosis* of bullous impetigo in neonates includes epidermolysis bullosa, bullous mastocytosis, herpetic infection, and early scalded skin syndrome. In older children, allergic contact dermatitis, burns, erythema multiforme, chronic bullous dermatosis of childhood, pemphigus, and bullous pemphigoid must be considered, particularly if the lesions do not respond to therapy.

Complications. Potential but very rare complications of either nonbullous or bullous impetigo include osteomyelitis, septic arthritis, pneumonia, and septicemia; positive blood culture results are rare in otherwise healthy children with localized lesions. Cellulitis has been reported in approximately 10% of patients with nonbullous impetigo but rarely follows the bullous form. Lymphangitis, suppurative lymphadenitis, guttate psoriasis, and scarlet fever occasionally follow streptococcal disease. There is no correlation between number of lesions and clinical involvement of the lymphatics or development of cellulitis in association with streptococcal impetigo.

Infection with nephritogenic strains of GABHS may result in acute poststreptococcal glomerulonephritis (Chapter 503.1). The clinical character of impetigo lesions is not predictive of the development of poststreptococcal glomerulonephritis. The most commonly affected age group is school-aged children 3–7 yr old. The latent period from onset of impetigo to development of poststreptococcal glomerulonephritis averages 18–21 days, which is longer than the 10-day latency period after pharyngitis. Poststreptococcal glomerulonephritis occurs epidemically after either pharyngeal or skin infection. Impetigo-associated epidemics have been caused by M groups 2, 49, 53, 55, 56, 57, and 60. Strains of GABHS that are associated with endemic impetigo in the United States have little or no nephritogenic potential. Acute rheumatic fever does not occur as a result of impetigo.

Treatment. Topical or systemic antibiotic treatment is superior to placebo or cleansing with 3% hexachlorophene soap. Furthermore, cleansing with 3% hexachlorophene soap adds little to no benefit over systemic antibiotics alone. Mupirocin is an ointment that is bactericidal by reversible inhibition of bacterial isoleucyl-transfer RNA synthetase. Applied topically three times daily for 7–10 days, it is equal to or greater in effectiveness, with fewer side effects, than oral erythromycin ethylsuccinate, 30–50 mg/kg/24 hr for 7–10 days. Rare instances of bacterial resistance to mupirocin have been reported, but most patients were treated irregularly or prophylactically for more than 2 wk. Topical fusidic acid may also be effective.

Systemic therapy with a β-lactamase–resistant oral antibiotic should be prescribed for patients with widespread involvement; when lesions are near the mouth, where topical medication may be licked off; or in cases of evidence of deep involvement, including cellulitis, furunculosis, abscess formation, or suppurative lymphadenitis. In areas without a high prevalence of *S. aureus* resistance to erythromycin, erythromycin ethylsuccinate (40 mg/kg/24 hr divided three to four times daily for 7 days) or erythromycin estolate (30 mg/kg/24 hr divided three to four times daily) is the preferred oral therapy. If erythromycin resistance is widespread in the community, alternative oral antibiotics that have been shown to be effective in children for treatment of impetigo include dicloxacillin; amoxicillin plus clavulanic acid, clindamycin, and a cephalosporin such as cephalexin, cefaclor, cefadroxil, cefprozil, or cefpodoxime. The choice among these various agents may be guided primarily by issues of cost, local availability, and compliance. The macrolides clarithromycin or azithromycin may be advantageous primarily in instances of intolerance to erythromycin but will not provide cure rates superior to those of erythromycin. No evidence suggests that a 10-day course of therapy is superior to a 7-day one. If a satisfactory clinical response is not achieved within 7 days, however, a culture should be taken by swabbing beneath the lifted edge of a crusted lesion. If a resistant organism is detected, an appropriate antibiotic should be given for an additional 7 days.

SUBCUTANEOUS TISSUE INFECTIONS

The principal determination for soft tissue infections is whether it is non-necrotizing or necrotizing; the former responds to antibiotic therapy alone, whereas the latter requires prompt surgical removal of all devitalized tissue in addition to antimicrobial therapy. Necrotizing soft tissue infections are potentially life-threatening conditions that are characterized by rapidly advancing local tissue destruction and systemic toxicity. Tissue necrosis distinguishes them from cellulitis; in cellulitis, an inflammatory infectious process involves subcutaneous tissue but does not destroy it. Necrotizing soft tissue infections characteristically present with a paucity of early cutaneous signs relative to the rapidity and degree of destruction of the subcutaneous tissues.

Cellulitis. Cellulitis is characterized by infection and inflammation of loose connective tissue, with limited involvement of the dermis and relative sparing of the epidermis. A break in the skin due to previous trauma, surgery, or an underlying skin lesion predisposes to cellulitis. Cellulitis is also more common in individuals with lymphatic stasis, diabetes mellitus, or immunosuppression.

ETIOLOGY. *Streptococcus pyogenes* and *S. aureus* are the most common etiologic agents. Occasionally, *Streptococcus pneumoniae*, group G or C streptococci, and in neonates, group B streptococci or rarely *Escherichia coli* are the causal organism. In patients who are immunocompromised or have diabetes mellitus, a number of other bacterial or fungal agents may be involved, notably *Pseudomonas aeruginosa; Aeromonas hydrophila* and occasionally other Enterobacteriaceae; *Legionella* spp; the Mucorales, particularly *Rhizopus* spp, *Mucor* spp, and *Absidia* spp; and *Cryptococcus neoformans*. Children with relapsed nephrotic syndrome may develop cellulitis due to *E. coli*. In children age 3 mo to 3–5 yr, *Haemophilus influenzae* type b was once an important cause of facial cellulitis, but its incidence has declined significantly since institution of immunization against this organism.

CLINICAL MANIFESTATIONS. Cellulitis presents clinically as an area of edema, warmth, erythema, and tenderness. The lateral margins tend to be indistinct because the process is deep in the skin, primarily involving the subcutaneous tissues in addition to the dermis. Application of pressure may produce pitting. Although distinction cannot be made with certainty in any particular patient, cellulitis as a result of *S. aureus* tends to be more localized and may suppurate, whereas infections due to *S. pyogenes* tend to spread more rapidly and may be associated with lymphangitis. Regional adenopathy and constitutional signs and symptoms of fever, chills, and malaise are common. Complications of cellulitis include subcutaneous abscess, bacteremia, osteomyelitis, septic arthritis, thrombophlebitis, endocarditis, and necrotizing fasciitis. Lymphangitis or glomerulonephritis also can follow infection with *S. pyogenes*.

DIAGNOSIS. Aspirates from the site of inflammation, skin biopsy, and blood cultures allow identification of the causal organism in approximately 25% of cases of cellulitis. Yield of the causative organism is approximately one third when the site of origin of the cellulitis is apparent, such as an abrasion or ulcer. An aspirate taken from the point of maximum inflammation yields the causal organism more often than does a leading-edge aspirate. Lack of success in isolating an organism stems primarily from the low number of organisms present within the lesion.

TREATMENT. Empirical therapy for cellulitis should be directed by the history of the illness, the location and character of the cellulitis, and the age and immune status of the patient. Cellulitis in a neonate should prompt a full sepsis work-up, followed by initiation of empirical therapy intravenously with a β-lactamase–stable antistaphylococcal antibiotic such as methicillin and an aminoglycoside such as gentamicin or a cephalosporin such as cefotaxime. Treatment of cellulitis in an infant or child younger than about 5 yr should provide coverage for *S. pyogenes* and *S. aureus* as well as *H. influenzae* type b and *S. pneumoniae*. The evaluation should include a blood culture, and if the infant is younger than 1 year, if signs of systemic toxicity are present, or if an adequate examination cannot be carried out, a lumbar puncture should also be performed. In most cases of cellulitis on an extremity, regardless of age, *S. aureus* and *S. pyogenes* are the cause and bacteremia is unlikely in an otherwise well-appearing child. Blood cultures should be obtained if sepsis is suspected. If fever, lymphadenopathy, and other constitutional signs are absent (e.g., white blood cell count < 15,000), treatment of cellulitis on an extremity may be initiated orally on an outpatient basis with a penicillinase-resistant penicillin such as dicloxacillin or cloxacillin or a first-generation cephalosporin such as cephalexin. If improvement is not noted or the disease progresses significantly within the first 24–48 hr of therapy, parenteral therapy is necessary. If fever, lymphadenopathy, or constitutional signs are present, therapy should be initiated parenterally. Oxacillin or nafcillin is effective in most cases, although if systemic toxicity is significant, consideration should be given to the addition of penicillin or clindamycin. Once the erythema, warmth, edema, and fever have decreased significantly, a 10-day course of treatment may be completed on an outpatient basis. Immobilization and elevation of an affected limb, particularly early in the course of therapy, may help to reduce swelling and pain.

Necrotizing Fasciitis. Necrotizing fasciitis is a subcutaneous tissue infection that involves the deep layer of superficial fascia but largely spares adjacent epidermis, deep fascia, and muscle.

ETIOLOGY. Relatively few organisms possess sufficient virulence to cause necrotizing fasciitis when acting alone. The most fulminant infections, associated with toxic shock syndrome and a high case-fatality rate, are caused by *S. pyogenes* (also see Chapter 168). Streptococcal necrotizing fasciitis in the absence of toxic shock-like syndrome may occur and is seldom fatal but may be associated with substantial morbidity. Necrotizing fasciitis can occasionally be caused by *S. aureus, Clostridium perfringens, Clostridium septicum, P. aeruginosa, Vibrio* spp, particularly *V. vulnificus,* and fungi of the order Mucorales, particularly *Rhizopus* spp, *Mucor* spp, and *Absidia* spp. Necrotizing fasciitis has also been reported on rare occasions to result from non–group A streptococci such as group B, C, F, or G streptococci, *S. pneumoniae,* or *H. influenzae* type b. Necrotizing fasciitis may be a polymicrobial infection. In most of these cases, a mixture of anaerobic bacteria and aerobic or facultative bacteria appear to act together to cause tissue necrosis. The most common aerobic or facultative bacteria are several species of hemolytic or nonhemolytic non–group A streptococci, *S. aureus, E. coli, Enterobacter* spp, and various other Enterobacteriaceae, and *Pseudomonas* spp. The anaerobes present are similar to those found in subcutaneous abscesses: *Bacteroides* spp, *Peptostreptococcus* spp, *Peptococcus* spp, *Prevotella* spp, *Porphyromonas* spp, *Clostridium* spp, and *Fusobacterium* spp. Infections due to any one organism or combination of organisms cannot be distinguished clinically from one another, although development of crepitance signals the presence of *Clostridium* spp or gram-negative bacilli such as *E. coli, Klebsiella, Proteus,* and *Aeromonas.*

EPIDEMIOLOGY. Necrotizing fasciitis may occur anywhere on the body; the most common locations, however, are the extremities, abdomen, and perineal region. Common predisposing conditions in neonates are omphalitis and balanitis after circumcision. The incidence of necrotizing fasciitis is highest in hosts with systemic or local tissue immunocompromise, such as those with diabetes mellitus, neoplasia, or peripheral vascular disease, and those recently having undergone surgery, those who abuse intravenous drugs, or those on immunosuppressive treatment, particularly with corticosteroids. The infection also can occur in healthy individuals after minor puncture wounds, abrasions, or lacerations; blunt trauma; surgical procedures, particularly of the abdomen, gastrointestinal or genitourinary tracts, or the perineum; or hypodermic needle injection. Since the mid-1980s, there has been a resurgence of fulminant necrotizing soft tissue infections due to *S. pyogenes,* which may occur in previously healthy individuals with little or no apparent compromise of immunologic or skin integrity. Necrotizing fasciitis due to *S. pyogenes* may occur after superinfection of varicella lesions. These children have tended to display onset, recrudescence, or persistence of high fever and signs of toxicity after the 3rd to 4th day of varicella.

CLINICAL MANIFESTATIONS. Necrotizing fasciitis begins with acute onset of local swelling, erythema, tenderness, and heat. Fever is usually present, and pain, tenderness, and constitutional signs are out of proportion to cutaneous signs, especially with involvement of fascia and muscle. Lymphangitis and lymphadenitis are usually absent. The infection advances along the superficial fascial plane, and initially there are few cutaneous signs to herald the serious nature and extent of subcutaneous tissue necrosis that is occurring. Skin changes may appear over 24–48 hr as nutrient vessels are thrombosed and cutaneous ischemia develops. Early clinical findings include ill-defined cutaneous erythema and edema, which extend beyond the area of erythema. Additional signs include formation of bullae filled initially with straw-colored and later bluish to hemorrhagic fluid, and darkening of affected tissues from red to purple to blue. Skin anesthesia and finally frank tissue gangrene and slough develop owing to the ischemia and necrosis. Vesiculation or bulla formation, ecchymoses, crepitus, anesthesia, and necrosis are ominous and indicative of advanced disease. Children with varicella lesions initially may show no cutaneous signs of superinfection with invasive *S. pyogenes* such as erythema or swelling. Significant systemic toxicity may accompany necrotizing fasciitis, including shock, organ failure, and death. Advance of the infection in this setting can be rapid, progressing to death within hours. In general, patients with involvement of the superficial or deep fascia and muscle tend to be more acutely and systemically ill and have more rapidly advancing disease than those with infection confined solely to subcutaneous tissues above the fascia. In an extremity, a *compartment syndrome* may develop and is manifest as tight edema, pain on motion, and loss of distal sensation and pulses. This is a surgical emergency.

DIAGNOSIS. Definitive diagnosis is made by surgical exploration, which should be undertaken as soon as the diagnosis is suspected. Necrotic fascia and subcutaneous tissue are gray and offer little resistance to blunt probing. Although MRI aids in delineating the extent and tissue planes of involvement, this procedure should not delay surgical intervention. Frozen section incisional biopsy specimen obtained early in the course of the infection can aid management by decreasing the time to diagnosis and helping establish margins of involvement. Gram stain of tissue can be particularly useful if chains of gram-positive cocci, indicative of infection with *S. pyogenes,* are seen.

TREATMENT. Early supportive care, surgical debridement, and parenteral antibiotic administration are mandatory. All devitalized tissue should be removed to freely bleeding edges, and repeat exploration is generally indicated within 24–36 hr to confirm that no necrotic tissue remains. This may need to be repeated on several occasions until devitalized tissue has ceased to form. Daily, meticulous wound care is also paramount.

Antibiotic therapy should be initiated parenterally as soon as possible with broad-spectrum agents against all potential pathogens. Most experts recommend initial empirical therapy with penicillin, ampicillin, or nafcillin; clindamycin; and an aminoglycoside for coverage against *S. pyogenes* and the broad spectrum of potential anaerobic and gram-negative pathogens. Clindamycin is often added to inhibit protein synthesis of new bacterial necrotizing toxins.

PROGNOSIS. The combined case fatality rate among children and adults with necrotizing fasciitis and toxic shock-like syndrome due to *S. pyogenes* has been approximately 60%. Death is less common in children, however, and in cases not complicated by toxic shock-like syndrome.

STAPHYLOCOCCAL SCALDED SKIN SYNDROME (RITTER DISEASE)

Clinical Manifestations. Staphylococcal scalded skin syndrome occurs predominantly in infants and children younger than 5 yr of age and includes a range of disease from localized bullous impetigo to generalized cutaneous involvement with systemic illness. Onset of the rash may be preceded by malaise, fever, irritability, and exquisite tenderness of the skin. Scarlatiniform erythema develops diffusely and is accentuated in flexural and periorificial areas. The conjunctivas are inflamed and occasionally become purulent. The brightly erythematous skin may rapidly acquire a wrinkled appearance, and in severe cases sterile, flaccid blisters, and erosions develop diffusely. Circumoral erythema is characteristically prominent, as is radial crusting and fissuring around the eyes, mouth, and nose. At this stage, areas of epidermis may separate in response to gentle shear force (Nikolsky sign). As large sheets of epidermis peel away, moist, glistening, denuded areas become apparent, initially in the flexures and subsequently over much of the body surface (Fig. 655–2). This may lead to secondary cutaneous infection, sepsis,

and fluid and electrolyte disturbances. The desquamative phase begins after 2–5 days of cutaneous erythema; healing occurs without scarring in 10–14 days. Patients may have pharyngitis, conjunctivitis, and superficial erosions of the lips, but intraoral mucosal surfaces are spared. Although some patients appear ill, many are reasonably comfortable except for the marked skin tenderness.

A presumed abortive form of the disease presents with diffuse, scarlatiniform, tender erythroderma, which is accentuated in the flexural areas but does not progress to blister formation. In these patients, Nikolsky sign may be absent. Although the exanthem is similar to that of streptococcal scarlet fever, strawberry tongue and palatal petechiae are absent. Staphylococcal scalded skin syndrome may be mistaken for a number of other blistering and exfoliating disorders, including bullous impetigo, epidermolysis bullosa, epidermolytic hyperkeratosis, pemphigus, drug eruption, erythema multiforme, and drug-induced toxic epidermal necrolysis. Toxic epidermal necrolysis can often be distinguished by a history of drug ingestion, the presence of Nikolsky sign only at sites of erythema, absence of perioral crusting, full-thickness epidermal necrosis, and a blister cleavage plane in the lowermost epidermis.

Etiology and Pathogenesis. Staphylococcal scalded skin syndrome is caused predominantly by phage group 2 staphylococci, particularly strains 71 and 55, which are present at localized sites of infection. Foci of infection include the nasopharynx and, less commonly, the umbilicus, urinary tract, a superficial abrasion, conjunctivae, and blood. The clinical manifestations of staphylococcal scalded skin syndrome are mediated by hematogenous spread, in the absence of specific antitoxin antibody of staphylococcal epidermolytic or exfoliative toxins A or B. The toxins have reproduced the disease in both animal models and human volunteers. Decreased renal clearance of the toxins may account for the fact that the disease is most common in infants and young children. Epidermolytic toxin A is heat stable and is encoded by bacterial chromosomal genes; epidermolytic toxin B is heat labile and is encoded on a 37.5-kb plasmid. Histopathologically, the site of blister cleavage is subcorneal through the granular layer. The epidermolytic toxins appear to produce the granular layer split by binding to desmoglein I within desmosomes. Evidence suggests that the toxins are members of the trypsin-like serine protease family and may exert their action through proteolysis.

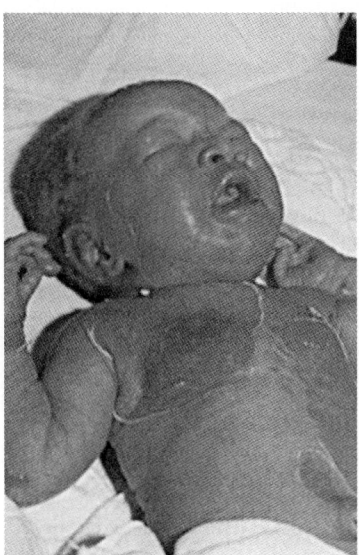

FIGURE 655–2. Infant with staphylococcal scalded skin syndrome. See also color section.

Diagnosis. Intact bullae are consistently sterile, unlike those of bullous impetigo, but cultures should be obtained from all suspected sites of localized infection and from the blood to identify the source for elaboration of the epidermolytic toxins. The subcorneal, granular layer split can be identified on skin biopsy; absence of an inflammatory infiltrate is characteristic. In cases that demand a rapid diagnosis, the exfoliated corneal layer can be seen on a frozen biopsy specimen of the desquamating epidermis. Scattered acantholytic cells, which are evident in the cleftlike bullae, can also be seen in a Tzanck preparation.

Treatment. Systemic therapy, either orally, in cases of localized involvement, or parenterally, with a semisynthetic penicillinase-resistant penicillin, should be prescribed because the staphylococci are usually penicillin resistant. Clindamycin may be added to inhibit bacterial protein (toxin) synthesis. The skin should be gently moistened and cleansed with Burow solution, Dakin solution, or isotonic saline. Application of an emollient provides lubrication and decreases discomfort. Topical antibiotics are unnecessary. Recovery is usually rapid, but complications such as excessive fluid loss, electrolyte imbalance, faulty temperature regulation, pneumonia, septicemia, and cellulitis may cause increased morbidity.

ECTHYMA (see Chapters 168 and 188)

This resembles nonbullous impetigo in onset and appearance but gradually evolves into a deeper, more chronic infection. The initial lesion is a vesicle or vesiculopustule with an erythematous base that erodes through the epidermis into the dermis to form an ulcer with elevated margins. The ulcer becomes obscured by a dry, heaped-up, tightly adherent crust that contributes to the persistence of the infection and scar formation. Lesions may be spread by autoinoculation, may be as large as 4 cm, and occur most frequently on the legs. Predisposing factors include pruritic lesions, such as insect bites, scabies, or pediculosis, which are subject to frequent scratching; poor hygiene; and malnutrition. Complications include lymphangitis, cellulitis, and rarely poststreptococcal glomerulonephritis. The causative agent is usually GABHS; *S. aureus* is also cultured from most lesions but is probably a secondary pathogen. Crusts should be softened with warm compresses and removed with an antibacterial soap. Systemic antibiotic therapy, as for impetigo, is indicated; almost all lesions are responsive to treatment with penicillin.

Ecthyma gangrenosa is a necrotic ulcer covered with a gray-black eschar. It is usually a sign of *P. aeruginosa* sepsis and usually occurs in immunosuppressed patients. Ecthyma gangrenosum occurs in up to 6% of patients with systemic *P. aeruginosa* infection but can also occur as a primary cutaneous infection by inoculation. The lesion begins as a red or purpuric macule that vesiculates and then ulcerates; there is a surrounding rim of pink to violaceous skin. The punched-out ulcer develops raised edges with a dense, black, depressed, crusted center. Lesions may be single or multiple; patients with bacteremia commonly have lesions in apocrine areas. Clinically similar lesions may also develop as a result of infection with other agents such as *S. aureus*, *A. hydrophila*, *Enterobacter* species, *Proteus* species, *Pseudomonas cepacia*, *Serratia marcescens*, *Aspergillus* species, Mucorales, *E. coli*, and *Candida* species. There is bacterial invasion of the adventitia and media of dermal veins but not arteries; the intima and lumina are spared. Blood cultures and skin biopsy for culture should be obtained, and empirical broad-spectrum, systemic therapy that includes coverage for *Pseudomonas* should be initiated as soon as possible.

BLASTOMYCOSIS-LIKE PYODERMA (PYODERMA VEGETANS)

This is an exuberant cutaneous reaction to bacterial infection, primarily in children who are malnourished and immunosup-

pressed. The organisms isolated most commonly from lesions are *S. aureus* and GABHS, but several other organisms have been associated with these lesions, including *P. aeruginosa*, *Proteus mirabilis*, diphtheroids, *Bacillus* species and *C. perfringens*. Hyperplastic, crusted plaques on the extremities are characteristic, sometimes forming from the coalescence of many pinpoint, purulent, crusted abscesses. Ulceration and sinus tract formation may develop, and additional lesions may appear at sites distant from the site of inoculation. Regional lymphadenopathy is common, but fever is not. Histopathologic examination reveals pseudoepitheliomatous hyperplasia and abscesses composed of neutrophils and/or eosinophils; giant cells are usually lacking. The differential diagnosis includes deep fungal infection, particularly blastomycosis and tuberculous and atypical mycobacterial infection. Underlying immunodeficiency should be ruled out, and the selection of antibiotics should be guided by susceptibility testing because the response to antibiotics is often poor.

BLISTERING DISTAL DACTYLITIS

This is a superficial blistering infection of the volar fat pad on the distal portion of the finger or thumb. More than one finger may be involved, as may the volar surfaces of the proximal phalanges, palms, and toes. Blisters are filled with a watery purulent fluid that contains polymorphonuclear leukocytes and chains of gram-positive cocci. Patients usually have no preceding history of trauma, and systemic symptoms are generally absent. Poststreptococcal glomerulonephritis has not occurred after blistering distal dactylitis. The infection is caused most commonly by GABHS but has also occurred as a result of infection with group B β-hemolytic streptococci and *S. aureus*. If left untreated, blisters may continue to enlarge and extend to the paronychial area. The infection responds to incision and drainage and a 10-day course of systemic penicillin or erythromycin therapy.

PERIANAL DERMATITIS

This presents most commonly in boys (70% of cases) between the ages of 6 mo and 10 yr as perianal dermatitis (90% of cases) and pruritus (80% of cases). The incidence of perianal dermatitis is not known precisely but ranges from 1/2,000 to 1/218 patient visits. The rash is superficial, erythematous, well marginated, nonindurated, and confluent from the anus outward. Acutely (<6 wk), the rash tends to be bright red, moist, and tender to touch. At this stage, a white pseudomembrane may be present. As the rash becomes more chronic, the perianal eruption may consist of painful fissures, a dried mucoid discharge, or psoriasiform plaques with yellow peripheral crust. In girls, the perianal rash may be associated with vulvovaginitis; the penis may be involved in boys. Approximately 50% of patients have rectal pain, most commonly described as burning inside the anus during defecation, and 33% have blood-streaked stools. Fecal retention is a frequent behavioral response to the infection. Patients may also have presented with guttate psoriasis. Although local induration or edema may occur, constitutional symptoms of fever, headache, and malaise are absent, suggesting that subcutaneous involvement, as in cellulitis, is absent. Familial spread of perianal dermatitis is common, particularly when family members bathe together or use the same water.

The *differential diagnosis* of perianal dermatitis includes psoriasis, seborrheic dermatitis, candidosis, pinworm infestation, sexual abuse, and inflammatory bowel disease. Differentiation from these other conditions can be accomplished by culturing a moderate to heavy growth of GABHS on 5% sheep blood agar. Perianal dermatitis may also be caused by *S. aureus*. Children with asymptomatic perianal colonization have light growth of GABHS on blood agar. Direct antigen studies for GABHS are also very sensitive (89%), but results may be falsely negative early in the course of the disease. Acute and convalescent sera for anti-streptolysin O or anti-DNase B are not helpful in making the diagnosis. The index case and family members should be cultured initially, and follow-up cultures to document bacteriologic cure after a course of treatment are also recommended.

Treatment with a single 10-day course of oral penicillin produces resolution of the dermatitis and symptoms in most patients; however, recurrence rates of 40–50% have been reported, emphasizing the need for close follow-up, including repeat culture. Erythromycin estolate and ethylsuccinate are excellent alternative treatments for those who are allergic to penicillin, who have not responded to a course of penicillin, or who are infected with *S. aureus*. Clindamycin has also been used successfully to treat recurrent perianal dermatitis. Mupirocin has been used in conjunction with oral antibiotics to treat recurrences but has not been evaluated as a single-drug therapy.

ERYSIPELAS (see Chapter 168)

FOLLICULITIS

This superficial infection of the hair follicle is most often caused by *S. aureus* (Bockhart impetigo); coagulase-negative staphylococci are the cause occasionally. The lesions are typically small, discrete, dome-shaped pustules with an erythematous base, located at the ostium of the pilosebaceous canals. Hair growth is unimpaired, and the lesions heal without scarring. Favored sites include the scalp, buttocks, and extremities. Poor hygiene, maceration, and drainage from wounds and abscesses can be provocative factors. Folliculitis can also occur as a result of tar therapy or occlusive wraps; the moist environment encourages bacterial proliferation. In HIV-infected patients, *S. aureus* may produce confluent erythematous patches with satellite pustules in intertriginous areas and violaceous plaques composed of superficial follicular pustules in the scalp, axillas, or groin. *Candida* may cause satellite follicular papules and pustules surrounding erythematous patches of intertrigo, and *Malassezia furfur* produces pruritic 2–3 mm erythematous, perifollicular papules and pustules on the back, chest, and extremities, particularly in patients with diabetes mellitus or on corticosteroids or antibiotics. Diagnosis is made by examining potassium hydroxide-treated scrapings from lesions. Detection of *Malassezia* may require a skin biopsy, demonstrating clusters of yeast and short, branching hyphae ("spaghetti and meatballs") in widened follicular ostia mixed with keratinous debris. *Malassezia* may be cultured on Sabouraud's dextrose agar supplemented with gentamicin, vancomycin, and olive oil.

The causative organism of folliculitis can be identified by Gram stain and culture of purulent material from the follicular orifice. *Treatment* for folliculitis includes topical antibiotic cleansers such as chlorhexidine or hexachlorophene. Topical antibiotic therapy is usually all that is required for mild cases, but more severe cases may require use of penicillinase-resistant systemic antibiotics such as dicloxacillin or cephalexin. In chronic recurrent folliculitis, daily application of a benzoyl peroxide lotion or gel may facilitate resolution.

Folliculitis caused by gram-negative organisms occurs primarily in patients with acne vulgaris treated long term with broad-spectrum systemic antibiotics. A superficial pustular form, caused by *Klebsiella, Enterobacter, E. coli,* or *P. aeruginosa,* occurs around the nose and spreads to the cheeks and chin. A deeper, nodular form of folliculitis on the face and trunk is caused by *Proteus.* Culture of infected follicles is necessary to establish the diagnosis. Treatment consists of incision and drainage of the deeper, larger cysts; topical neomycin or bacitracin; or selection of an oral antibiotic based on the sensitivity profile of the pathogenic organism. For severe, recalcitrant cases, 13-*cis*-retinoic acid, 1 mg/kg/24 hr, is helpful but should be administered only by experienced physicians because of side effects.

Sycosis barbae is a deeper, more severe recurrent inflammatory form of folliculitis caused by *S. aureus* that involves the entire depth of the follicle. Erythematous follicular papules and pustules develop on the chin, upper lip, and angle of the jaw, primarily in young black males. Papules may coalesce into plaques, and healing may occur with scarring. Affected individuals frequently are found to be *S. aureus* carriers. Treatment with warm saline compresses and topical antibiotics such as mupirocin generally clears the infection. More extensive, recalcitrant cases may require therapy with β-lactamase–resistant systemic antibiotics and elimination of *S. aureus* from sites of carriage.

Hot tub folliculitis is attributable to *P. aeruginosa,* predominantly serotype O-11. The lesions are pruritic papules and pustules or deeply erythematous to violaceous nodules that develop 8–48 hr after exposure and are most dense in areas covered by a bathing suit. Patients occasionally develop fever, malaise, and lymphadenopathy. The organism is readily cultured from pus. The eruption usually resolves spontaneously within 1–2 wk, often leaving postinflammatory hyperpigmentation, but topical agents with antipseudomonal activity, such as potassium permanganate and gentamicin cream, are sometimes necessary. Consideration should be given to use of systemic antibiotics (e.g., ciprofloxacin) in adolescent patients with constitutional symptoms. Immunocompromised children are susceptible to complications of pseudomonas folliculitis (e.g., cellulitis) and should avoid hot tubs.

FURUNCLES AND CARBUNCLES

These follicular lesions may originate from a preceding folliculitis or may arise initially as a deep-seated, tender, erythematous, perifollicular nodule. Although lesions are initially indurated, central necrosis and suppuration follow, leading to rupture and discharge of a central core of necrotic tissue and destruction of the follicle. Healing occurs with scar formation. Sites of predilection are the hair-bearing areas on the face, neck, axillae, buttocks, and groin. Pain may be intense if the lesion is situated in an area where the skin is relatively fixed, such as in the external auditory canal or over the nasal cartilages. Patients with furuncles usually have no constitutional symptoms; however, bacteremia may occasionally ensue. Rarely, lesions on the upper lip or cheek may lead to cavernous sinus thrombosis. Infection of a group of contiguous follicles, with multiple drainage points, accompanied by inflammatory changes in surrounding connective tissue is a carbuncle. Carbuncles may be accompanied by fever, leukocytosis, and bacteremia.

Etiology. The causative agent is usually *S. aureus,* which penetrates abraded perifollicular skin. Conditions predisposing to furuncle formation include obesity, hyperhidrosis, maceration, friction, and pre-existing dermatitis. Furunculosis is also more common in individuals with low serum iron levels, diabetes, malnutrition, HIV infection, or other immunodeficiency states. Recurrent furunculosis is frequently associated with carriage of *S. aureus* in the nares, axillae, or perineum or close contact with someone such as a family member who is a carrier. Other bacteria or fungi may occasionally cause furuncles or carbuncles; therefore, Gram stain and culture of the pus are indicated.

Treatment. This includes regular bathing with antimicrobial soaps and wearing of loose-fitting clothing, which minimizes predisposing factors for furuncle formation. Frequent application of a hot, moist compress may facilitate drainage of lesions. Large lesions may be drained by a small incision. Carbuncles and large or numerous furuncles should be treated with systemic penicillinase-resistant antibiotics such as cloxacillin orally or oxacillin parenterally. Penicillin-allergic patients can be treated with a cephalosporin, clindamycin, or erythromycin. Treatment of recurrent cases has been successful by colonization of the individual with a less virulent strain of *S. aureus* such as 502A.

The carriage state may be eliminated temporarily by application of mupirocin ointment for 5 days to the anterior nares. Attention to personal hygiene, use of an antibacterial soap, low-dose oral antistaphylococcal penicillin or clindamycin, and frequent handwashing may also be beneficial.

PITTED KERATOLYSIS

Pitted keratolysis occurs most frequently in humid tropical and subtropical climates, particularly in individuals whose feet are moist for prolonged periods, for example, as a result of hyperhidrosis, prolonged wearing of boots, or immersion in water. The lesions consist of 1–7 mm irregularly shaped superficial erosions of the horny layer on the soles, particularly at weight-bearing sites. Brownish discoloration of involved areas may be apparent. The condition is usually asymptomatic but frequently is malodorous. A rare, painful variant is manifested as thinned, erythematous to violaceous plaques in addition to the typical pitted lesions. The most likely etiologic agent is a species of *Corynebacterium*. *Actinomycetes*, *Dermatophilus*, and micrococci have also been isolated from lesions. Avoidance of moisture and maceration produces slow, spontaneous resolution of the infection. Therapeutic regimens that have been effective include topical application of 2% buffered glutaraldehyde, 20% formaldehyde solution (formalin) in Aquaphor, erythromycin, clindamycin, and the imidazoles.

ERYTHRASMA

This is a benign chronic superficial infection caused by *Corynebacterium minutissimum*. Predisposing factors include heat, humidity, obesity, skin maceration, and poor hygiene. Approximately 20% of patients have involvement of the toe webs. Other frequently affected sites are moist intertriginous areas such as the groin and axillas; the inframammary and perianal regions are involved occasionally. Sharply demarcated, irregularly bordered, brownish-red, slightly scaly patches are characteristic of the disease. Mild pruritus is the only constant symptom. *C. minutissimum* is a complex of related organisms that produce porphyrins that fluoresce brilliant coral-red under ultraviolet light. The diagnosis is readily made, and erythrasma is differentiated from dermatophyte infection and from tinea versicolor by Wood lamp examination. Bathing within 20 hr of Wood lamp examination, however, may remove the water-soluble porphyrins. Staining of skin scrapings with methylene blue or Gram stain reveals the pleomorphic, filamentous coccobacillary forms.

Most cases represent colonization, are asymptomatic, and require no therapy. Effective *treatment* can be achieved with topical erythromycin, clindamycin, miconazole, or Whitfield ointment or a 10–14 day course of oral erythromycin. Recurrence may be inhibited by frequent use of an antibacterial soap or an astringent such as 10–20% aluminum chloride in anhydrous ethyl alcohol.

ERYSIPELOID

This rare cutaneous infection is caused by inoculation of *Erysipelothrix rhusiopathiae* from contaminated animals, birds, fish, or their products. The localized cutaneous form is most common, characterized by well-demarcated diamond-shaped erythematous to violaceous patches at sites of inoculation. Local symptoms are generally not severe, constitutional symptoms are rare, and the lesions resolve spontaneously after weeks but can recur at the same site or develop elsewhere weeks to months later. The diffuse cutaneous form presents with lesions at several areas of the body in addition to the site of inoculation; it is also self-limited. The systemic form, caused by hematogenous spread, is accompanied by constitutional symptoms and may include endocarditis, septic arthritis, cerebral infarct and

abscess, meningitis, and pulmonary effusion. Diagnosis is confirmed by skin biopsy, which reveals the gram-positive organisms, and culture. The treatment of choice is parenteral erythromycin or penicillin.

TUBERCULOSIS OF THE SKIN (see Chapters 197 and 199)

Cutaneous tuberculosis infection occurs worldwide, particularly in association with HIV infection, malnutrition, and poor hygiene. Primary cutaneous tuberculosis is rare in the United States but occurs with the greatest frequency in infants and children; the overall incidence of cutaneous tuberculosis among those with all forms of tuberculosis in the United States is approximately 1–2%. All forms of cutaneous disease are caused by *Mycobacterium tuberculosis*, by *Mycobacterium bovis*, and occasionally by the bacillus Calmette-Guérin (BCG), an attenuated form of *M. bovis*; the manifestations caused by a given organism are indistinguishable from one another. After invasion of the skin, mycobacteria either multiply intracellularly within macrophages, leading to progressive disease, or are controlled by the host immune reaction.

A primary lesion, a *tuberculous chancre*, results when *M. tuberculosis* or *M. bovis* gains access to the skin or mucous membranes through trauma. Sites of predilection are the face, lower extremities, and genitals. The initial lesion develops 2–4 wk after introduction of the organism into the damaged tissue. A red-brown papule gradually enlarges to form a shallow, firm, sharply demarcated ulcer; satellite abscesses may be present. Some lesions acquire a crust resembling impetigo, and others become heaped up and verrucous at the margins. The primary lesion occurs in one third of cases as a painless ulcer on the conjunctiva, gingiva, or palate and occasionally as a painless acute paronychia. Painless regional adenopathy appears approximately 3–8 wk after inoculation and may be accompanied by lymphangitis, lymphadenitis, or perforation of the skin surface, forming scrofuloderma. Erythema nodosum develops in approximately 10% of cases. Untreated lesions heal with scarring within approximately 12 mo but may reactivate, may form lupus vulgaris, or rarely may progress to the acute miliary form.

M. tuberculosis or *M. bovis* can be cultured from the skin lesion and local lymph nodes, but acid-fast staining of histologic sections, particularly of a well-controlled infection, often does not reveal the organism. Clinically, the differential diagnosis is broad, including a syphilitic chancre; deep fungal or atypical mycobacterial infection; leprosy; tularemia; cat-scratch disease; sporotrichosis; nocardiosis; leishmaniasis; reaction to foreign substances such as zirconium, beryllium, silk or nylon sutures, talc, or starch; papular acne rosacea; and lupus miliaris disseminatum faciei. Spontaneous healing with scarring coincides with acquisition of immunity, at which time the skin lesions and infected nodes may become calcified. Antituberculous therapy is indicated (see Chapter 197).

Direct cutaneous inoculation of the tubercle bacillus into a previously infected individual with a moderate to high degree of immunity initially produces a small papule with surrounding inflammation. *Tuberculosis verrucosa cutis* (warty tuberculosis) forms when the papule becomes hyperkeratotic and warty, and several adjacent papules coalesce or a single papule expands peripherally to form a brownish-red to violaceous, exudative, crusted verrucous plaque. Irregular extension of the margins of the plaque produces a serpiginous border. Children have the lesion most commonly on the lower extremities after trauma and contact with infected material such as sputum or soil. Regional lymph nodes are involved only rarely. Spontaneous healing with atrophic scarring takes place slowly, over months to years; healing is also gradual with antituberculous therapy.

Lupus vulgaris is a rare, chronic, progressive form of cutaneous tuberculosis that develops in individuals with a moderate to high degree of tuberculin sensitivity induced by previous infection.

The incidence is greater in cool, moist climates, particularly in females. Lupus vulgaris develops as a result of direct extension from underlying joints or lymph nodes; through lymphatic or hematogenous spread; or rarely, by cutaneous inoculation with BCG vaccine. It most commonly follows cervical adenitis or pulmonary tuberculosis. Approximately 33% of cases are preceded by scrofuloderma, and 90% of cases present on the head and neck, most commonly on the nose or cheek; involvement of the trunk is uncommon. A typical solitary lesion consists of a brownish-red, soft papule that has an apple-jelly color when examined by diascopy. Expansion of the papule peripherally, or occasionally the coalescence of several papules, forms an irregular lesion of variable size and form. One or several lesions may develop, including nodules or plaques that are flat and serpiginous, hypertrophic and verrucous, or edematous in appearance. Spontaneous healing occurs centrally, and lesions characteristically reappear within the area of atrophy. Chronicity is characteristic, and persistence and progression of plaques over many years is common. Lymphadenitis is present in 40% of those with lupus vulgaris, and 10–20% have infection of the lungs, bones, or joints. Vegetative masses and ulceration involving the nasal, buccal, or conjunctival mucosa; the palate; the gingiva; or the oropharynx may cause extensive deformities. Squamous cell carcinoma, with a relatively high metastatic potential, may develop, usually after several years of the disease. After a temporary impairment in immunity, particularly after measles infection (i.e., *lupus exanthematicus*), multiple lesions may form at distant sites as a result of hematogenous spread from a latent focus of infection. The histopathology reveals a tuberculoid granuloma without caseation; organisms are extremely difficult to demonstrate. The differential diagnosis includes sarcoidosis, leprosy, atypical mycobacterial infection, blastomycosis, chromoblastomycosis, actinomycosis, leishmaniasis, tertiary syphilis, leprosy, hypertrophic lichen planus, psoriasis, lupus erythematosus, lymphocytoma, and Bower disease. Small lesions can be excised; antituberculous drug therapy usually halts further spread and induces involution.

Scrofuloderma results from enlargement, cold abscess formation, and breakdown of a lymph node, most frequently in a cervical chain, with extension to the overlying skin. Linear or serpiginous ulcers and dissecting fistulas and subcutaneous tracts studded with soft nodules may develop. Spontaneous healing may take years, eventuating in cordlike keloid scars; lupus vulgaris may also develop. Scrofuloderma of a cervical lymph node often originates in the larynx and was linked in the past to ingestion of milk containing *M. bovis*. Lesions may also originate from an underlying infected joint, tendon, bone, or epididymis. The differential diagnosis includes syphilitic gumma, deep fungal infections, actinomycosis, and hidradenitis suppurativa. The course is indolent, and constitutional symptoms are typically absent. Antituberculous therapy is usually effective.

Orificial tuberculosis presents on the mucous membranes and periorificial skin after autoinoculation of mycobacteria from sites of progressive infection; it is a sign of advanced internal disease and carries a poor prognosis. Lesions appear as yellowish or red, painful nodules that form punched-out ulcers with inflammation and edema of the surrounding mucosa. Treatment consists of identification of the source of infection and initiation of antituberculous therapy.

Miliary tuberculosis (hematogenous primary tuberculosis) rarely presents cutaneously, most commonly in infants and in individuals who are immunosuppressed after chemotherapy or infection with measles or HIV. The eruption consists of crops of symmetrically distributed, minute, erythematous to purpuric macules, papules, or vesicles. The lesions may ulcerate, drain, crust, and form sinus tracts or may form subcutaneous gummas, especially in malnourished children with impaired immunity. Constitutional signs and symptoms are common, and a leuke-

moid reaction or aplastic anemia may develop. Tubercle bacilli are readily identified in an active lesion. A fulminant course should be anticipated, and aggressive antituberculous therapy is indicated.

Single or multiple *metastatic tuberculous abscesses* (tuberculous gummas) may develop on the extremities and trunk by hematogenous spread from a primary focus of infection during a period of decreased immunity, particularly in malnourished and immunosuppressed children. The fluctuant, nontender, erythematous subcutaneous nodules may ulcerate and form fistulas.

Vaccination with BCG characteristically produces a papule approximately 2 wk after vaccination. The papule expands in size, typically ulcerates within 2–4 mo, and heals slowly with scarring. In approximately 1–2 per million vaccinations, a complication caused specifically by the BCG organism occurs, including regional lymphadenitis, lupus vulgaris, scrofuloderma, and subcutaneous abscess formation.

Tuberculids are skin reactions that exhibit tuberculoid features histologically but do not contain detectable mycobacteria. The lesions appear in a host who usually has moderate to strong tuberculin reactivity, has a history of previous tuberculosis of other organs, and usually shows a therapeutic response to antituberculous therapy. The cause of tuberculids is poorly understood. Most patients are in good health with no clear focus of disease at the time of the eruption. The most commonly observed tuberculid is the *papulonecrotic tuberculid*. Recurrent crops of symmetrically distributed, asymptomatic, firm, sterile, dusky-red papules appear on the extensor aspects of the limbs, the dorsum of the hands and feet, and the buttocks. The papules may undergo central ulceration and eventually heal, leaving sharply delineated, circular, depressed scars. The duration of the eruption is variable, but it usually disappears promptly after treatment of the primary infection. *Lichen scrofulosorum*, another form of tuberculid, is characterized by asymptomatic, grouped, pinhead-sized, often follicular pink or red papules that form discoid plaques, mainly on the trunk. Healing occurs without scarring.

Atypical mycobacterial infection may cause cutaneous lesions in children. *Mycobacterium marinum* is found in salt and freshwater and diseased fish; in the United States, it is most commonly acquired from tropical fish tanks and swimming pools. Traumatic abrasion of the skin serves as a portal of entry for the organism. Approximately 3 wk after inoculation, a single reddish papule develops and enlarges slowly to form a violaceous nodule or occasionally a warty plaque. The lesion occasionally breaks down to form a crusted ulcer or a suppurating abscess. Sporotrichoid erythematous nodules along lymphatics may also suppurate and drain. Lesions are most common on the elbows, knees, and feet of swimmers and the hands and fingers in aquarium-acquired infection. Systemic signs and symptoms are absent; regional lymph nodes occasionally become slightly enlarged but do not break down. Rarely, the infection becomes disseminated, particularly in an immunosuppressed host. A biopsy specimen of a fully developed lesion demonstrates a granulomatous infiltrate with tuberculoid architecture; intracellular organisms can usually be identified within the histiocytes with appropriate stains. The most effective antituberculous regimens include tetracycline, minocycline, and rifampin plus ethambutol. Application of heat to the affected site may be a useful adjunctive therapy. Spontaneous healing with scarring can be expected within several months to 2 yr (see Chapter 199).

Mycobacterium kansasii primarily causes pulmonary disease; skin disease is rare, often occurring in an immunocompromised host. Most commonly, sporotrichoid nodules develop after inoculation of traumatized skin. Lesions may develop into ulcerated, crusted, or verrucous plaques. The organism is relatively sensitive to antituberculous medications, which should be chosen on the basis of susceptibility testing.

M. scrofulaceum causes cervical lymphadenitis (scrofuloderma) in young children, typically in the submandibular region. Nodes enlarge over several weeks, ulcerate, and drain. The local reaction is nontender and circumscribed, constitutional symptoms are absent, and there generally is no evidence of lung or other organ involvement. Other atypical mycobacteria may cause a similar presentation, including *M. avium* complex, *M. kansasii*, and *M. fortuitum*. Treatment is accomplished by excision and antituberculous drugs (see Chapter 199).

Mycobacterium ulcerans causes a painless subcutaneous nodule after inoculation of abraded skin. Most infections occur in children in tropical rain forests. The nodule usually ulcerates, develops undermined edges, and may spread over large areas, most commonly on an extremity. Local necrosis of subcutaneous fat, producing a septal panniculitis, is characteristic. Ulcers persist for months to years before healing spontaneously with scarring and sometimes with lymphedema. Constitutional symptoms and lymphadenopathy are absent. Diagnosis is made by culturing the organism at 32–33°C. Treatment of choice is early excision of the lesion. Local heat therapy and oral chemotherapy may benefit some patients.

M. avium complex, composed of more than 20 subtypes, most commonly causes chronic pulmonary infection. Cervical lymphadenitis and osteomyelitis occur occasionally, and papules or purulent leg ulcers occur rarely by primary inoculation. Skin lesions may be an early sign of disseminated infection; the lesions may take various forms, including erythematous papules, pustules, nodules, abscesses, ulcers, panniculitis, and sporotrichoid spread along lymphatics. For treatment, see Chapter 199].

M. fortuitum complex is composed of two organisms: *M. fortuitum* and *M. chelonei*. These organisms cause disease in an immunocompetent host principally by primary cutaneous inoculation after traumatic injury, injection, or surgery. A nodule, abscess, or cellulitis develops 4–6 wk after inoculation. In an immunocompromised host, numerous subcutaneous nodules may form, break down, and drain. Treatment is based on identification and susceptibility testing of the organism.

Amren DP, Anderson AS, Wannamaker LW: Perianal cellulitis associated with group A streptococci. *Am J Dis Child* 1966;112:546.

Beyt BE Jr, Ortbals DW, Santa Cruz DJ: Cutaneous mycobacteriosis: Analysis of 34 cases with a new classification of the disease. *Medicine* 1980;60:95.

Bisno AL, Stevens DL: Streptococcal infections of skin and soft tissues. *N Engl J Med* 1996;334:240.

Brogan TV, Nizet V, Waldhausen JH, et al: Group A streptococcal necrotizing fasciitis complicating varicella: A series of ten patients. *Pediatr Infect Dis J* 1995; 14:588.

Darmstadt GL, Fleckman P, Jonas M, et al: Differentiation of cultured keratinocytes promotes adherence of *Streptococcus pyogenes. J Clin Invest* 1998;101:128.

Darmstadt GL, Lane AT: Impetigo: An overview. *Pediatr Dermatol* 1994;11:293.

Darmstadt GL, Mao-Qiang M, Saha SK, et al: Impact of topical oils on the skin barrier: possible implications for neonatal health in developing countries. *Acta Paediatr* 2002;9:1.

Darmstadt GL, Marcy SM: Skin and soft tissue infection. In Long SS, Prober CG, Pickering LK (editors): Principles and Practice of Pediatric Infectious Disease. New York, Churchill Livingstone, 1996.

Darmstadt GL, Mentele L, Podbielski A, et al: Role of group A streptococcal virulence factors in adherence to keratinocytes. *Infect Immunol* 2000;68:1215.

Darmstadt GL: Oral antibiotic therapy for uncomplicated bacterial skin infections in children. *Pediatr Infect Dis J* 1997;16:227.

Darmstadt GL: Skin and soft tissue infections. In Long SS, Prober CG, Pickering LK (editors): Principles and Practice of Pediatric Infectious Disease, 2nd ed. New York, Churchill Livingstone, 2002.

Darmstadt GL: Staphylococcal and streptococcal skin infections. In Harahap M (editor): Diagnosis and Treatment of Skin Infections. Oxford, Blackwell Science, 1997, p. 7–115.

Dillon HC Jr, Reeves MSA: Streptococcal immune responses in nephritis after skin infection. *Am J Med* 1974;56:333.

Doebbeling BN, Breneman DL, Neu HC, et al: Elimination of *Staphylococcus aureus* nasal carriage in health care workers: Analysis of six clinical trials with calcium mupirocin ointment. *Clin Infect Dis* 1993;17:466.

Ferrieri P, Dajani AS, Wannamaker LW, et al: Natural history of impetigo I. Site sequence of acquisition and familial patterns of spread of cutaneous streptococci. *J Clin Invest* 1972;51:2851.

Galen WK, Fischer G, Darmstadt GL: Bacterial Infections. In Schachner LA, Hansen RC (editors): *Pediatric Dermatology*, 3rd ed. New York, Churchill Livingstone, 2003, in press.

Gart GS, Forstall GJ, Tomecki KJ: Mycobacterial skin disease: Approaches to therapy. *Semin Dermatol* 1993;12:352.

Hayden GF: Skin diseases encountered in a pediatric clinic. *Am J Dis Child* 1985;139:36.

Koning S, van Suijlekom-Smit, Nouwen JL, et al: Fusidic acid cream in the treatment of impetigo in general practice: double blind randomized placebo controlled trial. *Br Med J* 2002;324:203–6.

Leyden JJ: Review of mupirocin ointment in the treatment of impetigo. *Clin Pediatr* 1992;31:549.

McCray MK, Esterly NB: Cutaneous eruptions in congenital tuberculosis. *Arch Dermatol* 1981;117:460.

Peterson CL, Vugia DJ, Meyers HB, et al: Risk factors for invasive group A streptococcal infections in children with varicella: Case-control study. *Pediatr Infect Dis J* 1996;15:151.

Sidbury R, Darmstadt GL: Microbiology. In Hoath SB, Maibach H (editors): *Neonatal Skin,* 2nd ed. New York, Marcel Dekker, 2002, in press.

Stevens DL: Invasive group A streptococcal infections: The past, present and future. *Pediatr Infect Dis J* 1994;13:561.

Tunnessen WW Jr: A survey of skin disorders seen in pediatric general and dermatology clinics. *Pediatr Dermatol* 1984;1:219.

Tunnessen WW Jr: Practical aspects of bacterial skin infections in children. *Pediatr Dermatol* 1985;2:255.

Chapter 656
Cutaneous Fungal Infections

TINEA VERSICOLOR

This common, innocuous, chronic fungal infection of the stratum corneum is caused by the dimorphic yeast *Malassezia furfur*. The synonyms *Pityrosporum ovale* and *P. orbiculare* were used previously to identify the causal organism.

Etiology. *M. furfur* is part of the indigenous flora, predominantly in the yeast form, and is found particularly in areas of skin that are rich in sebum production. Proliferation of filamentous forms occurs in the disease state. Predisposing factors include a warm, humid environment, excessive sweating, occlusion, high plasma cortisol levels, immunosuppression, malnourishment, and genetically determined susceptibility. The disease is most prevalent in adolescents and young adults.

Clinical Manifestations. The lesions vary widely in color. In whites, they typically are reddish brown, whereas in blacks they may be either hypopigmented or hyperpigmented. The characteristic macules are covered with a fine scale; they often begin in a perifollicular location, enlarge, and merge to form confluent patches, most commonly on the neck, upper chest, back, and upper arms (Fig. 656–1*A*). Facial lesions are not unusual in adolescents, and lesions occasionally appear on the forearms, dorsum of the hands, and pubis. There may be little or no pruritus. Involved areas do not tan after sun exposure. A papulopustular perifollicular variant of the disorder may occur on the back, chest, and sometimes the extremities.

Diagnosis. Examination with a Wood lamp discloses a yellowish-gold fluorescence. A potassium hydroxide (KOH) preparation of scrapings is diagnostic, demonstrating groups of thick-walled spores and myriad short, thick, angular hyphae, resembling spaghetti and meatballs (see Fig. 656–1*B*). Skin biopsy, including culture and special stains for fungi (e.g., periodic acid-Schiff), are often necessary to make the diagnosis in cases of primarily follicular involvement; organisms and keratinous debris can be seen within dilated follicular ostia.

Tinea versicolor must be distinguished from dermatophyte infections, seborrheic dermatitis, pityriasis alba, and secondary syphilis. Nonscaling pigmentary disorders, such as postinflammatory pigmentary change, may be mimicked if a patient has

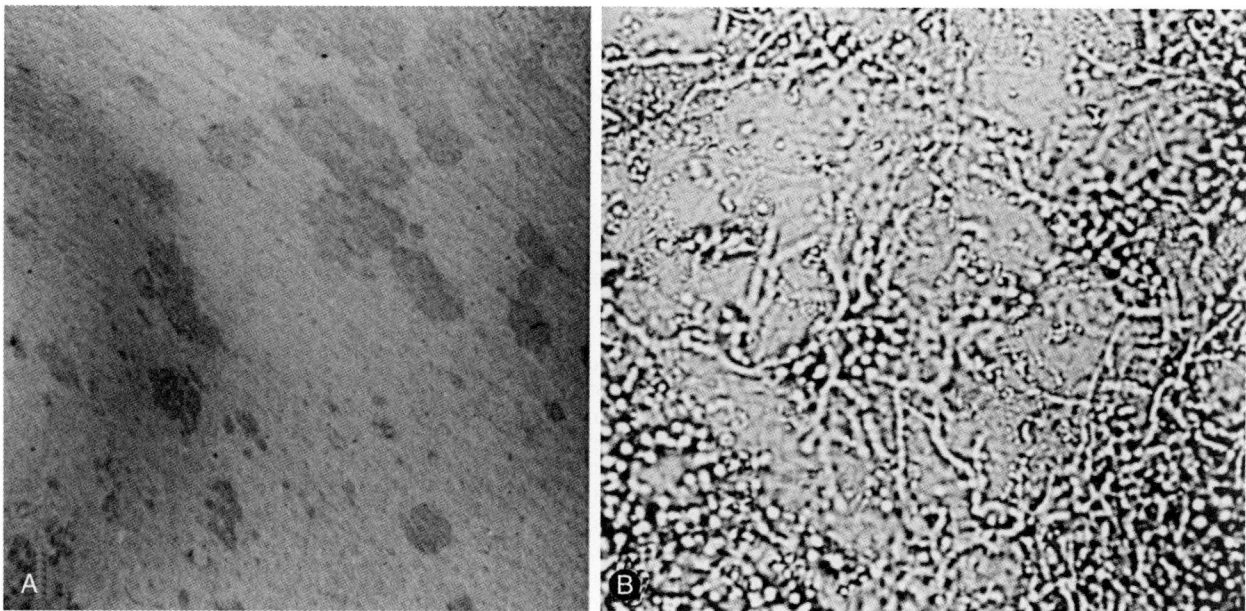

Figure 656–1. *A,* Hyperpigmented, sharply demarcated macules of varying sizes on the upper trunk characteristic of tinea versicolor. *B,* KOH preparation of *Malassezia furfur* demonstrating short, thick hyphae and clusters of spores.

removed the scales by scrubbing. Disseminated candidiasis must be differentiated from *M. furfur* folliculitis.

Treatment. Many therapeutic agents can be used to treat this disease successfully; however, the causative agent, a normal human saprophyte, is not eradicated from the skin, and the disorder recurs in predisposed individuals. Appropriate topical therapy may include one of the following: a selenium sulfide suspension applied for 5–10 min each day for 2 wk; 25% sodium hyposulfite or thiosulfate lotion applied twice daily for 2–4 wk; lotions, ointments, or creams containing 3–6% salicylic acid twice daily for 2–4 wk; or miconazole, clotrimazole, ketoconazole, or terbinafine cream twice daily for 2–4 wk. Recurrent episodes continue to respond promptly to these agents. Oral therapy may be more convenient and may be achieved successfully with ketoconazole or fluconazole, 400 mg, repeated in 1 wk, or itraconazole, 200 mg/24 hr for 5–7 days.

DERMATOPHYTOSES

Dermatophytoses are caused by a group of closely related filamentous fungi with a propensity for invading the stratum corneum, hair, and nails. The three principal genera responsible for infections are *Trichophyton, Microsporum,* and *Epidermophyton.*

Etiology. *Trichophyton* species cause lesions of all keratinized tissue, including skin, nails, and hair; *T. rubrum* is the most common dermatophyte pathogen overall. *Microsporum* species principally invade the hair, and the *Epidermophyton* species invade the intertriginous skin. Dermatophyte infections are designated by the word *tinea* followed by the Latin word for the anatomic site of involvement. The dermatophytes are also classified according to source and natural habitat. Fungi acquired from the soil are called *geophilic;* they infect humans sporadically, inciting an inflammatory reaction. Dermatophytes that are acquired from animals are *zoophilic;* transmission may be through direct contact or indirectly by infected animal hair or clothing. Infected animals frequently are asymptomatic. Dermatophytes acquired from humans are referred to as *anthropophilic;* these infestations range from chronic low-grade to acute inflammatory disease. *Epidermophyton* infections are transmitted only by humans, but

various species of *Trichophyton* and *Microsporum* can be acquired from both human and nonhuman sources.

Epidemiology. Host defense has an important influence on the severity of the infection. Disease tends to be more severe in individuals with diabetes mellitus, lymphoid malignancies, immunosuppression, and states with high plasma cortisol levels, such as Cushing syndrome. Some dermatophytes, most notably the zoophilic species, tend to elicit more severe, suppurative inflammation in humans. Some degree of resistance to reinfection is acquired by most infected persons and may be associated with a delayed hypersensitivity response. No relationship has been demonstrated, however, between antibody levels and resistance to infection. The frequency and severity of infection are also affected by the geographic locale, the genetic susceptibility of the host, and the virulence of the strain of dermatophyte. Additional local factors that predispose to infection include trauma to the skin, hydration of the skin with maceration, occlusion, and elevated temperature.

Occasionally, a secondary skin eruption referred to as a *dermatophytid* or *"id" reaction* appears in sensitized individuals and has been attributed to circulating fungal antigens derived from the primary infection. The eruption occurs most frequently on the fingers, hands, and arms and is characterized by grouped papules and vesicles and, occasionally, by sterile pustules. Symmetric urticarial lesions and a more generalized maculopapular eruption also can occur. Id reactions are most often associated with tinea pedis but also occur with tinea capitis; in the latter case, a generalized papulovesicular follicular eruption may occur.

Diagnosis. The important diagnostic procedures for the various dermatophyte diseases include examination of infected hairs with a Wood lamp, microscopic examination of KOH preparations of infected material, and identification of the etiologic agent by culture. Hairs infected with common *Microsporum* species fluoresce a bright blue-green; most *Trichophyton*-infected hairs do not fluoresce.

Clinical Manifestations. *Tinea capitis* is a dermatophyte infection of the scalp most often caused by *Trichophyton tonsurans*, occasionally by *Microsporum canis,* and much less commonly by other *Microsporum* and *Trichophyton* species. It is particularly common in black and Hispanic children age 4–14 yr. In *Microsporum* and some *Trichophyton* infections, the spores are distributed in a sheathlike fashion around the hair shaft (ectothrix infection), whereas *T. tonsurans* produces an infection within the hair shaft (endothrix). Endothrix infections may continue past the anagen phase of hair growth into telogen and are more chronic than infections with ectothrix organisms that persist only during the anagen phase. *T. tonsurans* is an anthropophilic species acquired most often by contact with infected hairs and epithelial cells that are on such surfaces as theater seats, hats, and combs. Dermatophyte spores may also be airborne within the immediate environment, and high carriage rates have been demonstrated in noninfected schoolmates and household members. *M. canis* is a zoophilic species that is acquired from cats and dogs.

The *clinical presentation* of tinea capitis varies with the infecting organism. The pattern produced by *Microsporum audouinii,* the most common cause of tinea capitis in the 1940s and 1950s, is characterized initially by a small papule at the base of a hair follicle. The infection spreads peripherally, forming an erythematous and scaly circular plaque *(ringworm)* within which the infected hairs become brittle and broken. Numerous confluent patches of alopecia develop, and patients may complain of severe pruritus. *M. audouinii* infection is no longer common in the United States. Endothrix infections such as those caused by *T. tonsurans* create a pattern known as "black-dot ringworm," characterized initially by many small circular patches of alopecia in which hairs are broken off close to the hair follicle. Another clinical variant presents with diffuse scaling with minimal hair loss secondary to traction; it strongly resembles seborrheic dermatitis, psoriasis, or atopic dermatitis. *T. tonsurans* may also produce a chronic and more diffuse alopecia (Fig. 656–2A). A severe inflammatory response produces elevated, boggy granulomatous masses *(kerions),* which are often studded with pustules (see Fig. 656–2B). Fever, pain, and regional adenopathy are common, and permanent scarring and alopecia may result. The zoophilic organism *M. canis* or the geophilic organism *Microsporum gypseum* also may cause kerion formation. *Favus,* a chronic form of tinea capitis that is rare in the United States, is caused by the fungus *Trichophyton schoenleinii.* Favus starts as yellowish-red papules at the opening of hair follicles. The papules expand and coalesce to form cup-shaped, yellowish, crusted patches that fluoresce dull green under a Wood lamp.

Tinea capitis can be confused with seborrheic dermatitis, psoriasis, alopecia areata, trichotillomania, and certain dystrophic hair disorders. When inflammation is pronounced, as in kerion, primary or secondary bacterial infection must also be considered. In adolescents, the patchy, moth-eaten type of alopecia associated with secondary syphilis may resemble tinea capitis. After prolonged tinea capitis has produced scarring, discoid lupus erythematosus and lichen planopilaris must also be considered in the differential diagnosis.

Microscopic examination of a KOH preparation of infected hair from the active border of a lesion discloses tiny spores surrounding the hair shaft in *Microsporum* infections and chains of spores within the hair shaft in *T. tonsurans* infections. Fungal elements usually are not seen in scales. A specific etiologic *diagnosis* of tinea capitis may be obtained by planting broken off infected hairs on Sabouraud medium with reagents to inhibit growth of other organisms; such identification may require 2 wk or more.

Oral administration of griseofulvin microcrystalline (15–20 mg/kg/24 hr) is the recommended *treatment* for all forms of tinea capitis; it may be necessary for 8–12 wk and should be terminated only after fungal culture results are negative. Adverse reactions to griseofulvin are rare but include nausea, vomiting, headache, blood dyscrasias, phototoxicity, and hepatotoxicity. Oral itraconazole is useful in instances of griseofulvin resistance, intolerance, or allergy. Itraconazole is given for 4–6 wk at a dosage of 3–5 mg/kg/24 hr with food, typically 100 mg on alternate days in children weighing 10–20 kg; 100 mg daily for children weighing 20–30 kg; 100 mg alternating with 200 mg for children weighing 30–50kg; and 200 mg/day for >50 kg. Capsules are preferable to the syrup, which may cause diarrhea. Terbinafine also appears to be effective at a dosage of 3–6 mg/kg/24 hr for 4–6 wk (<20 kg weight—62.5 mg/24 hr; 20–40 kg—125 mg/24 hr; adult dose—250 mg/24 hr) or possibly in pulse therapy, although it has limited activity against *M. canis.* Neither itraconazole nor terbinafine is approved by the Food and Drug Administration for treatment of dermatophyte infections in the pediatric population. Topical therapy alone is ineffective; it may be an important adjunct because it may decrease the shedding of spores. Asymptomatic dermatophyte carriage in family members is extremely common. One in three families have at least one member who is a carrier. Therefore, treatment of both patient and potential carriers with a sporicidal shampoo may hasten clinical resolution. For this purpose, vigorous shampooing with a 2.5% selenium sulfide or zinc pyrithione preparation is helpful. It is not necessary to shave the scalp.

Tinea corporis, infection of the glabrous skin, excluding the palms, soles, and groin, can be caused by most of the dermatophyte species, although *T. rubrum* and *T. mentagrophytes* are the most prevalent etiologic organisms. In children, infections with *M. canis* are also frequent. Tinea corporis can be acquired by direct contact with infected persons or by contact with infected scales or hairs deposited on environmental surfaces. *M. canis* infections are usually acquired from infected pets. Not infrequently, a single dermatophyte lesion is responsible for dissemination.

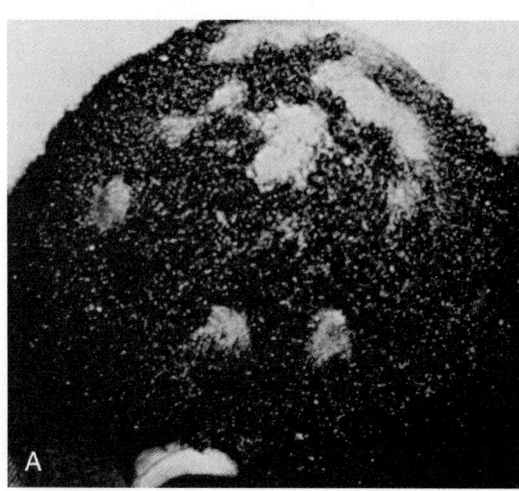
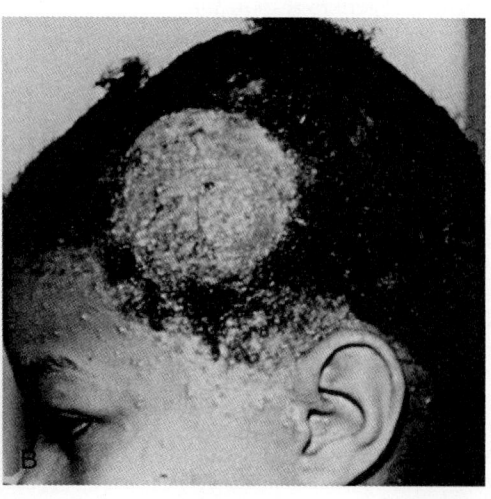

FIGURE 656–2. *A,* Patchy alopecia associated with tinea capitis. *B,* Elevated, boggy granuloma with multiple pustules (kerion) caused by inflammatory tinea capitis.

The most typical *clinical lesion* begins as a dry, mildly erythematous, elevated, scaly papule or plaque that spreads centrifugally as it clears centrally to form the characteristic annular lesion responsible for the designation ringworm (Fig. 656–3). At times, plaques with advancing borders may spread over large areas. Grouped pustules are another variant. Most lesions clear spontaneously within several months, but some may become chronic. Central clearing does not always occur, and differences in host response may result in wide variability in the clinical appearance, for example, granulomatous lesions called *Majocchi granuloma* due to penetration of organisms along the hair follicle to the level of the dermis, producing a fungal folliculitis and perifolliculitis, and the kerion-like lesions referred to as *tinea profunda*.

Many skin lesions, both infectious and noninfectious, must be differentiated from the lesions of tinea corporis. Those most frequently confused are granuloma annulare, nummular eczema, pityriasis rosea, psoriasis, seborrheic dermatitis, erythema chronicum migrans, and tinea versicolor. Microscopic examination of KOH wet mount preparations and cultures should always be obtained when fungal infection is considered. Tinea corporis usually does not fluoresce with a Wood lamp.

Tinea corporis usually responds to *treatment* with one of the topical antifungal agents (e.g., miconazole, clotrimazole, econazole, ketoconazole, terbinafine, naftifine) twice daily for 2–4 wk. In unusually severe or extensive disease, a course of therapy with oral griseofulvin microcrystalline may be required for several weeks. Itraconazole has produced excellent results in many cases with a 1–2 wk course of oral therapy.

Tinea cruris, infection of the groin, occurs most often in adolescent males and is usually caused by the anthropophilic species, *Epidermophyton floccosum* or *Trichophyton rubrum*, but occasionally by the zoophilic species *T. mentagrophytes*.

The initial *clinical lesion* is a small, raised, scaly, erythematous patch on the inner aspect of the thigh; this spreads peripherally, often developing numerous tiny vesicles at the advancing margin. It eventually forms bilateral, irregular, sharply bordered patches with hyperpigmented, scaly centers. In some cases, particularly in infections with *T. mentagrophytes*, the inflammatory reaction is more intense and the infection may spread beyond

the crural region. The penis is usually not involved in the infection, an important distinction from candidosis. Pruritus may be severe initially but abates as the inflammatory reaction subsides. Bacterial superinfection may alter the clinical appearance, and erythrasma or candidosis may coexist. Tinea cruris is more prevalent in obese persons and in those who perspire excessively and wear tight-fitting clothing.

The *diagnosis* is confirmed by culture and by demonstrating septate hyphae on a KOH preparation of epidermal scrapings. Tinea cruris must be differentiated from intertrigo, allergic contact dermatitis, candidosis, and erythrasma. Bacterial superinfection must be precluded when there is a severe inflammatory reaction.

Patients should be advised to wear loose cotton underwear. Topical *treatment* with an imidazole is recommended for severe infection, especially because these agents are effective in mixed candidal-dermatophytic infections. Pure dermatophytic infection may also be treated with tolnaftate.

Tinea pedis (athlete's foot), infection of the toe webs and soles of the feet, is uncommon in young children but occurs with some frequency in preadolescent and adolescent males. The usual etiologic agents are *T. rubrum, T. mentagrophytes*, and *E. floccosum*.

Most commonly, the lateral toe webs (third to fourth and fourth to fifth interdigital spaces) and the subdigital crevice are fissured, with maceration and peeling of the surrounding skin. Severe tenderness, itching, and a persistent foul odor are characteristic. These lesions may become chronic. This type of infection may involve overgrowth by bacterial flora, including *Micrococcus sedantarius, Brevibacterium epidermidis*, and gram-negative organisms. Less commonly, a chronic diffuse hyperkeratosis of the sole of the foot occurs with only mild erythema. In many cases, two feet and one hand are involved. This type of infection is more refractory to treatment and tends to recur. An inflammatory vesicular type of reaction may occur with *T. mentagrophytes* infection; this type is most common in young children. These lesions involve any area of the foot, including the dorsal surface, and are usually circumscribed. The initial papules progress to vesicles and bullae that may become pustular (Fig. 656–4). A number of factors, such as occlusive footwear and warm, humid weather, predispose to infection. Tinea pedis may be transmitted in shower facilities and swimming pool areas.

Tinea pedis must be differentiated from simple maceration and peeling of the interdigital spaces, which is common in children.

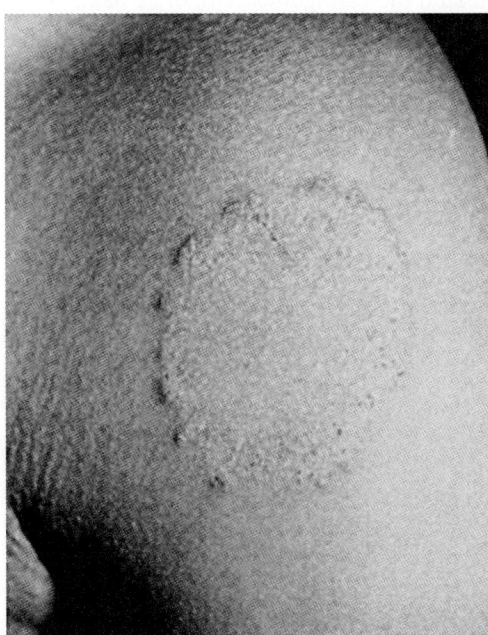

FIGURE 656–3. Circinate lesion of tinea corporis on the shoulder. Note the active papular border, scaling, and relative clearing centrally.

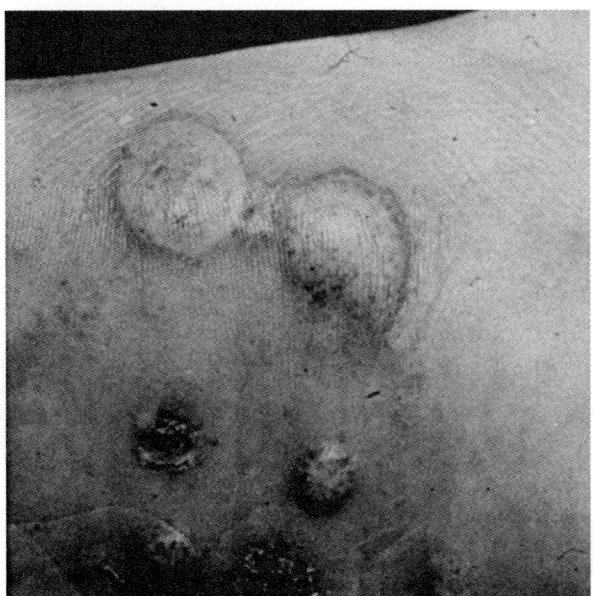

FIGURE 656–4. Multiple inflammatory bullae of tinea pedis.

Infection with *Candida albicans* and various bacterial organisms (erythrasma) may cause confusion or may coexist with primary tinea pedis. Contact dermatitis, dyshidrotic eczema, atopic dermatitis, and juvenile plantar dermatitis also simulate tinea pedis. Fungal mycelia can be seen on microscopic examination of a KOH preparation or by culture; the fourth toe web provides a high yield of infected scales; a blister top can also be used.

Treatment for mild infections includes simple measures such as avoidance of occlusive footwear, careful drying between the toes after bathing, and the use of an absorbent antifungal powder such as zinc undecylenate. Topical therapy with an azole, such as clotrimazole, miconazole, ketoconazole, or econazole is curative in most cases; each of these agents is also effective against candidal infection. Tolnaftate can be used in uncomplicated dermatophyte infections. Several weeks of therapy may be necessary, and low-grade, chronic infections, particularly those caused by *T. rubrum*, may be refractory. In such patients, oral griseofulvin therapy may effect a cure, but recurrences are common.

Tinea unguium is a dermatophyte infection of the nail plate; it occurs most often in patients with tinea pedis, but it may occur as a primary infection. It can be caused by a number of dermatophytes, of which *T. rubrum* and *T. mentagrophytes* are the most common.

The most superficial form of tinea unguium (i.e., white superficial onychomycosis) is due to *T. mentagrophytes*; it is manifested by irregular single or numerous white patches on the surface of the nail unassociated with paronychial inflammation or deep infection. *T. rubrum* generally causes a more invasive, subungual infection that is initiated at the lateral distal margins of the nail and is often preceded by mild paronychia. The middle and ventral layers of the nail plate, and perhaps the nail bed, are the sites of infection. The nail initially develops a yellowish discoloration and slowly becomes thickened, brittle, and loosened from the nail bed. In advanced infection, the nail may turn dark brown to black and may crack or break off.

Tinea unguium must be differentiated from various dystrophic nail disorders. Changes due to trauma, psoriasis, lichen planus, and eczema all can be confused with tinea unguium. Nails infected with *C. albicans* have several distinguishing features, most prominently pronounced paronychial swelling. Thin shavings taken from the infected nail, preferably from the deeper areas, should be examined microscopically with KOH and cultured. Repeated attempts may be required to demonstrate the fungus.

The long half-life of itraconazole in the nail has led to promising trials of intermittent short courses of therapy (e.g., double the normal dose for 1 wk of each month for 3–4 mo). Oral terbinafine also shows promise for the treatment of onychomycosis. Terbinafine once daily for 3–4 mo is more effective than itraconazole pulse therapy. Griseofulvin and application of topical fungistatic agents to the nail bed often are ineffective and are not recommended.

Tinea nigra palmaris is a rare but distinctive superficial fungal infection that occurs principally in children and adolescents. It is caused by the dimorphic fungus *Exophiala werneckii*, which imparts a gray-black color to the affected palm. The characteristic lesion is a well-defined hyperpigmented macule; scaling and erythema are rare, and the lesions are asymptomatic. Tinea nigra is often mistaken for a junctional nevus, melanoma, or staining of the skin by contactants. Treatment with Whitfield ointment, undecylenic acid ointment, miconazole, or tincture of iodine is most successful.

CANDIDAL INFECTIONS (CANDIDOSIS, CANDIDIASIS, AND MONILIASIS) (see Chapter 215)

The dimorphic yeasts of the genus *Candida* are ubiquitous in the environment, but *C. albicans* is the one that usually causes candi-

dosis in children. This yeast is not part of the indigenous skin flora, but it is a frequent transient on skin and may colonize the human alimentary tract and the vagina as a saprophytic organism. Certain environmental conditions, notably elevated temperature and humidity, are associated with an increased frequency of isolation of *C. albicans* from the skin. Many bacterial species inhibit the growth of *C. albicans*, and alteration of normal flora by the use of antibiotics may promote overgrowth of the yeast.

Oral Candidosis (Thrush). See Chapter 215.

Vaginal Candidosis. See Chapters 215 and 541. *C. albicans* is an inhabitant of the vagina in 5–10% of women, and vaginal candidosis is not uncommon in adolescent girls. A number of factors can predispose to this infection, including antibiotic therapy, corticosteroid therapy, diabetes mellitus, pregnancy, and the use of oral contraceptives. The infection is manifested by cheesy white plaques on an erythematous vaginal mucosa and by a thick white-yellow discharge. The disease may be relatively mild or may produce pronounced inflammation and scaling of the external genitals and surrounding skin with progression to vesiculation and ulceration. Patients often complain of severe itching and burning in the vaginal area. Before treatment is initiated, the diagnosis should be confirmed by microscopic examination and/or culture. The infection may be eradicated by insertion of nystatin or imidazole vaginal tablets, suppositories, creams, or foam. If these products are ineffective, the addition of oral nystatin tablets, 1–2 tablets tid for 14 days, may eliminate or decrease the candidal population in the gastrointestinal tract.

Congenital Cutaneous Candidosis. See Chapter 215.

Candidal Diaper Dermatitis. This is a ubiquitous problem in infants and, although relatively benign, is often frustrating because of its tendency to recur. Predisposed infants usually carry *C. albicans* in their intestinal tract, and the warm, moist, occluded skin of the diaper area provides an optimal environment for its growth. A seborrheic, atopic, or primary irritant contact dermatitis usually provides a portal of entry for the yeast.

The primary *clinical manifestation* consists of an intensely erythematous, confluent plaque with a scalloped border and a sharply demarcated edge. It is formed by the confluence of numerous papules and vesiculopustules; satellite pustules, those that stud the contiguous skin, are a hallmark of localized candidal infections. The perianal skin, inguinal folds, perineum, and lower abdomen are usually involved (Fig. 656–5). In males, the entire scrotum and penis may be involved with an erosive balanitis of the perimeatal skin; in females, the lesions may be found on the vaginal mucosa and labia. In some infants, the process is generalized, with erythematous lesions distant from the diaper area; in some cases, the generalized process may represent a fungal id (hypersensitivity) reaction.

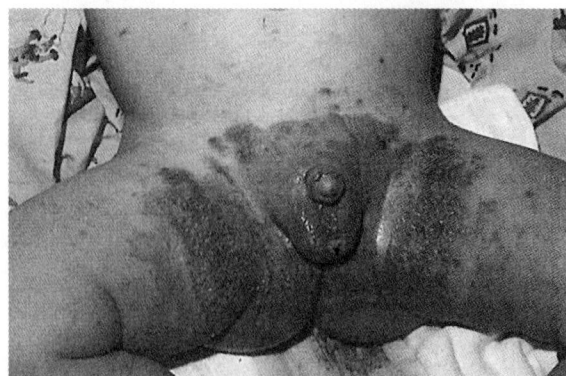

FIGURE 656–5. Erythematous confluent plaque with satellite pustules caused by candidal infection. See also color section.

The *differential diagnosis* includes other eruptions of the diaper area that may coexist with candidal infection. For this reason, it is important to establish a diagnosis by a KOH preparation or culture.

Treatment consists of applications of an anticandidal agent (nystatin, miconazole, clotrimazole, ketoconazole) with each diaper change or four times daily. Ointments are better tolerated than creams; lotions and creams may cause a burning sensation when applied to irritated skin, and powder may cake and cause erosion due to friction during movement. The combination of a corticosteroid and an antifungal agent is justified if inflammation is severe but may confuse the situation if the diagnosis is not firmly established. Corticosteroid should not be continued for more than a few days. Protection of the diaper area by an application of thick zinc oxide paste overlying the anticandidal preparation may be helpful; the paste is more easily removed with mineral oil than with soap and water. *Fungal id reactions* gradually abate with successful treatment of the diaper dermatitis or may be treated with a mild corticosteroid preparation. When recurrences of diaper candidosis are frequent, it may be helpful to prescribe a course of oral anticandidal therapy to decrease the yeast population in the gastrointestinal tract. Some infants seem to be receptive hosts for *C. albicans* and may reacquire the organism from a colonized adult.

Intertriginous Candidosis. This occurs most often in the axillae and groin, under the breasts, under pendulous abdominal fat folds, in the umbilicus, and in the gluteal cleft. Typical lesions are large, confluent areas of moist, denuded, erythematous skin with an irregular, macerated, scaly border. Satellite lesions are characteristic and consist of small vesicles or pustules on an erythematous base. With time, intertriginous candidal lesions may become lichenified, dry, scaly plaques. The lesions develop on skin subjected to irritation and maceration. Candidal superinfection is more likely to occur under conditions that lead to excessive perspiration, especially in obese children and in those with underlying disorders, such as diabetes mellitus. A similar condition, *interdigital candidosis*, commonly occurs in individuals whose hands are constantly immersed in water; fissures occur between the fingers and have red, denuded centers, with an overhanging white epithelial fringe. Similar lesions between the toes may be secondary to occlusive footwear. Treatment is the same as for other candidal infections.

Perianal Candidosis. Perianal dermatitis develops at sites of skin irritation as a result of occlusion, constant moisture, poor hygiene, anal fissures, and pruritus due to pinworm infestation. It may become superinfected with *C. albicans*, especially in children who are receiving oral antibiotic or corticosteroid medication. The involved skin becomes erythematous, macerated, and excoriated, and the lesions are identical to those of candidal intertrigo or candidal diaper rash. Application of a topical antifungal agent in conjunction with improved hygiene is usually effective. Underlying disorders such as pinworm infection must also be treated (see Chapter 270).

Candidal Paronychia and Onychia. See Chapter 653.

Candidal Granuloma. This is a rare response to an invasive candidal infection of skin. The lesions appear as crusted, verrucous plaques and hornlike projections on the scalp, face, and distal limbs. Affected patients may have single or numerous defects in immune mechanisms and are often refractory to topical therapy. A systemic anticandidal agent may be required for palliation or eradication of the infection.

Allen H, Honig P, Leyden J, et al: Selenium sulfide: Adjunctive therapy for tinea capitis. *Pediatrics* 1982;69:81.

Darmstadt GL, Dinulos JG, Miller Z: Congenital cutaneous candidiasis: clinical presentation, pathogenesis, and management guidelines. *Pediatrics* 2000;105:438.

Evans EG, Sigurgeirsson B: Double blind, randomized study of continuous terbinafine compared with intermittent itraconazole in treatment of toenail onychomycosis. *Br Med J* 1999;318:1031–5.

Faergemann J: Pityrosporum infections. *J Am Acad Dermatol* 1994;31:S18.

Friedlander SF, Aly R, Krafchik B, et al: Terbinafine in the treatment of *trichophyton* tinea capitis: a randomized, double-blind, parallel-group, duration-finding study. *Pediatrics* 2002;109:602–7.

Frieden IJ, Howard R: Tinea capitis: Epidemiology, diagnosis, treatment, and control. *J Am Acad Dermatol* 1994;31:S42.

Greer D: Treatment of symptom-free carriers in the management of tinea capitis. *Lancet* 1996;348:350.

Gupta AK, Adam P: Terbinafine pulse therapy is effective in tinea capitis. *Pediatr Dermatol* 1998;15:56.

Hubbard TW, de Triquet JM: Brush-culture method for diagnosing tinea capitis. *Pediatrics* 1992;90:416.

Jacobs AH, O'Connell BM: Tinea in tiny tots. *Am J Dis Child* 1986;140:1034.

Pomerantz AJ, Sabnis SS, McGrath GJ, et al: Asymptomatic dermatophyte carriers in the household of children with tinea capitis. *Arch Pediatr Adolesc Med* 1999;153:483.

Pong AL, McCuaig CC: Fungal infections, infestations, and parasitic infections in neonates. In Eichenfield LF, Frieden IJ, Esterly NB (editors): *Textbook of Neonatal Dermatology.* Philadelphia, WB Saunders, 2001, p. 223.

Rezabek GH, Friedman AD: Superficial fungal infections of the skin. Diagnosis and current treatment recommendations. *Drugs* 1992;43:674.

Rosenthal JR: Pediatric fungal infections from head to toe: What's new? *Curr Opin Pediatr* 1994;6:435.

Suarez S, Fallon-Friedlander S: Antifungal therapy in children: An update. *Pediatr Ann* 1998;27:177.

Zienicke HC, Korting HC, Lukacs K, et al: Dermatophytosis in children and adolescents: Epidemiological, clinical, and microbiological aspects changing with age. *J Dermatol* 1991;18:438.

Chapter 657
Cutaneous Viral Infections

WART (VERRUCA)

Human papillomaviruses (HPV) cause a spectrum of disease from warts to squamous cell carcinoma of the skin and mucous membranes, including the larynx (see Chapter 243). The incidence of all types of warts is highest in children and adolescents. HPV is spread by direct contact and autoinoculation, but transmission by fomites can occur. The clinical manifestations of infection develop 1 mo or longer after inoculation and depend on the HPV type, of which more than 70 are recognized; the size of the inoculum; the immune status of the host; and the anatomic site.

Clinical Manifestations. Cutaneous warts develop in 5–10% of children. *Common warts (verruca vulgaris),* caused most commonly by HPV types 2 and 4, occur most frequently on the fingers, dorsum of the hands, paronychial areas, face, knees, and elbows. They are well-circumscribed papules with a roughened, keratotic, irregular surface. When the surface is pared away, many black dots representing thrombosed dermal capillary loops are often visible. Periungual warts are often painful and may spread beneath the nail plate, separating it from the nail bed. *Plantar warts,* although similar to the common wart, are caused by HPV type 1 and are usually flush with the surface of the sole because of the constant pressure from weight bearing; they may be painful. Similar lesions (palmar) can also occur on the palms. They are sharply demarcated, often with a ring of thick callus. The surface keratotic material must sometimes be removed before the boundaries of the wart can be appreciated. Several contiguous warts (HPV type 4) may fuse to form a large plaque, the so-called *mosaic wart. Flat warts (verruca plana),* caused by HPV types 2, 3, and 10, are slightly elevated, minimally hyperkeratotic papules that usually remain less than 3 mm in diameter and vary in color from pink to brown. They may occur in profusion on the face, arms, dorsum of the hands, and knees. The distribution of several lesions along a line of cutaneous trauma is a helpful diagnostic feature. Lesions may be disseminated in the beard area by shaving and from the hairline onto the scalp by combing the hair. *Epidermodysplasia verruciformis*, caused primarily by HPV types 5 and 8, presents with many diffuse verrucous papules. Approximately 25% of cases are familial, occurring by autosomal recessive or X-linked inheritance, and 3–10% of patients have HPV-associated squamous cell carcinoma on sun-exposed skin.

Genital HPV infection occurs in nearly 40% of sexually active adolescents, most commonly as a result of infection with HPV types 6 and 11. *Condylomata acuminata (mucous membrane warts)* are moist, fleshy, papillomatous lesions that occur on the perianal mucosa (Fig. 657–1), labia, vaginal introitus, and perineal raphe and on the shaft, corona, and glans penis. Occasionally they obstruct the urethral meatus or the vaginal introitus. Because they are located in intertriginous areas, they may become moist and friable. When untreated, condylomata proliferate and become confluent, at times forming large cauliflower-like masses. Lesions can also occur on the lips, gingivae, tongue, and conjunctivae. Genital warts in children may occur after inoculation during birth through an infected birth canal, as a consequence of sexual abuse, or from incidental spread from cutaneous warts. A significant proportion of genital warts in children contain HPV types that are usually isolated from cutaneous warts. HPV infection of the cervix is a major risk factor for development of carcinoma, particularly if the infection is due to HPV types 16, 18, 31–33, 35, 39, 42, or 51–54. *Laryngeal (respiratory) papillomas* contain the same HPV types as in anogenital papillomas. Transmission is believed to occur from mothers with genital HPV infection to neonates who aspirate infectious virus during birth.

Pathology. The various types of warts differ in minor ways but share the basic changes of hyperplasia of the epidermal cells and vacuolation of the spinous keratinocytes, which may contain basophilic intranuclear inclusions (viral particles). Warts are confined to the epidermis and, contrary to the common misconception, do not have "roots." Parakeratosis, papillomatosis, and eosinophilic cytoplasmic inclusions, thought to represent altered keratohyalin, are additional variable histologic changes. Individuals with impaired cell-mediated immunity are particularly susceptible to HPV infection. Antibodies occur in response to infection but appear to have little protective effect.

Differential Diagnosis. Common warts are most often confused with molluscum contagiosum. Plantar and palmar warts may be difficult to distinguish from punctate keratoses, corns, and cal-

luses. In contrast to calluses, warts obliterate normal skin markings. Juvenile flat warts mimic lichen planus, lichen nitidus, angiofibromas, syringomas, milia, and acne. Condylomata acuminata may resemble condylomata lata of secondary syphilis.

Treatment. Various therapeutic measures are effective in the treatment of warts. More than 50% of warts disappear spontaneously within 2 yr, but failure to treat incurs the risk of spread to other sites. Warts are epidermal lesions and do not produce scarring unless they are managed surgically or treated in an overly aggressive fashion. Hyperkeratotic lesions (common, plantar, and palmar warts) are more responsive to therapy if the excess keratotic debris is gently pared with a scalpel until thrombosed capillaries are apparent; further paring induces bleeding. Treatment is most successful when done regularly and frequently (e.g., every 2 wk).

Common warts can be destroyed by applications of liquid nitrogen or cantharidin or by light electrodesiccation and curettage. Daily applications of 10–17% lactic acid and 10–17% salicylic acid in flexible collodion is a slow but painless method of removal that is effective in some patients. Recalcitrant warts may respond to 5% 5-*fluorouracil ointment* rubbed into lesions daily. Care must be taken to avoid contact with adjacent normal skin, which may cause undue irritation, erosion, or postinflammatory hyperpigmentation. Plantar and palmar warts may be treated with salicylic and lactic acids in collodion or 40% salicylic acid or urea plasters. After prolonged soaking in lukewarm water, keratotic debris can be removed by an emery board or pumice stone. Occlusive taping without medication for several weeks is also very effective. Condylomata respond best to weekly applications of 25% podophyllin in tincture of benzoin; the medication should be left on the warts for 4–6 hr and then removed by bathing. Condylomata localized to keratinized sites (e.g., buttocks) may not respond to podophyllin. Imiquimod (5% cream) applied three times weekly may be beneficial. Imiquimod is indicated for genital warts but is also helpful in other locations. A moist environment, and daily application may improve efficacy but increase the risk of irritation. Resistant lesions can usually be eradicated by weekly freezing with liquid nitrogen or by treatment with a carbon dioxide laser. Although intralesional injection of 1 million units of interferon-α or -β three times weekly for 3–4 wk appears to be effective against condylomata, this is not recommended because of a low incidence of effectiveness, high toxicity rate, and high cost. With all types of therapy, care should be taken to protect the surrounding normal skin from irritation.

MOLLUSCUM CONTAGIOSUM

The poxvirus that causes molluscum contagiosum is a large double-stranded DNA virus that replicates in the cytoplasm of host epithelial cells. The three types cannot be differentiated on the basis of clinical appearance, location of lesions, or a patient's age or sex. Type 1 virus causes most infections. The disease is acquired by direct contact with an infected person or from fomites and is spread by autoinoculation. School-aged children who are otherwise well and individuals who are immunosuppressed are affected most commonly. The incubation period is estimated to be 2 wk or longer.

Clinical Manifestations. Discrete, pearly, skin-colored, dome-shaped, smooth papules vary in size from 1–5 mm. They typically have a central umbilication from which a plug of cheesy material can be expressed (Fig. 657–2). The papules may occur anywhere on the body, but the face, eyelids, neck, axillas, and thighs are sites of predilection. They may be found in clusters on the genitals or in the groin of adolescents and may be associated with other venereal diseases in sexually active individuals. Lesions commonly involve the genital area in children but in most cases are not acquired by sexual transmission; search

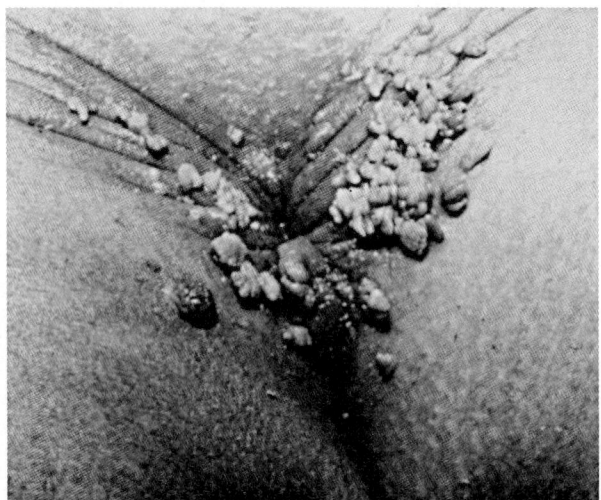

FIGURE 657–1. Condylomata acuminata in the perianal area of a toddler.

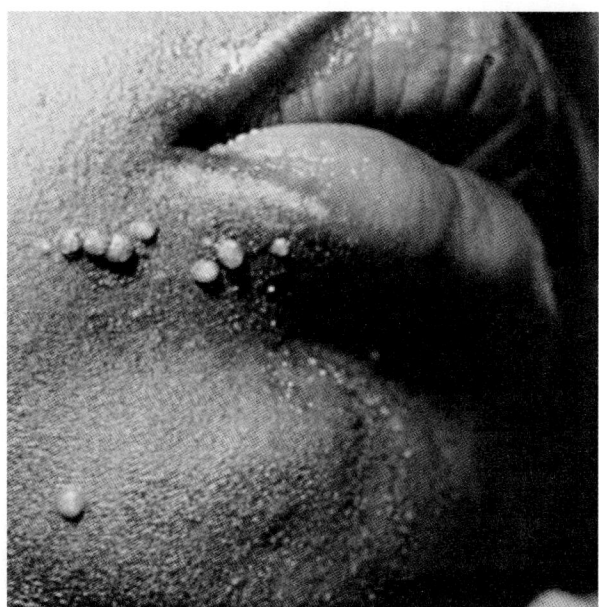

FIGURE 657–2. Grouped papules of molluscum contagiosum on the face.

should be undertaken, however, for other signs of sexual abuse. Lesions on the eyelid margin can produce unilateral conjunctivitis; rarely, lesions may appear on the conjunctiva or cornea. Mild surrounding erythema or an eczematous dermatitis may accompany the papules. Lesions on patients with AIDS tend to be large and numerous, particularly on the face; exuberant lesions may also be found in children with leukemia and other immunodeficiencies. Children with atopic dermatitis are susceptible to widespread involvement in areas of dermatitis.

Differential Diagnosis. This includes trichoepithelioma, basal cell carcinoma, ectopic sebaceous glands, syringoma, hidrocystoma, keratoacanthoma, and warty dyskeratoma. In individuals with AIDS, cryptococcosis may be indistinguishable clinically from molluscum contagiosum; rarely, coccidioidomycosis, histoplasmosis, or *Penicillium marneffei* infection masquerades with molluscum-like lesions in an immunocompromised host.

Pathology and Diagnosis. The epidermis is hyperplastic and hypertrophied, extending into the underlying dermis and projecting above the skin surface. The molluscum papule consists of a lobulated adhesive mass of virus-infected epidermal cells. Eosinophilic viral inclusion bodies (Henderson-Patterson or molluscum bodies) become more prominent as the cells move upward from the basal layer to the stratum corneum. The central plug of material, which is composed of virus-laden cells, may be shelled out from a lesion (see Treatment) and examined under the microscope with 10% potassium hydroxide or Wright or Giemsa stain. The rounded, cup-shaped mass of homogeneous cells, often with identifiable lobules, is diagnostic. Specific antibody against molluscum contagiosum virus is detectable in most infected individuals but is of uncertain immunologic significance. Cell-mediated immunity is thought to be important in host defense.

Treatment. Molluscum contagiosum is a self-limited disease; the average attack lasts 6–9 mo. However, lesions can persist for years, can spread to distant sites, and may be transmitted to others. Affected patients should be advised to avoid shared baths and towels until the infection is clear. Infection may spread rapidly and produce hundreds of lesions in children with atopic dermatitis or immunodeficiency. A brief 6–9 sec application of liquid nitrogen is very effective and, in most instances, is

a common treatment. The papules can also be destroyed by expressing the plug with a needle, a sharp curette, or a comedo extractor. Cantharidin 0.9% is a popular therapy and may be applied to each lesion without occlusion and frequently causes enough inflammation to facilitate spontaneous extrusion of the plug. Treatment of a few lesions is occasionally followed by resolution of the others. Sometimes, however, treatment with cantharidin results in formation of a rosette of new lesions encircling the site of treatment. Facial molluscum are more cosmetically upsetting to children and parents, and are more difficult to treat with destructive modalities such as liquid nitrogen or cantharidin. Tretinoin or imiquimod applied topically may be beneficial if not excessively irritating. Molluscum is an epidermal disease and should not be overtreated so that scarring results. A lesion-free period of 4 mo can be regarded as a cure.

Beutner KR: Cutaneous viral infections. *Pediatr Ann* 1993;22:247.
Darmstadt GL: Poxviridae (Molluscum contagiosum). In Long SS, Prober CG, Pickering LK (editors): *Principles and Practice of Pediatric Infectious Disease*, 2nd ed. New York, Churchill Livingstone, 2002.
Focht D, Spicer C, Fairchok M: The efficacy of duct tape vs cryotherapy in the treatment of verruca vulgaris (the common wart). *Arch Pediatr Adol Med* 2002;156:971–4.
Friedlander SF, Bradley JS: Viral infections. In Eichenfield LF, Frieden IJ, Esterly NB (editors): *Textbook of Neonatal Dermatology*. Philadelphia, WB Saunders, 2001, p. 201.
Gibbs S, Harvey I, Sterling J, et al: Local treatment for cutaneous warts: systematic review. *Br Med J* 2002;325:461–4.
Grussendorf-Conen EI, Jacobs S: Efficacy of imiquimod 5% cream in the treatment of recalcitrant warts in children. *Pediatr Dermatol* 2002;19:263–6.
Majewski S, Jablonska S: Human papillomavirus-associated tumors of the skin and mucosa. *J Am Acad Dermatol* 1997;36:659.
Schachner L, Hankin DE: Assessing child abuse in childhood condyloma acuminatum. *J Am Acad Dermatol* 1985;12:157.
Silverberg NB, Sidbury R, Mancini AJ: Childhood molluscum contagiosum: Experience with cantharidin in 300 patients. *J Am Acad Dermatol* 2000;43:503.

Chapter 658
Arthropod Bites and Infestations

ARTHROPOD BITES

Arthropod bites are a common affliction of children and occasionally pose a problem in diagnosis. A patient may be unaware of the source of the lesions or deny being bitten, making interpretation of the eruption difficult. In these cases, knowledge of the habits, life cycle, and clinical signs of the more common arthropod pests of humans may help lead to a correct diagnosis. The principal classes of arthropods that cause skin injury to humans are listed in Box 658–1. Some of the important dermatoses caused by arthropod bites and infestations are covered in this chapter; others are discussed in chapters addressing infectious organisms (see Part XVI).

Clinical Manifestations. The type of reaction that occurs after an arthropod bite depends on the species of insect and the age group and reactivity of the human host. Arthropods may cause injury to a host by various mechanisms, including mechanical trauma, such as the lacerating bite of a tsetse fly; invasion of host tissues, as in myiasis; contact dermatitis, as seen with repeated exposure to cockroach antigens; granulomatous reaction to retained mouth parts; transmission of systemic disease; injection of irritant cytotoxic or pharmacologically active substances, such as hyaluronidase, proteases, peptidases, and phospholipases in sting venom; and induction of anaphylaxis. Most reactions to arthropod bites, however, depend on antibody

BOX 658–1. Arthropods that Cause Human Skin Disease

Class Arachnida (four pairs of legs): mites, spiders, ticks
Class Chilopoda: centipedes
Class Diplopoda: millipedes
Class Insecta (three pairs of legs):
　　Order Diptera: mosquitoes, flies
　　Order Siphonaptera: fleas
　　Order Hymenoptera: ants, bees, wasps
　　Order Anoplura: lice
　　Order Hemiptera: bedbugs, kissing bugs
　　Order Coleoptera: beetles
　　Order Lepidoptera: butterflies, moths

formation to antigenic substances in saliva or venom. The type of reaction is determined primarily by the degree of previous exposure to the same or a related species of arthropod. When someone is bitten for the first time, no reaction develops. An immediate petechial reaction is occasionally seen, however, in newborn babies after a mosquito bite. After repeated bites, sensitivity develops, producing a pruritic papule approximately 24 hr after the bite; this is the most common reaction seen in young children. With prolonged, repeated exposure, a wheal develops within minutes after a bite, followed 24 hr later by papule formation; this combination of reactions is seen commonly in older children. By adolescence or adulthood, only a wheal may form, unaccompanied by the delayed papular reaction. Thus, adults may be unaffected in the same household as affected children. Ultimately, as a person becomes insensitive to the bite, no reaction occurs at all. This stage of nonreactivity is maintained only as long as the individual continues to be bitten regularly. Individuals in whom papular urticaria develops are in the transitional phase between development of primarily a delayed papular reaction and development of an immediate urticarial reaction.

Arthropod bites may occur as solitary, numerous, or profuse lesions, depending on the feeding habits of the perpetrator. For example, fleas tend to sample their host several times within a small localized area, whereas mosquitoes tend to attack a host at more randomly scattered sites. *Delayed hypersensitivity reactions* to insect bites, the predominant lesions in the young and uninitiated, are characterized by firm, persistent papules that may become hyperpigmented and are often excoriated and crusted. Pruritus may be mild or severe, transient or persistent. A central punctum is usually visible but may disappear as the lesion ages or is scratched. The *immediate hypersensitivity reaction* is characterized by an erythematous, evanescent wheal. If edema is marked, the wheal may be surmounted by a tiny vesicle. Certain beetles produce bullous lesions through the action of cantharidin, and hemorrhagic nodules and ulcers may be caused by various insects, including beetles and spiders. Bites on the lower extremities are more likely to be severe or persistent or become bullous than those located elsewhere. Complications of arthropod bites include development of impetigo, folliculitis, cellulitis, lymphangitis, and severe anaphylactic hypersensitivity reactions, particularly after the bite of certain Hymenoptera. The histopathologic changes are variable, depending on the arthropod, the age of the lesion, and the reactivity of the host. Acute urticarial lesions tend to show central vesiculation in which eosinophils are numerous. Papules most commonly show dermal edema and a mixed, superficial and deep perivascular inflammatory infiltrate, often including a number of eosinophils. At times, however, the dermal cellular infiltrate is so dense that a lymphoma is suspected. Retained mouth parts may stimulate a foreign body type of granulomatous reaction.

Papular urticaria occurs principally in the 1st decade of life, during the warmer months of the year. The most common cul-

prits are species of fleas, mites, bedbugs, gnats, mosquitoes, chiggers, and animal lice. Individuals with papular urticaria have predominantly transitional lesions in various stages of evolution between delayed-onset papules and immediate-onset wheals. The most characteristic lesion is an edematous redbrown papule; an individual lesion frequently starts as a wheal that in turn is replaced by a papule. A given bite may incite an id reaction at distant sites of quiescent bites in the form of erythematous macules, papules, or urticarial plaques. The disorder is characterized by a temporary arrest at a transitional phase; after a season or two, however, the reaction progresses from a transitional to a primarily immediate hypersensitivity urticarial reaction.

One of the most commonly encountered arthropod bites is that due to human, cat, or dog *fleas* (family Pulicidae). Eggs, which are generally laid in dusty areas and cracks between floorboards, give rise to larvae that then form cocoons. The cocoon stage can persist for up to 1 yr, and the animal emerges in response to vibrations from footsteps, accounting for the assaults that frequently befall the new owners of a recently reopened dwelling. Adult dog fleas can live without a blood meal for approximately 60 days. Attacks from fleas are more likely to occur when the fleas do not have access to their usual host; for example, cat or dog fleas are more voracious and problematic when one visits an area frequented by the pet than when the pet is encountered directly. Flea bites tend to be grouped in lines or irregular clusters. Fleas are often not seen on the body of a pet; diagnosis of flea bites, however, is aided by examination of debris from the animal's bedding material. The debris is collected by shaking the bedding into a plastic bag and examining the contents for fleas or their eggs, larvae, or feces.

Treatment. This is directed at alleviation of pruritus by oral antihistamines, cool compresses, and soothing lotions such as calamine, to which 0.25% menthol and 0.5% phenol can be added. Topical corticosteroid creams are rarely effective, and topical antihistamines are potent sensitizers and have no role in the treatment of insect bite reactions. A short course of systemic steroids may be helpful if many severe reactions occur, particularly around the eyes. Insect repellents containing diethyltoluamide (DEET) may afford moderate protection against mosquitoes, fleas, flies, chiggers, and ticks but are relatively ineffective against wasps, bees, and hornets. DEET must be applied to exposed skin and clothing to be effective. The most effective protection against mosquitoes, the human body louse, and other blood-feeding arthropods is use of DEET and permethrin-impregnated clothing; these measures are not effective, however, against the phlebotomine sandfly, which transmits leishmaniasis. Advocates of treatment with B-complex vitamins or thiamine hydrochloride maintain that these agents impart an offensive odor to sweat, warding off mosquitoes; this claim has not been substantiated by clinical trials.

An effort should be made to identify and eradicate the etiologic agent. Pets should be carefully inspected; crawl spaces, eaves, and other sites of the house or outbuildings frequented by animals and birds should be decontaminated; and baseboard crevices, mattresses, rugs, furniture, and animal sleeping quarters should be decontaminated. Agents that are effective for ridding the home of fleas include lindane, pyrethroids, and organic thiocyanates. Flea-infested pets may be treated with powders containing rotenone, pyrethroids, malathion, or methoxychlor.

INFESTATIONS

Scabies. Scabies is caused by burrowing and release of toxic or antigenic substances by the female mite *Sarcoptes scabiei* var. *hominis*. The most important factor that determines spread of scabies is the extent and duration of physical contact with an affected individual; the children and sexual partner of an affected individual are most at risk. Scabies is transmitted only rarely by fomites because the isolated mite dies within 2–3 days.

CLINICAL MANIFESTATIONS. In an immunocompetent host, scabies is frequently heralded by intense pruritus, particularly at night. The first sign of the infestation often consists of 1–2 mm red papules, some of which are excoriated, crusted, or scaling. Threadlike burrows are the classic lesion of scabies but may not be seen in infants. In infants, bullae and pustules are relatively common; the eruption may also include wheals, papules, vesicles, and a superimposed eczematous dermatitis; and the palms, soles (Fig. 658–1B), face, and scalp are often affected. In older children and adolescents, the clinical pattern is similar to that in adults, in whom preferred sites are the interdigital spaces, wrist flexors, anterior axillary folds, ankles, buttocks, umbilicus and belt line, groin, genitals in men, and areolas in women (see Fig. 658–1A); the head, neck, palms, and soles are generally spared. Red-brown nodules, most often located in covered areas such as the axillae, groin, and genitals, predominate in the less common variant called nodular

scabies. Untreated, scabies may lead to eczematous dermatitis, impetigo, ecthyma, folliculitis, furunculosis, cellulitis, lymphangitis, and id reaction. Children have been reported to develop glomerulonephritis as a result of streptococcal impetiginization of scabies lesions. In some tropical areas, scabies is the predominant underlying cause of pyoderma. A latent period of approximately 1 mo follows an initial infestation; thus, itching may be absent and lesions may be relatively inapparent in contacts who are asymptomatic carriers. On reinfestation, however, reactions to mite antigens are noted within hours.

ETIOLOGY AND PATHOGENESIS. An adult female mite measures approximately 0.4 mm in length, has four sets of legs, and has a hemispheric body marked by transverse corrugations, brown spines, and bristles on the dorsal surface. A male mite is approximately half her size and is similar in configuration. After impregnation on the skin surface, a gravid female exudes a keratolytic substance and burrows into the stratum corneum, often forming a shallow well within 30 min. She gradually extends this tract by 0.5–5 mm/24 hr along the boundary with the stratum granulosum. She deposits one to three oval eggs and numerous brown fecal pellets (scybala)

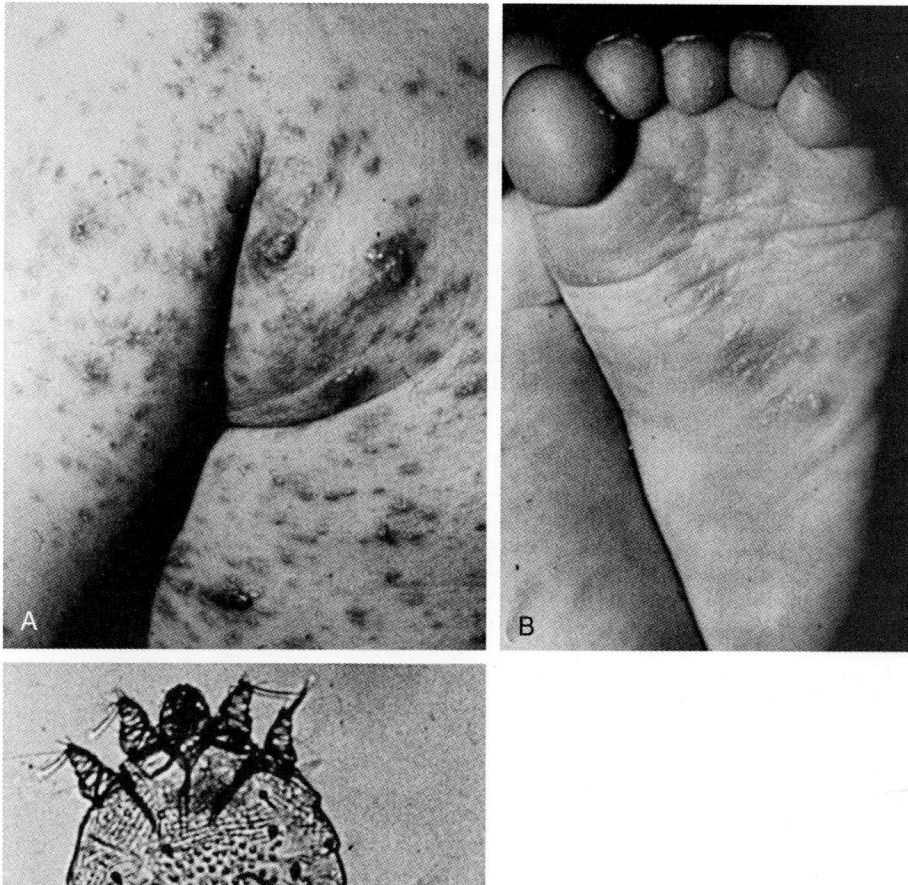

FIGURE 658–1. *A,* Eczematous dermatitis, papules, and nodules of human scabies. *B,* Vesiculopustular lesions of scabies on the soles of an infant. *C,* Human scabies mite obtained from scraping.

daily. When egg laying is completed, in 4–5 wk, she dies within the burrow. The eggs hatch in 3–5 days, releasing larvae that move to the skin surface to molt into nymphs. Maturity is achieved in about 2–3 wk. Mating occurs, and the gravid female invades the skin to complete the life cycle.

DIAGNOSIS. This can often be made clinically but is confirmed by microscopic identification of mites (see Fig. 658–1C), ova, and scybala in epithelial debris. Scrapings are most often positive when obtained from burrows, eczematous lesions, or fresh papules. A reliable method is application of a drop of mineral oil on the selected lesion, scraping of it with a No. 15 blade, and transfer of the oil and scrapings to a glass slide.

The *differential diagnosis* depends on the types of lesions present. Burrows are virtually pathognomonic for human scabies. Papulovesicular lesions are confused with papular urticaria, canine scabies, chickenpox, viral exanthems, drug eruptions, dermatitis herpetiformis, and folliculitis. Eczematous lesions may mimic atopic dermatitis and seborrheic dermatitis, and the less common bullous disorders of childhood may be suspected in infants with predominantly bullous lesions. Nodular scabies is frequently misdiagnosed as urticaria pigmentosa and Langerhans cell hysticocytosis. The histopathologic appearance of nodular scabies, consisting of a deep, dense, perivascular infiltrate of lymphocytes, histiocytes, plasma cells, and atypical mononuclear cells, may mimic malignant lymphoid neoplasms.

TREATMENT. Application of permethrin 5% cream (Elimite) or 1% lindane cream or lotion to the entire body from the neck down, with particular attention to intensely involved areas, is standard therapy. Scabies is frequently found above the neck in infants, however, also necessitating treatment of the scalp. The medication is left on the skin for 8–12 hr; if necessary, it may be reapplied in 1 wk for another 8–12 hr period. Because lindane is potentially neurotoxic, the vulnerability of small infants to percutaneous absorption dictates caution in prescribing it for them. Signs of lindane toxicity include nausea, vomiting, weakness, tremors, irritability, disorientation, seizures, and respiratory compromise. Systemic absorption and toxicity of lindane can be minimized by not applying the medication to warm, moist skin; not repeating an application within 7 days; and not using the medication on children who are underweight or malnourished or have extensive areas of inflamed, denuded, or secondarily infected skin. Permethrin 5% cream is a slightly more effective scabicide than lindane but is more expensive. It is poorly absorbed, rapidly metabolized by tissue esterases, and therefore of very low toxicity. For infants younger than 2 mo, alternative therapy includes 6% sulfur in petrolatum applied for three consecutive 24-hr periods. Topical sulfur ointment is messy and malodorous, stains clothing, and commonly causes irritant dermatitis. No controlled studies of its efficacy and safety have been published in recent years. Permethrin 5% cream is a better alternative for infants. Crotamiton cream or lotion is not recommended because of lack of efficacy and toxicity data.

Transmission of mites is unlikely more than 24 hr after treatment. Pruritus, which is due to hypersensitivity to mite antigens, may persist for a number of days and may be alleviated by a topical corticosteroid preparation. If pruritus persists for more than 2 wk after treatment, the patient should be reexamined for mites. Nodules are extremely resistant to treatment and may take several months to resolve. The entire family should be treated, as should caretakers of the infested child. Clothing, bed linens, and towels should be thoroughly laundered.

NORWEGIAN SCABIES. This variant of human scabies is highly contagious and occurs mainly in individuals who are mentally and physically debilitated, particularly those who are institutionalized and those with Down syndrome; in patients with poor cutaneous sensation, such as those with leprosy or syringomyelia; in patients who have severe systemic illness

such as leukemia or diabetes; and in immunosuppressed patients such as those with HIV infection. Affected individuals are infested by myriad mites that inhabit the crusts and exfoliating scales of the skin and scalp. The nails may become thickened and dystrophic; the subungual debris is densely populated by mites. The infestation is often accompanied by generalized lymphadenopathy and eosinophilia. On microscopic examination, one sees massive orthokeratosis and parakeratosis with numerous interspersed mites, psoriasiform epidermal hyperplasia, foci of spongiosis, and neutrophilic abscesses. Norwegian scabies is thought to represent a deficient host immune response to the organism. Management is difficult, requiring scrupulous isolation measures, removal of the thick scales, and repeated but careful applications of antiscabietic preparations. Ivermectin has been used successfully as single-dose therapy in refractory cases, particularly in HIV-infected patients; the Food and Drug Administration (FDA) has not approved it for treatment of scabies nor for any application in children younger than 5 yr.

CANINE SCABIES. This is caused by *S. scabiei* var. *canis*, the dog mite that is associated with mange. The eruption in humans, which is most frequently acquired by cuddling an infested puppy, consists of tiny papules, vesicles, wheals, and excoriated eczematous plaques. Burrows are not present because the mite infrequently inhabits human stratum corneum. The rash is pruritic and has a predilection for the arms, chest, and abdomen, the usual sites of contact with dogs. Onset is sudden and usually follows exposure by 1–10 days, possibly resulting from development of a hypersensitivity reaction to mite antigens. Recovery of mites or ova from scrapings of human skin is rare. The disease is self-limited because humans are not a suitable host; bathing and changing clothes are generally sufficient. Removal or treatment of the infested animal, however, is also necessary. Symptomatic therapy for itching is helpful. In rare cases in which mites are demonstrated in scrapings from an affected child, they can be eradicated by the same measures applicable to human scabies.

Other mites that occasionally bite humans include the *chigger* or harvest mite (*Eutrombicula alfreddugesi*), which prefers to live on grass, shrubs, vines, and stems of grain. Larvae have hooked mouthparts, which allow the chigger to attach to the skin, but not to burrow, to obtain a blood meal, most commonly on the lower legs. *Avian mites* may affect those who come into close contact with chickens or pet gerbils. Humans may occasionally be assaulted by avian mites that have infested a nest outside a window, an attic, heating vents, or an air conditioner. The dermatitis is variable, including grouped papules, wheals, and vesicular lesions on the wrists, neck, breasts, umbilicus, and anterior axillary folds. A prolonged investigation is often undertaken before the cause and source of the dermatitis are discovered.

Pediculosis. Three types of lice are obligate parasites of the human host: body or clothing lice (*Pediculus humanus corporis*), head lice (*Pediculus humanus capitis*), and pubic or crab lice (*Phthirus pubis*). Only the body louse serves as a vector of human disease (typhus, trench fever, relapsing fever). Body and head lice have similar physical characteristics; they are about 2–4 mm in length. Pubic lice are only 1–2 mm in length and are greater in width than length, giving them a crablike appearance. Female lice live for approximately 1 mo and deposit 3–10 eggs daily on the human host; body lice, however, generally lay eggs in or near the seams of clothing. The ova or nits are glued to hairs or fibers of clothing but not directly on the body. Ova hatch in 1–2 wk and require another week to mature; once the eggs hatch, the nits remain attached to the hair as empty sacs of chitin. Freshly hatched larvae die unless a meal is obtained within approximately 24 hr and every few days thereafter. Both nymphs and adult lice feed on human blood, injecting their salivary juices into the host and depositing their fecal matter on the skin. Symptoms of infestation do not appear immediately but develop as an individual becomes sensitized. *The hallmark of all types of pediculosis is pruritus.*

Pediculosis corporis is rare in children except under conditions of poor hygiene, especially in colder climates when the opportunity to change clothes on a regular basis is lacking. The parasite is transmitted mainly on contaminated clothing or bedding. The primary lesion is an intensely pruritic small red macule or papule with a central hemorrhagic punctum located on the shoulders, trunk, or buttocks. Additional lesions include excoriations, wheals, and eczematous, secondarily infected plaques. Massive infestation may be associated with constitutional symptoms of fever, malaise, and headache. Chronic infestation may lead to "vagabond's skin," which is manifested as lichenified, scaling, hyperpigmented plaques, most commonly on the trunk. Lice are found on the skin only transiently when they are feeding; at other times, they inhabit the seams of clothing. Nits are attached firmly to fibers in the cloth and may remain viable for up to 1 mo. Nits hatch when they encounter warmth from the host's body when the clothes are worn again. Therapy consists of improved hygiene and hot water laundering of all infested clothing and bedding; a uniform temperature of 65°C, wet or dry, for 15–30 min kills all eggs and lice. Alternatively, eggs hatch and nymphs starve if clothing is stored for 2 wk at 75–85°F. For people who are unable to change clothes, the clothes may be dusted while inside out with 10% lindane powder; the effect lasts for approximately 1 mo. Lindane lotion or permethrin cream applied for 8–12 hr can be used to eradicate any eggs and lice that happen to be on body hair.

Pediculosis capitis is an intensely pruritic infestation of lice in the scalp hair. Head-to-head contact as well as fomites are important modes of transmission. In summer months in many areas of the United States and in the tropics at all times of the year, shared combs, brushes, or towels have a more important role in louse transmission. Translucent 0.5-mm eggs are laid near the proximal portion of the hair shaft and become adherent to one side of the hair shaft. A nit cannot be moved along or knocked off the hair shaft with the fingers. Secondary pyoderma, after trauma due to scratching, may result in matting together of the hair and cervical and occipital lymphadenopathy. Hair loss does not result from pediculosis but may accompany the secondary pyoderma. Head lice are a major cause of numerous pyodermas of the scalp, particularly in tropical environments. Lice are not always visible, but nits are detectable on the hairs, most commonly in the occipital region and above the ears, rarely on beard or pubic hair. Dermatitis may also be noted on the neck and pinnae. An id reaction, consisting of erythematous patches and plaques, may develop, particularly on the trunk. For unknown reasons, head lice infrequently infest blacks.

Brushing and combing of the hair regularly helps to reduce the number of lice and eggs and helps to minimize the severity of the infestation. The *treatments* of choice are 0.5% malathion oris permethrin 1% cream rinse (Nix) applied for 10 min with a repeat application in 7–10 days. Alternative treatments include natural pyrethrin shampoos (RID; A-200 Pyrinate liquid, shampoo, or gel; R & C shampoo; Barc; Paratrol; Paranit; Triple X) and 1% lindane shampoo (Kwell) for 10 min with a repeat application in 7–10 days. Malathion 0.5% in isopropanol (Ovide lotion) is FDA approved for the treatment of head lice and should be applied to dry hair until hair and scalp are wet, and left on for 12 hours. Malathion may be useful in cases of pyrethrin or permethrin resistance. Malathion, like lindane shampoo, is not indicated for use in neonates and infants. The combination of permethrin plus oral trimethoprim-sulfamethoxazole is also highly effective and may be useful in hard to treat cases or recurrent infestations. All household members should be treated at the same time. Nits can be removed with a fine-toothed comb

after a 1:1 vinegar:water rinse or, if tenacious, after application of a creme rinse containing 8% formic acid, which dissolves the chitin attaching the nits to the hair shafts. Clothing and bed linens should be laundered in very hot water or dry-cleaned; brushes and combs should be discarded or coated with a pediculicide for 15 min and then thoroughly cleaned in boiling water.

Pediculosis pubis is transmitted by skin-to-skin or sexual contact with an infested individual; the chance of acquiring the lice by one sexual exposure is approximately 95%. The infestation is usually encountered in adolescents, although small children may occasionally acquire pubic lice on the eyelashes. Patients experience moderate to severe pruritus and may develop a secondary pyoderma from scratching. Excoriations tend to be shallower and the incidence of secondary infection is lower than in pediculosis corporis. Maculae ceruleae are steel-gray spots, usually less than 1 cm in diameter, which may appear in the pubic area and on the chest, abdomen, and thighs. Oval translucent nits, which are firmly attached to the hair shafts, may be visible to the naked eye or may be readily identified by a hand lens or by microscopic examination (Fig. 658–2). Grittiness, as a result of adherent nits, may sometimes be detected when the fingers are run through infested hair. Adult lice are difficult to detect because of their lower level of activity and smaller, translucent body compared with head or body lice. Because pubic lice may occasionally wander or be transferred to other sites on fomites, terminal hair on the trunk, thighs, axillary region, beard area, and eyelashes should be examined for nits. The coexistence of other venereal diseases should be considered.

Treatment by a 10-min application of a pyrethrin preparation is usually effective. Re-treatment may be required in 7–10 days. The shampoo form of lindane, which requires a 10-min application time, is an alternative choice, but lindane cream and lotion are no longer recommended for treatment of pubic lice. Infestation of eyelashes is eradicated by petrolatum applied three to five times/24 hr for 8–10 days. A less safe but effective alternative is 0.25% physostigmine ophthalmic ointment applied twice daily for 3 days. Clothing, towels, and bed linens

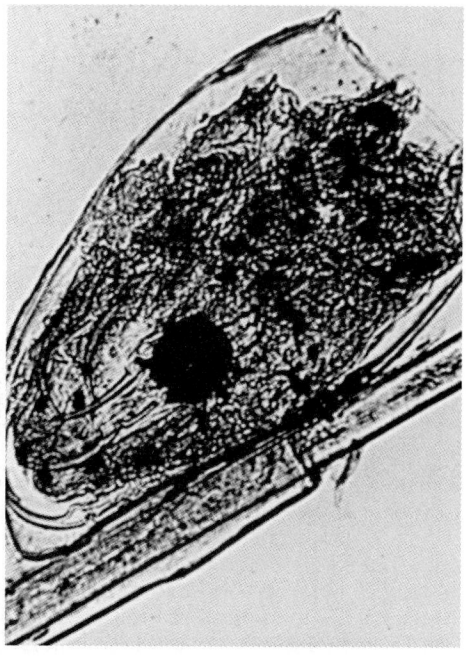

FIGURE 658–2. Intact nit on a human hair.

may be contaminated with nit-bearing hairs and should be thoroughly laundered or dry-cleaned.

Seabather's Eruption. Seabather's eruption is a severely pruritic dermatosis of inflammatory papules that develops within approximately 12 hr of bathing in salt water, primarily on body sites that were covered by a bathing suit. The eruption has been described primarily in waters of Florida and the Caribbean. Lesions, which may include pustules, vesicles, and urticarial plaques, are more numerous in those individuals who keep their bathing suit on for an extended period after leaving the water. The eruption may be accompanied by systemic symptoms of fatigue, malaise, fever, chills, nausea, and headache; approximately 40% of children younger than 16 yr had fever in one large series. Duration of the pruritus and skin eruption is 1–2 wk. Histopathologically, lesions consist of a superficial and deep perivascular and interstitial infiltrate of lymphocytes, eosinophils, and neutrophils. The eruption appears to be due to an allergic hypersensitivity reaction to venom from larvae of the thimble jellyfish *(Linuche unguiculata)*. Treatment is largely symptomatic; potent topical corticosteroids have been shown to provide relief to some patients.

Burkhart C: Fomite transmission with head lice: A continuing controversy. *Lancet* 2003;361:99–100.

Chew AL, Bashir SJ, Maibach HI: Treatment of head lice. *Lancet* 2000;356:523–4.

Gladstone HB, Darmstadt GL: Crusted scabies in an immunocompetent child treated with ivermectin. *Pediatr Dermatol* 2000;17:146.

Hipolito RB, Mallorca FG, Zuniga-Macaraig, et al: Head lice infestation: single drug versus combination therapy with one percent permethrin and trimethoprim/sulfamethoxazole. *Pediatrics* 2001;107:e30.

Keoki Williams, L, Reichert A, MacKenzie WR, et al: Lice, nits, and school policy. *Pediatrics* 2001;107:1011–4.

Lucky AW, Sayers P, Argus JD, et al: Avian mite bites acquired from a new source—pet gerbils. *Arch Dermatol* 2001;137:167–70.

Meinking TL, Entzel P, Villar ME, et al: Comparative efficacy of treatments for pediculosis capitis infestations. *Arch Dermatol* 2001;137:287–92.

Meinking TL, Taplin D, Hermida JL, et al: The treatment of scabies with ivermectin. *N Engl J Med* 1995;333:26.

Peterson C, Eichenfield L: Scabies. *Pediatr Ann* 1996;25:97.

Roberts R: Head lice. *N Eng J Med* 2002;346:1645–50.

Chapter 659
Acne

ACNE VULGARIS

Acne, particularly the comedonal form, occurs in approximately 80% of adolescents.

Pathogenesis. Lesions of acne vulgaris develop in sebaceous follicles, which consist of a large, multilobular sebaceous gland that drains its products into the follicular canal. The initial lesion of acne is a *comedo*, which is a dilated epithelium-lined follicular sac filled with lamellated keratinous material, lipid, and bacteria. An open comedo, known as a blackhead, has a patulous pilosebaceous orifice that permits visualization of the plug. An open comedo less commonly becomes inflammatory than a closed comedo or whitehead, which has only a pinpoint opening. An inflammatory papule or nodule develops from a comedo that has ruptured and extruded its follicular contents into the subadjacent dermis, inducing a neutrophilic inflammatory response. If the inflammatory reaction is close to the surface, a papule or pustule develops; if the inflammatory infiltrate develops deeper in the dermis, a nodule forms. Suppuration and an occasional

giant cell reaction to the keratin and hair are the cause of nodulocystic lesions; these are not true cysts but liquefied masses of inflammatory debris.

The primary pathogenetic alterations in acne are (1) abnormal keratinization of the follicular epithelium, resulting in impaction of keratinized cells within the follicular lumen, (2) increased sebaceous gland production of sebum, (3) proliferation of *Propionibacterium acnes* within the follicle, and (4) inflammation. At puberty, the sebaceous gland enlarges and sebum production increases in response to the increased activities of androgens of primarily adrenal origin. Comedonal acne, particularly of the central face, is frequently the first sign of pubertal maturation. The prevalence and severity of acne correlate with pubertal development and amount of sebum production. Initiation of acne in prepubertal children age 7–10 yr correlates significantly with the amount of wax esters in skin surface lipids and the concentration of serum androgenic steroid dehydroepiandrosterone sulfate (DHEA-S) secreted primarily by the adrenal glands. DHEA-S levels are not elevated, however, in the serum of many individuals with acne. DHEA-S may act locally, however, to stimulate sebum production by the sebaceous glands after being metabolized in hair follicle dermal papillae and sebaceous glands by 5α-reductase to more potent androgens such as 5α-dihydrotestosterone. Other sex steroid hormones such as testosterone and estradiol may also have a role in enhancing sebum production. A significant number of women with acne (25–50%), particularly those with relatively mild papulopustular acne, note that their acne flares approximately 1 wk before menstruation. The pathogenesis of this phenomenon is unknown.

Freshly formed sebum consists of a mixture of triglycerides, wax esters, squalene, and sterol esters. Normal follicular bacteria produce lipases that hydrolyze sebum triglycerides to free fatty acids; those of medium chain length (C8–C14) may be provocative factors in initiating an inflammatory reaction. Sebum also provides a favorable substrate for proliferation of bacteria. Sebaceous follicles are colonized by organisms of three types: an anaerobic diphtheroid, *P. acnes*; coagulase-negative *Staphylococcus epidermidis*; and a dimorphic yeast, *Pityrosporum ovale*. Each of these organisms possesses lipolytic enzymes; however, *P. acnes* appears to be largely responsible for the formation of free fatty acids. It is probable that bacterial proteases, hyaluronidases, and hydrolytic enzymes produce biologically active extracellular materials that increase the permeability of the follicular epithelium. Chemotactic factors released by the intrafollicular bacteria attract neutrophils and monocytes. Lysosomal enzymes from the neutrophils, released in the process of phagocytizing the bacteria, further disrupt the integrity of the follicular wall and intensify the inflammatory reaction.

Clinical Manifestations. Acne vulgaris is characterized by four basic types of lesions: open and closed comedones, papules, pustules, and nodulocystic lesions. One or more types of lesions may predominate; in its mildest form, which is often seen early in adolescence, lesions are limited to comedones on the central area of the face. Lesions may also involve the chest, upper back, and deltoid areas. A predominance of lesions on the forehead, particularly closed comedones, is often attributable to prolonged use of greasy hair preparations (pomade acne). Marked involvement on the trunk is most often seen in males. Lesions often heal with temporary postinflammatory erythema and hyperpigmentation; pitted, atrophic, or hypertrophic scars may be interspersed, depending on the severity, depth, and chronicity of the process. Diagnosis of acne is rarely difficult, although flat warts, folliculitis, and other types of acne may be confused with acne vulgaris.

Treatment. No evidence shows that early treatment, with the exception of isotretinoin, alters the course of acne. Acne can be controlled and severe scarring prevented, however, by judicious maintenance therapy that is continued until the disease process has abated spontaneously. Therapy must be individualized and aimed at preventing microcomedo formation through reduction of follicular hyperkeratosis, sebum production, the *P. acnes* population in follicular orifices, and free fatty acid production. Initial control takes at least 4–8 wk (Box 659–1). It is also important to address the potentially severe emotional impact of acne on adolescents.

The pediatrician must be aware of the frequently poor correlation between acne severity and psychosocial impact, particularly in adolescents. As adolescents become preoccupied with their appearance, offering treatment even to the youngster whose acne is mild may enhance self-image.

DIET. Little evidence shows that ingestion of particular foods can trigger acne flares. When a patient is convinced that certain dietary items exacerbate acne, it is prudent to omit those foods; however, it is unnecessary to impose unwarranted dietary restrictions.

CLIMATE. Climate appears to influence acne in that improvement frequently occurs during summer and flares are more common during winter. Remission during summer may relate, in part, to the relative absence of stress. Emotional tension and fatigue seem to exacerbate acne in many individuals; the mechanism is unclear but has been proposed to relate to an increased adrenocortical response.

CLEANSING. Cleansing with soap and water removes surface lipid and renders the skin less oily in appearance, but no evidence shows that surface lipid has a role in generating acne lesions. Only superficial drying and peeling are achieved by cleansing, and almost any mild soap or astringent is adequate. Repetitive cleansing can be harmful because it irritates and chaps the skin. Cleansing agents that contain abrasives and keratolytic agents, such as sulfur, resorcinol, and salicylic acid, may temporarily remove sebum from the skin surface. They exert a mild drying and peeling effect and suppress lesions to a limited degree. They do not, however, prevent microcomedones from forming. No evidence shows that preparations containing alcohol or hexachlorophene decrease acne because surface bacteria are not involved in the pathogenesis. Greasy cosmetic and hair preparations must be discontinued because they exacerbate pre-existing acne and cause further plugging of follicular pores. Manipulation and squeezing of facial lesions only ruptures intact lesions and provokes a localized inflammatory reaction.

BOX 659–1. Typical Treatment Regimens for Acne

COMEDONAL ACNE
Topical tretinoin, adapalene, or tazarotene applied daily
Salicylic acid
Azelaic acid

MILD PAPULOPUSTULAR ACNE
Benzoyl peroxide
Topical gel preparations of benzoyl peroxide with either clindamycin or erythromycin
Oral doxycycline or minocycline 75–100 mg twice daily plus topical retinoid

SEVERE PAPULOPUSTULAR OR NODULAR ACNE
Oral doxycycline or minocycline plus topical retinoid
Isotretinoin 1 mg/kg a day

From Webster GF: Acne vulgaris. *Br Med J* 2002;325:475–8.

TOPICAL THERAPY. The most effective topical preparations, particularly for comedones and papulopustular acne, include the benzoyl peroxide gels, retinoic acid, adapalene, and topical antibiotics. *Benzoyl peroxide* is an organic peroxide and oxidizing agent that dries and peels the skin, inhibits triglyceride hydrolysis and production of free fatty acids, is bacteriostatic for *P. acnes,* and causes follicular desquamation, disimpacting the follicle. Preparations are available in concentrations of 2.5%, 5%, and 10% prescription gels and 5% and 10% over-the-counter lotions. Benzoyl peroxide should be applied as a thin film, initially every other day, advancing over 2–3 wk to once-daily use as tolerated; the incidence of irritant or allergic contact dermatitis is 1%. Water-based gels are less irritating than alcohol-based ones, particularly for patients with atopic dermatitis or otherwise sensitive skin. Over-the-counter lotions are less effective than prescription gels.

Tretinoin (Retin-A), a derivative of retinoic acid, is the single most effective agent for treatment of comedonal acne. It affects keratinization in the sebaceous follicle by increasing turnover of epidermal cells and by decreasing the cohesiveness of the squamous cells; it thus aids in elimination of keratinous plugs. Erythema and peeling may be expected, particularly on initiation of therapy, and pustular flares from rupture of microcomedones are common. Flares may be minimized by starting treatment with benzoyl peroxide 2–3 wk before tretinoin. It may be applied once daily, 30 min after washing, in the form best tolerated (0.025% cream, 0.05% cream, 0.1% cream, 0.01% gel, 0.025% gel, and 0.05% liquid in increasing order of potency). Typically, 0.025% cream is prescribed initially; the strength of the formulation is increased sequentially until adequate control, without undue irritation, is achieved. Optimal results are not seen for 3–6 mo. Increased sensitivity to sunlight may occur, necessitating use of a sunscreen. Tazarotene an acetylinic retinoid (0.1% gel), is more effective in reducing noninflammatory lesions and equally effective in reducing inflammatory lesions as tretinoin (0.025%); it is equally effective as adapalene gel (0.1%). Erythema, burning, pruritus and peeling may be more common than with these other topical agents.

Adapalene (Differin gel), a derivative of naphthoic acid, is comedolytic and anti-inflammatory. A 0.1% gel may be more effective than 0.025% tretinoin gel and may have fewer side effects.

Topical antibiotics for use in patients with acne include clindamycin and erythromycin; they may be applied once or twice daily. Although not as effective as orally administered antibiotics or benzoyl peroxide, they serve as a useful therapeutic adjunct by inhibiting growth of *P. acnes.* The effectiveness of a topical antibiotic is enhanced by concurrent use of benzoyl peroxide or tretinoin. Use of topical erythromycin or clindamycin has occasionally resulted in the emergence of resistant bacteria. *Azelaic acid* (Azelex cream) has antimicrobial and keratolytic properties. A 20% cream is as effective as 0.05% tretinoin cream.

All topical preparations must be used for 4–8 wk before their effectiveness can be assessed. They may be used alone but frequently are more effective when used together. A popular and effective combination is use of benzoyl peroxide gel in the morning and tretinoin at night.

SYSTEMIC THERAPY. *Antibiotics,* especially tetracycline and its derivatives, are indicated for treatment of patients who cannot tolerate or have not responded to topical medications, who have moderate to severe inflammatory papulopustular and nodulocystic acne, and who have a propensity for scarring. The tetracyclines act by inhibiting bacterial lipases, causing a reduction in the concentration of free fatty acids; suppressing the normal follicular flora, mainly *P. acnes;* and inhibiting neutrophil chemotaxis and follicular inflammation.

Tetracycline, minocycline, and doxycycline have been shown to suppress granuloma formation, perhaps by inhibition of protein kinase C, an important membrane signal transducer. For most adolescent patients, therapy may be initiated with tetracycline, 1 g/24 hr, divided twice daily, for at least 6 wk, followed by a gradual decrease to the minimal effective dose. The drugs are best administered in combination with topical benzoyl peroxide or tretinoin but not topical antibiotics. Tetracycline absorption is inhibited by food, milk, iron supplements, aluminum hydroxide gel, and calcium-magnesium salts. It should be taken on an empty stomach 1 hr before or 2 hr after meals. Side effects of tetracycline include vaginal candidosis, particularly in those who take tetracycline concurrently with oral contraceptives; gastrointestinal irritation; phototoxic reactions, including onycholysis and brown discoloration of nails; esophageal ulceration; inhibition of fetal skeletal growth; and staining of growing teeth, precluding its use during pregnancy and in those younger than 9 yr. Oral antibiotics may decrease the effectiveness of oral contraceptive pills. Alternatives to tetracycline include erythromycin, minocycline, doxycycline, clindamycin, and occasionally trimethoprim-sulfamethoxazole. A possible complication of prolonged systemic antibiotic use is proliferation of gram-negative organisms, particularly *Enterobacter, Klebsiella, Escherichia coli, or Pseudomonas aeruginosa,* producing severe, refractory folliculitis.

Women who have acne and hormonal abnormalities, who are unresponsive to antibiotic therapy, or who are not candidates for isotretinoin therapy should be considered for a trial of *hormonal therapy.* An effective combination is an antiandrogen such as cyproterone acetate or spironolactone, given on days 5–15 of the menstrual cycle, and ethinyl estradiol, a synthetic estrogen used in oral contraceptives that is a potent inhibitor of sebum production, given on days 5–26. Two oral contraceptives are currently FDA approved for the treatment of acne. Topically applied antiandrogens without systemic side effects are currently under investigation.

Isotretinoin (13-*cis*-retinoic acid, Accutane) is indicated for moderate to severe nodulocystic acne that has not responded to conventional therapy or has recurred quickly after several successful courses of conventional therapy; for severe, scarring acne such as acne conglobata and acne fulminans; and for acne that is associated with severe psychologic disturbance. The recommended dosage is approximately 0.5–1.0 mg/kg/24 hr; younger male patients and those with primarily truncal lesions tend to require doses at the upper end of this range. Four months of therapy is required for most patients; a standard course in the United States lasts 16–20 wk. At the end of one course of isotretinoin, approximately 30% are cured, 35% need conventional topical and/or oral medications to maintain adequate control, and 25% have relapses and need an additional course of isotretinoin. Dosages below 0.5 mg/kg/24 hr, or a cumulative dose of less than 120 mg/kg, are associated with a significantly higher rate of treatment failure and relapse. If the disease process is not in remission 2 mo after the first course of isotretinoin, a second course should be considered. Isotretinoin reduces sebum excretion by 80% within 1 mo, converts sebaceous units to epithelial buds, decreases the population of *P. acnes,* decreases ductal cornification, and inhibits neutrophil chemotaxis and thus decreases the inflammatory response. Isotretinoin therapy does not alter gonadal or adrenal functions but induces a significant local decrease in 5α-dihydrotestosterone formation in the skin.

Isotretinoin use has many side effects. *It is highly teratogenic and is absolutely contraindicated in pregnancy;* pregnancy should be avoided for 1 mo after discontinuation of therapy. Two or three forms of birth control are required, as are monthly pregnancy tests. Concerns over cases of pregnancy despite warnings have prompted a manufacturer registration program, S.M.A.R.T. (System to Manage Accutane Related Teratogenicity) that requires physician enrollment and careful patient pregnancy screening in order to prescribe isotretinoin. Many patients also experience cheilitis, xerosis, periodic epistaxis, and blepharoconjunctivitis. Increased serum triglyceride and cholesterol levels are also common; it is important to rule out pre-existent liver disease and hyperlipidemia before initiating therapy and to check the triglyceride response 4 wk after commencing therapy. Less common but significant side effects include arthralgias, myalgias, depression, temporary thinning of the hair, paronychia, increased susceptibility to sunburn, formation of pyogenic granulomas, and colonization of the skin with *Staphylococcus aureus,* leading to impetigo, secondarily infected dermatitis, and scalp folliculitis. Rarely, hyperostotic lesions of the spine develop after more than one course of isotretinoin. Concomitant use of tetracycline and isotretinoin is contraindicated because either drug, but particularly when used together, can cause benign intracranial hypertension. Although no cause and effect relationship has been established, media attention to a possible link between isotretinoin and depression and/or suicide has mandated close attention to psychiatric well-being before and during isotretinoin prescription.

SURGICAL THERAPY. Intralesional injection of low-dose (3 mg/mL) midpotency glucocorticoids (e.g., triamcinolone) with a 30-gauge needle on a tuberculin syringe may hasten the healing of individual, painful nodulocystic lesions. Dermabrasion to minimize scarring should be considered only after the active process is quiescent.

DRUG-INDUCED ACNE

Pubertal and postpubertal patients who are receiving systemic corticosteroid therapy or potent topical steroids are predisposed to steroid-induced acne. This monomorphous folliculitis occurs primarily on the face, neck, chest (Fig. 659–1*A*), shoulders, upper back, arms, and, rarely, the scalp. Onset follows the initiation of steroid therapy by about 2 wk. The lesions are small erythematous papules or pustules that may erupt in profusion and are all in the same stage of development. Comedones may occur subsequently, but nodulocystic lesions and scarring are rare. Pruritus is occasional. The steroid appears to induce focal degeneration of the follicular epithelium, which incites a localized neutrophilic inflammatory response. Although steroid acne is relatively refractory if the medication is continued, the eruption may respond to use of tretinoin and a benzoyl peroxide gel. A prepubertal child with severe acne should be examined for endocrine disorders such as congenital adrenal hyperplasia. Studies of adrenal function are indicated in appropriate patients (see Chapter 571).

Other drugs that can induce acneiform lesions in susceptible individuals include isoniazid, phenytoin, phenobarbital, trimethadione, lithium carbonate, androgens (anabolic steroids), and vitamin B_{12}.

HALOGEN ACNE

Administration of medications containing iodides or bromides or, rarely, ingestion of massive amounts of vitamin-mineral preparations or iodine-containing "health foods" such as kelp may induce halogen acne. The lesions are often very inflammatory. Discontinuation of the provocative agent and appropriate topical preparations usually achieve reasonable therapeutic results.

CHLORACNE

Chloracne is due to external contact with, inhalation of, or ingestion of halogenated aromatic hydrocarbons, including polyhalogenated biphenyls, polyhalogenated naphthalenes (e.g., Halowax, which may be a component of wood preservatives and sealing compounds), and dioxins. Lesions are primarily comedonal; inflammatory lesions are infrequent but may include papules, pustules, nodules, and cysts. Healing occurs with atrophic or hypertrophic scarring. The face, postauricular regions, neck, axillae, genitals, and chest are involved most commonly. The nose is often spared. In cases of severe exposure, associated findings may include hepatitis, production of porphyrins, bulla formation on sun-exposed skin, hyperpigmentation, hypertrichosis, and palmar and plantar hyperhidrosis. Topical or oral retinoids may be effective; benzoyl peroxide and antibiotics are generally ineffective.

NEONATAL ACNE

Approximately 20% of normal neonates develop at least a few comedones within the 1st mo of life. Closed comedones predominate on the cheeks and forehead (see Fig. 659–1B); open comedones and papulopustules occur occasionally. The cause of neonatal acne is unknown but has been attributed to placental transfer of maternal androgens, hyperactive neonatal adrenal glands, and a hypersensitive neonatal end-organ response to androgenic hormones. Placental transfer of maternally ingested lithium and hydantoin may also cause acne in the neonate. The hypertrophic sebaceous glands involute spontaneously over a few months, as does the acne. If desired, the lesions can be treated effectively with topical tretinoin and/or benzoyl peroxide.

INFANTILE ACNE

Infantile acne usually presents at 3–16 mo of life, more commonly in boys than girls. Acne lesions are more numerous, pleomorphic, severe, and persistent than in neonatal acne. Open and closed comedones predominate on the face; papules and pustules occur frequently, but only occasionally do nodulocystic lesions develop. Pitted scarring is seen in 10–15%. The course may be relatively brief, or the lesions may persist for many months, although the eruption generally resolves by age 3 yr. Use of topical benzoyl peroxide gel and tretinoin usually clears the eruption within a few weeks; oral erythromycin is necessary occasionally. A history of severe acne in one or both parents is often elicited, and the child is at risk for development of severe acne in adolescence. A child with refractory acne warrants a search for an abnormal source of androgens such as a virilizing tumor or congenital adrenal hyperplasia.

TROPICAL ACNE

A severe form of acne occurs in tropical climates and is believed to be due to the intense heat and humidity; hydration of the pilosebaceous duct pore may accentuate blockage of the duct. Affected individuals tend to have an antecedent history of adolescent acne that is quiescent at the time of the eruption. Lesions occur mainly on the entire back, chest, buttocks, and thighs, with a predominance of suppurating papules and nodules. Secondary infection with *S. aureus* may be a complication. The eruption is refractory to acne therapy if the environmental factors are not eliminated.

ACNE CONGLOBATA

Acne conglobata is a chronic progressive inflammatory disease that occurs mainly in men, more commonly in whites than in blacks, but it may begin during adolescence. Patients usually have a history of pre-existing acne vulgaris. The principal lesion is the nodule, although one often finds a mixture of comedones with multiple pores, papules, pustules, nodules, cysts, abscesses, and subcutaneous dissection with formation of multichanneled sinus tracts. Severe scarring is characteristic. The face is relatively spared, but in addition to the back and chest, the buttocks, abdomen, arms, and thighs may be involved. Constitutional symptoms and anemia may accompany the inflammatory process. Coagulase-positive staphylococci and β-hemolytic streptococci are frequently cultured from lesions but do not appear to be involved primarily in the pathogenesis. Acne conglobata occasionally occurs in association with hidradenitis suppurativa and dissecting cellulitis of the scalp (as the follicular occlusion triad) and may be complicated by erosive arthritis and ankylosing spondyloarthritis. Endocrinologic studies are not revealing. Routine acne therapy is generally ineffective. Systemic therapy with a corticosteroid or sulfone may be required to suppress the intense inflammatory activity. Isotretinoin is the most effective form of therapy for some patients but may produce a flare after its initiation. Consequently, corticosteroids are often started before isotretinoin.

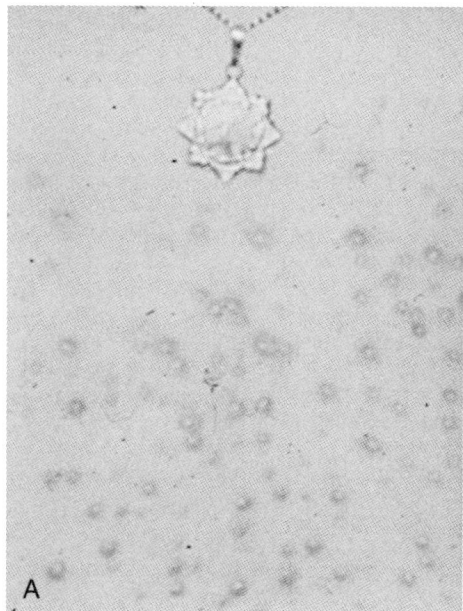 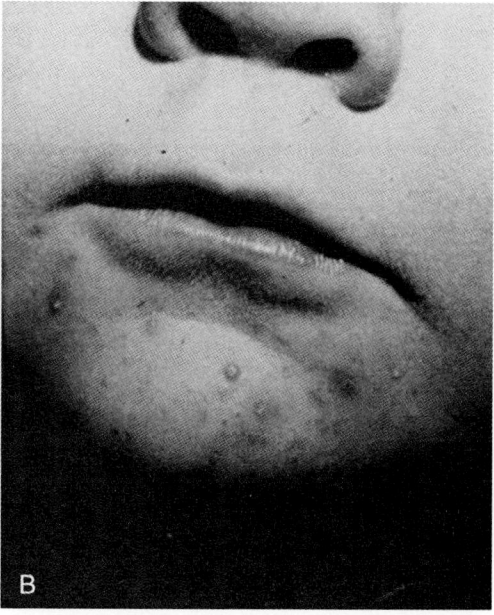

FIGURE 659–1. *A,* Monomorphous papular eruption of steroid acne. *B,* Acne in a male infant.

ACNE FULMINANS (ACUTE FEBRILE ULCERATIVE ACNE)

Acne fulminans is characterized by abrupt onset of extensive inflammatory, tender ulcerative acneiform lesions on the back and chest of male teenagers. The distinctive feature is the tendency for large nodules to form exudative, necrotic, ulcerated, crusted plaques. Lesions often spare the face and heal with scarring. A preceding history of mild papulopustular or nodular acne is noted in most patients. Constitutional symptoms and signs are common, including fever, debilitation, arthralgias, myalgias, weight loss, and leukocytosis. Blood cultures are sterile. Lesions of erythema nodosum sometimes develop on the shins. Osteolytic bone lesions may develop in the clavicle, sternum, and epiphyseal growth plates; affected bones appear normal or have slight sclerosis or thickening on healing. Salicylates may be helpful for the myalgias, arthralgias, and fever. Corticosteroids (1.0 mg/kg of prednisone) are started first; then approximately 1 wk later, isotretinoin (0.5 mg/kg) is added and continued for as long as inflammatory lesions persist, generally 3–4 mo. Dapsone may be effective if isotretinoin cannot be used. The corticosteroids are tapered over approximately 6 wk. Antibiotics are not indicated unless there is evidence of secondary infection. Compared with acne conglobata, acne fulminans presents in younger patients, is more explosive in onset, more commonly has associated constitutional symptoms and ulcerated crusted lesions, and less commonly has multiheaded comedones or involves the face.

Brown S, Shalita A: Acne vulgaris. *Lancet* 1998;351:1871.

Cunliffe WJ, Baron SE, Coulson LH: A clinical and therapeutic study of 29 patients with infantile acne. *Br J Dermatol* 2001;145:463–6.

Karvonen SL: Acne fulminans: Report of clinical findings and treatment of twenty-four patients. *J Am Acad Dermatol* 1993;28:572.

Lucky AW, Biro FM, Simbartl LA, et al: Predictions of severity of acne vulgaris in young adolescent girls: Results of a five-year longitudinal study. *J Pediatr* 1997;130:30.

Medical Letter: Is Accutane really dangerous? *Med Ltr* 2002:44:82

Medical Letter: Tazarotene (Tazorac) for acne. *Med Ltr* 2002:44:52

Sidbury R, Paller AS: The diagnosis and management of acne. *Pediatr Ann* 2000;29:17.

Webster GF: Acne vulgaris. *Br Med J* 2002;325:475–8.

Chapter 660
Tumors of the Skin

See also Chapters 497 and 641.

Epidermal Inclusion Cyst (Epidermoid Cyst). These are sharply circumscribed, dome-shaped, firm, freely movable, skin-colored nodules, often with a central dimple or punctum that is a plugged, dilated pore of a pilosebaceous follicle. Epidermoid cysts form most frequently on the face, neck, chest, or upper back and may periodically become inflamed and infected secondarily, particularly in association with acne vulgaris. The cyst wall may also rupture and induce an inflammatory reaction in the dermis. The wall of the cyst is derived from the follicular infundibulum; a mass of layered keratinized material that may have a cheesy consistency fills the cavity. Epidermoid cysts may arise from occlusion of pilosebaceous follicles, from implantation of epidermal cells into the dermis as a result of an injury that penetrates the epidermis, and from rests of epidermal cells. Multiple epidermoid cysts may be present in *Gardner syndrome* and the *nevoid basal cell carcinoma syndrome*. Excision of the cysts with removal of the entire sac and its contents is indicated, particularly if the cyst becomes recurrently infected. A fluctuant, infected cyst should first be incised, drained, and packed, and the patient should receive an antibiotic effective against *Staphylococcus aureus*. After the inflammation subsides, the cyst should be removed.

Milium. This is a pearly white or yellowish, firm, 1–2 mm subepidermal keratin cyst. Milia in newborns is discussed in Chapter 647. Secondary milia occur in association with subepidermal blistering diseases, chronic corticosteroid-induced atrophy, 5-fluorouracil therapy, or after dermabrasion. They are retention cysts caused by hyperproliferation of injured epithelium and are indistinguishable histopathologically from primary milia; those that develop after blistering usually arise from the eccrine sweat duct, but they may develop from the hair follicle, sebaceous duct, or epidermis. A milium body differs from an epidermoid cyst only in its small size.

Pilar Cyst (Trichilemmal Cyst). This is clinically indistinguishable from an epidermoid cyst. It presents as a smooth, firm, mobile nodule, predominantly on the scalp. These cysts occasionally develop on the face, neck, or trunk. The cyst may become inflamed and may occasionally suppurate and ulcerate. The cyst wall is composed of epithelial cells with indistinct intercellular bridges. The peripheral cell layer of the wall shows a palisade arrangement, which is not seen in an epidermoid cyst. No granular layer is present, the cyst cavity contains homogeneous eosinophilic keratinous material, and foci of calcification are seen in 25% of cases. The propensity to develop pilar cysts is inherited in an autosomal dominant manner; more than one cyst generally develops. Numerous pilar and epidermoid cysts, desmoid tumors, fibromas, lipomas, or osteomas may be associated with colonic polyposis or adenocarcinoma in Gardner syndrome. Pilar cysts shell out easily from the dermis.

Pilomatricoma. This is a benign tumor that presents as a 3–30 mm, firm, solitary, deep dermal or subcutaneous tumor on the head, neck, or upper extremities. The overlying epidermis is usually normal; the tumor may occasionally be located more superficially, however, tinting the overlying skin blue-red. Pilomatricomas may enlarge rapidly as a result of inflammation or hemorrhage and occasionally perforate the epidermis. Patients with both pilomatricoma and myotonic dystrophy are more likely to have several tumors and to have familial occurrence; in general, however, pilomatricomas are not hereditary. Histopathologically, irregularly shaped islands of epithelial cells are embedded in a cellular stroma. Calcium deposits are found in 75% of tumors. Pilomatricomas are caused by mutations in beta-catenin.

Trichoepithelioma. This is a smooth, round, firm, skin-colored 2–8 mm papule that is derived from immature hair follicles. Trichoepitheliomas generally occur singly on the face during childhood or early adulthood. Multiple trichoepitheliomas (*epithelioma adenoides cysticum*) are inherited autosomal dominantly, appear in childhood or at puberty, and gradually increase in number on the nasofacial folds, nose, forehead, and upper lip and occasionally on the scalp, neck, and upper trunk. Microscopically, these benign tumors are characterized by horn cysts composed of a fully keratinized center surrounded by basophilic cells in an adenoid network. Surgical excision is the therapy.

Eruptive Vellus Hair Cysts. These are asymptomatic, follicular, skin-colored, soft 1–3-mm papules on the chest. They may become crusted or umbilicated. Abnormal vellus hair follicles become occluded at the level of the infundibulum, resulting in retention of hairs within an epithelium-lined cystic dilatation of the proximal part of the follicle. Most cases are chronic, but spontaneous regression has been reported.

Steatocystoma Multiplex. This condition usually presents in adolescence or early adulthood with numerous soft to firm cystic nodules that are adherent to the underlying skin and are a few millimeters to 3 cm in diameter. When punctured, the cysts may drain oily or cheesy material. Sites of predilection include the sternal region, axillae, arms, and scrotal skin. The multiply folded cyst wall is lined on the luminal side with a thick, homogeneous, eosinophilic horny layer and lacks a granular layer. Flattened sebaceous gland lobules are often visible in the cyst wall, and lanugo hairs may be present in the cystic cavity.

Syringoma. These benign tumors are soft, small, skin-colored or yellowish-brown papules that develop on the face, particularly in the periorbital regions. Other sites of predilection include the axillae and umbilical and pubic areas. They often develop during puberty and are more frequent in females. Eruptive syringomas (eruptive hidradenoma) develop in crops over the anterior trunk during childhood or adolescence. A syringoma is derived from an intraepidermal sweat gland duct. They are of cosmetic significance only. Sparse lesions may be excised, but they are often too numerous to remove.

Infantile Digital Fibroma. This is a firm, smooth, erythematous or skin-colored nodule on the dorsal or lateral surfaces of the distal phalanges of the fingers and toes. More than 80% of tumors present in infancy; they may be present at birth. Lesions may be solitary or multiple and may present as "kissing" tumors on opposing digits. Generally, they are asymptomatic, but flexion deformity of the digits may occur. Clinically, the lesions resemble a fibroma, leiomyoma, angiofibroma, acquired digital fibrokeratoma, accessory digit, or mucous cyst. The diagnosis is confirmed by finding numerous spindle-shaped fibroblasts that contain small, dense, round eosinophilic cytoplasmic inclusion bodies composed of collections of actin microfilaments. A viral cause has been postulated. Local recurrence after simple excision of this tumor has been reported in 75% of patients. Because the tumor does not metastasize and may regress spontaneously within 2–3 yr, a course of expectant observation is advised. If functional impairment or flexion deformity of the digit becomes apparent, prompt full excision of the tumor is indicated.

Dermatofibroma (Histiocytoma). These benign dermal tumors may be pedunculated, nodular, or flat and are usually well circumscribed and firm but occasionally feel soft on palpation. The overlying skin is usually hyperpigmented, may be shiny or keratotic, and dimples when the tumor is pinched. Dermatofibromas range in size from 0.5–10 mm, arise most frequently on the limbs, and are usually asymptomatic but may occasionally be pruritic. They are composed of fibroblasts, young and mature collagen, capillaries, and histiocytes in varying proportions,

forming a nodule in the dermis that has poorly defined edges. The cause of these tumors is unknown, but trauma such as an insect bite or folliculitis appears to induce reactive fibroplasia. The differential diagnosis includes epidermal inclusion cyst, juvenile xanthogranuloma, hypertrophic scar, and neurofibroma. Dermatofibromas may be excised or left intact according to a patient's preference; they usually persist indefinitely but occasionally involute spontaneously.

Juvenile Xanthogranuloma. These are firm, dome-shaped, yellow, pink, or orange papules or nodules that vary in size from a few millimeters to approximately 4 cm in diameter. They usually present at birth or within the first several months of life; occasionally, they first appear in late childhood and, rarely, in adulthood. They are 10 times more common in white than in black individuals. Sites of predilection are the scalp, face, and upper trunk, where they may erupt in profusion or remain as solitary lesions. Nodular lesions may appear on the oral mucosa. Mature lesions are characterized histopathologically by a dermal infiltrate of lipid-laden histiocytes, admixed inflammatory cells, and Touton giant cells. The lesions may clinically resemble papulonodular urticaria pigmentosa, dermatofibromas, or xanthomas of hyperlipoproteinemia but can be distinguished from these entities histopathologically.

Affected infants are nearly always otherwise normal, and blood lipid values are not elevated. Café-au-lait macules are found on 20% of patients with juvenile xanthogranuloma. Xanthogranulomatous infiltrates occur occasionally in ocular tissues. This may result in glaucoma, hyphema, uveitis, heterochromia iridis, iritis, or sudden proptosis. Age younger than 2 years old, multiple lesions, and periocular location may heighten concerns for intraocular involvement. There appears to be an association among juvenile xanthogranuloma, neurofibromatosis, and childhood leukemia, most frequently juvenile chronic myelogenous leukemia. There is no need to remove these benign lesions because most of them regress spontaneously during the first few years. Residual pigmentation and atrophy, but not scarring, may result.

Lipoma. These benign collections of fatty tissue appear on the trunk, neck, and proximal portions of the limbs. They are soft, compressible, lobulated, subcutaneous masses that are movable against the overlying skin. Multiple lesions may occur occasionally, as in Gardner syndrome. Atrophy, calcification, liquefaction, or xanthomatous change may sometimes complicate their course. A lipoma is composed of normal fat cells surrounded by a thin connective tissue capsule. They represent a cosmetic defect and may be surgically excised. Multiple lipomas, identical to those that occur singly, are inherited in an autosomal dominant fashion and often appear by the 3rd decade in patients with *familial multiple lipomatosis*. Lipomas may appear intraabdominally, intramuscularly, and subcutaneously. *Congenital lipomatosis* presents during the first few months of life as large subcutaneous fatty masses on the chest, with extension into skeletal muscle. Congenital lipomatosis can also be a manifestation of Proteus syndrome. *Angiolipomas* usually present as numerous painful subcutaneous nodules on the arms and trunk.

Basal Cell Epithelioma (Basal Cell Carcinoma). Basal cell carcinoma is rare in children in the absence of a predisposing condition, such as nevoid basal cell carcinoma syndrome, xeroderma pigmentosum, nevus sebaceus of Jadassohn, arsenic intake, or exposure to irradiation. The lesions are pink, pearly, telangiectatic, smooth papules that enlarge slowly and may bleed or ulcerate. Sites of predilection are the face, scalp, and upper back. The differential diagnosis includes pyogenic granuloma, nevocellular nevus, epidermal inclusion cyst, closed comedo, dermatofibroma, and adnexal tumor. Depending on the site of occurrence and associated disease of the host, electrodesiccation and curettage or simple excision is usually curative. When the tumor is recurrent, larger than 2 cm in diameter, located on problematic anatomic areas such as the midface or ears, or is an aggressive histopathologic type, Mohs microscopically controlled surgery may be the most appropriate treatment.

Nevoid Basal Cell Carcinoma Syndrome (Basal Cell Nevus Syndrome, Gorlin Syndrome). This autosomal dominant syndrome maps to a gene on chromosome 9q22.3. This tumor suppressor gene is part of the hedgehog signaling pathway and is important in determining embryonic patterning and cell fate in a number of structures in the developing embryo. Mutations in human patched gene produce dysregulation of several genes involved in organogenesis and carcinogenesis. Consequently, the syndrome includes a wide spectrum of defects involving the skin, eyes, central nervous and endocrine systems, and bones. The predominant features are early onset basal cell carcinomas and mandibular cysts. Approximately 20% of those in whom a basal cell carcinoma develops before age 19 yr have this syndrome. Basal cell carcinomas appear between puberty and age 35 yr, erupting in crops of tumors that vary in size, color, and number and may be difficult to distinguish from other types of skin lesions. Sites of predilection are the periorbital skin, nose, malar areas, and upper lip, but the lesions can develop on the trunk and limbs and are not restricted to sun-exposed areas. Ulceration, bleeding, crusting, and local invasion can occur. Small milia, epidermal cysts, pigmented lesions, hirsutism, and palmar and plantar pits are additional cutaneous findings.

The facies of patients with this syndrome are characterized by temporoparietal bossing, prominent supraorbital ridges, a broad nasal root, ocular hypertelorism or dystopia canthorum, and prognathism. Keratinized cysts (odontogenic keratocysts) in the maxilla and mandible occur in most patients. They range in size from a few millimeters to several centimeters, may result in maldevelopment of the teeth, and cause pain, swelling of the jaw, facial deformity, bone erosion, pathologic fractures, and suppurating sinus tracts. Osseous defects such as anomalous rib development, spina bifida, kyphoscoliosis, and brachymetacarpalism occur in two thirds of patients, and ocular abnormalities including cataracts, glaucoma, coloboma, strabismus, and blindness occur in approximately one fourth. Some males have hypogonadism, with absent or undescended testes. Kidney malformations have also been reported. Neurologic manifestations include calcification of the falx, seizures, mental retardation, partial agenesis of the corpus callosum, hydrocephalus, and nerve deafness. The incidence of medulloblastoma, ameloblastoma of the oral cavity, fibrosarcoma of the jaw, teratoma, cystadenoma, cardiac fibroma, and ovarian fibroma is increased.

Treatment of these patients requires participation of various specialists according to individual clinical problems. Basal cell carcinomas should not be treated with irradiation. Most of the basal cell carcinomas have a clinically benign course, and it is often impossible to remove them all; those with an aggressive growth pattern and those on the central areas of the face, however, should be removed promptly. Oral retinoids are helpful in preventing the development of new tumors in some patients. Genetic counseling is also indicated.

Mucosal Neuroma Syndrome (Sippel Syndrome). Mucosal neuroma syndrome, an autosomal dominant trait, is characterized by an asthenic or marfanoid habitus with scoliosis, pectus excavatum, pes cavus, and muscular hypotonia. Patients have thick, patulous lips and soft tissue prognathism simulating acromegaly. Multiple mucosal neuromas or neurofibromas appear as pink, pedunculated or sessile nodules on the anterior third of the tongue, at the commissures of the lips, and on the buccal mucosa and palpebral conjunctiva. Various ophthalmologic defects and intestinal ganglioneuromatosis with recurrent diarrhea are additional common findings. There is a high incidence of medullary thyroid carcinoma associated with high calcitonin levels, pheochromocytoma, and hyperparathyroidism. Periodic screening tests for the associated malignant tumors are mandatory.

Chan EF, Gat U, McNiff JM, et al: A common skin tumor is caused by activating mutations in beta catenin. *Nat Genet* 1999;21:410.
Chang MW, Frieden IJ, Good W: The risk of intraocular juvenile xanthogranuloma: A survey of current practice and assessment of risk. *J Am Acad Dermatol* 1996;34:445.
Kimonis UE, Goldstein AM, Pastakia B, et al: Clinical manifestations in 105 persons with nevoid basal cell carcinoma syndrome. *Am J Med Genet* 1997;69:299.
Oro AE, Higgins KM, Ku Z, et al: Basal cell carcinomas in mice expressing sonic hedgehog. *Science* 1997;276:817.
Rotte JJ, de Vaan GA, Koopman RJ: Juvenile xanthogranuloma and acute leukemia: A case report. *Med Pediatr Oncol* 1994;23:57, 1994.
Wicking C, Bale AE: Molecular basis of the nevoid basal cell carcinoma syndrome. *Curr Opin Pediatr* 1997;9:630.

Chapter 661
Nutritional Dermatoses

Acrodermatitis Enteropathica. This is a rare autosomal recessive disorder caused by an inability to absorb sufficient zinc from the diet. Initial signs and symptoms usually occur during the first few months of life, often after weaning from breast to cow's milk. The cutaneous eruption consists of vesiculobullous, eczematous, dry, scaly, or psoriasiform skin lesions symmetrically distributed in the perioral, acral, and perineal areas and on the cheeks, knees, and elbows (Fig. 661–1). The hair often has a peculiar reddish tint, and alopecia of some degree is characteristic. Ocular manifestations include photophobia, conjunctivitis, blepharitis, and corneal dystrophy detectable by slit-lamp examination. Associated manifestations include chronic diarrhea, stomatitis, glossitis, paronychia, nail dystrophy, growth retardation, irritability, delayed wound healing, intercurrent bacterial infections, and superinfection with *Candida albicans*. Lymphocyte function and free radical scavenging are impaired. Without treatment, the course is chronic and intermittent but often relentlessly progressive. When the disease is less severe, only growth retardation and delayed development may be apparent.

The *diagnosis* is established by the constellation of clinical findings and detection of a low plasma zinc concentration. Histopathologic changes in the skin are nonspecific and include parakeratosis and pallor of the upper epidermis. The variety of manifestations of the syndrome may be due to the fact that zinc has a role in numerous metabolic pathways, including those of copper, protein, essential fatty acids, and prostaglandins, and zinc is incorporated into many zinc metalloenzymes.

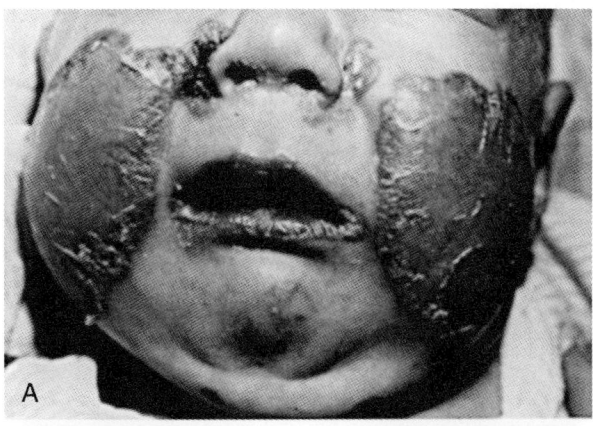

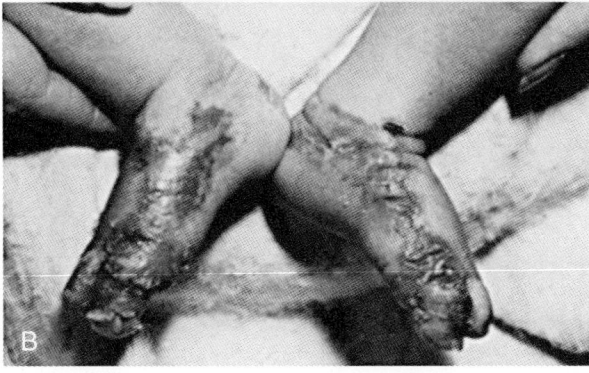

FIGURE 661–1. *A,* Psoriasiform facial lesions of zinc deficiency dermatitis. *B,* Similar lesions on the feet with secondary nail dystrophy.

Oral therapy with zinc compounds is the *treatment* of choice. Optimal doses range from 50 mg of zinc sulfate, acetate, or gluconate daily for infants up to 150 mg/24 hr for children; plasma zinc levels should be monitored, however, to individualize the dosage. Zinc therapy rapidly abolishes the manifestations of the disease. A syndrome resembling acrodermatitis enteropathica has been observed in patients with secondary zinc deficiency caused by long-term total parenteral nutrition without supplemental zinc or by chronic malabsorption syndromes. A rash similar to that of acrodermatitis enteropathica has also been reported in infants fed breast milk that is low in zinc and in those with maple syrup urine disease, organic aciduria, methylmalonic acidemia, biotinidase deficiency, essential fatty acid deficiency, severe protein malnutrition (e.g., kwashiorkor), and cystic fibrosis.

Essential Fatty Acid Deficiency. This causes a generalized, scaly dermatitis composed of thickened, erythematous, desquamating plaques. The eruption has been induced experimentally in animals fed a fat-free diet and has been observed in patients with chronic severe malabsorption such as in short-gut syndrome and in those sustained on a fat-free diet or fat-free parenteral alimentation. Linoleic (18:2 n-6) and arachidonic (20:4 n-6) acids are deficient, and an abnormal metabolite, 5,8,11-eicosatrienoic acid (20:3 n-9), is present in the plasma. Additional manifestations of essential fatty acid deficiency include alopecia, thrombocytopenia, and failure to thrive. The horny layer of the skin is cracked microscopically, the barrier function of the skin is disturbed, and transepidermal water loss is increased. Topical application of linoleic acid, which is present in sunflower seed and safflower oils, may ameliorate the clinical and biochemical skin manifestations. Appropriate nutrition should be provided.

Kwashiorkor. Severe protein and essential amino acid deprivation in association with adequate caloric intake can lead to kwashiorkor, particularly at the time of weaning to a diet that consists primarily of corn, rice, or beans (see Chapter 42.2). Cutaneous erythema develops first and, in mild cases in white children, progresses to fine desquamation along natural skin lines and on the shins, outer thighs, and back. In dark-skinned children, characteristic early findings include circumoral pallor, cutaneous depigmentation, and development of purple patches. As the disease advances, well marginated, slightly raised, purplish, waxy plaques appear, particularly in the diaper area and at sites of pressure such as the elbows, knees, and ankles and on the trunk. In severe cases, erosions and linear fissures develop. Sun-exposed skin is relatively spared, as are the feet and dorsal aspects of the hands. Nails are thin and soft, and hair is sparse, thin, and depigmented, sometimes displaying a flag sign of alternating light and dark bands that reflect alternating periods of adequate and inadequate nutrition. The cutaneous manifestations may closely resemble those of acrodermatitis enteropathica. The serum zinc level is often deficient, and in some cases, skin lesions of kwashiorkor heal more rapidly when zinc is applied topically.

Cystic Fibrosis (see Chapter 402). Five per cent to 10% of patients with cystic fibrosis develop protein-calorie malnutrition. Rash in infants with cystic fibrosis and malnutrition is rare but may appear by age 6 mo. The initial eruption consists of erythematous, scaling papules and progresses within 1–3 mo to extensive desquamating plaques. The rash is accentuated around the mouth and perineum and on the extremities (lower > upper). Alopecia may be present, but mucous membranes and nails are uninvolved.

Pellagra (see Chapter 44.5). This presents with edema, erythema, and burning of sun-exposed skin on the face, neck, and dorsal aspects of the hands, forearms, and feet. Lesions of pellagra may also be provoked by burns, pressure, friction, and inflammation. The eruption on the face frequently follows a butterfly distribution, and the dermatitis encircling the neck has been termed "Casal's necklace." Blisters and scales develop, and the skin increasingly becomes dry, rough, thickened, cracked, and hyperpigmented. Skin infections may be unusually severe. Pellagra develops in those with insufficient dietary intake or absorption of niacin and/or tryptophan. Administration of isoniazid, 6-mercaptopurine, or 5-fluorouracil may also produce pellagra. Nicotinamide supplementation and sun avoidance are the mainstays of therapy.

Scurvy (Vitamin C or Ascorbic Acid Deficiency) (see Chapter 44.9). This presents initially with follicular hyperkeratosis and coiling of hair on the upper arms, back, buttocks, and lower extremities. Perifollicular erythema and hemorrhage, particularly on the legs and advancing to involve large areas of hemorrhage, swollen, erythematous gums, stomatitis, and subperiosteal hematomas are also seen. The best method for confirmation of a clinical diagnosis of scurvy is a trial of vitamin C supplementation.

Vitamin A Deficiency (see Chapter 44.1). This deficiency presents initially with impairment of visual adaptation to the dark. Cutaneous changes include xerosis and hyperkeratosis and hyperplasia of the epidermis, particularly the lining of hair follicles and sebaceous glands. In severe cases, desquamation may be prominent.

Darmstadt GL: The skin and nutritional disorders in the newborn. *Eur J Pediatr Dermatol* 1998;8:221.

Darmstadt GL, Mao-Qiang M, Saha SK, et al: Impact of topical oils on the skin barrier: possible implications for neonatal health in developing countries. *Acta Paediatr* 2002;91:1.

Darmstadt GL, Schmidt CP, Wechsler DS, et al: Dermatitis as a presenting sign of cystic fibrosis. *Arch Dermatol* 1992;128:1358.

Hansen AE, Wiese HF, Boelsche AN, et al: Role of linoleic acid in infant nutrition. *Pediatrics* 1963;31:171.

Hansen RC, Lemen R, Revsin B: Cystic fibrosis manifesting with acrodermatitis enteropathica-like eruption. *Arch Dermatol* 1983;119:51.

Hendricks WM: Pellagra and pellagra-like dermatoses: Etiology, differential diagnosis, dermatopathology, and treatment. *Semin Dermatol* 1991;10:282.

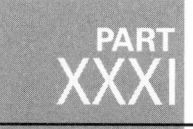

PART XXXI Bone and Joint Disorders

SECTION 1 *Orthopedic Problems*

Chapter 662

Growth and Development

George H. Thompson

Musculoskeletal disorders in children and adolescents are common; many can be managed safely and effectively by the pediatrician provided that an accurate diagnosis is established. The differential diagnosis of pediatric musculoskeletal disorders involves all diagnostic categories: congenital, developmental, acquired, infectious, inflammatory, mechanical, traumatic, neuromuscular, neoplastic, and psychogenic.

One must have a basic understanding of the effects of in utero positioning, the mechanism in which normal musculoskeletal growth occurs, and the relationships among skeletal growth, neurologic maturation, and normal developmental milestones.

In Utero Positioning. In the newborn, the imprint of the in utero position may be evident and confused with an abnormality. In utero positioning produces temporary joint and muscle contractures and affects the torsional alignment of the long bones, especially those of the lower extremities. Normal full-term newborns have 20–30 degree hip and knee flexion contractures. These resolve by 4–6 mo of age. The newborn hip externally rotates in extension 80–90 degrees and has limited internal rotation to 0–10 degrees. The lower leg frequently has inward rotation (internal tibial torsion), and the feet are supinated from their medial borders being wrapped against the posterolateral aspect of the opposite thigh. The top leg in the in utero position may show more changes than the bottom leg. The face may also be distorted, whereas the spine and upper extremities are less affected by the in utero position. The effects of in utero positioning, therefore, are physiologic in origin but may produce parental concerns. The child may be 3–4 yr old before the effects of the in utero position completely resolve.

Growth and Development. Each of the individual components of the skeletal system grow by different mechanisms. The long bones of the extremities (humerus, radius-ulna, femur, and tibia-fibula) have growth plates or physes at each end. Each contributes a varying proportion to the longitudinal growth of the individual bone as well as the extremity through a process termed *endochondral ossification*. The ends of each long bone are composed of the epiphyses. These are covered by articular cartilage and form the associated joints. Initially, the epiphyses are almost entirely cartilaginous and become progressively more ossified during growth. The articular cartilage also has growth potential, which contributes to the growth of the epiphysis. The perichondrial ring, which surrounds the physes, as well as the perichondrium around the epiphyses and periosteum, which surrounds the metaphysis and diaphyseal regions of the bone, contributes to appositional or circumferential growth.

Bones without physes, such as the pelvis, scapulae, carpals, and tarsals, grow by appositional bone growth from their surrounding perichondrium and periosteum. Other bones, such as the metacarpals, metatarsals, phalanges, and spine, grow by a combination of both appositional and endochondral ossification.

Trauma, infections, nutritional deficiencies (rickets), regional soft tissue processes, inborn errors of metabolism (mucopolysaccharidosis, mucolipidosis, Gaucher disease, and disorders of collagen or cartilage), and other metabolic processes may affect each of these growth processes, producing a distinct alteration in the particular growth function.

Developmental Milestones. Neurologic maturation, marked by the passage of motor milestones at regular intervals, is important for normal musculoskeletal development. The milestones for locomotion include independent sitting at 6 mo of age, crawling at 9 mo, walking without assistance at 12–15 mo, and running at 18 mo (see Chapters 10 through 12). There is a distinct relationship between skeletal form and gross motor function. Any process that produces a neurologic abnormality may cause a secondary delay in developmental milestones and an alteration of normal skeletal growth.

Chapter 663

Evaluation of the Child

George H. Thompson

The key to an accurate diagnosis is a careful history, a thorough physical examination, appropriate radiographic imaging, and, occasionally, laboratory testing. A glossary of common orthopedic terminology is provided in Table 663–1.

History. The history of the complaint is often the most important part of the evaluation. This is usually obtained from the parents or guardian, but the child, if old enough and cooperative, can also give useful information. The chief complaint is established first. This may include pain, deformity, joint stiffness, gait disturbance (limp, toe walking, in-toeing, out-toeing), swelling, or generalized muscle weakness. One must ascertain location and duration of symptoms; antecedent factors such as fever, trauma, radiation of pain, and neurologic symptoms; factors aggravating or alleviating the symptoms; and previous evaluations or treatment.

In children with chronic symptoms, the past medical history is also important. The prenatal or pregnancy history should be obtained (see Chapters 83.1, 85.5, and 89). This includes maternal diseases or illnesses, vaginal bleeding, oligohydramnios, ingestion of toxic substances or medications, and trauma. The birth history should determine the length of pregnancy; duration of labor; type of difficulty, if any, with delivery; birth presentation; birthweight; and Apgar score (see Chapters 85, 86, and 89). The condition of the child during the neonatal period is

TABLE 663–1. Glossary of Orthopedic Terminology

Term	Definition
Abduction	Movement away from the midline
Adduction	Movement toward and possibly across the midline
Anteversion	Increased angulation of the femoral head and neck with respect to the knee in the frontal plane
Apophysis	Bone growth center that is not a growth plate or physis and that has a strong muscle insertion (e.g., greater trochanter of femur)
Arthroplasty	Surgical reconstruction of a joint
Arthrotomy	Surgical incision into a joint
Calcaneus	Dorsiflexion of hindfoot
Cavovarus	High longitudinal or medial arch of foot with plantarflexed supinated forefoot and hindfoot varus
Cavus	High longitudinal arch of the foot (usually plantarflexed forefoot)
Dislocation	Complete loss of contact between two joint surfaces
Equinus	Plantarflexion of the forefoot, hindfoot, or entire foot
Extension	To straighten; the reverse of flexion
External or lateral rotation	Outward rotation away from the midline
Flexion	To bend
Internal or medial rotation	Inward rotation, toward the midline
Subluxation	Incomplete loss of contact between two joint surfaces
Valgum	Angulation of a bone or joint in which the apex is toward the midline; genu valgum results in knock-knee because the angulation of the knee is toward the midline
Varum	Angulation of a bone or joint away from the midline; genu varum results in bowleg because the angulation is away from the midline

important (see Chapter 86). In older infants and young children, evaluation of the presence and delay of developmental milestones for posture, locomotion, dexterity, social activities, and speech is important.

The family history may give clues to possible genetic disorders such as congenital syndromes, muscular dystrophy, skeletal dysplasias, and other disorders affecting the musculoskeletal system. It is important to inquire about specific problems, similar or not, on both the paternal and maternal sides of the family.

Physical Examination. The physical examination of a child with a musculoskeletal disorder must be thorough. It includes the careful evaluation of the musculoskeletal and neurologic systems as well as an appropriate general physical examination. Many common musculoskeletal disorders can be diagnosed by the history and physical examination alone. The examination of the musculoskeletal system includes four parts: observation, palpation, assessment of joint range of motion, and gait assessment in ambulatory children.

OBSERVATION. The first part of the musculoskeletal examination begins with inspection of the body. This must be accomplished by observing the child undressed. If the child can stand, posture, truncal alignment, and symmetry of the extremities can be evaluated. The skin is assessed for cutaneous lesions. The presence of café-au-lait spots may indicate neurofibromatosis, whereas a maculopapular rash may indicate juvenile rheumatoid arthritis. Infants or young children may be examined on their parent's lap so that they feel more secure and are more likely to be cooperative.

PALPATION. The involved joint, area of the extremity, or trunk that is of concern should be palpated for tenderness, masses, soft tissue swelling, and increased warmth. Abnormal joints should also be palpated for effusion, synovial thickening, increased warmth, and areas of tenderness.

JOINT RANGE OF MOTION. The range of motion of the involved joint or joints should be assessed and recorded. If the opposite joint is normal, this range should also be recorded for comparison purposes. It must be remembered that the range of motion of joints changes from infancy through childhood and into adolescence.

GAIT ASSESSMENT. Gait disturbances are one of the most common parental concerns in children. It is, therefore, important to have a thorough understanding of the development of normal gait. Human gait is dynamic, complex, and repetitive. The gait cycle is the time between right heel strike followed by left toe-off, left heel strike, and right toe-off and ends with right heel strike. The five events describe one gait cycle and include two phases: stance and swing. The stance phase is the period of time during which one of the two feet is on the ground. The swing phase is the portion of the gait cycle during which a limb is being advanced forward without ground contact.

Neurologic maturation is necessary for the development of gait and the normal progression of developmental milestones. The normal 1-yr-old child has a wide-based stance and rapid cadence with short steps. The elbows are flexed and reciprocal arm motion is not present. Foot strike occurs without initial heel strike. A 2-yr-old child shows increased velocity and step length and diminished cadence compared with a 1-yr-old. Most of the adult gait patterns are present in children by 3 yr of age, with changes of velocity, stride, and cadence continuing to 7 yr. The gait characteristics of a 7-yr-old child are similar to those of an adult.

Common gait disturbances include limp, torsional variations (in-toeing and out-toeing), and toe walking. In evaluating gait disturbance, it is important to observe the child walking and running. The child must be sufficiently undressed to allow visualization of the lower extremities and trunk during ambulation.

Limping. Limping is categorized into either painful (antalgic) or nonpainful (Trendelenburg gait) on the basis of the length of the stance phase. In a painful gait, the stance phase is shortened as the child decreases the time spent on the painful extremity. In a nonpainful gait, which is indicative of underlying proximal muscle weakness or hip instability, the stance phase is equal between the involved and uninvolved sides, but the child will lean or shift the center of gravity over the involved extremity for balance. If the disorder is bilateral, it produces a waddling gait. The differential diagnosis of limping is extensive. The vast majority of causes involve the lower extremity, but it must be remembered that spinal disorders, especially spinal cord or peripheral nerve disorders, can also produce limping and difficulty walking. Antalgic gaits are predominantly a result of trauma, infection, neoplasia, and rheumatologic disorders. Trendelenburg gaits are generally due to congenital, developmental, or muscular disorders. Thus, antalgic gaits are acute processes, whereas Trendelenburg gaits are chronic. The differential diagnosis of limping is presented in Table 663–2, and causes of limping according to age are seen in Table 663–3. Limping may also be due to nonskeletal disease such as testicular torsion, inguinal hernia, or appendicitis.

Torsional Variations. Torsional variations—in-toeing and out-toeing—are the most common gait disturbances that cause parents to seek advice from their pediatrician (see Chapters 664 and 665). Many do not require treatment because they are physiologic in origin and improve and resolve with normal growth and development. They produce significant anxiety and require the pediatrician to have a clear understanding of the cause and natural history to reassure the family. The common causes of in-toeing and out-toeing are presented in Table 663–4. The presence of in-toeing and out-toeing does not imply an abnormality of the foot but rather only the direction in which the foot is pointing during ambulation. The causes for torsional variations can occur from proximal (hip) to distal (foot) in the involved extremity. Some causes, such as clubfoot, are obvious, whereas others can be subtle.

Toe Walking. Toe walking or equinus gait is a less common cause of gait disturbance. It can be a normal finding in children up to 3 yr of age. Persistent toe walking thereafter or acquired toe walking at a later age is considered abnormal and requires careful evaluation. The common causes of unilateral and bilateral toe

TABLE 663-2. Differential Diagnosis of Limping

ANTALGIC	TRENDELENBURG
Congenital	*Developmental*
Tarsal coalition	DDH
	Leg-length discrepancy
Acquired	*Neuromuscular*
LCPD	Cerebral plasy
SCFE	Poliomyelitis
Trauma	
Sprains, strains, contusions	
Fractures	
Occult	
Toddler's fracture	
Abuse	
Neoplasia	
Benign	
Unicameral bone cyst	
Osteoid osteoma	
Malignant	
Osteogenic sarcoma	
Ewing sarcoma	
Leukemia	
Spinal cord tumors	
Infectious	
Septic arthritis	
Reactive arthritis	
Osteomyelitis	
Acute	
Subacute	
Diskitis	
Rheumatologic	
Juvenile rheumatoid arthritis	
Hip monoarticular synovitis (toxic transient synovitis)	

LCPD = Legg-Calvé-Perthes disease; SCFE = slipped capital femoral epiphysis; DDH = developmental dysplasia of the hip.
From Thompson GH: Gait disturbances. In Kliegman RM (editor): Practical Strategies of Pediatric Diagnosis and Therapy. Philadelphia, WB Saunders, 1996, pp 757–78.

walking are listed in Table 663–5. The differential diagnosis for persistent or acquired toe walking include (1) neuromuscular disorders, such as cerebral palsy, Duchenne muscular dystrophy, or spinal cord abnormalities (tethered cord); (2) congenital tendo-Achilles contracture; (3) leg-length discrepancy; and (4) habit.

NEUROLOGIC EVALUATION. A careful neurologic evaluation must be performed and includes muscle strength testing, sensory assessment, and evaluation of deep tendon and pathologic reflexes, such as the Babinski reflex. The pertinent negative and positive findings should be recorded. The neurologic

TABLE 663-4. Common Causes of In-Toeing and Out-Toeing

In-Toeing	Out-Toeing
Internal femoral torsion	External femoral torsion
Internal tibial torsion	External tibial torsion
Metatarsus adductus	Calcaneovalgus feet
Talipes equinovarus (clubfoot)	Hypermobile pes planus

From Thompson GH: Pediatric orthopedics (spine, hips, lower extremities, and feet). In Marcus RE (editor): Orthopedics. Los Angeles, Practice Management Information Corporation, 1991, pp 209–300.

TABLE 663-3. Common Causes of Limping According to Age

Age	Antalgic	Trendelenburg	Leg-Length Discrepancy

Toddler (1–3 yr)	Infection
	  Septic arthritis
	    Hip
	    Knee
	  Osteomyelitis
	  Diskitis
	Occult trauma
	  Toddler's fracture
	Neoplasia
		Hip dislocation (DDH)
		Neuromuscular disease
		  Cerebral palsy
		  Poliomyelitis
			⊖

Childhood (4–10 yr)	Infection
	  Septic arthritis
	    Hip
	    Knee
	  Osteomyelitis
	  Diskitis
	  Transient synovitis, hip
	LCPD
	Tarsal coalition
	Rheumatologic disorder
	JRA
	Trauma
	Neoplasia
		Hip dislocation (DDH)
		Neuromuscular disease
		  Cerebral palsy
		  Poliomyelitis
			⊕

Adolescence (11 + yr)	SCFE Rheumatologic disorder JRA Trauma: fracture, overuse Tarsal coalition Neoplasia		⊕

LCPD = Legg-Calvé-Perthes disease; JRA = juvenile rheumatoid arthritis; SCFE = slipped capital femoral epiphysis; DDH = developmental dysplasia of the hip; ⊖ = absent; ⊕ = present.
From Thompson GH: Gait disturbances. In Kliegman RM (editor): Practical Strategies of Pediatric Diagnosis and Therapy. Philadelphia, WB Saunders, 1996, pp 757–78.

evaluation should also assess the spine and identify the presence of deformity, such as scoliosis or kyphosis, as well as spinal mobility. The child's ability to forward flex and reverse the normal lumbar lordosis is a sign of normal mobility. Areas of tenderness and muscle spasm are determined by palpation.

Radiographic Assessment. Radiography is the principal method for the evaluation of the pediatric musculoskeletal system. This can include routine radiographs as well as special procedures such as technetium bone scans, CT, MRI, and ultrasonography.

ROUTINE RADIOGRAPHY. Routine radiographs are the first step and consist of anteroposterior and lateral views of the involved joint, bone, or area. Comparison views of the opposite side, if uninvolved, may be helpful in difficult situations but are usually not necessary. The type of radiographs for each anatomic area is discussed in the sections on specific disorders.

TABLE 663-5. Common Causes of Toe Walking (Equinus Gait)

Unilateral	Bilateral

Neuromuscular disorder
  Cerebral palsy (hemiplegia)
Leg-length discrepancy
  Hip dislocation (DDH)
	Neuromuscular disorder
	  Cerebral palsy (diplegia)
	  Duchenne muscular dystrophy
	  Tethered spinal cord
	Congenital tendo-Achilles contracture
	Habitual

DDH = Developmental dysplasia of the hip.
From Thompson GH: Gait disturbances. In Kliegman RM (editor): Practical Strategies of Pediatric Diagnosis and Therapy. Philadelphia, WB Saunders, 1996, pp 757–78.

TECHNETIUM BONE SCANS. These are particularly useful in looking for occult lesions when routine radiographs are normal. Common indications for bone scans include (1) early septic arthritis or osteomyelitis; (2) neoplasia, such as osteoid osteomas and leukemia; (3) metastatic lesions; (4) occult fractures, such as child abuse or a toddler fracture of the tibia; and (5) inflammatory disorders.

COMPUTED TOMOGRAPHY. Coronal and axial cross-section studies with CT can be beneficial in evaluating complex disorders of the spine, pelvis, and feet. It allows visualization of the bone anatomy and the relationship of bones to contiguous structures, which routine radiographs do not.

MAGNETIC RESONANCE IMAGING. This avoids ionizing radiation and is presumed not to produce biologically harmful effects. It produces excellent anatomic images of the musculoskeletal system, including the spinal cord and brain. It is especially useful for soft tissue lesions, allowing distinction among different muscles or muscle groups. Cartilage structures can be visualized, and different forms can be distinguished (articular cartilage of the knee can be distinguished from the fibrocartilage of the meniscus). MRI is helpful in visualizing joints that are unossified, which may occur in the shoulders, elbows, and hips of young infants. MRI distinguishes physiologic changes that occur in the bone marrow with respect to age and disease such as avascular necrosis. In children, MRI can be useful in the evaluation of (1) avascular necrosis of bone, especially the capital femoral epiphysis or femoral head; (2) bone and soft tissue neoplasms; (3) intra-articular abnormalities of the knee joint; (4) assessment of intraspinal pathologic conditions; and (5) deep tissue infections (fasciitis and myositis).

ULTRASONOGRAPHY. Ultrasonography has no ionizing radiation, no contrast material to be administered, and no biologically harmful effects and can be repeated as often as necessary. The equipment is portable; scans can be obtained in any plane. The disadvantages of ultrasonography include (1) bone is not penetrated, (2) static images are difficult to interpret, and (3) the results are operator dependent. The major indications for ultrasonography are (1) fetal studies of the extremities and spine, (2) developmental dysplasia of the hip, (3) joint effusions, (4) occult neonatal spinal dysraphism; (5) foreign bodies in soft tissues, and (6) popliteal cysts of the knee.

Laboratory Studies. Occasionally, hematologic tests are necessary in the evaluation of the pediatric musculoskeletal system. These may include a complete blood cell count, erythrocyte sedimentation rate, C-reactive protein determination, and blood culture for infectious disorders, such as septic arthritis or osteomyelitis. Rheumatoid factor, antinuclear antibodies, and human leukocyte antigen B27 screens are necessary for children with suspected rheumatologic disorders. Creatine kinase, aldolase, aspartate aminotransferase, and dystrophin testing are indicated in children with suspected disorders of striated muscle such as Duchenne or Becker muscular dystrophy.

Talking with Parents. Many problems are normal or physiologic variations that resolve with growth and development and require only observation. This is particularly true in torsional variations of the lower extremities, which can produce significant anxiety in the family. Establishing a strong rapport with the family is an important component in the patient-family-physician relationship. Active treatment is indicated when the disorder has the potential to produce disability and also when the treatment is effective in altering the natural history. In many instances, the treatment may not significantly improve the child's condition initially, but by altering the natural history, problems in adult life, such as degenerative osteoarthritis, will be avoided.

Several steps are helpful in establishing a working relationship with parents. The diagnosis should be accurate and accompanied by a clear explanation of the cause and natural history of the disorder. Treatment options, including observation, should be discussed along with the expected results, both short and long term. If observation is recommended, a follow-up evaluation should be performed to document resolution and give the family additional reassurance.

Finally, not all physiologic conditions resolve. A small percentage of these disorders may persist into adolescence. These may require treatment if problems are to be avoided in adult life. The longer a problem persists, the greater is the chance that the problem will not resolve and may require treatment.

Forero N, Okamura LA, Larson MA: Normal ranges of hip motion in neonates. *J Pediatr Orthop* 1989;9:391–95.

Kim MK, Karpas A: The limping child. *Clin Pediatr Emerg Med* 2002;3:129–37.

Kogan M, Smith J: Simplified approach to toe-walking. *J Pediatr Orthop* 2001;21:790–91.

Leet AI, Skaggs DL: Evaluation of the acutely limping child. *Am Fam Physician* 2000;61:1011–18.

Myers MR, Thompson GH: Imaging the child with a limp. *Pediatr Clin North Am* 1997;44:637–58.

Staheli LT: Normative data in pediatric orthopaedics. *J Pediatr Orthop* 1996;16:561–62.

Sutherland DH, Olsten R, Cooper L, et al: The development of gait. *J Bone Joint Surg Am* 1980;62A:336–53.

Thompson GH: Gait disturbances. In Kliegman RM (editor): *Practical Strategies in Pediatric Diagnosis and Therapy*, 2nd ed. Philadelphia, WB Saunders, 2003.

Todd FN, Lamoreaux LW, Skinner SR, et al: Variations in the gait of normal children: A graph applicable to the documentation of abnormalities. *J Bone Joint Surg Am* 1989;71A:196–204.

Chapter 664
The Foot and Toes

George H. Thompson

The foot and toes are important in stance and locomotion. Abnormalities affecting the foot can produce pain and abnormal shoe wear and can adversely affect function. The foot articulates with the lower end of the tibia. The ankle joint is a box joint, which allows foot dorsiflexion and plantarflexion with essentially no rotation. The talus articulates with the distal end of the tibia. Support is achieved through the medial malleolus of the tibia and the lateral malleolus of the distal fibula. The foot is divided into three regions: hindfoot, midfoot, and forefoot. The toes are a portion of the forefoot.

The hindfoot is composed of the talus and calcaneus. The latter forms the heel. The joint between these two bones is the talocalcaneal or subtalar joint. This joint has a gliding and rotatory motion, which allows inversion and eversion of the hindfoot. This is important for walking on uneven ground.

The midfoot is composed of the navicular, cuboid, and the three cuneiform bones. The midfoot and hindfoot articulate through the transverse tarsal joint (calcaneocuboid and talonavicular joints). This joint is important for midfoot rotation and for walking on uneven ground. Deformity or malalignment of subtalar, talonavicular, or calcaneocuboid joints can have a significant effect on the alignment and function of the foot and produces abnormal stress on the ankle joint.

The forefoot is composed of the metatarsals and toes. The 1st metatarsal is unique because it has a single physeal plate that is located proximally. The lateral four metatarsals have a single physis located distally. The great toe is composed of proximal and distal phalanges and a single interphalangeal joint. The lateral four toes have proximal, middle, and distal phalanges that articulate through a proximal interphalangeal joint and a distal interphalangeal joint. All phalanges have their physeal plates located proximally. Normal function of the foot and toes requires a coordinated action between the extrinsic muscles of the calf and intrinsic muscles of the foot.

664.1 ∎ Metatarsus Adductus

Congenital metatarsus adductus, a common problem among infants and young children, is also known as metatarsus varus if the forefoot is supinated as well as adducted. It occurs equally in males and females and is bilateral in approximately 50% of patients. There are hereditary tendencies; it tends to be more common in firstborn than in later children as a result of the increased molding effect from the primigravida uterus and abdominal wall. Approximately 10% of children with metatarsus adductus may have acetabular dysplasia. Careful examination of the hips is necessary in any child with metatarsus adductus. Pelvic radiographs are obtained in suggestive cases.

Clinical Manifestations. The forefoot is adducted and occasionally supinated. The hindfoot and midfoot are normal. The lateral border of the foot is convex, and the base of the 5th metatarsal appears prominent (Fig. 664–1). The medial border of the foot is concave. There is usually an increased interval between the 1st and 2nd toes, with the great toe being held in a greater varus position. Ankle dorsiflexion and plantarflexion are normal. Forefoot mobility can vary from flexible to rigid. This is assessed by stabilizing the hindfoot and midfoot in a neutral position with one hand and applying pressure over the 1st metatarsal head with the other. In the walking child with an uncorrected metatarsus adductus deformity, an in-toe gait and abnormal shoe wear may occur.

Radiographic Evaluation. Radiographs of the foot are not routinely necessary in metatarsus adductus because they do not demonstrate forefoot mobility. Anteroposterior (AP) and lateral weight-bearing or simulated weight-bearing radiographs are indicated when there is rigidity or failure of spontaneous improvement with growth. The AP radiographs demonstrate adduction of the metatarsals at the tarsometatarsal articulation and an increased intermetatarsal angle between the 1st and 2nd metatarsals. The lateral four metatarsals appear to have increased closeness and occasionally overlap at their base. The hindfoot and midfoot are normal.

Treatment. The treatment of metatarsus adductus is predominantly nonoperative. There are limited indications for surgery.

NONOPERATIVE. Most children with metatarsus adductus deformities respond to conservative treatment. The feet may be

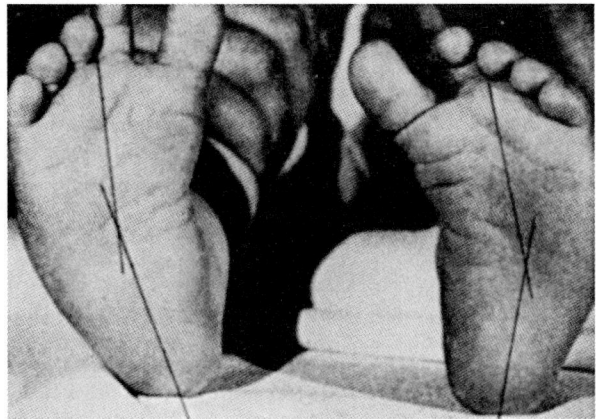

FIGURE 664–1. Metatarsus adductus. A line bisecting the hindfoot should pass through the second toe or between the second and third toes.

classified into three groups depending on forefoot flexibility. Type I feet are flexible and actively and passively overcorrect into mild abduction. Voluntary correction can be elicited by stimulating the peroneal musculature by stroking the lateral border of the foot. These feet usually require no treatment. Type II feet correct to the neutral position both passively and actively. These feet may benefit from an orthosis or corrective shoes such as straight or reverse last shoes. These are worn full-time (22 hr/day), and the condition is re-evaluated in 4–6 wk. If improvement occurs, treatment can be continued. If there is no improvement, serial plaster casts are necessary. Type III feet are rigid and do not correct to neutral. These feet are treated with serial casts. The best results are obtained when casting is initiated before 8 mo of age. Once correction has been achieved, orthoses or corrective shoes may be used for an additional 1–2 mo to maintain correction. Mild hallux varus, the "searching toe," may persist for several years after conservative correction and may be of concern to the parents. However, it eventually disappears with growth and the wearing of shoes.

OPERATIVE. Significant residual metatarsus adductus in children 4 yr of age and older may require surgical intervention. Children 4–6 yr of age usually require only a soft tissue release. Serial casting is performed postoperatively until forefoot correction has been obtained. This usually requires 2–3 mo. Children 6 yr of age or older require base of the metatarsal osteotomies or other osseous procedures to achieve satisfactory correction. The sequelae of mild residual metatarsus adductus are minimal.

664.2 ∎ Calcaneovalgus Feet

The calcaneovalgus foot is a relatively common finding in the newborn and is secondary to in utero positioning. A hyperdorsiflexed foot with forefoot abduction and increased heel valgus manifests this condition. It is usually associated with external tibial torsion. It is often unilateral but occasionally may be bilateral. In utero, the plantar surface of the foot was against the wall of the uterus, forcing it into a hyperdorsiflexed, abducted, and externally rotated position. The position also produces the external tibial torsion. When these two conditions are combined with the normal newborn increased external rotation of the hip (tight posterior capsule), it results in a lower extremity that appears excessively externally rotated.

Clinical Manifestations. The infant typically presents with an out-toe position of the involved extremity. The dorsum of the foot can easily be brought into contact with the anterior aspect of the lower leg; the forefoot is abducted, and the heel is in valgus. This should not be confused with the neonatal maturity classification of Dubowitz (see Chapter 86). External tibial torsion (20–50 degrees) is a common associated finding. Ankle motion shows normal or almost normal plantarflexion.

Three conditions must be distinguished from the calcaneovalgus foot: (1) congenital vertical talus, (2) posteromedial bow of the tibia, and (3) neuromuscular abnormalities with paralysis of the gastrocnemius muscle. The differentiation can usually be made during the physical examination.

Radiographic Evaluation. Anteroposterior and lateral simulated weight-bearing radiographs of the feet may be necessary to differentiate between the calcaneovalgus foot and a congenital vertical talus. In a calcaneovalgus foot, the radiographs are normal or there may be increased hindfoot valgus and forefoot abduction. If a posteromedial bow of the tibia is suspected, anteroposterior and lateral radiographs of the tibia and fibula are necessary.

Treatment. The typical calcaneovalgus foot requires no treatment. The hyperdorsiflexion of the foot resolves during the 1st 6 mo of life. The external tibial torsion, however, persists and follows the same natural history as internal tibial torsion.

Spontaneous improvement does not occur until the child begins to pull to stand and walk independently. It takes 6–12 mo thereafter for complete correction to occur. The majority of infants with calcaneovalgus feet and external tibial torsion have normally aligned feet and lower extremities by 2 yr of age.

664.3 Talipes Equinovarus (Clubfoot)

A clubfoot is a common foot deformity that involves not only the foot but also the entire lower leg. It can be classified into three groups: (1) congenital, (2) teratologic, and (3) positional. The congenital clubfoot is usually an isolated abnormality, whereas the teratologic form is associated with a neuromuscular disorder, such as myelodysplasia, arthrogryposis multiplex congenita, or a syndrome complex. The congenital form has also been called *idiopathic* or *neurogenic* on the basis of possible causes. The positional clubfoot is a normal foot that has been held in a deformed position in utero.

The *cause* of clubfoot is unknown. There are inheritance factors, and these are currently considered multifactorial with a major influence from a single autosomal dominant gene. Biopsy studies of the extrinsic muscles of the calf have indicated a probable neuromuscular cause. There are fiber type disproportions and increased neuromuscular junctions within these muscles. These findings are in contrast to previous etiologic theories in which deformity of the talus was believed to be the primary abnormality. Although the talus is certainly deformed with medial deviation of the head and neck, this is considered to be a secondary deformity.

Clinical Manifestations. The congenital form of clubfoot, which constitutes approximately 75% of all cases, is characterized by (1) the absence of other congenital abnormalities, (2) variable rigidity of the foot, (3) mild calf atrophy, and (4) mild hypoplasia of the tibia, fibula, and bones of the foot. It occurs more commonly in males (2:1) and is bilateral in 50% of cases. The probability for a random occurrence is approximately 1 in 1,000 births; within involved families, the probability is approximately 3% for subsequent siblings and 20–30% for offspring of involved parents.

Examination of the infant clubfoot demonstrates hindfoot equinus, hindfoot and midfoot varus, forefoot adduction, and variable rigidity. All these findings are secondary to the medial dislocation of the talonavicular joint. In the older child, the calf and foot atrophy are more obvious than in the infant, regardless of how well corrected or functional the foot. These findings are due to the causative aspects of clubfoot, not the method of treatment.

Radiographic Evaluation. Anteroposterior and lateral standing or simulated weight-bearing radiographs and maximum dorsiflexion lateral radiograph are used in the assessment of clubfeet. Non–weight-bearing radiographs are not helpful. Multiple different radiographic measurements can be made. The navicular bone, which is the primary site of deformity, does not ossify until 3 yr in the female and 4 yr in the male. This necessitates line measurements to determine the position of the unossified navicular bone and the overall alignment of the foot.

Treatment

NONOPERATIVE. Conservative treatment is initiated in all infants, although a significant proportion of children later require surgery. Nonoperative treatment includes taping, the use of malleable splints, and serial plaster casts. Taping and malleable splints are particularly useful in premature infants until they attain an appropriate size for casting. Serial plaster casts are the major method of nonoperative treatment. Before the cast is applied, the foot is gently manipulated toward the corrected position. The cast is then applied and changed at 1–2 wk intervals. Complete correction, both clinically and radi-

ographically, should be achieved by 3 mo of age. If this is accomplished, holding casts are then used for an additional 3–6 mo followed by orthoses or corrective shoes until the child is walking well. Failure to achieve clinical and radiographic correction by 3 mo of age is an indication for surgical treatment. Further attempts at conservative management may result in articular damage and a midfoot breech (rocker-bottom deformity).

OPERATIVE. The current method of surgical treatment is a complete soft tissue release. This is usually performed between 6 and 12 mo of age. Satisfactory long-term results can be expected in 80–90% of cases. Unsatisfactory results that require additional treatment are usually secondary to extrinsic muscle imbalance rather than incomplete correction. The use of tendon transfers and bone procedures, including arthrodeses (fusions), are primarily for salvage of recurrent clubfoot or incompletely corrected feet. Centralization of the tibialis anterior tendon has been particularly beneficial in young children with a dynamic pes varus, the most common residual abnormality. Triple arthrodeses are indicated in painful, deformed feet in adolescence.

664.4 Congenital Vertical Talus

Congenital vertical talus is an uncommon foot deformity with causes similar to those of talipes equinovarus. It must be distinguished from a calcaneovalgus foot, which is much more common. Typically, a congenital vertical talus is a rigid rocker-bottom deformity. The majority of these infants have an underlying disorder such as teratologic malformation (myelodysplasia and arthrogryposis multiplex congenita) or a syndrome such as trisomy 18.

Clinical Manifestations. The characteristic of a congenital vertical talus is a rocker-bottom foot. There is hindfoot equinovalgus, a convex plantar surface, forefoot abduction and dorsiflexion, and rigidity. A careful physical examination must be performed on all children to look for an underlying disorder or syndrome.

Radiographic Evaluation. Radiographic evaluation of a congenital vertical talus consists of an anteroposterior and lateral weight-bearing or simulated weight-bearing radiograph of the foot as well as a maximal plantarflexed lateral view. This typically reveals the vertically oriented talus, the dorsal displacement and abduction of the midfoot on the hindfoot, hindfoot valgus, and mobility.

Treatment. As in clubfeet, nonoperative treatment is the initial method of treatment of congenital vertical talus, although most cases later require surgical correction.

NONOPERATIVE. Serial casting after manipulation of the feet is performed beginning at birth. The forefoot is manipulated into equinus in an attempt to reduce the navicular onto the head of the talus. The success rate with nonoperative treatment is exceedingly low.

OPERATIVE. The operative management of congenital vertical talus is predominantly through a complete soft tissue release performed as a one-stage or two-stage procedure. Occasionally, in severe deformities, a naviculectomy may be necessary to realign the midfoot and hindfoot adequately. Fortunately, this is rarely necessary. In older children with persistent hindfoot valgus and pronation, a subtalar arthrodesis or a triple arthrodesis may be necessary to realign the foot and provide stability.

The goals of treatment of congenital vertical talus are pessimistic and include a plantigrade, pain-free foot that is able to wear shoes. Orthotic management is frequently necessary for a prolonged period postoperatively, if not for life, because of associated muscle weakness resulting from an underlying disorder.

664.5 Hypermobile Pes Planus (Flexible Flatfeet)

Hypermobile flatfeet or pronated feet are common sources of concern of parents. In general, these children are asymptomatic and have no functional limitations. Flatfeet are common in neonates and toddlers because of an associated laxity in the bone-ligament complexes of the feet and fat in the area of the medial longitudinal arch. These children usually demonstrate significant improvement by 6 yr of age. In the older child, flexible flatfeet are usually secondary to generalized ligamentous laxity, an autosomal dominant condition.

Clinical Manifestations. In the non–weight-bearing position in the older child with a flexible flatfoot, the normal medial longitudinal arch is present, but in the weight-bearing position, the foot becomes pronated with varying degrees of pes planus and heel valgus. Instead of weight-bearing over the lateral column of the foot, weight is shifted medially, producing pronation. Subtalar motion is normal or slightly increased. Loss of subtalar motion indicates a rigid flatfoot. Common causes of rigid flatfeet include a tendo-Achilles contracture, tarsal coalitions, neuromuscular abnormalities (cerebral palsy), and familial trait.

Radiographic Evaluation. Routine radiographs of asymptomatic flexible flatfeet are usually not indicated. Anteroposterior and lateral weight-bearing radiographs are obtained if there is rigidity or symptoms. On the anteroposterior radiograph, there is excessive heel valgus. The lateral view shows distortion of the normal straight line relationship between the long axis of the talus and the 1st metatarsal with either a sag of the talonavicular or naviculocuneiform joint, resulting in flattening of the normal medial longitudinal arch.

Treatment. The treatment of flexible flatfeet is conservative. Affected children do not have symptoms predictably. Therefore, modified shoes and orthoses do not significantly alter the clinical or radiographic appearance of the feet. It should be emphasized that the diagnosis of flexible flatfeet is usually not possible until after 6 yr of age. Treatment is indicated for abnormal shoe wear or symptoms not attributable to other causes. Feet that are symptomatic with vigorous physical activities usually respond readily to the use of a commercially available medial longitudinal arch support. Custom-made supports are much more expensive and, in most cases, not any more effective. Surgery, including subtalar joint inserts, is rarely indicated.

664.6 Tarsal Coalition

Tarsal coalition, also known as peroneal spastic flatfoot, is a relatively common foot disorder characterized by a painful, rigid flatfoot deformity and peroneal (lateral calf) muscle spasm but without true spasticity. It represents a congenital fusion or failure of segmentation between two or more tarsal bones. Any condition that alters the normal gliding and rotatory motion of the subtalar joint may produce the clinical appearance of a tarsal coalition. Thus, congenital malformations, arthritis or inflammatory disorders, infection, neoplasms, and trauma can be possible causes.

The most common tarsal coalitions occur at the medial talocalcaneal (subtalar) facet and between the calcaneus and navicular (calcaneonavicular) tarsal bones. Coalitions can be fibrous, cartilaginous, or osseous. Tarsal coalition occurs in approximately 1% of the general population; it appears to be inherited as a unifactorial autosomal dominant trait with nearly full penetrance. Approximately 60% of calcaneonavicular and 50% of the medial facet talocalcaneal coalitions are bilateral.

Clinical Manifestations. The onset of symptoms usually occurs during the 2nd decade of life. Although mild limitation of subta-lar motion and the flatfoot may have been present since early childhood, the onset of symptoms varies with the age at which the fibrous or cartilaginous bar begins to ossify and further decrease motion. The talonavicular coalition ossifies between 3 and 5 yr of age, the calcaneonavicular coalition between 8 and 12 yr, and the medial facet talocalcaneal coalition between 12 and 16 yr. The pain is typically felt laterally in the hindfoot and radiates proximally along the lateral malleolus and distal fibula (peroneal muscle spasm). Symptoms are frequently aggravated by sports or walking on uneven ground. Clinically, the foot is flat or pronated both in the weight-bearing and the non–weight-bearing positions. Subtalar and transverse tarsal joint motion is diminished or absent, and attempts at motion may produce pain.

Radiographic Evaluation. The diagnosis of a tarsal coalition is confirmed radiographically. Anteroposterior and lateral weight-bearing radiographs and an oblique radiograph of the foot should be obtained. Beaking of the anterior aspect of the talus on the lateral view is suggestive of a tarsal coalition. The oblique view demonstrates a calcaneonavicular coalition. Axial views through the hindfoot can be useful in the diagnosis of the medial facet talocalcaneal coalition. However, CT is the procedure of choice in the evaluation of coalitions, especially those involving the subtalar joint.

Treatment. The treatment of symptomatic tarsal coalitions varies according to the type of coalition, age of the patient, extent of the coalition, presence or absence of degenerative osteoarthritis, and degree of disability. The treatment may be nonoperative or operative. Nonoperative treatment may consist of cast immobilization, shoe inserts, or orthotics. Operative management consists of excision of the coalition and interposition of muscle (calcaneonavicular) and fat or split flexor hallucis longus tendon (medial facet talocalcaneal) to prevent hematoma formation and reossification of the coalition (Fig. 664–2). Resections are effective in relieving pain, improving subtalar motion, and allowing resumption of normal activities. However, if degenerative osteoarthritis is present, a triple arthrodesis may be necessary.

664.7 Cavus Feet

Cavus feet represent an exaggeration in the medial longitudinal arch associated with hindfoot varus and occasionally adduction of the forefoot. When the latter occurs, the deformity is called a *cavovarus deformity*. This type of deformity appears most commonly during the middle childhood years. Both idiopathic and neuromuscular types (hereditary motor-sensory neuropathies) may be seen. In either case, a cavovarus foot is usually a progressive deformity, leading to considerable compromise of foot function. These deformities tend to be rigid. The most important aspect of the evaluation of a patient with a cavovarus foot is to establish an accurate diagnosis. Possible causes include spinal cord disease and peripheral neuropathies, such as Charcot-Marie-Tooth disease.

Treatment. Aggressive treatment is usually necessary for moderate to severe cavus feet. This usually involves reconstructive surgery. Special shoes and shoe modifications are not helpful from a therapeutic standpoint but sometimes may be warranted to provide relief from abnormal pressure during weight-bearing. Surgical correction by soft tissue balancing and occasionally by osseous procedures is usually necessary.

664.8 Osteochondroses

Osteochondroses are pathologic processes that involve infarction, revascularization, resorption, and replacement of the

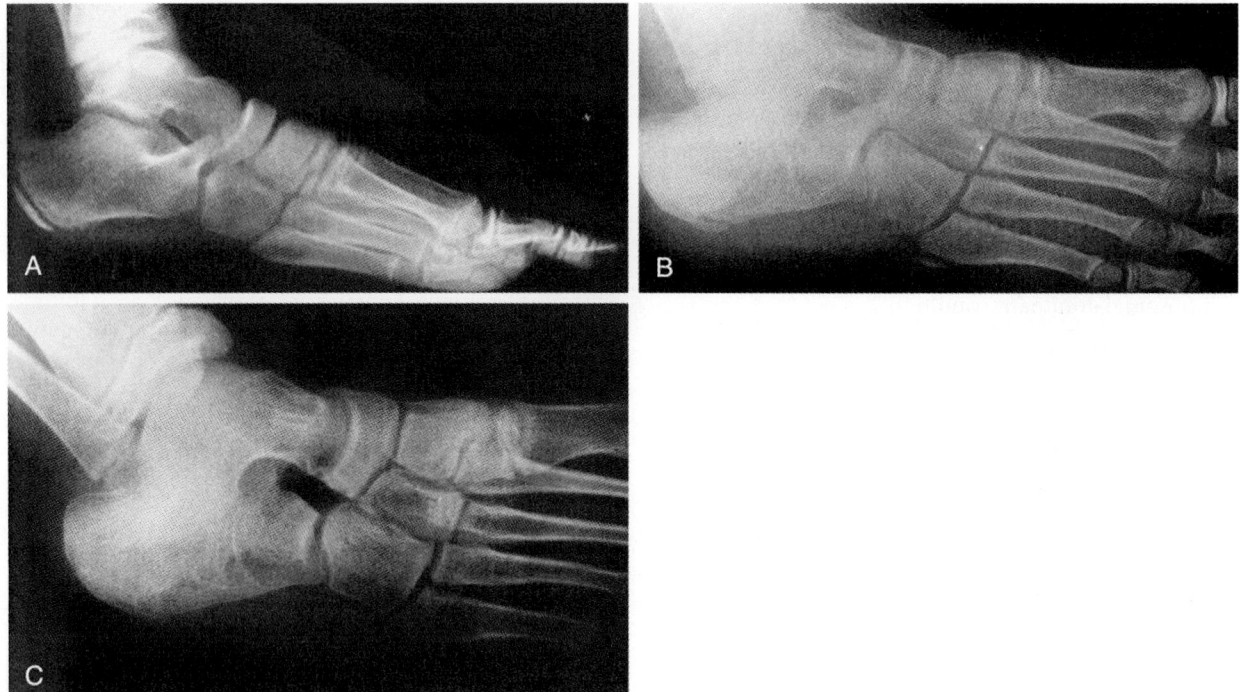

FIGURE 664–2. *A,* Standing lateral radiograph of the foot of a 12-yr-old girl with limited, painful subtalar joint motion. There is an extension of the anterior process of the calcaneus toward the navicular. This has been called the "anteater's nose" and is indicative of calcaneonavicular coalition. *B,* The oblique radiograph demonstrates the calcaneonavicular coalition. The small, unossified area in the center of the coalition is actually cartilaginous and will ultimately form a complete osseous bridge. *C,* Oblique radiograph after excision of the coalition and interposition of the extensor digitorum brevis muscle to prevent re-formation. This procedure restores subtalar joint motion and relieves discomfort.

affected bone. This is commonly termed *idiopathic avascular necrosis.* Both the tarsal navicular (*Köhler disease*) and the head or epiphysis of the 2nd metatarsal (*Freiberg disease*) may sustain avascular necrosis. These conditions are relatively uncommon and both produce pain, especially with activities. Symptomatic treatment is based on the severity of the child's complaint. Occasionally, a short-leg cast and a non–weight-bearing stance with crutches may be helpful in relieving symptoms.

As the older child enters the period of pubescent growth spurt, the fibrocartilaginous insertion of major muscle groups to bone is vulnerable to microfracture, resulting in inflammatory and healing responses. The usual site of microfractures in the foot is the attachment of the tendo-Achilles (heel cord) to the posterior aspect of the calcaneus. This produces another osteochondrosis: *Sever disease,* which is a common cause of heel pain. Symptoms wax and wane depending on the level of activity; and until skeletal maturity is achieved, the usual residual manifestation, if any, is bony enlargement at the tendon insertion site secondary to overgrowth during the healing response. Treatment is again symptomatic and includes the use of an anti-inflammatory agent and heel cord stretching.

664.9   Puncture Wounds of the Foot

For most puncture wound injuries, extensively cleansing the wound, ensuring prophylaxis for tetanus, and administering a broad-spectrum oral antibiotic are all that is needed. When infection occurs despite these measures, *Pseudomonas aeruginosa* and *Staphylococcus aureus* are the usual offending organisms. In pseudomonal osteomyelitis, the puncture usually injured the bone, cartilage, or joint. This is most common when the puncture wound is through the sole of a sneaker. The heat and per-

spiration and the material within the sneakers tend to promote the growth of this organism. Treatment of established infections includes wound debridement to remove necrotic tissue. Broad-spectrum antibiotics are administered, including methicillin and gentamicin, pending the outcome of the cultures. Subsequent antibiotic treatment is based on the results of these tests. After surgery, further microbial therapy is continued for 10–14 days. Most patients have a satisfactory response to this therapy.

664.10   Toe Deformities
ADOLESCENT BUNIONS

Adolescent bunions, a common pediatric foot deformity, are more common in girls (3:1); there is frequently a positive family history. There are both intrinsic and extrinsic factors associated with this deformity. The intrinsic factors include metatarsus primus varus, oblique 1st metatarsal-medial cuneiform articulation, short 1st metatarsal, and pes planus. Extrinsic factors include abnormal shoe wear (narrow toe box with an elevated heel) and a subtle underlying neurologic disorder, such as mild cerebral palsy.

Clinical Manifestations. An adolescent presenting with bunions requires careful evaluation. It must be determined whether it is the symptoms or the deformity, or both, that are of concern to the patient and the family. If pain is present, it must be ascertained whether it is due to activities and whether it produces functional limitation. It is also important to know what types of shoes are being worn when symptoms are present. When evaluating the foot, weight-bearing alignment, walking alignment, mobility of the 1st metatarsophalangeal joint, presence or absence of callus formation, and preferred shoe style must be determined.

Radiographic Evaluation. Anteroposterior and lateral weight-bearing radiographs of the feet are necessary in the assessment of adolescent bunions. This allows measurement of the (1) intermetatarsal angle, (2) hallux valgus angle, (3) distal metatarsal articular angle, (4) alignment of the 1st metatarsal-medial cuneiform joint, and (5) pes planus. The normal intermetatarsal angle between the long axes of the 1st and 2nd metatarsals is 10 degrees or less, and the normal hallux valgus angle is 25 degrees or less. A short 1st metatarsal can be diagnosed from these radiographs.

Treatment

NONOPERATIVE. Conservative management of adolescent bunions consists primarily of shoe modifications. It is important that footwear accommodate the width of the forefoot. Adolescents should be discouraged from wearing narrow-toed shoes with elevated heels. In the presence of a pes planus, an orthotic to restore the medial longitudinal arch may be beneficial.

OPERATIVE. The indications for surgical correction include an intermetatarsal angle between 12–18 degrees and failure of nonoperative management. The major indication for surgical treatment is symptoms, not cosmesis. Surgery rarely restores the foot to a completely normal appearance but is effective in narrowing the width of the forefoot, correcting the hallux valgus, improving weight-bearing alignment, and relieving symptoms. Surgery typically consists of a combination of a soft tissue and bone procedure. The osseous procedures are numerous and can be performed on the 1st metatarsal or medial cuneiform, or both.

CURLY TOES

The most common lesser toe deformity of childhood is curly toes. These represent a flexion deformity at the proximal interphalangeal joint with lateral rotation and varus alignment of the toe (Fig. 664–3). The 4th and 5th toes are the most commonly involved. Occasionally, the 2nd and 3rd toes are involved. The disorder is usually familial, bilateral, symmetric, and asymptomatic. The condition is secondary to short, tight flexor digitorum longus and flexor digitorum brevis tendons. The tightness in these tendons can be demonstrated by dorsiflexing the foot, which will increase the curling of the toes. Plantarflexion usually results in improvement. Radiographic evaluation of curly toe deformities is not necessary.

Treatment. In infants and young children, curly toe deformities should be observed because 25–50% resolve spontaneously. Taping or splinting is ineffective. At 3–4 yr of age, an open tenotomy of the toe flexor tendons can be performed. In older children and adolescents, a proximal interphalangeal joint fusion may be necessary.

OVERLAPPING FIFTH TOE

An overlapping 5th toe is a relatively common condition in which the 5th toe is adducted and overrides the 4th toe. It results in abnormal shoe wear and pain in approximately 50% of patients.

Examination of the 5th toe shows an extensor digitorum longus contracture. There is also a dorsal metatarsophalangeal joint contracture. The 5th toe is adducted, extended, and laterally rotated. It may be possible to realign the toe passively, but the corrected position cannot be maintained. Radiographs are not necessary in the evaluation of an overlapping fifth toe.

Treatment. Nonoperative treatment is ineffective; it can be corrected surgically. The most common procedure consists of a racket-shaped incision around the base of the toe. The extensor digitorum longus tendon is released along with the dorsal joint contracture. This allows the toe to be placed into its normal position.

POLYDACTYLY

Polydactyly is a relatively common deformity. It usually involves the 5th toe. It occurs in approximately 2 in 1,000 births. Approximately 30% of patients have a positive family history. It is important to assess for syndromes and other organ anomalies as well as other digit deformities such as polydactyly of the hand and syndactyly of adjacent toes. Duplication of the great toe is also possible. There may be associated metatarsal abnormalities.

Anteroposterior and lateral weight-bearing radiographs of both feet are obtained in the management of children with polydactyly. This demonstrates whether the duplication is articulated or rudimentary and whether there are metatarsal abnormalities.

Treatment. Rudimentary-type digits can be ligated at birth and allowed to autoamputate. Those that are articulated require excision at approximately 1 yr of age. The guidelines in polydactyly are to save the digit with best axial alignment, resect the projecting symptomatic toe, repair the capsule, balance the soft tissues, and shave any metatarsal prominences.

SYNDACTYLY

Syndactyly is a relatively common lesser toe condition. Cases of syndactyly are usually asymptomatic, and there may be a positive familial history. They can be classified into *zygosyndactyly* and *polysyndactyly*. In zygosyndactyly, there is complete or incomplete webbing. This usually occurs between the 2nd and 3rd toes. In polysyndactyly, there may be a duplication of the 5th toe, with a syndactyly between the 4th and 5th toes. Synostosis of the lateral metatarsals is common.

Treatment. Zygosyndactyly does not require treatment, but polysyndactyly may because of the associated anomalies.

HAMMER TOE

A hammer toe is similar to a curly toe except there is no malrotation of the involved toe. There is a flexion deformity at the proximal interphalangeal joint, and the metatarsophalangeal

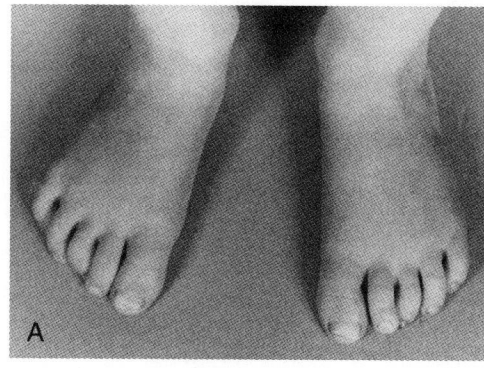
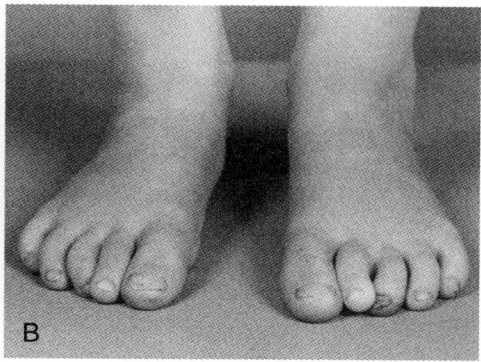

FIGURE 664–3. *A*, Bilateral curly toe deformities in a 4-yr old. There is flexion and varus rotation of the lateral three toes. *B*, The frontal view better demonstrates the curling of the toes, especially the third toes.

joint is extended. The metatarsal head may appear depressed. It is usually symmetric and bilateral, with the 2nd toe most commonly involved. The major problems with this deformity are painful calluses over the proximal phalangeal joint.

Treatment. Passive stretching and taping may be helpful in infants and young children. However, the majority requires surgical correction of the contracted flexor digitorum longus and flexor digitorum brevis tendons. Occasionally, tendon transfers are required.

MALLET TOE

Mallet toe is a flexion deformity at the distal interphalangeal joint. It may become symptomatic in adolescents as a result of a dorsal callosity or perhaps from nail bed irritation.

Treatment. Nonoperative treatment is usually ineffective. Correction is usually obtained by the release of the flexor digitorum longus tendon. Occasionally, in the adolescent, a distal interphalangeal joint fusion may be necessary.

CLAW TOE

Claw toes represent an extension contracture with dorsal subluxation of the metatarsophalangeal joint in association with flexion deformities of both the proximal and distal interphalangeal joints. They can occur idiopathically, but the majority is associated with a pes cavus deformity and is secondary to an underlying neurologic disorder, such as Charcot-Marie-Tooth disease. These deformities are complex and require careful assessment to determine the underlying cause.

Treatment. Claw toes are treated surgically, usually with soft tissue rebalancing and, occasionally, fusions of the proximal interphalangeal joint.

ANNULAR BANDS

Annular bands or constriction rings are relatively common congenital disorders that involve the toes and fingers. They may consist of simple constriction rings or rings with deformity of the distal part of the toe with swelling and lymphedema. Occasionally, the rings may be deep enough to have produced an amputation. Sometimes there will be an associated syndactyly with the adjacent toe. Annular bands of the lower extremity are frequently associated with clubfeet.

Treatment. The treatment of annular or constriction bands is predominantly observation. If there are deep rings with swelling and lymphedema, surgery may be necessary to relieve the congestion.

SUBUNGUAL EXOSTOSES

Subungual exostosis is an uncommon problem that primarily involves the great toe. It may simulate an ingrown toenail. On physical examination, there is a palpable mass beneath the toenail. The toe may appear irritated and similar to an infection; however, palpation reveals a mass rather than granulation tissue. Radiographs of the toe demonstrate exostosis of the distal phalanx.

Treatment. Subungual exostoses are managed by partial excision of the nail bed and removal of the underlying exostosis.

INGROWN TOENAIL

Ingrown toenails are relatively common in infants and young children and later in adolescents. These typically involve the medial and lateral borders of the great toe.

Treatment. Conservative treatment is usually effective. This consists of appropriate shoe modification, warm soaks, antibiotics,

elevation of the nail edge, and proper nail-cutting techniques. If this fails, surgery with wedge section of the involved border, including the nail matrix, is usually effective.

STUBBED GREAT TOE

Stubbed toes are common and in most patients heal spontaneously and rapidly. A Salter-Harris I fracture to the growth plate may occur, which also usually heals with minimal treatment.

Injuries associated with signs of nail bed bleeding or nail fold bleeding suggest the presence of an open fracture. The latter increases the risk for osteomyelitis, which may result in growth arrest of the distal phalanx of the great toe.

Persistent pain, bleeding, cellulitis, or pus drainage requires specific therapy for possible osteomyelitis, including oral or intravenous antistaphylococcal antibiotics, irrigation, and debridement.

664.11 Painful Foot

The causes of a painful foot can usually be determined from history and physical examination. The common causes are listed in Table 664–1. The specific treatment depends on the diagnosis and occasionally on the age of the child or adolescent.

664.12 Shoes

Clothing is worn for comfort, to enhance appearance, and for protection. Shoes should be selected on the same basis. Shoes are not corrective, and the foot does not need support for normal activities. The foot requires mobility to function normally. It has been demonstrated that populations that are predominantly barefoot have better feet than those that wear shoes. The best shoes for children are those that simulate the bare foot. They should be flexible, flat, and nonconstricting and made of material that "breathes." Shoes do not have to be expensive.

Because overuse foot symptoms are common, especially in the athletic adolescent, shock-absorbing shoes are a good choice. The thick-cushioned sole absorbs some of the shock of impact and thereby decreases discomfort.

Shoe modifications are sometimes appropriate for a specific problem. A lift may be prescribed if the limb is short, and a shoe insert may be helpful for the stiff and deformed foot or to distribute the weight load more evenly over the sole.

TABLE 664–1. Differential Diagnosis of Foot Pain by Age

0–6 Yr	6–12 Yr	12–20 Yr
Poor-fitting shoes	Poor-fitting shoes	Poor-fitting shoes
Foreign body	Sever disease	Stress fracture
Fracture	Enthesopathy (JRA)	Foreign body
Osteomyelitis	Foreign body	Ingrown toenail
Leukemia	Accessory navicular	Metatarsalgia
Puncture wound	Tarsal coalition	Plantar fasciitis
Drawing of blood	Ewing sarcoma	Osteochondroses
Dactylitis	Hypermobile flatfoot	(avascular necrosis)
JRA	Trauma (sprains, fractures)	Freiberg
	Puncture wound	Köhler
		Achilles tendinitis
		Trauma (sprains)
		Plantar warts
		Tarsal coalition

JRA = juvenile rheumatoid arthritis.

Metatarsus Adductus

Crawford AH, Gabriel KR: Foot and ankle problems. *Orthop Clin North Am* 1987;18:649–66.

Farsetti P, Weinstein SL, Ponseti IV: The long-term functional and radiographic outcomes of untreated and non-operatively treated metatarsus adductus. *J Bone Joint Surg Am* 1994;76A:257–65.

Calcaneovalgus Feet

Gibson DA: Torsional variations in the lower limbs of children. *Appl Ther* 1966;8:326–30.

Congenital Talipes Equinovarus (Clubfoot)

Cowell HR, Wein BK: Current concepts review: Genetic aspects of clubfoot. *J Bone Joint Surg Am* 1980;62A:1381–84.

Handelsman J, Badalamente MA: Neuromuscular studies in clubfoot. *J Pediatr Orthop* 1981;1:23–32.

Howard CB, Benson MKD: Clubfoot: Its pathological anatomy. *J Pediatr Orthop* 1993;13:654–59.

Ponseti IV: Current concepts review: Treatment of congenital club foot. *J Bone Joint Surg Am* 1992;74A:448–54.

Thompson GH, Simons GW III: Congenital talipes equinovarus (clubfeet) and metatarsus adductus. In Drennan JC (editor): *The Child's Foot and Ankle.* New York, Raven Press, 1992, pp 97–133.

Congenital Vertical Talus

Drennan JC: Instructional Course Lecture: Congenital vertical talus. *J Bone Joint Surg Am* 1995;77A:1916–23.

Duncan RD, Fixsen JA: Congenital convex pes valgus. *J Bone Joint Surg Br* 1999;81B:250–54.

Kodros SA, Dias LS: Single-stage correction of congenital vertical talus. *J Pediatr Orthop* 1999;19:42–48.

Sullivan JA: Pediatric flatfoot: Evaluation and management. *J Am Acad Orthop Surg* 1999;7:44–53.

Hypermobile Pes Planus (Flexible Flatfeet)

Akcali O, Tiner M, Ozaksoy D: Effects of lower extremity rotation on prognoses of flexible flatfoot in children. *Foot Ankle Int* 2000;21:72–74.

Black PR, Betts RP, Duckworth T, et al: The Viladot implant in flatfooted children. *Foot Ankle Int* 2000;21:478–81.

Giannini BS, Ceccarelli F, Benedetti MG, et al: Surgical treatment of flexible flatfeet in children: A four-year follow-up study. *J Bone Joint Surg Am* 2001;83:78–9.

Lin CJ, Lai KA, Kuan TS, et al: Correlating factors and clinical significance of flexible flatfeet in preschool children. *J Pediatr Orthop* 2001;21:378–82.

Mosca VS: Instructional Course Lecture: Flexible flatfoot and skewfoot. *J Bone Joint Surg Am* 1995;77:1937–45.

Staheli LT, Chew DE, Corbet M: The longitudinal arch: A survey of 882 feet in normal children and adults. *J Bone Joint Surg Am* 1987;69:426–28.

Staheli LT: Planovalgus foot deformity: Current Status. *J Am Podiatr Med Assoc* 1999;89:94–99.

Sullivan JA: Pediatric flatfoot: Evaluation and management. *J Am Acad Orthop Surg* 1999;7:44–53.

Tarsal Coalition

Blakemore LC, Cooperman DR, Thompson GH: The rigid flatfoot: Tarsal coalitions. *Foot Ankle Clin* 1998;3:609–31.

Bhone WH: Tarsal coalition. *Curr Opin Pediatr* 2001;13:29–35.

Cooperman DC, Janke BE, Gilmore A, et al: A three-dimensional study of calcaneonavicular tarsal coalitions. *J Pediatr Orthop* 2001;21:648–51.

Puncture Wounds of the Foot

Laughlin TJ, Armstrong DJ, Caporusso J: Soft-tissue and bone infections from puncture wounds in children. *West J Med* 1997;166:126–28.

Adolescent Bunions

Coughlin MJ: Roger A. Mann Award: Juvenile hallux valgus: Etiology and treatment. *Foot Ankle Int* 1995;16:682–97.

Thompson GH: Instructional Course Lecture: Bunions and deformities of the toes in children and adolescents. *J Bone Joint Surg Am* 1995;77:1924–36.

Curly Toes

Hamer AJ, Stanley D, Smith TW: Surgery for curly toe deformity: A double-blind, randomized, prospective trial. *J Bone Joint Surg Br* 1993;75:662–63.

Ross ERS, Menelaus MB: Open flexor tenotomy for hammer and curly toes in children. *J Bone Joint Surg Br* 1984;66:770–71.

Overlapping Fifth Toe

Black GB, Grogan DP, Bobechko WP: Butler arthroplasty for correction of the adducted fifth toe: A retrospective study of 36 operations between 1968 and 1982. *J Pediatr Orthop* 1985;5:439–41.

DeBoeck H: Butler's operation for congenital overriding of the fifth toe: Retrospective 1–7 year study of 23 cases. *Acta Orthop Scand* 1993;64:343–44.

Polydactyly

Morley SE, Smith PJ: Polydactyly of the feet in children: Suggestions for surgical management. *Br J Plast Surg* 2001;54:34–8.

Mubarak SJ, O'Brien TJ, Davids JR: Metatarsal epiphyseal bracket: Treatment by central physiolysis. *J Pediatr Orthop* 1993;13:5–8.

Nogami H: Polydactyly and polysyndactyly of the fifth toe. *Clin Orthop* 1986;204:216–65.

Venn-Watson EA: Problems in polydactyly of the foot. *Orthop Clin North Am* 1976;7:909–27.

Hammer Toe

Ross ER, Menelaus MB: Open flexor tenotomy for hammer toes and curly toes in childhood. *J Bone Joint Surg Br* 1984;66:770–71.

Mallet Toe

Tachdjian MO: *Pediatric Orthopedics.* Philadelphia, WB Saunders, 1992, pp 2670–2671.

Claw Toe

Coughlin MJ, Mann RA: Lesser toe deformities. In Mann RA (editor): *Surgery of the Foot.* St. Louis, CV Mosby, 1986, pp 132–148.

Myerson MS, Shereff MJ: The pathological anatomy of claw and hammer toes. *J Bone Joint Surg Am* 1989;71:45–49.

Annular Bands

Hennigan SP, Kuo KN: Resistant talipes equinovarus associated with congenital construction band syndrome. *J Pediatr Orthop* 2000;20:240–5.

McGuirk CK, Westgate MN, Holmes LB: Limb deficiencies in newborn infants. *Pediatrics* 2001;108:E64.

Tada K, Yanenobu K, Swanson A: Congenital constriction band syndrome. *J Pediatr Orthop* 1984;4:726–30.

Subungual Exostoses

Lokiec F, Ezra E, Krasin D, et al: A simple and efficient surgical technique for subungual exostosis. *J Pediatr Orthop* 2001;21:76–9.

Multhopp-Stephens H, Walling AK: Subungual (Dupuytren's) exostosis. *J Pediatr Orthop* 1995;15:582–84.

Ingrown Toenail

Kensinger DR, Guille JT, Horn D, et al: The stubbed great toe: Importance of early recognition and treatment of open fractures of the distal phalanx. *J Pediatr Orthop* 2001;21:31–34.

Reyzelman AM, Trumbello KA, Vayser DJ, et al: *Arch Fam Med* 2000;9:930–32.

Zuber TJ, Pfenninger JL: Management of ingrown toenails. *Am Fam Physician* 1995;52:181–190.

Shoes

Staheli LT: Instructional Course Lecture: Footwear for children. *Am Acad Orthop Surg* 1994;43:193–97.

Staheli LT: Psychosocial development and corrective shoe wear use in childhood. *J Pediatr Orthop* 1998;18:346–49.

Wenger DR, Mauldin D, Speck G, et al: Corrective shoes and inserts as treatment for a flexible flatfoot in infants and children. *J Bone Joint Surg Am* 1989;71:800–10.

Chapter 665
Torsional and Angular Deformities

George H. Thompson

665.1 Normal Developmental Alignment

The most common torsion and angular changes of the lower extremity are related to normal in utero positioning or acquired disorders.

In the typical in utero position, the hips are flexed, abducted, and externally rotated; the knees are flexed and the lower legs are internally rotated; and the feet are in slight equinus, supinated, and in contact with the posterolateral aspect of the opposite thigh. The combination of external rotation of the hip and internal rotation of the lower leg produces a bowed appearance of the lower extremities when the child begins to ambulate. This is not true bowing but rather a torsional combination. *Physiologic genu varum* or bowlegs resolves with 6–12 mo of independent ambulation.

Physiologic genu valgum or knock-knees is seen between 3 and 4 yr of age. This is true genu valgum and not the result of a torsional combination. This, too, resolves with growth, with the normal adult knee alignment obtained between 5 and 8 yr of age. The mean tibiofemoral angle at birth is 15 degrees of varus (Fig. 665–1). This decreases to approximately 10 degrees by 1 yr of age. Neutral alignment occurs between 18 and 20 mo of age. The maximal valgus of 12 degrees occurs at 3–4 yr of age. The values are similar for boys and girls. By 7 yr, the valgus alignment corrects to that of a normal adult (8 degrees in women; 7 degrees in men). Overall, 95% of developmental physiologic genu varum and genu valgum cases resolve with growth. This is also true for children with more pronounced physiologic varus or valgus, although some may not be completely corrected until adolescence.

TORSIONAL PROFILE

The torsional profile is beneficial in diagnosing and monitoring children with torsional variations (Fig. 665–2). The profile includes (1) foot progression angle, (2) hip rotation in extension, (3) thigh-foot angle, and (4) shape of the foot.

Foot Progression Angle. The foot progression angle represents the long axis of the foot with respect to the direction in which the child is walking (Fig. 665–3). Inward rotation is given a negative value, and outward rotation is given a positive value. A normal foot progression angle in children and adolescents is 10 degrees (range, –3 to 20 degrees). The foot progression angle serves only to define whether there is an in-toeing or out-toeing gait. The latter is considered abnormal when this angle exceeds 20 degrees.

Hip Rotation. Hip rotation in extension is assessed with the child prone, the thighs together, and the knees flexed 90 degrees (Fig. 665–4). In this position, the hip is in neutral alignment. As the lower leg is rotated outward, this produces internal rotation of the hip, whereas inward rotation produces external rotation. This is due to the anatomic shape of the proximal femur. The femoral neck normally has a 135-degree angle with the femoral shaft and 15 degrees of anterior rotation between femoral neck axis and the transcondylar axis of the distal femur. This angulation is known as femoral anteversion. By 1 yr of age there is approximately 45 degrees of internal and external rotation. Hip rotation should be symmetric. Asymmetric rotation may be indicative of a hip disorder, and radiographs of the pelvis are necessary.

Thigh-Foot Angle. With the child in the prone position for assessment of hip rotation, the long axis of the foot in the simulated weight-bearing position can be compared with the long axis of the thigh (Fig. 665–5). Inward rotation is given a negative value, and outward rotation is given a positive value. Inward rotation indicates internal tibial torsion, whereas outward rotation represents external tibial torsion. Infants have a mean angle of –5 degrees (range, –35 to 40 degrees) as a consequence of normal in utero position. In middle childhood through adult life, the mean thigh-foot angle is 10 degrees (range, –5 to 30 degrees).

Foot Shape. With the child still in the prone position, the shape of the foot is easily assessed (Fig. 665–6). This position is helpful in the assessment of metatarsus adductus or a calcaneovalgus foot. The mobility of the ankle and subtalar region can also be evaluated with the child in this position.

TORSIONAL DEFORMITIES

The common causes of in-toeing and out-toeing are presented in Table 663–4.

665.2 ▪ Internal Femoral Torsion

Internal femoral torsion is the most common cause of in-toeing in children 2 yr of age or older. It occurs more commonly in girls than boys (2:1). The majority of children with this condition have generalized ligamentous laxity. The cause of femoral torsion is controversial. Some believe that it is congenital and a result of persistent infantile femoral anteversion, whereas others believe it is acquired secondary to abnormal sitting habits.

Clinical Manifestations. Clinical features of internal femoral torsion demonstrate that the entire lower leg is inwardly rotated during gait. Characteristically, there will be 80–90 degrees of internal rotation of the hip in the prone position (torsional profile). External rotation, as a consequence, is limited to 0–10 degrees (Fig. 665–7). There will be features of generalized ligamentous laxity, including elbow and finger hyperextension, thumb hyperabduction, knee recurvatum, and hypermobile pes planus. Affected children commonly sit in the "television" or "W" style position. It is believed that this position allows the lower leg to act as a lever, thereby producing torsional changes in the "biologically plastic" femora. This condition is also called femoral anteversion, implying an abnormality of the proximal femur. However, the torsion actually occurs throughout the femoral shaft and results in a change in the normal alignment between the hip and the knee.

Radiographic Evaluation. Radiographic evaluation of internal femoral torsion is not routinely necessary, although a variety of radiographic techniques to measure femoral torsion have been described. CT and ultrasonography can assess the relationship between the proximal and distal femur. These studies are rarely indicated because the clinical measurements are equally accurate.

Treatment. The treatment of internal femoral torsion is predominantly by observation. Correction of abnormal sitting habits usually allows the torsion to resolve with normal growth and development. It takes 1–3 yr for complete correction to occur, depending on the age of the child when the sitting habits are corrected. The correction of sitting habits can be difficult in preschool-aged children and usually does not occur until they reach school age. The use of nighttime orthoses or daytime twister cables is of no value and may produce a compensatory external tibial torsion. The combination of internal femoral and compensatory external tibial torsion produces a pathologic genu valgum deformity. This can result in patellofemoral malalignment with patella subluxation or dislocation and pain.

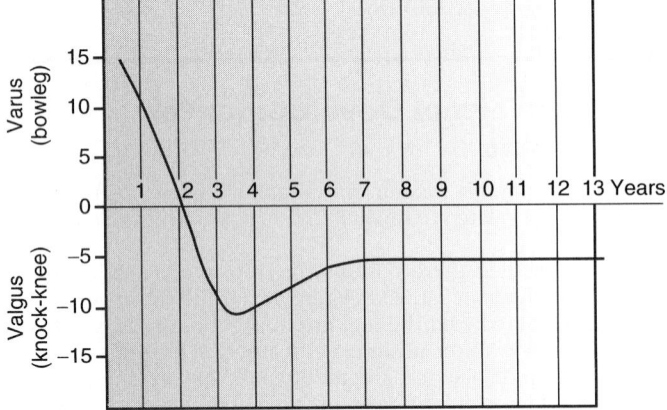

FIGURE 665–1. Graph demonstrating the normal development of the tibiofemoral or knee angle during growth. (Adapted from Salenius P, Vankka E: The development of the tibiofemoral angle in children. *J Bone Joint Surg Am* 1975;57A:259.)

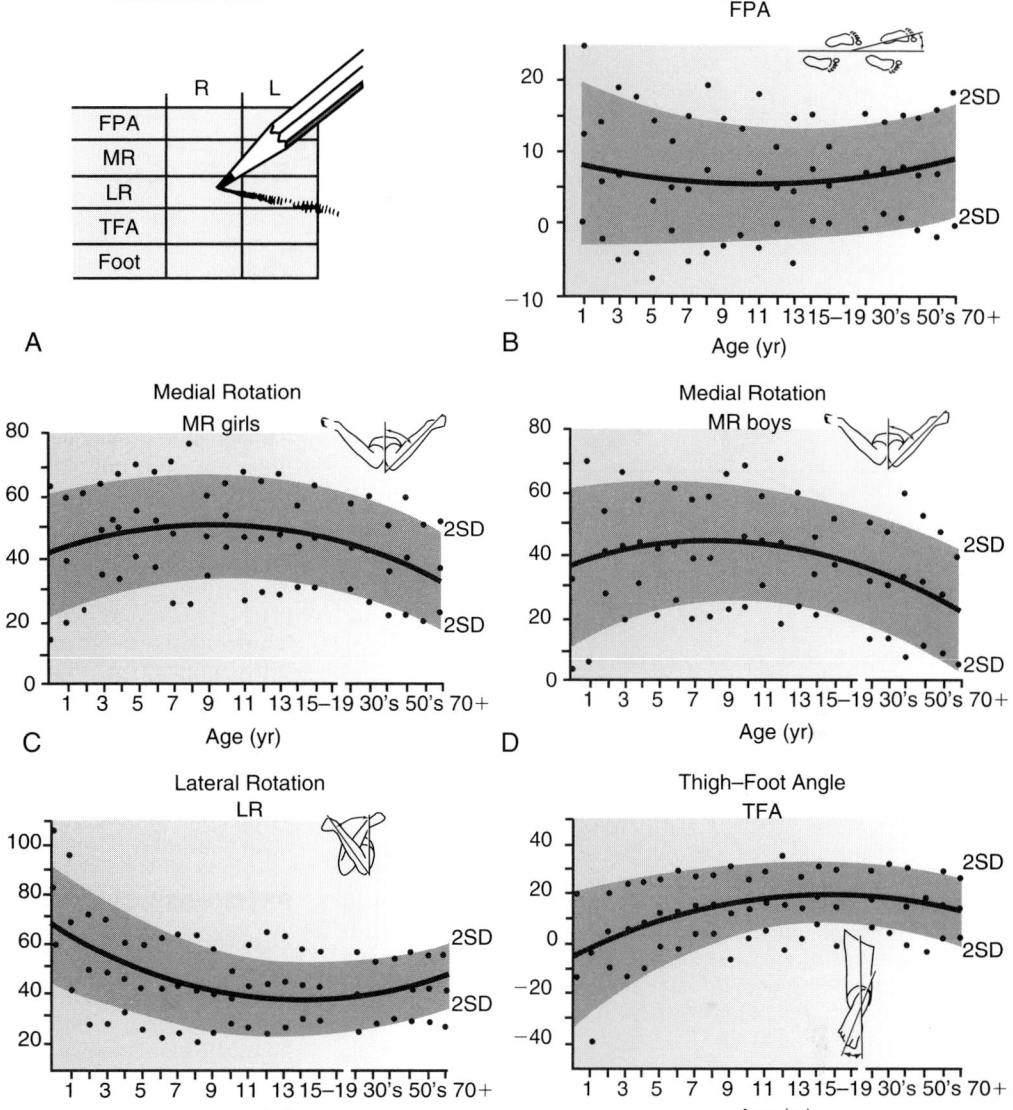

FIGURE 665–2. Range of normal values by age and sex with respect to the alignment of the lower extremity. *A*, Torsional profile. *B*, Foot progression angle (FPA) to determine the degree of in-toeing and out-toeing during ambulation. *C* and *D*, Medial (MR) or internal rotation of the hips in girls (*C*) and boys (*D*). *E*, Lateral (LR) or external rotation of the hips. *F*, Thigh-foot angle (TFA) to determine the degree of tibial torsion. Internal or medial tibial torsion is present if the angle is more than 20–30 degrees. (From Staheli LT: Torsional deformities. *Pediatr Clin North Am* 1986;33:1373.)

Children 10 yr of age or older may not have enough remaining musculoskeletal growth for spontaneous correction to occur, and surgical intervention may be necessary. The procedures advocated include proximal femoral varus derotation osteotomy and simple derotation osteotomy of either the proximal or the distal femur. Sufficient derotation is performed to allow equal internal and external hip rotation postoperatively.

665.3 Internal Tibial Torsion

Internal tibial torsion is the most common cause of in-toeing in children younger than 2 yr and is secondary to normal in utero positioning. This condition is commonly seen during the 2nd year of life and may be associated with metatarsus adductus.

Clinical Manifestations. The degree of tibial torsion can be measured by the prone thigh-foot angle (torsional profile).

Radiographic Evaluation. Radiographic assessment is of no value in this predominantly clinical disorder.

Treatment. Treatment of internal tibial torsion is by observation. This is a physiologic condition, and spontaneous resolution with

normal growth and development can be anticipated. Significant improvement usually does not occur until the child begins to pull to stand and walk independently. Thereafter, it takes 6–12 mo and occasionally longer for complete correction to occur. Night splints are of no value and should be avoided. Persistent internal tibial torsion in an older child or adolescent may require surgical derotation; however, this rarely occurs.

665.4 External Femoral Torsion

External femoral torsion, also known as femoral retroversion, is an uncommon disorder unless associated with a slipped capital femoral epiphysis (SCFE) (see Chapter 668.4).

Clinical Manifestations. The clinical examination of external femoral torsion shows excessive hip external rotation and limitation of internal rotation. Typically, the hip will externally rotate 70–90 degrees, whereas internal rotation is only 0–20 degrees (torsional profile). When idiopathic, it is usually a bilateral disorder. If the deformity is unilateral, especially in an obese older child or young adolescent, the presence of an SCFE must be considered.

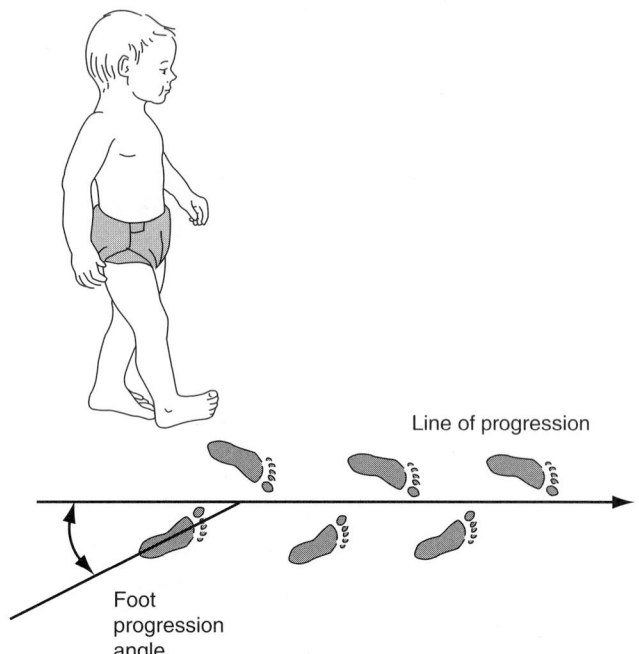

FIGURE 665–3. Foot progression angle. The long axis of the foot is compared with the direction in which the child is walking. If the long axis of the foot is directed outwardly, the angle is positive. If the foot is directed inwardly, the angle is negative and is indicative of in-toeing. (From Thompson GH: Gait disturbances. In Kliegman RM [editor]: *Practical Strategies in Pediatric Diagnosis and Therapy.* Philadelphia, WB Saunders, 1996.)

Radiographic Evaluation. Anteroposterior and Lauenstein (frog) lateral radiographs of the pelvis are necessary in any child or adolescent presenting with external femoral torsion, especially those who are obese or who have nontraumatic anterior thigh or knee pain (referred pain) or when the deformity is unilateral, to assess for a possible SCFE.

Treatment. The treatment of idiopathic external femoral torsion is usually observation because it ordinarily causes no significant functional impairment. An SCFE is treated surgically, and any proximal femoral retroversion improves with remodeling during subsequent growth.

Occasionally, persistent femoral retroversion after SCFE can produce functional impairment such as a severe out-toe gait and difficulty opposing one's knees in the sitting position. The latter can be disabling to adolescent females. Should this occur, a derotation osteotomy is beneficial.

665.5 External Tibial Torsion

External tibial torsion is a relatively common disorder and is frequently associated with a calcaneovalgus foot. It is secondary to a normal variation in in utero positioning.

Clinical Manifestations. External tibial torsion is indicated by an abnormally positive thigh-foot angle (torsional profile), typically 30–50 degrees. There is a calcaneovalgus foot (Fig. 665–8).

Radiographic Evaluation. Radiographic assessment for external tibial torsion is not necessary because there is no demonstrable radiographic abnormality.

Treatment. The treatment of external tibial torsion is observation. This condition follows the same clinical course as that of internal tibial torsion. Significant improvement does not occur during the 1st yr of life. However, with the onset of independent ambulation, spontaneous improvement begins to occur and is typically complete by 2–3 yr of age.

665.6 Genu Varum (Bowlegs)

The classification of genu varum is presented in Box 665–1. Physiologic genu varum and tibia vara (Blount disease) are the most common disorders.

PHYSIOLOGIC GENU VARUM

Physiologic bowlegs is a common torsional combination that is secondary to normal in utero positioning (Fig. 665–9). The tight posterior hip capsule results in an external rotation contracture. When it is combined with internal tibial torsion, it gives the clinical appearance of a bowleg deformity. Because it is physiologic, spontaneous resolution with normal growth and development can be anticipated. Significant improvement does occur during the 1st yr of life. By 2 yr of age, the majority of children have straight or neutrally aligned lower extremities.

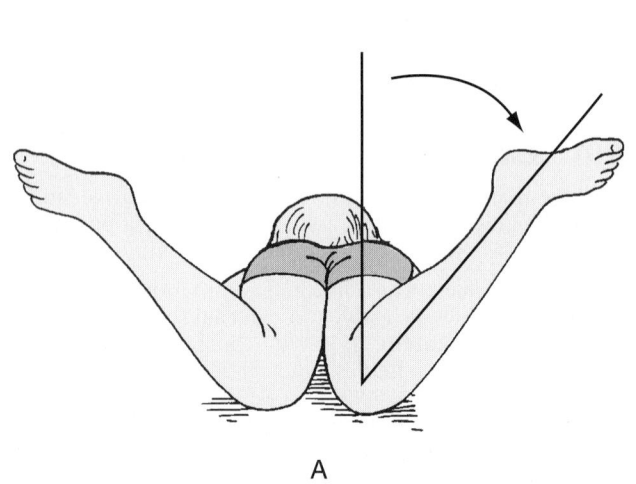

A

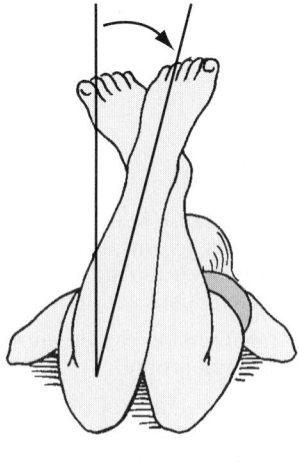

B

FIGURE 665–4. Hip rotation in extension. This is measured with the child in the prone position and the knee flexed 90 degrees. The lower leg is vertically oriented. This is considered the neutral position. On outward rotation *(A)*, the leg produces internal hip rotation; and on inward rotation *(B)*, the leg produces external hip rotation. (From Thompson GH: Gait disturbances. In Kliegman RM [editor]: *Practical Strategies in Pediatric Diagnosis and Therapy.* Philadelphia, WB Saunders, 1996.)

FIGURE 665–5. Thigh-foot angle. With the child in the prone position and the knees flexed and approximated, the long axis of the foot can be compared with the long axis of the thigh. The long axis of the foot bisects the heel and the second toe or lies between the second and third toes. External tibial torsion *(A)* produces excessive outward rotation. Normal alignment *(B)* is characterized by slight external rotation. Internal tibial torsion produces inward rotation of the foot and is a negative angle *(C)*. (From Thompson GH: Gait disturbances. In Kliegman RM, Nieder ML, Super DM [editors]: *Practical Strategies in Pediatric Diagnosis and Therapy.* Philadelphia, WB Saunders, 1996.)

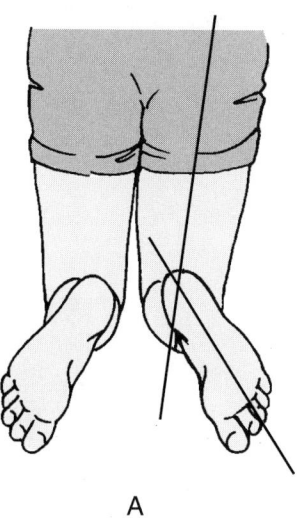
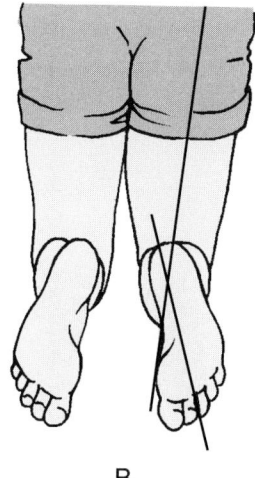
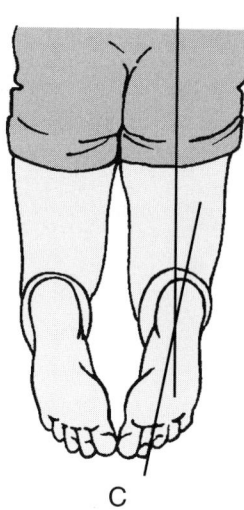

A   B   C

TIBIA VARA

Idiopathic tibia vara, or Blount disease, is an uncommon disorder characterized by abnormal growth of the medial aspect of the proximal tibial epiphysis, resulting in progressive varus angulation below the knee. Tibia vara can occur in any age group in a growing child and is classified as infantile (1–3 yr), juvenile (4–10 yr), and adolescent (11 yr or older). The juvenile and adolescent forms are commonly combined as late-onset tibia vara. All three groups share common characteristics, whereas the radiographic changes in the late-onset groups are less pronounced than those in the infantile form. Although the exact cause of tibia vara remains unknown, it appears to be secondary to growth suppression from increased compressive forces across the medial aspect of the knee.

Clinical Manifestations. The infantile form of tibia vara is the most common; its characteristics include female and black predominance, marked obesity, approximately 80% bilateral involvement, a prominent medial metaphyseal beak, internal tibial torsion, and leg-length discrepancy. The characteristics of the juvenile and adolescent forms (late-onset) include male and black predominance, marked obesity, normal or greater than normal height, approximately 50% bilateral involvement, slowly progressive genu varum deformity, pain rather than deformity as the primary initial complaint, no palpable proximal medial metaphyseal beak, minimal internal tibial torsion, mild medial collateral ligament laxity, and mild lower extremity length discrepancy. The differences among the three groups appear to be primarily due to age at onset, the amount of growth remaining, and the magnitude of the medial compression forces. The infantile group has the potential for the greatest deformity, and the adolescent group has the least.

Radiographic Evaluation. Children with tibia vara are usually assessed radiographically with an anteroposterior standing radiograph of both lower extremities and a lateral radiograph of the involved extremity. Positioning the child in weight-bearing stance allows maximal presentation of the clinical deformity. The metaphyseal-diaphyseal angle can be measured and is useful in distinguishing between physiologic genu varum and early tibia vara. The latter is difficult to diagnose radiographically before 2 yr of age. Fragmentation with a protuberant step deformity and beaking of the proximal medial tibial metaphysis are the major features of the infantile group. The changes in the proximal medial tibial metaphysis are less conspicuous in the late-onset forms, which are characterized by wedging of the medial portion of the epiphysis, a mild posteromedial articular depression, a serpiginous cephalad curved physis, and mild or no fragmentation or beaking of the proximal medial metaphysis (Fig. 665–10).

Occasionally, arthrography, MRI, or CT may be necessary to assess the meniscus, the articular surface of the proximal tibia, or the integrity of the proximal tibial physis. These tests are usually reserved for the more severe deformities.

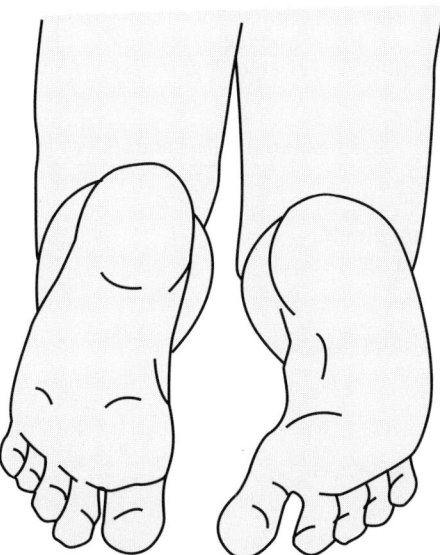

FIGURE 665–6. Foot shape. Using the same position for measurement of the thigh-foot angle, the shape of the foot can also be evaluated. In this illustration, the left foot has normal alignment, whereas the right foot demonstrates metatarsus adductus. (From Thompson GH: Gait disturbances. In Kliegman RM [editor]: *Practical Strategies in Pediatric Diagnosis and Therapy.* Philadelphia, WB Saunders, 1996.)

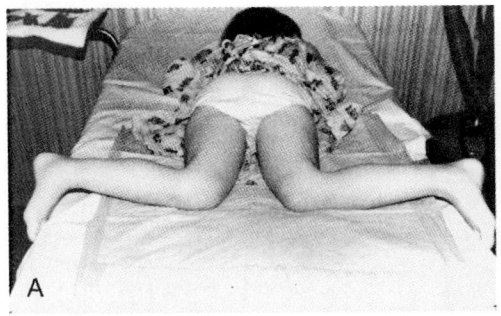

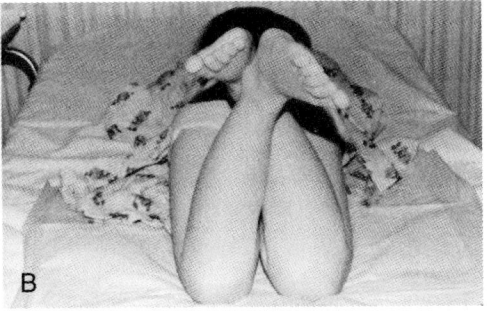

FIGURE 665–7. *A,* A 5-yr-old girl with bilateral internal femoral torsion. She has approximately 80 degrees of internal rotation bilaterally. *B,* External rotation is limited to approximately 15 degrees for a total arc of hip rotation of 90–95 degrees. (From Thompson GH: Gait disturbances. In Kliegman RM [editor]: *Practical Strategies in Pediatric Diagnosis and Therapy.* Philadelphia, WB Saunders, 1996.)

FIGURE 665–8. *A,* A 6-mo-old girl with an excessive external tibial torsion. This reverse, or anterior, thighfoot angle shows approximately 50 degrees of external tibial torsion. *B,* The same infant demonstrates a calcaneovalgus foot with forefoot abduction and increased hindfoot valgus. There is also hyperdorsiflexibility of the foot in the ankle mortise. (From Thompson GH: Gait disturbances. In Kliegman RM [editor]: *Practical Strategies in Pediatric Diagnosis and Therapy.* Philadelphia, WB Saunders, 1996.)

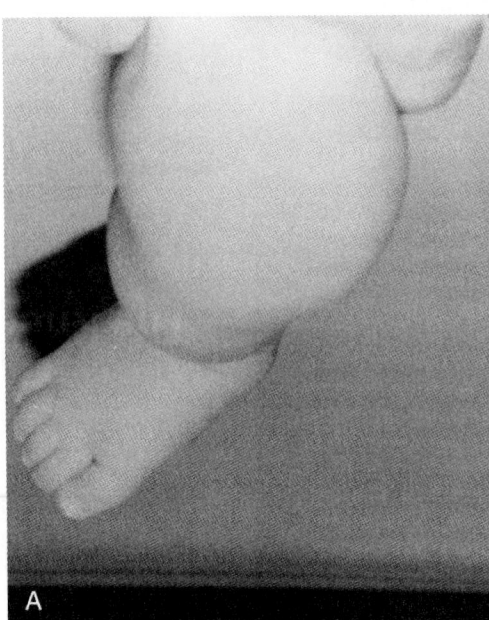

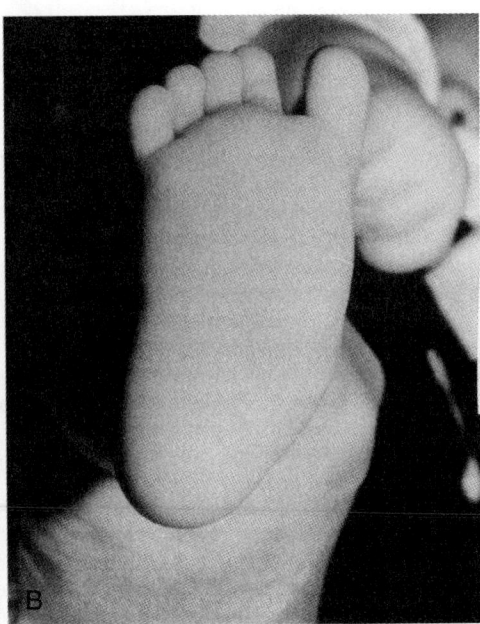

Treatment. The management of tibia vara may be both nonoperative and operative in the infantile form. Late-onset tibia vara is managed operatively.

NONOPERATIVE. Orthotic management can be considered for children with infantile tibia vara who are 3 yr of age or younger with mild deformities. In approximately 50% of children meeting these criteria, the deformity may be adequately corrected. A knee-ankle-foot orthosis should be used with a single medial upright, without a knee hinge. Pads and straps should be placed over the distal femur and proximal tibia to apply a valgus force. The orthosis should be worn 22–23 hr each day. A maximal trial of 1 yr of orthotic management is currently recommended. If complete correction is not obtained after 1 yr or if progression occurs during this time, a corrective osteotomy is indicated.

OPERATIVE. The indications for surgical treatment of infantile tibia vara include age of 4 yr or more, failure of orthotic management, and more severe deformities. Proximal tibial valgus osteotomy and associated fibular diaphyseal osteotomy are usually the procedures of choice (Fig. 665–11). In late-onset tibia vara, correction is also necessary to restore the mechanical axis of the knee. The same surgical options as presented for older children with infantile tibia vara are applicable in these age groups. A proximal tibial valgus osteotomy and diaphyseal fibular osteotomy are the most common procedures.

665.7 Genu Valgum (Knock-Knees)

The classification of genu valgum is presented in Box 665–2. Fortunately, the pathologic causes, with the exception of post-

traumatic disorders, are uncommon. As the spontaneous correction of physiologic bowlegs continues, there is typically an overcorrection, of variable degree, into mild genu valgum,

---

BOX 665–1. Classification of Genu Varum (Bowlegs)

PHYSIOLOGIC
ASYMMETRIC GROWTH

Tibia vara (Blount disease)
   Infantile
   Juvenile
   Adolescent
Focal fibrocartilaginous dysplasia
Physeal Injury
   Trauma
   Infection
   Tumor

METABOLIC DISORDERS

Vitamin D deficiency (nutritional rickets)
Vitamin D–resistant rickets
Hypophosphatasia

SKELETAL DYSPLASIA

Metaphyseal dysplasia
Achondroplasia
Enchondromatosis

Modified from Thompson GH: Angular deformities of the lower extremities. In Chapman MW (editor): *Operative Orthopedics,* 2nd ed. Philadelphia, JB Lippincott, 1993, pp 3131–164.

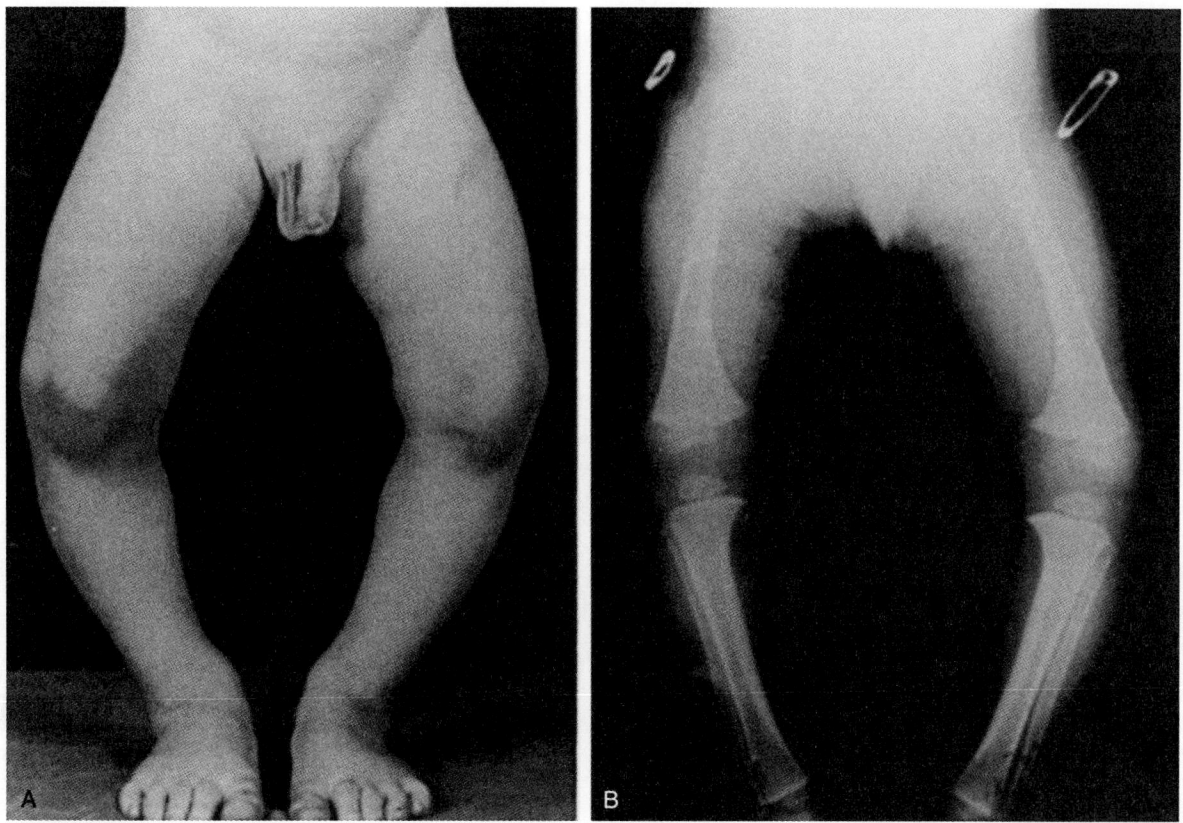

FIGURE 665–9. Infant with bilateral genu varum at 18 mo of age. This resolved spontaneously before 7 yr of age. *A,* Clinical photograph. *B,* Standing anteroposterior radiograph of the lower extremities. (From Tachdjian MO: *Pediatric Orthopedics,* 2nd ed. Philadelphia, WB Saunders, 1990.)

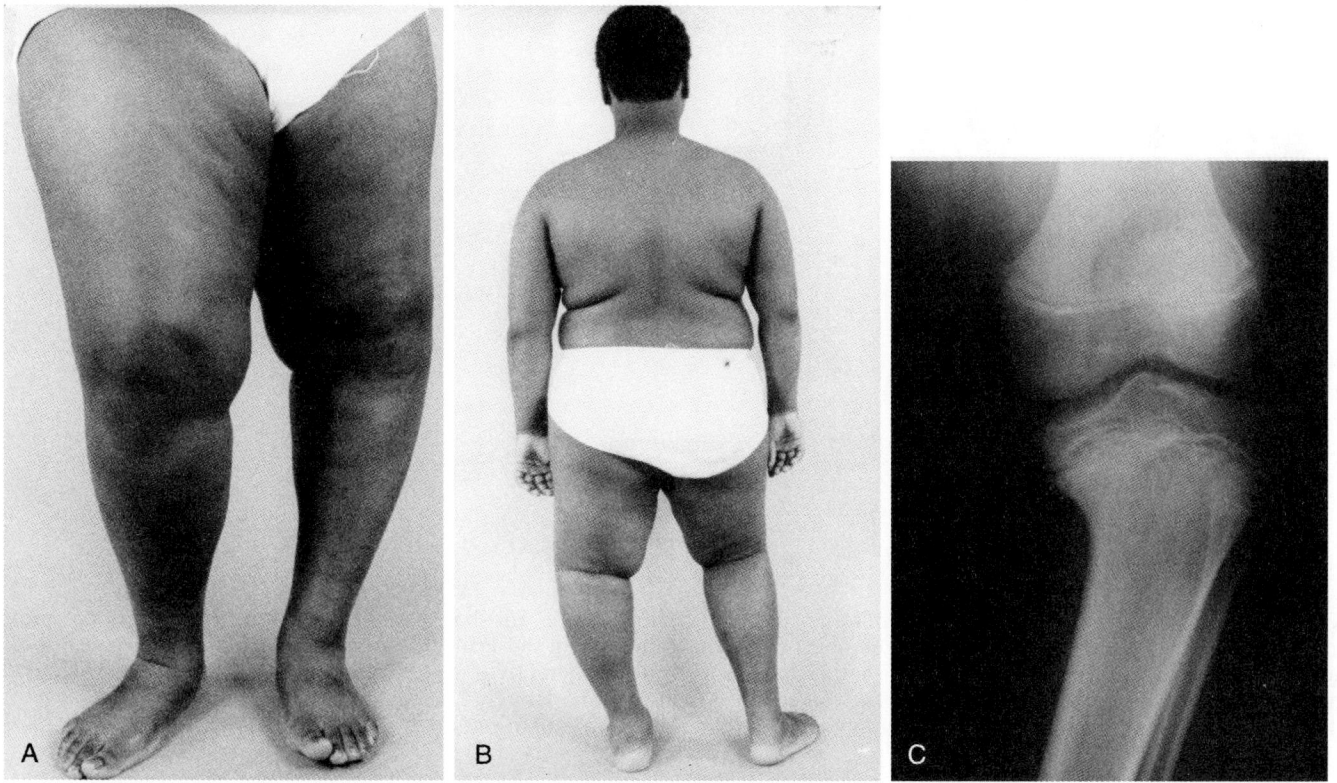

FIGURE 665–10. *A,* A 13-yr-old boy with late-onset, or adolescent, tibia vara. There is marked obesity and mild genu varum deformity of the left knee. *B,* Posterior view of the same child. *C,* Standing anteroposterior radiograph of the left knee demonstrating the tibia vara deformity but with less obvious changes than in the infantile form. The medial aspect of the proximal tibial epiphysis is narrow and the growth plate is irregular. The typical metaphyseal "beaking" is not present.

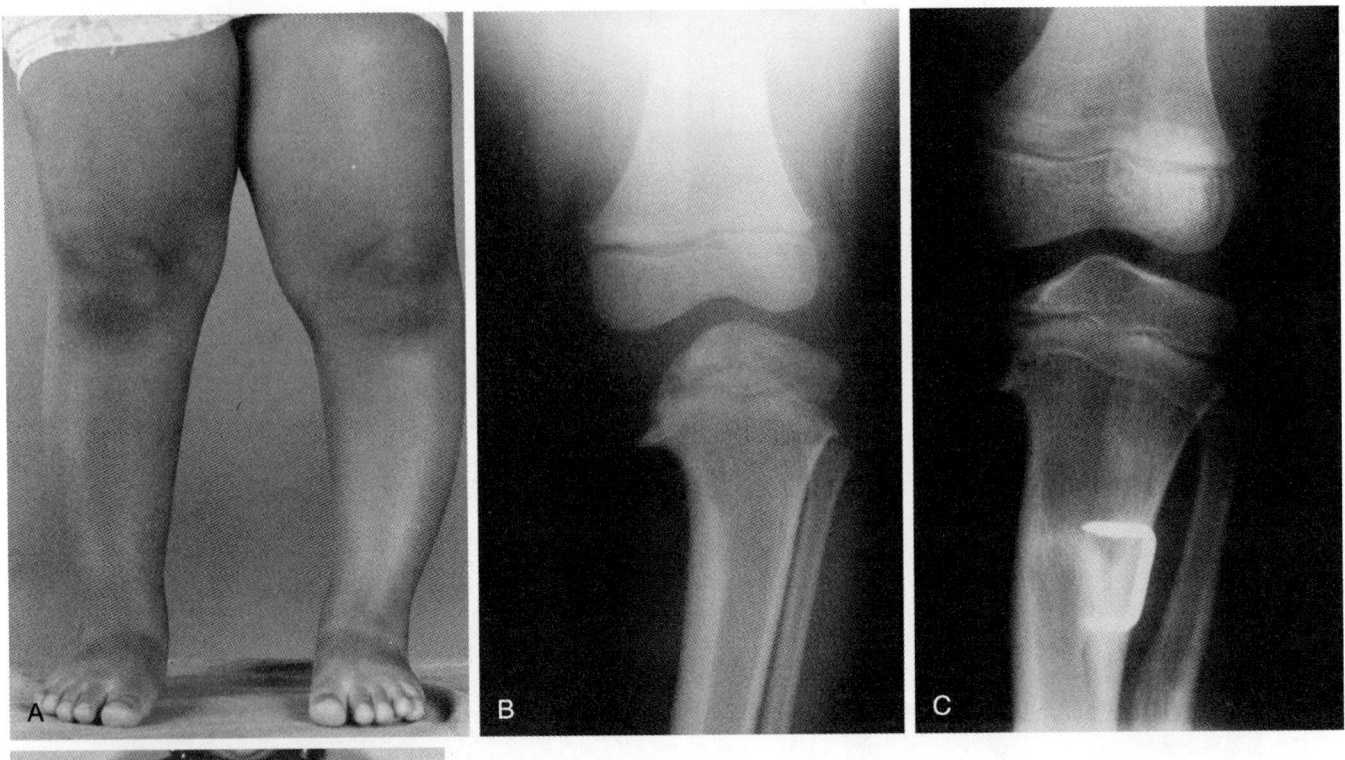

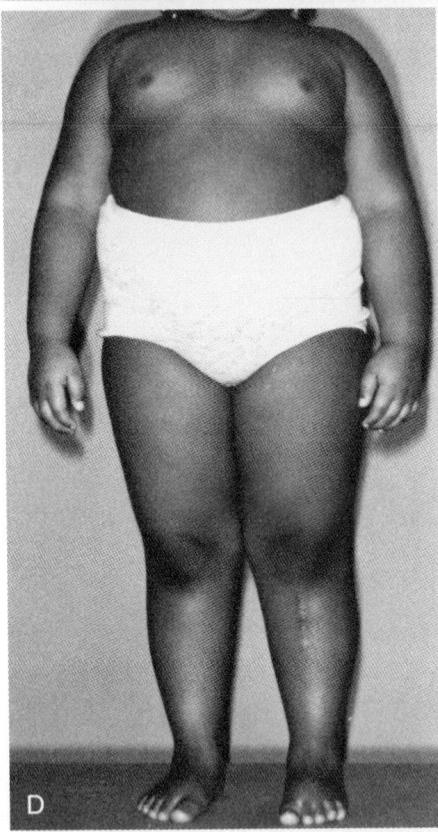

FIGURE 665–11. *A,* A 4-yr-old girl with infantile tibia vara. She is obese and has a moderate left genu varum deformity. *B,* Anteroposterior radiograph of the left knee demonstrating the genu varum deformity. There is narrowing and irregularity of the medial aspect of the proximal tibial epiphysis and beaking of the medial metaphysis. *C,* Repeat radiograph 2 yr after proximal tibial and diaphyseal fibular corrective osteotomy. The osteotomy is healed, and relatively normal growth is occurring in the proximal tibial epiphysis. *D,* Postoperative clinical photograph demonstrating symmetric alignment of the lower extremities.

or knock-knees. This physiologic angular variation is commonly seen between 3 and 5 yr of age. It is a true angular deformity that resolves spontaneously, with normal knee alignment being attained between 5 and 8 yr. Rarely is a knock-

knee orthosis indicated. Surgery may be required in adolescence for a persistent deformity. Options include medial physeal stapling, medial hemiepiphysiodesis, and corrective osteotomy.

PHYSIOLOGIC
ASYMMETRIC GROWTH
　Tibia valga
　Physeal injury
　Trauma after fracture of the proximal tibial metaphysis
　Infection
　Tumor

METABOLIC DISORDERS
　Renal osteodystrophy

SKELETAL DYSPLASIA
　Kniest syndrome

CONGENITAL ABNORMALITIES
　Congenital dislocation of the patella

NEUROMUSCULAR DISORDERS
　Cerebral palsy
　Myelodysplasia

From Thompson GH: Angular deformities of the lower extremities. In Chapman MW (editor): *Operative Orthopedics*, 2nd ed. Philadelphia, JB Lippincott, 1993, pp 3131–164.

665.8 Congenital Angular Deformities of the Tibia and Fibula

The differential diagnosis of congenital angular deformities of the lower leg (Box 665–3) includes posteromedial angulation, which is a benign process, and anterolateral angulation, which is a pathologic process.

Congenital Posteromedial Tibial Angulation (Bowing). This is an uncommon angular deformity that involves the distal one third of the tibia and fibula. There is a posteromedial bowing in association with a calcaneovalgus foot. The clinical appearance can be dramatic. The diagnosis is confirmed radiographically and shows the posteromedial angulation without other osseous abnormalities. A significant portion of the calcaneovalgus foot is due to the position of the distal tibia and ankle.

The *cause* of the congenital posteromedial bowing is unknown. The natural history is characterized by spontaneous resolution by 3–5 yr of age. However, there is residual shortening in the tibia and fibula. The fibula is usually slightly shorter than the tibia. The mean growth inhibition is 12–13% (range, 5–27%). The mean leg-length discrepancy at maturity is 4 cm (3–7 cm).

The *treatment* of congenital posteromedial bowing of the tibia and fibula is observation. All components of the deformity with the exception of leg-length inequality resolve with growth and development. The child should have periodic radiographic leg-length measurements to determine the degree of discrepancy and to predict the maximal discrepancy at maturity. This also

BOX 665–3. Differential Diagnosis of Congenital Angular Deformities of the Tibia and Fibula

POSTEROMEDIAL ANGULATION
ANTEROLATERAL ANGULATION
　Congenital pseudoarthrosis of the tibia
　Congenital longitudinal deficiency of the tibia (paraxial tibial hemimelia)
　Congenital longitudinal deficiency of the fibula (paraxial fibular hemimelia)

Modified from Thompson GH: Angular deformities of the lower extremities. In Chapman MW (editor): *Operative Orthopedics*, 2nd ed. Philadelphia, JB Lippincott, 1993, pp 3131–164.

allows information regarding the appropriate age for surgical intervention. Operative intervention for a defect other than leg-length discrepancy is rarely indicated. A corrective osteotomy may be necessary in patients with severe deformity that is not improving with growth and development. Patients with discrepancies greater than 5 cm may be candidates for tibial lengthening.

Congenital Anterolateral Tibial Angulation (Bowing). This type of bowing is associated with an underlying pathologic disorder (see Box 665–3). The diagnosis is made radiographically. *Congenital fibular hemimelia* represents a congenital absence of the fibula and usually the lateral portion of the foot, especially the fourth and fifth rays. *Congenital tibial hemimelia* represents a congenital absence of the tibia, either partial or total. Surgical reconstruction of these deformities is difficult, and most defects require amputation to achieve satisfactory function. *Congenital pseudoarthrosis* of the tibia is usually associated with neurofibromatosis. It represents a defect in the tibia that predisposes to pathologic fractures, which heal poorly. A variety of surgical techniques, including intramedullary rodding, electrical stimulation, and vascularized fibular transplants, have been used with varying success in this complex problem.

Internal and External Tibial and Femoral Torsion
Ruwe PA, Gage JR, Ozonoff MB, et al: Clinical determination of femoral anteversion: A comparison of established techniques. *J Bone Joint Surg Am* 1992;74A:820–30.
Staheli LT: Rotational problems in children. *Am Acad Orthop Surg Instr Course Lect* 1994;43:199–209.
Svenvingsen S, Terjesen T, Auflein M, et al: Hip rotation and in-toeing gait: A study of normal subjects from four years until adult age. *Clin Orthop* 1990;251:177–82.
Thompson GH: Gait disturbances. In Kliegman RM (editor): *Practical Strategies in Pediatric Diagnosis and Therapy*, 2nd ed. Philadelphia, WB Saunders, 2003.

Physiologic Genu Varum and Genu Valgum
Arazi M, Ogun TC, Memik R: Normal development of the tibiofemoral angle in children: A clinical study of 590 normal subjects from 3 to 17 years of age. *J Pediatr Orthop* 2001;21:264–67.
Cahuzac JPh, Vardon D, Sales de Gauzy J: Development of the clinical tibiofemoral angle in normal adolescents: A study of 427 normal subjects from 10 to 16 years of age. *J Bone Joint Surg Br* 1995;77B:729–32.
Do TT: Clinical and radiographic evaluation of bowlegs. *Curr Opin Pediatr* 2001;13:42–6.
Feldman MD, Schoenecker PL: Use of metaphyseal-diaphyseal angle in the evaluation of bowed legs. *J Bone Joint Surg Am* 1993;75:1602–9.
Heath CH, Staheli LT: Normal limits of knee angle in white children—genu varum and genu valgum. *J Pediatr Orthop* 1993;13:259–62.
Salenius P, Vankka E: The development of the tibiofemoral angle in children. *J Bone Joint Surg Am* 1975;57A:259–61.
Stevens PM, Maguire M, Dales MD, et al: Physeal stapling for idiopathic genu valgum. *J Pediatr Orthop* 1999;19:645–49.
Thompson GH: Angular deformities of the lower extremities in children. In Chapman MW (editor): *Operative Orthopedics*, 3rd ed. Philadelphia, JB Lippincott, 2001, pp 4287–4335.
Vankka E, Salenius P: Spontaneous correction of severe tibiofemoral deformity in growing children. *Acta Orthop Scand* 1982;53:567–70.

Tibia Vara
Davids JR, Blackhurst DW, Allen BL Jr: Radiographic evaluation of bowed legs in children. *J Pediatr Orthop* 2001;21:257–63.
Doyle BS, Volk G, Smith CI: Infantile Blount's disease: Long-term follow-up of surgically treated patients at skeletal maturity. *J Pediatr Orthop* 1996;16:469–76.
Greene WB: Instructional course lecture: Infantile tibia vara. *J Bone Joint Surg Am* 1993;75:130–43.
Henderson RC, Kemp GJ, Greene WB: Adolescent tibia vara: Alternatives for operative treatment. *J Bone Joint Surg Am* 1992;74:342–50.
Henderson RC, Kemp GJ, Hayes PRL: Prevalence of late-onset tibia vara. *J Pediatr Orthop* 1993;13:255–58.
Johnston CE II: Infantile tibia vara. *Clin Orthop* 1990;255:13–23.
Thompson GH, Carter JR: Late-onset tibia vara (Blount's disease): Current concepts. *Clin Orthop* 1990;255:24–35.
Zionts LE, Shean CJ: Brace treatment of early infantile tibia vara. *J Pediatr Orthop* 1998;18:102–9.

Congenital Posteromedial Tibial Bowing
Hofmann A, Wenger DR: Posteromedial bowing of the tibia: Progression of discrepancy in leg lengths. *J Bone Joint Surg Am* 1981;63:384–88.
Pappas AM: Congenital posteromedial bowing of the tibia and fibula. *J Pediatr Orthop* 1984;4:525–31.

Congenital Anterolateral Tibial Bowing
Truab JA, O'Connor W, Masso PD: Congenital pseudarthrosis of the tibia: A retrospective review. *J Pediatr Orthop* 1999;19:735–38.

Chapter 666
Leg-Length Discrepancy

George H. Thompson

Etiology. The common causes of leg (also called lower extremity)-length discrepancy are presented in Box 666–1.

Clinical Manifestations and Diagnosis. Signs and symptoms associated with leg-length discrepancy, other than limping, are usually related to the underlying cause. Approximately 65% of the growth of the entire lower extremity comes from the distal femoral (37%) and proximal tibial (28%) physes. Thus, growth disturbances around the knee can have the most adverse effect on leg length. Determination of the *skeletal, or bone, age* allows for a relatively accurate assessment of remaining growth. The *Gruelich and Pyle Atlas* (1950) remains the standard by which bone age is determined from an anteroposterior radiograph of the left hand and wrist. It is possible to estimate the *ultimate discrepancy at maturity* using growth-remaining tables such as the Moseley straight-line graph (Fig. 666–1) and the Green-Anderson table. The former, the most commonly used today, uses scanographic and bone age data to determine the ultimate discrepancy. It can also be used to follow the response of treatment. The clinical methods available are less accurate than the radiographic techniques, but they are useful. The most common clinical measurement is leveling the pelvis. Blocks of various thickness may be placed beneath the foot on the involved side until the iliac crests are level. The thickness indicates the amount of discrepancy.

Adult sitting height is approximately 52% of total height in the male and 53% in the female. Thus, two times the predicted length of the normal leg at maturity gives a close approximation of the *anticipated adult height*. This height plays an important role in determining equalization. Lengthening procedures are more applicable in predicted short adults, whereas shortening procedures are generally used for predicted normal height or taller

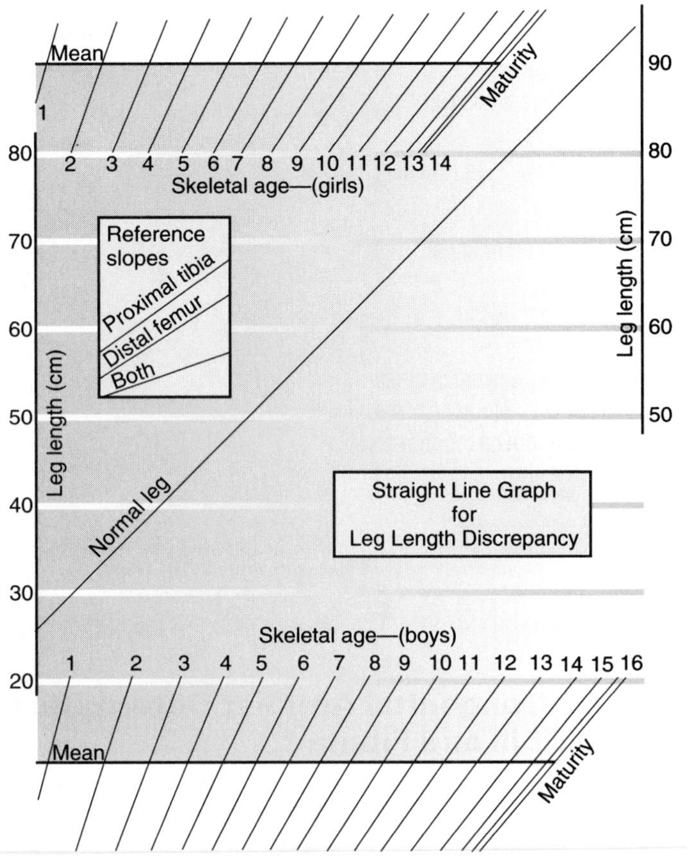

FIGURE 666–1. The Moseley straight-line graph for the assessment of leg-length inequalities. This allows simultaneous correlation of the normal leg, short leg, and bone age of the child. It will accurately predict lengths of each extremity at skeletal maturity. The reference slopes are used as a guide in determining when appropriate treatment should be performed.

individuals. In either case, acceptable body proportions must be maintained.

Children with *neuromuscular disorders* such as spastic hemiplegia benefit from 1–2 cm of shortening on the involved side to improve the swing phase of gait and increase toe clearance. Only extremities that are neurologically normal should be considered for equalization of leg lengths.

Angular deformities and coexistent joint abnormalities are important considerations in children with leg-length discrepancies. This is especially true when lengthening procedures are being considered. A child with a dysplastic acetabulum may subsequently experience a hip dislocation if femoral lengthening is attempted. Thus, any significant angular deformities or joint abnormalities should be corrected either before or simultaneously with leg-length equalization.

Radiographic Evaluation. Radiographic evaluations are the most accurate methods of assessing leg lengths. Four different types of radiographic techniques are available. The *teleoroentgenogram* is a single exposure of both lower extremities. Its primary indication is for young children, usually younger than 5 yr. There is a small amount of magnification error present, but it has the advantage of demonstrating any associated angular deformity. The *orthoroentgenogram* consists of three separate, slightly overlapping exposures of the hips, knees, and ankles on a long cassette. Bone length is measured directly on the radiograph. There is less magnification, and it is relatively accurate and demonstrates angular deformities. The *scanogram* is a simple, accurate method

---

BOX 666–1. Common Causes of Lower Extremity Length Discrepancies

CONGENITAL
Proximal femoral focal deficiency
Coxa vara
Hemiatrophy-hemihypertrophy (anisomelia)
Developmental dysplasia of the hip

DEVELOPMENTAL
Legg-Calvé-Perthes disease

NEUROMUSCULAR
Polio
Cerebral palsy (hemiplegia)

INFECTIOUS
Pyogenic osteomyelitis with physeal damage

TRAUMA
Physeal injury with premature closure
Overgrowth
Malunion (shortening)

TUMOR
Physeal destruction
Radiation-induced physeal injury
Overgrowth

Modified from Thompson GH: Gait disturbances. In Kliegman RM (editor): *Practical Strategies of Pediatric Diagnosis and Therapy.* Philadelphia, WB Saunders, 1996, pp 757–78.

of assessment. It consists of three narrow exposures of the hips, knees, and ankles on a standard cassette with a radiographic ruler laying next to the extremity. Thus, minimal magnification is present and accurate measurements can be made. However, angular deformities cannot be fully visualized and, if present, can lead to errors in measurement. CT is the most accurate technique and also shows angular deformity.

Treatment. The psychologic status of the child as well as that of the parents is an important consideration in treatment selection. Some equalization techniques are simple and safe, whereas others, especially lengthening procedures, are complex with high complication rates that require strict cooperation by the child and parents. Discrepancies of greater than 2 cm at skeletal maturity usually require treatment because these often cause the patient to limp. Equalization can be achieved by nonsurgical and surgical methods. In general, the goals are to maintain an appropriate adult height (5 ft 6 inches in males, 5 ft in females) and adequate body proportions. Shortening procedures are preferred, and lengthening procedures should be used cautiously.

ORTHOTICS AND PROSTHETICS. Orthotic devices are generally indicated for discrepancies between 2 and 3 cm in skeletally mature individuals. A heel lift is frequently all that is necessary to provide the patient with a normal gait. Because of normal pelvic rotation during the gait cycle, complete equalization is not necessary. The smallest lift that will allow the patient to walk without a limp is all that is necessary. Prostheses are necessary for severe discrepancies or uncorrectable deformities.

EXTREMITY SHORTENING PROCEDURES. Three procedures are used to shorten the longer extremity. *Epiphysiodesis* is indicated in children who have 5 cm or less predicted discrepancy at maturity, have adequate remaining growth for satisfactory correction, and have a predicted relatively normal, corrected adult height. It requires accurate timing to achieve equalization of the leg lengths at maturity. The disadvantages of epiphysiodesis include shortened stature, surgery on the unaffected extremity, the possibility of an angular growth deformity, and the irreversibility of the procedure itself. Percutaneous epiphysiodesis under fluoroscopic control is the most popular technique. This is an outpatient procedure that is effective and has a low complication rate. *Epiphyseal stapling* is performed to slow the rate of physeal growth. Three staples inserted extraperiosteally on each side of the physis are required to retard growth adequately. Once equalization has been achieved, the staples are removed, allowing normal growth to resume. Stapling on one side of the physis can be used to correct angular deformities around the knee. *Bone resection* is indicated for ultimate discrepancies of 5–6 cm in adults or adolescents who have inadequate remaining growth to undergo an epiphysiodesis. The femur can be shortened up to 6 cm and the tibia-fibula up to 3 cm before irreversible muscle weakness occurs.

EXTREMITY LENGTHENING PROCEDURES. The advantages of lengthening are equalization of significant leg-length discrepancies, maintenance of ultimate adult height, preservation of normal body proportions, surgery on the affected limb, correction of existing angular deformities, and elimination of orthoses. The disadvantages are that it is technically difficult to perform and has a significant complication rate. Common complications include pin tract infection, wound infection, hypertension, hip and knee subluxation, ankle equinus, loss of correction, delayed union, metal failure, and fatigue fractures after metal removal. *Transiliac or pelvic lengthening osteotomies* can provide a gain of up to 3 cm in length. These procedures are generally reserved for individuals with mild discrepancies who have ipsilateral shortening with acetabular dysplasia, an asymmetric pelvis, or possibly decompensated scoliosis. The callotasis technique allows progressive *lengthening of the femur or tibia.* An osteotomy is performed after application of an external fixator lengthening system. There is no initial lengthening. After

7–10 days, lengthening is begun at 1.0 mm/day (0.25 mm every 6 hr). This allows elongation of the forming callus. Significant lengthening of the bone can be achieved with this technique. Once the desired length has been achieved, the callus is allowed to consolidate. The lengthening device is removed after consolidation. The entire process requires approximately 1 mo per centimeter lengthened. The advantages of this procedure over previous lengthening techniques is that it requires only one procedure, allows greater lengthening, and has a lower complication rate. Occasionally, *a combination of a transiliac, femoral, or tibial diaphyseal lengthening and possibly leg-shortening procedures* such as epiphysiodesis is necessary to equalize leg lengths. The combination of femoral diaphyseal lengthening and contralateral epiphysiodeses is useful for discrepancies of 8–10 cm when a single lengthening is insufficient for complete correction.

Anderson M, Green WT, Messner M: Growth and predictions of growth in the lower extremities. *J Bone Joint Surg Am* 1963;45A:1–14.

Ballock RT, Weisner GL, Myers MT, et al: Current concepts. Hemihypertrophy: Concepts and controversies. *J Bone Joint Surg Am* 1997;79A:1731–38.

Dahl MT: Preoperative planning in deformity correction and limb lengthening surgery. *Am Acad Orthop Surg Instr Course Lect* 2000;49:503–9.

Gruelich WW, Pyle SI: *Radiographic Atlas of Skeletal Development of the Hand and Wrist,* 2nd ed. Stanford, CA, Stanford University Press, 1959.

Horton GA, Olney BW: Epiphysiodesis of the lower extremity: Results of the percutaneous technique. *J Pediatr Orthop* 1996;16:180–82.

Moseley CF: A straight line graph for leg-length discrepancies. *J Bone Joint Surg Am* 1977;59:174–79.

Paley D, Bhave A, Herzenberg JE, et al: Multiplier method for predicting limb-length discrepancy. *J Bone Joint Surg Am* 2000;82:1432–46.

Pritchett JW. Comparison of methods for prediction of lower-extremity growth. *J Bone Joint Surg Am* 2001;83A:1108–10.

Stanitski DF: Limb-length inequality: Assessment and treatment options. *J Am Acad Orthop Surg* 1999;7:143–53.

Yun AG, Severino R, Reinker K: Attempted limb lengthenings beyond twenty percent of the initial bone length: Results and complications. *J Pediatr Orthop* 2000;20:151–59.

Chapter 667
The Knee
George H. Thompson

The knee is a unique joint because the tibiofemoral articulation is constrained only by soft tissues rather than by geometric fit. The distal femur is cam-shaped, allowing it to have a gliding, hinged motion. The major constraints of the knee are the medial and lateral collateral ligaments, the anterior and posterior cruciate ligaments, and the medial and lateral menisci. Weight is transmitted through both the articular cartilage and the menisci. A second important area of the knee is the patellofemoral joint. It is the common site of problems especially in adolescence.

Pain around the knee is one of the most common presenting complaints in older children and adolescents. This may be insidious in onset or the result of trauma. *Accumulation of fluid* (effusion) in the knee indicates an abnormal intra-articular process. Fluid accumulating after injury is usually blood (hemarthrosis) and indicates a potentially serious injury to one or more of the ligaments or menisci or an occult fracture. Recurrent effusions may indicate a chronic internal derangement such as a meniscal tear. Unexplained accumulation of fluid may occur with arthritis (septic, viral, postinfectious, juvenile rheumatoid arthritis, systemic lupus erythematosus), hemorrhage secondary to hemophilia, and overactivity. Occasionally, this fluid requires aspiration to relieve discomfort and to help establish the diagnosis. The presence of fat globules in the blood aspirated from a hemarthrosis may indicate an occult fracture. The presence of purulent material indicates septic arthritis or osteomyelitis.

PEDIATRIC KNEE DISORDERS

Overuse syndromes, ligament injuries, and meniscal tears may occur in children and adolescents and are discussed later in this section (see Chapters 676.6 and 681).

667.1 Discoid Lateral Meniscus

Clinical Manifestations and Diagnosis. Each meniscus is semilunar or C-shaped, but occasionally the lateral meniscus persists as a solid disk of cartilage and is referred to as a discoid lateral meniscus. The normal meniscus is attached around its periphery and glides anteriorly and posteriorly with knee motion, but a discoid meniscus is less mobile and may be torn. Occasionally, there is no peripheral attachment around the posterolateral aspect of the meniscus, which may allow it to become displaced anteriorly with knee flexion, producing a loud click or clunk. A tear or anterior displacement is most likely to occur in late childhood or early adolescence (11–15 yr). Physical examination may show a mild effusion and a positive McMurray test in which the displacement of the meniscus is both palpable and audible. Anteroposterior radiography of the knee may show only widening of the lateral aspect of the knee joint. MRI or arthrography is required for definitive diagnosis.

Treatment. The treatment of discoid menisci is to excise tears and reshape the meniscus arthroscopically. Meniscal instability can occasionally be repaired or reconstructed concomitantly. Complete excision may be necessary if other procedures are unsuccessful.

667.2 Popliteal Cyst

Popliteal cyst (Baker cyst) is commonly seen during the middle childhood years. There is distention of the gastrocnemius and semimembranous bursa along the posterior aspect of the knee by synovial fluid from a tendon sheath or the knee joint. It is not associated with intra-articular pathologic conditions. Knee radiographs are normal. The diagnosis may be confirmed by ultrasonography or aspiration. *Treatment* is by observation, especially in children 10 yr of age and younger, because resolution over several years usually occurs. The only indications for surgical excision are the presence of symptoms or progressive enlargement.

667.3 Osteochondritis Dissecans

Osteochondritis dissecans commonly involves the knee and occurs when an area of bone adjacent to the articular cartilage becomes avascular and ultimately separates from the underlying bone. The exact cause is unknown, but trauma from the adjacent tibial spines is commonly implicated. The lateral portion of the medial femoral condyle is the most common site.

Clinical Manifestations and Diagnosis. The child or adolescent typically presents with a vague knee pain. Occasionally, a mild effusion may be present. With the knee fully flexed, it is possible to palpate the involved area directly on the articular cartilage of the medial femoral condyle. This is usually tender.

Anteroposterior, lateral, and tunnel radiographs of the knee are necessary to establish the diagnosis and to follow the disease process. In younger children, the overlying articular cartilage usually remains intact. As revascularization occurs, the bone heals spontaneously. With increasing age, the risk increases for articular cartilage fracture and separation of the bony fragment, producing a loose body. MRI is helpful in determining the integrity of the articular cartilage.

Treatment. In children 11 yr of age and younger, the treatment is primarily by observation. Periodic radiographs and occasionally

MRI may be necessary to assess the degree of healing. In adolescents 13 yr of age and older, especially those with a suspected loose body, arthroscopic surgical intervention may be necessary. This may consist of (1) excision of the loose body, (2) replacement and internal fixation, or (3) drilling of an intact lesion to promote revascularization and healing.

667.4 Osgood-Schlatter Disease

The patellar tendon inserts into the tibia tubercle, which is an extension of the proximal tibial epiphysis. This area is vulnerable to microfracture during late childhood or adolescence, especially in athletes, producing Osgood-Schlatter disease. It is most common in males. The natural history is usually benign. Physical examination demonstrates swelling, tenderness, and increased prominence of the tibia tubercle. Radiographs are usually necessary to rule out other lesions. Rest, restriction of activities, and, occasionally, a knee immobilizer may be necessary, combined with an isometric exercise program. Anti-inflammatory medications usually are not beneficial. Complete resolution of symptoms through physiologic healing (physeal closure) of the tibia tubercle usually requires 12–24 mo.

PATELLOFEMORAL DISORDERS

The patellofemoral joint depends on balance among the restraining ligaments, muscle forces, and the articular anatomy of the patellofemoral groove. The patella has a V-shaped bottom that guides it through the matching groove (trochlea) in the distal femur. The force of the muscles pulling through the quadriceps mechanism and the patellar tendon does not act in a straight line because the patellar tendon inclines in a slightly lateral direction with respect to the line of the quadriceps. This lateral movement, coupled with the movement of the restraining ligaments, tends to move the patella in a lateral direction. The vastus medialis muscle is necessary to counteract the laterally acting forces. An abnormality of any one or a group of these factors may make the patellofemoral joint function abnormally. The usual clinical manifestation is knee pain that is aggravated by vigorous activities.

667.5 Idiopathic Adolescent Anterior Knee Pain Syndrome

The idiopathic adolescent anterior knee pain syndrome is a common patellofemoral disorder that was previously known as *chondromalacia patellae*. The term was used to describe a deranged patellar articular surface. Evidence suggests that the articular surface is actually normal. The cause of the knee pain, which commonly occurs in early adolescence, is unknown.

Clinical Manifestations and Diagnosis. The anterior peripatellar knee pain is poorly localized. Symptoms are usually produced by vigorous physical activities such as running. Typically, there is no history of injury. The child does not complain of locking, giving way, or recurrent effusion. Gait, range of motion, alignment of the lower extremity, knee stability, patellar tracking, and areas of focal tenderness should be evaluated. The presence of patellofemoral crepitation is common in normal individuals and does not indicate underlying knee disease. Routine radiographs, including anteroposterior, lateral, and tunnel views, are not particularly helpful in evaluating the cause of adolescent anterior knee pain, except that they may eliminate other sources of pain.

Treatment. The treatment is predominantly conservative and may include flexibility exercises, strengthening exercises (isometric quadriceps), contrast therapies (ice and heat), orthoses, and medications (nonsteroidal anti-inflammatory drugs). A success rate of 70–90% can be anticipated. Rarely will arthroscopic evaluation of the knee and patellofemoral joint be necessary.

667.6 Patella Subluxation and Dislocation

Patella maltracking is usually due to a congenital deficiency or malalignment within the patellofemoral joint. This can consist of a high-riding patella (patella alta), genu valgum, hypoplasia of the lateral femoral condyle, ligamentous laxity, and malignant malalignment with internal femoral and external tibial torsion. Traumatic patella subluxation and dislocation can occur as a result of a direct blow to the patella along its medial aspect, but this is uncommon.

Clinical Manifestations and Diagnosis. Examination of a child with a maltracking patella that is predisposed to dislocation usually shows terminal subluxation of the patella when the knee is brought into full extension. There may be tenderness to palpation over the inferior surface of the lateral facet of the patella. Attempting to displace the patella laterally yields a subjective feeling of subluxation, resulting in the patient grabbing the examiner's hand. This has been termed the *apprehension sign*. The torsional profile should be performed for possible rotational abnormalities of the femur or tibia, or both. After an acute dislocation, there may be a hemarthrosis from capsular tearing or an osteochondral fracture.

Radiographs are necessary in the evaluation of patella subluxation or after an acute dislocation. They should include anteroposterior, lateral, and skyline tangential views of the patella to assess for an osteochondral fracture from the lateral femoral condyle or the patella.

Treatment. The majority of children presenting with acute patella dislocation can be treated nonoperatively. This normally consists of immobilization with the knee in extension for approximately 6 wk. The patient is started on isometric, straight leg-raising exercises as soon as possible. Once the immobilization is discontinued, the isometric exercise program should be continued until the knee is fully rehabilitated. Using this method, approximately 75% of patients do not have recurrent dislocations.

If patella subluxation is due to dynamic muscle imbalance, a specific muscle rehabilitation program, such as strengthening the vastus medialis, may be successful.

In children and adolescents with recurrent dislocations or failure of conservative management for patella subluxation, operative stabilization may be necessary. Depending on the disease, this may consist of an arthroscopic lateral release and, occasionally, a soft tissue reconstruction. The latter can be performed either proximally or distally depending on the age of the patient and the nature of the disease. Derotational osteotomies of the distal femur or proximal tibia, or both, are indicated if there is torsional malalignment.

Ahn JH, Shim JS, Hwang CH, et al: Discoid lateral meniscus in children: Clinic manifestations and morphology. *J Pediatr Orthop* 2001;21:812–16.

Bensahel H, Souchet P, Pennecot GF, et al: The unstable patella in children. *J Pediatr Orthop* 2000;9:265–70.

Davids JR: Pediatric knee: Clinical assessment and common disorders. *Pediatr Clin North Am* 1996;43:1067–90.

Heft F, Berguiristain J, Krauspe R, et al: Osteochondritis dissecans: A multicenter study of the European Pediatric Orthopaedic Society. *J Pediatr Orthop* 1999;8:231–45.

Kocher MS, DiCanzio J, Zurakowski D, et al: Diagnostic performance of clinical examination and selective magnetic resonance imaging in the evaluation of intraarticular knee disorders in children and adolescents. *Am J Sports Med* 2001;29:292–96.

Krause BPL, Williams JPR, Caterall A: The natural history of Osgood-Schlatter's disease. *J Pediatr Orthop* 1990;10:65–68.

Letts RM, Davidson D, Beaule P: Semitendinosus tenodesis for repair of recurrent dislocation of the patella in children. *J Pediatr Orthop* 1999;19:742–47.

Nietosvaara Y, Aalto K, Kallio PE: Acute patella dislocation in children: Incidence and associated osteochondral fractures. *J Pediatr Orthop* 1994;14:513–15.

Stanitski CL: Instructional course lecture: Anterior knee pain syndromes in the adolescent. *J Bone Joint Surg Am* 1993;75A:1407–16.

Vahasarja V, Kinnunen P, Lanning P, et al: Operative realignment of patellar malalignment in children. *J Pediatr Orthop* 1995;15:281–85.

Van Rhijn LW, Jansen EJ, Pruijs HE: Long-term follow-up of conservatively treated popliteal cysts in children. *J Pediatr Orthop* 2000;9:62–64.

Chapter 668
The Hip
George H. Thompson

The hip is a ball-and-socket (femoral head and acetabulum, respectively) joint that allows for geometric motion, including flexion, extension, abduction, adduction, and internal and external rotation. The bulk of the femoral head is composed of the capital femoral epiphysis (CFE). The femoral head and acetabulum have a trophic relationship and are interdependent for normal growth and development. When this relationship is interrupted, abnormal hip development follows. Muscle balance and activity related to appropriate gross motor function are essential to the normal development of the hip.

The blood supply to the CFE is unique. The retinacular vessels lie on the surface of the femoral neck but are intracapsular. They enter the epiphysis from the periphery. This makes the blood supply vulnerable to damage from septic arthritis, trauma, thrombosis, and other vascular insults. If the blood supply is lost, avascular necrosis or osteonecrosis may occur. This can result in deformity, either acutely or as a consequence to abnormal growth and development, and predisposes to abnormal hip function and degenerative osteoarthritis as an adult.

668.1 Developmental Dysplasia of the Hip

Developmental dysplasia of the hip (DDH) usually occurs in the neonatal period. The hips at birth are rarely dislocated but rather "dislocatable." Dislocations tend to occur after delivery and, thus, are postnatal in origin, although the exact time when dislocations occur is controversial. Because they are not truly congenital in origin, the term *developmental dysplasia of the hip* should be used. DDH is classified into two major groups: typical, in a neurologically normal infant, and teratologic, in which there is an underlying neuromuscular disorder, such as myelodysplasia, arthrogryposis multiplex congenita, or a syndrome complex. Teratologic dislocations are less common, occur in utero, and are therefore congenital.

Etiology. DDH has physiologic, mechanical, and postural etiologic factors.

The positive family history (20%) and the generalized ligamentous laxity are related factors. The majority of children with DDH have generalized ligamentous laxity, which can predispose to hip instability. Maternal estrogens and other hormones associated with pelvic relaxation result in further, although temporary, relaxation of the newborn hip joint. There is a 9:1 female predominance.

Approximately 60% of children with typical DDH are firstborns, and 30–50% were in the breech position. The frank breech position with the hips flexed and the knees extended is the position of highest risk. The breech position results in extreme hip flexion and limitation of hip motion. Increased hip flexion results in stretching of the already lax capsule and ligamentum teres. It also produces posterior uncoverage of the femoral head. Decreased hip motion leads to a lack of normal development of the cartilaginous acetabulum. There is also an association of congenital muscular torticollis (14–20%) and metatarsus adductus (1–10%) with DDH. The presence of either condition requires a careful examination of the hips.

Postnatal factors are also important determinants. Maintaining the hips in the position of adduction and extension may lead to dislocation. This puts the unstable hip under pressure because of the normal hip flexion and abduction contractures. An unstable femoral head, as a consequence, can be displaced from the acetabulum over several days or weeks.

Pathoanatomy. Because hips are not dislocated at birth, the components of the hip joint, excluding the hip capsule and ligamentum teres, are relatively normal. There may be some variations in the shape of the cartilaginous acetabulum, especially if the child was in a breech position in utero. If a dislocation is allowed to occur, acetabular dysplasia and maldirection, excessive femoral anteversion (torsion), and hip muscle contractures develop.

Clinical Manifestations. All neonates should be screened for DDH (Fig. 668–1). The Barlow test is the most important maneuver in examining the newborn hip. This provocative test to dislocate an unstable hip is performed by stabilizing the pelvis with one hand and then flexing and adducting the opposite hip and applying a posterior force (Fig. 668–2). If the hip is dislocatable, it is usually readily felt. After release of the posterior force, the hip usually relocates spontaneously. It has been estimated that only 1 in 100 newborn infants have clinically unstable hips (subluxation or dislocation), whereas only 1 in 800–1,000 of these infants eventually experience a true dislocation. The Ortolani test is a maneuver to reduce a recently dislocated hip. It is most likely to be positive in infants who are 1–2 mo of age because adequate time must have passed for the true dislocation to occur. In performing this test, the thigh is flexed and abducted and the femoral head is lifted anteriorly into the acetabulum (Fig. 668–2). If reduction is possible, the relocation will be felt as a "clunk," not an audible "click." After 2 mo of age, manual reduction of a dislocated hip is usually not possible because of the development of soft tissue contractures.

Limitation of hip abduction is indicative of soft tissue contractures and may indicate DDH. Conversely, hip abduction contractures may indicate dysplasia of the contralateral hip. An asymmetric number of thigh skinfolds and apparent shortening of an extremity and uneven knee levels when the supine infant's feet are placed together on the examining table with the hips and knees flexed (Galeazzi sign) indicate DDH with proximal displacement of the femoral head. Absent normal knee flexion contracture also occurs.

A common concern is the presence of audible *hip clicks* in infants. Hip clicks per se are not usually pathologic and are secondary to (1) breaking the surface tension across the hip joint, (2) snapping of gluteal tendons, (3) patellofemoral motion, or (4) femorotibial (knee) rotation.

In older or walking children, complaints of limping, waddling, increased lumbar lordosis, toe walking, and leg-length discrepancy may indicate an unrecognized DDH.

Radiographic Evaluation. Hip stability as well as acetabular development may be assessed accurately in neonates and young infants by dynamic ultrasonography. Radiographic evaluation in older infants and children includes anteroposterior and Lauenstein (frog) lateral radiographs of the pelvis. The ossific nucleus of the femoral head does not appear until 3–7 mo of age, and it may be further delayed in DDH. Line measurements are usually made to determine the relationship of the femoral head to the acetabulum (acetabular index, quadrant assessment, Shenton's line, and the center edge angle of Wiberg) (Fig. 668–3). Arthrography, CT, and MRI scans may be beneficial in

difficult cases, especially those involving older infants and children.

Treatment. The treatment of DDH should be individualized and depends on the patient's age and whether the hip is subluxated or dislocated.

BIRTH. When an unstable hip is recognized at birth, maintenance of the hip in the position of flexion and abduction ("human" position) for 1–2 mo is usually sufficient. This position maintains reduction of the femoral head and allows for tightening of the ligamentous structures as well as stimulation of normal growth and development. Methods that can be used to maintain the hip in this position include the Pavlik harness, Frejka splint, and a variety of abduction orthoses. Double and triple diapers, although controversial, are commonly used in newborns with dislocatable hips for 2–3 wk because the splints and harnesses usually do not initially fit satisfactorily. Treatment is continued until there is clinical stability of the hip and ultrasonographic or radiographic measurements are normal.

AGE 1–6 MONTHS. During this age, a true dislocation may develop. As a consequence, treatment is directed toward reduction of the femoral head into the acetabulum. The Pavlik harness is the treatment of choice in this age group. The harness attempts to place the hips in the human position by flexing them more than 90 degrees (preferably 100–110 degrees) and maintaining relatively full, but gentle abduction (50–70 degrees). This redirects the femoral head toward the acetabulum. Usually, spontaneous relocation of the femoral head occurs within 3–4 wk. The Pavlik harness is approximately 95% successful in dysplastic or subluxated hips and 80% successful in true dislocations. If reduction is achieved, use of the harness is continued until radiographic parameters have returned to normal. If a spontaneous reduction does not occur, a surgical closed reduction is indicated. This consists of (1) preliminary skin traction for 1–3 wk to bring the femoral head opposite the acetabulum, (2) percutaneous adductor tenotomy, (3) closed reduction, (4) arthrography to assess the concentricity of the reduction, and (5) application of a hip spica cast in the "human" position. Treatment is continued until the radiographic parameters are within normal limits.

AGE 6–18 MONTHS. In the older infant, surgical closed reduction is the major method of treatment. If at the time of reduction there is significant instability, an open reduction may be indicated. This can be through a medial or anterior approach.

AGE OF 18 MONTHS–8 YEARS. After 18 mo of age, the progressive deformities are so severe that open reduction followed by pelvic (innominate) osteotomy or femoral osteotomy, or both, is necessary to realign the hip. A femoral shortening derotation osteotomy is performed concomitantly if the reduction is tight, if there is excessive femoral anteversion, or if the child is 3 or 4 yr of age or older. Postoperatively, a hip spica cast is worn for 6–8 wk to allow healing. Thereafter, the child may be permitted to return to full activities gradually. Implanted metal is removed shortly after healing to prevent incorporation into the growing bone. Eighteen months of age is not an arbitrary age for these procedures. It has been demonstrated that approximately 25% of children who have a closed reduction performed between 9–12 mo of age, 50% who have one between 12–18 mo, and 75% who have one between 18 and 36 mo have residual acetabular dysplasia requiring a pelvic or femoral osteotomy at a later date.

Complications. The most important and severe complication of DDH is avascular necrosis of the CFE. This is an iatrogenic complication; reduction of the femoral head under pressure produces cartilaginous compression, and this can result in occlusion of the intra-articular, extraosseous epiphyseal vessels and produce CFE infarction, either partial or total. Revascularization follows, but abnormal growth and development may occur, especially if the physis is severely damaged. The hip is vulnerable to this complication before the development of the ossific

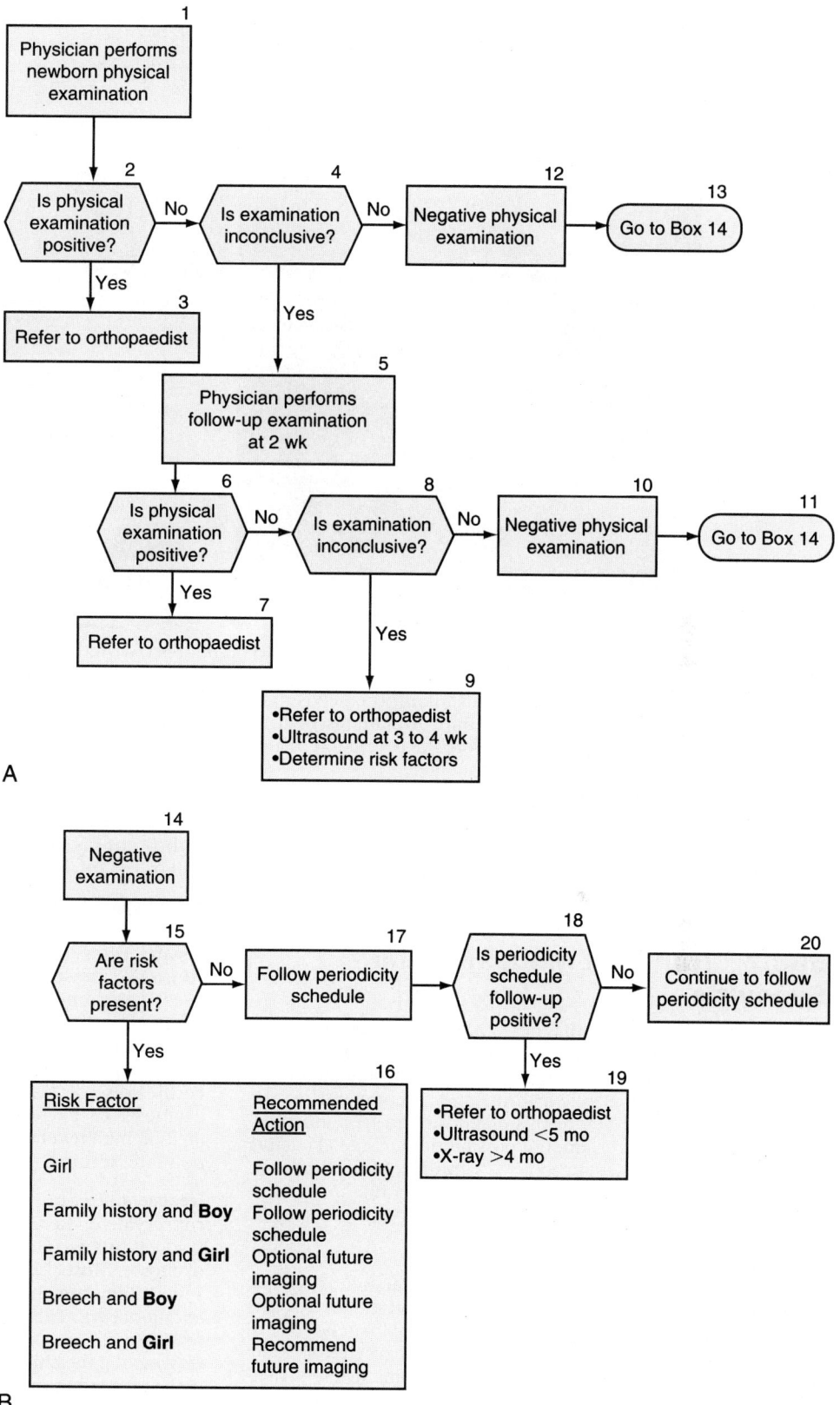

FIGURE 668–1. Screening for developmental hip dysplasia—clinical algorithm. (From Committee on Quality Improvement, Subcomitttee on Developmental Dysplasia of the Hip: Clinical Practice Guideline: Early detection of developmental dysplasia of the hip. *Pediatrics* 2000;105: 896–905.)

nucleus (4–6 mo). The management outlined previously is designed to minimize this complication; with appropriate use of these treatments, the incidence of avascular necrosis is 5–15%. Other potential complications in DDH include redislocation, residual subluxation, acetabular dysplasia, and postoperative complications, such as wound infections.

SEPTIC ARTHRITIS AND OSTEOMYELITIS

See Chapter 674 for a full discussion of septic arthritis and osteomyelitis. Diagnosis of septic arthritis and osteomyelitis is made by hip aspiration (arthrocentesis). This can be technically difficult and must always be performed under fluoroscopic

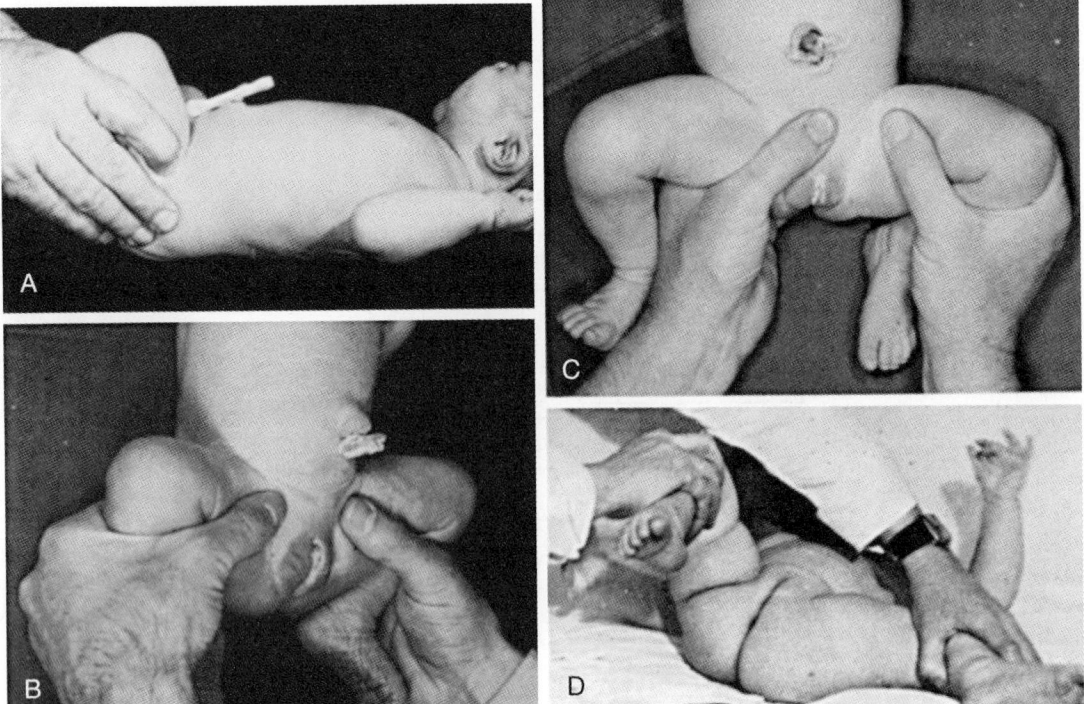

FIGURE 668–2. Newborn hip examination. *A,* The infant is laid on her back with the hips and knees flexed, and the examiner places the middle finger of each hand over each greater trochanter. *B,* The thumb of each hand is applied to the inner side of the thigh opposite the lesser trochanter. *C,* In a difficult infant, the pelvis may be steadied between a thumb over the pubis and fingers under the sacrum while the hip is tested (Barlow and Ortolani test) with the other hand. *D,* Limitation of hip abduction is also an early sign of developmental dislocation of the hip. Note the restriction in abduction of the right hip.

control. If no fluid is obtained from the hip joint, an arthrogram should be obtained, documenting that the hip joint has been entered.

668.2 Transient Monoarticular Synovitis

Transient synovitis of the hip is one of the more common causes of limping in a normal child. It is characterized by acute onset of pain, limp, and mild restriction of motion, especially abduction and internal rotation. Septic arthritis and osteomyelitis of the hip must be excluded before this diagnosis can be confirmed. The cause remains uncertain, but possibilities include (1) active or recent systemic viral syndrome, (2) trauma, and (3) allergic hypersensitivity. Biopsy specimens from the hip joint have demonstrated synovial hypertrophy secondary to nonspecific inflammatory reaction.

Clinical Manifestations. Transient monoarticular synovitis can occur in all age groups, but the mean age at onset is 6 yr; it occurs predominantly in the 3–8 yr age group. Approximately 70% of affected children have had a nonspecific upper respiratory tract infection 7–14 days before the onset of symptoms. There is usually an acute onset of symptoms with pain felt in the groin, anterior thigh, or knee; nontraumatic anterior thigh or knee pain may be referred from the hip. These children are usually ambulatory, and the hip is not held flexed, abducted, and laterally rotated unless a significant effusion is present. However, they walk with a painful, limping gait. They are usually afebrile or have a low-grade fever (temperature less than 38°C).

Laboratory values are usually normal, but occasionally a slight elevation in the erythrocyte sedimentation rate is seen.

Arthrocentesis produces normal results, although a joint effusion of 1–3 mL is common.

Radiographic Evaluation. Anteroposterior and Lauenstein (frog) lateral radiographs of the pelvis may be obtained and are usually normal. Ultrasonography of the hip may demonstrate a hip joint effusion. Ultrasound-guided hip joint fluid aspiration may be needed in some cases to determine if a septic hip is present. Technetium bone scan or MRI may be of value in ruling out the presence of other lesions, such as septic arthritis, tumor, fracture, slipped capital femoral epiphysis, or early Legg-Calvé-Perthes disease (LCPD). Transient monoarticular synovitis is a diagnosis of exclusion. High-risk criteria for septic arthritis include high fever and elevations of the erythrocyte sedimentation rate, serum C-reactive protein, and white blood cell counts.

Treatment. Treatment of monoarticular synovitis of the hip is conservative. Bed rest and no weight bearing until the pain resolves followed by limited activities thereafter is the treatment of choice. Most children are maintained on bed rest for less than 1 wk. They are then maintained on limited activities for 1–2 additional wk. This sometimes is difficult because children want to return to normal activities when their symptoms resolve. However, if the child is allowed to return to normal activities too early, exacerbation of symptoms may occur. Ibuprofen may shorten the duration of pain.

668.3 Legg-Calvé-Perthes Disease

LCPD is idiopathic osteonecrosis or avascular necrosis of the CFE, and the associated complications thereof, occurring in an immature, growing child. This osteochondrosis is caused by an interruption of the CFE blood supply. Its cause is unknown, but

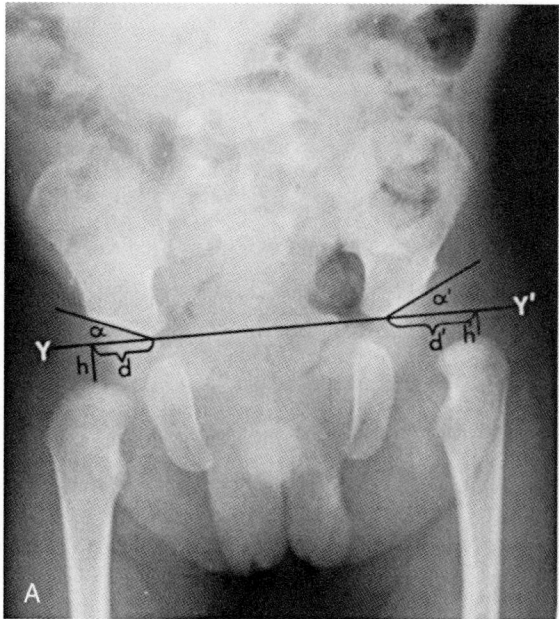 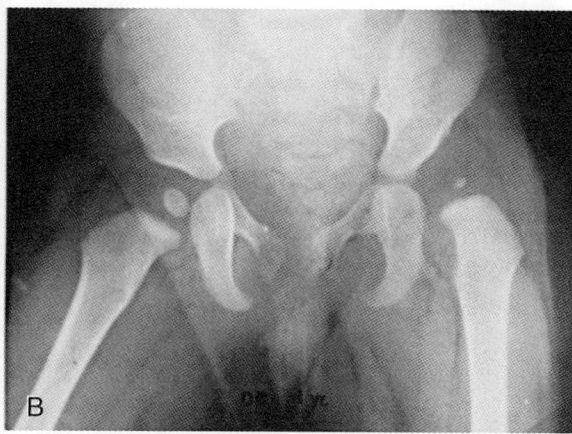

FIGURE 668–3. Pelvic radiographs demonstrating development dysplasia of the left hip. *A,* The Hilgenreiner method for identification of dysplasia of the hip before ossification of the capital femoral epiphysis; α' is greater than α, indicating greater obliquity of the acetabular roof. *d'* is greater than *d,* indicating lateral displacement of the femur. *h* is greater than *h',* indicating cephalad displacement of the femur. These relationships indicate dysplasia of the patient's left hip. *B,* Developmental dislocation of the left hip. The bony roof of the left acetabulum is quite oblique, and there is the beginning of a false acetabulum above its most lateral aspect. The left femur is displaced laterally and superiorly. The ossification center of the left capital femoral epiphysis is smaller than that of the right.

an association among protein C and protein S deficiency, thrombophilia, and hypofibrinolysis has been observed. It is primarily a disorder affecting males (4–5:1) and is bilateral in approximately 20% of children. Children with LCPD often have delayed bone age, disproportionate growth, and mild short stature.

Clinical Manifestations. The clinical onset of LCPD occurs between the ages of 2 and 12 yr (mean, 7 yr). Most children present with mild or intermittent pain in the anterior thigh and a limp. The classic presentation has been described as a "painless limp." The pertinent early physical findings include antalgic gait; muscle spasm with mild restriction of motion, especially abduction and internal rotation; proximal thigh atrophy; and mild shortness of stature.

Radiographic Evaluation. Anteroposterior and Lauenstein (frog) lateral radiographs of the pelvis should be obtained to establish the diagnosis (Fig. 668–4). The radiographic characteristics can be divided into five distinct stages representing a continuum of the disease process: (1) cessation of CFE growth, (2) subchondral fracture, (3) resorption (fragmentation), (4) reossification, and (5) healed or residual stage.

There are three radiographic classification systems of the extent of CFE involvement. Catterall developed a four-group classification on the basis of the appearance of the CFE at maximal resorption. Although this classification has been helpful in the retrospective analysis of results, it has limited prognostic value because it is difficult to apply in the earliest phases of the disease process. Salter-Thompson used two groups, and Herring and colleagues used three groups, depending on involvement or extent of involvement or the radiographic appearance of the lateral portion of the CFE. When intact, this area acts as a supporting column or pillar that shields the involved portion of the CFE from compression, which can produce collapse, deformity, and possible extrusion. Involvement results in a poorer prognosis.

The short-term prognosis relates to the femoral head deformity at the completion of the healing stage. Adverse risk factors include older age at clinical onset, extensive CFE involvement, loss of femoral head containment, reduced range of hip motion, and premature CFE closure. The long-term prognosis relates to the potential for osteoarthritis of the hip in adulthood. Older children with significant residual femoral head deformity are at risk for degenerative arthritis; the incidence is essentially 100% in children who are 10 yr of age or older at onset and who have residual femoral head deformity. This compares with a negligible risk in children who are 5 yr of age and younger at onset and 38% when onset occurs between 6 and 9 yr of age.

Two radiographic classifications evaluate the sphericity of the femoral head at the completion of the disease process, which correlates with the risk for degenerative osteoarthritis as an adult. In the Mose circle criteria, a transparent template with concentric circles is placed over the anteroposterior and Lauenstein lateral radiographs. If the variation of sphericity of the femoral head in the two views is 0–2 mm, the result is good; 2–3 mm, fair; and 3 mm or more, poor. Stulberg and colleagues' five-group classification is based on the shape of the femoral head and congruency with the acetabulum: class I, a spherical femoral head that is equal in size to the opposite uninvolved hip; class II, a spherical femoral head with coxa magna; class III, an oval femoral head with a congruent acetabulum; class IV, a flat femoral head with abnormalities of the femoral neck and acetabulum; and class V, a flat femoral head with a normal acetabulum. Classes I and II are spherical congruent hips; class III, a nonspherical congruent hip; and classes IV and V, incongruent hips.

Treatment. LCPD is a local, self-healing disorder. Prevention of femoral head deformity and secondary osteoarthritis are the only justifications for treatment. The treatment goals are (1) elimination of hip irritability; (2) restoration and maintenance of a good range of hip motion; (3) prevention of CFE collapse, extrusion,

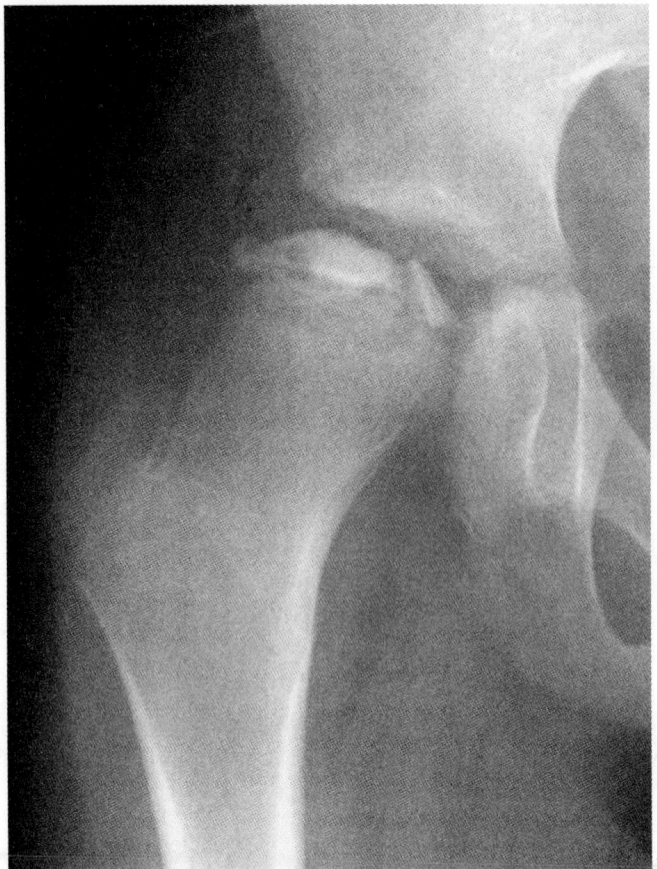

FIGURE 668–4. Anteroposterior radiograph of the right hip of an 8-yr-old boy with Legg-Calvé-Perthes disease. There is a collapsed yet dense capital femoral epiphysis with early fragmentation. The small medial triangle of the capital femoral epiphysis is uninvolved in the disease process.

or subluxation; and (4) attainment of a spherical femoral head at healing. Treatment uses the concept of containment (i.e., the femoral head is contained within the acetabulum so that the latter acts as a mold for the reossifying CFE). This may be accomplished by nonsurgical and surgical techniques.

OBSERVATION. Expectant observation is appropriate for all children younger than 6 yr at clinical onset regardless of the extent of CFE involvement. These children must be monitored closely, both clinically and radiographically.

INTERMITTENT SYMPTOMATIC TREATMENT. Temporary or periodic treatment with bed rest or abduction stretching exercises to maintain mobility can be used in conjunction with observation. Recurrent episodes of hip irritability with a temporary decrease in motion commonly occur during the phases of subchondral fracture and fragmentation, and the child may benefit from symptomatic treatment.

DEFINITIVE EARLY TREATMENT. Nonsurgical or surgical containment of the femoral head in the course of the disease is indicated when (1) the age at clinical onset is 6 yr or older (possibly 5 yr in girls), (2) the lateral portion of the CFE is involved, or (3) there is a loss of containment, as manifested by extrusion of the femoral head on anteroposterior radiograph.

Nonsurgical Containment. Abduction casts (Petrie) or orthoses can be used to contain the femoral head within the acetabulum. Containment is continued only until there is early radiographic subchondral reossification. Because this usually occurs 12–18 mo after clinical onset, nonsurgical containment methods can be limited to 18 mo or less with no adverse effect

on the outcome. The Atlanta Scottish Rite Hospital orthosis is the most widely used because it allows reciprocal motion and ambulation without crutches or external support. The success of nonsurgical containment has been challenged on the grounds that it does not alter the natural history of untreated LCPD.

Surgical Containment. A pelvic or femoral osteotomy can be used to contain the femoral head. The results of surgical containment appear to be better than those of nonsurgical containment; approximately 85% of patients have Stulberg class I, II, or III.

LATE SURGICAL MANAGEMENT FOR DEFORMITY. If significant femoral head deformity prevents reduction of the femoral head into the acetabulum, an alternative method must be considered. Several surgical procedures at least partially correct the various existing deformities, thereby alleviating the associated symptoms.

668.4 Slipped Capital Femoral Epiphysis

Slipped capital femoral epiphysis (SCFE) is the most common adolescent hip disorder. Its cause is unknown, but an endocrine basis has been suggested because SCFE is frequently accompanied by abnormalities of growth. Sex hormones, growth hormone, and other hormones alter the rate of growth in the CFE and the rate of skeletal growth. SCFE occurs in adolescents who are either obese and have delayed skeletal maturation or who are tall and thin and have had a recent growth spurt. In obese adolescents, a low level of sex hormones has been postulated, whereas in tall, thin individuals, an overabundance of growth hormone is implicated. SCFE can also occur as a complication of an underlying endocrine disorder such as hypothyroidism, pituitary disorders, pseudohypoparathyroidism, and others. When a SCFE occurs before puberty (10 yr of age or younger), an endocrine disorder (hypothyroidism, growth hormone deficiency) should be suspected.

Radiographic Evaluation. Anteroposterior and Lauenstein (frog) lateral radiographs of the pelvis are used for assessment of SCFE (Fig. 668–5). Both hips must be evaluated and compared. The earliest sign of SCFE is widening of the physis without slippage, a preslip condition. As slippage occurs, the CFE remains in the acetabulum and the femoral neck rotates predominantly anteriorly (although occasionally superiorly), resulting in a varus, retroverted femoral head and neck. The degree of slippage between the CFE and the femoral neck can be classified as mild (0–33%), moderate (34–50%), and severe (greater than 50%) by radiographic measurement techniques.

Diagnostic Classification. SCFE is classified as stable or unstable depending on the integrity between the CFE and femoral neck.

STABLE SLIPPED CAPITAL FEMORAL EPIPHYSIS. This is the most common type. Initially, the physis is wide but slippage has not occurred. There may be mild discomfort, but the physical examination is usually normal. Preslips are commonly seen in the opposite hip of an adolescent with a previous SCFE. The symptoms typically worsen as the slip develops and progresses. However, because there is continuity between the femoral neck and CFE, the symptoms are not severe, and the child is able to walk with a mildly antalgic, externally rotated gait (Fig. 668–6).

UNSTABLE SLIPPED CAPITAL FEMORAL EPIPHYSIS. In unstable SCFE, there are no or only mild antecedent symptoms such as pain or limp. Slippage then occurs suddenly, usually without trauma, and the pain is so severe that the child is usually unable to stand or bear weight even with external support on the involved extremity. The stability between the CFE and femoral neck is disrupted.

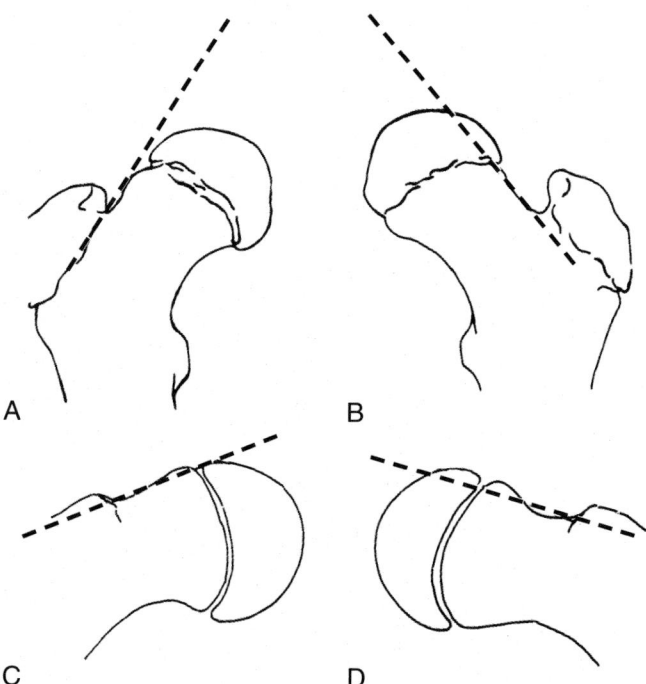

FIGURE 668–5. Slipped capital femoral epiphysis, anteroposterior view. A line superimposed on the superior femoral neck normally intersects part of the head (*B* and *D* are normal). With a slipped epiphysis, the line does not intersect the femoral head (*A* and *C*). Occasionally, the frog-leg view (*C* and *D*) is needed to demonstrate the slip. (From Chung S: Diseases of the developing hip joint. *Pediatr Clin North Am* 1986;33:1457.)

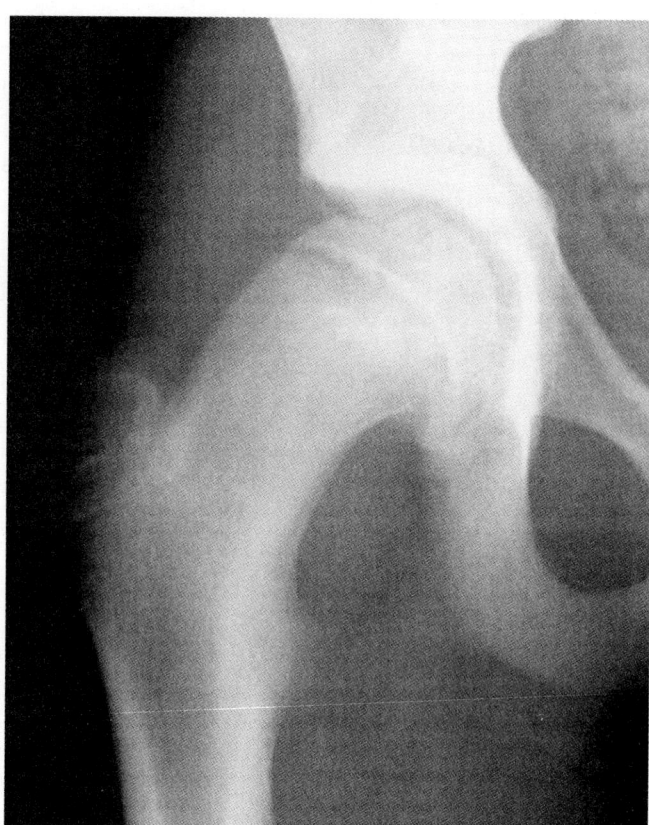

FIGURE 668–6. Anteroposterior radiograph of the right hip of a 13-yr-old boy with a moderately severe chronic (stable) slipped capital femoral epiphysis. Observe the physeal widening and the distorted relationship between the capital femoral epiphysis and femoral neck.

Clinical Manifestations. The physical findings in SCFE depend on the degree of slippage and the classification. In the unstable SCFE, the physical examination is limited as a result of severe pain with any attempted hip motion. In a stable SCFE, the patient has an antalgic gait and the affected extremity is externally rotated. Hip range of motion demonstrates a lack of internal rotation and increased external rotation. Also, as the hip is flexed, it becomes progressively externally rotated. Limitation of flexion and abduction may also be present if there is a severe varus deformity of the proximal femur. Twenty per cent of patients complain of knee pain only, although they have decreased hip rotation on physical examination. Adolescents, especially those who are obese, with nontraumatic anterior thigh or knee pain (referred pain) should be carefully evaluated for a SCFE.

Treatment. The goals of treatment for SCFE are to prevent further slippage and minimize complications. This is accomplished by performing an epiphysiodesis (closure) of the CFE. In situ pinning with one or two cannulated screws is the most popular technique. The screws can be inserted percutaneously under fluoroscopic control. Screw removal after CFE closure is controversial.

Complications. The two serious complications in SCFE are osteonecrosis and chondrolysis. Osteonecrosis or avascular necrosis occurs as a result of injury to the retinacular vessels. This can be due to forced manipulation of an acute or unstable SCFE, compression from intracapsular hematoma, or direct injury during surgery. Partial forms of osteonecrosis may also occur after internal fixation as a result of disruption of the intraepiphyseal blood vessels. Chondrolysis is a degeneration of the articular cartilage of the hip. Its cause is unclear, but it (1) is associated with more severe slips, (2) occurs more frequently among blacks and females, and (3) is associated with pins or screws protruding out of the femoral head.

Developmental Dysplasia of the Hip
Bialik V, Bialik GM, Blazer S, et al: Developmental dysplasia of the hip: A new approach to incidence. *Pediatrics* 1999;103:93–9.
Committee on Quality Improvement, Subcomitttee on Developmental Dysplasia of the Hip: Clinical Practice Guideline: Early detection of developmental dysplasia of the hip. *Pediatrics* 2000;105:896–905.
Castelein RM, Korte J: Limited hip abduction in the infant. *J Pediatr Orthop* 2001;21:668–70.
Guille JT, Pizzutillo PD, MacEwen GD: Developmental dysplasia of the hip from birth to six months. *J Am Acad Orthop Surg* 2000;8:232–42.
Grissom LE, Harcke HT: Ultrasonography and developmental dysplasia of the infant hip. *Curr Opin Pediatr* 1999;11:66–9.
Haynes DJ: Developmental dysplasia of the hip: Etiology, pathogenesis and examination and physical findings in the newborn. *Am Acad Orthop Surg Instr Course Lect* 2001;50:535–40.
Hennrikus WL: Developmental dysplasia of the hip: Diagnosis and treatment in children younger than 6 months. *Pediatr Ann* 1999;28:740–46.
Lerman JA, Emans JB, Millis MB, et al: Early failure of Pavlick harness treatment for developmental hip dysplasia: Clinical and ultrasound predictors. *J Pediatr Orthop* 2001;21:348–53.
Maxwell SL, Ruiz AL, Lappin KJ, et al: Clinical screening for developmental dysplasia of the hip in Northern Ireland. *BMJ* 2002;324:1031–33.
Moseley CF: Developmental hip dysplasia and dislocation: Management of the older child. *Am Acad Orthop Surg Instr Course Lect* 2001;50:547–53.
Vitale MG, Skaggs DL: Developmental dysplasia of the hip from six months to four years of age. *J Am Acad Orthop Surg* 2001;9:401–11.
Weintroub S, Grill F: Ultrasonography in developmental dysplasia of the hip. *J Bone Joint Surg Am* 2000;82:1004–18.
Willis RB: Developmental dysplasia of the hip: Assessment and treatment before walking age. *Am Acad Orthop Surg Inst Course Lect* 2001;50:541–5.

Transient Monoarticular Synovitis
Beach R: Minimally invasive approach to management of irritable hip in children. *Lancet* 2000;355:1202–3.

Hart JJ: Transient synovitis of the hip in children. *Am Fam Physician* 1996;54: 1587–91.

Kocher MS, Zurakowski D, Kasser JR: Differentiating between septic arthritis and transient synovitis of the hip in children: An evidence-based clinical prediction algorithm. *J Bone Joint Surg Am* 1999;81:1662–70.

Legg-Calvé-Perthes Disease

Catterall A: The natural history of Perthes disease. *J Bone Joint Surg Br* 1971;53B: 37–53.

Eldridge J, Dilley A, Austin H, et al: The role of protein C, protein S, and resistance to activated protein C in Legg-Perthes disease. *Pediatrics* 2001;107:1329–34.

Harel L, Kornreich L, Ashkenazi S, et al: Myer dysplasia in the differential diagnosis of hip disease in young children. *Arch Pediatr Adoles Med* 1999;153:943–45.

Herring JA, Neustadt JB, Williams JJ, et al: The lateral pillar classification of Legg-Calvé-Perthes disease. *J Pediatr Orthop* 1992;12:143–50.

Martinez AG, Weinstein SL, Dietz FR: The weight-bearing abduction brace for the treatment of Legg-Calvé-Perthes disease. *J Bone Joint Surg Am* 1992;74:12–21.

Meehan PL, Angel D, Nelson JM: The Scottish Rite abduction orthosis for the treatment of Legg-Perthes disease. *J Bone Joint Surg Am* 1992;74A:2–12.

Noonon KJ, Price CT, Kupiszewski SJ, et al: Results of femoral varus osteotomy in children older than 9 years of age with Perthes disease. *J Pediatr Orthop* 2001;21: 198–204.

Roy DR: Current concepts in Legg-Calvé-Perthes disease. *Pediatr Ann* 1999;28: 748–52.

Stulberg SD, Cooperman DR, Wallensten R: The natural history of Legg-Calvé-Perthes disease. *J Bone Joint Surg Am* 1981;63:1095–108.

Thompson GH, Price CT, Roy D, et al: Legg-Calvé-Perthes disease: Current concepts. *Am Acad Orthop Surg Instr Course Lect* 2002;51:367–84.

Slipped Capital Femoral Epiphysis

Burrow SR, Alman B, Wright JG: Short stature as a screening test for endocrinopathy in slipped capital femoral epiphysis. *J Bone Joint Surg Br* 2001;83B:263–68.

Dobbs MT, Weinstein SL: Natural history and long-term outcomes of slipped capital femoral epiphysis. *Am Acad Orthop Surg Instr Course Lect* 2001;50:571–75.

Loder RT: Unstable slipped capital femoral epiphyses. *J Pediatr Orthop* 2001;21: 694–99.

Loder RT, Aronsson DD, Dobbs MT, et al: Slipped capital femoral epiphysis. *Am Acad Orthop Surg Instr Course Lect* 2001;50:555–70.

Lubicky JP: Chondrolysis and avascular necrosis: Complications of slipped capital femoral epiphysis. *J Pediatr Orthop* 1996;5:162–67.

Reynolds RA: Diagnosis and treatment of slipped capital femoral epiphysis. *Curr Opin Pediatr* 1999;11:80–83.

Warner WC Jr, Beaty JH, Canale ST: Chondrolysis after slipped capital femoral epiphysis. *J Pediatr Orthop* 1996;5:168–72.

Chapter 669
The Spine

George H. Thompson

Abnormalities in the vertebral column are a common nontraumatic pediatric musculoskeletal problem. They may be present at birth or may develop during childhood or adolescence. Some disorders worsen with growth and may lead to an unacceptable appearance, alterations in pulmonary function, and early degenerative osteoarthritis of the spine. A simplified classification of the common spinal abnormalities is presented in Box 669–1.

In the anteroposterior (frontal) plane, the vertebral bodies of the normal spine are stacked squarely one on the other with little or no deviation from vertical alignment. The vertebral end-plates are parallel and the intervertebral disks are symmetric in height. In the sagittal plane, the spine has normal curvatures that provide balance and stability. The cervical and lumbar spine displays anterior convexity, termed *lordosis*; the thoracic spine and sacrum display posterior convexity and are *kyphotic*.

Alterations in normal spinal alignment that occur in the frontal plane are termed *scoliosis*. The majority of scoliotic deformities are idiopathic. Others can be congenital, associated with a neuromuscular disorder or syndrome, compensatory from a leg-length discrepancy, or caused by an intraspinal abnormality.

BOX 669–1. Classification of Spinal Deformities

SCOLIOSIS

Idiopathic

Infantile
Juvenile
Adolescent

Congenital

Failure of formation
  Wedge vertebrae
  Hemivertebrae
Failure of segmentation
  Unilateral bar
  Bilateral bar
Mixed

Neuromuscular

Neuropathic diseases
  Upper motor neuron
    Cerebral palsy
    Spinocerebellar degeneration (Friedreich ataxia, Charcot-Marie-Tooth disease)
    Syringomyelia
    Spinal cord tumor
    Spinal cord trauma
  Lower motor neuron
    Poliomyelitis
    Spinal muscular atrophy
Myopathic diseases
  Duchenne muscular dystrophy
  Arthrogryposis
  Other muscular dystrophies

Syndromes

Neurofibromatosis
Marfan syndrome

Compensatory

Leg-length discrepancy

KYPHOSIS

Postural Round-Back

Scheuermann Disease

Congenital Kyphosis

Adapted from the Terminology Committee, Scoliosis Research Society: A glossary of scoliosis terms. *Spine* 1976; 1:57.

669.1 Idiopathic Scoliosis

Etiology and Epidemiology. Idiopathic scoliosis is the most common form of scoliosis. It occurs in healthy, neurologically normal children; its cause is unknown. The incidence is only slightly greater in girls than in boys, but scoliosis is more likely to progress and require treatment in girls than in boys. There appears to be a genetic component, but the disorder is not transmitted in a pure mendelian fashion. The daughters of affected mothers are more likely than other children to have scoliosis, but identical twins are not uniformly affected. The magnitude of curvature in an affected individual is not related to the magnitude of curvature in relatives. Involved children also tend to show subtle changes in proprioception and vibratory sensation, suggesting that abnormalities of spinal cord posterior column function may have a causative role.

Idiopathic scoliosis can be divided into three groups on the basis of age at onset: infantile (birth–3 yr), juvenile (4–10 yr), and adolescent (11 yr and older). Adolescent idiopathic scoliosis is much more common than juvenile-onset scoliosis; infantile idiopathic scoliosis is extraordinarily rare.

Clinical Manifestations. A thorough history and physical examination is the first step in the evaluation of patients with suspected idiopathic scoliosis. Asymmetry of the posterior chest wall on forward bending (the Adams test) is the most striking and consistent abnormality in patients with scoliosis (Fig. 669–1). Rotation of the vertebral bodies within a curve toward the side of convexity of curvature displaces the attached ribs and overlying paraspinal musculature posteriorly on the convex side of the curve and creates a depression on the concave side. Associated findings include asymmetry in shoulder height, apparent leg-length discrepancy, flank asymmetry, and asymmetry of the anterior chest wall.

When the trunk is viewed from the side with the patient in the forward flexed position, the degree of *kyphosis* and *lordosis* can be evaluated. The upper region of the thoracic spine normally has a smooth, rounded curve that extends down to the midthoracic region. Flexible roundback that corrects easily when a child stands upright is common in adolescents. Sharp, abrupt, or accentuated forward angulation in the thoracic or thoracolumbar region is indicative of a kyphotic deformity. In the erect position, the lower lumbar spine is normally concave (lordotic). The magnitude of lordosis varies with age and among individuals of the same age. Children normally have less cervical lordosis and more lumbar lordosis than do adults or adolescents.

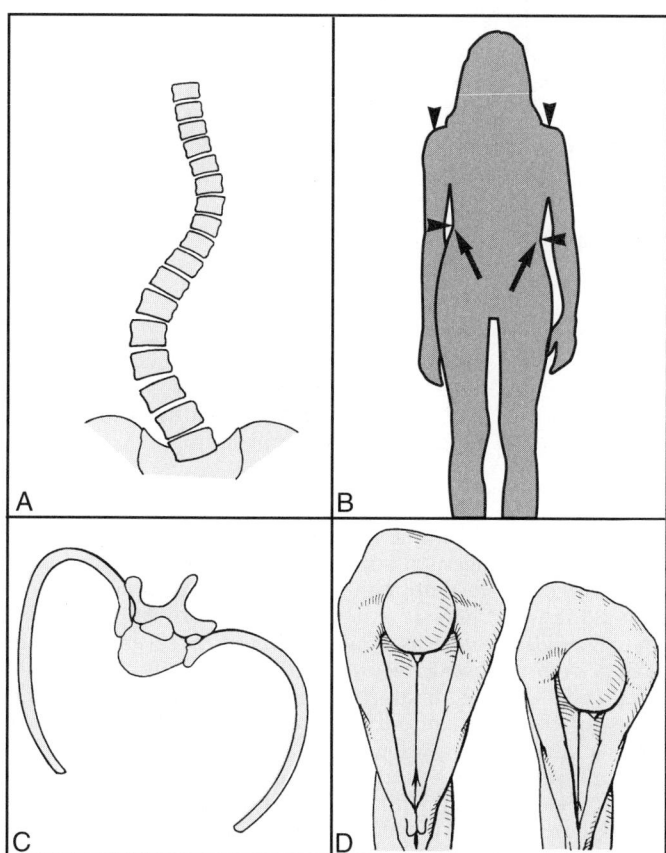

FIGURE 669–1. Structural changes in idiopathic scoliosis. *A,* As curvature increases, alterations in body configuration develop in both the primary and compensatory curve regions. *B,* Asymmetry of shoulder height, waistline, and elbow-to-flank distance are common findings. *C,* Vertebral rotation and associated posterior displacement of the ribs on the convex side of the curve are responsible for the characteristic deformity of the chest wall in scoliosis patients. *D,* In the school screening examination for scoliosis, the patient bends forward at the waist. Rib asymmetry of even a small degree is obvious. (From Scoles PV: Spinal deformity in childhood and adolescence. In Behrman RE, Vaughn VC III [editors]: *Nelson Textbook of Pediatrics,* Update 5. Philadelphia, WB Saunders, 1989.)

A careful neurologic evaluation is essential, especially in patients with apparent juvenile-onset scoliosis, atypical curve patterns, or back pain. The presence of café-au-lait spots, sacral dimpling, midline hairy patches, shoe size asymmetry, foot deformity, or a history of back pain or urinary incontinence suggests a nonidiopathic cause for the deformity.

School screening programs for early detection of scoliosis are common in North America. The forward bend test is the method employed; inclinometers to estimate the height of rib asymmetry are used in some centers. The sensitivity and specificity of the forward bend test depend on the skill of the examiner and the degree of curvature considered to be significant. Virtually all children with spinal curves greater than 20 degrees are identified by trained observers; unfortunately, a large number of normal children are identified as well. Estimates of the incidence of curvature greater than 20 degrees range from 0.1–1.0%, whereas positive screening rates run as high as 30%. In light of such information, the benefits of screening programs must be weighed against the costs of referral and the potential adverse effects of unnecessary radiographic examination.

Radiographic Evaluation. Radiographic examination is the reference standard for evaluation of patients with suspected spinal deformity. If there is clinical evidence of spinal deformity, standing posteroanterior (PA) and lateral standing radiographs of the entire spine should be obtained. Supine and side-bending radiographs are not necessary for initial assessment of scoliosis, kyphosis, or lordosis. The degree of curvature is determined by measuring the angular relationships between the most tilted vertebrae at either end of the apparent curve (the Cobb method). A line is drawn across the proximal end-plate of the superior end vertebra and the distal end-plate of the inferior end vertebra, and perpendicular lines are erected. The angle at the intersection of the perpendicular lines determines the degree of curvature. Another method to classify spinal curves is noted in Figure 669–2. The use of other imaging modalities, such as CT and MRI, should be reserved for cases in which nonidiopathic curvature is suspected.

Treatment. The risk for curve progression varies according to sex, age, menarchal status, and curve magnitude at initial discovery. Premenarchal girls with curves between 20 and 30 degrees have a significantly higher risk for progression than do girls 2 yr after menarche with similar curves; curve progression is likely in the first group and uncommon in the second. Boys with curvature of the same magnitude appear to have similar risks of progression when judged by other maturation standards. Curves less than 30 degrees rarely progress after skeletal maturation is complete; curves greater than 45 or 50 degrees often continue to progress during adult life.

The rationale for treatment of patients with idiopathic scoliosis is based on the assumption that patients with progressive scoliosis will acquire unacceptable deformities, premature degenerative joint disease, and progressive cardiorespiratory compromise and that treatment can positively affect these outcomes. Although there are conflicting data on the long-term outcome of untreated scoliosis, it appears reasonable to assume that patients with high-magnitude deformities will both look and feel different than their age- and sex-matched peers.

The generally accepted methods of treatment of progressive idiopathic adolescent scoliosis are bracing and surgical correction. There is no evidence that chiropractic treatment or exercise programs alter the outcome of scoliosis; transcutaneous electrical stimulation has been shown to have no effect. Most orthopedic surgeons recommend a trial of brace treatment for immature patients with curves less than 40 degrees. Although the efficacy of brace treatment has been questioned, current studies suggest a small decrease in the likelihood of progression for patients treated with bracing when compared with age-, sex-, and curve-matched peers followed by observation alone.

Criteria for Curve Classification

CURVE TYPE

Type	Proximal thoracic	Main thoracic	Thoracolumbar/ lumbar	Curve type
1	Non-structural	Structural (major*)	Non-structural	Main thoracic (MT)
2	Structural	Structural (major*)	Non-structural	Double thoracic (DT)
3	Non-structural	Structural (major*)	Structural	Double major (DM)
4	Structural	Structural (major*)	Structural	Triple major (TM)
5	Non-structural	Non-structural	Structural (major*)	Thoracolumbar/ lumbar (TL/L)
6	Non-structural	Structural	Non-structural (major*)	Thoracolumbar/ lumbar-main thoracic (TL/L-MT)

*Major = largest Cobb measurement, always structural; minor = all other curves with structural criteria applied.

LOCATION OF APEX (SRS definition)

Curve	Apex
Thoracic	T2-T11-12 disc
Thoracolumbar	T12-L1
	L1-2 disc-L4

MODIFIERS

Lumbar spine modifier	CSVL to lumbar apex	Modifiers	Thoracic sagittal profile T5-T12
A	CSVL between pedicles		− (Hypo) $<10°$ C
B	CSVL touches apical body(ies)		N (Normal) $10°-40°$
C	CSVL completely medial		+ (Hyper) $>40°$

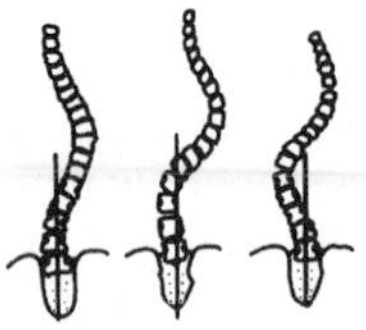

A B C

Curve type (1–6) + lumbar spine modifier (A, B or C) + thoracic sagittal modifier (−, N, or +)

SRS = Scoliosis Research Society, CSVL = center sacral vertical line.

FIGURE 669–2. Criteria for curve classification. (From Edgar M: A new classification of adolescent idiopathic scoliosis. *Lancet* 2002; 360:270–1, with permission.)

Bracing does not correct curvature; although improvement in Cobb angles is often noted during the active period of brace treatment, there are no studies that demonstrate consistent long-term maintenance of correction. A variety of spinal orthoses are employed; retrospective studies suggest little difference in outcome by brace type.

Surgical treatment is usually considered for patients with idiopathic curves greater than 45 degrees. Surgical treatment usually combines correction of deformity with permanently implanted internal fixation rods and posterior fusion of the involved vertebrae (Fig. 669–3). Occasionally, anterior spinal fusion and instrumentation may be indicated, especially in thoracolumbar and lumbar curves.

669.2 Congenital Scoliosis

Abnormalities of vertebral development during the first trimester of pregnancy often result in structural deformities of the spine that are evident at birth or become obvious in early childhood. Congenital scoliosis can be classified as (1) partial or complete failure of vertebral formation (wedge vertebrae or hemivertebrae), (2) partial or complete failure of segmentation (unsegmented bars), or (3) mixed. It may occur as an isolated deformity or in combination with other organ system malformations that are differentiating at the same time as the spine.

Congenital genitourinary malformations occur in 20% of children with congenital scoliosis. Unilateral renal agenesis is the most common abnormality. Duplication of ureters, horseshoe kidney, and genital anomalies also occur. Approximately 2% of children with associated genitourinary abnormalities have a silent, obstructive uropathy. Renal ultrasonography should be performed in all children with congenital scoliosis to assess for possible genitourinary problems. Other procedures, such as intravenous pyelography or MRI, may be necessary if the ultrasonogram is abnormal. Congenital heart disease occurs in 10–15% of children with congenital scoliosis.

A high percentage of patients with congenital scoliosis have associated defects of the spinal cord. *Spinal dysraphism* is the general term applied to such lesions; MRI studies suggest that they are present in as many as 40% of patients with congenital scoliosis. Spina bifida occulta is the most common and benign defect; myelomeningocele is the most severe. Other lesions include intradural and extradural lipomas, cysts and teratomas, and spinal cord tethers. In addition to spine asymmetry, physical examination in these patients often shows hairy patches, skin dimples, hemangiomas, and abnormalities of the feet and lower extremities. Asymmetric foot size, cavus feet, and calf atrophy strongly suggest the presence of spinal dysraphism in patients with congenital scoliosis. MRI is the procedure of choice for evaluating possible spinal dysraphism.

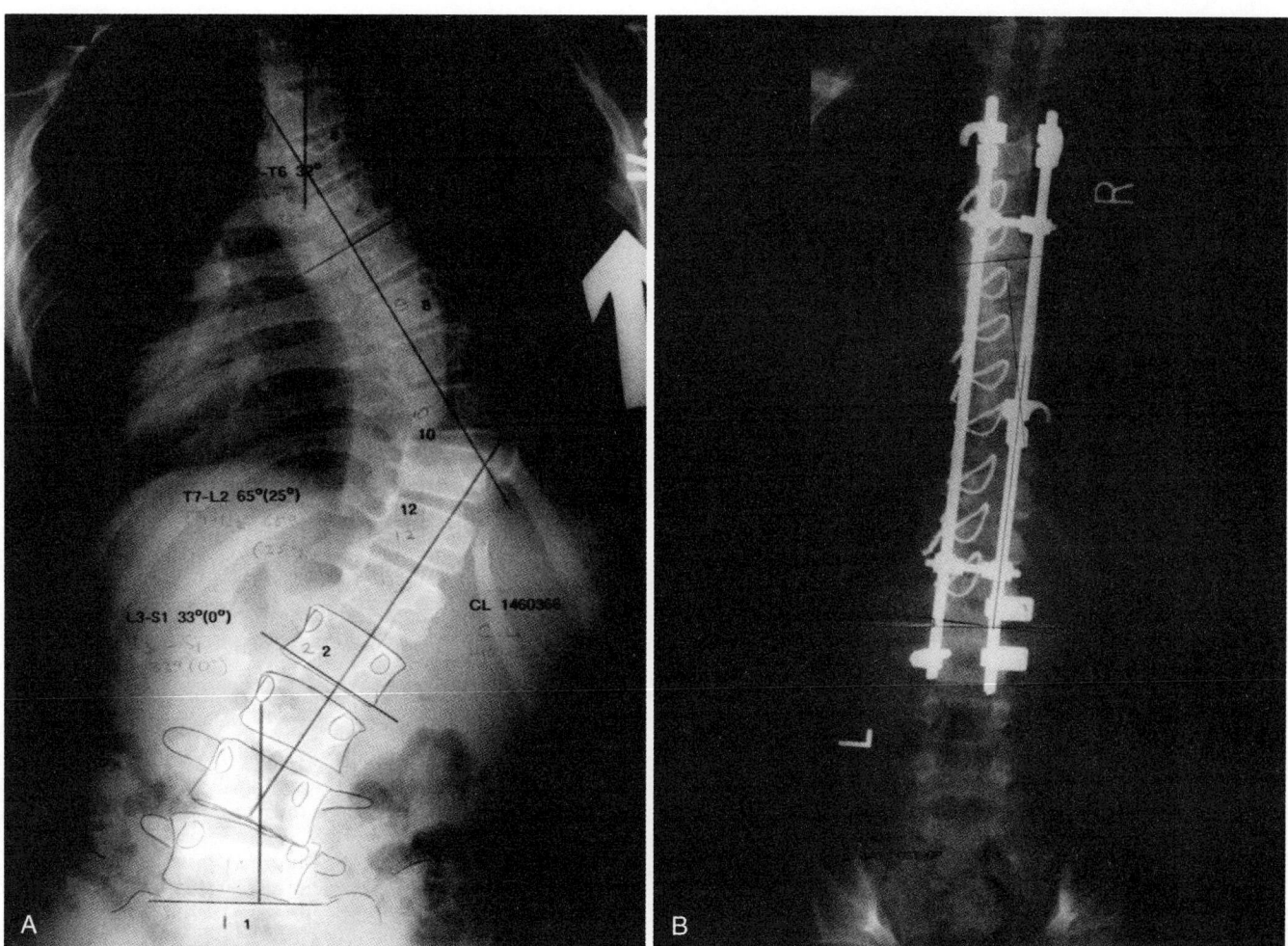

FIGURE 669–3. *A,* Preoperative standing posteroanterior radiograph of a 13-yr-old girl with a severe right thoracic section. Note the Cobb measurement technique. The numbers in parentheses indicate the degree of correction of the deformity on side-bending radiographs. *B,* Postoperative radiograph demonstrating a selective right thoracolumbar fusion and instrumentation from T3 to L2. Note the spontaneous improvement in the compensatory left lumbar curve after correction of the structural right thoracolumbar curve.

The risk for progression of spinal deformity in a child with congenital scoliosis depends on the growth potential of the malformed vertebra. Defects, such as block vertebra, have little growth potential and usually do not cause significant spinal deformity. Hemivertebrae may or may not cause significant deformity depending on location and their potential for growth. Unilateral unsegmented bars almost always produce progressive deformities. Approximately 25% of patients with congenital scoliosis do not demonstrate curve progression and do not require treatment. Most patients demonstrate some progression, and many require treatment. Patients are most at risk during periods of rapid growth before 2 and after 10 yr of age.

Early diagnosis and prompt treatment of progressive curves is essential. Orthotic treatment is of limited value because of the structural nature of congenital curvature. Often a combined anterior and posterior spinal fusion across the area of the deformity is required to halt progression and counteract the strong forces of growth. Anterior and posterior convex epiphysiodeses have been used to produce partial correction with growth. Hemivertebrae excision can also be considered. It is a serious mistake to defer treatment of progressive spinal curvatures while awaiting further spinal growth.

669.3 Neuromuscular Scoliosis, Genetic Syndromes, and Compensatory Scoliosis

Neuromuscular Scoliosis. Scoliosis is a common complication of many neuromuscular disorders of childhood. Muscle imbalance, soft tissue contracture, and progressive weakness predispose patients with disorders such as cerebral palsy, muscular dystrophies, and spinal muscular atrophy to scoliosis. In patients with myelodysplasia, structural malformations of the vertebral column complicate the problem. In general, the magnitude of the deformity depends on the severity of involvement, the pattern of weakness, and the progressive nature of the underlying disease process. Ambulatory patients with minimal involvement and cerebral palsy are much less likely to have significant spinal deformity than nonambulatory patients with profound involvement.

Progression of deformity in patients with neuromuscular scoliosis has serious consequences. Sitting and standing balance are altered, adversely affecting ambulation in marginal walkers and complicating seating support in nonambulators. Patients who must use their arms for trunk support lose a significant degree of independence. Severe curves decrease pulmonary reserve, compounding pre-existent respiratory problems.

Neuromuscular scoliosis can be treated safely and effectively in most instances, but the success of treatment depends on early recognition. Because scoliosis in most patients with neuromuscular disease progresses relentlessly once curvature begins, there is little reason to delay treatment once the deformity is identified. The forward bending test can be used for screening; the test may be performed in the sitting position for patients who cannot stand. Any asymmetry is an indication for radiographic evaluation. This should include posteroanterior and lateral standing radiographs of the entire spine. If the child or adolescent cannot stand, a sitting or supine (anteroposterior) radiograph is necessary.

The goal of treatment of neuromuscular scoliosis is to restore spinal alignment, stabilize respiratory function, and prevent progressive loss of independence. Nonambulatory patients are usually most comfortable, are more independent, and have better respiratory function when they are able to sit erect without external support. Unfortunately, options for treatment in neuromuscular scoliosis are limited. Orthotic management or bracing is usually not effective as definitive treatment in neuromuscular scoliosis. In young children, brace treatment may slow the rate of curve progression, allowing further spinal growth and delaying surgical intervention. For most patients with progressive deformity, surgery is necessary when treatment is indicated. Instrumentation systems provide effective correction and eliminate the need for external support in the postoperative period. Most patients may be out of bed immediately after surgery.

Syndromes. Children with certain syndromes are also at increased risk for spinal deformities. Common syndromes include neurofibromatosis and Marfan syndrome. These children require periodic evaluation and prompt referral for orthopedic evaluation at the first sign of a spinal deformity.

Compensatory Scoliosis. Leg-length inequality is a common cause of false-positive screening examinations (see Chapter 666). Discrepancies as small as 0.5 cm may produce asymmetry. The pelvis in such patients tilts toward the short side, producing a postural curve in the opposite direction. Because children with leg-length inequality may also have idiopathic or congenital scoliosis, careful evaluation is necessary. Any child with a lower extremity–length inequality should be referred for orthopedic evaluation.

669.4 Kyphosis (Round-Back)

The normal thoracic spine has a convex alignment in the sagittal plane, termed *kyphosis*. The normal radiographic range of kyphosis is 20–40 degrees; individuals with increased kyphotic alignment have the clinical sign of round-back. Round-back may be flexible or structural; structural round-back may be idiopathic or congenital in origin. Idiopathic round-back is sometimes referred to as Scheuermann disease.

FLEXIBLE KYPHOSIS

Round-back is a common concern of many parents of adolescents. They often are perceived by parents and teachers to sit and stand in a slouched position, and round-back is a common cause of referral from spine screening programs. Adolescents with postural round-back can correct the round-back appearance voluntarily in both the standing and prone positions. The overall angle of kyphosis may be increased on the standing lateral radiograph, but no vertebral abnormalities are present. A supine hyperextension lateral radiograph shows complete correction. It is commonly thought that such a posture leads to permanent deformity. Fortunately, there is no evidence that flexible round-back posture has adverse physical effects. A thoracic hyperextension exercise program may assist in strengthening the extensor muscles of the spine, but the patient has the ultimate responsibility for his or her posture. Orthotic treatment is not indicated for patients with flexible round-back.

STRUCTURAL KYPHOSIS

Scheuermann Disease (Idiopathic Kyphosis)

The term *Scheuermann kyphosis* is used for nonflexible (structural) kyphosis that develops during adolescence in previously normal children. Mild increases in structural kyphosis are equally common in girls and boys; the condition may worsen slightly more often in boys than in girls. The absolute incidence of the disorder is unknown because small degrees of structural kyphosis are neither clinically obvious nor significant. Cadaver studies indicate that the vertebral changes associated with structural round-back occur in 7–8% of the population. The cause is unclear, but histologic specimens obtained at the time of surgical correction of severe deformity suggest that a disordered pattern of endochondral ossification similar to that found in slipped capital femoral epiphysis and tibia vara may be responsible. This may be the result of increased pressure on the anterior vertebral growth plates in some individuals with severe flexible round-back, but the relationship has not been clearly established.

Clinical Manifestations. Patients with Scheuermann kyphosis present with thoracic kyphosis of greater degree and sharper contour than that seen in normal individuals. Unlike flexible round-back patients, affected individuals cannot actively correct the deformity. Many patients complain of occasional mild aching pain in the area of the kyphosis, but it is rarely severe or limiting. Careful neurologic examination is essential, but fortunately neurologic complications of Scheuermann kyphosis are rare.

Radiographic Evaluation. Radiographic assessment for kyphosis includes posteroanterior and lateral standing radiographs of the entire spine (Fig. 669–4). In addition to increased kyphotic angle, radiographic findings include (1) narrowing of disk space, (2) loss of the normal anterior height of the involved vertebra and elongation of the vertebral centrum, (3) wedging of 5 degrees or more in three or more vertebrae, and (4) irregularities of the end-plates, sometimes called *Schmorl nodes.*

Treatment. Treatment depends on the age of the patient, the degree of deformity, and the presence or absence of pain in the apical region. Scheuermann kyphosis appears to be primarily a cosmetic problem. There is little evidence that patients with kyphotic curves less than 70 or 80 degrees experience late progression, disabling pain, or neurologic compromise. Kyphotic deformities greater than 90 degrees are more likely to be aesthetically unacceptable, symptomatic, and progressive. There are few absolute guidelines for treatment, and decisions must be individualized. Mature patients with little or no pain and acceptable cosmetic alignment need no treatment. Immature patients with mild deformity may benefit from a hyperextension exercise program, whereas those with kyphotic deformities greater than 60 degrees require bracing if treatment is considered appropriate. Thoracic kyphosis usually requires a Milwaukee brace; in patients with thoracolumbar kyphosis, an underarm hyperextension orthosis can be used. Surgical treatment of Scheuermann disease is usually reserved for patients with severe and painful deformity who have completed growth. This usually involves a combination of anterior spinal release and fusion and posterior spinal fusion and instrumentation.

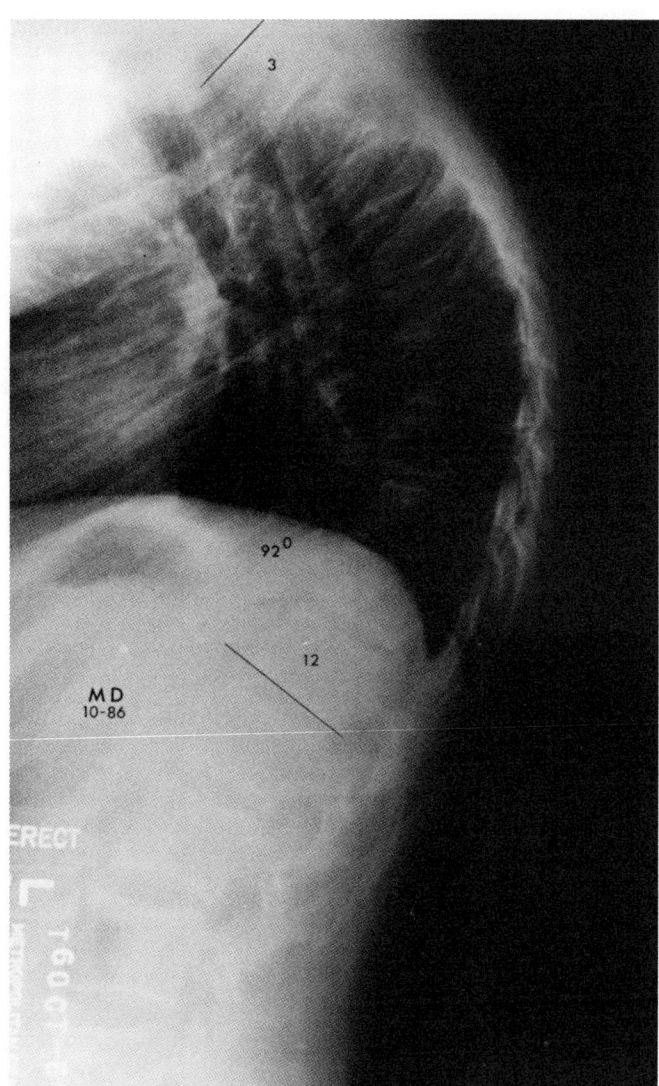

FIGURE 669–4. Standing lateral radiograph of a 14-yr-old boy with severe Scheuermann kyphosis. This measures 92 degrees between T3 and T12. Note the wedging of the vertebrae at T6, T7, T8, and T9. The normal thoracic kyphosis is 40 degrees or less.

Congenital Kyphosis

Congenital kyphosis, or kyphotic deformity, is the result of vertebral malformations that occur during the first trimester. The most common abnormalities are congenital failure of formation of all or part of the vertebral centrum and failure of anterior segmentation of the spine (anterior unsegmented bar). Severe deformities are usually recognized at birth and rapidly progress thereafter. The less obvious deformities may not become obvious until later in childhood. Progressive congenital kyphosis is a serious problem; paraplegia may develop as a result of compression of the spinal cord against the apex of the deformity. Patients with congenital kyphosis should be referred for specialty evaluation as soon as the deformity is recognized. Brace treatment is not effective. Surgical intervention is often necessary, and the results of surgery are best if performed before significant deformity has developed.

669.5 Back Pain in Children

Back pain in children is unusual and should be viewed with concern. In contrast to adults, in whom back pain is frequently mechanical or psychologic in origin, back pain in children is frequently due to organic causes, especially in preadolescent children. Back pain lasting more than a few days requires careful investigation. It has been reported that approximately 85% of children with back pain lasting more than 2 mo have a specific diagnosable lesion: 33% post-traumatic (occult fracture, spondylolysis); 33% developmental (kyphosis, scoliosis); and 18% infection or tumor. Only in the remaining 15% is the diagnosis nonspecific.

Clinical Manifestations. When confronted with a child with back pain, a careful history and physical evaluation are mandatory. The history includes the onset and duration of symptoms; antecedent factors; general health; family history; location, character, and radiation of pain; and neurologic symptoms, such as muscle weakness, sensory changes, and bowel or bladder dysfunction. Physical examination includes a complete musculoskeletal and neurologic evaluation. Spinal alignment, mobility, muscle spasm, and areas of tenderness are evaluated and recorded. The danger signs in childhood back pain include (1) persistent or increasing pain; (2) systemic symptoms, such as fever, malaise, or weight loss; (3) neurologic symptoms or findings; (4) bowel or bladder dysfunction; (5) young age, especially less than 4 yr (suspect tumor); and (6) painful left thoracic spine curvatures.

Radiographic and Laboratory Evaluation. Plain radiographs are the first diagnostic procedure to use in the evaluation of pediatric back pain, usually posteroanterior and lateral standing radiographs of the spine with right and left oblique views of the involved area. MRI or bone scans may be necessary depending on the location of the pain and the differential diagnoses. Laboratory studies, such as a complete blood cell count with differential, erythrocyte sedimentation rate (ESR), and tests for the juvenile forms of arthritis (juvenile rheumatoid arthritis and ankylosing spondylitis) may be necessary in certain cases (see Chapter 146). Cerebrospinal fluid should be evaluated if myelography is performed.

Differential Diagnosis. The differential diagnosis in pediatric back pain is extensive and is presented in Box 669–2.

669.6 Spondylolysis and Spondylolisthesis

Spondylolysis is the term used to refer to a defect in the pars interarticularis, the posterior plate of bone that connects the superior and inferior articular facets of a vertebral body. The abnormality most commonly occurs in the L5 vertebra and is sometimes associated with forward slip of the affected vertebra relative to the body of the first sacral vertebra, termed *spondylolisthesis*. Spondylolysis may be congenital or acquired. Cadaver studies indicate that 5–7% of the general population has pars interarticularis defects; asymptomatic spina bifida occulta at L5 or S1 often accompanies the lesion. Most individuals with congenital spondylolysis have little or no pain and do not acquire spondylolisthesis. In such a patient, the abnormality is usually noted as an incidental finding on radiographs made for other reasons. A small percentage of patients with spondylolysis acquire the lesion as a result of repetitive flexion exercises from activities such as gymnastics or diving. The lesion in such patients resembles a stress fracture and is more likely to be symptomatic. Spondylolisthesis, when present, is usually graded by the degree of slippage of one vertebra on the other: grade 1, less than 25%; grade 2, 25–50%; grade 3, 50–75%; grade 4, 75–100%; and grade 5, complete displacement.

Clinical Manifestations. Symptomatic patients with spondylolysis usually present with low back pain and hamstring muscle spasm. Radicular symptoms are not common. Urinary retention

BOX 669–2. Differential Diagnosis of Back Pain

INFLAMMATORY DISEASES

Diskitis (common before 6 yr)
Vertebral osteomyelitis (pyogenic, tuberculous)
Spinal epidural abscess
Pyelonephritis
Pancreatitis

RHEUMATOLOGIC DISEASES

Pauciarticular juvenile rheumatoid arthritis
Reiter syndrome
Ankylosing spondylitis
Psoriatic arthritis

DEVELOPMENTAL DISEASES

Spondylolysis (common in adolescents)
Spondylolisthesis (common in adolescents)
Scheuermann syndrome (common in adolescents)
Scoliosis (especially left thoracic)

MECHANICAL TRAUMA AND ABNORMALITIES

Hip-pelvic anomalies
Herniated disk
Overuse syndromes (common with athletic training and in gymnasts
   and dancers)
Vertebral stress fractures
Upper cervical spine instability

NEOPLASTIC DISEASES

Primary vertebral tumors (e.g., osteogenic sarcoma)
Metastatic tumor (e.g., neuroblastoma)
Primary spinal tumor (e.g., neuroblastoma, lipoma)
Malignancy of bone marrow (e.g., acute lymphocytic leukemia,
   lymphoma)
Benign tumors (e.g., eosinophilic granuloma, osteoid osteoma)

OTHER

After lumbar puncture
Conversion reaction
Juvenile osteoporosis

or incontinence are uncommon but, when present, imply serious compromise of the sacral nerve roots. Physical examination shows limitation of lumbar flexibility and tight hamstring muscles. When spondylolisthesis accompanies spondylolysis, lumbar lordosis is often reduced rather than accentuated, and sacral kyphosis is often present. The buttocks appear flattened and prominent, and the anterior abdominal wall is prominent. A palpable "step-off" at the lumbosacral area may be noted in patients with high-grade spondylolisthesis. The forward bend test for scoliosis should be performed because patients with spondylolysis may also have scoliosis. Careful neurologic examination is essential.

Radiologic Evaluation. Initial radiographic examination in patients with suspected disorders of the lumbosacral region should include anteroposterior, lateral, and oblique radiographs of the lumbosacral spine. Large cassette films of the spine should be obtained if there is a suspicion of scoliosis. When there is a history of urinary dysfunction or physical signs of nerve root compromise, MRI of the thoracolumbar spine should be performed.

Treatment. Treatment of spondylolysis depends on the presence of symptoms. Progressive slippage has been reported in children and adolescents with asymptomatic spondylolysis, and such patients should be re-examined at 6-mo intervals. Repeat radiographs are probably not necessary in the absence of symptoms or physical signs of progression. When indicated, a single standing lateral film of the lumbosacral junction provides information for routine follow-up. Patients with painful spondylolysis, especially when a stress fracture is suspected, may benefit from a period of immobilization in a body jacket or underarm orthosis. If this does not relieve pain, surgical intervention may be required to repair the defect or stabilize the affected vertebrae.

Progressive spondylolisthesis causes deformity and disability. Because surgical reduction of severe slip is difficult and carries significant risks, progressive slips are best treated before a severe deformity develops. Painful spondylolisthesis, or asymptomatic spondylolisthesis with greater than 25% slip, is usually treated by an in situ posterior spinal fusion regardless of the age of the patient.

669.7 ■ Disk Space Infection

Intervertebral diskitis is the term used for the association of back pain, progressive loss of intervertebral disk height, and erosion of adjacent vertebral end-plates usually in lumbar regions. The clinical findings and radiographic signs may be common manifestations of a number of underlying processes. Rarely, patients have severe back pain, high fever, and signs of bacteremia consistent with acute osteomyelitis. In most, the inflammatory process is much less severe, even though blood cultures (rarely) or aspirates of the involved area may occasionally yield bacteria. In some patients, there are few symptoms and signs and no evidence of systemic or local infection despite progressive radiographic changes. In these instances, the lesion may be of traumatic or rheumatic origin.

Clinical Manifestations. Symptoms in patients with intervertebral diskitis vary with age, and a high index of suspicion is required to establish the diagnosis. Very young children may simply be fussy and refuse to eat. Toddlers may cease walking. Older children and adolescents complain of back, abdominal, or pelvic pain. The physical findings in a child with a disk space infection are usually characteristic. The child maintains the spine in a straight, stiff, or splinted position and refuses to flex the lumbar spine. The normal lumbar lordosis is reversed, and there may be paravertebral muscle spasm. Fever is variable, and the systemic white blood cell count may be only mildly elevated. The ESR is usually elevated. The differential diagnosis includes vertebral body osteomyelitis which is associated with an older age at onset (7 vs 2 yr), longer duration of illness (33 vs 22 days), and the presence of fever, leukocytosis and bone destruction.

Radiographic Evaluation. The radiographic features vary according to the interval between the onset of symptoms and the diagnosis. Radiographic signs lag behind clinical symptoms. The characteristic findings of disk space (narrowing and irregularity of the adjacent vertebral body end-plates) are not often present at the time of initial presentation. Technetium bone scans and MRI scans become abnormal early in the disease and may establish the diagnosis in patients with suggestive symptoms and signs. MRI may show a paravertebral inflammatory mass in diskitis. MRI is most helpful in distinguishing diskitis from vertebral osteomyelitis.

Treatment. In patients with constitutional symptoms and signs suggestive of a bacterial cause, initial treatment should include a combination of immobilization and antibiotics. *Staphylococcus aureus* is the usual organism isolated in those patients with a clear bacterial cause, and appropriate antibiotic coverage should be initiated. Blood cultures may be helpful in identifying the organism. Aspiration needle biopsy of the disk space by CT guidance is not necessary and is usually reserved for children who do not respond to initial treatment with antibiotics. A minimum of 4–6 wk of antibiotic therapy should be used for patients with positive cultures, high white blood cell counts, or persistent elevation of the erythrocyte sedimentation rate. The appropriateness of antibiotics is less certain in patients with minimal symptoms, few signs, and normal laboratory studies. Immobilization alone may suffice in such cases. Surgical drainage is usually reserved for patients who do not respond to initial therapy or who have MRI evidence of abscess formation in the paravertebral area.

669.8 Intervertebral Disk Herniation

Intervertebral disk rupture is rare in children and uncommon in adolescents. In the United States, less than 1% of patients undergoing diskectomy are younger than 16 yr. The frequency of symptomatic intervertebral disk herniation is more common in Asiatic populations than in whites, perhaps because of the smaller size of the spinal canal.

Clinical Manifestations. Symptoms of intervertebral disk herniation in adolescents are similar to those in adults. The majority of affected patients report back pain; most have sciatic pain. About 30% complain of decreased sensation or paresthesia in the lower extremities. On physical examination, lumbar muscle spasm, scoliosis, and a decreased range of lumbar motion are common findings. A positive straight leg-raising test is present in most patients. Abnormal reflex patterns and lower extremity weakness are much less likely to be present in young patients than in adults. A history of trauma is occasionally present, and patients tend to be taller and slightly heavier than their peers. A positive family history of intervertebral disk disease is frequently present.

Radiographic Evaluation. Radiographs often show loss of lumbar lordosis and lumbar scoliosis. Loss of intervertebral disk height is rarely noted on plain films. MRI is currently the study of choice for localization of the lesion.

Treatment. Most symptoms respond to bed rest followed by gradual resumption of activities. When sciatic pain, loss of reflexes, or weakness persist, surgical excision of the intervertebral disk is indicated. Fusion is not necessary unless there is accompanying evidence of spinal instability. Good results can be expected about 75% of the time. The incidence of recurrent symptoms requiring repeat surgery is about 25%.

669.9 Tumors

Back pain may be the presenting complaint in children who have a tumor involving the vertebral column or the spinal cord. Other associated symptoms may include weakness of the lower extremities, scoliosis, and loss of sphincter control. Both benign and malignant tumors may occur; most are benign (see Chapter 493). Common benign tumors include osteoid osteomas, osteoblastoma, solitary bone cysts, and eosinophilic granuloma. Malignant tumors may be osseous (osteogenic or Ewing sarcoma), neurogenic (neuroblastoma), or metastatic in origin. Because the onset of symptoms usually precedes radiographic abnormality, radioisotope bone scans or MRI is necessary for localization and diagnosis. The treatment of tumors of the spinal column is complex and may involve a combination of surgery, radiotherapy, and chemotherapy. Side effects are common when combination therapy is required, and growth disturbances can be expected.

Idiopathic Scoliosis

Amato CR, Griggs S, McCoy B: Nighttime bracing with the Providence brace in adolescent girls with idiopathic scoliosis. *Spine* 2001;26:2006–12.

Ceballas T, Ferrer-Torrelles M, Castillo F, et al: Prognosis in infantile idiopathic scoliosis. *J Bone Joint Surg Am* 1980;62A:863–75.

Do T, Fras C, Burke S, et al: Clinical value of routine preoperative magnetic resonance imaging in adolescent idiopathic scoliosis: A prospective study of three hundred and twenty-seven patients. *Bone Joint Surg Am* 2001;83A:577–79.

Edgar M: A new classification of adolescent idiopathic scoliosis. *Lancet* 2002;360:270–71.

Figueiredo UM, James JIP: Juvenile idiopathic scoliosis. *J Bone Joint Surg Br* 1979;61B:36–42.

Goldberg CJ, Moore DP, Fogarty EE, et al: Adolescent idiopathic scoliosis: The effect of brace treatment on the incidence of surgery. *Spine* 2001;26:42–47.

Karol LA: Effectiveness of bracing in male patients with idiopathic scoliosis. *Spine* 2001;26:2001–5.

Killian JT, Mayberry S, Wilkinson L: Current concepts in adolescent idiopathic scoliosis. *Pediatr Ann* 1999;28:755–61.

Lantz CA, Chen J: Effects of chiropractic intervention on small scoliotic curves in younger subjects: A time series cohort design. *J Manipulative Physiol Ther* 2001;24:385–93.

Little DG, Song KM, Katz D, et al: Relationship of peak height velocity to other maturity indicators in idiopathic scoliosis in girls. *J Bone Joint Surg Am* 2000;82:685–93.

Lonstein JE, Carlson JM: The prediction of curve progression in untreated idiopathic scoliosis during growth. *J Bone Joint Surg Am* 1984;66A:1061–71.

Lonstein JE, Winter RB: The Milwaukee brace for the treatment of adolescent idiopathic scoliosis. *J Bone Joint Surg Am* 1994;76A:1207–21.

Miller NH: Cause and natural history of adolescent idiopathic scoliosis. *Orthop Clin North Am* 1999;30:343–52.

Nachemson AL, Peterson LE: Effectiveness of treatment with a brace for girls who have adolescent idiopathic scoliosis: A prospective controlled study based on data from the brace study of the Scoliosis Research Society. *J Bone Joint Surg Am* 1995;77A:815–22.

Noonan KJ, Weinstein SL, Jacobson WC, et al: Use of the Milwaukee brace for progressive idiopathic scoliosis. *J Bone Joint Surg Am* 1996;78A:557–67.

Reamy BV, Slakey JB: Adolescent idiopathic scoliosis: Review and current concepts. *Am Fam Physician* 2001;64:111–16.

Roach JW: Adolescent idiopathic scoliosis. *Orthop Clin North Am* 1999;30:353–65.

Rowe DE, Bernstein SM, Riddick MF, et al: A meta-analysis of the efficiency of non-operative treatments for idiopathic scoliosis. *J Bone Joint Surg Am* 1997;79A:664–74.

Shapiro G, Green DW, Fatica NS, et al: Medical complications in scoliosis surgery. *Curr Opin Pediatr* 2001;13:36–41.

Song KM, Little DG: Peak height velocity as a maturity factor for males with idiopathic scoliosis. *J Pediatr Orthop* 2000;20:286–88.

Yawn BP, Yawn RA, Hodge D, et al: A population-based study on school scoliosis screening. *JAMA* 1999;282:1427–32.

Congenital Scoliosis

Callahan BC, Georgopoulos G, Eilert RE: Hemivertebral excision for congenital scoliosis. *J Pediatr Orthop* 1997;17:96.

Deviren V, Bervin, S, Smith JA, et al: Excision of hemivertebrae in the management of congenital scoliosis involving the thoracic and thoracolumbar spine. *J Bone Joint Surg Br* 2001;83B:496–500.

Jaskwhich D, Ali RM, Patel TC, et al: Congenital scoliosis. *Curr Opin Pediatr* 2000;12:61–66.

Klemme WR, Polly DW Jr, Orchowski JR: Hemivertebral excision for congenital scoliosis in very young children. *J Pediatr Orthop* 2001;21:761–64.

McMaster MJ, Ohtsuka K: The natural history of congenital scoliosis: A study of 251 patients. *J Bone Joint Surg Am* 1982;64:1128–47.

Prahinski JR, Polly DW Jr, McHale KA, et al: Occult intraspinal anomalies in congenital scoliosis. *J Pediatr Orthop* 2000;20:59–63.

Suh SW, Sarwark JF, Vora A, et al: Evaluating congenital spine deformities for intraspinal anomalies with magnetic resonance imaging. *J Pediatr Orthop* 2001;21:525–31.

Thompson AG, Marks DS, Sayampanathan SR, et al: Long-term results of combined anterior and posterior convex epiphysiodesis for congenital scoliosis due to hemivertebrae. *Spine* 1995;20:1380–85.

Neuromuscular Scoliosis

Banta JV, Drummond DS, Ferguson RL: The treatment of neuromuscular scoliosis. *Am Acad Orthop Surg Instr Course Lect* 1999;48:551–62.

Bridwell KH, Baldus C, Iffrig TM, et al: Process measures and patient/parent evaluation of surgical management of spinal deformities in patients with progressive flaccid neuromuscular scoliosis (Duchenne's muscular dystrophy and spinal muscular atrophy). *Spine* 1999;24:1300–9.

McCarthy RE: Management of neuromuscular scoliosis. *Orthop Clin North Am* 1999;30:435–49.

Olafsson Y, Saraste H, Al-Dabbagh Z: Brace treatment in neuromuscular spine deformity. *J Pediatr Orthop* 1999;19:376–79.

Niethard FU, Heller KD: Neuromuscular scoliosis: Current concepts. *J Pediatr Orthop* 2000;9:215–16.

Yazici M, Asher MA, Hardacker JW: The safety and efficacy of Isola-Galveston instrumentation and arthrodesis in the treatment of neuromuscular spinal deformities. *J Bone Joint Surg Am* 2000;82:524–43.

Kyphosis—Scheuermann and Congenital

Ali RM, Green DW, Patel TC: Scheuermann's kyphosis. *Curr Opin Pediatr* 1999;11:70–75.

Lowe TG: Current concepts review: Scheuermann disease. *Orthop Clin North Am* 1999;30:475–87.

McMaster MJ, Singh H: Natural history of congenital kyphosis and kyphoscoliosis: A study of one hundred and twelve patients. *J Bone Joint Surg Am* 1999;81A:1367–83.

Sachs B, Bradford D, Winter R, et al: Scheuermann's kyphosis: Follow-up of Milwaukee brace treatment. *J Bone Joint Surg Am* 1987;69:50–57.

Wenger DR, Frick SL: Scheuermann's kyphosis. *Spine* 1999;24:2630–39.

Thompson GH, Blakemore LC: Kyphosis. In Fitzgerald RH Jr, Kaufer H, Malkani A (editors): *Orthopaedics.* St. Louis, CV Mosby, 2002, pp 1364–72.

Back Pain

Conrad EM III, Olszewski AD, Berger M, et al: Pediatric spine tumors with spinal cord compromise. *J Pediatr Orthop* 1992;12:454–60.

Feldman DS, Hedden DM, Wright JG: The use of bone scan to investigate back pain in children and adolescents. *J Pediatr Orthop* 2000;20:790–95.

King HA: Back pain in children. *Orthop Clin North Am* 1999;30:467–74.

Mason DE: Back pain in children. *Pediatr Ann* 1999;28:727–38.

Parisini P, DiSilvestre M, Greggi T, et al: Lumbar disc excision in children and adolescents. *Spine* 2001;26:1997–2000.

Richards BS, McCarthy RE, Akbarnia BA: Back pain in children and adolescents. *Am Acad Orthop Surg Instr Course Lect* 1999; 48:525–42.

Thompson GH: Back pain in children. *Am Acad Ortho Surg Instr Course Lect* 1994;43:221–30.

Thompson GH: Back pain. In Snyder RK (editor): *Essentials of Musculoskeletal Care.* Rosemont, IL, The American Academy of Orthopaedic Surgeons, 1997, pp 559–61.

Spondylolysis and Spondylolisthesis

Dubousset J: Treatment of spondylolysis and spondylolisthesis in children and adolescents. *Clin Orthop* 1997;337:77–85.

Lonstein JE: Spondylolisthesis in children: Cause, natural history, and management. *Spine* 1999;24:2640–48.

Saraste H: Long-term clinical and radiographical follow-up of spondylolysis and spondylolisthesis. *J Pediatr Orthop* 1987;7:631–38.

Seitsalo S, Osterman K, Hyvarinen H, et al: Severe spondylolisthesis in children and adolescents. *J Bone Joint Surg Br* 1990;72B:259–65.

Smith JA, Huss: Management of spondylolysis and spondylolisthesis in the pediatric and adolescent population. *Orthop Clin North Am* 1999;30:487–99.

Disk Space Infection

Brown R, Hussain M, McHugh K, et al: Discitis in young children. *J Bone Joint Surg Br* 2001;83B:106–11.

Fernandez M, Carroll CL, Baker CJ: Discitis and vertebral osteomyelitis in children: An 18-year review. *Pediatrics* 2000;105:1299–1304.

Chapter 670

The Neck

George H. Thomposn

Nonosseous and osseous abnormalities of the neck are relatively common in children. These are predominantly soft tissue, congenital, and neurologic in origin.

670.1 Torticollis

Torticollis (*torqueo*, "to twist" + *collum*, "neck") is the term applied to the clinical finding of a twisted neck. In most instances, the head is tipped toward one side and the chin rotated toward the other. Torticollis is a sign, not a disease, and may be the result of a wide range of underlying pathophysiologic processes. Torticollis that is present at birth may be the result of in utero positional (postural) effects or traumatic lesions of the sternomastoid muscle or of congenital abnormalities of the cervical spine. Torticollis in later childhood may be the result of trauma, inflammatory processes, spinal syrinx, or central nervous system neoplasia. The differential diagnosis of torticollis is extensive and is presented in Box 670–1.

Muscular torticollis is the most common variety and is presumed to result from injury to the sternocleidomastoid muscle during delivery. Large infants who have had difficult vertex deliveries as well as those who are breech or those with hip dysplasia are at special risk. In affected infants, normal rotation of the neck during delivery may produce bleeding within the substance of the sternocleidomastoid muscle (tumor) and a localized increase in pressure within the muscular compartment contained by the sternocleidomastoid fascia. Increased pressure produces focal ischemia; secondary fibrosis and contracture within the muscle result in the clinical finding of torticollis. Some infants have no tumor and may have torticollis secondary to in utero positioning.

BOX 670–1. Differential Diagnosis of Torticollis (Wryneck)

CONGENITAL

Muscular torticollis
Positional deformation
Hemivertebra (cervical spine)
Unilateral atlanto-occipital fusion
Klippel-Feil syndrome
Unilateral absence of sternocleidomastoid
Pterygium colli

TRAUMA

Muscular injury (cervical muscles)
Atlanto-occipital subluxation
Atlantoaxial subluxation
C2–3 subluxation
Rotary subluxation
Fractures

INFLAMMATION

Cervical lymphadenitis
Retropharyngeal abscess
Cervical vertebral osteomyelitis
Rheumatoid arthritis
Spontaneous (hyperemia, edema) subluxation with adjacent head and neck infection (rotary subluxation syndrome)
Upper lobe pneumonia

NEUROLOGIC

Visual disturbances (nystagmus, superior oblique paresis)
Dystonic drug reactions (phenothiazines, haloperidol, metoclopramide)
Cervical cord tumor
Posterior fossa brain tumor
Syringomyelia
Wilson disease
Dystonia musculorum deformans
Spasmus nutans

OTHER

Acute cervical disk calcification
Sandifer syndrome (gastroesophageal reflux, hiatal hernia)
Benign paroxysmal torticollis
Bone tumors (eosinophilic granuloma)
Soft tissue tumor
Hysteria

Swelling within the sternocleidomastoid muscle may be palpable in neonates with muscular torticollis; swelling diminishes shortly after birth, and the lesion may not be present in older infants. Contracture of the muscle results in the typical head tilt and rotation. In patients with a suggestive history and appropriate physical findings, programs of positioning and stimulation and gentle passive stretching exercises started within the first month of life often result in resolution. The parents should be instructed to rotate the chin gently toward the side of head tilt while simultaneously bringing the head to the upright position. As range of motion improves, the chin can be rotated past neutral and the head tilted toward the opposite side. Significant correction usually occurs within the first few months of life in patients with muscular torticollis. When deformity persists, the patient should be referred for orthopedic evaluation. Soft collars are not effective in treatment, and rigid devices produce secondary mandibular deformity. Surgical release of the sternocleidomastoid muscle is occasionally required in such patients and should be performed before the development of secondary facial asymmetry (plagiocephaly).

Congenital malformations of the cervical spine may also produce torticollis. Malformation or congenital cervical scoliosis result in deformity of the neck that will not respond to stretching exercise programs. Infants with torticollis, in whom there is no history of possible birth trauma and no evidence of a mass within the sternocleidomastoid muscle, should have anteroposterior and lateral cervical spine radiographs before a program of manipulation is recommended. At best, such infants respond minimally to stretching exercises; at worst, passive manipulation may injure the cervical spinal cord.

Torticollis arising later in childhood in previously normal children requires careful evaluation. The most common causes are minor cervical muscle trauma or inflammation of the cervical muscles secondary to upper respiratory illness. Inflammation of the head and neck region may produce a nontraumatic atlantoaxial subluxation. Most children with inflammatory torticollis do not have subluxation. Torticollis may be a manifestation of more serious abnormalities of the brain, especially a posterior fossa tumor, or spinal cord. Untreated torticollis in older children may result in loss of the normal rotational motion of the upper cervical spine or rotational subluxation of the upper cervical segments. The evaluation and treatment of suspected rotational fixation and subluxation in children is complex and should be performed by experienced specialists. Inflammatory torticollis responds to rest, anti-inflammatory agents, antibiotics if indicated, a soft collar, and, if needed, muscle relaxants (diazepam).

670.2 Klippel-Feil Syndrome

The clinical triad of short neck, low hairline, and restriction of neck motion in a patient with multiple coalitions of the cervical vertebrae defines this syndrome. There is an association of the Klippel-Feil triad with congenital abnormalities of the genitourinary tract, auditory system, spinal cord, and cardiovascular system, as well as with other abnormalities of the musculoskeletal system. **Sprengel anomaly** (congenital elevation of the scapula) is a common associated finding, and affected patients have a higher than expected incidence of scoliosis.

Affected children characteristically have low hairlines and short, sometimes webbed, necks. Decreased active and passive motion of the cervical spine is usually present, although the extent of restriction depends on the severity of the vertebral defects and may be difficult to detect in minimally affected patients. Torticollis may be present. Initial evaluation should include anteroposterior, lateral, and oblique views of the cervical spine. Flexion-extension lateral views, odontoid view, and CT may be necessary if instability is suspected. MRI is recommended for patients with neurologic deficits.

Thirty to 40% of patients with Klippel-Feil abnormality have structural abnormalities of the urinary tract. Double collecting systems, renal aplasia, horseshoe kidney, and recurrent pyelonephritis are common. Patients may die of uremia. The extent of the cervical abnormality correlates poorly with the severity of the underlying genitourinary abnormality, and thorough evaluation of the genitourinary tract is indicated in all patients.

670.3 Atlantoaxial Instability

Instability of the upper cervical spine in children is uncommon but potentially devastating. In the normal upper cervical spine, flexion and extension take place at the occiput-first cervical vertebra (C1) articulation and rotation occurs at the C1-2 joint. Neither joint is intrinsically stable, and both depend on the integrity of the ligaments and joint capsules that surround the joints to constrain motion. Developmental, traumatic, inflammatory, or metabolic lesions that affect the stability of the occiput-C1 or C1-2 joint have serious implications. Progressive myelopathy may develop in patients with chronic instability; acute impingement and death are possible in patients with severe instability.

Hypoplasia and Absence of the Odontoid Process. Rudimentary formation (os odontoideum) or absence of the odontoid process is well documented in disorders such as Morquio syndrome but

has been also reported in children with no demonstrable genetic or metabolic disorders. Absence of the odontoid may therefore be traumatic or congenital and is associated with varying degrees of upper cervical spine instability. In such patients, the proximal pole of the odontoid is absent and the base of the odontoid is rounded off below the arch of the first cervical vertebra, thereby resulting in C1-2 instability.

Symptoms vary depending on the degree of C1-2 instability. Preliminary evaluation should include controlled flexion and extension lateral radiographs of the cervical spine. MRI of the cervical spine performed in the neutral, flexed, and extended positions provides precise information on the size of the cervical canal, the position of the spinal cord within the canal, and the presence of spinal cord impingement. If available, anteroposterior and lateral tomography is also an excellent technique to identify small proximal ossicles. Transverse CT and sagittal reconstruction provide detailed information regarding the craniovertebral junction.

In normal asymptomatic patients without radiographic evidence of instability, restriction of contact sports and close observation is appropriate. In patients with Morquio syndrome, cervical stabilization should be considered even when such patients are asymptomatic and have little instability. In patients with cervical instability or abnormal neurologic findings, stabilization of the cervical spine is essential.

Down Syndrome. The association of trisomy 21 (Down syndrome) with instability of the upper cervical spine is well known; estimates of the incidence of instability range from 10–25%. Reported abnormalities include occipitoatlantal instability, atlantoaxial instability, occipitalization of the atlas, and os odontoideum. The number of patients with *symptoms* related to C1-2 instability or other anomalies of the cervical spine is much lower. A minority of Down syndrome patients with cervical instability have neurologic symptoms (see Chapter 70).

Patients with Down syndrome and upper cervical instability who have abnormal neurologic signs have highly variable manifestations. Obvious abnormalities such as incontinence, gait disturbances, and seizures may be the presenting symptoms in some patients, whereas others may be noted to have intermittent balance problems or decreased exercise tolerance. The incidence of instability increases with age. Unfortunately, significant neurologic injury, including quadriparesis or death, has been reported in previously asymptomatic patients.

The Orthopedic Section of the American Academy of Pediatrics has recommended screening of patients with Down syndrome with neurologic examination and lateral radiographs in the neutral, flexed, and extended positions. Patients with no neurologic abnormalities but with radiographic evidence of instability require further evaluation; at the least, they should be restricted from contact sports and followed periodically.

Patients with myelopathy and those with marked instability without myelopathy are candidates for cervical spine fusion. Decision-making is complicated by the lack of knowledge of the long-term outcome of patients with myelopathy treated nonoperatively and by the variability of outcome in patients treated surgically. Unfortunately, the results of surgical treatment of instability in Down syndrome are less predictable than that of instability in other conditions. Failure of fusion and graft resorption may occur, and the incidence of complications is high. It is not likely that preexistent myelopathic changes will improve. Based on these findings, it has been recommended that patients with instability and no neurologic abnormality be treated nonoperatively. When operative intervention is necessary, all parties must be aware of the high potential for serious complications.

The occurrence of sudden death in previously normal patients with Down syndrome and the documented development of instability with increasing age raise the issue of whether all patients with Down syndrome should be restricted from potentially dangerous activities. Given the incomplete state of knowledge at this time, this judgment appears best made on a case-by-case basis.

Torticollis

Celayir AC: Congenital muscular torticollis: Early and intensive treatment is critical: A prospective study. *Pediatr Int* 2000;42:504–7.

Chen CE, Ko JY: Surgical treatment of muscular torticollis above 6 years of age. *Arch Orthop Trauma Surg* 2000;120:149–51.

Cheng JC, Tang SP, Chen TM, et al: The clinical presentation and outcome of treatment of congenital muscular torticollis in infants—a study of 1086 cases. *J Pediatr Surg* 2000;35:1091–96.

Cheng JC, Wong MW, Tang SP, et al: Clinical determinants of the outcome of manual stretching in the treatment of congenital muscular torticollis in infants: A prospective study of eight hundred and twenty-one cases. *J Bone Joint Surg Am* 2001;83:679–87.

Davids J, Wenger D, Mubarak S: Congenital muscular torticollis: Sequela of intrauterine or perinatal compartment syndrome. *J Pediatr Orthop* 1993;13:141–47.

Gupta AK, Roy DR, Conlon ES: Torticollis secondary to posterior fossa tumors. *J Pediatr Orthop* 1996;16:505–7.

Mezue WC, Taha ZM, Bashir EM: Fever and acquired torticollis in hospitalized children. *J Laryngol Oncol* 2002;116:280–84.

O'Brien DF, Caird J, Kennedy M, et al: Posterior fossa tumours in childhood: Evaluation of presenting clinical features. *Ir Med J* 2001;94:52–3.

Tien YC, Su JY, Lin GT, Lin SY: Ultrasonographic study of the coexistence of muscular torticollis and dysplasia of the hip. *J Pediatr Orthop* 2001;21:343–47.

Klippel-Feil Syndrome

Herman MJ, Pizzutillo PD: Cervical spine disorders in children. *Orthop Clin North Am* 1999;30:457–66.

Pizzutillo PD, Woods M, Nicholson L, et al: Risk factors in Klippel-Feil syndrome. *Spine* 1994;19:2110–16.

Atlantoaxial Instability

Brockmeyer D: Down syndrome and craniovertebral instability. Topic review and treatment recommendations. *Pediatr Neurosurg* 1999:31:71–7.

Dai L, Yuan W, Ni B, et al: Os odontoideum: Etiology, diagnosis and management. *Surg Neurol* 2000;53:106–9.

Doyle JS, Lauerman WC, Wood KB, et al: Complications and long-term outcome of upper cervical spine arthrodesis in patients with Down syndrome. *Spine* 1996;21:1223–31.

Hensinger RN: Congenital anomalies of the cervical spine. *Clin Orthop* 1991;264:16–38.

Pueschel SM: Should children with Down syndrome be screened for atlantoaxial instability? *Arch Pediatr Adolesc Med* 1998;152:123–25.

Sarwark JF: Mucopolysaccharidoses, mucolipidoses, and homocystinuria. In Weinstein SL (editor): *The Pediatric Spine*. New York, Raven Press, 1994, pp 959–74.

Chapter 671
The Upper Limb
George H. Thompson

Upper limb disorders, with the exception of fractures, are less common in children and adolescents than are those involving the other areas of the musculoskeletal system.

SHOULDER

The shoulder joint is composed of the relatively small glenoid fossa of the scapula, which articulates with a proportionally larger hemispherical humeral head. The stability of the shoulder joint is provided by muscular and tendinous (rotator cuff) attachments. The shoulder has a relatively large range of motion because of this small articular surface and large muscle mass. Shoulder motion is a combination of glenohumeral and scapulothoracic motion.

671.1 Sprengel Deformity

Failure of the scapula to descend to its normal location is termed *Sprengel deformity.* The scapula is located at an abnormally high position with respect to the child's neck and thorax. This uncommon abnormality occurs with varying degrees of severity. Webbing of the skin between the neck and scapula and a low posterior hairline may be associated findings. In the severe form, a bone (omovertebral) may connect the scapula with the cervical spine and prevent scapulothoracic movement. There may also be associated muscle anomalies that further limit strength and stability of the shoulder girdle. In severe cases, the scapula is very high, producing a significant cosmetic deformity with markedly limited shoulder range of motion, particularly forward flexion and abduction. In the mild form, the scapula rides slightly high with less than normal motion. A Klippel-Feil anomaly (congenital fusion of one or more of the cervical spine vertebra) may also occur with Sprengel deformity.

Treatment. The best outcome in severe Sprengel deformity is achieved by surgically repositioning or, occasionally, partially resecting the scapula. An osteotomy of the clavicle is frequently necessary to bring the scapula to a more normal position. This improves the cosmetic appearance and increases shoulder motion, especially abduction.

671.2 Shoulder Dislocation

Traumatic dislocation of the shoulder is uncommon in childhood but increases in frequency during adolescence. Anterior dislocation is the most common type. It usually occurs when the shoulder is forced into abduction and external rotation. In young children, a Salter-Harris type II epiphyseal fracture is more likely to occur. Once a traumatic dislocation has occurred, there is damage to the anterior capsule and the associated musculature that may predispose to recurrent dislocation. The younger individuals are at the time of the initial dislocation, the more likely they are to experience recurrent dislocations.

Treatment. Closed reduction and immobilization in a shoulder immobilizer for 3–6 wk followed by rehabilitation is recommended for the first dislocation. Some favor early reconstruction rather than instituting conservative treatment because of the risk of recurrent dislocations.

ELBOW

The elbow joint is composed of three bones: the distal humerus, the proximal radius, and the ulna. There are three articulations: the radiohumeral, the ulnohumeral, and the proximal radioulnar. There are anterior and posterior indentations on the distal surface of the humerus: the anterior coronoid and the posterior olecranon fossa. These accept the coronoid and olecranon processes of the proximal ulna. It allows the elbow to flex 150 degrees and extend to neutral. The proximal radius is a relatively flat, circular structure that allows pronation and supination of the forearm to occur with approximately 90 degrees of motion at each. Abnormalities involving the elbow typically produce pain and loss of motion.

671.3 Nursemaid's Elbow

The radial head is not as bulbous in infants and young children as it is in older children. During early childhood, the annular ligament that passes around the neck of the proximal radius just below the radial head provides stability between the radius and ulna. When longitudinal traction is applied to the upper extremity with the elbow in extension, the annular ligament can slide over the radial head and become partially entrapped in the radiohumeral joint (Fig. 671–1). This is known as nursemaid's elbow or subluxation of the radial head. It represents a soft tissue interposition in the elbow joint. The subluxation of the annular ligament is initiated by either a jerk on the arm when the child

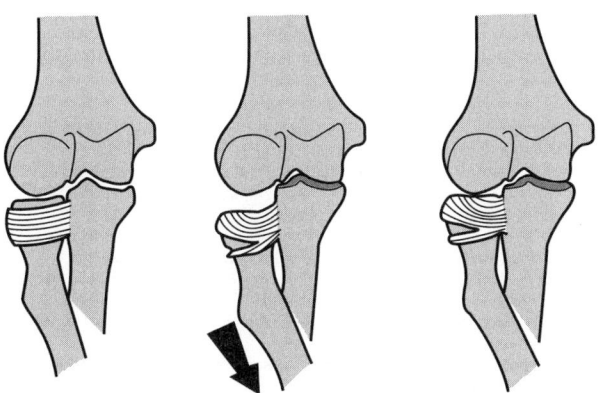

FIGURE 671–1. The pathology of nursemaid's, or pulled, elbow. The annular ligament is partially torn when the arm is pulled. The radial head moves distally and, when traction is discontinued, the ligament is carried into the joint. (From Rang M: *Children's Fractures,* 2nd ed. Philadelphia, JB Lippincott, 1983, p 193.)

falls while the hand is being held by a parent or when the child is forcibly lifted by the hand. It may also occur if the child falls and holds onto an object for support but allows longitudinal traction to be applied across the elbow. The hand typically is held in a pronated position, and the child may refuse to use the hand and may cry when the elbow is moved.

Treatment. Rotating the hand and forearm to a supinated position with pressure over the radial head usually reduces the annular ligament and restores full, normal use of the extremity. With reduction of the annular ligament, there is a palpable "click" felt along the lateral aspect of the elbow. Radiographs are not usually necessary to make the diagnosis. When a child is sent for radiographic evaluation before the annular ligament is reduced, this click may inadvertently occur during positioning.

The parents should be educated about the mechanism of injury and encouraged to avoid lifting or holding the child up by the hands or forearm. Once a subluxation has occurred, there is a propensity for recurrent episodes. Usually, there is sufficient development of the radial head to prevent subluxation of the annular ligament by 4 yr of age.

671.4   Panner Disease

Panner disease is an osteochondrosis that involves the ossific nucleus of the capitellum, the lateral aspect of the distal humeral epiphysis. This disorder is most common in adolescence and occurs predominantly in those engaged in sport activities that involve throwing. Adolescents complain of pain and may have crepitation and loss of motion, particularly pronation and supination.

The diagnosis can usually be made from anteroposterior and lateral radiographs of the elbow. Occasionally, oblique radiographs may be beneficial. Additional radiographic studies, such as MRI, may be helpful in identifying the extent of the lesion and determining whether the overlying articular cartilage is intact or disrupted.

Treatment. The treatment is usually conservative with restriction of activities. If the overlying articular cartilage is disrupted and joint fluid flows beneath the lesion, it may ultimately become a loose body. A loose osteocartilaginous fragment may be excised through an arthrotomy or arthroscopy. Occasionally, it is possible to repair the lesion by drilling it to allow for ingrowth of new blood vessels or by internal fixation with absorbable pins, which may allow the lesions to heal.

WRIST

The wrist is the articulation between the hand and the distal radius and ulna. The proximal row of carpal bones (scaphoid, lunate, and hamate) composes the articular surface of the hand. Anatomically, the distal radius has a 25-degree ulnar tilt and 12-degree volar angulation. The distal ulna is relatively flat, with the exception of the ulnar styloid, and has a small, triangle-shaped meniscus between its articulation with the hamate. There are three articulations: radiocarpal, ulnocarpal, and radioulnar. The wrist is not a common site for pediatric musculoskeletal disorders, with the exceptions of fractures involving the distal radius and ulna.

671.5   Ganglion

A synovial fluid-filled cyst around the wrist, a ganglion, is common in childhood. The usual site is the dorsum of the wrist near the radiocarpal joint; a common second site is over the volar radial aspect of the wrist. The disease is a defect in one of the joint capsules, which allows herniation of the synovium through the defect. If the synovium is ruptured, the fluid may be pumped into the soft tissues through the action of wrist motion; the fluid is subsequently walled off by reactive fibrous tissue.

Treatment. In children, ganglia are benign and tend to disappear over time. If a ganglion is sufficiently large, causes pain, or interferes with normal tendon functioning, aspiration of the cyst is sometimes helpful. Surgical excision of the cyst accompanied by removal of the tract that extends into the joint is curative.

671.6   Radial Clubhand

Absence of the radius, either total or partial, results in radial deviation of the hand and abnormal function. The ulna is usually hypoplastic as well as bowed, contributing to the shortness and deformity of the forearm and hand. This is an uncommon disorder but may be associated with a variety of other syndromes such as the VATER syndrome (vertebral defects, anal atresia, tracheoesophageal fistula with esophageal atresia, and radial and renal anomalies) or the Holt-Oram syndrome. Any child with a radial clubhand requires a careful evaluation for other disorders. The diagnosis is usually evident on physical examination, but radiographs show whether the radius is completely absent or whether there is a proximal remnant. Congenital absence of the thumb is a common accompaniment.

Treatment. The treatment of radial clubhand in infancy begins with serial casting or splinting in an attempt to center the carpus on the end of the ulna. Usually, a surgical procedure is ultimately necessary to centralize the hand adequately, provide stability, and place it into a position to maximize function. If the thumb is absent, a pollicization of the index finger can be performed to improve hand function.

HAND AND FINGERS

The hand and fingers are composed of the carpal and metacarpal bones proximally and the phalanges distally. The thumb has two phalanges (proximal and distal), whereas the fingers have three phalanges (proximal, middle, and distal). Thus, the thumb has an interphalangeal joint and the fingers have proximal and distal interphalangeal joints. The thumb and fingers articulate with the metacarpals at the metacarpophalangeal joints. The hand has a delicate balance among the intrinsic muscle system, a powerful extrinsic muscle system, fine sensory innervation, and specialized skin to allow it to be a highly mobile, sensitive, delicate, yet powerful appendage. Thumb and finger disorders, other than trauma, are relatively uncommon. When present, they tend to be due to congenital rather than developmental abnormalities.

671.7 Polydactyly

Extra digits, or polydactyly, occur as both simple and complex deformities. Skin tags and digit remnants are typically seen near the metacarpophalangeal joint of the small finger or the thumb. They do not have palpable bone in the base or possess voluntary motion and may simply be ligated or excised in the newborn period. Complex varieties require formal amputation, which is usually performed at approximately 1 yr of age. Syndromes in which polydactyly commonly occurs are listed in Box 671–1.

671.8 Syndactyly

Syndactyly also occurs in both simple and complex patterns. There should be concern about sharing of common important structures between the digits, such as the neurovascular bundle. There is also a tethering effect on the growth of the affected digits. Referral for delineation of specific disease and development of treatment strategies is indicated when the condition is recognized. Syndromes associated with syndactyly are presented in Box 671–2.

671.9 Congenital Trigger Thumb and Finger

A thickening in the tendon of the flexor hallucis longus (thumb) or the flexor digitorum longus (fingers) just below the first pulley of the digit may result in a triggering phenomenon. This thickening most likely is acquired rather than congenital. Each finger has a series of pulleys that prevent the tendons from bowstringing when flexed. This nodule may slide through the first pulley with a snapping, popping, or triggering sensation; this may or may not be painful. As the nodule enlarges because of the stimulation from triggering, it may ultimately be unable to pass beneath the pulley, resulting in a fixed flexion deformity of the interphalangeal joint of the thumb or the proximal interphalangeal joint and distal interphalangeal joints of the fingers. The nodule is typically palpable in the palm just proximal to the skin crease of the metacarpophalangeal joint. This is a clinical diagnosis and radiographs are not helpful.

Treatment. The treatment of a congenital trigger thumb or finger is a release of the first pulley. The normal excursion of the tendon does not allow the nodule to reach the next pulley. The release of the pulley does not cause bowstringing of the tendon.

Cleeman E, Flatow EL: Shoulder dislocations in the young patient. *Orthop Clin North Am* 2000;31:217–29.

Giele H, Giele C, Bower C, et al: The incidence and epidemiology of congenital upper limb anomalies: A total population study. *J Hand Surg Am* 2001;26:628–34.

Graham TJ, Ress AM: Finger polydactyly. *Hand Clin* 1998;14:49–64.

Lawton RL, Sambhu C, Mansat P, et al: Pediatric shoulder instability: Presentation, findings, treatment, and outcomes. *J Pediatr Orthop* 2002;22:52–61.

McAdams TR, Moneim MS, Omer GE Sr: Long-term follow-up of surgical release of the A1 pulley in childhood trigger thumb. *J Pediatr Orthop* 2002;22:41–43.

Moon WN, Suh WC, Kim IC: Trigger digits in children. *J Hand Surg Br* 2001;26:11–12.

Wang AA, Hutchinson DT: Longitudinal observation of pediatric hand and wrist ganglia. *J Hand Surg Am* 2001;26:599–602.

Watson S: The principles of management of congenital anomalies of the upper limb. *Arch Dis Child* 2000;83:10–17.

Chapter 672
Arthrogryposis
George H. Thompson

Arthrogryposis multiplex congenita refers to a symptom-complex characterized by multiple joint contractures present at birth. The involved muscles are replaced partially or completely by fat and fibrous tissue. This is not a single disease because there are approximately 150 different syndromes occurring with multiple congenital contractures that are categorized as arthrogryposis. Although most children who have this nonprogressive disorder survive, some die in infancy as a result of involvement of respiratory muscles. One major form (amyoplasia) of arthrogryposis multiplex congenita refers to the classic syndrome in which there is involvement of the upper and lower extremities. Amyoplasia accounts for approximately 40% of children who have multiple congenital contractures.

672.1 Amyoplasia

The cause of amyoplasia is unknown, but children with this disorder have a decreased number of anterior horn cells in the spinal cord, suggesting a neuropathic cause. Other studies have shown that the disorder may be myopathic in origin. In the latter instance, diminution of in utero movement may be the final common pathway leading to contractures. Every child presenting with multiple joint contractures should have a complete musculoskeletal evaluation and genetics consultation.

Clinical Manifestations. The distribution of involvement of multiple joint contractures is variable. The classic presentation involves the upper and lower extremities. The lower extremities are typically more involved than the upper extremities. Involvement of all four extremities is quadrimelic involvement. It is also possible that only the lower extremities or upper extremities (bimelic) may be involved. It is unusual to see only one extremity or a portion of one extremity (monomelic) involved.

The clinical features may include (1) adduction, internal rotation contractures of the shoulders; (2) fixed flexion or extension contractures of the elbow; (3) rigid volar flexion-ulnar deviation or dorsiflexion-radial deviation contractures of the wrists; (4) thumb and palm deformity; (5) rigid interpha-

---

BOX 671–1. Syndromes Associated with Polydactyly

Carpenter syndrome	Trisomy 13
Ellis–van Creveld syndrome	Orofaciodigital syndrome
Meckel-Gruber syndrome	Rubinstein-Taybi syndrome
Polysyndactyly	

BOX 671–2. Syndromes Associated with Syndactyly

Apert syndrome	Trisomy 21
Carpenter syndrome	Fetal hydantoin syndrome
de Lange syndrome	Laurence-Moon-Biedl
Holt-Oram syndrome	syndrome
Orofaciodigital	Fanconi panctyopenia
syndrome	Trisomy 13
Polysyndactyly	Trisomy 18

langeal joints of the thumb and fingers; (6) flexion, abduction, and external rotation hip contractures with dislocation of one or both hips; (7) fixed extension or flexion contractures of the knees; and (8) severe rigid bilateral clubfeet or congenital vertical tali.

Radiographic and Laboratory Evaluation. Radiographs should be obtained of the involved joints in all children presenting with multiple joint contractures. Screening radiographs of the spine and pelvis are almost always necessary for evaluation of possible spinal deformity and underlying hip dysplasia. Routine laboratory studies are usually not helpful in evaluating amyoplasia. If an underlying syndrome is suspected, such as congenital muscular dystrophy, creatine kinase determinations and chromosomal studies may be helpful.

Treatment. Correction of orthopedic deformities may be beneficial in maximizing walking or other functions. Each child must be treated individually with respect to potential rehabilitation and the possible treatment.

PHYSICAL THERAPY. Physical therapy with passive range of motion exercises can be beneficial in improving the range of motion in involved joints. However, it rarely completely corrects the existing contractures. Splinting (daytime or nighttime, or both) of the extremities may also improve joint range of motion. This is particularly useful in the hands and wrists. Postoperative splinting is important in maintaining alignment and preventing recurrence.

SERIAL CASTING. Serial casting can be helpful in further correcting soft tissue contractures after physical therapy has reached its maximal benefit. Serial casting is particularly useful in knee flexion contractures and in clubfeet. Casts are changed at weekly intervals, followed by a gentle manipulation of the involved area.

ORTHOSES. Orthotics can be beneficial in providing joint stability as well as maintaining alignment after satisfactory correction of contractures. The type of orthosis depends on the individual child's particular needs. It may be an ankle-foot orthosis if there is only ankle and foot involvement, a knee-ankle-foot orthosis if there is concomitant knee involvement, or a hip-knee-ankle-foot orthosis if there is involvement of all the joints of the lower extremities. Should scoliosis develop, a spinal orthosis such as a thoracolumbar spinal orthosis may be tried; it may slow the rate of progression and delay surgical intervention.

FRACTURE MANAGEMENT. Perinatal fractures commonly occur in children with arthrogryposis. These should be suspected if there is localized deformity, soft tissue swelling, erythema, or irritability. Rigid joints and hypotonia contribute to the increased incidence of fractures. These typically involve the shafts as well as the epiphyseal regions and should be managed with appropriate immobilization until adequate healing has occurred. It is important that radiographs be obtained in all children suspected of having a fracture before any physical therapy is initiated.

SURGERY. Surgery is usually necessary to achieve maximal correction of soft tissue contractures and joint deformities, reduce and stabilize dislocated hips, and correct foot deformities, and for partial correction and stabilization of spinal deformities.

Upper Extremities. Surgical treatment of upper extremity deformities depends on the type and degree of contracture as well as on the motor capabilities and functional needs of the patient. A child's compensatory or adaptive functioning of the upper extremities can be remarkable, and it is essential not to diminish function for cosmesis inadvertently. In bilateral involvement, it is preferable to have one extremity in extension and the other in flexion, but have them still be able to meet in the midline. This enhances function. Internal rotation contractures of the shoulder can be treated by soft tissue

releases and proximal humeral derotation osteotomies at a level proximal to the deltoid insertion. Extension contractures of the elbow may benefit from posterior capsulotomy and triceps tenotomy or lengthening to allow restoration of passive or active flexion. Active flexion can be partially restored with a transfer of the pectoralis muscle and its neurovascular bundle. Wrist deformities may be managed by tendon transfers, proximal row carpectomy, or shortening dorsal wedge radial osteotomies.

Lower Extremities. Most infants with clubfoot or vertical tali do not completely respond to passive stretching or serial casting. Complete soft tissue releases are usually required. Occasionally in a clubfoot, excision of the talus or talar decancellation may also be required to achieve a plantigrade foot.

Knee flexion contractures that are unresponsive to serial casting may benefit by a lengthening of the hamstring in association with a posterior knee capsulotomy. If this fails to correct the deformity to within 15–20 degrees of neutral, an extension osteotomy of the distal femur may be required. The value of walking with the knee extended is extremely beneficial. A recurrent flexion deformity may occur after an extension osteotomy if it is performed before adolescence. Knee extension contractures may also require treatment, especially if the child or adolescent is a nonambulator and cannot sit comfortably because of the extended position. Lengthening of the quadriceps mechanism may be beneficial.

Hip contractures may be improved by soft tissue releases. Occasionally, extension derotation osteotomies of the proximal femur may be helpful in completing the correction of the flexion, abduction, or external rotation contractures. Controversy exists as to whether bilateral dislocations of the hip should be reduced. If there is a unilateral dislocation, treatment is usually necessary to prevent leg-length discrepancy, pelvic obliquity, and possible scoliosis. Open reduction is accompanied by soft tissue releases, shortening derotation varus osteotomies of the proximal femurs, and pelvic osteotomies.

Scoliosis. Scoliosis is common in children with amyoplasia. The age at onset and patterns of deformity are variable. Orthotic management is usually effective only in slowing the rate of progression. In the majority of children, progression occurs slowly, and they ultimately require surgical intervention. Because of the associated soft tissue contractures, it is important that these curves not be allowed to become too severe because only partial correction will be obtained. Most children can be satisfactorily managed by a posterior spinal fusion and some type of segmental spinal instrumentation.

Axt MW, Niethard FU, Doderlein L, et al: Principles of treatment of the upper extremity in arthrogryposis multiplex congenita type I. *J Pediatr Orthop* 1997;6:179–85.

Ezaki M: Treatment of the upper limb in the child with arthrogryposis. *Hand Clin* 2000;16:703–11.

Hall JG: Arthrogryposis multiplex congenita: Etiology, genetics, classification, diagnostic approach, and general aspects. *J Pediatr Orthop* 1997;6:159–66.

Murray C, Fixsen JA: Management of knee deformity in classical arthrogryposis multiplex congenita (amyoplasia congenita). *J Pediatr Orthop* 1997;6:186–91.

Sells JM, Jaffe KM, Hall JG: Amyoplasia, the most common type of arthrogryposis: The potential for good outcome. *Pediatrics* 1996;97:225–31.

Shapiro F, Specht L: Current concepts review: The diagnosis and orthopaedic treatment of childhood spinal muscular atrophy, peripheral neuropathy, Friedreich ataxia and arthrogryposis. *J Bone Joint Surg Am* 1993;75A:1699–1714.

Sodergard J, Hakamies-Blomqvist L, Saino K, et al: Arthrogryposis multiplex congenita: Perinatal and electromyographic findings, disability, and psychosocial outcome. *J Pediatr Orthop* 1997;6:167–71.

Smith DW, Drennan JC: Arthrogryposis wrist deformities: Results of infantile serial casting. *J Pediatr Orthop* 2002;22:44–47.

Thompson GH: Arthrogryposis multiplex congenita. In Staheli LT (editor): *Pediatric Orthopaedic Secrets*. Philadelphia, Hanley & Belfus, 1998, pp 371–75.

Yingsakmongkol W, Kumar SJ: Scoliosis in arthrogryposis multiplex congenita: Results after nonsurgical and surgical treatment. *J Pediatr Orthop* 2000;20:656–61.

Chapter 673

Common Fractures

George H. Thompson

Fractures in children account for 10–15% of all childhood injuries. The skeletal system of children is anatomically, biomechanically, and physiologically different from that in adults. This results in different fracture patterns (including epiphyseal fractures), problems in diagnosis, and the use of management techniques.

The anatomic differences in the pediatric skeletal system include the presence of perosseous cartilage, physes, and a thicker, stronger, more osteogenic periosteum that produces callus more rapidly and in greater amounts. Biomechanically, the pediatric skeletal system can absorb more energy before deformation and fracture than can adult bone. This has been attributed to lower mineral content and the greater porosity of young bone. The increased porosity is caused by larger, more abundant haversian canals. This results in a lower modulus of elasticity and lower bending strength. As maturation occurs, the porosity decreases and the cortical bone becomes thicker and stronger.

Ligaments frequently insert into epiphyses. As a consequence, traumatic forces applied to an extremity may be transmitted to the physes. The strength of the physes is enhanced by interdigitating mammillary bodies and the perichondrial ring. Biomechanically, the physes are not as strong as the ligaments or metaphyseal bone. The physis is most resistant to traction and least resistant to torsional forces. The majority of injuries to the physes are secondary to rotational and angular forces.

The thick periosteum of a child's bones is a major determinant in whether a fracture becomes displaced. The thick periosteum may also act as an impediment to closed reduction because of the hinging phenomenon, or it may help stabilize a fracture after reduction.

Fracture Remodeling. Remodeling occurs by a combination of periosteal resorption and new bone formation. Thus, anatomic alignment in certain pediatric fractures is not always necessary. The major factors affecting fracture remodeling include the child's age, proximity of the fracture to a joint, and relationship of a residual deformity to the plane of the joint axis of motion. The amount of remaining growth provides the basis for remodeling: The younger the child, the greater is the remodeling potential. Fractures adjacent to a physis undergo the greatest amount of remodeling, provided that the deformity is in the plane of axis of motion for that joint. Fracture remodeling will be less effective in displaced intra-articular fractures, diaphyseal fractures, malrotation, and deformity not in the plane of joint axis of motion.

Overgrowth. Overgrowth, especially in long bones such as the femur, is due to physeal stimulation from the hyperemia associated with fracture healing. Femoral fractures in children younger than 10 yr frequently overgrow 1–3 cm. This is the reason for bayonet apposition of bone to compensate for the overgrowth that occurs over the next 1–2 yr. After 10 yr of age, overgrowth is less of a problem and anatomic alignment is recommended.

Progressive Deformity. Injuries to the physes can result in complete or partial closure. As a consequence, angular deformity or shortening, or both, can occur. The magnitude depends on the physis involved and the amount of growth remaining.

Rapid Healing. Fractures in children heal faster than do those in adults. This is due to children's growth potential and thicker, more metabolically active periosteum. As children approach adolescence and maturity, the rate of healing slows and becomes similar to that of an adult's.

673.1 Pediatric Fracture Patterns

Pediatric fracture patterns result, in part, from the anatomic, biomechanical, and physiologic characteristics of a child's skeletal system (Fig. 673–1). The majority of pediatric fractures can be managed by closed methods.

Complete. Complete fractures are the most common type and occur when both sides of the bone are fractured. These fractures

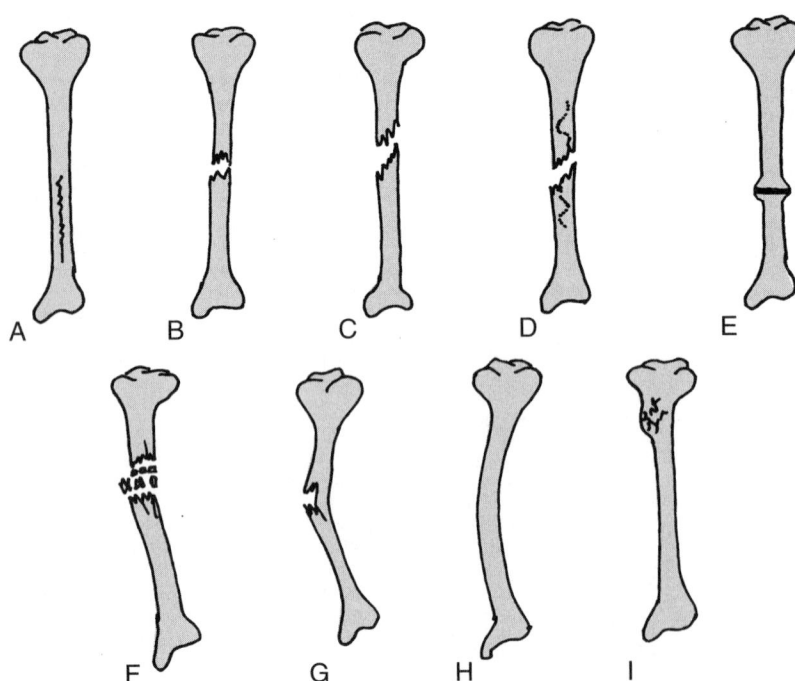

FIGURE 673–1. Illustration of fracture patterns. *A,* Longitudinal—fracture line parallel to bony axis. *B,* Transverse—fracture line perpendicular to bony axis. *C,* Oblique—fracture line at angle to bony axis. *D,* Spiral—fracture line runs curvilinear course to bony axis. *E,* Impacted—fractured bone ends compressed together. *F,* Comminuted—fragmentation of bone into three or more parts. *G,* Greenstick—bending of bone with incomplete fracture of convex side. *H,* Bowing—bony plastic deformation. *I,* Torus—buckling fracture. (From White N, Sty J: Radiological evaluation and classification of pediatric fractures. *Clin Ped Emerg Med* 2002;3:94–105.)

may be classified as spiral, transverse, oblique, or comminuted, depending on the direction of the fracture lines. Comminuted fractures are unusual in children.

Buckle or Torus Fracture. Compression of bone produces a buckle or torus fracture. These fractures typically occur in the metaphyseal areas in young children, especially in the distal radius. They are inherently stable and heal in 2–3 wk with simple immobilization.

Greenstick. When a bone is angulated beyond the limits of plastic deformation, a greenstick fracture may occur. This represents bone failure on the tension side and a plastic or bend deformity on the compression side. The energy was insufficient to result in a complete fracture.

Plastic Deformation or Bend Fractures. Traumatic bowing or bend deformities are caused by plastic deformation of bone. The bone was angulated beyond its limit of plastic deformation, but the energy was insufficient to produce a fracture. Thus, no fracture line is visible radiographically. It is most commonly seen in the ulna and, occasionally, the fibula.

Epiphyseal Fractures. Salter and Harris classified epiphyseal injuries into five groups: type I, separation through the physis, usually through the zones of hypertrophic and degenerating cartilage cell columns; type II, a fracture through a portion of the physis but extending through the metaphyses; type III, a fracture through a portion of the physis extending through the epiphysis and into the joint; type IV, a fracture across the metaphysis, physis, and epiphysis; and type V, a crush injury to the physis (Fig. 673–2). This classification allows generalized prognostic information regarding the risk for premature physeal closure and the indications for treatment. Type III and type IV epiphyseal fractures require anatomic alignment because of displacement of both the physis and the articular surface. Type V fractures are usually recognized in retrospect as a consequence of premature physeal closure. Type I and type II fractures usually can be managed by closed reduction techniques and do not require perfect alignment. A major exception is type II fractures of the distal femur. Fractures in this location have a poor prognosis unless almost anatomic alignment is obtained by either closed or open methods.

Child Abuse (see Chapter 35). Skeletal injury is common in nonaccidental trauma. Certain fractures have a high probability of child abuse that include metaphyseal lesions (bucket-handle or corner fractures), posterior rib fractures, scapular fractures, spinous process fractures, and sternal fractures. Multiple fractures (in different stages of healing), epiphyseal separations, vertebral body fractures, complex skull fracture, and digit fractures are moderately suspicious. Spiral femur fractures in nonambulatory infants and nonsupracondylar humerus fractures are also highly suggestive of nonaccidental trauma.

673.2 Clavicular Fractures

Fractures involving the junction of the middle and lateral aspects of the clavicle are common. These can be the result of birth injuries in newborns but are more typically the result of a fall on the outstretched arm or a direct blow to the clavicle. They are rarely associated with a neurovascular injury. Diagnosis is easily made by physical and radiographic evaluation. Anteroposterior radiograph of the clavicle and, occasionally, a cephalic view demonstrate the fracture. Typically, the fracture fragments are displaced and overlap 1–2 cm.

Treatment. The treatment of most clavicle fractures consists of an application of a figure-of-eight clavicle strap. This will extend the shoulders and minimize the amount of overlap of the fracture fragments. Rarely is anatomic alignment achieved, but this is not necessary. The fractures heal rapidly, usually in 3–6 wk. Commonly, a palpable mass of callus may be visible in thin children. This remodels satisfactorily in 6–12 mo.

673.3 Proximal Humerus Fractures

Salter-Harris type II fractures of the proximal humerus occur commonly in children and are due to a backward fall on the involved extremity with the elbow extended. Neurovascular injuries rarely occur. Diagnosis is made from anteroposterior and lateral radiographs of the shoulder or humerus.

Treatment. The treatment of these fractures is usually simple immobilization. Occasionally, a closed reduction may be necessary. A significant amount of deformity can be accepted because of the remodeling potential of this region; 80% of the growth of the humerus occurs from the proximal humeral epiphysis. A sling and swath and, occasionally, a coaptation splint may be necessary to provide satisfactory immobilization and comfort. In severely displaced fractures, closed reduction with immobilization may be necessary.

673.4 Distal Humerus Fractures

The distal humerus is one of the most common sites for fractures in children. These include separation of the distal humeral

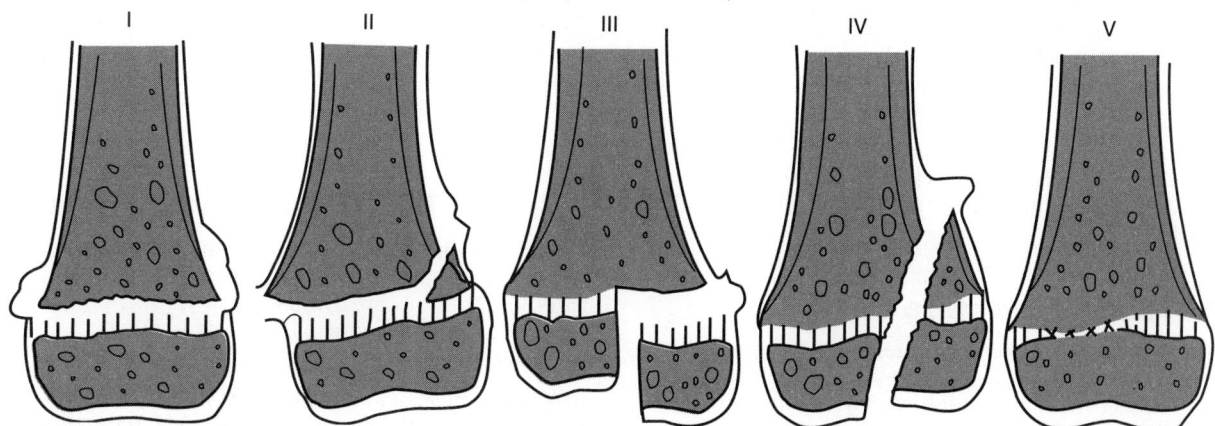

FIGURE 673–2. The types of growth plate injury as classified by Salter and Harris. (From an instructional course study, American Academy of Orthopaedic Surgeons, and Salter RB, Harris WR: Injuries involving the epiphyseal plate. *J Bone Joint Surg Am* 1963;45:587–622.)

epiphysis (transcondylar fracture), supracondylar fractures of the distal humerus, and epiphyseal fractures, such as the lateral condyle fractures. The transcondylar fracture occurs in neonates commonly as the result of child abuse. The other fractures are more likely to occur after a fall on the outstretched arm. Anterior and posterolateral radiographs of the involved extremity are necessary for the diagnosis. If the fracture is not visible but there is an altered relationship between the humerus and the radius and ulna or the presence of a posterior fat pad sign, a transcondylar fracture or an occult fracture should be suspected. Swelling and pain with attempted motion are the typical features of these fractures. Neurologic impairment may also occur, owing to close proximity of the median, ulnar, and radial nerves to these fractures.

Treatment. Treatment of fractures of the distal humerus is restoration of anatomic alignment. This is necessary to prevent deformity and to allow for normal growth and development. Closed reduction and frequently percutaneous internal fixation is necessary. Open reduction is necessary for fractures that cannot be reduced by closed methods.

673.5 Distal Radius and Ulna Fractures

Torus, or buckle, fractures of the distal radial metaphysis are among the most common fractures of childhood. They are usually the result of a simple fall on the hand with the wrist in dorsiflexion. This is an impacted fracture, and there is minimal soft tissue swelling or hemorrhage. It is common for a child to present 1–2 days later because the initial injury was believed to be only a sprain or contusion. The clinical characteristics are nonspecific, usually with mild tenderness to palpation directly over the fracture. Diagnosis is confirmed by anteroposterior and lateral radiographs of the wrist.

Treatment. Treatment of torus fractures of the distal radius and ulna is by a short-arm cast. Fractures are typically healed in 3–4 wk.

673.6 Phalangeal Fractures

Phalangeal fractures in children are usually the result of a direct blow to the finger. They are typically trapped in doors or struck by another object. If the distal phalanx is involved, there may be a subungual hematoma, which can be painful. This requires drainage. If the nail bed is bleeding, avulsed, or partially detached in association with a fracture, this is an open fracture and should be treated aggressively with irrigation, tetanus prophylaxis, and appropriate antibiotics. Occasionally, physeal involvement, especially Salter-Harris type II epiphyseal fracture, may occur. Anteroposterior and lateral radiographs of the digit confirm the fracture.

Treatment. The treatment of phalangeal fractures is usually by splint immobilization. Rarely is a closed reduction necessary. However, if there is angulation or malrotation, this procedure may be necessary.

673.7 Toddler Fracture

Toddler fractures represent a spiral fracture of the distal one third of the tibia. They are usually the result of simple falls while running or playing. They may also occur when stepping on an object on the floor. These fractures occur in children between 2–4 yr of age and, occasionally, up to 6 yr of age. Clinical features include pain, refusal to walk, minimal soft tissue swelling, a slight increase in warmth to palpation over the fracture, and

pain with palpation. These fractures may not be visible radiographically on anteroposterior and lateral radiographs of the tibia. Occasionally, oblique radiographs may reveal the fractures. The fracture can be detected by a technetium bone scan, but this is rarely necessary.

Treatment. Application of a long-leg cast in suspected cases relieves symptoms. Within 1–2 wk there is radiographic evidence of subperiosteal new bone formation. These fractures are usually healed within 3–4 wk.

673.8 Lateral Malleolar Fractures

A Salter-Harris type I separation of the distal fibular epiphysis is common in childhood. These fractures usually appear as ankle sprains. However, it must be remembered that ligaments are stronger than bone and that the epiphysis is more likely to separate than a ligament is to tear. Children present with soft tissue swelling and pain over the lateral malleolus. Careful palpation reveals that the bone is the site of greatest tenderness rather than the area over one of the three lateral ligaments. Anteroposterior, lateral, and mortise radiographs of the ankle are typically normal. The diagnosis can be confirmed by stress radiographs, but this is rarely necessary.

Treatment. Distal fibular epiphyseal separations require immobilization in a short-leg cast for 4–6 wk. Treatment is the same as that for a severe ankle sprain. This is why stress radiographs are rarely necessary. Follow-up radiographs show subperiosteal new bone formation in the metaphyseal region of the distal fibula.

673.9 Metatarsal Fractures

Fractures of the metatarsal shaft are usually the result of direct trauma to the dorsum of the foot. Children present with a history of injury followed by soft tissue swelling and, sometimes, ecchymosis. There is tenderness to palpation directly over the fracture. Diagnosis is obtained by anteroposterior and lateral radiographs of the foot.

Fractures of the tuberosity of the fifth metatarsal are also common. This has been termed *dancer's fracture*. It is an apophyseal avulsion fracture at the insertion of the peroneus brevis tendon. It typically occurs with the foot in an inverted position and the peroneal muscles contracting to realign the foot. The swelling, ecchymosis, and tenderness are limited to the tuberosity of the fifth metatarsal. Contraction of the peroneal musculature also increases discomfort. The diagnosis is confirmed radiographically.

Treatment. Metatarsal fractures are treated by a short-leg cast for 4–6 wk. Weight-bearing is allowed as tolerated. The one exception is the fifth metatarsal diaphyseal shaft fracture. This has an increased incidence of nonunion and should be treated by non–weight-bearing until there is radiographic evidence of early union.

673.10 Toe Phalangeal Fractures

Fractures of the lesser toes are common and are usually secondary to direct blows. They commonly occur when the child is barefoot. The toes are swollen, ecchymotic, and tender. There may be a mild deformity. Diagnosis is made radiographically. Bleeding suggests the possibility of an open fracture.

Treatment. The lesser toes usually do not require closed reduction unless significantly displaced. If necessary, reduction can usually be accomplished with longitudinal traction on the toe. Casting is not usually necessary. "Buddy" taping of the fractured toe to an adjacent stable toe usually provides satisfactory alignment and relief of symptoms. Crutches may be beneficial for several days until the soft tissue swelling and the discomfort decrease.

673.11 Operative Treatment

Certain pediatric fractures have better prognoses if the fractures are reduced, by either open or closed techniques, and then internally or externally stabilized (Table 673–1). Four to 5% of pediatric fractures require surgery. The common indications for operative stabilization in children and adolescents with open physes include (1) displaced epiphyseal fractures, (2) displaced intra-articular fractures, (3) unstable fractures, (4) fractures in the multiply injured child, and (5) open fractures.

The principles of surgical management of pediatric fractures are distinctly different from those of mature adolescents and adults. Multiple closed reductions of an epiphyseal fracture are contraindicated because they may cause repetitive damage to the germinal cells of the physis. Anatomic alignment at surgery is mandatory, especially for displaced intra-articular and epiphyseal fractures. When internal fixation is used, it should be simple (e.g., use of Kirschner wires, which can be removed as soon as the fracture is healed). Rigid fixation to allow immobilization of the extremity usually is not the goal; rather, stability sufficient to maintain anatomic alignment with supplemental immobilization, usually a plaster cast, is. Last, external fixators, when used, are removed as soon as possible and cast immobilization is substituted. The latter is indicated when soft tissue problems have been corrected or when the fracture is stable, or both.

Surgical Techniques. Three basic surgical techniques are used in the management of pediatric fractures. Open reduction and internal fixation may be required for displaced epiphyseal fractures, especially Salter-Harris types III and IV fractures, intra-articular fractures, and unstable fractures, such as those involving the forearm diaphysis, spine, and ipsilateral fractures of the femur and tibia (floating knee). Other indications include neurovascular injuries requiring repair and, occasionally, open fractures of the femur and tibia. Closed reduction and internal fixation is indicated for specific displaced epiphyseal, intra-articular, and unstable metaphyseal and diaphyseal fractures. Common indications include supracondylar fractures of the distal humerus, and phalangeal and femoral neck fractures. Anatomic alignment must be attained by a closed reduction

before this method can be used. Failure to obtain anatomic alignment is an indication for an open reduction.

The indications for external fixation in pediatric fractures include (1) severe grade II and grade III open fractures; (2) fractures associated with severe burn; (3) fractures with bone or extensive soft tissue loss that may require reconstructive procedures, such as free vascularized grafts, skin grafts, or other procedures; (4) fractures requiring distractions such as those with significant bone loss; (5) unstable pelvic fractures; (6) fractures in children with associated head injuries and spasticity; and (7) fractures associated with vascular or nerve repairs or reconstruction. The advantages of external fixation include rigid mobilization of the fractures, separation of the management of the fractured limb and associated wounds, and patient mobilization for treatment of other injuries and transportation for diagnostic and therapeutic procedures. The majority of complications with external fixation are pin tract infections and refracture after pin removal.

Bandyopandhyay S, Yen K: Non-accidental fractures in child maltreatment syndrome. *Clin Pediatr Emerg Med* 2002;3:145–52.

Beaty JH, Kasser JR (editors): *Rockwood and Wilkens' Fractures in Children*, 5th ed. Philadelphia, JB Lippincott, 2001.

Davidson JS, Brown DJ, Barnes SN, et al: Simple treatment for torus fractures of the distal radius. *J Bone Joint Surg Br* 2001;83:1173–75.

Della-Giustina K, Della-Giustina DA: Emergency department evaluation and treatment of pediatric orthopedic injuries. *Emerg Med Clin North Am* 1999;17:895–922.

Green NE, Swiontkowski MF (editors): *Skeletal Trauma in Children*, 3rd ed, vol 3. Philadelphia, WB Saunders, 2001.

Kocher MS, Waters PM, Micheli LJ: Upper extremity injuries in the pediatric athlete. *Sports Med* 2000;30:117–35.

Lane WC, Rubin DM, Monteith R, et al: Racial differences in the evaluation of pediatric fractures for physical abuse. *JAMA* 2002;288:1603–9.

Overly F, Steele DW: Common pediatric fractures and dislocations. *Clin Pediatr Emerg Med* 2002;3:106–17.

Salter RB, Harris WR: Injuries involving the epiphyseal plate. *J Bone Joint Surg Am* 1963;45:587–622.

Skaggs DL, Mirzayan R: The posterior fat pad sign in association with occult fracture of the elbow in children. *J Bone Joint Surg Am* 1999;81:1429–33.

Thompson GH, Haber LL: Upper extremity fractures in the pediatric patients. In Fitzgerald RH Jr, Kaufer H, Malkani A (editors): *Orthopaedics*. St. Louis, CV Mosby, 2002, pp 484–94.

White N, Sty J: Radiological evaluation and classification of pediatric fractures. *Clin Pediatr Emerg Med* 2002;3:94–105.

Chapter 674

Osteomyelitis and Suppurative Arthritis

Richard M. Lampe

Suppurative infections of bones and joints in children are important because of their potential to cause permanent disability. The frequency of skeletal infection is greater in infants and toddlers than in older children. Early recognition of osteomyelitis and suppurative arthritis (also called **septic arthritis**) in young patients before extensive infection develops and prompt institution of appropriate medical and surgical therapy minimize permanent damage. The risk is greatest if the physis (the growth plate of bone) or the synovium is damaged.

Etiology. Bacteria are the most common pathogens in acute skeletal infections. In osteomyelitis, *Staphylococcus aureus* is the most common infecting organism in all age groups, including newborns. Group B streptococcus and gram-negative enteric bacilli are also prominent pathogens in neonates; group A streptococcus is next in frequency but constitutes less than 10% of all cases. After 6 yr of age, most cases of osteomyelitis are caused by *S. aureus*,

---

TABLE 673–1. **Common Indications for Operative Stabilization**

Indication	Location
Displaced epiphyseal fractures (usually Salter-Harris types III and IV)	Lateral condyle Radial head Phalanx Distal femur Proximal tibia Distal tibia
Displaced intra-articular fractures	Radial neck Olecranon Femoral neck Patella
Unstable fractures	Distal humerus (supracondylar) Radius-ulna diaphysis Phalanx Spine
Multiply injured child (especially with associated head and neurologic injury)	Femoral diaphysis Tibial diaphysis Pelvis Spine
Open fractures	Upper and lower extremities Severe soft tissue injury

Adapted from Thompson GH, Wilber JH, Marcus RE: Internal fixation of fractures in children and adolescents: A comparative analysis. Clin Orthop 1984; 188:10–20.

streptococcus, or *Pseudomonas aeruginosa*. Cases of *Pseudomonas* are related almost exclusively to puncture wounds of the foot, with direct inoculation of *P. aeruginosa* from the foam padding of the shoe into bone or cartilage, which develops as osteochondritis. The microbial spectrum is diverse in suppurative arthritis, but *S. aureus* infection is most common. *Haemophilus influenzae* type b accounted for more than half of all cases of bacterial arthritis in infants before universal vaccination with conjugate vaccines but is now an uncommon cause. Group A streptococcus and *Streptococcus pneumoniae* (pneumococcus) historically cause 10–20% of cases. In sexually active adolescents gonococcus is a common cause of septic arthritis. Salmonella and *S. aureus* are the two most common causes of osteomyelitis in children with sickle cell anemia.

Infection with atypical mycobacteria can occur after penetrating injuries. Fungal infections usually occur as part of multisystem disseminated disease; *Candida* arthritis or osteomyelitis sometimes complicates bloodstream infection in neonates with indwelling vascular catheters. Primary viral infections of bones or joints are exceedingly rare, but arthralgia or arthritis accompanies many viral syndromes, suggesting immune-mediated pathogenesis.

A microbial etiology is confirmed in about three fourths of cases of osteomyelitis and two thirds of cases of suppurative arthritis. Prior antibiotic therapy and the inhibitory effect of pus on microbial growth may explain the low bacterial yield. Additionally some cases treated as bacterial arthritis are actually reactive arthritis (see Chapter 147) rather than primary infection.

Epidemiology. Osteomyelitis and suppurative arthritis are most common in young children. This is particularly true of arthritis, in which half of all cases occur by 2 yr of age and three fourths of all cases occur by 5 yr of age, compared with about one third and one half, respectively, for osteomyelitis among these age groups. Skeletal infections are consistently more common in boys than in girls, usually by a factor of 2:1. The behavior of boys may predispose to traumatic events. There appears to be no particular predilection for arthritis or osteomyelitis based on race, except for the increased incidence of skeletal infection in patients with sickle cell disease.

The majority of infections in otherwise healthy children are of hematogenous origin. Minor, closed trauma is a common preceding event in cases of osteomyelitis, occurring in about one third of patients. Infection of bones and joints can follow penetrating injuries or procedures such as arthroscopy, prosthetic joint surgery, intra-articular steroid injection, and orthopedic surgery, although this is uncommon. Impaired host defenses also increase the risk of skeletal infection.

Pathogenesis. The unique anatomy and circulation of the ends of long bones results in the predilection for localization of bloodborne bacteria. In the metaphysis, nutrient arteries branch into nonanastomosing capillaries under the physis, which make a sharp loop before entering venous sinusoids draining into the marrow. Blood flow in this area is sluggish and provides an ideal environment for bacterial seeding. Once a bacterial focus is established, phagocytes migrate to the site and produce an inflammatory exudate. The generation of proteolytic enzymes, toxic oxygen radicals, and cytokines results in decreased oxygen tension, decreased pH, osteolysis, and tissue destruction. As the inflammatory exudate progresses, pressure increases spread through the porous metaphyseal space via the haversian system and Volkmann canals into the subperiosteal space. Purulence beneath the periosteum may lift the periosteal membrane of the bony surface, further impairing blood supply to the cortex and metaphysis.

In newborns and young infants, transphyseal blood vessels connect the metaphysis and epiphysis, so it is common for pus from the metaphysis to enter the joint space. This extension through the physis has the potential to result in abnormal growth and bone or joint deformity. During the latter part of the first year of life, the physis forms, obliterating the transphyseal

blood vessels. Joint involvement once the physis forms may occur in joints where the metaphysis is intra-articular (e.g., hip, ankle, shoulder, and elbow) and subperiosteal pus ruptures into the joint space.

In later childhood the periosteum becomes more adherent, favoring pus to decompress through the periosteum. Once the growth plate closes in late adolescence, hematogenous osteomyelitis more often begins in the diaphysis and can spread to the entire intramedullary canal.

Suppurative arthritis primarily occurs as a result of hematogenous seeding of the synovial space. Less often, organisms enter the joint space by direct inoculation or extension from a contiguous focus. The synovial membrane has a rich vascular supply and lacks a basement membrane, providing an ideal environment for hematogenous seeding. The presence of bacterial endotoxin within the joint space stimulates cytokine production (tumor necrosis factor-α, interleukin-1) within the joint, triggering an inflammatory cascade. The cytokines stimulate chemotaxis of neutrophils into the joint space where proteolytic enzymes and elastases are released by neutrophils, damaging the cartilage. Proteolytic enzymes released from the synovial cells and chondrocytes also contribute to cartilage and synovium destruction. Bacterial hyaluronidase breaks down the hyaluronic acid in the synovial fluid, making the fluid less viscous and diminishing its ability to lubricate and protect the joint cartilage. Damage to the cartilage can occur through increased friction, especially for weight-bearing joints. The increased pressure within the joint space from accumulation of purulent material can compromise the vascular supply and induce pressure necrosis of the cartilage. Synovial and cartilage destruction results from a combination of proteolytic enzymes and mechanical factors.

Clinical Manifestations. The signs and symptoms of skeletal infection are highly dependent on the age of the patient. The earliest signs and symptoms are often subtle.

Neonates may exhibit pseudoparalysis or pain with movement of the affected extremity. Half of neonates do not have fever and may not appear ill. Older infants and children are more likely to have fever, pain, and localizing signs such as edema, erythema, and warmth. With involvement of the lower extremities, limp or refusal to walk is seen in approximately half of patients.

Erythema and edema of the skin and soft tissue overlying the site of infection is seen earlier in suppurative arthritis than in osteomyelitis, since the bulging infected synovium is usually more superficial whereas the metaphysis is located more deeply. Suppurative arthritis of the hip is an exception because of the deep location of the hip joint. Local swelling and redness with osteomyelitis may mean that the infection has spread out of the metaphysis into the subperiosteal space, representing a secondary soft tissue inflammatory response.

Long bones are principally involved in osteomyelitis (Table 674–1). The femur and tibia are equally affected and together constitute almost half of all cases. The bones of the upper extremities account for one fourth of all cases. Flat bones are less commonly affected. Joints of the lower extremity constitute three fourths of all cases of suppurative arthritis (Table 674–2). The elbow, wrist, and shoulder joints are involved in about one fourth of cases, and small joints are uncommonly infected.

There is usually only a single site of bone or joint involvement. Several bones or joints are infected in fewer than 10% of cases; notable exceptions are gonococcal infections and osteomyelitis in neonates, in whom two or more bones are involved in almost half of the cases.

Diagnosis. Aspiration of the infected site for Gram stain and culture when the history and physical findings indicate a strong likelihood of osteomyelitis or suppurative arthritis remains the definitive diagnostic technique and provides the optimal speci-

TABLE 674–1. Distribution of Affected Bones in Acute Hematogenous Osteomyelitis

Bone	No.	Per Cent
Tibia	107	24.3
Femur	105	23.8
Humerus	58	13.2
Fibula	26	5.9
Radius	17	3.9
Ulna	10	2.3
Vertebra	9	2.0
Foot bones	33	7.5
Pelvic bones	30	6.8
Hand bones	27	6.1
Chest bones	13	2.9
Head bones	6	1.4

Based on unpublished series of 372 patients with 441 infected bones.

men for culture to confirm the diagnosis. For suspected osteomyelitis, a steel needle is needed to penetrate the cortex into the metaphysis. If pus is encountered in the subperiosteal space, there is no need to go farther. Most large joint spaces are easy to aspirate, but the hip can pose technical problems; ultrasound guidance facilitates aspiration. If no fluid is obtained, contrast material is injected and a radiograph is obtained to ensure that the needle tip is in the joint cavity. Aspiration of joint or bone pus provides the best specimen for bacteriologic culture of infection. If gonococcus is suspected, cervical, anal, and throat cultures should also be obtained. A blood culture should be performed in all cases of suspected osteomyelitis or septic arthritis.

Synovial fluid analysis for cell count, differential, protein, and glucose has limited usefulness because noninfectious inflammatory diseases, such as rheumatic fever and rheumatoid arthritis, can also cause exuberant reaction with increased cells and protein and decreased glucose. Synovial fluid characteristics of suppurative arthritis can suggest infection but are not sufficiently specific to exclude infection.

There are no specific laboratory tests for osteomyelitis or suppurative arthritis. Tests such as white blood cell count and differential, erythrocyte sedimentation rate (ESR), and C-reactive protein (CRP) are very sensitive for bone and joint infections but are nonspecific and not helpful in distinguishing between skeletal infection and other inflammatory processes. The leukocyte count and ESR may be normal during the first few days of infection, and normal test results do not preclude the diagnosis of skeletal infection. Monitoring elevated ESR and CRP may be of value in response to therapy or identifying complications.

RADIOGRAPHIC EVALUATION. Radiologic studies play a crucial role in the evaluation of osteomyelitis and suppurative

TABLE 674–2. Distribution of Affected Joints in Acute Suppurative Arthritis

Joint	No.	Per Cent
Knee	309	39.6
Hip	173	22.2
Elbow	109	14.0
Ankle	104	13.3
Shoulder	37	4.7
Wrist	34	4.4
Sacroiliac	5	0.6
Interphalangeal	4	0.5
Metatarsal	3	0.4
Acromioclavicular	1	0.1
Sternoclavicular	1	0.1
Metacarpal	1	0.1

Based on unpublished series of 725 patients with 781 infected joints.

arthritis. Conventional radiographs, ultrasound, CT, MRI, and radionuclide studies may all contribute to establishing the diagnosis. Plain radiographs are often used for initial evaluation to exclude other causes such as trauma and foreign bodies. MRI has emerged as a very sensitive and specific test and is widely used for diagnosis.

Plain Radiographs. Within 72 hours of onset of symptoms of osteomyelitis, plain radiographs of the involved site using soft tissue technique, and compared to the opposite extremity if necessary, can show displacement of the deep muscle planes from the adjacent metaphysis caused by deep tissue edema. Lytic bone changes are not visible on radiographs until 30–50% of the bony matrix is destroyed. Tubular long bones do not show lytic changes for 7–14 days after onset of infection. Flat and irregular bones can take longer.

Plain films of suppurative arthritis may show widening of the joint capsule, soft tissue edema, and obliteration of normal fat lines. Plain films of the hip can show medial displacement of the obturator muscle into the pelvis (the obturator sign), lateral displacement or obliteration of the gluteal fat lines, and elevation of the Shenton line with a widened arc.

Ultrasonography. Ultrasound is helpful in detecting joint effusion and fluid collection in the soft tissue and subperiosteal regions and may guide localization for aspiration or drainage. Ultrasound is highly sensitive in the detection of joint effusion, particularly for the hip joint, where plain radiographs may be normal in more than 50% of cases of suppurative arthritis of the hip.

Computed Tomography and Magnetic Resonance Imaging. CT can demonstrate osseus and soft tissue abnormalities and is ideal for detecting gas in soft tissues. MRI is the best radiologic imaging technique for the identification of abscesses and for differentiation between bone and soft tissue infection. MRI provides precise anatomic detail of subperiosteal pus and accumulation of purulent debris in the bone marrow and metaphyses for possible surgical intervention. In acute osteomyelitis, purulent debris and edema appear dark with decreased signal intensity on T1 weighted images, with fat appearing bright (Fig. 674–1). The opposite is seen in T2 weighted images. The signal from fat can be diminished with fat suppression techniques to enhance visualization. Cellulitis and sinus tracts appear as areas of high signal intensity on T2 weighted images.

MRI appears to have comparable positive predictive value to radionuclide imaging in acute osteomyelitis. MRI is particularly useful in the evaluation of vertebral osteomyelitis and diskitis owing to the clear delineation between the vertebral body and cartilaginous disk.

Radionuclide Studies. Radionuclide imaging can be valuable to augment MRI, especially if multiple foci are suspected. Technetium-99 methylene diphosphonate (^{99m}Tc), which accumulates in areas of increased bone turnover, is the preferred agent of choice for radionuclide bone imaging (three-phase bone scan). Osteomyelitis causes increased vascularity, inflammation, and increased osteoblastic activity, resulting in an increased concentration of ^{99m}Tc. Any areas of increased blood flow or inflammation can cause increased uptake of ^{99m}Tc in the first phase (5–10 min) and second phase (2–4 hr), but osteomyelitis causes increased uptake of ^{99m}Tc in the third phase (24 hr). Three-phase imaging with ^{99m}Tc has excellent sensitivity (84–100%) and specificity (70–96%) in hematogenous osteomyelitis and can detect osteomyelitis within 24–48 hr after onset of symptoms. The sensitivity in neonates is much lower owing to poor bone mineralization. Advantages include infrequent need for sedation, lower cost, ability to image entire skeleton for detection of multiple foci, and ability to scan multiple times after one injection.

In suppurative arthritis, three-phase imaging with ^{99m}Tc shows symmetric uptake on both sides of the joint, limited to the bony structures adjacent to the joint. Radionuclide imaging is

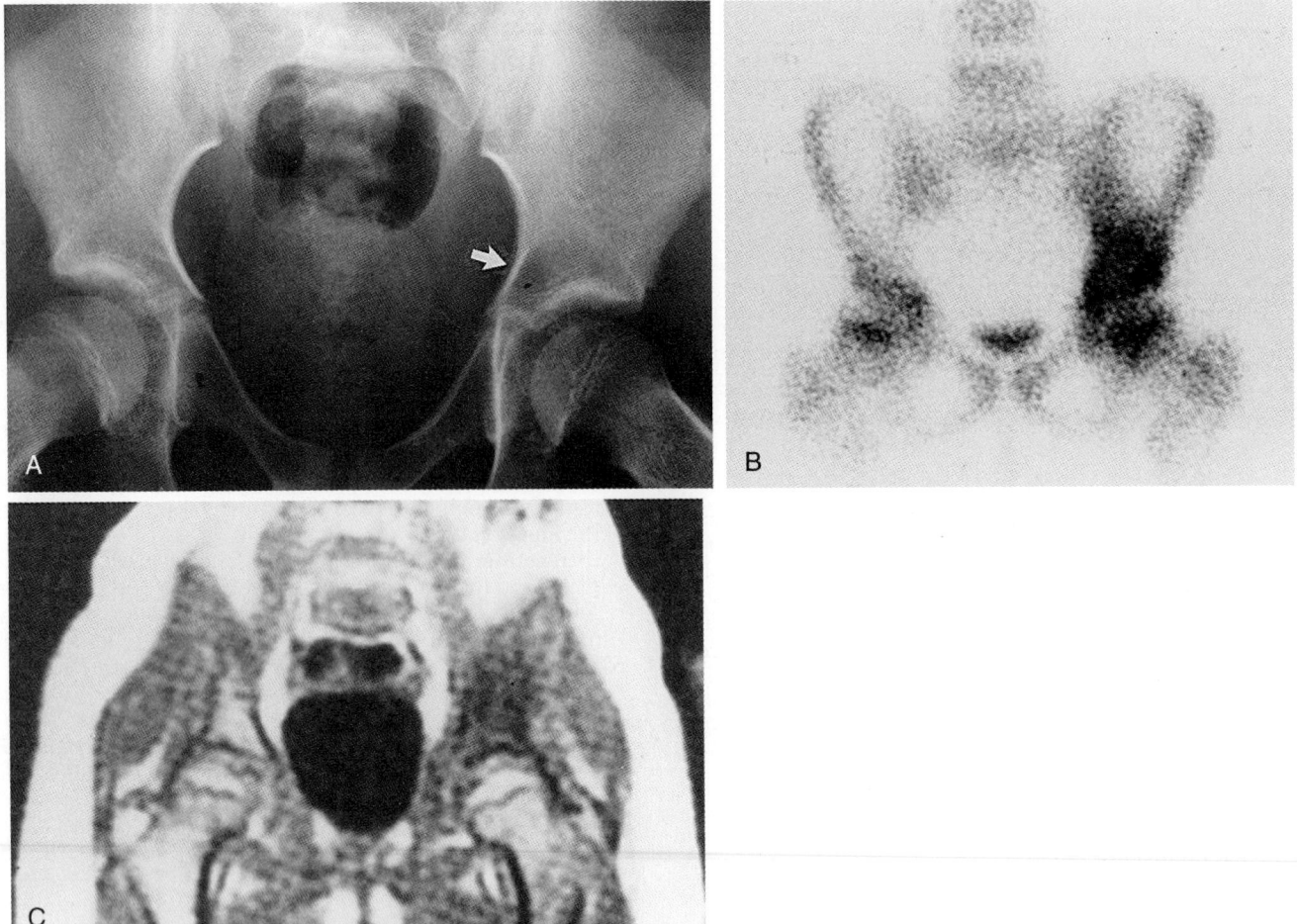

FIGURE 674–1. Pelvic osteomyelitis of the left iliac bone in a 12-yr-old girl with pain in the left hip region for 1–2 wk. *A,* Frontal radiograph of the pelvis shows mild demineralization of the acetabular portion of the iliac bone adjacent to the triradiate cartilage. There is very subtle periosteal reaction *(arrow)* along the margin of the sciatic notch. *B,* Technetium-99m bone scan shows increased uptake in the left iliac bone and mild increased uptake in the femoral head. *C,* Coronal MRI shows decreased signal from the marrow of the left iliac bone compared with the bright signal from the normal fatty marrow on the right. The femoral head is normal, and there is no joint effusion. Needle aspiration of the iliac bone yielded *Staphylococcus aureus;* the patient responded well to antimicrobial therapy. (From Markowitz RI: Diagnostic imaging. In Jenson HB, Baltimore RS [editors]: *Pediatric Infectious Diseases: Principles and Practice.* Norwalk, CT, Appleton & Lange, 1995.)

also useful to detect concomitant osteomyelitis and for evaluation of the sacroiliac joint.

DIFFERENTIAL DIAGNOSIS. The differential diagnosis of osteomyelitis includes trauma, both accidental and nonaccidental. Children with leukemia commonly have bone pain or joint pain as an early symptom. Neuroblastoma with bone involvement may be mistaken for osteomyelitis. Primary bone tumors need to be considered, but fever and other signs of illness are generally absent. Chronic recurrent multifocal osteomyelitis and synovitis, acne, pustulosis, hyperostosis, and osteitis (SAPHO) syndrome are rare conditions in children characterized by recurrent osteoarticular inflammation and different skin conditions, palmoplantar pustulosis, psoriasis, severe acne, neutrophilic dermatosis (Sweet syndrome), and pyoderma gangrenosum.

The differential diagnosis of suppurative arthritis depends on the joint or joints involved and the age of the patient. For the hip, toxic synovitis, Legg-Calvé-Perthes disease, slipped capital femoral epiphysis, psoas abscess, and proximal femoral, pelvic, or vertebral osteomyelitis and diskitis should be considered. For the knee, distal femoral or proximal tibial osteomyelitis, pauci-articular rheumatoid arthritis, and referred pain from the hip

should be considered. Other conditions such as trauma, cellulitis, pyomyositis, sickle cell disease, hemophilia, and Henoch-Schönlein purpura can mimic purulent arthritis. When several joints are involved, serum sickness, collagen vascular disease, rheumatic fever, and Henoch-Schönlein purpura should be considered. Reactive arthritis following a variety of bacterial and parasitic infections, streptococcal pharyngitis, or viral hepatitis can resemble acute suppurative arthritis (see Chapter 147).

Treatment. Optimal treatment of skeletal infections requires collaborative efforts of pediatricians, orthopedic surgeons, radiologists, and physiatrists.

ANTIBIOTIC THERAPY. The initial empirical antibiotic therapy is based on knowledge of likely bacterial pathogens at various ages, the results of the Gram stain of aspirated material, and additional considerations. In neonates, an antistaphylococcal penicillin, such as nafcillin or oxacillin (150–200 mg/kg/24 hr divided q6h IV), and a broad-spectrum cephalosporin, such as cefotaxime (150–200 mg/kg/24 hr divided q8h IV), provide coverage for the *S. aureus,* group B *Streptococcus,* and gram-negative bacilli. An aminoglycoside may be used in place of the cephalosporin, but aminoglycoside antibiotics have reduced antibacterial activity in sites with decreased oxygen tension and low pH, conditions that are present in tissue infections. If the neonate is a small premature infant or has a central vascular catheter, the possibility of nosocomial bacteria (*Pseudomonas aeruginosa* or coagulase-negative staphylococci) or fungi (*Candida*) should be considered.

In infants and children younger than 5 yr of age, the principal pathogens are *S. aureus*, streptococcus, and *H. influenzae* type b in children who have been vaccinated. Cefuroxime (200–300 mg/kg/24 hr divided q8h IV) provides coverage against these causes. After 5 yr of age and in the absence of special circumstances, virtually all cases of osteomyelitis are caused by gram-positive cocci; an antistaphylococcal antibiotic such as nafcillin (150–200 mg/kg/24 hr divided q6h) or cefazolin (100–150 mg/kg/24 hr divided q8h IV) can be used. In children older than 5 yr of age with suppurative arthritis, the bacterial causes are more varied and broader-spectrum drugs (a third-generation cephalosporin) are generally administered unless gram-positive cocci are seen in the Gram stain of synovial fluid.

Special situations dictate deviations from the usual empirical antibiotic selection. In patients with sickle cell disease with osteomyelitis, gram-negative enteric bacteria are common pathogens; a broad-spectrum cephalosporin such as cefotaxime or ceftriaxone is used in addition to an antistaphylococcal drug. Clindamycin (30–40 mg/kg/24 hr divided q6h IV) is a useful alternative drug for patients allergic to β-lactam drugs. In addition to good antistaphylococcal activity, clindamycin has broad activity against anaerobes and is useful for the treatment of infections secondary to penetrating injuries or compound fractures. Clindamycin and vancomycin (40 mg/kg/24 hr divided q6h IV) are alternatives when treating methicillin-resistant *S. aureus* infections. For immunocompromised patients, combination therapy is usually initiated, such as with vancomycin and ceftazidime, or with piperacillin-clavulanate and an aminoglycoside.

When the pathogen is identified, appropriate adjustments in antibiotics are made, if necessary. If a pathogen is not identified and a patient's condition is improving, therapy is continued with the antibiotic selected initially. If a pathogen is not identified and a patient's condition is not improving, re-aspiration or biopsy and the possibility of a noninfectious condition should be considered.

Duration of antibiotic therapy is individualized depending on organism isolated and clinical course. For infections caused by *S. aureus* or gram-negative bacillary infections, the minimum duration of antibiotics is 21 days, provided that (1) the patient shows prompt resolution of signs and symptoms (within 5–7 days) and (2) the ESR has normalized; a total of 4–6 wk of therapy may be required. For group A streptococcus, *S. pneumoniae*, or *H. influenzae* type b, antibiotics are given for a minimum of 10–14 days, using the same criteria. A total of 7 postoperative days of treatment is adequate for *Pseudomonas* osteochondritis when thorough curettage of infected tissue has been performed. Immunocompromised patients generally require prolonged courses of therapy, as do patients with mycobacterial or fungal infection.

Changing antibiotics from the intravenous route to oral administration when a patient's condition has stabilized, generally after 1 wk of intravenous therapy, may be considered. For the oral antibiotic regimen with β-lactam drugs for staphylococcal or streptococcal infection, a dosage two to three times that used for other infections is prescribed. The adequacy of the dose may be assessed by peak **serum bactericidal titers,** or **Schlichter titers,** 45–60 min after a dose of suspension or 60–90 min after a capsule or tablet. A serum bactericidal titer of 1:8 or more is considered desirable. The oral regimen decreases the risk of nosocomial infections related to prolonged intra-

venous therapy, is more comfortable for patients, and permits treatment outside the hospital if adherence to treatment can be assured. Alternatively, intravenous antibiotic therapy via a central venous catheter can be used for the completion of therapy at home.

SURGICAL THERAPY. Surgical management of skeletal infections has not been subjected to randomized prospective study comparing surgical procedures. When frank pus is obtained from subperiosteal or metaphyseal aspiration, a surgical drainage procedure is usually indicated. Surgical intervention is also often indicated after a penetrating injury and when a retained foreign body is possible.

Infection of the hip is considered a surgical emergency because of the vulnerability of the blood supply to the head of the femur. For joints other than the hip, daily aspirations of synovial fluid may be required. Generally, one or two subsequent aspirations suffice. If fluid continues to accumulate after 4–5 days, arthrotomy is needed. At the time of surgery, the joint is flushed with sterile saline solution. Antibiotics are not instilled, because they are irritating to synovial tissue and adequate amounts of antibiotic are achieved in joint fluid with systemic administration.

Treatment of chronic osteomyelitis consists of surgical removal of sinus tracts and sequestrum, if present. Antibiotic therapy is continued for several months or longer until clinical and radiographic findings suggest that healing has occurred.

PHYSICAL THERAPY. The major role of physical medicine is a preventive one. If a child is allowed to lie in bed with an extremity in flexion, limitation of extension may develop within a few days. The affected extremity should be kept in extension with sandbags, splints, or, if necessary, casts. Casts are also indicated when there is a potential for pathologic fracture. After 2–3 days, when pain is easing, passive range of motion exercises are started and continued until the child resumes normal activity. In neglected cases with flexion contractures, prolonged physical therapy is required.

Prognosis. When pus is drained and appropriate antibiotic therapy is given, the improvement in signs and symptoms is rapid. Failure to improve or worsening by 72 hr requires review of the appropriateness of the antibiotic therapy, the need for surgical intervention, or the correctness of the diagnosis. Acute-phase reactants may be useful as monitors. The serum CRP typically normalizes within 7 days after start of treatment, whereas the ESR typically rises for 5–7 days, then falls slowly, dropping sharply after 10–14 days. Failure of either of these acute-phase reactants to follow the usual course should raise concerns about the adequacy of therapy. Recurrence of disease and development of chronic infection after treatment occur in less than 10% of patients.

Because children are in a dynamic state of growth, sequelae of skeletal infections may not become apparent for months or years; therefore, long-term follow-up is necessary with close attention to range of motion of joints and bone length. Although firm data about the impact of delayed treatment on outcome are not available, it appears that initiation of medical and surgical therapy within 1 wk of onset of symptoms provides a better prognosis than delayed treatment.

Beretto-Piccoli BC, Sauvain MJ, Gal I, et al: Synovitis, acne, pustulosis, hyperostosis, osteitis (SAPHO) syndrome in childhood: A report of 10 cases and review of the literature. *Eur J Pediatr* 2000;159:594–601.

Bradley JS, Kaplan SL, Tan TQ, et al: Pediatric pneumococcal bone and joint infections. The Pediatric Multicenter Pneumococcal Surveillance Study Group (PMPSG). *Pediatrics* 1998;102:1376–82.

Burnett MW, Bass JW, Cook BA: Etiology of osteomyelitis complicating sickle cell disease. *Pediatrics* 1998;101:296–97.

Fernandez M, Carrol CL, Baker CJ: Discitis and vertebral osteomyelitis in children: An 18-year review. *Pediatrics* 2000;105:1299–304.

Gomez M, Maraqa N, Alvarez A, et al: Complications of outpatient parenteral antibiotic therapy in childhood. *Pediatr Infect Dis J* 2001;20:541–43.

Karwowska A, Davies HD, Jadavji T: Epidemiology and outcome of osteomyelitis in the era of sequential intravenous-oral therapy. *Pediatr Infect Dis J* 1998;17: 1021–26.

Kothari NA, Pelchavitz DJ, Meyer JS: Imaging of musculoskeletal infections. *Radiol Clin North Am* 2001;39:653–71.

Lew DP, Waldvogel FA: Osteomyelitis. *N Engl J Med* 1997;336:999–1007.

Nelson JD: Toward simple but safe management of osteomyelitis. *Pediatrics* 1997;99:883–84.

Nelson JD: Bugs, drugs and bones: A pediatric infectious disease specialist reflects on management of musculoskeletal infections. *J Pediatr Orthop* 1999;19:141–42.

Unkila-Kallio L, Kallio MJ, Eskola J, et al: Serum C-reactive protein, erythrocyte sedimentation rate, and white blood cell count in acute hematogenous osteomyelitis of children. *Pediatrics* 1994;93:59–62.

SECTION 2 *Sports Medicine*

Albert C. Hergenroeder and Joseph N. Chorley

Chapter 675

Epidemiology and Prevention of Injuries

Physical activity for youth is a national health priority. The Surgeon General's Healthy People 2010 Objectives emphasize moderate to vigorous physical activity on a regular basis for adolescents. Physical activity has favorable effects on hypertension, obesity, and serum lipid levels in youth. In adults, physical activity is associated with lower rates of cardiovascular disease, type 2 diabetes mellitus, osteoporosis, and colon and breast cancer.

Physicians should promote physical activity to their patients and make adjustments in the type of physical activity depending on their health status (Tables 675–1 through 675–3). Extra effort is needed to try to make physical activity part of the lifestyle for those with lower rates of physical activity and sports participation, including children with special health care needs, females, and those from lower socioeconomic groups. Coincident with promoting sports participation and physical activity, physicians have the responsibility of providing medical clearance for participation in physical activity and sports and for diagnosis and rehabilitation of injuries.

Having fun during sports participation should be a priority. Athletic success and having fun can occur together yet are not synonymous. Those who have not had success or fun may conclude they are not an athlete and eliminate exercise from their lifestyle. Youth sports programs should teach skills for life. Sports participation and physical activity can be associated with improved self-esteem, improved fitness, and the satisfaction of improving skills related to the sport. These benefits are more likely to occur when the demands of the sport match the physical, cognitive, emotional, and attitudinal resources of the youth. When the demands exceed these resources, frustration and reduced self-esteem can occur. This frustration can progress to clinical problems, such as falling grades, anxiety, and/or depression. The manifestations of the anxiety and depression are myriad and include unexplained fatigue, poor athletic performance, and musculoskeletal pain with no organic etiology. The physician should (1) rule out an underlying organic etiology; (2) review the athlete's training schedule; (3) review the athlete's nutritional intake, assuring adequate calories; and (4) if the evaluation reveals no organic etiology and overtraining appears to be the problem, recommend a reduction in training. Complete rest is not recommended; for most conditions some ongoing exercise training is prescribed, as long as the symptoms improve. The reduction in training, with some guidelines for criteria to gradually increase training if symptoms subside, gives the athlete a plan for returning to sports.

Some parents describe sports as a career pathway for their child. Playing on a Division I, select, or traveling team is in some parents' and coaches' minds a required step in the development of elite athletes who are "serious about their sport." The notion that there is one pathway to elite athletic status and that path includes beginning at a young age with intense, year-round training is misleading. Parents and coaches may believe that a given child has talent and requires more training and commitment to

TABLE 675–1. Classification of Sports by Contact

Contact or Collision	Limited Contact	Noncontact
Basketball	Baseball	Archery
Boxing*	Bicycling	Badminton
Diving	Cheerleading	Body building
Field hockey	Canoeing or kayaking	Bowling
Football	(white water)	Canoeing or kayaking (flat water)
Tackle	Fencing	Crew or rowing
Ice hockey†	Field events	Curling
Lacrosse	High jump	Dancing
Martial arts	Pole vault	Ballet
Rodeo	Floor hockey	Modern
Rugby	Football	Jazz
Ski jumping	Flag	Field events
Soccer	Gymnastics	Discus
Team handball	Handball	Javelin
Water polo	Horseback riding	Shot put
Wrestling	Racquetball	Golf
	Skating	Orienteering‡
	Ice	Power lifting
	In-line	Race walking
	Roller	Riflery
	Skiing	Rope jumping
	Cross-country	Running
	Downhill	Sailing
	Water	Scuba diving
	Skateboarding	Swimming
	Snowboarding	Table tennis
	Softball	Tennis
	Squash	Track
	Ultimate frisbee	Weight lifting
	Volleyball	
	Windsurfing or surfing	

Participation not recommended by the American Academy of Pediatrics.

†*The American Academy of Pediatrics recommends limiting the amount of body checking allowed for hockey players 15 years and younger to reduce injuries.*

‡*A race (contest) in which competitors use a map and compass to find their way through unfamiliar territory.*

From the American Academy of Pediatrics, Committee on Sports Medicine and Fitness: Medical conditions affecting sports participation. Pediatrics 2001;107:1205.

TABLE 675–2. Medical Conditions and Sports Participation*

Condition	May Participate
Atlantoaxial instability (instability of the joint between cervical vertebrae 1 and 2)	Qualified yes
Explanation: Athlete needs evaluation to assess risk of spinal cord injury during sports participation.	
Bleeding disorder	Qualified yes
Explanation: Athlete needs evaluation.	
Cardiovascular disease	
Carditis (inflammation of the heart)	No
Explanation: Carditis may result in sudden death with exertion.	
Hypertension (high blood pressure)	Qualified yes
Explanation: Those with significant essential (unexplained) hypertension should avoid weight and power lifting, body building, and strength training. Those with secondary hypertension (hypertension caused by a previously identified disease) or severe essential hypertension need evaluation. The National High Blood Pressure Education Working group defined significant and severe hypertension.	
Congenital heart disease (structural heart defects present at birth)	Qualified yes
Explanation: Those with mild forms may participate fully; those with moderate or severe forms or who have undergone surgery need evaluation. The 26th Bethesda Conference defined mild, moderate, and severe disease for common cardiac lesions.	
Dysrhythmia (irregular heart rhythm)	Qualified yes
Explanation: Those with symptoms (chest pain, syncope, dizziness, shortness of breath, or other symptoms of possible dysrhythmia) or evidence of mitral regurgitation (leaking) on physical examination need evaluation. All others may participate fully.	
Heart murmur	Qualified yes
Explanation: If the murmur is innocent (does not indicate heart disease), full participation is permitted. Otherwise, the athlete needs evaluation (see congenital heart disease and mitral valve prolapse).	
Cerebral palsy	Qualified yes
Explanation: Athlete needs evaluation.	
Diabetes mellitus	Yes
Explanation: All sports can be played with proper attention to diet, blood glucose concentration, hydration, and insulin therapy. Blood glucose concentration should be monitored every 30 minutes during continuous exercise and 15 minutes after completion of exercise.	
Diarrhea	Qualified no
Explanation: Unless disease is mild, no participation is permitted, because diarrhea may increase the risk of dehydration and heat illness. See fever.	
Eating disorders	Qualified yes
Anorexia nervosa	
Bulimia nervosa	
Explanation: Patients with these disorders need medical and psychiatric assessment before participation.	
Eyes	Qualified yes
Functionally one-eyed athlete	
Loss of an eye	
Detached retina	
Previous eye surgery or serious eye injury	
Explanation: A functionally one-eyed athlete has a best-corrected visual acuity of less than 20/40 in the eye with worse acuity. These athletes would suffer significant disability if the better eye were seriously injured, as would those with loss of an eye. Some athletes who previously have undergone eye surgery or had a serious eye injury may have an increased risk of injury because of weakened eye tissue. Availability of eye guards approved by the American Society for Testing and Materials and other protective equipment may allow participation in most sports, but this must be judged on an individual basis.	
Fever	No
Explanation: Fever can increase cardiopulmonary effort, reduce maximum exercise capacity, make heat illness more likely, and increase orthostatic tension during exercise. Fever may rarely accompany myocarditis or other infections that may make exercise dangerous.	
Heat illness, history of	Qualified yes
Explanation: Because of the increased likelihood of recurrence, the athlete needs individual assessment to determine the presence of predisposing conditions and to arrange a prevention strategy.	
Hepatitis	Yes
Explanation: Because of the apparent minimal risk to others, all sports may be played that the athlete's state of health allows. In all athletes, skin lesions should be covered properly, and athletic personnel should use universal precautions when handling blood or body fluids with visible blood.	
Human immunodeficiency virus infection	Yes
Explanation: Because of the apparent minimal risk to others, all sports may be played that the athlete's state of health allows. In all athletes, skin lesions should be covered properly, and athletic personnel should use universal precautions when handling blood or body fluids with visible blood.	
Kidney, absence of one	Qualified yes
Explanation: Athlete needs individual assessment for contact, collision, and limited-contact sports.	
Liver, enlarged	Qualified yes
Explanation: If the liver is acutely enlarged, participation should be avoided because of risk of rupture. If the liver is chronically enlarged, individual assessment is needed before collision, contact, or limited-contact sports are played.	
Malignant neoplasm	Qualified yes
Explanation: Athlete needs individual assessment.	
Musculoskeletal disorders	Qualified yes
Explanation: Athlete needs individual assessment.	
Neurologic disorders	
History of serious head or spine trauma, severe or repeated concussions, or craniotomy.	Qualified yes
Explanation: Athlete needs individual assessment for collision, contact, or limited-contact sports and also for noncontact sports if deficits in judgment or cognition are present. Research supports a conservative approach to management of concussion.	
Seizure disorder, well-controlled	Yes
Explanation: Risk of seizure during participation is minimal	
Seizure disorder, poorly controlled	Qualified yes
Explanation: Athlete needs individual assessment for collision, contact, or limited-contact sports. The following noncontact sports should be avoided: archery, riflery, swimming, weight or power lifting, strength training, or sports involving heights. In these sports, occurrence of a seizure may pose a risk to self or others.	
Obesity	Qualified yes
Explanation: Because of the risk of heat illness, obese persons need careful acclimatization and hydration.	
Organ transplant recipient	Qualified yes
Explanation: Athlete needs individual assessment.	
Ovary, absence of one	Yes
Explanation: Risk of severe injury to the remaining ovary is minimal.	

Table continued on following page

TABLE 675–2. **Medical Conditions and Sports Participation*** *Continued*

Condition	May Participate
Respiratory conditions	
Pulmonary compromise, including cystic fibrosis	Qualified yes
Explanation: Athlete needs individual assessment, but generally, all sports may be played if oxygenation remains satisfactory during a graded exercise test. Patients with cystic fibrosis need acclimatization and good hydration to reduce the risk of heat illness.	
Asthma	Yes
Explanation: With proper medication and education, only athletes with the most severe asthma will need to modify their participation.	
Acute upper respiratory infection	Qualified yes
Explanation: Upper respiratory obstruction may affect pulmonary function. Athlete needs individual assessment for all but mild disease. See fever.	
Sickle cell disease	Qualified yes
Explanation: Athlete needs individual assessment. In general, if status of the illness permits, all but high exertion, collision, and contact sports may be played. Overheating, dehydration, and chilling must be avoided.	
Sickle cell trait	Yes
Explanation: It is unlikely that persons with sickle cell trait have an increased risk of sudden death or other medical problems during athletic participation, except under the most extreme conditions of heat, humidity, and possibly increased altitude. These persons, like all athletes, should be carefully conditioned, acclimatized, and hydrated to reduce any possible risk.	
Skin disorders (boils, herpes simplex, impetigo, scabies, molluscum contagiosum)	Qualified yes
Explanation: While the patient is contagious, participation in gymnastics with mats; martial arts; wrestling; or other collision, contact, or limited-contact sports is not allowed.	
Spleen, enlarged	Qualified yes
Explanation: A patient with an acutely enlarged spleen should avoid all sports because of risk of rupture. A patient with a chronically enlarged spleen needs individual assessment before playing collision, contact, or limited-contact sports.	
Testicle, undescended or absence of one	Yes
Explanation: Certain sports may require a protective cup.	

**This table is designed for use by medical and nonmedical personnel. "Needs evaluation" means that a physician with appropriate knowledge and experience should assess the safety of a given sport for an athlete with the listed medical condition. Unless otherwise noted, this is because of variability of the severity of the disease, the risk of injury for the specific sports listed in Table 675–1, or both.*

From the American Academy of Pediatrics, Committee on Sports Medicine and Fitness: Medical conditions affecting sports participation. Pediatrics 2001;107:1206–7.

reach the elite status. Parents may experience achievement by proxy, with adult pride in the performance of their child. Positive, supportive behaviors include unconditional love and being an objective parent, manifest as enforcing medical recommendations, even against the will of the young athlete and the coach. Physicians' recommendations to reduce training are often challenged by young athletes, their parents, and coaches. An explanation of the diagnosis of a musculoskeletal injury, with anatomic models, to the youth and family, with the natural history of the injury if treated appropriately versus injury progression if the athlete continues with pain, is indicated. The physician can offer to talk to the coach on the athlete's behalf. The overriding principle that should guide return to play and rehabilitation recommendations is what is best for the short- and long-term health of the athlete. Behavior becomes pathologic when the parents' or coaches' goals take priority over the health and well-being of the child. When the parents give decisions to train and participate to the coach, exploitation and abuse can occur in an attempt to further the coach's career. The suggestion that parents and coaches do not have the athlete's health and well-being as the top priority is often met with resistance.

Year-round training may increase the risk of repetitive, overuse injuries and the risk of psychological burnout. This risk exists for children with talent in other activities, such as dance, drama, or singing. The overly focused athlete may have talent in other areas but will not be given the opportunity to discover this.

Coaches often require young athletes at some large high schools and elite youth teams to declare their allegiance to one sport, to the exclusion of all others. This is counter to the need for athletes to have time away from a sport, both physically and psychologically. There should not be an age at which the young athlete must declare his or her commitment to one sport.

In 2001, 65% of high school students participated in vigorous physical activity for 20 min or more on at least 3 of the previous 7 days. Fifty-five per cent of high school students played on school sports team in 2001, with 38% playing on teams outside of school. Approximately 30 million children and adoles-

cents participate in organized sports in the United States. Approximately 3 million injuries occur annually if injury is defined as time lost from the sport. Deaths in sports are rare, with the majority of nontraumatic deaths caused by cardiac diseases (see Chapter 428.6). There are three times more nontraumatic than traumatic deaths. The majority of traumatic deaths are caused by head and neck injuries. Within the same sport, injury rates for males and females are similar, with the exception of anterior cruciate ligament injuries, which are higher in females. The majority of sports injuries are sprains, strains, overuse injuries, contusions and, least of all, fractures. The potential for growth plate injury is a complication of appendicular trauma that distinguishes young athletes from adult athletes. An injury that might cause a ligament sprain in adults could cause a growth plate injury in a young athlete, because the growth plate is weaker than the ligament. A fracture of the growth plate (i.e., Salter-Harris type I injury) should be considered when there is point tenderness at the growth plate and the initial radiographic findings are normal (see Chapter 673). In addition, fracture rates in adolescence peak approximately 6 mo before peak height velocity in males and females. Peak accretion of bone mineral occurs approximately 6 mo after peak height velocity, suggesting that the increased fracture rate during early and mid adolescence may be related to a relative porosity of bone because bone mineralization, and presumably bone strength, may lag behind long bone growth, making long bones more susceptible to fracture. Overall, injury rates and injury severity in sports increase with age and pubertal development, related to the greater speed, strength, and intensity of competition.

Recognizing mechanisms of injury and enforcing rules that reduced the likelihood of that mechanism of injury, including penalizing dangerous play, have reduced catastrophic injury rates. Injury rates have also been reduced by removing environmental hazards, such as trampolines in gymnastics and stationary (vs breakaway) bases in softball, and by modifying heat injury rates in soccer tournaments by adding water breaks and reducing the playing time. Wearing equipment such as mouthguards can reduce dental injuries, yet they are not worn routinely by athletes in any sport except football. A common reason for re-injury is lack of rehabilitation of old injuries; appropriate rehabilitation reduces injury rates. Preseason training for high school athletes, with an emphasis on speed, agility, jump training, and flexibility is associated with lower injury rates in soccer and serious knee injuries in female athletes. Limited data and experience in implementing preseason programs exist to recommend broad implementation to prevent injuries. Pre-exercise stretching, alone, in otherwise healthy individuals, does not prevent injuries. One setting for implementing some of these prevention strategies and for detecting unrehabilitated injuries and medical problems that could impact participation in sports is the preparticipation sports examination (PSE).

Preparticipation Sports Examination. The PSE is performed with a directed history and a directed physical examination, including a screening musculoskeletal examination. It identifies possible problems in 1–8% of athletes and excludes less than 1% from participation. The PSE is not a substitute for the recommended comprehensive annual evaluation, which looks at behaviors that are potentially harmful to teens, such as sexual activity, drug use, suicide, and violence. The purposes of the PSE include detecting medical conditions that delay or disqualify athletic participation owing to a risk of injury or death; detecting previously undiagnosed medical conditions; detecting medical conditions that need further evaluation or rehabilitation before participation; providing guidance for sports participation for patients with health conditions; and meeting legal and insurance obligations. If possible, the PSE should be combined with the comprehensive annual health visit with emphasis on preventive health care (see Chapters 14 and 100). Another option is to perform the PSE and have the athlete complete a comprehensive screening questionnaire, such as the Guidelines for Adolescent Preventive Care (GAPS) form published by the American Medical Association (AMA). If problems are detected on the screening questionnaire, then a follow-up visit can be scheduled. This is less optimal because it relies on the sensitivity of a questionnaire, without an interview to detect health risk behaviors.

State requirements for how often a youth needs a PSE differ, ranging from annually to entry to a new school level (junior high, senior high, college). At a minimum, a focused, annual interim evaluation should be done on an otherwise healthy young athlete. The PSE is optimally performed 3–6 wk before the start of practice so that rehabilitation of old injuries and evaluation of potential health problems can be completed to minimize absence from practices or games.

HISTORY AND PHYSICAL EXAMINATION. The essential components of the PSE are the history and focused medical and musculoskeletal screening examinations. Identified problems require more investigation (Table 675–4). In the absence of symptoms, no screening laboratory tests are required.

Seventy-five per cent of significant findings are identified by the history; a standardized questionnaire given to the parent and athlete is important because the young athlete may not know or may forget important aspects of their history. The questionnaire should include questions about previous medical, surgical, cardiac, pulmonary, neurologic, dermatologic, visual, psychologic, musculoskeletal, and menstrual problems, as well as about heat illness, medications, allergies, immunizations, and diet. The most common identified problems are unrehabilitated injuries. An investigation of previous injuries including diagnostic tests, treatment, and present functional status is indicated. The most common musculoskeletal injuries identified are of the knee and ankle.

Sudden death during sports may result from undetected cardiac disease such as hypertrophic or other cardiomyopathies, anomalous coronary vessels, or a ruptured aorta in Marfan syndrome (see Chapter 690). In many cases the underlying heart disease is not suspected, and death is the first sign of heart disease (see Chapter 428.6). Chest radiographs, electrocardiograms (ECGs), and echocardiograms (ECHOs) are not recommended as screening tests. If there is a suspicion of heart disease, such as a history of syncope, presyncope, palpitations, excessive dyspnea with exercise, or a family history of a condition such as hypertrophic cardiomyopathy or prolonged QT or Marfan syndromes, then the evaluation should be complete and include a 12-lead ECG, an ECHO, a Holter or event capture monitor, and a stress test with ECG monitoring. Recommendations for participation with identified cardiac disease should be done in consultation with a cardiologist.

Disqualification and limitations for sports participation among various medical conditions are noted in Table 675–2. Classification of sports activities by type of demand is delineated in Table 675–3. Athletes may seek to participate in sports against medical advice and have done so successfully for professional sports. Section 504(a) of the Rehabilitation Act of 1973 prohibits discrimination against disabled athletes if they have capabilities/skills required to play a competitive sport. This was reinforced through the Americans with Disabilities Act of 1990. An amateur athlete has no absolute right to decide whether to participate in competitive sports. Participation in competitive

---

TABLE 675–3. Classification of Sports by Strenuousness

High to Moderate Intensity		
High to Moderate Dynamic and Static Demands	**High to Moderate Dynamic and Low Static Demands**	**High to Moderate Static and Low Dynamic Demands**
Boxing*	Badminton	Archery
Crew or rowing	Baseball	Auto racing
Cross-country skiing	Basketball	Diving
Cycling	Field hockey	Horseback riding (jumping)
Downhill skiing	Lacrosse	Field events (throwing)
Fencing	Orienteering	Gymnastics
Football	Race walking	Karate or judo
Ice hockey	Racquetball	Motorcycling
Rugby	Soccer	Rodeo
Running (sprint)	Squash	Sailing
Speed skating	Swimming	Ski jumping
Water polo	Table tennis	Water skiing
Wrestling	Tennis	Weight lifting
	Volleyball	

Low Intensity (Low Dynamic and Low Static Demands)

Bowling
Cricket
Curling
Golf
Riflery

*Participation not recommended by the American Academy of Pediatrics.
From the American Academy of Pediatrics, Committee on Sports Medicine and Fitness: Medical conditions affecting sports participation. Pediatrics 2001;107:1208.*

TABLE 675–4. Preparticipation Sports Examination

Component of the Physical Examination	Condition to be Detected
Vital signs	Hypertension, cardiac disease, brady/tachycardia
Height and weight	Obesity, eating disorders
Vision and pupil size	Legal blindness, absent eye, anisocoria
Lymph node	Infectious diseases, malignancy
Cardiac (performed standing and supine)	Heart murmur, prior surgery, rhythm
Pulmonary	Recurrent and exercise-induced bronchospasm, chronic lung disease
Abdominal	Organomegaly, abdominal mass
Skin	Contagious diseases (impetigo, herpes, staphylococcal, streptococcal)
Genitourinary	Varicocele, undescended testes, tumor
Musculoskeletal	Acute and chronic injuries, physical anomalies (scoliosis)

sports is considered a privilege, not a right. *Knapp v. Northwestern University* established that "difficult medical decisions involving complex medical problems can be made by responsible physicians exercising prudent judgment (which will be necessarily conservative when definitive scientific evidence is lacking or conflicting) and relying on the recommendations of specialist consultants or guidelines established by a panel of experts."

Chapter 676

Management of Musculoskeletal Injury

MECHANISM OF INJURY

Acute Injuries. The majority of musculoskeletal injuries are sprains, strains, and contusions. Often, the history of the injury is unclear and it is harder to evaluate the injury. More severe injuries, indicative of structural derangement, may have acute signs and symptoms such as immediate swelling, deformity, numbness or weakness, inability to continue playing, inability to walk without a limp, a loud painful pop, mechanical locking of the joint, or the sensation of instability when the athlete describes that at the time of the injury it felt like the bones moved in the wrong direction.

Overuse Injuries. Overuse injuries are caused by repetitive microtrauma that exceeds the body's rate of repair. This occurs in muscles, tendons, bone, bursas, cartilage, and nerves. Overuse injuries occur in all sports but more frequently in sports emphasizing repetitive motion (e.g., swimming, running, tennis, gymnastics). Parents' and coaches' excessively high expectations may add to the risk of an overuse injury in a young, eager-to-please athlete. Possible risks for or indicators of overuse or burnout include early specialization in a single sport, playing on a "select traveling team," practicing most days of the week without sufficient recovery period, loss of enjoyment, decreased performance, vague muscle soreness/stiffness, fatigue, dysphoria, and sleep disturbances. Factors can be categorized into extrinsic (training errors, poor equipment or workout surface) and intrinsic. Training error is the most frequently identified factor. At the beginning of the workout program, athletes may violate the "10% rule": Do not increase the duration or intensity of workouts more than 10% per week. Intrinsic factors include abnormal biomechanics (e.g., leg-length discrepancy, pes planus, pes cavus, tarsal coalition, valgus heel, external tibial torsion, femoral anteversion), muscle imbalance, inflexibility, and medical conditions (deconditioning, nutritional deficits, amenorrhea, obesity). The athlete should be asked about the specifics of his or her training. For example, runners should be asked about their shoes, orthotics or braces, running surface, pace, weekly mileage or time spent running per week, speed or hill workouts, duration of the current regimen, and previous injuries and rehabilitation. When causative factors are identified, they can be eliminated or modified so that after rehabilitation the athlete does not return to the same regimen and suffer re-injury.

For athletes engaged in excessive training that causes an overuse injury, curtailing all sports is not always feasible. A rehabilitation program designed to return athletes to their sport as soon as possible while minimizing exposure to re-injury is indicated. Early identification of an overuse injury requires less alteration of the workout regimen.

The *inflammatory response after injury* is manifested as pain, spasm, edema, and, if unabated, scarring. Pain and spasm cause decreased use of the affected area. Although reduced use may protect the area, continued nonuse causes atrophy and decreased flexibility, strength, endurance, and proprioception. Stiff, weak structures with poor proprioception do not function normally and are vulnerable to re-injury. The goals of treatment are to control pain and spasm to rehabilitate flexibility, strength, endurance, and proprioceptive deficits (Table 676–1).

INITIAL EVALUATION OF THE INJURED EXTREMITY

Initially, the examiner should determine the quality of the peripheral pulses and capillary refill rate as well as the gross motor and sensory function to assess for neurovascular injury. The first priorities are to maintain vascular and skeletal stability.

Criteria for immediate attention and rapid orthopedic consultation include vascular compromise (blood flow may be obstructed by a dislocated structure, so a skilled physician should reduce any obstructing dislocated joint); nerve compromise (peripheral nerve damage can be repaired after vascular and skeletal stability have been achieved); and open fracture (an open fracture should not be reduced immediately because of the risk of further contamination). The exposed wound should be covered with sterile saline-soaked gauze, and the injured limb should be padded and splinted. Pressure should be applied to any site of bleeding. Additional criteria include deep laceration over a joint, unreducible dislocation, grade III (complete) tear of a muscle-tendon unit, and displaced, significantly angulated fractures (depends on the bone involved, the degree of displacement and angulation, and neurovascular status of the extremity). After the neurovascular assessment, the management of acute musculoskeletal trauma should follow the RICE (rest, ice, compression, elevation) guidelines.

THE TRANSITION FROM IMMEDIATE MANAGEMENT TO RETURN TO PLAY

Rehabilitation of a musculoskeletal injury should begin on the day of the injury.

Phase 1: Limit further injury, control swelling and pain, and minimize strength and flexibility losses. This requires the use of an

TABLE 676–1. Staging of Overuse Injuries

Grade	Grading Symptoms	Treatment
I	Pain only after activity Does not interfere with performance or intensity Generalized tenderness Disappears before next session	Modification of activity, consider cross-training, home rehabilitation program
II	Minimal pain with activity Does not interfere with performance More localized tenderness	Modification of activity, cross-training, consider NSAIDs, home rehabilitation program
III	Pain interferes with activity and performance Definite area of tenderness Usually disappears between sessions	Significant modification of activity, strongly encourage cross-training, NSAIDs, home rehabilitation program, and outpatient physical therapy
IV	Pain with activities of daily living Pain does not disappear between sessions Marked interference with performance and training intensity	Discontinue activity temporarily, cross-training only, NSAIDs, home rehabilitation program and intensive outpatient physical therapy
V	Pain interferes with activities of daily living Signs of tissue injury (e.g., edema) Chronic or recurrent symptoms	Prolonged discontinuation of activity, cross-training only, NSAIDs, home rehabilitation program, and intensive outpatient physical therapy

NSAIDs = nonsteroidal anti-inflammatory drugs.

appropriate device such as crutches or a sling, ice, compression, elevation, and analgesia. Crutches, air stirrups for ankle sprains, slings for arm injuries, and elastic wraps (4 to 8 in) for compression are a reasonable inventory of office supplies. Ice in a plastic bag is placed directly on the skin for 20 min continuously, three to four times per day until the swelling resolves. Compression limits further bleeding and swelling but should not be so tight that it limits perfusion. Elevation of the extremity promotes venous return and limits swelling. Nonsteroidal anti-inflammatory drugs (NSAIDs) or acetaminophen is indicated for analgesia.

Pain-free isometric strengthening and range of motion should be initiated as soon as possible. Pain inhibits full muscle contraction; deconditioning results if the pain and resultant nonuse persist for days to weeks, thus delaying recovery. Education about the nature of the injury and the specifics of rehabilitation exercises including handouts with written instructions and drawings demonstrating the exercises are helpful.

Phase 2: Improve strength and range of motion (i.e., flexibility) while allowing the injured structures to heal. Protective devices are removed when the patient's strength and flexibility improve and activities of daily living are pain free. Flexibility can then be improved by a program of specific stretches, held for 15–20 sec for 3 to 5 repetitions, once or twice daily. A physical therapist or athletic trainer is invaluable in this treatment. Protective devices may need to be used for months during sports participation. Swimming, water jogging, and stationary cycling are good aerobic exercises that can allow the injured extremity to be rested or used pain free while maintaining cardiovascular fitness.

Phase 3: Achieve near normal strength and flexibility of the injured structures and further improve or maintain cardiovascular fitness. Strength and endurance are improved under controlled conditions using elastic bands and eventually free weights or exercise equipment. Proprioceptive training allows the athlete to redevelop a kinesthetic sense, which is critical to joint function and stability.

Phase 4: Return to exercise or competition without restriction. When the athlete has reached nearly normal flexibility, strength, proprioception, and endurance, he or she can start sports-specific exercises. The athlete will make the transition from the rehabilitation program to functional rehabilitation appropriate for the sport. Substituting sports participation for rehabilitation is inappropriate; rather, there should be progressive stepwise functional return to a full activity/play program. For instance, a basketball player recovering from an ankle injury might begin a walk-run-sprint-cut program before returning to competition. At any point in this progression if pain is experienced, the athlete needs to stop, apply ice, avoid running for 1–2 days, continue to do ankle exercises, and then resume running at a lower intensity and progress accordingly.

Relative Rest and Return-to-Play Guidelines. Relative rest means that the athlete can do whatever he or she wants as long as the injured structures do not hurt during or within 24 hr of the activity. Going beyond relative rest delays recovery.

DIFFERENTIAL DIAGNOSES OF MUSCULOSKELETAL PAIN

The presenting complaint of musculoskeletal pain can be caused by traumatic, rheumatologic, infectious, hematologic, psychologic, and oncologic processes. Symptoms such as fatigue, weight loss, rash, multiple joint complaints, fever, chronic or recent illness, and persistence of pain suggest diagnoses other than sports-related trauma. Incongruity between the patient's history and physical examination findings should lead to further evaluation. A normal review of systems with an injury history consistent with the physical findings suggests a sports-related etiology. Nonorganic causes are to be considered when the evaluation indicates the absence of identifiable organic disease yet the symptoms persist.

676.1 Growth Plate Injuries

Twenty per cent of pediatric sports injuries seen in the emergency department are fractures. Twenty-five per cent of those fractures involve an epiphysis (see Chapter 673). Growth in long bones occurs in three areas: the epiphyseal, or growth, plate, the articular surface (the cartilaginous covering of the bones), and the apophysis (the growth cartilage where major tendons attach to the bone). The growth plate can be acutely injured at the epiphysis (Salter-Harris fractures), the articular surface (osteochondritis dissecans), or the apophysis (avulsion fractures). Boys suffer about twice as many epiphyseal fractures as girls; the peak incidence of fracture is during peak height velocity (girls, 12 ± 2.5 yr; boys, 14 ± 2 yr).

The most common *epiphyseal injuries* are to the distal radius, followed by phalangeal and distal tibial fractures. Physeal injuries at the knee (distal femur and proximal tibia) are rare. Growth disturbance following a growth plate injury is a function of location, the part of the epiphysis fractured, and the vascular communication between the epiphysis and metaphysis. These factors influence the probability of physeal bar formation resulting in growth arrest at that growth plate. The areas making the largest contribution to longitudinal growth in the upper extremities are the proximal humerus and distal radius/ulna; in the lower extremities, they are the distal femur and the proximal tibia/fibula. Injuries to these areas are more likely to cause growth disturbance compared with epiphyseal injuries at the other end of these long bones. The part of the epiphysis fractured is described by the Salter-Harris classification system (see Fig. 673–2).

Osteochondritis dissecans (OCD) is avascular necrosis of the bone underlying the articular cartilage. The articular cartilage may flatten, soften, or break off. Some OCD lesions are asymptomatic (diagnosed on "routine" radiographs), whereas others are manifested as edema, pain, decreased range of motion, and mechanical symptoms (locking, popping, crepitus). Seventy-five per cent of OCD lesions are located on the medial side of the femoral notch on a non–weight-bearing surface and therefore may have minimal symptoms. Other joints where OCD lesions are identified are the ankle (talus) and elbow, usually involving the medial humeral epiphysis, capitellum, or radial head. OCD classically affects athletes in their second decade. The severity of the lesion is graded as follows: I—compression of the bone, cartilage intact; II—partial separation; III—loose fragment but still in place; and IV—loose fragment detached. Most grade I and II lesions heal spontaneously with protection of the injured joint from loading and torquing actions. If the lesion loosens, internal fixation or debridement may be required. The key to preventing complications is early diagnosis and treatment including no weight bearing or no traumatic activity until healing has occurred. Patients with OCD should be referred to an orthopedic surgeon.

Avulsion fractures occur when a forceful muscle contraction dislodges the apophysis from the bone. They occur most frequently around the hip, elbow, and ankle. Chronically increased traction at the muscle-apophysis attachment can lead to repetitive microtrauma, inflammation, and pain at the apophysis. The most common areas affected are the knee (*Osgood-Schlatter* and *Sindig-Larsen-Johannson disease*), the ankle (**Sever disease),** and the medial epicondyle (**Little League elbow).** Traction apophysitis of the knee and ankle can be potentially treated in a primary care setting, following the principles discussed under rehabilitation. The main goal of treatment is to minimize the intensity and frequency of pain and disability. Exercises that increase the strength, flexibility, and endurance of the muscles attached at the apophysis, using the relative rest principle, are appropriate. Symptoms can last for 12–24 mo if untreated. As growth slows, symptoms abate. Traction apophysitis of the elbow should be referred to a pediatric orthopedic surgeon.

676.2 Shoulder Injuries

An acute shoulder injury characterized by radiating symptoms down the arm should suggest the possibility that a coexisting neck injury has occurred. Neck pain and tenderness or limitation of cervical range of motion requires that the cervical spine be immobilized and that the athlete be transferred for further evaluation. If there is no neck pain or tenderness or limitation of motion of the cervical spine, then the shoulder is the site of the primary injury.

Acromioclavicular (AC) Separation. This injury most commonly occurs when an athlete falls or collides with another player or object and the point of contact is the distal clavicle. Patients have discrete tenderness at the AC joint and may have an apparent step-off between the distal clavicle and the acromion. If a humeral fracture is present, point tenderness is noted over the fracture. If a patient has crepitance, the arm should be immobilized in a sling and the patient transferred to the emergency department. AC separations in skeletally immature patients should be immobilized in a sling, and patients should be sent for radiographs because a Salter fracture of the distal clavicle may have occurred rather than an AC separation. Older (skeletally mature) athletes may not require radiography to evaluate a mild separation if the tenderness is discrete and over the AC joint. Salter fractures require consultation with an orthopedic surgeon. Assuming the radiographic results are negative, icing and pain-free range of motion exercises should be started. As the pain-free range improves, strengthening of the rotator cuff, deltoid, and trapezius muscles can start. When the AC joint is nontender and patients have sufficient strength to be functionally protected from a collision or fall and perform the maneuvers required for the sport, they can return to their sport. Surgery is not indicated for the majority of AC separations. Approximately 5% of AC separations are complicated by distal clavicular osteolysis, manifested as persistent pain for months and evidence of osteolysis radiographically. Distal claviculectomy is associated with alleviation of this persistent pain and full functional recovery.

Anterior Dislocation. The common mechanisms of injury are falling onto an outstretched hand with a straight arm or making contact with another player with the shoulder abducted to 90 degrees and forcefully rotated externally. An example of the latter is football players' tackling another player only with their arm. Patients complain of severe pain and that their shoulder "popped out of place" or "shifted." Patients with an unreduced anterior dislocation have a hollow region inferior to the acromion and a bulge in the anterior portion of the shoulder caused by anterior displacement of the humeral head. This differentiates it from a brachial plexus injury, but anterior dislocation can be complicated by injury to the brachial plexus manifest as a "stinger or burner" (see Head and Neck Injuries, later). Abnormal sensation of the lateral deltoid region (axillary nerve) and the extensor surface of the proximal forearm (musculocutaneous nerve) and the ability to contract the middle deltoid (resisted abduction) and biceps isometrically should be noted. An attempt to reduce the anterior dislocation is indicated, assuming no crepitance is present. Once the dislocation is reduced and radiographs (anteroposterior and West Point views) show a normal position, rehabilitation begins with isometric internal rotator strengthening. This can progress to elastic band exercises. The rotator cuff muscles are dynamic stabilizers of the shoulder anteriorly, and prevention of future anterior dislocations requires that their strength be restored. For 3 wk, no abduction beyond 10 degrees or external rotation beyond 90 degrees is allowed to permit anterior capsule healing. After 3 wk, as the internal rotator muscles strengthen, progressive strengthening of the rotator cuff muscles begins at greater degrees of abduction and external rotation. Patients can return to play when their strength, flexibility, and proprioception are equal to that of the uninvolved side so that they can protect the shoulder and perform the sports-specific activities pain free. Surgery is not recommended unless the shoulder has been dislocated at least three times and the patient has normal elasticity.

Patients with chronic shoulder pain may have symptoms due to repetitive stress, with some degree of *glenohumeral instability* causing inflammation in rotator cuff muscles and surrounding structures. Patients may have limitation of pain-free range of motion, a positive impingement sign, and reproduction of pain with resisted rotator cuff muscle testing. Rehabilitation consists of relative rest (including no throwing or whatever the causative activity is), icing, pain-free range of motion exercises, strengthening the rotator cuff muscles, and use of NSAIDs. Strengthening the rotator cuff muscles is critical because they are the dynamic stabilizers of the glenohumeral joint as the shoulder goes through a wide range of motion. As patients become pain free and range of motion and strength approach that of the uninvolved shoulder, they can begin functional rehabilitation, such as gently throwing a ball or swinging a racquet. If a patient continues to have pain despite these measures, another diagnosis should be considered, including a stress fracture of the proximal humerus (see later). More often, however, the athlete is not compliant with the treatment program and is exceeding the relative rest guideline. Weeks to months may often be required for an athlete to become pain free, with the length of recovery related to the duration of symptoms before starting on an appropriate rehabilitation program.

Proximal humeral stress fracture (epiphysiolysis) is a rare cause of proximal shoulder pain and is suspected when shoulder pain does not respond to routine measures. Gradual onset of deep shoulder pain occurs in a young (open epiphyseal plates) athlete involved in repetitive overhead motion, such as in baseball, tennis, or swimming, but with no history of trauma. Tenderness is noted over the proximal humerus; the diagnosis is confirmed by detecting a widened epiphyseal plate on plain radiographs or increased uptake on nuclear scan.

676.3 Elbow Injuries

Acute Injuries. The most common elbow dislocation is a posterior dislocation. The mechanism of injury is falling backward onto the outstretched arm with the elbow extended. Dislocation potentially compromises the brachial artery; rich collateral circulation makes distal arterial insufficiency unlikely. Intact radial and ulnar pulses are the best indicators of vascular integrity of the distal upper extremity. An obvious deformity is noted, with the olecranon process displaced prominently behind the distal humerus. Reduction is performed by gently applying longitudinal traction to the forearm with gentle upward pressure on the distal humerus. If reduction is not possible, the arm should be padded and placed in a sling and the patient transferred to the emergency department. Elbow injuries can compromise the radial, median, and ulnar nerves.

Supracondylar humeral fractures can result from the same mechanism of injury as elbow dislocations and can be complicated by coexisting injury to the brachial artery and, to a lesser extent, the median, radial, and ulnar nerves. A compartment syndrome may develop.

Chronic Injuries. Overuse injuries occur primarily in throwing sports and sports that require repetitive wrist flexion or extension or demand weight bearing on hands (gymnastics). "Little League elbow" is a broad term for several different elbow problems.

Overuse, poor technique, unrehabilitated injuries, and poor overall conditioning can lead to injury at the elbow and shoulder. In throwing overhand, medial stretching and lateral compressive forces are placed on the elbow. Repetitive stress is also placed on the flexor and extensor muscle groups' insertions located on the medial and lateral epicondyles, respectively.

Medial elbow pain is a common complaint of young throwers. The stage of bone maturation assists in formulation of the diagnosis. In preadolescents, who still have maturing secondary ossification centers, *traction apophysitis of the medial epicondyle* is likely. Patients have tenderness along the medial epicondyle; this is exacerbated by valgus stress or resisted wrist flexion. Treatment includes no throwing for 4–6 wk, pain-free strengthening, and stretching of the flexor/pronator group, followed by 1–2 wk of a progressive functional throwing program with accelerated rehabilitation. In adolescents, who have secondary ossification centers and whose epiphyseal plates have not fused, *avulsion fracture of the medial epicondyle* must be considered. In young adults, with fused epiphyses, the vulnerable structure is the *ulnar collateral ligament* (UCL). UCL tears are managed conservatively but may require surgery if the joint is unstable. Finally, *medial epicondylitis* is caused by overuse of the flexor-pronator muscle groups at their origin, the medial epicondyle, and occurs in sports requiring repetitive wrist flexion. Tenderness is felt over the medial epicondyle exacerbated by passive wrist extension or resisted wrist flexion. Treatment includes relative rest, analgesics, warm and cold modalities, stretching and strengthening wrist flexors, and counterforce bracing.

Lateral elbow compression during the throwing motion can cause problems at the radiocapitellar joint. *Panner disease* is osteochondrosis of the capitellum that presents between age 7–12 yr. *OCD* of the capitellum presents at age 13–16 yr. Although patients with both conditions present with insidious onset of lateral elbow pain exacerbated by throwing, patients with OCD have mechanical symptoms (popping and locking) and, more frequently, decreased range of motion. Patients with Panner disease have no mechanical symptoms and often have normal range of motion. The prognosis of Panner disease is excellent, and treatment consists of relative rest (no throwing), brief immobilization, and repeat radiographs in 6–12 wk to assess bone remodeling.

Lateral epicondylitis, or "tennis elbow," is caused by repetitive contraction of the extensor muscles at their origin on the lateral epicondyle. Tenderness is elicited over the lateral epicondyle, and pain is felt with passive wrist flexion and resisted wrist extension. Treatment includes relative rest. This injury may require a wrist splint worn during daily activity and at night. Treatment also includes analgesic medication, warm and cold modalities, stretching and strengthening wrist extensors, and counterforce bracing. Steroid injections help acutely, but, in the long-term, physiotherapy has the best results for healing. Functional rehabilitation, such as returning to playing tennis, should be gradual and progressive.

Other less common problems that cause elbow pain are ulnar neuropathy, triceps tendinitis and olecranon apophysitis, and loose bodies.

676.4 Back Injuries

Spondylolysis, a common cause of pain in athletes, is a stress fracture of the pars interarticularis (see Chapter 669.6). It can occur at any vertebral level but is most likely in the lower lumbar area. Besides direct trauma that causes an acute fracture, the mechanism of injury is either a congenital defect, which is exacerbated by lumbar extension loading, or a stress fracture due to repetitive extension loading. Ballet, weightlifting, gymnastics, and football are examples of sports in which repetitive extension loading of the lumbar spine occurs; however, it occurs in any activity where there is repetitive extension loading, including swimming. Patients often present with pain without a single precipitating event. However, there may be a precipitating injury. The diagnosis is often delayed. The pain is reproduced with lumbar extension while standing. The diagnosis is confirmed by finding a pars defect on an oblique lumbar spine radiograph. The defect is not easily seen on anteroposterior and lateral views. The diagnosis is established by single-photon emission CT or a traditional two-dimensional nuclear scan, the former being more sensitive. A plain CT scan can help in the identification of degree of bony involvement. *Spondylolisthesis* results from anterior displacement of the vertebral body. This is a known complication of untreated spondylolysis and is diagnosed by a lateral lumbar radiograph.

Facet syndrome has a similar history and physical examination findings as spondylolysis. It is caused by instability in the facet joint, posterior to the pars interarticularis and at the interface of the inferior and superior articulating processes. Facet syndrome can be established by identifying facet abnormalities on CT or by exclusion, requiring a nondiagnostic radiograph and nuclear scan to rule out spondylolysis.

Spondylolysis, spondylolisthesis, and facet syndrome are injuries posterior to vertebral bodies. Treatment of posterior element injuries is conservative, directed at reducing the extension loading activity, often for 6–12 mo. Extension loading activities include jogging, overhead weightlifting, landing from the vault in gymnastics, and ballet. Walking and cycling are appropriate exercises during rehabilitation. Bracing to reduce lordosis is advocated by some. Surgery is rarely required for spondylolisthesis. Increased emphasis is being placed on core strengthening exercises, first, then moving to exercises that attempt to increase the strength of the abdominal musculature and the flexibility of the lumbar extensor, hamstring, and quadriceps muscles.

Sciatica may be due to lumbar disk herniation or piriformis syndrome. It is unusual in early and middle pubertal athletes, yet not in older adolescent athletes. **Lumbar disk herniation** presents as back pain radiating to the buttocks or down the leg (often below the knee) (see Chapter 669.8). Physical examination findings include positive results of a straight-leg raising test, sciatica that worsens when the patient bends forward (i.e., lumbar flexion), and possibly reduced strength, sensation, or deep tendon reflexes in the leg. MRI has a 30% false-positive rate in diagnosing disk protrusion in adults; MRI confirms the clinical diagnosis. Assuming the herniation is not large, the pain is not intractable, and the neurologic deficit improves with therapy, the treatment of choice is analgesia, anti-inflammatory medication, and physical therapy. Bed rest or surgery is rarely necessary. Acute lumbar strain or contusion presents after a precipitating event, and the pain ranges from mild to disabling. Treatment includes analgesia, ultrasound with massage, and physical therapy, as tolerated. The natural history of acute back strain in adults is that 50% are better in 1 wk, 80% in 1 mo, and 90% in 2 mo, regardless of therapy. Treatment is as for disk herniation.

The **piriformis syndrome** is manifested as sciatica because the sciatic nerve passes through the piriformis muscle in 25% of individuals, and in the remainder it courses along the piriformis muscle. If the piriformis muscle is injured, the sciatic nerve can be secondarily involved and sciatica ensues. Patients may have some reproduction of sciatica with the straight-leg raising maneuver, but the pain is provoked with maneuvers that stretch or resist the piriformis muscle. The piriformis muscle is an external rotator of the hip. The "figure-of-four" test is done by externally rotating the ipsilateral hip by placing the foot on the contralateral quadriceps with the patient supine and then by bending the contralateral knee, causing stretch of the piriformis muscle. Pain would support the diagnosis of piriformis strain.

Sacroiliitis presents as lumbar pain that is usually chronic and without a history of trauma. Patients have a positive result of a **Patrick test,** which includes external rotation of the ipsilateral hip by placing the foot on the contralateral quadriceps with the patient in the supine position, placing one hand on the contralateral anterior-superior iliac spine, and then passively flexing the ipsilateral hip. A radiograph of the sacroiliac joints is indicated, and if results are positive, exploration for a rheumatologic disease (ankylosing spondylitis, juvenile rheumatoid arthritis, ulcerative colitis) is warranted. Treatment is with relative rest, nonsteroidal anti-inflammatory drugs, and physical therapy. Ankylosing spondylitis is more likely if the onset of lower back pain is before age 40 years, if there is morning stiffness that is associated with improvement with activity, and if the pain has a gradual onset and has lasted more than 3 months. Chronic back pain associated with stress can manifest as marked and widespread tenderness with superficial palpation, provoked by maneuvers such as pressure on the top of the head or allowing rotation of the spine and pelvis together; inconsistent performance on various tests; and loss of strength and sensation that do not fit a dermatomal pattern.

Less likely causes of sciatica are polyneuropathies and mass lesions that impinge on the sciatic nerve. Nerve conduction studies should be considered in these cases to establish the site of the nerve impingement and the site for further radiologic testing and other diagnostic tests. Other causes of lower back pain include infection (osteomyelitis, diskitis) and neoplasia (see Chapter 669.9). These should be considered in patients with fever, other constitutional signs, or lack of response to initial therapy. Osteomyelitis of the lower back is often, but not always, associated with fever. Suppurative organisms, for instance, are more likely to cause fever. Infection with *Mycobacterium tuberculosis* may present as lower back pain without fever. An epidural abscess is most likely to be associated with fever.

676.5 Hip and Pelvis Injuries

Hip and pelvis injuries represent a small percentage of sports injuries, but they are potentially severe and require prompt diagnosis. Hip pathology can present as knee pain and normal findings on knee examination.

Slipped capital femoral epiphysis (SCFE) usually presents in the 11–15 yr age range during the time of rapid linear bone growth (see Chapter 668.4). There is a higher incidence in males (4:1), in African-Americans, and obesity. Twenty-five per cent are bilateral but may not present synchronously. Pain and limitation of range of motion (especially internal hip rotation) are hallmarks. Radiographic examination shows the epiphysis displaced off the femur, which is described radiographically as "ice cream falling off the cone." If the condition is detected early, the epiphysis may show only slight widening. A bone scan or MRI may be required to diagnose an early or "preslip" SCFE. Non–weight bearing and urgent orthopedic referral are necessary.

Avulsion fractures occur in adolescents playing sports requiring sudden, explosive bursts of speed. Large muscles contract and create force greater than the strength of the attachment of the muscle to the apophysis. The most common sites of avulsion fractures (and the muscles that attach there) are the iliac crest (abdominal muscles), anterior superior iliac spine (sartorius), anterior inferior iliac spine (rectus femoris), lesser femoral trochanter (iliopsoas), and ischial tuberosity (hamstrings). Bilateral radiographs are required. When these fractures are nondisplaced or minimally displaced, healing occurs with conservative management in 4–12 wk. Surgery is reserved for displaced, large fracture fragments or failure of conservative management. Re-injury can occur with premature return to competition. Contact to the bone around the hip and pelvis causes exquisitely tender subperiosteal hematomas called *hip pointers*. Symptomatic care includes rest, ice, analgesia, and protection from re-injury.

A *stress fracture* may present as vague hip pain. If radiographs do not demonstrate a periosteal reaction consistent with a stress fracture, a bone scan or MRI may be required. Orthopedic consultation is necessary in femoral neck stress fractures because of their predisposition to nonunion. *Osteitis pubis* is an inflammation at the pubic symphysis that may be caused by excessive side-to-side rocking of the pelvis (hockey, roller-blading). Radiographic evidence (irregularity, sclerosis, widening of the pubic symphysis with osteolysis) may not be present until symptoms are present for 6–8 wk; bone scan and MRI are more sensitive to early changes. Relative rest for 6–12 wk may be required. *Legg-Calvé-Perthes disease* (avascular necrosis of the femoral head) also presents in childhood with insidious onset of limp and hip pain (see Chapter 668.3). Treatment allows remodeling of the femoral head by containing it within the acetabulum. Containment may necessitate the use of a brace or surgery.

676.6 Knee Injuries

The knee is the most common musculoskeletal site at which adolescents have complaints. Acute knee injuries that cause immediate disability are likely to be due to fracture, patellar dislocation, "internal derangement," or OCD. *Internal derangement* is a nonspecific term and includes injury to the cruciate and collateral ligaments, menisci (cartilage), fracture, or chondral lesions (see Chapter 667). The mechanism of injury is usually a weight-bearing event. After injury, if a player cannot bear weight within a few minutes, a fracture or internal derangement is more likely. If a player is able to bear weight and return to play after the injury, a serious injury is unlikely to have occurred.

Anterior cruciate ligament sprains occur from being hit directly, landing off balance from a jump, or quickly changing direction while running. *Posterior cruciate ligament sprains* occur from a direct blow to the region of the proximal tibia, such as might occur with a kick in martial arts or a dashboard injury. *Medial collateral ligament sprains* result from a valgus blow (directed inward) to the outside of the knee. *Lateral collateral ligament sprains* are unusual as isolated injuries. *Meniscal tears* occur by the same mechanisms as the anterior cruciate ligament sprains.

Patellar dislocations occur most often as a noncontact injury when the quadriceps muscles forcefully contract to extend the knee while the lower leg is externally rotated. The patella is almost always dislocated laterally, and this motion tears the medial patellar stabilizers, causing a rapidly enlarging medial hematoma. If a patient continually subluxates the patella or has hypermobile joints, little bleeding may ensue after a dislocation. Patellar dislocation is a great imitator of knee pathology and can present in a fashion similar to the causes of internal derangement mentioned earlier.

Physical Examination. The physician should inspect for hemarthrosis and obvious deformities; if these are present, the physician should assess neurovascular status and transfer the patient for emergency care. If no gross deformities are present and neurovascular integrity is intact, initial maneuvers include full passive extension and gentle valgus stress to the knee while the knee is in extension. The patient's ability to contract the vastus medialis obliques should be noted. Point tenderness is consistent with fracture or injury to the underlying structure; a medial meniscal tear may be manifest as tenderness along the medial joint line, however medial joint line tenderness is not specific for a medial meniscus tear. Presence of swelling in the first 24 hr is diagnostic of internal derangement. Limitation in either passive flexion or extension while rotating the tibia (the McMurray or modified McMurray tests) implies a meniscal injury, as do other maneuvers (Fig. 676–1). Ligament injury is manifested as pain or laxity with

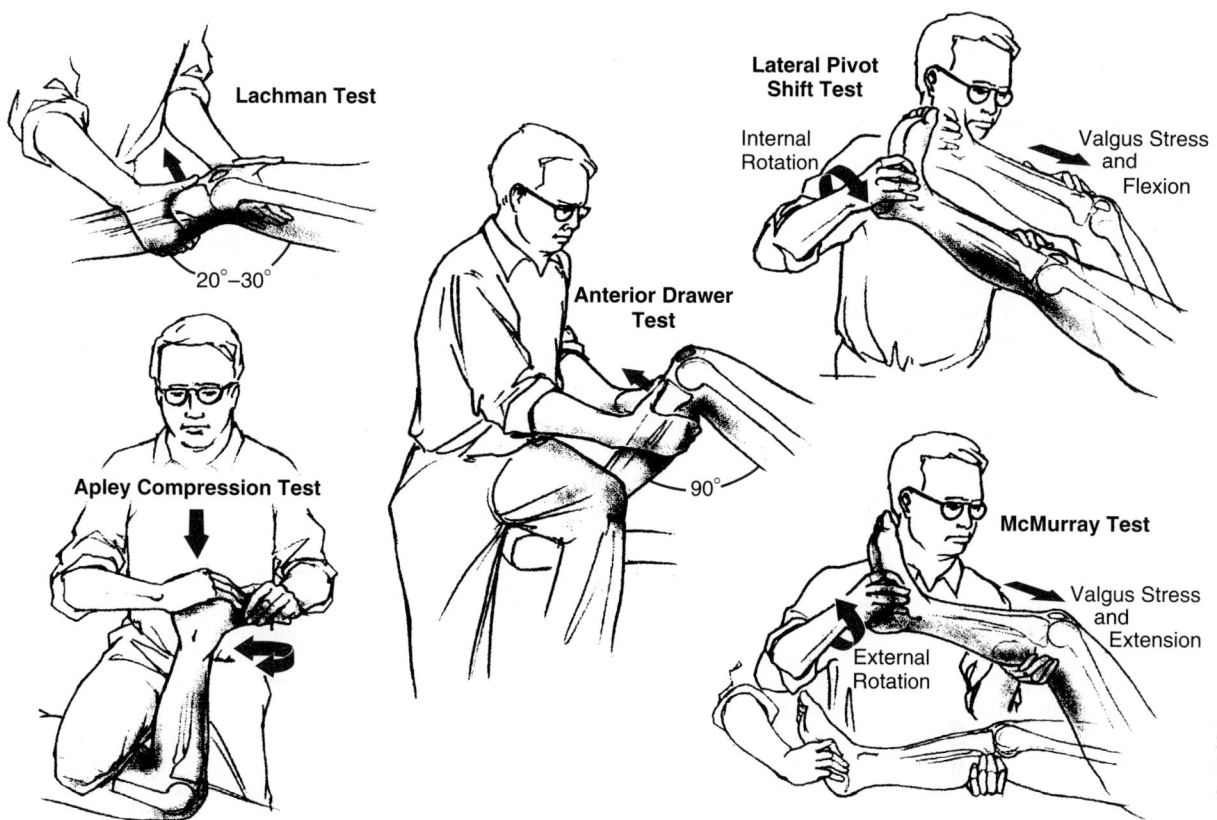

FIGURE 676–1. Examination maneuvers. Right knee shown. Examination maneuvers include the Lachman, anterior drawer, lateral pivot shift, Apley compression, and McMurray tests. The Lachman test, performed to detect anterior cruciate ligament (ACL) injuries, is conducted with the patient supine and the knee flexed 20–30 degrees. The anterior drawer test detects ACL injuries and is performed with the patient supine and the knee in 90 degrees of flexion. The lateral pivot shift test is performed with the patient supine, the hip flexed 45 degrees, and the knee in full extension. Internal rotation is applied to the tibia while the knee is flexed to 40 degrees under a valgus stress (pushing the outside of the knee medially). The Apley compression test, used to assess meniscal integrity, is performed with the patient prone and the examiner's knee over the patient's posterior thigh. The tibia is externally rotated while a downward compressive force is applied over the tibia. The McMurray test, used to assess meniscal integrity, is performed with the patient supine and the examiner standing on the side of the affected knee. (From Solomon DH, Simel DL, Bates DW, et al: Does this patient have a torn meniscus or ligament of the knee? *JAMA* 2001;286:1610.)

the appropriate maneuver. Gross laxity with passive maneuvers implies fracture. Patients with patellar dislocation have pain and apprehension when the examiner gently tries to push the patella laterally (the "apprehension sign"). If the patella is dislocated, reduction is indicated.

Initial Treatment of Acute Knee Injuries. If a patient cannot bear weight pain free or has clinical signs of instability, the knee should be immobilized, crutches given, and plain radiographs obtained. Straight-leg immobilizers offer no structural support. If any brace is used, a hinged brace is indicated. A brace with a lateral buttress is indicated for patients with acute patellar dislocation. Performing isometric quadriceps contractions pain free is necessary to maintain quadriceps strength and requires physical therapy. An elastic wrap or tubular stockinette can be applied for compression and the knee elevated throughout the day. Rehabilitation is indicated through a physical therapist or athletic trainer.

Treatment of Chronic Injuries. *Patellofemoral pain syndrome* (PFPS) is the most common cause of chronic anterior knee pain. It is worse going up stairs, after sitting for prolonged periods, or after squatting or running. The knee is usually stable, although the patient may complain of "giving way." In contrast to giving way from mechanical instability, such as with an ACL or meniscal tear in which the patient may fall to the ground, have

immediate pain, and develop effusion, the "giving way" of PFPS is usually due to quadriceps insufficiency or a transient pain causing the extensor mechanism to momentarily fail, yet the just-mentioned symptoms (e.g., falling to the ground) do not occur. The mechanism of PFPS includes a relatively weak vastus medialis muscle with hamstring and quadriceps muscle inflexibility and reduced endurance. The most common mechanism of injury is overuse. The diagnosis is confirmed with peripatellar tenderness.

Osgood-Schlatter disease is a traction apophysitis that is a variant of PFPS, with the injury occurring at the insertion of the patellar tendon on the tibial tuberosity. Osgood-Schlatter disease is treated like patellofemoral syndrome, with the addition of a protective Osgood-Schlatter pad, which protects the tibial tubercle from direct trauma. Patients should miss little if any time from sports. *Iliotibial band tendinitis* is the most common cause of chronic lateral knee pain. Generally it is not associated with swelling and instability. Tenderness should be elicited along the iliotibial band as it courses over the lateral femoral condyle or at its insertion at the Gerdy tubercle, along the lateral tibial plateau; tightness of the iliotibial band is also noted using the Ober test. Treatment principles follow those for patellofemoral syndrome, except the emphasis is on improving strength, flexibility, and endurance of the iliotibial band. As with any overuse injury, it is important to consider the kinetic chain and training errors in treating these conditions. If these are not corrected, it is likely that the condition will recur.

676.7 Shin Splints and Stress Fractures of the Lower Leg

Shin splints, presenting with pain along the medial tibia, is an overuse injury of the lower leg. The pain initially appears toward the end of exercise, and if exercise continues without rehabilitation, the pain worsens, occurs earlier in the exercise period, and lasts longer after exercise. Tenderness is elicited over a 5–15-cm area of the posterior tibialis muscle body (just medial to the tibia) but not over the bone. This is to be distinguished from a *tibial stress fracture,* in which the tenderness is more discrete (2–5 cm) over the tibia. The tenderness is worse with a stress fracture.

The diagnosis can be made by history and physical examination. Findings on plain radiographs of the tibia are normal with shin splints and in tibial stress fractures within the first few weeks of the injury. Afterward, the radiograph may demonstrate periosteal reaction if a stress fracture is present. A bone scan is the most sensitive test to diagnose stress fractures; it demonstrates discrete tracer uptake at the site(s) of the stress fracture. Increased uptake may be noted in the presence of shin splints but in a fusiform pattern along the periosteal surface. If results of the bone scan are normal, the diagnosis is likely to be shin splints.

The treatment of shin splints and tibial stress fractures is similar, involving relative rest, correcting training errors and kinetic chain dysfunction, and, possibly the use of appropriate running shoes (see Running, later). Fitness can be maintained with swimming, cycling, and water jogging, while following the relative rest guideline. After 7–10 days, patients can start on the walk-run program. If pain worsens, 2–3 pain-free days are required before resuming the walk-jog program. Ice should be used daily. Orthotics may be useful in patients who pronate. Stretching and strengthening the ankle dorsiflexors, plantarflexors, and everters can be useful. Analgesic medication can be used for shin splints but not routinely for stress fractures. Being pain free for 7–10 days is recommended before exercise walking is commenced; analgesics may mask the pain.

Stress fractures can occur in any bone in the lower extremity and are most common in the tibia and metatarsals. Stress fractures of the tarsal navicular, talus, proximal anterior third of the tibia, and femoral neck require consultation with an orthopedic surgeon.

676.8 Ankle Injuries

Ankle injuries are the most common acute athletic injury. Eighty-five per cent of ankle injuries are sprains, and 85% of those are inversion (foot planted with the lateral fibula moving toward the ground) injuries, 5% are eversion (foot planted with the medial malleolus moving toward the ground) injuries, and 10% are combined.

Examination and Injury Grading Scale. In obvious cases of fracture or dislocation, evaluating neurovascular status with as little movement as possible is the priority (Table 676–2). If no deformity is obvious, the next step is inspection for edema, ecchymosis, and anatomic variants. Key sites to palpate are the entire length of the fibula; the medial and lateral malleoli; the base of the fifth metatarsal; the anterior, medial, and lateral joint lines; and the navicular and the Achilles tendon complex. Assessment of active range of motion (patient alone) in dorsiflexion, plantarflexion, inversion, and eversion and of resisted range of motion is indicated. Passive movement in a pain-free range is seldom useful in the acute injury. The peroneal muscles are the

TABLE 676–2. Scheme for Grading Ankle Injuries

Severity	Signs and Symptoms	Disability
Grade I (mild)	Minimal swelling (clear definition of Achilles tendon), small area of tenderness, little or no hemorrhage, minimal decreased range of motion	Little or no limp with walking, minimal difficulty hopping (7–10 days' rest with optimal rehabilitation)
Grade II (moderate)	Moderate swelling (margin of Achilles tendon less defined), more generalized tenderness, some hemorrhage, decreased range of motion	Obvious limping with walking, unable to run, unable to hop, unable to do toe raise (2–4 wk rest with optimal rehabilitation)
Grade III (severe)	Diffuse swelling (no clear margins of Achilles tendon), widespread tenderness, hemorrhage evident, pronounced decreased range of motion	Unable to bear weight, involuntary guarding with examination (5–10 wk rest with optimal rehabilitation)

most often injured and best assessed in the plantarflexed foot with resisted eversion.

Provocative testing attempts to evaluate the integrity of the ligaments. In a patient with a markedly swollen, painful ankle, provocative testing is not helpful because of muscle spasm and involuntary guarding. The anterior drawer test assesses for anterior translation of the talus and competence of the anterior talofibular ligament (ATFL). The inversion stress test examines the competence of the ATFL and calcaneofibular ligament (Fig. 676–2). In the acute setting, the integrity of the tibiofibular ligaments and syndesmosis is examined by the syndesmosis squeeze test. The peroneal subluxation test applies pressure from behind the peroneal tendon with resisting eversion while plantar flexed. If results of either of these tests are abnormal, orthopedic consultation should be sought.

RADIOGRAPHS. Anteroposterior, lateral, and mortise views of the ankle are obtained when patients have pain in the area of the malleoli, are unable to bear weight, or have bone tenderness over the posterior distal tibia or fibula (Ottawa rules). A foot series should be obtained when patients have pain in the area of the midfoot, are unable to bear weight, or have bone tenderness over the navicular or fifth metatarsal. It is important to differentiate an avulsion fracture of the proximal fifth metatarsal from the Jones fracture of the more distal portion of the proximal fifth metatarsal. The former is treated as an ankle sprain; the latter fracture has an increased risk of nonunion and requires orthopedic consultation. The *talar dome fractures* are manifested as an

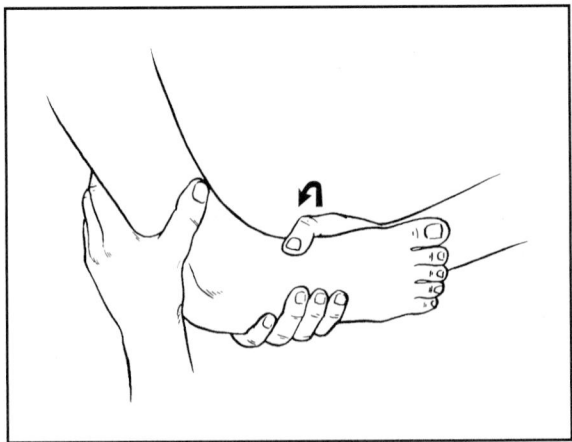

FIGURE 676–2. Inversion stress tilt test for ankle instability. (From Hergenroeder AC: Diagnosis and treatment of ankle sprains: A review. *Am J Dis Child* 1990;144:809.)

ankle sprain that does not improve. Radiographs on initial presentation may have subtle abnormalities. Inability to evert the ankle actively and pain over the peroneal retinaculum may indicate a *peroneal rupture or dislocation.* Children with signs restricted to the distal fibula are unlikely to have high risk fractures, which include all fractures except avulsion, buckle, and nondisplaced Salter-Harris I and II fractures of the distal fibula.

Rehabilitation. This should begin the day of injury; for those with pain with movement, isometric strengthening can be started. Important deficits to correct include loss of dorsiflexion, peroneal muscle weakness, and decreased proprioception. Until these deficits are restored, the ankle is vulnerable to re-injury. While standing on the uninjured side only, the athlete is instructed to hop five times as high as possible ("the five hop test"). When athletes are able to hop as high on the injured side without pain, they can return to sports.

Recurrent ankle injuries are more likely in patients who have not undergone complete rehabilitation. Ankle sprains are less likely in players wearing high-top shoes. Taping the ankle with adhesive tape provides no functional support. If functional support is needed, an ankle brace such as an air stirrup or canvas brace is indicated. Ankle sprains with residual functional instability after 9–12 mo of adequate rehabilitation may require surgery.

676.9 Foot Injuries

Sever disease (calcaneal apophysitis) occurs at the insertion of the Achilles tendon on the calcaneus. It is more common in boys (2:1); bilateral involvement occurs in 30%. Presentation is between age 8–13 yr. The chief complaint is activity-related heel pain. Tenderness is elicited at the insertion of the Achilles tendon into the calcaneus, and heel cords are tight. Treatment includes relative rest, ice, massage, stretching and strengthening of the Achilles' tendon, heel lifts (e.g., heel cups), and correcting abnormal foot morphology with orthotics or arch supports. With optimal management, symptoms improve in 4–8 wk. If there is no improvement, consideration should be given to less common causes of foot pain, including plantar fasciitis, tarsal coalitions, Achilles tendinitis, stress fractures, and OCD.

Chapter 677
Head and Neck Injuries

Head and neck injuries account for 90% of traumatic deaths and are the leading cause of permanent disability resulting from sports participation. The incidence of catastrophic neck injuries associated with incomplete neurologic recovery is less than 1/100,000. The incidence of sports-related catastrophic head and neck injuries has decreased secondary to improved equipment standards for helmets and enforcing rules to prohibit the use of the head as the point of initial contact when tackling.

Head Injury. Sixty-three per cent of mild traumatic head injuries in high school sports occur in football. The rate of mild traumatic brain injuries in the 10 most popular high school sports is (denominator = 100 player-seasons): football—3.7; wrestling—1.6; about 1.0 in girls and boys soccer and boys and girls basketball; 0.5 in softball and field hockey; 0.2 in baseball; and 0.1 in volleyball. The most common sequela of mild head injury is the *concussion,* a traumatically induced alteration of mental status not necessarily resulting in loss of consciousness. The constellation of complaints includes disturbance of vision and equilibrium, amnesia and other cognitive dysfunction, and headache (also see

Chapter 57.7). Multiple concussions can cause cognitive impairment, including impaired memory, attention, and planning activities and emotional lability and fatigue. Because of these potential problems, it is recommended that athletes with concussions avoid contact sports, the duration of this restriction depending on the number and severity of the concussions. Return to play guidelines after a concussion are given in Table 677–1.

An *epidural hematoma* is a rapidly accumulating hematoma between the dura and the cranium. Eighty-five per cent are associated with a skull fracture, and the most serious lacerate the middle meningeal artery. Most victims suffer loss of consciousness followed by a lucid, awake interval often associated with a severe headache. If untreated, this abruptly evolves to deterioration and death within 15–30 min. If treated appropriately, the outcome is generally excellent. A *subdural hematoma* occurs when an artery or bridging vein is torn between the dura and the brain parenchyma. It is the most frequent, identifiable

---

TABLE 677–1. Concussion Guidelines and Recommendations

Acute head injuries are usually divided into two categories:
1. Diffuse brain injuries—concussion and diffuse axonal injuries.
2. Focal brain injuries—all fractures and intracranial injuries.
It is not necessary to have loss of consciousness to have a concussion.* Several severity grading scales for concussion exist; one that is commonly used is the following:

Colorado Medical Society Guidelines

Grade	Confusion	Amnesia	Loss of Consciousness
I	+	–	–
II	+	+	–
III	+	+	+

Return-to-Play Criteria

Return-to-play criteria are based on prevention of the *second impact syndrome.* This syndrome is characterized by a loss of autoregulation of cerebral blood flow, manifest as a rapid increased intracranial pressure after a second head injury before full recovery from the initial head injury has occurred. Return to contact sports is based on the grade of the injury.

Recommendations for Return to Contact Sports Following a Concussion[†]

Grade	Minimum Time to Return	Time Asymptomatic[‡]
I	20 min	when examined
II	1 wk	1 wk
III	1 mo	1 wk

Recommendations for Return to Contact Sports After Repeated Concussions

Grade	Minimum Time to Return	Time Asymptomatic[‡]
I (2nd time)	2 wk	1 wk
II (2nd time)	1 mo	1 wk
I (× 3), II (× 2), III (× 2)	Season over	1 wk

In animal studies, there is evidence that there are microscopic changes in the brain after a concussion. These may not be evident in imaging studies, so the clinician must rely on history and neuropsychologic examination to follow a patient's progress. In college football players who experienced their first concussion, the neuropsychologic testing normalized in 5 days and symptoms of headache and memory resolved in 10 days.

The chronic effects of repetitive boxing injuries include cortical atrophy and a cavum septum pellucidum (identified radiographically). Whether this occurs in other sports in which head injuries are common (football, ice hockey, wrestling) or in which the head is used as part of the game (soccer) is debatable. However, there appears to be no danger in the young soccer player occasionally heading the ball.

[†]*Contact sports means any situation in which contact is possible, including practice.*

[‡]*A symptomatic athlete should not return to contact sports regardless of the initial diagnosis. Athletes with focal brain injuries are excluded from contact sports indefinitely. Patients with a neck injury can return to contact sports when they have full, pain-free range of motion, strength and sensation, and normal lordosis of the cervical spine.*

focal brain injury in sports and the most common cause of death in sports-related head injuries because it is also associated with cerebral contusion and edema. Patients may lose consciousness at the time of injury but recover in the acute setting. A *cerebral contusion,* bruising of the brain parenchyma, can present as focal symptoms at the site of injury (coup) or on the area opposite to the injury (contracoup). Cerebral contusions are often associated with skull fractures (see Chapter 57.7). Intracerebral hematoma is generally associated with severe head trauma and characterized by loss of consciousness and severe headache, if they regain consciousness. A subarachnoid hemorrhage is generally associated with loss of consciousness, severe headache, and rapidly deteriorating mental status. The latter has been associated with congenital arteriovenous malformations.

Neck Injuries. *Fracture with or without dislocation* is considered when a player has any head or neck injury or loss of consciousness and, more specifically, when the athlete has midline cervical pain, painful range of motion, or peripheral neurologic signs or symptoms after neck trauma. Patients should be immobilized and should have a full radiographic evaluation with anteroposterior, lateral, oblique, and open-mouth views before removing the neck immobilizer. If the radiographs are normal, patients should have flexion and extension radiographs to evaluate for ligamentous instability. If the patient cannot actively flex or extend the cervical spine, then CT is indicated. If patients have bilateral symptoms but normal findings on radiographs, a lesion impinging on the spinal cord, cord hematoma or edema, or stenotic cervical canal is possible and a non–contrast-enhanced MRI of the cervical spine is indicated. In adults following blunt trauma, a lower probability of cervical spine injury is associated with no midline cervical tenderness, no focal neurologic deficits, normal level of consciousness, no drugs or intoxicants, and no distracting painful injury elsewhere.

Transient quadriplegia (<36 hr) is manifested as sensory changes that may be associated with motor paresis involving both arms, both legs, or all four extremities. Functional spinal narrowing caused by congenital spinal stenosis, fused vertebrae, or a structural lesion that narrows the canal, such as disk herniation, is possible. These diagnoses are made by MRI. Players who have had a neck injury and functional spinal stenosis are at increased risk of permanent disability if they play contact sports. They must be excluded from contact sports.

Patients with a neck injury and an otherwise normal radiographic examination can return to contact sports when they have full, pain-free range of motion, strength and sensation, and normal lordosis of their cervical spine.

Brachial Plexus Injuries. The brachial plexus includes nerves originating from C5-T1 and emerging from the spinal column in the deep triangle of the neck. The upper trunk (C5-C6) can be contused or stretched during football when tackling with the shoulder or having the head forcefully flexed laterally. Manifestations include unilateral burning (known as a "burner" or "stinger"), paresthesia, and weakness in the arm, usually in a C5-C6 distribution manifested as the inability to forward flex or abduct the shoulder. These symptoms often resolve spontaneously within minutes. Bilateral symptoms, such as transient quadriplegia, are an indication to curtail participation until the patient is evaluated by MRI. If a player has recurrent "stingers," an MRI study of the cervical spine is indicated. Fifteen per cent of patients younger than age 21 yr with Down syndrome have atlantoaxial instability (AAI). Asymptomatic AAI has not been demonstrated to be a risk factor for symptomatic AAI, which is a rare condition in patients with Down syndrome. Special Olympics still require these radiographs in asymptomatic individuals with Down syndrome. All symptomatic patients, such as with evidence of upper motor neuron or posterior column dysfunction, need these radiographs.

Treatment. In the acute management of head and neck injuries, the principles of advanced life support are followed. Airway,

breathing, circulation, and other painful injuries/disability are the initial concerns (see Chapter 57.1). Other management principles include the following:

1. Assume a neck injury is present in an unconscious athlete and immobilize the cervical spine. Do not remove the helmet of an injured player with a suspected neck injury.

2. If access to a compromised airway is required, remove the face mask.

3. Do not use ammonia smelling salts. The noxious stimulant causes involuntary withdrawal, which may cause secondary injury to an unstable cervical spine.

4. Perform serial neurologic examinations. If the athlete is lucid, look for the signs indicative of a neck injury before the athlete is permitted to move. These include neck pain, painful range of motion, or bilateral neurologic signs.

Athletes with a suspected skull fracture, deteriorating mental status or worsening headache, focal neurologic deficits or seizure, loss of consciousness for more than 5 min, confusion lasting longer than 30 min, persistent emesis, more than one concussion in a practice/game, or inadequate postinjury supervision require transfer to an emergency department for evaluation and observation.

Chapter 678
Heat Injuries

After heart disease, the second most common cause of nontraumatic death is heat illness. One to two athletes per year in the United States die of this preventable form of sudden death. Heat illness is a continuum of clinical signs and symptoms that can be mild (heat stress) to fatal (heatstroke).

Seventy-five per cent of the energy produced by muscular contraction is manifest as heat, whereas 25% is converted into muscle work. Without proper heat dissipation mechanisms, intense exercise would elevate core body temperature by 1°C every 5 min and would approach heat stroke within 15–20 min of intense exercise. The body dissipates heat by radiation (60% heat transfer to the air), evaporation (20–25%), and convection (15%). With repeated exposure to heat for 8–12 days, the body acclimatizes. Children's ability to tolerate heat stress is not as effective as that of adults. Children have a lower sweat rate and slower acclimatization process, absorb greater ambient heat secondary to their higher surface area to body mass ratio, and produce more metabolic heat per mass unit.

Heat cramps, the most common heat injury, usually affect the calf and hamstring muscles. They respond to oral rehydration with electrolyte solution and with gentle stretching. *Heat syncope* is fainting after prolonged exercise attributed to poor vasomotor tone and depleted intravascular volume, and it responds to fluids, cooling, and supine positioning. *Heat edema* is mild edema of the hands and feet during initial exposure to heat; it resolves with acclimatization. *Heat tetany* is carpopedal tingling or spasms caused by heat-related hyperventilation. It responds to moving to a cooler environment and decreasing respiratory rate (or rebreathing by breathing into a bag).

Moderate heat injury is characterized by body temperature from 99–104°F. *Heat exhaustion* is manifested as headache, nausea, vomiting, dizziness, orthostasis, weakness, piloerection, and possibly syncope. The latter complaint should also suggest head trauma and cardiac conditions. Patients with moderate heat injury do not have serious central nervous system (CNS) dysfunction. *Treatment* includes moving to a cool environment, cooling the body with fans, removing excess clothing, and placing ice over the groin and axilla. If a patient is not able to tolerate oral rehydration, intravenous fluids are indicated. Patients should be monitored, including rectal temperature, for signs of heatstroke.

Severe heat injury is characterized by body temperature greater than 104°F and altered mental status. *Heatstroke* is a medical emergency; the mortality rate is 50%. Sports-related heatstroke is characterized by profuse sweating and is related to intense exertion, whereas "classic" heatstroke with dry, hot skin is of slower onset (days) in elderly or chronically ill persons exposed to summer heat waves. The physical response of a dehydrated athlete is to attempt to maintain the blood pressure by vasoconstriction, which makes it difficult to transfer heat peripherally. *Treatment* starts by addressing the airway, breathing, and circulation and proceeds to aggressive cooling using ice water baths, cooling fans, and removal of excess clothing. Intravenous fluid at a rate of 800 mL/m^2 in the first hour with dextrose/saline solution improves intravascular volume and the body's ability to dissipate heat. In a previously healthy individual, the risk of pulmonary and cerebral edema is minimal compared with the risk of uncorrected hypovolemia.

Heat-related illness can be prevented. The preparticipation sports examination should include screening questions to identify predisposing risk factors such as obesity, lack of physical conditioning, lack of acclimatization (usually requiring 8–10 exposures to the heat for 30–45 minutes), drugs/medications (amphetamines, LSD, alcohol, thyroid hormone, antihistamines, anticholinergics, haloperidol, phenothiazines, diuretics, laxatives, monoamine oxidase inhibitors, tricyclic antidepressants), excessive fluid/sweat loss (febrile illness, diarrhea, diabetes mellitus and insipidus, cystic fibrosis, dermatologic disorders with sweat gland dysfunction, some cyanotic congenital heart defects), inadequate intake (CNS disorder, mental retardation, or young age), or hypothalamic thermoregulatory dysfunction (malnutrition and eating disorders, prior heat injury).

Dehydration is common to all heat illness; therefore, measures to prevent dehydration may also prevent heat illness. Mild dehydration (2%) can decrease athletic performance and decrease normal thermoregulation. Thirst is not an adequate indicator of hydration status because it is initiated at 2–3% dehydration. Athletes are advised to be well hydrated before exercise and should drink every 20 min during exercise (5 oz for those weighing less than 40 kg, 9 oz for 60 kg, and 10–12 oz for those larger

than 60 kg). Free access to cold water, which is more efficiently absorbed than warm water, is effective and should be advocated to coaches. Scheduled breaks every 20–30 min with helmets off to get out of the heat can decrease the cumulative amount of heat exposure. Practices and competition should be scheduled in the early morning or late afternoon to avoid the hottest part of the day. Guidelines have been published about modification of activity related to the wet bulb temperature (Table 678–1). Proper clothing such as shorts and T-shirts without helmets can improve heat dissipation. Proper supervision by an individual who can recognize and treat early heat illness can prevent progression to more severe injury. Prepractice and postpractice weight can be helpful in determining the amount of fluid needed to be replaced (16 oz or ½ L/lb weight loss).

Water is adequate for exercise lasting less than 1 hr. Fluids with electrolyte and carbohydrate should be reserved for exercise lasting for more than 1 hr. However, if these drinks are not available, water intake should continue. Most commercially available sports drinks have 6–8% carbohydrate; experimenting with different drinks or diluting standard sports drinks can decrease the side effects of nausea, bloating, and abdominal pain. Salt pills should not be used because of their risk of causing hypernatremia and delayed gastric emptying.

Chapter 679

Female Athletes: Menstrual Problems and the Risk for Osteopenia

Special concerns are related to overtraining in young women and its effect on reproductive function and bone mineral status (see Chapter 107).

The majority of bone mass is acquired by the end of the 2nd decade. Sixty to 70% of adult bone mass is genetically determined, and the remaining is influenced by three controllable factors: exercise, calcium intake, and sex steroids, primarily estrogen. In general, exercise promotes bone mineralization in the majority of young women and is to be encouraged. In females with eating disorders and those who exercise to the point of excessive weight loss with amenorrhea or oligomenorrhea, exercise can be detrimental to bone mineral acquisition, resulting in reduced bone mineral content, or *osteopenia*.

Menstrual dysfunction, including amenorrhea or oligomenorrhea, can occur in women participating in any sport. The cause of the amenorrhea (amenorrhea will be used to refer to amenorrhea/oligomenorrhea here) must be established as for any other patient (see Chapter 107). In the absence of a pathologic cause, the diagnosis of hypothalamic amenorrhea is established by exclusion. It is characterized by reduced hypothalamic pulsatile release of gonadotropin-releasing hormone (GnRH) and, consequently, reduced serum gonadotropin concentrations. Athletes with amenorrhea have an increased risk of osteopenia and are at risk for stress fractures compared with their eumenorrheic athletic peers. This osteopenia is persistent, increasing their long-term risk for osteoporosis.

Young athletes with hypothalamic amenorrhea and without an eating disorder appear fit, typically have an estimated ideal body weight (eIBW) greater than 85%, and have training bradycardia (resting pulse in the range of 40–60 beats/min). There are three eating disorders that can present in the context of hypothalamic amenorrhea: (1) anorexia nervosa, manifest as weight less than 85% of eIBW with evidence of starvation

TABLE 678–1. Restraints on Activities at Different Levels of Heat Stress

WBGT		Restraints on Activities
°C	°F	
<24	<75	All activities allowed, but be alert for prodromes of heat-related illness in prolonged events
24.0–25.9	75.0–78.6	Longer rest periods in the shade; enforce drinking every 15 minutes
26–29	79–84	Stop activity of unacclimatized persons and other persons with high risk; limit activities of all others (disallow long-distance races, cut down further duration of other activities)
>29	>85	Cancel all athletic activities

WBGT is not air temperature. It indicates wet bulb globe temperature, an index of climatic heat stress that can be measured on the field by the use of a psychrometer. This apparatus, available commercially, is composed of three thermometers. One (wet bulb [WB]) has a wet wick around it to monitor humidity. Another is inside a hollow black ball (globe [G]) to monitor radiation. The third is a simple thermometer (temperature [T]) to measure air temperature. The heat stress index is calculated as WBGT = 0.7 WB temp + 0.2 G temp + 0.1 T temp.

It is noteworthy that 70% of the stress is due to humidity, 20% to radiation, and only 10% to air temperature.

From the American Academy of Pediatrics, Committee on Sports Medicine and Fitness: Climatic heat stress and the exercising child and adolescent. Pediatrics 2000; 106:159.

manifest as bradycardia, hypothermia, and orthostatic hypotension or orthostatic tachycardia; (2) bulimia nervosa, manifest as reduced or normal weight, with wider fluctuations of weight than would be expected based on their reported caloric intake and exercise; and (3) eating disorder not otherwise specified (EDNOS), with some of the features of either anorexia or bulimia nervosa, yet not meeting all criteria from the *Diagnostic and Statistical Manual for Mental Disorders*, 4th edition, for diagnosis of either (see Chapter 104).

The *treatment* of hypothalamic amenorrhea in the athlete involves lifestyle changes that result in reduced energy expenditure (i.e., exercise) and increased energy intake. The degree of recommended exercise reduction and increased caloric intake depends on the percent of eIBW. For example, if an athlete weighs 85–90% of eIBW and is exercising daily, then a reduction in exercise to 3 days a week and adding one or two dietary supplemental drinks (~250 kcal apiece) or snacks per day might be recommended. Generally, exercise is not recommend if the body weight is less than 85% of eIBW, although there are exceptions, especially if the athlete is eumenorrheic. Amenorrheic athletes who gain weight through reduced training and improved diet can resume menses spontaneously and increase their bone density. Gradually, their training is increased and their menstrual and nutritional status monitored. If the athlete is unable to gain weight with nutrition and medical counseling alone, then psychological consultation is sought. Estrogen replacement, usually in the form of low dose oral contraceptive pills, is recommended if the amenorrhea persists for 6 mo or more (see Chapter 108). Measuring bone mineral can help with the patient's decision if osteopenia is identified. If amenorrhea persists beyond 12 mo regardless of the bone density measurement, treatment with estrogen/progestin pills may be recommended (see Chapter 108). In making the decision to recommend estrogen/progestin pills in young women with hypothalamic amenorrhea one must consider (1) young women with anorexia nervosa and secondary amenorrhea have mean serum estradiol levels that approximate those of postmenopausal women and (2) osteopenia/osteoporosis is one of the more serious, long-term consequences of prolonged amenorrhea in adolescent athletes. The American Academy of Pediatrics Committee on Sports Medicine and Fitness recommends not providing estrogen replacement until age 16 yr. Premature use of estrogen could, theoretically, compromise adult height. There is a risk to delaying the start of estrogen/progestin therapy until epiphyseal growth is complete. The onset of anorexia nervosa before age 15 yr may affect bone size and density more than in those persons with onset after age 15 yr. Bone fragility is a function of bone size and density, which are both undergoing significant increases during puberty. A 15-yr-old with a bone age of 13 yr has achieved 96.4% of her adult height; one with a bone age of 14 yr has achieved 98.3% of her adult height; and one with a bone age of 15 yr has achieved 99% of her adult height. The mean height of females in North America is 163 cm at 15 yr of age. If estrogen therapy completely arrested height gain with the onset of therapy, then the female with a bone age of 15 yr at age 15 yr could potentially lose, on average, 1.6 cm of height if her potential adult height was 163 cm. More likely, height attainment would not be arrested and some height would still be achieved after estrogen therapy is initiated. Estrogen/progesterone replacement is recommended for females with amenorrhea at 15 yr of age and a bone age of 15 yr and considered for those with a bone age of 14 yr, depending on the degree of osteopenia and malnutrition.

Adequate calcium intake is important. The current recommended daily allowance for calcium is 1,200 mg Most adolescent females consume much less. An increase of calcium intake to 1,500 mg/day is suggested for women with amenorrhea. Increased calcium intake alone in adolescent females with anorexia nervosa may not improve bone density because of increased calcium excretion and decreased absorption.

Chapter 680
Ergogenic Aids

Also see Chapter 105.9.

Ergogenic aids are any substance used for performance enhancement beyond training alone. Most ergogenics are considered nutritional supplements and lack the regulatory supervision to ensure purity, drug interactions with prescription medications, long or short-term safety profile, a recommended therapeutic dose, or convincing research to substantiate claims.

Male and female high school students have reported lifetime prevalence use of anabolic steroids of 4.2% and 2.7%, respectively. Pediatricians should discourage this use. Anabolic steroids at supraphysiologic doses increase strength and lean muscle mass when combined with increased caloric intake and exercise. Some athletes "stack" multiple formulations at many times the therapeutic dose for presumed enhanced efficacy. Steroid "pro-hormones," such as dehydroepiandrosterone (DHEA) and androstenedione, are converted to estradiol more than testosterone and may have many of the same side effects as anabolic steroids. Short-term side effects of anabolic steroid use include liver toxicity (cholestatic jaundice, peliosis, hepatitis), endocrine abnormalities (gynecomastia, prostatic hypertrophy, hirsutism, impotence, decreased sperm count, testicular atrophy), hematologic changes (hypercoagulability, increased low-density lipoprotein and decreased high-density lipoprotein cholesterol), musculoskeletal problems (premature epiphyseal closure, muscle and tendon rupture), oncologic disorders (progression of prostate and breast cancer), dermatologic disorders (acne), and possibly psychiatric disorders. Anabolic steroid use should be suspected in an athlete with a rapid increase in lean mass and strength that is beyond that expected in normal development. Physical findings include gynecomastia, testicular shrinkage, jaundice, acne, and marked striae.

Creatine is a naturally occurring substance in the body that at the cellular level exists as phosphocreatine and theoretically increases muscle performance by faster rephosphorylation of adenosine diphosphate to adenosine triphosphate during brief high-intensity activities and as a lactic acid buffer during anaerobic activity. Because of the potential health risks (heat injury, gastrointestinal distress, renal disease) and lack of efficacy studies in adolescents, the American College of Sports Medicine recommends that creatine supplementation is not advised for those younger than 18 years of age.

γ-Hydroxybutyric acid (GHB) and its metabolites γ-butyrolactone (GBL) and 1,4-butanediol (BD) cause decreased mental status, altered sensorium, decreased respiratory drive, and coma. Although these drugs are taken primarily for recreational purposes, they have been used in some sports supplements. GHB, GBL, and BD have been linked to 122 serious illnesses and three deaths.

Chapter 681
Specific Sports and Associated Injuries

Gymnastics. Competitive gymnastics for females is a sport of adolescents. Participants are beginning the sport at 5–6 yr of age and achieving the highest level of competition in the mid teens, often retiring by age 20. A similar pattern occurs in males; however, their career, facilitated by pubertal development, including increasing strength, can extend into the 20s. Males tend to have more upper extremity injuries, and females have more lower extremity injuries. In addition to mechanical or traumatic injuries, female gymnasts tend to have delayed menarche and can have hypothalamic amenorrhea or oligomenorrhea, associated with low body weight. The typical body habitus of the elite gymnast manifest as reduced weight for height, coupled with amenorrhea or oligomenorrhea, would suggest that reduced bone density is a problem for female gymnasts. The bone density of gymnasts tends to be high. It is speculated that this is secondary to the impact forces on the lower extremities related to dismount from the vault. In spite of this increased bone density in female gymnasts, stress fractures are a significant problem. The short stature associated with male and female gymnasts is caused by selection bias and not the result of gymnastics training.

Common problems include acute, traumatic injuries, such as an ankle sprain, and chronic, overuse injuries, such as wrist and spine stress fractures. The incidence of injury increases with the level of skill and is greatest in the floor exercise. Wrist pain due to chronic upper extremity weight bearing can be caused by a distal radial stress Salter I fracture, which typically presents on the radial, dorsal aspect of the wrist, but can present on the ulnar aspect, and is worsened by passive extension and palpation. Other wrist injuries include triangular fibrocartilage complex (TFCC) tears, scaphoid fractures, dorsal ganglions, and carpal ligament injuries. Treatment in almost all cases involves immobilization for some period or time, application of ice, and administration of nonsteroidal anti-inflammatory drugs (NSAIDs). If pain persists, the correct diagnosis can be made by MRI or arthroscopic examination to rule out intra-articular tears, loose bodies, or ligamentous instability. The pediatrician should have a low threshold for referral to a hand specialist in a wrist injury that is not improving with rest. Ligamentous laxity may predispose to elbow or shoulder dislocation and ankle sprains. Spine problems include spondylolysis (pars interarticularis stress fracture) and spondylolisthesis (see Chapter 669.6) due to repetitive extension loading and need to be treated with relative rest, stretching, and possibly a thoracolumbosacral orthosis (TLSO). Re-introduction into gymnastics for all of these injuries can gradually occur, as long as the athlete stops whenever the pain recurs.

Swimming. Shoulder injury is the most common overuse injury of competitive swimmers. *Swimmer's shoulder* is a combination of subacromial bursitis and rotator cuff tendonitis usually of the supraspinatus and is manifested as shoulder pain and tenderness of the supraspinatus tendon. The onset may be insidious. Pain, due to subacromial bursitits, may be produced by the Hawkin impingement test, in which pain is provoked by passively forward flexing the humerus to 90 degrees and then internally rotating the humerus. Supraspinatus tendonitis produces pain with active abduction between 60 and 100 degrees and doing the "emptying the can" maneuver, in which the patient internally rotates the humerus at rest and then raises the arm in a plane halfway between forward flexion and abduction. Treatment includes ice, modification of stroke technique, rest, stretching, muscle strengthening of the rotator cuff and upper back muscles, physiotherapy, nonsteroidal anti-inflammatory agents (NSAIDs), and consideration of a subacromial bursa cortisone injection. Prevention includes avoiding overwork, proper technique, and strengthening and stretching exercises.

Baseball. Throwing injuries of the elbow and shoulder (especially among pitchers) are the most common baseball injuries. See Chapters 676.2 and 676.3. "Little League elbow" is due to repetitive valgus forces leading to stretching injury on the medial aspect of the elbow or compressive forces on the lateral aspect of the elbow. It has been suggested that these injuries can be prevented by preseason stretching and strengthening exercises; however, this has not been demonstrated in a prospective study. The most important consideration is limitation of the number of pitches and advising players, coaches, and athletes that they should stop immediately when they experience elbow pain and if it persists they need medical evaluation. It has been recommended that a young pitcher pitch no more than 200 pitches per week and play in no more than two games per week and that the maximum number of pitches per game be approximately six times the pitcher's age in years. Deaths in baseball are rare (4/year from 1973–1999) and are caused by chest wall trauma with the ball (commotio cordis) or head injury with the ball or bat. Protective equipment needs to be worn properly to try to prevent these injuries.

Ballet. This very demanding activity is associated with delayed menarche and eating disorders in female dancers (see Chapter 679). Acute injuries occur, most often of the lower extremities. As with any repetitive activity, overuse injuries are likely; the key is to make the correct diagnosis and also consider the kinetic chain dysfunction that may have contributed to that injury. A dancer may have an unrehabilitated ankle sprain, causing favoring of that leg, leading to a stress fracture of the contralateral tibia. Foot problems include metatarsal stress fractures, subungual hematomas, callus and bunion formation, sesamoiditis, and plantar fasciitis. There is no perfect ballet foot, although, theoretically, if the first and second rays are of equal length (manifest as the tips of the first two toes being equal) the dancer can go en pointe and distribute the weight more evenly. Going en pointe is a question that young ballet dancers and their parents may ask. An average age to go en pointe is 12 yr; however, a function test should be part of that decision: if the child can go en pointe, holding the position and not appearing unstable and weak and without pain, then he or she is probably ready to try dancing en pointe. Ankle problems include anterior and posterior impingement syndromes because of the extremes of range of motion in grand plié and en pointe, respectively. All other acute and overuse injuries of the lower extremity occur in dancers. Hip problems include both the medial snapping hip syndrome caused by the iliopsoas tendon's riding over the anterior hip capsule and tendinitis (piriformis, iliopsoas, rectus femoris). The piriformis syndrome occurs because of the repetitive external hip rotation required in ballet and can manifest as buttock and hip pain and sciatica. Spine problems include Scheuermann disease in males, idiopathic scoliosis in females, and spondylolysis.

Wrestling. Wrestlers have great fluctuations in weight to meet weight-matched competition standards. Such fluctuations are associated with fasting, dehydration, and then bingeing.

Wrestling holds may produce injury owing to various torques or forces applied to the extremities and spine; wrestling throws with subsequent falls may produce concussions, neck strain, or spinal cord injury. The two most common sites of injury are the shoulder and knee. "Stingers" and "burners" are due to a brachial plexopathy (see Football).

Shoulder subluxation is common. Patients are often aware of their shoulder's slipping in and out (see Chapter 676.2). Hand injuries are usually not severe and include recurrent metacarpophalangeal and proximal interphalangeal sprains. Treatment of hand injuries includes splinting and taping.

Knee injuries are common and potentially serious and include prepatellar bursitis, medial and lateral sprains, and medial and lateral meniscus tears (see Chapter 676.6). Prepatellar bursitis is caused by a traumatic impact to the mat or chronic trauma. Swelling occurs over the knee, and patients have no limitation of motion except full flexion. If the skin has been broken, a septic bursitis has to be considered. The physician must try to distinguish traumatic from infected bursitis, which may require aspiration of the bursa. Treatment of traumatic bursitis includes protective neoprene knee sleeves, NSAIDs, and bursectomy if there are several recurrences.

Dermatologic problems include herpes simplex (herpes gladiatorum), impetigo, staphylococcal furunculosis or folliculitis, superficial fungal infections, and contact dermatitis. The first two are contraindications to wrestling until the infection is non-infectious. If recurrent herpes infections occur, suppressive oral antiviral agents should be used.

Football. Football continues to be the sport with the highest number of injuries, the greatest number of participants (~1.5 million junior and senior high school participants and 75,000 college participants in 2001), and one of the sports with a high injury rate. In terms of the severity of injury, defined as days lost per injury, the average injury in football is less severe than many other sports. Most of the injuries are sprains, strains, and contusions that once treated appropriately result in minimal time away from football.

Although the majority of catastrophic sports injuries in the United States have occurred in football, these severe injuries are rare. (*Catastrophic* is defined as a fatal injury or a severe injury with or without permanent severe functional disability.) Between 1977 and 2001, 294 disabling injuries occurred in football, for an annual rate of 12/yr. Two hundred seventeen of these were to the cervical spine; the remainder were cerebral injuries. In 1999 there were 21 catastrophic injuries in high school and 3 in college football.

Head and neck football injuries include concussion, neck sprain, and brachial plexopathy. The latter is referred to as a "stinger" or "burner."

Lumbar spine injury manifested as low back pain may represent spondylolysis. Shoulder trauma can cause glenohumeral dislocation, the majority of which are anterior dislocations, acromioclavicular separations, and clavicular and humeral fractures.

Contusions to the arm and thigh muscles are common and may result in large hematomas if not treated aggressively. Assuming that there is no fracture, treatment includes ice and compression during most waking hours for the first few days to limit the expansion of the hematoma and then doing pain-free strengthening and stretching exercises until baseline function is achieved. Then return to contact can be approved. When the hematoma is allowed to persist and especially if there is a second hematoma into the first, myositis ossificans may develop. This requires surgical excision if the lesion causes functional limitations.

Knee injuries are the most common musculoskeletal complaint at the time of preseason examinations. Knee injuries are discussed in Chapter 676.6.

Ankle sprains occur, and the risk of re-injury may be reduced by rehabilitation and use of air stirrups for 6 mo. Turf toe, an injury to the first metatarsophalangeal joint, is caused by forceful dorsiflexion while playing on artificial turf in soft, light-weight, flexible shoes. Treatment of turf toe includes ice, NSAIDs, an orthotic to limit extension of the great toe, and rest. Corticosteroid injections are not beneficial. Turf toe can be a season- or career-limiting injury.

Hockey. Hockey is a collision sport associated with injuries caused by the puck or the stick hitting the player or by body contact with other players, the ice, or the boards, producing contusions, lacerations, fractures, sprains, or concussions. The risk for injury is reduced by proper equipment (helmets with face masks) and rules regarding dangerous body contact (checking from behind, high sticking, slashing, and fighting).

Specific hockey injuries include ankle sprains (dorsiflexion, eversion, and external rotation in contrast to the usual sprain of inversion in other sports), hip adductor strain, osteitis pubis, and various shoulder injuries from body contact. The latter include acromioclavicular sprain, dislocation, and clavicular fractures. The most serious injuries are to the head and neck.

Basketball and Volleyball. Common maneuvers of these two sports include using a ball with your hand, jumping, pivoting, running, and sudden stopping, which increase the risks for ankle, knee, and finger injury.

Knee overuse injuries include patellar tendonitis ("jumper's knee") and traction apophysitis (Osgood-Schlatter disease). As with other jumping sports, acute ligament sprains (medial collateral with or without anterior cruciate ligaments) can occur.

Ankle sprain is the most common injury and is usually caused by inversion with plantarflexion, placing the lateral ligaments at high tension. An avulsion fracture of the base of the fifth metatarsal at the insertion of the peroneus brevis tendon is another sequela of inversion ankle injuries. Achilles tendonitis is an overuse injury that may be exacerbated by rubbing of the tendon over high-top shoes. Foot pain may be due to retrocalcaneal bursitis, posterior tibial tendonitis, accessory tarsal navicular, calcaneal periostitis, plantar fasciitis, stress fracture of the tarsal navicular, Jones stress fracture of the fifth metatarsal, sesamoiditis, blisters, subungual hematoma, and paronychia.

Running. Running problems are due to an overuse (chronic repetitive motion) injury exacerbated by muscle imbalance, a minor skeletal deformity, or poor flexibility, strength or endurance, or proprioception. With each step while running, the foot impact ranges from three to eight times the athlete's body weight. Most problems ensue as the runner increases the distance or intensity of training. Minor variations (e.g., malalignment) in anatomy, which do not cause problems at rest, may predispose to injury at specific sites (patellofemoral stress, overpronation). Muscle fatigue, environmental temperature, and running surface (grass vs. unyielding concrete) also contribute to injuries. Prevention of injuries is possible by stretching and muscle-strengthening exercises for previous injuries and cross-training (bicycling, swimming) and adequate rest. Using good-quality running shoes that match an athlete's foot type is an essential first step. Gender-specific shoes are important because girls generally have a narrower rearfoot. Those who severely overpronate need a *motion control shoe* for maximum rearfoot and arch support in the midsole. Those who mildly overpronate need a *stability* shoe that has extra support in the medial midsole and some midsole cushion. Those who supinate need a *cushioned* shoe with more shock absorption in the midsole, more curved last, and minimal arch support.

Stress fractures of the femoral neck, inferior pubic rami, subtrochanteric area, proximal femoral shaft, proximal tibia, fibula, navicular, metatarsal, sesamoid, and calcaneal apophysis may occur. Stress fractures of all bones of the lower extremity can occur in runners. The most common are in the metatarsals, the tibia, and the fibula. Those that are the most worrisome in terms of risk of nonunion are in the anterior proximal tibia, the femoral neck, and the talus. Muscle strains frequently affect the hamstrings, followed by the quadriceps, hip adductors, soleus, and gastrocnemius muscles. Tendonitis involving the tendon and its sheath is common in the Achilles tendon, followed by the posterior tibial, peroneal, iliopsoas, and proximal hamstring tendons. Achilles tendonitis develops chronically, initially may get better during a run, is characterized by tenderness and crepitance if acute and nodularity if chronic, and must be distinguished from a retrocalcaneal bursitis. Treatment includes identification of underlying cause and temporary abstinence from running (begin cross-training), a ½-inch heel lift, heel cord stretching, and NSAIDs. Corticosteroid injection is not indicated.

Anterior knee pain is usually due to patellofemoral stress syndrome (runner's knee), which results from excessive dynamic, usually lateral, motion of the patellar tendon in relationship to the femoral intracondylar groove. Treatment includes stretching of the quadriceps and hamstring muscles and possibly the iliotibial band, quadriceps-strengthening exercises, ice, and relative rest. Foot orthotics may be indicated if there is no improvement with the aforementioned treatment. Posterior knee pain can be caused by gastrocnemius strain, whereas posteromedial pain may be due to proximal tibial stress fractures or semimembranosus or semitendinosus tendonitis and lateral knee pain may be due to iliotibial band syndrome and popliteus tendonitis. Iliotibial band syndrome may be a combination of a bursitis and tendonitis owing to mechanical friction of the band (an extension of the tensor fasciae latae) over the lateral femoral epicondyle.

Shin splints, or medial tibial stress syndrome (MTSS), is a descriptive term for pain over the anterior tibia and should be distinguished from tibial stress fractures and chronic compartment syndromes (see Chapter 676.7). MTSS usually occurs in new runners with overpronation. Treatment includes running on soft surfaces, proper shoe selection, and, possibly, orthotics, NSAIDs, and relative rest (or cross-training). Compartment syndromes involve the deep posterior or anterior compartments, producing local pain confined to the muscle (not to the bone). Classically, the pain will have onset at the same time during the run and will be relieved by rest. Pain usually prevents further training, thus limiting the risk of permanent nerve damage. Diagnosis is made by measurement of increased intracompartmental pressures during exercise.

Plantar fasciitis is an inflammation of the supporting structure of the longitudinal arch owing to repetitive cyclic loading with foot strike. Pain increases with the first step out of bed in the morning and with running and is located on the medial aspect of the heel. Treatment includes calf stretching, proper shoes, night splints, corticosteroid injection, relative rest, and ice massage of the heel. Calcaneal stress fracture must be considered especially in the amenorrheic distance runner.

Soccer. Injuries in soccer include abrasions, contusions, muscle strains, and ligament sprains (ankle, knee), owing partly to body-to-body contact, falls, running, and kicking. Hip problems include the "hip pointer" (iliac crest contusion), iliac crest apophysitis, and chronic groin pain (muscle strain, hernia, osteitis pubis). Femoral neck stress fractures, slipped femoral capital epiphysis, and avulsion fractures of the pelvis or femur are to be considered in the differential diagnosis yet are unusual causes of hip pain. All other lower and upper extremity injuries can occur in soccer.

Concussions occur in soccer. On the typical high school and college teams there would be approximately one concussion every three to four seasons and one concussion every season, respectively. The consensus is that heading, alone, does not lead to neurocognitive dysfunction. Concussion can lead to neurocognitive dysfunction, and concussions occur in soccer due to player/player, player/goal post, and player/ground contact. Proper heading technique should be taught in youth soccer; on long kicks, the receiving player traps the ball with the chest or leg, not the head; defenders kick the ball about 5 feet in front of their midfielders or forwards so the latter have to come to the ball and trap with their legs; players avoid heading the ball backward toward the goal (i.e., with cervical extension); referees, as with all sports, keep the game under control and penalize dangerous play; and guidelines for returning to play after a concussion should be followed. One study reported no evidence of impaired neurocognitive function or scholastic aptitude in college soccer players, with an average of 15 seasons of playing soccer and 28% of whom reported at least 1 concussion, compared with nonsoccer college athletes and student nonathletes.

Tennis. Lower extremity injuries occur twice as often as upper extremity injuries, and, overall, injury rates are similar for boys and girls. Common areas of injury in tennis include muscles and tendons of the elbow, shoulder, back, wrist, and abdomen. The risk for injury is increased by increased training; by unrehabilitated injuries with resultant deficits in flexibility, strength, and endurance; and by poor technique. Acute injuries of the lower extremities include ankle, knee, lower leg, and groin strains. Overuse injuries of the back and lower and upper extremities occur. The lower extremity injury patterns are related to the fact that for accomplished players, there are an average of eight direction changes per point, creating eccentric and concentric loads on the lower extremities. In the back, injuries are related to the marked and rapid load and direction change associated with serving; and the shoulder, elbow, and wrist are moving at velocities of up to 1700, 900, and 350 degrees/sec, respectively, in a repetitive fashion. Injuries can be related to improper equipment, such as a racquet that is too big, or to trying to learn techniques, such as hitting with top spin or with power before proper coordination and technique in basic strokes has been established. Overuse injuries include stress fractures of the humerus, ulna, and metacarpals and traction apophysitis of the calcaneus, tibial tubercle (Osgood-Schlatter disease), and medial humeral epicondyle.

Rotator cuff tendonitis is caused by repetitive overuse and may be related to anterior-posterior glenohumeral instability. Subluxation of the glenohumeral joint may also be present. Biceps tendonitis can present as anterior shoulder pain.

"Tennis elbow," or lateral epicondylitis, is due to repetitive overload of the wrist extensor/supinator mechanism, especially the extensor carpi radialis brevis (see Chapter 676.3). Medial epicondylitis is caused by repetitive overload of the wrist flexor/pronator muscle groups. This may secondarily involve the medial collateral ligament; however, the ligament is uncommonly the site of the primary injury. Nonunion of the medial and lateral humeral epicondyles is unusual. Medial epicondylar apophysitis may be associated with ulnar nerve dysfunction if there is an avulsion fracture. Olecranon apophysitis is similar to Osgood-Schlatter disease and is marked by pain at the olecranon with elbow extension.

Wrist problems include an enlarged dorsal ganglion cyst, radiocarpal joint capsular (impingement) synovitis, degenerative attrition (tears) of the triangular fibrocartilage complex, and fracture of the hook of the hamate.

Basic treatment includes relative rest, NSAIDs, application of ice, rehabilitation, learning proper mechanics, using properly sized racquets, protective counterforce bracing (elbow, wrist), strengthening exercises, and gradual return to tennis. Corticosteroid injections into the extensor/supinator muscle group for "tennis elbow" are not recommended because the outcome at 1 yr is poorer than for those treated with rehabilitation.

Skiing. Injuries are related to falls (concussions, contusion, lacerations) and ski-specific mechanisms. Overall injuries have declined, partly because of better equipment (boots, bindings, poles) and slope conditions. It has been recommended that children and adolescents wear helmets for skiing and snowboarding.

Thumb injuries resulting from falls with the thumb in abduction and hyperextension produce a sprain of the ulnar collateral ligament (skier's thumb). Complete tears with a 45-degree joint opening require surgical intervention, whereas smaller degrees of joint opening may be treated with a thumb spica cast for 4 wk. A Salter-Harris type III fracture may also be present; if the epiphyseal fracture is displaced, it requires open reduction and internal fixation.

Lower extremity injuries include fractures (often spiral) of the tibia ("boot top") and ankle and anterior cruciate ligament (ACL) sprains with or without tibial eminence fracture. Hemarthrosis is present in fractures and meniscal and ACL injuries. Some ACL sprains can be managed without surgery. However, for those that cannot, treatment of ACL sprains includes bracing, intra-articular reconstruction, and closed or open anatomic reduction of a tibial eminence fracture fragment.

American Academy of Pediatrics Committee on Sports Medicine and Fitness: Medical conditions affecting sports participation. *Pediatrics* 2001;107:1205–8.

Boutis K, Komar L, Jaramillo D, et al: Sensitivity of a clinical examination to predict need for radiography in children with ankle injuries: A prospective study. *Lancet* 2001;358:2118–21.

Christopher NC, Congeni J: Overuse injuries in the pediatric athlete: Evaluation, initial management, and strategies for prevention. *Clin Pediatr Emerg Med* 2002;3:118–28.

Committee on Sports Medicine and Fitness: Climatic heat stress and the exercising child and adolescent. *Pediatrics* 2000;106:158–59.

Committee on Sports Medicine and Fitness: Medical concerns in the female athlete. *Pediatrics* 2000;106:610–13.

Committee on Sports Medicine and Fitness: Medical conditions affecting sports participation. *Pediatrics* 2001;107:1205–9.

Heidt RS, Sweeterman LM, Carlonas Richelle L, et al: Avoidance of soccer injuries with preseason conditioning. *Am J Sport Med* 2000;28:659–62.

Hoffman JR, Mower WR, Wolfson AB, et al: Validity of a set of clinical criteria to rule out injury to the cervical spine in patients with blunt trauma. *N Engl J Med* 2000;343:94–99.

Maron BJ, Shirani J, Poliac LC, et al: Sudden death in young competitive athletes. *JAMA* 1996;276:199.

McClain LG, Reynolds S: Sports injuries in a high school. *Pediatrics* 1989;84:446.

McNally EG: Magnetic resonance imaging of the knee. *BMJ* 2002;325: 115–16.

The National Center for Catastrophic Sports Injury Research. Director, Frederick O. Mueller; Medical Director, Robert C. Cantu. www.unc.edu/depts/nccsi/

Powell JW, Barber-Foss KD: Traumatic brain injury in high school athletes. *JAMA* 1999;282:958–63.

Smidt N, van der Windt DAWM, Assendelft JJ, et al: Corticosteroid injections, physiotherapy, or a wait-and-see policy for lateral epicondylitis: A randomized controlled trial. *Lancet* 2002;359:657–62.

Solomon DH, Simel DL, Bates DW, et al: Does this patient have a torn meniscus or ligament of the knee? *JAMA* 2001;286:1610–20.

Speed CA: Corticosteroid injections in tendon lesions. *BMJ* 2001;323:382–86.

Tofler IR, Knapp PK, Drell MJ: The "achievement by proxy" spectrum: Recognition and clinical response to pressured and high-achieving children and adolescents. *J Am Acad Child Adolesc Psychiatry* 1999;38:213–16.

University Interscholastic League—Preparticipation Physical Evaluation, 2002. Search www.uil.utexas.edu/index.html. Go to Athletics, then to Athletic forms, then Preparticipation Physical Evaluation.

Warren WL, Bailes JE: On the field evaluation of athletic head injuries. *Clin Sports Med* 1998;17:13.

SECTION 3 *The Skeletal Dysplasias*

Chapter 682

General Considerations

William A. Horton and Jacqueline T. Hecht

The terms *skeletal dysplasias, bone dysplasias,* and *osteochondrodysplasias* refer to a genetically and clinically heterogeneous group of disorders of skeletal development and growth. Their prevalence is estimated to be about 1 in 4,000 births. They can be divided into the osteodysplasias typified by osteogenesis imperfecta (see Chapter 689) and the chondrodysplasias. The latter result from mutations of genes that are essential for skeletal development and growth. The clinical picture is dominated by skeletal abnormalities. The manifestations may be restricted to the skeleton, but in most cases nonskeletal tissues are also involved. The disorders may be lethal in utero or mild with features that go undetected.

The chondrodysplasias are distinguished from other forms of short stature by a disproportionality of skeletal manifestations. They are separated into individuals with predominantly short limbs and those with predominantly short trunks. Efforts to define the extent of clinical heterogeneity resulted in the delineation of more than 100 distinct entities. Many of these disorders result from mutations of a relatively small group of genes, the "chondrodysplasia genes."

An International Working Group on Bone Dysplasias named and classified these disorders based on genetic cause if known or on similarities of clinical and radiographic manifestations, which often imply a common pathogenesis and a common genetic basis, if the cause is unknown (Table 682–1). The classification differs from previous ones, which were based mainly on radiographic grounds. Disorders previously thought to be different were grouped together (e.g., pseudoachondroplasia, multiple epiphyseal dysplasia). By genetic definition, these are "allelic" disorders. In other instances, disorders believed to be related ended up in the different chondrodysplasia groups (e.g., achondrogenesis types Ia and II) because the mutant genes differ.

The better defined chondrodysplasia groups, such as the achondroplasia and type II collagenopathy groups, contain graded series of disorders that range from very severe to very mild. This may be true for other groups as more mutations are found and the full spectrum of clinical phenotypes associated with mutations of a given gene is defined. These disorders are clinical phenotypes distributed along spectra of phenotypic abnormality associated with mutations of particular genes. For mutations of some genes such as *COL2A1*, the distribution is fairly continuous, with clinical phenotypes merging into one another across a broad range. There is much less clinical overlap for mutations of some other genes, such as *FGFR3*, in which the distribution is discontinuous. Because most clinicians and most reference materials refer to the disorders as distinct entities, this vernacular continues to be used.

Although a few chondrodysplasias can be easily diagnosed, most require the analysis of information from the history, physical examination, skeletal radiographs, family history, and laboratory testing. The process involves recognizing complex patterns that are characteristic of the different disorders (Tables 682–2 and 682–3; Boxes 682–1 and 682–2). Comprehensive descriptions of disorders and references are at the On-Line Mendelian Inheritance in Man (OMIM) Internet site (see the references at the end of this chapter). OMIM numbers are given for disorders discussed in this and related chapters in this section.

Clinical Manifestations

GROWTH RELATED. The hallmark of the chondrodysplasias is disproportionate short stature. Although this refers to a disproportion between the limbs and the trunk, most disorders exhibit some shortening of both, and subtle degrees of disproportion may be difficult to appreciate, especially in premature, obese, or edematous infants. Disproportionate shortening of the limbs should be suspected if the upper limbs do not reach the mid pelvis in infancy or the upper thigh after infancy. Disproportionate shortening of the trunk is indicated by a short neck, small chest, and protuberant abdomen. Skeletal disproportion is usually accompanied by short stature (i.e., length and height below the 3rd percentile), but these measurements are occasionally within the low-normal range early in the course of certain conditions.

TABLE 682–1.

Gene Locus	Chromosome Location	Protein	Protein Function	Clinical Phenotype	OMIM	Disease Mechanism	Inherit
COL2A1	12q13.1-q13.3	Type II collagen α1 chain	Cartilage matrix protein	Achondrogenesis II	200610	Dominant negative	AD*
				Hypochondrogenesis	120140.0002	Dominant negative	AD*
				SED congenita	183900	Dominant negative	AD
				Kniest dysplasia	156550	Dominant negative	AD
				Late-onset SED		Dominant negative	AD
				Stickler dysplasia	108300	Haploinsufficiency	AD
SEDL	Xp22.2-p22.1	Sedlin	Intracellular transporter	X-linked SED tarda	313400	Loss of function	XLR
COL11A1	1p21	Type XI collagen α1 chain	Cartilage matrix protein	Stickler-like dysplasia	184840	Dominant negative	AD
COL11A2	6p21.3	Type XI collagen α2 chain	Cartilage matrix protein	Stickler-like dysplasia	215150	Loss of function	AR
COMP	19p12-p13.1	Cartilage oligomeric matrix protein	Cartilage matrix protein	Pseudoachondroplasia	177170	Dominant negative	AD
				MED	600969	Dominant negative	AD
COL9A2	1p32.2-p33	Type IX collagen α2 chain	Cartilage matrix protein	MED	600969	Dominant negative	AD
COL9A3	20q13.3	Type IX collagen α3 chain	Cartilage matrix protein	MED	600969	Dominant negative	AD
MATN3	2p24-p23	Matrilin 3	Cartilage matrix protein	MED	600969	Dominant negative	AD
COL10A1	6q21-q22.3	Type X collagen α1 chain	Hypertrophic cartilage matrix protein	Schmid metaphyseal chondrodyplasia	156500	Haploinsufficiency	AD
FGFR3	4p16.3	FGF receptor 3	Tyrosine kinase receptor for FGFs	Thanatophoric dysplasia I	187600	Gain of function	AD*
				Thanatophoric dysplasia II	187610	Gain of function	AD*
				Achondroplasia	100800	Gain of function	AD
				Hypochondroplasia	146000	Gain of function	AD
PTHR	3p21-p22	PTHrP receptor	G protein–coupled receptor for PTH and PTHrP	Jansen metaphyseal chondrodysplasia	156400	Gain of function	AD
DTDST	5q32-q33	DTD sulfate transporter	Transmembrane sulfate transporter	Achondrogenesis 1B	600972	Loss of function	AR*
				Atelosteogenesis II	256050	Loss of function	AR*
				Diastrophic dysplasia	222600	Loss of function	AR
SOX9	17q24.3-q25.1	SRY box 9	Transcription factor	Campomelic dysplasia	114290	Haploinsufficiency	AD
CBFA1	6p21	Core binding factor α subunit	Transcription factor	Cleidocranial dysplasia	119600	Haploinsufficiency	AD
LMX1B	9q34.1		Transcription factor	Nail-patella dysplasia	161200	Haploinsufficiency	AD
CTSK	1q21	Cathepsin K	Enzyme	Pyknodysostosis	265800	Loss of function	AR
RMPR	9p21-p12	Mitochondrial RNA–processing endoribonuclease	RNA-processing enzyme	CHH	250250	Loss of function	AR

*Usually lethal.

SED = spondyloepiphyseal dysplasia; MED = multiple epiphyseal dysplasia; DTD = diastrophic dysplasia; FGF = fibroblast growth factor; PTH = parathyroid hormone; PTHrP = parathyroid hormone–related protein; PTH = parathyroid hormone; SRY = sex-determining region of the Y chromosome; CHH = cartilage-hair hypoplasia.

There may also be disproportionate shortening of different segments of the limbs; the particular pattern may provide clues for specific diagnoses. Shortening is greatest in the proximal segments (upper arms and legs) in achondroplasia; this is termed *rhizomelic* shortening. Disproportionate shortening of the middle segments (forearms and lower legs) is called *mesomelic* shortening; *acromelic* shortening involves the hands and feet.

With some exceptions, there is a strong correlation between the age at onset and the clinical severity. Many of the so-called lethal neonatal chondrodysplasias are evident by the time routine fetal ultrasound examinations are performed at the end of the 1st trimester of gestation (see Box 682–1). Gestational standards exist for long-bone lengths; discrepancies are often detected between biparietal diameter of the skull and long-bone lengths. Many disorders become apparent around the time of birth; others manifest during the 1st yr of life. A number of disorders present in early childhood and a few in late childhood or later.

NON–GROWTH RELATED. Most patients also have problems unrelated to growth. Skeletal deformities, such as abnormal joint mobility, protuberances at and around joints, angular deformities, and so on, are common and usually symmetric. Skeletal abnormalities may adversely affect nonskeletal tissues. Impaired growth at the base of the skull and of vertebral pedicles reduces the size of the spinal canal in achondroplasia and

may contribute to spinal cord compression. Short ribs reduce thoracic volume, which may compromise breathing in patients with short trunk chondrodysplasias. Cleft palate is common to many disorders, presumably reflecting defective palatal growth.

Manifestations may be unrelated to the skeleton; they reflect expression of mutant genes in nonskeletal tissues. Examples include retinal detachment in spondyloepiphyseal dysplasia congenita, sex reversal in campomelic dysplasia, congenital heart malformations in Ellis-van Creveld syndrome, immune deficiency in cartilage-hair hypoplasia, and renal dysfunction in asphyxiating thoracic dystrophy. These nonskeletal problems provide valuable clues to specific diagnoses and must be managed clinically (see Table 682–3).

FAMILY AND REPRODUCTIVE HISTORY. A careful family history may identify relatives with the condition; a mendelian inheritance pattern may be elicited. Because the presentation may vary substantially in some disorders, features that might be related to the disorder should be identified. Special attention should be given to mild degrees of short stature, disproportion, deformities, and other manifestations such as precocious osteoarthritis because they may be overlooked by the family. Physical examination of relatives may be useful, as may the review of photographs, radiographs, and medical records of family members.

TABLE 682–2. Major Problems Associated with Skeletal Dysplasias

Problem	Example
Lethality[*]	Thanatophoric dysplasia
Associated anomalies[†]	Ellis–van Creveld syndrome
Short stature	Common to almost all
Cervical spine dislocations	Larsen syndrome
Severe limb bowing	Metaphyseal dysplasia, type Schmid
Spine curvatures	Metatropic dysplasia
Clubfeet	Diastrophic dysplasia
Fractures	Osteogenesis imperfecta
Pneumonias, aspirations	Campomelic dysplasia
Hydrocephalus	Achondroplasia
Joint problems (hips, knees)	Most skeletal dysplasias
Hearing loss	Common (greatest with cleft palate)
Myopia/cataracts	Stickler syndrome
Immune deficiency[‡]	Cartilage-hair hypoplasia
Sudden infant death syndrome	Achondroplasia (rare)
Pulmonary hypertension[§]	Achondroplasia
Poor body image	Variable, but common to all
Sex reversal	Campomelic dysplasia

[*]*Mostly due to severely reduced size of thorax.*
[†]*See Table 682–3.*
[‡]*At least four additional disorders, all involving the metaphyses, can have immunodeficiency.*
[§]*Uncommon.*

A reproductive history may reveal previous stillbirths, fetal losses, and other abnormal pregnancy outcomes resulting from a skeletal dysplasia. Pregnancy complications, such as polyhydramnios or reduced fetal movement, are common in bone dysplasias, especially neonatal lethal variants.

Even though most of the skeletal dysplasias are genetic, it is common to have no family history of the disorder. New mutations are common for autosomal dominant disorders, especially lethal disorders in the perinatal period (thanatophoric dysplasia, osteogenesis imperfecta). The majority of achondroplasia cases result from new mutations. Germ cell mosaicism, in which a parent has clones of mutant germ cells, has been observed in osteogenesis imperfecta and in other dominant disorders. A negative family history is common in recessive disorders.

RADIOGRAPHIC FEATURES. Radiographic evaluation for a chondrodysplasia should include plain films of the entire skeleton. Efforts should be made to identify which bones and which parts of bones (epiphyses, metaphyses, diaphyses) are most affected. If possible, films taken at different ages should be examined because the radiographic changes evolve with time. Films taken before puberty are generally more informative because pubertal closure of the epiphyses obliterates many of the signs needed for a radiographic diagnosis.

Diagnosis. If an infant or child is short with disproportionate features, a diagnosis is established by matching the observed clinical picture (defined primarily from clinical, family, and gestational histories; physical examination; and radiographic evaluation) with clinical phenotypes of well-documented disorders. Pediatricians should be able to gather most of this information and, in consultation with a radiologist, diagnose the common chondrodysplasias. There are a number of reference texts and online databases that provide information about the disorders and comprehensive lists of current references. For less common disorders and for infants and children whose phenotypes do not closely match well-established clinical phenotypes, consultation with experts in the bone dysplasia field is warranted.

Laboratory testing has not been useful in diagnosing chondrodysplasias. An exception is osteogenesis imperfecta, in which

TABLE 682–3. Associated Anomalies in Skeletal Dysplasias

Anomaly	Example
Heart defects	Ellis–van Creveld syndrome
Polydactyly	Short rib polydactyly, Majewski type
Cleft palate	Diastrophic dysplasia
Ear cysts	Diastrophic dysplasia
Hydrocephalus	Achondroplasia
Encephalocele	Dyssegmental dysplasia
Hemivertebrae	Dyssegmental dysplasia
Micrognathia	Campomelic dysplasia
Nail dysplasia	Ellis–van Creveld syndrome
Conical teeth, oligodontia	Ellis–van Creveld syndrome
Multiple oral frenulae	Ellis–van Creveld syndrome
Dentinogenesis imperfecta	Osteogenesis imperfecta
Pretibial skin dimples	Campomelic dysplasia
Cataracts, retinal detachment	Stickler syndrome
Intestinal atresia	Saldino-Noonan
Renal cysts	Saldino-Noonan
Campodactyly	Diastrophic dysplasia
Craniosynostosis	Thanatophoric dysplasia
Ichthyosis	Chondrodystrophica punctata
Hitchhiker thumb	Diastrophic dysplasia
Sparse scalp hair	Cartilage-hair hypoplasia
Hypertelorism	Robinow syndrome
Hypoplastic nasal bridge	Acrodysostosis
Clavicular agenesis	Cleidocranial dysplasia
Genital hypoplasia	Robinow syndrome
Tail	Metatropic dysplasia
Omphalocele	Beemer-Langer syndrome
Blue sclera	Osteogenesis imperfecta

BOX 682–1. Lethal Neonatal Dwarfism

USUALLY FATAL[*]
Achondrogenesis (different types)
Thanatophoric dyplasia
Short rib polydactyly, Majewski type
Short rib polydactyly, Saldino-Noonan type
Homozygous achondroplasia
Osteopetrosis (congenital form)
Campomelic dysplasia
Dyssegmental dysplasia, Silverman-Handmaker type
Osteogenesis imperfecta, type II
Hypophosphatasia (congenital form)
Chondrodysplasia punctata (rhizomelic form)

OFTEN FATAL
Asphyxiating thoracic dystrophy (Jeune syndrome)

OCCASIONALLY FATAL
Ellis–van Creveld syndrome
Diastrophic dysplasia
Metatropic dwarfism
Kniest dysplasia

[*]*A few prolonged survivors have been reported in most of these disorders.*

BOX 682–2. Usually Nonlethal Dwarfing Conditions Recognizable at Birth or Within First Few Months of Life

MOST COMMON
Achondroplasia
Osteogenesis imperfecta (types I, III, IV)
Spondyloepiphyseal dysplasia congenita
Diastrophic dysplasia
Ellis–van Creveld syndrome

LESS COMMON
Chondrodysplasia punctata (some forms)
Kniest dysplasia (not severe congenital forms)
Metatropic dysplasia
Langer mesomelic dysplasia

analysis of collagen synthesis by skin fibroblasts has helped establish a diagnosis. Osteogenesis imperfecta is not a chondrodysplasia, but it is frequently in the differential diagnosis, especially for newborns with severe skeletal deformities (see Chapter 689).

Molecular genetic testing for chondrodysplasias may be useful, especially for disorders in which recurrent mutations occur (typical achondroplasia has the same *FGFR3* mutation). Mutation testing for achondroplasia is available; however, the diagnosis can usually be made clinically. The greatest utility for testing may be for prenatal diagnosis for couples in whom both parents have typical (heterozygous) achondroplasia. They are at a 25% risk for the much more severe homozygous achondroplasia, which can be detected by mutation analysis. Another example is in disorders due to mutations of *DTDST*. These disorders are inherited in an autosomal recessive manner, and a limited number of mutant alleles have been found. If the mutations are identified in the patient, they should be detectable in the parents and potentially used for prenatal diagnosis. Nonetheless, most chondrodysplasia mutations tend to be dispersed throughout host genes. This phenomenon makes their detection more difficult and currently reduces the usefulness of such testing for diagnostic purposes.

Many of the chondrodysplasias have distinct histologic changes of the skeletal growth plate. Sometimes such tissues obtained at biopsy or discarded from a surgical procedure are helpful diagnostically. It is uncommon to make a diagnosis histologically if it was not already suspected on clinical grounds. An exception is for the lethal neonatal chondrodysplasias, in which an aborted fetus is macerated, thus making a clinical and radiographic assessment difficult.

Molecular Genetics. A number of chondrodysplasia genes have been identified (see Table 682–1). They encode several categories of proteins, including cartilage matrix proteins, transmembrane receptors, ion transporters, and transcription factors. The number of identified gene loci is much smaller than anticipated from the number of recognized clinical phenotypes. The vast majority of patients have disorders that map to fewer than 10 loci; mutations at two loci (*COL2A1* and *FGFR3*) account for more than half of all cases. There may be a limited number of genes whose function is critical to skeletal development, especially linear bone growth; mutations in these genes give rise to a wide range of chondrodysplasia clinical phenotypes.

Mutations at the *COL2A1* and *FGFR3* loci illustrate different genetic characteristics. *COL2A1* mutations are distributed throughout the gene with few instances of recurrence in unrelated persons. In contrast, *FGFR3* mutations are restricted to a few locations within the gene, and occurrence of new mutations at these sites in unrelated individuals is the rule. There is a strong correlation between clinical phenotype and mutation site for *FGFR3*, but not *COL2A1*, mutations.

Pathophysiology. Chondrodysplasia mutations act through different mechanisms. Most mutations involving cartilage matrix proteins cause disease when only one of the two copies (alleles) of the relevant gene is mutated. These mutations usually act through a *dominant negative mechanism* in which the protein products of the mutant allele interfere with the assembly and function of multimeric molecules that contain the protein products of both the normal and mutant alleles. The type II collagen molecule is a triple helix composed of three collagen chains, which are the products of the type II collagen gene, *COL2A1*. When chains from both normal and mutant alleles are combined to form triple helices, most molecules contain at least one mutant chain. It is not known how many mutant chains are required to produce a dysfunctional molecule but, depending on the mutation, it theoretically could be as few as one.

Mutations involving type X collagen differ from the model just described. They map to the region of the chain that is responsible for chain recognition; the chains must recognize each other before they can assemble into collagen molecules. Mutations are thought to disrupt this process. As a result, none of the mutant chains are incorporated into molecules. This mechanism is haploinsufficiency because the products of the mutant allele are functionally absent and the normal allele is insufficient for normal function. Mutations involving ion transport genes also act through a loss of function of the transporters. Alternatively, mutations of transmembrane receptors studied to date appear to act through a gain of function; the mutant receptors initiate signals in a constitutive manner independent of their normal ligands.

Regardless of genetic mechanism, the mutations ultimately disrupt endochondral ossification, the biologic process responsible for the development and linear growth of the skeleton. Indeed, a wide range of morphologic abnormalities of the skeletal growth plate, the anatomic structure in which endochondral ossification occurs, have been described in the chondrodysplasias.

Diagnosis and Treatment. The first step is to establish the correct diagnosis. This allows one to predict a prognosis and to anticipate the medical and surgical problems associated with a particular disorder. Establishing a diagnosis helps to distinguish between lethal disorders and nonlethal disorders in a premature or newborn infant (see Boxes 682–1 and 682–2). A poor prognosis for long-term survival may argue against initiating extreme lifesaving measures for thanatophoric dysplasia or achondrogenesis types Ib or II, whereas such measures may be indicated for infants with spondyloepiphyseal dysplasia congenita or diastrophic dysplasia, which have a good prognosis if the infant survives the newborn period.

Because there is no definitive therapy to normalize bone growth in any of the disorders, management is directed at preventing and correcting skeletal deformities, treating nonskeletal complications, genetic counseling, and helping patients and families learn to cope. Each disorder has its own unique set of problems, and consequently management must be tailored to each disorder. Medical information for a few disorders can be found at the Medical Information on Dwarfism website (see references at the end of the chapter).

There are a number of problems common to many chondrodysplasias for which general recommendations can be made. Children with most chondrodysplasias should avoid contact sports and other activities that cause injury or stress to joints. Good dietary habits should be established in childhood to prevent or minimize obesity in adulthood. Dental care should be started early to minimize crowding and malalignment of teeth. Children and relatives should be given the opportunity to participate in support groups, such as the Little People of America and Human Growth Foundation.

Two controversial approaches have been used to increase bone length. Surgical limb lengthening has been employed for a few disorders. Its greatest success has been in achondroplasia in which nonskeletal tissues tend to be redundant and easily stretched. The procedure is usually performed during adolescence. Injections of human growth hormone in pharmacologic doses comparable to those used to treat Turner syndrome have also been tried in several disorders; the results have been equivocal.

Apajasalo M, Sintonen H, Rautonen J, et al: Health-related quality of life patients with genetic skeletal dysplasias. *Eur J Pediatr* 1998;157:114.
Hall JG, Froster-Iskenius UG, Allanson JE: *Handbook of Normal Physical Measurements.* Oxford, Oxford University Press, 1989.
Horton WA: Molecular genetics of the human chondrodysplasias—1995. *Eur J Hum Genet* 1995;3:357.
Lachman RS: Neurologic abnormalities in the skeletal dysplasias: A clinical and radiological perspective. *Am J Med Genet* 1997;69:33.
Rimoin DL, Lachman RS: Chondrodysplasias. In Rimoin DL, Connor JM, Pyeritz RE (editors): *Emery and Rimoin's Principles and Practice of Medical Genetics,* 3rd ed. New York, Churchill Livingstone, 1996, p 2779.
Spranger J, Maroteaux P: The lethal osteochondrodysplasias. *Adv Hum Genet* 1995;19:1.

Spranger JW, Brill PW, Poznansk A: *Bone Dysplasias. An Atlas of Genetic Disorders of Skeletal Development*, 2nd ed. New York, Oxford University Press, 2002.

Taybi H, Lachman RS: *Radiology of Syndromes, Metabolic Disorders, and Skeletal Dysplasias*, 4th ed. New York, CV Mosby, 1996.

Online Resources
Medical Information on Dwarfism: http://www.lpaonline.org/resources.html
On-Line Mendelian Inheritance in Man (OMIM): http://www3.ncbi.nlm.nih.gov/omim

Chapter 683
Disorders Involving Cartilage Matrix Proteins

William A. Horton and Jacqueline T. Hecht

Some bone and joint disorders result from functional disturbances of cartilage matrix proteins. They fall into four groups corresponding primarily to the defective proteins: three collagens and the noncollagenous proteins COMP (cartilage oligomeric matrix protein) and matrilin 3. The clinical phenotypes differ between and within the groups, especially the spondyloepiphyseal dysplasia (SED) group. In some groups, there is substantial variation in clinical severity.

SPONDYLOEPIPHYSEAL DYSPLASIAS

The term *spondyloepiphyseal dysplasia* refers to a heterogeneous group of disorders characterized by shortening of the trunk and, to a lesser extent, the limbs. Severity ranges from achondrogenesis type II to the slightly less severe hypochondrogenesis (these two types are lethal in the perinatal period) to SED congenita and its variants, including **Kniest dysplasia** (which are apparent at birth and are usually nonlethal), to late-onset SED (which may not be detected until adolescence or later). The radiographic hallmarks are abnormal development of the vertebral bodies and of epiphyses, the extent of which corresponds to the clinical severity. All the SEDs result from heterozygous mutations of COL2A1; they are autosomal dominant disorders. The mutations are dispersed throughout the gene; there is a poor correlation between the mutation's location and the resultant clinical phenotype.

Lethal Spondyloepiphyseal Dysplasias. Achondrogenesis type II (OMIM 200610) is characterized by severe shortening of the neck and trunk and especially the limbs and by a large, soft head. Fetal hydrops and prematurity are common; infants are stillborn or die shortly after birth. Hypochondrogenesis (OMIM 12014002) refers to a clinical phenotype intermediate between achondrogenesis type II and SED congenita. It is typically lethal in the newborn period.

The severity of radiographic changes correlate with the clinical severity (Fig. 683–1). Both conditions produce short, broad tubular bones with cupped metaphyses. The pelvic bones are hypoplastic, and the cranial bones are not well mineralized. The vertebral bodies are poorly ossified in the entire spine in achondrogenesis type II and in the cervical and sacral spine in hypochondrogenesis. The pedicles are ossified in both.

Spondyloepiphyseal Dysplasia Congenita. The phenotype of this group, SED congenita (OMIM 183900), is apparent at birth. The head and face are usually normal, but a cleft palate is common. The neck is short and the chest is barrel shaped (Fig. 683–2). Kyphosis and exaggeration of the normal lumbar lordosis are common. The proximal segments of the limbs are shorter than the hands and feet, which often appear normal. Some infants have clubfoot or exhibit hypotonia.

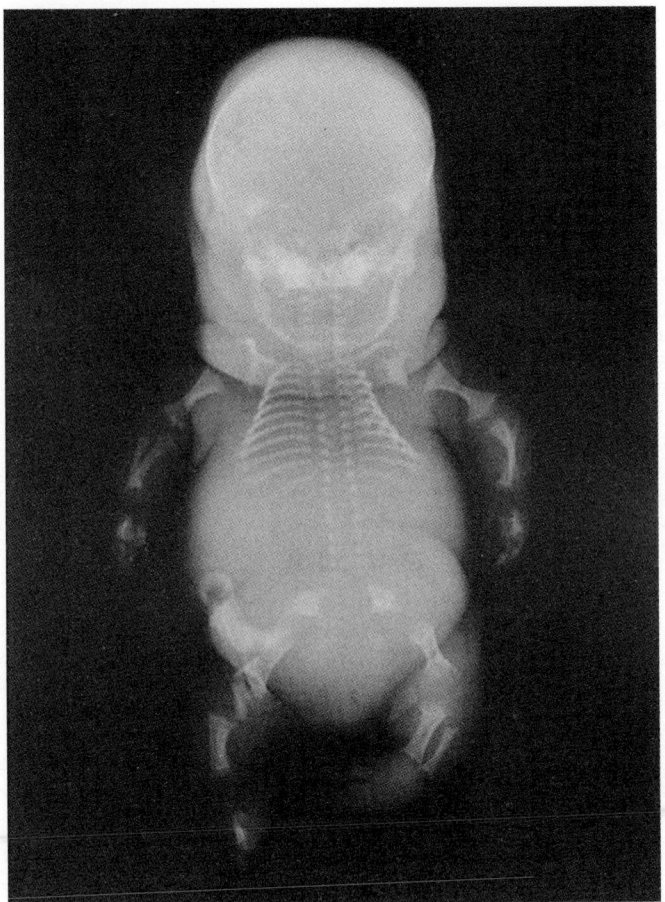

FIGURE 683–1. Stillborn with achondrogenesis type II. Note poor ossification of calvaria, vertebral bodies, and sacrum; hypoplasia of pelvic bones; and short tubular bones with cupped metaphyses.

Skeletal radiographs of the newborn reveal short tubular bones, delayed ossification of vertebral bodies, and proximal limb bone epiphyses (Fig. 683–3). Hypoplasia of the odontoid process; a short, square pelvis with a poorly ossified symphysis pubis; and mild irregularity of metaphyses are apparent.

Infants usually have normal developmental milestones; a waddling gait typically appears in early childhood. Childhood complications include respiratory compromise from spinal deformities and spinal cord compression due to cervicomedullary instability. The disproportionateness and shortening become progressively worse with age, and adult heights range from 95 to 128 cm. Myopia is typical; adults are predisposed to retinal detachment. Precocious osteoarthritis occurs in adulthood and requires surgical joint replacement.

Kniest Dysplasia. The Kniest dysplasia variant of SED (OMIM 156550) presents at birth with a short trunk and limbs associated with a flat face, prominent eyes, enlarged joints, cleft palate, and clubfoot. Radiographs show vertebral defects and short tubular bones with epiphyseal irregularities and metaphyseal enlargement that gives rise to a dumbbell appearance.

Motor development is often delayed because of the joint deformities, although intelligence is normal. Hearing loss and myopia commonly develop during childhood, and retinal detachment may occur as a late complication. Joint enlargement progresses during childhood and becomes painful; it is accompanied by flexion contractures and muscle atrophy, which may be incapacitating by adolescence.

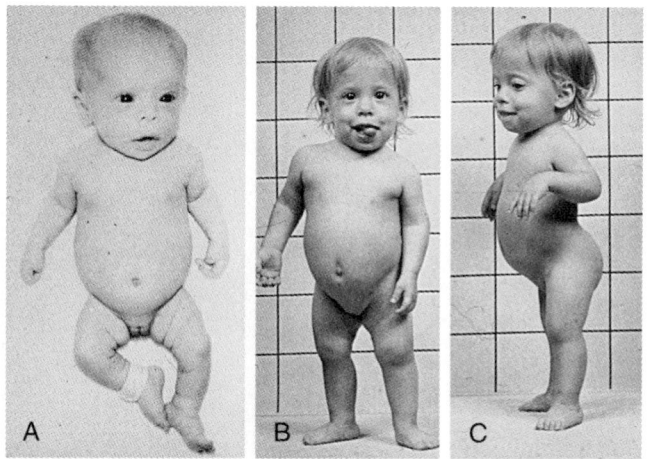

FIGURE 683–2. Spondyloepiphyseal dysplasia congenita is shown in infancy and early childhood. Note the short extremities, relatively normal hands, flat facies, and exaggerated lordosis.

Late-Onset Spondyloepiphyseal Dysplasia. This term refers to a mild to very mild clinical phenotype characterized by slightly short stature associated with mild epiphyseal and vertebral abnormalities on radiographs. It is typically detected during childhood or adolescence but may go unrecognized until adulthood when precocious osteoarthritis appears. This designation is nosologically distinct from SED tarda, which is clinically similar but results from mutation of the X-linked gene *SEDL*.

STICKLER DYSPLASIA (HEREDITARY OSTEOARTHRO-OPHTHALMOPATHY

Short stature is not a feature of Stickler dysplasia (OMIM 184840). It resembles SED because of its joint and eye manifestations. Mutations of genes encoding type XI collagen, which functionally interacts with type II collagen, have been identified in Stickler-like disorders (OMIM 184840, OMIM 215150). Stickler dysplasia is often identified in the newborn because of cleft palate and micrognathia (Pierre Robin anomaly). Infants typically have severe myopia and additional ophthalmologic complications, including choroidoretinal and vitreous degeneration; retinal detachment is common during childhood (Fig. 683–4). Sensorineural hearing loss may arise during adolescence, which is when symptoms of osteoarthritis may begin. Special attention must be given to the eye complications even in childhood.

SCHMID METAPHYSEAL DYSPLASIA

Schmid metaphyseal dysplasia (OMIM 156500) is one of several chondrodysplasias in which metaphyseal abnormalities dominate the radiographic features. It typically presents in early childhood with mild short stature, bowing of the legs, and a waddling gait (Fig. 683–5). Enlargement of joints, such as the wrist, may be found. Radiographs show flaring and irregular mineralization of the metaphyses of tubular bones of the proximal limbs (Fig. 683–6). Coxa vara is usually present and may

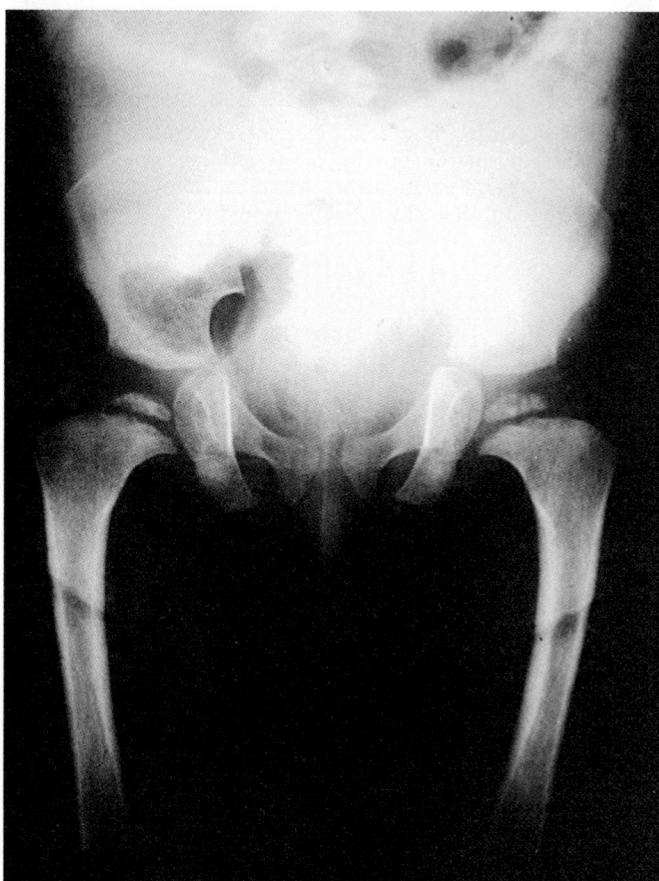

FIGURE 683–3. Radiograph of spondyloepiphyseal dysplasia congenita pelvis demonstrating squared pelvis, hypoplastic capital femoral epiphyses, and femoral necks that are wide and short.

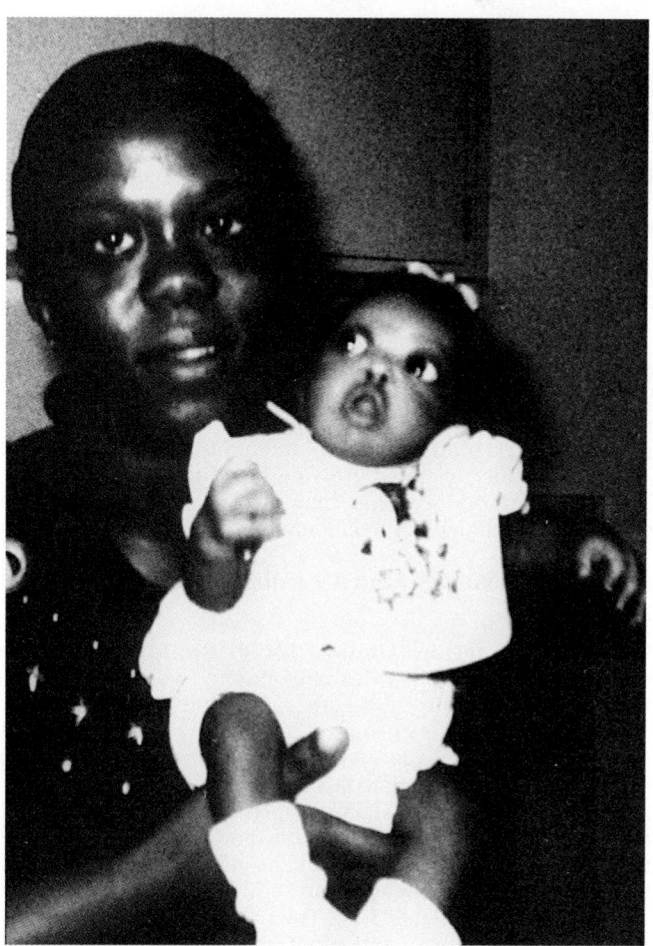

FIGURE 683–4. Stickler syndrome in mother and child. The facies are flat and the eyes are prominent.

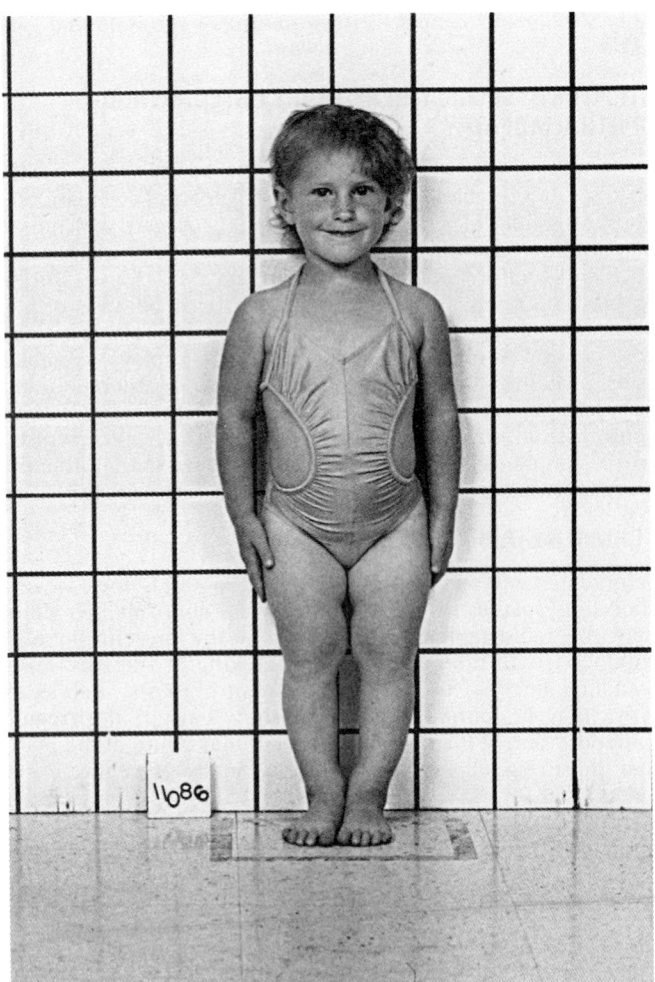

FIGURE 683–5. Female patient with metaphyseal dysplasia, type Schmid. The facies are normal and stature is mildly reduced. Mild tibia vara is present.

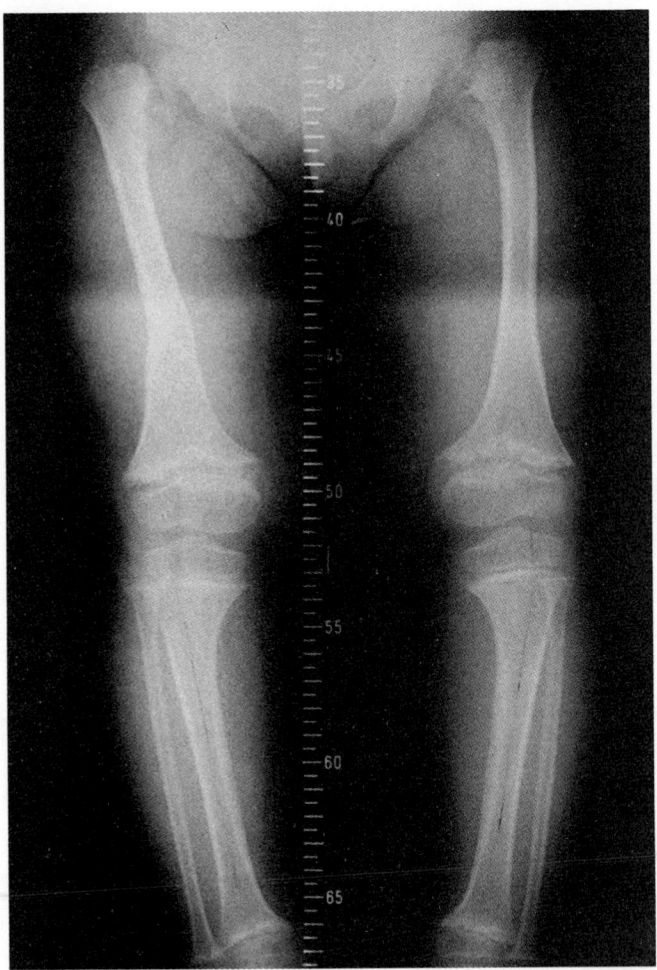

FIGURE 683–6. Radiograph of lower extremities in Schmid metaphyseal dysplasia showing short tubular bones and metaphyseal flaring and irregularities, abnormal capital femoral epiphyses, and femoral necks. The epiphyses are normal. Coxa vara is present.

require surgical correction. Short stature becomes more evident with age and affects the lower extremities more than the upper extremities; the manifestations are limited to the skeleton.

Schmid metaphyseal chondrodysplasia is due to heterozygous mutations of the gene encoding type X collagen; it is an autosomal dominant trait. The distribution of type X collagen is restricted to the region of growing bone in which cartilage is converted into bone. This may explain why radiographic changes are confined to the metaphyses.

PSEUDOACHONDROPLASIA AND MULTIPLE EPIPHYSEAL DYSPLASIA

Pseudoachondroplasia (OMIM 177170) and multiple epiphyseal dysplasia (MED) (OMIM 600969) are two distinct phenotypes that are grouped together because they result from mutations of the gene encoding COMP. The mutations are heterozygous in both; they are autosomal dominant traits. The clinical phenotypes are restricted to skeletal tissues.

Newborns with pseudoachondroplasia are average in size and appearance. Gait abnormalities and short stature mainly affect the limbs and become apparent in late infancy. The short stature becomes marked as the child grows and is associated with generalized joint laxity (Fig. 683–7). The hands are short, broad, and deviated in an ulnar direction; the forearms are bowed. Developmental milestones and intelligence are usually normal.

Lumbar lordosis and deformities of the knee develop during childhood; the latter frequently requires surgical correction. Pain is common in weight-bearing joints during childhood and adolescence, leading to osteoarthritis late in the second decade of life. Adults range in height from 105 to 128 cm.

Skeletal radiographs show distinctive abnormalities of vertebral bodies and of both epiphyses and metaphyses of tubular bones (Fig. 683–8).

The MED phenotype has skeletal abnormalities that predominantly affect the epiphyses as noted on radiographs. Two classic forms are a severe Fairbank type and a mild Ribbing type. Because of overlap in clinical features and because COMP mutations are found in both types, they may be considered clinical variants.

The more severe clinical phenotype has its onset during childhood, with mild short-limbed short stature, pain in weight-bearing joints, and a waddling gait. Radiographs show delayed and irregular ossification of epiphyses. More mildly affected individuals may not be recognized until adolescence or adulthood. Radiographic changes may be limited to the capital femoral epiphyses. In the latter case, mild MED must be distinguished from bilateral Legg-Perthes disease. Precocious osteoarthritis of hips and knees is the major complication in adults with MED. Adult heights range from 136 to 151 cm.

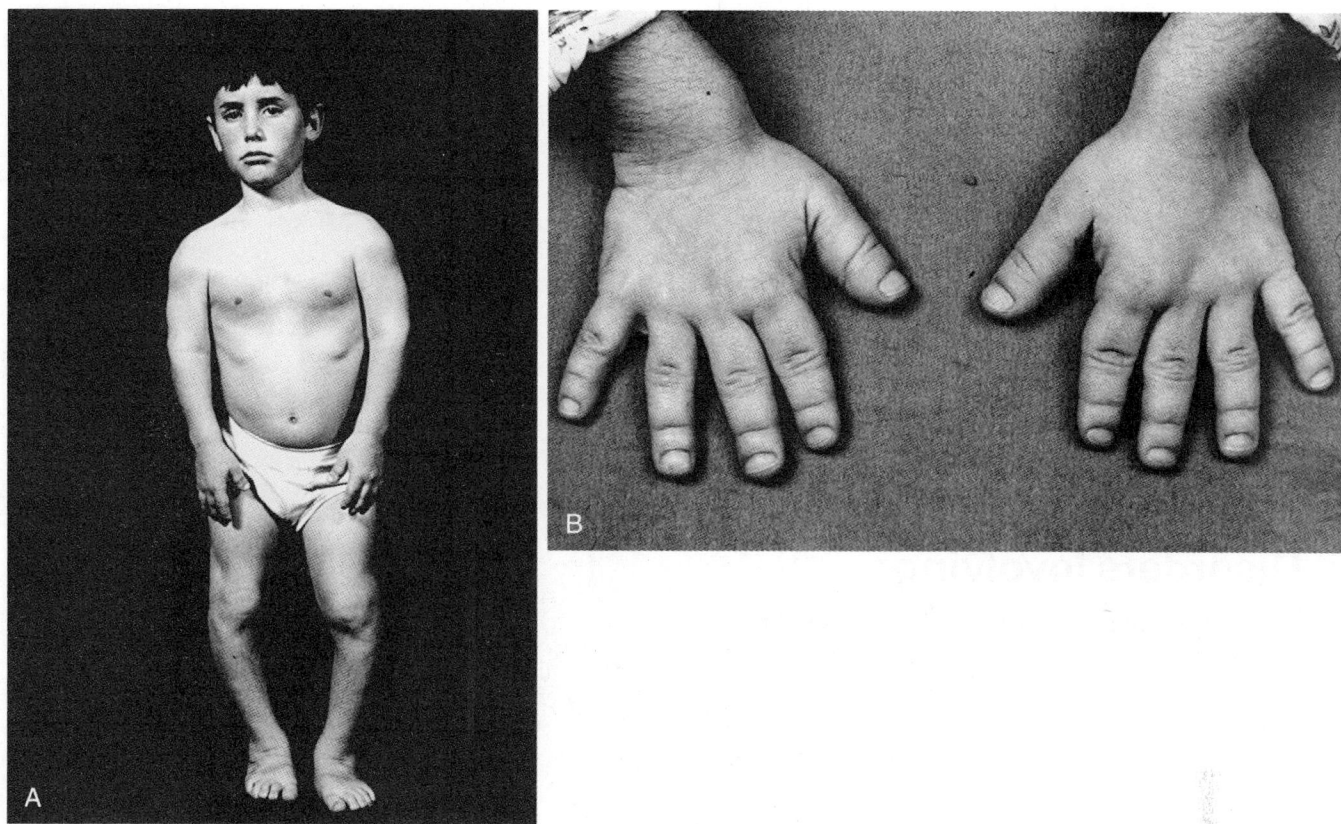

FIGURE 683–7. *A,* Pseudoachondroplasia in an adolescent male. The facies and head circumference are normal. There is shortening of all extremities and bowing of the lower extremities. *B,* Photograph of hands, demonstrating short stubby fingers.

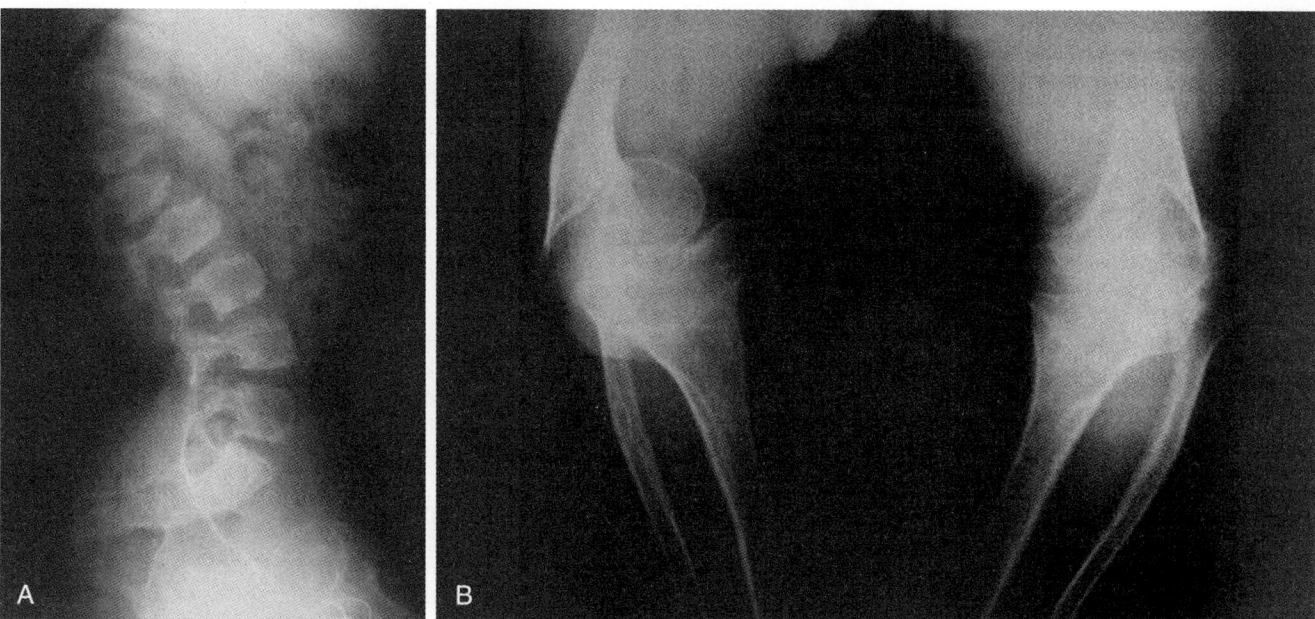

FIGURE 683–8. *A,* Lateral thoracolumbar spine radiograph of patient with pseudoachondroplasia showing central protrusion (tonguing) of the anterior aspect of upper lumbar and lower thoracic vertebrae. Note reduced vertebral body heights (platyspondyly) and secondary lordosis. *B,* Lower extremity radiograph of patient with pseudoachondroplasia showing large metaphyses, poorly formed epiphyses, and marked bowing of the long bones.

There are families with clinical and radiographic manifestations of MED that are not due to mutations of COMP. Some are linked to the gene encoding one of the type IX collagen chains. It has been suggested that COMP and type IX collagen interact functionally in cartilage matrix, thus explaining why mutations of different genes produce similar pictures. Mutations of the gene coding for another cartilage matrix protein, matrilin 3, have also been found in patients with MED.

Briggs MD, Mortier GR, Cole WG, et al: Diverse mutations in the gene for cartilage oligomeric matrix protein in a pseudoachondroplasia–multiple epiphyseal dysplasia disease spectrum. *Am J Hum Genet* 1998;62:311.

McKeand J, Rotta J, Hecht JT: Natural history study of pseudoachondroplasia. *Am J Med Genet* 1996;63:406.

Vikkula M, Metsaranta M, Ala-Kokko L: Type II collagen mutations in rare and common cartilage diseases. *Ann Med* 1994;26:107.

Winterpacht A, Hilbert M, Schwarze U, et al: Kniest and Stickler dysplasia phenotypes caused by collagen type II gene *(COL2A1)* defect. *Nat Genet* 1993;3:323.

Chapter 684

Disorders Involving Transmembrane Receptors

William A. Horton and Jacqueline T. Hecht

Disorders involving transmembrane receptors result from heterozygous mutations of genes encoding these receptors: *FGFR3* and *PTHR*. The mutations cause the receptors to become activated in the absence of physiologic ligands, which accentuates normal receptor function of negatively regulating bone growth. The mutations act by gain of negative function. In the *FGFR3* mutation group, in which the clinical phenotypes range from severe to mild, the severity appears to correlate with the extent to which the receptor is activated. Both *PTHR* and especially *FGFR3* mutations tend to recur in unrelated individuals.

ACHONDROPLASIA GROUP

The achondroplasia group represents a substantial percentage of patients with chondrodysplasias and contains thanatophoric dysplasia, the most common lethal chondrodysplasia with an incidence of 1 in 35,000 births; achondroplasia, the most common nonlethal chondrodysplasia with an incidence of 1 in 15,000 to 1 in 40,000 births, and hypochondroplasia. All three have mutations in a small number of locations in the *FGFR3* gene. There is a strong correlation between the mutation site and the clinical phenotype.

Thanatophoric Dysplasia. Thanatophoric dysplasia (TD) (OMIM 187600, OMIM 187610) presents before or at birth. In the former situation, ultrasonographic examination in mid gestation or later reveals a large head and very short limbs; the pregnancy is often accompanied by polyhydramnios and premature delivery. Very short limbs, short neck, long narrow thorax, and large head with midfacial hypoplasia dominate the clinical phenotype at birth (Fig. 684–1). The cloverleaf skull deformity known as **kleeblattschädel** is sometimes found. Newborns have severe respiratory distress because of their small thorax. Although this distress can be treated by intense respiratory care, the long-term prognosis is poor.

Skeletal radiographs distinguish two slightly different forms called TD I and TD II. In the more common TD I, radiographs show large calvariae with a small cranial base, marked thinning and flattening of vertebral bodies visualized best on lateral view, very short ribs, severe hypoplasia of pelvic bones, and very short and bowed tubular bones with flared metaphyses (Fig. 684–2). The femurs are curved and shaped like a telephone receiver. TD II differs mainly in that there are longer and straighter femurs.

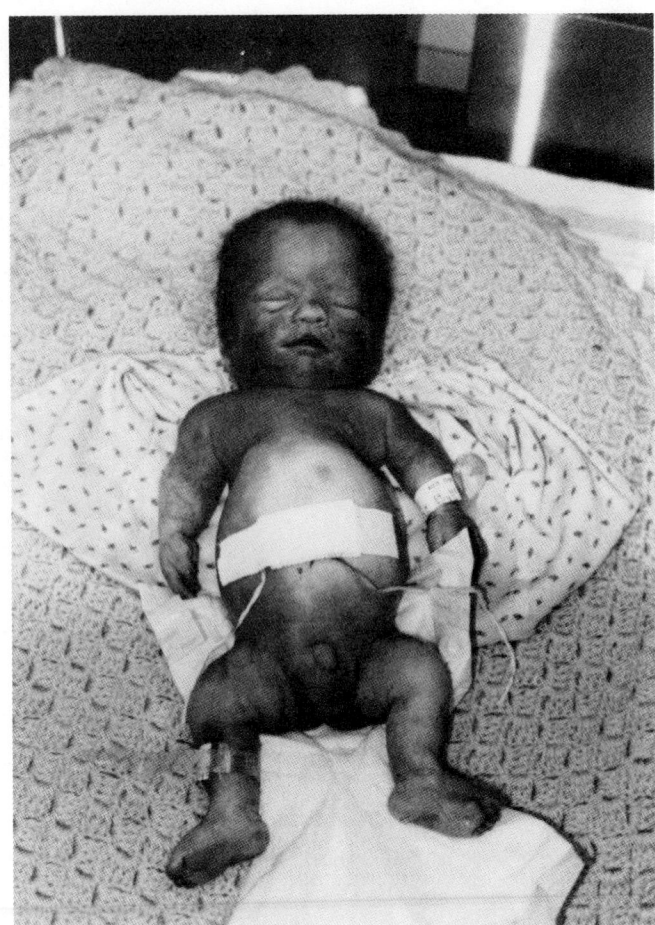

FIGURE 684–1. Stillborn infant with thanatophoric dysplasia. Limbs are very short, with upper limbs extending only two thirds of the way down the abdomen. The chest is narrow, exaggerating the protuberance of the abdomen. The head is relatively large.

The TD II clinical phenotype is associated with mutations that map to codon 650 of *FGFR3*, causing the substitution of a glutamic acid for the lysine. This activates the tyrosine kinase activity of a receptor that transmits signals to intracellular pathways. Mutations of the TD I phenotype map mainly to two regions in the extracellular domain of the receptor, where they substitute cysteine residues for other amino acids. Free cysteine residues are thought to form disulfide bonds promoting dimerization of receptor molecules, leading to activation and signal transmission.

TD I and TD II represent new mutations to normal parents. The recurrence risk is low. Because the mutated codons in TD are mutable for unknown reasons and because of the theoretical risk for germ cell mosaicism, parents are offered prenatal diagnosis for subsequent pregnancies.

Achondroplasia. Achondroplasia (OMIM 100800) is the prototype chondrodysplasia. It typically presents at birth with short limbs, a long narrow trunk, and a large head with midfacial hypoplasia and prominent forehead (Fig. 684–3). The limb shortening is greatest in the proximal segments, and the fingers often display a trident configuration. Most joints are hyperextensible, but extension is restricted at the elbow. A thoracolumbar gibbus is often found. Usually, birth length is slightly less than normal but occasionally plots within the low-normal range.

DIAGNOSIS. Skeletal radiographs confirm the diagnosis (Fig. 684–4). The calvarial bones are large, whereas the cranial base and facial bones are small. The vertebral pedicles are short

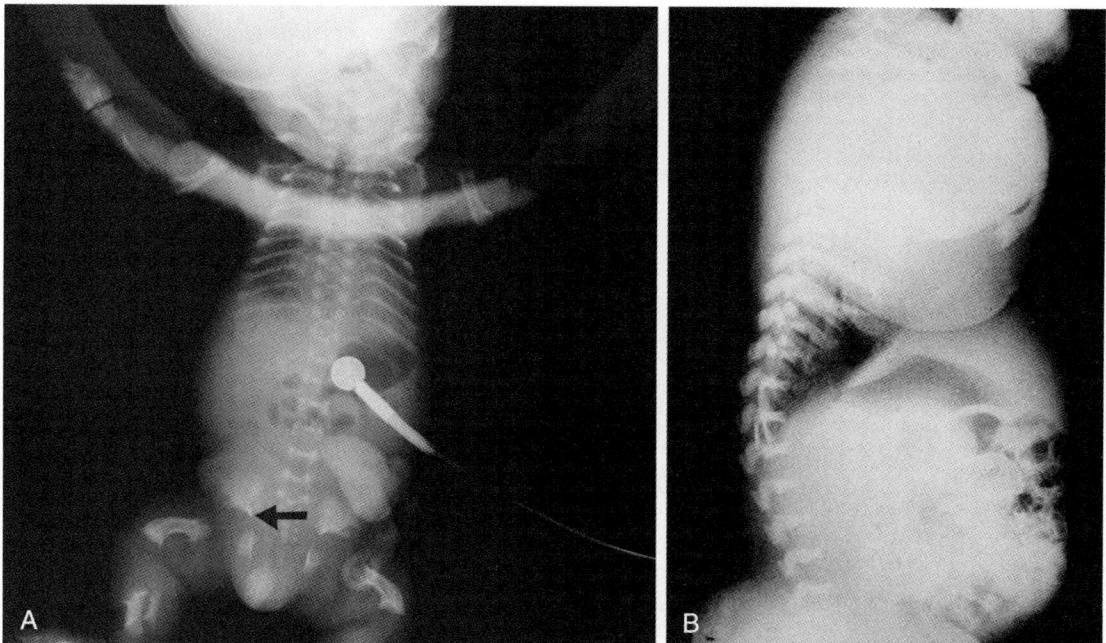

FIGURE 684–2. *A,* Neonatal radiograph of a child with thanatophoric dysplasia. Note medial acetabular spurs *(black arrow),* hypoplastic iliac bones, bowed femora with rounded protrusion of proximal femurs, hypoplastic thorax, and wafer-thin vertebral bodies. *B,* Lateral radiograph of the thoracolumbar spine in thanatophoric dysplasia, showing marked vertebral flattening and short ribs. Ossification defect of the central portion of the vertebral bodies is present.

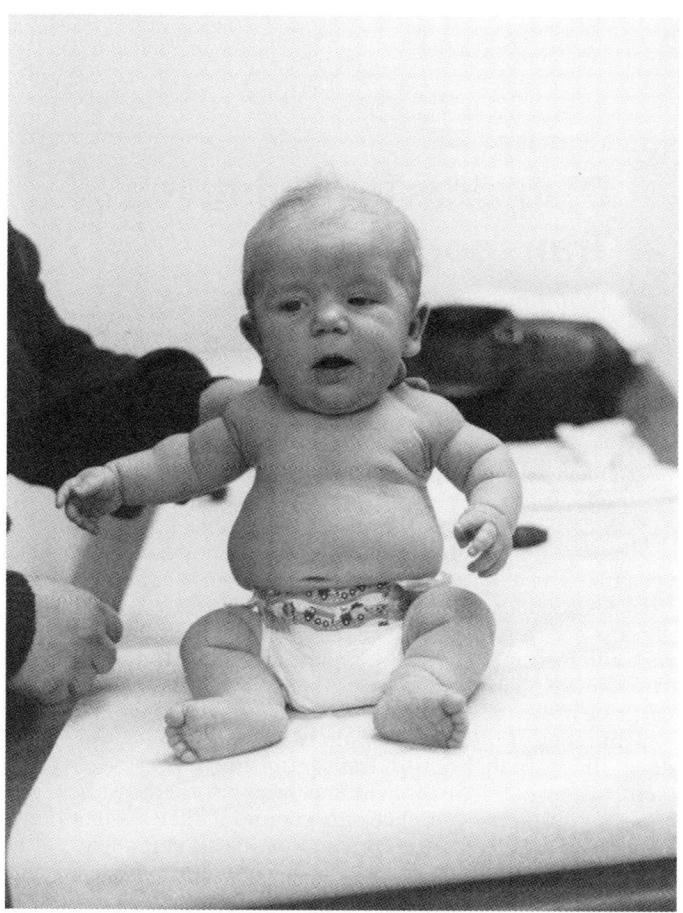

FIGURE 684–3. Infant with achondroplasia. The cranium is large and the forehead prominent. The nasal bridge is moderately flat, and the chest is small compared with the abdomen. Note medial arm and forearm creases, which reflect bowing at the sharpest concavity of the limbs.

throughout the spine as noted on a lateral radiograph. The interpedicular distance, which normally increases from the first to the fifth lumbar vertebrae, decreases in achondroplasia. The iliac bones are short and round, and the acetabular roofs are flat. The tubular bones are short with mildly irregular and flared metaphyses. The fibula is disproportionately long compared with the tibia.

CLINICAL MANIFESTATIONS. Infants usually exhibit delayed motor milestones, frequently not walking alone until 18–24 mo. This is due to hypotonia and mechanical difficulty balancing the large head on a normal-sized trunk and short extremities. Intelligence is normal unless central nervous system complications develop. As the child begins to walk, the gibbus usually gives way to an exaggerated lumbar lordosis.

Infants and children with achondroplasia progressively fall below normal standards for length and height. They can be plotted against standards established for achondroplasia. Adult heights typically range between 118 and 145 cm for males and between 112 and 136 cm for females. Surgical limb lengthening and human growth hormone treatment have been used to increase height; both are controversial.

There are several potential neurologic complications. Virtually all infants and children with achondroplasia have large heads, although only a fraction has true hydrocephalus. Head circumference should be carefully monitored using standards developed for achondroplasia, as should neurologic function in general. The spinal canal is stenotic, and spinal cord compression may occur at the foramen magnum and in the lumbar spine. The former most often presents in infants and small children; it may be associated with hypotonia, failure to thrive, quadriparesis, central and obstructive apnea, and sudden death. Surgical correction may be required for severe stenosis. Lumbar spinal stenosis usually does not present until early adulthood. Symptoms include paresthesias, numbness, and claudication in the legs. Loss of bladder and bowel control may be late complications.

Bowing of the legs is common and may need to be corrected surgically. Other common problems include dental crowding, articulation difficulties, obesity, and frequent episodes of otitis media, which may contribute to hearing loss.

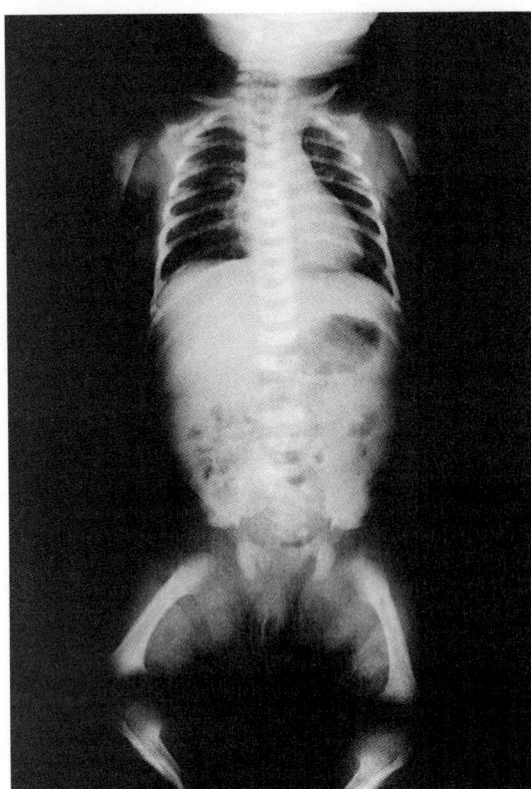

FIGURE 684–4. Radiograph of infant with achondroplasia, demonstrating interpedicular narrowing of the first through fifth lumbar vertebrae, short round iliac bones, and flat acetabular roofs. The tubular bones are short and show mild irregularities of the metaphyses.

GENETICS. All patients with typical achondroplasia have mutations at *FGFR3* codon 380. The mutation maps to the transmembrane domain of the receptor and is thought to stabilize receptor dimers that enhance receptor signals, the consequences of which inhibit linear bone growth. Achondroplasia behaves as an autosomal dominant trait; most cases arise from a new mutation to normal parents.

Because of the high frequency of achondroplasia among dwarfing conditions, it is relatively common for adults with achondroplasia to marry. Such couples have a 50% risk of transmitting their condition, heterozygous achondroplasia, to each offspring, as well as a 25% risk for homozygous achondroplasia. The latter condition exhibits intermediate severity between thanatophoric dysplasia and heterozygous achondroplasia and is usually lethal in the newborn period.

Hypochondroplasia. Hypochondroplasia (OMIM 146000) resembles achondroplasia but is milder. Usually, it is not apparent until childhood, when mild short stature affecting the limbs becomes evident. Children have a stocky build and slight frontal bossing of the head. Radiographic changes are mild and consistent with the mild achondroplastic phenotype. Complications are rare; some patients are never diagnosed. Adult heights range from 116 to 146 cm. An *FGFR3* mutation at codon 540 has been found in many patients with hypochondroplasia.

JANSEN METAPHYSEAL DYSPLASIA

Jansen metaphyseal chondrodysplasia (OMIM 156400) is a rare, dominantly inherited chondrodysplasia characterized by severe shortening of limbs associated with an unusual facial appearance. Sometimes it is accompanied by clubfoot and hypercalcemia. At birth, a diagnosis can be made from these clinical findings and radiographs that show short tubular bones with characteristic metaphyseal abnormalities that include flaring, irregular mineralization, fragmentation, and widening of the physeal space. The epiphyses are normal.

The joints become enlarged and limited in mobility with age. Flexion contractures develop at the knees and hips, producing a bent-over posture. Intelligence is normal, although there may be hearing loss.

Jansen metaphyseal chondrodysplasia is the only disorder due to mutations of *PTHR*. This G protein–coupled transmembrane receptor serves as a receptor for both *PTH* and *PTHrP*. Signaling through this receptor serves as a brake on the terminal differentiation of cartilage cells at a critical step in bone growth. Because the mutations activate the receptor, they enhance the braking effect and thereby slow bone growth.

American Academy of Pediatrics Committee on Genetics: Health supervision for children with achondroplasia. *Pediatrics* 1995;95:443.
Horton WA: Fibroblast growth factor receptor 3 and the human chondrodysplasias. *Curr Opin Pediatr* 1997;9:437.
Hunter AG, Bankier A, Rogers JG, et al: Medical complications of achondroplasia: A multicentre patient review. *J Med Genet* 1998;35:705.
Mogayzel PJ Jr, Carroll JL, Loughlin GM, et al: Sleep-disordered breathing in children with achondroplasia. *J Pediatr* 1998;132:667.
Pauli RM, Horton VK, Glinski LP, et al: Prospective assessment of risks for cervicomedullary-junction compression in infants with achondroplasia. *Am J Hum Genet* 1995;56:732.
Rousseau F, Bonaventure J, Legeai-Mallet L, et al: Clinical and genetic heterogeneity of hypochondroplasia. *J Med Genet* 1996;33:749.
Schipani E, Langman CB, Parfitt AM, et al: Constitutively activated receptors for parathyroid hormone and parathyroid hormone-related peptide in Jansen's metaphyseal chondrodysplasia. *N Engl J Med* 1996;335:708.
Tavormina P, Shiang R, Thompson L, et al: Thanatophoric dysplasia (types I and II) caused by distinct mutations in fibroblast growth factor receptor 3. *Nat Genet* 1995;9:321.

Chapter 685
Disorders Involving Ion Transporter

William A. Horton and Jacqueline T. Hecht

In order of decreasing severity, the disorders involving ion transporters include achondrogenesis type 1B, atelosteogenesis type II, and diastrophic dysplasia. They result from the functional loss of the sulfate ion transporter called *diastrophic dysplasia sulfate transporter* (DTDST), which is also referred to as SLC26A2 (solute carrier family 26, member 2). This protein transports sulfate ions into cells and is important for cartilage cells that add sulfate moieties to newly synthesized proteoglycans destined for cartilage extracellular matrix. Matrix proteoglycans are responsible for many of the properties of cartilage that allow it to serve as a template for skeletal development. The clinical manifestations result from defective sulfation of cartilage proteoglycans.

A number of mutant alleles have been found for the *DTDST* gene; they variably disturb transporter function. None is sufficient to cause disease alone; hence, the disorders are recessive traits requiring the presence of two mutant alleles. The phenotype is determined by the combination of mutant alleles; some alleles are present in more than one disorder.

Diastrophic Dysplasia (OMIM 22600). This well-characterized disorder is recognized at birth by the presence of very short extremities, clubfoot, and short hands with proximal displacement of the thumb producing a hitchhiker appearance (Fig. 685–1). The hands are usually deviated in an ulnar direction. Bony fusion of the metacarpophalangeal joints (sympha-

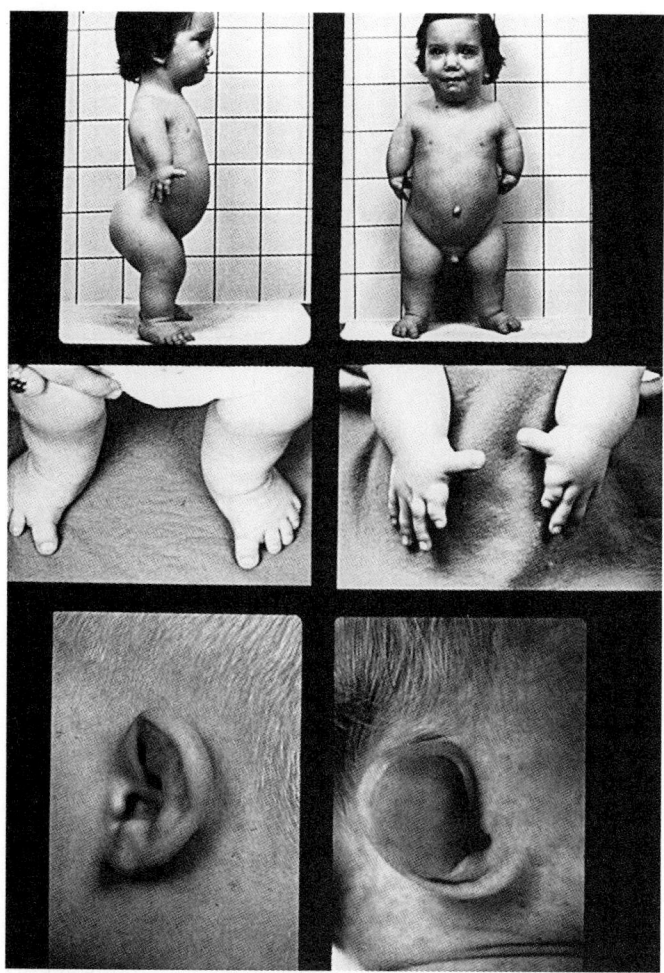

FIGURE 685–1. Child with diastrophic dysplasia. The extremities are dramatically shortened *(top).* Clubfoot is commonly observed *(middle left).* The fingers are short, especially the index finger; the thumb characteristically is proximally placed and has a hitchhiker appearance *(middle right).* The upper helix of the ears becomes swollen 3–4 wk postnatally *(lower left),* and this inflammation spontaneously resolves, leaving a cauliflower deformity of the pinnae *(lower right).*

langism) is common, as is restricted movement of many joints, including hips, knees, and elbows. The external ears frequently become inflamed soon after birth. The inflammation resolves spontaneously but leaves the ears fibrotic and contracted ("cauliflower" ear deformity). Many newborns have a cleft palate.

Radiographs reveal short and broad tubular bones with flared metaphyses and flat, irregular epiphyses (Fig. 685–2).

The capital femoral epiphyses are hypoplastic, and the femoral heads are broad. The ulnae and fibulae are disproportionately short. Carpal centers may be developmentally advanced; the first metacarpal is typically ovoid, and the metatarsals are twisted medially. There may be vertebral abnormalities, including clefts of cervical vertebral lamina and narrowing of the interpedicular distances in the lumbar spine.

Complications are primarily orthopedic and tend to be severe and progressive. The clubfoot deformity in the newborn resists usual treatments, and multiple corrective surgeries are common. Scoliosis typically develops during early childhood. It often requires multiple surgical procedures to control and sometimes compromises respiratory function in older children. Despite the orthopedic problems, patients typically have a normal life span and reach adult heights in the 105–130 cm range, depending on the severity of scoliosis. Growth curves are available for diastrophic dysplasia.

Some patients are mildly affected and exhibit slight short stature and joint contractures, no clubfoot or cleft palate, and correspondingly mild radiographic changes. The mild phenotype tends to recur within families. The recurrence risk for this autosomal recessive condition is 25%. Ultrasonographic examination can be employed for prenatal diagnosis, but if *DTDST* mutations can be identified in the parents, molecular genetic diagnosis is possible.

Achondrogenesis Type 1B (OMIM 600972) and Atelosteogenesis Type II (OMIM 256050).

Both of the conditions are rare recessive lethal chondrodysplasias. The most serious is achondrogenesis type 1B, which demonstrates a severe lack of skeletal development usually detected in utero or after a miscarriage. The limbs are extremely short, and the head is soft. Skeletal radiographs show poor to missing ossification of skull bones, vertebral bodies, fibulas, and ankle bones. The pelvis is hypoplastic, and the ribs are short. The femurs are short and exhibit a trapezoid shape with irregular metaphyses.

Infants with *atelosteogenesis type II* are stillborn or die soon after birth; prematurity is common. They exhibit very short limbs, especially the proximal segments. Clubfoot and dislocations of the elbows and knees may be detected. Hypoplasia of vertebral bodies, especially in the cervical and lumbar spine, is found on radiographs. The femora and humeri are hypoplastic and display a club-shaped appearance. The distal limb bones, including the ulna and fibula, are poorly ossified.

Both disorders carry a 25% recurrence risk and are potentially detectable in utero by mutation analysis if the mutant alleles are identified in the parents. Prenatal diagnosis should be possible with fetal ultrasonography.

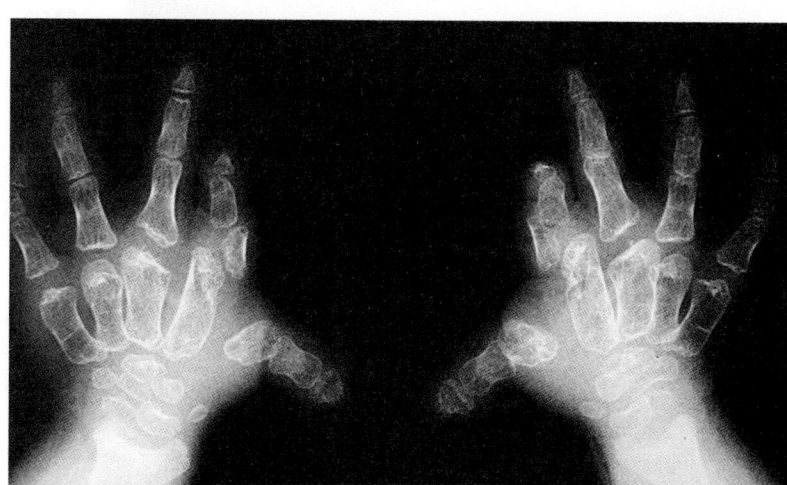

FIGURE 685–2. Radiograph of hands in diastrophic dysplasia. The metacarpals and phalanges are irregular and short. The first metacarpal is ovoid.

Hall BD: Diastrophic dysplasia: Extreme variability within a sibship. *Am J Med Genet* 1996;63:28.

Makitie O, Kaitila I: Growth in diastrophic dysplasia. *J Pediatr* 1997;130:641.

Newbury-Ecob R: Atelosteogenesis type 2. *J Med Genet* 1998;35:49.

Rossi A, Superti-Furga A: Mutations in the diastrophic dysplasia sulfate transporter (DTDST) gene *(SLC26A2):* 22 novel mutations, mutation review, associated skeletal phenotypes, and diagnostic relevance. *Hum Mutat* 2001;17:159.

Chapter 686
Disorders Involving Transcription Factors

William A. Horton and Jacqueline T. Hecht

There are three disorders involving transcription factors that result in bone dysplasias. One, campomelic dysplasia, is historically considered a chondrodysplasia. The other two, cleidocranial dysplasia and nail-patella syndrome, have been regarded as dysostoses, or abnormalities of single bones. The mutant genes that encode these transcription factors are *SOX9*, *CBFA1*, and *LMX1B*, respectively and are members of much larger gene families. For instance, *SOX9* is a member of the *SOX* family of genes related to the *SRY* (sex-determining region of the Y chromosome) gene; *CBFA1* belongs to the *runt* family of transcription factor genes, and *LMX1B* is one of the *LIM* homeodomain gene family. All three disorders are due to haploinsufficiency of the respective gene products; the disorders are dominant traits.

Campomelic Dysplasia. Apparent in newborn infants, campomelic dysplasia (OMIM 114290) is characterized by bowing of long bones (especially in the lower legs), short bones, respiratory distress, and other anomalies that include defects of the cervical spine, central nervous system, heart, and kidneys. Several cases of sex reversal of XY males have been reported. Radiographs confirm the bowing and often show hypoplasia of the scapulae and

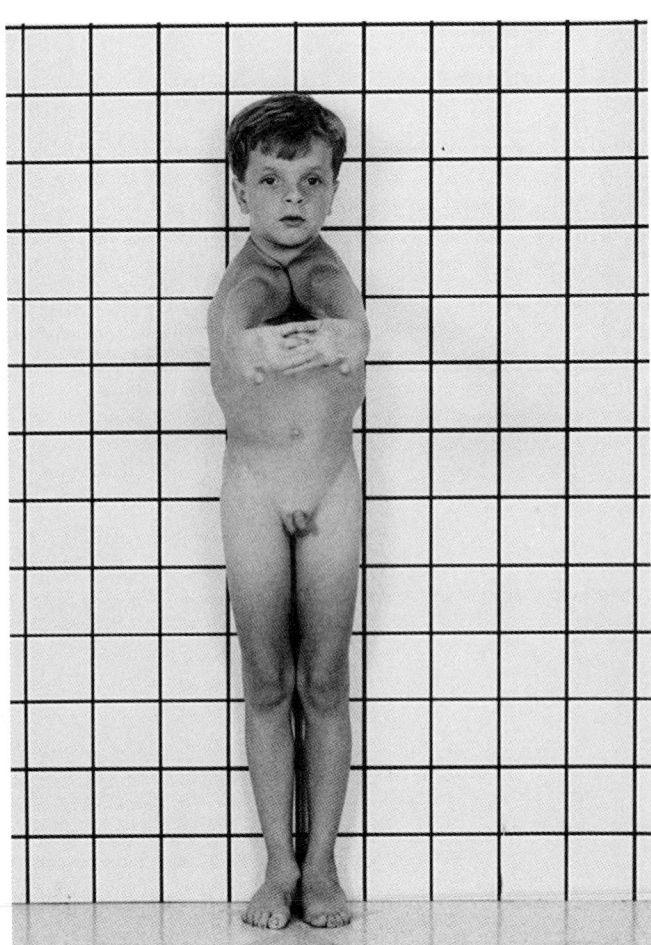

FIGURE 686–2. Cleidocranial dysplasia demonstrating approximation of the shoulder girdle in the midline. Note prominent high forehead and hypertelorism.

pelvic bones (Fig. 686–1). Affected infants usually die of respiratory distress in the neonatal period.

Cleidocranial Dysplasia. Cleidocranial dysplasia (OMIM 114290) is recognized in infants because of drooping shoulders, open fontanelles, prominent forehead, mild short stature, and dental abnormalities (Fig. 686–2). Radiographs reveal hypoplastic or absent clavicles, delayed ossification of the cranial bones with multiple ossification centers (wormian bones), and delayed ossification of pelvic bones. The course is usually uncomplicated except for dislocations, especially of the shoulders, and dental anomalies that require therapy.

Nail-Patella Syndrome. Dysplasia of the nails, absence or hypoplasia of the patella, abnormalities of the elbow, and spurs or "horns" extending from the iliac bones characterize the nail-patella syndrome (OMIM 119600), which is also called *osteo-onychodysostosis*. Some patients have nephritis that resembles chronic glomerulonephritis. There is a wide spectrum of severity; some patients present in early childhood, whereas others are asymptomatic as adults.

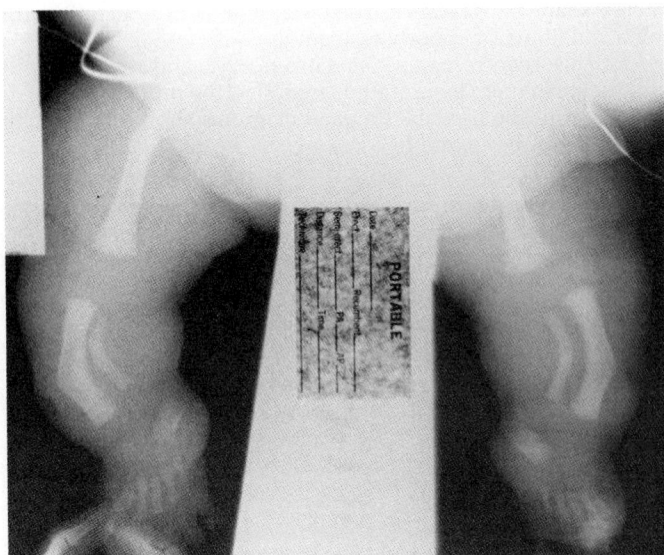

FIGURE 686–1. Radiograph of lower extremities of a child with campomelic dysplasia. Note bowed femurs, which are not particularly wide as compared with the thick bowed tibiae and fibulae.

Dryer SD, Zhou G, Baldini A, et al: Mutations in *LMX1B* cause abnormal skeletal patterning and renal dysplasia in nail patella syndrome. *Nat Genet* 1998;19:47.

Meyer J, Sudbeck P, Held M, et al: Mutational analysis of the *SOX9* gene in campomelic dysplasia and autosomal sex reversal: Lack of genotype/phenotype correlations. *Hum Mol Genet* 1997;6:91.

Mundlos S, Otto F, Mundlos C, et al: Mutations involving the transcription factor CBFA1 cause cleidocranial dysplasia. *Cell* 1997;89:773.

Chapter 687

Disorders Involving Defective Bone Resorption

William A. Horton and Jacqueline T. Hecht

Many bone dysplasias display increased bone density; most are rare. Osteopetrosis, which has many subtypes, and pyknodysostosis, and probably others in this category of bone dysplasias, result from defective bone resorption.

OSTEOPETROSIS

Two main forms of osteopetrosis have been delineated: a severe, autosomal recessive form (OMIM 259700) and a mild, autosomal dominant form (OMIM 166600). Disturbances of osteoclast function due to mutations in a gene encoding an osteoclast-specific subunit of the vacuolar proton pump *(TCIRG1)* are found in many patients with the recessive form. The dominant form of osteopetrosis has been genetically mapped to chromosome 1p21. The severe form is usually detected in infancy or earlier because of macrocephaly, hepatosplenomegaly, deafness, blindness, and severe anemia. Radiographs reveal diffuse bone sclerosis. Later films show a bone within a bone, which is characteristic. With time, infants typically fail to thrive and show psychomotor delay and worsening of cranial neuropathies and anemia. Dental problems, osteomyelitis of the mandible, and pathologic fractures are common. The most severely affected patients die during infancy; less severely affected individuals rarely survive beyond the 2nd decade. Those who survive beyond infancy usually have learning disorders but may have normal intelligence despite hearing and visual loss.

Clinical Manifestations. Most of the manifestations are due to failure to remodel growing bones. This leads to narrowing of cranial nerve foramina and encroachment on marrow spaces, which results in secondary complications, such as optic and facial nerve dysfunction, and anemia accompanied by compensatory extramedullary hematopoiesis in the liver and spleen.

The autosomal dominant form of osteopetrosis (Albers-Schönberg disease, osteopetrosis tarda, or marble bone disease) usually presents during childhood or adolescence with fractures and mild anemia and, less frequently, as cranial nerve dysfunction, dental abnormalities, or osteomyelitis of the mandible. Skeletal radiographs reveal a generalized increase in bone density and clubbing of metaphyses (Fig. 687–1). Alternating bands of lucent and dense bands produce a sandwich appearance to vertebral bodies. The radiographic changes are sometimes incidental findings in otherwise asymptomatic adolescents and adults.

Treatment. The basic defect is thought to involve osteoclast differentiation because bone marrow transplantation with reconstitution of osteoclasts from donor cells has been successful in some patients. Calcitriol and interferon gamma have been used with some benefit in some patients. Symptomatic care, such as dental care, transfusions for anemia, and antibiotic treatment of infections, is important for patients who survive infancy.

PYKNODYSOSTOSIS

An autosomal recessive bone dysplasia, pyknodysostosis (OMIM 265800) presents in early childhood as short limbs, characteristic facies, an open anterior fontanelle, a large skull with frontal and occipital bossing, and dental abnormalities.

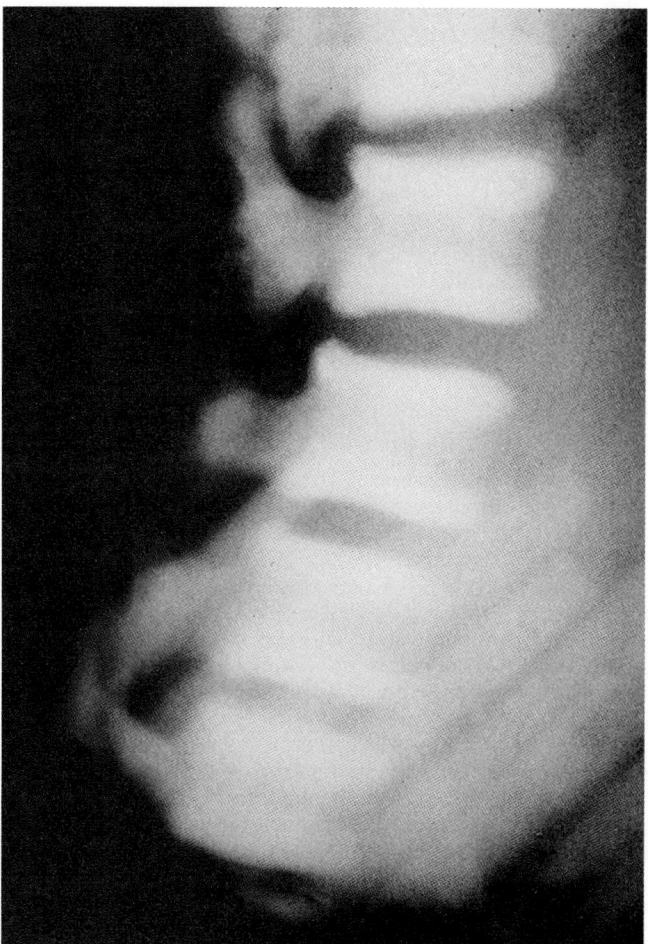

FIGURE 687–1. Lateral radiograph showing bone-in-bone appearance that is characteristic of osteopetrosis.

The hands and feet are short and broad, and the nails may be dysplastic. The sclerae may be blue. Minimal trauma often leads to fractures. Treatment is symptomatic and focused mainly on the management of dental problems and fractures. The prognosis is generally good, and patients typically reach heights of 130–150 cm.

Skeletal radiographs show a generalized increase in bone density. In contrast to many disorders in this group, the metaphyses are normal. Other changes include wide sutures and wormian bones in the skull, a small mandible, and hypoplasia of the distal phalanges.

Several mutations have been found in the gene encoding cathepsin K, a cysteine protease that is highly expressed in osteoclasts. The mutations predict loss of enzyme function, suggesting that there is an inability of osteoclasts to degrade bone matrix and remodel bones.

Charles JM, Key LL: Developmental spectrum of children with congenital osteopetrosis. *J Pediatr* 1998;132:371.

Frattini A, Orchard PJ, Sobacchi C, et al: Defects in TCIRG1 subunit of the vacuolar proton pump are responsible for a subset of human autosomal recessive osteopetrosis. *Nat Genet* 2000;25:343.

Gelb BD, Shi GP, Chapman HA, et al: Pycnodysostosis, a lysosomal disease caused by cathepsin K deficiency. *Science* 1996;273:1236.

Gerritsen EJ, Vossen JM, Fasth A, et al: Bone marrow transplantation for autosomal recessive osteopetrosis: A report from the Working Party on Inborn Errors of the European Bone Marrow Transplantation Group. *J Pediatr* 1994;125:896.

Key LL Jr, Rodriguiz RM, Willi SM, et al: Long-term treatment of osteopetrosis with recombinant human interferon gamma. *N Engl J Med* 1995;332:1594.

Chapter 688

Disorders for Which Defects Are Poorly Understood or Unknown

William A. Horton and Jacqueline T. Hecht

There are many chondrodysplasias, or chondrodysplasia clinical phenotypes, for which the genetic cause or basic mechanism is poorly understood or not known. Many illustrate features not found in other disorders and have historical significance in the evolution of chondrodysplasia nomenclature and classification.

Ellis-Van Creveld Syndrome. The Ellis-van Creveld syndrome (OMIM 225500), also known as *chondroectodermal dysplasia,* is a skeletal and an ectodermal dysplasia. The skeletal dysplasia presents at birth with short limbs, especially the middle and distal segments, accompanied by postaxial polydactyly of the hands and sometimes of the feet. Nail dysplasia and dental anomalies (including neonatal, absent, and premature loss of teeth, and upper lip defects) constitute the ectodermal dysplasia. Common manifestations also include atrial septum defects and other congenital heart defects.

Skeletal radiographs reveal short tubular bones with clubbed ends, especially the proximal tibia and ulna (Fig. 688–1). Carpal bones display extra ossification centers and fusion; cone-shaped epiphyses are evident in the hands. A bony spur is often noted above the medial aspect of the acetabulum.

Ellis-van Creveld syndrome is an autosomal recessive trait that occurs most often in the Amish. Mutations have been identified in a novel gene, *EvC,* although the function of its protein product is unknown. About 30% of patients die of cardiac or respiratory problems during infancy. Life span is otherwise normal; adult heights range from 109–152 cm.

Asphyxiating Thoracic Dystrophy. Asphyxiating thoracic dystrophy (OMIM 208500), or Jeune syndrome, is an autosomal recessive chondrodysplasia that resembles Ellis-van Creveld syndrome. Newborn infants present with a long, narrow thorax and respiratory insufficiency associated with pulmonary hypoplasia. Neonates often die. Other neonatal manifestations include slightly short limbs and postaxial polydactyly.

Skeletal radiographs show very short ribs with anterior expansion. Tubular limb bones are short with bulbous ends; cone-shaped epiphyses occur in hand bones. The iliac bones are short and square with a spur above the medial aspect of the acetabulum.

If infants survive the neonatal period, respiratory function usually improves as the rib cage grows. Progressive renal dysfunction frequently develops during childhood. Intestinal malabsorption and hepatic dysfunction have also been reported.

Short-Rib Polydactyly Syndromes. Four types of short-rib polydactyly syndrome (types I–IV) (OMIM 263530, 263520, 263510, 269860) have been described. All are lethal in the newborn period. Neonates present with respiratory distress, an extremely small thorax, very short extremities, polydactyly, and a variety of nonskeletal defects. Radiographs demonstrate very short ribs and tubular bones with changes characteristic for each type. All four types are autosomal recessive traits.

Cartilage-Hair Hypoplasia. Cartilage-hair hypoplasia (OMIM 250250) is also known as metaphyseal chondrodysplasia–McKusick type. It is recognized during the 2nd year because of growth deficiency affecting the limbs, accompanied by flaring of the lower rib cage, a prominent sternum, and bowing of the legs.

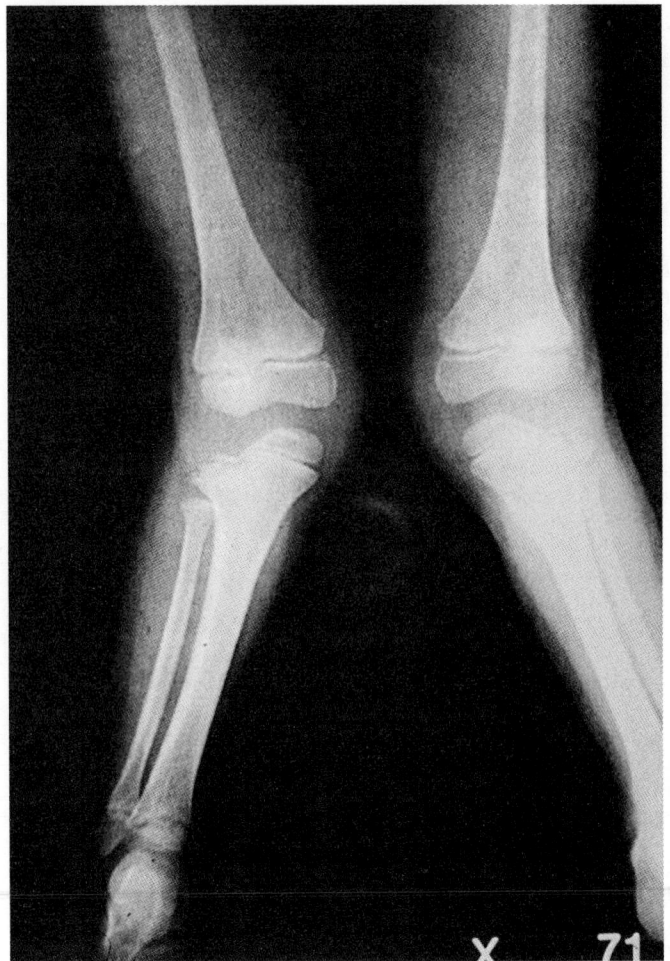

FIGURE 688–1. Radiograph of lower extremities in Ellis-van Creveld syndrome. Tubular bones are short, and proximal fibula is short. Ossification is retarded in lateral tibia epiphyses, causing a knock-knee deformity.

The hands and feet are short, and the fingers are very short with extreme ligamentous laxity. The hair is thin, sparse, and light colored, and nails are hypoplastic. The skin is hypopigmented.

Radiographs show short tubular bones with flared, irregularly mineralized and cupped metaphyses (Fig. 688–2). The knees are more affected than are the hips, and the fibula is disproportionately longer than the tibia. The metacarpals and phalanges are short and broad. Spinal radiographs reveal mild platyspondyly.

Nonskeletal manifestations associated with cartilage-hair hypoplasia include immune deficiency (T-cell abnormalities, neutropenia, leukopenia, and susceptibility to chickenpox; children also may have complications from smallpox and polio vaccinations), malabsorption, celiac disease, and Hirschsprung disease. Adults are at risk for malignancy, especially skin tumors and lymphoma. Adults reach heights of 107–157 cm.

Cartilage-hair hypoplasia shows autosomal recessive inheritance. Although rare, its highest prevalence is in the Amish and Finnish populations. It results from mutations of a gene coding for a large untranslated RNA component of an enzyme complex involved in processing mitochondrial RNA (RMRP). Loss of this gene product may interfere with processing of 5.8S ribosomal RNA, disturbing protein translation and control of mitosis.

Metatropic Dysplasia. There are at least two forms of metatropic dysplasia (OMIM 156530, 250600), an autosomal dominant and an autosomal recessive form. Regardless of type, newborn infants present with a long narrow trunk and short extremities.

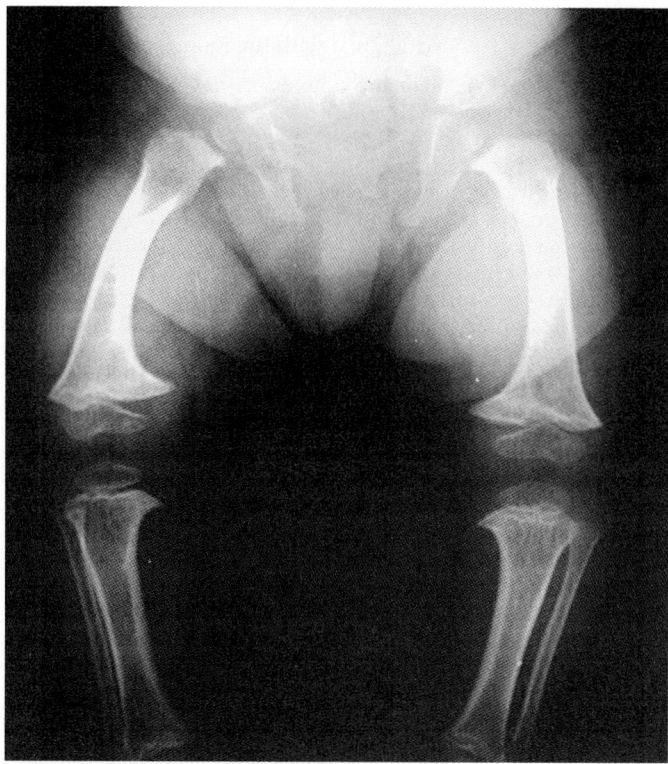

Figure 688–2. Radiograph of lower extremities in cartilage hair hypoplasia. The tubular bones are short and the metaphyses are flared and irregular. The fibula is disproportionately long compared with the tibia. The femoral necks are short.

A tail-like appendage sometimes extends from the base of the spine. Odontoid hypoplasia is common and may be associated with cervical instability. Kyphoscoliosis appears in late infancy and progresses through childhood, often becoming severe

enough to compromise cardiopulmonary function. The joints are large and become progressively restricted in mobility, except in the hands. Contractures often develop in the hips and knees during childhood. Although severely affected infants may die at a young age from respiratory failure, patients usually survive, although they may become disabled as adults from the progressive musculoskeletal deformities. Adult heights range from 110–120 cm.

Skeletal radiographs show characteristic changes dominated by severe platyspondyly and short tubular bones with expanded and deformed metaphyses that exhibit a dumbbell appearance (Fig. 688–3). The pelvic bones are hypoplastic and exhibit a halberd appearance because of a small sacrosciatic notch and a notch above the lateral margin of the acetabulum.

Spondylometaphyseal Dysplasia—Kozlowski Type. The Kozlowski type of spondylometaphyseal dysplasia (OMIM 184252) presents in early childhood with mild short stature involving mostly the trunk and a waddling gait. The hands and feet may be short and stubby. Radiographs show flattening of vertebral bodies. The metaphyses of tubular bones are widened and irregularly mineralized, especially at the proximal femur. The pelvic bones manifest mild hypoplasia.

Scoliosis may develop during adolescence. The disorder is otherwise uncomplicated, and manifestations are limited to the skeleton. Adults reach heights of 130–150 cm. The Kozlowski type of spondylometaphyseal dysplasia is an autosomal dominant trait.

Juvenile Osteochondroses. The juvenile osteochondroses are a heterogeneous group of disorders in which regional disturbances in bone growth cause noninflammatory arthropathies. They are summarized in Table 688–1. Some have localized pain and tenderness (Freiberg disease, Osgood-Schlatter disease, osteochondritis dissecans), whereas others present with painless limitation of joint movement (Legg-Calvé-Perthes disease, Scheuermann disease). Bone growth may be disrupted, leading to deformities. The diagnosis is usually confirmed radiographically, and treatment is symptomatic. The pathogenesis of these disorders is believed to involve ischemic necrosis of primary and

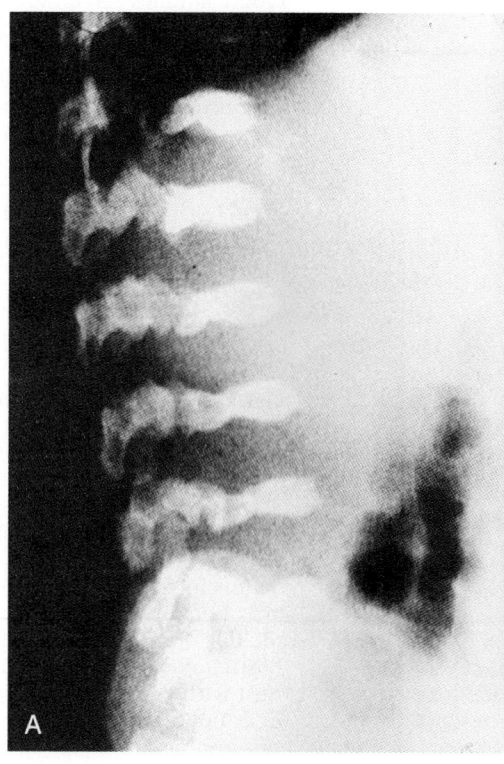
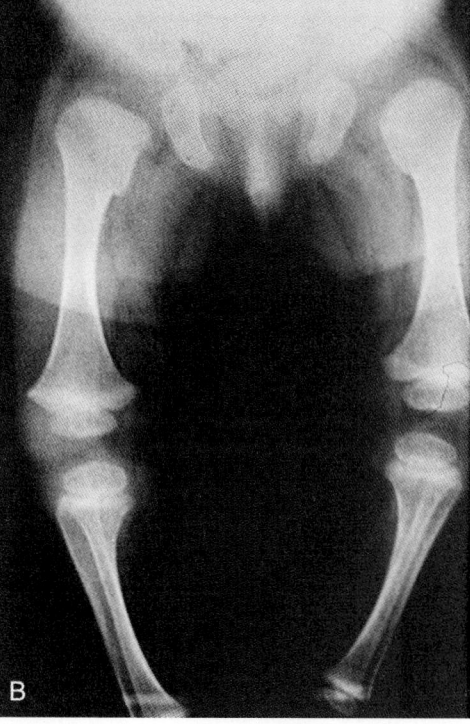

Figure 688–3. *A,* Radiograph of the lateral thoracolumbar spine in metatropic dysplasia showing severe platyspondyly. *B,* Radiograph of lower extremities in metatropic dysplasia showing short tubular bones with widened metaphyses. The femurs have a dumbbell appearance.

TABLE 688–1. Juvenile Osteochondroses

Eponym	Affected Region	Age at Presentation
Legg-Calvé-Perthes disease	Capital femoral epiphysis	3–12 yr
Osgood-Schlatter disease	Tibial tubercle	10–16 yr
Sever disease	Os calcaneus	6–10 yr
Freiberg disease	Head of second metatarsal	10–14 yr
Scheuermann disease	Vertebral bodies	Adolescence
Blount disease	Medial aspect of proximal tibial epiphysis	Infancy or adolescence
Osteochondritis dissecans	Subchondral regions of knee, hip, elbow and ankle	Adolescence

secondary ossification centers. Although familial forms have been reported, these disorders usually occur sporadically.

Beck M, Roubicek M, Rogers JG, et al: Heterogeneity of metatropic dysplasia. *Eur J Pediatr* 1983;140:231.

da Silva EO, Janovitz D, de Albuquerque SC: Ellis-van Creveld syndrome: Report of 15 cases in an inbred kindred. *J Med Genet* 1980;17:349.

Makitie O, Sulisalo T, de la Chapelle A, et al: Cartilage-hair hypoplasia. *J Med Genet* 1995;32:39.

Ruiz-Perez VL, Ide SE, Strom TM, et al: Mutations in a new gene in Ellis-van Creveld syndrome and Weyers acrodental dysostosis. *Nat Genet* 2000;24:283.

Ridanpaa M, van Eenennaam H, Pelin K, et al: Mutations in the RNA component of RNase MRP cause a pleiotropic human disease, cartilage-hair hypoplasia. *Cell* 2001;104:195.

Sharrard WJW: Abnormalities of the epiphyses and limb inequality. In Sharrard WJW (editor): *Paediatric Orthopaedics and Fracture*, 3rd ed. Oxford, Blackwell Scientific Publications, 1993, p 719.

Chapter 689
Osteogenesis Imperfecta

Joan C. Marini

Osteoporosis, a feature of both inherited and acquired disorders, classically demonstrates fragility of the skeletal system and a susceptibility to fractures of the long bones or vertebral compressions from mild or inconsequential trauma. Osteogenesis imperfecta (OI) (brittle bone disease), the most common genetic cause of osteoporosis, is a generalized disorder of connective tissue. The spectrum of OI is extremely broad, ranging from a form that is lethal in the perinatal period to a mild form in which the diagnosis may be equivocal in an adult.

Etiology. All types of OI are caused by structural or quantitative defects in type I collagen, the primary component of the extracellular matrix of bone and skin. In about 10% of clinically indistinguishable cases, no biochemical or molecular defect of collagen can be demonstrated. It is not clear whether these cases represent limitations in detection or genetic heterogeneity of the disorder.

Epidemiology. OI is an autosomal dominant disorder that occurs in all racial and ethnic groups. The incidence of OI that is detectable in infancy is about 1 in 20,000. There is a similar incidence of the mild form, OI type I.

Pathology. The collagen structural mutations cause OI bone to be globally abnormal. The bone matrix contains abnormal type I collagen fibrils and relatively increased levels of types III and V collagen. In addition, several noncollagenous proteins of bone

matrix are also reduced. The hydroxyapatite crystals deposited on this matrix are poorly aligned with the long axis of fibrils.

Pathogenesis. Type I collagen is a heterotrimer, composed of two α1(I) chains and one α2(I) chain. The chains are synthesized as procollagen molecules with short globular extensions on both ends of the central helical domain. The helical domain is composed of uninterrupted repeats of the sequence Gly-X-Y, where Gly is glycine, X is often proline, and Y is often hydroxyproline. The presence of glycine at every third residue is crucial to helix formation because its small side chain can be accommodated in the spatial constraints of the interior of the helical trimer. The chains are assembled into helices using crucial alignment sites in the carboxyl-terminal extension. Helix formation then proceeds linearly in a carboxyl to amino direction. Concomitant with helix assembly and formation, the chains are glycosylated at lysine residues.

The collagen structural defects are predominately of two types: 85% are point mutations causing substitutions of glycine residues by other amino acids, and 12% are single exon splicing defects. The clinically mild OI type I has a quantitative defect with mutations that cause one α1(I) allele to be functionally null. These patients make a reduced amount of normal collagen.

The relationship between genotype and phenotype remains elusive for the structural mutations. Lethal and nonlethal mutations occur with about equal frequency on both chains. For α2(I) mutations, lethal and nonlethal mutations occur in alternating regions along the chain. For mutations on the α1(I) chain, no model adequately predicts phenotype.

OI is an autosomal dominant disorder. A minority of OI cases with apparent recessive inheritance are caused by parental mosaicism and are also dominant.

Clinical Manifestations. OI has the triad of fragile bones, blue sclerae, and early deafness. OI was once divided into "congenita," the forms detectable at birth, and "tarda," the forms detectable later in childhood; this did not account for the variability of OI. The current classification divides OI into four types based on clinical and radiographic criteria.

TYPE I OSTEOGENESIS IMPERFECTA (MILD). This form is sufficiently mild that it is often found in large pedigrees. Many type I families have blue sclerae, recurrent fractures in childhood, and presenile hearing loss (30–60%). Both types I and IV are divided into A and B subtypes, depending on the absence (A) or presence (B) of dentinogenesis imperfecta. Other possible connective tissue abnormalities include easy bruising, joint laxity, and mild short stature compared with family members. Fractures result from mild to moderate trauma and decrease after puberty.

OSTEOGENESIS IMPERFECTA TYPE II (PERINATAL LETHAL). These infants may be stillborn or die in the 1st yr of life. Birthweight and length are small for gestational age. There is extreme fragility of the skeleton and other connective tissues. There are multiple intrauterine fractures of long bones, which have a crumpled appearance on radiographs. There is striking micromelia and bowing of extremities; the legs are held abducted at right angles to the body in the "frog-leg position." Multiple rib fractures create a beaded appearance and the small thorax contributes to respiratory insufficiency. The skull is large for body size with enlarged anterior and posterior fontanelles. Sclerae are dark blue-gray.

OSTEOGENESIS IMPERFECTA TYPE III (PROGRESSIVE DEFORMING). This is the most severe nonlethal form of OI and results in significant physical disability. Birthweight and length are often low normal. Fractures usually occur in utero. There is relative macrocephaly and triangular facies (Fig. 689–1). Postnatally, fractures occur from inconsequential trauma and heal with deformity. Disorganization of the bone matrix results in a "popcorn" appearance at the metaphyses (Fig. 689–2). The rib cage has flaring at the base, and pectal deformity is frequent.

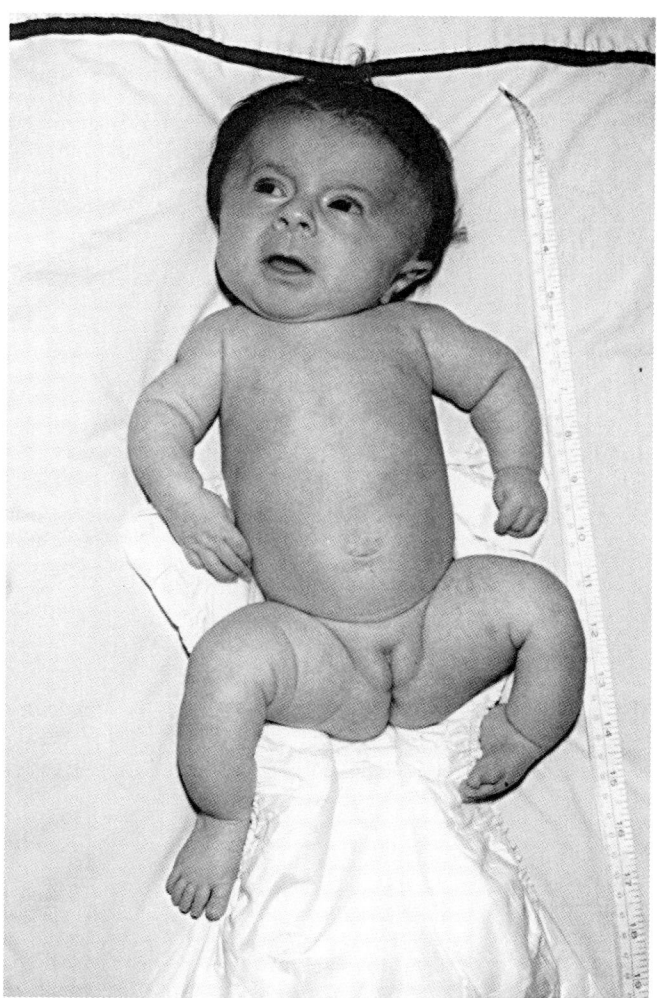

FIGURE 689–1. Infant with type III OI displays shortened bowed extremities, thoracic deformity, and relative macrocephaly.

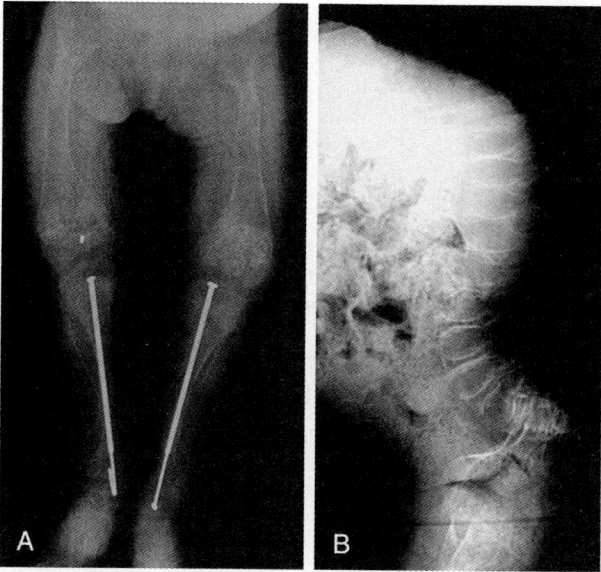

FIGURE 689–2. Typical features of type III OI radiographs in 6-yr-old child. *A,* Lower long bones are osteoporotic, with metaphyseal flaring, "popcorn" formation at growth plates, and placement of intramedullary rods. *B,* Vertebral bodies are compressed and osteoporotic.

Virtually all type III patients have scoliosis and vertebral compression. Growth falls below the curve by the first year; all type III patients have extreme short stature. Scleral hue ranges from white to blue.

OSTEOGENESIS IMPERFECTA TYPE IV (MODERATELY SEVERE). Patients with OI type IV may present at birth with in utero fractures or bowing of lower long bones. They may also present with recurrent fractures after ambulation. Most children have moderate bowing even with infrequent fractures. Children with OI type IV require orthopedic and rehabilitation intervention, but they are usually able to attain community ambulation skills. Fracture rates decrease after puberty. Radiographically, they are osteoporotic and have metaphyseal flaring and vertebral compressions. Patients with type IV have moderate short stature. Scleral hue may be blue or white.

OSTEOGENESIS IMPERFECTA TYPE V (HYPERPLASTIC CALLUS). There has been a proposal to distinguish as a distinct type a group of patients who are clinically within OI type IV. These patients have hyperplastic callus, calcification of the interosseus membrane of the forearm, and a radiodense metaphyseal band. Bone histology has a distinct meshlike appearance of the lamellae under polarized light. Collagen mutation screening is negative in this small group.

Laboratory Findings. The diagnosis is confirmed by collagen biochemical studies using fibroblasts cultured from a skin punch biopsy. Most collagen structural mutations cause a delay in helix formation, which results in overmodification of chains and the presence of broad or delayed bands on protein electrophoresis. In OI type I, the reduced amount of type I collagen results in an increase in the type III:type I collagen ratio detected by protein electrophoresis. Molecular techniques can identify the particular collagen mutation. This allows family members to be diagnosed using leukocyte DNA.

Severe OI can be detected prenatally by level II ultrasonography as early as 16 wk of gestation. OI and thanatophoric dysplasia may be confused. Fetal ultrasonography may not detect OI type IV and rarely detects OI type I. For recurrent cases, chorionic villus biopsy can be used for biochemical or molecular studies. Amniocytes produce false-positive biochemical studies but can be used for molecular studies in appropriate cases.

In the neonatal period, the normal to elevated alkaline phosphatase levels present in OI distinguish it from hypophosphatasia.

Complications. The morbidity and mortality of OI are cardiopulmonary. Recurrent pneumonias and transient cardiac failure occur in childhood, and cor pulmonale is seen in adults.

Neurologic complications include basilar invagination, brainstem compression, hydrocephalus, and syringohydromyelia. Most children with OI types III and IV have basilar invagination, but brainstem compression is infrequent. Basilar invagination is best detected with spiral CT of the craniocervical junction (Fig. 689–3).

Treatment. There is no cure for OI. For severe nonlethal OI, active physical rehabilitation in the early years allows children to attain a higher functional level than does orthopedic management alone. Children with OI type I and some with type IV are spontaneous ambulators. Children with type III and severe type IV benefit from long-leg plastic braces, gait aids, and a program of swimming and conditioning. Severely affected individuals require a wheelchair for community mobility but can acquire transfer and self-care skills. Teens with OI may require psychologic support with body image issues.

Orthopedic management of OI is aimed at fracture management and correction of deformity to enable function. Fractures

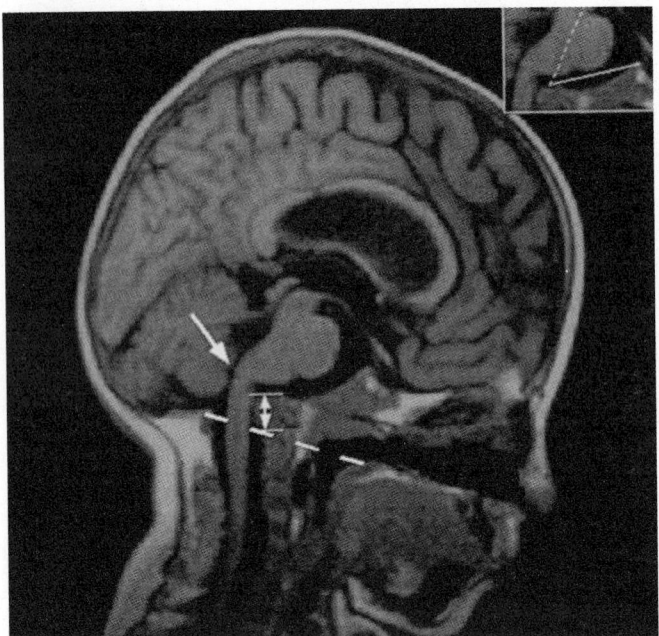

FIGURE 689–3. Typical features of basilar invagination shown in the sagittal MRI of an asymptomatic child with type III OI. There is invagination of the odontoid above the Chamberlain line causing compression and kinking at the pontomedullary junction *(arrow)*.

should be promptly splinted or cast; OI fractures heal well, and cast removal should be aimed at minimizing immobilization osteoporosis. Correction of deformity of the long bones requires an osteotomy procedure and placement of an intramedullary rod.

Treatments with calcium or fluoride supplements or calcitonin do not improve OI. Growth hormone improves bone histologic characteristics in growth-responsive children (usually types I and IV). Treatment with bisphosphonate drugs is effective in improving mobility and decreasing symptoms in many patients. Intravenous pamidronate or oral alendronate improves quality of life and inhibits bone resorption, thus increasing bone mineralization; these agents decrease fractures and bone pain, although the matrix still contains mutant type I collagen. The benefit for trabecular bone appears most promising, with increased vertebral bone density and height. The treatment effect may be independent of severity, mutation type, or age at onset of therapy. The effect of bisphosphonates on development and on the mechanical properties of cortical bone in long bones is under investigation.

Prognosis. OI is a chronic condition that limits both life span and functional level. Infants with OI type II usually die within months to a year of life. An occasional child with radiographic type II and extreme growth deficiency may survive to the teen years. Persons with OI type III have a reduced life span with clusters of mortality from pulmonary causes in early childhood, the teen years, and the 40s. OI types I and IV are compatible with a full life span.

Individuals with OI type III are usually wheelchair dependent. With aggressive rehabilitation, they may attain transfer skills and household ambulation. OI type IV children usually attain community ambulation skills either independently or with gait aids.

Genetic Counseling. OI is an autosomal dominant disorder, and the risk of an affected individual passing the gene to his or her offspring is 50%. An affected child usually has about the same severity of OI as the parent; however, there is variability of

expression and the child's condition can be either more or less severe than that of the parent.

The recurrence risk to an apparently unaffected couple of having a second child with OI is empirically noted to be 5–7%; this is the statistical chance that one parent has a germ line mosaicism. The collagen mutation in the unaffected parent is present in some germ cells and may be present in somatic tissues. If genetic testing reveals that a parent is a mosaic carrier, the risk of recurrence may be as high as 50%.

Antoniazzi F, Bertoldo F, Mottes M, et al: Growth hormone treatment in osteogenesis imperfecta with quantitative defect of type I collagen synthesis. *J Pediatr* 1996;129:432.
Åström E, Söderhäll S: Beneficial effect of long term intravenous bisphosphonate treatment of osteogenesis imperfecta. *Arch Dis Child* 2002;86:356–64.
Glorieux FH, Rauch F, Plotkin H, et al: Type V osteogenesis imperfecta: A new form of brittle bone disease. *J Bone Miner Res* 2000;15:1650.
Kuivaniemi H, Tromp G, Prockop DJ: Mutations in fibrillar collagens (types I, II, III, and XI), fibril-associated collagen (type IX), and network-forming collagen (type X) cause a spectrum of diseases of bone, cartilage and blood vessels. *Hum Mutat* 1997;9:300.
Lee YS, Low SL, Lim LA, et al: Cyclic pamidronate infusion improves bone mineralization and reduces fracture incidence in osteogenesis imperfecta. *Eur J Pediatr* 2001;160:641–4.
Marini JC, Gerber NL: Osteogenesis imperfecta: Rehabilitation and prospects for gene therapy. *JAMA* 1997;277:746.
Plotkin H, Rauch F, Bishop NJ: Pamidronate treatment of severe osteogenesis imperfecta in children under 3 years of age. *J Clin Endocrinol Metab* 2000;85:1846.
Smith R: Severe osteogenesis imperfecta: New therapeutic options? *BMJ* 2001;322:63–4.
Zacharin M, Bateman J: Pamidronate treatment of osteogenesis imperfecta—lack of correlation between clinical severity, age at onset of treatment, predicted collagen mutation and treatment response. *J Pediatr Endocrinol Metabol* 2002;15:163–74.

Chapter 690
Marfan Syndrome
Luther K. Robinson

Marfan syndrome is an autosomal dominantly inherited disorder with nearly complete penetrance but variable expressivity. The incidence of this disorder is about 1 per 5,000–10,000 births; nearly 30% of affected newborns represent sporadically occurring new mutations. Diagnosis of Marfan syndrome is based on clinical findings, some of which are age and maturation dependent (see Table 690–1).

Pathogenesis. Pathogenesis is related to abnormal biosynthesis of fibrillin-1, a 350-kd extracellular glycoprotein that is the major constituent of microfibrils that provide the scaffolding network of elastic fibers and have an anchoring function in nonelastic tissue such as aortic adventitia and the suspensory ligament of the eye. The fibrillin-1 *(FBN1)* locus resides within the long arm of chromosome 15 (15q21). More than 100 mutations distributed throughout *FBN1* have been described, each appearing to be unique to a given family. The relatively even distribution of mutations throughout *FBN1* likely contributes to the phenotypic variability of the disorder.

Clinical Manifestations. The diagnosis of the Marfan syndrome is based on the overall pattern of malformation (typically skeletal, cardiovascular, and ocular); many manifestations are age or maturation dependent. Tall stature may be present at birth and persist postnatally. Diminished subcutaneous fat may suggest failure to thrive in early infancy, but aggressive intervention (e.g., hyperalimentation) seldom is indicated. Hypotonia and ligamentous laxity may suggest developmental delays, but cognitive performance is normal for family. Neonatal (infantile,

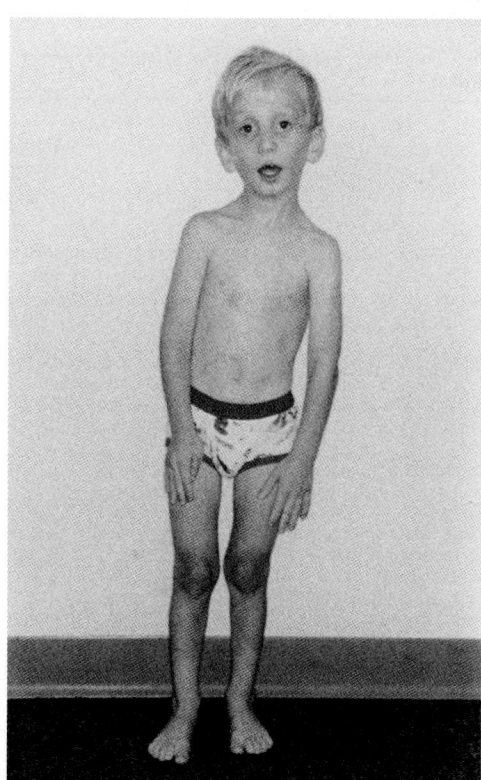

FIGURE 690–1. Marfan syndrome. Note the elongated facies, droopy lids, apparent dolichostenomelia, and mild scoliosis.

congenital) Marfan syndrome is more severe than cases observed in older children and may have clinical similarity to congenital contractural arachnodactyly (CCA), presenting as hypotonia, arachnodactyly, joint laxity and dislocations, and flexion contractures. The face is long, and the skin is lax with diminished recoil. The ears may appear large and pliant. Ocular examination may disclose megalocornea, iridodonesis, or frank lens dislocation. Cardiac examination often reveals murmurs of either mitral valve prolapse with regurgitation or aortic insufficiency, and aortic root dilatation may be documented echocardiographically. Older individuals display tall stature and a long, thin face with narrowness of the maxilla and dental crowding. Ocular abnormalities reflect the connective tissue defect and include blue sclerae, myopia, and suspensory ligament laxity with iridodonesis. Slit lamp examination as early as infancy may disclose lens dislocation, which may be congenital. Iridodonesis is a helpful clinical sign, but patients suspected of having Marfan syndrome should have ophthalmologic evaluations that include slit lamp examinations even in the absence of gross ocular abnormality.

Examination of the musculoskeletal system discloses dolichostenomelia (long thin limbs), and the arm span substantially exceeds the height. The lower segment (distance from pubis to heel) is increased in comparison with the upper segment (height minus lower segment) and contributes to a diminished upper segment/lower segment ratio (U_s/L_s). Hand findings are nonspecific and include long, thin fingers (arachnodactyly) that are hyperextensible. The thumb may be adducted across the narrow palm (Steinberg sign), and the thumb may appreciably overlap the fifth finger when encircling the wrist (wrist sign).

Long gracile ribs may contribute to various sternal anomalies including pectus excavatum ("funnel chest") or pectus carinatum ("pigeon breast"). The risk of scoliosis among adolescents is increased.

The connective tissue defect contributes to increased distensibility of lung parenchyma and dura and increases the risks of spontaneous pneumothorax and dural ectasia, respectively.

Progressive cardiovascular defects contribute to the substantial morbidity of Marfan syndrome. Echocardiography facilitates early detection of patients with cardiac complications. Progressive aortic root dilatation, whether or not accompanied by auscultatory evidence of aortic disease, occurs in 80–100% of cases and may be congenital. Some aortic root dilatation is seen in 90% of patients by age 20 yr.

In contrast to adults, frank aortic regurgitation is less common in children (seen in about 25% by age 20 yr), perhaps because the amount and duration of distention required to cause aortic dysfunction does not manifest until later life. Mitral valve prolapse (MVP) occurs as frequently as aortic dilatation and tends to be progressive, in contrast to the more static lesion of idiopathic MVP. MVP is usually present in most 8–10 yr old affected children; at this time it is asymptomatic and detected by echocardiography. Progressive MVP is the most common cause of morbidity in children with Marfan syndrome and may manifest as arrhythmias, heart failure, thromboemboli, or endocarditis. Mitral valve regurgitation is seen in about 50% of patients younger than 20 yr of age.

Diagnosis. Diagnosis of Marfan syndrome is based on clinical criteria (Table 690–1). In general, diagnosis of a sporadic or new mutation case requires that major manifestations of the disorder be present. In cases with an unequivocally affected first-degree relative, milder manifestations with at least one major malformation are supportive of the diagnosis. Tall stature with an abnormally U_s/L_s ratio or an increased span to height ratio (i.e., greater than 1.05) is the most consistent presenting feature. Echocardiography or MRI should show at least aortic root dilatation for age. Other abnormalities such as mitral valve prolapse, mitral regurgitation, or aortic regurgitation are supportive findings. A slit lamp examination is indicated in all suspected cases. Only 60–70% of patients who meet clinical criteria for Marfan syndrome have a known mutation in the fibrillin gene, whereas 12% of patients not meeting criteria have a gene mutation.

Laboratory evaluation should document a negative urinary cyanide nitroprusside test or specific amino acid studies to exclude cystathionine synthase deficiency (homocystinuria). Other conditions that should be excluded include idiopathic MVP, familial thoracic aneurysm (cystic medial necrosis/annuloaortic ectasia, Erdheim disease), congenital contractural arachnodactyly (CCA), Stickler (hereditary arthro-ophthalmopathy), pseudoxanthoma elasticum, and Shprintzen-Goldberg (craniosynostosis marfanoid habitus) syndrome. Although no genotype phenotype correlations have emerged, molecular genetic studies may be applicable to pedigrees with multiple affected family members.

Treatment. Therapy focuses on prevention of complications and genetic counseling. In view of the potential complexity of management required by some affected individuals, periodic referral to a multidisciplinary center with experience in the Marfan syndrome is advisable.

Pediatricians should work in concert with pediatric subspecialists to develop and coordinate a rational approach to expectant monitoring and treatment of potential complications. Yearly evaluations for such problems as cardiac valvular disease, scoliosis, joint dislocations, or ophthalmologic problems are imperative. Physical therapy may improve neuromuscular tone and strength in affected infants. Moderate nontraumatic physical activity such as bicycling or swimming should be encouraged as tolerated. Maximal exertion should be discouraged because of the stresses that increased cardiac output place on the aorta. Endocarditis prophylaxis should be instituted before dental or other invasive procedures.

TABLE 690–1. Diagnostic Criteria According to the Ghent Nosology[*]

Criterion	Major	Minor
Skeletal system		
Manifestations	Pectus carinatum or pectus excavatum requiring surgery, arm span to height ratio >1.05 or reduced US/LS <0.86 (adults), positive wrist and thumb sign, scoliosis >20° or spondylolisthesis, limited elbow extension (<170°), pes planus, protrusio acetabuli (radiography)	Facial appearance, joint hypermobility, pectus excavatum of moderate severity, highly arched palate
Involvement	4 of 7 major present	2 of 7 major present or 1 of 7 major and 2 of 4 minor present
Ocular system		
Manifestations	Ectopia lentis	Myopia, flat cornea, iris or ciliary muscle hypoplasia
Involvement	Ectopia lentis present	2 of 3 minor present
Cardiovascular system		
Manifestations	Aortic ascendens dilatation with or without aortic regurgitation and involving the sinuses of Valsalva; aorta ascendens dissection	Mitral valve prolapse, annulus mitralis calcification (age at onset, <40 yr), pulmonary artery dilatation, aorta descendens or aorta abdominalis dilatation or dissection (age at onset, <50 yr)
Involvement	1 of 2 major present	1 of 4 minor present
Pulmonary system		
Manifestations	None indicated	Pneumothorax, apical blebs (chest radiography)
Involvement	None indicated	1 of 2 minor present
Skin		
Manifestations	None indicated	Striae atrophicae (not associated with weight changes or pregnancy), recurrent or incisional herniae
Involvement	None indicated	1 of 2 minor present
Dura		
Manifestations	Lumbosacral dural ectasia by CT or MRI	None indicated
Involvement	Dural ectasia present	None indicated
Family		
Involvement	First degree family member independently fulfilling diagnostic criteria, mutation in *FBN1* known to cause Marfan syndrome	None indicated

[*]US/LS indicates the ratio of the upper segment (in meters) to the lower segment (in meters).
From Loeys B, et al: Genotype and phenotype analysis of 171 patients referred for molecular study of the fibrillin-1 gene FBN1 because of suspected Marfan syndrome. Arch Int Med 2001;161:2447–54.

β-Adrenergic blockade with agents such as propranolol or atenolol slows the progression of aortic dilatation and lessens the risk of catastrophic cardiac events. Acute aortic dissection may be managed by composite graft.

Optimal management of the pregnant adolescent has not been established. The risk that pregnancy will worsen cardiovascular abnormalities is of concern. Although substantial data are lacking, patients with minor cardiac manifestations and mild aortic root dilatation may tolerate pregnancy well and experience good maternal and fetal outcomes. Patients with aortic dilatation should be monitored echocardiographically at regular intervals. Although β-adrenergic blocking agents have not been shown to be teratogenic, the prenatally exposed fetus of a woman with Marfan syndrome should be monitored in the neonatal period for such drug-induced neonatal problems as hypotension, bradycardia, hypothermia, or hypoglycemia.

Prognosis. Longevity in the Marfan syndrome is diminished in comparison with population norms, primarily because of the increased risk of cardiovascular complications. Progressive dilatation of the aorta and aortic root may lead to aneurysm formation and dissection. These and other concerns pose not only medical but also psychologic stresses for the affected child and his or her parents, particularly during adolescence. Awareness of these issues and referral for support services may facilitate a positive perspective toward this condition.

Genetic Counseling. The heritable nature of the Marfan syndrome makes recurrence risk (genetic) counseling mandatory. As noted previously, 15–30% of cases are the first affected individuals in their families. Fathers of these sporadic cases have been, on average, 7–10 years older than fathers in the general population. This paternal age effect suggests that these cases represent new dominant mutations with minimal recurrence risks to the future offspring of the normal parents. Each child of an affected individual, however, has a 50% risk of inheriting the chromosome 15 with mutant *FBN1* allele and thus being affected. Recurrence risk counseling is best managed by professionals with expertise in the issues surrounding the chronic nature of this condition.

American Academy of Pediatrics Committee on Genetics: Health supervision of children with Marfan syndrome. *Pediatrics* 1996;98:978.

DePaepe A, Devereux RB, Dietz HC, et al: Revised criteria for Marfan syndrome. *Am J Med Genet* 1996;62;417.

Dietz HC, McIntosh I, Sakai LY, et al: Four novel *FBN1* mutations: Significance for mutant transcript level and EGF-like domain calcium binding in the pathogenesis of Marfan syndrome. *Genomics* 1993;17:468.

Franke U, Furthmayr H: Marfan's syndrome and other disorders of fibrillin. *N Engl J Med* 1994;330:1384.

Gross DM, Robinson LK, Smith LT, et al: Severe perinatal Marfan syndrome. *Pediatrics* 1989;84:83.

Loeys B, Nuytinck L, Delvaus I, et al: Genotype and phenotype analysis of 171 patients referred for molecular study of the fibrillin-1 gene *FBN1* because of suspected Marfan syndrome. *Arch Intern Med* 2001;161:2447–54.

Pereira L, Levran O, Ramirez F, et al: A molecular approach to stratification of cardiovascular risk in families with Marfan syndrome. *N Engl J Med* 1994;331:148.

Rossiter JP, Morales AJ, Repke JT, et al: A prospective longitudinal evaluation of pregnancy in the Marfan syndrome. *Am J Obstet Gynecol* 1995;173:1599.

Shores J, Berger KR, Murphy EA, Pyeritz RE: Progression of aortic dilatation and the benefit of long-term β-adrenergic blockade in Marfan's syndrome. *N Engl J Med* 1994;330:1335.

Sisk HE, Zahka KG, Pyeritz RE: The Marfan syndrome in early childhood: Analysis of 15 patients diagnosed at less than 4 years of age. *Am J Cardiol* 1983;52:353.

Van Karnebeek CDM, Naeff MSJ, Mulder BJM, et al: Natural history of cardiovascular manifestations in Marfan syndrome. *Arch Dis Child* 2001;84:129–37.

SECTION 4 *Metabolic Bone Disease*

Russell W. Chesney

Chapter 691
Bone Structure, Growth, and Hormonal Regulation

Also see Chapters 44.10, 44.11, 48.9, and 564.

Bone is a dynamic organ capable of rapid turnover, weight bearing, and withstanding the stresses of various physical activities. It is constantly being formed (modeling) and re-formed (remodeling). It is the major body reservoir for calcium, phosphorus, and magnesium. Disorders that affect this organ and the process of mineralization are designated metabolic bone diseases.

Because bone growth and turnover rates are high during childhood, many clinical features of metabolic bone diseases are more prominent in children than in adults.

The human skeleton consists of a protein matrix, largely composed of a collagen-containing protein, osteoid, on which is deposited a crystalline mineral phase. Although collagen-containing osteoid accounts for 90% of bone protein, other proteins are present, including osteocalcin, which contains γ-carboxyglutamic acid. Synthesis of osteocalcin is vitamin K and vitamin D dependent; and in high bone turnover states, serum osteocalcin values are often elevated.

The microfibrillar matrix of osteoid permits deposition of highly organized calcium phosphate crystals, including hydroxyapatite $[C_{10}(PO_4)_6 \bullet 6H_2O]$ and octacalcium phosphate $[Ca_8(H_2PO_4)_6 \bullet 5H_2O]$, plus less organized amorphous calcium phosphate, calcium carbonate, sodium, magnesium, and citrate. Hydroxyapatite is deep within bone matrix, whereas amorphous calcium phosphate coats the surface of newly formed or remodeled bone.

Bone growth occurs in children by the process of calcification of the cartilage cells present at the ends of bone. In accord with the prevailing extracellular fluid (ECF) calcium and phosphate concentrations, mineral is deposited in those chondrocytes or cartilage cells set to undergo mineralization. The main function of the vitamin D/parathyroid hormone (PTH)/endocrine axis is to maintain the ECF calcium and phosphate concentrations at appropriate levels to permit mineralization.

Other hormones also appear to regulate the growth and mineralization of cartilage, including growth hormone acting through insulin-like growth factors, thyroid hormones, insulin, and androgens, and estrogens during the pubertal growth spurt. By contrast, supraphysiologic concentrations of glucocorticoids impair cartilage function and bone growth and augment bone resorption.

Phosphate homeostasis is regulated by the kidneys, because intestinal phosphate absorption is nearly complete and renal excretion determines the serum level. Excessive intestinal phosphate absorption causes a fall in serum levels of ionized calcium and a rise in PTH secretion, resulting in phosphaturia, thus lowering the serum phosphate level and permitting the calcium level to rise. Hypophosphatemia blocks PTH secretion and promotes renal $1,25(OH)_2D$ synthesis. This latter compound also promotes greater intestinal phosphate absorption.

Rates of bone formation are coordinated with alterations in mineral metabolism at both the intestine and kidneys. Inadequate dietary intake or intestinal absorption of calcium causes a fall in serum levels of calcium and its ionized fraction. This serves as the signal for PTH synthesis and secretion, resulting in greater bone resorption to raise the serum calcium level, enhanced distal tubular reabsorption of calcium, and higher rates of synthesis by the kidneys of 1,25-dihydroxy-vitamin D $(1,25[OH]_2D)$, or calcitriol, the most active metabolite of vitamin D (Fig. 691–1). Calcium homeostasis thus is

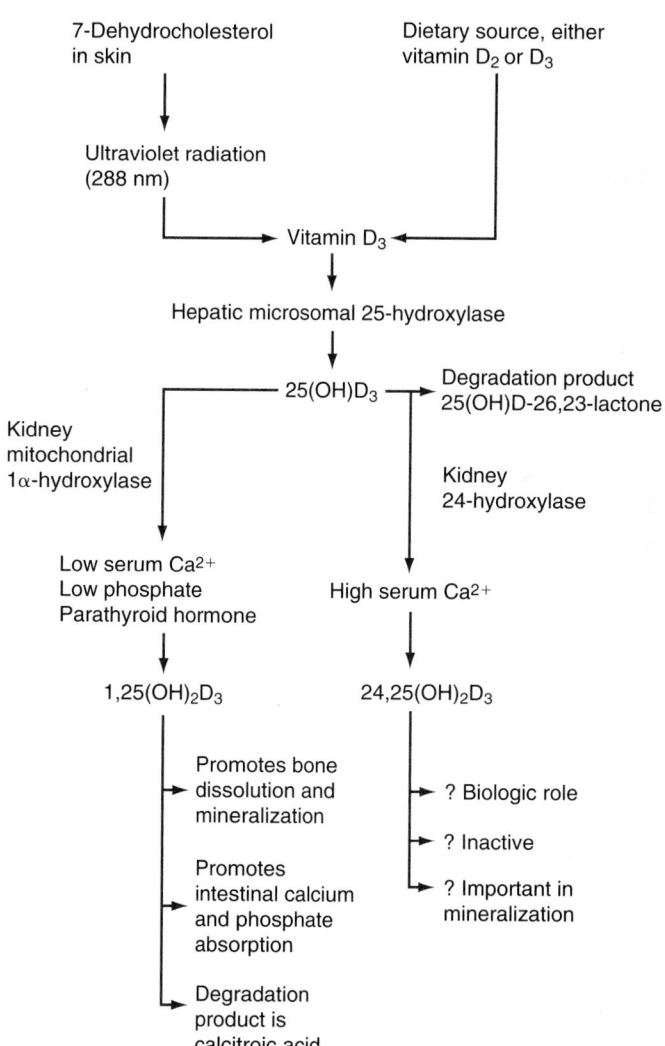

FIGURE 691–1. The metabolic pathway of vitamin D, indicating its conversion to the hormone $1,25(OH)_2D_3$ and to $24,25(OH)_2D_3$. Vitamin D_2 (ergosterol) of plant origin appears to undergo similar metabolic steps.

controlled at the intestine, because the availability of 1,25 $(OH)_2D$ ultimately determines the fraction of ingested calcium that is absorbed.

The growth pattern of bones is an acceleration of bone growth (length) of the limbs during prepubescence, increased growth (length) of the trunk (spine) during early adolescence, and increased bone mineral deposition in late adolescence. The use of dual-energy x-ray absorptiometry (DEXA) or quantitative computed tomography (QCT) permits measurement of both bone mineral content and bone density in healthy subjects and in children with metabolic bone disease.

An understanding of the metabolism of vitamin D is necessary to appreciate metabolic bone disease and rickets (see Fig. 691–1). The skin contains 7-dehydrocholesterol, which is converted to vitamin D_3 by ultraviolet radiation; other inactive vitamin D sterols are also produced (see Chapter 44.10). Vitamin D_3 is then transported in the bloodstream to the liver by a vitamin D–binding protein (DBP); DBP binds all forms of vitamin D. The plasma concentration of free or nonbound vitamin D is much lower than the level of DBP-bound vitamin D metabolites.

Vitamin D also can enter the metabolic pathway by ingestion of dietary vitamin D_2 (ergocalciferol) or vitamin D_3 (cholecalciferol), both of which are absorbed from the intestine because of the action of bile salts. After absorption, ingested vitamin D is transported by chylomicrons to the liver, where, along with skin-derived vitamin D_3, it is converted to 25-hydroxyvitamin D(25[OH]D) by the action of a hepatic microsomal enzyme requiring oxygen, NADPH, and magnesium to hydroxylate vitamin D at the 25th carbon atom. The 25(OH)D is next transported by DBP to the kidneys, where it undergoes further metabolism. 25(OH)D is the main circulat-

TABLE 691–1. Vitamin D Metabolic Values in Plasma of Normal Healthy Subjects

Metabolite	Plasma Value
Vitamin D_2	1–2 ng/mL
Vitamin D_3	1–2 ng/mL
25(OH) D_2	4–10 ng/mL
25(OH) D_3	12–40 ng/mL
Total 25(OH) D	15–50 ng/mL
24,25$(OH)_2D$	1–4 ng/mL
1,25$(OH)_2D$	
Infancy	70–100 pg/mL
Childhood	30–50 pg/mL
Adolescence	40–80 pg/mL
Adulthood	20–35 pg/mL

ing vitamin D metabolite in humans at a concentration of 20–80 ng/mL (Table 691–1). Because its synthesis is weakly regulated by feedback, its plasma level rises in summer and falls in winter. High vitamin D intake raises the plasma level of 25(OH)D to many times above normal, but the parent vitamin D itself is absorbed by adipose tissue.

In the kidneys, 25(OH)D undergoes further hydroxylation, depending on the prevailing serum concentration of calcium, phosphate, and PTH. If the calcium or phosphate level is reduced or the PTH level is elevated, the enzyme 25(OH)D-1-hydroxylase is activated and 1,25$(OH)_2D$ is formed. This metabolite circulates at a level that is only 0.1% of the level of 25(OH)D (see Table 691–1) and acts on the intestine to increase the active transport of calcium and stimulate phosphate absorption. Because 1α-hydroxylase is a mitochondrial

TABLE 691–2. Clinical Variants of Rickets and Related Conditions

Type	Serum Calcium Level	Serum Phosphorus Level	Alkaline Phosphatase Activity	Urine Concentration of Amino Acids	Genetics	Gene Defect Known
I. Calcium deficiency with secondary hyperparathyroidism (deficiency of vitamin D; low 25(OH)D and no stimulation of higher 1,25$(OH)_2D$ values)						
1. Lack of vitamin D						
a. Lack of exposure to sunlight	N or L	L	E	E		
b. Dietary deficiency of vitamin D	N or L	L	E	E		
c. Congenital	N or L	L	E	E		
2. Malabsorption of vitamin D	N or L	L	E	E		
3. Hepatic disease	N or L	L	E	E		
4. Anticonvulsive drugs	N or L	L	E	E		
5. Renal osteodystrophy	N or L	E	E	V		
6. Vitamin D–dependent type I	L	N or L	E	E	AR	Y
II. Primary phosphate deficiency (no secondary hyperparathyroidism)						
1. Genetic primary hypophosphatemia	N	L	E	N	XD	Y
2. Fanconi syndrome						
a. Cystinosis	N	L	E	E	AR	Y
b. Tyrosinosis	N	L	E	E	AR	Y
c. Lowe syndrome	N	L	E	E	XR	Y
d. Acquired	N	L	E	E		
3. Renal tubular acidosis, type II proximal	N	L	E	N		Y
4. Oncogenic hypophosphatemia	N	L	E	N		Y
5. Phosphate deficiency or malabsorption						
a. Parenteral hyperalimentation	N	L	E	N		
b. Low phosphate intake	N	L	E	N		
III. End-organ resistance to 1,25$(OH)_2D_3$						
1. Vitamin D–dependent type II (several variants)	L	L or N	E	E	AR	Y
IV. Related conditions resembling rickets						
1. Hypophosphatasia	N	N	L	Phosphoethanolamine elevated	AR	Y
2. Metaphyseal dysostosis						
a. Jansen type	E	N	E	N	AD	Y
b. Schmid type	N	N	N	N	AD	Y

N = normal; L = low; E = elevated; V = variable; X = X-linked; A = autosomal; D = dominant; R = recessive; Yes = Y.

enzyme that is tightly feedback regulated, the synthesis of $1,25(OH)_2D$ declines after serum calcium or phosphate values return to normal. Excessive $1,25(OH)_2D$ is converted to an inactive metabolite. In the presence of normal or elevated serum calcium or phosphate concentrations, the renal 25(OH)D-24-hydroxylase is activated, producing 24,25-dihydroxyvitamin D $(24,25[OH]_2D)$, which is a pathway for the removal of excess vitamin D, because the serum levels of $24,25(OH)_2D$ (1–5 ng/mL) become higher after ingestion of large amounts of vitamin D. Although hypervitaminosis D and production of inactive metabolites can occur after oral dosing (see Chapter 44.12), extensive skin exposure to sunlight does not usually produce toxic levels of $25(OH)D_3$, suggesting natural regulation of the production of this metabolite in cutaneous tissue.

Serum $1,25(OH)_2D$ levels are higher in children than in adults, are not as subject to seasonal variability, and peak in the 1st yr of life and again during the adolescent growth spurt. These values must be interpreted in light of the prevailing serum calcium, phosphate, and PTH values and with regard to the entire vitamin D metabolite profile.

Mineral deficiency prevents the normal process of bone mineral deposition. If mineral deficiency occurs at the growth plate, growth slows and bone age is retarded—a condition called rickets. Poor mineralization of trabecular bone resulting in a greater proportion of unmineralized osteoid is the condition of osteomalacia. Rickets is found only in growing children before fusion of the epiphyses, whereas osteomalacia is present at all ages. All patients with rickets have osteomalacia, but not all patients with osteomalacia have rickets. These conditions should not be confused with osteoporosis, a condition of equal loss of bone volume and mineral, caused in childhood by glucocorticoid administration, found in Turner and Klinefelter syndromes, following organ transplantation, or as an idiopathic condition.

Rickets may be classified as calcium-deficient or phosphate-deficient rickets. Because both calcium and phosphate ions constitute bone mineral, the insufficiency of either type in the ECF that bathes the mineralizing surface of bone results in rickets and osteomalacia. The two types of rickets are distinguishable by their clinical manifestations (Table 691–2). Rickets may also occur in the face of mineral deficiency, despite adequate vitamin D stores. True dietary calcium deficiency rickets is found in some parts of Africa but not in North America or Europe. A new form of phosphate-deficiency rickets may occur in infants given prolonged administrations of phosphate-sequestering aluminum salts as a treatment for colic or gastroesophageal reflux. This results in the phosphate depletion syndrome.

Chapter 692
Primary Chondrodystrophy (Metaphyseal Dysplasia)

In this condition, bowing of the legs, short stature, and a waddling gait appear in the absence of abnormalities of serum levels of calcium and phosphate, alkaline phosphatase activity, or vitamin D metabolites. *Metaphyseal chondrodysplasia (Jansen type)* is typified by cupped and ragged metaphyses, which develop mottled calcification at the distal ends of bone over time. Hypercalcemia, with serum values of 13–15 mg/dL, may

occur. The spine may also be deformed by the irregular growth of vertebrae. A defect in the parathyroid hormone receptor type I is associated with this syndrome. *Schmid type* of metaphyseal chondrodysplasia is less severe, although the radiographic appearance of the knees and extreme bowing of the lower limbs resemble signs seen in patients with familial hypophosphatemia. It is associated with defects in collagen type X. The hip abnormalities are more debilitating. Patients with both types of metaphyseal chondrodysplasia have lifelong short stature.

Metaphyseal dysostosis, or *Pyle disease,* results from defects in endochondral bone formation and metaphyseal modeling. The long ends of bones are splayed, resulting in an Erlenmeyer flask defect. Short stature is not present, and serum chemical levels are normal. Leonine features develop if the facial bones are involved.

No effective forms of treatment are available for the chondrodystrophies or dysostosis.

Chapter 693
Idiopathic Hypercalcemia

Excessive quantities of vitamin D used to enrich food or milk for infants can be associated with hypercalcemia. Although many infants may have been exposed to high levels of vitamin D, only a few develop hypercalcemia, failure to thrive, nephrolithiasis, and decline in renal function. These infants may have radiographic evidence of osteosclerosis and dense bones at the metaphyses. This disorder disappeared with reduction in the vitamin D content of milk but has been reported sporadically when errors in vitamin D formulation of milk have occurred. It may also be observed when growing premature infants are not appropriately weaned from specialized preterm formula enriched with calcium and vitamin D. In addition, at least three separate forms of hypercalcemia have been described.

Williams syndrome, or the elfin facies syndrome, consists of a constellation of manifestations of which hypercalcemia is an infrequent finding. The characteristic facial features include a small mandible, prominent maxilla, and upturned nose. The upper lip has a Cupid's bow curve. Small peglike teeth with numerous caries are common. Feeding problems and failure to thrive during the 1st yr of life are usual. Mild mental retardation and an unusual "cocktail party patter" personality are typical. The types of cardiac lesions found separately or together include supravalvular aortic stenosis, peripheral pulmonary stenosis, hypoplasia of the aorta, coronary artery stenosis, and atrial or ventricular septal defects. Sudden death may be secondary to arrhythmias or coronary artery disease. In hypercalcemic patients, nephrocalcinosis and sclerotic long bones are sometimes evident.

Williams syndrome is sporadic, and some children have hypervitaminosis D without evidence of increased maternal or infantile vitamin D intake. The fundamental defect is a mutation in the elastin gene. In most cases, the circulating values for vitamin D metabolites are normal. Patients with this disorder slowly excrete an infused calcium load and have evidence of increased production of 25(OH)D from vitamin D. Impaired calcitonin secretion to an infused calcium load has also been reported. Treatment is directed at cardiac, social, and educational problems.

Children may also have mild idiopathic hypercalcemia, which is usually transient. Phenotypic features of Williams syndrome are not found. These patients have hypercalciuria and sometimes nephrocalcinosis, possibly resembling infants who received excessive vitamin D. However, no evidence for abnormalities in vitamin D metabolism has been found.

Familial hypocalciuric hypercalcemia is an autosomal dominant condition in which affected children have asymptomatic hypercalcemia without hypercalciuria (see Chapters 564 and 567). Pancreatitis may occur in some families, and in a few kindreds neonates may present with life-threatening parathyroid hyperplasia. Instead of serum calcium levels of 12–15 mg/dL typically found in the parent, these infants have levels exceeding 18 mg/dL. All of these children have had mild parathyroid hyperplasia despite hypercalcemia, suggesting that the parathyroid gland does not respond appropriately to the signal of hypercalcemia. The gene for the calcium-sensing receptor in parathyroid, kidney, and other tissues is abnormal in families with familial benign hypocalciuric hypercalcemia. This gene is located on chromosome 3 in 90% of families, and the gene defect impairs the responsiveness of the calcium receptor to ionized calcium. Vitamin D metabolism is normal. Only the infants with serious hyperparathyroidism require an emergency parathyroidectomy. Although the serum magnesium level is elevated, it is not a serious concern.

If hypercalcemia persists in any of these conditions, therapy with bisphosphonates, which blocks bone resorption, has been useful in normalizing serum calcium values.

Chapter 694
Hypophosphatasia

Hypophosphatasia is an autosomal recessive disorder that radiographically resembles rickets and is defined by low serum alkaline phosphatase activity. It is an inborn error of metabolism in which activity of the tissue-nonspecific (liver/bone/kidney) alkaline phosphatase (TNSALP) is deficient. Single point mutations of the gene for alkaline phosphatase prevent the expression of the activity of this enzyme in vitro and indicate the necessity of this enzyme for normal skeletal mineralization. Missense mutations of the gene for the tissue nonspecific isoenzyme have been found, but other patients may have a regulatory defect involving this enzyme. Activity of the intestinal and placental enzyme is normal.

There is considerable heterogeneity in the severity of the disease. Some cases appear at birth, and diagnosis has even been made in utero by radiographic examination of a fetus. The disease may appear in a lethal neonatal or perinatal form *(congenital lethal hypophosphatasia)*, a severe infantile form, or a milder form occurring in childhood or late adolescence *(hypophosphatasia tarda)*. The lethal form is characterized by a moth-eaten appearance at the ends of the long bones, by severe deficiency of ossification throughout the skeleton, and by marked shortening of the long bones. Patients with the mild disease may present with bowing of the legs and variable statural shortening. Because calcium accumulation by mature chondrocytes does not occur, patients may appear to have rickets; hypercalcemia is common in the neonatal and infantile forms.

Unusual clinical manifestations include wormian bones in the calvaria, poor calcification of the frontal, parietal, and occipital bones, and premature loss of deciduous or permanent teeth, owing to hypoplasia of dental cementum. Because of the hypercalcemia in the infantile form, nephrocalcinosis is also found. In the childhood form, bone pain, frequent fractures, and milder skeletal deformities are evident, as well as premature tooth loss. The metaphyseal defect consists of irregular ossification, punched-out areas, and metaphyseal cupping.

In hypophosphatasia, large quantities of phosphoethanolamine are found in the urine because this compound cannot be degraded in the absence of TNSALP activity. Plasma inorganic pyrophosphate and pyridoxal–5-phosphate levels are also elevated for the same reason. Seizures in the lethal and infantile form of the disease may relate to impaired pyridoxine metabolism. Although no satisfactory therapy has been found, infusion of plasma rich in alkaline phosphatase activity has been helpful in healing bone in short-term studies. Bone marrow transplantation is successful using donors with normal TNSALP values. The clinical course of this condition often improves spontaneously as an affected child matures, although early death due to renal failure or flail chest leading to pneumonia may also occur in the severe infantile form of the disorder. Rare patients presenting identical clinical and radiographic patterns have normal serum alkaline phosphatase activities. Their disease has been labeled *pseudohypophosphatasia* and may represent the presence of a mutant alkaline phosphatase isozyme that reacts to artificial substrates in an alkaline environment (i.e., in a test tube) but not in vivo with natural substrates.

Chapter 695
Hyperphosphatasia

Excessive elevation of the bone isozyme of alkaline phosphatase in serum and significant growth failure characterize hyperphosphatasia. Osteoid proliferation in the subperiosteal portion of bone results in separation of the periosteum from the bone cortex. Bowing and thickening of the diaphyses are common, along with osteopenia. The disease usually has its onset by 2–3 yr of age, when painful deformity developing in the extremities leads to abnormal gait and sometimes fractures. Other common findings include pectus carinatum, kyphoscoliosis, and rib fraying. The skull is large, and the cranium is thickened (widened diploë) and may be deformed. Radiographically, the bony texture is variable; dense areas (showing a teased cotton-wool appearance) are interspersed with radiolucent areas and general demineralization. Long bones appear cylindrical, lose metaphyseal modeling, and contain pseudocysts showing a dense, bony halo.

In this autosomal recessive disorder, serum levels of both calcium and phosphate are normal, whereas urinary leucine amino acid peptidase activity and serum acid phosphatase levels are increased. This disorder is often called *juvenile Paget disease*, because, as in adult-onset Paget disease, calcitonin may reduce the rapid bone turnover found in this disorder; in children, the disorder is more generalized and symmetric. This disorder is distinct from Paget disease because histology of bone reveals a lack of normal cortical bone remodeling and an absence of the classic mosaic pattern of lamellar bone found in that adult condition. Hence, the term *juvenile Paget disease* is inappropriate.

Transient hyperphosphatasia occurs between 2 mo and 2 yr of age, has no associated manifestations other than some mild gastrointestinal symptoms, and is usually detected during routine (screening) laboratory evaluation for some unrelated complaint. Both liver and bone isoenzyme fractions are elevated;

there are no other manifestations of hepatic or bone dysfunction. The cause is unknown. Resolution usually occurs within 4–6 mo.

Familial hyperphosphatemia, an autosomal dominant trait, is another benign condition that is distinguished from the transient infantile form by persistent and asymptomatic elevations of serum alkaline phosphatase levels.

A more serious autosomal dominant variant, *expansile skeletal hyperplasia*, is characterized by early-onset deafness, premature loss of teeth, progressive hyperostotic widening of long bones causing painful phalanges in the hands, episodic hypercalcemia, and enhanced bone remodeling. A defect in the gene that encodes receptor activation of nuclear factor γB [NF-γB] is relevant. This gene appears to be necessary for osteogenesis, and the defect leads to increased activity in the skeleton of NF-γB.

Chapter 696
Familial Hypophosphatemia (Vitamin D–Resistant Rickets, X-Linked Hypophosphatemia)

The most commonly encountered non-nutritional form of rickets is familial hypophosphatemia. The usual mode of inheritance is X-linked dominant; some mothers of affected children exhibit clinical evidence of disease, such as bowing or short stature, whereas others show only fasting hypophosphatemia. Autosomal dominant and sporadic forms have also been reported.

Pathogenesis. Pathogenic mechanisms involve defects in the proximal tubular reabsorption of phosphate and in the conversion of 25(OH)D to 1,25(OH)$_2$D. The latter defect is evidenced by low-normal serum 1,25(OH)$_2$D levels despite hypophosphatemia and by the finding that further phosphate depletion of subjects with familial hypophosphatemia does not stimulate 1,25(OH)$_2$D synthesis as it does in normal subjects. Both a renal tubular reabsorption defect and reduced 1,25(OH)$_2$D synthesis are found in an animal model of this disease. In addition, oral phosphate supplementation alone cannot completely heal bone disease; the correction of osteomalacia requires 1,25(OH)$_2$D therapy. The activity of the Na$^+$-dependent phosphate transporter in the renal proximal tubule is reduced, resulting in excessive urinary phosphate excretion; however, this transporter protein is encoded on chromosome 5. Because the X-linked dominant disorder has an X-linked inheritance pattern, the abnormal gene found at Xp 22.1 is termed *PHEX* or *p*hosphate-regulating gene with *h*omologies to *e*ndopeptidases on the *X* chromosome. In the autosomal dominant form of hypophosphatemic rickets, mutations in the fibroblast growth factor, F6F23, are found. F6F23 appears to be a natural substrate for PHEX; and if F6F23 is not cleaved, it will diminish renal tubular phosphate transport and the synthesis of 1,25(OH)$_2$D.

Clinical Manifestations. Children with familial hypophosphatemia present with bowing of the lower extremities related to weight bearing at the age of walking. Tetany is not present, and the profound myopathy, rachitic rosary, and Harrison groove (pectus deformity) characteristic of calcium-deficient rickets are not evident (see Chapter 44.10). These children develop a waddling gait, smooth (rather than angular) bowing of the lower extremities, coxa vara, genu varum, genu valgum, and short stature. The adult height of untreated patients is 130–165 cm.

Pulp deformities and lesions of **intraglobular dentin** are characteristic tooth abnormalities, although enamel defects are found only occasionally. By contrast, calcium-deficient rickets usually results in enamel defects. Periapical infections are found in both forms of rickets. Therapy for metabolic bone disease does not correct the defect in intraglobular dentin in this condition.

Radiographic findings include metaphyseal widening and fraying and coarse-appearing trabecular bone. Cupping of the metaphysis occurs at the proximal and distal tibia and at the distal femur, radius, and ulna.

Laboratory Findings. Patients have a normal or slightly reduced serum calcium level (9–9.4 mg/dL; 2.24–2.34 mM), a moderately reduced serum phosphate level (1.5–3 mg/dL; 0.48–0.96 mM), elevated alkaline phosphatase activity, and no evidence of secondary hyperparathyroidism. Urinary phosphate excretion is large, despite hypophosphatemia, indicating a defect in renal tubular phosphate reabsorption possibly related to failure of PHEX to cleave and reduce F6F23 action. This disorder is typical of pure phosphate-deficient rickets, because aminoaciduria, glucosuria, bicarbonaturia, and kaliuria are never found. In potential obligate heterozygotes, who later develop disease, serum phosphate levels may remain normal for the first several months of life. The first laboratory abnormality is often a rise in serum alkaline phosphatase activity. The serum phosphate level probably remains normal for several months, because the glomerular filtration rate is quite low in neonates. Parathyroid hyperplasia with elevated serum parathyroid hormone (PTH) values is occasionally found, sometimes in sporadic cases.

Treatment. Oral phosphate supplements coupled with a vitamin D analogue to offset the secondary hyperparathyroidism that may accompany an oral phosphate load is the preferred treatment. Oral phosphate is usually given every 4 hr at least five times a day, because urinary excretion is constant and patients quickly become hypophosphatemic. Young children should receive 0.5–1 g/24 hr, whereas older children require 1–4 g/24 hr. Phosphate can be given as Joulie solution (dibasic sodium phosphate, 136 g/L, and phosphoric acid, 58.8 g/L), which contains 30.4 mg of phosphate/mL. Thus, a 5 mL dose given every 4 hr five times daily provides 760 mg of phosphate. This solution must be formulated by a pharmacist. A capsule form of phosphate (Neutra-Phos) is commercially available and provides 250 mg of phosphorus per capsule. Patient compliance is readily assessed because most of this dose is excreted in a 24-hr urine collection. The main side effect of oral phosphate therapy is diarrhea, which often improves spontaneously.

Providing a vitamin D analogue is important for complete bone healing and prevention of secondary hyperparathyroidism. Classically, vitamin D$_2$ was used at 2,000 IU/kg/24 hr, but more recently, dihydrotachysterol at a dosage of 0.02 mg/kg/24 hr or 1,25(OH)$_2$D at 50–65 ng/kg/24 hr has been effectively used. Hydrochlorothiazide may reduce the hypercalciuria evident after vitamin D therapy.

Familial hypophosphatemia was previously treated with 50,000–200,000 IU/24 hr (1.25–10 mg) of vitamin D$_2$, but this caused hypervitaminosis D with nephrocalcinosis, hypercalcemia, and permanent renal damage (see Chapter 44.12).

The term *vitamin D–resistant rickets* was used in the past to describe rickets in which patients failed to respond to a dose of vitamin D that would cure vitamin D deficiency. If appropriate doses of vitamin D or any of its metabolites fail to heal rickets, and if serum phosphate is not reduced, metaphyseal dysplasia should be considered (see Chapter 692).

With early diagnosis and good compliance, the bowing deformities can be minimized, and an adult height above 170 cm may be achievable. However, the influence of therapy on final height is controversial, because most patients remain short while in some studies good growth patterns are evident. For this reason trials of growth hormone therapy have been employed. Corrective osteotomies should always be deferred until rickets appears healed radiographically and until the serum alkaline phosphatase level is in the normal range. Surgery before bone healing may be followed by redevelopment of deformity and bowing. In some patients, aggressive medical management may obviate the need for surgical intervention. Patients undergoing osteotomy should stop taking all vitamin D preparations before surgery and should not start them again until they are again ambulating to avoid immobilization hypercalcemia. Because $1,25(OH)_2D$ has such a short half-life, it can be stopped just before surgery, whereas vitamin D_2 should be discontinued at least 1 mo before surgery. An additional advantage of $1,25(OH)_2D$ therapy is that it augments intestinal phosphate absorption and may improve phosphate balance. However, $1,25(OH)_2D$ should not be used without concomitant oral phosphate.

Certain patients have hypophosphatemia and hyperphosphaturia but no radiographic evidence of rickets. This condition, inherited as an autosomal dominant disorder, has been called *hypophosphatemic bone disease.* The serum concentrations of $1,25(OH)_2D$ are normal, and the renal tubular phosphate excretion defect is not as marked as in familial hypophosphatemic rickets, possibly because PHEX is normal and substrates other than F6F23 may influence phosphate transport. Short stature is not as prominent. Oral phosphate and $1,25(OH)_2D$ have been used to treat this disorder.

can be treated with a massive dose of vitamin D_2 (200,000–1 million IU/24 hr), the use of relatively low-dose $1,25(OH)_2D$ at 1–2 μg/24 hr heals this disorder. The gene for the enzyme 25(OH)D-1 α-hydroxylase is mutated and the enzyme activity reduced. The serum levels of $1,25(OH)_2D$ are low, despite hypocalcemia, hypophosphatemia, and elevated parathyroid hormone levels.

Some cases of vitamin D–dependent rickets fail to reverse after treatment with either high-dose vitamin D_2 or $1,25(OH)_2D$ at 1–2 μg/24 hr. Hypocalcemia, hypophosphatemia, aminoaciduria, and rickets persist in the presence of extremely high circulating levels of $1,25(OH)_2D$, usually above 180 pg/mL. Patients with hereditary $1,25(OH)_2D_3$-resistant rickets have (1) reduced or absent $1,25(OH)_2D_3$ binding to the human vitamin D nuclear receptor; (2) decreased affinity of this receptor for DNA so that transcription cannot occur; or (3) defective nuclear translocation or retention. An abnormal gene product is produced by the vitamin D receptor gene in these patients. A single amino acid substitution in an important DNA-binding site in the receptor may cause this disorder, thus preventing the binding of $1,25(OH)_2D$ and its receptor to the nucleus. Missense and truncation mutations of the DNA binding– or the steroid $(1,25[OH]_2D_3)$–binding portions of the vitamin D receptor have been found. This form of the disease, which is particularly prevalent among children of 1st-cousin marriages, is termed *vitamin D dependence, type II,* or *hereditary resistance to 1,25(OH)_2D.* Some patients have short stature and alopecia totalis. Rickets can sometimes be reversed by administration of 15–30 μg/24 hr of $1,25(OH)_2D$, but missing hair does not regrow.

Chapter 698
Oncogenous Rickets (Primary Hypophosphatemic Rickets Associated with Tumor)

Rickets associated with a tumor of mesenchymal origin that resolves on removal of the tumor is characterized by phosphaturia, hypophosphatemia, and, in adults, osteomalacia. Hemangiopericytomas are a common tumor type producing this syndrome. These tumors, which cause a phosphate-deficient form of rickets, are mostly benign, may become apparent only years after the development of rickets, and may be located in sites difficult to detect, such as the small bones of the hands and feet, the abdominal sheath, the nasal antrum, and the pharynx. This syndrome may also be associated with the epidermal nevus syndrome, neurofibromatosis (von Recklinghausen disease), and linear nevus syndrome.

In addition to hypophosphatemia and hyperphosphaturia, glycinemia and glycinuria are sometimes found in this form of rickets. These tumors elaborate massive amounts of F6F23, the phosphate-regulating gene product, which causes phosphaturia and impairs the conversion of 25(OH)D to $1,25(OH)_2D$. Serum 25(OH)D levels are normal, and serum $1,25(OH)_2D$ levels are low but rapidly rise to normal after tumor excision. Hypophosphatemia in this syndrome is

Chapter 697
Vitamin D–Dependent Rickets (Pseudovitamin D Deficiency, Hypocalcemic Vitamin D–Resistant Rickets)

Vitamin D–dependent rickets appears at age 3–6 mo in children who have been receiving dosages of vitamin D (400–600 IU/24 hr) that ordinarily prevent rickets (see Chapter 44.10). Serum calcium and phosphate levels are low, and alkaline phosphatase activity is elevated. This condition is a calcium-deficient form of rickets because patients have secondary hyperparathyroidism, aminoaciduria, glucosuria, renal tubular bicarbonate wasting, and renal tubular acidosis. These children also develop dental enamel hypoplasia. Although the rickets and biochemical features of this autosomal recessive disorder presumably caused by ectopic production by tumor cells of this specific fibroblast growth factor, which inhibits renal tubular reabsorption of phosphate. Surgery also cures the bone pain and myopathy, which, if untreated, may confine the child to a wheelchair. Children with acquired or late-appearing hypophosphatemic rickets should undergo bone radiographic examination or bone scan to search for tumors. If a tumor cannot be removed or is metastatic, treatment with 1,25(OH)$_2$D and oral phosphate or octreotide is often beneficial.

Chapter 699
Osteoporosis

Osteoporosis is a condition of multiple causes in which bone volume is reduced and increased fractures are evident. In contrast to osteomalacia with undermineralization and normal bone volume, histologic sections of bone in osteoporosis reveal a normal degree of mineralization but a reduction in the volume of bone, especially trabecular bone. Childhood osteoporosis may be primary, as in idiopathic juvenile osteoporosis, osteoporosis-pseudoglioma syndrome, and osteogenesis imperfecta, or secondary to conditions such as Klinefelter syndrome, Turner syndrome, leukemia, homocystinuria, or chronic glucocorticoid administration (Box 699–1). When no obvious secondary cause can be detected, idiopathic juvenile osteoporosis should be entertained if the following clinical features are evident: onset prior to puberty, long bone and lower back pain, fractures of the vertebrae, long bone and metatarsal fractures, washed-out appearance of the spine and long bones, and improvement after puberty. Trabecular bones such as the spine are particularly affected. In general, blood values of minerals, vitamin D metabolites, alkaline phosphatase, and parathyroid hormone are normal. DEXA evaluation shows markedly reduced bone mineral content and bone density. Although several modes of therapy (including oral calcium supplements, calcitriol, bisphosphonates, and calcitonin) have been used with some success, the effect of these treatments is difficult to gauge because spontaneous recovery may occur after puberty.

Osteoporosis-pseudoglioma is an autosomal recessive disorder manifested by variable age at onset, low bone mass, fractures in childhood, and abnormal eye development and is mapped to chromosome 11q12-13. The mutation is a loss of function in the gene for low-density lipoprotein receptor–related protein 5 *(LRP5).* Gain-of-function mutations in this gene produce increased bone density.

The life cycle implications of demineralization or osteoporosis in childhood on final bone mineral accretion should be understood—an important factor in the avoidance of post-menopausal osteoporosis in adults is the bone mass at the time of its decline (bone mass peaks at about 20 yr of age). For this reason, it is important to emphasize dietary vitamin D (400–800 IU daily), calcium intake (≥ 1200 mg daily), and weight bearing exercise to children and adolescents (see Chapter 679). Avoidance of cigarettes and alcohol is helpful. Dairy products, bony fish, green vegetables, and calcium-supplemented drinks (e.g., orange juice) form the major dietary sources of calcium. Adult-onset osteoporosis is also determined by as yet unidentified genetic factors that can influence

up to 75% of the variations in peak bone mass. Treatment with bisphosphonates of some secondary (particularly steroid-induced) and adult-onset osteoporosis has been quite successful (see Chapter 689).

BOX 699–1. Causes of Osteoporosis

ENDOCRINE DISEASES
Female hypogonadism
  Hyperprolactinemia
  Hypothalamic amenorrhea
  Anorexia nervosa
  Premature and primary ovarian failure
Male hypogonadism
  Primary gonadal failure (e.g., Klinefelter syndrome)
  Secondary gonadal failure (e.g., idiopathic hypogonadotropic hypogonadism)
  Delayed puberty
Hyperthyroidism
Hyperparathyroidism
Hypercortisolism
Growth hormone deficiency

GASTROINTESTINAL DISEASES
Subtotal gastrectomy
Malabsorption syndromes
Chronic obstructive jaundice
Primary biliary cirrhosis and other cirrhoses
Alactasia

BONE MARROW DISORDERS
Bone marrow transplant
Lymphoma
Leukemia
Hemolytic anemias
Systemic mastocytosis
Disseminated carcinoma

CONNECTIVE TISSUE DISEASES
Osteogenesis imperfecta
Ehlers-Danlos syndrome
Marfan syndrome
Homocystinuria

DRUGS
Alcohol
Heparin
Glucocorticoids
Thyroxine
Anticonvulsants
Gonadotropin-releasing hormone agonists
Cyclosporine
Chemotherapy

MISCELLANEOUS CAUSES
Cerebral palsy
Immobilization
Rheumatoid arthritis

From Finkelstein JS: Osteoporosis. In Andreoli TE (editor): *Cecil Essentials of Medicine,* 5th ed. Philadelphia, WB Saunders, 2001, p 657.

Boyden LM, Mao J, Belsky J, et al: High bone density due to a mutation in LDL-receptor related protein 5. *N Engl J Med* 2002;346:1513–21.
Chesney RW: A new form of rickets during infancy. *Arch Pediatr Adolesc Med* 1998;152:1168–69.
Mumm S, Jones J, Finnegan P, Whyte MP: Hypophosphatasia: Molecular diagnosis of Rathbun's original case. *J Bone Miner Res* 2001;16:1724–27.
Seikaly MG, Baum M: Thiazide diuretics arrest the progression of nephrocalcinosis in children with X-linked hypophosphatemia. *Pediatrics* 2001;108:1–4.
Seufert J, Ebert K, Muller J, et al: Octreotide therapy for tumor-induced osteomalacia. *N Engl J Med* 2001;345:1883–88.

Shulman RJ: Expanding role of bisphosphonate therapy in children. *J Pediatr* 1999;134:264–67.

Solomon CG: Bisphosphonates and osteoporosis. *N Engl J Med* 2002;346:642.

Thatcher TD, Fischer PR, Pettifor JM, et al: Case-control study of factors associated with nutritional rickets in Nigerian children. *J Pediatr* 2000;137:367–73.

White KE, Carn G, Lorenz-Depiereux B, et al: Autosomal-dominant hypophosphatemic rickets (ADHR) mutations stabilize FGF-23. *Kidney Int* 2001;60:2079–86.

Whyte MP, Hughes AE: Expansile skeletal hyperphosphatasia is caused by a 15-base pair tandem duplication in *TNFRSF11A* encoding RANK and is allelic to familial expansile osteolysis. *J Bone Miner Res* 2002;17:26–29.

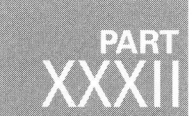
Chapter 700

Pediatric Radiation Injuries

Fred A. Mettler, Jr. and Madelyn M. Stazzone

Radiation injuries to children can usually be divided into four categories. The first is external exposure handling lost highly radioactive metallic sources used in industrial radiography. These exposures usually result in severe skin burns and sometimes bone marrow depression. A second type of injury occurs from internal incorporation of radioactive substances. The third type of injury results from accidents in radiation therapy. Radiation therapy normally has an accepted complication rate, but accidental overexposure can also result from miscalculations or machine malfunctions. Finally, potential neoplasms can occur years or decades after radiation exposure. Examples of these include a high rate of breast cancers in children treated for Hodgkin disease and thyroid cancer in children exposed to radioiodine around Chernobyl.

Radiation accidents involving children per se are rare. Between 1946 and 2000, about 150 fatalities worldwide could be attributed to radiation accidents, and only several of these occurred in children. The rarity of radiation injuries makes their recognition difficult. The public perception about radiation also makes management difficult because patients, their families, and medical staff are usually misinformed about the effects of radiation exposure.

When a radiation accident occurs, the pediatrician needs to be aware not only of the basic principles and management of the early phases of radiation injury but also of the later or delayed manifestations of radiation illness. In some accidents, children have presented with lethargy, nausea and vomiting, leukopenia, thrombocytopenia, or skin burns as manifestations of exposure to a highly radioactive source whose presence was not appreciated. Recognition of radiation exposure as the cause of these symptoms is often necessary for the exposure to be terminated.

Basic Principles. Ionizing radiation includes x-rays and gamma rays. These forms of radiation easily penetrate body tissues, depending on their energy, and can deposit their potentially harmful energy deep in the body. Particulate radiations include α particles and β particles. The α particles present a hazard only when they are inhaled, ingested, or deposited in an open wound, because they have extremely poor penetration capability and are unable to penetrate the outer layer of skin or even a sheet of paper. The β particles may penetrate as much as a few centimeters of tissue.

Although ionizing radiation is not appreciated by the human senses, it is easily detected, localized, and quantified through the use of various devices. If the radiation source is no longer present, recognition of radiation injury is made on the basis of history, the observed effects, and their temporal course.

Radiation was historically measured in three different units: the roentgen, rad, and rem. The roentgen is a unit of exposure based on the number of ion pairs produced in a volume of air.

The rad (radiation absorbed dose) is based on energy deposited per gram of tissue. The absorbed dose depends on the type of radiation and the size, shape, and composition of the object absorbing the radiation. A rem (roentgen equivalent in man) takes into account the biologic effects of various kinds of radiation. For x-rays and gamma rays, a rad and a rem are essentially equivalent. Most literature now uses international units. These include the gray (Gy), which is equal to 100 rads, and the sievert (Sv), which is equal to 100 rem. Radioactivity was historically expressed in units of curies (Ci). The international unit is the becquerel (Bq), and 1 curie equals 37 gigabecquerels (GBq).

Pathophysiology. Radiation injury involves energy deposited in a cell with subsequent formation of free radicals from water. Most of the free radicals that are formed recombine quickly because they are very reactive chemically, but they may occasionally interact with other nearby macromolecules.

At high radiation doses, parenchymal cells may die. The clinical effect may be insignificant if the cell is not critical to the survival of the individual. However, if a large number of cells are killed or they are essential, clinical symptoms become apparent. Not all cells in the body are equally radiosensitive. In general, rapidly dividing cells (e.g., the intestinal mucosa and bone marrow) are the most sensitive to cell killing by radiation, whereas cells that are slowly dividing or are nondividing (e.g., neurons) are quite resistant. Endothelial cells, arterioles, and capillaries have moderate radiosensitivity, and damage to these can reduce blood supply and result in effects months or several years after exposure.

At radiation doses less than 100 rads (1.0 Gy), most cell types survive, although they may be subject to transformation owing to faulty repair of DNA breaks, and there is the possibility of subsequent malignancy. Radiation-induced neoplasms (both benign and malignant) may occur after radiation exposure. Most leukemias (except chronic lymphocytic leukemia) can be induced by radiation and usually appear from 2–15 yr after exposure. Tumors of solid organs can also occur, although the tissues have varying sensitivity. The thyroid, female breast, and lung are among the most sensitive. Most solid tumors appear 10–50 yr after exposure. Thyroid and bone cancer may appear as early as 5 yr. Over a wide dose range, the risk of a radiation-induced tumor for many tissues is directly proportional to the radiation dose; however, for a given radiation dose, children appear to be at a 2- to 3-fold greater risk of subsequent tumors than adults. The wide use of CT scanning has raised concern about the possible induction of cancer in children in the future, but whether this will actually occur remains a matter of conjecture.

Although radiation principally affects DNA and although genetic effects of radiation have been observed in animals, hereditary effects of radiation exposure have not been observed in large epidemiologic studies over several generations (i.e., the Hiroshima and Nagasaki survivors). Concern about prenatal preconception radiation as a cause of childhood cancer has been shown to be unfounded.

WHOLE BODY IRRADIATION

Clinical Manifestations. Table 700–1 presents dose effect relationships for acute whole body penetrating radiation. A large single

TABLE 700–1. **Dose Effect Relationships After Acute Whole Body Irradiation from Gamma or X-rays**

Whole Body Absorbed Dose, Rads (Gy)	Findings
5 (0.05)	Asymptomatic
15 (0.15)	Asymptomtic (but chromosome aberrations may be present in cultured peripheral lymphocytes)
50 (0.5)	Asymptomatic (minor depression of white blood cells and platelets in a few persons)
100 (1.0)	Nausea and vomiting in approximately 10% of patients within 2 days of exposure
200 (2.0)	Nausea and vomiting in most persons exposed, with clear hematologic depression
400 (4.0)	Nausea, vomiting, and diarrhea within 48 hr; 50% mortality without medical treatment
600 (6.0)	100% mortality within 30 days from bone marrow failure without medical treatment
5,000 (50.0)	Cardiovascular collapse and central nervous system damage, with death in 24–72 hr

exposure of penetrating radiation can result in the *acute radiation syndrome*. The signs and symptoms of this syndrome result from damage to major organ systems that have different levels of radiation sensitivity, modulated by the rate at which the radiation exposure occurred. For example, 100 rads (1.0 Gy) delivered in 1 min would be symptomatic but 1 rad (0.01 Gy)/day for 100 days would not be symptomatic.

The *hematopoietic syndrome* occurs from acute whole body doses above 200 rads (2.0 Gy). A prodromal phase consists of nausea and vomiting within the first 12 hr, with symptoms usually lasting up to 48 hr. There follows a latent period of 2–3 wk during which patients may feel quite well. Although patients are asymptomatic, bone marrow impairment has occurred. The most obvious laboratory finding is lymphocyte depression (Table 700–2). Maximal bone marrow depression occurs approximately 30 days after exposure, when hemorrhage and infection can be major problems. If the bone marrow is not completely eradicated, a recovery phase then ensues. This radiation effect is similar to what occurs when whole body irradiation (given as 1,200 rads [12 Gy] in two treatments) is used to obliterate the bone marrow in leukemic children before bone marrow transplantation.

The *gastrointestinal syndrome* occurs from acute whole body doses above 800 rads (8 Gy). Prompt onset of nausea, vomiting, and diarrhea follows. There is a latent period of approximately 1 wk and then recurrence of gastrointestinal symptoms, sepsis, electrolyte imbalance, and, ultimately, death.

At dose levels over 3,000 rad (>30 Gy), the *cardiovascular/central nervous system (CNS) syndrome* predominates. Nausea, vomiting, prostration, hypotension, ataxia, and convulsions are almost immediate. Death usually occurs promptly.

TABLE 700–2. **Expected Outcome Based on Absolute Lymphocyte Count After Acute Penetrating Whole Body Irradiation**

Minimal Lymphocyte Count Within First 48 Hr After Exposure	Prognosis
1,000–3,000 normal range	No significant injury
1,000–1,500	Significant but probably nonlethal injury, good prognosis
500–1,000	Severe injury, fair prognosis
100–500	Very severe injury, poor prognosis
Under 100	Lethal without compatible bone marrow donor

Treatment. For the hematopoietic and gastrointestinal syndromes, treatment is supportive, involving transfusions, fluids, antibiotics, and antiviral agents. The cardiovascular/CNS syndrome is fatal within 1–14 days.

LOCALIZED IRRADIATION

Clinical Manifestations. Because localized exposure involves a small amount of tissue, systemic manifestations are less severe, and patients may survive even if local absorbed doses are very high. The hand is the most common site for accidental localized irradiation injuries, usually as a result of picking up or playing with lost radiation sources. The second most common site is the thigh and buttocks, predominantly from placing unsuspected highly radioactive radiography sources in the pockets. Most industrial radiography sources are easily capable of causing skin erythema or radiation burns from only a few minutes of direct contact.

There are several major differences between thermal burns and radiation burns. The effects of a thermal burn are present almost immediately, and patients invariably know what it was that burned them. If patients present with burnlike symptoms but no known cause, radiation should be suspected as the cause. Table 700–3 lists the findings expected after localized skin doses.

The penetrability of the radiation is an important factor in the outcome of local radiation injury. In cases of low-energy irradiation, recovery and skin grafting are possibilities, even after high absorbed skin doses. Gamma and x-rays, on the other hand, penetrate substantially and cause progressive obliterative endarteritis that may result in necrosis and gangrene. Very few initial symptoms occur in the first 12 hr unless the dose has been extremely high. Under these circumstances, patients may complain of hypersensitivity, tingling, or pain.

Erythema is similar to that seen with a first-degree burn. If erythema is seen within the first 48 hr, ulceration will probably occur. The erythema may come in waves. That is, it will be present, disappear, and return days or 1–3 wk later. Transepidermal injury is similar to a second-degree thermal burn. Blister formation may occur at 1–2 wk with doses in the range of 10,000 rads (100 Gy) and at 3 wk at dose levels of 3,000–5,000 rads (30–50 Gy).

Some tissues that may receive localized radiation exposure are relatively radiosensitive. These include the lens of the eye and the gonads. Cataract formation may occur with single gamma ray exposures in the range of 200–500 rads (2.0–5.0 Gy). Such cataracts usually take between 2 mo to several years to develop. Gonadal exposure has occurred in several accidental situations. Oligospermia may take up to 2 mo to develop. Transient infertility may result from doses as low as 15 rads (0.15 Gy), and permanent sterility may occur in men at dose levels between 300–600 rads (3.0–6.0 Gy). Both cataracts and infertility are common after whole body irradiation used to treat leukemia.

Treatment. Skin therapy is directed at prevention of infections. Treatment of localized injuries usually involves plastic surgery and grafting, if the radiation exposure was not very penetrating. The nature of the surgery depends on the dose at various depths

TABLE 700–3. **Skin Changes After Single Acute Exposure**

Absorbed Dose in Rads (Gy)	Findings
300 (3.0)	Threshold for erythema (100 keV diagnostic x-ray)
600 (6.0)	Threshold for erythema (10 MeV therapeutic x-ray)
1,500 (15.0)	Moist desquamation
2,000 (20.0)	Skin ulceration with slow healing
3,000 + (>30.0)	Gangrenous changes

in tissue and the location of the lesion. The full expression of radiation injury often is not apparent for 1–2 yr, owing to slow arteriolar narrowing that can cause delayed necrosis. After relatively penetrating radiation, amputation may be necessary because of obliterative changes in small vessels.

INTERNAL CONTAMINATION

Epidemiology. Accidents involving internal contamination are rare and generally are a result of misadministration in hospital settings or voluntary ingestion of unsuspected contaminated radioactive materials. Other relevant examples of potential internal contamination of children include that caused by breast-feeding mothers who have diagnostic nuclear medicine scans and radiation exposure of children when a parent or sibling receives a therapeutic dose of iodine 131. When such patients are allowed to go home, they will be excreting a moderate amount of activity through their urine (and to a lesser extent though saliva and sweat) for 1–2 wk, and it is best to have children use a separate bathroom and have their food prepared by somebody else, if possible, during this period. External exposure received by children as a result of radiation emanating directly from such a patient is not a problem, provided the children remain more than 3–6 feet away for about 5 days.

Clinical Manifestations. The hazards from internal contamination depend on the nature of the radionuclide (particularly in terms of its solubility in water, half-life, and radioactive emission), as well as the nature of the chemical compound. The signs and symptoms are similar to those described under whole body and local irradiation, depending on the dose and circumstances of ingestion.

Treatment. Internal contamination presents the physician with a dilemma. The most effective treatment requires knowledge of both the radionuclide and the chemical form, yet unless treatment is instituted very quickly, it rarely is effective. The general classes of treatment for internal contamination include removal, dilution, blocking, and chelation. Removal treatment involves cleaning a contaminated wound and performing stomach lavage or administration of cathartics in the case of ingestion. Administration of alginate-containing antacids (such as Gaviscon) also usually helps in removal by decreasing absorption in the gastrointestinal tract. An example of blocking therapy is the administration of potassium iodine or other stable iodine-containing compounds to patients with known internal contamination with radioactive iodine. The recommended dosage is 65 mg for children 3–18 yr old, 32 mg for children 1 mo–3 yr old, and 16 mg for infants younger than 1 mo old. The stable iodine effectively blocks the thyroid, although the effectiveness decreases rapidly as time increases after the contamination occurred. Another example of blocking therapy is the use of Prussian blue in cases of internal contamination by cesium. Dilution therapy is used in cases of tritium (radioactive hydrogen as water) contamination. Forcing fluids promotes excretion. Finally, cases of internal contamination with transuranic elements (e.g., americium and plutonium) may require chelation therapy with calcium diethylene triaminepentaacetic acid (DTPA).

EXTERNAL CONTAMINATION

The presence of external radioactive contamination on a patient's skin is not an immediate medical emergency. Management involves removing and controlling the spread of radioactive materials. If a patient has suspected surface contamination and no physical injuries, decontamination can be performed relatively easily. If there is substantial physical trauma or other life-threatening injuries that are combined with external contamination, only after the patient has been stabilized physiologically should surface decontamination proceed. In many

accident situations, essential medical care is inappropriately delayed by hospital emergency staff owing to fear of radiation or spread of contamination in the hospital.

Treatment of a patient who is externally contaminated and has other life-threatening injuries requires advance planning. The basic principles involved are as follows:

1. Bring the patient to a room where the traffic can be controlled.
2. While wearing protective clothing (universal precautions), remove the patient's clothing, and treat nonradiation life-threatening injuries first.
3. Call the hospital Radiation Safety Officer. Only after the patient is medically stable, wash potentially contaminated areas with washcloths, lukewarm water, and regular soap.
4. Get a complete blood cell count, ask the patient about nausea and vomiting, and consider possible therapy for internal contamination.

RADIATION THERAPY COMPLICATIONS AND ACCIDENTS

Radiation therapy uses high doses to kill malignant cells. Unfortunately, the sensitivity of normal cells is quite close to that of malignant cells, and to achieve significant cure rates, radiation oncologists also must accept a given percentage of serious complications (5–10%). This leaves little room for error either in calculations of dose or in the actual mechanical functioning of the machine. Radiation therapy protocols are reasonably standardized. Most regimens use about 5,000 rads (50 Gy) given in about 25 fractions over 5 wk. A treatment scheme that either uses doses much more than 10% higher than this or uses this dose with significantly fewer fractions poses a very high incidence of severe and potentially catastrophic complications.

The exact complications depend on the location of the treatment field. In children, because of the location of many childhood tumors, the CNS is commonly in the treatment field and suffers complications. Standard irradiation of the brain in children results in cortical atrophy in more than half of patients who received 2,000–6,000 rads (20–60 Gy); 26% have white matter changes (leukoencephalopathy), and 8% have calcifications (Fig. 700–1). The younger the age of the child at irradiation, the worse is the atrophy. Some patients also develop *mineralizing microangiopathy* (Fig. 700–2). Clinical findings after routine irradiation may include poor school performance and dysfunction of the pituitary and hypothalamus. As a result of overexposure to radiation, adverse effects may be severe and include lethargy, ataxia, spasticity, and progressive dementia. Radiation-induced changes of the brain are potentiated by methotrexate administered before, during, or after radiation therapy.

Cerebral necrosis is a serious and irreversible complication of radiation-induced vascular disease. It is usually diagnosed 1–5 yr after irradiation but can occur up to a decade later. Radiation-induced necrosis occurs with a moderate probability when radiation therapy schemes exceed 4,000 rads (40 Gy) in 10 fractions, 5,000 rads (50 Gy) in 20 fractions, or 6,000 rads (60 Gy) in 30 fractions or when individual fractions exceed 300 rads (3 Gy). The probability of necrosis is very high when treatment schemes exceed 5,000 rads (50 Gy) in 15 fractions, 6,000 rads (60 Gy) in 20 fractions, or 7,000 rads (70 Gy) in 30 fractions. Brain necrosis may be manifested by headache, increased intracranial pressure, seizures, sensory deficits, and psychotic changes.

Spinal cord irradiation may result in *radiation myelitis*, which may be either transient or permanent. Acute transient myelitis often appears 2–4 mo after irradiation. Patients with myelitis usually present with **Lhermitte sign,** a sensation of little electrical shocks in the arms and legs occurring with neck flexion or other movements that stretch the spinal cord.

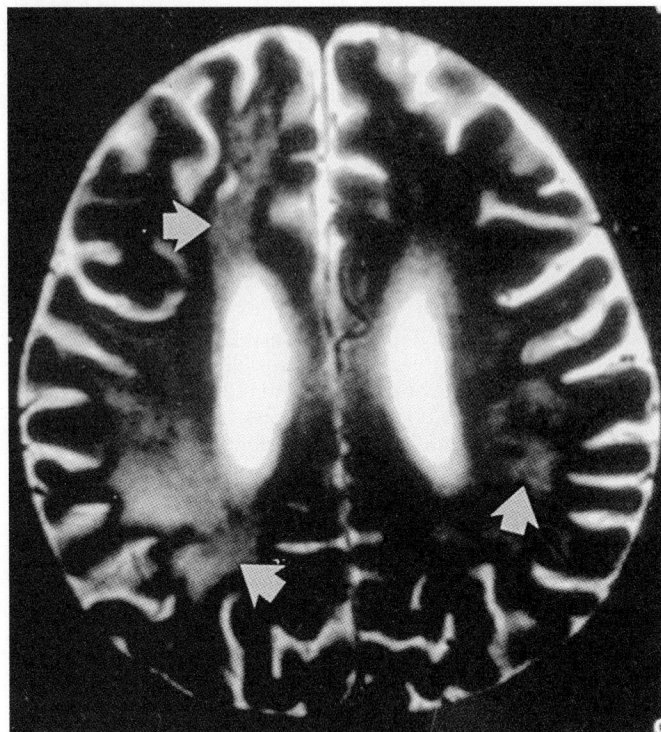

FIGURE 700–1. T2-weighted MRI of a child after radiotherapy shows white matter changes *(arrows)*.

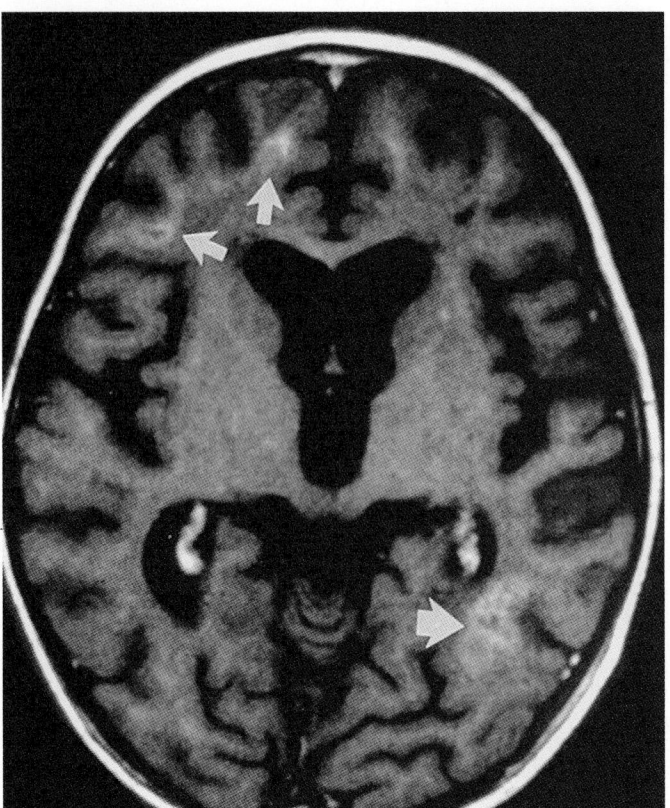

FIGURE 700–2. Generalized brain changes after radiotherapy. T1-weighted MRI of a child shows both central and cortical atrophy as well as high signal areas *(arrows)*, owing to mineralizing microangiopathy.

Reversal of transient myelopathy usually occurs between 8–40 wk and does not necessarily progress to late delayed necrosis.

Delayed myelopathy occurs after a mean latent period of 20 mo, but it can occur earlier if the total dose or dose per fraction is high. This is usually manifested by discontinuous deterioration and is irreversible. In the cervical and thoracic region, sensory dissociation develops, followed by spastic paresis and then flaccid paresis. In the lumbar cord, flaccid paresis is dominant. The mortality for high thoracic and cervical lesions reaches 70%, with death due to pneumonia and urinary tract infections. A 25–50% incidence of thoracic myelopathy occurs when treatment schemes exceed 6,000 rads (60 Gy) at 200 rads (2 Gy) per fraction, 4,000 rads (40 Gy) at 300 rads (3 Gy) per fraction, or 3,500 rads (35 Gy) at 400 rads (4 Gy) per fraction.

Irradiation also causes other effects specific to children. The *effect on growth* is most pronounced when children are younger than 6 yr and during their adolescent growth spurt. Scoliosis and hypoplasia of bones may occur if fractionated treatment schemes exceed 4,000 rads (40 Gy). Fractionated doses in excess of 2,500 rads (25 Gy) can result in slipped capital femoral epiphyses. An increase in the incidence of benign osteochondromas has also been reported after irradiation in children. Chest wall irradiation of girls with 1,500–2,000 rads (15–20 Gy) over 1 wk impairs breast development, and fractionated doses of 3,000–4,000 rads (30–40 Gy) cause fibrosis and atrophy of breast tissue. Virtually any tissues in a radiation therapy field may show disturbances in growth.

RADIATION CARCINOGENESIS

Radiation carcinogenesis is a potential late expression of radiation injury, and children are more sensitive to induction of tumors than adults. Breast cancer data from Hiroshima and Nagasaki indicate that per 100 rem (1.0 Sv), the relative risk in children is about 3.5 compared with 1.5 or so for women irradiated at 40 yr of age. Epidemiologic studies of children irradiated as infants for presumed thymic hyperplasia, of children treated with radiation for ringworm (tinea capitis) and for acne, and of children treated for hemangiomas and other disorders confirm that radiation can increase the risk of leukemia and cancer of the breast, thyroid, brain, skin, and other sites. Over 800 cases of thyroid cancer occurred in children around Chernobyl, mostly in children who were 0–2 yr of age at the time of the accident. There has been no increase in childhood leukemia or malformations in the Chernobyl children.

The incidence of second tumors is also increased in children who have received radiation therapy for childhood tumors, particularly neuroblastoma, retinoblastoma, and Hodgkin disease. A significant increase in soft tissue sarcomas has been noted in children treated for retinoblastoma, and genetic susceptibility has been implicated as well as radiation. In other large studies of children treated for childhood cancer, no increase in leukemia was observed, but there were increases in thyroid and breast cancer as well as bone sarcoma.

American Academy of Pediatrics: Risk of ionizing radiation exposure to children: A subject review. *Pediatrics* 1998;101:717.

Barrett I: Slipped capital femoral epiphysis following radiotherapy. *J Pediatr Orthop* 1985;5:263.

Furst C, Lundell M, Ahlback S, et al: Breast hypoplasia following irradiation of the female breast in infancy and early childhood. *Acta Oncol* 1989;28:519.

Goldwein J, Meadows J: Influence of radiation on growth in pediatric patients. *Clin Plast Surg* 1993;20:455.

Gusev I, Guskova AK, Mettler FA (eds): *Medical Management of Radiation Accidents*, 2nd ed. Boca Raton, FL, CRC Press, 2001.

Gutin PH, Leibel SA, Sheline GE: *Radiation Injury to the Nervous System*. New York, Raven Press, 1991.

Kasatkinan EP, Shilin DE, Rosenbloom AL, et al: Effects of low level radiation from Chernobyl accident in a population with iodine deficiency. *Eur J Pediatr* 1997; 156:916.

Mettler FA, Upton AC: *Medical Effects of Ionizing Radiation*, 2nd ed. Philadelphia, WB Saunders, 1995.

Robertson W, Butler M, D'Angio G, et al: Leg length discrepancy following irradiation for childhood tumors. *J Pediatr Orthop* 1991;11:284.

Scherer E, Streffer C, Trott KR (editors): *Radiopathology of Organs and Tissues.* New York, Springer-Verlag, 1991.

Schiebel-Jost P, Pfeil J, Niethard F, et al: Spinal growth after irradiation for Wilms tumor. *Int Orthop* 1991;15:387.

Shore R: Issues and epidemiological evidence regarding radiation induced thyroid cancer. *Radiat Res* 1992;131:98.

Sources and Effects of Ionizing Radiation, Report to the General Assembly 2000, United Nations Committee on the Effects of Atomic Radiation, Vienna, 2000.

Tokunaga M, Land C, Tukapka S, et al: Incidence of female breast cancer in atomic bomb survivors, 1950–1985. *Radiat Res* 1994;138:209.

Tucker MA, D'Angio G, Boice JD Jr, et al: Bone sarcomas linked to radiotherapy and chemotherapy in children. *N Engl J Med* 1987;317:588.

Tucker MA, Meadows AT, Morris-Jones P, et al: Therapeutic radiation at young age linked to secondary thyroid cancer. *Proc Am Soc Clin Oncol* 1986;5:827.

Wong FL, Boice JD Jr, Abramson DH, et al: Cancer incidence after retinoblastoma: Radiation dose and sarcoma risk. *JAMA* 1997;278:1262.

Chapter 701

Chemical Pollutants

Philip J. Landrigan and Joel A. Forman

Children today are at risk of exposure to more than 80,000 synthetic chemicals, most of which have been developed since World War II. They are especially likely to be exposed to the 2,863 high-production-volume (HPV) chemicals that are produced in amounts of 1 million pounds or more per year and are most widely dispersed in the environment. Fewer than half of the HPV chemicals have been tested for their potential hazards to health, and less than 10% have been assessed for their pediatric or developmental toxicity.

Children are uniquely vulnerable to chemical pollutants for several reasons:

1. They have proportionally greater exposures to many environmental pollutants than adults. Because they drink more water, eat more food, and breathe more air per kilogram of body weight, children are more heavily exposed to pollutants in water, food, and air. Children's hand-to-mouth behavior and their play close to the ground further magnify their exposures.

2. Children's metabolic pathways, especially in the first months after birth, are immature. In some instances, children are better able than adults to cope with environmental toxicants because they are unable to metabolize them to their active form. Commonly, however, children are less able to detoxify and excrete chemical pollutants.

3. Infants and children are growing and developing, and their developmental processes are uniquely sensitive to disruption by chemical pollutants. The disability resulting from exposures to chemicals during windows of early vulnerability can be severe and lifelong (Box 701–1).

4. Because children have many future years of life, they have time to develop multistage chronic diseases that may be triggered by early exposures.

CHEMICAL POLLUTANTS OF MAJOR CONCERN

Air Pollutants. Outdoor air pollutants of greatest concern are photochemical oxidants (especially ozone), oxides of nitrogen (NO_x), fine particulates, sulfur oxides, and carbon monoxide. These pollutants result principally from the combustion of fossil fuels. Automotive emissions are the major source of air pollution worldwide.

Elevated levels of air pollutants, especially elevations of ozone and NO_x, are associated with respiratory problems in children, including decreased pulmonary expiratory flow, wheezing, and

BOX 701–1. Examples of the Vulnerability of Infants and Children to Chemical Pollutants

Diethylstilbestrol and adenocarcinoma of the vagina
Thalidomide and phocomelia
Elevated risk of leukemia after prenatal exposure to trichloroethylene
Fetal alcohol syndrome
Neurobehavioral toxicity of low-dose exposure to lead
Increased risk of cancer after intrauterine exposure to nitrosamine, vinyl chloride, or ionizing radiation
Developmental neurotoxicity of organophosphate insecticides
Environmental tobacco smoke and the increased risk of sudden infant death syndrome and asthma

exacerbations of asthma. Fine particulate air pollution, even at low levels, is associated with slight increases in cardiopulmonary mortality and with an increased death rate from sudden infant death syndrome (SIDS).

Indoor air can also be an important source of respiratory irritation, because many children spend 80–90% of their time indoors. Indoor air pollution has become especially important in the United States since the energy crises of the 1970s, which led to the construction of tighter, more energy-efficient homes. Allergens in indoor air can contribute to respiratory problems and include cockroach, mite, mold, cat, and dog allergens. Some indoor molds produce chemical toxins called mycotoxins. Environmental tobacco smoke is another major contributor to exacerbations of childhood asthma.

Lead (see Chapter 703). Lead exposure occurs worldwide. Exposure is especially common in countries that still permit leaded gasoline. In the United States, pediatric blood lead levels have declined by more than 90% in the past 20 yr, principally as a result of removal of lead from gasoline. Nevertheless, the Centers for Disease Control and Prevention estimates that more than 900,000 children 1–6 yr of age still have blood lead levels of 10 μg/dL and higher. Prevalence is especially high among poor minority children in inner cities. Lead-based paint is the major source of exposure in the United States. Blood lead levels exceeding 10 μg/dL, and possibly even levels of 5–10 μg/dL, are associated with deficits in intellectual function, shortening of attention span, and increased risk of asocial behavior. The extent of injury is directly proportional to lead dose. Because intact lead-painted surfaces invariably break down, efforts to further reduce the number of lead poisoned children in the United States must focus on the identification and permanent removal of all lead-based paint, intact or not, from residences.

Mercury (see Chapter 702). Children may be exposed to either inorganic or organic mercury. Inorganic mercury produces dermatitis, gingivitis, stomatitis, tremor, and acrodynia. Organic or methyl mercury is fat soluble, readily penetrates the central nervous system (CNS), and produces a neurotoxic syndrome. Exposure to organic mercury occurs principally through consumption of fish that have accumulated mercury deposited in lakes and oceans as atmospheric fallout from combustion of coal; coal normally contains small quantities of mercury. Even low-dose exposure to organic mercury has been shown to be hazardous to the developing fetal brain, and pregnant women are therefore advised to curtail consumption of mercury containing fish such as tuna and swordfish. Although adverse neurologic effects have not been related to exposure from the preservative thimerosal, which contains ethyl mercury, thimerosal has been removed from routine childhood vaccines and maternal Rh vaccine (RhoGam) as a precautionary measure.

Asbestos. Between 1947 and 1973, asbestos was sprayed as insulation on classroom walls and ceilings in about 10,000 schools in the United States. Subsequent deterioration of this asbestos has released inhalable asbestos fibers into the air and thus poses a risk to children. Asbestos is a human carcinogen, and the two principal cancers caused by asbestos are lung cancer and mesothelioma. U.S. Federal law requires that all schools be inspected periodically for asbestos and the results made public. Removal is required only when asbestos is visibly deteriorating or is within the reach of children. In most cases, placement of barriers (dry walls or dropped ceilings) provides appropriate protection.

Environmental Tobacco Smoke. Smoking during pregnancy poses a hazard to the fetus (see Chapter 85). Infants born to women who smoke are, on the average, 10% smaller than infants born to nonsmoking women. Infants of parents who smoke have a higher risk of sudden infant death syndrome. Nicotine from tobacco smoke appears to be a developmental neurotoxin.

Passive smoking is also a hazard to children; 43% of children younger than 12 yr old in the United States live in a home with at least one smoker. Children exposed to environmental tobacco smoke have more lower respiratory illness, more middle-ear effusions, and more viral respiratory illnesses than unexposed children.

Pesticides. Pesticides are a diverse group of chemicals used to control insects, weeds, fungi, and rodents. Approximately 600 pesticides are registered with the U.S. Environmental Protection Agency.

Diet is a major route of children's exposure to pesticides; children are exposed to residues of multiple pesticides on fruit and vegetables. Children may also be exposed in homes or schools, on lawns, and in gardens. They may be exposed to pesticide drift from agricultural areas that have been sprayed. Children employed in agriculture or living in migrant farm camps are at risk of exposure to many pesticides.

Pesticides can cause a range of chronic toxic effects: polyneuropathy and CNS dysfunction (organophosphates), hormonal disruption and reproductive impairment (DDT, kepone, dibromochloropropane), cancer (aldrin, dieldrin, chlorphenoxy herbicides [2,4,5-T]), and pulmonary fibrosis (paraquat). Pesticide exposures to children can be reduced by minimizing applications to lawns, gardens, schools, and playgrounds; by adapting techniques of integrated pest management; and by reducing pesticide applications to food crops.

Children can be acutely overexposed to pesticides (see Chapter 704). The organophosphates and carbamates, both of which cause neurotoxicity through inhibition of acetylcholinesterase, cause the largest number of acute poisoning cases. Symptoms include meiosis (though not in all cases), excess salivation, abdominal cramping, vomiting, diarrhea, and muscle fasciculation. In severe cases, loss of consciousness, cardiac arrhythmias, and death by respiratory arrest occur. The war gas sarin is an organophosphate. See Chapter 704 for treatment of poisoning from drugs, chemicals, and plants.

PCBs, DDT, Dioxins, and Other Chlorinated Hydrocarbons. Chlorinated hydrocarbons are used as insecticides (DDT), plastics (polyvinyl chloride [PVC]), electrical insulators (polychlorinated biphenyls, [PCBs]), and solvents (trichloroethylene). Highly toxic dioxins and furans can be formed during synthesis of chlorinated herbicides or as by-products of plastic combustion. All of these materials are widely dispersed in the environment. DDT, PCBs, and dioxins are highly persistent.

The embryo, fetus, and young child are at particularly high risk of injury from PCBs, DDT, and dioxins. All these compounds are lipid soluble. They readily cross the placenta, and they accumulate in breast milk. Intrauterine exposure to PCBs has been repeatedly linked to persistent neurobehavioral dysfunction in children.

Fish from contaminated waters are a major source of children's exposure to PCBs. Children can be exposed in utero or through breast milk. To protect children and pregnant women in the United States against PCBs in fish, government agencies have issued fish consumption advisories for certain lakes and rivers. Combustion of medical wastes containing PVC and the bleaching of paper products with chlorine are major preventable sources of environmental dioxin and should be discouraged.

Endocrine Disruptors. A number of chemicals have been shown to adversely affect the endocrine systems of animals and humans, including diethylstilbestrol (DES), DDT, PCBs, and dioxins. Other chemicals are also suspected of possessing endocrine disruptor effects, including other pesticides and phthalates (plasticizers). Effects on wildlife include eggshell thinning in birds, sterility in seals, feminization and cryptorchidism in panthers, low hatching rates in alligators, and many others. In humans, endocrine disruption has been implicated in the epidemiologic observations of a trend toward earlier thelarche and menarche in girls, the increasing rates of testicular cancer and hypospadias, and decreasing sperm counts. The most clearly observed effects include adenocarcinoma of the vagina in women and cryptorchidism in men whose mothers took DES. The presence of elevated plasma phthalate esters has been associated with early thelarche in Puerto Rican girls. Some endocrine disruptors may also have adverse effects on brain development. Continuing research in this area is of particular importance because of the widespread human exposure to, and the long-term biopersistence of, many of these chemicals.

Environmental Carcinogens. Children may be exposed to carcinogenic pollutants in utero or after birth. Children appear more sensitive than adults to certain chemical carcinogens and also to radiation (see Chapter 700). The potential for in utero carcinogenesis was first recognized with the discovery that clear cell adenocarcinoma of the vagina could occur in women after intrauterine exposure to DES.

Several examples exist of carcinogenesis associated with exposures in the home and community. Children of asbestos workers and children who have grown up in communities near asbestos plants have been found to have a higher incidence of mesothelioma than unexposed populations. Children who grow up on farms have elevated rates of leukemia; pesticides are suspected of playing an etiologic role. Intrauterine exposure to trichloroethylene by way of contaminated drinking water has been associated with an increased incidence of leukemia among girls living near an industrial facility and industrial waste site.

The National Cancer Institute (NCI) reports that incidence rates of leukemia and cerebral glioma, the two most common forms of childhood malignancy, have been increasing for the past 3 decades, despite greatly improved therapy and declining death rates. The cumulative increase in incidence for glioma is now about 30%. Similar increases in incidence of childhood cancer have been seen in the United Kingdom. Research is ongoing to determine whether chemical pollutants in the environment have contributed to this reported increasing incidence of childhood cancer.

ROUTES OF EXPOSURE

Transplacental. Heavy metals and fat-soluble compounds such as PCBs and DDT readily cross the placenta. They may produce serious and irreversible toxic effects on the developing nervous, endocrine, and reproductive organs even at very low levels.

Water. About 200 chemicals have been found in various amounts in water supplies. Lead is especially common. In some older neighborhoods, lead in water derives from lead pipes. More commonly, it is dissolved (leached) from solder by soft, acidic water. The highest levels of lead occur in water that has been standing in pipes overnight; therefore, it is wise to run water for 2–3 min each morning before making up infant formula. Solvents and components of gasoline such as methyl tertiary-butyl ether (MTBE) and benzene are commonly encountered in ground water.

Air. Vehicular emissions are the major source of urban air pollution. Diesel exhaust is a human carcinogen. In rural areas, wood smoke can contribute to air pollution. Children living in the vicinity of smelters and chemical production plants can be exposed to toxic industrial emissions such as lead, benzene, and 1,3-butadiene.

Food. Many chemicals are intentionally added to food to improve appearance, taste, texture, or preservation. Many such chemicals have been poorly tested for potential toxicity. Residues of many pesticides are found in both raw and processed foods.

Work Clothes. Illnesses in children are at times traceable to contaminated dust from parents' work clothes; toxicity from lead, beryllium, dioxin, organophosphate pesticides, and asbestos has occurred. Prevention is achieved by providing facilities at work for changing and showering.

Schools. Children may be exposed in schools, kindergartens, and nurseries to lead paint, molds, asbestos, environmental tobacco smoke, pesticides, and hazardous arts and crafts materials. Substantial opportunities for prevention exist in the school environment, and pediatricians are often consulted for advice.

Child Labor. Four to 5 million children and adolescents in the United States work for pay, and child labor is widespread around the world. Working children are at high risk of physical trauma and injury. Also, they may be exposed to a wide range of toxic chemicals, including pesticides in agriculture and lawn work, asbestos in construction and building demolition, and benzene in pumping gasoline.

THE PHYSICIAN'S ROLE

Pediatricians should always be alert to the possibility that a chemical pollutant has caused disease in a child. In considering the origins of noninfectious disease, they should ask about the home environment, parental occupation, unusual exposures, and neighborhood factories. Especially when several unusual cases of disease or constellations of findings occur together, an environmental cause is possible. Any adolescent with a traumatic injury may have been injured at work.

The history is the single most important instrument for obtaining information on environmental exposures. Information about current and past exposures should routinely be sought through a few brief screening questions. Changes in patterns of exposure or new exposures may be especially important. If suspicious information is elicited, more detailed follow-up should be pursued. Referral to a pediatric environmental health specialty unit may be indicated. Accurate diagnosis of an environmental cause of disease can lead to better care of sick children and prevention of disease in other children.

American Academy of Pediatrics, Committee on Environmental Health: Environmental tobacco smoke: A hazard to children. *Pediatrics* 1997;99:639–42.

American Academy of Pediatrics, Committee on Environmental Health: Risk of ionizing radiation exposure to children: A subject review. *Pediatrics* 1998;101:717–19.

Centers for Disease Control and Prevention: Blood lead levels in young children—United States and selected states, 1996–1999. *MMWR Morbid Mortal Wkly Rep* 2000;49:1133–37.

Centers for Disease Control and Prevention: *National Report on Human Exposure to Environmental Chemicals.* Atlanta, Georgia, March 2001.

Colón I, Caro D, Bourdony CJ, et al: Identification of phthalate esters in the serum of young Puerto Rican girls with premature breast development. *Environ Health Perspect* 2000;108:895–900.

Environmental Defense Fund: *Toxic Ignorance: The Continuing Absence of Basic Health Testing for Top-Selling Toxic Chemicals in the United States.* Washington, DC, Environmental Defense Fund, 1997.

Etzel RA, Balk SJ (editors): *Handbook of Environmental Health for Children.* Elk Grove Village, IL, American Academy of Pediatrics, 1999.

Gilliland FD, Gerhane K, Rappaport EB, et al: The effects of ambient air pollution on school absenteeism due to respiratory illnesses. *Epidemiology* 2001;12:43–54.

Jacobson JL, Jacobson SW: Intellectual impairment in children exposed to polychlorinated biphenyls in utero. *N Engl J Med* 1996;335:783–89.

Lanphear BP: Cognitive deficits associated with blood lead concentrations < 10 μg/dL in US children and adolescents. *Public Health Rep* 2000;115:521–29.

Longnecker MP, Rogan WJ, Lucier G: The human health effects of DDT (dichlorodiphenyltrichloroethane) and PCBs (polychlorinated biphenyls) and an overview of organochlorines in public health. *Annu Rev Public Health* 1997;18:211–44.

Magnani C, Dalmasso P, Biggeri A, et al: Increased risk of malignant mesothelioma of the pleura after residential or domestic exposure to asbestos: A case-control study in Casale Monferrato, Italy. *Environ Health Perspect* 2001;109:915–19.

Paulozzi L, Erickson JD, Jackson RJ: Hypospadias trends in two American surveillance systems. *Pediatrics* 1997;100:831–34.

Paulson JA (editor): Children's Environmental Health. *Pediatr Clin North Am* 2001;48(5):xv–1337.

Rogan WJ, Dietrich KN, Ware JH, et al: The effect of chelation therapy with succimer on neuropsychological development in children exposed to lead. *N Engl J Med* 2001;344:1421–26.

Rosenstreich DL, Eggleston P, Kattan M, et al: The role of cockroach allergy and exposure to cockroach in causing morbidity among inner-city children with asthma. *N Engl J Med* 1997;336:1356–63.

Chapter 702
Heavy Metal Intoxication
Collin S. Goto

Metals are electropositive elements characterized by properties such as luster, malleability, and the ability to conduct electricity. Severe illness may result when humans are exposed to the group known as the heavy metals. These substances have an immense range of industrial applications, and the majority of human poisonings result from occupational and household exposures or consumption of contaminated food, water, or medicinal preparations.

Heavy metal intoxication tends to result in diverse multiorgan toxicity through widespread disruption of vital cellular functions. After ingestion, gastrointestinal, renal, hematologic, and nervous system toxicity are common. Cutaneous abnormalities are also seen, and inhalation of fumes and vapors may cause a severe pneumonitis. The protean manifestations of heavy metal intoxication can easily be misdiagnosed unless a meticulous history of environmental exposure is obtained. Among the most common causes of heavy metal intoxication, arsenic and mercury are discussed in this section. Lead poisoning is discussed in Chapter 703. Also see Chapters 706 and 713.

ARSENIC

Epidemiology. Arsenic exists in the following forms: elemental arsenic, arsine gas, inorganic arsenic salts, and organic arsenic compounds. Children may be poisoned after exposure to inorganic arsenic found in pesticides, herbicides, dyes, homeopathic medicines, and certain folk remedies from China, India, and Southeast Asia. Soil deposits may contaminate artesian well water. Occupational exposure may occur in industries such as glass manufacturing, pottery, electronic components, semiconductors, mining, smelting, and refining. Organic arsenic compounds may be found in seafood, pesticides, and some veterinary pharmaceuticals. In contrast to mercury, the organic forms of arsenic found in seafood are nontoxic.

Pharmacokinetics. Elemental arsenic is insoluble in water and bodily fluids and therefore is insignificantly absorbed and nontoxic. Inhaled arsine gas is rapidly absorbed through the lungs. The inorganic arsenic salts are well absorbed through the gastrointestinal tract and lungs. The organic arsenic compounds are well absorbed through the gastrointestinal tract.

After acute exposure, arsenic is rapidly distributed to all tissues. Inorganic arsenic is methylated and eliminated predominantly by the kidneys, with about 95% excreted in the urine and 5% excreted in the bile. The majority of the arsenic is eliminated in the first few days, with the remainder slowly excreted over a period of several weeks.

Pathophysiology. After exposure to arsine gas, absorbed arsine enters red blood cells (RBCs) and is oxidized to arsenic dihydride and elemental arsenic. Complexing of these derivatives with RBC sulfhydryl groups results in cell membrane instability and massive hemolysis. The inorganic arsenic salts poison enzymatic processes vital to cellular metabolism. Trivalent arsenic binds to sulfhydryl groups, resulting in decreased production of adenosine triphosphate through the inhibition of enzyme systems such as the pyruvate dehydrogenase and α-ketoglutarate complexes. Pentavalent arsenic may be biotransformed to trivalent arsenic or substituted for phosphate in the glycolytic pathway, resulting in uncoupling of oxidative phosphorylation.

Clinical Manifestations. Arsine gas is colorless, odorless, nonirritating, and highly toxic. Inhalation causes no immediate symptoms. After a latent period of 2–24 hr, massive hemolysis occurs, along with malaise, headache, weakness, dyspnea, nausea, vomiting, abdominal pain, hepatomegaly, pallor, jaundice, hemoglobinuria, and renal failure.

Gastrointestinal toxicity begins within minutes to hours of an acute ingestion of the inorganic arsenic salts, manifested by nausea, vomiting, abdominal pain, and diarrhea. Hemorrhagic gastroenteritis with extensive fluid loss and third spacing may result in hypovolemic shock. Cardiovascular toxicity includes QT interval prolongation, polymorphous ventricular tachycardia, congestive cardiomyopathy, pulmonary edema, and cardiogenic shock. Acute neurologic toxicity includes delirium, seizures, cerebral edema, encephalopathy, and coma. A delayed sensorimotor peripheral neuropathy may appear days to weeks after acute exposure, secondary to axonal degeneration. Early effects include painful dysesthesias, followed by diminished vibratory, pain, touch, and temperature sensation; decreased deep tendon reflexes; and, in the most severe cases, an ascending paralysis with respiratory failure mimicking Guillain-Barré syndrome. Other effects include fever, hepatitis, rhabdomyolysis, renal failure, hemolytic anemia, pancytopenia, and alopecia.

Subacute toxicity is characterized by prolonged fatigue, malaise, weight loss, headache, chronic encephalopathy, peripheral sensorimotor neuropathy, leukopenia, anemia, thrombocytopenia, chronic cough, and gastroenteritis. Transverse striae in the nails, known as Mees lines, become apparent 1–2 mo after exposure in about 5% of patients. Dermatologic findings include alopecia, oral ulceration, peripheral edema, a pruritic macular rash, and desquamation.

Chronic exposure to low levels of arsenic is usually from environmental or occupational sources. Well water contaminated with arsenic leached from ground mineral deposits has resulted in millions of cases of chronic arsenic toxicity in Bangladesh, Taiwan, Mexico, and other locations worldwide. Over the course of years, dermatologic lesions develop, including hyperpigmentation, hypopigmentation, hyperkeratoses (especially on the palms and soles), squamous and basal cell carcinomas, and Bowen disease. Encephalopathy and peripheral neuropathy may be present. In addition, hepatomegaly, hypersplenism, noncirrhotic portal fibrosis, and portal hypertension are known to occur. Blackfoot disease is an obliterative arterial disease of the lower extremities associated with chronic arsenic exposure in Taiwan.

Laboratory Findings. The diagnosis of arsenic intoxication is based on characteristic clinical findings, a history of exposure, and elevated urinary arsenic levels, which confirm the exposure. A spot urine arsenic level should be determined for sympto-

matic patients before chelation, although the result may be negative acutely. Because urinary excretion of arsenic is intermittent, definitive diagnosis depends on a 24-hr urine collection. Concentrations greater than 50 μg/L in a 24-hr urine collection are consistent with arsenic intoxication. Urine specimens must be collected in metal-free containers. Ingestion of seafood containing nontoxic arsenobetaine and arsenocholine can cause elevated urinary arsenic levels. Blood arsenic levels are rarely helpful because of their high variability and the rapid clearance of arsenic from the blood in acute poisonings. Elevated arsenic levels in the hair or nails must be interpreted cautiously because of the possibility of external contamination. Abdominal radiographs may demonstrate ingested arsenic, which is radiopaque.

Later in the course of illness, a complete blood cell count may show anemia, thrombocytopenia, and leukocytosis, followed by leukopenia, karyorrhexis, and basophilic stippling of RBCs. The serum levels of creatinine, bilirubin, and transaminases may be elevated; urinalysis may show proteinuria, pyuria, and hematuria; and examination of the cerebrospinal fluid may show elevated protein levels.

MERCURY

Epidemiology. Mercury exists in three forms: elemental mercury, inorganic mercury salts, and organic mercury. Elemental mercury is present in thermometers, sphygmomanometers, barometers, batteries, and some latex paints produced before 1991. Workers in industries producing these products may expose their children to the toxin when mercury is brought home on contaminated clothing. Vacuuming of carpet contaminated with mercury and breaking of mercury fluorescent light bulbs may result in elemental mercury vapor exposure. In addition, severe inhalation poisonings have resulted from attempts to separate gold from gold ore by heating mercury and forming a gold-mercury amalgam. Elemental mercury has also been used in folk remedies by Asian and Mexican populations for chronic stomach pain and by Latin Americans and Caribbean natives in occult practices (see Chapter 3). Dental amalgams containing elemental mercury release trace amounts of mercury that do not pose a credible risk to health. An expert panel for the National Institutes of Health has concluded that existing scientific evidence does not indicate that dental amalgams pose a health risk. They should not be replaced merely to decrease mercury exposure.

Inorganic mercury salts are found in pesticides, disinfectants, antiseptics, pigments, dry batteries, and explosives and as preservatives in some medicinal preparations.

Organic mercury in the diet, especially fish containing methyl mercury, is a major source of mercury exposure to the general population. Industries that may produce mercury-containing effluents include chlorine and caustic soda productions, mining and metallurgy, electroplating, chemical and textile manufacturing, paper and pharmaceutical manufacturing, and leather tanning. Mercury compounds in the environment are methylated to methyl mercury by soil and water microorganisms. Methyl mercury in the water rapidly accumulates in fish and other aquatic organisms, which are in turn consumed by humans. Well-known large outbreaks of methyl mercury intoxication include the incidents in Japan in the 1950s (from consumption of contaminated seafood) and in Iraq in 1971 (from consumption of grain treated with a methyl mercury fungicide).

Thimerosal is a mercury-containing preservative used in some vaccines. Thimerosal contains 49.6% mercury by weight and is metabolized to ethyl mercury and thiosalicylate. During an ongoing review of biologic products in response to the Food and Drug Administration (FDA) Modernization Act of 1997, the FDA determined that infants who received thimerosal-containing vaccines at multiple visits may have been exposed to more mercury than recommended by federal guidelines. As a precautionary measure, the American Academy of Pediatrics, American Academy of Family Physicians, Advisory Committee on Immunization Practices, and U.S. Public Health Service issued a joint recommendation in 1999 that thimerosal be removed from vaccines as quickly as possible. In the United States, thimerosal has been removed from all vaccines in the recommended childhood immunization schedule.

Pharmacokinetics. Inhaled elemental mercury vapor is 80% absorbed by the lungs and rapidly distributed to the central nervous system (CNS) because of its high lipid solubility. The elemental mercury is oxidized by catalase to the mercuric ion, which is the reactive form causing cellular toxicity. Elemental mercury liquid is poorly absorbed from the gastrointestinal tract, with less than 0.1% being absorbed. The half-life of elemental mercury in the tissues is about 60 days, with most of the excretion being in the urine.

Inorganic mercury salts are about 10% absorbed from the gastrointestinal tract and cross the blood-brain barrier to a lesser extent than elemental mercury. Mercuric salts are more soluble than mercurous salts and therefore produce greater toxicity. Elimination occurs primarily in the urine, with a half-life of about 40 days.

Methyl mercury is the most avidly absorbed of the organic mercury compounds, with about 90% absorbed from the gastrointestinal tract. Its lipophilic, short-chain alkyl structure enables methyl mercury to distribute rapidly across the blood-brain barrier and placenta. Methyl mercury is about 90% excreted in the bile, with the remainder being excreted in the urine. The half-life is 70 days.

Pathophysiology. After absorption, mercury is distributed to all tissues, particularly the CNS and kidneys. Mercury reacts with sulfhydryl, phosphoryl, carboxyl, and amide groups, resulting in disruption of enzymes, transport mechanisms, membranes, and structural proteins. Widespread cellular dysfunction or necrosis results in the multiorgan toxicity characteristic of mercury poisoning.

Clinical Manifestations. Five syndromes describe the clinical presentation of mercury poisoning:

Acute inhalation of elemental mercury vapor results in rapid onset of cough, dyspnea, chest pain, fever, chills, headaches, and visual disturbances. Gastrointestinal findings include metallic taste, salivation, nausea, vomiting, and diarrhea. Depending on the severity of the exposure, the illness may be self-limited or may progress to necrotizing bronchiolitis, interstitial pneumonitis, pulmonary edema, and death from respiratory failure. Younger children are more susceptible to pulmonary toxicity. Survivors may develop restrictive lung disease. Renal dysfunction and neurologic disturbances may develop subacutely.

Acute ingestion of inorganic mercury salts can present in a few hours with corrosive gastroenteritis manifested by oropharyngeal burns, nausea, hematemesis, severe abdominal pain, hematochezia, acute tubular necrosis, cardiovascular collapse, and death.

Chronic inorganic mercury intoxication produces the classic triad of tremor, neuropsychiatric disturbances, and gingivostomatitis. The syndrome may result from chronic exposure to elemental mercury, inorganic mercury salts, or certain organic mercury compounds, all of which may be metabolized to mercuric ions. The tremor starts as a fine intention tremor of the fingers that is abolished during sleep, but it may later involve the face and progress to choreoathetosis and spasmodic ballismus. Mixed sensorimotor neuropathy and visual disturbances may also be present. The neuropsychiatric disturbances include emotional lability, delirium, headaches, memory loss, insomnia, anorexia, and fatigue. Renal dysfunction ranges from asymptomatic proteinuria to nephrotic syndrome.

Acrodynia, or **pink disease,** is a rare idiosyncratic hypersensitivity reaction to mercury that occurs predominantly in children. The symptom complex includes generalized pain, paresthesias, and an acral rash that may spread to involve the face. It is typically pink, papular, and pruritic and may progress to desquamation and ulceration. Morbilliform, vesicular, and hemorrhagic variants have been described. Other important features include anorexia, apathy, and hypotonia, especially of the pectoral and pelvic girdles. Irritability, tremors, diaphoresis, insomnia, hypertension, and tachycardia may be present. The outcome is good after removal of the source of mercury exposure.

Methyl mercury intoxication is also referred to as **Minamata disease** after the widespread mercury poisoning that occurred at Minamata Bay in Japan after the ingestion of contaminated fish. Methyl mercury poisoning presents as delayed neurotoxicity after a latent period of weeks to months, characterized by ataxia; dysarthria; paresthesias; tremors; movement disorders; impairment of vision, hearing, smell, and taste; memory loss; progressive dementia; and death. Infants exposed in utero are the most severely affected, with low birthweight, microcephaly, profound developmental delay, cerebral palsy, deafness, blindness, and seizures.

Laboratory Findings. The diagnosis of mercury intoxication is based on characteristic clinical findings, a history of exposure, and elevated whole blood or urine mercury levels, which confirm the exposure. Levels less than 10 µg/L in whole blood and 20 µg/L in a 24-hr urine collection are considered normal. Although blood mercury levels may reflect acute exposure, they decrease as mercury redistributes into the tissues. Urine mercury levels are most useful for identifying chronic exposures, except in the case of methyl mercury, because methyl mercury undergoes minimal urinary excretion. Hair analysis for mercury is not reliable because hair reflects endogenous as well as exogenous mercury exposure (hair avidly binds mercury from the environment). Abdominal radiographs may demonstrate ingested radiopaque mercury.

Urinary markers of early nephrotoxicity include microalbuminuria, retinol-binding protein, β_2-microglobulin, and N-acetyl-β-D-glucosaminidase. Early neurotoxicity may be detected with neuropsychiatric testing and nerve conduction studies, whereas severe CNS toxicity is apparent on CT or MRI.

TREATMENT OF ARSENIC AND MERCURY INTOXICATION

The principles of management for arsenic and mercury intoxication include prompt removal from the source of poisoning, aggressive stabilization and supportive care, decontamination, and chelation therapy when appropriate. Once the diagnosis is suspected, the local poison control facility should be contacted and care coordinated with physicians who are familiar with the management of heavy metal poisoning.

Supportive care for patients exposed to arsine gas requires close monitoring for signs of hemolysis, including evaluation of the peripheral blood smear and urinalysis. Transfusion of packed RBCs may be necessary, as well as administration of intravenous fluids, sodium bicarbonate, and mannitol to prevent renal failure secondary to the deposition of hemoglobin in the kidneys. After inhalation of elemental mercury vapor, patients require careful monitoring of respiratory status, which may include pulse oximetry, arterial blood gas analysis, and chest radiography. Supportive care includes administration of supplemental oxygen and, in severe cases, intubation and mechanical ventilation.

Acute ingestion of inorganic arsenic and mercury salts results in hemorrhagic gastroenteritis, cardiovascular collapse, and multiorgan dysfunction. Fluid resuscitation, pressor agents, and transfusion of blood products may be required for management of cardiovascular instability. Severe respiratory distress, coma with loss of airway reflexes, intractable seizures, and respiratory paralysis are indications for intubation and mechanical ventilation. Renal function must be carefully monitored for signs of renal failure and the need for hemodialysis.

Gastrointestinal decontamination after ingestion of the inorganic arsenic and mercury salts has not been well studied. Because of the corrosive effects of these compounds, induced emesis is not recommended, and endoscopy may be considered before gastric lavage. Although arsenic and mercury are not well adsorbed to activated charcoal, its use is generally advocated, especially if co-ingestants are suspected. Whole bowel irrigation is used to remove any radiopaque material remaining in the gastrointestinal tract.

Chelation for acute arsenic and mercury poisoning is most effective when administered as soon as possible after the exposure. Chelation should be continued until 24-hr urinary arsenic or mercury levels return to normal (<50 μg/L for arsenic and <20 μg/L for mercury), the patient is symptom free, or the remaining toxic effects are believed to be irreversible. The efficacy of chelation in chronic exposures is reduced because heavy metal in the tissue compartment is relatively unexchangeable and some degree of irreversible toxicity has already occurred.

Dimercaprol, also known as 2,3-dimercaptopropanol or British antilewisite (BAL), is the chelator of choice if a patient cannot tolerate oral therapy. This is often the case in critically ill patients and after ingestion of the corrosive inorganic arsenic and mercury salts. BAL is available suspended in peanut oil and benzyl benzoate in 3-mL ampules at a concentration of 100 mg/mL for deep intramuscular (IM) injection. For arsenic poisoning, the recommended regimen of BAL is 2.5 mg/kg IM q6h for the first 2 days, 2.5 mg/kg IM q12h on the third day, then 2.5 mg/kg/day IM for 10 days. For severe arsenic poisoning, the dose of BAL is increased to 3 mg/kg IM q4h for 2 days, 3 mg/kg IM q6h on day 3, then 3 mg/kg IM q12h for 10 days. The dose of BAL for inorganic mercury poisoning is 5 mg/kg IM on the first day, then 2.5 mg/kg IM q12–24h for 10 days. The BAL–heavy metal complex is excreted in the urine and bile. A period of 5 days between courses of chelation is recommended. Adverse effects of BAL include pain at the injection site, hypertension, tachycardia, diaphoresis, nausea, vomiting, abdominal pain, a burning sensation in the oropharynx, and a feeling of constriction in the chest. BAL may cause hemolysis in glucose-6-phosphate dehydrogenase (G6PD)-deficient individuals. It is important to note that BAL is contraindicated for chelation of methyl mercury because BAL redistributes methyl mercury to the brain from other tissue sites, resulting in increased neurotoxicity.

Oral chelating agents are used to replace the painful BAL injections when the patient is stable enough to tolerate oral therapy and prolonged chelation is necessary. Succimer, also known as 2,3-dimercaptosuccinic acid (DMSA), is an orally administered water-soluble derivative of BAL. DMSA is available in 100-mg capsules. The recommended regimen of DMSA is 1,050 mg/m²/24 hr (or 30 mg/kg/24 hr) orally in three divided doses for 5 days, then 700 mg/m²/24 hr (or 20 mg/kg/24 hr) orally in two divided doses for 14 days. The DMSA–heavy metal complex is excreted in the urine and bile. A period of 2 wk between courses of chelation is recommended. Mild adverse effects include nausea, vomiting, diarrhea, loss of appetite, and transient elevations in liver enzyme levels. DMSA may also cause hemolysis in G6PD-deficient patients.

American Academy of Pediatics, Committee on Environmental Health. Technical report: Mercury in the environment: Implications for pediatricians. *Pediatrics* 2001;108:197–204.

Baum CR: Treatment of mercury intoxication. *Curr Opin Pediatr* 1999;11:265–68.

Centers for Disease Control and Prevention: Summary of the joint statement on thimerosal in vaccines. American Academy of Family Physicians, American Academy of Pediatricians, Advisory Committee on Immunization Practices, Public Health Service. *MMWR Morbid Mortal Wkly Rep* 2000;49:622–31.

Cullen NM, Wolf LR, St Clair D: Pediatric arsenic ingestion. *Am J Emerg Med* 1995; 432–35.

Kew J, Morris C, Aihie A, et al: Arsenic and mercury intoxication due to Indian ethnic remedies. *BMJ* 1993;306:506–7.

Kondo K: Congenital Minamata disease: Warnings from Japan's experience. *J Child Neurol* 2000;15:458–464.

Chapter 703
Lead Poisoning *Morri Markowitz*

Epidemiology. Lead exists in four isotopic forms and is classified as a metal. Chemically, its low melting point and ability to form stable compounds has made it useful for hundreds of products. Clinically, it is purely a toxicant; no organism has an essential function that is lead dependent. Medical knowledge pertaining to its toxicity has existed for more than 2,000 years. Nevertheless, its commercial attractiveness has resulted in the processing of millions of tons of lead ore. The result is widespread dissemination of lead in the human environment.

The threshold level at which lead causes biochemical, subclinical, or clinical disturbance has been redefined many times during the past 50 yr as a result of extensive research efforts. In clinical medicine, the blood lead level (BLL) is the gold standard for determining health effects. An ideal BLL is 0. However, since 1991, the Centers for Disease Control (CDC), followed by the American Academy of Pediatrics, has considered a BLL up to 10 μg/dL as being acceptable. This number is likely to decline with further research into the effects of lead.

Using 10 μg/dL as a reference point for children at risk for lead poisoning, public health measures have had remarkable success. In a major survey, the National Health and Nutrition Examination Survey II, conducted on a representative sample of the U.S. population between 1976 and 1980, showed greater than 85% of preschool-aged children had elevated BLLs; 98% of African-American preschoolers had elevated levels. Over the next 15 yr, government regulations resulted in the significant reduction of three main contributors to lead exposure: (1) the elimination of the use of tetraethyl leaded gasoline, (2) the banning of lead-containing solder to seal food and beverage containing cans, and (3) the application of a federal rule that limited the amount of lead allowed in paint intended for household use to less than 0.07% by weight. Continued surveillance by the CDC has shown that the prevalence of elevated BLLs has declined markedly and is now below 10% of preschoolers. Of these children, less than 10% have BLLs greater than 20 μg/dL. Children with levels high enough to be life threatening are rare, but deaths continue to occur. These estimates imply that there are still more than a half million U.S. children with elevated BLLs.

A closer analysis shows that the remaining cases of BLL elevations are not evenly distributed across the United States but vary considerably by state and county. Several factors have been identified that indicate increased risk of lead poisoning, including, in addition to preschool age, low socioeconomic status, living in older housing built primarily before 1960, urban location, and African-American race. The combination of these factors identifies a group of children of whom more than 20% still have elevated BLLs. Other high-risk groups include recent immigrants, including adoptees, from countries that still use leaded gasoline or ceramic ware with lead-containing glazes. Prevalence rates in many United States locations are unknown.

SOURCES OF EXPOSURE. Lead poisoning may occur in utero because lead readily crosses the placenta from maternal blood. The spectrum of toxicity is similar to that experienced by children after birth. The source of maternal blood lead content is either redistribution from endogenous stores, her skeleton, or newly acquired lead due to ongoing environmental exposure.

Although there are several hundred products that contain lead, such as batteries, cable sheathing, cosmetics, mineral supplements, plastics, and toys, the major source of exposure to U.S. children remains old lead-based paint; by estimates there are about 40 million households with some lead-based paint. As paint deteriorates it chalks, flakes, and turns to dust. Improper rehabilitation work of painted surfaces can result in dissemination of lead-containing dust throughout a home. The dust can coat all surfaces, including children's hands. All of these forms of lead can be ingested. If remodeling work is done by using heat to strip paint, then lead vapor concentrations in the room can reach levels sufficient to cause lead poisoning by way of inhalation.

Pathophysiology. The non-nutritive hand-to-mouth activity of young children provides the pathway for lead to enter the body in the majority of children. In nearly all cases lead is ingested either as a component of dust licked off of surfaces or in swallowed paint chips. Less commonly, water contaminated by its flow through lead pipes or brass fixtures is drunk or food is contaminated by contact with lead-glazed ceramic ware. Cutaneous contamination with inorganic lead compounds, as are found in pigments, does not result in a substantial amount of absorption. In contrast, organic lead compounds such as tetraethyl lead may penetrate through skin.

Once lead is in the intestine the percentage absorbed depends on several factors: particle size, pH, other material in the intestine, and nutritional status of essential elements. Large paint chips are difficult to digest and mainly are excreted. Fine dust can be dissolved more readily, especially in an acid medium. Lead eaten on an empty stomach is better absorbed than if taken with a meal. The presence of calcium and iron may decrease lead absorption by direct competition for binding sites. On the other hand, iron, and probably calcium, deficiency results in enhanced lead absorption, retention, and toxicity.

After absorption, lead is disseminated throughout the body by way of the blood. It circulates bound to erythrocytes; about 97% is bound on or in the red blood cell. The plasma fraction is too small to be measured by conventional techniques such as atomic absorption spectroscopy or anodic stripping voltammetry; it is, however, presumably the plasma portion that may enter cells and induce toxicity. In cells, lead has multiple effects. It binds to enzymes, particularly those with available sulfhydryl groups, changing the contour and diminishing function. The heme pathway, present in all cells, has three enzymes susceptible to lead inhibitory effects. The last enzyme in this pathway, ferrochelatase, enables protoporphyrin to chelate iron, thus forming heme. Protoporphyrin is readily measurable in red blood cells. Levels greater than 35 μg/dL are abnormal and are consistent with lead poisoning, iron deficiency, or recent inflammatory disease. Lack of heme affects multiple metabolic pathways. The accumulation of excess amounts of protoporphyrin and other heme precursors is toxic as well, independently of lead. Measurement of the erythrocyte protoporphyrin (EP) level is, therefore, a useful tool for monitoring biochemical lead toxicity. In general, EP levels begin to rise several weeks after BLLs have reached 20 μg/dL in a susceptible portion of the population and will be elevated in nearly all children with BLLs of more than 50 μg/dL. A decrease in EP levels also lags behind a decrease in BLLs by several weeks, because it depends on both cessation of further overproduction in marrow red cell precursors and cell turnover.

A second mechanism of lead toxicity is by way of its competition with calcium. Many calcium-binding proteins have a higher affinity for lead. Lead bound to these proteins may alter function, resulting in intracellular and intercellular communications breakdown. For example, neurotransmitter release is in part a calcium-dependent process that is adversely affected by lead.

Although these two mechanisms of toxicity may be reversible, a third way that lead may cause harm is by preventing the development of the normal tertiary structure in the brain. In immature mammals, the normal pruning process that results in elimination of multiple intercellular brain connections is inhibited by lead. This process is part of the timed developmental sequence that humans undergo as well. Failure to construct the appropriate tertiary brain structure during the first few years of life may, therefore, result in a permanent abnormality.

Clinical Manifestations. The BLL is the best studied measure of lead in children. Subclinical and clinical findings correlate with BLLs in populations. However, there is considerable inter-individual variability in this relationship. For instance, lead encephalopathy is more likely to be observed in children with BLLs greater than 100 μg/dL. Yet, one child may have no symptoms with a BLL of 300 μg/dL and another will be in the intensive care unit on life support for cerebral edema.

Several subclinical effects of lead have been demonstrated in cross-sectional epidemiologic studies. Hearing and height were inversely related to BLLs in children. In neither case does the lead effect reach a level that would bring an individual child to medical attention. Rather, as BLLs increased in the study population, a little more sound, at all frequencies, was needed to reach hearing threshold. Likewise, children with higher BLLs were slightly shorter than those with lower levels; for every 10 μg higher the BLL, the children were 1 cm shorter.

In addition, a number of longitudinal studies have followed cohorts of children from birth for as long as 20 yr and examined the relationship between BLLs and cognitive test scores over time. These studies were designed to address the question of whether lead causes or is a marker of cognitive deficits. In general, BLLs, expressed as either a level obtained at around 2 yr of age or a measure that integrates multiple BLLs drawn from a subject over time, are inversely related to cognitive test scores. On average, for each 1 μg/dL elevation in BLL the cognitive score is approximately a quarter to half a point lower. However, this relationship is not based on concurrent testing of lead and cognition. Rather it is the BLLs from early childhood that are predictors of the cognitive test results performed years later. This implies that the cognitive effects of lead are permanent.

Data from two studies challenge this implication. In the first, scores on the Bayley Scale of Mental Development were obtained repeatedly every 6 mo for the first 2 yr of life. Results correlated inversely with cord BLL, a measure of in utero exposure, but not with BLLs obtained concurrently at the time of developmental testing. However, after 2 yr of age all other cognitive tests performed on the cohort over the next 10 yr correlated with the BLLs at age 2 yr but not with cord BLLs. Thus, the effects of prenatal lead exposure on brain function were superseded by early childhood events and later BLLs. The second line of evidence is from an intervention study in which moderately lead-poisoned children, with initial BLLs of 20–55 μg/dL, were aggressively managed over 6 mo. Components of treatment included education regarding sources of lead and its abatement, nutritional guidance, multiple home and clinic visits, and, for a subset, chelation therapy. Average BLLs declined, and cognitive scores were again inversely related to the change in BLL. For every 1 μg/dL decrease in BLL, cognitive scores were one quarter point higher.

Behavior is also disturbed by lead. Hyperactivity is noted in young school-aged children with histories of lead poisoning or with concurrent elevations in BLL. Older children with higher bone lead content are more likely to be aggressive and to have behaviors that are predictive of later juvenile delinquency. Whether the behavioral effects of lead are reversible has only been examined in a single small study. Seven-year-old hyperactive children with BLLs in the 20s were randomized to receive a chelating agent (penicillamine), methylphenidate, or placebo. Teacher and parent ratings of behavior improved for the first two groups but not the placebo receivers. BLLs declined only in the chelated group.

Additional clinical signs and symptoms occur in the gastrointestinal and central nervous systems (CNS). Gastrointestinal symptoms include anorexia, abdominal pain, vomiting, and constipation, often occurring and recurring over a period of weeks. Children with BLLs of more than 20 µg/dL are twice as likely to have gastrointestinal complaints as those with lower BLLs. CNS symptoms are related to increasing cerebral edema and increased intracranial pressure. Headaches, change in mentation, lethargy, seizures, and coma leading to death are rarely seen at levels below 100 µg/dL but have been reported in children with a BLL as low as 70 µg/dL. The last reported death attributable to lead poisoning in the United States was in 2000 in a child with a BLL over 300 µg/dL. There is no clear cutoff for the appearance of hyperactivity in relation to BLL, but it is more likely to be observed in children who have reached 20 µg/dL.

Although not usually causing symptoms in children, other organs are affected by lead as well. At high levels, over 100 µg/dL, renal tubular dysfunction is observed. Lead induces a reversible Fanconi syndrome. Also at such BLL elevations, red cell survival is shortened and may contribute to anemia, although most cases of anemia in lead-poisoned children are due to other factors, such as iron deficiency and hemoglobinopathies.

Diagnosis

SCREENING. Approximately 99% of lead-poisoned children are identified by screening procedures rather than by clinical recognition of lead-related symptoms. Until 1997, universal screening by blood lead testing of all children at ages 12 and 24 mo was the standard. Because of the national decline in the prevalence of lead poisoning, this recommendation has been revised. Currently, targeted blood lead testing of high-risk populations is indicated. High risk is based on an evaluation of the likelihood of lead exposure. Departments of health are responsible for determining the local prevalence of lead poisoning as well as the percentage of housing built before 1950, the period of peak leaded paint use. When this information is available, informed screening guidelines for practitioners can be issued. For instance, in New York State, where a large percentage of housing is known to have been built before 1950, the Department of Health mandates that all children be tested for lead poisoning by blood analyses. In the absence of such data the practitioner should continue to test all children at 12 and 24 mo of age. In areas where the prevalence of lead poisoning and old housing is low, targeted screening may be performed based on a risk assessment. Three questions form the basis of a questionnaire (Box 703–1). Items that are pertinent to the locale or individual may be added. For example, if questioning determines that there is a lead-based industry in the child's neighborhood (e.g., a car battery factory) or that the child is a recent immigrant from a country that still uses leaded gasoline or the child has developmental delay, then blood lead testing would be appropriate. If feasible, venous sampling is always preferred to capillary sampling because the chances of false-positive and false-negative results are less.

INTERPRETATION OF BLOOD LEAD LEVELS. The current cutoff of a BLL of 10 µg/dL is an arbitrary and probably temporary point based on knowledge accumulated before 1991. Levels as low as 5 µg/dL may affect cognitive function, and older data support biochemical effects of lead occurring below this threshold as well.

A screening value at or above 10 µg/dL requires repeat testing for a diagnosis and to determine the intervention. The timing for the repeat evaluation depends on the initial value (Table 703–1). If the diagnostic (second) test confirms that the BLL is

elevated, then further testing will be required as per the recommended schedule (Table 703–2). **A confirmed venous BLL of 45 µg/dL or more requires prompt chelation therapy.**

OTHER TOOLS FOR ASSESSMENT. BLL determinations remain the gold standard for evaluating children, although techniques are available to measure lead in other tissues and body fluids. Experimentally, the method of x-ray fluorescence (XRF) allows direct and noninvasive assessment of bone lead stores. XRF methodology was used to evaluate a population that had long-term exposure to lead from a polluting battery recycling factory. The study found that the school-aged children had elevated bone lead levels but not BLLs. This is consistent with the slow turnover of lead in bone, measurable in years, in contrast to that in blood, measurable in weeks. It also indicates that children may have substantial lead in their bodies that will not be detected by routine blood lead testing. This stored lead may be released, resulting in toxic blood levels, if bone resorption rates suddenly increase, as occurs with immobilization of greater than a week and during pregnancy. Thus, children with histories of elevated BLLs are potentially at risk for recrudescence of lead toxicity long after ingestion has stopped and may pass this lead to the next generation. Currently, XRF methodology remains limited primarily for research uses.

Lead can also be measured in urine. Spontaneous excretion of lead, even in children with high BLLs, is usually low. Lead excretion may be stimulated by treatment with chelating agents, and this property is the basis of their use as a component of lead treatment. Urinary lead excretion has also been used to develop a test to identify children with lead burdens responsive to chelation therapy, the Lead Mobilization Test. In one version, a standardized protocol is employed that includes a fixed dose of the drug (500 mg/M² of CaNa₂EDTA given once intramuscularly, mixed 1:1 by volume with 1% procaine) followed by a timed urine collection of 6–8 hr that is analyzed for its lead content. Urine lead per dose of CaNa₂EDTA greater than or equal to 0.6 or urine lead levels greater than or equal to 200 µg/volume identifies children most likely to respond to a full course of treatment with an enhanced lead diuresis. Practical (collecting urine

---

BOX 703–1. Minimum Personal Risk Questionnaire

1. Does the child reside in or visit regularly a house that was built before 1950 (include settings such as daycare, babysitters or relatives).
2. Does the child reside in or visit regularly a house built before 1978 with recent or ongoing (past 6 mo) renovation.
3. Does the child have a sibling or playmate with lead poisoning.

From Centers for Disease Control and Prevention: *Screening Young Children for Lead Poisoning: Guidance for State and Local Public Health Officials.* Atlanta, CDC, 1997.

TABLE 703–1. Follow-up of Screening Test

If screening blood lead level is (µg/dL):	CDC Repeat *diagnostic* venous blood lead testing by:	AAP Repeat *diagnostic* venous blood lead testing by:
10–19	3 mo	1 mo
20–44	1 mo–1 wk (sooner the higher the lead)	1 wk
45–59	48 hr	48 hr
60–69	24 hr	48 hr
≥70	Immediately	Immediately

Adapted from Centers for Disease Control and Prevention: Screening Young Children for Lead Poisoning: Guidance for State and Local Public Health Officials. *Atlanta, CDC, 1997; and Committee on Environmental Health, American Academy of Pediatrics: Screening for elevated blood lead levels.* Pediatrics *1998;101:1072–78.*

TABLE 703–2. Follow-up of Diagnostic Test

If diagnostic blood lead test is (μg/dL):	Action
10–14	Repeat within 3 mo. Evaluate sources. Education: cleaning, hand-mouth
15–19	Repeat within 2 mo. Evaluate sources. Education: cleaning, hand-mouth. Department of health referral
20–44	Repeat within 1 mo. Evaluate sources. Education: cleaning, hand-mouth. Department of Health referral
≥45	Chelation therapy in addition to above
≥70	Immediate hospitalization and two-drug chelation in addition to evaluation, education, and referral

Data in part from Centers for Disease Control and Prevention: Screening Young Children for Lead Poisoning: Guidance for State and Local Public Health Officials. *Atlanta, CDC, 1997.*

on an infant for 6–8 hr in the office) and theoretical concerns (Is there a redistribution of lead after a single dose of chelating agent that may result in transient elevation in brain lead? Are there any data showing long term efficacy of children chelated on this basis?) have limited the use of this diagnostic test to a few experienced medical centers, and it is not recommended by the American Academy of Pediatrics.

Lead in hair is also measurable but is problematic, owing to concerns about contamination and interpretability.

Other tests are used as indirect assessments of lead exposure and accumulation. Radiographs of long bones may show dense bands at the metaphyses that may be difficult to distinguish from growth arrest lines but, if caused by lead, are indicative of months to years of exposure. For children with acute symptoms, when a BLL level result is not immediately available, a kidney-ureter-bladder view may be helpful; radiopaque flecks observed in the intestinal tract are consistent with very recent ingestion of lead-containing plaster or paint chips. The absence of radiographic findings does not rule out lead poisoning.

Because BLLs reflect recent ingestion or redistribution from other tissues but do not necessarily correlate with the body burden of lead or lead toxicity in an individual child, tests of lead effects may also be useful. After several weeks of lead accumulation and a BLL greater than 20 μg/dL, increases in erythrocyte protoporphyrin (EP) levels greater than 35 μg/dL may occur. An elevated EP level, not attributable to iron deficiency or recent inflammatory illness, is both an indicator of lead effect but also a useful test for assessing the success of the treatment; levels will begin to decrease a few weeks after successful interventions that reduce lead ingestion and increase lead excretion. Because EP is light sensitive, whole blood samples should be covered in aluminum foil (or equivalent) until analyzed.

Treatment. Once lead is in bone it is slowly released and is difficult to remove even with drugs. In addition, the cognitive/behavioral effects from lead may be irreversible. Thus, the main efforts in treating lead poisoning are to prevent it from occurring and to prevent further ingestion by already poisoned children. The main components of these efforts are the identification of environmental sources of lead exposure and their elimination, behavioral modification to reduce non-nutritive hand-to-mouth activity, and dietary counseling to ensure sufficiency of the essential elements calcium and iron. For the small minority of children in the United States with more severe lead poisoning, drug treatment is available that enhances lead excretion.

During health maintenance visits (see Chapter 5) a limited risk assessment is warranted that includes questions pertaining to the most common sources of lead exposure, namely, the condition of old paint, secondary occupational exposure via an adult living in the home, or proximity to an industrial source of pollution. If such a source is identified, its elimination will usu-

ally require assistance from public health and housing agencies as well as educational efforts aimed at the parents. Ideally, a family should move from a lead-contaminated dwelling until repairs are completed. In the interim, repeated washes of surfaces and the use of high-efficiency particle accumulator (HEPA) vacuum cleaners will help reduce exposure to lead-containing dust. Care in the selection of a contractor who is certified to perform lead abatement work is necessary. Sloppy work can cause dissemination of lead-containing dust and chips throughout a home or building and result in further elevation of a child's BLL. After the work is completed, dust wipe samples should be collected from floors and window sills and window wells to determine if the risk from lead has abated.

It is often observed that a single case of lead poisoning is discovered in a household with multiple family members, including other young children. This occurs despite a common source of exposure, such as peeling lead-based paint. The lack of accumulation in the other children, at least in part, is caused by differences in behavior. Parental efforts at reducing the hand-to-mouth activity of the affected child are necessary to decrease the risk of lead ingestion. Handwashing effectively removes lead; but in a home with lead-containing dust, lead rapidly accumulates on the child's hands after washing. Therefore, handwashing is best limited to the period immediately before nutritive hand-to-mouth activity is allowed to occur.

Because there is competition between lead and essential metals, it is reasonable to promote a healthy diet that is sufficient in calcium and iron content. The recommended daily intakes of these metals vary somewhat with age (see Chapter 40). In general, for children 1 yr of age and older a calcium intake of about 1 g/24 hr is sufficient. This is roughly the calcium content of a quart of milk (~1200 mg/qt) or calcium-fortified orange juice. Calcium absorption is vitamin D dependent. Although milk is vitamin D fortified, other nutritional sources of calcium are not. A multivitamin containing vitamin D may be prescribed for those children not drinking sufficient milk or who have inadequate sunshine exposure. Iron requirements also vary with age: 6 mg/24 hr for infants to 12 mg/24 hr for adolescents. It is more difficult to eat enough iron-containing foods to attain this intake than to ingest calcium, and iron deficiency is commonly observed in young lead-poisoned children. For children identified biochemically as being iron deficient, therapeutic iron at a daily dose of 5–6 mg/kg for 3 mo is appropriate. Iron absorption is enhanced when ingested with ascorbic acid (citrus juices). Whether doses of calcium and/or iron greater than the daily requirements offer any additional benefits to lead-poisoned children is under investigation but cannot be recommended at this time.

Drug treatment to remove lead is lifesaving for children with lead encephalopathy. Its role for nonencephalopathic children is to prevent symptom progression and further toxicity. Guidelines for selecting children for chelation are based on the BLL. A child with a venous BLL greater than or equal to 45 μg/dL should be treated. Four drugs are available in the United States: DMSA (succimer), $CaNa_2EDTA$ (versenate), BAL (dimercaprol), and penicillamine. DMSA and penicillamine can be given orally, whereas EDTA and BAL can only be administered parenterally. The choice of agent is guided by the severity of the lead poisoning, the effectiveness of the drug, and the ease of administration (Table 703–3). Children with BLLs between 44 and 70 μg/dL should be treated with a single drug, preferably DMSA. Those with BLLs of 70 μg/dL or greater require two-drug treatment: (1) $CaNa_2EDTA$ in combination with either DMSA or BAL for those without evidence of encephalopathy and (2) $CaNa_2EDTA$ and BAL for those with encephalopathy. Data on the combined treatment with $CaNa_2EDTA$ and DMSA for children with BLLs greater than 100 μg/dL are very limited.

Drug-related toxicities are generally minor and reversible. These include gastrointestinal distress, transient elevations in

TABLE 703–3. Chelation Therapy

Name	Synonym	Dose	Toxicity
Succimer	Chemet, DMSA	350 mg/m²/dose (**not 10 mg/kg**) q8h, PO, for 5 days; then q12h for 14 days	Gastrointestinal distress, rashes; elevated LFTs, depressed WBCs
Edetate	CaNa₂EDTA, versenate	1000–1500 mg/m²/24 hr; IV infusion, continuous or intermittent; IM divided q6h or q12h. For 5 days.	Proteinuria, pyuria, increasing BUN/creatinine—all rare. Hypercalcemia if too rapid an infusion. Tissue inflammation if infusion infiltrates
BAL	Dimercaprol, British AntiLewisite	300–500 mg/m²/24 h; **IM only** divided q4h. For 3–5 days. Only for blood lead level ≥ 70.	Gastrointestinal distress, altered mentation; elevated LFTs, hemolysis if G6PD deficiency; no concomitant iron therapy
D-Pen	Penicillamine	10 mg/kg/24 hr for 2 wk increasing to 25–40 mg/kg/24 hr; oral, divided q12h. For 12–20 wk.	Rashes, fever; blood dyscrasias, elevated LFTs, proteinuria. Allergic cross-reactivity with penicillin.

LFTs = Liver function tests; WBCs = white blood cells; BUN = blood urea nitrogen; G6PD = glucose-6-pyruvate dehydrogenase.
From Markowitz ME: Lead poisoning. Pediatr Rev 2000;21:327–35.

transaminase values, active urinary sediment, and neutropenia. The frequencies of these types of events are lowest for CaNa₂EDTA and DMSA and highest for BAL and penicillamine. All of the drugs are effective in reducing BLLs when given in sufficient doses over the recommended duration of time. However, these drugs may also increase lead absorption from the intestine and should be administered to children in lead-free environments. Some authorities also recommend the administration of a cathartic immediately before or concomitant with the initiation of chelation to eliminate the presence of lead already in the intestine.

None of these agents will remove all lead from the body. Within days to weeks after completion of a course of therapy the BLL rises, even in the absence of new ingestion. The presumed source of this rebound in the BLL is bone. Chelation is again indicated if the BLL rebounds to 45 µg/dL or greater. Children with initial BLLs greater than 70 µg/dL are likely to require more than one course. A minimum of 3 days between courses is recommended, if possible, to prevent treatment-related toxicities, especially kidney injury. Serial x-ray fluorescent measurements of bone lead content have shown that chelation with CaNa₂EDTA is associated with a decrease in bone lead levels; however, residual bone lead remains detectable even after multiple courses of treatment.

The indication for chelation therapy for children with BLL less than 45 µg/dL is less clear. Use of these drugs in children with BLLs between 20 and 44 µg/dL will result in transiently lowered BLLs, and in some this will be accompanied by reversal of lead-induced enzyme inhibition. However, very few of such children significantly increase their excretion of lead during chelation, raising the question of whether any long-term benefit is achieved. A study that enrolled 2-yr-old children with BLLs 20–44 µg/dL and randomized them to receive either DMSA or placebo found the following: BLLs decreased more in the first 6 mo after enrollment in the DMSA-treated group, but the levels converged by 1 yr of follow-up; cognitive test scores obtained at 4 yr of age were not statistically different between the groups. Thus, chelating all children with BLLs of 20–44 µg/dL is not recommended. However, it is possible that a subset of children may benefit. These might include children with persistently elevated BLLs. Another group may include children who can be shown to respond to a test dose of a chelating agent with an enhanced lead diuresis, an indication that the drug is effective at removing lead permanently from the body. Such children could be identified by administration of the Lead Mobilization Test. Data on cognitive outcomes are not available for either of these groups of children after chelation.

With successful intervention, BLLs decline, with the greatest fall in BLL occurring in the first 2 mo after therapy is initiated. Subsequently, the rate of change in BLL declines slowly, so that by 6–12 mo after identification the average child with moderate lead poisoning (BLL > 20 µg/dL) will have a BLL that is 50% lower. Children with more markedly elevated BLLs may take years to reach the acceptable threshold of 10 µg/dL even if all sources of lead exposure have been eliminated, behavior has been modified, and nutrition has been optimized. Thus, early screening remains the best way of avoiding the need for the treatment of lead poisoning.

Centers for Disease Control and Prevention: *Screening Young Children for Lead Poisoning: Guidance for State and Local Public Health Officials.* Atlanta, CDC, 1997.

Centers for Disease Control and Prevention: Update: Blood lead levels in young children—United States and selected states, 1996–1999. *MMWR Morbid Mortal Wkly Rep* 2000;49:1133–37.

Centers for Disease Control and Prevention: Fatal pediatric lead poisoning—New Hampshire, 2000. *MMWR Morbid Mortal Wkly Rep* 2001;50:457–59.

Chisolm JJ Jr, Kaplan E: Lead poisoning in childhood: Comprehensive management and prevention. *J Pediatr* 1968;73:942–50.

Committee on Drugs, American Academy of Pediatrics: Treatment guidelines for lead exposure in children. *Pediatrics* 1995;96:155–60.

Committee on Environmental Health, American Academy of Pediatrics: Screening for elevated blood lead levels. *Pediatrics* 1998;101:1072–78.

Gomar A, Hu H, Bellinger D, et al: Maternal bone lead as an independent risk factor for fetal neurotoxicity: A prospective study. *Pediatrics* 2002;110:116–18.

Lanphear BP, Dietrich K, Auinger P, et al: Cognitive deficits associated with blood lead concentrations <10 µg/dL in US children and adolescents. *Public Health Rep* 2000;115:521–29.

Markowitz ME: Lead poisoning. *Pediatr Review* 2000;21:327–35.

Rogan WJ, Dietrich KN, Ware JH, et al: The effect of chelation therapy with succimer on neuropsychological development in children exposed to lead. *N Engl J Med* 2001;344:1421–26.

Schwartz J: Low-level lead exposure and children's IQ: A meta-analysis and search for a threshold. *Environ Res* 1994;65:42–55..

Chapter 704

Poisonings: Drugs, Chemicals, and Plants (see also Chapter 713)

George C. Rodgers, Jr. and Nancy J. Matyunas

704.1 Epidemiology and Approach to Management

Of the more than 2 million human poisoning exposures reported annually to the Toxic Exposure Surveillance System (TESS) of the American Association of Poison Control Centers (AAPCC), more than 50% occurred in children 5 yr of age or younger. Almost all of these exposures are unintentional and reflect the propensity for children in this age group to put virtually anything in their mouths. See Chapters 57 and 701.

More than 90% of toxic exposures in children occur in the home, and most involve only a single substance. Ingestion is the most common route of poisoning exposure (76% of cases), with the dermal, ophthalmic, and inhalation routes each occurring in about 6% of cases. About 60% of cases involve nondrug products, most commonly cosmetics and personal care products, cleaning substances, plants, foreign bodies, and hydrocarbons. Pharmaceutical preparations comprise the remainder, with analgesics, cough and cold products, antimicrobial agents, and vitamins the most common categories. More than 75% of pediatric poisoning exposures can be managed without direct medical intervention, because either the product involved is not inherently very toxic or the quantity of the material involved is not sufficient to produce significant toxic effects. A partial list of nontoxic products commonly encountered by children is shown in Box 704–1. Death due to unintentional poisoning in young children is uncommon owing to increased product safety measures (e.g., child-resistant packaging), increased poison prevention education, early recognition of exposure, and improvements in medical management.

Poison prevention education should be an integral part of all well-child visits, even before a child is mobile. Counseling parents and other caregivers about potential poisoning risks, how to "poison-proof" a child's environment, and what to do if a poisoning occurs diminishes the likelihood of serious morbidity or mortality from an exposure. Poison prevention educational materials are available from both the American Academy of Pediatrics and regional poison control centers (1-800-222-1222 in the United States). See Chapter 5.

Poisoning exposures in children 6–12 yr of age are much less common (4% of exposures). Toxic exposures in adolescents are primarily intentional (suicide or abuse) or occupational. Pediatricians should be aware of the signs of drug abuse or suicidal ideation in this population and should aggressively intervene.

MANAGEMENT PLAN FOR POISONING AND OVERDOSE

History. Obtaining an accurate problem-oriented history is of paramount importance if a poisoning has occurred or is suspected. The following information should be obtained during the initial assessment:

DESCRIPTION OF TOXINS. Product names (brand, generic, or chemical) and ingredients, along with their concentrations, may be obtained from labels. Because many brand names that sound alike have very different ingredients, it is important to be precise. If the ingredient information is not readily available on the product, consultation with a poison control center can usually provide this information rapidly. Several characteristic toxic syndromes are described (Table 704–1). These may assist in identifying the offending agent.

BOX 704–1. Common Nontoxic Products

Abrasives
Antacids
Antibiotics
Ballpoint pen inks
Bathtub floating toys
Bath oil (castor oil and perfume)
Body conditioners
Bubble bath soaps (detergents)
Calamine lotion
Candles (beeswax or paraffin)
Caps (toy pistols, potassium chlorate)
Chalk (calcium carbonate)
Children's toy cosmetics
Clay (modeling)
Contraceptive agents
Corticosteroids
Cosmetics
Crayons (marked A.P. or C.P., gel)
Dehumidifying packets (silica or charcoal)
Deodorants—underarm
Fabric softeners
Fertilizers (if no insecticide or herbicides added)
Fishbowl additives
Glues and pastes
Golf ball (core may cause mechanical injury)
Grease
Hand lotions and creams
Hydrogen peroxide (medicinal 3%)
Incense
Indelible markers

Ink (black, blue—nonpermanent)
Iodophil disinfectants (unless allergic)
Laxatives
Lipstick
Lubricating oils (unless aspirated)
Magazines
Magic markers
Makeup
Matches
Mineral oil (unless aspirated)
Newspaper (chronic ingestion may result in lead poisoning)
Paint—indoor latex
Pencil lead (graphite, coloring)
Petroleum jelly (Vaseline)
Play-Doh
Polaroid picture coating fluid
Porous—tip ink marking pens
Putty
Rubber cement
Sachets
Shampoo
Shaving creams and lotions
Soap and soap products
Spackles
Suntan preparations
Sweetening agents (saccharin, aspartame)
Toothpaste (with and without fluoride)
Warfarin rodenticides (<0.5%)
Watercolor paints
Zinc oxide

MAGNITUDE OF EXPOSURE. Attempt to determine how much of the substance has been ingested. This can often be accomplished by counting the number of tablets or measuring the volume of liquid remaining. Because the toxicity of most agents is dose related, knowing the age or weight of the child aids in assessment. For inhalation, ocular, or dermal exposures, the concentration of the offending agent and the length of contact time with the material should be determined.

TIME OF EXPOSURE. For some products, toxic manifestations may be delayed for hours or days. Knowing the time lapse between exposure and the time to either medical

TABLE 704–1. Toxic Syndromes

Syndrome	Symptoms	Causes
Anticholinergic	Exocrine gland hyposecretion, thirst, flushed skin, mydriasis, hyperthermia, urinary retention, delirium, hallucinations, tachycardia, respiratory insufficiency	Belladonna alkaloids, jimsonweed, some mushrooms, antihistamines, tricyclic antidepressants, scopolamine
Cholinergic (muscarinic and nicotinic)	Exocrine gland hypersecretion, urination, nausea, vomiting, diarrhea, muscle fasciculations, miosis, weakness or paralysis, bronchospasm, tachycardia or bradycardia, convulsions, coma	Organophosphate and carbamate insecticides, some mushrooms, tobacco, black widow spider bites (severe)
Extrapyramidal	Tremor, rigidity, opisthotonos, torticollis, dysphonia, oculogyric crisis	Phenothiazines, haloperidol, metoclopramide
Hypermetabolic	Fever, tachycardia, hyperpnea, restlessness, convulsions, metabolic acidosis	Salicylates, some phenols, triethyltin, chlorophenoxy herbicides
Narcotic	Central nervous system depression, hypothermia, hypotension, hypoventilation, miosis	All narcotics, propoxyphene, heroin
Sympathomimetic	Excitation, psychosis, seizures, hypertension, tachypnea, hyperthermia, mydriasis	Amphetamines, phencyclidine, cocaine, crack cocaine, phenylpropanolamine, methylphenidate, theophylline, caffeine
Withdrawal	Abdominal cramps, diarrhea, lacrimation, sweating, "goose flesh," yawning, tachycardia, restlessness, hallucinations	Cessation of alcohol, barbiturates, benzodiazepines, narcotics

evaluation or the onset of symptoms may influence therapeutic intervention.

PROGRESSION OF SYMPTOMS. Knowing the nature and progression of symptoms is helpful for assessing the need for immediate life support, the prognosis, and the type of intervention that may need to be performed.

MEDICAL HISTORY. Underlying diseases may make a child more susceptible to the effects of a toxin. Concurrent drug therapy may also increase susceptibility, because certain drugs may interact with the toxin. Pregnancy is a common precipitating factor in adolescent suicide attempts and may influence the treatment plan.

DEMOGRAPHIC INFORMATION. This is particularly important to know if a parent or caregiver telephones the physician's office with a poisoning situation. Obtain the caller's telephone number and street address to allow for follow-up or to dispatch emergency personnel in the event phone contact is broken.

Initial Medical Care. If the patient is treated at home, follow-up assessment calls should be made approximately 0.5, 1, and 4 hr after exposure. Any change in the patient's condition may alter the decision to treat at home. Consultation with a poison control center for assistance in monitoring such patients should be considered. Poison control centers are staffed by nurses, pharmacists, and physicians specially trained to respond to and monitor poisoning exposures. If the patient requires hospital treatment, the probability of developing life-threatening symptoms dictates the mode of transportation used. After a decision to transport a patient is made, emergency department personnel should be notified so they can properly prepare. All product containers thought to be related to the exposure should be collected and transported with the patient. If the patient has vomited, the emesis should also be brought to the emergency department for possible toxicologic analysis.

Once the patient has arrived in the appropriate medical care setting, initial attention should focus on life support, with primary emphasis on cardiorespiratory care. Initial treatment of shock, dysrhythmias, and seizures is generally the same as for any other critically ill patient (see Chapter 57). Antidotes exist for only a few poisons (Table 704–2).

Preventing Absorption. Most toxins are rapidly absorbed from the gastrointestinal tract or through inhalation. Many may also be well absorbed upon dermal contact. Prompt action to remove the toxin and minimize contact with the absorptive surface is crucial and may prevent the development of major toxicity.

Dermal and ocular decontamination can be accomplished by flushing the affected area with tepid water. A minimum of 10 min is recommended for ocular exposures, although some chemicals, particularly alkaline corrosives, may require much longer periods of flushing. For dermal exposures, mild soap and water can be used.

For inhaled toxins, decontamination is generally accomplished by moving the patient to fresh air or, if necessary, administering oxygen. In addition to supportive care, a few specific antidotes are used for some specific inhaled toxins. These are listed in Table 704–2.

Several procedures are used to prevent absorption of a toxin from the stomach and gastrointestinal tract, and each has limitations and risks. The decision to use one particular method over another should be based on whether the technique chosen is likely to be of sufficient value to merit the risk of the procedure. Timing is a limitation because many toxins are rapidly absorbed from the stomach. A decontamination procedure instituted after the drug is absorbed poses a risk to the patient with no potential for benefit. In general, most liquid drug products are almost completely absorbed within 30 min of ingestion, and most solid dosage forms within 1–2 hr. Gastrointestinal decontamination beyond this time is unlikely to be of value.

EMESIS. The only emetic routinely used is syrup of ipecac, which contains two emetic alkaloids that work both in the central nervous system (CNS) and locally in the gastrointestinal tract to produce vomiting. The onset of emesis is usually 20–30 min after dosing, with vomiting occurring in 90–95% of patients. Several episodes of vomiting usually occur over a period of 1–2 hr. The recommended dose is 10 mL for infants 6–12 mo of age, 15 mL for children age 1–12 yr, and 30 mL for older children and adults. Ipecac should not be used in infants younger than 6 mo. Ipecac administration is followed by at least 8 oz of water or other clear fluid. At best, emesis with syrup of ipecac removes about one third of the stomach contents. Because of the delay in onset of emesis and poor yield, it should not be used as a general treatment for ingestions. Ipecac-induced emesis is contraindicated after the ingestion of caustics, hydrocarbons, and agents likely to cause the rapid onset of CNS or cardiovascular symptoms. The use of ipecac syrup has declined dramatically in the past 2 decades.

GASTRIC LAVAGE. This technique involves placing a tube into the stomach to aspirate contents, followed by flushing with aliquots of fluid, usually normal saline. Although gastric lavage has been widely used for many years, objective data do not document its efficacy, particularly in children, in whom only small-bore tubes can be used. Lavage is time consuming and, even under the best of circumstances, removes only a fraction of gastric contents. It should only be used in older children and only in select situations.

ACTIVATED CHARCOAL. The use of activated charcoal to prevent absorption of toxins has increased dramatically in the past 2 decades as data demonstrating its efficacy have accumulated. Activated charcoal is specially prepared to have a very large adsorptive surface area. Many, but not all, toxins are adsorbed onto its surface, preventing absorption from the gastrointestinal tract. Some toxins, including heavy metals, iron, lithium, hydrocarbons, cyanide, and low molecular weight alcohols, are not significantly bound to charcoal. In vitro, activated charcoal adsorbs about 1 g of toxin for each 10 g of charcoal; however, this relationship is generally not useful for clinical situations because the exact ingested dose is seldom known. The usual dose is 10–30 g for a child and 30–100 g for an adolescent or adult. Activated charcoal is commercially available mixed as a slurry in water or a solution of sorbitol, a cathartic. Flavoring may be added to improve palatability. In some serious poisonings, when life-threatening symptoms are present, repeated doses of activated charcoal may be useful to adsorb either toxin not bound by the first dose or toxin that may be recirculated through the gut. Under these circumstances, a cathartic should be used only with the first charcoal dose to prevent major fluid loss and dehydration. About 25% of patients receiving activated charcoal experience one episode of vomiting. Aspiration of activated charcoal into the lungs occasionally occurs. There is no evidence that aspiration of activated charcoal is more serious than aspiration of gastric contents alone. If charcoal is given through a gastric tube, placement of the tube should be carefully confirmed before activated charcoal is given, because instillation of charcoal directly into the lungs has disastrous effects.

CATHARTICS. Cathartics are commonly used in conjunction with activated charcoal to hasten the clearance of the charcoal-toxin complex, although no evidence shows that this is of value. Commonly used cathartics are sorbitol (maximum dose, 1 g/kg), magnesium sulfate (maximum dose, 250 mg/kg), and magnesium citrate (maximum dose, 250 mL/kg). Cathartics should be used with care in young children because of the risk of dehydration and electrolyte imbalance.

WHOLE BOWEL IRRIGATION. Whole bowel irrigation (WBI) involves instilling large volumes of a polyethylene glycol electrolyte solution (Colyte, GoLYTELY) into the stomach to cleanse the entire gastrointestinal tract. This technique has been

TABLE 704–2. Common Antidotes for Poisoning

Antidote	Use	Dose	Route	Adverse Effects/Warnings
N-Acetylcysteine (NAC, Mucomyst)	Acetaminophen; carbon tetrachloride and chloroform (experimental)	140 mg/kg loading, followed by 70 mg/kg q4h for 17 doses	PO	Nausea, vomiting IV form not available in USA
Atropine	Organophosphate and carbamate pesticides; bradycardia due to atrioventricular conduction defects	0.05 mg/kg repeated q5–10 min as needed. Dilute in 1–2 mL of NS for ET instillation.	IV/ET	Tachycardia, dry mouth, blurred vision, and urinary retention
BAL in oil (dimercaprol)	Arsenic, mercury, other metals	3–5 mg/kg/dose q4hr, for the first day; subsequent dosing depends on toxin	Deep IM	Local injection site pain and sterile abscess, nausea, vomiting, fever, salivation, nephrotoxicity
Benztropine (Cogentin)	Acute dystonic reactions	0.02–0.05 mg/kg/dose qd or bid (4 mg max)	IV/PO	Sedation, blurred vision, dry mouth, and tachycardia
Cyanide antidote kit	Cyanide	Amyl nitrite: 1 crushable ampule, inhale 30 sec of each min	Inhalation	Methemoglobinemia
	Hydrogen sulfide (nitrites only)	Sodium nitrite: 0.33 mL/kg of 3% solution if hemoglobin level not known, otherwise based on tables with product	IV	Methemoglobinemia
		Sodium thiosulfate: 1.6 mL (400 mg)/kg of 25% solution, may be repeated every 30–60 min to a maximum of 50 mL	IV	
Deferoxamine (Desferal)	Iron	Infusion of 15 mg/kg/hr (max 6 g/24 hr)	IV (preferred)	Hypotension (minimized by avoiding rapid infusion rates)
		IM: 90 mg/kg/dose q8h (max of 6 g/24 hr)	IM	
Digoxin-specific Fab antibodies (Digibind)	Digitalis glycosides (synthetic or natural)	One vial binds 0.6 mg of digitalis glycoside, ingested dose may be estimated from serum level (see table with product)	IV	Allergic reactions (rare), return of condition being treated with digitalis glycoside
Dimercaptosuccinic acid (succimer, DMSA, Chemet)	Lead and probably mercury, arsenic, and perhaps other metals	10 mg/kg/dose q8h for 5 days, then 10 mg/kg q12h for 14 days	PO	Nausea and vomiting; repeated courses may be needed
Diphenhydramine (Benadryl)	Extrapyramidal symptoms, acute dystonic reactions, allergic reactions	5 mg/kg divide q8h; 300 mg/24 hr max	IV/PO	Sedation or paradoxical agitation, ataxia
EDTA, calcium (calcium disodium, Versenate)	Lead, manganese, nickel, zinc, and perhaps chromium	1–1.5 g/m²/24 hr in divided doses q12h for 5 days	IV	Nausea, vomiting, fever, hypertension, arthralgias, allergic reactions, local inflammation, and nephrotoxicity (maintain adequate hydration)
Ethanol (ethyl alcohol)	Methanol, ethylene glycol	750 mg/kg loading dose followed by 80–150 mg/kg/hr infusion of 5% or 10% ethanol	IV/PO	Nausea, vomiting, sedation
Flumazenil (Romazicon)	Benzodiazepines	0.2 mg over 30 sec; if inadequate response, repeat q1min to 1 mg max	IV	Nausea, vomiting, facial flushing, agitation, headache, dizziness, seizures. Do not use for unknown or antidepressant ingestions *Note*: May not reverse respiratory depression
Fomepizole (4-methylpyrazole, Antizole)	Ethylene glycol; methanol	15 mg/kg load; 10 mg/kg q12h for 4 doses; 15 mg/kg q12h until level <20 mg/dL No specific dose for children.	IV	Infuse slowly over 30 min; increase doses to q4h if dialysis is concurrent
Glucagon	β-Blockers, calcium channel blockers, hypoglycemic agents	0.05 mg/kg bolus followed by infusion of 0.05 mg/kg/hr	IV	Hyperglycemia, nausea, and vomiting
Methylene blue	Methemoglobinemia	0.1–0.2 mL/kg of 1% solution, slow infusion, may be repeated q30–60 min	IV	Nausea, vomiting, headache, dizziness
Naloxone (Narcan)	Narcotics Clonidine (inconsistent response)	0.01 mg/kg; if no effect, give 0.1 mg/kg; may be repeated as needed; may give continuous infusion	IV	Acute withdrawal symptoms if given to addicted patients
Physostigmine (Antilirium)	Anticholinergic agents	0.02 mg/kg; slow push; may repeat q5–10 min to 2 mg max	IV/IM	Bradycardia, asystole, seizures, bronchospasm, vomiting, headache *Note*: Do not use with cyclic antidepressants
Pralidoxime (2-PAM, Protopam)	Organophosphate insecticides	25–50 mg/kg over 5–10 min (max 200 mg/min); can be repeated after 1–2 hr then q10–12 hr as needed	IV/IM	Nausea, dizziness, headache, tachycardia, muscle rigidity, and bronchospasm (rapid administration)
Pyridoxine (vitamin B₆)	Isoniazid, *Gyromitra* mushrooms Ethylene glycol (investigational)	Isoniazid: dose = dose of isoniazid Mushrooms: 25 mg/kg	IV	Uncommon

PO = oral; IV = intravenous; ET = endotracheal; IM = intramuscular; NS = normal saline.

successfully used to remove slowly absorbed products such as iron or sustained-release preparations. Whole bowel irrigation can be combined with the use of activated charcoal, if appropriate. It should be used with caution in young children because of the possibility of fluid and electrolyte imbalance.

Enhancing Elimination. Enhancing excretion is useful for only a few toxins. Dialytic techniques are not useful for drugs that are either highly protein bound or have a large volume of distribution. These techniques are also invasive and associated with risk. Certain procedures can be used for very specific agents.

DIURESIS. For most toxins, renal clearance is not proportionate to urine volume; thus diuresis alone does not increase elimination. Increasing the pH of the urine with intravenously administered bicarbonate increases the elimination of weak acids, such as salicylates and phenobarbital. Alternately, acidifying the urine to increase the elimination of weak bases such as amphetamine and phencyclidine is not clinically useful. This technique is termed *ion trapping*.

DIALYSIS. Hemodialysis and peritoneal dialysis have been used successfully to treat poisonings by select agents. Although hemodialysis is generally more efficient at removing toxins, peritoneal dialysis is often easier to perform in young children and may be sufficient. Few drugs or toxins are removed by dialysis in amounts sufficient to justify the risks and difficulty of dialysis. Examples of toxins for which dialysis may be useful include methanol, ethylene glycol, and large symptomatic ingestions of salicylate or theophylline.

HEMOPERFUSION. Hemoperfusion is a dialytic technique in which blood is passed through a column of activated charcoal or resin. It has been used successfully to treat large ingestions of salicylate, theophylline, and a few other selected agents. It is rarely used in small children because of the risks associated with its use.

Laboratory Evaluation. For some intoxications (e.g., salicylates, acetaminophen, iron, methanol, ethylene glycol), blood levels are integral to the treatment plan. For other intoxicants, qualitative measurement may assist in establishing a diagnosis but is not likely to change treatment. Examples include opioid toxicity, in which definitive treatment is based on symptoms not levels, or cyanide, in which treatment must be started rapidly and would be significantly delayed if the physician were to wait for laboratory confirmation. Comprehensive qualitative "drug screens" vary widely in their ability to detect toxins and generally add little information, particularly if the agent is known and a patient's symptoms are consistent with that agent. If a drug screen is ordered, it is important to know the specific drugs that can be identified by the test. Although drug screens can be done on any body fluid, urine is generally the best sample. The best way to use the laboratory is to discuss the case with a poison control center, medical toxicologist, or laboratory technologist and to provide appropriate samples and clinical data so that the most appropriate tests can be performed and properly interpreted.

American Academy of Clinical Toxicology and European Association of Poisons Centres and Clinical Toxicologists: Position statement: Ipecac syrup. *J Toxicol Clin Toxicol* 1997;35:699–709.
American Academy of Clinical Toxicology and European Association of Poisons Centres and Clinical Toxicologists: Position statement: Gastric lavage. *J Toxicol Clin Toxicol* 1997;35:711–19.
American Academy of Clinical Toxicology and European Association of Poisons Centres and Clinical Toxicologists: Position statement: Single-dose activated charcoal. *J Toxicol Clin Toxicol* 1997;35:721–41.
American Academy of Clinical Toxicology and European Association of Poisons Centres and Clinical Toxicologists: Position statement: Cathartics. *J Toxicol Clin Toxicol* 1997;35:743–52.
American Academy of Clinical Toxicology and European Association of Poisons Centres and Clinical Toxicologists: Position statement: Whole bowel irrigation. *J Toxicol Clin Toxicol* 1997;35:753–62.
American Academy of Clinical Toxicology and European Association of Poisons Centres and Clinical Toxicologists: Position statement and practice guidelines on the use of multiple-dose activated charcoal in the treatment of acute poisoning. *J Toxicol Clin Toxicol* 1999;37:731–51.
Bates N, Edwards N, Roper J, Volan G (editors): *Paediatric Toxicology: Handbook of Poisoning in Children.* New York, Stockton Press, 1993.
Bosse GM, Matyunas NJ: Delayed toxidromes. *J Emerg Med* 1999;17:679–90.
Burns MM: Activated charcoal as the sole intervention for treatment after childhood poisoning. *Curr Opin Pediatr* 2000;12:166–71.
Litovitz TL, Klein-Schwartz W, White S, et al: 2000 Annual report of the American Association of Poison Control Centers Toxic Exposure Surveillance System. *Am J Emerg Med* 2001;19:337–95.
Rodgers GC, Matyunas NJ (editors): *Handbook of Common Poisoning in Children*, 3rd ed. Chicago, American Academy of Pediatrics, 1994.
Shannon M: Ingestion of toxic substances in children. *N Engl J Med* 2000;342:186–91.
Spiller HA, Rodgers GC: Evaluation of administration of activated charcoal in the home. *Pediatrics* 2001;108:1–5.
Sugarman JM, Rodgers GC, Paul R: Utility of toxicology screening in a pediatric emergency department. *Pediatr Emerg Care* 1997; 13:194–7.
Woolf AD, Flynn E: Workplace toxic exposures involving adolescents aged 14 to 19 years. *Arch Pediatr Adolesc Med* 2000;154:234–8.

704.2 Acetaminophen

Acetaminophen is the most widely used analgesic and antipyretic, in part because of the finding of a relationship between Reye syndrome and salicylates. Consequently, acetaminophen is commonly available in the home, where it can be unintentionally ingested by young children or taken in an intentional overdose by adolescents.

Pathophysiology. Acetaminophen toxicity results from the formation of a highly reactive intermediate metabolite, *N*-acetyl-*p*-benzoquinoneimine (NAPQI). When therapeutic doses are administered, only a small amount (4%) of a dose is metabolized by hepatic cytochrome P450 enzymes to NAPQI, which is immediately conjugated with glutathione to form a harmless mercapturic acid conjugate. When hepatic stores of glutathione are depleted to less than 70% of normal, the NAPQI metabolite can combine with hepatic macromolecules to produce hepatocellular damage. The acute toxic dose of acetaminophen is generally considered to be more than 200 mg/kg in children younger than 12 yr. A single ingestion of more than 7.5 g is considered a minimum toxic dose in adolescents and adults. Repeated administration of acetaminophen at doses exceeding those recommended may lead to hepatic injury or failure in some children. Parents should be advised to follow closely the manufacturer's dosing guidelines and be aware of its presence in combination products.

Children younger than 6 yr are unlikely to develop significant toxicity after a single ingestion of even relatively large doses of acetaminophen. Nevertheless, at this time, children with a significant ingestion should have their plasma acetaminophen level measured and receive treatment with *N*-acetylcysteine (NAC) if the level falls within the toxic range on the nomogram. Adolescents have a higher incidence of toxic plasma levels after ingestion than do children. Even if a serious case of hepatotoxicity develops, the mortality rate is less than 0.5%. Patients who recover have no sequelae when observed 3–12 mo after the acute toxicity. Severely affected patients may require liver transplantation (see Chapter 349).

Clinical and Laboratory Manifestations. If untreated, patients who have acutely overdosed pass through four stages of toxicity (Table 704–3). Because early symptoms are nonspecific, physicians may fail to diagnose the ingestion without a good history or high index of suspicion. If a toxic ingestion is suspected, a plasma acetaminophen level should be measured 4 hr or more after ingestion. Measurement earlier than 4 hr after ingestion may be useful to determine if an ingestion has occurred, but cannot be used to determine the severity of an overdose. The level should be plotted on the Rumack-Matthew nomogram (Fig. 704–1) to determine whether antidotal treatment is indicated. The nomogram should only be used to evaluate the risk after acute exposure to regular release products. Liver function

<table>
<tr><td colspan="3">**TABLE 704-3. Stages in the Clinical Course of Acetaminophen Toxicity**</td></tr>
</table>

Stage	Time After Ingestion	Characteristics
I	1/2–24 hr	Anorexia, nausea, vomiting, malaise, pallor, diaphoresis
II	24–48 hr	Resolution of above; right upper quadrant abdominal pain and tenderness; elevated bilirubin, prothrombin time, hepatic enzymes; oliguria
III	72–96 hr	Peak liver function abnormalities; anorexia, nausea, vomiting, malaise may reappear
IV	4 days–2 wk	Resolution of hepatic dysfunction or complete liver failure

studies including enzymes, bilirubin, and prothrombin time should be followed daily in all patients with acetaminophen levels falling within the toxic range on the nomogram.

Treatment. After large acute overdose, when the need for antidotal treatment is anticipated and when treatment can be started

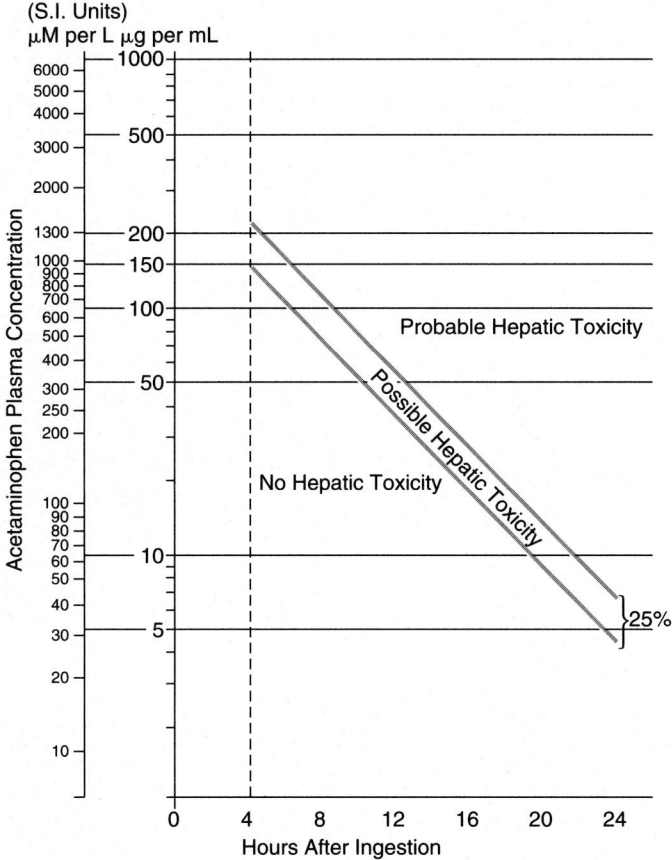

FIGURE 704–1. Rumack-Matthew nomogram for acetaminophen poisoning. Semilogarithmic plot of plasma acetaminophen levels versus time. *Cautions for the use of this chart:* (1) The time coordinates refer to time *after ingestion.* (2) Serum levels drawn before 4 hr may not represent peak levels. (3) The graph should be used only in relation to a single acute ingestion. (4) The lower *solid line* 25% below the standard nomogram is included to allow for possible errors in acetaminophen plasma assays and estimated time from ingestion of an overdose. (From Rumack BH, Hess AJ [eds]: Poisindex. Denver, 1995. Adapted from Rumack BH, Matthew H: Acetaminophen poisoning and toxicity. *Pediatrics* 1975;55:871.)

within 1–2 hr of the ingestion, activated charcoal administration should be considered. The antidote for acetaminophen poisoning is *N*-acetylcysteine (NAC or Mucomyst; see Table 704–2 for dosing). NAC serves as a precursor for glutathione synthesis, thus replenishing glutathione stores and preventing the reaction of NAPQI with hepatocytes. NAC therapy should be initiated as soon as possible after ingestion but may have value even if started 24–36 hr after the ingestion in severe cases. NAC is unpalatable and irritating to the gastrointestinal tract and should be diluted to a 5% solution with soda or fruit juice to minimize vomiting. Antiemetics may be used to control vomiting or NAC may be given directly into the stomach or upper intestine by tube. An intravenous preparation of NAC should soon be available in the United States; it is equally effective as oral NAC but given over a shorter time period. Physicians are encouraged to consult with a medical toxicologist or regional poison control center for cases involving subacute or chronic exposure or extended release products, because the Rumack-Matthew nomogram is not useful in making treatment decisions under these circumstances.

Anderson BJ, Holford NHG, Armishaw JC, et al: Predicting concentrations in children presenting with acetaminophen overdose. *J Pediatr* 1999;135:290–95.

Bond GR, Krenzelok EP, Normann SA, et al: Acetaminophen ingestion in childhood; Cost and relative risk of alternative referral strategies. *J Toxicol Clin Toxicol* 1994;32:513–25.

Caravati EM: Unintentional acetaminophen ingestion in children and potential for hepatotoxicity. *J Toxicol Clin Toxicol* 2000;38:291–96.

Cetaruk EW, Dart RC, Hurlbut KM, et al: Tylenol extended relief overdose. *Ann Emerg Med* 1997;30:104–8.

Heubi JE, Barbacci MB, Zimmerman HJ: Therapeutic misadventures with acetaminophen: Hepatotoxicity after multiple doses in children. *J Pediatr* 1998;132:22–7.

James LP, Wells E, Beard RH, et al: Predictors of outcome after acetaminophen poisoning in children and adolescents. *J Pediatr* 2002;140:522–26.

Luria JW, Ruddy R, Stephan M: Acute hepatic failure related to chronic acetaminophen intoxication. *Pediatr Emerg Care* 1996;12:291–93.

Perry HE, Shannon MW: Efficacy of oral versus intravenous *N*-acetylcysteine in acetaminophen overdose: Result of an open-label, clinical trial. *J Pediatr* 1998;132:149–52.

Rivers-Penera T, Gugig R, Davis J, et al: Outcome of acetaminophen overdose in pediatric patients and factors contributing to hepatotoxicity. *J Pediatr* 1997;130:300–4.

Rumack BH, Peterson RG: Acetaminophen overdose: Incidence, diagnosis and management in 416 patients. *Pediatrics* 1978;62:898–903.

Rumore MM, Blaiklock RG: Influence of age-dependent pharmacokinetics and metabolism of acetaminophen hepatotoxicity. *J Pharm Sci* 1992;81:203–7.

704.3 Salicylates

The incidence of salicylate poisoning has declined, particularly in young children, as the use of alternative antipyretics has increased. However, salicylate toxicity must still be considered in therapeutic situations as well as in cases of acute overdose. Methyl salicylate is the active ingredient in oil of wintergreen, a common component in rubefacients.

Pathophysiology. Salicylates directly or indirectly affect most organ systems by uncoupling oxidative phosphorylation, inhibiting Krebs cycle enzymes, and inhibiting amino acid synthesis. Various complex metabolic abnormalities result. Salicylates also decrease platelet adhesiveness and increase pulmonary capillary permeability. The acute toxic dose of salicylates is generally considered to be greater than 150 mg/kg.

Clinical and Laboratory Manifestations. The clinical presentation after acute poisoning differs significantly from chronic toxicity. Chronic toxicity results in signs and symptoms that are easily attributed to other causes, such as flu or other febrile illness. Young children are more susceptible to toxic effects because they are less able to buffer the acid load produced by salicylates.

After acute salicylate ingestion, nausea and vomiting occur secondary to gastric irritation. Salicylates directly stimulate the respiratory center, leading to hyperventilation and hyperpnea.

An increased respiratory rate results in respiratory alkalosis with compensatory alkaluria. Both potassium and sodium bicarbonate are excreted in the urine; however, early after exposure, the serum potassium concentration may be in the normal range. When sufficient potassium has been lost through the kidneys, an exchange of potassium for hydrogen ion occurs, and the urine becomes relatively acidic. This "paradoxical aciduria" occurs in the presence of a continued respiratory alkalosis. Dehydration and progressive metabolic acidosis, caused by the accumulation of lactic acid and other metabolic acids, eventually develop. Seriously poisoned patients are more than 5–10% dehydrated. Patients with chronic salicylate poisoning usually present with metabolic acidosis.

CNS changes are an important sign of serious toxicity. Agitation, restlessness, and confusion are common in children. Coma may develop secondary to cerebral edema. Pulmonary edema or hemorrhage may develop in more severe cases. Hyperglycemia or hypoglycemia, particularly in infants, has also been observed. Hepatotoxicity occurs after chronic exposure or very large acute ingestions. Death results from pulmonary edema and respiratory failure, cerebral edema, hemorrhage, severe electrolyte imbalance, or cardiovascular collapse.

Serial serum salicylate levels (obtained every 2–3 hr) should be monitored to evaluate for either continued absorption or impairment of excretion. The Done nomogram, once the standard tool for predicting salicylate toxicity after acute ingestion, is no longer used. After acute ingestion, patents with serum salicylate levels greater than 20 mg/dL should undergo continued observation and monitoring. Levels greater than 70 mg/dL may produce life-threatening effects. Patients with chronic salicylate toxicity may have a level within the therapeutic range (10–20 mg/dL). The level is low in relation to the severity of their illness, reflecting higher tissue concentrations of salicylate.

Urine pH and volume should be measured hourly in all seriously poisoned children. Plasma pH, glucose, potassium, and other electrolytes should be monitored at regular intervals. Clotting studies and liver function tests should be monitored in all severely poisoned patients.

Treatment. Initial treatment should include gastric decontamination, preferably with activated charcoal, if the patient presents soon after an acute ingestion. Salicylate tablets occasionally form into bezoars, which may be suspected if salicylate levels continue to rise many hours after ingestion or are persistently elevated. Gastric decontamination is usually not useful after chronic exposure.

Initial therapy focuses on rehydration and correction of electrolyte abnormalities (see Chapter 48). Large quantities of potassium and bicarbonate may be needed if symptoms have been present for some time after an acute ingestion or in the case of chronic salicylate poisoning, because body stores of these electrolytes may be severely depleted.

Urinary excretion of unmetabolized salicylate becomes an important route of elimination in overdose. Urinary clearance is affected by urine pH. Because metabolic acidosis produces a more acidic urine, a higher percentage of filtered salicylate remains in the un-ionized form, which is reabsorbed. Urinary salicylate elimination can be increased using ion trapping, increasing urine pH to convert a greater percentage of salicylate to the ionized form, which is then excreted in the urine. Each 1-unit increase in urine pH increases urinary salicylate clearance 4-fold. Urine pH should be raised to at least 7–7.5, using intravenous bicarbonate. It is important to remember that it may be impossible to alkalize the urine without adequately replenishing tissue stores of potassium. Acetazolamide (Diamox) should not be used to achieve urine alkalization.

In severe cases of salicylate intoxication, dialysis may be required both to remove salicylate and to correct electrolyte abnormalities. Indications for extracorporeal removal include serum levels more than 90 mg/dL, changes in neurologic status, respiratory or cardiovascular instability, refractory metabolic acidosis, severe hypokalemia, or renal failure. Hemodialysis is preferred over either peritoneal dialysis or charcoal hemoperfusion.

Brenner BE, Simon RR: Management of salicylate intoxication. *Drugs* 1982;24: 335–40.

Krause DS, Wolf BA, Shaw LM: Acute aspirin overdose: Mechanisms of toxicity. *Ther Drug Monit* 1992;14:441–51.

Leatherman JW, Schmitz PG: Fever, hyperdynamic shock, and multiple-system organ failure: A pseudo-sepsis syndrome associated with chronic salicylate intoxication. *Chest* 1991;100:1391–97.

Snodgrass W, Rumack BH, Peterson RG: Salicylate toxicity following therapeutic doses in young children. *J Toxicol Clin Toxicol* 1981;18:247–59.

Yip L, Dart RC, Gabow PA: Concepts and controversies in salicylate toxicity. *Emerg Med Clin North Am* 1994;12:351–64.

704.4 Ibuprofen

Ibuprofen is involved in a growing number of unintentional and intentional overdoses because of wider distribution and its increased use as an analgesic and antipyretic. Serious effects after overdose of ibuprofen are rare, occurring in fewer than 0.3% of cases reported to the AAPCC TESS database.

Pathophysiology. Prostaglandins are involved in a wide variety of physiologic processes. Ibuprofen inhibits prostaglandin synthesis, and this disruption produces the side effects reported with therapeutic use such as gastrointestinal irritation, reduced renal blood flow, and platelet dysfunction. The toxic mechanism of ibuprofen in acute overdose has not been well described. In children, doses less than 100 mg/kg do not cause toxicity, whereas doses greater than 400 mg/kg are capable of producing more serious effects, including seizures and coma.

Clinical and Laboratory Manifestations. Symptoms usually develop within 4 hr of ingestion and resolve within 24 hr. Common effects include nausea, vomiting, epigastric pain, drowsiness, lethargy, and ataxia. Anion gap metabolic acidosis, coma, transient apnea, renal failure, hypotension, and seizures are rare. Other reported effects include nystagmus, diplopia, headache, tinnitus, and transient deafness.

Symptoms may correlate with ibuprofen blood levels; however, data are limited and the test is not readily available. Renal function studies and acid-base balance should be monitored after ingestion of large doses.

Treatment. Good supportive care is essential because there is no antidotal therapy. Emesis is of little benefit, but activated charcoal can be administered. Extracorporeal removal methods have not been adequately evaluated and are not recommended.

Gunn VL, Taha SH, Liebelt EL, et al: Toxicity of over-the-counter cough and cold medications. *Pediatrics* 2001;108:E52.

Hall AH, Smolinske SC, Conrad FL, et al: Ibuprofen overdose: 126 cases. *Ann Emerg Med* 1986;15:1308–13.

Hall AH, Smolinske SC, Kulig KW, et al: Ibuprofen overdose: A prospective study. *West J Med* 1988;148:653–56.

Halpern SM, Fitzpatrick R, Volans GN: Ibuprofen toxicity: A review of adverse reactions and overdose. *Adverse Drug React Toxicol Rev* 1993;12:107–28.

Oker EE, Hermann L, Baum CR, et al: Serious toxicity in a young child due to ibuprofen. *Acad Emerg Med* 2000;7:821–23.

Perry SJ, Streete PJ, Volans GN: Ibuprofen overdose: The first two years of over-the-counter sales. *Hum Toxicol* 1987;6:173–78.

704.5 Antidepressants

The tricyclic antidepressants (TCAs) and the selective serotonin reuptake inhibitors (SSRIs) represent the two most common classes of antidepressants of toxicologic significance. Tricyclic antidepressants include amitriptyline, nortriptyline, and sinequan. SSRI agents include fluoxetine, sertraline, paroxetine, and citalopram.

TRICYCLIC ANTIDEPRESSANTS

Pathophysiology. These agents block the neuronal reuptake of norepinephrine, serotonin, and dopamine, in both the central and peripheral nervous systems. They also produce varying degrees of sedation, α-blocking, and anticholinergic effects. Inhibition of fast sodium channels in the myocardium leads to the development of cardiac dysrhythmias and myocardial depression. The potentially toxic dose of these agents in children ranges from 5–20 mg/kg.

Clinical and Laboratory Manifestations. The primary organ systems affected are the CNS and cardiovascular systems. Symptoms can develop as early as 30 min after ingestion, with serious symptoms usually developing within 6 hr of ingestion. The pattern of toxicity in children is slightly different from that described for adolescents and adults in that CNS effects occur more frequently in children than do cardiovascular effects. Drowsiness, lethargy, or coma have been reported in as many as one third of pediatric cases. Coma, when it occurs, usually resolves in a few hours, but may last longer than 24 hr. Seizures develop in about 15% of cases and can occur without warning. They are usually brief and resolve without treatment. Adolescents with comparable blood TCA levels suffer more significant toxicity than younger children.

Tachycardia, likely secondary to the anticholinergic actions of TCA, is the most common cardiovascular effect but does not usually compromise blood pressure. Hypertension may occur soon after ingestion but rarely requires treatment. Hypotension is uncommon but is a poor prognostic sign. Other cardiac findings include slowing of myocardial conduction, multifocal premature ventricular contractions, and ventricular tachycardia, flutter, or fibrillation. In addition to widening of the QRS complex, QT prolongation occurs with T-wave flattening or inversion, ST segment depression, right bundle branch block, and complete heart block.

Hypoventilation with respiratory arrest may occur without warning. Other reported effects include hyperthermia, choreiform movements, agitation, and twitching. An anticholinergic syndrome including mydriasis, disorientation, hallucinations, urinary retention, and diminished bowel sounds may be present.

The electrocardiogram (ECG) should be closely monitored for QRS widening and QT and QTc prolongation. QRS duration and axis deviation and the level of consciousness have been suggested as predictors of potential toxicity. ECG changes may not be useful predictors of toxicity in younger children because of normal variation. Blood levels of TCAs are not helpful in assessing or predicting the severity of the exposure but may aid in establishing a diagnosis.

Treatment. After general life support measures are instituted, including endotracheal intubation if indicated, efforts should be made to prevent absorption. Emesis is contraindicated because of the danger of aspiration from vomiting after the onset of CNS depression or seizures. Activated charcoal should be administered. Sodium bicarbonate in doses sufficient to achieve a serum pH of 7.45–7.55 should be administered to treat and prevent dysrhythmias. Lidocaine is used to treat dysrhythmias that are unresponsive to serum alkalization. Quinidine and procainamide should not be used because they further depress cardiac conduction. Hypotension may respond to standard fluid therapy, although vasopressors such as norepinephrine may be required. Severe, unresponsive hypotension is a poor prognostic sign. Hypertension usually is transient and does not require treatment. Seizures, if they require treatment, usually respond to benzodiazepine therapy. Physostigmine, once promoted as an "antidote" for TCA toxicity, is a dangerous agent that can cause seizures and dysrhythmias and should not be used. Because of the large volumes of distribution and high degree of plasma protein binding of TCAs, extracorporeal removal is not of value.

Asymptomatic children should be observed and the ECG monitored for at least 6 hr after exposure. If any manifestations of toxicity (e.g., a QRS interval > 0.10 msec, conduction defects, altered mental status, hypotension, or hypoventilation) develop, continue monitoring in an intensive care unit for 24 hr. Only completely asymptomatic children should be discharged after 6 hr of observation.

SELECTIVE SEROTONIN REUPTAKE INHIBITORS

These agents differ from TCAs in that they specifically inhibit reuptake of serotonin in the CNS. They have little or no effect on norepinephrine or dopamine reuptake and minimal, if any, anticholinergic or α-blocking effects.

Clinical Manifestations. These drugs have a wide therapeutic index so toxic effects are mild. The usual onset of symptoms is within 3 hr, with resolution of symptoms within 24 hr in treated patients. Most cases in children remain asymptomatic. Drowsiness or hyperactivity, agitation, and tachycardia are the most commonly reported effects. Nausea, vomiting, tremor, dizziness, and abdominal pain are less common. Life-threatening effects such as seizures and coma are rare but have been reported after very large ingestions. Cardiac conduction defects are not common. Adolescents have an increased incidence of symptoms, although they are still relatively minor. The toxic dose of these agents is not well defined.

A *serotonin syndrome* has been reported after accidental overdose of SSRIs as well as therapeutic use. It is an idiosyncratic reaction that includes confusion and disorientation, agitation, coma, hyperthermia, myoclonus, hyperreflexia, tremor, and muscle rigidity. Therapy is supportive, but awareness and recognition of the syndrome is important to prevent complications caused by inappropriate interventions.

Treatment. Gastrointestinal decontamination with activated charcoal is preferred over ipecac-induced emesis because of the potential for CNS depression. There is no specific therapy other than general supportive care.

Barbey JT, Roose SP: SSRI Safety in overdose. *J Clin Psychiatry* 1998;59(suppl 15):42–48.

James LP, Kearns GL: Cyclic antidepressant toxicity in children and adolescents. *J Clin Pharmacol* 1995;35:343–50.

Newton EH, Shih RD, Hoffman RS: Cyclic antidepressant overdose: A review of current management strategies. *Am J Emerg Med* 1994;12:376–79.

Shannon M, Liebelt EA: Toxicology reviews: Targeted management strategies for cardiovascular toxicity from tricyclic antidepressant overdose: The pivotal role for alkalinization and sodium loading. *Pediatr Emerg Care* 1998;14:293–98.

Spirko BA, Wiley JF: Serotonin syndrome: A new pediatric intoxication. *Pediatr Emerg Care* 1999;15:440–43.

704.6 Clonidine

Clonidine was first introduced for use as an antihypertensive but has found use in ADHD and tic syndromes in children (see Chapter 28). Increased use for pediatric indications has resulted in an explosion of acute poisoning and therapeutic misadventures.

Pathophysiology. The toxic effects of clonidine are a result of α_2-adrenergic receptor inhibition in the CNS. Children are very sensitive to the toxic effects of clonidine, with as little as 0.1 mg reported to produce significant toxicity. Serious toxicity has developed after sucking or chewing on a new or discarded topical patch preparation.

Clinical and Laboratory Manifestations. In clonidine naïve children, symptoms frequently develop within 1 hr of ingestion, thus rapid recognition and intervention is essential. Lethargy, miosis, bradycardia, and hypotension occur in all age groups. Apnea, respiratory depression, and coma are common findings in younger children. Serious symptoms usually resolve within

24 hr of ingestion. Serum clonidine levels are not readily available and not recommended.

Treatment. Immediate recognition of an exposure with transfer to a health care facility is of paramount importance. Gastric decontamination is usually of little value owing to the small quantities usually ingested and the rapid onset of serious symptoms. Aggressive supportive care is imperative. The ECG, vital signs, and blood gases are monitored as symptoms dictate. Naloxone (see Table 704–2) has been used with mixed success to reverse CNS and respiratory depression; however, its use should not replace supportive care. Because the duration of effect of naloxone is shorter than that of clonidine, administration by continuous infusion may be necessary. Extracorporeal removal techniques are not of value.

Erickson SJ, Duncan A: Clonidine poisoning—an emerging problem: Epidemiology, clinical features, management and preventative strategies. *J Paediatr Child Health* 1998;34:280–82.

Kappagoda C, Schell DN, Hanson RM, et al: Clonidine overdose in childhood: Implications of increased prescribing. *J Paediatr Child Health* 1998;34:508–12.

Tessa C, Mascalchi M, Matteucci L, et al: Permanent brain damage following acute clonidine poisoning in Munchausen by proxy. *Neuropediatrics* 2001;32:90–92.

704.7 Calcium Channel Blockers

Calcium channel blockers (CCBs) encompass a variety of chemical structures that produce various effects on the myocardium and the systemic vasculature. Specific agents include nifedipine, diltiazem, verapamil, amlodipine, and felodipine. They are available as regular-release and sustained-release preparations as well as in combination with diuretics and other antihypertensives. Their increasing therapeutic use has also increased the incidence of poisoning exposure.

Pathophysiology. The toxic effects of these drugs are an extension of their therapeutic effect in that they slow sinoatrial and atrioventricular nodal conduction and depress myocardial contractility. Inhibition of calcium influx into vascular smooth muscle cells results in arterial dilation and lowered blood pressure. CCBs affect both myocardial tissue and vascular smooth muscle; therefore, in overdose, either cardiac dysrhythmias or hypotension may occur or both effects may be evident. CCBs have a narrow therapeutic index; thus, any dose greater than the usual maximum daily therapeutic dose should be considered potentially toxic.

Clinical and Laboratory Manifestations. The onset of symptoms may occur within minutes of the ingestion of a regular release product or may be delayed several hours after the ingestion of a sustained-release product. Bradycardia and varying degrees of atrioventricular block are common. Hypotension develops secondary to dilation of vascular smooth muscle. Myocardial depression may lead to shock in severe cases. Confusion, agitation, or lethargy and possible coma may occur. Nausea and vomiting are common.

Careful blood pressure and electrocardiographic monitoring is essential. Although these agents block calcium channels, the serum calcium level is not affected. Hyperglycemia is also common, so serial serum glucose measurements should be followed. Blood levels of CCB are not readily available and are not useful in guiding therapy.

Treatment. After appropriate supportive care has been instituted, absorption should be prevented using activated charcoal if appropriate. Whole bowel irrigation should be considered if a sustained-release product has been ingested. Bradycardia and conduction disturbances are frequently unresponsive to atropine and often require the placement of a pacemaker. Isoproterenol may worsen hypotension and should not be used to treat bradycardia. Myocardial depression may contribute to

hypotension and should improve if conduction disturbances are reversed. Hypotension may be treated with fluids and vasopressors. Because many CCBs are available as sustained-release formulations, toxic effects may be prolonged if adequate gastrointestinal decontamination has not been performed.

Intravenous calcium may reverse myocardial depression, but it is not consistently effective. Calcium chloride is preferred over calcium gluconate because it contains a greater amount of calcium per gram. Because the duration of action of calcium salts is much shorter than that of CCBs, administration by continuous infusion may be necessary (see Table 704–2). Hypercalcemia does not produce clinical effects and is not a concern.

Glucagon improves cardiac conduction and contractility by promoting calcium ion influx through calcium channels indirectly (see Table 704–2). Its efficacy in the treatment of CCB overdose is not consistent. Other inotropic agents such as amiodarone have also been used with mixed success. High-dose infusion of regular insulin and glucose therapy has demonstrated some effectiveness; however, its use in children has not been examined. Extracorporeal elimination methods are not useful for removing CCBs.

Belson MG, Gorman SE, Sullivan K, et al: Calcium channel blocker ingestions in children. *Am J Emerg Med* 2000;18:581–86.

Gleyzer A, Traub S, Hoffman RS: Calcium channel blocker ingestions in children. *Am J Emerg Med* 2001;19:456–7.

Kerns W, Kline J, Ford MD: β-blocker and calcium channel blocker toxicity. *Emerg Med Clin North Am* 1994;12:365–89.

Lee DC, Greene T, Dougherty T, et al: Fatal nifedipine ingestions in children. *J Emerg Med* 2000;19:359–61.

704.8 Iron

Iron is one of the most common causes of childhood poisoning death. Iron-containing products are common in many homes and often resemble candy. The potential severity of exposure is based on the amount of elemental iron ingested. The amount of elemental iron ingested is calculated on the basis of the number of tablets ingested and the percentage of elemental iron in the salt. Ferrous sulfate contains 20%, ferrous gluconate 12%, and ferrous fumarate 33% elemental iron. Multiple vitamin products containing iron list on the label the amount of iron per tablet as elemental iron.

Pathophysiology. Iron is corrosive to the gastrointestinal mucosa. It also accumulates in the mitochondria and tissues to produce cellular damage and systemic toxicity. Iron causes venodilation and increased capillary permeability leading to hypotension. Reduced peripheral perfusion and mitochondrial damage result in lactic and citric acid accumulation, causing metabolic acidosis. Hepatic necrosis develops after serious poisoning, resulting in abnormal liver function tests and coagulopathies. Drowsiness and coma may develop as a result of hemodynamic instability or possibly a direct toxic effect of iron in the CNS. Greater than 60 mg/kg of elemental iron is generally considered a toxic dose.

Clinical and Laboratory Manifestations. Nausea, vomiting, diarrhea, and abdominal pain are the hallmark of iron poisoning and usually develop within 30 min–6 hr after ingestion. Hematemesis and bloody diarrhea may develop in more serious poisonings. The gastrointestinal signs may subside over 6–12 hr; however, careful observation is warranted because systemic toxicity due to cellular damage may ensue, particularly in patients with severe gastrointestinal signs, early hypotension, or drowsiness. Gastric scarring and pyloric stenosis can develop 2–4 wk after a large ingestion or in instances when iron tablets remain in prolonged contact with the gastrointestinal mucosa. Stenosis may be symptomatic and occasionally requires surgical intervention.

Serum iron levels should be obtained and evaluated in the context of symptoms. Iron levels should be obtained about 4 hr after ingestion. Serum iron levels less than 500 µg/dL, measured 4–8 hr after ingestion, indicate a low risk of significant toxicity. Levels greater than 500 µg/dL indicate significant toxicity is likely. Blood gas levels, serum glucose concentration, liver function tests, and coagulation studies should be monitored in patients with iron levels greater than 500 µg/dL.

Because iron is radiopaque, an abdominal radiograph may confirm the ingestion. Repeat radiographs may help with assessment of the efficiency of gastric decontamination methods. A negative result does not rule out iron ingestion because only undissolved tablets can be seen. Children's multiple vitamins are usually not visualized on radiography because of the low concentration of iron and the rapid dissolution of the tablets.

Treatment. Good supportive and symptomatic care is essential in cases of iron poisoning. Ipecac-induced emesis may be used to remove tablets from the stomach. Gastric lavage is not recommended in young children because of its inefficiency, particularly because of the large size of many iron tablets. Activated charcoal does not adsorb iron and should not be used. Whole bowel irrigation may be of benefit. If tablets adhere to the gastric mucosa, removal by endoscopic or surgical intervention (gastrotomy) or aggressive whole bowel irrigation has been attempted with mixed success.

Oral bicarbonate (2%), dilute Phospho-Soda (1:4), and magnesium hydroxide (milk of magnesia) react with iron to form less soluble, poorly absorbed iron salts, but this technique is of questionable clinical benefit. Complexation of iron in the gastrointestinal tract using oral deferoxamine is expensive, may increase iron absorption, and is generally not recommended.

Deferoxamine is a specific chelator of iron and is the antidote for moderate to severe iron intoxication (see Table 704–2 for dosing). Indications for deferoxamine include a serum iron level greater than 500 µg/dL, regardless of symptoms, or moderate to severe symptoms regardless of the serum iron level. It should be administered as a continuous intravenous infusion, continued until a patient is symptom free. The deferoxamine-iron complex may color the urine reddish (vin rosé), although this is an unreliable indicator of iron excretion.

Klein-Schwatrz W, Oderda GM, Gorman RL, et al: Assessment of management guidelines: Acute iron ingestion. *Clin Pediatr* 1990;29:316–21.
Mills KC, Curry SC: Acute iron poisoning. *Emerg Med Clin North Am* 1994;12: 397–413.
Morris CC: Recent trends in pediatric iron poisonings. *South Med J* 2000;93: 1229.
Schauben JL, Augenstein WL, Cox J, et al: Iron poisoning: Report of three cases and a review of therapeutic intervention. *J Emerg Med* 1990;8:309–19.
Tenenbein M: Whole bowel irrigation in iron poisoning. *J Pediatr* 1987;111: 142–45.
Tenenbein M: Hepatotoxicity in acute iron poisoning. *J Toxicol Clin Toxicol* 2001;39: 721–26.
Yatscoff RW, Wayne EA, Tenenbein M: An objective criterion for the cessation of deferoxamine therapy in the acutely iron poisoned patient. *J Toxicol Clin Toxicol* 1991;29:1–10.

704.9 Caustics

Pathophysiology. Caustics include acids and alkalis as well as a few common oxidizing agents such as bleach. Acids coagulate proteins, causing tissue necrosis. Alkalis digest and dissolve proteins, producing liquefaction necrosis with the risk of perforation if the injury is located in the intestinal tract. The severity of the chemical burn produced depends on the pH, the concentration of the agent, and the length of contact time. Agents with a pH below 2 or above 12 are most likely to produce significant injury.

Clinical Manifestations. Ingestion of caustic materials may produce oral burns visualized as reddened areas or whitish plaques.

Symptoms include pain, drooling, vomiting, or difficulty or refusal to swallow. Circumferential burns of the esophagus are prone to cause strictures on healing, which may require repeated dilation or surgical correction. Strong acids may sometimes produce scarring around the pylorus, leading to delayed onset of gastric obstruction. Caustics on the skin or in the eye can cause significant tissue damage.

Treatment. Initial treatment of caustic exposure includes thorough removal of the product from the skin or eye by flushing with water. Contaminated clothing should also be removed. Ingested agents should be rinsed from the oral cavity. Emesis and lavage are contraindicated. Activated charcoal should not be used, because it does not bind these agents. Patients should be evaluated for evidence of esophageal burns and, if symptoms are present, oral fluids or solids should be withheld. The absence of visible oral injury does not preclude significant esophageal lesions. Endoscopy should be performed in symptomatic patients or those in whom injury is highly suspect on the basis of history. The use of corticosteroids and esophageal stents is controversial. Prophylactic antibiotics do not improve outcomes.

Berkovits RNP, Bos CE, Wijburg FA, et al: Caustic injury of the oesophagus: Sixteen years experience, and introduction of a new model oesophageal stent. *J Laryngol Otol* 1996;110:1041–45.
Christensen HBT: Prediction of complications following unintentional caustic ingestion in children. Is endoscopy always necessary? *Acta Paediatr* 1995;84: 1177–82.
Gaudreault P, Parent M, McGuigan MA: Predictability of esophageal injury from signs and symptoms: A study of 378 children. *Pediatrics* 1983;71:767–70.
Harley EH, Collins MD: Liquid household bleach ingestion in children: A retrospective review. *Laryngoscope* 1997;107:122–25.
Penner GE: Acid ingestion: Toxicology and treatment. *Ann Emerg Med* 1980;9: 374–79.
Rothstein FC: Caustic injuries to the esophagus in children. *Pediatr Clin North Am* 1986;33:665–74.
Spitz L, Lakhoo K: Caustic ingestion. *Arch Dis Child* 1993;68:157–58.

704.10 Methanol and Ethylene Glycol

Methanol is commonly found in windshield washer fluids, fuel additives, liquid fuel canisters, and industrial solvents. Ethylene glycol is commonly found in car radiator antifreeze. Both solvents are well absorbed via inhalation or after skin contact; however, accidental ingestion is the most common route of exposure in children. The pathophysiology, clinical effects, and treatment of both chemicals are similar. Although each parent compound is capable of producing mild toxicity, it is the metabolites of each product that are responsible for the serious clinical effects that can follow exposure.

METHANOL

Pathophysiology. Methanol is metabolized in the liver by alcohol dehydrogenase to formaldehyde, which is further metabolized to formic acid by aldehyde dehydrogenase. Formic acid is metabolized through folate-dependent pathways to carbon dioxide and water. Toxicity is caused primarily by formic acid, which inhibits mitochondrial respiration. The development of serious toxic effects is delayed while formic acid is generated and accumulates in blood and tissues.

Clinical and Laboratory Manifestations. Drowsiness, mild inebriation, and gastric irritation, including nausea and vomiting, develop early after ingestion. The onset of serious effects, including profound metabolic acidosis and visual disturbances, is delayed up to 24 hr. Visual disturbances include blurred or cloudy vision, constricted visual fields, decreased acuity, and the "feeling of being in a snowstorm." Small children may not be able to describe these visual changes. Pupils may be dilated and unreactive to light, and retinal edema and optic disc hyperemia may be noted. Visual disturbances are usually reversible, but in significant poisonings, blindness has occasionally been permanent. An anion-gap metabolic acidosis develops; thus, serum electrolytes, pH, and acid-base balance should be monitored.

Children are usually discovered with an open container of product soon after an exposure, and determining if a significant exposure has occurred is usually a problem. Methanol blood measurements are usually available and can rule out an exposure; however, levels do not correlate well with toxicity. Formic acid levels may correlate more closely with toxicity; however, these levels are not routinely available. If methanol levels are not available, estimation of an osmolar gap has been recommended as a surrogate. Serum osmolarity is measured by the freezing point depression method and compared with a calculated serum osmolarity. The osmolar gap can be used to estimate the serum methanol level using the following formula:

$$\text{Osmolar gap} \times 3.2 = \text{Estimated methanol level (in mg/dL)}$$

ETHYLENE GLYCOL

Pathophysiology. Ethylene glycol is metabolized by alcohol dehydrogenase in the liver to glycoaldehyde, which is further converted to glycolic acid by aldehyde dehydrogenase. Glycolic acid is metabolized to glyoxylic acid and oxalic acid, which cause toxicity. The development of serious toxic effects is delayed while these acids are generated and accumulate in blood and tissues. Oxalic acid combines with serum and tissue calcium, causing hypocalcemia and the formation of calcium oxalate crystals.

Clinical and Laboratory Manifestations. Ethylene glycol toxicity is described as occurring in three stages; however, there is considerable overlap in the stages. Early symptoms occur 1–12 hr after ingestion and include gastric irritation, with nausea and vomiting, and CNS effects, including drowsiness and inebriation. Metabolic acidosis begins to develop. From 12–24 hr after ingestion, cardiac dysrhythmias, muscle pain, and tetany due to hypocalcemia may occur. Later in the clinical course, cardiac failure, seizures, cerebral edema, and renal failure occur. Renal failure is caused by the deposition of calcium oxalate crystals in renal tubules.

Ethylene glycol blood levels are not readily available, and results do not correlate well with toxicity. Glycolic acid and glyoxylic acid levels may correlate more closely with toxicity, but these levels are not routinely available. Sodium fluorescein is an additive in many commercial antifreeze products. It is renally excreted and may be visualized in urine up to 6 hr after ingestion when illuminated with Wood's lamp. This simple test may be used to confirm ethylene glycol ingestion in children; however, a negative test does not preclude a possible ingestion. Ethylene glycol levels can be estimated from an osmolar gap. The serum osmolarity is measured by the freezing point depression method and is compared with a calculated serum osmolarity. The osmolar gap can be used to estimate the serum ethylene glycol level using the following formula:

$$\text{Osmolar gap} \times 6.2 = \text{Estimated ethylene glycol level (in mg/dL)}$$

Calcium oxalate crystals are commonly seen in urine on microscopy but may not be evident early after exposure. Electrolytes, including calcium, should be monitored, as well as the ECG and renal function studies.

Methanol and Ethylene Glycol Treatment. Because methanol and ethylene glycol are rapidly absorbed, gastric decontamination is usually not of value. Activated charcoal does not bind either agent. Metabolic acidosis is treated with intravenous sodium bicarbonate at doses of 1–2 mEq/kg.

Ethanol is an antidote for both methanol and ethylene glycol poisoning because it is preferentially metabolized over methanol and ethylene glycol by alcohol dehydrogenase, thus preventing formation of toxic metabolites (see Table 704–2). The parent compounds are then excreted via the lungs and kidneys. Indications for ethanol therapy are a serum ethylene glycol level greater than 25 mg/dL or methanol level greater than 20 mg/dL, a significantly symptomatic patient, or ingestion of more than 0.4 mL/kg of 100% ethylene glycol or methanol. Assistance with ethanol dosing may be obtained through consultation with a medical toxicologist or poison control center. Fomepizole (see Table 704–2) is a potent competitive inhibitor of alcohol dehydrogenase that has been approved for use in both methanol and ethylene glycol poisoning. Like ethanol, it inhibits metabolism of methanol or ethylene glycol. Ease of dosing and lack of side effects are major advantages of fomepizole over ethanol. The high cost is a disadvantage. There is also very limited experience with this agent in children.

Hemodialysis effectively removes ethylene glycol, methanol, and their acid metabolites. It is also useful for correcting severe metabolic acidosis. The indications for hemodialysis are refractory metabolic acidosis, renal failure, or ethylene glycol or methanol blood levels exceeding 50 mg/dL. Both ethanol and fomepizole are removed by dialysis; thus, dosing of either must be increased during dialysis.

Brent J, McMartin K, Phillips S, et al: Fomepizole for the treatment of methanol poisoning. *N Engl J Med* 2001;8:424–29.

Brown MJ, Shannon MW, Woolf A, et al: Childhood methanol ingestion treated with fomepizole and hemodialysis. *Pediatrics* 2001;108:E77.

Church AS, Witting MD: Laboratory testing in ethanol, methanol, ethylene glycol and isopropanol toxicities. *J Emerg Med* 1997;15:687–92.

Casavant MJ: Fomepizole in the treatment of poisoning. *Pediatrics* 2001;107:170.

Glaser DS: Utility of the serum osmol gap in the diagnosis of methanol or ethylene glycol ingestion. *Ann Emerg Med* 1996;27:343–46.

Jacobsen D, McMartin KE: Antidotes for methanol and ethylene glycol poisoning. *J Toxicol Clin Toxicol* 1997;35:127–43.

Liu JJ, Daya MR, Carrasquillo O, et al: Prognostic factors in patients with methanol poisoning. *J Toxicol Clin Toxicol* 1998;36:175–81.

Shannon M: Toxicology reviews: fomepizole—a new antidote. *Pediatr Emerg Care* 1998;14:170–72.

704.11 Hydrocarbons

Hydrocarbons include a wide array of chemical substances found in thousands of commercial products. Many factors determine whether a particular product and exposure will produce systemic toxicity, local toxicity, or both.

Pathophysiology. The most important toxic effect of hydrocarbons is aspiration pneumonitis (see Chapter 385). Aspiration usually occurs at the time of ingestion, when coughing and gagging are common, but can be secondary to vomiting that commonly occurs after ingestion. The propensity of a hydrocarbon to cause aspiration pneumonitis is inversely proportional to its viscosity. Compounds with low viscosity, such as mineral spirits, naphtha, kerosene, gasoline, and lamp oil, spread rapidly across surfaces and cover large areas of the lungs when aspirated. Only small quantities (<1 mL) of low viscosity hydrocarbons need be aspirated to produce significant injury. Pneumonitis does not result from dermal absorption of hydrocarbons or from ingestion in the absence of aspiration.

Hydrocarbons can be absorbed after ingestion, inhalation, or dermal contact. Most hydrocarbons have anesthetic properties and can cause transient CNS depression. Several chlorinated solvents, most notably carbon tetrachloride, can produce hepatic toxicity. A few hydrocarbons have also been associated with renal toxicity. Benzene is known to cause cancer in humans after long-term exposure. The malignancy most commonly associated with benzene is acute myelogenous leukemia. Methylene chloride, found in some paint removers, is metabolized to carbon monoxide. Nitrobenzene, aniline, and related compounds can produce methemoglobinemia. Methemoglobin can be determined in the laboratory; its presence is also suggested if a drop of blood applied to filter paper remains brown as it dries. Methemoglobinemia is treated with the antidote methylene blue (see Table 704–2).

A number of volatile hydrocarbons, including toluene, propellants, refrigerants, and volatile nitrites, are commonly abused by inhalation. Some of these substances can sensitize the myocardium with the risk of dysrhythmias and sudden death. Chronic abuse of these agents can lead to cerebral atrophy, neuropsychological changes, peripheral neuropathy, and renal disease (see Chapter 105). All volatile hydrocarbons are lipid solvents and can cause defatting of the skin, producing local irritation or, with prolonged exposure, chemical burns.

Clinical and Laboratory Manifestations. Transient, mild CNS depression is common after hydrocarbon ingestion. Aspiration is characterized by coughing, which usually is the first clinical finding. Chest radiographs may be normal for as long as 8–12 hr after aspiration. Respiratory symptoms may remain mild or may rapidly progress to respiratory failure. Fever occurs and may persist for as long as 10 days after aspiration. Accompanying leukocytosis may be misleading because, in most cases of aspiration pneumonitis, no bacteria are present in the lungs. Chest radiographs may remain abnormal long after a patient is clinically normal and should not be used to guide acute treatment. Pneumatoceles may appear on the chest radiograph 2–3 wk after exposure. See Chapter 385.

Treatment. Emesis is contraindicated because of the risk of aspiration. Likewise, gastric lavage is contraindicated, except under special circumstances, because of the risk of vomiting and aspiration. Activated charcoal also is not useful, because it does not bind the common hydrocarbons. If hydrocarbon-induced pneumonitis develops, respiratory treatment is supportive. Corticosteroids should be avoided, because they are not effective and may be harmful. Prophylactic antibiotics should not be given because bacterial pneumonia occurs in only a very small percentage of cases. Respiratory failure has been successfully treated with both standard ventilation and with extracorporeal membrane oxygenation (ECMO).

Anas N, Nanasonthi V, Ginsburg CM: Criteria for hospitalizing children who have ingested products containing hydrocarbons. *JAMA* 1981;246:840–43.

Carder JR, Fuerst RS: Myocardial infarction after toluene inhalation. *Pediatr Emerg Care* 1997;13:117–19.

Chyka PA: Benefits of extracorporeal membrane oxygenation for hydrocarbon pneumonitis. *J Toxicol Clin Toxicol* 1996;34:357–63.

Edminster SC, Bayer MJ: Recreational gasoline sniffing: Acute gasoline intoxication and latent organolead poisoning. *J Emerg Med* 1985;3:365–70.

Flanagan RJ, Ruprah M, Meredith TJ, et al: An introduction to the clinical toxicology of volatile substances. *Drug Safety* 1990;5:359–83.

Gurwitz D, Kattan M, Levison H, et al: Pulmonary function abnormalities in asymptomatic children after hydrocarbon pneumonitis. *Pediatrics* 1978;62:789–94.

Meredith TJ, Ruprah M, Liddle A, et al: Diagnosis and treatment of acute poisoning with volatile substances. *Hum Toxicol* 1989;8:277–86.

704.12 Cholinesterase-Inhibiting Insecticides

The most commonly used insecticides are either organophosphates or carbamates. Both of these classes are inhibitors of cholinesterase enzymes. Nerve agents used in warfare are organophosphates. Most pediatric poisonings occur as the result of accidental exposure to insecticides in and around the home or farm.

Pathophysiology. Both organophosphates and carbamates bind to cholinesterase enzymes, preventing the degradation of acetylcholine, resulting in its accumulation at nerve synapses.

Enzymes affected include acetylcholinesterase or red blood cell cholinesterase, pseudocholinesterase (found in plasma), and neurotoxic esterase (found in the nervous system). If left untreated, organophosphates form a permanent bond to these enzymes, inactivating them. This process, called aging, occurs over the 2–3 days after exposure. Weeks to months are required for the body to regenerate inactivated enzymes. In contrast, carbamates form a temporary bond to the enzymes, allowing regeneration of the enzymes over several hours.

Clinical and Laboratory Manifestations. Clinical manifestations of organophosphate and carbamate toxicity relate to the accumulation of acetylcholine at peripheral nicotinic and muscarinic synapses and in the CNS. Muscarinic signs and symptoms include diaphoresis, emesis, urinary and fecal incontinence, tearing, drooling, bronchorrhea and bronchospasm, miosis, and hypotension and bradycardia. Nicotinic signs and symptoms include muscle weakness, fasciculations, tremors, hypoventilation, hypertension, tachycardia, and dysrhythmias. CNS effects include malaise, confusion, delirium, seizures, and coma. Symptoms caused by carbamate toxicity are usually less severe than those seen with organophosphates. A commonly used acronym for the most common symptoms is SLUDGE, which stands for **s**alivation, **l**acrimation, **u**rination, **d**efecation, **g**astrointestinal cramps, and **e**mesis.

Red blood cell cholinesterase and pseudocholinesterase levels can be readily measured in the laboratory. They may be useful in documenting an exposure but do not correlate well with symptoms. Significant symptoms do not generally occur until measured enzyme levels fall below 25% of normal. Red blood cell cholinesterase, although more difficult to measure, is a better reflection of the enzyme activity in the nervous system.

Treatment. Basic decontamination should be done on exposed persons. Activated charcoal can be used for gastric decontamination. Basic supportive care should be provided, including fluid and electrolyte replacement and intubation with artificial ventilation if necessary. Two antidotes are useful to treat poisoning with cholinesterase inhibitors: atropine and pralidoxime (2-PAM) (see Table 704–2). Atropine, which blocks the acetylcholine receptor, is useful for both organophosphates and carbamates. It is most effective at reversing the muscarinic and CNS effects. Often, large doses of atropine must be administered by continuous infusion. Pralidoxime chemically breaks the bond between the organophosphate and the enzyme, liberating the enzyme and degrading the organophosphate. Pralidoxime is only effective if used before the bond "ages" and becomes permanent. Pralidoxime is not necessary for carbamate poisonings because the bond between the insecticide and the enzyme degrades spontaneously. For significant organophosphate poisonings both antidotes are used and large doses of atropine may be necessary to achieve adequate reversal of symptoms. Without treatment, symptoms of organophosphate poisoning may persist for weeks, requiring continuous supportive care. Even with treatment, neurologic symptoms may occur and may persist.

Auito LA, et al: Life-threatening organophosphate-induced delayed polyneuropathy in a child after accidental chlorpyrifos ingestion. *J Pediatr* 1993;122:658–60.

Borowitz SM: Prolonged organophosphate toxicity in a twenty-six-month-old child. *J Pediatr* 1988;112:302–4.

Farrar HC, Wells TG, Kearns GL: Use of continuous infusion of pralidoxime for treatment of organophosphate in children. *J Pediatr* 1990;116:648–61.

Lifshitz M, Shahak E, Sofer S: Carbamate and organophosphate poisoning in young children. *Pediatr Emerg Care* 1999;15:102–3.

Morgan I: Carbamate insecticides. In Bates N, Edwards N, Roper J, Volan G (editors): *Paediatric Toxicology: Handbook of Poisoning in Children.* New York, Stockton Press, 1993, pp 114–16 and 255–59.

Rodgers GC, Matyunas NJ (editors): *Handbook of Common Poisoning in Children*, 3rd ed. Chicago, American Academy of Pediatrics, 1994, pp 200–3.

704.13 Toxic Gases

Although many industrial and naturally occurring gases pose a health risk by inhalation, only two, carbon monoxide (CO) and hydrogen cyanide, are considered in detail here. CO is a colorless, odorless gas produced during the combustion of any carbon-containing fuel. Hydrogen cyanide, as well as cyanide salts, is used in many industrial processes. It is also produced during combustion of many plastics and fabrics and is released during the metabolism of some chemicals, including the solvent acetonitrile and the drug nitroprusside.

Chlorine, chloramine, and hydrogen chloride are severe lung irritants and may cause a chemical pneumonitis. Nitrogen, propane, and methane are examples of simple asphyxiants.

CARBON MONOXIDE

Pathophysiology. CO toxicity develops through at least three mechanisms. First, it binds to hemoglobin, displacing oxygen, with an affinity for hemoglobin that is about 250 times that of oxygen. Second, CO impairs the ability of hemoglobin to release oxygen to tissues. Finally, CO also binds to cytochrome oxidase in tissues, impeding oxygen utilization. Although the relative contribution of each of these mechanisms to carbon monoxide toxicity is unclear, the net result is tissue hypoxia.

Clinical and Laboratory Manifestations. Symptoms of CO poisoning are generally proportionate to the concentration of carboxyhemoglobin in the blood. Carboxyhemoglobin levels can be measured in almost all hospital laboratories. Early symptoms are nonspecific and include headache, malaise, and nausea, which are often confused with the flu. At higher exposure levels, headaches become severe and dizziness, visual changes, and weakness may be present. Children may experience syncopal episodes as a first symptom. At high concentrations, coma, seizures, respiratory instability, and death may occur.

Treatment. In addition to general supportive care, treatment of CO poisoning requires the administration of high concentrations of oxygen. High concentrations of oxygen shorten the half-life of CO in the blood and tissues. Severely poisoned patients benefit from hyperbaric oxygen therapy. After a significant exposure, some patients may experience delayed-onset neurotoxicity, which may be permanent. Aggressive early treatment of patients with significant symptoms may diminish the risk of neurologic sequelae.

HYDROGEN CYANIDE

Pathophysiology. Cyanide produces toxicity by interfering with oxygen use in the cytochrome oxidase system, resulting in cellular hypoxia.

Clinical and Laboratory Manifestations. Clinical symptoms occur rapidly after significant exposure and include headache, agitation and confusion, loss of consciousness, convulsions, and cardiac dysrhythmias. Severe metabolic acidosis occurs rapidly. Death may occur. Cyanide levels can be measured in the blood, but tests are not readily available and levels do not correlate well with symptoms. Severe metabolic acidosis in a patient with suspected cyanide exposure (e.g., fire victims) should be assumed to be cyanide poisoning.

Treatment. The cornerstone of treatment is rapid administration of high concentrations of oxygen, together with the use of the Lilly Cyanide Antidote Kit. The kit includes nitrites (amyl nitrite and sodium nitrite) used to produce methemoglobin, which reacts with cyanide, forming cyanomethemoglobin. The kit also contains sodium thiosulfate, which is given to hasten the metabolism of cyanomethemoglobin to hemoglobin and the less toxic thiocyanate. Hydroxocobalamin (vitamin B_{12a}), which reacts with cyanide to produce cyanocobalamin (vitamin B_{12}), is

an alternative antidote, but is not currently available in the United States.

Barillo DJ, Goode R, Esch V: Cyanide poisoning in victims of fire: Analysis of 364 cases and review of the literature. *J Burn Care Rehabil* 1994;15:46–57.
Chou KJ, Fisher SL, Silver EJ: Characteristics and outcome of children with carbon monoxide poisoning with and without smoke exposure referred for hyperbaric oxygen therapy. *Pediatr Emerg Care* 2000;16:151–55.
Hardy KR, Thom SR: Pathophysiology and treatment of carbon monoxide poisoning. *J Toxicol Clin Toxicol* 1994;32:613–29.
Geller RJ, Ekins BR, Iknoian RC: Cyanide toxicity from acetonitrile-containing false nail remover. *Am J Emerg Med* 1991;9:268–70.
Meert KL, Heidemann SM, Sarnaik AP: Outcome of children with carbon monoxide poisoning treated with normobaric oxygen. *J Trauma* 1998;44:149–54.
Weaver LK, Hopkins RO, Chan KJ, et al: Carbon monoxide poisoning. *N Engl J Med* 2002;347:1057–67.
White SR: Pediatric carbon monoxide poisoning. In Penney DG (editor): *Carbon Monoxide Toxicity*. New York, CRC Press, 2000, pp 463–91.

704.14 Plants

Exposure to plants, both inside the home and outside in backyards and fields, is one of the most common causes of unintentional poisoning in children. Fortunately, ingestion of most plant parts (leaves, seeds, flowers) results in mild, self-limiting effects. The treatment is symptomatic and supportive. Box 704–2 contains a list of plants considered to be nontoxic. This means that the inherent toxicity of the product is so low that the ingestion of small to moderate quantities of plant material is unlikely to produce toxic symptoms. Table 704–4 contains information describing the effects after exposure to some toxic plants commonly found in and around the home and yard.

The potential toxicity of a particular plant is highly variable, depending on the part of the plant involved (flowers are generally less toxic than the root or seed), the time of year, the growing conditions of the plant, and the route of exposure. Assessment of the potential severity after a plant exposure is also complicated by the difficulty in properly identifying the plant. Many plants are known by several common names, and the common name of the same plant may vary between communities. Poison control centers have access to individuals able to assist in the proper identification of plants. They also keep current on the common poisonous plants in their service area and the seasons in which they are more abundant; thus, consultation with a poison control center is recommended if a potentially toxic plant is involved in the exposure. The literature describing plant exposure is often extrapolated from animal data or based on isolated case reports and thus is limited.

Gastrointestinal decontamination for potentially toxic ingestions includes the use of activated charcoal. Treatment is supportive and symptomatic.

BOX 704–2. Nontoxic Plants

African violet	Dracaena	Palm
Aluminum plant	Fern species	Peperomia
Aralia, false	(not asparagus fern)	Petunia
Aster	Fig	Poinsettia
Barberry	Gardenia	Poke berries
Begonia species	Geranium	Pyracantha
Boston fern	Hen and chicks	Rose
Carnation	Honeysuckle	Rubber plant
Chinese	Impatiens	Schefflera
evergreen	Jade plant	Snake plant
Christmas cactus	Kalanchoe	Spider plant
Coleus	Magnolia	Violet
Corn plant	Marigold	Wandering Jew
Dandelion	Mother-in-law's tongue	Yucca
Daylily	Nasturtium	
Dogwood	Norfolk Island pine	

TABLE 704–4. Common Poisonous Plants

Common Plant Name	Toxic Constituent	Symptoms or Special Treatment
Black nightshade Climbing nightshade Deadly nightshade Horse nettle Jimsonweed Potato/tomato (foliage & sprouts)	Anticholinergic alkaloids such as atropine and solanine	Anticholinergic syndrome; gastroenteritis
Asparagus fern Caladium Dumbcane Elephant ear Jack-in-the-pulpit Peace lily Philodendron Pothos Rhubarb (leaves) Skunk cabbage	Calcium oxalate crystals	Irritation and edema of mucous membranes, edema, gastroenteritis; large ingestions may cause hypocalcemia
Christmas pepper Hot pepper	Capsicum	Irritation and burning sensation of skin and mucous membranes
Foxglove Lily-of-the-valley Oleander	Cardiac glycosides	Irritation of mucous membranes, cardiac toxicity; severe intoxication may require dioxin-specific FAB fragments
Water hemlock	Cicutoxin	Grand mal seizures
Fall crocus	Colchicine	Gastroenteritis, cardiotoxicity
Poison hemlock	Conine	Salivation, nausea, vomiting, diarrhea, seizures, coma, respiratory paralysis
Cherry, apple, peach, apricot, chokecherry (seeds, pits, leaves)	Hydrocyanic acid-containing glycosides	Very large amounts may cause dyspnea, seizures, coma
Morning glory (seeds)	Lysergic acid monoethylamide	Gastroenteritis, hallucinations
Amaryllis Daffodil Narcissus (bulb)	Lycorine	Vomiting, diarrhea
Tobacco Cardinal flower	Nicotine	Salivation, gastroenteritis
May apple	Podophylloresin	Vomiting, diarrhea, drowsiness, peripheral neuropathy
Pokeweed (leaves, root)	Podophyllotoxin-like resins	Vomiting, sweating, colic, drowsiness
Castor bean (chewed seeds)	Ricin	Burning sensation of mouth, throat; gastroenteritis, hepatotoxicity, seizures
Yew	Taxine	Vomiting, abdominal pain, respiratory depression
Euphorbia Spurges	Unknown acrid principle	Mucous membrane irritation
Mistletoe (berries)	Viscotoxin, phoratoxin, lectins	Gastroenteritis, cardiovascular collapse

Bruneton J: *Toxic Plants Dangerous to Humans and Animals*, Secaucus, NJ, Lavoisier, 1999.
Krenzelok EP, Jacobsen TD, Aronis J: Those pesky berries—are they a source of concern? *Vet Hum Toxicol* 1998;40:101–3.
Lampe KF, McConn MA: *AMA Handbook of Poisonous and Injurious Plants*. Chicago, American Medical Association, 1985.
Turner NJ, Szczawinski AF: *Common Poisonous Plants and Mushrooms of North America*, Portland, OR, Timber Press, 1991.

Chapter 705
Nonbacterial Food Poisoning *Denise A. Salerno*
and Stephen C. Aronoff

705.1 Mushroom Poisoning

Consumption of wild mushrooms, a favorite pastime in Europe, is increasingly popular in the United States, with concomitant increases in fatal cases of mushroom poisoning.

Four clinical syndromes and seven classes of toxins are associated with wild mushroom poisoning. The clinical syndromes are divided according to the predominant system involved and the rapidity of onset of symptoms. The toxins produced by wild mushrooms are categorized as follows: cyclopeptides, monomethylhydrazine, muscarine, coprine, ibotenic acid, psilocybin, and unknown. Additionally, the edible wild mushroom *Tricholoma equestre* has been associated with delayed rhabdomyolysis, although the toxin has not been identified.

GASTROINTESTINAL: DELAYED ONSET

***Amanita* Poisoning.** Poisonings by species of *Amanita* and *Galerina* account for 95% of the fatalities due to mushroom intoxication, although the mortality rate for this group is 5–10%. Most species produce two classes of cyclopeptide toxins: (1) phalloidins, which are heptapeptides believed to be responsible for the early symptoms of *Amanita* poisoning; and (2) amanitotoxin, which is an octapeptide that inhibits RNA polymerase and subsequent production of messenger RNA. Cells with high turnover rates, such as those in the gastrointestinal mucosa, kidneys, and liver, are the most severely affected.

Histopathologically, *Amanita* poisoning causes cellular necrosis, which may occur throughout the gastrointestinal tract, the most heavily exposed site. Acute yellow atrophy of the liver and necrosis of the proximal renal tubules are found in lethal cases.

The *clinical course* produced by poisoning with *Amanita* or *Galerina* species is biphasic, after an initial 6–12 hr latent period. Nausea, vomiting, and severe abdominal pain ensue 6–24 hr after ingestion. Profuse watery diarrhea follows shortly thereafter and may last for 12–24 hr. During this time, as much as 9 L of fluid may be lost. From 24–48 hr after poisoning, jaundice, hypertransaminasemia (peaking at 72–96 hr), renal failure, and coma occur. Death occurs 4–7 days after the ingestion. A prothrombin time less than 10% of control is a poor prognostic factor.

Treatment of *Amanita* poisoning is both supportive and specific. Fluid loss from severe diarrhea during the early course of the illness is profound, requiring aggressive therapy for correction of this loss. In the late phase of the disease, management of renal and hepatic failure is also necessary.

Specific therapy for *Amanita* poisoning is designed to remove the toxin rapidly and to block binding at its target site. Oral activated charcoal and lactulose combined with fluid and electrolyte replacement are recommended as part of the initial treatment of children with *Amanita* poisoning. Forced diuresis should be avoided because this increases renal exposure. Intravenous penicillin G (250 mg/kg/24 hr) administered as a continuous infusion combined with silibinin, the water-soluble form of the flavolignone silymarin (in an intravenous dosage of 20–50 mg/kg/24 hr), acts synergistically to inhibit binding of both toxins and to interrupt enterohepatic recirculation of amanitotoxin. Hemodialysis and hemoperfusion are also recommended as part of the initial treatment for intoxicated children. Orthotopic liver transplantation is recommended for children in whom severe hepatic failure develops (see Chapter 349).

Monomethylhydrazine Intoxication. Species of *Gyromitra* contain monomethylhydrazine (CH_3NHNH_2), which inhibits central nervous system (CNS) enzymatic production of γ-aminobutyric acid (GABA). Monomethylhydrazine also oxidizes iron in hemoglobin, resulting in methemoglobinemia. Children with *Gyromitra* poisoning develop vomiting, diarrhea, hematochezia, and abdominal pain within 6–24 hr of ingestion of the toxin. Symptoms of CNS depression and seizures develop later in the clinical course. Hemolysis and methemoglobinemia are potential life-threatening complications of monomethylhydrazine poisoning. Severe methemoglobinemia may require dialysis.

Hypovolemia due to gastrointestinal fluid losses and seizures require supportive intervention. Pyridoxal phosphate, the coenzyme that catalyzes the production of GABA, can reverse the effects of monomethylhydrazine when administered in high doses. Pyridoxine hydrochloride (25 mg/kg) is administered intravenously at a frequency dependent on clinical improvement. Parenteral administration of methylene blue is indicated if the methemoglobin concentration exceeds 30%. Blood transfusions may be required for significant hemolysis.

AUTONOMIC NERVOUS SYSTEM: RAPID ONSET

Muscarine Poisoning. Mushrooms of the genera *Inocybe* and, to a lesser degree, *Clitocybe* contain muscarine or muscarine-related compounds. These quaternary ammonium derivatives bind to postsynaptic receptors, producing an exaggerated cholinergic response.

The *clinical manifestations* are characterized by the following hypercholinergic response: the onset of symptoms is rapid (30 min–2 hr after consumption) and consists of diaphoresis, excessive lacrimation, salivation, miosis, urinary and fecal incontinence, and vomiting. Respiratory distress caused by bronchospasm and increased bronchopulmonary secretions is the most serious complication. The symptoms subside spontaneously within 6–24 hr.

Atropine sulfate, the *specific antidote*, is administered intravenously (0.01 mg/kg; max 2 mg). This is repeated until the pulmonary symptoms resolve or the patient becomes overtly tachycardic.

Coprine Ingestion. *Coprinus atramentarius* and *Clitocybe clavipes* contain coprine. Like disulfiram (Antabuse), coprine inhibits the metabolism of acetaldehyde after ethanol ingestion. The clinical manifestations result from accumulation of acetaldehyde.

Coprine intoxication becomes apparent after ethanol ingestion and may occur up to 5 days after consuming the mushroom. Hyperemia of the face and trunk, tingling of the hands, metallic taste, tachycardia, and vomiting occur acutely. Hypotension may result from intense peripheral vasodilation.

The syndrome is typically self-limited and lasts only several hours. No specific antidote is available. If hypotension is severe, vascular re-expansion with isotonic parenteral solutions may be required. Small oral doses of propranolol have also been suggested.

CENTRAL NERVOUS SYSTEM: RAPID ONSET

Ibotenic Acid and Muscimol Intoxication. Although *Amanita muscaria* and *Amanita pantherina* may contain muscarine (see earlier), the toxins responsible for the CNS symptoms after ingestion of these mushrooms are muscimol and ibotenic acid. Muscimol, a hallucinogen, and ibotenic acid, an insecticide, have anticholinergic effects. From 30 min–3 hr after ingestion, CNS symptoms appear; obtundation, alternating lethargy and agitation, and, occasionally, seizures ensue. Nausea and vomiting are uncommon. If large amounts of muscarine are contained in the mushroom, symptoms of cholinergic crisis may also occur.

Specific therapy must be carefully selected. If an exaggerated cholinergic response is observed, atropine should be administered. Because ingestions of *A. muscaria* are frequently associated with anticholinergic findings, the acetylcholinesterase inhibitor physostigmine is used to reverse the delirium and coma. Seizures can be controlled with diazepam. Early treatment with ipecac (if the patient is conscious) and close observation are all that is required in most cases.

Indole Intoxication. Mushrooms belonging to the genus *Psilocybe* ("magic mushrooms") contain psilocybin and psilocin, two psychotropic compounds. Within 30 min after ingestion, patients experience euphoria and hallucinations, often accompanied by tachycardia and mydriasis. Fever and seizures have also been observed in children with psilocybin poisoning. These symptoms are short lived, usually lasting 6 hr after consumption of the mushroom. Severely agitated patients may respond to diazepam.

GASTROINTESTINAL: RAPID ONSET

Many mushrooms from various genera produce local gastrointestinal manifestations. The causative toxins are diverse and largely unknown. Within 1 hr of ingestion, patients develop acute abdominal pain, nausea, vomiting, and diarrhea. Symptoms may last from hours to days, depending on the species of mushroom.

Treatment is mainly supportive. Children with large fluid losses may require parenteral fluid therapy. It is imperative to differentiate ingestion of mushrooms of this class from ingestions of *Amanita* and *Galerina* species containing cyclopeptide toxins.

705.2 Solanine Poisoning

Solanine is a mixture of several related toxins found in "greened" and sprouted potatoes. Potatoes exposed to light and allowed to sprout produce a number of alkaloid glycosides containing the cholesterol derivative solanidine. Two of these glycosides, α-solanine and α-chaconine, are found in highest concentration in the peels of greened potatoes and in the sprouts. The solanine alkaloids bind to serum cholinesterase, suggesting a possible pathophysiologic mechanism.

Clinical manifestations of solanine intoxication occur within 7–19 hr after ingestion. The most common symptoms are vomiting and diarrhea; in more severe instances of poisoning, fever, generalized abdominal pain, coma, and hypovolemic shock occur.

Treatment of solanine poisoning is largely supportive. In the most severe cases, symptoms resolve within 11 days. Atropine treatment has not been evaluated.

705.3 Seafood Poisoning

Ciguatera Fish Poisoning. Major outbreaks of ciguatera fish poisoning have been reported in Florida, Hawaii, the Caribbean, South Pacific, and the Virgin Islands; however, with modern methods of transportation, the illness now occurs worldwide. Grouper is the most frequently identified source of the toxin, followed by snapper, kingfish, amberjack, dolphin, eel, and barracuda. Poisoning has also been associated with farm-raised salmon.

The source of this poisoning is the dinoflagellate *Gambierdiscus toxicus*, a microscopic unicellular organism found along coral reefs that produces high concentrations of ciguatoxin and maitotoxin. The toxins are passed along the food chain from small herbivorous fish that consume the dinoflagellate from the coral reefs to larger predatory fish and then to humans. These toxins are harmless in fish but produce distinct clinical symptoms in humans.

Ciguatoxin-1, a lipid with a molecular weight of approximately 1.1 kd, is odorless, colorless, tasteless, and is not destroyed by cooking or freezing. Ciguatoxin-1 increases the sodium permeability of excitable membranes, an action that is inhibited by calcium and tetrodotoxin.

The onset of *clinical manifestations* of ciguatoxin poisoning is rapid, usually occurring within 2–30 hr after ingesting contaminated fish. The illness is often biphasic. The earliest symptoms are diarrhea, vomiting, and abdominal pain; the second phase includes intense itching, rash on palms and soles, myalgias, and circumoral or extremity dysesthesias. The dysesthesia is characterized by reversal of hot and cold sensation. Tachycardia, bradycardia, and hypotension occur infrequently. Ciguatera fish poisoning is diagnosed based on clinical presentation, and the diagnosis is confirmed by testing the ingested fish for toxin.

Treatment of ciguatera fish poisoning is supportive. Gastric lavage is recommended to remove any remaining toxin. Intravenous fluids may be required for severe diarrhea, and parenteral administration of calcium can be used to treat hypotension. In a few patients with coma or prolonged symptoms, mannitol given within 24 hr of the onset of symptoms has successfully reversed the neurologic manifestations of intoxication. However, further studies are needed before a recommendation for mannitol therapy can be made. Gabapentin has reportedly been successful in treating the neurologic symptoms in a few patients. Most cases are self-limited; neurologic symptoms may last months. Death occurs in less than 0.1% of cases.

Scombroid (Pseudoallergic) Fish Poisoning. Epidemics have been associated with ingestion of members of the Scombresocidae or Scombridae families, notably albacore, mackerel, tuna, bonita, and kingfish. Nonscombroid fish and marine mammals, such as mahi-mahi (dolphin) and bluefish, have also been linked to outbreaks of poisoning.

Scombrotoxin, either histamine or the product of the action of the toxin on fish flesh, is responsible for the clinical syndrome. Histidine is found in high concentrations in the flesh of scombroid fish; the action of bacterial decarboxylases during putrification converts the histidine to histamine. Fish containing more than 20 mg of histamine per 100 g of flesh are toxic. In patients receiving isoniazid, a potent histaminase blocker, ingestion of fish flesh containing a lower concentration of histamine may be toxic.

The onset of *clinical manifestations* is acute and occurs within 10 min–2 hr after ingestion. The most common symptoms and signs include diarrhea, flushing, diaphoresis, urticaria, nausea, and headache. Abdominal pain, tachycardia, oral burning, dizziness, respiratory distress, and facial swelling also occur. The illness is usually self-limited, terminating within 8–10 hr.

Treatment is mainly supportive. Gastric lavage decreases continued absorption of histamine. With severe diarrhea, fluid replacement may be necessary. Antihistamines have been variably successful. Four patients with severe toxicity treated with cimetidine (a histamine blocker) responded rapidly. Because data are limited, cimetidine or ranitidine should be reserved for severe cases.

Paralytic Shellfish Poisoning. Filter-feeding mollusks, such as the black mussel and sea scallop, may become contaminated during dinoflagellate blooms or "red tides." The dinoflagellate *Ptychodiscus brevis* is often responsible for these red tides and contains several potent neurotoxins. Paralytic shellfish poisoning is a distinctive neurologic illness caused by 20 closely related heat-stable paralytic shellfish toxins. Saxitoxin is the most potent of the neurotoxins responsible for paralytic shellfish poisoning. This toxin prevents nerve conduction by inhibiting the sodium-potassium pump. Other toxins may be bioconverted to less toxic compounds. Consumption of bivalves, such as mussels, scallops, and clams, is the usual pathway of intoxication, although crustacea and fish have been implicated as well.

The onset of *clinical manifestations* of paralytic shellfish poisoning occurs rapidly, 30 min–2 hr after ingestion. Abdominal pain and nausea are common. Paresthesias are common and occur circumorally, in a stocking-glove distribution, or both. Perioral numbness or tingling, diplopia, ataxia, dysarthria, and the sensation of floating occur less commonly. Hot-cold reversal in temperature sensation is not unusual. In severe cases, respiratory failure from diaphragmatic paralysis may result.

No antidote for paralytic shellfish poisoning is known. Supportive care, including mechanical ventilation, may be needed. Although the symptoms are usually self-limited and short-lived, weakness and malaise may persist for weeks after ingestion.

Diarrhetic Shellfish Poisoning. Several outbreaks of diarrhetic shellfish poisoning have been reported in Europe after consumption of mussels, cockles, and other shellfish. The dinoflagellates *Dinophysis* and *Prorocentrum* produce okadaic acid and its derivatives, the dinophysistoxins. These compounds inhibit protein phosphatases. The intracellular accumulation of phosphorylated proteins causes increased fluid secretion by gut cells via calcium influx, mediated by cyclic adenosine monophosphate and prostaglandins.

Clinically, patients develop severe diarrhea. Care is supportive and directed at rehydration. The illness is self-limited, and recovery occurs in 3–4 days; few patients require hospitalization.

Amnesic Shellfish Poisoning. This entity was first reported in 1987 in Canada after a group of people developed severe gastroenteritis as well as neurologic symptoms, including memory loss, after eating mussels from Prince Edward Island. Subsequent cases have been identified after eating shellfish from the United States, Spain, and the United Kingdom. The responsible toxin, domoic acid, comes from a diatom, *Pseudo-nitzschia multiseries*, and is a potent glutamate agonist, disrupting neurochemical transmission in the brain. It also binds to glutamate receptors, which increase calcium influx, producing neuronal swelling in the hippocampal area of the brain and death.

The initial *clinical manifestations* are gastrointestinal. Memory loss is closely related to advanced age. Those patients younger than age 40 yr are more likely to only suffer from diarrhea, whereas those older than 50 yr suffer from short-term memory loss lasting months to years.

Mushroom Poisoning

Bedry R, Baudrimont I, et al: Brief report: Wild mushroom intoxication as a cause of rhabdomyolysis. *N Engl J Med* 2001;345:798.

Benjamin DR: Mushroom poisoning in infants and children: The *Amanita pantherina/muscaria* group. *Clin Toxicol* 1992;30:13.

Editorial: Mushroom poisoning. *Lancet* 1980;2:351.

Hanrahan JP, Gordon MA: Mushroom poisoning: Case reports and a review of therapy. *JAMA* 1984;251:1057.

Klein AS, Hart J, Brems JJ, et al: *Amanita* poisoning: Treatment and the role of liver transplantation. *Am J Med* 1989;86:187.

Litten W: The most poisonous mushrooms. *Sci Am* 1975;232:90.

McCormick DJ, Avbel AJ, Biggons RB: Nonlethal mushroom poisoning. *Ann Intern Med* 1979;90:332.

McDonald A: Mushrooms and madness: Hallucinogenic mushrooms and some psychopharmacological implications. *Can J Psychiatry* 1980;25:586.

Mitchell DH: *Amanita* mushroom poisoning. *Annu Rev Med* 1980;31:51.

Sabeel AI, Kurkus J, Lindholm T: Intensive hemodialysis and hemoperfusion treatment of *Amanita* mushroom poisoning. *Mycopathologia* 1995;131:107.

Solanine Poisoning

Editorial: Potato poisoning. *Lancet* 1979;2:681.

McMillan M, Thompson JC: An outbreak of suspected solanine poisoning in school boys: Examination of criteria of solanine poisoning. *Q J Med* 1979;48:227.

Ciguatera Fish Poisoning

Caplan CE: Ciguatera fish poisoning. *CMAJ* 1998;159:1394.

CDC: Ciguatera Fish Poisoning-Texas 1997. *JAMA* 1998;280:1394.

DiNubile MJ, Hokama Y: The ciguatera poisoning syndrome from farm-raised salmon. *Ann Intern Med* 1995;122:113.

Lange WR: Ciguatera fish poisoning. *Am Fam Physician* 1994;50:579.

Lawrence DN, Enriquez MB, Lumish RM, et al: Ciguatera fish poisoning in Miami. *JAMA* 1980;244:254.

Morris JG, Lewin P, Hargrett NT, et al: Clinical features of ciguatera fish poisoning. *Arch Intern Med* 1982;142:1090.

Palafox NA, Jain LG, Pinano AZ, et al: Successful treatment of ciguatera fish poisoning with intravenous mannitol. *JAMA* 1988;259:2740.

Perez CM, Vasquez PA, Perret CF: Treatment of ciguatera poisoning with gabapentin. *N Engl J Med* 2001;344:692.

Withers NW: Ciguatera fish poisoning. *Annu Rev Med* 1982;33:97.

Scombroid Fish Poisoning

Blakesley ML: Scombroid poisoning: Prompt resolution of symptoms with cimetidine. *Ann Emerg Med* 1983;12:104.

Gilbert RJ, Hobbs G, Murray CK, et al: Scombrotoxic fish poisoning: Features of the first 50 incidents to be reported in Britain (1976–9). *BMJ* 1980;281:71.

Hughes JM, Potter ME: Scombroid fish poisoning: From pathogenesis to prevention. *N Engl J Med* 1991;324:766.

Morrow JD, Margolies GR, Rowland J, et al: Evidence that histamine is the causative toxin of scombroid fish poisoning. *N Engl J Med* 1991;324:716.

Paralytic Shellfish Poisoning

Gessner BD, Middaugh JP: Paralytic shellfish poisoning in Alaska: A 20-year retrospective analysis. *Am J Epidemiol* 1995;141:766.

Hughes JM, Merson MH: Fish and shellfish poisoning. *N Engl J Med* 1976;295:1117.

Morris PD, Campbell DS, Taylor TJ, et al: Clinical and epidemiological features of neurotoxic shellfish poisoning in North Carolina. *Am J Public Health* 1991;81:471.

Popkiss MEE, Horstman DA, Harpur D: Paralytic shellfish poisoning: A report of 17 cases in Cape Town. *S Afr Med J* 1979;55:1017.

Shimizu Y, Yoshioka M: Transformation of paralytic shellfish toxins as demonstrated in scallop homogenates. *Science* 1981;212:547.

Whittle K, Gallacher S: Marine toxins. *BMJ* 2000;56:236.

Chapter 706

Biologic and Chemical Terrorism *Theodore J. Cieslak and Fred M. Henretig*

The events of September 11, 2001, and the subsequent outbreak of anthrax cases originating from exposure to contaminated mail should leave little doubt as to the ability of terrorists to execute an attack using biologic or chemical "weapons of mass destruction." Therefore, it is imperative that pediatricians be familiar with the clinical manifestations of diseases induced by biologic and chemical agents, many of which can be successfully treated if diagnoses are made early, therapy initiated promptly, and preventive measures instituted.

Etiology. Hundreds of biologic and chemical agents could theoretically be adapted for sinister use by terrorists. Attempts to ascertain which agents are most likely to be employed are fraught with difficulties. First, such analysis often depends on accurate intelligence, which is likely to be problematic. Second, many terrorists may choose to use weapons of opportunity, that is, agents that for some reason are readily available to some member of the terrorist group. Finally, the motives of terrorists are often obscure and difficult to predict. With these considerations in mind, a working group convened by the Centers for Disease Control and Prevention (CDC) elected to concentrate response efforts not necessarily on those agents most likely to be used but, rather, on those agents that, if used, would constitute the gravest potential threats to public health and security.

In the case of biologic agents, the CDC working group divided pathogens and toxins into three categories, with category A including diseases caused by those six agents posing the greatest threat. Viral hemorrhagic fevers are discussed in Chapter 246. This chapter focuses on the remaining diseases in category A: anthrax, plague, tularemia, smallpox, and botulism. In the case of chemical agents, a vast array of potentially harmful chemicals might conceivably be released by terrorists. Tank cars full of flammable industrial gases and liquids, corrosive industrial acids and bases, poisonous compounds such as cyanides and nitriles, pesticides, dioxins, and explosives traverse our railways and roads daily. In this chapter, however, the focus is on four classes of "military-grade" chemicals with a history of use in warfare, or manufactured specifically for use as weapons. These include the organophosphate-based nerve agents, vesicants, "blood agents" (cyanides), and certain "pulmonary agents."

Epidemiology and Pediatric-Specific Concerns. Large-scale attacks on civilian targets will almost certainly involve pediatric victims. Furthermore, pediatric patients may be more susceptible than adults to the effects of certain biologic and chemical agents. Thinner skin makes dermally active chemical agents, such as mustard, of greater risk to children than adults. A larger surface area per unit volume further increases the problem. Similarly, a small relative blood volume makes children more susceptible to the volume losses associated with enteric infections such as cholera and to gastrointestinal intoxications such as might be seen with exposure to the staphylococcal enterotoxins. A relatively high minute ventilation compared with adults increases the threat of agents delivered by way of the inhalational route. The fact that children live closer to the ground compounds this effect when heavier-than-air chemicals are involved. An immature blood-brain barrier may heighten the risk of central nervous system toxicity from nerve agents. Finally, developmental considerations make it less likely that a child would readily flee an area of danger, thereby increasing exposure to these various adverse effects. Also see Chapter 701.

In certain instances, children appear to have a unique susceptibility to potential agents that might be used by terrorists. Although adults generally suffer only a brief self-limited incapacitating illness after infection with Venezuelan equine encephalitis (VEE) virus, for example, young children are more likely to experience seizures, permanent neurologic sequelae, and even death. In the case of smallpox, waning immunity may disproportionately affect children. Vaccine-induced immunity to smallpox probably diminishes significantly after 3–10 yr. Although most adults are considered susceptible to smallpox, given that routine civilian immunization ceased in the early 1970s, older adults may enjoy some residual protection from death, if not from the development of disease. Today's children are among the first to grow up in a world without any individual or herd immunity to smallpox.

Children also may experience unique disease manifestations not seen in adults. In a study of melioidosis cases among children in Thailand, suppurative parotitis was observed as a characteristic presentation; this condition is not generally seen in adults with *Burkholderia pseudomallei* infection.

Pediatricians are likely to experience unique problems in managing childhood victims of biologic or chemical attack. Many of the drugs useful in treating such casualties are unfamiliar to pediatricians or have relative contraindications in childhood. The fluoroquinolones and tetracyclines are often mentioned as agents of choice in the treatment and prophylaxis of anthrax, plague, tularemia, brucellosis, and Q fever. Both are often avoided in children, although the risk of morbidity and mortality from biologic agent–induced diseases far outweighs the minor risks associated with short-term use of these agents. For example, ciprofloxacin received, as its first licensed pediatric indication, U.S. Food and Drug Administration (FDA) approval for use in the prophylaxis of anthrax after inhalational exposure (i.e., terrorism). Doxycycline is now licensed specifically in children for the same indication. Similarly, immunizations potentially useful in preventing biologic agent–induced diseases are often not approved for use in pediatric patients. The current anthrax vaccine is licensed only for those between 18–65 yr of age. The plague vaccine, currently out of production and probably ineffective against inhalational exposures, was only approved for 18–61 yr olds. The smallpox vaccine, a live vaccine employing vaccinia virus, can lead to fetal vaccinia and demise when given to pregnant women.

Moreover, many otherwise useful pharmaceuticals are not available in pediatric dosing regimens. The military distributes nerve agent antidote kits (NAAKs) consisting of autoinjectors designed for the rapid administration of atropine and pralidoxime. Many emergency departments and some ambulances stock these kits. The doses of agents contained in the NAAK are calculated for soldiers but are far in excess of those appropriate for young children. Similarly, although physical protection would not likely be useful in a civilian setting, it is noteworthy that commercially available devices such as gas masks are not typically available in pediatric sizes.

Finally, there may not be adequate numbers of pediatric hospital beds. In the event of a large-scale terrorist attack, as in the case with any large disaster, excess hospital bed capacity could potentially be provided at civilian and Department of Veterans Affairs hospitals under the auspices of the national disaster medical system. The system makes no specific provision for pediatric beds.

Clinical Manifestations. In the event of a terrorist attack, clinicians may be called on to make prompt diagnoses and render rapid life-saving treatment before the results of confirmatory diagnostic tests are available. Thus, although each potential agent of terrorism produces its own unique clinical manifestations, it is useful to consider their effects in terms of a limited number of distinct clinical syndromes. This will facilitate clinicians making prompt, rational decisions regarding empirical therapy. In general, casualties from a terrorist attack will develop symptoms immediately on exposure to an agent (or within the first several hours after exposure) or they will develop symptoms slowly over a period of days to weeks. In the former case, the sinister nature of the event is often obvious and the etiology more likely to be conventional or chemical in nature. Biologic agents, however, differ from conventional, chemical, and nuclear weapons (see Chapter 700) in that they have inherent incubation periods. Because of this, patients are likely to present far removed in time and place from the point of an unannounced exposure to a biologic agent. Thus, whereas traditional first responders such as firemen and paramedics may be at the forefront of a conventional or chemical terrorism response, the primary care physician is likely to constitute the first line of defense against the effects of a biologic agent.

With these considerations in mind, casualties can be categorized as either immediate or delayed in presentation. Within each of these categories, patients can be further classified as having primarily respiratory, neuromuscular, or dermatologic manifestations (Table 706–1). A limited number of agents may cause each particular syndrome, permitting institution of empiric therapy targeted at a short list of potential etiologies.

SUDDEN-ONSET NEUROMUSCULAR SYNDROME: NERVE AGENTS. The rapid onset of neuromuscular symptoms after an exposure should lead the clinician to consider nerve agent intoxication. The nerve agents (tabun, sarin, soman, and "VX") are organophosphate analogues of common pesticides that act as potent inhibitors of the enzyme acetylcholinesterase. They are hazardous via ingestion, inhalation, or cutaneous absorption.

The inhibition of cholinesterase by these compounds results in the accumulation of acetylcholine at neural and neuromuscular junctions, causing excess stimulation. The resultant cholinergic syndrome involves central, nicotinic, and muscarinic effects. Central effects include altered mental status progressing rapidly to lethargy and coma, as well as ataxia, convulsions, and respiratory depression. Nicotinic effects include muscle fasciculations and twitching, followed by weakness progressing to flaccid paralysis as the muscles fatigue. Muscarinic effects include miosis, visual blurring, profuse lacrimation, and watery rhinorrhea. Bronchospasm and increased bronchial secretions lead to cough, wheezing, dyspnea, and cyanosis. Cardiovascular manifestations include bradycardia, hypotension, and atrioventricular block. Flushing, sweating, salivation, nausea, vomiting, diarrhea, abdominal cramps, and urinary incontinence are also seen. In the absence of prompt intervention, death can quickly result from a combination of central effects and respiratory muscle paralysis.

DELAYED-ONSET NEUROMUSCULAR SYNDROME: BOTULISM. The delayed onset (hours to days after exposure) of neuromuscular symptoms is characteristic of botulism. Botulism occurs after exposure to one of seven related neurotoxins produced by certain strains of *Clostridium botulinum*, a strictly anaerobic spore-forming gram-positive bacillus commonly found in soil. Naturally occurring botulism (see Chapter 193) usually follows ingestion of preformed toxin (food poisoning) or results from intestinal toxin production (infantile form). Nonetheless, an aerosol exposure would likely result in a case of clinical botulism indistinguishable from that caused by natural exposures.

After exposure to botulinum toxin, clinical manifestations begin with bulbar palsies, causing patients to complain of ptosis, photophobia, and blurred vision from difficulty in accommodation. Symptoms can progress to include dysarthria, dysphonia, and dysphagia and, finally, a descending symmetric paralysis. Sensation and sensorium are not typically affected. In the absence of intervention, death often results from respiratory muscle failure.

TABLE 706–1. Diseases Caused by Agents of Chemical and Biologic Terrorism, Classified by Syndrome

	Neuromuscular Symptoms Prominent	Respiratory Symptoms Prominent	Dermatologic Findings Prominent
Sudden-onset	Nerve agents	Chlorine Phosgene Cyanide	Mustard Lewisite
Delayed-onset	Botulism	Anthrax Plague Tularemia	Smallpox

SUDDEN-ONSET RESPIRATORY SYNDROME: CHLORINE, PHOSGENE, AND CYANIDE. The acute onset of respiratory symptoms shortly after exposure should cause the clinician to consider a range of potential chemical agents. Nerve agents may, of course, affect respiration, but these effects are usually secondary to respiratory muscle paresis rather than pulmonary pathology per se. Moreover, this distinction should be readily evident clinically, because the nerve agent casualty will have generalized muscle involvement. In contrast, the toxic inhalants chlorine and phosgene produce respiratory distress without muscle involvement.

Chlorine is a dense, acrid, yellow-green gas that is heavier than air. After mild to moderate exposure, ocular and nasal irritation occur, followed by cough, a choking sensation, bronchospasm, and substernal chest tightness. Pulmonary edema, mediated by hydrochloric acid and free oxygen radical generation, follows moderate to severe exposures within 30 min to several hours. Hypoxemia and hypovolemia secondary to pulmonary edema are responsible for death in fatal cases.

Phosgene, like chlorine, is a common industrial compound that was used as a weapon on the battlefields of World War I. Its odor is sometimes said to resemble that of "new-mown hay." Similar to chlorine, phosgene is also thought to generate hydrochloric acid, contributing particularly to upper airway, nasal, and conjunctival irritation. Acylation reactions caused by the effects of phosgene on the pulmonary alveolar-capillary membrane lead to pulmonary edema. Phosgene lung injury may also be mediated, in part, by an inflammatory reaction associated with leukotriene production. Patients with mild to moderate exposures to phosgene may be asymptomatic, potentially causing victims to remain in a contaminated area. Pulmonary edema occurs 4–24 hr post exposure and is dose dependent, with heavier exposures causing earlier symptoms. Dyspnea may precede radiologic findings. In severe exposures, pulmonary edema may be so marked as to result in hypovolemia and hypotension. As in the case of chlorine, death results from hypoxemia and asphyxia.

Cyanide is a cellular poison with protean manifestations. Initially, however, cyanide toxicity is most likely to present as tachypnea and hyperpnea, progressing rapidly to apnea in cases with significant exposure. The efficacy of cyanide as a chemical terrorism agent is limited by its volatility in open air and relatively low lethality compared with nerve agents. Released in a closed room, however, cyanide could have devastating effects. Cyanide inhibits cytochrome a_3, interfering with normal mitochondrial oxidative metabolism and leading to cellular anoxia and lactic acidosis. In addition to respiratory distress, early findings among cyanide victims include tachycardia, flushing, dizziness, headache, diaphoresis, nausea, and vomiting. With greater exposure, seizures, coma, apnea, and cardiac arrest may follow within minutes. An elevated anion gap metabolic acidosis is typically present, and decreased peripheral oxygen utilization leads to an elevated mixed venous oxygen saturation value.

DELAYED-ONSET RESPIRATORY SYNDROME: ANTHRAX, PLAGUE, AND TULAREMIA. A delayed onset of respiratory symptoms (days after exposure) is characteristic of several infectious diseases that might be adapted for sinister use by terrorists. Among these are anthrax, plague, and tularemia.

Anthrax is caused by infection with the gram-positive spore-forming rod *Bacillus anthracis*. Its ability to form a spore enables the anthrax bacillus to survive for long periods in the environment and enhances its potential as a weapon.

The vast majority of naturally occurring anthrax cases are cutaneous, acquired by close contact with the hides, wool, bone, and other by-products of infected cattle, sheep, and goats. Cutaneous cases also may result from the intentional deployment of anthrax-contaminated fomites. Cutaneous anthrax is, however, quite amenable to therapy with a variety of antibiotics and is readily recognizable to experienced clinicians in endemic areas; it is thus rarely fatal. Common in parts of Asia and sub-Saharan Africa, only two cases of cutaneous anthrax had occurred in the United States in the 9 yr that preceded the cases in 2001. Gastrointestinal anthrax, which has never been described in the United States, can occur after the ingestion of contaminated meat. In the past, inhalational anthrax, or woolsorter's disease, was an occupational hazard of abattoir and textile workers. Now eliminated as a naturally occurring disease in the United States, it is this inhalational form of anthrax that poses the greatest threat. Following an inadvertent release in 1979 from a bioweapons facility at Sverdlovsk in the former Soviet Union, 66 of 77 known adult victims of inhalational anthrax died. In the bioterrorism attacks involving contaminated letters in the United States, 6 of 11 patients with inhalational anthrax have survived. Whether improved intensive care modalities, changes in antibiotic therapy, or earlier recognition accounts for this improved mortality rate remains to be determined.

Symptomatic inhalational anthrax typically begins 1–6 days after exposure, although incubation periods up to several weeks in length have been reported. The disease begins as a flulike illness, characterized by fever, myalgia, headache, and cough. A brief intervening period of improvement sometimes follows, but rapid deterioration then ensues; high fever, dyspnea, cyanosis, and shock mark this second phase. Hemorrhagic meningitis occurs in up to 50% of cases. Chest radiographs obtained late in the course of illness may reveal a widened mediastinum or prominent mediastinal lymphadenopathy; pleural effusions may also be seen. Gram stains of peripheral blood may demonstrate the organism at this stage. Prompt treatment is imperative; death occurs in as many as 95% of inhalational anthrax cases if such treatment is begun more than 48 hr after the onset of symptoms.

Whereas inhalational anthrax is a disease primarily of mediastinal lymphatic tissue, exposure to aerosolized **plague** bacilli typically leads to a primary pneumonia. Endemic plague is usually transmitted via the bites of fleas and is discussed in Chapter 186.3. The causative organism of all forms of human plague, *Yersinia pestis*, is a bipolar-staining, gram-negative facultative intracellular bacillus. An ability to survive within the macrophage aids its dissemination to distant sites after inoculation or inhalation. "Buboes," markedly swollen, tender regional lymph nodes in the distribution of a bite, are the hallmark feature of bubonic plague. Fever and malaise are typically present, and septicemia often develops as bacteria gain access to the circulation. Petechiae, purpura, and overwhelming disseminated intravascular coagulopathy (DIC) commonly occur, and 80% of bubonic plague victims will ultimately have positive blood cultures. Testimony to the extreme infectivity and lethality of plague is the fact that the "Black Death" eliminated one third of the population of Europe during the Middle Ages. The potential of bubonic plague as a weapon also was appreciated, as evidenced by its use in 1346 by invading Tatars against the garrison at Kaffa in the Ukraine.

Intentional aerosol dissemination of *Y. pestis* would likely result in a preponderance of pneumonic plague cases. Pneumonic plague may also arise secondarily after seeding of the lungs of septicemic patients. Symptoms include fever, chills, malaise, headache, and cough. Chest radiographs may reveal a patchy consolidation, and the classic clinical finding is one of blood-streaked sputum. DIC and overwhelming sepsis typically develop as the disease progresses. Untreated pneumonic plague has a fatality rate approaching 100%.

Tularemia is a highly infectious disease caused by the gram-negative coccobacillus *Francisella tularensis*. Naturally occurring tularemia is discussed in Chapter 189. The high degree of infectivity of *F. tularensis* (fewer than 10 organisms are thought necessary to produce infection via inhalation) as well as its survivability in the environment, contributes to its inclusion on the list of agents of concern. Several clinical forms of endemic tularemia are known, but inhalational exposure in a terrorist attack would likely lead to a plaguelike primary pneumonia or to typhoidal tularemia, manifest as a variety of nonspecific symptoms including fever, malaise, and abdominal pain.

SUDDEN-ONSET DERMATOLOGIC SYNDROME: MUSTARD AND LEWISITE. The development of skin lesions shortly after exposure is characteristic of the chemical vesicants. These compounds, often referred to as blistering agents, are cellular poisons and include the alkylating agent mustard and the organic arsenical lewisite. Tissue injury to rapidly reproducing cells begins within minutes of contact with these agents. In the case of mustard, clinical effects typically become evident several hours after exposure. In contrast, patients exposed to lewisite will feel immediate pain. In addition to cutaneous vesicle formation, the eyes and respiratory tract are also injured. Moreover, mustard exposure may lead to bone marrow suppression and both mustard and lewisite may produce significant gastrointestinal symptoms.

DELAYED-ONSET DERMATOLOGIC SYNDROME: SMALLPOX. The appearance of an exanthem, days to weeks after exposure, is likely to be a presenting feature of smallpox. Smallpox, caused by the variola virus, a member of the orthopoxvirus family, has an incubation period of 7–17 days. This would likely permit the wide dispersal of asymptomatic exposed persons, thus contributing to the spread of an outbreak. During the incubation period, virus replicates in the upper respiratory tract. A primary viremia ensues, during which time seeding of the liver and spleen occurs. A secondary viremia then develops, the skin is seeded, and the classic exanthem of smallpox appears.

Symptoms of smallpox begin abruptly during the phase of secondary viremia and include fever, rigors, vomiting, headache, backache, and extreme malaise. Within 2–4 days, macules appear on the face and extremities and then progress in synchronous fashion to papules, pustules, and finally scabs. As the scabs separate, survivors are often left with disfiguring, de-pigmented scars. The synchronous nature of the rash and its centrifugal distribution distinguish smallpox from chickenpox, which has a centripetal distribution. In the past, smallpox had a 30% mortality rate, with death typically resulting from visceral organ involvement.

Diagnosis. In some cases, the terrorist nature of a chemical or biologic attack may be obvious. This might be especially true in the case of a chemical attack when victims succumb in close temporal and geographic proximity to a dispersal device. Alternatively, terrorists may announce their attack. In other instances, however, the clinician may need to rely on epidemiologic clues to suspect an intentional release of chemical or biologic agents. The presence of large numbers of victims clustered in time and space should raise the clinician's index of suspicion, as should cases of unexpected death or unexpectedly severe disease. Diseases unusual in a given locale, in a given age group, or during a certain season likewise warrant further investigation. Simultaneous outbreaks of a disease in noncontiguous areas should cause one to consider an intentional release, as should outbreaks of multiple diseases in the same area. Conversely, even a single case of rare disorders such as anthrax or certain viral hemorrhagic fevers would be suspicious, and a single case of smallpox would almost certainly be the result of an intentional release. Finally, large numbers of dying animals might provide evidence of an unnatural aerosol release, as would evidence of a disparate attack rate between those known to be indoors and outdoors at a given time.

In a mass casualty setting, diagnoses may, of necessity, be made largely on clinical grounds. The diagnosis of nerve agent intoxication, for example, is based primarily on clinical recognition and the response to antidotal therapy. In addition, several simple rapid detection devices developed for military use are able to detect the presence of nerve agents. Some of these are commercially available and are stocked in certain emergency departments and public safety vehicles. "M8" and "M9" test papers, for example, detect nerve agents and mustard and are interpreted by means of a simple color change. Measurements of acetylcholinesterase in plasma or erythrocytes of nerve agent victims may be helpful in long-term prognostication, but correlation between cholinesterase levels and clinical effects is often poor, and the test is rarely available emergently.

Botulism should be suspected clinically among patients presenting with a symmetric, descending, flaccid paralysis. Although the differential diagnosis of botulism includes other uncommon neurologic disorders such as myasthenia gravis and the Guillain-Barré syndrome, the presence of multiple casualties with similar symptoms should facilitate discovery of a botulism outbreak.

Initially, the diagnosis of *cyanide poisoning* will also likely be made on clinical grounds in the face of the appropriate toxidrome. An unusually high anion gap metabolic acidosis and a greater than expected oxygen concentration in venous blood lend support to the clinical diagnosis. Elevated blood cyanide concentrations can confirm the clinical suspicion.

Anthrax should be suspected on finding gram-positive bacilli in skin biopsy material (in the case of cutaneous disease), blood smears, pleural fluid, or spinal fluid. Chest radiographs demonstrating a widened mediastinum in the context of fever and constitutional signs, and in the absence of another obvious explanation (e.g., blunt trauma or postsurgical infection), should also lead one to consider the diagnosis. Confirmation can be obtained by blood culture. State health laboratories and federal facilities at the CDC and at the U.S. Army Medical Research Institute of Infectious Diseases (USAMRIID) can confirm a diagnosis of anthrax by polymerase chain reaction and immunohistochemical assay.

A diagnosis of *plague* can similarly be suspected on finding bipolar "safety-pin"–staining bacilli in Gram or Wayson stains of sputum or aspirated lymph node material; confirmation is obtained by culturing *Y. pestis* from blood, sputum, or lymph node aspirate. The organism grows on standard blood or MacConkey TRA agars, but it is often misidentified by automated systems. *F. tularensis* grows poorly on standard media; its growth is enhanced on media containing cysteine. Because of its extreme infectivity, however, many laboratories prefer to make a diagnosis serologically using an enzyme-linked immunosorbent assay.

Smallpox should be suspected on clinical grounds and can be confirmed by culture or electron microscopy of scabs or vesicular fluid, although the manipulation of clinical material from suspected smallpox victims should be attempted only at public health laboratories able to employ maximum biocontainment precautions. Similar caution should be exercised with specimens from patients with various viral hemorrhagic fevers, a diagnosis that should be considered in those presenting with fever and a bleeding diathesis.

Prevention. Preventive measures should be considered in both a pre-exposure and a postexposure context. Pre-exposure protection against a chemical or biologic attack may consist of physical, chemical, or immunologic measures. Physical protection against primary attack often involves gas masks and protective suits; such equipment is used by the military and by certain hazardous materials response teams, but it is unlikely to be available to civilians at the precise moment when a release might occur. Medical personnel, however, must understand the principles of physical protection as they apply to infection control and the spread of contamination.

Pneumonic plague is spread through respiratory droplets. Droplet precautions, including the use of simple surgical masks, are thus warranted when caring for patients with plague. *Smallpox* is transmitted by droplet nuclei. Airborne precautions, including (ideally) a high-efficiency particulate air (HEPA) filter mask are warranted when caring for smallpox victims. Similarly, *viral hemorrhagic fever* patients should, in general, be managed using contact precautions. Most other biologic agent victims can be safely cared for while employing standard precautions. In the case of chemical agents, residual *mustard* or *nerve agent* on the skin or clothing of victims might potentially pose a hazard to medical personnel. Such victims, whenever possible, should thus have their clothing removed and be "decontaminated" using copious amounts of water before extensive medical care is rendered. Most other chemical agents are volatile enough that spread of agent among patients or from patient to caregiver is unlikely.

Pre-exposure chemical prophylaxis might conceivably be used on the basis of credible intelligence reports. For example, should officials deem that the threatened release of a specific biologic agent appears imminent, antibiotics might be distributed to a population preemptively. Obviously, opportunities to employ such a strategy are likely to be quite limited.

Licensed *vaccines* exist against anthrax and smallpox. Widespread use of either vaccine, however, is likely to be problematic, especially in children. The anthrax vaccine is licensed only for those persons age 18 yr and older. Moreover, the vaccine is given as a six-dose series over 18 mo and requires annual booster doses. These issues, coupled with a limited supply, make civilian employment of the current anthrax vaccine on a large scale unlikely.

Significant obstacles also exist to the widespread employment of smallpox vaccine, although public health officials have contemplated the resumption of a smallpox vaccination campaign. Whereas smallpox vaccine (prepared from vaccinia virus, an orthopoxvirus related to variola) was used safely and successfully in the past in even the youngest infants, it has a relatively high rate of serious complications in certain patients. Fetal vaccinia and demise can occur when pregnant women are vaccinated. Likewise, vaccinia gangrenosa, an often-fatal complication, can occur when immunocompromised persons are vaccinated. Another serious complication, eczema vaccinatum, occurs in those with pre-existing dermatoses. A severe vaccine-related encephalitis was well known during the era of widespread vaccination; because this occurs only in primary vaccinees, it would disproportionately affect pediatric patients. Autoinoculation can occur when virus present at the site of vaccination is manually transferred to other areas of skin or to the eye. Young children would presumably be at greater risk for such inadvertent transmission.

To manage these complications, vaccinia immune globulin (VIG) should be available when undertaking a vaccination campaign. VIG (0.6 mg/kg IM) may be given to vaccine recipients who experience severe complications or to significantly immunocompromised individuals exposed to smallpox, in whom vaccination would be unsafe. Stocks of current vaccine and of VIG are controlled by the CDC, and production of a new vaccine and VIG preparation has begun. In addition to a potential role in pre-exposure prophylaxis, it is thought that vaccination may be effective in postexposure prophylaxis if given within the first 4 days or so after exposure.

Anthrax vaccine might similarly be employed in a postexposure setting. Some authorities recommend three doses of this vaccine as an adjunct to postexposure chemoprophylaxis after documented exposure to aerosolized anthrax spores. Nonetheless, postexposure administration of oral antibiotics constitutes the mainstay of management for asymptomatic victims believed to have been exposed to anthrax, as well as to other bacterial agents such as plague and tularemia. Appropriate prophylactic regimens for various biologic exposures are provided in Table 706–2.

Treatment. Recommended therapies for overt diseases caused by various chemical and biologic agents are provided in Tables 706–2 and 706–3. It is quite likely, however, that the clinician attending to victims will need to make therapeutic decisions before the results of confirmatory diagnostic tests are available and in situations where the diagnosis is not known with certainty. In such cases, it is useful to note that many diseases and symptoms caused by chemical and biologic agents will resolve spontaneously, with only supportive care required. Chlorine and phosgene exposures can thus be successfully managed by providing meticulous attention to oxygenation and fluid balance. Mustard victims may require intensive multisystem support, but no specific antidote or therapy is available. Similarly, many viral diseases such as smallpox, most viral hemorrhagic fevers, and the equine encephalitides are managed supportively.

In addition to ensuring adequate oxygenation, ventilation, and hydration, the clinician may, in certain instances, need to provide specific empirical therapies on an urgent basis. Patients suffering from the sudden onset of severe neuromuscular symptoms may have nerve agent intoxication and should be promptly given atropine (0.05 mg/kg) for its antimuscarinic effects. Although atropine relieves bronchospasm and bradycardia, reduces bronchial secretions, and ameliorates the gastrointestinal effects of nausea, vomiting, and diarrhea, it does not improve skeletal muscle paralysis. Pralidoxime (also known as 2-PAM) cleaves the organophosphate moiety from cholinesterase and regenerates intact enzyme if "aging" has not occurred. The effect is most prominent at the neuromuscular junction and leads to improved muscle strength. Its prompt use (at a dose of 25 mg/kg) as an adjunct to atropine is recommended in all serious cases.

Both atropine and pralidoxime should ideally be administered intravenously in severe cases, although the intraosseous route may be acceptable. Some experts recommend that atropine be given intramuscularly in the presence of hypoxia to avoid arrhythmias associated with intravenous administration. Many EMS systems now stock military autoinjector kits consisting of atropine and 2-PAM for intramuscular injection. Kits containing pediatric doses are currently not available, although military kits (with 2 mg of atropine and 600 mg of pralidoxime) might be used in children older than 2–3 yr of age. Animal studies support the routine prophylactic administration of anticonvulsant doses of benzodiazepines, even in the absence of observable convulsive activity.

Delayed neuromuscular symptoms in the setting of terrorism might be due to botulism. Supportive care, with meticulous attention to ventilatory support, is the mainstay of botulism treatment. Such support may be necessary for several months, making the management of a large-scale botulism outbreak especially problematic in terms of medical resources. A licensed trivalent (types A, B, E) equine botulinum antitoxin is available through the CDC. Administration of this antitoxin is unlikely to reverse disease in symptomatic patients but may prevent further progression. A test dose should be administered before therapy, and patients reacting to this test dose should be desensitized. An investigational heptavalent despeciated (Fab$_2$) antitoxin, also produced in horses, is available through USAMRIID on a compassionate use protocol. In addition, a pentavalent (types A–E) investigational product, Botulism Immune Globulin Intravenous (Human), is available through the California Department of Health Services (510-540-2646), specifically for the treatment of infant botulism.

The rapid onset of respiratory symptoms may signal an exposure to chlorine, phosgene, cyanide, or a number of other toxic industrial chemicals. Although the mainstay of therapy in virtually all of these exposures consists of removal to fresh air and intensive supportive care, cyanide intoxication often requires the administration of specific antidotes, given in two stages.

TABLE 706–2. Critical Biologic Agents of Terrorism

Disease	Etiology	Clinical Findings	Incubation Period	Diagnostic Samples	Diagnostic Assay	Isolation Precautions*	Initial Treatment	Prophylaxis
Anthrax	*Bacillus anthracis*	Inhalational: febrile prodrome with rapid progression to mediastinal lymphadenitis, mediastinitis (chest x-ray: +/- infiltrates, widened mediastinum, pleural effusions); sepsis; shock; meningitis	1–5 days (up to 6 wk?)	Blood CSF Pleural fluid	Culture Gram stain ELISA PCR	Standard	Ciprofloxacin, 10–15 mg/kg (max 500 mg) IV q12h, or doxycycline, 2.2 mg/kg (max 100 mg) IV q12h[†]	Ciprofloxacin, 10–15 mg/kg (max 500 mg) PO q 12h × 60 days, or doxycycline 2.5 mg/kg (max 100 mg) PO q 12h × 60 days[‡]
		Cutaneous: papule progressing to vesicle, to ulcer, then to depressed black eschar, with marked edema		Skin biopsy	Immunohisto-chemical assay			
Plague	*Yersinia pestis*	Febrile prodrome with rapid progression to fulminant pneumonia with bloody sputum, sepsis, DIC	2–3 days	Blood, sputum, lymph node aspirate	Culture Gram or Wright-Giemsa stain ELISA, IFA Ag-ELISA	Pneumonic: droplet until patient treated for 3 days	Gentamicin, 2.5 mg/kg IV q8h[§], or doxycycline, 2.2 mg/kg IV (max 100 mg) IV q12h, or ciprofloxacin, 15 mg/kg (max 500 mg) IV q12h, or chloramphenicol, 25 mg/kg (max 1g) q6h	Doxycycline, 2.2 mg/kg (max 100 mg) PO q12h × 7 days, or ciprofloxacin, 20 mg/kg (max 500 mg) PO q12h × 7 days, or chloramphenicol, 25 mg/kg (max 1 g) PO q6h × 7 days
Smallpox	Variola virus	Febrile prodrome; synchronous vesicopustular eruption, predominately on face and extremities	7–17 days	Pharyngeal swab, scab material	ELISA, PCR Virus isolation	Airborne, droplet, contact	Supportive care	Vaccination within 4 days (consider vaccinia immunoglobulin: 0.6 mL/kg IM within 3 days of exposure for vaccine complications, immunocompromised persons)
Tularemia	*Francisella tularensis*	Pneumonic: abrupt onset of fever, fulminant pneumonia (chest x-ray: prominent hilar adenopathy)	2–10 days	Blood, sputum, serum	Culture‖ Serology: agglutination	Standard	Gentamicin, 2.5 mg/kg IV q8h[§], or doxycycline, 2.2 mg/kg (max 100 mg) IV q12h, or ciprofloxacin, 15 mg/kg (max 500 mg) IV q12h, or chloramphenicol, 15 mg/kg (max 1 g) IV q6h	Doxycycline, 2.2 mg/kg (max 100 mg) PO q12h, or ciprofloxacin 15 mg/kg (max 500 mg) PO q12h
		Typhoidal: fever, malaise, abdominal pain		Tissue	EM			
Botulism	*Clostridium botulinum* toxin	Afebrile; descending flaccid paralysis; cranial nerve palsies; sensation and mentation intact	1–5 days	Nasal swab?	Mouse bioassay, Ag-ELISA	Standard	CDC trivalent antitoxin (serotypes A, B, E), 1 vial (10 mL) IV DOD heptavalent antitoxin (serotypes A–G) (IND) California Dept of Health immunoglobulin (IND)	None
Viral hemorrhagic fevers	Arenaviradae (e.g., Lassa fever) Filoviradae (Ebola, Marburg)	Febrile prodrome; rapid progression to shock, purpura, bleeding diathesis	4–21 days	Serum, blood	Viral isolation Ag-ELISA RT-PCR Serology: Ab-ELISA	Contact, droplet; consider airborne if massive hemorrhage	Supportive care Ribavirin (arenaviruses): 30 mg/kg IV initially, 15 mg/kg IV q6h × 4 days, 7.5 mg/kg IV q8h × 6 days	None

*Brief definition of isolation precautions:
Standard: handwashing; gloves, masks, eye protection, face shields and nonsterile, fluid-resistant gowns for blood, body fluid exposure; appropriate handling of patient care equipment, linens, etc.; avoidance of needle-stick, sharps injury.
Airborne: standard, + private, negative-pressure room with external exhaust or HEPA-filtered recirculated air; special "fitted" and "sealing" respirator masks (e.g., N95).
Droplet: standard, + private room, "routine" mask within 3 feet of patient
Contact: standard, + private room; gloves at all times; handwashing after glove removal; gowns at all times, removed before leaving patient's room.
Adapted from American Academy of Pediatrics. Infection control for hospitalized children. In Pickering LK (editor): 2000 Redbook: Report of the Committee on Infectious Diseases, 25th ed. Elk Grove Village, IL. American Academy of Pediatrics, 2000, pp. 127–37.
[†] CDC recommended one or two additional antibiotics for inhalational anthrax in Fall 2001 outbreak: rifampin, vancomycin, penicillin or ampicillin, clindamycin, imipenem, or clarithromycin. Recommendations in future outbreaks may evolve rapidly, and frequent consultation with local health departments and CDC (1-770-488-7100; www.bt.cdc.gov) is encouraged.
[‡] Amoxicillin, 80 mg/kg/day divided q8h can be substituted if strain proves susceptible.
[§] Streptomycin, 15 mg/kg IM q12h may be substituted if available.
‖Laboratory must be notified that tularemia is suspected.
CSF = cerebrospinal fluid; ELISA = enzyme-linked immunosorbent assay; Ag = antigen; PCR = polymerase chain reaction; max = maximum dose; DIC = disseminated intravascular coagulation; IFA = immunofluorescent assay; EM = electron microscopy; DOD = Department of Defense; IND = investigational new drug; RT = reverse transcriptase.
From Henretig FH, Cieslak TJ, Eitzen EM: Biological and chemical terrorism. J Pediatr 2002; 141(3): 311–26. Used with permission.

TABLE 706–3. Critical Chemical Agents of Terrorism

Agent	Toxicity	Clinical Findings	Onset	Decontamination*	Management
Nerve agents: Tabun, Sarin, Soman, VX	Anticholinesterase: Muscarinic, nicotinic and CNS effects	Vapor: miosis, rhinorrhea, dyspnea; Liquid: Diaphoresis, vomiting; Both: coma, paralysis, seizures, apnea	Seconds: vapor; Minutes–hours: liquid	Vapor: fresh air, remove clothes, wash hair; Liquid: remove clothes, copious washing skin, hair with soap and water, ocular irrigation	ABCs; Atropine: 0.05 mg/kg IV†, IM‡ (min 0.1 mg, max 5 mg), repeat q2–5 min prn for marked secretions, bronchospasm; Pralidoxime: 25 mg/kg IV, IM§ (max 1 g IV; 2 g IM), may repeat within 30–60 min prn, then again q1h for one or two doses prn for persistent weakness, high atropine requirement; Diazepam: 0.3 mg/kg (max 10 mg) IV; lorazepam: 0.1 mg/kg IV, IM (max 4 mg); midazolam: 0.2 mg/kg (max 10 mg) IM prn seizures, or severe exposure
Vesicants: Mustard	Alkylation	Skin: erythema, vesicles; Eye: inflammation; Respiratory tract: inflammation	Hours	Skin: soap and water; Eyes: water (only effective if done within minutes of exposure)	Symptomatic care
Lewisite	Arsenical		Immediate pain		possibly BAL 3 mg/kg IM q4–6h for systemic effects of Lewisite in severe cases; Symptomatic care
Pulmonary agents: chlorine, phosgene	Liberate HCL, Alkylation	Eyes, nose, throat irritation (especially chlorine); Respiratory: bronchospasm, pulmonary edema (especially phosgene)	Minutes: eyes, nose, throat irritation, bronchospasm; Hours: pulmonary edema	Fresh air; Skin: water	Symptomatic care
Cyanide	Cytochrome oxidase inhibition: cellular anoxia, lactic acidosis	Tachypnea, coma, seizures, apnea	Seconds	Fresh air; Skin: soap and water	ABCs, 100% oxygen; Na bicarbonate prn metabolic acidosis; Na nitrite (3%): Dose (mL/kg) / Estimated Hgb (g/dL): 0.27 / 10; 0.33 / 12 (est. for average child); 0.39 / 14 (max 10 mL); Na thiosulfate (25%): 1.65 mL/kg (max 50 mL)

exposures:

Approximate Age	Approximate Weight	Number of Autoinjectors (each type)	Atropine Dose Range (mg/kg)	Pralidoxime Dose Range (mg/kg)
3–7 yrs	13–25 kg	1	0.08–0.13	24–46
8–14 yrs	26–50 kg	2	0.08–0.13	24–46
>14 yrs	>51 kg	3	0.11 or less	35 or less

*Decontamination, especially for patients with significant nerve agent or vesicant exposure; should be performed by health care providers garbed in adequate personal protective equipment. For emergency department staff, this consists of nonencapsulated, chemically resistant body suit, boots, and gloves with a full face air purifier mask/hood.

†Intraosseous route is likely equivalent to intravenous.

‡Atropine might have some benefit via endotracheal tube or inhalation, as might aerosolized ipratropium.

§Pralidoxime is reconstituted to 50 mg/mL (1 g in 20 mL water) for IV administration, and the total dose infused over 30 min, or may be given by continuous infusion (loading dose 25 mg/kg over 30 min, then 10 mg/kg/hr). For IM use, it might be diluted to a concentration of 300 mg/mL (1 g added to 3 mL water—by analogy to the US Army's Mark 1 autoinjector concentration), to effect a reasonable volume for injection. Each Mark 1 kit holds two autoinjectors, one each of atropine 2 mg (0.7 mL) and pralidoxime 600 mg (2 ml); while not approved for pediatric use, they might be considered as initial treatment in dire (especially prehospital) circumstances, for children with severe, life-threatening nerve agent toxicity who lack intravenous access, and for whom more precise, mg/kg IM dosing would be logistically impossible. Suggested dosing guidelines are offered; note potential excess of initial atropine and pralidoxime dose for age/weight.

ABCs = airway, breathing, and circulatory support; BAL = British antilewisite; CNS = central nervous system; Hgb = hemoglobin concentration; est. = estimated hemoglobin concentration; max = maximum; min = minimum; prn = as needed.

Adapted from Henretig FH, Cieslak TJ, Eitzen EM. Biological and chemical terrorism. J Pediatr 2002; 141(3):311–26. Used with permission.

A methemoglobin-forming agent such as sodium nitrite is administered first, because methemoglobin has high affinity for cyanide and causes it to dissociate from cytochrome oxidase. Nitrite dosing in children should be based on body weight to avoid excessive methemoglobin formation and nitrite-induced hypotension. For the same reasons, nitrites should be infused slowly over 5–10 min. A sulfur donor, such as sodium thiosulfate, is given next. This compound is used as a substrate by the hepatic enzyme rhodanese, which converts cyanide to thiocyanate, a less toxic compound excreted in the urine. Thiosulfate treatment itself is efficacious and relatively benign and, thus, may be used alone for mild to moderate cases. Sodium nitrite and sodium thiosulfate are packaged together in standard antidote kits, along with amyl nitrite, a sodium nitrite substitute that can be inhaled in prehospital settings where intravenous access is not available.

In cases in which the delayed onset of respiratory symptoms is potentially due to a terrorist attack, consideration should be given to the empirical administration of an antibiotic effective against anthrax, plague, and tularemia. Ciprofloxacin (10–15 mg/kg IV q12hr) or doxycycline (2.2 mg/kg IV q12hr) are reasonable choices. Although naturally occurring strains of *B. anthracis* are usually quite sensitive to penicillin G, these agents are chosen because penicillin-resistant strains of *B. anthracis* exist. Moreover, ciprofloxacin and doxycycline are effective against almost all known strains of *Y. pestis* and *F. tularensis*. Concerns about inducible β-lactamases in *B. anthracis* have led some experts to recommend one or two additional antibiotics in patients with inhalational anthrax. Rifampin, vancomycin, penicillin or ampicillin, clindamycin, imipenem, and clarithromycin are reasonable choices based on in vitro sensitivity data. Because *B. anthracis* relies on the production of two protein toxins, edema toxin and lethal toxin, for its virulence, drugs that act at the ribosome to disrupt protein synthesis (e.g., clindamycin and the macrolides) provide a theoretical advantage. Ciprofloxacin or doxycycline monotherapy is probably adequate in cases of cutaneous anthrax.

In patients in whom a diagnosis of plague or tularemia is established, streptomycin (15 mg/kg IM q12hr) or gentamicin (2.5 mg/kg IV/IM q8hr) is the preferred choice for therapy. In addition to doxycycline and ciprofloxacin, chloramphenicol (25 mg/kg IV q6hr) is an acceptable alternative. The latter should be employed in the 6% of pneumonic plague cases with concomitant meningitis. To be effective, therapy for pneumonic plague must be initiated within 24 hr of the onset of symptoms.

The management of vesicant-induced injury is similar to that required in burn victims and is largely symptomatic. Mustard victims will benefit from the application of soothing skin lotions such as calamine and the administration of analgesics. Early intubation of severely exposed patients is warranted to guard against edematous airway compromise. Oxygen and mechanical ventilation may be needed, and meticulous attention to hydration is of paramount importance. Lewisite victims can be managed in much the same manner as mustard victims. In addition, dimercaprol (British anti-Lewisite [BAL]) in oil, given intramuscularly, may help ameliorate the systemic effects of lewisite.

The management of symptomatic smallpox victims is also largely supportive, with attention to pain control, hydration status, and respiratory sufficiency again being of primary importance. The parenteral antiviral compound cidofovir, licensed for the treatment of cytomegalovirus retinitis in HIV-infected patients, has in vitro efficacy against variola and other orthopoxviruses. Its utility in treating smallpox victims is untested. Moreover, in the face of a large outbreak of disease, large-scale parenteral use of this drug would be problematic.

Franz DR, Jahrling PB, McClain DJ, et al: Clinical recognition and management of patients exposed to biological warfare agents. *Clin Lab Med* 2001;21:435–73.

Henretig FH, Cieslak TJ, Kortepeter MG, et al: Medical management of the suspected victim of bioterrorism: An algorithmic approach to the undifferentiated patient. *Emerg Med Clin North Am* 2002;20:351–64.
Henretig FH, Cieslak TJ, Eitzen EM: Biological and chemical terrorism. *J Pediatr* 2002;141:311–26.
Patt HA, Feigin RD: Diagnosis and management of suspected cases of bioterrorism: A pediatric perspective. *Pediatrics* 2002;109:685–92.
White SR, Henretig F, Dukes RG: Medical management of vulnerable populations and co-morbid conditions of victims of bioterrorism. *Emerg Med Clin North Am* 2002;20:365–92.

Chapter 707
Animal and Human Bites
Charles M. Ginsburg

It has been estimated that there are nearly 100 million dogs and cats in the United States, and all have the potential to inflict injury to a child. Animal bite injuries account for between 0.7–1% of visits to hospital emergency departments and free-standing emergency centers in the United States. The precise number of individuals who sustain a bite injury who seek medical attention in medical offices and primary care clinics has been estimated to exceed the number who seek care in emergency facilities.

Epidemiology. During the past 3 decades, there have been approximately 20 deaths per year in the United States from dog-inflicted injuries; 65% of these occurred in children who were younger than 11 yr of age. The breed of dog involved in the attacks on children varied; however, rottweilers, pit bulls, and German shepherds accounted for more than 50% of all fatal bite-related injuries. Unneutered male dogs account for approximately 75% of attacks; nursing dams often inflict injury to humans when children attempt to handle one of their puppies.

The majority of dog-related attacks occur in children between the ages of 6–11 yr of age, and males are attacked more often than females (1.5:1). Approximately two thirds of the attacks occur around the home, 75% of the biting animals are known by the child, and almost one half of the attacks are said to be unprovoked. By contrast, the 450,000 reported cat bites per year occur primarily in females and almost all are inflicted by known household animals. Rat bites and gerbil bites are not reportable conditions; therefore, there is a paucity of information available on the epidemiology of these injuries and the incidence of infection after rodent-inflicted bites or scratches.

Few data exist on the incidence and demographics of human bite injuries in pediatric patients; however, preschool-age and early school-age children appear to be the age groups at greatest risk to sustain an injury from a bite by a human. Human bites are the leading cause of injury in daycare centers in the United States.

Clinical Manifestations. Dog bite–related injuries can be divided into three, almost equal categories: abrasions, puncture wounds, and lacerations with or without an associated avulsion of tissue. The most common type of injury from cat and rat bites is a puncture wound. Human bite injuries are of two types, an occlusional injury that is incurred when the upper and lower teeth come together on a body part and, in older children and young adults, a clenched-fist injury that occurs when their fist, usually on their dominant hand, comes in contact with the tooth of another individual.

Diagnosis. Management of the victim of a bite should begin with a thorough history and physical examination. Careful attention should be paid to the circumstances surrounding the bite (type of animal, domestic or sylvatic, provoked or unprovoked, and location of the attack), a history of drug allergies, and the immunization status of the child and animal. During physical examination, meticulous attention should be paid to the type, size, and depth of the injury; the presence of foreign material in the wound; the status of underlying structures; and, in instances where the bite is on an extremity, the range of motion of the affected area. A diagram of the injury(s) should be recorded in the patient's medical record. A radiograph of the affected part should be obtained if there is likelihood that a bone or joint could have been penetrated or fractured or if foreign material is present. The possibility of a fracture or penetrating injury of the skull should be considered in individuals, particularly infants, who have sustained dog bite injuries to the face and head.

Complications. Infection is the most common complication of bite injuries, regardless of the species of biting animal. The decision to obtain material for culture from a wound depends on the species of the biting animal, the length of time that has transpired since the injury, the depth of the wound, the presence of foreign material contaminating the wound, and whether there is evidence of infection. Although potentially pathogenic bacteria have been isolated from up to 80% of dog bite wounds that are brought to medical attention within 8 hr after the bite, the infection rate for wounds receiving medical attention in less than 8 hr is small (2.5%–20%). Thus, unless they are deep and extensive, dog bite wounds that are less than 8 hr in duration do not need to be cultured unless there is evidence of contamination, early signs of infection, or the patient is immunocompromised. Species of *Capnocytophaga canimorsus*, uncommon pathogens in bite-inflicted injuries, have been isolated from nearly 5% of infected wounds in immunocompromised patients. By contrast, the infection rate in cat bite wounds that receive early medical attention is at least 50%; therefore, it is prudent to obtain material for culture from all but the most trivial cat-inflicted wounds and all other animal bite wounds that are not brought to medical attention within 8 hr, regardless of species of the biting animal.

The rate of infection after rodent bite injuries is not known. The majority of the oral flora of rats is similar to that of other mammals; however, approximately 50% and 25% of rats harbor strains of *Streptobacillus moniliformis* and *Spirillum minus*, respectively, in their oral flora. Each of these agents have the potential to cause infections manifested by fever, rash, and other systemic symptoms (i.e., **rat-bite fever**). In addition, *S. minus* is responsible for **sodoku,** which is characterized by fever, ulcerative lesions at the wound site, lymphadenopathy, and rash occurring days to weeks after the primary wound has healed.

All human bite wounds, regardless of the mechanism of injury, should be regarded as high risk for infection and cultured. Because of the large incidence of anaerobic infection after bite wounds, it is important to obtain material for anaerobic as well as aerobic cultures.

Treatment. After the appropriate material has been obtained for culture, the wound should be anesthetized, cleaned, and vigorously irrigated with copious amounts of normal saline. Irrigation with antibiotic-containing solutions provides no advantage over irrigation with saline alone and has the potential to cause local irritation of the tissues. Puncture wounds should be thoroughly cleansed and gently irrigated with a catheter or blunt-tipped needle; however, high-pressure irrigation should not be employed. Avulsed or devitalized tissue should be débrided and any fluctuant areas incised and drained.

Much controversy and few data exist to determine whether bite wounds should undergo primary closure or delayed primary closure (3–5 days) or be allowed to heal by secondary intention. Factors to be considered are the type, size, and depth of the wound; the anatomic location; the presence of infection; the time interval from the injury; and the potential for cosmetic disfigurement. Surgical consultation should be obtained for all patients with deep or extensive wounds, those involving the

bones and joints, and infected wounds that require open drainage. Although there is general agreement that infected wounds and those that are greater than 24 hr of age should not be sutured, there is disagreement and varying clinical experience about the efficacy and safety of closing wounds that are younger than 8 hr of age with no evidence of infection. All hand wounds are at high risk for infection, particularly if there has been disruption of the tendons or penetration of the bones; therefore, delayed primary closure is recommended for all but the most trivial bite wounds of the hands. In contrast to hand wounds, facial lacerations are at smaller risk for secondary infection because of the more luxuriant blood supply to this region. Many plastic surgeons advocate primary closure of facial bite wounds that have been brought to medical attention within 6 hr and have been thoroughly irrigated and debrided.

There are few studies that unequivocally demonstrate the efficacy of antimicrobial agents for prophylaxis of bite injuries; there is, however, a general consensus that antibiotics should be administered to all victims of human bites and all but the most trivial of dog, cat, and rat bite injuries, regardless of whether there is evidence of infection. The bacteriology of bite wound infections is primarily a reflection of the oral flora of the biting animal and, to a lesser extent, a reflection of the skin flora of the victim. Because each of the multitude of aerobic and anaerobic bacterial species that colonize the oral cavity of the biting animal has the potential to invade local tissue, multiply, and cause tissue destruction, the majority of bite wound infections are polymicrobial. Evidence suggests that there may be as many as five different species isolated from infected dog bite wounds.

Despite the large degree of homology in the bacterial flora of the oral cavity between humans, dogs, and cats, important differences exist between the biting species, and this is reflected in the type of wound infections that occur. The predominant bacterial species isolated from infected dog bite wounds are *Staphylococcus aureus* (20–30%), *Pasteurella multocida* (20–30%), *Staphylococcus intermedius* (25%), and *C. canimorsus*; approximately one half of dog bite wound infections contain mixed anaerobes. Similar species are isolated from infected cat bite wounds; however, *P. multocida* is the predominant species in at least 50% of cat bite wound infections. At least 50% or rats harbor strains of *Streptobacillus moniliformis* in their oropharynx, and approximately 25% harbor *S. minor*, an aerobic gram-negative organism. In human bite wounds, nontypable strains of *Haemophilus influenzae, Eikenella corrodens, S. aureus,* α-hemolytic streptococci, and β-lactamase–producing aerobes (about 50%) are the predominant species. Clenched fist injuries are particularly prone to infection by *Eikenella* (25%) and anaerobic bacteria (50%).

The choice between an oral and parenteral antimicrobial agent should be based on the severity of the wound, the presence and degree of overt infection, signs of systemic toxicity, and the immune status of the patient. Amoxicillin-clavulanate is an excellent choice for empirical oral therapy for human and animal bite wounds because of its activity against the majority of strains of bacteria that have been isolated from infected bite injuries. Similarly, ticarcillin-clavulanate or ampicillin and sulbactam are preferred for patients who require empirical parenteral therapy. Procaine penicillin remains the drug of choice for prophylaxis and treatment of rat-inflicted injuries. First-generation cephalosporins have limited activity against *P. multocida and E. corrodens* and, therefore, should not be used for prophylaxis or empirical initial therapy of bite wound infections. The therapeutic alternatives for penicillin-allergic patients are limited because the traditional alternative agents are generally inactive against one or more of the multiple pathogens that cause bite wound infections. Although erythromycin is commonly recommended as an alternative agent for penicillin-allergic patients who have suffered dog and cat bites, it has incomplete activity against strains of *P. multocida* and *S. monili-*

formis and is not effective against *E. corrodens*. Similarly, clindamycin and the combination trimethoprim-sulfamethoxazole have limited activity against strains of *P. multocida* and anaerobic bacteria, respectively. Azithromycin and the newer ketolide antibiotics may be considered because they have activity against aerobic and anaerobic bacteria that are present in infected bite wounds. Tetracycline is the drug of choice for penicillin-allergic patients who have sustained rat bite injuries.

Although the occurrence of tetanus after human or animal bite injuries is extremely rare, it is important to obtain a careful immunization history and to provide tetanus toxoid to all patients who are incompletely immunized or those in whom it has been longer than 10 yr since their last immunization. The need for postexposure rabies vaccine in victims of dog and cat bites is dependent on whether the biting animal is known to have been vaccinated and, most importantly, on the local experience with rabid animals in the community (see Chapter 251). The local health department should be consulted for advice in all instances where the vaccination status of the biting animal is unknown and instances where there is known endemic rabies in the community. Postexposure prophylaxis for hepatitis B should be considered in the rare instance in which an individual has sustained a human bite from an individual who is at high risk for hepatitis B.

All but the most trivial bite wounds of the hand should be immobilized in a position of function for 3–5 days, and patients with bite wounds of an extremity should be instructed to keep the affected extremity elevated for 24–36 hr or until the edema has resolved. All bite wound victims should be re-evaluated within 24–36 hr after the injury.

Prevention. It is not possible to prevent mammalian bite injuries; however, it is possible to reduce the risk of injury with anticipatory guidance. Parents should be routinely counseled during prenatal visits and routine health maintenance examinations about the risks of having potentially biting pets in the household; all should be cautioned against harboring exotic animals for pets. Additionally, parents should be made aware of the proclivity of certain breeds of dogs to inflict serious injuries and the protective instincts of nursing dams. All young children should be closely supervised, particularly when in the presence of animals and, from a very early age, taught to respect animals and to be aware of their potential to inflict injury.

Basic safety tips that should be taught to all children include the following:

- Do not disturb any animal that is sleeping or eating.
- Do not approach an unfamiliar animal.
- Do not disturb a dam that is caring for or feeding her puppies.
- Never run from a unaccompanied dog.
- Remain still if an unfamiliar animal approaches.
- Always allow a dog to see and sniff you before touching it.

Reduction of human bite injuries, particularly in daycare centers and schools, can be achieved by good surveillance of the children and having adequate supervisory personnel to child ratios.

Centers for Disease Control and Prevention: Dog bite–related fatalities—United States 1995–1996. *MMWR Morbid Mortal Wkly Rep* 1997;46:463.

Chapman S, Righetti J, Sung L: Preventing dog bites in children: Randomised controlled trial of an educational intervention. *BMJ* 2000;320:1512.

Cummings P: Antibiotics to prevent infection in patients with dog bite wounds: A meta-analysis of randomized trials. *Ann Emerg Med* 1994;23:535.

Dire DJ: Cat bite wounds: Risk factors for infection. *Ann Emerg Med* 1991;20:973.

Goldstein EJC: Bite wounds and infection. *Clin Infect Dis* 1992;14:663.

Goldstein EC, Citron DM, Richwald GA: Lack of in-vitro efficacy of oral forms of certain cephalosporins, erythromycin and oxacillin against *Pasteurella multocida*. *Antimicrob Agents Chemother* 1988;32:213.

Grossman JA, Adams JP, Kunec J: Prophylactic antibiotics in simple hand lacerations. *J Emerg Med* 1981;245:1055.

Raffin BJ, Freemark M: Streptobacillary rat-bite fever: A pediatric problem. *Pediatrics* 1979;64:214.

Sacks JJ, Lockwood R, Hornreich J, et al: Fatal dog attacks, 1989–1994. *Pediatrics* 1996;97:891.

Talan DA, Citron DM, Abrahamian FM, et al: Bacteriologic analysis of infected dog and cat bites. *N Engl J Med* 1999;340:85.

Chapter 708
Envenomations *Steve Holve*

The vast majority of bites and stings by spiders, snakes, and other venomous animals cause little more than local pain and do not require medical attention. However, pediatricians should be prepared to identify and treat those few individuals who present with severe envenomation. Children, unfortunately, are at greater risk for severe reactions because of their smaller volume for venom distribution.

Symptoms of envenomation may be either IgE mediated, such as anaphylaxis in response to Hymenoptera stings, or venom mediated, as with the bites of poisonous spiders or snakes or the sting of scorpions. Immediate hypersensitivity reactions are treated emergently as indicated in Chapter 137 on anaphylaxis. In moderate and severe envenomation, species-specific antivenin has been shown to ameliorate symptoms and prevent death, but the use of antivenin carries significant risks. Appropriate assessment of the risk:benefit ratio in the use of antivenin is therefore the most important skill a physician can possess in treating envenomation.

ANTIVENINS

Animal venoms are species-specific mixtures of polypeptides, proteolytic enzymes, glycoproteins, and vasoactive substances. In theory, for every venom an antivenin can potentially be produced. In the United States, only four antivenins approved by the Food and Drug Administration (FDA) are commercially available. For pit viper bites, horse serum–derived antivenin (Crotalidae), polyvalent, is available as well as a newly licensed sheep serum product, Crotalidae Polyvalent Immune Fab (ovine). In addition, horse serum–produced antivenin is available for coral snake *(Micrurus fulvius)* bites and black widow spider *(Latrodectus mactans)* bites. Other antivenins to more unusual species of snakes or scorpions are often available through local zoologic societies or the nearest poison control center.

All antivenins are animal-derived immunoglobulins that work by direct binding and neutralization of the proteins in venom. The animal origin of these products exposes patients to large amounts of foreign proteins that may cause both immediate and delayed hypersensitivity reactions.

Immediate hypersensitivity reactions (see Chapter 137), may be life threatening, and the incidence after administration of equine antivenin may be as high as 5–10%. Given the risk of anaphylaxis, antivenin should be given only in a setting in which full resuscitative measures including oxygen, endotracheal intubation, and epinephrine are available. Patients should be asked about medication allergies and previous exposure to antivenins. Skin testing using 0.02 mL of a 1:10 dilution of antivenin should be performed before intravenous infusion of antivenin. This testing should be performed only if antivenin is to be given, because fatal anaphylactic reactions have been reported with skin testing alone. A negative skin test response is reassuring, but the false-negative rate may be as high as 20%. Conversely, a positive skin test result does not preclude the use of antivenin, because the false-positive rate may be as high as 50%, but it does alert a clinician to the higher probability of a severe allergic reaction. In such instances, pretreatment with intravenous administration of diphenhydramine, 1 mg/kg, and methylprednisolone, 1–2 mg/kg, is required. Some toxicologists recommend pretreatment for all patients receiving antivenin.

If signs of immediate hypersensitivity develop during administration of antivenin, the infusion should be stopped until the patient is stabilized. If the severity of envenomation warrants continued infusion of antivenin, it may be resumed at a slower rate or simultaneously with administration of epinephrine. In such instances, consultation with the nearest toxicologist at a poison control center is advisable.

Delayed hypersensitivity or *serum sickness* (see Chapter 138) develops in up to 65% of patients who receive equine-derived antivenin and in 15% of patients who receive ovine-derived products. Serum sickness results from deposition of antigen-antibody complexes on endothelial surfaces. It usually develops 5–21 days after exposure and may last for weeks. It is most commonly manifested as urticaria, pruritus, arthralgia, and malaise but rarely may present as immune complex glomerulonephritis, neuritis, or myocarditis. Intradermal skin tests have not been shown to predict the risk of serum sickness accurately. Prophylactic use of antihistamines and corticosteroids may reduce the risk of serum sickness and is definitely of benefit if symptoms develop.

SNAKEBITE

Of the more than 3,000 known species of snakes, only 200 are poisonous to humans. Of poisonous snakes, 90% are members of one of three families: the Hydrophidae, or poisonous sea snakes; the Elapidae, which includes the cobras, mambas, and coral snakes; and the Viperidae, or true vipers.

In the United States, 95% of poisonous snakebites are by the Crotalidae, or pit vipers, which are a subfamily of the true vipers. Pit vipers may be identified by their triangular heads, elliptical eyes, and the identifiable pit between the eyes and nose (Fig. 708–1). Members of the pit viper family in this country include the rattlesnakes, cottonmouths, and copperheads.

The other native poisonous snakes in the United States are the coral snakes, which are found in Texas and the Southeast and are members of the Elapidae family. Coral snakes are small and

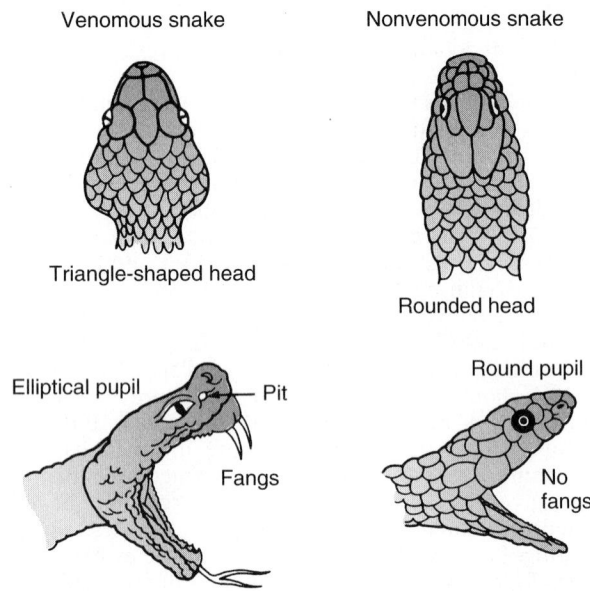

FIGURE 708–1. Identification of venomous snakes. (Modified from Rosen P, et al [editors]: *Emergency Medicine*, 3rd ed. St. Louis, CV Mosby, 1992.)

have a small, rounded head and brightly colored bands of black and red separated by more narrow yellow bands. The rhyme "red on yellow, kill a fellow; red on black, venom lack" serves to differentiate the coral snake from the similar-appearing but nonpoisonous scarlet king snake.

Epidemiology. Approximately 45,000 snakebites are reported in the United States each year; only 8,000 are inflicted by venomous snakes. Most snakebites are in young males and involve alcohol intoxication and a history of the victim's foolishly trying to capture or play with the snake. Despite these many bites, only 12–15 deaths are recorded each year. Unfortunately, children, because of their smaller body mass for venom distribution, are far more likely to have a serious systemic reaction to envenomation and account for more than half of the fatalities.

Pathogenesis. Snake venom is a mixture of polypeptides, proteolytic enzymes, and toxins, which are species specific. Venom from the Elapidae and the Hydrophidae is primarily neurotoxic and has a curare-like effect by blocking neurotransmission at the neuromuscular junction. Death due to envenomation results from respiratory depression. Crotalidae venom is cytolytic, causing tissue necrosis, vascular leak, and coagulopathies. Death from pit viper bites results from hemorrhagic shock, adult respiratory distress syndrome, and renal failure.

Clinical Manifestations. Pit viper bites usually occur on the extremities; pain and swelling occur at the site within minutes. As the venom moves proximally, edema and ecchymosis advance and, in severe cases, bulla formation and tissue necrosis ensue. Systemic symptoms include nausea, vomiting, diaphoresis, weakness, tingling around the face, and muscle fasciculations. Rarely, patients may present in shock with generalized edema or cardiac arrhythmias. Complex clotting abnormalities often occur.

Bites of most Elapidae, including the coral snakes, are minimally painful because the venom has no cytotoxin. However, lack of immediate symptoms should not be mistaken for the absence of serious envenomation. The venom of the coral snake is primarily neurotoxic, and symptoms can rapidly progress in a few hours from mild drowsiness to cranial nerve palsies, weakness, and death from respiratory failure.

Treatment. The first task is to determine if the bite was by a poisonous snake and if envenomation occurred. If the snake has been killed, it should be brought to the emergency department for identification. More than 80% of snakebites in the United States are by nonpoisonous snakes; these bites cause minimal pain and no swelling and require only local wound care.

If the bite is by a venomous snake, immediate care is directed toward decreasing lymphatic flow to limit the spread of venom into the circulation. Immobilization of the extremity, pressure at the site of envenomation, and a proximal tourniquet accomplish this goal. The tourniquet should be loose enough to insert a finger and allow arterial blood flow, because ischemia only exacerbates local tissue damage. Similarly, applying ice to the bite site or using excision and suction is believed to cause more tissue damage than benefit and should be avoided.

On arrival at the emergency department, the patient should have a large-bore intravenous line inserted and blood for baseline laboratory studies should be obtained. Initial blood tests should include type and crossmatch because a progressive coagulopathy may make later typing impossible. Other needed tests include complete blood cell and platelet counts; prothrombin and partial thromboplastin times; fibrinogen and fibrin degradation products; and blood urea nitrogen, creatinine, and creatine phosphokinase levels. These studies need to be repeated at intervals, depending on the severity of envenomation. Baseline vital signs and measurement of the circumference of the bitten extremity should be obtained, and demarcation of ecchymosis and swelling should be marked on the limb so progression can be monitored. The wound should be cleansed and tetanus toxoid given if appropriate.

The decision to use antivenin depends on the severity and progression of symptoms. In general, rattlesnake envenomation requires antivenin and copperhead bites do not, with cottonmouth bites falling between these extremes. The severity of envenomation is commonly graded on a four-point scale (Table 708–1). Most pit viper envenomations cause symptoms within 2 hr and almost always within 6 hr; if symptoms are not present, the bite may be presumed to have been "dry" and a grade 0 envenomation. A grade 1 envenomation with only localized swelling requires nothing more than pain control and careful observation. Unfortunately, children, because of their smaller size, are far more likely to have severe envenomation, and more than 75% of children have a grade 2 or 3 envenomation, which requires antivenin.

Antivenin is most effective if delivered within 4 hr of the bite and is of little value if administration is delayed beyond 12 hr. As discussed earlier, antivenin poses a small but significant risk of an immediate hypersensitivity reaction with an apparent greater risk in equine-derived products compared with ovine-derived antivenin. Antivenin (Crotalidae) polyvalent is administered in increments of 5 vials and repeated as needed to neutralize circulating venom, as measured by normalization of clotting parameters and a halt in the progression of swelling of the affected limb. Children often require more antivenin than a similarly envenomated adult because of their small volume-to-venom ratio. The recently licensed Crotalidae Polyvalent Immune Fab (ovine) appears to have the advantage of rarely causing immediate hypersensitivity and far less risk of serum sickness but has a shorter half-life and may require re-dosing. The choice of antivenin product, the rapidity of administration, and the volume of antivenin administered are best decided in consultation with a toxicologist.

Any person who has been bitten by a coral snake should be administered 3 to 5 vials of antivenin (*M. fulvius*) prophylactically. After being bitten by a coral snake, victims may be asymptomatic for hours before suffering paralysis and respiratory failure. Antivenin is effective only if given before symptoms develop and is ineffective in reversing them once they have occurred.

Prognosis. Despite the potential for mortality and severe morbidity with poisonous snakebites, both can be minimized by early and judicious use of appropriate antivenin. Even extremities with marked tissue necrosis will return to full function with the resolution of swelling, and only rarely is delayed skin grafting required.

ARACHNID ENVENOMATION

The arachnids contain the largest number of known venomous species. More than 20,000 venomous spiders have been identified, but most are of no danger to humans because they lack either potent venom or fangs capable of penetrating the human skin. In the United States, the only significant morbidity is caused by spiders in two genera, *L. mactans* (the black widow spider) and *Loxosceles* (the fiddleback or brown recluse spider).

Latrodectism. The black widow is found throughout the United States, though more commonly in the South. The black widow is glossy black and has bright red or orange markings on the ventral surface of the abdomen, although only the species *L. mactans* has the classic hourglass markings. Females have a body length of 1.5 cm and a leg span of 4–5 cm. Males of the species are approximately half the size of females and pose no threat to humans because their fangs are too short to penetrate the skin. The black widow is commonly found in protected places such as under rocks or in woodpiles, outhouses, and stables.

PATHOGENESIS. The venom of the black widow contains a potent neurotoxin, α-latrotoxin, which binds to presynaptic neuronal membranes, causing dramatic release of acetylcholine and norepinephrine at the neuromuscular junction. The outpouring of these neurotransmitters results in excessive muscle depolarization and autonomic hyperactivity.

CLINICAL MANIFESTATIONS. The bite causes both local and systemic effects. A pinprick sensation is usually felt at the bite, which develops into a pale area of 2–3 mm with a red border. Within an hour, dull, crampy pain is felt around the site and gradually extends throughout the body. In the past, it was claimed that upper extremity bites present with chest tightness and grunting respirations whereas lower extremity bites present with abdominal pain and boardlike rigidity; however, either may occur regardless of bite location. In addition to the severe muscle cramping, most children have nausea, vomiting, and diaphoresis, along with agitation and hypertension. In extremely rare instances, symptoms may progress to respiratory arrest and death.

Because of presentation with a painful, boardlike abdomen, a bite from the black widow spider can mimic acute appendicitis or peritonitis. A key point in the differential diagnosis is that most patients with black widow bites are hypertensive and agitated and tend to move about, seeking a comfortable position, whereas patients with a surgical abdomen are often hypotensive and try to lie still and avoid movement. Many past reports of deaths from black widow bites were related to patients' mistakenly taken to surgery for a presumed acute abdomen. Therefore, obtaining an accurate history and making the correct diagnosis are the most important steps in managing black widow spider bites.

TREATMENT. Muscle cramping and agitation are the main causes of discomfort and can usually be well controlled with intravenous opiates for pain and benzodiazepines for muscle relaxation. Calcium infusions and dantrolene were previously used for muscle cramping; however, neither is efficacious and they are no longer recommended.

Use of antivenin versus symptomatic treatment in black widow bites is determined by the knowledge that without treatment all symptoms will resolve in 24–48 hr but that symptoms can be excruciating. Conservative measures should be tried first before using antivenin if satisfactory pain control is not achieved. A decision tree for treatment is shown in Figure 708–2.

If antivenin is used, an intradermal test dose should be given and all precautions as listed in the earlier antivenin section should be followed. The risk of anaphylaxis is less than that associated with snake antivenin and is less than 1%. One vial of antivenin is usually sufficient, and symptoms of envenomation subside rapidly within 1–3 hr. As with other antivenin products, serum sickness may develop in 5–21 days.

TABLE 708–1. Classification of Envenomation Severity

Grade 0	No envenomation
Grade 1	Minimal envenomation (local swelling and pain without progression)
Grade 2	Moderate envenomation (swelling, pain, or ecchymosis progressing beyond the site of injury; mild systemic or laboratory manifestations)
Grade 3	Severe envenomation (marked local response, severe systemic findings, and significant alteration in laboratory findings)

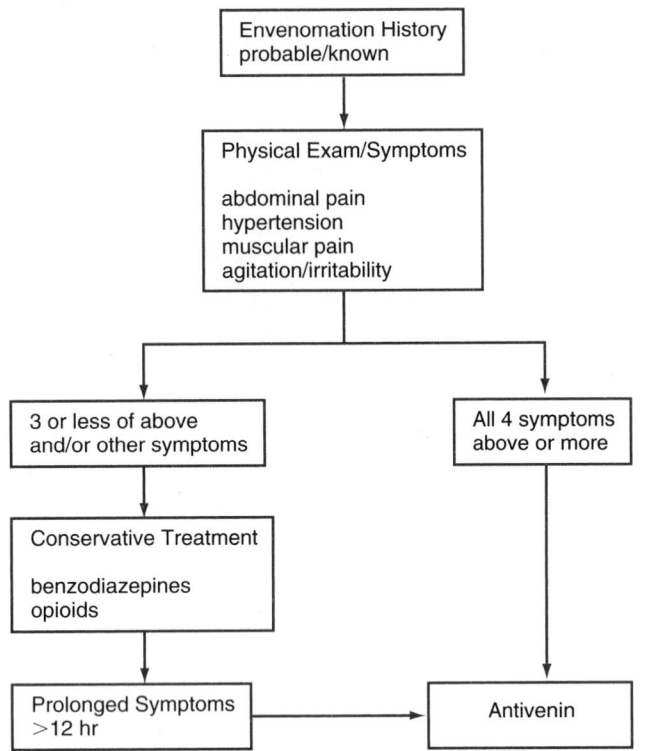

FIGURE 708–2. Decision process for treating pediatric black widow spider envenomation. (Courtesy of Robin Woestman, Loma Linda Children's Hospital, Loma Linda, CA.)

In addition to systemic symptoms of the bite, a hemorrhagic blister forms within 1–2 days. As the blister sloughs, it leaves the characteristic necrotic ulcer of brown recluse spider bites. Most ulcers remain at 1–2 cm but can enlarge up to 15 cm in diameter and involve the full thickness of the skin and some underlying tissue.

TREATMENT AND PROGNOSIS. The outcome in brown recluse spider bites is excellent, and most bites resolve with supportive care alone. Patients with systemic symptoms or significant hemolysis should be admitted to the hospital for pain control and monitoring. Hydration and maintenance of urine output are essential if there is significant hemoglobinuria. Treatment of the ulcerative skin lesions is also supportive, with local wound care. Pain usually subsides in a few days, although complete skin healing requires weeks. Hyperbaric oxygen to promote wound healing, dapsone for leukocyte inhibition, and cyproheptadine, a platelet aggregation inhibitor, all have been recommended to prevent enlargement of skin ulcers; however, none has proven beneficial. In rare instances, large necrotic ulcers require delayed skin grafting.

SCORPION BITES

More than 1,000 species of scorpions are found worldwide; all of them are capable of delivering venom through a stinger located at the end of a six-segment tail. Of medical importance are the small number of species that belong to the family Butidae, which produce venom that is neurotoxic to humans. Among the most toxic species are those of the *Buthus (Leiurus)* in India and the Middle East, *Tityus* in Brazil and Trinidad, and *Centruroides* in Mexico and the desert Southwest of the United States. The majority of stings, even by toxic species, cause only a painful local reaction. However, given their small size, infants and young children who are stung are at risk for severe autonomic dysfunction, multisystem organ failure, and even death.

Pathogenesis. Scorpion venoms vary by species, but all have hyaluronidase, serotonin, histamine releasers, and neurotoxins, of which the latter are the most important component. These neurotoxins can bind to the presynaptic membranes, causing release of acetylcholine and stimulation of both the sympathetic and parasympathetic nervous systems.

Clinical Manifestations. The only medically significant scorpion species in the United States is *Centruroides elixicada*, which is found in the Southwest. Most stings cause an immediate local reaction that can vary from mild burning to severe pain. Severe envenomation causes autonomic dysfunction within a few hours of the sting. Symptoms include agitation, irritability, salivation, blurred vision, and tremulousness with signs of hypertension, tachycardia, tachypnea, and nystagmus. Rarely, in small children or infants, respiratory failure, convulsions, or coma may occur. In these cases, if a history of a sting is not elicited, a diagnosis of encephalitis may be entertained and the correct diagnosis of scorpion envenomation obscured by the fact that children with severe *Centruroides* envenomation may have mild cerebrospinal fluid pleocytosis.

Envenomation by other scorpion species may have specific features. Stings by *Tityus* species in South America are a major cause of pancreatitis, and envenomation by *Buthus* can cause severe hypertension, direct toxic myocarditis, and life-threatening myocardial ischemia.

Treatment. Localized pain can be treated with application of ice and analgesics; pain usually markedly diminishes within 24 hr. For *C. elixicada*, severe envenomation with autonomic instability requires hospital admission for sedation and observation. Symptoms usually resolve within 24–48 hr. If cardiopulmonary compromise occurs, consideration should be given to adminis-

Loxoscelism. Although the bite of a number of spiders can result in mild tissue reactions, only species of the genus *Loxosceles* can cause significant skin necrosis. Members of this genus are commonly known as the "fiddleback spider" because of the brown violin-shaped marking on the thorax or as the "brown recluse spider" because of their predilection for living in dark, undisturbed places such as woodpiles, closets, and basements.

EPIDEMIOLOGY. All species are dull colored and have a small body measuring 1 cm and legs extending up to 5 cm. The species with the most potent bite, *Loxosceles reclusa*, is found most commonly in the river country of mid America but is also found in the South. Other less potent *Loxosceles* species are found throughout the United States, although their numbers decrease with more northern latitudes.

CLINICAL MANIFESTATIONS. The venom of the brown recluse contains hyaluronidase, or spreading factor, and sphingomyelinase D, a protein that lyses cell walls. The bite is often unnoticed or felt only as a pinprick. It typically occurs when a spider is unknowingly trapped against the skin while the victim is putting on clothes; thus, the bite is often on the upper arm, lateral thorax, inner thigh, or rarely on the hands or face. Within 2 hr, a painful, sinking blue macule with a halo of inflammation occurs at the bite site, followed by systemic symptoms that include fever, chills, nausea, and vomiting. In a minority of cases, but more commonly in small children, hemolysis can occur. The hemolysis is presumed secondary to toxin action because Coombs test results are negative and the coagulation system is not activated as measured by platelet counts, fibrin split products, and prothrombin time. In extremely rare instances, massive hemolysis can occur and may lead to disseminated intravascular coagulopathy or renal failure.

tering antivenin. *Centruroides*-specific antivenin is not FDA approved but is available by contacting the Arizona Poison Control Center at (520) 626-6016. It is prepared from goat serum and poses the same small risk of immediate anaphylaxis and later serum sickness as other antivenins produced from horse serum. The use of antivenin, if warranted, leads to complete resolution of symptoms within 1–2 hr. Antivenin for other scorpion species is available in countries where those species are found or through zoologic societies.

HYMENOPTERA STINGS

The insect order of Hymenoptera includes the ants, bees, and wasps, which are characterized by the presence of a stinger at the end of the abdomen through which venom is injected. They are found throughout the United States and worldwide.

Hymenoptera venom, a mixture of proteins and vasoactive substances, is not very potent; most stings cause only local reactions that can be treated with application of cold compresses and analgesics. However, 1–4% of the population is sensitized to Hymenoptera venom and is at risk for immediate hypersensitivity reactions. Each year, 50–150 people in the United States die of anaphylaxis caused by Hymenoptera stings.

Any Hymenoptera envenomation that presents as urticaria, angioedema, wheezing, or hypotension should be treated aggressively for an immediate hypersensitivity reaction with intravenous fluids, oxygen, and epinephrine (see Chapter 137). In the past, any child who sustained a Hymenoptera sting and who had a systemic reaction and a positive result of a skin prick test with Hymenoptera venom was advised to have desensitization with venom-specific immunotherapy. Reports suggest that the clinical course of most children with venom sensitivity is much less severe than previously thought. Fewer than 20% of children with systemic reactions from an initial sting will have systemic reactions with subsequent stings. Evaluating IgE levels, radioallergosorbent testing (RAST), or results of skin prick tests with Hymenoptera venom are not predictive of future systemic reactions.

Children with large local reactions should receive corticosteroids and antihistamines. Children who have systemic reactions including wheezing do not require venom immunotherapy but should carry an emergency kit with epinephrine. Children who have had a life-threatening immediate hypersensitivity reaction should carry an epinephrine kit with them at all times and should undergo venom immunotherapy. More than 95% of these patients have lifelong protection after 3–5 years of immunotherapy.

MARINE ENVENOMATION

Stingrays. Although found only in tropical and subtropical waters, stingrays cause more human envenomations than any other marine vertebrate. The stinging spines on their whiplike tails are retroserrated, and therefore they commonly cause a jagged laceration along with envenomation.

Minor punctures may resemble cellulitis, whereas more severe envenomations may cause marked tissue destruction and necrosis. Regardless of the appearance of the lesion, stingray envenomation is intensely painful for 24–28 hr. Systemic manifestations include nausea and vomiting and, more rarely, paralysis, hypotension, bradycardia, and seizures.

Treatment begins with thorough cleaning of the wound and tetanus prophylaxis. Because stingray toxins are heat labile, immersion in hot water denatures the protein elements of the venom and decreases pain. Additional analgesia should be provided as needed. Superinfection with aerobic and anaerobic organisms, including *Vibrio* species, is common, and antibiotic prophylaxis should be considered.

Scorpionfish. Members of the family Scorpaenidae include the zebrafish, scorpionfish, and stonefish; all have venomous spines

that become erect on stimulation. Envenomation by the Scorpaenidae causes immediate pain that may last for hours or days. Victims may suffer intense local tissue destruction in which superinfections are common. Systemic manifestations include vomiting, abdominal pain, headache, delirium, seizures, and cardiorespiratory failure. Therapy is similar to that for stingray envenomations. Envenomations with severe systemic symptoms benefit from antivenin administration.

Coelenterate Envenomations. Members of the phylum Cnidaria are common to the oceans of the world. Cnidarian species all share a common anatomic feature: minuscule capsules (cnidae) that contain a highly folded tubule that everts on contact, thereby injecting the venom.

Envenomation causes an immediate stinging sensation that may be associated with paresthesias, pruritus, and local edema. In more severe envenomations, systemic signs may include nausea and vomiting, myalgias, headache, and, more rarely, seizures, coma, and cardiorespiratory collapse. Most lethal envenomations have been attributed to the Pacific box jellyfish, *Chironex fleckeri*, which is indigenous to the waters off Australia, and the Atlantic Portuguese man-of-war, *Physalia physalis*.

Treatment of these envenomations begins in the ocean; the wounds should be rinsed in seawater because fresh water may lyse venom-producing cells (nematocysts), leading to further envenomation. Irrigation of the sting site with vinegar, rubbing alcohol, or baking soda is beneficial because it inhibits nematocyst discharge. Visible tentacle fragments should be removed with forceps, and microscopic fragments may be removed by gently shaving the affected area. Antihistamines and corticosteroids are indicated for swelling and urticaria.

Seabather's Eruption. Seabather's eruption is an intensely pruritic vesicular or maculopapular eruption that primarily affects the skin surfaces covered by swimwear. It is caused by exposure to the larvae of two species of the phylum Cnidaria: the sea anemone, *Edwardsiella lineata*, which is found off the coast of the northeastern United States; and the thimble jellyfish, *Linuche unguiculata*, which is the principal cause of seabather's eruption in Florida and the Caribbean.

Epidemics of seabather's eruption occur during summer months in which there are large quantities of larvae in the water. An intensely pruritic rash begins within 4–24 hr of exposure and may persist for days or weeks. Associated symptoms may include fever, chills, headache, malaise, conjunctivitis, and urethritis. Antihistamines are the mainstay of treatment, although corticosteroids, either applied topically or given systemically, may be beneficial in severe cases.

Antivenins

Boyer L, Seifert S, Cain J: Recurrence phenomena after immunoglobulin therapy for snake envenomations: Guidelines for clinical management with crotaline Fab antivenom. *Ann Emerg Med* 2001;37:196–201.
Dart R, McNally J: Efficacy, safety and use of snake antivenoms in the United States. *Ann Emerg Med* 2001;37:181–88.

Snakebites

Davidson T, Schafer S: Rattlesnake bites: Guidelines for aggressive treatment. *Postgrad Med* 1994;96:107.
Gaar G: Assessment and management of coral and other exotic snake envenomations. *J Fla Med Assoc* 1996;83:178–82.
Gold BS, Dart RC, Barish RA: Bites of venomous snakes. *N Engl J Med* 2002;347: 347–56.
McKinney P: Out of hospital and interhospital management of crotaline snakebite. *Ann Emerg Med* 2001;37:168–74.

Arachnid and Insect Envenomations

Anderson PC: Spider bites in the United States. *Dermatol Clin* 1997;15: 307–14.
Hauk P, Friedl K, Kaufmehl K, et al: Subsequent insect stings in children with hypersensitivity to Hymenoptera. *J Pediatr* 1995;126:185–90.
Muller U: New developments in the diagnosis and treatment of Hymenoptera venom allergy. *Int Arch Allergy Immunol* 2001;124:447–53.

Sofer S, Shahak E, Gueron M: Scorpion envenomation and antivenom therapy. *J Pediatr* 1994;124:973–78.

Woestman R, Perkin R, Van Stralen D: The black widow: Is she deadly to children? *Pediatr Emerg Care* 1996;12:360–68.

Marine Envenomations

Brown C, Shepherd S: Marine trauma, envenomations and intoxications. *Emerg Med Clin North Am* 1992;10:385–408.

Williams GC: Stinging seas. *Calif Wild* 2000;53(4):12–17.

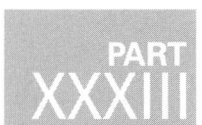
Laboratory Medicine, Drug Therapy, and Reference Tables

Chapter 709

Laboratory Testing in Infants and Children *John F. Nicholson and*

Michael A. Pesce

Because of genetic heterogeneity, biologic and environmental variability, and inhomogeneity of subclinical health status, normal values for many laboratory tests do not show a gaussian bell-shaped distribution curve. As a result, the population mean and the standard deviation (SD) are frequently less useful than the range of normal values, generally given as the 95% normal range, that is, the range of values obtained in testing a normal population minus the lowest 2.5% and the highest 2.5%. The serum sodium concentration in children, which is tightly controlled physiologically, has a distribution that is essentially gaussian; the mean value ±2 SD gives a range very close to that actually observed in 95% of children (Table 709–1). Alternatively, the serum creatine kinase level, which is subject to diverse influences and is not actively controlled, does not show a gaussian distribution, as evidenced by the lack of agreement between the range actually observed and that predicted by the mean value ±2 SD.

A refinement of referencing that is used with increasing frequency is reporting the value obtained together with the percentile of normal values into which the value obtained falls. This method is useful when one is testing for risk factors such as in determination of serum cholesterol. A further modification that is necessary for many tests performed in infants and children is calculating the age-related adjustment of the normal range. Both age adjustment and the use of percentiles are illustrated in the normal values for serum cholesterol in Table 726–6. A final modification needed for reporting normal ranges is referencing to the Tanner stage of sexual maturation, which is most useful in assessing pituitary and gonadal function.

Accuracy and Precision of Laboratory Tests. Technical accuracy is an important consideration in interpreting the results of a laboratory test. Because of improvements in methods of analysis and elimination of analytic interferences, the accuracy of most tests is limited primarily by their precision. **Accuracy** is a measure of the nearness of the test result to the actual value, whereas **precision** is a measure of the reproducibility of a result. No test can be more accurate than it is precise. Analysis of precision by repetitive measurements of a single sample gives rise to a gaussian distribution with a mean and SD. The estimate of precision is the coefficient of variation (CV):

$$CV = \frac{SD}{Mean} \times 100$$

The CV is not likely to be constant over the full range of values obtained in clinical testing, but it is about 5% in the normal range. The CV is generally not reported but is always known by the laboratory. It is particularly important in assessing the significance of changes in laboratory results. For example, a common situation is the need to assess hepatotoxicity incurred as a result of administration of a therapeutic drug and reflected in the serum alanine aminotransferase (ALT) value. If serum ALT increases from 25 U/L to 40 U/L, is the change significant? The CV for ALT is 7%. Using the value obtained plus or minus 2 × CV to express the extremes of imprecision, it can be seen that a value of 25 U/L is unlikely to reflect an actual concentration greater than 29 U/L, and a value of 40 U/L is unlikely to reflect an actual concentration of less than 34 U/L. Therefore, the change in the value as obtained by testing is likely to reflect a real change in circulating ALT levels. Continued monitoring of ALT is indicated even though both values for ALT are within normal limits. "Likely" in this case is only a probability. Inherent biologic variability is such that the results of two successive tests may suggest a trend that will disappear on further testing.

The precision of a test may also be indicated by providing confidence limits for a given result. Ordinarily, 95% confidence limits are used, indicating that it is 95% certain that the value obtained lies between the two limits reported. Confidence limits are calculated using the mean and SD of replicate determinations:

$$95\% \text{ Confidence limits} = Mean \pm t \times SD$$

where t is a constant derived from the number of replications. In most cases t = 2.

Sensitivity, Accuracy, and Testing Purpose. There are some circumstances in which sensitivity and accuracy of an analysis are reduced or increased as functions of clinical purpose. For example, ion exchange chromatography of plasma amino acids for the diagnosis of inborn errors of metabolism is usually performed at a sensitivity that allows measurement of all the amino acids with a single set of standards. The range of values is roughly 20–800 μmol/L, and accuracy is poor at values of 20 μmol/L or less. The detection of homocysteine in this type of analysis suggests an inborn error of methionine metabolism. Adjusting the analysis to achieve greater sensitivity, one can accurately measure homocysteine in normal plasma (3–12 μmol/L). This more sensitive test is used in the assessment of cobalamin status and in the analysis of risk factors for atherosclerotic cardiovascular disease.

Predictive Value of Laboratory Tests. Predictive value (PV) theory deals with the usefulness of tests as defined by their sensitivity

TABLE 709–1. Gaussian and Nongaussian Laboratory Values in 458 Normal Schoolchildren Aged 7–14 Yr

	Serum Sodium (mM/L)	Serum Creatine Kinase (U/L)
Mean	141	68
SD	1.7	34
Mean ± 2 SD	138–144	0–136
Actual 95% range	137–144	24–162

SD = standard deviation.

(ability to detect a disease) and specificity (ability to define absence of a disease).

$$\text{Sensitivity} = \frac{\text{Number positive by test}}{\text{Total number positive}} \times 100$$

$$\text{Specificity} = \frac{\text{Number negative by test}}{\text{Total number without disease}} \times 100$$

$$\text{PV of a positive test result} = \frac{\text{True positive results}}{\text{Total positive results}} \times 100$$

$$\text{PV of a negative test result} = \frac{\text{True negative results}}{\text{Total negative results}} \times 100$$

The problems addressed by PV theory are false-negative and false-positive test results. Both are major considerations in interpreting screening tests in general and neonatal screening tests specifically.

Testing for human immunodeficiency virus (HIV) seroreactivity serves to illustrate some of these considerations. If it is assumed that approximately 1,100,000 of 284,000,000 residents of the United States are infected with HIV (prevalence = 0.39%) and that 90% of those infected demonstrate antibodies to HIV, we can consider the usefulness of a simple test with 99% sensitivity and 99.5% specificity. If the entire population of the United States were screened, it would be possible to identify most of those infected with HIV.

$$1,100,000 \times 0.9 \times 0.99 = 980,100 \ (89.1\%)$$

There will be 119,900 false-negative test results. Even with a 99.5% specificity, the number of false-positive test results would be larger than the number of true-positive results:

$$284,000,000 \times 0.005 = 1,420,000$$

There will be 281,480,000 true-negative results.

PV of positive test result =

$$\frac{980,100}{(980,100 + 1,420,000)} \times 100 = 41\%$$

PV of negative test result =

$$\frac{281,480,000}{(281,480,000 + 119,900)} \times 100 = 99.96\%$$

Given the high cost associated with follow-up of false-positive test results, the anguish produced by a false-positive result, and the lack of effective therapy, it is easy to see why universal screening for HIV seropositivity received a low priority immediately after the introduction of testing for HIV infection.

By contrast, we can consider the screening of 100,000 individuals from groups at increased risk for HIV in whom the overall prevalence of disease is 10%, all other considerations being unchanged.

$$\text{True-positive results} = 0.9 \times 0.99 \times 10,000 = 8,910$$

$$\text{False-positive results} = 0.005 \times 90,000 = 450$$

$$\text{False-negative results} = 10,000 - 8,910 = 1,090$$

$$\text{PV of positive test result} = \frac{8,910}{8,910 + 450} \times 100 = 95\%$$

$$\text{PV of negative test result} = \frac{89,500}{89,550 + 1,090} \times 100 = 99\%$$

These two hypothetical testing strategies illustrate that the diagnostic efficiency of testing heavily depends on the prevalence of the disease being tested for, even if the test is a superior one such as the test for HIV antibodies. Because the treatment of pregnant women infected with HIV is effective in preventing vertical transmission of the infection, screening has now been expanded to all pregnant women. The proven effectiveness of current therapy to prevent neonatal infection has intensified screening for HIV early in pregnancy even though the risk of maternal infection is relatively low.

Neonatal Screening Tests. Almost all the diseases detected in neonatal screening programs have a very low prevalence, and the tests are, for the most part, quantitative rather than qualitative. In general, the strategy is to use the initial screening test to separate a highly suspect group of patients from normal infants (i.e., to increase the prevalence) and then to follow this suspect group aggressively. This strategy is illustrated by a scheme used in screening newborns for congenital hypothyroidism, the prevalence of which is 25/100,000 liveborn infants. The initial test performed is for thyroxine in whole blood, and infants with the lowest 10% of test results are considered suspect. If all infants with hypothyroidism were in the suspect group, the prevalence of disease in this group would be 250/100,000 infants. The original samples obtained from the suspect group are retested for thyroxine and are tested for thyroid-stimulating hormone. This second round of testing results in an even more highly suspect group composed of 0.1% of the infants screened and having a prevalence of hypothyroidism of 25,000/100,000 subjects. This final group is aggressively pursued for further testing and treatment. Even with a 1,000-fold increase in prevalence, 75% of the population aggressively tested is euthyroid. The justifications advanced for the program are that treatment is easy and effective and that the alternative if undetected and untreated—long-term custodial care—is both unsatisfactory and expensive.

At its inception neonatal screening was driven by the selection of genetic diseases whose clinical manifestations developed postnatally such as phenylketonuria, galactosemia, and homocystinuria. The diseases could be treated effectively by simple means instituted shortly after birth. The screening tests are microbiologic assays that are disease specific.

Tandem mass spectrometry (MSMS) is a technically advanced method in which many compounds are initially separated by molecular weight. Each compound is then fragmented to allow identification. The process requires roughly 2 min per sample and can detect 20 or more inborn errors of metabolism. The effects of prematurity, neonatal illness, and of intensive neonatal management on metabolites in blood complicate interpretation of results. The predictive value of a positive screening result is likely to be less than 10%; that is, 90% of positive results are not indicative of a genetic disorder of metabolism. Nonetheless, MSMS permits diagnoses to be made before clinical illness develops. MSMS is not directed toward diseases defined as treatable but toward all the diseases, each of which is rare, that the technique can identify (Box 709–1). As of this writing at least 19 states use MSMS for neonatal screening, 4 more are in the process of implementing MSMS, and at least 10 more states are considering its use.

More common diseases have also become targets for neonatal screening programs. Congenital hypothyroidism was selected for screening because of its frequency and its ease of treatment. Sickle cell disease, easily detected, can be treated more effectively if diagnosed before clinical signs appear. Results of neonatal screening for cystic fibrosis (CF) show that there are clear benefits from preclinical diagnosis but also that there are some inherent difficulties of genetic screening for complex autosomal recessive diseases that are common and caused by a rather large number of mutations of a single gene. The definitive diagnostic test for CF is the measurement of concentrations of sodium and chloride in sweat, a test that is not practical during the first weeks of life. Neonates with CF generally have elevations in whole blood trypsinogen. This allows the definition of a group of neonates with high risk for CF. Performance of DNA analysis for common mutations that cause CF can reduce the suspect group to achieve a higher likelihood of disease among them and a manageable number of infants on whom to perform sweat tests. The problems include (1) uncommon mutations are not included in the screening panel (thus cases of CF caused by them can be missed); (2) common mutations that cause clinically innocent elevations of whole blood trypsinogen in heterozygous neonates will be false positives that will alarm parents; and (3) CF with normal sweat test results is rare but is likely to be missed. Congenital adrenal hyperplasia, another common disorder, is now included in neonatal screening programs. In this instance, the most common disorders are not life threatening but the life-threatening disorders commonly threaten life in the neonatal period.

The expansion of the menu of screening tests presents a significant additional cost to society in that screening programs generally attempt to identify all affected neonates and, in so doing, follow-up a significant percentage of false-positive screening results. The fact that an infant is called back suggests that the infant is "not right" to the parents. This suggestion is not automatically dismissed when the initial screening result is determined to be a false positive. For this reason, screening programs engender substantial need for effective counseling for parents whose infants are called back for follow-up testing.

Testing in Differential Diagnosis. The use of laboratory tests in differential diagnosis satisfy PV theory because a correct differential diagnosis should result in a relatively high prevalence of the disease under consideration. An example of testing in differential diagnosis is the measurement of urinary vanillylmandelic acid (VMA) for diagnosis of neuroblastoma. A simple spot test for VMA is not useful in general screening programs because of the low prevalence of neuroblastoma (3 cases/100,000) and the low sensitivity of the test (69%). Even though the specificity of urinary VMA is 99.6%, testing of 100,000 children would produce 2 true-positive test results, 400 false-positive results, and 1 false-negative result. The PV of a positive result in this setting is 0.5%, and the PV of a negative result is 99.99%, not much different from the assumption that neuroblastoma is not present at all. Testing for urinary VMA in a 3-yr-old child with an abdominal mass, however, gives a useful result because the prevalence of neuroblastoma is at least 50% in 3-yr-old children with abdominal masses. If 100 such children are tested and the prevalence of neuroblastoma in the group is assumed to be 50%, a satisfactory PV is obtained.

PV of positive test result =

$$\frac{0.69 \times 50}{0.69 \times 50 + (0.004 \times 50)} \times 100 = 99\%$$

PV of negative test result =

$$\frac{0.996 \times 50}{0.996 \times 50 + (0.31 \times 50)} \times 100 = 76\%$$

Here a test with a low sensitivity is powerful in differential diagnosis because the PV of a positive result is almost 100% in the setting of high prevalence.

SEROLOGIC TESTS FOR LYME DISEASE. Using laboratory testing as a means to refine a differential diagnosis poses problems, as exemplified by serologic testing for Lyme disease, which is a tick-borne infection by *Borrelia burgdorferi* that has various manifestations in both early and late stages of infection (see Chapter 204). Direct demonstration of the organism is difficult, and serologic test results for Lyme disease are not reliably positive in young patients presenting early with erythema chronicum migrans. These results become positive after a few weeks of infection and remain positive for years. In an older population being evaluated for late-stage Lyme disease, some individuals will have recovered from either clinical or subclinical Lyme disease and some will have active Lyme disease, with both groups having true-positive serologic test results. Of those individuals without Lyme disease, some will have true-negative serologic test results but a significant percentage will have antibodies to other organisms that cross-react with *B. burgdorferi* antigens.

This set of circumstances gives rise to a number of problems. First, the protean nature of Lyme disease makes it difficult to ensure a high prevalence of disease in subjects to be tested. Second, the most appropriate antibodies to be detected are imperfectly defined, leading to a wide variety of entry tests with varying rates of false positivity and false negativity. Third, the natural history of the antibody response to infection and the difficulty of demonstrating the causative organism directly combine to make the laboratory diagnosis of early Lyme disease difficult. Fourth, in the diagnosis of late-stage Lyme disease in older subjects, the laboratory diagnosis is plagued by misleading positive (either false-positive or true-positive but not clinically relevant) results of the entry test, typically an enzyme-linked immunosorbent assay, that uses whole *B. burgdorferi* organisms. A review of 788 patients referred to a specialty clinic with the diagnosis of Lyme disease revealed that the diagnosis was correct in 180 patients, that 156 patients had true seropositivity without active Lyme disease, and that 452 had never had Lyme disease, even though 45% of them were seropositive by at least one test before referral.

The two-step approach, similar to that used in HIV testing, is commonly used: (1) a screening test that has high sensitivity (e.g., ELISA) and excellent negative predictive value; followed by (2) a confirmatory test for verification of positive screening tests that is very specific (e.g., Western blot to detect antibodies to selected bacterial antigens). Negative screening tests and negative verification tests are reported as negative. Positive verification tests are reported as positive. However, standardization of the testing

TABLE 709–2. Laboratory Profile as a Review of Systems

Laboratory Test	Assessment Facilitated by Tests
Complete blood cell count and platelets	Nutrition, status of formed elements
Complete urinalysis	Renal function/genitourinary tract inflammation
Albumin and cholesterol	Nutrition
ALT, bilirubin, GGT	Liver function
BUN, creatinine	Renal function, nutrition
Sodium, potassium, chloride, bicarbonate	Electrolyte homeostasis
Calcium and phosphorus	Calcium homeostasis

ALT = alanine aminotransferase; GGT = γ-glutamyltransferase; BUN = blood urea nitrogen.

procedures is difficult in North America where only one pathogenic strain of *B. burgdorferi* is found and is more difficult elsewhere in the Northern Hemisphere where as many as three pathogenic strains are present. Identification of microbial DNA in body fluids by polymerase chain reaction is definitive but invasive.

LABORATORY SCREENING AS A REVIEW OF SYSTEMS. Screening profiles (Table 709–2), used as a technical review of systems or to establish a baseline, facilitate patient care in specific circumstances, including the following: (1) an illness is clearly present, but a specific diagnosis is elusive; (2) a patient requires intensive care for any clinical problem; and (3) treatment is indicated that employs a new drug in postmarketing evaluation or a drug known to have systemic adverse effects.

RISK FACTORS AND PREDICTIVE VALUE. When a given laboratory value within the spectrum of the reference range is considered a risk factor, it is generally true that, in the absence of clinical manifestations, the value has no predictive worth as an indicator of disease and has little worth in predicting the likelihood of future disease in any individual case.

American Academy of Pediatrics and American Thyroid Association: Newborn screening for congenital hypothyroidism. *Pediatrics* 1987;80:745–49.

Clayton EW: Issues in state newborn screening programs. *Pediatrics* 1992;90:641–46.

Farrell PM, Kosrok MR, Rock MJ, et al: Early diagnosis of cystic fibrosis through neonatal screening prevents severe malnutrition and improves long-term growth. *Pediatrics* 2001;107:1–13.

Galen RS, Gambino SR: *Beyond Normality.* New York, Academic Press, 1975.

Hu LT, Klempner MS: Update on the prevention, diagnosis, and treatment of Lyme disease. *Adv Intern Med* 2001;46:247–75.

National Newborn Screening and Genetics Resource Center (website): http://genes-r-us.uthscsa.edu

Steere AC, Taylor E, McHugh GL, et al: The overdiagnosis of Lyme disease. *JAMA* 1993;269:1812–6.

Zytkovicz TH, Fitzgerald EF, Marsden D, et al: Tandem mass spectrometric analysis for amino, organic, and fatty acid disorders in newborn dried blood spots: A two-year summary from the New England Newborn Screening Program. *Clin Chem* 2001;47:1945–55.

always be used. Refer to Figures 710–1 and 710–2 for estimations related to dosages.

In preparing the reference range listings, a number of abbreviations, symbols, and codes were used (Table 710–1).

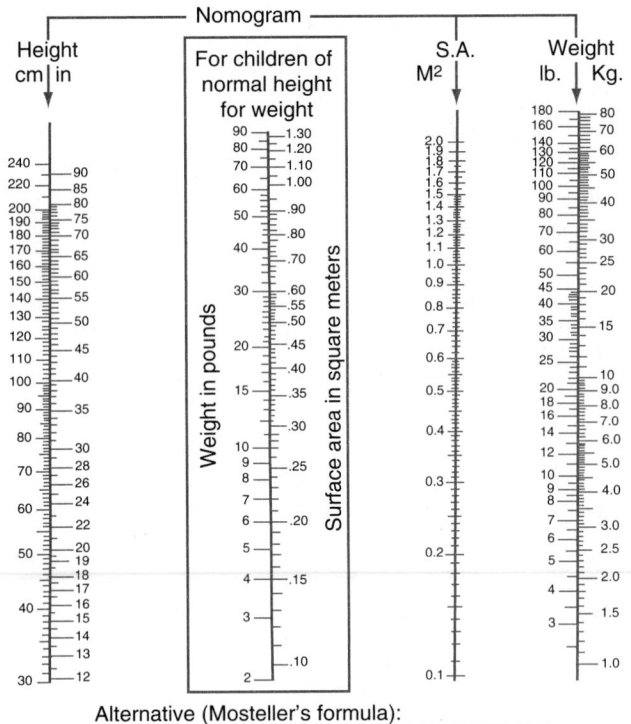

Alternative (Mosteller's formula):

$$\text{Surface area (m}^2) = \sqrt{\frac{\text{Height (cm)} \times \text{Weight (kg)}}{3600}}$$

FIGURE 710–1. Nomogram for estimation of surface area. The surface area is indicated where a straight line that connects the height and weight levels intersects the surface area column; or, if the patient is roughly of average size, from the weight alone *(enclosed area)*. (Nomogram modified from data of E. Boyd by CD West.) (See also Briars G, Bailey B: Surface area estimation: Pocket calculator v nomogram. *Arch Dis Child* 1994;70:246.)

Chapter 710

Reference Ranges for Laboratory Tests and Procedures *John F. Nicholson and*

Michael A. Pesce

In the following tables, the reference ranges apply to infants, children, and adolescents when possible. For many analyses, however, separate reference ranges for children and adolescents are not well delineated. When interpreting a test result, the reference range supplied by the laboratory performing the test should

TABLE 710–1. Prefixes Denoting Decimal Factors

Prefix	Symbol	Factor
Mega	M	10^6
Kilo	k	10^3
Hecto	h	10^2
Deka	da	10^1
Deci	d	10^{-1}
Centi	c	10^{-2}
Milli	m	10^{-3}
Micro	μ	10^{-6}
Nano	n	10^{-9}
Pico	p	10^{-12}
Femto	f	10^{-15}

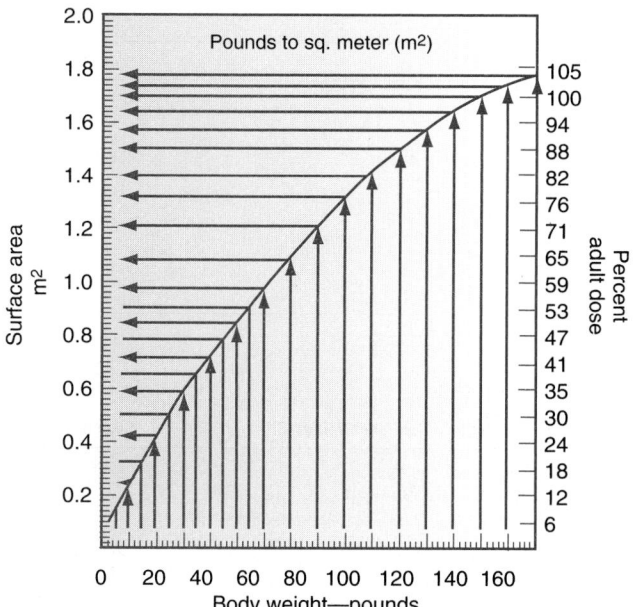

FIGURE 710–2. Relationship between body weight in pounds, body surface area, and adult dosage. The surface area values correspond with those set forth by Crawford and associates (1950). Note that the 100% adult dose is for a patient weighing about 140 lb and having a surface area of about 1.7 m². (From Talbot NB, et al: *Metabolic Homeostasis—A Syllabus for Those Concerned with the Care of Patients.* Cambridge, Harvard University Press, 1959.)

TABLE 710–2. Abbreviations

Ab	Absorbance
AU	Arbitrary unit
cap	Capillary
CH_{50}	Dilution required to lyse 50% of indicator red blood cell; indicates complement activity
CKBB	Brain isoenzyme of creatine kinase
CKMB	Heart isoenzyme of creatine kinase
Cr	Creatinine
CSF	Cerebrospinal fluid
D	Day, days
F	Female
g	Gram
hr	Hour, hours
Hb	Hemoglobin
HbCO	Carboxyhemoglobin
hpf	High-power field
IU	International unit of hormone activity
L	Liter
M	Male
mEq/L	Milliequivalents per liter
min	Minute, minutes
mm^3	Cubic millimeter, microliter (μL)
mmHg	Millimeters of mercury
mo	Month, months
mol	Mole
mOsm	Milliosmole
MW	Relative molecular weight
nm	Nanometer (wavelength)
Pa	Pascal
pc	Postprandial
RBC	Red blood cell(s), erythrocyte(s)
RT	Room temperature
s	Second, seconds
SD	Standard deviation
U	International unit of enzyme activity
V	Volume
WBC	White blood cell(s)
WHO	World Health Organization
wk	Week, weeks
yr	Year, years

TABLE 710–3. Symbols

>	Greater than
≥	Greater than or equal to
<	Less than
≤	Less than or equal to
±	Plus/minus
≅	Approximately equal to

TABLE 710–4. Abbreviations for Specimens

S	Serum
P	Plasma
(H)	Heparin
(LiH)	Lithium heparin
(E)	Ethylenediaminetetraacetic acid (EDTA)
(C)	Citrate
(O)	Oxalate
W	Whole blood
U	Urine
F	Feces
CSF	Cerebrospinal fluid
AF	Amniotic fluid
(NaC)	Sodium citrate
(NH_4H)	Ammonium heparinate

TABLE 710–5. Key to Comments

30°, 37°	Temperature of enzymatic analysis (Celsius)
a	Values obtained are significantly method-dependent
b	Values in older males are higher than those in older females
c	Values in older females are higher than those in older males
d	Atomic absorption
e	Borate affinity chromatography
f	Cation-exchange chromatography
g	Ektachem, proprietary analytic system of Johnson & Johnson Clinical Diagnostics, Inc.
i	Electrophoresis
j	Enzymatic assay
k	Enzyme-amplified immunoassay
l	Fluorometric method
m	Fluorescence-activated cell sorting (FACS)
n	Fluorescence polarization
o	Gas chromatography
p	High-performance liquid chromatography (HPLC)
q	Indirect fluorescent antibody (IFA) assay
r	Ion-selective electrode
s	Nephelometry
t	Optical density
u	Radial immunodiffusion (RID)
v	Radioimmunoassay (RIA)
w	Spectrophotometry

REFERENCE LABORATORY VALUES

TABLE 710–6. Reference Ranges

I. Analyses of Blood

A. Formed Elements, Indices, and Coagulation Factors

Analyte or Procedure	Specimen	Reference Values (USA)		Conversion Factor	Reference Values (SI)	Comments
Activated partial thromboplastin time (APTT)	P(C)	25–35s Infants <90 s		×1	25–35 s Infants <90 s	
Clotting time Lee-White, 37°C	W	Glass tubes 5–8 min (5–15 min at RT) Silicone tubes about 30 min prolonged			Glass tubes 5–8 min (5–15 min at RT) Silicone tubes about 30 min prolonged	
Coagulation factor assays Factor I, see *Fibrinogen* Factor II	P(C)	0.5–1.5 U/mL or 60–150% of normal		×1	0.5–1.5 kU/L *or* 60–150 AU	
Factor IV, see *Calcium* Factor V		0.5–2.0 U/mL or 60–150% of normal		×1	0.5–2.0 kU/L *or* 60–150 AU	
Factor VII		65–135% of normal		×1	65–135 AU	
Factor VIII		60–145% of normal		×1	60–145 AU	
Factor VIII antigen		50–200% of normal		×1	50–200 AU	
Factor IX		60–140% of normal		×1	60–140 AU	
Factor X		60–130% of normal		×1	60–130 AU	
Factor XI		65–135% of normal		×1	65–135 AU	
Factor XII		65–150% of normal		×1	65–150 AU	
Factor XIII (fibrin stabilizing factor, FSF)	W(C,O)	Minimal hemostatic level 0.02–0.05 U/mL 1–2% of normal		×1,000 ×1	20–50 U/L or 1–2 AU	
Fibrin degradation products (D-dimer)	P(C)	Adults 68–494 µg/L Mean 207		×1	68–494 µg/L Mean 207	(Pittet et al)
Fibrinogen	(NaC)	Newborn: 125–300 mg/dL Adult: 200–400		×0.01	1.25–3.00 g/L 2.00–4.00	

Erythrocytes:

Erythrocyte count (RBC count)	W(E)	Millions of cells/mm³(µL)			×10¹² cells/L	
		Cord blood	3.9–5.5		3.9–5.5	
		1–3 d (cap)	4.0–6.6	×1	4.0–6.6	
		1 wk	3.9–6.3		3.9–6.3	
		2 wk	3.6–6.2		3.6–6.2	
		1 mo	3.0–5.4		3.0–5.4	
		2 mo	2.7–4.9		2.7–4.9	
		3–6 mo	3.1–4.5		3.1–4.5	
		0.5–2 yr	3.7–5.3		3.7–5.3	
		2–6 yr	3.9–5.3		3.9–5.3	
		6–12 yr	4.0–5.2		4.0–5.2	
		12–18 yr, M	4.5–5.3		4.5–5.3	
		F	4.1–5.1		4.1–5.1	

Hematocrit (HCT, Hct) Calculated from MCV and RBC count (electronic displacement or laser)	W(E)	% of packed red cells (V red cells/V whole blood cells × 100)			Volume fraction (V red cells/V whole blood)	
		1 d (cap)	48–69%	×0.01	0.48–0.69	
		2 d	48–75%		0.48–0.75	
		3 d	44–72%		0.44–0.72	
		2 mo	28–42%		0.28–0.42	
		6–12 yr	35–45%		0.35–0.45	
		12–18 yr, M	37–49%		0.37–0.49	
		F	36–46%		0.36–0.46	
		18–49 yr, M	41–53%		0.41–0.53	
		F	36–46%		0.36–0.46	

Hemoglobin (Hb)	W(E)	g/dL			mmol/L	MW Hb = 64,500
		1–3 d (cap)	14.5–22.5	×0.155	2.25–3.49	
		2 mo	9.0–14.0		1.40–2.17	
		6–12 yr	11.5–15.5		1.78–2.40	
		12–18 yr, M	13.0–16.0		2.02–2.48	
		F	12.0–16.0		1.86–2.48	
		18–49 yr, M	13.5–17.5		2.09–2.27	
		F	12.0–16.0		1.86–2.48	
	P(H)	See *Blood, chemical elements*				

Erythrocyte indices (RBC indices): Mean corpuscular hemoglobin (MCH)		pg/cell			fmol/cell	
		Birth	31–37	×0.0155	0.48–0.57	
		1–3 d (cap)	31–37		0.48–0.57	
		1 wk–1 mo	28–40		0.43–0.62	
		2 mo	26–34		0.40–0.53	
		3–6 mo	25–35		0.39–0.54	
		0.5–2 yr	23–31		0.36–0.48	
		2–6 yr	24–30		0.37–0.47	
		6–12 yr	25–33		0.39–0.51	
		12–18 yr	25–35		0.39–0.54	
	W(E)	18–49 yr	26–34		0.40–0.53	

TABLE 710–6. Reference Ranges *Continued*

Analyte or Procedure	Specimen	Reference Values (USA)		Conversion Factor	Reference Values (SI)		Comments
Mean corpuscular hemoglobin concentration (MCHC)	W(E)	% Hb/cell or g Hb/dL RBC			mmol Hb/L RBC		
		Birth	30–36	×0.155	4.65–5.58		
		1–3 day (cap)	29–37		4.50–5.74		
		1–2 wk	28–38		4.34–5.89		
		1–2 mo	29–37		4.50–5.74		
		3 mo–2 yr	30–36		4.65–5.58		
		2–18 yr	31–37		4.81–5.74		
		>18 yr	31–37		4.81–5.74		
Mean corpuscular volume (MCV)	W(E)	µm³			fL		
		1–3 d (cap)	95–121	×1	95–121		
		0.5–2 yr	70–86		70–86		
		6–12 yr	77–95		77–95		
		12–18 yr, M	78–98		78–98		
		F	78–102		78–102		
		18–49 yr, M	80–100		80–100		
		F	80–100		80–100		
Erythrocyte sedimentation rate (ESR) Westergren, modified		mm/hr		×1	mm/hr		
		Child	0–10		0–10		
		Adult M, <50	0–15		0–15		
	W(E)	F, <50	0–20		0–20		
Wintrobe		Child	0–13		0–13		
		Adult M,	0–9		0–9		
		F,	0–20		0–20		
ZETA		41–54%			41–54 AU		
Leukocyte count (WBC)	W(E)	×1,000 cells/mm³ (µL)			×10⁹ cells/L		
		Birth	9.0–30.0	×1	9.0–30.0		
		24 hr	9.4–34.0		9.4–34.0		
		1 mo	5.0–19.5		5.0–19.5		
		1–3 yr	6.0–17.5		6.0–17.5		
		4–7 yr	5.5–15.5		5.5–15.5		
		8–13 yr	4.5–13.5		4.5–13.5		
		Adult	4.5–11.0		4.5–11.0		
Leukocyte differential	W(E)	%			Number fraction		
Myelocytes		0		×0.01	0		
Neutrophils—"bands"		3–5			0.03–0.05		
Neutrophils—"segs"		54–62			0.54–0.62		
Lymphocytes		25–33			0.25–0.33		
Monocytes		3–7			0.03–0.07		
Eosinophils		1–3			0.01–0.03		
Basophils		0–0.75			0–0.0075		
		Cells/mm³ (µL)			×10⁶ cells/L		
Myelocytes		0		×1	0		
Neutrophils—"bands"		150–400			150–400		
Neutrophils—"segs"		3,000–5,800			3,000–5,800		
Lymphocytes		1,500–3,000			1,500–3,000		
Monocytes		285–500			285–500		
Eosinophils		50–250			50–250		
Basophils		15–50			15–50		

			Age				
Lymphocyte Subsets	W(E)	*2–3 mo*	*4–8 mo*	*12–23 mo*	*24–59 mo*		in (Denny et al)
Median lymphocytes, total		5.68 × 10⁹/L	5.99 × 10⁹/L	5.16 × 10⁹/L	4.06 × 10⁹/L		
5th–95th centiles		2.92–8.84	3.61–8.84	2.18–8.27	2.40–5.89		
Median CD3 lymphocytes		4.03 × 10⁹/L	4.27 × 10⁹/L	3.33 × 10⁹/L	3.04 × 10⁹/L		
5th–9th centiles		2.07–6.54	2.28–6.45	1.46–5.44	1.61–4.23		
Median CD4 lymphocytes		2.83 × 10⁹/L	2.95 × 10⁹/L	2.07 × 10⁹/L	1.80 × 10⁹/L		
5th–95th centiles		1.46–5.11	1.69–4.60	1.02–3.60	0.90–2.86		
Median CD8 lymphocytes		1.41 × 10⁹/L	1.45 × 10⁹/L	1.32 × 10⁹/L	1.18 × 10⁹/L		
5th–95th centiles		0.65–2.45	0.72–2.49	0.57–2.23	0.63–1.91		
Median % lymphocytes		66	64	59	50		
5th–95th centiles		55–78	45–79	44–72	38–64		
Median % CD3 lymphocytes		72	71	66	72		
5th–95th centiles		60–87	57–84	53–81	62–80		
Median % CD4 lymphocytes		52	49	43	42		
5th–95th centiles		41–64	36–61	31–54	35–51		
Median % CD8 lymphocytes		25	24	25	30		
5th–95th centiles		16–35	16–34	16–38	22–38		

Analyte or Procedure	Specimen	Reference Values (USA)		Conversion Factor	Reference Values (SI)		Comments
Osmotic fragility test (RBC fragility) pH 7.4, 20°C	W(H)	%NaCl (g/dL)	% Hemolysis		NaCl (g/L)	Hemolyzed fraction	
		0.30	97–100	×0.01 (hemolyzed fraction)	3.0	0.97–1.00	
		0.35	90–99		3.5	0.90–0.99	
		0.40	50–95		4.0	0.50–0.95	
		0.45	5–45		4.5	0.05–0.45	
		0.50	0–6		5.0	0.00–0.06	
		0.55	0		5.5	0.00	
Osmotic fragility test (sterile incubation) at 37°C		%NaCl (g/dL)	% Hemolysis		NaCl (g/L)	Hemolyzed fraction	
		0.20	95–100	×0.01 (hemolyzed fraction)	2.0	0.95–1.00	
		0.30	85–100		3.0	0.85–1.00	
		0.35	75–100		3.5	0.75–1.00	
		0.40	65–100		4.0	0.65–1.00	
		0.45	55–95		4.5	0.55–0.95	
		0.50	40–85		5.0	0.40–0.85	

Table continued on following page

REFERENCE LABORATORY VALUES

TABLE 710–6. **Reference Ranges** *Continued*

REFERENCE LABORATORY VALUES

Analyte or Procedure	Specimen	Reference Values (USA)		Conversion Factor	Reference Values (SI)		Comments
		0.55	15–70		5.5	0.15–0.70	
		0.60	0–40		6.0	0.00–0.40	
		0.65	0–10		6.5	0.00–0.10	
		0.70	0–5		7.0	0.00–0.05	
		0.85	0		8.5	0.00	
Partial thromboplastin time (PTT) Nonactivated Activated, see *Activated partial thromboplastin time*	W(NaC)	60–85 s (platelin)			60–85 s		
Platelet count (thrombocyte count)	W(E)	×10³/mm³ (µL) Newborn 84–478 (after 1 wk, same as adult) Adult 150–400		×10⁶	×10⁹/L 84–478 150–400		(Buck)
Prothrombin time (PT) One-stage (Quick)	W(NaC)	In general, 11–15 s (varies with type of thromboplastin) Newborn prolonged by 2–3 s International normalized ratio (INR) used only for patients receiving Coumarin		×1	11–15 s Newborn prolonged by 2–3 s INR used only for patients receiving Coumarin		
		Clinical problem	Target INR		Clinical problem	Target INR	
		Deep venous thrombosis	2.0–3.0		Deep venous thrombosis	2.0–3.0	
		Prosthetic heart valve	2.5–3.0		Prosthetic heart valve	2.5–3.0	
Two-stage modified (Ware and Seegers)	W(NaC)	18–22 s			18–22 s		
RBC count, see *Erythrocyte count* RBC fragility, see *Osmotic fragility*							
Red cell volume	W(H)	M 20–36 mL/kg F 19–31		×0.001	M 0.020–0.036 L/kg F 0.019–0.031		
Reticulocyte count	W(E,H,O)	Adults 0.5–1.5% of erythrocytes or 25,000–75,000/mm³ (µL)		×0.01 ×10⁶	0.005–0.015 (number fraction) or 25,000–75,000 × 10⁶/L Number fraction		
			%				
	W (capillary)	1 day	0.4–6.0	×0.01	0.004–0.060		
		7 day	<0.1–1.3		<0.001–0.013		
		1–4 wk	<1.0–1.2		<0.001–0.012		
		5–6 wk	<0.1–2.4		<0.001–0.024		
		7–8 wk	0.1–2.9		0.001–0.029		
		9–10 wk	<0.1–2.6		<0.001–0.026		
		11–12 wk	0.1–1.3		0.001–0.013		
Sedimentation rate, see *Erythrocyte* *sedimentation rate*							
Sickle cell tests Sodium metabisulfite Dithionite test	W (E,H,O) W (E,H,O)	Negative Negative					
Sucrose hemolysis and sugar-water tests for paroxysmal noctural hemoglobinuria (PNH)	W (C,O)	≤5% lysis 6–10% lysis questionable		×0.01	Lysed fraction ≤0.05 Lysed fraction 0.06–0.10 questionable		
Thrombin time	W (NaC)	Control time ± 2 s when control is 9–13 s			Control time ± 2 s when control is 9–13 s		
Thromboplastin time, activated, see *Activated partial thromboplastin* *time (APTT)*							
Tourniquet test		<5–10 petechiae in 2.5 cm circle on forearm (halfway between systolic and diastolic pressure for 5 min); 0–8 petechiae in 6 cm circle (50 mm Hg for 15 min); 10–20 petechiae in 5 cm circle (80 mm Hg)			<5–10 petechiae in 2.5 cm circle on forearm (halfway between systolic and diastolic pressure for 5 min); 0–8 petechiae in 6 cm circle (50 mm Hg for 15 min); 10–20 petechiae in 5 cm circle (80 mm Hg)		
WBC, see *Leukocyte*							
B. Chemical Elements							
Acetone Semiquantitative Quantitative	S,P(O)	Negative (<3 mg/dL) 0.3–2.0 mg/dL		×0.1722	Negative (<0.5 mmol/L) 0.05–0.34 mmol/L		
Adrenocorticotropic hormone (ACTH)	P(H)		pg/mL		ng/L		
		Cord:	130–160	×1	130–160		
		1–7 day postnatal	100–140		100–140		
		Adults 0800 hr	25–100		25–100		
		1800 hr	<50		<50		
Alanine aminotransferase (ALT, SGPT)	S	0–5 day	6–50 U/L	×1	6–50 U/L		37°bw
		1–19 yr	5–45		5–45		(Lockitch, et al, 1988a)
Albumin	P	Premature 1 day	1.8–3.0 g/dL	×10	18–30 g/L		g (Meites)
		Full term <6 day	2.5–3.4		25–34		
		<5 yr	3.9–5.0		39–50		
		5–19 yr	4.0–5.3		40–53		
Aldolase	S	10–24 mo	3.4–11.8 U/L	×1	3.4–11.8 U/L		j (Visnapu et al)
		25 mo–16 yr	1.2–8.8		1.2–8.8		
Aldosterone	S,P(H,E)	Supine					(Esoterix Endocrinology) *Ad lib* sodium intake
		Premature infants					
		26–28 wk	5–635 ng/dL	×0.0277	0.14–17.6 nmol/L		
		31–35 wk	19–141		0.53–3.9		
		Full-term infants					
		3 day	7–184 ng/dL		0.19–5.1 nmol/L		
		1 wk	5–175		0.14–4.8		
		1–12 mo	5–90		0.14–2.5		

TABLE 710–6. Reference Ranges *Continued*

Analyte or Procedure	Specimen	Reference Values (USA)		Conversion Factor	Reference Values (SI)	Comments
		Children	Supine			
		1–2 yr	7–54 ng/dL		0.19–1.5 nmol/L	
		2–10 yr	3–35		0.1–0.97	
		10–15 yr	2–22		0.1–0.6	
Alkaline phosphatase, see *Phosphatase alkaline*						
Amino acids, plasma, quantitative	P(H)					(Shapira, et al)

	Premature 0–6 wk µmol/L	Full-term 0–1 mo µmol/L	1–24 mo µmol/L	2–18 yr µmol/L	Adult µmol/L	×1	0–6 wk µmol/L	0–1 mo µmol/L	1–24 mo µmol/L	2–18 yr µmol/L	Adult µmol/L
1-Methylhistidine	4–28	0–43	0–44	0–42	72–124		4–28	0–43	0–44	0–42	72–124
3-Methylhistidine	5–33	0–5	0–5	0–5	0		5–33	0–5	0–5	0–5	0
Alanine	212–504	131–710	133–439	152–547	177–583		212–504	131–710	133–439	152–547	177–583
Arginine	34–96	6–140	12–133	10–140	15–128		34–96	6–140	12–133	10–140	15–128
Asparagine	90–295	29–132	21–95	23–112	35–74		90–295	29–132	21–95	23–112	35–74
Aspartic acid	24–50	20–129	0–23	1–24	1–25		24–50	20–129	0–23	1–24	1–25
Citrulline	20–87	10–45	3–35	1–46	12–55		20–87	10–45	3–35	1–46	12–55
Cystathionine	5–10	0–3	0–5	0–3	0–3		5–10	0–3	0–5	0–3	0–3
Cystine	15–70	17–98	16–84	5–45	5–82		15–70	17–98	16–84	5–45	5–82
Ethanolamine	–	0–115	0–4	0–7	0–153		–	0–115	0–4	0–7	0–153
Glutamic acid	107–276	62–620	10–133	5–150	10–131		107–276	62–620	10–133	5–150	10–131
Glutamine	248–850	376–709	246–1182	254–823	205–756		248–850	376–709	246–1182	254–823	205–756
Glycine	298–602	232–740	81–436	127–341	151–490		298–602	232–740	81–436	127–341	151–490
Histidine	72–134	30–138	41–101	41–125	0–8		72–134	30–138	41–101	41–125	0–8
Hydroxylysine	0	0–7	0–7	0–2	0		0	0–7	0–7	0–2	0
Hydroxyproline	tr–80	0–91	0–63	3–45	0–53		tr–80	0–91	0–63	3–45	0–53
Isoleucine	23–85	26–91	31–86	22–107	30–108		23–85	26–91	31–86	22–107	30–108
Leucine	151–220	48–160	47–155	49–216	72–201		151–220	48–160	47–155	49–216	72–201
Lysine	128–255	92–325	52–196	48–284	0–39		128–255	92–325	52–196	48–284	0–39
Methionine	37–91	10–60	9–42	7–47	10–42		37–91	10–60	9–42	7–47	10–42
Ornithine	77–212	48–211	22–103	10–163	48–195		77–212	48–211	22–103	10–163	48–195
Phenylalanine	98–213	38–137	31–75	26–91	35–85		98–213	38–137	31–75	26–91	35–85
Phosphoethanolamine	5–35	3–27	0–6	0–69	0–40		5–35	3–27	0–6	0–69	0–40
Phosphoserine	10–45	7–47	1–20	1–30	2–14		10–45	7–47	1–20	1–30	2–14
Proline	92–310	110–417	52–298	59–369	97–329		92–310	110–417	52–298	59–369	97–329
Sarcosine	0	0–625	0	0–9	0		0	0–625	0	0–9	0
Serine	127–248	99–395	71–186	69–187	58–181		127–248	99–395	71–186	69–187	58–181
Taurine	151–411	46–492	15–143	0–170	54–210		151–411	46–492	15–143	0–170	54–210
Threonine	150–330	90–329	24–174	35–226	60–225		150–330	90–329	24–174	35–226	60–225
Tryptophan	28–136	0–60	23–71	0–79	10–140		28–136	0–60	23–71	0–79	10–140
Tyrosine	147–420	55–147	22–108	24–115	34–112		147–420	55–147	22–108	24–115	34–112
Valine	99–220	86–190	64–294	74–321	119–336		99–220	86–190	64–294	74–321	119–336
α-Aminoadipic acid	0	0	0	0	0–6		0	0	0	0	0–6
α-Aminobutyric acid	14–52	8–24	3–26	4–31	5–41		14–52	8–24	3–26	4–31	5–41
β-Alanine	0	0–10	0–7	0–7	0–12		0	0–10	0–7	0–7	0–12
β-Aminoisobutyric acid	0	0	0	0	0		0	0	0	0	0
γ-Aminobutyric acid	0	0–2	0	0	0		0	0–2	0	0	0

Analyte or Procedure	Specimen	Reference Values (USA)		Conversion Factor	Reference Values (SI)	Comments
Aminolevulinic acid (ALA)	S	15–23 µg/dL (lower in child)		×0.076	1.1–1.8 µmol/L	
Ammonia	W	<30 day	21–95 µmol/L	×1	<30 day · 21–95 µmol/L	(Diaz et al)
		1–12 mo	18–74		1–12 mo · 18–74	
		1–14 yr	17–68		1–14 yr · 17–68	
		>14 yr	19–71		>14 yr · 19–71	
Amylase	S,P	1–19 yr	30–100 U/L % Pancreatic	×1	30–100 U/L % Pancreatic fraction	(Lockitch et al, 1988a) (Gillard et al)
Isoenzymes	S,P(H)	Cord—8 mo	0–34%	×0.01	0–0.34	
		9 mo–4 yr	5–56%		0.05–0.56	
		5–19 yr	23–59%		0.23–0.59	
Androstenedione	S	Tanner Age	Male			(Esoterix Endocrinology)
		1 <9.8 yr	8–50 ng/dL	×0.03492	0.28–1.75	
		2 9.8–14.5	31–65		1.08–2.27	
		3 10.7–15.4	50–100		1.75–3.49	
		4 11.8–16.2	48–140		1.68–4.89	
		5 12.8–17.3	65–210		2.27–7.33	
		Adult 18–40	75–205		2.62–7.16	
	S	Tanner Age	Female			
		1 <9.2 yr	8–50 ng/dL	×0.03492	0.28–1.75	
		2 9.2–13.7	42–100		1.47–3.49	
		3 10.0–14.4	80–190		2.79–6.63	
		4 10.7–15.6	77–225		2.69–7.86	
		5 11.8–18.6	80–240		2.79–8.38	
		Adult 18–40	60–245		2.10–8.56	
		Postmenopausal	30–120		1.05–4.19	
Anion gap (sodium – [chloride + bicarbonate])	P(H)	7–16 mEq/L		×1	7–16 mEq/L	
Anti-deoxyribonuclease B titer (anti-DNase B titer)	S	Age	Upper limit of normal	×1	Age · Upper limit of normal	(Kaplan et al)
		4–6 yr	240–480 U		4–6 yr · 240–480 U	
		7–12 yr	480–800 U		7–12 yr · 480–800 U	
Antidiuretic hormone (hADH, vasopressin)	P(E)	Plasma osmolarity mOsm/kg	Plasma ADH pg/mL		Plasma ADH ng/L	
		270–280	<1.5	×1	<1.5	
		280–285	<2.5		<2.5	
		285–290	1–5		1–5	
		290–295	2–7		2–7	
		295–300	4–12		4–12	

Table continued on following page

TABLE 710–6. **Reference Ranges** *Continued*

Analyte or Procedure	Specimen	Reference Values (USA)		Conversion Factor	Reference Values (SI)		Comments
Antistreptolysin-O titer (ASO titer)	S	Age 2–5 yr 6–9 yr 10–12 yr	Upper limit of normal 120–160 Todd units 240 Todd units 320 Todd units		Age 2–5 yr 6–9 yr 10–12 yr	Upper limit of normal 120–160 Todd units 240 Todd units 320 Todd units	(Kaplan et al)
α-1-Antitrypsin	S	0–5 day 143–440 mg/dL 1–9 yr 147–245 9–19 yr 152–317		×0.01	1.43–4.40 g/L 1.47–2.45 1.52–3.17		(Lockitch et al, 1988b)
Apolipoproteins A-1	S	2–12 mo 133 ± 27 mg/dL 2–10 yr 143 ± 18		×0.01	1.33 ± 0.27 g/L 1.43 ± 0.18		(Baroni et al)
B	S	2–12 mo 73 ± 16 mg/dL 2–10 yr 78 ± 17		×0.01	0.73 ± 0.16 g/L 0.78 ± 0.17		
CII	S	2–12 mo 47.0 ± 16 mg/L 2–10 yr 41.0 ± 16		×1	47.0 ± 16 mg/L 41.0 ± 16		
CIII	S	2–12 mo 76.0 ± 29 mg/L 2–10 yr 69.0 ± 22		×1	76.0 ± 29 mg/L 69.0 ± 22		
E	S	2–12 mo 41.0 ± 9 mg/L 2–10 yr 39.0 ± 10		×1	41.0 ± 9 mg/L 39.0 ± 10		
Lipoprotein(a)	S	2–12 mo 42.0 ± 36 mg/L 2–10 yr 64.0 ± 57		×1	42.0 ± 36 mg/L 64.0 ± 57		
		6–16 yr Median: 19 mg/dL Range: 11–95 mg/dL		×10	6–16 yr Median: 190 mg/L Range: 110–950 mg/L		By immunoturbimetry (Laskowska-Klita et al)
Ascorbic acid, see *Vitamin C* Aspartate aminotransferase (AST, SGOT)	S	0–5 day 35–140 U/L 1–9 yr 15–55 10–19 yr 5–45		×1	35–140 U/L 15–55 5–45		37° b (Lockitch et al, 1988b)
Base excess	W(H)		mmol/L Newborn (–10)–(–2) Infant (–7)–(–1) Child (–4)–(+2) Thereafter (–3)–(+3)	×1	mmol/L (–10)–(–2) (–7)–(–1) (–4)–(+2) (–3)–(+3)		
Bicarbonate	S,P	Arterial 21–28 mmol/L Venous 22–29		×1	21–28 mmol/L 22–29		
Bile acids, total	S, fasting S, 2 hr pc F	0.3–2.3 µg/mL 1.8–3.2 µg/mL 120–225 mg/24 hr		×1 ×1	0.3–2.3 mg/L 1.8–3.2 mg/L 120–225 mg/L		
Bilirubin, total	S,P		Premature mg/dL	Full-term mg/dL	Premature µmol/L	Full-term µmol/L	
	S	Cord blood <2.0 0–1 day <8.0 1–2 day <12.0 2–5 day <16.0 >5 day <20.0	<2.0 <6.0 <8.0 <12.0 <10	×17.10	<34 <137 <205 <274 <340	<34 <103 <137 <205 <171	
Bilirubin, conjugated	S	0–0.2 mg/dL		×17.10	0–3.4 µmol/L		
Bleeding time (BBT) Ivy		Normal 2–7 min Borderline 7–11 min		×1	2–7 min 7–11 min		
Simplate (G-D)		2.75–8 min			2.75–8 min		
Blood volume	W(H)	M 52–83 mL/kg F 50–75 mL/kg		×0.001	M 0.052–0.083 L/kg F 0.050–0.075 L/kg		
Brucellosis, agglutinins	S	≤1:8		×1	≤1:8		
C-peptide of insulin	S	Children 0.4–2.2 ng/mL 8:00 AM fasting		×1	0.4–2.2 µg/L		(Esoterix Endocrinology)
C-reactive protein	S	Cord blood 52–1,330 ng/mL 2–12 yr 67–1,800		×1	52–1,330 µg/L 67–1,800		k (Unten and Hokama)
C-reactive protein (high sensitivity)	S	Values: geometric mean in mg/L (mean ± 2 SD)		×1	Values: geometric mean in mg/L s (mean ± 2 SD)		(Chenillot et al)
		Males	Females		Males	Females	
		5–14y: 0.37 mg/L (0.17–1.07) 15–28y: 0.47 mg/L (0.31–1.38) 29–75y: 0.98 mg/L (0.34–1.90)	0.38 mg/L (0.17–1.10) 0.62 mg/L (0.20–1.90) 0.98 mg/L (0.31–3.13)		5–14y: 0.37 mg/l (0.17–1.07) 15–28y: 0.47 mg/l (0.17–1.38) 29–75y: 0.98 mg/l (0.34–2.85)	0.38 mg/l (0.17–1.10) 0.62 mg/l (0.20–1.90) 0.98 mg/l (0.31–3.13)	
Calcitonin	S,P(H,E)	Male	Female	×0.28	Male	Female	(Nichols Institute Diagnostics)
		3–26 pg/mL Higher in newborn infants	2–17 pg/mL		0.8–7.2 pmol/L	0.6–4.7 pmol/L	
Calcium, ionized (Ca)	S,P(H), W(H)		mg/dL		mmol/L		
		Cord blood 5.0–6.0 Newborn, 3–24 hr 4.3–5.1 24–48 hr 4.0–4.7 Thereafter 4.8–4.92 *or* 2.24–2.46 mEq/L		×0.25 ×0.5	1.25–1.50 1.07–1.27 1.00–1.17 1.12–1.23 1.12–1.23		
Calcium, total	S		mg/dL		mmol/L		
		Cord blood 9.0–11.5 Newborn, 3–24 hr 9.0–10.6 24–48 7.0–12.0 4–7 d 9.0–10.9 Child 8.8–10.8 Thereafter 8.4–10.2		×0.25	2.25–2.88 2.3–2.65 1.75–3.0 2.25–2.73 2.2–2.70 2.1–2.55		
Carbon dioxide, partial pressure (Pco₂)	W(H)		mmHg		kPa		
		Newborn 27–40 Infant 27–41 Thereafter, M 35–48 F 32–45		×0.1333	3.6–5.3 3.6–5.5 4.7–6.4 4.3–6.0		

TABLE 710–6. Reference Ranges *Continued*

Analyte or Procedure	Specimen	Reference Values (USA)				Conversion Factor	Reference Values (SI)			Comments
Carbon dioxide, total (tco₂)	S,P (H)		mmol/L				mmol/L			
		Cord	14–22			×1	14–22			
		Premature	14–27				14–27			
		Newborn	13–22				13–22			
		Infant	20–28				20–28			
		Child	20–28				20–28			
		Thereafter	23–30				23–30			
Carbon monoxide (carboxyhemoglobin)	W(E)	Nonsmokers	<2% HbCO			×0.01	HbCO fraction <0.02			
		Smokers	<10%				<0.10			
		Lethal	>50%				>0.5			
Carnitine	P		μmol/L					μmol/L		(Schmidt-Sommerfeld, et al)
		Age	Total	Free			Age	Total	Free	
		1 day	36.4 ± 10.8	20.1 ± 6.7		×1	1 day	36.4 ± 10.8	20.1 ± 6.7	
		2–7 day	25.2 ± 4.1	14.9 ± 3.0			2–7 day	25.2 ± 4.1	14.9 ± 3.0	
		8–28 day	36.7 ± 10.5	27.6 ± 9.7			8–28 day	36.7 ± 10.5	27.6 ± 9.7	
		29 day–1 yr	47.6 ± 7.7	35.5 ± 6.5			29 day–1 yr	47.6 ± 7.7	35.5 ± 6.5	
		1–6 yr	54.4 ± 9.9	41.7 ± 7.9			1–6 yr	54.4 ± 9.9	41.7 ± 7.9	
		6–10 yr	56.2 ± 11.4	41.4 ± 10.0			6–10 yr	56.2 ± 11.4	41.4 ± 10.0	
		10–17 yr	53.4 ± 9.5	39.4 ± 8.7			10–17 yr	53.4 ± 9.5	39.4 ± 8.7	
		22–60 yr	54.0 ± 12.6	39.1 ± 8.6			22–60 yr	54.0 ± 12.6	39.1 ± 8.6	
β-Carotene	S		μg/dL				μmol/L			
		Infant	20–70			×0.0186	0.37–1.30			
		Child	40–130				0.74–2.42			
		Thereafter	60–200				1.12–3.72			
Catecholamines, fractionated	P(E)	Norepinephrine								
			pg/mL							
		Supine	100–400			×5.911	591–2,364 pmol/L			
		Standing	300–900				1,773–5,320			
		Epinephrine	pg/mL							
		Supine	<70			×5.458	<382 pmol/L			
		Standing	<100				<546			
		Dopamine	<30 pg/mL			×6.528	<196 pmol/L			
		(no postural change)					(no postural change)			
Ceruloplasmin	S	0–5 day	5–26 mg/dL			×10	50–260 mg/L			CS (Lockitch et al, 1988b)
		1–19 yr	20–46 mg/dL				200–460 mg/L			
Chloride	S,P(H)	Cord blood	96–104 mmol/L			×1	96–104 mmol/L			
		Newborn	97–110				97–110			
		Thereafter	98–106				98–106			
Cholesterol, total	S	1–3 yr	45–182 mg/dL			×0.0259	1.15–4.70 mmol/L			j (Lockitch et al, 1988a)
		4–6 yr	109–189				2.80–4.80			
	S		Male			×0.0259	Male			(Mayo Laboratories)
			Percentiles					Percentiles		
		Age	5	75	95		Age	5	75	95
		6–9 yr	126	172	191 mg/dL		6–9 yr	3.26	4.45	4.94 mmol/L
		10–14 yr	130	179	204		10–14 yr	3.36	4.63	5.28
		15–19 yr	114	167	198		15–19 yr	2.95	4.32	5.12
			Female				Female			
			Percentiles					Percentiles		
		Age	5	75	95			5	75	95
		6–9 yr	122	173	209 mg/dL		6–9 yr	3.16	4.47	5.41 mmol/L
		10–14 yr	124	174	217		10–14 yr	3.21	4.50	5.61
		15–19 yr	125	175	212		15–19 yr	3.23	4.53	5.48
Chorionic gonadotropin	S,P(E)	Child and male undetectable								(Abbott)
β-Subunit (β-hCG)		F, post-conception	mIU/mL			×1	IU/L			
		1–2 wk	9–130				9–130			
		2–3 wk	75–2,600				75–2,600			
		3–4 wk	850–20,800				850–20,800			
		4–5 wk	4,000–100,200				4,000–100,200			
		5–10 wk	11,500–289,000				11,500–289,000			
		10–14 wk	18,300–137,000				18,300–137,000			
Complement components										
Total hemolytic complement activity (CH₅₀)	P(E)	75–160 U/mL				×1	75–160 IU/L			
Total complement decay rate (functional)	P(E)	~10–20%				×0.01	~0.10–0.20 (fraction of decay rate) > 0.50			
		Deficiency >50%					(fraction of decay rate)			
Classic pathway components										
C1q	S		mg/dL				mg/L			
		Cord blood	1.0–14.9			×10	10–149			
		1 mo	2.2–6.2				22–62			
		6 mo	1.2–7.6				12–76			
		Adult	5.1–7.9				51–79			
C1r	S	2.5–3.8 mg/dL				×10	25–38			
C1s (C1 esterase)	S	2.5–3.8 mg/dL				×10	25–38			
C2	S		mg/dL				mg/L			
		Cord blood	1.6–2.8			×10	16–28			
		1 mo	1.9–3.9				19–39			
		6 mo	2.4–3.6				24–36			
		Adult	1.6–4.0				16–40			
C3	S		mg/dL				mg/L			s (Meites)
		Cord blood	57–116			×10	570–1,160			
		1–3 mo	53–131				530–1,310			
		3 mo–1 yr	62–180				620–1,800			

Table continued on following page

REFERENCE LABORATORY VALUES

TABLE 710–6. **Reference Ranges** *Continued*

Analyte or Procedure	Specimen	Reference Values (USA)		Conversion Factor	Reference Values (SI)	Comments
C4	S	1 yr–10 yr Adult mg/dL	77–195 83–177	×10	770–1,950 830–1,770 mg/L	s (Meites)
C5	S	Cord blood 1–3 mo 3 mo–10 yr Adult mg/dL	7–23 7–27 7–40 15–45	×10	70–230 70–270 70–400 150–450 mg/L	
C6	S	Cord blood 1 mo 6 mo Adult mg/dL	3.4–6.2 2.3–6.3 2.4–6.4 3.8–9.0	×10	34–62 23–63 24–64 38–90 mg/L	
C7	S	Cord blood 1 mo 6 mo Adult 4.9–7.0 mg/dL	1.0–4.2 2.2–5.2 3.7–7.1 4.0–7.2	×10 ×10	10–42 22–52 37–71 40–72 49–70 mg/L	
C8	S	4.3–6.3 mg/dL		×10	43–63 mg/L	
C9	S	4.7–6.9 mg/dL		×10	47–69 mg/L	
Alternative pathway components C4 binding protein	S	18.0–32.0 mg/dL		×10	180–320 mg/L	
Factor B (C3 proactivator) RID	P(E)	mg/dL Cord blood 1 mo 6 mo Adult	 7.8–15.8 6.2–28.6 16.9–29.3 14.7–33.5	×10	mg/L 78–158 62–286 169–293 147–335	
Nephelometry	S	Newborn Adult mg/dL	14–33 mg/dL 20–45	×10	140–330 mg/L 200–450 mg/L	
Properdin	S	Cord blood 1 mo 6 mo Adult	1.3–1.7 0.6–2.2 1.3–2.5 2.0–3.6	×10	13–17 6–22 13–25 20–36	
Regulatory protein b1H-globulin (C3b inactivator accelerator)	S	mg/dL Cord blood 1 mo 6 mo Adult	 26–42 24–56 33–61 40–72	×10	mg/L 260–420 240–560 330–610 400–720	
C1 inhibitor (esterase inhibitor)	P(E)	17.4–24.0 mg/dL		×10	174–240 mg/L	
Complement decay rate (functional)	S	<20% decay Deficiency >50% decay		×0.01	<0.20 (fractional decay) >0.50 (fractional decay)	
C3b inactivator (KAF)	S	mg/dL Cord blood 1 mo 6 mo Adult	 1.8–2.6 1.5–3.9 2.3–4.3 2.6–5.4	×10	mg/L 18–26 15–39 23–43 26–54	
S protein	S	41.8–60.0 mg/dL		×10	418–600 mg/L	
Copper	S	0–5 d 1–9 yr 10–14 yr 15–19 yr	9–46 µg/dL 80–150 80–121 64–160	×0.157	1.4–7.2 µmol/L 12.6–23.6 12.6–19.0 11.3–25.2	cd (Lockitch, et al., 1988c)
Corticobinding globulin (CBG), see *Transcortin*						
Cortisol	S,P(H)	µg/dL Newborn Adults, 0800 hr 1600 hr 2000 hr	 1–24 5–23 3–15 ≤50% of 0800 hr	×27.59 ×0.01	nmol/L 28–662 138–635 82–413 Fraction of 0800 hr ≤0.50	
Creatine kinase	S	Cord blood 5–8 hr 24–33 hr 72–100 hr Adult	70–380 U/L 214–1,175 130–1,200 87–725 5–130	×1	70–380 U/L 214–1,175 130–1,200 87–725 5–130	30°b (Jedeikin et al)
Creatine kinase isoenzymes	S	 Cord blood 5–8 hr 24–33 hr 72–100 hr Adult	% MB 0.3–3.1 1.7–7.9 1.8–5.0 1.4–5.4 0–2%	%BB 0.3–10.5 3.6–13.4 2.3–8.6 5.1–13.3 0		
Creatinine Jaffe, kinetic, or enzymatic	S,P	mg/dL Cord blood Newborn Infant Child Adolescent Adult M F	 0.6–1.2 0.3–1.0 0.2–0.4 0.3–0.7 0.5–1.0 0.6–1.2 0.5–1.1	×88.4	µmol/L 53–106 27–88 18–35 27–62 44–88 53–106 44–97	
Jaffe, manual	S,P	0.8–1.5 mg/dL		×88.4	70–133 µmol/L	
Creatinine clearance (endogenous)	S,P, and U	Newborn 40–65 mL/min/1.73 m² <40 yr, M 97–137 F 88–128 Decreases ~6.5 mL/min/decade				

TABLE 710–6. Reference Ranges *Continued*

Analyte or Procedure	Specimen	Reference Values (USA)			Conversion Factor	Reference Values (SI)		Comments
Cyclic AMP	P(E)	Male ng/mL 5.6–10.9 Female 3.6–8.9			×3.04	Male nmol/L 17–33 Female 11–27		
Dehydroepiandrosterone	S	Tanner	Age	Male	×0.0347			(Esoterix Endocrinology)
		1	<9.8 yr	31–345 ng/dL		1.07–11.96 nmol/L		
		2	9.8–14.5	110–495		3.81–17.16		
		3	10.7–15.4	170–585		5.89–20.28		
		4	11.8–16.2	160–640		5.55–22.19		
		5	12.8–17.3	250–900		8.67–31.21		
			Adult	160–800		5.55–27.74		
			Female					
		1	<9.2 yr	31–345 ng/dL		1.07–11.96 nmol/L		
		2	9.2–13.7	150–570		5.20–19.76		
		3	10.0–14.4	200–600		6.93–20.80		
		4	10.7–15.6	200–780		6.93–24.27		
		5	11.8–18.6	215–850		7.45–29.47		
		Adult	Follicular	160–800		5.55–27.74		
			Luteal	160–800		5.55–27.74		
Dehydroepiandrosterone sulfate (DHEA-sulfate) (DHEA-S)	S	Tanner	Age	Male	×0.026			(Esoterix Endocrinology)
		1	<9.8 y	13–83 µg/dL		0.34–2.16 µmol/L		
		2	9.8–14.5	42–109		1.09–2.83		
		3	10.7–15.4	48–200		1.25–5.2		
		4	11.8–16.2	102–385		2.65–10.01		
		5	12.8–17.3	120–370		3.12–9.62		
			21–30 y	100–460		2.60–11.96		
		Tanner	Age	Female				
		1	<9.2 yr	19–144 µg/dL		0.49–2.96 µg/dL		
		2	9.2–13.7	34–129		0.88–3.35		
		3	10.0–14.4	32–226		0.83–8.48		
		4	10.7–15.6	58–260		1.51–6.76		
		5	11.8–18.6	44–248		1.14–6.45		
			21–30 y	76–255		1.98–6.63		
Deoxycorticosterone	S				×0.03026			(Esoterix Endocrinology)
		Newborn	Very high			Very high		
		1–12 mo	7–49 ng/dL			0.2–1.5 nmol/L		
		Prepubertal (2–10 yr)	2–34 ng/dL			0.1–1 nmol/L		
		Pubertal and adult	2–19 ng/dL			0.1–0.6 nmol/L		
11-Desoxycortisol Specific compound S	S				×0.02886			(Esoterix Endocrinology)
		Full-term 3 day	13–147			0.38–4.24		
		Full-term 1–12 mo	<10–156			<0.29–4.50		
		Prepub. child. (8:00 AM)	20–155			0.58–4.47		
		Pubertal and adult (8:00 AM)	12–158			0.35–4.56		
Dihydrotestosterone (DHT)	S	Tanner	Age	Male	×0.03443			(Esoterix Endocrinology)
		1	<9.8	<3 ng/dL		<0.10 nmol/L		
		2	9.8–14.5	3–17		0.10–0.59		
		3	10.7–15.4	8–33		0.28–1.14		
		4	11.8–16.2	22–52		0.76–1.79		
		5	12.8–17.3	24–65		0.83–2.24		
			Adult	30–85		1.03–2.93		
	S	Tanner	Age	Female	×0.03443			
		1	<9.2 yr	<3 ng/dL		<0.10 nmol/L		
		2	9.2–13.7	5–12		0.17–0.41		
		3	10.0–14.4	7–19		0.24–0.65		
		4	10.7–15.6	4–13		0.14–0.45		
		5	11.8–18.6	3–18		0.10–0.62		
		Adult	Follicular	4–22		0.14–0.76		
			Luteal	4–22		0.14–0.76		
Disaccharide absorption test	S	Change in glucose from fasting value			×0.055	Change in glucose from fasting value		
		Normal	>30 mg/dL			Normal	>1.67 mmol/L	
		Inconclusive	20–30			Inconclusive	1.11–1.67	
		Abnormal	<20			Abnormal	<1.11	
Electrophoresis, hemoglobin, see *Hemoglobin electrophoresis*								
Epinephrine, see *Catecholamines, fractionated*								

Erythropoietin
  RIA
  Hemagglutination
  Bioassay
	S	<5–20 mU/mL
		25–125
		5–18
					×1	<5–20 U/L
						25–125
						5–18		

Estradiol	S	Tanner	Age	Male	×36.71			(Esoterix Endocrinology)
		1	<9.8 yr	0.5–1.1 ng/dL		18–40 pmol/L		
		2	9.8–14.5	0.5–1.6		18–59		
		3	10.7–15.4	0.5–2.5		18–92		
		4	11.8–16.2	1.0–3.6		37–132		
		5	12.8–17.3	1.0–3.6		37–132 29–128		
			Adult	0.8–3.5				
			Female					
		1	<9.2 yr	0.5–2.0 ng/dL		18–73 pmol/L		
		2	9.2–13.7	1.0–2.4		37–88		
		3	10.0–14.4	0.7–6.0		26–220		
		4	10.7–15.6	2.1–8.5		77–312		
		5	11.8–18.6	3.4–17		125–624		
		Adult	Follicular	3–10		110–367		
			Luteal	7–30		257–1,100		

Table continued on following page

REFERENCE LABORATORY VALUES

TABLE 710–6. **Reference Ranges** *Continued*

Analyte or Procedure	Specimen	Reference Values (USA)		Conversion Factor	Reference Values (SI)	Comments
Estriol (E_3), free	S	Weeks of gestation	µg/L		nmol/L	
		25	3.5–10.0	×3.47	12.1–34.7	
		28	4.0–12.5		13.9–43.4	
		30	4.5–14.0		15.6–48.6	
		32	5.0–16.0		17.4–55.5	
		34	5.5–18.5		19.1–64.2	
		36	7.0–25.0		24.3–86.8	
		37	8.0–28.0		27.8–97.2	
		38	9.0–32.0		31.2–111.0	
		39	10.0–34.0		34.7–118.0	
		40–41	10.5–25.0		36.4–86.8	
Estriol (E_3), total	S	Pregnancy (wk)	ng/mL		nmol/L	
		24–28	30–170	×3.467	104–590	
		28–32	40–220		140–760	
		32–36	60–280		208–970	
		36–40	80–350		280–1210	
		Adult, M and nonpregnant F	<2		<7	
Estrogens, total	S		pg/mL		ng/L	
		Child	<30	×1	<30	
		M	40–115		40–115	
		F, cycle—days				
		1–10 day	61–394		61–394	
		11–20 day	122–437		122–437	
		21–30 day	156–350		156–350	
		Prepubertal	≤40		≤40	
Free fatty acids	S	Premature				(Meites)
		10–55 day	0.15–0.71 mmol/L	×1	0.15–0.71 mmol/L	(Bonnefont et al)
	W	1–12 mo	0.5–1.6 mmol/L	×1	0.5–1.6 mmol/L	
		1–7 yr	0.6–1.5		0.6–1.5	
		7–15 yr	0.2–1.1		0.2–1.1	
Ferritin	S		ng/mL		µg/L	
		Newborn	25–200	×1	25–200	
		1 mo	200–600		200–600	
		2–5 mo	50–200		50–200	
		6 mo-15 yr	7–140		7–140	
		Adult, M	15–200		15–200	
		F	12–150		12–150	
α-Fetoprotein (AFP)	S	Pregnancy Wk	Median ng/mL		Median µg/L	
		15	34	×1	34	
		16	38		38	
		17	44		44	
		18	49		49	
		19	56.5		56.5	
		20	66		66	
Folate	S	Newborn 7.0–32 ng/mL		×2.265	15.9–72.4 nmol/L	
		Thereafter 1.8–9			4.1–20.4	
	W(E)	150–450 ng/mL RBCs			340–1020 nmol/L cells	
Follicle stimulating hormone (FSH)	S	Tanner Age	Male			(Esoterix Endocrinology)
		1 <9.8 yr	0.26–3.0 mIU/mL	×1	0.26–3.0 U/L	
		2 9.8–14.5	1.8–3.2		1.8–3.2	
		3 10.7–15.4	1.2–5.8		1.2–5.8	
		4 11.8–16.2	2.0–9.2		2.0–9.2	
		5 12.8–17.3	2.6–11.0		2.6–11.0	
		Adult	2.0–9.2		2.0–9.2	
		Tanner Age	Female			
		1 <9.2 yr	1.0–4.2 mIU/mL		1.0–4.2 U/L	
		2 9.2–13.7	1.0–10.8		1.0–10.8	
		3 10.0–14.4	1.5–12.8		1.5–12.8	
		4 10.7–15.6	1.5–11.7		1.5–11.7	
		5 11.8–18.6	1.0–9.2		1.0–9.2	
		Adult Follicular	1.8–11.2		1.8–11.2 mIU/mL	
		Midcycle	6–35		6–35	
		Luteal	1.8–11.2		1.8–11.2	
		Postmenopause	30–120		30–120	
Fructosamine	S	0–3 yr	1.56–2.27 mmol/L	×1	1.56–2.27 mmol/L	w (De Schepper et al)
		3–6 yr	1.73–2.34		1.73–2.34	
		6–9 yr	1.82–2.56		1.82–2.56	
		9–15 yr	2.02–2.63		2.02–2.63	
Galactose	S	Newborn	0–20 mg/dL	×0.0555	0–1.11 mmol/L	
	P	5 mo–17 yr	0.0–0.5 mg/dL		0.0–0.03 mmol/L	j (Pesce and Boudorian, 1982a)
Galactose-1-PO_4	W(H)	5 mo–17 yr	0–44 µg/g Hb	×0.0038	0–0.17 µmol/g Hb	l (Pesce and Boudorian, 1982b)
Galactose-1-PO_4 uridylyltransferase	W(H)	18–26 U/g Hb		×1	18–26 U/g Hb	(Pesce and Boudorian, 1977c)
Gastrin	S	Newborn	20–300 pg/mL	×1	20–300 ng/L <10–125	
		Children	<10–125			a (Esoterix Endocrinology)
Glucagon	P(E)	Children and adults (fasting)	50–150 pg/mL	×1	50–150 ng/L	(Esoterix Endocrinology)
Glucose	S		mg/dL		mmol/L	
		Cord blood	45–96	×0.0555	2.5–5.3	
		Premature	20–60		1.1–3.3	
		Neonate	30–60		1.7–3.3	
		Newborn				

TABLE 710–6. **Reference Ranges** *Continued*

Analyte or Procedure	Specimen	Reference Values (USA)		Conversion Factor	Reference Values (SI)		Comments
		1 day	40–60	×0.0555	2.2–3.3		
		>1 day	50–90		2.8–5.0		
		Child	60–100		3.3–5.5		
		Adult	70–105		3.9–5.8		
	W(H)	Adult	65–95		3.6–5.3		
Glucose, 2 hr post	S	<120 mg/dL		×0.0555	<6.7 mmol/L		
Glucose tolerance test (GTT)	S		mg/dL			mmol/L	(American Diabetes Association)
Oral dose, adult: 75 g Child: 1.75 g/kg of ideal weight up to maximum of 75			Normal Diabetic	×0.0555		Normal Diabetic	
		Fasting	70–105 ≥126			3.9–5.8 ≥7.0	
		60 min	120–170 ≥200			6.7–9.4 ≥11	
		90 min	100–140 ≥200			5.6–7.8 ≥11	
		120 min	70–120 ≥200			3.9–6.7 ≥11	
Glucose-6-phosphate dehydrogenase (G6PD) in erythrocytes Bishop, modified	W(E,H,C)	Adult			Adult		
		3.4–8.0 U/g Hb		×0.0645	0.22–0.52 mU/mol Hb		
		98.6–232 U/10^{12}RBC		×10^{-3}	0.10–0.23 nU/10^{6}RBC		
		1.16–2.72 U/mL RBC		×1	1.16–2.72 kU/L RBC		
		Newborn: 50% higher			Newborn: 50% higher		
Gammaglutamyltranspeptidase (GGT, GGTP)	S	Cord blood	37–193 U/L	×1	37–193 U/L		37°b (Knight and Haymond)
		0–1 mo	13–147		13–147		
		1–2 mo	12–123		12–123		
		2–4 mo	8–90		8–90		
		4 mo–10 yr	5–32		5–32		
		10–15 yr	5–24		5–24		
Growth hormone (hGH) somatotropin	S,P(E,H)						(Esoterix Endocrinology)
		Newborn					
		1 day	5–53 ng/mL	×1	5–53 µg/L		
		1 wk	5–27		5–27		
		1–12 mo	2–10		2–10		
	Fasting, at rest	Child	<0.7–6 ng/mL		<0.7–6 µg/L		
		Adult	<0.7–6		<0.7–6		
Ham's test, see *Acidified serum test*							
Haptoglobin	S	0–1 mo	<5.8–196 mg/dL	×0.01	<0.058–1.960 g/L		(Davis et al)
		1 mo–19 yr	22–164		0.220–1.640		
Hemoglobin total	W	See *Blood, formed elements*					
	P(H)	<10 mg/dL		×0.155	<1.55 µmol/L		
		<3 mg/dL with butterfly setup and 18-gauge needle			<0.47 µmol/L with butterfly setup and 18-gauge needle		
HDL Cholesterol	S	1–13 yr	35–84 mg/dL	×0.0259	0.9–2.15 mmol/L		ac (Meites)
		14–19 yr	35–65		0.90–1.65		
Glycohemoglobin hemoglobin A$_{1c}$	W(H)		% of total Hb		Fraction of total Hb		
		1–5 yr	2.1–7.7	×0.01	0.021–0.077		f (Meites)
		5–16 yr	3.0–6.2		0.030–0.062		
Total glycohemoglobin	W(H)	4–16 yr	6.0–10.0%		0.060–0.100		e (Meites)
Hemoglobin A	W (E,C,H)	>95%		×0.01	Fraction of Hb: >0.95		
Hemoglobin A$_2$ (HbA$_2$)	W(E,O)				Mass fraction		
		Adult: 1.5–3.5% (2 SD)			0.015–0.035 (2SD)		
		Lower in infants <1 yr					
Hemoglobin (Hb) electrophoresis	W(H,E,C)				Mass fraction		
		HbA >95%		×0.01	HbA >0.95		
		HbA2 1.5–3.5%			HbA2 0.015–0.035		
		HbF <2%			HbF <0.02		
Hemoglobin F	W(E)		%HbF		Mass fraction		
Alkali denaturation		1 day	63–92	×0.01	0.63–0.92		
		5 day	65–88		0.65–0.88		
		3 wk	55–85		0.55–0.85		
		6–9 wk	31–75		0.31–0.75		
		3–4 mo	<2.0–59		<0.02–0.59		
		6 mo	<2–9		<0.02–0.09		
		Adult	<2		<0.02		
Hemoglobin H (HbH) Isopropanol precipitation	W (H,E,C)	No precipitation at 40 min			No precipitation at 40 min		
Homocysteine	P	2 mo–18 yr	3.3–11.3 µmol/L	×1	3.3–11.3 µmol/L		(Vilaseca et al)
17-Hydroxyprogesterone (17-OHP)	S	Premature infants					(Esoterix Endocrinology)
		26–28 wk, day 4: 124–841 ng/dL		×0.03029	3.76–25.5 nmol/L		
		31–35 wk, day 4: 26–568			0.79–17.2		
		Full-term infants					
		3 day	7–77 ng/dL		0.2–2.33 nmol/L		
		1–12 mo					
		Male					
		Peak values of 40–200 ng/dL between 30 and 60 day			Peak values of 1.21 to 6.1 nmol/L between 30 and 60 day		
		Female	13–106 ng/dL				
		Prepubertal children			0.39–3.21 nmol/L		
		3–90 ng/dL			0.09–2.73 nmol/L		
		Tanner Age Male					
		1 <9.8 yr 3–90 ng/dL			0.09–2.73 nmol/L		
		2 9.8–14.5 5–115			0.15–3.48		
		3 10.7–15.4 10–138			0.30–4.18		

TABLE 710–6. **Reference Ranges** *Continued*

Analyte or Procedure	Specimen	Reference Values (USA)			Conversion Factor	Reference Values (SI)	Comments
		4	11.8–16.2	29–180		0.88–5.45	
		5	12.8–17.3	24–175		0.73–5.30	
		Adult		27–199		0.82–6.03	
		Tanner	Age	Female			
		1	<9.2 yr	3–82 ng/dL		0.09–2.48 nmol/L	
		2	9.2–13.7	11–98		0.33–2.97	
		3	10.0–14.4	11–155		0.33–4.69	
		4	10.7–15.6	18–230		0.55–6.97	
		5-	11.8–18.6	20–265		0.61–8.03	
		Adult	Follicular	15–70		0.45–2.12	
			Luteal	35–290		1.06–8.78	
β-Hydroxybutyrate		1–12 mo	0.1–1.0 mmol/L		×1	0.1–1.0 mmol/L	(Bonnefont et al)
		1–7 yr	<0.1–0.9			<0.1–0.9	
		7–15 yr	<0.1–0.3			<0.1–0.3	
Hypoxanthine	W	Age					(Jung et al)
		12–36 hr	2.7–11.2 µmol/L		×1	2.7–11.2 µmol/L	
		3 day	1.3–7.9			1.3–7.9	
		5 day	0.6–5.7			0.6–5.7	
Immunoglobulin A (IgA)	S	Cord blood	1.4–3.6 mg/dL		×10	14–36 mg/L	s (Meites)
		1–3 mo	1.3–53			13–530	
		4–6 mo	4.4–84			44–840	
		7 mo–1 yr	11–106			110–1060	
		2–5 yr	14–159			140–1590	
		6–10 yr	33–236			330–2360	
		Adult	70–312			700–3120	
Immunoglobulin D (IgD)	S	Newborn: none detected				None detected	
		Thereafter: 0–8 mg/dL			×10	0–80 mg/L	
Immunoglobulin E (IgE)	S	M 0–230 IU/mL			×1	0–230 kIU/L	
		F 0–170				0–170	
Immunoglobulin G (IgG)	S	Cord blood	636–1606 mg/dL		×0.01	6.36–16.06 g/L	s (Meites)
		1 mo	251–906			2.51–9.06	
		2–4 mo	176–601			1.76–6.01	
		5–12 mo	172–1069			1.72–10.69	
		1–5 yr	345–1236			3.45–12.36	
		6–10 yr	608–1572			6.08–15.72	
		Adult	639–1349			6.39–13.49	

IgG Subclasses	S	(mg/dL)				×10			(mg/L)				(Mayo Medical Laboratories 2001)

Age	IgG1	IgG2	IgG3	IgG4	IgG1	IgG2	IgG3	IgG4
Cord	435–1084	143–453	27–146	<47	4350–10840	1430–4530	70–1460	<470
1–7 day	381–937	117–382	21–115	<44	3810–9370	1170–3820	10–1150	<440
8–14 day	327–790	92–310	16–85	<40	3270–7900	920–3100	160–850	<400
3–4 wk	218–496	40–167	4–23	<33	2180–4960	400–1670	40–230	<330
2 mo	194–480	35–164	4–36	<30	1940–4800	350–1640	40–360	<300
3 mo	167–447	28–157	4–52	<24	1670–4470	280–1570	40–520	<240
4 mo	143–394	23–147	4–65	<14	1430–3940	230–1470	40–650	<140
5 mo	158–392	24–132	6–68	<13	1580–3920	240–1320	60–680	<130
6 mo	175–390	24–115	8–72	<11	1750–3900	240–1150	80–720	<110
7 mo	190–388	25–100	10–75	<10	1900–3880	250–1000	100–750	<100
8 mo	200–417	26–123	10–76	<16	2000–4170	260–1230	100–760	<160
9 mo	211–450	26–149	10–77	<22	2110–4500	260–1490	100–770	<220
10–12 mo	241–543	28–221	10–80	<39	2410–5430	280–2210	100–800	<390
13–20 mo	281–692	30–343	10–88	<68	2810–6920	300–3430	100–880	<680
21–36 mo	310–729	46–387	10–96	<77	3100–7290	460–3870	100–960	<770
3 yr	348–773	72–441	10–105	<87	3480–7730	720–4410	100–1050	<870
4 yr	370–804	88–455	11–108	<97	3700–8040	880–4550	110–1080	<970
5 yr	375–835	94–468	12–111	<106	3750–8350	940–4680	120–1110	<1060
6 yr	380–866	100–481	14–115	<115	3800–8660	1000–4810	140–1150	<1150
7 yr	385–896	105–494	16–118	<124	3850–8960	1050–4940	160–1180	<1240
8 yr	390–927	111–507	18–122	<133	3900–9270	1110–5070	180–1220	<1330
9 yr	395–958	117–520	19–125	<142	3950–9580	1170–5200	190–1250	<1420
10 yr	400–989	123–534	21–129	<151	4000–9890	1230–5340	210–1290	<1510
11 yr	405–1020	128–547	23–132	<160	4050–10200	1280–5470	230–1320	<1600
12 yr	410–1051	134–560	25–136	<169	4100–10510	1340–5600	250–1360	<1690
13 yr	415–1081	140–573	27–139	<178	4150–10810	1400–5730	270–1390	<1780
14 yr	419–1102	145–582	28–141	<184	4190–11020	1450–5820	280–1410	<1840
≥15 yr	423–1112	149–586	29–142	<187	4230–11120	1490–5860	290–1420	<1870

Analyte or Procedure	Specimen	Reference Values (USA)		Conversion Factor	Reference Values (SI)	Comments
Immunoglobulin M (IgM)	S	Cord blood	6.3–25 mg/dL	×10	63–250 mg/L	s (Meites)
		1–4 mo	17–105		170–1050	
		5–9 mo	33–126		330–1260	
		10–1 y	41–173		410–1730	
		2–8 yr	43–207		430–2070	
		9–10 yr	52–242		520–2420	
		Adult	56–352		560–3520	
Insulin (12 hr fasting)	S	Newborn	3–20 uU/mL	×1.0	3–20 mU/L	
		Thereafter	7–24		7–24	
Insulin with oral glucose tolerance test	S	Min	uU/mL		mU/L	
		0	7–24	×1	7–24	
		30	25–231		25–231	
		60	18–276		18–276	
		120	16–166		16–166	
		180	4–38		4–38	

TABLE 710–6. Reference Ranges *Continued*

Analyte or Procedure	Specimen	Reference Values (USA)				Conversion Factor	Reference Values (SI)				Comments
Insulin-like growth factor 1 (IGF-1)	S	*Infants*	Term (40 wk gestation)		Preterm (<40 wk gestation)		×1	Term		Preterm (birth = 40 wk)		(Esoterix Endocrinology)
			Range (ng/mL)	Mean (ng/mL)	Range (ng/mL)	Mean (ng/mL)		Range (µg/L)	Mean (µg/L)	Range (µg/L)	Mean (µg/L)	
		Birth	15–109	59	21–93	51		15–109	59	21–93	51	
		2 mo	15–109	55	23–163	81		15–109	55	23–163	81	
		4 mo	7–124	50	23–171	74		7–124	50	23–171	74	
6 mo			7–93	41	15–132	61		7–93	41	15–132	61	
		12 mo	15–101	56	15–179	77		15–101	56	15–179	77	
		Children and young adults	Male		Female			Male		Female		
			(ng/mL)	(ng/mL)	(ng/mL)	(ng/mL)		(µg/L)	(µg/L)	(µg/L)	(µg/L)	
		1–2 yr	30–122	76	56–144	100		30–122	76	56–144	100	
		3–4 yr	54–178	116	74–202	138		54–178	116	74–202	138	
		5–6 yr	60–228	144	82–262	172		60–228	144	82–262	172	
		7–8 yr	113–261	187	112–276	194		113–261	187	112–276	194	
		9–10 yr	123–275	199	140–308	224		123–275	199	140–308	224	
		11–12 yr	139–395	267	132–376	254		139–395	267	132–376	254	
		13–14 yr	152–540	346	192–640	416		152–540	346	192–640	416	
		15–16 yr	257–601	429	217–589	403		257–601	429	217–589	403	
		17–18 yr	236–524	380	176–452	314		236–524	380	176–452	314	
		19–20 yr	281–510	371	217–475	323		281–510	371	217–475	323	
		21–30 yr	155–432	289	87–368	237		155–432	289	87–368	237	
Interleukin 6	P	Adults	<12.5 pg/mL				×1	<12.5 ng/L				(Krafte-Jacobs et al)
		Children	7 ± 1					7 ± 1				
Iron	S	All ages	22–184 µg/dL				×0.1791	4–33 µmol/L				(Lockitch et al, 1988c)
Iron-binding capacity, total (TIBC)	S	Infant 100–400 µg/dL					×0.179	17.90–71.60 µmol/L				
		Thereafter 250–400						44.75–71.60				
Ketone bodies, qualitative	S	Negative					×1	Negative				(Bonnefont et al)
Ketone bodies, quantitative	W	1–12 mo	0.1–1.5 mmol/L					0.1–1.5 mmol/L				Sum of acetone, β-hydroxybutyrate and acetoacetate
		1–7 yr	0.15–2.0					0.15–2.0				
		7–15 yr	<0.1–0.5					<0.1–0.5				
LDL-Cholesterol (LDLC)	S,P(E)		mg/dL				×0.0259	mmol/l				
			M	F				M	F			
		Cord blood	10–50	10–50				0.26–1.30	0.26–1.30			
		1–9 yr	60–140	60–150				1.55–3.63	1.55–3.89			
		10–19 yr	50–170	50–170				1.30–4.40	1.30–4.40			
		20–29 yr	60–175	60–160				1.55–4.53	1.55–4.14			
		30–39 yr	80–190	70–170				2.07–4.92	1.81–4.40			
		40–49 yr	90–205	80–190				2.33–5.31	2.07–4.92			
		Recommended (desirable) range for adults <130 mg/dL						1.68–4.53				
L+-Lactate	W	1–12 mo	1.1–2.3 mmol/L				×1	1.1–2.3 mmol/L				(Bonnefont et al)
		1–7 yr	0.8–1.5					0.8–1.5				
		7–15 yr	0.6–0.9					0.6–0.9				
D-Lactate	P(H)	6 mo–3 yr	0.0–0.3 mmol/L				×1	0.0–0.3 mmol/L				j (Rosenthal and Pesce)
Lactate dehydrogenase	S	<1 yr	170–580 U/L				×1	170–580 U/L				37° a (Meites)
		1–9 yr	150–500					150–500				
		10–19 yr	120–330					120–330				
Isoenzymes	S		% of Total Activity									
			1–6 yr	7–19 yr								
		LD1	20–38	20–35								
		LD2	27–38	31–38								
		LD3	16–26	19–28								
		LD4	5–16	7–13								
		LD5	3–13	5–12								
Lead	W(H)		*m*g/dL				×0.0483	*m*mol/L				
		Child	<10					<0.48				
		Adult	<40					<1.93				
		Toxic	≥100					≥4.83				
Lipase	P,S	1–18 yr	3–32 U/L				×1	3–32 U/L				(Soldin et al, 1995)
Lipoprotein electrophoresis	S	Distinct β band; negligible chylomicron and pre–β-bands										
Long-acting thyroid stimulating hormone (LATS)	S	Undetectable						Undetectable				
Luteinizing hormone (LH)	S	Tanner	Age	Male			×1					(Esoterix Endocrinology)
		1	<9.8 yr	0.02–0.3 mIU/mL				0.02–0.3 U/L				
		2	9.8–14.5	0.2–4.9				0.2–4.9				
		3	10.7–15.4	0.2–5.0				0.2–5.0				Referred to WHO 2nd International Standard
		4–5	11.8–17.3	0.4–7.0				0.4–7.0				
		Adult		1.5–9				1.5–9				
		Tanner	Age	Female								
		1	<9.2 yr	0.02–0.18 mIU/mL				0.02–0.18 U/L				
		2	9.2–13.7	0.02–4.7				0.02–4.7				
		3	10.0–14.4	0.10–12.0				0.10–12.0				
		4–5	10.7–15.6	0.4–11.7				0.4–11.7				
		Adult	Follicular	29				2–9				
			Midcycle	18–49				18–49				
			Luteal	2–11				2–11				
Magnesium	P(H)	0–6 day	1.2–2.6 mg/dL				×0.411	0.48–1.05 mmol/L				w (Meites)
		7 d–2 yr	1.6–2.6					0.65–1.05				
		2–14 yr	1.5–2.3					0.60–0.95				

REFERENCE LABORATORY VALUES

Table continued on following page

TABLE 710–6. **Reference Ranges** *Continued*

Analyte or Procedure	Specimen	Reference Values (USA)			Conversion Factor	Reference Values (SI)			Comments
Methemoglobin (MetHb)	W(E,H,C)	0.06–0.24 g/dL or 0.78 ± 0.37% of total Hb			× 155 × 0.01	9.3–37.2 µmol/L 0.0078 ± 0.0037 (mass fraction)			
Methylmalonic acid	S	4–14 yr	0.03–0.26 µmol/L		× 1	0.03–0.26 µmol/L			(Straczek et al)
Microsomal antibodies, thyroid, see *Thyroid microsomal antibodies*									
Myoglobin	S	6–85 ng/mL			× 1	6–85 µg/L			
Osmolality	S	Child, adult 275–295 mOsmol/kg H₂O							
Oxygen, partial pressure (Po₂)	W(H), arterial		mmHg		× 0.133		kPa		
		Birth	8–24			1.1–3.2			
		5–10 min	33–75			4.4–10.0			
		30 min	31–85			4.1–11.3			
		>1 hr	55–80			7.3–10.6			
		1 day	54–95			7.2–12.6			
		Thereafter	83–108			11–14.4			
		(decreases with age)							
Oxygen saturation	W(H), arterial		% Saturation				Fraction saturated		
		Newborn	85–90%		× 0.01	0.85–0.90			
		Thereafter	95–99%			0.95–0.99			
Po₂, see *Oxygen, partial pressure*									
Po₂ at half saturation (Po₂[0.5] or P₅₀)	W(H), arterial	25–29 mm Hg			× 0.133	3.3–3.9 kPa			
Parathyroid hormone (PTH) Intact (IRMA)	S	Cord blood 2 yr—Adult	≤3.0 pg/mL 9–65		× 0.1053	≤0.32 pmol/L 0.95–6.8			(Nichols Institute Diagnostics)
pH	W(H), arterial		pH				H⁺ concentration		
		Premature (48 hr)	7.35–7.50				31–44 nmol/L		
		Birth, full term	7.11–7.36				43–77		
		5–10 min	7.09–7.30				50–81		
		30 min	7.21–7.38				41–61		
		>1 hr	7.26–7.49				32–54		
		1 day	7.29–7.45				35–51		
		Thereafter	7.35–7.45				35–44		
		Must be corrected for body temperature							
Phenylalanine	S	Premature	2.0–7.5 mg/dL		× 60.54	120–450 µmol/L			
		Newborn	1.2–3.4			70–210			
		Thereafter	0.8–1.8			50–110			
Phosphatase, acid prostatic (RIA)	S	<3.0 ng/mL			× 1	<3.0 µg/l			
Roy Brower, and Hayden 37°C		0.11–0.60 U/L			× 1	0.11–0.60 U/L			
Phosphatase, alkaline	S	1–9 yr	145–420 U/L		× 1	1–9 yr	145–420 U/L		37°C aw (Lockitch et al, 1988a)
		10–11 yr	130–560			10–11 yr	130–560		
			Male	Female			Male	Female	
		12–13 yr	200–495	105–420		12–13 yr	200–495	105–420	
		14–15 yr	130–525	70–230		14–15 yr	130–525	70–230	
		16–19 yr	65–260	50–130		16–19 yr	65–260	50–130	
Phospholipids, total	S,P(E)		mg/dL				g/L		
		Newborn	75–170		× 0.01	0.75–1.70			
		Infant	100–275			1.00–2.75			
		Child	180–295			1.80–2.95			
		Adult	125–275			1.25–2.75			
Phosphorus, inorganic	S,P(H)	0–5 day	4.8–8.2 mg/dL		× 0.3229	1.55–2.65 mmol/L			w (Meites)
		1–3 yr	3.8–6.5			1.25–2.10			
		4–11 yr	3.7–5.6			1.20–1.80			
		12–15 yr	2.9–5.4			0.95–1.75			
		16–19 yr	2.7–4.7			0.90–1.50			
Plasma volume	P(H)	M 25–43 mL/kg F 28–45			× 0.001	M 0.025–0.043 L/kg F 0.028–0.045			
Potassium	S	<2 mo	3.0–7.0 mmol/L		× 1	3.0–7.0 mmol/L			r (Meites) Increased by hemolysis; serum values systematically higher than plasma values
		2–12 mo	3.5–6.0			3.5–6.0			
		>12 mo	3.5–5.0			3.5–5.0			
	P(H)	3.5–4.5 mmol/L				3.5–4.5 mmol/L			
Prealbumin (transthyretin)	P	2–6 mo	142–330 mg/L		× 1	142–330 mg/L			s (Sherry et al.)
		6–12 mo	120–274			120–274			
		1–3 yr	108–259			108–259			
Progesterone	S	Tanner	Age	Male	× 0.03180				(Esoterix Endocrinology)
		1	<9.8 yr	<10–33 ng/dL		<0.32–1.05 nmol/L			
		2	9.8–14.5	<10–33		<0.32–1.05			
		3	10.7–15.4	<10–48		<0.32–1.53			
		4	11.8–16.2	10–108		0.32–3.43			
		5	12.8–17.3	21–82		0.67–2.61			
			Adult	13–97		0.41–3.08			
		Tanner	Age	Female					
		1	<9.2 yr	<10–33 ng/dL		<0.32–1.05 nmol/L			
		2	9.2–13.7	10–55		<0.32–1.75			
		3	10.0–14.4	10–450		0.32–14.31			
		4	10.7–15.6	10–1300		0.32–41.34			
		5	11.8–18.6	10–950		0.32–30.21			
		Adult	Follicular	15–70		0.48–2.23			
			Luteal	200–2500		6.36–79.50			

TABLE 710–6. **Reference Ranges** *Continued*

Analyte or Procedure	Specimen	Reference Values (USA)		Conversion Factor	Reference Values (SI)		Comments
Prolactin	S	Male	Female	×0.0426	Male	Female	(Esoterix Endocrinology)
		3–18	3–24 ng/mL		0.13–0.77	0.13–1.02 nmol/L	
		Higher in newborn infants			Higher in newborn infants		
Protein, total	S		g/dL			g/L	(Meites)
		Premature	4.3–7.6	×10		43–76	
		Newborn	4.6–7.4			46–74	
		1–7 yr	6.1–7.9	×10		61–79	
		8–12 yr	6.4–8.1			64–81	
		13–19 yr	6.6–8.2			66–82	
Protein electrophoresis	S		g/dL			g/L	
		Albumin					
		Premature	3.0–4.2	×10		30–42	
		Newborn	3.6–5.4			36–54	
		Infant	4.0–5.0			40–50	
		Thereafter	3.5–5.0			35–50	
		α1-Globulin					
		Premature	0.1–0.5			1–5	
		Newborn	0.1–0.3			1–3	
		Infant	0.2–0.4			2–4	
		Thereafter	0.2–0.3			2–3	
		α2-Globulin					
		Premature	0.3–0.7			3–7	
		Newborn	0.3–0.5			3–5	
		Infant	0.5–0.8			5–8	
		Thereafter	0.4–1.0			4–10	
		β-Globulin					
		Premature	0.3–1.2			3–12	
		Newborn	0.2–0.6			2–6	
		Infant	0.5–0.8			5–8	
		Thereafter	0.5–1.1			5–11	
		γ-Globulin					
		Premature	0.3–1.4			3–4	
		Newborn	0.2–1.0			2–10	
		Infant	0.3–1.2			3–12	
		Thereafter	0.7–1.2			7–12	
		Higher in blacks			Higher in blacks		
Pyruvate	W	7–17 yr	0.076 ± 0.026 mmol/L	×1	0.076 ± 0.026 mmol/L		(Pianosi et al)
Renin (renin activity, plasma; PRA)	P(E)		ng/mL/hr			µg/L/hr	
		0–3 yr	<16.6	×1		<16.6	
		3–6 yr	<6.7			<6.7	
		6–9 yr	<4.4			<4.4	
		9–12 yr	<5.9			<5.9	
		12–15 yr	<4.2			<4.2	
		15–18 yr	<4.3			<4.3	
		Normal sodium diet					
		Supine	0.2–2.5			0.2–2.5	
		Upright	0.3–4.3			0.3–4.3	
		Low sodium diet					
		Upright	2.9–24			2.9–24	
Retinol-binding protein (RBP)	S	0–5 day	0.8–4.5 mg/dL	×10		8–45 mg/L	s (Lockitch, et al, 1988b)
		1–9 yr	1.0–7.8			10–78	
		10–13 yr	1.3–9.9			13–99	
		14–19 yr	3.0–9.2			30–92	
Reverse triiodothyronine (rT3)	S		ng/dL			nmol/L	
		1–5 yr	15–71	×0.0154		0.23–1.1	
		5–10 yr	17–79			0.26–1.2	
		10–15 yr	19–88			0.29–1.36	
		Adults	30–80			0.46–1.23	
Selenium	S	0–5 day	5.7–9.4 µg/dL	×0.127		0.72–1.20 µmol/L	d (Lockitch et al, 1988c)
		1–9 yr	9.6–16.1			1.22–2.05	
		10–19 yr	10.3–18.5			1.31–2.35	
Sodium	S,P (LiH,NH₄H)		mmol/L			nmol/L	
		Newborn	134–146	×1		134–146	
		Infant	139–146			139–146	
		Child	138–145			138–146	
		Thereafter	136–146			136–146	
Somatomedin C, see *Insulin-like growth factor 1*							
T3, see *Triiodothyronine*							
T4, see *Thyroxine*							
Testosterone	S	Tanner	Age	Male	×0.03467		(Esoterix Endocrinology)
		1	<9.8 yr	<3–10 ng/dL		<0.1–0.35 nmol/L	
		2	9.8–14.5	18–150		0.62–5.20	
		3	10.7–15.4	100–320		3.47–11.10	
		4	11.8–16.2	220–620		7.63–21.50	
		5	12.8–17.3	350–970		12.14–3363	
			Adult	350–1030		12.14–35.71	
		Tanner	Age	Female			
		1	<9.2 yr	<3–10 ng/dL		<0.1–0.35 nmol/L	
		2	9.2–13.7	7–28		0.24–0.97	

Table continued on following page

TABLE 710–6. **Reference Ranges** *Continued*

Analyte or Procedure	Specimen	Reference Values (USA)			Conversion Factor	Reference Values (SI)			Comments
		3	10.0–14.4	15–35		0.52–1.21			
		4	10.7–15.6	13–32		0.45–1.11			
		5	11.8–18.6	20–38		0.69–1.32			
			Adult	10–55		0.35–1.91			
Testosterone, free	S	Male	pg/mL	% Free		Male	pmol/L	Fraction free	(Esoterix Endocrinology)
		Cord	5–22	2.0–4.4	×3.4673		17–76	0.02–0.044	
		1–15 day	1.5–31	0.9–1.7			5.2–107	0.009–0.017	
		1–3 mo	3.3–18	0.4–0.8			11.4–62	0.004–0.008	
		3–5 mo	0.7–14	0.4–1.1			2.4–49	0.004–0.011	
		5–7 mo	0.4–4.8	0.4–1.0			1.4–16.6	0.004–0.011	
		1–10 yr	0.15–0.6	0.4–0.9			0.5–2.1	0.004–0.009	
		Pubertal	not defined				not defined		
		Adult	52–280	1.5–3.2			180–971	0.015–0.032	
		Female	pg/mL	% Free		Female	pmol/l	Fraction free	
		Cord	4–16	2.0–3.9			13.9–55	0.02–0.039	
		1–15 day	0.5–2.5	0.8–1.5			1.7–8.7	0.008–0.015	
		1–3 mo	0.1–1.3	0.4–1.1			0.3–4.5	0.004–0.011	
		3–5 mo	0.3–1.1	0.5–1.0			1.1–3.8	0.005–0.01	
		5–7 mo	0.2–0.6	0.5–0.8			0.7–2.1	0.005–0.008	
		1–10 yr	0.15–0.6	0.4–0.9			0.5–2.1	0.004–0.009	
		Pubertal	not defined				not defined		
		Adult	1.1–6.3	0.8–1.4			3.8–21.8	0.008–0.014	
Thiamine (vitamin B₁)	S	0–2.0 μg/dL			×37.68	0.0–75.4 nmol/L			
Thyroglobulin	S	Cord blood	14.7–101.1 ng/mL		×1	14.7–101.1 μg/L			(Nichols Institute Diagnostics)
		Birth–35 mo	10.6–92.0			10.6–92.0			
		3–11 yr	5.6–41.9			5.6–41.9			
		12–17 yr	2.7–21.9			2.7–21.9			
Thyroid microsomal antibodies	S	Nondetectable (hemagglutination)				Nondetectable (hemagglutination) or			
Thyroid thyroglobulin	S	or <1:10				<1:10			
Tanned RBC agglutination test		Children ≤ 1:4 dilution				≤1:4 dilution			
		Thereafter ≤1:10				≤ 1:10			
Thyroid stimulating hormone	S	Premature (28–36 wk)							(Nichols Institute Diagnostics)
		1st wk of life	0.7–27.0 mIU/L		×1	0.7–27.0 mIU/L			
		Term infants							
		Birth–4 d	1.0–38.9			1.0–28.9			
		2–20 wk	1.7–9.1			1.7–9.1			
		5 mo–20 yr	0.7–6.4			0.7–6.4			
Thyroid uptake of radioactive iodine	Activity over thyroid gland	2 hr	<6%		×0.01	2 hr <0.06			
		6 hr	3–20%			6 hr 0.03–0.20			
		24 hr	8–30%			24 hr 0.08–0.30			
Thyroid uptake of ⁹⁹ᵐTc04	Activity over thyroid gland	After 24 hr	0.4–3.0%		×0.01	Fractional uptake 0.004–0.03			
Thyrotropin releasing hormone (hTRH)	P	5–60 pg/mL			×2.759	14–165 pmol/L			
Thyroxine binding globulin (TBG)	S		mg/dL			mg/L			
		Cord blood	1.4–94		×10	14–94			
		1–4 wk	1.0–9.0			10–90			
		1–12 mo	2.0–7.6			20–76			
		1–5 yr	2.9–5.4			29–54			
		5–10 yr	2.5–5.0			25–50			
		10–15 yr	2.1–4.6			21–46			
		Adult	1.5–3.4			15–34			
Thyroxine, total	S	Full-term infants			×12.9	Full-term infants			(Esoterix Endocrinology)
		1–3 day	8.2–19.9 μg/dL			1–3 d	106–256 nmol/L		
		1 wk	6.0–15.9			1 wk	77–205		
		1–12 mo	6.1–14.9			1–12 mo	79–192		
		Prepubertal children				Prepubertal children			
		1–3 yr	6.8–13.5 μg/dL			1–3 yr	88–174 nmol/L		
		3–10 yr	5.5–12.8			3–10 yr	71–165		
		Pubertal children and adults				Pubertal children and adults			
			4.2–13.0 μg/dL				54–167 nmol/L		
Thyroxine, free	S	Newborn infants			×12.9	Full-term infants			(Esoterix Endocrinology)
		3 day	2.0–4.9 ng/dL			3 d	26–631 pmol/L		
		Infants				Infants			
			0.9–2.6 ng/dL				12–33 pmol/L		
		Prepubertal children				Prepubertal children			
			0.8–2.2 ng/dL				10–28 pmol/L		
		Pubertal children and adults				Pubertal children and adults			
			0.8–2.3 ng/dL				10–30 pmol/L		
Thyroxine, total	W	Newborn screen (filter paper) 6.2–22 μg/dL			×12.9	80–283 nmol/L			
Transcortin	S	M	1.5–2.0 mg/dL		×10	15–20 mg/L			
		F, Follicular	1.7–2.0			17–20			
		Luteal	1.6–2.1			16–21			
		Postmenopausal	1.7–2.5			17–25			
		Pregnancy							
		21–28 wk	4.7–5.4			47–54			
		33–40 wk	5.5–7.0			55–70			

TABLE 710–6. Reference Ranges *Continued*

Analyte or Procedure	Specimen	Reference Values (USA)	Conversion Factor	Reference Values (SI)	Comments
Transferrin isoforms (test for congenital disorders of glycosylation)	S	Mono-oligosaccharide ≤0.074 Di-oligosaccharide 0.075–0.109 Indeterminate A-oligosaccharide ≤0.022 Di-oligosaccharide	×1	Mono-oligosaccharide ≤0.074 Di-oligosaccharide 0.075–0.109 Indeterminate A-oligosaccharide ≤0.022 Di-oligosaccharide	(Mayo Medical Laboratories)
Transferrin (siderophilin)	S	95–385 mg/dL	×0.01	0.95–3.85 g/L	(Davis et al)

Triglycerides	S, after ≥12 hr fast	**mg/dL**
		    M F
		Cord blood 10–98 / 10–98
		0–5 yr 30–86 / 32–99
		6–11 yr 31–108 / 35–114
		12–15 yr 36–138 / 41–138
		16–19 yr 40–163 / 40–128
		20–29 yr 44–185 / 40–128
		Recommended (desirable) levels
			×0.01	**g/L**
				    M F
				0.10–.98 / 0.10–0.98
				0.30–0.86 / 0.32–0.99
				0.31–1.08 / 0.35–1.14
				0.36–1.38 / 0.41–1.38
				0.40–1.63 / 0.40–1.28
				0.44–1.85 / 0.40–1.28	

Recommended (desirable)		For adults
		  Male 40–160 mg/dL
		  Female 35–135
				For adults
				  Male 0.40–1.60 g/l
				  Female 0.35–1.35	

Triidothyronine, free	S	**pg/dL** Cord blood 20–240 1–3 day 200–610 6 wk 240–560 Adult (20–50 yr) 230–660	×0.01536	**pmol/L** 0.3–3.7 3.1–9.4 3.7–8.6 3.5–10.0	
Triiodothyronine resin uptake test (T3RU)	S	Newborn 26–36% Thereafter 26–35%	×0.01	Fractional uptake 0.26–0.36 0.26–0.35	
Triiodothyronine, total	S	**ng/dL** Cord blood 30–70 Newborn 75–260 1–5 yr 100–260 5–10 yr 90–240 10–15 yr 80–210 Thereafter 115–190	×0.0154	**nmol/L** 0.46–1.08 1.16–4.00 1.54–4.00 1.39–3.70 1.23–3.23 1.77–2.93	
Troponin I	S	Mean 0.311 ng/mL 95% Confidence limits 0.088–1.12 ng/mL	×1	Mean 0.311 µg/L 95% Confidence limits 0.088–1.12 µg/L	(Thiru et al) a
Troponin T	S	Full-term newborn Median: 0 ng/mL Range: 0–0.14 ng/mL	×1	Full-term newborn Median: 0 µg/L Range: 0–0.14 µg/L	k (Mäkikallio et al)
Tyrosine	S	**mg/dL** Premature 7.0–24.0 Newborn 1.6–3.7 Adult 0.8–1.3	×0.0552	**mmol/L** 0.39–1.32 0.088–0.20 0.044–0.07	
Urea nitrogen	S.P	**mg/dL** Cord blood 21–40 Premature (1 wk) 3–25 Newborn 3–12 Infant/child 5–18 Thereafter 7–18	×0.357	**mmol urea/L** 7.5–14.3 1.1–9 1.1–4.3 1.8–6.4 2.5–6.4	
Uric acid	S	1–5 yr 1.7–5.8 mg/dL 6–11 yr 2.2–6.6 M 12–19 yr 3.0–7.7 F 12–19 yr 2.7–5.7	×59.48	100–350 µmol/L 130–390 180–460 160–340	j (Meites)
Vitamin A (retinol)	S	1–6 yr 20–43 µg/dL 7–12 yr 25–48 13–19 yr 26–72	×0.0349	0.70–1.5 µmol/L 0.9–1.7 0.9–2.5	p (Lockitch, et al, 1988c)
Vitamin B, see *Thiamine*					
Vitamin B₂, see *Riboflavin*					
Vitamin B₆	P(E)	3.6–18 ng/mL	×4.046	14.6–72.8 nmol/L	
Vitamin B₁₂	S	Newborn 175–800 pg/mL Thereafter 140–700	×0.738	129–590 pmol/L 103–157	
Vitamin C	P(O,H,E)	0.6–2.0 mg/dL	×56.78	34–113 µmol/L	
Vitamin D, 25-hydroxy	S	1–30 day 1.9–33.4 ng/mL 31 d–1 yr 7.4–53.3	×1	1.9–33.4 µg/L 7.4–53.3	(Soldin et al, 1997)
Vitamin D₃, 1,25-dihydroxy (calcitriol)	S	25–45 pg/mL	×2.4	60–108 nmol/L	
Vitamin E (tocopherol)	S	1–6 yr 3.0–9.0 mg/L 7–19 yr 4.4–10.4	×2.32	7–21 µmol/L 10–24	p (Lockitch, et al, 1988c)
Xylose absorption test	S	**mg/dL**		**mmol/L**	
0.5 g/kg in H₂O, 25 g maximum		Child, 1 hr >20	×0.0667	>1.33	

Table continued on following page

TABLE 710–6. Reference Ranges *Continued*

Analyte or Procedure	Specimen	Reference Values (USA)		Conversion Factor	Reference Values (SI)	Comment
Zinc	S	Adult, 2 hr	>25		>1.67	d (Lockitch et al, 1988c)
		1–19 yr	64–118 µg/dL	×0.1530	9.8–18.1 µmol/L	

C. Analyses of Blood for Drugs of All Classes

Antibiotics	Specimen	Peak		Trough		Conversion Factor	SI Peak		SI Trough		Comment
		Therapeutic	Toxic	Therapeutic	Toxic		Therapeutic	Toxic	Therapeutic	Toxic	
Amikacin	S	20–25 µg/mL	>30	1–4 µg/mL	>8	×1.708	34–43 µmol/L	>51	1.7–6.8	>14	kn (Taylor and Caviness)
Chloramphenicol	S	10–20 µg/mL	>25			×3.095	31–62 µmol/L	>77			k (Taylor and Caviness)
Gentamicin	S	6–10 µg/mL	>12	0.5–2.0	>2.0	×2.064	12–21 µmol/L	>25	1.0–4.1	>4.1	kn (Taylor and Caviness)
Netilmicin	S	6–10 µg/mL	>12	0.5–2.0	>2	×2.103	13–21 µmol/L	>25	1.1–4.2	>4.2	kn (Taylor and Caviness)
Tobramycin	S	6–10 µg/mL	>12	0.5–2.0	>2	×2.139	13–21 µmol/L	>26	1.1–4.3	>4.3	kn (Taylor and Caviness)
Vancomycin	S	30–40 µg/mL	>60	5–10	>20	×0.303	9.1–12.1 µmol/L	>18.2	1.5–3.0	>6.1	kn (Syva)

Other Drugs	Specimen	Reference Values (USA)		Conversion Factor	Reference Values (SI)	Comment
Acetaminophen	S,P(H,E)	Therapeutic	10–30 µg/mL	×6.62	66–200 µmol/L	n
		Toxic	>200		>1,300	
Amphetamine	S,P(H,E)	Therapeutic	20–30 ng/mL	×7.396	150–220 nmol/L	
		Toxic	>200		>1,500	
Amitriptyline (includes nortriptyline)	S	Therapeutic	100–250 ng/mL	×1	100–250 µg/L	(Syva)
Nortriptyline (only)		Therapeutic	50–150 ng/mL	×1	50–150 µg/L	
Caffeine	S,P	Therapeutic for neonatal apnea 5–20 µg/mL		×5.150	26–103 µmol/L	k (Syva)
Carbamazepine	S,P(H,E) at trough	Therapeutic	4–10 µg/mL	×4.233	17–42 µmol/L	kn
		Toxic	>12		>51	
Chloral hydrate	S	As trichloroethanol		×6.694	13–80 µmol/L	
		Therapeutic	2–12 µg/mL			
		Toxic	>20		>134	
Diazepam	S,P(H,E) at trough	Therapeutic	100–1,000 ng/mL	×3.512	350–3500 nmol/L	
		Toxic	>5,000		>17,500	
Digitoxin	S,P(H,E) 6 hr post dose	Therapeutic	20–35 ng/mL	×1.307	26–46 nmol/L	n
		Toxic	>45		>59	
Digoxin	S,P(H,E)		ng/mL		nmol/L	kn
	12 hr post dose					
		Therapeutic				
		CHF	0.8–1.5	×1.281	1–1.9	
		Arrhythmias	1.5–2.0		1.9–2.6	
		Toxic				
		Child	>2.5		>3.2	
		Adult	>3.0		>3.8	
Diphenylhydantoin, see *Phenytoin*						
Doxepin (includes desmethyldoxepine)	S,P	Therapeutic	110–250 ng/mL	×1	110–250 µg/L	(Syva)
Ethanol	W(O),S	Toxic	50–100 mg/dL	×0.2171	11–22 nmol/L	
		Depression of CNS >100			>22	
Ethosuximide	S,P(H,E) at trough	Therapeutic	40–100 µg/mL	×7.084	280–700µmol/L	kn
		Toxic	>150		>1,060	
Imipramine (includes desipramine)	S	Therapeutic	150–250 ng/mL	×1	150–250 µg/L	k (Syva)
Lithium	S,P (not LiH)	12 hr after dose				
		Therapeutic	0.6–1.2 mmol/L	×1	0.6–1.2 mmol/L	
		Toxic	>2 mmol/L		>2 mmol/L	
Lysergic acid diethylamide	P(E)	After hallucinogenic dose			After hallucinogenic dose	
	U	0.005–0.009 µg/mL		×3089	15.5–27.8 nmol/L	
		0.001–0.050 µg/mL			3.1–155 nmol/L	
Methotrexate	S,P	After high-dose therapy			After high-dose therapy	kn
		Toxic >5 µmol/L at 24 hr		×1	Toxic >5 µmol/l at 24 hr	
		Toxic >1 µmol/L at 48 hr			Toxic >1 µmol/l at 48 hr	
Paraldehyde	S,P(H,E)	Sedative	10–100 µg/mL	×7.567	75–750 µmol/L	(Koren et al)
		Anticonvulsant	100–200		>750–1,500	
		Toxic	>200		>1,500	
		Lethal	>500		>3,750	
Phenacetin	P(E)	Therapeutic 1–20 µg/mL		×5.580	5.6–110 µmol/L	
		Toxic	50–250		280–1,400	
Phenobarbital	S,P(H,E) at trough		µg/mL		µmol/L	kn
		Therapeutic	15–40	×4.306	65–170	
		Toxic				
		Slowness, ataxia, nystagmus	35–80		150–345	
		Coma with reflexes	65–117		280–504	
		Coma without reflexes	>100		>430	
Phensuximide (both parent and N-desmethyl metabolite)	S,P(H,E)	Therapeutic	40–60 µg/mL	×5.71	228–343 µmol/L	
Phenytoin	S,P(H,E)	Therapeutic	10–20 µg/mL	×3.964	40–80 µmol/L	
Primidone	S,P(H,E) at trough	Therapeutic	5–12 µg/mL	×4.582	23–55 µmol/L	(Taylor and Caviness)
		Toxic	>15		>69	
		Toxic (neonatal)	>20		>92	
Procainamide	S,P(H,E)	Therapeutic	4–10 µg/mL	×4.25	17–42 µmol/L	
		Toxic	>10–12 µg/mL		>42–51 µmol/L	

TABLE 710–6. Reference Ranges *Continued*

Analyte or Procedure	Specimen	Reference Values (USA)		Conversion Factor	Reference Values (SI)	Comments
		(Also consider concentration of metabolite *N*-acetylprocainamide [NAPA].)				
Propranolol	S,P(H,E) at trough	Therapeutic 50–100 ng/mL		×3.856	190–380 nmol/L	
Quinidine	S,P(H,E)	Therapeutic	2–5 µg/mL	×3.083	6.2–15.5µmol/L	
		Toxic	>6		>18.5	
Salicylate	S,P(H,E) at trough	Therapeutic	15–30 mg/dL	×0.0724	1.1–2.2 mmol/L	
		Toxic	>30		>18.5	
Theophylline	S,P(H,E)		µg/mL	µmol/L	kn	
		Therapeutic				
		Bronchodilator	10–20	×5.550	56–110	
		Neonatal apnea	5–10		28–56	
		Toxic	>20		>110	
Valproic acid	S,P(H,E) at trough	Therapeutic	50–100 µg/mL	×6.934	350–700 µmol/L	
		Toxic	>100		>700	

II. Analyses of Urine
A. Formed Elements

Analyte or Procedure	Specimen	Reference Values (USA)	Conversion Factor	Reference Values (SI)	Comments
Sediment casts	U	Hyaline occasional (0–1) casts/hpf RBC not seen WBC not seen Tubular epithelial not seen Transitional and squamous epithelial not seen		Hyaline occasional (0–1) casts/hpf RBC not seen WBC not seen Tubular epithelial not seen Transitional and squamous epithelial not seen	

Cells		RBC 0–2/hpf
		WBC
		  Males 0–3/hpf
		  Females and children 0–5/hpf
		Epithelial few; more frequent in newborn
		Bacterial: unspun: no organisms per oil immersion field
		Spun: <20 organisms/hpf
				RBC 0–2/hpf
				WBC
				  Males 0–3/hpf
				  Females and children 0–5/hpf
				Epithelial few; more frequent in newborn
				Bacterial: unspun: no organisms per oil immersion field
				Spun: <20 organisms/hpf	

Specific gravity	U U, 24 hr	Adult 1.002–1.030 After 12 hr fluid restriction >1.025 1.015–1.025		Adult 1.002–1.030 After 12 hr fluid restriction >1.025	

Urine volume	U, 24 hr		mL/24 hr		L/24 hr	
		Newborn	50–300	×0.001	0.050–0.300	
		Infant	350–550		0.350–0.550	
		Child	500–1000		0.500–1.000	
		Adolescent	700–1400		0.700–1.400	
		Thereafter, M	800–1800		0.800–1.800	
		F	600–1600		0.600–1.600	
		(varies with intake and other factors)				

B. Chemical Elements

Analyte or Procedure	Specimen	Reference Values (USA)		Conversion Factor	Reference Values (SI)	Comments
Acetone, semiquantitative	U	Negative			Negative	
Albumin	U	4–16 yr 3.35–18.3 mg/24 hr/1.73 m²				(Meites)
Aldosterone	U	Newborn:				
		1–3 days:	20–140 µg/g Cr	×0.3139	6.28–43.94 nmol/mmol Cr	
			0.5–5 µg/24 hr	×2.775	1.39–13.88 nmol/day	
		Prepubertal:				
		4–10 years	4–22 µg/g Cr	×0.3139	1.26–6.91 nmol/mmol Cr	
			1–8 µg/24 hr	×2.775	2.78–22.20 nmol/day	
		Adults:	1.5–20 µg/g Cr	×0.3139	0.47–6.28 nmol/mmol Cr	
			3–19 µg/24 hr	×2.775	8.32–52.72 nmol/day	
Amino acids, urine, quantitative	U			×0.1131		

	Premature 0–6 wk µmol/g Cr	Full-term 0–1 mo µmol/g Cr	1–24 mo µmol/g C	2–18 yr µmol/g C	Adult µmol/g C	0–6 wk mmol/mol Cr	0–1 mo mmol/mol Cr	1–24 mo mmol/mol Cr	2–18 yr mmol/mol Cr	Adult mmol/mol Cr	(Shapira, et al)
1-Methylhistidine	170–880	96–499	106–1275	170–1688	170–1680	19–100	11–56	12–144	19–191	19–190	
3-Methylhistidine	420–1340	189–680	147–391	182–365	160–520	48–152	21–77	17–44	21–41	18–59	
Alanine	1320–4040	982–3055	767–6090	231–915	240–670	149–457	11–346	87–689	26–103	27–76	
Anserine	–	0–3	0–5	0	0	0	0	0–1	0	0	
Arginine	190–820	35–214	38–165	31–109	10–90	21–93	4–24	4–19	4–12	1–10	
Asparagine	1350–5250	185–1550	252–1280	72–332	99–470	153–594	21–175	29–145	8–38	11–53	
Aspartic acid	580–1520	336–810	230–685	0–120	60–240	66–172	38–92	26–77	0–14	7–27	
Carnosine	260–370	97–665	203–635	72–402	10–90	29–42	11–75	23–72	8–45	1–10	
Citrulline	240–1320	27–181	22–180	10–99	8–50	27–149	3–20	2–20	1–11	1–6	
Cystathionine	260–1160	16–147	33–470′	0–26	20–50	29–131	2–17	4–53	0–3	2–6	
Cystine	480–1690	212–668	68–710′	25–125	43–210	54–191	24–76	8–80	3–14	5–24	
Ethanolamine	–	840–3400	0–2230	0–530	0–520	0	95–385	0–252	0–60	0–59	
Glutamic acid	380–3760	70–1058	54–590	0–176	39–330	43–425	8–120	6–67	0–20	4–37	
Glutamine	520–1700	393–1042	670–1562	369–1014	190–510	59–192	44–118	76–177	42–115	21–58	
Glycine	7840–23600	5749–16423	3023–11148	897–4500	730–4160	887–2669	650–1858	342–1261	101–509	83–470	
Histidine	1240–7240	908–2528	815–7090	644–2430	460–1430	140–819	103–286	92–802	73–275	52–162	
Hydroxylysine	–	10–125	10–97	40–102	40–90	0	1–14	1–11	5–12	5–10	
Hydroxyproline	560–5640	40–440	0–4010	0–3300	0–26	63–638	5–50	0–454	′0–373	0–3	
Isoleucine	250–640	125–390	38–642	10–126	16–180	28–72	14–44	4–73	1–14	2–20	
Leucine	190–790	78–195	70–570	30–500	30–150	21–89	9–22	8–64	3–57	3–17	
Lysine	1860–16460	270–1850	189–850	153–634	145–634	210–1862	31–209	21–96	17–72	16–72	
Methionine	500–1230	342–880	174–1090	16–114	38–210	57–139	39–100	20–123	2–13	4–24	
Ornithine	260–3350	118–554	55–364	31–91	20–80	29–379	13–63	6–41	4–10	2–9	
Phenylalanine	920–2280	91–457	175–1340	61–314	51–250	104–258	10–52	20–152	7–36	6–28	
Phosphoethanolamine	80–340	0–155	108–533	18–150	20–100	9–38	0–18	12–60	2–17	2–11	

Table continued on following page

TABLE 710–6. Reference Ranges *Continued*

Analyte or Procedure	Specimen	Reference Values (USA)						Reference Values (SI)			Comment
Phosphoserine		500–1690	150–339	112–304	70–138	40–510	57–191	17–38	13–34	8–16	5–58
Proline		1350–10460	370–2323	254–2195	0	0	153–1183	42–263	29–248	0	0
Sarcosine		0	0–56	30–358	0–26	0–80	0	0–6	3–40	0–3	0–9
Serine		1680–6000	1444–3661	845–3190	362–1100	240–670	190–679	163–414	96–361	41–124	27–76
Taurine		5190–23620	1650–6220	545–3790	639–1866	380–1850	587–2671	187–703	62–429	72–211	43–209
Threonine		840–5700	445–1122	252–1528	121–389	130–370	95–645	50–127	29–173	14–44	15–42
Tryptophan		0	0	0–93	0–108	0–70	0	0	0–11	0–12	0–8
Tyrosine		1090–6780	220–1650	333–1550	122–517	90–290	123–767	25–187	38–175	14–58	10–33
Valine		180–890	113–369	99–316	58–143	27–260	20–101	13–42	11–36	7–16	3–29
α-Aminobutyric acid		50–710	8–65	30–136	0–77	0–90	6–80	1–7	3–15	0–9	0–10
α-Aminoadipic acid		70–460	0–180	45–268	2–88	40–110	8–52	0–20	5–30	0–10	5–12
β-Alanine		1020–3500	25–288	0–297	0–65	0–130	115–396	3–33	0–34	0–7	0–15
β-Aminoisobutyric acid		50–470	421–3133	802–4160	291–1482	10–510	6–53	48–354	91–470	33–168	1–58
γ-Aminoisobutyric acid		20–260	0–15	0–105	15–30	0–32	2–29	0–2	0–12	2–3	0–4

Analyte or Procedure	Specimen	Reference Values (USA)		Conversion Factor	Reference Values (SI)		Comment
Aminolevulinic acid (ALA)	U	1.3–7.0 mg/24 hr		×7.626	9.9–53.4 µmol/24 hr		
Ammonia	U	500–1,200 mgN/24 hr		0.0714	36–86 mmol/24 hr		
Bilirubin	U	Negative			Negative		
Calcium, total	U	Ca in Diet	mg/24 hr		mmol/24 hr		
		Ca free	5–40	×0.025	0.13–1.0		
		Low to average	50–150		1.25–3.8		
		Average (20 mmol/24 hr)	100–300		2.5–7.5		
Catecholamines, fractionated	U	Norepinephrine	µg/24 hr	×5.911	nmol/24 hr		
		0–1 yr	0–10		0–59		
		1–2 yr	0–17		0–100		
		2–4 yr	4–29		24–171		
		4–7 yr	8–45		47–266		
		7–10 yr	13–65		77–384		
		Thereafter	15–80		87–473		
	U	Epinephrine	µg/24 hr		nmol/24 hr		
		0–1 yr	0–2.5	×5.458	0–13.6		
		1–2 yr	0–3.5		0–19.1		
		2–4 yr	0–6.0		0–32.7		
		4–7 yr	0.2–10		1.1–55		
		7–10 yr	0.5–14		2.7–76		
		Thereafter	0.5–20		2.7–109		
		Dopamine	µg/24 hr		nmol/24 hr		
		0–1 yr	0–85	×6.528	0–555		
		1–2 yr	10–140		65–914		
		2–4 yr	40–260		261–1697		
		Thereafter	65–400		424–2611		
Catecholamines, total, free	U		µg/24 hr		µg/24 hr		
		0–1 yr	10–15	×1	10–15		
		1–5 yr	15–40		15–40		
		6–15 yr	20–80		20–80		
		Thereafter	30–100		30–100		
Chloride	U	Infant	2–10 mmol/24 hr	×1	2–10 mmol/24 hr		
		Child	15–40		15–40		
		Thereafter	110–250		110–250		
		(varies greatly with chloride intake)					
Copper	U	5–18 yr 0.36–7.56 mg/mol creatinine		×15.7	6–119 µmol/mol creatinine		cd (Lockitch et al, 1988c)
Coproporphyrin	U	34–234 µg/24 hr		×1.5	51–351 nmol/24 hr		
Cortisol free	U		µg/24 hr		nmol/day		
		Child	2–27	×2.759	5.5–74		
		Adolescent	5–55		14–152		
		Adult	10–100		27–276		
Creatinine	U	Premature	8.1–15.0 mg/kg/24 hr	×8.84	72–133 µmol/kg/24 hr		aw (Meites)
		Full term	10.4–19.7		92–174		
		1.5–7 yr	10–15		88–133		
		7–15 yr	5.2–41		46–362		
Cyclic AMP	U	<3.3 mg/24 hr or <1.64 mg/g creatinine		×3.040	<10 µmol/24 hr <600 µmol cAMP/mol creatinine		
Estradiol, urinary	U	Adult male	0–6 µg/24 hr	×3.671	Adult male	0–22 nmol/day	
		Adult female			Adult female		
		Follicular	0–3 µg/24 hr		Follicular	0–11 nmol/day	
		Ovulatory peak	4–14		Ovulatory peak	15–51	
		Luteal	4–10		Luteal	15–37	
Estriol (E3), total	U		mg/24 hr		µmol/24 hr		
		Pregnancy (wk)					
		30	6–18	×3.467	21–62		
		35	9–28		31–97		
		40	13–42		45–146		
		Decrease of >40% of previous value suggests fetus at risk			Fraction of previous value of <0.60 suggests fetus at risk		
Estrogens, total	U, 24 hr		µg/24 hr		µg/24 hr		
		Child	<10	×1	<10		
		Adult male	5–25		5–25		
		Adult female					
		Preovulation	5–25		5–25		
		Ovulation	28–100		28–100		
		Luteal peak	22–80		22–80		
		Pregnancy	<45,000		<45,000		
		Postmenopausal	<10		<10		

TABLE 710–6. Reference Ranges *Continued*

Analyte or Procedure	Specimen	Reference Values (USA)		Conversion Factor	Reference Values (SI)	Comments
Ferric chloride test	U	Negative			Negative	
Galactose	U	Newborn	≤60 mg/dL	×0.0555	≤3.33 mmol/L	
		Thereafter	<14 mg/24 hr	×0.00555	<0.08 mmol/24 hr	
Glucose						
Quantitative, enzymatic	U	<0.5 g/24 hr		×5.55	<2.8 mmol/24 hr	
Qualitative	U	Negative			Negative	
Hemoglobin (Hb)	U	Negative			Negative	
Homovanillic acid	U, 24 hr	0–1 yr	<32.2 mg/g Cr	×0.62	<20 mmol/mol Cr	p (Meites)
		2–4 yr	<22		<14	
		5–19 yr	<14		<8	
5-Hydroxyindole acetic acid (5-HIAA)	U	3–8 yr				(Nichols Institute Reference Laboratories)
		0.4–5.6 mg/24 hr		×8.8	3.5–49.3 μmol/24 hr	
		1.2–16.2 mg/g Cr		×0.5917	0.71–9.6 mmol/mol Cr	
		9 yr and older				
		0.9–7 mg/24 hr		×8.8	7.9–61.9 μmol/24 hr	
		1.3–8.7 mg/g Cr		×0.5917	0.78–5.15 mmol/mol Cr	
Hydroxyproline, free and bound	U	3 day	33–112 μmol/24 hr	×1	33–112 μmol/24 hr	w (Meites)
		10 day	148–225		148–225	
		20 day	229–310		229–310	
17-Hydroxycorticosteroids (17-OHCS)	U		mg/24 hr		μmol/24 hr	(Conversion based on hydrocortisone, MW = 362)
		0–1 yr	0.5–1.0	×2.76	1.4–2.8	
		Child	1.0–5.6		2.8–15.5	
		Adult, M	3.0–10.0		8.2–27.6	
		F	2.0–8.0		5.5–22	
		or 3–7 mg/g Cr		×0.312	or 0.9–2.5 mmol/mol Cr	
17-Ketogenic steroids (17-KGS)	U		mg/24 hr		μmol/24 hr	(Conversion based on dehydroepiandros-terone, MW = 288)
		0–1 yr	<1.0	×3.467	<3.5	
		1–10 yr	<5		<17	
		11–14 yr	<12		<42	
		Thereafter, M	5–23		17–80	
		F	3–15		10–52	
Ketone bodies, qualitative	U	Negative			Negative	
17-Ketosteroid (17-KS), total	U		mg/24 hr		μmol/24 hr	Zimmerman reaction (conversion based on dehydroepiandrosterone, MW=288)
		14d–2 yr	<1	×3.467	<3.5	
		2–6 yr	<2		<7	
		6–10 yr	1–4		3.5–14	
		10–12 yr	1–6		3.5–21	
		12–14 yr	3–10		10–35	
		14–16 yr	5–12		17–42	
		Thereafter,				
		M 18–30 yr	9–22		31–76	
		M >30 yr	8–20		28–70	
		F	6–15		21–52	
Lead	U, 24 hr	<80 μg/L		×0.00483	<0.39 μmol/L	
Magnesium	U, 24 hr	1–6 mo		×1		
		(breast milk)	0.04–1.55 mmol/L		0.04–1.55 mmol/L	
		(formula)	0.04–1.40		0.04–1.40	
Metanephrines, total	U, 24 hr	<1 yr	<15.9 μmol/g Cr	×0.1131	<1.80 mmol/mol Cr	(Meites)
		1–2 yr	<14.8		<1.67	
		3–4 yr	<12.8		<1.45	
		5–8 yr	<11.7		<1.32	
		9–13 yr	<10.5		<1.19	
Methylmalonic acid	U	6–12 wk	0–57 mg/g Cr	×0.9579	0–55 mmol/mol Cr	o (Meites)
Mucopolysaccharides	U	<2 yr	<50 μg/g Cr	×0.1131	<5.7 mg/mmol Cr	(Meites)
		2–4 yr	<25		<2.8	
		4–15 yr	<20		<2.3	
Myoglobin	U	Negative			Negative	
Niacin (nicotinic acid)	U	0.3–1.5 mg/24 hr		×8.113	2.43–12.17 μmol/24 hr	
Occult blood	U	Negative			Negative	
Organic acids	U	Adult				(Hoffman et al)
Lactic		115–407 μmol/g Cr		×0.1132	13–46 mmol/mol Cr	
2-Hydroxyisobutyric		Not detected			Not detected	
Glycolic		159–486			18–55	
3-Hydroxybutyric		Not detected–18			Not detected–2.0	
3-Hydroxyisobutyric		36–168			4.1–19	
2-Hydroxyisovaleric		Not detected			Not detected	
3-Hydroxyisovaleric		61–221			6.9–25	
Methylmalonic		Not detected			Not detected	
4-Hydroxybutyric		2.7–51			0.3–5.8	
Ethylmalonic		3.57–37			0.4–4.2	
Succinic		4.4–141			0.5–16	
Fumaric		1.8–7			0.2–0.8	
Glutaric		5.3–23			0.6–2.6	
3-Methylglutaric		Not detected			Not detected	
Adipic		7–309			0.8–35	
Pyruvic		23–70			2.6–7.9	
Pyroglutamic		8–557			0.9–63	
2-Oxoisovaleric		Not detected			Not detected	

Table continued on following page

REFERENCE LABORATORY VALUES

TABLE 710–6. Reference Ranges *Continued*

Analyte or Procedure	Specimen	Reference Values (USA)		Conversion Factor	Reference Values (SI)	Comments
Acetoacetic		Not detected			Not detected	
Mevalonic		0.5–1.9			0.06–0.22	
2-Hydroxyglutaric		7–460			0.8–52	
3-Hydroxy-3-methyl-glutaric		Not detected–88			Not detected–10	
p-Hydroxyphenylacetic		31–195			3.5–22	
2-Oxoisocaproic		Not detected			Not detected	
Suberic		Not detected–26			Not detected–2.9	
Orotic		Not detected			Not detected	
cis-Aconitic		24–389			2.7–44	
Homovanillic		8–49			0.9–5.5	
Azeleic		11–137			1.3–5.5	
Isocitric		318–743			36–84	
Citric		619–1998			70–226	
Sebacic		Not detected			Not detected	
4-Hydroxyphenyllactic		1.8–23			0.2–2.6	
2-Oxoglutaric		35–654			4–74	
5-Hydroxyindoleacetic		Not detected–64			Not detected–72	
Succinylacetone		Not detected			Not detected	
Orotic acid	U	0–20.1 mg/g Cr		× 0.7247	0–14.6 mmol/mol Cr	aw (Meites)
Osmolality	U	50–1400 mOsmol/kg H$_2$O, depending on fluid intake. After 12 hr fluid restriction >850 mOsmol/kg H$_2$O			50–1400 mOsmol/kg H$_2$O, depending on fluid intake. After 12 hr fluid restriction >850 mOsmol/kg H$_2$O	
	U, 24 hr	300–900 mOsmol/kg H$_2$O			300–900 mOsmol/kg H$_2$O	
pH and Acidity	U		pH		H$^+$ concentration	
		Newborn/neonate	5–7		0.1–10 µmol/L	
		Thereafter	4.5–8 (average 6)		0.01–32 µmol/L (average 1.0 µmol/L)	
Phenylalanine	U	10 days–2 wk	1–2 mg/24 hr	× 6.054	6–12 µmol/24 hr	
		3–12 yr	4–18		24–110	
		Thereafter	trace–17		trace–103	
Phenylpyruvic acid, qualitative	U	Negative by FeCl$_3$ test			Negative by FeCl$_3$ test	
Porphobilinogen (PBG)						
Quantitative	U	0–2.0 mg/24 hr		× 4.42	0–8.8 µmol/24 hr	
Qualitative	U	Negative			Negative	
Potassium	U, 24 hr	2.5–125 mmol/L varies with diet			2.5–125 mmol/L varies with diet	
Pregnanetriol	U		mg/24 hr		µmol/24 hr	
		2 wk–2 yr	0.02–0.2	× 2.972	0.06–0.6	
		2–5 yr	<0.5		<1.5	
		5–15 yr	<1.5		<4.5	
		>15 yr	<2.0		<5.9	
Protein, total	U, 24 hr	1–14 mg/dL		× 10	10–140 mg/L	
		50–80 mg/24 hr (at rest)		× 1	50–80 mg/24 hr	
		<250 mg/24 hr after intense exercise			<250 mg/24 hr after intense exercise	
Electrophoresis		Average % Total Protein			Fraction of Total	
		Albumin	37.9	× 0.01	0.379	
		α1-Globulin	27.3		0.273	
		α2-Globulin	19.5		0.195	
		β-Globulin	8.8		0.088	
		γ-Globulin	3.3		0.033	
Riboflavin (vitamin B$_2$)	U		µg/g Cr		µmol/mol Cr	
		1–3 yr	500–900		150–270	
		4–6 yr	300–600	× 0.3	90–180	
		7–9 yr	270–500		81–150	
		10–15 yr	200–400		60–1200	
		Adult	80–269		24–81	
Sodium	U, 24 hr	40–220 (diet-dependent)			40–220	
Thiamine (vitamin B$_1$)	U, acidified with HCl		µg/g Cr		µmol/mol Cr	
		1–3 yr	176–200	× 0.426	75–85	
		4–6 yr	121–400		52–170	
		7–9 yr	181–350		77–149	
		10–12 yr	181–300		77–128	
		13–15 yr	151–250		64–107	
		Thereafter	66–129		28–55	
Vanillylmandelic acid (VMA)	U	0–1 yr	<18.8 mg/g Cr	× 0.5709	<11 mmol/mol Cr	p (Meites)
		2–4 yr	<11		<6	
		5–19 yr	<8		<5	
Xylose absorption test 0.5 g/kg to 25 g maximum	U, 5 hr	Child	16–33% of ingested dose	× 0.01	Fraction ingested dose 0.16–0.33	
		Adult	g/5 hr		mmol/5 hr	
		5 g dose	>1.2	× 6.66	>8.00	
		25 g dose	>4.0		>26.64	
Zinc	U	5–18 yr 10.1–95.9 mg/mol Cr		× 0.0153	0.15–1.47 mmol/mol Cr	d (Lockitch, et al, 1988c)

III. Analysis of Feces
A. Chemical Elements

Analyte or Procedure	Specimen	Reference Values (USA)		Conversion Factor	Reference Values (SI)	Comments
α-1-Antitrypsin	F	<1 yr (breast milk)	<4.4 mg/g solid			u (Meites)
		(formula)	<2.9			
		6 mo–44 yr (cow's milk, regular diet)	<1.7 mg/g solid			
Bile acids, total	F	120–225 mg/24 hr		× 1	120–225 mg/24 hr	
Calcium, total	F	Avg. 0.64 g/24 hr		× 25	16 mmol/24 hr	

TABLE 710–6. Reference Ranges *Continued*

Analyte or Procedure	Specimen	Reference Values (USA)			Conversion Factor	Reference Values (SI)	Comments
Coproporphyrin	F, 24 hr	<30 µg/g dry weight 400–1,200 µg/24 hr			×1.5	<45 nmol/g dry weight 600–1,800 nmol/dry	
Fat, fecal	F, 72 hr collection			g/24 hr		g/24 hr	
		Infant, breast-fed		<1	×1	<1	
		0–6 yr		<2		<2	
		Adult		<7		<7	
		Adult (fat-free diet)		<4		<4	
		Coefficient of fat absorption		(%)	×0.01	Absorbed fraction	
		Infant, breast-fed		>93		>0.93	
		Infant, formula-fed		>83		>0.83	
		>1 yr		≥95		≥0.95	
Occult blood	F	Negative (<2 mL blood/24 hr in ~ 100–200 g stool)				Negative	
pH and Acidity	F	pH 7.0–7.5				H⁺ concentration 31–100 nmol/L	

IV. Analyses of Cerebrospinal Fluid
A. Formed Elements

Analyte or Procedure	Specimen	Reference Values (USA)		Conversion Factor	Reference Values (SI)	Comments
Cell count	CSF		cells/mm³ (µL)	×10⁶	×10⁶ cells/L	
		Premature	0–25 mononuclear		0–25	
			0–10 polymorphonuclear		0–10	
			0–1000 RBC		0–1000	
		Newborn	0–20 mononuclear		0–20	
			0–10 polymorphonuclear		0–10	
			0–800 RBC		0–800	
		Neonate	0–5 mononuclear		0–5	
			0–10 polymorphonuclear		0–10	
			0–50 RBC		0–50	
		Thereafter	0–5 mononuclear		0–5	
		(Numbers of cells in very young infants are greater than those in older individuals' CSF, without substantial implication for growth and development in most instances)				
Leukocyte differential count	CSF		%		Fraction	
		Lymphocytes	62 ± 34	×0.01	0.62 ± 0.34	
		Monocytes	36 ± 20		0.36 ± 0.20	
		Neutrophils	2 ± −5		0.02 ± 0.05	
		Histiocytes	0-rare		0-rare	
		Ependymal cells*	0-rare		0-rare	
		Eosinophils	0-rare		0-rare	
		*Includes pia-arachnoid mesothelial cells.				
Cerebrospinal fluid pressure	CSF		70–180 mm water		70–180 mm water	
Cerebrospinal fluid volume	CSF	Child	60–100 mL ×0.001		0.06–0.10 L	
		Adult	100–160		0.1–0.16	

B. Chemical Elements

Analyte or Procedure	Specimen	Reference Values (USA)		Conversion Factor	Reference Values (SI)	Comments
Amino acids in CSF	CSF					f (Dickinson and Hamilton)
Taurine		6.3 ± 1.8 µmol/L		×1	6.3 ± 1.8 µmol/L	
Aspartic acid		0.9 ± 0.5			0.9 ± 0.5	
Threonine		25 ± 10			25 ± 10	
Serine + asparagine		38 ± 23			38 ± 23	
Glutamine		509 ± 144			509 ± 144	
Proline		0.6			0.6	
Glutamic acid		7.0 ± 4.9			7.0 ± 4.9	
Glycine		6.6 ± 1.8			6.6 ± 1.8	
Alanine		23 ± 9.4			23 ± 9.4	
Valine		14 ± 5.5			14 ± 5.5	
Half cystine		0.2			0.2	
Methionine		2.6 ± 1.6			2.6 ± 1.6	
Isoleucine		4.4 ± 1.3			4.4 ± 1.3	
Leucine		11 ± 3.6			11 ± 3.6	
Tyrosine		9.1 ± 5.0			9.1 ± 5.0	
Phenylalanine		9.2 ± 5.8			9.2 ± 5.8	
Ornithine		5.7 ± 1.8			5.7 ± 1.8	
Lysine		19 ± 6.6			19 ± 6.6	
Histidine		13 ± 4.4			13 ± 4.4	
Arginine		20 ± 5.8			20 ± 5.8	
Calcium, total	CSF	2.1–2.7 mEq/L or 4.2–5.4 mg/dL		×0.50 ×0.25	1.05–1.35 mmol/L 1.05–1.35	
Chloride	CSF	118–132 mmol/L		×1	118–132 mmol/L	
Glucose	CSF	Adult	40–70 mg/dL	×0.0555	2.2–3.9 mmol/L	
Hypoxanthine	CSF	0–1 mo	1.8–5.5 µmol/L	×1	1.8–5.5 µmol/L	(Jung et al)
Total protein column	CSF, lumbar	8–32 mg/dL		×10	80–320 mg/L	
Turbidimetry	CSF, lumbar		mg/dL		mg/L	
		Premature	40–300		400–3,000	
		Newborn	45–120		450–1,200	
		Child	10–20		100–200	
		Adolescent	15–20		150–200	
		Thereafter	15–45		150–450	
Electrophoresis	CSF		% of Total		Fraction of Total	
		Prealbumin	2–7	×0.01	0.02–0.07	
		Albumin	56–76		0.56–0.76	
		α1-Globulin	2–7		0.02–0.07	
		α2-Globulin	4–12		0.04–0.12	
		β-Globulin	8–18		0.08–0.18	
		γ-Globulin	3–12		0.03–0.12	

Table continued on following page

REFERENCE LABORATORY VALUES

TABLE 710–6. Reference Ranges *Continued*

Analyte or Procedure	Specimen	Reference Values (USA)	Conversion Factor	Reference Values (SI)	Comments
V. Analyses of Other Body Fluids					
A. Chemical Analyses					
1. AMNIONIC FLUID					
Amniotic fluid analysis Ab450nm	AF	28 wk 0–0.048 A 40 wk 0–0.02 A	×1	0–0.048 A 0–0.02 A	t
Bilirubin	AF	28 wk <0.075 mg/dL (or Ab450 <0.048) 40 wk <0.025 mg/dL (or Ab450 <0.02)	×17.10	<1.3 µmol/L (or Ab450 <0.048) <0.43 µmol/L (or Ab450 <0.02)	
Creatinine	AF	After 37 wk gestation >2.0 mg/dL	×88.4	After 37 wk gestation >180 µmol/L	
Estriol (E3), free	AF	ng/mL (95% range) Wk 16–20 1.0–3.2 20–24 2.1–7.8 24–28 2.1–7.8 28–32 4.0–13.6 32–36 3.6–15.5 36–38 4.6–18.0 38–40 5.4–19.8	×3.47	nmol/L (95% range) 3.5–11.1 7.3–27.1 7.3–27.1 13.9–47.2 12.5–53.8 16.0–62.5 18.7–68.7	
α-Fetoprotein (AFP)	AF	Wk Amniotic Fluid (Mean ISD) µg/mL 15 13.5 ± 3.42 16 11.7 ± 3.38 17 10.3 ± 3.03 18 9.5 ± 3.22 19 7.1 ± 2.86 20 5.7 ± 2.45			
Lecithin/sphingomyelin (L/S) ratio	AF	2.0–5.0 indicates probable fetal lung maturity (>3.0 in infants or diabetic mothers)		2.0–5.0 indicates probable fetal lung maturity (>3.0 in infants of diabetic mothers)	
Lecithin phosphorus	AF	>0.10 mg/dL indicates probable adequate fetal lung maturity	×0.3229	>0.032 mmol/L indicates probable adequate fetal lung maturity	
2. SWEAT Chloride	Sweat	Normal <40 mmol/L Indeterminate 45–60 Cystic fibrosis >60	×1	<40 mmol/L 40–60 >60	(Gibson et al)
Sodium	Sweat	Normal <40 mmol/L Indeterminate 40–60 Cystic fibrosis >60	×1	<40 mmol/L 40–60 >60	(Gibson et al)

REFERENCE LABORATORY VALUES

Abbott Laboratories, Diagnostic Division, Abbott Park, IL, 1996.

American Diabetes Association: Report of the Expert Committee on the Diagnosis and Classification of Diabetes Mellitus. *Diabetes Care* 1997;20:1183.

Baroni S, Scribano D, Valentini P, et al: Serum apolipoproteins A1, B, CII, CIII, E, and lipoprotein (a) in children. *Clin Biochem* 1996;29:603.

Bonnefont JP, Specola NB, Vassault A, et al: The fasting test in children: Application to the diagnosis of pathological hypo- and hyperketotic states. *Eur J Pediatr* 1990;150:80.

Buck ML: Anticoagulation with warfarin in infants and children. *Ann Pharmacother* 1996;30:1316.

Chenillot O, Henny J, Steinmetz J, et al: High-sensitivity C-Reactive protein: Biological variations and reference limits. *Clin Chem Lab Med* 2000;38:1003–11.

Davis ML, Austin C, Messner BL, et al: IFCC-standardized pediatric reference intervals for 10 serum proteins using the Beckman Array 360 System. *Clin Biochem* 1996;29:489.

De Schepper J, Derde MP, Goubert P, Gorus F: Reference values for fructosamine concentrations in children's sera: Influence of protein concentration, age and sex. *Clin Chem* 1988;34:2444–47.

Denny T, Yogev R, Gelman R, et al: Lymphocyte subsets in healthy children during the first five years of life. *JAMA* 1992;267:1484.

Diaz J, Tornel PL, Martinez P: Reference intervals for blood ammonia in healthy subjects, determined by microdiffusion. *Clin Chem* 1995;41:1048.

Dickinson JC, Hamilton PB: The free amino acids of human spinal fluid determined by ion exchange chromatography. *J Neurochem* 1966;13:1179.

Esoterix Endocrinology, Calabasas Hills, CA 91301.

Gibson LE, di Sant'Agnese PA, Schwachman H: Procedure for the quantitative iontophoretic sweat test for cystic fibrosis. Rockville, MD, Cystic Fibrosis Foundation, 1985, pp 1–4.

Gillard BK, Simbala JA, Goodglick L: Reference intervals for amylase isoenzymes in serum and plasma of infants and children. *Clin Chem* 1983;29:1119.

Hoffman G, Aramaki S, Blum-Hoffman E, et al: Quantitative analysis for organic acids in biological samples: Batch isolation followed by gas chromatographic-mass spectrometric analysis. *Clin Chem* 1989;35:587.

Instructions for Authors: Systeme International (SI) conversion factors for selected laboratory components. *JAMA* 1999;281:19.

Jedeikin R, Makela SK, Shennan AT, et al: Creatine kinase isoenzymes in serum from cord blood and the blood of healthy full-term infants during the first three postnatal days. *Clin Chem* 1982;28:317.

Jung D, Lun L, Zinsmeyer J, et al: The concentration of hypoxanthine and lactate in the blood of healthy and hypoxic newborns. *J Perinat Med* 1985;13:43.

Kaplan EL, Rothermel CD, Johnson DR: Antistreptolysin O and anti-deoxyribonuclease B titers: Normal values for children ages 2 to 12 in the United States. *Pediatrics* 1998;101:86.

Knight JA, Haymond RE: γ-Glutamyltransferase and alkaline phosphatase activities compared in serum of normal children and children with liver disease. *Clin Chem* 1981;27:48.

Koren G, Butt W, Rajchgot P, et al: Intravenous paraldehyde for seizure control in neonates. *Neurology* 1986;36:108.

Krafte-Jacobs B, Bock GH: Circulating erythropoietin and interleukin-6 concentrations increase in critically ill children with sepsis and septic shock. *Crit Care Med* 1996;24:1455.

Laskowska-Klita T, Szymczak E, Radomyska B: Serum homocysteine and lipoprotein (a) concentrations in hypercholesterolemic and normocholesterolemic children. *Clin Pediatr* 2001;40:149–54.

Lockitch G, Halstead AC, Albersheim S, et al: Age and sex specific pediatric reference intervals for biochemistry analytes as measured on the Ektachem-700 analyzer. *Clin Chem* 1988a;34:1622.

Lockitch G, Halstead AC, Quigley G, MacCallum C: Age and sex specific pediatric reference intervals: Study design and methods illustrated by measurement of serum proteins with the Behring LN nephelometer. *Clin Chem* 1988b;34:1618.

Lockitch G, Halstead AC, Wadsworth L, et al: Age and sex specific pediatric reference intervals and correlations for zinc, copper, selenium, iron, vitamins A and E, and related proteins. *Clin Chem* 1988c;34:1625.

Mäkikallio K, Vuolteenaho O, Jouppila P, et al: Association of severe placental insufficiency and systemic venous pressure rise in the fetus with increased neonatal cardiac troponin T levels. *Am J Obstet Gynecol* 2000;183:726–31.

Mayo Medical Laboratories, Rochester, MN 55905

Meites S (editor): *Pediatric Clinical Chemistry, Reference (Normal) Values*, 3rd ed. Washington, DC, American Association for Clinical Chemistry, 1989.

Nichols Institute Diagnostics, San Juan Capistrano, CA 92675

Pesce MA, Bodourian S, Harris RC, Nicholson JF: Enzymatic micromethod for measuring galactose-1-phosphate uridylyltransferase in erythrocytes. *Clin Chem* 1977c;23:1711.

Pesce MA, Bodourian S, Nicholson JF: A new microfluorometric method for the measurement of galactose-1-phosphate in erythrocytes. *Clin Chem Acta* 1982b;118:177.

Pesce MA, Boudorian S: Clinical significance of plasma galactose and erythrocyte galactose-1-phosphate measurements in transferase-deficient galactosemia and in individuals with below-normal transferase activity. *Clin Chem* 1982a;28:301.

Pianosi P, Seargeant L, Haworth JC: Blood lactate and pyruvate concentrations, and their ratio during exercise in healthy children: Developmental perspective. *Eur J Appl Physiol* 1995;71:518.

Pittet JL, de Moerloose P, Reber G, et al: VIDAS D-dimer: Fast quantitative ELISA for measuring D-dimer in plasma. *Clin Chem* 1996;42:410.

Rosenthal P, Pesce MA: Long-term monitoring of D-lactic acidosis in a child. *J Pediatr Gastroenterol Nutr* 1985;4:674.

Schmidt-Sommerfeld E, Werner D, Penn D: Carnitine plasma concentrations in 353 metabolically healthy children. *Eur J Pediatr* 1988;147:356.

Shapira E, Blitzer MG, Miller JB, Africk DK: *Biochemical Genetics. A Laboratory Manual.* New York, Oxford University Press, 1989.

Sherry B, Jack RM, Weber A, Smith AL: Reference interval for prealbumin for children two to 36 months old. *Clin Chem* 1988;34:1878.

Soldin SJ, Bailey J, Beatey J, et al: Pediatric reference ranges for lipase. *Clin Chem* 1995;41:593.

Soldin SJ, Hicks JM, Bailey J, et al: Pediatric reference ranges for 25 hydroxy vitamin D during the summer and winter. *Clin Chem* 1997;43:S200.

Straczcek J, Felden F, Dousset B, et al: Quantification of methymalonic acidin serum measured by capillary gas chromatography-mass spectrometry astert.-butyldimethylsilyl derivatives. *J Chromatogr* 1993;620:1.

Syva Company: *TDM Serum Sample Guide.* Palo Alto, CA, 1986.

Taylor WJ, Caviness MHD (editors): *A Textbook for the Clinical Application of Therapeutic Drug Monitoring.* Irving, TX, Abbott Laboratories, Diagnostic Division, 1986.

Thiru YN, Pathan N, Bignall S, et al: A myocardial cytotoxic process is involved in the cardiac dysfunction of meningococcal septic shock. *Crit Care Med* 2000;28:2979–83.

Unten SK, Hokama Y: Enzyme immunoassay for C-reactive protein analysis. *J Clin Lab Anal* 1987;1:205.

Vilaseca MA, Moyano D, Ferrer I, et al: Total homocysteine in pediatric patients. *Clin Chem* 1997;43:690.

Visnapu LA, Karlson LK, Dubinsky EJ, et al: Pediatric reference ranges for serum aldolase. *Am J Clin Pathol* 1989;91:476.

TABLE 710–7. **Composition of Commonly Used Oral and Parenteral Solutions (Raymond Adelman and Michael Solhaug)**
(See related conversion Tables 710–8 to 710–10)

Fluid	CHO g/dL	Prot*	Calories per L	Na mEq/L	K mEq/L	Cl mEq/L	$HCO_3^†$ mEq/L	Ca mEq/L	$P^‡$ mEq/L	Mg mEq/L	Osm§ mOsm/kg H_2O
Oral											
Apple juice¶	11.9	0.1	480		0.4	26		3	4.5		700
Coca cola¶	10.9		435	4.3	0.1		13.4				656
Ginger ale¶	9.0		360	3.5	0.1		3.6				565
Grape juice	16.6	0.2	672	0.4	30		32				1027
Grapefruit juice¶ (canned, sugar added)	17.8	0.6	736	0.2	35			6.5			591
Milk	4.9	3.5	670	22	36	28	30	60	54		260*
Orange juice¶	10.4	0.7	444	0.2	49		50				654
Pepsi-Cola	12		480	6.5	0.8		7.3				—
Pineapple juice (canned)¶	13.5	0.4	556	0.2	38			7.5	9		783
Prune juice¶	19	0.4	776	0.9	60			7	20		—
Root beer¶				3.5	3.9						588
Seven-Up¶	8.0		320	7.5	0.2			0.3			564
Tomato juice (canned, salted)¶	4.3		172	100	59	150	10	3	18		592
Gatorade	5.9		250	21	2.5	17			6.8		377
Hydra-lyte	2.5		100	84	10	59	15	<1	<1		300
Lytren	7.0		280	30	25	25	36	4	5	4	267**
Pedialyte	5.0		200	30	20	30	28	4		4	387
Rhydrate	2.5	0	100	75	25	65	30	0	0	0	305
Resol Solution	2.0	0	83	50	20	50	34	4	5	4	269
Ricelyte Oral Sol. (rice syrup solids)	3.0	0	140	50	25	45	34	0	0	0	200
Parenteral											
CHO‡‡ in H_2O	5–10		200–400								266–532
Isotonic saline	0–5		0–200	154		154					292–558
½ isotonic saline	2.5–5		100–200	77		77					280–415
3% (M/2) saline				513		513	513				969
5% saline				855		855	855				1616
M/6 sodium lactate				167			167				
5% sodium bicarbonate				595			595				
Lactated Ringer's solution	0–5–10		0–20 0–40 0	130	4	109	28	3			261–531–801
Modified Butler 1 (a)	5		200	25	20	22	23		3	3	360
Modified Butler 2 (b)	5–10		200–400	56	25	49	26		12	5	423–719**
Talbot (c)	5		200	40	35	40	20		15		409
Human plasma protein fraction (d)		5		130	2	50	50				
Blood‡‡		3		95	4	50	40		2	1–2	
Dextran 10% (low mol. wt.) (e)	5		200								
Dextran 10% in saline (f)				154		154					
Dextran 6% (high mol. wt.) (g)	5–10		200–400								
Dextran 6% in saline (h)				154		154					
Mannitol 20%§§											

Available Additives

Glucose 50%	0.5 g/mL
Sodium chloride	2.5 and 5 mEq/mL
Sodium acetate	2 and 4 mEq/mL
Sodium lactate	5 mEq/mL
Sodium bicarbonate	0.5 (4.2%) mEq/mL and 0.9 (7.5%)mEq/mL
Potassium acetate	2 and 4 mEq/mL

Table continued on following page

TABLE 710–7. Composition of Commonly Used Oral and Parenteral Solutions (Raymond Adelman and Michael Solhaug)
(see related conversion Tables 710–8 to 710–10) *Continued*

Fluid	CHO g/dL	Prot*	Calories per L	Na mEq/L	K mEq/L	Cl mEq/L	HCO$_3$† mEq/L	Ca mEq/L	P‡ mEq/L	Osm§ Mg mEq/L	mOsm/kg H$_2$O
Potassium chloride	2 and 3 mEq/mL										
Potassium phosphate	4.4 mEq/mL of potassium and 3 mM/ml phosphate										
Calcium gluconate 10%	9.3 mg (0.465 mEq/mL) elemental calcium										
Calcium chloride 10%	27.3 mg (1.4 mEq/mL) elemental calcium										
Ammonium chloride	5 mEq/mL										
Magnesium sulfate	0.8 mEq/mL, 1 mEq/mL, and 4 mEq/mL available as the 10%, 12.5%, and 50% solutions										

Selected Commercial Preparations in the United States (possible slight variations in composition from values in table)

(a)	Ionosol MB in D$_5$W (A); Isolyte P with 5% Dextrose (M)
(b)	Ionosol B in D$_5$W (A); Electrolyte #2 with 10% Invert Sugar (C,M); 10% Travert in electrolyte #2 (B)
(c)	Ionosol T in D$_5$W (A); Isolyte M (M)
(d)	Plasmatein (A); Plasmanate (C)
(e) (f)	LMD 10% (A); Dextran 40 (C,M); Rheomacrodex (P); Gentran 40 (B)
(g) (h)	Dextran 70 (A); Macrodex (P); Gentran 75 in 10% Travert (B)
(A, Abbott; B, Baxter; C, Cutter; M, McGraw; P, Pharmacia)	

*Protein or amino acid equivalent.
†Actual or potential bicarbonate, such as acetate, lactate, citrate.
‡Calculated according to valence of 1.8.
§Osmolality except for values shown (**), which are osmolarity (in mOsm/L).
¶Composition varies slightly, depending on source.
**See § above.
††Glucose (dextrose, fructose, or invert sugar).
‡‡Red cell contents not included in calculations.
§§Also available: mannitol 5%, 10%, 15%, and 20%.
Sources: Pennington JAT (editor): Bowes & Church's Food Values of Portions Commonly Used, *17th ed. Philadelphia, Lippincott Williams & Wilkins, 1997; Olin BR (editor): Facts and Comparisons. Philadelphia, JB Lippincott, 1993; Murray BN, Peterson LJ: Unpublished observations. Additional Values in Wendland BE, Arbus GS: Oral fluid therapy: Sodium and potassium content and osmolality of some commercial soups, juices and beverages. Can Med Assoc J 1979, 121:564.*

TABLE 710–8. Method for Conversion of Milligrams to Milliequivalents per Liter (or to Millimoles per Liter)

mg = milligrams   mL = milliliter
g = grams   1 mL = 1.000027 cc

dL = deciliter = 100 mL

$$mEq/L \text{ (milliequivalents per liter)} = \frac{mg/L}{\text{equivalent weight}}$$

$$\text{Equivalent weight} = \frac{\text{atomic weight}}{\text{valence of element}}$$

For example: A sample of blood serum contains 10 mg of Ca in 1 dL (100 mL) The valence of Ca is 2, and the atomic weight is 40. The equivalent weight of Ca is therefore 40 ÷ 2, or 20. The milliequivalents of Ca per liter are 10 (mg/dL) × 10 (dL/L) ÷ 20, or 5 milliequivalents per liter.

$$mM/L \text{ (millimoles per liter)} = \frac{mg/L}{\text{molecular weight}}$$

Vol. % (volume per cent) = mM/L × 2.24 for a gas whose properties approach that of an ideal gas, such as oxygen or nitrogen. For carbon dioxide, the factor is 2.226.

TABLE 710–9. Factors for Conversion of Concentration Expressed in Milliequivalents per Liter to Milligrams per Deciliter (100 mL), and Vice Versa, for Common Ions that Occur in Physiologic Solutions

Element or Radical	mEq/L to mg/dL		mg/dL to mEq/L	
Sodium	1	2.30	1	.4348
Potassium	1	3.91	1	.2558
Calcium	1	2.005	1	.4988
Magnesium	1	1.215	1	.8230
Chloride	1	3.55	1	.2817
Bicarbonate (HCO$_3^-$)	1	6.1	1	.1639
Phosphorus valence 1	1	3.10	1	.3226
Phosphorus valence 1.8	1	1.72	1	.5814
Sulfur valence 2	1	1.60	1	.625

Example: to convert milliequivalents of magnesium per liter to milligrams per deciliter (100 mL), multiply by the factor 1.215; to convert milligrams of potassium per deciliter (100 mL) to milliequivalents per liter, multiply by the factor 0.2558.

TABLE 710–10. Milliequivalents and Milligrams of Cations and Anions Present in a Millimole of Salts Commonly Used in Physiologic Solutions

Salt	mg/mmol Salt	Cation	mEq/mmol Salt	mg/mmol Salt	Anion	mEq/mmol Salt	mg/mmol Salt
Sodium chloride (NaCl)	58.5	Na$^+$	1	23.0	Cl$^-$	1	35.5
Potassium chloride (KCl)	74.6	K$^+$	1	39.1	Cl$^-$	1	35.5
Sodium bicarbonate (NaHCO$_3$)	84.0	Na$^+$	1	23.0	HCO$_3^-$	1	61.0
Sodium lactate (CH$_3$CHOHCOONa)	112.0	Na$^+$	1	23.0	CH$_3$CHOHCOO$^-$	1	89.0
Potassium phosphate monobasic (K$_2$HPO$_4$)	174.2	K$^+$	1	78.2	HPO$_4^{2-}$	2	96.0
Potassium phosphate dibasic (KH$_2$PO$_4$)	136.1	K$^+$	1	39.1	H$_2$PO$_4^-$	1	97.0
Calcium chloride, anhydrous (CaCl$_2$)	111.0	Ca^{2+}	2	40.0	Cl$_2^{2-}$	2	71.0
Calcium chloride dihydrate (CaCl$_2$·2H$_2$O)	147.0	Ca^{2+}	2	40.0	Cl$_2^{2-}$	2	71.0
Magnesium chloride, anhydrous (MgCl$_2$)	95.2	Mg^{2+}	2	24.3	Cl$_2^{2-}$	2	71.0
Magnesium chloride hexahydrate (MgCl$_2$·6H$_2$O)	203.3	Mg^{2+}	2	24.3	Cl$_2^{2-}$	2	71.0
Ammonium chloride (NH$_4$Cl)	53.5	NH$_4^+$	1	18.0	Cl$^-$	1	35.5

TABLE 710–11. Food Composition for Short Method of Dietary Analysis (Lewis A. Barness and John S. Curran)*

Food and Approximate Measure	Weight g	Food Energy kcal	Protein g	Fat g	Carbohydrate g	Calcium mg	Iron mg	Vitamin A IU	Thiamine mg	Riboflavin mg	Niacin mg	Ascorbic Acid mg
Milk, cheese, cream; related products												
Cheese: blue, cheddar (1 cu in, 17 g), cheddar process (1 oz), Swiss (1 oz) cottage (from skim) creamed (1/2 c)	30	105	6	9	1	165	0.2	345	0.01	0.12	Trace	0
	115	120	16	5	3	105	0.4	190	0.04	0.28	0.1	0
Cream: half-and-half (cream and milk) (2 tbsp) For light whipping add 1 pat butter	30	40	1	4	2	30	Trace	145	0.01	0.04	Trace	Trace
Milk: whole (3.5% fat) (1 c) fluid, nonfat (skim) and buttermilk (from skim)	245	160	9	9	12	285	0.1	350	0.08	0.42	0.1	2
	245	90	9	Trace	13	300	Trace	—	0.10	0.44	0.2	2
Milk beverage (1 c): cocoa, chocolate drink made with skim milk. For malted milk add 4 tbsp half-and-half (270 g)	245	210	8	8	26	280	0.6	300	0.09	0.43	0.3	Trace
Milk desserts, custard (1 c) 248 g, ice cream (8 fl oz) 142 g		290	8	17	29	210	0.4	785	0.07	0.34	0.1	1
Cornstarch pudding (248 g), ice milk (1 c) 187 g		280	9	10	40	290	0.1	390	0.08	0.41	0.3	2
White sauce, med (1/2 c)	130	215	5	16	12	150	0.2	610	0.06	0.22	0.3	Trace
Egg: 1 Large	50	80	6	6	Trace	25	1.2	590	0.06	0.15	Trace	0
Meat, Poultry, Fish, Shellfish, Related Products												
Beef, lamb, veal: lean and fat, cooked, inc. corned beef (3 oz) (all cuts)	85	245	22	16	0	10	2.9	25	0.06	0.19	4.2	0
lean only, cooked; dried beef (2+ oz) (all cuts)	65	140	20	5	0	10	2.4	10	0.05	0.16	3.4	0
Beef, relatively fat, such as steak and rib, cooked (3 oz)	85	350	18	30	0	10	2.4	60	0.05	0.14	3.5	0
Liver: beef, fried (2 oz)	55	130	15	6	3	5	5.0	30,280	0.15	2.37	9.4	15
Pork, lean and fat, cooked (3 oz) (all cuts)	85	325	20	24	0	10	2.6	0	0.62	0.20	4.2	0
lean only, cooked (2+ oz) (all cuts)	60	150	18	8	0	5	2.2	0	0.57	0.19	3.2	0
ham, light cure, lean and fat, roasted (3 oz)	85	245	18	19	0	10	2.2	0	0.40	0.16	3.1	0
Luncheon meats: bologna (2 sl), pork sausage, cooked (2 oz), frankfurter (1), bacon, broiled or fried crisp (3 sl)	85	185	9	16	—	5	1.3	—	0.21	0.12	1.7	0
Poultry												
Chicken: flesh only, broiled (3 oz)	85	115	20	3	0	10	1.4	80	0.05	0.16	7.4	0
fried (2+ oz)	75	170	24	6	1	10	1.6	85	0.05	0.23	8.3	0
Turkey, light and dark, roasted (3 oz)	85	160	27	5	0	—	1.5	—	0.03	0.15	6.5	0
Fish and shellfish												
Salmon (3 oz) (canned)	85	130	17	5	0	165	0.7	60	0.03	0.16	6.8	0
Fish sticks, breaded, cooked (3–4)	75	130	13	7	5	10	0.3	—	0.03	0.05	1.2	0
Mackerel, halibut, cooked	85	175	19	10	0	10	0.8	515	0.08	0.15	6.8	0
Bluefish, haddock, herring, perch, shad, cooked (tuna canned in oil, 20 g)	85	160	19	8	2	20	1.0	60	0.06	0.11	4.4	0
Clams, canned; crab meat, canned; lobster; oyster, raw; scallop; shrimp, canned	85	75	14	1	2	65	2.5	65	0.10	0.08	1.5	0
Mature Dry Beans and Peas, Nuts, Peanuts, Related Products												
Beans: white with pork and tomato, canned (1 c) Red (128 g), lima (96 g), cowpeas (125 g), cooked (1/2 c)	260	320	16	7	50	140	4.7	340	0.20	0.08	1.5	5
Nuts: almonds (12), cashews (8), peanuts (12), peanut butter (1 tbsp), pecans (12), English walnuts (2 tbsp), coconut (1/4 c)	15	125	8	—	25	35	2.5	5	0.13	0.06	0.7	—
		95	3	8	4	15	0.5	5	0.05	0.9	—	
Vegetables and Vegetable Products												
Asparagus, cooked, cut spears (2/3 c)	115	25	3	Trace	4	25	0.7	1,055	0.19	0.20	1.6	30
Beans: green (1/2 c) cooked 60 g; canned 120 g		15	1	Trace	3	30	0.4	340	0.04	0.06	0.3	8
Lima, immature, cooked (1/2 c)	80	90	6	1	16	40	2.0	225	0.14	0.08	1.0	14

Table continued on following page

TABLE 710–11. Food Composition for Short Method of Dietary Analysis (Lewis A. Barness and John S. Curran)* *Continued*

Food and Approximate Measure	Weight g	Food Energy kcal	Protein g	Fat g	Carbohydrate g	Calcium mg	Iron mg	Vitamin A IU	Thiamine mg	Riboflavin mg	Niacin mg	Ascorbic Acid mg
Broccoli spears, cooked (²/₃ c)	100	25	3	Trace	4	90	0.8	2,500	0.09	0.20	0.8	90
Brussels sprouts, cooked (²/₃ c)	85	30	3	Trace	5	30	1.0	450	0.07	0.12	0.7	75
Cabbage (110 g); cauliflower, cooked (80 g); and sauerkraut, canned (150 mg) (reduce ascorbic acid value by one third for kraut) (²/₃ c)		20	1	Trace	4	35	0.5	80	0.05	0.05	0.3	37
Carrots, cooked (²/₃ c)	95	30	1	Trace	7	30	0.6	10,145	0.05	0.05	0.5	6
Corn, 1 ear, cooked (140 g); canned (130 g) (¹/₂ c)		75	2	Trace	18	5	0.4	315	0.06	0.06	1.1	6
Leafy greens: collards (125 g); dandelions (120 g), kale (75 g), mustard (95 g), spinach (120 g), turnip (100 g cooked, 150 g canned) (²/₃ c cooked and canned)		30	3	Trace	5	175	1.8	8,570	0.11	0.18	0.8	45
Peas, green (¹/₂ c)	80	60	4	1	10	20	1.4	430	0.22	0.09	1.8	16
Potatoes, baked, boiled (100 g), 10 pc. French fried (55 g) (for fried, add 1 tbsp cooking oil)		85	3	Trace	30	10	0.7	Trace	0.08	0.04	1.5	16
Pumpkin, canned (¹/₂ c)	115	40	1	1	9	30	0.5	7,295	0.03	0.06	0.6	6
Squash, winter, canned (¹/₂ c)	100	65	2	1	16	30	0.8	4,305	0.05	0.14	0.7	14
Sweet potato, canned (¹/₂ c)	110	120	2	—	27	25	0.8	8,500	0.05	0.05	0.7	15
Tomato, 1 raw, ²/₃ c canned, ²/₃ c juice	150	35	2	Trace	7	14	0.8	1,350	0.10	0.06	1.0	29
Tomato catsup (2 tbsp)	35	30	1	Trace	8	10	0.2	480	0.04	0.02	0.6	6
Other, cooked (beets, mushrooms, onions, turnips) (¹/₂ c)	95	25	1	—	5	20	0.5	15	0.02	0.10	0.7	7
Other, commonly served raw, cabbage (¹/₂ c, 50 g), celery (3 sm stalks, 40 g), cucumber (¹/₄ med, 50 g), green pepper (¹/₂, 30 g), radishes (5, 40 g)		10	Trace	Trace	2	15	0.3	100	0.03	0.03	0.2	20
carrots, raw (¹/₂ carrot)	25	10	Trace	Trace	2	10	0.2	2,750	0.02	0.02	0.2	2
lettuce leaves (2 lg)	50	10	1	Trace	2	34	0.7	950	0.03	0.04	0.2	9
Fruits and Fruit Products												
Cantaloupe (¹/₂ med)	385	60	1	Trace	14	25	0.8	6,540	0.08	0.06	1.2	63
Citrus and strawberries: orange (1), grapefruit (¹/₂), juice (¹/₂ c), strawberries (¹/₂ c), lemon (1), tangerine (1)		50	1		13	25	0.4	165	0.08	0.03	0.3	55
Yellow, fresh: apricots (3), peach (2 med); canned fruit and juice (¹/₂ c) or dried, cooked, unsweetened: apricot, peaches (¹/₂ c)		85	—	—	22	10	1.1	1,005	0.01	0.05	1.0	5
Other, dried: dates, pitted (4), figs (2), raisins (¹/₄ c)	40	120	1	—	31	35	1.4	20	0.04	0.04	0.5	—
Other, fresh apple (1), banana (1), figs (3), pear (1)		80	—	—	21	15	0.5	140	0.04	0.03	0.2	6
Grain Products												
Enriched and whole grain: bread (1 sl, 23 g), biscuit (¹/₂), cooked cereals (¹/₂ c), prepared cereals (1 oz), graham crackers (2 lg), macaroni, noodles, spaghetti (¹/₂ c, cooked), pancake (1, 27 g), roll (¹/₂ c), waffle (¹/₂, 38 g)		65	2	1	16	20	0.6	10	0.09	0.05	0.7	
Unenriched bread (1 sl, 23 g), cooked cereal (¹/₂ c), macaroni, noodles, spaghetti (¹/₂ c), popcorn (¹/₂ c), pretzel sticks, small (15), roll (¹/₂)		65	2	1	16	10	0.3	5	0.02	0.02	0.3	
Desserts												
Cake, plain (1 pc), doughnut (1). For iced cake or doughnut add value for sugar (1 tbsp). For chocolate cake add chocolate (30 g)	45	145	2	5	24	30	0.4	65	0.02	0.05	0.2	
Cookies, plain (1)	25	120	1	5	18	10	0.2	20	0.01	0.01	0.01	—
Pie crust, single crust (¹/₇ shell)	20	95	1	6	8	3	0.3	0	0.04	0.03	0.3	—
Flour, white, enriched (1 tbsp)	7	25	1	Trace	5	1	0.2	0	0.03	0.02	0.2	0
Fats and Oils												
Butter, margarine (1 pat, ¹/₂ tbsp)	7	50	Trace	6	Trace	1	0	230	—	—	—	—

Food and approximate measure											
Fats and oils, cooking (1 tbsp), French dressing (2 tbsp)	125	0	14	0	0	0	0	0	0	0	0
Salad dressings, mayonnaise type (1 tbsp)	80	Trace	9	1	2	0.1	45	Trace	Trace	Trace	0
Sugars, Sweets											
Candy, plain (1/2 oz), jam and jelly (1 tbsp), syrup (1 tbsp), gelatin dessert, plain (1/2 c), beverages, carbonated (1 c)	60	0	0	14	3	0.1	Trace	Trace	Trace	Trace	Trace
Chocolate fudge (1 oz), chocolate syrup (3 tbsp)	125	2	1	30	15	0.6	10	Trace	0.02	0.1	Trace
Molasses (1 tbsp), caramel (1/2 oz)	40	Trace	Trace	8	20	0.3	Trace	Trace	Trace	Trace	Trace
Sugar (1 tbsp)	45	0	0	12	0	Trace	0	0	0	0	0
Miscellaneous											
Chocolate, bitter (1 oz)	145	3	15	8	20	1.9	20	0.01	0.07	0.4	0
Sherbet (1/2 c)	130	1	1	30	15	Trace	55	0.01	0.03	Trace	2
Soups											
Bean, pea (green) (1 c)	150	7	4	22	50	1.6	495	0.09	0.06	1.0	4
Noodle, beef, chicken (1 c)	65	4	2	7	10	0.7	50	0.03	0.04	0.9	Trace
Clam chowder, minestrone, tomato, vegetable (1 c)	90	3	2	14	25	0.9	1,880	0.05	0.04	1.1	3

*See related conversion Tables 710–8 to 710–10.
From Wilson ED, Fisher KH, Fuqua ME: Principles of Nutrition, 2nd ed. New York, John Wiley & Sons, 1965, pp 528–533.

TABLE 710–12. Nutritive Value of Baby Foods (Per Serving)*

Food	Serving g	Energy kcal	Protein g	Fat g	Carbohydrate g	Sodium mg	Calcium mg	Iron mg	Vitamin A IU	Thiamine mg	Riboflavin mg	Niacin mg	Ascorbic Acid mg
Cereals													
Barley	2.4	9	0.3	0.1	1.8	1	19	1.1		0.07	0.07	0.9	0
High protein	2.4	9	0.9	0.1	1.1	1	17	1.8		0.06	0.07	0.8	0
Mixed	2.4	9	0.3	0.1	1.8	1	18	1.5		0.06	0.07	0.8	0
Oatmeal	2.4	10	0.3	0.2	1.7	1	18	1.8		0.07	0.06	0.9	0
Rice	2.4	9	0.2	0.1	1.9	1	20	1.8		0.06	0.05	0.8	0
Dinners, Jar													
Beef and egg noodle	213	122	5.4	4.0	15.7	37	18	0.9	1,400	0.06	0.08	1.2	3
Chicken and noodles, jr.	213	109	4.1	3.0	16.1	36	36	0.8	1,900	0.06	0.07	1.1	3
Macaroni and ham, jr.	213	127	6.8	2.9	18.0	101	159	0.8	1,100	0.12	0.21	1.7	5
Turkey and rice, jr.	213	104	3.8	2.9	15.3	33	50	0.6	2,200	0.02	0.06	0.6	3
Spaghetti, tomato, beef, jr.	213	135	5.4	2.7	21.6	42	39	1.1	1,500	0.14	0.15	2.3	5
Fruits													
Applesauce, jr.	213	79	0.1	0.0	21.9	5	10	0.4	20	0.03	0.06	0.1	81
Applesauce, apricots, jr.	220	104	0.5	0.5	27.3	6	13	0.6	745	0.03	0.07	0.3	39
Bananas, tapioca, jr.	220	147	0.8	0.4	39.1	21	17	0.7	100	0.03	0.04	0.5	57
Peaches	220	157	1.3	0.4	41.6	10	11	0.6	400	0.03	0.07	1.4	42
Pears	213	93	0.6	0.2	24.7	4	18	0.5	70	0.03	0.06	0.4	47
Meats, Poultry													
Beef	99	105	14.3	4.9	0	65	8	1.6	100	0.01	0.16	3.3	2
Chicken	99	148	14.6	9.5	0	50	54	1.0	200	0.01	0.16	3.4	2
Ham	99	123	14.9	6.6	0	66	5	1.0	30	0.14	0.19	2.8	2
Lamb	99	111	15.0	5.2	2.5	73	7	1.6	30	0.02	0.20	3.2	2
Turkey	99	128	15.2	7.0	0	72	28	1.3	600	0.02	0.25	3.4	2
Egg Yolks	94	191	9.4	16.3	0.9	37	72	2.6	1,200	0.07	0.25	1.45	1
Vegetables													
Beans	206	51	2.5	0.3	11.8	3	133	2.2	900	0.04	0.21	0.7	17
Beets	128	43	1.7	0.1	9.8	106	18	0.4	40	0.01	0.06	0.2	4
Carrots	213	67	1.7	0.4	15.4	104	49	0.8	25,000	0.05	0.09	1.1	12
Mixed	213	88	3.1	0.8	17.4	77	24	0.9	9,000	0.06	0.07	1.4	5
Peas	213	113	7.0	1.1	19.0	15	34	1.9	700	0.15	0.13	2.0	9
Squash	213	51	1.8	0.4	12.0	3	50	0.7	4,000	0.02	0.14	0.8	17
Sweet potatoes	220	113	2.4	0.3	30.7	49	35	0.8	15,000	0.06	0.08	0.8	21

*See related conversion Tables 710–6 to 710–8.
Data from Pennington JAT (editor): Bowes and Church's Food Values of Portions Commonly Used, 15th ed. New York, Harper & Row, 1989.

TABLE 710–13. Equivalent Temperature Readings (Celsius and Fahrenheit)

C	F	C	F	C	F	C	F
0	32.0	37.2	99	39.2	102.6	41.2	106.2
20	68.0	37.4	99.3	39.4	102.9	41.4	106.5
30	86.0	37.6	99.7	39.6	103.3	41.6	106.9
31	87.8	37.8	100.1	39.8	103.7	41.8	107.2
32	89.6	38	100.4	40.0	104	42	107.6
33	91.4	38.2	100.8	40.2	104.4	43	109.4
34	93.2	38.4	101.2	40.4	104.7	44	111.2
35	95.0	38.6	101.5	40.6	105.1	100	212
36	96.8	38.8	101.8	40.8	105.4		
37	98.6	39	102.2	41.0	105.8		

To convert Celsius (centigrade) readings to Fahrenheit, multiply by 1.8 and add 32. To convert Fahrenheit readings to Celsius, subtract 32 and divide by 1.8.

Chapter 711
Principles of Drug Therapy

Michael D. Reed and Peter Gal

Clinical pharmacology is concerned with the integration of the pharmacokinetic and pharmacodynamic profile of a drug to optimize drug therapy. **Pharmacokinetics** is the quantitative evaluation of each component of disposition of a compound, that is, the processes of absorption, distribution, metabolism, and excretion. The ability to estimate the pharmacokinetic parameters of a drug accurately permits the determination of the dose and dose interval to achieve a defined target concentration, desired pharmacologic effect, or both. A drug concentration in a specific body fluid is, in theory, a reflection of the drug concentration in tissue, reflecting its concentration at its site of action, the receptor. The concentration of a drug in blood (or other body fluid), however, is not necessarily equal to the concentration of the drug in tissue or at its receptor site. It is important to appreciate the challenges involved in determining drug concentrations in body fluids, including physical access of that body fluid, available volume that can be safely removed, and the sensitivity and specificity of available laboratory methodology.

Pharmacodynamics involves the correlation of pharmacologic response to a measured drug concentration in blood (or other body fluid). The pharmacologic or toxicologic effects of most drugs are a result of their interaction with micromolecular and macromolecular components of cells. Rational prescribing of drugs depends on a fundamental understanding of the pharmacokinetic and pharmacodynamic profile of the drug, and studies show that drugs dosed using pharmacokinetic/pharmacodynamic dosing approaches have better response rates and less toxicity. Understanding the effect of age is essential to understanding pediatric drug therapy, because age is one of the most important variables that influences the processes responsible for disposition of a drug and action in children.

Influence of Age on Drug Therapy. Drugs administered orally must cross many physiologic membranes before entering the systemic circulation and being distributed to their site of action.

GASTROINTESTINAL ABSORPTION. Although certain xenobiotics and nutrients are absorbed by active transport or facilitated diffusion, most drugs are absorbed from the gastrointestinal tract by passive diffusion. A number of important patient variables can affect the rate and extent of gastrointestinal absorption of a drug, including pH-dependent diffusion; the presence, absence, and type of gastric contents; gastric emptying time; and gastrointestinal motility. These physiologic processes reflect a clear but highly variable dependence on a patient's age (Table 711–1). Despite the clear maturational changes observed in the functional capacity of these processes and their importance to intestinal drug absorption, the overall bioavailability of most orally administered medications in neonates and young infants is adequate. Whenever possible, the oral route for drug administration is preferred.

ALTERNATIVE ROUTES OF DRUG ABSORPTION. Another common means of extravascular drug administration in infants and children, other than the oral route, is the intramuscular route. Drugs administered intramuscularly should be water soluble at physiologic pH to prevent precipitation and the resultant decreased, delayed, or erratic absorption from the injection site. Lipid solubility of a drug favors diffusion into the capillaries. Blood flow to and from the injection site should be adequate to ensure absorption into the systemic circulation. This physiologic requirement may be compromised in seriously ill infants and children with poor peripheral perfusion resulting from low cardiac output and respiratory disease.

The skin is another important but often overlooked organ for the absorption of various therapeutic agents and environmental chemicals. This is exemplified by the toxic effects noted in newborn infants exposed to hexachlorophene, aniline-containing disinfectant solutions, and hydrocortisone. The percutaneous absorption of a compound is directly related to the degree of skin hydration and inversely related to the thickness of the stratum corneum. The full-term newborn's integument is a more effective functional barrier than the skin of a premature infant. More importantly, however, the ratio of the newborn's skin surface area to body weight is approximately three times greater than that of an adult. Therefore, the amount of drug absorbed into the systemic circulation (bioavailability) for an identical percutaneous dose of a drug is approximately three times greater in an infant than in an adult. These characteristics of skin make topical creams and patch formulation of drugs important means of drug delivery in infants with adequate perfusion.

The effects of maturational changes on the bioavailability of a drug are unpredictable. A prolonged gastric emptying time and irregular intestinal peristaltic activity can lead to erratic rates of drug absorption, reducing the amount of drug absorbed, blunting or delaying the peak serum concentration, or both. Reducing the rate or amount of total drug absorbed into the body (or both) can be therapeutically important, leading to inadequate dosing, whereas blunting or delaying a drug's peak serum concentration may be of only minor clinical significance. The extent to which maturational changes influence gastrointestinal drug absorption also depends on the specific drug formulation administered. Solid dosage forms (tablets, capsules) must dissolve into solution before the drug can cross cell membranes. Most drugs administered to infants and young children are available in a liquid formulation, including some as a suspension. In general, the rate of absorption is faster after administration of a liquid dosing formulation (liquid > suspension) as compared with solid formulations (capsule ≥ tablet > sustained/delayed-release tablet).

TABLE 711–1. Physiologic Factors That Influence the Oral Absorption of Medications

Parameter	Neonate	Infant	Child
Gastric acid secretion	Reduced	Normal	Normal
Gastric emptying time	Decreased	Increased	Increased
Intestinal motility	Reduced	Normal	Normal
Biliary function	Reduced	Normal	Normal
Microbial flora	Acquiring	Adult pattern	Adult pattern

DRUG DISTRIBUTION. Understanding the distribution characteristics of the drug in the body is important when selecting the dose. Although the distribution volume, the **V_d or the apparent volume of distribution,** of a drug does not denote any real physiologic volume, an estimate of this pharmacokinetic parameter provides insight into the total amount of drug present in the body relative to its concentration in blood and thus the tissue distribution. Knowledge of the V_d of a drug is important when selecting an initial loading dose or designing an optimal drug dosage regimen to attain a pre-selected target concentration. The value of the V_d for a number of drugs differs markedly among newborns (premature vs. full-term), infants, and children as compared with adults. These differences are a result of many important age-dependent variables, including the composition and size of body water compartments, protein binding characteristics, and hemodynamic factors, including cardiac output, regional blood flow, and membrane permeability. The absolute amounts and distribution of body water and fat depend on a child's age and are well characterized. Changes in body water compartment sizes and water distribution account for the differences observed in the V_d in infants and children.

The extent to which a drug is bound to circulating plasma proteins directly influences the distribution characteristics of the drug. Only the free, unbound drug can be distributed from the vascular space into other body fluids and tissues, where it binds to its receptor and stimulates a response. Drug binding to plasma proteins depends on a number of age-related variables, including the absolute amount of proteins available, their respective number of available binding sites, the affinity constant of the drug for the protein, the influence of pathophysiologic conditions, and the presence of endogenous substances, which may compete for protein binding (protein displacement interactions). These and other clinically important variables can affect drug protein binding relative to age. The extent to which a drug is bound to protein markedly influences its V_d and body clearance (Cl) as well as intensity of pharmacologic effects.

Albumin, α_1-acid glycoprotein, and lipoproteins are the most important circulating proteins responsible for drug binding in plasma. The absolute concentration of these proteins is influenced by age, nutrition, and disease. Basic drugs bind mainly to albumin, α_1-acid glycoprotein, and lipoprotein, whereas acidic and neutral compounds bind primarily to albumin. Serum albumin and total protein concentrations are decreased during infancy, approaching adult values by the age of 10–12 mo. A similar pattern of maturation is observed with α_1-acid glycoprotein; concentrations appear to be approximately three times lower in neonatal plasma compared with those in maternal plasma, achieving values comparable to those of adults by 12 mo of age.

In addition to drugs, several endogenous substances presenting in human plasma may bind to plasma proteins and compete for available drug-binding sites. During the neonatal period, free fatty acids, bilirubin, and 2-hydroxybenzoylglycine compete for albumin binding sites and influence the resultant balance between free and bound drug concentrations. Clinically significant protein binding displacement reactions occur only when a drug is more than 80–90% protein bound, the Cl of a drug is limited, and its apparent V_d is small, usually less than 0.15 L/kg. It is prudent to assess a drug's potential for displacement of bilirubin from protein-binding sites before its administration to premature and newborn infants.

DRUG METABOLISM. The moment a drug molecule is present within the body, the process of its removal begins. The overall rate of drug removal is described by the pharmacokinetic parameter clearance (Cl), or body Cl. A drug's body Cl is the summation of all clearance mechanisms involved in removing that compound from the body (see later under "Clearance"). The primary organ for drug metabolism is the liver, although the kidney, intestine, lung, adrenals, blood (phosphatases, esterases), and skin can also biotransform certain compounds. For most drugs (lipophilic weak acids or weak bases), biotransformation to more polar, water-soluble compounds facilitates their elimination from the body through the bile, kidney, or lung. Although the biotransformation of most drugs results in pharmacologically weaker or inactive compounds, parent compounds may be transformed into active metabolites or intermediates (e.g., theophylline to caffeine, carbamazepine to 10,11-carbamazepine epoxide). Conversely, pharmacologically inactive parent compounds or prodrugs may be converted to an active moiety (e.g., chloramphenicol succinate to active chloramphenicol base, cefuroxime axetil to active cefuroxime) before subsequent biotransformation and body elimination.

Drug metabolism within the hepatocyte involves two primary enzymatic processes: phase I, or nonsynthetic, and phase II, or synthetic, reactions. **Phase I reactions** include oxidation, reduction, hydrolysis, and hydroxylation reactions, whereas **phase II reactions** primarily involve conjugation with glycine, glucuronide, or sulfate. Most drug-metabolizing enzymes are located in the smooth endoplasmic reticulum of cells. Of these mixed-function oxidase systems, the cytochrome (CYP) P450 system has been studied in greatest detail. The **CYP450 enzyme system** is a supergene family with more than 13 primary enzymes and a number of isozymes of specific gene families. The specific subfamilies, or isozymes, most responsible for human drug metabolism involve CYP450 1A2, 2D6, 2C19, and 3A4. At birth, the concentration of drug-oxidizing enzymes in fetal liver (corrected for liver weight) is similar to that in adult liver. The activity of these oxidizing enzyme systems is reduced, however, which is reflected by a prolonged body elimination for drugs that depend on oxidation pathways in newborns (e.g., phenytoin, diazepam). Postnatally, the hepatic cytochrome P450 mono-oxygenase system appears to mature rapidly; metabolic activity similar to or in excess of the adult value is achieved by approximately 6 mo of age. An understanding of the substrates for specific isozymes and the effects certain drugs may have on isozyme activity (e.g., induction, inhibition) allows the clinician to predict the possibility of clinically important metabolic-based drug-drug interactions. Substrates, inducers, and inhibitors of specific isozymes important in human drug metabolism are summarized in Table 711–2.

The activity of certain hydrolytic enzymes, including blood esterases, is also reduced during the neonatal period. Blood esterases are important for the metabolic clearance of cocaine, and the reduced activity of these plasma esterases in the newborn may account for the delayed metabolism of cocaine in neonates.

Because elimination of metabolites is reduced in preterm and full-term infants, accumulation of active metabolites not considered clinically relevant in older infants, children, and adults may occur in infants. Such is the case with the *N*-methylation of theophylline to caffeine. This pathway becomes more important in neonates because theophylline is less readily metabolized, making it more available for *N*-methylation. Caffeine itself is normally metabolized before elimination, but in preterm infants with immature liver enzymes the compound is mainly eliminated by the kidneys. This renal elimination is slow because of the immaturity of renal function in young infants, resulting in the potential for marked caffeine accumulation and toxicity if caffeine concentrations collected before steady-state are not appropriately interpreted.

Understanding the sequence of maturation of processes of drug metabolism is important when developing dosage recommendations for drugs that undergo extensive hepatic metabolism. An example of the consequences of failing to appreciate these processes is the tragedy that occurred after the administration of usual doses of chloramphenicol (75–100 mg/kg/24 hr) to premature and newborn infants (fatal gray-baby syndrome) and the resultant beneficial use of this compound in the same

TABLE 711–2. Important Cytochrome P450 Isozymes in Human Drug Metabolism: Isozyme Substrates, Inhibitors, and Inducers

Isoenzyme	Polymorphism	Substrates	Inhibitors	Inducers
1A2	Possible	Acetaminophen, caffeine, clomipramine, clozapine, imipramine, phenacetin, propranolol, tacrine, theophylline	Fluvoxamine, quinolones (e.g., ciprofloxacin)	Cruciferous vegetables, omeprazole, aromatic hydrocarbons, smoking
2C9	Yes	Diclofenac, ibuprofen, phenytoin, tolbutamide, S-warfarin	Fluconazole, isoniazid, itraconazole(?), ketoconazole(?), sulfaphenazole	Rifampin
2C19	Yes	Amitriptyline, citalopram, diazepam, imipramine, mephobarbital, olmeprazole, propranolol	Fluconazole, fluvoxamine, fluoxetine, omeprazole	Rifampin
2D6	Yes	Amitriptyline, citalopram, clomipramine, codeine, desipramine, dextromethorphan, doxepin, encainide, flecainide, fluoxetine, haloperidol, imipramine, loratadine, metoprolol, nortriptyline, paroxetine, perphenazine, propafenone, propranolol, risperidone, thioridazine, timolol, tramadol	Cimetidine, fluoxetine, norfluoxetine, nefazodone (plus metabolites), paroxetine, perphenazine, propoxyphene, quinidine, sertraline, thioridazine	
2E1	No	Acetaminophen, alcohol, chlorzoxazone, dapsone	Disulfiram, isoniazid	Ethanol, isoniazid
3A4	Possible	Alfentanil, alprazolam, amiodarone, amitriptyline, astemizole, carbamazepine, cisapride, cyclosporine, dapsone, diazepam, diltiazem, disopyramide, erythromycin, ethinylestradiol, imipramine, indinavir, lidocaine, loratadine, lovastatin, midazolam, nifedipine, nefazodone, progesterone, quinidine, ritonavir, saquinovir, tacrolimus (FK-506), terfenadine, testosterone, triazolam, verapamil	Cimetidine, citalopram, diltiazem, ethynylestradiol, fluconazole, fluvoxamine, fluoxetine, indinavir, norfluoxetine, itraconazole, ketoconazole, macrolides (clarithromycin, erythromycin), metronidazole, nefazodone, naringenin, ritonavir	Carbamazepine, dexamethasone, phenobarbital, phenytoin, rifampin

patient population when the dose was appropriately adjusted (15–50 mg/kg/24 hr) to compensate for the decreased hepatic ability for glucuronidation. Chloramphenicol glucuronide is the primary metabolite of chloramphenicol, which is then excreted through the kidneys.

The ultimate ability of children to metabolize drugs may be genetically modulated. Pharmacogenetic predisposition to slow drug metabolism along certain enzymatic pathways can provide important clues to patients at risk for drug toxicity. This is a rapidly developing area of research, and it is reasonable to anticipate future clinical applications for pharmacogenetic and pharmacogenomic knowledge about drug metabolism.

DRUG EXCRETION. The amount of drug that is filtered by the glomerulus per unit of time depends on the functional ability of the glomerulus, on the integrity of renal blood flow, and on the extent of drug-protein binding. The amount of drug filtered is inversely related to the degree of protein binding. Only the free drug is filtered by the glomerulus and excreted. Although highly variable, renal blood flow averages 12 mL/min at birth, approaching the adult value by 5–12 mo of age. The glomerular filtration rate is 2–4 mL/min in full-term infants, increases to 8–20 mL/min by 2–3 days of life, and approaches the adult value by 3–5 mo of age. Before 34 wk of gestation, glomerular filtration is markedly reduced and increases slowly.

PHARMACOKINETICS

Basic Concepts. Pharmacokinetics is the mathematical expression of the time course of drug movement in the body. It is clinically useful only when integrated with the pharmacodynamic characteristics of the drug. Because the pharmacologic effects of most drugs are reversible, the time of onset, intensity, and duration of effect of a drug are proportional to the amount of drug in the body at any point in time. Pharmacokinetic-based methods can be used to predict drug concentration at any time after a dose is administered and can facilitate calculation of a drug dose to achieve a desired concentration. Recognition that the pharmacologic effects, toxicologic effects, or both correlate best with its concentration in a biologic fluid (blood) rather than the absolute dose administered is the foundation of applied clinical pharmacokinetics.

The **biodisposition** of most drugs used clinically is best described using the principles of linear or first-order pharmaco-

kinetics—that is, the serum concentration or, more appropriately, the amount of drug in the body is directly proportional to the dose administered. For example, if the dose of a drug that follows linear pharmacokinetics is doubled, its resultant concentration in blood (at steady state) also doubles. This characteristic of proportionality, combined with appropriate patient monitoring, is often used clinically to make adjustments in drug dosing (see later, "Individualization of Drug Dose"). In contrast, some drugs, such as phenytoin, salicylate, and alcohol, exhibit saturation kinetics; their elimination pathways become "saturated," and the resultant drug concentration in the blood changes disproportionately to the dose administered. Under usual clinical conditions, these drugs exhibit linear (first-order) elimination characteristics at low doses (low serum concentrations) but, as the amount of drug in the body increases with increasing dose, their elimination pathways become saturated. Such drugs are often called drugs that follow the principles of zero-order, or Michaelis-Menten, kinetics. The classic principles of elimination half-life ($t_{1/2}$) and Cl do not apply to drugs that exhibit zero-order kinetics. Describing more drug disposition profiles in pediatric patients, where sampling volumes and frequency must be limited has been made more feasible through newer pharmacokinetic research techniques, such as optimal sampling theory.

DRUG ABSORPTION AND BIOAVAILABILITY. To be effective, a drug must be absorbed from its site of administration into the systemic circulation, from where it is distributed to its site of action and eliminated from the body. Bioavailability is a measure of the amount of drug absorbed into the systemic circulation over a finite period. With few exceptions (prodrugs), a drug administered intravenously is 100% bioavailable. The bioavailability of a drug is most often described as a fraction of the amount absorbed after extravascular drug administration relative to intravenous (IV) drug administration. Bioavailability is calculated as the ratio of the area under the drug concentration time curve (AUC) determined after extravascular drug administration to the drug AUC obtained after intravenous administration (i.e., AUC oral/AUC IV).

The absorption profile of a drug is a composite that depends on both the bioavailability (amount) and the rate of absorption into the systemic circulation. The rate and extent of drug absorption are influenced by a number of physicochemical and patient-related factors. For example, the presence of food in the stomach and duodenum can decrease the rate but generally does not affect the overall extent of absorption of many orally administered drugs. The clinical relevance of this interaction depends on whether the drug's efficacy is related to its peak serum concentration (decreased rate would blunt the peak concentration) or the total amount of drug in the body. Appreciating the rate of drug absorption can be important in anticipating the onset of toxicologic symptoms in cases of drug overdose. In contrast, a disease or a drug interaction that results in a decrease in drug bioavailability would be expected to influence a patient's response to therapy. The concurrent administration of phenytoin and enteral tube feedings can markedly decrease phenytoin bioavailability. Such drug-food interactions may be easily overlooked as a cause of therapeutic failure.

VOLUME OF DISTRIBUTION. The V_d is the hypothetical volume of fluid in which a drug is distributed; it is a proportionality constant that relates the amount of drug in the body to its serum concentration. The apparent V_d is expressed by the equation $V_d = D/C_p$, where C_p is the peak concentration of drug following administration of the dose D. The V_d may be used to calculate the initial or loading dose (LD) of a drug needed to achieve a desired serum concentration (C_p). V_d may also be used to select an appropriate bolus dose to increase from a known subtherapeutic concentration to a target therapeutic concentration. If a desired C_p is selected and an age-appropriate "average" V_d is known or obtained from the literature, a dose necessary to obtain that concentration can be easily calculated:

$$LD = C_p \ (mg/L) \times V_d \ (L/kg) \times patient's \ body \ weight \ (kg)$$

Furthermore, it is apparent from this relationship that drug elimination from the body, or drug clearance, does not influence the initial or loading dose of a drug. For example, although a drug may be eliminated from the body only through the kidneys, the initial dose is the same for patients with normal renal function as for those with compromised or no renal function. The first dose of drug achieves an equilibrium concentration between body fluids and tissues.

ELIMINATION HALF-LIFE. The **elimination half-life ($t_{1/2}$)** of a drug is the time required for any given concentration in blood (or other biologic fluid) to decrease to half of the initial value, that is, the time required for half the amount of drug present in the fluid to be cleared. The $t_{1/2}$ can be determined as

$$t_{1/2} = 0.693/Kd$$

where Kd is equal to the slope of the terminal portion of the natural log of the linear serum concentration versus time curve. The $t_{1/2}$ depends on both the Cl and V_d of the drug. A more useful formula for $t_{1/2}$, which reflects these important relationships, is

$$t_{1/2} = (0.693)(V_d)/Cl$$

Thus, a change in $t_{1/2}$ does not necessarily reflect a change in body Cl of a drug. This dependence of $t_{1/2}$ on V_d is exemplified by the influence of extracorporeal membrane oxygenation (ECMO) on drug disposition. For most drugs, ECMO-induced changes are due to an increase in drug V_d rather than any change in drug Cl. Nevertheless, despite this important distinction, the $t_{1/2}$ is often used clinically to adjust dosing intervals, primarily because it can easily be calculated in the clinic or at the patient's bedside. The $t_{1/2}$ of a drug can also be used to determine the time necessary to achieve the steady-state concentration, that is, the point at which the amount of drug administered (dose) is equivalent to the amount of drug cleared from the body. After three half-lives, 87.5% of a drug's steady-state concentration is achieved; after four half-lives, it is 93.8%; and after five half-lives, it is 100%. When integrated with a target concentration strategy, the $t_{1/2}$ of a drug is often used to determine a drug's dosage interval.

CLEARANCE. **Clearance (Cl)** is the pharmacokinetic parameter that estimates the theoretical volume from which a drug is removed per unit of time. The body clearance of a drug reflects the amount of drug removed or eliminated from the body per unit of time, whereas renal Cl reflects the amount of drug cleared by the kidneys per unit of time. Total body Cl is the summation of all Cl mechanisms for a given drug (Cl_{renal}, $Cl_{hepatic}$, Cl_{lung}). The body Cl can be calculated as

$$Cl = (0.693)(V_d)/t_{1/2}$$

with the preferred mathematical method of drug dose/AUC where the dose is corrected for bioavailability. Knowledge of the Cl of a drug is fundamental when determining the need for a drug and how often its dose must be repeated to maintain a given serum concentration. It is the most important pharmacokinetic parameter for determining the steady-state drug concentration for a given dose rate. Changes in organ function responsible for the removal of a drug from the body are reflected as a change in the drug Cl. A drug's body Cl is influenced by the integrity of blood flow and by the functional ability of the organs involved in removing the drug from the body.

Individualization of Drug Dose. The clinical response to an average or usual recommended dose of drug can vary considerably, even when the dose is administered relative to a patient's body weight, surface area, and stage of maturation. This variation is a result of interindividual differences in drug pharmacokinetics and pharmacodynamics and a number of biologic variables, including genetic differences in drug metabolism or drug receptors, and concurrent pathophysiology. Individual variability with respect to drug efficacy and possibly toxicity frequently necessitates the adjustment of dosage regimens for specific patients, especially when prescribing drugs with a low therapeutic index. For some drugs the dose may be adjusted according to the patient's immediate and readily quantifiable clinical response. For other drugs, dosage adjustment may be guided more appropriately by combining clinical response with measuring the concentration of drug in plasma or serum. Such an approach to therapy is often called a **target concentration strategy**, where a drug's pharmacologic or toxicologic response can be directly related to a specific serum concentration range. It is important to recognize that the therapeutic ranges described for drugs reflect a continuum of concentrations along which increasing percentages of patients can be expected to have a clinical response and toxicity (pharmacodynamic curves), and it is the tradeoff between benefit and risk that each clinician must use to decide whether targeting the lower or upper region of the therapeutic range or even exceeding the therapeutic range is optimal. Close attention to the pharmacologic actions and physiologic responses is necessary for this optimal target concentration strategy.

Reported therapeutic concentration ranges for drugs are usually determined from studies of only a limited number of patients, mostly adults, and these therapeutic ranges represent an average (mean) value, and therefore only 49% of the population is encompassed within the two standard deviations that surround this mean value. Thus, the clinical monitoring of serum drug concentrations serves only as a guide to pharmacologic intervention and dose adjustment. Serum drug concentration values must be interpreted individually for each patient. For example, one patient may have a complete clinical response when the serum concentration of drug X is within the "low" portion of the therapeutic range or window. Conversely, the next patient, with the same disease of similar severity requiring the same drug X, may require a serum drug concentration above or below the reported therapeutic concentration range to achieve the same degree of positive therapeutic response. Toxicity, however, may limit how much above the therapeutic range the serum drug concentration may safely be raised. Therefore, therapeutic ranges for serum drug concentrations serve only as guidelines for therapy. Drug efficacy must be assessed by clinical response.

Serum drug concentration-time values or profiles may also be compared with previously determined patient-specific values or literature reports to assess patient compliance with a prescribed drug regimen. More commonly, the determination of a drug concentration in biologic fluid helps to achieve an optimal therapeutic regimen while reducing the likelihood of drug toxicity. Finally, the determination of a drug concentration in a biologic fluid provides a means to assess the influences, if any, of disease process or drug interaction on a drug's disposition profile.

Therapeutic drug monitoring is not appropriate, necessary, or practical for all drugs. Drugs with well-defined and easily recognizable and monitored pharmacodynamic effects do not warrant routine monitoring (diuresis with diuretics, lowering of blood pressure by an antihypertensive). For therapeutic drug monitoring to be of clinical value, a clear concentration-response or concentration-toxicity relationship should be identifiable. Patient age and the extent or severity of disease can influence the relationships among drug concentration, efficacy, and toxicity. Unfortunately, a clear relationship between a specific serum drug concentration and effect is available for only a limited number of drugs in contrast to the large number of drugs with "recommended" therapeutic ranges.

A number of variables should be considered when designing strategies to monitor therapy using a serum drug concentration. When measuring a drug's concentration in blood, the pharmacokinetic characteristics of that drug must be recalled so that blood samples can be obtained at appropriate times in relation to administration of the drug. This permits proper interpretation of drug concentrations and therapeutic effects and helps avoid serious therapeutic errors. Peak drug concentrations in blood usually do not refer to the highest concentration achieved in blood with that drug but usually to the postdistribution peak drug concentration. Thus, a lag time often exists between the time of drug administration and the time that is recommended to obtain the "peak" blood sample. Also, most clinical determinations of drug concentrations in biologic fluids routinely measure (report) the total drug concentration in that fluid (free drug concentration plus concentration of drug bound to protein equals total drug concentration). This approach assumes a constant ratio of free to bound drug at various concentrations and under differing pathophysiologic conditions, which may not always be true; thus, caution must be exercised in its extrapolation. For example, clinically important imbalances between free and total drug concentrations have been observed with the drug phenytoin in critically ill trauma patients and in patients with severe renal disease. As a result, many laboratories are now beginning to report both free *and* total serum concentrations of drugs or have these results available on request. Despite these differences, it is generally unusual for an imbalance in this ratio to be clinically significant, except for those drugs whose protein binding, under normal circumstances, is more than 90%.

Chronopharmacology is the effect of biologic rhythms on drug disposition and response. Many drugs are influenced pharmacokinetically and pharmacodynamically by this phenomenon. It is important to be aware of these situations and to time doses and blood sample collections appropriately.

ADDITIONAL CONSIDERATIONS

Method of Drug Administration. It is often assumed that intravenous administration of a drug is rapid and complete. Neither is always true. The length of time necessary to infuse the total dose of an intravenously administered drug depends on a number of factors, including the flow rate of the primary intravenous fluid, the dead space of the system into which the drug is injected, and the total volume in which the drug is diluted. Because most standard intravenous fluid delivery systems, including their tubing, are designed for adult use, they contain a large volume/unit of length. This introduces a relatively large dead space factor, which causes substantial infusion delays when operated at the slow flow rates necessary for infants and children. Even intravenous infusion systems designed for pediatric patients can have problems and limitations that may confound drug therapy management and require clinician awareness.

Several steps can be taken to minimize problems with intravenous drug administration to small infants and children. These include the following: standardization and documentation of the total administration time; documentation of the volume and content of the solution used to "flush" an intravenous dose; standardization of specific infusion techniques (infusion duration, volumes) for drugs with a narrow therapeutic index; standardization of dilution and infusion volumes for drugs given by intermittent IV injection; avoidance of attaching lines for drug infusion to a central hub with other solutions infused concurrently at widely disparate rates; preferential use of large-gauge cannula; maintenance of the recommended solution at a specified height above the infusion site for use with a gravity-based controller; and the use of low-volume tubing and the most distal sites for access of the drug into an existing intravenous line.

Drug-Drug Interactions. When two or more drugs are administered to the same patient, the pharmacokinetic and pharmacodynamic properties of each agent may be modified by their combined interaction. Drugs may interact by a number of different mechanisms; these may be classified on the basis of pharmaceutics, pharmacokinetics, pharmacodynamics, or a combination thereof. These interactions may result in unpredictable clinical effects or toxicologic responses. Pharmaceutic interactions include those resulting in drug inactivation when compounds are mixed together physically prior to patient administration as in syringes, infusion tubing, or parenteral fluid preparations.

Pharmacokinetic interactions can occur when the disposition characteristics of one compound (absorption, distribution, metabolism, excretion, or a combination thereof) are influenced by those of another. This type of interaction may involve one or more aspects of the pharmacokinetic profile of the drug. One drug may reduce the rate but not the overall extent of absorption, or a compound may displace a drug from its protein binding sites while concomitantly retarding its elimination from the body. Metabolic-based drug-drug interactions can occur whenever two compounds compete for the same metabolic site (see Table 711–2).

Drugs may interact pharmacodynamically and compete for the same receptor or physiologic system, thus altering a patient's response to drug therapy. The number of known, clinically important drug interactions, combined with the ever-increasing number of available pharmacologic agents, emphasizes the need to critically assess the possibility or presence of drug-drug interactions in any patient receiving multiple drugs.

Drugs in Human Milk. Almost all drugs administered to lactating women are secreted to some extent into their milk and may be ingested by the nursing infant. In general, drug use should be as minimal as possible during lactation; a few drugs have been reported to affect the nursing infant adversely. Obviously, it is not possible or desirable for lactating women to stop taking needed medications. If a question exists about the amount of drug a breast-feeding infant may be receiving or about possible drug effects on the infant, a sample of the mother's milk can be analyzed. Furthermore, up-to-date and specific information regarding breast milk distribution of medications and, most importantly, the amount a nursing infant would actually receive (absorb) can be obtained by consulting a clinical pharmacy/pharmacology service.

Prescribing Medications. Factors such as taste, smell, color, consistency, dosing frequency, and cost affect the degree to which patients comply with their therapeutic drug regimen. Prescribing generically equivalent medications can sometimes reduce the cost of a drug. Such prescribing should be done only when it is clearly known that the generic brand affords equivalent bioavailability, bioeffectiveness, and patient acceptability. Unfortunately, complete bioequivalence data are not available for all drugs and, when in doubt, the prescribing physician should consult with the pharmacist.

A prescription issued by the prescribing physician should always direct the dispensing of just enough drug to treat the patient, leaving only a small amount of drug left over after the prescribed course of therapy has been completed. This small residual allows for some drug in case of doses accidentally spilled or lost. Parents should be instructed to discard all remaining doses of a prescribed medication after the completed course of therapy to protect against accidental poisoning or improper self-medication at a later date. Patient medication instructions on the prescription should state the specific number of doses the patient should receive each day and the total duration of therapy (number of days of therapy). The number of times the prescribing physician allows the prescription to be refilled should be noted on the prescription label; if no refills are to be permitted, this should also be specified on the written prescription.

Compliance with the Prescribed Regimen. Little is known about the many factors that determine the degree of compliance with a physician's instructions, but it is clear that many patients frequently do not take medication consistently or in the manner intended or prescribed. Moreover, patients frequently take home remedies or medications not recommended or prescribed by their physician. A child's compliance with a prescribed therapeutic regimen is usually only as good as that of the parents. Compliance can often be maximized by carefully educating the family about the nature of the child's illness, the action of the medications prescribed, and the importance of following the instructions precisely. Often, if the instructions are written down clearly and in detail for the family and if the regimen results in minimal interference with the daily living schedule (particularly parental sleeping habits), compliance with the therapeutic regimen is improved. Collaboration between prescribing physician and dispensing pharmacist can often identify compliance problems and improve compliance through patient education.

Avent ML, Ransom JL, Kumar N, et al: Intravenous drug delivery in the newborn: Vigilance in approach and application. *J Neonatol* 1994;1:9.

Berlin CM Jr: Advances in pediatric pharmacology and toxicology. *Adv Pediatr* 2001;48:439–64.

Choonara I, Gill A, Nunn A: Drug toxicity and surveillance in children. *Br J Clin Pharmacol* 1996;42:407–10.

Gal P, Reed M. Therapeutic drug monitoring in the newborn. In Polin RA, Fow WW (editors): *Fetal and Neonatal Physiology,* 2nd ed. Philadelphia, WB Saunders, 1997.

Gilman JT, Gal P: Pharmacokinetic and pharmacodynamic data collection in children and neonates: A quiet frontier. *Clin Pharmacokinet* 1992;23:1–9.

Kearns GL, Reed MD: Clinical pharmacokinetics in infants and children: A reappraisal. *Clin Pharmacokinet* 1989;17(Suppl 1):29–67.

Leeder JS: Pharmacogenetics and pharmacogenomics. *Pediatr Clin North Am* 2001;48:765–81.

Reed MD: Optimal sampling theory: An overview of its application to pharmacokinetic studies in infants and children. *Pediatrics* 1999;104:627–32.

Tange SM, Grey VL, Senecal PE: Therapeutic drug monitoring in pediatrics: A need for improvement. *J Clin Pharmacol* 1994;34:200–14.

TenEick AP, Nakamura H, Reed MD: Drug-drug interactions in pediatric psychopharmacology. *Pediatr Clin North Am* 1998;45:1233–64.

Wilson JT, Kearns GL, Murphy D, et al: Paediatric labelling requirements: Implications for pharmacokinetic studies. *Clin Pharmacokinet* 1994;26:308–25.

Chapter 712

Medications

Peter Gal and Michael D. Reed

TABLE 712–1. General Medications

Drug (Trade Names, Formulations)	Indications (Mechanism of Action) and Dosing	Comments (Cautions, Adverse Events, Monitoring)
Abciximab ReoPro Intravenous solution, 2 mg/mL in 5-mL vials.	**Inhibit platelet aggregation through inhibiting the glycoprotein IIb/IIIa receptor pathway. Used in combination with IVIG and aspirin to accelerate regression of coronary aneurysms in Kawasaki disease. In adults, used for preventing platelet aggregation with various acute coronary syndromes and procedures.** *Children and adults:* Loading dose 0.25 mg/kg, followed by an infusion of 0.125 μg/kg/min for 12 hr.	*Adverse events:* Bleeding.
Acarbose Precose. Tablet: 25, 50, 100 mg.	**Treatment of type 2 diabetes mellitus, treatment of postprandial hypoglycemia in children after Nissen fundoplication.** *Children:* 12.5 to 50 mg with each feed. *Adults:* Initial 25 mg tid at the start of each meal; titrate to response (max: 100 mg tid).	*Adverse events:* Flatulence, abdominal pain, diarrhea.
Acetaminophen Analgesic, non-narcotic; antipyretic. Tempra; Tylenol; multiple generic and brand-name products. Caplet: 160, 325, 500 mg. Capsule: 325, 500 mg. Drops: 100 mg/mL (15 mL); 120 mg/2.5 mL (35 mL). Granules, premeasured packs: 30 mg (32 s). Suppositories: 120, 325 mg. Combination products with acetaminophen include cough and cold preparations and with codeine.	**Mild to moderate pain** (inhibits prostaglandin synthesis in CNS and peripheral pain impulse generation). **Fever** (inhibits hypothalamic heat regulation center). *Infants and children* <12 yr: 10–15 mg/kg/dose q4–6h. *Children* >12 yr and adults: 325–650 mg q4–6 hr or 1,000 mg 3–4 times daily. Maximum: 5 doses/24 hr (children) or 4 g/24 hr (adults) administered PO or PR.	*Cautions:* Overdose can cause fatal hepatic necrosis. Treat acute overdoses with acetylcysteine. Chronic concurrent use with enzyme inhibitors, especially alcohol, can lead to hepatic necrosis. Avoid aspartame-containing products in patients with phenylketonuria (e.g., chewable tablets).

TABLE 712–1. General Medications *Continued*

Drug (Trade Names, Formulations)	Indications (Mechanism of Action) and Dosing	Comments (Cautions, Adverse Events, Monitoring)
Acetazolamide Diuretic, carbonic anhydrase inhibitor. Dazamide; Diamox. Capsule, sustained release: 500 mg. Injection: 500 mg/5 mL. Tablet: 125, 250 mg.	**Hydrocephalus due to communicating intraventricular hemorrhage** (carbonic anhydrase inhibition decreases CSF production). *Neonates:* 25 mg/kg/24 hr to start and increase to bid, tid, and qid over 4–7 days. **Glaucoma** (carbonic anhydrase inhibition decreases formation of aqueous humor). *Children:* 8–30 mg/kg/24 hr PO divided q6–8h or 20–40 mg/kg/24 hr IV divided q6h. **Epilepsy, as adjunct to other drugs in refractory seizures** (uncertain mechanism). *Children and adults:* 8–30 mg/kg/24 hr in 1–4 divided doses (max: 1 g/24 hr). **Edema** (diuretic). *Children:* 5 mg/kg/24 hr IV or PO. *Adults:* 250–375 mg/24 hr IV or PO.	*Caution:* Used in combination with furosemide for hydrocephalus. Reduce dose and extend dosing interval if renal function is compromised. Avoid if patient has sulfa allergy. IM very painful because of alkaline pH of drug. *Adverse events:* Metabolic acidosis, hypochloremia, hypokalemia, nausea, anorexia, drowsiness, fatigue, muscle weakness, renal calculi.
Acetylcysteine Antidote, acetaminophen; mucolytic agent. Mucomyst; Mucosil; Mucosol. Solution, as sodium: 10% [100 mg/mL] (4, 10, 30 mL); 20% [200 mg/mL] (4, 10, 30, 100 mL)	**Mucolytic** (free sulfhydryl group opens up disulfide bonds in mucoproteins, lowering viscosity). Dose is based on 10% solution or diluted 20% solution (1:1) for inhalation. *Infants:* 2–4 mL tid–qid. *Children:* 6–10 mL tid–qid. *Adolescents:* 10 mL tid–qid. **Acute acetaminophen overdose** (provides alternative metabolic pathway for conjugation of toxic metabolites, restoring normal glutathione levels). *Children and adults:* 140 mg/kg loading dose, followed by 70 mg/kg q4h for 17 doses. Repeat dose if emesis occurs within 1 hr of administration.	*Cautions:* Give a bronchodilator 10–15 min before nebulized Mucomyst to avoid bronchospasm. Follow treatment with chest percussion and suction to manage increased secretions. Dilute nebulized doses with saline or sterile water and oral solutions with soft drinks or orange juice. Prepare inhaled as 1:1 and PO as 1:3 solutions. *Adverse events:* Stomatitis nausea, vomiting, urticaria. *Monitoring:* Check acetaminophen concentration no earlier than 4 hr post overdose. Give complete acetylcysteine course regardless of acetaminophen concentrations.
Adenosine Antiarrhythmic agent, miscellaneous. Adenocard. Injection, preservative free: 3 mg/mL (2 mL).	**Paroxysmal supraventricular tachycardia (PSVT)** treatment (slows conduction time through the AV node). *Neonates and children:* 0.05 mg/kg IV push, then increase bolus doses by 0.05 mg/kg q 2 min until a clinical response occurs or a maximum dose of either 0.25 mg/kg or 12 mg is achieved. *Adults:* 6 mg IV push, if no response in 2 min, give 12 mg IV push. May repeat 12 mg IV bolus if needed.	*Cautions:* Use a peripheral IV site. May cause bronchoconstriction in asthmatics. Methylxanthines (e.g., theophylline or caffeine) antagonize adenosine effects so higher adenosine doses are needed Contraindicated in 2nd or 3rd degree AV block or sick sinus syndrome. *Adverse events:* Heart block, flushing, chest palpitations, bradycardia, hypotension, dyspnea, headache, dizziness, nausea. *Monitoring:* Continuous ECG, blood pressure, respirations.
Albumin, human Blood product derivative; plasma volume expander. Albuminar; Albumisol; Albutein; Buminate; Plasbumin. Injection: 5% [50 mg/mL] (50, 250, 500, 1,000); 25% 250 mg/mL] (10, 20, 50, 100 mL).	**Plasma volume expansion and treatment of hypovolemia** (increase intravascular oncotic pressure and mobilize fluid from interstitium to intravascular space). *Neonates:* 0.5–1 g/kg/dose (max 1 g/kg/24 hr). *Infants and children:* 0.5–1 g/kg/dose (max 6 g/kg/24 hr). *Adults:* 25 g/dose (max 250 g/24 hr).	*Cautions:* 25% albumin may increase risk of IVH in preterm infants so 5% is preferred in these cases. Infusion should be over at least 2 hr in neonates. Infusion may be over 30–60 min for hypovolemia. *Adverse events:* Precipitation of heart failure, pulmonary edema, hypertension, tachycardia due to volume overload. Immune reactions (e.g., fever, chills, rash). Increased mortality in critically ill patients. *Monitoring:* Vital signs.
Albuterol Adrenergic agonist agent; β₂-adrenergic agonist agent; bronchodilator; sympathomimetic. Proventil; Ventolin; Volmax. Aerosol, oral: 90 µg/spray [200 inhalations] (17 g). Capsule, microfine for inhalation, as sulfate (Rotacaps): 200 µg. Solution, inhalation, as sulfate: 0.083% [0.83 mg/mL] (3 mL); 0.5% [5 mg/mL] (20 mL). Syrup, as sulfate (strawberry flavor): 2 mg/5 mL (480 mL). Tablet, as sulfate: 2, 4 mg. Tablet, extended release: 4 mg.	**Bronchodilator** (β₂-agonist). **Inhalation dose:** *Neonates, infants, children, and adults:* **Metered dose inhaler (MDI):** 1–2 puffs prn, or 5 min before exercise or tid–qid. **Rotohaler:** 1–2 capsules prn, or q4–6h, or before exercise. **Nebulizer solution:.** *Neonates:* 0.1–0.5 mg/kg/dose prn or q2–6h. *Children:* 1.25–2.5 mg prn or q4–6h. *Adults:* 1.25–5 mg prn or q4–6h **PO:** *Neonates:* 0.1–0.3 mg/kg/dose q6–8h. *Children:* <6 yr: *0.1–0.2 mg/kg/dose tid.* 6–12 yr: *2 mg/dose tid–qid* >12 yr: *2–4 mg tid–qid.*	*Cautions:* Increased use or lack of effect may indicate loss of asthma control requiring medical attention. Better to use prn or before exercise. *Adverse events:* Hyperglycemia, hypokalemia, tachycardia, palpitations, nervousness, CNS stimulation, insomnia, tremor. *Monitoring:* Evaluate clinical response and pulmonary function, e.g., peak flowmeter (patient should achieve >80% of personal best peak expiratory flow rate after use). *Comments:* May mix albuterol nebulizer solution with cromolyn or ipratropium nebulizer solutions. Give MDI doses with an extender device.
Alfentanil hydrochloride Analgesic, narcotic; general anesthetic. Alfenta Injection. Injection, preservative free: 500 µg/mL (2, 5, 10, 20 mL).	**Analgesia, anesthesia** (narcotic analgesic). *Neonates, infants, and children <12 yr:* 5–15 µg/kg IV injected over 3–5 min or 0.5–3 µg/kg/min continuous infusion (limited experience and doses poorly established). *Adults:* IV continuous infusion 0.5–1.5 µg/kg/min.	*Cautions:* Bolus doses of 9–15 µg/kg caused chest wall rigidity in 9 of 20 newborns, compromising respiration in 4 patients. Use a skeletal muscle relaxant concurrently. Avoid in patients with increased intracranial pressure or severe respiratory depression. *Adverse events:* Bradycardia, hypotension, increased intracranial pressure, antidiuretic hormone release. *Comment:* Dose based on lean weight for obese patients.
Alglucerase Enzyme, glucocerebrosidase. Ceredase Injection. Injection: 10 units/mL (5 mL); 80 units/mL (5 mL).	**Enzyme replacement therapy for type I Gaucher disease** (replaces the missing enzyme β-glucosidase needed to break down and thus avoid accumulation of glucosyl ceramide-laden macrophages in bone liver and spleen).	*Adverse events:* Fever, chills, abdominal discomfort, nausea, vomiting, local IV site. *Monitoring:* Resolution of anemia, thrombocytopenia, bleeding tendencies, and hepatosplenomegaly (within 6 mo). Improved bone mineralization (usually noted at 80–104 wk of therapy).

Table continued on following page

TABLE 712–1. General Medications *Continued*

Drug (Trade Names, Formulations)	Indications (Mechanism of Action) and Dosing	Comments (Cautions, Adverse Events, Monitoring)
	20–60 units/kg IV infused over 1–2 hr. Typically repeated q 2 wk but varies from q 2 days to q 4 wk depending on response.	
Allopurinol Anti-gout agent; uric acid–lowering agent. Lopurin; Zyloprim. Tablet: 100, 300 mg.	**Prevent attacks of gouty arthritis and nephropathy.** **Prevent cancer chemotherapy-induced hyperuricemia** (inhibits xanthine oxidase thus preventing conversion of hypoxanthine to uric acid). *Children* ≤ 10 yr: 10 mg/kg/24 hr in 2–3 divided doses. *Children >10 yr and adults:* 200–600 mg/24 hr in 2–3 divided doses. **Gout, chemotherapy-induced hyperuricemia.** 600–800 mg/24 hr in 2–3 divided doses starting 1–2 day before chemotherapy and continue for 3 days. Renal impairment: CrCl 10–50: reduce dose to 50%, CrCl <10: reduce dose to 30% of suggested.	*Cautions:* Discontinue at first sign of rash. *Adverse events:* Rashes including erythema multiforme, renal impairment, hepatitis, peripheral neuropathy, and vasculitis *Monitoring:* Uric acid levels decrease in 1–2 days with maximum effect seen in 1–3 wk.
Alprazolam Antianxiety agent. Benzodiazepine. Xanax. Tablet: 0.25, 0.5, 1, 2 mg.	**Treatment of anxiety or panic attacks** (not certain but may be mediated through γ-aminobutyric acid). *Children:* 0.005–0.02 mg/kg/dose tid. *Adults:* 0.25–0.5 mg bid–tid, max: 4 mg/24 hr (anxiety) and 10 mg/24 hr (panic).	*Cautions:* Abrupt discontinuation results in withdrawal reactions including seizures. Safety not established in children <18 yr. Pregnancy risk factor D. *Adverse events:* Drowsiness, confusion, sedation.
Alprostadil Prostaglandin. Prostin VR Pediatric Injection. Injection: 500 μg/mL (1 mL).	**Maintain patency of the ductus arteriosus in cyanotic heart lesions.** Direct vasodilation of ductus smooth muscle. *Neonates and infants:* 0.05–0.1 μg/kg/min as continuous IV infusion, may gradually increase to maximum of 0.4 μg/kg/min or wean as low as 0.005 μg/kg/min depending on response.	*Adverse events:* Apnea, bradycardia, hypotension, tachycardia, flushing, seizure-like activity, cortical hyperostosis (with >6 mo use), diarrhea, gastric-outlet obstruction (if ≥ 5 days use). *Monitoring:* Therapeutic response includes increase in systemic blood pressure, improved oxygen saturation or Po$_2$, and less acidosis on blood pH. Discontinue immediately if severe apnea or bradycardia.
Aluminum acetate Topical skin product. Acid Mantle; Bluboro; Boropak; Domeboro; PediBoro. Powder, to make topical solution: 1 packet/pint of water = 1:40 solution. Solution, otic: Aluminum acetate 1:10 with acetic acid 2% (60 mL). Tablet: 1 tablet/pint = 1:40 dilution.	**Astringent wet dressing for relief of inflammatory conditions of the skin; prophylaxis of swimmer's ear.** *Children and adults:* Otic: Instill 4–6 drops q2–3h initially then q4–6h until itching or burning resolves. Topical: Soak the affected area in the solution for 15–30 min 2–4 times daily.	*Adverse events:* Local irritation.
Aminocaproic acid Hemostatic agent. Amicar. Injection: 250 mg/mL (20, 96, 100 mL). Syrup (raspberry flavor): 250 mg/mL (480 mL). Tablet: 500 mg.	**Treatment of excessive bleeding resulting from systemic hyperfibrinolysis** (inhibits activation of plasminogen). *Children:* PO, IV load 100–200 mg/kg, maintenance 100 mg/kg q6h or 33.3 mg/kg/hr continuous infusion. Traumatic hyphema: 100 mg/kg q4h (max 30 g/24 hr). *Adults:* Load 5 g over 1 hr, then 1–1.25 g/hr until bleeding stops (max: 30 g/24 hr).	*Cautions:* Avoid in disseminated intravascular coagulation and hematuria of the upper urinary tract. Contains benzyl alcohol, so avoid in neonates <1500 g. *Adverse events:* Hypotension, bradycardia, arrhythmias, dizziness, headache, nasal congestion. *Monitoring:* D-dimer or fibrin split products, activated clotting time (target 180–200 sec), serum potassium (especially if renal function decreased).
Aminophylline (Theophylline equivalent listed in brackets.) Bronchodilator; respiratory stimulant; theophylline derivative. Aminophyllin; Phyllocontin; Somophyllin; Truphylline. Injection, IV (Aminophyllin): 25 mg/mL [19.7 mg/mL] (10, 20 mL). Liquid, oral: 105 mg/5 mL [90 mg/5 mL] (240 mL). Suppository, rectal (Truphylline): 250 mg [197.5 mg], 500 mg [395 mg]. Tablet (Aminophyllin): 100 mg [79 mg], 200 mg [158 mg]. Tablet, controlled release [12 hr] (Phyllocontin): 225 mg [178 mg]. Tablet, enteric coated: 100 mg [79 mg], 200 mg [158 mg]. See *Theophylline* for oral dosing.	**Apnea of prematurity, ventilator weaning in neonates, bronchodilator, weak pulmonary anti-inflammatory effects.** Increase contractility and decrease fatigability of diaphragm and respiratory muscles, weak bronchodilator, CNS stimulation, decrease airway responsiveness to stimuli. Exact mechanisms for these effects remain controversial. *Neonates* (for apnea of prematurity, ventilator weaning, or bronchospasm): Loading dose: 6 mg/kg IV or PO. Maintenance dose: 2.5–3 mg/kg/dose q12 hr IV or PO. **Asthma chronic therapy (see *Theophylline*).** Use in acute therapy is of questionable value. If used as continuous IV infusion: *Children:* 6 wk–6 mo: 0.5 mg/kg/hr. 6 mo–1 yr: 0.7 mg/kg/hr. 1–9 yr: 1 mg/kg/hr. 9–12 yr: 0.9 mg/kg/hr. 12 yr–adult: 0.7 mg/kg/hr.	*Cautions:* May cause or worsen arrhythmias, seizures, or gastroesophageal reflux. Theophylline clearance is modified by numerous disease states and drugs requiring dosing adjustments guided by serum theophylline concentrations. Clearance is reduced by viral illnesses, fever >102°F for >24 hr, cor pulmonale, and drugs that inhibit P450 enzymes (cimetidine, verapamil, macrolides, quinolones); reduce dose by 50%. *Adverse events:* Feeding intolerance in neonates or gastrointestinal discomfort in children and adults, nausea, vomiting, CNS irritability, agitation, tachycardia, and tachyarrhythmias. *Monitoring:* Theophylline blood levels correlate with clinical effects and toxicity. Target levels are somewhat controversial. *Neonates:* 6–15 mg/L (65% of neonates will not have apnea eliminated until levels exceed 10 mg/L if continuous electronic monitoring is performed. Levels above 10 mg/L are needed for ventilator weaning. Levels of 5–15 mg/L are sufficient for bronchodilation). *Children:* Theophylline alone is ineffective for acute asthma. For chronic asthma, theophylline levels of 5–15 mg/L are effective, but levels should exceed 10 mg/L for prevention of exercise-induced bronchospasm.
Amiodarone hydrochloride Antiarrhythmic agent, class III. Cordarone. Tablet: 200 mg.	**Management of resistant, life-threatening ventricular arrhythmias or PSVT unresponsive to less toxic agents** (class III antiarrhythmic agent, prolongs action potential and refractory period in myocardial tissue).	*Cautions:* Use benzyl alcohol–free product in neonates. Minimize risk of torsades de pointes by correcting low potassium and magnesium. Inhibits cytochrome P450 enzymes, so many drugs that are metabolized will have markedly increased levels and effects including

TABLE 712–1. General Medications *Continued*

Drug (Trade Names, Formulations)	Indications (Mechanism of Action) and Dosing	Comments (Cautions, Adverse Events, Monitoring)
Injection: 50 mg/mL (3 mL); Cordarone contains benzyl alcohol and polysorbate (Tween) 80. Injection, benzyl alcohol-free and polysorbate-free: 15 mg/mL (10 mL); Amio-Aqueous contains an aqueous acetate buffer; available via orphan drug status or compassionate use from the manufacturer Academic Pharmaceuticals, Inc. (847) 735-1170.	**Oral dose:** *Infants and children:* <*1 yr:* 600–800 mg/1.73 m^2/24 hr in two divided doses. >*1 yr:* 10–20 mg/kg/24 hr in two divided doses for 10 days, then 5–10 mg/kg/24 hr. *Adults:* 800 mg/24 hr in two divided doses. Cut all doses in half, i.e., one dose per day after 1–4 wk of treatment or arrhythmias are controlled. **IV dose:** *Infants and children:* load 5 mg/kg over 1 hr, then continuous infusion of 5–15 µg/kg/min. *Adults:* 150 mg over 10 min, then 0.5 mg/min.	theophylline, phenytoin, warfarin, other antiarrhythmics, methotrexate, and cyclosporine. *Adverse events:* Proarrhythmia (may be bradyarrhythmias or tachyarrhythmias or heart block); fatigue, malaise, nightmares, behavioral changes; hypothyroidism, hyperglycemia, elevated triglycerides, skin color changes (slate blue), photosensitivity, rash, liver toxicity (may be fatal or just increased liver enzymes), pulmonary toxicity (potentially fatal) includes pulmonary fibrosis, interstitial pneumonitis, hypersensitivity pneumonitis (present as cough, fever, dyspnea, chest radiographic changes), photophobia, thrombocytopenia. *Monitoring:* Pulmonary, liver, and thyroid function tests; chest radiograph, ECG, eye examination, and clinical signs and symptoms of toxicity. Amiodarone concentration: 2–4 µmol/L.
Amitriptyline hydrochloride Antidepressant, tricyclic; antimigraine agent. Elavil; Emitrip; Endep. Injection: 10 mg/mL (10 mL) Tablet: 10, 25, 50, 75, 100, 150 mg.	**Depression (increases CNS concentrations of serotonin and norepinephrine by inhibiting reuptake).** *Children:* 1–1.5 mg/kg/24 hr divided tid. *Adolescent:* 30–100 mg at bedtime or divided bid (max 200 mg/24 hr). *Adults:* 30–100 mg q 24 hr (max 300 mg/24 hr). **Analgesic for neuropathic or chronic pain or migraine prophylaxis.** *Children:* 0.1 mg/kg at bedtime and advance over 2–3 wk to effect. Maximum: 2 mg/kg at bedtime. *Adolescents:* 25 mg divided bid and increase dose to effect or max: dose: 200 mg/24 hr. *Adults:* start 25 mg at bedtime and increase to effect or max: dose: 300 mg/24 hr.	*Cautions:* Cardiac conduction abnormalities may occur, monitor ECG. Do not discontinue abruptly because withdrawal syndrome may occur. *Adverse events:* Dry mouth, constipation, weight gain, postural hypotension, drowsiness, confusion, headache, visual disturbance. *Monitoring:* Amitriptyline concentrations: therapeutic 100–250 ng/mL; nortriptyline concentrations: therapeutic 50–150 ng/mL.
Ammonium chloride Metabolic alkalosis, treatment agent: urinary acidifying agent. Generic. Injection: 26.75% [5 mEq/mL] (20 mL). Tablet: 500 mg. Tablet enteric coated: 500 mg.	**Systemic or urinary acidification (dissociation of ammonium and chloride then replacement of bicarbonate ions by chloride ions).** *Children:* 75 mg/kg/24 hr IV divided q6h (max: daily dose: 6 g). *Adults:* 1.5 g/dose IV q6h.	*Adverse events:* Hyperchloremia, hyperammonemia, hyperkalemia.
Amrinone lactate Adrenergic agonist agent. Inocor. Injection: 5 mg/mL (20 mL).	**Treatment of low cardiac output states (increase cellular levels of cyclic AMP).** *Neonates:* 0.75 mg/kg IV bolus over 2–3 min then 3–5 µg/kg/min continuous infusion IV. *Infants and children:* 0.75 mg/kg IV bolus over 2–3 min then 5–10 µg/kg/min continuous infusion. *Adults:* 0.75 mg/kg IV bolus over 2–3 min then 5–10 µg/kg/min.	*Cautions:* Increased cardiac output may cause excess diuresis if diuretic doses are not adjusted. May repeat bolus doses if clinical response is inadequate. *Adverse events:* Hypotension, arrhythmias, thrombocytopenia.
Antihemophilic factor, human Antihemophilic agent; blood product derivative. Alphanate; Hemofil M; Humate-P; Koate-HP; Koate-HS; Monoclate-P; Profilate OSD. Injection (approximate factor VIII activity per vial): 200, 250, 500, 750, 1,000, 1,250, 1,500 units; exact potency labeled on each vial.	**Factor VIII deficiency in hemophilia (provides factor VIII).** *All patients:* Units required = weight (kg) × 0.5 × desired increase factor VIII (% of normal). *Adverse events:* Tachycardia, allergy, blood-borne viral infections.	*Monitoring:* Plasma antihemophilic factor levels
Antipyrine and benzocaine Otic agent, analgesic; otic agent, ceruminolytic. Allergan Ear Drops; Aurafair; Auralgan; Aurodex; Auroto; Oto; Otocalm Ear Solution, otic: antipyrine 5.4% and benzocaine 1.4% (10, 15 mL).	**Temporary relief of ear pain and inflammation (topical anesthetic and anti-inflammatory).** *All patients:* Fill ear canal, and then moisten cotton pledget and place into meatus. May repeat q1–2h until pain relief. Limit use to about 3 days.	*Adverse events:* Stinging, methemoglobinemia.
Antithrombin III **Thrombate III**	**Antithrombin III deficiency due to disseminated intravascular coagulation or shock and surgery complications. Treatment of thrombosis in ATIII deficiency.** *All patients:* Dose (IU) = (120 − patient ATIII) × wt (kg).	*Monitoring:* Check ATIII levels: maintain between 80% and 120%.
Antivenin (Crotalidae) polyvalent Antivenom. Generic. Injection: Lyophilized serum, diluent (10 mL); one vacuum vial to yield 10 mL of antivenom.	**Antivenom for snake bite from North and South American crotalids, i.e., rattlesnake, copperhead, cottonmouth, tropical moccasins, fer-de-lance, bushmaster.** Dosing based on severity of bite—mild: 5 vials, moderate: 10 vials, severe: > 15 vials.	*Cautions:* Sensitivity reactions, including anaphylaxis (treat with epinephrine and antihistamine and brief holding of dose).
Arginine hydrochloride Diagnostic agent, growth hormone function; metabolic alkalosis, treatment agent. R-Gene. Injection: 10% [0.475 mEq chloride/mL] (500 mL).	**Pituitary function test (stimulates pituitary release of growth hormone and prolactin).** *Children:* 500 mg/kg over 30 min. *Adults:* 300 mL over 30 min.	*Adverse events:* Flushing, headache, hyperglycemia, hyperkalemia, metabolic acidosis. *Monitoring:* Plasma growth hormone concentrations.
Ascorbic acid Nutritional supplement; urinary acidifying agent; vitamin, water soluble.	**Scurvy.** *Children:* 100–300 mg/24 hr. *Adults:* 100–250 mg bid.	*Adverse events:* Gastrointestinal upset, renal stones.

Table continued on following page

MEDICATIONS

TABLE 712–1. General Medications *Continued*

Drug (Trade Names, Formulations)	Indications (Mechanism of Action) and Dosing	Comments (Cautions, Adverse Events, Monitoring))
Ascorbicap; C-Crystals; Cecon; Cetane; Cevalin; Ce-Vi-Sol; Dull-C; Flavorcee; Vita-C. Capsule, timed-release: 500 mg. Crystals: 4 g/teaspoonful (1,000 g). Injection: 250 mg/mL (2 mL, 30 mL), 500 mg/mL (1, 2, 50 mL). Lozenge: 60 mg. Powder: 4 g/teaspoonful (1,000 g). Solution, oral: 35 mg/0.6 mL (50 mL), 100 mg/mL (50 mL). Syrup: 500 mg/5 mL (5, 10, 120, 480 mL). Tablet: 25, 50, 100, 250, 500, 1,000 mg. Tablet, chewable: 100, 250, 500, 1,000 mg. Tablet, timed release: 500, 1,000, 1,500 mg.	**Urinary acidification.** *Children:* 500 mg q6h. *Adults:* 4–12 g/24 hr in 3–4 divided doses.	
Asparaginase Antineoplastic agent, miscellaneous. Elspar. Injection: 10,000 units/vial.	**Cancer chemotherapy (inhibits protein synthesis to deprive cancer cells of asparagine).** *Children and adults:* Doses may vary depending on specific protocol being used: 6,000 units/m² IM, 3 times/wk for 3 wk as part of combination therapy. High-dose IM therapy: 25,000 units/m²/dose q wk × 9 doses. IV therapy: 1,000 units/kg/24 hr for 10 days; or 200 units/kg/24 hr × 28 days.	*Cautions:* Stop drug if any signs of renal failure or pancreatitis occur. Be prepared to treat anaphylaxis at each dose. *Adverse events:* Myelosuppression (WBC and platelets; is mild and rare) onset, 7 days; nadir, 14 days; recovery, 21 days. Hepatotoxicity, pancreatitis, gastrointestinal upset, azotemia, hyperglycemia, coagulopathy.
Aspirin Analgesic, non-narcotic; anti-inflammatory agent; antiplatelet agent; antipyretic; nonsteroidal anti-inflammatory agent (NSAID), oral; salicylate. Anacin; A.S.A.; Ascriptin; Aspergum; Bayer Aspirin; Bufferin; Easprin; Ecotrin; Empirin; Gensan; Halfrin; Measurin, ZORprin. Suppository, rectal: 60, 120, 125, 130, 195, 200, 300, 325, 600, 650, 1,200 mg. Tablet: 325, 500, 650 mg. Tablet, buffered: 325 mg with aluminum hydroxide 75 mg and magnesium hydroxide 75 mg; 325 mg with aluminum hydroxide 150 mg and magnesium hydroxide 150 mg; 500 mg with aluminum hydroxide 33 mg and magnesium hydroxide 150 mg. Chewable: 75, 81 mg. Chewing gum: 227 mg. Controlled release: 800 mg. Enteric coated (delayed release): 80, 165, 325, 500, 650, 975 mg. Timed release: 650 mg. Tablet, with caffeine: 400 mg and caffeine 32 mg; 500 mg and caffeine 32 mg.	**Pain, inflammation, fever (prostaglandin synthesis inhibition).** *Children:* 10–15 mg/kg/dose q4–6h. *Adults:* 650–1,000 mg/dose q4–6 hr (max: 4 g/24 hr). **Kawasaki disease (acute phase).** *Children:* 80–100 mg/kg/24 hr divided q6h. **Rheumatic fever.** 60–100 mg/kg/24 hr divided q6h.	*Cautions:* Contraindicated in children <16 yr with chickenpox or flu-like symptoms due to risk of Reye syndrome. Discontinue if hearing loss or tinnitus occurs. *Adverse events:* Bleeding from gums or gastrointestinal tract, gastric ulcers, bronchospasm in asthmatics, hearing loss, and tinnitus. *Monitoring:* Check serum concentration 2 hr after a dose for Kawasaki disease (target 150–300 µg/mL) or rheumatic fever (target: 250–400 µg/mL).
Astemizole Antihistamine. Hismanal. Tablet: 10 mg.	**Allergy and rhinitis (competitive H₁-receptor blocker).** *Children:* <6 yr: 0.2 mg/kg once daily. 6–12 yr: 5 mg once daily. >12 yr and adults: 10–30 mg/24 hr.	*Cautions:* Syncopal episodes may be a marker of arrhythmias including QT interval prolongation leading to fatal arrhythmias. Discontinue if ECG shows QT prolongation, syncopal episode, or drugs that impair hepatic metabolism (e.g., erythromycin, ketoconazole) are added.
Atenolol Antianginal agent; antihypertensive; β-adrenergic blocker. Tenormin. Injection: 0.5 mg/mL (10 mL). Tablet: 25, 50, 100 mg.	**Hypertension, arrhythmias (competitive β₁-blocker).** *Children:* 0.8–1.5 mg/kg/24 hr (max: 2 mg/kg/24 hr). *Adults:* 25–200 mg/24 hr PO, 5 mg IV over 5 min.	*Cautions:* Avoid abrupt discontinuation, taper over 1–2 wk. *Adverse events:* Bradycardia, lethargy, headache, constipation, wheezing, dyspnea.
Atorvastatin calcium Lipitor. Tablet: 10, 20, 40 mg.	**Hypercholesterolemia, including homozygous familial hypercholesterolemia (inhibit HMG-CoA reductase).** *Children >6 yr:* 10–80 mg/24 hr. *Adults:* 10–80 mg/24 hr.	*Adverse events:* Dyspepsia, flatulence, pancreatitis, hepatitis, myalgia, arthralgia. *Monitoring:* Plasma lipid profile.
Atracurium besylate Neuromuscular blocker agent, nondepolarizing; skeletal muscle relaxant, paralytic. Tracrium. Injection: 10 mg/mL (5, 10 mL).	**Neuromuscular blocker for muscle paralysis (binds to cholinergic receptor sites to block neural transmission).** *Children:* <2 yr: 0.3–0.4 mg/kg as needed. >2 yr to adults: 0.4–0.5 mg/kg then 1 mg/kg 20 to 45 min after each initial block to maintain effect. Continuous IV infusion: 0.4–0.8 mg/kg/hr.	*Cautions:* Make sure airway and respiratory support are secure before use. Contains benzyl alcohol; neonatal use should be limited. Does not have sedative or analgesic properties, so adjunct sedative/analgesic should be used. *Monitoring:* Muscle twitch response to peripheral nerve stimulator.
Atropine sulfate Anticholinergic agent; anticholinergic agent, ophthalmic; antidote, organophosphate poisoning; antispasmodic agent, gastrointestinal; bronchodilator; ophthalmic agent, mydriatic. Atropair Ophthalmic; Atropine-Care Ophthalmic; Atropisol Ophthalmic; Isopto Atropine Ophthalmic; I-Tropine Ophthalmic; Ocu-Tropin. Ophthalmic injection: 0.05 mg/mL (5 mL); 0.1 mg/mL (5, 10 mL); 0.3 mg/mL (1, 30 mL); 0.4 mg/mL (1, 20,	**Preoperative medication to inhibit secretions and salivation (blocks action of acetylcholine and antagonizes histamine and serotonin).** *Neonates and children:* <5 kg: 0.2 mg/kg 30 min preop then q4–6h. >5 kg: 0.1–0.2 mg/kg/dose (max: 0.4 mg/dose). *Adults:* 0.4–0.6 mg IV or SC 30 min preoperatively. **Treatment of sinus bradycardia.** *Neonates and children:* 0.02 mg/kg (minimum dose: 0.1 mg); IV or intratracheal (max: 0.5 mg);	*Cautions:* Avoid in narrow angle glaucoma, gastrointestinal obstruction, thyrotoxicosis, and tachycardia. *Adverse events:* Tachycardia, palpitations, delirium, ataxia, dry hot skin, tremor, impaired vision.

TABLE 712–1. General Medications *Continued*

Drug (Trade Names, Formulations)	Indications (Mechanism of Action) and Dosing	Comments (Cautions, Adverse Events, Monitoring)
30 mL); 0.5 mg/mL (1, 5, 30 mL); 0.8 mg/mL (0.5, 1 mL); 1 mg/mL (1, 10 mL). Ointment, ophthalmic: 0.5% (3.5 g); 1% (3.5 g). Solution, ophthalmic: 0.5% (1, 5 mL); 1% (1, 2, 5, 15 mL); 2% (1, 2 mL). Tablet: 0.4 mg. Tablet, soluble: 0.4, 0.6 mg.	may repeat 5 min later, one time. *Adults:* 0.5–1 mg every 5 min (maximum total dose: 2 mg). **Antidote to organophosphate poisoning.** 0.02–0.05 mg/kg q 10–20 min until atropine effect (tachycardia, mydriasis, fever), then q1–4h for at least 24 hr.	
Attapulgite Antidiarrheal. Children's Kaopectate; Diasorb; Donnagel; Kaopectate Advanced Formula; Kaopectate Maximum Strength Caplets; K-Pec; Parepectolin; Rheaban. Caplet: 750 mg. Liquid: 600 mg activated attapulgite/15 mL (180, 240, 360, 480 mL); 750 mg activated attapulgite/15 mL (120 mL). Suspension: 600 mg/15 mL. Tablet, chewable: 300, 600, 750 mg.	**Uncomplicated diarrhea (absorbent action).** *Children:* *3–6 yr:* 300–750 mg/dose (max: 7 doses). *6–12 yr:* 600–1,500 mg/dose (max: 7 doses). *>12 yr and adults:* 1,200–3,000 mg/dose (max: 7 doses).	*Caution:* Do not use for diarrhea due to dysentery, enterocolitis, or toxigenic bacteria.
Auranofin Gold compound. Ridaura. Capsule: 3 mg [gold 29%].	**Treatment of active stage of rheumatoid or psoriatic arthritis (immunomodulating effect).** *Children:* Initial dose: 0.1 mg/kg/24 hr; usual maintenance dose: 0.15 mg/kg/24 hr in 1–2 doses (max: 0.2 mg/kg/24 hr). *Adults:* 6 mg/24 hr in 1–2 doses (max: 9 mg/24 hr in 1–3 doses).	*Adverse events:* Itching, skin rash, stomatitis, conjunctivitis, proteinuria, alopecia, glossitis, leukopenia, thrombocytopenia, hematuria, anemia, agranulocytosis, eosinophilia, peripheral neuropathy, interstitial pneumonitis, angioedema, hepatotoxicity. *Monitoring:* Discontinue if WBC <4,000/mm^3 or granulocytes <1,500/mm^3 or platelets <100,000/mm^3.
Aurothioglucose Gold compound. Solganal. Suspension, sterile: 50 mg/mL [gold 50%] (10 mL).	**Treatment of active rheumatoid or psoriatic arthritis (immunomodulator).** *Children:* 0.25 mg/kg/dose wk 1, increase 0.25 mg/kg/dose every wk to maintenance dose 0.75–1.0 mg/kg/dose weekly (max: 25 mg/dose, total 20 doses). *Adults:* 10 mg wk 1, then 25 mg wk 2 and 3, then 50 mg/wk until cumulative dose 1 g given.	*Cautions:* Administer by deep IM injection. *Adverse events:* Same as for auranofin.
Azatadine maleate Antihistamine. Optimine. Tablet: 1 mg.	**Treatment of allergy, allergic rhinitis, and urticaria (antihistamine, anticholinergic).** *Children <12 yr:* Not recommended. *Children >12 yr and adults:* 1–2 mg twice daily.	*Adverse events:* Sedation, dry mouth, thickened bronchial secretions
Azathioprine Immunosuppressant agent. Imuran. Injection, as sodium: 100 mg (10 mL). Tablet: 50 mg.	**Prevent transplant rejection.** *Children and adults:* initial 2–5 mg/kg/24 hr IV or PO, maintenance 1–3 mg/kg/24 hr. **Treatment of autoimmune diseases, e.g., lupus, arthritis, nephrotic syndrome.** (Inhibit synthesis of DNA, RNA, and proteins. Antagonize purine metabolism.) *Adults:* 1 mg/kg/24 hr × 6–8 wk.	*Cautions:* Chronic use causes increased risk of lymphoma and skin cancer. May cause irreversible bone marrow suppression. Reduce dose to 25% of normal if concurrent allopurinol used. *Adverse events:* Fever, chills, nausea, vomiting, diarrhea, thrombocytopenia, leukopenia, hepatotoxicity, rash.
Baclofen Skeletal muscle relaxant, nonparalytic. Lioresal. Injection, intrathecal: 0.5 mg/mL (20 mL); 2 mg/mL (5 mL). Tablet: 10, 20 mg.	**Spasticity associated with MS or spinal cord lesions. Trigeminal neuralgia (inhibits transmission of monosynaptic and polysynaptic reflexes at the spinal cord level).** *Children: 2–7 yr:* 10–15 mg/24 hr divided q8h and titrate up q 3 days (max: 40 mg/24 hr PO). *Adults:* 5 mg q8h and gradually increase by 5 mg q 3 days (max: 80 mg/24 hr PO). Intrathecal (adults only).	*Caution:* Avoid abrupt discontinuation, slowly titrate to discontinue. *Adverse events:* Drowsiness, vertigo, psychiatric reactions, ataxia, hypotonia.
Beclomethasone Adrenal corticosteroid; anti-inflammatory agent; corticosteroid, inhalant (oral); corticosteroid, nasal; glucocorticoid. Beclovent Oral Inhaler, Beconase AQ Nasal Inhaler, Beconase Nasal Inhaler, Vancenase AQ Inhaler, Vanceril Oral Inhaler. Inhalation: Nasal (Beconase, Vancenase): 42 μg/inhalation [200 metered doses] (16.8 g). Oral (Beclovent, Vanceril): 42 μg/inhalation [200 metered doses] (16.8 g). Spray, aqueous, nasal (Beconase AQ, Vancenase AQ): 42 μg/inhalation [200 metered doses] (25 g).	**Asthma (oral inhalation), rhinitis (nasal aerosol) (anti-inflammatory, immune modulator).** *Adults and children (inhaler):* 1–2 inhalations 2–4 times daily (maximum dose children: 10 puffs, adults: 20 puffs daily). *Adults and children (nasal spray):* 1 spray in each nostril 2–4 times daily	*Adverse events: Candida* in mouth, burning and irritation of nasal mucosa, cough, hoarseness, headache. *Monitoring:* Inhaled corticosteroids should be administered via an extender device for better lung delivery and less local toxicity.
Benzocaine Local anesthetic, oral; local anesthetic, topical. Americaine; Anbesol Maximum Strength; Babee Teething Lotion: BiCOZENE; chigger tox; Dermaplast; Foille Plus; Hurricaine; Orabase-B; Orabase Gel; Orabase-O, Ora Jel Brace-Aid Oral Anesthetic; Ora Jel Maximum Strength; Ora Jel Mouth-Aid; Rhulicaine; Solar Caine; Unguentine.	**Temporary relief of pain associated with minor skin injuries (local anesthetic).** *Children and adults:* Apply to affected area as needed.	*Adverse events:* Local irritation or sensitization.

Table continued on following page

MEDICATIONS

TABLE 712–1. General Medications *Continued*

Drug (Trade Names, Formulations)	Indications (Mechanism of Action) and Dosing	Comments (Cautions, Adverse Events, Monitoring)
Topical: Aerosol: 5% (97.5 mL, 105 mL) 20% (20, 60, 120 g). Cream: 5% (30, 454 g); 6% (28.4 g). Gel 15% (7 g). Liquid: with benzyl benzoate and soft soap (30 mL). Lotion: 8% (90 mL). Ointment: 5% (3.5, 30 g).		
Benzonatate Topical anesthetic. Tessalon Perles.	**Relief of nonproductive cough (topical anesthetic action).** *Children <10 yr:* Not indicated. *Children >10 yr and adults:* 100 mg tid or q4h to maximum of 600 mg/24 hr.	*Adverse events:* Sedation, numbness, dizziness, headache.
Benzoyl peroxide Acne products, topical skin product. Benzoxyl; Benzac W; Clear by Design; Clearasil; Dermo Xyl; Desquam-X; Loroxide; Oxy-5; Panoxyl; Panoxyl-AQ; Persa-Gel; Phiso AC-BP; Vanoxide. Cleansing bar: 5% (120 g); 10% (120 g). Cleansing lotion: 5% (120 mL, 150 mL, 240 mL); 10% (120 mL, 150 mL). Cream: 5% (30 g); 10% (30 g, 45 g). Facial mask: 5%. Gel: 2.5% (45 g, 60 g, 90 g); 5% (45 g, 60 g, 90 g, 120 g); 10% (45 g, 60 g, 90 g, 120 g). Lotion: 5% (30 mL, 42.5 mL, 60 mL); 5.5% (25 mL); 10% (30 mL, 42.5 mL, 60 mL). Stick: 10%.	**Acne treatment (keratolytic and comedolytic effects and kill anaerobic bacteria).** *Children and adults:* Apply sparingly 1–3 times daily for 15 min. May increase strength and duration of exposure as tolerated.	*Adverse events:* Contact dermatitis, local irritation, stinging, or erythema.
Benztropine mesylate Anticholinergic agent: antidote, drug-induced dystonic reactions; anti-Parkinson agent. Cogentin. Injection: 1 mg/mL (2 mL). Tablet: 0.5 mg, 1 mg, 2 mg.	**Parkinsonism, drug-induced extrapyramidal reaction (block striatal cholinergic receptors).** *Children >3 yr:* 0.02–0.05 mg/kg/dose 1–2 times daily. *Adults:* 1–4 mg/24 hr 1–2 times daily.	*Adverse events:* Tachycardia, drowsiness, nervousness, hallucinations, dry mouth, blurred vision, mydriasis.
Benzylpenicilloyl-polylysine Diagnostic agent, penicillin allergy skin test. Pre-Pen. Injection: 0.25 mL.	**Adjunct to assessing the risk of penicillin hypersensitivity (elicits type 1 urticarial reactions by IgE-mediated reaction).** *Children and adults:* Scratch technique uses a 20-gauge needle to make a 3–5 mm scratch on dermis; apply a small drop of solution to scratch and rub it in gently with applicator. Intradermal injection of 0.1–0.2 mL of Pre-Pen and 0.9% saline in 2 sites at least 1 inch apart.	*Monitoring:* Scratch test is positive if a pale wheal of 5–15 mm or more occurs within 10 min. Intradermal test is positive in 5–15 min. Discontinue antihistamines before performing tests (hydroxyzine and diphenhydramine for at least 4 days, astemizole for 6–8 wk).
Beractant Lung surfactant. Survanta. Suspension: 200 mg (8 mL).	**Prophylaxis and treatment of respiratory distress syndrome in premature infants (replace deficiency of endogenous surfactant).** *Neonates:* 4 mL/kg via endotracheal tube. May repeat q6h to a total of 4 doses. Rotate infant to right, then left and administer ½ dose on each side over 2–3 sec.	*Adverse events:* Bradycardia, hypotension, oxygen desaturation, pulmonary air leaks, airway obstruction, pulmonary hemorrhage, hypocarbia. *Monitoring:* Heart rate, oxygen saturation, and frequent arterial blood gases. Adjust ventilator to minimize episodes of hyperoxia and hypocarbia.
Betamethasone Adrenal corticosteroid; anti-inflammatory agent; corticosteroid, systematic; corticosteroid, topical; glucocorticoid. Alphatrex Topical; Betalene Topical; Betatrex Topical; Beta Val Topical; Celestone Oral, Celestone Phosphate Injection; Celestone Soluspan; Cel-U-Jec Injection; Diprolene AF Topical; Diprolene Topical; Diprosone Topical; Maxivate Topical; Psorion Topical; Selestoject Injection; Teledar Topical; Uticort Topical; Valisone Topical. Base (Celestone): Syrup: 0.6 mg/5 mL. Tablet: 0.6 mg. Benzoate (Uticort): Cream, emollient base: 0.025% (60 g). Gel, topical: 0.025% (15 g, 60 g). Lotion: 0.025% (60 mL). Dipropionate (Alphatrex, Diprosone, Maxivate, Tela Dar): Aerosol, topical: 0.1% (85 g). Cream: 0.05% (15, 45 g). Lotion: 0.05% (20, 30, 60 mL). Ointment, topical: 0.05% (15, 45 g). Diproprionate (Psorion): Cream: 0.05% (15, 45 g). Dipropanate, augmented (Diprolene, Diprolene AF): Cream, emollient base: 0.05% (15 g, 45 g). Gel, topical: 0.05% (15, 45 g). Lotion: 0.05% (30, 60 mL). Ointment, topical: 0.05% (15, 45 g).	**Systemic use to stimulate fetal lung maturation in preterm labor. Topical use to treat inflammatory dermatoses.** *Children and adults:* Topical application of thin film to affected area 2–4 times daily. *Pregnant female:* 12 mg IM q24h for 2 doses.	*Adverse events:* Maternal pulmonary edema and hypertension, headache.

TABLE 712–1. General Medications *Continued*

Drug (Trade Names, Formulations)	Indications (Mechanism of Action) and Dosing	Comments (Cautions, Adverse Events, Monitoring)
Valerate (Betatrex, Beta-Val, Valisone): Cream: 0.01% (15, 60 g); 0.1% (15, 45, 110, 430 g). Lotion: 0.1% (20 mL, 60 mL). Ointment, topical: 0.1% (15 g, 45 g). Powder for compounding: 5, 10 g. Sodium phosphate (Celestone Phosphate, Selestoject): Injection: Equivalent to 3 g/mL (5 mL). Sodium phosphate and acetate (Celestone Soluspan): Injection, suspension: 6 mg/mL [3 mg betamethasone and betamethasone sodium phosphate and 3 mg betamethasone acetate per mL] (5 mL).		
Bethanechol Cholinergic agent. Duvoid; Myotonachol, Urecholine. Injection: 5 mg/mL (1 mL). Tablet: 5, 10, 25, 50 mg.	**Treatment of nonobstructive urinary retention or gastroesophageal reflux (stimulate cholinergic receptors in smooth muscle in urinary and gastrointestinal tracts).** *Children:* 0.3–0.6 mg/kg/24 hr divided into 3–4 doses. *Adults:* 10–50 mg 2–4 times/24 hr.	*Adverse events:* Hypotension, abdominal cramps, diarrhea, vomiting, salivation, urinary frequency, bronchial constriction, sweating.
Biotin Biotinidase deficiency; treatment agent; vitamin, water soluble. Biotin Forte; Biotin Forte Extra Strength; Bio-Tn; d-Biotin. Tablet: 300, 400, 600, 800 μg; 2.5, 3, 5, 10 mg.	**Treatment of primary biotinidase deficiency or nutritional biotin deficiency, component of vitamin B complex (required for various metabolic functions).** *Children and adults:* Biotin deficiency: 5–20 mg once/24 hr. Biotinidase deficiency: 5–10 mg once daily.	
Bisacodyl Laxative, stimulant. Bisacodyl Uniserts; Bisco-Lax; Carter's Little Pills; Clysodrast V; Dulcagen; Dulcolax; Fleet laxative. Enema: 10 mg/30 mL. Powder: 1.5 mg with tannic acid 2.5 g per packet (25 s, 50 s). Suppository, rectal: 5, 10 mg. Tablet, enteric coated: 5 mg.	**Treatment of constipation (direct smooth muscle irritation to stimulate gastrointestinal peristalsis).** *Children:* <2 yr: 5 mg rectal suppository. >2 yr: 10 mg rectal suppository. >6 yr: 5–10 mg PO at bedtime or before breakfast. *Adults:* 5–30 mg PO dose, 10 mg rectal suppository.	*Adverse events:* Fluid and electrolyte imbalance, abdominal cramps.
Bismuth subsalicylate Antidiarrheal, gastrointestinal agent, gastric or duodenal ulcer treatment. Bismatrol; Pepto-Bismol. Liquid: 262 mg/15 mL (120 mL, 240 mL, 360 mL, 480 mL); 524 mg/15 mL (120, 240, 360 mL). Tablet, chewable: 262 mg.	**Treatment of diarrhea or gastrointestinal ulcer (adsorbs extra water and toxins in large intestine and kills bacterial pathogens).** *Children or adults:* Up to 8 doses/24 hr. *3–6 yr:* 1/3 tablet or 5 mL. *6–9 yr:* 2/3 tablet or 10 mL. *9–12 yr:* 1 tablet or 15 mL. *Adults:* 2 tablets or 30 mL.	*Cautions:* Avoid in patients with influenza or chickenpox because of salicylate content. *Adverse events:* Discoloration of tongue, grayish-black stools.
Bleomycin Antineoplastic agent, antibiotic type. Blenoxane. Powder for injection: 15 units.	**Palliative treatment for several cancers and sclerosing agent for malignant effusions (inhibit synthesis of DNA).** *Children and adults:* 10–20 units/m²/dose IV, IM, SC (0.25–0.5 unit/kg) 1–2 times per wk in combination regimens.	*Cautions:* Reduce dose in renal dysfunction. *Adverse events:* Interstitial pneumonitis, pulmonary fibrosis, nonproductive cough, phlebitis, leukopenia, thrombocytopenia, stomatitis, vomiting, alopecia, hyperkeratosis of hand and nails, desquamation, Raynaud phenomenon; avoid oxygen use.
Bretylium Antiarrhythmic agent, class III. Bretylol. Injection: 50 mg/mL (10 mL, 20 mL); 100 mg/mL. Injection, premixed in D₅W: 1 mg/mL (500 mL); 2 mg/mL (250 mL); 4 mg/mL (250, 500 mL).	**Treatment of serious or life-threatening arrhythmias (inhibits release of norepinephrine at postganglionic nerve endings).** *Children:* 2–5 mg/kg IV or IM, may repeat q 10–20 min to maximum 30 mg/kg. *Adults:* Initial dose 5 mg/kg, then 10 mg/kg q 15–30 min to maximum 35 mg/kg. Note: Cardioversion/defibrillation must be attempted before and after each dose of bretylium.	*Adverse events:* Hypotension, increased premature ventricular contractions, bradycardia, nasal congestion, sweating, hiccups. *Monitoring:* ECG, blood pressure.
Brompheniramine Antihistamine. Bromarest, Bromphen Elixir, Chlorphed, Cophene-B Injection, Dehist Injection, Dimetane Oral, Nasahist B Injection, ND-Stat Injection, Oraminic II Injection, Sinusol-B Injection, Veltane Tablet. Elixir: 2 mg/5 mL with alcohol 3% (120, 480, 4,000 mL). Injection: 10 mg/mL (10 mL). Tablet: 4, 8, 12 mg. Tablet, sustained release: 8, 12 mg.	**Treatment of allergic symptoms, e.g., rhinitis and urticaria (competes with histamine for H₁-receptor sites).** *Children:* <6 yr: 0.125 mg/kg/dose q6h (max: 8 mg/24 hr) PO. 6–12 yr: 2–4 mg/dose q6–8h (max: 16 mg/24 hr) PO. *Adults:* 4–8 mg/dose q4–6h (max: 24 mg/24 hr) PO. IV, IM, SC route: <12 yr: 0.5 mg/kg/24 hr divided q6h. >12 yr: 10 mg/dose (max: 40 mg/24 hr).	*Adverse events:* Sedation, dry mouth.
Budesonide Adrenal corticosteroid; anti-inflammatory agent; corticosteroid, nasal, glucocorticoid. Rhinocort. Aerosol: 50 μg released per actuation to deliver ~32 μg to patient via nasal adapter [200 metered doses] (7 g). Pulmicort Turbohaler (dry powder inhaler). Inhalation powder 200 μg/inhalation.	**Treatment of chronic rhinitis or asthma (suppress inflammation).** *Children >6 and adults:* Rhinocort nasal spray 2 puffs in each nostril twice daily or 4 puffs in each nostril once daily. *Children >6 yr:* Pulmicort Turbohaler 1–2 inhalations bid. *Adults:* 1–4 inhalations bid.	*Adverse events:* Oral thrush, dysphonia (minimize by rinsing mouth after dose).

Table continued on following page

TABLE 712–1. General Medications *Continued*

Drug (Trade Names, Formulations)	Indications (Mechanism of Action) and Dosing	Comments (Cautions, Adverse Events, Monitoring)
Bumetanide Antihypertensive; diuretic, loop. Bumex Injection: 0.25 mg/mL (2, 4, 10 mL). Tablet: 0.5, 1, 2 mg.	**Management of edema or fluid overload states (prevent sodium and chloride reabsorption at the ascending loop of Henle and proximal tubule).** PO, IV, IM: *Neonates:* 0.01–0.05 mg/kg/dose q 24–48h. *Infants and children:* 0.015–0.1 mg/kg/dose q6–24h (max: 10 mg/24 hr). *Adults:* 0.5–2 mg/dose (max: 10 mg/24 hr).	*Adverse events:* Electrolyte depletion, dehydration.
Bupivacaine Local anesthetic, injectable. Marcaine, Sensorcaine, Sensorcaine-MPF Bupivacaine. Injection: Preservative free: 0.25% [2.5 mg/mL]; 0.5% [5 mg/mL]; 0.75% [7.5 mg/mL]. With preservative: 0.25% [2.5 mg/mL]; 0.5% [5 mg/mL]. Bupivacaine and epinephrine [2:2 million] injection: Preservative free: 0.25% [2.5 mg/mL]; 0.5% [5 mg/mL]; 0.75% [7.5 mg/mL]. With preservative: 0.25% [2.5 mg/mL]; 0.5% [5 mg/mL]. Bupivacaine in dextrose [8.25% injection (spinal)]: Preservative free: 0.75% [7.5 mg/mL].	**Local anesthetic (block initiation and conduction of nerve impulses by decreasing permeability of neuron to sodium ions).** Caudal Block *Children:* 1–3.7 mg/kg. *Adults:* 15–30 mL of 0.25% or 0.5%. Epidural Block *Children:* 1.25 mg/kg/dose. *Adults:* 10–20 mL of 0.25% or 0.5%. Peripheral nerve block: 5 mL dose of 0.25% (12.5 mg) or 0.5% (25 mg); max: 400 mg/24 hr. Sympathetic nerve block: 20–50 mL of 0.25% (no epinephrine).	*Cautions:* Excess doses may result in seizures, bradyarrhythmias, metabolic acidosis, apnea, and methemoglobinemia. Avoid epinephrine for nerve block near end artery since risk of necrosis.
Bupropion Antidepressant. Wellbutrin. Tablet: 75, 100 mg.	**Depression, attention deficit disorder, smoking cessation (block serotonin activity and norepinephrine reuptake).** *Children:* Anecdotal experience had benefits at 75–100 mg 2–3 times/24 hr. *Adults:* Begin 100 mg twice daily and may gradually increase to maximum of 450 mg/24 hr.	*Adverse events:* Agitation, insomnia, headache, psychosis, confusion, anxiety, seizures, akathisia, fever, chills, dry mouth, constipation, nausea, vomiting
Busulfan Antineoplastic agent, alkylating agent. Myleran. Tablet: 2 mg.	**Treatment of chronic myelogenous leukemia (CML) or as part of marrow ablation conditioning before bone marrow transplant (interferes with DNA alkylation).** *Children:* (for CML remission) 0.06–0.12 mg/kg/24 hr; titrate dose to keep leukocyte count >40,000/mm³; (for BMT conditioning) 1 mg/kg/dose q6h for 16 doses. *Adults:* (for CML remission) 0.06 mg/kg/24 hr.	*Adverse events:* Severe pancytopenia, leukopenia, thrombocytopenia, and bone marrow suppression (onset, 7–10 days; nadir, 14–21 days; recovery, 28 days). *Monitoring:* CBC with differential and platelet count (discontinue if WBC <20,000/mm³). Hemoglobin, liver function tests.
Caffeine, citrated Central nervous system stimulant, nonamphetamine; respiratory stimulant. Tablet: 65 mg [anhydrous caffeine 32.5 mg], caffeine citrate, caffeine benzoate.	**Treatment of apnea of prematurity (stimulate central inspiratory drive and sensitivity to carbon dioxide).** *Neonates:* PO or IV (citrate or benzoate). Dose as caffeine base: loading dose 10 mg/kg. Maintenance dose: 5–10 mg/kg/24 hr as 1 or 2 doses/24 hr.	*Cautions:* Sodium benzoate displaces bilirubin from binding and should be avoided in neonates with elevated indirect bilirubin. *Adverse events:* Tachycardia, agitation, irritability, gastric irritation. *Monitoring:* Caffeine concentrations: therapeutic >10 µg/mL; toxic >50 µg/mL.
Calcifediol 25-hydroxycholecalciferol; 25-hydroxyvitamin D₃; vitamin D analog. Calderol. Capsule: 20, 50 µg.	**Treatment of metabolic bone disease associated with chronic renal failure (regulates serum calcium homeostasis as a vitamin D analog).** *Infants:* 5–7 µg/kg/24 hr. *Children and adults:* 20–100 µg/kg daily or every other day titrated to obtain normal serum calcium and phosphate levels.	*Cautions:* Avoid in hypercalcemia, hypervitaminosis D, malabsorption states. Ensure adequate calcium intake during use. *Adverse events:* Hypercalcemia, gastrointestinal intolerance.
Calcitriol Vitamin D analog; 1,25 dihydroxycholecalciferol, vitamin, fat soluble. Calcijex, Rocaltrol. Capsule: 0.25, 0.5 µg. Injection: 1 µg/mL (1 mL); 2 µg/mL (1 mL).	**Treatment of hypocalcemia and metabolic bone disease, reduce elevated parathyroid hormone levels, decrease severity of psoriatic lesions in psoriatic vulgaris (regulate serum calcium homeostasis and increase calcium absorption).** *Premature infants* (hypocalcemia): 0.05 µg/kg/24 hr IV or 1 µg/24 hr PO. *Children:* 0.01–0.08 µg/kg/24 hr. *Adults:* 0.25–1 µg/24 hr.	*Adverse events:* Hypercalcemia, vitamin D toxicity.
Calcium salts (PO and IV) Calcium carbonate Elemental calcium listed in brackets. Antacid; calcium salt; electrolyte supplement, oral Alka-Mints, Cal-Plus, Mylanta, Os-Cal, Tums. Capsule: 1,500 mg [600 mg].. Liquid: 1,000 mg/5 mL (360 mL). Cardiac Arrest Lozenge: 600 mg [240 mg]. Powder: 6.5 g/packet [2.6]. Suspension, oral: 1,250 mg/5 mL [500 mg]. Tablet: 650 mg [260 mg], 1,500 mg [600 mg] Tablet, chewable.	**Hypocalcemic tetany, cardiac disturbances of hyperkalemia (moderate nerve and muscle performance).** Hypocalcemic Tetany *Neonates:* 2.4 mEq/kg/24 hr in divided doses (if due to citrated blood transfusion give 0.45 mEq/dL transfused blood). *Infants and children:* 10 mg/kg over 5–10 min (may repeat in 6–8 hr) followed by infusion with maximum of 200 mg/kg/24 hr. *Adults:* 4.5–16 mEq repeated until response. *Infants and children:* 20 mg/kg IV and may repeat in 10 min. *Adults:* 2–4 mg/kg repeated every 10 min as needed.	*Caution:* Make sure of IV access site to avoid severe IV burns; bradycardia. *Adverse events:* Constipation, hypercalcemia, milk-alkali syndrome. *Monitoring:* Continuous ECG; serum calcium, potassium, and magnesium levels.

Calcium Content of Salts

Salt	Mg of Calcium/g of Salt (Elemental)	mEq Ca²⁺/g of Salt
Ca carbonate	400	20
Ca chloride	270	13.5
Ca glubionate	64	3.2
Ca gluceptate	82	4.1
Ca gluconate	90	4.5
Ca lactate	130	6.5
Ca phosphate	390	19.3

TABLE 712–1. General Medications *Continued*

Drug (Trade Names, Formulations)	Indications (Mechanism of Action) and Dosing	Comments (Cautions, Adverse Events, Monitoring)
Calcium chloride Calcium salt, electrolyte supplement, parenteral. Cal Plus. Elemental calcium listed in brackets. Injection: 10% = 100 mg/mL [27.2 mg/mL] (10 mL) (1.4 mEq calcium/mL).	**Prevention of calcium depletion, relief of acid indigestion (source of calcium and neutralizes acid).** *Children:* *<6 mo:* 400 mg/24 hr. *6–12 mo:* 600 mg/24 hr. *1–5 yr:* 800 mg/24 hr. *6–10 yr:* 800–1,200 mg/24 hr. *>10 yr and adult:* 1,000–1,500 mg/24 hr.	
Calcium glubionate Calcium Salt; Electrolyte Supplement, Oral. Neo-Calglucon. Syrup: 1.8 g/5 mL [115 mg/5 mL] (480 mL) (1.2 mEq calcium/mL).		
Capsaicin Analgesic, topical; topical skin product. R-Gel, Zostrix-HP Topical, Zostrix Topical. Cream: 0.025% (45, 90 g); 0.075% (30, 60 g). Gel: 0.025% (15, 30 mL).	**Topical treatment of pain associated with postherpetic neuralgia, rheumatoid arthritis, osteoarthritis, diabetic neuropathy, and postsurgical pain (induces release of substance P depleting peripheral nerves and preventing reaccumulation).** *Children >2 yr and adults:* Apply to affected area at least 3–4 times daily.	*Adverse events:* Local itching, stinging, burning, and erythema.
Calfactant Infasurf Intratracheal suspension of calf lung surfactant (35 mg phospholipids, 0.65 mg proteins, 0.26 mg SP-B/mL)	**Prophylaxis or treatment of respiratory distress syndrome, treatment of persistent pulmonary hypertension.** *Neonates:* 3 mL/kg/dose 1–4 times q12h *Children and adults:* Not indicated	*Caution:* Monitor ventilator status closely; may require rapid weaning within minutes of the dose. *Adverse events:* Bradycardia, airway obstruction, and cyanosis.
Captopril Angiotensin-converting enzyme (ACE) inhibitors; antihypertensive. Capoten. Tablet: 12.5, 25, 50, 100 mg.	**Management of hypertension and treatment of heart failure (ACE inhibitor).** *Premature newborns:* 0.01 mg/kg q8–12h. *Neonates:* Initial 0.05–0.1 mg/kg/dose q8–24h and titrate upward to response (max: 0.5 mg/kg/dose q6–24h). *Infants:* Initial 0.15–0.3 mg/kg/dose; and titrate upward (max: 6 mg/kg/24 hr in 1–4 divided doses). *Children:* Initial 0.3–0.5 mg/kg/dose and titrate upward (max: 6 mg/kg/24 hr divided into 2–4 doses). *Older children:* Initial 6.25–12.5 mg/kg/dose q12–24h then titrate (max: 6 mg/kg/24 hr in 2–4 doses). *Adolescents and adults:* Initial 12.5–25 mg/dose and titrate (max: 450 mg/24 hr).	*Cautions:* Use with caution in renal artery stenosis or patients with volume depletion. *Adverse events:* Cough, angioedema, oliguria, hyperkalemia.
Carbamazepine Anticonvulsant, miscellaneous. Epitol, Tegretol. Suspension, oral (citrus-vanilla flavor): 100 mg/5 mL (450 mL). Tablet: 200 mg. Tablet, chewable: 100 mg. Tegretol XR: 100, 200, 400 mg (sustained-release product).	**Treatment of generalized tonic-clonic and partial seizures, pain relief in trigeminal neuralgia and diabetic neuropathy, bipolar disorders (limit influx of sodium ions across cell membranes or other unknown mechanisms).** *Children:* *<6 yr:* initial 5 mg/kg/24 hr in 2–4 divided doses; may increase q 5–7 days by 5 mg/kg based on effect or toxicity and serum concentration. *6–12 yr:* initial 10 mg/kg/24 hr in 2–4 divided doses; increase by 100 mg or 5 mg/kg/24 hr at weekly intervals until therapeutic levels are achieved (usual dose: 800–1,200 mg/24 hr). *Adults:* Initial 200 mg twice daily; increase by 200 mg at weekly intervals until therapeutic levels are achieved (usual dose 1.6 to 2.4 g/24 hr in 3–4 divided doses).	*Caution:* Avoid in patients with bone marrow depression; may cross-react in patients with tricyclic antidepressant hypersensitivity. *Adverse events:* Sedation, dizziness, fatigue, ataxia, confusion, nausea, vomiting, blurred vision, nystagmus, bone marrow depression, leukopenia, neutropenia, thrombocytopenia, pancytopenia, aplastic anemia, hepatitis, hypersensitivity reactions. *Monitoring:* Serum concentrations correlate with clinical response (6–12 μg/mL), and neurologic and visual toxicity (>8 μg/mL but particularly >12 μg/mL). Drug dosing requirements will increase over first 4 wk because of hepatic enzyme induction by carbamazepine. Monitor serum concentrations to increase doses appropriately.
Carbamide peroxide Otic agent, ceruminolytic. Auro Ear Drops, Gly-Oxide Oral, Proxigel Oral, Murine Ear Drops. Gel, oral: 11% (36 g). Solution, oral: 10% in glycerin (15, 22.5, 30, 60 mL). Otic: 6.5% in glycerin (15, 30 mL).	**Relief of minor inflammation of oral mucosa including gums and lips, and removal of ear wax (release of hydrogen peroxide, which inhibits bacteria and softens ear wax).** *Children and adults:* *Gel:* Gently massage on affected area 4 times daily. *Oral solution:* Apply several drops to affected area 4 times daily for up to 7 days. (expectorate 2–3 min after each use). *Otic solution:* Tilt head sideways and instill 5–10 drops bid for up to 4 days. Keep drops in ear canal for several minutes by tilting head and placing cotton in ear.	*Adverse events:* Local irritation.

MEDICATIONS

Table continued on following page

TABLE 712–1. General Medications *Continued*

Drug (Trade Names, Formulations)	Indications (Mechanism of Action) and Dosing	Comments (Cautions, Adverse Events, Monitoring)
Carbinoxamine and pseudoephedrine Antihistamine/decongestant combination. Carbiset Tablet; Carbodec Syrup; Rondec Drops. Drops: carbinoxamine maleate 2 mg and pseudo-ephedrine hydrochloride 25 mg/mL (30 mL with dropper). Syrup: carbinoxamine maleate 4 mg and pseudo-ephedrine hydrochloride 60 mg/5 mL (120, 480 mL). Tablet: Film-coated: carbinoxamine maleate 4 mg and pseudoephedrine hydrochloride 60 mg. Sustained release: carbinoxamine maleate 8 mg and pseudoephedrine hydrochloride 120 mg.	**Temporary relief of nasal congestion, runny nose, sneezing, and allergy symptoms (antihistamine as H_1-blocker, and decongestant as α- and β-receptor stimulant).** *Children:* Dose 4 times daily: *1–3 mo:* $1/4$ dropper (0.25 mL). *3–6 mo:* $1/2$ dropper (0.5 mL). *6–9 mo:* $3/4$ dropper (0.75 mL). *9–18 mo:* 1 dropper (1.0 mL). *18 mo–6 yr:* 2.5 mL syrup. *6–12 yr:* 5 mL syrup or 1 tablet. *Children >12 yr and adults:* 1 tablet 4 times daily, or 1 sustained-release tablet twice/24 hr.	*Cautions:* Avoid in narrow angle glaucoma, coronary artery disease, gastrointestinal or genitourinary obstruction, or monoamine oxidase inhibitor therapy. *Adverse events:* Hypertension, tachycardia, drowsiness, sedation, thickening of bronchial secretions.
Carboplatin Antineoplastic agent, alkylating agent. Paraplatin powder for injection, lyophilized: 50, 150, 450 mg.	**Treatment of multiple tumors including pediatric brain tumor and neuroblastoma (platination of DNA interferes with DNA function).** *Children:* Solid tumor: 300–600 mg/m² IV once q 4 wk. Brain tumor: 175 mg/m² IV once wk for 4 wk (2 wk recovery period between courses). *Adults:* 360 mg/m² IV once q 4 wk.	*Adverse events:* Neutropenia, leukopenia, thrombocytopenia, peripheral neuropathy, ototoxicity, abnormal liver and renal function, alopecia, nausea, vomiting. *Monitoring:* Neutrophil and platelet count affect dose selection as follows: platelets <50,000/mm³ or neutrophils <500/mm³: give 75% of recommended dose (nadir: 14–21 days post dose).
Carmustine Antineoplastic agent, alkylating agent (nitrosourea). BiCNU powder for injection: 100 mg/vial packaged with 3 mL of absolute alcohol for use as a sterile diluent.	**Treatment of cancers including brain tumor, Hodgkin disease and non-Hodgkin lymphoma, and multiple myeloma (inhibits key enzymatic reactions involved in DNA synthesis).** *Children:* 200–250 mg/m² IV q 4–6 wk as a single dose. *Adults:* 150–200 mg/m² IV q 6 wk as a single dose.	*Adverse events:* Nausea, vomiting, myelosuppression (nadir 4–6 wk post dose), alopecia, stomatitis, anorexia, diarrhea, dizziness, ataxia, pulmonary fibrosis, hepatic and renal dysfunction, retinitis, optic neuritis.
Carnitine Dietary supplement. Carnitor, Vitacarn. Capsule: 250 mg. Injection: 1 g/5 mL (5 mL). Liquid (cherry flavor): 100 mg/mL (10 mL). Tablet: 330 mg.	**Treatment of carnitine deficiency and improve utilization of IV fat emulsions by premature infants (facilitates long-chain fatty acid entry into the mitochondria and required in energy metabolism).** *Premature infants:* 8–16 mg/kg/24 hr IV infusion. *Children:* 50–100 mg/kg/24 hr in 2–3 divided doses PO, 50 mg/kg/dose q4–6h IV (max: 300 mg/kg/24 hr). *Adults:* 0.33–1 g/dose 2–3 times daily PO, 50 mg/kg/dose q4–6h (max: 300 mg/kg/24 hr).	*Adverse events:* Nausea, vomiting, abdominal cramps, body odor.
Carvedilol Coreg. Tablet: 3.125, 6.25, 12.5, 25 mg.	**β-Receptor blocker with vasodilator activity, used to treat congestive heart failure or hypertension.** *Children:* Initial dose 0.08 mg/kg and gradual increase dose over 2–3 mo based on response to maximum 0.5 mg/kg/24 hr divided q12h.	*Caution:* May cause AV block, arrhythmias, bradycardia, or worsen asthma or heart failure. *Drug interactions:* May cause excessive hypotension when used with other antihypertensives.
Cascara sagrada Laxative, stimulant. Liquid, aromatic fluid extract: 5, 120 mL. Tablet: 325 mg.	**Temporary relief of constipation (direct chemical irritation of gastrointestinal mucosa).** *Infants:* 1.25 mL once daily. *Children 2–11 yr:* 2.5 mL once daily. *>12 yr and adults:* 5 mL once daily.	*Cautions:* Fecal impaction, gastrointestinal obstruction, gastrointestinal bleeding. Onset of effect 6–10 hr, so give at bedtime. *Adverse events:* Gastrointestinal cramps, urine discolored red or brown.
Castor oil Laxative, Stimulant. Alphamul, Emulsoil, Fleet, Purge. Emulsion, oral; Liquid, oral: 100% (60, 120, 480 mL).	**Bowel or rectal evacuation for surgery (stimulates peristalsis).** *Infants <2 yr:* 1–5 mL single dose. *Children 2–11 yr:* 5–15 mL. *>12 yr and adults:* 15–60 mL	*Adverse events:* Electrolyte disturbances, abdominal cramps.
Charcoal Adsorbent, antidote. Actidose-Aqua, Actidose with Sorbitol, Charcocaps.	**Emergency treatment of poisoning by certain drugs and chemicals; gastrointestinal dialysis to promote elimination of certain drugs and toxins; treat diarrhea (adsorb toxic substance; interfere with entero-hepatic recycling of certain drugs).** *Children and adults:* 1–2 g/kg or 5–10 times the weight of the ingested poison (limit sorbitol to 1–2 times daily); may repeat doses q2–6h.	*Adverse events:* Constipation, black stools.
Chloral hydrate Hypnotic; sedative. Noctec; capsules: 250, 500 mg. Syrup: 250, 500 mg/5 mL. Suppository: 324, 500, 648 mg.	**Short-term sedative/hypnotic (mechanism unknown).** *Neonates:* 25 mg/kg/dose. *Infants and children:* 25–100 mg/kg/dose. *Adults:* 250–1,000 mg/dose. Doses may be repeated q6–8h. Lower-end doses cause sedation; higher-end doses cause hypnosis.	*Cautions:* Repeat doses in neonates may cause accumulation of active metabolite trichloroethanol (TCE), which can cause hepatic toxicity and bilirubin displacement.

TABLE 712–1. General Medications *Continued*

Drug (Trade Names, Formulations)	Indications (Mechanism of Action) and Dosing	Comments (Cautions, Adverse Events, Monitoring)
Chlorambucil Antineoplastic alkylating agent. Leukeran, 2-mg tablet.	**Management of various cancers including Hodgkin and non-Hodgkin lymphoma, and chronic lymphocytic leukemia; and nephrotic syndrome (alkylation interferes with DNA replication and RNA transcription).** *Children and adults:* 0.1–0.2 mg/kg/24 hr for 3–6 wk. Longer treatment doses are adjusted based on blood counts.	*Adverse events:* Bone marrow suppression (onset, 7 days; nadir, 10–14 days; recovery, 28 days); rashes, hyperuricemia, nausea, vomiting, diarrhea, oral ulceration, pulmonary fibrosis, hepatic necrosis, peripheral neuropathy.
Chlorothiazide Diuretic. Generic tablets: 250, mg 500 mg; suspension: 250 mg/5 mL; powder for injection: 500 mg.	**Treatment of fluid overload states and hypertension (inhibits sodium reabsorption in distal tubule).** *Neonates and infants <6 mo:* PO: 20–40 mg/kg/24 hr divided q12h; IV: 2–8 mg/kg/24 hr divided q12h. *Infants >6 mo and children:* PO: 20 mg/kg/24 hr in 2 divided doses; IV: 4 mg/kg/24 hr. *Adults:* PO: 500 mg–2 g/24 hr in 1–2 doses; IV: 500–1,000 mg/24 hr.	*Adverse events:* Hypokalemia, hypochloremic alkalosis, hyperglycemia, hyperlipidemia, hypercalcemia, hyperuricemia, leukopenia, prerenal azotemia.
Chlorpheniramine maleate Antihistamine, generic. Capsule: 12 mg; timed-release capsule: 6, 8, 12 mg; syrup: 2 mg/5 mL; tablet: 4, 8, 12 mg; chewable tablet: 2 mg; timed-release tablet: 8, 12 mg.	**Treat allergic symptoms (compete with histamine for H_1-receptor sites).** *Children: 2–6 yr:* 1 mg q4–6h. *6–12 yr:* 2 mg q4–6h or sustained-release 8 mg at bedtime. *>12 yr and adults:* 4 mg q4–6h or sustained-release 12 mg at bedtime.	*Adverse events:* Drowsiness, excitation or hyperactivity (in children), dry mouth, blurred vision.
Chlorpromazine Phenothiazine. Thorazine. Capsule: 30, 75, 150, 200, 300 mg. Oral concentrate: 30 mg/mL, 100 mg/mL. Suppository: 25, 100 mg. Syrup: 10 mg/5 mL. Tablet: 10, 25, 50, 100, 200 mg. Injection: 25 mg/mL.	**Treatment of psychosis, mania, Tourette syndrome, behavioral problems, nausea, and vomiting (blocks postsynaptic mesolimbic dopaminergic receptors in the brain, strong α-adrenergic blocking effect).** *Children >6 mo:* PO: 0.5–1 mg/kg/dose q4–6h; rectal: 1 mg/kg/dose q6–8 h; IM or IV: 0.5–1 mg/kg/dose q6–8h. *Adults:* Psychosis: PO: 30–800 mg/24 hr in 1–4 divided doses (start low and titrate up to effect); IV or IM: 25 mg initial dose and titrate up to effect (maximum: 400 mg/dose q4–6h). Nausea or vomiting: PO: 10–25 mg q4–6h. IM or IV: 25–50 mg q4–6 h. Rectal: 50–100 mg q6–8h.	*Adverse events:* Hypotension, tachycardia, arrhythmias, pseudoparkinsonism, tardive dyskinesia, akathisia, dystonias, constipation, nasal congestion, dry mouth, malignant hyperpyrexia. *Monitoring:* Chlorpromazine concentrations: therapeutic 50–300 ng/mL; toxic >750 ng/mL.
Chlorpropamide Sulfonylurea. Diabinese. Tablet: 100, 250 mg.	**Control blood sugar in non–insulin-dependent diabetes mellitus (type II) (stimulate insulin release from pancreatic islet cells).** *Adults:* Initial 250 mg once daily, may increase to response by 125 mg q 3–5 days to response (max: 750 mg/24 hr).	*Adverse events:* Gastrointestinal problems, photosensitivity, hepatotoxicity, hyponatremia, SIADH.
Chlorthalidone Thiazide diuretic. Hygroton. Tablet: 20, 25, 100 mg.	**Treatment of fluid overload and mild hypertension (inhibits sodium and chloride reabsorption in the cortical-diluting segment of the ascending loop of Henle).** *Children:* 1–2 mg/kg once daily. *Adults:* 25–100 mg once daily.	*Adverse events:* Photosensitivity, fluid and electrolyte imbalance, hypokalemia.
Chlorzoxazone Skeletal muscle relaxant. Parafon Forte, Paraflex. Tablet: 250, 500 mg.	**Symptomatic relief of muscle spasm and pain (depress polysynaptic reflexes at spinal cord and subcortical levels).** *Children:* 20 mg/kg/24 hr in 3–4 divided doses. *Adults:* 250–500 mg 3–4 times daily.	*Adverse events:* Drowsiness.
Cholestyramine resin Antilipemic agent. Questran. Powder: 4 g resin/9 g powder.	**Management of elevated cholesterol (forms a nonabsorbable complex with bile salts and low-density lipoprotein-cholesterol).** *Children:* 240 mg/kg/24 hr in 3 divided doses. *Adults:* 4 g/dose 1–6 times daily.	*Adverse events:* Hyperchloremic acidosis, constipation, nausea, vomiting, abdominal pain and distention, malabsorption of fat-soluble vitamins.
Choline magnesium trisalicylate Nonsteroidal anti-inflammatory agent (NSAID). Trilisate. Liquid: 500 mg salicylate/5 mL. Tablet: 500, 750, 1,000 mg.	**Management of arthritis disorders (inhibit prostaglandin synthesis).** *Children:* 30–60 mg/kg/24 hr in 3–4 divided doses. *Adults:* 500–1,500 mg/dose 1–3 times daily.	*Cautions:* Avoid in patients with suspected influenza or varicella infections due to risk for Reye syndrome; avoid in asthmatics and others at risk for serious hypersensitivity reactions. *Adverse events:* Gastrointestinal intolerance, tinnitus, hepatotoxicity, pulmonary edema. *Monitoring:* Salicylate concentrations: anti-inflammatory 150–300 µg/mL; analgesic or antipyretic effect 30–50 µg/mL.
Chorionic gonadotropin Gonadotropin, ovulation stimulator. Chorex, Choron, Pregnyl. Powder for injection 200, 500, 1,000, 2,000 units/mL (10 mL).	**Treatment of hypogonadotropic hypogonadism; cryptorchidism; induce ovulation (stimulate production of gonadal steroid hormones; substitute for luteinizing hormone to stimulate ovulation).**	*Adverse events:* Mental depression, tiredness, precocious puberty, premature closure of the epiphyses.

Table continued on following page

MEDICATIONS

TABLE 712–1. **General Medications** *Continued*

Drug (Trade Names, Formulations)	Indications (Mechanism of Action) and Dosing	Comments (Cautions, Adverse, Events, Monitoring)
	Children: *Prepubertal cryptorchidism:* 1,000–2,000 units/m^2/dose 3 times/wk for 3 wk or 500 units 3 times/wk for 4–6 wk. *Hypogonadotropic hypogonadism:* 500–1,000 units/dose 3 times/wk for 3 wk; or 4,000 units 3 times/wk for 6–9 mo then taper to 2,000 units 3 times/wk for 3 mo. *Adults (menotropin dose):* 5,000 units 3 times/wk for 4–6 mo.	
Cimetidine Histamine-2 antagonist. Cimetidine. Tablet: 200, 300, 400, 800 mg. Liquid: 300 mg/5 mL. Injection: 150 mg/mL.	**Short-term treatment and long-term prophylaxis of gastroesophageal reflux disease and gastrointestinal ulcers and hyperacidity (competitive inhibition of histamine at H$_2$ receptors).** *Neonates:* PO, IV, IM: 5–10 mg/kg/24 hr divided q8–12h. *Infants:* PO, IV, IM: 10–20 mg/kg/24 hr divided q6–12h. *Children:* PO, IV, IM: 20–40 mg/kg/24 hr divided q6h. *Adults:* 300 mg q6h (prolong dosing interval for creatinine clearance below 40 mL/min).	*Cautions:* Potent enzyme inhibitor thus may cause toxic accumulation of drugs that are metabolized (e.g., antidepressants, anticonvulsants, theophylline, warfarin, cisapride). *Adverse events:* Dizziness, drowsiness, bradycardia. *Monitoring:* Target gastric pH $\geq$ 5.
Cisapride Prokinetic gastrointestinal agent. Propulsid. Tablet: 10 mg.	**Treatment of gastroesophageal reflux, gastroparesis, and refractory constipation (enhances release of acetylcholine at myenteric plexus).** *Neonates–Children:* 0.15–0.3 mg/kg/dose 3–4 times daily. *Adults:* 10–20 mg 4 times daily. Give doses 15–30 min before meals.	*Cautions:* High doses or combination with enzyme inhibitors (e.g., erythromycin, cimetidine) may cause QT-interval prolongation predisposing to torsades de pointes. *Adverse events:* Tachycardia, prolonged QT interval, headache, anxiety, insomnia, gastrointestinal cramping, flatulence, diarrhea. *Monitoring:* ECG baseline and early treatment.
Cisplatin Antineoplastic agent, alkylating agent. Platinol. Injection, aqueous: 1 mg/mL. Powder for injection: 10 mg , 50 mg.	**Treatment of multiple tumor types (inhibit DNA synthesis).** *Children and adults:* 37–75 mg/m^2 once q 2–3 wk or 50–120 mg/m^2 once q 21–28 days (administer over 4–6 hr). Adjust dose in renal impairment: CrCl 10–50 mL/min = 75% of dose; CrCl <10 mL/min = 50% of dose.	*Adverse events:* Nausea vomiting (lasts up to 1 wk post dose), myelosuppression (onset, 10 days; nadir, 14–23 days; recovery, 21–39 days), acute renal failure, chronic nephropathy (sodium, magnesium, and water wasting; hyperuricemia), peripheral neuropathy (irreversible), ototoxicity (high-frequency hearing loss), extravasation injury, elevated liver enzymes, alopecia, optic neuritis, arrhythmias.
Citrate solutions Alkalinizing agent. Bicitra (sodium citrate 500 mg and citric acid 334 mg/5 mL = 1 mEq sodium + 1 mEq bicarbonate equivalent per mL). Polycitra (sodium citrate 500 mg and citric acid 334 mg and potassium citrate 550 mg/5 mL = 1 mEq sodium + 1 mEq potassium + 2 mEq bicarbonate equivalent per mL).	**Treatment of chronic metabolic acidosis (citrate salts are oxidized in the body to form bicarbonate).** *Neonates, infants, and children:* 2–3 mEq/kg/24 hr in 3–4 divided doses with water after meals. *Adults:* 15–30 mL with water after meals and at bedtime.	*Adverse events:* Hypernatremia, hyperkalemia, metabolic alkalosis.
Clomipramine Antidepressant. Anafranil. Capsule: 25, 50, 75 mg.	**Treatment of obsessive-compulsive disorder and panic attacks (affects serotonin and norepinephrine uptake).** *Children:* Start 25 mg/24 hr and gradually increase to response (max: 200 mg/24 hr). *Adults:* Start 25 mg/24 hr and dose to response (max: 250 mg/24 hr).	*Adverse events:* Dizziness, drowsiness, dry mouth, constipation, nausea, weight gain, nervousness, anxiety, seizures, hypotension, arrhythmias, parkinsonian syndrome, insomnia.
Clonazepam Benzodiazepine. Klonopin. Tablets: 0.5, 1, 2 mg.	**Prophylaxis of seizure types: absence, Lennox-Gastaut, akinetic, myoclonic (depress nerve transmission in the motor cortex).** *Children:* 0.01–0.3 mg/kg/24 hr in 2–3 divided doses, then increase by 0.5 mg/24 hr q 3–5 days to response (max: 0.3 mg/kg/24 hr). *Adults:* Initial dose 0.1 mg bid; then 0.2–2.4 mg/24 hr in 2–4 divided doses.	*Adverse events:* Tachycardia, chest pain, drowsiness, fatigue, impaired memory and coordination, depression, blurred vision, nausea, vomiting, dry mouth, hypersalivation, anorexia, bronchial hypersecretion, respiratory depression, physical and psychological dependence. *Monitoring:* Clonazepam concentrations: therapeutic 20–80 ng/mL; toxic >80 ng/mL; loss of efficacy with prolonged use (tachyphylaxis). *Cautions:* Taper doses gradually to avoid sympathetic overactivity symptoms.
Clonidine α-Adrenergic agonist. Catapres. Tablet 0.1, 0.2, 0.3 mg. Transdermal patch 0.1, 0.2, 0.3 mg/24 hr.	**Treatment of hypertension; attention deficit disorder (ADD); narcotic withdrawal; aid in diagnosis of pheochromocytoma and growth hormone deficiency (stimulates α_2- adrenoreceptors in the brainstem).** *Neonates:* Narcotic withdrawal: 1 μg/kg q6–8h to start and may titrate to targeted abstinence score (max: 2 μg/kg/dose q4h). *Children:* ADD: initial 0.05 mg/24 hr, increase q 3–7 days by 0.05 mg/24 hr given in 3–4 divided doses to response (max: 0.4 mg/24 hr). Hypertension: 5–10 μg/kg/24 hr in 2–4 divided doses (max: 0.9 mg/24 hr). Clonidine tolerance test for growth hormone release: 4 μg/kg × 1 dose. *Adults:* hypertension oral: 0.2–2.4 mg/24 hr in 2–4 doses titrated to response; transdermal: 0.1–0.3 mg/24 hr titrated to effect.	*Adverse events:* Drowsiness, dizziness, dry mouth, constipation, hypotension.

TABLE 712–1. General Medications *Continued*

Drug (Trade Names, Formulations)	Indications (Mechanism of Action) and Dosing	Comments (Cautions, Adverse Events, Monitoring)
Clorazepate Benzodiazepine. Tranxene. Tablet 3.75, 7.5, 15 mg.	**Anxiety and panic disorders; adjunct in management of partial seizures (facilitate transmission of inhibitory neurotransmitter, γ-aminobutyric acid [GABA]).** *Children: 9–12 yr:* 3.75–7.5 mg/dose bid (max: 60 mg/24 hr). *>12 yr and adults:* 7.5 mg/dose bid–tid (max: 90 mg/24 hr). *Adults:* 7.5–15 mg/dose bid–qid.	*Adverse events:* Drowsiness, confusion, depression, blurred vision.
Clozapine Clozaril, generic. Tablets: 25, 100 mg.	**Atypical antipsychotic, dibenzepin chemical group.** *Children:* Start at 6.25 mg bid, increase by 6.25 mg/24 hr weekly as needed. Typical dose: 50–300 mg/24 hr. *Adults:* Start 25 mg q 24 hr and titrate up by 25–50 mg/24 hr to 450–500 mg/24 hr divided tid at 2 wk. Further dose increases should not exceed 100 mg/wk (max: 900 mg/24 hr).	*Caution:* Agranulocytosis, sometimes fatal, has been reported in 1.3% of patients. Thus white blood cell (WBC) counts must be done at baseline and every wk for the first 6 mo of treatment, then every other wk. WBC counts must be checked every other week thereafter. If clozapine is discontinued, check WBC weekly for the next 4 wk. *Adverse events:* Seizures, orthostatic hypotension, extrapyramidal symptoms (less often than typical antipsychotics), hyperglycemia, dizziness, drowsiness, headache, tremor, excessive salivation (especially during sleep) *Drug interactions:* Clozapine levels may increase with concurrent use of enzyme inhibitors. Clozapine is highly protein bound and may displace other highly protein bound drugs (e.g., warfarin).
Codeine Narcotic analgesic. Generic, combination products. Injection. Tablet.	**Treatment of mild to moderate pain and cough (inhibition of ascending pain pathways; central action in medulla to suppress cough).** *Children:* Pain: 0.5–1 mg/kg/dose q4–6h (max: 60 mg/dose). Cough: 1–1.5 mg/kg/24 hr divided q4–6h. *Adults:* Pain: 15–60 mg/dose q4–6h as needed. Cough: 10–20 mg/dose q4–6h (max: 120 mg/24 hr).	*Adverse events:* Drowsiness, constipation, nausea, anorexia, vomiting, sedation, dizziness.
Colchicine Anti-inflammatory/anti-gout agent. Generic. Injection: 0.5 mg/mL.. Tablet: 0.5, 0.6 mg.	**Management of familial Mediterranean fever, acute and chronic gouty arthritis (decrease leukocyte motility and phagocytosis in joints).** *Children:* Prophylaxis of familial Mediterranean fever: *<5 yr:* 0.5 mg/24 hr. *>5 yr:* 1–1.5 mg/24 hr in 2–3 divided doses. *Adults:* gouty arthritis: PO: 0.5–0.6 mg q2h to symptom relief or gastrointestinal toxicity (max: 8 mg/24 hr). IV: 1–3 mg load then 0.5 mg/dose q6h until response (max: 4 mg/24 hr).	*Caution:* Reduce dose by 50% if CrCl <10 mL/min. *Adverse events:* Nausea, vomiting, diarrhea, abdominal pain.
Colfosceril palmitate Lung surfactant. Exosurf. Intratracheal suspension, 108 mg/10 mL.	**Neonatal respiratory distress syndrome (RDS) (replaces deficient surfactant, lowers surface tension at air-fluid interface in alveoli).** *Neonates:* 5 mL/kg/dose as prophylaxis or rescue therapy for RDS (max: 4 doses, although no proven benefit for >2 doses).	*Caution:* Administer via sideport using special endotracheal tube adaptor with ½ dose with head and torso tilted to left and ½ dose head and torso tilted to right; give each half over 1–2 min. *Adverse events:* Pulmonary hemorrhage, overventilation (causing hyperoxia and hypocarbia), PDA.
Corticotropin, ACTH Adrenal corticosteroid. Acthar. Injection, repository: 40, 80 units/mL. Tablet: 5, 10, 25 mg.	**Infantile spasms; diagnostic agent in adrenocortical insufficiency; acute exacerbations of multiple sclerosis; severe muscle weakness in myasthenia gravis (stimulates adrenal cortex to release adrenal steroids, androgenic substances, and a small amount of aldosterone).** *Children:* Inflammation or immunosuppression: IV, IM, SC (aqueous): 1.6 units/kg/24 hr or 50 units/m² divided q6–8h; IM (gel): 0.8 unit/kg/24 hr or 25 units/m²/day divided q12–24h. Infantile spasms: 5–160 units/kg/24 hr has been used for 1 wk–12 mo as IM gel (prednisone 2 mg/kg/24 hr has equal efficacy). *Adults:* Acute exacerbations of MS: 80–120 units/24 hr for 2–3 wk.	*Caution:* May mask signs of infection; do not administer live vaccines; may exacerbate heart failure or hypertension. *Adverse events:* Insomnia, nervousness, increased appetite, indigestion, diabetes mellitus, joint pain, epistaxis, mood swings, pancreatitis, esophagitis, muscle wasting, bone growth suppression, opportunistic infections.
Cortisone acetate Adrenal corticosteroid. Cortone. Injection: 50 mg/mL. Tablet: 5, 10, 25 mg.	**Management of adrenocortical insufficiency (replacement).** *Children:* PO: 0.5–0.75 mg/kg/24 hr divided q8h; IM: 0.25–0.35 mg/kg/24 hr. *Adults:* PO, IM: 20–300 mg/24 hr in 1–2 doses.	*Cautions:* Avoid in active fungal infection and most other serious infections except shock or meningitis. *Adverse events:* Insomnia, nervousness, pseudotumor cerebri, headache, increased appetite, peptic ulcer, diabetes mellitus, edema, hypertension, cataracts, glaucoma, and hypokalemia. *Comment:* See comparison of corticosteroids under *Hydrocortisone.*

Table continued on following page

MEDICATIONS

TABLE 712–1. **General Medications** *Continued*

Drug (Trade Names, Formulations)	Indications (Mechanism of Action) and Dosing	Comments (Cautions, Adverse Events, Monitoring)
Cosyntropin Adrenal corticosteroid. Cortrosyn. Powder for injection: 0.25 mg.	**Diagnosis of primary versus secondary adrenocortical deficiency (stimulates adrenal cortex to release adrenal steroids).** *Neonates:* 0.015 mg/kg/dose. *Children <2 yr:* 0.125 mg. *Children >2 yr and adults:* 0.25 mg. Give dose in early morning	*Adverse events:* Flushing, mild fever, pruritus, pancreatitis. *Monitoring:* Measure plasma cortisol before and exactly 30 min after dose. Normal response is serum cortisol increase >7 µg/dL (>193 nmol/L), or peak response increase >18 µg/dL (497 nmol/L).
Cromolyn sodium Mast cell stabilizer. Intal, Gastrocrom, NasalCrom, Crolom, ophthalmic solution. Capsule (oral): 100 mg. Inhalation: 20 mg. Metered dose inhaler: 800 µg/spray. Nebulizer solution: 10 mg/mL (2 mL). Nasal solution: 40 mg/mL. Ophthalmic solution: 4%	**Prevention of chronic symptoms of asthma, rhinitis, conjunctivitis, systemic mastocytosis, food allergy, and inflammatory bowel disease (prevents mast cell release of histamine and leukotrienes).** *Children and adults:* Asthma: 1–2 puffs (MDI) or 2 mL (nebulizer solution) 3–4 times daily. Rhinitis: 1 spray each nostril 3–4 times daily. Conjunctivitis: 1–2 drops 4–6 times daily. Mastocytosis, food allergy: *Children:* 100 mg/dose qid (max: 40 mg/kg/24 hr). *Adults:* 200 mg/dose qid (max: 400 mg/dose qid).	*Adverse events:* Hoarseness and coughing (mainly with powder for inhalation), burning and stinging at administration site.
Crotamiton Scabicidal Eurax. Cream: 10%. Lotion: 10%.	**Treatment of scabies (mechanism unknown).** *Infants, children, and adults:* Wash area thoroughly, towel dry, apply a thin layer, and massage drug into skin. Repeat application in 24 hr. Take a cleansing bath 48 hr after final application. May repeat in 7 days if needed.	*Adverse events:* Local irritation.
Cyanocobalamin, vitamin B$_{12}$ Nutritional supplement. Generic. Injection: 100, 1,000 µg/mL. Tablet: 25, 50, 100, 250, 500, 1,000 µg.	**Pernicious anemia, vitamin B$_{12}$ deficiency (coenzyme for various metabolic functions).** Pernicious anemia: *Children:* 30–50 µg/24 hr to total dose 1,000–5,000 µg, and then follow with 100 µg mo. *Adults:* 100 µg/24 hr for 6–7 days, then 100 µg/mo. Vitamin B$_{12}$ deficiency: *Children:* 100 µg/24 hr for 10–15 days then once or twice/wk for several mo. *Adults:* 30 µg/24 hr for 5–10 days then 100–200 µg/mo.	*Monitoring:* Serum B$_{12}$ levels (normal: 150–750 pg/mL). Some reports of neuropsychiatric problems have been reported with levels <300 pg/mL.
Cyclizine Antinauseant. Marezine. Injection: 50 mg/mL. Tablet: 50 mg.	**Prevent and treat motion-related nausea, vomiting, and vertigo; control postoperative nausea and vomiting (mechanism unknown).** *Children 6–12 yr:* PO: 25 mg/dose up to 3 times / 24 hr as needed. *Adults:* PO: 50 mg up to q4–6h (30 min before travel); max: 200 mg/24 hr; IM 50 mg q4–6h as needed.	*Adverse events:* Drowsiness, dry mouth, headache, diplopia, urinary retention.
Cyclopentolate Mydriatic. Cyclogyl, AK-Pentolate. Ophthalmic solution: 0.5%, 1%, 2%.	**Diagnostic procedures requiring mydriasis and cycloplegia (prevents the muscles of the ciliary body and iris from responding to cholinergic stimulation).** *Infants:* 1 drop 0.5% into each eye 5–10 min before examination. *Children and adults:* 1 drop 0.5% or 1% in eye 40–50 min before procedure (may repeat 1 drop in 5 min if necessary); may use 2% if heavily pigmented iris.	*Caution:* Avoid in narrow angle glaucoma. *Adverse events:* Tachycardia, CNS stimulation, psychosis, agitation, local burning. *Monitoring:* Cycloplegia and mydriasis begin in 15–60 min and last up to 24 hr (reduce to 3–6 hr with pilocarpine).
Cyclophosphamide Antineoplastic alkylating agent. Cytoxan; Neosar. Powder for injection: 0.1, 0.2, 0.5, 1.0, 2.0 g. Tablet: 25, 50 mg.	**Management of various cancers including Hodgkin disease, malignant lymphomas, leukemias, etc.; nephrotic syndrome; systemic lupus erythematosus (SLE); rheumatoid arthritis (RA); and rheumatoid vasculitis (interferes with normal function of DNA by alkylation).** *Children and adults with no hematologic problems:* Induction: IV: 40–50 mg/kg (1.5–1.8 g/m2) in divided doses over 2–5 days. PO: 1–5 mg/kg/24 hr. Maintenance: IV: 10–15 mg/kg (350–550 mg/m^2) q 7–10 days or 3–5 mg/kg twice/wk. PO: *Children:* 2–5 mg/kg twice/wk. *Adults:* 1–5 mg/kg/24 hr. *Children:* SLE: 500–750 mg/m^2/mo. Juvenile RA/vasculitis: IV 10 mg/kg q 2 wk. Bone marrow transplant conditioning: IV 50 mg/kg/24 hr for 3–4 days.	*Cautions:* Maintain high fluid intake to avoid hemorrhagic cystitis and consider administration of mesna. *Adverse events:* Cardiotoxicity with high doses, pericardial effusion, congestive heart failure, alopecia, nausea, vomiting, taste distortion, stomatitis, anorexia, hemorrhagic cystitis, leukopenia (onset: 7 days; nadir: 8–15 days; recovery: 21 days), thrombocytopenia, hepatotoxicity, jaundice, renal toxicity, secondary malignancy.

TABLE 712–1. General Medications *Continued*

Drug (Trade Names, Formulations)	Indications (Mechanism of Action) and Dosing	Comments (Cautions, Adverse Events, Monitoring)
	Nephrotic syndrome: PO: 2–3 mg/kg/24 hr (when steroids fail, use for up to 12 wk). Adjust doses for: Renal function: CrCl 25–50 mL/min: decrease 50% CrCl <25 mL/min: avoid use. For decreased bone marrow function: reduce dose 33–50%.	
Cyproheptadine hydrochloride Antihistamine. Generic, Periactin. Syrup: 2 mg/5 mL. Tablet: 4 mg.	**Treatment of allergic symptoms (H$_1$-receptor and serotonin antagonist).** *Children 2–6 yr:* 2 mg/dose q8–12h. *>7 yr and adults:* 4 mg/dose q8–12h (max: 0.5 mg/kg/24 hr).	*Adverse events:* Drowsiness, sedation, thickened bronchial secretions, bronchospasm, appetite stimulation, and photosensitivity.
Cysteine Nutritional supplement. Generic. Injection: 50 mg/mL.	**Supplement to crystalline amino acid solutions to meet amino acid nutritional requirements during parenteral nutrition (replace deficiency, also enhances solubility of calcium and phosphate in TPN solutions).** *Neonates and infants:* Add 40 mg cysteine to 1 g of amino acids (typically results in 20–100 mg/kg/24 hr of cysteine).	*Adverse events:* Metabolic acidosis, azotemia, elevated blood urea nitrogen, nausea.
Cytarabine HCl, Ara-C Antineoplastic, antimetabolite. Cytosar-U (powder for injection: 0.1, 0.5, 1, 2 g). Tarabine PFS. Injection: 20 mg/mL.	**Used in combination therapy to treat leukemias and lymphomas (inhibits DNA polymerase to inhibit DNA synthesis, works in S-phase of cell division).** *Children and adults:* (doses depend on individual protocols). *Typical dose:* Induction: IV 100–200 mg/m^2/24 hr for 5–10 days or until remission. Maintenance: IV 70–200 mg/m^2/24 hr for 2–5 days at monthly intervals; IM, SC: 1–1.5 mg/kg single dose at 1–4 wk intervals. IT: 5–75 mg/m^2 q 2–7 days until CNS findings normalize (concentration should not exceed 100 mg/mL).	*Adverse events:* Fever, rash, oral/anal ulcerations, nausea, vomiting, diarrhea, mucositis, liver dysfunction, bleeding, myelosuppression (onset 4–7 days, nadir 14–18 days, recovery 21–28 days), alopecia, conjunctivitis (administer corticosteroid eye drops around-the-clock before, during, and after high dose Ara-C), dizziness, headache, neuritis (prevent CNS toxicities with pyridoxine administration on days of high-dose Ara-C administration).
Dacarbazine Antineoplastic agent. DTIC-Dome, generic. Injection: 100, 200, 500 mg.	**Treatment of various tumors (alkylating agent and possibly some antimetabolite activity).** *Children:* Solid tumors: 200–470 mg/m^2/24 hr over 5 days q 21–28 days; neuroblastoma: 800–900 mg/m^2 on day 1 of combination therapy q 3–4 wk. Hodgkin disease: 375 mg/m^2 on days 1 and 15 of combination treatment; repeat q 28 days. *Adults:* Hodgkin disease: 150 mg/m^2/24 hr for 5 days; repeat q 4 wk.	*Adverse events:* Pain and burning at infusion site, nausea and vomiting, leukopenia (onset: 7 days; nadir: 10–14 days; recovery: 21–28 days), weakness, polyneuropathy, paresthesias, elevated liver enzymes, sinus congestion, alopecia, metallic taste.
Dactinomycin Antineoplastic agent. Actinomycin D, Cosmegen. Powder for injection: 0.5 mg.	**Treatment of various tumor types (binds to guanine portion of DNA blocking replication and transcription of the DNA template).** *Children >6 mo and adults:* 15 μg/kg/24 hr or 400–600 μg/m^2/24 hr for 5 days; may repeat every 3–6 wk.	*Adverse events:* Myelosuppression (onset: 7 days; nadir: 14–21 days; recovery: 21–28 days), fatigue, malaise, fever, alopecia, skin eruptions, acne, severe nausea and vomiting, diarrhea, mucositis, stomatitis, hypocalcemia, hyperuricemia.
Danaparoid Orgaran Injection: 750 anti-Xa units in 0.6 mL.	**Antithrombotic agent, acts by inhibiting anti-Xa and anti-IIa effects (anti Xa/anti-IIa activity >22). Low molecular weight heparinoid consisting mainly of heparan sulfate. Use for heparin-induced thrombocytopenia (cross-reactivity with heparin antibodies is <10%, compared with >90% for low molecular weight heparin).** *Children:* Loading dose: 30 U/kg, maintenance dose: 1.2–2.0 U/kg/hr. *Adults:* Treatment: Loading dose *<50 kg:* 1,500 U; *50–90 kg:* 2,250 U; *>90 kg:* 3,000 U. Follow loading dose with 400 U/hr for 4 hr, then 300 U/h for 4 hr, then maintenance dose 150–200 U/hr. Prophylaxis: *<50 kg:* 750 U q12 hr; *50–90 kg:* 1500 U q8h; *>90 kg:* 1,500 U q12 h.	*Monitoring:* Check plasma anti-Xa levels, target 0.5–0.8 U/mL for treatment, target 0.2–0.4 U/mL for prophylaxis. Monitoring traditional clotting studies (e.g., PT, APTT, ACT) is not beneficial as no effect is seen. *Adverse events:* Bleeding (risk is lower than with unfractionated heparin).
Dantrolene sodium Skeletal muscle relaxant. Dantrium. Capsule: 25, 50, 100 mg. Powder for injection: 20 mg.	**Treatment of spasticity associated with upper motor neuron disorders such as spinal cord injury, stroke, cerebral palsy or multiple sclerosis; also used to treat malignant hyperthermia (interferes with release of calcium ion from the sarcoplasmic reticulum).**	*Cautions:* Should not be used where spasticity is used to maintain posture or balance; avoid in patients with active liver disease. *Adverse events:* Drowsiness, fatigue, dizziness, confusion, blurred vision, seizures, diarrhea, stomach cramps, nausea, vomiting, pleural effusion with pericarditis, hepatitis.

Table continued on following page

MEDICATIONS

TABLE 712–1. General Medications *Continued*

Drug (Trade Names, Formulations)	Indications (Mechanism of Action) and Dosing	Comments (Cautions, Adverse Events, Monitoring)
	Spasticity: *Children:* 0.5 mg/kg/dose twice daily; increase frequency q 4–7 days to 3–4 times daily; then increase dose by 0.5 mg/kg to maximum of 3 mg/kg/dose 2–4 times daily. *Adults:* Start 25 mg/24 hr and increase dose by 25 mg or frequency q 4–7 days to maximum of 100 mg 2–4 times daily. Hyperthermia: *Children and adults:* Oral: 4–8 mg/kg/24 hr in 4 divided doses given 1–2 days before surgery (prophylaxis), or for 1–3 days post surgery (post-crisis follow-up). IV: 2.5 mg/kg starting 1.5 hr before surgery and run over 1 hr (prophylaxis) or 1 mg/kg/dose and repeated as needed (crisis); max: 10 mg/kg.	
Daunorubicin hydrochloride Antineoplastic. Cerubidine. Powder for injection: 20 mg.	**Treatment of acute nonlymphocytic leukemia (ANLL) and myeloblastic leukemia (inhibition of DNA and RNA synthesis).** *Children:* Remission induction for acute lymphocytic leukemia (combination therapy): 25–45 mg/m² on day 1 every wk for 4 cycles (max: total 300 mg/m²). *Adults:* 30–60 mg/m²/24 hr for 3–5 days; repeat dose in 3–4 wk; total cumulative dose should not exceed 400–600 mg/m² (lower end if prior cardiotoxic drugs or chest irradiation).	*Caution:* Avoid in patients with heart failure or arrhythmias. Irreversible cardiotoxicity may occur if total dose exposure exceeds: 550 mg/m² in adults, 400 mg/m² if chest irradiation, 300 mg/m² in children >2 yr, 10 mg/kg in children <2 yr. *Adverse events:* Alopecia, red discoloration of urine, nausea, vomiting, diarrhea, gastrointestinal ulceration, stomatitis, myelosuppression (onset, 7 days; nadir, 14 days; recovery, 21–28 days), extravasation-related tissue ulceration and necrosis, congestive heart failure, hyperuricemia, hepatotoxicity. *Monitoring:* Serum bilirubin and aspartate aminotransferase (AST) (to adjust doses for hepatic impairment): bilirubin 1.2–3 mg/dL or AST 60–180 IU: reduce dose to 75%; bilirubin 3.1–5 mg/dL or AST >180 IU: reduce dose to 50%; bilirubin >5 mg/dL: omit use.
Deferoxamine mesylate Chelating agent. Desferal. Powder for injection: 500 mg.	**Treatment of acute iron intoxication or secondary chronic iron overload (forms complex with iron to form ferrioxamine, which is removed by kidneys).** *Children:* Acute iron intoxication: IM: 90 mg/kg/dose q8h. IV: 15 mg/kg/hr (max: 6 g/24 hr). Chronic iron overload: IV: 15 mg/kg/hr (max: 12 g/24 hr). SC: 20–40 mg/kg/24 hr over 8–12 hr via portable infusion device. *Adults:* Acute iron intoxication: IM: 1 g STAT, then 0.5 g q4h (max: 6 g/24 hr). IV: 15 mg/kg/hr (max: 6 g/24 hr). Chronic iron overload: IM: 0.5–1 g/24 hr. SC: infuse 1–2 g/24 hr over 8–24 hr.	*Caution:* Contraindicated in patients with primary hemochromatosis. *Adverse events:* Local pain and induration, flushing, hypotension, tachycardia, fever, hearing loss, blurred vision, cataracts. *Monitoring:* Serum ferritin, iron, total iron binding capacity. Audiometry and eye examination with chronic use.
Desipramine hydrochloride Antidepressant, tricyclic. Norpramin, Pertofrane. Tablet: 10, 25, 50, 75, 100, 150 mg. Capsule: 25, 50 mg.	**Treatment of depression, attention deficit disorder, neuropathic pain (increases synaptic concentrations or serotonin and norepinephrine by inhibiting reuptake).** *Children 6–12 yr:* 1–3 mg/kg/24 hr (max: 5 mg/kg/24 hr). *Adolescents:* Initial 25–50 mg/24 hr, gradually increase (max: 150 mg/24 hr). *Adults:* Initial 75 mg/24 hr, gradually increase (max: 300 mg/24 hr).	*Cautions:* Abrupt discontinuation can result in withdrawal symptoms; tablets contain tartrazine (may be problem for asthmatics), contraindicated in narrow angle glaucoma. *Adverse events:* Dizziness, drowsiness, headache, blurred vision, dry mouth, constipation, increased appetite, cardiac arrhythmias, and hypotension. *Monitoring:* Desipramine concentrations: therapeutic 100–300 ng/mL, toxic >300 ng/mL; check ECG.
Desmopressin acetate Vasopressin analog. DDAVP, Stimate. Injection: 4 µg/mL. Nasal solution: 0.1 mg/mL.	**Treatment of diabetes insipidus, control of bleeding in certain types of hemophilia, primary nocturnal enuresis (enhances reabsorption of water in the kidneys, dose-dependent increase in factor VIII and plasminogen activator).** *Children:* Diabetes insipidus: *3 mo–12 yr:* PO: 0.05 mg initially then titrate to response. IV: 5 µg/24 hr in 1–2 doses. Hemophilia: *>3 mo:* IV: 0.3 µg/kg, may repeat dose if needed, use 30 min before procedure. Nocturnal enuresis: *>6 yr:* 20 µg at bedtime. *Children >12 yr and adults:* Diabetes insipidus: PO: 0.05 mg twice daily then titrate to response. IV, SC: 2–4 µg/24 hr.	*Cautions:* Avoid using in patients with type IIB or platelet-type von Willebrand disease, hemophilia A with factor VII levels <5% or hemophilia B. *Adverse events:* Facial flushing, headache, dizziness, increased blood pressure, hyponatremia, water intoxication. *Monitoring:* Serum electrolytes, plasma and urine osmolality, urine output, factor VIII antigen levels, activated partial thromboplastin time, factor VII activity level.

TABLE 712–1. General Medications *Continued*

Drug (Trade Names, Formulations)	Indications (Mechanism of Action) and Dosing	Comments (Cautions, Adverse Events, Monitoring)
Dexamethasone Adrenal corticosteroid. Decadron. Aerosol: Oral 84 µg/activation, nasal 84 µg/spray. Cream: 0.1%, 0.04%. Injection: 4, 8, 10, 16, 20, 24 mg/mL. Ophthalmic ointment: 0.05%. Ophthalmic suspension: 0.1, 0.5%. Oral solution: 0.5 mg/5 mL. Tablet: 0.25, 0.5, 0.75, 1, 1.5, 2, 4, 6 mg. Elixir: 0.5 mg/5 mL.	Intranasal: 5–40 µg/24 hr in 1–3 doses. Hemophilia: IV: 0.3 µg/kg. Intranasal: <50 kg = 150 µg, >50 kg = 300 µg. Enuresis: PO: 0.2–0.4 mg at bedtime. **Systemically and locally for acute and chronic inflammation; allergic, neoplastic and autoimmune diseases; cerebral edema, septic shock, *Haemophilus influenzae* meningitis, diagnostic agent (decreases inflammation and suppresse normal immune response).** *Neonates:* Airway edema or extubation: IV: 0.25 mg/kg every 12 hr for 3–4 doses (start >4 hr before scheduled extubation). Bronchopulmonary dysplasia: IV, PO: 0.25 mg/kg/dose q12h for 6 doses then taper over 1 to 6 wk (regimens may begin as early as day 1). *Children:* Airway edema or extubation: PO, IM, IV: 0.5–2 mg/kg/24 hr divided q6h (begin 24 hr before extubation and continue for 4–6 doses post extubation). Antiemetic (chemotherapy-induced): IV: 10 mg/m² first dose then 5 mg/m²/dose q6h as needed (start before chemotherapy). Anti-inflammatory: PO, IM, IV: 0.08–0.3 mg/kg/24 hr divided q6–12h. Bacterial meningitis: IV: 0.6 mg/kg/24 hr divided q6h for days 1–4 of antibiotics. Cerebral edema: PO, IM, IV: loading dose 1–2 mg/kg, then 1–1.5 mg/kg/24 hr divided q4–6h. taper over 1 to 6 wk Inhalation: 2 puffs 3–4 times daily. Nasal spray: 1–2 sprays in each nostril twice daily. Physiologic replacement: PO, IM, IV: 0.03–0.15 mg/kg/24 hr divided q6–12h. *Adults:* Anti-inflammatory: PO, IM, IV: 0.5–9 mg/24 hr divided q6–12h. Antiemetic: Same as for children. Cerebral edema: IV: 10 mg STAT, then 4 mg q6h. Diagnosis of Cushing syndrome: 1 mg at 11 P.M., draw plasma cortisol at 8 A.M. the following day. Shock: IV: 1–6 mg/kg (max: 40 mg) and may repeat q2–6h. *Children and adults:* Ophthalmic: Ointment: apply q3–4h to conjunctival sac as thin coating; suspension: instill 2 drops into conjunctival sac every hr during day and every other hr at night. Gradually taper doses when inflammation resolves. Topical: Apply 1–4 times daily.	*Caution:* Dexamethasone use for neonates with bronchopulmonary dysplasia has been associated with increased incidence of cerebral palsy, and this risk should be weighed against potential benefits. *Adverse events:* Insomnia, nervousness, increased appetite, hypertension, hyperglycemia, gastrointestinal hyperacidity (stress ulcer risk), cataracts, adrenal suppression, poor growth. *Comment:* See comparison of corticosteroids under *Hydrocortisone.*
Dextran Plasma volume expander. Dextran 40 (low molecular weight): Gentran; LMD. Dextran 70 (high molecular weight): Gentran; Macro Dex.	**Blood volume expander in shock or impending shock (similar to albumin).** *Children:* Max: 20 mL/kg on day 1, then 10 mL/kg/24 hr for not more than 5 days. *Adults:* 500–1,000 mL at a rate of 20–40 mL/min (max: 10 mL/kg/24 hr for 5 days).	*Adverse events:* (Primarily associated with excessive doses)—pulmonary edema, bleeding due to impaired platelet function.
Dextroamphetamine CNS stimulant. Generic, Dexedrine, Adderall. Tablet: 5, 10 mg. Sustained-release capsule: 5, 10, 15 mg.	**Treatment of attention deficit disorder, narcolepsy, and exogenous obesity (blocks reuptake of dopamine and norepinephrine from the synapse).** *Children 6–12 yr:* Narcolepsy and attention deficit disorder: Initial 5 mg/24 hr, may increase by 5 mg/24 hr at weekly intervals to response (max: 60 mg/24 hr). *>12 yr and adults:* Initial 20 mg/24 hr, may increase at 10-mg increments weekly (max: 60 mg/24 hr).	*Caution:* Avoid concurrent use of monoamine oxidase inhibitors. *Adverse events:* Hypertension, tachycardia, palpitations, arrhythmias, insomnia, agitation, irritability, nervousness, headache, depression, tremor, exacerbation of tics and movement disorders, mydriasis, physical and psychological dependence, anorexia, nausea, diarrhea, abdominal cramps, growth suppression. *Monitoring:* Blood pressure, growth, CNS activity.
Dextromethorphan Antitussive. Robitussin, generics. Liquid: 7.5 mg/5 mL. Lozenge: 5 mg.	**Symptomatic relief of coughs, best when cough is nonproductive (depresses the medullary cough center).** *Children 2–6 yr:* 2.5–7.5 mg q4–8h or extended-release 15 mg q12h (max: 30 mg/24 hr).	*Adverse events:* (Mainly with overdose)—drowsiness, dizziness, respiratory depression, blurred vision, nausea, gastrointestinal upset, constipation.

Table continued on following page

MEDICATIONS

TABLE 712–1. **General Medications** Continued

Drug (Trade Names, Formulations)	Indications (Mechanism of Action) and Dosing	Comments (Cautions, Adverse Events, Monitoring)
	6–12 yr: 10–15 mg q4–8h or extended-release 30 mg twice daily (max: 60 mg/24 hr). *>12 yr and adults:* 10–30 mg q4–8h or extended-release 60 mg twice daily (max: 120 mg/24 hr).	
Diazepam Benzodiazepine. Generic, Valium. Tablet: 2, 5, 10 mg. Oral solution: 5 mg/mL. Injection: 5 mg/mL.	**Treatment of anxiety, panic disorders, status epilepticus, alcohol withdrawal; provide sedation; skeletal muscle relaxant (thought to increase neuroinhibitory action of γ-aminobutyric acid).** *Infants and children:* Status epilepticus: IV: 0.05–0.3 mg/kg/dose given over 2–3 min; may repeat q 30 min to maximal total dose of 5–10 mg. Rectal: 0.5 mg/kg, then 0.25 mg/kg in 10 min if needed. Sedation: PO: 0.2–0.3 mg/kg (max: 10 mg); IM, IV: 0.04–0.3 mg/kg (max: 0.6 mg/kg/8 hr). *Adults:* Status epilepticus: IV: 5–10 mg q 30 min (max: 30 mg/8 hr). Anxiety, sedation, muscle relaxant: PO, IM, IV: 2–10 mg 2–4 times daily.	*Adverse events:* Hypotension, bradycardia, cardiac arrest (with IV dose), drowsiness, ataxia, fatigue, confusion, impaired coordination, paradoxical excitement, amnesia, blurred vision, diplopia, sweating, dry mouth, constipation or diarrhea, increased or decreased appetite, hiccups, physical and psychological dependence. *Monitoring:* Desired clinical endpoints and toxic endpoints should be monitored; doses to achieve effects vary considerably between patients.
Diazoxide Antihypertensive. Hyperstat, injection: 15 mg/mL. Proglycem, oral suspension: 50 mg/mL. Capsule: 50 mg.	**Emergency lowering of blood pressure, treatment of hyperinsulinemic hypoglycemia related to islet cell tumors or nesidioblastosis (smooth muscle relaxation, inhibit insulin release from the pancreas).** Hypertension: *Children and adults:* 1–3 mg/kg; may repeat in 5–15 min, dose every 4–24 hr. Hyperinsulinemic hypoglycemia: *Newborns and infants:* PO: 8–15 mg/kg/24 hr divided q8–12h (start on low end). *Children and adults:* PO: 3–8 mg/kg/24 hr divided q8–12h (start on low end).	*Adverse events:* Hypotension, dizziness, weakness, nausea, vomiting.
Dibucaine Local anesthetic. Nupercainal. Cream: 0.5%. Ointment: 1%.	**Temporary relief of pain and itching due to hemorrhoids and minor skin irritation or damage (block initiation and conduction of nerve impulses).** *Children and adults:* Topical: Apply gently to affected area (children 7.5 g/24 hr, adults 30 g/24 hr). Rectal: Insert with rectal applicator morning, evening, and after each bowel movement.	*Adverse events:* Local irritation, contact dermatitis.
Diclofenac sodium Nonsteroidal anti-inflammatory agent. Cataflam, tablets: 50 mg. Voltaren, tablets: 25, 50, 75 mg. Ophthalmic solution: 0.1%.	**Treatment of mild to moderate acute or chronic pain; postoperative inflammation after cataract extraction (inhibit prostaglandin synthesis).** PO: *Children:* 2–3 mg/kg/24 hr in 2–4 divided doses. *Adults:* 100–200 mg/24 hr in 2–4 divided doses. Ophthalmic: 1 drop in affected eye qid for 2 wk, to begin 24 hr after cataract surgery.	*Adverse events:* Dizziness, headache, fluid retention, indigestion, abdominal pain, peptic ulcer, gastrointestinal bleeding, renal impairment.
Dicyclomine Anticholinergic agent. Antispas, Bentyl, generic. Capsule: 10, 20 mg. Tablet: 20 mg. Syrup: 10 mg/5 mL. Injection: 10 mg/mL.	**Treatment of functional disturbances of gastrointestinal motility, e.g., irritable bowel syndrome (block the actions of acetylcholine).** *Infants >6 mo:* PO: 5 mg/dose tid–qid. *Children:* 10 mg tid–qid. *Adults:* 40 mg qid (start at ½ dose and gradually increase; IM: Use 20 mg qid). *Cautions:* Avoid in narrow angle glaucoma, gastrointestinal obstruction, urinary tract obstruction, and myasthenia gravis.	*Adverse events:* Tachycardia, palpitations, nervousness, irritability, confusion, muscle hypotonia, blurred vision, photophobia, urinary retention, nausea, vomiting, constipation, dry mouth, urticaria, pruritus.
Digoxin Cardiac glycoside. Lanoxin, generic. Capsule: 50, 100, 200 µg. Elixir: 50 µg/mL. Tablet: 125, 250, 500 µg. Injection: 100, 250 µg/mL.	**Treatment of systolic heart failure and supraventricular tachyarrhythmias (increase intracellular calcium through inhibition of sodium/potassium ATPase pump; suppression of AV node conduction).** *Neonate:* 10–30 µg/kg IV load, then 5–10 µg/kg/24 hr maintenance dose. *1 mo–2 yr:* 30 µg/kg load, then 10–15 µg/kg/24 hr maintenance dose. *2–10 yr:* 30 µg/kg load, then 5–10 µg/kg/24 hr maintenance dose. *Child >10 yr:* 10 µg/kg load, then 2–5 µg/kg/24 hr maintenance dose. *Adult:* 10–15 µg/kg load, then 0.1 to 0.5 mg/24 hr maintenance dose. Adjust doses for reduced renal function: CrCl 10–50 mL/min: reduce dose to 25–75%;	*Cautions:* Contraindicated in AV block, idiopathic hypertrophic subaortic stenosis, or constrictive pericarditis. *Adverse events:* Anorexia, nausea, vomiting, diarrhea, feeding intolerance, bradycardia, arrhythmias, lethargy, depression, vertigo, blurred vision, diplopia, photophobia, yellow or green vision. *Monitoring:* Efficacy and toxicity are closely related to serum concentrations and dosing should be guided by measuring serum digoxin concentrations: therapeutic: 0.8–2 ng/mL; toxic: >2–2.5 ng/mL. Digoxin-like immune substances (DLIS) may falsely elevate digoxin levels in neonates and children, so pretreatment digoxin levels can be obtained and subtracted from treatment levels or samples can be run through a free-level filter to remove DLIS before assay. Check post-distribution levels (drawn at least 6–8 hr post dose) at steady-state (2–4 wk) or if ECG or clinical signs of toxicity. Check ECG, serum electrolytes, calcium, and

TABLE 712–1. General Medications *Continued*

Drug (Trade Names, Formulations)	Indications (Mechanism of Action) and Dosing	Comments (Cautions, Adverse Events, Monitoring)
	CrCl <10 mL/min: reduce dose to 10–25% of normal.	magnesium. Check heart rate.
Digoxin Immune Fab Digoxin antidote. Digibind. Powder for injection: 38 mg.	**Treatment of digitalis intoxication from digoxin or digitoxin (binds with molecules of unbound digoxin or digitoxin and is renally cleared).** *Infants, children, and adults:* Dose is based on amount of digoxin or digitoxin ingested or estimated total body load (TBL) based on post-distributive serum concentration: TBL Digoxin = concentration (ng/mL) $\times$ 5.6 $\times$ weight (kg)/1,000. TBL Digoxin = mg ingested $\times$ 0.8. TBL Digitoxin = concentration (ng/mL) $\times$ 0.56 $\times$ wt (kg)/1,000. TBL Digitoxin = mg ingested. Dose Digoxin Immune Fab (mg) = TBL Digoxin $\times$ 76. Dose Digoxin Immune Fab (# vials) = TBL/0.5.	*Adverse events:* Worsening of heart failure or atrial fibrillation, hypokalemia, facial swelling, and redness. *Monitoring:* ECG, digoxin serum concentrations will greatly increase with digoxin immune Fab and do not reflect body stores or correlate with clinical toxicity.
Dihydrotachysterol Vitamin D analog. Hytakerol, generic. Capsule: 0.125 mg. Tablet: 0.125 mg. Solution: 0.2 mg/mL, 0.2 mg/5 mL.	**Treatment of hypocalcemia associated with hypoparathyroidism and renal osteodystrophy (stimulates calcium and phosphate intestinal absorption).** *Neonates:* 0.05–0.1 mg/24 hr. *Infants and young children:* 1–5 mg/24 hr for 4 days then 0.5–1.5 mg/24 hr. *Older children and adults:* 0.75–2.5 mg/24 hr for 4 days, then 0.2–1 mg/24 hr (max: 1.5 mg/24 hr). Renal osteodystrophy: 0.1–0.6 mg/24 hr.	*Adverse events:* Hypercalcemia, hypercalciuria, elevated serum creatinine.
Diltiazem Calcium channel blocker. Cardizem, Dilacor. Tablet: 30, 60, 90, 120 mg. Capsule (sustained-release): 60, 90, 120, 180, 240, 300 mg. Injection: 5 mg/mL.	**Treatment of hypertension and atrial tachyarrhythmias (inhibit calcium ions from entering the "slow channels" during depolarization).** *Children:* PO: 1.5–2 mg/kg/24 hr in 3–4 divided doses. *Adolescents and adults:* PO: 90–480 mg/24 hr in 3–4 divided doses as tablets or 1–2 doses as sustained-release capsules. IV: 0.25 mg/kg load, then 5–15 mg/hr continuous infusion.	*Cautions:* Diltiazem is a hepatic enzyme inhibitor and may cause accumulation and toxicity for concurrently used drugs which are metabolized. *Adverse events:* Hypotension, bradycardia, edema, AV block, dizziness, nausea, vomiting.
Dimenhydrinate Antihistamine. Dramamine, generic. Capsule: 50 mg Injection: 50 mg/mL. Tablet: 50 mg. Liquid: 12.5 mg/4 mL.	**Treatment of nausea, vomiting, and vertigo associated with motion sickness (competes with histamine for H₁-receptor).** *Children:* *2–5 yr:* 12.5–25 mg q6–8h (max: 75 mg/24 hr). *6–12 yr:* 25–50 mg q6–8h (max: 150 mg/24 hr). *Adults:* 50–100 mg q4–6h (max: 400 mg/24 hr).	*Adverse events:* Drowsiness, dizziness, hypotension, tachycardia.
Dimercaprol BAL. Injection: 100 mg/mL.	**Antidote to gold, arsenic, and mercury poisoning and adjunct to edetate calcium disodium in lead poisoning (chelates with heavy metals to form nontoxic stable compounds).** *Children and adults:* Mild arsenic and gold poisoning: 2.5 mg/kg/dose IM q6h for 2 days, then q12h on day 3, then q24h for 10 days. Severe arsenic or gold poisoning: 3 mg/kg/dose q4h for 2 days, then q6h on day 3, then q12h for 10 days. Mercury poisoning: 5 mg/kg load, then 2.5 mg/kg/dose 1–2 times/day for 10 days. Lead poisoning: Mild: 4 mg/kg load, then 3 mg/kg/dose q4h for 2–7 days. Severe: 4 mg/kg/dose q4h for 2–7 days.	*Adverse events:* Hypertension, tachycardia, convulsions, nausea, vomiting, fever, headache, nervousness, blepharospasm, nephrotoxicity. *Monitoring:* Specific heavy metal levels, urine pH should be kept alkaline
Diphenhydramine Benadryl, generic. Capsule or tablet: 25, 50 mg. Injection: 10 mg/mL, 50 mg/mL. Syrup or elixir: 12.5 mg/5 mL. Cream or lotion: 1%.	**Antihistamine (competitive inhibitor of H₁-receptor).** *Children:* 5 mg/kg/24 hr divided q6h as needed IM, IV, PO (max: 300 mg/24 hr). *Adults:* 10–50 mg/dose q4h as needed (max: 400 mg/24 hr). *Topical:* Apply 3–4 times daily.	*Adverse events:* Hypotension, tachycardia, drowsiness, paradoxical excitement, thickened bronchial secretions, dry mouth.
Diphenoxylate and Atropine Lomotil. Tablet, oral solution.	**Antidiarrheal (diphenoxylate inhibits excessive gastrointestinal motility, atropine is to prevent abuse).** *Children:* *2–5 yr:* 4 mL (2 mg diphenoxylate) tid. *5–8 yr:* 4 mL qid. *8–12 yr:* 4 mL 5 times daily. *Adults:* 15–20 mg/24 hr in 3–4 divided doses.	*Adverse events:* Nervousness, dizziness, drowsiness, headache, dry mouth, urinary retention, blurred vision, paralytic ileus.

Table continued on following page

TABLE 712–1. **General Medications** *Continued*

Drug (Trade Names, Formulations)	Indications (Mechanism of Action) and Dosing	Comments (Cautions, Adverse Events, Monitoring)
Disopyramide Norpace. Capsule: 100, 150 mg.	**Treatment of ventricular arrhythmias and atrial tachyarrhythmias (antiarrhythmic class 1a, decreases myocardial excitability and conduction velocity).** *Children:* *<1 yr:* 10–30 mg/kg/24 hr divided q6h. *1–4 yr:* 10–20 mg/kg/24 hr divided q6h. *4–12 yr:* 10–15 mg/kg/24 hr divided q6h. *12–18 yr:* 6–15 mg/kg/24 hr divided q6h. *Adults:* 100–200 mg q6h.	*Cautions:* Avoid in 2nd- or 3rd-degree AV block; will worsen heart failure, urinary retention, glaucoma, and some arrhythmias. *Adverse events:* Urinary retention/hesitancy, dry mouth, fatigue, malaise, constipation, cholestasis, elevated liver enzymes. *Monitoring:* Creatinine clearance (decrease dose to q8h if 30–40 mL/min, q12h if 15–30 mL/min, q24h if <15 mL/min). ECG, blood pressure, signs of heart failure. Blood levels (therapeutic range: atrial arrhythmias 2.8–3.2 µg/mL, ventricular arrhythmias 3.3–7.5 µg/mL).
Dobutamine Dobutrex. Injection.	**Treatment of hypotension (stimulates β_1-adrenergic receptors).** *Neonates:* 2–20 µg/kg/min. *Children and adults:* 2.5–40 µg/kg/min constant infusion.	*Cautions:* Avoid in patients with IHSS, atrial fibrillation or flutter, or sulfite sensitivity. *Adverse events:* Tachycardia, ectopic heartbeats, angina, palpitations, tachyarrhythmias, tingling sensation, paresthesias, and leg cramps.
Docusate Colace, Surfak, generic. Capsule, liquid, syrup (may be combined with casanthrol).	**Stool softener, laxative (reduces surface tension of oil-water interface of stool).** *<3 yr:* 10–40 mg/24 hr in 1–4 doses. *3–6 yr:* 20–60 mg/24 hr in 1–4 doses. *6–12 yr:* 40–150 mg/24 hr. *> 12 yr and adults:* 50–400 mg/24 hr.	*Adverse events:* Diarrhea, abdominal cramping.
Dolasetron mesylate Anzemet. Tablet: 50, 100 mg. Injection.	**Prevention and treatment of chemotherapy and postoperative nausea and vomiting (5-HT$_3$ receptor antagonist).** *Children >2 yr and adults:* IV, PO: 1.8 mg/kg (max: 100 mg) as single dose 30 min before chemotherapy; 0.35 mg/kg (max: 12.5 mg) given 15 min before stopping anesthesia for postoperative nausea.	*Adverse events:* Hypotension, headache, tachycardia, dizziness.
Dopamine Intropin. Injection.	**Treatment of hypotension and shock (stimulates dopaminergic receptors and adrenergic receptors).** *Neonates, children, and adults:* 1–20 µg/kg/min IV infusion rate (mL/hr) = 6 × weight (kg) × desired dose (µg/kg/min)/mg drug per 100 mL IV fluid.	*Cautions:* Contains sulfites. *Adverse events:* Tachycardia, ectopic beats, ventricular arrhythmias, tissue necrosis with extravasation, vasoconstriction, gangrene of extremities, excess urine output (doses <5 µg/kg/min), oliguria (doses >10 µg/kg/min).
Dornase alpha Pulmozyme. Inhalation solution: 1 mg/mL.	**Management of cystic fibrosis to improve pulmonary function (DNA enzyme which reduces viscosity of mucus).** *Neonates, children, and adults:* 2.5 mL 1–2 times daily, nebulized with Pulmo-Aide or Pari-Proneb compressor.	*Adverse events:* Pharyngitis, voice alteration, cough, rhinitis, hemoptysis.
Doxacurium Nuromax. Injection: 1 mg/mL.	**Skeletal muscle paralysis (neuromuscular blockade by competing with acetylcholine for neuromuscular receptor).** *Children 2–12 yr:* Initial 30–50 µg/kg, then 5–10 µg/kg/dose every 1–2 hr. *Adults:* Initial 50 µg/kg, then 5–10 µg/kg/dose every 1–2 hr.	*Adverse events:* Skeletal muscle weakness, hypotension. *Monitoring:* Peripheral nerve stimulator.
Doxapram Dopram. Injection: 20 mg/mL.	**Treatment of apnea of prematurity refractory to methylxanthines (respiratory and CNS stimulant).** *Neonates:* Initial 2.5–3 mg/kg followed by infusion of 1 mg/kg/hr (max: 2.5 mg/kg/hr). *Caution:* Contains benzyl alcohol (recommended doses deliver 5.4–27 mg/kg/24 hr).	*Adverse events:* Hypertension, tachycardia, arrhythmias, CNS stimulation, irritability, seizures, hyperpyrexia, vomiting, increased gastric residuals, hyperglycemia.
Doxepin Adapin, Sinequan. Tricyclic antidepressant. Capsule: 10, 25, 50, 75, 100, 150 mg. Oral concentrate: 10 mg/mL. Cream: 5%.	**Treatment of depression, analgesic for neuropathic pain (increase synaptic concentrations of serotonin and norepinephrine).** *Children:* 1–3 mg/kg/24 hr. *Adolescent:* 25–50 mg/24 hr to start, max: 100 mg/24 hr. *Adults:* 30–150 mg/24 hr to start, max: 300 mg/24 hr (single dose max: 150 mg).	*Caution:* Contraindicated for narrow-angle glaucoma. *Adverse events:* Sedation, drowsiness, dizziness, headache, dry mouth, constipation, increased appetite, weight gain, urinary retention, difficult urination, blurred vision, hypotension, arrhythmias. *Monitoring:* ECG, doxepin concentrations: therapeutic 30–150 ng/mL, toxic >500 ng/mL.
Doxorubicin hydrochloride Adriamycin, Rubex. Injection: 2 mg/mL. Powder for injection.	**Antineoplastic used for various tumor types (inhibit DNA and RNA synthesis).** *Children:* 35–75 mg/m^2/dose repeat every 21 days; or 20–30 mg/m^2 repeat every wk; or 60–90 mg/m^2 given as continuous infusion over 96 hr q 3–4 wk. *Adults:* 60–75 mg/m^2/dose every 21 days. *Liver disease:* reduce dose: bilirubin 1.2–3 (reduce by 50%), bilirubin >3 (reduce by 75%).	*Caution:* Contraindicated if patient has congestive heart failure, cardiomyopathy, received a total dose of 550 mg/m^2 (400 mg/m^2 if prior or concurrent daunorubicin, idarubicin, mitoxantrone, cyclophosphamide, irradiation to cardiac area). *Adverse events:* Cardiotoxicity, alopecia, hyperpigmentation of nail bed, hyperuricemia, stomatitis, esophagitis, mucositis, nausea, vomiting, thrombocytopenia (onset, 7 days; nadir, 10–14 days; recovery, 21–28 days), lacrimation, extravasation tissue necrosis, phlebitis.
Dronabinol, tetrahydrocannabinol Marinol. Capsule: 2.5, 5, 10 mg.	**Antiemetic for cancer chemotherapy (inhibits the vomiting center).** *Children and adults:* 5 mg/m^2/dose q2–4h starting 1–3 hr before chemotherapy (max: 15 mg/m^2/dose).	*Adverse events:* Drowsiness, difficulty concentrating, mood change, hallucinations. *Monitoring:* Monitor for abuse.

TABLE 712–1.   General Medications *Continued*

Drug (Trade Names, Formulations)	Indications (Mechanism of Action) and Dosing	Comments (Cautions, Adverse Events, Monitoring)
Droperidol Inapsine. Injection: 2.5 mg/mL.	**Antiemetic, antipsychotic (alters the action of dopamine in the CNS and has α-adrenergic blockade).** *Children 2–12 yr:* IV, IM: 0.05–0.06 mg/kg/dose q4–6h as needed for nausea. *Adults:* IV, IM: 2.5–5 mg/dose q3–4h as needed.	*Adverse events:* Hypotension, tachycardia, extrapyramidal reactions, confusion, memory loss.
D-Xylose Xylo-pfan. Powder for oral solution.	**Diagnostic agent used to evaluate intestinal disorders due to disease or injury (mechanism not understood).** *Children:* 500 mg/kg as 5–10% solution; max: 25 g. *Adults:* 5–25 g as 10% solution followed by 200–400 mL of water.	*Adverse events:* Nausea, vomiting, cramping, intestinal bloating. *Monitoring:* Blood and urinary D-Xylose concentrations.
Edetate calcium disodium Calcium Disodium Versenate. Injection: 200 mg/mL.	**Antidote for acute and chronic lead poisoning (chelating agent).** *Children and adults:* 500 mg/m²/dose once daily.	*Cautions:* Contraindicated in severe renal failure and patients with active tuberculosis or healed calcified tubercular lesions. *Adverse events:* Arrhythmias, hypotension, seizures, headache, chills, skin eruptions, hypomagnesemia, hypokalemia, hypocalcemia, hyperuricemia, vomiting, diarrhea, abdominal cramps, back pain, muscle cramps, paresthesia, tetany, nephrotoxicity, respiratory arrest. *Monitoring:* 24-hr urine collection after first dose for ratio lead excretion/mg calcium EDTA (positive test >0.5–0.6); blood lead level.
Edetate disodium Chealamide, Disotate, generic. Injection: 150 mg/mL.	**Emergency treatment of hypercalcemia and digitalis-induced ventricular dysrhythmias (chelating agent).** *Children:* 40–70 mg/kg/24 hr slow infusion over 3–4 hr; administer for 5 days then 5 days off drug. *Adults:* 50 mg/kg/dose for 5 days, then 2 days off, then restart for total of 15 doses. *Digitalis arrhythmias (children and adults):* 15 mg/kg/hr continuous infusion (max: 60 mg/kg/24 hr).	*Cautions:* Contraindicated in severe renal failure and tuberculosis. *Adverse events:* Arrhythmias, hypotension, seizures, headache, chills, hypokalemia, hypocalcemia, hypomagnesemia, hyperuricemia, vomiting, diarrhea, abdominal cramps, dysuria, back pain, nephrotoxicity.
Edrophonium chloride Reversol, Tensilon, Enlon. Injection: 10 mg/mL.	**Diagnosis of myasthenia gravis, differentiation of cholinergic crisis from myasthenia crisis, reversal of nondepolarizing neuromuscular blockers, treatment of paroxysmal atrial tachycardia (inhibits destruction of acetylcholine by acetylcholinesterase).** *Infants:* IM: 0.5–1 mg; IV: 0.1 mg followed by 0.4 mg (if no response). *Children:* diagnosis (initial): IM: <34 kg: 1 mg; >34 kg: 5 mg IV: 0.04 mg/kg over 1 min followed by 0.16 mg/kg given within 45 sec (if no response); max:: 10 mg total. Titration of oral anticholinesterase therapy: IV 0.04 mg/kg given 1 hr after oral intake of treatment drug; if strength improves increase dose of neostigmine or pyridostigmine. *Adults:* Diagnosis: IM: Initial 10 mg; if cholinergic reaction occurs, give 2 mg in 30 min to rule out false-negative reaction. IV: 2 mg given over 15 sec, 8 mg given 45 sec later (if no response). Titration of oral anticholinesterase therapy: IV 1–2 mg given 1 hr after an oral dose. Increase oral dose if strength improves.	*Adverse events:* Arrhythmias, hypotension, nausea, vomiting, diarrhea, stomach cramps, excess sweating, urinary frequency, lacrimation, diplopia, miosis, laryngospasm, bronchospasm, respiratory paralysis.
Enalapril/Enalaprilat Vasotec. Oral (enalapril): 2.5, 5, 10, 20 mg. Injection (enalaprilat): 1.25 mg/mL. Extemporaneous formulations are available.	**Treatment of hypertension and congestive heart failure (angiotensin-converting enzyme inhibition).** *Neonate:* PO: 0.1 mg/kg/24 hr in 1–2 doses (may increase to 0.4 mg/kg/24 hr for congestive heart failure or adequate hypertension response). IV: 5–10 μg/kg/dose every 8–24 hr. *Infants and children:* PO: 0.1–0.5 mg/kg/24 hr in 1–2 doses. IV: 5–10 μg/kg/dose q8–24h. *Adolescent and adults:* PO: 2.5–5 mg/24 hr and titrate to max 40 mg/24 hr in 2 doses. IV: 0.625–1.25 mg/dose q6h (max: 20 mg/24 hr). *Caution:* Avoid or adjust dose in patients with renal impairment (CrCl 10–50 mL/min, give 75% of dose; CrCl <10 mL/min, give 50% of dose).	*Adverse events:* Hypotension, tachycardia, syncope, fatigue, dizziness, headache, cough, hyperkalemia, hypoglycemia. *Comments:* Lower doses if concurrent diuretics or reduced renal function, concurrent indomethacin may blunt response.

Table continued on following page

TABLE 712–1. General Medications *Continued*

Drug (Trade Names, Formulations)	Indications (Mechanism of Action) and Dosing	Comments (Cautions, Adverse Events, Monitoring)
Enoxaparin sodium Lovenox. Injection: 30 mg/0.3 mL.	**Prophylaxis and treatment of venous thromboembolism (low molecular weight heparin with activity against factor Xa and IIa).** *Neonates and children:* SC: 1 mg/kg q8–12h. *Adults:* SC: 30 mg twice daily or 1 mg/kg twice daily (depends on indication).	*Adverse events:* Thrombocytopenia and hemorrhage (less than unfractionated heparin). *Monitoring:* Dose to heparin plasma level (anti-factor Xa assay) mid-interval 0.5–1.0 U/mL, or trough 0.3–0.7 U/mL
Epinephrine Adrenalin. Injection: 0.01 mg/mL, 0.1 mg/mL, 1 mg/mL. Suspension: 5 mg/mL. Aerosol MDI, inhalation solution, ophthalmic solution, topical solution.	**Treatment of cardiac arrest, bronchospasm, anaphylactic reactions, open-angle glaucoma (stimulates α, β_1, and β_2 receptors).** *Neonates:* IV, intratracheal: 0.01–0.03 mg/kg (0.1–0.3 mL/kg of 1:10,000 solution) q 3–5 min. *Infants and children:* SC: 0.01 mg/kg (0.01 mL/kg/dose of 1:1,000 solution, or 0.005 mL/kg/dose of suspension). IV: 0.01 mg/kg (0.1 mL/kg of 1:10,000 solution) (max: 1 mg). IT: 0.1 mg/kg/dose (0.1 mL/kg of 1:1,000 solution) (max: 0.2 mL/kg). Continuous infusion: 0.1–1 µg/kg/min per response. Nebulization: 0.25–0.5 mL of 2.25% racemic epinephrine diluted in 3 mL normal saline. Ophthalmic: instill 1–2 drops in eye(s) 1–2 times daily. *Adults:* IV: 1–5 mg q 3–5 min. IT: 1 mg initial; max: 12.5 mg/dose. IM, SC: 0.1–0.5 mg q 10–15 min. Continuous infusion: 1–10 µg/min. Ophthalmic: Instill 1–2 drops in eye(s) 1–2 times daily.	*Adverse events:* Tachycardia, hypertension, nervousness, restlessness, irritability, headache, tremor, weakness, nausea, vomiting, acute urinary retention.
Epoetin alfa, erythropoietin, EPO Epogen, Procrit. Injection: Preservative-free vial 2,000, 3,000, 4,000, 10,000 U/mL. Preserved 10,000 U/mL.	**Anemia associated with prematurity, end-stage renal disease, zidovudine-treated HIV-infected patients, cancer patients receiving chemotherapy (induces erythropoiesis).** Administer IV, SC. *Neonates:* 100–500 units/kg/dose q 1–2 days for 10–21 days. *Children and adults:* Cancer patients: 150 units/kg/dose 3 times/wk (may increase to 300 units/kg/dose). Hemodialysis patients: 50–100 units 3 times/wk. Zidovudine-treated patients: 100 units/kg/dose 3 times/wk.	*Caution:* Uncontrolled hypertension, neutropenia in newborns must have adequate iron stores and may require oral or intravenous iron supplement. *Adverse events:* Hypertension, edema, headache, fever, rash, arthralgias, hypersensitivity. *Monitoring:* Serum iron, reticulocyte count, hematocrit (reduce dose or stop EPO if hematocrit above 40), blood pressure.
Ergocalciferol Calciferol, Drisdol, generic. Tablet, capsule: 50,000 units. Liquid: 8,000 units/mL. Injection: 500,000 units/mL (1 µg = 40 units).	**Treatment of refractory rickets, hypophosphatemia, hypoparathyroidism (vitamin D analog stimulates calcium and phosphate absorption).** *Premature infants:* 10–20 µg/24 hr. Renal failure: *Children:* 100–1,000 µg/24 hr. *Adults:* 500 µg/24 hr. Hypoparathyroidism: *Children:* 1.25–5 mg/24 hr. *Adults:* 0.625–5 mg/24 hr. Rickets: *Children:* 75–125 µg/24 hr. *Adults:* 0.25–1.5 mg/24 hr.	*Adverse events:* Hypercalcemia, weakness, lethargy, hypertension, arrhythmias, mild acidosis, hypercholesterolemia, nausea, vomiting, constipation, nephrocalcinosis, photophobia. *Monitoring:* Serum calcium and phosphorus, alkaline phosphatase, bone radiography.
Ergotamine Cafatine, Cafergot. Tablet: 1 mg/2 mg. Aerosol: 9 mg/mL. Suppository: 2 mg.	**Prevent or abort vascular headaches, e.g., migraine or cluster headache (ergot alkaloid α-adrenergic blocker).** *Older children and adolescents:* 1 mg SL or PO at onset of attack and q30 min to relief (max: 3 mg per attack). *Adults:* 1–2 mg SL or PO, may repeat q30 min to maximum of 6 mg (maximal dose/wk: 10 mg).	*Caution:* Reduce dose by 50% if patient is taking chronic methysergide. *Adverse events:* Tachypnea, vasospasm, nausea, vomiting, diarrhea, leg cramps, muscle weakness, paresthesias.
Esmolol Brevibloc. Injection: 10 mg/mL.	**Antiarrhythmic, antihypertensive (β-blocker, class II antiarrhythmic).** *Children:* 100–500 µg/kg over 1 min then continuous infusion 200–1,000 µg/kg/min. *Adults:* 500 µg/kg over 1 min then 50–200 µg/kg/min.	*Caution:* Contraindicated in sinus bradycardia, heart block, uncompensated heart failure. *Adverse events:* Hypotension, bradycardia, Raynaud phenomenon, dizziness, confusion, lethargy, bronchoconstriction
Ethacrynic acid Edecrin. Tablet: 25, 50 mg. Injection.	**Diuretic (act at ascending loop of Henle).** *Children:* PO: 1–3 mg/kg/24 hr. IV: 0.5–1 mg/kg/dose q8–24h. *Adults:* PO: 25–400 mg/24 hr. IV: 0.5–1 mg/kg/dose q8–24h.	*Adverse events:* Hypotension, fluid and electrolyte depletion, hyperuricemia, ototoxicity, tinnitus.

TABLE 712–1. General Medications *Continued*

Drug (Trade Names, Formulations)	Indications (Mechanism of Action) and Dosing	Comments (Cautions, Adverse Events, Monitoring)
Ethosuximide Zarontin. Capsule: 250 mg. Syrup: 250 mg/5 mL.	**Anticonvulsant for treatment of absence, myoclonic, and akinetic epilepsy (increased seizure threshold).** *Children:* *<6 yr:* Start 15 mg/kg/24 hr in 2 doses; increase q 4–7 days to therapeutic level, usually 15–40 mg/kg/24 hr in 2 doses. Max: 1.5 g/24 hr. *>6 yr and adults:* Start 250 mg twice daily; increase by 250 mg/24 hr q 4–7 days up to therapeutic level or 1.5 g/24 hr.	*Adverse events:* Sedation, lethargy, nausea, vomiting, anorexia, abdominal pain, leukopenia, thrombocytopenia, aplastic anemia. *Monitoring:* Ethosuximide concentrations: therapeutic 40–100 μg/mL; toxic 150 μg/mL.
Etoposide, VP-16 VePesid. Capsule: 50 mg. Injection: 20 mg/mL.	**Antineoplastic for treatment of various cancers (inhibits mitotic activity).** *Children:* IV: 150 mg/m^2/24 hr for 3 days for 2–3 cycles for acute myelocytic leukemia remission or brain tumor; 160 mg/m^2/24 hr for 4 days for bone marrow transplant conditioning. *Adults:* IV: 50–100 mg/m^2/24 hr for 3–5 days per course. PO = IV dose × 2 to nearest 50 mg.	*Adverse events:* Hypotension, tachycardia, fever, headache, chills, alopecia, rash, urticaria, nausea, vomiting, diarrhea, mucositis, myelosuppression, anemia (nadir, 7–14 days), thrombocytopenia (nadir, 9–16 days), peripheral neuropathy, bronchospasm.
Factor IX complex (human) Konyne 80, Proplex, Profilnine. Injection.	**Antihemophilic agent to control bleeding in patients with factor IX deficiency, i.e., hemophilia B or Christmas disease, or with inhibitors to factor VIII, i.e., hemophilia A (replacement of deficient factor).** *Children and adults:* 20–25 units/kg/dose up to q24h; factor VIII–inhibitor patients: 75–100 units/kg/dose up to q6h.	*Adverse events:* Flushing, fever, headache, chills, urticaria, thrombosis (with high doses), tingling, tightness of head and neck.
Famotidine Pepcid. Tablet: 20, 40 mg. Injection.	**Treatment of gastric and duodenal ulcer and control of gastric pH in critically ill patients (blocks H$_2$-receptors).** *Infants and children:* PO, IV: 1–2 mg/kg/24 hr in 1–2 doses; max: 40 mg/24 hr. *Adults:* PO: 40 mg/24 hr at bedtime; IV: 20 mg q12h.	*Cautions:* Reduce dose for renal function: CrCl 30–50 mL/min give 50% of dose; CrCl <30 mL/min give 25% of dose. *Adverse events:* Gastrointestinal discomfort, thrombocytopenia, increased liver enzymes.
Fat emulsion Intralipid, Liposyn. Injection: 10%, 20%.	**Source of essential fatty acids and calories (nutritional supplement with parenteral nutrition).** *Premature infants:* start 0.5 g/kg/24 hr and increase by 0.5 g/kg/24 hr as tolerated to 3 g/kg/24 hr. *Infants and children:* start 0.5–1 g/kg/24 hr and increase at 0.5 g/kg/24 hr increments as tolerated to maximum of 3–4 g/kg/24 hr. *Adolescents and adults:* 1 g/kg/24 hr and increase as tolerated to maximum of 2.5 g/kg/24 hr.	*Cautions:* Fat calories should not exceed 60% of total daily calories. Contraindicated in patients with severe egg or soybean allergies. *Adverse events:* Hyperlipidemia, hepatomegaly, dyspnea, and hypoxemia may occur if infused too quickly or excessive dose. *Monitoring:* Serum triglycerides.
Felbamate Felbatol. Tablet: 400, 600 mg. Oral suspension: 600 mg/5 mL.	**Adjunctive therapy primarily used for refractory generalized and partial seizures associated with Lennox-Gastaut syndrome (anticonvulsant with unknown mechanism of action).** *Children: 2–14 yr:* Start 15 mg/kg/24 hr in 3–4 doses, increase weekly by 15 mg/kg/24 hr to maximum of 45 mg/kg/24 hr or 3,600 mg (whichever is less). *> 14 yr:* Start 1,200 mg/24 hr in 3–4 doses; increase weekly by 1,200 mg/24 hr to max 3,600 mg/24 hr.	*Caution:* Over 30 cases each of hepatic failure and aplastic anemia with multiple fatalities have been reported. *Adverse events:* Headache, insomnia, somnolence, fatigue, behavioral changes, depression, ataxia, anorexia, nausea, vomiting, diarrhea, thrombocytopenia, granulocytopenia, leukopenia, agranulocytosis, aplastic anemia, hepatitis, acute liver failure. *Monitoring:* Interacts with phenytoin, carbamazepine, and valproate; monitor drug levels if felbamate added.
Fentanyl citrate Duragesic, Sublimaze. Injection, transdermal, oral lozenge.	**Relief of pain, sedation, preoperative medication, anesthesia adjunct (narcotic analgesic, binds to opium receptors).** *Neonates and infants:* IV: 1–4 μg/kg/dose; may repeat every 2–4 hr or continuous infusion 0.5–5 μg/kg/hr. *Children 1–12 yr:* Pain: IM, IV: 1–3 μg/kg/dose, may repeat q 30–60 min; continuous infusion 1–5 μg/kg/hr; Oralet 5–15 μg/kg. *Children >12 yr and adults:* Pain: IV, IM: 0.5–1 μg/kg/dose; may repeat in 30–60 min. Transdermal: 25–100 μg/hr system as needed for relief. PO: 5 μg/kg or 400 μg (whichever is less). Anesthesia: IV, IM: 2–50 μg/kg.	*Cautions:* Rapid IV infusion may result in skeletal muscle and chest wall rigidity with impaired ventilation and respiratory distress; physical dependence may occur in 3–5 days. *Adverse events:* Hypotension, bradycardia, CNS depression, constipation, biliary tract spasm, nausea, vomiting, urinary tract spasm, respiratory depression.
Fexofenadine Allegra. Capsule: 60 mg. Tablet: 30, 60, 180 mg.	**Antihistamine with selective peripheral H$_1$-receptor activity. Treat seasonal allergic rhinitis and chronic idiopathic urticaria.** *Children <12 yr:* 30 mg bid. *Children >12 yr and adults:* 60 mg bid, or 180 mg q24h.	*Adverse events:* Very good safety profile; toxicity is rare even with overdoses (mainly dizziness, drowsiness, and dry mouth).

Table continued on following page

MEDICATIONS

TABLE 712–1. **General Medications** Continued

Drug (Trade Names, Formulations)	Indications (Mechanism of Action) and Dosing	Comments (Cautions, Adverse Events, Monitoring)
Filgrastim, G-CSF Neupogen. Injection: 300 µg/mL.	Granulocyte colony-stimulating factor; reduces duration of neutropenia (stimulates the production, maturation, and activation of neutrophils). *Neonates:* 5 µg/kg/dose daily for 3–6 doses. *Children and adults:* 5–10 µg/kg/dose daily for up to 14 days, may discontinue if absolute neutrophil count remains >1,000/mm^3 for 3 consecutive days.	*Cautions:* Malignancy with myeloid characteristics. *Adverse events:* Hypotension, vasculitis, fever, exacerbation of pre-existing skin disorders, increased uric acid, thrombocytopenia, medullary pain (dose-related and mostly located in lower back, iliac crest, and sternum), hematuria, proteinuria.
Flecainide Tambocor. Tablet: 50, 100, 150 mg. Extemporaneous formulation.	Treatment of supraventricular tachycardia and ventricular arrhythmias (antiarrhythmic class 1c, slows conduction in cardiac tissue). *Children:* Initial 1–3 mg/kg/24 hr in 3 divided doses; may increase up to 12 mg/kg/24 hr. *Adults:* Initial 100 mg q12h; may increase by 100 mg/24 hr q 4 days to max 400 mg/24 hr.	*Caution:* Decrease dose by 25–50% in renal failure; avoid in 2nd- or 3rd-degree heart block. *Adverse events:* Bradycardia, heart block, worsening arrhythmias, congestive heart failure, dizziness, visual disturbances, headache, fatigue, asthenia, nausea, constipation, abdominal pain, elevated liver enzymes, paresthesias, and tremor. *Monitoring:* Serum trough concentrations (therapeutic 0.2–1 µg/mL).
Fludarabine, FAMP Fludara. Injection powder.	Treatment of B-cell chronic lymphocytic leukemia and acute lymphocytic leukemia unresponsive to previous therapy (antineoplastic, antimetabolite). *Children:* 10 mg/m^2 over 15 min, followed by 30.5 mg/m^2/24 hr by continuous infusion for 5 days. *Adults:* 20–25 mg/m^2 over 30 min for 5 days.	*Adverse events:* Neurotoxicity (primarily progressive demyelinating encephalopathy with mental status deterioration), somnolence, weakness, seizures, metabolic acidosis, hyperuricemia, hyperphosphatemia, hyperkalemia, hypocalcemia, nausea, vomiting, diarrhea, stomatitis, metallic taste, myelosuppression (WBC nadir, 8 days; platelet nadir, 16 days; recovery, 5–7 wk), pneumonitis, dyspnea, nonproductive cough, interstitial pneumonitis, hearing loss, reversible hepatotoxicity.
Fludrocortisone acetate Florinef. Tablet: 0.1 mg.	Partial replacement therapy for adrenal insufficiency (mineralocorticoid with glucocorticoid activity). *Infants and children:* 0.05–0.1 mg/24 hr. *Adults:* 0.05–0.2 mg/24 hr.	*Adverse events:* Hypertension, edema, congestive heart failure, convulsions, headache, acne, rash, bruising, hypokalemia, HPA-axis (adrenal) suppression, peptic ulcer, muscle weakness.
Flumazenil Romazicon. Injection.	Benzodiazepine antagonist to reverse sedative effects (antagonize benzodiazepine effects on γ-aminobutyric acid/benzodiazepine receptor complex). *Children:* 0.005–0.01 mg/kg load, then as continuous infusion 0.005–0.01 mg/kg/hr (maximal cumulative dose: 1 mg).	*Caution:* Avoid if benzodiazepine is used to manage potentially life-threatening conditions, e.g., status epilepticus, increased intracranial pressure. *Adverse events:* Arrhythmias, hypotension or hypertension, seizures, acute withdrawal symptoms (if patient dependent on benzodiazepine or tricyclic antidepressant).
Flunisolide AeroBid, Nasalide. Metered-dose inhaler: 250 µg/puff. Nasal spray: 25 µg/actuation.	Treatment of asthma and rhinitis (inhaled steroid, anti-inflammatory). *Children and adults:* Oral inhalation: 2–4 puffs twice daily; nasal spray: 1–2 sprays in each nostril bid–tid.	*Adverse events:* Candidal infections of nose and throat, dysphonia, sore throat, bitter taste, nasal irritation, headache, dizziness, short-term growth retardation.
Fluocinolone acetonide Fluonid, Synalar, generic. Topical cream, ointment, shampoo, solution, oil: 0.01–0.025%.	Inflammation and corticosteroid-responsive dermatoses (topical adrenocorticosteroid, anti-inflammatory). *Children and adults:* Apply a thin layer bid–qid.	*Adverse events:* Acne, hypopigmentation, allergic dermatitis, skin atrophy, folliculitis, secondary infection, HPA-axis suppression, growth retardation.
Fluocinonide Fluonex, Lidex, generic. Cream, gel, ointment, solution: 0.05%.	Inflammation and corticosteroid-responsive dermatoses (topical adrenocorticosteroid, anti-inflammatory). *Children and adults:* Apply a thin layer 2–4 times qid.	*Adverse events:* Acne, hypopigmentation, allergic dermatitis, skin atrophy, folliculitis, secondary infection, HPA-axis suppression, growth retardation.
Fluoride Generic. Oral drops, topical gel, lozenge, tablet, topical rinse, oral solution.	Prevention of dental caries (promotes remineralization, increase resistance to acid dissolution). Dental rinse or gel: *Children:* 5–10 mL after brushing. *Adults:* 10 mL after brushing.	*Adverse events:* Gastrointestinal upset if swallowed, stannous fluoride may stain teeth.
Fluorometholone Flarex, FML. Ophthalmic ointment 0.1%. Ophthalmic suspension: 0.1, 0.25%.	Inflammatory conditions of the eye (ophthalmic glucocorticoid, anti-inflammatory). *Children >2 yr and adults:* Ointment: Apply 3 times daily in mild to moderate cases and q4h in severe cases. Drops: instill 1–2 drops into conjunctival sac every hr while awake and q2h at night until response, then q4–8h.	*Adverse events:* Local stinging and burning, increased intraocular pressure.
Fluorouracil Adrucil, Efudex, Fluoroplex. Injection, topical solution, cream.	Cancer chemotherapy (antineoplastic antimetabolite that inhibits thymidylate synthase leading to thymidine depletion). *Children and adults:* IV: 12 mg/kg/24 hr (max: 800 mg/24 hr) for 4–5 days then 6 mg/kg every other day for 4 doses. Repeat in 4 wk. Cream or solution 5%: Apply to entire affected area bid.	*Adverse events:* Arrhythmias, hypotension, heart failure, cerebellar ataxia, somnolence, alopecia, skin pigmentation, pruritic maculopapular rash, photosensitivity, erythrodysesthesias of hands and feet, loss of nails, hyperpigmentation of nail beds, nausea, vomiting, diarrhea, gastrointestinal hemorrhage, esophagitis, stomatitis, hepatotoxicity, conjunctivitis, myelosuppression (WBC and platelets: onset, 7–10 days; nadir, 9–14 days; recovery, 21 days).
Fluoxetine hydrochloride Prozac. Capsule: 10, 20 mg.	Treatment of depression and obsessive-compulsive disorders (antidepressant, inhibits CNS serotonin uptake).	*Caution:* Avoid in patients on monoamine oxidase inhibitors. *Adverse events:* Headache, nervousness, insomnia, anxiety, mania, suicidal ideation, tremor, nausea, anorexia, diarrhea,

MEDICATIONS

TABLE 712–1. General Medications *Continued*

Drug (Trade Names, Formulations)	Indications (Mechanism of Action) and Dosing	Comments (Cautions, Adverse Events, Monitoring)
Liquid: 20 mg/5 mL.	*Children 5–18 yr:* Initial 5–10 mg/24 hr then titrate slowly to effect (max: 20 mg/24 hr). *Adults:* Initial 20 mg/24 hr then slowly increase daily dose in 20 mg increments to effect (max: 80 mg/24 hr).	constipation, dry mouth, weight loss. *Monitoring:* Serum concentrations of fluoxetine (therapeutic: 100–800 ng/mL), norfluoxetine (therapeutic: 100–600 ng/mL).
Fluticasone Flonase, Flovent. Nasal solution: 50 μg/spray. Metered-dose inhaler (MDI): 44, 110, 220 μg/spray. Rotadisk: 50, 100, 250 μg/dose.	**Treatment of allergic rhinitis and chronic asthma (inhaled corticosteroid).** *Children and adults:* Nasal spray: 1–2 sprays in each nostril once daily. MDI: 88–880 μg bid (depending on asthma severity and need for systemic corticosteroids). Rotadisk: 50–1,000 μg bid (depending on asthma severity and need for systemic corticosteroids).	*Adverse events:* Dysphonia, oral thrush, adrenal suppression, growth suppression, cataracts.
Fluvoxamine Luvox, generic. Tablet: 25, 50, 100 mg.	**Serotonin reuptake inhibitor; treatment of depression, obsessive-compulsive disorder (OCD).** *Children <12 yr:* Start 25 mg/hr increase by 25 mg/24 hr q 4–7 days to effect or maximum of 200 mg/24 hr. Divide into 2 daily doses if >50 mg/24 hr needed. *Children >12 yr:* Start 25 mg/24 hr; increase by 25 mg/24 hr q 4–7 days to effect or maximum of 300 mg/24 hr. Divide into 2 daily doses if >50 mg/24 hr needed. *Adults:* Start 50 mg/24 hr; increase by 50 mg/24 hr q 4–7 days to effect or maximum of 300 mg/24 hr. If more than 100 mg/24 hr is needed, divide into 2 doses/24 hr.	*Caution:* Do not abruptly discontinue doses or withdrawal syndrome may occur over several days. Taper dose by 25–50 mg/24 hr q 5–7 days. *Adverse events:* Somnolence, headache, dry mouth, nausea, constipation. *Drug interactions:* Inhibits cytochrome 2D6 liver enzymes; drugs such as methadone and phenothiazines may have increased levels when used concurrently.
Folic acid Generic. Injection. Tablet: 0.4, 0, 8, 1 mg. Extemporaneous formulation.	**Treatment of folate deficiency anemias, i.e., megaloblastic, macrocytic (cofactor for normal erythropoiesis).** *Neonates to 6 mo:* PO: 25–35 μg/24 hr. *6 mo–3 yr:* 50 μg/24 hr. *4–6 yr:* 75 μg/24 hr. *7–10 yr:* 100 μg/24 hr. *11–14 yr:* 150 μg/24 hr. *>15 yr and adults:* 200 μg/24 hr. Folate deficiency: 1 mg/24 hr.	*Caution:* Large folate doses may mask hematologic effects of vitamin B_{12} deficiency while allowing the neurologic consequences to progress.
Fosphenytoin Cerebyx Injection: 10 mL vials contain 750 mg fosphenytoin (500 mg phenytoin), 2-mL vials contain 150 mg fosphenytoin.	**Treatment of acute seizures (may substitute or intravenous phenytoin).** *Children and adults:* Loading dose is 15–20 mg/kg phenytoin dosing equivalents (maximum rate: 150 mg/min). May substitute IV or IM for phenytoin maintenance doses. Each 1.5 mg fosphenytoin = 1 mg phenytoin dosing equivalent.	*Cautions:* Same as phenytoin. *Drug interactions:* Same as phenytoin.
Furosemide Lasix, generic. Injection: 10 mg/mL. Oral solution: 10 mg/mL, 40 mg/mL. Tablet: 20, 40, 80 mg.	**Diuretic (inhibits sodium and chloride reabsorption at the ascending loop of Henle and distal tubule).** *Premature infants:* 0.5–2 mg/kg IV or 1–4 mg/kg PO q12–48h (dose to response). *Infants and children:* 1–2 mg/kg IV or 1–4 mg/kg PO q6–24h or continuous infusion (start at 0.05 mg/kg/hr and adjust dose to response). *Adults:* 10–600 mg/24 hr in 1–4 divided doses; or continuous infusion 0.05 mg/kg/hr (adjust dose to effect).	*Adverse events:* Dehydration, electrolyte loss, hyperuricemia, photosensitivity, ischemic hepatitis, hypercalciuria, renal stones, ototoxicity (IV infusion rate >4 mL/min), gastrointestinal intolerance.
Gabapentin Neurontin. Capsule: 100, 300, 400 mg.	**Adjunct to treatment of partial and secondarily generalized seizures; treatment of neuropathic pain (mechanism not certain).** *Children 2–12 yr:* 15–35 mg/kg/24 hr in 3 divided doses (max: 50 mg/kg/24 hr). *Children >12 yr and adults:* Start 300 mg daily, then daily increase by 300 mg to 900–3,600 mg/24 hr in 3 divided doses.	*Adverse events:* Somnolence, dizziness, fatigue, depression, hyperactivity, aggression, dyspepsia, constipation, nausea, weight gain, diplopia.
Gamma globulin *See Immune globulin* **Gentian violet** Generic. Topical solution: 1%, 2%.	**Treatment of cutaneous and mucocutaneous infections (kills *Candida*, staphylococcal species, and some vegetative gram-positive bacteria).** *Infants:* Apply 3 or 4 drops of a 0.5% solution under tongue or on lesion after feedings. *Children and adults:* Apply 0.5–2% with cotton to lesion bid–tid for 3 days.	*Caution:* Do not swallow. *Adverse events:* Burning, local irritation or sensitivity reactions.

Table continued on following page

TABLE 712–1. General Medications *Continued*

Drug (Trade Names, Formulations)	Indications (Mechanism of Action) and Dosing	Comments (Cautions, Adverse Events, Monitoring)
Glucagon Powder for injection.	**Treatment of hypoglycemia (stimulates hepatic glycolysis and gluconeogenesis).** *Neonates:* 0.3 mg/kg/dose (max: 1 mg) IV, IM, SC. *Children:* 0.025–0.1 mg/kg/dose (max: 1 mg); may repeat in 20 min. *Adults:* 0.5–1 mg; may repeat in 20 min as needed.	*Adverse events:* Nausea, vomiting, hypersensitivity reactions.
Glycopyrrolate Robinul, generic. Injection: 0.2 mg/mL. Tablet: 1 mg.	**Inhibits salivation and excessive secretions of the respiratory tract; bronchodilator, adjunct to treatment of peptic ulcer, reversal of muscarinic effects on cholinergic agents (anticholinergic).** *Children:* Control of secretions: PO: 40–100 µg/kg/dose tid–qid. IM, IV: 4–10 µg/kg/dose q3–4h. Preoperative IM: 4.4–8.8 µg/kg/dose 30–60 min before procedure.	*Adverse events:* Tachycardia, nervousness, headache, insomnia, drowsiness, dry mouth, constipation, nausea, urinary retention, blurred vision.
Gold sodium thiomalate Myochrysine, generic. Injection: 25 mg/mL.	**Treatment of rheumatoid arthritis (mechanism unknown).** *Children:* Test dose: 10 mg IM; followed by 1 mg/kg IM q wk for 20 wk; then 1 mg/kg/dose q 2–4 wk (max: 50 mg/dose). *Adults:* Test dose: 10 mg IM; then 25–50 mg/wk; then 25–50 mg IM every 2–4 wk once response is noted.	*Cautions:* Patient should be sitting or lying for 10 min after the dose; avoid in patients with systemic lupus erythematosus or blood dyscrasias. *Adverse events:* Headache, flushing, seizures, exfoliative dermatitis, erythema nodosum, hives, alopecia, loss of nails, stomatitis, gingivitis, glossitis, conjunctivitis, eosinophilia, leukopenia, thrombocytopenia, hematuria, proteinuria, nephrotic syndrome, pulmonary fibrosis and interstitial pneumonitis, hepatotoxicity, peripheral neuropathy. *Monitoring:* Gold serum concentrations (therapeutic 1–3 µg/mL).
Gonadorelin Factrel, Lutrepulse. Injection.	**Evaluate gonadotropin regulation in precocious or delayed puberty, treat primary hypothalamic amenorrhea (stimulates release of luteinizing hormone).** *Children:* IV (HCl salt) 100 µg. *Children >12 yr and adults:* IV, SC: 100 µg during days 1–7 of menstrual cycle.	*Adverse events:* Flushing, lightheadedness, headache, abdominal discomfort. *Monitoring:* Plasma luteinizing hormone and follicle-stimulating hormone.
Granisetron Kytril. Injection: 1 mg/mL. Tablet: 1 mg.	**Antiemetic (selective 5-HT$_3$ antagonist).** *Children >2 yr and adults:* IV 10–20 µg/kg 15–30 min before chemotherapy; may repeat 2–3 doses in 24 hr. PO: 1 mg bid starting 1 hr before chemotherapy.	*Adverse events:* Arrhythmias, bradycardia, transient blood pressure changes, agitation, anxiety, liver enzyme elevations.
Guaifenesin, Glycerol Guaiacolate Generic. ± Codeine, dextromethorphan, phenylpropanolamine, or phenylephrine. Syrup, tablet, capsule, liquid.	**Temporary control of cough (expectorant).** *Children <2 yr:* 12 mg/kg/24 hr in 6 divided doses. *2–5 yr:* 50–100 mg q4h (max: 600 mg/24 hr). *6–11 yr:* 100–200 mg q4h (max: 1,200 mg/24 hr). *>12 yr and adults:* 200–400 mg q4h (max: 2.4 g/24 hr).	*Caution:* Monitor doses and toxicities of other drugs in combination products.
Guanethidine Ismelin. Tablet: 10, 25 mg.	**Treatment of moderate to severe hypertension (acts as false neurotransmitter).** *Children:* 0.2 mg/kg/24 hr; may increase by 0.2 mg/kg/24 hr every wk to maximum of 3 mg/kg/24 hr. *Adults:* Initial 10 mg/24 hr; increase weekly to maximum of 25–50 mg/24 hr.	*Adverse events:* Palpitations, chest pain, peripheral edema, fatigue, headache, drowsiness, confusion, constipation, anorexia, urinary frequency, nocturia, paresthesias, visual disturbances, orthostatic hypotension.
Guanfacine HCl Tenex. Tablet: 1 mg.	**Treatment of hypertension and attention deficit disorder (ADD) (stimulate α$_2$-receptors in the brainstem)** *Children:* ADD: 1 mg/24 hr. *Adults:* 1 mg/24 hr; may increase q 4 wk to maximum of 3 mg/24 hr.	*Adverse events:* Somnolence, dizziness, dry mouth, constipation, gastrointestinal upset.
Haloperidol Haldol, generic. Oral concentrate: 2 mg/mL. Tablet: 0.5, 1, 2, 5, 10, 20 mg. Injection.	**Treatment of severe behavioral problems including psychoses and Tourette disorder (competitive blocker of dopamine receptors).** *Children 3–12 yr:* PO: start 0.25–0.5 mg/24 hr in 2–3 divided doses, then increase weekly by 0.25–0.5 mg daily based on response to max 0.15 mg/kg/24 hr. *6–12 yr:* IM: 1–3 mg/dose q4–8h (max: 0.15 mg/kg/24 hr). *Adults:* PO: 0.5–5 mg 2–3 times daily. IM: 2–5 mg q4–8h.	*Adverse events:* Drowsiness, restlessness, anxiety, extrapyramidal symptoms, dystonia, akathisia, pseudoparkinsonism, tardive dyskinesia, neuroleptic malignant syndrome, seizures, constipation, weight gain, swelling of breasts, hypotension, tachycardia, arrhythmias, urinary retention, blurred vision, rental pigmentation, cholestatic liver disease, agranulocytosis, leukopenia. *Monitoring:* Plasma concentrations (therapeutic 5–15 ng/mL, toxic >42 ng/mL).
Heparin (unfractionated) Generic Injection.	**Prophylaxis and treatment of thromboembolism (potentiates actions of antithrombin III).** *Neonates, infants, and children:* Thrombosis and ECMO: load 50 units/kg IV bolus, and 15–35 units/kg/hr continuous IV infusion maintenance dose (adjust to target activated partial thromboplastin time [APTT] or heparin level). Catheter patency: 0.5–1 unit/mL. *Adults:* load 70–100 units/kg IV push, 15–25 units/kg/hr continuous IV infusion (target	*Caution:* Avoid if severe thrombocytopenia, intracranial hemorrhage, bacterial endocarditis. *Adverse events:* Bleeding from various sites, e.g., urine, gums, nose; bruising, thrombocytopenia, thrombosis. *Monitoring:* APTT (therapeutic, 1.5–2.5 times baseline; toxic >2.5 times baseline); plasma heparin concentration (anti-factor X assay: therapeutic 0.3–0.7 units/mL).

TABLE 712–1. General Medications *Continued*

Drug (Trade Names, Formulations)	Indications (Mechanism of Action) and Dosing	Comments (Cautions, Adverse Events, Monitoring)
	APTT or heparin level); SC: 5,000 units q8–12h for prophylaxis.	
Histrelin Supprelin. Injection.	**Central idiopathic precocious puberty (gonadotropin-releasing hormone analog).** *Children:* SC: 10 μg/kg once daily. *Adult female:* 100 μg/24 hr for endometriosis.	*Adverse events:* Anxiety, depression, irritability, insomnia, headaches.
Homatropine hydrobromide Isopto Homatropine, generic. Ophthalmic solution: 2%, 5%.	**Producing cycloplegia and mydriasis for refraction, treatment of uveitis (anticholinergic).** *Children:* For mydriasis: 1 drop of 2% solution before procedure; may repeat every 10 min as needed. Uveitis: 1 drop 2% solution bid–tid. *Adults:* Mydriasis: 1–2 drops of 2% or 5% solution before procedure; may repeat every 10 min. Uveitis: 1–2 drops of 2% or 5% solution bid–tid.	*Adverse events:* Blurred vision, photophobia, local stinging, and respiratory congestion.
Human growth hormone Humatrope, Nutropin, Protropin. Injection.	**Treatment of growth failure due to inadequate growth hormone secretion (replacement therapy).** *Children:* Humatrope: 0.06 mg/kg (0.15 IU/kg) 3 times/wk. Nutropin: 0.043 mg/kg/24 hr. Protropin: 0.1 mg/kg (0.26 IU/kg) 3 times/wk.	*Adverse events:* Local lipoatrophy, hypothyroidism, pain in hip or knee.
Hyaluronidase Wydase. Injection: 150 units/mL.	**Treatment of extravasation, enhance absorption of fluids administered by hypodermoclysis (hydrolysis of hyaluronic acid to modify permeability of connective tissue).** *Neonates, infants, children:* inject using 25–26 g needle (total 1 mL, 150 U) SC or intradermal at 5 sites (0.2 mL to each) at the leading edge of the extravasation.	*Adverse events:* Tachycardia, hypotension, erythema.
Hydralazine Generic. Injection: 20 mg/mL. Tablet. Extemporaneous formulations.	**Treatment of hypertension, adjunct treatment of congestive heart failure with nitrates (direct vasodilation of arterioles).** *Neonates:* IV: 0.1–0.5 mg/kg/dose q6–8h. PO: 0.25–1 mg/kg/dose q6–8h. *Infants and children:* IM, IV start 0.1–0.2 mg/kg/dose q4–6h and titrate to effect (max: 3.5 mg/kg/24 hr). PO: 0.75–1 mg/kg/24 hr in 2–4 divided doses (max: 7.5 mg/kg/24 hr). *Adults:* IM, IV: 10–20 mg/dose every 4–6 hr (max 40 mg/dose). PO: 10–25 mg/dose qid and titrate to effect (max: 300 mg/24 hr).	*Adverse events:* Palpitations, flushing, tachycardia, headache, nausea, vomiting, anorexia, diarrhea, lupus-like syndrome, arthralgias, and peripheral neuropathy (related to pyridoxine deficiency).
Hydrochlorothiazide Generic. Oral solution: 50 mg/5 mL. Tablet: 25, 50, 100 mg. Combination products (e.g., spironolactone).	**Treatment of hypertension and fluid overload (edema) states, e.g., bronchopulmonary dysplasia, congestive heart failure; prevention of recurrent renal calcium stones (diuretic inhibits sodium reabsorption in distal tubule).** *Neonates and infants:* 2–4 mg/kg/24 hr in 2 divided doses. *Infants >6 mo and children:* 2 mg/kg/24 hr in 2 divided doses. *Adults:* 12.5–100 mg/24 hr.	*Adverse events:* Hypokalemia, hypochloremia, hypomagnesemia, hyperglycemia, hyperuricemia, hyperlipidemia, pancreatitis, leukopenia, thrombocytopenia, aplastic anemia, hepatitis, intrahepatic cholestasis, prerenal azotemia.
Hydrocortisone Generic. Cream, ointment, gel, lotion, injection, oral suspension, rectal foam	**Treatment of adrenal insufficiency, congenital adrenal hyperplasia, shock, corticosteroid-responsive dermatoses, adjunctive treatment of ulcerative colitis (anti-inflammatory, glucocorticoid).** *Neonates, infants, young children:* Adrenal insufficiency: 1–2 mg/kg IV bolus, then 25–150 mg/24 hr divided q6h. Congenital adrenal hyperplasia: IV 0.5–0.7 mg/kg/24 hr start, then 0.3–0.4 mg/kg/24 hr maintenance therapy; give doses as 1/4 in AM, 1/4 at noon, and 1/2 at night. Shock: IV: 35–50 mg/kg, then 50–150 mg/kg/24 hr divided q6h for 48–72 hr. *Infants and older children:* Adrenal insufficiency: 1–2 mg/kg IV bolus, then 150–250 mg/24 hr divided q6–8h. Anti-inflammatory: IV, IM: 1–5 mg/kg/24 hr in 1–2 doses; PO: 2.5–10 mg/kg/24 hr divided q6–8h. Shock: IV: 50 mg/kg/dose q4h. Status asthmaticus: IV: 1–2 mg/kg/dose q6h.	*Caution:* Abrupt withdrawal may cause acute adrenal insufficiency. *Adverse events:* Hypertension, hyperglycemia, hypokalemia, euphoria, insomnia, headache, Cushing syndrome, peptic ulcer, cataracts, immunosuppression, skin and muscle atrophy, acne, edema.

Relative Potency of Corticosteroids

Drug	Anti-inflammatory Effect (mg)	Sodium-Retaining Effect (mg)
Hydrocortisone	100	100
Cortisone	80	80
Prednisolone	20	100
Prednisone	20	100
Methylprednisolone	16	0
Triamcinolone	16	0
Dexamethasone	2	0
Desoxycorticosterone	0	2

Table continued on following page

TABLE 712–1. General Medications *Continued*

Drug (Trade Names, Formulations)	Indications (Mechanism of Action) and Dosing	Comments (Cautions, Adverse Events, Monitoring)
Hydromorphone Dilaudid, generic. Injection. Tablet: 2, 4 mg. Syrup: 1 mg/5 mL. Suppository: 3 mg.	*Adults:* Anti-inflammatory: IV, IM, PO: 15–240 mg/dose q12h. Shock: IV: 0.5–2 g q2–6h. Rectal: 1 Application 1–2 times/24 hr for 2–3 wk. Topical: Apply 3–4 times/24 hr. **Analgesic, antitussive (narcotic).** *Children 6–12 yr:* Cough: PO: 0.5 mg q3–4h as needed. Pain: PO: 0.03–0.08 mg/kg/dose q4–6h as needed. IV: 0.015 mg/kg/dose q4–6h as needed. *Children >12 yr and adults:* Cough: PO: 1 mg every 3–4 hr as needed. Pain: PO, IV, IM, SC: 1–4 mg/dose q4–6h as needed.	*Caution:* Tablet and syrup contain tartrazine, which may exacerbate asthma; do not discontinue abruptly after continuous use. *Adverse events:* Sedation, drowsiness, confusion, restlessness, headache, tachycardia, hypotension, physical and psychological addiction, nausea, vomiting, constipation, stomach cramps, decreased urination, ureteral spasm, respiratory depression, shortness of breath, miosis, antidiuretic hormone release, sensitivity reactions (due to histamine release). *Comment:* IV, IM hydromorphone 1.5 mg = morphine 10 mg; oral hydromorphone 7.5 mg = morphine 30 mg (acute) or 60 mg (chronic).
Hydroxocobalamin, vitamin B$_{12}$ Codroxomin, Hybalamin, others. Injection.	**Treatment of pernicious anemia, vitamin B$_{12}$ deficiency, increased vitamin B$_{12}$ requirements (replacement therapy).** *Children:* 100 µg/24 hr IM to total 1 mg over 2 wk, then 30–50 µg/mo. *Adults:* 30 µg/24 hr for 5–10 days, then 100–200 µg/mo.	*Comment:* May require co-administration of folate.
Hydroxychloroquine Plaquenil sulfate. Tablet: 200 mg. Extemporaneous formulations.	**Suppression or chemoprophylaxis of malaria; treatment of systemic lupus erythematosus and rheumatoid arthritis (interferes with digestive vacuole function within sensitive malarial parasites, impairs complement-dependent antigen-antibody reactions).** *Children:* Chemoprophylaxis of malaria: 5 mg/kg once wk (begin 1–2 wk before exposure and continue for 4 wk after leaving high-risk area). Acute malaria attack: 10 mg/kg initial dose followed by 5 mg/kg in 6–8 hr on day 1, 400 mg once on day 2 and day 3. *Adults:* Malaria prophylaxis: 400 mg once wk (timing as above). Acute malaria attack: Day 1: 800 mg, then 400 mg in 6–8 hr; day 2: 400 mg once; day 3: 400 mg once. Rheumatoid arthritis and lupus erythematosus: 400 mg once daily, may increase by 200 mg if inadequate response in 4–12 wk, reduce to 200–400 mg/24 hr once response occurs and long-term maintenance is needed.	*Caution:* Avoid in porphyria or psoriasis. *Adverse events:* Headache, confusion, agitation, insomnia, nightmares, psychosis, visual field defects, retinitis, blindness, bone marrow suppression, thrombocytopenia, liver failure, anorexia, nausea, vomiting, diarrhea, lichenoid dermatitis, bleaching of hair, itching, ototoxicity. *Monitoring:* Ophthalmologic exams for visual field changes
Hydroxyurea Mylocel tablets, Hydrea, generic. Tablet: 1,000 mg. Capsule: 500 mg.	**Cancer chemotherapy, sickle cell anemia (interfere with DNA synthesis during S-phase of cell division).** *Children:* 1,500–3,000 mg/m^2 q 4–6 wk. *Adults:* Cancer chemotherapy: 80 mg/kg every third day, or 20–30 mg/kg/24 hr sickle cell anemia: 10–20 mg/kg/24 hr.	*Adverse events:* Drowsiness, headache, hallucinations, seizures, nausea, vomiting, mucositis, stomatitis, myelosuppression (onset, day 7; nadir, day 10; recovery, day 21), alopecia, maculopapular rash, dry skin, erythema of face and hands, hepatitis, increased blood urea nitrogen and creatinine, hyperuricemia.
Hydroxyzine Generic. Injection, syrup, tablet, capsule.	**Treatment of allergy, itching, anxiety, and nausea and adjunct for chronic pain management (H$_1$-receptor blocker).** PO, IM: *Children:* 0.6 mg/kg/dose q6h. *Adults:* 10–100 mg/dose tid–qid.	*Caution:* May worsen narrow-angle glaucoma, prostatic hypertrophy, bladder neck obstruction, asthma, and chronic obstructive pulmonary disease. *Adverse events:* Hypotension, drowsiness, dizziness, headache, dry mouth, urinary retention, pain at injection site.
Hyoscyamine (with atropine, scopolamine, and phenobarbital) Donnatal, generic. Capsule, elixir, tablet.	**Treatment of irritable bowel, spastic colon, spastic bladder, and renal colic (anticholinergic).** *Children:* Donnatal 0.1 mL/kg/dose q4h (max: 5 mL). *Adults:* 1–2 tablets (or 5–10 mL) tid–qid. *Caution:* Contraindicated in narrow-angle glaucoma, myasthenia gravis, gastrointestinal and genitourinary obstruction.	*Adverse events:* Tachycardia, palpitations, headache, drowsiness, nervousness, dry mouth, constipation, dysphagia, paralytic ileus, blurred vision, nasal congestion.
Ibuprofen Generic. Suspension: 100 mg/5 mL. Tablet: 200, 300, 400, 600, 800 mg.	**Treatment of pain, fever, rheumatoid arthritis (nonsteroidal anti-inflammatory, inhibit prostaglandin synthesis).** *Children:* Pain, fever: 5–10 mg/kg/dose q6–8h. Juvenile rheumatoid arthritis: 30–50 mg/kg/24 hr in 4 divided doses.	*Adverse events:* Abdominal cramps, heartburn, nausea, gastrointestinal bleeding and perforation, fluid retention, edema, hypertension, tachycardia, acute renal failure.

TABLE 712–1. General Medications *Continued*

Drug (Trade Names, Formulations)	Indications (Mechanism of Action) and Dosing	Comments (Cautions, Adverse Events, Monitoring)
Idarubicin Idamycin. Injection.	*Adults:* 400–800 mg/dose tid–qid (max: 3.2 g/24 hr). **Combination chemotherapy for acute myelocytic and lymphocytic leukemia (AML and ALL) (inhibits DNA and RNA synthesis).** *Children:* ALL: 10–12 mg/m^2 IV once daily for 3 days per treatment course. *Adults:* AML: 8–12 mg/m2 IV daily for 3 days per treatment course.	*Adverse events:* Headache, infection, hemorrhage, mucositis, stomatitis, alopecia, rash, urticaria, nausea, vomiting, diarrhea, leukopenia (nadir, 8–19 days), thrombocytopenia (nadir, 10–15 days), myocardial toxicity (arrhythmias, cardiomyopathy, heart failure, ECG changes). *Monitoring:* Maximal lifetime dose = 137.5 mg/m^2. Lower dose by 25% if severe mucositis present or serum creatinine >2 mg/dL; lower dose by 50% if bilirubin >2.5 mg/dL; do not give dose if bilirubin >5 mg/dL.
Ifosfamide Ifex. Injection.	**Cancer chemotherapy (alkylating agent).** *Children:* IV: 1,200–1,800 mg/m^2/24 hr for 5 days q 21–28 days; or 5 g/m^2 as single IV infusion. *Adults:* 700–2,000 mg/m^2/24 hr for 5 days q 21–28 days; or 5 g/m^2 as single IV infusion.	*Adverse events:* Alopecia, nausea, vomiting, stomatitis, hemorrhagic cystitis (administer MESNA for uroprotection), hematuria, renal damage, somnolence, confusion, hallucinations, coma, polyneuropathy, depressive psychosis, elevated liver enzymes, myelosuppression (onset, day 7; nadir, 10–14 days), pulmonary fibrosis, nasal stuffiness, cardiotoxicity.
Imipramine Tofranil, generic. Injection, capsule, tablet.	**Treatment of depression, enuresis, pain (tricyclic antidepressant, increase synaptic concentrations of norepinephrine and serotonin).** *Children:* Depression: start 1.5 mg/kg/24 hr; may increase by 1 mg/kg/24 hr q 3–4 days (max: 5 mg/kg/24 hr). Enuresis: >6 yr, 10–25 mg at bedtime. Cancer pain: 0.2–0.4 mg/kg at bedtime; may increase dose 50% q 3–4 days (max: 3 mg/kg). *Adolescents:* PO: start 25–50 mg/24 hr; may gradually increase to maximum of 200 mg/24 hr. *Adults:* PO: 25 mg tid–qid; may increase dose gradually to maximum of 300 mg/24 hr; IM: Initial up to 100 mg in divided doses.	*Adverse events:* Arrhythmias, postural hypotension, drowsiness, sedation, confusion, headache, dry mouth, constipation, urinary retention, increased liver enzymes, seizures, urinary retention. *Monitoring:* Imipramine concentrations (therapeutic: imipramine and desipramine 150–250 ng/mL, toxic >1,000 ng/mL).
Immune globulin, intravenous (IVIG) Gamimune, Sandoglobulin, generic. Injection.	**Immunodeficiency syndrome, idiopathic thrombocytopenic purpura, acute bacterial or viral infections in immunocompromised or neutropenic patients, Kawasaki disease, Guillain-Barré syndrome, demyelinating polyneuropathy (replacement therapy or interference with Fc receptors in the reticulo-endothelial system for autoimmune diseases).** *Neonates:* 500–750 mg/kg once. *Children and adults:* Immunodeficiency syndrome: 100–400 mg/kg/ dose q 2–4 wk. Chronic lymphocytic leukemia: 400 mg/kg/ dose q 3 wk. Idiopathic thrombocytopenic purpura: 1,000 mg/kg/dose for 2–5 consecutive days then q 3–6 wk. Kawasaki disease: 2 g/kg single dose. Cytomegalovirus infection: 500 mg/kg/dose every other day for 7 doses. Severe systemic infection: 500–1,000 mg/kg/wk. Polyneuropathy: 1 g/kg/24 hr for 2 consecutive days each mo.	*Caution:* Doses should be based on ideal body weight (not total body weight). *Adverse events:* Flushing, tachycardia, chills, nausea, dyspnea, fever, hypersensitivity reactions, headache, aseptic meningitis.
Indomethacin Indocin, generic (oral forms). Capsule: 25, 50 mg. Suspension: 25 mg/5 mL. Injection.	**Closure of the patent ductus arteriosus (PDA) in neonates, treatment of rheumatoid disorders, acute gouty arthritis, pain (NSAID, prostaglandin inhibition), hereditary hypokalemic salt-losing renal tubulopathies.** *Neonates:* IV: 0.10–0.25 mg/kg/dose q12h for 3–6 doses. Inflammatory rheumatoid disorders: *Children:* 1–2 mg/kg/24 hr in 2–4 doses (max: 4 mg/kg/24 hr). *Adults:* 25–50 mg/dose 2–3 times/24 hr (max: 200 mg/24 hr).	*Caution:* Avoid in premature neonates with necrotizing enterocolitis, poor renal function, or active bleeding, and all patients with active gastrointestinal bleeding. *Adverse events:* Confusion, dizziness, headache, nausea, vomiting, abdominal pain, gastrointestinal bleeding, ulcers, gastrointestinal perforation, bone marrow suppression, impaired platelet aggregation, oliguria, renal failure, hypertension, edema, hyperkalemia. *Monitoring:* Indomethacin (concentrations in PDA closure): therapeutic 1–3 µg/mL.
Insulin *Rapid-acting:* Lispro, Regular, Semilente; *Intermediate-acting:* NPH, Lente; *Long-acting:* Ultralente; *Combination products* (e.g., Novolin 70/30, contains Lente 70 units, Regular 30 units). Humulin, Novolin (human insulin, preferred form); beef insulin, pork insulin.	**Treatment of insulin-dependent diabetes mellitus and non–insulin-dependent diabetes not adequately controlled with oral hypoglycemic agents (replacement therapy).** *Neonates:* Regular insulin 0.01–0.1 units/kg/hr continuous infusion, or SC 0.1–0.2 units/kg every 6–12 hr.	*Caution:* Check for drugs that increase or decrease insulin effect, do not change insulin types or brands once patient is regulated since dosing requirements will then change, start new patients on human insulin if possible. *Adverse events:* Hypoglycemia (and associated symptoms of dizziness, weakness, paresthesias, numbness of mouth, fatigue, mental confusion, hunger, nausea, visual problems),

Table continued on following page

TABLE 712–1. General Medications *Continued*

Drug (Trade Names, Formulations)	Indications (Mechanism of Action) and Dosing	Comments (Cautions, Adverse Events, Monitoring)
Injection.	*Children and adults:* 0.5–1 unit/kg/24 hr. Adjust doses to blood glucose and hemoglobin A_{1C} results. *Adolescents (during growth spurt):* 0.8–1.2 units/kg/24 hr. Diabetic ketoacidosis: Continuous infusion IV: 0.1 unit/kg/hr adjusted to serum glucose. Hyperkalemia: Try calcium gluconate and $NaHCO_3$ first, then dextrose 50% 0.5–1 mL/kg and regular insulin 1 unit per 4–5 g dextrose.	hypokalemia. *Monitoring:* Blood glucose (teach patient to monitor at home and make insulin dosing corrections per results), hemoglobin A_{1C}, urine glucose, and acetone.
Interferon alfa-2a Roferon-A. Injection.	**In children treat hemangiomas of infancy and pulmonary hemangiomas (inhibits cellular growth, alters cellular differentiation).** *Infants and children:* SC: 1–3 million units/m²/24 hr. *Adults:* 3–20 million units/m²/dose/24 hr to 3 times/wk depending on the indication.	*Adverse events:* Tachycardia, arrhythmias, hypotension, edema, CNS depression, confusion, fatigue, dizziness, and flu-like symptoms (begin 2–6 hr after dose and last up to 24 hr).
Ipecac syrup Generic. Syrup: 70 mg/mL.	**Induces vomiting to treat certain toxic ingestions (stimulates medullary chemoreceptor trigger zone).** *Children:* May repeat dose in 20 min one time. *6–12 mo:* 5–10 mL followed by 20 mL/kg of water *1–12 yr:* 15 mL followed by 20 mL/kg of water *>12 yr and adults:* 30 mL followed by 300 mL of water.	*Cautions:* Do not use if: patient is unconscious, absent gag reflex, seizures, ingestion of strong bases or acids or volatile oils. Do not confuse with ipecac fluid extract, which is 14 times more potent. *Adverse events:* Lethargy, persistent vomiting, diarrhea.
Ipratropium Atrovent. Nebulization solution: 0.02%. Metered-dose inhaler (MDI): 18 µg/puff. Nasal spray: 0.3%, 0.6%.	**Bronchodilator, treatment of rhinitis (anticholinergic).** *Neonates:* Nebulized 100 µg/dose or MDI 1–2 puffs tid–qid. *Infants and children:* Nebulized 125–250 µg or MDI 1–2 puffs 3–6 times/24 hr. *Adults:* Nebulized 500 µg or MDI 2 puffs tid–qid. Nasal spray for rhinitis: 1–2 sprays in each nostril bid–tid.	*Adverse events:* Dry mouth, nervousness, dizziness, headache, blurred vision, urinary retention.
Iron Iron dextran complex (injection). Ferrous sulfate, gluconate, etc. (oral).	**Treatment of iron deficiency, hypochromic, microcytic anemia (replacement therapy).** Injection: IM, IV: Give 0.25–0.5 mL test dose 1 hr before starting iron dextran therapy Dose (mL/kg) = Hgb (normal - actual) × 0.0476 + 1 mL/5 kg max: <5 kg = 25 mg, 5–10 kg = 50 mg >10 kg = 100 mg. PO (mg iron): *Children:* Prophylaxis: 1–2 mg/kg/24 hr. Deficiency: 3–6 mg/kg/24 hr in 1–3 divided doses. *Adults:* Prophylaxis 60 mg/24 hr. Deficiency: 60 mg 2–4 times/24 hr.	*Adverse events:* (Oral) Gastrointestinal irritation, nausea, constipation, dark stools: (IV, IM) hypotension, flushing, dizziness, fever, headache, metallic taste, arthralgia, anaphylaxis. *Monitoring:* Hemoglobin (normal <15 kg = 12 mg%, >15 kg = 14.8 mg%), reticulocyte count, serum ferritin.
Isoetharine Generic. Metered-dose inhaler (MDI), inhalation solution.	**Bronchodilator (β-agonist stimulation).** *Children:* Nebulize 0.01 mL/kg of 1% solution. *Adults:* Nebulize 0.5–1 mL of 0.5–1% solution; MDI 1–2 puffs q4h as needed.	*Adverse events:* Tachycardia, headache, tremor, excitement, restlessness, nausea.
Isoproterenol Generic. Injection, sublingual tablets, nebulizer solution, metered-dose inhaler (MDI).	**Asthma or chronic obstructive pulmonary disease, ventricular arrhythmias due to AV node block, low-output shock states (stimulate β₁- and β₂-receptors).** *Neonates, infants, and children:* IV infusion 0.05–2 µg/kg/min. *Children:* MDI 1–2 puffs every 4 hr as needed; nebulize 0.01 mL of 1% solution; SL tablets 5–10 mg every 3–4 hr (max: 30 mg/24 hr). *Adults:* MDI 1–2 puffs 4–6 times/24 hr; nebulize 0.25–0.5 mL of 1% solution; SL tablets 10–20 mg q3–4h (max: 60 mg/24 hr); IV infusion 2–20 µg/min.	*Adverse events:* Tachycardia, palpitations, chest pain, nervousness, restlessness, anxiety, headache, insomnia, tremor, gastrointestinal distress, nausea, paradoxical bronchospasm.
Kaolin and pectin Generic. Oral suspension.	**Treatment of uncomplicated diarrhea (absorbent action).** *Children:* *3–6 yr:* 15–30 mL/dose. *6–12 yr:* 30–60 mL/dose. *>12 yr:* 60–120 mL/dose.	*Cautions:* Some products contain bismuth subsalicylate and may cause bleeding disorders. Avoid in dysentery, toxigenic diarrheas.
Ketamine Ketalar. Injection: 10 mg/mL, 50 mg/mL, 100 mg/mL.	**Anesthesia for short procedures (direct action on cortex and limbic system to produce dissociative anesthesia).** *Children:* Give 30 min before procedure. PO: 6–10 mg/kg; IM: 3–7 mg/kg; IV: 0.5–2 mg/kg. *Adults:* 3–8 mg/kg; IV: 1–4.5 mg/kg (supplemental doses are ¹/₃ of initial dose).	*Adverse events:* Hypertension, tachycardia, hypotension, bradycardia, increased cerebral blood flow and intracranial pressure, hallucinations, delirium, tonic-clonic movements, increased metabolic rate, hypersalivation, nausea, vomiting, respiratory depression, apnea, increased airway resistance, cough, emergence reactions.

TABLE 712–1. General Medications *Continued*

Drug (Trade Names, Formulations)	Indications (Mechanism of Action) and Dosing	Comments (Cautions, Adverse Events, Monitoring)
Ketorolac Acular. Ophthalmic. Toradol. Tablet, injection.	Treatment of pain; ocular itching with conjunctivitis (NSAID, inhibits prostaglandin). *Children 2–16 yr:* IM, IV: 0.4–1 mg/kg/dose PO: 1 mg/kg/dose q6h if needed. *Adults:* IM: 60 mg; IV: 30 mg up to q6h as needed. Ophthalmic: 1 drop in eye 4 times/24 hr for up to 7 days.	*Adverse events:* Edema, somnolence, dizziness, headache, dyspepsia, nausea, diarrhea, gastrointestinal pain, gastrointestinal bleeding, peptic ulcer, impaired platelet aggregation, oliguria, acute renal failure, dyspnea, wheezing, pain at injection site.
Labetalol Normodyne, Trandate. Injection: 5 mg/mL. Tablet: 100, 200, 300 mg.	Treatment of mild to severe hypertension (blocks α- and β-adrenergic receptors). *Children:* PO: Start 4 mg/kg/24 hr in 2 doses, then gradually increase (max: 40 mg/kg/24 hr). IV: Start 0.2–1 mg/kg/dose (max: 20 mg/dose), continuous IV infusion 0.4–1 mg/kg/hr (max: 3 mg/kg/hr). *Adults:* PO: 100 mg bid; may increase every 2–3 days (max: 2.4 g/24 hr). IV: Start 20 mg; repeat boluses 40 mg q 10 min (max: total dose 300 mg), continuous IV infusion 2 mg/min and titrate to response.	*Adverse events:* Orthostatic hypotension, congestive heart failure, conduction disturbance, bradycardia, drowsiness, fatigue, headache, dry mouth, nasal congestion, bronchospasm.
Lactulose Generic. Syrup: 10 g/15 mL.	Treatment of constipation, hepatic encephalopathy (osmotic effect on stool in colon, acidification of stool promotes NH_4^+ elimination). *Infants:* 2.5–10 mL/24 hr in 3–4 doses. *Children:* 40–90 mL/24 hr in 3–4 doses. *Adults:* 30–45 mL/dose 3–4 times/24 hr.	*Adverse events:* Flatulence, abdominal discomfort, diarrhea, nausea, vomiting. *Monitoring:* Target 2–3 soft stools per day, serum ammonia.
Lamotrigine Lamictal. Tablet: 25, 100, 150, 200 mg. Chewable dispersible tablet: 2, 5, 25 mg.	Treatment of partial seizures (blocks sodium channels and inhibits presynaptic release of glutamate and aspartate). *Children 2–12 yr:* 0.6 mg/kg/24 hr in 1–2 doses for 2 wk, then 1.2 mg/kg/24 hr in 2 doses for 2 wk, then 5–15 mg/kg/24 hr in 2 doses per response (max: 400 mg/24 hr). *If patient is on valproate:* 0.15 mg/kg/24 hr in 1–2 doses for 2 wk, then 0.3 mg/kg/24 hr in 2 doses for 2 wk, then 1–5 mg/kg/24 hr in 2 doses (max: 200 mg/24 hr). *Adults:* Start 50 mg/24 hr for 2 wk, then 100 mg/24 hr, then increase by 100 mg/24 hr at weekly intervals to response (max: 500 mg/24 hr). If patient is on *valproate:* 25 mg every other day for 2 wk, then 25 mg/24 hr for 2 wk, then increase by 25 mg/24 hr every wk to response (max: 150 mg/24 hr).	*Caution:* Serious rashes (potentially fatal) can occur and are particularly common in children and especially if doses are increased too quickly. Slow increase in dosing is especially important for patients on valproic acid. *Adverse events:* Dizziness, sedation, headache, agitation, exacerbation of seizures, rashes (maculopapular or erythematous eruptions), angioedema, photosensitivity, nystagmus, amblyopia, nausea, vomiting.
Lansoprazole Prevacid. Capsule: 15, 30 mg.	Treatment of gastric or duodenal ulcer (proton pump inhibitor). *Children:* *Adults:* 15–30 mg/24 hr.	
Leucovorin Wellcovorin, generic. Tablet: 5, 15 mg. Injection.	Antidote for folic acid antagonists, e.g., methotrexate, treatment of folate-deficient megaloblastic anemias of infancy, nutritional folate deficiency when oral folate cannot be used (reduced form of folic acid so conversion is not necessary, replacement therapy). *Children and adults:* Methotrexate rescue: IV: 10 mg/m² to start then 10 mg/m² PO q6h for 72 hr; increase dose to 100 mg/m² q3h if 24 hr after methotrexate dose the serum creatinine is increased by >50%, or methotrexate serum level is >5 × 10⁻⁶ M (continue until level <1 × 10⁻⁸ M). High-dose methotrexate rescue: IV 100–1000 mg/m²/dose Intrathecal methotrexate: IV 12 mg/m² as single dose Megaloblastic anemia of infancy: IM 3–6 mg/24 hr.	*Adverse events:* Rash, itching erythema. *Monitoring:* Plasma methotrexate levels (a leukovorin dosing nomogram is available based on methotrexate levels at various times after the dose.)
Leuprolide Lupron. Injection.	Treatment of precocious puberty, prostate cancer (decreases levels of luteinizing hormone and follicle-stimulating hormone). 0.15–0.3 mg/kg/dose q 28 days (min: 7.5 mg); SC: 20–45 µg/kg/24 hr. *Adults:* Prostate cancer: IM: 7.5 mg/dose/mo; SC: 1 mg/24 hr.	*Adverse events:* Weight gain, hot flashes, depression, nausea, vomiting, gastrointestinal bleeding, myalgia, bone pain, weakness, blurred vision, estrogenic effects.

Table continued on following page

TABLE 712–1. General Medications *Continued*

Drug (Trade Names, Formulations)	Indications (Mechanism of Action) and Dosing	Comments (Cautions, Adverse Events, Monitoring)
Levothyroxine Synthroid, generic. Injection, tablet.	**Thyroid replacement therapy.** PO: *0–6 mo:* 8–10 µg/kg/24 hr. *6–12 mo:* 6–8 µg/kg/24 hr. *1–5 yr:* 5–6 µg/kg/24 hr. *6–12 yr:* 4–5 µg/kg/24 hr. *>12 yr:* 2–3 µg/kg/24 hr. *Adults:* 12.5–50 µg/24 hr (max: 200 µg/24 hr). IV, IM: 50–75% of PO dose. Myxedema coma: 200–500 µg for one dose. Thyroid suppression therapy: 2–6 µg/kg/24 hr for 7–10 days.	*Adverse events:* Tachycardia, cardiac arrhythmias, hypertension, nervousness, headache, insomnia, hair loss, increased appetite, weight loss, tremor, sweating.
Lidocaine Generic. Injection. Topical (alone or in combination with prilocaine [EMLA]).	**Treatment of ventricular arrhythmias, local anesthetic (class 1B antiarrhythmic, blocks initiation and conduction of impulses).** *Children and adults:* Topical: Apply to affected area (max: 3 mg/kg/dose) at least 2 hr apart. Local anesthetic injection: doses as needed, max: 4.5 mg/kg not closer than 2 hr apart. Arrhythmias: *Children:* Load 1 mg/kg (may repeat q 5–10 min to maximum of 3 mg/kg), IV continuous infusion: 20–50 µg/kg/min ($^1/_2$ dose if liver disease or poor cardiac output). *Adults:* Load 1–1.5 mg/kg (may repeat to maximum of 3 mg/kg), IV continuous infusion: 2–4 mg/min ($^1/_2$ dose for liver disease or heart failure). ET route: 2–2.5 times IV dose. Pre-hospital post–myocardial infarction: 300 mg IM.	*Caution:* Avoid lidocaine with epinephrine preparations for arrhythmias. *Adverse events:* Arrhythmias, heart block, lethargy, coma, seizures, nausea, vomiting, paresthesias, blurred vision, diplopia, local skin irritation or rash. *Monitoring:* Lidocaine serum levels (therapeutic 1–5 µg/mL, toxic >6 µg/mL).
Liothyronine Cytomel (oral), Triostat (injection), generic.	**Replacement therapy in hypothyroidism.** *Neonates, infants, and children <3 yr:* Congenital hypothyroidism (cretinism): PO: 5 µg/24 hr initially then may increase 5 µg q 3 days to maximum of 20 µg/24 hr (50 µg/ 24 hr for children age 1–3 yr). Hypothyroidism: *Children:* 5 µg/24 hr; increase by 5 µg q 1–2 wk (usual 15–20 µg/24 hr). *Adults:* Start 5 µg/24 hr; increase by 5 µg/24 hr q 1–2 wk to 25 µg then by 12.5–25 µg q 1–2 wk to maximum of 100 µg/24 hr.	*Adverse events:* Palpitations, tachycardia, hypertension, nervousness, insomnia, headache, hair loss, diarrhea, abdominal cramps, tremor, sweating. *Monitoring:* Thyroid function, T_3, thyroid-stimulating hormone.
Lithium Generic. Syrup: 300 mg/5 mL. Tablet: 300 mg. Capsule: 150, 300, 600 mg.	**Management of acute mania, bipolar disorders, and depression (alters cation exchange across cell membranes).** *Children:* 15–60 mg/kg/24 hr in 3–4 doses (start low and increase at weekly intervals). *Adolescents:* 600–1,800 mg/24 hr in 3–4 doses at regular intervals. *Adults:* 300 mg 3–4 times/24 hr to start; may gradually increase per blood levels (max 2.4 g/24 hr). **May use twice-daily dosing if sustained-release product used.** *Renal impairment:* CrCl 10–50 mL/min 50–75% of normal dose; CrCl <10 mL/min 25–50% of normal dose.	*Adverse events:* Polydipsia, nausea, diarrhea, impaired taste, bloated feeling, weight gain, tremor, muscle twitching, weakness, fatigue, diabetes insipidus, nonspecific nephron atrophy, renal tubular acidosis, leukocytosis, vision problems, hypothyroidism, goiter, skin eruptions, acne. *Monitoring:* Serum lithium concentrations are essential to proper use of lithium, must be drawn 8–12 hr after a dose (therapeutic: acute mania 0.6–1.2 mEq/L, protection against future episodes 0.6–1 mEq/L; toxic >1.5 mEq/L; seizures >2.5 mEq/L. Watch for accumulation during salt loss and dehydration states.
Lomustine, CCNU CeeNu. Capsule: 10, 40, 100 mg.	**Treatment of various cancers (alkylating agent, inhibits DNA and RNA synthesis).** *Children:* 75–100 mg/m² as single dose every 6 wk. *Adults:* 100–130 mg/m² as single dose every 6 wk.	*Adverse events:* Nausea, vomiting, myelosuppression (onset, 14 days; nadir, 4–5 wk; recovery, 6 wk), neurotoxicity, stomatitis, diarrhea, anemia, alopecia, hepatotoxicity, renal failure, pulmonary fibrosis (with cumulative doses >600 mg). *Monitoring:* Reduce dose if CrCl <50 mL/min, or platelet and WBC counts remain low beyond 6 wk.
Loperamide Imodium, generic. Liquid: 1 mg/5 mL. Tablet: 2 mg. Capsule: 2 mg.	**Treatment of acute and chronic diarrhea (directly inhibits intestinal peristalsis).** *Children:* *2–5 yr:* 1 mg tid. *6–8 yr:* 2 mg bid. *8–12 yr:* 2 mg tid. *Adults:* 4 mg initially, then 2 mg after each loose stool (max: 16 mg/24 hr).	*Adverse events:* Sedation, fatigue, dizziness, nausea, vomiting, constipation.
Loratadine Tablet: 10 mg. Claritin. Syrup: 1 mg/mL.	**Treatment of allergic symptoms (antihistamine, H_1-receptor antagonist).** *Children >3 yr:* <30 kg 5 mg/24 hr, >30 kg 10 mg/24 hr. *Adults:* 10 mg/24 hr.	*Caution:* Prolonged QT intervals may occur if combined with drugs that inhibit liver enzymes; watch for drug interactions. *Adverse events:* Somnolence, fatigue, anxiety, depression, headache.

TABLE 712–1.   **General Medications** *Continued*

Drug (Trade Names, Formulations)	Indications (Mechanism of Action) and Dosing	Comments (Cautions, Adverse Events, Monitoring)
Lorazepam Ativan, generic. Injection. Tablet: 0.5, 1, 2 mg. Oral solution: 2 mg/mL.	**Treatment for anxiety, sedation, and seizures; adjunct to antiemetic therapy (benzodiazepine, increase action of γ-aminobutyric acid).** Antiemetic therapy: *Children:* IV 0.04–0.08 mg/kg/dose q6h as needed. Anxiety/sedation: *Neonates:* IV: 0.1–0.4 mg/kg/dose q4–6h as needed. *Infants and children:* IV: 0.05–0.1 mg/kg/dose q4–8h. *Adults:* PO: 1–10 mg/24 hr in 2–3 divided doses. Insomnia: *Adults:* 2–4 mg at bedtime. Status epilepticus: *Neonates:* IV: 0.05–0.2 mg/kg/dose over 2–5 min; may repeat in 10–15 min. *Infants and children:* IV: 0.1 mg/kg load over 2–5 min; may give additional 0.05 mg/kg bolus in 10–15 min. *Adolescents:* IV: 0.07 mg/kg/dose over 2–5 min; may repeat in 10–15 min. *Adults:* IV: 4 mg/dose over 2–5 min; may repeat in 10 min.	*Caution:* Do not discontinue abruptly after long-term use to avoid possible abstinence symptoms. *Adverse events:* Several cases of myoclonus have been reported in neonates, tachycardia, drowsiness, depression, confusion, paradoxical excitement, blurred vision, and diplopia.
Magnesium citrate, citrate of magnesia Generic. Solution: 300 mL.	**Evacuation of bowel (osmotic retention of fluid and increased peristalsis).** *Children <6 yr:* 2–4 mL/kg. Children 6–12 yr: 100–150 mL. *>12 yr and adults:* 150–300 mL.	*Adverse events:* Hypermagnesemia, hypotension, abdominal cramps, muscle weakness, CNS depression. *Monitoring:* Toxicity related to serum magnesium levels (>3 mg/dL, depressed CNS; >5 mg/dL, somnolence and depressed deep tendon reflexes; >12 mg/dL, respiratory paralysis and heart block).
Magnesium gluconate Generic. Tablet: 500 mg.	**Magnesium replacement therapy.** *Children:* 10–20 mg/kg/dose elemental magnesium qid. *Adults:* 300 mg elemental magnesium qid.	*Adverse events:* Hypermagnesemia (see *Magnesium citrate*). *Monitoring:* Serum magnesium concentration (normal: children, 1.5–1.9 mg/dL; adults, 2.2–2.8 mg/dL).
Magnesium oxide Generic. Tablet: 400, 420, 500 mg. Capsule: 140 mg.		
Magnesium hydroxide, milk of magnesia Generic. Liquid, tablet.	**Short-term treatment of constipation (osmotic retention of fluid promotes peristalsis).** *Children:* *<2 yr:* 0.5 mL/kg/dose. *2–5 yr:* 5–15 mL once daily. *6–12 yr:* 15–30 mL once daily. *>12 yr and adults:* 30–60 mL once daily.	*Adverse events:* (see *Magnesium citrate*).
Magnesium sulfate Generic. Granules: 40 mEq/5 g. Injection: 50% solution.	**Treatment of hypomagnesemia, and seizures associated with acute nephritis in children, also used as a cathartic (cofactor for many enzymes in the body and is important in calcium and potassium hemostasis).** Hypomagnesemia: *Neonates:* IV: 25–50 mg/kg/dose q8h for 2–3 doses. *Children:* PO: 100–200 mg/kg/dose qid; IM, IV: 25–50 mg/kg/dose q6h for 3–4 doses. *Adults:* PO: 3 g q6h for 4 doses; IM, IV: 1 g q6h for 4 doses. Daily maintenance magnesium: *Neonates, infants, and children:* IV: 30–60 mg/ kg/24 hr. *Adolescents:* IV: 42–54 mg/kg/24 hr. *Adults:* IV: 0.5–3 g/24 hr. Infuse IV doses over 2–4 hr (max: 125 mg/kg/hr). Management of seizures and hypertension: *Children:* IM, IV: 20–100 mg/kg/dose q4–6h as needed. Cathartic: *Children:* PO: 0.25 g/kg/dose. *Adults:* PO: 10–30 g.	*Caution:* Magnesium may accumulate to toxic levels in renal insufficiency. *Adverse events:* (see *Magnesium citrate*).
Manganese Injection: 0.1 mg/mL.	**Trace element added to parenteral nutrition (cofactor in many enzyme systems).** *Infants:* 2–10 µg/kg/24 hr in TPN solutions. *Adults:* 150–800 µg/24 hr in TPN solutions.	*Monitoring:* Reference manganese plasma level is 4–14 µg/L.
Mannitol Generic. Injection.	**Promotion of diuresis, reduction of increased intracranial pressure.** *Children and adults:* IV: 200 mg/kg test dose; initial, 0.5–1 g/kg; maintenance, 0.25–0.5 g/kg q4–6h.	*Adverse events:* Circulatory overload, congestive heart failure, headache, chills, seizures, fluid and electrolyte imbalance. *Monitoring:* After test dose evaluate urine output of at least 1 mL/kg/hr (children) or 30–50 mL/hr (adults) for 2–3 hr; for increased intracranial pressure maintain serum osmolality 310–320 mOsm/kg.

Table continued on following page

TABLE 712–1.   General Medications *Continued*

Drug (Trade Names, Formulations)	Indications (Mechanism of Action) and Dosing	Comments (Cautions, Adverse Events, Monitoring)
Mechlorethamine, nitrogen mustard Mustargen Hydrochloride. Injection.	**Cancer chemotherapy (alkylating agent, inhibits DNA and RNA synthesis).** *Children:* As part of MOPP regimen, IV 6 mg/m² on days 1 and 8 of 28-day regimen. *Adults:* IV: 0.4 mg/kg (12–16 mg/m²) as single monthly dose.	*Caution:* Extravasation should be treated promptly with sterile sodium thiosulfate (¹/₆ M) and apply cold compress for 6–12 hr. *Adverse events:* Nausea, vomiting, diarrhea, severe myelosuppression (onset, 4–7 days; nadir, 14 days; recovery, 21 days), ototoxicity, precipitation of herpes zoster, alopecia, hyperuricemia.
Meclizine Generic. Tablet, capsule.	**Prevention and treatment of motion sickness, and treatment of vertigo (anticholinergic and CNS depressant effects).** *Children and adults:* PO: 25–50 mg taken 1 hr before travel for motion sickness; 25–100 mg/24 hr in divided doses for vertigo.	*Adverse events:* Drowsiness, headache, fatigue, dry mouth, increased appetite, weight gain
Medium chain triglycerides MCT Oil. Oil: 14 g/15 mL.	**Dietary supplement for those who cannot digest long-chain fats, ketogenic diet for seizure disorders (nutritional supplement).** *Infants:* 0.5 mL every other feed and may advance by 0.5 mL q 2–3 days as tolerated. *Children:* Ketogenic diet for seizures: 50–70% of total calories (usually about 40 mL with each meal); cystic fibrosis: 1 tablespoon tid. *Adults:* 15 mL tid–qid.	*Adverse events:* Nausea, vomiting, abdominal pain, ketosis.
Medrysone HMS Liquefilm. Ophthalmic solution.	**Treatment of conjunctivitis (inhibits inflammatory response).** *Children and adults:* Ophthalmic: Instill 1 drop in conjunctival sac bid–qid (may use q1–2h for 1–2 days).	*Adverse events:* Local stinging and burning, increased intraocular pressure, cataracts.
Melphalan Alkeran. Injection. Tablet: 2 mg.	**Cancer chemotherapy (alkylating agent, inhibits DNA and RNA synthesis).** *Children:* IV: 10–35 mg/m²/dose q 21–28 days; high-dose: 140–220 mg/m² before bone marrow transplantation. PO: 4–20 mg/m²/24 hr for 1–21 days. *Adults:* IV 16 mg/m²/dose q 2 wk for 4 doses monthly. PO: 0.15 mg/kg/24 hr for 7 days or 0.25 mg/kg/24 hr for 4 days, repeat q 4–6 wk.	*Adverse events:* Myelosuppression (onset, 7 days; nadir, 8–10 days and 27–32 days; recovery, 42–50 days), secondary malignancy, alopecia, vesiculation of skin, syndrome of inappropriate secretion of antidiuretic hormone, nausea, vomiting, diarrhea, stomatitis, hemorrhagic cystitis, pulmonary fibrosis, interstitial pneumonitis, vasculitis.
Meperidine Generic. Injection, syrup: 50 mg/5 mL. Tablet: 50, 100 mg.	**Narcotic analgesic, adjunct to anesthesia (binds to opiate receptors in CNS).** *Children:* IM, IV, SC: 1–1.5 mg/kg/dose q3–4h. *Adults:* IM, IV, SC: 50–100 mg/dose q3–4h as needed (equipotent oral dose is 3 times IV dose).	*Caution:* Scheduled use may result in metabolite accumulation in diminished renal function, which may lead to CNS stimulation or seizures. *Adverse events:* Hypotension, weakness, tiredness, headache, anorexia, stomach cramps, hallucination, paradoxical excitation, seizures, physical and psychological dependence. *Comment:* Equianalgesic dose to morphine 10 mg IV is meperidine 100 mg IV, IM, or 300 mg PO.
Mephenytoin Mesantoin. Tablet: 100 mg.	**Treatment of tonic-clonic and partial seizures (decreases sodium ion influx across cell membranes)** *Children:* 3–15 mg/kg/24 hr in 3 divided doses. *Adults:* Start 50–100 mg/24 hr; then increase weekly by 50–100 mg (max: 800 mg/24 hr).	*Adverse events:* Drowsiness, slurred speech, psychiatric changes, confusion, nausea, vomiting, constipation, leukopenia, hepatitis, blurred vision, nystagmus, photophobia, and lymphadenopathy. *Monitoring:* Total mephenytoin level (25–40 μg/mL).
Mephobarbital Mebaral. Tablets: 32, 50, 100 mg.	**Sedative, treatment of epilepsy (increases seizure threshold).** *Children:* 4–10 mg/kg/24 hr in 2–4 doses. *Adults:* 200–600 mg/24 hr in 2–4 doses.	*Adverse events:* Drowsiness, lethargy, confusion, mental depression, paradoxical excitement, psychological and physical dependence, constipation, nausea, vomiting. *Monitoring:* Phenobarbital concentrations (therapeutic 10–40 μg/mL).
Mercaptopurine Purinethol. Injection, tablet. Extemporaneous formulations.	**Treatment of leukemias and non-Hodgkin lymphoma (antimetabolite, blocks purine synthesis).** *Children:* PO: Induction: 2.5–5 mg/kg once daily; maintenance: 1.5–2.5 mg/kg/24 hr. IV continuous infusion: 50 mg/m²/hr for 24–48 hr *Adults:* PO: Induction: 2.5–5 mg/kg once daily; maintenance: 1.5–2.5 mg/kg/24 hr. *Renal function CrCl <50 mL/min:* dose every 48 hr.	*Adverse events:* Hepatotoxicity (cholestasis and necrosis), nausea, anorexia, vomiting, diarrhea, stomach pain, stomatitis, mucositis, rash, hyperpigmentation, myelosuppression (onset, 7–10 days; nadir, 14 days; recovery, 21 days), renal toxicity, hyperuricemia, eosinophilia, drug fever
Mesna Mesnex. Injection: 100 mg/mL.	**Protects against hemorrhagic cystitis from ifosfamide and cyclophosphamide therapy (binds and detoxifies urotoxic metabolites via active sulfhydryl group).** *Children and adults:* IV: 20% w/w of ifosfamide or cyclophosphamide dose started 15 min before alkylating agent dose, and repeat same mesna dose at 3, 6, 9, and 12 hr after alkylating agent dose. PO: 40% w/w of alkylating agent in 3 doses 4 hr apart.	*Adverse events:* Hypotension, headache, nausea, vomiting, bad taste in mouth, limb pain. *Monitoring:* Urinalysis.
Metaproterenol, orciprenaline Alupent, Metaprel, generic.	**Bronchodilator (stimulates β₂-receptors).** *Children:*	*Caution:* Some generic nebulizer solutions contain sulfites that may exacerbate asthma.

TABLE 712–1. **General Medications** *Continued*

Drug (Trade Names, Formulations)	Indications (Mechanism of Action) and Dosing	Comments (Cautions, Adverse Events, Monitoring)
Metered-dose inhaler (MDI). Inhalation solution. Tablet: 10, 20 mg. Syrup: 10 mg/5 mL.	PO: *<2 yr:* 0.4 mg/kg/dose tid–qid. *2–6 yr:* 1.3–2.6 mg/kg/24 hr divided q6h. *6–9 yr:* 10 mg/dose qid. *>9 yr and adults:* 20 mg/dose tid–qid. MDI: 2–3 puffs q4h. Nebulizer: *Infants and children:* 0.01–0.02 mL/kg of 5% solution q4–6h. *Adolescents and adults:* 0.3 mL of 5% solution q4–6h.	*Adverse events:* Tremor, nervousness, overactivity, tachycardia, hypotension, headache. *Comment:* Dilute nebulizer solution in 2.5 mL normal saline.
Methadone Dolophine, generic. Injection: 10 mg/mL. Tablet: 5, 10 mg. Oral solution: 5 mg/mL.	**Management of severe pain, narcotic detoxification (binds to opiate receptors in CNS).** *Neonates (abstinence syndrome):* 0.05–0.2 mg/kg/dose q12h; then adjust/taper based on abstinence scores. *Children:* Analgesia: IV, IM, PO: 0.1 mg/kg/dose q4h for 2–3 doses, then q6–12h as needed. Narcotic abstinence: Start 0.05–0.1 mg/kg/dose q6h and taper per abstinence scores. *Adults:* IV, IM, SC, PO. Analgesia: 2.5–20 mg q6–8h. Detoxification: 15–40 mg/24 hr.	*Adverse events:* Weakness, drowsiness, dizziness, nausea, vomiting, constipation, ileus. *Monitoring:* Methadone accumulates with repeated doses and patients should be monitored for excess CNS depression.
Metformin Glucophage. Tablet: 500, 850, 100 mg.	**Treatment of type 2 diabetes; increases insulin sensitivity and improves glucose tolerance; hypoglycemic effect.** *Children 10–16 yr:* Start with 500 mg bid with meals; increase in 500-mg increments weekly to response (max: 2,000 mg/24 hr). *Adults:* Start with 850 mg q24h or 500 mg bid; titrate by 500 mg once/wk or 850 mg q 2 wk to response or maximum dose 2550 mg/24 hr.	*Caution:* Avoid use if creatinine clearance <60 mL/min, serum creatinine >1.5 mg/dL (males) or >1.4 mg/dL (females). Monitor for lactic acidosis. Discontinue for any process that may predispose to metabolic acidosis or renal dysfunction until the situation is resolved. Avoid alcohol. *Adverse events:* Nausea, vomiting, diarrhea, indigestion, flatulence.
Methimazole Tapazole. Tablet: 5, 10 mg.	**Treatment of hyperthyroidism (blocks iodine synthesis in the thyroid gland, inhibits synthesis of thyroid hormone).** *Children:* Start 0.4 mg/kg/24 hr, then maintenance 0.2 mg/kg/24 hr. *Adults:* Start 5 mg/kg q8h; maintenance dose: 5–15 mg/24 hr (max: 60 mg/24 hr).	*Adverse events:* Fever, rash, leukopenia, agranulocytosis, SLE-like syndrome, nausea, vomiting, stomach pain, loss of taste, cholestatic jaundice, constipation, weight gain. *Monitoring:* Thyroid function tests for hypothyroidism or hyperthyroidism.
Methocarbamol Robaxin, generic. Injection: 100 mg/mL. Tablet: 500, 750 mg.	**Treatment of muscle spasm (skeletal muscle relaxant through CNS depressive effects).** *Children:* Treatment of tetanus: IV: 15 mg/kg/dose q6h for 3 days only. *Adults:* IV: 1–2 g q6h. PO: 1.5 g tid–qid for 2–3 days, then decrease to 4–4.5 g/24 hr.	*Adverse events:* Syncope, bradycardia, hypotension, drowsiness, dizziness, headache, nausea, metallic taste.
Methohexital Brevital. Injection.	**Induction and maintenance of general anesthesia (ultra-short-acting barbiturate).** *Children:* IM (preoperative): 5–10 mg/kg/dose; IV: (induction) 1–2 mg/kg/dose. Rectal: 20–35 mg/kg/dose. *Adults:* IV (induction): 50–120 mg, then 20–40 mg q 4–7 min.	*Adverse events:* Apnea, respiratory depression, hiccups, laryngospasm, hypotension, skeletal muscle twitching and rigidity, tremor, seizures, headache, nausea, vomiting.
Methotrexate Generic. Injection. Tablet: 2.5 mg.	**Treatment of neoplasms, psoriasis, rheumatoid arthritis (antimetabolite, inhibition of DNA and purine synthesis).** *Children:* Juvenile rheumatoid arthritis: PO, IM: 5–15 mg/m²/wk as a single dose. Antineoplastic: PO, IM: 7.5–30 mg/m² q 1–2 wk; IV: 10–33 g/m² bolus dose or infused over 6–42 hr. *Adults:* Rheumatoid arthritis: PO: 7.5 mg once wk. Psoriasis: PO, IM: 10–25 mg/dose once/wk. Antineoplastic: PO, IM, IV: 25–50 mg/m²/wk. Reduced renal function: CrCl 61–80 mL/min = reduce 25%. CrCl 51–60 mL/min = reduce 33%. CrCl 10–50 mL/min = reduce dose by 50–70%.	*Caution:* Avoid if severe renal or hepatic dysfunction. *Adverse events:* Hepatotoxicity, nephropathy, vasculitis, malaise, fatigue, encephalopathy, headache, seizures, chills, fever, cystitis, stomatitis, enteritis, nausea, vomiting, diarrhea, alopecia, photosensitivity, increase or decrease in skin pigmentation, urticaria, arthralgia, hyperuricemia, myelosuppression (onset, 7 days; nadir, 10 days; recovery, 21 days). *Monitoring:* Methotrexate concentrations (toxic if >1 × 10⁻⁷ mol/L for more than 40 hr. Ensure adequate hydration and urinary alkalinization.
Methsuximide Celontin. Capsule: 150, 300 mg.	**Control of absence seizures, and adjunct in partial complex seizure management (increases seizure threshold, suppresses nerve transmission).** *Children:* 10–15 mg/kg/24 hr divided in 3–4 doses; may increase at weekly intervals (max: 30 mg/kg/24 hr). *Adults:* Start 300 mg/24 hr; may increase by 300 mg/24 hr at weekly intervals (max: 1,200 mg/24 hr).	*Adverse events:* Dizziness, drowsiness, lethargy, headache, ataxia, aggressiveness, depression, anorexia, nausea, vomiting, hiccups, agranulocytosis, aplastic anemia, leukopenia, thrombocytopenia. *Monitoring:* Methsuximide concentrations (therapeutic 10–40 μg/mL, toxic >4 μg/mL).

Table continued on following page

TABLE 712–1. **General Medications** *Continued*

Drug (Trade Names, Formulations)	Indications (Mechanism of Action) and Dosing	Comments (Cautions, Adverse Events, Monitoring)
Methyldopa Aldomet, generic. Injection: 50 mg/mL. Tablet: 125, 250, 500 mg. Oral suspension: 250 mg/5 mL.	**Treatment of hypertension (false α-neurotransmitter metabolite stimulates inhibitory α-adrenergic receptors).** *Children:* PO: Start 10 mg/kg in 2–4 doses; may increase q 2 days (max: 65 mg/kg/24 hr or 3 g/24 hr). IV: Start 2–4 mg/kg/dose; may increase to 5–10 mg/kg/dose per response (max: 65 mg/kg/24 hr). *Adults:* PO: Start 250 mg 3 times/24 hr; may increase to max 3 g/24 hr. IV: 0.25–1 g q6h (max: 4 g/24 hr). Renal dysfunction: Extend interval.	*Caution:* Tolerance to effects occurs, so chronic use requires concurrent diuretic. *Adverse events:* Drowsiness, mental depression, headache, dry mouth, fever, chills, vertigo, fluid retention, edema, hepatocellular injury, cholestatic liver disease, cirrhosis, pancreatitis, nausea, vomiting, diarrhea, hemolytic anemia, positive Coombs test, leukopenia, thrombocytopenia, paresthesias, weakness, hypotension, bradycardia. *Monitoring:* Blood pressure, liver enzymes, Coombs test (direct).
Methylene blue Urolene Blue. Injection: 10 mg/mL. Tablet: 65 mg.	**Antidote for cyanide poisoning and drug-induced methemoglobinemia (promotes conversion of methemoglobin to hemoglobin, combines with cyanide to form cyan-methemoglobin).** *Children and adults:* Methemoglobinemia: IV: 1–2 mg/kg; may repeat after 1 hr if needed. NADPH-methemoglobin reductase deficiency: PO: 1–1.5 mg/kg/24 hr (given with 5–8 mg/kg/24 hr of ascorbic acid).	*Caution:* Avoid in glucose-6-phosphate dehydrogenase deficiency and renal insufficiency. *Adverse events:* Urine and feces turn blue-green, anemia.
Methylphenidate Ritalin, generic. Tablet: 5, 10, 20 mg. Tablet, sustained release: 20 mg.	**Attention deficit disorder (ADD), narcolepsy, adjunct for pain management (CNS stimulant).** *Children >5 yr:* 0.3–0.6 mg/kg/dose (max: 2 mg/kg/24 hr). *Adults:* 10 mg bid–tid (max: 60 mg/24 hr).	*Cautions:* Avoid in patients with motor tics, Tourette syndrome, or marked agitation or psychosis. May become addictive if used in high doses at frequent intervals. *Adverse events:* Nervousness, insomnia, agitation, anorexia, disorders, tics, growth retardation (controversial and minimal if real), addiction (not a concern with typical ADD dosing).
Methylprednisolone Solu-Medrol (injection). Depo-Medrol (injection, IM). Medrol (tablets), generic. Topical ointment.	**Anti-inflammatory and immunosuppressant glucocorticoid used in allergic, inflammatory, and neoplastic disorders, and acute spinal cord injury.** *Children:* Anti-inflammatory and immunosuppressant: PO, IM, IV: 0.5–2 mg/kg/24 hr divide q6–12h. Lupus nephritis: IV: 30 mg/kg every other day for 6 doses. Acute spinal cord injury: 30 mg/kg over 15 min, followed in 45 min by continuous infusion of 5.4 mg/kg/hr for 23 hr. PO: 2–60 mg/24 hr in 1–4 doses. IV: 40–250 mg q4–6h. IM: 10–80 mg/24 hr.	*Caution:* Avoid if live virus vaccine given or tuberculosis or fungal infection present. *Adverse events:* Hypertension, edema, nervousness, agitation, psychosis, pseudomotor cerebri, headache, mood swing, delirium, euphoria, hyperglycemia, hypokalemia, alkalosis, HPA-axis (adrenal) suppression, Cushing syndrome, skin atrophy, bruising, hyperpigmentation, peptic ulcer disease, muscle weakness, bone loss, joint pain, growth retardation, cataracts, glaucoma, immunosuppression. *Comment:* See comparison of corticosteroids under *Hydrocortisone.*
Metoclopramide Reglan, generic. Injection: 5 mg/mL. Tablet: 5, 10 mg. Oral solution: 10 mg/mL. Syrup: 5 mg/5 mL.	**Treatment of diabetic gastroparesis, gastroesophageal reflux, and nausea associated with chemotherapy and surgery (blocks dopamine receptors in chemoreceptor trigger zone, enhances gastrointestinal motility and gastroduodenal sphincter tone).** *Neonates infants, and children:* Gastroesophageal reflux: IV, PO: 0.033–0.1 mg/kg/dose q8h. *Children:* Postoperative antiemetic: IV: 0.1–0.2 mg/kg/dose q6–8h as needed. Chemotherapy antiemetic: PO, IV: 1–2 mg/kg/dose q2–4h (pre-treat with diphenhydramine to avoid extrapyramidal reactions). *Adults:* Antiemetic: PO, IV: 1–2 mg/kg/dose q2–4h. Gastroesophageal reflux: PO: 10–15 mg qid. Renal dysfunction: Decrease dose.	*Cautions:* May precipitate seizures, cause acute dystonic reactions, and worsen asthma (if sulfite-containing formulation). In elderly, chronic use is associated with increased risk and earlier onset of Parkinson disease (pediatric studies lacking). *Adverse events:* Weakness, drowsiness, diarrhea, prolactin stimulation, breast tenderness, extrapyramidal reactions; IV administration is associated with an intense feeling of anxiety and restlessness followed by drowsiness. *Comment:* Administer oral doses 30 min before meals and at bedtime. *Monitoring:* Creatinine clearance: CrCl 40–50 mL/min: give 75% of recommended dose; CrCl <40 mL/min: give 50% of recommended dose; CrCl <10 mL/min: give 25% of recommended dose.
Metolazone Zaroxolyn, Mykrox. Tablet.	**Treatment of fluid overload states (diuresis, inhibits sodium reabsorption at distal tubules).** *Children:* 0.2–0.4 mg/kg/24 hr in 1–2 doses. *Adults:* 2.5–20 mg/24 hr.	*Adverse events:* Fluid and electrolyte imbalance, hyperglycemia, hypocalcemia, hypomagnesemia, nausea, vomiting, blood dyscrasias.
Metoprolol Lopressor. Injection: 1 mg/mL. Tablet: 50, 100 mg.	**Treatment of hypertension, tachyarrhythmias, idiopathic hypertrophic subaortic stenosis, migraine prophylaxis (selective blocker of β_1-receptors).** *Children:* PO: 1–5 mg/kg/24 hr. *Adults:* PO: 100–450 mg/24 hr in 2–3 doses; IV: 5 mg q 2 min for 3 doses.	*Adverse events:* Mental depression, tiredness, weakness, bradycardia, reduced peripheral circulation, worsens diabetes mellitus, worsens asthma, insomnia, nightmares.

TABLE 712–1. **General Medications** *Continued*

Drug (Trade Names, Formulations)	Indications (Mechanism of Action) and Dosing	Comments (Cautions, Adverse Events, Monitoring)
Mexilitene Mexitil, generic. Capsule: 150, 200, 250 mg. Extemporaneous formulation.	**Treatment of ventricular arrhythmias, neuropathic pain (class 1B antiarrhythmic).** *Children:* 1.4–5 mg/kg/dose q8h. *Adults:* 200 mg q8h (max: 1,200 mg/24 hr). Renal dysfunction: CrCl <10 mL/min: give 50% of dose.	*Adverse events:* Atrial and ventricular arrhythmias, bradycardia, hypotension, confusion, dizziness, nervousness, tremor, ataxia, numbness of fingers or toes, weakness, blurred vision, tinnitus, increased liver enzymes, gastrointestinal discomfort. *Monitoring:* Mexiletine concentrations: therapeutic 0.5–2 µg/mL, toxic >2 µg/mL.
Midazolam Versed. Injection: 1 mg/mL, 5 mg/mL. Extemporaneous formulation.	**Sedation, anticonvulsant (benzodiazepine, increase γ-aminobutyric acid).** *Neonates:* IV: Continuous infusion 0.15–0.5 µg/ kg/min for sedation; IV bolus 0.05–0.15 mg/ kg q2–4h. *Infants and children:* Status epilepticus: IV load 0.15 mg/kg followed by continuous infusion 1 µg/kg/min. Sedation: IV: 0.05–0.2 mg/kg load, then either same dose q1–2h or continuous infusion 1–2 µg/kg/min. Intranasal: 2.5 mg (0.5 mL) in each naris (total, 5 mg) using 5 mg/mL injection. *>12 yr:* 0.5 mg q 3–4 min to effect. *Adults:* 0.5–2 mg q 2 min to effect (usually 2–5 mg).	*Adverse events:* Several cases of myoclonus and prolonged movement disorders have been reported in neonates treated with midazolam. Withdrawal reactions may occur if abrupt discontinuation. Sedation, amnesia, paradoxical excitation, blurred vision, diplopia, nasal burning, apnea, respiratory depression noted.
Mitomycin Mutamycin. Injection.	**Cancer chemotherapy (antibiotic type alkylating agent inhibits DNA and RNA synthesis).** *Children and adults:* Depends on protocol; typically IV 3 mg/m²/24 hr for 5 days q4–6 wk; up to 40–50 mg/m² single dose for bone marrow transplant.	*Adverse events:* Nausea, vomiting, myelosuppression (onset, 21 days; nadir, 36 days; recovery, 42–56 days), tingling of extremities, paresthesias, alopecia, fingernail discoloration, mouth ulcers, cardiac failure (doses >30 mg), interstitial pneumonitis, pulmonary fibrosis.
Mitoxantrone, DHAD Novantrone. Injection.	**Cancer chemotherapy (anthracycline analog inhibits DNA and RNA synthesis throughout entire cell cycle).** Acute nonlymphocytic leukemias: *Children <2 yr:* 0.4 mg/kg/24 hr for 3–5 days. *>2 yr and adults:* 8–12 mg/m²/24 hr for 5 days. Solid tumors: *Children:* 18–20 mg/m² q 3–4 wk or 5–8 mg/m² weekly. *Adults:* 12–14 mg/m² q 3–4 wk (max: total 80–120 mg/m²).	*Adverse events:* Cardiotoxicity (less than other anthracyclines), seizures, headache, fever, elevated liver enzymes, renal failure, conjunctivitis, myelosuppression (onset, 7–10 days; nadir, 14 days; recovery, 21 days).
Molindone hydrochloride Moban. Tablet: 5, 10, 25, 50, 100 mg. Oral concentrate: 20 mg/mL.	**Management of psychotic disorder (actions similar to chlorpromazine but more extrapyramidal effects and less sedation).** *Children:* *3–5 yr:* 1–2.5 mg/kg/24 hr in 4 doses. *5–12 yr:* 0.5–1 mg/kg/24 hr in 4 doses. *Adults:* 50–225 mg/24 hr.	*Adverse events:* Extrapyramidal effects, akathisia, dyskinesias, constipation, blurred vision, orthostatic hypotension, seizures, neuroleptic malignant syndrome, dry mouth, weight gain, galactorrhea, urinary retention, agranulocytosis, leukopenia, retinal pigmentation.
Montelukast Singulair. Tablet: 4 (chewable), 5 (chewable), 10 mg.	**Prophylaxis and chronic treatment of asthma (leukotriene receptor blocker for LTD4).** *Children 2–5 yr:* 4 mg once daily in evening. *Children: 6–14 yr:* 5 mg once daily in the evening. *>15 yr and adults:* 10 mg once daily in the evening.	*Adverse events:* Headache, dizziness, dyspepsia, fatigue, elevated liver enzymes.
Morphine Generic. Injection, oral solution, suppository. Tablet, sustained-release (SR). Tablet, controlled-release (CR). Tablet.	**Relief of moderate to severe pain (narcotic analgesic).** *Neonates:* IV, IM, SC. Analgesia: 0.05–0.2 mg/kg/dose q 2–4 hr; continuous infusion 0.025–0.05 mg/kg/hr. *Infants and children:* IV, IM, SC: 0.1–0.2 mg/kg/ dose q 2–4 hr; PO: 0.2–0.5 mg/kg/dose q4–6h. *Adolescents >12 yr:* IV: 3–4 mg; may repeat in 5 min if needed. *Adults:* PO: 10–30 mg q4h or CR tablet 15–30 mg q8–12h. IV, IM, SC: 2.5–20 mg/dose q2–6h as needed or continuous infusion 0.8–10 mg/hr.	*Cautions:* May develop physical dependence after >5–7 days continuous use; if so, taper dose. Some preparations contain sulfites. *Adverse events:* Hypotension, bradycardia, nausea, vomiting, constipation, sedation, confusion, decreased urination, respiratory depression.
Mupirocin Bactroban. Ointment: 2%.	**Topical treatment of impetigo and other gram- positive skin infections (inhibit bacterial protein and RNA synthesis).** *Children and adults:* Apply to affected area 4–5 times daily. Intranasal (eliminate nasal carriage of *Staphylococcus aureus*): Apply small amount bid–qid for 5–14 days.	*Adverse events:* Stinging and irritation at application site.
Muromonab-CD3, OKT3	**Treatment of acute allograft rejection in renal transplant patients (coats circulating T lymphocytes facilitating their opsonization by the reticuloendothelial system, and promotes removal of all CD3 molecules from T lymphocyte antigen receptor complex).**	*Cautions:* Severe first-dose reactions may occur; recommend methylprednisolone 1 mg/kg IV 2–6 hr before first OKT3 dose and hydrocortisone 100 mg IV 30 min after each OKT3 dose and as needed.

Table continued on following page

MEDICATIONS

TABLE 712–1. General Medications *Continued*

Drug (Trade Names, Formulations)	Indications (Mechanism of Action) and Dosing	Comments (Cautions, Adverse Events, Monitoring)
Orthoclone OKT3. Injection: 5 mg/5 mL.	*Children <12 yr:* 0.1 mg/kg/24 hr for 10–14 days; or if <30 kg, give 2.5 mg/24 hr for 10–14 days. *>12 yr and adults:* 5 mg/24 hr for 10–14 days.	*Adverse events:* Shortness of breath, pulmonary edema, fever, chills, trembling, nausea, vomiting, diarrhea, headache, stiff neck, photophobia, flu-like symptoms. *Monitoring:* OKT3 serum trough levels (if maintained near 1µg/mL then CD3 counts remain low).
Mycophenolate mofetil CellCept. Capsule: 250 mg.	**Prevent rejection of allograph transplants, used in conjunction with other drugs (active metabolite MPA inhibits T- and B-cell proliferation, T-cell generation, and antibody secretion).** *Children:* 600 mg/m²/dose bid. *Adults:* 1,000 mg/dose bid.	*Adverse events:* Hypertension, insomnia, dizziness, fever, headache, bone marrow suppression, tremor, back pain, myalgia, dyspnea, cough, pharyngitis, hematuria, renal tubular necrosis, lymphoproliferative disease.
Nadolol Corgard. Tablet: 20, 40, 80, 120, 160 mg.	**Antiarrhythmic, antihypertensive, and migraine prophylaxis: (nonselective β-adrenergic receptor antagonist).** *Children:* 0.5–2.5 mg/kg PO q24h for supraventricular tachycardia. *Adults:* 40 mg q24h; titrate upward to desired effect (usual dose: 40–80 mg/24 hr up to 640 mg/24 hr).	*Cautions:* Should not be used in patients with asthma, bronchoconstriction, or uncontrolled heart failure. Adjust dose with renal dysfunction (CrCl <50 mL/min). *Adverse effects:* Bradycardia, heart failure, bronchospasm. *Drug interactions:* Other hypotensive drugs, diuretics. Antagonizes β-sympathomimetic drugs (e.g., albuterol).
Nalbuphine Nubain. IV, IM, SQ: 10 mg/mL.	**Analgesic (opiate agonist with partial opiate antagonistic activity for treatment of moderate to severe pain).** *Children ≥1 yr:* 0.1–0.2 mg/kg IV, IM, SC, q3–4h. Maximal single dose: 20 mg; maximal daily dose: 160 mg.	*Cautions:* Like most opiate analgesics may stimulate histamine release and cause CNS and respiratory depression. Use with caution in hepatic disease or with other respiratory depressants. Dependence potential. *Adverse effects:* Hypotension, sedation, respiratory depression. Naloxone reverses effects.
Naloxone Narcan, generic. Injection: 0.4 mg/mL. Injection neonate: 0.02 mg/mL.	**Opiate antagonist: antagonizes all opiate receptors—used in the treatment of opiate excess (overdose, poisoning).** *Neonates and children:* 0.1 mg/kg IV (max dose: 2 mg). If no response, repeat q 2–3 min until desired effect. May give by continuous IV infusion.	*Cautions:* May precipitate acute opiate withdrawal. Duration of effect of many opiates may be longer than naloxone requiring individualized naloxone dosing. Administer via IV push.
Naproxen Aleve, Anaprox, Naprosyn, generic. Tablet: 220, 250, 275, 375, 550 mg. Suspension: 125 mg/5 mL.	**Nonsteroidal anti-inflammatory drug for the treatment of mild to moderate pain, inflammation, fever (inhibits prostaglandin synthesis).** *Neonates:* Do not use owing to probably negative effects on renal function. *Children:* 5–7 mg/kg PO q8–12h. *Adults:* 250–375 mg PO q8–12h (max: 1,250 mg/24 hr).	*Cautions:* Gastrointestinal upset/irritation, reversible interference with platelet aggregation. Do not administer to infants <3 mo of age. *Adverse effects:* Dizziness, gastrointestinal irritation, rash, age-related decreased renal function.
Nedocromil Tilade. Aerosol: 1.75 mg/activation.	**Chronic treatment of asthma/allergic disorders. Mast cell stabilizer (also stabilizes other cells to mediator release—neutrophils, eosinophils, platelets), nonsteroidal.** *Children and adults:* 1–2 puffs 2–4 times/24 hr. Dose titrated to clinical response.	*Cautions:* Only effective as chronic therapy. Produces no bronchodilatation. *Adverse effects:* Dysphonia, chest irritation/pain.
Neostigmine Prostigmin, generic. Tablet: 15 mg (as bromide). Injection: 0.25, 0.5, 1 mg/mL (as methylsulfate).	**Treatment of myasthenia gravis, reversal of nondepolarizing neuromuscular blocking agents (NDNM). Competitively inhibits acetylcholine esterase augmenting effects of endogenous acetylcholine.** *Children:* 0.01–0.04 mg/kg IV, IM, SC q2–4h; titrate dose to desired effect. To reverse NDNM 0.025–1 mg/kg/dose (max adult dose: 5 mg).	*Cautions:* Patients with asthma/bronchospasm, bradycardia. Does not antagonize succinylcholine. *Adverse effects:* Bradycardia, abdominal cramps, urinary frequency.
Niacin Nicobid, generic. Tablet: 25, 50, 100, 250, 500 mg. Tablet, timed-release: 150, 250, 500, 750 mg. Capsule, timed-release: 125, 250, 300, 400, 500 mg. Elixir: 50 mg/5 mL. Injection: 100 mg/mL.	**Vitamin supplementation (vitamin B₃), hyperlipidemia, vasodilator.** *Children:* IV, IM, SC, PO titrated to desired effect (max: 10 mg/kg/24 hr).	*Cautions:* Titrate dose upward and administer IV slowly to avoid/minimize flushing. *Adverse effects:* Flushing, tachycardia, dizziness, hyperuricemia. *Drug interactions:* Augments hypotensive effects of antihypertensives.
Nifedipine Adalat, Procardia, generic. Capsule (liquid filled): 10, 20 mg. Tablet, timed-release: 30, 60, 90 mg. Capsule, timed-release: 30, 60, 90 mg.	**Antihypertensive, antiarrhythmic calcium channel antagonist.** *Infants and children:* Hypertensive emergency 0.25–0.5 mg/kg/dose PO/SL: q4–6h (max: 10 mg). Hypertropic cardiomyopathy: 0.2–0.3 mg/kg PO q8h. *Adults:* 10 mg/dose titrated to effect (max: 120–180 mg/24 hr).	*Caution:* Do not crush or break timed-release tablet. *Adverse effects:* Profound, acute hypotension, flushing, dizziness. More rapid effect if drug is administered without food. Concurrent grapefruit juice may increase bioavailability and effects. *Drug interactions:* Cimetidine, cyclosporine, phenytoin, possibly digoxin. *Comment:* Preferred route is oral, not SL. Clinical effects due to swallowing. Capsule content approximates 10 mg in 0.34 mL and 20 mg in 0.45 mL.
Nitric oxide Nitroprusside Nipride, generic. Injection: 10 mg/mL, 25 mg/mL.	**Antihypertensive, congestive heart failure: controlled, titratable blood pressure control.** *Children and adults:* 0.3–0.5 µg/kg/min; titrate dose to desired effect; rarely requires >6 µg/kg/min (probable max: 8 µg/kg/min).	*Cautions:* Metabolized to thiocyanate/cyanide, which accumulates with renal dysfunction. *Adverse effects:* Profound hypotension, tachycardia, thyroid suppression, acidosis, seizures. Cyanide toxicity—metabolic acidosis, pink skin methemoglobinemia.

TABLE 712–1. General Medications *Continued*

Drug (Trade Names, Formulations)	Indications (Mechanism of Action) and Dosing	Comments (Cautions, Adverse Events, Monitoring)
		Administer by continuous IV infusion. Protect solution from direct light. Thiosulfate co-administration prevents toxicity (10 mg thiosulfate for each 1 mg nitroprusside).
Norepinephrine bitartrate Levophed. Injection: 1 mg/mL base.	**Hypotension/shock. Sympathomimetic/ adrenergic agonist.** *Children:* 0.05–0.1 µg/kg/min; titrate dose to desired effect (max dose: 2 µg/kg/min).	*Cautions:* Extravasation may cause severe tissue necrosis. Administer into large vein by continuous IV infusion. Ensure patient fluid status. May cause profound vasoconstriction. *Adverse effects:* Hypertension, cardiac arrhythmias, headache. Drug dose based on norepinephrine base.
Nortriptyline Aventyl, Pamelor, generic. Capsule: 10, 25, 50, 75 mg. Solution: 10 mg/5 mL.	**Tricyclic antidepressant, nocturnal enuresis: central synaptic norepinephrine/serotonin reuptake inhibitor.** *Children:* Nocturnal enuresis: 10–20 mg/24 hr; titrate upward to maximum of 40 mg/24 hr. Depression: 1–3 mg/kg PO/24 hr (bedtime) titrated to effect. May give in divided doses q6h (usual max dose: 150 mg/24 hr).	*Cautions:* Avoid in patients with cardiac conduction abnormalities, cardiac disease. Slow dose adjustment in patients with hepatic dysfunction. *Adverse effects:* Anticholinergic effects (dry mouth, tachycardia, blurred vision, urinary retention), sedation. *Drug interactions:* Clonidine, MAO inhibitors.
Octreotide Sandostatin. Injection: 0.05, 0.1, 0.2, 0.5, 1 mg/mL.	**Antisecretory somatostatin analog.** *Children:* Secretory diarrhea: 1–10 µg/kg IV, SC q12 hr; titrate dose to effect. May give via continuous IV infusion *Adults:* For treatment of vasoactive intestinal peptide secreting tumors: 100–150 µg IV, SC q12h.	*Cautions:* Continuous long-term use (months) may cause cholelithiasis, hypothyroidism. *Adverse effects:* Flushing, dizziness, hypo/hyperglycemia. Infuse IV over 20–30 min, IV push over 3 min.
Olanzapine Zyprexa Tablet: 2.5, 5, 7.5, 10, 15, 20 mg.	**Atypical antipsychotic, monaminergic antagonist with high affinity for serotonin, dopamine, histamine, muscarinic, and α_1-adrenergic receptors. Actual mechanism of action is unknown.** *Children:* Start 2.5–5 mg q24h; titrate weekly by 2.5–5 mg to 15–20 mg/24 hr as q24h dosing. *Adults:* Start 5–10 mg/24 hr; increase by 5 mg weekly to response (max: 20 mg/24 hr).	*Adverse events:* Postural hypotension, somnolence, tremor, dizziness, akathisia, asthenia, dry mouth, constipation, dyspepsia, increased appetite, weight gain, hyperglycemia, amenorrhea and vaginitis in females.
Olsalazine Dipentum. Capsule: 10, 20, 250 mg.	**Inflammatory bowel disease, anti-inflammatory drug, 5-aminosalicylic acid derivative.** *Adults:* 500 mg q12h.	*Cautions:* Administer with food. *Adverse effects:* Headache, cramps, diarrhea, dizziness, rash, cholestasis.
Omeprazole Prilosec. Capsule: 10, 20 mg.	**Gastric acid hypersecretion/ulcer disease. Proton pump inhibitor of parietal cell hydrogen ion secretion.** *Children:* 0.6–0.7 mg/kg PO q24h. Dose titrated to desired gastric pH. *Adults:* Usual 20–40 mg/24 hr PO.	*Caution:* Drug granules in capsule must be swallowed whole; do not chew *Drug interactions:* May decrease diazepam, phenytoin clearance. May reduce itraconazole, digoxin absorption.
Ondansetron Ondansetron. Tablet: 4, 8 mg. Injection: 2 mg/mL.	**Antiemetic. Treatment of nausea/vomiting associated with cancer chemotherapy/ surgery and other causes (drug toxicity). Selective serotonin-3 receptor antagonist.** *Infants and children:* 0.15 mg/kg IV q8h; may give as continuous IV infusion 0.45 mg/kg/24 hr (max: 24–32 mg/24 hr). Child PO dose for mild to moderate nausea/vomiting: 4–8 mg q8–12h).	*Adverse effects:* Headache, chest pain. Does not cause dystonia/sedation. *Comment:* Oral bioavailability ~50%. Doses given ~30 min before starting chemotherapy.
Oxcarbazepine Trileptal. Tablet (film-coated): 150, 300, 600 mg. Suspension: 300 mg/5 mL.	**Used for seizure disorders (except absence).** *Children 3–17 yr:* Start 8–10 mg/kg/24 hr divided bid (max: 600 mg/24 hr); increase over 2 wk to 30–45 mg/kg/24 hr divided bid per response. *Adults:* Start at 600 mg/24 hr divided bid, then gradually increase over 2–4 wk to 1,200 mg/24 hr divided bid (max: 2,400 mg/24 hr).	*Cautions:* Cut dose in half if creatinine clearance <30 mL/min. Toxicities are mainly CNS (headache, somnolence, dizziness, etc), diplopia, gastrointestinal (nausea, vomiting, diarrhea) and hyponatremia.
Oxybutynin Ditropan, generic. Tablet: 5 mg. Syrup: 5 mg/5 mL.	**Urinary antispasmodic. Relaxes smooth muscle by antagonizing acetylcholine.** *Children:* 0.2 mg/kg PO q6–12h (max: 5 mg PO q8h). *Adults:* 5 mg per dose up to 4 times daily.	*Cautions:* Patients with renal and/or liver disease. *Adverse effects:* Tachycardia, drowsiness, sedation, dry mouth, blurred vision. *Drug interactions:* Additive anticholinergic effects/CNS depression, e.g., antihistamines.
Oxycodone (Various brands, generic). Tablet: 5 mg.	**Analgesic. Opiate analgesic for the treatment of moderate to severe pain.** *Children:* 0.05–0.15 mg/kg PO q4–6h (max: 5 mg). *Adults:* 5 mg per dose PO q4–6h (max: 5 mg.)	*Cautions:* Like most opiate analgesics may stimulate histamine release and may cause CNS and respiratory depression. Use with caution in hepatic disease or with other respiratory depressants. Dependence potential. *Adverse effects:* Hypotension, sedation, respiratory depression. Naloxone reverses effects.
Pamidronate disodium Aredia. Injection: 30, 60, 90 mg.	**Treatment of hypercalcemia, Paget disease. Osteogenesis Imperfecta, Osteopenia Bisphosphonate derivative binds to bone inhibiting osteoclast-mediated calcium resorption. Dose based on serum calcium concentration.** *Children:* 1 mg/kg/24 hr for consecutive days q 3 mo; 10–40 mg/m² over 5–8 hr q mo. *Adults:* Serum calcium 12–13.5 mg/dL: 60–90 mg; serum calcium >13.5 mg/dL: 90 mg. Wait	*Cautions:* Leukopenia, thrombophlebitis. Drug incompatible with calcium containing IV solutions. *Adverse effects:* Hypertension, syncope, hypocalcemia, hypophosphatemia, hypothyroidism, bone pain.

Table continued on following page

TABLE 712–1. General Medications *Continued*

Drug (Trade Names, Formulations)	Indications (Mechanism of Action) and Dosing	Comments (Cautions, Adverse Events, Monitoring)
	7 days to assess full effect of dose before re-treatment. Paget disease: 30 mg/24 hr for 3 consecutive days.	
Pancreatin Various brands. Capsule, tablet, timed-release capsule, powder.	**Pancreatic enzyme replacement. Individual products contain different amounts of lipase, amylase, and protease.** *Children and adults:* Dose titrated to desirable stool frequency and consistency.	*Cautions:* Excessive dosing may lead to impaction; inadequate dosing may lead to steatorrhea. Exogenous pancreatic enzymes inactivated by gastric acid; use microencapsulated forms when possible. *Drug interactions:* Reduction of gastric acid (e.g., H_2-receptor antagonists/omeprazole/antacids) may enhance effectiveness. *Adverse effects:* Rash, abdominal complaints, constipation, hyperuricemia, allergy.
Pancuronium Pavulon, generic. Injection: 1 mg/mL, 2 mg/mL.	**Anesthetic/skeletal muscle relaxant. Nondepolarizing neuromuscular antagonist.** *Children and adults:* 0.04–0.1 mg/kg IV q20–30 min. Dose titrated to desired effects.	*Cautions:* Ventilation must be supported during neuromuscular blockade. Dose adjustment with renal dysfunction. *Adverse effects:* Tachycardia, hypertension, prolonged muscle weakness. *Drug interactions:* Possible augmented muscle weakness with aminoglycosides, anesthetics, and colistin.
Papaverine hydrochloride Cerespan, Pavabid, generic. Capsule: 150 mg. Tablet, time-released. Injection.	**Vasodilator, antimigraine. Generalized smooth muscle relaxant. Common pediatric use for preservation of arterial catheters to prolong function.** *Children:* 30 mg papaverine plus 250 units heparin per 250 mL IV solution (0.45–0.9% NaCl) infused.	*Cautions:* Avoid in neonates because may cause cerebral vasodilatation predisposing to CNS hemorrhage. *Adverse effects:* Flushing, tachycardia, hypotension, dizziness. *Drug interactions:* Additive hypotensive effect.
Paraldehyde Paral, generic. Liquid: 1 g/mL.	**Anticonvulsant, sedative. Generalized CNS depressant used as adjunct treatment for refractory status epilepticus, alcohol withdrawal.** *Children:* 0.15 mL/kg/dose PO, PR. May repeat once in 4–6 hr. IM formulation not available in United States. *Adults:* 5–10 mL per dose.	*Cautions:* May give IM but inject remote from nerves owing to risk of damage. Use glass syringe/tubing because drug reacts with plastic. Rectal route preferred to IM route. Mix rectal solution 2:1 in oil (e.g., olive oil). *Adverse effects:* Sedation, gastric irritation, thrombophlebitis.
Paregoric Generic. Liquid: 2 mg morphine equivalent per 5 mL.	**Antidiarrheal, analgesic. Camphorated tincture of opium.** *Children:* 0.25–0.5 mL/kg PO q6–12h. *Adults:* 5–10 mL PO q6–12h. Neonatal abstinence syndrome: dose titrated to desired effect.	*Comments:* Each 5 mL of paregoric contains 2 mg morphine equivalent, 20 mg camphor, 20 mg benzoic acid. Final alcohol content 45%.
Paroxetine Paxil. Tablets: 10, 20, 40 mg Oral suspension: 10 mg/5 mL.	**Serotonin reuptake inhibitor. Effective for treatment of depression, obsessive-compulsive disorder, panic disorder, and social anxiety disorder.** *Children:* Start 10 mg q24h; increase at weekly intervals by 10 mg/24 hr to maximum 60 mg/24 hr. *Adults:* Start 20 mg q24h, increase by 10 mg/24 hr at weekly intervals to response or maximum 60 mg q 24 hr.	*Cautions:* Do not discontinue abruptly or withdrawal syndrome may occur. Taper by 10 mg/24 hr every 5–7 days to avoid problems. Avoid use with monamine oxidase inhibitors except in extreme situations. *Adverse events:* Somnolence, dizziness, insomnia, tremor, nervousness, decreased appetite, asthenia, nausea, constipation. *Drug interactions:* Paroxetine inhibits the cytochrome 2D6 isoenzyme and may interact with phenothiazines and type 1C antiarrhythmics. Concurrent use with thioridazine may elevate thioridazine levels causing prolonged QTc intervals and predispose to torsades de pointes.
Pegaspargase Oncaspar. Injection.	**Antineoplastic agent used in combination for induction of acute lymphoblastic leukemia. Also called PEG-L-asparaginase.** *Children and adults:* IM, IV: 2,500 units/m^2 q 14 days. Dose usually dictated by specific protocol.	*Cautions:* Hepatotoxic, allergic reactions. Contraindicated in patients with pancreatitis, significantly hemorrhagic events associated with L-asparaginase. *Drug interactions:* Possible interactions with methotrexate, vincristine, corticosteroids.
Pemoline Cylert. Tablet: 18.75, 37.5, 75 mg. Tablet, chewable: 37.5 mg.	**Central nervous system stimulant used in the treatment of attention deficit disorder. Structurally unique from methylphenidate.** *Children:* 1 mg/kg/24 hr PO as single dose each morning. Titrate to effect 0.5 mg/kg/24 hr q 1–2 wk. Usual max dose 3 mg/kg/24 hr (~112.5 mg/24 hr).	*Cautions:* Insomnia, anorexia, weight loss. *Adverse effects:* Central nervous system stimulation, seizures, hypertension, increased liver function studies, hepatitis, movement disorders. *Drug interactions:* Possible with other central nervous system stimulants, sympathomimetics.
Penicillamine Cuprimine, Depen. Capsule: 12, 250 mg. Tablet: 250 mg.	**Metal chelating agent with affinity for copper (Wilson disease) and lead. Also used as an adjunct for the treatment of severe rheumatoid arthritis.** **Wilson disease:** Dose titrated to maintain >1 mg/24 hr urinary copper excretion. *Infants and children:* 20 mg/kg/24 hr PO q6–12h (max: 1 g/24 hr). *Adults:* 1 g/24 hr PO q6–12h (max: 2 g). **Lead intoxications** *Infants and children:* 30–40 mg/kg/24 hr PO q8–12h (max: 1.5 g/24 hr). *Adults:* 1–1.5 g/24 hr PO q8–12h.	*Cautions:* Cross allergen in patients allergic to penicillin. Do not administer with food or iron/zinc compounds. *Adverse effects:* Rash, pruritus, nausea, vomiting, anemia, bone marrow suppression, nephrotic syndrome, systemic lupus erythematosus–like syndrome. *Drug interactions:* Other metals, iron, gold, mercury, antimalarials.

TABLE 712–1. General Medications *Continued*

Drug (Trade Names, Formulations)	Indications (Mechanism of Action) and Dosing	Comments (Cautions, Adverse Events, Monitoring)
Pentazocine Talwin. Tablet: 50 mg with 50 mg naloxone (parenteral deterrent). Injection: 30 mg/mL.	**Rheumatoid arthritis** *Children:* 3 mg/kg/24 hr PO q12h, increasing by 3 mg/kg/24 hr q 2–3 mo to max 10 mg/kg/24 hr. **Opiate analgesic of the benzo orphan type for** **the treatment of moderate to severe pain.** *Children >14 yr of age and adults:* 50 mg PO q3–4h; titrate to effect to 100 mg dose not to exceed 600 mg/24 hr. May give IM or IV reducing oral dose by one third.	*Cautions:* Generalized CNS depressant possesses weak antagonistic action and may precipitate opiate withdrawal. *Adverse effects:* CNS depression, nausea, vomiting, respiratory depression, histamine release.
Pentobarbital Nembutal, generic. Capsule: 50, 100 mg. Elixir: 18.2 mg/5 mL. Suppository: 30, 60, 120, 200 mg. Injection.	**Short-acting barbiturate used as an** **anticonvulsant, sedative/hypnotic, anesthetic.** **Sedation** *Children:* 2–6 mg/kg/24 hr PO, IM q6h. May give rectally dosed by body weight: 4.5–10 kg: 30 mg; 10–18 kg: 30–60 mg; 18–36 kg: 60 mg; 36–50 kg: 60–120 mg. **Pentobarbital coma** *Children:* Loading dose 10–15 mg/kg IV slowly over 1–2 hr monitoring blood pressure and heart rate. Maintenance infusion 1 mg/kg/hr increasing up to 5 mg/kg/hr to maintain burst suppression on EEG.	*Cautions:* Hypotension in hypovolemic patients; injectables contain propylene glycol. *Adverse effects:* Arrhythmias, bradycardia, hypotension, respiratory depression, laryngospasm, dependence. *Drug interactions:* May increase metabolism of many hepatically cleared drugs; oral contraceptives, griseofulvin, corticosteroids. *Monitoring:* Pentobarbital concentrations: Sedation 1–5 µg/mL; coma 20–40 µg/mL.
Pentoxifylline Trental. Tablet, timed-release: 400 mg.	**Used in the treatment of peripheral vascular** **disease (Raynaud syndrome) and** **investigationally in reducing tumor** **necrosis factor, neutrophil adhesion, and** **platelet aggregation.** *Children:* Antiplatelet effect in Kawasaki disease: 20 mg/kg/24 hr PO q8h. *Adults:* 400 mg PO tid.	*Cautions:* Administer with meals to reduce gastrointestinal upset. *Adverse effects:* Hypotension, tachycardia, dizziness, nausea, vomiting. *Drug interactions:* Cimetidine, possible augmenting of warfarin, heparin effects.
Phenazopyridine Pyridium, generic. Tablet: 100, 200 mg.	**Urinary anesthetic for possible symptomatic** **relief of urinary burning and itching** **associated with urologic procedures or** **urinary tract infection.** *Children:* 12 mg/kg/24 hr PO q8h. *Adults:* 100–200 mg PO q6–8h.	*Caution:* Discolors urine to orange or red. *Adverse effects:* Headache, rash, methemoglobinemia. Administer with food to decrease gastrointestinal side effects.
Phenobarbital Generic. Elixir: 15 mg/5 mL; 20 mg/5 mL. Tablet: 8, 15, 30, 60, 100 mg. Injection: 30 mg/mL, 60 mg/mL, 130 mg/mL.	**Barbiturate CNS depressant used as a sedative,** **hypnotic, anticonvulsant, anesthetic.** **Anticonvulsant: loading dose** *Children and adults:* 15–20 mg/kg PO, IV. **Maintenance dose** *Neonates:* 3–4 mg/kg/24 hr PO, IV, q12–24h. *Children:* 5–6 mg/kg/24 hr PO, IV, q12–24h. *Adults:* 1–3 mg/kg/24 hr PO, IV, q12–24h. **Sedation** *Children:* 2 mg/kg per dose. **Hyperbilirubinemia** *Children:* 3–8 mg/kg/24 hr PO, IV q12–24h. *Adults:* 90–180 mg/24 hr PO, IV q12–24h.	*Cautions:* Dose titrated to desired effect. Administer IV ≤30 mg/min in infants and children and ≤60 mg/min in adults. *Adverse effects:* Hypotension, drowsiness, respiratory depression, paradoxical hyperactivity. *Drug interactions:* May increase metabolism of many hepatically cleared drugs; oral contraceptives, griseofulvin, corticosteroids. Certain drugs may interfere with phenobarbital metabolism: valproic acid, chloramphenicol, felbamate. *Target serum concentrations:* 15–40 µg/mL; coma (acute) > 60 µg/mL. *Monitoring:* Phenobarbital concentrations: sedation 15–40 µg/mL; coma >60 µg/mL.
Phenoxybenzamine Dibenzyline. Capsule: 10 mg.	**α-Adrenergic receptor antagonist used for** **symptomatic treatment of pheochromocytoma.** *Children:* 0.2–2 mg/kg/24 hr PO q24h. Titrate dose to desired effect (e.g., blood pressure). *Adults:* 10 mg per dose PO q12h; titrate dose to effect.	*Cautions:* Long-acting α-receptor antagonist. *Adverse effects:* Postural hypotension, syncope, dizziness. *Drug interactions:* Sympathomimetics.
Phentolamine Regitine. Injection: 5 mg/mL.	**α-Adrenergic antagonist used in the diagnosis/** **treatment of pheochromocytoma and for** **extravasation of drugs with α-adrenergic** **effects (e.g., dopamine, dobutamine,** **epinephrine, norepinephrine, phenylephrine).** Pheochromocytoma Diagnosis: *Children:* 0.05–0.1 mg/kg/dose (usual max dose: 5 mg). *Adults:* 5 mg per dose. Preoperatively: *Children:* 0.05–0.1 mg/kg/dose q1–2h titrating to effect and needed duration. Usual max dose: 5 mg. **Extravasation** 5–10 mg in 10 mL 0.95 normal saline. Infiltrate area with small volume using 27–30 gauge needle not to exceed total dose of 0.1 mg/kg.	*Cautions:* Short-acting α-receptor antagonist. *Adverse effects:* Hypotension, dizziness, gastritis. *Drug interactions:* Sympathomimetics.
Phenylephrine hydrochloride Neo-Synephrine, generic. Injection: 10 mg/mL. Nasal drops/spray: 0.16–1%. Eye drops.	**α-Adrenergic receptor agonist, peripheral** **vasoconstrictor; used in treatment of** **hypotension in shock and in many nasal** **decongestants.** **Nasal decongestant** *Infants:* 1–2 drops per naris q3–4h 0.16% solution. *Children 1–6 yr:* 1–2 drops/spray per naris q3–4h 0.125% solution.	*Cautions:* Patients with hypertension. Injection contains sulfites. Rebound nasal stuffiness with prolonged nasal use/abuse. *Adverse effects:* Hypertension, angina, bradycardia, restlessness, necrosis if IV infiltrates. *Drug interactions:* Sympathomimetics, α-receptor antagonists, monoamine oxidase inhibitors.

Table continued on following page

TABLE 712–1. General Medications *Continued*

Drug (Trade Names, Formulations)	Indications (Mechanism of Action) and Dosing	Comments (Cautions, Adverse Events, Monitoring)
	6–12 yr: 1–2 drops/spray q3–4h 0.25% solution. *>12 yr and adults:* 1–2 drops/spray per naris q3–4h 0.25–0.5% solution. **Hypotension/shock** *Children:* 5–20 µg/kg per dose IV q10–15 min. May give by continuous IV infusion 0.1–0.5 µg/kg/min titrated to desired effects (e.g., blood pressure). *Adults:* 0.1–0.5 mg/dose q10–15 min continuous IV infusion 100–180 µg/min titrating to desired effect. **Paroxysmal supraventricular tachycardia** *Children:* 5–10 µg/kg IV over 20–30 sec. *Adults:* 0.25–0.5 mg IV over 20–30 sec.	
Phenytoin Dilantin; generic (use cautiously). Capsule, slow (extended) release: 30, 100 mg. Capsule, prompt release: 30, 100 mg. Suspension: 125 mg/5 mL. Injection: 50 mg/mL.	**Anticonvulsant and antiarrhythmic.** **Status epilepticus: loading dose** *Neonate:* 15–20 mg/kg IV; do not exceed 0.5 mg/ kg/min. *Children and adults:* 15–18 mg/kg IV; do not exceed 1–3 mg/kg/min. **Maintenance dose** *Neonate:* 5 mg/kg/24 hr PO, IV q12–24h. *Children 0.5–6 yr:* 8–10 mg/kg/24 hr *7–9 yr:* 6–8 mg/kg/24 hr PO, IV q12–24h *10–16 yr:* 6–7 mg/kg/24 hr PO, IV q12–24h. *Adults:* 300–600 mg/24 hr q12–24h. **Arrhythmias: loading dose** *Children and adults:* 1.25 mg/kg IV q5 min until desired effect or total dose 15 mg/kg. **Maintenance dose** *Children:* 5–10 mg/kg/24 hr q8–12h. *Adults:* 250 mg per dose q6–8h.	*Cautions:* Infuse slowly IV; variable oral bioavailability; chewable tablet most consistent. Must shake oral suspension very well before use. Follows saturation (Michaelis-Menten) pharmacokinetics. Certain disease states (renal failure, acute head trauma) may lead to imbalance between free and protein-bound drug. *Adverse effects:* Lethargy, dizziness, nystagmus, hypotension, hirsutism, gingival hyperplasia, rash, Stevens-Johnson syndrome, hepatitis, thrombophlebitis. *Drug interactions:* May increase metabolism of certain hepatically cleared drugs; oral contraceptives, griseofulvin, corticosteroids, cyclosporin; highly protein bound and may cause displacement interaction. *Monitoring:* Phenytoin concentrations: therapeutic 8–20 µg/mL. If necessary, measure free drug concentration: therapeutic 1–2 µg/mL.
Physostigmine Antilirium. Injection, ophthalmic solution, and ointment.	**Competitive antagonist of acetylcholine.** **Unlike neostigmine, crosses the blood-** **brain barrier with central effects. Used** **with extreme caution in the reversal of** **anticholinergic effects.** *Children:* 0.001–0.03 mg/kg/dose IM, IV, SQ, repeated q15–20 min to desired effect (max total dose: 2 mg). *Adults:* 0.5–2 mg IM, IV, SQ repeated q15–20 min until desired effect.	*Cautions:* Patients with bradycardia, cardiac dysrhythmias, asthma, ulcer disease. Should be used as an antidote only in life-threatening situations by experienced individuals. *Adverse effects:* Palpitations, restlessness, excessive salivation, secretions, muscle fasciculations, bronchospasm.
Phytonadione AquaMEPHYTON, Mephyton. Tablet: 5 mg. Injection.	**Vitamin K₁ for nutritional supplementation** **and treatment of hemorrhagic disease of** **the newborn or from warfarin-like** **compound anticoagulant toxicity.** *Children:* 1–2 mg/dose IM, IV, SQ dosed to effect; PO dose may increase to 2.5 to 5 mg. *Adults:* 10 mg/24 hr IM, IV, SQ; 5–25 mg/24 hr PO. Higher doses may be required for reversal of warfarin-like anticoagulant toxicity.	*Cautions:* Infuse slowly IV (over 15–30 min) to avoid flushing. Multiple doses may be needed for prolonged period depending on type of coumarin anticoagulant. *Adverse effects:* Flushing, hypotension
Piroxicam Feldene. Capsule: 10, 20 mg.	**Nonsteroidal anti-inflammatory agent used as** **an analgesic and in therapy for rheumatoid** **disorders.** *Children:* 0.2–0.3 mg/kg q 24 hr PO (max dose: 15 mg/kg/24 hr). *Adults:* 10–20 mg q24h.	*Cautions:* Limited data in infants and children, may require more frequent daily dosing in pediatrics. Administer with food/milk to decrease gastrointestinal side effects. Do not use in young infants. *Adverse effects:* Dizziness, gastrointestinal upset, nausea/vomiting, ulcer, hepatitis, decreased renal function.
Polyethylene glycol-electrolyte solution Golytely, Colovage, Colyte. Powder for reconstitution.	**Bowel lavage solution used before bowel** **radiology or in poisonings.** *Children:* 25–40 mL/kg/hr up to 1.5–2 L/hr until rectal effluent clear; usual max dose 4 L for x-ray may go much higher if used for poisonings (e.g., iron). *Adults:* 2,400 mg q10–20 min until 4 L consumed. May go higher for poisonings.	*Caution:* In patients with bowel disease (colitis) or obstruction. *Adverse effects:* Nausea, cramps, bloating.
Poractant alfa Curosurf Intratracheal suspension of porcine lung extract, surfactant (80 mg phospholipids, 1 mg protein, 0.3 mg SP-B/mL).	**Prophylaxis or treatment of respiratory distress** **syndrome, treatment of persistent pulmonary** **hypertension.** *Neonates:* 2.5 mL/kg (200 mg/kg) for dose #1, may repeat dose of 1.25 mL/kg (100 mg/kg) 2 times q12h *Children and adults:* Not indicated.	*Caution:* Monitor ventilator status closely; may require rapid weaning within minutes of the dose. *Adverse events:* Bradycardia, airway obstruction, and cyanosis.
Pralidoxime Protopam (2-PAM). Tablet: 500 mg. Injectable.	**Acetylcholinesterase reactivator used in the** **treatment of organophosphate poisoning;** **possible treatment of toxicity from** **cholinergic drugs.** *Children:* 20–50 mg/kg/dose IM, IV repeated in 1–2 hr if muscle weakness has not been	*Caution:* As antidote for organophosphate poisoning; use in combination with atropine. Excessive dosing may cause cholinergic effects. Too-rapid IV administration associated with tachycardia, laryngospasm. Infuse IV over 15–30 min. *Adverse effects:* Hypertension, dizziness, nausea, muscle weakness/rigidity.

TABLE 712–1. General Medications *Continued*

Drug (Trade Names, Formulations)	Indications (Mechanism of Action) and Dosing	Comments (Cautions, Adverse Events, Monitoring)
	relieved; when desired effect obtained dose q12h. *Adults:* 1–2 g IM, IV q5–6h (dose based on clinical response).	
Prazosin Minipress, generic. Capsule: 1, 2, 5 mg.	**Competitive antagonist of postsynaptic α-adrenergic receptors used in the treatment of hypertension/heart failure.** *Children:* 0.1 mg/kg/24 hr PO q6h titrating dose to desired blood pressure. Usual max dose: 0.4 mg/kg/24 hr or 15 mg total dose. Consider additive/synergistic combinations with diuretics. *Adults:* 3 mg/24 hr PO q8–12h, titrating dose to desired blood pressure. Usual dose range: 3–15 mg/24 hr.	*Caution:* Profound hypotension may occur after first dose ("first-dose phenomenon") more common in fluid- and/or salt-depleted patients. *Adverse effects:* Syncope, palpitations, dizziness, fluid retention. *Drug interactions:* Other hypotensive drugs (diuretics, β-receptor antagonists).
Prednisolone DeltaCortef, Hydeltrasol, Predalone, generic. Tablet: 5 mg. Suspension. Injection.	**Glucocorticosteroid used in the treatment of inflammatory disorders including allergic, respiratory, rheumatic, endocrine, and neoplastic disorders.** **Asthma** *Children:* 0.5–4 mg/kg/24 hr PO, IV q6–12h. *Adulst:* 5–60 mg/24 hr PO, IV. **Anti-inflammatory** *Children:* 0.1–2 mg/kg/24 hr PO, IV q6h–q day.	*Cautions:* Dose titrated to desired effect; use shortest treatment course to avoid side effects. May slow growth, increase salt retention. *Adverse effects:* Edema, hypertension, psychosis, Cushing syndrome. HPA-axis (adrenal) suppression, peptic ulcer. *Drug interactions:* Barbiturate, phenytoin, rifampin. *Comment:* See comparison of corticosteroids under *Hydrocortisone.*
Prednisone Deltasone, Liquid Pred, generic. Tablet: 1, 2.5, 5, 10, 20, 50 mg. Syrup: 5 mg/5 mL. Injection.	**Glucocorticosteroid used in the treatment of inflammatory disorders including allergic, respiratory, rheumatic, endocrine, and neoplastic disorders.** **Asthma** *Children:* 0.5–4 mg/kg/24 hr PO, q6–12h. *Adults:* 5–60 mg/24 hr PO. **Anti-inflammatory** *Children:* 0.1–2 mg/kg/24 hr PO, IV q6–24h.	*Cautions:* Dose titrated to desired effect; use shortest treatment course to avoid side effects. May slow growth, increase salt retention. *Adverse effects:* Edema, hypertension, psychosis, Cushing syndrome. HPA-axis (adrenal) suppression, peptic ulcer. *Drug interactions:* Barbiturate, phenytoin, rifampin. *Comment:* See comparison of corticosteroids under *Hydrocortisone.*
Primidone Mysoline, generic. Tablet: 50, 250 mg. Suspension: 250 mg/5 mL.	**Anticonvulsant used in the treatment of generalized tonic-clonic, complex partial and focal seizures.** *Neonate:* 12–20 mg/kg/24 hr PO, q8–12h. *Children:* 10–25 mg/kg/24 hr PO q8–12h. *Children >8 yr and adults:* 125–1,500 mg/24 hr PO q8–12h (usual max: 2 g/24 hr).	*Caution:* Partially metabolized to phenobarbital and PEMA. *Adverse effects:* Sedation, ataxia, rash. *Drug interactions:* Valproate, griseofulvin, phenytoin. *Monitoring:* PEMA concentrations: therapeutic 5–12 µg/mL.
Procainamide Pronestyl, Procan. Tablet and capsule: 250, 375, 500 mg. Tablet, sustained-release: 250, 500, 750, 1,000 mg. Injection.	**Class Ia antiarrhythmic; ventricular tachycardia, premature ventricular contractions, paroxysmal atrial tachycardia, atrial fibrillation.** **Loading dose** *Children:* 3–6 mg/kg/dose IV over 5 min not to exceed 100 mg/dose; repeat q5–10 min as needed to max 15 mg/kg total dose. Do not exceed 500 mg in 30 min. **Maintenance dose** *Children:* 15–50 mg/kg/24 hr PO q3–6h; 20–30 mg/kg/24 hr IM, IV; not to exceed 4 g/24 hr; continuous IV infusion 20–80 µg/kg/min, usual max 2 g/24 hr. *Adults:* 250–500 mg/dose q3–6h (max: 2–4 g/24 hr).	*Caution:* Causes positive antinuclear antibody reaction, general cardiodepressant. Metabolized to active NAPA. *Adverse effects:* Hypotension, arrhythmias, AV block, confusion, agranulocytosis, systemic lupus erythematosus–like syndrome, fever, rash. *Drug interactions:* Cimetidine, β-antagonists, anticholinergic agents. *Monitoring:* Procainamide concentrations: therapeutic 4–10 µg/mL. Sum of procainamide and NAPA: therapeutic 10–30 µg/mL.
Procarbazine Capsule: 50 mg.	**Antineoplastic used in the treatment of Hodgkin lymphoma, bronchogenic carcinoma.** **Hodgkin disease** *Children:* 1.5–3 mg/kg/24 hr (50–100 mg/m²) PO, q24hr for 10–14 days per 28-day cycle. **Bone marrow transplant preparation** 12.5 mg/kg/dose. **Neuroblastoma and medulloblastoma** *Children:* 100–200 mg/m²/dose per protocol.	*Caution:* Dose based on disease-based protocol and concurrent drugs. Avoid alcohol (causes disulfiram-like reaction). Possesses some MAO inhibitory activity. *Adverse effects:* CNS depression, confusion, ataxia, marrow suppression, alopecia, flu-like syndrome. *Drug interactions:* Alcohol, tricyclic antidepressants, phenothiazines, tyramine-containing foods sympathomimetics.
Prochlorperazine Compazine, generic. Tablet: 5, 10, 25 mg. Capsule, sustained-release: 10, 15, 30 mg. Injection. Suppository: 2.5, 5, 25 mg. Syrup: 5 mg/5 mL.	**Piperazine-type phenothiazine antiemetic. Use should be avoided in children.** *Children:* 0.4 mg/kg/24 hr PO; rectal, q6–8 hr; 0.1–0.15 mg/kg/24 hr IM q8–12h. *Adults:* 5–10 mg/dose PO tid–qid.	*Caution:* Acute dystonic reaction common in children. *Adverse effects:* Sedation, extrapyramidal reactions, photosensitivity, cholestatic jaundice. *Drug interactions:* Additive CNS effects, α-receptor antagonists.
Promethazine Phenergan; generic. Tablet: 12.5, 25, 50 mg. Syrup. Suppository. Injection.	**Phenothiazine with primary antihistaminic activity used in the treatment of nausea, vomiting, motion sickness, allergy.** **Motion sickness** *Children:* 0.5 mg/kg PO, 30–60 min before departure; then q8–12h as needed.	*Caution:* Potentiates anticholinergic effects *Adverse effects:* Sedation, hypotension, extrapyramidal reactions, blurred vision. *Drug interactions:* Additive sedative effects.

Table continued on following page

TABLE 712–1. General Medications *Continued*

Drug (Trade Names, Formulations)	Indications (Mechanism of Action) and Dosing	Comments (Cautions, Adverse Events, Monitoring)
	Sedation-antiemetic *Children:* 0.25–1 mg/kg/dose IM, IV, rectal, q4–6h as needed.	
Propafenone Rythmol. Tablet: 150, 225, 300 mg.	**Class 1c antiarrhythmic agent. Effective against pediatric SVT.** *Children:* 200–600 mg/m²/24 hr divided q8h *Adults:* 150 mg q8h (450 mg/24 hr). May titrate at 3–5 day intervals to 300 mg q8h (max: 900 mg/24 hr).	*Cautions:* May worsen or cause arrhythmias, heart failure, or angina. Also causes dizziness, fatigue, nausea, vomiting, and constipation. *Drug interactions:* Increases digoxin levels (dose-related), cyclosporin, and theophylline.
Propantheline bromide ProBanthine, generic. Tablet: 7.5, 15 mg.	**Synthetic anticholinergic antispasmodic used as adjunctive therapy for gastrointestinal or bladder spasm, irritable bowel.** *Children:* 1.5–3 mg/kg/24 hr PO, q4–8h. Dose to desired effect.	*Caution:* Avoid in patients with decreased bowel motility. *Adverse effects:* Sedation, tachycardia, dry mouth, blurred vision, mydriasis.
Propofol Diprivan. Injection.	**Nonbarbiturate sedative, hypnotic, general anesthetic.** **Sedation** *Children:* 1.5–3 mg/kg/dose IV over 1–2 min. **Continuous sedation** (mechanical ventilation). *Children:* 5.5 mg/kg for 30 min; increase to 6 mg/kg for 30 min; increase to 8 mg/kg for 1 hr; increase to 10 mg/kg for 1 hr; increase to final infusion rate of 12.5 mg/kg/hr.	*Caution:* Dose titration regimen to permit adequate sedation-accommodating drugs complex. Pharmacokinetics. Single-use vials in lipid emulsion. *Adverse effects:* Hypotension, bradycardia, hyperlipidemia, questionable metabolic acidosis.
Propoxyphene Darvon. Capsule. Tablet.	**Analgesic for mild to moderate pain. Binds opiate receptors. Less dependence liability than codeine.** *Children:* 2–3 mg/kg/24 hr PO q4–6h. Titrate dose to desired effect. *Adults:* Hydrochloride 65 mg/dose PO, q4–6h (max dose: 390 mg); napsylate salt 100 mg PO, q4–6h (max dose: 600 mg).	*Caution:* Weak opiate agonist with limited abuse potential. *Adverse effects:* Sedation, dizziness, nausea, vomiting, constipation, dependence.
Propranolol Inderal, generic. Tablet: 10, 20, 40, 60, 80 mg. Solution: 4 mg/mL, 8 mg/mL, and concentrate 80 mg/mL. Injection: 1 mg/mL. Sustained-release capsule: 60, 80, 120, 160 mg.	**Nonselective β-adrenergic receptor antagonist (β₁ and β₂).** *Neonates:* 0.25 mg/kg/dose PO q6–8h; titrate to desired response, increasing dose slowly (max dose 5 mg/kg/24 hr). IV: 0.01 mg/kg over 10–15 min; titrate to desired effect (max dose: 1 mg/kg/24 hr). **Arrhythmias/hypertension** *Children:* 0.5–1 mg/kg/24 hr PO q6–8h titrated upward to 2–5 (mg/kg/24 hr, over 3–5 days). *IV dose:* 0.01–0.1 mg/kg/dose infused over 10–15 min as needed (max dose: 1 mg infants; 3 mg children). *Adults:* 40–80 mg/24 hr, titrating to response; range 40–320 mg/24 hr PO q6–8h. **Thyrotoxicosis** *Neonates:* 2 mg/kg/24 hr PO q6–8h; titrate to response. *Children:* 2–4 mg/kg/24 hr PO q6–8h; titrate to response. **Migraine prophylaxis** *Children:* 0.6–2 mg/kg/24 hr PO q6–8h (usual max: 4 mg/kg/24 hr).	*Caution:* Drug undergoes substantial first-pass metabolism explaining huge difference between IV and PO doses. Use cautiously IV and in patients with congestive heart failure, asthma, chronic obstructive pulmonary disease. Monitor heart rate for drug effect. *Adverse effects:* Decreased cardiac contractility, hypotension, bradycardia, hypoglycemia, bronchospasm.
Propylthiouracil (PTU) Generic. Tablet: 50 mg.	**Antithyroid that inhibits thyroid hormone synthesis by interfering with incorporation of iodine.** *Neonates:* 5–10 mg/kg/24 hr PO q8h and titrate to effect. *Children:* 5–7 mg/kg/24 hr PO q8h titrate to effect. *Adults:* 300–450 mg/24 hr PO q8h increasing to 600–1,200 mg/24 hr.	*Caution:* Marked drug effect usually requires 24–36 hr. *Adverse effects:* Vertigo, rash, blood dyscrasias, hepatitis, arthralgia, interstitial pneumonitis.
Protamine sulfate Generic. Injection: 10 mg/mL.	**Heparin antidote, neutralizing its anticoagulant effect.** 1 mg protamine neutralizes 90 USP units of lung-derived heparin and 115 USP units of intestinal-derived heparin. Protamine dose calculated on duration of time since last heparin dose using heparin elimination half-life (~1 hr) to determine estimated heparin body stores.	*Caution:* Calculate dose carefully as protamine excess can cause anticoagulation. Monitor partial thromboplastin time with use. *Adverse effects:* Hypotension, dyspnea, hypersensitivity.
Pseudoephedrine Generic. Tablet: 30, 60 mg; timed-release: 120 mg. Capsule: 60 mg; timed-release: 120 mg. Syrup: 15 mg/mL.	**Indirectly acting sympathomimetic used as a nasal decongestant/symptoms of common cold.** *Infants and children:* 4 mg/kg/24 hr PO, q6–12h. *Adults:* 60 mg/dose PO, q6–8h; max: 240 mg/24 hr.	*Caution:* In patients with hypertension, heart disease. *Adverse effects:* Tachycardia, headache, nervousness, tremor. *Drug interactions:* Monoamine oxidase inhibitors, propranolol, pressors.
Pyridostigmine Mestinon. Tablet: 60 mg; sustained-release 180 mg. Syrup: 60 mg/5 mL. Injection: 5 mg/mL.	**Cholinesterase inhibitor used in the treatment of myasthenia gravis; reversal of neuro-muscular blocking agents.** **Myasthenia gravis** *Children:* 0.05–0.15 mg/kg/dose IM, IV; max dose	*Caution:* In patients with asthma, cardiac dysfunction/arrhythmias, peptic ulcer. *Adverse effects:* Bradycardia, AV block, seizures, headache, diarrhea, abdominal cramping, salivation, urinary frequency, muscle weakness, miosis, lacrimation,

TABLE 712–1. **General Medications** *Continued*

Drug (Trade Names, Formulations)	Indications (Mechanism of Action) and Dosing	Comments (Cautions, Adverse Events, Monitoring)
	10 mg; titrate to desired effect; PO dose 7 mg/kg/24 hr in 5–6 divided doses. *Adults:* 2 mg IM, IV q2–3h; PO dose 60 mg per dose q8h; titrate to desired effect. **Reversal of neuromuscular blocking agents.** *Children:* 0.1–0.25 mg/kg/dose IM, IV; titrate to effect; may need to co-administer atropine/ glycopyrrolate. *Adults:* 10–20 mg per dose with atropine/ glycopyrrolate.	increased bronchial secretions.
Pyridoxine Nestrex, generic. Tablet: 25, 50, 100 mg; sustained-release: 100 mg. Injection: 100 mg/mL.	**Vitamin B$_6$ used for dietary or drug-induced (e.g., isoniazid, hydralazine) deficiency and B$_6$-dependent seizures.** **Pyridoxine-dependent seizures.** *Children:* 50–100 mg PO, IM, IV; maintenance dose 50–100 mg/24 hr. **Dietary deficiency.** *Children:* 5–15 mg/24 hr for 3–4 wk then 2.5–5 mg/24 hr. *Adults:* 10–20 mg/24 hr for 3–4 wk. **Drug-induced neuritis.** *Children:* 1 mg/kg/24 hr PO, IM, IV, q day. *Adults:* 100–200 mg/24 hr PO, IM, IV, q day.	*Caution:* May decrease serum phenobarbital and phenytoin concentrations. Large IV doses may precipitate seizures. *Adverse effects:* Nausea, decreased folic acid, liver function tests.
Quetiapine Seroquel. Tablet: 25, 100, 200, 300 mg.	**Atypical antipsychotic. Antagonist of serotonin, dopamine, and α$_1$- and α$_2$-adrenergic receptors.** *Children:* Start 12.5 mg bid, then increase in 25–50 mg increments to 300–400 mg/24 hr divided in 2–3 doses. *Adults:* Start 25 mg bid, then increase in 25–50 mg increments q 2–3 days to response, 300–400 mg/24 hr divided in 2–3 doses (max: 800 mg/24 hr).	*Adverse events:* Somnolence, dizziness, headache, constipation, dry mouth, dyspepsia, postural hypotension, tachycardia.
Quinidine Quinaglute, Quinidex, generic. Tablet (sulfate): 200, 300 mg; sustained-release: 300 mg. Sustained-release gluconate: 324 mg. Injection, gluconate: 80 mg/mL.	**Myocardial depressant used in the treatment of arrhythmias: supraventricular tachycardia, paroxysmal ventricular tachycardia, premature atrial/ventricular contractions.** *Children:* 2 mg/kg PO, IM, IV test dose to exclude idiosyncrasy: 20–50 mg/kg/24 hr sulfate salt q4h PO; gluconate salt 2–10 mg/kg/dose q3–6h IV. *Adults:* 199–600 mg/dose sulfate salt q4–6h PO; 324–972 mg/dose q8–12h gluconate salt; 200–400 mg/dose sulfate IV; titrate to effect.	*Caution:* First-dose syncope; 267 mg quinidine gluconate = 200 mg quinidine sulfate. Infuse IV slowly <10 mg/min. *Adverse effects:* Syncope, hypotension, heart block, fever, abdominal discomfort, bone marrow suppression, thrombocytopenia, idiopathic thrombocytopenic purpura, cinchonism. *Drug interactions:* Verapamil, cimetidine, phenytoin, phenobarbital, rifampin, digoxin.
Ranitidine Zantac, generic. Tablet/capsule: 150, 300 mg. Syrup: 15 mg/mL. Injection: 25 mg/mL. Effervescent granules and tablet: 150 mg.	**H$_2$-receptor antagonist competitively inhibits gastric acid secretion in gastric/peptic ulcer disease/stress ulcer prophylaxis, gastroesophageal reflux disease.** *Neonates:* 1.5–2 mg/kg/24 hr PO, IV q12h; continuous 24 hr IV infusion 0.04 mg/kg/hr (max: 1 mg/kg/24 hr). *Children:* 1–5 mg/kg/24 hr PO, IM, IV q6–8h; continuous 24 hr IV infusion 2–5 mg/kg/24 hr. *Adults:* 150 mg/dose PO q12 hr or 300 mg PO qhs; 50–100 mg/dose IM, IV q6–8h.	*Caution:* Dose may be titrated to desired gastric pH from gastric aspirate. *Adverse effects:* Headache, mental confusion, pain at injection site. *Comment:* Very few if any clinically important drug-drug interactions.
Risperidone Risperdal. Tablet: 0.25, 0.5, 1, 2, 3, 4 mg Oral liquid: 1 mg/mL.	**Atypical antipsychotic.** *Children:* Start 0.25 mg bid; increase per response to 3 mg bid. *Adolescents and adults:* Start 1 mg bid; increase to 3 mg bid or response.	*Caution:* May cause QT prolongation and increase risk of sudden cardiac death; monitor ECG and avoid concurrent use with other drugs that prolong QT interval. *Adverse events:* Dizziness, drowsiness, agitation, headache, tachycardia, constipation, dry mouth, orthostatic hypotension, weight gain.
Riboflavin Generic. Tablet: 25, 50, 100 mg.	**Vitamin used in supplementation and deficiency states.** Deficiency: *Children:* 2.5–10 mg/24 hr PO, q8–12h. *Adults:* 5–30 mg/24 hr PO, q8–12h.	*Adverse effects:* Extremely rare. *Drug interaction:* Probenecid.
Rocuronium Zemuron. Injection: 10 mg/mL.	**Anesthetic/skeletal muscle relaxant, nondepolarizing neuromuscular blocking agent.** *Children and adults:* 0.6–1.2 mg/kg/initial dose: subsequent doses administered as needed 0.2 mg/kg q 20–30 min. Continuous IV infusion 10–12 µg/kg/min.	*Cautions:* Ventilation must be supported during neuromuscular blockade. Dose adjustment with hepatic dysfunction. *Adverse effects:* Tachycardia, hypotension, prolonged muscle weakness, bronchospasm. *Drug interactions:* Possible augmented muscle weakness with aminoglycosides, anesthetics, colistin.
Salmeterol Serevent. Aerosol canister.	**Long-acting β$_2$-adrenergic agonist (~8–12+ hr), bronchodilator used in the treatment of reversible airways disease. Excellent in patients with nocturnal asthma.** *Children and adults:* 1 (21 µg)–2 puffs, aerosol q12h; titrate to desired effect.	*Caution:* Not for use in acute asthma attack. *Adverse effects:* Tachycardia, palpitations, headache, nervousness, muscle tremor, cough, airway irritation.

Table continued on following page

MEDICATIONS

TABLE 712–1. General Medications *Continued*

Drug (Trade Names, Formulations)	Indications (Mechanism of Action) and Dosing	Comments (Cautions, Adverse Events, Monitoring)
Sargramostim Leukine, Prokine. Injection: 250, 500 μg.	**Granulocyte-macrophage (GM-CSF) colony-stimulating factor for acceleration of myeloid recovery from chemotherapy/marrow insult.**	*Caution:* Monitor blood cell count to define duration of therapy *Adverse effects:* Tachycardia, hypotension, flushing, fluid retention, fever, malaise, bone pain, myalgia, rigors, dyspnea.
Scopolamine Transderm Scōp, generic. Transdermal patch.	**Anticholinergic agent used for control of secretions, postoperative antiemetic and motion sickness.** **Postoperative emesis** *Children:* 6 μg/kg/dose IM, IV, SC q6–8h. *Adults:* 0.3–0.65 mg/dose IM, IV, SC q6–8h. **Motion sickness** *Children and adults:* One patch behind the ear at least 4 hr before movement.	*Caution:* Narrow-angle glaucoma, ileus. Use patch cautiously in children younger than age 12 yr. *Adverse effects:* Tachycardia, disorientation, sedation, psychosis, dry mouth, constipation, urinary retention, blurred vision. *Drug interactions:* Other anticholinergic compounds, may interfere with gastrointestinal absorption of certain drugs.
Senna Senokot, X-Prep, generic. Syrup: 218 mg/5 mL. Tablet: 187 mg, 217 mg, 600 mg. Granules: 326 mg/teaspoon.	**Stimulant cathartic for short-term treatment of constipation, bowel preparation before radiology.** *Children:* 10–20 mg/kg/dose PO, q12–24h.	*Caution:* Avoid prolonged use (>1 wk), dependence. *Adverse effects:* Abdominal cramping, diarrhea, fluid and electrolyte imbalance.
Sertraline Zoloft. Tablets: 25, 50, 100 mg Oral solution (concentrate): 20 mg/mL.	**Antidepressant. Serotonin reuptake inhibitor. Treatment of depression, obsessive-compulsive disorder, panic disorder, post-traumatic stress disorder, attention deficit disorder.** *Children 6–12 years:* Start 25 mg q24h; increase by 25 mg weekly to response, dose q24h (max: 200 mg/24 hr). *Children >12 years and adults:* Start 50 mg q24h, increase 25–50 mg weekly to response, dose q24h (max: 200 mg/24 hr).	*Caution:* Do not discontinue abruptly or withdrawal symptoms (SSRI discontinuation syndrome) may occur. Taper maximum 50 mg/24 hr every 5–7 days. *Adverse events:* Insomnia, somnolence, headache, dry mouth, nausea, diarrhea.
Simethicone Mylicon, Gas-X, generic. Chewable tablet: 40, 80, 125 mg. Capsule: 125 mg. Drops: 40 mg/0.6 mL.	**Antiflatulent for symptomatic relief of colic, excessive gas.** *Children <2 yr:* 20 mg/dose PO q4–6h. *Children 2–12 yr:* 40 mg/dose q6h. *Children >12 yr and adults:* 40–120 mg PO q6h, dose titrated to effect.	*Comments:* Very safe drug with rare adverse effects. Dose may be titrated to desired effect by increasing dose or more frequent doses per day. Avoid gas-producing and gastrointestinal irritant foods.
Sodium polystyrene sulfonate Kayexalate, generic. Powder for suspension.	**Ion-exchange resin that removes potassium for sodium for the treatment of hyperkalemia.** *Children:* 4 g/kg/24 hr PO, q4–8h; Rectal: 4–12 g/kg/24 hr PR q2–6h. *Adults:* 15 g/dose PO, q6–12h.	*Cautions:* Follow serum potassium closely. Do not mix with potassium containing liquids (e.g., orange juice). *Adverse effects:* Abdominal cramping, bloating, hypokalemia.
Sodium thiosulfate Tinver, generic. Injection: 100 mg/mL, 250 mg/mL.	**Cyanide (nitroprusside) and cisplatin antidote. Provides an extra sulfur to rhodanese enzyme to enhance cyanide detoxification.** **Nitroprusside:** *Children and adults:* 1 g sodium thiosulfate for every 100 mg nitroprusside administered. May infuse in same IV. **Cisplatin:** *Adults:* 12 g IV infused over 6 hr before or concurrent with cisplatin infusion. Alternate: 9 g/m² IV bolus followed by 1.2 g/m²/hr for 6 hr before or during cisplatin infusion.	*Caution:* Rapid IV infusion may cause hypotension. *Adverse effects:* Very unusual. Hypotension, local irritation at infusion site.
Sotalol Betapace. Tablet: 80, 120, 160 mg.	**Class III antiarrhythmic. Treat supraventricular and ventricular arrhythmias.** *Children:* 2–8 mg/kg/24 hr divided q8–12h. *Adults:* Start 80 mg q12hr and titrate q 3–4 days to response (max: 640 mg/24 hr).	*Cautions:* Proarrhythmic effects, worsen congestive heart failure or diabetes. Reduce dose for declining renal function (1/2 dose for CrCl < 60 mL/min, 1/3 dose for CrCl < 30 mL/min. Extend interval to decrease dose).
Spironolactone Aldactone, generic. Tablet: 25, 50, 100 mg.	**Competitive aldosterone antagonist used as a mild, potassium-sparing diuretic, antihypertensive, in chronic liver disease.** *Neonates:* 1–3 mg/kg/24 hr PO divided q12–24h. *Children:* 1.5–3.3 mg/kg/24 hr PO divided q8–24h. *Adults:* 25–200 mg per dose PO q12–24h.	*Caution:* Careful monitoring of serum potassium/potassium intake. Suspension may be made with crushed tablets in water/glycerin. *Adverse effects:* Lethargy, hyperkalemia, gynecomastia, nausea, rash.
Streptokinase Streptase. Injection.	**Thrombolytic agent used in the treatment of deep-vein thrombosis, stroke, catheter patency.** Thrombosis: 3,500–4,000 units infused IV over 30 min followed by 1,000–1,500 units IV continuous infusion. Clotted catheter: 10,000–25,000 units in normal saline the volume of the catheter instilled into catheter for ~1 hr then removed (aspirated).	*Caution:* Recent strep infection may reduce efficacy. *Adverse effects:* Bleeding bronchospasm, flushing, rash. *Drug interactions:* Anticoagulants, antiplatelet drugs.
Succimer Chemet. Capsule: 100 mg.	**Metal chelator that forms water-soluble salts with lead, mercury, and arsenic.** *Children/adults:* 10 mg/kg/dose PO q8h for 5 days then 10 mg/kg/dose PO q12h for 14 days.	*Caution:* Maintain adequate hydration. Capsule may be opened and beads sprinkled onto soft food. *Adverse effects:* Headache, dizziness, nausea, abdominal cramping, flu-like symptoms.
Succinylcholine Anectine. Injection.	**Neuromuscular blocking agent.** *Children:* 1–2 mg IV initial dose; maintenance 0.3–0.6 mg/kg IV q 5–10 min dose titrated to level of skeletal muscle relaxation.	*Caution:* In patients with hyperkalemia, severe trauma, increased intraocular or intracranial pressure. *Adverse effects:* Bradycardia, hypotension, malignant hyperthermia, hyperkalemia, bronchospasm.

TABLE 712–1. **General Medications** *Continued*

Drug (Trade Names, Formulations)	Indications (Mechanism of Action) and Dosing	Comments (Cautions, Adverse Events, Monitoring)
	Adults: 0.6 mg/kg up to 150 mg IV initial dose; maintenance dose: 0.04–0.07 mg/kg IV q 5–10 min titrated to effect.	*Drug interactions:* Muscle depressants/relaxants.
Sucralfate Carafate. Tablet: 1 g. Suspension: 1 g/10 mL.	**Aluminum salt of sulfated sucrose in the presence of acid forms a paste-like substance that adheres to damaged mucosa.** *Children:* 40–80 mg/kg/24 hr PO divided q6–8h. Stomatitis 5–10 mL swish/spit or swallow q6h. *Adults:* 1 g per dose PO q4–6h.	*Caution:* May use topically for stomatitis. *Adverse effects:* Headache, constipation, abdominal cramping, rash. *Drug interactions:* Decreases absorption of phenytoin, tetracycline, ketoconazole, theophylline, digoxin, cimetidine.
Sufentanil Sufenta. Injection.	**Opioid analgesic used in anesthesia and for pain management.** *Children:* 10–25 µg/kg IV initial dose titrated to desired effect with 25–50 µg/kg. *Adults:* 0.5–8 µg/kg initial dose with maintenance 10–50 µg/kg.	*Caution:* In patients with head trauma or concurrent monoamine oxidase inhibitors adverse effect profiles of all opiates are potentiated. *Adverse effects:* Bradycardia, vasodilatation, nausea, vomiting, blurred vision, respiratory depression, addiction potential. *Drug interactions:* CNS/respiratory depressants.
Sulfasalazine Azulfidine, generic. Tablet: 500 mg.	**Anti-inflammatory 5-aminosalicylic acid derivative combined with sulfonamide used in the treatment of inflammatory bowel disease.** *Children:* Initial 40–75 mg/kg/24 hr PO divided q4–6h not to exceed 6 g/24 hr; maintenance 30–50 mg/kg/24 hr PO divided q6–8h. *Adults:* 1 g per dose PO q6–8h (max dose: 6 g/24 hr).	*Caution:* Hypersensitivity to sulfa drugs. *Adverse effects:* Rash, dizziness, headache, nausea, bone marrow suppression. *Drug interactions:* Decreases folate and digoxin absorption.
Tacrolimus Prograf. Injection. Capsule: 1 mg, 5 mg. Extemporaneous preparation.	**Prevent graft versus host disease in organ transplant (immunosuppressant).** *Children:* PO: 0.15 mg/kg every 12 hr; IV continuous infusion: 0.05–0.1 mg/kg/24 hr. *Adults:* PO: 0.075–0.15 mg/kg q12h; IV continuous infusion: 0.05–0.1 mg/kg/24 hr.	*Adverse events:* Hypertension, headache, insomnia, abdominal and back pain, fever, asthenia, pruritus, hypo/hyperkalemia, hypomagnesemia, hyperglycemia, nausea, vomiting, diarrhea, anemia, leukocytosis, liver damage, nephrotoxicity, dyspnea, pleural effusion, peripheral edema. *Monitoring:* Tacrolimus trough concentrations: Therapeutic: 9.8–19.4 ng/mL using whole-blood ELISA assay; 0.5–1.5 ng/mL using serum high-pressure liquid chromatography.
Teniposide, VM-26 Vumon. Injection: 10 mg/mL.	**Treatment of acute lymphocytic leukemia (ALL) and lung cancer (inhibits cells from entering mitosis).** *Children:* IV: Start 130 mg/m^2/wk, increase at 3 wk to 150 mg/m^2, and at 6 wk to 180 mg/m^2. *Adults:* ALL 250 mg/m^2 wk for 4–8 wk.	*Caution:* Increases intracellular accumulation of methotrexate and thus toxicity. *Adverse events:* Nausea, vomiting, diarrhea, mucositis, myelosuppression, alopecia, rash, fever, hemorrhage, peripheral neuropathy. *Comment:* Down syndrome patients should be started at half the usual dose.
Terbutaline sulfate Brethine, generic. Injection. Tablet: 2.5, 5 mg. Metered-dose inhaler (MDI).	**Bronchodilator (β$_2$-receptor agonist).** *Children <12 yr:* PO: 0.05 mg/kg/dose (max: 5 mg) q8h. SC: 0.005–0.01 mg/kg/dose (max: 0.4 mg); may repeat in 15–20 min. *Children ≥12 yr and adults:* PO: 2.5–5 mg/dose q6–8h. SC: 0.25 mg/dose; may repeat in 15 min. *Children and adults:* MDI 1–2 puffs q6–8h as needed.	*Adverse events:* Tachycardia, arrhythmias, flushing, headache, nervousness, tremor, hypokalemia, muscle cramps, paradoxical bronchospasm.
Terfenadine Seldane. Tablet: 60 mg.	**Treatment of allergic symptoms (antihistamine).** *Children:* *3–6 yr:* 15 mg bid. *6–12 yr:* 30 mg bid. *>12 yr and adults:* 60 mg twice/24 hr.	*Caution:* QT interval prolongation and fatal arrhythmias may occur if combined with drugs that inhibit liver enzymes. *Adverse events:* Drowsiness, fatigue. *Drug interactions:* Azole antifungals, macrolides, cimetidine may prolong QT interval and produce dysrhythmias.
Testosterone Generic. Injection.	**Androgen replacement in male hypogonadism and delayed puberty (replacement therapy).** *Children:* IM **Male hypogonadism:** Initiation of prepubertal growth and delayed puberty: 40–50 mg/m^2/dose monthly; terminal growth phase: 100 mg/m^2/dose twice monthly. *Adults:* Hypogonadism: IM 50–400 mg q 2–4 wk.	*Caution:* May accelerate bone maturation without producing compensating gain in linear growth. *Adverse events:* Acne, bladder irritability, aggressive behavior, depression, sleeplessness, headache, hirsutism, hepatic dysfunction.
Tetanus antitoxin Injection.	Prevention or treatment of tetanus when tetanus immune globulin unavailable. *Children and adults:* SC, IM. Prophylaxis: <30 kg 1,500 units; >30 kg 3,000–5,000 units. Treatment: Inject 10,000–40,000 units into wound and 40,000–100,000 units IV.	*Adverse events:* Serum sickness, urticaria, skin eruptions, allergic reactions.
Tetanus immune globulin Hyper-Tet. Injection.	**Prophylaxis and treatment of tetanus.** Prophylaxis: *Children:* 4 units/kg. *Adults:* 250 units IM. Treatment: *Children:* 500–3,000 units. *Adults:* 3,000–6,000 units (infiltrate some of dose around wound).	*Adverse events:* Allergic reactions.

Table continued on following page

MEDICATIONS

TABLE 712–1. **General Medications** *Continued*

Drug (Trade Names, Formulations)	Indications (Mechanism of Action) and Dosing	Comments (Cautions, Adverse Events, Monitoring)
Theophylline Generic. Syrup, solution, elixir, capsule, tablet (sustained-release forms also). (See under *Aminophylline* for intravenous dosing.)	**Treatment of apnea of prematurity, symptoms of reversible airway disease (affects intracellular transport of calcium, phosphodiesterase inhibitor, weak anti-inflammatory agent).** *Neonates:* Apnea, bronchodilation: loading dose 6–10 mg/kg; maintenance dose: 2–4 mg/kg/dose q12h. *Infants and children:* *6 wk–6 mo:* 10 mg/kg/24 hr. *6 mo–1 yr:* 12–18 mg/kg/24 hr. *1–9 yr:* 20–24 mg/kg/24 hr. *9–12 yr:* 16 mg/kg/24 hr. *12–16 yr:* 13 mg/kg/24 hr. *Adults:* 10 mg/kg/24 hr. (Dosing may be increased for smokers and enzyme-inducing drugs; decrease dose if enzyme inhibitors, liver disease, heart failure, or hypothyroid.)	*Cautions:* May cause or worsen arrhythmias, seizures, or gastroesophageal reflux. Theophylline clearance is modified by numerous disease states and drugs requiring dosing adjustments guided by serum theophylline concentrations. Clearance is reduced by viral illnesses, fever >102°F for >24 hr, cor pulmonale, and drugs that inhibit P450 enzymes (cimetidine, verapamil, macrolides, quinolones); reduce dose by 50%. *Adverse events:* Tachycardia, nervousness, hyperactivity, difficulty concentrating, irritability, agitation, headache, nausea, vomiting, abdominal pain, feeding intolerance, frequent urination, seizures and arrhythmias at toxic levels. *Monitoring:* Theophylline concentrations: therapeutic: neonatal apnea: 6–15 µg/mL; prevent intubation or promote extubation: 10–20 µg/mL; bronchodilation: 5–20 µg/mL; toxic >20 µg/mL.
Thiamine Generic. Injection. Tablet: 50, 100, 250, 500 mg.	**Nutritional supplement, treatment of beriberi and Wernicke encephalopathy (essential coenzyme in carbohydrate metabolism).** Beriberi: *Children:* IM, IV: 10–25 mg/24 hr; or PO: 10–50 mg/24 hr for 2 wk, then 5–10 mg/24 hr for 1 mo. *Adults:* IM, IV: 5–30 mg tid for 2 wk, then oral 5–30 mg/24 hr for 1 mo. Wernicke: IM, IV: 100 mg/24 hr until consuming a balanced diet.	*Adverse events:* Cardiovascular collapse with repeated IV doses, angioedema, rash, tingling.
Thioguanine 6-TG. Tablet: 40 mg.	**Treatment of leukemias (purine analog inhibits synthesis and utilization of purine nucleotides).** *Children <3 yr:* Acute nonlymphocytic leukemia: PO: 3.3 mg/kg/24 hr in 2 doses for 4 days. *Children >3 yr and adults:* PO: 2–3 mg/kg once daily (rounded to nearest 20 mg) until remission.	*Adverse events:* Myelosuppression (onset, 7–10 days; nadir, 14 days; recovery, 21 days), nausea, vomiting, diarrhea, anorexia, stomatitis, hyperuricemia, unsteady gait.
Thiopental Pentothal Sodium. Injection.	**Anesthesia induction and maintenance, intractable seizures, increased intracranial pressure (ultra-short-acting barbiturate).** *Neonates:* Anesthesia: 3–4 mg/kg; seizures: 2–3 mg/kg IV; repeat doses 1 mg/kg as needed. *Infants and children:* IV anesthesia: 5–8 mg/kg; seizures: 2–3 mg/kg; increased intracranial pressure: 1.5–5 mg/kg; repeated as needed. *Adults:* IV: 25–250 mg as needed for effect. Sedation: Rectal. *Children:* 5–10 mg/kg/dose. *Adults:* 3–4 g/dose.	*Adverse events:* Cramping, diarrhea, rectal bleeding, hypotension, myocardial depression, prolonged somnolence and recovery, emergence delirium, respiratory depression, coughing, bronchospasm, laryngospasm, hiccups, sneezing. *Monitoring:* Thiopental concentrations: Therapeutic: hypnosis: 1–5 µg/mL; anesthesia: 7–130 µg/mL; coma: 30–100 µg/mL.
Thioridazine Mellaril, generic. Oral concentrate: 30, 100 mg/mL. Oral suspension: 25 mg/5 mL, 100 mg/5 mL. Tablet: 10, 15, 25, 50, 100, 150, 200 mg.	**Treatment of psychosis, neurosis, and severe behavior problems in children (phenothiazine, block dopamine receptors in the brain).** *Children >2 yr:* 0.5–3 mg/kg/24 hr in 2–3 doses. *Children >12 yr and adults:* 25–800 mg/24 hr in 2–4 doses.	*Adverse events:* Pseudoparkinsonism, tardive dyskinesia, akathisia, dystonias, dizziness, neuroleptic malignant syndrome, impaired temperature regulation, orthostatic hypotension, pigmentary retinopathy, cholestatic jaundice, leukopenia, agranulocytosis, urinary retention, constipation, dry mouth, gastrointestinal upset, hyperpigmentation, photosensitivity.
Thiotepa Thioplex. Injection.	**Cancer chemotherapy (alkylating agent, inhibit DNA, RNA, and protein synthesis).** *Children:* IV (depends on protocol): regular dose: 25–65 mg/m² q 3–4 wk; high dose: 300 mg/m²/24 hr for 3 doses. *Adults:* IV continuous infusion 15–35 mg/m² over 48 hr.	*Adverse events:* Myelosuppression (onset, 7–10 days; nadir, 14 days; recovery, 28 days), dizziness, fever, headache, anorexia, nausea, vomiting, alopecia, rash, pruritus, hyperuricemia, hematuria, hemorrhagic cystitis, stomatitis.
Thiothixene Navane, generic. Injection. Capsule: 1, 2, 5, 10, 20 mg. Oral concentrate: 5 mg/mL.	**Management of psychosis (phenothiazine, block CNS dopamine receptors).** *Children <12 yr:* 0.25 mg/kg/24 hr in divided doses. *Children >12 yr and adults:* PO: 6–60 mg/24 hr in 3 doses; IM: 4 mg 2–4 times/24 hr (max: 30 mg/24 hr).	*Adverse events:* Orthostatic hypotension, pseudoparkinsonism, tardive dyskinesia, akathisia, dystonias, constipation, urinary retention, dry mouth, stomach pain, nasal congestion, pigmentary retinopathy, agranulocytosis, leukopenia, neuroleptic malignant syndrome, impaired temperature regulation, finger tremor, cholestatic jaundice.
Thrombin, topical Thrombinar, Thrombogen, Thrombostat. Powder.	**Hemostasis for minor bleeding from capillaries and venules (catalyze the conversion of fibrinogen to fibrin).** *Children and adults:* Apply topically as solution 1,000–2,000 units/mL directly to site.	*Adverse events:* Allergy.
Tiagabine Gabitril Tablet: 2, 4, 12, 16, 20 mg.	**Treatment of partial seizures. Used as adjunctive, add-on therapy.** γ-Aminobutyric acid reuptake inhibitor. *Infants and children:* 1.5 mg/kg/24 hr in 2–4 divided doses.	*Cautions:* CNS problems including dizziness, drowsiness, ataxia, tremor, and muscle weakness; also may cause nonconvulsive status epilepticus.

TABLE 712–1. General Medications *Continued*

Drug (Trade Names, Formulations)	Indications (Mechanism of Action) and Dosing	Comments (Cautions, Adverse Events, Monitoring)
Timolol Timoptic. Ophthalmic solution, ophthalmic gel, tablet.	*Adolescents and adults:* Start at 4 mg once daily; increase by 4–8 mg q wk until response (max: 56 mg/24 hr). **Treat elevated intraocular pressure (block β_1- and β_2-receptors, and decrease aqueous humor production).** *Children:* (Only ophthalmic use) instill 0.25% solution 1 drop twice daily, may increase to 0.5% solution if response inadequate, may decrease to once daily if controlled. *Adults:* Same ophthalmic dose as children.	*Adverse events:* Bronchospasm, bradycardia, hypotension, visual disturbance, conjunctivitis, keratitis.
Tissue plasminogen activator, TPA Alteplase, Retavase. Injection.	**Thrombolytic therapy (enhance conversion of plasminogen to plasmin).** *Neonates:* 0.1–0.5 mg/kg/hr for 3–10 hr. *Children:* 0.1–0.6 mg/kg/hr for 6 hr. *Adults:* 100 mg infused as 60 mg in first hr, 20 mg in 2nd hr, 20 mg in 3rd hr.	*Caution:* Initiate heparin concurrently to avoid thrombosis and thrombotic emboli. *Adverse events:* Bleeding, arrhythmias (related to post-1st myocardial infarction reperfusion). *Monitoring:* D-Dimer, fibrinogen, bleeding time.
Tolazoline Priscoline. Injection: 25 mg/mL.	**Treatment of persistent pulmonary hypertension (α-adrenergic blocker and histamine release).** *Neonates:* IV: 1–2 mg/kg load, then 1–2 mg/kg/hr continuous infusion.	*Adverse events:* Hypotension, flushing, tachycardia, increases secretions from respiratory and gastrointestinal tract, gastrointestinal bleeding and perforation, oliguria, pulmonary hemorrhage, thrombocytopenia. *Monitoring:* Preductal and postductal oxygen saturation, arterial blood gases.
Tolmetin sodium Tolectin, generic. Tablet: 200, 600 mg. Capsule: 400 mg.	**Treatment of rheumatoid arthritis including JRA (NSAID, prostaglandin inhibition).** *Children >2 yr:* 15–30 mg/kg/24 hr in 3–4 doses. Analgesia: 5–7 mg/kg/dose. *Adults:* 400–600 mg 3 times/24 hr (max dose: 2 g/24 hr).	*Adverse events:* Gastrointestinal upset, peptic ulcer disease, hypertension, edema, dizziness, headache, acute renal failure, tinnitus.
Topiramate Topamax. Capsule: 15, 25 mg. Tablet: 25, 100, 200 mg.	**Treatment of seizure disorders. Broad spectrum of seizure types covered and multiple mechanisms proposed.** *Children 2–16 years:* Start 1–3 mg/kg/24 hr PO qhs for 1 wk; titrate dose increases every 1–2 wk by 1–3 mg/kg/24 hr dosed bid; typical dose 5–10 mg/kg/24 hr divided q12h. Capsules may be sprinkled on food to administer. *Adults:* Start 25–50 mg PO q24h; increase by 25–50 mg/24 hr q wk (max dose: 1,600 mg/24 hr). Reduce dose by 50% if CrCl <60 mL/min.	*Cautions:* If used with other carbonic anhydrase inhibitors, additive effects may predispose to renal stones.
Tranexamic acid Cyklokapron. Injection: 100 mg/mL. Tablet: 500 mg.	**Use in hemophilia patients during and after tooth extractions to reduce or prevent hemorrhage (competitively inhibits activation of plasminogen).** *Children and adults:* IV: 10 mg/kg immediately before surgery then oral 25 mg/kg/dose 3–4 times/24 hr for 2–8 days.	*Adverse events:* Hypotension, thromboembolic complications (including CNS), thrombocytopenia, nausea, vomiting, diarrhea. *Comment:* Decrease dose in renal impairment (CrCl 50–80 mL/min give 50% of dose; CrCl 10–50 mL/min give 25% of dose; CrCl <10 mL/min give 10% of dose).
Trazodone Desyrel, generic. Tablet: 50, 100, 150, 300 mg.	**Antidepressant (inhibit serotonin reuptake, α-adrenergic blockade).** *Children 6–18 yr:* Start 1.5–2 mg/kg/24 hr in 3 doses; may increase q 3–4 days (max: 6 mg/kg/24 hr). *Adolescents:* Start 25–50 mg/24 hr; may increase gradually (max: 150 mg) in 2–3 doses. *Adults:* Start 50 mg tid; may increase by 50 mg q 3 days to effect (max: 600 mg/24 hr).	*Adverse events:* Headache, confusion, dizziness, dry mouth, nausea, bad taste in mouth, constipation, blurred vision, muscle tremors, hypotension, tachycardia. *Drug interactions:* Fluoxetine may increase levels. *Monitoring:* Trazodone concentrations (limited correlation with clinical effectiveness): therapeutic 0.5–2.5 μg/mL; toxic >4 μg/mL.
Tretinoin Retin-A. Cream: 0.025%, 0.05%, 0.1%. Topical gel: 0.01%, 0.025%. Topical liquid: 0.05%.	**Treatment of acne vulgaris, photo-damaged skin, and some skin cancers (inhibits microcomedone formation and eliminates lesions).** *Children >12 yr:* Apply weaker formulation once daily at bedtime. Increase as needed.	*Adverse events:* Excessive skin dryness, erythema, scaling, and local stinging and burning; photosensitivity (use sun block), initial acne flare-up.
Triamcinolone Generic. Injection (Amcort). Oral (Aristocort). Topical (Aristocort). Metered-dose inhaler (MDI) (Azmacort). Nasal spray (Nasacort).	**Treatment of inflammatory and allergic conditions (corticosteroid).** *Children 6–12 yr:* IM: 0.03–0.2 mg/kg q 1–7 days. MDI: 2 puffs 2–4 times/24 hr). Intranasal: 1 spray in each nostril 1–2 times/24 hr. Injection: Intra-articular, intrabursal, or tendon sheath 2.5–15 mg (repeat as needed). *Children >12 yr and adults:* MDI: 2–4 puffs 2–4 times/24 hr; intranasal: 2 sprays in each nostril once daily (max: 4 sprays/24 hr). Intra-articular, intrasynovial; 2.5–40 mg; PO: 40–100 mg/24 hr in 1–4 doses. Topical: Apply thin film bid–tid.	*Adverse events:* Atrophy of tissue at local application site, fatigue, cataracts, osteoporosis, oral candidiasis (with MDI), poor growth. *Comment:* See comparison of corticosteroids under *Hydrocortisone.*

Table continued on following page

MEDICATIONS

TABLE 712–1. **General Medications** *Continued*

Drug (Trade Names, Formulations)	Indications (Mechanism of Action) and Dosing	Comments (Cautions, Adverse Events, Monitoring)
Triamterene Dyrenium. Capsule: 50, 100 mg (combination drugs, e.g., with hydrochlorothiazide).	**Diuretic to treat edema or hypertension (competes with aldosterone for receptor sites in distal renal tubules).** *Children:* PO: 2–4 mg/kg/24 hr in 1–2 doses (max: 6 mg/kg/24 hr). *Adults:* 100–300 mg/24 hr in 1–2 doses.	*Caution:* Do not use in patients with renal failure; avoid concurrent potassium supplements to avoid hyperkalemia. *Adverse events:* Constipation, nausea, headache, fatigue, hyperkalemia, hyponatremia, hyperchloremic metabolic acidosis.
Trientine Syprine. Capsule: 250 mg.	**Treatment of Wilson disease in patients intolerant to penicillamine (chelating agent).** *Children <12 yr:* 500–1,500 mg/24 hr in 2–4 doses. *Children >2 yr and adults:* 750–2,000 mg/24 hr in 2–4 doses.	*Comment:* Take 1 hr before or 2 hr after meals. Do not break capsule in any way and take with full glass of water. If capsule breaks, wash area of skin where contents touch thoroughly with water. *Adverse events:* Iron-deficiency anemia, malaise, epigastric pain, thickening and fissuring of skin, muscle cramps, systemic lupus erythematosus.
Trifluoperazine Stelazine. Oral concentrate: 10 mg/mL. Tablet: 1, 2, 5, 10 mg. Injection.	**Treatment of psychosis (phenothiazine, block dopamine in the CNS).** *Children 6–12 yr:* PO: 1 mg 1–2 times/24 hr, gradually increase to effect (max: 15 mg/24 hr); IM: 1 mg twice daily. *>12 yr and adults:* PO: 1–2 mg bid; IM: 1–2 mg q4–6h as needed (max: 10 mg/24 hr).	*Adverse events:* Hypotension, tachycardia, arrhythmias, pseudoparkinsonism, tardive dyskinesia, akathisia, dystonias, constipation, nasal congestion, dry mouth, malignant hypertension.
Trimethaphan camsylate Arfonad. Injection.	**Treatment of hypertensive emergencies (adrenergic and cholinergic blocker).** *Children:* 50–150 µg/kg/min. *Adults:* 0.5–2 mg/min.	*Adverse events:* Anorexia, nausea, dry mouth, ileus, urinary retention, cycloplegia, itching, urticaria, apnea, hypotension.
Trimethobenzamide Tigan, generic. Capsule: 100, 250 mg. Rectal suppository: 100, 200 mg. Injection: 100 mg/mL.	**Control of nausea and vomiting (inhibits CNS stimulation of chemoreceptor trigger zone).** *Children:* PO, rectal: 15–20 mg/kg/24 hr in 3–4 doses. *Adults:* PO: 250 mg tid–qid. IM, rectal: 200 mg tid–qid.	*Adverse events:* Drowsiness, dizziness, headache, diarrhea, muscle cramps.
Tromethamine THAM. Injection: 0.3 M (1 mEq THAM = 3.3 mL).	**Correction of metabolic acidosis (combines with hydrogen ions to form bicarbonate and buffer).** *Neonates, infants, children, and adults:* Dose (mL of 0.3 M solution) = Weight (kg) × base deficit; or 1–2 mEq/kg/dose.	*Adverse events:* Apnea, hypoglycemia, hyperkalemia, tissue irritation, or necrosis if direct contact.
Tropicamide Mydriacyl. Ophthalmic solution 0.5%, 1%.	**Short-acting mydriatic agent (blocks sphincter muscle of iris and ciliary body from responding to cholinergic stimulation).** *Children and adults:* Cycloplegia: Instill 1–2 drops of 1% solution; may repeat in 5 min. Mydriasis: Instill 1–2 drops of 0.5% solution 15–20 min before examination.	*Adverse events:* Tachycardia, drowsiness, headache, dry mouth, blurred vision, photophobia.
Tubocurarine Injection.	**Neuromuscular blocker used in anesthesia (block acetylcholine receptors).** *Neonates:* Start 0.3 mg/kg; maintenance: 0.1 mg/kg/dose. *Children:* Start 0.2–0.5 mg/kg, then 0.04–0.1 mg/kg/dose maintenance. *Adults:* Start 6–9 mg, then 3–4.5 mg maintenance.	*Adverse events:* Hypotension, prolonged respiratory depression.
Urokinase Abbokinase. Injection.	**Thrombolytic agent for treatment of recent onset thrombosis (activates plasminogen conversion to plasmin).** *Neonates, infants, children, and adults:* IV load 4,400 units/kg, maintenance dose 4,000–10,000 units/kg/hr. Occluded IV catheter: fill entire volume of catheter with urokinase 5,000 units/mL and leave in lumen for 1–4 hr.	*Adverse events:* Bleeding, hematoma, allergic reactions, bronchospasm. *Monitoring:* D-Dimer, fibrin degradation products, activated coagulation time.
Ursodiol, ursodeoxycholic acid Actigall. Capsule: 300 mg. Extemporaneous formulations.	**Gallbladder stone dissolution, reversal of TPN-induced cholestasis in neonates (decrease cholesterol content of bile).** *Neonates:* 10–18 mg/kg/24 hr PO divided into 1–3 doses per day. *Infants:* 30 mg/kg/24 hr 0.8–12h. *Adults:* 300 mg at bedtime for 6–12 mo.	*Adverse events:* Diarrhea, dyspepsia, biliary pain, rhinitis, pruritus, headache.
Valproic acid and derivatives Depakene, generic, Depakote. Depakote delayed-release tablet, capsule sprinkle: 125, 250, 500 mg. Depakene capsule: 250 mg. Syrup: 250 mg/5 mL. Injection.	**Treatment of simple and complex generalized and partial seizures (block sodium and slow T channels).** *Neonates:* Refractory seizures: load 20 mg/kg orally, then 10 mg/kg/dose q12h. *Children and adults:* Seizures: 10–15 mg/kg/24 hr in 2–3 doses; then increase weekly by 5–10 mg/kg/24 hr to effect; may need up to 100 mg/kg/day in 3–4 divided doses, especially if used with concurrent enzyme inducers (e.g., phenytoin, carbamazepine).	*Caution:* Hepatic failure with fatalities have been reported, especially if patient is younger than age 2 yr or receiving other anticonvulsants. If used in neonates, monitor serum ammonia. *Adverse events:* Drowsiness, irritability, confusion, malaise, headache, tremor, sensorineural hearing loss, hyperammonemia, hepatotoxicity, nausea, vomiting, diarrhea, pancreatitis, thrombocytopenia, increased appetite, weight gain. *Monitoring:* Valproate concentrations: therapeutic 50–100 µg/mL; toxic >150 µg/mL.

TABLE 712–1. **General Medications** *Continued*

Drug (Trade Names, Formulations)	Indications (Mechanism of Action) and Dosing	Comments (Cautions, Adverse Events, Monitoring)
Vasopressin Pitressin. Injection: 20 pressor units/mL.	**Treatment of diabetes insipidus; prevention and treatment of postoperative abdominal distention; treatment of acute gastrointestinal hemorrhage (antidiuretic hormone analog).** *Children:* Diabetes insipidus: IM, SC: 2.5–10 units/dose 2–4 times/24 hr. Gastrointestinal hemorrhage: IV continuous infusion 0.002–0.01 units/kg/min. *Adults:* Diabetes insipidus: IM, SC: 5–10 units/dose 2–4 times/24 hr. Gastrointestinal hemorrhage: IV continuous infusion 0.2–0.4 units/min.	*Adverse events:* Increased blood pressure, bradycardia, arrhythmias, fever, flatulence, abdominal cramps, nausea, vomiting, tremor, sweating, circumoral pallor, water intoxication.
Vecuronium Norcuron. Injection.	**Adjunct to anesthesia, neuromuscular blocker (blocks acetylcholine from binding to motor end-plates).** *Neonates:* 0.03–0.15 mg/kg/dose q1–2h as needed. *Infants >7 wk–12 mo:* 0.05–0.1 mg/kg qh as needed. *Children 1 yr–adults:* 0.05–0.1 mg/kg qh as needed.	*Adverse events:* Tachycardia, hypotension, flushing, bradycardia, circulatory collapse, hypersensitivity reactions.
Venlafaxine Effexor. Tablet: 25, 37.5, 50, 75, 100 mg.	**Treatment of depression, obsessive-compulsive disorder, attention deficit disorder (serotonin and norepinephrine reuptake inhibitor).** *Children:* 25–200 mg/24 hr; start low and titrate up every 4–7 days. *Adults:* Start 75 mg/24 hr; titrate q 4–7 days to effect or maximum of 375 mg/24 hr.	*Caution:* Taper slowly (max: 25 mg/24 hr q 5–7 days) if stopping drug to avoid withdrawal syndrome. *Adverse events:* Headache, somnolence, dizziness, insomnia, nervousness, nausea, dry mouth, constipation, blurred vision.
Verapamil Calan, Isoptin, generic. Sustained-release capsule: 120, 180, 240, 360 mg. Sustained-release tablet: 120, 180, 240 mg. Tablet: 40, 80, 120 mg. Injection.	**Calcium-channel antagonist used in the treatment of hypertension and supraventricular dysrhythmias.** Doses in infants and young children not well established: *Infants:* 0.1–0.2 mg/kg and children 0.1–0.3 mg/kg per dose IV repeated to desired effect. *Children:* 4–8 mg/kg/24 hr PO q6–8h; usual dose 5 mg/kg/24 hr. *Adults:* 240–480 mg/24 hr PO divided q6–8 hr; q12h with extended-release products. May sprinkle contents of capsule onto soft food without affecting absorption.	*Caution:* Adjust dose in renal disease. Avoid IV use in neonates/young infants, or those with heart failure. *Adverse effects:* Hypotension, bradycardia, heart block, dizziness, seizure, abdominal discomfort. Avoid in newborns due to several reports of fatality due to heart block. *Drug interactions:* May increase concentrations of caffeine, digoxin, carbamazepine, cyclosporine; decreased concentrations with rifampin, phenobarbital.
Vigabatrin Sabril (not available in USA, available in Canada, Mexico, Europe, and other countries). Tablet: 500 mg. Dry powder sachet.	**Effective against infantile spasms, partial seizures, and other seizure types. Mechanism is γ-aminobutyric acid transaminase inhibitor.** *Children:* 40–150 mg/kg/24 hr in 1–2 doses.	*Caution:* May cause bilateral visual field deficits, do baseline eye examination and then every 6 months. CNS depression, psychiatric reactions, behavioral problems, and gastrointestinal intolerance may occur.
Vinblastine sulfate Alkaban-AQ; Velban; generic. Injection.	**Treatment of several cancers (bind to mitotic spindle to inhibit metaphase).** *Children:* IV Hodgkin disease: 2.5–6 mg/m²/24 hr q 1–2 wk for 3–6 wk (max: 12.5 mg/m²/wk). *Adults:* 3.7–18.5 mg/m²/24 hr q 7–10 days.	*Adverse events:* Alopecia, nausea, vomiting, abdominal cramps, constipation, diarrhea, stomatitis, myelosuppression (onset, 4–7 days; nadir, 4–10 days; recovery, 17 days), tachycardia, orthostatic hypotension, dermatitis, photosensitivity, muscle pain, paresthesias, urinary retention, hyperuricemia, peripheral neuropathy (loss of deep tendon reflexes, headache, weakness).
Vincristine Oncovin, generic. Injection.	**Treatment of various cancers (bind to mitotic spindle to inhibit metaphase).** *Children: <10 kg or BSA <1 m²:* 0.05 mg/kg once/wk. *>10 kg or BSA >1 m²:* 1–2 mg/m² once/wk. *Adults:* 0.4–1.4 mg/m² once/wk.	*Adverse events:* Constipation, paralytic ileus, depression, confusion, insomnia, headache, jaw pain, optic atrophy, blindness, loss of deep tendon reflexes in legs, numbness, tingling, pain, stocking-and-glove paresthesias, footdrop, wristdrop, syndrome of inappropriate secretion of antidiuretic hormone, photophobia, hyperuricemia, stomatitis, phlebitis, myelosuppression (onset, 7 days; nadir, 10 days; recovery, 21 days).
Vitamin A Aquasol A, generic. Injection. Oral drops. Capsule.	**Treatment or prevention of deficiency; supplementation in patients with measles (co-factor for many biochemical processes) and improve growth in children with HIV or malaria. Prevention of bronchopulmonary dysplasia in neonates.** *Neonates:* 4,000 IU IM 3 times/wk, or 2,000 IU IM every other day. *Children:* Vitamin A deficiency with xerophthalmia: *1–8 yr:* PO: 5,000 units/24 hr for 5 days; IM: 5000–15,000 units/24 hr for 10 days. *>8 yr and adults:* PO: 500,000 units/24 hr for 3 days, then 50,000 units/24 hr for 14 days, then 20,000 units/24 hr for 2 months.	*Adverse events:* Irritability, vertigo, lethargy, fever, headache, hypercalcemia.

Table continued on following page

MEDICATIONS

TABLE 712–1. **General Medications** *Continued*

Drug (Trade Names, Formulations)	Indications (Mechanism of Action) and Dosing	Comments (Cautions, Adverse Events, Monitoring)
	Vitamin A deficiency without corneal changes: *Children <1 yr:* IM: 100,000 units q 4–6 mo. *>1 yr:* IM: 200,000 units q 4–6 mo. *>8 yr and adults:* IM: 100,000 units/24 hr for 3 days, then 50,000 units/24 hr for 14 days. Prophylaxis of patients at risk and supplementation in measles: PO dose q 4–6 mo. *Children <1 yr:* 100,000 units. *>1 yr:* 200,000 units. Improve growth in children with HIV or malaria or diarrheal disease: *Infants <1 yr:* 100,000 units q24h for 2 doses, then 100,000 units (one dose) at 4 and 8 mo. *Children >1 yr:* 200,000 units q24h for 2 doses, then 200,000 units (one dose) at 4 and 8 mo.	
Vitamin E Generic. Capsule, oral drops, tablet, cream, ointment.	**Nutritional supplement (antioxidant).** *Neonates, premature infants:* 25–50 units/24 hr. *Children:* 1 unit/kg/24 hr; sickle cell anemia: 450 units/24 hr; cystic fibrosis: 100–400 units/24 hr; β-thalassemia: 750 units/24 hr. *Adults:* 60–75 units/24 hr.	*Adverse events:* Rare.
Warfarin Coumadin, generic. Tablet: 1, 2, 2.5, 4, 5, 7.5, 10 mg.	**Anticoagulant that antagonizes hepatic vitamin K synthesis depleting vitamin K–dependent clotting factors II, VII, IX, and X.** *Children:* Initial dose 0.2 mg/kg once PO then usual dose approximates 0.1 mg/kg/24 hr PO. Dose titrated to desired prothrombin time and INR targets. Avoid large loading doses because complete anticoagulant effect depends on elimination half-lives of the target clotting factors. Full effects may not be observed until 2–3 days after a warfarin dose adjustment negating rapid dose changes. *Caution:* Younger infants require higher doses (typical mean dose 0.3 mg/kg/24 hr). Avoid foods with high vitamin K content (green leafy vegetables).	*Adverse effects:* Bleeding, skin necrosis, hemoptysis. *Drug interactions:* Aspirin, barbiturates, carbamazepine, cimetidine, omeprazole, phenytoin, rifampin, vitamin K, ritonavir, delavirdine.
Xylometazoline Otrivin. Nasal solution: 0.05%, 0.1%.	**Symptomatic relief of nasal congestion (stimulates α-adrenergic receptors to produce vasoconstriction).** *Children 2–12 yr:* Instill 2–3 drops 0.05% solution in each nostril q8–10h. *Children >12 yr and adults:* Instill 2–3 drops 0.1% solution in each nostril every 8–10 hr.	*Caution:* Do not use for more than 4 consecutive days or exceed recommended dosage because it may cause rebound congestion and chemical pneumonitis and create dependence. *Adverse events:* Palpitations, headache, dizziness, drowsiness, sweating, blurred vision.
Zafirlukast Accolate. Tablet: 20 mg.	**Leukotriene D₄ and E₄ antagonist inhibiting the effect of slow-reactive substance(s) of anaphylaxis (SRS-A) on bronchial smooth muscle. Not effective in reversing acute bronchoconstriction, although therapy can be continued in acute attacks.** *Children 7–11 yr:* 20 mg/24 hr PO divided q12h. *Adolescents and adults:* 40 mg/24 hr PO divided q12h. Administer doses 1 hr before or 2 hr after meals.	*Caution:* Based on mechanism of action this drug is effective for prophylaxis and does not reverse bronchoconstriction. *Adverse effects:* Headache, nausea, dyspepsia, elevated liver function tests. *Drug interactions:* Blocks CYP 2C9 and 3A4 hepatic isozymes; macrolides, theophylline, carbamazepine, terfenadine, astemizole.
Zileuton Zyflo. Tablet: 600 mg.	**5-Lipoxygenase inhibitor inhibiting the formation of leukotrienes LTB1, LTC1, LTD1, and LTE1. Not effective in reversing acute bronchoconstriction, although therapy can be continued in acute attacks.** *Adolescents and adults:* 2,400 mg/24 hr PO divided q6h.	*Caution:* Based on mechanism of action this drug is effective for prophylaxis and does not reverse bronchoconstriction. *Adverse effects:* Chest pain, headache, nausea, dyspepsia, elevated liver function tests. *Drug interactions:* Macrolides, theophylline, propranolol, warfarin, terfenadine, astemizole.
Zinc supplements Generic. Injection, liquid, tablets.	**Prevention and treatment of zinc deficiency (replacement therapy).** Zinc deficiency: Oral: *Infants and children:* 0.5–1 mg/kg/24 hr in 1–3 doses. *Adults:* 25–50 mg/dose tid. TPN supplement: *Preterm infants:* 400 μg/kg/24 hr. *Infants <3 mo:* 250 μg/kg/24 hr. *Infants >3 mo:* 100 μg/kg/24 hr. *Children:* 50 μg/kg/24 hr.	*Adverse events:* Rare, but if excessive doses are used may cause copper deficiency.
Ziprasidone Geodon Capsule: 20, 40, 60, 80 mg.	**Atypical antipsychotic.** *Children:* Start 5 mg/24 hr; increase q48h to response. Dose bid. *Adults:* Start 20 mg bid; increase q48h to response (max: 80 mg bid).	*Caution:* May prolong QTc intervals and predispose to arrhythmia (especially torsades de pointes); avoid concurrent use of drugs that may also prolong QTc interval. *Adverse events:* Agitation, anxiety, dizziness, drowsiness, headache, insomnia, tachycardia, constipation, dry mouth, orthostatic hypotension, weight gain. *Drug interactions:* CYP3A4 inhibitors will decrease clearance and predispose to toxicity. Enzyme inducers will increase clearance and may increase dose requirements.

MEDICATIONS

TABLE 712–1. General Medications *Continued*

Drug (Trade Names, Formulations)	Indications (Mechanism of Action) and Dosing	Comments (Cautions, Adverse Events, Monitoring)
Zonisamide Zonegran. Capsules (gelatin): 100 mg.	**Treat seizure disorders. Mechanism uncertain.** *Children:* Start 2–4 mg/kg/24 hr; then increase by 2–5 mg/kg/24 hr q2–4days to response, usually 4–20 mg/kg/24 hr. *Adults:* Start with 100 mg/24 hr; may increase by 100 mg/24 hr every 2 wk to maximum of 600 mg/24 hr.	*Cautions:* Children are predisposed to hypohidrosis and hyperthermia with this drug. Most common side effects are drowsiness, rash, and renal stones

TABLE 712–2. Antibacterial Medications (Antibiotics)

Drug (Trade Names, Formulations)	Indications (Mechanism of Action) and Dosing	Comments
Amikacin sulfate Amikin. Injection: 50 mg/mL, 250 mg/mL.	**Aminoglycoside antibiotic active against gram-negative bacilli, especially *Escherichia coli, Klebsiella, Proteus, Enterobacter, Serratia,* and *Pseudomonas.*** *Neonates:* Postnatal age ≤7 days: 1,200–2,000 g: 7.5 mg/kg q12–18h IV or IM; >2,000 g: 10 mg/kg q12h IV or IM; postnatal age >7 days: 1,200–2,000 g IV or IM: 7.5 mg/kg q8–12hr IV or IM; >2,000 g: 10 mg/kg q8h IV or IM. *Children:* 15–25 mg/kg/24 hr divided q8–12h IV or IM. *Adults:* 15 mg/kg/24 hr divided q8–12h IV or IM.	*Cautions:* Anaerobes, *Streptococcus* (including *S. pneumoniae*) are resistant. May cause ototoxicity and nephrotoxicity. Monitor renal function. Drug eliminated renally. Administered IV over 30–60 min. *Drug interactions:* May potentiate other ototoxic and nephrotoxic drugs. *Target serum concentrations:* Peak 25–40 mg/L; trough <10 mg/L.
Amoxicillin Amoxil, Polymox. Capsule: 250, 500 mg. Tablet: chewable: 125, 250 mg. Suspension: 125 mg/5 mL, 250 mg/5 mL. Drops: 50 mg/mL.	**Penicillinase-susceptible β-lactam: gram-positive pathogens except *Staphylococcus, Salmonella, Shigella, Neisseria, E. coli,* and *Proteus mirabilis.*** *Children:* 20–50 mg/kg/24 hr divided q8–12h PO. Higher dose of 80–90 mg/kg/24 hr PO for otitis media. *Adults:* 250–500 mg q8–12h PO. Uncomplicated gonorrhea: 3 g with 1 g probenecid PO.	*Cautions:* Rash, diarrhea, abdominal cramping. Drug eliminated renally. *Drug interaction:* Probenecid.
Amoxicillin-clavulanate Augmentin. Tablet: 250, 500, 875 mg. Tablet, chewable: 125, 200, 250, 400 mg. Suspension: 125 mg/5 mL, 200 mg/5 mL, 250 mg/5 mL, 400 mg/5 mL.	**β-Lactam (amoxicillin) and β-lactamase inhibitor (clavulanate) enhances amoxicillin activity against penicillinase-producing bacteria: *S. aureus* (not methicillin-resistant organism), *Streptococcus, Haemophilus influenzae, Moraxella catarrhalis, E. coli, Klebsiella, Bacteroides fragilis.*** *Neonates:* 30 mg/kg/24 hr divided q12h PO. *Children:* 20–45 mg/kg/24 hr divided q8–12h PO. Higher dose 80–90 mg/kg/24 hr PO for otitis media.	*Cautions:* Drug dosed on amoxicillin component. May cause diarrhea, rash. Drug eliminated renally. *Drug interaction:* Probenecid. *Comment:* Higher dose may be active against penicillin tolerant/resistant *S. pneumoniae.*
Ampicillin Polycillin, Omnipen. Capsule: 250, 500 mg. Suspension: 125 mg/5 mL, 250 mg/5 mL, 500 mg/5 mL. Injection.	**β-Lactam with same spectrum of antibacterial activity as amoxicillin.** Neonates: Postnatal age ≤7 days ≤2,000 g: 50 mg/kg/24 hr IV or IM q12hr (meningitis: 100 mg/kg/24 hr divided q12h IV or IM); >2,000 g: 75 mg/kg/24 hr divided q8h IV or IM (meningitis: 150 mg/kg/24 hr divided q8h IV or IM). Postnatal age >7 days <1200 g: 50 mg/kg/24 hr IV or IM q12h (meningitis: 100 mg/kg/24 hr divided q12h IV or IM); 1,200–2,000 g: 75 mg/kg/24 hr divided q8h IV or IM (meningitis: 150 mg/kg/24 hr divided q8h IV or I M); >2,000 g: 100 mg/kg/24 hr divided q6h IV or IM (meningitis: 200 mg/kg/24 hr divided q6h IV or IM). *Children:* 100–200 mg/kg/24 hr divided q6h IV or IM (meningitis: 200–400 mg/kg/24 hr divided q4–6h IV or IM). *Adults:* 250–500 mg q4–8h IV or IM.	*Cautions:* Less bioavailable than amoxicillin causing greater diarrhea. *Drug interaction:* Probenecid.
Ampicillin-sulbactam Unasyn. Injection.	**β-Lactam (ampicillin) β-lactamase inhibitor (sulbactam) enhances ampicillin activity against penicillinase-producing bacteria: *S. aureus, Streptococcus, H. influenzae, M. catarrhalis, E. coli, Klebsiella, B. fragilis.***	*Cautions:* Drug dosed on ampicillin component. May cause diarrhea, rash. Drug eliminated renally. *Note:* Higher dose may be active against penicillin-tolerant/resistant *S. pneumoniae.* *Drug interaction:* Probenecid.

Table continued on following page

MEDICATIONS

TABLE 712–2. Antibacterial Medications (Antibiotics) *Continued*

Drug (Trade Names, Formulations)	Indications (Mechanism of Action) and Dosing	Comments
	Children: 100–200 mg/kg/24 hr divided q4–8h IV or IM. *Adults:* 1–2 g q6–8h IV or IM (max daily dose: 8 g).	
Azithromycin Zithromax. Tablet: 250 mg. Suspension: 100 mg/5 mL, 200 mg/5 mL.	**Azalide antibiotic with activity against *S. aureus, Streptococcus, H. influenzae, Mycoplasma, Legionella, Chlamydia trachomatis.*** *Children:* 10 mg/kg PO on day 1 (max: 500 mg) followed by 5 mg/kg PO q24h for 4 days. Group A *Streptococcus* pharyngitis: 12 mg/kg/ 24 hr PO (max: 500 mg) for 5 days. *Adults:* 500 mg PO day 1 followed by 250 mg for 4 days. Uncomplicated *C. trachomatis* infection: single 1 g dose PO.	*Note:* Very long half-life permitting once-daily dosing. No metabolic-based drug interactions (unlike erythromycin and clarithromycin), limited gastrointestinal distress. Shorter-course regimens (e.g., 1–3 days) under investigation. Three-day therapy (10 mg/kg/24 hr × 3 days) and single-dose therapy (30 mg/kg): use with increasing frequency (not for streptococcus pharyngitis).
Aztreonam Azactam. Injection.	**β-Lactam (monobactam) antibiotic with activity against gram-negative aerobic bacteria, Enterobacteriaceae, and *Pseudomonas aeruginosa.*** *Neonates:* Postnatal age ≤7 days ≤2,000 g: 60 mg/ kg/24 hr divided q12h IV or IM; >2,000 g: 90 mg/ kg/24 hr divided q8h IV or IM; postnatal age >7 days <1,200 g: 60 mg/kg/24 hr divided q12h IV or IM; 1,200–2,000 g: 90 mg/kg/24 hr divided q8h IV or IM; >2,000 g: 120 mg/kg/24 hr divided q6–8h IV or IM. *Children:* 90–120 mg/kg/24 hr divided q6–8h IV or IM. For cystic fibrosis up to 200 mg/kg/24 hr IV. *Adults:* 1–2 g IV or IM q8–12h (max 8 g/24 hr).	*Cautions:* Rash, thrombophlebitis, eosinophilia. Renally eliminated. *Drug interaction:* Probenecid.
Carbenicillin Geopen Injection. Geocillin oral tablet.	**Extended-spectrum penicillin (remains susceptible to penicillinase destruction) active against *Enterobacter*, indole-positive *Proteus*, and *Pseudomonas.*** *Neonates:* Postnatal age ≤7 days ≤2,000 g: 225 mg/kg/24 hr divided q8h IV or IM; >2000 g: 300 mg/kg/24 hr divided q6h IV or IM; >7 days: 300–400 mg/kg/24 hr divided q6h IV or IM. *Children:* 400–600 mg/kg/24 hr divided q4–6h IV or IM.	*Cautions:* Painful given intramuscularly; rash; each gram contains 5.3 mEq sodium. Interferes with platelet aggregation at high doses, increases in liver transaminase levels. Renally eliminated. Oral tablet for treatment of urinary tract infection only. *Drug interaction:* Probenecid.
Cefaclor Ceclor. Capsule: 250, 500 mg. Suspension: 125 mg/5 mL, 187 mg/5 mL, 250 mg/5 mL, 375 mg/5 mL.	**Second-generation cephalosporin active against *S. aureus, Streptococcus* including *S. pneumoniae, H. influenzae, E. coli, Klebsiella*, and *Proteus.*** *Children:* 20–40 mg/kg/24 hr divided q8–12h PO (max dose: 2 g). *Adults:* 250–500 mg q6–8h PO.	*Cautions:* β-Lactam safety profile (rash, eosinophilia) with high incidence of serum sickness reaction. Renally eliminated. *Drug interaction:* Probenecid.
Cefadroxil Duricef, Ultracef. Capsule: 500 mg. Tablet: 1,000 mg. Suspension: 125 mg/5 mL, 250 mg/5 mL, 500 mg/5 mL.	**First-generation cephalosporin active against *S. aureus, Streptococcus, E. coli, Klebsiella*, and *Proteus.*** *Children:* 30 mg/kg/24 hr divided q12h PO. (max dose: 2g). *Adults:* 250–500 mg q8–12h PO.	*Cautions:* β-Lactam safety profile (rash, eosinophilia). Renally eliminated. Long half-life permits q12–24h dosing. *Drug interaction:* Probenecid.
Cefazolin Ancef, Kefzol. Injection.	**First-generation cephalosporin active against *S. aureus, Streptococcus, E. coli, Klebsiella*, and *Proteus.*** *Neonates:* Postnatal age ≤7 days 40 mg/kg/24 hr divided q12h IV or IM; >7 days 40–60 mg/kg/ 24 hr divided q8h IV or IM. *Children:* 50–100 mg/kg/24 hr divided q8h IV or IM. *Adults:* 0.5–2 g q8h IV or IM (max dose: 12 g/24 hr).	*Caution:* β-Lactam safety profile (rash, eosinophilia). Renally eliminated. Does not adequately penetrate CNS. *Drug interaction:* Probenecid.
Cefdinir Omnicef. Capsule: 300 mg. Oral suspension: 125 mg/5 mL.	**Extended-spectrum, semi-synthetic cephalosporin.** *Children 6 mo–12 yr:* 14 mg/kg/24 hr in 1 or 2 doses PO (max: 600 mg/24 hr). *Adults:* 600 mg q24h PO.	*Cautions:* Reduce dosage in renal insufficiency (creatinine clearance <60 mL/min). Avoid taking concurrently with iron-containing products and antacids because absorption is markedly decreased; take at least 2 hr apart. *Drug interaction:* Probenecid. *Adverse events:* Diarrhea, nausea, vaginal candidiasis
Cefepime Maxipime. Injection.	**Expanded-spectrum, fourth-generation cephalosporin active against many gram-positive and gram-negative pathogens, including many multi-drug-resistant pathogens.** Children: 100–150 mg/kg/24 hr q8–12h IV or IM. Adults: 2–4 g/24 hr q12h IV or IM.	*Cautions:* β-Lactam safety profile (rash, eosinophilia). Renally eliminated. *Drug interaction:* Probenecid.
Cefixime Suprax. Tablet: 200, 400 mg. Suspension: 100 mg/5 mL.	**Third-generation cephalosporin active against *Streptococcus, H. influenzae, M. catarrhalis, N. gonorrhoeae, S. marcescens*, and *P. vulgaris.* No antistaphylococcal or antipseudomonal activity.** *Children:* 8 mg/kg/24 hr divided q12–24h PO. *Adults:* 400 mg/24 hr divided q12–24h PO.	*Cautions:* β-Lactam safety profile (rash, eosinophilia). Renally eliminated. Does not adequately penetrate CNS. *Drug interaction:* Probenecid.

TABLE 712–2. Antibacterial Medications (Antibiotics) *Continued*

Drug (Trade Names, Formulations)	Indications (Mechanism of Action) and Dosing	Comments
Cefoperazone sodium Cefobid. Injection.	**Third-generation cephalosporin active against many gram-positive and gram-negative pathogens.** *Neonates:* 100 mg/kg/24 hr divided q12h IV or IM. *Children:* 100–150 mg/kg/24 hr divided q8–12h IV or IM. *Adults:* 2–4 g/24 hr divided q8–12h IV or IM (max dose: 12 g/24 hr).	*Cautions:* Highly protein bound cephalosporin with limited potency reflected by weak antipseudomonal activity. Variable gram-positive activity. Primarily hepatically eliminated in bile. *Drug interaction:* Disulfiram-like reaction with alcohol.
Cefotaxime sodium Claforan. Injection.	**Third-generation cephalosporin active against gram-positive and gram-negative pathogens. No antipseudomonal activity.** *Neonates:* ≤7 days: 100 mg/kg/24 hr divided q12h IV or IM; >7 days: <1,200 g 100 mg/kg/24 hr divided q12h IV or IM; >12,000 g: 150 mg/kg/24 hr divided q8h IV or IM. *Children:* 150 mg/kg/24 hr divided q6–8h IV or IM (meningitis: 200 mg/kg/24 hr divided q6–8h IV). *Adults:* 1–2 g q8–12h IV or IM (max: 12 g/24 hr).	*Cautions:* β-Lactam safety profile (rash, eosinophilia). Renally eliminated. Each gram of drug contains 2.2 mEq sodium. Active metabolite. *Drug interaction:* Probenecid.
Cefotetan disodium Cefotan. Injection.	**Second-generation cephalosporin active against *S. aureus, Streptococcus, H. influenzae, E. coli, Klebsiella, Proteus,* and *Bacteroides.* Inactive against *Enterobacter.*** *Children:* 40–80 mg/kg/24 hr divided IV or IM q12h. *Adults:* 2–4 g/24 hr divided q12h IV or IM (max: 6 g/24 hr).	*Cautions:* Highly protein-bound cephalosporin, poor CNS penetration; β-lactam safety profile (rash, eosinophilia), disulfiram-like reaction with alcohol. Renally eliminated (~20% in bile).
Cefoxitin sodium Mefoxin. Injection.	**Second-generation cephalosporin active against *S. aureus, Streptococcus, H. influenzae, E. coli, Klebsiella, Proteus,* and *Bacteroides.* Inactive against *Enterobacter.*** *Neonates:* 70–100 mg/kg/24 hr divided q8–12h IV or IM. *Children:* 80–160 mg/kg/24 hr divided q6–8h IV or IM. *Adults:* 1–2 g q6–8h IV or IM (max dose: 12 g/24 hr).	*Cautions:* Poor CNS penetration; β-lactam safety profile (rash, eosinophilia). Renally eliminated. Painful given intramuscularly. *Drug interaction:* Probenecid.
Cefpodoxime proxetil Vantin. Tablet: 100 mg, 200 mg. Suspension: 50 mg/5 mL, 100 mg/5 mL.	**Third-generation cephalosporin active against *S. aureus, Streptococcus, H. influenzae, M. catarrhalis, N. gonorrhoeae, E. coli, Klebsiella,* and *Proteus.* No antipseudomonal activity.** *Children:* 10 mg/kg/24 hr divided q12h PO. *Adults:* 200–800 mg/24 hr divided q12h PO (max dose: 800 mg/24 hr). Uncomplicated gonorrhea: 200 mg PO as single-dose therapy.	*Cautions:* β-Lactam safety profile (rash, eosinophilia). Renally eliminated. Does not adequately penetrate CNS. Increased bioavailability when taken with food. *Drug interaction:* Probenecid; antacids and H-2 receptor antagonists may decrease absorption.
Cefprozil Cefzil. Tablet: 250, 500 mg. Suspension: 125 mg/5 mL, 250 mg/5 mL.	**Second-generation cephalosporin active against *S. aureus, Streptococcus, H. influenzae, E. coli, M. catarrhalis, Klebsiella,* and *Proteus.*** *Children:* 30 mg/kg/24 hr divided q8–12h PO. *Adults:* 500–1,000 mg/24 hr divided q12h PO (max dose: 1.5 g/24 hr).	*Cautions:* β-Lactam safety profile (rash, eosinophilia). Renally eliminated. Good bioavailability; food does not affect bioavailability. *Drug interaction:* Probenecid.
Ceftazidime Fortaz, Ceptaz, Tazicef, Tazidime. Injection.	**Third-generation cephalosporin active against gram-positive and gram-negative pathogens including *Pseudomonas aeruginosa.*** *Neonates:* Postnatal age ≤7 days: 100 mg/kg/24 hr divided q12h IV or IM; >7 days ≤1,200 g: 100 mg/kg/24 hr divided q12h IV or IM; >1,200 g: 150 mg/kg/24 hr divided q8h IV or IM. *Children:* 150 mg/kg/24 hr divided q8h IV or IM (meningitis: 150 mg/kg/24 hr IV divided q8h). *Adults:* 1–2 g q8–12h IV or IM (max: 8–12 g/24 hr).	*Cautions:* β-Lactam safety profile (rash, eosinophilia). Renally eliminated. Increasing pathogen resistance developing with long-term, widespread use. *Drug interaction:* Probenecid.
Ceftizoxime Cefizox. Injection.	**Third-generation cephalosporin active against gram-positive and gram-negative pathogens. No antipseudomonal activity.** *Children:* 150 mg/kg/24 hr divided q6–8h IV or IM. *Adults:* 1–2 g q6–8h IV or IM (max dose: 12 g/24 hr).	*Cautions:* β-Lactam safety profile (rash, eosinophilia). Renally eliminated. *Drug interaction:* Probenecid.
Ceftriaxone sodium Rocephin. Injection.	**Third-generation cephalosporin active against gram-positive and gram-negative pathogens. No antipseudomonal activity. Very potent and β-lactamase stable.** *Neonates:* 50–75 mg/kg q24h IV or IM. *Children:* 50–75 mg/kg q24h IV or IM (meningitis: 75 mg/kg dose 1 then 80–100 mg/kg/24 hr divided q12–24h IV or IM). *Adults:* 1–2 g q24h IV or IM (max dose: 4 g/24 hr).	*Cautions:* β-Lactam safety profile (rash, eosinophilia). Eliminated via kidney (33–65%) and bile; can cause sludging. Long half-life and dose-dependent protein binding favors q24h rather than q12h dosing. Can add 1% lidocaine for IM injection.

Table continued on following page

TABLE 712–2. Antibacterial Medications (Antibiotics) *Continued*

Drug (Trade Names, Formulations)	Indications (Mechanism of Action) and Dosing	Comments
Cefuroxime (cefuroxime axetil for oral administration) Ceftin, Kefurox, Zinacef. Injection. Suspension: 125 mg/5 mL. Tablet: 125, 250, 500 mg.	**Second-generation cephalosporin active against *S. aureus, Streptococcus, H. influenzae, E. coli, M. catarrhalis, Klebsiella*, and *Proteus.*** *Neonates:* 40–100 mg/kg/24 hr divided q12h IV or IM. *Children:* 200–240 mg/kg/24 hr divided q8h IV or IM; PO administration: 20–30 mg/kg/24 hr divided q8h PO. *Adults:* 750–1,500 mg q8h IV or IM (max dose: 6 g/24 hr).	*Cautions:* β-Lactam safety profile (rash, eosinophilia). Renally eliminated. Food increases PO bioavailability. *Drug interaction:* Probenecid.
Cephalexin Keflex, Keftab. Capsule: 250, 500 mg. Tablet: 500 mg, 1 g. Suspension: 125 mg/5 mL, 250 mg/5 mL, 100 mg/mL drops.	**First-generation cephalosporin active against *S. aureus, Streptococcus, E. coli, Klebsiella*, and *Proteus.*** *Children:* 25–100 mg/kg/24 hr divided q6–8h PO. *Adults:* 250–500 mg q6h PO (max dose: 4 g/24 hr).	*Cautions:* β-Lactam safety profile (rash, eosinophilia). Renally eliminated. *Drug interaction:* Probenecid.
Cephradine Velosef. Capsule: 250, 500 mg. Suspension: 125 mg/5 mL, 250 mg/5 mL.	**First-generation cephalosporin active against *S. aureus, Streptococcus, E. coli, Klebsiella*, and *Proteus.*** *Children:* 50–100 mg/kg/24 hr divided q6–12h PO. *Adults:* 250–500 mg q6–12h PO (max dose: 4 g/24 hr).	*Cautions:* β-Lactam safety profile (rash, eosinophilia). Renally eliminated. *Drug interaction:* Probenecid.
Chloramphenicol Chloromycetin. Injection. Capsule: 250 mg. Ophthalmic, otic solutions. Ointment.	**Broad-spectrum protein synthesis inhibitor active against many gram-positive and gram-negative bacteria, *Salmonella*, vancomycin-resistant *Enterococcus faecium, Bacteroides*, other anaerobes, *Mycoplasma, Chlamydia*, and *Rickettsia; Pseudomonas* usually resistant.** *Neonates:* Initial loading dose 20 mg/kg followed 12 hr later by: postnatal age ≤7 days: 25 mg/kg/24 hr q24h IV; >7 days: ≤2,000 g: 25 mg/kg/24 hr q24h IV; >2,000 g: 50 mg/kg/24 hr divided q12h IV. *Children:* 50–75 mg/kg/24 hr divided q6–8h IV or PO (meningitis: 75–100 mg/kg/24 hr IV divided q6h). *Adults:* 50 mg/kg/24 hr divided q6h IV or PO (max dose: 4 g/24 hr).	*Cautions:* Gray-baby syndrome (from too-high dose in neonate), bone marrow suppression, aplastic anemia (monitor hematocrit, free serum iron). *Drug interactions:* Phenytoin, phenobarbital, rifampin may decrease levels. *Target serum concentrations:* Peak 20–30 mg/L; trough 5–10 mg/L.
Ciprofloxacin Cipro. Tablet: 100, 250, 500, 750 mg. Injection. Ophthalmic solution and ointment. Otic suspension. Oral suspension: 250 and 500 mg/5 mL.	**Quinolone antibiotic active against *P. aeruginosa, Serratia, Enterobacter, Shigella, Salmonella, Campylobacter, Neisseria gonorrhoeae, H. influenzae, M. catarrhalis*, some *S. aureus*, and *Streptococcus.*** *Neonates:* 10 mg/kg q12h PO or IV. *Children:* 15–30 mg/kg/24 hr divided q12h PO or IV; cystic fibrosis: 20–40 mg/kg/24 hr divided q8–12h PO or IV. *Adults:* 250–750 mg q12h; 200–400 mg IV q12h PO (max dose: 1.5 g/24 hr).	*Cautions:* Concerns of joint destruction in juvenile animals not seen in humans; tendonitis, superinfection, dizziness, confusion, crystalluria, some photosensitivity. *Drug interactions:* Theophylline, magnesium-, aluminum-, or calcium-containing antacids, sucralfate, probenecid, warfarin, cyclosporine.
Clarithromycin Biaxin. Tablet: 250, 500 mg. Suspension: 125 mg/5 mL, 250 mg/5 mL.	**Macrolide antibiotic with activity against *S. aureus, Streptococcus, H. influenzae, Legionella, Mycoplasma*, and *C. trachomatis.*** *Children:* 15 mg/kg/24 hr divided q12h PO. *Adults:* 250–500 mg q12h PO (max dose: 1 g/24 hr).	*Cautions:* Adverse events less than erythromycin; gastrointestinal upset, dyspepsia, nausea, cramping. *Drug interactions:* Same as erythromycin: astemizole carbamazepine, terfenadine cyclosporine, theophylline, digoxin, tacrolimus.
Clindamycin Cleocin. Capsule: 75, 150, 300 mg. Suspension: 75 mg/5 mL. Injection. Topical solution, lotion, and gel. Vaginal cream.	**Protein synthesis inhibitor active against most gram-positive aerobic and anaerobic cocci except *Enterococcus.*** *Neonates:* Postnatal age ≤7 days <200 g: 10 mg/kg/24 hr divided q12h IV or IM; >2000 g: 15 mg/kg/24 hr divided q8h IV or IM; >7 days <1,200 g: 10 mg/kg/24 hr IV or IM divided q12h; 1,200–2,000 g: 15 mg/kg/24 hr divided q8h IV or IM; >2,000 g: 20 mg/kg/24 hr divided q8h IV or IM. *Children:* 10–40 mg/kg/24 hr divided q6–8h IV, IM, or PO. *Adults:* 150–600 mg q6–8h IV, IM, or PO (max dose: 5 g/24 hr IV or IM or 2 g/24 hr PO).	*Cautions:* Diarrhea, nausea, *C. difficile*–associated colitis, rash. Administer slow IV over 30–60 min. Topically active as an acne treatment.
Cloxacillin sodium Tegopen. Capsule: 250, 500 mg. Suspension: 125 mg/5 mL.	**Penicillinase-resistant penicillin active against *S. aureus* and other gram-positive cocci except *Enterococcus* and coagulase-negative staphylococci.** *Children:* 50–100 mg/kg/24 hr divided q6h PO. *Adults:* 250–500 mg q6h PO (max dose: 4 g/24 hr).	*Cautions:* β-Lactam safety profile (rash, eosinophilia). Primarily hepatically eliminated; requires dose reduction in renal disease. Food decreases bioavailability. *Drug interaction:* Probenecid.
Co-trimoxazole (trimethoprim-sulfamethoxazole; TMP-SMZ) Bactrim, Cotrim, Septra, Sulfatrim. Tablet: SMZ 400 mg and TMP 80 mg. Tablet DS: SMZ 800 mg and TMP 160 mg. Suspension: SMZ 200 mg and TMP 40 mg/5 mL. Injection.	**Antibiotic combination with sequential antagonism of bacterial folate synthesis with broad antibacterial activity: *Shigella, Legionella, Nocardia, Chlamydia, Pneumocystis carinii.* Dosage based on TMP component.** *Children:* 6–20 mg TMP/kg/24 hr or IV divided q12h PO.	*Cautions:* Drug dosed on TMP (trimethoprim) component. Sulfonamide skin reactions: rash, erythema multiforme, Stevens-Johnson syndrome, nausea, leukopenia. Renal and hepatic elimination; reduce dose in renal failure. *Drug interactions:* Protein displacement with warfarin, possibly phenytoin, cyclosporine.

TABLE 712–2. Antibacterial Medications (Antibiotics) *Continued*

Drug (Trade Names, Formulations)	Indications (Mechanism of Action) and Dosing	Comments
	P. carinii pneumonia: 15–20 mg TMP/kg/24 hr divided q12h PO or IV. *P. carinii* prophylaxis: 5 mg TMP/kg/24 hr or 3 times/wk PO. *Adults:* 160 mg TMP q12h PO.	
Demeclocycline Declomycin. Tablet: 150, 300 mg. Capsule: 150 mg.	**Tetracycline active against most gram-positive cocci except *Enterococcus*, many gram-negative bacilli, anaerobes, *Borrelia burgdorferi* (Lyme disease), *Mycoplasma*, and *Chlamydia*.** *Children:* 8–12 mg/kg/24 hr divided q6–12h PO. *Adults:* 150 mg PO q6–8h. Syndrome of inappropriate antidiuretic hormone secretion: 900–1,200 mg/24 hr or 13–15 mg/kg/24 hr divided q6–8h PO with dose reduction based on response to 600–900 mg/24 hr.	*Cautions:* Teeth staining, possibly permanent (if administered <8 yr of age) with prolonged use; photosensitivity, diabetes insipidus, nausea, vomiting, diarrhea, superinfections. *Drug interactions:* Aluminum-, calcium-, magnesium-, zinc- and iron-containing food, milk, dairy products may decrease absorption.
Dicloxacillin Dynapen, Pathocil. Capsule: 125, 250, 500 mg. Suspension: 62.5 mg/5 mL.	**Penicillinase-resistant penicillin active against *S. aureus* and other gram-positive cocci except *Enterococcus* and coagulase-negative staphylococci.** *Children:* 12.5–100 mg/kg/24 hr divided q6h PO. *Adults:* 125–500 mg q6h PO.	*Cautions:* β-Lactam safety profile (rash, eosinophilia). Primarily renally (65%) and bile (30%) elimination. Food may decrease bioavailability. *Drug interaction:* Probenecid.
Doxycycline Vibramycin, Doxy. Injection. Capsule: 50, 100 mg. Tablet: 50, 100 mg. Suspension: 25 mg/5 mL. Syrup: 50 mg/5 mL.	**Tetracycline antibiotic active against most gram-positive cocci except *Enterococcus*, many gram-negative bacilli, anaerobes, *Borrelia burgdorferi* (Lyme disease), *Mycoplasma*, and *Chlamydia*.** *Children:* 2–5 mg/kg/24 hr divided q12–24h PO or IV (max dose: 200 mg/24 hr). *Adults:* 100–200 mg/24 hr divided q12–24h PO or IV.	*Cautions:* Teeth staining, possibly permanent (<8 yr of age) with prolonged use; photosensitivity, nausea, vomiting, diarrhea, superinfections. *Drug interactions:* Aluminum-, calcium-, magnesium-, zinc-, iron-, kaolin-, and pectin-containing products, food, milk, dairy products may decrease absorption. Carbamazepine, rifampin, barbiturates may decrease half-life.
Erythromycin E-Mycin, Ery-Tab, Ery-C, Ilosone. Estolate 125, 500 mg. Tablet EES: 200 mg. Tablet base: 250, 333, 500 mg. Suspension: estolate 125 mg/5 mL, 250 mg/5 mL, EES 200 mg/5 mL, 400 mg/5 mL. Estolate drops: 100 mg/mL. EES drops: 100 mg/2.5 mL. Available in combination with sulfisoxazole (Pediazole), dosed on erythromycin content.	**Bacteriostatic macrolide antibiotic most active against gram-positive organisms, *Corynebacterium diphtheriae*, and *Mycoplasma pneumoniae*. May also be used to promote gastrointestinal motility and improve feeding intolerance in preterm infants.** *Neonates:* Postnatal age ≤7 days: 20 mg/kg/24 hr divided q12h PO; >7 days <1,200 g: 20 mg/kg/24 hr divided q12h PO; >1,200 g: 30 mg/kg/24 hr divided q8h PO (give as 5 mg/kg/dose q6h to improve feeding intolerance). *Children:* Usual max dose 2 g/24 hr. Base: 30–50 mg/kg/24 hr divided q6–8h PO. Estolate: 30–50 mg/kg/24 hr divided q8–12h PO. Stearate: 20–40 mg/kg/24 hr divided q6h PO. Lactobionate: 20–40 mg/kg/24 hr divided q6–8h IV. Gluceptate: 20–50 mg/kg/24 hr divided q6h IV: usual max dose 4 g/24 hr IV. *Adults:* Base: 333 mg PO q8h; estolate/stearate/base: 250–500 mg q6h PO.	*Cautions:* Motilin agonist leading to marked abdominal cramping, nausea, vomiting, diarrhea. Associated with hypertrophic pyloric stenosis in young infants. Many different salts with questionable tempering of gastrointestinal adverse events. Rare cardiac toxicity with IV use. Dose of salts differ. Topical formulation for treatment of acne. *Drug interactions:* Antagonizes hepatic CYP 450 3A4 activity: astemizole, carbamazepine, terfenadine, cyclosporine, theophylline, digoxin, tacrolimus, carbamazepine.
Gentamicin Garamycin. Injection. Ophthalmic solution, ointment, topical cream.	**Aminoglycoside antibiotic active against gram-negative bacilli, especially *E. coli, Klebsiella, Proteus, Enterobacter, Serratia*, and *Pseudomonas*.** *Neonates:* Postnatal age ≤7 days 1,200–2,000 g: 2.5 mg/kg q12–18h IV or IM; >2,000 g: 2.5 mg/kg q12h IV or IM; postnatal age >7 days 1,200–2,000 g: 2.5 mg/kg q8–12h IV or IM; >2,000 g: 2.5 mg/kg q8h IV or IM. *Children:* 2.5 mg/kg/24 hr divided q8–12h IV or IM. Alternatively may administer 5–7.5 mg/kg/24 hr IV once daily. *Intrathecal:* Preservative-free preparation for intraventricular or intrathecal use: neonate: 1 mg/24 hr; children: 1–2 mg/24 hr IT; adults: 4–8 mg/24 hr. Adults: 3–6 mg/kg/24 hr divided q8h IV or IM.	*Cautions:* Anaerobes, *S. pneumoniae*, other *Streptococcus* are resistant. May cause ototoxicity and nephrotoxicity. Monitor renal function. Drug eliminated renally. Administered IV over 30–60 min. *Drug interactions:* May potentiate other ototoxic and nephrotoxic drugs. *Target serum concentrations:* Peak 6–12 mg/L; trough <2 mg/L with intermittant daily dose regimens only.
Imipenem-cilastatin Primaxin. Injection.	**Carbapenem antibiotic active against broad-spectrum gram-positive cocci and gram-negative bacilli including *P. aeruginosa* and anerobes. No activity against *Stenotrophomonas maltophilia*.** *Neonates:* Postnatal age ≤7 days <1,200 g: 20 mg/kg q18–24h IV or IM; >1,200 g: 40 mg/kg divided q12h IV or IM; postnatal age >7 days 1,200–2,000 g: 40 mg/kg q12h IV or IM; >2,000 g: 60 mg/kg q8h IV or IM.	*Cautions:* β-Lactam safety profile (rash, eosinophilia), nausea, seizures. Cilastatin possesses no antibacterial activity; reduces renal imipenem metabolism. Primarily renally eliminated. *Drug interaction:* Possibly ganciclovir.

Table continued on following page

TABLE 712–2. **Antibacterial Medications (Antibiotics)** *Continued*

Drug (Trade Names, Formulations)	Indications (Mechanism of Action) and Dosing	Comments
	Children: 60–100 mg/kg/24 hr divided q6–8h IV or IM. *Adults:* 2–4 g/24 hr divided q6–8h IV or IM (max dose: 4 g/24 hr).	
Linezolid Zyvox. Tablet: 400, 600 mg. Oral suspension: 100 mg/ 5 mL. Injection: 100 mg/5mL.	**Oxazolidinone antibiotic active against gram-positive cocci (especially drug-resistant organisms), including** ***Staphylococcus, Streptococcus, Enterococcus faecium,*** **and** ***E. fecalis.*** **Interferes with protein synthesis by binding to 50S ribosome subunit.** *Children:* 10 mg/kg q12h IV or PO. *Adults:* Pneumonia: 600 mg q12h IV or PO; skin infections: 400 mg q12h IV or PO.	*Adverse events:* Myelosuppression, pseudomembranous colitis, nausea, diarrhea, headache. *Drug interaction:* Probenecid.
Loracarbef Lorabid. Capsule: 200 mg. Suspension: 100 mg/5 mL, 200 mg/5 mL.	**Carbacephem very closely related to cefaclor (second-generation cephalosporin) active against** ***S. aureus, Streptococcus, H. influenzae, M. catarrhalis, E. coli, Klebsiella,*** **and** ***Proteus.*** *Children:* 30 mg/kg/24 hr divided q12h PO (max dose: 2 g). *Adults:* 200–400 mg q12h PO (max dose: 800 mg/24 hr).	*Cautions:* β-Lactam safety profile (rash, eosinophilia). Renally eliminated. *Drug interaction:* Probenecid.
Meropenem Merrem. Injection.	**Carbapenem antibiotic active against broad-spectrum gram-positive cocci and gram-negative bacilli including** ***P. aeruginosa*** **and anerobes. No activity against** ***Stenotrophomonas maltophilia.*** *Children:* 60 mg/kg/24 hr divided q8h IV meningitis: 120 mg/kg/24 hr [max 6 g/24 hr] q8h IV. *Adults:* 1.5–3 g q8h IV.	*Cautions:* β-Lactam safety profile; appears to possess less CNS excitation than imipenem. 80% renal elimination. *Drug interaction:* Probenecid.
Metronidazole Flagyl, Metro-IV, generic. Topical gel, vaginal gel. Injection. Tablet: 250, 500 mg.	**Highly effective in the treatment of infections due to anaerobes.** *Neonates:* <1,200 g: 7.5 mg/kg q 48 hr PO or IV; postnatal age ≤7 days 1,200–2,000 g: 7.5 mg/kg/24 hr q 24 hr PO or IV; 2,000 g: 15 mg/kg/24 hr divided q12h PO or IV; postnatal age >7 days 1,200–2,000 g: 15 mg/kg/24 hr divided q12h PO or IV; >2,000 g: 30 mg/kg/24 hr divided q12h PO or IV. *Children:* 30 mg/kg/24 hr divided q6–8h PO or IV. *Adults:* 30 mg/kg/24 hr divided q6h PO or IV (max dose: 4 g/24 hr).	*Cautions:* Dizziness, seizures, metallic taste, nausea, disulfiram-like reaction with alcohol. Administer IV slow over 30–60 min. Adjust dose with hepatic impairment. *Drug interactions:* Carbamazepine, rifampin, phenobarbital may enhance metabolism; may increase levels of warfarin, phenytoin, lithium .
Mezlocillin sodium Mezlin. Injection.	**Extended-spectrum penicillin active against** ***E. coli, Enterobacter, Serratia,*** **and** ***Bacteroides;*** **limited antipseudomonal activity.** *Neonates:* Postnatal age ≤7 days: 150 mg/kg/24 hr divided q12h IV; >7 days: 225 mg/kg divided q8h IV. *Children:* 200–300 mg/kg/24 hr divided q4–6h IV; cystic fibrosis 300–450 mg/kg/24 hr IV. *Adults:* 2–4 g/dose q4–6h IV (max dose: 12 g/24 hr).	*Cautions:* β-Lactam safety profile (rash, eosinophilia); painful given intramuscularly; each gram contains 1.8 mEq sodium. Interferes with platelet aggregation with high doses; increases noted in liver function test results. Renally eliminated. Inactivated by β-lactamase enzyme. *Drug interaction:* Probenecid.
Mupirocin Bactroban. Ointment.	**Topical antibiotic active against** ***Staphylococcus*** **and** ***Streptococcus.*** Topical application: Nasal (eliminate nasal carriage) and to the skin 2–4 times per day.	*Caution:* Minimal systemic absorption as drug metabolized within the skin.
Nafcillin sodium Nafcil, Unipen. Injection. Capsule: 250 mg. Tablet: 500 mg.	**Penicillinase-resistant penicillin active against** ***S. aureus*** **and other gram-positive cocci except** ***Enterococcus*** **and coagulase-negative staphylococci.** *Neonates:* Postnatal age ≤7 days 1,200–2,000 g: 50 mg/kg/24 hr divided q12h IV or IM; >2,000 g: 75 mg/kg/24 hr divided q8h IV or IM; postnatal age >7 days 1,200–2,000 g: 75 mg/kg/ q8h; >2,000 g: 100 mg/kg divided q6–8h IV (meningitis: 200 mg/kg/24 hr divided q6h IV). *Children:* 100–200 mg/kg/24 hr divided q 4–6 hr IV. *Adults:* 4–12 g/24 hr divided q4–6h IV (max dose: 12 g/24 hr).	*Cautions:* β-Lactam safety profile (rash, eosinophilia), phlebitis; painful given intramuscularly; oral absorption highly variable and erratic (not recommended). *Adverse effect:* Neutropenia.
Nalidixic acid NegGram. Tablet: 250, 500, 1,000 mg. Suspension: 250 mg/5 mL.	**First-generation quinolone effective for short-term treatment of lower urinary tract infections caused by** ***E. coli, Enterobacter, Klebsiella,*** **and** ***Proteus.*** *Children:* 50–55 mg/kg/24 hr divided q6h PO; suppressive therapy 25–33 mg/kg/24 hr divided q6–8h PO. *Adults:* 1 g q6h PO; suppressive therapy: 500 mg q6h PO.	*Cautions:* Vertigo, dizziness, rash. Not for use in systemic infections. *Drug interactions:* Liquid antacids.

TABLE 712–2. **Antibacterial Medications (Antibiotics)** *Continued*

Drug (Trade Names, Formulations)	Indications (Mechanism of Action) and Dosing	Comments
Neomycin sulfate Mycifradin, generic. Tablet: 500 mg. Topical cream, ointment. Solution: 125 mg/5 mL.	**Aminoglycoside antibiotic used for topical application or orally before surgery to decrease gastrointestinal flora (nonabsorbable) and hyperammonemia.** *Infants:* 50 mg/kg/24 hr divided q6h PO. *Children:* 50–100 mg/kg/24 hr divided q6–8h PO. *Adults:* 500–2,000 mg/dose q6–8h PO.	*Cautions:* In patients with renal dysfunction because small amount absorbed may accumulate. *Adverse events:* Primarily related to topical application, abdominal cramps, diarrhea, rash. Aminoglycoside ototoxicity and nephrotoxicity if absorbed.
Nitrofurantoin Furadantin, Furan, Macrodantin. Capsule: 50, 100 mg. Extended-release capsule: 100 mg. Macrocrystal: 50, 100 mg. Suspension: 25 mg/5 mL.	**Effective in the treatment of lower urinary tract infections caused by gram-positive and gram-negative pathogens.** *Children:* 5–7 mg/kg/24 hr divided q6h PO (max dose: 400 mg/24 hr); suppressive therapy 1–2.5 mg/kg/24 hr divided q12–24h PO (max dose: 100 mg/24 hr). Adults: 50–100 mg/24 hr divided q6h PO.	*Cautions:* Vertigo, dizziness, rash, jaundice, interstitial pneumonitis. Do not use with moderate to severe renal dysfunction. *Drug interactions:* Liquid antacids.
Ofloxacin Ocuflox 0.3% ophthalmic solution: 1, 5, 10 mL. Floxin 0.3% otic solution: 5, 10 mL.	**Quinolone antibiotic for treatment of conjunctivitis or corneal ulcers (ophthalmic solution); and otitis externa and chronic suppurative otitis media (otic solution) caused by susceptible gram-positive, gram-negative, anaerobic bacteria, or *Chlamydia trachomatis*.** *Child >1–12 yr:* Conjunctivitis: 1–2 drops in affected eye(s) q2–4h for 2 days, then 1–2 drops qid for 5 days. Corneal ulcers: 1–2 drops q 30 min while awake and at 4 hours at night for 2 days, then 1–2 drops hourly for 5 days while awake, then 1–2 drops q6h for 2 days. Otitis externa (otic solution): 5 drops into affected ear bid for 10 days. Chronic suppurative otitis media: treat for 14 days. *Child >12 yr and adults:* *Ophthalmic solution doses same as for younger children.* Otitis externa (otic solution): Use 10 drops bid for 10 or 14 days as for younger children.	*Adverse events:* Burning, stinging, eye redness (ophthalmic solution), dizziness with otic solution if not warmed.
Oxacillin sodium Prostaphlin. Injection. Capsule: 250, 500 mg. Suspension: 250 mg/5 mL.	**Penicillinase-resistant penicillin active against *S. aureus* and other gram-positive cocci except *Enterococcus* and coagulase-negative staphylococci.** *Neonates:* Postnatal age ≤7 days 1,200–2,000 g: 50 mg/kg/24 hr divided q12h IV; >2,000 g: 75 mg/kg/24 hr IV divided q8h IV; postnatal age >7 days <1,200 g: 50 mg/kg/24 hr IV divided q12h IV; 1,200–2,000 g: 75 mg/kg/24 hr divided q8h IV; >2,000 g: 100 mg/kg/24 hr IV divided q6h IV. *Infants:* 100–200 mg/kg/24 hr divided q4–6h IV. *Children:* PO 50–100 mg/kg/24 hr divided q4–6h IV. *Adults:* 2–12 g/24 hr divided q4–6h IV (max dose: 12 g/24 hr).	*Cautions:* β-Lactam safety profile (rash, eosinophilia). Moderate oral bioavailability (35–65%). Primarily renally eliminated. *Drug interaction:* Probenecid. *Adverse effect:* Neutropenia.
Penicillin G Injection. Tablets.	**Penicillin active against most gram-positive cocci; *S. pneumoniae* (resistance is increasing), group A *Streptococcus*, and some gram-negative bacteria (e.g., *N. gonorrhoeae*, *N. meningitidis*).** *Neonates:* Postnatal age ≤7 days 1,200–2,000 g: 50,000 units/kg/24 hr divided q12h IV or IM (meningitis: 100,000 units/kg/24 hr divided q12h IV or IM); >2,000 g: 75,000 units/kg/24 hr divided q8h IV or IM (meningitis: 150,000 units/kg/24 hr divided q8h IV or IM); postnatal age >7 days ≤1,200 g: 50,000 units/kg/24 hr divided q12h IV (meningitis: 100,000 units/kg/24 hr divided q12h IV); 1,200–2,000 g: 75,000 units/kg/24 hr q8h IV (meningitis: 225,000 units/kg/24 hr divided q8h IV); >2,000 g: 100,000 units/kg/24 hr divided q6h IV (meningitis: 200,000 units/kg/24 hr divided q6h IV). *Children:* 100,000–250,000 units/kg/24 hr divided q4–6h IV or IM (max: 400,000 units/kg/24 hr). *Adults:* 2–24 million units/24 hr divided q4–6h IV or IM.	*Cautions:* β-Lactam safety profile (rash, eosinophilia), allergy, seizures with excessive doses particularly in patients with marked renal disease. Substantial pathogen resistance. Primarily renally eliminated. *Drug interaction:* Probenecid.
Penicillin G, benzathine Bicillin. Injection.	**Long-acting repository form of penicillin effective in the treatment of infections responsive to persistent, low penicillin concentrations (1–4 wk), e.g., group A *Streptococcus* pharyngitis, rheumatic fever prophylaxis.**	*Cautions:* β-Lactam safety profile (rash, eosinophilia), allergy. Administer by IM injection only. Substantial pathogen resistance. Primarily renally eliminated. *Drug interaction:* Probenecid.

Table continued on following page

MEDICATIONS

TABLE 712–2. Antibacterial Medications (Antibiotics) *Continued*

Drug (Trade Names, Formulations)	Indications (Mechanism of Action) and Dosing	Comments
Penicillin G, procaine Crysticillin. Injection.	*Neonates >1,200 g:* 50,000 units/kg IM once. *Children:* 300,000–1.2 million units/kg q 3–4 wk IM (max: 1.2–2.4 million units/dose). *Adults:* 1.2 million units IM q 3–4 wk. **Repository form of penicillin providing low penicillin concentrations for ~12 hr.** *Neonates >1,200 g:* 50,000 units/kg/24 hr IM. *Children:* 25,000–50,000 units/kg/24 hr IM for 10 days (max: 4.8 million units/dose). Gonorrhea: 100,000 units/kg (max: 4.8 million units/24 hr) IM once with probenecid 25 mg/kg (max dose: 1 g). *Adults:* 0.6–4.8 million units q12–24h IM.	*Cautions:* β-Lactam safety profile (rash, eosinophilia), allergy. Administer by IM injection only. Substantial pathogen resistance. Primarily renally eliminated. *Drug interaction:* Probenecid.
Penicillin V Pen VK, V-Cillin K. Tablet: 125, 250, 500 mg. Suspension: 125 mg/5 mL, 250 mg/5 mL.	**Preferred oral dosing form of penicillin, active against most gram-positive cocci;** *S. pneumoniae* **(resistance is increasing), other** *Streptococcus,* **and some gram-negative bacteria (e.g.,** *N. gonorrhoeae,* *N. meningitidis***).** *Children:* 25–50 mg/kg/24 hr divided q4–8h PO. *Adults:* 125 mg–500 mg q6–8h PO (max dose: 3 g/24 hr).	*Cautions:* β-Lactam safety profile (rash, eosinophilia), allergy, seizures with excessive doses particularly in patients with renal disease. Substantial pathogen resistance. Primarily renally eliminated. Inactivated by penicillinase. *Drug interaction:* Probenecid.
Pentamidine isethionate Pentam. Injection. Aerosol.	**Antiprotozoal agent effective in the prevention and treatment of** *P. carinii* **infections.** *Children: P. carinii* treatment 4 mg/kg/24 hr q24h IV or IM (preferred) for 14 days. Prophylaxis: 4 mg/kg IV or IM q 2–4 wk; aerosol adjusted to minute ventilation (4–8 mg/kg/dose) up to 300 mg/dose. Visceral leishmaniasis: 4 mg/kg/ 24 hr IV or IM for 14 days. *Adults: P. carinii* treatment 4 mg/kg/24 hr IV or IM (preferred) for 14 days. Prophylaxis: 300 mg/dose q 3–4 wk.	*Cautions:* Hypotension, hypoglycemia, cardiac arrhythmias, pain at injection site, nephrotoxicity; cough/bronchospasm with aerosol; 33–66% renally eliminated. *Drug interactions:* Other nephrotoxins (e.g., aminoglycosides, amphotericin B, cyclosporine).
Piperacillin Pipracil. Injection.	**Extended-spectrum penicillin active against** *E. coli, Enterobacter, Serratia, P. aeruginosa,* **and** *Bacteroides.* *Neonates:* Postnatal age ≤7 days 150 mg/kg/24 hr divided q8–12h IV; >7 days; 200 mg/kg divided q6–8r IV. *Children:* 200–300 mg/kg/24 hr divided q4–6h IV; cystic fibrosis: 350–500 mg/kg/24 hr IV. *Adults:* 2–4 g/dose q4–6h (max dose: 24 g/24 hr) IV.	*Cautions:* β-Lactam safety profile (rash, eosinophilia); painful given intramuscularly; each gram contains 1.9 mEq sodium. Interferes with platelet aggregation/serum sickness-like reaction with high doses; increases in liver function tests. Renally eliminated. Inactivated by penicillinase. *Drug interaction:* Probenecid.
Piperacillin-tazobactam Zosyn. Injection.	**Extended-spectrum penicillin (piperacillin) combined with a β-lactamase inhibitor (tazobactam) active against** *S. aureus, H. influenzae, E. coli, Enterobacter, Serratia, Acinetobacter, P. aeruginosa,* **and** *Bacteroides.* *Children:* 300–400 mg/kg/24 hr divided q6–8 h IV or IM. *Adults:* 3.375 g q6–8h IV or IM.	*Cautions:* β-Lactam safety profile (rash, eosinophilia); painful given intramuscularly; each gram contains 1.9 mEq sodium. Interferes with platelet aggregation, serum sickness–like reaction with high doses, increases in liver function test results. Renally eliminated. *Drug interaction:* Probenecid.
Quinupristin/dalfopristin Synercid. IV injection: powder for reconstitution, 10 mL contains 150 mg quinupristin, 350 mg dalfopristin.	**Streptogramin antibiotic (quinupristin) active against vancomycin-resistant** *E. faecium* **(VRE) and methicillin-resistant** *S. aureus.* **Not active against** *E. faecalis.* *Children and adults:* VRE: 7.5 mg/kg q8h IV for VRE; skin infections: 7.5 mg/kg q12h IV.	*Adverse events:* Pain, edema, or phlebitis at injection site, nausea, diarrhea. *Drug interactions:* Synercid is a potent inhibitor of CYP3A4.
Sulfadiazine Tablet: 500 mg.	**Sulfonamide antibiotic primarily indicated for the treatment of lower urinary tract infections due to** *E. coli, P. mirabilis,* **and** *Klebsiella.* Toxoplasmosis: *Neonates:* 100 mg/kg/24 hr divided q12h PO with pyrimethamine 1 mg/kg/24 hr PO (with folinic acid). *Children:* 120–200 mg/kg/24 hr divided q6h PO with pyrimethamine 2 mg/kg/24 hr divided q12h PO ≥ 3 days then 1 mg/kg/24 hr (max dose: 25 mg/24 hr) with folinic acid. Rheumatic fever prophylaxis: ≤30 kg: 500 mg/24 hr q24h PO; >30 kg: 1 g/24 hr q24h PO.	*Cautions:* Rash, Stevens-Johnson syndrome, nausea, leukopenia, crystalluria. Renal and hepatic elimination; avoid use with renal disease. Half-life ~10 hr. *Drug interactions:* Protein displacement with warfarin, ?phenytoin, methotrexate.
Sulfamethoxazole Gantanol. Tablet: 500 mg. Suspension: 500 mg/5 mL.	**Sulfonamide antibiotic used for the treatment of otitis media, chronic bronchitis, and lower urinary tract infections due to susceptible bacteria.** *Children:* 50–60 mg/kg/24 hr divided q12h PO. *Adults:* 1 g/dose q12h PO (max dose: 3 g/24 hr).	*Cautions:* Rash, Stevens-Johnson syndrome, nausea, leukopenia, crystalluria. Renal and hepatic elimination; avoid use with renal disease. Half-life ~ 12 hr. Initial dose often a loading dose (doubled). *Drug interactions:* Protein displacement with warfarin, ?phenytoin, methotrexate.

TABLE 712–2. Antibacterial Medications (Antibiotics) *Continued*

Drug (Trade Names, Formulations)	Indications (Mechanism of Action) and Dosing	Comments
Sulfisoxazole Gantrisin. Tablet: 500 mg. Suspension: 500 mg/5 mL. Ophthalmic solution, ointment.	**Sulfonamide antibiotic used for the treatment of otitis media, chronic bronchitis, and lower urinary tract infections due to susceptible bacteria.** *Children:* 120–150 mg/kg/24 hr divided q4–6h PO (max dose: 6 g/24 hr). *Adults:* 4–8 g/24 hr q divided q4–6h PO.	*Cautions:* Rash, Stevens-Johnson syndrome, nausea, leukopenia, crystalluria. Renal and hepatic elimination; avoid use with renal disease. Half-life ~ 7–12 hr. Initial dose often a loading dose (doubled). Drug interactions: Protein displacement with warfarin, ?phenytoin, methotrexate.
Ticarcillin Ticar. Injection.	**Extended-spectrum penicillin active against *E. coli, Enterobacter, Serratia, P. aeruginosa,* and *Bacteroides.*** *Neonates:* Postnatal age ≤7 days <2,000 g: 150 mg/kg/24 hr divided q8–12h IV; >7 days: <2,000 g: 225 mg/kg/24 hr divided q8h IV; >7 days <1,200 g: 150 mg/kg/24 hr divided q12h IV; 1,200–2,000 g: 225 mg/kg/24 hr divided q8h IV; >2,000 g: 300 mg/kg/24 hr divided q6–8h IV. *Children:* 200–400 mg/kg/24 hr divided q4–6h IV; cystic fibrosis: 400–600 mg/kg/24 hr IV. *Adults:* 2–4 g/dose q4–6h IV (max dose: 24 g/24 hr).	*Cautions:* β-Lactam safety profile (rash, eosinophilia); painful given intramuscularly; each gram contains 5–6 mEq sodium. Interferes with platelet aggregation; increases in liver function tests. Renally eliminated. Inactivated by penicillinase. *Drug interaction:* Probenecid.
Ticarcillin-clavulanate Timentin. Injection.	**Extended-spectrum penicillin (ticarcillin) combined with a β-lactamase inhibitor (clavulanate) active against *S. aureus, H. influenzae, Enterobacter, E. coli, Serratia, P. aeruginosa, Acinetobacter,* and *Bacteroides.*** *Children:* 280–400 mg/kg/24 hr q4–8h IV or IM. *Adults:* 3.1 g q4–8h IV or IM (max dose: 18–24 g/24 hr).	*Cautions:* β-Lactam safety profile (rash, eosinophilia); painful given intramuscularly; each gram contains 5–6 mEq sodium. Interferes with platelet aggregation; increases in liver function tests. Renally eliminated. *Drug interaction:* Probenecid.
Tobramycin Nebcin, Tobrex. Injection. Ophthalmic solution, ointment.	**Aminoglycoside antibiotic active against gram-negative bacilli, especially *E. coli, Klebsiella, Enterobacter, Serratia, Proteus,* and *Pseudomonas.*** *Neonates:* Postnatal age ≤7 days, 1,200–2,000 g: 2.5 mg/kg q12–18h IV or IM; >2,000 g: 2.5 mg/kg q12h IV or IM; postnatal age >7 days, 1,200–2,000 g: 2.5 mg/kg q8–12h IV or IM; >2,000 g: 2.5 mg/kg q8h IV or IM. *Children:* 2.5 mg/kg/24 hr divided q8–12h IV or IM. Alternatively may administer 5–7.5 mg/kg/24 hr IV. Preservative-free preparation for intraventricular or intrathecal use: neonate: 1 mg/24 hr; children: 1–2 mg/24 hr; adults: 4–8 mg/24 hr. *Adults:* 3–6 mg/kg/24 hr divided q8h IV or IM.	*Cautions:* S. pneumoniae, other Streptococcus, and anaerobes are resistant. May cause ototoxicity and nephrotoxicity. Monitor renal function. Drug eliminated renally. Administered IV over 30–60 min. *Drug interactions:* May potentiate other ototoxic and nephrotoxic drugs. *Target serum concentrations:* Peak 6–12 mg/L; trough <2 mg/L.
Trimethoprim Proloprim, Trimpex. Tablet: 100, 200 mg.	**Folic acid antagonist effective in the prophylaxis and treatment of *E. coli, Klebsiella, Proteus mirabilis,* and *Enterobacter* urinary tract infections; *P. carinii* pneumonia.** *Children:* For urinary tract infection: 4–6 mg/kg/24 hr divided q12h PO. *Children >12 yr and adults:* 100–200 mg q12h PO. *P. carinii* pneumonia (with dapsone): 15–20 mg/kg/24 hr divided q6h for 21 days PO.	*Cautions:* Megaloblastic anemia, bone marrow suppression, nausea, epigastric distress, rash. *Drug interactions:* Possible interactions with phenytoin, cyclosporine, rifampin, warfarin.
Vancomycin Vancocin, Luphocin. Injection. Capsule: 125 mg, 250 mg. Suspension.	**Glycopeptide antibiotic active against most gram-positive pathogens including *Staphylococcus* (including methicillin-resistant *S. aureus* and coagulase-negative staphylococci), *S. pneumoniae* including penicillin-resistant strains, *Enterococcus* (resistance is increasing), and *Clostridium difficile*–associated colitis.** *Neonates:* Postnatal age ≤7 days, <1,200 g: 15 mg/kg/24 hr divided q24h IV; 1,200–2,000 g: 15 mg/kg/24 hr divided q12–18h IV; >2,000 g: 30 mg/kg/24 hr divided q12h IV; postnatal age >7 days, <1,200 g: 15 mg/kg/24 hr divided q24h IV; 1,200–2,000 g: 15 mg/kg/24 hr divided q8–12h IV; >2,000 g: 45 mg/kg/24 hr divided q8h IV. *Children:* 45–60 mg/kg/24 hr divided q8–12h IV; *Clostridium difficile*–associated colitis; 40–50 mg/kg/24 hr divided q6–8h PO. Adults: 0.5–1 g IV q12h IV.	*Cautions:* Ototoxicity and nephrotoxicity particularly when co-administered with other ototoxic and nephrotoxic drugs. Infuse IV over 45–60 min. Flushing (red-man syndrome) associated with rapid IV infusions, fever, chills, phlebitis (central line is preferred). Renally eliminated. *Target serum concentrations:* Peak (1 hr after 1 hr infusion) 30–40 mg/L; trough 5–10 mg/L.

TABLE 712–3. Antimycobacterial Medications

Drug (Trade Names, Formulations)	Indications (Mechanism of Action) and Dosing	Comments
Cycloserine Seromycin. Capsule: 250 mg.	**Adjunctive antituberculous agent less effective than isoniazid or streptomycin.** *Children:* 10–20 mg/kg/24 hr PO divided q12h. *Adults:* 250–500 mg per dose PO q12h (max daily dose: 1,000 mg).	*Cautions:* Headache, dizziness, confusion, psychosis, seizures, photosensitivity, folate/vitamin B_{12} deficiency. Primarily renally eliminated. *Drug interactions:* Phenytoin, additive CNS effects with isoniazid.
Ethambutol HCl Myambutol. Tablet: 100, 400 mg.	**For use in combination with other agents.** *Children:* 15 mg/kg/24 hr PO q24h. *Adults:* 15 mg/kg/24 hr PO q24h (max dose: 2.5 g/24 hr).	*Cautions:* Optic neuritis, decreased visual acuity, headache, dizziness, rash, peripheral neuropathy.
Ethionamide Trecator-SC. Tablet: 250 mg.	**For use in combination with other agents. Consider co-administration of vitamin B_6.** *Children:* 15–20 mg/kg/24 hr PO divided q8–12h (max: 1,000 mg/24 hr). *Adults:* 500–1,000 mg PO q8–24h.	*Cautions:* Gastrointestinal upset, hepatotoxicity, vitamin B_6 deficiency, dizziness, headache, metallic taste, optic neuritis.
Isoniazid INH, Nydrazid. Tablet: 50, 100, 300 mg. Syrup: 50 mg/5 mL. Injection.	**For use in combination with other agents.** *Children:* 10–20 mg/kg/24 hr PO divided q12–24h (max: 300 mg/24 hr); prophylaxis dose 10 mg/kg/24 hr. *Adults:* 5 mg/kg/24 hr PO once daily; usual maximum dose: 300 mg/24 hr. Twice weekly therapy (after 3 mo daily therapy): *Children:* 20–40 mg/kg/dose (max: 900 mg) twice weekly. *Adults:* 15 mg/kg/dose (max: 900 mg) twice weekly.	*Cautions:* Dizziness, seizures, rash, pellagra, gastrointestinal upset, peripheral neuropathy (may give vitamin B_6 1–2 mg/kg/24 hr without effect on antituberculous activity), hepatotoxicity. *Drug interactions:* Increase serum concentrations of phenytoin, carbamazepine.
Kanamycin Injection.	**Aminoglycoside antibiotic used in combination with other agents.** *Children:* 15 mg/kg/24 hr IM or IV divided q12h. *Adults:* 1 g/24 hr IM or IV (max: dose 1 g/24 hr).	*Cautions:* Aminoglycoside adverse effect profile (ototoxicity, and nephrotoxicity).
Pyrazinamide Tablet: 500 mg.	**For use in combination with other agents.** *Children:* 15–40 mg/kg/24 hr PO divided q12–24h (max: 2 g/24 hr). *Adults:* 15–30 mg/kg/24 hr PO divided q6–24h (max: 2 g/24 hr).	*Cautions:* Photosensitivity, gastrointestinal upset, hyperuricemia, arthralgia, hepatotoxicity (especially doses >30 mg/kg/24 hr).
Rifabutin Mycobutin. Capsule: 150, 300 mg. Injection. Extemporaneous liquid formulation.	**Treatment (in combination with other antimycobacterial agents) and prevention of infections with *Mycobacterium avium* complex.** Inhibits DNA-dependent RNA polymerase. *Infants and children:* Treatment (preliminary guidelines): 5–7 mg/kg/24 hr PO once daily. Prophylaxis: 5 mg/kg/24 hr PO once daily. *Adults:* 300 mg PO once daily.	*Cautions:* Dosing information in pediatrics is evolving. Fever, headache, confusion, gastrointestinal upset, increased liver function tests, anemia, neutropenia may cause orange-red discoloration of secretions of urine, tears, sweat. *Drug interactions:* May enhance metabolism of many drugs: warfarin, corticosteroids, opiates, oral contraceptives.
Rifampin Rifadin, Rimactane. Capsule: 150, 300 mg. Injection. Extemporaneous liquid formulation.	**For use in combination with other agents.** *Children:* 10–20 mg/kg/24 hr PO or IV divided q12–24h. *Adults:* 10 mg/kg/24 hr PO or IV once daily (max: 600 mg/24 hr). Twice weekly therapy (after 3 mo daily therapy): *Children:* 10–20 mg/kg/dose (max: 600 mg) PO twice weekly. *Adults:* 10 mg/kg/dose (max: 600 mg) PO twice weekly.	*Cautions:* Hepatotoxicity, influenza-like syndrome, rash, pruritus, leukopenia, arthralgia; may cause orange-red discoloration of urine, tears, sweat. *Drug interactions:* Induces hepatic enzymes decreasing effect/concentrations of opiates, anticoagulants, barbiturates, carbamazepine, phenytoin, azole antifungals, cyclosporine, corticosteroids.
Rifapentine Priftin. Tablets: 150 mg.	**Treatment of pulmonary tuberculosis in combination with other drugs.** *Children >12 yr and adults:* 600 mg at intervals >72 hours for 2 mo; then 600 mg q wk for 4 mo.	*Cautions:* Red-orange discoloration of body fluids as with rifampin. Administer concomitant pyridoxine (vitamin B_6) to avoid neuropathy. *Drug Interactions:* Same as rifampin.
Streptomycin Generic. Injection.	**Aminoglycoside antibiotic used in combination with other agents.** *Neonates:* 10–20 mg/kg/24 hr IM q24h. *Children:* 20–40 mg/kg/24 hr IM divided q12h not to exceed 1 g/24 hr. *Adults:* 15 mg/kg/24 hr IM q24h, not to exceed 1 g/24 hr.	*Cautions:* Aminoglycoside adverse effect profile (ototoxicity and nephrotoxicity).

TABLE 712–4. Antifungal Medications

Drug (Trade Names, Formulations)	Indications (Mechanism of Action) and Dosing	Comments
Amphotericin B Lipid Complexes Abelcet (ABLC); Ambisome (liposome); Amphotec (ABCD). Injection.	**Polyene effective against a broad spectrum of fungi: *Candida, Aspergillus, Coccidioides, Histoplasma, Sporothrix, Blastomyces.*** Available as the traditional colloidal suspension and newer lipid-complex/liposomal formulations. Lipid formulations permit higher doses with increased patient tolerance.	*Cautions:* Hypotension, fever, chills, flushing; pre-medicate with meperidine and acetaminophen. Drug augments potassium and magnesium excretion requiring aggressive monitoring and supplementation. Lipid formulations markedly attenuate renal toxicity. *Drug interactions:* Concurrent nephrotoxic drugs.

MEDICATIONS

TABLE 712–4. Antifungal Medications *Continued*

Drug (Trade Names, Formulations)	Indications (Mechanism of Action) and Dosing	Comments
	Children and adults: 2.5–5 mg/kg IV infused over 1–2 hr q24h; may use higher doses of 7.5–10 mg/kg/24 hr if indicated and if tolerated.	
Caspofungin Cancidas. Powder for infusion: 50, 70 mg.	**Antifungal active against *Aspergillus*.** *Children:* 1–2 mg/kg/24 hr as single daily dose (dosing and use in pediatrics still investigational). *Adults:* Loading dose 70 mg day 1, then 50 mg q24h; infuse over 1 hr.	*Caution:* Reduce daily dose to 35 mg for moderate hepatic insufficiency
Clotrimazole Lotrimin, Gyne-Lotrimin. Troche, topical cream, vaginal tablets, and cream.	**Topical imidazole active against *Cryptococcus*, *Aspergillus*, *Candida*, and *Coccidioides* for the treatment of oropharyngeal, skin, vaginal infections.** *Children and adults:* 1 troche dissolved 5–6 times daily; vaginal cream/tablet: 100–200 mg qhs; topical cream: apply twice daily.	*Cautions:* Minimal adverse effects, nausea, skin irritation. Topical/troche ineffective for systemic infections.
Econazole nitrate Spectazole. Topical cream: 1%.	**Topical agent effective in the treatment of tinea corporis, cruris, pedis, and cutaneous candidiasis.** *Children and adults:* Apply over affected areas once daily.	*Cautions:* Minimal adverse effects—skin irritation.
Fluconazole Diflucan. Tablet: 50, 100, 150, 200 mg. Suspension: 10 mg/mL, 40 mg/mL. Injection.	**Imidazole effective against *Cryptococcus* and *Candida* infections of the oropharynx, vagina, meningitis.** *Neonates:* Thrush: 6 mg/kg IV or PO q24h for 1st day then 3 mg/kg/24 hr q24h for 14–21 days. Systemic infections: 6–12 mg/kg/24 hr IV or PO q72h for postnatal age <14 days or once daily for postnatal age >14 days. *Children:* 6–12 mg/kg/24 hr IV or PO q24h; cryptococcal meningitis: 12 mg/kg/24 hr 1st day then 6–12 mg/kg/24 hr IV or PO q24h.	*Cautions:* Dizziness, rash, nausea, abdominal pain, elevated liver function tests, superinfection with *C. krusei*. Reduce dose with reduced renal function. *Drug interactions:* Warfarin, oral antidiabetic agents, astemizole, cisapride, cyclosporine, phenytoin, rifampin, terfenadine, zidovudine.
Flucytosine Ancobon, 5FC. Capsule: 250, 500 mg.	**Used in combination with amphotericin B (resistance develops rapidly) against *Candida*, *Cryptococcus*, and *Aspergillus* infections.** *Neonates:* 50–100 mg/kg/24 hr PO divided q12–24hr. *Children and adults:* 100–150 mg/kg/24 hr PO divided q6–8h. Monitor blood levels.	*Cautions:* Confusion, rash, nausea, vomiting, bone marrow suppression with sustained serum concentrations >100 mg/L, elevation results of liver function tests. *Drug interactions:* Aluminum and magnesium salts delay absorption rate.
Griseofulvin Fulvicin, Grisactin. Microsize capsule: 125, 250 mg. Suspension: 125 mg/5 mL. Tablet: UF 250 mg, 500 mg. Ultra-microsize PG tablet: 125, 165, 250, 330 mg.	**Treatment of tinea infections of the hair, nails, and skin due to *Microsporum*, *Epidermophyton*, and *Trichophyton*.** Ultra-microsize formulation has almost complete absorption whereas absorption of microsize is variable (40–80%). *Children:* Microsize 10–20 mg/kg/24 hr PO divided q12–24h; ultra-microsize: 5–10 mg/kg/24 hr PO divided q12h. *Adults:* Microsize 500–1,000 mg/24 hr PO divided q12–24h; ultra-microsize: 330–375 mg/24 hr PO divided q12h.	*Cautions:* Headache, nausea, diarrhea, rash, photosensitivity. Administration with a fatty meal increases oral absorption. *Drug interactions:* Warfarin, phenobarbital, oral contraceptives, ?phenytoin.
Itraconazole Sporanox. Capsule: 100 mg.	**Synthetic triazole active against *Candida*, *Aspergillus*, *Cryptococcus*, and *Histoplasma*.** Limited dosing data in pediatrics. *Children:* 3–5 mg/kg/24 hr PO once daily; doses as high as 5–10 mg/kg/24 hr have been used. *Adults:* 200–400 mg/24 hr PO divided q12h; serious infections: 600 mg/24 hr q8h for 3–4 days then 200–400 mg/24 hr.	*Cautions:* Hypertension, nausea, headache, dizziness, rash, hepatitis. Food increases bioavailability. *Drug interactions:* Carbamazepine, isoniazid, rifampin, phenytoin, phenobarbital, cyclosporin. Antacids/H$_2$ antagonists decrease bioavailability.
Miconazole Micatin, Monistat. Topical cream, vaginal tablet, lotion, powder. Injection.	**Imidazole active against *Cryptococcus*, *Candida*, *Coccidioides*, and *Pseudallescheria boydii* for topical or IV use in superficial infections.** *Neonates:* 5–15 mg/kg/24 hr IV divided q8–24h. *Children:* 20–40 mg/kg/24 hr IV divided q8h; vaginal cream/tablet 100–200 mg qhs; topical cream: apply twice daily. *Adults:* 200 mg stat then 1.2–3.6 g/24 hr IV divided q8h. *Bladder irrigation:* 200 mg in 25 mL saline.	*Cautions:* Dizziness, nausea, hyperlipidemia, tremors, rash, hives. Mostly used for the treatment of topical infections.

Table continued on following page

MEDICATIONS

TABLE 712–4. **Antifungal Medications** *Continued*

Drug (Trade Names, Formulations)	Indications (Mechanism of Action) and Dosing	Comments
Natamycin Natacyn. Ophthalmic suspension: 5%.	**Fungal eye infections, e.g., blepharitis, conjunctivitis, keratitis caused by susceptible organisms (e.g., *Candida*, *Aspergillus*, *Cephalosporium*, *Fusarium*, and *Penicillium*).** Fungicidal by altering membrane permeability. *Children and adults:* Keratitis: Instill 1 drop into conjunctival sac every 1–2 hr for 3–4 days, then may reduce to 6–8 doses/24 hr. Blepharitis and conjunctivitis: instill 1 drop 4–6 times daily.	
Nystatin Mycostatin, Nilstat.	**Polyene effective against many yeasts and molds.** Oral candidiasis: *Neonates:* 100,000 units qid. *Infants:* 200,000 units qid. *Children and adults:* 400,000–600,000 units qid. Topical: Apply bid–qid.	*Cautions:* Minimal adverse effects with topical application, nausea, skin irritation. Tablet ineffective for systemic infections.
Terbinafine Lamisil. Tablet: 250 mg.	**Onychomycosis and tinea pedis.** *Children <20 kg:* 62.5 mg PO q24h (fingernails for 6 wk, toenails for 12 wk, tinea for 2 wk) *Children 20–40 kg:* 125 mg PO q24h (fingernails for 6 wk, toenails for 12 wk, tinea for 2 wk). *Children >40 kg and adults:* 250 mg PO q24h (fingernails for 6 wk, toenails for 12 wk, tinea for 2 wk).	*Cautions:* Administer with food for slightly increased bioavailibility (~20%) *Drug Interactions:* May interfere with CYP2D6 (tricyclic antidepressants, selective serotonin reuptake inhibitors, select β-blockers. Metabolism increased by enzyme inducers.

TABLE 712–5. **Antiviral Medications**

Drug (Trade Names, Formulations)	Indications (Mechanism of Action) and Dosing	Comments
Acyclovir Zovirax. Capsule: 200 mg. Tablet: 400, 800 mg. Suspension: 200 mg/5 mL. Injection. Ointment.	**Herpes simplex (HSV) encephalitis, mucosal, cutaneous, genital infections; herpes zoster, varicella-zoster, cytomegalovirus (CMV) prophylaxis.** *Neonates:* HSV encephalitis: 60 mg/kg/24 hr IV divided q8h. *Children and adults:* 15 mg/kg/24 hr IV divided q8–12h. HSV infection in immunocompromised host: *Children and adults:* 15–30 mg/kg/24 hr IV divided q8h. HSV encephalitis/varicella infection/CMV prophylaxis in immunocompromised host: *Children and adults:* 30 mg/kg/24 hr IV divided q8h. Oral dosing for HSV/zoster infection: *Children and adults:* 1,200 mg/24 hr divided q4–8h (max pediatric dose: 80 mg/24 hr).	*Cautions:* Headache, dizziness, rash, bone marrow suppression. Poor oral bioavailability—best given in frequent daily doses (e.g., q4h). Primarily renally eliminated. 4.2 mEq Na/g of acyclovir. *Drug interaction:* Probenecid, zidovudine.
Amantadine Symmetrel. Capsule: 100 mg. Syrup: 50 mg/5 mL.	**Prophylaxis and treatment (all ages) of influenza A infections.** Prophylaxis or treatment: *Children 1–9 yr or <40 kg:* 5 mg/kg/24 hr PO divided q12h (max: 150 mg/24 hr). *Children >9 yr and >40 kg and adults:* 200 mg/ 24 hr PO divided q12h.	*Cautions:* Anticholinergic effects, and may potentiate other anticholinergic medications. Drowsiness, dizziness, confusion, hypotension, urinary retention. Renally eliminated; reduce dose with renal impairment. No dosage reduction necessary for hepatic impairment. Not removed by hemodialysis.
Famciclovir Famvir. Tablet: 500 mg.	**Oral prodrug formulation of penciclovir used in the treatment of acute herpes zoster. Limited data in pediatrics.** *Adults:* 500 mg PO q8h for 7 days.	*Cautions:* Headache, dizziness, nausea, adjust dose in renal insufficiency (e.g., penciclovir). Rate of absorption, not overall bioavailability, reduced if taken with food.
Foscarnet Foscavir. Injection.	**Treatment of CMV infections, retinitis, and acyclovir-resistant HSV mucocutaneous infection, and herpes zoster.** CMV retinitis: IV infusion rate 60 mg/kg/hr. *Children and adults:* Induction therapy: 180 mg/kg/24 hr IV divided q8h; maintenance therapy: 90–120 mg/kg/24 hr IV once daily. Acyclovir-resistant HSV infection: *Children and adults:* 120 mg/kg/24 hr divided q8–12h.	*Cautions:* Hypertension, dizziness, seizures, decreased electrolytes (Ca, Mg, K), genitourinary complications, bronchospasm, nephrotoxicity. Adjust dose with renal dysfunction. IV infusion dilution for peripheral venous administration 12 mg/mL; central venous administration 24 mg/mL.
Ganciclovir Cytovene. Injection.	**Treatment of CMV infections including retinitis.** CMV retinitis: *Children and adults:*	*Cautions:* Headache, seizures, hypertension, nausea, marrow suppression, renal/liver toxicity, rash, photophobia. Primarily renally eliminated.

TABLE 712–5. **Antiviral Medications** *Continued*

Drug (Trade Names, Formulations)	Indications (Mechanism of Action) and Dosing	Comments
Capsule: 250 mg.	Induction therapy: 10 mg/kg/24 hr IV (over 1–2 h) divided q12h for 14–21 days; maintenance therapy: 5–6 mg/kg/24 hr IV once daily. CMV disease and prophylaxis (solid organ transplant): Induction: 10 mg/kg/24 hr IV divided q12h for 7–14 days then 5–6 mg/kg/24 hr IV once daily.	*Drug interactions:* Probenecid, immunosuppressants. *Comment:* Oral dose form very poor bioavailability (5–6%).
Idoxuridine (IDU) Herplex. Ophthalmic solution: 1%.	**Topical therapy for herpes simplex keratitis.** *Children and adults:* Apply ointment 5 times daily and ophthalmic solution (1 drop) to affected eye(s) 7–10 times daily and at bedtime.	*Cautions:* Local irritation, pruritus, ocular edema.
Interferon alfa-2b Intron A. Powder for injection, lyophilized 3, 5, 10, 18, 25, and 50 million IU per vial. Solution for injection: 3, 5, 10, 18, and 25 million IU per vial.	**Chronic hepatitis B and chronic hepatitis C, and some neoplastic diseases.** *Adults:* Chronic hepatitis B dose: 5 million IU daily or 10 million IU 3 times/wk for total dose 30–35 million IU/wk SC or IM for 16 wk. Chronic hepatitis C dose: 3 million IU SC or IM 3 times weekly for 6 mo. *Children:* Safety and efficacy in children <18 yr not established.	*Cautions:* Flu-like symptoms and photosensitivity are common. Alanine aminotransferase often increases > 2 times baseline at 8–12 wk, especially in responders, and therapy should be continued if this occurs.
Interferon beta-1a/Interferon beta-1b Avonex/ Betaseron. Powder for injection, lyophilized: 33 µg (6.6 mIU)/ 0.3 mg (9.6 mIU).	**Unlabeled use as antiviral agent for herpes of the lips or genitals, and acute non-A/non-B hepatitis. Labeled use is for relapsing-remitting multiple sclerosis.** *Adults:* 30 µg IM once weekly or 0.25 mg SC every other day. *Children:* Safety and efficacy in children <18 yr of age has not been established.	*Cautions:* Flu-like symptoms occur in up to 75% of patients. Photosensitivity is common.
Oseltamivir Tamiflu. Capsule: 75 mg. Suspension: 12 mg/mL.	**Use for prophylaxis or treatment of influenza A and B infections.** Acts by inhibiting influenza virus neuraminidase. *Children:* >1 yr: 30 mg q12h PO up to 15 kg; 45 mg q12h PO 16–23 kg; 60 mg q12h PO >23–40 kg and 75 mg PO q12h >40 kg. *Adults:* Treatment with 150 mg/24 hr divided q12h for 5 days (must be started within 2 days of onset of symptoms). Prophylaxis with 75 mg once daily for up to 6 wk if high risk of exposure.	*Cautions:* Most common adverse reactions include nausea, vomiting, and diarrhea.
Ribavirin Virazole. Powder for aerosol.	**Aerosol therapy for RSV infections, particularly for patients with underlying conditions, including bronchopulmonary dysplasia and/or congenital heart diseases.** *Children and adults:* Use SPAG-2 small particle generator at 20 mg/mL concentration for continuous aerosolization 12–18 hr per day. High-dose/short-duration aerosol administration under investigation.	*Cautions:* Rash, irritation, hypotension; drug may precipitate in ventilation tubing; use in well-ventilated areas, minimize staff contact. Best results when initiated early in clinical course.
Rimantadine Flumadine. Tablet: 100 mg. Syrup: 50 mg/5 mL.	**Prophylaxis (all ages) and treatment (>13 yr) of influenza A infections.** Prophylaxis only: *Children 1–9 yr or <40 kg:* 5 mg/kg/24 hr PO divided q12h (max: 150 mg/24 hr). *Children 10–13 yr:* 100 mg PO divided q12h. Prophylaxis or treatment: *Adolescents >13 yr and adults:* 200 mg/24 hr PO divided q12h.	*Cautions:* Anticholinergic effects, and may potentiate other anticholinergic medications. Drowsiness, dizziness, confusion, hypotension, urinary retention. Hepatically metabolized; reduce dosage to one-half usual dose for persons with severe liver disease or CrCl ≤10 mL/min.
Trifluridine Viroptic. Ophthalmic solution: 1%.	**Treatment of herpes simplex keratitis.** *Children and adults:* Instill 1 drop into affected eye(s) q2h while awake and at bedtime for up to 21 days.	*Cautions:* Local irritation, pruritus, ocular edema.
Vidarabine (Ara-A) Vira-A. Injection. Ophthalmic ointment.	**Herpes simplex and varicella zoster infections.** HSV infections: *Neonates:* 15–30 mg/kg/24 hr IV infusion over 18–24 hr. *Children and adults:* 15 mg/kg/24 hr IV once daily over 12 hr. Herpes zoster/varicella zoster infections: *Children and adults:* 10 mg/kg/24 hr IV once daily over 12 hr.	*Cautions:* Bone marrow suppression, disorientation, ataxia, seizures, syndrome of inappropriate secretion of antidiuretic hormone. Metabolites primarily renally eliminated. *Drug interactions:* Marrow suppressants.
Zanamivir Relenza. Blisters of powder for inhalation: 5 mg.	**Treatment of influenza infections type A and B via selective inhibition of influenza virus neuraminidase.** *Children and adolescents ≥ 7 yr:* 2 inhalations (10 mg) q12h for 5 days. Day 1 administer 2 doses provided dosing interval is >2 hr.	*Cautions:* Administer with caution to patients with hyperreactive airway disease because bronchospasm may occur from the powder. If the patient uses a bronchodilator, pretreatment before the zanamivir dose is advised. May cause nausea, diarrhea, nasal symptoms, and sinusitis in a small proportion of patients. Best results if therapy is started within 2 days of onset of symptoms.

Table continued on following page

MEDICATIONS

TABLE 712–6. Antiretroviral-HIV Medications

Drug (Trade Names, Formulations)	Indications (Mechanism of Action) and Dosing	Comments
Abacavir Ziagen. Tablet: 300 mg. Oral solution: 20 mg/mL.	**Nucleoside reverse transcriptase inhibitor for treatment of HIV-1 infection.** *Children > 3 mo and < 50 kg:* 8 mg/kg q12h (using oral solution). *Children >50 kg:* 20 mg/kg q12h or 15 mg/kg q8h (use capsules). *Adults:* 300 mg q12h.	*Cautions:* Nausea and vomiting 5–15%, diarrhea 5–10%; hypersensitivity reactions within first 6 wk of therapy.
Amprenavir Agenerase. Capsules: 50, 150 mg. Oral solution: 15 mg/mL.	**Protease inhibitor for treatment of HIV-1 infection.** *Children 4–12 yr or <50 kg:* 20 mg/kg bid or 15 mg/kg tid (max daily dose: 2,400 mg) as capsules; or 22.5 mg/kg bid or 17 mg/kg tid as oral solution. *Adolescents 13–16 yr and > 50 kg:* 1,200 mg bid. *Adults:* 1,200 mg bid. Reduce dose with moderate or severe liver impairment.	*Cautions:* May exacerbate diabetes mellitus or cause new-onset diabetes. Nausea, vomiting, diarrhea, rash, and taste disorders are also seen in > 3% of patients. Product provides relatively high doses of vitamin E. *Drug interactions:* Inhibits CYP3A4 liver enzymes and may cause toxic levels of warfarin, anticonvulsants, antiarrhythmics, calcium channel blockers, etc. Amprenavir is highly metabolized by cytochrome P450, and elimination may be altered by enzyme inhibitors or enzyme inducers.
Didanosine Videx, DDI. Chewable buffered tablet: 25, 50, 100, 150 mg. Buffered powder packet: 100, 167, 250 mg. Capule, delayed release: 125, 200, 250, 400 mg.	**Purine analog—intracellular metabolite inhibits viral RNA-directed DNA polymerase.** *Infants <90 days:* 100 mg/m²/24 hr PO divided q12h. *Children:* 180–300 mg/m²/24 hr PO divided q12h. *Adolescents (>13 yr) and adults <60 kg:* 125 mg PO q12h (buffered oral solution 167 mg PO q12h. *>60 kg:* 200 mg PO q12h (buffered oral solution 250 mg PO q12h). Administer on an empty stomach 1 hr before or 2 hr after a meal to decrease food effect.	*Cautions:* Headache (~30%), diarrhea, pancreatitis, peripheral neuropathy, optic neuritis, liver dysfunction. Renally eliminated. Food decreases bioavailability up to 50%. Tablets dissolved in water stable for 1 hr (4 hr in buffered solution). *Drug interactions:* Antacids/gastric acid antagonists may increase bioavailability; possible decreased absorption of ciprofloxacin, ganciclovir, ketoconazole, itraconazole.
Efavirenz Sustiva. Capsule: 50, 100, 200 mg.	**Non-nucleoside reverse transcriptase inhibitor used in combination with other antiretroviral agents to treat HIV-1 infection.** *Adolescents and adults:* 600 mg/24 hr, at bedtime. *Children ≥3 yr:* 10–<15 kg = 200 mg; 15–<20 kg = 250 mg; 20–<25 kg = 300 mg; 25–<32.5 kg = 350 mg; 32.5–<40 kg = 400 mg; ≥40 kg = 600 mg (give all doses once daily). Do not administer with fatty foods because absorption is increased 50%, but may administer with regular meals or without food.	*Cautions:* Combining with nelfinavir causes rash in 40% of pediatric patients. Severe CNS and psychiatric symptoms, including depression, may occur, especially if psychiatric or drug abuse history. False-positive screening tests for cannabinoid have been observed, but confirmatory tests are accurate. *Drug interactions:* Efavirenz induces CYP3A4 liver enzymes and may increase clearance of drugs metabolized by this pathway (e.g., warfarin, ethinyl estradiol) and several other HIV drugs. Drugs that induce CYP3A4 (e.g., phenobarbital, rifampin, rifabutin) will increase clearance of efavirenz. Drug also inhibits CYPs 2C9 and 2C19.
Indinavir Crixivan. Capsule: 100, 200, 333, 400 mg.	**Protease inhibitor for combination use with nucleoside analogs and other protease inhibitors. Evolving experience with neonatal and pediatric dosing.** *Children:* 1,500 mg/m²/24 hr PO divided q8h (max single dose: 800 mg). *Adults:* 2,400 mg/24 hr PO divided q8h. Chemoprophylaxis after high-risk exposure given in combination with zidovudine and lamivudine. Administer on an empty stomach 1 hr before or 2 hr after a meal to decrease food effect.	*Cautions:* Nephrolithiasis, nausea, hyperbilirubinemia, headache, diabetes. Reduce dose by ~25% with mild to moderate liver dysfunction. *Drug interactions:* Didanosine decreases absorption; rifampin reduces levels; ketoconazole, ritonavir, and other protease inhibitors decrease indinavir metabolism. Do not co-administer astemizole, cisapride, terfenadine.
Lamivudine Epivir, 3TC. Tablet: 150 mg. Solution: 5 mg/mL, 10 mg/mL.	**Reverse transcriptase inhibitor used in combination with zidovudine and/or other anti-HIV drugs. Evolving experience with neonatal and pediatric dosing.** *Infants, children and adolescents:* 8 mg/kg/24 hr PO divided q12h (max dose: 300 mg). *Adults:* 300 mg/24 hr PO divided q12h. Suggested chemoprophylaxis regimen for occupational exposure: lamivudine, 150 mg PO q12h, with zidovudine, 200 mg PO q8h, and indinavir, 800 mg PO q8h.	*Cautions:* Headache, psychomotor disorders, nausea, feeding problems, abdominal pain, pancreatitis, neutropenia, musculoskeletal pain. Adjust dose in patients with creatinine clearance <30 mL/min. Medication may be administered with or without food. *Drug interactions:* Trimethoprim/sulfamethoxazole may increase 3TC levels.
Nelfinavir Viracept. Tablet: 250 mg. Suspension: 250 mg/ 5 g powder.	**Protease inhibitor as monotherapy or preferably in combination with nucleoside analogs and other protease inhibitors. Evolving experience with neonatal and pediatric dosing.** *Neonates:* 30 mg/kg/24 hr PO divided q8h under study. *Children and adolescents:* 60–135 mg/kg/24 hr PO divided q8h. *Adults:* 750 mg/dose PO q8h or 1250 mg PO q12h. Administer with a meal to optimize absorption; avoid acidic food or drink (e.g., orange juice). Tablet can be dissolved in water to administer as a solution.	*Cautions:* Many adverse effects including hypertension, headaches, dizziness, diarrhea, anemia, leukopenia, hepatitis, iritis, dyspnea, sweating. *Drug interactions:* Rifampin, phenobarbital, carbamazepine reduce levels; ketoconazole, ritonavir, indinavir, and other protease inhibitors decrease nelfinavir metabolism. Nelfinavir inhibits CYP3A4 activity. Do not co-administer astemizole, cisapride, terfenadine. May interfere with oral contraceptives.
Nevirapine Viramune. Tablet: 200 mg. Suspension: 50 mg/5 mL.	**Non-nucleosides reverse transcriptase inhibitor specific for HIV-1 transcriptase (not HIV-2) or human polymerase. Evolving experience with neonatal and pediatric dosing.**	*Cautions:* Severe rash, Stevens-Johnson syndrome, headache, nausea, diarrhea, increased liver function tests. May give with or without food.

TABLE 712–6. Antiretroviral-HIV Medications *Continued*

Drug (Trade Names, Formulations)	Indications (Mechanism of Action) and Dosing	Comments
	Neonates: 5 mg/kg/24 hr PO for 14 days, then 240 mg/m^2/24 hr PO divided q12h for 14 days, then 400 mg/m^2/24 hr PO divided q12h. *Children:* 240 mg/m^2/24 hr PO divided q12h for 14 days; if tolerated, increase dose to maximum dose 400 mg/m^2/24 hr PO divided q12h, or 400 mg/24 hr. *Adolescents and adults:* 200 mg PO q24h for 14 days; if tolerated, 200 mg/dose q12h.	*Drug interactions:* Nevirapine induces hepatic CYP450 3A activity and decreases indinavir, saquinavir concentrations; rifampin decreases nevirapine serum levels; cimetidine, macrolides block metabolism.
Ritonavir Norvir. Capsule: 100 mg. Solution: 80 mg/mL.	**Protease inhibitor often effective against saquinavir and zidovudine-resistant virus; ritonavir-resistant strains often cross-resistant with other agents.** *Children:* 400 mg/m^2/24 hr PO divided q12h; titrate upward in 50 mg/m^2 per dose increments to 800 mg/m^2/24 hr PO q12h. *Adolescents and adults:* 400–600 mg per dose PO q12h. Administer dose with food to enhance . bioavailability	*Cautions:* Headache, nausea, taste aversion, pancreatitis, elevated serum lipids, elevated liver function tests, hypoglycemia, rash. *Drug interactions:* Ritonavir is a substrate and has affinity for many hepatic CYP450 enzymes that may lead to many important drug interactions (e.g., protease inhibitors, antiarrhythmics, antidepressants, cisapride). Ritonavir metabolism is influenced by enzyme inducers and inhibitors
Saquinavir Invirase, hard gelatin capsule. Mesylate capsule: 200 mg. Gelatin liquid-filled (Fortovase) capsule: 200 mg.	**Protease inhibitor. Dosing information in neonates, infants, and children is evolving.** $\geq$ *16 yr:* Liquid filled (Fortovase base): 1200 mg q8h PO, hard gelatin capsule (Inverase-mesylate salt): 600 mg q8h PO) Administration with a high-fat meal enhances bioavailability. Concurrent grapefruit juice may increase bioavailability.	*Cautions:* Photosensitivity, changes in blood pressure, confusion, ataxia, nausea, elevated liver function tests, rash, marrow suppression, bleeding. *Drug interactions:* Rifampin, phenobarbital, carbamazepine decreases serum levels; saquinavir may decrease metabolism of calcium channel antagonists; azoles (e.g., ketoconazole), macrolides, indinavir, ritonavir may increase levels.
Stavudine Zerit; d4T. Capsule: 15, 20, 30, 40 mg. Powder for oral suspension.	**Nucleoside analog reverse transcriptase inhibitor. Dosing information in neonates and infants is evolving.** *Children <30 kg:* 2 mg/kg/24 hr PO divided q12h. *Adolescents and adults:* 30–60 kg 30 mg per dose PO q12h; >60 kg 40 mg per dose PO q12h.	*Cautions:* Peripheral neuropathy, headache, nausea, pancreatitis, elevated liver function tests, rash. Primary renal elimination. *Drug interactions:* Other drugs associated with peripheral neuropathy (e.g., cisplatin, gold, isoniazid).
Zalcitabine Hivid; ddc. Tablet: 0.375, 0.75 mg.	**Nucleoside analog reverse transcriptase inhibitor. Dosing information in neonates, infants, and children is evolving.** *Children:* 0.01 mg/kg PO q8h. *Adolescents and adults:* 0.75 mg PO q8h. Doses best taken 1 hr before or 2 hr after a meal.	*Cautions:* Cumulative dose-related peripheral neuropathy, pancreatitis. Cardiac dysfunction, lactic acidosis, marrow suppression, hepatitis, jaundice, rash. Primary renal elimination. *Drug interactions:* Magnesium and aluminum antacids, metoclopramide may decrease absorption; other drugs associated with peripheral neuropathy (e.g., cisplatin, gold, isoniazid).
Zidovudine Retrovir, AZT, ZDV. Capsule: 100 mg. Tablet: 300 mg. Syrup: 50 mg/5 mL. Injection.	**Nucleoside analog reverse transcriptase inhibitor. Dosing information in premature neonates is evolving.** *Neonates:* 8 mg/kg/24 hr PO divided q6h; 6 mg/kg/24 hr IV divided q6h. *Children 6 wk–12 yr:* 480 mg/m^2/24 hr PO divided 8h; 360 mg/m^2/24 hr IV divided q6h; continuous infusion 20 mg/m^2/hr. *Children >12 yr and adults:* 200 mg per dose PO q8h or 300 mg per dose PO q12h; 1–2 mg/kg per dose IV q4h.	*Cautions:* Headache, seizure, lactic acidosis, diarrhea, bone marrow suppression, cholestatic hepatitis, rash. Primarily renal elimination. Infuse IV over 1 hr at a final concentration of 4 mg/mL. *Drug interactions:* Rifampin may increase metabolism; cimetidine, fluconazole, valproic acid may decrease metabolism.

TABLE 712–7. Antiparasitic Medications

Drug (Trade Names, Formulations)	Indications (Mechanism of Action) and Dosing	Comments
Atovaquone Mepron. Suspension: 750 mg/5 mL.	**Alternative therapy for mild to moderate *Pneumocystis carinii* pneumonia in patients intolerant of trimethoprim/sulfamethoxazole. Very limited experience with the drug in children.** Treatment of *P. carinii* pneumonia: *Children <13 y:* limited data, 40 mg/kg/24 hr PO q12h. *Adolescents and adults:* 750 mg PO q12h. Prophylaxis of *P. carinii: Children <13 yr,* limited data, 40 mg/kg/24 hr PO q12h. *Adolescents and adults:* 1500 mg PO qd. Toxoplasmosis prophylaxis: *Adolescents and adults:* 1500 mg PO qd. Administer doses with food.	*Cautions:* Dizziness, fever, rash, elevations in liver enzymes, neutropenia. Drug absorption increased when co-administered with food. *Drug interaction:* Rifampin may decrease levels.
Chloroquine phosphate Aralen, generic. Tablet: 250 mg (contains 150 mg base) and 500 mg (contains 300 mg base). Injection.	**Effective in the suppression and treatment of malaria and extraintestinal amebiasis. Dose drug on base equivalent.** Malaria prophylaxis: *Children:* 5 mg/kg/wk PO (max: 300 mg/dose). *Adults:* 300 mg/wk PO.	*Cautions:* Hypotension, headache, confusion, psychotic episodes, rash, peripheral neuropathy, blood dyscrasias, retinopathy, tinnitus. Administer with meals to decrease gastrointestinal upset. Liquid may be prepared from tablets using strong flavoring agent (cherry or chocolate) to mask bitter taste.

Table continued on following page

TABLE 712–7. Antiparasitic Medications

Drug (Trade Names, Formulations)	Indications (Mechanism of Action) and Dosing	Comments
	Acute malaria treatment: *Children:* 10 mg/kg PO initial dose (max dose: 600 mg); 5 mg/kg 6 hr later then 5 mg/kg PO once daily for 2 days. IM 5 mg/kg initial dose, 5 mg/kg 6 hr later (max IM dose: 10 mg/kg/24 hr). *Adults:* 600 mg PO initially, 300 mg 6 hr later then 300 mg PO once daily for 2 days. Extraintestinal amebiasis: *Children:* 10 mg/kg PO daily for 2–3 wk (max daily dose: 300 mg). *Adults:* 600 mg PO once daily for 2 days then 300 mg once daily for 2–3 wk.	
Furazolidone Furoxone. Tablet: 100 mg. Suspension: 50 mg/15 mL.	**Effective in the treatment of protozoal diarrhea, enteritis.** *Infants >1 mo and children:* 5–9 mg/kg/24 hr PO divided q6h (max daily dose: 400 mg). *Adults:* 100 mg/dose PO q6h.	*Cautions:* May cause hemolytic anemia in infants <1 mo of age; caution in glucose-6-phosphate dehydrogenase deficiency, hypotension, nausea, vomiting, hypoglycemia, hypersensitivity reactions, pulmonary infiltration. *Drug interactions:* Monoamine oxidase inhibitors; disulfiram-like alcohol reaction.
Lindane Kwell, Scabene. Lotion: 1%. Shampoo: 1%.	**Topical treatment for scabies, head lice (*Pediculus capitis*), crab lice (*Pediculus pubis*).** *Scabies:* Apply thin layer to affected area, remove (by showering) in 6–8 hr in children and after 18–24 hr in adults. *Pediculosis:* Shampoo with adequate amount (15–30 mL) and lather for 5 min then rinse thoroughly and comb.	*Cautions:* Dermal absorption may cause seizures, dizziness, hepatitis, blood dyscrasias. Do not apply to denuded/inflamed skin; avoid contact to eyes/mucous membranes.
Mebendazole Vermox, generic. Chewable tablet: 100 mg.	**Treatment of ascariasis (roundworm), hookworm, enterobiasis (pinworm), trichuriasis (whipworm).** *Children and adults:* Pinworm: 100 mg PO once; may repeat in 2 wk. Hookworm/roundworm/whipworm: 100 mg PO q12h for 3 consecutive days; 2nd course, if needed, in 3–4 wk. Capillariasis: 200 mg PO q12h for 3 wk.	*Cautions:* Very well tolerated; dizziness, nausea, rash, leukopenia, transient elevation in liver function tests. Enhanced absorption when administered with food. Tablets may be chewed or swallowed whole.
Metronidazole Flagyl, Metro-IV, generic. Topical gel, vaginal gel. Tablet: 250, 500 mg. Injection.	**Effective in the treatment of anaerobic and protozoal infections particularly, amebiasis, giardiasis, trichomoniasis.** Amebiasis: *Children:* 35–50 mg/kg/24 hr PO divided q8h. *Adults:* 500–750 mg per dose PO q8h. Other parasitic infections *Children:* 15–30 mg/kg/24 hr PO divided q8h. *Adults:* 250 mg per dose PO q8h; alternate dose 2 g single-dose therapy.	*Cautions:* Dizziness, seizures, metallic taste, nausea, disulfiram-like reaction with alcohol. Administer IV slowly over 30–60 min. *Drug interactions:* Carbamazepine, rifampin, phenobarbital may enhance metabolism; may increase levels of warfarin, phenytoin, lithium.
Niclosamide Niclocide. Chewable tablet: 500 mg.	**Effective in the treatment of tapeworm infections (beef, fish, dog/cat, and dwarf tapeworms). Drug active against intestinal cestodes only.** Beef and fish tapeworm: *Children:* 40 mg/kg PO once (max dose: 2 g). *Adults:* 2 g PO once. May repeat in 7 days. Dwarf tapeworm: *Children:* 40 mg/kg q24h PO for 7 days (max daily dose: 2 g). *Adults:* 2 g q24h PO for 7 days.	*Cautions:* Dizziness, headache, rash, alopecia, abdominal pain, nausea. Patients should chew tablets completely. *Drug interactions:* Hepatic enzyme inducers may enhance metabolism (e.g., carbamazepine, rifampin, phenobarbital).
Pentamidine isethionate Pentam, Nebupent. Inhalation, injection.	**For the treatment and prevention of *Pneumocystis carinii* pneumonia usually in patients intolerant of trimethoprim/sulfamethoxazole.** *Pneumocystis carinii* pneumonia treatment: *Infants (> 4 mo) children, and adults:* 4 mg/kg/24 hr IM or IV for 14–21 days. *Pneumocystis carinii* prophylaxis: *Children and adults:* 4 mg/kg/dose IM, IV q 2–4 wk. Aerosol once/mo using Respigard II nebulizer: *Infants:* Use dose formula (2.27 mg/kg pentamidine) × [nebulizer output (L/min)] × patient body weight (kg) divided by alveolar ventilation (L/min). *Children >5 yr:* 300 mg per dose q 4 wk. *Adults:* 300 mg q 4 wk.	*Cautions:* Hypotension, tachycardia, dizziness, hypoglycemia, nausea, marrow suppression, pain at injection site, nephrotoxicity, irritation of airway, cough, bronchospasm with aerosol. Adjust dose with renal dysfunction. IV route preferred. *Drug interactions:* Other nephrotoxins (aminoglycosides, vancomycin, amphotericin B, cyclosporine).
Permethrin Elimite, Nix. Cream: 5%. Creme rinse: 1%.	**Topical treatment for scabies, head lice (*Pediculus capitis*), crab lice (*Pediculus pubis*).** Head lice: *Children and adults:* wash areas, rinse, apply creme rinse liberally, leave on hair for 10 min,	*Cautions:* Dermal absorption unlikely. Do not apply to denuded/inflamed skin; avoid contact to eyes/mucous membranes. May cause rash.

TABLE 712–7. **Antiparasitic Medications** *Continued*

Drug (Trade Names, Formulations)	Indications (Mechanism of Action) and Dosing	Comments
	rinse and comb. May repeat treatment in 7 days. Scabies: *Children and adults:* Apply and leave on for 8–16 hr before removing with water.	
Piperazine citrate Vermizine, generic. Tablet: 250 mg.	**Alternative therapy for pinworm and roundworm.** Pinworm: *Children and adults:* 65 mg/kg/24 hr PO once daily for 7 days; may repeat course in 7 days. Roundworm: *Children and adults:* 75 mg/kg/24 hr PO once daily for 2 days (max dose: 3.5 g/24 hr); may repeat course in 7 days.	*Cautions:* Neurotoxicity, dizziness, seizures, tremor, visual disturbances, allergic reactions.
Praziquantel Biltricide. Tablet: 600 mg.	**Effective in all stages of schistosomiasis and many intestinal tapeworm and trematode infestations.** Schistosomiasis: *Children and adults:* 20 mg/kg/dose PO q8h for 1 day. May be effective at lower dose (20 mg/kg PO q12h for 1 day). Other trematodes: *Children and Adults:* 75 mg/kg/24 hr PO divided q8h for 1–2 days. Tapeworm: *Children and adults:* 5–10 mg/kg as a single dose.	*Cautions:* Central nervous system depression, dizziness, fever, rash, abdominal pain, eosinophilia. *Drug interaction:* Alcohol may increase CNS depression.
Primaquine phosphate Tablet: 26 mg (15 mg base).	**Effective in the prevention and treatment of malaria. Dose drug on base equivalent.** *Children:* 0.3 mg base/kg/24 hr PO once daily for 14 days (max daily dose: 15 mg). *Adults:* 15 mg PO once daily for 14 days.	*Cautions:* Pruritus, abdominal complaints, anemia, methemoglobinemia. Caution in patients with G6PD or NADH methemoglobin reductase deficiency.
Pyrantel pamoate Antiminth; Pin-Rid. Capsule: 180 mg. Liquid: 50, 144 mg/mL. Suspension: 50 mg/mL.	**Treatment of ascariasis (roundworm) hookworm, enterobiasis (pinworm), and trichostrongyliasis infections.** *Children and adults:* Pinworm, roundworm, trichostrongyliasis: 100 mg PO once; may repeat in 2 wk. Hookworms, roundworms, or whipworms: 11 mg/kg PO single dose (max dose: 1 g); may repeat in 2 wk for pinworm infestation. Hookworms: 11 mg/kg PO once daily for 3 consecutive days (max dose: 1 g/24 hr).	*Cautions:* Rash, elevation in liver function tests, abdominal cramps, dizziness, headache. *Drug interaction:* Possible antagonism of piperazine activity.
Pyrimethamine Daraprim. Tablet: 25 mg.	**Prophylaxis and in combination with other drugs for the treatment of malaria in combination with sulfa in treatment of toxoplasmosis and in combination with dapsone for prophylaxis against *P. carinii* infection in HIV patients.** Malaria prophylaxis: Begin drug 2 wk before entering endemic areas. Use for malaria decreasing owing to increased resistance and adverse effects. *Children:* 0.5 mg/kg once wk (max dose: 25 mg). Chloroquine-resistant malaria (with quinine and sulfa). Toxoplasmosis (with sulfadiazine): *Children:* 2 mg/kg/24 hr PO divided q12h for 2–3 days then 1 mg/kg/24 hr PO q24 hr, with sulfadiazine for 6 mo then 1 mg/kg/24 hr PO q24hr, 3 times/wk (max daily dose: 25 mg/24 hr). *Adults:* 50–75 mg plus 1–4 g sulfadiazine PO 3 times/wk. *Toxoplasma gondii* prophylaxis: *Infants >1 mo:* 1 mg/kg/24 hr PO q24h plus dapsone. *Adolescents and adults:* 50 mg PO once weekly plus dapsone. *Pneumocystis carinii* prophylaxis: *Adolescents and adults:* 50–75 mg PO once wk plus dapsone.	*Cautions:* Administer folinic acid (5–10 mg/kg 3 times/wk) to prevent hematologic toxicity; seizures, headache, photosensitivity, rash, folic acid deficiency, marrow suppression, tremor. Tablets may be crushed to prepare an extemporaneous suspension formulation.
Quinine Quinamm, generic. Capsule: 65, 200, 300, 325 mg. Tablet: 162.5, 260 mg.	**Antimalarial agent with decreasing effectiveness as resistance increasingly develops.** Chloroquine-resistant malaria: *Children:* 30 mg/kg/24 hr PO divided q8h for 3–7 days with another antimalarial agent. *Adults:* 650 mg per dose PO q8h for 3–7 days with another antimalarial agent.	*Cautions:* Glucose-6-phosphate dehydrogenase hemolysis, flushing, tachycardia, fever, headache, rash, nausea, tinnitus, cinchonism. *Drug interactions:* Interferes with digoxin disposition; aluminum-containing antacids decrease absorption.

Chapter 713

Herbal Medicines

Kathi J. Kemper and Paula Gardiner

Herbs and other dietary supplements are the most commonly used complementary therapies for children and adolescents. Several billion dollars are spent on these products each year in the United States. In a survey conducted in the late 1990s by the Puget Sound Pediatric Research Network, approximately one third of parents reported having given their child products containing *Echinacea* to prevent or treat upper respiratory tract infections. In other surveys, 20–30% of children or adolescents report using herbs or other dietary supplements such as creatine, androstenedione, and protein powders. Rates are higher among children with chronic, incurable, or recurrent conditions such as cystic fibrosis, cancer, arthritis, inflammatory bowel disease, and recurrent otitis media. Because physicians have not routinely asked patients and families about their use of these products, only 40% of patients who use herbs have talked with their physician about their use.

Herbal products are widely perceived as being safe because they are natural. They are also frequently considered as having low therapeutic efficacy, owing to a paucity of publications about them in scientific journals. However, conventional wisdom about herbs may be mistaken, resulting in risks to patients and providers.

Although as a general rule most herbs are safer and less costly than most medications, herbal products can cause serious toxicity. Acute hepatic toxicity and death may result from ingestion of even small amounts of *Amanita* mushrooms; overdoses of other herbs, such as digitalis, ephedra, and pennyroyal can cause life-threatening complications. Despite its historical use for spiritual and medicinal purposes, chronic use of tobacco has become a leading cause of morbidity and mortality in the past century. Although they may not cause problems with one-time use, chronic use of other herbs, such as *Aristolochia*, coltsfoot, and comfrey can cause severe hepatic or renal damage and cancer. As with medications, even when an herb is safe when used correctly, it can cause mild or severe toxicity when used incorrectly. For example, tea tree oil is safe when applied to mild fungal infections of the skin but can cause stinging and irritation when applied to eczema; if taken orally, it can cause coma in small children and animals. Furthermore, some persons are more sensitive to adverse effects than others; although most persons note only bad breath or body odor when taking garlic supplements, others report severe gastrointestinal distress after eating even moderate amounts of garlic. Similarly, although peppermint is a commonly used and usually benign gastrointestinal spasmolytic (included in after-dinner mints and teas and increasingly used to ease discomfort during colonoscopy), it can exacerbate gastroesophageal reflux in other patients.

The potency of herbal products is far less consistent than pharmaceutical medications. Because of natural variability, herbal products may contain widely varying concentrations of active ingredients; variations of 10- to 1,000-fold have been reported for several popular herbs by independent consumer testing groups. Labels are not required to reflect accurate content or concentrations of ingredients. Herbal products may be unintentionally contaminated with pesticides, animal wastes, or the wrong herb that was misidentified during harvesting. Products from developing countries may contain toxic levels of mercury, cadmium, or lead, either from unintentional contamination during manufacturing or from intentional additions by producers who believe these metals have therapeutic value. Thirty to 40% of Asian patent medicines include potent pharmaceuticals such as analgesics, antibiotics, hypoglycemic agents, or corticosteroids; typically, the labels for these products are not written in English and do not note the inclusion of pharmaceutical agents.

Even when herbal products contain known amounts of standardized ingredients and are used correctly, they may cause serious interactions with other medications. For example, St. John's wort can enhance elimination of digoxin, protease inhibitors, and numerous antibiotics, leading to subtherapeutic serum levels of these important medications; it can also increase the risk of serotonin syndrome in patients taking antidepressant medications. Ginkgo increases the risk of bleeding in patients taking anticoagulants. Licorice may enhance the anti-inflammatory effects and adverse effects of glucocorticoid medications. Ma huang (ephedra) increases the cardiovascular and sympathetic nervous system effects of a number of medications such as decongestants.

In the United States, herbal products are not regulated like medications. The 1994 Dietary Supplement and Health Education (DSHEA) Act allows herbal products to be marketed without prior testing for efficacy or safety. Products may contain little or none of the herb on the label, and they may contain other herbs. Product labels may make "structure-function" claims but may not claim to prevent or treat specific medical conditions. For example, a label may claim that a product "promotes a healthy immune system" but it may not claim to cure the common cold. The U.S. Food and Drug Administration (FDA) can only begin the process of restricting sales of certain products after receiving reports of adverse effects. As with medications, adverse reactions to herbs should be reported to the FDA's MedWatch program (https://www.accessdata.fda.gov/scripts/medwatch/); failure to do so limits the FDA's ability to monitor and manage the clinical and public health risks of these products.

Some herbal products may be helpful adjunctive treatments for common childhood problems. For example, one study documented that 3–4 oz/day of an herbal tea (containing chamomile, fennel, vervain, licorice, and balm-mint) was significantly more effective than a placebo tea as a treatment for infant colic. Numerous studies have documented the wound healing properties of topical aloe vera. Other studies have proven that ginger is an effective antiemetic. Kava kava, gotu kola, hops, lemon balm, lavender and passion flower, and valerian have mild anxiolytic and/or sedative effects. Herbal ear drops provide mild analgesia for mild to moderate otitis media.

As with medications, most herbs have undergone far more testing in adult than in pediatric populations. Typically, herbalists recommend that teenagers use adult doses, children 7–12 yr of age use half of the adult dose, children 3–6 yr of age use one fourth of the adult dose, and herbs be used only cautiously, if at all, in children 2 yr of age or younger. Herbs used for common conditions and the toxicity of selected herbs are described in Tables 713–1 through 713–4 and resources for information on herbal medicine are listed in Box 713–1.

TABLE 713–1.   Herbs for Asthma

Herb or Combination	RCTs?	Demonstrated Benefit?	Adverse Effects/Drug Interactions	Purported Mechanism
Coffee/tea	None recently in children	Epidemiologic data suggest fewer symptoms in coffee drinkers	Tachycardia, insomnia, jitteriness, decreased appetite; potential interaction with β-agonist	Methylxanthines Increased intracellular cAMP Bronchodilator
Shinpi-To	None in children	Yes, in historical data	Unknown. Potential interaction with leukotriene blockers	Blocks 5-lipo-oxygenase and phospholipase A_2
Saiboku-To	Yes in adults	Yes, corticosteroid-sparing in adults	Unknown. Potential increase in corticosteroid adverse effects	Inhibits 11 β-hydroxylase (blocks steroid breakdown) Blocks 5-lipo-oxygenase Inhibits platelet-activating factor
Ma huang (*Ephedra sinica*)	Yes	Yes	Cardiovascular and central nervous system toxicity, deaths reported, potential interaction with β-agonists	β- Agonist Bronchodilator
Licorice (*Glycyrrhiza glabra*)	No	Case series suggest corticosteroid-sparing effects	Pseudohyperaldosteronism, hypertension, peripheral edema, potential increase in corticosteroid adverse effects	Inhibits 11 β-hydroxylase and cortisol breakdown
Coleus forskolii	No	Case series in adults	Unknown	Decreased cAMP metabolism Bronchodilator
Tylophora indica	Yes in adults	Yes	Unknown	Unknown
Ginkgo biloba	No	Yes in pilot study	Unknown	Platelet-activating factor antagonist Antioxidant
Onions (*Allium cepa*)	No	In vitro and animal data support use	Hypersensitivity is rare	Blocks leukotriene synthesis
Bee pollen	No	No	Anaphylaxis	Unknown

RCT = randomized controlled trials; cAMP = cyclic adenosine monophosphate.
From Kemper KJ, Lester MR: Alternative asthma therapies: An evidence-based review. Contemp Pediatr *1999;16:162–95.*

TABLE 713–2.   Commonly Used Sedative Herbs

Sedative Herbs	Scientific Studies	Potential Adverse Effects or Interactions	Adult Dose
German chamomile	In controlled trials, chamomile and its constituents have positive effects as a mild sedative.	*Adverse effects:* Allergic reactions *Pregnancy and lactation:* no known adverse effects in pregnancy, lactation, and childhood *Drug interactions:* none known	*Tea:* 150 mL of boiling water over 3 g fresh flower heads, steep for 5–10 min; 3 × day.
Hops (*Humulus lupulus*)	Historical and anecdotal use. Controlled trials have used hops/valerian combinations; these show improvements in sleep with the combination.	*Adverse effects:* allergic reactions, skin irritation *Pregnancy and lactation:* no data available *Drug interactions:* sedative activity increases the sleeping time induced by pentobarbital	*Tea:* 0.5 to 1 g dried hops before bed, typically in combination with valerian
Kava kava (*Piper methysticum*)	Randomized controlled trials in adults demonstrate anxiolytic effects.	*Adverse effects:* drowsiness, lethargy; slowed reaction time; withdrawal syndrome; chronic use may lead to yellow, dry skin and red eyes *Pregnancy and lactation:* insufficient information available *Drug interactions:* may potentiate sedative and anxiolytic effects of other herbs and medications	60–120 mg kava lactones up to 300 mg of kava lactones daily to dried root/rhizome: 1.5–3.0 g/day in divided doses
Lavender (*Lavandula*)	Animal data and adult case series and controlled trials suggest anticonvulsant and sedative effects.	*Adverse effects:* allergies with topical use; toxic if large doses taken internally *Pregnancy and lactation:* historically contraindicated during pregnancy owing to possible emmenagogue effects; no documented adverse effects *Drug interactions:* may potentiate sedative and anticonvulsant effects of other drugs	*Massage aromatherapy:* 1–10 mL of the essential oil can be added to 25 mL of a carrier oil. *Bath soak:* add ¼–½ cup of dried lavender flowers to the hot bath water.
Lemon balm (*Melissa officinalis*)	Animal data suggest sedative hypnotic effects. All RCTs have examined lemon balm/valerian combinations; most show enhanced sleep quality.	*Adverse effects:* allergic reactions are possible *Pregnancy and lactation:* insufficient data; generally recognized as safe *Drug interactions:* none known	*Tea:* 2–3 g of dried herb, steeped in water; usually combined with valerian or lavender
Passionflower (*Passiflora alata*)	Case reports and historical use; most often combined with other herbs such as valerian. *Drug interactions:* none known .	*Adverse effects:* allergic reactions are possible *Pregnancy and lactation:* insufficient data;	*Tea:* 0.25–1 g (about 1 tsp. of crushed dried flowers per cup water) *Solid extract:* 150–300 mg (sold in capsules) daily
Valerian (*Valeriana officinalis*)	Randomized double-blind placebo controlled studies in adults show decreased sleep latency and improved sleep quality.	*Adverse effects:* headaches, insomnia *Pregnancy and lactation:* insufficient data *Drug interactions:* sedative activity increases the sleeping time induced by pentobarbital	*Tea:* 2–3 g of fresh or dried root per cup; 1–3 × day. *Capsules:* 400 mg before bed

From Gardiner P, Kemper KJ: Herbs for sleep problems. Contemp Pediatr *2002;19(2):69–87* and Gardiner P, Kemper KJ: Herbs in pediatric and adolescent medicine. Pediatr Rev *2000;21:44–57.*

TABLE 713–3. Herbs for Skin Conditions

Action	Herb/Supplement for Topical Use
Soothing/emollient	Aloe, calendula
Anti-inflammatory	Aloe, chamomile, evening primrose oil (PO), lemon balm
Antiviral	Aloe vera, calendula, chamomile, lemon balm
Antibacterial	Aloe vera, calendula, chamomile, lavender, lemon balm, tea tree oil
Antifungal	Lavender, tea tree oil

From Gardiner P, Coles D, Kemper KJ: The skinny on herbal remedies for dermatologic disorders. Contemp Pediatr 2001;18:103–4, 107–10, 112–14.

TABLE 713–4. Potentially Toxic Herbs

Herb	Toxic Constituents	Typical Uses	Potential Acute Adverse Effects	How to Treat Overdose
Aconitum (monkshood, wolfsbane)	Di-ester alkaloids: hypaconitine and aconitine (aconitine increases permeability for sodium ions and slows down repolarization leading to paralysis of the nerve)	Facial neuralgia and sciatica Headache and migraines Rheumatic pain, arthritis, gout Pericarditis sicca	Nausea, vomiting, and hypersalivation CNS: paresthesias, muscular weakness dizziness, ataxia, seizures, and coma Cardiac: bradycardia, hypotension, rhythm disorders	Supportive care Dioxin-specific antibodies, unless history excludes cardiac glycosides Do not give ipecac Activated charcoal and gastric emptying may help Avoid type 1 antiarrhythmics
Artemisia absinthium (wormwood)	Thujone and isothujone—neurotoxins	Anorexia Dyspeptic conditions Liver and gallbladder disorders	Mental status changes: restlessness, vertigo, tremors, agitation and seizures, headache Vomiting, stomach and intestinal cramps Rhabdomyolysis and renal failure	Supportive care Benzodiazepines
Atropa belladonna (deadly nightshade)	Alkaloids: hyoscyamine (the L-isomer of atropine	Gastrointestinal complaints Cardiac insufficiency and arrhythmia Asthma	Anticholinergic reaction: tachycardia, hyperthermia, mydriasis, urinary and bowel retention, restlessness Nervous system and respiratory depression	Gastric lavage Physostigmine given in consultation with poison specialist External cooling if temperature >102°F Benzodiazepines Hydration
Digitalis purpurea (foxglove)	Cardioactive glycosides: purpurea glycoside, digitoxin gitoxin,	Ulcers, boils, headaches, abscesses, paralysis, cardiac insufficiency	Nausea and vomiting, headache, loss of appetite Cardiac rhythm disorders Central nervous system: stupor, confusion, visual disorders, depression, psychosis, hallucinations	Supportive care Gastric lavage Activated charcoal Treat the symptoms
Ephedra sinica (ma huang) Common names: Miner's tea Mexican tea Desert herb	Alkaloids: ephedrine, pseudoephedrine (stimulates sympathomimetic receptors and the central nervous system)	Decongestant for upper respiratory infection Asthma Weight loss Stimulant	Cardiac: hypertension, cardiomyopathy, myocardial infarction, arrhythmias Central nervous system: dizziness, restlessness, headaches, anxiety, hallucinations, tremors, seizures, psychosis, strokes Nausea and vomiting Contraindicated if diabetic or has hypertension, angle-closure glaucoma, anxiety, prostate adenoma, thyroid disease, pheochromocytoma	Activated charcoal Benzodiazepine for seizures and sedation Vasodilators for hypertension Lidocaine and β blockers for arrhythmias External cooling if temperature >102°F Hydration therapy
Lobelia inflata (lobelia)	Piperidine alkaloid: L-Lobeline (stimulates nicotinic receptors)	Expectorant Asthma Spasmolytic Emetic To induce mental clarity and a feeling of well-being	Gastrointestinal: nausea and vomiting, abdominal pain, diarrhea Central nervous system: anxiety and headache, dizziness, tremors, seizures, paresthesias, euphoria Cardiac: arrhythmias, bradycardia, transient increase in blood pressure, decreased respiratory rate In overdose, lobeline may cause hypotension Diaphoresis, muscle fasciculations and weakness, tremors, respiratory depression Dermatitis	Supportive care Gastric emptying Activated charcoal Benzodiazepines
Mentha pulegium (pennyroyal)	Pennyroyal oil has a hepatotoxic effect. Acute poisoning is not found with proper administration of the designated therapeutic use of pennyroyal leaf. However, drug is not recommended owing to hepatotoxicity.	Insect repellent Respiratory illness Digestive disorders Emmenagogue Abortifacient Wound treatment Gout	Uterine contractions, Gastrointestinal: nausea, vomiting, abdominal pain, hepatitis Neurotoxin: delirium, dizziness, convulsions, seizures, paralysis, encephalopathy, and coma Renal failure and hypertension Shock and disseminated intravascular coagulation Contraindicated in pregnancy	Supportive care N-acetylcysteine

TABLE 713–4. Potentially Toxic Herbs *Continued*

Herb	Toxic Constituents	Typical Uses	Potential Acute Adverse Effects	How to Treat Overdose
Pausinystalia yohimbe (yohimbe)	Indole alkaloids Yohimbe: α_2-adrenoreceptor antagonist	Sexual disorders Exhaustion Improve muscle function	Adverse reactions: dizziness, headache, anxiety, hypertension, indigestion, rash, insomnia, tachycardia, tremor, vomiting, hallucinations, nervousness, paresthesias, hypothermia, salivation, mydriasis, diarrhea, palpations, and tachycardia Contraindicated in kidney and liver disease	Gastric emptying Activated charcoal Antiarrhythmics Hydration
Phytolacca americana (pokeweed, American nightshade)	Triterpene saponins (irritate mucous membranes) Lectins (toxic)	Anti-inflammatory Arthritis Cancer treatment Emetic and cathartic Rheumatism	Dizziness, somnolence, nausea, vomiting, diarrhea, tachycardia, hemorrhagic gastritis, hypotension, lymphocytosis, headache, respiratory depression, seizures	Hydration therapy, electrolyte correction gastric emptying activated charcoal electrolyte replacement Emesis should not be induced if patient is experiencing symptoms of overdose.
Stramonium folium (jimson weed)	Alkaloids: hyoscyamine (the L-isomer of atropine)	Asthma and cough Diseases of the autonomic nervous system	In high doses leads to restlessness, mania, hallucinations, delirium Overdose: tachycardia, mydriasis, flushing, dry mouth, decreased sweating, miction, constipation	Supportive care Gastric lavage Decreasing temperature Physostigmine Benzodiazepines
Viscum album (mistletoe)	Alkaloids Viscotoxins (*Viscum album*) cause hypotension, bradycardia, and arterial vasoconstriction Lectins	Antineoplastic adjuvant Antihypertensive Nervous disorders—calmative agent Rheumatism Antispasmodic	Fever, headaches, nausea, vomiting, diarrhea, bradycardia, angina, change in blood pressure, seizures, confusion, hallucination, allergic reactions, miosis, mydriasis, chills, coma Two reported deaths in the past 35 yr; most ingestions lead to mild reactions	Supportive therapy Data inconclusive for inducing emesis Activated charcoal

From Gardiner P, Kemper KJ: Herbs for sleep problems. Contemp Pediatr *2002;2:69–87: and Gardiner P, Kemper KJ: Herbs in pediatric and adolescent medicine*. Pediatr Rev *2000;21: 44–57.*

BOX 713–1. Resources for Herbal Medicine

BOOKS
- Blumenthal M: *Herbal Medicine, Expanded German Commission E Monographs.* American Botanical Council, 2000. Austin, Tx
- Newall C: *Herbal Medicine: A Guide for Health Care Professionals.* Pharmaceutical Press, 1996. London, Eng
- *PDR for Herbal Medicines.* Medical Economics Company, 2000.

PERIODICALS
- *Prescribers Letter.* Therapeutic Research Center, email: mail@pletter.com (209-472-2240) CME credit available
- *Review of Natural Products.* Facts and Comparisons (1-800-223-0554)

DATABASES
- Natural Medicine Comprehensive Database: http://www.naturaldatabase.com
- International Bibliographic Information On Dietary Supplements (IBIDS) http://ods.od.nih.gov/databases/ibids.html
- Micromedex Internet Health Care Series: www.micromedex.com
- ConsumerLabs: www.consumerlabs.com

WEBSITES

Government
- NIH Office of Dietary Supplements: http://dietary-supplements.info.nih.gov/index.aspx
- FDA MEDWATCH, monitoring program for reporting adverse effects: http://www.fda.gov/medwatch (1-800-FDA-1088)

Information on Herbs
- American Botanical Council: http://www.herbalgram.org
- Longwood Herbal Task Force: www.mcp.edu/herbal
- HERBMED: http://www.herbmed.org
- The Natural Pharmacist: http://www.tnp.com

Toxicology Information
- Toxicology Information Resource Center: http://www.ornl.gov/TechResources/tirc/hmepg.html
- TOXLINE and TOXNET, from the National Library of Medicine: http://sis.nlm.nih.gov/Tox/ToxMain.html

Boyer EW, Kearney S, Shannon MW, et al: Poisoning from a dietary supplement administered during hospitalization. *Pediatrics* 2002;109:E49.

Buck ML, Michel RS: Talking with families about herbal therapies. *J Pediatr* 2000;136:673–78.

Chan E, Gardiner P, Kemper KJ: At least it's natural...Herbs and dietary supplements in ADHD. *Contemp Pediatr* 2000;9:116–30.

Gardiner P, Kemper KJ: Peripheral brain: Herbs in pediatric and adolescent medicine. *Pediatr Rev* 2000;21:44–57.

Gardiner P, Conboy LA, Kemper KJ: Herbs and adolescent girls: Avoiding the hazards of self-treatment. *Contemp Pediatr* 2000;3:133–54.

Gardiner P, Coles D, Kemper KJ: The skinny on herbal remedies for dermatologic disorders. *Contemp Pediatr* 2001;18:103–4,107–10, 112–14.

Gardiner P, Kemper KJ: Herbs for sleep problems. *Contemp Pediatr* 2002;2:69–87.

Haller CA, Benowitz NL: Adverse cardiovascular and central nervous system events associated with dietary supplements containing ephedra alkaloids. *N Engl J Med* 2000;343:1833–8.

Kemper KJ: Otitis media—what to do when parents don't want antibiotics or tubes. *Contemp Pediatr* 2002;4:47–60.

Kemper KJ, Lester MR: Alternative asthma therapies: An evidence-based review. *Contemp Pediatr* 1999;16:162–95.

Kemper KJ and Longwood Herbal Task Force: Shark cartilage, cat's claw and other complementary cancer therapies. *Contemp Pediatr* 1999;11:102–26.

Thomassoni AJ, Simone K: Herbal medicines for children: An illusion of safety? *Curr Opin Pediatr* 2001;13:162–9.

Weizman Z, Alkrinawi S, Goldfarb D, et al: Efficacy of herbal tea preparation in infantile colic. *J Pediatr* 1993;122:650–2.

Index

Note: Page numbers followed by the letter b refer to boxes, those followed by f refer to figures, and those followed by t refer to tables.

INDEX